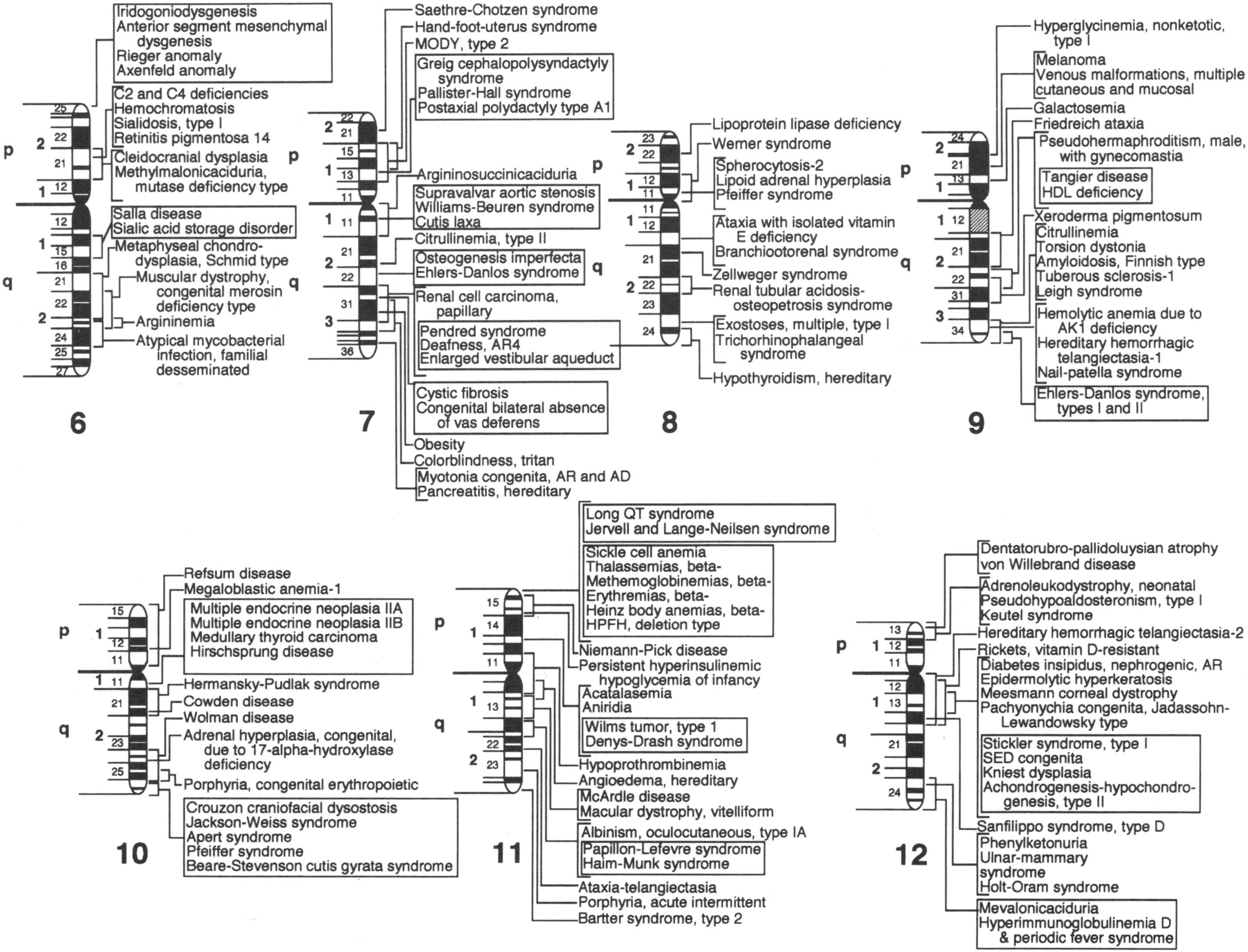

6
Iridogoniodysgenesis
Anterior segment mesenchymal dysgenesis
Rieger anomaly
Axenfeld anomaly
C2 and C4 deficiencies
Hemochromatosis
Sialidosis, type I
Retinitis pigmentosa 14
Cleidocranial dysplasia
Methylmalonicaciduria, mutase deficiency type
Salla disease
Sialic acid storage disorder
Metaphyseal chondrodysplasia, Schmid type
Muscular dystrophy, congenital merosin deficiency type
Argininemia
Atypical mycobacterial infection, familial desseminated
7
Saethre-Chotzen syndrome
Hand-foot-uterus syndrome
MODY, type 2
Greig cephalopolysyndactyly syndrome
Pallister-Hall syndrome
Postaxial polydactyly type A1
Argininosuccinicaciduria
Supravalvar aortic stenosis
Williams-Beuren syndrome
Cutis laxa
Citrullinemia, type II
Osteogenesis imperfecta
Ehlers-Danlos syndrome
Renal cell carcinoma, papillary
Pendred syndrome
Deafness, AR4
Enlarged vestibular aqueduct
Cystic fibrosis
Congenital bilateral absence of vas deferens
Obesity
Colorblindness, tritan
Myotonia congenita, AR and AD
Pancreatitis, hereditary
8
Lipoprotein lipase deficiency
Werner syndrome
Spherocytosis-2
Lipoid adrenal hyperplasia
Pfeiffer syndrome
Ataxia with isolated vitamin E deficiency
Branchiootorenal syndrome
Zellweger syndrome
Renal tubular acidosis-osteopetrosis syndrome
Exostoses, multiple, type I
Trichorhinophalangeal syndrome
Hypothyroidism, hereditary
9
Hyperglycinemia, nonketotic, type I
Melanoma
Venous malformations, multiple cutaneous and mucosal
Galactosemia
Friedreich ataxia
Pseudohermaphroditism, male, with gynecomastia
Tangier disease
HDL deficiency
Xeroderma pigmentosum
Citrullinemia
Torsion dystonia
Amyloidosis, Finnish type
Tuberous sclerosis-1
Leigh syndrome
Hemolytic anemia due to AK1 deficiency
Hereditary hemorrhagic telangiectasia-1
Nail-patella syndrome
Ehlers-Danlos syndrome, types I and II
10
Refsum disease
Megaloblastic anemia-1
Multiple endocrine neoplasia IIA
Multiple endocrine neoplasia IIB
Medullary thyroid carcinoma
Hirschsprung disease
Hermansky-Pudlak syndrome
Cowden disease
Wolman disease
Adrenal hyperplasia, congenital, due to 17-alpha-hydroxylase deficiency
Porphyria, congenital erythropoietic
Crouzon craniofacial dysostosis
Jackson-Weiss syndrome
Apert syndrome
Pfeiffer syndrome
Beare-Stevenson cutis gyrata syndrome
11
Long QT syndrome
Jervell and Lange-Neilsen syndrome
Sickle cell anemia
Thalassemias, beta-
Methemoglobinemias, beta-
Erythremias, beta-
Heinz body anemias, beta-
HPFH, deletion type
Niemann-Pick disease
Persistent hyperinsulinemic hypoglycemia of infancy
Acatalasemia
Aniridia
Wilms tumor, type 1
Denys-Drash syndrome
Hypoprothrombinemia
Angioedema, hereditary
McArdle disease
Macular dystrophy, vitelliform
Albinism, oculocutaneous, type IA
Papillon-Lefevre syndrome
Haim-Munk syndrome
Ataxia-telangiectasia
Porphyria, acute intermittent
Bartter syndrome, type 2
12
Dentatorubro-pallidoluysian atrophy
von Willebrand disease
Adrenoleukodystrophy, neonatal
Pseudohypoaldosteronism, type I
Keutel syndrome
Hereditary hemorrhagic telangiectasia-2
Rickets, vitamin D-resistant
Diabetes insipidus, nephrogenic, AR
Epidermolytic hyperkeratosis
Meesmann corneal dystrophy
Pachyonychia congenita, Jadassohn-Lewandowsky type
Stickler syndrome, type I
SED congenita
Kniest dysplasia
Achondrogenesis-hypochondrogenesis, type II
Sanfilippo syndrome, type D
Phenylketonuria
Ulnar-mammary syndrome
Holt-Oram syndrome
Mevalonicaciduria
Hyperimmunoglobulinemia D & periodic fever syndrome

The Metabolic & Molecular Bases of Inherited Disease

eighth edition

EDITORS

Charles R. Scriver, M.D.C.M.
Alva Professor of Human Genetics, Professor of Pediatrics, Faculty of Medicine, Professor of Biology, Faculty of Science, McGill University; Director (retired), deBelle Laboratory of Biochemical Genetics and Biochemical Genetics Clinical Unit, McGill University–Montreal Children's Hospital Research Institute, McGill University Health Centre, Montreal, Quebec, Canada

Arthur L. Beaudet, M.D.
Henry and Emma Meyer Professor and Chair, Department of Molecular and Human Genetics, Professor, Departments of Pediatrics and Molecular and Cellular Biology, Baylor College of Medicine, Houston, Texas

William S. Sly, M.D.
Alice A. Doisy Professor of Biochemistry and Molecular Biology, Chair, Edward A. Doisy Department of Biochemistry and Molecular Biology, Professor of Pediatrics, St. Louis University School of Medicine, St. Louis, Missouri

David Valle, M.D.
Professor of Pediatrics and Molecular Biology, Howard Hughes Medical Institute, McKusick-Nathans Institute of Genetic Medicine. The Johns Hopkins University School of Medicine, Baltimore, Maryland

ASSOCIATE EDITORS

Barton Childs, M.D.
Emeritus Professor of Pediatrics, The Johns Hopkins University School of Medicine, Baltimore, Maryland

Kenneth W. Kinzler, Ph.D.
Professor of Oncology, The Johns Hopkins University School of Medicine, Baltimore, Maryland

Bert Vogelstein, M.D.
Investigator, Howard Hughes Medical Institute, Clayton Professor of Oncology and Pathology, The Johns Hopkins University School of Medicine, Baltimore, Maryland

The Metabolic & Molecular Bases of Inherited Disease

eighth edition

VOLUME III

EDITORS

Charles R. Scriver, M.D.C.M.
Arthur L. Beaudet, M.D.
William S. Sly, M.D.
David Valle, M.D.

ASSOCIATE EDITORS

Barton Childs, M.D.
Kenneth W. Kinzler, Ph.D.
Bert Vogelstein, M.D.

McGRAW-HILL
Medical Publishing Division

New York St. Louis San Francisco Auckland Bogotá Caracas Lisbon London Madrid Mexico City
Milan Montreal New Delhi San Juan Singapore Sydney Tokyo Toronto

McGraw-Hill
A Division of The McGraw-Hill Companies

The Metabolic and Molecular Bases of Inherited Disease, 8th Edition

1234567890 KGPKGP 09876543210

ISBNs
0-07-913035-6
0-07-136319-X (vol. 1)
0-07-136320-3 (vol. 2)
0-07-136321-1 (vol. 3)
0-07-136322-X (vol. 4)
This book was set in Times Roman by Progressive Information Technologies, Inc.
The editors were Martin J. Wonsiewicz, Susan R. Noujaim, and Peter J. Boyle;
the production supervisor was Richard Ruzycka; the text designer was José R. Fonfrias;
the cover designer was Elizabeth Schmitz; Barbara Littlewood prepared the index.
Quebecor Printing/Kingsport was printer and binder.
This book is printed on acid-free paper.

Library of Congress Cataloging-in-Publication Data

The metabolic and molecular bases of inherited disease / editors,
Charles R. Scriver ... [et al.].–8th ed.
p.; cm.
Includes bibliographical references and index.
ISBN 0-07-913035-6 (set)
1. Metabolism, Inborn errors of 2. Medical genetics. 3. Pathology, Molecular. I. Scriver, Charles R.
[DNLM: 1. Hereditary Diseases. 2. Metabolic Diseases. 3. Metabolism, Inborn Errors.
WD 200 M5865 2001]
RC627.8 . M47 2001
616′.042–dc21

00-060957

INTERNATIONAL EDITION
ISBNs 0-07-116336-0
0-07-118833-9 (vol. 1)
0-07-118834-7 (vol. 2)
0-07-118835-5 (vol. 3)
0-07-118836-3 (vol. 4)

CONTENTS

VOLUME I

PART 1
INTRODUCTION

PART 2
PERSPECTIVES

PART 5
CHROMOSOMES

PART 6
DIAGNOSTIC APPROACHES

PART 7
CARBOHYDRATES

VOLUME II

PART 8
AMINO ACIDS

PART 11
PURINES AND PYRIMIDINES

PART 12
LIPIDS

VOLUME III

PART 16
LYSOSOMAL DISORDERS

PART 17
VITAMINS

PART 18
HORMONES

PART 19
BLOOD

PART 20
IMMUNE AND DEFENSE SYSTEMS

PART 21
MEMBRANE TRANSPORT DISORDERS

VOLUME IV

PART 22
CONNECTIVE TISSUE

PART 23
CARDIOVASCULAR SYSTEM

PART 24
KIDNEY

PART 25
MUSCLE

Color plates appear between pages 1296 and 1297.

CONTRIBUTORS

Lauri A. Aaltonen, M.D. [34]*
Senior Fellow, Academy of Finland, Dept. of Medical Genetics, Haartman Institute, Finland
Lauri.aaltonen@helsinki.fi

Frank Accurso, M.D. [201]
Dept. of Pediatrics, University of Colorado School of Medicine; Director, The Mike McMorris Cystic Fibrosis Center, The Children's Hospital, Denver, Colorado
accurso.frank@tchden.org

Milton B. Adesnik, Ph.D. [16]
Professor of Cell Biology, Dept. of Cell Biology, New York University School of Medicine, New York, New York
Adesnm01@popmail.med.nyu.edu

Björn A. Afzelius, M.D. [187]
Professor Emeritus, Wenner-Gren Institute, Stockholm University, Arrhenius Laboratories, Stockholm, Sweden
Bjorn.Afzelius@zub.su.se

Naji Al-Dosari, M.D. [57]
Duke University, Durham, North Carolina
naji@acpub.duke

Rando L. Allikmets, Ph.D. [243]
Dept. of Ophthalmology, Columbia University, New York, New York
rla22@columbia.edu

Robert J. Alpern, M.D. [195]
Dean, Southwestern Medical School, Ruth W. and Milton P. Levy, Sr., Chair in Molecular Nephrology, Atticus James Gill Chair in Medical Science, Div. of Nephrology, UT Southwestern Medical Center at Dallas, Dallas, Texas
Robert.alpern@email.swmed.edu

Wallace L.M. Alward, M.D. [242]
Dept. of Opthalmology and Visual Sciences, University of Iowa College of Medicine, Iowa City, Iowa
wallace-alward@uiowa.edu

Joanna S. Amberger, M.D. [1]
McKusick-Nathans Institute of Genetic Medicine, Johns Hopkins University School of Medicine, Baltimore, Maryland
joanna@peas.welch.jhu.edu

Donald C. Anderson, M.D. [188]
Professor, Dept. of Pediatrics, Baylor College of Medicine, Vice President and Chief Scientific Officer, Pharmacia & Upjohn, Kalamazoo, Michigan
donald.c.anderson@pnu.com

Karl E. Anderson, M.D. [124]
Professor of Preventive Medicine and Community Health, Internal Medicine, and Pharmacology and Toxicology, Dept. of Preventive Medicine and Community Health, University of Texas Medical Branch, Galveston, Texas
karl.anderson@utmb.edu

Mary E. Anderson, Ph.D. [96]
Assistant Professor, Dept. of Microbiology and Molecular Cell Sciences, University of Memphis, Memphis, Tennessee
Mary@mmcs.memphis.edu

Generoso Andria, M.D. [152]
Professor of Pediatrics, Department of Pediatrics, Federico II University, Naples, Italy

Stylianos E. Antonarakis, M.D., D.Sc. [13, 172]
Professor and Director of Medical Genetics, Div. of Medical Genetics, University of Geneva Medical School, Geneva, Switzerland
stylianos.antonarakis@medicine.unige.ch

Irwin M. Arias, M.D. [125]
Professor and Chairman, Dept. of Physiology, Tufts University, Boston, Massachusetts
irwin.arias@tufts.edu

Gerd Assmann, M.D., F.R.C.P [118, 122, 142]
Professor of Medicine, Director, Institute for Clinical Chemistry and Lab Medicine, Director, Institute for Arteriosclerosis Research, Westfälische Wilhelms-University, Münster, Germany
assmann@uni-muenster.de

Arleen D. Auerbach, Ph.D. [31]
Associate Professor, Laboratory of Human Genetics and Hematology, The Rockefeller University, New York, New York
auerbac@rockvax.rockefeller.edu

Perti Aula, M.D. [141, 200]
Professor of Medical Genetics, Medical Genetics Dept., University of Helsinko, Haartman Institute, Haartmaninkatu, Finland
Perti.aula@helsinki.fi

Salvatore Auricchio, M.D. [75]
Professor, Dept. di Pediatria, Università Federico II Napoli, Italy

Andrea Ballabio, M.D. [149, 166, 225]
Professor of Medical Genetics, Second University of Naples, Director, Telethon Institute of Genetics and Medicine (TIGEM), Naples, Italy
ballabio@tigem.it

Peter G. Barth [130]
Professor of Pediatric Neurology, University of Amsterdam Academic Medical Centre, Emma Children's Hospital and Clinical Chemistry, Amsterdam, The Netherlands
p.g.barth@amc.uva.nl

Stephen B. Baylin, M.D. [58]
Professor of Oncology and Medicine, Associate Director for Research, The Johns Hopkins Oncology Center, Baltimore, Maryland
sbaylin@jhmi.edu

Philip A. Beachy, M.D. [205]
Professor of Molecular Biology and Genetics, Howard Hughes Medical Institute, The Johns Hopkins University School of Medicine, Baltimore, Maryland
pbeachy@jhmi.edu

Arthur L. Beaudet, M.D. [1, 229]
Henry and Emma Meyer Professor and Chair, Dept. of Molecular and Human Genetics, Professor, Depts. of Pediatrics and Molecular and Cellular Biology, Baylor College of Medicine, Houston, Texas
abeaudet@bcm.tmc.edu

Michael A. Becker, M.D. [106]
Professor of Medicine
Dept. of Medicine University of Chicago School of Medicine, Chicago, Illinois
mbecker@medicine.bsd.uchicago.edu

*The numbers in brackets following each contributor's name refer to chapters written or co-written by that contributor.

David M.O. Becroft, M.D. [113]
Dept. of Obstetrics and Gynecology, University of Auckland School of Medicine, Auckland, New Zealand
David.Genevieve.Becroft@extra.co.nz

Lenore K. Beitel, Ph.D. [161]
Research Scientist, Lady Davis Institute for Medical Research, Sir M.B. Davis–Jewish General Hospital, Montreal, Quebec, Canada
mdtm001@musica.mcgill.ca

John W. Belmont, M.D., Ph.D. [185]
Dept. of Molecular and Human Genetics, Baylor College of Medicine, Houston, Texas
jbelmont@bcm.tmc.edu

Merrill D. Benson, M.D. [209]
Professor of Medicine, Pathology and Medical Genetics, Dept. of Medical and Molecular Genetics, Indiana University School of Medicine, Indianapolis, Indiana
mdbenson@iupui.edu

Wolfgang Berger, M.D. [239]
Max-Planck-Institute for Molecular Genetics, Berlin, Germany
berger@molgen@mpg.de

Michel Bergeron, M.D. [196]
Professor of Physiology, Dept. of Physiology, Université de Montréal, Montreal, Quebec, Canada
Bergermi@ere.umontreal.ca

Sten Erik Bergstrom, M.D. [187]
Dept. of Pediatrics, Huddinge University Hospital, Stockholm, Sweden

Ernest Beutler, M.D. [127, 146, 182]
Chairman, Dept. of Molecular and Experimental Medicine, Scripps Clinic and Research Foundation, La Jolla, California
beutler@scripps.edu

Daniel G. Bichet, M.D. [163]
Professor of Medicine, University of Montreal, Director, Clinical Research Unit, Hopital du Sacre-Coeur de Montreal, Montreal, Quebec, Canada
D-Binette@crhsc.umontreal.ca

Sandra H. Bigner, M.D. [57]
Professor of Pathology, Dept. of Pathology, Duke University Medical Center, Durham, North Carolina
Bigne002@mc.duke.edu

David F. Bishop, Ph.D. [124]
Professor of Human Genetics, Dept. of Human Genetics, Mount Sinai School of Medicine, New York, New York
David.bishop@mssm.edu

Ingemar Björkhem, M.D., Ph.D. [123]
Professor and Head Physician, Dept. of Medical Laboratory Sciences and Technology, Division of Clinical Chemistry, Karolinska Institutet, Huddinge University Hospital, Huddinge, Sweden
Ingemar.Bjorkhem@chemlab.hs.sll.se

E. Joan Blanchette-Mackie, M.D. [145]
Chief, Sect. of Lipid Cell Biology, Laboratory of Cell Biochemistry and Biology, National Institute of Diabetes and Digestive and Kidney Diseases, Bethesda, Maryland
eb78u@nih.gov

Nenad Blau, M.D., Ph.D. [78]
Associate Professor, Div. of Clinical Chemistry and Biochemistry, Dept. of Pediatrics, University Children's Hospital, Zurich, Switzerland
blau@access.unizh.ch

Kirsten Muri Boberg, M.D., Ph.D. [123]
Dept. of Clinical Chemistry, Rikshospitalet, Oslo, Norway
kirsten.boberg@online.no

Sir Walter F. Bodmer, M.D., Ph.D., F.R.C.Path, F.R.S. [11]
Imperial Cancer Research Fund Laboratories, University of Oxford, Institute of Molecular Medicine, John Radcliffe Hospital, Oxford, United Kingdom
walter.bodmer@hertford.ox.ac.uk

C. Richard Boland, M.D. [32]
Professor of Medicine; Chief, Gastroenterology, University of California, San Diego, La Jolla, California
CRBOLAND@UCSD.EDU

Dirk Bootsma, M.D. [28]
Dept. of Cell Biology and Genetics, Erasmus University, Rotterdam, The Netherlands
Bootsma@gen.fgg.eur.nl

Thomas H. Bothwell, M.D., D.Sc. [127]
Emeritus Professor of Medicine, Honorary Professorial Research Fellow, Faculty of Medicine, University of Witwatersrand, Medical School, Johannesburg, South Africa
014jozo@chiron.wits.ac.za

G. Steven Bova, M.D. [56]
Assistant Professor, Depts. of Pathology, Urology and Oncology, Johns Hopkins Hospital, Pelican Laboratory, Baltimore, Maryland
gbov@jhmi.edu

Bernard Brais, M.D., MPhil, Ph.D. [216]
Direction de L'IREP, Centre de recherche du CHUM, Hopital Notre-Dame, Montreal, Quebec, Canada

David S. Bredt, M.D., Ph.D. [168]
Associate Professor of Physiology, Dept. of Physiology, University of California, San Francisco
bredt@phy.ucsf.edu

Jan L. Breslow, M.D. [121]
Frederick Henry Leonhardt Professor, Director, Laboratory of Biochemical Genetics and Metabolism, The Rockefeller University, New York, New York
breslow@rockvax.rockefeller.edu

Martijn H. Breuning, M.D. [248]
Dept. of Clinical Genetics, Centre for Human and Clinical Genetics, Leiden University Medical Centre, Leiden, The Netherlands M.H.Breuning@kgc.azl.nl

H. Bryan Brewer, Jr., M.D. [118, 122]
Chief, Molecular Disease Branch, National Heart, Lung, and Blood Institute, Bethesda, Maryland
bryan@mdb.nhlbi.nih.gov

Garrett M. Brodeur, M.D. [21, 60]
Div. of Oncology, Children's Hospital of Philadelphia, Philadelphia, Pennsylvania
brodeur@email.chop.edu

Dieter Brömme, Ph.D. [137]
Associate Professor of Human Genetics, Mount Sinai School of Medicine, New York, New York
brommd01@doc.mssm.edu

Michael D. Brown [105]
Assistant Professor, The Center for Molecular Medicine, Emory University School of Medicine, Atlanta, Georgia
mdbrown@gen.emory.edu

Michael S. Brown, M.D. [120]
Regental Professor, Johnson Center for Molecular Genetics, University of Texas Southwestern Medical Center, Dallas, Texas
mike.brown@utsouthwestern.edu

George J. Broze, Jr., M.D. [175]
Professor of Medicine, Cell Biology and Physiology, Washington University School of Medicine, Barnes-Jewish Hospital at Washington University, St. Louis, Missouri
gbroze@im.wustl.edu

John D. Brunzell, M.D. [117]
Professor of Medicine, Program Director, General Clinical Research Center, Dept. of Medicine, University of Washington School of Medicine, Seattle, Washington
brunzell@u.washington.edu

Saul W. Brusilow, M.D. [85]
Professor of Pediatrics Emeritus, The Johns Hopkins Hospital, Baltimore, Maryland
sbru@jhmi.edu

Manuel Buchwald, O.C., Ph.D., F.R.S.C. [31]
Professor, Molecular and Medical Genetics, University of Toronto, Chief of Research and Director, Research Institute, Hospital for Sick Children, Toronto, Ontario, Canada
Manuel.Buchwald@sickkids.on.ca

Peter H. Byers, M.D. [205]
Professor, Dept. of Pathology and Medicine, Dept. of Pathology, University of Washington, Seattle, Washington
pbyers@u.washington.edu

Daniel P Cahill, M.D., Ph.D. [22]
Dept. of Oncology, The Johns Hopkins University School of Medicine, Baltimore, Maryland

Paul Cairns, M.D. [54]
Fox Chase Cancer Center, Philadelphia, Pennsylvania 19111

Giovanna Camerino, Ph.D. [62]
Professor Biologia Generale E Genetica Medica, Universitá Di Pavia, Pavia, Italy
camerino@unipv.it

Hubert Carchon, Ph.D. [74]
Assistant Professor, University of Leuven, Centre for Metabolic Disease, Leuven, Belgium
hubert.carchon@med.kuleuven.ac.be

Eugene D. Carstea, M.D. [145]
Director, Saccomanno Research Institute, St. Mary's Hospital and Medical Center, Grand Junction, Colorado
gcarstea@stmarygj.com

Webster K. Cavenee, M.D. [36]
Director, Ludwig Institute for Cancer Research, University of California, San Diego, La Jolla, California

Aravinda Chakravarti, Ph.D. [251]
Henry J. Knott Professor and Director, McKusick-Nathans Institute of Genetic Medicine, Johns Hopkins University School of Medicine, Baltimore, Maryland
aravinda@jhmi.edu

Arlene B. Chapman, M.D. [215]
Associate Professor of Medicine, Director, Hypertension and Renal Disease Research Center, Emory University School of Medicine, Atlanta, Georgia
arlene_chapman@emory.org

Robert W. Charlton, M.D. [127]
Emeritus Professor, University of Witwatersrand Medical School, Johannesburg, South Africa
014jozo@chiron.wits.ac.za

Christiane Charpentier, Ph.D. [66]
Biologist, INSERM-Paris France, Metabolic/Diabetes Unit-Dept. of Pediatrics, Hopital Necker Enfants Malades, Paris, France
Elisabeth.saudubray@nck.ap_hop_paris.fr

Yuan-Tsong Chen, M.D., Ph.D. [71]
Professor of Pediatrics and Genetics, Chief, Div. of Medical Genetics, Duke University Medical Center, Durham, North Carolina
chen0010@mc.duke.edu

Russell W. Chesney, M.D. [194]
Le Bonheur Professor and Chair, Dept. of Pediatrics, Le Bonheur Children's Medical Center, University of Tennessee, Memphis, Tennessee
rchesney@utmem.edu

Barton Childs, M.D. [2, 3, 4]
Emeritus Professor of Pediatrics, The Johns Hopkins University School of Medicine, Baltimore, Maryland

Kathleen R. Cho, M.D. [53]
Associate Professor, Depts. of Pathology and Internal Medicine, University of Michigan Medical School, Ann Arbor, Michigan
kathcho@umich.edu

Streamson C. Chua, Jr. [157]
Dept. of Medicine, Columbia University College of Physicians and Surgeons, New York, New York

David T. Chuang, Ph.D. [87]
Associate Professor, Dept. of Biochemistry, University of Texas Southwestern Medical Center, Dallas, Texas
david.chuang@utsouthwestern.edu

Dominic W. Chung, Ph.D. [171]
Dept. of Biochemistry School of Medicine, University of Washington, Seattle, Washington
chung@u.washington.edu

Carmen Cifuentes-Diaz, Ph.D. [231]
Laboratoire de Neurogénétique Molécularie, INSERM, GENOPOLE, Evry, France
c.diaz@genopole.inserm.fr

James E. Cleaver, M.D. [28]
Dept. of Dermatology, University of California at San Francisco Cancer Center, San Francisco, California
jcleaver@cc.ucsf.edu

J.B. Clegg [181]
Institute of Molecular Medicine, John Radcliffe Hospital, Oxford, United Kingdom

Bruce E. Clurman, M.D. [23]
Assistant Professor, Fred Hutchinson Cancer Research Center, Seattle, Washington
bclurman@fhcrc.org

Anne-Marie Codori, Ph.D. [49]
Dept. of Psychiatry and Behavioral Sciences, The Johns Hopkins University School of Medicine, Baltimore, Maryland

Joy D. Cogan, M.D. [162]
Research Assistant Professor of Pediatric Genetics, Div. of Genetics, Vanderbilt University School of Medicine, Nashville, Tennessee
joy.cogan@mcmail.vanderbilt.edu

Francis S. Collins, M.D., Ph.D. [39]
National Human Genome Research Institute, Bethesda, Maryland
Fc23@nih.gov

Mary Ellen Conley, M.D. [184]
St. Jude Children's Research Hospital, University of Tennessee School of Medicine, Memphis, Tennessee
maryellen.conley@stjude.org

David N. Cooper, Ph.D. [13]
Professor of Human Molecular Genetics, Institute of Medical Genetics, University of Wales College of Medicine, Cardiff, Wales, United Kingdom
cooperdn@cardiff.ac.uk

Valerie Cormier-Daire, M.D., Ph.D. [99]
Dept. of Medical Genetics, Hopital Necker Enfants Malades, Paris, France
cormier@necker.fr

Richard G.H. Cotton, Ph.D., D.Sc. [1, 78]
Professor, Mutation Research Centre, Director, Mutation Research Centre, St. Vincent's Hospital, Fitzroy, Victoria, Australia
cotton@ariel.ucs.unimelb.edu.au

Fergus J. Couch, M.D. [47]
Assistant Professor, Dept. of Laboratory Medicine and Pathology, Mayo Foundation and Clinic, Rochester, Minnesota
Couch.Fergus@mayo.edu

Diane Wilson Cox, M.D., Ph.D. [219]
Professor and Chair, Dept. of Medical Genetics, Genetics Sect. Head, Child Health, Capital Health Authority, Dept. of Medical Genetics, University of Alberta, Edmonton, Alberta, Canada
diane.cox@ualberta.ca

Rody P. Cox, M.D., Ph.D. [86]
Professor of Internal Medicine, Dept. of Internal Medicine, University of Texas, Southwestern Medical Center, Attending Physician, Parkland Memorial Hospital and St. Paul University Hospital, Dallas, Texas
rcox@mednet.swmed.edu

William J. Craigen, M.D., Ph.D. [14]
Dept. of Molecular and Human Genetics, Baylor College of Medicine, Houston, Texas
wcraigen@bcm.tmc.edu

Donnell J. Creel, Ph.D. [220]
Research Professor, Moran Eye Center, University of Utah School of Medicine, Salt Lake City, Utah
Donnell.creel@hsc.utah.edu

Frans P.M. Cremers, Ph.D. [236]
Associate Professor, Dept. of Human Genetics University Medical Center Nymegen, Nymegen, The Netherlands
F.Cremers@Antrg.azn.nl

Valeria Cizewski Culotta, Ph.D. [126]
Associate Professor, Dept. of Environmental Health Sciences, Johns Hopkins University, School of Hygiene and Public Health, Baltimore, Maryland
vculotta@JHSPH.edu

Garry R. Cutting, M.D. [201]
Professor of Pediatrics and Medicine, McKusick-Nathan Institute of Genetic Medicine, The Johns Hopkins University, Baltimore, Maryland
gcutting@jhmi.edu

Christopher J. Danpure, Ph.D. [133]
Professor of Molecular Cell Biology, MRC Laboratory for Molecular Cell Biology, University College London, London, United Kingdom
c.danpure@ucl.ac.uk

Earl W. Davie, Ph.D. [169]
Dept. of Biochemistry School of Medicine, University of Washington, Seattle, Washington

Alessandra d'Azzo, Ph.D. [152]
Professor, Member, Dept. of Genetics, St. Jude Children's Research Hospital, Memphis, Tennessee
sandra.dazzo@stjude.org

Samir S. Deeb, Ph.D. [117, 238]
Research Professor of Medicine and Genetics, Dept. of Genetics, University of Washington School of Medicine, Seattle, Washington
deeb@genetics.washington.edu

Robert J. Desnick, Ph.D., M.D. [124, 137, 139, 144, 150]
Professor and Chairman, Human Genetics, Professor of Pediatrics; Attending Physician, Dept. of Human Genetics, Mount Sinai School of Medicine, New York, New York
rjdesnick@mcvax.mssm.edu

Harry C. Dietz, M.D. [206]
Associate Investigator, Howard Hughes Medical Institute, Professor, Dept. of Pediatrics, Medicine and Molecular Biology and Genetics, McKusick-Nathan Institute of Genetic Medicine, Johns Hopkins University School of Medicine, Baltimore, Maryland
hdietz@jhmi.edu

Mary C. Dinauer, M.D., Ph.D. [189]
Novz Letzter Professor of Pediatrics and Medical and Molecular Genetics, Riley Hospital for Children, Indiana University School of Medicine, Director, Herman B. Wells Center for Pediatric Research, Indianapolis, Indiana
mdinauer@iupui.edu

Jiahuan Ding, M.D., Ph.D. [101]
Director, Molecular Diagnostics, Senior Scientist, Associate Professor, Baylor University, Waco, Texas, Institute of Metabolic Disease, Baylor University Medical Center, Dallas, Texas
j.ding@baylordallas.edu

Michael J. Dixon, M.D. [246]
Professor of Dental Genetics, School of Biological Sciences, Dept. of Dental Medicine and Surgery, University of Manchester, Manchester, United Kingdom
mdixon@fs1.scg.man.ac.uk

Patricia A. Donohoue, M.D. [159]
Associate Professor, Dept. of Pediatrics, Div. of Endocrinology, University of Iowa Hospitals, Dept. of Pediatrics, The Children's Hospital of Iowa, Iowa City, Iowa
patricia-donohoue@uiowa.edu

Thaddeus P. Dryja, M.D. [235]
Professor of Ophthalmology, Harvard Medical School, Dept. of Ophthalmology, Massachusetts Eye and Ear Infirmary, Boston, Massachusetts
dryja@helix.mgh.harvard.edu

Louis Dubeau, M.D., Ph.D. [51]
Professor, Dept. of Pathology, USC/Norris Comprehensive Cancer Center, Keck School of Medicine of USC, Los Angeles, California
ldubeau@hsc.usc.edu

Thomas D. DuBose, Jr., M.D. [195]
Peter T. Bohan Professor and Chair, Dept. of Internal Medicine, Professor of Molecular and Integrative Physiology, University of Kansas School of Medicine, Kansas City, Kansas
tdubose@kumc.edu

Jacques E. Dumont, M.D., Ph.D. [158]
Professor of Biochemistry, Head, Institut de Recherche interdisciplinaire, Faculté de Medecine, Université Libre de Bruxelles, Brussels, Belgium
jedumont@ulb.ac.be

Marinus Duran, M.D. [128]
Academic Medical Center, Laboratory Genetic Metabolic Diseases, University of Amsterdam, Amsterdam, The Netherlands
m.duram@amc.uva.nl

Michael J. Econs, M.D. [197]
Associate Professor of Medicine and Medical and Molecular Genetics, Indiana University School of Medicine, Indianapolis, Indiana
mecons@iupui.edu

Lora Hedrick Ellenson, M.D. [52]
Associate Professor and Director, Div. of Gynecologic Pathology, Weill Medical College of Cornell University, New York, New York
lhellens@med.cornell.edu

Nathan A. Ellis, M.D. [59]
Associate Member, Dept. of Human Genetics, Memorial Sloan-Kettering Cancer Center, New York, New York
n-ellis@ski.mskcc.org

Lynne W. Elmore, Ph.D. [59]
Research Associate, Dept. of Pathology, School of Medicine, Virginia Commonwealth University, Richmond, Virginia
LWElmore@hsc.vcu.edu

Charis Eng, M.D., Ph.D. [45]
Assoc. Professor of Medicine and Human Cancer Genetics, The Ohio State University; Hon. Fellow, CRC, Human Cancer Genetics Research Group, Univ. of Cambridge, United Kingdom; Director, Clinical Cancer Genetics Program, Ohio State University, Columbus, Ohio
Eng-1@medctr.osu.edu

Christine M. Eng, M.D. [150]
Associate Professor, Dept. of Molecular and Human Genetics, Baylor College of Medicine, Houston, Texas
ceng@bcm.tmc.edu

Charles J. Epstein, M.D. [63]
Professor of Pediatrics, Co-Director, Program of Human Genetics, Chief, Div. of Medical Genetics, Dept. of Pediatrics, University of California at San Francisco, California
cepst@itsa.ucsf.edu

Charles T. Esmon, Ph.D. [170]
Head, Cardiovascular Biology Research Program, Oklahoma Medical Research Foundation, Investigator, Howard Hughes Medical Institute, Oklahoma Medical Research Foundation, Oklahoma City, Oklahoma
charles-esmon@omrf.ouhsc.edu

Lindsay A. Farrer, Ph.D. [234]
Genetics Program, Boston University School of Medicine, Boston, Massachusetts
farrer@neugen.bu.edu

Eric R. Fearon, M.D. [26]
Div. of Molecular Medicine and Genetics, University of Michigan Medical Center, Ann Arbor, Michigan
fearon@umich.edu

Andrew P. Feinberg, M.D., M.P.H. [18]
King Fahd Professor of Medicine, Oncology and Molecular Biology and Genetics, Johns Hopkins Medical School, Baltimore, Maryland
afeinberg@jhu.edu

Anthony H. Fensom, Ph.D. [143]
Prince Philip Laboratory, Guy's Hospital, London, United Kingdom

Wayne A. Fenton, Ph.D. [94, 155]
Dept. of Genetics, Yale University School of Medicine, New Haven, Connecticut
wayne.fenton@yale.edu

Malcolm A. Ferguson-Smith, F.R.S. [62]
Professor, Dept. of Clinical Veterinary Medicine, University of Cambridge, Centre for Veterinary Science, Cambridge, United Kingdom

Clair A. Francomano, M.D. [210]
National Center for Human Genome Research, National Institutes of Health, Bethesda, Maryland
clairf@nhgri.nih.giv

Deborah L. French, Ph.D. [177]
Assistant Professor of Medicine and Immunobiology, Div. of Hematology, Mount Sinai School of Medicine, New York, New York
dfrench@mssm.edu

Frank E. Frerman, Ph.D. [95, 103]
Professor of Pediatrics, Dept. of Pediatrics, University of Colorado Health Science Center, Denver, Colorado
Frank.frerman@uchsc.edu

Carol Freund, Ph.D. [240]
Dept. of Clinical Bioethics, National Institutes of Health, Bethesda, Maryland
cfreund@nih.gov

Theodore Friedmann, M.D. [107]
Dept. of Pediatric/Molecular Genetics, University of California, San Diego, Center for Molecular Genetics, La Jolla, California
tfriedmann@ucsd.edu

Tony Frugier, MSc [231]
Laboratoire de Neurogénétique Moléculaire, INSERM, GENOPOLE, Evry, France
t.frugier@genopole.inserm.fr

Elaine Fuchs, Ph.D. [221]
Amgen Professor of Basic Sciences, HHMI, Dept. of Molecular Genetics and Cell Biology, University of Chicago, Chicago, Illinois
lain@midway.uchicago.edu

Lars Fugger, M.D., Ph.D. [12]
Professor, Dept. of Clinical Immunology, Aarhus University Hospital, Aarhus, Denmark
fugger@inet.uni2.dk

T. Mary Fujiwara, MSc [163]
Assistant Professor, Depts. of Human Genetics and Medicine, McGill University, Div. of Medical Genetics, Montreal General Hospital, Montreal, Quebec, Canada
fujiwara@bagel.epi.mcgill.ca

Toshiyuki Fukao, M.D., Ph.D. [102]
Department of Pediatrics, Gifu University School of Medecine, Gifu, Japan
toshi-gif@umin.ac.jp

William A. Gahl, M.D., Ph.D. [199, 200]
Head, Sect. on Human Biochemical Genetics, Heritable Disorders Branch, National Institute of Child Health and Human Development, Bethesda, Maryland
bgahl@helix.nih.gov

David Gailani, M.D. [175]
Assistant Professor of Pathology and Medicine, Director, Clinical Coagulation Laboratory, Vanderbilt Hospital, Hematology/Oncology Div., Vanderbilt University, Nashville, Tennessee
dave.gailani@mcmail.vanderbilt.edu

Hans Galjaard, M.D., Ph.D. [152]
Professor of Clinical Genetics, Dept. of Clinical Genetics, Erasmus University Medical Faculty, Rotterdam, The Netherlands
galjaard@algm.azr.nl

Carlos A. Garcia, M.D. [227]
Professor, Dept. of Psychiatry and Neurology, Tulane University Health Sciences Center, New Orleans, Louisiana
cgarcia2@tulane.edu

Paolo Gasparini, M.D. [191]
Medical Genetics Service, IRCCS-Ospedale CSS, San Giovanni Rotondo, Foggia, Italy
genetcss@fg.nettuno.it

Richard A. Gatti, M.D. [29]
Professor, Dept. of Pathology, School of Medicine, University of California, Los Angeles, Los Angeles, California
rgatti@mednet.ucla.edu

Bruce D. Gelb, M.D. [137]
Associate Professor of Pediatrics and Human Genetics, Mount Sinai School of Medicine, New York, New York
gelbb01@doc.mssm.edu

James L. German, III, M.D. [30]
Professor, Dept. of Pediatrics, Weill Medical College of Cornell University, New York, New York
jlg2003@mail.med.cornell.edu

Gregory G. Germino, M.D. [215]
Associate Professor of Medicine, Div. of Nephrology, Johns Hopkins University School of Medicine, Baltimore, Maryland
ggermino@welch.jhu.edu

Ali Gharavi, M.D. [211]
Assistant Professor of Medicine, Mount Sinai School of Medicine, New York, New York; Visiting Assistant Professor, Dept. of Genetics, Yale University School of Medicine, New Haven, Connecticut
ali.gharavi@yale.edu

K. Michael Gibson, Ph.D. [91]
Director, Biochemical Genetics Laboratory, Associate Professor, Dept. of Molecular and Medical Genetics, Biochemical Genetics Lab, Oregon University Health Sciences, Portland, Oregon
gibsonm@ohsu.edu

Volkmar Gieselmann, M.D. [148]
Professor and Director, Biochemisches Institut, Christian-Albrechts-Universitat Zu Kiel, Kiel, Germany
office@biochem.uni-kiel.de

Rachel H. Giles, Ph.D. [248]
Dept. of Immunology, University Medical Center Utrecht, Utrecht, The Netherlands
R.Giles@lab.azu.nl

David Ginsburg, M.D. [178]
Warner-Lambert/Parke-Davis Professor of Medicine and Human Genetics, Investigator, Howard Hughes Medical Institute, The University of Michigan Medical Center, Ann Arbor, Michigan
ginsburg@umich.edu

Jonathan David Gitlin, M.D. [126]
Helene B. Roberson Professor of Pediatrics, Professor of Pathology and Immunology, Director, Division of Pediatric Immunology and Rheumatology, Washington University School of Medicine, St. Louis Children's Hospital, St. Louis, Missouri
gitlin@kidsal.wustl.edu

Richard Gitzelmann, M.D. [70]
Professor Emeritus, Div. of Metabolic and Molecular Pediatrics, University Children's Hospital, University of Zurich, Zurich, Switzerland

M. Goedert, M.D., Ph.D. [234]
MRC Laboratory of Molecular Biology, Cambridge, England, United Kingdom
mg@mrc-lmb.cam.ac.uk

Joseph L. Goldstein, M.D. [120]
Paul J. Thomas, Professor of Genetics and Chair, Dept. of Molecular Genetics, University of Texas Southwestern Medical Center, Dallas, Texas
joseph.goldstein@utsouthwestern.edu

Peter N. Goodfellow, B.Sc., D.Phil. [62]
Senior Vice President, Discovery Biopharmaceutical Research and Development, SmithKline Beecham, Harlow, Essex, United Kingdom
peter_n_goodfellow@sbphrd.com

Stephen I. Goodman, M.D. [95, 103]
Chief, Sect. of Genetics, Metabolism, and Birth Defects, Professor of Pediatrics, Dept. of Pediatrics, School of Medicine, University of Colorado Health Science Center, Denver, Colorado
stephen.goodman@uchsc.edu

Paul Goodyer, M.D. [191]
Professor of Pediatrics, McGill University, Montreal Children's Hospital, Nephrology Dept., Montreal, Quebec, Canada
paul.goodyer@muhc.mcgill.ca

Jerome L. Gorski, M.D. [247]
Professor of Pediatrics and Human Genetics, Director, Div. of Pediatric Genetics, Div. of Clinical Genetics, Dept. of Pediatrics, University of Michigan, Ann Arbor, Michigan
jlgorski@umich.edu

André Gougoux, M.D. [196]
Professor of Medicine, CHUM (Pavillon Notre Dame), Université de Montréal, Montreal, Quebec, Canada

Stephen J. Gould, Ph.D. [129]
Associate Professor, Dept. of Biological Chemistry, The Johns Hopkins University School of Medicine, Baltimore, Maryland
sgould@jhmi.edu

Gregory A. Grabowski, M.D. [146]
Director, Div. and Program in Human Genetics, Children's Hospital Research Foundation, Cincinnati, Ohio
grabg0@chmcc.org

Denis M. Grant, Ph.D. [9]
Genetics and Genomic Biology Programme, Research Institute, Hospital for Sick Children, Toronto, Ontario, Canada
grant@sickkids.on.ca

Roy A. Gravel, Ph.D. [94, 153]
Professor, Cell Biology and Anatomy, University of Calgary, Calgary, Alberta, Canada
rgravel@ucalgary.ca

Eric D. Green, M.D., Ph.D [10]
Chief, Genome Technology Branch, Director, NIH, Intramural Sequencing Center, National Human Genome Research Institute, Bethesda, Maryland
egreen@nhgri.nih.gov

Daniel L. Greenberg, M.D. [169]
Dept. of Medicine, University of Washington Medical Center, Division of Hematology, Seattle, Washington
robin@u.washington.edu

James E. Griffin, M.D. [160]
Professor of Internal Medicine, Diana and Richard C. Strauss Professor in Biomedical Research, University of Texas Southwestern Medical Center, Dallas, Texas
jgrif2@mednet.swmed.edu

Markus Grompe, M.D. [79]
Dept. of Molecular/Medical Genetics and Dept. of Pediatrics, Oregon Health Sciences University, Portland, Oregon
grompem@ohsu.edu

James Gusella, M.D. [40]
Molecular Neurogenetics Unit, Massachusetts General Hospital, Charlestown, Massachusetts

David H. Gutmann, M.D., Ph.D. [39]
Associate Professor, Director, Neurofibromatosis Program, St. Louis Children's Hospital, Dept. of Neurology, Washington University, St. Louis, Missouri
gutmannd@neuro.wustl.edu

Daniel A. Haber, M.D., Ph.D. [38]
Associate Professor of Medicine, Harvard Medical School, Director, Center for Cancer Risk Analysis, Massachusetts General Hospital Cancer Center, Lab of Molecular Genetics, Charlestown, Massachusetts
haber@helix.mgh.harvard.edu

Theodora Hadjistilianou, M.D. [36]
Associate Professor, Dept. of Ophthalmology, University of Siena School of Medicine, Siena, Tuscany, Italy

Judith G. Hall, M.D. [15]
Dept. of Pediatrics, British Columbia Children's Hospital, Vancouver, British Columbia, Canada
judyhall@interchange.ubc.ca

Ada Hamosh, M.D., M.P.H. [1, 90]
Associate Professor of Pediatric, McKusick-Nathans Institute of Genetic Medicine, The Johns Hopkins University School of Medicine, Johns Hopkins Hospital, Baltimore, Maryland
ahamosh@jhmi.edu

Folker Hanefeld, M.D. [84]
Professor of Pediatrics and Child Neurology, Georg-August-Universitat, Zentrum Kinderheilkunde, Abt. Padiatrie, Schwerpunkt Neuropadiatrie, Germany

Isabel Hanson, M.D. [240]
Molecular Medicine Center, Western General Hospital, Edinburgh, United Kingdom
isabel.hanson@ed.ac.uk

Jean-Pierre Hardelin [254]
Unite de Genetique des Deficits Sensoriels, Institut Pasteur, Paris, France

Peter S. Harper, M.D. [217]
Professor and Consultant in Medical Genetics, University of Wales College of Medicine, Heath Park Institute of Medical Genetics, Cardiff, United Kingdom
harperps@cardiff.ac.uk

Curtis C. Harris, M.D. [59]
Chief, Laboratory of Human Carcinogenesis, National Cancer Institute, Bethesda, Maryland
Curtis_Harris@NIH.GOV

Klaus Harzer, M.D. [134]
Professor, Neurochemical Laboratory, University of Tübingen, Institut für Hirnforschung, Tübingen, Germany
hirnforschung@uni-tuebingen.de

Richard J. Havel, M.D. [114, 115]
Professor Emeritus, Cardiovascular Research Institute, University of California School of Medicine, San Francisco, California
dargank@curi.ucsf.edu

J. Ross Hawkins, Ph.D. [62]
Principal Scientist of Development Incyte Genomics, Ltd. Cambridge, United Kingdom
Ross.Hawkins@incyte.com

Michael R. Hayden, M.D., ChB, Ph.D., FRCP(C), FRSC [223]
Professor of Medical Genetics, Centre for Molecular Medicine and Therapeutics, University of British Columbia, Vancouver, British Columbia, Canada
mrh@cmmt.ubc.ca

Vincent J. Hearing, M.D. [220]
Laboratory of Cell Biology, National Institutes of Health, Bethesda, Maryland

Jacqueline T. Hecht, Ph.D. [210]
Dept. of Pediatrics, University of Texas Medical School, Houston, Texas
jhecht@ped1.med.uth.tmc.edu

Peter Hechtman, Ph.D. [82]
Associate Professor of Biology, Human Genetics, and Pediatrics, McGill University, Dept. of Biochemical Genetics, Montreal Children's Hospital, Montreal, Quebec, Canada
Peter@uww.debelle.mcgill.ca

James F. Hejtmancik, M.D., Ph.D. [241]
National Eye Institute, National Institutes of Health, Bethesda, Maryland
f3h@helix.nih.gov

Raoul C. M. Hennekam, Ph.D., M.D. [248, 249]
Pediatrician and Clinical Geneticist, Dept. of Pediatrics and Institute for Human Genetics, Academic Medical Center, University of Amsterdam, Amsterdam, The Netherlands
r.c.hennekam@amc.uva.nl

Meenhard Herlyn, Ph.D. [44]
Professor, The Wistar Institute, Philadelphia, Pennsylvania
herlynm@wistar.upenn.edu

Michael S. Hershfield, M.D. [109]
Dept. of Medicine and Biochemistry, Duke University Medical Center, Durham, North Carolina
msh@biochem.duke.edu

Hugo S.A. Heymans [130]
Professor of Pediatrics, Director and Chairman. Emma Children's Hospital and Clinical Chemistry, University of Amsterdam Academic Medical Centre, Amsterdam, The Netherlands
h.s.heymans@amc.uva.nl

Howard H. Hiatt, M.D. [73]
Professor of Medicine, Harvard Medical School, Senior Physician, Div. of General Medicine, Dept. of Medicine, Brigham and Women's Hospital, Boston, Massachusetts
hhiatt@partners.org

D.R. Higgs [181]
Institute of Molecular Medicine, John Radcliffe Hospital, Oxford, United Kingdom
drhiggs@molbiol.ox.ac.uk

Katherine A. High, M.D. [173]
William H. Bennett Professor of Pediatrics, UPENN School of Medicine, Director of Research, Hematology Div., Director, Hematology and Coagulation Laboratories, Children's Hospital of Philadelphia, Philadelphia, Pennsylvania
high@email.chop.edu

Adrian V. S. Hill, D.Phil., D.M. [7]
Professor of Human Genetics, Wellcome Trust Centre for Human Genetics, Headington, Oxford, United Kingdom
adrian.hill@imm.ox.ac.uk

Akira Hirono, M.D., Ph.D. [182]
Research Associate, Okinaka Memorial Institute for Medical Research, Tokyo, Japan
Ncc01353@nifty.nc.jp

Rochelle Hirschhorn, M.D. [135]
Professor of Medicine and Cell Biology, Chief, Div. of Medical Genetics, Dept. of Medicine, New York University School of Medicine, New York, New York
hirscr01@mcrcr0.med.nyu.edu

Helen H. Hobbs, M.D. [120]
Professor, Depts. of Internal Medicine and Molecular Genetics, The University of Texas Southwestern Medical Center at Dallas, Dallas, Texas
helen.hobbs@utsouthwestern.edu

Jan H.J. Hoeijmakers, M.D. [28]
Dept. of Cell Biology and Genetics, Erasmus University, Rotterdam, The Netherlands
hoeijmakers@gen.fgg.eur.nl

Sandra L. Hofmann, M.D., Ph.D. [154]
Associate Professor of Internal Medicine, Hamon Center for Therapeutic Oncology Research, University of Texas Southwestern Medical Center, Dallas, Texas
hofmann@simmons.swmed.edu

Jeffrey M. Hoeg, M.D. [118]
Chief, Section on Molecular Biology, Molecular Disease Branch, National Institutes of Health, Bethesda, Maryland
Deceased 7/21/98.

Michael D. Hogarty, M.D. [21]
Div. of Oncology, The Children's Hospital of Philadelphia, Philadelphia, Pennsylvania
hogartym@email.chop.edu

Edward J. Hollox, Ph.D. [76]
Institute of Genetics, University of Nottingham, Queens Medical Centre Nottingham, United Kingdom
Ed.Hollox@Nottingham.ac.uk

Edward W. Holmes, M.D. [110]
Vice Chancellor and Dean, School of Medicine, University of California, San Diego, California

John B. Holton, Ph.D. [72]
Emeritus Consultant Clinical Scientist, Clinical Biochemistry, Southmead Hospital, Bristol, United Kingdom

John J. Hopwood, Ph.D. [149]
Professor & Head, Lysosomal Diseases Research Unit, Dept. of Chemical Pathology, Women's and Children's Hospital, North Adelaide, South Australia
john.hopwood@adelaide.edu.au

Ourania Horaitis, B.Sc. [1]
Co-ordinator, HUGO Mutation Database Initiative, Mutation Research Centre, St. Vincent's Hospital, Fitzroy, Melbourne, Victoria, Australia
horaitis@ariel.ucs.unimelb.edu.au

D. Jonathan Horsford, B.Sc. [240]
Program in Developmental Biology, Hospital for Sick Children, Toronto, Ontario, Canada
djhors@sickkids.on.ca

Arthur L. Horwich, M.D. [85]
Professor of Genetics and Pediatrics, Investigator, HHMI, Yale School of Medicine/HHMI, New Haven, Connecticut
horwich@csb.yale.edu

James R. Howe, M.D. [35]
Assistant Professor, Dept. of Surgery, University of Iowa College of Medicine, Iowa City, Iowa
James_howe@uiowa.edu

Ralph H. Hruban, M.D. [50]
Professor of Pathology and Oncology, The Johns Hopkins University, School of Medicine, Dept. of Oncology and Pathology, Baltimore, Maryland
rhruban@jhmi.edu

Chien-an A. Hu, Ph.D. [81]
Research Associate, McKusick-Nathans Institute of Genetic Medicine, Johns Hopkins University School of Medicine, Baltimore, Maryland
cahu@welch.jhu.edu

Lynn D. Hudson, Ph.D. [228]
Acting Chief, Lab of Developmental Neurogenetics, National Institute of Neurologic Disorders and Stroke, National Institutes of Health, Bethesda, Maryland
hudsonl@ninds.nih.gov

Donald E. Hultquist [180]
Associate Chair, Dept. of Biological Chemistry, University of Michigan Medical School, Ann Arbor, Michigan
hultquis@umich.edu

Keith Hyland, Ph.D. [78]
Associate Professor, Baylor University, Associate Professor, University of Texas Southwestern Medical Center, Senior Research Scientist, Baylor University Medical Center, Institute of Metabolic Diseases, Dallas, Texas
k.hyland@baylordallas.edu

Akitada Ichinose, M.D., Ph.D. [171]
Professor and Chairman, Dept. of Molecular Pathological Biochemistry, Yamagata University School of Medicine, Yamagata, Japan
aichinos@med.id.yamagata-u.ac.jp

Yiannis A. Ioannou, Ph.D. [150]
Associate Professor, Dept. of Human Genetics, Mount Sinai School of Medicine, New York, New York
yiannis.ioannou@mssm.edu

William B. Isaacs, Ph.D. [56]
Professor of Urology and of Oncology, Dept. of Urology, The Johns Hopkins University School of Medicine, Baltimore, Maryland
wisaacs@mail.jhmi.edu

Dirk Isbrandt, M.D. [84]
Research Scientist, Universitat Hamburg, Zentrum fur Molekulare Neurobiologie Hamburg, Institut fur Neurale Signalverarbeitung, Hamburg, Germany
isbrandt@uni-hamburg.de

Jaak Jaeken, M.D., Ph.D. [74, 112, 148]
Professor of Pediatrics, University of Leuven; Director, Center for Metabolic Disease, University Hospital Gasthuisberg, Leuven, Belgium
Jaak.jacken@uz.kuleuven.ac.be

Ernst R. Jaffe, M.D. [180]
Distinguished University Professor of Medicine Emeritus, Albert Einstein College of Medicine, Bronx, New York
(Deceased)

Cornelis Jakobs, Ph.D. [91, 132]
Associate Professor, Head Metabolic Unit, Dept. of Clinical Chemistry, Vrije Universiteit Medical Centre, Amsterdam, The Netherlands
C.Jakobs@AZVU.nl

Anu Jalanko, Ph.D. [141]
Senior Scientist, Dept. of Human Molecular Genetics, National Public Health Institute, Helsinki, Finland
Anu.jalanko@ktl.fi

Joanna C. Jen, M.D. [204]
Assistant Professor, Dept. of Neurology, UCLA School of Medicine, Los Angeles, California
jjen@ucla.edu

Gerardo Jimenez-Sanchez, M.D., Ph.D. [3,4]
McKusick-Nathans Institute of Genetic Medicine, Johns Hopkins University School of Medicine, Baltimore, Maryland
gjimenez@jhmi.edu

H.A. Jinnah, M.D., Ph.D. [107]
Assistant Professor, Dept. of Neurology, Johns Hopkins Hospital, Baltimore, Maryland
hjinnah@welch.jhu.edu

Hans Joenje, Ph.D. [31]
Senior Scientist, Dept. Clinical and Human Genetics, Free University Medical Center, Amsterdam, The Netherlands
H.Joenje.HumGen@med.vu.nl

Jean L. Johnson, M.D. [128]
Assistant Research Professor, Dept. of Biochemistry, Duke University Medical Center, Durham, North Carolina
jean_johnson@biochem.duke.edu

Keith J. Johnson, Ph.D. [217]
Professor of Genetics, Head, Div. of Molecular Genetics, Institute of Biomedical and Life Sciences, University of Glasgow, Glasgow, United Kingdom
K.Johnson@bio.gla.ac.uk

Michael V. Johnston, M.D. [90]
Professor of Neurology and Pediatrics, The Johns Hopkins University School of Medicine, Kennedy Krieger Institute, Baltimore, Maryland
johnston@kennedykrieger.org

Michael M. Kaback, M.D. [153]
Professor, Depts. of Pediatrics and Reproductive Medicine, University of California, San Diego, Children's Hospital and Health Center, San Diego, California
mkaback@ucsd.edu

Steven E. Kahn, M.B., Ch.B. [67]
Associate Professor of Medicine, University of Washington, Staff Physician, VA Puget Sound Health Care System, Seattle, Washington
skahn@u.washington.edu

Muriel I. Kaiser-Kupfer, M.D. [241]
Chief, Ophthalmic Genetics, National Eye Institute, Bethesda, Maryland
kaiserm@box-k.nih.gov

Anne Kallioniemi, M.D. [20]
Cancer Genetics Branch, National Human Genome Research Institute, Bethesda, Maryland

Werner Kalow, M.D. [9]
Professor Emeritus, Dept. of Pharmacology, University of Toronto, Toronto, Ontario, Canada
w.kalow@utoronto.ca

Naoyuki Kamatani, M.D. [108]
Professor and Director, Institute of Rheumatology, Tokyo Women's Medical University, Tokyo, Japan
kamatani@ior.twmu.ac.jp

Alexander Kamb, Ph.D. [44]
Chief Scientific Officer, Arcaris, Inc., Salt Lake City, Utah
kamb@arcaris.com

John P. Kane, M.D., Ph.D. [114, 115]
University of California, San Francisco, California
Kane@itsa.ucsf.edu

Hitoshi Kanno, M.D., Ph.D. [182]
Assistant Professor, Dept. of Biochemistry, Nihon University School of Medicine, Tokyo, Japan
hikanno@med.nihon-u.ac.jp

Josseline Kaplan [237]
Unite de Recherches sur les Handicaps, Genetiques de L'Enfant, INSERM, Hôpital des Enfants Malades, Paris, Cedex, France

George Karpati, M.D., FRCP(C), FRS(C) [216]
Director, Neuromuscular Research, Dept. Neurology/Neurosurgery, Montreal Neurological Institute, McGill University, Montreal, Quebec, Canada
mcgk@musica.mcgill.ca

Seymour Kaufman, Ph.D. [77]
Emeritus Chief, Laboratory of Neurochemistry, National Institute of Mental Health, National Institutes of Health, Bethesda, Maryland
kaufman@codon.nih.gov

Haig H. Kazazian, Jr., M.D. [172]
Chairman, Dept. of Genetics, University of Pennsylvania School of Medicine, Philadelphia, Pennsylvania
kazazian@mail.med.upenn.edu

Mark T. Keating, M.D. [203]
Professor of Medicine and Human Genetics, Eccles Institute of Human Genetics, University of Utah/Howard Hughes Medical Institute, Eccles Institute of Human Genetics, Salt Lake City, Utah
mark@howard.genetics.utah.edu

Richard I. Kelley, M.D., Ph.D. [249]
Associate Professor of Pediatrics, Johns Hopkins University, Director of Metabolism, Kennedy Krieger Institute, Baltimore, Maryland
kelle_ri@jhuvms.hcf.jhu.edu

Scott E. Kern, M.D. [50]
Associate Professor of Oncology, Johns Hopkins University School of Medicine, Baltimore, Maryland
sk@jhmi.edu

Keith Kerstann, M.A. [105]
The Center for Molecular Medicine, Emory University School of Medicine, Atlanta, Georgia
kkersta@gen.emory.edu

Richard A. King, M.D. [220]
Professor, University of Minnesota, Minneapolis, Minnesota
kingx002@tc.umn.edu

Kenneth W. Kinzler, Ph.D. [17, 27, 48]
Professor of Oncology, The Johns Hopkins University School of Medicine, Baltimore, Maryland
kinzlke@jhmi.edu

D. Richard Klausner, M.D. [41]
Director, National Cancer Institute, Bethesda, Maryland
Klausner@helix.nih.gov

Michael Koenig, M.D. [232]
Professor of Medical Genetics, University of Louis Pasteur, Strasbourg; Adjunct Director of the Genetics Diagnosis Laboratory, Institute de Genetique et de Biologie Moleculaire et Cellulaire, CNRS-INSERM-ULP, Illkirch, Strasbourg, France
mkoenig@igbmc.u-strasbg.fr

Thomas Kolter, Ph.D. [134]
Kekule-Institut für Organische Chemie und Biochemie, der Reinnischen Friedrich-Wilhelms Universität Bonn, Bonn, Germany
kolter@snchemie1.chemie.uni-bonn.de

Stuart Kornfeld, M.D. [138]
Professor of Medicine, Div. of Hematology-Oncology, Dept. of Medicine, Washington University School of Medicine, St. Louis, Missouri
skornfel@im.wustl.edu

Kenneth H. Kraemer, M.D. [28]
Research Scientist, Basic Research Laboratory, National Cancer Institute, Bethesda, Maryland
kraemerk@nih.gov

Jan P. Kraus, Ph.D. [88]
Professor of Pediatrics and Cellular/Structural Biology, Dept. of Pediatrics, University of Colorado School of Medicine, Denver, Colorado
jan.kraus@uchsc.edu

Michael Krawczak, M.D. [13]
Professor, Institute of Medical Genetics, University of Wales College of Medicine, Cardiff, Wales, United Kingdom
krawczak@cardiff.ac.uk

Berry Kremer, M.D., Ph.D. [223]
Professor, Dept. of Neurology, University Medical Center Nijmegen, The Netherlands
h.kremer@czzoneu.azn.nl

Anjli Kukreja, Ph.D. [69]
Research Associate, Weill College of Medicine, Cornell University, New York
anjlik@hotmail.com

Bert N. La Du, Jr., M.D., Ph.D. [92]
Emeritus Professor of Pharmacology, Dept. of Pharmacology, University of Michigan Medical School, Ann Arbor, Michigan
bladu@umich.edu

Marie Lambert, M.D. [79]
Service de genetique medicale, Centre de recherche, Ste-Justine Hospital, Montreal, Quebec, Canada
lamberma@medclin.umontreal.ca

Risto Lappatto, M.D., Ph.D. [111]
Consultant Pediatrician, University of Helsinki, Helsinki, Finland
Risto.Lapatto@helsinki.fi

Agne Larsson, M.D., Ph.D. [96]
Professor of Pediatrics, Chairman, Dept. of Pediatrics, Children's Hospital, Karolinska Institutet, Huddinge University Hospital, Stockholm Sweden
agne.larsson@klinvet.ki.se

David H. Ledbetter, Ph.D. [65]
Professor and Chair, Dept. of Human Genetics, The University of Chicago, Chicago, Illinois
dhl@genetics.uchicago.edu

Rudolph L. Leibel, M.D. [157]
Chief, Division of Molecular Genetics, Co-Director, Naomi Berrie Diabetes Center, Professor of Pediatrics and Medicine, Columbia University College of Physicians & Surgeons, New York, New York
RL232@columbia.edu

Eran Leitersdorf, M.D. [123]
Professor of Medicine, Dorothy and Maurice Bucksbaum Chair in Molecular Genetics, Head, Center for Research, Prevention, and Treatment of Atherosclerosis, Dept. of Medicine, Hadassah University Hospital, Jerusalem, Israel
eran1@hadassah.org.il

Christoph Lengauer, M.D. [22]
The Johns Hopkins Oncology Center, Baltimore, Maryland
lengauer@jhmi.edu

Thierry Levade, Ph.D. [143]
Laboratoire de Biochemie, Maladies Metaboliques, CJF INSERM, Institut Louis Bugnard, Toulouse, France

Jacqueline Levilliers [254]
Unite de Genetique des Deficits Sensoriels, Institut Pasteur, Paris, France

Harvey L. Levy, M.D. [80, 88, 193]
Associate Professor of Pediatrics, Harvard Medical School, Senior Associate in Medicine and Genetics, Children's Hospital, Boston, Massachusetts
levy_h@al.tch.harvard.edu

Richard Alan Lewis, M.D. [243]
Professor, Dept. of Ophthalmology, Medicine, Pediatrics and Molecular Human Genetics, Baylor College of Medicine, Houston, Texas
rlewis@bcm.tmc.edu

Roland Libau, M.D. [12]
Postdoctoral Fellow, Dept. of Microbiology and Immunology, Stanford University School of Medicine, Stanford, California

Uri A. Liberman, M.D., Ph.D. [165]
Professor of Physiology and Medicine, Head, Dept. of Endocrinology and Metabolism, Rabin Medical Center, Beilinson Campus, Sackler School of Medicine, Tel-Aviv University, Petach-Tikvah, Israel
uliberman@clalit.org.il

Richard P. Lifton, M.D. [211]
Associate Investigator, Howard Hughes Medical Institute, Chair, Dept. of Genetics, Professor of Genetics, Internal Medicine & Molecular Biophysics, Yale University School of Medicine, New Haven, Connecticut
richard.lifton@yale.edu

W. Marston Linehan, M.D. [41]
Chief, Urologic Oncology Branch, National Cancer Institute, Bethesda, Maryland
Wml@nih.gov

Thomas Linke, M.D. [143]
Institute fur Organisch Chemie, Bonn, Germany

A. Thomas Look, M.D. [19]
Dept. of Experimental Oncology, St. Jude Children's Research Hospital, Memphis, Tennessee
Thomas.look@stjude.org

Marie T. Lott, M.A. [105]
Research Specialist, Supervisor, Center for Molecular Medicine, Emory University School of Medicine, Atlanta, Georgia
mtlott@gen.emory.edu

James R. Lupski, M.D., Ph.D. [65, 227, 243]
Cullen Professor of Molecular and Human Genetics and Professor of Medicine, Dept. of Molecular and Human Genetics, Baylor College of Medicine, Houston, Texas
jlupski@bcm.tmc.edu

Andreas Lux, Ph.D. [212]
Research Associate, Dept. of Genetics, Duke University Medical Center, Durham, North Carolina

Samuel E. Lux, IV, M.D. [183]
Robert A. Stranahan Professor of Pediatrics, Harvard Medical School Chief, Div. of Hematology/Oncology, Children's Hospital, Boston, Massachusetts
lux@genetics.med.harvard.edu

Lucio Luzatto, M.D., Ph.D. [179]
Scientific Director, Instituo Nazionale per la Ricerca sul Cancro, Genova, Italy
luzzatto@hp380.ist.unige.it

Stanislas Lyonnet, M.D., Ph.D. [251]
Professor of Genetics, University of Paris, Dept. de Genetique et Unite, INSERM, Hospital Necker-Enfants Malades, Paris, France
lyonnet@necker.fr

Mack Mabry, M.D. [58]
Div. of Radiology, The Johns Hopkins Hospital, Baltimore, Maryland

Mia MacCollin, M.D. [40]
Assistant Professor of Neurology, Massachusetts General Hospital, Charlestown, Massachusetts
maccollin@helix.mgh.harvard.edu

Noel Keith Maclaren, M.D. [69]
Professor of Pediatrics, Director, Juvenile Diabetes, Weill College of Medicine, Cornell University, New York
NKMaclaren@aol.com

Edward R. B. McCabe, M.D., Ph.D [97, 167]
Professor and Executive Chair, Dept. of Pediatrics UCLA School of Medicine; Physician-in-Chief, Mattel Children's Hospital at UCLA, Los Angeles, California
emccabe@pediatrics.medsch.ucla.edu

Hugh O. McDevitt, M.D. [12]
Professor of Microbiology and Immunology, Stanford University School of Medicine, Stanford, California
hughmcd@stanford.edu

Roderick R. McInnes, M.D., Ph.D. [80, 240]
University of Toronto Tanenbaum Chair in Molecular Medicine, Professor of Pediatrics and Molecular Genetics, University of Toronto, Head, Program in Developmental Biology, Research Institute, Hospital for Sick Children, Toronto, Ontario, Canada
mcinnes@sickkids.on.ca

Victor A. McKusick, M.D. [1]
Professor , McKusick-Nathans Institute of Genetic Medicine, Johns Hopkins University School of Medicine, Baltimore, Maryland
McKusick@peas.welch.jhu.edu

Roger E. McLendon, M.D. [57]
Associate Professor; Director of Anatomic Pathology Services; Chief, Sect. of Neuropathology, Duke University Medical Center, Durham, North Carolina
roger.mclendon@duke.edu

Michael J. McPhaul, M.D. [160]
Professor, Dept. of Internal Medicine, Div. of Endocrinology and Metabolism, University of Texas Southwestern Medical Center, Dallas, Texas
mcphaul@pop3.utsw.swmed.edu

Robert W. Mahley, M.D., Ph.D. [119]
Director, Gladstone Institute of Cardiovascular Disease, Professor of Pathology and Medicine, University of California, San Francisco
rmahley@gladstone.ucsf.edu

David Malkin, M.D. [37]
Associate Professor of Pediatrics, University of Toronto, Program in Cancer and Blood Research, Research Institute, Hospital for Sick Children, Toronto, Ontario, Canada
David.malkin@sickkids.on.ca

Ned Mantei, Ph.D. [75]
Professor, Swiss Federal Institute of Technology, Institute for Cell Biology, Zurich, Switzerland
mantei@cell.biol.ethz.ch

Douglas A. Marchuk, Ph.D. [212]
Assistant Professor, Dept. of Genetics, Duke University Medical Center, Durham, North Carolina
march004@mc.duke.edu

Sandrine Marlin [254]
Unite de Genetique des Deficits Sensoriels, Institut Pasteur, Paris, France

Karen L. Marsh, Ph.D. [246]
University of Manchester, School of Biological Sciences, Manchester, United Kingdom

George M. Martin, M.D. [8]
Professor of Pathology, Adjunct Professor of Genetics, Director, Alzheimer's Disease Research Center, Attending Pathologist, Medical Center, University of Washington School of Medicine, Seattle, Washington
gmmartin@u.washington.edu

Martín G. Martín, M.D. [190]
Dept. of Pediatrics, Gastroenterology, UCLA School of Medicine, Los Angeles, California
mmartin@mednet.ucla.edu

Paula Martin, Ph.D. [214]
Dept. of Biochemistry, University of Oulu, Finland
paula.martin@oula.fi

Stephen J. Marx, M.D. [43, 165]
Chief, Genetics and Endocrinology Sect., National Institutes of Health, Bethesda, Maryland
stephenm@intra.niddk.nih.gov

Gert Matthijs, Ph.D. [74]
Assistant Professor, Center for Human Genetics, University Hospital of Leuven, Centre for Human Genetics, Leuven, Belgium
gert.matthijs@med.kuleuven.ac.be

Atul Mehta, M.D. [179]
Consultant Hematologist, Dept. of Hematology, Royal Free Hospital, London, United Kingdom
atul.mehta@rfh.nthames.nhs.uk

Judith Melki, M.D., Ph.D. [231]
Neurogénétique Moléculaire, INSERM, GENOPOLE, Evry, France
j.melki@genopole.inserm.fr

Paul S. Meltzer, M.D., Ph.D. [20]
Sect. of Molecular Cytogenetics, Lab of Cancer Genetics, National Institutes of Health, Bethesda, Maryland

Claude J. Migeon, M.D. [159]
Professor of Pediatrics, Div. of Pediatric Endocrinology, The Johns Hopkins University School of Medicine, Baltimore, Maryland
cmigeon@welchlink.welch.jhu.edu

Tetsuro Miki, Ph.D. [33]
Geriatric Research Education and Clinical Center, University of Washington, Seattle, Washington

Beverly S. Mitchell [109]
Wellcome Professor of Cancer Research, University of North Carolina, Lineberger Comprehensive Cancer Center, Chapel Hill, North Carolina

Grant A. Mitchell, M.D. [79, 102]
Div. of Medical Genetics, Hopital Ste-Justine, Montreal, Quebec, Canada
mitchell@justine.umontreal.ca

Shiro Miwa, M.D. [182]
Director, Okinaka Memorial Institute for Medical Research, Tokyo, Japan

Maria Judit Molnar, M.D., Ph.D. [216]
Dept. of Neurology, Medical University of Debrecen, National Institute of Psychiatry and Neurology, Budapest, Hungary
molnarm@jaguar.dote.hu

Jill A. Morris, Ph.D. [145]
Senior Research Biologist, Dept. of Pharmacology, Merck Research Laboratories, West Point, Pennsylvania
jill_morris@merck.com

Ann B. Moser, BA [131]
Kennedy Krieger Institute, Baltimore, Maryland
mosera@kennedykrieger.org

Hugo W. Moser, M.D. [131, 143]
Professor of Neurology and Pediatrics, Johns Hopkins University, Director of Neurogenetics, Kennedy Krieger Institute, Baltimore, Maryland
moser@kennedykrieger.org

Björn Mossberg, M.D., Ph.D. [187]
Chief Physician, Dept. of Respiratory Medicine and Allerology, Huddinge University Hospital Stockholm, Sweden
bjorn.mossberg@lungall.hs.sll.se

Arno G. Motulsky, M.D., D.Sc. [127, 238]
Professor Emeritus Active of Medicine and Genetics, Attending Physician, University of Washington Hospital, Div. of Medical Genetics, Dept. of Medicine, University of Washington, Seattle, Washington
agmot@u.washington.edu

S. Harvey Mudd, M.D. [88]
Guest Scientist, Laboratory of Molecular Biology, National Institute of Mental Health, National Institutes of Health, Bethesda, Maryland
sbm@codon.nih.gov

Maximilian Muenke, M.D. [245, 250]
Chief, Medical Genetics Branch, National Human Genome Research Institute, National Institutes of Health, Bethesda, Maryland
muenke@nih.gov

Joseph Muenzer, M.D., Ph.D. [136]
Associate Professor of Pediatrics, Dept. of Pediatrics, University of North Carolina at Chapel Hill, North Carolina
muenzer@css.unc.edu

Arnold Munnich, M.D., Ph.D. [99, 237]
Professor, Dept. of Pediatrics, INSERM, Hopital des Enfants Malades, Hopital Necker, Paris, France
munnich@necker.fr

Jun Nakura, M.D., Ph.D. [33]
Department of Geriatric Medicine, School of Medicine, Ehime University, Ehime, Japan
nakura@ m.ehime-u.ac.jp

Eiji Nanba, M.D. [151]
Associate Professor, Gene Research Center, Tottori University, Yonago, Japan
enanba@grape.med.tottori-u.ac.jp

William M. Nauseef, M.D. [189]
Professor, Inflammation Program and Dept. of Medicine, University of Iowa, Iowa City, Iowa
william-nauseef@uiowa.ed

Barry D. Nelkin, Ph.D. [58]
Associate Professor of Oncology, Johns Hopkins University School of Medicine, Baltimore, Maryland
bnelkin@jhmi.edu

Edward B. Neufeld, Ph.D. [145]
National Heart, Lung, and Blood Institute, Bethesda, Maryland
neufelde@mail.nih.gov

Elizabeth F. Neufeld, Ph.D. [136]
Professor and Chair Biological Chemistry, Dept. of Biological Chemistry, UCLA School of Medicine, Los Angeles, California
eneufeld@mednet.ucla.edu

Peter E. Newburger, M.D. [189]
Professor of Pediatrics and Molecular, Genetics/Microbiology; Director, Pediatric Hematology/Oncology, University of Massachusetts Medical School, Worcester, Massachusetts
peter.newburger@ummed.edu

Peter J. Newman, Ph.D. [177]
Senior Investigator, Vice President and Assoc. Director for Research, The Blood Center, Milwaukee, Wisconsin
pjnewman@bcsew.edu

Irene F. Newsham, Ph.D. [36]
Dept. of Anatomy and Pathology, Medical College of Virginia, Richmond, Virginia
inewsham@hsc.vcu.edu

Jeffrey L. Noebels, M.D., Ph.D. [230]
Professor of Neurology, Neuroscience, and Molecular and Human Genetics, Dept. of Neurology, Baylor College of Medicine, Houston, Texas
jnoebels@bcm.tmc.edu

Josette Noël, M.D. [196]
Assistant Professor, Dept. of Physiology, Université de Montréal, Montreal, Quebec, Canada
josette.noel@umontreal.ca

Lawrence M. Nogee, M.D. [218]
Associate Professor, Dept. of Pediatrics, Div. of Neonatology, Johns Hopkins University School of Medicine, Baltimore, Maryland
lnogee@welch.jhu.edu

Virginia Nunes, Ph.D. [191]
Medical and Molecular Genetics Center, L'Hospitalet de Llobregat, Barcelona, Catalunya, Spain
vnunes@iro.es

Robert L. Nussbaum, M.D. [252]
Chief, Genetic Diseases Research Branch, National Human Genome Research Institute, Bethesda, Maryland
rlnuss@nhgri.nih.gov

William S. Oetting, M.D. [220]
Assistant Professor, University of Minnesota, Minneapolis, Minnesota
bill@lenti.med.umn.edu

Harry T. Orr, M.D. [226]
University of Minnesota, Institute of Human Genetics, Minneapolis, Minnesota
harry@lenti.med.umn.edu

Akihiro Oshima, M.D. [151]
Visiting Investigator, Dept. of Veterinary Science, National Institute of Infectious Diseases, Tokyo, Japan
oshima@nih.go.jp

Manuel Palacín, M.D. [191]
Professor, Biochemistry and Molecular Biology, Faculty of Biology, Dept. of Biochemistry and Physiology, University of Barcelona, Barcelona, Spain
mnpalacin@porthos.bio.ub.es

Cristina Panozzo, Ph.D. [231]
Laboratoire de Neurogénétique Moléculaire, INSERM, GENOPOLE, Evry, France
c.panozzo@genopole.inserm.fr

Lucie Parent, M.D. [196]
Associate Professor, Dept. of Physiology, Université de Montréal, Montreal, Quebec, Canada
lucie.parent@umontreal.ca

Peter Parham, Ph.D. [12]
Professor of Structural Biology and of Microbiology and Immunology, Stanford University, Stanford, California
Peropa@leland.stanford.edu

Morag Park, M.D. [25]
Molecular Oncology Group, Royal Victoria Hospital, Montreal, Quebec, Canada
morag@lan1.molonc.mcgill.ca

Keith L. Parker, M.D., Ph.D. [159]
Professor of Internal Medicine and Pharmacology, Dept. of Internal Medicine, UT Southwestern Medical Center, Dallas, Texas
kparke@mednet.swmed.edu

Ramon Parsons, M.D., Ph.D. [45]
Assistant Professor, Columbia Institute of Cancer Genetics, Columbia University, New York, New York
rep15@columbia.edu

Marc C. Patterson, M.D. [145]
Consultant, Div. of Child and Adolescent Neurology, Mayo Clinic, Rochester, Minnesota
mpatterson@mayo.edu

Leena Peltonen, M.D., Ph.D. [141, 154]
Professor and Chair of Human Genetics, Dept. of Human Genetics, UCLA School of Medicine, Los Angeles, California
lpeltonen@mednet.ucla.edu

Peter G. Pentchev, Ph.D. [145]
Chief, Sect. of Cellular and Molecular Pathophysiology, Developmental and Metabolic Neurology Branch, National Institutes of Neurological Disorders and Stroke, Bethesda, Maryland
peter.pentchev@xtra.co.nz

Isabelle Perrault, M.D. [237]
Unite de Recherches sur les Handicaps, Genetiques de L'Enfant, INSERM, Hôpital des Enfants Malades, Paris, France

Gloria M. Petersen, Ph.D. [49]
Professor of Clinical Epidemiology, Consultant, Mayo Foundation, Mayo Clinic, Rochester, New York
peterg@mayo.edu

Christine Petit [254]
Unite de Genetique des Deficits Sensoriels, Institut Pasteur, Paris, France
cpetit@pasteur.fr

Fred Petrij, M.D. [248]
Clinical Genetics Registrar, Dept. of Clinical Genetics, Erasmus University, Rotterdam, The Netherlands
petrij@kgen.azr.nl

James M. Phang, M.D. [81]
Chief, Metabolism and Cancer Susceptibility Sect., Basic Research Laboratory, Div. of Basic Sciences, National Cancer Institute, Frederick, Maryland
phang@mail.ncifcrf.gov

John A. Phillips, III, M.D. [162]
Professor of Pediatrics and Biochemistry, Div. of Medical Genetics, Vanderbilt University School of Medicine, Nashville, Tennessee
john.phillips@mcmail.vanderbilt.edu

Joram Piatigorsky, Ph.D. [241]
Chief, Laboratory of Molecular and Developmental Biology, National Eye Institute, Bethesda, Maryland
joramp@intra.nei.nih.gov

Leonard Pinsky, M.D. [161]
Professor, Depts. of Medicine, Human Genetics, Biology and Pediatrics, McGill University, Lady Davis Institute for Medical Research, Sir M.B. Davis–Jewish General Hospital, Montreal, Quebec, Canada
rrosenzw@ldi.jgh.mcgill.ca

Eleanor S. Pollak, M.D. [173]
Assistant Professor of Pathology and Laboratory Medicine, Hospital of the University of Pennsylvania, Associate Director, Clinical Coagulation Laboratory, The Children's Hospital of Philadelphia, Philadelphia, Pennsylvania
pollak@mail.med.upenn.edu

Bruce A.J. Ponder, Ph.D., F.R.C.P. [42]
CRC Professor of Oncology, University of Cambridge, Cambridge Institute for Medical Research, Cambridge, United Kingdom
bajp@mole.bio.cam.ac.uk

Mortimer Poncz, M.D. [177]
Professor of Pediatrics, University of Pennsylvania Medical Center, Philadelphia, Pennsylvania

Daniel Porte, Jr., M.D. [67]
Professor of Medicine, University of California San Diego; Staff Physician, VA San Diego Health Care System, San Diego, California
dporte@ucsd.edu
poncz@email.chop.edu

Steven M. Powell, M.D. [55]
Assistant Professor of Medicine, Div. of Gastroenterology, University of Virginia Health Systems, Charlottesville, Virginia
SMP8N@virginia.edu

James M. Powers, M.D. [131]
Dept. of Pathology, University of Rochester Medical Center, Rochester, New York

Richard L. Proia, Ph.D. [153]
Chief, Genetics of Development and Disease Branch, National Institute of Diabetes and Digestive and Kidney Diseases, National Institutes of Health, Bethesda, Maryland
proia@nih.gov

Kathleen P. Pratt, Ph.D. [171]
Instructor, Department of Biochemistry, University of Washington, Seattle
kpratt@u.washington.edu

Stanley B. Prusiner, M.D. [224]
Director, Institute for Neurodegenerative Diseases, Professor of Neurology and Biochemistry, Dept. of Neurology, University of California, San Francisco, California

Louis J. Ptáček, M.D. [204]
Associate Professor, Associate Investigator, Dept. of Neurology Human Genetics, Howard Hughes Medical Institute, University of Utah, Salt Lake City, Utah
ptacek@genetics.utah.edu

Jennifer M. Puck, M.D. [185]
Head Chief, Immunologic Genetics Sect., National Human Genome Research Institute, Genetics and Molecular Biology Branch, Bethesda, Maryland
jpuck@nhgri.nih.gov

Leena Pulkkinen, Ph.D. [222]
Jefferson Institute of Molecular Medicine, Dept. of Dermatology and Cutaneous Biology, Jefferson Medical College, Thomas Jefferson University, Philadelphia, Pennsylvania
leena.pulkkinen@mail.tju.edu

Reed E. Pyeritz, M.D., Ph.D. [206]
Professor of Human Genetics, MCP Hahnemann School of Medicine, Philadelphia, Pennsylvania
pyeritz@yahoo.com

Kari O. Raivio, M.D. [111]
Professor of Perinatal Medicine, School of Medicine, University of Helsinki, Helsinki, Finland
kari.raivio@helsinki.fi

Stanley C. Rall, Jr., Ph.D. [119]
Investigator, Gladstone Institute of Cardiovascular Disease, San Francisco, California

Bonnie W. Ramsey, M.D. [201]
Dept. of Pediatrics, University of Washington School of Medicine, Children's Hospital Regional Medical Center, Seattle, Washington
bramsey@u.washington.edu

Ahmed Rasheed [57]
Research Assistant Professor, Duke University Medical Center, Durham, North Carolina
a.rasheed@duke.edu

Gerald V. Raymond, M.D. [129]
Assistant Professor, Neurology, Kennedy Krieger Institute, Johns Hopkins University School of Medicine, Baltimore, Maryland
raymond@kennedykrieger.org

Andrew P. Read, MA, Ph.D., FRC Path, FmedSci [244]
Professor of Human Genetics, Dept. of Medical Genetics, St. Mary's Hospital, University of Manchester, Manchester, United Kingdom
andrew.read@man.ac.uk

Jonathan J. Rees, MBBS, FRCP [46]
Professor and Chairman, Dept. of Dermatology, The University of Edinburgh, Edinburgh, Scotland, United Kingdom
Jonathan.rees@ed.ac.uk

Samuel Refetoff, M.D. [158]
Professor of Medicine and Pediatrics, Director, Endocrinology Laboratory, Depts. of Medicine and Pediatrics and the J.P. Kennedy Jr. Mental Retardation Research Center, The University of Chicago, Chicago, Illinois
refetoff@medicine.bsd.uchicago.edu

Arnold J.J. Reuser, Ph.D. [135]
Associate Professor of Cell Biology, Erasmus University Rotterdam, Dept. of Clinical Genetics, Rotterdam, The Netherlands
reuser@ikg.fgg.eur.nl

William B. Rizzo, M.D. [98]
Professor of Pediatrics, Human Genetics, Biochemistry, and Molecular Biophysics, Dept. of Pediatrics, Medical College of Virginia, Virginia Commonwealth University, Richmond, Virginia
wrizzo@hsc.vcu.edu

James M. Roberts, M.D. [23]
Div. of Basic Sciences, Fred Hutchinson Cancer Research Center, Seattle, Washington 98104

Brian H. Robinson, Ph.D. [100]
Professor, Depts. of Biochemistry and Pediatrics, Program Head, Metabolism, Senior Scientist, Genetics and Genomic Biology, Hospital for Sick Children, Toronto, Ontario, Canada
bhr@sickkids.on.ca

Charles R. Roe, M.D. [101]
Institute of Metabolic Disease, Baylor University Medical Center, Dallas, Texas
cr.roe@baylordallas.edu

Hans-Hilger Ropers, M.D., Ph.D. [236, 239]
Professor, Dept. of Human Genetics, Max-Planck-Institute fuer Molekulare Genetik, Berlin, Germany
Ropers@molgen.mpg.de

Michael Rosenbaum, M.D. [157]
Associate Professor of Clinical Pediatrics and Clinical Medicine, Div. of Molecular Genetics, Russ Berrie Research Center, Columbia University College of Physicians and Surgeons, New York, New York
mr475@columbia.edu

David S. Rosenblatt, M.D. [94, 155]
Professor of Human Genetics, Medicine, Pediatrics, and Biology, Director, Div. of Medical Genetics, McGill University Health Centre, Royal Victoria Hospital, Montreal, Quebec, Canada
mc74@musica.mcgill.ca

Agnes Rötig, Ph.D. [99]
Dept. of Genetics, INSERM, Hopital Necker, Paris, France
roetig@necker.fr

Jayanta Roy Chowdhury, M.D., M.R.C.P. [125]
Professor of Medicine and Molecular Genetics, Dept. of Medicine and Molecular Genetics, Albert Einstein College of Medicine at Yeshiva University, Bronx, New York
chowdhur@aecom.yu.edu

Namita Roy Chowdhury, Ph.D. [125]
Professor of Medicine and Molecular Genetics, Albert Einstein College of Medicine, Bronx, New York

Jean-Michel Rozet, M.D. [237]
Unite de Recherches sur les Handicaps, Genetiques de L'Enfant, INSERM, Hôpital des Enfants Malades, Paris, France

Edward M. Rubin, M.D., Ph.D. [121]
Head, Genome Sciences Dept., Lawrence, Berkeley Laboratory, University of California at Berkeley, Berkeley, California
emrubin@lbl.gov

Charles M. Rudin, M.D. [24]
Assistant Professor of Medicine, University of Chicago Medical Center, Chicago, Illinois
crudin@medicine.bsd.uchicago.edu

Elena I. Rugarli, M.D. [225]
Researcher, Telethon Institute of Genetics and Medicine (TIGEM), Milan, Italy
rugarli@tigem.it

David W. Russell, Ph.D. [160]
Eugene McDermott Distinguished Professor of Molecular Genetics, University of Texas Southwestern Medical Center Dallas, Texas
russell@utsw.swmed.edu

Pierre Rustin, Ph.D. [99]
Dept. of Genetics, INSERM, Hopital Des Enfants-Malades, Paris, France
rustin@necker.fr

David D. Sabatini, M.D., Ph.D. [16]
Frederick L. Ehrman Professor and Chairman, Dept. of Cell Biology, New York University School of Medicine, New York, New York
Sabatd01@popmail.med.nyu.edu

Richard L. Sabina, Ph.D. [110]
Associate Professor of Biochemistry, Dept. of Biochemistry, Medical College of Wisconsin, Milwaukee, Wisconsin
sabinar@mcw.edu

J. Evan Sadler, M.D., Ph.D. [174]
Professor, Depts. Of Medicine, Biochemistry and Molecular Biophysics; Investigator, Howard Hughes Medical Institute, Washington University School of Medicine, St. Louis, Missouri
esadler@im.wustl.edu

Amrik S. Sahota, Ph.D., F.A.C.M.G. [108]
Dept. of Genetics, Nelson Biological Laboratories, Rutgers University, Piscataway, New Jersey
sahota@nel-exchange.vutgers.edu

Mika Saksela, M.D. [111]
Research Associate, Children's Hospital, University of Helsinki, Helsinki, Finland
Mika.Saksela@Helsinki.fi

Julian R. Sampson, M.D. [233]
Professor of Medical Genetics Institute of Medical Genetics, University of Wales, College of Medicine, Cardiff, United Kingdom
wmgjrs@cardiff.ac.uk

Konrad Sandhoff, Ph.D. [134, 143, 153]
Director and Professor of Biochemistry, Kekule-Institut fur Organische Chemie und Biochemie, Universitat Bonn, Bonn, Germany
sandhoff@uni-bonn.de

Michael C. Sanguinetti, Ph.D. [203]
University of Utah, Eccles Institute of Human Genetics, Salt Lake City, Utah
mike.sanguinetti@hci.utah.edu

Silvia Santamarina-Fojo, M.D, Ph.D. [118]
Chief, Section on Cell Biology, Molecular Disease Branch, National Institutes of Health, Bethesda, Maryland
silvia@mdb.nhlbi.nih.gov

Carmen Sapienza, Ph.D. [15]
Professor of Pathology and Laboratory Medicine, Associate Director, Fels Institute for Cancer Research, Temple University School of Medicine, Philadelphia, Pennsylvania
sapienza@unix.temple.edu

Shigeru Sassa, M.D., Ph.D. [124]
Emeritus Head, Laboratory of Biochemical Hematology, The Rockefeller University, New York, New York
sassa@rockvax.rockefeller.edu

Jean-Marie Saudubray, M.D. [66]
Director of the Metabolic/Diabetes Unit, Professor, Dept. of Pediatrics, Hopital Necker Enfants Malades, Paris, France
Elisabeth.saudubray@nck.ap_hop_paris.fr

Alan J. Schafer, Ph.D. [253]
Vice President Genetics, Incyte Genomics, Cambridge, United Kingdom
alan.schafer@incyte.com

Gerard Schellenberg, Ph.D. [33]
Veterans Affairs Medical Center, Seattle, Washington
zachdad@u.washington.edu

Detlev Schindler, M.D. [139]
Director, Cell Culture, Biochemistry and Flowcytometry Div.; Associate Professor of Human Genetics, Dept. of Human Genetics, University of Wuerzburg, Wuerzburg, Germany
schindler@biozentrum.uni-wuerzburg.de

Jerry A. Schneider, M.D. [199]
Professor of Pediatrics; Benard L. Maas Chair in Inherited Metabolic Disease, Dean for Academic Affairs, Office of the Dean, School of Medicine, University of California, San Diego School of Medicine, La Jolla, California
jschneider@ucsd.edu

Edward H. Schuchman, Ph.D. [144]
Professor of Human Genetics, Dept. of Human Genetics, Mount Sinai School of Medicine, Member, Institute for Gene Therapy and Molecular Medicine, New York, New York
schuchman@msvax.mssm.edu

C. Ronald Scott, M.D. [89]
Professor, Dept. of Pediatrics, University of Washington School of Medicine, Seattle, Washington
crscott@u.washington.edu

Charles R. Scriver, M.D.C.M. [1, 5, 77]
Alva Professor of Human Genetics, Professor of Pediatrics, Faculty of Medicine, Professor of Biology, Faculty of Science, McGill University; McGill University-Montreal Children's Hospital Research Institute, McGill University Health Centre, Montreal, Quebec, Canada
mc77@musica.mcgill.ca

Udo Seedorf, M.D. [142]
Institut fur Klinische Chemie and Laboratoriumsmedizin, Zentrallaboratorium Westfalische Wilhelms-Universitat, Munster, Germany
seedorfu@uni-muenster.de

Christine E. Seidman, M.D. [213]
Investigator, Howard Hughes Medical Institute
Professor Medicine and Genetics, Director, Cardiovascular Genetics Center, Dept. of Medicine, Brigham and Women's Hospital, Harvard Medical School, Boston, Massachusetts
cseidman@rascal.med.harvard.edu

Jonathan G. Seidman, Ph.D. [213]
Henrietta B. and Frederick H. Bugher Professor of Cardiovascular Genetics, Investigator, Howard Hughes Medical Institute, Harvard Medical School, Boston, Massachusetts

Giorgio Semenza, M.D. [75]
Professor, Dept. of Biochemistry, Swiss Institute of Technology, Laboratorium fur Biochemie, Zurich, Switzerland; Professor, Dept. of Chemistry and Medical Biochemistry, University of Milan, Milan, Italy
giorgio.semenza@unimi.it
semenza@bc.biol.ethz.ch

Gul N. Shah, Ph.D. [208]
Assistant Research Professor, Edward A. Doisy Dept. of Biochemistry and Molecular Biology, Saint Louis University School of Medicine, St. Louis, Missouri
shahgn@slu.edu

Lisa G. Shaffer, Ph.D. [65]
Associate Professor, Dept. of Molecular and Human Genetics, Baylor College of Medicine, Houston, Texas
lshaffer@bcm.tmc.edu

Larry J. Shapiro, M.D. [166]
W.H. and Marie Wattis Distinguished Professor, Chairman, Dept. of Pediatrics, University of California Medical Center, San Francisco, California
Lshapiro@peds.ucsf.edu

Val C. Sheffield, M.D., Ph.D. [242]
Professor of Pediatrics, Associate Investigator, Howard Hughes Medical Institute, Dept. of Pediatrics, Div. of Medical Genetics, University of Iowa Hospital and Clinic, Iowa City, Iowa
Val-sheffield@uiowa.edu

Stephanie L. Sherman, Ph.D. [64]
Dept. of Genetics Emory University School of Medicine, Atlanta, Georgia
ssherman@genetics.emory.edu

Vivian E. Shih, M.D. [87]
Professor of Neurology, Harvard Medical School, Director, Amino Acid Disorder Laboratory/Metabolic Disorders Unit, Massachusetts General Hospital, Charlestown, Massachusetts
vshih@partners.org

John M. Shoffner, M.D. [104]
Director, Molecular Medicine, Molecular Medicine Laboratory, Children's Healthcare of Atlanta, Atlanta, Georgia
john.shoffner@choa.org

David Sidransky, M.D. [54]
Dept. of Otolaryngology-HNS, The Johns Hopkins University School of Medicine, Baltimore, Maryland
dsidrans@jhmi.edu

Olli Simell, M.D. [83, 192]
Professor of Pediatrics, Dept. of Pediatrics, University of Turku, Turku, Finland
Olli.simell@utu.fi

H. Anne Simmonds, Ph.D. [108]
Purine Research Unit, Guy's Hospital, London Bridge, London, United Kingdom
anne.simmonds@kcl.ac.uk

Ola H. Skjeldal, M.D., Ph.D. [132]
Div. of Pediatrics, Ullevaal University Hospital, Oslo, Norway
ola.skjeldal@klinmed.uio.no

William S. Sly, M.D. [1, 138, 208]
Alice A. Doisy Professor of Biochemistry and Molecular Biology, Chair, Edward A. Doisy Dept. of Biochemistry and Molecular Biology, Professor of Pediatrics, St. Louis University School of Medicine, St. Louis, Missouri
slyws@slu.edu

C. Wayne Smith, M.D. [188]
Head, Sect. of Leukocyte Biology; Professor, Depts. of Pediatrics, Microbiology and Immunology, Sect. of Leukocyte Biology, Children's Nutrition Research Center, Baylor College of Medicine Houston, Texas
cwsmith@bcm.tmc.edu

Kirby D. Smith, Ph.D. [131]
Professor of Pediatrics, Kennedy Krieger Institute, McKusick-Nathans Institute of Genetic Medicine, The Johns Hopkins University School of Medicine, Baltimore, Maryland
smithk@mail.jhmi.edu

Oded Sperling, Ph.D. [198]
Professor and Chairman of Clinical Biochemistry, Dept. of Clinical Biochemistry, Rabin Medical Center, Petah-Tikva, Israel
odeds@post.tau.ac.il

Allen M. Spiegel, M.D. [164]
Director, National Institute of Diabetes and Digestive and Kidney Diseases, Bethesda, Maryland
allens@amb.niddk.nih.gov

Peter H. St. George-Hyslop, M.D. [234]
Professor, Dept. of Medicine, Center for Research in Neurodegenerative Diseases, University of Toronto, Toronto, Ontario, Canada
p.hyslop@utoronto.ca

Beat Steinmann, M.D. [70]
Professor, Div. of Metabolism and Molecular Pediatrics, University Children's Hospital, Zurich, Switzerland
beat.steinmann@kispi.unizh.ch

Sylvia Stöckler-Ipsiroglu, M.D. [84]
Dept. of Pediatrics, University Hospital Vienna, Laboratory for Inherited Metabolic Diseases, Wahringergurtel, Vienna, Austria

Edwin M. Stone, M.D., Ph.D. [242]
Dept. of Ophthalmology and Visual Sciences, University of Iowa College of Medicine, Iowa City, Iowa
edwin-stone@viowa.edu

Pietro Strisciuglio, M.D. [152]
Associate Professor of Pediatrics, Dept. of Pediatrics, "Magna Graecia", Catanzaro, Italy
strisciuglio_unicz@libero.it

Sharon F. Suchy, Ph.D. [252]
Staff Scientist, Genetic Disease Research Branch, National Human Genome Research Instit, Bethesda, Maryland
suchy@nhgri.nih.gov

Kathleen E. Sullivan, M.D., Ph.D. [186]
Assistant Professor of Pediatrics, Children's Hospital of Philadelphia, Philadelphia, Pennsylvania

Andrea Superti-Furga, M.D. [202]
Div. of Metabolism and Molecular Pediatrics, University of Zurich, Universitaets-Kinderklinik, Zurich, Switzerland
asuperti@access.unizh.ch

Kinuko Suzuki, M.D. [145, 147, 153]
Professor of Pathology and Lab Medicine, Dept. of Pathology and Lab Medicine, School of Medicine, University of North Carolina at Chapel Hill
kis@med.unc.edu

Kunihiko Suzuki, M.D. [147, 153]
Director Emeritus, Neuroscience Center, Professor of Neurology and Psychiatry, School of Medicine,
University of North Carolina at Chapel Hill, North Corolina
Kuni.Suzuki@attglobal.net

Yoshiyuki Suzuki, M.D. [147, 151]
Professor and Director, Nasu Institute for Developmental Disabilities, Clinical Research Center, International University of Health and Welfare, Otawara, Japan
suzukiy@iuhw.ac.jp

Dallas M. Swallow, Ph.D. [76]
Professor of Human Genetics, The Galton Laboratory, Dept. of Biology, University College London, London, United Kingdom
dswallow@hgmp.mrc.ac.uk

Lawrence Sweetman, Ph.D. [93]
Professor, Institute of Biomedical Studies, Baylor University; Director, Mass Spectrometry Lab, Institute of Metabolic Disease, Baylor University Medical Center, Dallas, Texas
l.sweetman@baylordallas.edu

Alan Richard Tall, M.D. [121]
Tilden Weger Bieler Professor of Medicine, Dept. of Medicine, Div. of Molecular Medicine, Columbia University College of Physicians and Surgeons, New York, New York
art1@columbia.edu

Robert M. Tanguay, Ph.D. [79]
Laboratoire de genetique cellulaire et developpementale, Pavillon Charles-Eugene Marchand, Université Laval, Ste-Foy, Quebec, Canada
robert.tanguay@rsvs.ulaval.ca

Robin G. Taylor, Ph.D. [80]
Dept. of Genetics, The Hospital for Sick Children Research Institute, Toronto, Canada
rgtaylor@alumni.haas.org

Simeon I. Taylor, M.D., Ph.D. [68]
Lilly Research Fellow, Lilly Research Laboratories, Indianapolis, Indiana

Harriet S. Tenenhouse, Ph.D. [197]
Professor of Pediatrics and Human Genetics, Auxiliary Professor of Biology, Div. of Medical Genetics,
McGill University, Montreal Children's Hospital Research Institute, Montreal, Quebec, Canada
mdht@www.debelle.mcgill.ca

Jess G. Thoene, M.D. [199]
Karen Gore Professor; Director, Hayward Genetics Center, Human Genetics Program, Tulane University School of Medicine, New Orleans, Louisiana
jthoene@mailhost.tcs.tulane.edu

George H. Thomas, Ph.D. [140]
Professor of Pediatrics, Pathology and Medicine, The Johns Hopkins University School of Medicine, Director of Kennedy Krieger Institute Genetics Laboratory Baltimore, Maryland
thomasg@kennedykrieger.org

Craig B. Thompson, M.D. [24]
Abramson Family Cancer Research Institute, University of Pennsylvania, Philadelphia, Pennsylvania
drt@mail.med.upenn.edu

Beat Thöny, Ph.D. [78]
Associate Professor, Division of Clinical Chemistry & Biochemistry, Div. of Chemistry and Biochemistry, University of Zurich, Zurich, Switzerland
bthony@kispi.unizh.ch

Roland Tisch, Ph.D. [12]
Postdoctoral Fellow, Dept. of Microbiology and Immunology, Stanford University School of Medicine, Stanford, California

Jay A. Tischfield, Ph.D. [108]
MacMillan Professor and Chair, Dept. of Genetics, Rutgers University, Professor of Pediatrics and Psychiatry, Robert Wood Johnson Medical School, Piscataway, New Jersey

John A. Todd, M.D. [6]
Professor, Dept. of Medical Genetics, Cambridge University; Institute for Medical Research, Addenbrooke's Hospital, Cambridge, United Kingdom
john.todd@cimr.cam.ac.uk

Douglas M. Tollefsen, M.D., Ph.D. [176]
Professor of Medicine, Hematology Div., Washington University Medical School, St. Louis, Missouri
tollefsen@im.wustl.edu

Eileen P. Treacy, M.D. [5]
Associate Professor of Human Genetics and Pediatrics; Director, Biochemical Genetics Unit, Div. of Medical Genetics, Dept. of Biochemical Genetics, Montreal Children's Hospital, Montreal, Quebec, Canada
mcet@musica.mcgill.ca

Jeffrey M. Trent, M.D., Ph.D. [20]
Chief, Lab of Cancer Genetics, National Human Genome Research Institute, Bethesda, Maryland
jtrent@nih.gov

Mark A. Trifiro, Ph.D. [161]
Associate Professor, Dept. of Medicine, McGill University; Associate Physician, Dept. of Medicine, Lady Davis Institute for Medical Research, Sir Mortimer B. Davis Jewish General Hospital, Montreal, Canada, Quebec
mdtm@musica.mcgill.ca

Karl Tryggvason, M.D. [214]
Div. Matrix Biology, Dept. of Medical Biochemistry and Biophysics, Karolinska Institut, Stockholm, Sweden
karl.tryggvason@mbb.ki.se

William T. Tse, M.D., Ph.D. [183]
Children's Hospital/Dana-Farber Cancer Institute, Div. of Hematology/Oncology, Boston, Massachusetts
William_tse@dfci.harvard.edu

Edward G.D. Tuddenham, M.D. [172]
Professor, MRC/CSC, Hammersmith Hospital, London, United Kingdom
etuddenh@rpms.ac.uk

Eric Turk, Ph.D. [190]
Dept. of Physiology, UCLA School of Medicine, Los Angeles, California
eturk@mednet.ucla.edu

Linda A. Tyfield, M.D. [72]
Consultant Clinical Scientist, Hon. Sr. Research Fellow, Dept. of Child Health, University of Bristol, Molecular Genetics Unit, The Lewis Laboratories, Southmead Hospital, Bristol, United Kingdom
linda.tyfield@bristol.ac.uk

Jouni Uitto, M.D., Ph.D. [222]
Jefferson Institute of Molecular Medicine, Dept. of Dermatology and Cutaneous Biology, Jefferson Medical College, Philadelphia, Pennsylvania
jouni.uitto@mail.tju.edu

Gerd M. Utermann, M.D. [116]
Professor and Chair, Institute for Medical Biology and Human Genetics, Leopold-Franzens University of Innsbruck, Innsbruck, Austria
Gerd.Utermann@uibk.ac.at

David Valle, M.D. [1, 3, 4, 5, 81, 83, 129]
Professor of Pediatrics Genetics and Molecular Biology, Investigator Howard Hughes Medical Institute, McKusick-Nathans Institute of Genetic Medicine, The Johns Hopkins University, Baltimore, Maryland
dvalle@jhmi.edu

Georges Van den Berghe, M.D. [70, 112]
Professor, Dept. of Biochemistry and Cellular Biology, University of Louvain Medical School, Director of Research, Laboratory of Physiological Chemistry, Christian de Duve Institute of Cellular Pathology, Brussels, Belgium
vandenberghe@bchm.ucl.ac.be

Peter van Endert, M.D. [12]
Postdoctoral Fellow, Dept. of Microbiology and Immunology, Stanford University School of Medicine, Stanford, California

Albert H. van Gennip, M.D. [113]
Laboratory Genetic Metabole Diseases, Academic Medical Center, University of Amsterdam, Amsterdam, The Netherlands

Veronica van Heyningen, D.Phil., F.R.S.E. [240]
Head of Cell and Molecular Genetics Sect., MRC Human Genetics Unit, Western General Hospital, Edinburgh, Scotland, United Kingdom
v.vanheyningen@hgu.mrc.ac.uk

Marie T. Vanier, M.D., Ph.D. [145]
Directeur de Recherche INSERM, Lyon-Sud Medical School, Oullins, France
vanier@univ-lyonl.fr

André B.P. Van Kuilenburg, M.D. [113]
Laboratory Genetic Metabole Diseases, Academic Medical Center, University of Amsterdam, Amsterdam, The Netherlands

Emile Van Schaftingen, M.D., Ph.D. [74]
Professor of Biochemistry, Laboratory of Physiological Chemistry, ICP, Universite Catholique de Louvain, Brussels, Belgium
vanschaftingen@bchm.ucl.ac.be

Gilbert Vassart, M.D., Ph.D. [158]
Head, Dept. of Medical Genetics, Institut de Recherche Interdisciplinaire, Universite Libre de Bruxelles, Brussels, Belgium
gvassart@ulb.ac.be

Bert Vogelstein, M.D. [17, 27, 48]
Investigator, Howard Hughes Medical Institute, Clayton Professor of Oncology and Pathology, The Johns Hopkins University School of Medicine, Baltimore, Maryland
vogelbe@welch.jhu.edu

Arnold von Eckardstein, M.D. [122]
Institut für Klinische Chemie und Laboratoriumsmedizin, Zentrallaboratorium, Westfälische Wilhelms-Universität Münster, Münster, Germany
vonecka@uni-muenster.de

Kurt von Figura, Ph.D. [84, 148]
Director and Professor, Institute of Biochemistry II Zentrum Biochemie und Molekulare Zellbiologie Georg-August-Universitat Gottingen, Gottingen, Germany
kfigura@gwdg.de

Tom Vulliamy, Ph.D. [179]
Clinical Scientist, Honorary Lecturer, Dept. of Hematology, Imperial College of School of Medicine, Hammersmith Hospital, London, United Kingdom
t.vulliamy@ic.ac.uk

Douglas C. Wallace, Ph.D. [105]
Robert W. Woodruff, Professor of Molecular Genetics, Professor and Director, Center for Molecular Medicine, Emory University School of Medicine, Atlanta, Georgia
dwallace@gen.emory.edu

John H. Walter, M.D. [72]
Consultant Pediatrician, Willink Biochemical Genetics Unit, Royal Manchester Children's Hospital, Pendlebury, Manchester, United Kingdom
john@jhwalter.demon.co.uk

Ronald J.A. Wanders, Ph.D. [130, 132]
Professor of Clinical Enzymology and Inherited Diseases, University of Amsterdam Academic Medical Centre, Emma Children's Hospital and Clinical Chemistry, Amsterdam, The Netherlands
wanders@amc.uva.nl

Stephen T. Warren, Ph.D. [64]
Rollins Research Center, Emory University School of Medicine, Atlanta, Georgia
swarren@bimcore.emory.edu

Paul A. Watkins, M.D., Ph.D. [131]
Associate Professor, Neurology, Dept. of Neurogenetics, Kennedy Krieger Institute, Johns Hopkins University, Baltimore, Maryland
watkins@kennedykrieger.org

Sir David J. Weatherall, M.D., FRS [181]
Regius Professor of Medicine, Institute of Molecular Medicine, John Radcliffe Hospital, Headington, Oxford, United Kingdom
janet.watt@imm.ox.ac.uk

Barbara L. Weber, M.D. [47]
Professor of Medicine and Genetics; Director, Breast Cancer Program; Assoc. Director, Cancer, Control and Population Science, University of Pennsylvania Cancer Center, Philadelphia, Pennsylvania
weberb@mail.med.upenn.edu

Dianne R. Webster, Ph.D [113]
National Testing Center, Lab Plus Auckland Hospital, Auckland, New Zealand

Lee S. Weinstein, M.D. [164]
Investigator, Metabolic Disease Branch, National Institute of Diabetes and Digestive Kidney Diseases, Bethesda, Maryland

Michael J. Welsh, M.D. [201]
Investigator, Howard Hughes Medical Institute, Dept. of Internal Medicine, University of Iowa College of Medicine, Iowa City, Iowa
mjwelsh@blue.weeg.uiowa.edu

David A. Wenger, Ph.D. [147]
Professor of Neurology and Biochemistry and Molecular Pharmacology, Jefferson Medical College, Philadelphia, Pennsylvania
David.wenger@mail.tju.edu

Jeffrey A. Whitsett, M.D. [218]
Div. of Pulmonary Biology, Children's Hospital Medical Center, Cincinnati, Ohio
jeff.whitsett@chmcc.org

Michael P. Whyte, M.D. [207]
Professor of Medicine, Pediatrics, and Genetics, Div. of Bone and Mineral Diseases, Washington University School of Medicine, Barnes-Jewish Hospital, Medical Scientific Director, Center for Metabolic Bone Disease and Molecular Research, Shriners Hospital for Children, St. Louis, Missouri
mwhyte@shrinenet.org

Andrew O.M. Wilkie, M.D., F.R.C.P. [245]
Senior Research Fellow in Clinical Science, Wellcome Trust, Institute of Molecular Medicine, John Radcliffe Hospital, Headington, Oxford, United Kingdom
awilkie@worf.molbiol.ox.ac.uk

Douglas Wilkin, Ph.D. [210]
Medical Genetics Branch, National Human Genome Research Institute, Bethesda, Maryland

Huntington F. Willard, Ph.D. [61]
Henry Wilson Payne Professor and Chairman of Genetics, Director, Center for Human Genetics, Case Western Reserve University School of Medicine, Cleveland, Ohio
hfw@po.cwru.edu

Julian C. Williams, M.D., Ph.D. [93]
Associate Professor of Pediatrics, USC School of Medicine, Head, Div. Of Med. Genetics, Children's Hospital LA, Med. Dir., Dept. of Pathology and Laboratory Medicine Genetics Laboratories, Los Angeles, California
jwilliams@chlais.usc.edu

Jean D. Wilson, M.D. [160]
Charles Cameron Sprague Distinguished Chair in Biomedical Science, Clinical Professor of Internal Medicine, Dept. of Internal Medicine, University of Texas Southwestern Medical Center, Dallas, Texas
jwils1@mednet.swmed.edu

Jerry A. Winkelstein, M.D. [186]
Dept. of Pediatrics, Johns Hopkins University School of Medicine, Baltimore, Maryland
jwinkels@welchlink.welch.jhu.edu

Barry Wolf, M.D., Ph.D. [156]
Associate Chair for Research, Head, Div. of Pediatric Research, Professor, Div. of Human Genetics, University of Connecticut School of Medicine, Director of Pediatric Research, Connecticut Children's Medical Center, Hartford, Connecticut
bwolf@hsc.vcu.edu

Allan W. Wolkoff, M.D. [125]
Professor, Albert Einstein College of Medicine, Liver Research Center Bronx, New York
wolkoff@aecom.yu.edu

W.G. Wood [181]
Institute of Molecular Medicine, John Radcliffe Hospital, Oxford, United Kingdom

Ronald G. Worton, C.M., Ph.D., F.R.S.C. [216]
CEO and Scientific Director, Ottawa General Hospital Research Institute, University of Ottawa, Ottawa, Ontario, Canada
rworton@ogh.on.ca

Ernest M. Wright, D.Sc. [190]
Professor and Chair, Dept. of Physiology, UCLA School of Medicine, Los Angeles, California
ewright@mednet.ucla.edu

Charles John Yeo, M.D. [50]
Professor and Attending Surgeon, Dept. of Surgery and Oncology, The Johns Hopkins Hospital, Baltimore, Maryland
cyeo@jhmi.edu

Chang-En Yu, M.D., Ph.D. [33]
Veterans Affairs Puget Sound Health Care System, Seattle Div. and the Dept. of Medicine, University of Washington, Seattle, Washington
changeyu@u.washington.edu

Berton Zbar, M.D. [41]
Chief, Laboratory of Immunology, National Cancer Institute-Frederick Cancer, Research Facility, Frederick, Maryland
zbar@mail.ncifcrf.gov

Huda Y. Zoghbi, M.D. [226, 255]
Professor, Dept. of Pediatrics and Molecular and Human Genetics; Investigator Howard Hughes Medical Institute, Baylor College of Medicine, Houston, Texas
hzoghbi@bcm.tmc.edu

PREFACE TO THE EIGHTH EDITION

Following "the new synthesis" of Mendelism and Darwinism, Theodosins Dobzhansky stated that biology makes sense only in the light of evolution.[1] A corollary to that opinion would say that medicine without biology does not make sense. This book, now in its eighth edition, presents evidence that biology, as we come to know it in the era of genomics, is helping to make better sense of medicine.

In its first edition,[2] this book, then known as *The Metabolic Basis of Inherited Disease* (MBID), focused almost exclusively on the Mendelian diseases falling into the category known as "inborn errors of metabolism." For the next five editions, MBID served as a medical companion to human biochemical genetics which had its own seminal text.[3] Then, to acknowledge the increasing relevance of molecular biology and molecular genetics, for the seventh edition we changed its title to: *The Metabolic and Molecular Bases of Inherited Disease* (*MMBID*). There were further changes in the seventh edition: complex genetic traits were increasingly recognized, cancer being a notable new section of the book, and even more so in the CD-ROM update of the print edition. Chromosomal disorders had appeared in the sixth edition and they increased their presence in the seventh, along with a chapter dedicated to imprinting.

The eighth edition of MMBID, now appearing in the first year of the twenty-first century, contains new chapters on the history of the inborn errors of metabolism (Chapter 3), their impact on health (Chapter 4) and their response to treatment (Chapter 5). This edition further reveals how genetics is contributing to the understanding of complex traits and birth defects as well as the Mendelian diseases with nominal pathways of metabolism or development. It is not surprising then that MMBID-8 should have chapters on aging and hypertension or on Hirschsprung disease, for example. In brief, this book is becoming a "textbook of medicine," as predicted by one reviewer of an earlier edition.[4]

Five questions formulated as such by Victor McKusick among others have been of abiding interest in medicine since at least the time of Osler: (1) What is the problem? (2) How did it happen? (3) What is the cause? (4) What can be done? (5) Will it happen again? The questions address the corresponding issues of diagnosis, pathogenesis, ultimate and proximal cause, treatment and prevention, and inherited risks of recurrence. As for cause, the theme of special interest shared by every entity discussed in this book is *mutation*: mutation that modifies phenotype, contributes to pathogenesis of the disease and, in various ways, identifies a key component in a "pathway" or "network" responsible for homeostasis and functional integrity.

MMBID-8 is being published as genome projects, both human and nonhuman, yield information and knowledge about the organization and nucleotide sequences of genomes. The allied field of research, now called genomics, has been called "a journey to the center of biology."[5] Comparative genomics reveals that homeostasis of energy metabolism and many aspects of intermediary metabolism are encoded in genes with a very long evolutionary history (see Chapter 4). Moreover, a number of the human disorders can be analyzed functionally in yeast in a manner some will call "biochemical genomics"[6] and there is a corresponding database cross-referencing human and yeast phenotypes.[7] Accordingly, Dobzhansky's angle of vision is increasingly validated.

At the same time, the genomes of *C. elegans* and *Drosophila* are telling us that development of multicellular organisms is controlled by the major portion of the corresponding genomes and each organism has particular programs for particular body plans. New sections and chapters in MMBID-8 are devoted to various disorders of development in *H. sapiens*.

It follows that biology is indeed a shared language for medicine.[8] However, shared language does not preclude particular language to deal with variant phenotypes (the diseases), their clinical consequences, and the specialization in clinical expertise required to address them. In recognition of this, the book contains material in the particular languages of counseling, testing and screening, and treatment; indeed, in a language increasingly accessed on Web sites by patients who want to know. The particular language extends beyond phenotype, counseling, and so on; it reaches the patient. Every patient who has one of the so-called "single-gene" diseases described in this book has an "orphan" disease; furthermore, because of biological individuality, each patient has his or her own private (orphan) form of unhealth. In other words, this book is an ultimate guidebook for *individualized medicine*.

MMBID-8 will contribute to an instauration of the clinician-investigator, a colleague who has been much marginalized by successes in the basic science and molecular and cellular biology and the corresponding contributions to medical science. The original editions of MBID were written largely by clinician-investigators; or by basic scientists who still retained a familiarity with patients or did research that was patient-oriented and disease-oriented.[9] However, in the more recent editions of MMBID, the chapters themselves and the majority of the references cited in them were more often than not authored by persons doing basic research, sometimes rather remote from the patient's primary problem. But, as the "genome project" moves from its structural to a functional phase and into biochemical- and pharmacogenomics, the editors of MMBID recognize a need for the return of the clinician-investigator. The latter must share equal status with the basic scientist so that science can be translated quickly into benefits for patients. That is why some chapters in MMBID-8 (e.g., 66 and 99) are devoted to clinical algorithms.

The prefaces to MBID-6 and MMBID-7 described how the editors chose material for Chapters and Parts of these editions. In the seventh edition, we said: "If there is an identifiable molecular explanation for the disease — and it affects a dynamic phenotype, metabolic or otherwise — then it is a candidate for inclusion .... The expansion of topics here is selective and obviously not inclusive of all possibilities." Although MMBID-8 has not changed its title, it has changed in many other ways. It has three new associate editors (Barton Childs, Kenneth Kinzler, and Bert Vogelstein), new chapters have appeared (the total is now 255) and the number of authors now exceeds 500. That the printed and bound book exceeds 7000 pages is not really a surprise, but it is an abiding reason to have portable and online versions of the book.

A survey undertaken by some of the editors, by some of our readers and owners of the seventh edition showed that 70% used the book at least once per week. Half those persons believed the book should grow beyond its original domain; that content of MMBID-7 was appropriate; and over 90% of the readers welcomed the prospect of a Web version.

The editors intend to keep MMBID-8 "user friendly;" and also to keep it up to date. We hope a portable version of MMBID-8 will be available for those who wish to have something they can carry home; there will be a Web version. In this latter format, MMBID will become a "continuous book," able to update all material and to incorporate new topics as they become pertinent to our stated mission. Accordingly, as more and more scientific print literature goes "on line" in one format or another, MMBID will do likewise;

the web version will allow MMBID to reincarnate itself through a long and healthy life.

So much seems to change between editions of MMBID; for example, a new team — Susan Noujaim, Peter Boyle, Marty Wonsiewicz, and others at McGraw-Hill — have translated formidable stacks of typescript into a book agreeable to the publisher. On the other hand, stability can still be found in the life of this book; the editors are still working with the same colleagues: Lynne Prevost and Huguette Rizziero (CRS), Grace Watson (AB), Elizabeth Torno (WS), Sandy Muscelli (DV); while Kathy Helwig helped the new editors (BC, KK, and BV). The process of reading manuscripts and proofs was yet again lightened by the tolerant support of our families and by colleagues at the places of business.

REFERENCES

1. Dobzhansky TH: "Nothing in biology makes sense except in the light of evolution." *Am Biol Teach* **35**:125, 1973.
2. Stanbury JB, Wyngaarden JB, Fredrickson DS (eds.): *The Metabolic Basis of Inherited Disease*. McGraw-Hill Book Co., New York. 1960.
3. Harris H: The principles of human biochemical genetics. *Frontiers of Biology* (Neuberger A, Tatum EL (eds.), Vol. 19. North Holland Pub. Co., London, 1970. North-Holland Research Monographs.
4. Childs B: Book Review. *The Metabolic Basis of Inherited Disease*. 6th ed. 2 volumes. Scriver CR, Beaudet AL, Sly WS, Valle D (eds.). *Am J Hum Genet* **46**:848, 1990.
5. Lander ES, Weinberg RA: Genomics: Journey to the center of biology. *Science* **287**:1777, 2000.
6. Carlson M: The awesome power of yeast biochemical genomics. *Trends Genet* **16**:49, 2000.
7. Bassett DE Jr., Boguski MS, Spencer F, Reeves R, Kim SH, Weaver T, Hieter P: Genome cross-referencing and XREFdb: Implications for the identification and analysis of genes mutated in human disease. *Nat Genet* **15**:339, 1997.
8. Scriver CR: American Pediatric Society Presidential Address 1995. Disease, war and biology: Language for medicine — and pediatrics. *Pediatric Res* **38**:819, 1995.
9. Goldstein JL, Brown MS: The clinical investigator: Bewitched, bothered, and bewildered — but still beloved. Editorial. *J Clin Invest* **99**:2803, 1997.

PREFACE TO THE SEVENTH EDITION

The sixth edition of *The Metabolic Basis of Inherited Disease* experienced "transition, transformation, and challenge." Transition continues in the seventh edition with the arrival of many new authors. Challenge remains, like the mountain whose peak is never in view while the climb proceeds. And there is transformation again, not least with the title: *The Metabolic and* Molecular *Bases of Inherited Disease*. The new word is significant.

A reviewer of the sixth edition reminds us of the original plan for the book: to present "the pertinent clinical, biochemical, and genetic information concerning those metabolic anomalies grouped under Garrod's engaging term 'inborn errors of metabolism.' "[1] The term *molecular* is a belated but natural homecoming for Garrod. During his lifetime, Garrod's views grew to encompass inherited susceptibility to any disease originating in our chemical individuality. These ideas emerged fully developed, for their time, in Garrod's second book. *The Inborn Factors in Disease*. That we have been slow to perceive the reach of his thinking is a theme of his recent biographer.[2] To accept it and put it to use requires the means to test its validity. Molecular analysis of the genetic variation causing or predisposing to disease provides the opportunity. The inborn errors of metabolism are simply our most obvious illustrations of the genetic variation that affects health and the molecular underpinnings of that variation. A corresponding analysis of multifactorial diseases is the obvious next step in the understanding of disease.[3] Need we say that MMBID-7 is nothing less than a textbook of molecular medicine, encompassing the diseases about which we know most? We predict that the "classic" textbooks of medicine in the future will look more and more like MMBID.

Change in the title of MBID did something else: it solved a problem the editors created for themselves in MBID-6, again commented on by the above-mentioned reviewer.[1] When we included topics not overtly "metabolic" in the sixth edition, for example, Down and fragile X syndromes, primary ciliary dyskinesia, collagen disorders and the muscular dystrophies, we moved well beyond the canonical theme of inborn errors of *metabolism*. The nonmetabolic topics are further expanded in this edition because they conform to a *logic of disease*, as it is called by Barton Childs in Chapter 2. The manifestations of any "genetic" disease are explained by a process (pathogenesis) that originates in part or in full form an intrinsic cause (mutation); and, since genotype is one of the determinants of the phenotype (disease), it follows that diagnosis, treatment, and counseling should be motivated form the genetic point of view because the disease involves both the patient and his or her family.

If there is an identifiable molecular explanation for the disease — and it affects a dynamic phenotype, metabolic or otherwise — then it is a candidate for inclusion in the seventh edition. The expansion of topics here is selective and obviously not inclusive of all possibilities. If this were the case, the table of contents would resemble the McKusick catalog, *Mendelian Inheritance in Man*! Nevertheless, yet a further 32 chapters are new to this edition of MBID while 31 others were introduced in the sixth edition; new ideas appear again and again in virtually all "old" chapters. Will it be three volumes — or more — for the eighth edition? (A CD-ROM format is under serious consideration for the next edition.) The Summary Table, immediately preceding Chapter 1, surveys the information in MMBID-7.

In the first section of the book, the following major new themes appear:

- A logic of disease based on genetic and evolutionary concepts that challenges conventional medical thinking (Chapter 2).
- Mutational mechanisms, including dynamic mutations (elastic or unstable DNA) (Chapter 3) and the methods to detect them (Chapter 1).
- Pharmacogenetics (Chapter 4) as a classical illustration of multifactorial disease (with ultimate and proximate causes) and of the "idiosyncratic reaction to drugs" — to recall Garrod's felicitous phrase.
- Diagnostic algorithms for the patient with an inborn error of metabolism (Chapter 5).
- Mapping of genes (genomics) (Chapter 6), along with an increased awareness that mutant gene expression may involve more than conventional Mendelian inheritance: for example, imprinting and mosaicism (Chapter 7).
- How cellular organelles, protein targeting and posttranslational modification, and the HLA complex affect expression of "genetic" disease (the subjects of Chapters 8 and 9, respectively).
- Cancer appears as a major theme for the first time in this edition (Chapters 10 to 15). Cancers are products of genetic damage. Modified events in pathways release cells from the normal controls of replication and growth. The cascades of events controlled by proto-oncogenes are counterparts of Garrod's pathways of metabolism. Because cancers can involve constitutional mutations, somatic mutations, or both, they further expand the conceptual boundaries of the book.
- Processes of inactivation harbored on the X chromosome (Chapter 16) and knowledge about the testis-determining factor and primary sex reversal (Chapter 17) are topics new to the section on chromosomes, itself an innovation of the sixth edition.

An awesome expansion of information continues in old and new chapters. The new chapters include, for example, insulin gene defects (Chapter 22); a completely new look at nonketotic hyperglycinemia (Chapter 37); diseases of the mitochondrial genome (Chapter 46); the apolipoprotein (a) molecule and its association with heart disease (Chapter 58); oxalosis as a peroxisomal disorder (Chapter 75); lysosomal enzyme activator proteins (Chapter 76); Pompe disease as a disease of lysosome function (Chapter 77) rather than a disease of carbohydrate metabolism; Lowe syndrome, separated from the Fanconi syndrome, following positional cloning of the gene (Chapter 123); Marfan syndrome, a disease of fibrillin dysfunction (Chapter 135); the muscular dystrophies (Chapters 140 and 141), and hypertrophic cardiomyopathy (Chapter 142). All is not new; in recognition of tradition, the spelling of *alcaptonuria* has reverted to *alkaptonuria* (Chapter 39).

A new section on disease of the eye (Chapters 143 to 146) includes retinitis pigmentosis, choroideremia, and disorders of color vision and crystallins. Discussions of epidermolysis bullosa (Chapter 149). Huntington disease (Chapter 152), and prion-related diseases (Chapter 153) reflect emerging molecular information on diseases of skin and brain. Chapter 154, the last in the book, catches recent developments involving half a dozen diseases.

The authors of chapters about particular diseases were asked to remember the needs of physicians and families, and they provide up-to-date information on diagnosis, treatment, and counseling. (These aspects are dealt with an even greater depth in a book that functions as our companion — the excellent *Inborn Metabolic*

Diseases: Diagnosis and Treatment, edited by J. Fernandes, J-M. Saudubray, and K. Tada.)

Some 200 authors wrote for MBID-6; 302 have written for MMBID-7; they have achieved the continuing transformation of this text. While so much seems to change overnight in molecular biology and genetics, stability can be found in the life of this book. Gail Gavert, Mariapaz Ramos-Englis, J. Dereck Jeffers, Peter McCurdy, and their colleagues have translated formidable stacks of typescript into a book agreeable to the publisher. The editors are still working with the same colleagues: Lynne Prevost and Huguette Rizziero (CRS), Grace Watson (AB), Elizabeth Torno (WS), and Sandy Muscelli (DV), Loy Denis was again our editorial coordinator until the last stages of this edition; her successor is Catherine Watson. The process of reading manuscripts and proofs was lightened by the tolerant support of our families and by colleagues at the place of business.

As this edition went to press, Harry Harris died. A giant in our field, his imprint is apparent everywhere in the book.

REFERENCES

1. Childs B: Book Review: *The Metabolic Basis of Inherited Disease*, 6th ed. *Am J Hum Genet* **66**:848, 1990.
2. Bearn AG: *Archibald Garrod and the Individuality of Man*. New York, Oxford University Press, 1993, 227 pp.
3. King RA, Rutter JI, Motulsky AG: *The Genetic Basis of Common Diseases*. New York, Oxford University Press, 1993, 978 pp.

PREFACE TO THE SIXTH EDITION

This edition of *The Metabolic Basis of Inherited Disease* marks a transition, a changing of the guard, as it were, among the editors. The sixth edition also reflects a transformation in the field of endeavor it encompasses; and there is a challenge too — for future editions. Transitions can be difficult and transformations sometimes produce unhappy results; neither need be the case here. Challenges can invigorate.

THE TRANSITION

Stanbury-Wyngaarden-'n-Fredrickson, collectively, were one famous "author" known to everyone in the field. This extraordinary editorial organism piloted the novel and timely book they had introduced and then edited through four successful editions. By a remarkable fision — or was it fusion? — the fifth edition was placed under the care of Stanbury-Wyngaarden-'n-Fredrickson, Goldstein 'n Brown. Now that giant has stepped aside, handing the challenge to a new team. The new editors have discovered how great the former ones were — if they hadn't known it before. Very large shoes had to be filled!

THE TRANSFORMATION

The sixth edition has many new features, notably the evidence of molecular genetics in one chapter after another. If *The Metabolic Basis of Inherited Disease* has had an abiding rationale, it was that the cause of all diseases listed in it was Mendelian and the diseases (so-called inborn errors of metabolism) were exceptions to be treasured for their illumination of human biology and for the insight they gave into pathogenesis of disease. But always there was a feeling that one did not understand cause as well as one should because not much was known about the genes. That situation is changing. There are new data about loci and structures of numerous normal genes and about the mutations affecting the phenotype encoded by them.

With 31 new chapters, the book is approximately one-third larger than it was. Accordingly, this edition appears for the first time in a two-volume format. It is a change undertaken with reluctance, but size of type, weight of paper, and the like had been adapted to the limit in the previous edition to accommodate the mass of information presented there. We elected to revise and print all chapters instead of using a précis of some, as in the last edition. Authors were encouraged to focus on up-to-date material and to use previous editions as archives of older material. But the wealth of new information neutralized contraction of the old. Hence the option taken here; to divide the book into two volumes, between separate covers.

New topics in the sixth edition include the following: There is a formal discussion of gene mapping and the medical use of genome markers (Chapter 6). Down syndrome (Chapter 7) and fragile X syndrome (Chapter 8) illustrate how any genetic disorder can eventually accommodate to our views of molecular genetics. They are the thin edge of the wedge toward understanding a great deal about human genetic disease and the editors introduce these chapters with some trepidation, realizing they could well be the very thin edge of a very big wedge — one of our challenges for future editions. One new chapter (122) covers the lactose deficiency polymorphism. This disorder does not fit the paradigm of a rare inborn error because it is so common; on the other hand, it does represent a Mendelian disadaptive phenotype for some individuals. There is a whole new section on peroxisomal diseases (Chapters 57–60) and Chapter 3 covers organelle biogenesis. Contiguous gene syndromes appear in this edition for the first time. The retinoblastoma story (Chapter 9) began as a contiguous gene syndrome; the new chapter encompasses this and analogous phenomena. Chapter 5 on oncogenes is new. The genes for retinoblastoma, chronic granulomatosus disease, and Duchenne muscular dystrophy are now known through techniques of "reverse" or "indirect" genetics. They are harbingers of what is to come in other diseases and they are topics developed at some length in this edition. Two appendices to Chapter 1, experiments in this edition, list: (1) the Mendelian disorders that can be diagnosed at the DNA level through oligonucleotide probes or by tightly linked markers that associate with alleles encoding mutant gene products; useful probes and their sources are catalogued in this appendix; (2) the mapped loci and their chromosomal assignments in the most current version of Victor McKusick's famous catalog available as we went to press. Perhaps a future edition will also catalog what we know about the mutant alleles at the loci encoding disease. Meanwhile the summary table grows in Chapter 1. It was introduced for the first time in the fifth edition and it is continued here for two reasons: first to show, in a simple manner, the growth of subject material between the last and present editions; second, to show how the white spaces in the fifth edition table are being filled in.

THE CHALLENGE

The future holds the potential for a separate chapter delineating the biochemical basis of each variant listed in McKusick's *Mendelian Inheritance in Man.* If this is the case, there will be many hundred chapters in subsequent editions of MBID. In addition, most monogenic disorders are not monogenic but modified through other loci by definable biochemical mechanisms; and most diseases are caused by polygenic and multifactorial mechanisms which also have a biochemical basis. Cytogenetic disorders have a biochemical basis as well, and in some instances the phenotypes may be determined by one or a few loci. These all represent effects of the constitutional genotypes on the phenotype, but there is also the role of somatic mutation in the pathogenesis of malignancies whether inherited or sporadic. With the explosion of information virtually assured, the challenge of how to focus and mold future editions is a daunting one.

This book has not grown unattended. In addition to the herculean efforts of some 200 authors and their assistants, others assured a safe passage during the development of the book, notably Dereck Jeffers and Gail Gavert at McGraw-Hill; Loy Denis, who served as coordinator for the editors and authors; and our own assistants: Lynne Prevost and Huguette Rizziéro (CRS), Grace Watson (AB), Elizabeth Torno (WS), and Sandy Muscelli (DV). But especially we thank our extraordinary predecessors for their nurture and care of a book many of us have come to admire and need. If this edition meets with the approval of its former editors, we will have partially done the job we acquired; the readers will ultimately decide whether it was done satisfactorily.

Last, an acknowledgment to our families; they know more about this book than they bargained for . . .!

Charles R. Scriver
Arthur L. Beaudet
William S. Sly
David Valle

The Metabolic & Molecular Bases of Inherited Disease

eighth edition

PART 16

LYSOSOMAL DISORDERS

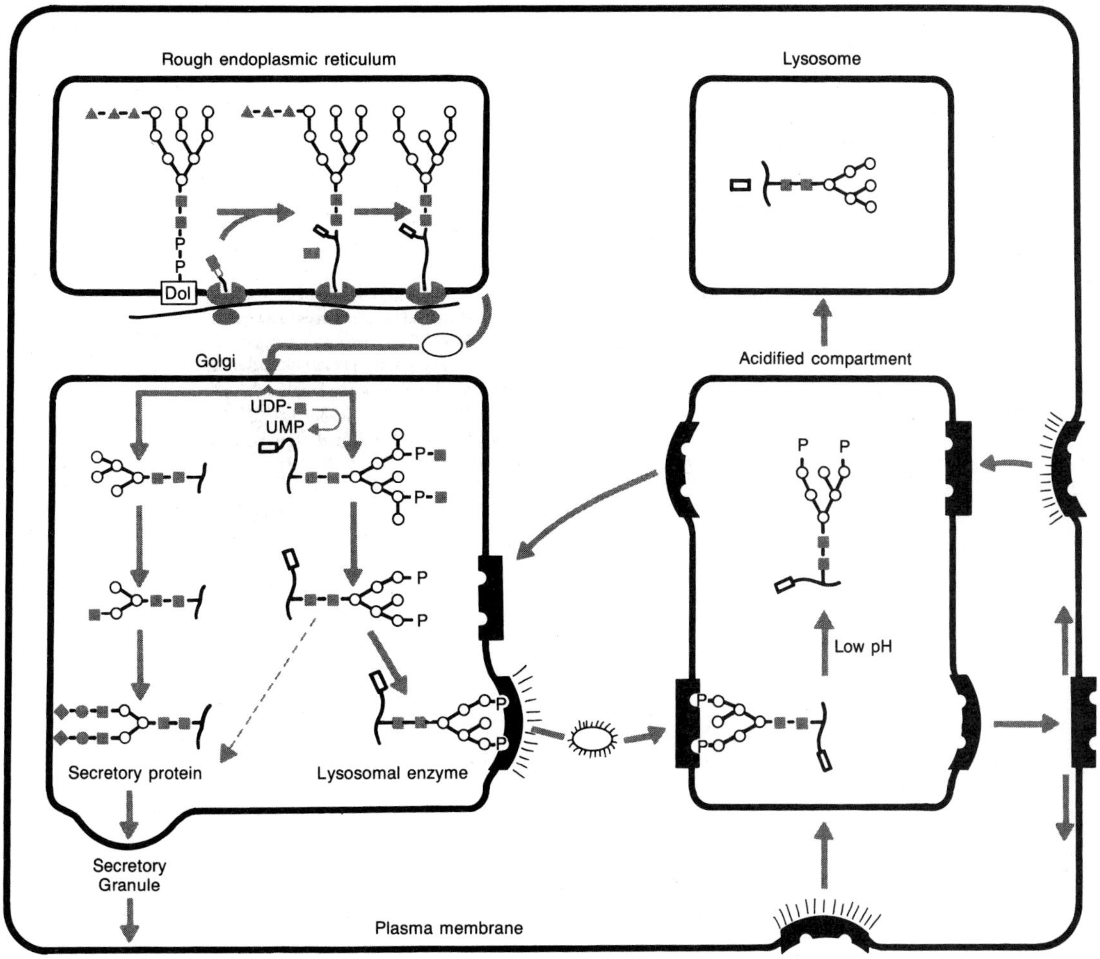

CHAPTER 134

Sphingolipid Activator Proteins

Konrad Sandhoff ▪ Thomas Kolter ▪ Klaus Harzer

1. **The lysosomal degradation of sphingolipids with short hydrophilic head groups is dependent on small nonenzymic glycoproteins, called sphingolipid activator proteins (SAPs), including saposins and the G_{M2} activator protein.**
2. **Two genes code for all established and putative SAPs known so far. One gene on human chromosome 5, consisting of 4 exons and 3 introns, encodes the G_{M2} activator protein; a second gene on chromosome 10, consisting of 15 exons and 14 introns, codes for the SAP precursor, which is processed to 4 homologous activator proteins or saposins, SAP-A, SAP-B, SAP-C, and SAP-D.**
3. **The mature human G_{M2} activator consists of a polypeptide chain of 162 amino acids and carries one *N*-linked carbohydrate chain on Asn 32. It is a membrane-active protein that binds structurally related glycosphingolipids and stimulates their degradation by a specific interaction with *β*-hexosaminidase A. This activator is essential for the hydrolysis of ganglioside G_{M2} and glycolipid G_{A2} in vivo.**
4. **Four point mutations have been identified so far in the G_{M2} activator gene in AB variant of G_{M2} gangliosidosis. They result in premature degradation of the G_{M2} activator and cause a pronounced neuronal storage of ganglioside G_{M2} and glycolipid G_{A2}. The clinical course and pathologic findings observed in AB variant closely resemble those of Tay-Sachs disease.**
5. **The SAP precursor (prosaposin), with a total of 524 amino acids and 5 *N*-glycosylation sites, contains 4 homologous domains, each of about 80 amino acids. A major proportion of the precursor pool is exported to the cell surface and then imported into the lysosomal compartment, where it is processed to the mature glycoproteins SAP-A, SAP-B, SAP-C, and SAP-D. The occurrence of SAP precursor in body fluids and its neurotrophic properties indicate that its function is not restricted to being the precursor of the mature intracellular SAPs.**
6. **In vitro, SAP-A stimulates glucosylceramidase and galactosylceramidase in the presence of detergents. The degradation of galactosylceramide is also stimulated by SAP-A in cultured cells.**
7. **SAP-B is a nonspecific glycolipid-binding protein that stimulates the hydrolysis of about 20 glycolipids by different enzymes, in particular the hydrolysis of sulfatide by arylsulfatase A.**
8. **So far, six different mutations have been identified in the stretch of the SAP precursor gene coding for SAP-B. They result in a loss of the mature SAP-B, causing the accumulation of sulfatide and some other sphingolipids. The clinical course of the disease resembles that of juvenile metachromatic leukodystrophy, with certain exceptions.**
9. **In vitro, SAP-C stimulates the hydrolysis of glucosylceramide by glucosylceramidase, galactosylceramide by galactosylceramidase, and sphingomyelin by acid sphingomyelinase. In vivo, SAP-C is essential for the degradation of glucosylceramide. The glycoprotein factor has been proposed to bind to, and thereby activate, glucosylceramidase. It is a membrane-active protein that solubilizes lipids. Deficiency of SAP-C results in a juvenile variant of Gaucher disease, with pronounced accumulation of glucosylceramide in the reticuloendothelial system. SAP-C seems to have a role also in galactolipid breakdown.**
10. **SAP-D is required for the degradation of ceramide by acid ceramidase in vivo.**
11. **A SAP precursor deficiency due to a homozygous mutation in the initiation codon was found in a boy who died at 16 weeks and his fetal sib. The complete absence of the SAP precursor and the four mature SAPs results in a generalized accumulation of ceramide, glucosylceramide, galactosylceramide, sulfatide, lactosylceramide, digalactosylceramide, ganglioside G_{M3}, and so forth. The symptoms of the disease resembled those of Gaucher (type 2) more than those of Farber disease.**
12. **It is hypothesized that sphingolipid activator proteins are essential for the degradation of intralysosomal vesicles containing former components of the plasma membrane.**
13. **Intracellular routing of SAP precursor and of the G_{M2} activator protein is only in part dependent on mannose-6-phosphate residues. Their endocytosis occurs in a carbohydrate-independent manner. Cellular uptake of the SAP precursor and lysosomal delivery is mediated by the low-density lipoprotein receptor-related protein (LRP).**
14. **Mice with disrupted genes for SAP precursor and G_{M2} activator have been developed as authentic models for known human diseases.**

INTRODUCTION AND HISTORY

The lysosomal degradation of sphingolipids is accomplished by the stepwise action of specific acid exohydrolases. Several of these enzymes need the assistance of small nonenzymic glycoprotein cofactors to attack their lipid substrates. In 1964, Mehl and Jatzkewitz discovered the first such "sphingolipid activator protein," which stimulated degradation of sulfatides by arylsulfatase A[1–3] by solubilizing the lipid.[4] However, activator proteins for degradation of ganglioside G_{M1} by *β*-galactosidase[5,6] and of globotriaosylceramide by *α*-galactosidase A[7] were later described which turned out to be identical with the sulfatide activator protein.[8–11] Then, the identity of a sphingomyelinase activator protein (A_2 activator[12]) with this factor was demonstrated by Edman degradation.[13] Various names were given to this protein (e.g., activator of cerebroside sulfatase,[3] G_{M1} activator protein,[6] SAP-1,[14] and saposin B[15,16]). In this article, we use the designation SAP-B.

An activator protein stimulating the activity of glucosylceramidase toward the natural and synthetic substrates was initially described by Ho and O'Brien.[17] In contrast to SAP-B, this factor seems to stimulate the enzyme directly by binding to it.[18–20] Subsequently, such factors were purified by different laboratories from Gaucher spleen (factor P,[21] heat stable factor,[22,23] sphingolipid activator protein A_1[12]), normal and Gaucher brain,[24] normal human spleen,[12,22] bovine spleen (coglucosidase[25]), and guinea pig liver.[26] All of the human factors seem to be identical based on cDNA analysis and Edman degradation.[27–29] The protein to which this human cDNA corresponds, but also including the protein's nonhuman functional counterparts from guinea pig,[26] bovine spleen,[30] and other sources, is called saposin C or SAP-2, and in this chapter is referred to as SAP-C.

The physiological importance of sphingolipid activator proteins became clear when the AB variant of G_{M2} gangliosidosis could be attributed to the deficiency of a specific activator protein required for degradation of ganglioside G_{M2} by β-hexosaminidase A.[31,32] Like SAP-B, G_{M2} activator protein (G_{M2} activator) forms water-soluble 1:1 complexes with the lipid substrate and thus accelerates its degradation by the enzyme.[33] However, in contrast to SAP-B, it also specifically interacts with β-hexosaminidase A.[34] G_{M2} activator was shown to be clearly different from SAP-B.[35,36] The G_{M2} activator described earlier by Hechtman and LeBlanc[37,38] had a low specific activity and differed in its physicochemical properties from that deficient in AB variant.

When sequence data of the sphingolipid activator proteins became available, it turned out that only two genes code for all activators known so far. One gene, located on q31 of human chromosome 5,[39,212] carries the genetic information for the G_{M2} activator, and a second on region q21 of chromosome 10[40–42] encodes the SAP precursor (prosaposin), which is processed to four homologous proteins (SAPs, saposins), including SAP-B (saposin B) and SAP-C (saposin C).[27–29,43]

Because the number of identified patients is still small, the full clinical spectrum for each of the activator deficiencies remains uncertain. In the case of defects in the SAP precursor gene, only patients with isolated SAP-B, SAP-C, or SAP precursor deficiencies have been described to date.

Structure formulas, required activator proteins, and the diseases associated with their deficiency are given in Fig. 134-1;[196] recent advances in the biochemistry of sphingolipidoses are summarized in reference 218.

G_{M2} ACTIVATOR

Biochemistry and Molecular Biology

Properties. The G_{M2} activator protein consists of a polypeptide chain of 162 amino acids and carries one *N*-linked carbohydrate chain on Asn 32.[44] The molecular mass obtained by gel filtration (23.5 kDa[45] or 25 kDa[46]) is in agreement with the value found by denaturing SDS gel electrophoresis (21.5 kDa)[45] and that calculated for the polypeptide chain without carbohydrate (17.6 kDa),[44] indicating a monomeric structure of the protein. Its isoelectric point at pH 4.8[45,46] is due to a predominance of acidic amino acids.[44,46] Its eight cysteine residues[44] form disulfide bridges,[206] which might contribute to its biologically active tertiary structure[221] as well as to its unusual stability toward heat (stable up to 60°C), and to proteases such as trypsin and chymotrypsin.[44,46] The G_{M2} activator has been heterologously expressed in *E. coli*. The recombinant, carbohydrate-free protein has a higher molecular specific activity than the carbohydrate containing G_{M2} activator purified from human postmortem tissues.[47]

Specificity and Mechanism of Action. G_{M2} activator protein stimulates the degradation of ganglioside G_{M2}, of glycolipid G_{A2}, and, to a minor extent, of globoside by β-hexosaminidase A, but not that by β-hexosaminidase B.[45,46] It accelerates the hydrolysis of lipids but not that of water-soluble synthetic substrates. It is essential for the degradation of G_{M2} and G_{A2} in vivo. In the AB variant of G_{M2} gangliosidosis, the deficiency of G_{M2} activator[31] results in an accumulation of ganglioside G_{M2} and glycolipid G_{A2} but not of globoside as in variant O (deficiency of β-hexosaminidase β-chain).[48]

The following model for the action of G_{M2} activator protein has been suggested:[33] The surface-active G_{M2} activator binds and lifts a single G_{M2} molecule from a lipid aggregate or lipid bilayer and forms a water-soluble 1:1 protein-lipid complex. β-Hexosaminidase A binds to this complex, cleaves the G_{M2} molecule to yield ganglioside G_{M3}, and releases the activator-lipid complex. The activator reinserts the G_{M3} molecule into the membrane and binds another G_{M2} molecule.

The affinity of G_{M2} activator for lipids (dissociation constants of about 3.5 μM and 450 μM for G_{M2} and G_{A2}, respectively[45]) is mainly due to hydrophobic interactions.[33,45] The protein also recognizes the sialic acid and the terminal *N*-acetylgalactosamine residue of G_{M2}.[45] Reduction or methylation of the carboxyl group in the sialic acid residue prevents the stimulatory action of the G_{M2} activator on the degradation of the lipids.[49] In the absence of enzyme, G_{M2} activator is able to transfer sphingolipids from donor liposomes to acceptor liposomes.[33] Only molecules of the outer leaflet are accessible to it. The presence of the sialic acid and *N*-acetylgalactosamine residues of G_{M2} seems to be important for a high transfer rate (the rates decrease in the order, $G_{M1} > G_{M2} > G_{D1a} > G_{M3} > G_{A2}$). According to a recent in vitro study, binding affinity decreases in the order $G_{M2} > G_{T1b} > G_{M1} > G_{b4} > G_{M3} > G_{A2}$.[50] Transfer of lipids between membranes occurs also at neutral pH.[50] Binding of G_{M2} activator to a wide variety of negatively charged glycosphingolipids has been found in gel filtration experiments.[51]

The G_{M2} activator only stimulates the degradation of G_{M2} and G_{A2} by β-hexosaminidase A, although in the presence of suitable detergents, β-hexosaminidase A and B are both able to degrade these lipids.[45,46] The G_{M2} activator-G_{M2} complex, as well as the G_{M2} activator alone, can act as a competitive inhibitor for the degradation of water-soluble synthetic substrates specific for the active site on the α chain of β-hexosaminidase A.[34] This suggests a specific interaction between G_{M2} activator and β-hexosaminidase A. Such interaction would also explain why the degradation of ganglioside G_{D1a}-GalNAc is not stimulated by G_{M2} activator in spite of the fact that it is a substrate for β-hexosaminidase A and can be transferred from donor to acceptor liposomes by G_{M2} activator.[52] When the G_{D1a}-GalNAc-G_{M2} activator complex binds to β-hexosaminidase A, the bond susceptible to the enzyme is probably too distal to enter the active site on the α chain. Retardation of β-hexosaminidase A by an affinity column using recombinant G_{M2} activator also indicates an interaction between the enzyme and the activator.[53] In contrast to these results, a stimulation of G_{D1a}-GalNAc degradation by G_{M2} activator has been reported.[54]

From the data available, the mechanism of action of G_{M2} activator is still not completely clear. G_{D1a}-GalNAc has the same terminal GalNAcβ1-4Gal(3-2αNeuAc) structure as G_{M2}. However, the linkage susceptible to β-hexosaminidase A is 6 to 8 Å away from the membrane surface instead of 2.2 Å as in G_{M2},[52] when using glycolipids integrated into liposomes as substrates. Because G_{D1a}-GalNAc is degraded by β-hexosaminidase A without G_{M2} activator, it would be sufficient if G_{M2} activator lifts ganglioside G_{M2} a few angstroms out of the membrane (Fig. 134-2). This view is supported by the observation that derivatives of ganglioside G_{M2}, with drastically shortened fatty acid chains and increased water solubility, are degraded by β-hexosaminidase A in the absence of G_{M2} activator or detergents.[52] β-Hexosaminidase A is a water-soluble enzyme that acts on substrates of the membrane surface. Like a razor blade, it recognizes and cleaves all substrates (e.g., G_{D1a}-GalNAc) that stick out far enough into the aqueous phase. However, glycosphingolipid substrates with oligosaccharide head groups too short to be reached by the active site of the enzyme cannot be degraded. Their degradation requires a second component, the G_{M2} activator. This specialized

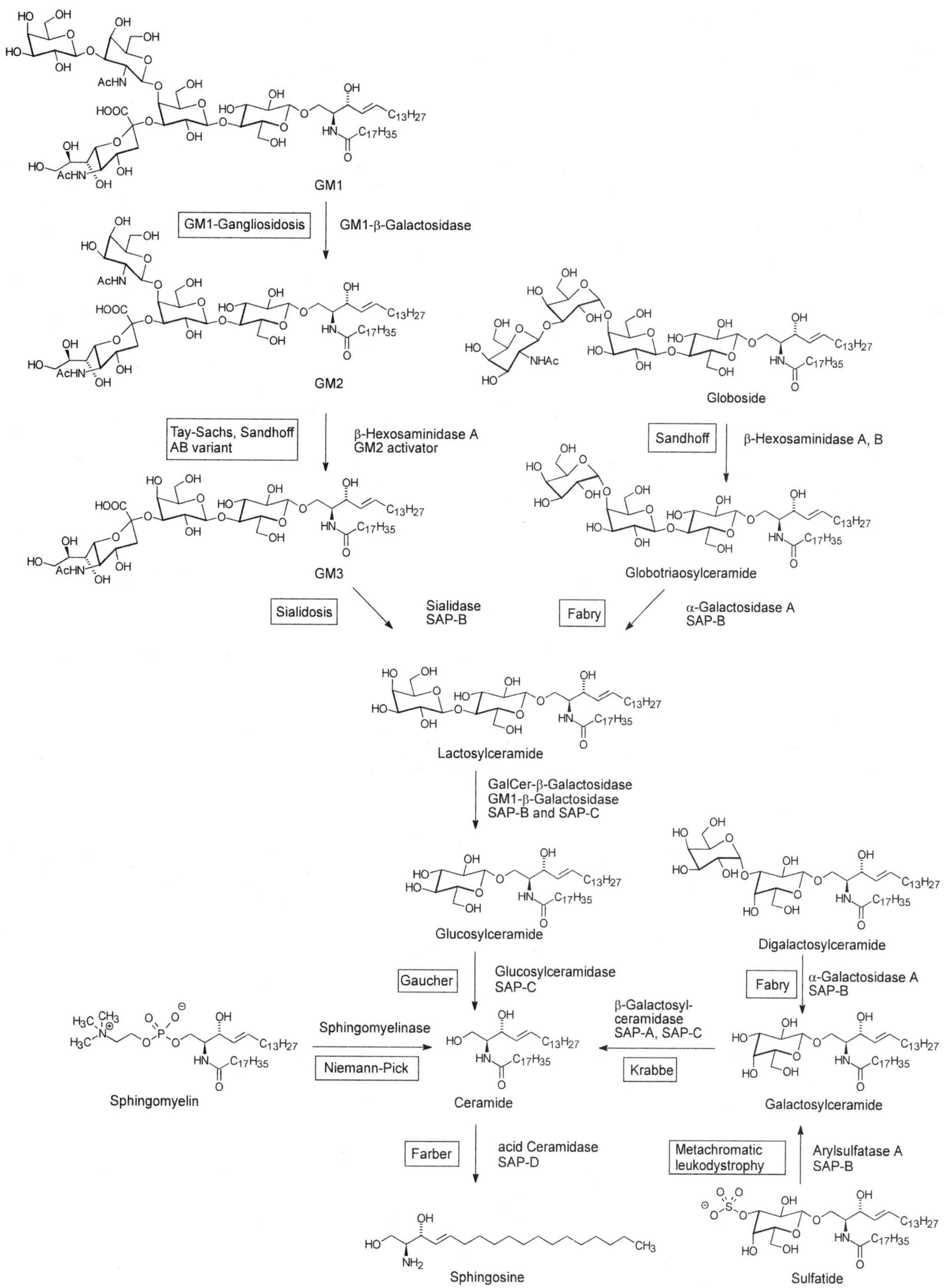

Fig. 134-1 Degradation of selected sphingolipids in the lysosomes of the cells.[196] The eponyms of individual diseases are given. Only those activator proteins that are required for the respective degradation step in vivo are indicated. Heterogeneities within the lipid portion of molecular species are not shown.

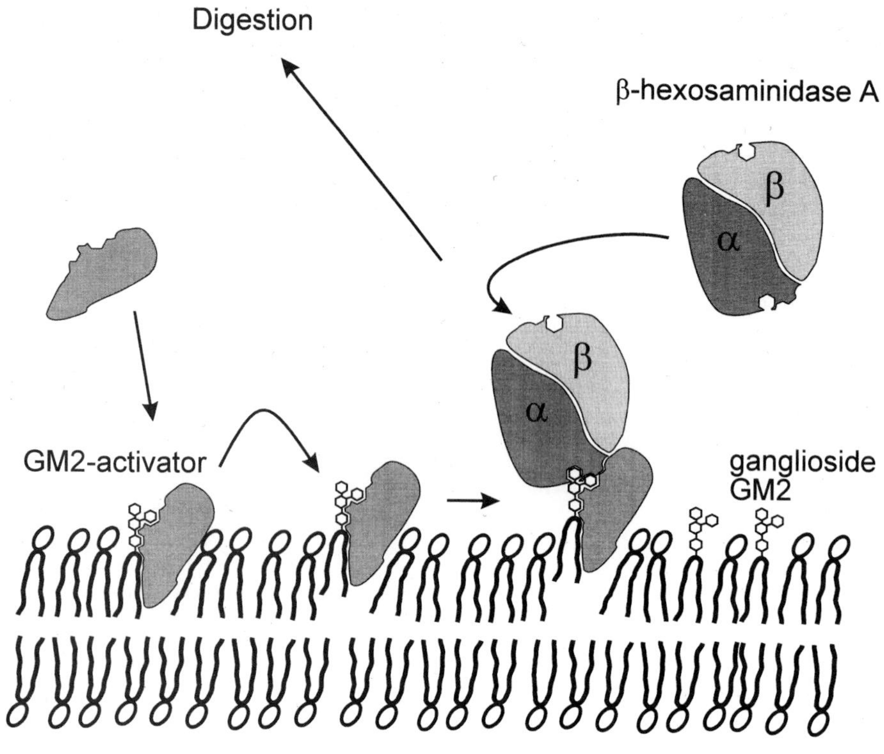

Fig. 134-2 Model for the G_{M2} activator-stimulated degradation of ganglioside G_{M2} by human β-hexosaminidase A (modified from reference 194). Water-soluble β-hexosaminidase A does not degrade membrane-bound ganglioside G_{M2}, which has a short carbohydrate chain, in the absence of G_{M2} activator or appropriate detergents. The G_{M2} activator binds one molecule of ganglioside G_{M2} and lifts it out of the membrane. The activator-lipid complex can be recognized by water-soluble β-hexosaminidase A which cleaves the lipid substrate.

glycosphingolipid binding protein forms a complex with the substrate (e.g., ganglioside G_{M2}), lifts it from the membrane, and presents it to the β-hexosaminidase A for degradation. This view is in accordance with the results of physical-chemical measurements at phosphatidylcholine monolayers. The G_{M2} activator inserts into this model membrane up to a lateral pressure of 25 mN/m which is in the range of the values found in some, but not all, naturally occurring membranes.[210] Also, microcalorimetrical experiments indicate a membrane activity of the G_{M2} activator.

According to an alternative model,[55] the G_{M2} activator acts by modifying the *N*-acetylgalactosamine-sialic acid interaction within the oligosaccharide moiety. This view is not supported by the observation that the G_{M2} activator is not required for the degradation of G_{M2} derivatives with truncated alkyl chains or the degradation of G_{D1a}-GalNAc. In both cases, the structure of the trisaccharide head group should be identical with that of ganglioside G_{M2}. Moreover, glycolipid G_{A2}, where this interaction cannot take place, is a storage compound in G_{M2} activator deficiency and recombinant G_{M2} activator protein is able to restore defective G_{A2} degradation in AB-variant fibroblasts.[56] Also the mouse G_{M2} activator stimulates hydrolysis of G_{A2} by mouse hexosaminidase A and, to a lesser extent, also by hexosaminidase B.[181] Furthermore, G_{A2} is a storage compound in G_{M2} activator knockout mice.[201] This cannot be explained by the model introduced by Wu et al.[55]

Genomic and mRNA Structure. The gene of the G_{M2} activator has been mapped to human chromosome 5 using an enzyme-linked immunosorbent assay (ELISA) to identify the human protein in human-mouse somatic-cell hybrids.[39] Later on it was mapped to 5q32-33 and a nonfunctional pseudogene was identified on chromosome 3.[60,61] The gene covers a region of at least 15 kb.[57] The protein-coding region is interrupted by three introns. The 2.4-kb cDNA codes for a preproprotein of 193 amino acids.[57,58] The signal peptide for the entry to the rough endoplasmic reticulum (23 amino acids) and the mature protein (162 amino acids) are connected by an 8-amino acid propeptide which is missing in the mature protein.[44,59–62]

Biosynthesis. The G_{M2} activator was localized in the lysosomes.[63] Processing studies on cultured human skin fibroblasts revealed that the G_{M2} activator protein is synthesized as a 24-kDa precursor which was found only in the medium of the cultured fibroblasts.[64] Only the mature form of 21 to 22.5 kDa was detected in cells, which suggests rapid processing following biosynthesis. In human epidermal keratinocytes, the G_{M2} activator is synthesized as a 22-kDa precursor bearing a single high-mannose *N*-linked oligosaccharide chain on a peptide backbone of 18 kDa.[65] Processing of the *N*-glycan gives rise to a high mannose type of 22 kDa, a complex type of 24 kDa, and a multiantennary type of 25 to 27 kDa. Approximately one-third of the precursor population is secreted and consists to more than 90 percent of the 24-kDa form. Intracellular activator is processed to a mature protein of 20 kDa with a 17-kDa peptide bearing a multiantennary *N*-glycan without phosphate residues. The existence of an alternatively spliced G_{M2} activator protein[66] could not be confirmed in this study. Tunicamycin treatment revealed that nonglycosylated activator is delivered to the lysosomes with essentially the same kinetics as in nontreated cells. These data suggest also a mannose-6-phosphate independent transport of the activator to the lysosomes.[65] This observation is in agreement with the finding that recombinant, nonglycosylated activator is efficiently endocytosed by fibroblasts from AB variant patients.[47] Two mechanisms are also reported for the recapture of extracellular G_{M2} activator by fibroblasts.[67]

G_{M2} Activator Deficiency

Clinical Aspects. The clinical and pathologic findings in G_{M2} activator deficiency (AB variant of G_{M2} gangliosidosis) are similar to those in Tay-Sachs disease (TSD; B variant; see Chap. 153 on the G_{M2} gangliosidoses). Therefore, a summary for classical TSD is given first. By the age of about 3 to 8 months, motor and other abilities, such as smiling, grasping, rolling over, and head control (if ever achieved), start to be lost. Nystagmus and a startle response to sound are often noted. Free sitting and walking are not achieved, and muscle weakness increases to hypotonia. Macular cherry-red spots and the beginning of optic atrophy appear in the eye fundi. Myoclonus to sound, epileptic fits, or generalized seizures commence at about 1 year of age, and psychomotor regression and blindness become evident. Slowed waves in the electroencephalograms are superimposed with sharp spikes and waves. Muscle hypotonia goes along with some limb hypertonicity and very brisk tendon reflexes. The Babinski sign is positive, and macrocephaly develops. Dementia, convulsive phases, dysphagia, decerebrate spastic ("frog") posturing, respiratory tract infections, and distress mark the downhill course. Death occurs in 90 percent of cases between the ages of 1 and 4 years. Neuropathologically, severe cortical nerve-cell losses are seen, with most of the remaining cortical neurons (and those outside the central nervous system) being swollen. Widespread cortical gliosis and secondary demyelination are also seen.[68]

In G_{M2} activator deficiency (nine cases[48,68–73,78]; clinical data on two proven cases were supplied by Dr. R. Stephens and Ms. E.P. Young from the Hospital for Sick Children, Great Ormond Street, London, and one case by Dr. J.M. Gigonnet and Dr. M.T. Vanier, Hôpitaux de Lyon), many of these signs were present, but some were milder. In contrast to TSD, all of these patients have been non-Jewish. The disease ran, from onset until death, from 11 to about 19, 14 to 27, 6 to 32, 5 to 37, unknown age to 39, about 8 to about 40 (three), and 5 to about 65 months, suggesting a slightly delayed onset and course in comparison with classical TSD. In at least two patients, head control and free sitting were still possible after the age of 1 year, and one patient transiently had achieved incomplete walking. Decreased visual attentiveness and horizontal nystagmus were sometimes observed. Cherry-red (or cherry-black, in a black girl) macular spots were present in all nine patients, but in at least one patient with late-developing dementia, vision was still present at age 2.[69,73] Large head circumference was noted in only three patients. In one case, in which death occurred at 37 months, there was neither excessive response to noise nor any seizure activity. Neuropathologically, substantial macrocephaly and nerve cell losses were absent, and cortical gliosis and demyelination were similar to, or less pronounced than, in TSD. The ubiquitous neuronal lipid storage (shown also in rectal biopsies from two cases) was, however, accompanied by clear astrocytic storage in one case. In this patient, cerebellar atrophy was more distinct than cerebral atrophy, and it was more distinct than cerebellar atrophy in classical TSD. Except for hepatomegaly in one patient,[78] visceromegaly was absent, as were other symptoms not associated with TSD.

Molecular Defects. Only a few cases of G_{M2} activator deficiency have been analyzed so far at the molecular level.[31,63,74,75] In most cases, no cross-reactive material was found in cultured skin fibroblasts or tissue samples of the patients. However, fibroblasts of one patient synthesized a precursor protein with an elevated size (26.5 kDa instead of 24 kDa) and secreted it into the medium.[64] A single amino acid substitution of Cys 107 to Arg 107 was the cause of a total G_{M2} activator deficiency. This mutation abolishes the correct formation of a disulfide bridge, which is important for the structure[221] and stability of the protein, and thus may cause a rapid degradation of the protein.[76,59] In a second case, a single amino acid substitution of Arg 169 to Pro 169 led to complete deficiency of the protein in the patient's cells.[77]

A Saudi Arabian child with consanguineous parents was homozygous for a 3-bp deletion 262–264 resulting in the loss of Lys88.[78] The earliest sign of G_{M2A} deficiency was a mild motor weakness beginning at 8 months of age. The offspring of a consanguineous Spanish mating was homozygous for a single-base deletion in codon 137 (Δ410A) that caused a frameshift in the G_{M2A} gene (fsH137).[78] The frameshift resulted in substitution of 33 amino acids, the loss of another 24 amino acid residues, and a termination codon at residue 170.

Cultured fibroblasts of both of the above deletion patients produced normal levels of G_{M2}-activator mRNA. Pulsed-chase labeling of cultured fibroblasts indicated premature degradation of both the mutant and the truncated G_{M2} activator in the endoplasmic reticulum or the Golgi apparatus. Heterologous expression of the two mutant proteins revealed residual activities of 3 percent and 8 percent, respectively. However, in biosynthetic studies no mature protein could be detected within the lysosomes.[78]

Pathobiochemistry. Despite the presence of β-hexosaminidases A and B, the degradation of ganglioside G_{M2} and glycolipid G_{A2}, but not of globoside, is blocked in G_{M2} activator deficiency, resulting in an accumulation of these lipids (15 percent and 2.8 percent, respectively, of brain tissue dry weight).[48] G_{D1a}-GalNAc, a minor storage material in variant O (Sandhoff disease) and variant B (Tay-Sachs disease) of G_{M2} gangliosidosis, is not elevated in AB variant.[52]

Diagnosis. ELISA is a fast and simple method to determine the amount of G_{M2} activator in tissue samples, cultured fibroblasts, and body fluids.[63] The concentrations of G_{M2} activator in normal human serum and urine, in single experiments, were 48 ng and 600 ng protein per milliliter, respectively. The values found in normal liver, spleen, brain, and placenta ranged from 50 to 120 ng/mg of protein. The extremely high values found in kidney (800 ng/mg protein) are due to elevated biosynthesis of G_{M2} activator mRNA in epithelial cells of the collecting duct.[214] In tissues from G_{M2} gangliosidosis patients of variant B (Tay-Sachs disease) and variant O, its level is elevated by a factor of 2 to 10.[63,74]

Because some mutations may only affect the activity but not the biosynthesis and the stability of G_{M2} activator, immunochemical methods will not detect all cases of G_{M2} activator deficiency. All types of G_{M2} gangliosidosis can be diagnosed by combining loading tests with the determination of β-hexosaminidase A activity.[79] Cultured skin fibroblasts of the patients are supplemented with radiolabeled ganglioside G_{M2} or, even better, with ganglioside G_{M1}.[151] After 24 h the cells are harvested and the fraction of G_{M2} degraded per hour and milligrams of cell protein is determined. Only 10 to 20 percent of normal β-hexosaminidase A activity is sufficient for a normal degradation rate.[79,80] In cases of G_{M2} activator deficiency almost no G_{M2} degradation is observed despite normal β-hexosaminidase A activity.[81] When G_{M2} activator protein is added to the medium of cultured skin fibroblasts from such a patient, it is taken up by the cells and the catabolism of ganglioside G_{M2} is normalized.[32]

SAP PRECURSOR (PROSAPOSIN)

Molecular Biology and Biosynthesis

Genomic and mRNA Structure. The cDNA of the human SAP precursor encodes a polypeptide chain of 524 amino acids (without those encoded by exon 8, see below) starting with a typical signal peptide for entering the ER and containing four homologous domains of some 80 amino acids each (see Fig. 134-3).[27–29,43] These domains correspond to mature SAP-A,[82] SAP-B,[13,44] SAP-C,[83] and SAP-D[43] isolated from human tissues. The degree of identity between these proteins ranges from 23 to 39 percent, with 15 amino acids being conserved in all 4 proteins, among them all 6 cysteine residues and an *N*-glycosylation signal.

The SAP precursor gene covers a region of at least 17 kb[84,85] on segment q21-q23 of chromosome 10.[41,42] The gene was mapped to chromosome 10q22.1 by fluorescence *in situ* hybridization.[86] Additional fine localization was done using a new polymorphism.[223] The positions of its 14 introns, of the cysteine residues, and of the *N*-glycosylation sites show some regularities, supporting the assumption that the SAP precursor gene arose by sequential duplication of an ancestral gene coding for only one SAP domain. Exon 8 consists of only nine base pairs, which code for three amino acids near the C-terminus of SAP-B.[84,87] The mRNAs found include some lacking the nine bases of exon 8, some with only the last six bases, and some with all nine bases of exon 8.[28,87] A physiological significance of the

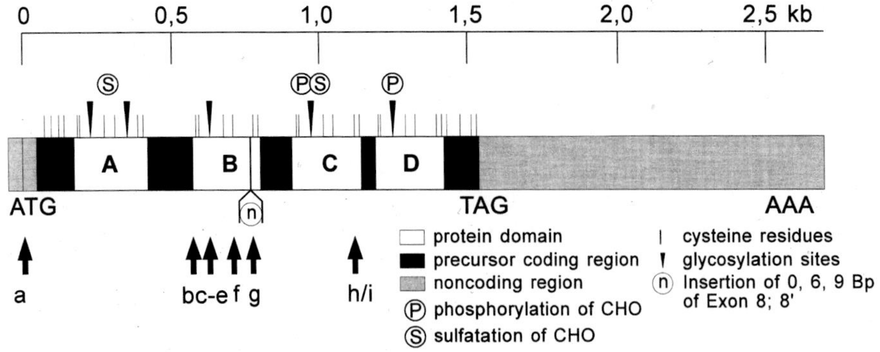

Fig. 134-3 Structure of the SAP precursor cDNA.[194] The cDNA of SAP precursor codes for a sequence of 524 amino acids (or of 527 amino acids[84]), including a signal peptide of 16 amino acids. The four domains on the precursor, A-D, correspond to the mature proteins found in human tissues: SAP-A is also known as saposin A; SAP-B is also known as saposin B or SAP-1 or sulfatide-activator; SAP-C is also known as SAP-2 or saposin C or glucosylceramidase activator protein; SAP-D is also known as saposin D or component C. The positions of the cysteine residues are marked by vertical bars and the positions of the *N*-glycosylation sites by arrow heads. CHO = carbohydrates. The position of the known mutations leading to diseases are given: a = A1T (Met1Leu);[90] b = g-t-transversion within the 3′ acceptor splice site between intron e and exon 6;[180] c = C650T (Thr217Ile);[173,174] d = A643C (Asn215His);[213] e = C645A (Asn215Lys);[219] f = G722C (Cys241Ser);[84] g = 33-bp insertion after G777 (11 additional amino acids after Met259);[172,175] h = G1154T (Cys385Phe);[184] i = T1155G (Cys385Gly).[185]

Gln-Asp-Gln insertion in the SAP-B domain of SAP precursor has been studied.[88] While synthetic peptides containing an α-helix, with and without the amino acid insertion, showed different binding affinities for G_{M1}-ganglioside, sulfatide, and sphingomyelin in vitro,[228] expression of the three different SAP precursor cDNAs[88] in baby hamster kidney cells yielded three correctly processed mature SAP-B isoforms. Compared to each other in loading experiments on SAP precursor-deficient human fibroblasts, these isoforms exerted identical activating effects upon sulfatide and globotriaosylceramide degradation.

Biosynthesis and Processing. Early biosynthetic studies on SAP-B[89] revealed a 65-kDa protein which is probably generated by cotranslational glycosylation of the 53-kDa polypeptide at all five potential glycosylation sites.[28] The oligosaccharide moieties are modified in the Golgi apparatus to yield a precursor protein of 70 kDa containing complex-type oligosaccharide chains. The 70-kDa precursor is secreted even in the absence of ammonium chloride[90] and has been found in human milk.[91,92] Its size can be reduced to a 53-kDa form by *N*-glycanase treatment. The 70-kDa precursor is transported to the lysosomes and proteolytically processed to intermediate forms of 35 to 53 kDa and then to the mature polypeptide chains of 13 kDa. Final trimming of the carbohydrate portion yields 8- to 11-kDa forms. This last step does not take place in G_{M1} gangliosidosis because of the deficiency of lysosomal β-galactosidase. Similar studies using an anti-SAP-C antiserum revealed the same results, except that no 35-kDa intermediates were detected.[93] Most lysosomal enzymes reach the lysosomes via the mannose-6-phosphate pathway. This mechanism is largely blocked in I-cell disease (mucolipidosis II), in which the formation of the mannose-6-phosphate signal is impaired due to a defect in the phosphotransferase. Studies on cultured I-cell fibroblasts suggest that the SAP precursor might be transported by the same mechanism. In I-cell fibroblasts, only low levels of cross-reactive material were found with antisera against SAP-B[94] or SAP-C,[95] and the low activity of glucosylceramidase in such cells has been attributed to the deficiency of SAP-C and not of the enzyme.[96] The SAP precursor, but no mature SAP-B, was detected within I-cell fibroblasts, and large amounts of the precursor were found in the culture medium.[89,97] On the other hand, when SAP precursor from normal cells was added to the medium of control skin fibroblasts, it was taken up by the cells and processed to the mature proteins.[89] The uptake of mature SAP-C by cultured neuroblastoma cells could be inhibited by mannose-6-phosphate and a pentamannosyl-phosphate.[98]

Biosynthesis and processing of SAP precursor in cultured human skin fibroblasts were restudied using polyclonal anti-SAP-C antibodies.[99] The SAP precursor bears phosphate residues on noncomplex carbohydrate chains linked to the SAP-C and -D domains as well as sulfate residues on complex carbohydrate chains on the SAP-A, -C, and, possibly, on the SAP-D domain. SAP precursor with high mannose-carbohydrate chains is converted from a 65-kDa to a 73-kDa form in the Golgi apparatus bearing complex carbohydrates and processed to forms of 30 to 50 kDa. Proteolytic processing starts at the stage of early endosomes. Normal fibroblasts internalized SAP precursor secreted from I-cell fibroblasts nearly as efficiently as SAP precursor secreted from normal fibroblasts. Moreover, deglycosylated SAP precursor is taken up by mannose-6-phosphate receptor double knockout mouse fibroblasts more efficiently than the glycosylated protein. These data suggest that targeting of SAP precursor from the Golgi to the lysosomes is only in part dependent on mannose-6-phosphate residues, while endocytosis occurs in a carbohydrate-independent manner.

SAP-B[100–102] and SAP-C[103,104] were localized in the lysosomes by various biochemical, immunochemical, and electron microscopic techniques. In some lysosomes the labeling of SAP-C by the immunogold technique was most prominent around the perimeter of the matrix, suggesting an association between SAP-C and lysosomal membrane components.[103] The proteolytic processing of SAP precursor has been studied in detail in mammalian and insect cells.[105] Among other proteases, cathepsin D is involved in the proteolytic processing of SAP precursor into the mature SAPs.[106]

Biochemistry

A structural motif known as SAP-like domain has been found in several lipid-binding proteins including the SAPs.[107] It is characterized by three intradomain disulfide linkages and a subset of conserved amino acid residues with hydrophobic side chains. Saposin-like proteins (SAPLIP) carry out diverse functions on a common backbone structure. The three-dimensional structure of a SAP-like domain has been solved by NMR-spectroscopy:[108] the structure of porcine NK-lysin is characterized by five amphiphilic α-helices folded into a single globular domain. Also, sequence homology of saposin-like proteins with plant aspartic proteases has been reported in which C- and amino-terminal halves of the domains have been swapped. According to this, these proteins have been called "swaposins."[109] There is evidence that the precursor of pulmonary surfactant protein B contains three SAP-like domains.[225]

SAP-A (Saposin A). ***Properties and Possible Function.*** SAP-A consists of 84 amino acids and is *N*-glycosylated on Asn 21 and Asn 42.[82] SDS-PAGE of native SAP-A revealed a molecular mass of 16 kDa, which is reduced to 10 kDa after total deglycosylation with *N*-glycanase. In vitro, SAP-A stimulates glucosylceramidase and galactosylceramidase by a similar mechanism but to a lower extent than SAP-C.[82,110] No SAP-A deficiency has been characterized so far except for that in SAP precursor deficiency (see "SAP Precursor Deficiency" below) in which galactosylceramidase shows very low activity in a liposomal assay system.[111] It was suggested that SAP-A and SAP-C may act synergistically,[20] at least on β-glucosylceramidase. In vitro, recombinant SAP-A binds to glucosylceramidase without activating the enzyme in physiological concentrations.[112] In cultured skin fibroblasts derived from the original patients with SAP precursor deficiency, the impaired galactosylceramide degradation could be partially restored by the addition of SAP-A, SAP-C, or a mixture of these activators to the culture medium. Because galactosylceramide degradation is apparently normal in cells derived from a patient with SAP-C deficiency, SAP-A seems to be involved in galactosylceramide degradation in living cells.[211] Compare also the SAP-C section for information on the specificity of SAP-A and SAP-C.

SAP-B (Sulfatide Activator; SAP-1). ***Properties.*** Edman degradation[13,44] of human SAP-B revealed a polypeptide chain of 80 amino acids carrying one *N*-linked complex type carbohydrate chain on Asn 21.[113] The molecular mass found by gel filtration (20 to 22 kDa)[3,6,7,114] is about twice the value calculated from the sequence (8.9 kDa without carbohydrate) and obtained by SDS-PAGE (8 to 11 kDa),[89,114] suggesting a homodimeric structure. The 13-kDa forms found in G_{M1} gangliosidosis are due to impaired processing of the carbohydrate chain due to a defective acid β-galactosidase.[94] The isoelectric point of SAP-B is at pH 4.1 to 4.3.[3,6] From the sequence data, three amphiphilic α-helices were predicted for each subunit which most likely build up the hydrophobic lipid-binding site of SAP-B.[27,43] SAP-B from pig kidney has been purified, characterized,[115,116] and three intrachain disulfide bonds have been identified.[117,118] These cross-linkages and the compact folding of the protein may be the reason for its unusual stability toward extreme pH (pH 1.4 to 12), heat (up to 95°C), and proteases (trypsin and chymotrypsin).[6,7]

Specificity and Mechanism of Action. Under in vitro conditions, SAP-B stimulates the degradation of sulfatide, seminolipid (a sulfoglycerolipid), and, to a minor extent, their diacetylated forms, 3-sulfogalactosylsphingosine (psychosine sulfate) and lyso-seminolipid.[119] In vitro, it accelerates the degradation of ganglioside G_{M1} by β-galactosidase,[5,6] of globotriaosylceramide by α-galactosidase A,[7] and of sphingomyelin by sphingomyelinase.[12,13] In addition to sulfatides, ganglioside G_{M1}, globotriaosylceramide, and sphingomyelin, SAP-B binds to phosphatidylserine and galactosylceramide,[4] to gangliosides G_{M2} and G_{M3}, and to glycolipid G_{A1}.[14] It stimulates the degradation of glycolipid G_{A1} by β-galactosidase[120,121] and of gangliosides G_{D1a}, G_{T1b}, and G_{M3} by lysosomal sialidase.[122] SAP-B has also been shown to stimulate the hydrolysis of about 20 natural or chemically modified glycolipids, among them glycerolipids, by six enzymes of human, plant, or bacterial origin.[123]

The mode of action proposed for SAP-B[4] resembles in several aspects that for the G_{M2} activator: SAP-B binds to single-lipid molecules from micelles or membranes and lifts them as water-soluble 1:1 complexes.[4,121,124] These complexes serve as substrates for the subsequent enzymatic reactions. The enzyme cleaves the terminal group from the activator-bound substrate molecules. The shortened lipids are replaced by new substrate molecules and the cycle starts again.

To explain the broad lipid specificity of SAP-B, a triple binding domain model for the interaction of lipids with this protein has been proposed.[125] According to this proposal, the hydrophobic ceramide moiety binds to a hydrophobic domain in SAP-B which might be built up by six amphiphilic helices (three from each subunit of SAP-B) as in serum albumin.[126] The negative charge of the sulfate group (in sulfatide) or of the sialic acid residues (in G_{M1}) interacts with a positively charged group on SAP-B, and hydroxyl groups of the carbohydrate portion of the glycolipid form hydrogen bonds with a complementary structure on the activator protein. If at least two such interactions are possible, the lipid is bound.

Experimental data largely support this model. Both the acyl residue in the ceramide moiety and the nature of the carbohydrate chain are important for recognition of a lipid by SAP-B.[121] SAP-B only stimulates the degradation of sulfatide and G_{M1} derivatives with acyl chains of at least 6 and 8 carbon atoms, respectively. Sulfatide and G_{M1} derivatives with shorter acyl chains are more water soluble, less tightly bound to lipid phases, and therefore directly recognized by the catabolic enzymes and degraded.[121] Lipids with less than three hexoses are transferred from donor to acceptor liposomes at very low rates compared to complex lipids ($G_{D1a} > G_{M1} > G_{M2} >$ sulfatide $>$ galactosylceramide $> G_{M3}$), and glucosylceramide is not transferred at all. On the other hand, a negative charge of the lipid is not essential because methylation of the sialic acid carboxyl group in G_{M1}[127] or its reduction to an alcohol[121] has no effect on the degradation rate of the lipid in the presence of SAP-B.

In contrast to the G_{M2} activator protein and SAP-C (see below), no specific interaction of SAP-B with an enzyme has been observed.

SAP-C (Glucosylceramidase Activator; SAP-2). ***Properties.*** Human SAP-C consists of a polypeptide chain of 80 amino acids carrying one complex type or hybrid type *N*-linked carbohydrate chain on Asn 22.[83,128] The carbohydrate chain is heterogeneous,[83,100,128,129] but has no influence on the activator activity of SAP-C.[128,130] The molecular mass determined by SDS-PAGE ranges from 5 to 12 kDa, depending on the degree of glycosylation and on experimental details.[25,128,129,131] Gel filtration of native SAP-C revealed a mass of 20 kDa,[21,24,25] which is about twice the value calculated from the amino acid sequence (8.9 kDa without carbohydrate[83]), indicating a homodimeric structure. Its isoelectric point is at pH 4.3 to 4.4.[25] SAP-C is described as a heat-stable (up to 95°C)[21,129] but pronase-labile[21,25,132] protein. Like in SAP-B, the six cysteine residues[83] per monomer stabilize the protein by forming intramolecular disulfide bridges. The positions of the disulfide bridges in SAP-B and SAP-C have been identified by mass spectrometry.[118] A sample of SAP-C has also been obtained by chemical synthesis.[133]

Recently, peptides from various regions of the SAP-C domain have been used to localize regions that mediate the binding of SAP-C to glucosylceramidase and the activation of this enzyme. Glucocerebrosidase activation sites (residues 27 to 34 and 41 to 49) and binding sites (residues 6 to 27 and 45 to 60) on SAP-C have been identified by this approach.[134] Also a SAP-C:glucocerebrosidase complex with a stoichiometry of 4:2 has been postulated. In another study, two functional domains, each comprising a binding site adjacent to or partially overlapping with an activation site, were determined within amino acid sequences 6 to 34 and 41 to 60.[135]

Specificity and Mechanism of Action. In vitro, SAP-C stimulates the activity of lysosomal glucosylceramidase against lipid- and water-soluble synthetic substrates.[17] It also activates galactosylceramidase[24,132,136] and sphingomyelinase.[12,132,136] Unlike G_{M2} activator and SAP-B, SAP-C apparently does not bind to lipid or synthetic substrates,[18] but forms complexes with membrane-associated enzymes and thereby activates them.[18,20,137,138] When the lipid substrates of glucosylceramidase, galactosylceramidase, and sphingomyelinase are incorporated into liposomal membranes, the degradation rates in the absence or presence of SAP-C are nearly independent of diluting the incubation volume with buffer.[139] This suggests that all molecules involved are membrane-bound and that the enzymatic reaction takes place at least in part on the membrane surface. SAP-B and SAP-C stimulated the degradation of lactosylceramide by G_{M1}-β-galactosidase and galactosylceramide in a detergent-free liposomal system.[140] While

SAP-B formed water-soluble complexes with lactosylceramide that were recognized by G_{M1}-β-galactosidase, SAP-C more efficiently stimulated lactosylceramide degradation by galactosylceramidase occurring exclusively on liposomal surfaces. These findings explain why the deficiency in only one β-galactosidase or one sphingolipid activator protein does not block lactosylceramide catabolism and therefore does not result in the lysosomal accumulation of this lipid.

In the presence of phosphatidylserine SAP-C was reported to form 1:1 complexes with glucosylceramidase.[18,137] On the other hand, ultracentrifugation studies revealed that rat liver glucosylceramidase (56 kDa) forms high-molecular-weight aggregates (190 kDa) in the presence of human SAP-C and phosphatidylserine[19] or G_{M1},[141] and is thereby activated by a factor of 25. Human glucosylceramidase does not strictly require SAP-C to form such aggregates.[19] This may explain why acidic phospholipids, such as phosphatidic acid, phosphatidylserine, and phosphatidylinositol, efficiently activate this enzyme toward glucosylceramide or synthetic substrates even in the absence of SAP-C[18,137–139,142] by lowering the K_m values and raising the V_{max} values.[22,139] Addition of SAP-C stimulates the enzyme by further lowering the K_m values and raising the V_{max} values.[25,141] Kinetic experiments revealed an apparent K_d for the binding of SAP-C to the enzyme of about 0.1 mM and excluded cooperativity in this binding.[18]

Acidic phospholipids and SAP-C seem to bind at different sites on glucosylceramidase, thereby promoting conformational changes leading to aggregate formation and to the activation of the enzyme. Recently, it was shown that the binding of those effectors had synergistic stimulatory effects on the enzyme.[20,110] SAP-C is also able to solubilize lipids.[208]

The placental factor described by Vaccaro and coworkers[143] might be different from SAP-C. It seemed to be tightly bound to the enzyme because it was separated from it only by hydrophobic chromatography. It stimulates the degradation of glucosylceramide (but not of water-soluble synthetic substrates) by glucosylceramidase, probably by promoting the binding of the enzyme to substrate micelles.[144] Their subsequent studies[145,146] were important in showing that SAP-A, C, and D acquire hydrophobic properties on acidification, while the hydrophilicity of SAP-B remains apparently unchanged. At acidic pH values needed for binding, SAP-C and D destabilize the phospholipid membranes of large unilamellar vesicles composed of phosphatidylcholine, phosphatidylserine, and cholesterol, while SAP-A and B minimally affected the bilayer integrity.[145] They also demonstrated that glucosylceramide inserted in large unilamellar vesicles was degraded seven- to eightfold more slowly than glucosylceramide inserted in small unilamellar vesicles. A partial stimulation of glucosylceramide hydrolysis was observed by the addition of SAP-A or SAP-C, which could be enhanced by the addition of both activator proteins. SAP-B and SAP-D had no effect. SAP-C increased the rate of hydrolysis of both the artificial water-soluble substrate and the lipid substrate while SAP-A only stimulated degradation of the sphingolipid. This study indicates that SAP-C is responsible for the membrane binding of glucosylceramidase, while SAP-A stimulation might be related to its effect on the conformation of the enzyme.[146] For a more detailed study of SAP-C specificity, taking into account the lysosomal lipid composition, compare references 142 to 146 and 208 with the paragraph about the topology of lysosomal digestion.

SAP-D (Saposin D). ***Properties and Possible Function.*** SAP-D[147] contains 78 amino acids and carries one *N*-linked carbohydrate chain on Asn 20.[43] Its molecular mass on SDS-PAGE is 10 kDa and it was found to contain 16 percent carbohydrate.[147] In vitro, SAP-D showed some stimulatory activity on a crude sphingomyelinase preparation.[147]

SAP-D stimulates the lysosomal degradation of ceramide by acid ceramidase in vivo. This was established in feeding studies with SAP precursor-deficient human fibroblasts; in these cells SAP-D reduces the amount of accumulated ceramide.[148] Also a crude preparation of ceramidase was stimulated fourfold by SAP-D in an in vitro assay at acid pH.[149]

In vitro results indicate that acid sphingomyelinase is also stimulated by SAP-B and SAP-C.[12,13,83] This stimulation is not necessary for the in vivo degradation of sphingomyelin by this enzyme.[148,150] Also the SAP precursor knockout mice show no sphingomyelin accumulation.[205]

SAP Precursor. ***Properties and Possible Function.*** Studies about the pH-dependent conformational properties of the SAP domains indicated that acidic pH triggers the exposure of hydrophobic domains of SAP-A, SAP-C, and SAP-D but has no effect on the hydrophilicity of SAP-B.[145] This pH-dependent change in domain hydrophobicity was paralleled by the pH-dependent binding of SAP-C and SAP-D to large unilamellar phospholipid vesicles and the destabilization of phospholipid membranes, while SAP-A and SAP-B minimally interacted with the vesicles and membranes. With chimeric proteins constructed of sequence fragments of SAP-B and SAP-C, the neurotrophic and acid glucosylceramidase-activating properties were localized on the SAP-C domain. SAP-C amino acid residues 22 to 31 were identified to have neurotrophic effects, and the activating site of SAP-C was assigned to residues 47 to 62.[135]

SAP precursor (prosaposin) may have functions of its own. Native human SAP precursor and recombinant SAP precursor (obtained from *Spodoptera frugiperda* cells after transfection with baculovirus containing a full-length cDNA coding for human SAP precursor) show stimulatory activity for degradation of glucosylceramide by β-glucosidase and of G_{M1} ganglioside by β-galactosidase.[152,153] The SAP precursor (prosaposin) and SAPs A, B, C, and D bind gangliosides and transfer them from donor liposomes to erythrocyte ghost membranes.[152] SAP precursor, purified from human milk, shows neurotrophic activity to protect hippocampal CA1 neurons from ischemic damage in vivo[224] and to promote regeneration of transected sciatic nerve.[222] Part of this activity seemed to be mediated through an 18-amino-acid sequence located in the amino-terminal hydrophilic region of the rat SAP-C domain.[154] In addition, SAP precursor stimulated neurogenesis and increased choline acetyltransferase activity in NS20Y neuroblastoma cells.[155] This effect was mediated by a 12-amino-acid peptide that is also located in the amino-terminal portion of SAP-C, but which does not overlap with the region responsible for the neurotrophic effect on hippocampal CA1 neurons. Moreover, the neuroblastoma cell studies identified a high-affinity binding site indicative of receptor-ligand interaction initiating a signal transduction cascade and resulting in neuronal differentiation.[155] A putative receptor for SAP precursor has been partially purified from baboon brain by affinity chromatography using a SAP-C column. A molecular weight of 55 kDa and G-protein association have been reported for this receptor.[207] A more comprehensive study revealed that the SAP precursor can be taken up by cells by at least three independent receptor mechanisms, the low-density lipoprotein receptor-related protein (LRP), the mannose-6-phosphate receptor, and the mannose receptor.[186]

SAP precursor, but no mature SAP, was detected in human secretory fluids such as CSF, semen, milk,[91] pancreatic juice, and bile.[156] Its amount in milk changed in a characteristic way during the lactating period. SAP precursor was released from human platelets in response to stimulation by thrombin. Using antisera against human SAP-B and bovine SAP-C, the relative amounts of SAP precursor, intermediate forms, and mature SAPs were analyzed in different rat tissues.[157] Skeletal muscle, heart, and brain contain mainly precursor forms, while mature forms dominate in spleen, lung, liver, and kidney. SAP precursor, SAP-C and peptides containing the neurotrophic sequence located in the SAP-C domain were able to increase sulfatide concentrations in primary and transformed Schwann cells, suggesting that SAP precursor binds to a receptor that initiates signal transduction to promote myelin lipid synthesis and prolong cell survival in these cell types.[158] This might explain the deficiency of myelin observed in SAP precursor-deficient mice and humans. Binding studies using[125] I-labeled SAP precursor and a radiolabeled SAP precursor-derived peptide suggest a single class of specific binding sites with a K_d of 2.5 nM and 18.3 nM, respectively. In PC12 cells, binding leads to protein tyrosine phosphorylation including phosphorylation of MAPK, suggesting the involvement of MAPK, in signal transduction by SAP precursor.[159]

The rat sulfated glycoprotein I (SGP-1) is homologous to human SAP precursor (70 percent identity) and is believed to be the rat equivalent,[160] although definite proof is still lacking. SGP-1 is secreted as an uncleaved protein into the seminiferous tubule by Sertoli cells. Here, and in the efferent duct, high concentrations of the protein were found (60 to 110 μg/ml), whereas the serum level was low (1.5 μg/ml).[161] SGP-1 is believed to be involved in the degradation of lipids in residual bodies and/or in the modification of membrane lipids during sperm maturation. Cross-reactive material to anti-SGP-1 antiserum was found in the lysosomes of Sertoli cells. However, western blot analysis showed only unprocessed SGP-1 but no smaller fragments.[161] Although a lipid-binding function of a putative SAP-B domain of SGP-1 was proposed to depend on the inclusion or exclusion of exon 8 in the alternatively spliced SGP-1 mRNAs similar to the SAP precursor mRNAs,[226] the effect on lipid binding of the three amino acids encoded by exon 8 seems negligible according to studies with the SAP precursor.[88] In a murine equivalent of the SAP precursor (if different from murine SGP-1), expression of an mRNA homologous to that of prosaposin was high in brain, Sertoli cells, corpus luteum, and present in a 12.5-day-old embryo in brain stem and genital ridge.[162] The investigation of the tissue distribution of rat SPG-1 revealed its prevalent occurrence in specialized cells lining fluid compartments.[163]

Another homologous protein having a function outside the cell is the human pulmonary surfactant-associated protein SP-B.[164,165] It is synthesized as a precursor of some 40 kDa, which is processed to yield a small peptide of 6 to 14 kDa. Lung surfactant is composed of phospholipids and small apoproteins and has the function of reducing the surface tension in lung alveoli. The cDNA of SP-B codes for three protein domains homologous to those of prosaposin, the second of which corresponds to mature SP-B.

SAP DEFICIENCIES

SAP-B (Sulfatide Activator; SAP-1) Deficiencies

Clinical Aspects. The clinical findings in SAP-B deficiency are similar to those in metachromatic leukodystrophy (MLD; see Chap. 148 on metachromatic leukodystrophy), but not in all instances. Therefore, a summary of the three main forms of MLD is given first.

Late infantile MLD begins between 1 and 2 years of age, with a tendency to fall, gait disability, and psychomotor retardation. Ataxia, pes equinovarus, spasticity, muscle atrophy, rare epileptic fits, a reduced nerve-conduction velocity, neuroimaged leukodystrophy, a moderately increased CSF protein content, an increased urinary excretion of sulfatide, spastic quadriparesis, dementia (though incomplete for a long time), and decerebration mark the downhill course, with death occurring before 5 years of age.

Juvenile MLD runs a similar course, but the symptoms start between 3 and 10 years of age and culminate in death between 10 and 20 years.

Adult MLD is extremely variable. Psychotic histories can often be misleading and are followed by subtle signs of motor disability and vegetative (e.g., gallbladder) dysfunction, ataxia, spastic paresis, and only late identification of leukodystrophy by neuroimaging. Nerve-conduction velocity and CSF protein content may remain almost unremarkable. Neuropathologically, the degree of demyelination is variable, with the lesions in the central and peripheral nervous system showing metachromatically stained macrophages. In the peripheral myelin lesions, storage material is also present in the Schwann cells.

In SAP-B deficiency (nine cases[166–171,180,213,219]), some of the main signs of MLD were present in eight of the nine patients studied. However, the clinical features of the infantile patient described with developmental delay, muscle hypotonia, and seizures[169] were not characteristic of late infantile MLD. Between onset of symptoms at 6 months of age and death at 28 months, the only signs suggestive of a leukodystrophy were pallid optic disks and posturing with back hyperextension. The infant's neuroimaged brain atrophy, depressed deep tendon reflexes, absence of spasticity, brief seizures, and tongue fasciculation were more suggestive of a neuronal disease. Neuropathologically there were, however, clear signs of MLD. In addition, most cortical neurons had a ballooned cytoplasm, and neuronal loss was severe in the brain stem. In keeping with MLD, macrophages and kidney tubuli were filled with metachromatic material.

The early juvenile SAP-B-deficient patient[170] met the even more specific criteria for childhood MLD. His parents were first cousins, and he had a sister (not studied) with the same disease. He became symptomatic at 18 months and was still alive but in a poor, wheelchair-bound condition at 7 years. Additional signs were the sluggish reaction to light of his dilated pupils, a reduced swallowing reflex, and several generalized seizures. His weak tendon reflexes and early loss of speech were less typical of MLD, but spastic quadriparesis with positive Babinski sign was typical of MLD. A rectal biopsy taken at age 4 years suggested heterogeneous sphingolipid storage. Submucosal macrophages were filled with metachromatic material (ultrastructure of sulfatide storage), while neurons were crowded with nonmetachromatic, but periodic acid-Schiff-positive material (ultrastructure of membranous bodies of the gangliosidosis type), and endothelial cells showed pleomorphic depositions.

The juvenile SAP-B-deficient sibs[166] had first-cousin parents and started their clinical course at 4.5 (the girl) and 6 (the boy) years of age. The girl's early symptoms included gnashing of her teeth and wringing of her hands. She stopped being able to ride her bicycle, and her mental state regressed. Right-sided floppiness and a focal seizure were noted. By the age of 6 she had stopped walking and talking and had generalized motor seizures. Increased muscle tone, contracted arms, exaggerated reflexes, a reduced nerve-conduction velocity, and a borderline high CSF protein were her MLD-like findings. The boy started his course with a generalized seizure, and he began to forget things. By 11 years of age he had lost his intellectual functions. By 19 years, he was uncommunicative, nonambulatory, and incontinent. Hyperreflexia and extreme spasticity were observed. There have been no subsequent reports.

The adult SAP-B-deficient patient[167,168,172] had consanguineous parents. Signs included an ataxic gait, intellectual deterioration, muscle hypertonicity, a strongly reduced nerve-conduction velocity, a distinctly increased CSF protein, metachromasia in peripheral nerves, high urinary sulfatide levels, and neuroimaged periventricular signs of demyelination, as in MLD. However, she was only 1 year of age when her psychomotor retardation was first noted. Her full-scale IQ was 40 at age 15 years and had decreased more rapidly than her motor skills. By age 21, she was dysarthric, suggesting pseudobulbar involvement. Her height, weight, and head circumference were below the third percentile, and her eye fundi showed macular grayness. While her arms displayed spastic crossing and forced grasping, her legs showed weak muscle tone, with absent reflexes and sensory disturbance. Some ambulation was still possible, but she required assistance. She became severely demented, had lost the ability to speak, had swallowing problems, and became incontinent before she died at age 22. Postmortem findings have not been reported.

Molecular Defects. Defects of SAP-B analyzed so far (see Fig. 134-3) could be attributed to homoallelic point mutations that destroyed the glycosylation site,[171,173,174,213,219] substituted a cysteine residue,[87] or generated a new splice site that leads to a 33-base insertion into the mRNA.[172,175] A G-to-T transversion within the acceptor splice site between intron e and exon 6 abolished normal RNA splicing.[180] These mutations allow normal biosynthesis and processing of the precursor. However, these mutated SAP-B molecules seem to be rapidly degraded after they are released from the precursor because they are not detectable in such cell lines.[169,170,171,176] A homoallelic A643C transversion generates a stable but inactive gene product, Asn215His, lacking the glycosylation site.[213] A homoallelic C → A transversion in the same, highly conserved codon (Asn215Lys) was recently described.[219]

Pathobiochemistry. The discovery of patients with SAP-B deficiency provided strong evidence for the in vivo function of this protein. The genetic defect of SAP-B leads to variant forms of MLD (see "Clinical Aspects" above) but with a nearly normal arylsulfatase A level.[170,176] In addition to sulfatide,[170,171] increased amounts of globotriaosylceramide and digalactosylceramide were excreted with the urine of three patients.[9,180] The degradation of externally added sulfatide or globotriaosylceramide by cultured skin fibroblasts is nearly totally blocked[170,171,176] but can be raised by adding SAP-B to the culture medium.[176,177] Loading of these cells with ganglioside G_{D1a} led to elevated levels of G_{M3} and, to a lower extent, of lactosylceramide, but not of G_{M1}.[177] These findings emphasize a role of SAP-B in the degradation of sulfatide by arylsulfatase A, of globotriaosylceramide and digalactosylceramide by α-galactosidase A, and possibly of G_{M3} by acid sialidase.[178] The stimulation of the α-galactosidase A-catalyzed degradation of globotriaosylceramide by SAP-B has been demonstrated in a detergent-free liposomal system.[179]

The g → 12t transversion within the acceptor splice site between intron e and exon 6 of the SAP precursor gene[180] led to abnormal splicing of exon 6 during mRNA maturation. One of the two detectable shortened mRNAs encoded a SAP precursor with apparently normal biosynthesis and processing, except that no mature SAP-B was detectable. The second mRNA bearing a complete deletion of exon 6 encoded a polypeptide of only 60 kDa, which was not further processed nor transported beyond the endoplasmic reticulum.

An A643C transversion in the SAP precursor gene of a 4-year-old MLD patient led to the exchange of Asn215 to His and to the elimination of the glycosylation site in SAP-B.[213] The mutation had no effect on intracellular transport, maturation, and stability of the modified SAP precursor.

Transfection of fibroblasts of a patient with SAP-B deficiency (due to a point mutation destroying its glycosylation site) with a cDNA construct for the SAP precursor restored normal SAP-B levels in the cells and normalized their sulfatide catabolism.[171]

Diagnosis. Analysis of the lipid pattern in urine sediment of patients may provide the first evidence for SAP-B deficiency (see "Pathobiochemistry" above). More confident results may be obtained by the determination of the SAP-B level in urine, fibroblast extracts, or tissue samples by ELISA.[169–171,176] Glycosylation defects within the SAP-B domain, however, might appear immunologically normal. Direct determination of SAP-B activity in biologic samples is difficult because high protein concentrations inhibit the assay.[182] Like the G_{M2} activator deficiency, sulfatide loading tests, together with the determination of arylsulfatase A activity, may provide a valuable tool to verify an initial diagnosis of SAP-B deficiency.[79,170,171,177]

SAP-C (Gaucher Activator; SAP-2) Deficiency

Clinical and Pathological Aspects. The clinical findings in SAP-C deficiency (Gaucher activator deficiency) are thought to be similar to those in Gaucher disease type 3 (see Chap. 146), which is a juvenile visceromegalic and neuronopathic disease. Gaucher disease type 3 is a variable disease, with most patients showing splenohepatomegaly by the age of 1 year. Growth retardation, delayed skeletal maturation, hematologic signs of hypersplenism, Gaucher cells in the bone marrow, and increased serum acid phosphatase are early signs. Psychomotor development is retarded and is usually evident by 1 year of age. Oculomotor problems, electroencephalographic abnormalities (observed more frequently than epileptic seizures), ataxia, and spastic paraparesis are frequent neurologic signs. Skeletal complications are experienced by more than 50 percent of patients. After a dementing process (either low- or high-grade), death usually occurs within the first three (mostly the second) decades of life, but sometimes later. In SAP-C deficiency (two cases[12,183]) the patients' histories contained the main signs of Gaucher disease type 3, as outlined above. In addition, one patient (data from Dr. P. Wyss, Basel) started walking late and was never able to stand up from a sitting position. At the age of 4 years she displayed a shuffling and clumsy gait, spoke incompletely, and despaired of her disabilities. The parents noticed her thick belly and weak hip muscles, and her doll-like face showed brownish pigment spots. In her ocular fundi, irregular pigmentation was seen. Neurologic and electromyographic findings indicated atrophic muscles with muscle weakness accentuated in the pelvic girdle. She showed spasticity and seizures before death at 14 years of age. For the second patient, a complete study is now available.[227] The boy developed normally until age 8 years when epileptic fits started. At 10 years focal adversive seizures became generalized. He presented intention tremor, discrete ptosis, and bilateral abducens nerve paresis. The spleen was massively (6 cm below costal margin), and the liver slightly, enlarged. Bone marrow smears contained some Gaucher cells. Platelet counts were normal, but serum acid phosphatase activity was elevated. During the next years the neurologic signs increased with myoclonic jerks, frequent generalized seizures, slurred speech, ocular apraxia with horizontal nystagmus (but vertical gaze still unimpaired), loss of motor and intellectual abilities, progressive bilateral pyramidal tract syndrome, and slight cerebellar signs. At age 13 he presented complete supranuclear gaze paralysis, severe ataxia, and tremor. Palpebral flutter was elicited on his speech attempts, but exogenous stimuli elicited myoclonus, which also existed continuously. Additional clonic seizures occurred daily and could also be elicited by intermittent photic stimuli. EEG showed slow disorganized background and increase of paroxysmal occipital discharge; nocturnal EEG yielded a few vertex spikes, no spindles, and minor intercritical multifocal paroxysms also in extraoccipital regions; cyclic sleep organization was preserved. The boy died with bronchopneumonia in an epileptic status at age 15.5 years. Different antiepileptic therapy strategies never had any effect. Gaucher-like skeletal and skin abnormalities were always absent. Hypersplenic sequelae were low with only one transient pancytopenic and anemic phase that was documented. On pathologic examination, Gaucher cells were widespread in different organs, but they were absent in the cerebral perivascular spaces. The brain was remarkable for varying rates of nerve cell losses in different regions, most striking in the dentate nuclei. General demyelination was absent, but, locally, the hili of the dentate nucleus were severely, and the pyramidal tracts slightly, demyelinated. However, throughout the central nervous system many of the remaining neurons were enlarged and filled with PAS-positive material, the changes peaking in the spinal cord motoneurons. Further features were focally ballooned dendrites of Purkinje cells and some axon spheroids and neuronophagic nodules in different brain regions. Ultrastructurally, neuronal storage cytosomes reflected the cerebral lipid storing process. The membrane-bound inclusions contained lamellae stacked loosely or densely with parallel bilayers. Other inclusions had an electron-dense granular center and peripheral concentric or radial lamellae. Lipofuscin cytosomes were also frequent. Extracerebral neuronal storage was seen in the enteric plexus nerve cells.

Molecular Defects. In the two analyzed cases, SAP-C deficiency was attributed to point mutations (see Fig. 134-3) substituting the same cysteine residue by phenylalanine[184] and glycine,[185] respectively, on one of the alleles. No other SAP proteins seem to be affected, suggesting a normal biosynthesis and processing of the precursor. However, in both patients it seems that no prosaposin mRNA is transcribed from the other allele.[184,185] The mutated SAP-C molecules, if of normal antigenicity, are probably degraded because no cross-reactive material to anti-SAP-C antiserum was detected in fibroblasts or tissues of the patients.[12,183]

Pathobiochemistry. In vivo, SAP-C seems to be essential for the degradation of glucosylceramide. Its genetic defect causes accumulation of the lipid (also in the brain[227]) leading to a variant form of Gaucher disease (see "Clinical and Pathological Aspects" above). In the liver and spleen, a large accumulation of glucosylceramide, but not of other lipids, is found, while the level of glucosylceramidase is normal.[183] Sphingomyelin catabolism seems to be unaffected. A possible involvement of SAP-C in galactosylceramide catabolism[211] has to be clarified.

Diagnosis. SAP-C deficiency is a Gaucher-like disease with nearly normal glucosylceramidase activity. The diagnosis may be verified by an immunochemical analysis of extracts of tissue samples or cultured skin fibroblasts from the patient[12,183] or by molecular biology studies.[184]

SAP Precursor Deficiency

Clinical Aspects. The clinical findings for the first known case of SAP precursor deficiency (combined SAP deficiency, SAPD, prosaposin deficiency) were similar to those in Gaucher disease type 2 (see Chap. 146), which is an infantile, acute neuronopathic, visceromegalic disease, with death usually occurring within the first 2 years of life. The first clue that the prosaposin gene was affected came from the Adelaide Children's Hospital findings that the patient[187] and his affected fetal sib[103] were deficient in immunoreactive SAP-C (SAP-2). The following account of the patient's extremely acute postnatal downhill course is modified from the original paper.[187] Directly after birth, the patient showed hyperkinetic or cloniform motor abnormalities. Fasciculations of his elongated tongue and periauricular muscles, a spontaneous Babinski sign, reduced patellar tendon reflexes, and an exaggerated Moro reflex were observed. Low blood glucose and calcium levels were both corrected, and a generalized clonic seizure required anticonvulsant treatment. Tonic paroxysms, often starting from the mouth, persisted. The mother noted the baby's deep, hoarse cry. Endotracheal ventilation was also started. Computed tomography of the brain at age 3 weeks showed multicentric hypodense areas, which, however, at reexamination of CT scans were not strongly suggestive of hypomyelination. A scan at patient age 99 days showed only slight frontal hypomyelination but slight general brain atrophy. Massive hepatosplenomegaly suggested a storage disease, and storage macrophages resembling Gaucher cells were observed in a bone marrow smear at the age of 5 weeks. Enzyme studies with leukocytes showed a profound deficiency of β-galactosylceramidase (as in Krabbe disease) activity. The ultrastructure of liver, nerve, and skin biopsies confirmed that it was a lysosomal storage disease. Among the abundant vesicular inclusions and additional membranous bodies in the liver sinusoidal cells (Fig. 134-4), there were only a few structures suggestive of Gaucher disease. Following serial convulsive attacks, death occurred from respiratory and circulatory failure at the age of 16 weeks. The parents did not want an autopsy performed. In the amniotic fluid cells from the mother's next pregnancy, ceramide catabolism was found to be affected (see "Pathobiochemistry") similarly to the fibroblasts from the propositus, and the parents elected to terminate the pregnancy. Biochemical and ultrastructural signs for the fetus were almost identical to those for the propositus.[111]

Molecular Defect. The total deficiency of the SAP precursor in the siblings was due to a homoallelic mutation in the initiation codon (see Fig. 134-3).[90] As a result of this mutation, all four SAP

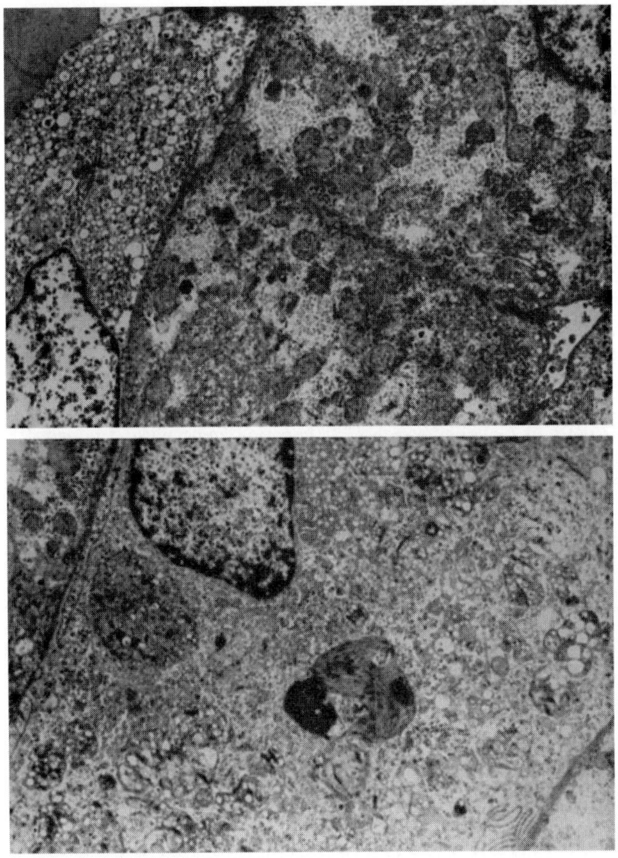

Fig. 134-4 Liver biopsy from SAP precursor-deficient patient. ***Upper panel*****: Sinusoidal cell (at the left of two hepatocytes) crowded with vesicular inclusions.** ***Lower panel*****: Sinusoidal cells with additional membranous inclusions (×10,600). (*****Courtesy of Dr. Roggendorf, Würzburg, Germany.*****)**

proteins, A to D, derived from this precursor were deficient. The parents of the sibs with this SAP precursor-deficient disorder (SAPD)[187] are fourth cousins. They are healthy, but they both carry the mutant allele, indicating a recessive inheritance.[90]

Skin fibroblast cells from the two original patients deficient in the SAP precursor have now been SV40-transformed to keep them available for further studies in the future. Biochemical and immunological anomalies are unchanged as compared to the untransformed cells.[188]

Pathobiochemistry. In cultured skin fibroblasts from the SAPD sibs, reduced activities of glucosylceramidase, galactosylceramidase, and ceramidase were observed,[187] and elevations of ceramide, glucosylceramide, lactosylceramide, sulfatide, and ganglioside G_{M3}, but not sphingomyelin, were found in their organ tissues.[111,150] For both the SAPD child and fetus, no SAP precursor, mature SAP-B, SAP-C, or intermediate forms were detected in the cultured cells or media with anti-SAP-B and anti-SAP-C serums.[90] After loading the cells with sphingomyelin and glucosylceramide, ceramide accumulated in the cells,[187] indicating an impaired catabolism of the latter lipid. Loading studies with labeled ganglioside G_{M1} revealed an impaired ganglioside G_{M3} degradation, and there was a greatly reduced incorporation of label into the biosynthetic products, phosphatidylcholine, and sphingomyelin.[178] Loading studies[150] with sulfatide, globotriaosylceramide, lactosylceramide, and galactosylceramide[211] showed similar pathologic results.[150] These studies indicate that there were defects at multiple sites in the sphingolipid catabolic pathway, which is not unexpected given the simultaneous deficiency of all four SAP proteins. Of particular note was the impaired catabolism of ceramide in SAPD, which points to the involvement of SAP protein in this degradative step.[148,188]

Diagnosis. SAP precursor deficiency can be diagnosed with immunochemical methods. However, a definite proof of a SAP precursor defect can only be obtained by the demonstration of a molecular defect or by performing processing studies using antiserums against more than one SAP protein.

REGULATION OF BIOSYNTHESIS

The high levels of SAP-C (SAP-2) found in Gaucher spleen[189] draw attention to a possible regulation of the expression of the SAP precursor gene. Only a few observations may support the hypothesis that a high load of sphingolipids leads to a compensatory increase in the biosynthesis of SAPs. Taniike et al.[190] observed an elevation in the level of lysosomal SAP-B after loading fibroblasts from a patient with MLD with sulfatide. An elevated level of mRNA of SAP precursor was also observed in B cells of Gaucher patients.[191] Injecting mice with conduritol B epoxide, an inhibitor of glucosylceramidase, led to an increase of liver glucosylceramide and SAP-C.[192] Injection of glucosylceramide also raised the SAP-C level in the liver. However, it cannot be ruled out that the elevated levels of SAP proteins in various sphingolipidoses are also due to codeposition of these proteins together with the lipid storage material because very high levels of SAP-B and SAP-C were found not only in Gaucher spleen, but also in Tay-Sachs brain.[189] The suppression of prosaposin synthesis has been related to the abnormal stratum corneum formation in patients with atopic skin through lower activation of glucocerebrosidase.[193] Surprisingly, the storage material in the infantile neuronal ceroid lipofuscinoses is mainly composed of SAP-A and SAP-D.[215–217]

ACTIVATOR PROTEINS AND THE TOPOLOGY OF LYSOSOMAL DIGESTION

According to a model of the topology of endocytosis and lysosomal digestion[194] introduced in 1992, the degradation of plasma membrane-derived lipids occurs on the surface of intraendosomal and intralysosomal vesicles. This model is of relevance for the mechanism of sphingolipid activator proteins because lipid composition and diameter of vesicles drastically influence the activator protein-dependent degradation of sphingolipids.

It is generally assumed that components of the plasma membrane reach the lysosomal compartment by endocytic membrane flow via the early and late endocytic reticulum.[195] After a series of vesicle budding and fusion events through the endosomal compartment, the membrane fragments enter the lysosomal compartment as part of the lysosomal membrane. Because the inner leaflet of the lysosomal membrane is protected by a thick glycocalix composed of glycoproteins, this view cannot explain how degradation of former plasma membrane components can specifically occur without destruction of the lysosomal membrane.

In an alternative model for the topology of endocytosis, components of the plasma membrane pass through the endosomal compartment as intraendosomal vesicles that become intralysosomal vesicles or membrane structures on reaching the lysosomes (Fig. 134-5).[194] The vesicles are initially formed in the early endosome by selective invagination (budding-in) of endosomal membranes enriched for components of the plasma membrane. The surrounding endosome then passes along the endocytic pathway by the normal, successive events of membrane fission and fusion. The intraendosomal vesicles, however, are carried along as passengers. When the vesicle reaches the lysosome, glycoconjugates originating from the outer leaflet of the plasma membrane face the lysosol on the outer leaflet of intralysosomal vesicles and are thus accessible for the degrading enzymes. In this model, there is no glycocalix blocking the action of hydrolases. This hypothesis is supported by a series of observations.[196,197]

In vitro studies have been carried out to understand the mechanism of action of sphingolipid-activator proteins. However, in most of the studies, the specific lipid composition of the lysosome, as well as the vesicle-bound nature of the lipid substrate, have not been taken into account. Moreover, only data on the total lipid composition of lysosomes are available and not on the composition of intralysosomal vesicles, which have to be assumed to serve as the real substrates for activator protein-dependent degradation. Experiments using unilamellar liposomes of a size that correspond to the size of intralysosomal vesicles observed to date, indicate that the presence of negatively charged lipids is required for degradation of sulfatide by arylsulfatase A in the presence of SAP-B, of glucosylceramide by glucocerebrosidase in the presence of SAP-C, and of ceramide by acid ceramidase in the presence of SAP-D. Degradation experiments have been performed using phosphatidylcholine liposomes dotted with bis(monoacylglycero)phosphate or dolicholphosphate. These negatively charged lipids occur in the lysosomes and were selected to mimic the in vivo situation as closely as possible. Glucosylceramide incorporated into phosphatidylcholine liposomes was hydrolyzed at a very slow rate by glucosylceramidase, even in the presence of SAP-C. The insertion of negatively charged lysosomal lipids like bis(monoacylglycero)phosphate, dolicholphosphate, or phosphatidylinositol stimulated the hydrolysis up to thirtyfold.[208] Also, the stimulatory effect of SAP-D on ceramide hydrolysis is highly dependent on the presence of bis(monoacylglycero)phosphate or another negatively charged phospholipid in a

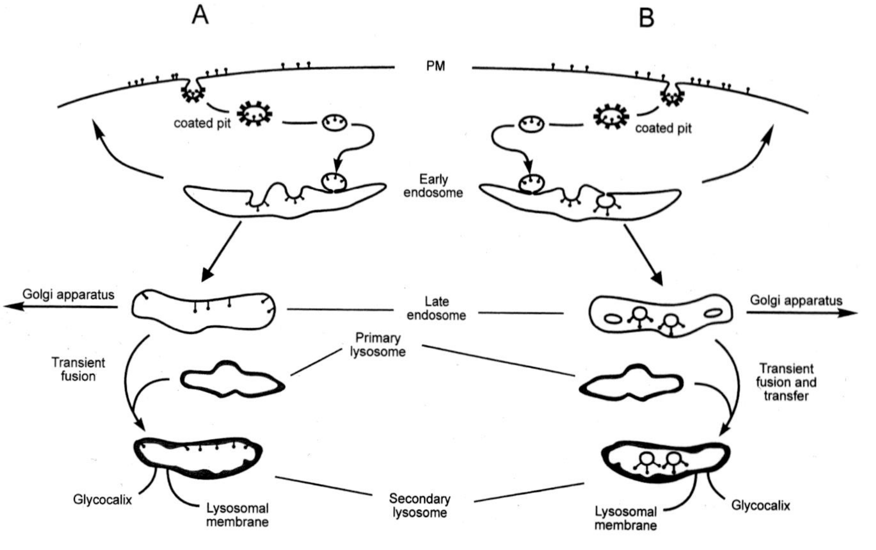

Fig. 134-5 Two models for the topology of endocytosis and lysosomal digestion of glycosphingolipids (GSLs) derived from the plasma membrane.[196] Molecules in the membrane are subjected to a sorting process which directs some of them to the lysosomal compartment, others to the Golgi apparatus, and yet others back to the plasma membrane. Conventional model (*A*): degradation of GSLs derived from the plasma membrane occurs selectively within the lysosomal membrane. Alternative model for the topology of endocytosis and digestion of GSLs (*B*): during endocytosis, glycolipids of the plasma membrane become incorporated into the membranes of intraendosomal vesicles (multivesicular bodies). The vesicles are transferred into the lysosomal compartment when the late endosome fuses with primary lysosomes. PM = plasma membrane; • = glycosphingolipid.

detergent-free liposomal assay system.[209] The rate of ceramide hydrolysis is not strongly affected by the size of unilamellar phospholipid vesicles in the range of 50 to 200 nm.

ANIMAL MODELS

Animal models are valuable for the study of pathogenesis and approaches to therapy of sphingolipid storage diseases. In the recent past, mouse models for the different variant forms of the G_{M2} gangliosidoses, including G_{M2} activator deficiency, have been developed (see reference 198 for a review). While the phenotype of these variants is only slightly different in humans, the animal models show drastic differences in severity and course of the diseases. The reason for this is the specificity of sialidase, which is different between mouse and human. The animals deficient in the SAP precursor gene developed a clinical, pathologic, and biochemical phenotype, closely resembling that of the human disease.

G_{M2} Activator Deficiency

The cDNA[199] and gene[200,201] of the G_{M2} activator from mice have been characterized. Like the human gene, the gene of the G_{M2} activator consists of four exons. The intron-exon borders are conserved between human and mouse. The mouse model for G_{M2} activator[201] deficiency expresses an intermediate phenotype between the mouse models of the other variants of G_{M2}-gangliosidosis, Tay-Sachs, and Sandhoff mice. They demonstrate an age-dependent onset of severe motor defects, but have a normal life span. Storage of ganglioside G_{M2} and, to a lesser extent, G_{A2} occurs in restricted regions of the brain. They correspond to the affected regions in hexa $-/-$ mice (piriform, entorhinal cortex, amygdala, hypothalamic nuclei). Storage occurred predominantly in large pyramidal neurons in the middle layer with little storage in the spinal cord and the visceral organs. A major difference between the G_{M2} activator and the β-hexosaminidase α-chain knockout mice was the additional storage of glycolipid G_{A2} in the cerebellar neurons and glial cells of the G_{M2} activator knockout mice. Impaired motor coordination detected in the G_{M2} activator knockout mice can be correlated to significant storage in this portion of the brain. The low level of G_{A2} storage in the mice indicates that the β-hexosaminidase-mediated degradation of G_{A2} can proceed in the absence of the activator protein, albeit at a reduced rate. The lipid storage pattern observed in G_{M2} activator-deficient mice indicates that the G_{M2} activator also facilitates the degradation of G_{A2} at least in this species.

SAP Precursor Deficiency

The SAP precursor from mouse tissue has been characterized by cDNA sequencing. It is homologous to the human protein but contains 31 additional amino acids between the domains of SAP-C and SAP-D.[202] Also the mouse gene[203] of the SAP precursor, including promoter organization,[220] has been characterized. It consists of 15 exons and 14 introns. As in the humans,[88] mouse exon 8 is alternatively spliced in transcribed mRNAs in a tissue-specific manner. The SAP precursor gene was mapped to mouse chromosome 10 by analysis of interspecies crosses. Psap, as well as the genes of the homologous pulmonary surfactant proteins 2 and 4, map to the 10q21-q23 region.[204]

A mouse model for SAP precursor deficiency has been developed.[205] SAP precursor-deficient mice developed a clinical, pathologic, and biochemical phenotype closely resembling that of the human disease. Mice surviving birth and therefore exhibiting a later-onset phenotype developed rapidly progressive neurologic signs around 20 days and died at 35 to 38 days. Unlike in the human disease, they had no organomegaly. At day 30, severe hypomyelination and PAS-positive storage materials were found throughout the nervous system. The storage materials were also seen in abnormal cells in the liver and spleen. Most prominently lactosylceramide, and additionally ceramide, glucosylceramide, galactosylceramide, sulfatide, and globotriaosylceramide were abnormally increased in the brain, liver, and kidney, and their catabolism was abnormally slow in cultured fibroblasts.

ACKNOWLEDGMENT

Work in the authors' laboratories was supported by the Deutsche Forschungsgemeinschaft.

REFERENCES

1. Mehl E, Jatzkewitz H: Eine Cerebrosidsulfatase aus Schweineniere. *Hoppe Seyler's Z Physiol Chem* **339**:260, 1964.
2. Jatzkewitz H, Stinshoff K: An activator of cerebroside sulfatase in human normal liver and in cases of congenital metachromatic leukodystrophy. *FEBS Lett* **32**:129, 1973.
3. Fischer G, Jatzkewitz H: The activator of cerebroside sulfatase: Purification from human liver and identification as a protein. *Hoppe Seyler's Z Physiol Chem* **356**:605, 1975.
4. Fischer G, Jatzkewitz H: The activator of cerebroside sulfatase-A. Model of the activation. *Biochim Biophys Acta* **528**:69, 1978.
5. Li Y-T, Mazzotta Y, Wan C-C, Orth R, Li S-C: Hydrolysis of Tay-Sachs ganglioside by β-hexosaminidase A of human liver and urine. *J Biol Chem* **248**:7511, 1973.
6. Li S-C, Li Y-T: An activator stimulating the enzymic hydrolysis of sphingoglycolipids. *J Biol Chem* **251**:1159, 1976.
7. Gärtner S, Conzelmann E, Sandhoff K: Activator protein for the degradation of globotriaosylceramide by human α-galactosidase. *J Biol Chem* **258**:12378, 1983.
8. Inui K, Emmett M, Wenger DA: Immunological evidence for the deficiency in an activator protein for sulfatide sulfatase in a variant form of metachromatic leukodystrophy. *Proc Natl Acad Sci U S A* **80**:3074, 1983.
9. Li S-C, Kihara H, Serizawa S, Li Y-T, Fluharty AL, Mayes JS, Shapiro LJ: Activator protein required for the enzymatic hydrolysis of cerebroside sulfate. *J Biol Chem* **260**:1867, 1985.
10. Vogel A, Fürst W, Abo-Hashish MA, Lee-Vaupel M, Conzelmann E, Sandhoff K: Identity of the activator proteins for the enzymatic hydrolysis of sulfatide, ganglioside G_{M1} and globotriaosylceramide. *Arch Biochem Biophys* **259**:627, 1987.
11. Banks MN, Herbert SJ, Wynn CH: Activator proteins for sulphatide hydrolysis and G_{M1}-ganglioside hydrolysis — Probable identity on the basis of their co-purification, properties, ligand binding and immunochemical interactions. *Glycoconj J* **4**:157, 1987.
12. Christomanou H, Aignesberger A, Linke RP: Immunochemical characterization of two activator proteins stimulating enzymic sphingomyelin degradation in vitro: Absence of one of them in a human Gaucher disease variant. *Biol Chem Hoppe Seyler* **367**:879, 1986.
13. Kleinschmidt T, Christomanou H, Braunitzer G: Complete amino-acid sequence of the naturally occurring A2 activator protein for enzymic sphingomyelin degradation: Identity to the sulfatide activator protein (SAP 1). *Biol Chem Hoppe Seyler* **369**:1361, 1988.
14. Wenger DA, Inui K: Studies on the sphingolipid activator protein for enzymatic hydrolysis of G_{M1} ganglioside and sulfatide, in Barranger JA, Brady RO (eds): *Molecular Basis of Lysosomal Storage Disorders*. New York, Academic, 1984, p 61.
15. O'Brien JS, Kishimoto Y: Saposin proteins: Structure, function and role in human lysosomal storage disorders. *FASEB J* **5**:301, 1991.
16. Hiraiwa M, Kishimoto Y: Saposins and their precursor, prosaposin: multifunctional glycoproteins. *Trends Glycosci Glycotechnol* **8**:341, 1996.
17. Ho MW, O'Brien JS: Gaucher's disease: Deficiency of "acid" β-glucosidase and reconstitution of enzyme activity in vitro. *Proc Natl Acad Sci U S A* **68**:2810, 1971.
18. Berent SL, Radin NS: Mechanism of activation of glucocerebrosidase by co-β-glucosidase (glucosidase activator protein). *Biochim Biophys Acta* **664**:572, 1981.
19. Prence E, Chakravorti S, Basu A, Clark LS, Glew RH, Chambers JA: Further studies on the activation of glucocerebrosidase by a heat-stable factor from Gaucher spleen. *Arch Biochem Biophys* **236**:98, 1985.
20. Fabbro D, Grabowski GA: Human acid β-glucosidase. Use of inhibitory and activating monoclonal antibodies to investigate the enzymes catalytic mechanism and saposin A and C binding sites. *J Biol Chem* **266**:15021, 1991.
21. Ho MW, O'Brien JS, Radin NS, Erickson JS: Glucocerebrosidase — Reconstitution of activity from macromolecular components. *Biochem J* **131**:173, 1973.

22. Peters SP, Coyle P, Coffee CJ, Glew RH, Kuhlenschmidt MS, Rosenfeld L, Lee YC: Purification and properties of a heat-stable glucocerebrosidase activating factor from control and Gaucher spleen. *J Biol Chem* **252**:563, 1977.
23. Basu A, Glew RH, Daniels LB, Clark LS: Activators of spleen glucocerebrosidase from control and patients with various forms of Gaucher's disease. *J Biol Chem* **259**:1714, 1984.
24. Wenger DA, Roth S: Isolation of an activator protein for glucocerebrosidase in control and Gaucher disease brain. *Biochem Int* **5**:705, 1982.
25. Berent SL, Radin NS: β-Glucosidase activator protein from bovine spleen ("coglucosidase"). *Arch Biochem Biophys* **208**:248, 1981.
26. Sano A, Radin NS, Johnson LJ, Tarr GE: The activator protein for glucosylceramide β-glucosidase from Guinea pig liver. *J Biol Chem* **263**:19597, 1988.
27. O'Brien JS, Kretz KA, Dewji N, Wenger DA, Esch F, Fluharty AL: Coding of two sphingolipid activator proteins (SAP-1 and SAP-2) by same genetic locus. *Science* **241**:1098, 1988.
28. Nakano T, Sandhoff K, Stümper J, Christomanou H, Suzuki K: Structure of full-length cDNA coding for sulfatide activator, a co-β-glucosidase and two other homologous proteins: Two alternate forms of the sulfatide activator. *J Biochem* **105**:152, 1989.
29. Rorman EG, Grabowski GA: Molecular cloning of a human co-β-glucosidase cDNA: Evidence that four sphingolipid hydrolase activator proteins are encoded by single genes in humans and rats. *Genomics* **5**:486, 1989.
30. Sano A, Mizuno T, Kondoh K, Hineno T, Ueno S, Kakimoto Y, Morita N: Saposin-C from bovine spleen: Complete amino acid sequence and relation between the structure and its biological activity. *Biochim Biophys Acta* **1120**:75, 1992.
31. Conzelmann E, Sandhoff K: Deficiency of a factor necessary for stimulation of hexosaminidase A-catalyzed degradation of ganglioside G_{M2} and glycolipid G_{A2}. *Proc Natl Acad Sci U S A* **75**:3979, 1978.
32. Sonderfeld S, Conzelmann E, Schwarzmann G, Burg J, Hinrichs U, Sandhoff K: Incorporation and metabolism of ganglioside G_{M2} in skin fibroblasts from normal and G_{M2} gangliosidosis subjects. *Eur J Biochem* **149**:247, 1985.
33. Conzelmann E, Burg J, Stephan G, Sandhoff K: Complexing of glycolipids and their transfer between membranes by the activator protein for lysosomal ganglioside G_{M2} degradation. *Eur J Biochem* **123**:455, 1982.
34. Kytzia H-J, Sandhoff K: Evidence for two different active sites on human hexosaminidase A: Interaction of G_{M2} activator protein with hexosaminidase A. *J Biol Chem* **260**:7568, 1985.
35. Li S-C, Nakamura T, Ogamo A, Li Y-T: Evidence for the presence of two separate protein activators for the enzymic hydrolysis of G_{M1} and G_{M2} gangliosides. *J Biol Chem* **254**:10592, 1979.
36. Fürst W, Vogel A, Lee-Vaupel M, Conzelmann E, Sandhoff K: Glycosphingolipid activator proteins, in Freysz L, Dreyfus H, Massarelli R, Gatt S (eds): *Enzymes of Lipid Metabolism II*. New York, Plenum, 1986, p 315.
37. Hechtman P: Characterization of an activating factor required for hydrolysis of G_{M2} ganglioside catalyzed by hexosaminidase A. *Can J Biochem* **55**:315, 1977.
38. Hechtman P, LeBlanc D: Purification and properties of the hexosaminidase A—Activating protein from human liver. *Biochem J* **167**:693, 1977.
39. Burg J, Conzelmann E, Sandhoff K, Solomon E, Swallow DM: Mapping of the gene coding for the human G_{M2} activator protein to chromosome 5. *Ann Hum Genet* **49**:41, 1985.
40. Kao F-T, Law ML, Hartz J, Jones C, Zhang X-L, Dewji N, O'Brien JS, Wenger DA: Regional localization of the gene coding for sphingolipid activator protein SAP-1 on human chromosome 10. *Somat Cell Mol Genet* **13**:685, 1987.
41. Inui K, Kao F-T, Fujibayashi S, Jones C, Morse HG, Law ML, Wenger DA: The gene coding for a sphingolipid activator protein, SAP-1, is on human chromosome 10. *Hum Genet* **69**:197, 1985.
42. Fujibayashi S, Kao F-T, Jones C, Morse H, Law M, Wenger DA: Assignment of the gene for human sphingolipid activator-2 (SAP-2) to chromosome 10. *Am J Hum Genet* **37**:741, 1985.
43. Fürst W, Machleidt W, Sandhoff K: The precursor of sulfatide activator protein is processed to three different proteins. *Biol Chem Hoppe Seyler* **369**:317, 1988.
44. Fürst W, Schubert J, Machleidt W, Meyer HE, Sandhoff K: The complete amino-acid sequences of human ganglioside G_{M2}-activator protein and cerebroside sulfate activator protein. *Eur J Biochem* **192**:709, 1990.
45. Conzelmann E, Sandhoff K: Purification and characterization of an activator protein for the degradation of glycolipids G_{M2} and G_{A2} by hexosaminidase A. *Hoppe Seyler's Z Physiol Chem* **360**:1837, 1979.
46. Li S-C, Hirabayashi Y, Li Y-T: A protein activator for the enzymic hydrolysis of G_{M2} ganglioside. *J Biol Chem* **256**:6234, 1981.
47. Klima H, Klein A, van Echten G, Schwarzmann G, Suzuki K, Sandhoff K: Over-expression of a functionally active human G_{M2}-activator protein in *Escherichia coli*. *Biochem J* **292**:571, 1993.
48. Sandhoff K, Harzer K, Wässle W, Jatzkewitz H: Enzyme alterations and lipid storage in three variants of Tay-Sachs disease. *J Neurochem* **18**:2469, 1971.
49. Handa S, Nakamura K: Modification of sialic acid carboxyl group of ganglioside. *J Biochem* **95**:1323, 1984.
50. Smiljanicgeorgijev N, Rigat B, Xie B, Wang W, Mahuran DJ: Characterization of the affinity of the G_{M2} activator protein for glycolipids by a fluorescence dequenching assay. *Biochim Biophys Acta* **1339**:192, 1997
51. Hama Y, Li YT, Li SC: Interaction of G_{M2} activator protein with glycosphingolipids. *J Biol Chem* **272**:2828, 1997.
52. Meier EM, Schwarzmann G, Fürst W, Sandhoff K: The human G_{M2} activator protein: A substrate specific cofactor of hexosaminidase A. *J Biol Chem* **266**:1879, 1991.
53. Yadao F, Hechtman P, Kaplan F: Formation of a ternary complex between G_{M2} activator protein, G_{M2} ganglioside and hexosaminidase A. *Biochim Biophys Acta* **1340**:45, 1997.
54. Li S, Wu Y, Sugiyama E, Taki T, Kasama T, Casellato R, Sonnino S, Li Y: Specific recognition of *N*-acetylneuraminic acid in the G_{M2} epitope by human G_{M2} activator protein. *J Biol Chem* **270**:24246, 1995.
55. Wu YY, Lockyer JM, Sugiyama E, Pavlova NV, Li YT, Li SC: Expression and specificity of human G_{M2} activator protein. *J Biol Chem* **269**:16276, 1994.
56. Bierfreund U, Lemm T, Hoffmann A, Uhlhorn-Dierks G, Childs RA, Yuen CT, Feizi T, et al: Recombinant G_{M2}-activator protein stimulates the in vivo degradation of G_{A2} in G_{M2} gangliosidosis AB variant fibroblasts but shows no detectable binding of G_{A2} in an in vitro assay. *Neurochem Res* **24**:295, 1999.
57. Klima H, Tanaka A, Schnabel D, Nakano T, Schröder M, Suzuki K, Sandhoff K: Characterization of full-length cDNA and the gene coding for the human G_{M2}-activator protein. *FEBS Lett* **289**:260, 1991.
58. Schröder M, Klima H, Nakano T, Kwon H, Quintern LE, Gärtner S, Suzuki K, Sandhoff K: Isolation of a cDNA encoding the human G_{M2} activator protein. *FEBS Lett* **251**:197, 1989.
59. Xie B, Wang W, Mahuran DJ: A Cys138-to-Arg substitution in the G_{M2} activator protein is associated with the AB variant form of G_{M2} gangliosidosis. *Am J Hum Genet* **50**:1046, 1992.
60. Swallow DM, Islam I, Fox MF, Povey S, Klima H, Schepers U, Sandhoff K: Regional localization of the gene coding for the G_{M2} activator protein (G_{M2A}) to chromosome 5q32-33 and confirmation of the assignment of G_{M2AP} to chromosome 3. *Ann Hum Genet* **57**:187, 1993.
61. Xie B, Kennedy JL, McInnes B, Auger D, Mahuran D: Identification of a processed pseudogene related to the functional gene encoding the G_{M2} activator protein: Localization of the pseudogene to human chromosome 3 and the functional gene to human chromosome 5. *Genomics* **14**:796, 1992.
62. Klima H, Klein A, van Echten G, Schwarzmann G, Suzuki K, Sandhoff K: Over-expression of a functionally active human G_{M2}-activator protein in *Escherichia coli*. *Biochem J* **292**:571, 1993.
63. Banerjee A, Burg J, Conzelmann E, Carroll M, Sandhoff K: Enzyme-linked immunosorbent assay for the ganglioside G_{M2}-activator protein: Screening of normal human tissues and body fluids, of tissues of G_{M2} gangliosidosis, and for its subcellular localization. *Hoppe Seyler's Z Physiol Chem* **365**:347, 1984.
64. Burg J, Banerjee A, Sandhoff K: Molecular forms of G_{M2}-activator protein: A study on its biosynthesis in human skin fibroblasts. *Biol Chem Hoppe Seyler* **366**:887, 1985.
65. Glombitza GJ, Becker E, Kaiser HW, Sandhoff, K: Biosynthesis, processing, and intracellular transport of G_{M2} activator protein in human epidermal keratinocytes. The lysosomal targeting of the G_{M2} activator is independent of a mannose-6-phosphate signal. *J Biol Chem* **272**:5199, 1997.
66. Wu YY, Sonnino S, Li Y, Li S: Characterization of an alternatively spliced G_{M2} activator protein, GM2A protein. *J Biol Chem* **271**:10611, 1996.
67. Rigat B, Wang W, Leung A, Mahuran DJ: Two mechanisms for the recapture of extracellular G_{M2} activator protein: Evidence for a major secretory form of the protein. *Biochemistry* **36**:8325, 1997.

68. Adachi M, Schneck L, Volk BW: Progress in investigations of sphingolipidoses. *Acta Neuropathol (Berl)* **43**:1, 1978.
69. Kolodny EH, Wald I, Moser HW, Cogan DG, Kuwabara T: G_{M2}-gangliosidosis without deficiency in the artificial substrate cleaving activity of hexosaminidases A and B [Abstract]. *Neurology* **23**:427, 1973.
70. De Baecque CM, Suzuki K, Rapin I, Johnson AB, Whethers DL, Suzuki K: G_{M2}-gangliosidosis, AB variant. Clinicopathological study of a case. *Acta Neuropathol (Berl)* **33**:207, 1975.
71. Goldman JE, Yamanaka T, Rapin I, Adachi M, Suzuki K, Suzuki K: The AB variant of G_{M2}-gangliosidosis: Clinical, biochemical, and pathological studies of two patients. *Acta Neuropathol (Berl)* **52**:189, 1980.
72. Hechtman P, Gordon BA, Ng Ying Kin NMK: Deficiency of the hexosaminidase A activator protein in a case of G_{M2} gangliosidosis; variant AB. *Pediatr Res* **16**:217, 1982.
73. Harrell LS: Tay-Sachs disease (amaurotic familial idiocy) in a non-Jewish male: A case report. *J Am Osteopath Assoc* **66**:303, 1966.
74. Hirabayashi Y, Li Y-T, Li S-C: The protein activator specific for the enzymic hydrolysis of G_{M2} ganglioside in normal human brain and in brains of three types of G_{M2} gangliosidosis. *J Neurochem* **40**:168, 1983.
75. Kytzia H-J, Hinrichs U, Maire I, Suzuki K, Sandhoff K: Variant of G_{M2}-gangliosidosis with hexosaminidase A having a severely changed substrate specificity. *EMBO J* **2**:1201, 1983.
76. Schröder M, Schnabel D, Suzuki K, Sandhoff K: A mutation in the gene of glycolipid-binding protein (G_{M2}-activator) that causes G_{M2}-gangliosidosis variant AB. *FEBS Lett* **290**:1, 1991.
77. Schröder M, Schnabel D, Hurwitz R, Young E, Suzuki K, Sandhoff K: Molecular genetics of G_{M2}-gangliosidosis AB variant: A novel mutation and expression in BHK cells. *Hum Genet* **92**:437, 1993.
78. Schepers U, Glombitza GJ, Lemm T, Hoffmann A, Chabàs A, Ozand P, Sandhoff K: Molecular analysis of a G_{M2}-activator deficiency in two patients with G_{M2}-gangliosidosis AB variant. *Am J Hum Genet* **59**:1048, 1996.
79. Leinekugel P, Michel S, Conzelmann E, Sandhoff K: Quantitative correlation between the residual activity of β-hexosaminidase A and arylsulfatase A and the severity of the resulting lysosomal storage disease. *Hum Genet* **88**:513, 1992.
80. Conzelmann E, Sandhoff K: Partial enzyme deficiencies: Residual activities and the development of neurological disorders. *Dev Neurosci* **6**:58, 1983–84.
81. Sandhoff K, Conzelmann E, Neufeld EF, Kaback MM, Suzuki K: The G_{M2} gangliosidoses, in Scriver C, Beaudet AL, Sly WS, Valle D (eds): *The Metabolic Basis of Inherited Diseases*, 6th ed, vol. 2, chap. 72. New York, McGraw-Hill, 1989, p 1807.
82. Morimoto S, Martin BM, Yamamoto Y, Kretz KA, O'Brien JS, Kishimoto Y: Saposin A: Second cerebrosidase activator protein. *Proc Natl Acad Sci U S A* **86**:3389, 1989.
83. Kleinschmidt T, Christomanou H, Braunitzer G: Complete amino-acid sequence and carbohydrate content of the naturally occurring glucosylceramide activator protein (A_1 activator) absent from a new human Gaucher disease variant. *Biol Chem Hoppe Seyler* **368**:1571, 1987.
84. Holtschmidt H, Sandhoff K, Fürst W, Kwon HY, Schnabel D, Suzuki K: The organization of the gene for the human cerebroside sulfate activator protein. *FEBS Lett* **280**:267, 1991.
85. Rorman EG, Scheinker V, Grabowski GA: Structure and evolution of the human prosaposin chromosomal gene. *Genomics* **13**:312, 1992.
86. Bar-Am I, Avivi L, Horowitz M: Assignment of the human prosaposin gene (PSAP) to 10q22.1 by fluorescence in situ hybridization. *Cytogenet Cell Genet* **72**:316, 1996.
87. Holtschmidt H, Sandhoff K, Kwon HY, Harzer K, Nakano T, Suzuki K: Sulfatide activator protein: Alternative splicing generates three messenger RNAs and a newly found mutation responsible for a clinical disease. *J Biol Chem* **266**:7556, 1991.
88. Henseler M, Klein A, Glombitza GJ, Suzuki K, Sandhoff K: Expression of the three alternative forms of the sphingolipid activator protein precursor in baby hamster kidney cells and functional assays in a cell culture system. *J Biol Chem* **271**:8416, 1996.
89. Fujibayashi S, Wenger DA: Biosynthesis of the sulfatide/G_{M1} activator protein (SAP-1) in control and mutant cultured skin fibroblasts. *Biochim Biophys Acta* **875**:554, 1986.
90. Schnabel D, Schröder M, Fürst W, Klein A, Hurwitz R, Zenk T, Weber J, Harzer K, Paton B, Poulos A, Suzuki K, Sandhoff K: Simultaneous deficiency of sphingolipid activator proteins 1 and 2 is caused by a mutation in the initiation codon of their common gene. *J Biol Chem* **267**:3312, 1992.
91. Kondoh K, Hineno T, Sano A, Kakimoto Y: Isolation and characterization of prosaposin from human milk. *Biochem Biophys Res Commun* **181**:286, 1991.
92. Patton S, Carson GS, Hiraiwa M, O'Brien JS, Sano A: Prosaposin, a neurotrophic factor: Presence and properties in milk. *J Dairy Sci* **80**:264, 1997.
93. Wenger DA, Fujibayashi S: Studies of SAP-1 and SAP-2 in cultured skin fibroblasts, in Freysz L, Dreyfus H, Massarelli R, Gatt S (eds): *Enzymes of Lipid Metabolism II*. New York, Plenum, 1986, p 339.
94. Inui K, Wenger DA: Biochemical, immunological, and structural studies on a sphingolipid activator protein (SAP-1). *Arch Biochem Biophys* **233**:556, 1984.
95. Fujibayashi S, Wenger DA: Studies on a sphingolipid activator protein (SAP-2) in fibroblasts from patients with lysosomal storage diseases, including Niemann-Pick disease type C. *Clin Chim Acta* **146**:147, 1985.
96. Varon R, Kleijer WJ, Thompson EJ, d'Azzo A: Evidence for the deficiency of β-glucosidase-activating factor in fibroblasts of patients with I-cell disease. *Hum Genet* **62**:66, 1982.
97. Ranieri E, Paton B, Poulos A: Preliminary evidence for a processing error in the biosynthesis of Gaucher activator in mucolipidosis disease types II and III. *Biochem J* **233**:763, 1986.
98. Datta SC, Snider RM, Radin NS: Uptake by neuroblastoma cells of glucosylceramide, glucosylceramide glucosidase, its stimulator protein, and phosphatidylserine. *Biochim Biophys Acta* **877**:387, 1986.
99. Vielhaber G, Hurwitz R, Sandhoff K: Biosynthesis, processing, and targeting of sphingolipid activator protein (SAP) precursor in cultured human fibroblasts. Mannose 6-phosphate receptor-independent endocytosis of SAP precursor. *J Biol Chem* **272**:32438, 1997.
100. Mraz W, Fischer G, Jatzkewitz H: The activator of cerebroside sulphatase — Lysosomal localization. *Hoppe Seyler's Z Physiol Chem* **357**:1181, 1976.
101. Tamaru T, Fujibayashi S, Brown WR, Wenger DA: Immunocytochemical localization of sphingolipid activator protein-1, the sulfatide/G_{M1} activator, to lysosomes in human liver and colon. *Histochemistry* **86**:195, 1985.
102. Taniike M, Inui K, Shinoda K, Okada S, Shiotani Y, Yabuuchi H: Correlation of subcellular localization of disease-specific inclusions and sphingolipid activator protein-1 (SAP-1) in sulfatide sulfatase-deficient fibroblasts. *Acta Histochem Cytochem* **21**:565, 1988.
103. Paton BC, Hughes JL, Harzer K, Poulos A: Immunocytochemical localization of sphingolipid activator protein 2 (SAP-2) in normal and SAP-deficient fibroblasts. *Eur J Cell Biol* **51**:157, 1990.
104. Chiao Y-B, Chambers JP, Glew RH, Lee RE, Wenger DA: Subcellular localization of the heat-stable glucocerebrosidase activator substance in Gaucher spleen. *Arch Biochem Biophys* **186**:42, 1978.
105. Leonova T, Qi X, Bencosme A, Ponce E, Sun Y, Grabowski GA: Proteolytic processing patterns of prosaposin in insect and mammalian cells. *J Biol Chem* **271**:17312, 1996.
106. Hiraiwa M, Martin BM, Kishimoto Y, Conner GE, Tsuji S, O'Brien JS: Lysosomal proteolysis of prosaposin, the precursor of saposins (sphingolipid activator proteins): Its mechanism and inhibition by ganglioside. *Arch Biochem Biophys* **341**:17, 1997.
107. Munford RS, Sheppard PO, O'Hara PJ: Saposin-like proteins (SAPLIP) carry out diverse functions on a common backbone structure. *J Lipid Res* **36**:1653, 1995.
108. Liepinsh E, Andersson M, Ruysschaert JM, Otting G: Saposin fold revealed by the NMR structure of NK-lysin. *Nature Struct Biol* **10**:793, 1997
109. Ponting CP, Russell RB: Swaposins: Circular permutations within genes encoding saposin homologues. *Trends Biochem Sci* **20**:179, 1995.
110. Morimoto S, Kishimoto Y, Tomich J, Weiler S, Ohashi T, Barranger JA, Kretz KA, O'Brien JS: Interaction of saposin, acidic lipids, and glucosylceramidase. *J Biol Chem* **265**:1933, 1990.
111. Bradová V, Smid F, Ulrich-Bott B, Roggendorf W, Paton BC, Harzer K: Prosaposin deficiency: Further characterization of the sphingolipid activator protein-deficient sibs. Multiple glycolipid elevations (including lactosylceramidosis), partial enzyme deficiencies and ultrastructure of the skin in this generalized sphingolipid storage disease. *Hum Genet* **92**:143, 1993.
112. Qi X, Leonova T, Grabowski GA: Functional human saposins expressed in *Escherichia coli*. Evidence for binding and activation properties of saposin C with acid β-glucosidase. *J Biol Chem* **269**:16746, 1994.
113. Yamashita K, Inui K, Totani K, Kochibe N, Furukawa M, Okada S: Characteristics of asparagine-linked sugar chains of sphingolipid activator protein 1 purified from normal human liver and G_{M1} gangliosidosis (type 1) liver. *Biochemistry* **29**:3030, 1990.

114. Mitsuyama T, Gasa S, Nojima T, Taniguchi N, Makita A: Purification and properties of galactosylceramide sulfatase activator from human liver. *J Biochem* **98**:605, 1985.
115. Fluharty AL, Katona Z, Meek WE, Frei K, Fowler AV: The cerebroside sulfate activator from pig kidney: Purification and molecular structure. *Biochem Med Metabol Biol* **47**:66, 1992.
116. Fluharty AV, Meek WE, Katona Z, Tsay KK: The cerebroside sulfate activator from pig kidney: Derivatization, cerebroside sulfate binding, and metabolic correction. *Biochem Med Metabol Biol* **47**:86, 1992
117. Stevens RL, Faull KF, Conklin KA, Green BN, Fluharty AL: Porcine cerebroside sulfate activator: Further structural characterization and disulfide identification. *Biochemistry* **32**:4051, 1993.
118. Vaccaro AM, Salvioli R, Barca A, Tatti M, Ciaffoni F, Maras B, Siciliano R, Zappacosta F, Amoresano A, Pucci P: Structural analysis of saposin C and B — Complete localization of disulfide bridges. *J Biol Chem* **270**:9953, 1995.
119. Fischer G, Reiter S, Jatzkewitz H: Enzyme hydrolysis of sulphosphingolipids and sulphoglycerolipids by sulfatase A in the presence and absence of activator protein. *Hoppe Seyler's Z Physiol Chem* **359**:863, 1978.
120. Inui K, Wenger DA: Properties of a protein activator of glycosphingolipid hydrolysis isolated from the liver of a patient with G_{M1} gangliosidosis, type 1. *Biochem Biophys Res Commun* **105**:745, 1982.
121. Vogel A, Schwarzmann G, Sandhoff K: Glycosphingolipid specificity of the human sulfatide activator protein. *Eur J Biochem* **200**:591, 1991.
122. Fingerhut R, Vanderhorst GTJ, Verheijen FW, Conzelmann E: Degradation of ganglioside by the lysosomal sialidase requires an activator protein. *Eur J Biochem* **208**:623, 1992.
123. Li S-C, Sonnino S, Tettamanti G, Li Y-T: Characterization of a nonspecific activator protein for the enzymatic hydrolysis of glycolipids. *J Biol Chem* **263**:6588, 1988.
124. Fischer G, Jatzkewitz H: The activator of cerebroside sulfatase: Binding studies with enzyme and substrate demonstrating the detergent function of the activator protein. *Biochim Biophys Acta* **481**:561, 1977.
125. Wynn C: A triple-binding-domain model explains the specificity of the interaction of a sphingolipid activator protein (SAP-1) with sulphatide, G_{M1}-ganglioside and globotriaosylceramide. *Biochem J* **240**:921, 1986.
126. Brown JR, Shockley P: Serum albumin: Structure and characterization of its ligand binding sites, in Jost PC, Hayes-Griffith O (eds): *Lipid-Protein Interactions*. New York, Wiley, 1982, p 25.
127. Li S-C, Serizawa S, Li Y-T, Nakamura K, Handa S: Effect of modification of sialic acid on enzymic hydrolysis of gangliosides G_{M1} and G_{M2}. *J Biol Chem* **259**:5409, 1984.
128. Sano A, Radin NS: The carbohydrate moiety of the activator protein for glucosylceramide β-glucosidase. *Biochem Biophys Res Commun* **154**:1197, 1988.
129. Peters SP, Coffee CJ, Glew RH, Lee RE, Wenger DA, Li S-C, Li Y-T: Isolation of heat-stable glucocerebrosidase activator from the spleens of three variants of Gaucher's disease. *Arch Biochem Biophys* **183**:290, 1977.
130. Paton BC, Poulos A: Analysis of the multiple forms of Gaucher spleen sphingolipid activator protein 2. *Biochem J* **254**:77, 1988.
131. Christomanou H, Kleinschmidt T: Isolation of two forms of an activator protein for the enzymic sphingomyelin degradation from human Gaucher spleen. *Biol Chem Hoppe Seyler* **366**:245, 1985.
132. Wenger DA, Sattler M, Roth S: A protein activator of galactosylceramide β-galactosidase. *Biochim Biophys Acta* **712**:639, 1982.
133. Weiler S, Carson W, Lee Y, Teplow DB, Kishimoto Y, O'Brien JS, Barranger JA, Tomich JM: Synthesis and characterization of a bioactive 82-residue sphingolipid activator protein, saposin C. *J Mol Neurosci* **4**:161, 1993.
134. Weiler S, Kishimoto Y, O'Brien JS, Barranger JA, Tomich JM: Identification of the binding and activating sites of the sphingolipid activator protein, saposin C, with glucocerebrosidase. *Protein Sci* **4**:756, 1995.
135. Qi X, Qin W, Sun Y, Kondo K, Grabowski GA: Functional organization of saposin C. Definition of the neurotrophic and acid beta-glucosidase activation regions. *J Biol Chem* **271**:6874, 1996.
136. Poulos A, Ranieri E, Shankaran P, Callahan JW: Studies on the activation of the enzymic hydrolysis of sphingomyelin liposomes. *Biochim Biophys Acta* **793**:141, 1984.
137. Ho MW: Specificity of low molecular weight glycoprotein effector of lipid glycosidase. *FEBS Lett* **53**:243, 1975.
138. Ho MW, Rigby M: Glucocerebrosidase: Stoichiometry of association between effector and catalytic proteins. *Biochim Biophys Acta* **397**:267, 1975.
139. Sarmientos F, Schwarzmann G, Sandhoff K: Specificity of human glucosylceramide β-glucosidase towards synthetic glucosylsphingolipids inserted into liposomes — Kinetic studies in a detergent-free assay system. *Eur J Biochem* **160**:527, 1986.
140. Zschoche A, Fürst W, Schwarzmann G, Sandhoff K: Hydrolysis of lactosylceramide by human galactosylceramidase and G_{M1}- β-galactosidase in a detergent-free system and ist stimulation by sphingolipid activator proteins, sap-B and sap-C. *Eur J Biochem* **222**:83, 1994.
141. Basu A, Glew RH: Characterization of the activation of rat liver β-glucosidase by sialosylgangliotetraosylceramide. *J Biol Chem* **260**:13067, 1985.
142. Ho MW, Light ND: Glucocerebrosidase: Reconstitution from macromolecular components depends on acidic phospholipids. *Biochem J* **136**:821, 1973.
143. Vaccaro AM, Muscillo M, Gallozzi E, Salvioli R, Tatti M, Suzuki K: An endogenous activator protein in human placenta for enzymic degradation of glucosylceramide. *Biochim Biophys Acta* **836**:157, 1985.
144. Vaccaro AM, Muscillo M, Salvioli R, Tatti M, Gallozzi E, Suzuki K: The binding of glucosylceramidase to glucosyl ceramide is promoted by its activator protein. *FEBS Lett* **216**:190, 1987.
145. Vaccaro AM, Ciaffoni F, Tatti M, Salvioli R, Barca A, Tognozzi D, Scerch C: pH-dependent conformational properties of saposins and their interactions with phospholipid membranes. *J Biol Chem* **270**:30576, 1995.
146. Vaccaro AM, Tatti M, Ciaffoni F, Salvioli R, Barca A, Scerch C: Effect of saposins A and C on the enzymatic hydrolysis of liposomal glucosylceramide. *J Biol Chem* **272**:16862, 1997.
147. Morimoto S, Martin BM, Kishimoto Y, O'Brien JS: Saposin D: A sphingomyelinase activator. *Biochem Biophys Res Commun* **156**:403, 1988.
148. Klein A, Henseler M, Klein C, Suzuki K, Harzer K, Sandhoff K: Sphingolipid activator protein D (sap-D) stimulates the lysosomal degradation of ceramide in vivo. *Biochem Biophys Res Commun* **200**:1440, 1994.
149. Azuma N, O'Brien JS, Moser HW, Kishimoto Y: Stimulation of acid ceramidase activity by saposin D. *Arch Biochem Biophys* **311**:354, 1994.
150. Paton BC, Schmid B, Kustermann-Kuhn B, Poulos A, Harzer K: Additional biochemical findings in a patient and fetal sib with a genetic defect in the sphingolipid activator protein (SAP) precursor, prosaposin. Evidence for a deficiency in SAP-1 and for a normal lysosomal neuraminidase. *Biochem J* **285**:481, 1992.
151. Sango K, Yamanaka S, Hoffmann A, Okuda Y, Grinberg A, Westphal H, McDonald MP, Crawley JN, Sandhoff K, Suzuki K, Proia RL: Mouse models of Tay-Sachs and Sandhoff diseases differ in neurologic phenotype and ganglioside metabolism. *Nat Genet* **11**:170, 1995.
152. Hiraiwa M, O'Brien JS, Kishimoto Y, Galdzicka M, Fluharty AL, Ginns EI, Martin BM: Isolation, characterization, and proteolysis of human prosaposin, the precursor of saposins (sphingolipid activator proteins). *Arch Biochem Biophys* **304**:110, 1993.
153. Hiraiwa M, Soeda S, Kishimoto Y, O'Brien JS: Binding and transport of gangliosides by prosaposin. *Proc Natl Acad Sci U S A* **89**:11254, 1992.
154. Kotani Y, Matsuda S, Wen TC, Sakanaka M, Tanaka J, Maeda N, Kondoh K, Ueno S: Sano: A hydrophilic peptide comprising 18 amino acid residues of the prosaposin sequence has neurotrophic activity in vitro and in vivo. *J Neurochem* **66**:2197, 1996.
155. O'Brien JS, Carson GS, Seo H-C, Hiraiwa M, Weiler S, Tomich JM, Barranger JA, Kahn M, Azuma N, Kishimoto Y: Identification of the neurotrophic sequence of prosaposin. *FASEB J* **9**:681, 1995.
156. Hineno T, Sano A, Kondoh K, Ueno S-I, Kakimoto Y, Yoshida K-I: Secretion of sphingolipid hydrolase activator precursor, prosaposin. *Biochem Biophys Res Commun* **176**:668, 1991.
157. Sano A, Hineno T, Mizuno T, Kondoh K, Ueno S-I, Kakimoto Y, Inui K: Sphingolipid hydrolase activator proteins and their precursors. *Biochem Biophys Res Commun* **165**:1191, 1989.
158. Hiraiwa M, Taylor EM, Campana WM, Darin SJ, O'Brien JS: Cell death prevention, mitogen-activated protein kinase stimulation, and increased sulfatide concentrations in Schwann cells and oligodendrocytes by prosaposin and prosaptides. *Proc Natl Acad Sci U S A* **94**:4778, 1997.
159. Campana WM, Hiraiwa M, Addison KC, O'Brien JS: Induction of MAPK phosphorylation by prosaposin and prosaptide in PC12 cells. *Biochem Biophys Res Commun* **229**:706, 1996.

160. Collard MW, Sylvester SR, Tsuruta JK, Griswold MD: Biosynthesis and molecular cloning of sulfated glycoprotein 1 secreted by rat Sertoli cells: Sequence similarity with the 70-kilodalton precursor to sulfatide/G_{M1} activator. *Biochemistry* **27**:4557, 1988.
161. Sylvester SR, Morales C, Oko R, Griswold MD: Sulfated glycoprotein-1 (saposin precursor) in reproductive tract of the male rat. *Biol Reprod* **41**:941, 1989.
162. Levy H, Or A, Eyal N, Wilder S, Widgerson M, Kolodny EH, Zimran A, Horowitz M: Molecular aspects of Gaucher disease. *Dev Neurosci* **13**:352, 1991.
163. Morales CR, El-Alfy M, Zhao Q, Igdoura SA: Expression and tissue distribution of rat sulfated glycoprotein-1 (prosaposin). *J Histochem Cytochem* **44**:327, 1996.
164. Patthy L: Homology of the precursor of pulmonary surfactant-associated protein SP-B with prosaposin and sulfated glycoprotein 1. *J Biol Chem* **266**:6035, 1991.
165. Glasser SW, Korfhagen TR, Weaver T, Pilot-Matias T, Fox JL, Whitsett JA: cDNA and deduced amino acid sequence of human pulmonary surfactant-associated proteolipid SPL (Phe). *Proc Natl Acad Sci U S A* **84**:4007, 1987.
166. Shapiro LJ, Aleck KA, Kaback MM, Itabashi H, Desnick RJ, Brand N, Stevens RL, Fluharty AL, Kihara H: Metachromatic leukodystrophy without arylsulfatase A deficiency. *Pediatr Res* **13**:1179, 1979.
167. Hahn AF, Gordon BA, Gilbert JJ, Hinton GG: The AB-variant of metachromatic leukodystrophy (postulated activator protein deficiency). Light and electron microscopic findings in a sural nerve biopsy. *Acta Neuropathol (Berl)* **55**:281, 1981.
168. Hahn AF, Gordon BA, Feleki V, Hinton GG, Gilbert JJ: A variant form of metachromatic leukodystrophy without arylsulfatase deficiency. *Ann Neurol* **12**:33, 1982.
169. Wenger DA, DeGala G, Williams C, Taylor HA, Stevenson RE, Pruitt JR, Miller J, Garen PD, Balentine JD: Clinical, pathological, and biochemical studies on an infantile case of sulfatide/G_{M1} activator protein deficiency. *Am J Med Genet* **33**:255, 1989.
170. Schlote W, Harzer K, Christomanou H, Paton BC, Kustermann-Kuhn B, Schmid B, Seeger J, Beudt U, Schuster I, Langenbeck U: Sphingolipid activator protein 1 deficiency in metachromatic leucodystrophy with normal arylsulphatase A activity-A clinical, morphological, biochemical, and immunological study. *Eur J Pediatr* **150**:584, 1991.
171. Rafi MA, Amini S, Zhang X, Wenger DA: Correction of sulfatide metabolism after transfer of prosaposin cDNA to cultured cells from a patient with SAP-1 deficiency. *Am J Hum Genet* **50**:1252, 1992.
172. Zhang X-L, Rafi MA, DeGala G, Wenger DA: Insertion in the mRNA of a metachromatic leukodystrophy patient with sphingolipid activator protein-1 deficiency. *Proc Natl Acad Sci U S A* **87**:1426, 1990.
173. Rafi MA, Zhang X-L, DeGala G, Wenger DA: Detection of a point mutation in sphingolipid activator protein-1 mRNA in patients with a variant form of metachromatic leukodystrophy. *Biochem Biophys Res Commun* **166**:1017, 1990.
174. Kretz KA, Carson GS, Morimoto S, Kishimoto Y, Fluharty AL, O'Brien JS: Characterization of a mutation in a family with saposin B deficiency: A glycosylation site defect. *Proc Natl Acad Sci U S A* **87**:2541, 1990.
175. Zhang XL, Rafi MA, Degala G, Wenger DA: The mechanism for a 33-nucleotide insertion in messenger RNA causing sphingolipid activator protein (SAP-1)-deficient metachromatic leukodystrophy. *Hum Genet* **87**:211, 1991.
176. Stevens RL, Fluharty AL, Kihara H, Kaback MM, Shapiro LJ, Marsh B, Sandhoff K, Fischer G: Cerebroside sulfatase activator deficiency induced metachromatic leukodystrophy. *Am J Hum Genet* **33**:900, 1981.
177. Conzelmann E, Lee-Vaupel M, Sandhoff K: The physiological roles of activator proteins for lysosomal glycolipid degradation, in Salvayre R, Douste-Blazy L, Gatt S (eds): *Lipid Storage Disorders: Biological and Medical Aspects*. New York, Plenum, 1988, p 323.
178. Schmid B, Paton BC, Sandhoff K, Harzer K: Metabolism of G_{M1} ganglioside in cultured skin fibroblasts: Anomalies in gangliosidoses, sialidoses, and sphingolipid activator protein (SAP, saposin) 1 and prosaposin deficient disorders. *Hum Genet* **89**:513, 1992.
179. Kase R, Bierfreund U, Klein A, Kolter T, Itoh K, Suzuki M, Hashimoto Y, Sandhoff K, Sakuraba H: Only sphingolipid activator protein B (SAP-B or saposin B) stimulates the degradation of globotriaosylceramide by recombinant human lysosomal alpha-galactosidase in a detergent-free liposomal system. *FEBS Lett* **393**:74, 1996.
180. Henseler M, Klein A, Reber M, Vanier MT, Landrieu P, Sandhoff K: Analysis of a splice site mutation in the SAP precursor gene of a patient with metachromatic leukodystrophy. *Am J Hum Genet* **58**:65, 1996.
181. Yuziuk JA, Bertoni C, Beccari T, Orlacchio A, Wu YY, Li SC, Li YT: Specificity of mouse G_{M2} activator protein and β-N-acetylhexosaminidases A and B. Similarities and differences with their human counterparts in the catabolism of GM2. *J Biol Chem* **273**:66, 1998.
182. Conzelmann E, Sandhoff K: Activator proteins for lysosomal glycolipid hydrolysis, in Ginsburg V (ed): *Methods in Enzymology*, vol 138. Orlando, FL, Academic Press, 1987, p 792.
183. Christomanou H, Chabas A, Pampols T, Guardiola A: Activator protein deficient Gaucher's disease. *Klin Wochenschr* **67**:999, 1989.
184. Schnabel D, Schröder M, Sandhoff K: Mutation in the sphingolipid activator protein 2 in a patient with a variant of Gaucher disease. *FEBS Lett* **284**:57, 1991.
185. Rafi MA, de Gala G, Zhang X, Wenger DA: Mutational analysis in a patient with a variant form of Gaucher disease caused by SAP-2 deficiency. *Somat Cell Mol Genet* **19**:1, 1993.
186. Hiesberger T, Huttler S, Rohlmann A, Schneider W, Sandhoff K, Herz J: Cellular uptake of saposin (SAP) precursor and lysosomal delivery by the low density lipoprotein receptor-related protein (LRP). *EMBO J* **17**:4617, 1998.
187. Harzer K, Paton BC, Poulos A, Kustermann-Kuhn B, Roggendorf W, Grisar T, Popp M: Sphingolipid activator protein (SAP) deficiency in a 16-week-old atypical Gaucher disease patient and his fetal sibling: Biochemical signs of combined sphingolipidoses. *Eur J Pediatr* **149**:31, 1989.
188. Chatelut M, Harzer K, Christomanou H, Feunteun J, Pieraggi M, Paton BC, Kishimoto Y, O'Brien JS, Basile JP, Thiers JC, Salvayre R, Levade T: Model SV40-transformed fibroblast lines for metabolic studies of human prosaposin and acid ceramidase deficiencies. *Clin Chim Acta* **262**:1, 1997.
189. Morimoto S, Yamamoto Y, O'Brien JS, Kishimoto Y: Distribution of saposin proteins (sphingolipid activator proteins) in lysosomal storage diseases. *Proc Natl Acad Sci U S A* **87**:3493, 1990.
190. Taniike M, Inui K, Shinoda K, Okada S, Shiotani Y, Yabuuchi H: Correlation of subcellular localization of disease-specific inclusions and sphingolipid activator protein-1 (SAP-1) in sulfatide sulfatase-deficient fibroblasts. *Acta Histochem Cytochem* **21**:565, 1988.
191. Reiner O, Dagan O, Horowitz M: Human sphingolipid activator protein-1 and sphingolipid activator protein-2 are encoded by the same gene. *J Mol Neurosci* **1**:225, 1989.
192. Datta SC, Radin NS: Glucosylceramide and the level of the glucosidase-stimulating proteins. *Lipids* **21**:702, 1986.
193. Chang-Yi C, Kusuda S, Seguchi T, Takahashi M, Aisu K, Tezuka T: Decreased level of prosaposin in atopic skin. *J Invest Dermatol* **109**:319, 1997.
194. Fürst W, Sandhoff K: Activator proteins and topology of lysosomal sphingolipid catabolism. *Biochim Biophys Acta* **1126**:1, 1992.
195. Griffiths G, Hoflack B, Simons K, Mellman I, Kornfeld S: The mannose-6-phosphate receptor and the biogenesis of lysosomes. *Cell* **52**:329, 1988.
196. Sandhoff K, Kolter T: Topology of glycosphingolipid degradation. *Trends Cell Biol* **6**:98, 1996.
197. Burkhardt JK, Hüttler S, Klein A, Möbius W, Habermann A, Griffiths G, Sandhoff K: Accumulation of sphingolipids in SAP precursor (prosaposin) deficient fibroblasts occurs as intralysosomal membrane structures and can be completely reversed by treatment with human SAP precursor. *Eur J Biochem* **73**:10, 1997.
198. Kolter T, Sandhoff K: Glycosphingolipid degradation and animal models of G_{M2}-gangliosidoses. *J Inherit Metab Dis* **21**:548, 1998.
199. Yamanaka S, Johnson ON, Lyu MS, Kozak CA, Proia RL. Titel. *Genomics* **24**:601, 1994.
200. Bertoni C, Apolloni MG, Stirling JL, Li SC, Li YT, Orlacchio A, Beccari T: Structural organization and expression of the gene for the mouse G_{M2} activator protein. *Mamm Genome* **8**:90, 1997
201. Liu Y, Hoffmann A, Grinberg A, Westphal H, McDonald MP, Miller KM, Crawley JN, Sandhoff K, Suzuki K, Proia RL: Mouse model of G_{M2} activator deficiency manifests cerebellar ganglioside storage and motor impairment. *Proc Natl Acad Sci U S A* **94**:8138, 1997.
202. Tsuda M, Sakiyama T, Endo H, Kitagawa T: The primary structure of mouse saposin. *Biochem Biophys Res Commun* **184**:1266, 1992.
203. Zhao Q, Hay N, Morales CR: Structural analysis of the mouse prosaposin (SGP-1) gene reveals the presence of an exon that is alternatively spliced in transcribed mRNAs. *Mol Reprod Dev* **48**:1, 1997
204. Kozak CA, Adamson MC, Horowitz M: Genetic mapping of the mouse prosaposin gene (Psap) to mouse chromosome 10. *Genomics* **23**:508, 1994.

205. Fujita N, Suzuki K, Vanier MT, Popko B, Maeda N, Klein A, Henseler M, Sandhoff K, Nakayasu H, Suzuki K: Targeted disruption of the mouse sphingolipid activator protein gene: A complex phenotype, including severe leukodystrophy and wide-spread storage of multiple sphingolipids. *Hum Mol Genet* **5**:711, 1996.
206. Schütte CG, Lemm T, Glombitza GJ, Sandhoff K: Complete localization of disulfide bonds in G_{M2} activator protein. *Protein Sci* **7**:1, 1998.
207. Hiraiwa M, Campana WM, Martin BM, O'Brien JS: Prosaposin receptor: Evidence for a G-Protein-associated receptor. *Biochem Biophys Res Commun* **240**:415, 1997.
208. Wilkening G, Linke T, Sandhoff K: Lysosomal degradation on vesicular membrane surfaces: enhanced glucosylceramide degradation by lysosomal anionic lipids and activators. *J Biol Chem* **273**:30271, 1998.
209. Linke T, Wilkening G, Sandhoff K: Stimulation of ceramide hydrolysis by acidic phospholipids and activator proteins in a detergent-free assay system. (Manuscript in preparation.)
210. Giehl A, Lemm T, Bartelsen O, Sandhoff K, Blume A: Interaction of the G_{M2} activator protein with phospholipid-ganglioside bilayer membranes and with monolayers at the air-water interface. *Eur J Biochem* **261**:650, 1999.
211. Harzer K, Paton BC, Christomanou H, Chatelut M, Levade T, Hiraiwa M, O'Brien JS: Saposins (sap) A and C activate the degradation of galactosylceramide in living cells. *FEBS Lett* **417**:270, 1997.
212. Heng HH, Xie B, Shi XM, Tsui LC, Mahuran DJ: Refined mapping of the G_{M2} activator protein (G_{M2A}) locus to 5q31.3-33.1, distal to the spinal muscular atrophy locus. *Genomics* **18**:429, 1993.
213. Wrobe D, Henseler M, Huettler S, Pascual Pascual SI, Chabas A, Sandhoff K: A non-glycosylated and functionally deficient mutant (N215H) of the sphingolipid activator protein B (SAP-B) in a novel case of metachromatic leukodystrophy (MLD). *J Inherit Metab Dis* **23**:63, 2000.
214. Schepers U, Lemm T, Herzog V, Sandhoff K: Characterization of regulatory elements in the 5′-flanking region of the G_{M2} activator gene-transcriptional up-regulation reveals increased amounts of G_{M2} activator protein in kidney epithelial cells Manuscript submitted.
215. Tyynelä J, Palmer DN, Baumann M, Haltia M: Storage of saposins A and D in infantile neuronal ceroid lipofuscinosis. *FEBS Lett* **330**:8, 1993.
216. Haltia M, Tyynelä J, Baumann M, Henseler M, Sandhoff K: Immunological studies on sphingolipid activator proteins in the neuronal ceroid-lipofuscinoses. *Gerontology* **41(Supp 2)**:239, 1995.
217. Tyynelä J, Baumann M, Henseler M, Sandhoff K, Haltia M: Sphingolipid activator proteins in neuronal ceroid-lipofuscinoses: an immunological study. *Acta Neuropathol (Berl)* **89**:391, 1995.
218. Kolter T, Sandhoff K: Recent advances in the biochemistry of sphingolipidoses. *Brain Pathol* **8**:79, 1998.
219. Gatti R, Regis S, Corsolini F, Caroli F, Keulemans JLM, van Diggelen OP: An Asn>Lys substitution in a conserved residue of saposin B leading to the loss of the single *N*-glycosylation site in a patient with metachromatic leukodystrophy and normal arylsulfatase A activity [Abstract]. *11th ESGLD Workshop*, Sept. 18-21, 1997, Bad Deutsch-Altenburg, Austria.
220. Sun Y, Jin P, Grabowski GA: The mouse prosaposin locus: promoter organization. *DNA Cell Biol* **16**:23, 1997.
221. Xie B, Rigat B, Smijanic-Georgijev N, Deng H, Mahuran D: Biochemical characterization of the Cys138Arg substitution associated with the AB variant form of G_{M2} gangliosidosis: Evidence that Cys138 is required for the recognition of the G_{M2} activator/G_{M2} ganglioside complex by beta-hexosaminidase A. *Biochemistry* **37**:814, 1998.
222. Kotani Y, Matsuda S, Sakanaka M, Kondoh K, Ueno S, Sano A: Prosaposin facilitates sciatic nerve regeneration in vivo. *J Neurochem* **66**:2019, 1996.
223. Cormand B, Montfort M, Chabas A, Vilageliu L, Grinberg D: Genetic fine localization of the beta-glucocerebrosidase (GBA) and prosaposin (PSAP) genes: Implications for Gaucher disease. *Hum Genet* **100**:75, 1997.
224. Sano A, Matsuda S, Wen TC, Kotani Y, Kondoh K, Ueno S, Kakimoto Y, Yoshimura H, Sakanaka M: Protection by prosaposin against ischemia-induced learning disability and neuronal loss. *Biochem Biophys Res Commun* **204**:994, 1994.
225. Zaltash S, Johansson J: Secondary structure and limited proteolysis give experimental evidence that the precursor of pulmonary surfactant protein B contains three saposin-like domains. *FEBS Lett* **423**:1, 1998.
226. Zhao Q, Bell AW, El-Alfy M, Morales CR: Mouse testicular sulfated glycoprotein-1: Sequence analysis of the common backbone structure of prosaposins. *J Androl* **19**:165, 1998.
227. Pàmpols T, Pineda M, Girós ML, Ferrer I, Cusi V, Chabás A, Sanmarti FX, Vanier MT, Christomanou H: Neuronopathic juvenile glucosylceramidosis due to sap-C deficiency: Clinical course, neuropathology and brain lipid composition, in this Gaucher disease variant. (Manuscript in preparation.)
228. Lamontagne S, Potier M: Modulation of human saposin B sphingolipid-binding specificity by alternative splicing. A study with saposin B-derived synthetic peptides. *J Biol Chem* **269**:20528, 1994.

CHAPTER 135

Glycogen Storage Disease Type II: Acid α-Glucosidase (Acid Maltase) Deficiency

Rochelle Hirschhorn ▪ Arnold J.J. Reuser

1. **Glycogen storage disease type II (GSDII), also termed acid maltase deficiency (AMD) or Pompe disease, is an inherited disorder of glycogen metabolism resulting from defects in activity of the lysosomal hydrolase acid α-glucosidase in all tissues of affected individuals. The disorder is transmitted as an autosomal recessive trait.**
2. **The clinical presentation of GSDII encompasses a range of phenotypes, all of which include varying degrees of myopathy but differ with respect to age of onset, extent of organ involvement, and rate of progression to death. The most severe is the classic infantile-onset disease, described by Pompe and delineated prior to discovery of the deficiency of acid maltase, with prominent cardiomegaly, hypotonia, hepatomegaly, and death due to cardiorespiratory failure, usually before 2 years of age. At the other extreme is a slowly progressive proximal myopathic adult-onset disease with onset as late as the second to sixth decade and involvement essentially only of skeletal muscle. Between these two extremes there is a heterogeneous group, variously termed childhood, juvenile, or muscular variant, generally with onset after early infancy, a predominance of skeletal muscle involvement, usually without cardiac involvement, and a more slowly progressive course as compared with classic infantile-onset Pompe disease. Progressive proximal muscle weakness including major impairment of respiratory function dominates the picture and death results usually from respiratory failure.**
3. **The enzyme deficiency results in intralysosomal accumulation of glycogen of normal structure in numerous tissues. The accumulation is most marked in cardiac and skeletal muscle and in hepatic tissues of infants with the generalized disorder. In late-onset GSDII, intralysosomal accumulation of glycogen is virtually limited to skeletal muscle and is of lesser magnitude. Electromyographic abnormalities suggestive of the diagnosis include pseudomyotonic discharges and irritability, but in juvenile- and adult-onset patients, the abnormalities can vary in different muscles. CAT scans can reveal the site(s) of affected muscles. Most patients have elevated blood plasma levels of creatine kinase (CK) and elevations in hepatic enzymes, particularly in adult-onset patients, can be found.**
4. **The clinical diagnosis is confirmed by virtual absence (infantile-onset) or markedly reduced activity (late-onset) of acid α-glucosidase in muscle biopsies and cultured fibroblasts. Purified lymphocytes and lymphoid cell lines also exhibit the enzyme abnormalities, but have been less extensively used for diagnosis, and misdiagnosis may occur with imperfectly fractionated peripheral blood lymphocytes. Assay of unfractionated leukocytes is not reliable in most laboratories unless combined with use of antibodies. In general, the amount of residual enzyme activity correlates inversely with the severity of disease.**
5. **Prenatal diagnosis has been made by determination of acid α-glucosidase deficiency in cultured amniotic cells and chorionic villus biopsies. DNA analysis is of supportive diagnostic value and provides a means for definitive carrier detection.**
6. **Both the human cDNA and structural gene have been isolated, characterized, and used to analyze mutations. The cDNA for human acid α-glucosidase is over 3.6 kb, with 2859 nucleotides (nt) of coding sequence, a 3′ untranslated region of 550 bp, and a 5′ untranslated region of at least 218 bp. The coding region predicts 952 amino acids in a nonglycosylated protein of 105.37 kDa, with an amino-terminal signal sequence for synthesis within the ER. The enzyme is extensively modified posttranslationally by glycosylation within the ER at all seven predicted sites, subsequent remodeling of the asparagine-linked carbohydrate and phosphorylation of mannose residues, providing the mannose-6-phosphate recognition marker for targeting to lysosomes. The enzyme is additionally modified by both amino- and C-terminal proteolytic cleavage, primarily within lysosomes. The structural gene contains 20 exons in approximately 20 kb of genomic DNA and has been localized to human chromosome 17q25 and designated GAA.**
7. **The disorder is genetically heterogeneous, with missense, nonsense, and splice-site mutations, partial deletions, and insertions described in the relatively small number of patients analyzed. A few mutations have been described that are common in particular ethnic groups, including Chinese and African-Americans. Additionally a single mutation is responsible for adult-onset disease in over half of Caucasian adult-onset patients.**
8. **Definitive therapy is not currently available, although supportive measures, particularly of respiratory function, can have a significant impact on patients with the late-onset disease. Dietary therapy has been used in late-onset patients. Trials of enzyme replacement therapy have begun. The first published results of a phase 2 trial with recombinant human α-glucosidase from milk of transgenic**

A list of standard abbreviations is located immediately preceding the index in each volume. Additional abbreviations used in this chapter include: AMD = acid maltase deficiency; CblC = cobalamin C; CK = creatine kinase; 4MUG = 4-methylumbelliferyl--D-glucopyranoside; GSDII = glycogen storage disease type II; TK = thymidine kinase.

rabbits have shown some therapeutic effects. Possibilities for gene therapy are under investigation.

9. **There are several naturally occurring animal models of the infantile- and late-onset disease. Knockout mice have now also been developed. Ameliorative effects of enzyme therapy have been described in knockout mice and in a quail model.**
10. **There is a second syndrome associated with intravacuolar accumulation of glycogen but normal acid α-glucosidase activity, characterized by prominent cardiac abnormalities, involvement of skeletal muscle, and variable mental retardation. This syndrome may encompass more than one mode of inheritance. The X-linked inherited Danon disease is caused by a primary deficiency of the lysosomal membrane protein LAMP-2.**

HISTORICAL BACKGROUND

More than 50 years ago, Pompe described a 7-month-old female child who died suddenly with idiopathic hypertrophy of the heart.[1] Although the syndrome had been described previously, Pompe made the critical observation that there was massive accumulation of glycogen within vacuoles, not only in the heart, but in all tissues examined. As is often the case, a similar observation was reported in the same year.[2] Over the next two decades, additional clinical manifestations of idiopathic cardiomegaly associated with storage of glycogen were defined, including muscular weakness with marked hypotonia, hepatomegaly, macroglossia, and marked cardiomegaly, with death before 1 year of age.[3] Discovery of the metabolic basis of the disorder in 1963 was made possible by a series of discoveries in two apparently unrelated areas of biochemistry and cell biology. First, delineation of the normal pathway for glycogen metabolism allowed for a classification of diseases due to pathologic glycogen metabolism. The Coris' investigations led to the classification of what was then called "Pompe disease" as glycogen storage disease type II (GSDII), the most severe of the glycogen storage disorders.[4] In GSDII, in contrast to several of the other glycogen storage disorders, no defect in the described pathway of glycogen degradation could be found, and the stored glycogen was of normal structure. At the same time, de Duve identified and characterized a new organelle, the lysosome, as a membrane-bound vacuole containing a variety of hydrolytic enzymes, all active at acid pH and capable of degrading various bonds found in macromolecules. Based on these two advances, Hers and coworkers, in two brief manuscripts that have had a profound conceptual impact,[5,6] described an α-glucosidase present in lysosomes, active at acid pH and capable of releasing glucose from glycogen as well as maltose. They also demonstrated that this acid α-1,4-glucosidase, or acid maltase, was absent in tissues from four infants with classic Pompe disease, and in a fifth infant who also had early onset of severe muscular disease but without prominent cardiomegaly. Because the major site of glycogen storage and metabolism is within the cytoplasm, these discoveries revealed an unexpected role for lysosomes in degradation of glycogen, presumably following "autophagy" of intracytoplasmic glycogen. Hers made the prediction, now fulfilled, that "it can be expected that other deposition diseases might be explained on the basis of the absence of other lysosomal enzymes." Acid α-glucosidase deficiency was thus the first of the approximately 40 lysosomal storage disorders now described.

The discovery that genetic deficiency of acid α-glucosidase (acid maltase) was the metabolic basis of disease in GSDII, and that the enzyme deficiency could be detected in multiple cell types, provided a specific diagnostic test. As a result, over the next decade, patients with acid α-glucosidase deficiency and only skeletal muscle involvement were described with childhood- and adult-onset forms of the disease.[7–15,52] The clinical spectrum of GSDII, also alternatively designated as acid maltase deficiency (AMD), was expanded to include these additional presentations.[16–18]

CLINICAL MANIFESTATIONS

The clinical presentation of GSDII encompasses a range of phenotypes, all of which include varying degrees of myopathy but differ with respect to age of onset, extent of organ involvement, and rate of progression to death. The most severe is the classic infantile-onset disease, described by Pompe and delineated prior to discovery of the deficiency of acid maltase, with prominent cardiomegaly, hypotonia, and death prior to 1 to 2 years of age. At the other extreme is a slowly progressive myopathic adult-onset disease with onset as late as the second to sixth decade and involvement essentially only of skeletal muscle. Between these two extremes there is a heterogeneous group, variously termed childhood, juvenile, or muscular variant, generally with onset after early infancy, a predominance of skeletal muscle involvement, usually without cardiac involvement, and a more slowly progressive course as compared with classic infantile-onset Pompe disease.[16–22] It should be noted that all case histories not confirmed by enzyme diagnosis could represent a second more recently delineated vacuolar glycogen storage disorder with superficially similar clinical manifestations and histopathologic features but not due to deficiency of acid maltase (see "Vaculoar Glycogen Storage Disease Without α-Glucosidase Deficiency: Danon Disease" below).

Infantile-Onset Disease

Infantile-onset GSDII can present in two different forms: the classic Pompe disease and the less common muscular variant (Table 135-1).[5,16–35,63,64] The classic disorder described by Pompe[1] has been the most frequently reported in infancy and presents within the first few months of life with marked cardiomegaly, striking hypotonia, rapidly progressive weakness, macroglossia, and less marked hepatomegaly (Fig. 135-1*A*). Patients often present with feeding difficulties and respiratory problems frequently complicated by pulmonary infection. The diagnosis is often first suspected either because of the prominent cardiomegaly on chest x-ray films or the "floppy baby" appearance. Based on findings in the animal models of the disorder, the feeding problems could reflect esophageal involvement in addition to the macroglossia, although there are no physiological data in humans (other than storage of glycogen) to support this hypothesis. X-ray and echocardiography, as well as examination at autopsy, reveal a markedly enlarged heart with increased thickness of the walls of both ventricles and of the interventricular septum with marked diminution in size of the ventricular cavities (Fig. 135-1*B,E*). The cardiomegaly is progressive. Left ventricular thickening increases over time, and eventually there is obstruction to left ventricular outflow.[33] EKG often shows a shortened PR interval and large QRS complexes.[29]

Table 135-1 Clinical Features in GSDII (Acid Maltase Deficiency)* (% of Total (#) of Patients with Each Clinical Feature)

Clinical Feature	Infantile (78) % total	Juvenile (24) % total	Adult (27) % total
Age of onset			
<2 years	99	58	0
2–15 years	1	42	0
>15 years	0	0	100
Muscular weakness	96	100	100
Cardiomegaly	95	4	0
Hepatomegaly	82	29	4
Macroglossia	62	8	4

*Adapted from references 19 and 20. The original table based the classification of infantile vs. juvenile on the presence or absence of cardiomegaly. The one patient with cardiomegaly in the juvenile category (4%) had only mild changes. In a similar summary in reference 17, each patient is presented graphically, enabling more detailed correlations in individual patients.

Macroglossia, hepatomegaly, and weakness of respiratory muscles are common. Despite the profound general muscle weakness, manifested as hypotonia and flaccidity, muscles are generally firm and even hypertrophic in appearance. There is generalized glycogen deposition predominantly in cardiac, skeletal, smooth muscle, and liver (Fig. 135-1*C,D*), and also in renal tubular epithelium and central nervous system, including anterior horn cells and neurons of brain stem nuclei. However, mental

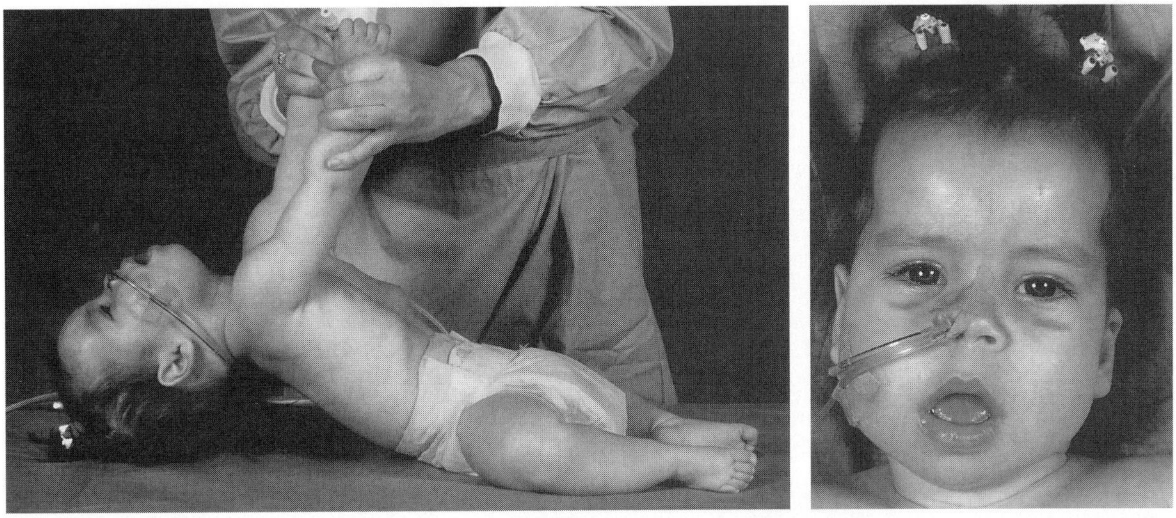

A

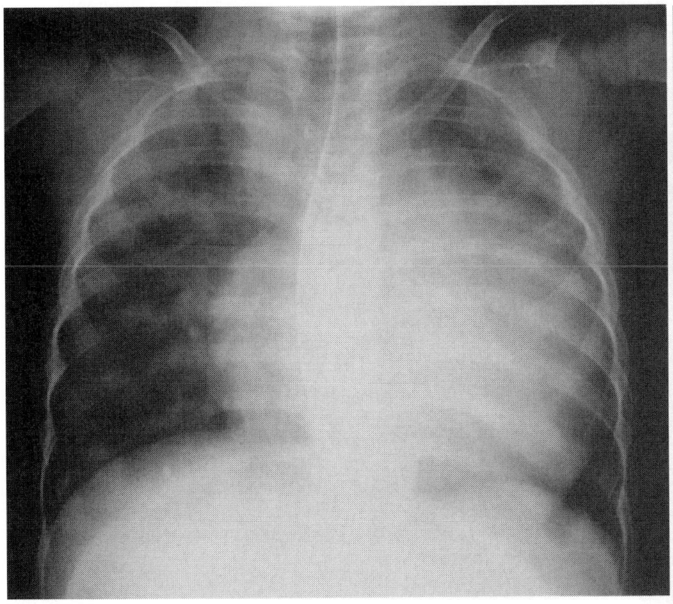

B

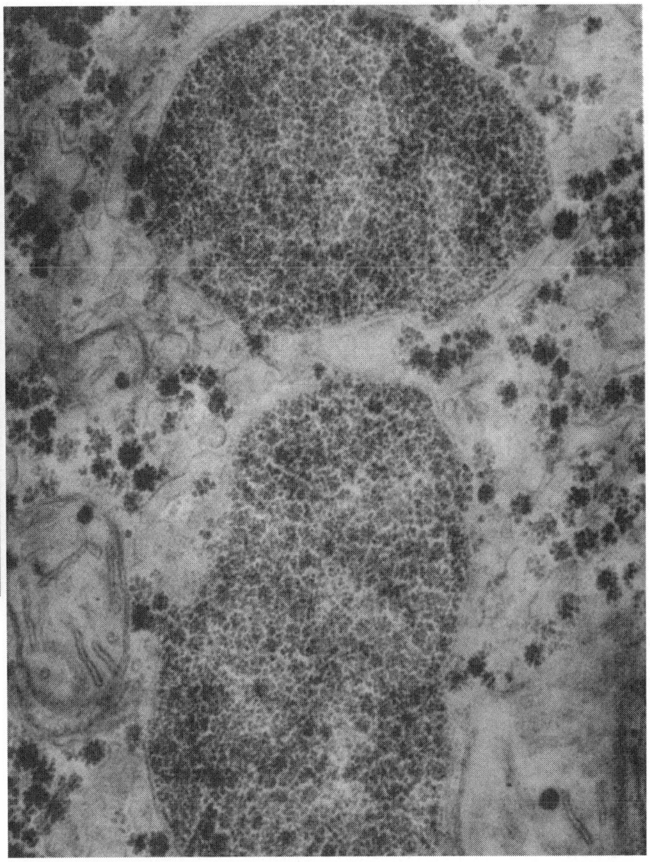

C

Fig. 135-1 Infantile-onset GSDII. ***A,*** **An 8-month-old baby girl was diagnosed at 2 months of age because of floppiness, poor feeding, and delayed developmental milestones (note the head-lag and the frog-like posture of the legs). Upon clinical investigation, generalized muscle weakness, cardiac enlargement, and macroglossia were noted. The liver was palpable at 3 cm below the costal margin. The finding of complete acid α-glucosidase deficiency in cultured skin fibroblasts established the diagnosis.** ***B,*** **Chest roentgenogram of a 4-month-old female infant with generalized glycogen storage disease type II. The massive heart dominates the film.** ***C,*** **Electron micrograph of a portion of a hepatic parenchymal cell from a liver biopsy of a patient with acid α-glucosidase deficiency. Two vacuoles filled with glycogen are seen at magnification ×69,000. A membrane can be followed around most of the periphery of the vacuoles. (*From Baudhuin P, Hers HG, Loeb H,* Lab Invest *13:1139, 1964. Used with permission.*)** ***D,*** **The muscle biopsy shows massive accumulation of glycogen in virtually all fibers (5 μM sections fixed with glutaraldehyde and stained with PAS). (*Courtesy of Dr. Ans T. van der Ploeg and Dr. M. Christa B. Loonen, Sophia Children's Hospital, Rotterdam.*)** ***E,*** **The heart of a patient at autopsy (age at death was 5 months). The heart is greatly enlarged, with thickened ventricles, due to extensive glycogen infiltration. There is some endocardial thickening.**

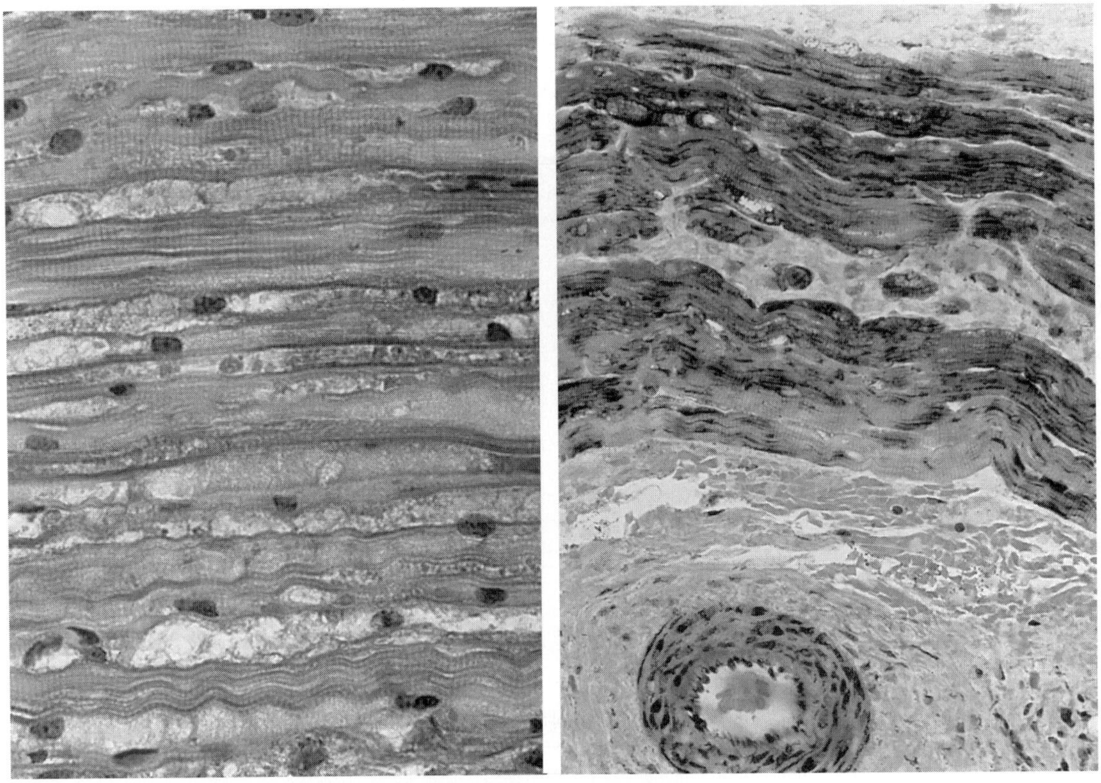

D

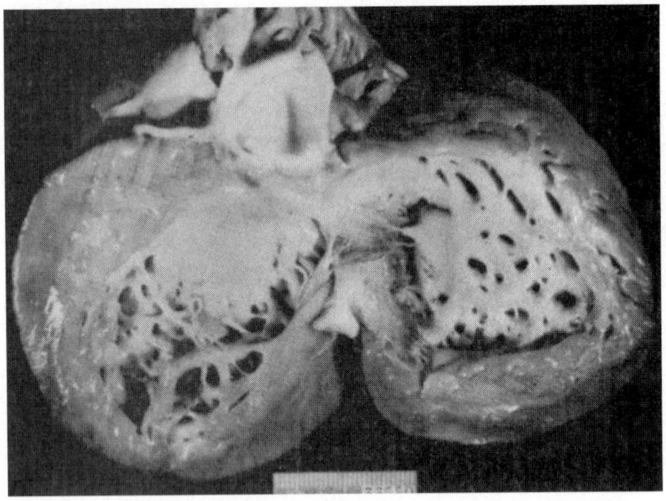

E

Fig. 135-1 (Continued)

development is grossly normal, and the rare report of mental retardation does not exceed the frequency of mental retardation in the general population. The course is rapidly progressive with death usually before 1 to 2 years of age due to cardiorespiratory failure.[17–21]

Infantile-Onset Non-classic

It is also clear that some patients with onset in early infancy (within the first 6 months of life) can present with a predominance of muscular symptoms without cardiomegaly. Thus, one of the first five patients diagnosed by Hers did not have apparent cardiomegaly.[5] In a review by Engel et al., 5 of 20 patients presenting in the first few months of life had profound muscular weakness but did not have cardiomegaly.[17] There is, however, an overall correlation of increasing age of onset with absence of cardiomegaly, even in cases with onset within the first 6 months of life (see Table 135-1).[17] Hepatomegaly and macroglossia are less common in this group, although macroglossia can be the first recognized abnormality. While some of these early-onset infants with predominance of skeletal muscle symptoms died before 1 year of age, several survived beyond 2 years. This less classic presentation of infantile-onset GSDII is often classified as childhood, juvenile, or muscular variant in reviews despite the early age of onset. Such cases may be missed and misdiagnosed as suffering from other disorders, including Werdnig-Hoffmann disease or a progressive muscular dystrophy.

Childhood- and Juvenile-Onset Disease

The childhood- or juvenile-onset disease overlaps clinically with both the classic and muscular variant of the infantile onset disorder (Table 135-1).[5,7–13,16–22,36–51] There is ambiguity in the literature as to the use of the term infantile-onset as compared with juvenile- or childhood-onset. Some authors use the designations only with reference to age of onset, while most authors classify as juvenile or childhood all cases with skeletal muscle involvement only (muscular variant), as well as cases with onset after 6 to 12 months of age and a somewhat slower progression. Essentially, the classification is arbitrary and there is a continuous spectrum with overlap in age of onset, organ involvement, and rate of progression. There is, in general, correlation of later age of onset with both absence of cardiac involvement and slower progression, but this may not apply to individual cases. In summary, of patients presenting before the age of 2, over 80 percent had both cardiomegaly and muscular weakness, while the remainder exhibited muscular symptoms without cardiac manifestations (Table 135-1). Of patients presenting after the age of 2, virtually all had skeletal muscle involvement without obvious cardiomegaly. Additionally, it has been proposed that there is a subset of childhood-onset patients with predominantly involvement of skeletal muscle but with presence of left ventricular hypertrophy without outflow obstruction (A. Slonim, personal communication). The course of childhood, juvenile-onset disease is more slowly progressive than classic infantile-onset disease, although age of onset does not necessarily correlate with age at death. The syndrome can present as delayed motor milestones (if age of onset is early enough), followed by progressive proximal muscle weakness with involvement of respiratory muscles. Cardiomegaly, hepatomegaly, and macroglossia can be seen but are infrequent. Muscle weakness is predominantly proximal. Lordosis and/or kyphosis/scoliosis may be prominent, even requiring surgical intervention, and a local pseudohypertrophy can be seen.[47] The disorder can be misdiagnosed as a muscular dystrophy. Death usually occurs because of respiratory failure before the end of the third decade.

Adult-Onset Disease

Adult-onset GSDII can present clinically as a slowly progressive proximal myopathy (see Fig. 135-2) or with symptoms dominated by respiratory insufficiency.[13–22,52–88] Symptoms of the underlying disease may not begin until the second to sixth decade of life. In all cases reported to date, there is absence of cardiomegaly. In some cases, patients were athletically active during adolescence, documenting the lack of earlier symptomatology.[69,79] In most patients, the clinical picture is dominated by slowly progressive proximal muscle weakness with truncal involvement and greater involvement of the lower than the upper limbs. Not all muscles even in the same area are equally affected. Disproportionate atrophy of the paraspinal muscles seen on CT scanning may be diagnostically suggestive in cases presenting with predominance of low back pain.[82] With the increasing weakness there is disappearance of deep tendon reflexes. The disorder has frequently been misdiagnosed as polymyositis and mistakenly treated with steroids. The disorder may be confused with scapuloperoneal syndromes; in one case, the disorder presented as rigid spine syndrome.[88] Initial myopathic symptoms may be subtle and have included exercise-induced urinary incontinence.[83] In approximately one-third of cases, weakness of the respiratory muscles, particularly the diaphragm, may predominate, with initial

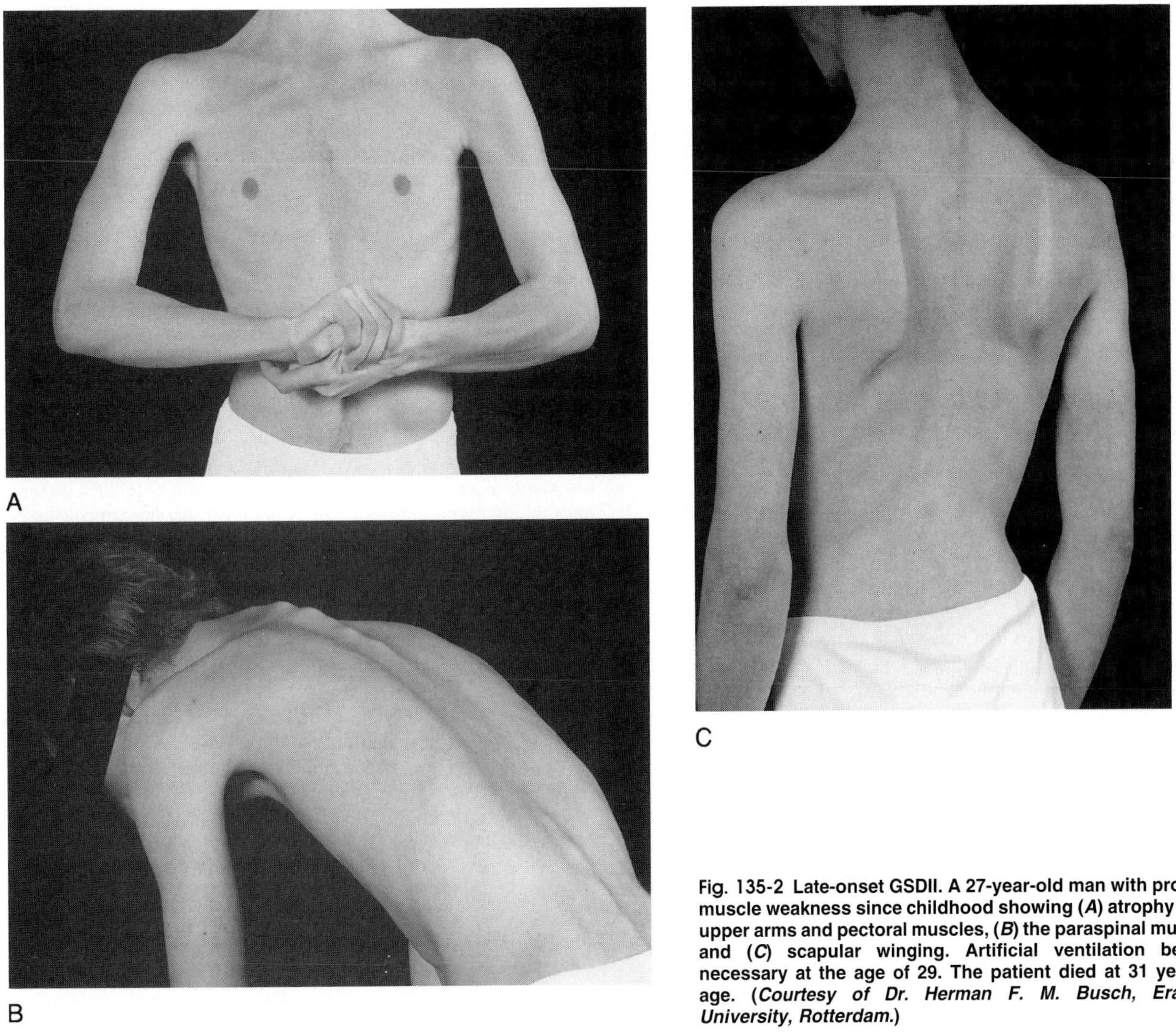

A

B

C

Fig. 135-2 Late-onset GSDII. A 27-year-old man with proximal muscle weakness since childhood showing (*A*) atrophy of the upper arms and pectoral muscles, (*B*) the paraspinal muscles, and (*C*) scapular winging. Artificial ventilation became necessary at the age of 29. The patient died at 31 years of age. (*Courtesy of Dr. Herman F. M. Busch, Erasmus University, Rotterdam.*)

symptoms including somnolence, morning headache, orthopnea, and exertional dyspnea. The onset of respiratory involvement may be very subtle, presenting as obstructive sleep apnea.[86] Other patients may present initially with respiratory failure,[59,66,71–73,77] although it is possible that the respiratory symptoms had been preceded by unrecognized progressive muscular weakness.[88–90,95,96] Acute respiratory failure may be precipitated by infections and patients can survive with appropriate support and live for over a decade longer with adequate supportive measures. Vital capacity is diminished, most markedly in the supine position, but this diminution usually follows onset of muscular weakness. All published case histories of adult-onset disease have been recently reviewed.[87] Death in patients with either presentation usually results from respiratory failure, and the appearance preterminally of signs of pulmonary hypertension and cardiac failure may further obfuscate the correct diagnosis.[424]

Clinical Laboratory Studies: Electromyography, Serum Enzymes, Skeletal Muscle Biopsy, Glycogen Content and Imaging

Electromyography reveals a myopathic pattern in all types, although in the later-onset disease, some muscles may appear normal. Myotonic discharges but without clinical myotonia (pseudomyotonic discharges) are common. Conduction times for motor and sensory nerves are normal.[17–20,30]

Serum CK is elevated, with the highest increase of up to tenfold in infantile-onset patients. CK is usually also elevated in adult-onset patients, but to a lesser degree, and may even be normal, but can be the basis for investigations leading to the diagnosis.[250a] Hepatic enzymes may be elevated, particularly in late-onset patients, and may truly reflect elevation of enzymes released from muscle.[96] There are no abnormalities of glucose metabolism, including normal responses to epinephrine and glucagon administration. There is a normal rise in venous lactate on ischemic exercise, consistent with a normal pathway for phosphorolytic glycogen breakdown.[20]

Muscle biopsy shows the presence of vacuoles that stain positively for glycogen (PAS), as well as for the lysosomal enzyme acid phosphatase. The vacuoles in infantile-onset patients also contain acid mucins or glycolipids. Increased acid phosphatase staining may be seen without obvious vacuolization. Increased glycogen is also seen freely dispersed as well as within vacuoles. There is an increase of over tenfold in glycogen content. Some authors have reported preferential involvement of type I fibers, but this selectivity is not a constant feature.[40–42] Type 2B fiber deficiency, indicative of type 2 motor neuron dysfunction in the spinal cord, has been documented, consistent with a neurologic component to the muscle dysfunction. The EM appearance has been reviewed extensively by Engel.[17] There is a diminishing gradient of severity of involvement with increasing age of onset. In adult-onset patients there is a wide variation in the pathology of different muscles so that biopsies of some muscles may appear either normal or atrophic, lacking diagnostic features of the disease. Vacuolization is more common in severely affected muscles. It now appears that the detection of glycogen by EM is a result of the presence of the proteins, including glycogenin, now known to be an integral part of the glycogen molecule. Quantitative determinations of glycogen content of muscle range from normal to threefold elevated.

Noninvasive procedures may increasingly aid in clinical investigations and particularly may in the future become more significant for evaluation of efficacy of proposed therapeutic interventions. Echocardiography is now an accepted adjunct for evaluating cardiac involvement and future studies may reveal cardiac involvement in patients with the muscular variant. CT and MRI scans[82,89–91] may be helpful in determining involvement of specific muscles with high glycogen content that are most likely to provide a morphologically diagnostic biopsy, presumably because excessive deposition results in high x-ray absorption on CT and high signal intensity on MRI. Cerebral abnormalities have been reported using MRI in an infantile-onset case with a classic presentation and muscle biopsy (although the diagnosis was not confirmed by enzyme assay and theoretically could represent Danon disease).[91] Other abnormalities of muscle are visible by CT scan and are particularly useful in delineating the muscle involvement in adult-onset disease.[82,90] In vivo assessment of muscle and liver glycogen concentrations can be precisely made by MRS based on natural abundance ^{13}C (natural abundance nuclear magnetic resonance spectroscopy or MRS).[97,98] PET scanning's role awaits implementation and evaluation.

The final diagnosis must rest on determination of deficiency of acid α-glucosidase activity in appropriate cell types (muscle or fibroblasts) and more recently can be further aided by definition of mutations. These aspects are discussed more fully below.

Pathology at Autopsy

Examination of tissue at autopsy has been performed in patients with all types of presentations.[20,27,28,36,54,61,79,81] Microscopic and biochemical examination of tissues from infantile-onset patients with classic disease reveals marked accumulation of glycogen in liver, heart, and skeletal muscle, with an over tenfold increase in glycogen content of muscle and a threefold increase in liver. The glycogen accumulation is predominantly intralysosomal, largely as beta particles, but is also cytoplasmic. There is also widespread accumulation of glycogen in numerous additional tissues, including smooth muscle, endothelial cells, kidney, lymphocytes, the eye (sparing pigmented cells of the iris and retina), skin, and cultured fibroblasts. The accumulation of glycogen in the nervous system is more marked in the spinal cord and brain stem, with relative sparing of cortical neurons. Glycogen accumulation is prominent in Schwann cells, spinal neurons (including anterior horn cells and motor nuclei of the brain stem and spinal ganglia), myenteric plexus, astrocytes, oligodendroglia, endothelial cells, and pericytes.[28]

In adult-onset patients, there are minimal to absent changes in any tissue other than skeletal muscle. Glycogen content is within normal limits in liver,[19,61,67,80b,81] and is variably elevated in skeletal muscle, ranging from normal to moderately elevated in different muscles from the same patient. Changes in cerebral vasculature have been reported in a few cases of childhood- and adult-onset disease.[54,80b,80c]

Additional Clinical and Pathologic Findings Possibly Associated with Acid α-Glucosidase Deficiency

Several additional clinical abnormalities have been described in more than one patient. These abnormalities could be part of the syndrome or be chance occurrences of a second disorder, particularly to be expected in consanguineous families. The reports of a patient with GSDII and cobalamin C (CblC) disease, or combined with deficiency of debrancher enzyme, appear to be in the latter category.[34,35] Cleft lip and/or palate was noted in at least three case histories of both infantile- and juvenile-onset patients (including one of the first cases reported by Hers),[5,37,55] and was recently serendipitously identified in two additional cases. A contiguous gene defect due to deletions including both the gene for GSDII and a contiguous gene have now been excluded in these two patients.[335] The enzyme deficiency could increase susceptibility to action of a linked or unlinked gene resulting in midline abnormalities of development. Alternatively, the association may be coincidental or represent a pleiotropic effect, possibly secondary to the macroglossia. One author (RH) has seen histories in three cases describing poorly defined "facial dysmorphism" at birth which appeared to disappear during the first months of life, but that in one case, was the initial feature leading to further investigations and eventual diagnosis of GSDII. This facial dysmorphism may reflect a combination of laxity of facial muscles and macroglossia. Perinatal death may also occur and in at least one case was documented as occurring in an infant with GSDII (reference 335 and unpublished observation [R. Hirschhorn]).

Vascular pathology, particularly in the brain, and including aneurysm formation, may be a feature of later-onset GSDII.[67,80c,81] This is consistent with vacuolar accumulation of glycogen in blood vessel walls observed in autopsies of other patients.[54,80b,80c,81] Autopsy of one such patient with manifestations of intracerebral vascular abnormality revealed numerous small aneurysms of cerebral and cerebellar small arteries as well as vacuolar degeneration of small and large arteriolar walls.[81] Although in several of these cases there were other contributing factors, including hypertension and family history of aneurysms, in one case no such contributing factors were described. These observations suggest that neurologic symptoms due to abnormalities of cerebral vasculature may be a feature of later-onset disorder. Primary lower motor neuron abnormalities and bulbar involvement have also been suggested in adult-onset patients.[60] An adult-onset patient with a 10-year history of mild progressive proximal weakness presented with what was considered to be prominent bulbar involvement, manifested as difficulty with swallowing, breathlessness, and coughing.[92] Alternatively, these manifestations could simply reflect major involvement of muscles of the upper digestive tract, and respiratory muscles with hypoxia because the symptoms were ameliorated following adequate ventilation. Epilepsy and dementia, reported in a single adult-onset case but not in her three affected sibs, may well be a coincidental finding.[93] A neurogenic component in the skeletal muscular dysfunction is supported by the accumulation of glycogen in peripheral nervous tissues, as discussed above. Lastly, unusual presentations with cardiomegaly but absence of muscle weakness have been described.[17,51] One patient with childhood onset of disease and cardiomegaly but no involvement of skeletal muscle had acid α-glucosidase activity that was only moderately reduced (43 percent of normal) but with a diminished affinity for substrate (fivefold increased K_m).[51] While patients with only cardiac symptoms could represent yet another clinical presentation of GSDII, it is also possible that these are cases of the more recently delineated syndrome of GSDII with normal acid maltase and coincidental occurrence of a normal variant of the acid maltase enzyme (see "Lysosomal Glycogen Storage Disease without α-Glucosidase Deficiency" below). Alternatively, specific mutations at the acid maltase locus, such as mutations altering K_m, may be more deleterious when expressed in cardiac than in skeletal muscle.

Clinical Genetics: Mode of Inheritance, Frequency, Heterozygotes

The disorder is inherited as an autosomal recessive trait, as evidenced by equal numbers of male and female patients as well as affected sibs of both sexes, occurrence of consanguineous matings, and absence of clinical abnormalities in the parents. In addition, healthy parents of affected children (obligate heterozygotes) usually have diminished acid α-glucosidase activity (see also "Heterozygote Detection" below under "α-Glucosidase in Patients").

There is currently debate as to the frequency of the disorder in western nations and estimates have ranged from 1/300,000 to 1/40,000. Based on the data presented in Chap. 71, the frequency of affected is 1/300,000, but more recent data suggest that this may be an underestimate. In some regions, the frequency appears to be much greater, based on the carrier frequency. In southern China and in Taiwan, infantile-onset GSDII is the most common of the glycogen storage disorders; it is estimated that between 0.5 and 1 percent of the population are carriers, with an approximate estimated frequency of affected children of 1 in 50,000.[99]

A recent estimate of frequency of GSDII in the Dutch population was based on results of testing 3000 newborns for the three mutations previously found to be common in patients with GSDII in the Dutch population (IVS 1(−13T > G), del exon18 and 525delT). The prior data as to the frequency of these mutations among disease alleles allowed for calculation of the proportion of disease alleles that would be ascertained by the screen for the three mutations and therefore calculation of carrier frequency for all disease alleles.[100,100a] This resulted in an estimated frequency of infantile onset disease of 1/138,000 with, however, very wide confidence intervals (95 percent CI of 1/43,000 to 1/536,000). The frequency of adult-onset disease was considerably greater (1/57,000), resulting in an overall frequency of 1/40,000 (95 percent CI of 1/18,000 to 1/100,000). These frequencies appeared to agree with the prevalence at birth of GSDII in the Dutch population.[100b]

A similar recent study directed at determining carrier frequency in a New York population reported three carriers among 928 randomly selected normal individuals, based on testing for seven mutations[101] (and see "Mutations" below). Two carried "null" mutations while the third carried a mutation found only in adult-onset disease. The sample contained an ethnically diverse population and consisted of 25 percent African-American, 42 percent Hispanic, 6 percent Asian, 10 percent Caucasian, and 17 percent individuals of unknown extraction. The authors stated that, based on their study of 74 patients with GSDII, the seven mutations would detect 29 percent of disease alleles. Based on the results of the screening, the authors reported an extrapolated carrier frequency of 1 in 100, with a calculated incidence of disease of 1 in 40,000. However, recalculation of these data, based on recent knowledge as to the ethnic distribution of the mutations included in the screening, provides an interesting alternative interpretation. Two of the three carriers identified were among the 233 African-Americans tested and both were carriers for the mutations that are common and virtually limited to this ethnic group. The mutation present in one of the carriers is very common in African-Americans (Arg854X; 50 percent of mutant alleles), whereas the mutation present in the second carrier also occurs in African-American patients (Met318Thr). An additional mutation that was included in the screen was found once in an African-American. Therefore, three of the mutations screened for account for 57 percent of disease alleles in a group of African-American patients (21/37 alleles), with the remaining disease alleles in African-Americans different from the mutations included in the "screen" (reference 330 and R. Hirschhorn, unpublished observation). With these considerations, the carrier frequency in the African-American population tested in this report is approximately 1/58 (2/233 × 2), predicting a disease frequency of 1/14,000 among African-Americans. The third carrier was heterozygous for the leaky IVS 1 mutation that is conditional for adult-onset disease and present in approximately 50 to 65 percent of adult-onset Caucasian patients, heterozygous with a null allele (see "Mutations"). Because the IVS 1 splice mutation is always heterozygous with an "infantile-onset" mutation, and to date has only been reported in Caucasian populations, additional data is required to estimate frequency of adult-onset disease based on this study.

In summary, the incidence of the disease may vary in different ethnic groups and for the different clinical forms. The frequency of infantile-onset disease in a diverse outbred Caucasian population remains to be determined, but is at least 1/100,000 to 1/200,000. The highest frequency of infantile-onset disease may be among African-Americans (1/14,000) and among Chinese (1/40,000 to 1/50,000). The frequency of infantile-onset disease among individuals of Dutch descent is lower (1/137,000) but still greater than initial estimates. Additional ethnic variation as to the frequency of infantile-onset disease is likely. The frequency of late-onset disease in Caucasian populations may be as high as 1/60,000. These observations as to the possible importance of ethnic derivation and incidence of adult-onset mutations must be kept in mind in the course of counseling patients and their families, particularly with respect to calculation of risk estimates for infantile and/or late-onset disease in offspring of a known carrier and an unrelated individual.

Heterozygous carriers are considered healthy. However, occurrence of periorbital swelling after infusion of hydroxyethyl starch was reported in an individual who, based on enzyme assay, appeared to be a carrier for a deficiency allele.[102] Detection of carriers by measurement of enzyme activity does not appear to be reliable. Earlier studies as to use of lymphocytes stimulated to divide have not been evaluated in a large group. DNA-based methods should now provide a means for carrier detection within families.

Prenatal diagnosis is discussed separately following discussion of molecular pathology, because prenatal diagnosis now may include molecular as well as enzymatic assays.

The disease is usually clinically similar in sibs, although some degree of intrafamilial variation between affected sibs has been reported.[69,84] This may reflect segregation of more than two mutant α-glucosidase alleles in the same family. Alternatively, the variation may be due to segregation of unlinked modifying genes or to environmental factors. Families have been reported with both the adult- and infantile-onset forms of the disease in the same family.[103–107] This was shown in a Dutch family to reflect allelic diversity of mutations, demonstrated by segregation of the mutant alleles in cell hybrids in the one family studied, and more recently by mutational analysis. Thus, the grandparental adult-onset patient carried two different mutant alleles, the most common adult-onset mutation IVS 1(−13T > G) (conditional for late-onset disease) and the single nucleotide deletion T525 (conditional in homozygosity for classic Pompe). The son inherited the total deficiency allele (delT525). This mutation has a high frequency in the Dutch population (see "Mutations" below) and an apparently chance mating of the son with an unrelated carrier for the same total deficiency allele resulted in the offspring with infantile-onset disease and homozygosity for the total deficiency allele delT525.

ACID α-GLUCOSIDASE (ACID MALTASE)

Several landmark papers demonstrated that acid α-glucosidase is a lysosomal enzyme that catalyzes the hydrolysis of α-1,4- and α-1,6-glucosidic linkages at acid pH, leading to the complete hydrolysis of its natural substrate glycogen, a branched chain polymer of glucose[5,6,108–110] (see Chap. 71 for a discussion of glycogen metabolism and structure of glycogen). Early studies demonstrated that acid α-glucosidase is synthesized and processed along a pathway common to many soluble lysosomal enzymes, involving extensive posttranslational modification of both the protein and of attached oligosaccharides.[111–113] While this is the major pathway for acid α-glucosidase, there is evidence for differences in processing compared to most lysosomal enzymes and/or for alternative pathways with different localization in tissues such as intestines and kidney (see "Lysosomal and Nonlysosomal Localization" below). Combined biochemical and molecular biologic studies have provided evidence that the unprocessed enzyme is catalytically inactive; identified the active site as homologous to the active site of mammalian sucrase-isomaltase, maltase-glucoamylase, glucosidase II, neutral α-glucosidase C, and α-glucosidases of lower species, despite differences in substrate specificity (family 31 glycosyl hydrolases); and demonstrated that proteolytic processing results in increased activity for the natural substrate, glycogen, as compared with low-molecular-weight substrates.

Biochemistry of Purified Enzyme: Physical and Kinetic Properties

Acid α-glucosidase has been isolated with varying degrees of purity from a variety of tissues from different species, including murine, bovine, canine, chicken, quail, and human liver; rat and human kidney; human heart; human placenta; rabbit muscle; and human urine.[5,6,108–132] The most successful purification procedures in these early studies took advantage of two different properties of the enzyme. First, α-glucosidase is retarded on Sephadex G100, presumably reflecting binding to the α-1,6 linkages present in Sephadex, and can be eluted efficiently with the substrate maltose, providing an "affinity" purification.[109] Second, the enzyme is N-glycosylated with high-mannose-type oligosaccharides and therefore binds to and can be eluted from concanavalin A Sepharose with methyl-manno- or methyl-glucopyranoside. Early studies of these purified preparations were significant for defining the kinetic properties of acid α-glucosidase as well as the gross physical characteristics. More recently, in preparation for providing sufficient human enzyme for therapeutic purposes, several forms of recombinant human acid α-glucosidase were produced in genetically modified bacteria—CHO, BHK, and COS cells—and were purified from media and cell lysates.[133–136,139] In addition, recombinant human enzyme has been produced and purified in the milk of genetically engineered mice (see "Therapy" below for details).[137–139]

The enzyme was initially reported to have a molecular mass of approximately 100 kDa and to be glycosylated. The enzyme hydrolyzes α-1,4-glucosidic linkages in high-molecular-weight α-glucans, including its natural substrate glycogen and soluble starch, as well as low-molecular-weight natural and artificial substrates, including maltose, maltotriose to maltooctaose,[125] 4-methylumbelliferyl α-D-glucopyranoside (4MUG), 6-bromo-2-naphthyl α-D-glucopyranoside, and p-nitrophenyl α-D-glucopyranoside. The enzyme also hydrolyzes α-1,6-glucosidic linkages in isomaltose to a lesser extent, and catalyzes trans-glucosylation reactions. The activity of the enzyme for isomaltose and for trans-glucosylation is intrinsic to the acid α-glucosidase, and is not due to contaminating enzymes. Thus, tissues from children with Pompe disease are devoid of both the α-1,4 and the α-1,6 hydrolytic, as well as the trans-glucosylation, activity.[108] There is one report that acid α-glucosidase from rabbit muscle hydrolyzes the α-1,2 and α-1,3 linkages in nigerose and kojibiose.[125] This is an interesting observation that probably reflects the structural homology between lysosomal acid α-glucosidase and other human α-glucosidases (isozymes) and between α-glucosidases from other species that have somewhat differing substrate specificities although they share extensive homology (see "Additional Isozymes with α-Glucosidase Activity; Homology Relationships" below, and Table 135-3). Different glycogen substrates are hydrolyzed at rates that appear to be inversely related to size of the glycogen.[127] Because lysosomal glycogen is formed by disulfide bridges between lower-molecular-weight material, an enzyme that reduces such thiol bonds may play a role in hydrolysis of intralysosomal glycogen.[127] The approximate average relative affinities (K_m) and maximal velocities (V_{max}) for the most frequently utilized substrates are summarized in Table 135-2. As noted above, there may be species differences in kinetic parameters that are not indicated in Table 135-2. The enzyme is active at acid pH, with a pH optimum of 4.0 to 5.0, and with slight differences for the different substrates. More recently, recombinant human acid α-glucosidase has been purified and characterized from several different sources (CHO, BHK, and COS cells and milk of genetically engineered mice).[133–139] These studies, also discussed in "Therapy," have confirmed the conclusions as to size, pH optima, and substrate specificities obtained from older studies of purified enzyme. Alternative methods of purification that are designed for commercial preparation of large amounts of enzyme for therapeutic purposes are now being developed.

There are several activators and inhibitors of acid α-glucosidase. Inhibitors include turanose, castanospermine, acarbose,

Table 135-2 Kinetic Properties of Lysosomal Acid α-Glucosidase

Substrate	K_m	Relative V_{max}
Glycogen*	10–30 (mg/ml)	100
Maltose	3–11 (mM)	100
4MUG†	0.9 (mM)	10
Isomaltose	40 (mM)	3

*Different types of glycogen have been used; higher K_m indicates lower affinity.
†4-Methylumbelliferyl α-D-glucopyranoside

conduritol beta-epoxide, and nojirimycine and its derivatives.[109,110,125,132,140–148] Several, if not all, of the currently available inhibitors are not specific for acid α-glucosidase; they also inhibit several of the neutral isozymes of α-glucosidase and the intestinal glycosidases. Nonabsorbable inhibitors are currently being used in the therapy of diabetes.[144] Development of more specific inhibitors as therapeutic agents is an area of current investigation. Conduritol beta-epoxide is a site-specific inactivator, covalently binding to the catalytic site of acid α- and β-glucosidases, and possibly other glucosidases. From the early studies, TRIS and low concentrations of turanose appeared to be the most specific inhibitors of the lysosomal acid α-glucosidase; more recently, both compounds were reported to inhibit other glucosidase isozymes, possibly at different concentrations. Polyclonal antibodies raised to purified acid α-glucosidase can inhibit the hydrolysis of glycogen, probably by steric hindrance, while not affecting the activity for low-molecular-weight substrates.[121,243,250] The enzyme is inactivated at alkaline pH, but reportedly can be protected by the presence of sulfhydryl reagents. Monovalent cations and/or albumin activate the enzyme. There is a report on a naturally occurring, heat-stable, approximately 25-kDa protein activator of the enzyme, but further characterization of this activator is required.[149]

Molecular Analysis of the Transcribed Human Acid α-Glucosidase

Both the cDNA and the structural gene for human acid α-glucosidase have been isolated and analyzed.[150–155] Several insights have become apparent from combined molecular biologic studies of the cDNA and biochemical analysis, including more precise definition of proteolytic processing and sites for glycosylation and phosphorylation.[150–159,164,174] In addition, the molecular biology has provided unexpected insight into homology relationships of the catalytic site to other glucosidases (see below).

The cDNA for human acid α-glucosidase is over 3.6 kb, with 2859 nucleotides (nt) of coding sequence (including the initiating methionine [ATG] and the codon for termination of translation), predicting 952 amino acids in a nonglycosylated protein of 105.37 kDa (see Fig. 135-3).[151–152] The sequence of the cDNA is in GenBank accession numbers M34424 and Y00839; the latter begins with numbering from the initiation of translation (ATG), and all numbering of mutations in the cDNA use the numbering in Y00839. The two accessions differ only as to which polymorphic amino acid is present at several sites (see below). The remainder of the cDNA consists of a 3′ untranslated region of 550 bp following the termination codon and a 5′ untranslated region preceding the ATG of at least 218 bp as determined from the largest (3.627 kb) cDNA isolated. Primer extension results suggest that there is an additional 220 bp of 5′ untranslated mRNA. The sequence predicts seven potential sites for N-linked glycosylation (Asn-X-Ser/Thr; excluding X = proline), at codons 140, 233, 390, 470, 652, 882, and 925. Molecular biologic studies, discussed in detail below, indicate that all these sites can be glycosylated, and that there must be at least two glycosylation sites that are phosphorylated.[164] The theoretical size of a fully glycosylated but noncleaved precursor would therefore be approximately 119 kDa (see Fig. 135-3).

Posttranslational Modification: Proteolytic Processing

Early pulse-chase experiments showed that acid α-glucosidase, like other lysosomal enzymes, is extensively modified posttranslationally by glycosylation and subsequent phosphorylation of mannose residues, providing the mannose-6-phosphate recognition marker for targeting to lysosomes, as well as by proteolytic cleavage, primarily within lysosomes.[111,112,126,130,157,158,160] These studies identified a precursor form of approximately 110 kDa, a small proportion of which is secreted. The 110-kDa protein is further proteolytically processed to species of 95, 76, and 70 kDa, as estimated on SDS gels.

Analysis of the cDNA reveals that lysosomal acid α-glucosidase is synthesized as a precursor calculated to be 105 kDa with a very hydrophobic N-terminus containing amino acid sequence with homology to signal sequences that direct cotranslational translocation of proteins to the ER. Pulse-chase studies of acid α-glucosidase produced in COS (monkey kidney) cells transfected with a normal cDNA, combined with amino acid sequence analysis of intermediate protein species, demonstrate that cleavage of the acid α-glucosidase signal peptide occurs at the second potential cleavage site, between glycine at codon 28 and histidine at codon 29, as determined by analysis of the secreted enzyme. However, unlike most other lysosomal enzymes, this signal sequence is cleaved at a point following transport into the ER, initially remaining membrane attached, confirming the early reports of a membrane-associated species.[158,162] This membrane attachment could explain the localization of acid α-glucosidase to plasma membranes in some cell types (see "Lysosomal and Nonlysosomal Localization" below). Following removal of the signal peptide, the precursor enzyme is further processed proteolytically within late endosomes and/or lysosomes. Processing occurs both at the N- and C-terminal ends, resulting in three major species of 95, 76, and 70 kDa, the latter two corresponding to the major species found in purified enzyme.[151,157,158] The

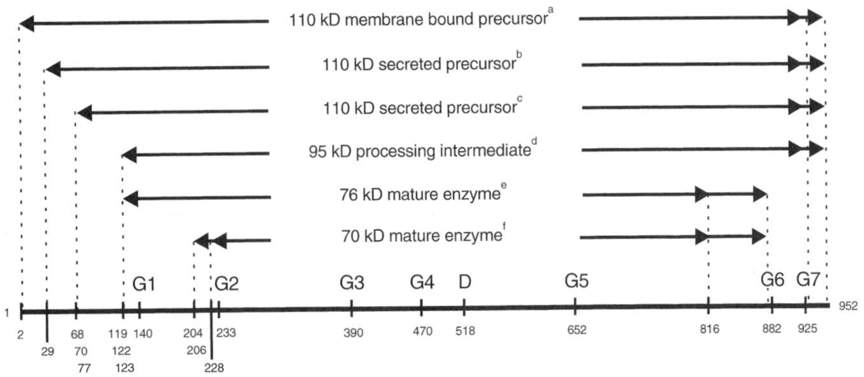

Fig. 135-3 Processing of α-glucosidase. The sites of proteolytic processing, of N-linked glycosylation, and of catalytic amino acid of the translated acid α-glucosidase (G1 to G7 = site of N-linked glycosylation, D = catalytic amino acid) are indicated. *A*, A 110-kDa membrane-bound precursor intracellular in human α-glucosidase cDNA transfected COS-1 cells. *B*, A 110-kDa secreted precursor from human α-glucosidase cDNA transfected BHK cells. *C*, A 110-kDa secreted precursor from human urine, human α-glucosidase cDNA transfected CHO cells, and milk of mice carrying a human GAA transgene. *D*, A 95-kDa processing intermediate from human placenta and from human α-glucosidase cDNA transfected BHK cells. *E*, A 76-kDa mature enzyme from human placenta, from human α-glucosidase cDNA transfected BHK and CHO cells, and from milk of mice carrying a human GAA transgene. *F*, A 70-kDa mature enzyme from human placenta and from human α-glucosidase cDNA transfected BHK cells.

various steps of proteolytic processing are summarized schematically in Fig. 135-3. The N-terminal processing sites were identified precisely by Edman degradation of the purified molecular species. The C-terminal sites are uncertain, but their location is roughly known by deduction. Following cleavage of the signal peptide, processing occurs first at the N-terminus to generate the 95-kDa species, with the first amino acid predominantly glycine at codon 123. The 76-kDa mature enzyme is generated by C-terminal proteolytic cleavage of the 95-kDa species, because the N-terminal amino acids of the 95- and 76-kDa species are identical. The site of the C-terminal cleavage is between codons 816 and 882, based on amino acid sequence analysis of a peptide derived from the 76-kDa species and on the effect exerted by deletion of the sixth glycosylation site.[164] Thus, deletion of either of the two C-terminal glycosylation sites at codons 882 and 925 reduces the size of the 95-kDa species by the expected 2 kDa, but has no effect on the size of the 76-kDa mature enzyme, indicating that codon 882 is not present in the 76-kDa enzyme protein.[164] Additional N-terminal proteolytic processing generates the 70-kDa species of mature enzyme, with alanine at codon 204 predominating as the N-terminal amino acid, but with additional proteolysis apparently occurring 2 and 24 amino acids downstream of the major site. Trace amounts of additional high-molecular-weight short-lived species, predominantly of approximately 100 kDa, were also reported in these and earlier studies, and appear to indicate an intermediate N-terminal proteolytic step, possibly occurring at Ala 70, as found in the precursor enzyme excreted in urine.[126,151] A similarly complex proteolytic processing of lysosomal α-glucosidase occurs in cow, quail, chicken, dog, and mouse, but there are species-specific differences in the sizes of the intermediate- and end-products.[109,129,131,390,398] Studies with brefeldin A, blocking exit of the enzyme from the Golgi, indicate that processing occurs in a post-Golgi compartment. The N- and C-terminal proteolytic processing steps either occur at different intracellular sites or by the action of different enzymes. Thus, leupeptin, the inhibitor of serine-thiol proteases, delays conversion of a usually transitory 100-kDa intermediate to the 95-kDa intermediate and blocks further conversion to the 76-kDa species. By contrast, treatment with ammonium chloride only blocks conversion of the 95- to 76-kDa species.[158] All the major molecular species of acid α-glucosidase seen in pulse-chase experiments are also found in enzyme preparations purified to apparent homogeneity. However, the proteolytically processed 76- and 70-kDa mature forms are the major species found in such purified preparations of acid α-glucosidase, consistent with an estimated 2-h half-life of the precursor[156] and a longer half-life of the mature enzyme, estimated as 5 to 8 days.[255]

Proteolytic processing is required for catalytic activity and for increasing the activity toward glycogen as substrate relative to that for low-molecular-weight substrates.[126,158] The membrane-bound precursor, retaining the signal peptide, is enzymatically inactive, as shown by inability to bind the catalytic site inhibitor conduritol beta-epoxide.[146,158] Consistent with these results, recombinant enzyme, synthesized in bacteria and presumably not processed, is not enzymatically active, as determined using 4MUG as substrate, although the enzyme retains antigenic sites.[139] (Alternatively, the lack of enzymatic activity of the recombinant enzyme expressed in bacteria could be due to lack of appropriate glycosylation that may also be required for enzyme activity in vitro.) Further proteolytic processing progressively increases the activity of the enzyme expressed in COS cells for glycogen relative to the artificial substrate 4MUG. There is a sevenfold increase in the relative activity of the 76-/70-kDa species for glycogen as compared with the 110-kDa precursor (lacking the signal peptide), with intermediate values for the 95-kDa species.[158] Earlier studies of purified species had demonstrated that although proteolytic processing of the enzyme is accompanied by increases in relative activity for glycogen as compared with maltose, this increase is not due to alterations in K_m.[126] Other biochemical studies had shown that the 76- and 70-kDa species are both enzymatically active.[130] The finding that proteolytic processing appears to be required for optimal activity for the natural substrate glycogen could reflect a conformational change that allows for more efficient access of the large substrate glycogen to a possible additional substrate binding site and/or the catalytic site.[157] Biochemical studies are consistent with a single catalytic/substrate site.[132] Additional 10- to 25-kDa species have been found in preparations of the purified enzyme.[111,123,124] While these lower-molecular-weight species could be contaminants, they could also either indicate copurification of a 25-kDa activator protein that has been described but not further investigated, or represent proteolytically cleaved fragments from acid α-glucosidase that remain noncovalently attached under nondenaturing conditions.[149]

Posttranslational Modification: N-Linked Glycosylation

Molecular studies indicated that all seven potential glycosylation sites are utilized.[164] Conservative substitution of glutamine for asparagine at any of six of these sites results in a reduction in size of the protein species by approximately 2 kDa, consistent with loss of a site that is normally glycosylated. However, there is no alteration in total activity, processing, or localization. By contrast, deletion of the site at codon 233 allows for normal synthesis but reduces total activity to 20 percent of normal, delays transport to the Golgi, and interferes with further lysosomal localization and maturation of the enzyme.[164] Treatment of the cells with tunicamycin, to prevent glycosylation at all sites, renders the enzyme unstable, and prevents transport of the enzyme. These combined results suggest either that glycosylation of the site at codon 233 is essential for stability, further localization, and maturation, or that substitution of glutamine at that site results in an unstable protein. The estimation of five glycosylated sites in the 76-kDa enzyme and four in the 70-kDa enzyme is consistent with prior biochemical determinations of four to five glycosylated sites in the mature (76- and 70-kDa) enzyme,[165] and suggests that all potential glycosylation sites in the mature enzyme are utilized. None of the single mutations at glycosylation sites resulted in rerouting of enzyme to the secretory pathway.

Differences in the extent of glycosylation of the two major species in purified enzyme have been reported, presumably resulting from removal of oligosaccharides within lysosomes. The total hexose content of the 76-kDa species has been reported to be almost twice that of the 70-kDa species, a difference that cannot be accounted for by differences in glycosylation sites.[130] Nonglycosylated as well as glycosylated species of both the 76- and 70-kDa forms have also been reported.[122] These results indicate that some oligosaccharides are removed from the enzyme within lysosomes. The oligosaccharide chains appear to be predominantly of the simple high-mannose type, although some oligosaccharides of complex type are also found.[164,165] The formation of complex-type chains is induced by a relatively slow intracellular transport, as in mucin-secreting HT-29 M6 colon carcinoma cells and by preventing acid α-glucosidase from exiting the *trans*-Golgi reticulum with brefeldin A.[156,158,159]

Posttranslational Modification: Phosphorylation of Mannose Residues

The high-mannose oligosaccharides of lysosomal enzymes are phosphorylated in the Golgi by the sequential action of two enzymes, as described in Chaps. 16 and 138. Pulse-chase experiments using radiolabeled phosphate reveal phosphorylation of the proteolytically processed mature acid α-glucosidase.[112] By contrast, the enzyme purified from tissues containing predominantly mature forms of the enzyme does not contain mannose-6-phosphate residues.[163] These findings are consistent with rapid dephosphorylation of the mature enzyme within lysosomes (seen with other lysosomal enzymes). At least two of the glycosylation sites within the mature 76-kDa enzyme are phosphorylated because individual deletion of each of four of the five sites present within the 76-kDa protein (codons 140, 390, 470, and 652) by substitution of glutamine for asparagine did not prevent phosphorylation of the mature enzyme.[164] As discussed previously, substitution at the glycosylation site at codon 233 results in an enzyme with markedly diminished stability and impaired maturation, leading to a reduction in the phosphorylated 76-kDa species.

A small proportion of the newly synthesized enzyme escapes targeting to lysosomes and is found in the extracellular milieu as a high-molecular-weight enzyme. This "precursor" enzyme, as well as the "precursor" excreted in urine, are phosphorylated and can be taken up by cells via mannose-6-phosphate receptors for delivery to lysosomes. While both the precursor from urine and that released from cells are rapidly taken up by different cell types (high-uptake enzyme), the mature dephosphorylated enzyme is taken up by many cell types very slowly[126] (see "Therapy" below). While the major steps of posttranslational processing of acid α-glucosidase have been delineated, the precise details of several intermediate steps, as well as possible tissue and/or species variation, remain to be elucidated.

Charge Heterogeneity of Purified Enzyme Resulting from Processing and/or Normal Genetic Variation (Allozymes or Normal Allelic Variants)

Isoelectric focusing of purified enzyme and staining for either protein or enzymatic activity reveals multiple different forms. The bulk of the evidence indicates that the charge differences reflect the different protein species produced by proteolytic processing rather than differences in carbohydrate structure or other posttranslational modifications such as, for example, amidation or SH reactions.[163] However, in human enzyme purified from tissues of more than a single individual (and possibly also in other species), some of the heterogeneity could reflect the presence of different allozymes (normal allelic variants) present in the normal population (see "Normal Biochemical and Molecular Genetic Variation" below).

Lysosomal and Nonlysosomal Localization

The initial studies clearly demonstrated that acid α-glucosidase is localized to lysosomes and is targeted to lysosomes via mannose-6-phosphate receptors. However, the pathway for targeting of specific lysosomal enzymes appears to be dependent on both the enzyme and the tissue, with at least two alternative mechanisms for lysosomal targeting.[166–171] There is evidence that acid α-glucosidase is targeted to lysosomes by a mannose-6-phosphate-independent pathway,[168] as well as by both the 215-kDa cation-independent and 45-kDa cation-dependent mannose-6-phosphate receptors. In addition, the enzyme can be localized to other subcellular sites in some tissues by an unidentified mechanism. Acid α-glucosidase has been detected immunochemically at the cell surface in microvillar membranes of intestines,[166,171] a human colon carcinoma cell line,[169,170] and kidney proximal tubule epithelial cells.[167] In these polarized cells, acid α-glucosidase is localized to the apical surface and most of the acid α-glucosidase secreted is at the apical surface, in contrast to secretion of most other lysosomal enzymes at the basolateral surface. The precursor form of the acid α-glucosidase is found at the brush border, as determined using monoclonal antibodies that distinguish between precursor and mature enzyme. This brush-border enzyme cannot be displaced by incubation with mannose-6-phosphate.[170] These observations suggest that acid α-glucosidase is sorted in a mannose-6-phosphate-independent fashion, and in some cell types, in a manner apparently unique among lysosomal enzymes. It is now apparent that the signal peptide of acid α-glucosidase is not cleaved cotranslationally and in some cells could therefore sort to the plasma membrane, as does the homologous brush-border enzyme sucrase-isomaltase. Acid α-glucosidase is also found at the cell surface of COS cells transfected with a cDNA for the enzyme.[157]

The sorting and targeting of acid α-glucosidase in muscle cells has not been critically investigated with respect to precise transport and localization. Such studies could be relevant for understanding the pathophysiology of the different mutations responsible for the deficiency disorder, particularly with respect to patients with adult-onset disease and considerable residual activity. Additionally, such studies would be relevant to trials of enzyme replacement therapy.

Catalytic Mechanism, Site, and Homology: General Overview

Lysosomal acid α-glucosidase can be classified as belonging to the very large group of enzymes classified as glycosyl hydrolases. The general mechanism for hydrolysis of the glycosidic bond uses general acid catalysis, requiring two critical residues: a proton donor within hydrogen-bonding distance of the glycosidic oxygen and a nucleophile/base. These enzymes are further classified into two groups based on whether the product of catalysis retains or inverts the original stereochemical α- or β-anomeric configuration of the substrate. In retaining enzymes, the nucleophilic catalytic base is close to the sugar anomeric carbon. The glycosyl hydrolases are further subdivided into "families," based on the nature of the carbohydrate substrates hydrolyzed (as in EC classifications) and on sequence homologies.[172] Homologies can either be to similar enzymes (isozymes) in the same species (paralogs) or to similar enzymes in different species (orthologs).

Lysosomal acid α-glucosidase retains the original α-anomeric configuration (retaining mechanism) and, based on homology, is the prototypic enzyme of "family 31" glycosyl hydrolases that includes enzymes from mammals to plants.[173] While the ProDom database lists several orthologs but only one human paralog (sucrase-isomaltase), it is apparent (based on published analysis and additional unpublished analysis by the authors of this review and as discussed under homologies) that at least four additional human α-glucosidases that have been cloned are human paralogs belonging to the same family 31 glycosyl hydrolases that includes lysosomal acid α-glucosidase. Several clear orthologs of acid α-glucosidase (murine and quail) have also been cloned, as well as an increasing number of related α-glucosidases from various species. The evolutionary tree remains to be elucidated.

Catalytic Site

The active site of human acid α-glucosidase, as determined by isolation and amino acid sequence analysis of a peptide binding the active site inhibitor conduritol β-epoxide, is contained in codons 513 to 524 (DGMWIDMNEPSN).[174] These results indicate that Asp518 is the essential carboxylate. Evidence consistent with these predictions has been provided for the human enzyme by in vitro mutagenesis of the putative active site and determination of loss of binding of the active site inhibitor conduritol β-epoxide and of enzymatic activity. Thus, mutation of the essential carboxylate Asp 518 to asparagine, glutamic acid, or glycine reduces enzymatic activity to 4 to 10 percent of normal, as determined by expression of mutant cDNA in COS cells. Substitution of Trp 516 by Arg also reduces activity to approximately 15 percent of normal. Substitution of Asp 513 by glutamic acid also reduces enzyme activity to 25 percent of normal, but this reduction appears to reflect abnormalities in routing, processing, and maturation of the mutant enzyme, as evidenced by absence of secreted enzyme and of the 76-kDa mature form.[174] The experimentally determined catalytic site conforms to the consensus sequence derived by analysis of sequence homology of paralogous and orthologous cloned α-glucosidase genes and determination of a consensus "signature" sequence ([GF][LIVMF]WXDM[NSA]E).[173]

Biochemistry and Homology Based on Analysis of Sequence: Additional Human α-Glucosidases (Isozymes) that are Paralogs of Lysosomal Acid α-Glucosidase

Table 135-3 summarizes the paralogs. There are several additional isozymes of human α-glucosidase (enzymes that exhibit

Table 135-3 Human α-Glucosidases Isozymes (Paralogs Belonging to Human Family 31 Glucosyl Hydrolases)

	Acid α-glucosidase GAA	Sucrase-isomaltase S-I	Maltase-glucoamylase	Glucosidase II GANAB	Neutral α-glucosidase C GNAC
pH optimum	3.0–4.0	5.0–5.5	5.0–5.5	7.5 (broad)	7.5 (broad)
Tissue	ubiquitous	small intestines	small intestines, PMN, kidney	ubiquitous	ubiquitous?
Intracellular localization	lysosomes	brush border	brush border	endoplasmic reticulum	?
Protein	monomer, processed to 95, 75 & 70 kDa	2 catalytic sites cleaved from cell & into 2 subunits	2 catalytic sites	heterodimer with a second protein for ER retention	monomer
mRNA size	3.6	6.0	6.5	3.9	>3.5
Amino acids	952	1,827	1,857	944	914
Chromosome	17q25	3q25-26	7q35-36	11q11-14	15q15-22
Homology to GAA (% similarity)	100	41/57	55/52	45	47

α-1,4-glucosidase activity) but that are coded for by different genetic loci. Definite orthologs of each of these human isozymes have been described in other mammalian species.[175–210] The α-glucosidase isozymes additional to lysosomal acid α-glucosidase can be divided into two broad groups. The first group includes two apparently ubiquitous isozymes: neutral α-glucosidase C (GANC) and glucosidase II (also previously called neutral α-glucosidase AB in earlier publications and designated as GANAB on the human gene map). The second group consists of enzymes with limited tissue expression and includes intestinal sucrase-isomaltase, intestinal maltase-glucoamylase, and an as-yet-uncloned α-glucosidase expressed in lamellar bodies (Table 135-3). Recent cloning and analysis of the genes for these various isozymes have greatly clarified the earlier biochemical studies, and, on the basis of homology, indicate that four of these additional isozymes all belong to the same family 31 glycosyl hydrolases that includes lysosomal acid α-glucosidase.[172,173,173a] Such homologous enzymes in a single species coded for by separate genetic loci are currently defined as paralogous genes, in contrast to related genes in different species that are defined as orthologous genes. The paralogous human α-glucosidases differ in their specific substrate specificities, pH optima, and tissue localization. The molecular bases for the differences in substrate specificity and pH optima are not yet elucidated, while the differences in tissue expression undoubtedly reflect undefined differences in promoter or intronic regions.

The two different ubiquitous α-glucosidase isozymes were originally designated neutral α-glucosidase AB and neutral α-glucosidase C based on their relative mobilities in starch gel electrophoresis and greater activity at neutral pH.[175] These two human isozymes differ (AB vs. C) with respect to molecular weight, isoelectric point, substrate specificity, chromosomal localization, and presence of normal genetic variations. By biochemical analysis, neutral α-glucosidase C has a molecular weight of 92 ± 10 kDa and a pI of 5.5, and releases glucose from glycogen as well as from low-molecular-weight artificial and natural substrates containing α-1,4-glucosidic linkages.[178] The gene is localized to the long arm of chromosome 15 (15q21) and was officially designated GANC on the human gene map.[177] The enzyme also shows a genetic biochemical polymorphism, and there are four different alleles segregating in the normal population.[176] One of these alleles is unusual in that it is "silent" (no detectable enzyme activity), with an estimated gene frequency of 0.174, predicting that 3 percent of the population will be homozygous-deficient for α-glucosidase C. The possible physiological significance of this apparent loss of α-glucosidase C activity is not known. While variation in neutral α-glucosidase C does not appear to play a role in the gross clinical variation of GSDII,[179] it remains possible that presence of the null allele could vary phenotype within the three different clinical forms despite apparently identical acid α-glucosidase genotype.

It is now clear, based on biochemical and (more compellingly) genetic evidence, that α-glucosidase AB (GANAB) is synonymous with the glycoprotein-processing enzyme glucosidase II present in the endoplasmic reticulum.[178,180–186,207,208] Biochemical studies had indicated that α-glucosidase AB has a native molecular weight of > 150 kDa, and hydrolyzed α-1,4 linkages but not in glucose oligosaccharides larger than maltose.[178] Extensive biochemical studies of glucosidase II have shown that glucosidase II can also hydrolyze α-1,4 linkages in maltose (but not any larger α-glucan), as was found for GANAB. However, glucosidase II is primarily responsible for catalyzing the hydrolysis of the α-1,3 linkages of the second and third of the three terminal glucose residues present on the dolichol intermediate transferred en bloc to asparagine residues for N-linked glycosylation. Consistent with the identity of glucosidase II and GANAB, cells deficient for glucosidase II (as defined by specific enzyme assay) are also deficient for GANAB (as defined by electrophoresis and *in situ* enzyme detection), and both activities are restored by introduction of the gene for glucosidase II.[181,182,208] The enzyme is the most prominent neutral α-glucosidase isozyme detected in most tissues when 4MUG is used as substrate.[178,183–186] The gene for α-glucosidase AB or glucosidase II has been localized to the long arm of chromosome 11 (designated GANAB on the human gene map).[122,180] Based on studies in nonhuman species, glucosidase II is a heterodimer consisting of a catalytic unit and a second subunit that contains the ER localization signal.

The sequence of the cDNA is now known for both human glucosidase II and human neutral α-glucosidase C (GANC). The encoded glucosidase II catalytic subunit[207–210] predicts a protein of 944 amino acids with homology to acid α-glucosidase (32 percent identity, 45 percent similarity) and very high homology to glucosidase II from other mammalian species.[177,178,210] The cloned noncatalytic beta subunit containing the ER retention signal accounts for the biochemically determined higher molecular weight of the native enzyme than that predicted by the catalytic unit alone. The cloned neutral α-glucosidase C predicts a protein of 914 amino acids and a molecular weight of 104 kDa with similar homology as glucosidase II to acid α-glucosidase (32 percent identity and 47 percent similarity) (reference 210 and R. Hirschhorn, unpublished observations). The homology is extensive and includes the amino terminus as well as the middle portion encompassing the catalytic site and a second more 3′ signature sequence for family 31 glycosyl hydrolases. The homology of the two neutral isozymes is greater to each other (50 percent identity, 69 percent similarity) than to other α-glucosidases, primarily because of homology in the 5′ end (reference 210 and R. Hirschhorn, unpublished observations).

Additional apparently high-molecular-weight neutral α-glucosidase isozymes have been purified from brush border of intestines, kidney, urine, and cell-surface membranes of neutrophils.[187–203] The two genes that code for these enzymes have now been cloned. The first is sucrase isomaltase, which is a duplicated/fused gene with two catalytic sites and expression limited to intestines. Sucrase-isomaltase has been shown to have homology with acid α-glucosidase (39 percent identity and 41 percent similarity; 40 percent identity, 57 percent similarity).[151,204,205] The second gene is maltase-glucoamylase, which is also a duplicated/fused gene with homology of both the maltase and glucoamylase to acid α-glucosidase (41 percent identity and 55 percent similarity; 38 percent identity and 52 percent similarity). Maltase-glucoamylase is primarily expressed in the intestines, but is also expressed in kidney and PMNs.[206] The enzyme also appears to be a differentiation marker in neutrophils.[197] It is now apparent that maltase-glucoamylase is the α-glucosidase present in PMNs that interferes with simple diagnosis of GSDII using peripheral blood cells. The earlier biochemical data are consistent with these conclusions. These earlier biochemical studies first defined the presence in neutrophils, intestines, kidney, and urine of an isozyme with a pH optimum overlapping that for lysosomal acid α-glucosidase and the ability to cleave substrates commonly used to determine acid α-glucosidase activity. Based on studies using antibodies, comparison of electrophoretic mobility, native molecular weights of purified enzymes, and of ability to hydrolyze substrates from maltose to glycogen, with greater activity for oligomers of three to five residues, the intestinal enzyme was thought to be identical to the α-glucosidase expressed in kidney and PMNs.[187–200] The cloning of maltase-glucoamylase may provide the means to identify a substrate or inhibitor that would differentiate between the lysosomal acid α-glucosidase and the confounding maltase-glucoamylase present in PMNs.

In summary, the cloning of several human α-glucosidases has clarified the relationships of several of the α-glucosidase isozymes that have previously been described biochemically and genetically. In addition to lysosomal acid α-glucosidase, these enzymes include sucrase-isomaltase,[205] maltase-glucoamylase,[206] glucosidase II (GANAB),[207–209] and neutral α-glucosidase C (GANC) (reference 210 and R. Hirschhorn, unpublished observations). In addition to overall homology relative to the lysosomal enzyme, ranging from 45 to 57 percent (similarity), these enzymes share homology at the catalytic site and at a region within the sequence defined as a second "signature" for family 31 glycosyl hydrolases. The two intestinal enzymes are duplicated/fused genes with two separate catalytic sites that differ as to their substrate affinities. All of these related enzymes differ as to their specific substrate specificities and pH optimum as well as to their chromosomal, tissue and subcellular localization. The most significant finding with respect to diagnosis of GSDII has been the identification of intestinal maltase-glucoamylase as the enzyme in PMNs that interferes with diagnosis of GSDII using peripheral blood cells (Table 135-3).

α-Glucosidase of Lung Lamellar Bodies

There is at least one additional isozyme of α-glucosidase that has not yet been definitively characterized. Lamellar bodies of lung, specialized organelles that contain surfactant, contain an acid α-glucosidase with pH optimum and substrate specificity similar to the lysosomal enzyme.[211] However, the lamellar body isozyme is coded for by a different genetic locus, because lung from a child with acid α-glucosidase deficiency contained normal amounts of the lamellar body-specific enzyme.[212] The lamellar body α-glucosidase is not glycosylated and does not cross-react with antibody to the lysosomal enzyme. Nonetheless, the enzyme may be ancestrally related, because a cDNA for acid α-glucosidase hybridized to an additional mRNA in lung that is considerably larger than the mRNA for acid α-glucosidase detected.[213] It is not certain whether this isozyme is expressed in any other tissues, such as intestines. The lamellar body α-glucosidase enzyme has not been purified, and its size is unknown.

Orthologs of Acid α-Glucosidase in Multiple Species: Sequence-Based Homology

Computer-based analysis revealed homology of α-glucosidases from vertebrates, including mammals and birds, and extending to *C. elegans*, lower eukaryotes such as yeast, prokaryotes, and plants.[151,204, 205,207, 214–228] The highest region of homology is in the region of the catalytic site with a second region also highly homologous and conserved. The evolutionary tree appears to have branched early to result in the paralogs found in humans.

Two clear direct ancestors (orthologs) of acid α-glucosidase have been cloned from mice and quail.[227,228] The murine acid α-glucosidase shows very high homology (85 percent). Quail exhibit two α-glucosidases, both with greatest homology to the lysosomal α-glucosidase. Only one of the two quail α-glucosidases is deficient in GSDII of quail. The second enzyme normally represents a minor proportion of total acid α-glucosidase activity and is expressed primarily in early development. There is no evidence for a second acid α-glucosidase in humans, but this has not been examined critically for a developmentally controlled second gene in humans or in other species additional to quail.

CHARACTERIZATION OF α-GLUCOSIDASE IN PATIENTS WITH GSDII

Enzymatic Diagnosis

Lysosomal acid α-glucosidase is present in all tissues of the body, as well as in fibroblasts, amniotic cells, chorionic villi, lymphocytes, EBV-transformed B-cell lines, and urine. Enzyme activity in patients has been determined in different tissues and cell types, but, for diagnostic purposes, it has been determined primarily in muscle,[51,65,195,230,233,237,238,245,250a,256,262,270,272] fibroblasts,[23, 24, 63, 64, 232, 236, 239, 242, 247, 250, 250a, 252, 264–266] lymphocytes,[229,235,248,250a,252,258] leukocytes,[195,196,233,234,240,248,259,260] EBV-transformed B-cell lines,[196,300] and urine.[232,241,244,246,252,267] These assays have measured hydrolysis of several different substrates, including (most commonly) glycogen (of varying size), the α-1,4-linked glucose disaccharide maltose, and the artificial substrate 4MUG. Transglucosylation and hydrolysis of the α-1,6-linked disaccharide isomaltose has been measured infrequently.[5,230]

Measurement of acid α-glucosidase activity in muscle tissue and cultured fibroblasts most reliably and clearly demonstrates absence of enzyme activity in infantile-onset cases. Therefore, assays of these tissues should also most clearly reflect true residual activity in juvenile- and adult-onset patients. Of these two methods, the fibroblasts seem preferable because the assays are more sensitive and obtaining the tissue is less invasive for the patient. Mixed leukocytes and urine are not suitable for definitive diagnosis by simple enzyme assay with artificial 4MUG (i.e., without use of antibody in the assay) substrate because of the presence of maltase-glucoamylase ("renal" isozyme) in both neutrophils and urine, as discussed above. However, several investigators have used urine and mixed leukocytes for diagnosis in combination with antibody to lysosomal acid α-glucosidase to differentiate between activity due to the lysosomal enzyme and that due to nonrelevant isozymes. Lymphocytes separated from blood also show the enzyme deficiency, but could be less routinely reliable because of residual contamination with granulocytes. EBV-transformed B-cell lines also exhibit the deficiency, but normally express considerably lower activity (as well as mRNA) than do fibroblasts, making the measurement of residual enzyme activity more difficult. It is the opinion of one author (RH) that when assays of lymphocytes that do not show enzyme deficiency, the presence or absence of the enzyme should be confirmed by assay of muscle, fibroblasts, or EBV-transformed B cells. In

Table 135-4 Relative Enzyme Activity (% Normal Activity) in Fibroblasts and Muscle of GSDII Patients with Different Clinical Phenotypes*

	Infantile	Juvenile	Adult
Fibroblasts			
Average (n)	0.5 (11)	4.0 (3)	1) 18.0 (13/16)
Range	(0.2–0.9)	(1.5–5.0)	(14.7–39.5)
			2) 1.6 (3/16)
			(0.8–3.0)
Muscle			
Average (n)	"0" (3)	5.0 (5)	7.7 (10)
Range		(2.4–8.1)	(2.9–11.9)

*Adapted from references containing values for large numbers of patients assayed in the same laboratory.[245,265] There was a clear separation of values for three of the adult-onset patients from the 13 others tested and values for these 3 patients are tabulated separately.[265]

summary, it seems that the most reliable definitive diagnosis can be made with muscle or fibroblasts, using maltose or 4MUG as the substrate.

In general, infantile-onset patients have undetectable enzyme activity in muscle tissue obtained by biopsy and very low activity in fibroblasts, whereas most adult-onset patients exhibit substantial residual enzyme activity. Juvenile-onset patients exhibit intermediate but overlapping values (Table 135-4).[22,63,64,250,265,300] While most juvenile- and adult-onset patients have activity that is reduced to a lesser extent than in infantile cases, rare late-onset patients have enzyme activity that is not clearly distinguishable from that in infantile-onset patients. At the opposite extreme, and more significant for diagnosis, residual enzyme activity can overlap with activity found in healthy carriers of the disease and with the lower end of values found in normals. There is also considerable overlap in residual enzyme activity between the juvenile- and adult-onset groups, suggesting that the amount of residual activity is not the sole determinant of the clinical phenotype. Additionally, the occurrence of possible "pseudodeficiency" alleles segregating in the normal population may contribute to discordance between the biochemical and clinical phenotype. An allele with very low activity for MUG was serendipitously discovered in an obligate heterozygote who was asymptomatic in early adulthood.[271] Homozygosity or heterozygosity for the GAA2 allele (see "Posttranslational Processing" above and "Normal Biochemical and Molecular Variation" below) causes a "pseudodeficiency" when assayed with the usual concentrations of glycogen.[175,250a,290–292]

There are at least two different explanations for cases in which the degree of enzyme deficiency does not correlate with clinical severity. As a relatively trivial explanation applicable to many inherited metabolic disorders, the enzyme activity in vitro may not correlate with the activity in vivo because enzyme assays utilize conditions that are different from those found in vivo. In addition, many of the determinations of acid α-glucosidase utilize maltose and artificial substrates rather than the natural substrate glycogen. Even when glycogen is used, it is often not of the same molecular weight and structure as that found in lysosomes, and acid α-glucosidase activity has been shown to be inversely proportional to the size of the glycogen substrate. As a more fundamental consideration, acid α-glucosidase apparently must be proteolytically processed for full activity on the natural substrate glycogen and localized to lysosomes in order to prevent intralysosomal accumulation of glycogen. There could be subtle tissue-specific differences in these processes that modulate the residual activity per organ.[272] Mutations that result in defects in processing and localization could therefore account for some of the lack of correlation of clinical severity and quantitative enzyme activity. (Correlations of genotype and biochemical and clinical phenotypes are discussed in "Molecular Pathology" below.)

Heterozygote Detection

Parents of affected patients (obligate heterozygotes) usually show reduced α-glucosidase activity. Several groups have specifically investigated the feasibility of detecting heterozygotes.[229,230,244,253] All previous studies are summarized in reference 253. There is significant overlap between values in obligate heterozygotes and the normal population; sufficient studies to define the extent of overlap precisely have not been performed. In individual families, it may be possible to identify heterozygotes, but at this time DNA-based detection would seem more appropriate and definitive within families. (Anecdotally, we have seen heterozygotes who carry a common infantile-onset mutation reported by established laboratories as having normal acid α-glucosidase activity in lymphocytes.)

Abnormal Metabolites

Nonglycogen polysaccharide storage has been reported in tissues, as well as urinary excretion of glucose-containing oligosaccharides.[274–279]

Qualitative Studies (Biosynthesis, Processing, and Localization)

A series of experiments sought to address the issues of the relationship between residual enzyme activity and functional enzyme activity by examining the processing and localization of newly synthesized enzyme in patients with infantile-, juvenile-, and adult-onset disease.[51,156,160,161,250,254,255,257,265,272,273] A variety of abnormalities have been described, including diminished synthesis, abnormalities in exit from the ER and Golgi complex, targeting to lysosomes, and processing, as well as in catalytic activity and protein precipitable by antibody. The largest of these studies also included *in situ* localization.[265] One study demonstrated a difference in the posttranslational processing of acid α-glucosidase in cultured fibroblasts compared to muscle of the same patient.[272] Because many, if not most, of the patients are likely to be genetic compounds, the results could represent the combined effects of different abnormalities in the products of the two different mutant alleles. Similar analysis of activity and processing of individual recombinant mutant alleles could be additionally informative for attempts at correlation of genotype and biochemical and clinical phenotype. However, such studies have not explained the adult-onset phenotype of a patient (GM1935) who exhibits extremely low residual enzyme activity.[64,265,300,302,305] The presence of extensive genetic heterogeneity has also been inferred based on variation with respect to the presence or absence of inactive enzyme protein, as detected by reaction with antibodies. Most, but not all, infantile-onset patients studied from Europe, South Africa, and America have not had substantial amounts of enzyme protein that is catalytically inactive, indicating that the mutation(s) result in either unstable proteins, unstable mRNA, or absence of transcription or translation.[63,64,111,120–122,243,250,252,257,263,264,301] By contrast, normal amounts of enzyme protein that is catalytically inactive appear to be very common in China, where all seven infantile-onset patients studied exhibited protein precipitable by antibody.[273] In a study from Japan, it was convincingly demonstrated quantitatively that five of six patients, including two infantile-onset patients, had normal amounts of catalytically inactive enzyme protein.[262] These observations suggest that there may be only a few common mutations segregating in these populations. It is now known that 80 percent of mutant alleles carry the same mutation in China, and that this mutation may be responsible for the immunoreactive protein (see "Molecular Pathology" below). In adult-onset patients, enzyme protein detected by antibody has been found, but usually only in proportion to the residual enzyme activity.[63,250,255] Consistent with these findings, many adult patients have now been identified as heterozygous for the frequent IVS

1(−13T > G.) leaky splice-site mutation in combination with a nonfunctional null allele, resulting in a net reduction of synthesis of residual normal acid α-glucosidase (see "Molecular Pathology" below). It should be noted that in all such studies the different antibodies used, and the effect of different mutations on antigenic sites recognized by these antibodies, can affect the results obtained.

MOLECULAR BIOLOGY OF THE NORMAL AND THE MUTANT GENE FOR ACID α-GLUCOSIDASE (GAA)

Chromosomal Localization

The human gene for acid α-glucosidase was initially localized to the distal portion of the long arm of human chromosome 17 and designated GAA on the human gene map.[280–287] The gene is genetically linked to the locus for thymidine kinase (TK) in both humans and mice.[285–287] There has been some ambiguity in the precise regional localization, but the gene has been definitely mapped to the terminal portion of the long arm of human chromosome 17 (17q25.2–q25.3), distal to, but with the same localization as, Tk.[288] This localization has been confirmed by two other groups.

Structural Gene

The structural gene for acid α-glucosidase (containing the introns or intervening DNA as well as the exons) and the cDNA have been isolated and analyzed.[150–155] The analysis of the cDNA has provided insight into the biochemistry of acid α-glucosidase and has been discussed in the earlier section dealing with biochemistry of the normal enzyme. The isolation of both the cDNA and structural gene allows definition of the specific mutations in patients. Molecular definition of the genetic heterogeneity should provide insight into the basis for the clinical and biochemical heterogeneity of the disorder, and should facilitate diagnosis.

The structural gene is approximately 20 kb and contains 20 exons (see Fig. 135-4).[153–155] The first exon has only a 5′ untranslated sequence and is separated by an approximately 2.7-kb intron from the second exon that contains 33 nt of 5′ noncoding sequence, followed by the initiation ATG. A region in IVS 1 has been identified that markedly reduces the level of mRNA transcription.[321] The second and the last exons are quite large (578 and 607 bp). The remaining exons range from 85 to 187 bp. The large second exon codes for the signal peptide, the Pro-sequence of the acid α-glucosidase precursor, and the first 61 amino acids of the 76-kDa precursor. The evolutionarily conserved catalytic site domain is contained in exons 10 and 11. Except at the 5′ donor site in IVS 19, the splice-site junctions conform to the consensus splice-site sequences. Mutations at approximately half the splice sites would potentially result in disruption of the reading frame. The last exon contains 60 bp of coding sequence and the 3′ untranslated sequence.

The sequence preceding exon 1 has been determined, and the region required to promote transcription of the DNA into mRNA (promoter region) has been defined.[152–155] A 400-bp fragment upstream of the first (noncoding) exon is sufficient to promote expression. This region has characteristics of a housekeeping gene because it has a high content of guanines and cytosines (GC-rich; 80 percent), with at least four potential binding sites for the transcription factor Sp1, but no obvious CAAT or TATA boxes.

Normal Biochemical and Molecular Genetic Variation (Polymorphisms)

It is increasingly apparent from studies of many genetic disorders that normal genetic variation can play a significant role in determining the phenotype resulting from a single mutation. Prior to the isolation of the cDNA and structural gene for acid α-glucosidase, inherited normal biochemical variants (allozymes) of human acid α-glucosidase had been described.[175,289–294] There are three common allelic forms of human acid α-glucosidase (designated GAA1, GAA2, and GAA4) segregating in the general population. These reflect a normal biochemical genetic polymorphism. The alleles are codominantly expressed and their products can be differentiated by differences in isoelectric point and/or mobility in starch gel. Because of segregation of the three alleles, six common phenotypes are generated. The gene frequencies of the three alleles are 0.92, 0.03, and 0.06, respectively, for GAA1, GAA2, and GAA4, predicting that almost 20 percent of the population is heterozygous for these normal polymorphisms. Both of the rarer allozymes have a more basic pI with approximate pI (assuming a pI for GAA1 of 4.4) of GAA2 = 4.45 and GAA4 = 4.5. The rarest of the three allozymes (GAA2) was initially discovered because it exhibits lower affinity for the high-molecular-weight polysaccharide substrate starch, which is used as a support medium in electrophoresis, and thus it migrates more rapidly to the anode despite its pI, which would predict the reverse migration pattern. Although the GAA2 allozyme has a normal K_m for low-molecular-weight substrates, it has diminished affinity for the α-glucosidic linkages of starch (explaining the more rapid migration), as well as for the α-1,6 linkages in Sephadex.[175] The GAA2 allozyme also has a lower-than-normal affinity for high-molecular-weight glucose polymers, including glycogen (tenfold higher K_m).[290] Despite the markedly reduced affinity of the GAA2 allozyme for glycogen, homozygosity for the GAA2 allozyme was apparently without discernible deleterious effects in one individual, at least into early adolescence. Although a second homozygous adult was ascertained because of muscle weakness, a muscle biopsy was reportedly normal and the symptoms ascribed to coexisting chronic alcoholism.[291]

The molecular bases for the GAA2 allozyme and the GAA4 allozyme have been identified.[292,293] The GAA2 allozyme is due

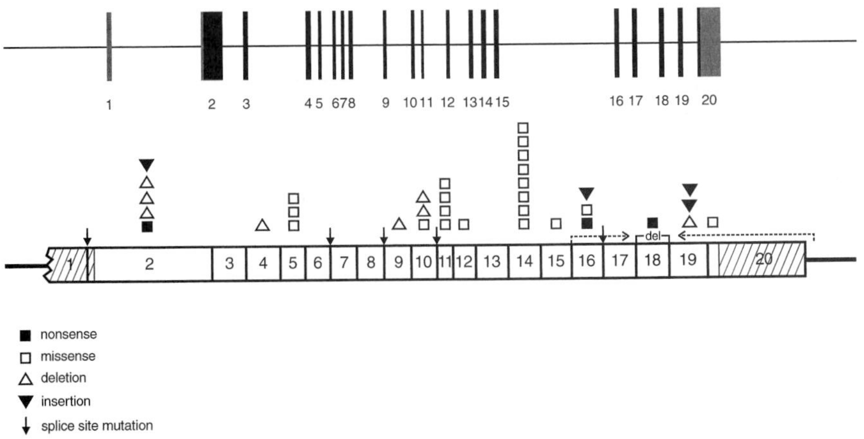

Fig. 135-4 *Top*: Genomic structure of human GAA. Bars represent exons and horizontal lines represent introns. Gray represents untranslated sequence and black represents coding sequence. *Bottom*: Distribution of different types of deleterious mutations found in patients with GSDII. (Only exons are indicated, with arrows representing mutations at splice sites.) (See Table 135-7.)

Table 135-5 Normal Genetic Variation: Single-Nucleotide Polymorphisms (SNPs) in the Coding Region and 3′UT

Nucleotide change	Amino acid change	Location (exon)	Predicted heterozygosity (approximate)	References (see footnotes)
271G/A*	Asp91Asn	2	0.08	292
324C/T	Cys108	2	0.39	152
596G/A	Arg199His	3	0.44	152
642C/T	Ser214	3	0.23	152
668 A/G	His223Arg	3	0.44	152
921 A/T¶	Ala307	5	¶	306, 330
1203 A/G	Gln401	8	0.45	152
1374 C/T	Tyr458	9	0.11	305, 306
1581 G/A	Arg527	11	0.40	152
1726G/A§	*Gly576Ser*	*12*	*? Pakistani*	325
*1917 G/A***	*Val639*	*14*	*? Turkish*	329
2065 G/A†	Glu689Lys	15	0.30	293, 310, 331
2133 A/G	Thr711	15	0.42	152
2154 T/C¶	Val718	15	?	330
2238G/C‡	*Trp746Cys*	*16*	?	310
2338 A/G	Ile780Val	17	0.42	152
2446 G/A¶	Val816Ile	17	0.15	305, 307
2553 A/G	Gly851	18	0.50	152
2780 C/T¶	Thr927Ile	19	0.13	305, 307
2808 C/T	*Asp936*	*20*	*?*	22
2862G/A	—	20 (UT)	0.18	305
ins2998G	—	20 (UT)		151
2951G/A	—	*20 (UT)*		*unpublished*

Italics with annotations or "?" either indicates changes that could be deleterious, changes that may be limited to the original ethnic group from which the patient derived (Pakistani for 1726G/A and Turkish for 1917G/A), or that have not been published in a full peer-reviewed manuscript.

*Type 2 biochemical polymorphism (GAA*2), alters K_m for glycogen; see text for additional references.

†Type 4 biochemical polymorphism (GAA*4), more common in Asians; see text for additional references.

‡Low activity (10–15% normal) only seen once on an allele downstream of a deletion and could in theory be deleterious by itself.

§Found downstream of a nonsense mutation in a Pakistani patient, not formally tested, and could be deleterious.

¶May have higher frequency in individuals of African descent, particularly for the 2154C/T, which has not been seen to date in Caucasians (RH).

**There is a typographical error in the published manuscript and the correct bp number is in this table and the Web site.

to an Asp91Asn substitution (see Table 135-5), consistent with the more basic pI of the GAA2 enzyme. The GAA4 allozyme is due to a Glu689Lys amino acid substitution. Despite the very nonconservative nature of the amino acid substitution, there is no effect upon enzyme activity for low-molecular-weight substrates and migration in starch gels is indistinguishable from the common allozyme, suggesting normal affinity for high-molecular-weight substrates. This allele has a high frequency in Chinese populations.[331] A fourth allozyme, GAA3, migrates slightly faster in starch gel than the common GAA1 allozyme, and therefore could have an altered K_m for high-molecular-weight substrates. This allozyme has been reported from Malaysia, predominantly in individuals of Indian descent, and could have been missed in population surveys for the other allozymes. The molecular basis for this allozyme is unknown.

With the isolation of the cDNA and structural gene, additional genetic variation has been uncovered. Over 20 reported single nucleotide polymorphisms (SNPs or alternate base pairs at a single site) have been reported in the 2659 bp of the coding region of normals, a frequency grossly similar to that reported at other different loci. Almost half of the alternative bases in the acid α-glucosidase cDNA result in amino acid substitutions, while the remainder are silent (Table 135-5). These normal variants could potentially interact with mutations to modulate the resulting phenotype. Two of these amino acid substitutions (Asp91Asn and Glu689Lys), as discussed in more detail above, correspond to previously described biochemical polymorphisms, for which allele frequencies have been determined by biochemical methods and agree with the allele frequencies determined by DNA-based methods.[175,289,292,293] The Glu689Lys or GAA4 polymorphism is linked to the common infantile-onset mutation in Taiwan.[331] Both the Val816Ile and Thre927Ile substitutions reportedly are not deleterious because they are common normal variants.[305,307] In contrast, the Trp746Cys substitution could be a deleterious mutation because it diminishes activity to 10 percent of normal for low-molecular-weight substrates, although activity for glycogen has not been evaluated.[310] Similarly, the Gly576Ser substitution, reported in only one individual downstream of a deleterious mutation, has not been tested for effect on activity.[325] This substitution could be a normal variant found only in specific ethnic groups, but the substitution occurs at a highly conserved amino acid and requires further clarification before being considered a normal variant. Several of these amino acid substitutions are in linkage disequilibrium. Thus Ile816 and Ile927 are commonly linked in African-American individuals.[307] Our unpublished data indicates that Arg199 is in disequilibrium with His223 and His199 with Arg223.

There is additional normal variation in introns, some of which has been detected as restriction fragment length polymorphisms (RFLPs), all resulting from the presence in normal individuals of alternative base pairs within introns that alter sites for restriction enzymes.[287,295–299] Nine of the more fully characterized RFLPs

Table 135-6 Restriction Fragment Length Polymorphisms at the Acid α-Glucosidase Locus (GAA)*

Enzyme	Location/Probe	Sizes	Gene Frequency	Het†
*Xba*I‡	IVS 2	2.0	0.72	0.40
		1.5	0.28	
*Pst*I C‡	1506–1857	1.55	0.74	0.38
		1.35	0.26	
*Sac*I B	1857–2520	3.8	0.05	0.08
		3.4	0.95	
*Pst*I A	1857–2520	4.9	0.07	0.13
		4.4	0.93	
*Pst*I B	2520–3236	3.8	0.26	0.38
		3.6	0.73	
*Rsa*I	2520–3236	3.9	0.21	0.38
		3.7	0.79	
*Sac*I A	3236–3406	5.5	0.12	0.23
		5.3	0.88	
		3.3	0.01	
*Hind*III	1506–end	5.6	0.05	0.09
		5.3	0.95	
*Taq*I	1506–end	10.0	0.94	0.12
		9.0	0.06	

*See text for two additional RFLPs
†Frequency of heterozygotes in the population
‡Detectable by PCR and enzyme digestion
2520–3236 = cDNA probe detecting exons 18–20
1857–2520 = cDNA probe detecting exons 13–17
1506–1857 = cDNA probe detecting exons 10–13

are listed in Table 135-6.[154,295–299] Additional RFLPs detected by *Stu*I89 and *Eco*RI88 have also been reported. Furthermore, direct sequence analysis of PCR-amplified DNA revealed additional intronic single-nucleotide changes and insertions. We have observed more than 10 polymorphisms in more than one individual that are in the intronic areas close to exons, although the number of individuals examined for most is small. These include IVS 2 − 67G/C; IVS 2 − 39G/T; IVS 2 − 4G/C (the basis for the reported *Xba*I RFLP[299]); IVS 4 − 48C/T; IVS 4 + 7 ins 7 bp[322]; IVS 9 − 19C/G;[313] IVS 10 − 52A/C; IVS 13 + 21 G/A; IVS 14 + 20 A/G;[328] IVS 16 + 20 A/G; IVS 16 + 24 T/C. Several of the polymorphisms are at sites that suggest a possible effect on splicing efficiency. Additional alterations have been seen in single individuals. Although allele frequencies have been determined for the RFLPs, the molecular basis is unknown for most. Conversely, allele frequencies in a diverse and/or a defined population have not been published for most of the non-RFLP single-nucleotide changes.

Molecular Pathology (Mutations)

Significant advances have been made during the past several years in different areas related to the molecular pathology of acid α-glucosidase deficiency. The number of mutations identified is increasing rapidly and has already quadrupled since the seventh edition of this book, with over 40 mutations identified and published to date (Table 135-7). These are catalogued and regularly updated at several sites on the Internet including www.eur.nl/fgg/ch1/pompe/mutation.htm (curated by the authors of this chapter).

Initial Southern and northern analyses detected multiple different abnormalities in size and amount of mRNA and in DNA restriction fragments,[300] consistent with a high frequency of nonmissense mutations. However, approximately half of mutations now reported are missense mutations, with the remainder consisting of nonsense, splice site, small deletions and insertions, and large deletions. The apparent preponderance of missense mutations may reflect emphasis in initial studies on analysis of cDNA. With the increasing use of mutation detection based on PCR amplification of genomic DNA, the spectrum of mutations has shifted to mutations that affect mRNA stability, such as nonsense, splice site, and small frameshifting insertions and/or deletions that result in premature termination, consistent with the earlier results of northern and Southern blotting. Frequent occurrence of these types of mutation is not surprising because casual perusal of the coding sequence reveals multiple regions for polymerase transcription errors as well as areas with repeats that typically surround small deletions/insertions. Most of the deletions are small, but a very large, approximately 9-kb, deletion extending past the 3′ end of the gene and mediated by recombination involving the frequent repetitive Alu sequence has been identified. The next largest deletion of approximately 0.5 kb (extending from IVS 17 to IVS 18) apparently reflects recombination at direct repeats. Additional deletions may be found because the second mutation in a number of patients has defied detection by PCR-based techniques.[327,333]

The mutations are spread throughout the gene although there appears to be a higher concentration of missense mutations in exon 11 (containing the catalytic site), exon 14, a second area of evolutionary conservation, and in exon 5. The concentration of missense mutations in exon 14 suggests a functional significance for this region that contains a "signature sequence" for acid α-glucosidase and related enzymes.[226,328] Nonetheless, the concentration may be spurious because specific screening for this exon in a large number of patients identified four of these mutations. The screening was done because of the high degree of homology with related enzymes. Similarly, the area of the catalytic site was an initial site of concentrated screening. Surprisingly, mutations in exons 18 to 20 appear important, despite this area being lost during the processing to mature enzyme (see Fig. 135-3). Perhaps these mutations interfere with processing necessary for acquisition of full activity for the natural substrate or result in misfolding in the ER with an unstable protein that is degraded.

Most mutations to date have been described in one or two patients. However, several mutations are very frequent, either in the general population or in specific ethnic groups (Table 135-8). The most common mutation with the widest distribution appears to be a leaky splice-site mutation found in over half of adult-onset Caucasian patients (allele frequency of 0.67 to 0.46).[311,313,317] In two specific ethnic groups, a single mutation accounts for the majority of infantile-onset disease. In Chinese patients from Taiwan, the Asp645Glu mutation has an allele frequency of 0.8,[331] while among Africans and African-Americans the Arg854X nonsense mutation has an allele frequency of 0.5.[330] Based on identical haplotypes for the several single nucleotide polymorphic changes in the cDNA, both the Asp645Glu and Arg854X mutations in these populations appear to have derived from a common founder. The origin of the Arg854X mutations was traced back as most likely arising in the north-central part of Africa. A del525T and delexon18 are very common in the Dutch population and not considerably less frequent in a random Caucasian population (allele frequencies of 0.34 vs. 0.04 to 0.09 for del525T and 0.23 vs. 0.01 to 0.06 for delex18).[316,332] It would seem likely that these two mutations also arose by founder effect in Dutch individuals, although both mutations occur within sequence contexts that would suggest that they could also recur independent of a common founder. Several mutations have been reported in three or more patients including Gly309Arg (quite common in Dutch and surrounding populations), Cys647W (in French Canadians and Portuguese), and del482/483 CC (in French). A group of Turkish patients had only a limited number of mutations, with the double insertion in exon 19 mutation (2741AG > CAGG) found in more than one patient (see Table 135-7 for references). While the prevalence of these mutations in specific populations presumably results from a founder effect, it should be noted that several of the missense and nonsense mutation are C > T or G > A substitutions at CpG dinucleotides, a hotspot for mutation. These mutations can, therefore, be expected to also be independently recurrent. Thus, the Asp645Glu mutation

Table 135-7 Mutations in Patients with GSDII*

NT Change		Exon	Amino Acid	Reference
Missense Mutations				
896	T→G	5	Leu299Arg	313
925	G→A	5+	Gly309Arg	327
953	T→C	5	Met318Thr	304
1441	T→C	10	Trp481Arg	333
1555	A→G	11	Met519Val	312
1561	G→A	11+	Glu521Lys	303
1585/6	TC→GT	11	Ser529Val	319
1634	C→T	11	Pro545Leu	309, 329a
1696	T→C	12	Ser566Pro	329
1927	G→A	14+	Gly643Arg	306, 329
1933	G→C	14	Asp645His	314
1933	G→A	14+	Asp645Asn	328
1935	C→A	14	Asp645Glu	302, 305, 307, 308, 331
1941	C→G	14	Cys647Trp	310, 328
1942	G→A	14+	Glu648Ser	328
2014	C→T	14+	Arg672Trp	328
2015	G→A	14+	Arg672Gln	328
2173	C→T	15+	Arg725Trp	306
2303	C→G	16	Pro768Arg	329
2846	T→A	20	Val949Asp	330
Nonsense Mutations				
118	C→T	2+	Arg 40X	325
172	C→T	2	Gln 58X	335
2237	G→A	16+	Trp746X	323
2560	C→T	18+	Arg854X	305, 322
Splice Site Mutations				
−13	t→g	IVS 1	Δ exon 2	311, 313, 315, 317, 321
−22	t→g	IVS 6	Δ exon 6	322, 329a
+1	g→a	IVS 8		333
+1	g→c	IVS10	Δ exon 0	311
+2	t→c	IVS16	Δ 16bp exon 16	324
Insertions/Deletions				
+258 C		2	Pro86→SHIFT	323
Δ271 G		2	Phe90→SHIFT	329a
Δ379/380TG		2	Trp126→SHIFT	327
Δ482/483 CC		2	Phe160→SHIFT	326
Δ525 T		2	Thr175→SHIFT	309, 315–317, 321
Δ766–785		4	Gln255→SHIFT	323, 328
Δ1411–1414 GAGA		9	Asn470→SHIFT	320
Δ1441T		10	Val480→SHIFT	333
Δ13nt 1456–1468		10	Thr485→SHIFT	310
Ins 2242 G		16	Gly747→SHIFT	323, 328
Ins 2432 C		17	Leu811→SHIFT	329a
ΔIVS17-IVS18		18	Δ exon 18	310, 315, 316, 317, 318, 332
Δ2707–2709		19	ΔLys903	313
InsC2741/InsG2743		19	Pro913→SHIFT	329
ins 18nt2775		19	ins/dup 6 aa	323
ΔIVS15→ex20		16–20	Δex16→ 20Alu/Alu	334

**Mutations and references are only to mutations found in patients, shown to be deleterious, and in full manuscripts. This table therefore does not include:*
(1) 1204 T→ C;TRP402ARG in exon 8 reported in cloning as a deleterious mutation but not reported in any patient[157]
(2) 1432 G→ A;Gly478Arg in exon 9 (reported in a review only[22])
(3) 1556 T→ C;Met519Thr in exon 11 (reported in a review only[22])
+ = C→T or G→A mutation at CpG "hot spot" for mutations
A mutation database can be found at www.eur.nl/fgg/ch1/pompe/mutation.htm (curated by the authors of this chapter). *This database currently includes mutations that are only listed in the footnote to this table.*

has recurred independently on different chromosomal backgrounds in Chinese and in an African-American.

In general, the nature and properties of the mutations correlate with the clinical and biochemical phenotype. Several mutations can be considered to be mutations conditional for late-onset disease, based on presence of the mutation in adult- or juvenile-onset patients either in homozygosity or heteroallelic with a null mutation present in infantile-onset patients. These adult-onset mutations include the leaky IVS 1 splice-site mutation (only found in late-onset patients heteroallelic with a null mutation),

Table 135-8 Frequent Mutations in GSDII Patients

Mutation*	Ethnic Group	Allele Frequency	Phenotype†
IVS 1–13 t > g (splice)	Caucasian	0.4–0.6	Juvenile/Adult
Asp645Glu	Taiwanese	0.8	Infantile
Arg854X	Afro American	0.5	Infantile
del525T	Dutch	0.34‡	Infantile
"del exon 18"	Dutch	0.23‡	Infantile

*Several additional mutations appear to be common in specific populations, although allele frequencies have not been as extensively defined. These are Gly309Arg (quite common in Dutch and surrounding populations), Cys647W (in French Canadians), the S566P mutation and the double insertion insC2741/insG2743 (in Turkish patients).

†If the mutation in homozygosity results in infantile-onset disease, the phenotype has been classified as an infantile onset. Such mutations are also present in adult- and juvenile-onset patients but heteroallelic with the "leaky" IVS 1 mutation that confers the late-onset phenotype.

‡These two mutations are not uncommon in random U.S. Caucasian GSDII patients, but with considerably lower frequency (0.04–0.09 for del 525T and 0.01–0.06 for del ex 18).[316,317,332]

Pro545Leu (homozygous in an adult-onset), Arg672Trp, Arg672Gln, Arg725Trp, IVS 6 − 22t > g and possibly Ser529Val (where the second mutation is as yet undefined), and an IVS 10 splice-site mutation (only found in an adult-onset heterozygous with the IVS 1 mutation). The remainder of mutations can be classified as infantile-onset, null mutations because they have been found in infantile-onset patients. For many of these infantile mutations, determination of residual activity or residual protein delivered to lysosomes following transient expression has been consistent with the presumed severely deleterious nature of mutations classified as infantile. This definition of mutation type, depending primarily on the clinical phenotype of patients in whom the mutations have been found, may in the future be found to be incomplete, as illustrated by the Asp645Glu mutation discussed below. However, classification of mutations as adult, based on in vitro experiments such as measurement of residual normal transcripts for splice-site mutations and determination of enzyme activity following transient expression of mutant cDNAs, has given ambiguous results for some mutations.

Although genotypes correlate with biochemical phenotypes, and gross clinical phenotype-genotype correlations can be made, it is clear that there are unanswered questions. Patients have been described in whom there is apparent divergence between genotype and either clinical or experimental biochemical phenotype. With increasing frequency, the IVS 1(−13T > G) mutation is found in patients ranging from childhood/juvenile-onset to onset after the fifth decade of life. The mutation present on the second allele does not appear to explain this wide variation in phenotype and there may be modifying genes. Two missense mutations, Asp645Glu and Gly643Arg, as discussed below, are not easily classified and appear to represent divergence of phenotype and genotype. For many of the multiple different mutations, too few patients have been identified as carrying them to attempt to correlate clinical and molecular findings.

Genetic mechanisms that can result in divergence of genotype and phenotype include somatic mosaicism, presence of second interacting intragenic mutations, differences in intragenic background (normal polymorphisms), differential leakiness of the common splice-site mutation, and linked or unlinked modifying genes. The most dramatic example of divergence is provided by the phenotypic differences between individuals bearing the conservative Asp645Glu missense mutation. This mutation in homozygosity is the commonest cause of infantile-onset disease in China. However, the same mutation is found in an adult-onset African-American patient, heterozygous with the R854X nonsense mutation that in homozygosity is the most frequent cause of infantile-onset disease in African-Americans. These two patients differ in genetic background as to normal polymorphisms that cause amino acid substitutions, which may explain the differences in phenotype. Alternatively, somatic mosaicism in the adult-onset patient has to be considered as the basis for the milder-than-expected phenotype. While *de novo* mutations, either in parental germ cells or during embryogenesis and thereby resulting in mosaicism, are rare in autosomal recessive disorders, such events have been reported, particularly in disorders with a high carrier frequency.[310] Moreover, a *de novo* mutation, probably arising in a parental germ cell, has been reported in GSDII.[310] If the *de novo* mutation arises during embryogenesis it could result in somatic mosaicism and adult-onset rather than infantile-onset disease. Unfortunately, parents of patients with late-onset disease are often not available for studies that would reveal such mosaicism. A possible second similar example of apparent divergence of phenotype and genotype is the Gly643Arg mutation, originally reported in an adult-onset patient heterozygous with Arg725Trp and now found in heterozygosity in an infantile-onset patient. Transient expression of the two mutations (Gly643Arg and Arg725Trp) gave essentially identical results of low, barely detectable amounts of residual enzyme expression and therefore would not have predicted that the Gly643Arg mutation would be found in infantile-onset patients.[306,329] Similarly, inability to detect activity by transient transfection has been reported for Arg672Trp and Arg672Gln, classified by the clinical definition used above as mutations specific for adult- or juvenile-onset disease.[328] These observations suggest that either differences in genetic background or other undetected mutations play a role for these mutations or that the currently used methods for measuring residual enzyme activity by overexpression following transient transfection and using substrates other than the natural substrate glycogen do not correlate with in vivo residual enzyme activity.

Possible nongenetic reasons for the divergence seen in some patients between clinical phenotype and genotype include trivial factors such as misclassification because of incomplete definition of age at onset or inability of current methods to experimentally measure residual activity of mutations that reflects in vivo residual activity. Environmental factors such as diet and exercise could also play a role.

PRENATAL DIAGNOSIS

Pompe disease was one of the first disorders for which prenatal diagnosis was attempted.[99,325,336–351] Initially diagnosis was attempted by enzyme analysis of amniotic fluid or microscopy of amniotic cells, neither of which is now widely used.[336–341] Subsequently, enzyme analysis of amniotic cells, and additionally (for the past 15 years), direct enzyme analysis of uncultured chorionic villi, primarily using 4MUG as substrate, have been the methods of choice. Some investigators also assay cultured chorionic villus cells, particularly when only small amounts of tissue are available. Worldwide several hundred prenatal diagnoses have been made successfully. Special measures were recommended by some investigators to eliminate the possible interference of neutral α-glucosidase activity, for example by using antibodies[345,348] or maltose as substrate[349] instead of 4MUG. However, when using 4MUG at pH 4.0, complete deficiency of α-glucosidase activity (< 2 percent of normal) was found in all recently reported affected pregnancies, either using chorionic villi or amniocytes,[351] indicating the reliability of the simple and rapid 4MUG assay. The use of uncultured chorionic villi has major advantages because of the early stage of sampling (12th week of pregnancy) and the rapid diagnosis (within 1 day). Additionally, the much higher α-glucosidase activity in villi compared to amniocytes facilitates the interpretation in cases of heterozygosity and low activity. Contamination of chorionic villus samples with maternal tissue has been a matter of concern. Therefore, it is important that villi are selected and prepared for direct enzyme assay by experienced hands, making the risk seem very small.

With increasing knowledge about mutations at the GAA locus and advancing expertise with mutation detection, a prenatal enzyme diagnosis may be confirmed by DNA analysis.[325,351] DNA-based diagnosis without knowledge of the specific mutation(s) may also be feasible by linkage analysis of RFLPs. Mutation analysis may be particularly useful in the diagnosis of rare cases with ambiguous results of enzyme assay. Such a situation may be anticipated when the fetus is at risk for juvenile- or adult-onset disease with residual α-glucosidase activity or when one of the parents has very low enzyme activity (e.g., 10 percent of normal) and possibly late-onset disease. In principle, mutation analysis also allows for the detection of carriers in affected families and the screening for some of the more frequent mutations in their partners. In populations with a tradition of consanguineous marriage, this could effectively lead to finding couples at risk before a first affected child is born (see "Heterozygote Detection" above).

THERAPY

Effective therapy is currently not available, although supportive therapy can have a major impact in the childhood-, juvenile- and adult-onset disease. A controlled feeding regimen or diet may help to prevent a decline in the net protein balance and counteract the observed increased muscle protein breakdown.[352] High-protein diets have been reported to have a positive effect, as have diets rich in branched chain amino acids.[352–360] However, only 25 percent of the patients reported to have followed a high-protein diet showed either improvement of respiratory or skeletal muscle function. An objective evaluation of the effects remains difficult.[352] The high-protein diet is often combined with prescription of ephedrine (HPET). Ventilatory support, which provides ameliorative therapy, has also been utilized, particularly in late onset patients. Respiratory support of late-onset patients during the night with an oscillating bed, cuirass respirator, or mouth cap may improve the quality of life. It can have dramatic effects during a period of respiratory decompensation due to a complicating infectious process, with a return to the prior clinical status after appropriate therapy. Inspiratory muscle training has also been attempted. Ventilatory support in the most severe conditions requires respirator support via tracheostomy. However, this carries the risk of the patient becoming respirator dependent.

Enzyme replacement therapy (ERT) aims at correcting the metabolic basis of GSDII directly; in principle, it should be feasible for all clinical subtypes. However, because there is accumulation of glycogen in nervous tissue in the infantile-onset disease, it is possible that administration of enzyme would ameliorate the major manifestations of disease but, because of its inability to cross the blood-brain barrier, would over time unmask progressive neurologic impairment. The natural course of the disease indicates a minimal risk for this to occur in juvenile- and adult-onset disease. The major requirements for ERT include availability of sufficient quantities of nonimmunogenic and stable enzyme that will be taken up by the major organs affected by the glycogen storage (i.e., heart, muscle, and liver). Enzyme replacement therapy for GSDII was attempted very soon after the discovery of the enzymatic defect, but these trials were limited in duration and amount of enzyme administered, and also used either highly immunogenic foreign proteins or "low-uptake" forms of the acid α-glucosidase.[361–363] Acid α-glucosidase from the fungus *Aspergillus niger* was administered in short trials to at least three children with infantile-onset disease, with evidence for uptake into liver with diminution of glycogen in the two cases treated with the largest amount of enzyme. However, the glycogen storage in skeletal muscle was not corrected and the terminally ill patients developed an immunologic response to the foreign protein. A limited trial with purified "low-uptake" human enzyme from placentas was undertaken with similarly negative results.[363]

The elucidation of the significance of mannose-6-phosphate receptor-mediated endocytosis and the basis for "high-uptake" enzyme required for efficient uptake of enzyme into lysosomes has given new impetus to investigations of enzyme replacement therapy for lysosomal storage disorders such as GSDII. Several studies have documented uptake of enzyme and/or reduction of glycogen content of cultured fibroblasts and muscle cells on incubation with acid α-glucosidase.[268,270,364–369] Perfusion of rat heart with "high-uptake" enzyme (containing the mannose-6-phosphate recognition marker) but not with unphosphorylated enzyme resulted in significant uptake of enzyme.[370] Moreover, in vivo administration of phosphorylated acid α-glucosidase to mice apparently led to uptake of enzyme in heart and skeletal muscle while the uptake of unphosphorylated enzyme was less efficient.[371] In addition, lysosomal enzymes appeared to be able to cross the transendothelial barrier.[372]

With the cloning of the acid α-glucosidase cDNA and gene, it has become feasible to produce human recombinant acid α-glucosidase on a large scale in genetically engineered CHO cells, in the milk of transgenic animals, in bacteria, and in insect cells.[133–139] Enzyme from CHO cells and in milk undergoes the proper posttranslational modification to be potentially useful for ERT. Overexpression and secretion by CHO cells was obtained by placing the acid α-glucosidase cDNA under transcriptional control of the human polypeptide chain elongation factor 1α gene promoter, or by cloning it in tandem with the dihydrofolate reductase gene allowing for methotrexate-induced amplification.[133,136] The enzyme harvested from the cell culture media is the 110-kDa precursor (see "Posttranslational Processing" above) and bears mannose-6-phosphate residues facilitating uptake by cultured fibroblast and muscle cells from humans and quails with GSDII. The enzyme is transported to lysosomes and diminishes the lysosomal glycogen storage.[133,136,369] When administered intravenously to guinea pig, it leads to increase of acid α-glucosidase activity in liver, heart, and possibly skeletal muscle.[133] Most promising, this human recombinant enzyme, when given intravenously to 4-week-old acid α-glucosidase-deficient quails (every 2 to 3 days for 18 days) resulted in an increase of acid α-glucosidase activity in most tissues and in a decrease to normal of glycogen content in heart and liver.[374] Similar short-term treatment of GSDII knockout mice with this recombinant enzyme resulted in significant correction of the enzyme deficiency in most organs, but not in brain.[138,373]

The production of recombinant human acid α-glucosidase in the mammary gland of mice was accomplished by placing either the acid α-glucosidase cDNA or gene under the control of a mammary gland-specific bovine α_{S1}-casein gene promoter.[137,138] The genomic construct worked far better than the cDNA and can result in production of more than 1 mg/ml human acid α-glucosidase. The milk enzyme resembles the natural acid α-glucosidases from human urine and the human recombinant precursor produced in CHO cells in physical and biochemical parameters.[137,138] The enzyme is taken up in a mannose-6-phosphate-dependent manner by cultured fibroblasts, and depletes the lysosomal glycogen deposit in cells of patients. When injected intravenously, the recombinant enzyme corrects the acid α-glucosidase deficiency in heart and skeletal muscle of knockout mice. The combination of the bovine α_{S1}-casein gene promoter and the human acid α-glucosidase gene is universally functional and is being utilized for industrial production of human recombinant acid α-glucosidase in rabbit milk. Additionally, this latter enzyme has proved its therapeutic potential by correcting the enzyme deficiency in virtually all tissues of GSDII knockout mice (except brain) and by reducing the lysosomal glycogen storage.[373] Clinical trials in humans have begun for enzyme derived from rabbit milk and from CHO cells. The first report of the trial with the transgenic enzyme has just been published and covers a period of 36 weeks in which four patients with classical early-onset GSDII were treated with weekly doses of initially 15–20 and later 40 mg recombinant enzyme per kg body weight.[425] The therapeutic effects obtained include increase of α-glucosidase activity in skeletal muscle and improvement of muscle morphology and function. The cardiac size decreased significantly and the cardiac function improved. Respiratory insufficiency may be prevented when treatment is started early. Survival appears to be prolonged since the patients are at the writing of this review 1.5–2 years old, which is beyond the mean age of survival of patients with classical infantile-onset GSDII.

In contrast to ERT, which has to be administered repeatedly, gene therapy eventually aims at providing a permanent endogenous source of enzyme for the affected tissues. However, all of the problems present for gene therapy with the currently available vectors and methods of administration apply equally to GSDII as for other autosomal recessive disorders. Nonetheless, initial studies demonstrating that this approach could be applicable to GSDII have been reported. The human acid α-glucosidase cDNA was transferred with a retroviral vector to enzyme-deficient myoblasts in culture and intracellular targeting of enzyme to lysosomes was obtained with an increase of activity to thirtyfold the normal level followed by digestion of glycogen. Moreover, the enzyme was secreted and able to correct distant untransfected cells via mannose-6-phosphate receptor-mediated endocytosis. Additionally, correction was obtained by fusion of transduced myoblasts with neighboring untransduced myotubes.[375] Similar results were reported with adenovirus vector transduced fibroblasts and muscle cells.[376,377] The feasibility of adenoviral vector mediated gene transfer was further tested *in vivo* by intracardiac and intramuscular injections in newborn rats. Expression of recombinant human acid α-glucosidase was obtained in both organs at levels of 1 mg/mg tissue and correct lysosomal localization was suggested by the presence of mature 76-kDa enzyme.[376] Local correction of enzyme deficiency and reduction of glycogen storage was reported in muscle of Japanese quail with GSDII following intramuscular injection of an adenovirus vector containing human acid α-glucosidase cDNA.[378]

These preliminary studies illustrate the use of *ex vivo* and *in vivo* approaches to gene therapy directed at muscle cells. Two different scenarios that can be considered for application of gene therapy in GSDII include the direct approach, whereby the gene is delivered *in vivo* to the target tissues, and the indirect approach, in which myoblasts (or other cells to provide *in vivo* enzyme) are first treated *ex vivo* and than reimplanted to obtain a lasting effect, with spreading of enzyme from the site of transplant to more distant parts of the body. Other methods of gene delivery continue to be investigated.[379,380] More recent results report the use of a modified adenoviral vector encoding human acid α-glucosidase that has been targeted to the liver.[378a] A single intravenous dose applied to mice resulted in high-level expression in the liver from which organ precursor α-glucosidase was secreted and distributed via the circulation to heart and skeletal muscle where it reduced the lysosomal glycogen content. Clinical application in patients with GSDII is not possible with the currently available adenoviral vectors because of potentially lethal toxicity, even with a single injection. Additionally, repeated doses are required to sustain the correction of the lysosomal glycogen storage and these are currently precluded by the occurrence of immune responses.

Bone marrow transplantation, presumably to provide enzyme secreted by the normal cells continuously, has been attempted in humans and cattle with acid α-glucosidase deficiency. However, the results do not appear promising. In a human trial, engraftment of the haploidentical transplant was apparently transitory, no enzyme could be detected in muscle cells, and the patient died of complications of the transplant.[381] This result was noted not to be surprising, given the biology of acid α-glucosidase deficiency.[382] In cattle, natural hematopoietic chimeras were created, but there was no apparent effect on the course of the disease.[383]

ANIMAL MODELS

There are several naturally occurring animal models of GSDII, including Brahman and Shorthorn cattle, Lapland dog, Japanese quail, cats, and sheep.[384–400] Several different mouse models were recently made by targeted disruption of the acid α-glucosidase gene in mouse embryonic stem cells,[138,401,402] and currently provide the most widely available and useful animal models. Comparisons between the animal models and the human disease phenotypes are hampered by the very different physiology of the species and by the concomitant differences in lengths of gestation period, time to maturity, and average normal life span.[401] When cardiac involvement is taken as a measure, the Lapland dog,[385,386] the sheep model,[399] a subpopulation of affected Shorthorn cattle,[396,398] and the knockout mouse[401,402,402] appear to be most analogous to the human infantile-onset disorder. In Brahman cattle,[394] in the majority of Shorthorn breed,[396,398] and in the Japanese quail model,[387,388,391] there is no obvious cardiac involvement, although PAS-positive vacuoles are present in cardiomyocytes. Combined with survival to young adulthood, these latter models are clinically most similar to the human juvenile- or adult-onset disease. However, when the relative life span of the species is taken as a measure, age of onset and death occurs in all animal models later than in the human infantile disease.

Other than by clinicopathologic criteria, the various naturally occurring models can be compared by biochemical-genetic criteria. Affected Lapland dogs produce a near normal quantity of acid α-glucosidase but without enzymatic activity.[131] Information on the acid α-glucosidase synthesis in Shorthorn cattle is inconclusive because enzyme activity in mononuclear blood cells is less than 5 percent of normal while the mRNA content is normal, consistent with a missense mutation that could either be completely null or retain some residual activity. By contrast, acid α-glucosidase mRNA and protein are undetectable in Brahman cattle,[398] and the enzyme activity is less than 1 percent of normal, similar to that found in a subset of humans with infantile-onset disease. Similar presence or absence of enzymatic protein but absence of enzyme activity is also seen in the human infantile-onset disorder. However, it is now clear that the presence or absence of enzyme protein is a function of the specific mutation in humans and presumably in the naturally occurring models. The presence or absence of enzyme activity would be expected to be a more significant measure of comparison with the human. The Japanese quail model is complicated by the existence in this species of two acidic α-glucosidases (termed by the authors as GAAI and GAAII) as well as two neutral α-glucosidases. The two acidic and the neutral "embryonic" isozymes hydrolyze 4MUG as well as the natural substrates maltose and glycogen. The "adult" neutral isozyme only displays activity towards the artificial 4MUG substrate.[378,403,404] This adult neutral isozyme is probably the quail equivalent of glucosidase II, the ER enzyme responsible for trimming of glucose from asparagine-linked carbohydrates, while it can be speculated that the embryonic neutral α-glucosidase could be an ortholog of the mammalian neutral α-glucosidase C. A characteristic feature of the embryonic α-glucosidase is down-regulation from day 3 before hatching (when this isozyme accounts for about 80 percent of the total neutral activity) to day 21 after hatching (when the relative activity is less than 5 percent).[389,403,404] Affected quail have virtually undetectable mRNA levels for the so-called GAAI isozyme which is considered to be the "authentic" homologue of human acid α-glucosidase. This gene was cloned by screening a quail liver cDNA library with degenerate primers to two conserved regions of the human and mouse GAA gene and the α-glucosidase gene from tetrahymena. However, a second acid α-glucosidase cDNA (GAAII) was cloned by screening a quail cDNA library from ovarian large follicles with an RT-PCR product from cultured skin fibroblast mRNA and found to be overexpressed in affected animals. Because both gene products have activity for 4MUG, maltose, and glycogen it was speculated that the GAAII gene product accounts for the 13 to 16 percent residual acid α-glucosidase activity of affected animals and explains the delay of clinical manifestations.[227] Interestingly, however, the same speculation was made concerning the contribution of the "embryonic" isozyme to the clinical course.

Combining all information presently available on the GAAII gene product and the "embryonic" isozyme initially would suggest that the two isozymes (embryonic neutral and GAAII) are in fact the same. However, comparison of predicted protein sequence of the two quail cloned acid α-glucosidases reveals that both have highest homology to the human lysosomal acid α-glucosidase and not to either the human neutral α-glucosidase C[210] or glucosidase II, suggesting that there are four different gene products in the quail. Surprisingly, the quail acid α-glucosidase I, deficiency of which is presumed to be responsible for the glycogen storage disease, has lesser overall homology to human acid α-glucosidase as compared to the quail acid α-glucosidase II still present in diseased animals (31/46 vs. 52/68 percent identity/similarity). At present it is uncertain whether the residual α-glucosidase activity by itself can be taken as a comparative measure to classify the Japanese quail as a model for adult-onset GSDII. Additional experiments would be needed to resolve these questions.

The three mouse models that were recently described differ in the way the GAA gene was disrupted, that is, by insertion of a neogene cassette in either exon 13 or exon 6, and by removal of exon 6 via Cre/lox-mediated recombination.[401,402] However, they are biochemically identical, as demonstrated by a total lack of acid α-glucosidase mRNA, protein, and activity in all organs tested, and progressive lysosomal glycogen accumulation in heart, skeletal muscle, and other tissues detectable from the first weeks after birth. They reach adulthood and produce litters. Nevertheless, the exon 6-inserted and exon 6-deleted mice develop differently. The former have markedly reduced locomotor activity by 3.5 weeks of age, whereas the latter don't show these abnormalities up to 6.5 months of age.[402] The exon 13-inserted mice were not subjected to locomotor testing. Therefore, it is unclear to which exon 6 model they compare. The majority of exon 13-inserted mice survive beyond 1 year, but have then developed muscle weakness, affecting the hind limbs in particular, and cardiomegaly.[402a] Clinical heterogeneity is observed among littermates in all of the three mouse models. Intra- and interlinear variability of phenotype may relate to differences in genetic background. Pure strains have not yet been obtained. The knockout mouse model mimics infantile-onset GSDII by genetic, biochemical, and pathologic criteria, but adult-onset disease by clinical course, age of onset, and age of death. As for the naturally occurring animal models, the question remains whether to consider the relative age of the species, or the absolute length of the pathogenic process for clinical subtyping. Overall, the observations in knockout mice suggest the presence of modifying genes.[402b]

As noted in the description of clinical manifestations, the animal models have given valuable clues to the pathologic process. Vomiting due to accumulation of glycogen in the esophageal musculature and dilatation of the lower esophagus is the major clinical symptom in the Lapland dog and may parallel the frequent feeding difficulties reported in the human disorder.[385,386,405,406] Furthermore, the observed involvement of vascular smooth muscle cells in Lapland dog, quail, cattle, and knockout mice[402a] may translate into the occurrence of aneurysms of the basal artery in human adult disease. Storage in smooth muscle cells could also explain deficient bladder functions in late-onset GSDII. By contrast, neurologic manifestations of excitement and hyperesthesia are reportedly very prominent in the Brahman cattle, but are not know in humans.[394]

The value of animal models for development of therapeutic interventions is evident and the first successful applications have been reported (see "Therapy" above).

LYSOSOMAL GLYCOGEN STORAGE DISEASE WITHOUT α-GLUCOSIDASE DEFICIENCY (Danon Disease)

Several cases of cardiomyopathy with vacuolar storage of glycogen but with normal activity of acid α-glucosidase have been reported.[407,423] The clinical picture is of a hypertrophic cardiomyopathy, with clinical signs of skeletal muscle myopathy and with mental retardation in most cases. Arrhythmias, including Wolff-Parkinson-White, are common. There is no other organomegaly reported. CK enzyme can be elevated tenfold. Age of onset has been primarily in late adolescence. A neonatal form has also been reported. The pathological hallmark of the disease is intracytoplasmic vacuoles containing autophagic material and glycogen in skeletal and cardiac muscles. Since glycogen is not always increased in the disease, it is not a typical glycogen storage disease. The syndrome appears to be heterogeneous, with defects at more than one locus resulting in different modes of inheritance. A review of 10 pedigrees leaves open X-linked dominant and autosomal dominant inheritance, but favors an X-linked dominant mode.[407] Danon disease is considered X-linked. At the writing of this review, Danon disease was just reported to be caused by a deficiency of a major lysosomal membrane protein, LAMP-2.[426] In 10 unrelated patients, mutations in the LAMP-2 gene, which maps to the X chromosome, have been found which all caused a complete LAMP-2 deficiency. The importance of LAMP-2 is supported by the phenotype of LAMP-2-deficient mice.[427] These mice are characterized by an extensive accumulation of autophagic vacuoles in liver, pancreas, spleen, kidney, and skeletal and heart muscle. Cardiac myocytes display ultrastructural abnormalities accompanied by severe reduction of heart contractility. The phenotypic alterations in LAMP-2-deficient mice clearly go beyond the pathology described so far in the human cases of Danon disease in that they include autophagic lesions in nonmuscular tissues including neutrophilic leukocytes, hepatocytes, and acinar gland cells in pancreas. It remains to be determined if similar alterations can be found in human patients or if these alterations represent mouse-specific functions of LAMP-2.

REFERENCES

1. Pompe J-C: Over idiopatische hypertrophie van het hart. *Ned Tijdschr Geneeskd* **76**:304, 1932.
2. Putschar M: Uber angeborene Glykogenspeicher-Krankheit des Herzens. "Thesaurismosis glycogenica" (v. Gierke). *Beitr Pathol Anat Allg Pathol* **90**:222, 1932.
3. Di Sant Agnese P, Andersen DH, Mason HH: Glycogen storage disease of the heart. *Pediatrics* **6**:607, 1950.
4. Cori GT: Glycogen structure and enzyme deficiencies in glycogen storage disease. *Harvey Lect* **8**:145, 1954.
5. Hers HG: Alpha-glucosidase deficiency in generalized glycogen-storage disease (Pompe's disease). *Biochem J* **86**:11, 1963.
6. Lejeune N, Thines-Sempoux D, Hers HG: Tissue fractionation studies: Intracellular distribution and properties of alpha-glucosidases in rat liver. *Biochem J* **86**:16, 1963.
7. Courtecuisse V, Royer P, Habib R, Monnier C, Demos J: Glycogenose musculaire par deficit d'alpha-1-4-glucosidase simulant une dystrophie musculaire progressive. *Arch Fr Pediatr* **22**:1153, 1965.
8. Zellweger H, Brown BI, McCormick WF, Tu J: A mild form of muscular glycogenosis in two brothers with alpha-1,4-glucosidase deficiency. *Ann Pediatr* **205**:413, 1965.
9. Isch F, Juif J G, Sacrez R, Thiebaut F: Muscular glycogenosis of myopathic form caused by acid maltase deficiency. *Pediatrie* **21**:71, 1966.
10. Smith J, Zellweger H, Afifi AK: Muscular form of glycogenosis type II (Pompe). *Neurology* **17**:537, 1967.
11. Roth JC, Williams HE: The muscular variant of Pompe's disease. *J Pediatr* **71**:567, 1967.
12. Swaiman K, Kennedy WR: Late infantile acid maltase deficiency. *Arch Neurol* **18**:642, 1968.
13. Engel AG, Dale AJD: Autophagic glycogenosis of late onset with mitochondrial abnormalities: Light and electron microscopic observations. *Mayo Clin Proc* **43**:233, 1968.
14. Hudgson P, Gardner-Medwin D, Worsfold M, Pennington RJT, Walton JN: Adult myopathy from glycogen storage disease due to acid maltase deficiency. *Brain* **91**:435, 1968.
15. Engel AG: Acid maltase deficiency of adult life. *Trans Am Neurol Assoc* **94**:250, 1969.
16. Engel AG, Seybold ME, Lambert EH, Gomez MR: Acid maltase deficiency: Comparison of infantile, childhood, and adult types. *Neurology* **20**:382, 1970.

17. Engel AG, Gomez MR, Seybold ME, Lambert EH: The spectrum and diagnosis of acid maltase deficiency. *Neurology* **23**:95, 1973.
18. Sugimoto, Engel AG, Seybold ME, Lambert EH, Gomez MR: Acid maltase deficiency: Comparison of infantile, childhood, and adult types. *Neurology* **20**:382, 1970.
19. Hers H-G, van Hoof F, de Barsy T: Glycogen storage diseases, in Scriver CR, Beaudet AL, Sly WS, Valle D (eds): *The Metabolic Basis of Inherited Disease,* 6th ed, vol 1. New York, McGraw-Hill, 1989, p 425.
20. Di Mauro S: Metabolic myopathies, in Vinken PJ, Bruyn GW, Ringel SP (eds): *Handbook of Clinical Neurology: Diseases of Muscle Part II,* vol 41. Amsterdam, Elsevier North-Holland, 1979, p 175.
21. Engel AG, Hirschhorn R: Acid maltase deficiency, in: Engel AG, Franzini-Armstrong C (eds): *Myology: Basic and Clinical*, 2nd ed, vol. 2. New York, McGraw-Hill, 1994, p 1533.
22. Reuser AJJ, Kroos MMP, Hermans MMP, Bijvoet AGA, Verbeet MP, Van Diggelen OP, Kleijer WJ, Van der Ploeg AT: Glycogenosis type II (acid maltase deficiency). *Muscle Nerve* **S3**:61, 1995.
23. Nitowsky HM, Grunfeld A: Lysosomal alpha-glucosidase in type II glycogenosis; activity in leukocytes and cell cultures in relation to genotype. *J Lab Clin Med* **69**:472, 1967.
24. Dancis J, Hutzler J, Lynfield J, Cox RP: Absence of acid maltase in glycogenosis type 2 (Pompe's disease) in tissue culture. *Am J Dis Child* **117**:108, 1969.
25. Hogan GR, Gutmann L, Schmidt R, Gilbert E: Pompe's disease. *Neurology* **19**:894, 1969.
26. Baudhuin PHG, Gers HG, Loeb H: An electron microscopic and biochemical study of type II glycogenosis. *Lab Invest* **13**:1139, 1964.
27. Gambetti P, DiMauro S, Baker L: Nervous system in Pompe's disease: Ultrastructure and biochemistry. *J Neuropathol Exp Neurol* **30**:412, 1971.
28. Martin JJ, De Barsy T, Van Hoof F, Palladini G: Pompe's disease: An inborn lysosomal disorder with storage of glycogen. A study of brain and striated muscle. *Acta Neuropathol (Berl)* **23**:229, 1973.
29. Gillette PC, Nihill MR, Singer DB: Electrophysiological mechanism for the short PR interval in Pompe disease. *Am J Dis Child* **128**:622, 1974.
30. Lenard HG, Schaub J, Keutel J, Osang M: Electromyography in type II glycogenosis. *Neuropaediatrie* **5**: 410, 1974.
31. Sakurai I, Tosaka A, Mori Y, Imura S, Aoki K: Glycogenosis type II (Pompe). The fourth autopsy case in Japan. *Acta Pathol Jpn* **24**:829, 1974.
32. Potter JL, Robinson HB, Kramer JD, Schafer IA: Apparent normal leukocyte acid maltase activity in glycogen storage disease type II (Pompe's disease). *Clin Chem* **26**:1914, 1980.
33. Seifert BL, Snyder MS, Klein AA, O'Loughlin JE, Magid MS, Engle MA: Development of obstruction to ventricular outflow and impairment of inflow in glycogen storage disease of the heart: Serial echocardiographic studies from birth to death at 6 months. *Am Heart J* **123**:239, 1992.
34. Wijburg FA, Rosenblatt DS, Oorthuys JWE, Van't Hek LGFM, Poorthuis BJHM, Sanders MK, Schutgens RBH: Clinical and biochemical observations in a patient with combined Pompe disease and cblC mutation. *Eur J Pediatr* **151**:127, 1992.
35. Tsao CY, Boesel CP, Wright FS: A hypotonic infant with complete deficiencies of acid maltase and debrancher enzyme. *J Child Neurol* **9**:90, 1994.
36. Martin JJ, De Barsy T, De Schrijver T, Leroy JG, Palladini G: Acid maltase deficiency (type II glycogenosis): Morphological and biochemical study of a childhood phenotype. *J Neurol Sci* **30**:155, 1976.
37. Tanaka K, Shimazu S, Oya N, Tomisawa M, Kusunoki T, Soyama K, Ono E: Muscular form of glycogenosis type II (Pompe's disease). *Pediatrics* **63**:124, 1979.
38. Nakagawa M, Nakazato O, Osame M, Nakashima H, Igata A: Muscle type acid maltase deficiency. An intermediate case between childhood type and adult type. *Rinsho Shinkeigaku* **22**:57, 1982.
39. Olgunturk R, Bilgic A, Caglar M, Sinangil F: Acid maltase deficiency in adolescence: Report of an unusual case. *Turk J Pediatr* **24**:115, 1982.
40. Matsuishi T, Terasawa K, Yoshida I, Yano E, Yamashita F, Hidaka T, Ishihara O, Yoshino M, Nonaka I, Kurokawa T, Nakamura Y: Vacuolar myopathy with type 2 A fiber atrophy and type 2 B fiber deficiency. A case of childhood form acid alpha-1,4-glucosidase deficiency. *Neuropediatrics* **13**: 173, 1982.
41. Horoupian DS, Kini KR, Weiss L, Follmer R: Selective vacuolar myopathy with atrophy of type II fiber. Occurrence in a childhood case of acid maltase deficiency. *Arch Neurol* **35**: 175, 1978.
42. Papapetropoulos T, Paschalis C, Manda P: Myopathy due to juvenile acid maltase deficiency affecting exclusively the type I fibres. *J Neurol Neurosurg Psychiatry* **47**:213, 1984.
43. Matsuishi T, Yoshino M, Terasawa K, Nonaka I: Childhood acid maltase deficiency. A clinical, biochemical and morphologic study of three patients. *Arch Neurol* **41**: 47, 1984.
44. Temple JK, Dunn DW, Blitizer MG, Shapira E: The "muscular variant" of Pompe disease: Clinical, biochemical and histologic characteristics . *Am J Med Genet* **21**: 597, 1985.
45. Origuchi Y, Itai Y, Matsumoto S, Matsuishi T: Quantitative histological study of the sural nerve in a child with acid maltase deficiency (glycogenosis type II). *Pediatr Neurol* **2**:346, 1986.
46. Danon MJ, DiMauro S, Shanske S, Archer FL, Miranda AF: Juvenile-onset acid maltase deficiency with unusual familial features. *Neurology* **36**:818, 1986.
47. Iancu TC, Lerner A, Shiloh H, Bashan N, Moses S: Juvenile acid maltase deficiency presenting as paravertebral pseudotumour. *Eur J Pediatr* **147**:372, 1988.
48. Wong KS, Lai C, Ng HK: Late-onset acid maltase deficiency in a Chinese girl. *Clin Exp Neurol* **28**:210, 1991.
49. DiFiore MT, Manfredi R, Marri L, Zucchini A, Azzaroli L, Manfredi G: Acid maltase deficiency in childhood early diagnosis and clinical follow-up of late-onset glycogen storage disease type II. *Acta Neurol* **15**:258, 1993.
50. Kim DG, Jung K, Lee MK, Hyun IG, Lim HJ, Song HG, Chi JG: A case of juvenile form Pompe's disease manifested as chronic alveolar hypoventilation. *J Korean Med Sci* **8**:221, 1993.
51. Suzuki Y, Tsuji A, Omura K, Nakamura G, Awa S, Kroos M, Reuser AJJ: K_m mutant of acid alpha-glucosidase in a case of cardiomyopathy without signs of skeletal muscle involvement. *Clin Genet* **33**:376, 1988.
52. Engel AG: Acid maltase deficiency in adults: Studies in four cases of a syndrome which may mimic muscular dystrophy or other myopathies. *Brain* **93**:599, 1970.
53. Kolmel HW, Assmus H, Seiler D: Myopathy due to acid maltase deficiency. Pompe's disease in adolescence and adult. *Arch Psychiatr Nervenkr* **218**:93, 1974.
54. Martin JJ, De Barsy T, Den Tandt WR: Acid maltase deficiency in non-identical adult twins: A morphological and biochemical study. *J Neurol* **213**:105, 1976.
55. Schlenska GK, Heene R, Spalke G, Seiler D: The symptomatology, morphology and biochemistry of glycogenosis type II (Pompe) in the adult. *J Neurol* **212**:237, 1976.
56. Gullotta F, Stefan H, Mattern H: Pseudodystrophische muskelglykogenose im erwachsenenalter (Saure-maltase-mangel-syndrom). *J Neurol* **213**:199, 1976.
57. Pongratz D, Schlossmacher I, Koppenwallner C, Hubner G: An especially mild myopathic form of glycogenosis type II. Problems of clinical and light microscopic diagnosis. *Pathol Eur* **11**:39, 1976.
58. Domanic N, Akman N, Ozand P, Muftuoglu AU: Heterogenous glycogen storage disease in one family. *Hum Hered* **26**:217, 1976.
59. Lightman NI, Schooley RT: Adult-onset acid maltase deficiency: Case report of an adult with severe respiratory difficulty. *Chest* **72**:250, 1977.
60. Karpati G, Carpenter S, Eisen A, Aube M, DiMauro S: The adult form of acid maltase (alpha-1,4-glucosidase) deficiency. *Ann Neurol* **1**:276, 1977.
61. DiMauro S, Stern LZ, Mehler M, Nagle RB, Payne C: Adult onset acid maltase deficiency: A postmortem study. *Muscle Nerve* **1**:27, 1978.
62. Bertagnolio B, DiDonato S, Peluchetti D, Rimoldi M, Storchi G, Cornelio F: Acid maltase deficiency in adults: Clinical, morphological and biochemical study of three patients. *Eur Neurol* **17**:193, 1978.
63. Beratis NG, LaBadie GU, Hirschhorn K: Characterization of the molecular defect in infantile and adult acid alpha-glucosidase deficiency fibroblasts. *J Clin Invest* **62**:1264, 1978.
64. Beratis NG, LaBadie GU, Hirschhorn K: Genetic heterogeneity in acid alpha-glucosidase deficiency. *Am J Hum Genet* **35**:21, 1983.
65. Askanas V, Engel WK, DiMauro S, Brooks BR, Mehler M: Adult-onset acid maltase deficiency: Morphologic and biochemical abnormalities reproduced in cultured muscle. *N Engl J Med* **294**:573, 1976.
66. Rosenow EC, Engel AE: Acid maltase deficiency in adults presenting as respiratory failure. *Am J Med* **64**:485, 1978.
67. Miyamoto Y, Etoh Y, Ryuichiro J, Noda K, Ohya I, Morimatsu Y: Adult-onset maltase deficiency in siblings. *Acta Pathol Jpn* **35**: 1533, 1985.

68. Trend PS, Wiles CM, Spencer GT, Morgan-Hughes JA, Lake BD, Patrick AD: Acid maltase deficiency in adults (diagnosis and management in five cases). *Brain* **108**:845, 1985.
69. Swash M, Schwartz MS, Apps MCP: Adult onset acid maltase deficiency: Distribution and progression of clinical and pathological abnormality in a family. *J Neurol Sci* **68**:61, 1985.
70. Lenders MB, Martin JJ, de Barsy T, Ceyterick C, Marchau M: Acid maltase deficiency in adults. *Acta Neurol Belg* **86**:152, 1986.
71. Vilchez JJ, Budin J, Lainez JM, Cabello A: Insuficiencia respiratoria por paralisis diafragmatica en un efficit de maltasa acida. *Arch Neurobiol* **49**:153, 1986.
72. Sivak ED, Salanga VD, Wilbourn AJ, Mitsumoto H, Golish J: Adult-onset acid maltase deficiency presenting as diaphragmatic paralysis. *Ann Neurol* **9**:613, 1981.
73. Lissac J, Fardeau M, Contamin F, Poenaru L, Der Agopian P, Salmona J: Acid maltase deficiency with diaphragmatic paralysis and respiratory insufficiency in adults [Letter]. *Nouv Presse Med* **11**:3797, 1982.
74. Akamatsu A, Nomoto R, Nagao H, Murakami H, Nonaka I, Tara M, Kato M: Adult form acid maltase deficiency—A case report. *Jpn J Med* **21**:203, 1982.
75. McComas CF, Schochet S Jr, Morris H, Romansky SG, Gutmann L: The constellation of adult acid maltase deficiency: Clinical, electrophysiologic, and morphologic features. *Clin Neuropathol* **2**:182, 1983.
76. Brunel D, Fanjoux J, Raphael JC, Goulon M: A new case of acid maltase deficiency. Treatment by artificial respiration at home [Letter]. *Presse Med* **13**:2322, 1984.
77. Keunen RW, Lambregts PC, Op de Coul AA, Joosten EM: Respiratory failure as initial symptom of acid maltase deficiency. *J Neurol Neurosurg Psychiatry* **47**:549, 1984.
78. Pongratz D, Kotzner H, Hubner G, Deufel T, Wieland OH: Adult form of acid maltase deficiency presenting as progressive spinal muscular atrophy. *Dtsch Med Wochenschr* **109**:537, 1984.
79. Wolf RE, Mark EJ, McNeely BU: Case record of the Massachusetts General Hospital. *N Engl J Med* **315**:694, 1986.
80. Isaacs H, Savage N, Badenhorst M, Whistler T: Acid maltase deficiency: A case study and review of the pathophysiological changes and proposed therapeutic measures. *J Neurol Neurosurg Psychiatry* **49**:1011, 1986.
80a. Sivak ED, Ahmad M, Muzaffar A, Hanson MR, Mitsumoto H, Wilbourn AJ: Respiratory insufficiency in adult-onset acid maltase deficiency. *South Med J* **80**:205, 1987.
80b. Van der Walt JD, Swash M, Leake J, Cox EL: The pattern of involvement of adult-onset acid maltase deficiency at autopsy. *Muscle Nerve* **10**:272, 1987.
80c. Matsuoka Y, Senda Y, Hirayama M, Matsui T, Takahashi A: Late-onset acid maltase deficiency associated with intracranial aneurysm. *J Neurol* **235**:371, 1988.
81. Kretzschmar HA, Wagner H, Hubner G, Danek A, Witt TN, Mehraein P: Aneurysms and vacuolar degeneration of cerebral arteries in late-onset acid maltase deficiency. *J Neurol Sci* **98**:169, 1990.
82. Cinnamon J, Slonim AE, Black KS, Gorey MT, Scuderi DM, Hyman RA: Evaluation of the lumbar spine in patients with glycogen storage disease: CT demonstration of patterns of paraspinal muscle atrophy. *AJNR Am J Neuroradiol* **12**:1099, 1991.
83. Chancellor AM, Warlow CP, Webb JN, Lucas MG, Besley GT, Broadhead DM: Acid maltase deficiency presenting with a myopathy and exercise induced urinary incontinence in a 68 year old male [Letter]. *J Neurol Neurosurg Psychiatry* **54**:659, 1991.
84. Barohn RJ, McVey AL, DiMauro S: Adult acid maltase deficiency. *Muscle Nerve* **16**:672, 1993.
85. Moufarrej NA, Bertorini TE: Respiratory insufficiency in adult-type acid maltase deficiency. *South Med J* **86**:560, 1993.
86. Margolis ML, Howlett P, Goldgerg R, Eftychiadis A, Levine S: Obstructive sleep apnea syndrome in acid maltase deficiency. *Chest* **105**:947, 1994.
87. Felice KJ, Alessi AG, Grunnet ML: Clinical variability in adult-onset acid maltase deficiency: Report of affected sibs and review of literature. *Medicine* **74**:131, 1995.
88. Fadic R, Waclawik AJ, Brooks BR, Lotz BP: The rigid spine syndrome due to acid maltase deficiency. *Muscle Nerve* **20**:364, 1997.
89. Arai Y, Osawa M, Shishikura K, Suzuki H, Saito K, Fukuyama Y, Suige H: Computed tomography and magnetic resonance imaging of affected muscle in childhood acid α-glucosidase deficiency: A case report. *Brain Dev* **15**:147, 1993.
90. de Jager AEJ, Vliet TM, Ree TC, Oosterink BJ, Loonen MCB: Muscle computer tomography in adult-onset acid maltase deficiency. *Muscle Nerve* **3**:398, 1998.
91. Lee CC, Chen CY, Chou TY, Chen FH, Lee CC, Zimmerman RA: Cerebral MR manifestations of Pompe disease in an infant. *AJNR Am J Neuroradiol* **17**:321, 1996.
92. Barnes D, Hughes RAC: Adult-onset maltase deficiency with prominent bulbar involvement and ptosis. *J R Soc Med* **86**:50, 1993.
93. Prevett M, Enevoldson TP, Duncan JS: Adult onset acid maltase deficiency associated with epilepsy and dementia: A case report. *J Neurol Neurosurg Psychiatry* **55**:509, 1992.
94. Ullrich K, Grobe H, Korinthenber R, von Bassewitz DB: Severe course of glycogen storage disease type II (Pompe's disease) without development of cardiomegalia. *Pathol Res Pract* **181**:627, 1986.
95. Wokke JH, Ausems MG, van den Boogaard MJ, Ippel EF, van Diggelen O, Kroos MA, Boer M, Jennekens FG, Reuser AJJ, Ploos van Amstel HK: Genotype-phenotype correlation in adult-onset acid maltase deficiency. *Ann Neurol* **38**:450, 1995.
96. DiFiore MT, Manfredi R, Marri L, Zucchini A, Azzaroli L, Manfredi G: Elevation of transaminases as an early sign of late-onset glycogenosis type II [Letter]. *Eur J Pediatr* **152**:784, 1993.
97. Shulman RG, Rothman DL, Price TB: Nuclear magnetic resonance studies of muscle and applications to exercise and diabetes. *Diabetes* **45(Suppl 1)**:893, 1996.
98. Cox IJ: Development and applications of in vivo clinical magnetic resonance spectroscopy. *Prog Biophys Mol Biol* **65**:45, 1996.
99. Lin CY, Hwang B, Hsiao KJ, Jin YR: Pompe's disease in chinese and the prenatal diagnosis by determination of alpha-glucosidase activity. *J Inherit Metab Dis* **10**:11, 1987.
100. Ausems MGEM, Verbiest J, Hermans MMP, Kroos MA, Beemer FA, Wokke JHJ, Sandkuijl LA, Reuser AJJ, Van der Ploeg AT: Frequency of glycogen storage disease type II in the Netherlands: Implications for diagnosis and genetic counselling. *Eur J Hum Genet* **7**:713, 1999.
100a. Kroos MA, Van der Kraan M, Van Diggelen OP, Kleijer WJ, Reuser AJJ, Van den Boogaard MJ, Ausems MGEM, Ploos van Amstel HK, Poenaru L, Nicolino M, Wevers R: Glycogen storage disease type II: Frequency of three common mutant alleles and their associated clinical phenotypes studied in 121 patients. *J Med Genet* **32**:836, 1995.
100b. Ausems MGEM, Ten Berg K, Kroos MA, Van Diggelen OP, Wevers RA, Poorthuis BJHM, Niezen-Koning KE, Van der Ploeg AT, Beemer FA, Reuser AJJ, Sandkuijl LA, Wokke JHJ: Glycogen storage disease type II: Birth prevalence agrees with predicted genotype frequency. *Commun Genet* **2**:91, 1999.
101. Martiniuk F, Chen A, Mack A, Arvanitopoulos E, Chen Y, Rom WN, Codd WJ, Hanna B, Alcabes P, Raben N, Plotz P: Carrier frequency for glycogen storage disease type II in New York and estimates of affected individuals born with the disease. *Am J Med Genet* **79**:69, 1998.
102. Kiehl P, Metze D, Kresse H, Reimann S, Kraft D, Kapp A: Decreased activity of acid alpha-glucosidase in a patient with persistent periocular swelling after infusions of hydroxyethyl starch. *Br J Dermatol* **138**:672, 1998.
103. Koster JF, Busch HFM, Slee RG, Van Weerden TW: Glycogenosis type II: The infantile- and late-onset acid maltase deficiency observed in one family. *Clin Chim Acta* **87**:451, 1978.
104. Busch HFM, Koster JF, Van Weerden TW: Infantile and adult onset acid maltase deficiency occurring in the same family. *Neurology* **29**:415, 1979.
105. Loonen MCB, Busch HFM, Koster JF, Martin JJ, Niermeijer MF, Schram AW, Brouwer-Kelder B, Mekes W, Slee RG, Tager JM: A family with different clinical forms of acid maltase deficiency (glycogenosis type II): Biochemical and genetic studies. *Neurology* **31**:1209, 1981.
106. Hoefsloot LH, Van Der Ploeg AT, Kroos MA, Hoogeveen-Westerveld M, Oostra BA, Reuser AJJ: Adult and infantile glycogenosis type II in one family, explained by allelic diversity. *Am J Hum Genet* **46**:45, 1990.
107. Kroos MA, Van der Kraan M, Van Diggelen OP, Kleijer WJ, Reuser AJJ: Two extremes of the clinical spectrum of glycogen storage disease type II in one family: A matter of genotype. *Hum Mutat* **9**:17, 1997.
108. Brown BI, Brown DH, Jeffrey PL: Simultaneous absence of alpha-1-4-glucosidase and alpha-1-6-glucosidase activities (pH 4) in tissues of children with type II glycogen storage disease. *Biochemistry* **9**:1423, 1970.
109. Auricchio F, Bruni CB: Purification of an acid alpha-glucosidase by dextran-gel filtration. *Biochem J* **105**:35, 1967.

110. Auricchio F, Bruni CB, Sica V: Further purification and characterization of the acid alpha-glucosidase. *Biochem J* **108**:161, 1968.
111. Hasilik A, Neufeld EF: Biosynthesis of lysosomal enzymes in fibroblasts: Synthesis as precursors of higher molecular weight. *J Biol Chem* **285**:4937, 1980.
112. Hasilik A, Neufeld EF: Biosynthesis of lysosomal enzymes in fibroblasts; phosphorylation of mannose residues. *J Biol Chem* **285**:4946, 1980.
113. Kornfeld S: Trafficking of lysosomal enzymes in normal and disease states. *J Clin Invest* **77**:1, 1986.
114. Bruni CB, Auricchio F, Covelli I: Alpha-glucosidase glucohydrolase from cattle liver. *J Biol Chem* **244**:4735, 1969.
115. Jeffrey PL, Brown DH, Brown BI: Studies of lysosomal alpha-glucosidase. I. Purification and properties of the rat liver enzyme. *Biochemistry* **9**:1403, 1970.
116. Jeffrey PL, Brown DH, Brown BI: Studies of lysosomal alpha-glucosidase. II. Kinetics of action of the rat liver enzyme. *Biochemistry* **9**:1416, 1970.
117. Bruni CB, Sica V, Auricchio F, Covelli I: Further kinetic and structural characterization of the lysosomal alpha-D-glucoside glucohydrolase from cattle liver. *Biochim Biophys Acta* **212**:470, 1970.
118. Palmer TN: The substrate specificity of acid alpha-glucosidase from rabbit muscle. *Biochem J* **124**:701, 1971.
119. Palmer TN: The maltase, glucoamylase and transglucosylase activities of acid alpha-glucosidase from rabbit muscle. *Biochem J* **124**:713, 1971.
120. De Barsy T, Jacquemin P, Devos P, Hers H: Rodent and human acid alpha-glucosidase: Purification, properties and inhibition by antibodies; Investigation in type II glycogenosis. *Eur J Biochem* **31**:156, 1972.
121. Koster JF, Slee RG: Some properties of human liver acid alpha-glucosidase. *Biochim Biophys Acta* **482**:89, 1977.
122. Murray AK, Brown BI, Brown DH: The molecular heterogeneity of purified human liver lysosomal alpha-glucosidase (acid alpha-glucosidase). *Arch Biochem Biophys* **185**:511, 1978.
123. Chambers JP, Williams JC: Acid alpha-glucosidase from human heart. *Enzyme* **29**:109, 1983.
124. Martiniuk F, Honig J, Hirschhorn R: Further studies of the structure of human placental acid alpha-glucosidase. *Arch Biochem Biophys* **231**:454, 1984.
125. Matsui H, Saski M, Takemasa E, Kaneta T, Chiba S: Kinetic studies on the substrate specificity and active site of rabbit muscle acid alpha-glucosidase. *J Biochem* **96**:993, 1984.
126. Oude Elferink RPJ, Brouwer-Kelder EM, Surya I, Strijland A, Kroos M, Reuser AJJ, Tager JM: Isolation and characterization of a precursor form of lysosomal alpha-glucosidase from human urine. *Eur J Biochem* **139**:489, 1984.
127. Calder PC, Geddes R: Regulation of lysosomal glycogen metabolism: Studies of the actions of mammalian acid alpha-glucosidases. *J Biochem* **21**:569, 1989.
128. Nakasone S, Ohshita T, Iwamasa T: Heterogeneity of pig lysosomal acid alpha-glucosidase: Affinity to sephacryl S-200 gel and tissue distribution. *Biochem J* **279**:719, 1991.
129. Sips HJ, Reuser AJJ, Van Der Veer E: Synthesis and intracellular localization of chick acid alpha-glucosidase in chick erythrocyte-human fibroblast heterokaryons. *Exp Cell Res* **162**:555, 1986.
130. Tsuji A, Suzuki Y: Biosynthesis of two components of human acid alpha-glucosidase. *Arch Biochem Biophys* **259**:234, 1987.
131. Walvoort HC, Slee RG, Sluis KJ, Koster JF, Reuser AJ: Biochemical genetics of the Lapland dog model of glycogen storage disease type II (acid alpha-glucosidase deficiency). *Am J Med Genet* **19**:589, 1984.
132. Onodera S, Matsui H, Chiba S: Single active site mechanism of rabbit liver acid alpha-glucosidase. *J Biochem* **105**:611, 1989.
133. Van Hove JLK, Yang HW, Wu J-Y, Brady R, Chen Y-T: High-level production of recombinant human lysosomal acid alpha-glucosidase in Chinese hamster ovary cells which targets to heart muscle and corrects glycogen accumulation in fibroblasts from patients with Pompe disease. *Proc Natl Acad Sci U S A* **93**:65, 1996.
134. Wu JY, Van Hove JL, Huang YS, Chen YT: Expression of catalytically active human multifunctional glycogen-debranching enzyme and lysosomal acid alpha-glucosidase in insect cells. *Biochem Mol Biol Int* **39**:755, 1996.
135. Van Hove JLK, Yang HW, Oliver LM, Pennybacker MF, Chen Y-T: Purification of recombinant human precursor acid alpha-glucosidase. *Biochem Mol Biol Int* **43**:613, 1997.
136. Fuller M, Van der Ploeg A, Reuser AJ, Anson DS, Hopwood JJ: Isolation and characterisation of a recombinant, precursor form of lysosomal acid alpha-glucosidase. *Eur J Biochem* **234**:903, 1995.
137. Bijvoet AG, Kroos MA, Pieper FR, de Boer HA, Reuser AJ, van der Ploeg AT, Verbeet MP: Expression of cDNA-encoded human acid alpha-glucosidase in milk of transgenic mice. *Biochim Biophys Acta* **1308**:93, 1996.
138. Bijvoet AGA, Kroos MA, Pieper FR, Vander Vliet M, De Boer HA, Van der Ploeg AT, Verbeet MP, Reuser AJJ: Recombinant human acid alpha-glucosidase: High level production in mouse milk, biochemical characteristics, correction of enzyme deficiency in GSDII KO mice. *Hum Mol Genet* **7**:1815, 1998.
139. Martiniuk F, Tzall S, Chen A: Recombinant human acid alpha-glucosidase generated in bacteria: Antigenic, but enzymatically inactive. *DNA Cell Biol* **11**:701, 1992.
140. Saul R, Ghidoni JJ, Molyneux RJ, Elbein A: Castanospermine inhibits alpha-glucosidase activities and alters glycogen distribution in animals. *Proc Natl Acad Sci U S A* **82**:93, 1985.
141. Schmidt DD, Frommer W, Junge B, Muller L, Wingender W, Schafer D: Alpha-glucosidase inhibitors. New complex oligosaccharides of microbial origin. *Naturwissenschaften* **64**:535, 1977.
142. Lullmann-Rauch R: Lysosomal glycogen storage mimicking the cytological picture of Pompe's disease as induced in rats by injection of an alpha-glucosidase inhibitor I Alterations in liver. *Virchows Arch B Cell Pathol Incl Mol Pathol* **38**:89, 1981.
143. Lullmann-Rauch R: Lysosomal glycogen storage mimicking the cytological picture of Pompe's disease as induced in rats by injection of an alpha-glycosidase inhibitor II Alterations in kidney, adrenal gland, spleen and soleus muscle. *Virchows Arch B Cell Pathol Incl Mol Pathol* **39**:187, 1982.
144. Konishi Y, Okawa Y, Hosokawa S, Fujimori K, Fuwa H: Lysosomal glycogen accumulation in rat liver and its in vivo kinetics after a single intraperitoneal injection of acarbose, an alpha-glucosidase inhibitor. *J Biochem* **107**:197, 1990.
145. Wisselaar HA, Van Dongen JM, Reuser AJJ: Effects of *N*-hydroxyethyl-1-deoxynojirimycin (BAY m 1099) on the activity of neutral- and acid alpha-glucosidases in human fibroblasts and HepG2 cells. *Clin Chim Acta* **182**:41, 1989.
146. Grabowski GA, Osiecki-Newman K, Dinur T, Fabbro D, Legler G, Gatt S, Desnick RJ: Human acid beta glucosidase: Use of conduritol B epoxide derivatives to investigate the catalytically active normal and Gaucher disease enzymes. *J Biol Chem* **261**:8263, 1986.
147. Hirsh AJ, Yao SYM, Young JD, Cheeseman CI: Inhibition of glucose absorption in the rat jejunum: A novel action of alpha-d-glucosidase inhibitors. *Gastroenterology* **113**:205, 1997.
148. Lebovitz HE: Alpha-glucosidase inhibitors. *Endocrinol Metab Clin North Am* **26**:539, 1997.
149. Radin NS, Shukka A, Shukla GS, Sano A: Heat-stable protein that stimulates acid alpha-glucosidase. *Biochem J* **264**:845, 1989.
150. Martiniuk F, Mehler M, Pellicer A, Tzall S, LaBadie G, Hobart C, Ellenbogen A, Hirschhorn R: Isolation of a cDNA for human acid alpha glucosidase and detection of genetic heterogeneity for mRNA in three alpha glucosidase deficient patients. *Proc Natl Acad Sci U S A* **83**:9641, 1986.
151. Hoefsloot LH, Hoogeveen-Westerveld M, Kroos MA, Van Beeumen J, Reuser AJJ, Oostra BA: Primary structure and processing of lysosomal alpha glucosidase; homology with the intestinal sucrase-isomaltase complex. *EMBO J* **7**:1697, 1988.
152. Martiniuk F, Mehler M, Tzall S, Meredith G, Hirschhorn R: Sequence of the cDNA and 5′ flanking region for human acid alpha glucosidase, detection of an intron in the 5′ untranslated leader sequence, definition of 18 base pair polymorphisms and additional differences with previous cDNA and amino acid sequences. *DNA Cell Biol* **9**:85, 1990.
153. Hoefsloot LH, Hoogeveen-Westerveld M, Reuser AJJ, Oostra BA: Characterization of the human lysosomal alpha glucosidase gene. *Biochem J* **272**:493, 1990.
154. Martiniuk F, Bodkin M, Tzall S, Hirschhorn R: Isolation and partial characterization of the structural gene for human acid alpha glucosidase (GAA). *DNA Cell Biol* **10**:283, 1991.
155. Tzall S, Martiniuk F: Identification of the promoter region and transient expression for human acid alpha glucosidase in deficient cells. *Biochem Biophys Res Commun* **176**:1509, 1991.
157. Hoefsloot LH, Willemsen R, Kroos MA, Hogeveen-Westerveld M, Hermans MMP, Van der Ploeg AT, Oostra BA, Reuser AJJ: Expression and routing of human lysosomal alpha glucosidase in transiently transfected mammalian cells. *Biochem J* **272**:485, 1990.

158. Wisselaar HA, Kroos MA, Hermans MMP, van Beeumen J, Reuser AJJ: Structural and functional changes of lysosomal acid alpha-glucosidase during intracellular transport and maturation. *J Biol Chem* **268**:2223, 1993.
159. Franci C, Egea G, Arribas R, Reuser AJJ, Real FX: Lysosomal alpha-glucosidase: Cell specific processing and altered maturation in HT-29 colon cancer cells. *Biochem J* **314**:33, 1996.
160. Oude Elferink RPJ, Van Doorn-Van Wakeren J, Strijand A, Reuser AJJ, Tager JM: Biosynthesis and intracellular transport of alpha-glucosidase and cathepsin D in normal and mutant human fibroblasts. *Eur J Biochem* **153**:55, 1985.
161. Van Der Horst GTJ, Hoefsloot EH, Kroos MA, Reuser AJJ: Cell-free translation of human lysosomal alpha-glucosidase: Evidence for reduced precursor synthesis in an adult patient with glycogenosis type II. *Biochim Biophys Acta* **910**:123, 1987.
162. Tsujii A, Suzuki Y: The precursor of acid alpha-glucosidase is synthesized as a membrane-bound enzyme. *Biochem Int* **15**:945, 1987.
163. Henken RD, Chambers JP, Williams JC: The molecular basis for charge heterogeneity in human acid-alpha glucosidase. *Biochim Biophys Acta* **829**:44, 1985.
164. Hermans MMP, Wisselaar HA, Kroos MA, Oostra BA, Reuser AJJ: Human lysosomal alpha-glucosidase: Functional characterization of the glycosylation sites. *Biochem J* **289**:681, 1993.
165. Mutsaers JHGM, Van Halbeek H, Vliegenthart JFG, Tager JM, Reuser AJJ, Kroos M, Galjaard H: Determination of the structure of the carbohydrate chains of acid alpha-glucosidase from human placenta. *Biochim Biophys Acta* **911**:244, 1987.
166. Fransen JAM, Ginsel LA, Cambier PH, Klumperman J, Oude Elferink RPJ, Tager JM: Immunocytochemical demonstration of the lysosomal enzyme alpha glucosidase in the brush border of human intestinal epithelial cells. *Eur J Cell Biol* **47**:72, 1988.
167. Oude-Elferink RPJ, Fransen JAM, Klumperman J, Ginsel LA, Tager JM: Secretion of a precursor form of lysosomal alpha glucosidase from the brush border of human kidney proximal tubule cells. *Eur J Cell Biol* **50**:299, 1989.
168. Tsuji A, Omura K, Suzuki Y: Intracellular transport of acid alpha-glucosidase in human fibroblasts: Evidence for involvement of phosphomannosyl receptor-independent system. *J Biochem (Tokyo)* **104**:276, 1988.
169. Klumperman J, Fransen JAM, Boekestijn TC, Elferink RPJO, Matter K, Hauri HP, Tager JM, Ginsel LA: Biosynthesis and transport of lysosomal alpha-glucosidase in the human colon carcinoma cell line Caco-2: Secretion from the apical surface. *Cell Sci* **100**:339, 1991.
170. Klumperman J, Fransen JAM, Tager JM, Ginsel LA: The cation-independent mannose 6-phosphate receptor is not involved in the polarized secretion of lysosomal alpha-glucosidase from Caco-2 cells. *Eur J Cell Biol* **57**:147, 1992.
171. Willemsen R, Brunken R, Sorber CWJ, Hoogeveen AT, Wisselaar HA, Van Dongen JM, Reuser AJJ: A quantitative immunoelectron-micoscopic study on soluble, membrane-associated with membrane-bound lysosomal enzymes in human intestinal epithelial cells. *Histochem J* **23**:467, 1991.
172. Henrissat B: Glycosidase families. *Biochem Soc Trans* **26**:153, 1998.
173. http://protein.toulouse.infra.fr/prodom.html.
173a. Family 31 glycosyl hydrolases: www.expasy.ch/cgi-bin/lists? glygosid. txt
174. Hermans MMP, Kroos MA, van Beeumen J, Oostra BA, Reuser AJJ: Human lysosomal alpha-glucosidase: Characterization of the catalytic site. *J Biol Chem* **266**:13507, 1991.
175. Swallow DM, Corney G, Harris H, Hirschhorn R: Acid alpha-glucosidase: A new polymorphism in man demonstrable by "affinity" electrophoresis. *Ann Hum Genet* **38**:391, 1975.
176. Martiniuk F, Hirschhorn R: Human neutral alpha-glucosidase C: Genetic polymorphism including a "null" allele. *Am J Hum Genet* **32**:497, 1980.
177. Martiniuk F, Hirschhorn R, Smith M: Assignment of the gene for human neutral alpha-glucosidase C to chromosome 15. *Cytogenet Cell Genet* **27**:168, 1980.
178. Martiniuk F, Hirschhorn R: Characterization of neutral isozymes of human alpha-glucosidase: Difference in substrate specificity, molecular weight and electrophoretic mobility. *Biochem Biophys Acta* **658**:248, 1981.
179. Van Der Ploeg AT, Kroos MA, Swallow DM, Reuser AJJ: An investigation of the possible influence of neutral alpha-glucosidases on the clinical heterogeneity of glycogenosis type II. *Ann Hum Genet* **53**:185, 1989.
180. Martiniuk F, Smith M, Ellenbogen A, Desnick RH, Astrin K, Mitra J, Hirschhorn R: Assignment of the gene for neutral alpha-glucosidase AB to chromosome 11. *Cytogenet Cell Genet* **35**:110, 1983.
181. Martiniuk F, Ellenbogen A, Hirschhorn R: Identity of neutral alpha-glucosidase AB and the glycoprotein processing enzyme glucosidase II: Biochemical and genetic studies. *J Biol Chem* **260**:1238, 1985.
182. Martiniuk F, Pellicer A, Hirschhorn R: Transient expression of human neutral alpha glucosidase AB (glucosidase II) in enzyme-deficient mouse lymphoma cells. *J Biol Chem* **260**:14351, 1985.
183. Burns DM, Touster O: Purification and characterization of glucosidase II, an endoplasmic reticulum hydrolase involved in glycoprotein biosynthesis. *J Biol Chem* **257**:9990, 1982.
184. Saxena S, Shailubhai K, Dong-Yu B, Vijay IK: Purification and characterization of glucosidase II involved in N-linked glycoprotein process in bovine mammary gland. *Biochem J* **247**:563, 1987.
185. Alonso JM, Santacecilia A, Chinchetru MA, Calvo P: Characterization of the maltase activity of glucosidase II from rat liver. *Biol Chem Hoppe-Seyler* **374**:977, 1993.
186. Hentges A, Bause E: Affinity purification and characterization of glucosidase II from pig liver. *J Biol Chem* **378**:1031, 1997.
187. De Burlet G, Sudaka P: Purification de la maltase neutre renale humaine. *Biochimie* **58**:621, 1976.
188. De Burlet G, Sudaka P: Proprietes catalytiques de l'alpha-glucosidase neutre du rein humain. *Biochimie* **59**:7, 1977.
189. De Burlet G, Vannier C, Giudicelli J, Sudaka P: Neutral alpha-glucosidase from human kidney: Molecular and immunological properties. Relationship with intestinal glucoamylase. *Biochimie* **61**:1177, 1980.
190. Giudicelli J, Emiliozzi R, Vannier C, De Burlet G, Sudaka P: Purification by affinity chromatography and characterization of a neutral alpha-glucosidase from horse kidney. *Acta Biochim Biophys* **612**:85, 1980.
191. Reiss U, Sacktor B: Kidney brush border membrane maltase: Purification and properties. *Arch Biochem Biophys* **209**:342, 1981.
192. Giudicelli J, Boudouard M, Delque P, Vannier C, Sudaka P: Horse kidney neutral alpha-glucosidase: Purification of the detergent-solubilized enzyme; comparison with the proteinase-solubilized forms. *Biochim Biophys Acta* **831**:59, 1985.
193. Pereira B, Sivakami S: Neutral maltase/glucoamylase from rabbit renal cortex. *Biochem J* **261**:43, 1989.
194. Nishinaka H, Minamiura N, Matoba K, Furusawa M, Yamamoto T: On the origin of alpha-glucosidase in human urine. *J Histochem Cytochem* **30**:1186, 1982.
195. Dreyfus JC, Alexandre Y: Electrophoretic characterization of acidic and neutral amylo α-1,4-glucosidase (acid maltase) in human tissues and evidence for two electrophoretic variants in acid maltase deficiency. *Biochem Biophy Res Commun* **48**:914, 1972.
196. Dreyfus JC, Poenaru L: Alpha glucosidases in white blood cells with reference to the detection of acid alpha-1,4-glucosidase deficiency. *Biochem Biophys Res Commun* **85**:615, 1978.
197. Jean-Marie P, Giudicelli J, Delque P, Cassuto J, Sudaka P, Ayraud N: Neutral maltase: A marker of cell differentiation in human myeloid leukaemias? *Br J Haematol* **52**:641, 1982.
198. Stio M, Vanni P, Ferrini PR, Giachetti E, Bosi A, Pinzauti G: Neutral maltase of human granulocytes: Localization on the extracytoplasmic side of the plasma membrane and some properties. *Biochem Med Metab Biol* **40**:186, 1988.
199. Bayer PD, Vittori C, Sudaka P, Giudicelli J: Purification and properties of neutral maltase from human granulocytes. *Biochem J* **263**:647, 1989.
200. Noren O, Sijostrom H, Cowell GM, Jranum-Jensen J, Hansen OC, Welinder KG: Pig intestinal microvillar maltase-glucoamylase. *J Biol Chem* **261**:12306, 1986.
200a. Lukomskaya IS, Voznyi VY, Lanskaya IM, Podkidisheva EI: Use of β-maltosides (p-nitrophenyl-β-D-maltoside and 4-methylumbelliferyl-β-d-maltoside) as substrates for the assay of neutral alpha-glucosidase from human kidney and urine. *Clin Chim Acta* **244**:145, 1996.
201. Quaroni A, Semenza G: Partial amino acid sequences around the essential carboxylate in the active sites of the intestinal sucrase-isomaltase complex. *J Biol Chem* **11**:3250, 1976.
202. Hu C, Spiess M, Semenza G: The mode of anchoring and precursor forms of sucrase-isomaltase and maltase-glucoamylase in chicken intestinal brush-border membrane: Phylogenetic implications. *Biochim Biophys Acta* **896**:275, 1987.

203. Brown BI, Brown DH: The subcellular distribution of enzymes in Type II glycogenosis and the occurrence of an oligo alpha-1,4-glucan glucohydrolase in human tissues. *Biochim Biophys Acta* **110**:124, 1965.
204. Barnes AK, Wynn CH: Homology of lysosomal enzymes and related proteins: Prediction of posttranslational modification sites including phosphorylation of mannose and potential epitopic and substrate binding sites in the alpha- and beta-subunits of hexosaminidases, alpha-glucosidase, and rabbit and human isomaltase. *Protein Struct Funct Genet* **4**:182, 1988.
205. Chantret I, Lacasa M, Chevalier G, Ruf J, Islam I, Mantei N, Edwards Y, Swallow D, Rousset M: Sequence of the complete cDNA and the 5′ structure of the human sucrase-isomaltase gene. Possible homology with a yeast glucoamylase. *Biochem J* **285**:915, 1992.
206. Nichols BL, Eldering J, Avery S, Hahn D, Quaroni A, Sterchi E: Human small intestinal maltase-glucoamylase cDNA cloning. *J Biol Chem* **273**:3076, 1998.
207. Trombetta ES, Simons JF, Helenius A: Endoplasmic reticulum glucosidase II is composed of a catalytic subunit, conserved from yeast to mammals, and a tightly bound noncatalyic HDEL-containing subunit. *J Biol Chem* **271**:27509, 1996.
208. Flura T, Brada D, Ziak M, Roth J: Expression of a cDNA encoding the glucose trimming enzyme glucosidase II in CHO cells and molecular characterization of the enzyme deficiency in a mutant mouse lymphoma cell line. *Glycobiology* **7**:617, 1997.
209. Genbank accession numbers AJ000332 and KIAA0088.
210. Huie ML, Hirschhorn R: Computer-assisted cloning of neutral alpha glucosidase C. *Am J Hum Genet* **635**:1036A, 1998.
211. De Vries ACJ, Schram AW, Van Den Berg M, Tager JM, Batenburg JJ, Van Golde LMG: An improved procedure for the isolation of lamellar bodies from human lung. Lamellar bodies free of lysosomes contain a spectrum of lysosomal-type hydrolases. *Biochim Biophys Acta* **922**:259, 1987.
212. De Vries ACJ, Schram AW, Tager JM, Baternburg JJ, van Golde MG: A specific acid alpha-glucosidase in lamellar bodies of the human lung. *Biochim Biophys Acta* **837**:230, 1985.
213. Newgard CB, Norkiewicz B, Hughes SD, Frenkel RA, Coats WS, Martiniuk F, Johnston JM: Developmental expression of glycogenolytic enzymes in rabbit tissues: Possible relationship to fetal lung maturation. *Biochim Biophys Acta* **1090**:333, 1991.
214. Dohmen RJ, Strasser AW, Dahlems UM, Holleberg CP: Cloning of the Schwanniomyces occidentalis glucoamylase gene (GAM1) and its expression in Saccharomyces cerevisiae. *Gene* **95**:111, 1990.
215. Naim HY, Niermann T, Kleinhans U, Hollenberg CP, Strasser AWM: Striking structural and functional similarities suggest that intestinal sucrase-isomaltase, human lysosomal alpha glucosidase and Schwanniomyces occidentalis glucoamylase are derived from a common ancestral gene. *FEBS Lett* **294**:109, 1991.
216. Kinsella BT, Hogan S, Larkin A, Cantwell BA: Primary structure and processing of the Candida tsukubaensis alpha-glucosidase. Homology with the rabbit intestinal sucrase-isomaltase complex and human lysosomal alpha glucosidase. *Eur J Biochem* **202**:657, 1991.
217. Kimura A, Takata M, Sakai H, Matsui, Takai N, Takayanagi T, Nishimura I, Uozumi T, Chiba S: Complete amino acid sequence of crystalline alpha-glucosidase from *Aspergillus niger. Biosci Biotech Biochem* **56**:1368, 1992.
218. Parker GF, Roberts DB: AGI, a previously unreported *D. melanogaster* alpha-glucosidase: Partial purification, characterization, and cytogenetic mapping. *Biochem Genet* **3–4**:117, 1996.
219. Shariful Alam MD, Nakashima S, Deyashiki Y, Banno Y, Hara A, Nozawa Y: Molecular cloning of a gene encoding acid alpha-glucosidase from tetrahymena pyriformis. *J Eur Microbiol* **43**:295, 1996.
219a. Sugimoto M, Suzuki Y: Molecular cloning, sequencing, and expression of a cDNA encoding alpha-glucosidase from mucor javanicus. *J Biochem* **119**:500, 1996.
220. Alam S, Nakashima S, Deyashiki Y, Banno Y, Hara A, Nozawa Y: Molecular cloning of a gene encoding acid alpha-glucosidase from *Tetrahymena pyriformis*. *J Eukaryot Microbiol* **43**:295, 1996.
221. Tibbot BK, Skadsen RW: Molecular cloning and characterization of a giberellin-inducible, putative alpha-glucosidase gene from barley. *Plant Mol Biol* **30**:229, 1996.
222. Nakamura A, Nishimura I, Yokoyama A, Lee DG, Hikada M, Masaki H, Kimura A, Chiba S, Uozumi T: Cloning and sequencing of an alpha-glucosidase gene from *Aspergillus niger* and its expression in *A. nidulans*. *J Biotechnol* **53**:75, 1997.
223. Sugimoto M, Furui S, Suzuki Y: Molecular cloning and characterization of a cDNA encoding alpha-glucosidase from spinach. *Plant Mol Bio* **33**:765, 1997.
224. Matsui H, Iwanami S, Ito H, Honma M, Chiba S: Cloning and characterization of a cDNA encoding alpha-glucosidase from sugar beet. *Biosci Biotechnol Biochem* **61**:875, 1997.
225. Taylor MA, George LA, Ross HA, Davies HV: cDNA cloning and characterization of an alpha-glucosidase gene from potato (Solanum tuberosum L). *Plant J* **13**:419, 1998.
226. Frandsen TP, Svensson B: Plant alpha-glucosidases of the glycoside hydrolase family 31. Molecular properties, substrate specificity, reaction mechanism, and comparison with family members of different origin. *Plant Mol Biol* **37**:1, 1998.
227. Kunita R, Nakabayashi O, Wu JY, Hagiwara Y, Mizutani M, Pennybacker M, Chen YT, Kikuchi T: Molecular cloning of acid alpha-glucosidase cDNA of Japanese quail. *Biochim Biophys Acta* **1362**:269, 1997.
228. Ding JH, Yang BZ, Reuser AJJ, Roe CR: Cloning and sequence analysis of Mus Musculus acid alpha-glucosidase. SWISS-PROT accession number P70699, 1996.
229. Hirschhorn K, Nadler HL, Waithe WI, Brown BI, Hirschhorn R: Detection of heterozygotes for Pompe's disease by lymphocyte stimulation. *Science* **166**:1632, 1969.
230. Engel AG, Gomez MR: Acid maltase levels in muscle in heterozygous acid maltase deficiency and in non-weak and neuromuscular disease controls. *J Neurol Neurosurg Psychiatry* **33**:801, 1970.
231. Salafsky IS, Nadler HL: Alpha-1,4 glucosidase activity in Pompe's disease. *J Pediatr* **79**:794, 1971.
232. Salafsky IS, Nadler HL: A fluorometric assay of alpha-glucosidase and its application in the study of Pompe's disease. *J Lab Clin Med* **81**:450, 1972.
233. Angelini C, Engel AG: Comparative study of acid maltase deficiency: Biochemical differences between infantile, childhood, and adult types. *Arch Neurol* **26**:344, 1972.
234. Koster JF, Slee RG, Hulsmann WC: The use of leucocytes as an aid in the diagnosis of a variant of glycogen storage disease type II (Pompe's disease). *Eur J Clin Invest* **2**:467, 1972.
235. Kelleter R, Seiler D: Glycogen breakdown in human lymphocytes: Activities of phosphorylase and alpha-1-4 glucosidases. *Clin Chim Acta* **42**:57, 1972.
236. Koster JF, Slee RG, Hulsmann WC, Niermeijer MF: The electrophoretic pattern and activities of acid and neutral maltase of cultivated fibroblasts and amniotic fluid cells from controls and patients with the variant of glycogen storage disease type II (Pompe's disease). *Clin Chim Acta* **40**:294, 1972.
237. Angelini C, Engel AG: Comparative study of acid maltase deficiency: Biochemical differences between infantile, childhood, and adult types. *Arch Neurol* **26**:344, 1972.
238. Angelini C, Engel AG: Subcellular distribution of acid and neutral alpha-glucosidases in normal, acid maltase deficient, and myophosphorylase deficient human skeletal muscle. *Arch Biochem Biophys* **156**:350, 1973.
239. Angelini C, Engel AG, Titus JL: Adult acid maltase deficiency: Abnormalities in fibroblasts cultured from patients. *N Engl J Med* **287**:948, 1972.
240. Broadhead DM, Butterworth J: Pompe's disease: Diagnosis in kidney and leukocytes using 4-methylumbelliferyl-alpha-d-glucopyranoside. *Clin Genet* **13**:504,1978.
241. Salafsky IS, Nadler HL: Deficiency of acid alpha-glucosidase in the urine of patients with Pompe's disease. *J Pediatr* **82**:294, 1973.
242. Seiter CW, Summer GK: Glycogen metabolism in human skin fibroblasts. Influence of maltase on the activity of acid alpha-1,4,-glucosidase. *Proc Soc Exp Biol Med* **149**:945, 1975.
243. Koster JF, Slee RG, Van Der Klei-Van Moorsel JM, Rietra PJGM, Lucas CJ: Physico-chemical and immunological properties of acid alpha-glucosidase from various human tissues in relation to glycogenosis type II (Pompe's disease). *Clin Chim Acta* **68**:49, 1976.
244. Mehler M, DiMauro S: Late-onset acid maltase deficiency: Detection of patients and heterozygotes by urinary enzyme assay. *Arch Neurol* **33**:692, 1976.
245. Mehler M, DiMauro S: Residual acid maltase activity in late-onset acid maltase deficiency. *Neurology* **27**:178, 1977.
246. Soyama K, Ono E, Shimada N, Tanaka K, Kusunoki T: Urinary alpha-glucosidase analysis for the detection of the adult form of Pompe's disease. *Clin Chim Acta* **77**:61, 1977.

247. Butterworth J, Broadhead DM: Diagnosis of Pompe's disease in cultured skin fibroblasts and primary amniotic fluid cells using 4-methylumbelliferyl-alpha-d-glucopyranoside as substrate. *Clin Chim Acta* **78**:335, 1977.
248. Broadhead DM, Butterworth J: Alpha-glucosidase in Pompe's disease. *J Inherit Metab Dis* **1**:153, 1978.
249. Bienvenu J, Carrier H, Freycon F, Mathieu M: Heterogeneite de la glycogenose par deficit en alpha-1,4-glucosidase: Etude enzymatique dans trois families. *Clin Chim Acta* **84**:277, 1978.
250. Reuser AJJ, Koster JF, Hoogeveen A, Galjaard H: Biochemical, immunological, and cell genetic studies in glycogenosis type II. *Am J Hum Genet* **30**:132, 1978.
250a. Ausems MGEM, Lochman P, Van Diggelen OP, Ploos van Amstel HK, Reuser AJJ, Wokke JHJ: A diagnostic protocol for adult-onset glycogen storage disease type II. *Neurology* **52**:851, 1999.
251. De Barsy T, Ferriere F, Fernandez-Alvarez E: Uncommon case of type II glycogenosis. *Acta Neuropathol (Berl)* **47**:245, 1979.
252. Bienvenu J, Mathieu M: Immunochemical studies of human acid alpha-1,4-glucosidase in type II glycogenosis. *Enzyme* **26**:182, 1981.
253. Loonen MCB, Schram AW, Koster JF, Niermeijer MF, Busch HFM, Martin JJ, Brouwer-Kelder B, Mekes W, Slee RG, Tager JM: Identification of heterozygotes for glycogenosis 2 (acid maltase deficiency). *Clin Genet* **19**:55, 1981.
254. Steckel F, Gieselmann V, Waheed A, Hasilik A, Von Figura K, Oude Elferink RPJ, Kalsbeek R, Tager JM: Biosynthesis of acid alpha-glucosidase in late-onset forms of glycogenosis type II (Pompe's disease). *FEBS Lett* **150**:69, 1982.
255. Reuser AJJ, Kroos M: Adult forms of glycogenosis type II: A defect in an early stage of acid alpha-glucosidase realization. *FEBS Lett* **146**:361, 1982.
256. Miranda AF, Shanske S, Hays AP, DiMauro S: Immunocytochemical analysis of normal and acid maltase-deficient muscle cultures. *Arch Neurol* **42**:371, 1985.
257. Reuser AJJ, Kroos M, Oude Elferink RPJ, Tager JM: Defects in synthesis, phosphorylation, and maturation of acid alpha-glucosidase in glycogenosis type II. *J Biol Chem* **260**:8336, 1985.
258. Kuriyama M, Kohriyama T, Iwamasa T, Hiwatari R, Osame M, Igata A: Lymphocyte alpha-glucosidase in late-onset glycogenosis type II. *Arch Neurol* **46**:460, 1989.
259. Kohriyama T, Kuriyama M, Hiwatari R, Osame M, Igata A: Partial characterization of leucocyte alpha-glucosidase in late onset glycogenosis type II. *Tohoku J Exp Med* **157**:355, 1989.
260. Kuriyama M, Hiwatari RI, Osame M, Igata A: Leucocyte alpha-1,4- and alpha-1, 6-glucosidase activities towards oligosaccharides in late onset glycogenosis type II. *Tohoku J Exp Med* **161**:343, 1990.
261. Shin YS, Endres W, Unterreithmeier J, Rieth M, Schaub J: Diagnosis of Pompe's disease using leukocyte preparations. Kinetic and immunological studies of 1,4-alpha-glucosidase in human fetal and adult tissues and cultured cells. *Clin Chim Acta* **148**:9, 1985.
262. Ninomiya N, Matsuda I, Matsuoka T, Iwamasa T, Nonaka I: Demonstration of acid alpha-glucosidase in different types of Pompe disease by use of an immunochemical method. *J Neurol Sci* **66**:129, 1984.
263. Henkel RD, Dreesman GR, Kennedy RC, Howell RR, Williams JC: Detection of human acid alpha-glucosidase in fibroblasts using monoclonal antibodies in a biotin-avidin amplified ELISA. *Hybridoma* **4**:351, 1985.
264. Iwamasa T, Nashiro K, Ohshita T, Matsuda I: Subcellular distribution of acid alpha-glucosidase in fibroblasts and of antigenically cross-reactive material in Pompe's disease fibroblasts. *Histochem J* **18**:613, 1986.
265. Reuser AJJ, Kroos M, Willemsen R, Swallow D, Tager JM, Galjaard H: Clinical diversity in glycogenosis type II: Biosynthesis and in situ localization of acid alpha-glucosidase in mutant fibroblasts. *J Clin Invest* **79**:1689, 1987.
266. TagerJM, Oude Elferink RPJ, Reuser A, Kroos MA, Ginsel LA, Fransen JAM, Klumperman J: Alpha-glucosidase deficiency (Pompe's disease). *Enzyme* **38**:280, 1987.
267. Tsuji A, Yang RC, Omura K, Imabayashi T, Suzuki Y: A simple differential immunoprecipitation assay of urinary acid and neutral alpha-glucosidases for glycogenosis II. *Clin Chim Acta* **167**:313, 1987.
268. Van der Ploeg AT, Kroos MA, Van Dongen J, Visser WJ, Bolhuis PA, Loonen MCB, Reuser AJJ: Breakdown of lysosomal glycogen in cultured fibroblasts from glycogenosis type II patients after uptake of acid alpha-glucosidase. *J Neurol Sci* **79**:327, 1987.
269. Usuki F, Ishiura S, Nonaka I, Sugita H: Alpha-glucosidase isoenzymes in normal and acid maltase-deficient human skeletal muscles. *Muscle Nerve* **2**:365, 1988.
270. Van der Ploeg AT, Bolhuis PA, Wolterman RA, Visser JW, Loonen MCB, Busch HFM, Reuser AJJ: Prospect for enzyme therapy in glycogenosis II variants: a study on cultured muscle cells. *J Neurol* **235**:392, 1988.
271. Nishimoto J, Inui K, Okada S, Ishigami W, Hirota S, Yamano T, Yabuuchi H: A family with pseudodeficiency of acid alpha-glucosidase. *Clin Genet* **33**:254, 1988.
272. Willemsen R, Van der Ploeg AT, Busch HFM, Zondervan PE, Van Noorden CJ, Reuser AJJ: Synthesis and in situ localization of lysosomal alpha-glucosidase in muscle of an unusual variant of glycogen storage disease type II. *Ultrastruct Pathol* **17**:515, 1993.
273. Lin C, Lee S, Chang Z, Su S, Hwang B, Han S: Preparation of monoclonal antibodies against acid alpha-glucosidase for study of Chinese glycogenosis type II patients. *Hybridoma* **11**:493, 1992.
274. Wolfe HJ, Cohen RB: Nonglycogen polysaccharide storage in glycogenosis type 2. *Arch Pathol* **86**:579, 1968.
275. Lennartson G, Lundblad A, Lundsten J, Svensson S, Hager A: Glucose-containing oligosaccharides in the urine of patients with glycogen storage disease type II and type III. *Eur J Biochem* **83**:325, 1978.
276. Blom W, Luteyn JC, Kelhot-Dijkman HH, Huijmans JGH, Loonen MCB: Thin-layer chromatography oligosaccharides in urine as a rapid indication for the diagnosis of lysosomal acid maltase deficiency (Pompe's disease). *Clin Chim Acta* **134**:221, 1983.
277. Kuriyama M, Hiwatari R, Ariga T, Sakano Y, Abe J, Osame M, Igata A: Neutral oligosaccharides in the urine of a patient with glycogen storage disease type II. *J Biochem* **98**:1041, 1985.
278. Giros ML, Alvarez L: Hepatic glycogenosis with defects in the glycogen breakdown pathway: Urinary oligosaccharide profile. *J Inherit Metab Dis* **14**:311, 1991.
279. Jay V, Christodoulou J, Mercer-Connolly A, McInnes RR: "Reducing body"-like inclusions in skeletal muscle in childhood-onset acid maltase deficiency. *Acta Neurophathol (Berl)* **85**:111, 1992.
280. Solomon E, Swallow D, Burgess S, Evans L: Assignment of the human acid alpha-glucosidase gene to chromosome 17 using somatic cell hybrids. *Ann Hum Genet* **42**:273, 1979.
281. Weil D, Van Cong N, Gross M-S, Frezal J: Localisation du gene de l'alpha-glucosidase acide (alpha-GLU) sur le segment q21-qter du chromosome 17 par l'hybridation cellulaire interspecifique. *Hum Genet* **52**:249, 1979.
282. D'Ancona GG, Wurm J, Croce CM: Genetics of type II glycogenosis: Assignment of the human gene for acid alpha-glucosidase to chromosome 17. *Proc Natl Acad Sci U S A* **76**:4526, 1979.
283. Solomon E, Barker DF: Report of the committee on the genetic constitution of chromosome 17. *Cytogenet Cell Genet* **51**:319, 1989.
284. Halley DJJ, Konings A, Hupkes P, Galjaard H: Regional mapping of the human gene for lysosomal alpha-glucosidase by in situ hybridization. *Hum Genet* **67**:326, 1984.
285. De Jonge AJ, De Smit S, Kroos MA, Reuser AJJ: Cotransfer of syntenic human genes into mouse cells using isolated metaphase chromosomes or cellular DNA. *Hum Genet* **69**:32, 1985.
286. Martiniuk F, Hirschhorn R, D'Eustachio P: Linkage of acid alpha-glucosidase (GAA) and thymidine kinase (Tk-1) to esterase-3 (Es-3) on mouse chromosome 11. *Mamm Genome* **1**:267, 1991.
287. Haines JL, Ozelius LJ, McFarlane H, Menon A, Tzall S, Martiniuk F, Hirschhorn R, Gusella JF: A genetic linkage map of chromosome 17. *Genomics* **8**:1, 1990.
288. Kuo WL, Hirschhorn R, Huie ML, Lau C, Hirschhorn K: Localization and ordering of acid alpha-glucosidase (GAA) and thymidine kinase (TK1) by fluorescence *in situ* hybridization. *Hum Genet* **97**:404, 1996.
289. Nickel BE, McAlpine PJ: Extension of human acid alpha-glucosidase polymorphism by isoelectric focusing in polyacrylamide gel. *Ann Hum Genet* **46**:97, 1982.
290. Beratis NG, LaBadie GU, Hirschhorn K: An isozyme of acid alpha-glucosidase with reduced catalytic activity for glycogen. *Am J Hum Genet* **32**:137, 1980.
291. Swallow DM, Kroos M, Van der Ploeg AT, Griffiths B, Islam I, Marenah CB, Reuser AJJ: An investigation of the properties and possible clinical significance of the lysosomal alpha-glucosidase GAA2 allele. *Ann Hum Genet* **53**:177, 1989.
292. Martiniuk F, Bodkin M, Tzall S, Hirschhorn R: Identification of the base pair change responsible for a human acid alpha glucosidase allele with lower "affinity" for glycogen (GAA2) and transient gene expression in deficient cells. *Am J Hum Genet* **47**:440, 1990.

293. Huie ML, Menaker M, McAlpine PJ, Hirschhorn R: Identification of an E689K substitution as the molecular basis of the human acid alpha glucosidase type 4 allozyme (GAA*4). *Annal Hum Genet* **60**:365, 1996.
294. Teng YS, Tan SG: Acid alpha-glucosidase in Malaysians: Population studies and the occurrence of a new variant. *Hum Hered* **29**:2, 1979.
295. Tzall S, Martiniuk F, Hirschhorn R: Further characterization of Sac I RFLPs at the acid alpha glucosidase (GAA) locus. *Nucleic Acids Res* **18**:1930, 1990.
296. Tzall S, Martiniuk F, Adler A, Hirschhorn R: Identification of an *Rsa*I RFLP at the acid alpha glucosidase (GAA) locus. *Nucleic Acids Res* **18**:1661, 1990.
297. Tzall S, Martiniuk F, Ozelius L, Gusella J, Hirschhorn R: Further characterization of *Pst*I RFLPs at the acid alpha glucosidase (GAA) locus. *Nucleic Acids Res* **19**:1727, 1991.
298. Tzall S, Martiniuk F, Hirschhorn R: Identification of *Taq*I and *Hind*III RFLPs at the acid alpha glucosidase (GAA) locus. *Nucleic Acids Res* **19**:1727, 1991.
299. Hoefsloot LH, Hoogeveen-Westerveld M, Oostra BA, Reuser AJJ: An XbaI restriction site polymorphism in the acid alpha glucosidase gene (GAA). *Nucleic Acids Res* **19**:682, 1991.
300. Martiniuk F, Mehler M, Tzall S, Meredith G, Hirschhorn R: Extensive genetic heterogeneity in patients with acid alpha glucosidase deficiency as detected by abnormalities of DNA and mRNA. *Am J Hum Genet* **47**:73, 1990.
301. Van der Ploeg AT, Hoefsloot LH, Hoogeveen-Westerveld M, Petersen EM, Reuser AJJ: Glycogenosis type II: Protein and DNA analysis in five South African families from various ethnic origins. *Am J Hum Genet* **44**:787, 1989.
302. Martiniuk F, Mehler M, Bodkin M, Tzall S, Hirschhorn K, Zhong N, Hirschhorn R: Identification of the mutation from an adult onset patient with glycogenosis type II expressing only one allele. *DNA Cell Biol* **10**:681, 1991.
303. Hermans MMP, de Graaff E, Kroos MA, Wisselaar HA, Oostra BA, Reuser AJJ: Identification of a point mutation in the human lysosomal alpha glucosidase gene causing infantile glycogenosis Type II. *Biochem Biophys Res Commun* **179**:919, 1991.
304. Zhong N, Martiniuk F, Tzall S, Hirschhorn R: Identification of a missense mutation in one allele of a patient with Pompe's disease and use of endonuclease digestion of PCR amplified RNA to demonstrate lack of mRNA expression from the second allele. *Am J Hum Genet* **49**:635, 1991.
305. Hermans MMP, de Graaff E, Kroos MA, Wisselaar HA, Willemsen R, Oostra BA, Reuser AJJ: The conservative substitution Asp645Glu in lysosomal alpha glucosidase affects transport and phosphorylation of the enzyme in an adult patient with glycogen-storage disease type II. *Biochem J* **289**:687,1993.
306. Hermans MMP, Kroos MA, deGraaff E, Oostra BA, Reuser AJJ: Two mutations affecting the transport and maturation of lysosomal alpha-glucosidase in an adult case of glycogen storage disease type II. *Hum Mutat* **2**:268,1993.
307. Hermans MMP, Svetkey LP, Oostra BA, Chen YT, Reuser AJJ: The loss of a polymorphic glycosylation site caused by Thr-927 → Ile is linked to a second polymorphic Val-816 → Ile substitution in lysosomal alpha-glucosidase of American Blacks. *Genomics* **16**:300, 1993.
308. Shieh JJ, Wang LY, Lin Cy: Point mutation in Pompe disease in Chinese. *J Inherit Metab Dis* **17**:145, 1994.
309. Hermans MMP, De Graaf E, Kroos MA, Mohkamsing S, Eussen BJ, Joosse M, Willemsen R, Kleijer WJ, Oostra BA, Reuser AJJ: The effect of a single base pair deletion (del T525) and a C1634T missense mutation (pro545leu) on the expression of lysosomal alpha-glucosidase in patients with glycogen storage disease type II. *Hum Mol Genet* **12**:2213, 1994.
310. Huie ML, Chen A, Grix A, Sklower-Brooks S, Hirschhorn R: A de novo 13 nt deletion, a missense mutation and a deletion of exon 18 in two patients with infantile onset GSD II. *Hum Mol Genet* **3**:1081, 1994.
311. Huie ML, Chen AS, Tsujino S, Shanske S, DiMauro S, Engel AG, Hirschhorn R: Aberrant splicing in adult onset glycogen storage disease type II (GSDII): Molecular identification of an IVS1 (−13T6G) mutation in a majority of patients and a novel IVS10 (+1GT6CT) mutation. *Hum Mol Genet* **3**:2231, 1994.
312. Huie ML, Hirschhorn R, Chen A, Martiniuk F, Zhong N: A mutation at the catalytic site (M519V) in glycogen storage disease type II (Pompe's disease). *Hum Mutat* **4**:291, 1994.
313. Boerkoel CF, Exelbert R, Nicastri C, Nichols RC, Miller FW, Plotz PH, Raben, N: Leaky splicing mutation in the acid maltase gene is associated with delayed onset of glycogenosis type II. *Am J Hum Genet* **56**:887, 1995.
314. Lin CY, Shieh JJ: Identification of a de novo point mutation resulting in infantile form of Pompe disease. *Biochem Biophys Res Commun* **208**:886, 1995.
315. Wokke JHJ, Ausems MGEM, Van den Boogaard MJH, Ippel EF, Van Diggelsen O, Kroos MA, Boer M, Jennekens FGI, Reuser AJJ, van Amstel HKP: Genotype-phenotype correlation in adult-onset acid maltase deficiency. *Ann Neurol* **38**:450, 1995.
316. Van der Kraan M, Kroos MA, Joosse M, Bijvoet AGA, Verbeet MP, Kleijer WJ, Reuser AJJ: Deletion of exon 18 is a frequent mutation in glycogen storage disease type II. *Biochem Biophys Res Commun* **203**:1535, 1994.
317. Kroos MA, Van Der Kraan M, Van Diggelen OP, Kleijer WP, Reuser AJJ, et al.: Glycogen storage disease type II: Frequency of three common mutant alleles and their associated clinical phenotypes studied in 121 patients. *Med Genet* **32**:836, 1995.
318. Ausems MGEM, Kroos MA, Van Kraan M, Smeitink JAM, Kleijer WJ, HK Ploos van Amstel, Reuser AJJ: Homozygous deletion of exon 18 leads to degradation of the lysosomal acid alpha-glucosidase precursor and to the infantile form of glycogen storage disease type II. *Clin Genet* **49**:325, 1996.
319. Tsunoda H, Ohshima T, Tohyama J, Sasaki M, Sakuragawa N, Martiniuk F: Acid alpha-glucosidase deficiency: Identification and expression of a missense mutation (S529V) in a Japanese adult phenotype. *Hum Genet* **97**:496, 1996.
320. Shieh J-J, Lin C-Y: Identification of a small deletion in one allele of patients with infantile form of glycogen storage disease type II. *Biochem Biophys Res Commun* **219**:322, 1996.
321. Raben N, Nichols RC, Martiniuk F, Plotz PH: A model of mRNA splicing in adult lysosomal storage disease (glycogenosis type II). *Hum Mol Genet* **5**:995, 1996.
322. Adams EM, Becker JA, Griffith, Segal A, Plotz PH, Raben N: Glycogenosis Type II: A juvenile-specific mutation with an unusual splicing pattern and a shared mutation in African Americans. *Hum Mutat* **10**:128, 1997.
323. Beesley CE, Child AH, Yacoub MY: The identification of five novel mutations in the lysosomal acid alpha-(1,4)-glucosidase gene from patients with glycogen storage disease type II. *Hum Mutat* **11**:413, 1998.
324. Hermans MMP, van Leenen D, Kroos D, Reuser AJJ: Mutation detection in glycogen storage disease type II by RT-PCR and automated sequencing. *Biochem Biophys Res Commun* **241**:414, 1997.
325. Kroos MA, Waitfield AE, Joosse M, Winchester B, Reuser AJJ, MacDermot KD: A novel acid alpha-glucosidase mutation identified in a Pakistani family with glycogen storage disease type II. *J Inherit Metab Dis* **20**:556, 1997.
326. Nicolino M, Puech JP, Letourneur F, Fardeau M, Kahn A, Poenaru L: Glycogen storage disease type II (acid maltase deficiency): Identification of a novel small deletion (delCC482+483) in French patients. *Biochem Biophys Res Commun* **235**:138, 1997.
327. Kroos MA, van Leenen D, Verbiest J, Reuser AJ, Hermans MM: Glycogen storage disease type II: Identification of a dinucleotide deletion and a common missense mutation in the lysosomal alpha-glucosidase gene. *Clin Genet* **53**:379, 1998.
328. Huie ML, Tsujino S, Sklower Brooks S, Engel A, Elias E, Bonthron DT, Beesley C, Shanske S, DiMauro S, Goto YI, Hirschhorn R: Glycogen storage disease type II: Identification of four novel missense mutations (D645N, G648S, R672W, R672Q) and two insertions/deletions in the acid-glucosidase locus of patients of differing phenotype. *Biochem Biophys Res Commun* **244**:921, 1998.
329. Hermans MMP, Kroos MA, Smeitink JAM, van der Ploeg AT, Kleijer WJ, Reuser AJJ: glycogen storage disease type II: Genetic and biochemical analysis of novel mutations in infantile patients from Turkish ancestry. *Hum Mutat* **11**:209, 1998.
329a. Vorgerd M, Burwinkel B, Reichmann H, Malin JP, Kilimann MF: Adult-onset glycogen storage disease type II: Phenotypic and allelic heterogeneity in German patients. *Neurogenetics* **1**:205, 1998.
330. Becker JA, Vlach J, Raben N, Nagaraju, Adams EM, Hermans MM, Reuser AJJ, Books SS, Tiffit CJ, Hirschhorn R, Huie ML, Nicolino M, Plotz PH: The African origin of the common mutation in African-American patients with glycogen storage disease type II (GSDII). *Am J Hum Genet* **62**:991, 1998.
331. Shieh J-J, Lin C-Y: Frequent mutation in Chinese patients with infantile type of GSDII in Taiwan: Evidence for a founder effect. *Hum Mutat* **11**:306, 1998.

332. Hirschhorn R, Huie ML: Frequency of mutations for glycogen storage disease type II in different populations: The del525T and delexon18 mutations are not generally "common" in Caucasian populations. *J Med Genet* **36**:85, 1999.
333. Raben N, Lee E, Lee L, Hirschhorn R, Plotz P: Novel mutations in African American patients with Pompe disease. *Hum Mutat Mutation In Brief 209 Online*, 1998.
334. Huie ML, Shanske AL, Kasper JS, Marion RW, Hirschhorn R: A large Alu-mediated deletion identified by PCR, as the molecular basis for glycogen storage disease type II (GSDII). *Hum Genet* **104**:94, 1999.
335. Huie ML, Kasper JS, Arn PH, Greenberg CR, Hirschhorn R: Increased occurrence of cleft lip in glycogen storage disease type II (GSDII): Exclusion of a contiguous gene syndrome in two patients by presence of intragenic mutations (including a novel nonsense mutation Gln58Stop). *Am J Med Genet*, **85**:5, 1999.
336. Nadler HL: Patterns of enzyme development using cultivated human fetal cells from amniotic fluid. *Biochem Genet* **2**:119, 1968.
337. Nadler HL, Messina AM: In utero detection of type-II glycogenosis (Pompe's disease). *Lancet* **2**:1277, 1969.
338. Cox RP, Douglas G, Hutzler J, Lynfield J, Dancis J: In utero detection of Pompe's disease. *Lancet* **1**:893, 1970.
339. Nadler HL, Bigley RH, Hug G: Prenatal detection of Pompe's disease. *Lancet* **2**:369, 1970.
340. Hug G, Schubert WK, Soukup S: Prenatal diagnosis of type II glycogenosis. *Lancet* **1**:1002, 1970.
341. Hug G, Soukup S, Ryan M, Chuck G: Rapid prenatal diagnosis of glycogen-storage disease type II by electron microscopy of uncultured amniotic fluid cells. *N Engl J Med* **310**:1018, 1984.
342. Niermeijer MF, Koster JF, Jahodova M, Fernandes J, Heukels-Dully MJ, Galjaard H: Prenatal diagnosis of type II glycogenosis (Pompe's disease) using microchemical analyses. *Pediatr Res* **9**:498, 1975.
343. Fensom AH, Benson PF, Blunt S, Brown SP, Coltart TM: Amniotic cell 4-methylumbelliferyl alpha-glucosidase activity for prenatal diagnosis of Pompe's disease. *J Med Genet* **13**:148, 1976.
344. Besancon AM, Castelnau L, Nicolesco H, Dumez Y, Poenaru L: Prenatal diagnosis of glycogenosis type II (Pompe's disease) using chorionic villi biopsy. *Clin Genet* **27**:479, 1985.
345. Grubisic A, Shin YS, Meyer W, Endres W, Becker U, Wischerath H: First trimester diagnosis of Pompe's disease (glycogenosis type II) with normal outcome: Assay of acid alpha-glucosidase in chorionic villous biopsy using antibodies. *Clin Genet* **30**:398, 1986.
346. Shin YS, Rieth M, Tausenfreund J, Endres W: First trimester diagnosis of glycogen storage disease Type II and Type III. *J Inherit Metab Dis* **12(Suppl 2)**:289, 1989.
347. Hug G, Chen Y-T, Kay HH, Bossen EH: Chorionic villus ultrastructure in Type II glycogen storage disease (Pompe's disease). *N Engl J Med* **324**:342, 1991.
348. Wei C, Yeh G, Chen H, Wang L, Lin C: Enzyme inhibitory assay using monoclonal antibody against acid alpha-D-glucosidase in prenatal diagnosis to identify homozygotes of Pompe's disease. *Acta Paediatr* **33**:104, 1992.
349. Park HK, Kay HH, McConkie-Rosell A, Lanman J, Chen Y-T: Prenatal diagnosis of Pompe's disease (type II glycogenosis) in chorionic villus biopsy using maltose as a substrate. *Prenat Diagn* **12**:169, 1992.
350. Minelli A, Piantanida M, Simoni G, Rossella F, Romitti L, Brambati B, Danesino D: Prenatal diagnosis of metabolic diseases on chorionic villi obtained before the ninth week of pregnancy. *Prenat Diagn* **12**:959, 1992.
351. Kleijer WJ, Van der Kraan M, Kroos MA, Groener JE, Van Diggelen OP, Reuser AJJ, Van der Ploeg AT: Prenatal diagnosis of glycogen storage disease type II: Enzyme assay or mutation analysis? *Pediatr Res* **38**:103, 1995.
352. Bodamer OAF, Leonard JV, Halliday D: Dietary treatment in late-onset acid maltase deficiency. *Eur J Pediatr* **156**:S39, 1997.
353. Slonim AE, Coleman RA, McElligot MA, Najjar J, Hirschhorn K, Labadie GU, Mrak R, Evans OB, Shipp E, Presson R: Improvement of muscle function in acid maltase deficiency by high-protein therapy. *Neurology* **33**:34, 1983.
354. Margolis ML, Hill R: Acid maltase deficiency in an adult (evidence for improvement in respiratory function with high-protein dietary therapy). *Am Rev Respir Dis* **134**:328, 1986.
355. Umpleby AM, Wiles CM, Trend PS, Scobie IN, Macleod AF, Spencer GT, Sonksen PH: Protein turnover in acid maltase deficiency before and after treatment with a high protein diet. *J Neurol Neurosurg Psychiatry* **50**:587, 1987.
356. Demey HE, Van Meerbeeck JP, Vandewoude MFJ, Prove AM, Martin JJ, Bossaert LL: Respiratory insufficiency in acid maltase deficiency: The effect of high protein diet. *J Parenter Enter Nutr* **13**:321, 1989.
357. Padberg GW, Wintzen AR, Giesberts MAH, Sterk PJ, Molenaar AJ, Hermans J: Effects of high-protein diet in acid maltase deficiency. *J Neurol Sci* **90**:111, 1989.
358. Umpleby AM, Trend PS, Chubb D, Conaglen JV, Williams CD, Hesp R, Scobie IN, Wiles CM, Spencer G, Sonksen PH: The effect of a high protein diet on leucine and alanine turnover in acid maltase deficiency. *J Neurol Neurosurg Psychiatry* **52**:954, 1989.
359. Mobarhan S, Pintozzi RL, Damle P, Friedman H: Treatment of acid maltase deficiency with a diet high in branched chain amino acids. *J Parenter Enter Nutr* **14**:210, 1990.
360. Ferrer X, Coquet M, Saintarailles J, Ellie E, Deleplanque B, Desnuelle C, Levade T, Lagueny A, Julien J: Myopathy in adults caused by acid maltase deficiency. A trial of treatment with high protein diet. *Rev Med Interne* **13**:149, 1992.
361. Hug J, Schubert WK: Lysosomes in type II glycogenosis. Changes during administration of extract from *Aspergillus niger*. *J Cell Biol* **35**:C1, 1967.
362. Lauer RM, Mascarinas T, Racela AS, Diehl AM, Brown BI: Administration of a mixture of fungal glucosidases to a patient with type II glycogenosis (Pompe's disease). *Pediatrics* **42**:672, 1968.
363. De Barsy T, Jacquemin P, Van Hoof F, Hers HG: Enzyme replacement in Pompe's disease: An attempt with purified human alpha glucosidase, in Desnick RJ, Bernlohr R, Krivit W (eds): *Enzyme Therapy in Genetic Diseases*. Baltimore, MD, Williams & Wilkins, 1973, p 184.
364. Di Marco PN, Howell JM, Dorling PR: Bovine glycogenosis type II. Uptake of lysosomal alpha-glucosidase by cultured skeletal muscle and reversal of glycogen accumulation. *FEBS Lett* **190**:301, 1985.
365. Howell JM, Di Marco PN, Dorling PR: Enzyme replacement therapy in muscle cultures: Bovine generalised glycogenosis type II. *Muscle Nerve* **9(5S)**:187, 1986.
366. Van Der Ploeg AT, Bolhuis PA, Wolterman RA, Visser JW, Loonen MCB, Busch HFM, Reuser AJJ: Prospect for enzyme therapy in glycogenosis II variants: A study on cultured muscle cells. *J Neurol* **235**:392, 1988.
367. Reuser AJ, Kroos MA, Ponne NJ, Wolterman R, Loonen M, Busch, HF, Visser WJ, Bolhuis PA: Uptake and stability of human and bovine acid alpha-glucosidase in cultured fibroblasts and skeletal muscle cells from glycogenosis type II patients. *Exp Cell Res* **155**:178, 1984.
368. Van der Ploeg AT, Loonen MCB, Bolhuis PA, Busch HMF, Reuser AJJ, Galjaard H: Receptor-mediated uptake of acid alpha-glucosidase corrects lysosomal glycogen storage in cultured skeletal muscle. *Pediatr Res* **24**:90, 1988.
369. Yang HW, Kikuchi T, Hagiwara Y, Mizutani M, Chen Y-T, Van Hove JLK: Recombinant human acid alpha-glucosidase corrects acid alpha-glucosidase-deficient human fibroblasts, quail fibroblast, and quail myoblasts. *Pediatr Res* **43**:374, 1998.
370. Van der Ploeg AT, Van Der Kraaij AMM, Willemsen R, Kroos MA, Loonen MCB, Koster JF, Reuser AJJ: Rat heart perfusion as model system for enzyme replacement therapy in glycogenosis type II. *Pediatr Res* **28**:344, 1988.
371. Van der Ploeg AT, Kroos MA, Willemsen R, Brons NHC, Reuser AJJ: Intravenous administration of phosphorylated acid alpha-glucosidase leads to uptake of enzyme in heart and skeletal muscle of mice. *J Clin Invest* **87**:513, 1991.
372. Willemsen R, Wisselaar HA, Van der Ploeg AT: Plasmalemmal vesicles are involved in transendothelial transport of albumin, lysosomal enzymes and mannose-6-phosphate receptor fragments in capillary endothelium. *Eur J Cell Biol* **51**:235, 1990.
373. Bijvoet AGA, Van Hirtum H, Kroos MA, Van de Kamp EHM, Schoneveld O, Visser P, Brakenhoff JPJ, Weggeman M, Van Corven EJ, Van der Ploeg AT, Reuser AJJ: Human acid α-glucosidase from rabbit milk has therapeutic effect in mice with glycogen storage disease type II. *Hum Mol Genet* **8**:2145, 1999.
374. Kikuchi T, Wen Yang H, Pennybacker M, Ichihara N, Mizutani M, Van Hove JLK, Chen Y-T: Clinical and metabolic correction of Pompe disease by enzyme therapy in acid maltase-deficient quail. *J Clin Invest* **101**:827, 1998.
375. Zaretsky JZ, Candotti F, Boerkoel C, Adams EM, Yewdell JW, Blaese MR, Plotz PH: Retroviral transfer of acid alpha-glucosidase cDNA to enzyme-deficient myoblasts results in phenotypic spread of the genotypic correction by both secretion and fusion. *Hum Gene Ther* **8**:1555, 1997.

376. Pauly DF, Matelis LA, Lawrence JH, Byrne BJ, Kessler PD: Complete correction of acid alpha-glucosidase deficiency in Pompe disease fibroblasts in vitro, and lysosomally targetted expression in neonatal rat cardiac and skeletal muscle. *Gene Ther* **5**:473, 1998.
377. Nicolino MP, Puech J-P, Kremer EJ, Reuser AJJ, Mbebi C, Verdiere-Sahuque M, Kahn A, Poenaru L: Adenovirus-mediated transfer of acid alpha-glucosidase gene into fibroblasts from patients with glycogen storage disease type II leads to high level expression of enzyme and corrects glycogen accumulation. *Hum Mol Genet* **7**:1695, 1998.
378. Tsjunino S, Kinoshita N, Tashiro T, Ikeda K, Ichihara N, Kikuchi H, Hagiwara Y, Mizutani M, Kikuchi T, Sakuragawa N: Adenovirus-mediated transfer of human acid maltase gene reduces glycogen acccumulation in skeletal musscle of Japanese quail with acid maltase deficiency. *Hum Gene Ther* **9**:1609, 1998.
378a. Amalfitano A, McVie-Wylie AJ, Hu H, Dawson TL, Raben N, Plotz P, Chen YT: Systemic correction of the muscle disorder glycogen storage disease type II after hepatic targeting of a modified adenovirus vector encoding human acid α-glucosidase. *Proc Natl Acad Sci U S A* **96**:8861, 1999.
379. Ryman BE, Jewkes RF, Jeyasingh K: Potential applications of liposomes to therapy. *Ann N Y Acad Sci* **308**:281, 1978.
380. Williams JC, Murray AK: Enzyme replacement in Pompe disease with an alpha glucosidase low-density lipoprotein complex, in Desnick RJ (ed): *Enzyme Therapy in Genetic Diseases*:2 New York, Alan R. Liss, 1980, p 415.
381. Watson JG, Gardner-Medwin D, Goldfinch ME, Pearson ADJ: Bone marrow transplantation for glycogen storage disease type II (Pompe's disease). *N Engl J Med* **314**:385, 1986.
382. Hoogerbrug PM, Wagemaker G, van Bekkum DW, Reuser AJJ, Van der Ploeg AT: Bone marrow transplantation for Pompe's disease. *N Engl J Med* **315**:65, 1986.
383. Howell JM, Dorling PR, Shelton JN, Taylor EG, Palmer DG, Di Marco PN: Natural bone marrow transplantation in cattle with Pompe's disease. *Neuromusc Disord* **6**:449, 1991.
384. Walvoort HC: Glycogen storage diseases in animals and their potential value as models of human disease. *J Inherit Metab Dis* **55**:3, 1983.
385. Walvoort HC, Slee RG, Koster JF: Canine glycogen storage disease type II. A biochemical study of an acid alpha-glucosidase-deficient Lapland dog. *Biochim Biophys Acta* **715**:63, 1982.
386. Walvoort HC, Dormans JAMA, van den Ingh TSGAM: Comparative pathology of the canine model of glycogen storage disease type II (Pompe's disease). *J Inherit Metab Dis* **8**:38, 1985.
387. Nunoya T, Tajima M, Mizutani M: A new mutant of Japanese quail (*Coturnix coturnix japonica*) characterized by generalized glycogenosis. *Lab Anim* **17**:138, 1983.
388. Higuchi I, Nonaka I, Usuki F, Ishiura S, Sugita H: Acid maltase deficiency in the Japanese quail: Early morphological event in skeletal muscle. *Acta Neuropathol (Berl)* **73**:32, 1987.
389. Usuki F, Ishiura S, Higuchi I, Sugita H: Reappearance of embryonic neutral alpha-glucosidase isoenzyme in acid maltase-deficient muscle of Japanese quail. *Exp Neurol* **100**:394, 1988.
390. Suhara Y, Ishiura S, Tsukahara T, Sugita H: Mature 98,000-dalton acid alpha glucosidase is deficient in Japanese quails with acid maltase deficiency. *Muscle Nerve* **12**:670, 1989.
391. Fujita T, Nonaka I, Sugita H: Japanese quail and human acid maltase deficiency: A comparative study. *Brain Dev* **13**:247, 1991.
392. Richards RB, Edwards JR, Cook RD, White RR: Bovine generalized glycogenosis. *Neuropathol Appl Neurobiol* **3**:45, 1977.
393. Howell JM, Dorling PR, Cook RD, Robinsin WF, Bradley S, Gawthorne JM: Infantile and late onset form of generalized glycogenosis type II in cattle. *J Pathol* **134**:266, 1981.
394. O'Sullivan BM, Healy PJ, Fraser IR, Nieper RE, Whittle RJ, Sewell CA: Generalized glycogenosis in Brahman cattle. *Aust Vet J* **57**:227, 1981.
395. Dorling PR, Howell JM, Gawthorne JM: Skeletal muscle alpha glucosidases in bovine generalized glycogenosis type II. *Biochem J* **198**:409, 1981.
396. Howell JM, Dorling PR, Cook RD, Robinson WF, Bradley S, Gawthorne JM: Infantile and late onset form of generalized glycogenosis type II in cattle. *J Pathol* **134**:266, 1981.
397. Healy P, Nicholls P, Martiniuk F, Tzall S, Hirschhorn R, Howell MJ: Evidence of molecular heterogeneity for generalised glycogenosis between and within breeds of cattle. *Aust Vet J* **72**:309, 1995.
398. Wisselaar HA, Hermans MMP, Visser WJ, Kroos MA, Oostra BA, Aspden W, Harrison B, Hetzel DJS, Reuser AJJ, Drinkwater RD: Biochemical genetics of glycogenosis type II in Brahman cattle. *Biochem Biophys Res Commun* **190**:941, 1993.
398a. Reichmann KG, Twist JO, Thistlethwait EJ: Clincal, diagnostic and biochemical features of generalised glycogenosis type II in Brahman cattle. *Aust Vet J* **70**:405, 1993.
399. Manktelow BW, Hartley WJ: Generalized glycogen storage disease in sheep. *J Comp Pathol* **85**:139, 1975.
400. Sandstrom B, Westman J, Ockerman PA: Glycogenosis of the central nervous system in the cat. *Acta Neuropathol (Berl)* **14**:194, 1969.
401. Bijvoet AGA, Van der Kamp EHM, Kroos MA, Ding J-H, Yang BZ, Visser P, Bakker CE, Verbeet MPH, Oostra BA, Reuser AJJ, Van der Ploeg AT: Generalized glycogen storage and cardiomegaly in a knockout mouse model of Pompe disease. *Hum Mol Genet* **7**:53, 1998.
402. Raben N, Nagaraju K, Lee E, Kessler P, Byrne B, Lee L, LaMarca M, King C, Ward J, Sauer B, Plotz P: Targeted disruption of the acid alpha-glucosidase gene in mice causes an illness with critical features of both infantile and adult human glycogen storage disease type II. *J Biol Chem* **273**:19086, 1998.
402a. Bijvoet AGA,Van Hirtum H, Vermey M, Van Leenen D, Van der Ploeg AT, Mooi WJ Reuser AJJ: Pathologic features of glycogen storage disease type II highlighted in the knockout mouse model. *J Pathol* **89**:416, 1999.
402b. Raben N, Nagaraju K, Lee E, Plotz P: Modulation of disease severity in mice with targeted disruption of the acid alpha-glucosidase gene. *Neuromuscul Disord* **10**:283, 2000.
403. Usuki F, Ishiura S, Sugita H: Isolation and characterization of three alpha-glucosidases from the Japanese quail. *J Biochem* **99**:985, 1986.
404. Usuki F, Ishiura S, Sugita H: Developmental study of alpha-glucosidases in Japanese quails with acid maltase deficiency. *Muscle Nerve* **9**:537, 1986.
405. Walvoort HC, Vannes JJ, Stokhof AA, Wolvekamp WT: Canine glycogen storage disease type II: A clinical study of 4 affected Lapland dogs. *J Am Anim Hosp Assoc* **20**:279, 1984.
406. King TS, Anderson JR, Wraight EP, Hunter JO, Cox TM: Skeletal muscle weakness and dysphagia caused by acid maltase deficiency: nutritional consequences of coincident celiac sprue. *Jpn J Parenter Enteral Nutr* **21**:46, 1997.
407. Verloes A, Massin M, Lombet J, Grattagliano B, Soyeur D, Rigo J, Koulischer L, Van Hoof F: Nosology of lysosomal glycogen storage disease without in vitro acid maltase deficiency: Delineation of a neonatal form. *Am J Med Genet* **72**:135, 1997.
408. Danon MJ, Oh SJ, Di Mauro S, Manaligod JRR, Eastwood A, Naidu S, Schliselfeld LH: Lysosomal glycogen storage disease with normal acid maltase. *Neurology* **31**:51, 1981.
409. Riggs JE, Schochet SS, Gutmann L, Shanske S, Neal WA, Di Mauro S: Lysosomal glycogen storage disease without acid maltase deficiency. *Neurology* **33**:873, 1983.
410. Hartz ZHS, Servidei S, Peterson PL, Chang CH, Di Mauro S: Cardiomyopathy, mental retardation and autophagic vacuolar myopathy. *Neurology* **37**:1065, 1987.
411. Byrne E, Dennett X, Crotty B, Trounce I, Sands JM, Hawkins R, Hammond J, Anderson S, Haan EA, Pollard A: Dominantly inherited cardioskeletal myopathy with lysosomal glycogen storage and normal acid maltase levels. *Brain* **109**:523, 1986.
412. Bru P, Pellissier JF, Gatau-Pelanchon J, Faugere G, deBarsy T, Levy S, Gerard JR: Glycogenose lysosomiale cardio-musculaire de l'adulte sans deficit enzymatique connu. *Arch Mal Coeur* **1**:109, 1988.
413. Tachi N, Tachi M, Sasaki K, Tomita H, Wakai S, Annaka S, Minami R, Tsurui S, Sugie H: Glycogen storage disease with normal acid maltase: Skeletal and cardiac muscles. *Pediatr Neurol* **5**:60, 1989.
414. Ullrich K, Von Bassewitz D, Shin J, Korinthenberg R, Sewell S, Von Figura K: Lysosomal glycogen storage disease without deficiency of acid alpha-glucosidase. *Prog Clin Biol Res* **306**:163, 1989.
414a. Kashio N, Usuki F, Akamine T, Nakagawa S, Higuchi I, Nakahara K, Okada A, Osame M, Murata F: Cardiomyopathy, mental retardation, and autophagic vacuolar myopathy abnormal MRI findings in the head. *J Neurol Sci* **105**:1, 1991.
415. Itoh M, Asano Y, Shimohira M, Iwakawa Y, Goto Y, Nonaka I: A patient with lysosomal glycogen storage disease with normal acid maltase [Japanese]. *No To Hattatsu* **25**:459, 1993.
416. Dworzak F, Casazza F, Mora M, De Maria R, Gronda E, Baroldi G, Rimoldi M, Morandi L, Cornelio F: Lysosomal glycogen storage with normal acid maltase: A familial study with successful heart transplant. *Neuromuscul Disord* **4**:243, 1994.

417. Katsumi Y, Tokonami F, Matsui M, Aii H, Nonaka I: A case of glycogen storage disease with normal acid maltase accompanied with the abnormal platelet function [Japanese]. *Rinsho Shinkeigaku* **34**:827, 1994.
418. Usuki F, Takenaga S, Higuchi I, Kashio N, Nakagawa M, Osame M: Morphologic findings in biopsied skeletal muscle and cultured fibroblasts from a female patient with Danon's disease (lysosomal glycogen storage disease without acid maltase deficiency). *J Neurol Sci* **127**:54, 1994.
419. Dworzak F, Mora M, Borroni C, Cornelio F, Blasevich F, Cappellini A, Tagliavini F, Bertagnolio B: Generalized lysosomal storage in Yunis Varon syndrome. *Neuromuscul Disord* **5**:423, 1995.
420. Murakami N, Goto Y, Itoh M, Katsumi Y, Wada T, Ozawa E, Nonaka I: Sarcolemmal indentation in cardiomyopathy with mental retardation and vacuolar myopathy. *Neuromuscul Disord* **5**:149, 1995.
421. Usuki F, Osame M: Lysosomal glycogen storage disease without acid maltase deficiency [Review]. *Nippon Rinsho* **53**:3050, 1995.
422. Katsumi Y, Fukuyama H, Ogawa M, Matsui M, Tokonami F, Aii H, Sugie H, Murakami N, Nonaka I: Cerebral oxygen and glucose metabolism in glycogen storage disease with normal acid maltase: Case report. *J Neurol Sci* **140**:46, 1996.
423. Tse HF, Shek TW, Tai YT, Lau YK, Ma L: Case report: Lysosomal glycogen storage disease with normal acid maltase: An unusual form of hypertrophic cardiomyopathy with rapidly progressive heart failure. *Am J Med Sci* **312**:182, 1996.
424. D'Aguzzi A, Scherer TA: Decompensated cor pulmonale as the first manifestation of adult-onset myopathy. *Respiration* **65**:317,1998.
425. Van den Hout H, Reuser AJJ, Vulto AG, Loonen MCB, Cromme-Dijkhuis A, Van der Ploeg AT: Recombinant human α-glucosidase from rabbit milk in Pompe patients. *Lancet* **356**:397, 2000.
426. Nishino I, Fu J, Tanji K, Yamada T, Shimojo S, Koori T, Mora M, Riggs JE, Oh S, Koga Y, Sue CM, Murakami N, Shanske S, Byrne E, Bonilla E, Nonaka I, DiMauro S, Hirano M: Primary LAMP-2 deficiency causes X-linked vacuolar cardiomyopathy and myopathy (Danon disease). *Nature*, **406**:906, 2000.
427. Tanaka Y, Guhde G, Suter A, Eskelinen EL, Hartmann D, Lüllmann-Rauch R, Janssen PML, Blanz J, Von Figura K, Saftig P: Accumulation of autophagic vacuoles and cardiomyopathy in LAMP-2-deficient mice. *Nature* **406**:902, 2000.

CHAPTER 136

The Mucopolysaccharidoses

Elizabeth F. Neufeld ▪ Joseph Muenzer

1. **The mucopolysaccharidoses (MPS) are a group of lysosomal storage disorders caused by deficiency of enzymes catalyzing the degradation of glycosaminoglycans (mucopolysaccharides). Depending on the enzyme deficiency, the catabolism of dermatan sulfate, heparan sulfate, keratan sulfate, chondroitin sulfate, or hyaluronan may be blocked, singly or in combination. Lysosomal accumulation of glycosaminoglycan molecules results in cell, tissue, and organ dysfunction. Glycosaminoglycan fragments generated by alternative pathways are excreted in urine. There are 11 known enzyme deficiencies that give rise to 7 distinct MPS. Table 136-1 presents the affected enzymes and glycosaminoglycans, and the corresponding syndromes and subtypes.**
2. **The stepwise degradation of glycosaminoglycans requires four exoglycosidases, five sulfatases, and one nonhydrolytic transferase. Endoglycosidases also participate in the degradation. The genes and cDNAs encoding most of these enzymes have been cloned, leading to elucidation of their primary structure, to production of recombinant enzymes, and to identification of mutations causing disease.**
3. **The MPS share many clinical features, although in variable degrees. These include a chronic and progressive course, multisystem involvement, organomegaly, dysostosis multiplex, and abnormal facies. Hearing, vision, airway, cardiovascular function, and joint mobility may be affected. Profound mental retardation is characteristic of MPS IH (Hurler syndrome), the severe form of MPS II (Hunter syndrome), and all subtypes of the MPS III (Sanfilippo syndrome), but normal intellect may be retained in other MPS. The bony lesions of MPS IV (Morquio syndrome) are specific to that disorder. There is clinical similarity between different enzyme deficiencies, and, conversely, a wide spectrum of clinical severity within any one enzyme deficiency. Supportive management—with particular attention to respiratory and cardiovascular complications, loss of hearing and vision, communicating hydrocephalus, and spinal cord compression—can greatly improve the quality of life for patients and their families.**
4. **The MPS are rare diseases. They are transmitted in an autosomal recessive manner except for MPS II, which is X-linked. Mutations underlying any one MPS are very heterogeneous, but one or a few mutant alleles may predominate in specific populations. Most are point mutations or small changes in the gene, although major DNA rearrangements and large deletions occur in MPS II. Correlation of disease severity with genotype is sometimes possible, but the effect of missense mutations is generally difficult to predict.**
5. **Enzyme assays are available for diagnosis, including prenatal diagnosis, of all the MPS. Identification of heterozygotes on the basis of enzyme activity is generally difficult or insufficiently accurate. Because of the heterogeneity of mutations, diagnosis and carrier testing by DNA analysis requires knowledge of the mutant alleles in the family under consideration.**
6. **There are numerous animal models of MPS. In addition to the models derived from mutations that have occurred naturally in dogs, cats, rats, mice, and goats, there are several mouse models created by targeted disruption of the corresponding mouse gene. The biochemical and pathologic features of these animal models is generally quite similar to those of their human counterparts, but the clinical presentations may be milder.**
7. **The MPS have long been considered potentially amenable to therapy by exogenously supplied enzyme. The success of bone marrow transplantation in altering the course of some MPS demonstrated that enzyme from donor hematopoietic cells could reduce glycosaminoglycan storage in somatic tissues of the recipient. Unfortunately, the variable neurologic benefit and the high risk associated with bone marrow transplantation limit the value of this form of therapy. Enzyme replacement is under active development, while gene therapy is at a much earlier stage. The animal models of MPS are proving extremely useful for developing and testing novel therapies.**

The mucopolysaccharidoses (MPS) are a family of heritable disorders, caused by deficiency of lysosomal enzymes needed to degrade glycosaminoglycans (or "mucopolysaccharides," an older name). The undegraded or partially degraded glycosaminoglycans are stored in lysosomes (Fig. 136-1) and/or excreted in urine. MPS I through VII involve the deficiency of 1 of 10 enzymes needed for the stepwise degradation of dermatan sulfate, heparan sulfate, keratan sulfate, or chondroitin sulfate, singly or in combination; a recent addition to this family of disorders, MPS IX, involves hyaluronan. The disorders are chronic and progressive, and usually display a wide spectrum of clinical severity within one enzyme deficiency. The classification and major features of the MPS are summarized in Table 136-1.

The reader is referred to earlier publications for comprehensive reviews of clinical and pathologic aspects of the MPS,[1–6] and of the discoveries that led to our understanding of the biochemical basis of this group of disorders.[7,8] The chapter in the previous edition of this book[9] was written just as the MPS were entering the era of molecular genetics. Since then, the genes encoding all but one of the enzymes underlying the known MPS have been cloned and numerous mutations have been identified in each disorder. The enzymes have been produced in recombinant systems. MPS have been discovered in animals or created by homologous recombination. The availability of molecular tools and of animal models has energized efforts to develop effective therapy.

ENZYMES OF GLYCOSAMINOGLYCAN DEGRADATION

Understanding the normal pathways of glycosaminoglycan catabolism has been closely tied to the elucidation of enzyme deficiencies in the MPS. The role of many of the enzymes became apparent only through the consequences of their absence. Figures

A list of standard abbreviations is located immediately preceding the index in each volume. An additional abbreviation used in this chapter is: BMT = bone marrow transplantation.

Table 136-1 **Classification of the Mucopolysaccharidoses**

Number	Eponym	MIM number	Chromosome locus	Major clinical manifestations	Enzyme deficiency	Glycosaminoglycan affected
MPS IH	Hurler	252800	4p16.3	Corneal clouding, dysostosis multiplex, organomegaly, heart disease, mental retardation, death in childhood	α-L-Iduronidase	Dermatan sulfate, heparan sulfate
MPS IS	Scheie	252800	4p16.3	Corneal clouding, stiff joints, normal intelligence and life span	α-L-Iduronidase	Dermatan sulfate, heparan sulfate
MPS IH/S	Hurler-Scheie	252800	4p16.3	Phenotype intermediate between IH and IS	α-L-Iduronidase	Dermatan sulfate, heparan sulfate
MPS II (severe)	Hunter (severe)	309900	Xq28	Dysostosis multiplex, organomegaly, no corneal clouding, mental retardation, death before 15 years	Iduronate sulfatase	Dermatan sulfate, heparan sulfate
MPS II (mild)	Hunter (mild)	309900	Xq28	Normal intelligence, short stature, survival to adulthood and often longer	Iduronate sulfatase	Dermatan sulfate, heparan sulfate
MPS IIIA	Sanfilippo A	252900	17q25.3	Profound mental deterioration, hyperactivity, relatively mild somatic manifestations; milder forms known to exist	Heparan *N*-sulfatase (sulfamidase)	Heparan sulfate
MPS IIIB	Sanfilippo B	252920	17q21	Phenotype similar to IIIA	α-*N*-Acetyl-glucosaminidase	Heparan sulfate
MPS IIIC	Sanfilippo C	252930	Not Known	Phenotype similar to IIIA	Acetyl-CoA:α-glucosaminide acetyltransferase	Heparan sulfate
MPS IIID	Sanfilippo D	252940	12q14	Phenotype similar to IIIA	N-Acetylglucosamine 6-Sulfatase	Heparan sulfate
MPS IVA	Morquio A	253000	16q24.3	Distinctive skeletal abnormalities, corneal clouding, odontoid hypoplasia; milder forms known to exist	Galactose 6-sulfatase (*N*-acetylgalactosamine 6-sulfatase)	Keratan sulfate, chondroitin 6-sulfate
MPS IVB	Morquio B	253010	3p21.33	Spectrum of severity as in IVA	β-Galactosidase	Keratan sulfate
MPS V	No longer used			—	—	—
MPS VI	Maroteaux-Lamy	253200	5q13-q14	Dysostosis multiplex, corneal clouding, normal intelligence; survival to teens in severe form; milder forms exist	*N*-Acetylgalactosamine 4-sulfatase (arylsulfatase B)	Dermatan sulfate
MPS VII	Sly	253220	7q21.11	Dysostosis multiplex, hepatosplenomegaly; wide spectrum of severity, including fetal and neonatal form	β-Glucuronidase	Dermatan sulfate, heparan sulfate chondroitin 4-, 6-sulfates
MPS VIII	No longer used			—	—	—
MPS IX	—	601492	3p21.2-p21.3	Periarticular soft tissue masses; short stature	Hyaluronidase	Hyaluronan

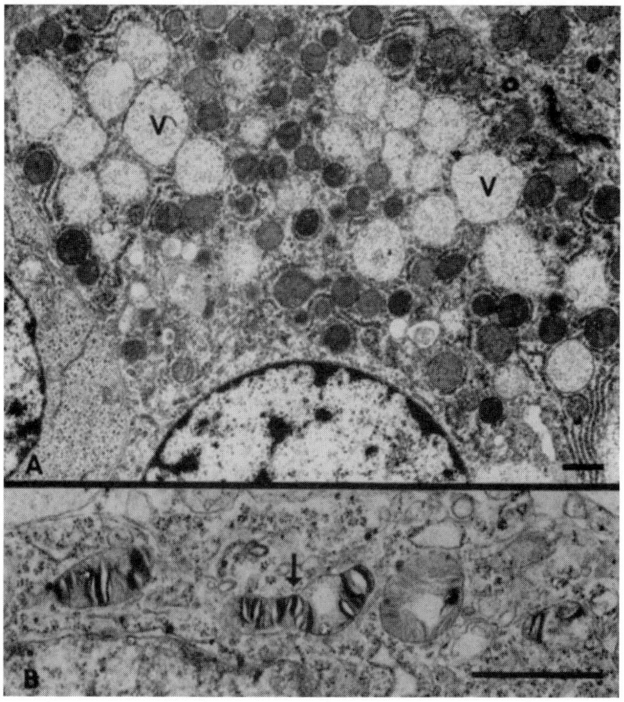

Fig. 136-1 Characteristic appearance of cells in mucopolysaccharidoses. *Upper panel*: large vacuoles (V) that may appear empty or contain fine granular material, in a hepatocyte from a Hurler patient. *Lower panel*: inclusion bodies (arrow), named zebra bodies for their striated appearance, in a cerebral neuron of a Hunter patient. The vacuoles are lysosomes engorged with stored glycosaminoglycans, whereas the zebra bodies are thought to contain glycolipids as well. The bars represent 1 μM. (*Courtesy of Dr. A. J. Garvin, Medical University of South Carolina, Charleston, SC*.)

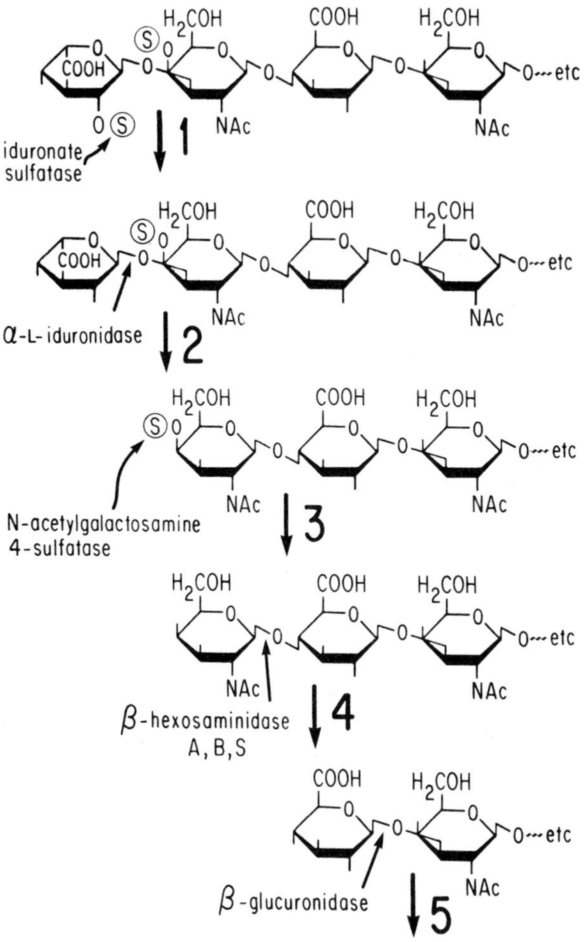

Fig. 136-2 Stepwise degradation of dermatan sulfate. The deficiency diseases corresponding to the numbered reactions are: 1 = MPS II, Hunter syndrome; 2 = MPS I, Hurler, Hurler-Scheie, and Scheie syndromes; 3 = MPS VI, Maroteaux-Lamy syndrome; 4 = Sandhoff disease for β-hexosaminidase A and B; there are knockout mice in which all three isoenzymes are deficient, but no comparable disease in humans; 5 = MPS VII, Sly syndrome. This drawing depicts all structures known to occur within dermatan sulfate, and does not imply that they occur in equal proportion. For instance, L-iduronic acid occurs much more frequently than glucuronic acid and only a few of the α-L-iduronic residues are sulfated.

136-2 to 136-5 illustrate the pathways of lysosomal degradation of dermatan sulfate, heparan sulfate, keratan sulfate, chondroitin sulfate, and hyaluronan, as well as the enzyme deficiencies in the MPS. The glycosaminoglycans themselves are lysosomal degradation products derived by proteolytic removal of the protein core of proteoglycans—the macromolecular forms in which these molecules exist at the cell surface or in the extracellular matrix (with the exception of hyaluronan, which has no protein core).

Most of the enzyme deficiencies were discovered in the 1970s, after which interest turned to purification of the normal enzymes and elucidation of their synthesis and transport to lysosomes. Better understanding of the primary structure of the enzyme proteins has come from isolation of the cDNAs in which they are encoded. More detailed studies became possible with the availability of recombinant forms of the enzymes. These studies of normal enzymes provide the background for understanding the effects of disease-producing mutations.

Enzymes of Dermatan Sulfate Catabolism

Dermatan sulfate consists of sulfated *N*-acetylgalactosamine alternating with uronic acid residues. The latter are predominantly L-iduronic acid, some of which are sulfated; there are also occasional glucuronic acid residues.[10] Degradation proceeds stepwise from the nonreducing end, as shown schematically in Fig. 136-2, by the sequential action of three exo-glycosidases (α-L-iduronidase, β-glucuronidase, and β-hexosaminidase) and two sulfatases (iduronate 2-sulfatase and *N*-acetylgalactosamine 4-sulfatase). An endoglycosidase, hyaluronidase, may also participate to a limited extent in the degradation process by cleaving next to the occasional glucuronic acid residues.

Glycosidases

α-L-Iduronidase, the enzyme that is deficient in MPS I, hydrolyzes terminal α-L-iduronic acid residues of dermatan sulfate (Fig.136-2, reaction 2) and of heparan sulfate (see below). Originally studied as "Hurler corrective factor,"[11] the enzyme was purified and characterized from human[12–15] and animal tissues.[16,17] Its distribution in porcine tissues has been determined.[18] The protein sequences deduced from the nucleotide sequences of cDNA encoding human,[19] canine,[17] and murine[20] α-L-iduronidase have a high degree of homology, and predict proteins of 653, 655, and 634 amino acids, respectively. Biosynthesis experiments in cultured fibroblasts had established that the enzyme is made in precursor form, processed intracellularly to a shorter form with the loss of about 100 amino acids, and that it has the mannose-6-phosphate marker for targeting to lysosomes.[17,19,21,22] The active enzyme exists in monomeric form. Analysis of the carbohydrate residues of recombinant human α-L-iduronidase secreted by overexpressing CHO cells[23,24] showed that although all six glycosylation sites are utilized, the mannose-6-phosphate marker is carried only on sites 3 and 6.[25] The recombinant enzyme is efficiently endocytosed by the mannose-6-phosphate receptor, with half-maximal uptake at 0.7 nM.[23] Although α-L-iduronidase has not yet been crystallized, the three-dimensional structure of its active site has been predicted.[26]

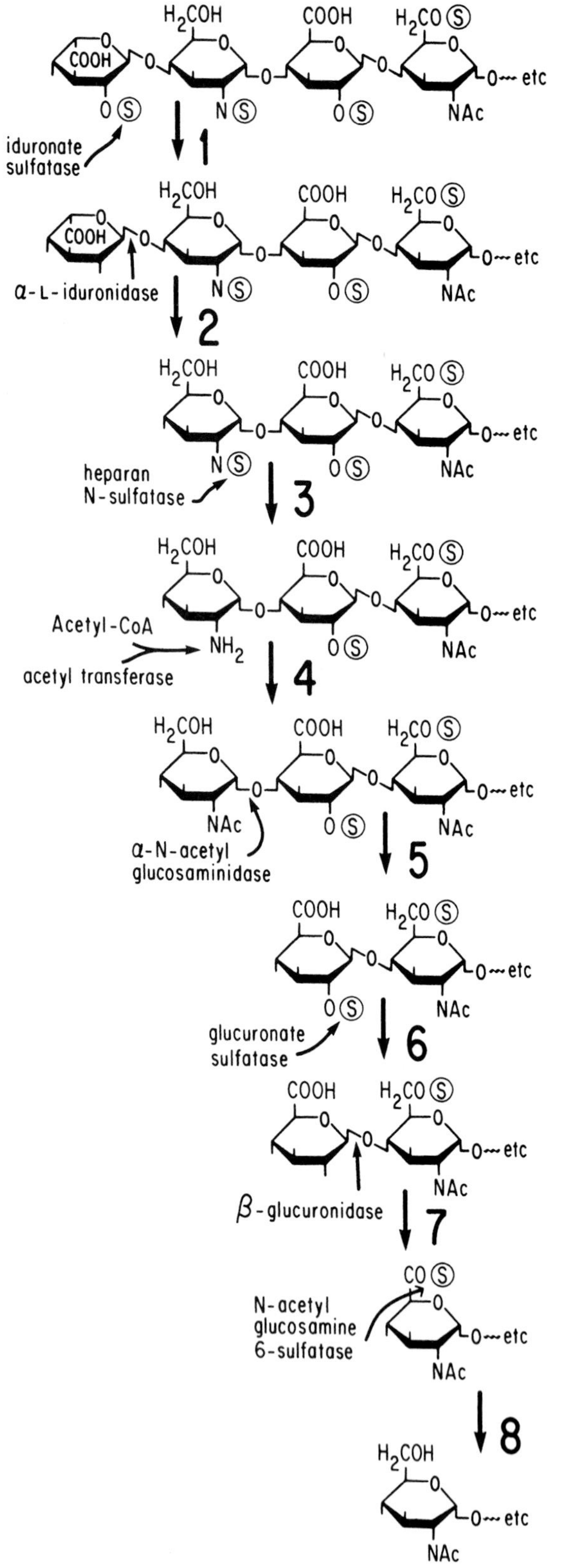

Fig. 136-3 Stepwise degradation of heparan sulfate. The deficiency diseases corresponding to the numbered reactions are: 1 = MPS II, Hunter syndrome; 2 = MPS I, Hurler, Hurler-Scheie, and Scheie syndromes; 3 = MPS III A, Sanfilippo syndrome type A; 4 = MPS III C, Sanfilippo syndrome type C; 5 = MPS III B, Sanfilippo syndrome type B; 6 = no deficiency disease yet known; 7 = MPS VII, Sly syndrome; 8 = MPS III D, Sanfilippo syndrome type D. The drawing depicts all structures known to occur within heparan sulfate, and does not imply that they occur stoichiometrically. For example, very few of the glucuronic acid residues are sulfated.

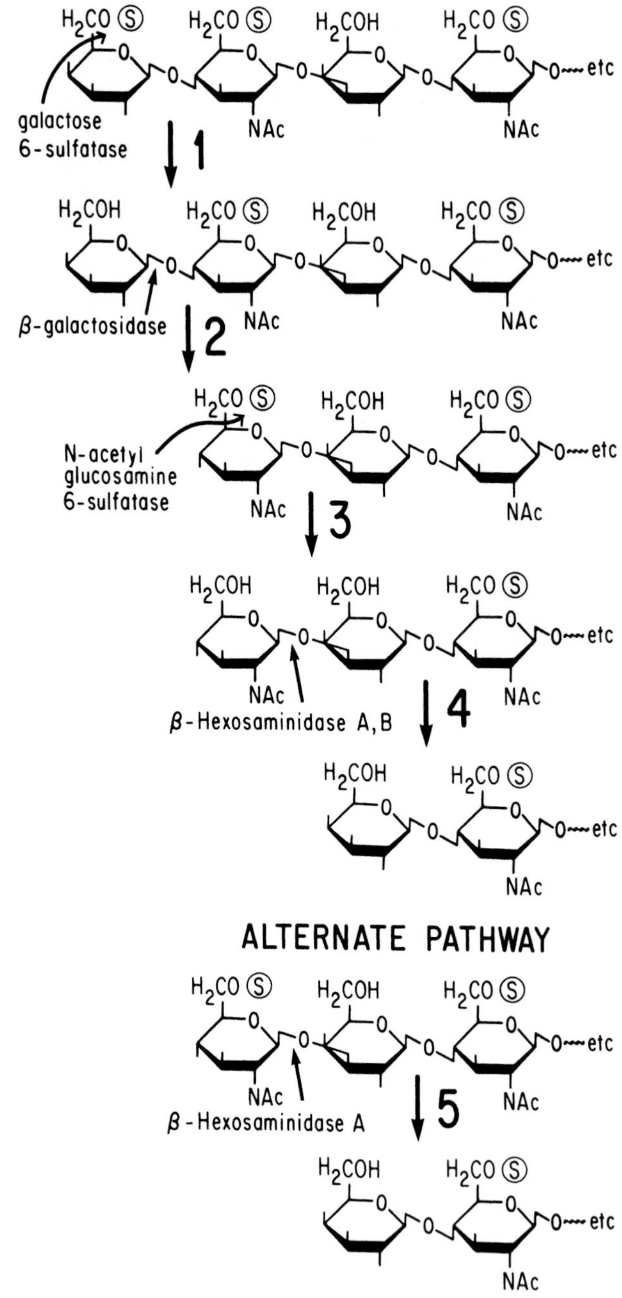

Fig. 136-4 Stepwise degradation of keratan sulfate. The deficiency diseases corresponding to the numbered reactions are 1 = MPS IV A, Morquio syndrome type A; 2 = MPS IV B, Morquio syndrome type B; 3 = MPS III D, Sanfilippo syndrome type D; 4 = Sandhoff disease; and 5 = Tay-Sachs and Sandhoff disease. The alternate pathway releases intact *N*-acetylglucosamine 6-sulfate, a departure from the usual stepwise cleavage of sulfate and sugar residues.

β-Glucuronidase, the enzyme deficient in MPS VII, removes the glucuronic acid residues present in dermatan sulfate (Fig. 136-2, reaction 5) as well as in heparan sulfate, chondroitin sulfate, and hyaluronan (see below). It was the first of the lysosomal enzymes of glycosaminoglycan degradation to be studied at a molecular level. It has been purified to homogeneity from a number of mammalian sources (reviewed in reference 27). It has a dual localization in some tissues, particularly rodent liver, where it also occurs in microsomes with the protein egasyn, to which it binds through the C-terminus.[28] The active enzyme is a tetramer of subunits of 75 kDa, which are synthesized in precursor form and proteolytically processed.[29] Studies of β-glucuronidase have figured prominently in the elucidation of lysosomal enzyme

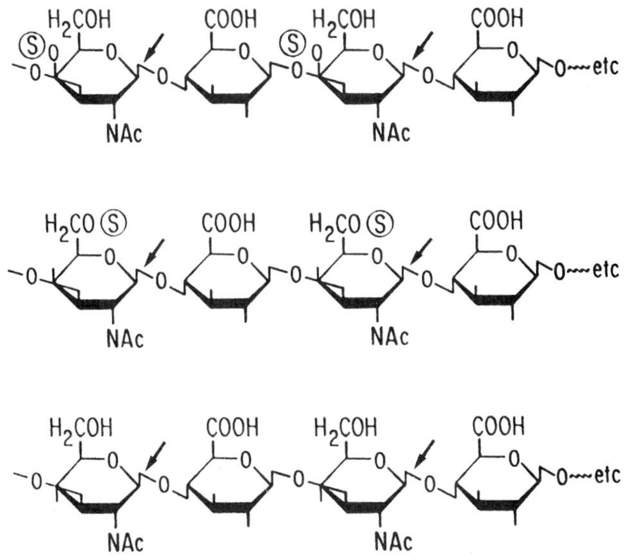

Fig. 136-5 Endoglycosidase degradation of chondroitin sulfate and hyaluronan. Arrows show potential sites for hyaluronidase cleavage of chondroitin 4-sulfate (top), chondroitin 6-sulfate (middle), and hyaluronan (bottom) into oligosaccharide fragments. The oligosaccharides are hydrolyzed further by stepwise action of *N*-acetylgalactosamine 4-sulfatase or 6-sulfatase (for oligosaccharides derived from chondroitin 4- or 6-sulfate), β-hexosaminidase A or B, and β-glucuronidase.

transport,[30] for it was the recognition marker of this enzyme that was first identified as mannose-6-phosphate.[31] Full-length cDNAs encoding proteins of 651 (human) and 648 (rodent) amino acids have been sequenced and expressed.[32–34] Of the four potential glycosylation sites, all are used in the human enzyme but sites 2 and 3 are preferentially phosphorylated.[35] The crystallographic structure of human β-glucuronidase has been determined at a resolution of 2.6 Å.[36]

β-Hexosaminidase has been viewed as the glycosidase required for removal of the *N*-acetylgalactosamine residues of dermatan sulfate (see Fig. 136-2, reaction 4). Yet patients with Sandhoff disease (Chap. 153), who lack both major isoenzymes of β-hexosaminidase (A and B), show only modest glycosaminoglycan storage in tissues[37] and cultured fibroblasts.[38] This apparent paradox has been resolved by study of knockout mice deficient in β-hexosaminidase. Only when all three isoenzymes, A, B, and S, were lacking did the mice have a frank mucopolysaccharidosis.[39,40] This indicates that the S isoenzyme, an unstable protein of low abundance, which normally may have little physiological function, can participate in the degradation of dermatan sulfate in the absence of isoenzymes A and B.

Sulfatases

Two distinct sulfatases are required for the degradation of dermatan sulfate: iduronate 2-sulfatase and *N*-acetylgalactosamine 4-sulfatase. They are part of a family of homologous proteins that includes all sulfatases studied to date, and they carry the common posttranslational modification of a cysteine residue in the catalytic site to 2-amino-3-oxopropionic acid.[41] This modification is required for catalytic activity of all sulfatases, and its absence underlies the disorder known as multiple sulfatase deficiency (Chap. 149).

Iduronate sulfatase, the enzyme deficient in MPS II, specifically removes the sulfate group from the 2- position of L-iduronic acid present in dermatan sulfate (Fig. 136-2, reaction 1) and in heparan sulfate (see below). It was originally studied as the "Hunter corrective factor,"[42] which is understood today to be a secreted form of iduronate sulfatase with the mannose-6-phosphate recognition marker for lysosomal targeting. The enzyme has been purified to homogeneity from a number of human tissues.[43] The sequence deduced from the human cDNA indicates a protein of 550 amino acids (including a 25-amino acid signal sequence) and seven potential *N*-glycosylation sites,[44] while the murine cDNA, which is 85 percent homologous, predicts a protein of 564 amino acids and six potential *N*-glycosylation sites.[45] Some proteolytic processing occurs in lysosomes. Overexpression in cultured human fibroblasts leads to poor processing.[46] Recombinant human enzyme secreted by CHO cells has properties similar to the naturally occurring enzyme, including endocytosis into fibroblasts by the mannose-6-phosphate receptor.[47]

Desulfation of *N*-acetylgalactosamine 4-sulfate is a property of arylsulfatase B, the enzyme deficient in Maroteaux-Lamy syndrome. The enzyme has been purified to homogeneity from human[48,49] and feline[48] tissues. Its biosynthesis, studied in skin fibroblasts, indicates the phosphorylation of mannose residues and proteolytic cleavage characteristic of lysosomal enzymes.[50,51] The human[52,53] and feline[54] cDNAs encoding the enzyme have been cloned and expressed; the sequence deduced for the human protein has 533 amino acids, 46 of which are in the signal peptide. Recombinant human[55] and feline[56] *N*-acetylgalactosamine 4-sulfatases secreted by CHO cells have properties similar to the naturally occurring enzymes, including endocytosis by the mannose-6-phosphate receptor.[55] Crystallographic studies have been performed at 2.5 Å resolution;[57] these reveal the catalytic mechanism by which the 2-amino 3-oxo-propionic acid (derived from cysteine 91) can form a sulfate ester intermediate.

Hyaluronidase

The enzymes described above are exoglycosidases and exosulfatases; they can hydrolyze linkages only at the nonreducing termini and must act sequentially to degrade the glycosaminoglycan. Hyaluronidase, described in greater detail below, is an endoglycosidase (endohexosaminidase), which can cleave dermatan sulfate internally between *N*-acetylgalactosamine and the occasional adjoining glucuronic acid residues. Although the fragments of dermatan sulfate found in urine of MPS patients are probably generated by hyaluronidase, the role of the enzyme in the normal lysosomal degradation of dermatan sulfate is not known. Cleavage by hyaluronidase followed by excretion of the resulting fragments may be considered an alternative catabolic route when the primary pathway is blocked; it appears to be limited to certain tissues and probably does not occur in fibroblasts.[58]

Enzymes of Heparan Sulfate Catabolism

Heparan sulfate ("heparitin" in the older literature) consists of glucuronic acid and L-iduronic acid residues, some of which are sulfated, alternating with α-linked glucosamine residues. The latter are either sulfated or acetylated on the amino group and may be sulfated on the 6-hydroxyl.[59] Although heparan sulfate shares with heparin a similarity in name and in carbohydrate composition, it is not an effective anticoagulant. While we consider the common features of heparan sulfate in generic fashion, there is considerable variation in the degree and type of sulfation, as well as in the proportion of glucuronic acid and L-iduronic acid, both between different species of heparan sulfate and within a single heparan sulfate chain.[59] This permits different species of heparan sulfate (which are synthesized and transported to the cell surface or extracellular matrix as proteoglycans) to fulfill diverse biologic functions such as binding and activation of growth factors.[60]

Heparan sulfate is degraded stepwise, as shown schematically in Fig. 136-3, by the action of three glycosidases, three, or perhaps four, sulfatases, and one enzyme that is not a hydrolase but an acetyltransferase. It has been suggested that these enzymes function cooperatively in a complex, allowing the product of one enzyme to be passed efficiently to the next enzyme in the pathway.[61]

Glycosidases. Terminal L-iduronic acid and glucuronic acid residues of heparan sulfate are cleaved by α-L-iduronidase and β-glucuronidase, respectively (Fig. 136-3, reactions 2 and 7).

These enzymes have been discussed above in the context of dermatan sulfate degradation. Individuals with α-L-iduronidase deficiency (MPS I) or β-glucuronidase deficiency (MPS VII) are therefore blocked in the degradation of heparan sulfate as well as of dermatan sulfate.

α-*N*-acetylglucosaminidase, the enzyme deficient in MPS IIIB, is required for the removal of the *N*-acetylglucosamine residues that exist in heparan sulfate or are generated during lysosomal degradation of this polymer by the action of acetyl-CoA transferase (Fig.136-3, reaction 5). It has been purified to homogeneity from human[62–64] and animal[65] sources. The enzyme is active as both monomer and oligomer. Its biosynthesis includes the processing steps characteristic of lysosomal enzymes.[66] The cDNA sequence predicts a protein of 743 amino acids including the signal peptide.[64,65]

Sulfatases. Iduronate sulfatase is required for the desulfation of 2-sulfated iduronic acid residues in heparan sulfate (Fig.136-3, reaction 1). This enzyme has been discussed in the context of dermatan sulfate degradation. Patients with iduronate sulfatase deficiency (MPS II) are blocked in the catabolism of both dermatan sulfate and heparan sulfate.

Glucuronate 2-sulfatase, the last of the lysosomal enzymes of glycosaminoglycan degradation to be discovered,[67] is not yet associated with any known deficiency disease. It has been purified and characterized from human liver[68] and shown to act on the rare sulfated glucuronic acid residue[69,70] present in heparan sulfate (Fig. 136-3, reaction 6). Glucuronate sulfatase is present in fibroblasts of patients with MPS II and is, therefore, distinct from iduronate sulfatase. The gene encoding this enzyme has not yet been cloned.

Heparan *N*-sulfatase, the enzyme deficient in MPS IIIA, is specific for sulfate groups linked to the amino group of glucosamine (Fig. 136-3, reaction 3). Technically, such groups are sulfamate rather than sulfate, and the enzyme may therefore be designated "sulfamate sulfohydrolase" or simply "sulfamidase." The human enzyme has been purified and characterized.[71] The cDNA sequence predicts a protein of 502 amino acids, including a 20-amino acid signal peptide.[72] Recombinant human heparan *N*-sulfatase has been purified from secretions of overexpressing CHO cells and shown to have properties similar to those of liver enzyme, including endocytosis by the mannose-6-phosphate receptor.[73]

N-acetylglucosamine 6-sulfatase (Fig. 136-3, reaction 8) is deficient in MPS IIID. The enzyme was originally thought to be specific for the 6-sulfated *N*-acetylglucosamine residues of heparan sulfate, which are in α-linkage, and was thought to be inactive toward the same residues in keratan sulfate, which are in β-linkage.[74] However, the earlier data have been reinterpreted, as described in the section on keratan sulfate degradation. The sulfatase can desulfate the 6-sulfated *N*-acetylglucosamine present in α- or in β-linkage, or even as a free monosaccharide.[75–77] The human liver enzyme has been purified and characterized.[76,78] The cDNA sequence predicts a protein of 552 amino acids. Recombinant caprine enzyme, purified from secretions of overexpressing CHO cells, has properties similar to the human enzyme, including uptake by the mannose-6-phosphate receptor.[79]

Acetyltransferase. Perhaps the most intriguing of the catabolic enzymes is acetyl-CoA:α-glucosaminide *N*-acetyltransferase, the enzyme deficient in MPS IIIC.[80] It is the only known lysosomal enzyme that is not a hydrolase. It catalyzes the acetylation of the glucosamine amino groups that have become exposed by the action of heparan *N*-sulfatase but that cannot be hydrolyzed directly (see Fig. 136-3, reaction 4). Free glucosamine can be substituted in vitro for the glycosaminoglycan substrate.[81,82] Although the enzyme has been purified to only a modest degree,[83,84] much has been learned about its mechanism of action.[85] On the cytoplasmic side, the enzyme (which is in the lysosomal membrane) acetylates itself by transfer of acetyl groups from acetyl-CoA; this half-reaction occurs at a neutral pH. On the luminal side, where the pH is acidic, the enzyme transfers its acetyl group to a glucosamine residue. A histidine is implicated at the active site.[86] The two-step mechanism, proposed on the basis of kinetic studies, has been confirmed by genetic evidence; cells from one group of MPS IIIC patients can catalyze the first half-reaction but not the second, whereas cells from the other group lack all activity.[87] The cDNA encoding this interesting enzyme has not yet been isolated.

Heparanase. Heparanase (probably a family of enzymes[88]) is an endoglucuronidase that may also participate in the catabolism of heparan sulfate by cleaving the polymer into smaller fragments, some of which are released in urine.[89] As in the case of dermatan sulfate cleavage by hyaluronidase, cleavage of heparan sulfate by endoglucuronidase provides an alternative pathway that reduces the amount of glycosaminoglycan stored in tissues of patients with MPS I, II, III, or VII. On the other hand, the fragments of heparan sulfate released by heparanase may themselves be deleterious, because heparan sulfate is a bioactive substance that acts as a co-factor for FGF binding to and activation of the FGF receptor.[60,90] Therefore, it is possible that heparan sulfate fragments entering the extracellular matrix compete with the binding of growth factors to the resident heparan sulfate proteoglycan.

Enzymes of Keratan Sulfate Catabolism

Keratan sulfate is the only glycosaminoglycan that contains no uronic acid. Instead, galactose residues, mostly sulfated, alternate with sulfated *N*-acetylglucosamine residues. Inability to degrade keratan sulfate gives rise to MPS IV, the Morquio syndrome. The unique clinical manifestations of this disorder are attributable to the restricted tissue distribution of keratan sulfate (corneas and cartilage), in contrast to the much wider distribution of dermatan sulfate and heparan sulfate. Like the other two glycosaminoglycans, keratan sulfate is degraded sequentially from the nonreducing end by the action of glycosidases and sulfatases, as shown in Fig. 136-4.

Glycosidases. The galactose residues of keratan sulfate are removed by β-galactosidase (Fig. 136-4, reaction 2). β-Galactosidase is a well-characterized lysosomal enzyme;[91] the sequence of its cDNA predicts a protein of 677 amino acids, including a 23-amino acid signal peptide.[92–94] Newly made β-galactosidase undergoes the processing characteristic of lysosomal enzymes, but in addition undergoes aggregation to a multimer of approximately 1600 kDa.[95] The normal enzyme hydrolyzes terminal β-linked galactose residues found in G_{M1} ganglioside, glycoproteins, and oligosaccharides, as well as in keratan sulfate. Total absence of β-galactosidase activity results in G_{M1} gangliosidosis (Chap. 151), whereas MPS IVB results from mutations that selectively impair catalytic activity toward keratan sulfate. β-Galactosidase activity is also impaired in galactosialidosis, a combined deficiency of β-galactosidase and sialidase activities caused by a primary deficiency of a third protein, the "protective protein/cathepsin A," the three proteins entering into large enzymatically active complexes (Chap. 152).

β-Hexosaminidase, most commonly known for its deficiency in Tay-Sachs disease and Sandhoff disease (Chap. 153), has been discussed above in the context of dermatan sulfate degradation. Its role in the degradation of keratan sulfate is unique in that it can participate in two alternative reactions. One is the conventional removal of a terminal *N*-acetylglucosamine residue, which can be catalyzed by both the A and B (and perhaps S) isoenzymes of β-hexosaminidase (Fig. 136-4, reaction 4). But, in addition, the A (but not the B) isoenzyme can remove *N*-acetylglucosamine 6-sulfate *en bloc*[96] (Fig. 136-4, reaction 5). The 6-sulfated amino sugar is thought to occupy the binding site for anionic substrates, which is also used by G_{M2} ganglioside.[97] There is evidence that this one-step removal of sulfated *N*-acetylglucosamine occurs in vivo,[98] but the relative contribution of the two alternative reactions to the normal degradation of keratan sulfate is not known.

Sulfatases. The sulfatase that cleaves the 6-sulfate from galactose residues (Fig. 136-4, reaction 1) is deficient in patients with MPS IVA. This enzyme also removes 6-sulfate residues from the *N*-acetylgalactosamine residues of chondroitin sulfate C; for historic reasons, it is named after the latter activity. *N*-Acetylgalactosamine 6-sulfatase has been purified to homogeneity;[99] its cDNA encodes 522 amino acids, including a 26-amino acid signal sequence, and bears marked similarity to other sulfatases.[100] It has been suggested that *N*-acetylgalactosamine 6-sulfatase associates in a large aggregate with β-galactosidase, neuraminidase, and cathepsin A/protective protein.[101] Recombinant human *N*-acetylgalactosamine 6-sulfatase has properties similar to those of the naturally occurring enzyme, including endocytosis via the mannose-6-phosphate receptor.[102]

The *N*-acetylglucosamine 6-sulfatase that catalyzes reaction 3 in the degradation of keratan sulfate (Fig. 136-4) is the same enzyme that catalyzes reaction 8 in the degradation of heparan sulfate (Fig. 136-3). It is lacking in patients with MPS IIID (see above). But patients with MPS IIID do not excrete keratan sulfate because β-hexosaminidase A can bypass the block (reaction 5 in Fig. 136-4); instead, they excrete *N*-acetylglucosamine 6-sulfate in urine in addition to heparan sulfate.[98,103,104]

Enzymes of Chondroitin Sulfate and Hyaluronan Degradation

Chondroitin 4- and 6-sulfate can be broken down by a combination of enzymes acting in stepwise fashion. These include β-glucuronidase, β-hexosaminidase, *N*-acetylgalactosamine 4-sulfatase (arylsulfatase B), and *N*-acetylgalactosamine 6-sulfatase; each was discussed above. In addition, the endohexosaminidase, hyaluronidase, can cleave at the *N*-acetylgalactosamine residues (Fig. 136-5, arrows), bypassing the blocks in chondroitin sulfate degradation created by the enzyme deficiencies in MPS IVA, MPS VI, MPS VII, and Sandhoff disease.

Hyaluronan (formerly called hyaluronic acid) is such a large macromolecule that some fragmentation by the hyaluronidase is probably important for its degradation. Absence of hyaluronidase has recently been discovered in one patient, who showed lysosomal storage of glycosaminoglycan.[105] The enzyme deficiency has been designated MPS IX.[106] While hyaluronidases comprise a family of enzymes with similar activity, the plasma enzyme and lysosomal enzymes are believed to be identical.[107] The reaction product is primarily a tetrasaccharide. The cDNA encoding plasma hyaluronidase was cloned and found to encode a protein of 435 amino acids.[108] It is not clear whether the enzyme uses the mannose-6-phosphate targeting system.[109]

Comments on Enzyme Deficiencies

Glycosaminoglycan Storage and Excretion. The type of glycosaminoglycans stored or excreted by MPS patients can generally be predicted from the enzyme deficiency and from the glycosaminoglycan synthesized by a particular tissue. With respect to fine structure, the prediction is that the nonreducing terminus of the stored glycosaminoglycan would be the residue that is the normal substrate for the missing enzyme. This was documented in several cases; for instance, MPS II fibroblasts, lacking iduronate sulfatase, accumulate dermatan sulfate with the predicted 2-sulfated iduronic acid termini;[110,111] urinary heparan sulfate fragments from patients with Sanfilippo syndrome A, B, and C have the expected glucosamine *N*-sulfate, *N*-acetylglucosamine, and unsubstituted glucosamine, respectively, at the nonreducing termini.[112] As pointed out above, endoglycosidases may bypass the block; thus the absence of massive chondroitin sulfate storage and excretion in MPS IV, VI, and VII may be explained by the ability of hyaluronidase to release small fragments. In an unusual reaction, β-hexosaminidase A can remove a sulfated sugar when the sulfatase is absent. The low-molecular-weight compounds generated by these endocleavages and the sulfated hexosamine released by the β-hexosaminidase A reaction are excreted in urine,[104] but are missed in routine analyses that are geared toward the larger polymers.

The earlier literature contains several reports of patients with urinary excretion of glycosaminoglycans other than those listed in Table 136-1. Some of these reports may reflect analytical errors. A report of *N*-acetylglucosamine 6-sulfatase deficiency with combined excretion of heparan sulfate and keratan sulfate, originally thought to represent a new disease entity (MPS VIII), was subsequently retracted,[113] and the classification of MPS VIII was declared void.[114] The next disorder to be described[105] was therefore designated MPS IX.

Glycosphingolipid Accumulation. In addition to glycosaminoglycans, gangliosides G_{M2} and G_{M3} accumulate in brains of MPS patients[115–118] and of animal models.[20,119,120] These lipids are thought to be stored in zebra bodies (see Fig. 136-1B), which are reminiscent of the lysosomal inclusions seen in sphingolipidoses. The accumulation of the gangliosides is puzzling because their degradation does not involve the enzymes of glycosaminoglycan catabolism. Some enzymes of ganglioside catabolism may be inhibited secondary to glycosaminoglycan accumulation; the inhibition of ganglioside sialidase may be particularly relevant.[121] It may be significant that ganglioside accumulation has been found in the brains of patients with MPS I, MPS II (severe), and MPS IIIA, IIIB, and IIID, all of whom show mental retardation, but not in the brain of a patients with MPS IS, whose intelligence was normal.[116,117]

CLINICAL MANIFESTATIONS AND MANAGEMENT

Mucopolysaccharidosis I (Hurler, Scheie, and Hurler-Scheie Syndromes)

Deficiency of α-L-iduronidase can result in a wide range of clinical involvement, with three major recognized clinical entities—Hurler and Scheie syndromes representing phenotypes at the two ends of the clinical spectrum, and the Hurler-Scheie syndrome representing a phenotype of intermediate clinical severity.[1,2,4,9] In addition, there are patients who do not fit precisely into any of these three clinical entities.[122–124] The clinical phenotypes are not distinguishable biochemically by routine diagnostic procedures, because they all have the following features: excessive urinary dermatan and heparan sulfate excretion; absence of α-L-iduronidase activity; and accumulation of glycosaminoglycan in cultured fibroblasts that is correctable by uptake of α-L-iduronidase. Mutation analysis now permits the classification of some patients (see below), but in most cases, assignment to the subtype of MPS I can be made only on the basis of clinical criteria, including the rate of progression of symptoms.

MPS IH (Hurler). Although the Hurler syndrome has been the prototype for the description of mucopolysaccharidoses, this may be misleading because it is not representative of all mucopolysaccharidoses; it is representative only of the severe end of a clinical spectrum (Fig. 136-6). It is a progressive disorder with multiple organ and tissue involvement that leads to death in childhood. An infant with Hurler syndrome appears normal at birth but may have inguinal or umbilical hernias. Diagnosis of Hurler syndrome is commonly made between 4 and 18 months of age; a combination of skeletal deformities, recurrent ear and nose infections, inguinal and umbilical hernias, coarse facial features, hepatosplenomegaly, and enlarged tongue first prompt medical attention.[125] Fatal cardiomyopathy with autopsy-confirmed endocardial fibroelastosis has been a presenting feature for some MPS I infants less than 1 year old.[126,127] The cardiac failure may precede the recognition of a storage disorder because the earliest manifestations of MPS IH may be subtle or nonspecific. Patients with Hurler syndrome may be unusually large in infancy, but a deceleration of growth commonly occurs between 6 and 18

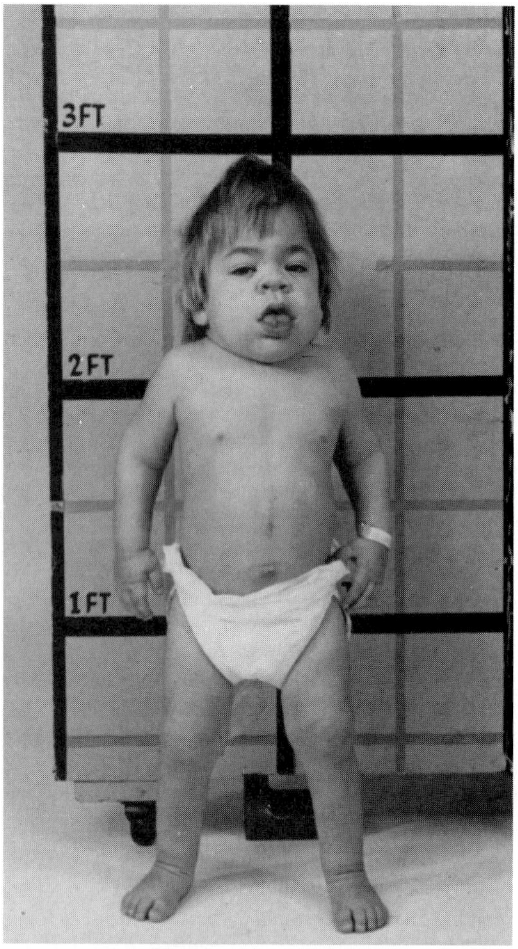

Fig. 136-6 MPS IH (Hurler syndrome) in a 4-year-old boy. Diagnosis was made at the age of 15 months, at which time he had developmental delay, hepatomegaly, and skeletal involvement. At the time of the picture, the patient had short stature, an enlarged tongue, persistent nasal discharge, stiff joints, and hydrocephalus. Verbal language skills consisted of four to five words. The patient had a severe hearing loss and wore hearing aids. He was able to learn sign language, which greatly improved communication. A ventriculoperitoneal shunt was placed after progressive ventricular enlargement was observed and elevated central nervous system pressure measured under anesthesia. He died after a respiratory arrest occurred while he was riding the school bus shortly before his seventh birthday. Two to 3 months before his death he had a rapid decline of muscle tone resulting in progressive breathing problems, poor head control, and inability to walk. His father described him as a happy child who didn't complain and was a joy to be around.

months, with a maximum stature of 110 cm reported. Developmental delay is usually apparent by 12 to 24 months, with a maximum functional age obtainable of 2 to 4 years followed by progressive deterioration. Most children with Hurler syndrome develop only limited language skills because of the developmental delay, chronic hearing loss, and enlarged tongue. Some degree of hearing loss is probably universal, usually due to a combination of conductive and neurosensory problems; hearing aids are helpful in some children. Most Hurler children have recurring upper-respiratory tract and ear infections, noisy breathing, and persistent, copious nasal discharge. Progressive clouding of the cornea also begins during the first year of life, and glaucoma may occur in some patients.[128] The communicating hydrocephalus in Hurler syndrome is usually associated with increased intracranial pressure; shunting procedures are beneficial for most children. Obstructive airway disease, respiratory infection, and cardiac complications are the usual causes of death. Severe diffuse coronary artery disease can occur early in the course of Hurler syndrome; selective coronary angiography underestimates the extent of disease.[129,130]

Radiologic changes seen in Hurler syndrome typify the constellation of skeletal abnormalities in mucopolysaccharidoses known as dysostosis multiplex.[1,2,131] The skull is large, with thickened calvarium, premature closure of lamboid and sagittal sutures, shallow orbits, enlarged J-shaped sella, and abnormal spacing of the teeth with dentigerous cysts. Anterior hypoplasia of lumbar vertebrae with kyphosis is seen early. The diaphyses of the long bones are enlarged, with irregular appearances of the metaphyses. Epiphyseal centers are not well developed. The pelvis is usually poorly formed, with small femoral heads and coxa valga. Clavicles are short, thickened, and irregular. The ribs have been described as oar-shaped, narrowed at their vertebral ends, and flat and broad at their sternal ends. Phalanges are shortened and trapezoidal in shape, with widening of the diaphysis.

MPS IH/S (Hurler-Scheie). This classification is used to describe a clinical phenotype that is intermediate between the Hurler and Scheie syndromes. It is characterized by progressive somatic involvement, including dysostosis multiplex, with little or no intellectual dysfunction (Fig. 136-7).

Corneal clouding, joint stiffness, deafness, and valvular heart disease can develop by the early to mid-teens and cause significant impairment and loss of function. Some patients with MPS IH/S have micrognathia, which creates a characteristic facies. Pachymeningitis cervicalis, compression of the cervical cord due to mucopolysaccharide accumulation in the dura, occurs in MPS IH/S, but communicating hydrocephalus appears to be uncommon in patients with normal intelligence. Spondylolisthesis of the lower spine leading to spinal cord compression can occur in MPS IH/S as well as in MPS IS patients. The onset of symptoms is usually observed between 3 and 8 years, and survival to adulthood is common. Cardiac involvement and upper airway obstruction contribute to clinical mortality.

MPS IS (Scheie). This mild form of MPS I is characterized by joint stiffness, aortic valve disease, corneal clouding, and few other somatic features (Fig. 136-8). The facial features are characteristically coarse, but intelligence and stature are normal. The joint involvement is prominent in the hands with a claw-hand deformity. MPS IS patients can have a stiff painful foot, pes cavus, and genu valgum. The joint deformity in the hands and feet[132] coupled with the development of carpal-tunnel syndrome can lead to limitation of function. Ophthalmologic manifestations include glaucoma and retinal degeneration that, in addition to the severe corneal clouding, may contribute to significant visual impairment. Obstructive airway disease causing sleep apnea develops in some patients, necessitating tracheostomy, which has been beneficial.[133] Aortic valvular disease, with stenosis and/or regurgitation, occurs due to buildup of mucopolysaccharide deposits on valves and chordae tendineae. Valve replacement has been beneficial in MPS IS and MPS IH/S.[134,135] Compression of the cervical cord by thickened dura, pachymeningitis cervicalis, with resulting myelopathy can occur in MPS IS, although less commonly than in MPS IH/S. Deafness has been reported in some patients, but the etiology is unknown. The onset of significant symptoms is usually after the age of 5 years, with the diagnosis commonly made between 10 and 20 years of age.

Mucopolysaccharidosis II (Hunter Syndrome)

The Hunter syndrome comprises two recognized clinical entities, mild and severe, but these may represent two ends of a wide spectrum of clinical severity.[2,136–139] The mild and severe forms of Hunter syndrome are separated on clinical grounds because iduronate sulfatase activity appears equally deficient in both forms; however, mutation analysis can be helpful in many cases (see below). The severe form of Hunter syndrome has features similar to Hurler syndrome, except for the lack of corneal clouding

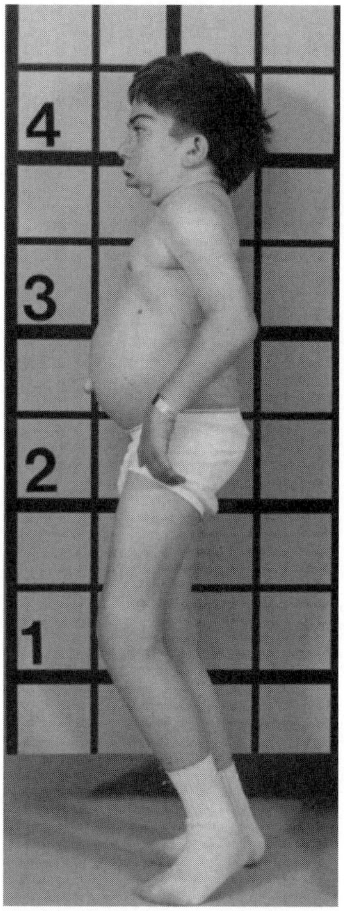

Fig. 136-7 MPS IH/S (Hurler-Scheie syndrome) in a 14.5-year-old boy. The patient demonstrates short stature, stiff joints, micrognathia, corneal clouding, umbilical hernia, hepatosplenomegaly, a systolic murmur, and normal intelligence. Diagnosis was made at the age of 1 year based on skeletal abnormalities consistent with MPS. At age 10, during attempted endotracheal intubation for carpal tunnel surgery, the patient had a respiratory arrest. Progressive joint restriction and corneal clouding had been the major clinical problems until the age of 16, when the symptoms of obstructive apnea and congestive heart failure developed. Nasal continuous positive airway pressure while sleeping dramatically relieved the obstructive apnea, alleviating the need for a tracheostomy. He had increasing visual loss with development of glaucoma, which was difficult to treat. He graduated from high school at age 19 and attended college. He died at age 21 from complications of open-heart surgery 4 days after an aortic valve replacement. Valvuloplasty (aortic and mitral) procedures prior to the attempt at valve replacement had some clinical benefit.

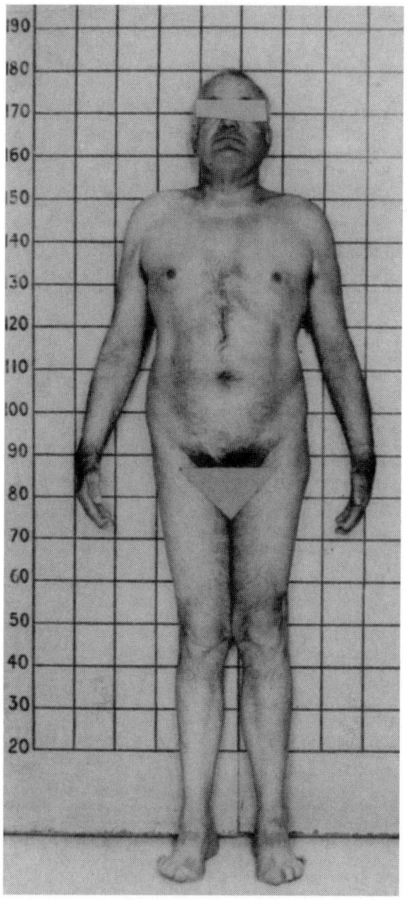

Fig. 136-8 MPS IS (Scheie syndrome) in a highly intelligent man who retired from the practice of law at the age of 74 years. He was 20 years younger when the picture was taken. Stiff joints, particularly claw hands and deformed feet (first noticed at age 7), and visual impairment due to corneal clouding (first recorded by an ophthalmologist at age 13), pigmentary retinopathy, and glaucoma were physically limiting features. He also has had carpal tunnel syndrome, genu valgum, hypertrichosis, inguinal hernia, "broad-mouth" facies, and aortic regurgitation. The normal stature is noteworthy. Deafness, beginning in his 40s, was profound by age 75, when he was also blind. He lived to the age of 78. A sister, 13 years younger, is similarly affected.

and slower progression of somatic and central nervous system involvement. The mild form is analogous to Hurler/Scheie or Scheie syndrome, with a longer life span, a slower progression of somatic deterioration, and retention of intelligence. The occurrence of a pebbly, ivory-colored skin lesion over the back, upper arms, and lateral aspects of the thigh is unique to the Hunter syndrome, but its presence does not correlate with the severity of the disease.

The Hunter syndrome is inherited in an X-linked recessive manner, males generally do not reproduce, and therefore affected females are not expected. Nevertheless, there are a few girls with well-documented Hunter syndrome, generally of the mild form.[140–143] These affected girls are heterozygotes in whom some additional genetic event has prevented the expression of the normal allele (see "Molecular Genetics" below).

MPS II (Severe). The severe type of Hunter syndrome is characterized by coarse facial features, short stature, skeletal deformities, joint stiffness, and mental retardation (Fig. 136-9). The onset of the disease usually occurs between 2 and 4 years of age with progressive neurologic and somatic involvement.[139] Patients can have severe retinal degeneration, but corneas characteristically remain clear. Chronic diarrhea, due to autonomic nervous system involvement and perhaps also to mucosal dysfunction, is a troublesome problem in many of the younger patients. Recurrent ear infections and progressive hearing impairment occur in most patients. Moderate to severe communicating hydrocephalus probably exacerbates the central nervous system deterioration with increased intracranial pressure after the age of 7 to 10 years. The communicating hydrocephalus may be present at the time of diagnosis and progress slowly over many years. Extensive neurologic involvement, similar to that of late stages of Sanfilippo syndrome, precedes death, which usually occurs between 10 and 15 years, although it may occur earlier. The usual causes of death are obstructive airway disease and cardiac failure due to valvular dysfunction, myocardial thickening, pulmonary hypertension, coronary artery narrowing, and myocardial disease.

Some of the most severely affected Hunter patients have additional features including Hurler-like symptoms, early onset of seizures, and ptosis. This atypical phenotype is caused by large

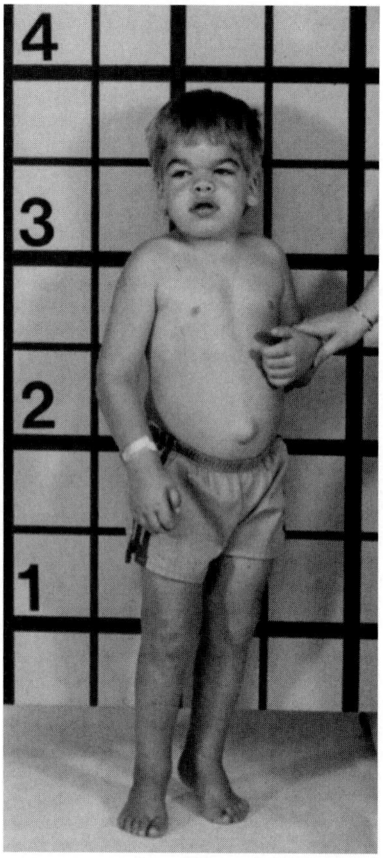

Fig. 136-9 Severe MPS II (Hunter syndrome) in a 6-year-old boy. Diagnosis was suspected at 1 year of age because of facial appearance, but a urine mucopolysaccharide screen was negative. Enzymatic diagnosis was made at age 22 months after a family history of a maternal uncle with mental retardation and coarse facial features became known to the parents. At the time the picture was taken, the patient had hepatomegaly, joint stiffness, severe hearing loss, developmental delay, recurrent ear infections, and hyperactivity. From about 1 to 7 years of age, he was hyperactive to the point of being uncontrollable and required less than 2 h of sleep per night. At age 8, he had an unsteady gait, refused to eat solid foods, and had significant loss of overall skills. For the next 4 years, his functioning level was stable with decreased hyperactivity. By age 13, he could no longer walk, had severe joint involvement, and had weight loss due to progressive problems with swallowing. His chronic nasal discharge and frequent ear infections have much improved since the age of 10. He was never toilet trained, and has had severe constipation for the last 7 years, requiring frequent enemas. Now 18 years old, he has limited movement with poor trunk support, as well as minimal awareness of his surroundings. He constantly chews on his hands and soft objects. A gastrostomy tube was recently placed to supplement feeding.

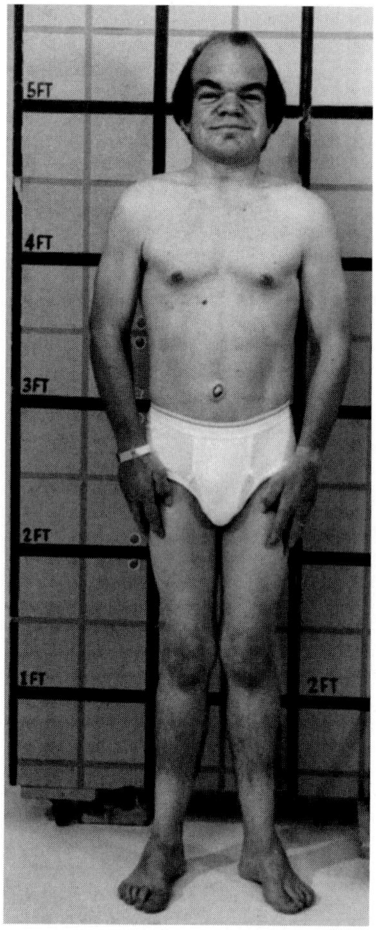

Fig. 136-10 Mild MPS II (Hunter syndrome) in a 28-year-old man. At the age of 13, when the diagnosis was made, he had joint stiffness, coarse facial features, heart murmur, and normal intelligence. The patient has had surgery for inguinal hernia and carpal tunnel syndrome. Two maternal uncles and a nephew also have Hunter syndrome. He is married and has two healthy daughters. He has a very active career as a minister and counselor. Now 42 years old, he is healthy, but develops wheezing with upper respiratory infections, requiring treatment.

deletions that include iduronate sulfatase and contiguous genes[144,145] (see "Molecular Genetics" below).

MPS II (Mild). A milder form of Hunter syndrome is characterized by preservation of intelligence and survival into adulthood, but with obvious somatic involvement (Fig. 136-10).[137,138] Somatic features similar to those seen in severely affected Hunter patients can develop in these patients, but at a reduced rate of progression. Hearing impairment is probably universal, and hearing aids are beneficial. Carpal tunnel syndrome and joint stiffness are common and can result in loss of function. Cervical myopathy due to a narrowed spinal canal and cord compression may be more common than generally recognized.[146] Discrete corneal opacities detectable only by slit-lamp examination have been observed.[147] Electroretinography gives evidence of retinal dysfunction, but to a much lesser extent than in the severe form.[148] Chronic papilledema has been reported in patients with mild Hunter syndrome without raised intracranial pressure,[149,150] perhaps due to deposition of glycosaminoglycans within the sclera, causing compression of the optic nerve at the intrascleral level. Some patients with mild Hunter syndrome have survived into the fifth and sixth decades of life, with the longest known survival to age 87;[151] however, death may occur in early adulthood or even in the late teens, usually from airway obstruction and cardiac failure.

Mucopolysaccharidosis III (Sanfilippo Syndrome)

Patients with Sanfilippo syndrome make up a biochemically diverse, but clinically similar, group, classified into four types based on the enzyme deficiency. Heparan *N*-sulfatase is deficient in type A, α-*N*-acetylglucosaminidase in type B, acetyl-CoA : α-glucosaminide acetyltransferase in type C, and *N*-acetyl glucosamine 6-sulfatase in type D. The four enzymes are required for the degradation of heparan sulfate (Fig. 136-3). Phenotypic variation exists among MPS III patients but to a lesser degree than in the other MPS, possibly because very mild forms of MPS III may be more difficult to recognize.

The Sanfilippo syndrome is characterized by severe central nervous system degeneration, but only mild somatic disease (Figs. 136-11 and 136-12). Such disproportionate involvement of the central nervous system is unique among the MPS. Onset of clinical features usually occurs between 2 and 6 years in a child who

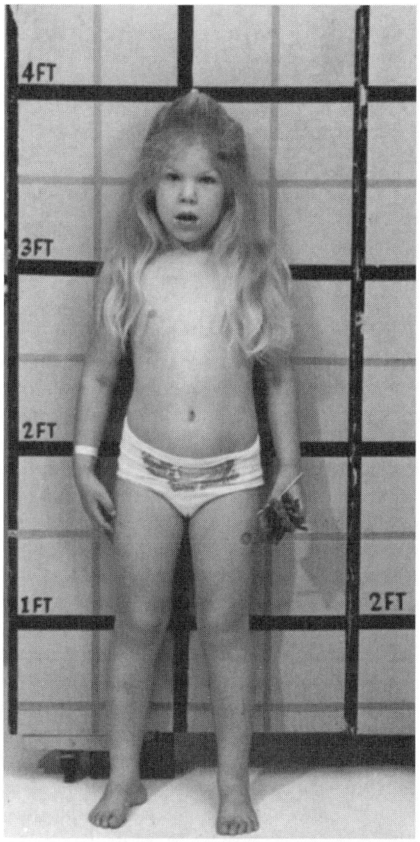

Fig. 136-11 MPS IIIA (Sanfilippo syndrome, type A) in a 7-year-old girl. The patient had normal developmental skills until about 5 years of age, at which time she was toilet trained, was able to feed and dress herself, and spoke in complete sentences. She was learning to read and write. At the time of the picture, she had a normal physical appearance with mild hepatomegaly, but showed a significant loss of function. At age 11, she was able to feed herself and functioned at a 3- to 4-year-old level. Her language skills were limited, but she was usually able to communicate her needs. She remained toilet trained up to the age of 13. She had minimal deterioration in skills from age 9 to 14, but rapid decline over the next 18 months. She stopped talking at the age of 14. At 15.5 years, her mental abilities were less than those of a year-old infant, but she was able to ride a tricycle, use a spoon, and drink from a cup. With her decline in function, she had outbursts of aggressive behavior that could result in significant harm to others, although previously her hyperactivity was not a major problem. Now 20 years old, she requires constant custodial care, but is still able to feed herself and no longer has behavior outbursts. She still recognizes her parents and enjoys taking walks. She had a severely affected older brother, whose disease progressed more rapidly during childhood. He died accidentally before his seventeenth birthday after choking on a rubber glove.

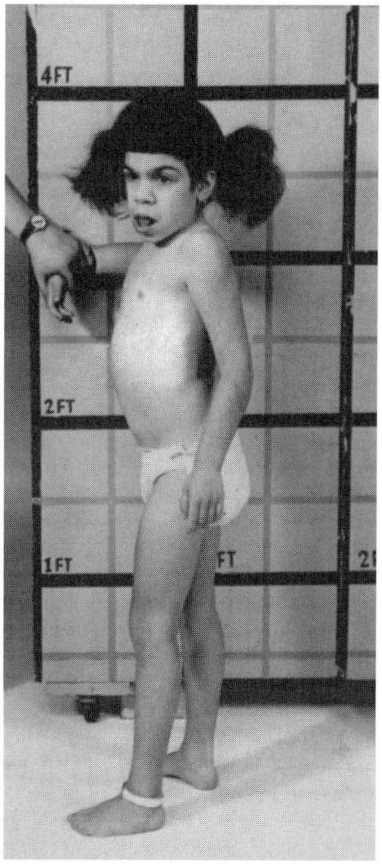

Fig. 136-12 MPS IIIB (Sanfilippo syndrome type B) in a 7-year-old girl. Enzymatic diagnosis was made at 14 months of age, when the child presented with slight coarsening of facial features, increased body hair, and a family history of an older brother with MPS IIIB who had been diagnosed at 3.5 years of age. At the time of the picture, the patient had mild hepatomegaly, cardiomegaly, severe hearing loss, recurrent ear infections, hirsutism, marked hyperactivity, and aggressive behavior that limited her ability to interact with other children; she had no language skills, but was able to feed herself. She attended a special school, and generally was a happy child. At age 15.5 years, she stopped walking and required a gastrotomy tube for nutritional support because she refused to eat. During the year before her death, shortly before she reached age 17, she was severely neurologically impaired and no longer recognized her family. Her brother, who died at age 16 due to severe neurologic disease, had a more rapidly progressing disease during childhood.

previously appeared normal, but may occur earlier or later. Presenting features can include hyperactivity with aggressive behavior, delayed development, coarse hair, hirsutism, sleep disorders, and mild hepatosplenomegaly (the latter is found in young patients, but is uncommon in teenagers and adults with MPS III). There may be a significant delay in the diagnosis of MPS III after the onset of symptoms due to the mild somatic and radiographic features and to a high incidence of false negative results in the urinary screening test for excess mucopolysaccharides. Coarse facial features are not a prominent component of Sanfilippo syndrome, and some patients have normal features as adults. Skeletal involvement is minimal, with only mild dysostosis multiplex, usually normal stature for age, and mild joint stiffness which rarely causes loss of function. Recurrent and sometimes severe diarrhea is unexplained, but usually improves in older children. Speech development is often delayed, with poor articulation and content, and some patients may never learn to speak. Severe hearing loss is common in the moderate to severely affected patient. Seizures commonly occur in the older patient, but are usually easily controlled. Early onset of puberty occurs in many MPS III patients.[152]

Severe neurologic degeneration occurs in most patients by 6 to 10 years of age, accompanied by rapid deterioration of social and adaptive skills. Cranial CT at the onset of mental deterioration demonstrates mild to moderate cortical atrophy in most patients. Progression to severe cortical atrophy occurs in the late stages of the disease. Patients can be very withdrawn and lose contact with the environment as a result of the progressive dementia. Sleep disturbances and insomnia are common.[153] Severe behavior problems are usual and can include poor attention span, uncontrollable hyperactivity, temper tantrums, destructive behavior, and physical aggression. Profound mental retardation and behavior problems often occur in patients with normal physical strength, making treatment particularly difficult. Pharmacologic management of the behavior problems gives variable results;[154] behavior modification may occasionally be effective.[155]

It is difficult to distinguish individual patients with any of the four types of the Sanfilippo syndrome on clinical grounds because there is significant clinical heterogeneity in each disorder. Overall, type A is the most severe, with earlier onset, more rapid progression of symptoms, and shorter survival, while type B patients have been known to remain functional into the third or even fourth decades.[156] However, there are adult patients with type A,[157] as well as severe patients with type B (Muenzer, personal observation). A particularly grave form of type A Sanfilippo syndrome occurs in the Cayman Islands.[158] Severe and mild forms of Sanfilippo syndrome have been reported even within the same family.[159] The type C and D forms of MPS III also appear to be clinically heterogeneous.

Mucopolysaccharidosis IV (Morquio Syndrome)

Morquio syndrome is caused by defective degradation of keratan sulfate. Two enzyme deficiencies resulting in Morquio syndrome are recognized, each with a wide spectrum of clinical manifestations: a deficiency of *N*-acetylgalactosamine 6-sulfatase in MPS IVA and of β-galactosidase in MPS IVB (Fig. 136-4). Both types of Morquio syndrome are characterized by short-trunk dwarfism, fine corneal deposits, a skeletal (spondyloepiphyseal) dysplasia distinct from that in the other MPS, and preservation of intelligence.

The predominant clinical features of Morquio syndrome are those related to the skeleton and their effects on the central nervous system[160,161] (Fig. 136-13). As in most mucopolysaccharidoses, patients with Morquio syndrome appear normal at birth. The appearance of genu valgum, kyphosis, growth retardation with short trunk and neck, and waddling gait with a tendency to fall are early symptoms of Morquio syndrome. Holzgreve et al.[160] report that the first symptoms caused by the disease in 11 patients with MPS IVA occurred between 1 and 3 to 4 years of age, although the diagnosis of Morquio syndrome was not made until 3 to 15 years of age. Typical skeletal anomalies of Morquio syndrome include dwarfism with short trunk; platyspondylia; odontoid hypoplasia; kyphosis; hyperlordosis; scoliosis; ovoid deformities of the vertebrae; genu valgum; ulnar deviation of the wrist; valgus deformity of the elbow; inclinations of distal ends of radius and ulna toward each other; deformities of metacarpals and short phalanges; epiphyseal deformities of the tubular bones; widened metaphyses; and osteoporosis.[1,4] Joints tend to be hypermobile secondary to ligamentous laxity, but decreased joint mobility can occur in the large joints (especially hips and knees, and sometimes elbows).

Odontoid hypoplasia is a universal clinical finding with grave medical consequences for patients with Morquio syndrome.[162] The instability of the hypoplastic odontoid process with ligamentous laxity can result in life-threatening atlantoaxial subluxation. Cervical myelopathy can develop early in patients with the severe form of Morquio syndrome. Patients with the severe form may not survive beyond their twenties or thirties. Paralysis from the myelopathy, restrictive chest wall movement, and valvular heart disease all contribute to their shortened life span. Surgery to stabilize the upper cervical spine, usually by spinal fusion, can be lifesaving.[163,164] Atlantoaxial instability and subsequent subluxation and quadriparesis have also been reported in one patient each with MPS I[165] and MPS VII.[166]

Extraskeletal manifestations of Morquio syndrome may include hearing impairment, mild corneal clouding, hepatomegaly, upper airway obstruction, cardiac valvular lesions, and small teeth with abnormally thin enamel and frequent caries formation.[161,167] Unusual facial features (coarsening of facies, prognathism, and broad mouth) are commonly found.

MPS IVB, β-galactosidase deficiency, was initially considered to be the mild form of Morquio syndrome because in the first patients described, the progression of skeletal dysplasias and stunting of growth were less pronounced than in MPS IVA.[168,169] However, subsequent reports have described patients with MPS IVB whose clinical disease was as severe as that seen in the severe form of MPS IVA.[170,171] In addition, patients with a mild form of MPS IVA have been reported, having almost normal stature, mild skeletal abnormalities with dysplastic hips, corneal clouding, and absent keratosulfaturia.[172–177] Nelson and Thomas[177] reported

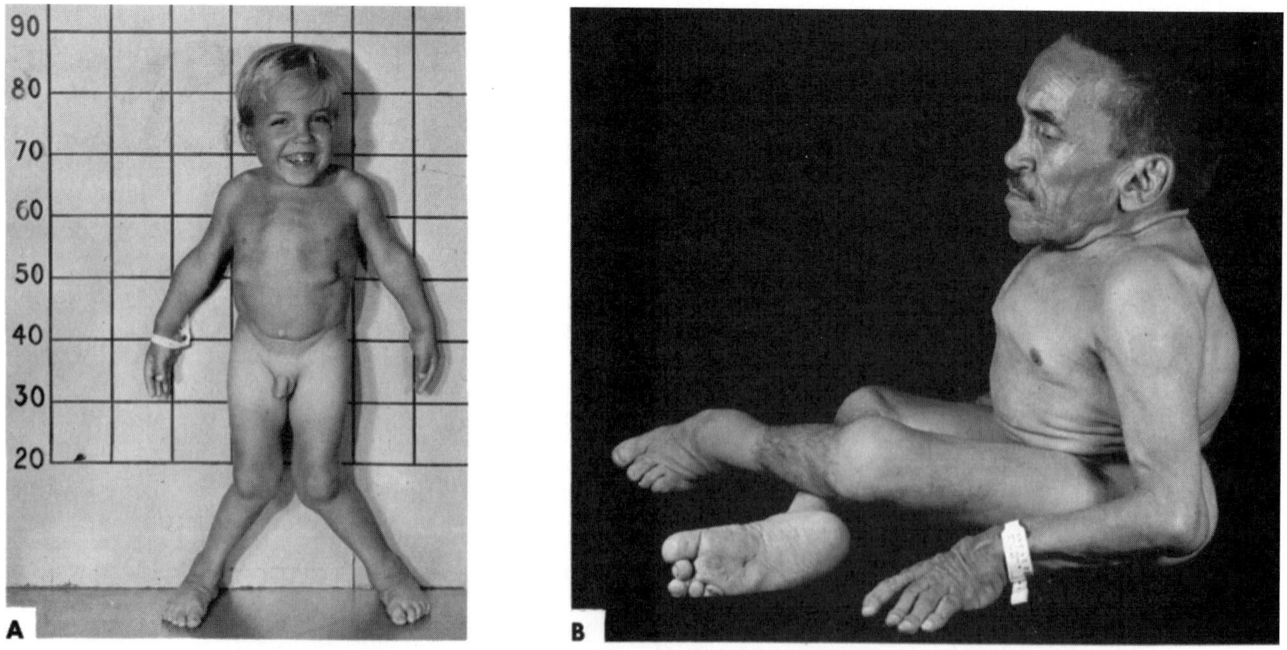

Fig. 136-13 MPS IV (Morquio syndrome). *A*, Clinically and radiologically this 8.5-year-old boy shows the skeletal deformities typical of the Morquio syndrome. The mother noted flaring of the lower ribs at birth, flat feet at age 3 years, and a small size at age 4, when the diagnosis was made. *B*, At the age of 55, when this picture was taken, this man showed pectus carinatum, bilateral genu valgum, diffuse corneal clouding, atlantoaxial subluxation, and bilateral sensorineural deafness. A protuberance of the chest was first noted at age 2. He attended a school for the handicapped and performed well academically. He worked all his life in his brother's architectural firm. He died of cardiorespiratory failure at the age of 69. A similarly affected brother died at age 24. Both patients are described in references 1 and 4.

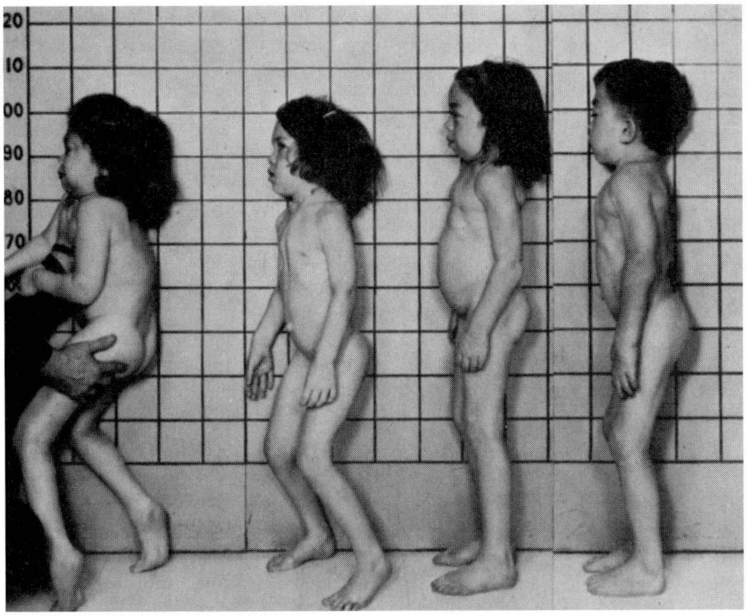

Fig. 136-14 MPS VI (Maroteaux-Lamy syndrome). These four sibs, all with the severe form of MPS VI, were aged 14, 9, 13, and 11 years (from left to right) at the time of the picture.[1] In the oldest sib, noisy breathing was noted at 2 years of age and flexion contractures at the knees at 4 years. She was a good student. At the age of 9, generalized weakness slowly developed to the point at which she could not feed herself, but she remained alert. She was hospitalized at age 11 for her first episode of congestive heart failure and died at age 15.5 years. The three other sibs have followed a similar course.

that patients with a mild form of MPS IVA had odontoid dysplasia, but did not have atlantoaxial instability. Therefore it is apparent that each enzyme deficiency has a wide spectrum of clinical manifestations.

Mucopolysaccharidosis VI (Maroteaux-Lamy Syndrome)

Maroteaux-Lamy syndrome was first recognized in 1963 by Maroteaux and coworkers[178] as a Hurler-like syndrome, but with preservation of intelligence and excretion of dermatan sulfate unaccompanied by heparan sulfate. Milder forms of MPS VI have been recognized since the initial description of the disorder.[4] All forms of Maroteaux-Lamy syndrome are caused by deficiency of *N*-acetylgalactosamine 4-sulfatase (arylsulfatase B).

Mental development is usually normal in patients with Maroteaux-Lamy syndrome, although physical and visual impairments may impede psychomotor performance. Although mental retardation has been reported in two families with arylsulfatase B deficiency,[179,180] it is not clear that the retardation was caused by the MPS.

The somatic involvement in the severe form of Maroteaux-Lamy syndrome is similar to that in Hurler syndrome (Fig. 136-14). An enlarged head and a deformed chest may be present at birth. Umbilical and/or inguinal hernias are common. Growth can be normal for the first few years of life but seems to virtually stop after the age of 6 or 8 years, with the ultimate height of severely affected patients ranging from 110 to 140 cm. Corneal opacities are easily detected by slit-lamp examination. Obvious corneal clouding develops in some patients and can result in visual impairment. Restriction of joint movement (knee, hip, and elbow) develops in the first years of life, and the children assume a crouched stance. Claw-hand deformities are seen in children secondary to flexion contractures of the fingers. Nerve entrapment syndromes, particularly of the carpal tunnel, are common and can be improved with surgery. The facies can remain relatively mildly affected in some patients, but others assume the coarseness characteristic of Hurler syndrome. Hepatomegaly is always present after the age of 6 years, and an enlarged spleen is found in half the patients.[181] The skin usually is described as "tight," and mild hirsutism is found. The typical severe MPS VI patient at the end of the first decade of life has a shortened trunk with protuberant abdomen and prominent lumbar lordosis. Aortic and mitral valvular dysfunction due primarily to thickened calcified stenotic valves are the most prominent cardiac involvement in the milder phenotypes.[182] Successful single and double (aortic and mitral) valve replacements have been reported in MPS VI.[183] Acute infantile cardiomyopathy has been reported in two MPS VI infants as a presenting feature of the disorder.[184,185] Most reported patients with the severe form of MPS VI have died of heart failure in the second to third decades.

The skeletal changes associated with the severe Maroteaux-Lamy syndrome are similar to radiographic findings of Hurler syndrome and are striking examples of dysostosis multiplex. The pelvic changes are particularly severe, with acetabulum hypoplasia and small flared iliac wings. The prominent radiologic features also include macrocephaly with a large sella, ovoid deformity of vertebral bodies, a hood-shaped deformity or blunt anterior hypoplasia of vertebral bodies of L1 or L2, epiphyseal dysplasia of the proximal femur, an elongated femoral neck in a valgus position, and irregular diaphyseal distension of tubular bones.

Spinal cord compression from thickening of the dura in the upper cervical spinal canal with resultant myelopathy is a frequent occurrence in patients with the milder forms of MPS VI. A 41-year-old woman with a mild-to-intermediate form of MPS VI had an insidious development of compressive cervical myelopathy with resulting spastic tetraparesis.[186] There was substantial improvement following laminectomy and excision of the markedly thickened dura (5 mm). The spinal cord compression with resultant myelopathy may be associated with developmental abnormalities of the vertebral bodies and dural thickening. The compression myelopathy associated with a kyphoscoliotic deformity of thoracolumbar spine in a 10-year-old patient with MPS VI has been described.[187]

Mucopolysaccharidosis VII (Sly Syndrome)

β-Glucuronidase deficiency was first recognized in a patient with a phenotype reminiscent of MPS IH or MPS II.[188] The patient had an unusual facies, protruding sternum, hepatosplenomegaly, umbilical hernia, thoracolumbar gibbus, marked vertebral deformities, and moderate mental deficiency (Fig.136-15). Granulocytes showed striking coarse metachromatic granules. Fine corneal opacities were not noted until 8 years of age. Moderate mental retardation was evident by age 3 but appeared not to be progressive. In addition, neurologic regression did not occur after 3 to 4 years of age. Radiographic changes of dysostosis multiplex were moderately severe. Since the description of the original patient, many patients with β-glucuronidase deficiency have been reported (reviewed in references 189 to 191). The patients have

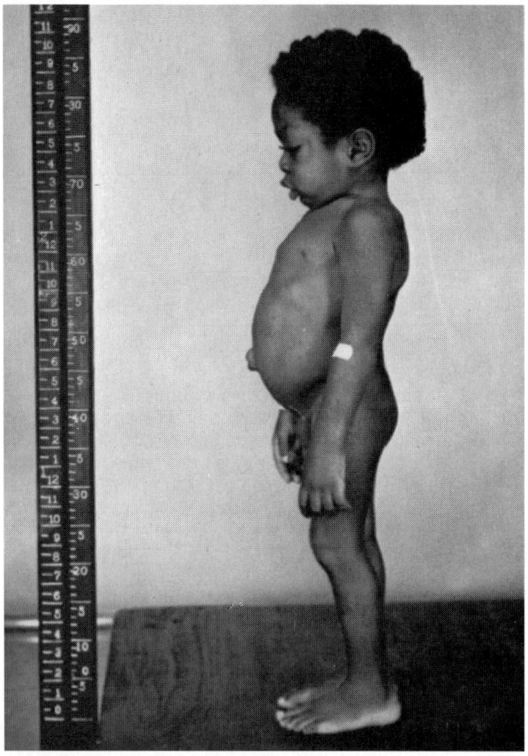

Fig. 136-15 MPS VII (Sly syndrome). This is the original patient with β-glucuronidase deficiency.[188] Aged 3 years at the time this picture was taken, he showed flared ribs, pigeon breast, hepatosplenomegaly, and umbilical hernia. During childhood and adolescence, his major problems were orthopedic. Progressive kyphoscoliosis was treated with a body brace. Because of odontoid hypoplasia, he wore a neck brace to stabilize his neck. Progressive deformity of the hips made walking painful for several years, and he had to use a cane or walker when on his feet for prolonged periods. Mental retardation was moderate but nonprogressive. Despite these limitations, he attended special school regularly, was happily adjusted, and appeared to be enjoying life until he died unexpectedly following a meal at age 20. Autopsy revealed aspiration but did not definitively establish the cause of death.

presented with a wide range of clinical severity ranging from nonimmune hydrops fetalis to mild disease in adults. The severe neonatal form may be the most common type of the Sly syndrome. It is characterized by hydrops fetalis, dysostosis multiplex, dysmorphic features, and clinical and pathologic findings of a lysosomal storage disease.[191–197] The neonatal form itself is heterogeneous, ranging from death *in utero* to mild or no hydrops at birth. A review of other pregnancies among mothers of MPS VII patients suggests an increased number of spontaneous abortions.[191] The neonatal form of β-glucuronidase deficiency is one of the few lysosomal storage diseases with clinical manifestations *in utero* or at birth.[198]

Most patients presenting beyond the neonatal period have increased urinary glycosaminoglycans and dysostosis multiplex, but with variable onset and severity of other clinical features. MPS VII patients who present as infants or young children (severe form) have typical Hurler features such as hepatomegaly, inguinal and/or umbilical hernias, moderate skeletal abnormalities, repeated episodes of pneumonia in the first years of life, short stature, and developmental delay. Corneal clouding has been a variable finding. A mild form of later onset (after 4 years of age) is characterized by progressive skeletal involvement with normal intelligence and typically no corneal clouding.[189,190,199] As in most MPS disorders, a spectrum of clinical severity occurs in MPS VII, with the neonatal and the mild forms representing two ends of a clinical spectrum. In retrospect, the first MPS VII patient described (Fig. 136-15) had an intermediate phenotype.

Mucopolysaccharidosis IX (Hyaluronidase Deficiency)

Only one patient has been reported to date with mucopolysaccharidosis IX.[105] Major findings were bilateral nodular soft-tissue periarticular masses, with transient episodes of painful swelling of the masses and generalized cutaneous swelling that resolved spontaneously within 3 days. She has mildly dysmorphic craniofacial features with acquired short stature and normal joint movement and intelligence. Pelvic radiography revealed multiple bilateral nodular, intra-articular soft-tissue masses, and acetabular erosions. These manifestations are presumably consequences of the inability to degrade the hyaluronan that is normally found in high concentration in cartilage and synovial fluid.

Management of the Mucopolysaccharidoses

Because most MPS patients are not candidates for specific therapies, management consists of supportive care and treatment of complications, even as specific therapies are being developed (see below). The progressive nature of organ involvement in MPS patients dictates the need for continual evaluation of their clinical status.[200] Systematic evaluation of hearing, vision, and joint function coupled with treatment of specific problems can lead to improved quality of life by minimizing the handicapping effects of diffuse systemic disease.

Hydrocephalus. Ventricular enlargement is known to occur in patients with MPS and may be due to the combination of cortical atrophy secondary to central nervous system degeneration or a defect in cerebrospinal fluid reabsorption.[201–205] The defective reabsorption of cerebrospinal fluid in MPS is presumably due to thickening of the meninges and dysfunction of the pacchionian granulation in the arachnoid villi. Thickened meninges and ventricular enlargement are common findings at autopsy in MPS. The communicating hydrocephalus that occurs in MPS is usually only slowly progressive, with clinical symptoms that are difficult to distinguish from the primary neurologic disease. Acute symptoms such as vomiting and papilledema due to communicating hydrocephalus are uncommon.[204]

Computerized tomography (CT) studies on 12 patients with MPS showed that the development of hydrocephalus was variable and suggested that shunting procedures are sometimes indicated to improve quality of life.[203] Noncontrast cranial CT studies showed mild to severe hydrocephalus in 32 of 42 MPS patients (MPS I, II, and III) ranging in age from 18 months to 26 years[5] (Muenzer J, unpublished data). Ventricular enlargement was unsuspected in most patients at the time of initial evaluation. All patients with ventricular enlargement had mental retardation, the degree of enlargement correlating with severity of retardation, whereas only 2 of the 10 patients with normal CT scans had mental retardation. Two patients with Hurler syndrome, who were less than 2 years of age, had minimally abnormal CT scans and mild developmental delay. The eight MPS patients with normal CT scans and normal intelligence represented only two MPS types: Hurler/Scheie and mild Hunter syndromes. The ventricular enlargement in Hurler and severe Hunter syndromes is usually associated with increased central nervous system pressure and a communicating hydrocephalus as demonstrated by lumbar cisternography. The CT scans in the older patients with Sanfilippo syndrome showed ventricular enlargement with evidence of diffuse cortical atrophy. No evidence of papilledema was found in MPS patients with hydrocephalus and documented increased intracranial pressure when examined under anesthesia.

Ventriculoperitoneal shunting in MPS patients with moderate to severe hydrocephalus is generally palliative. The degree to which hydrocephalus contributes to the neurologic deterioration in MPS is unknown. Few patients have had shunts implanted at the onset of their hydrocephalus; early recognition of hydrocephalus and shunting may provide a better outcome. The presence of increased central nervous system pressure and progressive ventricular enlargement can be used as indications for a shunting procedure. The ventricular enlargement in patients with Sanfilippo syndrome is probably secondary to cortical atrophy, and it is generally thought that shunting would not be beneficial. However, a recent report indicated that shunting alleviated some extreme behavioral disturbances in six Sanfilippo patients[206] and the issue deserves further study.

Vision. Corneal clouding is common in MPS I, MPS IV, MPS VI, and MPS VII, and can lead to significant visual disability.[207–209] Corneal transplantation has been performed, but the long-term outcome is not always successful.[210,211] Patients with clear grafts may still have poor vision because of associated retinal and/or optic nerve disease. Glaucoma is a complication in several of the MPS.[128,212–216] The trabecular meshwork is usually engorged with glycosaminoglycans, and the sclera and cornea are thickened, causing shallow anterior chambers.

Retinal degeneration commonly occurs in MPS I, II, and III, resulting in decreased peripheral vision and night blindness.[148] A night-light may help reduce sleep disturbances.

Hearing. Deafness, usually of combined conductive and neurosensory origin, occurs commonly in MPS.[217–220] The deafness has been attributed to three causes: frequent middle ear infections, deformity of the ossicles, and probable abnormalities of the inner ear. Auditory brain-stem response is abnormal in a nonspecific way, probably reflecting a mixture of middle ear, cochlear, eighth-nerve, and lower-brain-stem anomalies (Pikus AT, Muenzer J, unpublished data). Ventilating tubes can minimize the long-term sequelae of the frequent episodes of acute otitis media and chronic middle ear effusions that are commonplace in most MPS patients. Most MPS patients have significant hearing loss and would benefit from hearing aids. Aggressive audiologic management strategies are needed to maintain the highest quality of life.

Joint Stiffness. Joint stiffness is a common feature of all MPS, except for Morquio syndrome, in which there is ligamentous laxity. Limitation of motion and joint stiffness can cause significant loss of function. The abnormal joint function probably results from a combination of metaphyseal deformities and thickened joint capsules secondary to glycosaminoglycan accumulation and fibrosis. Range-of-motion exercises appear to offer some benefits in preserving joint function, and should be started early. Once significant limitation has occurred, increased range of motion may not be achieved, although further limitation may be minimized. The indications of physical therapy and its benefits in MPS should be further studied.

Carpal Tunnel Syndrome. Carpal tunnel syndrome is a very common complication in MPS, but most patients lack typical symptoms (pain, tingling, or numbness) until severe compression occurs.[221–223] Because of the high incidence of carpal tunnel syndrome and the minimal subjective complaints, routine electromyographic/nerve conduction velocity testing is recommended.[223] The loss of thumb function due to carpal tunnel syndrome can be a significant handicap in combination with the skeletal dysplasia, which can also lead to decreased hand movement. Surgical decompression of the median nerve has resulted in complete restoration of motor hand activity in some and partial improvements in others.[223,224] Clearly, to obtain the best outcome, nerve decompression should be undertaken in an early stage of involvement, prior to severe nerve damage.

Obstructive Airway Disease. A narrowed trachea, thickened vocal cords, redundant tissue in the upper airway, and an enlarged tongue all contribute to airway obstruction.[225–228] Intermittent obstruction in the severely involved MPS patients is common and may lead to sleep apnea.[229] Obstructive apnea has been reported in two patients with Scheie syndrome who had loud snoring and daytime sleepiness.[133] Tracheostomy can produce a dramatic symptomatic improvement in patients with obstructive apnea. Obstructive sleep apnea in a 23-year-old man with MPS II who had diffuse airway obstruction, daytime hypersomnolence, snoring, and alveolar hypoventilation was successfully treated with high pressure nasal continuous positive airway pressure and supplemental oxygen.[230] Obstructive airway disease is probably common in the severely involved MPS patients, but sleep studies to determine the extent of airway compromise are not routinely performed.[229,231] Tonsillectomy and adenoidectomy are frequently performed in patients with MPS to correct eustachian tube dysfunction and decrease airway obstruction. Treatment of tracheal lesions by laser excision may benefit some MPS patients.[232]

Anesthesia. Patients with MPS present major anesthesia risks.[233–240] In Morquio syndrome in particular, but also in MPS I, II, and VI, the atlantoaxial joint is unstable, requiring careful positioning and avoidance of hyperextension of the neck. Induction of anesthesia can be difficult because of inability to maintain an adequate airway. Visualization can be limited during intubation, and smaller than anticipated endotracheal tubes may be required. Recovery from anesthesia may be slow, and postoperative airway obstruction is common. Death has been reported as a result of anesthesia complication. MPS patients should undergo general anesthesia only in centers staffed with anesthesiologists experienced in these disorders.

Cardiovascular Disease. Clinical evidence of heart disease occurs in most patients with MPS who have moderate to severe somatic disease (reviewed in reference 134). Valvular disease, myocardial thickening, systemic and pulmonary hypertension, and narrowing of the coronary arteries with ischemia, if not infarction, all contribute to congestive heart failure and instances of sudden cardiovascular collapse. Arterial narrowing of the abdominal aorta and visceral and renal arteries probably contributes to the development of systemic hypertension.[241] Mitral regurgitation is the most common valvular disease in MPS IH and MPS II severe, while aortic valvular disease is more likely to occur in MPS IH/S, MPS IS, MPS IV, and MPS VI. Valve replacement has been reported in MPS IH/S, MPS IS, and MPS VI.[135] Cardiac evaluation at regular intervals with echocardiography is useful in the treatment of patients through serial monitoring of ventricular function and size. Bacterial endocarditis prophylaxis should be advised for the MPS patient with cardiac abnormalities.

Spinal Cord Compression. Spinal cord compression commonly occurs in MPS IV, but has been reported in all MPS disorders except MPS III and MPS IX. Spinal cord compression can occur from subluxation due to atlantoaxial instability with odontoid hypoplasia, and from increased soft tissue around the dens.[162,242] The fibrous tissue around the dens may be secondary to the cervical instability. Reduced exercise tolerance may be the earliest symptom of a cervical myelopathy in MPS.

To optimize the timing of surgical stabilization in MPS IV, MRI of the cervical spine is recommended at the time of diagnosis and at regular intervals thereafter. Surgery to stabilize the surgical spine in MPS IV by posterior fusion can be life saving. However, if cord compression is severe, with a significant anterior soft tissue mass, transoral anterior decompression followed by posterior fusion may be required.[162] Progressive cord compression with resulting cervical myelopathy due to dura thickening is common in the mild forms of MPS I, MPS II, and MPS VI, but may not be recognized until severe disease develops.[146]

Progressive lumbar gibbus or kyphosis is commonly seen in all MPS disorders except MPS III.[243] The rate of progression and degree of lumbar kyphosis is variable, with the deformity measuring over 90° in some MPS I children.[244] Neurologic complications are uncommon because the location of the deformity (apex usually located at L2) is normal below the conus. Posterior spinal fusion is effective in stopping the progressive spinal deformity.

GENETICS

Incidence

The MPS are rare disorders, and epidemiologic data are scarce (Table 136-2). The number of diagnosed cases as a fraction of live births (or of male live births for MPS II) in a specified period and in a given geographic area are provided by Lowry et al.[245] for all MPS in British Columbia in the years 1952–1986 and by Nelson[246] for all MPS in Northern Ireland in the years 1958–1985. Other surveys have focused on specific MPS: MPS II in Israel, 1967–1975,[247] MPS II in the United Kingdom, 1955–1974,[248] and MPS III in the Netherlands, 1945–1969.[249] The numbers of cases presented in Table 136-2 are thought to be underestimates due to incomplete ascertainment. The apparent incidence of MPS IH and MPS II cases in British Columbia dropped precipitously after 1972,[245] causing a downward revision of earlier estimates.[250] This drop may have resulted, in part, from emergence of accurate biochemical tests for prenatal diagnosis. The study of Sanfilippo syndrome in the Netherlands found 40 probands out of 6 million births (1/150,000) between 1945 and 1969, but this result, not very different from those of the British Columbia and Northern Ireland surveys, was corrected for an ascertainment probability of 0.488 to give 1/73,000.[249] To further correct for incomplete ascertainment, Van de Kamp[249] calculated the incidence of Sanfilippo syndrome in the Netherlands from the incidence of phenylketonuria (known from neonatal screening) and the ratio of Sanfilippo patients to PKU patients in institutions for the mentally retarded. This treatment of the data assumed that patients with the two diseases would have been institutionalized in the same proportion during the period studied. The resulting value for the apparent incidence of Sanfilippo syndrome, 1/24,000 births, is the one generally quoted (see, for example, references 9 and 106), but because of the method used to derive it, it is not directly comparable to other published data on MPS incidence.

There are population differences in the frequency of particular MPS; for instance, Table 136-2 shows MPS II to be more common in Israel and MPS IV in Northern Ireland. Other studies show Sanfilippo syndrome type B to be the most prevalent in Greece[251] and type A in England.[252] The apparent rarity of MPS VII may be due to frequent fetal or neonatal lethality.[192] It is likely that the true incidence of the MPS will become known only when progress in therapy will make it desirable to institute early screening.

Molecular Genetics

Genes encoding most of the glycosaminoglycan degradative enzymes were cloned and characterized in the 1990s. Elucidation of each normal DNA structure has been followed by a profusion of studies identifying mutations. Although the situation is somewhat different for each MPS, a few generalizations can be made. Mutations underlying any one MPS are very numerous, but one or a few mutations may sometimes predominate in particular geographic or ethnic population; others may recur because of mutational hot spots. Some mutations can be clearly classified as null (i.e., resulting in no enzyme activity whatsoever); these include major DNA deletions and rearrangements, frameshifts, mutations in splice-site consensus regions, and nonsense codons. Two null alleles (or one in the case of MPS II) are expected to lead to severe disease, but a milder disease would result if one allele permits residual activity. The clinical effect of missense mutations can generally be predicted only on the basis of prior experience with those mutations. Even knowledge of the enzyme structure and catalytic site may not help in predicting the effect of missense mutations, as many amino acid substitutions act by preventing transport of the newly made protein out of the endoplasmic reticulum rather than by interfering with catalysis.

MPS I. The gene encoding α-L-iduronidase (*IDUA*) spans 19 kb and includes 14 exons.[253] It has been localized to chromosome 4p16.3, close to the Huntington disease gene.[254,255] Based on

Table 136-2 Incidence of the Mucopolysaccharidoses

MPS	Geographic area	Incidence per live births: Total	Male	Reference
MPS IH	British Columbia	1/144,000		245
	Northern Ireland	1/76,000		246
MPS IH/S	Northern Ireland	1/280,000		246
MPS IS	British Columbia	1/1,300,000		245
	Northern Ireland	< 1/840,000		246
MPS II	Israel		1/34,000	247
	United Kingdom		1/132,000	248
	British Columbia		1/111,000	245
	Northern Ireland		1/72,000	246
MPS III				
A:B:C, 6:2:3	Netherlands	1/73,000*		249
A only	British Columbia	1/324,000		245
A:B, 2:1	Northern Ireland	1/280,000		246
MPS IVA	British Columbia	1/216,000		245
	Northern Ireland	1/76,000		246
MPS VI	British Columbia	1/1,300,000		245
	Northern Ireland	< 1/840,000		246
MPS VII	British Columbia	1/1,300,000		250
	Northern Ireland	1/840,000 (hydrops fetalis)		246

*The actual data showed 1/150,000, but were corrected for an estimated ascertainment of 0.488.[249]

linkage disequilibrium between haplotypes of the *IDUA* gene and MPS I mutations, Scott et al.[256,257] postulated the existence of some common alleles. Indeed two major alleles, W402X and Q70X, and a minor allele, P533R, account for over half the MPS I alleles in the Caucasian population. None of these alleles produce functional enzymes, and singly or in combination give rise to the severe form of α-L-iduronidase deficiency, or MPS IH. The relative frequency of the W402X and Q70X alleles varies in different parts of Europe,[258–260] while the P533R allele is relatively frequent in Sicily.[261] These European alleles were not found in Israeli Arab MPS IH patients[262] nor in MPS I Japanese patients,[263] both groups having their own unique alleles. In addition to the common mutations, there are numerous mutations that occur in one or a few families. A comprehensive 1995 review[264] listed 46 disease-producing mutations and 30 nonpathologic polymorphisms, a number that will no doubt keep growing as more populations are studied. The increase is expected to be primarily in the number of mutations that are null, for which there is no theoretical limit.

On the other hand, mutations causing the attenuated clinical phenotypes of MPS IS or MPS IH/S are expected to be limited. An interesting mutation that results in Scheie syndrome is a base substitution in intron 7 that creates a new splice site and produces a frameshift; because the old splice site is not obliterated, some normal enzyme can be made.[265,266] The level of α-L-iduronidase programmed by this allele in cultured fibroblasts is only 0.13 percent of normal;[267] assuming that α-L-iduronidase expression in fibroblasts is representative of the patient's tissues, this shows that only a trace of enzyme is needed to overcome the worst features of MPS I. Most other alleles that lead to MPS IS or MPS IH/S carry missense mutations.[268,269] Exceptions are Y343X, a premature termination codon that is used as an acceptor splice site, thereby creating an in-frame deletion,[270,271] and X654G, which predicts an extension of the enzyme at the carboxyl end.[269] The R89Q substitution found in MPS IS and MPS IH/S patients[266] is of interest for several reasons: it occurs at a position which on theoretical grounds has been implicated in catalysis;[26] its deleterious effect may be potentiated by a polymorphism, A361T;[266,272] and it occurs among Japanese as well as Caucasian MPS I patients.[263] Because it is a CpG mutation, it probably arose independently in different parts of the world. It is of interest that in the Japanese population, although not in the other groups studied, MPS IH/S is the result of compound heterozygosity of two mutations (704ins5 and R89Q), which, in homozygous form, would give rise to MPS IH and MPS IS, respectively, as McKusick et al. had postulated in 1972.[273]

MPS II. The Hunter syndrome is the only X-linked MPS. Its locus has been mapped to Xq28. The human gene encoding iduronate sulfatase (*IDS*) contains nine exons spread over 24 kb.[274,275] An IDS-like pseudogene, comprised of copies of exons 2 and 3 and intron 7, is located about 20 kb from the active gene.[276] The neighboring DNA is generally gene-rich, with a number of genes immediately proximal and distal to the iduronate sulfatase locus.[145,276]

As soon as *IDS* cDNA became available to probe Southern blots, it was appreciated that some MPS II patients had major deletions or rearrangements of the *IDS* gene.[44,277–279] All of them had severe disease. A recurring rearrangement is due to recombination between the intron 7 region of the gene and a homologous region near exon 3 of the pseudogene, with inversion of the intervening DNA.[280,281] The recombination is precise, with bases neither lost nor gained in the process.[281] It has been suggested that this recombination starts with double-stranded breaks.[282] A different rearrangement, found in one patient, was identified as replacement of exons 4 through 7 by a fragment of the pseudogene.[283] Two partial deletions were found in yet another patient, one within the *IDS* gene and the second within the adjoining W gene.[284] Very large deletions of the *IDS* locus may extend to adjoining genes, including the FMR1 and FMR2 genes, resulting in a contiguous gene syndrome.[145,285] This may explain unusual phenotypes of some very severely affected Hunter patients; early onset of seizures, for instance, has been attributed to deletion of FMR2.[145]

The large deletions and rearrangements are seen in only a fifth of Hunter patients.[286] The majority have point mutations—missense, nonsense, frameshift, altered splice sites—or small deletions or insertions.[286–294] An unusual mutation is that of a 178-bp deletion that abolishes the promoter region with resulting loss of expression.[295] The small mutations, of which 80 have already been described, may result in either mild or severe forms of Hunter syndrome. As discussed above, correlating genotype and phenotype is not always simple, and the issue is further compounded in the case of Hunter syndrome by the lack of well-defined and universally accepted criteria for classifying the disease as severe or mild. About half of the base substitutions occurs at CpG dinucleotides[292] and may therefore have arisen independently in unrelated families. A change at one particularly mutagenic codon, R468W, was reported in a mildly affected U.S. patient[296] and in a severely affected Japanese patient,[294] while R468Q, R468L, and R468G have all been reported only in severely affected patients.[286,294,297] New mutations have been found to occur predominantly in male meioses, so that the new mutants are more likely to be heterozygous mothers than affected males.[278,292]

The Hunter syndrome has been diagnosed in female patients, but it is a rare occurrence. The simultaneous presence of two mutant alleles is improbable because affected MPS II males generally do not reproduce. Therefore, the disease is most likely to occur in heterozygotes because of nonrandom inactivation of the X chromosome. In the first such reported case, an X:5 translocation disrupted one *IDS* allele at the chromosome breakpoint and left the other allele on the intact but inactivated X chromosome.[140,298,299] Analysis of the methylation of the *IDS* gene in cells of a female Hunter patient with a normal karyotype showed that the paternal allele, carrying a *de novo* mutation, was active whereas the normal maternal allele was inactive;[300] her particularly severe developmental delay was explained by the mutation being a deletion that extended from the *IDS* to the *FMR1* locus.[301] In another case, it was the maternal allele carrying the R468Q mutation that was expressed, whereas the normal paternal allele was inactive.[142] An unusual case of nonrandom inactivation was found in a pair of identical twins, one of whom was unaffected while the other one had a mild form of Hunter syndrome;[143] because the mutation was a frameshift early in the gene,[302] it must be presumed that the normal allele retained some activity to protect the affected twin from severe disease.

MPS IIIA. The gene encoding heparan *N*-sulfatase (*MPS3A*) spans about 11 kb, includes 8 exons,[303] and is localized to chromosome 17q25.3.[72] More than three dozen disease-producing mutations, as well as several polymorphisms, have already been found.[72,304–308] Most of these are of the missense type, with a few premature terminations and small deletions. The predominant mutations vary in different groups: R245H was found to be the most common among Australian, Dutch, and German,[305] R74C among Polish,[306] S66W among Italian, especially Sardinian,[307] and 1091delC among Spanish[308] patients. It is likely that these concentrations in particular geographic groups represent founder effects.

MPS IIIB. The gene encoding α-*N*-acetylglucosaminidase (*NAGLU*) spans 8.5 kb, comprises 6 exons, and is localized on chromosome 17q21.[64,65] A number of mutations have been found already, but most of them are private mutations, indicating great molecular heterogeneity of this very rare MPS.[65,309,310]

MPS IIIC and IIID. The molecular tools for studying Sanfilippo syndrome type C have yet to be developed. The finding of a 14;21 Robertsonian translocation in two sibs affected with MPS IIIC and a normal karyotype in their unaffected sib led to the suggestion that chromosome 14 or 21 might include the gene(s) encoding acetyl-CoA:α-glucosaminide acetyltransferase, even though there is a high (1/8) probability that the association is a chance occurrence.[311]

The cDNA encoding *N*-acetylglucosamine 6-sulfatase has been isolated[312] and used to assign the Sanfilippo D locus to chromosome 12q14.[313]

MPS IVA. The gene encoding *N*-acetylgalactosamine 6-sulfatase (*GALNS*) spans 40 to 50 kb, comprises 14 exons,[314,315] and has been localized to chromosome 16q24.3.[316,317] The number of mutations identified is rapidly approaching 100.[318–326] These are primarily single-base changes or small deletions; however, large deletions detectable on Southern blots have been reported in a few patients.[318,325] In one instance, the deletion extended into the gene encoding adenine phosphoribosyltransferase, so that the patient suffered from deficiency of both enzymes. Most mutations occur only in single cases among Japanese, European, Australian, Indian, and Pakistani patients, but two mutations, I113F and T312S, are recurring, particularly among patients from Northern Ireland and patients from Australia thought to be of British-Irish descent based on their names.[323,326] This distribution of the two mutant alleles suggests a founder effect and may explain the relatively high incidence of MPS IVA reported for Northern Ireland (Table 136-2). The T312S allele permits residual activity and confers a mild clinical phenotype.[326]

A number of polymorphic haplotypes have been described,[327,328] which might be useful for heterozygote detection even when the disease-producing mutation has not been identified.

MPS IVB. Mutations in the gene encoding β-galactosidase that underlie the Morquio syndrome type B (MPS IVB) must affect the enzyme in such a way as to prevent degradation of keratan sulfate without inhibiting the degradation of G_{M1} ganglioside and causing G_{M1} gangliosidosis (MIM 230500; see Chap. 151). Several missense mutations have been described in this rare form of the Morquio syndrome.[329,330]

MPS VI. The gene encoding *N*-acetylgalactosamine 4-sulfatase (*ARSB*) is comprised of 8 exons[331] and is localized to chromosome 5q13-q14.[332] More than 30 mutations have been reported, most of which were found in single families. Mutations which in homozygosity give rise to the severe form of Maroteaux-Lamy syndrome include frameshift[333–335] and nonsense mutations,[336] clearly null mutations. Missense mutation, on the other hand, can give rise to severe, intermediate, or mild disease.[337–341] To understand the effect of the mutations on clinical phenotype, Litjens et al.[341] examined the level of enzyme activity produced by Chinese hamster ovary cells stably transfected with mutagenized cDNA, but found only imperfect correspondence. As discussed for other MPS, genotype/phenotype correlation for missense mutations in MPS VI is not reliable enough for prognosis or counseling.

MPS VII. The human gene encoding β-glucuronidase (*GUSB*) spans 21 kb and is subdivided into 12 exons;[342] it is localized to chromosome 7q21.11.[343] The human genome includes multiple unprocessed pseudogenes and/or closely related genes on several other chromosomes,[344,345] requiring special precautions in designing primers to study the gene itself.

The index patient (Fig. 136-15), whose clinical phenotype was one of intermediate severity, was shown to be a compound heterozygote with a missense allele and a nonsense allele.[344] More than three dozen additional mutations have been identified, mostly missense, but also nonsense, frameshift, and splice site, but with no recorded large deletions or insertions.[191,345–353] Some of the mutations are associated with mild forms of the disease, or even with pseudodeficiency, whereas others are associated with the very severe (fetal or neonatal) form of the disease. As is true of the other MPS, the clinical phenotype cannot be deduced from inspection of missense mutations. A surprising complication was found in attempts to determine the effect of mutations on β-glucuronidase activity by expressing mutagenized cDNA in cultured mammalian cells; the level of activity obtained for some mutant enzyme was very high, approaching or even exceeding the normal level.[344,349] Because β-glucuronidase is active as a tetramer, it was suggested that overexpression drove the oligomerization of the mutant enzyme, allowing it to acquire catalytic activity.[349]

MPS IX. The human gene encoding hyaluronidase (*HYAL1*) has been mapped to chromosome 3p21.2-p21.3.[354] Elucidation of mutations in hyaluronidase deficiency is expected to follow shortly.

BIOCHEMICAL AND MOLECULAR DIAGNOSIS

Differential Diagnosis

Analysis of urinary glycosaminoglycans was the earliest method available for diagnosis of the MPS and remains useful as a preliminary diagnostic test. Numerous methods have been devised, ranging from semiquantitative spot tests to precise qualitative and quantitative measurements (critically reviewed in references 3, 6, 355, and 356). Identification of urinary glycosaminoglycans can help to discriminate between broad classes of mucopolysaccharidoses but not to distinguish between subgroups. Spot tests are quick, inexpensive, and useful for preliminary evaluation, but are subject to both false positive and false negative results. The reliability of the results depends largely on the testing laboratory.[357,358] A rapid semiquantitative method is based on metachromasia of glycosaminoglycan-dye complexes in solution.[359,360] It has been suggested that quantitative measurements alone may miss some MPS patients, who have a normal level but an abnormal distribution of glycosaminoglycans.[356] The current development of therapies, all of which ought to be initiated before irreversible damage has set in (see below), has shown a need for screening large numbers of infants in order to identify those affected with MPS. Substances other than glycosaminoglycans, such as the lysosomal membrane-associated protein LAMP-1, are also excreted in excess in the MPS and therefore may serve as the basis for such tests.[361]

Definitive diagnosis is established by enzyme assays[362,363] (reviewed in reference 9). Because lysosomal enzymes are present in all cells except mature erythrocytes, the deficiency can be determined in a variety of cells and body fluids. Cultured fibroblasts, leukocytes, or serum are generally used, the choice depending on the particular enzyme and the preference of the testing laboratory; some diagnostic laboratories post procedures for sample preparation and shipment on their Web sites. The glycosidases can be easily assayed with chromogenic (p-nitrophenyl) or fluorogenic (4-methylumbelliferyl) substrates. Though equally reliable, assays for sulfatases and for the *N*-acetyltransferase that rely on radioactive substrates are relatively inconvenient and often eschewed by diagnostic laboratories. Fluorogenic substrates have been synthesized to replace the radioactive ones for MPS IIIA,[364,365] MPS IIIC,[366] and MPS IVA,[367] leaving MPS II as the only MPS for which a radioactive enzyme assay is required at the present time.

Prenatal Diagnosis

Prenatal diagnosis is routinely carried out on cultured cells from amniotic fluid or chorionic villus biopsies using the same enzymatic assays as for cultured fibroblasts. Some difficulty has been reported with MPS I diagnosis because of low α-L-iduronidase in normal chorionic villi, but it may be accomplished by taking appropriate precautions.[368] Confirmation with cultured cells is recommended when borderline results are obtained with the uncultured material. Measurement of radiolabeled [^{35}S]glycosaminoglycan accumulation by cultured cells[369] may also be used for prenatal diagnosis of MPS (except for MPS IV). The technique is useful when the enzyme deficiency at risk cannot be established in time or in cases of pseudodeficiency.[370]

Cell-free amniotic fluid may be used for measurement of iduronate sulfatase activity for prenatal diagnosis of the Hunter syndrome,[371] but the user should be aware of possible maternal contribution that may mask an enzyme deficiency in the fetus. β-Glucuronidase deficiency has been reported in amniotic fluid surrounding an MPS VII fetus with hydrops fetalis.[372] We are not aware of other enzymes that would be usefully measured in amniotic fluid. Measurement of glycosaminoglycans in amniotic fluid is generally unreliable.

The Hunter syndrome occasionally poses a problem in prenatal diagnosis if the fetus is a heterozygous female. Skewed distribution of cells expressing the mutant allele may give test results resembling those of an affected male fetus.[373,374] This may cause some concern as there are well-documented instances of Hunter syndrome in heterozygous females (see above). But affected females are exceedingly rare, and it is far more likely that abnormal results for a heterozygous female fetus are due to sampling of chorionic villus or to overgrowth of one type of cell in amniocyte culture.

Carrier Testing

Carrier testing is the service most frequently requested by MPS families, second only to demands for effective therapy. It is now possible to provide definite information on carrier status, provided the mutation is known in the family under consideration. When the mutation is not known, it may be necessary to use older methods, with the limitations discussed earlier.[9] One such method takes advantage of the origin of hair roots from a very small number of cells and the resulting mosaicism of iduronate sulfatase in hair roots of Hunter heterozygotes.[375,376] It is also possible to assay enzymes under conditions carefully designed to insure linearity of reaction rate.[377] The results are most reliable when the enzyme activity is in the low range (positive identification of the carrier) and least reliable when the activity is in the normal range because there is considerable overlap between the normal and heterozygous ranges. These biochemical tests will be superseded by molecular tests as mutation analysis becomes less costly and more generally applicable.

Molecular Diagnosis

Any consideration of DNA-based tests must consider the great heterogeneity of mutations underlying each of the MPS (see above). It is essential that the mutant allele be identified for the specific family before molecular diagnosis is undertaken for members at risk. Because so many patients are compound heterozygotes, both mutant alleles must be known for carrier testing of the autosomal MPS. Once the mutant allele(s) has been identified (by the mutation itself or by an intragenic polymorphism), molecular diagnosis may be easier and require less material, which is particularly important for prenatal diagnosis. However, until mutation analysis becomes more readily available, diagnosis should be established by enzyme assay. On the other hand, DNA-based diagnosis is the only definitive test for determining carrier status.

ANIMAL MODELS

Animal models are available for most of the MPS (Table 136-3). Most are naturally occurring mutations that arose spontaneously in existing animal colonies, or that were discovered in pets brought in by their owners. Such naturally occurring models include canine[378] and feline[379] MPS I; canine[380] MPS II; canine[381] MPS IIIA; caprine[382] MPS IIID; feline[383,384] and murine (rat)[385] MPS VI; and canine,[386,387] feline,[388] and murine[389] MPS VII. MPS IIIB has been described in the emu,[390] but the affected birds also appear to have a gangliosidosis.[391–393] Characterization of the mutant enzymes and genes in the animal MPS disorders, as well as of the pathologic consequences,[17,56,120,394–399] have generally proceeded in much the same way as for the human MPS. Application of homologous recombination technology ended dependence on chance discoveries of naturally occurring mutants; several mouse models of MPS have already been generated by targeted disruption of mouse genes encoding lysosomal enzymes of glycosaminoglycan degradation.[400–403]

The biochemistry and pathology of MPS in animal models are usually very close to those in their human counterpart; however, the clinical manifestations, although generally similar to the manifestations of the human disorders, may progress more slowly. For example, dogs affected with MPS I have a clinical course that

Table 136-3 **Animal Models of Mucopolysaccharidoses**

MPS	Species	Reference	Mutation	Reference
MPS I	Canine	378	IVSI+IG > A	394
	Feline	379	Not yet available	—
	Murine*	401	Targeted disruption of exon 6	401
MPS II	Canine	380	Not known	—
	Murine	403	Targeted disruption of exons 4 and 5	403
MPS IIIA	Canine	381	Not known	—
MPS IIIB	Avian (emu)	390	Not known	—
	Murine	402	Targeted disruption of exon 6	402
MPS IIID	Caprine	382	R102X	396
MPS VI	Feline	383	L476P	56
	Feline		D520N	398
	Murine (rat)	385	c.507insC	397
	Canine	484	Not known	—
	Murine	400	Targeted disruption of exon 5	400
MPS VII	Canine	386	R166H	399
	Feline	388	E351K	485
	Murine	389	c.1470delC	395

*Murine refers to mouse unless "rat" is specified.

is more reminiscent of MPS IH/S than of MPS IH even though they are homozygous for a null (splice site) mutation. Mice affected with MPS VII, also homozygous for a null (frameshift) mutation, have a progressive disease with 50 percent survival beyond 150 days,[404] although human patients with two null alleles would probably have an early lethal form of the disease. Knockout mice with MPS I, IIIB, and VI live well into adulthood and are fertile.[400–402,405] The generally good health of young animals with MPS makes them excellent subjects for the development of therapy, as is discussed in the following section.

DEVELOPMENT OF THERAPY FOR THE MPS

The discovery of lysosomal storage disease by Baudhuin and colleagues was accompanied by the optimistic prediction that such disorders should be treatable with exogenous enzymes, which would reach lysosomes by the process of endocytosis.[406] Hope was stimulated by the finding that enzyme replacement worked extremely well in cell culture. The catabolism of glycosaminoglycans in fibroblasts derived from MPS patients could be restored to normal by addition of specific "corrective factors" to the culture medium.[407] The factors were later identified as the missing lysosomal enzymes that have a mannose-6-phosphate recognition marker for efficient, receptor-mediated endocytosis into fibroblasts.[8,31]

These observations are the foundation for development of therapy for the MPS. The relevant enzyme can be administered directly (enzyme replacement), or it can be administered indirectly either by transplanted donor tissue (bone marrow transplantation) or by autologous cells genetically modified to express the enzyme (gene therapy) in order to clear the patient's lysosomal deposits. In the case of bone marrow transplantation (BMT), it is believed that donor-derived cells can provide enzyme not only by secretion but also by direct contact with recipient cells.[408–410] The issues are the same for all approaches: Can enzyme be provided to affected tissues in sufficient quantity to make a significant impact on the clinical progression of the disease, and for disorders with a major central nervous system component, will therapeutic enzyme reach the brain?

Enzyme Replacement

Correcting defective glycosaminoglycan catabolism in cultured cells by enzyme replacement was accomplished three decades ago, although understood as such only some years later. But scaling up to test the procedure in animal models presented a major problem. Purification from tissues usually yielded the desired enzyme in minute amounts and without the mannose-6-phosphate targeting signal. This difficulty was surmounted only after isolation of cDNAs made it possible to produce recombinant enzymes. Fortunately, cultured mammalian cells, stably transfected to overexpress lysosomal enzymes, secrete substantial quantities of these enzymes with the mannose-6-phosphate marker intact; it is then a simple matter to purify the enzymes from the culture medium.[23,24,47,55,73,79,102,411]

Animal models have proved extremely useful for testing enzyme replacement therapy. Tests have been conducted with recombinant β-glucuronidase in MPS VII mice,[412–414] with α-L-iduronidase in MPS I dogs,[415,416] and with arylsulfatase B in MPS VI cats.[417,418] In all instances, there was a rapid clearance of the enzyme from circulation. Most of the enzyme went to the liver, which was quickly cleared of vacuolation, but spleen and kidney were also readily cleared. With a sufficient dose of enzyme, even brain[413] and bone[418] showed improvement. Not surprisingly, treatment begun in the neonatal period for the MPS VI and MPS VII animals was more effective therapeutically than treatment begun later.[413,418] MPS VII mice treated from birth performed normally in the Morris water maze test and retained normal auditory function,[414] while MPS VI cats had reduced skeletal dysplasia.[418] Marked slowing of disease progression was seen in an MPS I dog which was not started on therapy until the age of 52 months.[416] Although antibodies developed against the α-L-iduronidase, acute anaphylactoid reaction was readily prevented by premedication with antihistamine and slow infusion of the enzyme.[415] However, if a high titer of antibodies were to develop, it could cause loss of efficacy of the therapeutic enzyme.[419]

Experience gained with enzyme replacement in the MPS I dog permitted initiation of a human clinical trial of recombinant α-L-iduronidase for MPS I patients; early results demonstrate reduction of hepatosplenomegaly, decrease in urinary glycosaminoglycans, and clinical changes with improved joint range of motion, decreased pain, and improved endurance and activity.[420] If the promising preliminary results are maintained over a longer term, recombinant α-L-iduronidase is likely to become a pharmaceutic for treatment of MPS I. It is expected that clinical trials will be undertaken for other MPS when the recombinant enzymes can be produced in sufficient amounts.

Bone Marrow Transplantation

Early clinical trials — administration of plasma, leukocytes, fibroblasts, or amnion — failed to make any lasting improvement in the clinical picture, probably because these procedures provided only an insignificant quantity of enzyme.[9] In 1981, Hobbs et al.[421] reported that allogeneic BMT for a 9-year-old boy with Hurler syndrome could dramatically improve the somatic features of the disease. Since then our understanding of the benefits and limitations of BMT has come both from extensive clinical experience with MPS patients and from numerous experimental studies in animal models.

Studies in Animal Models. MPS I dogs transplanted at 5 months with bone marrow from unaffected littermates were followed for 20 months.[422–425] Urinary excretion of glycosaminoglycans and lysosomal storage were reduced; clinical problems such as lameness, skeletal dysplasia, cardiac changes, and corneal clouding were alleviated, and disease progression was slowed by BMT.

Early reports of BMT for feline MPS VI showed resolution of facial dysmorphology and clearing of the corneas,[426,427] but corneal clearing did not occur in a later study.[428] Clinical improvement was seen only in one of 8 MPS VI rats treated at birth with BMT, even though all the animals showed significant biochemical and pathologic changes.[429] These variable results may be attributed to the amount of enzyme that can be transferred from the donor bone marrow-derived hematopoietic cells to the recipient's deficient tissues; this amount, marginal at best, may be influenced by such factors as degree of chimerism achieved.

BMT treatment of MPS VII mice was effective in increasing life span to normal and decreasing storage in numerous tissues;[430] the effect was even greater when the procedure was performed in newborn mice.[431,432] However, when the procedure was carried out in the newborn period, there was significant radiation-induced neuronal damage and growth retardation.[431] A combination of enzyme replacement from birth, followed by bone marrow transplantation at 6 weeks (at which time further enzyme administration was discontinued), had long-term positive effects as great as enzyme therapy alone; in addition, corneas were cleared, and the mice did not develop antibodies to the enzyme.[404] These results point to future strategies for therapy of human MPS that combine several approaches in order to maximize their effectiveness.

Clinical Experience. Since the original report,[421] more than 200 MPS patients (mostly MPS I) have received allogeneic bone marrow and, more recently, stem cell transplants.[433–441] Early experiments showed promising biochemical results. Urinary and cerebrospinal fluid glycosaminoglycan levels usually decreased to normal over a period of a few months. Hepatic α-L-iduronidase activity was 3 to 10 percent of normal in the first year after BMT.[435] Both Kupffer cells and hepatocytes were cleared of glycosaminoglycans in transplanted MPS I, MPS II, and MPS VI patients, as measured by light and electron microscopy, but only the Kupffer cells were cleared in patients with MPS III.[442]

Successful and stable bone marrow engraftment in the MPS IH patients has resulted in significant clinical improvement of the somatic disease and increased long-term survival.[441,443–449] Resolution or improvement has been noted for hepatosplenomegaly, joint stiffness, facial appearance, obstructive sleep apnea, cardiac disease, communicating hydrocephalus, and hearing loss.

In contrast to the improvement seen in most somatic tissues after BMT, the skeletal[244,450,451] and ocular anomalies[452] were not corrected. Although skeletal anomalies may have been less severe in some MPS IH patients after BMT, most have developed dysostosis multiplex. In part due to the increased survival after BMT, MPS IH patients have developed increasing pain and stiffness of hips and knees, carpal tunnel syndrome, spinal cord compression, and progression of the thoracolumbar kyphosis. Invasive orthopedic procedures, including femoral osteotomies, acetabular reconstruction, and posterior spinal fusions, have been necessary for many patients post-BMT in an attempt to maintain function and gait.[244,451,453] The ocular status and retinal function in MPS patients after BMT have not normalized and may have declined.[452] Although corneal clouding has improved or resolved in some MPS patients,[439,454] most have no change or worsened corneal clouding and ocular status after BMT.[452] Despite early improvement in retinal function as measured by electroretinography, longer follow-up suggests progressive retinal decline after BMT.[452] The somatic changes seen in MPS IH have also been seen in the small number of other MPS patients who received BMT.[433,434,455–457]

The neuropsychologic outcomes have varied widely after BMT. Some patients have maintained their rate of learning with low-normal intelligence.[438–441,454,458] MPS IH patients transplanted before 24 months of age and with a baseline Mental Developmental Index greater than 70 have had an improved long-term outcome. The microglia of the central nervous system, which are of bone marrow origin, are thought to be the source of enzyme in the brain after BMT.[459,460] Neuropsychologic function may be lower either when the donor is a carrier or the recipient's engraftment is less than complete.[440] The long-term survival with preservation of intellectual functioning in some MPS IH patients with null mutations rules out inadvertent selection of patients with the milder forms of MPS I and supports a direct effect of BMT on the central nervous system.[437–439,441] Preservation of intellectual function did not occur in patients with severe MPS II or MPS III,[458,461] but the cause of this failure is not clear because most of these patients had been transplanted after 24 months of age.

The clinical outcome of BMT in the MPS patients has varied considerably. Factors that affect the outcome of BMT include the type of the MPS disorder, the genotype of the donor, the degree of clinical involvement, and the age at the time of transplantation. Failure to achieve stable engraftment and graft-versus-host disease has been a significant barrier to successful BMT for many MPS patients.[438,440,462]

Although BMT has significantly modified the natural history of the disease and improved survival in some MPS patients, the procedure is not curative. Somatic disease is generally improved, except for the skeleton and eyes, but neurologic outcomes have varied. BMT is a major procedure that carries a high risk of morbidity and mortality from poor engraftment and graft-versus-host disease. It should be used only in carefully selected cases with extensive pretransplantation clinical assessment and counseling, and with systematic long-term monitoring of the results.

Gene Therapy

The first stage of development has been to construct viral vectors carrying the gene (or rather, the cDNA) encoding the enzyme, and to demonstrate that cells transduced with these vectors can express high levels of the enzyme and become donors of corrective enzyme in vitro. The next stage has been to test the therapeutic effect of the transduced cells in vivo in animal models of MPS. The third stage is clinical trials with human MPS patients.

Expression of enzyme in deficient fibroblasts after transduction with a retroviral construct carrying the corresponding cDNA has been shown for MPS I,[463] MPS II,[464] MPS IIIA,[465] MPS VI,[466] and MPS VII.[467,468] Successful transduction and enzyme expression in hematopoietic cells has also been shown for bone marrow progenitor cells (CD34+) from Hurler patients[469,470] and fetal liver cells from MPS VII mice.[471] Transduced fibroblasts can secrete α-L-iduronidase for uptake by neuronal and glial cells,[472] and transduced CD34+ cells can secrete α-L-iduronidase for uptake into MPS I fibroblasts[470] and macrophages.[469]

Vector-modified cells have been introduced into animals affected with MPS to determine their ability to provide enzyme to cells of the host. Several months after transduced bone marrow cells were administered to lethally irradiated MPS VII mice, the liver and spleen were free of storage material, even though only a very low level of β-glucuronidase was expressed at that time.[473,474] Retroviral vector-corrected fibroblasts injected directly into MPS VII mouse brain cleared stored material near the injected site.[475] Other strategies to get the gene into the central nervous system have been to provide it in a herpes virus vector by corneal inoculation[476] or in an adenoviral vector by intravenous injection.[477] Some expression of β-glucuronidase was demonstrated histochemically in a limited number of central nervous system cells in both these instances of direct in vivo gene therapy.

"Neo-organs" represent a novel approach to ensure long-term survival of genetically modified cells that secrete the therapeutic enzyme. The cells are embedded into collagen lattices, which are surgically implanted into the peritoneal cavity, where they become vascularized to form the neo-organs. This approach has been used for delivery of β-glucuronidase to MPS VII mice[478] and dogs.[479] In both cases, β-glucuronidase was found in liver and spleen at a level that was low but sufficient to normalize the histology. The effect was long lasting — five months in the mouse and a year in the dog. Because migration of fibroblasts from the neo-organs and reinfection with helper virus were ruled out, the results showed that the secreted enzyme could be taken up at distant sites.[479] The delivery of human α-L-iduronidase from neo-organs to liver and spleen was also observed in mice, but a therapeutic effect could not be measured because the mice used were not deficient in α-L-iduronidase.[480]

Clinical trials are being undertaken very cautiously[481,482] and without expectation that they would provide effective therapy at this time. Gene therapy for the MPS suffers from the major problems of the gene therapy field as a whole: inefficient delivery and transient expression of the gene.[483] We can expect that, as better vectors are developed, they will be applied to MPS. Gene therapy for the MPS should be considered as promising but still in the very early stages of development.

REFERENCES

1. McKusick VA: *Heritable Disorders of Connective Tissue*. St. Louis, MO, CV Mosby, 1972.
2. Spranger J: The systemic mucopolysaccharidoses. *Ergeb Inn Med Kinderheilkd* **32**:165, 1972.
3. Sly WS: The mucopolysaccharidoses, in Bondy PD, Rosenberg LE (eds): *Metabolic Control and Disease*, Philadelphia, Saunders, 1980, p 545.
4. McKusick VA, Neufeld EF: The mucopolysaccharide storage diseases, in Stanbury JB, Wyngaarden JB, Fredrickson DS, Goldstein JL, Brown MS (eds): *The Metabolic Basis of Inherited Disease*, 5th ed. New York, McGraw-Hill, 1983, p 751.
5. Muenzer J: Mucopolysaccharidoses. *Adv Pediatr* **33**:269, 1986.
6. Whitley CB: The mucopolysaccharidoses, in Beighton P (ed): *McKusick's Heritable Disorders of Connective Tissue*, 5th ed. St. Louis, CV Mosby, 1993, p 367.
7. McKusick VA: The William Allan Memorial Award Lecture: Genetic nosology: Three approaches. *Am J Hum Genet* **30**:105, 1978.
8. Neufeld EF: Lessons from genetic disorders of lysosomes. *Harvey Lect* **75**:41, 1979.

9. Neufeld EF, Muenzer J: The mucopolysaccharidoses, in Scriver CR, Beaudet AL, Sly WS, Valle D (eds): *The Metabolic and Molecular Bases of Inherited Disease*, 7th ed. New York, McGraw-Hill, 1995, p 2465.
10. Roden L: Structure and metabolism of connective tissue proteoglycans, in Lennarz WJ (ed): *The Biochemistry of Glycoproteins and Proteoglycans*. New York, Plenum, 1980, p 267.
11. Barton RW, Neufeld EF: The Hurler corrective factor. Purification and some properties. *J Biol Chem* **246**:7773, 1971.
12. Rome LH, Garvin AJ, Neufeld EF: Human kidney alpha-L-iduronidase: Purification and characterization. *Arch Biochem Biophys* **189**:344, 1978.
13. Clements PR, Brooks DA, Saccone GT, Hopwood JJ: Human alpha-L-iduronidase. 1. Purification, monoclonal antibody production, native and subunit molecular mass. *Eur J Biochem* **152**:21, 1985.
14. Schuchman EH, Guzman NA, Desnick RJ: Human alpha-L-iduronidase. I. Purification and properties of the high uptake (higher molecular weight) and the low uptake (processed) forms. *J Biol Chem* **259**:3132, 1984.
15. Schuchman EH, Guzman NA, Takada G, Desnick RJ: Human alpha-L-iduronidase. II. Comparative biochemical and immunologic properties of the purified low and high uptake forms. *Enzyme* **31**:166, 1984.
16. Ohshita T, Sakuda H, Nakasone S, Iwamasa T: Purification, characterization and subcellular localization of pig liver alpha-L-iduronidase. *Eur J Biochem* **179**:201, 1989.
17. Stoltzfus LJ, Sosa-Pineda B, Moskowitz SM, Menon KP, Dlott B, Hooper L, Teplow DB, et al: Cloning and characterization of cDNA encoding canine alpha-L-iduronidase. mRNA deficiency in mucopolysaccharidosis I dog. *J Biol Chem* **267**:6570, 1992.
18. Sakuda H, Kusaba A, Ohshita T, Iwamasa T: Tissue and cellular distribution of alpha-L-iduronidase in the pig. *J Histochem Cytochem* **38**:785, 1990.
19. Scott HS, Anson DS, Orsborn AM, Nelson PV, Clements PR, Morris CP, Hopwood JJ: Human alpha-L-iduronidase: cDNA isolation and expression. *Proc Natl Acad Sci U S A* **88**:9695, 1991.
20. Clarke LA, Nasir J, Zhang H, McDonald H, Applegarth DA, Hayden MR, Toone J: Murine alpha-L-iduronidase: cDNA isolation and expression. *Genomics* **24**:311, 1994.
21. Myerowitz R, Neufeld EF: Maturation of alpha-L-iduronidase in cultured human fibroblasts. *J Biol Chem* **256**:3044, 1981.
22. Taylor JA, Gibson GJ, Brooks DA, Hopwood JJ: Alpha-L-iduronidase in normal and mucopolysaccharidosis-type-I human skin fibroblasts. *Biochem J* **274**:263, 1991.
23. Kakkis ED, Matynia A, Jonas AJ, Neufeld EF: Overexpression of the human lysosomal enzyme alpha-L-iduronidase in Chinese hamster ovary cells. *Protein Expr Purif* **5**:225, 1994.
24. Unger EG, Durrant J, Anson DS, Hopwood JJ: Recombinant alpha-L-iduronidase: Characterization of the purified enzyme and correction of mucopolysaccharidosis type I fibroblasts. *Biochem J* **304**:43, 1994.
25. Zhao KW, Faull KF, Kakkis ED, Neufeld EF: Carbohydrate structures of recombinant human alpha-L-iduronidase secreted by Chinese hamster ovary cells. *J Biol Chem* **272**:22758, 1997.
26. Durand P, Lehn P, Callebaut I, Fabrega S, Henrissat B, Mornon JP: Active-site motifs of lysosomal acid hydrolases: Invariant features of clan GH-A glycosyl hydrolases deduced from hydrophobic cluster analysis. *Glycobiology* **7**:277, 1997.
27. Paigen K: Mammalian beta-glucuronidase: Genetics, molecular biology, and cell biology. *Prog Nucl Acid Res Mol Biol* **37**:155, 1989.
28. Medda S, Chemelli RM, Martin JL, Pohl LR, Swank RT: Involvement of the carboxyl-terminal propeptide of beta-glucuronidase in its compartmentalization within the endoplasmic reticulum as determined by a synthetic peptide approach. *J Biol Chem* **264**:15824, 1989.
29. Erickson AH, Blobel G: Carboxyl-terminal proteolytic processing during biosynthesis of the lysosomal enzymes beta-glucuronidase and cathepsin D. *Biochemistry* **22**:5201, 1983.
30. Neufeld EF: Lessons from genetic disorders of lysosomes. *Harvey Lect* **75**:41, 1981.
31. Kaplan A, Achord DT, Sly WS: Phosphohexosyl components of a lysosomal enzyme are recognized by pinocytosis receptors on human fibroblasts. *Proc Nat Acad Sci U S A* **74**:2026, 1977.
32. Nishimura Y, Rosenfeld MG, Kreibich G, Gubler U, Sabatini DD, Adesnik M, Andy R: Nucleotide sequence of rat preputial gland beta-glucuronidase cDNA and in vitro insertion of its encoded polypeptide into microsomal membranes. *Proc Nat Acad Sci U S A* **83**:7292, 1986.
33. Oshima A, Kyle JW, Miller RD, Hoffmann JW, Powell PP, Grubb JH, Sly WS, et al.: Cloning, sequencing, and expression of cDNA for human beta-glucuronidase. *Proc Nat Acad Sci U S A* **84**:685, 1987.
34. Powell PP, Kyle JW, Miller RD, Pantano J, Grubb JH, Sly WS: Rat liver beta-glucuronidase. cDNA cloning, sequence comparisons and expression of a chimeric protein in COS cells. *Biochem J* **250**:547, 1988.
35. Shipley JM, Grubb JH, Sly WS: The role of glycosylation and phosphorylation in the expression of active human beta-glucuronidase. *J Biol Chem* **268**:12193, 1993.
36. Jain S, Drendel WB, Chen ZW, Mathews FS, Sly WS, Grubb JH: Structure of human beta-glucuronidase reveals candidate lysosomal targeting and active-site motifs. *Nat Struct Biol* **3**:375, 1996.
37. Applegarth DA, Bozoian G: Mucopolysaccharide storage in organs of a patient with Sandhoff's disease. *Clin Chim Acta* **39**:269, 1972.
38. Cantz M, Kresse H: Sandhoff disease: Defective glycosaminoglycan catabolism in cultured fibroblasts and its correction by beta-*N*-acetylhexosaminidase. *Eur J Biochem* **47**:581, 1974.
39. Sango K, McDonald MP, Crawley JN, Mack ML, Tifft CJ, Skop E, Starr CM, et al.: Mice lacking both subunits of lysosomal beta-hexosaminidase display gangliosidosis and mucopolysaccharidosis. *Nat Genet* **14**:348, 1996.
40. Suzuki K, Sango K, Proia RL, Langaman C: Mice deficient in all forms of lysosomal beta-hexosaminidase show mucopolysaccharidosis-like pathology. *J Neuropathol Exper Neurol* **56**:693, 1997.
41. Schmidt B, Selmer T, Ingendoh A, von Figura K: A novel amino acid modification in sulfatases that is defective in multiple sulfatase deficiency. *Cell* **82**:271, 1995.
42. Cantz M, Chrambach A, Bach G, Neufeld EF: The Hunter corrective factor. Purification and preliminary characterization. *J Biol Chem* **247**:5456, 1972.
43. Bielicki J, Freeman C, Clements PR, Hopwood JJ: Human liver iduronate-2-sulphatase. Purification, characterization and catalytic properties. *Biochem J* **271**:75, 1990.
44. Wilson PJ, Morris CP, Anson DS, Occhiodoro T, Bielicki J, Clements PR, Hopwood JJ: Hunter syndrome: Isolation of an iduronate-2-sulfatase cDNA clone and analysis of patient DNA. *Proc Natl Acad Sci U S A* **87**:8531, 1990.
45. Daniele A, Faust CJ, Herman GE, Di Natale P, Ballabio A: Cloning and characterization of the cDNA for the murine iduronate sulfatase gene. *Genomics* **16**:755, 1993.
46. Froissart R, Millat G, Mathieu M, Bozon D, Maire I: Processing of iduronate 2-sulphatase in human fibroblasts. *Biochem J* **309**:425, 1995.
47. Bielicki J, Hopwood JJ, Wilson PJ, Anson DS: Recombinant human iduronate-2-sulphatase: Correction of mucopolysaccharidosis-type II fibroblasts and characterization of the purified enzyme. *Biochem J* **289**:241, 1993.
48. McGovern MM, Vine DT, Haskins ME, Desnick RJ: Purification and properties of feline and human arylsulfatase B isozymes. Evidence for feline homodimeric and human monomeric structures. *J Biol Chem* **257**:12605, 1982.
49. Gibson GJ, Saccone GT, Brooks DA, Clements PR, Hopwood JJ: Human *N*-acetylgalactosamine-4-sulphate sulphatase. Purification, monoclonal antibody production and native and subunit M_r values. *Biochem J* **248**:755, 1987.
50. Steckel F, Hasilik A, von Figura K: Biosynthesis and maturation of arylsulfatase B in normal and mutant cultured human fibroblasts. *J Biol Chem* **258**:14322, 1983.
51. Taylor JA, Gibson GJ, Brooks DA, Hopwood JJ: Human *N*-acetylgalactosamine-4-sulphatase biosynthesis and maturation in normal, Maroteaux-Lamy and multiple sulphatase-deficient fibroblasts. *Biochem J* **268**:379, 1990.
52. Schuchman EH, Jackson CE, Desnick RJ: Human arylsulfatase B: MOPAC cloning, nucleotide sequence of a full-length cDNA, and regions of amino acid identity with arylsulfatases A and C. *Genomics* **6**:149, 1990.
53. Peters C, Schmidt B, Rommerskirch W, Rupp K, Zühlsdorf M, Vingron M, Meyer HE, et al.: Phylogenetic conservation of arylsulfatases. cDNA cloning and expression of human arylsulfatase B. *J Biol Chem* **265**:3374, 1990.
54. Jackson CE, Yuhki N, Desnick RJ, Haskins ME, O'Brien SJ, Schuchman EH: Feline arylsulfatase B (ARSB): Isolation and expression of the cDNA, comparison with human ARSB, and gene localization to feline chromosome A1. *Genomics* **14**:403, 1992.
55. Anson DS, Taylor JA, Bielicki J, Harper GS, Peters C, Gibson GJ, Hopwood JJ: Correction of human mucopolysaccharidosis type VI fibroblasts with recombinant *N*-acetylgalactosamine-4-sulphatase. *Biochem J* **284**:789, 1992.
56. Yogalingam G, Litjens T, Bielicki J, Crawley AC, Muller V, Anson DS, Hopwood JJ: Feline mucopolysaccharidosis type VI. Characterization

of recombinant *N*-acetylgalactosamine 4-sulfatase and identification of a mutation causing the disease. *J Biol Chem* **271**:27259, 1996.
57. Bond CS, Clements PR, Ashby SJ, Collyer CA, Harrop SJ, Hopwood JJ, Guss JM: Structure of a human lysosomal sulfatase. *Structure* **5**:277, 1997.
58. Klein U, von Figura K: Characterization of dermatan sulfate in mucopolysaccharidosis VI. Evidence for the absence of hyaluronidase-like enzymes in human skin fibroblasts. *Biochim Biophys Acta* **630**:10, 1980.
59. Kjellén L, Lindahl U: Proteoglycans: Structures and interactions [published erratum, *Annu Rev Biochem* 61:following viii, 1992]. *Annu Rev Biochem* **60**:443, 1991.
60. Conrad HE: *Heparin-binding proteins*. New York, Academic Press, 1998.
61. Freeman C, Hopwood JJ: Human alpha-L-iduronidase. Catalytic properties and an integrated role in the lysosomal degradation of heparan sulphate. *Biochem J* **282**:899, 1992.
62. von Figura K: Human alpha-*N*-acetylglucosaminidase. 1. Purification and properties. *Eur J Biochem* **80**:523, 1977.
63. Sasaki T, Sukegawa K, Masue M, Fukuda S, Tomatsu S, Orii T: Purification and partial characterization of alpha-*N*-acetylglucosaminidase from human liver. *J Biochem (Tokyo)* **110**:842, 1991.
64. Weber B, Blanch L, Clements PR, Scott HS, Hopwood JJ: Cloning and expression of the gene involved in Sanfilippo B syndrome (mucopolysaccharidosis III B). *Hum Mol Genet* **5**:771, 1996.
65. Zhao HG, Li HH, Bach G, Schmidtchen A, Neufeld EF: The molecular basis of Sanfilippo syndrome type B. *Proc Natl Acad Sci U S A* **93**:6101, 1996.
66. von Figura K, Hasilik A, Steckel F, van de Kamp J: Biosynthesis and maturation of alpha-*N*-acetylglucosaminidase in normal and Sanfilippo B fibroblasts. *Am J Hum Genet* **36**:93, 1984.
67. Shaklee PN, Glaser JH, Conrad HE: A sulfatase specific for glucuronic acid 2-sulfate residues in glycosaminoglycans. *J Biol Chem* **260**:9146, 1985.
68. Freeman C, Hopwood JJ: Human liver glucuronate 2-sulphatase. Purification, characterization and catalytic properties. *Biochem J* **259**:209, 1989.
69. Bienkowski MJ, Conrad HE: Structural characterization of the oligosaccharides formed by depolymerization of heparin with nitrous acid. *J Biol Chem* **260**:356, 1985.
70. Freeman C, Hopwood JJ: Glucuronate-2-sulphatase activity in cultured human skin fibroblast homogenates. *Biochem J* **279**:399, 1991.
71. Freeman C, Hopwood JJ: Human liver sulphamate sulphohydrolase. Determinations of native protein and subunit M_r values and influence of substrate aglycone structure on catalytic properties. *Biochem J* **234**:83, 1986.
72. Scott HS, Blanch L, Guo XH, Freeman C, Orsborn A, Baker E, Sutherland GR, et al.: Cloning of the sulphamidase gene and identification of mutations in Sanfilippo A syndrome. *Nat Genet* **11**:465, 1995.
73. Bielicki J, Hopwood JJ, Melville EL, Anson DS: Recombinant human sulphamidase: Expression, amplification, purification and characterization. *Biochem J* **329**:145, 1998.
74. Kresse H, Paschke E, von Figura K, Gilberg W, Fuchs W: Sanfilippo disease type D: Deficiency of *N*-acetylglucosamine-6-sulfate sulfatase required for heparan sulfate degradation. *Proc Natl Acad Sci U S A* **77**:6822, 1980.
75. Hopwood JJ, Elliott H: *N*-acetylglucosamine 6-sulfate residues in keratan sulfate and heparan sulfate are desulfated by the same enzyme. *Biochem Int* **6**:141, 1983.
76. Freeman C, Clements PR, Hopwood JJ: Human liver *N*-acetylglucosamine-6-sulphate sulphatase. Purification and characterization. *Biochem J* **246**:347, 1987.
77. Shilatifard A, Cummings RD: Sulphate release from keratan sulphate and heparan sulphate by bovine *N*-acetylglucosamine-6-sulphate sulphatase. *Glycobiology* **5**:291, 1995.
78. Freeman C, Hopwood JJ: Human liver *N*-acetylglucosamine-6-sulphate sulphatase. Catalytic properties. *Biochem J* **246**:355, 1987.
79. Litjens T, Bielicki J, Anson DS, Friderici K, Jones MZ, Hopwood JJ: Expression, purification and characterization of recombinant caprine *N*-acetylglucosamine-6-sulphatase. *Biochem J* **327**:89, 1997.
80. Klein U, Kresse H, von Figura K: Sanfilippo syndrome type C: Deficiency of acetyl-CoA: alpha-glucosaminide *N*-acetyltransferase in skin fibroblasts. *Proc Natl Acad Sci U S A* **75**:5185, 1978.
81. Hopwood JJ, Elliott H: The diagnosis of the Sanfilippo C syndrome, using monosaccharide and oligosaccharide substrates to assay acetyl-CoA: 2-amino-2-deoxy-alpha-glucoside *N*-acetyltransferase activity. *Clin Chim Acta* **112**:67, 1981.
82. Pallini R, Leder IG, di Natale P: Sanfilippo type C diagnosis: Assay of acetyl-CoA: Alpha-glucosaminide *N*-acetyltransferase using [^{14}C]glucosamine as substrate and leukocytes as enzyme source. *Pediatr Res* **18**:543, 1984.
83. Freeman C, Clements PR, Hopwood JJ: Acetyl-CoA:alpha-glucosaminide *N*-acetyl transferase: Partial purification from human liver. *Biochem Int* **6**:663, 1983.
84. Bame KJ, Rome LH: Acetyl-CoA: Alpha-glucosaminide *N*-acetyltransferase from rat liver. *Methods Enzymol* **138**:607, 1987.
85. Bame KJ, Rome LH: Acetyl coenzyme A: Alpha-glucosaminide *N*-acetyltransferase. Evidence for a transmembrane acetylation mechanism. *J Biol Chem* **260**:11293, 1985.
86. Bame KJ, Rome LH: Acetyl-coenzyme A: Alpha-glucosaminide *N*-acetyltransferase. Evidence for an active site histidine residue. *J Biol Chem* **261**:10127, 1986.
87. Bame KJ, Rome LH: Genetic evidence for transmembrane acetylation by lysosomes. *Science* **233**:1087, 1986.
88. Bame KJ, Robson K: Heparanases produce distinct populations of heparan sulfate glycosaminoglycans in Chinese hamster ovary cells. *J Biol Chem* **272**:2245, 1997.
89. Kindler A, Klein U, von Figura K: Characterization of glycosaminoglycans stored in mucopolysaccharidosis III A: Evidence for a generally occurring degradation of heparan sulfate by endoglycosidases. *Hoppe Seyler's Z Physiol Chem* **358**:1431, 1977.
90. Ornitz DM, Herr AB, Nilsson M, Westman J, Svahn CM, Waksman G: FGF binding and FGF receptor activation by synthetic heparan-derived di- and trisaccharides. *Science* **268**:432, 1995.
91. Distler JJ, Jourdian GW: Beta-galactosidase from bovine testes. *Methods Enzymol* **50**:514, 1978.
92. Oshima A, Tsuji A, Nagao Y, Sakuraba H, Suzuki Y: Cloning, sequencing, and expression of cDNA for human beta-galactosidase. *Biochem Biophys Res Commun* **157**:238, 1988.
93. Morreau H, Galjart NJ, Gillemans N, Willemsen R, van der Horst GT, d'Azzo A: Alternative splicing of beta-galactosidase mRNA generates the classic lysosomal enzyme and a beta-galactosidase-related protein. *J Biol Chem* **264**:20655, 1989.
94. Yamamoto Y, Hake CA, Martin BM, Kretz KA, Ahern-Rindell AJ, Naylor SL, Mudd M, et al.: Isolation, characterization, and mapping of a human acid beta-galactosidase cDNA. *DNA Cell Biol* **9**:119, 1990.
95. Paschke E, Niemann R, Strecker G, Kresse H: Aggregation properties of beta-galactosidase of human urine and degradation of its natural substrates by a purified preparation of the enzyme. *Biochim Biophys Acta* **704**:134, 1982.
96. Kresse H, Fuchs W, Glössl J, Holtfrerich D, Gilberg W: Liberation of *N*-acetylglucosamine-6-sulfate by human beta-*N*-acetylhexosaminidase A. *J Biol Chem* **256**:12926, 1981.
97. Kytzia HJ, Sandhoff K: Evidence for two different active sites on human beta-hexosaminidase A. Interaction of GM2 activator protein with beta-hexosaminidase A. *J Biol Chem* **260**:7568, 1985.
98. Fuchs W, Beck M, Kresse H: Intralysosomal formation and metabolic fate of *N*-acetylglucosamine 6-sulfate from keratan sulfate. *Eur J Biochem* **151**:551, 1985.
99. Glössl J, Truppe W, Kresse H: Purification and properties of *N*-acetylgalactosamine 6-sulphate sulphatase from human placenta. *Biochem J* **181**:37, 1979.
100. Tomatsu S, Fukuda S, Masue M, Sukegawa K, Fukao T, Yamagishi A, Hori T, et al.: Morquio disease: Isolation, characterization and expression of full-length cDNA for human *N*-acetylgalactosamine-6-sulfate sulfatase. *Biochem Biophys Res Commun* **181**:677, 1991.
101. Pshezhetsky AV, Potier M: Association of *N*-acetylgalactosamine-6-sulfate sulfatase with the multienzyme lysosomal complex of beta-galactosidase, cathepsin A, and neuraminidase. Possible implication for intralysosomal catabolism of keratan sulfate. *J Biol Chem* **271**:28359, 1996.
102. Bielicki J, Fuller M, Guo XH, Morris CP, Hopwood JJ, Anson DS: Expression, purification and characterization of recombinant human *N*-acetylgalactosamine-6-sulphatase. *Biochem J* **311**:333, 1995.
103. Hopwood JJ, Elliott H: Isolation and characterization of *N*-acetylglucosamine 6-sulfate from the urine of a patient with Sanfilippo type D syndrome and its occurrence in normal urine. *Biochem Int* **6**:831, 1983.
104. Hopwood JJ, Elliott H: Urinary excretion of sulphated *N*-acetylhexosamines in patients with various mucopolysaccharidoses. *Biochem J* **229**:579, 1985.

105. Natowicz MR, Short MP, Wang Y, Dickersin GR, Gebhardt MC, Rosenthal DI, Sims KB, et al.: Clinical and biochemical manifestations of hyaluronidase deficiency. *N Engl J Med* **335**:1029, 1996.
106. OMIM, Online Mendelian Inheritance in Man, at Johns Hopkins University, Baltimore, MD, 1998.
107. Kreil G: Hyaluronidases — A group of neglected enzymes. *Protein Sci* **4**:1666, 1995.
108. Frost GI, Csòka TB, Wong T, Stern R: Purification, cloning, and expression of human plasma hyaluronidase. *Biochem Biophys Res Commun* **236**:10, 1997.
109. Natowicz MR, Wang Y: Plasma hyaluronidase activity in mucolipidoses II and III: Marked differences from other lysosomal enzymes. *Am J Med Genet* **65**:209, 1996.
110. Bach G, Eisenberg F Jr, Cantz M, Neufeld EF: The defect in the Hunter syndrome: Deficiency of sulfoiduronate sulfatase. *Proc Natl Acad Sci U S A* **70**:2134, 1973.
111. Sjoberg I, Fransson LA, Matalon R, Dorfman A: Hunter's syndrome: A deficiency of L-idurono-sulfate sulfatase. *Biochem Biophys Res Commun* **54**:1125, 1973.
112. Toma L, Dietrich CP, Nader HB: Differences in the nonreducing ends of heparan sulfates excreted by patients with mucopolysaccharidoses revealed by bacterial heparitinases: A new tool for structural studies and differential diagnosis of Sanfilippo's and Hunter's syndromes. *Lab Invest* **75**:771, 1996.
113. Di Ferrante N: *N*-acetylglucosamine-6-sulfate sulfatase deficiency reconsidered. *Science* **210**:448, 1980.
114. McKusick V: *Mendelian Inheritance in Man*. Baltimore, MD, Johns Hopkins, 1986.
115. Constantopoulos G, McComb RD, Dekaban AS: Neurochemistry of the mucopolysaccharidoses: Brain glycosaminoglycans in normals and four types of mucopolysaccharidoses. *J Neurochem* **26**:901, 1976.
116. Constantopoulos G, Dekaban AS: Neurochemistry of the mucopolysaccharidoses: Brain lipids and lysosomal enzymes in patients with four types of mucopolysaccharidosis and in normal controls. *J Neurochem* **30**:965, 1978.
117. Constantopoulos G, Eiben RM, Schafer IA: Neurochemistry of the mucopolysaccharidoses: Brain glycosaminoglycans, lipids and lysosomal enzymes in mucopolysaccharidosis type III B (alpha-*N*-acetylglucosaminidase deficiency). *J Neurochem* **31**:1215, 1978.
118. Jones MZ, Alroy J, Rutledge JC, Taylor JW, Alvord EC Jr, Toone J, Applegarth D, et al.: Human mucopolysaccharidosis IIID: Clinical, biochemical, morphological and immunohistochemical characteristics. *J Neuropathol Exp Neurol* **56**:1158, 1997.
119. Constantopoulos G, Shull RM, Hastings N, Neufeld EF: Neurochemical characterization of canine alpha-L-iduronidase deficiency disease (model of human mucopolysaccharidosis I). *J Neurochem* **45**:1213, 1985.
120. Jones MZ, Alroy J, Boyer PJ, Cavanagh KT, Johnson K, Gage D, Vorro J, et al.: Caprine mucopolysaccharidosis-IIID: Clinical, biochemical, morphological and immunohistochemical characteristics. *J Neuropathol Exp Neurol* **57**:148, 1998.
121. Baumkötter J, Cantz M: Decreased ganglioside neuraminidase activity in fibroblasts from mucopolysaccharidosis patients. Inhibition of the activity in vitro by sulfated glycosaminoglycans and other compounds. *Biochim Biophys Acta* **761**:163, 1983.
122. Roubicek M, Gehler J, Spranger J: The clinical spectrum of alpha-L-iduronidase deficiency. *Am J Med Genet* **20**:471, 1985.
123. Colavita N, Orazi C, Fileni A, Leone PC, Ricci R, Segni G: A further contribution to the knowledge of mucopolysaccharidosis I H/S compound. Presentation of two cases and review of the literature. *Australas Radiol* **30**:142, 1986.
124. Jellinger K, Paulus W, Grisold W, Paschke E: New phenotype of adult alpha-L-iduronidase deficiency (mucopolysaccharidosis I) masquerading as Friedreich's ataxia with cardiopathy. *Clin Neuropathol* **9**:163, 1990.
125. Cleary MA, Wraith JE: The presenting features of mucopolysaccharidosis type IH (Hurler syndrome). *Acta Paediatr* **84**:337, 1995.
126. Donaldson MD, Pennock CA, Berry PJ, Duncan AW, Cawdery JE, Leonard JV: Hurler syndrome with cardiomyopathy in infancy. *J Pediatr* **114**:430, 1989.
127. Stephan MJ, Stevens EL Jr, Wenstrup RJ, Greenberg CR, Gritter HL, Hodges GF, Guller B: Mucopolysaccharidosis I presenting with endocardial fibroelastosis of infancy. *Am J Dis Child* **143**:782, 1989.
128. Nowaczyk MJ, Clarke JT, Morin JD: Glaucoma as an early complication of Hurler's disease. *Arch Dis Child* **63**:1091, 1988.
129. Braunlin EA, Hunter DW, Krivit W, Burke BA, Hesslein PS, Porter PT, Whitley CB: Evaluation of coronary artery disease in the Hurler syndrome by angiography. *Am J Cardiol* **69**:1487, 1992.
130. du Cret RP, Weinberg EJ, Jackson CA, Braunlin EA, Boudreau RJ, Kuni CC, Carpenter BM, et al.: Resting Tl-201 scintigraphy in the evaluation of coronary artery disease in children with Hurler syndrome. *Clin Nucl Med* **19**:975, 1994.
131. Grossman H, Dorst JP: The mucopolysaccharidoses and mucolipidoses, in HJ Kaufman (ed): *Prog Pediatr Radiol* **4**: 495, 1973.
132. Hamilton E, Pitt P: Articular manifestations of Scheie's syndrome. *Ann Rheum Dis* **51**:542, 1992.
133. Perks WH, Cooper RA, Bradbury S, Horrocks P, Baldock N, Allen A, Van't Hoff W, et al.: Sleep apnea in Scheie's syndrome. *Thorax* **35**:85, 1980.
134. Pyeritz RE: Cardiovascular manifestations of heritable disorders of connective tissue. *Prog Med Genet* **5**:191, 1983.
135. Butman SM, Karl L, Copeland JG: Combined aortic and mitral valve replacement in an adult with Scheie's disease. *Chest* **96**:209, 1989.
136. Young ID, Harper PS, Archer IM, Newcombe RG: A clinical and genetic study of Hunter's syndrome. 1. Heterogeneity. *J Med Genet* **19**:401, 1982.
137. Young ID, Harper PS, Newcombe RG, Archer IM: A clinical and genetic study of Hunter's syndrome. 2. Differences between the mild and severe forms. *J Med Genet* **19**:408, 1982.
138. Young ID, Harper PS: Mild form of Hunter's syndrome: Clinical delineation based on 31 cases. *Arch Dis Child* **57**:828, 1982.
139. Young ID, Harper PS: The natural history of the severe form of Hunter's syndrome: A study based on 52 cases. *Dev Med Child Neurol* **25**:481, 1983.
140. Mossman J, Blunt S, Stephens R, Jones EE, Pembrey M: Hunter's disease in a girl: Association with X:5 chromosomal translocation disrupting the Hunter gene. *Arch Dis Child* **58**:911, 1983.
141. Clarke JT, Willard HF, Teshima I, Chang PL, Skomorowski MA: Hunter disease (mucopolysaccharidosis type II) in a karyotypically normal girl. *Clin Genet* **37**:355, 1990.
142. Sukegawa K, Song XQ, Masuno M, Fukao T, Shimozawa N, Fukuda S, Isogai K, et al.: Hunter disease in a girl caused by R468Q mutation in the iduronate-2-sulfatase gene and skewed inactivation of the X chromosome carrying the normal allele. *Hum Mutat* **10**:361, 1997.
143. Winchester B, Young E, Geddes S, Genet S, Hurst J, Middleton-Price H, Williams N, et al.: Female twin with Hunter disease due to nonrandom inactivation of the X-chromosome: A consequence of twinning. *Am J Med Genet* **44**:834, 1992.
144. Wraith JE, Cooper A, Thornley M, Wilson PJ, Nelson PV, Morris CP, Hopwood JJ: The clinical phenotype of two patients with a complete deletion of the iduronate-2-sulphatase gene (mucopolysaccharidosis II — Hunter syndrome). *Hum Genet* **87**:205, 1991.
145. Timms KM, Bondeson ML, Ansari-Lari MA, Lagerstedt K, Muzny DM, Dugan-Rocha SP, Nelson DL, et al.: Molecular and phenotypic variation in patients with severe Hunter syndrome. *Hum Mol Genet* **6**:479, 1997.
146. Vinchon M, Cotten A, Clarisse J, Chiki R, Christiaens JL: Cervical myelopathy secondary to Hunter syndrome in an adult. *AJNR Am J Neuroradiol* **16**:1402, 1995.
147. Spranger J, Cantz M, Gehler J, Liebaers I, Theiss W: Mucopolysaccharidosis II (Hunter disease) with corneal opacities. Report on two patients at the extremes of a wide clinical spectrum. *Eur J Pediatr* **129**:11, 1978.
148. Caruso RC, Kaiser-Kupfer MI, Muenzer J, Ludwig IH, Zasloff MA, Mercer PA: Electroretinographic findings in the mucopolysaccharidoses. *Ophthalmology* **93**:1612, 1986.
149. Beck M: Papilloedema in association with Hunter's syndrome. *Br J Ophthalmol* **67**:174, 1983.
150. Beck M, Cole G: Disc oedema in association with Hunter's syndrome: Ocular histopathological findings. *Br J Ophthalmol* **68**:590, 1984.
151. Hobolth N, Pedersen C: Six cases of a mild form of Hunter syndrome in five generations. Three affected males with progeny. *Clin Genet* **20**:121, 1978.
152. Tylki-Szymanska A, Metera M: Precocious puberty in three boys with Sanfilippo A (mucopolysaccharidosis III A). *J Pediatr Endocrinol Metab* **8**:291, 1995.
153. Colville GA, Watters JP, Yule W, Bax M: Sleep problems in children with Sanfilippo syndrome. *Dev Med Child Neurol* **38**:538, 1996.
154. Cleary MA, Wraith JE: Management of mucopolysaccharidosis type III. *Arch Dis Child* **69**:403, 1993.
155. Nidiffer FD, Kelly TE: Developmental and degenerative patterns associated with cognitive, behavioural and motor difficulties in the

Sanfilippo syndrome: An epidemiological study. *J Ment Defic Res* **27**:185, 1983.
156. van de Kamp JJ, Niermeijer MF, von Figura K, Giesberts MA: Genetic heterogeneity and clinical variability in the Sanfilippo syndrome (types A, B, and C). *Clin Genet* **20**:152, 1981.
157. Lindor NM, Hoffman A, O'Brien JF, Hanson NP, Thompson JN: Sanfilippo syndrome type A in two adult sibs. *Am J Med Genet* **53**:241, 1994.
158. Matalon R, Deanching R, Nakamura F, Bloom A: A recessively inherited lethal disease in a Caribbean isolate — A sulfamidase deficiency. *Pediatr Res* **14**:524, 1980.
159. Di Natale P: Sanfilippo B disease: A re-examination of a sibship after 12 years. *J Inherit Metab Dis* **14**:23, 1991.
160. Holzgreve W, Grobe H, von Figura K, Kresse H, Beck H, Mattei JF: Morquio syndrome: Clinical findings in 11 patients with MPS IVA and 2 patients with MPS IVB. *Hum Genet* **57**:360, 1981.
161. Northover H, Cowie RA, Wraith JE: Mucopolysaccharidosis type IVA (Morquio syndrome): A clinical review. *J Inherit Metab Dis* **19**:357, 1996.
162. Hughes DG, Chadderton RD, Cowie RA, Wraith JE, Jenkins JP: MRI of the brain and craniocervical junction in Morquio's disease. *Neuroradiology* **39**:381, 1997.
163. Skeletal Dysplasia Group: Instability of the upper cervical spine. *Arch Dis Child* **64**:283, 1989.
164. Stevens JM, Kendall BE, Crockard HA, Ransford A: The odontoid process in Morquio-Brailsford's disease. The effects of occipitocervical fusion. *J Bone Joint Surg Br* **73**:851, 1991.
165. Brill CB, Rose JS, Godmilow L, Sklower S, Willner J, Hirschhorn K: Spastic quadriparesis due to C1–C2 subluxation in Hurler syndrome. *J Pediatr* **92**:441, 1978.
166. Pizzutillo PD, Osterkamp JA, Scott CI Jr, Lee MS: Atlantoaxial instability in mucopolysaccharidosis type VII. *J Pediatr Orthop* **9**:76, 1989.
167. John RM, Hunter D, Swanton RH: Echocardiographic abnormalities in type IV mucopolysaccharidosis. *Arch Dis Child* **65**:746, 1990.
168. O'Brien JS, Gugler E, Giedion A, Wiessmann U, Herschkowitz N, Meier C, Leroy J: Spondyloepiphyseal dysplasia, corneal clouding, normal intelligence and acid beta-galactosidase deficiency. *Clin Genet* **9**:495, 1976.
169. Arbisser AI, Donnelly KA, Scott CI Jr, DiFerrante N, Singh J, Stevenson RE, Aylesworth AS, et al.: Morquio-like syndrome with beta galactosidase deficiency and normal hexosamine sulfatase activity: Mucopolysaccharidosis IVB. *Am J Med Genet* **1**:195, 1977.
170. van Gemund JJ, Giesberts MA, Eerdmans RF, Blom W, Kleijer WJ: Morquio-B disease, spondyloepiphyseal dysplasia associated with acid beta-galactosidase deficiency. Report of three cases in one family. *Hum Genet* **64**:50, 1983.
171. van der Horst GT, Kleijer WJ, Hoogeveen AT, Huijmans JG, Blom W, van Diggelen OP: Morquio B syndrome: A primary defect in beta-galactosidase. *Am J Med Genet* **16**:261, 1983.
172. Fujimoto A, Horwitz AL: Biochemical defect of non-keratan-sulfate-excreting Morquio syndrome. *Am J Med Genet* **15**:265, 1983.
173. Hecht JT, Scott CI Jr, Smith TK, Williams JC: Mild manifestations of the Morquio syndrome [Letter]. *Am J Med Genet* **18**:369, 1984.
174. Beck M, Glossl J, Grubisic A, Spranger J: Heterogeneity of Morquio disease. *Clin Genet* **29**:325, 1986.
175. Nelson J, Broadhead D, Mossman J: Clinical findings in 12 patients with MPS IV A (Morquio's disease). Further evidence for heterogeneity. Part I: Clinical and biochemical findings. *Clin Genet* **33**:111, 1988.
176. Nelson J, Kinirons M: Clinical findings in 12 patients with MPS IV A (Morquio's disease). Further evidence for heterogeneity. Part II: Dental findings. *Clin Genet* **33**:121, 1988.
177. Nelson J, Thomas PS: Clinical findings in 12 patients with MPS IV A (Morquio's disease). Further evidence for heterogeneity. Part III: Odontoid dysplasia. *Clin Genet* **33**:126, 1988.
178. Maroteaux P, Leveque B, Marie J, Lamy M: Une nouvelle dysostose avec elimination urinaire de chondoitin-sulfate B. *Presse Med* **71**:1849, 1963.
179. Taylor HR, Hollows FC, Hopwood JJ, Robertson EF: Report of a mucopolysaccharidosis occurring in Australian aborigines. *J Med Genet* **15**:455, 1978.
180. Vestermark S, Tonnesen T, Andersen MS, Guttler F: Mental retardation in a patient with Maroteaux-Lamy. *Clin Genet* **31**:114, 1987.
181. Spranger JW, Koch F, McKusick VA, Natzschka J, Wiedemann HR, Zellweger H: Mucopolysaccharidosis VI (Maroteaux-Lamy's disease). *Helv Paediatr Acta* **25**:337, 1970.
182. Tan CT, Schaff HV, Miller FA Jr, Edwards WD, Karnes PS: Valvular heart disease in four patients with Maroteaux-Lamy syndrome. *Circulation* **85**:188, 1992.
183. Marwick TH, Bastian B, Hughes CF, Bailey BP: Mitral stenosis in the Maroteaux-Lamy syndrome: A treatable cause of dyspnea. *Postgrad Med J* **68**:287, 1992.
184. Miller G, Partridge A: Mucopolysaccharidosis type VI presenting in infancy with endocardial fibroelastosis and heart failure. *Pediatr Cardiol* **4**:61, 1983.
185. Hayflick S, Rowe S, Kavanaugh-McHugh A, Olson JL, Valle D: Acute infantile cardiomyopathy as a presenting feature of mucopolysaccharidosis VI. *J Pediatr* **120**:269, 1992.
186. Young R, Kleinman G, Ojemann RG, Kolodny E, Davis K, Halperin J, Zalneraitis E, et al.: Compressive myelopathy in Maroteaux-Lamy syndrome: Clinical and pathological findings. *Ann Neurol* **8**:336, 1980.
187. Wald SL, Schmidek HH: Compressive myelopathy associated with type VI mucopolysaccharidosis (Maroteaux-Lamy syndrome). *Neurosurgery* **14**:83, 1984.
188. Sly WS, Quinton BA, McAlister WH, Rimoin DL: Beta glucuronidase deficiency: Report of clinical, radiologic, and biochemical features of a new mucopolysaccharidosis. *J Pediatr* **82**:249, 1973.
189. Lee JE, Falk RE, Ng WG, Donnell GN: Beta-glucuronidase deficiency. A heterogeneous mucopolysaccharidosis. *Am J Dis Child* **139**:57, 1985.
190. Sewell AC, Gehler J, Mittermaier G, Meyer E: Mucopolysaccharidosis type VII (beta-glucuronidase deficiency): A report of a new case and a survey of those in the literature. *Clin Genet* **21**:366, 1982.
191. Vervoort R, Islam MR, Sly WS, Zabot MT, Kleijer WJ, Chabas A, Fensom A, et al.: Molecular analysis of patients with beta-glucuronidase deficiency presenting as hydrops fetalis or as early mucopolysaccharidosis VII. *Am J Hum Genet* **58**:457, 1996.
192. Nelson A, Peterson L, Frampton B, Sly WS: Mucopolysaccharidosis VII (beta-glucuronidase deficiency) presenting as nonimmune hydrops fetalis. *J Pediatr* **101**:574, 1982.
193. Irani D, Kim HS, El-Hibri H, Dutton RV, Beaudet A, Armstrong D: Postmortem observations on beta-glucuronidase deficiency presenting as hydrops fetalis. *Ann Neurol* **14**:486, 1983.
194. Kagie MJ, Kleijer WJ, Huijmans JG, Maaswinkel-Mooy P, Kanhai HH: Beta-glucuronidase deficiency as a cause of fetal hydrops. *Am J Med Genet* **42**:693, 1992.
195. Stangenberg M, Lingman G, Roberts G, Ozand P: Mucopolysaccharidosis VII as cause of fetal hydrops in early pregnancy. *Am J Med Genet* **44**:142, 1992.
196. Nelson J, Kenny B, O'Hara D, Harper A, Broadhead D: Foamy changes of placental cells in probable beta glucuronidase deficiency associated with hydrops fetalis. *J Clin Pathol* **46**:370, 1993.
197. Molyneux AJ, Blair E, Coleman N, Daish P: Mucopolysaccharidosis type VII associated with hydrops fetalis: Histopathological and ultrastructural features with genetic implications. *J Clin Pathol* **50**:252, 1997.
198. Machin GA: Hydrops revisited: Literature review of 1,414 cases published in the 1980s. *Am J Med Genet* **34**:366, 1989.
199. de Kremer RD, Givogri I, Argarana CE, Hliba E, Conci R, Boldini CD, Capra AP: Mucopolysaccharidosis type VII (beta-glucuronidase deficiency): A chronic variant with an oligosymptomatic severe skeletal dysplasia. *Am J Med Genet* **44**:145, 1992.
200. Wraith JE: The mucopolysaccharidoses: A clinical review and guide to management. *Arch Dis Child* **72**:263, 1995.
201. Fowler GW, Sukoff M, Hamilton A, Williams JP: Communicating hydrocephalus in children with genetic inborn errors of metabolism. *Childs Brain* **1**:251, 1975.
202. Yatziv S, Epstein CJ: Hunter syndrome presenting as macrocephaly and hydrocephalus. *J Med Genet* **14**:445, 1977.
203. Watts RW, Spellacy E, Kendall BE, du Boulay G, Gibbs DA: Computed tomography studies on patients with mucopolysaccharidoses. *Neuroradiology* **21**:9, 1981.
204. Shinnar S, Singer HS, Valle D: Acute hydrocephalus Hurler's syndrome. *Am J Dis Child* **136**:556, 1982.
205. Van Aerde J, Campbell A: Hydrocephalus and shunt placement [Letter]. *Am J Dis Child* **137**:187, 1983.
206. Robertson SP, Klug GL, Rogers JG: Cerebrospinal fluid shunts in the management of behavioural problems in Sanfilippo syndrome (MPS III). *Eur J Pediatr* **157**:653, 1998.
207. Sugar J: Corneal manifestations of the systemic mucopolysaccharidoses. *Ann Ophthalmol* **11**:531, 1979.
208. Maumenee IH: The eye in connective tissue diseases. *Prog Clin Biol Res* **82**:53, 1982.

209. Alhadeff JA, Tennant L, O'Brien JS: Altered isoenzyme patterns of liver alpha-L-fucosidase in cystic fibrosis. *Clin Genet* **10**:63, 1976.
210. Schwartz MF, Werblin TP, Green WR: Occurrence of mucopolysaccharide in corneal grafts in the Maroteaux-Lamy syndrome. *Cornea* **4**:58, 1985.
211. Naumann G: Clearing of cornea after perforating keratoplasty in mucopolysaccharidosis type VI (Maroteaux-Lamy syndrome) [Letter]. *N Engl J Med* **312**:995, 1985.
212. Quigley HA, Goldberg MF: Scheie syndrome and macular corneal dystrophy. An ultrastructural comparison of conjunctiva and skin. *Arch Ophthalmol* **85**:553, 1971.
213. Spellacy E, Bankes JL, Crow J, Dourmashkin R, Shah D, Watts RW: Glaucoma in a case of Hurler disease. *Br J Ophthalmol* **64**:773, 1980.
214. Cantor LB, Disseler JA, Wilson FMd: Glaucoma in the Maroteaux-Lamy syndrome. *Am J Ophthalmol* **108**:426, 1989.
215. Cahane M, Treister G, Abraham FA, Melamed S: Glaucoma in siblings with Morquio syndrome. *Br J Ophthalmol* **74**:382, 1990.
216. Mullaney P, Awad AH, Millar L: Glaucoma in mucopolysaccharidosis 1-H/S. *J Pediatr Ophthalmol Strabismus* **33**:127, 1996.
217. Hayes E, Babin R, Platz C: The otologic manifestations of mucopolysaccharidoses. *Am J Otol* **2**:65, 1980.
218. Peck JE: Hearing loss in Hunter's syndrome — Mucopolysaccharidosis II. *Ear Hear* **5**:243, 1984.
219. Bredenkamp JK, Smith ME, Dudley JP, Williams JC, Crumley RL, Crockett DM: Otolaryngologic manifestations of the mucopolysaccharidoses. *Ann Otol Rhinol Laryngol* **101**:472, 1992.
220. Ruckenstein MJ, Macdonald RE, Clarke JT, Forte V: The management of otolaryngological problems in the mucopolysaccharidoses: A retrospective review. *J Otolaryngol* **20**:177, 1991.
221. Wraith JE, Alani SM: Carpal tunnel syndrome in the mucopolysaccharidoses and related disorders. *Arch Dis Child* **65**:962, 1990.
222. Haddad FS, Jones DH, Vellodi A, Kane N, Pitt MC: Carpal tunnel syndrome in the mucopolysaccharidoses and mucolipidoses. *J Bone Joint Surg Br* **79**:576, 1997.
223. Van Heest AE, House J, Krivit W, Walker K: Surgical treatment of carpal tunnel syndrome and trigger digits in children with mucopolysaccharide storage disorders. *J Hand Surg (Am)* **23**:236, 1998.
224. Pronicka E, Tylki-Szymanska A, Kwast O, Chmielik J, Maciejko D, Cedro A: Carpal tunnel syndrome in children with mucopolysaccharidoses: Needs for surgical tendons and median nerve release. *J Ment Defic Res* **32**:79, 1988.
225. Brama I, Gay I, Feinmesser R, Springer C: Upper airway obstruction in Hunter syndrome. *Int J Pediatr Otorhinolaryngol* **11**:229, 1986.
226. Sasaki CT, Ruiz R, Gaito R Jr, Kirchner JA, Seshi B: Hunter's syndrome: A study in airway obstruction. *Laryngoscope* **97**:280, 1987.
227. Peters ME, Arya S, Langer LO, Gilbert EF, Carlson R, Adkins W: Narrow trachea in mucopolysaccharidoses. *Pediatr Radiol* **15**:225, 1985.
228. Myer CMD: Airway obstruction in Hurler's syndrome — Radiographic features. *Int J Pediatr Otorhinolaryngol* **22**:91, 1991.
229. Shapiro J, Strome M, Crocker AC: Airway obstruction and sleep apnea in Hurler and Hunter syndromes. *Ann Otol Rhinol Laryngol* **94**:458, 1985.
230. Ginzburg AS, Onal E, Aronson RM, Schild JA, Mafee MF, Lopata M: Successful use of nasal-CPAP for obstructive sleep apnea in Hunter syndrome with diffuse airway involvement. *Chest* **97**:1496, 1990.
231. Semenza GL, Pyeritz RE: Respiratory complications of mucopolysaccharide storage disorders. *Medicine (Baltimore)* **67**:209, 1988.
232. Adachi K, Chole RA: Management of tracheal lesions in Hurler syndrome. *Arch Otolaryngol Head Neck Surg* **116**:1205, 1990.
233. Baines D, Keneally J: Anaesthetic implications of the mucopolysaccharidoses: A fifteen-year experience in a children's hospital. *Anaesth Intensive Care* **11**:198, 1983.
234. Kempthorne PM, Brown TC: Anaesthesia and the mucopolysaccharidoses: A survey of techniques and problems. *Anaesth Intensive Care* **11**:203, 1983.
235. Brown TC: The airway in mucopolysaccharidoses [Letter]. *Anaesth Intensive Care* **12**:178, 1984.
236. Sjøgren P, Pedersen T, Steinmetz H: Mucopolysaccharidoses and anaesthetic risks. *Acta Anaesthesiol Scand* **31**:214, 1987.
237. Nicolson SC, Black AE, Kraras CM: Management of a difficult airway in a patient with Hurler-Scheie syndrome during cardiac surgery. *Anesth Analg* **75**:830, 1992.
238. Wilder RT, Belani KG: Fiberoptic intubation complicated by pulmonary edema in a 12-year-old child with Hurler syndrome. *Anesthesiology* **72**:205, 1990.
239. Walker RW, Darowski M, Morris P, Wraith JE: Anaesthesia and mucopolysaccharidoses. A review of airway problems in children. *Anaesthesia* **49**:1078, 1994.
240. Moores C, Rogers JG, McKenzie IM, Brown TC: Anaesthesia for children with mucopolysaccharidoses [Comment]. *Anaesth Intensive Care* **24**:459, 1996.
241. Taylor DB, Blaser SI, Burrows PE, Stringer DA, Clarke JT, Thorner P: Arteriopathy and coarctation of the abdominal aorta in children with mucopolysaccharidosis: Imaging findings. *AJR Am J Roentgenol* **157**:819, 1991.
242. Parsons VJ, Hughes DG, Wraith JE: Magnetic resonance imaging of the brain, neck and cervical spine in mild Hunter's syndrome (mucopolysaccharidoses type II). *Clin Radiol* **51**:719, 1996.
243. Levin TL, Berdon WE, Lachman RS, Anyane-Yeboa K, Ruzal-Shapiro C, Roye DP Jr: Lumbar gibbus in storage diseases and bone dysplasias. *Pediatr Radiol* **27**:289, 1997.
244. Tandon V, Williamson JB, Cowie RA, Wraith JE: Spinal problems in mucopolysaccharidosis I (Hurler syndrome). *J Bone Joint Surg Br* **78**:938, 1996.
245. Lowry RB, Applegarth DA, Toone JR, MacDonald E, Thunem NY: An update on the frequency of mucopolysaccharide syndromes in British Columbia [Letter]. *Hum Genet* **85**:389, 1990.
246. Nelson J: Incidence of the mucopolysaccharidoses in Northern Ireland. *Hum Genet* **101**:355, 1997.
247. Schaap T, Bach G: Incidence of mucopolysaccharidoses in Israel: Is Hunter disease a "Jewish disease"? *Hum Genet* **56**:221, 1980.
248. Young ID, Harper PS: Incidence of Hunter's syndrome. *Hum Genet* **60**:391, 1982.
249. Van De Kamp JJP: A clinical and genetical study of 75 patients in the Netherlands, in *Doctoral Thesis*. S'Gravenhage, JH Pasmans, 1979.
250. Lowry RB, Renwick DH: Relative frequency of the Hurler and Hunter syndromes. *N Engl J Med* **284**:221, 1971.
251. Michelakakis H, Dimitriou E, Tsagaraki S, Giouroukos S, Schulpis K, Bartsocas CS: Lysosomal storage diseases in Greece. *Genet Couns* **6**:43, 1995.
252. Whiteman P, Young E: The laboratory diagnosis of Sanfilippo disease. *Clin Chim Acta* **76**:139, 1977.
253. Scott HS, Guo XH, Hopwood JJ, Morris CP: Structure and sequence of the human alpha-L-iduronidase gene. *Genomics* **13**:1311, 1992.
254. Scott HS, Ashton LJ, Eyre HJ, Baker E, Brooks DA, Callen DF, Sutherland GR, et al.: Chromosomal localization of the human alpha-L-iduronidase gene (IDUA) to 4p16.3. *Am J Hum Genet* **47**:802, 1990.
255. MacDonald ME, Scott HS, Whaley WL, Pohl T, Wasmuth JJ, Lehrach H, Morris CP, et al.: Huntington disease-linked locus D4S111 exposed as the alpha-L-iduronidase gene. *Somat Cell Mol Genet* **17**:421, 1991.
256. Scott HS, Litjens T, Hopwood JJ, Morris CP: A common mutation for mucopolysaccharidosis type I associated with a severe Hurler syndrome phenotype. *Hum Mutat* **1**:103, 1992.
257. Scott HS, Litjens T, Nelson PV, Brooks DA, Hopwood JJ, Morris CP: Alpha-L-iduronidase mutations (Q70X and P533R) associate with a severe Hurler phenotype. *Hum Mutat* **1**:333, 1992.
258. Bunge S, Kleijer WJ, Steglich C, Beck M, Zuther C, Morris CP, Schwinger E, et al.: Mucopolysaccharidosis type I: Identification of 8 novel mutations and determination of the frequency of the two common alpha-L-iduronidase mutations (W402X and Q70X) among European patients. *Hum Mol Genet* **3**:861, 1994.
259. Gort L, Chabas A, Coll MJ: Analysis of five mutations in 20 mucopolysaccharidosis type I patients: High prevalence of the W402X mutation. *Hum Mutat* **11**:332, 1998.
260. Voskoboeva EY, Krasnopolskaya XD, Mirenburg TV, Weber B, Hopwood JJ: Molecular genetics of mucopolysaccharidosis Type I: Mutation analysis among the patients of the former Soviet Union. *Mol Genet Metab* **65**:174, 1998.
261. Gatti R, Di Natale P, Villani GR, Filocamo M, Muller V, Guo XH, Nelson PV, et al.: Mutations among Italian mucopolysaccharidosis type I patients. *J Inherit Metab Dis* **20**:803, 1997.
262. Bach G, Moskowitz SM, Tieu PT, Matynia A, Neufeld EF: Molecular analysis of Hurler syndrome in Druze and Muslim Arab patients in Israel: Multiple allelic mutations of the IDUA gene in a small geographic area. *Am J Hum Genet* **53**:330, 1993.
263. Yamagishi A, Tomatsu S, Fukuda S, Uchiyama A, Shimozawa N, Suzuki Y, Kondo N, et al.: Mucopolysaccharidosis type I: Identification of common mutations that cause Hurler and Scheie syndromes in Japanese populations. *Hum Mutat* **7**:23, 1996.

264. Scott HS, Bunge S, Gal A, Clarke LA, Morris CP, Hopwood JJ: Molecular genetics of mucopolysaccharidosis type I: Diagnostic, clinical, and biological implications. *Hum Mutat* **6**:288, 1995.
265. Moskowitz SM, Tieu PT, Neufeld EF: Mutation in Scheie syndrome (MPS IS): A G → A transition creates new splice site in intron 5 of one IDUA allele. *Hum Mutat* **2**:141, 1993.
266. Scott HS, Litjens T, Nelson PV, Thompson PR, Brooks DA, Hopwood JJ, Morris CP: Identification of mutations in the alpha-L-iduronidase gene (IDUA) that cause Hurler and Scheie syndromes. *Am J Hum Genet* **53**:973, 1993.
267. Ashton LJ, Brooks DA, McCourt PA, Muller VJ, Clements PR, Hopwood JJ: Immunoquantification and enzyme kinetics of alpha-L-iduronidase in cultured fibroblasts from normal controls and mucopolysaccharidosis type I patients. *Am J Hum Genet* **50**:787, 1992.
268. Clarke LA, Scott HS: Two novel mutations causing mucopolysaccharidosis type I detected by single strand conformational analysis of the alpha-L-iduronidase gene. *Hum Mol Genet* **2**:1311, 1993.
269. Tieu PT, Bach G, Matynia A, Hwang M, Neufeld EF: Four novel mutations underlying mild or intermediate forms of alpha-L-iduronidase deficiency (MPS IS and MPS IH/S). *Hum Mutat* **6**:55, 1995.
270. Tieu PT, Menon K, Neufeld EF: A mutant stop codon (TAG) in the IDUA gene is used as an acceptor splice site in a patient with Hurler syndrome (MPS IH). *Hum Mutat* **3**:333, 1994.
271. Lee-Chen GJ, Lee-Wang TR: Mucopolysaccharidosis type I: Identification of novel mutations that cause Hurler/Scheie syndrome in Chinese families. *J Med Genet* **34**:939, 1997.
272. Scott HS, Nelson PV, Litjens T, Hopwood JJ, Morris CP: Multiple polymorphisms within the alpha-L-iduronidase gene (IDUA): Implications for a role in modification of MPS-I disease phenotype. *Hum Mol Genet* **2**:1471, 1993.
273. McKusick VA, Howell RR, Hussels IE, Neufeld EF, Stevenson RE: Allelism, non-allelism, and genetic compounds among the mucopolysaccharidoses. *Lancet* **1**:993, 1972.
274. Wilson PJ, Meaney CA, Hopwood JJ, Morris CP: Sequence of the human iduronate 2-sulfatase (IDS) gene. *Genomics* **17**:773, 1993.
275. Flomen RH, Green EP, Green PM, Bentley DR, Giannelli F: Determination of the organisation of coding sequences within the iduronate sulphate sulphatase (IDS) gene. *Hum Mol Genet* **2**:5, 1993.
276. Timms KM, Lu F, Shen Y, Pierson CA, Muzny DM, Gu Y, Nelson DL, et al.: 130 kb of DNA sequence reveals two new genes and a regional duplication distal to the human iduronate-2-sulfate sulfatase locus. *Genome Res* **5**:71, 1995.
277. Wehnert M, Hopwood JJ, Schroder W, Herrmann FH: Structural gene aberrations in mucopolysaccharidosis II (Hunter). *Hum Genet* **89**:430, 1992.
278. Beck M, Steglich C, Zabel B, Dahl N, Schwinger E, Hopwood JJ, Gal A: Deletion of the Hunter gene and both DXS466 and DXS304 in a patient with mucopolysaccharidosis type II. *Am J Med Genet* **44**:100, 1992.
279. Froissart R, Blond JL, Maire I, Guibaud P, Hopwood JJ, Mathieu M, Bozon D: Hunter syndrome: Gene deletions and rearrangements. *Hum Mutat* **2**:138, 1993.
280. Steen-Bondeson ML, Dahl N, Tonnesen T, Kleijer WJ, Seidlitz G, Gustavson KH, Wilson PJ, et al.: Molecular analysis of patients with Hunter syndrome: Implication of a region prone to structural alterations within the IDS gene. *Hum Mol Genet* **1**:195, 1992.
281. Bondeson ML, Dahl N, Malmgren H, Kleijer WJ, Tonnesen T, Carlberg BM, Pettersson U: Inversion of the IDS gene resulting from recombination with IDS-related sequences is a common cause of the Hunter syndrome. *Hum Mol Genet* **4**:615, 1995.
282. Lagerstedt K, Karsten SL, Carlberg BM, Kleijer WJ, Tonnesen T, Pettersson U, Bondeson ML: Double-strand breaks may initiate the inversion mutation causing the Hunter syndrome. *Hum Mol Genet* **66**:627, 1997.
283. Birot AM, Bouton O, Froissart R, Maire I, Bozon D: IDS gene-pseudogene exchange responsible for an intragenic deletion in a Hunter patient. *Hum Mutat* **8**:44, 1996.
284. Karsten SL, Lagerstedt K, Carlberg BM, Kleijer WJ, Zaremba J, Van Diggelen OP, Czartoryska B, et al.: Two distinct deletions in the IDS gene and the gene W: A novel type of mutation associated with the Hunter syndrome. *Genomics* **43**:123, 1997.
285. Birot AM, Delobel B, Gronnier P, Bonnet V, Maire I, Bozon D: A 5-megabase familial deletion removes the IDS and FMR-1 genes in a male Hunter patient. *Hum Mutat* **7**:266, 1996.
286. Hopwood JJ, Bunge S, Morris CP, Wilson PJ, Steglich C, Beck M, Schwinger E, et al.: Molecular basis of mucopolysaccharidosis type II: Mutations in the iduronate-2-sulphatase gene. *Hum Mutat* **2**:435, 1993.
287. Jonsson JJ, Aronovich EL, Braun SE, Whitley CB: Molecular diagnosis of mucopolysaccharidosis type II (Hunter syndrome) by automated sequencing and computer-assisted interpretation: Toward mutation mapping of the iduronate-2-sulfatase gene. *Am J Hum Genet* **56**:597, 1995.
288. Sukegawa K, Tomatsu S, Fukao T, Iwata H, Song XQ, Yamada Y, Fukuda S, et al.: Mucopolysaccharidosis type II (Hunter disease): Identification and characterization of eight point mutations in the iduronate-2-sulfatase gene in Japanese patients. *Hum Mutat* **6**:136, 1995.
289. Popowska E, Rathmann M, Tylki-Szymanska A, Bunge S, Steglich C, Schwinger E, Gal A: Mutations of the iduronate-2-sulfatase gene in 12 Polish patients with mucopolysaccharidosis type II (Hunter syndrome). *Hum Mutat* **5**:97, 1995.
290. Villani GR, Balzano N, Grosso M, Di Natale P: Mutation analysis in Hunter patients. *Pediatr Med Chir* **18**:71, 1996.
291. Olsen TC, Eiken HG, Knappskog PM, Kase BF, Mansson JE, Boman H, Apold J: Mutations in the iduronate-2-sulfatase gene in five Norwegians with Hunter syndrome. *Hum Genet* **97**:198, 1996.
292. Rathmann M, Bunge S, Beck M, Kresse H, Tylki-Szymanska A, Gal A: Mucopolysaccharidosis type II (Hunter syndrome): Mutation "hot spots" in the iduronate-2-sulfatase gene. *Am J Hum Genet* **59**:1202, 1996.
293. Gort L, Coll MJ, Chabas A: Mutations in the iduronate-2-sulfatase gene in 12 Spanish patients with Hunter disease. *Hum Mutat* **1(Suppl)**:566, 1998.
294. Isogai K, Sukegawa K, Tomatsu S, Fukao T, Song XQ, Yamada Y, Fukuda S, et al.: Mutation analysis in the iduronate-2-sulphatase gene in 43 Japanese patients with mucopolysaccharidosis type II (Hunter disease). *J Inherit Metab Dis* **21**:60, 1998.
295. Timms KM, Huckett LE, Belmont JW, Shapira SK, Gibbs RA: DNA deletion confined to the iduronate-2-sulfatase promoter abolishes IDS gene expression. *Hum Mutat* **11**:121, 1998.
296. Crotty PL, Braun SE, Anderson RA, Whitley CB: Mutation R468W of the iduronate-2-sulfatase gene in mild Hunter syndrome (mucopolysaccharidosis type II) confirmed by in vitro mutagenesis and expression. *Hum Mol Genet* **1**:755, 1992.
297. Whitley CB, Anderson RA, Aronovich EL, Crotty PL, Anyane-Yeboa K, Russo D, Warburton D: Caveat to genotype-phenotype correlation in mucopolysaccharidosis type II: Discordant clinical severity of R468W and R468Q mutations of the iduronate-2-sulfatase gene. *Hum Mutat* **2**:235, 1993.
298. Roberts SH, Upadhyaya M, Sarfarazi M, Harper PS: Further evidence localising the gene for Hunter's syndrome to the distal region of the X chromosome long arm. *J Med Genet* **26**:309, 1989.
299. Wilson PJ, Suthers GK, Callen DF, Baker E, Nelson PV, Cooper A, Wraith JE, et al.: Frequent deletions at Xq28 indicate genetic heterogeneity in Hunter syndrome. *Hum Genet* **86**:505, 1991.
300. Clarke JT, Greer WL, Strasberg PM, Pearce RD, Skomorowski MA, Ray PN: Hunter disease (mucopolysaccharidosis type II) associated with unbalanced inactivation of the X chromosomes in a karyotypically normal girl [Comment]. *Am J Hum Genet* **49**:289, 1991.
301. Clarke JT, Wilson PJ, Morris CP, Hopwood JJ, Richards RI, Sutherland GR, Ray PN: Characterization of a deletion at Xq27-q28 associated with unbalanced inactivation of the nonmutant X chromosome [Comment]. *Am J Hum Genet* **51**:316, 1992.
302. Goldenfum SL, Young E, Michelakakis H, Tsagarakis S, Winchester B: Mutation analysis in 20 patients with Hunter disease. *Hum Mutat* **7**:76, 1996.
303. Karageorgos LE, Guo XH, Blanch L, Weber B, Anson DS, Scott HS, Hopwood JJ: Structure and sequence of the human sulphamidase gene. *DNA Res* **3**:269, 1996.
304. Blanch L, Weber B, Guo XH, Scott HS, Hopwood JJ: Molecular defects in Sanfilippo syndrome type A. *Hum Mol Genet* **6**:787, 1997.
305. Weber B, Guo XH, Wraith JE, Cooper A, Kleijer WJ, Bunge S, Hopwood JJ: Novel mutations in Sanfilippo A syndrome: Implications for enzyme function. *Hum Mol Genet* **6**:1573, 1997.
306. Bunge S, Ince H, Steglich C, Kleijer WJ, Beck M, Zaremba J, van Diggelen OP, et al.: Identification of 16 sulfamidase gene mutations including the common R74C in patients with mucopolysaccharidosis type IIIA (Sanfilippo A). *Hum Mutat* **10**:479, 1997.
307. Di Natale P, Balzano N, Esposito S, Villani GR: Identification of molecular defects in Italian Sanfilippo A patients including 13 novel mutations. *Hum Mutat* **11**:313, 1998.

308. Montfort M, Vilageliu L, Garcia-Giralt N, Guidi S, Coll MJ, Chabas A, Grinberg D: Mutation 1091delC is highly prevalent in Spanish Sanfilippo syndrome type A patients. *Hum Mutat* **12**:274, 1998.
309. Schmidtchen A, Greenberg D, Zhao HG, Li HH, Huang Y, Tieu P, Zhao HZ, et al.: NAGLU mutations underlying Sanfilippo syndrome type B. *Am J Hum Genet* **62**:64, 1998.
310. Zhao HG, Aronovich EL, Whitley CB: Genotype-phenotype correspondence in Sanfilippo syndrome type B. *Am J Hum Genet* **62**:53, 1998.
311. Zaremba J, Kleijer WJ, Huijmans JG, Poorthuis B, Fidzianska E, Glogowska I: Chromosomes 14 and 21 as possible candidates for mapping the gene for Sanfilippo disease type IIIC. *J Med Genet* **29**:514, 1992.
312. Robertson DA, Freeman C, Nelson PV, Morris CP, Hopwood JJ: Human glucosamine-6-sulfatase cDNA reveals homology with steroid sulfatase. *Biochem Biophys Res Commun* **157**:218, 1988.
313. Robertson DA, Callen DF, Baker EG, Morris CP, Hopwood JJ: Chromosomal localization of the gene for human glucosamine-6-sulphatase to 12q14. *Hum Genet* **79**:175, 1988.
314. Nakashima Y, Tomatsu S, Hori T, Fukuda S, Sukegawa K, Kondo N, Suzuki Y, et al.: Mucopolysaccharidosis IV A: Molecular cloning of the human *N*-acetylgalactosamine-6-sulfatase gene (GALNS) and analysis of the 5′-flanking region. *Genomics* **20**:99,1994.
315. Morris CP, Guo XH, Apostolou S, Hopwood JJ, Scott HS: Morquio A syndrome: Cloning, sequence, and structure of the human *N*-acetylgalactosamine 6-sulfatase (GALNS) gene. *Genomics* **22**:652, 1994.
316. Masuno M, Tomatsu S, Nakashima Y, Hori T, Fukuda S, Masue M, Sukegawa K, et al.: Mucopolysaccharidosis IV A: Assignment of the human *N*-acetylgalactosamine-6-sulfate sulfatase (GALNS) gene to chromosome 16q24. *Genomics* **16**:777, 1993.
317. Baker E, Guo XH, Orsborn AM, Sutherland GR, Callen DF, Hopwood JJ, Morris CP: The Morquio A syndrome (mucopolysaccharidosis IVA) gene maps to 16q24.3. *Am J Hum Genet* **52**:96, 1993.
318. Tomatsu S, Fukuda S, Uchiyama A, Hori T, Nakashima Y, Kondo N, Suzuki Y, et al.: Molecular analysis by Southern blot for the *N*-acetylgalactosamine-6-sulphate sulphatase gene causing mucopolysaccharidosis IVA in the Japanese population. *J Inherit Metab Dis* **17**:601, 1994.
319. Ogawa T, Tomatsu S, Fukuda S, Yamagishi A, Rezvi GM, Sukegawa K, Kondo N, et al.: Mucopolysaccharidosis IVA: Screening and identification of mutations of the *N*-acetylgalactosamine-6-sulfate sulfatase gene. *Hum Mol Genet* **4**:341, 1995.
320. Tomatsu S, Fukuda S, Cooper A, Wraith JE, Yamada N, Isogai K, Kato Z, et al.: Two new mutations, Q473X and N487S, in a Caucasian patient with mucopolysaccharidosis IVA (Morquio disease). *Hum Mutat* **6**:195, 1995.
321. Tomatsu S, Fukuda S, Cooper A, Wraith JE, Rezvi GM, Yamagishi A, Yamada N, et al.: Mucopolysaccharidosis type IVA: Identification of six novel mutations among non-Japanese patients. *Hum Mol Genet* **4**:741, 1995.
322. Fukuda S, Tomatsu S, Cooper A, Wraith JE, Kato Z, Yamada N, Isogai K, et al.: Mucopolysaccharidosis IVA (Morquio A): Three novel small deletions in the *N*-acetylgalactosamine-6-sulfate sulfatase gene. *Hum Mutat* **8**:187, 1996.
323. Tomatsu S, Fukuda S, Cooper A, Wraith JE, Rezvi GM, Yamagishi A, Yamada N, et al.: Mucopolysaccharidosis IVA: Identification of a common missense mutation I113F in the *N*-acetylgalactosamine-6-sulfate sulfatase gene. *Am J Hum Genet* **57**:556, 1995.
324. Bunge S, Kleijer WJ, Tylki-Szymanska A, Steglich C, Beck M, Tomatsu S, Fukuda S, et al.: Identification of 31 novel mutations in the *N*-acetylgalactosamine-6-sulfatase gene reveals excessive allelic heterogeneity among patients with Morquio A syndrome. *Hum Mutat* **10**:223, 1997.
325. Fukuda S, Tomatsu S, Masuno M, Ogawa T, Yamagishi A, Rezvi GM, Sukegawa K, et al.: Mucopolysaccharidosis IVA: Submicroscopic deletion of 16q24.3 and a novel R386C mutation of *N*-acetylgalactosamine-6-sulfate sulfatase gene in a classical Morquio disease. *Hum Mutat* **7**:123, 1996.
326. Yamada N, Fukuda S, Tomatsu S, Muller V, Hopwood JJ, Nelson J, Kato Z, et al.: Molecular heterogeneity in mucopolysaccharidosis IVA in Australia and Northern Ireland: Nine novel mutations including T312S, a common allele that confers a mild phenotype. *Hum Mutat* **11**:202, 1998.
327. Iwata H, Tomatsu S, Fukuda S, Uchiyama A, Rezvi GM, Ogawa T, Hori T, et al.: Mucopolysaccharidosis IVA: Polymorphic haplotypes and informative RFLPs in the Japanese population. *Hum Genet* **95**:257, 1995.
328. Rezvi GM, Tomatsu S, Fukuda S, Yamagishi A, Cooper A, Wraith JE, Iwata H, et al.: Mucopolysaccharidosis IVA: A comparative study of polymorphic DNA haplotypes in the Caucasian and Japanese populations. *J Inherit Metab Dis* **19**:301, 1996.
329. Oshima A, Yoshida K, Shimmoto M, Fukuhara Y, Sakuraba H, Suzuki Y: Human beta-galactosidase gene mutations in Morquio B disease. *Am J Hum Genet* **49**:1091, 1991.
330. Ishii N, Oohira T, Oshima A, Sakuraba H, Endo F, Matsuda I, Sukegawa K, et al.: Clinical and molecular analysis of a Japanese boy with Morquio B disease. *Clin Genet* **48**:103, 1995.
331. Modaressi S, Rupp K, von Figura K, Peters C: Structure of the human arylsulfatase B gene. *Biol Chem Hoppe-Seyler* **374**:327, 1993.
332. Litjens T, Baker EG, Beckmann KR, Morris CP, Hopwood JJ, Callen DF: Chromosomal localization of ARSB, the gene for human *N*-acetylgalactosamine-4-sulphatase. *Hum Genet* **82**:67, 1989.
333. Litjens T, Morris CP, Robertson EF, Peters C, von Figura K, Hopwood JJ: An *N*-acetylgalactosamine-4-sulfatase mutation (delta G238) results in a severe Maroteaux-Lamy phenotype. *Hum Mutat* **1**:397, 1992.
334. Isbrandt D, Arlt G, Brooks DA, Hopwood JJ, von Figura K, Peters C: Mucopolysaccharidosis VI (Maroteaux-Lamy syndrome): Six unique arylsulfatase B gene alleles causing variable disease phenotypes. *Am J Hum Genet* **54**:454, 1994.
335. Isbrandt D, Hopwood JJ, von Figura K, Peters C: Two novel frameshift mutations causing premature stop codons in a patient with the severe form of Maroteaux-Lamy syndrome. *Hum Mutat* **7**:361, 1996.
336. Villani GRD, Balzano N, Di Natale P: Two novel mutations of the arylsulfatase B gene in two Italian patients with severe form of mucopolysaccharidosis. *Hum Mutat* **11**:410, 1998.
337. Wicker G, Prill V, Brooks D, Gibson G, Hopwood J, von Figura K, Peters C: Mucopolysaccharidosis VI (Maroteaux-Lamy syndrome). An intermediate clinical phenotype caused by substitution of valine for glycine at position 137 of arylsulfatase B. *J Biol Chem* **266**:21386, 1991.
338. Jin WD, Jackson CE, Desnick RJ, Schuchman EH: Mucopolysaccharidosis type VI: Identification of three mutations in the arylsulfatase B gene of patients with the severe and mild phenotypes provides molecular evidence for genetic heterogeneity. *Am J Hum Genet* **50**:795, 1992.
339. Voskoboeva E, Isbrandt D, von Figura K, Krasnopolskaya X, Peters C: Four novel mutant alleles of the arylsulfatase B gene in two patients with intermediate form of mucopolysaccharidosis VI (Maroteaux-Lamy syndrome). *Hum Genet* **93**:259, 1994.
340. Simonaro CM, Schuchman EH: *N*-acetylgalactosamine-4-sulfatase: Identification of four new mutations within the conserved sulfatase region causing mucopolysaccharidosis type VI. *Biochim Biophys Acta* **1272**:129, 1995.
341. Litjens T, Brooks DA, Peters C, Gibson GJ, Hopwood JJ: Identification, expression, and biochemical characterization of *N*-acetylgalactosamine-4-sulfatase mutations and relationship with clinical phenotype in MPS-VI patients. *Am J Hum Genet* **58**:1127, 1996.
342. Miller RD, Hoffmann JW, Powell PP, Kyle JW, Shipley JM, Bachinsky DR, Sly WS: Cloning and characterization of the human beta-glucuronidase gene. *Genomics* **7**:280, 1990.
343. Schwartz CE, Stanislovitis P, Phelan MC, Klinger K, Taylor HA, Stevenson RE: Deletion mapping of plasminogen activator inhibitor, type I (PLANH1) and beta-glucuronidase (GUSB) in 7q21-q22. *Cytogenet Cell Genet* **56**:152, 1991.
344. Shipley JM, Klinkenberg M, Wu BM, Bachinsky DR, Grubb JH, Sly WS: Mutational analysis of a patient with mucopolysaccharidosis type VII, and identification of pseudogenes. *Am J Hum Genet* **52**:517, 1993.
345. Vervoort R, Lissens W, Liebaers I: Molecular analysis of a patient with hydrops fetalis caused by beta-glucuronidase deficiency, and evidence for additional pseudogenes. *Hum Mutat* **2**:443, 1993.
346. Tomatsu S, Sukegawa K, Ikedo Y, Fukuda S, Yamada Y, Sasaki T, Okamoto H, et al.: Molecular basis of mucopolysaccharidosis type VII: Replacement of Ala619 in beta-glucuronidase with Val. *Gene* **89**:283, 1990.
347. Tomatsu S, Fukuda S, Sukegawa K, Ikedo Y, Yamada S, Yamada Y, Sasaki T, et al.: Mucopolysaccharidosis type VII: Characterization of mutations and molecular heterogeneity. *Am J Hum Genet* **48**:89, 1991.
348. Wu BM, Sly WS: Mutational studies in a patient with the hydrops fetalis form of mucopolysaccharidosis type VII. *Hum Mutat* **2**:446, 1993.

349. Wu BM, Tomatsu S, Fukuda S, Sukegawa K, Orii T, Sly WS: Overexpression rescues the mutant phenotype of L176F mutation causing beta-glucuronidase deficiency mucopolysaccharidosis in two Mennonite siblings. *J Biol Chem* **269**:23681, 1994.
350. Vervoort R, Islam MR, Sly W, Chabas A, Wevers R, de Jong J, Liebaers I, et al.: A pseudodeficiency allele (D152N) of the human beta-glucuronidase gene. *Am J Hum Genet* **57**:798, 1995.
351. Islam MR, Vervoort R, Lissens W, Hoo JJ, Valentino LA, Sly WS: Beta-glucuronidase P408s, P415l mutations: Evidence that both mutations combine to produce an MPS VII allele in certain Mexican patients. *Hum Genet* **98**:281, 1996.
352. Vervoort R, Buist NR, Kleijer WJ, Wevers R, Fryns JP, Liebaers I, Lissens W: Molecular analysis of the beta-glucuronidase gene: Novel mutations in mucopolysaccharidosis type VII and heterogeneity of the polyadenylation region. *Hum Genet* **99**:462, 1997.
353. Vervoort R, Gitzelmann R, Bosshard N, Maire I, Liebaers I, Lissens W: Low beta-glucuronidase enzyme activity and mutations in the human beta-glucuronidase gene in mild mucopolysaccharidosis type VII, pseudodeficiency and a heterozygote. *Hum Genet* **102**:69, 1998.
354. Csòka TB, Frost GI, Heng HH, Scherer SW, Mohapatra G, Stern R: The hyaluronidase gene HYAL1 maps to chromosome 3p21.2-p21.3 in human and 9F1-F2 in mouse, a conserved candidate tumor suppressor locus. *Genomics* **48**:63, 1998.
355. Pennock CA: A review and selection of simple laboratory methods used for the study of glycosaminoglycan excretion and the diagnosis of the mucopolysaccharidoses. *J Clin Pathol* **29**:111, 1976.
356. Piraud M, Boyer S, Mathieu M, Maire I: Diagnosis of mucopolysaccharidoses in a clinically selected population by urinary glycosaminoglycan analysis: A study of 2,000 urine samples. *Clin Chim Acta* **221**:171, 1993.
357. Berry HK: Screening for mucopolysaccharide disorders with the Berry spot test. *Clin Biochem* **20**:365, 1987.
358. de Jong JG, Hasselman JJ, van Landeghem AA, Vader HL, Wevers RA: The spot test is not a reliable screening procedure for mucopolysaccharidoses. *Clin Chem* **37**:572, 1991.
359. Whitley CB, Draper KA, Dutton CM, Brown PA, Severson SL, France LA: Diagnostic test for mucopolysaccharidosis. II. Rapid quantification of glycosaminoglycan in urine samples collected on paper matrix. *Clin Chem* **35**:2074, 1989.
360. de Jong JG, Heijs WM, Wevers RA: Mucopolysaccharidoses screening: Dimethylmethylene blue versus alcian blue. *Ann Clin Biochem* **31**:267, 1994.
361. Meikle PJ, Brooks DA, Ravenscroft EM, Yan M, Williams RE, Jaunzems AE, Chataway TK, et al.: Diagnosis of lysosomal storage disorders: Evaluation of lysosome-associated membrane protein LAMP-1 as a diagnostic marker. *Clin Chem* **43**:1325, 1997.
362. Hall CW, Liebaers I, Di Natale P, Neufeld EF: Enzymic diagnosis of the genetic mucopolysaccharide storage disorders. *Methods Enzymol* **50**:439, 1978.
363. Kresse H, von Figura K, Klein U, Glossl J, Paschke E, Pohlmann R: Enzymic diagnosis of the genetic mucopolysaccharide storage disorders. *Methods Enzymol* **83**:559, 1982.
364. Karpova EA, Voznyi Ya V, Keulemans JL, Hoogeveen AT, Winchester B, Tsvetkova IV, van Diggelen OP: A fluorimetric enzyme assay for the diagnosis of Sanfilippo disease type A (MPS IIIA). *J Inherit Metab Dis* **19**:278, 1996.
365. Kleijer WJ, Karpova EA, Geilen GC, Keulemans JL, Huijmans JG, Tsvetkova IV, Voznyi Ya V, et al.: Prenatal diagnosis of Sanfilippo A syndrome: experience in 35 pregnancies at risk and the use of a new fluorogenic substrate for the heparin sulphamidase assay. *Prenat Diagn* **16**:829, 1996.
366. Voznyi YV, Karpova EA, Dudukina TV, Tsvetkova IV, Boer AM, Janse HC, van Diggelen OP: A fluorimetric enzyme assay for the diagnosis of Sanfilippo disease C (MPS III C). *J Inherit Metab Dis* **16**:465, 1993.
367. van Diggelen OP, Zhao H, Kleijer WJ, Janse HC, Poorthuis BJ, van Pelt J, Kamerling JP, et al.: A fluorimetric enzyme assay for the diagnosis of Morquio disease type A (MPS IV A). *Clin Chim Acta* **187**:131, 1990.
368. Young EP: Prenatal diagnosis of Hurler disease by analysis of alpha-iduronidase in chorionic villi. *J Inherit Metab Dis* **15**:224, 1992.
369. Fratantoni JC, Neufeld EF, Uhlendorf BW, Jacobson CB: Intrauterine diagnosis of the Hurler and Hunter syndromes. *N Engl J Med* **280**:686, 1969.
370. Gatti R, Borrone C, Filocamo M, Pannone N, Di Natale P: Prenatal diagnosis of mucopolysaccharidosis I: A special difficulty arising from an unusually low enzyme activity in mother's cells. *Prenat Diagn* **5**:149, 1985.
371. Liebaers I, Di Natale P, Neufeld EF: Iduronate sulfatase in amniotic fluid: An aid in the prenatal diagnosis of the hunter syndrome. *J Pediatr* **90**:423, 1977.
372. Piraud M, Froissart R, Mandon G, Bernard A, Maire I: Amniotic fluid for screening of lysosomal storage diseases presenting in utero (mainly as non-immune hydrops fetalis). *Clin Chim Acta* **248**:143, 1996.
373. Kleijer WJ, Moody PD, Liebaers I, van de Kamp JJ, Niermeijer MF: Prenatal monitoring for the Hunter syndrome: The heterozygous female fetus. *Clin Genet* **15**:113, 1979.
374. Cooper A, Thornley M, Wraith JE: First-trimester diagnosis of Hunter syndrome: Very low iduronate sulphatase activity in chorionic villi from a heterozygous female fetus [Comment]. *Prenat Diagn* **11**:731, 1991.
375. Nwokoro N, Neufeld EF: Detection of hunter heterozygotes by enzymatic analysis of hair roots. *Am J Hum Genet* **31**:42, 1979.
376. Yutaka T, Fluharty AL, Stevens RL, Kihara H: Iduronate sulfatase analysis of hair roots for identification of Hunter syndrome heterozygotes. *Am J Hum Genet* **30**:575, 1978.
377. Zlotogora J, Bach G: Heterozygote detection in Hunter syndrome. *Am J Med Genet* **17**:661, 1984.
378. Shull RM, Munger RJ, Spellacy E, Hall CW, Constantopoulos G, Neufeld EF: Canine alpha-L-iduronidase deficiency. A model of mucopolysaccharidosis I. *Am J Pathol* **109**:244, 1982.
379. Haskins ME, Jezyk PF, Desnick RJ, McDonough SK, Patterson DF: Alpha-L-iduronidase deficiency in a cat: A model of mucopolysaccharidosis I. *Pediatr Res* **13**:1294, 1979.
380. Wilkerson MJ, Lewis DC, Marks SL, Prieur DJ: Clinical and morphologic features of mucopolysaccharidosis type II in a dog: Naturally occurring model of Hunter syndrome. *Vet Pathol* **35**:230, 1998.
381. Fischer A, Carmichael KP, Munnell JF, Jhabvala P, Thompson JN, Matalon R, Jezyk PF, et al.: Sulfamidase deficiency in a family of dachshunds: A canine model of mucopolysaccharidosis IIIA (Sanfilippo A). *Pediat Res* **44**:74, 1998.
382. Thompson JN, Jones MZ, Dawson G, Huffman PS: *N*-acetylglucosamine 6-sulphatase deficiency in a Nubian goat: A model of Sanfilippo syndrome type D (mucopolysaccharidosis IIID). *J Inherit Metab Dis* **15**:760, 1992.
383. Jezyk PF, Haskins ME, Patterson DF, Mellman WJ, Greenstein M: Mucopolysaccharidosis in a cat with arylsulfatase B deficiency: A model of Maroteaux-Lamy syndrome. *Science* **198**:834, 1977.
384. Di Natale P, Annella T, Daniele A, Spagnuolo G, Cerundolo R, de Caprariis D, Gravino AE: Animal models for lysosomal storage diseases: A new case of feline mucopolysaccharidosis VI. *J Inherit Metab Dis* **15**:17, 1992.
385. Yoshida M, Noguchi J, Ikadai H, Takahashi M, Nagase S: Arylsulfatase B-deficient mucopolysaccharidosis in rats. *J Clin Invest* **91**:1099, 1993.
386. Haskins ME, Desnick RJ, DiFerrante N, Jezyk PF, Patterson DF: Beta-glucuronidase deficiency in a dog: A model of human mucopolysaccharidosis VII. *Pediatr Res* **18**:980, 1984.
387. Haskins ME, Aguirre GD, Jezyk PF, Schuchman EH, Desnick RJ, Patterson DF: Mucopolysaccharidosis type VII (Sly syndrome). Beta-glucuronidase-deficient mucopolysaccharidosis in the dog. *Am J Pathol* **138**:1553, 1991.
388. Gitzelmann R, Bosshard NU, Superti-Furga A, Spycher MA, Briner J, Wiesmann U, Lutz H, et al.: Feline mucopolysaccharidosis VII due to beta-glucuronidase deficiency. *Vet Pathol* **31**:435, 1994.
389. Birkenmeier EH, Davisson MT, Beamer WG, Ganschow RE, Vogler CA, Gwynn B, Lyford KA, et al.: Murine mucopolysaccharidosis type VII. Characterization of a mouse with beta-glucuronidase deficiency. *J Clin Invest* **83**:1258, 1989.
390. Giger U, Shivaprasad H, Wang P, Jezyk P, Patterson D, Bradley G: Mucopolysaccharidosis type IIIB (Sanfilippo B syndrome) in emus [Abstract]. *Vet Pathol* **34**:5, 1997.
391. Bermudez AJ, Johnson GC, Vanier MT, Schröder M, Suzuki K, Stogsdill PL, Johnson GS, et al.: Gangliosidosis in emus (*Dromaius novaehollandiae*). *Avian Dis* **39**:292, 1995.
392. Freischutz B, Tokuda A, Ariga T, Bermudez AJ, Yu RK: Unusual gangliosidosis in emu (*Dromaius novaehollandiae*). *J Neurochem* **68**:2070, 1997.
393. Bermudez AJ, Freischutz B, Yu RK, Nonneman D, Johnson GS, Boon GD, Stogsdill PL, et al.: Heritability and biochemistry of gangliosidosis in emus (*Dromaius novaehollandiae*). *Avian Dis* **41**:838, 1997.

394. Menon KP, Tieu PT, Neufeld EF: Architecture of the canine IDUA gene and mutation underlying canine mucopolysaccharidosis I. *Genomics* **14**:763, 1992.
395. Sands MS, Birkenmeier EH: A single-base-pair deletion in the beta-glucuronidase gene accounts for the phenotype of murine mucopolysaccharidosis type VII. *Proc Natl Acad Sci U S A* **90**:6567, 1993.
396. Cavanagh KT, Leipprandt JR, Jones MZ, Friderici K: Molecular defect of caprine *N*-acetylglucosamine-6-sulphatase deficiency. A single base substitution creates a stop codon in the 5′ region of the coding sequence. *J Inherit Metab Dis* **18**:96, 1995.
397. Kunieda T, Simonaro CM, Yoshida M, Ikadai H, Levan G, Desnick RJ, Schuchman EH: Mucopolysaccharidosis type VI in rats: Isolation of cDNAs encoding arylsulfatase B, chromosomal localization of the gene, and identification of the mutation. *Genomics* **29**:582, 1995.
398. Yogalingam G, Hopwood JJ, Crawley A, Anson DS: Mild feline mucopolysaccharidosis type VI. Identification of an *N*-acetylgalactosamine-4-sulfatase mutation causing instability and increased specific activity. *J Biol Chem* **273**:13421, 1998.
399. Ray J, Bouvet A, DeSanto C, Fyfe JC, Xu D, Wolfe JH, Aguirre GD, et al.: Cloning of the canine beta-glucuronidase cDNA, mutation identification in canine MPS VII, and retroviral vector-mediated correction of MPS VII cells. *Genomics* **48**:248, 1998.
400. Evers M, Saftig P, Schmidt P, Hafner A, McLoghlin DB, Schmahl W, Hess B, et al.: Targeted disruption of the arylsulfatase B gene results in mice resembling the phenotype of mucopolysaccharidosis VI. *Proc Natl Acad Sci U S A* **93**:8214, 1996.
401. Clarke LA, Russell CS, Pownall S, Warrington CL, Borowski A, Dimmick JE, Toone J, et al.: Murine mucopolysaccharidosis type I: targeted disruption of the murine alpha-L-iduronidase gene. *Hum Mol Genet* **6**:503, 1997.
402. Li HH, Yu WH, Zhao KW, Rozengurt N, Lyons KM, Anagnostaras SG, Neufeld EF: A mouse model for Sanfilippo syndrome type B. *Am J Hum Genet* **63**:A15, 1998.
403. Muenzer J: Unpublished data, 1998.
404. Sands MS, Vogler C, Torrey A, Levy B, Gwynn B, Grubb J, Sly WS, et al.: Murine mucopolysaccharidosis type VII: Long-term therapeutic effects of enzyme replacement and enzyme replacement followed by bone marrow transplantation. *J Clin Invest* **99**:1596,1997.
405. Russell C, Hendson G, Jevon G, Matlock T, Yu J, Aklujkar M, Ng KY, et al.: Murine MPS I: Insights into the pathogenesis of Hurler syndrome. *Clin Genet* **53**:349, 1998.
406. Baudhuin P, Hers HG, Loeb H: An electron microscopic and biochemical study of Type II glycogen. *Lab Invest* **13**:1139, 1964.
407. Fratantoni JC, Hall CW, Neufeld EF: The defect in Hurler and Hunter syndromes. II. Deficiency of specific factors involved in mucopolysaccharide degradation. *Proc Natl Acad Sci U S A* **64**:360, 1969.
408. Olsen I, Dean MF, Muir H, Harris G: Acquisition of beta-glucuronidase activity by deficient fibroblasts during direct contact with lymphoid cells. *J Cell Sci* **55**:211, 1982.
409. Olsen I, Oliver T, Muir H, Smith R, Partridge T: Role of cell adhesion in contact-dependent transfer of a lysosomal enzyme from lymphocytes to fibroblasts. *J Cell Sci* **85**:231, 1986.
410. Di Natale P, Annella T, Daniele A, Negri R, Nitsch L: Cell-to-cell contact between normal fibroblasts and lymphoblasts deficient in lysosomal enzymes. *Biochim Biophys Acta* **1138**:143, 1992.
411. Grubb JH, Kyle JW, Cody LB, Sly WS: Large scale purification of phosphorylated recombinant human beta-glucuronidase from over-expressing mouse L cells. *FASEB J* **7**:A1255, 1993.
412. Vogler C, Sands M, Higgins A, Levy B, Grubb J, Birkenmeier EH, Sly WS: Enzyme replacement with recombinant beta-glucuronidase in the newborn mucopolysaccharidosis type VII mouse. *Pediatr Res* **34**:837, 1993.
413. Sands MS, Vogler C, Kyle JW, Grubb JH, Levy B, Galvin N, Sly WS, et al.: Enzyme replacement therapy for murine mucopolysaccharidosis type VII. *J Clin Invest* **93**:2324, 1994.
414. O'Connor LH, Erway LC, Vogler CA, Sly WS, Nicholes A, Grubb J, Holmberg SW, et al.: Enzyme replacement therapy for murine mucopolysaccharidosis type VII leads to improvements in behavior and auditory function. *J Clin Invest* **101**:1394, 1998.
415. Shull RM, Kakkis ED, McEntee MF, Kania SA, Jonas AJ, Neufeld EF: Enzyme replacement in a canine model of Hurler syndrome. *Proc Natl Acad Sci U S A* **91**:12937, 1994.
416. Kakkis ED, McEntee MF, Schmidtchen A, Neufeld EF, Ward DA, Gompf RE, Kania S, et al.: Long-term and high-dose trials of enzyme replacement therapy in the canine model of mucopolysaccharidosis I. *Biochem Mol Med* **58**:156, 1996.
417. Crawley AC, Brooks DA, Muller VJ, Petersen BA, Isaac EL, Bielicki J, King BM, et al.: Enzyme replacement therapy in a feline model of Maroteaux-Lamy syndrome. *J Clin Invest* **97**:1864, 1996.
418. Byers S, Nuttall JD, Crawley AC, Hopwood JJ, Smith K, Fazzalari NL: Effect of enzyme replacement therapy on bone formation in a feline model of mucopolysaccharidosis type VI. *Bone* **21**:425, 1997.
419. Brooks DA, King BM, Crawley AC, Byers S, Hopwood JJ: Enzyme replacement therapy in Mucopolysaccharidosis VI: Evidence for immune responses and altered efficacy of treatment in animal models. *Biochim Biophys Acta* **1361**:203, 1997.
420. Kakkis E, Muenzer J, Tiller G, Waber L, Belmont J, Passage M, Izykowski B, et al.: Recombinant alpha-l-iduronidase replacement therapy in mucopolysaccharidosis I: Results of a human clinical trial. *Am J Hum Genet* **63**:A25, 1998.
421. Hobbs JR, Hugh-Jones K, Barrett AJ, Byrom N, Chambers D, Henry K, James DC, et al.: Reversal of clinical features of Hurler's disease and biochemical improvement after treatment by bone-marrow transplantation. *Lancet* **2**:709, 1981.
422. Shull RM, Walker MA: Radiographic findings in a canine model of mucopolysaccharidosis I. Changes associated with bone marrow transplantation. *Invest Radiol* **23**:124, 1988.
423. Gompf RE, Shull RM, Breider MA, Scott JA, Constantopoulos GC: Cardiovascular changes after bone marrow transplantation in dogs with mucopolysaccharidosis I. *Am J Vet Res* **51**:2054, 1990.
424. Breider MA, Shull RM, Constantopoulos G: Long-term effects of bone marrow transplantation in dogs with mucopolysaccharidosis I. *Am J Pathol* **134**:677, 1989.
425. Constantopoulos G, Scott JA, Shull RM: Corneal opacity in canine MPS I. Changes after bone marrow transplantation. *Invest Ophthalmol Vis Sci* **30**:1802, 1989.
426. Gasper PW, Thrall MA, Wenger DA, Macy DW, Ham L, Dornsife RE, McBiles K, et al.: Correction of feline arylsulphatase B deficiency (mucopolysaccharidosis VI) by bone marrow transplantation. *Nature* **312**:467, 1984.
427. Wenger DA, Gasper PW, Thrall MA, Dial SM, LeCouteur RA, Hoover EA: Bone marrow transplantation in the feline model of arylsulfatase B deficiency. *Birth Defects Orig Article Ser* **22**:177, 1986.
428. Aguirre G, Raber I, Yanoff M, Haskins M: Reciprocal corneal transplantation fails to correct mucopolysaccharidosis VI corneal storage. *Invest Ophthalmol Vis Sci* **33**:2702, 1992.
429. Simonaro CM, Haskins ME, Kunieda T, Evans SM, Visser JW, Schuchman EH: Bone marrow transplantation in newborn rats with mucopolysaccharidosis type VI: Biochemical, pathological, and clinical findings. *Transplantation* **63**:1386, 1997.
430. Birkenmeier EH, Barker JE, Vogler CA, Kyle JW, Sly WS, Gwynn B, Levy B, et al.: Increased life span and correction of metabolic defects in murine mucopolysaccharidosis type VII after syngeneic bone marrow transplantation. *Blood* **78**:3081, 1991.
431. Sands MS, Barker JE, Vogler C, Levy B, Gwynn B, Galvin N, Sly WS, et al.: Treatment of murine mucopolysaccharidosis type VII by syngeneic bone marrow transplantation in neonates. *Lab Invest* **68**:676, 1993.
432. Sands MS, Erway LC, Vogler C, Sly WS, Birkenmeier EH: Syngeneic bone marrow transplantation reduces the hearing loss associated with murine mucopolysaccharidosis type VII. *Blood* **86**:2033, 1995.
433. Krivit W, Pierpont ME, Ayaz K, Tsai M, Ramsay NK, Kersey JH, Weisdorf S, et al.: Bone-marrow transplantation in the Maroteaux-Lamy syndrome (mucopolysaccharidosis type VI). Biochemical and clinical status 24 months after transplantation. *N Engl J Med* **311**:1606, 1984.
434. McGovern MM, Ludman MD, Short MP, Steinfeld L, Kattan M, Raab EL, Krivit W, et al.: Bone marrow transplantation in Maroteaux-Lamy syndrome (MPS type 6): Status 40 months after BMT. *Birth Defects* **22**:41, 1986.
435. Whitley CB, Ramsay NK, Kersey JH, Krivit W: Bone marrow transplantation for Hurler syndrome: Assessment of metabolic correction. *Birth Defects Orig Article Ser* **22**:7, 1986.
436. Hugh-Jones K: Psychomotor development of children with mucopolysaccharidosis type 1-H following bone marrow transplantation. *Birth Defects* **22**:25, 1986.
437. Whitley CB, Belani KG, Chang PN, Summers CG, Blazar BR, Tsai MY, Latchaw RE, et al.: Long-term outcome of Hurler syndrome following bone marrow transplantation. *Am J Med Genet* **46**:209, 1993.
438. Peters C, Balthazor M, Shapiro EG, King RJ, Kollman C, Hegland JD, Henslee-Downey J, et al.: Outcome of unrelated donor bone marrow

transplantation in 40 children with Hurler syndrome. *Blood* **87**:4894, 1996.
439. Vellodi A, Young EP, Cooper A, Wraith JE, Winchester B, Meaney C, Ramaswami U, et al.: Bone marrow transplantation for mucopolysaccharidosis type I: Experience of two British centres. *Arch Dis Child* **76**:92, 1997.
440. Peters C, Shapiro EG, Anderson J, Henslee-Downey PJ, Klemperer MR, Cowan MJ, Saunders EF, et al.: Hurler syndrome: II. Outcome of HLA-genotypically identical sibling and HLA-haploidentical related donor bone marrow transplantation in fifty-four children. The Storage Disease Collaborative Study Group. *Blood* **91**:2601, 1998.
441. Guffon N, Souillet G, Maire I, Straczek J, Guibaud P: Follow-up of nine patients with Hurler syndrome after bone marrow transplantation [Comment]. *J Pediatr* **133**:119, 1998.
442. Resnick JM, Krivit W, Snover DC, Kersey JH, Ramsay NK, Blazar BR, Whitley CB: Pathology of the liver in mucopolysaccharidosis: Light and electron microscopic assessment before and after bone marrow transplantation. *Bone Marrow Transplant* **10**:273, 1992.
443. Malone BN, Whitley CB, Duvall AJ, Belani K, Sibley RK, Ramsay NK, Kersey JH, et al.: Resolution of obstructive sleep apnea in Hurler syndrome after bone marrow transplantation. *Int J Pediatr Otorhinolaryngol* **15**:23, 1988.
444. Christiansen SP, Smith TJ, Henslee-Downey PJ: Normal intraocular pressure after a bone marrow transplant in glaucoma associated with mucopolysaccharidosis type I-H. *Am J Ophthalmol* **109**:230, 1990.
445. Navarro C, Dominguez C, Costa M, Ortega JJ: Bone marrow transplant in a case of mucopolysaccharidosis I Scheie phenotype: Skin ultrastructure before and after transplantation. *Acta Neuropathol (Berl)* **82**:33, 1991.
446. Krivit W, Shapiro EG: Bone marrow transplantation for storage diseases, in Desnick RJ (ed): *Treatment of Genetic Disease*. New York, Churchill-Livingstone, 1991, p 203.
447. Viñallonga X, Sanz N, Balaguer A, Miro L, Ortega JJ, Casaldaliga J: Hypertrophic cardiomyopathy in mucopolysaccharidoses: Regression after bone marrow transplantation. *Pediatr Cardiol* **13**:107, 1992.
448. Gatzoulis MA, Vellodi A, Redington AN: Cardiac involvement in mucopolysaccharidoses: Effects of allogeneic bone marrow transplantation. *Arch Dis Child* **73**:259, 1995.
449. Papsin BC, Vellodi A, Bailey CM, Ratcliffe PC, Leighton SE: Otologic and laryngologic manifestations of mucopolysaccharidoses after bone marrow transplantation. *Otolaryngol Head Neck Surg* **118**:30, 1998.
450. Field RE, Buchanan JA, Copplemans MG, Aichroth PM: Bone-marrow transplantation in Hurler's syndrome. Effect on skeletal development. *J Bone Joint Surg Br* **76**:975, 1994.
451. Masterson EL, Murphy PG, O'Meara A, Moore DP, Dowling FE, Fogarty EE: Hip dysplasia in Hurler's syndrome: Orthopaedic management after bone marrow transplantation [Comment]. *J Pediat Orthop* **16**:731, 1996.
452. Gullingsrud EO, Krivit W, Summers CG: Ocular abnormalities in the mucopolysaccharidoses after bone marrow transplantation. Longer follow-up. *Ophthalmology* **105**:1099, 1998.
453. Krivit W, Shapiro E, Hoogerbrugge PM, Moser HW: State of the art review. Bone marrow transplantation treatment for storage diseases. Keystone. January 23, 1992. *Bone Marrow Transplant* **10(Suppl 1)**:87, 1992.
454. Hoogerbrugge PM, Brouwer OF, Bordigoni P, Ringden O, Kapaun P, Ortega JJ, O'Meara A, et al.: Allogeneic bone marrow transplantation for lysosomal storage diseases. The European Group for Bone Marrow Transplantation [Comment]. *Lancet* **345**:1398, 1995.
455. Bergstrom SK, Quinn JJ, Greenstein R, Ascensao J: Long-term follow-up of a patient transplanted for Hunter's disease type IIB: A case report and literature review. *Bone Marrow Transplant* **14**:653, 1994.
456. Li P, Thompson JN, Hug G, Huffman P, Chuck G: Biochemical and molecular analysis in a patient with the severe form of Hunter syndrome after bone marrow transplantation. *Am J Med Genet* **64**:531, 1996.
457. Yamada Y, Kato K, Sukegawa K, Tomatsu S, Fukuda S, Emura S, Kojima S, et al.: Treatment of MPS VII (Sly disease) by allogeneic BMT in a female with homozygous A619V mutation. *Bone Marrow Transplant* **21**:629, 1998.
458. Shapiro EG, Lockman LA, Balthazor M, Krivit W: Neuropsychological outcomes of several storage diseases with and without bone marrow transplantation. *J Inherit Metab Dis* **18**:413, 1995.
459. Unger ER, Sung JH, Manivel JC, Chenggis ML, Blazar BR, Krivit W: Male donor-derived cells in the brains of female sex-mismatched bone marrow transplant recipients: A Y-chromosome specific in situ hybridization study. *J Neuropathol Exp Neurol* **52**:460, 1993.
460. Krivit W, Sung JH, Shapiro EG, Lockman LA: Microglia: The effector cell for reconstitution of the central nervous system following bone marrow transplantation for lysosomal and peroxisomal storage diseases. *Cell Transplant* **4**:385, 1995.
461. McKinnis EJ, Sulzbacher S, Rutledge JC, Sanders J, Scott CR: Bone marrow transplantation in Hunter syndrome. *J Pediatr* **129**:145, 1996.
462. Peters C, Shapiro EG, Krivit W: Hurler syndrome: Past, present, and future [Editorial; Comment]. *J Pediatr* **133**:7, 1998.
463. Anson DS, Bielicki J, Hopwood JJ: Correction of mucopolysaccharidosis type I fibroblasts by retroviral-mediated transfer of the human alpha-L-iduronidase gene. *Hum Gene Ther* **3**:371, 1992.
464. Braun SE, Aronovich EL, Anderson RA, Crotty PL, McIvor RS, Whitley CB: Metabolic correction and cross-correction of mucopolysaccharidosis type II (Hunter syndrome) by retroviral-mediated gene transfer and expression of human iduronate-2-sulfatase. *Proc Natl Acad Sci U S A* **90**:11830, 1993.
465. Bielicki J, Hopwood JJ, Anson DS: Correction of Sanfilippo A skin fibroblasts by retroviral vector-mediated gene transfer. *Hum Gene Ther* **7**:1965, 1996.
466. Fillat C, Simonaro CM, Yeyati PL, Abkowitz JL, Haskins ME, Schuchman EH: Arylsulfatase B activities and glycosaminoglycan levels in retrovirally transduced mucopolysaccharidosis type VI cells. Prospects for gene therapy. *J Clin Invest* **98**:497, 1996.
467. Wolfe JH, Schuchman EH, Stramm LE, Concaugh EA, Haskins ME, Aguirre GD, Patterson DF, et al.: Restoration of normal lysosomal function in mucopolysaccharidosis type VII cells by retroviral vector-mediated gene transfer. *Proc Natl Acad Sci U S A* **87**:2877, 1990.
468. Taylor RM, Wolfe JH: Cross-correction of beta-glucuronidase deficiency by retroviral vector-mediated gene transfer. *Exp Cell Res* **214**:606, 1994.
469. Fairbairn LJ, Lashford LS, Spooncer E, McDermott RH, Lebens G, Arrand JE, Arrand JR, et al.: Long-term in vitro correction of alpha-L-iduronidase deficiency (Hurler syndrome) in human bone marrow. *Proc Natl Acad Sci U S A* **93**:2025, 1996.
470. Huang MM, Wong A, Yu X, Kakkis E, Kohn DB: Retrovirus-mediated transfer of the human alpha-L-iduronidase cDNA into human hematopoietic progenitor cells leads to correction in trans of Hurler fibroblasts. *Gene Ther* **4**:1150, 1997.
471. Casal ML, Wolfe JH: Amphotropic and ecotropic retroviral vector viruses transduce midgestational murine fetal liver cells in a dual-chambered cocultivation system. *Gene Ther* **4**:39, 1997.
472. Stewart K, Brown OA, Morelli AE, Fairbairn LJ, Lashford LS, Cooper A, Hatton CE, et al.: Uptake of alpha-(L)-iduronidase produced by retrovirally transduced fibroblasts into neuronal and glial cells in vitro. *Gene Ther* **4**:63, 1997.
473. Wolfe JH, Sands MS, Barker JE, Gwynn B, Rowe LB, Vogler CA, Birkenmeier EH: Reversal of pathology in murine mucopolysaccharidosis type VII by somatic cell gene transfer. *Nature* **360**:749, 1992.
474. Marechal V, Naffakh N, Danos O, Heard JM: Disappearance of lysosomal storage in spleen and liver of mucopolysaccharidosis VII mice after transplantation of genetically modified bone marrow cells. *Blood* **82**:1358, 1993.
475. Taylor RM, Wolfe JH: Decreased lysosomal storage in the adult MPS VII mouse brain in the vicinity of grafts of retroviral vector-corrected fibroblasts secreting high levels of beta-glucuronidase [Comment]. *Nat Med* **3**:771, 1997.
476. Wolfe JH, Deshmane SL, Fraser NW: Herpesvirus vector gene transfer and expression of beta-glucuronidase in the central nervous system of MPS VII mice. *Nat Genet* **1**:379, 1992.
477. Ohashi T, Watabe K, Uehara K, Sly WS, Vogler C, Eto Y: Adenovirus-mediated gene transfer and expression of human beta-glucuronidase gene in the liver, spleen, and central nervous system in mucopolysaccharidosis type VII mice. *Proc Natl Acad Sci U S A* **94**:1287, 1997.
478. Moullier P, Bohl D, Heard JM, Danos O: Correction of lysosomal storage in the liver and spleen of MPS VII mice by implantation of genetically modified skin fibroblasts [Comment]. *Nat Genet* **4**:154, 1993.
479. Moullier P, Bohl D, Cardoso J, Heard JM, Danos O: Long-term delivery of a lysosomal enzyme by genetically modified fibroblasts in dogs. *Nat Med* **1**:353, 1995.
480. Salvetti A, Moullier P, Cornet V, Brooks D, Hopwood JJ, Danos O, Heard JM: In vivo delivery of human alpha-l-iduronidase in mice implanted with neo-organs. *Hum Gene Ther* **6**:1153, 1995.
481. Braun SE, Pan D, Aronovich EL, Jonsson JJ, McIvor RS, Whitley CB: Preclinical studies of lymphocyte gene therapy for mild Hunter syndrome (mucopolysaccharidosis type II). *Hum Gene Ther* **7**:283, 1996.

482. Whitley CB, McIvor RS, Pan D, Stroncek DF, Aronovich EL, Burger SR, McCullough J: Clinical trial of gene therapy for a mannose-6-phosphate receptor-mediated lysosomal storage disease, mucopolysaccharidosis type II (Hunter syndrome). *Am J Hum Genet* **61**:A359, 1997.
483. Verma IM, Somia N: Gene therapy—Promises, problems and prospects [News]. *Nature* **389**:239, 1997.
484. Neer TM, Dial SM, Pechman R, Wang P, Oliver JL, Giger U: Clinical vignette. Mucopolysaccharidosis VI in a miniature pinscher. *J Vet Intern Med* **9**:429, 1995.
485. Fyfe JC, Kurzhals RL, Giger U, Haskins ME, Patterson DF, Wang P, Wolfe JH, et al.: A missense mutation causing beta-glucuronidase deficiency in feline MPS VII. *Am J Hum Genet* **59**:A197, 1996.

CHAPTER 137

Pycnodysostosis: Cathepsin K Deficiency

Bruce D. Gelb ■ Dieter Brömme ■ Robert J. Desnick

1. **Pycnodysostosis, an inborn error of bone matrix degradation, results from the deficient activity of the lysosomal protease, cathepsin K, in the osteoclasts of affected individuals. The enzymatic defect leads to a reduced ability of osteoclasts to remove organic bone matrix, which causes defective bone growth and remodeling. Partially degraded collagen fibrils are found in lysosomes within osteoclasts that are actively resorbing bone.**
2. **The disorder is transmitted as an autosomal recessive trait by the gene encoding cathepsin K, localized to chromosomal region 1q21. The human cathepsin K cDNA and genomic sequences have been isolated, characterized, and used to analyze the mutations causing pycnodysostosis. All identified defects have been point mutations in the coding region, which obliterate the collagenolytic activity of the mature enzyme.**
3. **Clinical manifestations include short stature, a typical dysmorphic appearance, generalized osteosclerosis, dysplastic bones including hypoplasia of the distal phalanges, clavicles, and various craniofacial bones, as well as pathologic fractures and dental abnormalities. Associated complications include osteomyelitis of the jaw, upper airway obstruction, growth hormone deficiency, and myelophthisis. Life span is normal, although disability secondary to the orthopedic problems may cause premature demise.**
4. **Diagnosis is usually made by clinical and radiologic examinations. Demonstration of cathepsin K gene defects confirms the diagnosis. Prenatal diagnosis can be accomplished by demonstration of the specific cathepsin K mutation(s) in chorionic villi or cultured amniotic cells, or by linkage analysis for couples known to be cathepsin K mutation carriers.**
5. **Therapy is directed at preventing or ameliorating the orthopedic, dental, and medical complications. Surgical intervention may be necessary for patients with significant upper airway obstruction. Growth hormone repletion may improve linear growth for individuals with growth hormone deficiency.**

Pycnodysostosis, an osteosclerotic skeletal dysplasia, results from the defective activity of cathepsin K, a lysosomal cysteine protease. The disorder, which is inherited as an autosomal recessive trait, results from the decreased capacity of osteoclasts to degrade organic bone matrix during bone growth and remodeling. Ultrastructural studies of osteoclasts from affected individuals show typical multinucleated cells with mitochondria, a ruffled border, and pathologic vacuoles containing undegraded collagen fibrils. The decreased rate of bone degradation results in the accumulation of bone mass as well as abnormal bone morphology due to perturbed skeletogenesis. Clinically, the cardinal features include short stature, diffuse bone sclerosis of the long and the flat bones, and a bone dysplasia with hypoplastic mandible, delayed cranial suture closure, short phalanges, and hypoplastic clavicles, as well as numerous dental abnormalities, such as hypodontia, delayed eruption, and enamel hypoplasia. The disease can be differentiated from osteopetrosis by the lack of cranial nerve compressions, generally normal hematopoiesis, and the dysplastic bone features. The most frequent complications associated with pycnodysostosis are orthopedic, including pathologic fractures, nonunion of fractures, and spondylolisthesis. Additional problems include dental caries, osteomyelitis of the jaw, and upper airway obstruction. Life span may be normal and affected females can carry pregnancies to term. Heterozygous carriers have no apparent phenotype.

HISTORICAL ASPECTS

The osteosclerotic disorder, now known as pycnodysostosis, was first described in Spain in 1956 by Collado-Otero.[1] The report, entitled *Una forma mas de distrofia osea*, received little attention. The disorder was rediscovered independently by two groups in 1962.[2,3] In France, Maroteaux and Lamy described a brother and sister, aged 4 years and 18 months, respectively, with short stature, osteosclerosis, loss of the angle of the mandible, delayed cranial suture closure, short fingers with irregular nails, and pathologic fractures.[2] They designated this clinical constellation as pycnodysostosis, combining the Greek word πυκνός meaning dense with *dysostosis* referring to the abnormally developed bone. By studying several additional cases, they recognized that the disorder was inherited as an autosomal recessive trait, and noted the particularly high incidence of parental consanguinity. They also distinguished this disorder from osteopetrosis (Albers-Schönberg disease) by the absence of the cranial nerve compression that occurs in osteopetrosis. Andrén, Dymling, Hogeman, and Wendeberg independently described similar findings in two Swedish adult monozygotic twin sisters, designating the disorder *osteopetrosis acro-osteolytica*.[3] They also examined the calcium and phosphorus metabolism, finding that the skeletal accretion rates were decreased, and bone biopsies were performed that had nonspecific histologic findings. In a review of pycnodysostosis, Sedano and coworkers found several earlier case reports in the literature[4] that had been erroneously diagnosed as osteopetrosis, citing the 1923 publication by Montanari as the earliest recognition of the disease entity.[5]

While the original clinical descriptions were thorough, a few additional aspects of the phenotype were delineated in subsequent reports. For example, several studies documented the dental abnormalities associated with pycnodysostosis. These abnormalities include delayed eruption, persistence of primary teeth, hypodontia, enamel hypoplasia, and malposition of teeth.[4] Osteomyelitis of the jaws, predominantly affecting the mandible, has been reported in a limited number of adults.[6] These infections are often complications of dental extractions and generally prove difficult to treat; surgical intervention was required in several cases and there have been at least two fatalities. Several patients have been reported with evidence of myelophthisis, generally presenting with anemia, thrombocytopenia, and secondary hepatosplenomegaly caused by extramedullary hematopoiesis.[7–11] These findings, in a small percentage of pycnodysostosis patients, established that clinically apparent bone marrow impingement does not unequivocally differentiate pycnodysostosis from osteopetrosis. To date, however, no patients with pycnodysostosis have been found to have cranial nerve compression. Recently, two groups documented growth hormone deficiency in patients with pycnodysostosis.[12,13] Treatment with growth hormone resulted in significant acceleration in linear growth.

The underlying defect resulting in pycnodysostosis was discovered in 1996 by Gelb and coworkers using a positional cloning strategy to identify the causative gene.[14] The chromosomal locus of the pycnodysostosis gene was first identified in 1995 by two research groups who used large families with multiple affected individuals to perform genetic linkage studies.[15,16] The diseased locus was assigned to a 4-cM region at chromosomal band 1q21.[15] Using additional polymorphic DNA markers, Gelb and coworkers were able to refine the critical region to 2 cM.[17] They then established a physical map for the pycnodysostosis critical region using yeast artificial chromosome clones, and excluded several candidate genes, including the cysteine protease cathepsin S, which had previously been mapped to 1q21.[14] The cathepsin S gene was considered an excellent candidate for this disease because cysteine cathepsins had been implicated in the degradation of organic bone matrix by osteoclasts.[18–21] Cathepsin S activity, however, was normal in pycnodysostosis patients.[14] Efforts to identify another cathepsin candidate led to cathepsin K, which was recently cloned and highly expressed in osteoclasts.[22,23] The cathepsin K gene was mapped into the pycnodysostosis critical region near the cathepsin S gene.[14] Subsequently, cathepsin K cDNAs were reverse-transcribed from lymphoblast RNA, amplified by PCR, and sequenced, identifying three significant mutations among three unrelated pycnodysostosis families. Expression in mammalian cells of a mutation which predicted the substitution of a tryptophan codon for the stop codon, resulted in no immunologically detectable protein despite an adequate transcript level, thereby providing the final proof that cathepsin K gene defects caused pycnodysostosis.[14]

Although rare, pycnodysostosis attained considerable attention when Maroteaux and Lamy argued persuasively that the famous French painter Henri de Toulouse-Lautrec had this disorder.[24] Toulouse-Lautrec had short stature and suffered femoral fractures after minor falls on two separate occasions during childhood. Born into an aristocratic French family, his skeletal disorder appears to have played a role in his choice of avocation as well as his artistic vision. No diagnosis was made during his life, and no radiologic studies were performed prior to his death in 1901. Preceding the first descriptions of pycnodysostosis as a disease entity, a number of authors had speculated about Toulouse-Lautrec's correct diagnosis, proposing such entities as osteogenesis imperfecta,[25] achondroplasia,[26] pseudoachondroplasia,[27] and polyepiphysial dysplasia.[28] Maroteaux and Lamy noted several aspects about Toulouse-Lautrec's disorder which strongly suggested the diagnosis of pycnodysostosis. His parents were first cousins and he seems to have had at least three affected cousins whose parents (siblings of Toulouse-Lautrec's father and mother) were also first cousins, highly suggestive of autosomal recessive inheritance. In addition to his short stature, the two pathological fractures which he sustained would be consistent with this diagnosis, but too few for a patient with osteogenesis imperfecta. Finally, pictures of Toulouse-Lautrec from early childhood clearly document the increased size of his head, a common finding in pycnodysostosis. While the retrospective diagnosis of Maroteaux and Lamy has been generally accepted, some have questioned their conclusion.[29] In particular, Frey, the author of a recent biography of Toulouse-Lautrec,[30] provided photographic evidence that the artist's chin was neither small nor recessed, and that his fingers were not short.[29,31] Missing from Frey's critique, however, was the concept of phenotypic heterogeneity, which is clearly observed for pycnodysostosis, even among affected members of the same family.[32] That is, some features of this disorder, such as osteosclerosis, appear to be invariably present, but others, such as finger length, show variability ranging from the classic phenotype to nearly normal. The preponderance of evidence still suggests that, among the currently defined skeletal dysplasias, pycnodysostosis is the most likely diagnosis of the disorder that afflicted Toulouse-Lautrec. Definitive proof could be obtained from roentgenograms of his skeleton but, as Maroteaux wrote, "the remains of Toulouse-Lautrec deserve to rest in peace."[33]

CLINICAL MANIFESTATIONS

Skeletal Anomalies

Adult height is reduced in pycnodysostosis with observed values ranging from 135 to 160 cm in males and 117 to 152 cm in females. While short stature is unquestionably a principal feature of this skeletal dysplasia, the high prevalence of lower extremity fractures, the substantial percentage of cases reported from developing regions of the world where nutrition may not be optimal, and a possible role of growth hormone deficiency (see below) suggest that nongenetic factors are also relevant in determining height at maturity in affected individuals. Almost no serial height data are available from pycnodysostosis patients, but inspection of the growth curves derived from cross-sectional data suggests that growth velocity is subnormal. Birth length appears to be normal or nearly normal. There also is disproportion with relatively well conserved truncal length compared to leg length such that the upper/lower ratio is increased (Fig. 137-1).[32]

The hands and feet are typically short and broad with short digits, particularly affecting the terminal phalanges, which show distal flaring (Fig. 137-2). The nails are often dystrophic.[34] The

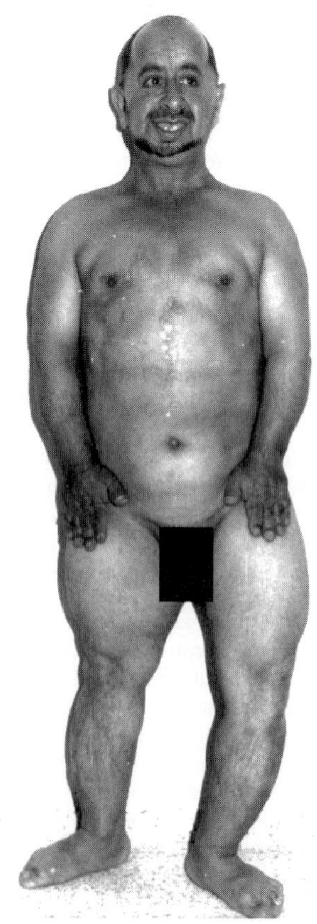

Fig. 137-1 A 48-year-old man with pycnodysostosis. This patient has short stature with short limbs and brachydactyly, as well as some typical facial features including micrognathia, beaked nose, and prominent forehead.

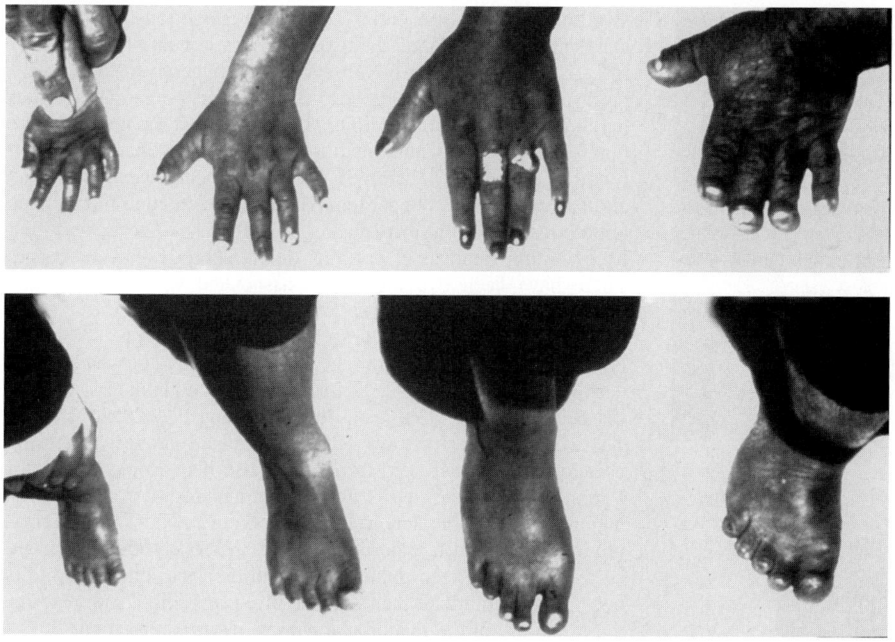

Fig. 137-2 Hands and feet from four related patients with pycnodysostosis. Brachydactyly is present in all patients and splaying of the distal phalanges is most apparent in the oldest patient on the right. The phenotypic variability is also shown, as the hand of the third patient is nearly normal in appearance.

limbs are short, and bowing of the legs may be observed due to previous fractures. The clavicles are typically hypoplastic at their acromial end. The spine also may be deformed with kyphosis, scoliosis, or increased lumbar lordosis.[34]

On roentgenographic examination, the most striking feature is the pervasive increase in bone density (Fig. 137-3).[32,34] This finding is confirmed by quantitative computerized tomography of the trabecular bone of the lumbar spine showing values of 250 to 300 percent of normal-for-age values and dual-photon x-ray densitometry which reveals lumbar spinal densities of 140 to 160 percent and femoral neck densities of 105 to 170 percent of normal control values, respectively.[35] The medullary canals are visualized in all patients, but are somewhat narrowed by the osteosclerosis, a radiologic feature which distinguishes this disorder from osteopetrosis in which the marrow space becomes obliterated.[36] Widening of the distal portion of the femurs (Erlenmeyer-flask deformity) is variably present. The distal phalanges are notably hypoplastic, often disappearing at the ungual tufts. This feature has been termed acro-osteolysis, which might be a misnomer because evidence for a lytic process does not exist. Vertebral anomalies also have been noted occasionally, including coxa valga and incomplete segmentation at C1-C2 and at L5-S.[32,34] Serial roentgenograms of one patient documented the loss of the horns of the hyoid bone during childhood.[37]

Blood chemistries, including alkaline phosphatase, serum calcium, and serum phosphorus as well as levels of the bone-related hormones (parathyroid hormone, osteocalcin, calcitonin) are normal.[3,11–13,35,38,39]

Craniofacial/Dental Abnormalities

In patients with pycnodysostosis, the head tends to be large with frontal and occipital bulging (Fig. 137-1). The anterior and posterior fontanels are usually open beyond the appropriate age of closure. Failure of cranial suture fusion may be detected on palpation.[34] Mild-to-moderate exophthalmos may be noted. The nose is often prominent and beak-like.[4] The lower portion of the face often has a full appearance, but the chin is generally small with retrognathia. The ears are normal in shape and position.

Roentgenograms of the skull reveal the same osteosclerotic changes noted throughout the appendicular skeleton.[34] The orbital rims and the base of the skull tend to be particularly dense.[4,40] The skull is typically dolichocephalic with frontal and occipital bossing. Any and all of the cranial sutures may be open, and the anterior and posterior fontanels may be patent. Wormian bones are observed frequently. The paranasal sinuses are hypoplastic or absent and the mastoid air cells often fail to pneumatize. The facial bones, maxilla, and mandible are generally hypoplastic. The angle of the mandible is obliterated, an apparently invariant and pathognomonic sign of this disorder.[4,34,40]

Inspection of the mouth reveals a high-arched palate with a deep groove in nearly all patients.[40] Macroglossia also has been noted in some patients, probably being relative to the small mandible in these patients.

Numerous quantitative and qualitative dental abnormalities are found in patients with pycnodysostosis, including retention of deciduous teeth, delayed eruption of permanent teeth, and hypodontia, which was found in a majority of patients.[4,40] The teeth may be small (microdontia) and have enamel hypoplasia, hypercementosis, obliteration of the pulp chamber, and/or hypoplasia of the dental roots. The teeth are usually malpositioned and crowded due to the presence of small alveolar arches. Malocclusion with an anterior crossbite is often noted.[40] Dental caries are frequently problematic, attributed to the difficulties in maintaining good dental hygiene when the teeth are overcrowded.

Orthopedic Abnormalities

Patients are prone to pathologic fractures, most commonly of the long bones. Edelson and colleagues reviewed the orthopedic findings in 14 related patients, ranging in age from $1\frac{1}{2}$ to 50 years.[32] Among 11 patients greater than 4 years of age, evidence of fractures was found in one or both tibiae in all but one individual. Femoral fractures were evident in all five teenage and adult patients, tending to be more severe in the older adults. Bilateral subtrochanteric femoral fractures occurred sequentially in a 50-year-old woman, a striking finding because this type of fracture constituted only 5 percent of femoral neck fractures in a large series.[41] A survey of the long bones of the upper extremities revealed humeral, radial, or ulnar fractures in three adult patients.[32] These transverse stress fractures of the long bones of the upper and lower extremities healed, but tended not to obliterate the fracture lines, which is an abnormal finding.

Defects in the spine also are common in pycnodysostosis. Among eight related patients who were 9 years of age or older, lumbar spondylolysis was present in all, affecting L4 and L5 in six cases and L5 only in two.[32] In a 1989 review of the pycnodysostosis literature, Currarino identified six cases of spondylolysis at L5, one at L4, and two at L4 and L5 (including a 4-month-old patient).[42] At least one case of spondylolisthesis,

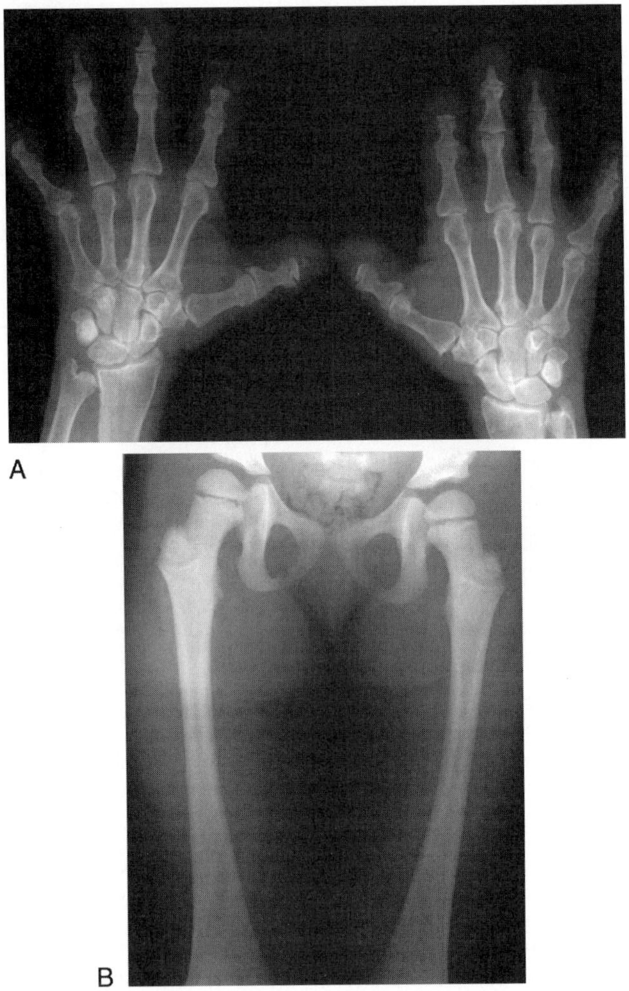

A

B

Fig. 137-3 Roentgenograms of two patients with pycnodysostosis. *A*, Anterior-posterior view of the hands of an 82-year-old women. Brachydactyly is apparent as is acro-osteolysis affecting the therminal phalanges. This latter finding is variable with greater severity of the second than fourth fingers in this patient. *B*, Anterior-posterior view of the femurs and pelvis of 6-year-old girl. Generalized osteosclerosis with narrowing of the medullary space is apparent.

Grade I at L5, has been observed.[32] Spondylolysis also can be observed in the cervical spine, usually at C2.[32,42] For example, a $2\frac{1}{2}$-year-old boy presented with spondylolysis at C2 and C3 after minor trauma. A year later, after minimal orthopedic treatment secondary to poor compliance, the C3 lesion had healed but the C2 spondylolytic lesion remained with some mild cervical instability.[32]

A radiologic skeletal survey in 14 related patients identified several other fracture sites.[32] These included a metatarsal stress fracture with nonunion, a calcaneal stress fracture, three clavicular fractures, and four scapular fractures, generally through the base of the coracoid process, with nonunion in all instances. Whether fracture healing is adequate in patients with pycnodysostosis is not clear. It appears that the majority of fractures will heal, but the risk of nonunion is increased.[32,43] In addition, the persistence of radiolucent fracture lines and the minimal increase in uptake of technetium pyrophosphate at fracture sites during bone scans has been cited as evidence that fracture healing is reduced in pycnodysostosis.[32]

Infectious Complications

Osteomyelitis of the jaw is a complication of pycnodysostosis that has been reported in several individuals, nearly all adults, who presented with draining intra- or extraoral fistulae, pain, and facial swelling, often a few months after dental extractions.[6,44,45] Dental caries and/or periodontal disease, perhaps secondary to the crowding of teeth frequently observed in pycnodysostosis, may predispose to these infections.[44] The primary site of the osteomyelitis has been the mandible, although rare cases involving the maxilla alone or in combination with the mandible have been reported. Aggressive therapy is required to cure these infections and has included curettage, removal of sequestra, and intravenous antibiotics. Persistent or recurrent infections have occurred, often necessitating removal of portions of the necrotic, infected bone. There have been two mortalities associated with osteomyelitis of the jaw: a patient who had a sequestrectomy and died 5 days later of unknown causes[6] and a noncompliant patient with maxillary osteomyelitis who returned with meningitis and deteriorated despite antibiotic therapy.[45] Three cases of mandibular osteomyelitis occurred after fractures sustained during dental extractions.[6] These pathologic fractures tend not to heal properly, forming pseudoarthroses that need to be stabilized. The proclivity toward osteomyelitis of the jaw is not believed to result from a fundamental immunologic deficit, but rather from the poor vascularization observed in osteosclerotic bone.[44] Moreover, adult bones are less well-vascularized than those of children and the mandible is less well-vascularized than the maxilla, providing a rationale for the proclivity of the mandibular infections in adult patients.

Hematologic Abnormalities

The vast majority of patients have normal peripheral blood smears despite imaging studies and bone biopsies routinely demonstrating impingement on the marrow cavity. A small number of patients have had myelophthisis, presenting as microcytic anemia, thrombocytopenia, and hepatosplenomegaly.[7–11] Examination of the bone marrow in three such cases revealed hypoplasia with fibrosis.[7,9,11] One young girl[9] with signs of myelophthisis had an older brother who also was affected by the skeletal dysplasia but had a normal peripheral blood smear. Moreover, the myelophthisis in the girl resolved spontaneously (X. Rialland, personal communication), which suggests that stochastic or environmental factors may be responsible in part for the development of bone marrow failure in pycnodysostosis.

Upper Airway Obstruction

The upper airway tends to be anatomically narrow due to an abnormally elongated soft palate with low-lying uvula, glossoptosis, and retrognathia.[46–48] In several patients, upper airway obstruction has been clinically significant, resulting in obstructive sleep apnea, chronic CO_2 retention, pulmonary hypertension, and right heart failure.[47–49] Adenoidal and/or tonsillar hyperplasia has not been a striking feature in these patients, although a 3-year-old girl with mild obstruction benefited from adenoidectomy.[46] One patient with severe obstruction and right heart failure was treated surgically by shortening of the soft palate with subsequent resolution of the obstruction and complications.[47]

Growth Hormone Deficiency

Two reports describing five children and two adults[12,13] and unpublished data from four children (F. Griegg, Mount Sinai School of Medicine, New York, NY; K. Araki, Kochi Medical School, Kochi, Japan; W. Riley, Driscoll Children's Hospital, Corpus Christi, Texas; personal communications) have revealed that growth hormone deficiency may accompany pycnodysostosis. In the most extensive study,[12] three of four children and two adults with pycnodysostosis were shown to have low basal growth hormone levels and inadequate responses to provocative testing with clonidine and glucagon. Circulating IGF-I levels also were low. All patients had normal glucose tolerance, thyroid function, and serum cortisol levels. Computerized tomographic scans of the head revealed normal hypothalamic-pituitary regions except in one child, who had a partially empty sella with mild cortical atrophy. Two children, who were treated with growth hormone (15 U/m^2/week divided into daily subcutaneous doses), experienced

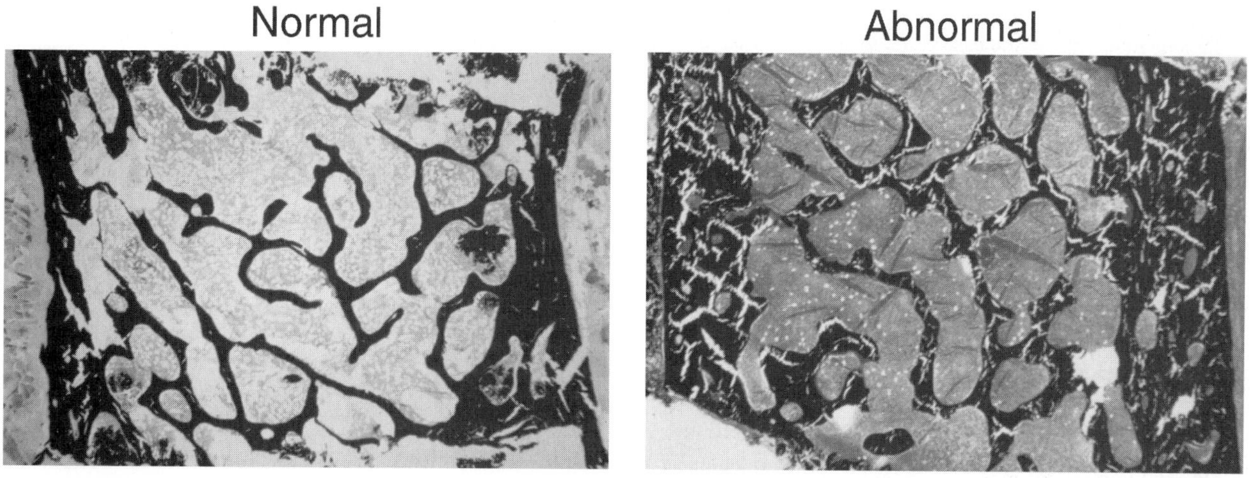

Fig. 137-4 Light micrographs comparing pycnodysostosis and normal bone. Bone biopsies taken from a normal individual (left) and a child with pycnodysostosis (right) demonstrate that both cortical and trabecular bone are excessively thick in pycnodysostosis. The marrow space is narrowed but the cellular elements are preserved in the disorder (von Kossa staining; ×12.5 magnification). (*Courtesy of Michael Klein, Mount Sinai School of Medicine, New York, NY.*)

significant acceleration in growth after 1 year. Bone age, which was delayed prior to therapy, did not accelerate. One patient[13] was treated with growth hormone for 2 years and showed continued growth acceleration, increasing in height from −4.8 standard deviations prior to therapy to −4.4 and −3.8 after 1 and 2 years of therapy, respectively. While growth hormone therapy appears to accelerate linear growth in pycnodysostosis patients with growth hormone deficiency, no data are available to demonstrate that heights at maturity will be increased. In addition, there is no explanation for the growth hormone deficiency. Because the sella turcica appears to be normal in most patients and the remainder of the pituitary function is normal, either cathepsin K deficiency directly affects growth hormone metabolism or feedback to the hypothalamic-pituitary axis in these patients with inadequate bone resorption results in down-regulation of growth hormone production and secretion.

PATHOLOGY

Bone

Both cortical and trabecular bone are increased in thickness, based on light microscopic studies (Fig. 137-4).[38,39,43,50,51] The cortical bone is organized normally into osteons and lamellae, but the increased numbers of fragmented osteons, as well as the predominance of lacunae in interstitial lamellae which lack osteocytes (due to osteocyte death), suggest an increased overall age of the bone elements. The trabeculae are composed of relatively normal lamellar bone, but are sclerotic. The marrow cavity is typically smaller than normal but contains normal hematopoietic cellular elements. The quantity of trabeculae covered by osteoid is reduced, and the lining osteoblasts are generally inactive.[38,39,43,50] Dynamic bone histomorphometry, performed by administering tetracycline 14 and 7 days prior to the bone biopsy, revealed decreased rates of Haversian and cortical-endosteal bone formation as well as decreased formation of new bone centers.[43,51] The number of osteoclasts is increased as is the number of nuclei per osteoclast.[38] The cartilage growth plate also is abnormal.[52,53] The cartilage is narrow and, rather than being organized into columns, contains small islands with short, thick primary trabeculae. The zone of provisional calcification is narrow.

Ultrastructural studies performed by Everts and coworkers[54] revealed activated osteoclasts apposed to bone surface in Howship's lacunae (Fig. 137-5). Pycnodysostosis osteoclasts have typical ruffled borders facing the subosteoclastic space, beneath which is bone undergoing demineralization. Everts and colleagues noted the presence of cytoplasmic vacuoles in the osteoclasts that contained cross-banded structures, which strongly suggested the presence of collagen fibrils. Because collagen fibrils are never observed in osteoclasts in normal bone, they correctly concluded that the fundamental defect in pycnodysostosis was the abnormal degradation of collagen by osteoclasts.[54] The ultrastructure of the growth plate also is deranged, with the majority of chondrocytes

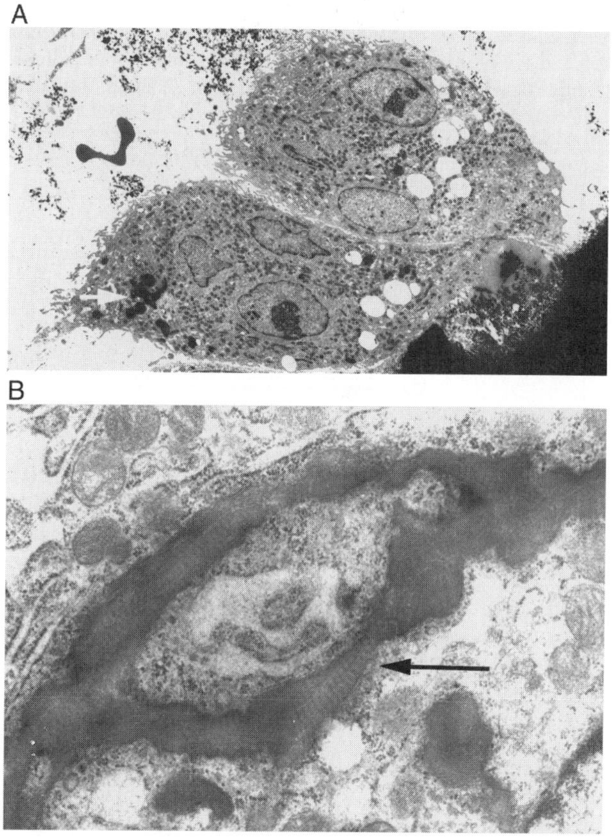

Fig. 137-5 Electron micrographs of an osteoclast from an individual with pycnodysostosis. *A,* The osteoclast is attached to the mineralized bone surface (black material in the lower right corner) which it is actively degrading. Within the osteoclast, there are numerous vacuoles containing collagen fibrils (white arrow) (×3200). *B,* High-power electron micrograph of collagen-containing vacuole. A striated collagen fibril is indicated (black arrow) (×30,000). (*Courtesy of Vincent Everts, University of Amsterdam, Amsterdam.*)

having cytoplasmic vacuoles containing granular and irregular lamellar structures.[52,53] While based on only a single observation, this finding suggests that cathepsin K may play a role in endochondral bone formation.

Nonskeletal Tissues

The only information concerning nonosseous tissues in pycnodysostosis comes from the limited report of an autopsy of a 21-month-old boy who died after aspirating gastric contents.[46] The only nonosseous tissues examined were the liver and spleen, which were both normal by light microscopy.

THE BIOCHEMISTRY OF CATHEPSINS AND CATHEPSIN K

Nomenclature of Cathepsins

The word *kathepsin* (from the Greek word καθέψειν, which means "to digest") was coined by Willstätter and Baumann in 1929 to describe a newly discovered group of intracellular acid proteases. The diversity of proteolytic mechanisms among such proteases, which had not been recognized at that time, has led to their subclassification according to the critical residue in the active site: cysteine proteases (cathepsins B, L, S, H, K, C, O, and W), aspartic proteases (cathepsins D and E), and serine protease (cathepsins A and G). The first mammalian cysteine proteases to be identified (cathepsins B, L, and H) were ubiquitous housekeeping lysosomal proteases with no or little substrate specificity, but the more recently identified members of this protease family (cathepsins S, K, and W) do exhibit (nonoverlapping) tissue specificity and defined in vivo substrate specificity. For example, cathepsin S is specifically expressed in lymphatic tissues and is responsible for the cleavage of the invariant chain in the MHC-class II complexes in antigen-presenting cells, whereas cathepsin K is predominantly expressed in osteoclasts and constitutes the critical protease in bone resorption.

Mechanism and Substrate Specificity of Cysteine Proteases

Cysteine cathepsins possess an active-site nucleophilic cysteine residue, which forms a covalent bond with the carbonyl carbon of the scissile bond (i.e., the bond to be cleaved) of the bound substrate. A histidine residue that, together with the active cysteine, forms the so-called ion-pair, completes the active site of cysteine proteases. The ion-pair is stabilized by an asparagine residue, also in the active site, which is completely conserved among the papain family of cysteine proteases. The mechanism of peptide hydrolysis by cysteine proteases is depicted in Fig. 137-6.

Whereas the catalytic site is responsible for the cleavage of a peptide bond in the substrate, the binding region of the active site provides the substrate specificity of the protease. Schechter and Berger defined seven sites of interaction between amino acid residues of the substrate with binding sites in the protease. Residues in the substrate on the N-terminal side of the scissile bond are termed P1, P2, etc., while residues on the C-terminal end are termed P1′, P2′, etc. The subsites (or binding pockets) in the protease which bind these N-terminal and C-terminal residues are designated S1, S2, etc., and S1′, S2′, etc., respectively. Whereas the S2 subsites in all papain-like cysteine proteases for which the three-dimensional structures have been solved are accurately described as binding pockets, the other subsites more closely resemble shallow crevices on the surface of the protease. The well-defined structural properties of the S2 subsite define the primary substrate specificity of papain-like cathepsins.

Expression of Recombinant Cathepsin K

The human cathepsin K prepropeptide has been expressed by two research groups using the baculovirus system.[55–57] Cathepsin K

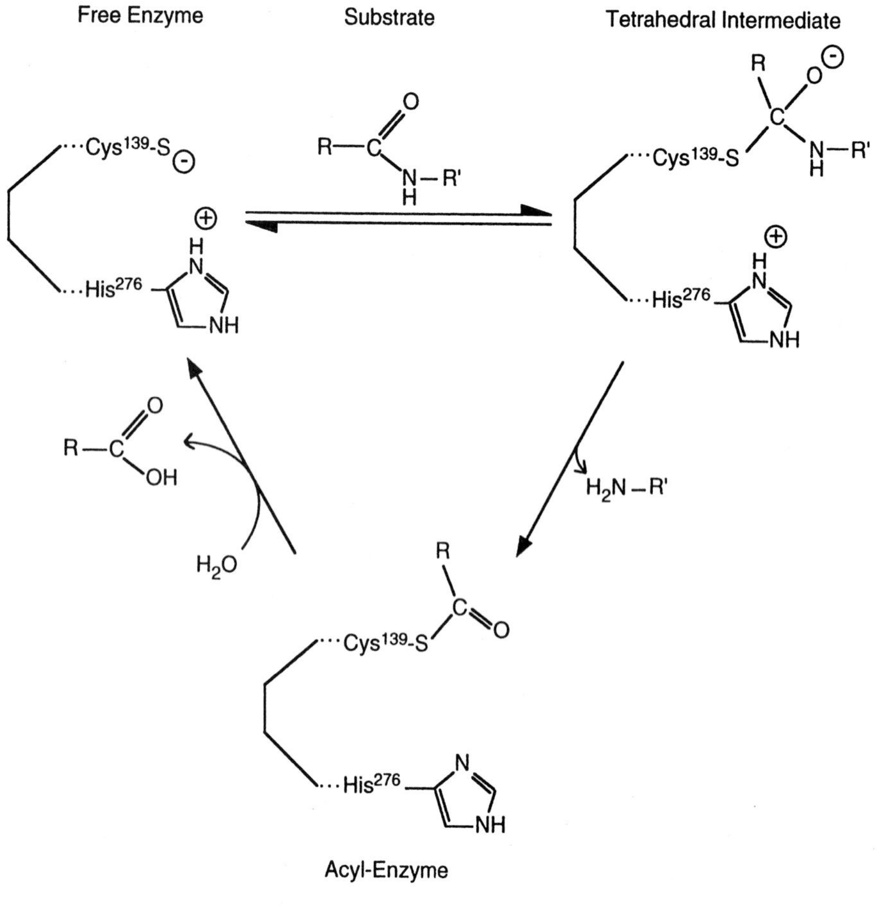

Fig. 137-6 Mechanism of peptide hydrolysis by cysteine cathepsins. An acylation reaction between free cathepsin (upper left-hand side) with its Cys-His dipole and the target protein at the sessile bond results in an unstable tetrahedral intermediate (upper right-hand side) with subsequent release of the C-terminal peptide from the target protein, leaving an acyl-enzyme. A subsequent deacylation reaction results in the release of the N-terminal peptide of the target protein and restoration of free cathepsin.

proenzyme was collected from supernatant and amino terminal sequencing confirmed that the isolated 37-kDa protein was the proform of cathepsin K. Matrix-assisted laser desorption ionization-mass spectrometric (MALDI-MS) analysis of the proform indicated that approximately 3 percent of the mass was due to glycosylation, whereas electrospray mass spectrometry (ESMS) and MALDI-MS analyses of the mature protein revealed that it was not glycosylated, indicating glycosylation occurred at the consensus *N*-glycosylation site in the pro region.[57] In addition, these studies showed that six of the eight Cys residues in the mature enzyme were in disulfide linkages.[57] The cathepsin K proenzyme was catalytically inactive but could be activated either by pepsin[55] or by prolonged incubation at low pH and elevated temperature under reducing conditions.[56] Incubation of the cathepsin K proenzyme with either activated cathepsin K or B failed to result in activation. Procathepsin K in which the active cysteine had been mutated could not autoactivate at pH 4.0, but was processed to the mature form by the wild-type cathepsin K enzyme, suggesting that cathepsin K is autocatalytic at low pH *in vitro* and possibly in vivo.[57] The activation of the proform resulted in the generation of a 29-kDa peptide which was a monomer. N-terminal sequencing of the mature enzyme autoprocessed at pH 4.0 showed a mixture of N-termini of Gly^{113}, Arg^{114}, and Ala^{115}.[57] N-terminal sequencing and MALDI-MS of the propeptides revealed a variety of cleavage sites but preferential cleavage at Glu^{19}, Ser^{98}, and Glu^{110}.

Cathepsin K enzymatic activity was characterized biochemically using fluorescent and natural substrates. Using benzyloxycarbonyl methylcoumarylamide dipeptides (Z-P_2-R-MCA), Brömme and coworkers showed that the order of the substrate preference at the P_2 position for cathepsin K was $L \gg F > V \gg R$, most similar to the substrate specificity for cathepsin S.[55] The catalytic efficiency (k_{cat}/K_m) of cathepsin K towards these dipeptide substrates was comparable to cathepsins S and B, but approximately one order of magnitude less than cathepsin L. Using Z-FR-MCA as substrate, Brömme and coworkers established that the pH-activity curve for cathepsin K had an optimum at pH 6.1 with a bell-shaped profile ($pK_1 = 4.00$ and $pK_2 = 8.13$).[55] The pH-stability assay with cathepsin K revealed that the recombinant enzyme had approximately 50 percent residual activity after 1 h at pH 6.5, ranking it as more stable than cathepsin L, but less stable than cathepsin S.[55]

The inhibitor profile for cathepsin K was typical for a member of the papain superfamily of cysteine proteases.[55,56] The active enzyme was strongly inhibited by generalized cysteine cathepsin inhibitors such as E-64 and cystatin as well as by serine/cysteine protease inhibitors such as leupeptin and calpeptin. As expected, specific serine and aspartic protease inhibitors, as well as metalloproteinase inhibitors, had no effect on cathepsin K activity.

The proteolytic properties of baculovirus-expressed cathepsin K against protein substrates has also been assessed in vitro.[55] Cathepsin K was elastolytic with a maximal activity at pH 5.5 and had an activity that exceeded those of cathepsins L and S as well as elastase. Cathepsin K also was strongly collagenolytic with maximal degradation of type I collagen in the pH range from 5.0 to 6.0. The primary cleavage site of type I collagen apparently occurs in the telopeptide region and, possibly, within the N-terminal portion of the triple helix. This cleavage specificity is in sharp contrast with the tissue collagenases (metalloproteinases) which cleave the α monomers into $\frac{3}{4}$ and $\frac{1}{4}$ fragments. Cathepsin K displayed strong gelatinase activity over a pH range from 5.0 to 7.0. Cathepsin K also was shown to cleave osteonectin, a component of organic bone matrix, at least in two sites, one with the dipeptide Leu-Arg at positions P_2-P_1.[56]

Three-Dimensional Structure of Human Cathepsin K

Two groups succeeded in obtaining crystal structures for mature human cathepsin K complexed with the inhibitor E-64, or APC3328.[58,59] The cathepsin K crystal had approximate dimensions of 55 Å × 35 Å × 37 Å and was arranged in two domains separated by an active site cleft. The active cysteine (Cys^{139}) was at the N-terminus of a long α-helix in the domain containing the N-terminus and was separated by 3.65 Å from the active histidine (His^{276}) with which it is believed to form a thiolate-imidazolium ion pair. His^{276} and the third member of the active triad, Asn^{296}, were in the C-terminal domain and formed a hydrogen bond at 2.8 Å. Based on the data obtained with the APC3328 inhibitor, McGrath and coworkers showed that there was a nucleophilic attack of the Cys^{139} $S\gamma$ on the position corresponding to the carbonyl carbon of P1 and that the attack occurred on the *si* face, in contrast to serine, aspartyl-, and metalloproteinases, which all attack the *re* face of their substrates.[59] The S2 pocket contacted the P2 substrate residue which, for cathepsin K, was preferentially leucine. The derived structure showed a good fit for a Leu in the P2 position as well as sufficient space for the β-branched Val in P2, but a fit with Phe at P2 that is poor relative to that found for the S2 structures of cathepsins B, S, and L. These predictions based on the S2-P2 structure were consistent with the substrate-specificity data derived for these cathepsins with synthetic dipeptide substrates.[55] The S3 pocket was constituted primarily by Tyr^{201} and Asp^{196} and appeared to immobilize the P3 residue in a pincer grasp. Comparison of the three-dimensional structure of cathepsin K with that for human cathepsin B, actinidin, and papain, the three other members of the papain superfamily for which such information is available, revealed closest structural homology with actinidin (root mean square deviation of 0.72 Å) and lowest homology with human cathepsin B (root mean square deviation of 1.13 Å), although all shared substantial similarity in overall folding.[58] In fact, cathepsin B was significantly different from all other known members of the papain family because it alone is a dipeptidyl carboxypeptidase, a property attributed to a unique 10-amino acid loop overlying its active site.[58]

THE MOLECULAR GENETICS OF CATHEPSIN K

Gene Assignment

The locus for human cathepsin K was assigned to chromosomal band 1q21 by fluorescence *in situ* hybridization (FISH), as well as by genetic and physical mapping. Gelb and coworkers fluorescently labeled the human cathepsin K cDNA and showed that it hybridized to 1q21 on human metaphase chromosome preparations.[60] In addition, genetic mapping of pycnodysostosis placed the cathepsin K gene between chromosome 1 polymorphic markers *D1S2344* and *D1S2343/D1S2345*, a region of about 2 cM at 1q21.[17] Two markers within this region, *D1S498* and *D1S2347*, never recombined with disease and had been placed on the 1996 Genethon human genetic linkage map at no recombination distance from *D1S2343* and *D1S2345*. Finally, the gene was mapped physically using yeast and P1 artificial chromosomes (YACs and PACs, respectively).[14,60] A sequence-tagged site (STS) marker for cathepsin K was amplified from two YAC clones, 947e1 and 978e4, from the Centre d'Etude Polymorphism Humaine (CEPH) megaYAC library. STS markers for two other genes that had previously been mapped to 1q21 by FISH, cathepsin S and MCL1, also were amplified from the same two YACs. These YACs were part of a contig that placed the polymorphic marker *D1S498* immediately telomeric to MCL1. STSs for cathepsins K and S were amplified from the same PAC, 74e16.[60] Because PAC insert sizes range from 100 to 150 kb, these two cathepsin genes, each around 10 kb in length, lie in close proximity to one another. The combination of the genetic and physical mapping data provide the following order: *D1S2344*-[cathepsin K-cathepsin S]-MCL1-*D1S498-D1S2347*-[*D1S2343-D1S2345*].

The Cathepsin K cDNA

The cathepsin K cDNA was cloned originally from a rabbit osteoclast library[61] and subsequently from cDNA libraries from several human tissues, including bone, spleen, and macrophages,[22,23,62,63] as well as from mouse bone and heart.[64,65] The 1670-bp human cDNA has 5′ and 3′ untranslated regions of 99 and 566 bp, respectively, and an open reading frame of 987 bp encoding a 329-residue polypeptide with a predicted unglycosylated $M_r = 36{,}963$. The predicted protein sequence had the typical prepropeptide organization of cysteine proteases of the papain family, including a 15-amino acid signal sequence and a 99-residue pro piece, predicting unglycosylated masses of 35,308 and 23,494 for the propeptide and mature enzyme, respectively. The predicted signal sequence had typical features including a four-residue central hydrophobic domain (VLLL), an α-helix-breaking proline residue at position minus 6 from the putative cleavage site, and an alanine residue at position minus 1.

Compared to the mature enzyme region, the proregions of the related cysteine cathepsins of the papain superfamily are poorly conserved with imperfect sequence alignment and lower degrees of amino acid homology. For instance, cathepsin K and L were 60 percent homologous across the mature enzyme region, but only 38 percent homologous in the proregion.[22] Despite this relative lack of conservation in the proregion, Vernet and coworkers were able to identify a relatively well-conserved seven amino acid propeptide motif, G-x-N-x-F-x-D, among the members of the papain family of cysteine proteases.[66] They demonstrated by site-directed mutagenesis that significant alterations of residues 1, 3, 5, and 7 in that motif in papain resulted in complete loss of enzymatic function secondary to improper protein folding.[66] This domain shows variability among the papain family members and exists in cathepsin K as A-M-N-H-L-G-D (conserved residues in bold) with the alanine in position 1 also being found in cathepsins L and H and the leucine residue in position 5 being present in cathepsin S.

The cathepsin K mature region is highly conserved with the other cysteine cathepsins of the papain family, the highest level of homology being with cathepsins L and S (60 percent and 58 percent, respectively).[22] The catalytic triad within the active site contains active cysteine, histidine, and asparagine residues which are conserved completely among all papain family members, and are present in cathepsin K at positions 139, 276, and 296, respectively. The other invariably conserved residues among the papain family also were found in cathepsin K (N^{133} in the putative oxyanion-binding pocket, G^{179}, G^{180}, and W^{292}).

Analysis of the predicted amino acid sequence of human cathepsin K revealed two possible *N*-glycosylation sites, one in the proregion (N^{103}-D^{104}-T^{105}) and the other in the mature enzyme (N^{161}-L^{162}-S^{163}). The latter site may not be used, however, as it is followed immediately by a proline residue and is not completely conserved, being present in the orthologous site in the rabbit cathepsin K gene, but not in the mouse or chicken genes. In fact, the putative proregion *N*-glycosylation site was the only one conserved among all four cathepsin K orthologues as well as with the highly homologous human cathepsin S.[64]

Consistent with its involvement in bone resorption, cathepsin K was highly expressed in osteoclasts and in osteoclastomas.[22,62] Quantitation of cathepsin K sequences in an human osteoclast cDNA library confirmed the abundance, which was at least one order of magnitude greater than those for cathepsins B, L, and S.[67] Lower levels of expression were detected in heart, lung, skeletal muscle, colon, ovary, and placenta.[22,62] *In situ* hybridization of bone histologic sections with an antisense cathepsin K cDNA probe revealed intense signals from osteoclasts and chondroclasts, lower levels in some mononuclear cells in the bone marrow, but none from other bone cells such as osteoblasts, osteocytes, and chondrocytes.[67,68]

The Cathepsin K Gene

Structural Organization. Genomic clones containing the human cathepsin K gene have been isolated and characterized (Fig. 137-7).[60,69] The approximately 11-kb gene comprises 8 exons ranging in size from 103 to 665 bp. Exon 1 contains the entire 5′ untranslated region save one additional base in exon 2. Exon 2 contains the translation initiation ATG, all codons for the signaling prepeptide, and a portion of the propeptide; exon 4 encodes the C-terminus of the propeptide and the N-terminus of the mature enzyme; and exon 8 contains the stop codon. This exonic organization is highly homologous to those for the cathepsin S and L genes. The seven introns range from 86 bp to approximately 1500 bp.[60] The exon-intron boundary sequences conformed to the GT/AG rule except for the 5′ splicing donor site of exon 3, which contained the sequence TGgc, a pattern observed in approximately 1 percent of such sites. Rood and coworkers identified four *Alu* repetitive elements within introns, one in intron 4, and three in intron 5.[69] A highly polymorphic dinucleotide repeat sequence was also noted in intron 1.[69]

The cathepsin K transcription initiation site was determined by 5′ rapid amplification of cDNA ends (RACE), ribonuclease protection, and primer extension analyses. Using osteoclast mRNA, Rood and coworkers amplified a 49-bp 5′ UTR and verified its validity using a ribonuclease protection assay.[69] Gelb and coworkers performed primer extension analyses using brain and lung RNA, and identified three initiation sites that correspond to 5′ UTR lengths of 40, 102, and 169 bp.[60] These results suggest the presence of multiple initiation sites, a common finding among genes lacking TATA sequences in their promoter regions.

Regulatory Elements. The 5′ flanking region of the human cathepsin K gene lacks the canonical TATA and CAAT box sequences. Sequence analysis of this region revealed several putative regulatory elements including two SP1 sequences (one of which was 3′ to the 5′-most putative transcription initiation site), two AP1, two AP3, four PEA3, two H-APF-1, an Ets-1, and a Pu.1 site.[69] The H-APF-1 sites are particularly noteworthy as they bind IL-6, a cytokine with an established role in stimulation of osteoclast activity.[70,71] In addition, H-APF-1 elements have been found during sequence analysis of the 5′ flanking regions of the human and mouse tartrate-resistant acid phosphatase genes, which also are highly expressed in osteoclasts.[72,73] The Pu.1 element, which lies approximately 850 bp 5′ to the transcription initiation sites, is the consensus sequence for Pu.1, a transcription factor of the Ets family with an established role in macrophage/monocyte differentiation.[74] Because osteoclasts derive from the same progenitors in the bone marrow, Pu.1 may be relevant for the tissue-specific expression of cathepsin K.

Indirect evidence from in vitro studies indicates that retinoic acid, estrogen, and the oncogene, v-Jun, regulate cathepsin K transcription in osteoclasts.[75–77] Isolated rabbit osteoclasts were exposed to all-*trans*-retinoic acid in tissue culture, resulting in activation as measured by a bone pit assay and an increase in steady state cathepsin K transcript levels, which was not blocked by cycloheximide but was blocked by actinomycin D. It was also documented that mature osteoclasts expressed message for two retinoic acid receptors, RARα and RXRβ.[75] Conversely, mature

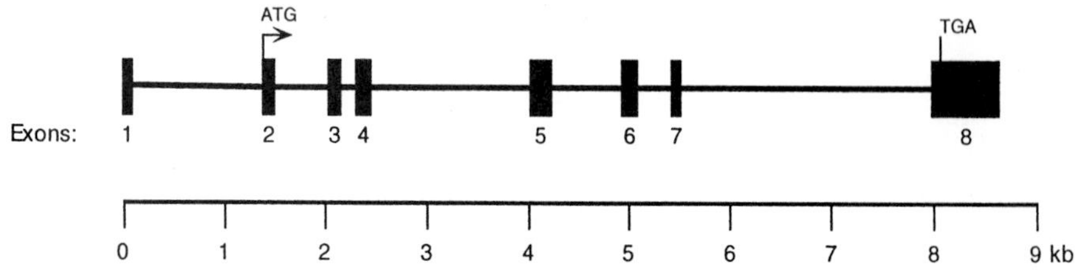

Fig. 137-7 Genomic organization of the human cathepsin K gene. The eight exons are shown as black boxes with the translation initiation ATG and TGA stop codons indicated. The thick black lines indicate the seven introns. The cumulative size of the cathepsin K genomic sequence is shown on the scale.

rabbit osteoclasts formed fewer pits after incubation with 10 nM 17β-estradiol and there was also a decrease in steady state cathepsin K message levels which could be blocked by actinomycin D, but not cycloheximide.[76] Chicken embryo fibroblasts were transformed with v-Jun and a clone representing an avian homologue of cathepsin K was isolated.[77] Northern analysis revealed that cathepsin K message levels were overexpressed by approximately tenfold in transformed cells, a relatively specific phenomenon because parallel experiments using several other oncogenes (v-Src, v-Ha-Ras, c-Fos, and Myc) failed to elicit similar up-regulation of cathepsin K.

The 3′ Flanking Region. The 3′ flanking region of the human cathepsin K gene was analyzed by Rood and coworkers.[69] Two putative polyadenylation signals were identified and, based on the presence of a CATTCA motif 20 bp downstream, the more 3′ polyadenylation signal was deemed likely to be the correct one. Examination of the four published human cathepsin K cDNA sequences failed to reveal a consensus (suggesting that some may not be full-length) but the cDNA with the longest 3′ UTR had the poly(A) addition immediately after that CATTCA sequence.[63]

MOLECULAR PATHOLOGY OF PYCNODYSOSTOSIS

The establishment of cathepsin K gene defects as the underlying cause of pycnodysostosis and the delineation of the genomic organization of the gene has permitted investigation of the molecular lesions causing this disorder. To date, all cathepsin K gene defects are point mutations in the coding sequence of either the proregion or the mature enzyme. Expression of several missense mutants has revealed that all obliterate cathepsin K's collagenase activity and most eliminate its proteolytic properties entirely.

Cathepsin K Gene Defects

Ten cathepsin K gene defects have been identified in patients with pycnodysostosis (Fig. 137-8). These mutations have been of three types: nonsense, missense, and stop codon changes.[14,78,79] Two proregion mutations have been found, both in an American Caucasian family of Northern European descent with two children affected by pycnodysostosis.[78] One proregion mutation, carried by the mother, was K52X, a severe nonsense mutation predicted to eliminate the mature enzyme. The paternal mutation in this family was G79E, which affected the sixth residue in the relatively conserved G-x-N-x-F-x-D motif (see above). Molecular modeling of G79E using nine amino acid residues, with the mutated residue occupying the central position, predicted significant alterations in the conformation and surface electrostatic potential near the C-terminal aspartate residue. Because the proregions of cysteine cathepsins have a documented role in protein folding, the perturbations on the pro piece introduced by the G79E mutation presumably caused improper folding of the cathepsin K proenzyme, resulting in the loss of protease activity. The G79E mutant allele was expressed in *Pichia pastores*, and the results of the expression studies were consistent with this prediction. Despite the production of immunologically detectable proenzyme protein, which included a mature region with the normal cathepsin K primary structure, no mature protein or enzymatic activity was detected, strongly implicating a perturbation in the secondary structure of the mature protein caused by the G79E substitution in the propeptide.

Eight mutations have been identified in the coding sequence of the mature enzyme,[14,78,79] including two nonsense defects, Q190X and R241X, which predict termination of the protein prior to the active histidine. Because the active histidine forms an ion pair with the active cysteine, which is critical for substrate proteolysis, both truncated proteins have no activity. Five cathepsin K missense mutations in the mature region have been detected: G146R, Y212C, A277E, A277V, and R312G.[14,78] The expression of these five mutant cathepsin K polypeptides in *Pichia pastores* resulted in immunologically detectable precursor proteins derived from all constructs.[78] However, the 30-kDa mature protein was not detected after treatment of the mutant precursors with pepsin (which activates wild-type cathepsin K), and fluorescent enzyme assays using Z-LR-MCA revealed no detectable protease activity for the G146R, A277E, A277V, and R312G mutant proteins. These results were compared qualitatively to the effects of the particular mutation on the three-dimensional structure of cathepsin K. Gly^{146} lies deep within the active site cleft so the substitution of the large, charged Arg residue in the G146R mutant enzyme was expected to have significant adverse effects upon this protein. The A277E and A277V mutations altered another residue in the active site, Ala^{277}. This alanine residue is immediately next to the invariably conserved His^{276} residue that forms the ion pair with the active cysteine (Cys^{139}) to effect protein catalysis. Moreover, the Ala^{277} residue is highly conserved among the papain family members, existing as either an alanine or a glycine residue in nearly all instances.[80] It was anticipated that the replacement of Ala^{277} by a charged residue in the A277E mutation would obliterate protease activity, but these expression studies revealed that even the A277V change, which appeared to introduce a less drastic alteration, resulted in a precursor protein that was unable to autoactivate and was unstable in the presence of pepsin. Thus, the obliterative effects of the A277V mutation suggest that there is little tolerance

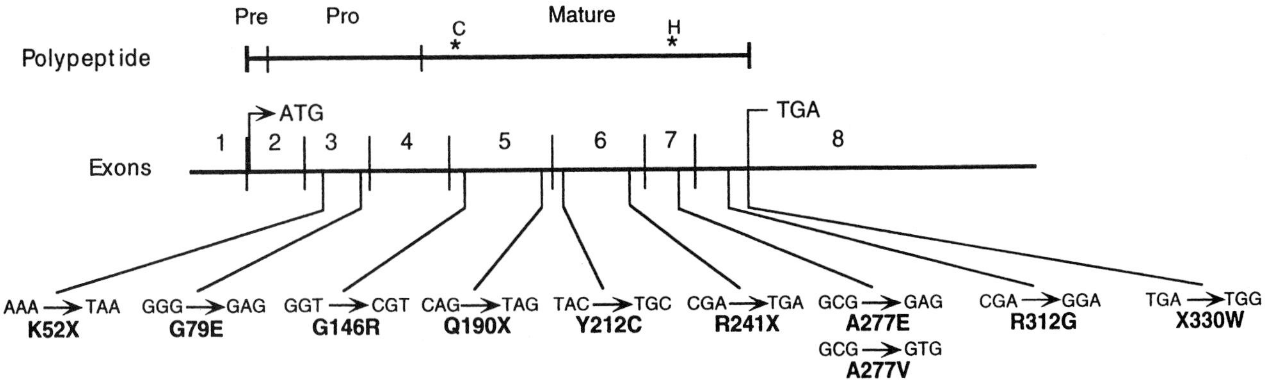

Fig. 137-8 Pycnodysostosis mutations in the cathepsin K gene. DNA changes to codons and their predicted effects on the cathepsin K protein are indicated above and positioned on the cathepsin K gene, which is divided into eight exons. The initiation and stop codons are indicated in exons 2 and 8, respectively. The effects of these mutations on the cathepsin K prepropeptide are shown below. The positions of the cysteine, histidine, and asparagine residues, which form the active triad in the active cleft, are indicated on the normal polypeptide.

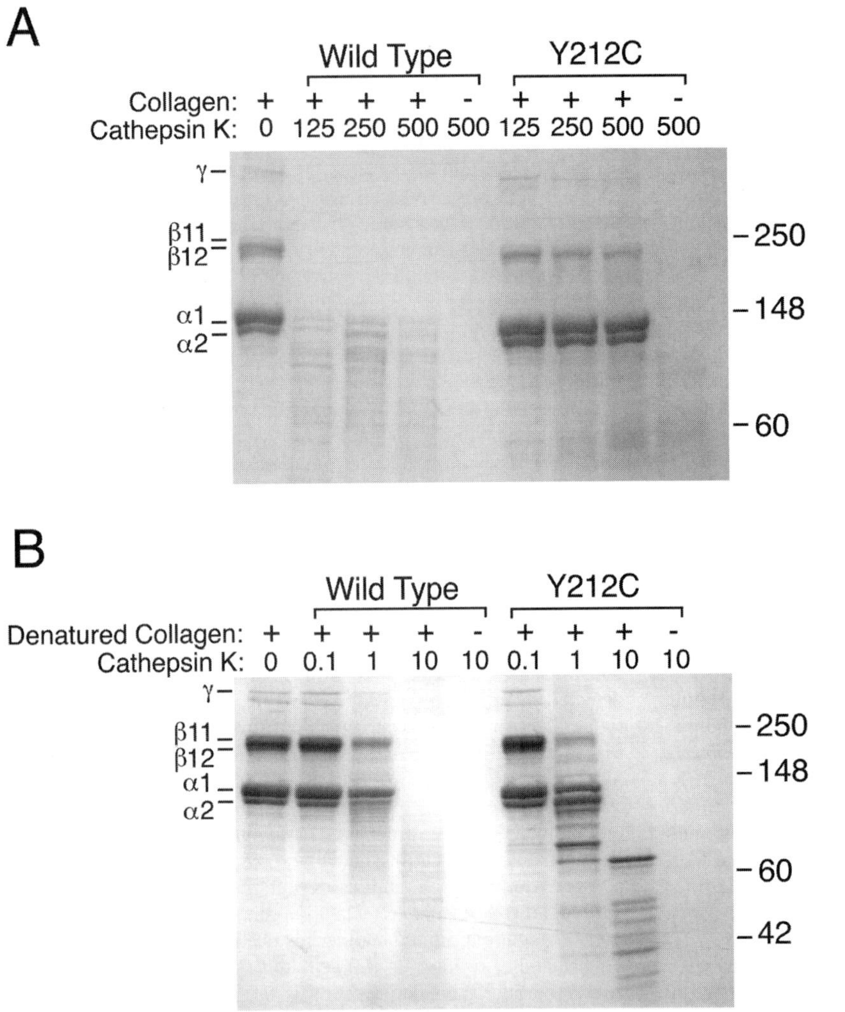

Fig. 137-9 SDS-PAGE of type I collagen (soluble calf skin collagen) after digestion with recombinant wild-type and Y212C cathepsin K enzymes. *A,* Collagenase activity. Digestion of soluble calf skin collagen at 28°C and pH 5.5 for 12 h by wild-type and Y212C cathepsin K enzymes is shown. The presence (+) or absence (−) of collagen and the concentration of the cathepsin K in nM are indicated. *B,* Gelatinase activity. Digestion of denatured soluble calf skin collagen by wild-type and Y212C cathepsin K enzymes is shown. The presence (+) or absence (−) of gelatin and the concentration of the cathepsin K in nM are indicated. Molecular mass standards (kDa) are indicated in the right margin and the collagen proteins are labeled in the left margin.

for larger amino acid side groups at this critical position in the active cleft.

The effects of the fourth missense mutation with no residual activity, R312G, are less obvious. The Arg[312] residue does not lie within the active site; instead, it resides on the surface. Based on the three-dimensional structure of human procathepsin L,[81] Arg[312] would not be expected to interact with the pro piece, so the R312G lesion presumably affects the precursor protein structure directly. The Arg[312] residue is conserved among approximately two-thirds of the papain family members, never existing as a glycine residue,[80] and the R312G mutation eliminates a positive charge, all consistent with the conclusion that this mutation significantly disrupts the surface structure of the cathepsin K proenzyme in this region.

The Y212C mutant had residual protease activity against the Z-LR-MCA substrate.[78] Biochemical characterization of the Y212C protein revealed that its catalytic efficiency (k_{cat}/K_m) was 34 percent of wild-type and that its pH activity curve was very similar to that of wild-type, but that the mutant protein was highly unstable at pH 5.5 and 6.5. Most revealingly, the Y212C enzyme had minimal activity against type I collagen but continued to exhibit substantial gelatinase activity (Fig. 137-9). The fact that the Y212C enzyme is still capable of degrading denatured proteins (gelatin) as well as a synthetic dipeptide favored by wild-type cathepsin K suggests that the structural deformation caused by the Y212C mutation prevents engagement of the type I collagen substrate. The Tyr[212] residue lies on the surface of the mature protein, not in the active site. This residue is completely conserved among the six known human cysteine cathepsins, except for cathepsin H in which it exists as a phenylalanine residue, and is never a cysteine residue among any papain family member.[80] Because the Y212C mutation introduces a thiol group that might form a novel disulfide bridge or disrupt existing ones, it suggests that the structural deformation perturbs the function of the mature enzyme towards its most critical substrate, type I collagen. Finally, the Y212C mutation has been observed in only a single pycnodysostosis patient who was heteroallelic for it and the severe nonsense mutation, R241X. Therefore, it remains to be seen if an individual harboring two Y212C alleles would also manifest the typical pycnodysostosis phenotype.

Finally, a mutation in the stop codon X330W was described in the large Israeli-Arab kindred used for the initial linkage studies by Gelb and coworkers.[14] While this mutation was predicted to result in the elongation of the C-terminus of the enzyme by 19 additional amino acids, transient expression of the X330W mutation in mammalian 293 cells resulted in no immunologically detectable protein despite good steady state transcript levels.[14] This was interpreted to mean that the X330W mutant protein is highly unstable.

Genotype/Phenotype Correlations

No rigorous genotype/phenotype correlations have been performed for pycnodysostosis and the predominance of incomplete clinical descriptions in the literature make such correlations difficult. An aspect of the phenotype for which there is sufficient data to permit a comparison is linear height. Compilation of data from several published reports reveals that most, but not all, pycnodysostosis patients have short stature, but the degree ranges widely. Moreover, substantial differences were encountered even when comparing the heights of individuals within the same family (obviating some concerns about environmental factors).[32] Comparison of hand and foot sizes reveals substantial intrafamilial variability,[32] and the facial appearance can also vary within families from near normal to the classic dysmorphic appearance with micrognathia, full lips, bulbous nose, malar hypoplasia, and broad forehead (Desnick and Gelb, personal observations). Given this phenotypic heterogeneity within families and between individuals who have cathepsin K mutations that obliterate enzyme function, the prediction of clinical severity for young children diagnosed with pycnodysostosis is difficult and may depend on as-yet-unidentified modifying genes and environmental factors.

To date, all of the reported cathepsin K mutations result in enzymes that cannot degrade type I collagen, and all but one eliminate any protease function. Thus, patients with pycnodysostosis can be considered to have no cathepsin K activity. Examination of carrier individuals has failed to document any phenotype, particularly an effect on bone density. One might speculate, then, on the existence of an allelic disorder in which patients inherit cathepsin K mutation(s) resulting in diminished, but measurable, collagenolytic capacity. Individuals with 5 to 10 percent residual cathepsin K activity in their osteoclasts might have increased bone density, perhaps manifesting only as a resistance to osteopenia and osteoporosis, but little of the dysplastic features associated with pycnodysostosis. The identification of such an entity must await the examination of candidate individuals or the creation of relevant animal models.

PATHOPHYSIOLOGY

The cathepsin K deficiency in pycnodysostosis results in derangements of bone growth and remodeling, which stem from abnormal function of osteoclasts. To understand the pathophysiology of pycnodysostosis, the normal biology of osteoclasts is reviewed briefly and the current information about the dysfunction in those cells associated with cathepsin K deficiency is discussed. Readers desiring more in-depth information about osteoclasts are referred to the several recent reviews (see references 82–84).

Osteoclasts are multinucleated giant cells with 10 to 20 nuclei per cell.[85] They derive from hematopoietic cells,[86–90] specifically from granulocyte-macrophage colony-forming units,[91] and are a member of the monocyte/macrophage family, sharing substantial similarity with macrophages, which are also polykaryons. Several features, however, distinguish osteoclasts from macrophages, including the presence of calcitonin receptors,[92,93] abundant levels of tartrate-resistant acid phosphatase,[94] cellular polarization with a ruffled border,[85] and the capacity to resorb mineralized bone and degrade bone matrix.[82,83] Osteoclasts are rare bone cells, generally located on endosteal surfaces within the Haversian system and on the periosteal surfaces beneath the periosteum, attached to bone at sites of bone turnover.[83] Ultrastructurally, they are rich in mitochondria, lysosomes, and perinuclear Golgi complexes.[95] The ruffled border is comprised of projections of the plasma membrane from the cell surface facing the bone. It is surrounded by the sealing zone, which is closely apposed to the bone and above which is the clear zone, an organelle-free region rich in actin-like filaments. The bone lying beneath the ruffled border is subjected to degradation, forming resorption lacunae.[83]

The surface of bone is invested with a thin layer of nonmineralizing collagen,[96] which is removed by the matrix metalloproteinase, and collagenase, which is synthesized and secreted either by osteoblasts[97–100] or by osteoclasts.[101–103] After this collagenolysis, osteoclasts are able to attach to the cleaned bone surface via their integrin receptors $\alpha_V\beta_3$ (vitronectin receptor), $\alpha_2\beta_1$, and $\alpha_V\beta_1$.[104,105] The vitronectin receptor binds the RGD (Arg-Gly-Asp) recognition motif of the extracellular matrix, especially osteopontin. Following attachment, the osteoclasts seal off the subosteoclastic space and become activated, leading to an increase in intracellular calcium and increased acidification of intracellular vacuoles.[106,107]

The first step in bone remodeling by activated, attached osteoclasts is the removal of the inorganic mineral from the bone underlying the subosteoclastic space.[108] This demineralization is accomplished by acidification of the subosteoclastic space to about pH 4.5,[109] requiring a massive efflux of protons driven by a vacuolar H^+-ATPase pump.[110,111] The vacuolar H^+-ATPase pump is abundantly expressed in activated osteoclasts and localizes to the ruffled border. To maintain intracellular pH despite this loss of H^+ ions, osteoclasts utilize the carbonic anhydrase II transporter at their apical surface to exchange intracellular HCO_3^- for extracellular Cl^- ions.[112,113]

The second step in bone remodeling by osteoclasts is the proteolytic removal of organic matrix, which has been exposed by the demineralization process. Type I collagen constitutes 90 percent of this matrix,[114] which has been shown to be degraded at low pH by the fluid from the subosteoclastic space.[115] Because matrix metalloproteinases are inactivated at low pH, the primary candidates for this collagenolytic activity were cysteine cathepsins. Nonspecific cysteine cathepsin inhibitors were shown to inhibit organic matrix degradation by osteoclasts,[18–21] and early studies showed the presence of cathepsins B and L in the resorption lacunae.[116–118]

With the recent discovery that cathepsin K is highly expressed in osteoclasts, efforts are now directed toward understanding its role in organic matrix degradation. Cathepsin K message has been localized by *in situ* hybridization to osteoclasts that are actively degrading bone, while no message was detected in other cell types such as osteoblasts, osteocytes, and most hematopoietic marrow cells.[68] Studies with cathepsin K antisense oligonucleotides revealed significant inhibition of the synthesis of cathepsin K protein, and bone resorption was reduced 30 to 50 percent as measured by pit number and depth in a standard in vitro bone pit assay.[119] Interestingly, use of the nonspecific cysteine cathepsin inhibitor, E-64, resulted in a similar degree of inhibition in that assay, further evidence that cathepsin K is the central cysteine protease in bone matrix degradation.

Immunohistochemical localization of cathepsin K using specific anticathepsin K antibodies revealed the expected presence of immunoreactive material in osteoclasts, primarily within cytoplasmic vacuoles and at the ruffled border in one study,[68] but clustered at the apical surface in another study.[67] A small number of mononuclear cells, perhaps representing osteoclast precursors, were also shown to have immunoreactivity, whereas osteoblasts, osteocytes, and bone marrow cells were negative.[67] Further studies are needed to clarify whether, as anticipated, cathepsin K is present in the subosteoclastic space as well as in lysosomes within the osteoclast. It is worth noting that the mannose-6-phosphate pathway, which is used for targeting vesicles from the Golgi complex to lysosomes in most cell types, has been implicated for transporting vesicles to the plasma membrane in osteoclasts, suggesting that substantial secretion of cathepsin K into the subosteoclast space does occur.[120]

The clinical and histologic findings in pycnodysostosis document in an unequivocal fashion that cathepsin K is critical for bone growth and remodeling. When deficient, osteoclastic activity becomes inadequate, although not absent. Histologic and ultrastructural studies confirm that osteoclastogenesis is normal in the absence of cathepsin K activity. Moreover, osteoclasts are able to attach to the bone surface, become activated, and demineralize bone. The cathepsin K deficiency then impedes proper removal of organic matrix. Recent confocal microscopic studies have revealed that the normal pathway for removing matrix proteins liberated from the subosteoclastic space is through endocytosis at the ruffled membrane and subsequent transcytosis of the vacuoles to the basolateral membrane where the material is secreted into the extracellular space.[121,122] Thus, the observation of collagen fibrils within vacuoles in pycnodysostosis osteoclasts[54] suggests that the degradation of collagen is inadequate but that the endocytotic pathway attempts to take up the large fragments released from the matrix and dispose of them through the transcytotic mechanism. It is unclear which enzymes are initiating the release of the collagen fibrils from the matrix. Because the presence of cathepsin K in the subosteoclastic space seems highly probable and because cathepsin K appears to clip the collagen in or near the telopeptide domain, one imagines that this protease has a central role in initiating collagen release and proteolysis. In the absence of that activity, other proteases, such as cathepsin L, which has activity towards this substrate,[123] may be recruited for this function. In addition, prior studies have shown that additional proteolysis of collagenous remnants normally occurs after the retraction of osteoclasts from the resorption lacunae, most likely by matrix metalloproteinases.[21,124] Thus, incomplete matrix degradation by the osteoclasts may be compensated to some degree by this custodial function.

The processes of bone accretion and degradation are linked in a complex and not completely understood fashion. Substantial information is available about the control of osteoclastogenesis and osteoclast activation by osteoblasts.[83,125] Osteoblasts produce several factors that have been implicated in this crosstalk including stimulatory factors such as interleukin (IL)-1, IL-6,[126] IL-11,[127,128] and macrophage colony-stimulating factor (M-CSF),[129] and inhibitory ones such as transforming growth factor-β and nitric oxide.[130,131] Considerably less is known about mechanisms by which osteoclasts might influence osteoblastogenesis and the rate of bone synthesis. A striking histologic feature of bone in pycnodysostosis is the paucity of osteoblasts that are actively synthesizing new bone. While sensible from a teleological point of view, the actual mechanism(s) by which the inadequate bone matrix degradation by osteoclasts results in this decreased synthesis remain obscure.

DIAGNOSIS

Clinical Evaluation

The diagnosis of pycnodysostosis is made from the clinical and radiologic features. The cardinal clinical signs include short stature, typical dysmorphic facial appearance, and bony abnormalities such as delayed suture closure, short splayed distal phalanges, and pathologic fractures. The observation of such features prompts radiologic skeletal surveys that reveal the generalized increase in bone density with narrowed but preserved medullary cavities in the long bones and dysplastic features of the craniofacial, clavicular, and long bones. The loss of the angle of the mandible, a constant feature, is particularly noteworthy. Differential diagnosis includes osteopetrosis (Albers-Schönberg disease), osteogenesis imperfecta, sclerosteosis, endosteal hyperostosis (Worth type), progressive diaphyseal dysplasia (Camurati-Engelmann syndrome), cleidocranial dysplasia, and mandibuloacral dysplasia.[4,34] Osteopetrosis shares the osteosclerotic features with pycnodysostosis as well as some associated features such as pathologic fractures and osteomyelitis of the jaw.[4,34,36] In osteopetrosis, however, the degree of the osteosclerosis is greater, such that the bone marrow cavity is usually obliterated, resulting in pancytopenia and signs of extramedullary hematopoiesis, and the cranial foramina are narrowed, causing nerve compression which results in blindness and deafness. Moreover, the dysplastic skeletal features of pycnodysostosis are not present in osteopetrosis. Osteogenesis imperfecta is noted in the differential diagnosis of pycnodysostosis because of the shared feature of pathologic fractures. The two entities differ significantly, however, as osteogenesis imperfecta is associated with far greater risk for such fractures, with osteopenia, and, for most forms, with normal stature.[4,34,36] Sclerosteosis, an autosomal recessive disorder similar to van Buchem syndrome, is characterized by increased bone density and hyperostosis, but there are usually anomalies of the digits.[132] Endosteal hyperostosis (Worth type) is an autosomal dominant condition characterized by reduction in marrow space, and a widened and deep mandible with an increased gonial angle.[133] Affected individuals tend to have cranial nerve involvement and elevated serum alkaline phosphatase levels. Progressive diaphyseal dysplasia is another osteosclerotic bone disorder, principally involving the diaphyses of the tubular bones.[36] Affected patients, however, have a tall, asthenic habitus and may suffer from a variety of other symptoms such as muscular weakness, a waddling gait, and leg pains which are not encountered among pycnodysostosis patients. In addition, the inheritance of progressive diaphyseal dysplasia is autosomal dominant. Cleidocranial dysplasia, another autosomal dominant skeletal disorder, shares several features with pycnodysostosis such as short stature, persistent cranial sutures and fontanels, as well as clavicular hypoplasia.[36] Patients with cleidocranial dysplasia, however, do not have osteosclerosis and their dysmorphic features are rather different. Mandibuloacral dysplasia also has several features in common with pycnodysostosis: mandibular hypoplasia, persistent cranial sutures, Wormian bones, hypoplastic clavicles, hypoplasia of the distal phalanges (or acro-osteolysis), and autosomal recessive inheritance.[36,134] The features of mandibuloacral dysplasia, however, do not include short stature or osteosclerosis, and patients may manifest joint stiffness, atrophic skin over the hands and feet, and alopecia which are not observed in pycnodysostosis. In sum, pycnodysostosis is a distinct disease entity that can generally be differentiated by physical examination and radiologic studies from other disorders with overlapping skeletal features.

Individuals who are heterozygous for a cathepsin K mutation cannot be discerned clinically. To date, no differences in the heights, bone densities, or the appearance of the heterozygous carriers have been detected. The only means of identifying such individuals is by inference in a pedigree, or by molecular studies, such as mutation and haplotype analyses.

Prenatal Diagnosis

There are no reports of the prenatal diagnosis of pycnodysostosis. Biochemical studies of cathepsin K activity are not diagnostically useful because that activity is tissue-specific. Thus, assaying the chorionic villi or amniotic fluid cells is not useful. Ultrasonographic monitoring might detect some of the cardinal defects of pycnodysostosis, such as the loss of the angle of the mandible and clavicular hypoplasia,[135–137] while other aspects of the phenotype, such as cranial suture and fontanel changes, are probably normal during the fetal period. The degree of bone thickening *in utero* has not been established, but is likely quite mild. Because newborn and young infants with pycnodysostosis are often nearly normal in length, fetal length determinations also suffer from a lack of sensitivity and are not specific. Finally, there are fundamental issues concerning the desirability of making a prenatal determination for this disorder, which are discussed below in "Genetic and Family Counseling."

TREATMENT

Medical Management

The primary issues in the care of patients with pycnodysostosis are the management of the orthopedic, dental, and medical complications. Treatment is directed at preventing or ameliorating complications because no therapy has been devised to restore cathepsin K activity in osteoclasts. Nearly all patients suffer several bone fractures, but most heal with standard orthopedic management.[32] Complaints of symptoms referable to the neck or lower back should be investigated radiologically because spondylolysis of the cervical and lumbar spine has been documented in several patients. Because of the tendency for pathologic fractures, physical activities should be curtailed and contact sports avoided.

Patients with pycnodysostosis require attentive, prophylactic dental care. The tendency for dental caries and osteomyelitis of the jaw after extractions should be noted in planning dental care.

Extractions, which may be necessary due to the small oral cavity, may result in mandibular fracture. Routine use of antibiotics after extractions should be considered. There are no reports of orthodontic intervention for the correction of the dental malposition. Given the density of the underlying bone and the primary defect in bone remodeling, such efforts might prove challenging.

Upper airway obstruction has resulted in complications, even severe right heart failure, in a number of patients. Given this tendency, efforts should be made to elicit symptoms and signs of obstructive sleep apnea during history taking and physical examination. It is important to recall that obstruction can occur despite minimal hyperplasia of the adenoids and tonsils. Surgical intervention to shorten the soft palate has been successful in at least one instance.[47] Young patients undergoing any surgical procedure with general anesthesia require careful airway management.

Short stature associated with pycnodysostosis is one of the least acceptable features for patients and families. Recent studies documenting the presence of growth hormone deficiency in several patients and showing an apparent response in such individuals to repletion therapy suggest that intervention might be beneficial. It must be emphasized, however, that the number of treated subjects was small and that a lack of long-term follow-up precludes concluding that ultimate adult height was improved. Growth hormone therapy has been well tolerated without documented side effects, but the cost is high, and to be effective, daily injections must be continued for a long period of time. Until additional data are reported for growth hormone therapy in this disease, no firm conclusions about advisability can be reached. Attempts at increasing final height through invasive orthopedic procedures, such as the distraction technique of Ilizarov, which have proven effective for some skeletal dysplasias,[138,139] have not been reported for pycnodysostosis, and might prove hazardous given the imperfect bone healing which has been noted in the disorder.

The hematologic complications of pycnodysostosis due to impingement on the marrow space are rare, and the factors that place an individual patient at risk have not been elucidated. Routine monitoring of complete blood counts will detect patients developing myelophthisis, and the observation of hepatosplenomegaly should prompt further evaluation for this complication. Information about prognosis and therapeutic efficacy is scant, but the myelophthisis resolved spontaneously in one patient and responded to oral prednisone therapy in another.

The psychological impact of pycnodysostosis on affected individuals and families should be considered. The combination of short stature and dysmorphic appearance, which both become more evident through childhood and adolescence, may impact adversely on some individuals.[140,141] The limited morbidity associated with this disorder and the potential for full and productive lives may lessen the psychosocial impact relative to some other inherited disorders.

Genetic and Family Counseling

Pycnodysostosis is inherited as an autosomal recessive trait and appears to be fully penetrant. On average, one-quarter of the offspring born to two cathepsin K-mutation carriers have the disease. The prevalence of carriers in the population has not been established, but appears to be less than 1 in 500. Like all rare autosomal recessive disorders, disease prevalence is higher among couples who are consanguineous, which is relevant in more than 30 percent of cases of pycnodysostosis.[4]

At present, the only available therapy is preventive. Molecular evaluation of families in which at least one affected offspring has been identified may permit surveillance of future pregnancies by ultrasonographic and/or molecular studies. No data are currently available on the sensitivity of anatomic evaluation of fetuses by ultrasound, nor have any prenatal diagnoses been reported. Molecular studies suggest that this disorder is genetically homogeneous and disease-causing cathepsin K mutations have been found in all affected families studied (Gelb, unpublished data). Tightly linked polymorphic DNA markers also are available for evaluations in which one or both cathepsin K mutations have not been identified. Despite the potential for prenatal diagnostics, many couples may prefer to proceed with pregnancies of affected fetuses as the acceptability of this disorder with normal psychomotor development, potentially normal life span, and only moderate dysmorphism appears to be high. For at-risk couples lacking prior molecular workup, specific questioning about consanguinity should be considered as counseling for the genetic risk of other autosomal recessive traits will depend upon the response. Unless consanguinity is practiced in the community, counseling for heterozygotes, such as sibs identified during molecular studies, should stress the relatively low risk for having affected offspring (less than 1 in 2000).

Potential Therapy for the Cathepsin K Deficiency

Restoration of some cathepsin K activity in osteoclasts would be beneficial for pycnodysostosis, restoring growth potential for young children and normalizing bone remodeling in postpubertal adolescents and adults, which would diminish the risk for pathologic bone fractures. While no therapy is currently available, two potential therapies can be envisioned. First, allogeneic bone marrow transplantation would provide normal osteoclast progenitors. Successful engraftment, even if partial, and even if donated by a carrier, would restore some cathepsin K activity to nearly all osteoclasts because they are polykaryons arising from fusion of several immature cells. While bone marrow transplantation for HLA-matched related donors has been used successfully in disorders such as sickle cell disease,[142–144] the morbidity and mortality of this therapy may preclude its usefulness for pycnodysostosis in which patients typically have a normal life span and mild disability. Such a measure, however, could be considered for the rare patient with a significant complication, for example, myelophthisis, which would potentially be reversible if cathepsin K activity in osteoclasts could be partially restored.

Gene therapy for cathepsin K deficiency must await the same development in technology required for several other disorders, that is, an ability to isolate and transfect totipotent hematopoietic stem cells, achieve sustained gene expression, and at least partially repopulate the bone marrow. Efforts directed at achieving this specifically for pycnodysostosis are unlikely because the disorder is so rare, but adaptation of techniques from other bone marrow-targeting studies may render this feasible in the future.

ACKNOWLEDGMENTS

The authors express their thanks to the physicians who provided information about their pycnodysostosis patients for this review, as well as to the following for their expert assistance: Robert J. Gorlin, D.D.S, Michael Klein, M.D., and David L. Rimoin, M.D., Ph.D. This work was supported in part by a grant from the March of Dimes Birth Defects Foundation, grants (R29 AR44231 to BDG and 5 R37 DK34045 to RJD) from the National Institutes of Health, a grant from the National Center for Research Resources for the Mount Sinai General Clinical Research Center (5 M01 RR00071), and a grant for the Mount Sinai Child Health Research Center (5 P30 HD 28822).

REFERENCES

1. Collado-Otero F: Una forma mas de distrofia osea. *Acta Pediatr Esp* **14**:1, 1956.
2. Maroteaux P, Lamy M: La pycnodysostose. *Presse Med* **70**:999, 1962.
3. Andren L, Dymling JF, Hogeman KE, Wendeberg B: Osteopetrosis acro-osteolytica: A syndrome of osteopetrosis, acro-osteolysis and open sutures of the skull. *Acta Chir Scand* **124**:496, 1962.
4. Sedano HP, Gorlin RJ, Anderson VE: Pycnodysostosis: Clinical and genetic considerations. *Am J Dis Child* **116**:70, 1968.
5. Montanari U: Acondroplasia e disostosi cleidocrania digitale. *Chir Organi Mov* **7**:379, 1923.

6. van Merkesteyn JPR, Bras J, Vermeeren JIJF, van der Sar A, Statius van Eps LW: Osteomyelitis of the jaws in pycnodysostosis. *J Oral Maxillofac Surg* **16**:615, 1987.
7. Balthazar E, Smith EH, Moskowitz H: Pycnodysostosis: An unusual case. *Brit J Radiol* **45**:304, 1972.
8. Santhanakrishnan BR, Panneerselvam S, Ramesh S, Panchatcharam M: Pycnodysostosis with visceral manifestation and rickets. *Clin Pediatr* **25**:416, 1986.
9. Le Bouedec S, Pellier I, Rialland X, Granry JC: Forme familiale de pycnodysostose avec manifestations hématolgiques chez un enfant. *Arch Pédiatr* **2**:456, 1995.
10. Kozlowski K, Yu JS: Pycnodysostosis: A variant form with visceral manifestations. *Arch Dis Child* **47**:804, 1972.
11. Kumar R, Misra PK, Singhal R: An unusual case of pycnodysostosis. *Arch Dis Child* **63**:558, 1988.
12. Soliman AT, Rajab A, Al Salmi I, Darwish A, Asfour M: Defective growth hormone secretion in children with pycnodysostosis and improved linear growth after growth hormone treatment. *Arch Dis Child* **75**:242, 1996.
13. Darcan S, Akisü M, Taneli B, Kendir G: A case of pycnodysostosis with growth hormone deficiency. *Clin Genet* **50**:422, 1996.
14. Gelb BD, Shi GP, Chapman HA, Desnick RJ: Pycnodysostosis, a lysosomal disease caused by cathepsin K deficiency. *Science* **273**:1236, 1996.
15. Gelb BD, Edelson JG, Desnick RJ: Linkage of pycnodysostosis to chromosome 1q21 by homozygosity mapping. *Nat Genet* **10**:235, 1995.
16. Polymeropoulos MH, Ortiz de Luna RI, Ide SE, Torres R, Rubenstein J, Francomano CA: The gene for pycnodysostosis maps to human chromosome 1cen-q21. *Nat Genet* **10**:238, 1995.
17. Gelb BD, Spencer E, Obad S, Edelson JG, Fauré S, Weissenbach J, Desnick RJ: Pycnodysostosis: Refined linkage and radiation hybrid analyses reduce the critical region to 2 cM at 1q21 and map two candidate genes. *Hum Genet* **98**:141, 1996.
18. Everts V, Delaissé J-M, Korper W, Niehof A, Vaes G, Beerstsen W: Degradation of collagen in the bone-resorbing compartment underlying the osteoclast involves both cysteine-proteinases and matrix metalloproteinases. *J Cell Physiol* **150**:221, 1992.
19. Delaissé J-M, Eeckhout Y, Vaes G: Inhibition of bone resorption in culture by inhibitors of thiol proteinases. *Biochem J* **192**:365, 1980.
20. Delaissé J-M, Eeckhout Y, Vaes G: In vivo and in vitro evidence for the involvement of cysteine proteinases in bone resorption. *Biochem Biophys Res Commun* **125**:441, 1984.
21. Everts V, Delaissé J-M, Korper W, Beertsen W: Involvement of matrix metalloproteinases and cysteine proteinases in degradation of bone matrix, in Davidovitch Z (ed.): *The Biological Mechanisms of Tooth Rruptions, Resorption and Replacement by Implants*. Boston, Harvard Society for the Advancement of Orthodontics, 1994, p 85.
22. Brömme D, Okamoto K: Human cathepsin O2, a novel cysteine protease highly expressed in osteoclastomas and ovary: Molecular cloning, sequencing and tissue distribution. *Biol Chem Hoppe-Seyler* **376**:379, 1995.
23. Shi G-P, Chapman HA, Bhairi SM, DeLeeuw C, Reddy VY, Weiss SJ: Molecular cloning of human cathepsin O, a novel endoproteinase and homologue of rabbit OC2. *FEBS Lett* **357**:129, 1995.
24. Maroteaux P, Lamy M: The malady of Toulouse-Lautrec. *JAMA* **191**:715, 1965.
25. Seedorff KS: *Osteogenesis Imperfecta: Study of Clinical Features and Heredity Based on 55 Danish Families Comprising 180 Affected Persons*. Copenhagen, Ejnar Munksgaards Forlag, 1949.
26. Sejournet G: La maladie de Toulouse-Lautrec. *Presse Med* **63**:1866, 1955.
27. Krabbe KH: La maladie de Henri de Toulouse-Lautrec. *Acta Psychiat Neurol Scand* **108**:211, 1956.
28. Lévy G: Reflexions sur la maladie de Toulouse-Lautrec. *Sem Hop Paris* **33**:2691, 1957.
29. Frey JB: What dwarfed Toulouse-Lautrec? *Nat Genet* **10**:128, 1995.
30. Frey J: *Toulouse-Lautrec: A life*. New York, Viking Press, 1994.
31. Frey J: Toulouse-Lautrec's diagnosis (letter). *Nat Genet* **11**:363, 1995.
32. Edelson JG, Obad S, Geiger R, On A, Artul HJ: Pycnodysostosis: Orthopedic aspects with a description of 14 new cases. *Clin Orthop* **280**:263, 1992.
33. Maroteaux P: Toulouse-Lautrec's diagnosis (letter). *Nat Genet* **11**:362, 1995.
34. Elmore SM: Pynodysostosis: A review. *J Bone Joint Surg* **49A**:153, 1967.
35. Karkabi S, Reis ND, Linn S, Edelson G, Tzehoval E, Zakut V, Dolev E, et al: Pycnodysostosis: Imaging and laboratory observations. *Calcif Tissue Int* **53**:170, 1993.
36. Taybi H, Lachman RS: *Radiology of syndromes, metabolic disorders, and skeletal dysplasias*, 4th ed. New York, Mosby, 1996.
37. Theander G: Partial disappearance of the hyoid bone in pycnodysostosis. *Acta Radiol* **19**:237, 1978.
38. Beneton MNC, Harris S, Kanis JA: Paramyxovirus-like inclusions in two cases of pycnodysostosis. *Bone* **8**:211, 1987.
39. Cabrejas ML, Fromm GA, Roca JF, Mendez MA, Bur GE, Ferreyra ME, Demarchi C, et al: Pycnodysostosis: some aspects concerning kinetics of calcium metabolism and bone pathology. *Am J Med Sci* **271**:215, 1976.
40. Muto T, Michiya H, Taira H, Murase H, Kanazawa M: Pycnodysostosis: Report of a case and review of the Japanese literature, with emphasis on oral and maxillofacial findings. *Oral Surg Oral Med Oral Pathol* **72**:449, 1991.
41. Roth VG: Pycnodysostosis presenting with bilateral subtrochanteric fractures. *Clin Orthop* **117**:247, 1976.
42. Currarino G: Primary spondylolysis of the axis vertebra (C2) in three children, including one with pycnodysostosis. *Pediatr Radiol* **19**:535, 1989.
43. Soto RJ, Mautalen CA, Hojman D, Codevilla A, Pique J, Pangaro JA: Pycnodysostosis: Metabolic and histologic studies. *Birth Defects Orig Art Ser* **5**:109, 1969.
44. Iwu CO: Bilateral osteomyelitis of the mandible in pycnodysostosis. A case report. *Int J Oral Maxillofac Surg* **20**:71, 1991.
45. Zachariades N, Koundouris I: Maxillofacial symptoms in two patients with pycnodysostosis. *J Oral Maxillofac Surg* **42**:819, 1984.
46. Nielsen EL: Pycnodysostosis: Six cases with new symptoms and an autopsy. *Acta Paediatr Scand* **63**:437, 1974.
47. Aronson DC, Heymans HS, Bijlmer RP: Cor pulmonale and acute liver necrosis, due to upper airway obstruction as part of pycnodysostosis. *Eur J Pediatr* **141**:251, 1984.
48. Yousefzadeh DK, Agha AS, Reinertson J: Radiographic studies of upper airway obstruction with cor pulmonale in a patient with pycnodysostosis. *Pediatr Radiol* **8**:45, 1979.
49. Fitzgerald T: Pycnodysostosis with right heart failure due to hypoplastic mandible and chronic upper airway obstruction. *Brit J Radiol* **61**:322, 1988.
50. Meredith SC, Simon MA, Laros GS, Jackson MA: Pycnodysostosis: a clinical, pathological, and ultramicroscopic study of a case. *J Bone Joint Surg* **60A**:1122, 1978.
51. Sarnsethsiri P, Hitt OK, Eyring EJ, Frost HM: Tetracycline-based study of bone dynamics in pycnodysostosis. *Clin Orthop* **74**:301, 1971.
52. Stanescu R, Stanescu V, Maroteaux P: Anomalies ultrastructurales des chondrocytes de la pycnodysostose. *Nouv Presse Med* **4**:2647, 1975.
53. Stanescu V, Stanescu R, Maroteaux P: Pathogenic mechanisms in osteochondrodysplasias. *J Bone Joint Surg Am* **66**:817, 1984.
54. Everts V, Aronson DC, Beertsen W: Phagocytosis of bone collagen by osteoclasts in two cases of pycnodysostosis. *Calcif Tissue Int* **37**:25, 1985.
55. Brömme D, Okamoto K, Wang BB, Biroc S: Human cathepsin O2, a matrix protein-degrading cysteine protease expressed in osteoclasts. *J Biol Chem* **271**:2126, 1996.
56. Bossard MJ, Tomazek TA, Thompson SK, Amegadzie BY, Hanning CR, Jones C, Kurdyla JT, et al.: Proteolytic activity of human osteoclast cathepsin K. *J Biol Chem* **271**:12517, 1996.
57. McQueney MS, Amegadzie BY, D'Alessio K, Hanning CR, McLaughlin MM, McNulty D, Carr SA, et al.: Autocatalytic activation of human cathepsin K. *J Biol Chem* **272**:13955, 1997.
58. Zhao B, Janson CA, Amegadzie BY, D'Alessio K, Griffin C, Hanning CR, Jones C, et al.: Crystal structure of human osteoclast cathepsin K complex with E-64 [letter]. *Nat Struct Biol* **4**:109, 1997.
59. McGrath ME, Klaus JL, Barnes MG, Brömme D: Crystal structure of human cathepsin K complexed with a potent inhibitor [letter]. *Nat Struct Biol* **4**:105, 1997.
60. Gelb BD, Shi G-PP, Heller M, Weremowicz S, Morton C, Desnick RJ, Chapman HA: Structure and chromosomal assignment of the human cathepsin K gene. *Genomics* **41**:258, 1997.
61. Tezuka K, Tezuka Y, Maejima A, Sato T, Nemoto K, Kamioka H, Hakeda Y, et al.: Molecular cloning of a possible cysteine proteinase predominantly expressed in osteoclasts. *J Biol Chem* **269**:1106, 1994.
62. Inaoka T, Bilbe G, Osamu I, Tezuka K-I, Kumegawa M, Kokubo T: Molecular cloning of human cDNA for cathepsin K: Novel cysteine proteinase predominantly expressed in bone. *Biochem Biophys Res Commun* **206**:89, 1995.

63. Li Y-P, Alexander M, Wucherpfennig AL, Yelick P, Chen W, Stashenko P: Cloning and complete coding sequence of a novel human cathepsin expressed in giant cells of osteoclastomas. *J Bone Miner Res* **10**:1197, 1995.
64. Gelb BD, Moissoglu K, Zhang J, Brömme D, Desnick RJ: Cathepsin K: Isolation and characterization of the murine cDNA and genomic sequence, the homolog of the pycnodysostosis gene. *Biochem Mol Med* **59**:200, 1996.
65. Rantakokko J, Aro HT, Savontaus M, Vuorio E: Mouse cathepsin K: cDNA cloning and predominant expression of the gene in osteoclasts, and in some hypertrophying chondrocytes during mouse development. *FEBS Lett* **393**:307, 1996.
66. Vernet T, Berti PJ, de Montigny C, Musil R, Tessier DC, Menard R, Magny M-C, et al.: Processing of the papain precursor. *J Biol Chem* **270**:10838, 1995.
67. Drake FH, Dodds RA, James IE, Connor JR, Debouck C, Richardson S, Lee-Rykaczewski E, et al.: Cathepsin K, but not cathepsins B, L, or S, is abundantly expressed in human osteoclasts. *J Biol Chem* **271**:12511, 1996.
68. Littlewood-Evans A, Kokubo T, Ishibashi O, Inaoka T, Wlodarski B, Gallagher JA, Bilbe G: Localization of cathepsin K in human osteoclasts by in situ hybridization and immunohistochemistry. *Bone* **20**:81, 1997.
69. Rood JA, Van-Horn S, Drake FH, Gowen M, Debouck C: Genomic organization and chromosome localization of the human cathepsin K gene (CTSK). *Genomics* **41**:169, 1997.
70. Udagawa N, Takahashi N, Katagiri T, Tamura T, Wasa S, Findlay DM, Marine TJ, et al.: Interleukin (IL)-6 induction of osteoclast differentiation depends on IL-6 receptors expressed on osteoblastic cells but not on osteoclast progenitors. *J Exp Med* **182**:1461, 1995.
71. de la Mata J, Uy HL, Guise TA, Story B, Boyece BF, Mundy GR, Roodman GD: Interleukin-6 enhances hypercalcemia and bone resorption mediated by parathyroid hormone-related protein in vivo. *J Clin Invest* **95**:2846, 1995.
72. Reddy SV, Scarcez T, Windle JJ, Leach RJ, Hundley JE, Chirgwin JM, Chou JY, et al.: Cloning and characterization of the 5′-flanking region of the mouse tartrate-resistant acid phosphatase gene. *J Bone Miner Res* **8**:1263, 1993.
73. Reddy SV, Hundley JE, Alantara O, Linn R, Leach RJ, Boldt DH, Roodman GH: Characterization of the mouse tartrate-resistant acid phosphatase (TRAP) gene promoter. *J Bone Miner Res* **10**:601, 1995.
74. Zhang D, Hetherington C, Chen H, Tenen DG: The macrophage transcripton factor Pu.1 directs tissue-specific expression of the macrophage colony-stimulating factor receptor. *Mol Cell Biol* **14**:373, 1994.
75. Saneshige S, Mano H, Tezuka K-I, Kakudo S, Mori Y, Honda Y, Itabashi A, et al.: Retinoic acid directly stimulates osteoclastic bone resorption and gene expression of cathepsin K/OC-2. *Biochem J* **309**:721, 1995.
76. Mano H, Yuasa T, Kameda T, Miyazawa K, Nakamaru Y, Shiokawa M, Mori Y, et al.: Mammalian mature osteoclasts as estrogen target cells. *Biochem Biophys Res Commun* **223**:637, 1996.
77. Hadman M, Gabos L, Loo M, Sehgal A, Bos TJ: Isolation and cloning of JTAP-1: a cathepsin like gene upregulated in response to V-Jun induced cell transformation. *Oncogene* **12**:135, 1996.
78. Hou W-S, Brömme D, Zhao Y, Mehler E, Dushey C, Weinstein H, Sa Miranda C, et al.: Cathepsin K: Characterization of novel mutations in the pro and mature polypeptide regions causing pycnodysostosis. *J Clin Invest* **103**:731, 1999.
79. Johnson MR, Polymeropoulos MH, Vos HL, Ortiz-de-Luna RI, Francomano CA: A nonsense mutation in the cathepsin K gene observed in a family with pycnodysostosis. *Genome Res* **6**:1050, 1996.
80. Berti PJ, Storer AC: Alignment/phylogeny of the papain superfamily of cysteine proteases. *J Mol Biol* **246**:273, 1995.
81. Colombe R, Grochulski P, Sivaramen J, Menard R, Mort JS, Cygler M: Structure of human procathepsin L reveals the molecular basis of inhibition by the prosegment. *EMBO J* **15**:5492, 1996.
82. Teitelbaum SL, Tondravi MM, Ross FP: Osteoclasts, macrophages, and the molecular mechanisms of bone resorption. *J Leukoc Biol* **61**:381, 1997.
83. Roodman GD: Advances in bone biology: The osteoclast. *Endocr Rev* **17**:308, 1996.
84. Hall TJ, Chambers TJ: Molecular aspects of osteoclast function. *Inflamm Res* **45**:1, 1996.
85. Lucht U: Osteoclasts — ultrastructure and function, in the reticuloendothelial system. A comprehensive treatise, in Carr I, Daems WT (eds.): *Morphology*. New York, Plenum, 1980, p 705.
86. Walker DG: Congenital osteoporosis in mice cured by parabiotic union with normal siblings. *Endocrinology* **91**:916, 1972.
87. Walker DG: Osteopetrosis cured by temporary parabiosis. *Science* **180**:875, 1973.
88. Kahn AJ, Simmons DJ: Investigation of the cell lineage in bone using a chimera of chick and quail embryonic tissue. *Nature* **258**:325, 1975.
89. Coccia PF, Krivit W, Cervenka J, Lawson C, Kersey JH, Kim TH, Nesbit ME, et al: Successful bone marrow transplantation for infantile malignant osteopetrosis. *N Engl J Med* **302**:701, 1980.
90. Shioi A, Ross FP, Teitelbaum SL: Enrichment of generated murine osteoclasts. *Calcif Tissue Int* **55**:387, 1994.
91. Kurihara N, Chenu C, Civin CI, Roodman GD: Identification of committed mononuclear precursors for osteoclast-like cell formed in long-term marrow cultures. *Endocrinology* **126**:2733, 1990.
92. Goldring SR, Gorn AH, Yamin M, Krane SM, Wang JT: Characterization of the structural and functional properties of cloned calcitonin receptor cDNAs. *Hormone Metab Res* **25**:477, 1993.
93. Ikegame M, Rakopoulos M, Zhou H, Houssami S, Martin TJ, Moseley JM, Findlay DM: Calcitonin receptor isoforms in mouse and rat osteoclasts. *J Bone Miner Res* **10**:59, 1995.
94. Minkin C: Bone acid phosphatase: Tartrate-resistant acid phosphatase as a marker of osteoclast function. *Calcif Tissue Int* **34**:141, 1982.
95. Holtrop MD, King GJ: The ultrastructure of the osteoclast and its functional implications. *Clin Orthop* **123**:177, 1977.
96. Chow JMW, Chambers TJ: An assessment of the prevalence of organic material on bone surface. *Calcif Tissue Int* **50**:118, 1992.
97. Chambers TJ, Fuller K: Bone cells predispose bone surfaces to resorption by exposure of mineral to osteoclastic contact. *J Cell Sci* **76**:155, 1985.
98. Chambers TJ, Darby JA, Fuller K: Mammalian collagenase predisposes bone surfaces to osteoclastic resorption. *Cell Tiss Res* **241**:671, 1985.
99. Otsuka K, Sodek J, Limeback HF: Collagenase synthesis by osteoblast-like cells. *Calcif Tissue Int* **36**:722, 1984.
100. Meikle MC, Bord S, Hembry RM, COmpston J, Croucher PI, Reynolds JJ: Human osteoblasts in culture synthesize collagenase and other matrix metalloproteinases in response to osteotropic hormones and cytokines. *J Cell Sci* **103**:1093, 1992.
101. Sato T, del-Carmen-Ovejero M, Hou P, Heegaard AM, Kumegawa M, Foged NT, Delaisse JM: Identification of the membrane-type matrix metalloproteinase MT1-MMP in osteoclasts. *J Cell Sci* **110**:589, 1997.
102. Delaisse JM, Eeckhout Y, Neff L, Francois-Gillet C, Henriet P, Su Y, Vaes G, et al.: (Pro)collagenase (matrix metalloproteinase-1) is present in rodent osteoclasts and in the underlying bone-resorbing compartment. *J Cell Sci* **106**:1071, 1993.
103. Blavier L, Delaisse JM: Matrix metalloproteinases are obligatory for the migration of preosteoclasts to the developing marrow cavity of primitive long bones. *J Cell Sci* **108**:3649, 1995.
104. Nesbitt S, Nesbit A, Helfich M, Horton MA: Biochemical characterization of human osteoclast integrins. Osteoclasts express av b 3, a2 b1, and av b1 integrins. *J Biol Chem* **268**:16737, 1993.
105. Flores ME, Norgard M, Heinegard D, Reinholt FP, Anderson G: RGD-directed attachment of isolated rat osteoclasts to osteopontin, bone sialoprotein, and fibronectin. *Exp Cell Res* **201**:526, 1992.
106. Shankar G, Davison I, Helfrich MH, Mason WT, Horton MA: Integrin receptor-mediated mobilization of intracellular calcium in rat osteoclasts. *J Cell Sci* **105**:61, 1993.
107. Hashizume Y, Araki S, Sawada K, Yamada K, Katayama K: Adhesive substrates influence acid-productive activities of cultured rabbit osteoclasts: Cultured osteoclasts with large vacuoles have enhanced acid-productive activities. *Exp Cell Res* **218**:452, 1995.
108. Blair HC, Kahn AJ, Crouch EC, Jeffrey JJ, Teitelbaum SL: Isolated osteoclasts resorb the organic and inorganic components of bone. *J Cell Biol* **102**:1164, 1986.
109. Fallon MD: Bone resorbin fluid from osteoclasts is acidic: An in vitro micropuncture study, in Cohn CV, Fujita T, Potts J JT, Talmadge RV (eds.): *Endocrine Control of Bone and Calcium Metabolism*. Amsterdam, Elsevier, 1984, p 305.
110. Blair HC, Teitelbaum SL, Ghiselli R, Gluck S: Osteoclastic bone resorption by a polarized vacuolar proton pump. *Science* **245**:855, 1989.
111. Bartkiewicz M, Hernando N, Reddy SV, Roodman GD, Baron R: Characterization of the osteoclast vacuolar H(+)-ATPase β-subunit. *Gene* **160**:157, 1995.
112. Anderson RE, Schraer H, Gay CV: Ultrastructural immunocytochemical localization of carbonic anhydrase in normal and calcitonin treated chick osteoclasts. *Anat Rec* **204**:9, 1982.

113. Teti A, Blair HC, Teitelbaum SL, Tan H, Koziol CM, Schlesinger PH: Cytoplasmic pH regulation and chloride/bicarbonate exchange in avian osteoclasts. *J Clin Invest* **83**:227, 1991.
114. Robey PG, Boskey AL: The biochemistry of bone, in Marcus R, Feldman D, Kelsey J (eds.): *Osteoporosis*. San Diego, Academic Press, 1996, p 95.
115. Teitelbaum SL, Grosso LE, Lacey DL, Tan H, McCort DW, Jeffrey JJ, Teitelbaum SL: Extracellular matrix degradation at acid pH: Avian osteoclast collagenase isolation and characterization. *Biochem J* **290**:873, 1993.
116. Goto T, Kiyoshima T, Moroi R, Tsukuba T, Nishimura Y, Himeno M, Yamamoto K, et al.: Localization of cathepsins B,D, and L in the rat osteoclast by immuno-light and -electron microscopy. *Histochem* **101**:33, 1994.
117. Sasaki T, Ueno-Matsuda E: Cysteine-proteinase localization in osteoclasts: An immunochemical study. *Cell Tiss Res* **271**:177, 1993.
118. Rifkin BR, Vernillo AT, Kleckner AP, Auszmann JM, Rosenberg LR, Zimmerman M: Cathepsin B and L activities in isolated osteoclasts. *Biochem Biophys Res Commun* **179**:63, 1991.
119. Inui T, Ishibashi O, Inaoka T, Origane Y, Kumegawa M, Kokubo T, Yamamura T: Cathepsin K antisense oligodeoxynucleotide inhibits osteoclastic bone resorption. *J Biol Chem* **272**:8109, 1997.
120. Blair HC, Teitelbaum SL, Schimke PA, Konsek JD, Koziol CM, Schlesinger PH: Receptor-mediated uptake of mannose-6-phospate bearing glycoprotein by isolated chicken osteoclast. *J Cell Physiol* **137**:476, 1988.
121. Nesbitt SA, Horton MA: Trafficking of matrix collagens through bone-resorbing osteoclasts. *Science* **276**:266, 1997.
122. Salo J, Lehenkari P, Mulari M, Metsikkö K, Väänänen HK: Removal of osteoclast bone resorption products by transcytosis. *Science* **276**:270, 1997.
123. Maciewicz RA, Etherington DJ, Kos J, Turk V: Collagenolytic cathepsins of rabbit spleen: A kinetic analysis of collagen degradation and inhibition by chicken cystatin. *Collagen Rel Res* **7**:295, 1987.
124. Heersche JNM: Mechanism of osteoclastic bone resorption: A new hypothesis. *Calcif Tissue Res* **26**:81, 1978.
125. Martin TJ, Ng KW: Mechanisms by which cells of the osteoblast lineage control osteoclast formation and activity. *J Cell Biochem* **56**:357, 1994.
126. Feyen JH, Elford P, Di Padova FE, Trechsel U: Interleukin-6 is produced by bone and modulated by parathyroid hormone. *J Bone Miner Res* **4**:633, 1989.
127. Girasole G, Passeri G, Jilka RL, Manolagas SC: Interleukin-11: A new cytokine critical for osteoclast development. *J Clin Invest* **93**:1516, 1994.
128. Romas E, Udagawa N, Hilton DJ, Martin TJ, Ng KW: Osteotrophic factors regulate interleukin-11 production by osteoblasts. *J Bone Miner Res* **10**:S142, 1995.
129. Weir EC, Horowitz MC, Baron R, Centrella M, Kacinski BM, Insogna KL: Macrophage colony-stimulating factor release and receptor expression in bone cells. *J Bone Miner Res* **8**:1507, 1993.
130. Mundy GR: The effects of TGF-beta on bone. *Ciba Found Symp* **157**:137, 1991.
131. Lowik CW, Nibbering PH, van de Ruit M, Papoulos SE: Inducible production of nitric oxide in osteoblast-like cells and in fetal mouse bone explants is associated with suppression of osteoclastic bone resorption. *J Clin Invest* **93**:1465, 1994.
132. Hansen HG: Sklerosteose, in Opitz H, Schmid F (eds.): *Handbuch der Kinderheilkunde*. Berlin, Springer, 1967, p 351.
133. Gorlin RJ, Glass L: Autosomal dominant osteosclerosis. *Radiology* **125**:547, 1977.
134. Young LW, Radebaugh JF, Rubin P, Sensenbrenner JA, Fiorelli G: New syndrome manifested by mandibular hypoplasia, acroosteolysis, stiff joints and cutaneous atrophy (mandibuloacral dysplasia) in two unrelated boys. *Birth Defects Orig Art Ser* **VII**:291, 1971.
135. Gordienko IY, Grechanina EY, Sopko NI, Tarapurova EN, Mikchailets LP: Prenatal diagnosis of osteochondrodysplasias in high risk pregnancy. *Am J Med Genet* **63**:90, 1996.
136. Hassan J, Sepulveda W, Teixeira J, Garrett C, Fisk NM: Prenatal sonographic diagnosis of cleidocranial dysostosis. *Prenat Diagn* **17**:770, 1997.
137. Sharony R, Browne C, Lachman RS, Rimoin DL: Prenatal diagnosis of the skeletal dysplasias. *Am J Obstet Gynecol* **169**:668, 1993.
138. Cattaneo R, Villa A, Catagni M, Tentori L: Strategies for limb lengthening in achondroplasia using the Ilizarov method—The experience of the hospital of Lecco, Italy. *Basic Life Sci* **48**:381, 1988.
139. Bell DF, Boyer MI, Armstrong PF: The use of the Ilizarov technique in the correction of limb deformities associated with skeletal dysplasia. *J Pediatr Orthop* **12**:283, 1992.
140. Stabler B, Clopper RR, Siegel PR, Stoppani C, Compton PG: Academic achievement and psychological adjustment in short children. *J Dev Behav Pediatr* **14**:1, 1994.
141. Zimet GD, Owens R, Dahms W, Cutler M, Litvene M, Cuttler L: Psychosocial outcome of children evaluated for short stature. *Arch Pediatr Adolesc Med* **151**:1017, 1997.
142. Johnson FL, Look AT, Gockerman J, Ruggiero MR, Dalla-Pozza, Billings FT: Bone-marrow transplantation in a patient with sickle-cell anemia. *N Engl J Med* **311**:780, 1984.
143. Vermylen C, Fernandez-Robles E, Ninane J, Cornu G: Bone marrow transplantation in five children with sickle cell anaemia. *Lancet* **1**:1427, 1988.
144. Walters MC, Patience M, Leisenring W, Eckman JR, Scott JP, Mentzer WC, Davies SC, et al: Bone marrow transplantation for sickle cell disease [see comments]. *N Engl J Med* **335**:369, 1996.

CHAPTER 138

I-Cell Disease and Pseudo-Hurler Polydystrophy: Disorders of Lysosomal Enzyme Phosphorylation and Localization

Stuart Kornfeld ▪ William S. Sly

1. I-cell disease (mucolipidosis II, or ML-II) and pseudo-Hurler polydystrophy (mucolipidosis III, or ML-III) are related genetic diseases, with rare occurrence and autosomal recessive inheritance.

2. I-cell disease shows many of the clinical and radiographic features of Hurler syndrome but presents earlier and does not show mucopolysacchariduria. There is severe progressive psychomotor retardation, and death usually occurs in the first decade. Pseudo-Hurler polydystrophy is milder and presents later, and survival into adulthood is possible.

3. In both diseases, there is abnormal lysosomal enzyme transport in cells of mesenchymal origin. In these cells, newly synthesized lysosomal enzymes are secreted into the extracellular medium instead of being targeted correctly to lysosomes. Affected cells show dense inclusions filled with storage material, and lysosomal enzymes are present at elevated levels in the serum and body fluids of affected patients.

4. In normal cells, targeting of lysosomal enzymes to lysosomes is mediated by receptors that bind mannose 6-phosphate recognition markers on the enzymes. The recognition marker is synthesized in a two-step reaction in the Golgi complex, and it is the enzyme that catalyzes the first step in this process, UDP-*N*-acetylglucosamine:lysosomal enzyme *N*-acetylglucosaminyl-1-phosphotransferase, which is defective in ML-II and ML-III.

5. The phosphotransferase is a low-abundance, membrane-bound enzyme complex of three subunits ($\alpha_2\beta_2\gamma_2$) that are the products of two genes. Biochemical studies suggest that the enzyme possesses two domains, one of which is associated with its catalytic activity and the other with the specific recognition of lysosomal enzymes.

6. A variety of defects have been described in the genes encoding phosphotransferase. Fibroblasts from four patients with ML-II had no detectable transcript for the α/β subunit, and two patients with ML-III, complementation group A, had greatly reduced levels of this transcript. Both groups had the transcript for the γ-subunit gene. Patients from three families with ML-III, complementation group C, had a frameshift mutation in the γ-subunit gene. Their mutant enzyme is catalytically active but is defective in recognizing lysosomal enzymes as substrates.

7. While all cells and tissues of affected individuals are deficient in phosphotransferase activity, not all cells are deficient in lysosomal enzyme content. This indicates that some cell types have mannose 6-phosphate-independent pathway(s) that function in the transport of lysosomal enzymes. The nature of the alternate pathway(s) in these cell types is unknown.

8. Diagnosis of ML-II and ML-III can be made biochemically by estimation of serum lysosomal enzyme levels. The characteristic pattern of enzyme deficiencies in fibroblasts also can be used, as can the ratio of extracellular to intracellular enzyme activities. The phosphotransferase activity also can be measured. In general, ML-II and ML-III must be distinguished on clinical criteria and on progression of the disease. Prenatal diagnosis is reliable, and carrier detection is also possible.

9. There is no definitive treatment.

In 1967, a disease was described that resembled the Hurler syndrome but lacked mucopolysacchariduria and presented earlier.[1,2] One exceptional feature of this newly recognized condition was the presence of numerous phase-dense inclusions in the cytoplasm of fibroblasts from affected individuals (Fig. 138-1). These cells were termed *inclusion cells* (abbreviated *I-cells*), and the disease subsequently was termed *I-cell disease.*[3] Such inclusions also were seen in cells from patients with another condition, *pseudo-Hurler polydystrophy,* that was milder clinically and presented later than I-cell disease.[4,5] This was the first indication of a relationship between these two conditions.

By the early 1970s, a number of biochemical defects had been observed in I-cell disease. These included a deficiency of multiple lysosomal enzymes in cultured fibroblasts[3,6–8] and their presence in the culture medium at abnormally high levels.[8,9] The sera and body fluids of I-cell disease patients also showed elevated levels of lysosomal enzymes.[10] Hickman and Neufeld made key

A list of standard abbreviations is located immediately preceding the index in each volume. Nonstandard abbreviations used in this chapter include: SRP = signal-recognition particle; MPR = mannose 6-phosphate receptor; Man-6-P = mannose 6-phosphate; CI-MPR = cation-independent mannose 6-phosphate/IGF-II receptor; CD-MPR = cation-dependent mannose 6-phosphate receptor.

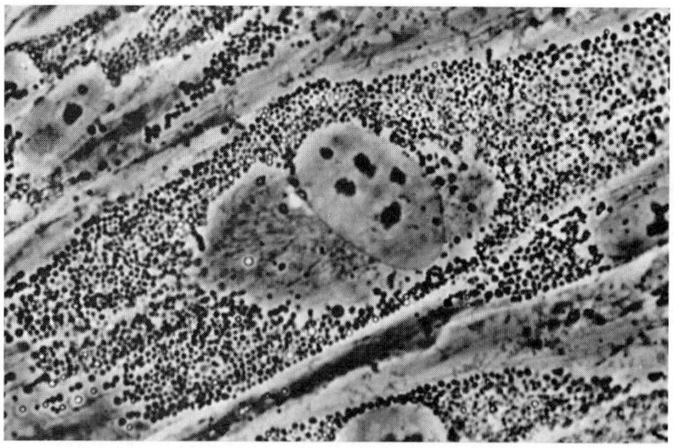

Fig. 138-1 Cultured skin fibroblasts from a patient with I-cell disease. Note the dense inclusions, from which the disease acquired its name, present throughout the cytoplasm. Magnification ×740. (Photograph kindly provided by Jules Leroy, University of Antwerp.)

observations that I-cell disease fibroblasts were capable of endocytosis of the lysosomal enzymes secreted by normal cells but that normal cells were incapable of internalizing the enzymes secreted by I-cell disease fibroblasts.[8] These observations suggested that lysosomal enzymes contained a recognition marker for uptake and transport to lysosomes and that enzymes from I-cell fibroblasts lacked this marker. The idea of a recognition marker subsequently was confirmed, and it was identified ultimately as mannose 6-phosphate, a sugar phosphate for which there was no precedent on mammalian glycoproteins.[11–13] The biosynthetic pathway by which mannose 6-phosphate is added to lysosomal enzymes was later elucidated, and I-cell disease (and pseudo-Hurler polydystrophy) cells were shown to be defective in the first enzyme in this pathway (UDP-*N*-acetylglucosamine:lysosomal enzyme *N*-acetylglucosaminyl-1-phosphotransferase).[14,15]

The term *mucolipidosis* was coined by Spranger and Wiedemann to denote diseases that combined clinical features common to both the mucopolysaccharidoses and the sphingolipidoses.[16] In this classification, I-cell disease was designated *ML-II*, and pseudo-Hurler polydystrophy was designated *ML-III* (the relationship between them was not yet realized). This classification is not ideal because I-cell disease and pseudo-Hurler polydystrophy are fundamentally different from other known lysosomal storage diseases. However, the terms *ML-II* and *ML-III* are so well established in the literature that they will be used in this chapter as synonyms for *I-cell disease* and *pseudo-Hurler polydystrophy*, respectively. The first example of ML-II in a cat was reported in 1996.[17]

CLINICAL MANIFESTATIONS

Mucolipidosis II (I-Cell Disease)

I-cell disease is characterized by severe psychomotor retardation and by many of the clinical features and radiologic changes that are seen in the Hurler syndrome[18] (Fig. 138-2). However, the earlier onset of signs and symptoms, the absence of excess mucopolysacchariduria, and the more rapidly progressive course leading to death between 5 and 8 years of age allow clinical differentiation of ML-II from the Hurler syndrome (see Chap. 136). As in Hurler syndrome, patients have coarse facial features and severe skeletal abnormalities that include kyphoscoliosis, anterior beaking and wedging of the vertebral bodies, a lumbar gibbus deformity, widening of the ribs, and proximal pointing of the metacarpals.[19–22] Birth weight and length are often below normal, and the clinical features of the disease may be obvious at birth.[23] Neonates with I-cell disease usually show coarse facial features, craniofacial abnormalities, and restricted joint movement

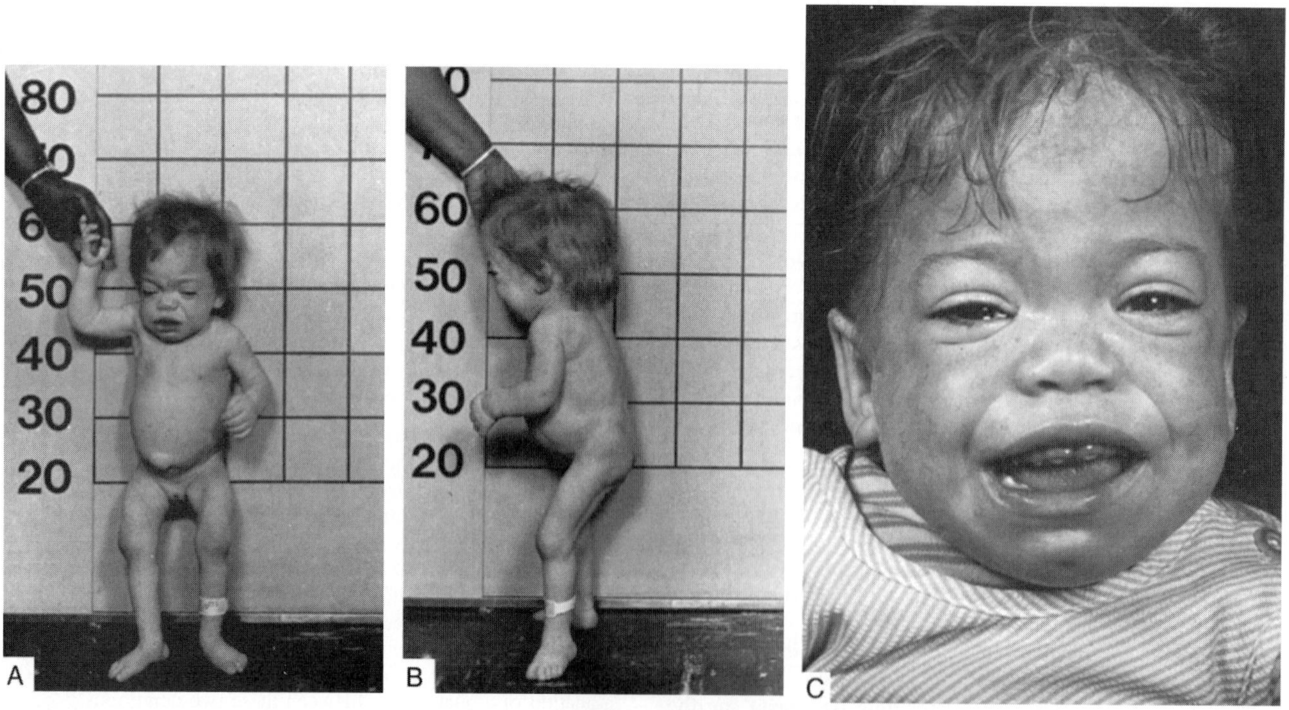

Fig. 138-2 I-cell disease (ML-II) in a 27-month-old child. Although abnormalities in appearance were noted by the parents at 2 months, the patient was diagnosed as having Down syndrome and later Hurler syndrome. At 27 months, I-cell disease was diagnosed on clinical and biochemical bases. The patient showed severe dysostosis multiplex, mental retardation, hepatomegaly, cardiomegaly, recurrent upper respiratory infections, umbilical hernias, and diastasis recti abdominis—all progressive. Corneal clouding was apparent on slit-lamp examination and subsequently became grossly evident. *A,B.* Front and side views showing coarse facies, prominent abdomen, umbilical hernia, joint contractures, and upper lumbar kyphosis. *C.* Detail of facies showing characteristic gingival hyperplasia.

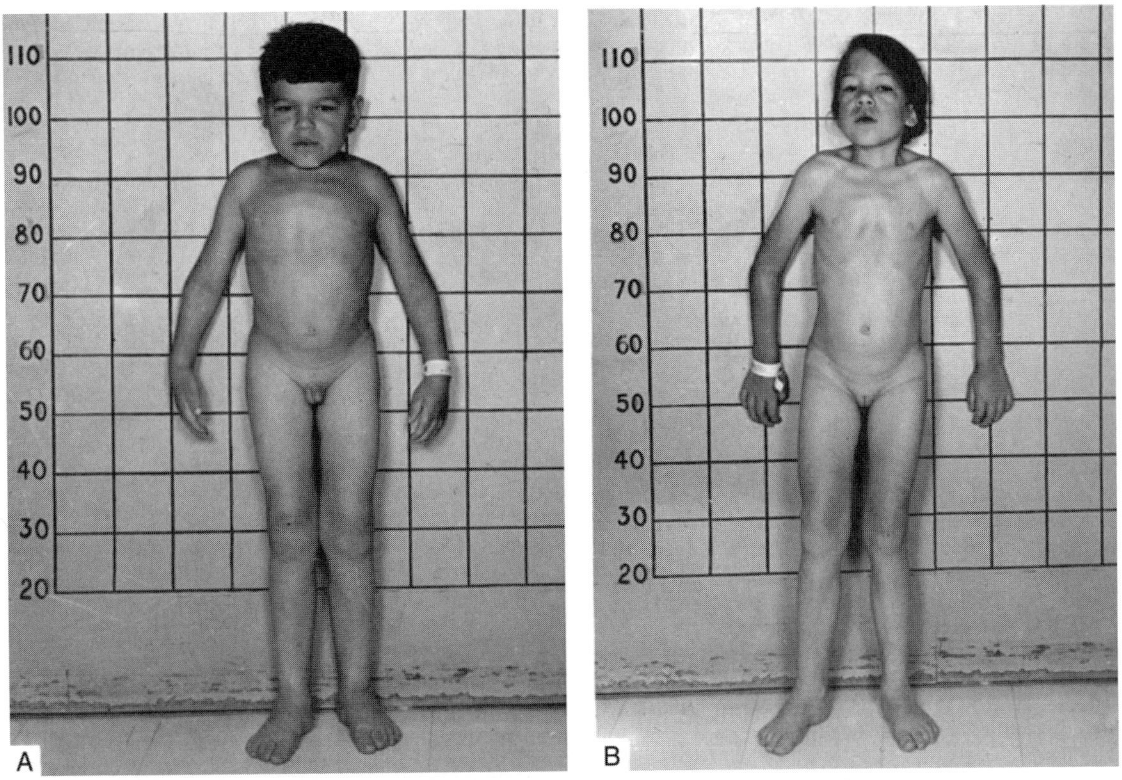

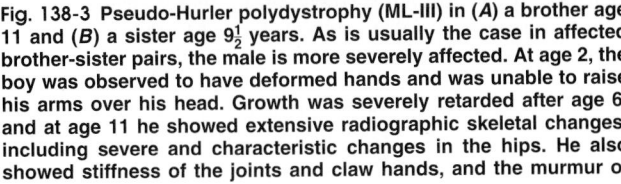

Fig. 138-3 Pseudo-Hurler polydystrophy (ML-III) in (*A*) a brother age 11 and (*B*) a sister age 9½ years. As is usually the case in affected brother-sister pairs, the male is more severely affected. At age 2, the boy was observed to have deformed hands and was unable to raise his arms over his head. Growth was severely retarded after age 6, and at age 11 he showed extensive radiographic skeletal changes, including severe and characteristic changes in the hips. He also showed stiffness of the joints and claw hands, and the murmur of aortic regurgitation was present. At this age there was no corneal clouding, even by slit-lamp examination, but by age 17, clouding was clearly evident. The sister showed similar abnormalities at age 3½ to 4 years, and there was evidence of a corneal haze on slit-lamp examination. At age 13, the murmur of aortic regurgitation was present. In both individuals, IQ was estimated to be about 70. Attempts at correction of severe bilateral hip disease by hip replacement were only partially successful.

despite generalized hypotonia. Presenting features also may include congenital hip dislocation, fractures, hernias, and bilateral talipes equinovarus.[24,25] Striking gingival hyperplasia is a unique clinical feature that distinguishes ML-II from the Hurler syndrome.[23,24,26,27]

The clinical course is characterized by progressive failure to thrive and by developmental delay. The facial features become characteristic, with a high forehead, puffy eyelids, prominent epicanthal folds, flat nasal bridge, anteverted nostrils, gingival hyperplasia, and macroglossia. Psychomotor retardation is usually obvious by 6 months. Linear growth decelerates during the first year and stops during the second year. Joint immobility progresses, with development of claw-hand deformities and kyphoscoliosis. Head size remains unchanged. Abdominal protuberance with hepatomegaly is prominent, as are umbilical and inguinal hernias. Splenomegaly is minimal. Respiratory infections are frequent, as are bouts of otitis media. Corneal haziness is common, and corneal opacities are evident on slit-lamp examination as diffuse stromal granularities. Cardiomegaly and cardiac murmurs are common, and aortic insufficiency is not infrequent.[23,28]

Mental retardation is somewhat variable but usually severe and slowly progressive. However, Okada et al. pointed out that motor development was more severely retarded than mental development in the 21 patients whose clinical courses they summarized.[28] Cardiorespiratory complications usually led to death between the fifth and eighth year of life, but there are now several reports of patients surviving into their teens.[28,29]

Mucolipidosis III (Pseudo-Hurler Polydystrophy)

ML-III is a much milder disorder with later onset of clinical signs and symptoms (2 to 4 years). The clinical course is also more slowly progressive, permitting survival into adulthood.[30,31] Affected patients (Fig. 138-3) share many clinical feature with patients with the mild to moderately severe forms of mucopolysaccharidosis types I and VI (see Chap. 136). However, unlike patients with MPS I and MPS VI, patients with ML-III have no mucopolysacchariduria. Stiffness of the hands and shoulders suggestive of rheumatoid arthritis is one of the most common early manifestations.[32] These symptoms make it difficult for patients to dress themselves without assistance. By 4 to 6 years of age, most patients have claw-hand deformities, scoliosis, and short stature. Progressive destruction of the hip joints is one of the most disabling features of ML-III, and it often leads to a characteristic waddling gait. Occasional patients with a very mild form of the disease may present with isolated involvement of the hip and spine.[33] Carpal tunnel syndrome is seen frequently. Mild coarsening of the facial features and thickening of the skin become apparent after the sixth year. Although visual complaints are uncommon and corneas usually appear clear, slit-lamp examination usually reveals stromal granularities by the seventh year. Traboulsi and Maumenee concluded that ML-III patients develop a characteristic triad of ophthalmologic findings that includes corneal clouding, mild retinopathy, and hyperopic astigmatism.[34] Cardiac valvular involvement, evidenced by the murmur of aortic insufficiency, is usual by the end of the first decade, but symptomatic cardiac insufficiency is rare. Puberty is normal. The skeletal dysplasia in the hands, hips, elbows, and shoulders is slowly progressive through the first two decades. Radiographic findings of dysostosis multiplex are moderately severe, and certain pelvic and vertebral changes are considered characteristic of ML-III. These findings include low iliac wings with hypoplastic bodies, flattening and irregularity of the proximal femoral epiphyses with valgus deformity of the femoral necks, underdevelopment of the posterior parts of the vertebral bodies of the dorsal spine, and hypoplasia of the anterior third of the vertebral bodies of the lumbar spine.[35] For reasons that are unclear, the radiologic changes appear consistently more severe in affected males than in affected females.

Nearly 50 percent of reported patients have some learning disability or mental retardation.[30] Subclinical central nervous system abnormalities may be detected with the use of electrophysiologic techniques.[36] Although patients are known to survive into the eighth decade,[31] relatively little is known with certainty about the life expectancy or the natural course of the illness beyond the third decade.

PATHOLOGY

Mucolipidosis II

A characteristic feature of ML-II is the presence of numerous membrane-bound vacuoles containing electron-lucent or fibrillogranular material in the cytoplasm of mesenchymal cells, especially fibroblasts. These are the inclusion bodies for which the disease was named. The contents of such vacuoles have not been well characterized but probably include oligosaccharides, mucopolysaccharides, and lipids.[37–40] Pathologic changes have been observed in mesenchymal cells of tissues of a 15-week-old fetus[41] and in placenta at the fourteenth week of pregnancy.[42,43]

The skeletal system is very seriously affected, and the radiologic features described earlier correlate well with abnormalities of bone structure seen on microscopic examination.[44–46] Abnormalities of cartilage structure also have been seen in patients with I-cell disease.[44,47] All this appears to indicate impaired production or maintenance of extracellular matrix by several types of mesenchymal cells.

The central nervous system shows essentially normal morphology except for the presence of lamellar bodies in spinal ganglia neurons[48] and in the anterior horn cells of one patient.[49] Only minimal alterations were seen in the peripheral nervous system.[49] However, magnetic resonance imaging (MRI) of the cranium in a patient with I-cell disease showed ventriculomegaly with frontal lobe atrophy and bifrontal leukomalacia, indicating that morphologic abnormalities in the central nervous system may occur in some patients.[50] Skeletal muscle fibers appear normal by light and electron microscopy, but satellite cells have some vacuoles.[49] Consistent with this observation, it has been noted that myoblasts in culture show the I-cell defect both biochemically and morphologically and are slower to fuse than normal myoblasts.[51] Once myotubes are formed, however, they do not exhibit the morphologic or biochemical defects. There is one report of a deficiency of type I muscle fibers, in the absence of denervation, in a quadriceps muscle biopsy of an ML-II patient, suggesting a developmental disruption of motor unit organization.[52] Such features may be correlated with the neuromuscular disability of patients with I-cell disease.

The muscular tissue of the heart appears normal, but heart valves show impressive thickening due to the presence of numerous vacuolated fibroblasts.[44,49] In liver, damage to fibroblasts in the periportal spaces is visible, while Kupffer cells and hepatocytes are essentially normal.[44,49] In the kidney, the glomerular podocytes, which are thought to represent mesenchymal cells, are the most severely affected.[49,53] In one study, the podocytes were essentially normal in the longest surviving patient (10 years), while patients who died at earlier ages (2 weeks to 4 years) showed heavy vacuolation.[49] It is not clear what the functional significance of this finding is, but it appears to represent the only histologic difference in visceral organs between ML-II patients who die in infancy or early childhood and those who survive well into the first decade of life.[49]

ML-II patients often have repeated upper respiratory infections. Examination of one patient showed no radiographic abnormality of the trachea, but at autopsy, the base of the tongue, epiglottis, larynx, and trachea were thickened with balloon cells filled with acid mucopolysaccharide and mucolipids.[54]

Mucolipidosis III

The pathology of ML-III is not as well documented as that of ML-II. Fibroblasts cultured from ML-III patients show inclusion bodies similar to those of ML-II cells, although these may not be as prominent.[5,55] We are not aware of any reports of autopsy studies of ML-III patients.

NORMAL PATHWAYS OF BIOSYNTHESIS AND TRANSPORT OF LYSOSOMAL ENZYMES

The biosynthesis of lysosomal enzymes possessing the mannose 6-phosphate marker uses the common cellular machinery for the synthesis of glycoproteins as well as two specific enzymes involved in the formation of the mannose 6-phosphate residues (Fig. 138-4). Lysosomal enzymes, together with many membrane proteins and proteins destined for secretion, are synthesized on endoplasmic reticulum–bound ribosomes (see Chap. 16). Such proteins have a so-called signal sequence that mediates their interaction with a signal-recognition particle (SRP).[56,57] The nascent protein-SRP complex then binds to the SRP-recognition protein (docking protein), and the nascent protein is translocated into the lumen of the endoplasmic reticulum, with subsequent cleavage of the signal peptide.[56,57] As is the case with most other glycoproteins, lysosomal enzymes are modified in the endoplasmic reticulum by the addition of high-mannose oligosaccharides donated by a dolichol pyrophosphate intermediate.[58] These oligosaccharides are then subjected to the typical trimming reactions that have been shown to occur in the endoplasmic reticulum, and the nascent glycoproteins are then transferred to the Golgi apparatus, where further trimming and modification take place. In the Golgi, the lysosomal enzymes are specifically modified by the addition of the mannose 6-phosphate marker. This marker is generated through the concerted action of two enzymes[59–62] (Fig. 138-5). The first step in the process is the addition of an α-*N*-acetylglucosamine 1-phosphate residue to the six position of a mannose on the high-mannose oligosaccharide on the lysosomal enzyme. This gives rise to a phosphodiester intermediate. The enzyme catalyzing the reaction is UDP-*N*-acetylglucosamine:lysosomal enzyme *N*-acetylglucosaminyl-1-phosphotransferase (termed *phosphotransferase*). The second step of the process involves removal of the *N*-acetylglucosamine residue, catalyzed by the enzyme *N*-acetylglucosamine 1-phosphodiester-*N*-acetylglucosaminidase, to expose the mannose 6-phosphate marker. This enzyme initially was called a phosphodiesterase, but mechanistic studies showed it to be a glycosidase.[63] Both enzymes are multisubunit proteins. Bovine phosphotransferase has been purified as a complex of M_r 540,000 composed of three different subunits ($\alpha_2\beta_2\gamma 2$) that are the products of two genes, one encoding the 166-kDa α and 51-kDa β subunits and the other encoding the 56-kDa γ subunit[64] (W. Canfield, personal communication). Phosphodiester *N*-acetylglucosaminidase is a tetramer composed of two disulfide-linked homodimers with subunits of M_r 68,000.[65] It is the product of a single gene.[65a]

Recognition of Lysosomal Enzymes by the Phosphotransferase

In addition to catalyzing the first step in the synthesis of the mannose 6-phosphate recognition marker, phosphotransferase is also responsible for the specificity of the process. It is this enzyme that specifically selects lysosomal enzymes from the large number of other glycoproteins present in the lumen of the Golgi apparatus for phosphorylation.[60,66] The affinity of phosphotransferase for lysosomal enzymes is 100 to 150 times greater than its affinity for nonlysosomal glycoproteins.[66,67] The oligosaccharide units of lysosomal enzymes, however, are not significantly different from those of other glycoproteins that are poor substrates for the

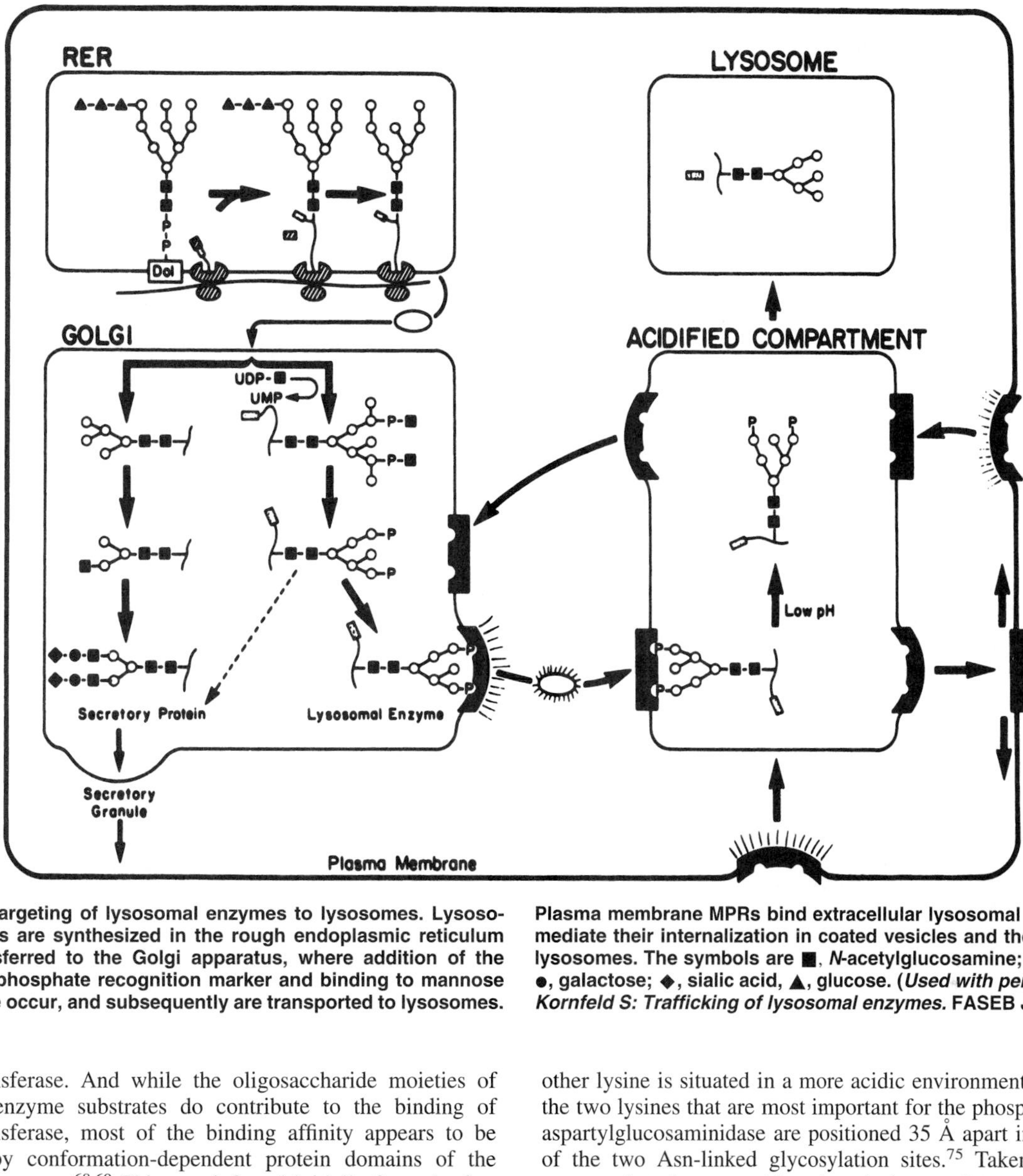

Fig. 138-4 Targeting of lysosomal enzymes to lysosomes. Lysosomal enzymes are synthesized in the rough endoplasmic reticulum (RER), transferred to the Golgi apparatus, where addition of the mannose 6-phosphate recognition marker and binding to mannose 6-phosphate occur, and subsequently are transported to lysosomes. Plasma membrane MPRs bind extracellular lysosomal enzymes and mediate their internalization in coated vesicles and their transfer to lysosomes. The symbols are ■, *N*-acetylglucosamine; ○, mannose; ●, galactose; ◆, sialic acid, ▲, glucose. (*Used with permission from Kornfeld S: Trafficking of lysosomal enzymes.* FASEB J *1:462, 1979.*)

phosphotransferase. And while the oligosaccharide moieties of lysosomal enzyme substrates do contribute to the binding of phosphotransferase, most of the binding affinity appears to be generated by conformation-dependent protein domains of the lysosomal enzymes.[68,69] This was inferred initially from the fact that deglycosylated lysosomal enzymes are potent inhibitors of phosphotransferase, and this inhibition is relieved by heat treatment or proteolysis of the deglycosylated enzymes.[68]

The first insight into the nature of the recognition domain came from studies of chimeric proteins derived from human cathepsin D and pepsinogen.[70–72] Although these two aspartyl proteases share 45 percent identity in amino acid sequence, pepsinogen is a secretory protein, whereas cathepsin D is a lysosomal enzyme. These studies revealed that substitution of residues from two noncontinuous regions of the carboxyl lobe of cathepsin D (lysine 203 and amino acids 265-293, particularly lysines 265 and 293) into the pepsinogen backbone was sufficient to generate an efficient phosphotransferase recognition domain. When localized to the homologous position in the crystal structure of porcine pepsinogen, these residues were found to be in direct apposition on the surface of the molecule. This region represents a portion of a more extended recognition site on the surface of cathepsin D.[71,72] Studies of other lysosomal enzymes have confirmed that selected lysine residues are the critical components of the phosphotransferase binding site.[73–77]

In the case of cathepsin D and cathepsin L, the two lysines that serve as the major determinants of the phosphorylation signal are positioned 34 Å apart, with the lysine closest to the glycosylated asparagine being located in a basic microenvironment, while the other lysine is situated in a more acidic environment.[77] Similarly, the two lysines that are most important for the phosphorylation of aspartylglucosaminidase are positioned 35 Å apart in the vicinity of the two Asn-linked glycosylation sites.[75] Taken together, it appears that the recognition domain is a surface patch with the critical elements being lysine residues that are correctly spaced relative to each other and to the carbohydrate unit. The conformational nature of the recognition domain explains the failure to detect amino acid sequence identity between lysosomal enzymes.

Mannose 6-Phosphate Receptors

Following acquisition of the mannose 6-phosphate marker, lysosomal enzymes can be recognized by specific receptors that direct their transfer to lysosomes. Two such mannose 6-phosphate receptors (MPR) are known.[78,79] One of the receptors is a large molecule with an M_r of approximately 275,000, whereas the other receptor has a subunit M_r of approximately 46,000.[80–83] Both are type I integral membrane glycoproteins with three structural domains: an N-terminal extracytoplasmic domain, a single transmembrane region, and a C-terminal cytoplasmic domain (Fig. 138-6). The extracytoplasmic domain of the large receptor consists of 15 contiguous repeating elements, each of which is homologous to and similar in size to the extracellular domain of the small receptor. This indicates that both receptors were derived from a common ancestor, with the large receptor arising from multiple duplications of a single ancestral gene.

The large receptor binds 2 moles of mannose 6-phosphate (Man-6-P), whereas the small receptor binds 1 mole of Man-6-P

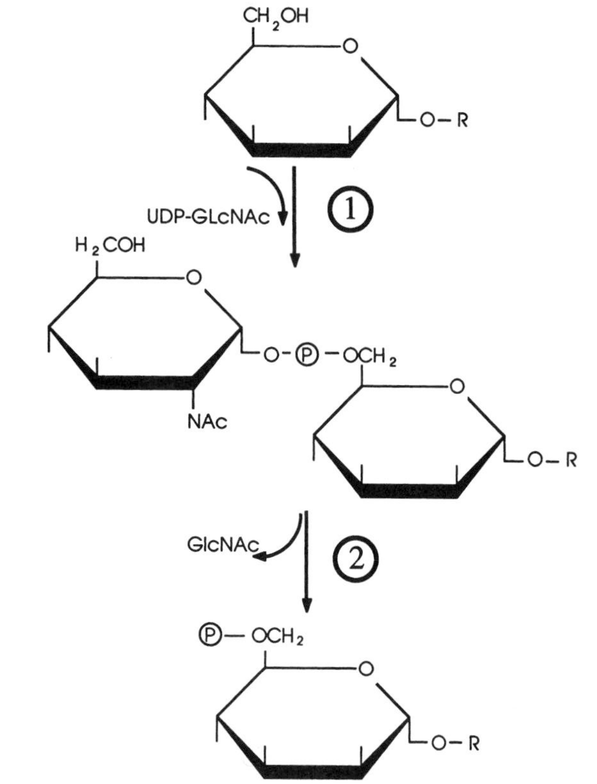

Fig. 138-5 The biosynthesis and mannose 6-phosphate recognition marker. R represents the oligosaccharide on the nascent lysosomal enzyme. Reaction 1 is catalyzed by UDP-*N*-acetylglucosamine:lysosomal enzyme *N*-acetylglucosaminyl-1-phosphotransferase. Reaction 2 is catalyzed by *N*-acetylglucosamine 1-phosphodiester-*N*-acetylglucosaminidase.

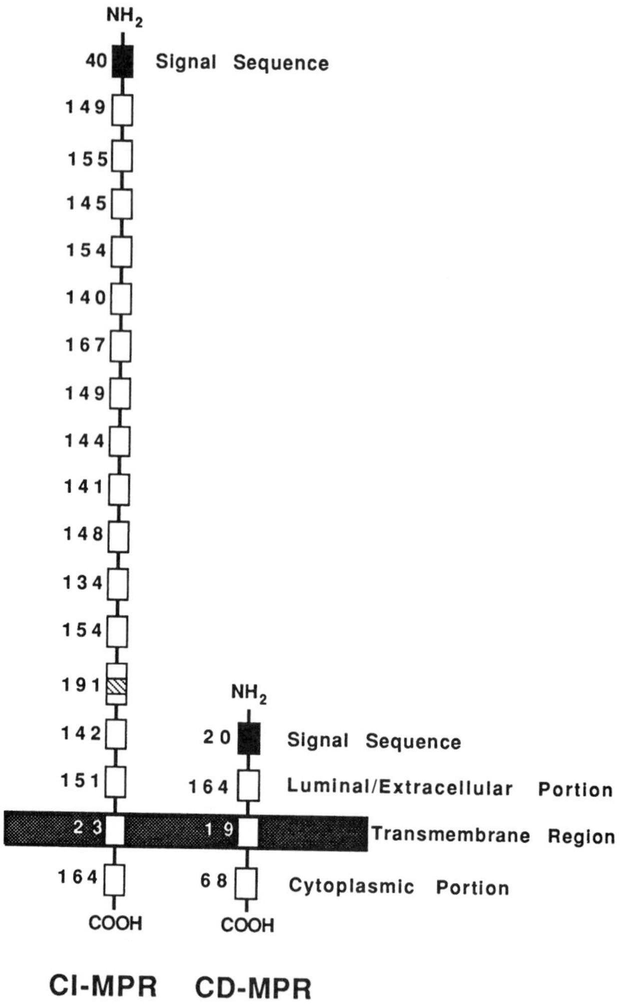

Fig. 138-6 A diagram of the cation-independent MPR and cation-dependent MPR. The number of amino acids in each domain is shown.[80–83] The extracellular domain of the CD-MPR is homologous to each of the repeating units of the extracellular portion of CI-MPR. The hatched region in repeat number 13 of the CI-MPR represents the sequence that is similar to sequences found in the collagen-binding domain in the fibronectin receptor, in bovine seminal fluid protein, and in factor XII.[80,81]

per subunit, or 2 moles of Man-6-P per dimer, which is the major form of the receptor in the membrane.[84–86] The binding of Man-6-P by the large receptor does not require divalent cations, and thus this receptor has been termed the *cation-independent MPR (CI-MPR)* to distinguish it from the other receptor, which does require divalent cations for optimal ligand binding.[87–89] The latter receptor is referred to as the *cation-dependent MPR (CD-MPR)*. However, the divalent cation dependence of the small receptor is species-specific, with the bovine and murine forms requiring divalent cations,[89,90] while the human and porcine forms apparently do not.[91–93] The CI-MPR from human, bovine, and rat sources also binds nonglycosylated polypeptide hormone insulin-like growth factor II with high affinity.[94–100] For this reason, the CI-MPR also has been termed the *Man-6-P/IGF-II receptor*. The binding site for insulin-like growth factor II has been localized to repeating domain 11,[101–103] whereas the two binding sites for Man-6-P are on repeating domains 3 and 9.[104] Interestingly, the chicken and frog receptors lack the high-affinity insulin-like growth factor II binding site,[105,106] and domain 11 of the chicken receptor is less conserved than the other repeating domains when compared with the human sequence.[107]

The three-dimensional structure of the extracytoplasmic domain of the bovine CD-MPR complexed to Man-6-P has been solved, providing insight into the mechanism of lysosomal enzyme binding.[108] The extracellular domain crystallized as a dimer, with each monomer folding into a nine-stranded flattened β barrel that bears a striking resemblance to avidin (Fig. 138-7). The distance of 40 Å between the two ligand-binding sites accommodates single Man-6-P residues from two oligosaccharides but not a single diphosphorylated oligosaccharide. This is consistent with the report that the CD-MPR exhibits a higher affinity for lysosomal enzymes that have multiple oligosaccharides containing one phosphomonoester, whereas the CI-MPR preferentially binds lysosomal enzymes enriched in oligosaccharides with two phosphomonoesters.[109]

There is considerable evidence that both receptors function in the targeting of newly synthesized lysosomal enzymes. Gene disruption experiments in mice have revealed that animals expressing only one of the MPRs are viable in the appropriate genetic background, whereas mice lacking both MPRs survive at a low frequency and only for a few postnatal weeks.[110–114] This indicates that each receptor can functionally compensate for the loss of the other, although the compensation is only partial because animals lacking one or the other receptor have elevated levels of plasma lysosomal enzymes.[112,113] Similarily, cultured fibroblasts that are deficient in either MPR are partially impaired in intracellular lysosomal enzyme sorting, and overexpression of the remaining MPR fails to fully compensate for the lack of the other receptor.[103,111,112,114–117] In these experiments, the secretion of lysosomal enzymes is greatest in the absence of the CI-MPR, indicating that this receptor is the more efficient of the two in mediating sorting. Further, it has been shown in in vitro experiments that saturating amounts of the CI-MPR bind essentially all the Man-6-P-containing glycoproteins secreted by MPR-negative

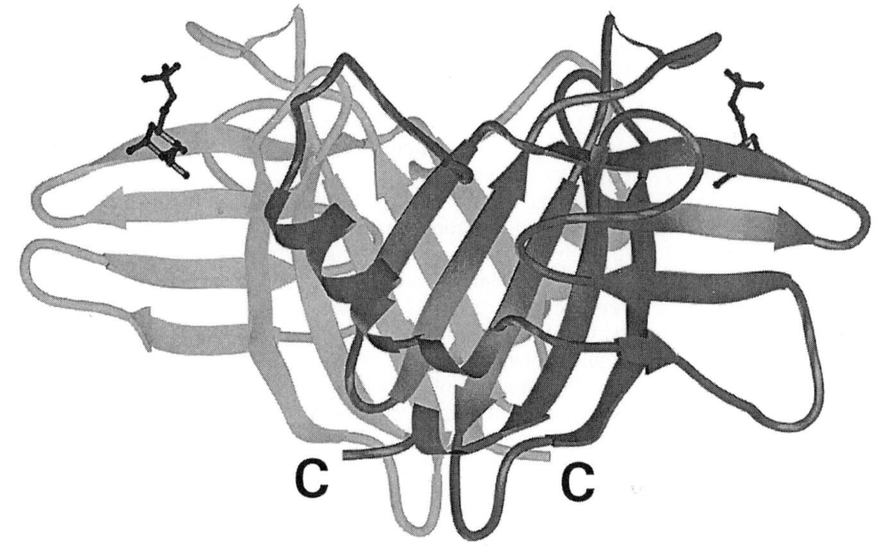

Fig. 138-7 Ribbon diagram of the bovine CD-MPR dimer. There are two CD-MPR monomers within the asymmetric unit. The ligand, Man-6-P, is also shown (ball and stick model).[108]

cells, whereas the CD-MPR binds only a subset of these ligands.[118] The fact that overexpression of the CI-MPR in CD-MPR-negative fibroblasts fails to completely correct the excess secretion of lysosomal enzymes indicates that additional factors influence the efficiency of sorting in the cell.

While lysosomal enzymes acquire the Man-6-P recognition marker in the cis region of the Golgi,[119] the major site for lysosomal enzyme sorting is believed to be the last Golgi compartment, which has been variously termed the *trans Golgi network* (TGN), the *trans Golgi reticulum,* the *trans tubular network,* and the *GERL* (Golgi endoplasmic reticulum lysosome).[120] Binding of lysosomal enzymes to the MPRs is followed by incorporation of the complexes into clathrin-coated vesicles that exit the Golgi and subsequently fuse with acidic prelysosomal/endosomal compartments (see Fig. 138-4). The low pH of these compartments induces the lysosomal enzymes to dissociate from the receptors.[121] The lysosomal enzymes are then packaged into lysosomes, while the receptors recycle to the Golgi to mediate further rounds of transport or move to the plasma membrane.

The Endocytic Pathway

In some cell types such as fibroblasts, lysosomal enzymes may be transported from the extracellular milieu to lysosomes through receptor-mediated endocytosis[78,122,123] (see Fig. 138-4). These cells possess a cell surface CI-MPR that comprises 10 to 20 percent of the total cellular complement of this receptor. Following internalization in endocytic vesicles, the lysosomal enzymes dissociate from the receptors in a prelysosomal/endosomal acidic compartment; the lysosomal enzymes are then packaged into lysosomes, while the receptors recycle and can participate in further rounds of endocytosis. Both pools of receptors, cell surface and intracellular, are in fairly rapid equilibrium.[78,122,123] Although the CD-MPR is present on the cell surface and undergoes rapid internalization, it functions inefficiently in the uptake of lysosomal enzymes because it binds ligand poorly at the cell surface.[90,124]

The determinants on the MPRs required for rapid endocytosis from the cell surface and efficient lysosomal enzyme sorting in the Golgi are located on the cytoplasmic tails of these proteins.[78] In the case of the CI-MPR, the sequence Tyr-Lys-Tyr-Ser-Lys-Val, representing residues 24 to 29 of the 163 amino acid cytoplasmic tail, serves as the internalization signal.[125,126] The last four residues of this sequence, particularly the Tyr at position 26 and the Val at position 29, account for most of the activity. This sequence contains the critical elements present in the internalization signal of many membrane proteins that undergo rapid endocytosis, namely, an aromatic (Tyr) residue in the N-terminal position separated from a bulky hydrophobic/aromatic residue in the C-terminal position by two amino acids.[125,127] The CD-MPR contains three internalization sequences in its cytoplasmic tail, including a phenylalanine-based motif, a tyrosine-based motif, and a di-leucine motif.[128,129] Both receptors require a conserved casein kinase II site followed by the di-leucine motif at the C-terminus of the cytoplasmic tail to mediate efficient lysosomal enzyme sorting in the Golgi.[129–132] Within the casein kinase II site it is the cluster of acidic residues that is required for sorting rather than phosphorylation of the serine residue. In addition, the tyrosine-based motif also contributes to the efficiency of sorting by the CI-MPR.[133] It is presumed that these protein motifs within the cytoplasmic tails of the receptors interact with the Golgi and plasma membrane adaptor complexes that are components of the clathrin-coated pits.[134,135]

The transport pathway from the cell surface to lysosomes was discovered first and was thought originally to be the major route of delivery of newly synthesized acid hydrolases to lysosomes. It was suggested that the enzymes were first delivered to the extracellular environment and then reinternalized for delivery to lysosomes.[8] It is now clear that, in most cell types, the bulk of lysosomal enzymes is transported to lysosomes by the intracellular pathway. Transport of enzymes from the plasma membrane accounts for only a small portion of total delivery.[136] Nonetheless, the ability of I-cell disease fibroblasts to internalize normal lysosomal enzymes by this pathway was a key factor in identifying the defect in these cells.

Alternate Pathways to Lysosomes

One unexplained feature of the ML-II and ML-III syndromes is the fact that not all cells are deficient in lysosomal enzyme content,[137,138] even though all cells and tissues so far examined have been shown to be deficient in the phosphotransferase activity. Many cell types (including hepatocytes, Kupffer cells, and leukocytes) and several organs (including liver, spleen, kidney, and brain) have nearly normal levels of intracellular lysosomal enzymes. These observations suggest that there is an alternate pathway for lysosomal enzymes to be transported to lysosomes that does not require the mannose 6-phosphate recognition marker. In fact, a mannose 6-phosphate-independent targeting system has been demonstrated in several mammalian cell types[123,139–141] and in a number of other species.[142,143] Another mechanism that may be used by specific cell types is the internalization of lysosomal enzymes present at high concentration in the serum of ML-II and ML-III patients by cell surface receptors that recognize carbohydrates, such as galactose, *N*-acetylglucosamine, mannose, and L-fucose, present in the enzymes.[138]

Another interesting fact is that two lysosomal enzymes are present at nearly normal levels in ML-II and ML-III fibroblasts. These are β-glucocerebrosidase, a membrane-associated enzyme,[144] and acid phosphatase, an enzyme that is synthesized as a transmembrane glycoprotein and then proteolyzed to a soluble form on arrival in the lysosome.[145] It has been demonstrated that both these proteins, along with the lysosomal membrane proteins, are targeted to lysosomes by a pathway that does not require phosphorylation.[123,146] In the case of acid phosphatase and the lysosomal membrane proteins, the signal for lysosomal targeting is contained in the cytoplasmic tails of these proteins.[147,148]

PRIMARY BIOCHEMICAL DEFECT IN ML-II AND ML-III

The identification of mannose 6-phosphate as the recognition marker that mediates the internalization of acid hydrolases by fibroblasts[11–13] and the observation that I-cell disease fibroblasts are defective in the incorporation of ^{32}P into several lysosomal enzymes[149,150] suggested that these cells were defective in the synthesis of this marker. With the development of assays for phosphotransferase and phosphodiester-*N*-acetylglucosaminidase, it was shown that the first enzyme in the pathway, the phosphotransferase, was deficient in both I-cell disease and pseudo-Hurler polydystrophy.[14,15] No patients have been found who lack the second enzyme.

Phosphotransferase Assay

The assay for phosphotransferase is sensitive and reliable. The original assay used [^{32}P]UDP-GlcNAc as the donor substrate and α-methylmannose or purified lysosomal enzymes as the acceptor substrates.[151] Using this assay, with α-methylmannose as the acceptor, it was shown that in fibroblasts from I-cell patients the phosphotransferase was absent or barely detectable, whereas in cells from ML-III patients there was residual activity of from 2 to 20 percent of normal levels.[152] In a study of Japanese I-cell disease patients, there was less than 2 to 13 percent of control activity.[28] In this study, the patients had a somewhat mild I-cell phenotype, and the severity of the clinical phenotype did not correlate with the level of enzyme activity.[34] Fibroblasts of parents of affected individuals (obligate heterozygotes) have a lower level of activity than is found in fibroblasts of normal individuals.[153]

The assay using ^{32}P-labeled substrate is inconvenient, however, in that the donor substrate is not commercially available, and it is therefore necessary to synthesize and purify it. In addition, the substrate has a limited shelf life due to the half-life of the isotope. [^{3}H or ^{14}C]UDP-GlcNAc also can be used in the assay. These substrates are commercially available and have long half-lives. However, the use of these substrates initially resulted in assays with high backgrounds and therefore low sensitivity. The assay has since been modified to improve the sensitivity and reliability using these commercially available substrates, and the results obtained with the modified assay are reported to be comparable with those seen using the ^{32}P-labeled substrate.[154,155]

It should be noted that when assayed with artificial acceptors such as α-methylmannoside, the less common variant of ML-III patients (group C of the complementation groups discussed below) will show normal levels of activity. This is also true of obligate heterozygotes of this variant.

Complementation Studies/Heterogeneity of ML-II and ML-III

Clinical variability has long been observed in patients with ML-II and ML-III. In an effort to understand the basis of this variability, complementation analyses of fibroblasts from many patients were initiated. In these studies, fibroblasts from individual patients were fused with cells from other patients using polyethylene glycol as a fusogen. Complementation of pairs of fibroblasts was indicated by the increased intracellular lysosomal enzyme activity of the heterokaryons compared with the unfused homokaryon mixtures and by the disappearance of the abnormal forms of these enzymes (see "Other Biochemical Defects" below).[156–158] Complementation also has been monitored by measuring the phosphotransferase activity of the heterokaryons.[159]

One such study of ML-III patient fibroblasts showed the existence of three complementation groups (groups A, B, and C), although one of these groups (group B) was represented by a single cell line.[156] Complementation also was observed among ML-II fibroblasts, although this was less conclusive than that seen with ML-III fibroblasts,[157] and in another study, several instances of complementation between ML-II and ML-III fibroblasts were seen.[158] These complementation studies indicate genetic heterogeneity, consistent with the finding that phosphotransferase is a multisubunit enzyme.[64]

Biochemical evidence for heterogeneity also emerged from kinetic studies of phosphotransferase activity. During the development of the phosphotransferase assay, it was noticed that while most ML-III patients were defective in enzyme activity, whether this was measured using lysosomal enzymes or artificial substances as the acceptor substrates, enzyme from one sibship (GM3391) had normal activity toward α-methylmannoside despite very low activity with lysosomal enzymes.[152] This prompted the hypothesis that the phosphotransferase possessed two distinct domains, a catalytic domain and a domain that was important in specific recognition of lysosomal enzymes.

Further studies have supported this hypothesis. Careful analysis of the kinetic parameters and of the temperature sensitivity of the residual activity of a number of ML-III fibroblasts has shown the existence of two types of defects.[159–162] In one group (group A), the catalytic activity of the enzyme is reduced both with artificial substrates and with lysosomal enzymes. The affinity of the residual activity for the lysosomal enzymes is normal, however, and activity can be somewhat normalized by assaying at 23°C rather than at 37°C.[159–162] The group C mutation appears to result in an enzyme that is defective in recognition of lysosomal enzymes but which has normal activity toward the artificial substrates.[152,159–162] Thus the enzyme in group A fibroblasts has a defective catalytic domain, whereas in group C fibroblasts the domain that recognizes the lysosomal enzymes is defective. This model for lysosomal enzyme recognition by phosphotransferase is shown in Fig. 138-8. The molecular size of phosphotransferase from fibroblasts of a number of these patients has been estimated by a radiation inactivation technique.[163,164] Phosphotransferase from patients with ML-II and the group A type of ML-III was significantly smaller (151–174 kDa) than the normal enzyme (225–278 kDa), whereas the enzyme from the group C patients was very large, ranging from 321 to 547 kDa. However, the values for the normal enzyme do not agree with those obtained for the purified bovine enzyme.[64]

A subset of ML-II fibroblast lines showed restoration of phosphotransferase activity to almost normal levels when the cells were grown in the presence of 80 mM sucrose.[165] One possible explanation is that the sucrose stabilized the defective phosphotransferase in the responding cells.

Genetic Defects in ML-II and ML-III

Phosphotransferase is a complex of three subunits ($\alpha_2\beta_2\gamma_2$) that are the product of two genes, one encoding the α and β subunits and the other encoding the γ subunit[64] (W. Canfield, personal communication). The human gene for α/β contains 22 exons spanning 80 kb on chromosome 12p.[166] It encodes a precursor molecule that undergoes proteolytic cleavage to give rise to the 928 amino acid α and 328 amino acid β subunits that contain 18 and 3 potential Asn-linked glycosylation sites, respectively. The gene for the γ subunit on chromosome 16p encodes a mature protein of 281 amino acids with 2 potential Asn-linked glycosylation sites.[167]

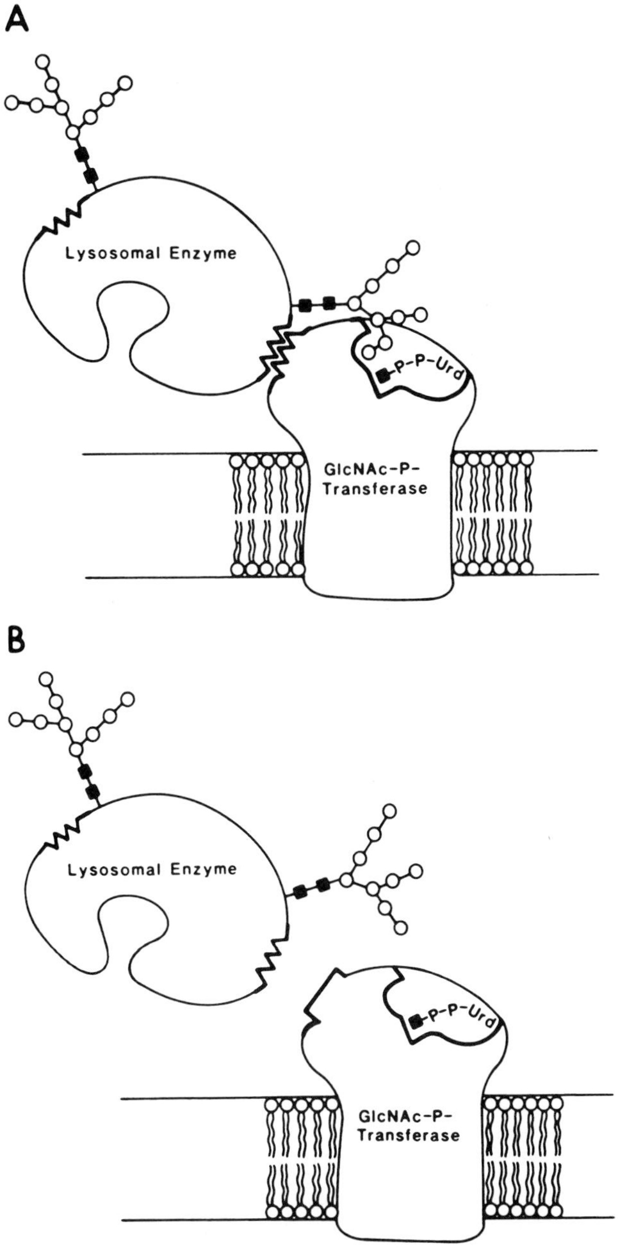

Fig. 138-8 A model for the recognition of lysosomal enzymes by *N*-acetylglucosaminylphosphotransferase. *A.* Enzyme from normal individuals. The proposed protein domain of the lysosomal enzyme that is recognized by the phosphotransferase is represented as ⌇. *B.* Phosphotransferase from individuals with the variant form of ML-III, where the defect appears to be in the recognition of lysosomal enzymes rather than in the catalytic site (*Used with permission from Kornfeld S: Trafficking of lysosomal enzymes.* FASEB J *1:462, 1987.*)

Fibroblasts from four patients with ML-II had no detectable transcripts for the α/β subunit.[166] Amplification of the individual exons showed them to be present, suggesting that the molecular defects in ML-II are point mutations or small deletions. The fibroblasts of two patients with ML-III, complementation group A, had greatly reduced levels of the α/β transcript.[166] This would account for the low level of phosphotransferase activity present in the cells of these patients. The transcript for the γ subunit was present in both instances. In three families with ML-III, complementation group C, an insertion of a single cytosine at codon 167 of the γ-subunit gene was present, resulting in a frameshift with a premature translation termination predicted 107 bp downstream from the insertion.[167] Since this mutation results in a phosphotransferase that is catalytically active but impaired in the ability to recognize lysosomal enzymes as acceptors, it seems likely that the γ-subunit functions in substrate recognition.

Other Biochemical Defects in ML-II and ML-III

While it is now clear that the primary defect in the ML-II and ML-III syndromes is the deficiency of phosphotransferase activity, cells from these patients also exhibit a number of secondary defects. The cells are deficient in the activities of a large number of lysosomal enzymes due to the hypersecretion of these proteins.[3,6–9] In addition, it has been reported that many of the lysosomal enzymes synthesized by the cells show abnormal electrophoretic patterns.[168,169] This may be explained in two ways. First, the sugar side chains are qualitatively different. The addition of mannose 6-phosphate to the oligosaccharide units of the newly synthesized lysosomal enzymes prevents mannose trimming and subsequent complex-type glycosylation of that particular side chain.[170] In the absence of this addition (as in I-cell disease), the nonphosphorylated high-mannose units undergo trimming by mannosidases and become further processed to complex-type units; the result is that the enzymes in these cells differ from their normal counterparts. They show greater "terminal" glycosylation (galactose and sialic acid addition) and thus have more negative charge. Second, polypeptides are also different. Lysosomal enzymes are normally synthesized as preproenzymes; they are proteolytically processed initially in the endoplasmic reticulum by removal of the signal sequence.[171] Later they undergo further proteolytic modification in the lysosome.[172] This lysosomal processing may be related to activation of some enzymes or to stabilization in the acidic environment of the lysosome. In the absence of proper targeting to the lysosome, this processing does not occur. As a result, the enzymes secreted from these cells have higher molecular weights than those normally found for the same enzymes in lysosomes.

Several studies have shown excessive accumulation of free (nonpeptide) cystine in lysosomes of ML-II fibroblasts.[173–176] Such storage is also seen in fibroblasts from patients with benign and nephropathic cystinosis, another inherited lysosomal storage disease (see Chap. 200). It has been suggested that the cystine transport protein that mediates cystine egress from lysosomes may not be processed properly in I-cell lysosomes that lack a full contingent of hydrolytic enzymes. The relationship between the defects in these two cell types is not clear.

Another interesting secondary defect in I-cell disease fibroblasts is the abnormally high content of sialic acid of these cells that seems to confer increased sensitivity to freezing.[177] It has been demonstrated that neuraminidase treatment of the cells prior to preservative freezing in liquid nitrogen enables the cells to adapt more easily to thawing and subsequent subculture.[178]

Several years ago it was reported that β-glucosidase activities were deficient in ML-II fibroblasts when assayed in the absence of detergents but normal when tested in the presence of detergents.[179] It was hypothesized that the decreased β-glucosidase activity was due to the deficiency of an activator protein that could be replaced by detergents in the in vitro assays. Several other activator proteins are known for lysosomal enzymes, and these appear to be located in lysosomes. Inui and colleagues have provided immunologic evidence for a partial deficiency of activator protein for the hydrolysis of G_{M1} ganglioside and sulfatide in skin fibroblasts, liver, and brain of ML-II patients.[180,181] An activator protein that activates β-glucocerebrosidase, β-galactocerebrosidase, and sphingomyelinase also has been shown to be abnormal in ML-II and ML-III fibroblasts.[182,183] All these findings suggest that activator proteins may be targeted to the lysosome in a mannose 6-phosphate-dependent manner and that lysosomal enzymes that are not affected by the primary defect in ML-II and ML-III may exhibit lower enzyme activity than in normal cells due to impaired targeting of their activator proteins.

DIAGNOSIS

Homozygotes

Biochemical confirmation of the diagnosis of ML-II and ML-III can be made in two ways. First, the activities of lysosomal enzymes in serum or in cultured fibroblasts can be measured. In general, a 10- to 20-fold increase in serum β-hexosaminidase, iduronate sulfatase, and arylsulfatase A is diagnostic of these disorders.[30,184,185] If cultured fibroblasts are available, the characteristic pattern of lysosomal enzyme deficiencies may be used, as can the ratio of extracellular to intracellular enzyme activities.[7,30,186,187] The assay of lysosomal enzyme activities in white blood cells is not reliable for this diagnosis because of their mannose 6-phosphate-independent targeting pathway.[188,189] Second, the level of phosphotransferase activity in white blood cells or in cultured fibroblasts can be measured directly.[153,155] As discussed earlier, this assay can now be performed reliably using commercially available substrates.[154,155]

ML-II cannot be distinguished from ML-III on the basis of residual lysosomal enzyme activity or localization, since these are similar in the two disorders.

Prenatal Diagnosis

Prenatal diagnosis of ML-II has been made following amniocentesis using the elevated lysosomal enzyme activity of amniotic fluid and the decreased activity of lysosomal enzymes in cultured amniotic cells as criteria for diagnosis.[41,190–192] This method is considered reliable but usually gives a late second trimester diagnosis (20-22 weeks of pregnancy). However, there is one report of a prenatal diagnosis of ML-II using amniotic fluid obtained at 11 weeks of gestation.[193] There have been two other first trimester prenatal diagnoses of ML-II, following lysosomal enzyme determination on trophoblast biopsy material obtained at 10 weeks of gestation.[194] While it was possible to make the diagnosis on the basis of fresh biopsy material, the authors of the report concluded that diagnosis was more reliable when made on cultured material. Even with the 2- to 4-week delay for cell culture following chorionic villus biopsy, this procedure may be more acceptable than amniocentesis to couples at risk for ML-II. Ben-Yoseph et al. have reported that it is possible to perform phosphotransferase assays on chorionic villi obtained at 9 weeks of gestation.[195] Electron microscopy of chorionic villi has also been used to obtain a rapid diagnosis of ML-II in three prenatal assessments of pregnancies known to be at risk for the disorder.[196] Marked vacuolation in chorionic villus cells was observed in the samples from fetuses that were subsequently proven to have ML-II.

A case of fetal ML-II has been diagnosed in a pregnancy at risk for the disorder by monitoring the serum hexosaminidase level of the mother during pregnancy and comparing this with those of controls not at risk for this disorder.[197] While this preliminary observation needs further investigation, it may be of use as a simple means of early diagnosis of ML-II.[197]

One important complicating factor in the prenatal diagnosis of ML-II is the heterogeneity in lysosomal enzyme expression. It is therefore important to examine carefully the index case fibroblasts in every case.

Heterozygote Identification

Fibroblasts and white blood cells from parents of patients (obligate heterozygotes) have intermediate levels of phosphotransferase activity.[153] These obligate heterozygotes also have somewhat elevated levels of serum β-hexosaminidase compared with normal individuals. The use of these two criteria has allowed the scoring of individuals at risk for the carrier state.[153,155]

It should be stressed that heterozygotes for the complementation group C variant of ML-III (see above) will show normal activity and kinetic parameters when assayed using α-methylmannoside as acceptor substrate.

TREATMENT

There is no specific or definitive treatment for I-cell disease or mucolipidosis III. Generally, the same principles apply that are discussed for the mucopolysaccharidoses (see Chap. 136). Symptomatic treatment of frequent respiratory infections with antibiotics is important. Physical therapy may slow the progression of joint immobility in ML-III patients. Two patients with I-cell disease responded to a limited extent to bone marrow transplantation.[198,199] Although progressive hip disability may require total hip replacement in ML-III, results of long-term follow-up of treated patients are not documented in the literature.

Dr. S. E. Kopits (personal communication, May 1988) indicated that he has had no success with any form of corrective hip reconstruction with prepubertal ML-III patients. Based on his experience, he advises patients to defer hip surgery until after puberty. Total hip replacement has been effective in postpubertal patients with ML-III.

ACKNOWLEDGMENTS

This chapter was authored by Drs. Elizabeth Neufeld and Victor McKusick in the fifth edition and Drs. Catherine Nolan and William Sly in the sixth edition. We gratefully acknowledge the fine example their chapters provided and the clinical illustrations (Figs. 138-1, 138-2, and 138-3) used from their chapters.

REFERENCES

1. Leroy JG, DeMars RI: Mutant enzymatic and cytological phenotypes in cultured human fibroblasts. *Science* **157**:804, 1967.
2. DeMars RI, Leroy JG: The remarkable cells cultured from a human with Hurler's syndrome: An approach to visual selection for in vitro genetic studies. *In Vitro* **2**:107, 1967.
3. Tondeur M, Vamos-Hurwitz E, Mockel-Pohls S, Dereume JP, Cremer N, Loeb H: Clinical, biochemical, and ultrastructural studies in a case of chondrodystrophy presenting the I-cell phenotype in culture. *J Pediatr* **79**:366, 1971.
4. Maroteaux P, Lamy M: La pseudopolydystrophie de Hurler. *Presse Med* **55**:2881, 1966.
5. Taylor HA, Thomas GH, Miller CS, Kelly TE, Siggers D: Mucolipidosis III (pseudo-Hurler polydystrophy): Cytological and ultrastructural observations of cultured fibroblast cells. *Clin Genet* **4**:388, 1973.
6. Lightbody J, Weissmann U, Hadorn B, Herschkowitz N: I-cell disease: Multiple lysosomal-enzyme defect. *Lancet* **1**:451, 1971.
7. Leroy JG, Jo M, McBrinn MC, Zielke K, Jacob J, O'Brien JS: I-cell disease: Biochemical studies. *Pediatr Res* **6**:752, 1972.
8. Hickman S, Neufeld EF: A hypothesis for I-cell disease: Defective hydrolases that do not enter lysosomes. *Biochem Biophys Res Commun* **49**:922, 1972.
9. Wiesmann UN, Lightbody J, Vasella F, Herschkowitz N: Multiple enzyme deficiency due to enzyme leakage. *New Engl J Med* **284**:109, 1971.
10. Wiesmann U, Vasella F, Herschkowitz N: I-cell disease: Leakage of lysosomal enzymes into extracellular fluids. *New Engl J Med* **285**:1090, 1971.
11. Kaplan A, Achord DT, Sly WS: Phosphohexosyl components of a lysosomal enzyme are recognized by pinocytosis receptors on human fibroblasts. *Proc Natl Acad Sci USA* **74**:2026, 1977.
12. Natowicz MR, Chi MM-Y, Lowry OH, Sly WS: Enzymatic identification of mannose 6-phosphate on the recognition marker for receptor-mediated pinocytosis of β-glucuronidase by human fibroblasts. *Proc Natl Acad Sci USA* **76**:4322, 1979.
13. Distler J, Hieber V, Sahagian G, Schmickel R, Jourdian GW: Identification of mannose 6-phosphate in glycoproteins that inhibit the assimilation of β-galactosidase by fibroblasts. *Proc Natl Acad Sci USA* **76**:4235, 1979.
14. Reitman AL, Varki A, Kornfeld S: Fibroblasts from patients with I-cell disease and pseudo-Hurler polydystrophy are deficient in uridine 5′-diphosphate-*N*-acetylglucosamine: Glycoprotein *N*-acetylglucosaminyl-phosphotransferase activity. *J Clin Invest* **67**:1574, 1981.
15. Hasilik A, Waheed A, von Figura K: Enzymatic phosphorylation of lysosomal enzymes in the presence of UDP-*N*-acetylglucosamine:

Absence of the activity in I-cell fibroblasts. *Biochem Biophys Res Commun* **98**:761, 1981.

16. Spranger JW, Wiedemann HR: The genetic mucolipidoses. *Humangenetik* **9**:113, 1970.
17. Bosshard NU, Hubler M, Arnold S, Briner J, Spycher MA, Sommerlade H-J, von Figura K, Gitzelmann R: Spontaneous mucolipidosis in a cat: An animal model of human I-cell disease. *Vet Pathol* **33**:1, 1996.
18. Leroy JG, Spranger JW, Feingold M, Dopitz JM: I-cell disease: A clinical picture. *J Pediatr* **79**:360, 1971.
19. Taber P, Gyepes MT, Philippant M, Ling S: Roentgenographic manifestations of Leroy's I-cell disease. *AJR* **118**:213, 1973.
20. Patriquin HB, Kaplan P, Kind HP, Gideon A: Neonatal mucolipidosis II (I-cell disease): Clinical and radiologic features in three cases. *AJR* **129**:37, 1977.
21. Lemaitre L, Remy J, Farriaux JP, Dhondt JL, Walbaum R: Radiological signs of mucolipidosis II or I-cell disease. *Pediatr Radiol* **7**:97, 1978.
22. Herman TE, McAlister WH: Neonatal mucolipidosis II (I-cell disease) with dysharmonic epiphyseal ossification and butterfly vertebral body. *J Perinatol* **16**:400, 1996.
23. Spritz RA, Doughty RA, Spackman TJ, Murnane MJ, Coates PM, Koldovksy O, Zackai EH: Neonatal presentation of I-cell disease. *J Pediatr* **93**:954, 1978.
24. Cipolloni C, Boldrini A, Dontiett, Maiorana A, Coppa GB: Neonatal mucolipidosis II (I-cell disease): Clinical, radiological and biochemical studies in a case. *Helv Paediatr Acta* **35**:85, 1980.
25. Michels VV, Dutton RV, Caskey CT: Mucolipidosis II: Unusual presentation with a congenital angulated fracture. *Clin Genet* **21**:225, 1982.
26. Whelan DT, Chang PL, Cockshott PW: Mucolipidosis II. The clinical, radiological and biochemical features in three cases. *Clin Genet* **24**:90, 1983.
27. Taylor NG, Shuff RY: I-cell disease: An unusual cause of gingival enlargement. *Br Dent J* **176**:106, 1994.
28. Okada S, Owada M, Sakiyama T, Yutaka T, Ogawa M: I-cell disease: Clinical studies of 21 Japanese cases. *Clin Genet* **28**:207, 1985.
29. Satoh Y, Sakamoto K, Fujibayashi Y, Uchiyama T, Kajiwara N, Hatano M: Cardiac involvement in mucolipidosis: Importance of non-invasive studies for detection of cardiac abnormalities. *Jpn Heart J* **24**:149, 1983.
30. Kelly TE, Thomas GH, Taylor HA: Mucolipidosis III (pseudo-Hurler polydystrophy): Clinical and laboratory studies in a series of 12 patients. *Johns Hopkins Med J* **137**:156, 1975.
31. Umehara F, Matsumoto W, Kuriyama M, Sukegawa K, Gasa S, Osame M: Mucolipidosis III (pseudo-Hurler polydystrophy): Clinical studies in aged patients in one family. *J Neurol Sci* **146**:167, 1997.
32. Brik R, Mandel H, Aizin A, Goldscher D, Ziegler M, Bialik V, Berant M: Mucolipidosis III presenting as a rheumatological disorder. *J Rheumatol* **20**:133, 1993.
33. Freisinger P, Padovani JC, Maroteaux P: An atypical form of mucolipidosis III. *J Med Genet* **29**:834, 1992.
34. Traboulsi E, Maumenee IH: Ophthalmologic findings in mucolipidosis III (pseudo-Hurler polydystrophy). *Am J Ophthalmol* **102**:529, 1986.
35. Spranger JW, Langer LO Jr, Wiedemann H-R: *Bone Dysplasias: An Atlas of Constitutional Disorders of Skeletal Development*. Philadelphia, Saunders, 1974, p 183.
36. Toscano E, Perretti A, Balbi P, Silvestro E, Andria G, Parenti G: Detection of subclinical central nervous system abnormalities in two patients with mucolipidosis III by the use of motor and somatosensory evoked potentials. *Neuropediatrics* **29**:40, 1998.
37. Dawson G, Matalon R, Dorfman A: Glycosphingolipids in cultured human skin fibroblasts: II. Characterization and metabolism in fibroblasts from patients with inborn errors of glycosphingolipid and mucopolysaccharide metabolism. *J Biol Chem* **247**:5951, 1972.
38. Hieber V, Distler J, Jourdian GW, Schmickel R: Accumulation of 35S-mucopolysaccharides in cultured mucolipidosis cells. *Birth Defects* **6**:307, 1975.
39. Thomas GH, Tiller GE Jr, Reynolds LW, Miller CS, Bace JW: Increased levels of sialic acid associated with sialidase deficiency in I-cell disease (mucolipidosis II) fibroblasts. *Biochem Biophys Res Commun* **71**:188, 1976.
40. Strecker G, Peers MC, Michalski JC, Hondi-Assah T, Fournet B, Spik G, Montreuil J, Farriaux J-P, Maroteaux P, Durand P: Structure of nine sialyloligosaccharides accumulate in urine of 11 patients with three different types of sialidosis: Mucolipisosis II and two new types of mucolipidosis. *Eur J Biochem* **75**:390, 1977.
41. Aula P, Rapola J, Autio S, Raivio K, Karjalainen O: Prenatal diagnosis and fetal pathology of I-cell disease (mucolipidosis type II). *J Pediatr* **87**:221, 1975.
42. Erickson RP, Pfleuger OH, Sandman R, Hall BD: Placental pathology in ML II. Selected abstracts: Diseases of connective tissue. *Birth Defects* **11**(6):365, 1975.
43. Rapola J, Aula P: Morphology of the placenta in fetal I-cell disease. *Clin Genet* **11**:107, 1977.
44. Martin JJ, Leroy JG, Farriaux JP, Fontaine G, Desnick RJ, Cabello A: I-cell disease (mucolipidosis II). *Acta Neuropathol (Berl)* **33**:285, 1975.
45. Babcock DS, Bove KE, Hug G, Dignan PSJ, Soukup S, Warren NS: Fetal mucolipidosis II (I-cell disease): Radiologic and pathologic correlation. *Pediatr Radiol* **16**:32, 1986.
46. Pazzaglia UE, Beluffi G, Castello A, Coci A, Zatti G: Bone changes of mucolipidosis II at different ages: Postmortem study of three cases. *Clin Orthop* **276**:283, 1992.
47. Nogami H, Oohira A, Suzuki F, Tsuda K: Cartilage of I-cell disease. *Pediatr Res* **15**:330, 1981.
48. Nagashima K, Sakakibara K, Endo H, Konishi Y, Nakamura N, Suzuki Y, Abe T: I-cell disease (mucolipidosis II): Pathological and biochemical studies of an autopsy case. *Acta Pathol Jpn* **27**:251, 1977.
49. Martin JJ, Leroy JG, Van Eygen M, Ceuterick C: I-cell disease: A further report on its pathology. *Acta Neuropathol (Berl)* **64**:234, 1984.
50. Breningstall GN, Tubman DE: Magnetic resonance imaging in a patient with I-cell disease. *Clin Neurol Neurosurg* **96**:161, 1994.
51. Shanske S, Miranda AF, Penn AS, Dimauro S: Mucolipidosis II (I-cell disease): Studies of muscle biopsy and muscle cultures. *Pediatr Res* **15**:1334, 1981.
52. Kula RW, Shafiq SA, Sher JH, Qazi QH: I-cell disease (mucolipidosis II): Differential expression in satellite cells and mature muscle fibers. *J Neurol Sci* **63**:75, 1984.
53. Castagnaro M, Alroy J, Ucci AA, Jaffe R: Lectin histochemistry and ultrastructure of kidneys from patients with I-cell disease. *Arch Pathol Lab Med* **111**:285, 1987.
54. Peters ME, Arya S, Langer LO, Gilbert EF, Carlson R, Adkins W: Narrow trachea in mucopolysaccharidoses. *Pediatr Radiol* **15**:225, 1985.
55. Stein H, Berman ER, Lioni N, Merin S, Sleskin J, Cohen T: Pseudo-Hurler polydystrophy (mucolipidosis III): A clinical, biochemical, and ultrastructural study. *Isr J Med Sci* **10**:463, 1974.
56. Walter P, Johnson AE: Signal sequence recognition and protein targeting to the endoplasmic reticulum membrane. *Annu Rev Cell Biol* **10**:87, 1994.
57. Rapoport TA, Jungnickel B, Kutay U: Protein transport across the eukaryotic endoplasmic reticulum and bacterial inner membrane. *Annu Rev Biochem* **65**:271, 1996.
58. Kornfeld R, Kornfeld S: Assembly of asparagine-linked oligosaccharides. *Annu Rev Biochem* **54**:631, 1985.
59. Reitman ML, Kornfeld S: UDP-*N*-Acetylglucosamine: Glycoprotein *N*-acetylglucosamine-1-phosphotransferase. *J Biol Chem* **256**:4275, 1981.
60. Waheed A, Hasilik A, von Figura K: UDP-*N*-acetylglucosamine: Lysosomal enzyme precursor *N*-acetylglucosamine-1-phosphotransferase. *J Biol Chem* **257**:12322, 1982.
61. Varki A, Kornfeld S: Identification of a rat liver α-*N*-acetylglucosaminyl phosphodiesterase capable of removing "blocking" α-*N*-acetylglucosamine residues from phosphorylated high mannose oligosaccharides of lysosomal enzymes. *J Biol Chem* **255**:8398, 1980.
62. Waheed A, Hasilik A, von Figura K: Processing of the phosphorylated recognition marker in lysosomal enzymes. *J Biol Chem* **256**:5717, 1981.
63. Varki A, Sherman N, Kornfeld S: Demonstrations of the enzymatic mechanisms of α-*N*-acetyl-d-glucosamine-1-phosphodiester *N*-acetylglucosaminidase (formerly called α-*N*-acetylglucosaminylphosphodiesterase) and lysosomal α-*N*-acetylglucosaminidase. *Arch Biochem Biophys* **222**:145, 1983.
64. Bao M, Booth JL, Elmendorf BJ, Canfield WM: Bovine UDP-*N*-acetylglucosamine: Lysosomal-enzyme *N*-acetylglucosamine-1-phosphotransferase: I. Purification and subunit sturcture. *J Biol Chem* **271**:31437, 1996.
65. Kornfeld R, Bao M, Brewer K, Noll C, Canfield WM: Purification and multimeric structure of bovine *N*-acetylglucosamine-1-phosphodiester α-*N*-acetylglucosaminidase. *J Biol Chem* **273**:23203, 1998.

65a. Kornfeld R, Bao M, Brewer K, Noll C, Canfield WM: Molecular cloning and functional expression of two splice forms of human *N*-acetylglucosamine-1-phosphodiester α-*N*-acetylglucosaminidase. *J Biol Chem* **274**:32778, 1999.
66. Reitman ML, Kornfeld S: Lysosomal enzyme targeting: *N*-acetylglucosaminylphosphotransferase selectively phosphorylates native lysosomal enzymes. *J Biol Chem* **256**:11977, 1981.
67. Bao M, Elmendorf BJ, Booth JL, Drake RR, Canfield WM: Bovine UDP-*N*-acetylglucosamine: Lysosomal-enzyme *N*-acetylglucosamine-1-phosphotransferase: II. Enzymatic characterization and identification of the catalytic subunit. *J Biol Chem* **271**:31446, 1996.
68. Lang L, Reitman ML, Tang J, Roberts RM, Kornfeld S: Lysosomal enzyme phosphoryation: Recognition of a protein-dependent determinant allows specific phosphorylation of oligosaccharides present on lysosomal enzymes. *J Biol Chem* **259**:14663, 1984.
69. Little LE, Alcouloumre M, Drotar AM, Herman S, Robertson R, Yeh RY, Miller AL: Properties of *N*-acetylglucosamine-1-phosphotransferase from human lymphoblasts. *Biochem J* **248**:151, 1987.
70. Baranski TJ, Faust PL, Kornfeld S: Generation of a lysosomal enzyme targeting signal in the secretory protein pepsinogen. *Cell* **63**:281, 1990.
71. Baranski TJ, Koelsch G, Hartsuck JA, Kornfeld S: Identification and molecular modeling of a recognition domain for lysosomal enzyme targeting. *J Biol Chem* **266**:23233, 1991.
72. Baranski TJ, Cantor AB, Kornfeld S: Lysosomal enzyme phosphorylation: I. Protein recognition determinants in both lobes of procathepsin D mediate its interaction with UDP-GlcNAc:lysosomal enzyme *N*-acetylglucosamine-1-phosphotransferase. *J Biol Chem* **267**:23342, 1992.
73. Cuozzo JW, Sahagian GG: Lysine is a common determinant for mannose phosphorylation of lysosomal proteins. *J Biol Chem* **269**:14490, 1994.
74. Cuozzo JW, Tao K, Wu QL, Young W, Sahagian GG: Lysine-based structure in the proregion of procathepsin L is the recognition site for mannose phosphorylation. *J Biol Chem* **270**:15611, 1995.
75. Tikkanen R, Petola M, Oinonen C, Rouvinen J, Peltonen L: Several cooperating binding sites mediate the interaction of a lysosomal enzyme with phosphotransferase. *EMBO J* **16**:6684, 1997.
76. Nishikawa A, Gregory W, Frenz J, Cacia J, Kornfeld S: The phosphorylation of bovine DNase I Asn-linked oligosaccharides is dependent on specific lysine and arginine residues. *J Biol Chem* **272**:19408, 1997.
77. Cuozzo JW, Tao K, Cygler M, Mort JS, Sahagian GG: Lysine-based structure responsible for selective mannose phosphorylation of cathepsin D and cathepsin L defines a common structural motif for lysosomal enzyme targeting. *J Biol Chem* **273**:21099, 1998.
78. Kornfeld S: Structure and function of the mannose 6-phosphate/insulin-like growth factor II receptors. *Annu Rev Biochem* **61**:307, 1992.
79. Hille-Rehfeld A: Mannose 6-phosphate receptors in sorting and transport of lysosomal enzymes. *Biochim Biophys Acta* **1241**:177, 1995.
80. Oshima A, Nolan CM, Kyle JW, Grubb JH, Sly WS: The human cation-independent mannose 6-phosphate receptor. *J Biol Chem* **263**:2553, 1988.
81. Lobel P, Dahms NM, Kornfeld S: Cloning and sequence analysis of the cation-independent mannose 6-phosphate receptor. *J Biol Chem* **253**:2563, 1988.
82. Pohlmann R, Nagel G, Schmidt B, Stein M, Lorkowski G, Krentler C, Cully J, Meyer HE, Grzeschik K-H, Mersmann G, Hasilik A, von Figura K: Cloning of a cDNA encoding the human cation-dependent mannose 6-phosphate specific receptor. *Proc Natl Acad Sci USA* **84**:5575, 1987.
83. Dahms NM, Lobel P, Breitmeyer J, Chirgwin JM, Kornfeld S: 46 kDa mannose 6-phosphate receptor: Cloning, expression, and homology to the 215 kd mannose 6-phosphate receptor. *Cell* **50**:181, 1987.
84. Tong PY, Gregory W, Kornfeld S: Ligand interactions of the cation-independent mannose 6-phosphate receptor: The stoichiometry of mannose 6-phosphate binding. *J Biol Chem* **264**:7962, 1989.
85. Tong PY, Kornfeld S: Ligand interactions of the cation-dependent mannose 6-phosphate receptor: Comparison with the cation-independent mannose 6-phosphate receptor. *J Biol Chem* **264**:7970, 1989.
86. Nadimpalli SK, Schmidt B, von Figura K, Hille E: Antibodies against the cytoplasmic tail can differentiate between the quaternary forms of the M_r 46,000 mannose 6-phosphate receptor. *FEBS Lett* **280**:61, 1991.
87. Sahagian GG, Distler J, Jourdian JW: Characterization of a membrane-associated receptor from bovine liver that binds phosphomannosyl residues of bovine testicular β-galactosidase. *Proc Natl Acad Sci USA* **78**:4289, 1981.
88. Steiner AW, Rome LH: Assay and purification of a solubilized membrane receptor that binds the lysosomal enzyme α-l-iduronidase. *Arch Biochem Biophys* **214**:681, 1982.
89. Hoflack B, Kornfeld S: Purification and characterization of a cation-dependent mannose 6-phosphate receptor from murine P388D1 macrophages and bovine liver. *J Biol Chem* **260**:12008, 1985.
90. Ma Z, Grubb JH, Sly WS: Cloning, sequencing, and functional characterization of the murine 46 kDa mannose 6-phosphate receptor. *J Biol Chem* **266**:10589, 1991.
91. Junghans U, Waheed A, von Figura K: The "cation-dependent" mannose 6-phosphate receptor binds ligands in the absence of divalent cations. *FEBS Lett* **237**:81, 1988.
92. Baba T, Watanabe K, Arai Y: Isolation and characterization of the 36-kDa D-mannose 6-phosphate receptor from porcine testis. *Carbohydr Res* **177**:153, 1988.
93. Watanabe H, Grubb JH, Sly WS: The overexpressed human 46-kDa mannose 6-phosphate receptor mediates endocytosis and sorting of β-glucuronidase. *Proc Natl Acad Sci USA* **87**:8036, 1990.
94. Morgan DO, Edman JC, Standring DN, Fried VA, Smith MC, Roth RA, Rutter WJ: Insulin-like growth factor II receptor as a multi-functional binding protein. *Nature* **329**:301, 1987.
95. MacDonald RG, Pfeffer SR, Coussens L, Tepper MA, Brocklebank CM, Mole JE, Anderson JK, Chen E, Czech MP, Ullrich A: A single receptor binds both insulin-like growth factor II and mannose 6-phosphate. *Science* **239**:1134, 1988.
96. Tong PY, Tollefsen SE, Kornfeld S: The cation-independent mannose 6-phosphate receptor binds insulin-like growth factor II. *J Biol Chem* **263**:2585, 1988.
97. Roth RA, Stover C, Hari J, Morgan DO, Smith MC, Sara V, Fried VA: Interactions of the receptor for insulin-like growth factor II with mannose 6-phosphate receptor. *Biochem Biophys Res Commun* **149**:600, 1987.
98. Waheed A, Braulke T, Junghans U, von Figura K: Mannose 6-phosphate/insulin like growth factor II receptor: The two types of ligands bind simultaneously to one receptor at different sites. *Biochem Biophys Res Commun* **152**:1248, 1988.
99. Kiess W, Blickenstaff GD, Sklar MM, Thomas CL, Nissley SP, Sahagian GG: Biochemical evidence that the type II insulin-like growth factor receptor is identical to the cation-independent mannose 6-phosphate receptor. *J Biol Chem* **263**:9339, 1988.
100. Nolan CM, Kyle JW, Watanabe H, Sly WS: Binding of insulin-like growth factor II (IGF-II) by human cation-independent mannose 6-phosphate receptor/IGF-II receptor expressed in receptor-deficient mouse L cells. *Cell Regul* **1**:197, 1990.
101. Dahms NM, Wick DA, Brzycki-Wessell MA: The bovine mannose 6-phosphate/insulin-like growth factor II receptor: Localization of the insulin-like growth factor II binding site to domains 5–11. *J Biol Chem* **269**:3802, 1994.
102. Garmroudi F, MacDonald RG: Localization of the insulin-like growth factor II (IGF-II) binding/cross-linking site of the IGF-II/mannose 6-phosphate receptor to extracellular repeats 10–11. *J Biol Chem* **269**:26944, 1994.
103. Schmidt B, Kiecke-Siemsen C, Waheed A, Braulke T, von Figura K: Localization of the insulin-like growth factor II binding site to amino acids 1508–1566 in repeat 11 of the mannose 6-phosphate/insulin-like growth factor II receptor. *J Biol Chem* **270**:14975, 1995.
104. Dahms NM, Rose PA, Molkentin JD, Zhang Y, Brzycki, MA: The bovine mannose 6-phosphate/insulin-like growth factor II receptor: The role of arginine residues in mannose 6-phosphate binding. *J Biol Chem* **268**:5457, 1993.
105. Canfield WM, Kornfeld S: The chicken liver cation-independent mannose 6-phosphate receptor lacks the high affinity binding site for insulin-like growth factor II. *J Biol Chem* **264**:7100, 1989.
106. Clairmont KB, Czech MP: Chicken and *Xenopus* mannose 6-phosphate receptors fail to bind insulin-like growth factor II. *J Biol Chem* **264**:16390, 1989.
107. Zhou M, Zhongmin MA, Sly, WS: Cloning and expression of the cDNA of chicken cation-independent mannose-6-phosphate receptor. *Proc Natl Acad Sci USA* **92**:9762, 1995.
108. Roberts DL, Weix DJ, Dahms NM, Kim JJ: Molecular basis of lysosomal enzyme recognition: Three-dimensional structure of the cation-dependent mannose 6-phosphate receptor. *Cell* **93**:639, 1998.
109. Munier-Lehmann H, Mauxion F, Bauer U, Lobel P, Hoflack B: Re-expression of the mannose 6-phosphate receptors in receptor-deficient fibroblasts: Complementary function of the two mannose 6-phosphate

receptors in lysosomal enzyme targeting. *J Biol Chem* **271**:15166, 1996.
110. Filson AJ, Louvi A, Efstratiadis A, Robertson EJ: Rescue of the T-associated maternal effect in mice carrying null mutations in Igf-2 and Igf2r, two reciprocally imprinted genes. *Development* **118**:731, 1993.
111. Koster A, Saftig P, Matzner U, von Figura K, Peters C, Pohlmann R: Targeted disruption of the M_r 46000 mannose 6-phosphate receptor gene in mice results in misrouting of lysosomal proteins. *EMBO J* **12**:5219, 1993.
112. Ludwig T, Ovitt CE, Bauer U, Hollinshead M, Remmler J, Lobel P, Ruther U, Hoflack B: Targeted disruption of the mouse cation-dependent mannose 6-phosphate receptor results in partial missorting of lysosomal enzymes. *EMBO J* **12**:5225, 1993.
113. Wang ZQ, Fung MR, Barlow DP, Wagner EF: Regulation of embryonic growth and lysosomal targeting by the imprinted *Igf2/Mpr* gene. *Nature* **372**:464, 1994.
114. Ludwig T, Eggenschwiler J, Fisher P, D'Ercole AF, Davenport ML, Efstratiadis A: Mouse mutants lacking of the type 2 IGF receptor (IGF2R) are rescued from perinatal lethality in *Igf2* and *Igf1r* null backgrounds. *Dev Biol* **177**:517, 1996.
115. Ludwig T, Munier-Lehmann H, Bauer U, Hollinshead M, Ovitt C, Lobel P, Hoflack B: Differential sorting of lysosomal enzymes in mannose 6-phosphate receptor-deficient fibroblasts. *EMBO J* **13**:3430, 1994.
116. Pohlmann R, Wendland M, Boeker C, von Figura K: The two mannose 6-phosphate receptors transport distinct complements of lysosomal proteins. *J Biol Chem* **270**:27311, 1995.
117. Kasper D, Dittmer F, von Figura K, Pohlmann R: Neither type of mannose 6-phosphate receptor is sufficient for targeting of lysosomal enzymes along intracellular routes. *J Cell Biol* **134**:615, 1996.
118. Sleat DE, Lobel P: Ligand binding specificities of the two mannose 6-phosphate receptors. *J Biol Chem* **272**:731, 1997.
119. Lazzarino DA, Gabel CA: Biosynthesis of the mannose 6-phosphate recognition marker in transport-impaired mouse lymphoma cells: Demonstration of a two-step phosphorylation. *J Biol Chem* **263**:10118, 1988.
120. Griffiths G, Simons K: The trans Golgi network: Sorting at the exit site of the Golgi complex. *Science* **234**:438, 1986.
121. Gonzalez-Noriega A, Grubb JH, Talkad V, Sly WS: Chloroquine inhibits lysosomal enzyme pinocytosis and enhances lysosomal enzyme secretion by impairing receptor recycling. *J Cell Biol* **85**:839, 1980.
122. Creek KE, Sly WS: The role of the phosphomannnosyl receptor in the transport of acid hydrolases to lyosomes, in Dingle JT, Dean RT, Sly WS (eds): *Lysomes in Biology and Pathology*, vol 7. Amsterdam, Elsevier, 1984, p 63.
123. Kornfeld S, Mellman I: The biogenesis of lysosomes. *Annu Rev Cell Biol* **5**:483, 1989.
124. Stein M, Zijderhand-Bleekemoen JE, Geuze H, Hasilik A, von Figura K: *M*r 46,000 mannose 6-phosphate specific receptor: Its role in targeting of lysosomal enzymes. *EMBO J* **6**:2677, 1987.
125. Canfield WM, Johnson KF, Ye RD, Gregory W, Kornfeld S: Localization of the signal for rapid internalization of the bovine cation-independent mannose 6-phosphate/insulin-like growth factor-II receptor to amino acids 24–29 of the cytoplasmic tail. *J Biol Chem* **266**:5682, 1991.
126. Jadot M, Canfield WM, Gregory W, Kornfeld S: Characterization of the signal for rapid internalization of the bovine mannose 6-phosphate/insulin-like growth factor II receptor. *J Biol Chem* **267**:11069, 1992.
127. Trowbridge IS, Collawn JF, Hopkins CR: Signal-dependent membrane protein trafficking in the endocytic pathway. *Annu Rev Cell Biol* **9**:129, 1993.
128. Johnson KF, Chan W, Kornfeld S: The cation-dependent mannose 6-phosphate receptor contains two internalization signals in its cytoplasmic domain. *Proc Natl Acad Sci USA* **87**:10010, 1990.
129. Denzer K, Weber B, Hille-Rehfeld A, von Figura K, Pohlmann R: Identification of three internalization sequences in the cytoplasmic tail of the 46 kDa mannose 6-phosphate receptor. *Biochem J* **326**:497, 1997.
130. Johnson KF, Kornfeld S: A his-leu-leu sequence near the carboxyl terminus of the cytoplasmic domain of the cation-dependent mannose 6-phosphate receptor is necessary for the lysosomal enzyme sorting function. *J Biol Chem* **267**:17110, 1992.
131. Mauxion F, Le Borgne R, Munier-Lehmann H, Hoflack B: A casein kinase II phosphorylation site in the cytoplasmic domain of the cation-dependent mannose 6-phosphate receptor determines the high affinity interaction of the AP-1 Golgi assembly proteins with membranes. *J Biol Chem* **271**:2171, 1996.
132. Chen HJ, Yuan J, Lobel P: Systematic mutational analysis of the cation-independent mannose 6-phosphate/insulin-like growth factor II receptor cytoplasmic domain: An acidic cluster containing a key aspartate is important for function in lysosomal enzyme sorting. *J Biol Chem* **272**:7003, 1997.
133. Johnson KF, Kornfeld S: The cytoplasmic tail of the Man-6-P/IGF-II receptor has two signals for lysosomal enzyme sorting in the Golgi. *J Cell Biol* **119**:249, 1992.
134. Pearse BMF, Robinson MS: Clathrin, adaptors and sorting. *Annu Rev Cell Biol* **6**:151, 1990.
135. Kirchhausen T, Bonifacino JS, Riezman H: Linking cargo to vesicle formation. *Curr Opin Cell Biol* **9**:488, 1997.
136. Vladutiu GD, Rattazzi, M: Excretion-re-uptake route of β-hexosaminidase in normal and I-cell disease cultured fibroblasts. *J Clin Invest* **63**:595, 1979.
137. Owada M, Neufeld EF: Is there a mechanism for introducing acid hydrolases into liver lysosomes that is independent of mannose 6-phosphate recognition? *Biochem Biophys Res Commun* **105**:814, 1982.
138. Waheed A, Pohlmann R, Hasilik A, von Figura K, van Elsen A, Leroy JG: Deficiency of UDP-*N*-acetylglucosamine: Lysosomal enzyme *N*-acetylglucosamine-1-phosphotransferase in organs of I-cell patients. *Biochem Biophys Res Commun* **105**:1052, 1982.
139. Rijnboutt S, Kal AJ, Geuze HJ, Aerts H, Strous GJ: Mannose 6-phosphate-independent targeting of cathepsin D to lysosomes in HepG2 Cells. *J Biol Chem* **266**:23586, 1991.
140. Dicioccio RA, Miller AL: Phosphorylation and subcellular location of α-l-fucosidase in lymphoid cells from patients with I-cell disease and pseudo-Hurler polydystrophy. *Glycobiology* **3**:489, 1993.
141. Glickman JN, Kornfeld S: Mannose 6-phosphate-independent targeting of lysosomal enzymes in I-cell disease B lymphoblasts. *J Cell Biol* **123**:99, 1993.
142. Cardelli JA, Golumbeski GS, Dimond RL: Lysosomal enzymes in *Dictyostelium discoideum* are transported at distinctly different rates. *J Cell Biol* **102**:1264, 1986.
143. Klionsky DJ, Banta LM, Emr SD: Intracellular sorting and processing of a yeast vacuolar hydrolase: The proteinase A propeptide contains vacuolar targeting information. *Mol Cell Biol* **8**:2105, 1988.
144. Aerts JMFG, Brul S, Donker-Koopman WE, van Weely S, Murray GJ, Barranger JA, Tager JM, Schram AW: Efficient routing of glucocerebrosidase to lysosomes requires complex oligosaccharide chain formation. *Biochem Biophys Res Commun* **141**:452, 1986.
145. Waheed A, Gottschalk S, Hille A, Krentler C, Pohlmann R, Braulke T, Hauser H, Geuze H, von Figura K: Human lysosomal acid phosphatase is transported as a transmembrane protein to lysosomes in transfected baby hamster kidney cells. *EMBO J* **7**:2351, 1988.
146. Barriocanal JG, Bonifacino JS, Yuan L, Sandoval IV: Biosynthesis, glycosylation, movement through the Golgi system, and transport to lysosomes by an *N*-linked carbohydrate-independent mechanism of three lysosomal integral membrane proteins. *J Biol Chem* **261**:16755, 1986.
147. Peters C, Braun M, Weber B, Wendland M, Schmidt B, Pohlman R, Waheed A, von Figura K: Targeting of a lysosomal membrane protein: A tyrosine-containing endocytosis signal in the cytoplasmic tail of lysosomal acid phosphatase is necessary and sufficient for targeting to lysosomes. *EMBO J* **9**:3497, 1990.
148. Williams MA, Fukuda M: Accumulation of membrane glycoproteins in lysosomes requires a tyrosine residue at a particular position in the cytoplasmic tail. *J Cell Biol* **111**:955, 1990.
149. Bach G, Barsal R, Cantz M: Deficiency of extracellular hydrolase phosphorylation. *Biochem Biophys Res Commun* **91**:976, 1979.
150. Hasilik A, Neufeld EF: Biosynthesis of lysosomal enzymes in fibroblasts: Phosphorylation of mannose residues. *J Biol Chem* **255**:4946, 1980.
151. Reitman ML, Lang L, Kornfeld S: UDP-*N*-acetylglucosamine: Lysosomal enzyme *N*-acetylglucosamine-1-phosphotransferase. *Methods Enzymol* **107**:163, 1984.
152. Varki A, Reitman ML, Kornfeld S: Identification of a variant of mucolipidosis III (pseudo-Hurler polydystrophy): A catalytically active *N*-acetylglucosaminylphosphotransferase that fails to phosphorylate lysosomal enzymes. *Proc Natl Acad Sci USA* **78**:7773, 1981.
153. Varki A, Reitman ML, Vannier A, Kornfeld S, Grubb JH, Sly WS: Demonstration of the heterozygous state for I-cell disease and pseudo-Hurler polydystrophy by assay of *N*-acetylglucosaminyl phosphotransferase in white blood cells and fibroblasts. *Am J Hum Genet* **34**:719, 1982.

154. Ben-Yoseph Y, Baylerian MS, Nadler HL: Radiometric assays of *N*-acetylglucosaminylphosphotransferase and α-*N*-acetylglucosaminyl phosphodiesterase with substrates labeled in the glucosamine moiety. *Anal Biochem* **142**:297, 1984.
155. Mueller OT, Little LE, Miller AL, Lozzio CB, Shows TB: I-cell disease and pseudo-Hurler polydystrophy: Heterozygote detection and characteristics of the altered *N*-acetylglucosaminephosphotransferase in genetic variants. *Clin Chim Acta* **150**:175, 1985.
156. Honey NK, Mueller OT, Little LE, Miller AL, Shows TB: Mucolipidosis II is genetically heterogeneous. *Proc Natl Acad Sci USA* **79**:7420, 1982.
157. Shows TB, Mueller OT, Honey NK, Wright CE, Miller AL: Genetic heterogeneity of I-cell disease is demonstrated by complementation of lysosomal enzyme processing mutants. *Am J Med Genet* **12**:343, 1982.
158. Mueller OT, Honey NK, Little LE, Miller AL, Shows TB: Mucolipidosis II and III: The genetic relationship between two disorders of lysosomal enzyme biosynthesis. *J Clin Invest* **72**:1016, 1983.
159. Ben-Yoseph Y, Pack BA, Mitchell DA, Elwell DG, Potier M, Melancon SB, Nadler HL: Characterization of the mutant N-acetylglucosaminylphosphotransferase in I-cell disease and pseudo-Hurler polydystrophy: Complementation analysis and kinetic studies. *Enzyme* **35**:106, 1986.
160. Lang L, Takahashi T, Tang J, Kornfeld S: Lysosomal enzyme phosphorylation in human fibroblasts. *J Clin Invest* **76**:2191, 1985.
161. Little LE, Mueller OT, Honey NK, Shows TB, Miller AL: Heterogeneity of *N*-acetylglucosamine 1-phosphotransferase within mucolipidosis III. *J Biol Chem* **261**:733, 1986.
162. Ben-Yoseph Y, Mitchell DA, Yager RM, Wei JT, Chen TH, Shih LY: Mucolipidoses II and III variants with normal *N*-acetylglucosamine 1-phosphotransferase activity toward alpha-methylmannoside are due to nonallelic mutations. *Am J Hum Genet* **50**:137, 1992.
163. Ben-Yoseph Y, Potier M, Pack BA, Mitchell DA, Melancon SB, Nadler HL: Molecular size of *N*-acetylglucosaminyl-phosphotransferase and α-*N*-acetylglucosaminyl phosphodiesterase as determined *in situ* in Golgi membranes by radiation inactivation. *Biochem J* **235**:883, 1986.
164. Ben-Yoseph Y, Potier M, Mitchell DA, Pack BA, Melancon SB, Nadler HL: Altered molecular size of *N*-acetylglucosamine-1-phosphotransferase in I-cell disease and pseudo-Hurler polydystrophy. *Biochem J* **248**:697, 1987.
165. Okada S, Inui K, Furukawa M, Midorikawa M, Nishimoto J, Yabuuchi H, Kato T, Watanabe M, Gasa S, Makita A: Biochemical heterogeneity in I-cell disease: Sucrose-loading test classifies two distinct subtypes. *Enzyme* **38**:267, 1987.
166. Canfield W, Bao M, Pan J, D'Souza A, Brewer K, Pan H, Roe B, Raas-Rothschild A: Mucolipidosis II and mucolipidosis IIIA are caused by mutations in the GlcNAc-phosphotransferace α/β gene on chromosome 12. *Am J Hum Genet* **63**:A15, 1998.
167. Raas-Rothschild A, Cormier-Daire V, Bao M, Genin E, Salomon R, Brewer K, Zeigler M, Mandel H, et al: Truncation of the UDP-*N*-acetylglucosamine: Lysosomal enzyme *N*-acetylglucosamine-1-phosphotransferase γ-subunit gene causes variant mucolipidosis III (pseudo-Hurler polydystrophy). *J Clin Invest*, **105**:673, 2000.
168. Vladutiu GD, Rattazzi MC: Abnormal lysosomal hydrolases excreted by cultured fibroblasts in I-cell disease (mucolipidosis II). *Biochem Biophys Res Commun* **67**:956, 1975.
169. Honey NK, Miller AL, Shows TB: The mucolipidoses: Identification by abnormal electrophoretic patterns of lysosomal hydrolases. *Am J Med Genet* **9**:239, 1981.
170. Goldberg D, Gabel C, Kornfeld S: Processing of lysosomal enzyme oligosaccharide units, in Dingle JT, Dean RT, Sly WS (eds): *Lysosomes in Biology and Pathology*, vol 7. New York, Elsevier, 1994, pp 45–62.
171. Skudlarek MD, Novak EK, Swank RT: Processing of lysosomal enzymes in macrophages and kidney, in Dingle JT, Dean RT, Sly WS (eds): *Lysosomes in Biology and Pathology*, vol 7. New York, Elsevier, 1984, pp 17–43.
172. Hasilik A, von Figura K: Processing of lysosomal enzymes in fibroblasts, in Dingle JT, Dean RT, Sly WS (eds): *Lysosomes in Biology and Pathology*, vol 7. New York, Elsevier, 1984, pp 3–16.
173. Tietze F, Butler JD: Elevated cystine levels in cultured skin fibroblasts from patients with I-cell disease. *Pediatr Res* **13**:1350, 1979.
174. Steinherz R, Makov N, Narinsky R, Meidan B, Kohn G: Comparative study of cystine clearance in cystinotic and I-cell fibroblasts upon exposure to cystine dimethyl ester. *Enzyme* **32**:126, 1984.
175. Greene AA, Jonas AJ, Harms E, Smith ML, Pellett OL, Bump EA, Miller AL, Schneider JA: Lysosomal cystine storage in cystinosis and mucolipidosis type II. *Pediatr Res* **19**:1170, 1985.
176. Tietze F, Rome LH, Butler JD, Harper GS, Gahl WA: Impaired clearance of free cystine from lysosome enriched granular fractions of I-cell disease patients. *Biochem J* **237**:9, 1986.
177. Sly WS, Lagwinska E, Schlesinger S: Enveloped virus acquires the membrane defect when passaged in fibroblasts from I cell disease patients. *Proc Natl Acad Sci USA* **73**:2443, 1976.
178. Vladutiu GD, Fike RM, Amigone VT: Influence of sialic acid on cell surface properties in I cell disease fibroblasts. *In Vitro* **17**:588, 1981.
179. Varon R, Kleijer JW, Thompson EJ, D'Azzo A: Evidence for the deficiency of β-glucosidase-activating factor in fibroblasts of patients with I-cell disease. *Hum Genet* **62**:66, 1982.
180. Inui K, Emmett M, Wenger DA: Immunological evidence for deficiency in an activator protein for sulfatide sulfatase in a variant form of metachromatic leukodystrophy. *Proc Natl Acad Sci USA* **80**:3074, 1983.
181. Inui K, Wenger DA: Biochemical, immunological and structural studies on a sphingolipid activator protein (SAP-1). *Arch Biochem Biophys* **233**:556, 1984.
182. Fujibayashi S, Wenger DA: Studies on a sphingolipid activator protein (SAP-2) in fibroblasts from patients with lysosomal storage diseases, including Niemann-Pick disease type C. *Clin Chim Acta* **146**:147, 1985.
183. Ranieri E, Paton B, Poulos A: Preliminary evidence for a processing error in the biosynthesis of Gaucher activator in mucolipidosis disease types II and III. *Biochem J* **233**:763, 1986.
184. Herd JK, Dvorak AD, Wiltse HE, Eisen JD, Kress BC, Miller AL: Mucolipidosis type III: Multiple elevated serum and urine enzyme activities. *Am J Dis Child* **132**:1181, 1978.
185. Liebaers I, Neufeld EF: Iduronate sulfatase activity in serum, lymphocytes and fibroblasts: Simplified diagnosis of the Hunter syndrome. *Pediatr Res* **10**:733, 1976.
186. Hall CW, Liebaers I, DiNatale P, Neufeld EF: Enzymatic diagnosis of the genetic mucopolysaccharide storage disorders. *Methods Enzymol* **50**:439, 1978.
187. Lie KK, Thomas GH, Taylor HA, Sensenbrenner JA: Analysis of *N*-acetyl-β-d-glucosaminidase in mucolipidosis II (I-cell disease). *Clin Chim Acta* **45**:243, 1978.
188. Kato E, Yokoi T, Taniguchi N: Lysosomal acid hydrolases in lymphocytes of I-cell disease. *Clin Chim Acta* **95**:285, 1979.
189. Tanaka T, Kobayashi M, Fukuda T, Tsuzi Y, Usui T: I-cell disease: Nine lysosomal enzyme levels in lymphocytes and granulocytes. *Hiroshima J Med Sci* **28**:190, 1979.
190. Huijing F, Warren RJ, McLeod AGW: Elevated activity of lysosomal enzymes in amniotic fluid of a fetus with mucolipidosis II (I-cell disease). *Clin Chim Acta* **44**:453, 1973.
191. Matsuda I, Arashuma S, Mitsuyama T, Oka Y, Ikeuchi T, Kaneko Y, Ishikawa M: Prenatal diagnosis of I-cell disease. *Hum Genet* **30**:69, 1975.
192. Gehler J, Cantz M, Stoeckenius M, Spranger J: Prenatal diagnosis of mucolipidosis II (I-cell disease). *Eur J Pediatr* **122**:201, 1976.
193. Poenaru L, Mezard C, Akli S, Oury J-F, Dumez Y, Boue J: Prenatal diagnosis of mucolipidosis type II on first trimester amniotic fluid. *Prenatal Diagn* **10**:231, 1990.
194. Poenaru L, Castelnau L, Dumez Y, Thepot F: First trimester prenatal diagnosis of mucolipidosis II (I-cell disease) by chorionic biopsy. *Am J Hum Genet* **36**:1379, 1984.
195. Ben-Yoseph Y, Mitchell DA, Nadler HL: First trimester prenatal evaluation for I-cell disease by *N*-acetylglucosamine-1-phosphotransferase assay. *Clin Genet* **33**:38, 1988.
196. Carey WF, Jaunzems A, Richardson M, Fong BA, Chin SJ, Nelson PV: Prenatal diagnosis of mucolipidosis II: Electron microscopy and biochemical evaluation. *Prenat Diagn* **19**:252, 1999.
197. Hug G, Bove KE, Soukup S, Ryan M, Bendon R, Babcock D, Warren NS, Dignan PS: Increased serum hexosaminidase in a woman pregnant with a fetus affected by mucolipidosis II (I-cell disease). *N Engl J Med* **311**:988, 1984.
198. Kurobane I, Inoue S, Gotoh Y-H, Kato S, Tamura M, Narisawa K, Tada K: Biochemical improvement after treatment by bone marrow transplantation in I-cell disease. *Tohoku J Exp Med* **150**:63, 1986.
199. Imaizumi M, Gushi K, Kurobane I, Inoue S, Suzuki J, Koizumi Y, Suzuki H, et al: Long-term effects of bone marrow transplantation for inborn errors of metabolism: A study of four patients with lysosomal storage diseases. *Acta Paediatr Jpn* **36**:30, 1994.

CHAPTER 139

α-N-Acetylgalactosaminidase Deficiency: Schindler Disease

Robert J. Desnick ▪ Detlev Schindler

1. Schindler disease is a recently recognized autosomal recessive disorder caused by the deficient activity of α-*N*-acetylgalactosaminidase, a lysosomal hydrolase previously known as α-galactosidase B. The enzymatic defect results in the accumulation of sialylated and asialoglycopeptides, as well as glycosphingolipids and oligosaccharides with α-*N*-acetylgalactosaminyl residues.

2. The disease is clinically heterogeneous; three major phenotypes have been identified. Type I disease is an infantile-onset neuroaxonal dystrophy. The disease has been described in three related infants, two sibs, and a distant cousin. It is characterized by normal development for the first 8 to 15 months of life, followed by a rapid neurodegenerative course resulting in severe psychomotor retardation, cortical blindness, myoclonus, seizures, and a decorticate state by 3 to 4 years of age. Type II disease is an adult-onset disorder characterized by angiokeratoma corporis diffusum and mild intellectual impairment. To date, three affected adults in two unrelated consanguineous families have been identified. Type III disease, described in two sibs and an unrelated child, is an intermediate and variable form with manifestations ranging from seizures and moderate psychomotor retardation in infancy to a milder autistic presentation with speech and language delay, and marked behavioral difficulties in early childhood.

3. Morphologic examination of a cortical brain biopsy from a type I patient revealed abundant "spheroids" in terminal and preterminal axons, the characteristic pathology of a neuroaxonal dystrophy. The type I patients had no histologic evidence of lysosomal pathology, whereas the type II patients had prominent cytoplasmic vacuoles in granulocytes, monocytes, and lymphocytes. Ultrastructural examination of skin from the type II patients revealed numerous cytoplasmic vacuoles containing amorphous or filamentous material in endothelial cells of blood and lymphatic vessels, sweat gland cells, and axons. In contrast, only peripheral blood cells have been examined in type III disease and no vacuolation was observed by electron microscopy.

4. Diagnosis of affected homozygotes and heterozygous carriers can be made by determination of the α-*N*-acetylgalactosaminidase activity in various sources. Affected individuals have abnormal urinary oligosaccharide and glycopeptide profiles. Prenatal diagnosis is feasible by demonstration of the enzymatic defect in chorionic villi or cultured amniocytes.

5. The α-*N*-acetylgalactosaminidase gene has been localized to the chromosomal region 22q13.1 → 13.2. The full-length cDNA and the entire 14-kb gene encoding α-*N*-acetylgalactosaminidase have been isolated and sequenced. Comparison of the human α-*N*-acetylgalactosaminidase and α-galactosidase A genes revealed remarkable homology of their predicted amino acid sequences and positions of their intron-exon junctions, which suggests that they evolved by duplication and divergence from a common ancestral gene. Characterization of the mutations in the α-*N*-acetylgalactosaminidase gene causing the three subtypes revealed a nonsense (E193X) and several missense mutations (S160C, E325K, R329W, and E367K). Transient expression of the type I E325K and the type II R329W alleles revealed that both mutant enzyme subunits were synthesized, but were unstable, the E325K glycopeptide having a shorter half-life. Consistent with this finding, no enzyme protein was immunologically detectable in cultured fibroblasts from either the type I or type II probands who were homoallelic for these mutations.

6. The murine α-*N*-acetylgalactosaminidase gene is highly homologous to the human sequence and was used to produce knockout mice which have α-*N*-acetylgalactosaminidase deficiency, and which pathologically have lysosomal accumlation of substrates with α-*N*-acetylgalactosaminyl residues in neural and visceral tissues with the notable occurrence of "spheroids" in the spinal cord which resemble those seen in Seitelberger disease.

The deficient activity of the lysosomal exoglycosidase, α-*N*-acetylgalactosaminidase (also known as α-galactosidase B), recently was identified in three phenotypically distinct disorders: an infantile neuroaxonal dystrophy (designated type I); a milder, adult-onset disorder characterized by angiokeratoma corporis diffusum, mild intellectual impairment, and peripheral neuroaxonal degeneration (designated type II); and an intermediate and variable form with manifestations ranging from epilepsy and mental retardation in infancy to autistic behavior evident in early childhood (designated type III). All three disease subtypes have very low levels of α-*N*-acetylgalactosaminidase activity, have identical patterns of urinary glycopeptide accumulation, and are inherited as autosomal recessive traits.

Type I disease, first identified in two German brothers of consanguineous descent by Schindler and colleagues,[1–8] is a severe neurodegenerative disorder characterized by early normal development followed by the rapid retrogression of developmental milestones. The affected brothers were cortically blind, had myoclonus, and were profoundly retarded and neurologically impaired by 3 to 4 years of age. A distant cousin, a maternal third cousin and paternal fourth cousin of the original probands (designated 3rd/4th cousin), who also was homoallelic for the same type I mutations, presented with severe

A list of standard abbreviations is located immediately preceding the index in each volume. Additional abbreviations used in this chapter include: $GbOse_5Cer$ = globopentaosylceramide; $GbOse_3Cer$ = globotriaosylceramide; HTF = *Hpa*II tiny fragments.

convulsions, was psychomotor retarded, and died at 1.5 years during a prolonged grand mal seizure. In contrast, type II disease, first described in a 46-year-old consanguineous Japanese woman by Kanzaki and associates,[9,10] was initially reported as an adult-onset form of diffuse angiokeratoma with glycopeptiduria. Following the identification of deficient α-*N*-acetylgalactosaminidase activity as the enzymatic defect,[11] subsequent investigations of the Japanese proband revealed mild intellectual impairment and peripheral neuroaxonal degeneration.[12] Subsequently, two consanguineous Spanish siblings with similar manifestations were reported.[13] Type III disease was first reported in two Dutch sibs; the older infant presented with seizures beginning at 11 months and had evidence of mild psychomotor retardation at 3.8 years of age, while a 3-year-old brother with the enzyme deficiency only had mild clinical involvement.[14,15] More recently, a 7-year-old male of Italian, French, and Albanian ancestry was described who was autistic, thereby expanding the clinical manifestations of the type III phenotype[16] (I. Maire, personal communication).

Limited information is available on the pathologic and biochemical abnormalities in the three subtypes, as the only deceased patient had no autopsy. However, the recent availability of the cDNA and genomic sequences encoding α-*N*-acetylgalactosaminidase[17,18] has permitted the identification of the specific molecular defects in all patients. Of note, the E325K allele that was homoallelic in the German type I infants occurred as one of the mutations in the heteroallelic Dutch and Italian/French/Albanian type III children.[15,19,20] Thus, the clinical spectrum and the morphologic, biochemical, and molecular pathologies of this disease are evolving.

Although there are few recognized cases, this disease is an important "experiment of nature" for several reasons. First, it is the only inherited neuroaxonal dystrophy in which the specific biochemical and molecular defects are known. Presumably, the inherited neuroaxonal dystrophies represent a family of inborn errors involving neuroaxonal transport.[21] That the deficient activity of lysosomal α-*N*-acetylgalactosaminidase leads to neuroaxonal pathology implicates a role for this glycosidase and the lysosomal apparatus in neuroaxonal transport. Second, the occurrence of distinct morphologic findings in the severe infantile type I and milder, later-onset type II patients is unique among lysosomal disorders. Although both type I and type II patients have essentially no α-*N*-acetylgalactosaminidase activity, the characteristic lysosomal inclusions have been observed only in the late-onset type II patients. Limited information is available on the type III probands, but no vacuolated lymphocytes were observed by electron microscopy. That certain mutations in the α-*N*-acetylgalactosaminidase gene cause lysosomal pathology, whereas others do not, is intriguing and suggests that different mutations may alter specific structural domains with unique functions or, alternatively, that modifying factors are responsible for the phenotypic heterogeneity.

Finally, α-*N*-acetylgalactosaminidase is of particular interest because it is a recently recognized member of the lysosomal complex containing α-neuraminidase, β-galactosidase, and the "protective protein" (see Chap. 152). The presence of α-*N*-acetylgalactosaminidase in this complex presumably permits the sequential hydrolysis of *O*-linked oligosaccharides from mucins and various sialylated glycopeptides. That the same sialoglycopeptides accumulate in sialidosis (α-neuraminidase deficiency), galactosialidosis (protective protein deficiency), and the subtypes of Schindler disease,[22] suggests that a completely functional complex is required for the degradation of these *O*-linked glycopeptides. Thus, further characterization of this disease and α-*N*-acetylgalactosaminidase may provide insights into the role of this lysosomal enzyme in neuroaxonal transport, functional domains of the enzyme important for neuroaxonal transport or enzymatic hydrolysis, and the organization of lysosomal enzymes in complexes or "catabolons" for the sequential degradation of certain glycoconjugates.

In the sixth edition of this text,[5] α-*N*-acetylgalactosaminidase deficiency had only been described in type I patients. At that time, this entity was designated by the eponym *Schindler disease*, rather than α-*N*-acetylgalactosaminidase deficiency, which is more cumbersome to use and difficult to recall. Subsequently, the adult-onset type II patients and the type III children were reported, extending the clinical spectrum of the disease. Although the important contributions of Kanzaki, van Diggelen, Chabás, Maire, and others are fully acknowledged, the Schindler disease eponym has been retained for information retrieval and for easier recall.

HISTORICAL ASPECTS

Although this disorder is one of the most recently described, its history is interesting and instructive. Key to the recognition of this entity were physician suspicion, phenotypic clues, and diligent pursuit of the pathologic and biochemical defects. The history of the investigations that led to the delineation of the first type I and II patients is described in the seventh edition of this text.[23] Briefly, Dr. Detlev Schindler, a human geneticist at the University of Wurzburg, recognized the first patients with type I disease in 1985. He sought to define the nature of the metabolic defect in these patients, and in 1987, together with Otto van Diggelen, a biochemist at Erasmus University in Rotterdam, they identified the enzymatic defect as α-*N*-acetylgalactosaminidase deficiency. The subsequent examination of a cortical brain biopsy revealed that the type I disease was a neuroaxonal dystrophy.[3]

The clinical spectrum of this disease was expanded in 1988, when Kanzaki and coworkers described the first type II patient,[9] and then again in 1994, when de Jong et al. reported the first type III patients.[14] Kanzaki's group described a 46-year-old Japanese woman with diffuse angiokeratoma corporis diffusum and glycoaminoaciduria.[9,10,24] Recognizing that the proband's angiokeratoma and sialoglycopeptiduria could be due to the deficient activity of α-*N*-acetylgalactosaminidase, one of us (R.J.D.) contacted Dr. Kanzaki to obtain urine and cultured cells from the proband. Analysis of the urinary glycopeptides from the Japanese proband revealed structures identical to those of the German infantile-onset patients.[22,24,25] Moreover, the demonstration of deficient α-*N*-acetylgalactosaminidase activity in the Japanese proband confirmed the suspicion that she had a milder, adult-onset form of the disease.[11] A second type II family was reported in 1994 by Chabás and coworkers.[13] They described a 42-year-old man and his 38-year-old sister, products of consanguineous marriage, who had angiokeratoma corporis diffusum, lymphedema, and α-*N*-acetylgalactosaminidase deficiency.

de Jong and his colleagues further delineated the clinical heterogeneity of α-*N*-acetylgalactosaminidase deficiency when they reported a 2-year-old girl with epilepsy, mild mental retardation, and α-*N*-acetylgalactosaminidase deficiency.[14] She was identified by routine urinary metabolic screening which revealed oligosaccharide and glycopeptide patterns identical to those of the type I and type II patients. A younger brother, one of twins, also had α-*N*-acetylgalactosaminidase deficiency and developmental delay. More recently, a 7-year-old male of French, Italian, and Albanian descent, who presented with speech and language delay and prominent autistic behavior, was found to have α-*N*-acetylgalactosaminidase deficiency[16] (I. Maire, personal communication). These children delineated a distinct, intermediate phenotype, designated type III disease, because they have onset in infancy or early childhood of mild developmental delay and/or behavioral manifestations rather than the severe neurodegenerative process experienced by the type I patients. Thus, the clinical spectrum of α-*N*-acetylgalactosaminidase deficiency now includes infantile, late infantile/juvenile, and adult-onset subtypes with a broad spectrum of symptoms, presumably related to the nature of the underlying mutations in the α-*N*-acetylgalactosaminidase gene, which encode altered glycopeptides with differing amounts of residual function.

CLINICAL MANIFESTATIONS

Type I Disease

The first cases of type I α-*N*-acetylgalactosaminidase deficiency were recognized in two German brothers, the consanguineous offspring of fourth cousins of German descent.[1–4] The clinical course experienced by these patients was characterized by three stages: (a) apparently normal development in the first 9 to 12 months; (b) a period of developmental delay followed by rapid regression starting in the second year of life; and (c) increasing neurologic impairment resulting by 3 to 4 years of age in cortical blindness, spasticity, myoclonus, decorticate posturing, and profound psychomotor retardation.

Both affected brothers were the products of normal pregnancies, labors, and deliveries. Their early development was normal. They both sucked vigorously, had reactive smiles at 6 weeks, and began play activity at 2 to 3 months of life. They rolled over at 4 months, sat at 6.5 months, and bottle-fed themselves by 7 and 9 months, respectively (Fig. 139-1). The older affected brother crawled at 9.5 months and from 12 to 15 months of life developed the ability to walk independently for short distances, climb on chairs, use a spoon, and say up to 10 different words. The younger sib was more developmentally impaired. He was never able to stand from a sitting position, to crawl, or to learn any words.

Sudden falling episodes and startle reactions at 12 months signaled clinical onset of the disease in the older brother. In the younger sib, grand mal seizures began at 8 months and occurred 5 times over the next 6 months. Maximal development was achieved at 15 months in both brothers. Thereafter, each experienced rapid regression, the younger brother deteriorating at a faster rate. Both developed strabismus, nystagmus, optic atrophy, muscular hypotonia, and frequent myoclonic movements. By 3 to 4 years of age, both brothers exhibited profound psychomotor retardation and spasticity, were immobile, and had decorticate postures, cortical blindness, and little, if any, contact with the environment.

The physical findings of the affected brothers were essentially identical after 4 to 5 years of age. Both had decorticate posturing, marked flexion contractures of the joints, and frequent myoclonus (Fig. 139-2). They had no voluntary movements and were essentially unresponsive to stimuli. They did not appear to hear or see. The older brother was normocephalic, and his height and weight were at the fiftieth percentile for age. In contrast, the younger brother had a head circumference which was −1 SD for height, a height at the third percentile, and a weight below the third percentile for age. Neurologic examination of both sibs revealed symmetric hyperreflexia, muscular hypotonia and hypertonia,

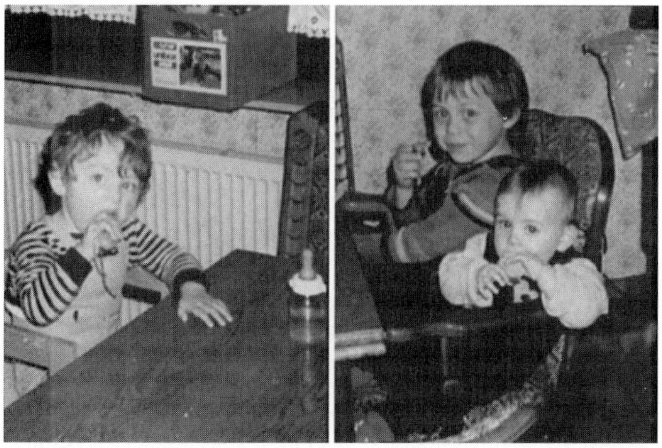

Fig. 139-1 The affected sibs with type I disease at 2.3 years (left) and at 1 year (right).

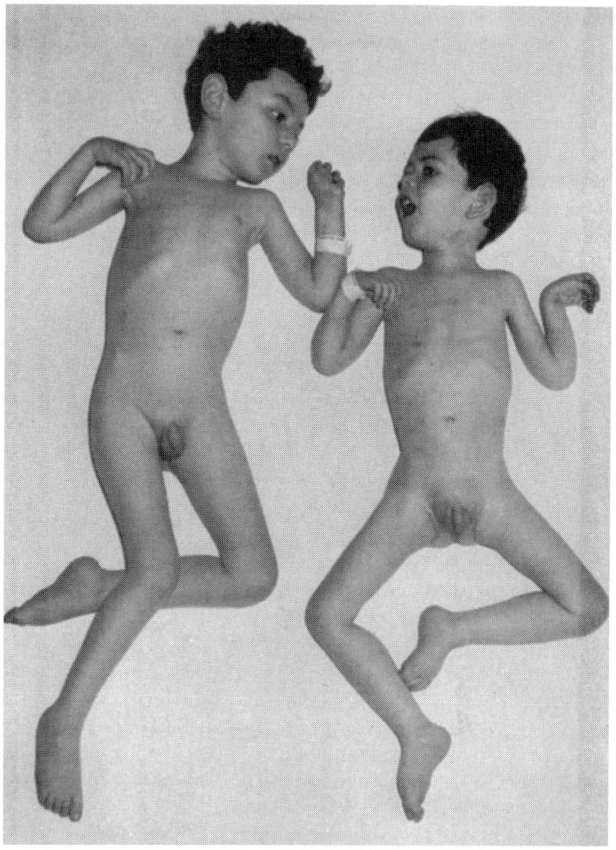

Fig. 139-2 The affected sibs at 5 years 3 months (left) and at 4 years (right). (*From Schindler et al.[3] Used with permission.*)

rigidity, reduced muscle mass, and bilateral optic atrophy. Their developmental skills were at the newborn level. There were no other visceral signs of a storage disease; their facies were normal, there were no macular, corneal, or lenticular lesions, nor were organomegaly, dysostosis multiplex, or dermatologic abnormalities present. At 11 and 12 years of age, the brothers remain in a similar vegetative state with essentially no contact with their environment. They have extremely reduced muscle and bone masses and severe contractures at all extremities. They are also incontinent, dependent on tube feeding, and require frequent nasopharyngeal suctioning. They have survived several episodes of intercurrent pneumonias, primarily because of the diligent nursing efforts of their parents.

Routine laboratory studies, including complete blood counts and blood and cerebrospinal fluid chemistries, were all within normal limits. The older brother's blood group was A; the younger brother's was O. Skeletal X-ray studies revealed systemic, diffuse, severe osteopenia and bilateral subluxation of the hips. Brain CT and MRI studies showed marked atrophy of the cerebellum, brain stem, and cervical spinal cord. The optic tracts, cranial nerves, and cerebral gray and white matter were hypotrophic; the generalized atrophy also involved the supratentorial cortical structures. These findings were consistent with an overall reduced cerebral glucose metabolism compared to normal values for age, seen on positron emission tomography (PET) using 2-[^{18}F]fluoro-2-deoxy-D-glucose (Fig. 139-3).[26] Regional cerebral glucose metabolism decreased directly with the degree of brain atrophy seen on MRI. Supratentorial cortical regions showed asymmetrical hypometabolism, whereas infratentorial structures (cerebellar hemispheres, brain stem, mesencephalon, and hypothalamus), which were predominantly affected by the atrophic process, revealed a more distinct, symmetrical hypometabolism. There was a moderate relative increase of regional glucose metabolism in the lentiform nucleus and the head of the caudate similar to that

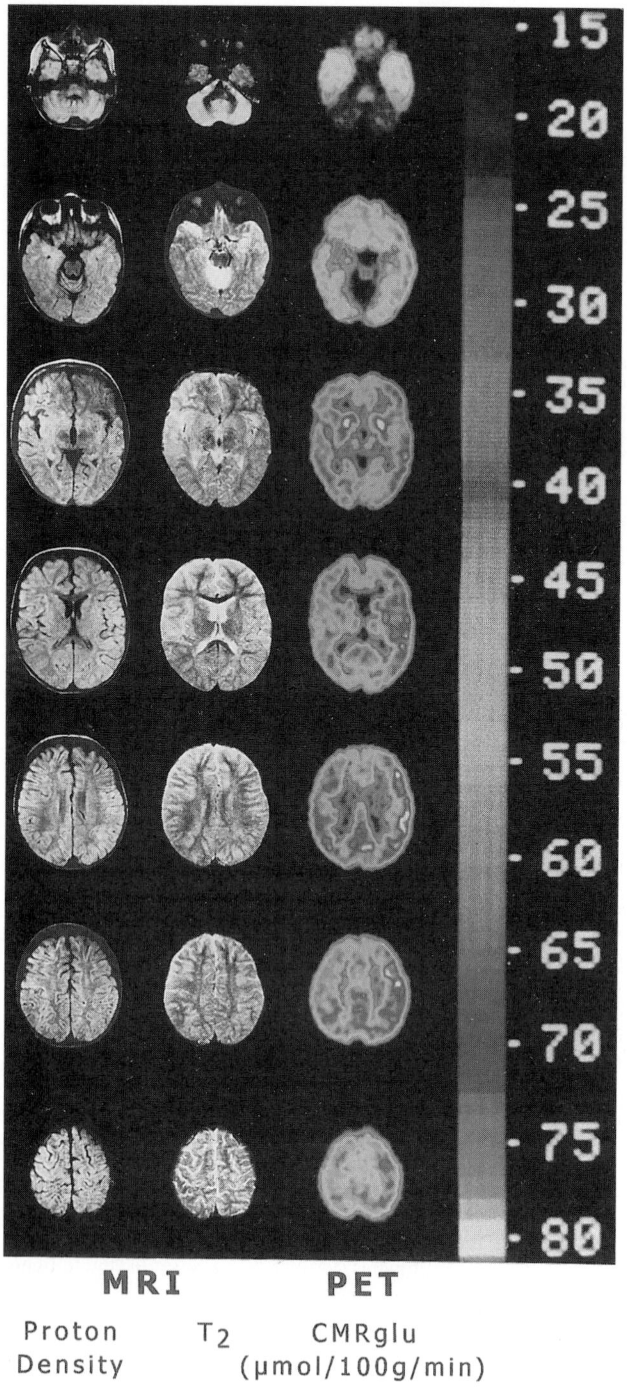

Fig. 139-3 MRI axial plane sections and corresponding representative transaxial FDG-PET scans of the younger German sib with type I disease at age 4 years showing the degree and distribution of brain atrophy. (*From Rudolf et al.*[26] *Used with permission.*)

described in other neurodegenerative disorders associated with active epilepsy. The EEG showed diffuse dysfunction with multifocal irritative features, such as isolated spikes and spike-wave complexes. Quantitative EEG and brain mapping revealed marked slowing, especially in the central, parietal, and occipital regions. Brain stem auditory, somatosensory, and visual-evoked potentials showed low amplitude, delayed responses, or both, but suggested some informational processing.

An infant cousin of the affected German sibs was diagnosed after he was deceased.[15] This patient was the consanguineous product of an uneventful pregnancy and developed normally for the first 6 months of life. At 7 months, he experienced several grand mal seizures, most occurring during febrile episodes associated with respiratory tract infections. Little or no development was noted from 15 to 18 months of age and he died unexpectedly at 18 months of life from apnea during a prolonged convulsion. The diagnosis of α-*N*-acetylgalactosaminidase deficiency was made on plasma and cultured fibroblasts from skin preserved shortly after his death when the relationship to the first patients was recognized. However, no autopsy was performed.

Type II Disease

Type II α-*N*-acetylgalactosaminidase deficiency was initially described in a 46-year-old Japanese female with angiokeratoma corporis diffusum and glycopeptiduria.[9–12] A disseminated petechiae-like eruption was first noted on the proband's lower torso at about 28 years of age. The eruption spread slowly over her body, including her face and extremities, essentially in a distribution typical to that of hemizygotes with Fabry disease (see Chap. 150). She was the product of a first-cousin marriage, and there was no family history of individuals with similar dermatologic findings. The proband was married, had two normal children, and worked in a hospital as a nurse's aide.

At diagnosis, she had a slightly coarse facies with an enlarged nasal tip, depressed nasal bridge, and thick lips. Dermatologic examination revealed dry skin, which was densely peppered with tiny, deep red to purple maculopapules ranging in diameter from <1 to 3 mm. The lesions were distributed over her entire body, including the face and fingers, but they were denser on the axillae, breasts, lower aspects of the abdomen, groin, buttocks (Fig. 139-4), and upper aspects of the thighs. Similar telangiectasias were noted on the lips, and on the oral and pharyngeal mucosa. Dilated blood vessels were also present on the ocular conjunctiva, and were observed with a corkscrew-like tortuosity in the fundi. No retinal hemorrhages, macular changes, or corneal opacities were present. Endoscopic examination revealed telangiectasia on the gastric mucosa. There was no organomegaly,

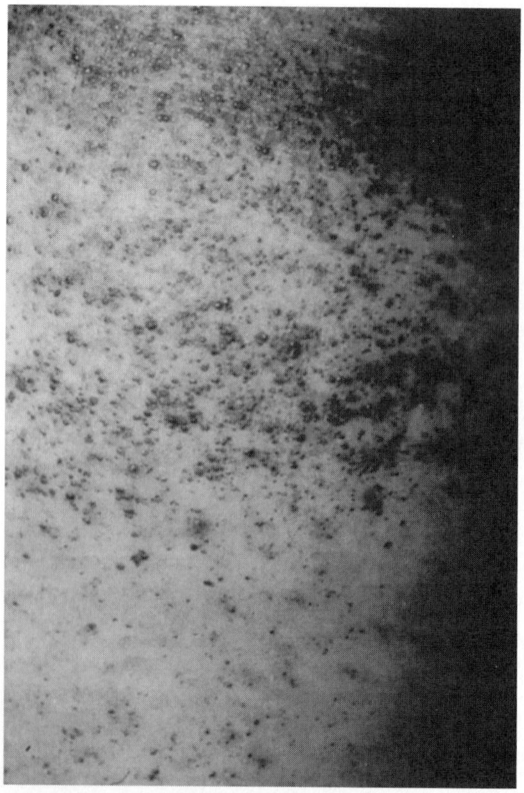

Fig. 139-4 Distribution and density of angiokeratoma on the back thigh of the Japanese proband with type II disease. (*From Kanzaki et al.*[12] *Used with permission.*)

lymphadenopathy, or skeletal abnormality. The neurologic examination was within normal limits, although the patient had a dull affect and was mentally slow.

Routine laboratory studies were all normal, including complete blood cell counts and liver enzymes, serum urea nitrogen, creatinine, electrolytes, blood glucose, and serum protein. The patient's blood group was A_1. Urinalysis was negative for glucose and protein; the urinary amino acids and acid mucopolysaccharides were within normal limits. Results of various endocrine studies, a chest radiograph, and a skeletal X-ray survey also were normal. Cardiac examination revealed a normal sinus rhythm, and the electrocardiographic findings were normal both at rest and with exercise.

Psychometric evaluation revealed a low intelligence quotient (IQ 70) using the Wechsler adult intelligence scale. Verbal IQ was 66 and performance IQ was 83. The EEG and CT findings of the brain were unremarkable. MRI of the brain revealed a few small lacunar infarctions; no gross atrophy of the parenchyma was observed. Nerve conduction studies of the right peroneal nerve, where the patient complained of numbness, revealed normal conduction amplitude and velocity in the motor fibers. However, there was a marked decrease in amplitude (0.5 μV; normal = 1.2 to 9 μV) with normal velocity in the sensory fibers. Similar results were obtained from the right median nerve. Electromyographic findings of the muscles innervated by these nerves were normal. These results were indicative of peripheral neuroaxonal degeneration.

Recently, Chabás et al. reported two adult sibs with type II disease, the offspring of consanguineous Spanish parents.[13] At diagnosis, the 42-year-old male had slightly coarse facies with thick lips and an enlarged nasal tip. Lymphedema of his lower extremities, first noted at 10 to 14 years of age, was progressive, and hyperkeratosis developed. Subsequently, the patient noted punctate red cutaneous lesions between his umbilicus and upper thighs. A skin biopsy showed angiectases in the upper dermis indicative of angiokeratoma corporis diffusum. At age 30, the patient had a pain crisis in his right leg and paresthesias in his left arm, the latter probably due to the carpal tunnel syndrome.

On physical examination, pertinent findings included a left ventricular hypertrophy with normal heart rate and rhythm, tortuosity of the conjunctival and retinal vessels, and a diffuse haziness in the corneal epithelium. Neurologic examination showed normal muscle mass and tonus, and symmetric reflexes. Nerve conduction studies of motor fibers in the right peroneal nerve and the median nerves were normal, as was the conduction of sensory fibers in the left median nerve. Psychometric evaluation revealed an intelligence quotient in the lower normal range (IQ = 84) with normal verbal IQ, but decreased performance IQ. Laboratory test results, including hepatic and renal function studies, were normal. The patient's blood type was A. Urinary sediment analysis for glycolipids was normal.

His 38-year-old sister's course was similar, as she had progressive lymphedema and mild angiokeratoma corporis diffusum involving her abdomen, breasts, and gingival mucosa. She also had tortuosity of her conjunctival vessels and blood group A. Other studies were not performed.

Type III Disease

Three children with α-*N*-acetylgalactosaminidase deficiency from two unrelated families were described with an intermediate phenotype, designated type III disease[14,16] (I. Maire, personal communication). In a Dutch family, two sibs were affected. The older female was essentially well until she experienced severe asymmetric convulsions at 11 months of age. She had a high fever, which precipitated uncontrollable grand mal seizures, and attacks of apnea and bradycardia, which required admission to an intensive care unit. Although the fever and convulsions responded to medication, a few days after detubation she developed pneumonia, a high fever, sepsis, and multiple organ failure from which she slowly recovered. Psychomotor retardation was noted later. She walked by herself and spoke only single words at 21 months. On examination at age 2, mild psychomotor retardation and strabismus were observed. At 2.4 years of age, she had four convulsions, mostly associated with fever, despite treatment with antiepileptic drugs. She did not have dysmorphic features, organomegaly, cutaneous lesions, or vacuolated lymphocytes. A CT scan of the brain appeared normal at age 2. The diagnosis was made by the characteristic urinary oligosaccharide and glycopeptide patterns and by the demonstration of α-*N*-acetylgalactosaminidase deficiency in fibroblasts and leukocytes.

Her younger brother was also affected. At 9 months of age, his developmental performance was reported to be within normal limits, but probably less advanced than that of his twin sister.[14] At age 4 years, he had some developmental delay, particularly in language skills, but neurologic tests had not been performed.[15] Of interest, the mother was an effectively treated epileptic, and epilepsy also occurred in the father's family.

A third patient with type III disease was recently recognized in France[16] (I. Maire, personal communication). This patient was the only child of unrelated parents of French, Italian, and Albanian descent. Pregnancy, labor, and delivery were uneventful. The boy's early development was reportedly normal; however, he sat alone at 9 months and walked independently at 18 months. His parents sought medical advice when the boy reached age 2 as he neither spoke nor engaged or interacted with others. On physical examination, at age 6, he had no dysmorphic features, organomegaly, skeletal or cutaneous abnormalities, or abnormal neurologic findings. Weight, height, and head circumference were at −0.5 SD for age. He was characterized as having a restless attitude, diminished attention span, emotional instability and irritability, and fits of anger with stereotyped and ritualistic behavior. His intellectual development was impaired and he only had rudimentary syntax. These behavioral findings led to the diagnosis of autism.

Brain MRI and spinal X-rays were unremarkable. Psychometric evaluation was difficult because of his behavior. His intelligence quotient was markedly decreased (IQ = 48), with a verbal IQ of 58 and a performance IQ of 46. Routine laboratory studies, including complete blood cell counts, blood glucose, serum electrolyte and protein concentration, and liver enzymes, were all within normal limits. Vacuolated lymphocytes were not found in blood smears. Serum and urinary amnio acid profiles were normal, as were the urinary organic acids.

PATHOLOGY

Type I Disease

In the type I probands, the major pathologic finding was the remarkable neuropathology (Fig. 139-5), which characterized the disease as a neuroaxonal dystrophy.[3] Of equal note was the absence of the visceral abnormalities typically observed in most lysosomal storage diseases. In fact, light and electron microscopic studies of peripheral blood cells, aspirated and biopsied bone marrow, conjunctiva, jejunal mucosa, muscle, liver, and sural nerve of the type I probands were all essentially normal. The absence of storage material in these visceral tissues was not surprising, because similar findings occur in Tay-Sachs disease, in which the lysosomal deposits are almost exclusively observed in neural cells. The ultrastructural observation of alterations in autonomic axons of the myenteric plexus from a rectal biopsy first raised the possibility of neuronal pathology. The abnormal material was "tubular" and appeared to be free in the cytoplasm of dystropic axons (Fig. 139-6). These changes were not uniformly observed in other axons and were initally considered possibly due to nonspecific axonal degeneration. Subsequently, a neocortical biopsy from the older sib revealed innumerable abnormal structures[27] (Figs. 139-5*A* and 139-5*B*). These structures stained intensely with toluidine blue, ranged up to 50 μm in greatest dimension, and were distributed throughout the neocortex without

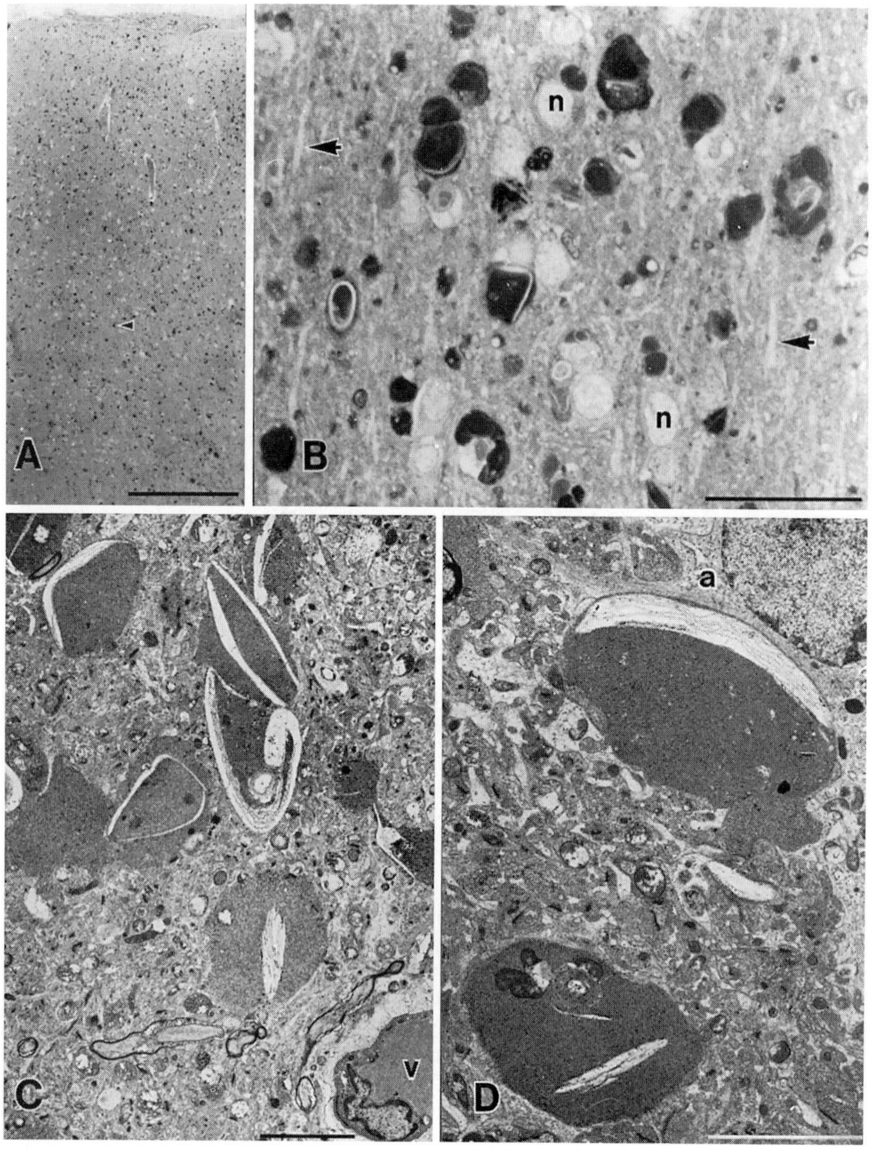

Fig. 139-5 Spheroids in neocortical biopsy: *A,* Abundance, and uniform distribution of spheroids (darkest dots, arrowhead) throughout cortex; plane of section normal to pial surface (top); semithin section, toluidine blue, ×45, bar = 500 μm. *B-D,* Spheroids occupy neuropil and display characteristic numbers, density, dimensions, configurations, and content of various organelles and optically empty acicular clefts: *B,* Pale neuronal nuclei (n) and apical dendrites (arrows) give orientation; semithin section, toluidine blue, ×634, bar = 50 μm. *C,* Profiles of at least 11 spheroids lie in neocortical neuropil near a small blood vessel (v); ×3840, bar = 5 μm. *D,* Two dense spheroids in neuropil that is otherwise morphologically normal; one spheroid apposes an astrocytic perikaryon (a); ×6240, bar = 5 μm. (*From Wolfe et al.*[27] *Used with permission.*)

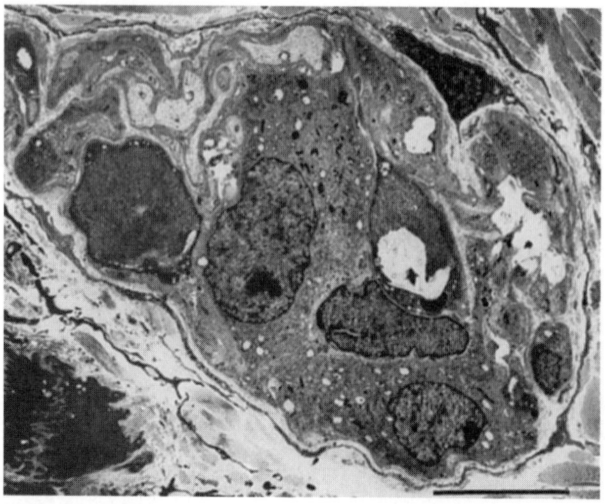

Fig. 139-6 Rectal myenteric ganglion: Two axonal spheroids with electron-lucent clefts in autonomic ganglion cells in the myenteric plexus of a rectal biopsy; ×7000, bar = 10 μm. (*From Schindler et al.*[3] *Used with permission.*)

apparent laminar or columnar organization; they became rare at the corticomedullary junction, and were not identified in deeper white matter. They displayed rounded, polygonal, or faceted contours and had heterogeneous contents. Many contained conspicuous acicular clefts with circular, ovoid, crescentic, boomerang-shaped, jagged, or spicular profiles (Fig. 139-5*B*).

By electron microscopy, the abnormal structures in the neocortical neuropil comprised membranous arrays and organelles, bound externally by a plasma membrane facing an epithelial interspace (Figs. 139-5*C* and 139-5*D*). The occurrence of these structures surrounded by gyres of compact myelin, and the presence of presynaptic elements, defined them as preterminal and terminal axonal spheroids, respectively, the neuropathologic hallmark of the neuroaxonal dystrophies. The ultrastructure of these membranous axonal spheroids was complex and heterogeneous. Three components predominated: (a) the tubulovesicular array, an elaborate membranous maze of ramifying irregular tubules; (b) the lamelliform array, comprising aperiodically angulated, sharply defined membranes describing loops, whorls, meandering profiles, and semiparallel arrays, and (c) acicular clefts, conspicuous by light and electron microscopy (Figs. 139-5*C* and 139-5*D*). Various other axoplasmic elements also occurred in variable numbers in many spheroids, including mitochondria,

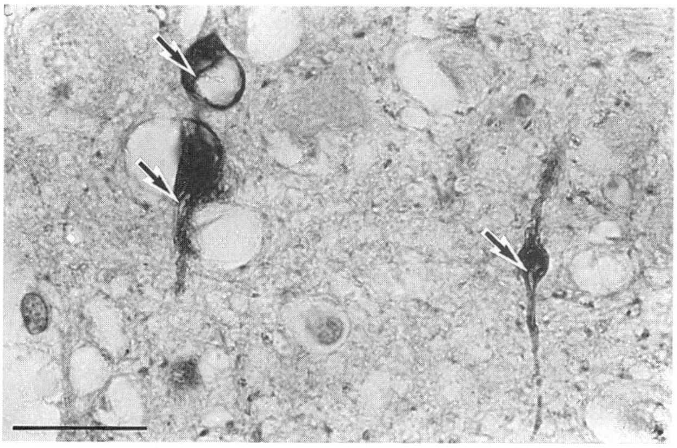

Fig. 139-7 Axonal spheroids in neocortical neuropil are GABAergic and strongly immunoreact with peroxidase-linked antibodies to glutamic acid decarboxylase (anti-GAD). Semithin section, hematoxylin-eosin counterstain; ×1386, bar = 20 μm. (*From Schindler et al., unpublished data.*)

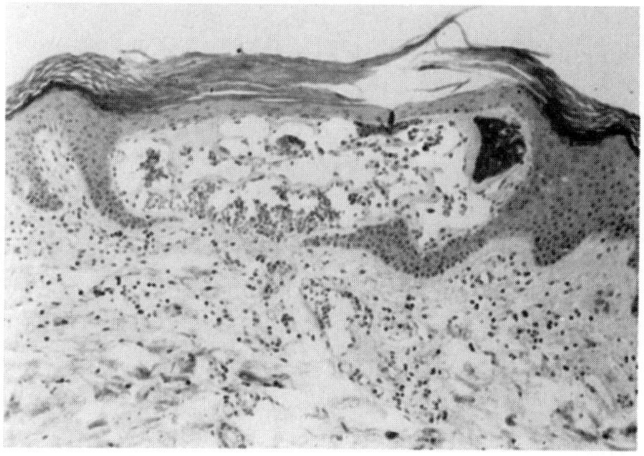

Fig. 139-8 Histopathology of a skin lesion from the Japanese type II proband showing hyperkeratosis of the epidermis and dilated capillaries in the upper dermis (semithin section, hematoxylin-eosin counterstain, ×60). (*From Kanzaki et al.*[12] *Used with permission.*)

compound lipid droplets, glycogen particles, granulated vesicles, rare microtubules, and small heterogeneous dense bodies. Compared to adjacent normal preterminal axons, telodendria, and perikaryal cytoplasm, the cytoplasmic matrix in the axonal speroids was diffusely electron-dense, pervaded by osmiophilic amorphous or finely granular material. Unambiguous neurofilaments were not observed, consistent with the nonargyrophilic nature of the spheroids. Neurons appeared normal in number, laminar distribution, and perikaryal and dendritic contour. Meganeurites, or profiles suggestive of storage, were not identified in neurons or in any other cell type in the neocortical biopsy. Astrocytosis was not observed.

Based on the neocortical findings, the rectal biopsies from the affected type I sibs were reexamined in greater detail. Membranous axonal spheroids were identified in the myenteric plexus and ganglionic neuropil from both siblings.[27,28] The autonomic axonal spheroids displayed the same basic ultrastructure as the central spheroids described above.

A particularly striking finding was that the neocortical axonal spheroids occurred in GABAergic neurons,[29] as demonstrated by their detection with antibodies to glutamic acid decarboxylase (anti-GAD) (Fig. 139-7). Long-term persistence of axonal spheroids in GABAergic neurons and GABAergic cell loss has been related to defective GABAergic circuits.[30] Mental retardation, movement disorders, and other motor deficits, as well as seizures, are secondary to defects in inhibitory GABAergic neurotransmission or occur following selective dropout of these inhibitory neurons, or both.[31] It is likely that the selective compromise of the inhibitory GABAergic connectivity is an important factor underlying the brain dysfunction in this disease.

Notably, high-magnification electron microscopy of various cell types, including cultured fibroblasts from the affected brothers, revealed the presence of inclusions with lamellar, filamentous, and granular material in single membrane-bound organelles. This observation, of pleomorphic inclusion bodies and the demonstration of *Helix pomatia* lectin-positive inclusions in cultured fibroblasts,[2] clearly demonstrated that lysosomal storage does occur in type I disease, although only in fibroblasts to date.

It is notable that very similar axonal spheroids have been observed in Seitelberger disease,[32–36] Hallervorden-Spatz disease,[21,37,38] and other forms of inherited neuroaxonal dystrophy. Plasma, lymphoblasts, and/or fibroblasts from over 10 unrelated patients with Seitelberger disease, diagnosed by ultrastructural examination, were not deficient in α-*N*-acetylgalactosaminidase activity.[3] Because the clinical, pathologic, and ultrastructural manifestations in Seitelberger disease are similar to those in Schindler disease, it is likely that some patients diagnosed with infantile neuroaxonal dystrophy actually had type I disease.

Type II Disease

In Giemsa-stained peripheral blood smears from the proband with type II disease, small cytoplasmic vacuoles were observed in granulocytes, monocytes, and lymphocytes. These vacuoles did not stain positive with periodic acid-Schiff, alcian blue, or toluidine blue. Histopathologic examination of the skin lesions showed localized hyperkeratosis and dilated thin-walled blood vessels[11,12] (Fig. 139-8). Dilated lymphatic vessels were observed in the mid dermis as well as the upper dermis.

Ultrastructural examination of both involved and uninvolved skin revealed numerous cytoplasmic vacuoles in several cell types, including endothelial cells in blood and lymphatic vessels, pericytes, fibroblasts, fat cells, Schwann cells, axons, arrector smooth-muscle cells, and eccrine sweat gland cells. They were most prominent in vascular endothelial cells (Fig. 139-9) and the

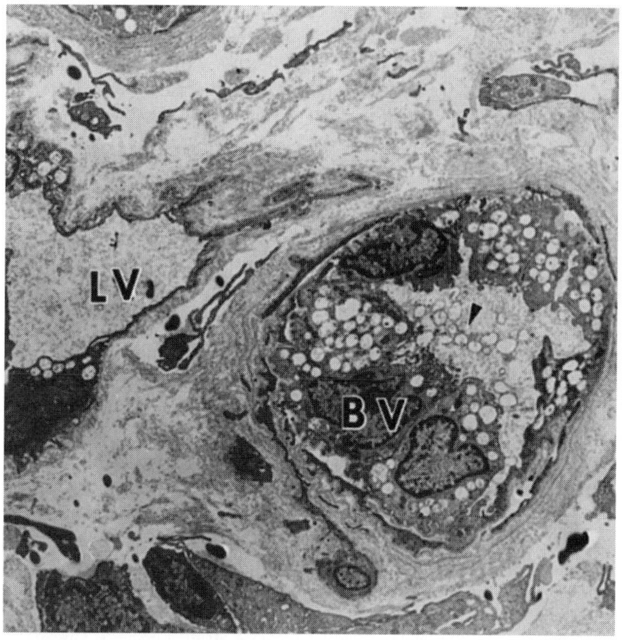

Fig. 139-9 Electron micrograph showing numerous vacuoles in endothelial cells of blood vessels (BV) and dilated lymphatic vessels (LV) from the Japanese type II proband (×2000). (*From Kanzaki et al.*[12] *Used with permission.*)

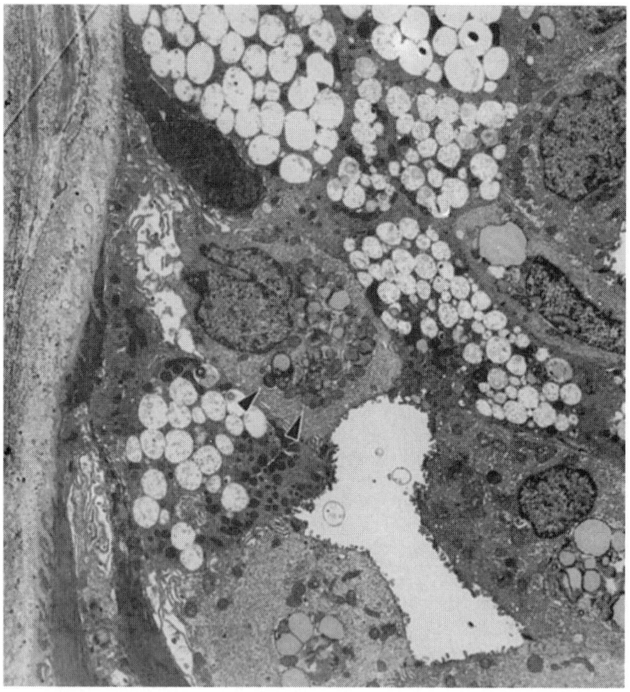

Fig. 139-10 Electron micrograph of the secretory portion of eccrine sweat gland cells showing numerous vacuoles in cytoplasm. Arrowheads point to vacuoles containing electron-dense lamellated structures (×2000). (*From Kanzaki et al.*[12] *Used with permission.*)

secretory portion of sweat gland cells (Fig. 139-10). These clear membrane-lined vacuoles were empty or contained filamentous material. Electron-dense multilayered structures were observed only in vacuoles of the sweat gland cells. Vascular endothelial cells of the kidney had similar lysosomal vacuolization as those in skin, but the epithelial cells appeared normal. Similar, but smaller, vacuoles also were observed in peripheral leukocytes.

Type III Disease

To date, the pathologic examination of type III disease has been limited to peripheral blood cells. In the Dutch sibs, histologic and electron microscopic examination of lymphocytes, granulocytes, and monocytes were normal and no vacuolation was observed.[14] Similar findings were noted in the French type III patient.[16]

THE METABOLIC DEFECT

Nature of the Accumulated Glycoconjugates

The deficient activity of α-*N*-acetylgalactosaminidase (EC 3.2.1.49) in all disease subtypes leads to an accumulation of glycoconjugates with terminal α-*N*-acetylgalactosaminyl moieties in various tissues and fluids. Table 139-1 lists some of the major α-*N*-acetylgalactosaminyl-containing glycoconjugates detected in normal human tissues. α-*N*-Acetylgalactosaminyl residues occur in *O*-linked and *N*-linked glycopeptides and glycoproteins (e.g., mucins, blood group A substances), in glycosphingolipids (e.g., Forssman glycolipid), and in proteoglycans (e.g., cartilage keratan sulfate II).[39–41] Potentially, each of these compounds can be the source of substrates that accumulate in this disease. However, the nature and concentrations of the accumulating glycoconjugate substrates in tissues of patients with α-*N*-acetylgalactosaminidase deficiency remain the subject of investigation, because all of the identified patients with this disease are living (except for a type I patient diagnosed retrospectively and not autopsied[15]), and the only sources available for analysis have been urine, blood, tissue biopsies, and cultured cells.

Glycopeptides and Glycoproteins. Glycopeptides and glycoproteins with *O*-linked oligosaccharide moieties accumulate in patients with α-*N*-acetylgalactosaminidase deficiency.[22,24,25,42] Various structures containing *O*-linked α-*N*-acetylgalactosaminyl moieties are shown in Table 139-1. The mucins most commonly contain a Galβ(1 → 3)Gal*N*Acα(1 → O)Ser/Thr core structure and additional *N*-acetylneuraminyl, fucosyl, *N*-acetylglucosaminyl and/or galactosyl residues.[43–46] In addition, a variety of *N*-linked glycopeptides and glycoproteins contain α-*N*-acetylgalactosaminyl moieties, including the predominant *N*-linked glycopeptide structure in human erythrocytes, which has a complex-type triantennary oligosaccharide composed of 20 to 30 residues with a terminal A blood group trisaccharide.[39]

High-resolution thin-layer chromatography of the excreted urinary glycopeptides accumulated in patients with all three subtypes revealed four major compounds that were identified by comigration with known standards[1,3,10,13,14,22] (Fig. 139-11); these glycopeptides were further characterized by structural analyses.[24,25,42,47,48] For example, the structure of the tetrasaccharide monopeptide below was determined at high resolution without prior derivatization from urine of the two type I-disease siblings by electrospray mass spectrometry.[42] The structures of the accumulated glycopeptides are shown in Table 139-2.

The type I proband who was blood group A-positive also excreted the blood group A trisaccharide at a concentration about fivefold greater than that in age-matched normal urines[1] (Table 139-2). The urine from the type I and II patients also contained the dipeptide tetrasaccharide, NeuNAcα(2 → 3)Galβ(1 → 3)[NeuNAcα(2 → 6)]GalNAcα(1 → O)-Thr-Pro.[24,25,47] In addition, amino acid analysis of the peptide moiety of this urinary sialoglycopeptide from the type I patients revealed threonine, serine, proline, glycine, and glutamic acid in a molar ratio of 6.3 : 2.7 : 2.6 : 1.7 : 1.0.[25] It is assumed that the structures of the excreted glycopeptides and oligosaccharides in the type III patients are identical to those in the type I and II patients. However, the amounts of the accumulating glycopeptides and oligosaccharides in the urine of patients with each subtype (except type I) have not been reported, nor have the nature and concentrations of the glycopeptides and/or oligosaccharides accumulating in tissues been reported.

The structures of the accumulated sialoglycopeptides in the urines of the type I and II patients were remarkably similar to those excreted by patients with sialidosis (isolated α-neuraminidase deficiency)[49] and galactosialidosis (combined α-neuraminidase and β-galactosidase deficiencies) due to mutations in the gene encoding the protective protein.[50] The fact that most of the same sialoglycopeptides accumulate in these disorders suggests that *O*-linked sialoglycopeptides of the mucin type are hydrolyzed by the α-neuraminidase/β-galactosidase/protective protein complex, which also appears to contain α-*N*-acetylgalactosaminidase.[51,52] It is intriguing to speculate that mutations in any one of the enzymes can alter the ability of this complex to degrade substrates that would normally be sequentially hydrolyzed by each of these exoglycosidases (see below).

Glycosphingolipids. Glycosphingolipids with α-*N*-acetylgalactosaminyl residues include those with blood group A activity and the Forssman glycolipid. The blood group A glycosphingolipids are characterized by the terminal blood group A-specifying trisaccharide, GalNAcα(1 → 3)Gal(2← 1)αFuc.[53] They contain varying numbers of internal Galβ(1 → 3)GlcNAcβ(1 → 3) (type I) and/or Galβ(1 → 4)GlcNAcβ(1 → 3) (type 2) units and the core structure, Galβ(1 → 4)Glcβ(1 → 1′)Cer.[39,54,55] In humans, Forssman antigen has been detected in low amounts in normal lung and was increased fivefold in lung carcinomas, regardless of blood type.[56,57] Forssman antigen also has been found in intestinal mucosal carcinoma, but not in normal mucosal cells.[58] The complete chemical synthesis of this neutral glycosphingolipid has been accomplished.[59]

Table 139-1 Various Glycoconjugates Containing α-N-Acetylgalactosaminyl Residues

	Structure	Trivial Name	References
O-Linked Glycopeptides:	Galβ(1→3)GalNAcα(1→O)-Ser/Thr		39,40
	NeuAcα(2→6)GalNAcα(1→O)-Ser/Thr		40
	NeuAcα(2→3)Galβ(1→3)GalNAcα(1→O)-Ser/Thr		40
	Fucα(1→2)Galβ(1→3)GalNAcα(1→O)-Ser/Thr		39,43
	Fucα(1→2)Galβ(1→4)GlcNAcβ(2→6)\ GalNAcα(1→O)-Ser/Thr Fucα(1→2)Galβ(1→3)/		43
	Galβ(1→4)\ GlcNAcβ(2→6)\ Fucα(1→2)/ GalNAcα(1→O)-Ser/Thr Galβ(1→3)/	SSEA-1 determinant	43
	NeuAcα(2→6)\ GalNAcα(1→3)\ GalNAcα(1→O)-Ser/Thr Galβ(1→3)/ Fucα(1→2)/	Blood group A mucin	39
N-Linked Glycopeptides:	GalNAcα(1→3)\ R↓ Galβ(1→4)[GlcNAcβ(1→3)Galβ(1→4)]ₙGlcNAcβ(1→2)Manα(1→6)\ Fucα(1→6)\ Fucα(1→2)/ R↓ Manβ(1→4)GlcNAcβ(1→4)GlcNAc Asn Fucα(1→2)Galβ(1→4)[GlcNAcβ(1→3)(1→3)Galβ(1→4)]ₙGlcNAcβ(1→2)Manα(1→3)/ NeuACGalβ(1→4)GlcNAcβ(1→6)\ / [GlcNAcβ(1→3)Galβ(1→4)]ₙGlcNAcβ(1→4)	Blood group AHi glycopeptide	39
Glycosphinogolipids:	GalNAcα(1→3)\ Galβ(1→3)GlcNAcβ(1→3)Galβ(1→4)Glcβ(1→1′)Cer Fucα(1→2)/	A^a Type 1 chain	53–55
	GalNAcα(1→3)\ Galβ(1→4)GlcNAcβ(1→3)Galβ(1→4)Glcβ(1→1′)Cer Fucα(1→2)/	A^a Type 2 chain	53–55
	GalNAcα(1→3)GalNAcβ(1→3)Galα(1→4)Galβ(1→4)Glcβ(1→1′)Cer	Forssman antigen	56–59
Mucopolysaccharide:	R—β(1→3)Galβ(1→4)GlcNAcβ(1→6)\ GalNAcα(1→O)-Ser/Thr NeuAcα(2→3) Galβ(1→3)/	Keratan sulfate, type II	41

R = Peptide portion of proteoglycan.

The individual neutral glycosphingolipids in plasma, erythrocytes, urinary sediment, and a cortical biopsy from the type I German sibs were quantitatively analyzed and were found to be within their respective normal ranges.[3] The metabolism of the endogenous neutral glycosphingolipids in cultured fibroblasts from the type I patients has been investigated in greater detail using [^{14}C]galactose to label these compounds metabolically.[60] There were no significant differences in glycosphingolipid biosynthesis or degradation in the cultured cells from the type I patients and normal individuals. High-resolution thin-layer chromatographic analysis of the individual glycolipids revealed virtually identical steady state compositions. Forssman glycosphingolipid was not detected in normal or type I disease fibroblasts using a very sensitive immuno-overlay technique with monoclonal anti-Forssman antibody.[60] The addition of α-N-acetylgalactosaminyl-containing glycolipids including [ceramide-^{3}H]Forssman glycosphingolipid, the more water-soluble fluorescent C_6-NBD-lyso-Forssman glycolipid, and the blood group A derivative neoglycolipid, GalNAc(Fuc)GalPEN [^{14}C]Ac, to cell extracts or cultured fibroblasts from the type I patients resulted in the accumulation of these substrates, consistent with the enzymatic defect.

The degradation of blood group A glycosphingolipid, A-6-2, Gal*N*Acα(1 → 3)(Fucα(1 → 2)(Gal*β*(1 → 4)Glc*N*Ac*β*(1 → 3) Gal*β* (1 → 4)Glc*β*(1 → 1′)Cer, [^{3}H]-labeled in its ceramide moiety, also has been studied in cultured fibroblasts from patients with α-N-acetylgalactosaminidase deficiency.[61] In normal cells, the expected metabolites included various less-polar products and some lipids resulting from reuse of the the liberated sphingosine, mainly sphingomyelin and phosphatidylcholine. In α-N-acetylgalactosaminidase-deficient cells, blood group glycolipid A-6-2 was not degraded. It has been estimated that approximately 0.5 mg of the blood group glycolipids are degraded per day.[61] Thus, a significant amount of blood group A-active glycolipids would accumulate in blood type A or AB patients. Although overt neutral glycosphingolipid accumulation was not detected in cultured fibroblasts, plasma, erythrocytes, urinary sediment, or cerebral cortex from the blood type A type I patient, it is possible that individual α-N-acetylgalactosaminyl-containing glycosphingolipids, including the blood group A glycolipids, may accumulate in various tissues and cause disease pathology. However, disease manifestations due to such glycosphingolipid accumulation may be insignificant, but the analysis of the tissue glycolipids in type I patients is required to provide this information.

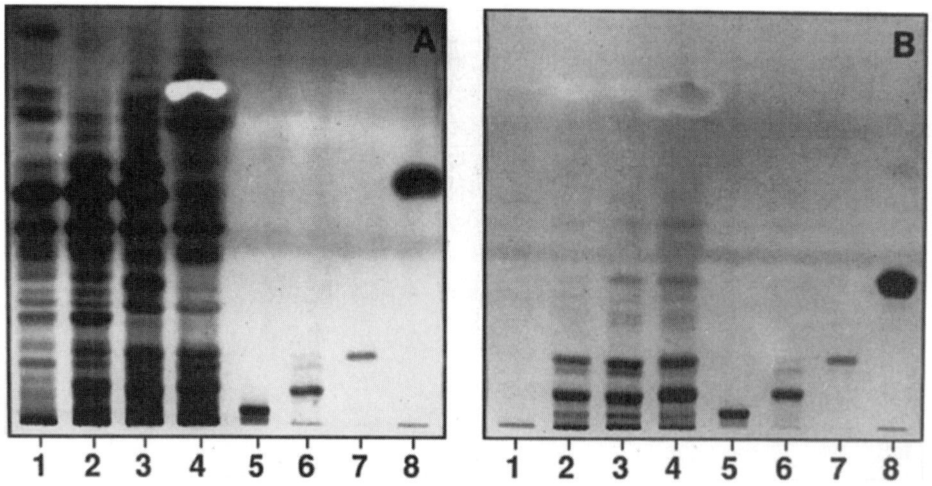

Fig. 139-11 Thin-layer chromatographic profiles of urinary oligosaccharides (A) and glycopeptides (B) from a normal individual (lane 1), the affected brothers with type I disease (lanes 2 and 3), and the Japanese female with type II disease (lane 4). The four major abnormal glycopeptide bands in the patients' urine comigrated with the glycopeptide standards, NeuNAcα(2 → 3)Galβ(1 → 3)[NeuNAcα(2 → 3)Galβ(1 → 4)GlcNAcα(2 → 6)]GalNAcα(1 → O)-Ser/Thr (lane 5), NeuNAcα(2 → 3)Galβ(1 → 3)[Neu-NAcα(2 → 6)]GalNAcα(1→O)-Ser/Thr (lane 6), NeuNAcα(2→3)Galβ(1→3)GalNAcα(1→O)-Ser/Thr (lane 7), GalNAc (lane 8A), and GalNAcα(1 → O)-Ser/Thr (lane 8B). (*From Schindler et al.*[22] *Used with permission.*)

Glycosaminoglycans. A keratan sulfate type II mucopolysaccharide containing an *O*-linked α-*N*-acetylgalactosaminyl residue has been identified in normal human skeletal cartilage.[41] To date, the accumulation of this mucopolysaccharide in skeletal cartilage from α-*N*-acetylgalactosaminidase-deficient patients has not been investigated. In addition, the urinary glycosaminoglycans in patients with all three disease subtypes were not increased, and the glycosaminoglycan metabolism in cultured fibroblasts from type I patients was normal when assayed by [^{35}S]sulfate pulse-chase studies.[3]

α-*N*-Acetylgalactosaminidase: The Enzymatic Defect

The deficient activity of lysosomal α-*N*-acetylgalactosaminidase is the specific enzymatic defect in types I, II, and III Schindler disease.[1–5,7,11,12] Initially, the enzymatic defect was identified in the type I patients by determining the pNP-αGalNAc activity in plasma, leukocytes, and cultured fibroblasts from the affected sibs and other family members.[1,2] Using this assay, the affected type I sibs had apparent residual activities of less than 2 percent of the respective normal mean values, and their heterozygous parents had reduced activities at the lower end of the normal range. Subsequent assays performed with the more sensitive fluorogenic substrate, 4-methylumbelliferyl-α-D-*N*-acetylgalactosaminide (4MU-αGalNAc),[3,62] detected 0.5 to 2 percent residual activity in plasma, cultured fibroblasts, or cultured lymphoblasts from the affected type I, II, and III patients and provided significantly improved heterozygote discrimination[3,11–14,63] (Table 139-3).

Immunologic studies have been conducted to further characterize the nature of the enzymatic defect in the patients with type I, II, and III probands using monospecific rabbit antihuman α-*N*-acetylgalactosaminidase antibodies raised against the homogeneous lung enzyme (see "Purification" under "Human α-*N*-Acetylgalactosaminidase" below).[3,11] Immunoblotting studies revealed two bands of cross-reactive immunologic material (CRIM), estimated to be 48 and 117 kDa, respectively, in the purified enzyme preparation. The same two bands were present in fibroblast extracts from obligate heterozygotes and normal individuals (Fig. 139-12), consistent with the occurrence of monomeric and homodimeric forms of the normal enzyme (see "Physical Properties" under "Human α-*N*-Acetylgalactosaminidase" below). Immunoblotting revealed the absence of detectable enzyme protein in fibroblast extracts from patients with all three subtypes;[3,11,15] that neither immunoreactive band was detectable

Table 139-2 Accumulated Urinary Compounds in Types I and II Schindler Disease

Oligosaccharide	
Blood group A trisaccharide*	Ga1NAα(1 → 3) Gal (2← 1) αFuc
Glycopeptides	
1	GalNAcα (1 → O)-Ser/Thr
2	NeuNAcα (2 → 3) Galβ (1 → 3) GalNAcα (1 → O)-Ser/Thr
2a	Galβ(1 → 3) [NeuNAcα (2 → 6] GalNAcα(1 → O)-Ser/Thr
3	NeuNAcα(2 → 3) Galβ (1 → 3) [NeuNAcα (2 → 6)] GalNAcα (1 → O)-Ser/Thr Pro
3a	NeuNAcα (2 → 3) Galβ (1 → 3) [NeuNAcα (2 → 6)] GalNAcα (1 → O)-Thr/Thr Pro
4	NeuNAcα (2 → 3) Galβ (1 → 3) [NeuNAcα (2 → 3)] GalNAcβ (1 → 4) GlcNAcβ (1 → 6) GlcNAcα (1 → O)-Ser/Thr
4a	Galβ (1 → 3) [NeuNAcα (2 → 3] Galβ (1 → 3) [Galβ (1 → 4) GlcNAcβ (1 → 6)] GalNAcα (1 → O)-Ser/Thr
4b	NauNAcα(2 → 3) Galβ (1 → 3) [Galβ (1 → 4) GlcNAcβ (1 → 6)] GalNAcα (1 → O)-Ser/Thr
5	(NeuNAc)$_2$ (Galβ (1 → 4) GlcNAc)$_2$ Galβ (1 → 3) GlcNAcα(1 → O)-Ser/Thr

Only in patients with blood group A.[1,25]
Glycine and glutamic acid also have been found on this glycopeptide.[25,47,48]

Table 139-3 α-*N*-Acetylgalactosaminidase Activity in Schindler Disease Subtypes

Source	*Plasma* (Percent of Normal Enzyme Activity)	*Lymphoblasts*	*Fibroblasts*
Type I disease			
German family[3,5]			
Affected homozygote, sib	0.5	0.5	0.7
Affected homozygote, sib	1.1	0.7	1.2
Normal, brother	120.0	77.8	69.3
Heterozygote, mother	53.0	31.5	24.2
Heterozygote, father	53.0	29.4	41.2
Heterozygote, maternal uncle	54.9	39.8	—
Affected homozygote, cousin	1.1	—	1.0
Type II disease			
Japanese family[11,12]			
Affected homozygote	1.1	0.4	0.7
Normal husband	93.4	117.0	—
Heterozygote, son	65.2	39.1	23.2
Heterozygote, daughter	64.1	22.0	—
Heterozygote, sib	26.0	36.4	45.2
Heterozygote, sib	55.4	19.6	51.7
Heterozygote, sib	49.0	32.6	67.5
Spanish family[13]			
Affected homozygote, sib	0.5	—	0.7
Affected homozygote, sib	—	—	1.6
Type III disease			
Dutch family[14]			
Affected homozygote, sib	4.0	—	5.0
Affected homozygote, sib	3.0	—	—
Normal sister	104.0	—	—
Heterozygote, mother	32.0	—	—
Heterozygote, father	26.0	—	—
French family[16]			
Affected homozygote	—	—	2.0
Normal individuals*			
	(nmol/h/ml)	(nmol/h/mg protein)	
Mean ± 1 SD	18.4 ± 5.1	44.5 ± 11.2	213.5 ± 56.1
Range	10.9 – 30.0	21.7 – 63.4	141.3 – 350.7
n	104	50	34

*Assayed with mM 4MU-α-GalNAc.

suggested that the two enzyme forms were encoded by the same gene (see Fig. 139-12). These findings also indicated that the enzymatic deficiency in all three subtypes resulted from different mutations that impaired enzyme synthesis or stability, consistent with the fact that only a small amount (<2 percent) of α-*N*-acetylgalactosaminidase activity was detected in cells from the affected patients.

Human α-*N*-Acetylgalactosaminidase

Previously, human α-*N*-acetylgalactosaminidase was known as lysosomal α-galactosidase B.[64–70] The confusion concerning the substrate specificity of this enzyme originally resulted from the use of artificial substrates in the identification and determination of the enzymatic defect in Fabry disease.[71–75] In 1970, Kint[71] was the first to use *p*-nitrophenyl-α-D-galactopyranoside (pNP-αGal) and 4-methylumbelliferyl-α-D-galactopyranoside (4MU-αGal) to demonstrate the marked, but not total, deficiency of α-galactosidase activity in hemizygotes with Fabry disease (see Chap. 150). Kint[71,76,77] and others[72–75,78–80] subsequently demonstrated that two enzymes cleaved the synthetic, water-soluble pNP-αGal and 4MU-αGal substrates. One enzyme, designated α-galactosidase A, was thermolabile and inhibited by myoinositol, while the other, designated α-galactosidase B, was thermostable, had a higher K_m toward artificial galactosides, and was not inhibited by myoinositol. α-Galactosidase A was deficient in Fabry disease, whereas α-galactosidase B was responsible for the residual α-galactosidase activity in Fabry hemizygotes when water-soluble substrates were used.[71–75,81,82]

Electrophoretic and isoelectric focusing studies revealed multiple forms of α-galactosidase A in various sources from normal individuals, the major components having pI values of 4.3 to 5.1.[79,83–85] In contrast, only a single form of α-galactosidase B was observed with a pI value of about 4.4.[79,83–85] Neuraminidase treatment of normal α-galactosidase A or B in crude tissue extracts and in purified preparations converted the multiple α-galactosidase A forms to a single activity band at pI 5,[83,86] whereas the migration of α-galactosidase B was not altered by neuraminidase treatment.[74,83,85–89] These and other findings initially suggested that α-galactosidases A and B were enzyme forms with similar substrate specificities that differed in their glycosylation.[73,74,76,77,89] In addition, partially purified human α-galactosidase B was shown to hydrolyze, albeit very inefficiently, the natural glycosphingolipid substrate, globotriaosylceramide, when incubated in the presence of a heat-stable glycoprotein activator.[87,90]

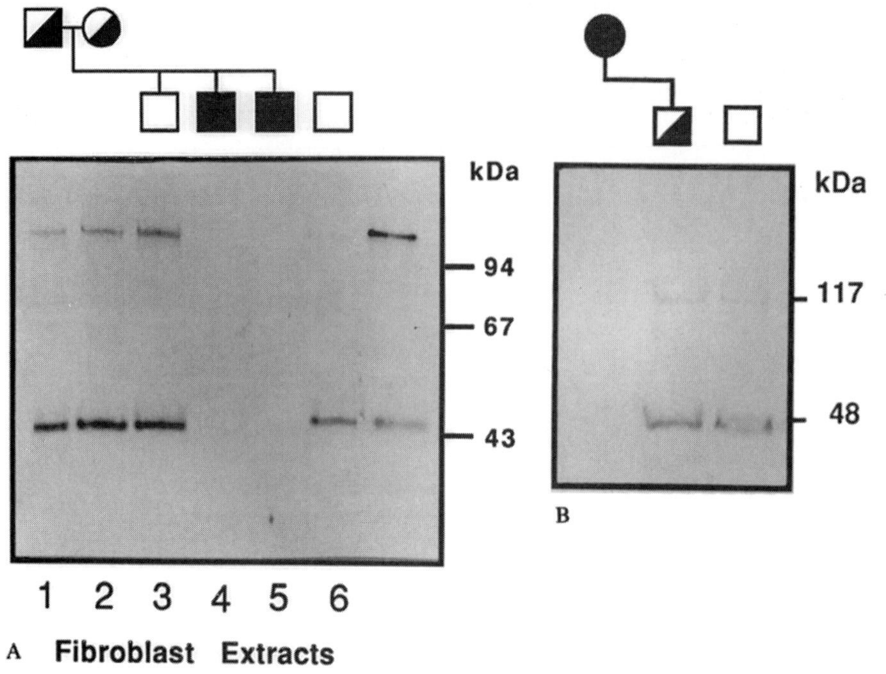

Fig. 139-12 Immunoblot of human α-*N*-acetylgalactosaminidase. ***A*, Fibroblast extracts from family members with type I disease: father (lane 1), mother (lane 2), unaffected brother (lane 3), and affected brothers (lanes 4 and 5), a normal individual (lane 6), and purified lung enzyme (lane 7). *B*, Fibroblast extracts from the Japanese family members with type II disease: proband (lane 1), her son (lane 2), and a normal individual (lane 3). Note that both the 48- and 117-kDa enzyme bands are absent in the type I and II probands. (*A from Schindler et al.*[3] *and B from Kanzaki et al.*[11] *Used with permission.*)**

However, subsequent studies of these enzymes[64,79,85,91] demonstrated kinetic, structural, and immunologic differences, which indicated that they were not glycoforms, but were distinct proteins.

In 1977, Dean et al.[65,66] and Schram et al.[64] independently showed that α-galactosidase B actually was an α-*N*-acetylgalactosaminidase that was competitively inhibited by α-*N*-acetylgalactosamine. Purified α-galactosidase B was shown to have a higher affinity for α-*N*-acetylgalactosaminides ($K_m \approx 1$ mM) than for α-galactosides ($K_m \approx 20$ mM), as well as the same physical properties (e.g., thermostability and pH optimum) as human α-*N*-acetylgalactosaminidase purified from liver.[92] Thus, it was concluded that α-galactosidase B was actually an α-*N*-acetylgalactosaminidase. This enzyme was not a focus of interest or investigation until it was found deficient in type I Schindler disease.[1–5]

Purification. Table 139-4 summarizes the purification and physical properties of human α-*N*-acetylgalactosaminidase isolated from various sources. The enzyme has been purified to homogeneity from placenta,[79,85] liver,[90,92] spleen,[93] and lung.[94] The purification strategy was similar to that for α-galactosidase A (see Chap. 150). Concanavalin A Sepharose chromatography was typically employed as a first step to enrich the glycoprotein fraction from crude tissue extracts. DEAE-cellulose chromatography afforded additional purification and nearly complete separation of α-*N*-acetylgalactosaminidase from α-galactosidase A, the latter being eluted at a lower salt concentration.[70,79,83,94,95] Hydroxylapatite chromatography completely separated the two enzymes and provided a significant purification step.[83,90,94] Gel filtration[85,90] or chromatography using ampholyte displacement,[90] SP-Sephadex,[85] or butyl agarose[85] has been used as a final purification step. However, affinity chromatography on α-galactosylamine coupled to Sepharose provided the most efficient purification step for both α-*N*-acetylgalactosaminidase and α-galactosidase A. The former can be specifically eluted with *N*-acetylgalactosaminide,[93,94] whereas both can be selectively eluted with D-galactose.[83]

Physical Properties. Human α-*N*-acetylgalactosaminidase is a relatively thermostable enzyme.[64,67,79,83,92] At 50°C, the half-life for the enzyme at pH 4.8 to 7.0 is greater than 2 h.[64,67,70,75,82,92,96] The enzyme has been estimated to have a native molecular weight of 90 to 117 kDa by gel filtration[64,69,70,74,79,93] (see Table 139-4).

Table 139-4 Purification and Properties of Human α-*N*-Acetylgalactosaminidase

Source	Specific Activity (nmol/h/mg)	Substrate	pH Optimum	pI	K_m (mM)	Molecular Weight: Native (kDa)	Molecular Weight: Subunit (kDa)	Reference
Placenta	67,000	4MU-αGal	4.5	4.4		150		79
Placenta	271,000	4MU-αGal	4.4	4.4	13.0	117	47.7	85
Liver	4,580	pNP-αGalNAc	4.3					92
Liver	4,740	pNP-αGalNAc			1.0	110		64, 69
Liver	14,800	4MU-αGal		4.9	11.7			86
Liver	394,000	4MU-αGal	4.8	4.5	6.8	90		70, 90
Liver	2,900,000	oNP-αGalNAc	4.3		1.3	90		70, 90
Lung	370,000	4MU-αGal	4.6	4.6		117	45	94
Liver	7	4MU-αGal	4.6	4.3	4.0	90		74
Liver	251,000	4MU-αGal					46.8	93

The subunit molecular weights of the enzyme from human placenta and liver have been reported to be 47.7 kDa and 46.8 kDa, respectively.[85,93] SDS polyacrylamide gel electrophoresis of homogeneous α-*N*-acetylgalactosaminidase from human lung revealed species of ≈48 and ≈117 kDa.[17] When the purified lung enzyme was subjected to native polyacrylamide gel electrophoresis, only a single species of ≈117 kDa was detected. Immunoblotting of the purified enzyme or crude human fibroblast extracts (after SDS gel electrophoresis) with rabbit antihuman lung α-*N*-acetylgalactosaminidase antibodies demonstrated two immunoreactive species of 48 and 117 kDa, respectively. Notably, both species were present in immunoblots of normal human fibroblasts, but neither was detected in fibroblasts from the patients with type I, II, or III disease,[3,11,15,97] suggesting that both species were encoded by a single gene (see Fig. 139-12). Microsequencing of both the 48- and 117-kDa species revealed identical *N*-terminal amino acid sequences. Subsequent tryptic mapping of the 48- and 117-kDa species determined that the maps were identical and that the 117-kDa species was the homodimeric form of the 48-kDa species.[17] These findings indicated that the enzyme is a homodimer which is highly resistant to denaturation. Evidence for the homodimeric structure also is based on biosynthetic studies of α-*N*-acetylgalactosaminidase in human fibroblasts.[98,99] Further support for the homodimeric structure is inferred from studies of the porcine enzyme, which was a dimer with native and subunit molecular weights of 102 and 52 kDa, respectively.[100]

***N*-Linked Oligosaccharide Structures.** The carbohydrate content and oligosaccharide moieties present in the human enzyme have been reported.[85,98,101] The human placental enzyme contained 5 percent neutral sugars and 0.3 percent sialic acid.[85] Analysis of the radiolabeled oligosaccharides from immunoprecipitated human fibroblast α-*N*-acetylgalactosaminidase revealed high-mannose-type oligosaccharide structures ($Man_{8-9}GlcNAc$) on both precursor and processed enzyme forms; only the precursor had phosphorylated mannose residues.[98] The virtual absence of complex-type oligosaccharide moieties containing terminal sialic acid residues was supported by the previously mentioned neuraminidase studies, which did not alter the pI of the enzyme.[83]

More recently, the structures of the *N*-linked oligosaccharides on the purified secreted forms of α-*N*-acetylgalactosaminidase overexpressed in Chinese hamster ovary cells were determined.[101] The structures were liberated by hydrazinolysis and were analyzed by HPLC resolution and digestion by a series of exoglycosidases. Hydrazinolysis liberated neutral (46.1 percent), monosialyl (21.3 percent), disialyl (6.2 percent), trisialyl (1.6 percent), monophosphoryl (17.1 percent), diphosphoryl (5.5 percent), and monosialyl monophosphoryl oligosaccharides (2.2 percent). The neutral fraction contained six types—high mannose, hybrid, and mono-, bi-, tri- and tetra-antennary complex-type oligosaccharides—in which $Man_{5-6}GlcNac_2$, $GalGlcNAcMan_6GlcNAcFucGlcNAc$, 2,6-branched $Gal_3GlcNAc_3Man_3GlcNAcFucGl$-cNAc, and $Gal_2GlcNAc_2Man_3GlcNAc(Fuc)_{0-1}GlcNAc$ were predominant. The sialic acid residues were exclusively α2,3-linked, and the desialylated oligosaccharides predominantly had structures of fucosylated and fully galactosylated di-, 2,4 and 2,6-branched tri-, and tetraantennary structures. Phosphate groups were exclusively in the monoester form. The major dephosphorylated oligosaccharides were $Man_{6-7}GlcNAc_2$ and $GalGlcNAcMan_6GlcNAcGlc$-NAc. The monosialyl monophosphoryl oligosaccharides had core structures of $GalGlcNAcMan_6GlcNAc(Fuc)_{0-1}GlcNAc$. When compared to the oligosaccharide structures on the secreted recombinant human α-galactosidase A, which is evolutionarily related and highly homologous, both enzymes' oligosaccharides had similar phosphorylation patterns. However, α-*N*-acetylgalactosaminidase contained more sialylated structures (8.5 vs. 28.9 percent of total oligosaccharides), indicating that the recombinant enzyme had more complete complex-type structures.

Kinetic Properties. Human lysosomal α-*N*-acetylgalactosaminidase had an acidic pH optimum of about 4.6 for various synthetic chromogenic or fluorogenic substrates (Table 139-5). The apparent K_m values for the enzyme toward synthetic α-galactosides were high, approximately 12 to 20 mM for 4MU-αGal and 20 to 30 mM for pNP-αGal. In contrast, the enzyme's affinity for the α-*N*-acetylgalactosamine glycon was about tenfold lower, with apparent K_m values for oNP-α-*N*-acetylgalactosaminide (oNP-αGalNAc) ranging from 1 to 2 mM. The apparent K_m toward the fluorogenic substrate, 4MU-αGalNAc, for the purified human lung enzyme was 1.6 mM.[63] Neither pNP-αGalNAc nor 4MU-αGalNAc was hydrolyzed by purified human α-galactosidase A.[63] For purified human liver α-*N*-acetylgalactosaminidase, the turnover number using oNP-αGalNAc as substrate was calculated to be 6600 min^{-1} using a molecular weight for the native enzyme of 110 kDa.[84] The apparent K_m of human liver α-*N*-acetylgalactosaminidase toward the Forssman glycosphingolipid (globopentaosylceramide; GbOse5Cer) was 0.59 mM with a V_{max} of 1.6×10^5 nmol/h/mg at the pH optimum, 3.9 (see Table 139-5). Other possible natural substrates, including *O*-linked glycopeptides with terminal α-*N*-acetylgalactosaminyl residues, have not been used to characterize the kinetic properties of this enzyme. Moreover, kinetic studies of the human enzyme have been limited to characterization of its exoglycosidase activity. Use of substrates with internal α-*N*-acetylgalactosaminyl moieties could definitively determine if the enzyme can also function as an endoglycosidase.

α-*N*-Acetylgalactosaminidase hydrolysis of globotriaosylceramide ($GbOse_3Cer$), the primary glycosphingolipid substrate for human α-galactosidase, occurs at an extremely low rate, if at all, in vitro. α-*N*-Acetylgalactosaminidase did not cleave $GbOse_3Cer$ in cultured fibroblasts or tissues from Fabry hemizygotes,[75,91] and minimal, if any, hydrolysis was detected using

Table 139-5 Kinetic Properties of Human α-*N*-Acetylgalactosaminidase

Source	Substrate	pH Optimum	K_m (mM)	V_{max} (nmol/h/mg	Reference
Liver	4MU-αGal	4.8	6.8	1.1×10^6	65,90
Liver	oNP-αGalNAc	4.3	1.3	3.6×10^6	65,90
Liver	$GbOse_5$*	4.4	3.7	5.5×10^5	65
Liver	$GbOse_5Cer$	3.9	0.59	1.6×10^5	65,90
Liver	$GbOse_3Cer$	4.3	0.35	1.1×10^4	65,90
Placenta	4MU-αGal	4.4	13.0		83
Lung	4MU-αGalNAc	4.5	0.37		63
Liver	pNP-αGalNAc	4.3	3.1		92

*$GbOse_5$ = Forssman glycosphingolipid globopentaosylceramide; $GbOse_3Cer$ = globotriaosylceramide, Gal(α1 → 4)Glc(β1 → 1)Cer.

radiolabeled $GbOse_3Cer$ and/or highly purified enzyme[65,84] (see Table 139-5). Inhibitors can be used to discriminate α-*N*-acetylgalactosaminidase and α-galactosidase activities in assays with chromogenic or fluorogenic α-galactosides. α-*N*-Acetylgalactosaminidase activity is inhibited about 95 percent by 100 mM *N*-acetylgalactosamine (GalNAc), while it has no effect on α-galactosidase A activity.[102] Conversely, 500 mM myoinositol inhibits about 50 percent of α-galactosidase A activity without affecting the activity of α-*N*-acetylgalactosaminidase.[79,96] The K_i of α-*N*-acetylgalactosaminidase for GalNAc was 3.1 mM with pNP-αGalNAc.[92]

For comparison, purified α-*N*-acetylgalactosaminidase from porcine and bovine liver had a pH optimum of 4.3 to 4.7.[103,104] The bovine α-*N*-acetylgalactosaminidase specifically cleaved pNP-αGalNAc with a K_m of 6.5 mM and had a K_i of 10 mM with GalNAc.[103] Additionally, partially purified α-*N*-acetylgalactosaminidases from bovine liver and ox spleen cleaved the terminal α-*N*-acetylgalactosaminyl residues that were *O*-linked to serine or threonine in desialylated ovine and bovine submaxillary mucins.[103,105]

Biosynthetic Studies. Early studies of the biosynthesis and processing of human α-*N*-acetylgalactosaminidase indicated that the enzyme was synthesized in cultured fibroblasts as a 65-kDa precursor and then was processed to a 48-kDa mature form.[98] Subsequent biosynthetic studies in cultured fibroblasts using normal and mutant cell lines indicated that the normal enzyme precursor was 52 kDa and that the 65-kDa polypeptide was not a glycoprotein like the other lysosomal enzymes, and probably was not related to α-*N*-acetylgalactosaminidase.[99] After a 4-h pulse labeling and 17-h chase, the 52-kDa precursor glycopolypeptide was completely replaced by a mature enzyme subunit of ≈49 kDa. Treatment of both the 52-kDa precursor and the 49-kDa mature polypeptides with endoglycosidase F resulted in the formation of a deglycosylated 42-kDa species. These findings indicated that after cleavage of a signal peptide, the enzyme subunit was normally modified by carbohydrate (rather than proteolytic) processing, thereby accounting for the 3-kDa difference between the precursor and the mature enzyme subunits.

Notably, the E325K mutation (see below) in type I patients did not interfere with the synthesis of the 52-kDa precursor. However, the mutant precursor apparently was not phosphorylated and disappeared during the 17-h chase. Because the mutant precursor was not detected in the media, the absent conversion to the immunologically detectable mature enzyme subunit suggested that the mutation in the type I patients caused an unstable precursor polypeptide that was subject to rapid intracellular degradation. These results presumably were limited by the sensitivity of immunodetection, because recent biosynthetic studies of the E325K type I enzyme expressed in COS-1 cells indicated that the mature 48-kDa enzyme subunit was synthesized, but unstable.[106] Similar findings were observed for the biosynthesis of the mature mutant R329W enzyme subunit expressed in COS-1 cells, but the Japanese type II mutant polypeptide was slightly more stable than the German type I polypeptide.[106] Interestingly, studies of cultured fibroblasts from a Dutch type III patient revealed normal synthesis of the precursor and the production of a small amount of mature enzyme subunit.[15]

MOLECULAR GENETICS OF α-*N*-ACETYLGALACTOSAMINIDASE

Our understanding of human α-*N*-acetylgalactosaminidase and the three disease subtypes has been greatly advanced by the isolation of the full-length cDNA and entire genomic sequences encoding this lysosomal glycosidase.[17,18] The full-length cDNA sequence provided the primary structure of the enzyme precursor, including the signal peptide, and the genomic sequence permitted characterization of the structural organization and regulatory elements of this housekeeping gene.

Gene Assignment

The gene encoding human α-*N*-acetylgalactosaminidase was originally assigned to chromosome 22 by somatic cell hybridization techniques.[107,108] The human enzyme, detected by the use of antihuman α-*N*-acetylgalactosaminidase antibodies,[107] segregated in human-mouse and human-Chinese hamster hybrid clones with human chromosome 22 and with human mitochondrial aconitase, an enzyme previously assigned to chromosome 22.[108] Subsequently, the locus for human α-*N*-acetylgalactosaminidase was regionally localized to 22q13 → qter using somatic cell hybrids containing human X;22 and 1;22 reciprocal translocations.[109] Recently, the gene assignment was refined further to the region 22q13.1 → 13.2 using somatic cell hybrids with additional chromosome 22 rearrangements.[110]

The α-*N*-Acetylgalactosaminidase cDNA

The full-length pAGB-3 cDNA encoding human α-*N*-acetylgalactosaminidase was isolated, sequenced, and expressed in COS-1 cells.[17] Authenticity was established by colinearity of the cDNA's predicted amino acid sequence with 129 microsequenced residues of the purified protein. The 2158-bp cDNA had a 344-bp 5′ untranslated region, a 1236-bp open reading frame that encoded 411 amino acids, a 514-bp 3′ untranslated region, and a 64-bp poly(A) tract. An upstream, inframe ATG occurred at nucleotide −192, but there were inframe termination codons at nucleotide positions −141, −135, and −120, indicating that the ATG at −192 was nonfunctional. A single consensus polyadenylation signal (AATAAA) at nt 1729–1734 and a consensus recognition sequence (CACTG) for the U4 small, nuclear, ribonucleoprotein were located 16 and 65 bp upstream from the poly(A) tract, respectively.

Analysis of the deduced amino acid sequence of the full-length cDNA indicated a signal peptide sequence of 17 residues, because Leu-18 was the N-terminal residue of the microsequenced mature enzyme. When the weight-matrix method of von Heijne[111] was used to predict the peptidase cleavage site, the preferred site, between Ala-13 and Gln-14, had a score of 4.34, whereas cleavage after Met-17 had a score of 2.38. The predicted molecular mass of the 394-residue mature, unglycosylated enzyme subunit (M_r = 44,700) was consistent with that (42 kDa) estimated by NaDod-SO_4/PAGE of the deglycosylated species above. These findings suggested that the mature glycoprotein subunit had at least two *N*-linked oligosaccharide chains, although there were six putative *N*-glycosylation sites at asparagine residues 124, 177, 201, 359, 385, and 391.

For transient expression, the full-length cDNA was subcloned into the eukaryotic expression vector p91023(B) and the construct was transfected into COS-1 cells. Compared with the endogenous mean α-*N*-acetylgalactosaminidase activity in mock transfected COS-1 cells (mean: 35 U/mg; range: 23 to 50 U/mg; n = 6) when assayed 72 h after transfection, the cells had a mean activity of 600 U/mg (range: 104 to 2400 U/mg; n = 6), or about 17 times the endogenous activity. The expressed human enzyme protein, which had a subunit molecular weight of ≈48 kDa, was detected by immunoblot analysis using rabbit-antihuman α-*N*-acetylgalactosaminidase antibodies, whereas the endogenous monkey enzyme was visible as a faint band at ≈40 kDa or was undetectable.

Northern hybridization analyses revealed two transcripts of about 2.2 and 3.6 kb in total, cytoplasmic or poly(A)+ RNA, which were present in similar amounts. A cap site was determined to be at nucleotide −347 by primer extension of total placental RNA using two overlapping oligonucleotide probes. The 3.6-kb transcript resulted from a second AATAAA polyadenylation signal that was 1366 bp downstream (nt 3100–3105) of the first polyadenylation hexamer identified in the pAGB-3 cDNA. A 3.6-kb cDNA encoding α-*N*-acetylgalactosaminidase was isolated from a human retinal library and was identical to the originally cloned cDNA sequence with the exception of an additional 125 bp of 5′ untranslated and 1379 bp of 3′ untranslated sequence. The

3.6-kb cDNA confirmed the alternative use of polyadenylation hexamers in producing two mRNA transcripts and also indicated that the α-*N*-acetylgalactosaminidase gene had at least two transcriptional start sites, since its 5′ untranslated region extended 125 bp upstream from the previously identified cap site.

Computer-assisted searches of nucleic acid and protein databases revealed no significant nucleotide or amino acid sequence similarities between α-*N*-acetylgalactosaminidase and that of any other DNA or protein sequence, except for human α-galactosidase A.[72,112] Comparison of the nucleic acid and deduced amino acid sequences of the full-length α-*N*-acetylgalactosaminidase and α-galactosidase A cDNAs revealed 55.8 and 46.9 percent overall homology, respectively.

Tsuji et al. reported a similar human α-*N*-acetylgalactosaminidase cDNA sequence, pcD-HS1204, which differed from pAGB-3 by a 70-bp insertion at nucleotide 957 and by several nucleotide substitutions (nucleotides 493, 494, 524, 614, and 667).[51] The 70-bp insert consisted of three inverted repeats (nucleotides 919–926, 919–936, and 919–944) and a direct repeat (nucleotides 940–957) from nucleotides 919 to 957 of the pAGB-3 coding sequence. Subsequent sequencing of the region, including pAGB-3 codons 254 to 351 in the genomic clone gAGB-1,[17] revealed a 2048-bp sequence containing a 1754-bp intron between pAGB-3 nucleotides 957 and 958. The intronic sequence did not have the 70-bp insertion in either orientation, but it did contain two *Alu*-repetitive sequences in reverse orientation. Expression of the pcD-HS1204 sequence did not produce α-*N*-acetylgalactosaminidase activity, consistent with the fact that this clone contained an artifact.[113] Three subsequently isolated clones, pcD-HS1207, pcD-1225, and pcD-HS1237, contained insert sequences that were essentially identical to pAGB-3, which expressed α-*N*-acetylgalactosaminidase, further confirming that pAGB-3 was the authentic α-*N*-acetylgalactosaminidase cDNA sequence.[113]

The α-*N*-Acetylgalactosaminidase Gene

Structural Organization. Genomic clones containing the entire α-*N*-acetylgalactosaminidase gene have been isolated and characterized.[18] Clone gAGB-1 contained the entire 13,709-bp genomic sequence, which was completely sequenced.[18] The α-*N*-acetylgalactosaminidase gene contained 9 exons, which ranged in length from 95 to 2028 bp, with exon 1 containing the 344-nucleotide 5′ untranslated region and the codons for the first 6 amino acids of the 17-residue signal peptide. The 8 introns ranged in length from 304 to 2684 bp. All splice junctions followed the GT/AG rule[114] and were consistent with the 5′ and 3′ consensus sequences for splice junctions of RNA polymerase II transcribed genes.[115] Putative lariat branch points were identified between −40 and −18 nucleotides from the 3′ splice junction for all 8 introns by similarity to the less well-conserved consensus sequence (C/T)N(C/T)T(A/G)A(A/C/T).[116] The α-*N*-acetylgalactosaminidase genomic sequence also confirmed the presence of two polyadenylation hexamers of AATAAA whose alternative use resulted in the 2.2- or 3.6-kb α-*N*-acetylgalactosaminidase transcripts.[17]

Regulatory Elements. Computer-assisted analysis of the α-*N*-acetylgalactosaminidase 1432-bp 5′ flanking region identified three Sp1 binding sites, one antisense site at nt −364 and two antisense sites at nt −410 and −596, respectively, and three GC boxes (at −23, −68, and −257) from the A of the translational start site.[117] Two CAAT-like elements were identified at nt −644 and −678,[118] whereas TATA-like elements were not found. The 5′ flanking region was GC-rich (≈56 percent), but there was no HTF island. The CpG:GpC ratio was 0.625, whereas typical HTF islands have ratios greater than 1.0.[117,119] The absence of a TATA box and the high GC content are known features in the promoter regions of other housekeeping genes.[120] Imperfect inverted repeats were identified at nucleotides −436 to −455 and at −355 to −374, which could pair with a predicted ΔG of −34.8 kcal/mol.[18] The structure predicted by this pairing may be important to promoter function. Further evaluation of these putative promoter elements requires footprinting and functional assays with deletion/mutation mapping.

***Alu*-Repetitive Elements.** Six *Alu*-repetitive elements[121] were identified in the 14-kb genomic sequence: one each in the 5′ flanking region and intron 1, and two each in introns 6 and 7. All six were in the reverse orientation. The homology of these repetitive elements with the consensus 300-nucleotide sequence ranged from 54.1 to 87.4 percent. When categorized in "subfamilies" according to the classification of Jurka and Smith,[122] *Alu*-1 in the 5′ flanking region belonged to the older "J" subfamily, and 10 of the 15 diagnostic positions were identical to the 7SL RNA sequence. The other five *Alu* elements were homologous to the older "a" branch of the more modern "S" subfamily. Comparison of the *Alu* elements to each other revealed a divergence of 18.6 to 53.1 percent, suggesting that each *Alu* element resulted from a separate retroposon event. Of the 24 CpG dinucleotides in the consensus sequence, the number in each of the six *Alu* elements that presumably underwent spontaneous deamination of 5-methylcytosine to thymidine ranged from 11 to 18.

The α-Galactosidase Gene Family. As noted above, human α-*N*-acetylgalactosaminidase and α-galactosidase A had similar biochemical properties, and the subsequent isolation of their respective full-length cDNAs revealed remarkable identity (46.9 percent) of their predicted amino acid sequences.[17,112] The highly homologous amino acid sequences suggested that the genes encoding these two lysosomal glycosidases evolved from a common ancestral sequence.[17] Indeed, comparison of the organization of the α-*N*-acetylgalactosaminidase gene with that of α-galactosidase A[18,123] indicated that six of the eight α-*N*-acetylgalactosaminidase introns (2 through 7) interrupted the coding sequence at positions identical to those of all six introns in the α-galactosidase A genomic sequence[18] (Fig. 139-13). The amino acid identity between the homologous α-*N*-acetylgalactosaminidase exons 2 through 7 and α-galactosidase A exons 1 through 6 ranged from 46.2 to 62.7 percent (49.2 to 66.1

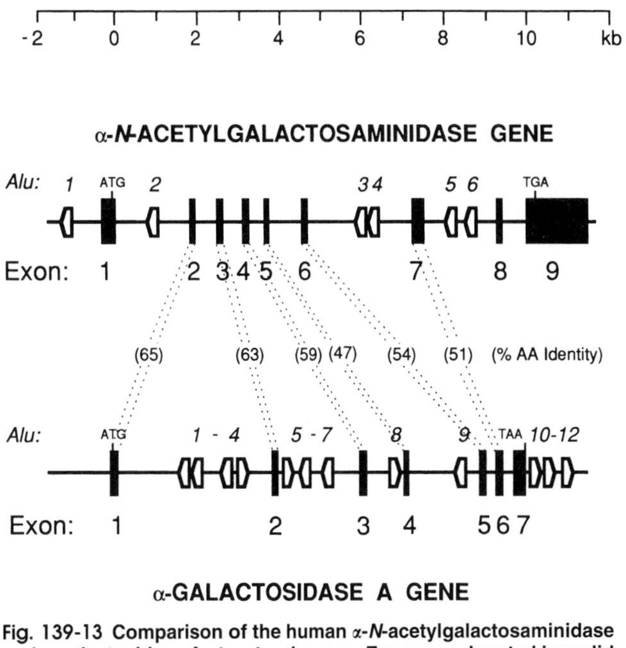

Fig. 139-13 Comparison of the human α-*N*-acetylgalactosaminidase and α-galactosidase A structural genes. Exons are denoted by solid rectangles. Pentagons indicate the positions and orientations of the *Alu* repeat elements. Dashed lines denote homologous exons, and the percent amino acid identity is indicated in parentheses. (*From Wang and Desnick.*[18] *Used with permission.*)

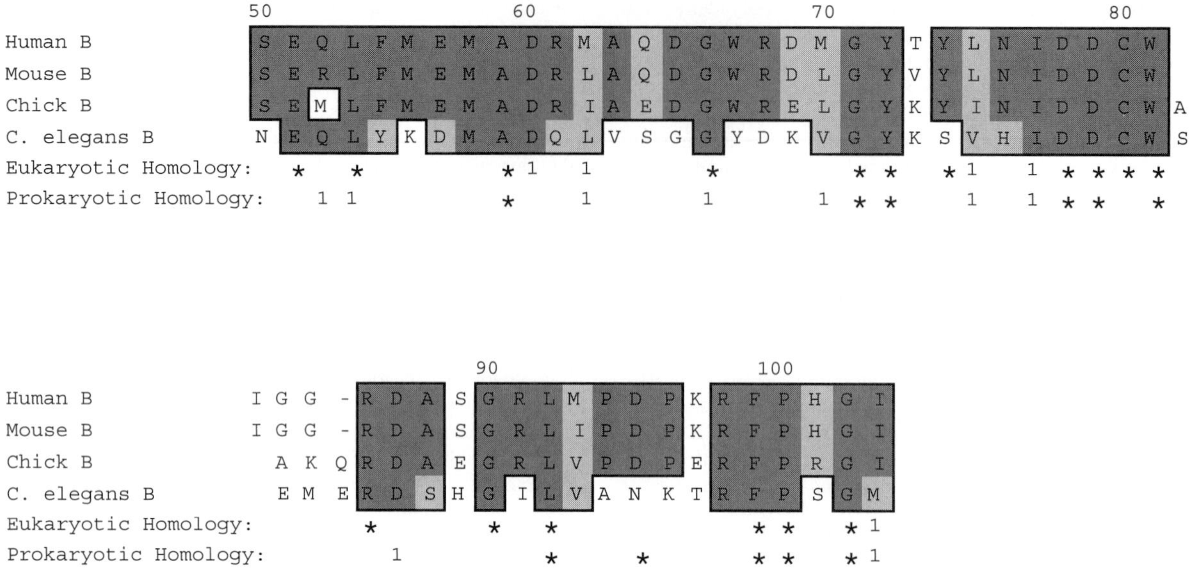

Fig. 139-14 Comparison of amino acid sequences in the "α-galactoside signature" region deduced from the full-length cDNAs encoding mouse, human, chicken, and *C. elegans* α-*N*-acetylgalactosaminidase as well as of α-galactosidase A sequences from 29 eukaryotic and prokaryotic species.[138] This region corresponds to the residues 51 to 103 and 65 to 117 in the human α-*N*-acetylgalactosaminidase and human α-galactosidase A cDNAs, respectively. The darker-shaded identical and the lighter-shaded isofunctional residues encoded by the α-*N*-acetylgalactosaminidase genes are boxed. If the α-galactosidase A residues in 20 of the 22 eukaryotic species, or in 3 or more of the 7 prokaryotic species, were identical or isofunctional, they were indicated by a star or a plus, respectively, under the corresponding α-*N*-acetylgalactosaminidase residue. Gaps were introduced for optimal alignment.

percent isofunctional similarity), with only a few single amino acid gaps.[18,123] In contrast, the homology between α-*N*-acetylgalactosaminidase exons 8 and 9 and α-galactosidase A exon 7 dropped significantly to 15.8 percent, with multiple gaps. Intriguingly, the divergence between the two coding regions occurred at nucleotide 957 of the α-*N*-acetylgalactosaminidase cDNA, which is the last nucleotide in α-*N*-acetylgalactosaminidase exon 7. The homologous intron placement and remarkable amino acid identity of the six exonic sequences were consistent with the two genes having had a common origin. Presumably, they were duplicated from a common ancestral gene and underwent subsequent divergence to acquire their specific functions.[124] Lack of homology between α-*N*-acetylgalactosaminidase and α-galactosidase A after α-*N*-acetylgalactosaminidase exon 7 suggests that this position may represent the 3′ boundary of the common ancestral gene. A similar mechanism has been proposed for the evolution of the β-hexosaminidase α and β chains[125] and the functional acid β-glucosidase gene and its adjacent pseudogene.[126]

Additional support for the notion that α-*N*-acetylgalactosaminidase and α-galactosidase A have evolved from a common ancestral gene is derived from the amino acid homology of the human, mouse, chicken, and *C. elegans* α-*N*-acetylgalactosaminidase cDNAs[18,127,128] with the α-galactosidase A cDNAs from human and more than 30 other species.[129] Comparison of these sequences suggests that α-*N*-acetylgalactosaminidase exons 2 through 7 were conserved functional domains common to both α-*N*-acetylgalactosaminidases and α-galactosidases. For example, a predicted amino acid sequence known as the "α-galactosidase signature" was highly homologous over a region of 50 residues in the four α-*N*-acetylgalactosaminidases and all reported α-galactosidase cDNAs (Fig. 139-14). Subsequent structure/function and crystallographic studies should permit further assessment of the catalytic functions of these "α-galactosidase-specific" domains that have been conserved in evolution.

The Mouse α-*N*-Acetylgalactosaminidase cDNA and Gene. For structure/function analysis and for the generation of a mouse model of α-*N*-acetylgalactosaminidase deficiency, the mouse α-*N*-acetylgalactosaminidase cDNA and genomic sequences were isolated and characterized.[129–131] The cDNA had an open reading frame of 1245 bp encoding a 415-amino-acid polypeptide which included a 17-residue signal peptide. The cDNA had 81 percent nucleotide and 81.8 percent predicted amino acid identity with the human α-*N*-acetylgalactosaminidase cDNA sequence. Northern analysis revealed a single transcript of about 1.9 kb. The functional integrity of this cDNA was demonstrated by transient expression in COS-1 cells. Using the murine α-*N*-acetylgalactosaminidase cDNA as a probe, genomic clones were isolated and characterized. The mouse α-*N*-acetylgalactosaminidase genomic sequence also was isolated.[129–131] The murine gene spanned ≈10 kb and had 9 exons. Nucleotide identity between the human and mouse α-*N*-acetylgalactosaminidase exons ranged from 67.4 to 89.5 percent, with the homology higher for exons 2 to 7 than for 1, 8, and 9. Moreover, there was strong homology between the murine exonic sequences for α-*N*-acetylgalactosaminidase and α-galactosidase A, ranging from 25 to 62 percent, with the identity being greatest for α-*N*-acetylgalactosaminidase exons 2 to 7 than for exons 1, 8, and 9. Although the identities between the two murine sequences were lower than those with their corresponding human sequences, these findings further support the evolution of the α-galactosidase gene family described above.

MOLECULAR PATHOLOGY

Characterization of the Mutations Causing α-*N*-Acetylgalactosaminidase Deficiency

The mutations causing the three subtypes of α-*N*-acetylgalactosaminidase deficiency have been determined for each of the affected probands.[15,19,20,106] RT-PCR of total RNA from cultured fibroblasts from the German type I sibs generated a cDNA that had a G-to-A transition of cDNA nucleotide 973, which predicted the substitution of an evolutionarily conserved glutamic acid (E) by a lysine (K) at residue 325 in exon 8 (designated E325K).[19] Dot-blot hybridization of genomic DNA from the probands and first-degree relatives with normal and E325K-specific oligonucleotides indicated that the probands were homoallelic for this mutation, which occurred at a CpG dinucleotide. Subsequently, a 3rd/4th cousin of the original type I probands from the same village in Germany was retrospectively diagnosed.[15] Analysis of genomic DNA from cultured fibroblasts revealed that the affected cousin also was homoallelic for the E325K mutation. This finding was instructive, as it had been suggested that the originally described German type I probands had inherited two recessive diseases, α-*N*-acetylgalactosaminidase deficiency and infantile neuroaxonal dystrophy.[28] However, the finding of a 3rd/4th cousin who had both diseases strongly supports homozygosity for a single recessive gene as the cause of both the enzyme deficiency and the neuroaxonal dystrophy, unless the two causative genes were adjacent or tightly linked. The odds that two recessive traits that were not closely linked would cosegregate in two affected sibs, their normal sib, and their 3rd/4th cousin are remote.

In the Japanese and Spanish probands with type II disease, different mutations were identified in the α-*N*-acetylgalactosaminidase gene. In the cDNA from the consanguineous Japanese type II proband, generated by RT-PCR of total RNA from cultured fibroblasts, a C-to-T transition occurred at cDNA nucleotide 985, which predicted the substitution of an evolutionarily conserved arginine (R) by a tryptophan (W) substitution at position 329 in exon 8 (designated R329W).[106] This mutation, which also occurred at a CpG dinucleotide, was confirmed by dot-blot hybridization analysis with allele-specific oligonucleotides.[106] The two consanguineous Spanish siblings with type II disease were homoallelic for a G-to-T transversion at cDNA nucleotide 579 in exon 5 that predicted a glutamic acid (E) to termination codon (X) at position 193 (designated E193X). The E193X nonsense mutation would truncate the mutant polypeptide after residue 192, presumably rendering the truncated enzyme inactive and unstable. In fact, the enzyme precursor was not detected in biosynthetic studies of the enzyme in cultured fibroblasts from these patients.[15]

The mutations in the recently identified type III patients who have intermediate phenotype were determined by directly amplifying each of the exons from genomic DNA and sequencing. Of note, the Dutch and French/Italian/Albanian type III patients each had one E325K mutant allele, the lesion found in the three type I probands, and second new mutations. The determination of whether the E325K lesion was inherited from a common ancestor requires haplotype analysis. The second mutant allele in the Dutch sibs was a C-to-G transversion of cDNA nucleotide 478, which predicted the substitution of an evolutionarily conserved serine (S) by a cysteine (C) at position 160 in exon 4 (designated S160C). A small amount of the mature enzyme polypeptide was detectable on immunoblots of radiolabeled fibroblasts from an affected Dutch sib.[15] The French/Italian/Albanian patient was heteroallelic for the E325K mutation and another missense mutation, a G-to-A transition of cDNA nucleotide 1099 in codon 367 in exon 8 predicting the substitution of an evolutionarily conserved glutamic acid (E) by a lysine (K) (designated E367K).[20]

Transient Expression of the α-*N*-Acetylgalactosaminidase Mutations. Further characterization of the type I E325K and type II R329W mutations was performed by transient expression of the mutant cDNAs in COS-1 cells. Immunoblot analysis of extracts of COS-1 cells transfected with the E325K and R329W expression constructs revealed the presence of the mutant proteins with subunit molecular weights of ≈48 kDa.[19,106] However, neither mutant protein expressed 4MU-αGalNAc activity above endogenous COS-1 levels, whereas the normal cDNA expressed immunologically detectable protein, which had α-*N*-acetylgalactosaminidase activity that was 17 times greater than that in mock-transfected COS-1 cells. To date, the type II E193X nonsense and type III S160C and E367K missense alleles have not been expressed, so it is not known whether they produce mutant proteins with residual activity.

The fact that fibroblast extracts from the type I (homoallelic for E325K) and type II patients (homoallelic for E329W or E193X) were CRIM-negative[3,11,12,15,16] suggested that these mutations rendered their enzyme polypeptides unstable, such that the mutant polypeptides were rapidly degraded in cultured cells and, presumably, in vivo. The detection of immunoreactive type I and II mutant polypeptides expressed in COS-1 cells most likely reflects the "pulsed" synthesis of the altered human polypeptides, which were then degraded as a result of instability and/or the inability of the polypeptide subunits to associate into the more stable dimeric form. Thus, the classification of a mutation as CRIM-negative based on studies of the patient's cells or tissues does not imply that the enzyme is not synthesized. Biosynthetic studies, performed by Hu et al.[99] in cultured fibroblasts, indicated that the E325K 52-kDa precursor was synthesized, but not phosphorylated. In contrast, biosynthetic studies performed in transfected COS-1 cells indicated that the enzyme was rapidly synthesized as the 48-kDa precursor and was then translationally glycosylated to an ≈53-kDa form (A.M. Wang and R.J. Desnick, unpublished results). Subsequently, the glycopeptide precursor subunit was processed to an ≈50- to 51-kDa mature form. The half-life of the normal enzyme was about 30 h. In contrast, biosynthetic studies of the expressed E325K and R329W polypeptides revealed similar processing, but reduced half-lives of about 11 and 19 h, respectively. These studies indicated that the two mutations expressed glycopeptides that were unstable, the half-life of the type I E325K subunit being less than that of the type II R329W glycopeptide. Further studies are required to determine why these lesions, which are only three residues apart, cause such different phenotypes.

Genotype/Phenotype Correlations. It is intriguing to speculate on the nature of the mutations causing the remarkably distinct subtype phenotypes. The only significant pathology observed on histologic and ultrastructural examination of tissues from the type I sibs was in axons and cultured fibroblasts.[2,3,27] In contrast, the type II probands had morphologic evidence of lysosomal accumulation in the endothelial cells of blood and lymphatic vessels, in circulating blood cells, and in cutaneous axons.[10–12] Only peripheral blood cells were examined in the type III probands and no vacuolated cells were observed.[14,16] These observations suggest the possibility of different domains on the enzyme responsible for its function in neuroaxonal transport or lysosomal hydrolysis, or the action of modifying factors. That a major site of α-*N*-acetylgalactosaminidase hydrolysis is in neuronal cells is supported by the demonstration (using the α-*N*-acetylgalactosaminide-specific *Vicia villosa* lectin) of terminal α-*N*-acetylgalactosaminyl residues on the surface of nonpyramidal multipolar neurons in the cerebral cortex of humans.[132] That there is no ultrastructural evidence for accumulation in other tissues of the type I probands suggests that their mutations in the α-*N*-acetylgalactosaminidase gene result in mutant homodimers that can hydrolyze substrates in lysosomes but cannot function in neuroaxonal transport. This may relate to the mutant enzyme's ability to function in the protective protein complex[51,52] but its inability to perform its function in neuroaxonal transport (see "Molecular Pathology" above). It is also conceivable that an alternative pathway or enzymatic activity is present in certain cell types for the hydrolysis of α-*N*-acetylgalactosaminyl residues. For example, there may be an endo-α-*N*-acetylgalactosaminidase, such as that found in microorganisms,[133,134] which can hydrolyze certain α-*N*-acetylgalactosaminyl linkages, thereby limiting the substrates that accumulate in this disease. Alternatively, α-*N*-acetylgalactosaminyl substrates may occur in relatively low abundance or only in certain cell types.

Secondary Structure Analyses. Computer-assisted secondary structural predictions of the amino acid sequence in the regions of the E325K and R329W mutations were performed using the algorithm of Garnier et al.[135] Compared with the predicted secondary structure of the normal sequence, the glutamic acid to lysine substitution in the German type I patients extended a

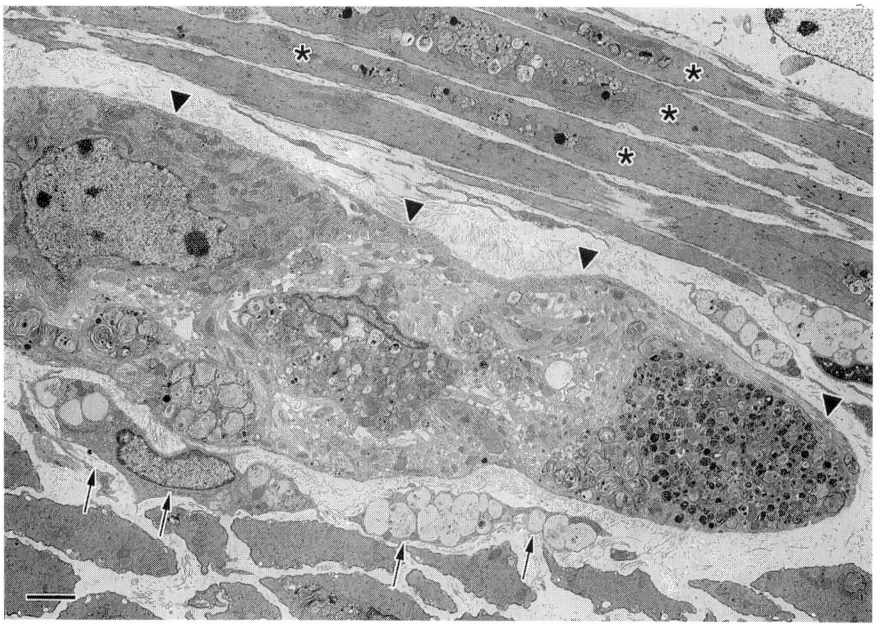

Fig. 139-15 Tunica muscularis of the small intestine of an α-*N*-acetylgalactosaminidase-deficient mouse. A ganglion of the myenteric plexus occupies the center of the micrograph (triangles). Abnormal storage is seen in several cell types: myenteric plexus neurons contain numerous single-membrane-bound laminated whorls admixed with electron-dense bodies. Similar inclusions are present in the cytoplasm of smooth muscle cells (asterisks). Interstitial fibroblasts (arrows) contain many secondary lysosomes distended by flocculent filamentous and vesicular material. Scale bar, 2 μm.

β-pleated sheet region upstream of the amino acid substitution and created a region of α-helicity around and including the mutation. The Japanese R329W mutation in the type II patient predicted a shortening of β-pleated sheet downstream of the amino acid substitution. The Dutch type III S160C mutation predicted that the adjacent (amino-terminal) turn involving three residues (155 to 157) was increased to include five residues (154 to 158). The French type III E367K mutation predicted the replacement of a β-turn-β structure with a 15-residue β-pleated sheet.

Murine α-*N*-Acetylgalactosaminidase Deficiency

Using gene-targeting techniques, mice with α-*N*-acetylgalactosaminidase deficiency have been generated.[130] The murine α-*N*-acetylgalactosaminidase genomic sequence was used to construct a replacement-type vector for homologous recombination. After transfection of embryonic stem cells and positive/negative selection, homologous recombination was detected in about 1 in 40 surviving cells. A positive clone was injected into blastocysts, which then were transplanted in pseudopregnant females. Following germ line transmission through chimeric mice, the animals were bred to homozygosity. The homozygous mice with no detectable α-*N*-acetylgalactosaminidase activity appeared normal, were fertile, bred, lived a normal life span, and appeared to have no clinically evident neurologic disease.

However, the pathology of the α-*N*-acetylgalactosaminidase-deficient mice was remarkable. Histologically, two main lesions were identified: (a) widespread lysosomal storage of abnormal material in the central nervous system and other organs[136] and (b) focal axonal swellings or "spheroids" in the central nervous system.

Lysosomal storage was histologically observed in numerous cell types in the central nervous system and in various organs. These storage vacuoles were predominantly found in interstitial or mesenchymal cells in the brain, dorsal root ganglia, parasympathetic ganglia, gastrointestinal tract, kidney, skin, and uterus. Neuronal storage varied from minimal to profound and was greatest in the submucosal and myenteric plexus of the gastrointestinal tract; less in the dorsal root, trigeminal, and parasympathetic ganglia; and least in the central nervous system. Perivascular macrophages, either within the neuroparenchyma or in the subarachnoid space, consistently contained the most storage material. In the kidney, there was marked enlargement and vacuolation of glomerular podocytes and mesangial cells, and abnormal storage was present in the collecting duct epithelium. In the gastrointestinal tract, there was marked lysosomal storage in the smooth muscle cells of the tunica muscularis.

Ultrastructurally, the inclusions were detected in a variety of cell types including neurons of the central and peripheral nervous systems, epithelial cells and fibroblasts of the choroid plexus, vascular endothelium, cutaneous vascular smooth muscle cells, and satellite, perineurial, and endoneurial cells of sensory and enteric ganglia (Fig. 139-15). The enlarged lysosomes contained flocculent, particulate material, concentric lamellar figures, multivesicular bodies and/or dense bodies.

The second histologic finding was the occurrence of axonal spheroids. On light microscopy, a survey of the central nervous system revealed normal architecture, and the number of neurons appeared to be within normal limits. However, axonal spheroids were found rarely in the brain, but were sporadically observed throughout the entire length of the spinal cord in a distribution limited to the dorsal gray and white matter. The spheroids were rounded, ovoid, or irregular structures with diameters up to 50 μm; they stained weakly eosinophilic with hematoxylin and eosin, and light blue with toluidine blue. Their content varied from homogenous to complex, but commonly they contained dark punctate material interspersed with finely granular material. Electron microscopy showed densely packed tubulovesicular arrays with multiple acicular clefts, which were either empty or contained lamellar material. Mitochondria and other organelles also were observed within these structures. Some spheroids were surrounded by an attenuated myelin sheath indicative of their axonal origin while others had synapses on their perimeter or were continuous with a neuritic process (Fig. 139-16).

The murine model appears to mimic the unique pathology of the human disease. However, in the absence of autopsied human material only preliminary comparisons can be made. Most notably, the axonal spheroids in the spinal cords of the knockout mice had remarkable ultrastructural similarity to the cortical spheroids in type I disease and to those observed in the central nervous system of infantile neuroaxonal dystrophy (Seitelberger disease).[32,33,36,137] The spheroids in these disorders share a common and characteristic ultrastructural morphology (that is, tubulovesicular arrays with acicular clefts) that differs from those in other lysosomal storage disorders or nonspecific spheroids secondary to other neuropathologic processes. The latter, nonspecific spheroids contain an aggregate of light and dense bodies, vesicular profiles,

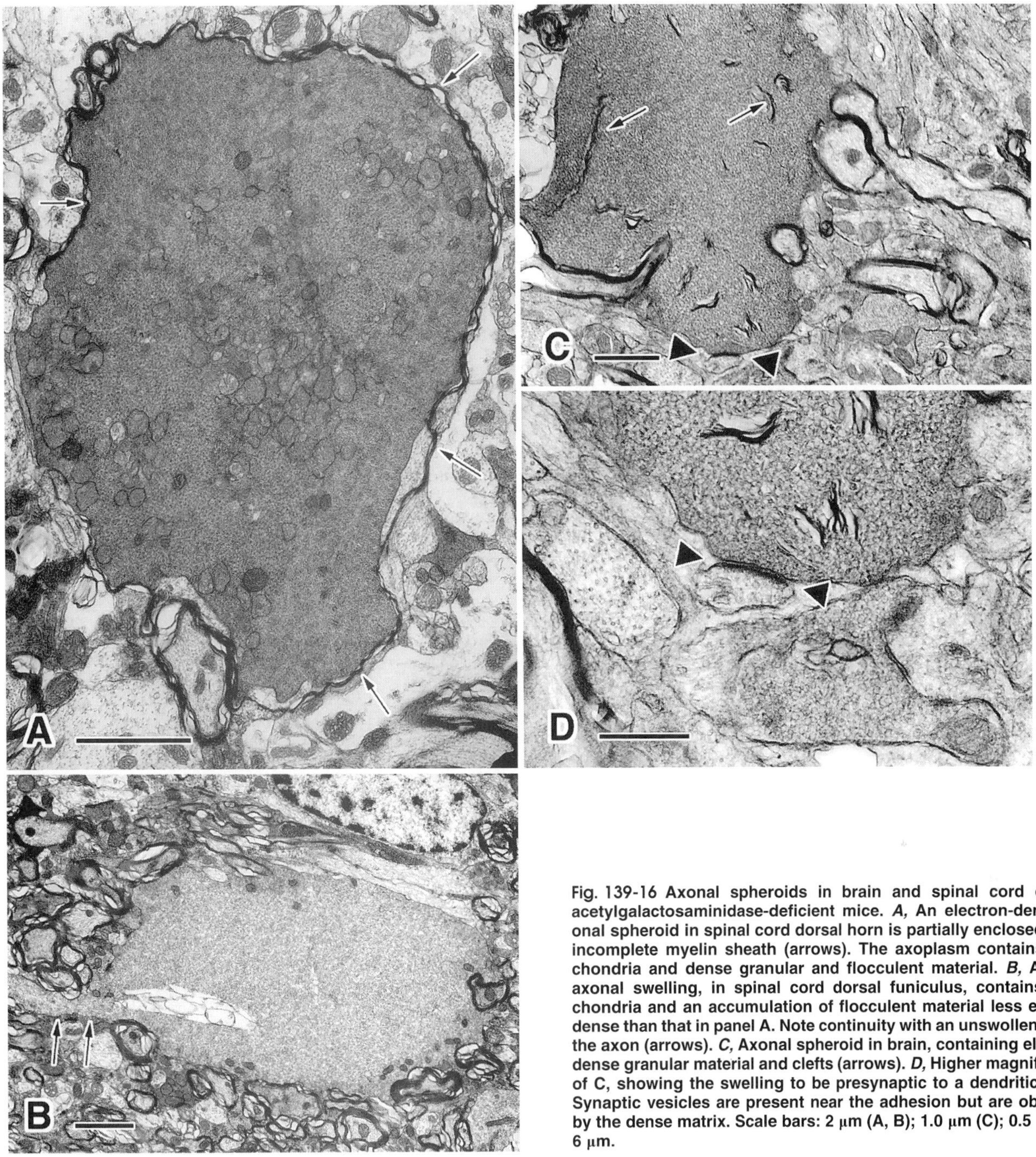

Fig. 139-16 Axonal spheroids in brain and spinal cord of α-*N*-acetylgalactosaminidase-deficient mice. *A,* An electron-dense axonal spheroid in spinal cord dorsal horn is partially enclosed by an incomplete myelin sheath (arrows). The axoplasm contains mitochondria and dense granular and flocculent material. *B,* Another axonal swelling, in spinal cord dorsal funiculus, contains mitochondria and an accumulation of flocculent material less electron dense than that in panel A. Note continuity with an unswollen part of the axon (arrows). *C,* Axonal spheroid in brain, containing electron-dense granular material and clefts (arrows). *D,* Higher magnification of C, showing the swelling to be presynaptic to a dendritic spine. Synaptic vesicles are present near the adhesion but are obscured by the dense matrix. Scale bars: 2 μm (A, B); 1.0 μm (C); 0.5 μm (D). 6 μm.

and other components. Although the distribution of spheroids in type I disease has not yet been determined, in Seitelberger disease (infantile neuroaxonal dystrophy) spheroids are found in large numbers in the spinal cord and medulla and less so in the cerebrum. Thus, the preponderance of spheroids in the spinal cord in these animals was not unexpected.

The widespread lysosomal storage in these mice is similar to that observed in various cells of type II patients.[12,13] The histologic and ultrastructural characteristics of the stored material in the mice were consistent with oligosaccharide, glycopeptide, and glycolipid accumulation. In contrast, no lamellar figures were observed in the human subtypes, supporting the biochemical finding of little, if any, glycolipid accumulation in various human sources. That the knockout model had pathology similar to its human counterpart should permit investigation of the role of α-*N*-acetylgalactosaminidase in neuroaxonal transport and facilitate future evaluation of various neuron-targeted therapeutic strategies, including gene therapy.

DIAGNOSIS

Biochemical Evaluation

Children who experience developmental regression, myoclonus, and/or grand mal seizures in the first or second years of life, who have clinical manifestations compatible with type I disease, and who have no visceral evidence of a metabolic disorder should be considered for biochemical evaluation. The finding of cortical, cerebellar and/or brain stem atrophy on CT scans or MRI is compatible with a neuroaxonal dystrophy. The ultrastructural demonstration of the characteristic "tubulovesicular" material in dystrophic axons in the myenteric plexus of biopsied rectum should suggest this diagnosis. Individuals with angiokeratoma corporis diffusum and moderate intellectual impairment should be evaluated for type II disease. An initial screening may include the histochemical and/or ultrastructural examination of peripheral blood elements, bone marrow, or a skin biopsy. The demonstration of clear cytoplasmic vacuoles or the ultrastructural finding of enlarged lysosomes containing filamentous material would be consistent with the diagnosis of type II disease. The recent discovery of the Dutch and French/Italian/Albanian probands with type III disease has expanded the diagnostic indications for this disease. Children with significant speech and language delay and with autistic behavior should be evaluated for type III disease.

For all subtypes, initial biochemical screening can be performed by analysis of the urinary oligosaccharide and glycopeptide profiles (see Fig. 139-11) or by determination of the α-*N*-acetylgalactosaminidase activity in plasma, isolated leukocytes, and/or cultured lymphoblasts or fibroblasts, using the commercially available chromogenic substrate, pNP-αGalNAc,[1,2] or the more sensitive fluorogenic substrate, 4MU-αGalNAc (see Table 139-3).[3,62] Prenatal diagnosis can be accomplished by determining the α-*N*-acetylgalactosaminidase activity in chorionic villi obtained at 9 to 10 menstrual weeks or in cultured amniocytes obtained by amniocentesis at about 15 to 16 menstrual weeks. Knowledge of the mutations causing Schindler disease in a given family or at-risk couple permits molecular-based prenatal diagnostic studies.

Genetic Counseling

Genetic counseling should be provided to all families in which the diagnosis of an affected individual is made. All three disease subtypes are inherited as autosomal recessive traits. The recurrent risk in an affected fetus for each subsequent pregnancy of a carrier couple is 25 percent. Normal sibs of affected individuals have a 67 percent chance of being carriers. At-risk individuals in each family should have diagnostic enzyme determinations to identify all possible carriers. Identification of heterozygous carriers of the disease-causing gene is most reliably performed with the synthetic fluorogenic 4MU-αGalNAc substrate[3,4,11,62] (see Table 139-3).

TREATMENT

There is no specific treatment for the subtypes of this disease and appropriate supportive care should be implemented as indicated.

ACKNOWLEDGMENTS

The authors express their appreciation to Drs. Otto van Diggelen, Irene Maire, and Claire Gay for recent information on their patients; Drs. Ori Brenner and Victor Friedrich for the murine knockout pathology; Dr. Lela Simonaro for determination of the type III mutations in the French patient; Dr. David Bishop for his contributions to the biochemical section of this chapter; Dr. Kenneth H. Astrin for his assistance in preparation of this chapter; Dr. Anne Wang for her contributions to the previous edition of this text; and the nursing staff of the General Clinical Research Center (GCRC) at the Mount Sinai School of Medicine for their expert nursing care of the type I patients. This chapter was supported in part by grants from the National Institutes of Health, including a research grant (MERIT Award 5 R01 DK34045), a grant (2 M01 RR00071) for the Mount Sinai General Clinical Research Center from the National Center for Research Resources, and a grant (P30 HD28822) for the Mount Sinai Child Health Research Center.

REFERENCES

1. van Diggelen OP, Schindler D, Kleijer WJ, Huijmans JMG, Galjaard H, Linden HU, Peter-Katalinic J, Egge H, Dabrowski U, Cantz M: Lysosomal α-*N*-acetylgalactosaminidase deficiency: A new inherited metabolic disease. *Lancet* **2**:804, 1987.
2. van Diggelen OP, Schindler D, Willemsen R, Boer M, Kleijer WJ, Huijmans JMG, Blom W, et al.: α-*N*-Acetylgalactosaminidase deficiency, a new lysosomal storage disorder. *J Inherit Metab Dis* **11**:349, 1988.
3. Schindler D, Bishop DF, Wolfe DE, Wang AM, Egge H, Lemieux RU, Desnick RJ: Neuroaxonal dystrophy due to lysosomal α-*N*-acetylgalactosaminidase deficiency. *N Engl J Med* **320**:1735, 1989.
4. Desnick RJ, Wang AM: Schindler disease: An inherited neuroaxonal dystrophy due to α-*N*-acetylgalactosaminidase deficiency. *J Inherit Metab Dis* **13**:549, 1990.
5. Desnick RJ, Bishop DF: Fabry Disease: a-Galactosidase deficiency; Schindler disease: α-*N*-acetylgalactosaminidase deficiency, in Scriver CR, Beaudet AL, Sly WS, Valle D (eds): *The Metabolic Basis of Inherited Disease* (6th ed). New York, McGraw-Hill, 1989, p 1751.
6. Desnick RJ, Schindler D: Alpha-N-acetylgalactosaminidase deficiency, in Buyse M, (ed): *Birth Defects Encyclopedia*. Boston, Blackwell Scientific, 1990, p 92.
7. Desnick RJ, Wang AM: α-*N*-Acetylgalactosaminidase deficiency: Schindler disease, in Scriver CR, Beaudet AL, Sly WS, Valle D (eds): *The Metabolic and Molecular Bases of Inherited Disease* vol. 2 (7th ed). New York, McGraw-Hill, 1995, p 2509.
8. Schindler D, Wang AM, Desnick RJ: Infantile neuroaxonal dystrophy due to deficient α-*N*-acetylgalactosaminidase activity, in Asbury AK, Budka H, Sluga E (eds): *Sensory Neuropathies*. Wien, Springer, 1995, p 133.
9. Kanzaki T, Yokota M, Mizuno N, Matsumoto Y, Hirabayashi Y: Clinical and ultrastructural studies of a novel angiokeratoma corporis diffusum. *Clin Res* **36**:177A, 1988.
10. Kanzaki T, Yokota M, Mizuno N, Matsumoto Y, Hirabayashi Y: Novel lysosomal glycoaminoacid storage disease with angiokeratoma corporis diffusum. *Lancet* **1**:875, 1989.
11. Kanzaki T, Wang AM, Desnick RJ: Lysosomal α-*N*-acetylgalactosaminidase deficiency, the enzymatic defect in angiokeratoma corporis diffusum with glycopeptiduria. *J Clin Invest* **88**:707, 1991.
12. Kanzaki T, Yokota M, Irie F, Hirabayashi Y, Wang AM, Desnick RJ: Angiokeratoma corporis diffusum with glycopeptiduria due to deficient lysosomal α-*N*-acetylgalactosaminidase activity. *Arch Dermatol* **129**:460, 1993.
13. Chabás A, Coll MJ, Aparicio M, Rodriguez Diaz E: Mild phenotypic expression of α-*N*-acetylgalactosaminidase deficiency in two adult siblings. *J Inherit Metab Dis* **17**:724, 1994.
14. de Jong J, van den Berg C, Wijburg H, Willemsen R, van Diggelen O, Schindler D, Hoevenaars F, Wevers R: Alpha-*N*-acetylgalactosaminidase deficiency with mild clinical manifestations and difficult biochemical diagnosis. *J Pediatr* **125**:385, 1994.
15. Keulemans JLM, Reuser AJJ, Kroos MA, Willemsen R, Hermans MMP, van den Ouweland AMW, de Jong JGN, et al.: Human α-*N*-acetylgalactosaminidase (α-NAGA) deficiency: New mutations and the paradox between genotype and phenotype. *J Med Genet* **33**:458, 1996.
16. Gay C, Maire I, Piraud M, Blanchon YC, Lauras B, Desnick RJ: Schindler disease, α-*N*-acetylgalactosaminidase deficiency presenting as autism. In review.
17. Wang AM, Bishop DF, Desnick RJ: Human α-*N*-acetylgalactosaminidase: Molecular cloning, nucleotide sequence, and expression of a full-length cDNA. *J Biol Chem* **265**:21859, 1990.
18. Wang AM, Desnick RJ: Structural organization and complete sequence of the human α-*N*-acetylgalactosaminidase gene: Homology with the α-galactosidase A gene provides evidence for evolution from a common ancestral gene. *Genomics* **10**:133, 1991.
19. Wang AM, Schindler D, Desnick RJ: Schindler disease: The molecular lesion in the α-*N*-acetylgalactosaminidase gene that causes an infantile neuroaxonal dystrophy. *J Clin Invest* **86**:1752, 1990.
20. Simonaro L, Maire I, Gay C, Desnick RJ: Schindler type III disease: Identification and characterization of the disease-causing mutations in the α-*N*-acetylgalactosaminidase gene. In review.
21. Griffin JW, Watson DF: Axonal transport in neurological disease. *Ann Neurol* **23**:3, 1988.
22. Schindler D, Kanzaki T, Desnick RJ: A method for the rapid detection of urinary glycopeptides in α-*N*-acetylgalactosaminidase deficiency and other lysosomal storage diseases. *Clin Chim Acta* **190**:81, 1990.
23. Desnick RJ, Ioannou YA, Eng CM: α-Galactosidase A deficiency: Fabry disease, in Scriver CR, Beaudet AL, Sly WS, Valle D (eds): *The Metabolic and Molecular Bases of Inherited Disease* vol. 2 (7th ed). New York, McGraw-Hill, 1995, p 2741.
24. Hirabayashi Y, Matsumoto Y, Matsumoto M, Toida T, Iida N, Matsubara T, Kanzaki T, et al.: Isolation and characterization of major urinary amino acid *O*-glycosides and a dipeptide *O*-glycoside from a

new lysosomal storage disorder (Kanzaki disease). Excessive excretion of serine- and threonine-linked glycan in the patient urine. *J Biol Chem* **265**: 1693, 1990.

25. Linden H-U, Klein RA, Egge H, Peter-Katalinic J, Dabrowski J, Schindler D: Isolation and structural characterization of sialic acid-containing glycopeptides of the *O*-glycosidic type from the urine of two patients with a hereditary deficiency in α-*N*-acetylgalactosaminidase activity. *Biol Chem Hoppe-Seyler* **370**: 661, 1989.
26. Rudolf J, Grond M, Schindler D, Heiss W-D, Desnick RJ: Cerebral glucose metabolism in Type I α-*N*-acetylgalactosaminidase deficiency, an inherited neuroaxonal dystrophy. *J Child Neurol* **14**:543, 1999.
27. Wolfe DE, Schindler D, Desnick RJ: Neuroaxonal dystrophy in infantile α-*N*-acetylgalactosaminidase deficiency. *J Neurol Sci* **132**: 44, 1995.
28. Wolfe DE: Infantile neuroaxonal dystrophy associated with α-*N*-acetylgalactosaminidase deficiency: On relating axonal spheroids to a lysosomal deficiency, in Asbury AK, Budka H, Sluga E (eds): *Sensory Neuropathies*. Wien, Springer, 1995, p 197.
29. Nieuwenhuys R: *Chemoarchitecture of the brain*. Berlin, Springer, 1985, p 44.
30. Walkley SU, Baker HJ, Rattazzi MC, Haskins ME, Wu J-Y: Neuroaxonal dystrophy in neuronal storage disorders: Evidence for major GABAergic neuron involvement. *J Neurol Sci* **104**: 1, 1991.
31. Walkley SU: Pathobiology of neuronal storage disease. *Int Rev Neurobiol* **29**: 191, 1988.
32. Seitelberger F: Eine unbekannte Form von infantiler Lipoid-Speicher-Krankheit des Gehirns. Proceedings of the First International Congress of Neuropathology (Rome, Sept. 8–13, 1952). Torino, Rosenberg & Sellier 1952, p 323.
33. Seitelberger F, Jellinger K: Neuroaxonal dystrophy and Hallervorden-Spatz disease, in Goldensohn ES, Appel SH (eds): *Scientific Approaches to Clinical Neurology* vol. 2. Philadelphia, Lea and Febiger, 1977, p 1052.
34. Cowen D, Olmstead EV: Infantile neuroaxonal dystrophy. *J Neuropathol Exp Neurol* **22**: 175, 1963.
35. Hedley-Whyte ET, Gilles FH, Uzman BG: Infantile neuroaxonal dystrophy. *Neurology* **18**: 891, 1968.
36. de Leon GA, Mitchell MH: Histological and ultrastructural features of dystrophic isocortical axons in infantile neuroaxonal dystrophy (Seitelberger a & disease.). *Acta Neuropathol (Berl)* **66**: 89, 1985.
37. Indravasu S, Dexter RA: Infantile neuroaxonal dystrophy and its relationship to Hallervorden-Spatz disease. *Neurology* **18**: 693, 1968.
38. Park BE, Netsky MG, Betsill WL: Pathogenesis of pigment and spheroid formation in Hallervorden-Spatz syndrome and related disorders. *Neurology* **25**: 1172, 1975.
39. Hakomori S-I: Blood group ABH and Ii antigens of human erythrocytes: Chemistry, polymorphism, and their developmental change. *Semin Hematol* **18**: 39, 1981.
40. Berger E, Buddecke E, Kamerling JP, Kobatu A, Paulson JC, Vliegenthart JFG: Structure, biosynthesis and functions of glycoprotein glycans. *Experientia* **38**: 1129, 1982.
41. Poole AR: Proteoglycans in health and disease: Structure and functions. *Biochem J* **236**: 1, 1986.
42. Peter-Katalinic J, Williger K, Egge H, Green B, Hanisch F-G, Schindler D: The application of electrospray mass spectrometry for structural studies on a tetrasaccharide monopeptide from the urine of a patient with α-*N*-acetylgalactosaminidase deficiency. *J Carbohydr Chem* **13**: 447, 1994.
43. Lamblin G, Lhermitte M, Klein A, Roussel P, van Halbeek H, Vliegenthart JFG: Carbohydrate chains from human bronchial mucus glycoproteins: A wide spectrum of oligosaccharide structures. *Biochem Soc Trans* **12**: 591, 1984.
44. Feizi T, Gooi HC, Childs RA, Picarel JK, Uemura K, Loomes LM, Thorpe SJ, Hounsell EF: Tumor-associated and differentiation antigens on the carbohydrate moieties of mucin-type glycoproteins. *Biochem Soc Trans* **12**: 591, 1984.
45. Takasaki S, Yamashita K, Kobat A: The sugar chain structures of ABO blood group active glycoproteins obtained from human erythrocyte membrane. *J Biol Chem* **253**: 6086, 1978.
46. Lloyd KO, Kabat EA: Immunological studies on blood groups, XLI. Proposed structures for the carbohydrate portions of blood group A, B, H, Lewis[a] and Lewis[b] substances. *Proc Natl Acad Sci U S A* **61**: 1470, 1968.
47. Hirabayashi Y, Kanzaki T: Defects in the metabolism of the *O*-linked oligosaccharides of glycoproteins. *Trends Glycosci Glycotechnol* **2**: 93, 1990.
48. Williger K, Peter-Katalinic J, Schindler D, Hanisch F-G, Egge H: Structures of *O*-glycopeptides from urine of a patient with α-*N*-acetylgalactosaminidase deficiency. *Biol Chem Hoppe-Seyler* **373**: 853, 1992.
49. Lecat D, Lemmonier M, Derappe C, Lhermitte M, Halbeek H, Dorland L, Vliengenthart JFG: The structure of sialyl-glycopeptides of the *O*-glycosidic types, isolated from sialidosis (mucolipidosis I) urine. *Eur J Biochem* **140**: 415, 1984.
50. Takahashi Y, Nakamura Y, Yamaguchi S, Orii T: Urinary oligosaccharide excretion and severity of galactosialidosis and sialidosis. *Clin Chim Acta* **203**: 199, 1991.
51. Tsuji S, Yamauchi T, Hiraiwa M, Isobe T, Okuyama T, Sakimura K, Takahashi Y, Mishizawa M, Uda Y, Miyatake T: Molecular cloning of a full-length cDNA for human α-*N*-acetylgalactosaminidase (α-galactosidase B). *Biochem Biophys Res Commun* **163**: 1498, 1989.
52. Warner TG, Louie A, Potier M: Photolabeling of the α-neuraminidase/β-galactosidase complex from human placenta with a photoreactive neuraminidase inhibitor. *Biochem Biophys Res Commun* **173**: 13, 1990.
53. Rege VP, Painter TJ, Watkins WM, Morgan WTJ: Three new trisaccharides obtained from human blood group A, B, H and Le[a] substances: Possible sugar sequences in the carbohydrate chains. *Nature* **200**: 532, 1963.
54. Makita A, Taniguchi N: Glycosphingolipids, in Wiegandt H (ed): *Glycolipids*. New York, Elsevier, 1985, p 1.
55. Breimer ME, Jovall P-A: Structural characterization of a blood group A heptoglycosylceramide with globoseries structure. The major glycolipid based blood group A antigen of human kidney. *FEBS Lett* **179**: 165, 1985.
56. Yoda Y, Ishibashi T, Makita A: Isolation, characterization, and biosynthesis of Forssman antigen in human lung and lung carcinoma. *J Biochem* **88**: 1887, 1980.
57. Taniguchi N, Yokosawa N, Narita M, Mitsuyama T, Makita A: Expression of Forssman antigen synthesis and degradation in human lung cancer. *J Natl Can Inst* **67**: 577, 1981.
58. Hakomori S, Wang S-M, Young WWJ: Isoantigenic expression of Forssman glycolipid in human gastric and colonic mucosa: Its possible identity with "A-like antigen" in human cancer. *Proc Natl Acad Sci U S A* **74**: 3023, 1977.
59. Paulsen H, Bünsch A: Synthese der pentosaccharid-kette des Forssman-antigens. *Carbohydr Res* **100**: 143, 1982.
60. Klima B, Pohlentz G, Schindler D, Egge H: An investigation into the glycolipid metabolism of α-*N*-acetylgalactosaminidase-deficient fibroblasts using native and artificial glycolipids. *Biol Chem Hoppe-Seyler* **373**: 989, 1992.
61. Asfaw B, Schindler D, Ledvinová J, Cerny B, Smid F, Conzelmann E: Degradation of blood group A glycolipid A-6-2 by normal and mutant human skin fibroblasts. *J Lipid Res* **39**: 1768, 1998.
62. Szweda R, Spohr U, Lemieux RU, Schindler D, Bishop DF, Desnick RJ: Synthesis of 4-methylumbelliferyl glycosides for the detection of α- and β-D-galactopyranosaminidases. *Can J Chem* **67**: 1388, 1989.
63. Schindler D, Wang AM, Bishop DF, Desnick RJ: A fluorescence-based assay for the determination of α-*N*-acetylgalactosaminidase activity and the identification of homozygotes and heterozygotes for α-*N*-acetylgalactosaminidase deficiency. *Enzyme*, in review.
64. Schram AW, Hamers MN, Tager JM: The identity of α-galactosidase B from human liver. *Biochim Biophys Acta* **482**: 138, 1977.
65. Dean KJ, Sung S-SJ, Sweeley CC: The identification of α-galactosidase B from human liver as an α-*N*-acetylgalactosaminidase. *Biochem Biophys Res Commun* **77**: 1411, 1977.
66. Dean KJ, Sung S-SJ, Sweeley CC: Purification and partial characterization of human liver α-galactosidases: Is α-galactosidase B an α-*N*-acetylgalactosaminidase? *Fed Proc* **36**: 731, 1977.
67. Schram AW, Hamers MN, Brouwer-Kelder B, Donker-Koopman WE, Tager JM: Enzymological properties and immunological characterization of α-galactosidase isozymes from normal and Fabry human liver. *Biochim Biophys Acta* **482**: 125, 1977.
68. Schram AW: *Studies on Human α-Galactosidase, N-acetyl-α-Galactosaminidase and α-Glucosidase in Relation to Lysosomal Storage Diseases*. PhD Thesis, University of Amsterdam, 1978.
69. Schram AW, de Groot PG, Hamers MN, Brouwer-Kelder B, Donker-Koopman WE, Tager JM: Further characterization of two forms of *N*-acetyl-α-galactosaminidase from human liver. *Biochim Biophys Acta* **525**: 410, 1978.
70. Bishop DF, Dean KJ, Sweeley CC, Desnick RJ: Purification and characterization of human α-galactosidase isozymes: Comparison of tissue and plasma forms and evaluation of purification methods, in Desnick RJ (ed): *Enzyme Therapy in Genetic Diseases*. New York, A.R. Liss, 1980, p 17.

71. Kint JA: Fabry's disease: α-galactosidase deficiency. *Science* **167**:1268, 1970.
72. Beutler E, Kuhl W: Biochemical and electrophoretic studies of a-galactosidase in normal man, in patients with Fabry's disease, and in Equidae. *Am J Hum Genet* **24**:237, 1972.
73. Wood S, Nadler HL: Fabry's disease: Absence of an α-galactosidase isozyme. *Am J Hum Genet* **24**:250, 1972.
74. Ho MW, Beutler S, Tennant L, O'Brien JS: Fabry's disease: Evidence for a physically altered α-galactosidase. *Am J Hum Genet* **24**:256, 1972.
75. Romeo G, Childs B, Migeon B: Genetic heterogeneity of α-galactosidase in Fabry's disease. *FEBS Lett* **27**:161, 1972.
76. Kint JA: On the existence and the enzymatic interconversion of α-galactosidase in human organs. *Arch Int Phys Biochem* **79**:633, 1971.
77. Kint JA, Huys A: Effect of bacterial neuraminidase on the isoenzymes of acid hydrolases of human brain and liver. Proceedings of the International Symposium on Glycolipids, Glycoproteins and Mucopolysaccharides of the Nervous System. New York, 1972, p 273.
78. Desnick RJ, Allen KY, Desnick SJ, Raman MK, Bernlohr RW, Krivit W: Fabry's disease: Enzymatic diagnosis of hemizygotes and heterozygotes. Alpha-galactosidase activities in plasma, serum, urine, and leukocytes. *J Lab Clin Med* **81**:157, 1973.
79. Beutler E, Kuhl W: Purification and properties of human α-galactosidases. *J Biol Chem* **247**:7195, 1972.
80. Beutler E, Kuhl W: Fabry's disease: Structural or regulatory mutation? *J Lab Clin Med* **78**:987a, 1971.
81. Kano I, Yamakawa T: The properties of α-galactosidase remaining in kidney and liver of patients with Fabry's disease. *Chem Phys Lipids* **13**:283, 1974.
82. Salvayre R, Maret A, Negre A, Douste-Blazy L: Properties of multiple molecular forms of α-galactosidase and α-*N*-acetylgalactosaminidase from normal and Fabry leukocytes. *Eur J Biochem* **100**:377, 1979.
83. Bishop DF, Desnick RJ: Affinity purification of α-galactosidase A from human spleen, placenta, and plasma with elimination of pyrogen contamination. Properties of the purified splenic enzyme compared to other forms. *J Biol Chem* **256**:1307, 1981.
84. Dean KJ, Sweeley CC: Studies on human liver α-galactosidases. I. Purification of α-galactosidase A and its enzymatic properties with glycolipid and oligosaccharide substrates. *J Biol Chem* **254**:9994, 1979.
85. Kusiak JW, Quirk JM, Brady RO, Mook JE: Purification and properties of the two major isozymes of α-galactosidase from human placenta. *J Biol Chem* **253**:184, 1978.
86. Romeo G, Dimatteo G, d'Urso M, Li S-C, Li Y-T: Characterization of human α-galactosidase A and B before and after neuraminidase treatment. *Biochim Biophys Acta* **391**:349, 1975.
87. Beutler E, Guinto E, Kuhl W: Variability of α-galactosidase A and B in different tissues of man. *Am J Hum Genet* **25**:42, 1973.
88. Sorensen SA, Hasholt L: α-Galactosidase isozymes in normal individuals, and in Fabry hemizygotes and heterozygotes. *Ann Hum Genet* **43**:313, 1980.
89. Mapes CA, Sweeley CC: Interconversion of the A and B forms of ceramide trihexosidase from human plasma. *Arch Biochem Biophys* **158**:297, 1973.
90. Dean KJ, Sweeley CC: Studies on human liver α-galactosidases. II. Purification and enzymatic properties of α-galactosidase B (α-*N*-acetylgalactosaminidase). *J Biol Chem* **254**:10001, 1979.
91. Rietra PJGM, van den Bergh FAJTM, Tager JM: Properties of the residual α-galactosidase activity in the tissues of a Fabry hemizygote. *Clin Chim Acta* **62**:401, 1975.
92. Callahan JW, Lassila EL, den Tandt WR, Philippart M: Alpha-*N*-acetylgalactosaminidase: Isolation, properties and distribution of the human enzyme. *Biochem Med* **7**:424, 1973.
93. Wilkinson F: PhD Thesis, Michigan State University, 1988.
94. Calhoun DH, Bishop DF, Bernstein HS, Quinn M, Hantzopoulos P, Desnick RJ: Fabry disease: Isolation of a cDNA clone encoding human alpha-galactosidase A. *Proc Natl Acad Sci U S A* **82**:7364, 1985.
95. Romeo G, D'Urso M, Pisacane A, Blum E, De Falco A, Ruffilli A: Residual activity of a-galactosidase A in Fabry's disease. *Biochem Genet* **13**:615, 1975.
96. Crawhall JC, Banfalvi M: Fabry's disease: Differentiation between two forms of α-galactosidase by myoinositol. *Science* **177**:527, 1972.
97. Schachern PA, Shea DA, Paparella MM, Yoon TH: Otologic histopathology of Fabry's disease. *Ann Otol Rhinol Laryngol* **98**:359, 1989.
98. Sweeley CC, LeDonne NC Jr, Robbins PW: Post-translational processing reactions involved in the biosynthesis of lysosomal α-*N*-acetylgalactosaminidase in cultured human fibroblasts. *Arch Biochem Biophys* **223**:158, 1983.
99. Hu P, Reuser AJJ, Janse HC, Kleijer WJ, Schindler D, Sakuraba H, Tsuji A, Suzuki Y, van Diggelen OP: Biosynthesis of human α-*N*-acetylgalactosaminidase: Defective phosphorylation and maturation in infantile a-NAGA deficiency. *Biochem Biophys Res Commun* **175**:1097, 1991.
100. Sung S-SJ, Sweeley CC: Purification and partial characterization of porcine liver α-*N*-acetylgalactosaminidase. *J Biol Chem* **255**:6589, 1980.
101. Matsuura F, Ohta M, Ioannou YA, Desnick RJ: Human α-galactosidase A: Characterization of the *N*-linked oligosaccharides on the intracellular and secreted glycoforms overexpressed by Chinese hamster ovary cells. *Glycobiology* **8**:329, 1998.
102. Mayes JS, Scheerer JB, Sifers RN, Donaldson ML: Differential assay for lysosomal α-galactosidases in human tissues and its application to Fabry's disease. *Clin Chim Acta* **112**:247, 1981.
103. Weissmann B, Hinrichsen DF: Mammalian α-acetylgalactosaminidase. Occurrence, partial purification, and action on linkages in submaxillary mucins. *Biochemistry* **8**:2034, 1969.
104. Weissmann B, Friederici D: Occurrence of a mammalian α-*N*-acetyl-D-galactosaminidase. *Biochim Biophys Acta* **117**:498, 1966.
105. Werries E, Wollek E, Gottschalk A, Buddecke E: Separation of *N*-acetyl-α-glucosaminidase and *N*-acetyl-α-galactosaminidase from ox spleen. Cleavage of the *O*-glycosidic linkage between carbohydrate and polypeptide in ovine and bovine submaxillary glycoprotein by *N*-acetyl-α-galactosaminidase. *Eur J Biochem* **10**:445, 1969.
106. Wang AM, Kanzaki T, Desnick RJ: The molecular lesion in the α-*N*-acetylgalactosaminidase gene that causes angiokeratoma corporis diffusum with glycopeptiduria. *J Clin Invest* **94**:839, 1994.
107. de Groot PG, Hamers MN, Westerveld A, Schram AW, Meera Khan P, Tager JM: A new immunochemical method for the quantitative measurement of specific gene products in man-rodent somatic cell hybrids. *Hum Genet* **44**:295, 1978.
108. de Groot PG, Westerveld A, Meera Khan P, Tager JM: Localization of a gene for human α-galactosidase B (= *N*-acetyl-α-D-galactosaminidase) on chromosome 22. *Hum Genet* **44**:305, 1978.
109. Geurts van Kessel AHM, Westerveld A, de Groot PG, Meera Khan P, Hagemeijer A: Regional localization of the genes coding for human ACO2, ARSA, and NAGA on chromosome 22. *Cytogenet Cell Genet* **28**:169, 1980.
110. Budarf M, McDermid H, Wang AM, Desnick RJ, Emmanuel B: Localization of the NAGA gene to 22q13.1Æ13.2 in somatic cell hybrids. In review.
111. von Heijne G: A new method for predicting signal sequence cleavage sites. *Nucleic Acids Res* **14**:4683, 1986.
112. Kornreich R, Desnick RJ, Bishop DF: Nucleotide sequence of the human α-galactosidase A gene. *Nucleic Acids Res* **17**:3301, 1989.
113. Yamauchi T, Hiraiwa M, Kobayashi H, Uda Y, Miyatake T, Tsuji S: Molecular cloning of two species of cDNAs for human α-*N*-acetylgalactosaminidase and expression in mammalian cells. *Biochem Biophys Res Commun* **170**:231, 1990.
114. Breathnach R, Chambon P: Organization and expression of eucaryotic split genes coding for proteins. *Ann Rev Biochem* **50**:349, 1981.
115. Mount SM: A catalog of splice junction sequences. *Nucleic Acids Res* **10**:459, 1982.
116. Reed R, Maniatis T: The role of the mammalian branchpoint sequence in pre-mRNA splicing. *Genes Dev* **2**:1268, 1988.
117. Dynan WS, Tjian R: Control of eukaryotic messenger RNA synthesis by sequence specific DNA-binding proteins. *Nature* **316**:774, 1985.
118. Benoist C, Chambon P: In vivo sequence requirements of the SV40 early promotor region. *Nature* **290**:340, 1981.
119. Lindsay S, Bird AP: Use of restriction enzymes to detect potential gene sequences in mammalian DNA. *Nature* **327**:336, 1987.
120. Bird AP: CpG-rich islands and the function of DNA methylation. *Nature* **321**:209, 1986.
121. Deininger PL, Jolly DJ, Rubin CM, Friedmann T, Schmid CW: Basic sequence studies of 300 nucleotide renatured repeated human cDNA clones. *J Mol Biol* **151**:17, 1981.
122. Jurka J, Smith T: A fundamental division in the Alu family of repeated sequences. *Proc Natl Acad Sci U S A* **85**:4775, 1988.
123. Bishop DF, Kornreich R, Desnick RJ: Structural organization of the human α-galactosidase A gene: Further evidence for the absence of a 3′ untranslated region. *Proc Natl Acad Sci U S A* **85**:3903, 1988.
124. Maeda N, Smithies O: The evolution of multi-gene families: Human haptoglobin genes. *Ann Rev Genet* **20**:81, 1986.

125. Proia RL: Gene encoding the human β-hexosaminidase chain: Extensive homology of intron placement in the α- and β-chain genes. *Proc Natl Acad Sci U S A* **85**:1883, 1988.
126. Horowitz M, Wilde S, Horowitz Z, Reiner O, Gelbart T, Beutler E: The human glucocerebrosidase gene and pseudogene: Structure and evolution. *Genomics* **4**:87, 1989.
127. Zhu A, Goldstein J: Cloning and functional expression of a cDNA encoding coffee bean α-galactosidase. *Gene* **140**:227, 1994.
128. Wilson R, Ainscough R, Anderson K, Baynes C, Berks M, Bonfield J, Burton J, et al.: 2.2 Mb of contiguous nucleotide sequence from chromosome III of *C. elegans* [see comments]. *Nature* **368**:32, 1994.
129. Wang AM, Ioannou YA, Zeidner KM, Desnick RJ: Murine α-*N*-acetylgalactosaminidase: Isolation, and expression of full-length cDNA and genomic organization. *Mol Genet Metab* **65**:165, 1998.
130. Wang AM, Stewart CL, Desnick RJ: α-*N*-Acetylgalactosaminidase: Characterization of the murine cDNA and genomic sequences and generation of mice by targeted gene disruption. *Am J Hum Genet* **53**:99, 1993.
131. Herrmann T, Schindler D, Tabe H, Onodera O, Igarashi S, Polack A, Zehnpfennig D, Tsuji S: Molecular cloning, structural organization, sequence, chromosomal assignment and expression of the mouse alpha-*N*-acetylgalactosaminidase gene. *Gene* **211**:205, 1998.
132. Nakagawa F, Schulte BA, Spicer SS: Selective cytochemical demonstration of glycoconjugate-containing terminal *N*-acetylgalactosamine on some brain neurons. *J Comp Neurol* **243**:280, 1986.
133. Kobata A, Takasaki S: Endo-β-galactosidase and endo-α-*N*-acetyl-D-galactosaminidase from *Diplococcus pneumoniae*. *Methods Enzymol* **50**:560, 1978.
134. Umemoto J, Bhavanandan VP, Davidson EA: Purification and properties of an endo-α-*N*-acetyl-D-galactosaminidase from *Diplococcus pneumoniae*. *J Biol Chem* **252**:8609, 1977.
135. Garnier J, Osguthorpe DJ, Robson B: Analysis of the accuracy and implication of simple methods for predicting the secondary structure of globular proteins. *J Mol Biol* **120**:97, 1978.
136. Wang AM, Simonaro C, Brenner O, Friechrich V, Stewart CL, Desnick RJ: Schindler disease: Generation of a murine model by targeted disruption of the α-*N*-acetylgalactosaminidase gene. In review.
137. Seitelberger F: Neuroaxonal dystrophy: Its relation to aging and neurological disease, in Vinken PJ, Bruyn GW, Klawans HL (eds): *Handbook of Clinical Neurology*, vol. 49 (Rev Ser 5). Amsterdam, Elsevier Science Publishers, 1986, p 391.
138. Benson DA, Boguski MS, Lipman DJ, Ostell J, Ouellette BFF: GenBank. *Nucleic Acids Res* **26**:1, 1998.

CHAPTER 140

Disorders of Glycoprotein Degradation: α-Mannosidosis, β-Mannosidosis, Fucosidosis, and Sialidosis

George H. Thomas

1. Most, if not all, glycoproteins are synthesized by one of two pathways. The glycosyl transferase pathway synthesizes oligosaccharides linked O-glycosidically to serine or threonine, whereas the dolichol, lipid-linked pathway synthesizes oligosaccharides linked N-glycosidically to asparagine. Ultimately, the oligosaccharides are degraded in lysosomes by a group of exoglycosidases acting at the nonreducing termini, and by endo-β-N-acetylglycosaminidase and aspartylglucosaminidase at the reducing end. Specific deficiencies of these enzymes result in glycoprotein or oligosaccharide storage diseases. Four such human disorders are discussed in this chapter.
2. Human α-mannosidosis (MIM 248500) is one of two disorders of glycoprotein catabolism associated with abnormal levels and excretion of small mannose-rich oligosaccharides. The more severe (infantile or type I) phenotype includes rapidly progressive mental retardation, hepatosplenomegaly, severe dysostosis multiplex, and often death between 3 and 12 years of age. The milder (juvenile-adult or type II) phenotype, accounting for approximately 10–15 percent of cases, is characterized by a milder and more slowly progressive course with survival into adulthood. While patients are generally placed into one of these two groups, there may in fact be a continuum of clinical findings rather than a clear separation. The biochemical alterations in α-mannosidosis result from a deficiency of the lysosomal enzyme α-mannosidase. The gene that codes for the precursors of the subunits of this enzyme and maps to human chromosome 19p13.2–q12 has been isolated and sequenced. The mode of inheritance is autosomal recessive.
3. Human β-mannosidosis (MIM 248510), a more recently described disorder of oligosaccharide catabolism, results from a deficiency of β-mannosidase activity and is associated with increased storage and excretion of Man(β1 → 4)GlnNAc. The clinical phenotype, based on the 13 patients described to date, remains unclear. The most severe findings include status epilepticus, severe quadriplegia, and death by 15 months, while the mildest findings have been limited to the presence of angiokeratomas. To date, the most frequent findings have been mental retardation, respiratory infections, and hearing losses with associated speech impairments. In keeping with data showing an autosomal mode of inheritance, the responsible gene has been mapped to human chromosome 4q21–25. A composite cDNA, consisting of an 87-nucleotide 5′-untranslated region, a 2640-nucleotide coding region, and a 556-nucleotide untranslated region, codes for a 3.7-kb transcript. The enzyme, a lysosomal protein, has a molecular mass of 100 kDa.
4. Fucosidosis (MIM 230000) is an autosomal recessive disorder resulting from a deficiency of the lysosomal hydrolase α-fucosidase. While at least two phenotypes have been described in this disorder, recent data suggest that individual patients may actually represent a continuum within a wide spectrum of severity. The more severely affected patients have, within the first year of life, the onset of psychomotor retardation, coarse facies, growth retardation, dysostosis multiplex, neurologic retardation, and increase in sweat sodium chloride. In contrast, the milder phenotypes are characterized by the presence of angiokeratoma, longer survival, and more normal levels of sweat sodium chloride. The enzyme defect results in the accumulation and excretion of a variety of glycoproteins, glycolipids, and oligosaccharides containing fucoside moieties. Although the disorder is panethnic, the majority of patients have been from Italy or the southwestern part of the United States. A high frequency of consanguinity has been seen in affected families. The gene (*FUCA1*) that codes for the common subunit that makes up the multiple forms of α-fucosidase has been isolated sequenced, and mapped to chromosome 1p24. At least 23 mutations causing fucosidosis have been reported. Of these, only four result in an amino acid substitution, with the remaining mutations presumed to result in unstable or defective mRNA, e.g. premature stop codons, frameshifts, defective splicing, large deletions.
5. Sialidosis (MIM 256550), the final disorder reviewed in this chapter, is also an autosomal recessive lysosomal storage disorder. Type I sialidosis, the milder form of this disorder, is characterized by the development of ocular cherry-red spots and generalized myoclonus in the second or third decade of life. Additional findings, reported in more than 50 percent of patients, include seizures, hyperreflexia, and ataxia. Type II sialidosis is distinguished from this milder

A list of standard abbreviations is located immediately preceding the index in each volume. Nonstandard abbreviations used in this chapter include: *FUCA1* = gene symbol for α-fucosidase; *FUCA1P* = gene symbol for α-fucosidase pseudogene; *FUCA2* = gene symbol for locus influencing plasma fucosidase levels; *MANB* = gene symbol for α-mannosidosis locus.

form by the early onset of a progressive, rather severe, mucopolysaccharidosis-like phenotype with visceromegaly, dysostosis multiplex, and mental retardation. Both forms of the disease result from deficiency of the neuraminidase that normally cleaves terminal α2 → 3 and α2 → 6 sialyl linkages of several oligosaccharides and glycopeptides that are found in increased amounts in tissues and fluids of affected patients. The gene coding for this neuraminidase maps to human chromosome 6p21 in the region containing the HLA locus. A 1.9-kb cDNA, containing an open reading frame of 1245 nucleotides, is predicted to code for a protein containing 415 amino acids. Direct evidence that this gene is responsible for isolated deficiencies of sialidase is provided by the detection of mutations in this locus in at least nine sialidosis patients.

6. **No definitive treatment is currently available for these lysosomal enzyme deficiencies. Identification of affected fetuses by biochemical analysis is reliable and has been demonstrated for each of these abnormalities by means of chorionic villus samples or cultured amniotic fluid cells.**

This chapter primarily considers lysosomal storage diseases involving well-defined loci that cause defects in the degradation of the sugar side chains of cellular glycoproteins. Glycoproteins are characterized by the presence of oligosaccharide chains covalently attached to a peptide backbone. These include peptides linked with oligosaccharides through the hydroxyl groups of serine or threonine or through the free amino group of asparagine. Proteoglycans and oligosaccharides linked to collagen and basement membrane proteins are considered separately in Chaps. 136 and 206, respectively. Genetic defects in degradation may be restricted to glycoproteins or may involve other macromolecules. This is because certain oligosaccharide linkages are found in glycolipids and proteoglycans as well as in glycoproteins. Hence, a deficiency of a single lysosomal enzyme may result in accumulation of more than one class of oligosaccharide-containing macromolecules (Table 140-1).

The glycoprotein storage diseases considered here conform to the general conceptual framework of lysosomal storage diseases. Each demonstrates deficiency of a lysosomal hydrolase, accumulation and urinary excretion of the substrates ordinarily degraded by that enzyme, a progressive clinical course, and considerable variation of the phenotype associated with different defects at a single locus. In addition, these disorders often manifest clinical features that usually would be considered part of the mucopolysaccharidosis phenotype, such as coarse facies, dysostosis multiplex, and/or abnormal eye findings.

In addition to collagen and mucopolysaccharides, mammalian tissues contain two major groups of glycoproteins with distinct structural differences and separate synthetic pathways (Table 140-2). The biosynthesis and structure of glycoproteins are reviewed in greater detail elsewhere.[1–5] The oligosaccharides are synthesized as the proteins make the transit from the rough endoplasmic reticulum (ER) to the smooth ER and through the Golgi apparatus. The protein portions of the glycoproteins are synthesized on membrane-bound polysomes. The sugar nucleotide synthetic pathway involves the transfer to the growing oligosaccharide chain of single sugars from sugar nucleotides. Oligosaccharides synthesized by this pathway are found linked to protein through an O-glycosidic linkage of N-acetylgalactosamine (GalNAc) to serine or threonine. There is extensive diversity of the oligosaccharide structures within this category.[1] A specific example of an O-glycosidic oligosaccharide is the blood group megalosaccharide, shown in Fig. 140-1. The oligosaccharides of glycolipids that are synthesized by this pathway and related structures found on lipids are discussed in Chap. 150. Most of the degradative defects to be discussed involve structures of the N-glycosidic type discussed below, but defective degradation of the O-glycosidic oligosaccharides is involved in some instances.

The dolichol pathway for synthesis of oligosaccharides utilize lipid-linked intermediates.[2,4,5] A complex pathway is involved to produce the structure shown in Fig. 140-2. This structure is thought to be the common intermediate that is transferred to the peptide backbone. The entire oligosaccharide structure is linked to the protein through an N-glycosidic linkage of GalNAc to asparagine.[4] Once transferred to the protein, the oligosaccharide structure undergoes a series of trimming and elongation steps that result in a final structure of either the "high-mannose" or the "complex" type.[4] These changes are summarized in Fig. 140-3, where structure A represents the final lipid intermediate, shown in detail in Fig. 140-2. Structure B represents a typical high-mannose oligosaccharide unit, and structure C represents a typical complex oligosaccharide unit. Again, there is extensive diversity in the detail of oligosaccharide structures.[1,4] See Chapter 16 for a more detailed discussion of the biosynthesis and structure of these glycoproteins.

Table 140-1 Disorders of Glycoprotein Degradation

Disorder	Chap. No.	Glycoproteins	Glycolipids
Mucolipidosis II and III	138	Generalized	Defect
Schindler disease	139	Probable	Unknown
α-Mannosidosis	140	Major	None
β-Mannosidosis	140	Major	?None
α-Fucosidosis	140	Major	Present
Sialidosis	140	Major	?Minimal
Aspartylglucosaminuria	141	Major	None
G_{M1} gangliosidosis	151	Present	Major
Galactosialidosis	152	Major	?Minimal
G_{M2} gangliosidosis (Sandhoff)	153	Present	Major

Table 140-2 Characteristics of Synthesis and Structure of Glycoproteins

Sugar Nucleotide Pathway	Dolichol Pathway
1. Sequential transfer of single sugars	1. Use of dolichol-linked intermediates
2. O-Glycosidic linkage of GalNAc to serine or threonine	2. N-Glycosidic linkage of GlcNAc to asparagine
3. Tunicamycin resistance	3. Tunicamycin sensitivity
4. Examples: blood group substance and submaxillary mucins	4. High-mannose, complex subtypes
	5. Examples: thyroglobulin and IgM

DEGRADATION OF GLYCOPROTEINS

Because glycoproteins occur widely, both within cells and on cell surfaces,[6] normal cellular metabolism and turnover involve the degradation of large amounts of these materials. There is, moreover, considerable cellular and biochemical evidence indicating that this catabolism normally occurs completely inside the lysosomes of a wide variety of cell types. As illustrated by the diseases discussed in this chapter, an interruption or blockage at any step in the degradation of the glycan portions of the glycoproteins can cause lysosomal alterations resulting in cellular pathology and, ultimately, clinical disease.[7–12]

The protein backbones of the glycoproteins are degraded from both the end and internal sites by a series of lysosomal proteases and peptidases. This process contrasts with the normal bidirectional degradation of the oligosaccharide portion of the molecules, which is accomplished by the ordered removal of sugars from the

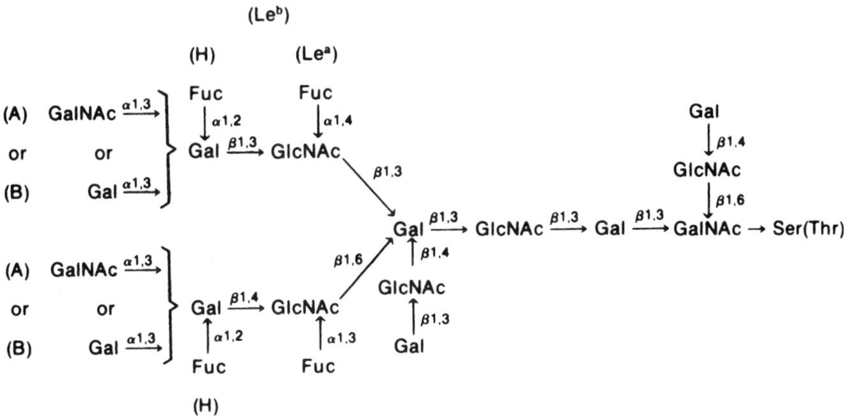

Fig. 140-1 Composite megalosaccharide proposed for blood group substance. *(From Kornfeld and Kornfeld,[1] as modified from Feizi et al. J Immunol 106:1578, 1971.)*

nonreducing ends and, to a lesser extent, cleavages at the reducing end of the Asn-linked oligosaccharides.[13] Cleavage from the nonreducing termini of the oligosaccharide is carried out by a number of exoglycosidases catalyzing the sequential removal of single sugars from the oligosaccharide branches. The lysosomal enzymes involved in these steps include neuraminidase (sialidase), β-galactosidase, β-N-acetylhexosaminidase, β-mannosidase, α-mannosidase, and α-fucosidase.

The additonal pathway for Asn-linked oligosaccharides involves the ordered removal of fucose and N-acetylglucosamine from the protein-oligosaccharide linkage region, i.e., the reducing end of the oligosaccharide. The last enzyme step, the action of a reducing-end β-N-acetylglucosaminidase (chitobiase), results in the cleavage of the chitobiose linkage, GlcNAc($\beta 1 \rightarrow 4$)GlcNAc, between two N-acetylglucosamine residues.[14–17] This chitobiose core, normally found adjacent to the asparagine in oligosaccharides synthesized by the dolichol pathway, is exposed by aspartylglucosaminidase, which cleaves the amide bond between chitobiose and asparagine at the reducing end of the oligosaccharide (Chap. 141).[18–21] Prior to this step, any fucose at the 6-position of the terminal GlcNAc must be cleaved by α-fucosidase. As a result, the enzymatic hydrolysis of the di-N-acetylchitobiose core is the last step in the ordered disassembly of the core region of the Asn-linked glycoprotein. A composite, complex type N-glycosidic oligosaccharide and the proposed hydrolytic steps required for its degradation are shown in Fig. 140-4.

A deficiency of any one of the required lysosomal enzymes results in cellular accumulation and urinary excretion of products of partial degradation of the oligosaccharides. The metabolites that accumulate are the result of defects in and/or interactions of three major types of hydrolysis previously discussed, i.e., single sugar removal from the nonreducing end, endoglycosidic hydrolysis at the chitobiose linkage, and hydrolysis of the glycoasparagine linkage.[13]

Although these incompletely digested products are discussed further as part of the review of abnormalities in each specific disease, some of the findings are summarized in Fig. 140-5. The stored materials in these lysosomal diseases appear to be products of incomplete degradation of known oligosaccharide structures and are compatible with the metabolites one would expect to result from specific enzyme deficiencies. Almost all of the storage disease structures are known to occur within typical high-mannose or complex glycoproteins.[6] Whereas mannosidosis and sialidosis patients have alterations in oligosaccharides and aspartylglucosaminuria patients accumulate only glycopeptides, both oligosaccharides and glycopeptides accumulate in the tissues and fluids of fucosidosis patients.

Finally, although several animals afflicted with inherited disorders of glycoprotein metabolism have been found to be valuable as models for their human disease counterparts, one must be aware of the differences in glycoprotein catabolism among species.[13] Specifically, humans and rats have a lysosomal chitobiase,[14–17] whereas most other animals (dogs, cats, goats, sheep, and cattle) either lack or have low levels of this activity.[13,16,17,22] Thus, while humans suffering from defects in oligosaccharide metabolism accumulate and excrete oligosaccharides that bear, at their reducing end, a single N-acetylglucosamine residue, most animals having similar disorders but lacking chitobiase accumulate compounds that have a bis-N-acetylglucosamine (chitobiose) residue.[22] The presence or absence of the intact GlcNAc($\beta 1 \rightarrow 4$)GlcNAc moiety at the reducing end of the various storage materials is, therefore, correlated with the presence or absence of chitobiase activity.[13]

HISTORY OF CLINICAL DISORDERS

In the late 1960s, individuals with phenotypes resembling certain inherited mucopolysaccharidoses but lacking mucopolysacchariduria were described in the medical literature.[23–25] These patients were found variously to have features suggestive of one of the mucopolysaccharidoses, the lipomucopolysaccharidoses, or the mucolipidoses. It was, however, soon recognized that these individuals actually had a new group of disorders resulting from inherited defects in lysosomal enzymes responsible for the catabolism of glycoproteins (Table 140-3).

Several of the patients were ultimately found to have α-mannosidosis, a disorder first described by Öckerman in 1967.[26] In the same year, Jenner and Pollitt described a brother and sister with mental retardation and large quantities of urinary aspartylglucosamine,[27] later shown to result from a deficiency of aspartylglucosaminidase.[28] See Chap. 141 for a detailed discussion of this disorder. In 1968 fucosidosis was described by Durand

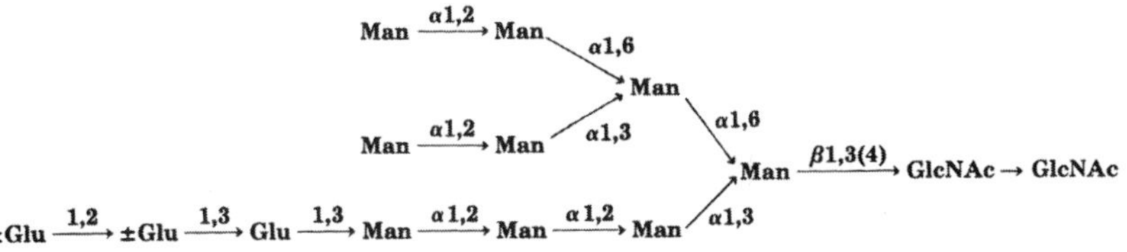

Fig. 140-2 Proposed structure of the lipid-linked oligosaccharide precursor in glycoprotein synthesis. *(From S. Kornfeld, J Biol Chem, 253:7762, 1978. Used by permission.)*

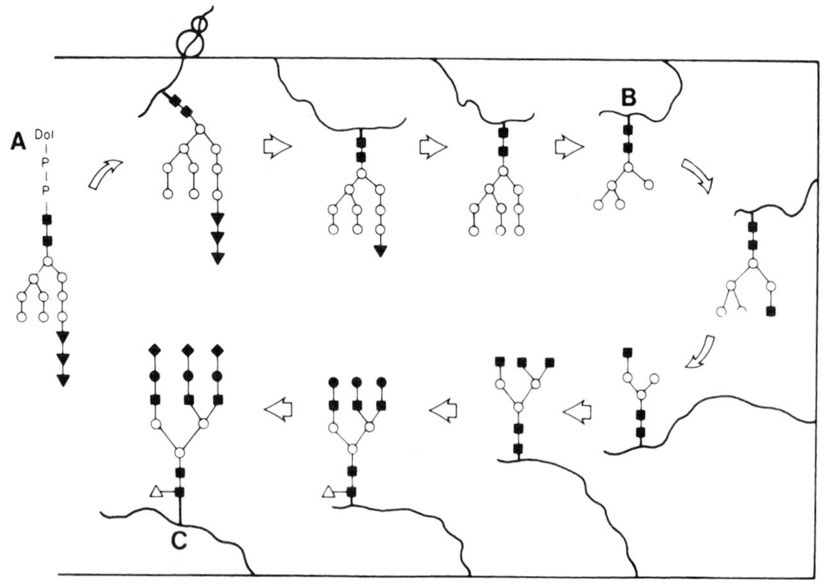

Fig. 140-3 Proposed sequence for the synthesis of complex oligosaccharides. Dol = dolichol. The symbols are: ■ = GlcNAc; ○ = Man; ▼ = Glc; ● = Gal; ◆ = SA; △ = Fuc. The precursor, shown in detail in Fig. 140-2, is indicated as A; B indicates a high-mannose structure; and C indicates a complex structure. (*With modification from S. Kornfeld, J Biol Chem, 253:7771, 1978. Used by permission.*)

et al.,[29] and the defect in α-fucosidase was concomitantly reported by Van Hoff and Hers.[30]

Sialidosis, resulting from a deficiency of neuraminidase (sialidase), was not clarified until 1977;[31,32] the original patient having been classified earlier as having lipomucopolysaccharidosis[23] and mucolipidosis I.[24] This was soon followed by the recognition that a deficiency of neuraminidase was also responsible for the cherry-red spot–myoclonus syndrome.[33–35] The clinical and biochemical relationship between sialidosis and galactosialidosis that also resulted in early confusion has also since been resolved (Chap. 152).

The last disease to be described in this group of disorders, β-mannosidosis, was first identified in goats having a rapidly fatal neurologic disease.[36] The human counterpart of this disease was simultaneously reported in 1986 by Cooper et al.[37] and by Wenger and colleagues.[38] Since this time, additional patients have been described.[39–43] Several disorders having alterations not only in glycopeptides and/or oligosaccharides but also in other compounds are discussed elsewhere in this text. These disorders include Schindler disease (Chap. 139), G_{M1} gangliosidosis (Chap. 151), G_{M2} gangliosidosis type 2 (Chap. 153), and galactosialidosis (Chap. 152).

Other early case reports, now included within the spectrum of inborn errors of oligosaccharide catabolism, are reviewed in a text on the lysosomal storage diseases.[44] A small book entitled *Genetic Errors of Glycoprotein Metabolism*, published in 1982, documents many of the early investigations into this group of disorders, with chapters on sialidosis,[7] fucosidosis,[8] and α-mannosidosis.[9] The reader is also referred to several excellent reviews covering topics relevant to glycoproteins. These include discussions of biosynthesis and function[4,6] and normal degradation[13] and overviews of inborn errors of glycoproteins.[11,12]

The genes responsible for the enzymes involved in each of the above disorders have now been mapped, characterized, and sequenced. See Table 140-4 for an overview of these data. As outlined in Table 140-5, at least one, and in most cases more, mutations have been identified in each of the clinical forms of these disorders.

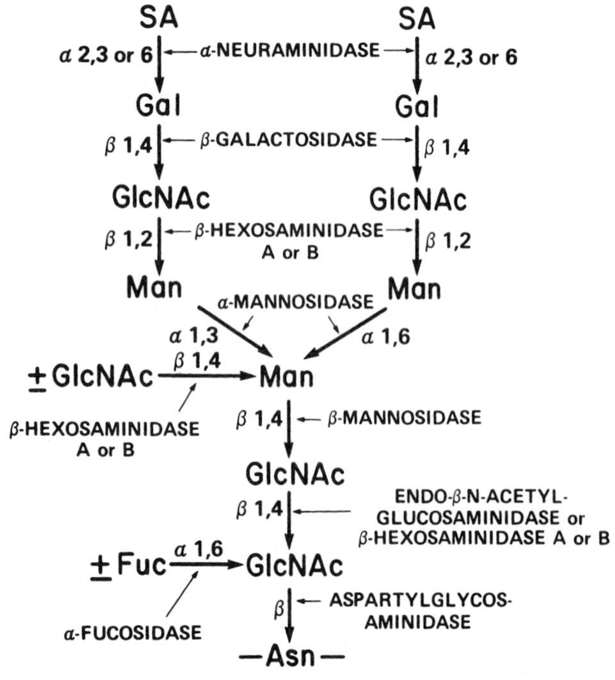

Fig. 140-4 Probable steps in degradation of complex oligosaccharide structure.

α-MANNOSIDOSIS

Clinical Features

To date, reports of at least 90 cases of α-mannosidosis have appeared in the medical literature.[26,45–83] This includes 67 patients reported up to 1982 and reviewed by Chester et al.[9] plus an additional 23 patients described since.[63,65–83] Among other things, these reports document that, like many lysosomal diseases, this disorder is characterized by a rather wide range of clinical phenotypes (see Fig. 140-6; Tables 140-3, 140-6). The more severely affected patients, found in the infantile age group, are considered to have the "type I" form of this disorder, while a milder form of the disorder occurring in juveniles and adults is designated "type II."[9,53]

Virtually all type I and type II patients have mental retardation, facial coarsening, and some degree of dysostosis multiplex (see Fig. 140-6; Tables 140-3, 140-6). It should be noted, however, that these features have been reported to be very mild in some patients.[68,77,80] Additional findings include recurrent bacterial infections, which may be related to a defect in leukocyte

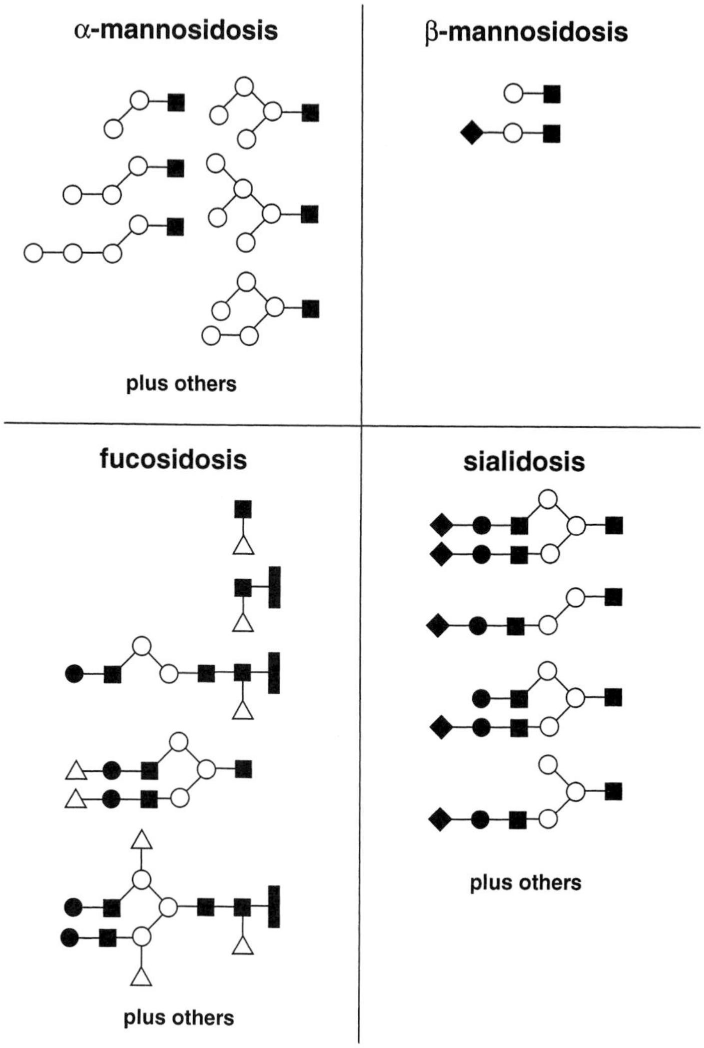

Fig. 140-5 Graphic summary of major storage and/or urinary products in the four glycoprotein storage diseases reviewed in this chapter. ■ = GlcNAc; ○ = Man; ▼ = Glc; ● = Gal; ◆ = SA; △ = Fuc; ▮ = asparagine.

chemotaxis.[72] Other findings include deafness, hepatomegaly, hernias, and lenticular or corneal opacities. The ocular findings are distinctive and include posterior opacities in a spokelike pattern in the lens and superficial opacities in the cornea (Fig. 140-7).[54,57,73] The skeletal dysplasia[55] includes thickening of the calvaria in the majority of patients. The vertebral bodies are prominently involved, with ovoid configurations, flattening, and beaking appearance, sometimes in association with gibbus deformity. Patients with the more severe infantile, or type I, phenotype suffer from rapid mental deterioration, obvious hepatosplenomegaly, more severe dysostosis multiplex than seen in type II, and often death between 3 and 10 years of age.

In contrast, individuals with the milder juvenile-adult, or type II, form of the disorder are characterized by more normal early development, with mental retardation becoming apparent only during childhood or adolescence. Hearing loss is particularly prominent in type II patients. Dysostosis multiplex is milder than that found in type I individuals, and patients often survive into adulthood. Destructive synovitis,[65,67] hydrocephalus,[74] spastic paraplegia,[69] pancytopenia,[75] and hyperphagia[81] have also been reported in type II patients. MRI studies of the head in three patients demonstrated bony changes, verticalization of the chiasmatic sulcus, cerebellar atrophy, and white matter signal changes.[70] The clinical course of mannosidosis is often described as being gradual, sometimes with imperceptible progression.[64,76,77,80] While there may be a continuum of phenotypes rather than a clear separation, it is nevertheless possible in most cases to distinguish type I from type II patients. See, for example, the comparison of the clinical, biochemical, and radiographic findings in the two forms of the disease by Bennett et al.[80]

One of the more useful laboratory findings is the presence of vacuolated lymphocytes in almost all α-mannosidosis patients. While there is no evidence of mucopolysacchariduria, urine from both type I and II patients, when examined by thin-layer chromatography, is characterized by abnormal oligosaccharide patterns.[80] Decreased serum IgG can occur, and a decreased PR interval on EKG has been reported.[78]

Treatment

One patient with α-mannosidosis underwent bone marrow transplantation (at 7 years of age) and died 18 weeks later from bronchopneumonia. While there was some evidence of enzymatic correction at autopsy, there was no evidence of decreased neuronal vacuolization.[79] A kidney transplant has also been carried out on a 23-year-old type II mannosidosis patient with end-stage renal failure. Three years after the transplant, the graft was functioning well with no evidence of renal deposits. The clinical course of the mannosidosis at the time of the report was stated to be "silent," while the patient's quality of life was said to be good.[84]

In an animal study, Walkley et al.[85] examined the efficacy of bone marrow transplantation as a means of enzyme replacement. Three kittens lacking α-mannosidase received bone marrow transplants at ages 8, 10, and 12 weeks of age using normal sibs as donors. While clinical evidence of cerebellar disease was seen in two of the three treated cats, these animals showed little or no progression of neurologic signs 1–2 years after the transplants. In

Table 140-3 Major Features of α-Mannosidosis, β-Mannosidosis, Fucosidosis, and Sialidosis

Disorders	Onset	Facial Findings	Dysostosis Multiplex	Neurologic Findings	Organomegaly	Eye Findings	Hemologic Findings	Other Findings
α-Mannosidosis								
Type I	3–12 mos.	Coarse	+++	MR (severe)	+++	Cataracts, corneal opacities	Vacuolated lymphocytes	Hearing loss
Type II	1–4 yrs.	Coarse	++	MR	++	Cataracts, corneal opacities	Vacuolated lymphocytes	Hearing loss (severe)
β-Mannosidosis								
	1–6 yrs.	Dysmorphic (mild)	+/−	MR	−	Normal	Normal	Angiokeratomas
Fucosidosis								
Type I	3–18 mos.	Coarsening (mild)	++	MR, seizures	++		Vacuolated lymphocytes	↑sweat NaCl
Type II	1–2 yrs.	Coarsening (mild)	++	MR	++	Tortuous conjunctival vessels	Vacuolated lymphocytes	Angio keratomas (anhidrosis)
Sialidosis								
Type I	8–25 yrs.	Normal	−	Myoclonus seizures	−	Cherry-red spot, ↓acuity	Vacuolated lymphocytes (rarely)	Neuropathy & ↓deep tendon reflexes
Type II								
Congenital	In utero	Coarse	+++	MR	+++	?	Vacuolated lymphocytes	Hydrops, ascites, stillbirth
Infantile	0–12 mos.	Coarse	+++	MR	+/−	Cherry-red spot	Vacuolated lymphocytes	Renal involvement
Juvenile	2–20 yrs.	Coarsening (mild)	++	MR, myoclonus	−	Cherry-red spot, ↓acuity	Vacuolated lymphocytes	Angiokeratomas

MR = mental retardation

contrast, the untreated affected cats became severely impaired. The authors provided evidence that the bone marrow transplantation (at least in kittens) restored significant levels of the missing enzyme within neurons of the central nervous system.[85]

Pathology

Pathologic studies of biopsy[86] and autopsy[45,69,74,87] material are available. Light microscopy of the liver demonstrates granular or foamy cytoplasm in the hepatocytes. Periodic acid–Schiff (PAS) staining varies with the histochemical extraction procedure. Electron microscopy (EM) studies show the presence of multiple vacuoles in hepatocytes and Kupffer cells, often with a reticulogranular pattern, although many other types of inclusions are observed. Examination of the central nervous system reveals marked and widespread ballooning of the nerve cells. The cytoplasm has an empty or vacuolated appearance. EM again demonstrates membrane-bound vacuoles with a predominantly reticulogranular pattern.

Table 140-4 Genes Involved in Glycoprotein Disorders

	Map location	Gene size	Exons (No.)	cDNA (ORF) Nucleotides
α-Mannosidase	19p13–q12	22 kb	24	3030*
β-Mannosidase	4q21–q25	NR	NR	3293*
α-Fucosidase	1p34	23 kb	8	1383**
Sialidase	6p21	3.5 kb	6	1245**

See discussion under "Gene Structure" of each gene for details and references. NR = not reported at time of review; ORF = open reading frame; * cDNA; ** ORF

Biochemical Storage

Although it is known that mannose-rich compounds accumulate in the various tissues of α-mannosidosis patients,[26,88] few studies have been carried out on material from these sources. Instead, most of the analyses to date have been of mannose-rich fractions isolated from the urine of affected individuals. Early investigations established that the chemical structure of the three major urinary metabolites are as follows:[89]

1. Man(α1 → 3)Man(β1 → 4)GlcNAc
2. Man(α1 → 2)Man(α1 → 3)Man(β1 → 4)GlcNAc
3. Man(α1 → 2)Man(α1 → 2)Man(α1 → 3) Man(β1 → 4)GlcNAc

Subsequently, Strecker et al.[90] and Yamashita et al.[91] isolated and characterized several additional urinary mannose-containing oligosaccharides. Although the two groups found identical structures for several of the newly discovered compounds, they found different compositions for others.[90,91]

Since then, 17 mannose-rich oligosaccharides have been isolated and identified from pooled urine of two mannosidosis patients.[92,93] Three of these compounds are identical to the major metabolites noted above, 13 are identical to those reported previously by Yamashita et al.,[91] and one represented a newly discovered compound.

Each of the oligosaccharides isolated from the urine of mannosidosis patients has a single GlcNAc residue at the reducing end, not the GlcNAc(β1 → 4)GlcNAc core expected from the hydrolysis of Asn-linked glycoproteins. This finding appears to result from the enzymatic digestion of the chitobiose core found in glycoproteins and their oligosaccharide products by an endo-N-

Table 140-5 Human Mutations Known or Presumed to Be Responsible for Glycoprotein Disorders

Disease	Nucleotide	Amino Acid	Genotype	Reference
Sialidosis				
	1258G → T	H337X	compound	379
	401T → G	L91R	compound	379
	1337delC	Frameshift	compound	379
	7insACTC	Frameshift	homozygous	389
	779T → A	F260Y	compound	389
	1088T → C	L303P	compound	389
α-Mannosidosis				
	212A → T	H71L	homozygous	102
β-Mannosidosis				
	IVS-2A → G	Splicing	homozygous	186
Fucosidosis*				
	188C → T	S63L	homozygous	293
	758delA	Frameshift	homozygous	291
	1201G → T	G401X	homozygous	290
	1030ins66	In-frame insertion	homozygous	294
	IVS5+1G → A	Splicing	homozygous	292
	229C → T	Q77X	heterozygous	288, 289
	1145G → A	W382X	heterozygous	289
	633C → A	Y211X	homozygous	289
	421del C	Frameshift	homozygous	289
	794del C	Frameshift	homozygous	289
	646del A	Frameshift	heterozygous	289
	340del10	Frameshift	homozygous	295
	549G → A	W183X	homozygous	295
	14C → G	P5R	homozygous	295
	1988insT	Frameshift	homozygous	295
	985A → T	N329Y	homozygous	295
	1123G → T	E375X	homozygous	287
	179G → A	G60D	homozygous	286
	451delAA	Frameshift	heterozygous	286
	del exons 7&8	del 2 exons	homozygous	286
	1264C → T	Q422X	heterozygous	288
	1264C → T	Q422X	homozygous	240

*Reviewed by Willems et al.[399]

acetyl-β-glucosaminidase.[14,15] In addition, although the most abundant urinary compound, Man(α1 → 3)Man(β1 → 4)GlcNAc, appears to be derived from incomplete digestion of complex glycans, it lacks the expected mannose residue linked (α1 → 6) to the core mannose residue.[91] The absence of this compound appears to be due to the presence of a lysosomal (α1 → 6) mannosidase that remains active in affected patients lacking the major α-mannosidase.[94–96]

Comparative studies have demonstrated that the urinary oligosaccharides differ in bovine, feline, and human mannosidoses.[97] One study suggests that this is due to differences in the metabolic pathways — i.e., cattle and cats lack the endo-N-acetyl-β-glucosaminidase found in humans — and there are differences in the severity of the enzyme defects.[98]

The Enzyme and the Enzyme Defect

For some time, α-mannosidase activity has been known to exist in a variety of tissues.[9] The enzyme became of interest to human medical geneticists following the report of a patient who lacked this enzyme and accumulated mannose-rich oligosaccharides.[26]

Mannosidase activity in normal tissue results from the combined actions of Golgi membrane mannosidase(s) having a neutral pH optimum[99] and a lysosomal form of the enzyme (EC 3.2.1.24).[100] The lysosomal form is characterized by an acidic pH optimum; broad substrate specificity, including synthetic compounds, e.g., p-nitrophenyl-α-mannoside; and sensitivity to swainsonine. While early investigations suggested that this lysosomal enzyme existed in two major forms, designated "A" and "B,"[101] later studies have indicated a more complex pattern.[102]

Previously, the enzyme in fibroblasts was reported to be synthesized as a precursor of ~110-kDa, with subsequent proteolytic processing to two subunits of 63 to 67 kDa and 40 to 46 kDa.[103] Similarly, it was reported that mannosidase A in human liver consisted of equimolar numbers of 26- and 62-kDa subunits, whereas the B form contained the 26-kDa subunit and variable numbers of the 58- and 62-kDa subunits.[104] Subsequently, Tsuji and Suzuki,[105] using placental tissue, detected only 65- and 27-kDa subunits and provided evidence that differences reported in the early preparations might be due to proteolytic degradation. Although they differ in their molecular mass and subunit compositions, the A and B subunits are immunologically indistinguishable.[104] It is believed, therefore, that these two forms of the enzyme are coded for by a single locus.[104]

In a more recent study of human placenta, Nilssen et al.[102] reinvestigated the structure of this enzyme. While they agree that α-mannosidase is coded for by a single locus, their evidence indicates that the precursor is processed first into three (not two) glycoproteins, of 70, 42, and 15 kDa. It is suggested that the smallest, and previously unreported, 15-kDa peptide was missed in the early studies due to technical difficulties of the methods utilized. Evidence is also presented that the 70-kDa glycoprotein, found in both this and the earlier studies, is further processed into three more peptides joined together by disulfide bridges.

The molecular and genetic relationships of the various forms of the neutral and acidic mannosidases have not been completely elucidated; however, it is known that mannosidosis patients lack the acidic forms of the enzyme but retain the neutral enzyme(s).[9,106] Genetic heterogeneity is suggested by reports of some α-mannosidosis patients who have high residual mannosidase activity.[61,107–110] In the majority of these patients, the residual enzyme appears to have increased heat lability and a marked increase in the K_m against certain artificial substrates. In addition, there have been reports that the mutant enzyme is activated by cobalt and to varying degrees by zinc.[53,111] Immunologic studies of this residual material have yielded conflicting results. Specifically, antibodies against human liver α-mannosidase fail to react with this material, while rabbit anti–human placenta and anti–pig kidney mannosidase antibodies yield positive reactions.[53,112,113]

Several investigators have found an accumulation of acid mannosidase activity in media in which mannosidosis fibroblasts have been cultured.[103,114–116] These findings were interpreted by one group as suggesting that "the defect in mannosidosis is expressed only after the enzyme has been delivered to lysosomes and presumably undergone some form of processing here."[116] Later, evidence was presented that mannosidosis fibroblasts do not synthesize acid-mannosidase and that the enzyme secreted by these cells is not related immunologically to lysosomal mannosidase.[104]

Inheritance and Incidence

The data provided both by reports of families containing both male and female offspring affected with mannosidosis and by the results of molecular mapping clearly indicate that this disorder is inherited in an autosomal recessive manner (MIM 248500).[9,117] Therefore, for each pregnancy of a carrier couple, the risk of having an affected child is 25 percent.

Gene Assignment

Early studies of mouse-human hybrids indicated that the gene encoding acidic α-mannosidase is located on human chromosome 19.[118,119] Additional studies of mouse-human hybrids containing rearranged or deleted human chromosomes provided evidence that the gene locus is located on the central region of this chromosome,

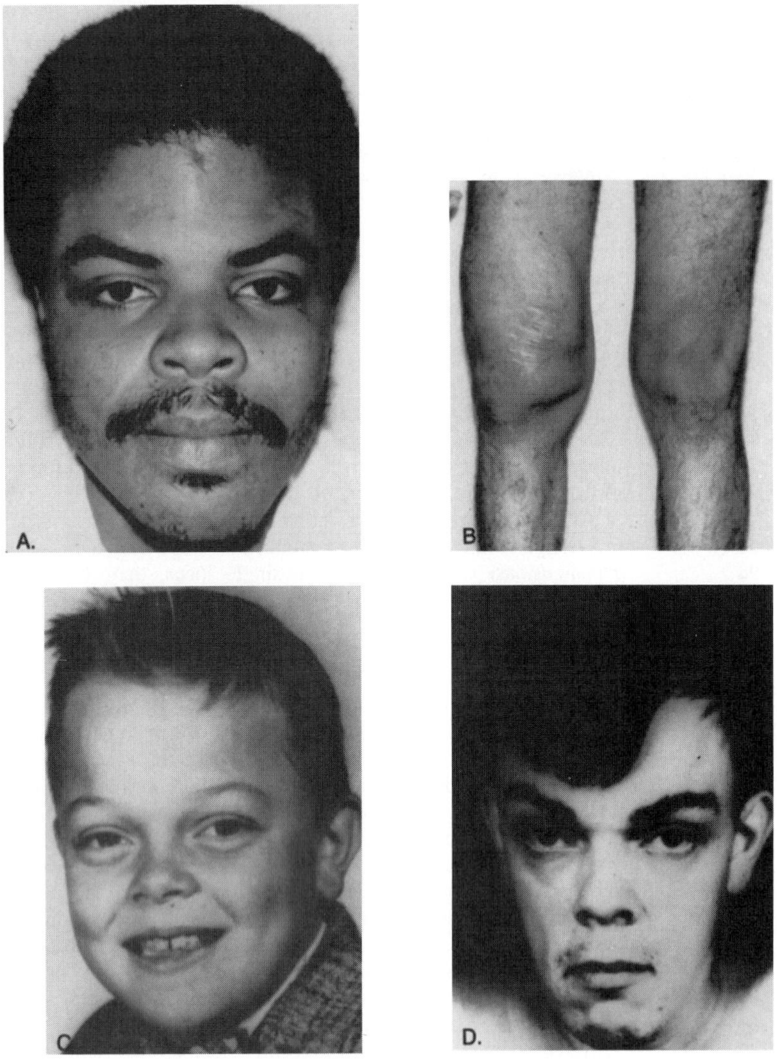

Fig. 140-6 Clinical features of α-mannosidosis. (A, B) Twenty-two-year-old male with α-mannosidosis type II, showing facial appearance and destructive synovitis of the knees. (C, D) Patient with α-mannosidosis at the ages of 12 and 30 years. (*C and D are from Montgomery, Thomas, and Valle.[66] Used by permission of The Johns Hopkins Medical Journal.*)

i.e., 19p13–q13[120,121] or, more recently, 19p13.2–q12.[122] Using a panel of human/rodent somatic cell hybrids, Bachinski et al.[123] showed that the DNA fragment responsible for α-mannosidase activity maps to the long arm of human chromosome 19 [proximal to *D19S7* and peptidase D [*PEPD*]). Subsequently, Nebes and Schmidt,[124] using degenerate oligonucleotide primers to generate a cDNA probe, isolated a full-length cDNA by plaque hybridization. From this they deduced the amino acid sequence of a protein believed to be human lysosomal α-mannosidase B. In agreement with the above data, this cDNA mapped to the *MANB* locus on the long arm of chromosome 19. While some of the sequence data was later shown to be incorrect (see below), expression studies provided direct evidence that this putative cDNA did in fact code for a protein with α-mannosidase activity.[125]

Gene Structure

Emiliani et al.[126] purified human lysosomal α-mannosidase in sufficient quantities to permit partial amino acid sequencing. Analysis of the N-terminal residue of a 30-kDa polypeptide of this material directly confirmed that the cDNA isolated by Nebes and Schmidt[124] does in fact code for human α-mannosidase. Sequence analysis of cDNA isolated from several human tissues by Liao et al.,[127] however, demonstrated sequence differences when compared to the data originally published by Nebes and Schmidt.[124] Sequence discrepancies were also noted by Wakamatsu et al.[128] and Riise et al.[129] Most if not all of these differences have subsequently been reported to have been due to errors in the original published sequence, which the authors later revised;[130] thus, the sequences reported by Liao et al.[127] Waksmatsu et al.,[128] and Riise et al.[129] represent the correct data (GenBank U60885).

Liao et al[127] cloned 3.0- and 3.6-kb cDNAs by RT-PCR of mRNA from human spleen. When expressed in *Pichia pastoris*, the shorter of the two cDNAs (containing 2964 bp) encodes a protein having all the characteristics of α-mannosidase previously isolated from human liver. Expression studies with the 3.6-kb product failed to yield enzyme activity. Northern blot analysis demonstrated the presence of a 3-kb RNA transcript in all human tissues examined: A minor amount of the 3.6-kb product was also identified in several tissues. Similar sequence results were obtained on overlapping fragments obtained by PCR of human fibroblast and human lung cDNA by Nilssen et al.[102] Northern blot analysis by this group, however, revealed a single transcript of ~3.5 kb in all tissues examined.

Wakamatsu et al.[128] and Riise et al.,[129] using human *MANB* cDNAs as probes, isolated and sequenced the entire human MANB gene. Both groups found the gene to consist of 24 exons spanning approximately 21 to 22 kb and that it appears to be controlled by a 5′ flanking sequence similar to that found previously in other lysosomal enzymes (see Table 140-4). Based on their data, Riise et al.[129] concluded that the processed mRNA product of this gene should contain 3443 bp which agrees well with the 3.5-kb mRNA found earlier by Nebes and Schmidt.[124]

In parallel investigations, murine,[131,132] feline,[133] and bovine[134] cDNAs have been isolated and sequenced. The deduced amino acid of the mouse α-mannosidase shows 75 percent[132] to 76

Table 140-6 Clinical Features Specifically Noted in α-Mannosidosis Patients

Clinical Abnormality	After 1982*		Before 1982**	
	n	%	*n*	%
Mental retardation	23/23	100	53/55	96
Hearing loss	21/23	91	39/47	83
Coarse facies	15/23	65	60/61	98
Recurrent infections	14/23	61	32/48	66
Dysostosis multiplex	13/23	56	55/59	93
Delayed motor development	12/23	52	41/45	91
Impaired speech	11/23	48	30/33	91
Hepatomegaly	8/23	35	25/54	46
Ocular changes	5/23	22	21/61	34
Macrocephaly	3/23	13	7/21	33
Hernia	2/23	9	22/31	71

*Data from 23 patients (refs. [63,65–71,76,77,79–83]) published after 1981 review by Chester et al.[9] Numbers and percentages for each feature are minimum estimates, i.e., symptoms are considered to be positive only if specifically noted in published reports.
**Data abstracted from 1982 review of 67 patients by 1982 by Chester et al.,[9] including only patients in which the feature was noted to be present or absent. See the original report for more details and complete references for case reports prior to 1982.

percent[133] identity to the human enzyme, while the feline is 81 percent identical.[133] The authenticity of the isolated murine cDNA was demonstrated by expression in *Pichia pastoris*[131] or COS[132] cells. Northern blot analysis showed a major transcript (~3.0–3.5 kb) in all tissues examined.[131,132] As was found in human tissue, the bovine gene is organized into 24 exons.[134]

Mutations

The first detailed description of a mutation associated with α-mannosidosis was found in two children of consanguineous parents.[102] These sibs, of Palestinian origin, were found to be homozygous for a 212A → T transversion resulting in a His → Leu substitution (see Table 140-4). While direct expression studies were not carried out in this family, evidence that this alteration is the cause of the disease in these sibs is provided by the fact that the mutation was not detected in a large number of controls and that the alteration occurs in a conserved position of the gene in several species.[102]

The results of a mutational analysis of six type II α-mannosidosis patients have also appeared in abstract form.[135] With PCR followed by SSCP analysis, a total of three missense mutations were identified in four of these individuals. Three patients were found to be homozygous and one heterozygous for the mutations believed to be responsible for the presence of mannosidosis in these individuals. No mutation was identified by the PCR/SSCP analysis in the remaining two patients. While this was not directly proven, it was concluded that the missense mutations detected in the MANB gene of these patients resulted in their disease.

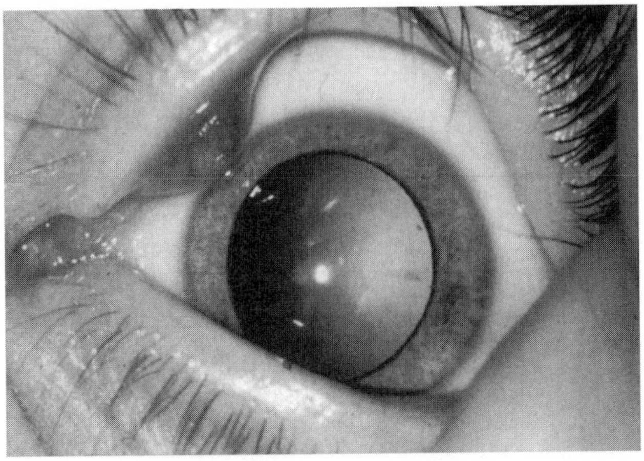

Fig. 140-7 Spoke-like cataracts in a 3-year-old patient with α-mannosidosis. (*From Wong et al.*[83] *Reprinted by permission of Wiley-Liss, Inc, a subsidiary of John Wiley & Sons, Inc.*)

Laboratory Diagnosis

Patients affected with α-mannosidosis excrete increased amounts of several oligosaccharides, the major one being Man(α1 → 3)Man(β1 → 4)GlcNAc.[89,136] Increased amounts of this and related compounds can most easily be demonstrated by any one of several thin-layer chromatography techniques widely utilized for the detection of inherited oligosaccharide disorders (Fig. 140-8).[137–140] For a detailed discussion of these methods of urinary screening, see the review by Sewell.[141] High-performance chromatography of oligosaccharides in urine[142] and fibroblasts[143] has also been described. As do individuals affected with other errors of glycoprotein degradation, α-mannosidosis patients have an abnormal pattern of oligosaccharide excretion.

Although its significance is currently unclear, the report that two sibs with mannosidosis, as well as 16 aspartylglucosaminuria patients, have elevated serum dolichol levels[144,145] suggests that the measurement of this compound might also be a useful screening tool. Once a urinary oligosaccharide pattern suggestive of α-mannosidosis is demonstrated, the diagnosis can be confirmed or excluded by direct measurement of α-mannosidase activity in any one of several tissues, e.g., white blood cells, fibroblasts, and cultured amniotic fluid cells. Direct measurement of α-mannosidase in plasma has been less reliable than the assay of cellular enzyme levels, probably because of forms of mannosidase enzymes in plasma that are not decreased in mannosidosis patients.[9] Evidence, has been presented however, that if the pH is carefully selected, e.g., pH 4.0, plasma can also be utilized for the diagnosis of α-mannosidosis.[146]

Prenatal Diagnosis

There are several reports of the successful prenatal diagnosis of mannosidosis. These include a report of an affected fetus, later confirmed,[147] and experience with two families in which two fetuses were affected while a third was found to be free of the disease.[148] Activity of α-mannosidase has been demonstrated in trophoblast biopsy material,[149] and a first-trimester diagnosis using chorionic villi has been reported.[150] It should be noted, however, that α-mannosidase activity in chorionic villi has been found to be less than one-third of that found in cultured amniotic fluid cells,[151] emphasizing the importance of good normal control data. Although these studies were carried out with no serious difficulties, the presence of both residual activity and forms of α-mannosidase not affected in mannosidosis patients must be taken into account in interpreting the results of a prenatal study for this disorder.[108]

Animal Models

There are at least three unrelated animal models for human α-mannosidosis. The best known one, bovine mannosidosis, is an autosomal inherited disorder found in Aberdeen Angus cattle.[152,153] The disorder has also been described in a number of related breeds of cattle, e.g., Red Angus, Murray Grey, Galloway, and shorthorns.[154] The disease in these animals is characterized by ataxia, incoordination, tremor, and aggressive behavior. Like humans with mannosidosis, animals affected with the bovine form of this disorder have reduced levels of the acidic form of α-D-mannosidase.[153] It has been estimated that in the absence of genetic testing, approximately 400 Angus calves born in Australia each year would be affected with this disorder.[155] The actual prevalence of α-mannosidosis in Angus cattle in Australia, however, has been reduced as the result of an industry-sponsored

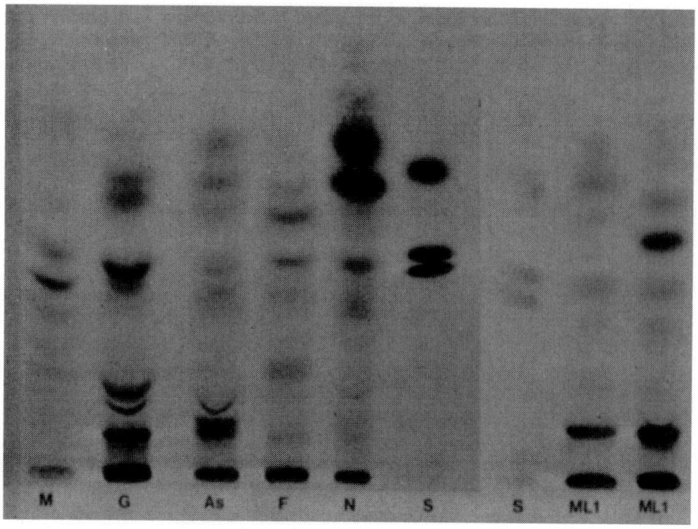

Fig. 140-8 Thin-layer chromatogram of urine with orcinol detection. M = α-mannosidosis; G = G_{M1} gangliosidosis; AS = aspartylglucosaminuria; F = fucosidosis; N = normal control; S = standard mixture of fructose, lactose, and reffinose; ML1 = sialidosis. (*From Sewell.*[137] *Used by permission.*)

disease control effort.[155] Additionally, α-mannosidosis has been found in a domestic short-hair cat having similar clinical findings, i.e., multiple skeletal deformities, retarded growth, ataxia, intention tremors, and deficiency of α-mannosidase activity.[156,157] More recently this disorder has been described in Persian cats.[158–162]

β-MANNOSIDOSIS

Clinical Features

A deficiency of β-mannosidase was first described in goats having severe neurologic disease associated with dysmyelination of the central nervous system and early death.[36] Numerous medical geneticists, aware of the disorder in goats, searched for a comparable human condition; however, the first such case was not discovered until 1986.[37,38] As of this time, there are reports of at least 13 cases in ten families.[37–43,163–165] Based on these early case reports, the clinical findings in humans do not appear to be as severe as those in the affected goats. The most consistent clinical finding in the human patients has been mental retardation, which has been reported in all but two patients.[163,164] Additional common findings include respiratory infections and hearing losses, noted in over 60 percent of reported cases (see Tables 140-3, 140-7). Coarse facies, corneal changes, hepatosplenomegaly, dysostosis multiplex, or vacuolated lymphocytes have not been reported in any β-mannosidosis patients (see Fig. 140-9). For this reason, this may be an underdiagnosed disorder. In contrast to the mild clinical findings, however, all patients suffer from complete deficiencies in β-mannosidase and the resulting biochemical alterations (see Table 140-3).

The most severely affected patient had status epilepticus at 12 months of age, severe quadriplegia, and death at 15 months.[41] In contrast, a much milder phenotype has been reported in two adult brothers, with mental retardation, angiokeratomas, and few other clinical findings.[37] A 22-year-old female, also having angiokeratomas but in this case associated with normal intelligence, has also been described.[164] The latter patient was, however, reported to be "somewhat introverted and scantly communicative."[164] Finally, a 14-year-old male lacking β-mannosidase has been described, with bilateral thenar amyotrophy and a progressive demyelinating peripheral neuropathy. While intelligence testing indicated a global IQ of 102, the patient was clinically depressed; his family was concerned about his apathy at an early age.[163]

Given the clinical heterogeneity in the small number of patients described to date, it is difficult to define precisely the phenotype associated with this condition (see Table 140-7). Interpretation of the clinical features is also complicated by the fact that one patient coincidentally was also affected with Sanfilippo A mucopolysaccharidosis,[38] while another also had ethanolaminuria.[43] Complementation studies indicate that the combined presence of β-mannosidosis and Sanfilippo A mucopolysaccharidosis resulted not from a common factor affecting both enzymes but rather from two independent mutations.[166]

While most β-mannosidosis patients have been reported to be normal for the first few months of life, all but two of the 13 patients described to date have eventually displayed mental retardation. Mild facial dysmorphism was reported in some patients, although this usually has not been as severe or as characteristic as that seen in patients with the various forms of the mucopolysaccharidoses. Skeletal abnormalities occur[40] but are not usual and do not include dysostosis multiplex. Hepatosplenomegaly has not been noted in any of the reported patients. Upper and lower respiratory tract infections, ear infections, and hearing loss have been reported frequently. Behavior has sometimes been described as aggressive, unstable, depressed, and/or introverted. CT scan of the brain is usually normal, but atrophy was observed in the most severely affected patient.[41] Angiokeratomas have been reported in two adult brothers in one family[37] and in an unrelated female in a second family.[164]

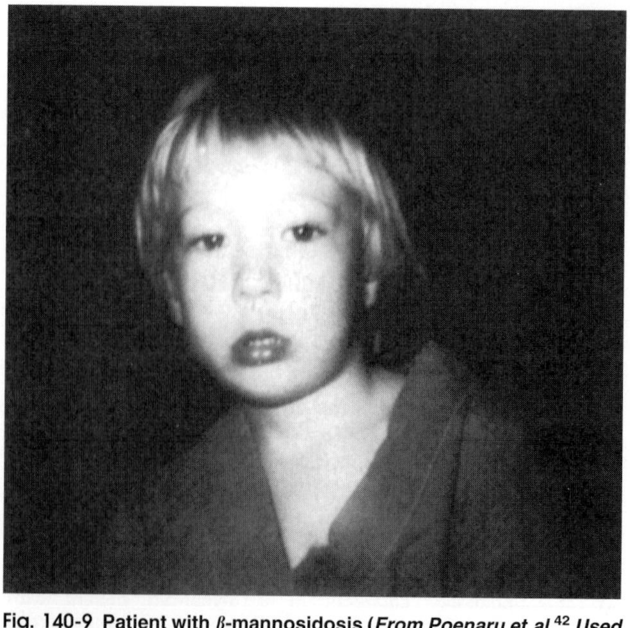

Fig. 140-9 Patient with β-mannosidosis (*From Poenaru et al.*[42] *Used by permission.*)

Table 140-7 Clinical Features Specifically Noted in More Than 10 Percent of 13 Patients with β-Mannosidosis*

Clinical Abnormality	Patients n	%
Mental retardation	11	85
Respiratory infection	8	62
Hearing loss	8	62
Speech impairment	5	38
Facial dysmorphism	4	31
Angiokeratoma	3	23
Hypotonia	3	23
Skeletal abnormalities	2	15

*Number and percentage for presence of each feature are minimum estimates; i.e., symptoms are considered to be absent unless specifically noted to be present in original report. Data from references 37–43,163,164,165.

Pathology

Very little pathologic information is available from mannosidosis patients. Cytoplasmic vacuoles were reported in a skin biopsy but not in lymphocytes or bone marrow cells in one patient.[37] Slight vacuolization and granulation of bone marrow cells were reported in another patient.[40]

Biochemical Storage

A disaccharide containing mannose and N-acetylglucosamine, shown to be Man(β1 → 4)GlcNAc,[38,39] is the major abnormal component found in the urine of β-mannosidosis patients. Quantitative analyses carried out by Tjoa et al.[167] detected 65 and 73 mg of this compound per millimole of creatinine in the urine of two affected sibs. These values are much higher than those found in the urine of controls (< 0.02 mg) and of patients with related inborn errors of metabolism (trace to 5.1 mg per millimole of creatinine).[167,168] Cultured fibroblasts from sibs with β-mannosidosis contained 52 and 68 nmol Man(β1 → 4)GlcNAc per milligram of protein.[169]

A sialylated compound, sialyl(α2 → 6)Man(β1 → 4)GlcNAc, has also been detected approximately 10 percent of the concentration of Man(β1 → 4)GlcNAc in the urine of these patients.[170,171] This compound is believed to result from the enzymatic sialylation of the major storage compound. A urinary carbohydrate-urea conjugate has also been found in these patients.[170]

The Enzyme and the Enzyme Defect

Elevations of short nondegraded oligosaccharides of the type described above are compatible with the expected effects of a deficiency of lysosomal β-mannosidase. This enzyme, the last exoglycosidase involved in the sequential degradation of oligosaccharides, normally cleaves the β-mannoside linkage at the interbranching core of these compounds. β-Mannosidase has been partially characterized in tissues from a variety of mammalian sources, including goats[172,173] and guinea pigs.[174] Additionally, the properties of this enzyme have been studied in a variety of human tissues and fluids, including urine,[175] serum,[175,176] fibroblasts,[177] leukocytes,[178] and placenta.[179] The results of the initial investigations of this enzyme were summarized in a review by Percheron et al.[180] These investigations showed the enzyme to have an optimum pH of 4.2 to 4.5, an apparent K_m with p-nitrophenyl-β-mannopyranoside of 2.2 to 2.8 mM, and a molecular mass of 90 to 110 kDa.[180] Enzyme inhibition occurs in the presence of sucrose.[181] In a purified preparation from human placenta, the enzyme was found to be a lysosomal protein with a molecular mass of 110 kDa containing high-mannose oligosaccharide side chains deficient in sialic acid.[179] After gel electrophoresis, this enzyme appeared to show several peptides of lower molecular mass, ranging from 57 to 98 kDa.[179] Further biochemical studies have been carried out on enzyme purified from human urine by Guadalupi et al.[182] Using this source, this group of investigators isolated two forms of the enzyme, which they designated β-mannosidase A and B. Sodium dodecyl sulfate-polyacrylamide gel electrophoresis analysis suggested that the A band consists of three subunits (75 kDa, 49 kDa, and 37 kDa) and the B band of one 75-kDa and two 49-kDa peptides. Similar results were obtained with enzyme obtained from human kidney.[182] Both forms of the human urine enzyme displayed optimal activity at pH 4.3.

Inheritance and Incidence

All data indicate that β-mannosidosis is inherited as an autosomal recessive disorder (MIM 248510).[117] Evidence supporting this conclusion includes the following: affected sibs in three of the families,[37,39,40] first-cousin parents in two families,[39,43] and existence of both affected males and affected females.[37–43] Additionally, the parents, while clinically unaffected, have reduced levels of β-mannosidase activity suggestive of heterozygosity. Autosomal inheritance is, of course, also compatible with the evidence that the gene is located on human chromosome 4 (see "Gene Assignment").

Because β-mannosidosis in humans has been described in only a relatively few patients and may be underdiagnosed, the incidence of this disorder remains unclear. Although many of the parents of reported patients have European backgrounds, the actual distribution of this disorder is unknown. Parental origins have been reported to be Hindu,[37] Turkish,[39] Czechoslovakian gypsy,[40] Jamaican-Irish,[41] "European,"[42] and black African.[163]

Gene Assignment

Early, indirect evidence suggested that the gene for β-mannosidase was on human chromosome 4. This conclusion was based in part on the observation that in mice a locus for β-mannosidase had been linked to the *Adh-3* locus.[183] Evidence that the *Adh-3*, as well as at least two other genes, showed homology between mouse chromosome 3 and human chromosome 4 indicated that this chromosome might be the location for the human β-mannosidase gene.[117] This conclusion was also in agreement with data showing that β-mannosidase mapped to bovine chromosome 6, shown previously to paint with human chromosome 4.[184] Direct evidence that this is indeed the case was supplied by Southern blot hybridization with a bovine probe of a panel of 24 human-rodent hybrid cell lines containing DNA from individual human chromosomes.[185] The gene was further localized to human 4q21–q25 in a similar manner using a PCR-generated human probe against human-rodent cell hybrids containing various deletions of chromosome 4 (Table 140-4).[186]

Gene Structure

The production of a monoclonal antibody against bovine β-mannosidase facilitated a four-step purification of this enzyme.[187] Using peptide sequence data obtained from this purified material, Chen et al.[185] cloned and characterized a cDNA coding for the entire bovine kidney β-mannosidase. This composite cDNA contains 3852 nucleotides encoding 879 amino acids. The deduced amino acid sequence matches the sequence determined by direct analysis of the purified enzyme. Similar results with the caprine gene were obtained by Leipprandt et al.[188] Using PCR primers based initially on the bovine and later on goat data, this group isolated, sequenced, and characterized a cDNA for the caprine enzyme. This cDNA also appeared to code for an 879-amino-acid protein with 95.2 percent identity to the predicted bovine sequence.[188]

The first full-length human β-mannosidase cDNA was sequenced by Alkhayat et al. in 1998 (Gen Bank U60337).[186] They found the composite human cDNA to consist of an 87-nucleotide 5′-untranslated region, a 2640-nucleotide coding region, and a 566-nucleotide untranslated region. Northern blot analysis of multiple tissues indicated the product of this gene to be a 3.7-kb transcript.[186] As with the caprine and bovine genes, this cDNA was predicted to encode 879 amino acids, starting with the predicted signal sequence, and to have 75 percent amino acid sequence identity with those of these animals (Table 140-4).[186]

Mutations

The first mutation responsible for human β-mannosidosis[186] was identified in a previously described Czech gypsy family.[40] The affected siblings (a severely affected female and her less severely affected brother) were found to be homozygous for an A → G transition 2 bp upstream of a splice acceptor site (Table 140-5).[186] This alteration, which results in activation of a cryptic site as well as in exon skipping, was predicted to give rise to two short protein products.[186]

Laboratory Diagnosis

Patients suffering from β-mannosidosis may be identified by the detection of abnormal patterns of urinary oligosaccharides by thin-layer chromatography. For this analysis, small amounts of urine are separated on silica-coated plates.[189] Solvent systems commonly utilized for the detection of β-mannosidosis include butanol–acetic acid–water (2:1:1 v/v)[39–41,190] and/or propanol–acetic acid–water (85:1:15 v/v).[39,40] The hexose-containing compounds are detected with an orcinol-sulfuric acid spray followed by heat. The major abnormal compound excreted in β-mannosidosis coincides with lactose with the first of these solvents but is separated from this compound with the second.[39–41] Many of the standard urinary oligosaccharide screening methods fail to identify β-mannosidosis patients;[141] however, a new method of HPLC has demonstrated abnormalities.[142] Finally, one β-mannosidosis patient has been reported to have elevated levels of ethanolamine in the plasma and urine.[43] Although the significance of this observation remains unknown, it is of interest that the original patient with ethanolaminosis was first believed to have had symptoms suggestive of a lysosomal storage disease.[191]

A more definitive method of diagnosing this disorder is based on the measurement of β-mannosidase in leukocytes or fibroblasts. This enzyme activity is most easily measured with one of two synthetic substrates, 4-methylumbelliferyl-β-D-mannopyranoside[177] or p-nitrophenyl-β-D-mannopyranoside.[42] The assay conditions,[42,176,179,190,192] as well as normal values and findings in affected families,[39–43] have been described in sufficient detail to permit the introduction of this procedure by any experienced biochemical laboratory.

Prenatal Diagnosis

To date, we are aware of at least two attempts at prenatal diagnosis for β-mannosidosis. In a study carried out with the original family reported by Wenger et al.,[38] both cultured amniotic fluid cells and cells from CVS had normal enzyme levels, indicating an unaffected fetus, which was confirmed after birth (D. Wenger, personal communication). Similar results were reported by Kleijer et al., who found heterozygote levels of enzyme in both chorionic villi and amniotic fluid cells from a fetus at risk for β-mannosidosis.[193] On the basis of this and experiences with other inherited disorders of oligosaccharide metabolism, it would be expected that if one had sufficient normal data, one should be able to carry out a prenatal diagnosis of this disorder. This suggestion is also supported by the isolation of the involved β-mannosidase from human placenta[179] and by detailed analysis of human chorionic β-mannosidase.[194]

Animal Models

Before the discovery of β-mannosidosis in humans in 1986, the disease had been documented in goats.[36,195,196] More recently, β-mannosidosis has been described in 12 Salers calves.[197] In contrast to the relatively mild course of the human disorder, the disease in both animals is much more severe: a fatal disorder involving demyelination and/or dysmyelination.[195,197] It has been postulated[198] that the differences in the severity of this disorder in humans and in the animal model may be the result of differences in the types and/or metabolism of abnormal materials stored in goats,[36] cattle,[199] and humans.[170,171]

FUCOSIDOSIS

Clinical Features

There are a large number of reports of patients with fucosidosis.[8,200–203] While a careful comparison of these cases indicates repetitive reporting of some patients,[204–232] a review of 77 cases published in 1991 provided an appendix of clinical findings up to that time (Table 140-8).[201] Traditionally, two phenotypes have been identified: a more severe infantile form referred to as type I and a milder form designated type II (Table 140-3). The clinical findings of the 77 cases compiled in the 1991 review[201] suggests, however, that this may be a somewhat arbitrary classification, there being, in fact, a continuum of severity.[201] Moreover, the description of a patient with mild initial symptoms but a rapidly fatal outcome adds to this complexity.[202] Additionally, mild and severe forms of the disease have been found within the same sibship[203] and among patients homozygous for the same mutation, e.g., the common Gln → stop mutation at codon 422.[201] The latter data not only complicate the classification of patients but also suggest that the clinical findings result from not only the fucosidase deficiency but also nongenetic factors and/or modifier genes.

In spite of these shortcomings, the classification of most patients into either the type I or the type II subgroup has been found to be helpful in many cases. Patients with the more severe phenotype (type I) typically have onset of psychomotor retardation within the first year of life, coarse facies, growth retardation, dysostosis multiplex, and neurologic deterioration. The sodium chloride content of sweat is increased markedly in this form of the disorder. While hepatosplenomegaly, cardiomegaly, seizures, and infections also frequently occur, these findings are more variable.

The milder (type II) phenotype is associated with onset of psychomotor retardation between 1 and 2 years of age. The coarse facies, growth retardation, dysostosis multiplex, and neurologic signs are similar to or slightly milder than those in type I. The major features that distinguish this milder phenotype from the more severe one are the presence of angiokeratoma (Fig. 140-10), longer survival, and more normal sweat sodium chloride values, although anhidrosis may be present. As noted previously, the best clinical picture of this disorder is provided by the comprehensive

Table 140-8 Clinical Features in 77 Patients Affected with Fucosidosis

Clinical Abnormality	Patients n	%
Mental retardation	73	95
Neurologic deterioration	68	88
Coarse facies	61	79
Growth retardation	60	78
Recurrent infections	60	78
Kyphoscoliosis	51	66
Dysostosis multiplex	45	58
Angiokeratoma	40	52
Joint contractures	37	48
Seizures	29	38
Visceromegaly	23	30
Hearing loss	9	12
Hernia	7	9
Loss of visual acuity	5	6

Number and percentage of patients are minimum estimates. Symptoms were regarded as being absent if their presence was not clearly indicated. (*From Willems et al.*[201] *by permission of* American Journal of Medical Genetics)

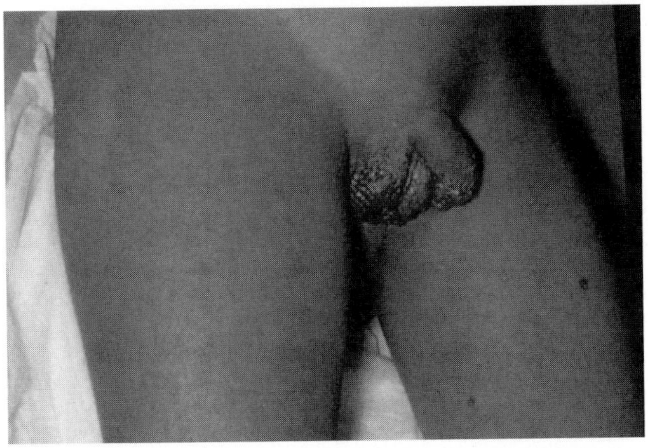

Fig. 140-10 Angiokeratoma in patient with fucosidosis type II. (*From Fleming et al.*[203] *Used by permission of Blackwell Science Ltd.*)

review of 77 patients published in 1991.[201] The major findings of this review are summarized in Table 140-8.

The angiokeratomas that occur in fucosidosis are essentially indistinguishable from those seen in Fabry disease, both in appearance and in distribution.[203,206,213,233–236] Angiokeratomas were found in about one-third of patients under age 10, 75 percent of these between ages 10 and 20, and about 85 percent of those over age 20.[201] Stature is substantially reduced in virtually all patients, but head circumference is usually normal.[201] The ocular findings in fucosidosis are not prominent, but tortuosity of conjunctival vessels occurs and a pigmentary retinopathy has been described.[235,237] Neuroradiologic findings have included abnormalities of the globus pallidus, thalamus, and internal capsules.[238,239] At least one patient suffered from a rapidly progressive dystonia that was initially focal but later became bilateral.[240] The skeletal findings are those of a mild dysostosis multiplex.[215,226] Changes in the vertebrae are prominent, with ovoid configuration and beaking. The acetabula are often deformed and sclerotic. The shafts of the long bones may be widened. Vacuolated lymphocytes have been present where examined. For 44 patients with a recorded age of death, 43 percent died before age 10 and 41 percent after age 20.[201]

Treatment

An allogeneic bone marrow transplant has been reported in an 8-month-old child who was shown to lack fucosidase following the diagnosis in his older brother.[241] Eighteen months after the transplant there was evidence of mild neurodevelopmental delay; however, the patient's MRI scan was reported to show improvement. His older, untreated affected sib was reported to have shown far greater developmental delay at the same age.

Pathology

Postmortem examination of type I patients[204,223] has revealed enlargement of the brain, heart, liver, spleen, and pancreas. The adrenal glands are atrophic. The gallbladder is described as strawberry-like. Biopsy studies of affected liver indicate the presence of foamy cytoplasm in some hepatocytes and Kupffer cells. Ultrastructural studies indicate the presence of vacuoles with heterogeneous content, some appearing empty, some having reticular formation, and some displaying lamellar structure.[205,207] Ultrastructural studies of biopsy material from the brain indicate a similar heterogeneity in the appearance of storage vacuoles.[205] There is a striking vacuolization of the epithelial cells of the sweat glands[213,216,234] and of the conjunctiva.[216]

Biochemical Storage

It was recognized from the earliest report[29] that fucosidosis probably represented faulty degradation of both sphingolipids and polysaccharides. The major glycolipid accumulating is the H-antigen glycolipid, Fuc(α1 $\rightarrow$ 2)Gal(β1 $\rightarrow$ 4)GlcNAc-α-Gal-ceramide.[242,243] There is major accumulation of glycolipid in liver but only minor storage in brain. Studies of the oligosaccharides found in the tissues and urine of fucosidosis patients have indicated the presence of a decasaccharide, Fuc(α1 $\rightarrow$ 2) Gal(β1 $\rightarrow$ 4) GlcNAc(β1 $\rightarrow$ 2) Man[Fuc(α1 $\rightarrow$ 2) Gal(β1 $\rightarrow$ 4) GlcNAc(β1 $\rightarrow$ 2)Man](α1 $\rightarrow$ 3/6)Man(β1 $\rightarrow$ 4)GlcNAc, and a disaccharide, Fuc(α1 $\rightarrow$ 6)GlcNAc[243,244] (see Fig. 140-5). Subsequent studies[245–248] identified numerous other oligosaccharides and glycoasparagines in the urine and tissues of fucosidosis patients. In one study,[249] 22 glycopeptides were identified in the urine of a patient but the presence of the decasaccharide could not be confirmed. All of the glycopeptides contained a fucosyl residue on the GlcNAc, which is linked to asparagine. In the most definitive study to date,[25] fucosylglycoasparagines have been separated from urine by reverse-phase HPLC and their structures determined by 400-MHz ^{1}H-NMR analysis.[250] The results of this study, which extend and agree well with previous reports, also confirm that the linkage of α(1 $\rightarrow$ 6)fucose to GlcNAc is a common feature of all the abnormal metabolites found in the urine of fucosidosis patients.[250]

There is a suggestion that fucosidosis type I and type II can be distinguished by the pattern of urinary excretion.[251] Oligosaccharide is the predominant as the storage material accumulated in the brain of patients. The suggestion that increased keratan sulfate is present in the urine in fucosidosis requires further study.[252]

The relationships of blood group substances to the stored material in fucosidosis deserve special mention. These substances are determined by oligosaccharide chains linked to proteins or lipids. The H, Lea, and Leb antigens are determined by the presence of fucosyltransferases. On the one hand, the genotype at these loci may determine the exact nature of the stored material in fucosidosis patients; on the other hand, the presence of fucosidosis may increase the expression of these antigens.[213,253] Data are still insufficient to determine if blood type affects the clinical course of fucosidosis.

The Enzyme and the Enzyme Defect

Human α-fucosidase, a lysosomal enzyme, cleaves fucose from the nonreducing end of a variety of oligosaccharides, glycoproteins, and glycolipids. Moreover, it can hydrolyze fucose linked by α1 $\rightarrow$ 2, α1 $\rightarrow$ 3, α1 $\rightarrow$ 4, or α1 $\rightarrow$ 6 bonds, usually to galactose or N-acetylglucosamine.[254]

Human tissue α-L-fucosidase is composed of multiple forms of a common subunit of approximately 50 to 60 kDa,[8,254] and there is evidence of two related protein bands of 51 and 56 kDa.[255] Deglycosylation of fucosidase does not affect its catalytic properties or conformation; however, it does change its pH optimum and decrease its thermostability.[256] The enzyme has been purified from a variety of tissues and its kinetic, electrophoretic, and immunologic properties studied extensively, as reviewed elsewhere.[254] Evidence from interconversion studies suggests that the various forms of fucosidase are partly explained by the existence of monomer, dimer, and tetramer forms. Evidence suggesting the possible existence of differences in the common subunit or protein[257] has been reviewed.[8,254] Although it is not clear whether the subunits differ with respect to polypeptides, carbohydrates, or both,[254] cloning studies of the human fucosidase gene provide evidence for only one structural gene.[258–260]

Detailed kinetic studies have revealed four active sites per tetrameric complex, which suggests that the enzyme is predominantly a homotetramer.[261] While Johnson and coworkers[262,263] found a mature 50-kDa subunit that appeared to be processed from a 53-kDa glycosylated precursor, Wauters et al.[264] reported evidence for the processing of a 51-kDa precursor molecule to a mature 59- to 61-kDa end product, which they suggested was due to glycosylation.

Several studies have provided molecular evidence of the presence of heterogeneity among fucosidosis patients. In one investigation in which a polyclonal antibody was used, liver from a single fucosidosis patient lacked detectable α-fucosidase protein.[265] In a larger study, fibroblasts from 8 of 11 fucosidosis patients were also found to have no detectable fucosidase enzyme protein, whereas two patients synthesized the 53-kDa precursor but had none of the mature processed enzyme.[262] The cells of the remaining patient in this study contained small amounts of cross-reacting material. Investigations carried out on lymphoid cells from fucosidosis patients showed that these cells synthesized reduced amounts of α-fucosidase that was catalytically inefficient and secreted more rapidly than that of controls.[266–268]

Inheritance and Incidence

As is the case with the other errors of glycoprotein metabolism, fucosidosis is an autosomal recessive disease (MIM 230000).[117] Although the disorder is panethnic, the majority of reported patients have been from Italy and the United States.[201] In Italy, many of the patients have been concentrated in the Reggio Calabria area,[200] whereas in the United States the majority of patients have been descendants of the early Spanish settlers in the southwestern part of the country (D. Wenger, personal communication). Evidence suggesting that fucosidosis does not occur with a high frequency in any population is provided by Willems et al.,[201] who were able to identify only 77 fucosidosis patients in a combined literature search and international survey. Consanguinity was reported in 40 percent of the 45 families identified in this review, again indicating that this is a rare autosomal recessive disorder.[201]

Gene Assignment

Early investigations demonstrated that the expression of human α-fucosidase activity in cell hybrids was correlated with the presence or absence of chromosome 1.[269,270] This chromosomal assignment is supported by family studies showing a linkage between electrophoretic polymorphisms of fucosidase and the Rh locus, known to be on chromosome 1.[271] Analysis of hybrid cell lines containing different rearrangements of human chromosome 1 indicates that enzyme activity is correlated with the presence or absence of material containing band p34 of this chromosome.[272] The grain distribution of *in situ* hybridization studies in which a cDNA clone was used further localized the *FUCA1* locus to the distal region of 1p34.[273] In at least the two families examined in this study,[274] the restriction fragment length polymorphion (RFLP) score of a linkage analysis of two RFLPs in the *FUCA1* gene and the fucosidosis mutation provides further evidence that defects in this gene are responsible for fucosidosis.

The latter observation is important because Southern blot analysis had previously shown that *FUCA1* cDNA also hybridizes to the short arm of chromosome 2.[274] Subsequently, part of this sequence was cloned, and initial studies suggested that it had the properties of a processed pseudogene.[275] This was confirmed when it was shown to be 80 percent identical to that of fucosidase cDNA but to lack an open reading frame.[276] This pseudogene, now designated *FUCA1P*, has been mapped to 2q31–q32 by *in situ* hybridization.[277] This localization was confirmed by the demonstration of tight linkage of this gene with the α1 chain of type III collagen (*COL3A1*), which had been mapped to 2q24–q34.[277]

Eiberg et al.[278] have also shown that a second locus (*FUCA2*) that influences plasma fucosidase activity is linked to the plasminogen gene, now known to be on chromosome 6[279] at either band q26 or band q27.[280,281] The latter gene, which is not involved in α-fucosidosis, may involve a regulatory rather than a structural gene. It must, however, be considered if one measures α-fucosidase activity in serum, because an individual with this normal variant might be misdiagnosed as an affected individual.

Gene Structure

A partial cDNA clone was first isolated from a human hepatoma library (GenBank M10355).[282] This clone demonstrated extensive colinearity of nucleotide and amino acid sequence with the 347-amino-acid region that was included. Subsequently, larger cDNA clones containing the complete coding sequence and a poly (A) region were isolated.[258,259] The open reading frame is predicted to encode a protein of 461 amino acids consisting of a 22-amino-acid signal peptide and a processed mature enzyme of 439 amino acids.[259] Finally, such a full-length cDNA has been isolated and its expression demonstrated in transfected COS cells.[260] The gene structure for human fucosidase includes eight exons spanning 23 kb (Table 140-4).[276] A cDNA encoding rat liver α-fucosidase[283] showed 82 percent nucleotide sequence identity with that reported in an incomplete human sequence.

Mutations

The isolation of a cDNA encoding α-fucosidase, followed by the publication of the sequence of the 8 exons found in this gene,[276] has enabled several groups of investigators to identify and characterize a variety of mutations (Table 140-5). These alterations are responsible for the occurrence of fucosidosis in several unrelated families with different ethnic backgrounds. To date, at least 13 mutations in the *FUCA1* gene have been described. These include five different base changes resulting in premature stop codons,[284–290] four different single-base deletions,[289,291] a two-base deletion resulting in a frameshift,[286] a large deletion involving two exons,[201,286,292] a base substitution resulting in defective splicing,[292] base changes resulting in amino acid substitutions,[286,293] and a homozygous 66-bp insertion in exon 6 of yet another patient.[294] The detection of five additional novel mutations in another six patients extends the evidence for the presence of genetic heterogeneity in this disorder.[295] In addition, an A to G transition in exon 5 resulting in the replacement of Gln by Avg (Q281R) has been found to be a common polymorphism in the human fucosidase gene.[296] Although this mutation affects the electrophoretic mobility of the enzyme, it does not appear to be a disease-causing mutation.[296]

With the exception of one mutation causing a premature stop defect, found in at least eight families,[284,285] most of the other known mutations have been found in isolated families, confirming that fucosidosis results from a large number of different mutations.[286,295] The mutation that has repeatedly been observed involves a Gln to stop mutation (GAA → TAA) at codon 422 (Q422X) and causes loss of an *Eco*RI restriction enzyme site, which is convenient for molecular diagnosis.[285] Of the known mutations, only a few yield an amino acid substitution;[286] the others involve mutations that are presumed to result in unstable or defective mRNA. This observation suggests that mutations resulting in amino acid substitutions in α-fucosidase might often retain enough enzymatic activity to prevent clinically evident disease or, alternatively, to result in a clinical phenotype sufficiently different not to be identified as a variant of fucosidosis.

Laboratory Diagnosis

Urine samples from individuals suffering from either type I or type II fucosidosis contain excessive amounts of several fucoglycoconjugates. These include a variety of both fucoglycopeptides[249] and fucooligosaccharides,[297,298] the former being present in higher amounts than the latter.[8]

The presence of increased levels of the fucose-containing glycoconjugates can be detected most easily by thin-layer chromatography (see Fig. 140-7).[137–140,299] For routine screening, urine from suspected patients is usually analyzed by one of the general screening techniques suitable for the detection of not only fucosidosis but also the related inborn errors of glycoprotein metabolism: mannosidosis, aspartylglycosaminuria, and sialidosis. On chromatographic separation and staining (with orcinol, for example) any abnormal levels of oligosaccharides are revealed by the distinctive chromatographic patterns of the staining material.[137–140,299] Details of these methods have been reviewed.[141] A method based on the simultaneous detection of both urinary oligosaccharides and glycopeptides,[300] a modified thin-layer chromatography method,[300] or analysis by HPLC[142] may represent improved screening techniques for this disorder.

As in aspartylglucosaminuria, urine samples from fucosidosis patients also yield an abnormal pattern when stained with ninhydrin followed by heating at an elevated temperature.[301,302] Under these conditions, fucosidosis urine yields a blue spot similar to that seen in aspartylglucosamine urine.

The most direct and precise means of diagnosing fucosidosis is based on the enzymatic assay of α-L-fucosidase in any available cell type, e.g., white blood cells and cultured fibroblasts. Routinely, the enzyme assay is based on the cleavage of either p-nitrophenyl-α-L-fucopyranoside (colorimetric) or 4-methylumbelliferyl-α-L-fucopyranoside (fluorimetric) at an acidic pH.[303,304]

Although the determination of fucosidase activity is one of the most reliable means of establishing the presence or absence of fucosidosis, its use is complicated by the fact that some apparently normal individuals have extremely low levels of this enzyme in serum or plasma.[305,306] Because of this normal variability, results obtained with these samples must be interpreted with great care. See the review by Willems et al. for a more detailed discussion of atypical patients and potential misdiagnosis.[201] DiCioccio et al.[307] have provided data that suggest that the measurement of both fucosidosis activity and protein concentration by ELISA may yield more definitive clinical results.

Prenatal Diagnosis

Normal cultured amniotic fluid cells have been reported to contain higher levels of fucosidase activity than cultured skin fibroblasts. Although there has been a report of at least one diagnostic error concerning a pregnancy involving twins at risk for fucosidosis,[210] at this time it appears that an experienced laboratory should be able to carry out this diagnostic procedure.[308] Indeed, a number of reports describe the successful diagnosis of both affected[200] and nonaffected[217] fetuses in pregnancies being monitored with special reference to fucosidosis. It has been suggested that DNA analysis should be considered in families seeking prenatal diagnosis for this disorder,[201] but this can be considered only when the molecular lesion in the specific family at risk has been established by previous studies or when linkage analysis is informative.

Animal Models

A deficiency of α-L-fucosidase activity was found in white blood cells and fibroblasts obtained from two Springer Spaniel dogs having progressive ataxia, proprioceptive deficits, dysphagia, and wasting.[309] These findings were similar to those described earlier in Springer Spaniels that had a progressive disorder but in which the enzyme defect was not established.[310] Fucosidosis has also been described in a Springer Spaniel having a malabsorption syndrome but lacking neurologic abnormalities.[311]

Additional reports of Springer Spaniels having fucosidosis suggest that this may be a relatively common inherited disorder in this breed of dogs,[312] including those found in the United States.[313] Detailed studies have demonstrated less than 5 percent residual fucosidase and an accumulation of fucose-containing glycoasparagines in the brains of dogs affected with this disorder.[314,315] These findings indicate that canine fucosidosis is indeed a valid animal model for human fucosidosis. Correction of the fucosidase enzyme deficiency by allogeneic bone marrow transplantation following total lymphoid irradiation was demonstrated by using this animal model.[316–318]

The cDNA coding for the canine α-fucosidase has been isolated and sequenced by Occhiodoro and Anson.[319] Both the cDNA and the predicted amino acid sequence of its product show high homology (82.6 percent and 84 percent, respectively) to the human homologues.[319] Skelly et al.[320] found the gene to span 12 kb and to consist of 12 exons. The transcript was predicted to code for either 466[319] or 465[320] amino acids, including a signal peptide.

SIALIDOSIS

Clinical Features

In an early review, Lowden and O'Brien[321] suggested that patients suffering from isolated neuraminidase deficiencies could be divided into at least two groups. Using a clinical classification, the less affected patients, i.e., those lacking physical changes (normosomatic), are referred to as having sialidosis type I. The more severely affected (dysmorphic) patients having obvious physical changes are designated as having sialidosis type II. Because of the rather broad spectrum of severely affected patients, Lowden and O'Brien[321] further divided the type II disease into infantile and juvenile sialidosis. Later, Young et al.[322] added yet another category, designated "congenital sialidosis," to the type II subgroup. All forms of the disease result from recessively inherited deficiencies of the neuraminidase that normally cleaves terminal $\alpha 2 \rightarrow 3$ and $\alpha 2 \rightarrow 6$ sialyl linkages of several oligosaccharides and glycopeptides. As would be expected, increased amounts of these compounds are found in tissues and fluids of affected patients.

Because sialidosis type I, the milder form of the disorder, lacks most of the physical changes seen in the type II patients, it was considered the normosomatic form of the disorder in the original classification by Lowden and O'Brien.[321] For the first 20 to 30 years of life, individuals with this form are generally normal in terms of both development and appearance. Type I patients generally come to medical attention as a result of the development of gait abnormalities, concerns regarding visual acuity, or both (Tables 140-3, 140-9). It is also at this time that the presence of ocular cherry-red spots is often noted (Fig. 140-11). The onset of this milder form of the disorder, while variable, generally occurs during the second or third decade of life.

This milder (type I) form of the disease, also referred to as the "cherry-red spot–myoclonus" syndrome, has been described in at least 27 patients;[33–35,323–333] see Table 140-9 for a summary of the most common findings noted in these reports. The visual handicap, which is progressive, is often associated with impaired color

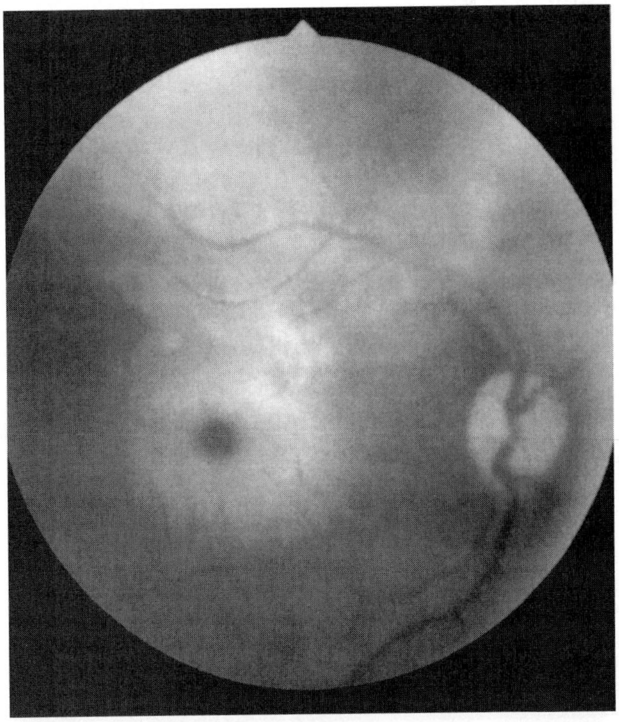

Fig. 140-11 Cherry-red spot in patient with sialidosis Type I. (*From Federico et al.*[313] *Reproduced with permission of S. Karger AG, Basel.*)

Table 140-9 Clinical Features Specifically Noted in More Than 10% of 27 Patients with Sialidosis Type I*

Clinical Abnormality	Patients n	%
Cherry red spot	27/27	100
Myoclonus	23/27	85
Visual defects	19/27	70
Ataxia	16/27	59
Hyperreflexia	14/27	52
Seizures	13/27	48
Dysarthria	9/27	33
Nystagmus	8/27	30
Hypotonia	5/27	19
Lens/corneal opacity	4/27	15

Data include those taken, in part, from a review of 23 patients referenced in 140-2 of Federico et al.[333] plus 3 sibs[332] and an isolated case[333] not included in the original review.

*Numbers and percentages for each feature are minimum estimates; i.e., symptoms are considered to be positive only if specifically noted in published reports.

Table 140-11 Clinical Features Specifically Noted in More than 10% of 12 Patients Designated as Having the Infantile-[281] or Childhood-Onset[298] Form of Sialidosis type II*

Clinical Abnormality	Patients n	%
Coarse facies	12/12	100
Dysostosis multiplex	12/12	100
Developmental delay	11/12	92
Short stature	9/12	75
Hepatomegaly	9/12	75
Cherry-red spots	8/12	67
Splenomegaly	6/12	50
Myoclonus	6/12	50
Lens opacities	6/12	50
Corneal opacities	5/12	42
Ataxia	3/12	25

*Numbers and percentages for each feature are minimum estimates, i.e., symptoms are considered to be positive only if specifically noted in published reports. Data include those taken, in part, from the review of 12 patients referenced in Table 140-2 by Young et al.[322]

vision[324,327] and/or night blindness.[35] The ocular cherry-red spot, while a consistent finding, is sometimes described as being atypical. Punctate lenticular opacities have been described in several patients.[34,324,326] The myoclonus, which is generalized and frequently debilitating, is poorly controlled by medication. Additionally, the myoclonus has been reported to be exacerbated by stimuli, smoking,[326] and menstrual cycle.[327] Nystagmus, ataxia, and grand mal seizure have also been reported. As the disease progresses, the myoclonus may interfere with walking, sitting, and other physical activities. Visual acuity also continues to decrease over the course of the disorder. A detailed discussion of the clinical and electrophysiological aspects of the myoclonus in sialidosis and other diseases is available.[334]

Sialidosis type II is distinguished from the milder form of the disorder by much earlier onset of the symptoms, the presence of abnormal somatic features, and more rapid progression of the disease process (Table 140-3). As noted above, type II disease has generally been subdivided into congenital (Table 140-10) and infantile (Table 140-11) forms (Fig. 140-12). While Lowden and O'Brien[321] also included a juvenile form of the disease in their classification, many of the patients in this subgroup may in fact suffer from a form of galactosialidosis[322,330] (see Chap. 152).

Sialidosis type II patients classified as having the infantile-onset[321] or childhood-onset[322] form of the disorder include those who are relatively normal or minimally abnormal at birth.[31,32,322,323,335–343] While there is a continuum of severity in this group, all patients develop a progressively severe, mucopolysaccharidosis-like phenotype, visceromegaly, dysostosis multiplex, and mental retardation. Additional clinical findings, also usually present at an early age, include coarse facial features, increased head size, and short stature. Cherry-red spots and myoclonus are observed in older children, and survival to the second decade has been reported for at least some infantile-onset patients. See Table 140-11 for a listing of the most common clinical findings in this group of patients.

Table 140-10 Clinical Features Specifically Noted in More Than 10% of 11 Patients with the Congenital Form of Sialidosis Type II*

Clinical Abnormality	Patients n	%
Hepatosplenomegaly	11/11	100
Hydrops/Ascites	9/11	82
Coarse facies	3/11	27
Dysostosis multiplex	2/11	18
Proteinuria	2/11	18
Edema	2/11	18

*Numbers and percentages for each feature are minimum estimates, i.e., symptoms are considered to be positive only if specifically noted in published reports. Data from references [322,341,342,344–347].

In contrast to the above patients, who are normal at birth, at least 11 patients from a total of seven families have been described with severe clinical abnormalities present at birth.[341,342,344–347] See the discussion by Young et al.[322] and Table 140-10 for a review of the major findings in these patients. Patients with this so-called congenital form of sialidosis type II present with hydrops fetalis and/or neonatal ascites, with stillbirth or death at an early age. Facial edema, inguinal hernias, hepatosplenomegaly, stippling of the epiphyses, and periosteal cloaking may be present at birth. In addition to the patients included in this group, at least one distinctive family displaying severe renal involvement has been described.[338] It should be noted, however, that a number of patients classified as having one of the forms of sialidosis type II have also been found to have nephrosis.[348]

Both the biochemical and the clinical diagnosis of the various forms of sialidosis are complicated by the existence of not only the isolated neuraminidase deficiency described here but also a clinically similar disorder resulting from a combined deficiency of neuraminidase and β-galactosidase, designated "galactosialidosis" (see Chap. 152). Because of the existence of similar infantile and congenital phenotypes in both of these disorders, it is often difficult to determine whether neuraminidase deficiency is isolated or occurs in combination with β-galactosidase deficiency.[322,338,344–347] Biochemical studies, somatic cell hybridization, and genetic mapping have, however, clearly established that sialidosis and galactosialidosis result from mutations of different genes and are thus two distinct disorders.[7,321–323,349] Additional information regarding the clinical and biochemical relationships of these two disorders is discussed in detail in Chap. 152.

Pathology

Pathologic descriptions and/or reports of EM findings in tissues of sialidosis patients have appeared in several clinical reports[34,324,327,335,337,344] or reviews.[7,321] Vacuolated lymphocytes and bone marrow foam cells are prominent in the type II but absent in the type I form of the disorder. Liver biopsies demonstrate vacuolization that is prominent in Kupffer cells but less impressive in hepatocytes. Vacuolization is also observed in nerve biopsies,

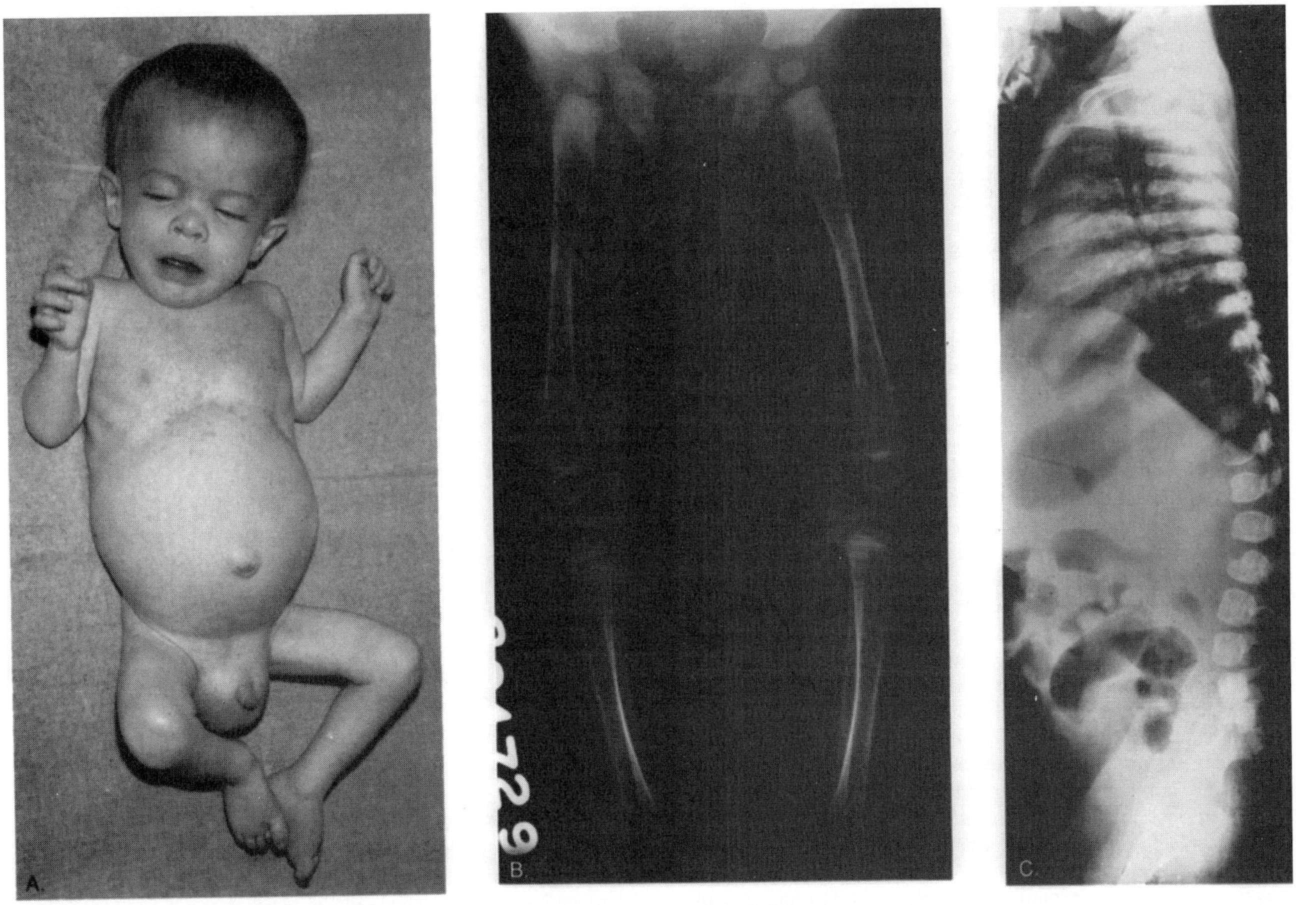

Fig. 140-12 Clinical features of infantile sialidosis. (A) Abdominal distension, hydroceles, and abnormal facial appearance at 11 months of age. (B, C) Dysostosis multiplex at 15 months of age. (*From Aylsworth et al.*[344] *Used by permission.*)

tissue fibroblasts, myenteric plexus neurons, and brain biopsy material. EM changes include membrane-bound vacuoles, which have been variously described as containing reticulogranular material, electron-dense bodies, floccular material, lamellar inclusions, and lipofuscin.

Biochemical Storage

Much of the early information concerning the biochemical alterations resulting from the deficiency of the lysosomal neuraminidase (sialidase) is based on the characterization of oligosaccharides isolated from the urine of sialidosis patients.[350–352] In general, these findings have been confirmed and extended as new techniques of analysis became available.[353–355] Most of the compounds found in excessive amounts in the urine of these patients contain N-acetylglucosamine at the reducing end and N-acetylneuraminic acid at the nonreducing terminus. Similar compounds have been found in the abdominal ascites fluid of a child with the severe infantile form of this disorder.[356] The neuraminic acid is linked to galactose via either $\alpha(2 \rightarrow 6)$ (70 percent) or $\alpha(2 \rightarrow 3)$ (30 percent) linkages.[354] The structures of these various compounds are closely related and are believed to originate from the sugar side chains of glycoproteins as a result of the action of an endo-N-acetylglucosaminidase. Concentrations of urinary oligosaccharides are correlated with the clinical severity of the affected patients; they are 3.5 times higher in infantile-type sialidosis patients than in late-type patients.[354] Comparative studies of oligosaccharides excreted by galactosialidosis and sialidosis patients have yielded conflicting results. Takahashi et al.[354] found excessive galactosyl-terminated oligosaccharides in galactosialidosis patients, while these compounds were not detected by van Pelt et al.[355,357]

Glycopeptides and/or oligosaccharides having similar structures are also stored in tissues and cultured fibroblasts from sialidosis patients. Sialidosis fibroblasts cultured in the presence of radiolabeled acetylmannosamine accumulate excessive levels of labeled sialic acid covalently bound to anionic conjugates.[358,359] Further analysis showed the labeled sialic acid to be present in at least nine distinct sialyl-containing compounds. Analysis of these compounds indicated that they are sialyloligosaccharides derived from complex N-aspartyl-linked glycoproteins.[360] Similar findings have been found with radioactively labeled fetuin endocytosed by sialidosis cells.[361]

The primary structures of the sialyloligosaccharides in sialidosis I fibroblasts (sialylated mono-, di-, and triantennary N-glycosidic N-acetyllactosamine oligosaccharides having Man(β1 $\rightarrow$ 4)GlcNAc at the reducing end) are consistent with those expected for a neuraminidase deficiency.[362] A comparative study of the storage materials of galactosialidosis and sialidosis fibroblasts revealed only quantitative differences, in spite of the additional β-galactosidase deficiency in the latter cells.[363] As noted previously, however, differences between these two groups of patients have been found in urine by at least one group.[354]

Together, these data indicate that lysosomal neuraminidase normally cleaves terminal $2 \rightarrow 3$ and $2 \rightarrow 6$ sialyl linkages of several oligosaccharides and glycoproteins.[364–366] In addition, evidence has been presented that this lysosomal enzyme also cleaves sialic acid from G_{M3} ganglioside in the presence of cholate.[367] This activity appears to be distinct from that of a second G_{M3} ganglioside sialidase, present in membranes, that is stimulated by Triton X-100.[367] It has therefore been suggested that the cholate-stimulated G_{M3} sialidase activity is a genuine activity found in normal cells and absent in sialidosis patients.[367] Evidence supporting this suggestion includes the report that a purified placental sialidase liberated sialic acid residues not only from oligosaccharides and glycoproteins but also from gangliosides, at least in the presence of detergents.[368,369] Additional evidence indicating that ganglioside as well as sialyloligosaccharide catabolism may be impaired in sialidosis is provided by the report of elevated levels of gangliosides in autopsy tissues of a patient affected with this disorder.[370]

The Enzyme and the Enzyme Defect

Evidence from investigations carried out over the last 20 years, clearly indicates that there are at least three human neuraminidases. Based on differences in subcellular localizations, pH optima, and substrate preferences, these enzymes are designated cytosolic, plasma membrane, and lysosomal. It is now well established that it is the lysosomal α-neuraminidase that is lacking in sialidosis patients. Both the clinical and the research efforts involving this enzyme, however, have been complicated by the fact that it is unstable, i.e., is quickly destroyed by freezing, sonication, solubilization, and most purification procedures.[371,372]

Most of the early information regarding the properties of this enzyme was obtained with crude preparations of cultured skin fibroblasts from either normal controls[371–373] or individuals affected with one of the sialidoses.[35,321,371] The lysosomal neuraminidase, active against various glycoprotein and oligosaccharide substrates, has also been isolated from human placenta and extensively characterized in the laboratories of Galjaard[374–376] and Hiraiwa.[368,369] A suggestion[377] that human neuraminidase was the processed product of prosaposin has not been supported by additional data, which demonstrated that the results of the earlier study were most likely due to a component of immunoglobulin G that cross-reacts with antisaposin antibodies.[378]

Based on an analysis of the cDNA that codes for this enzyme, it was predicted that the protein would consist of 415 amino acids, including a signal sequence, a central hydrophobic core, and a more polar c-terminal domain.[379] (See "Gene Structure" below for more details.) The mass of this protein was predicted to be 45.467 kDa, which would be reduced to 40.435 kDa upon removal of the signal sequence.[379] Assuming glycosylation at all three potential sites, the size of the processed protein, following removal of the signal sequence, was estimated to be 45 kDa. Direct evidence supporting this figure has been obtained by western blot analysis in a study that demonstrated the presence of two major bands (44 and 46 kDa), which, after deglycosylation, yielded a single 40-kDa protein.[379]

Neuraminidase exists as a multienzyme complex consisting of neuraminidase, β-galactosidase, and a "protective protein." Subsequent studies showed that the amino acid sequence of the protective protein has homologies with carboxypeptidase[380] and deamidase.[381] Enzyme studies using isolated protective protein demonstrated that in fact it has both lysosomal carboxypeptidase[382,383] and cathepsin A–like activity.[384] (See Galjaard et al.[385] and Chap. 152 for a detailed discussion of these findings.)

Both the mild (type I) and the severe (type II) forms of sialidosis result from inherited deficiencies of the enzyme. An inherited primary deficiency of neuraminidase was first demonstrated in the severe (type II) form of sialidosis.[31,32] Shortly thereafter, several investigators[33–35,324] described a similar deficiency in a milder clinical disorder, the so-called cherry-red spot–myoclonus syndrome, now classified as sialidosis type I. Deficiencies of this enzyme have been demonstrated with a variety of both natural (sialyllactose, sialylhexosaccharides, and fetuin) and synthetic (3-methoxyphenyl-N-acetyl neuraminic acid and 4-methylumbelliferyl-α-D-N-acetylneuraminic acid) substrates.

In addition to people with the primary neuraminidase deficiency discussed in this chapter, there are also patients with a similar clinical disorder who suffer from a combined deficiency of neuraminidase and β-galactosidase. Current evidence indicates that the combined deficiency results from the loss of a protective (cathepsin A–like) protein required to interact with the galactosidase and neuraminidase complex.[349,385,386] (See Chap. 152 for a detailed review of this form of the disorder.)

Inheritance and Incidence

To date, all of the clinical forms of sialidosis appear to be inherited in an autosomal recessive manner (MIM 256550).[117] The presence of consanguinity and affected sibs, as well as the absence of affected individuals in different generations of the same family, support this conclusion.[7] Intermediate neuraminidase levels in parents of affected patients[321] and gene-mapping studies[387] also provide direct evidence that the enzyme deficiencies in these individuals result from an autosomal recessive inherited primary enzyme defect involving neuraminidase. Although the genetic relationships of the various clinical forms of the sialidosis remain uncertain, ethnic predilections of at least some of the forms appear to differ. The majority of type I patients have been Italian.

Gene Assignment

Mueller et al.[387] provided evidence that the expression of the glycoprotein-specific α-neuraminidase, absent in sialidosis patients, requires the products of more than one gene for normal expression. There is now much data that indicate that at least three proteins (cathepsin A, β-galactosidase, and neuraminidase) are required to form an active multienzyme complex.[349] While early complementation analysis indicated that the neuraminidase deficiency in a sialidosis type II patient was caused by a structural gene on Chromosome 10pter,[387] other data linked the gene to the HLA locus on the short arm of human chromosome 6.[388] FISH analysis, with probes prepared from the neuraminidase cDNA clones isolated by Bonten et al.[379] and Pshezhetsky et al.[389] directly localized this gene to 6p21, the region known to contain the HLA locus (Table 140-4).[379]

In contrast, the combined galactosidase/neuraminidase deficiencies found in galactosialidosis patients result from mutations in the gene coding human protective protein/cathepsin A[349] located on chromosome 20.[387] Decreased carboxypeptidase/protective protein in a patient with a ring chromosome 20 suggests that the gene is located on the distal segment of the long arm of this chromosome.[390] From these and other data, it is clear that sialidosis patients and individuals with combined deficiencies of neuraminidase and β-galactosidase suffer from two distinct and separate genetic disorders.

Gene Structure

The human cDNA that codes for α-neuraminidase and is responsible for the various forms of sialidosis was independently isolated and characterized by Bonten et al.[379] and Pshezhetsky et al. (GenBank AF040958).[389] Based on expected homologies with sialidases from different animal species, both Bonten et al.[379] and Pshezhetsky et al.[389] identified putative human neuraminidase cDNA clones in dbEST data bases. Both groups found the 1.9-kb cDNA to contain an open reading frame of 1245 nucleotides that was predicted to code for a protein containing 415 amino acids, including a signal sequence.[379] There were three potential Asn-linked glycosylation sites. While the predicted amino acid sequence has extensive homology with many other neuraminidases, both studies demonstrated that transient expression of the cDNA clone restored activity in human fibroblasts lacking lysosomal acid sialidase activity. Moreover, expression studies showed that the enzyme product was compartmentalized in lysosomes and had the expected acidic pH optimum.[379] Milner et al.[391] reported what is apparently the same gene to be ~3.5 kb long and to consist of six exons (See Table 140-5).

Mutations

Evidence that the gene described above is responsible for most, if not all, forms of isolated deficiencies of neuraminidase is provided by the findings of three independent mutations of the gene in type I sialidosis sibs and a type II sialidosis patient by Bonten et al.[379] A similar number of alterations was found in six additional patients by Pshezhetsky et al. (Table 140-5).[389] Expression studies of the mutagenized cDNA of the type found by Bonten provided direct evidence that the mutations in the first report resulted in nonfunctional enzyme.[379]

Laboratory Diagnosis

Like patients with the other inherited disorders of glycoprotein catabolism, sialidosis patients excrete increased amounts of several oligosaccharides (see Fig. 140-8)[350,392] and sialylglycopeptides[393] derived from glycoproteins. Because the metabolic block in these individuals results in inability to cleave the terminal sialic acid residues, the accumulated complex sugars are rich in sialic acid. Although detailed analysis of the accumulated oligosaccharides is too time-consuming for routine clinical diagnosis, several useful screening tests based on the demonstration of abnormal patterns and/or amounts of these compounds by thin-layer chromatography have been described[137–140] and reviewed.[141] Following application of the urine samples, the thin-layer plates are developed in an appropriate solvent and then stained. Staining with orcinol, utilized for the detection of other disorders of glycoprotein degradation, is usually suitable for the routine detection of the abnormal pattern of urinary oligosaccharide characteristic of this group of disorders. When desired, the sialic acid–containing oligosaccharides can also be specifically localized with resorcinol.[140] Alternatively, one can simultaneously examine urine samples for both oligosaccharides and glycopeptides.[300] Urine samples from both type I and type II patients,[321] as well as from newborns with the congenital or hydropic form of this disorder,[346] yield abnormal patterns when these techniques are applied.

The definitive diagnosis of sialidosis is based on the direct measurement of sialidase activity in appropriate fresh tissue samples, i.e., fibroblasts, cultured amniotic fluid cells, or white blood cells. In contrast to the procedure with tissue samples for most other lysosomal enzymes, care must be taken to ensure that the tissue to be examined has not been frozen or exposed to prolonged sonication.[372] Although several substrates can be utilized for this enzyme assay, the substrate of choice appears to be 4-methylumbelliferyl-β-N-acetylneuraminic acid.[394] The use of this sensitive substrate is particularly important with white blood cells, because these cells contain only about one-tenth of the sialidase activity found in cultured fibroblast cells. One group recommends not using leukocytes for diagnosis.[373] It may be difficult to distinguish sialidosis patients from galactosialidosis patients if intermediate levels of β-galactosidase are observed. In these patients, measuring of neuraminidase levels in the parents as well as complementation testing of the cells of the patient might be useful. Measurement of carboxypeptidase activity should also distinguish galactosialidosis patients who lack this activity from sialidosis patients who have normal levels of this enzyme.[382]

Prenatal Diagnosis

Neuraminidase activity is readily detectable in fresh, normal, cultured amniotic fluid cells as well as in chorionic villi samples.[151] These cells must be handled with special care, because enzyme activity is quickly destroyed by freezing, sonication, or exposure to temperatures of 37°C.[372] If possible, the enzyme activity should be determined with a sensitive assay, i.e., a fluorescent technique based on enzymatic cleavage of 4-methylumbelliferyl-β-N-acetylneuraminic acid.[395] To date, there have been at least three reports of successful prenatal diagnostic procedures for families at risk for various forms of sialidosis. These included both affected and unaffected fetuses in a family at risk for congenital sialidosis[345] and an unaffected pregnancy in a family at risk for sialidosis type II.[395]

Animal Models

A strain of mice (SM/J) has been shown to have a deficiency of neuraminidase in some but not all tissues.[396] Specifically, although there is a decrease in the levels of neuraminidase in liver, the enzyme levels in other tissues were either normal or only slightly diminished. Additionally, no increase in the sialic acid content of the liver was demonstrated in these animals. It was therefore suggested that this strain of mice may not be a good model for the various types of human sialidosis.[117] More recently, however, transient expression of a cDNA encoding mouse lysosomal enzyme was found to correct the sialidase deficiencies in both human sialidosis and SM/J fibroblasts.[397] Direct evidence that a point mutation in the sialidase gene in the SM/J mouse is responsible for the partial deficiency has been presented by Rottier et al.[398] These data, combined with the finding of a high degree of homology and similar linkages of the enzyme in question to the histocompatibility locus in mice and humans, indicate that the SM/J mouse is a model for the human disorder.[397,398]

REFERENCES

1. Kornfeld R, Kornfeld S: Structure of glycoproteins and their oligosaccharide units, in Lennarz WJ (ed): *The Biochemistry of Glycoproteins and Proteoglycans*. New York, Plenum, 1980.
2. Struck DK, Lennarz EJ: The function of saccharide-lipids in synthesis of glycoproteins, in Lennarz WJ (ed): *The Biochemistry of Glycoproteins and Proteoglycans*. New York, Plenum, 1980, p 35.
3. Schachter H, Roseman S: Mammalian glycosyltransferases: Their role in the synthesis and function of complex carbohydrates and glycolipids, in Lennarz WJ (ed): *The Biochemistry of Glycoproteins and Proteoglycans*. New York, Plenum, 1980, p 85.
4. Kornfeld R, Kornfeld S: Assembly of asparagine-linked oligosaccharides. *Annu Rev Biochem* **54**:631, 1985.
5. Waechter CJ, Scher MG: Biosynthesis of glycoproteins, in Margolis RU, Margolis RK (eds): *Complex Carbohydrates of Nervous Tissue*. New York, Plenum, 1979, p 75.
6. Berger EG, Buddecke E, Kamerling JP, Kobata A, Paulson JC, Vliegenthart JFG: Structure, biosynthesis and functions of glycoprotein glycans. *Experientia* **38**:1129, 1982.
7. O'Brien JS: Sialidosis, in Durand P, O'Brien JS (eds): *Genetic Errors of Glycoprotein Metabolism*. Berlin, Springer-Verlag, 1982, p 3.
8. Durand P, Rossanna G, Borrone G: Fucosidosis, in Durand P, O'Brien JS (eds): *Genetic Errors of Glycoprotein Metabolism*. Berlin: Springer-Verlag, 1982, p 49.
9. Chester MA, Lundblad A, Öckerman P-A, Autio S: Mannosidosis, in Durand P, O'Brien JS (eds): *Genetic Errors of Glycoprotein Metabolism*. Berlin, Springer-Verlag, 1982, p 89.
10. Aula P, Autio S, Ravio KO, Rapola J: Aspartylglucosaminuria, in Durand P, O'Brien JS (eds): *Genetic Errors of Glycoprotein Metabolism*. Berlin, Springer-Verlag, 1982, p 123.
11. Cantz M, Ulrich-Bott B: Disorders of glycoprotein degradation. *J Inherit Metab Dis* **13**:523, 1990.
12. Warner TG, O'Brien JS: Genetic defects in glycoprotein metabolism. *Annu Rev Genet* **17**:395, 1983.
13. Aronson NN Jr, Kuranda MJ: Lysosomal degradation of Asn-linked glycoproteins. *FASEB J* **3**:2615, 1989.
14. DeGasperi R, Li Y-T, Li S-C: Presence of two endo-β-N-acetylglucosaminidases in human kidney. *J Biol Chem* **264**:9329, 1988.
15. Brassart D, Baussant T, Wieruszeski J-M, Strecker G, Montreuil J, Michalski J-C: Catabolism of N-glycosylprotein glycans: Evidence for a degradation pathway of sialylglyco-asparagines resulting from the combined action of the lysosomal aspartylglucosaminidase and endo-N-acetyl-β-D-glucosaminidase: A 400 MHz 1H-NMR study. *Eur J Biochem* **169**:131, 1987.
16. Aronson NN Jr, Backes M, Kuranda MJ: Rat liver chitobiase: Purification, properties, and role in the lysosomal degradation of Asn-linked glycoproteins. *Arch Biochem Biophys* **272**:290, 1989.
17. Fisher KJ, Aronson NN Jr: Cloning and expression of the cDNA sequence encoding the lysosomal glycosidase di-N-acetylchitobiase. *J Biol Chem* **267**:19607, 1992.
18. Baumann M, Peltonen L, Aula P, Kalkkinen N: Isolation of human hepatic 60 kDa aspartylglycosaminidase consisting of three non-identical polypeptides. *Biochem J* **262**:189, 1989.
19. Kaartinen V, Williams JC, Tomich J, Yates JR III, Hood LE, Mononen I: Glycosaparaginase from human leukocytes: Inactivation and covalent modification with diazo-oxonorvaline. *J Biol Chem* **266**:5860, 1991.
20. Tollersrud OK, Aronson NN Jr: Comparison of liver glycosylasparaginases from six vertebrates. *Biochem J* **282**:891, 1990.
21. Enomaa N, Heiskanen T, Halila R, Sormunen R, Seppala R, Vihinen M, Peltonen L: Human aspartylglucosaminidase. A biochemical and

immunocytochemical characterization of the enzyme in normal and aspartylglucosaminuria fibroblasts. *Biochem J* **286**:613, 1992.
22. Sonz Z, Li S-C, Li Y-T: Absence of endo-β-N-acetylglucosaminidase activity in the kidneys of sheep, cattle and pig. *Biochem J* **248**:145, 1987.
23. Spranger J, Wiedemann H-R, Tolksdorf M, Graucob E, Caesar R: Lipomucopolysaccharidose: Eine neue speicherkrankheit. *Z Kinderheilk* **103**:285, 1968.
24. Spranger JW, Wiedemann H-R: The genetic mucolipidoses: Diagnosis and differential diagnosis. *Humangenetik* **9**:113, 1970.
25. van Hoff F, Hers HG: The abnormalities of lysosomal enzymes in mucopolysaccharidoses. *Eur J Biochem* **7**:34, 1968.
26. Öckerman P-A: A generalised storage disorder resembling Hurler's syndrome. *Lancet* **2**:239, 1967.
27. Jenner FA, Pollitt RJ: Large quantities of 2-acetamido-1(β-1-aspartamido)-1,2-dideoxyglucose in the urine of mentally retarded siblings. *Biochem J* **103**:48, 1967.
28. Pollitt RJ, Jenner FA, Merskey H: Aspartylglycosaminuria: An inborn error of metabolism associated with mental defect. *Lancet* **2**:253, 1968.
29. Durand P, Borrone G, Della Cella G, Philipart M: Fucosidosis. *Lancet* **1**:1198, 1968.
30. van Hoff F, Hers HG: Mucopolysaccharidosis by absence of α-fucosidase. *Lancet* **1**:1198, 1968.
31. Cantz M, Gehler J, Spranger J: Mucolipidosis I: Increased sialic acid content and deficiency of an α-N-acetylneuraminidase in cultured fibroblasts. *Biochem Biophys Res Commun* **74**:732, 1977.
32. Spranger J, Gehler J, Cantz M: Mucolipidosis I-A sialidosis. *Am J Med Genet* **1**:21, 1977.
33. O'Brien JS: Neuraminidase deficiency in the cherry-red spot–myoclonus syndrome. *Biochem Biophys Res Commun* **79**:1136, 1977.
34. Rapin I, Goldfisher S, Katzman R, Engel J, O'Brien JS: The cherry-red spot–myoclonus syndrome. *Ann Neurol* **3**:234, 1978.
35. Thomas GH, Tipton RE, Ch'ien LT, Reynolds LW, Miller CS: Sialidase (α-N-acetyl neuraminidase) deficiency: The enzyme defect in an adult with macular cherry-red spots and myoclonus without dementia. *Clin Genet* **13**:369, 1978.
36. Jones MZ, Dawson G: Caprine β-mannosidosis: Inherited deficiency of β-D-mannosidase. *J Biol Chem* **256**:5185, 1981.
37. Cooper A, Sardharwalla IB, Roberts MM: Human β-mannosidase deficiency. *N Engl J Med* **315**:1231, 1986.
38. Wenger DA, Sujansky E, Fennessey PV, Thompson JN: Human β-mannosidase deficiency. *N Engl J Med* **315**:1201, 1986.
39. Dorland L, Duran M, Hoefnagels FET, Berg JN, Fabery de Jonge H, Van Eeghen-Cransberg K, Van Sprang FJ, Van Diggelen OP: β-Mannosidosis in two brothers with hearing loss. *J Inherit Metab Dis* **11**:255, 1988.
40. Kleijer WJ, Hu P, Thoomes R, Boer M, Hujimans JGM, Blom W, van Diggelen OP, Seemanova E, Macek M: β-Mannosidase deficiency: Heterogeneous manifestation in the first female patient and her brother. *J Inherit Metab Dis* **13**:867, 1990.
41. Cooper A, Wraith JE, Savage WJ, Thornley M, Noronha MJ: β-Mannosidase deficiency in a female infant with epileptic encephalopathy. *J Inherit Metab Dis* **14**:18, 1991.
42. Poenaru L, Akli S, Rocchiccioli F, Eydoux P, Zamet P: Human β-mannosidosis: A 3-year-old boy with speech impairment and emotional instability. *Clin Genet* **41**:331, 1992.
43. Wijburg H, de Jong J, Wevers R, Bakkeren J, Trijbels F, Sengers R: β-Mannosidosis and ethanolaminuria in a female patient. *Eur J Pediatr* **151**:311, 1992.
44. Hers HG, Van Hoof F: *Lysosomes and Storage Diseases*. New York, Academic, 1973.
45. Kjellman B, Gamstorp I, Brun A, Öckerman P-A, Palmgren B: Mannosidosis: A clinical and histopathologic study. *J Pediatr* **75**:366, 1969.
46. Autio S, Nordén NE, Öckerman P-A, Riekkinen P, Rapola J, Louhimo T: Mannosidosis: Clinical, fine-structural and biochemical findings in three cases. *Acta Paediatr Scand* **62**:555, 1973.
47. Nordén NE, Öckerman P-A, Szabo L: Urinary mannose in mannosidosis. *J Pediatr* **82**:686, 1973.
48. Tsay GC, Dawson G, Matalon R: Excretion of mannose-rich complex carbohydrates by a patient with α-mannosidase deficiency (mannosidosis). *J Pediatr* **84**:865, 1974.
49. Farriaux JP, Legouis I, Humbel R, Dhondt JL, Richard P, Strecker G, Fourmaintraux A, Ringel J, Fontaine G: La mannosidose: A propos de 5 observations. *Nouv Presse Med* **4**:1867, 1975.
50. Loeb H, Tondeur M, Toppet M, Cremer N: Clinical, biochemical and ultrastructural studies of an atypical form of mucopolysaccharidosis. *Acta Paediatr Scand* **58**:220, 1969.
51. Booth CW, Chen KK, Nadler HL: Mannosidosis: Clinical and biochemical studies in a family of affected adolescents and adults. *J Pediatr* **88**:821, 1976.
52. Aylsworth AS, Taylor HA, Stuart CF, Thomas GH: Mannosidosis: Phenotype of a severely affected child and characterization of α-mannosidase activity in cultured fibroblasts from the patient and his parents. *J Pediatr* **88**:814, 1976.
53. Desnick RJ, Sharp HL, Grabowski GA, Brunning RD, Quie PG, Sung JH, Gorlin RJ, Ikonne JU: Mannosidosis: Clinical, morphologic, immunologic, and biochemical studies. *Pediatr Res* **19**:985, 1976.
54. Murphree AL, Beaudet AL, Palmer EA, Nichols BL: Cataract in mannosidosis. *Birth Defects* **12**:319, 1976.
55. Spranger J, Gehler J, Cantz M: The radiographic features of mannosidosis. *Radiology* **119**:401, 1976.
56. Yunis JJ, Lewandowski RC, Sanfilippo SJ, Tsai MY, Foni I, Bruhl HH: Clinical manifestations of mannosidosis — a longitudinal study. *Am J Med* **61**:841, 1976.
57. Arbisser AI, Murphree AL, Gardia CA, Howell RR: Ocular findings in mannosidosis. *Am J Ophthalmol* **82**:465, 1976.
58. Vidgoff J, Lovrien EW, Beals RK, Buist NRM: Mannosidosis in three brothers — a review of the literature. *Medicine* (Baltimore) **56**:335, 1977.
59. Kistler JP, Lott IT, Kolodny EH, Friedman RB, Nersasian R, Schnur J, Mihm MC, Dvorak AM, Dickersin R: Mannosidosis: New clinical presentation, enzyme studies, and carbohydrate analysis. *Arch Neurol* **34**:45, 1977.
60. Milla PJ, Black IE, Patrick AD, Hugh-Jones K, Oberholzer V: Mannosidosis: Clinical and biochemical study. *Arch Dis Child* **52**:937, 1977.
61. Bach G, Kohn G, Lasch EE, El Massri M, Ornoy A, Sekeles E, Legum C, Cohen MM: A new variant of mannosidosis with increased residual enzymatic activity and mild clinical manifestation. *Pediatr Res* **12**:1010, 1978.
62. Gordon BA, Carson R, Haust MD: Unusual clinical and ultrastructural features in a boy with biochemically typical mannosidosis. *Acta Paediatr Scand* **69**:787, 1980.
63. Mitchell ML, Erickson RP, Schmid D, Hieber V, Poznanski AK, Hicks SP: Mannosidosis: Two brothers with different degrees of disease severity. *Clin Genet* **20**:191, 1981.
64. Autio S, Louhimo T, Helenius M: The clinical course of mannosidosis. *Ann Clin Res* **14**:93, 1982.
65. Patton MA, Barnes IC, Young ID, Harper PS, Pennock CA: Mannosidosis in two brothers: Prolonged survival in the severe phenotype. *Clin Genet* **22**:284, 1982.
66. Montgomery TR, Thomas GH, Valle DL: Mannosidosis in an adult. *Johns Hopkins Med J* **151**:113, 1982.
67. Weiss SW, Kelly WD: Bilateral destructive synovitis associated with alpha mannosidase deficiency. *Am J Surg Pathol* **7**:487, 1983.
68. Warner TG, Mock AK, Nyhan WL, O'Brien JS: α-Mannosidosis: Analysis of urinary oligosaccharides with high performance liquid chromatography and diagnosis of a case with unusually mild presentation. *Clin Genet* **25**:248, 1984.
69. Kawai H, Nishino H, Nishida Y, Yoneda K, Yoshida Y, Inui T, Masuda K, Saito S: Skeletal muscle pathology of mannosidosis in two siblings with spastic paraplegia. *Acta Neuropathol* (Berlin) **68**:201, 1985.
70. Dietemann L, Filippi de la Palavesa MM, Tranchant C, Kastler B: MR findings in mannosidosis. *Neuropathology* **32**:485, 1990.
71. Margollicci M, Bartalini G, Balestri P, Fois A: Direct transfer in vitro of α-D-mannosidase activity from normal lymphocytes to fibroblasts of a patient with α-mannosidosis. *J Inherit Metab Dis* **13**:277, 1990.
72. Quie PG, Cates KL: Clinical conditions associated with defective polymorphonuclear leukocyte chemotaxis. *Am J Pathol* **88**:711, 1977.
73. Letson RD, Desnick RJ: Punctate lenticular opacities in type II mannosidosis. *Am J Ophthalmol* **85**:218, 1978.
74. Halperin JL, Landis DMD, Weinstein LA, Lott IT, Kolodny EH: Communicating hydrocephalus and lysosomal inclusions in mannosidosis. *Arch Neurol* **41**:777, 1984.
75. Press OW, Fingert H, Lott IT, Dickersin CR: Pancytopenia in mannosidosis. *Arch Intern Med* **143**:1268, 1983.
76. Noll RB, Kulkarni R, Netzloff ML: Development in patients with mannosidosis. *Arch Neurol* **43**:157, 1986.
77. Noll RB, Netzloff ML, Kulkarni R: Long-term follow-up of biochemical and cognitive functioning in patients with mannosidosis. *Arch Neurol* **46**:507, 1989.

78. Mehta J, Desnick RJ: Abbreviated PR interval in mannosidosis. *J Pediatr* **92**:599, 1978.
79. Will A, Cooper A, Hatton C, Sardharwalla IB, Evans DIK: Bone marrow transplantation in the treatment of α-mannosidosis. *Arch Dis Child* **62**:1044, 1987.
80. Bennett JK, Dembure PP, Elsas LJ: Clinical and biochemical analysis of two families with type I and type II mannosidosis. *Am J Med Genet* **55**:21, 1995.
81. Owayed A, Clarke JTR: Hyperphagia in patients with α-mannosidosis type II. *J Inherit Metab Dis* **20**:727, 1997.
82. Kawai H, Yoneda K, Takeda M, Nishida Y, Nishino H, Masuda K, Saito S: Isozyme pattern of leukocyte α-D-mannosidase in patients with mannosidosis. *Jpn J Hum Genet* **33**:1, 1988.
83. Wong LTK, Vallance H, Savage A, Davidson AGF, Applegarth D: Oral zinc therapy in the treatment of α-mannosidosis. *Am J Med Genet* **46**:410, 1993.
84. Segoloni GP, Colla L, Messina M, Stratta P: Renal transplantation in a case of mannosidosis. *Transplantation* **61**:1654, 1996.
85. Walkley SU, Thrall MA, Dobrenis K, Huang M, March PA, Siegel DA, Wurzelmann S: Bone marrow transplantation corrects the enzyme defect in neurons of the central nervous system in a lysosomal storage disease. *Proc Natl Acad Sci* USA **91**:2970, 1994.
86. Monus Z, Konyar E, Szabo L: Histomorphologic and histochemical investigations in mannosidosis. *Virchows Arch B Cell Pathol* **26**:159, 1977.
87. Sung JH, Hayano M, Desnick RJ: Mannosidosis: Pathology of the nervous system. *J Neuropathol Exp Neurol* **36**:807, 1977.
88. Öckerman P-A: Mannosidosis: Isolation of oligosaccharide storage material from brain. *J Pediatr* **75**:360, 1969.
89. Nordén NE, Lundblad A, Svenson S, Autio S: Characterization of two mannose-containing oligosaccharides isolated from the urine of patients with mannosidosis. *Biochemistry* **13**:871, 1974.
90. Strecker G, Fournet B, Bouquelet S, Montreuil J, Dhondt JL, Farriaux JP: Étude chimique des mannosides urinaires excrétés au cours de la mannosidose. *Biochimie* **58**:579, 1976.
91. Yamashita K, Tachibana Y, Mihara K, Okada S, Yabuuchi H, Kobata A: Urinary oligosaccharides of mannosidosis. *J Biol Chem* **255**:5126, 1979.
92. Matsuura F, Nunez HA, Grabowski GA, Sweeley CC: Structural studies of urinary oligosaccharides from patients with mannosidosis. *Arch Biochem Biophys* **207**:337, 1981.
93. Jardine I, Matsuura F, Sweeley CC: Electron ionization mass spectra of reduced and parmethylated urinary oligosaccharides from patients with mannosidosis. *Biomed Mass Spectrom* **11**:562, 1984.
94. Al Daher S, DeGasperi R, Daniel P, Hall N, Warren CD, Winchester B: The substrate-specificity of human lysosomal α-D-mannosidase in relation to genetic α-mannosidosis. *Biochem J* **277**:743, 1991.
95. Michalski C, Haeuw J-F, Wieruszeski J-M, Montreuil J, Strecker G: *In vitro* hydrolysis of oligomannosyl oligosaccharides by the lysosomal α-D-mannosidases. *J Biochem* **189**:369, 1990.
96. DeGasperi R, Daniel PF, Warren CD: A human lysosomal α-mannosidase specific for the core of complex glycans. *J Biol Chem* **267**:9706, 1992.
97. Abraham D, Blakemore WF, Jolly RD, Sidebotham R, Winchester B: The catabolism of mammalian glycoproteins. *Biochem J* **215**:573, 1973.
98. DeGasperi R, Al Daher S, Daniel PF, Winchester BG, Jeanloz RW, Warren CD: The substrate specificity of bovine and feline lysosomal α-D-mannosidases in relation to α-mannosidosis. *J Biol Chem* **266**:16556, 1991.
99. Tabas I, Kornfeld S: Purification and characterization of a rat liver Golgi α-mannosidase capable of processing asparagine-linked oligosaccharides. *J Biol Chem* **254**:11655, 1979.
100. Opheim DJ, Touster O: Lysosomal α-D-mannosidase of rat liver. *J Biol Chem* **253**:1017, 1978.
101. Carroll M, Dance N, Masson PK, Robinson D, Winchester BG: Human mannosidosis—the enzyme defect. *Biochem Biophys Res Commun* **49**:579, 1972.
102. Nilssen O, Berg T, Riise HMF, Ramachandran U, Evjen G, Hansen GM, Malm D, Tranebjaerg L, Tollersrud OK: α-Mannosidosis: Functional cloning of the lysosomal α-mannosidase cDNA and identification of a mutation in two affected siblings. *Hum Mol Genet* **6**:717, 1997.
103. Pohlmann R, Hasilik A, Cheng S, Pemble S, Winchester B, von Figura K: Synthesis of lysosomal α-mannosidase in normal and mannosidosis fibroblasts. *Biochem Biophys Res Commun* **115**:1083, 1983.
104. Cheng SH, Malcolm S, Pemble S, Winchester B: Purification and comparison of the structures of human liver acidic α-D-mannosidases A and B. *Biochem J* **233**:65, 1986.
105. Tsuji A, Suzuki Y: Purification of human placental acid α-mannosidase by an immunological method. *Biochem Int* **15**:483, 1987.
106. Taylor HA, Thomas GH, Aylsworth A, Stevenson RE, Reynolds LW: Mannosidosis: Deficiency of a specific α-mannosidase component in cultured fibroblasts. *Clin Chim Acta* **59**:93, 1975.
107. Beaudet AL, Nichols BL: Residual altered α-mannosidase in human mannosidosis. *Biochem Biophys Res Commun* **68**:292, 1976.
108. Poenaru L, Miranda C, Dreyfus J-C: Residual mannosidase activity in human mannosidosis. Characterization of the mutant enzyme. *Am J Hum Genet* **32**:354, 1980.
109. Burditt L, Chotai K, Halley D, Winchester B: Comparison of the residual acidic α-D-mannosidase in three cases of mannosidosis. *Clin Chim Acta* **104**:201, 1980.
110. Tsvetkova IV, Rosenfeld EL, Prigozina IG: An unusual case of mannosidosis with severe deficiency of acid mannosidase in leukocytes and high residual enzymatic activity in skin fibroblasts. *Clin Chim Acta* **107**:37, 1980.
111. Hultberg B, Masson PK: Activation of residual acidic α-mannosidase activity in mannosidosis tissues by metal ions. *Biochem Biophys Res Commun* **67**:1473, 1980.
112. Mersmann G, Buddecke E: Evidence for material from mannosidase fibroblasts cross reacting with anti-acidic α-mannosidase antibodies. *FEBS Lett* **73**:123, 1977.
113. Burditt LJ, Chotai KA, Winchester BG: Evidence that the mutant enzyme in fibroblasts of a patient with mannosidosis does not crossreact with antiserum raised against normal acidic α-mannosidase. *FEBS Lett* **91**:186, 1978.
114. Hultberg B, Masson PK: Normal extracellular excretions of acidic α-mannosidase activity by mannosidosis fibroblast cultures. *Biochim Biophys Acta* **481**:573, 1977.
115. Halley DJJ, Winchester BG, Burditt LJ, d'Azzo A, Robinson D, Galjaard H: Comparison of the α-mannosidase in fibroblast cultures from patients with mannosidosis and mucolipidosis II and from controls. *Biochem J* **187**:541, 1980.
116. Ben-Yoseph Y, Defranco CL, Charrow J, Hahn LC, Nadler HL: Apparently normal extracellular acidic α-mannosidase in fibroblast cultures from patients with mannosidosis. *Am J Hum Genet* **34**:100, 1982.
117. McKusick VA, Francomano CA, Antonarakis SE: *Mendelian Inheritance in Man—Catalogs of Autosomal Dominant, Autosomal Recessive, and X-Linked Phenotypes* 11th ed. Baltimore, Johns Hopkins University Press, 1994.
118. Champion MJ, Shows TB: Mannosidosis: Assignment of the lysosomal α-mannosidase B gene to chromosome 19 in man. *Proc Natl Acad Sci USA* **74**:2968, 1977.
119. Ingram PH, Bruns GAP, Regina VM, Eisenman RE, Gerald PS: Expression of α-D-mannosidase in man-hamster somatic cell hybrids. *Biochem Genet* **15**:455, 1977.
120. Brook JD, Shaw DJ, Meredith L, Bruns GAP, Harper PS: Localization of genetic markers and orientation of the linkage group of chromosome 19. *Hum Genet* **68**:282, 1984.
121. Martinvik F, Ellenbogen A, Hirschhorn K, Hirschhorn R: Further localization of the gene for human acid alpha glucosidase (GAA), peptidase D (PEPD) and α-mannosidase B (MANB) by somatic cell hybridization. *Hum Genet* **69**:109, 1985.
122. Kaneda Y, Hayes H, Uchida T, Yoshida MC, Okada Y: Regional assignment of five genes on human chromosome 19. *Chromosoma* **95**:8, 1987.
123. Bachinski LL, Krahe R, White BF, Wieringa B, Shaw D, Korneluk R, Thompson LH, Johnson K, Siciliano MJ: An informative panel of somatic cell hybrids for physical mapping on human chromsome 19q. *Am J Hum Genet* **52**:375, 1993.
124. Nebes VL, Schmidt MC: Human lysosomal alpha-mannosidase: Isolation and nucleotide sequence of the full-length cDNA. *Biochem Biophys Res Commun* **200**:239, 1994.
125. Wang W, Nebes VL, Schmidt MC, Barranger JA: Expression of human lysosomal alpha-mannosidase activity in transfected murine cells and human alpha-mannosidase deficient fibroblasts. *Biochem Biophys Res Commun* **224**:619, 1996.
126. Emiliani C, Martino S, Stirling JL, Maras B, Orlacchio A: Partial sequence of the purified protein confirms the identity of cDNA coding for human lysosomal α-mannosidase B. *Biochem J* **305**:363, 1995.
127. Liao YF, Lal A, Moreman KW: Cloning, expression, purification, and characterization of the human broad specificity lysosomal acid α-mannosidase. *J Biol Chem* **271**:28348, 1996.
128. Wakamatsu N, Gotoda Y, Saito S, Kawai H: Characterization of the human MANB gene encoding lysosomal α-D-mannosidase. *Gene* **198**:351, 1997.

129. Riise HMF, Berg T, Nilssen O, Romeo G, Tollersrud OK, Ceccherini I: Genomic structure of the human lysosomal α-mannosidase gene (MANB). *Genomics* **42**:200, 1997.
130. Nebes VL, Schmidt MC: Erratum. *Biochem Biophys Res Commun* **232**:583, 1997.
131. Merkle RK, Zhang Y, Ruest PJ, Lal A, Liao YF, Moremen KW: Cloning, expression, purification, and characterization of the murine lysosomal acid α-mannosidase. *Biochim Biophys Acta* **1336**:132, 1997.
132. Beccari T, Appolloni MG, Costanzi E, Stinchi S, Stirling JL, Della Fazia MA, Servillo G, Viola MP, Orlacchio A: Lysosomal α-mannosidases of mouse tissues: Characteristics of the isoenzymes, and cloning and expression of a full-length cDNA. *Biochem J* **327**:45, 1997.
133. Berg T, Tollersrud OK, Walkley SU, Siegel D, Nilssen O: Purification of feline lysosomal α-mannosidase, determination of its cDNA sequence and identification of a mutation causing α-mannosidosis in Persian cats. *Biochem J* **328**:863, 1997.
134. Tollersrud OK, Berg T, Healy P, Evjen G, Ramachandran U, Nilssen O: Purification of bovine lysosomal α-mannosidase, characterization of its gene and determination of two mutations that cause α-mannosidosis. *Eur J Biochem* **246**:410, 1997.
135. Gotoda Y, Wakamatsu N, Nishida Y, Abramowicz MJ, Neves VL, Kawai H: Structural organization, sequence, and mutation analysis of MANB gene encoding the human lysosomal α-mannosidase. *Am J Hum Genet* **59**: A260, 1996.
136. Nordén NE, Lundblad A: A mannose-containing trisaccharide isolated from urines of three patients with mannosidosis. *J Biol Chem* **248**:6210, 1973.
137. Sewell AC: An improved thin-layer chromatographic method for urinary oligosaccharide screening. *Clin Chim Acta* **92**:411, 1979.
138. Sewell AC: Urinary oligosaccharide excretion in disorders of glycolipid, glycoprotein, and glycogen metabolism. *Eur J Pediatr* **134**:183, 1980.
139. Sewell AC: Simple laboratory determination of excess oligosacchariduria. *Clin Chem* **27**:243, 1981.
140. Holmes EW, O'Brien JS: Separation of glycoprotein-derived oligosaccharides by thin-layer chromatography. *Anal Biochem* **93**:167, 1979.
141. Sewell AC: Urinary oligosaccharides, in Hommes FA (ed): *Techniques in Diagnostic Human Biochemical Genetics*. New York, Wiley-Liss, 1991, p 219.
142. Hommes FA, Varghese M: High-performance liquid chromatography of urinary oligosaccharides in the diagnosis of glycoprotein degradation disorders. *Clin Chim Acta* **203**:211, 1991.
143. Blom HJ, Andersson HC, Krasnewich DM, Gahl WA: Pulsed amperometric detection of carbohydrates in lysosomal storage disease fibroblasts: A new screening technique for carbohydrate storage diseases. *J Chromatogr* **533**:11, 1990.
144. Salaspuro M, Salmela K, Humaloja K, Autio S, Arvio M, Palo J: Elevated level of serum dolichol in aspartylglucosaminuria. *Life Sci* **47**:627, 1990.
145. Humaloja K, Roine RP, Salmela K, Halmesmäki E, Jokelainen K, Salaspuro M: Serum dolichols in different clinical conditions. *Scand J Clin Lab Invest* **51**:705, 1991.
146. Prence EM, Natowicz MR: Diagnosis of α-mannosidosis by measuring α-mannosidase in plasma. *Clin Chem* **38**:501, 1992.
147. Maire I, Zabot MT, Mathieu M, Cotte J: Mannosidosis: Tissue culture studies in relation to prenatal diagnosis. *J Inherit Metab Dis* **1**:19, 1978.
148. Poenaru L, Girard S, Thèpot F, Madelenat P, Huraux-Rendu C, Vinet M-C, Dreyfus J-C: Antenatal diagnosis in three pregnancies at risk for mannosidosis. *Clin Genet* **16**:428, 1979.
149. Poenaru L, Kaplan L, Dumez J, Dreyfus JC: Evaluation of possible first trimester prenatal diagnosis in lysosomal diseases by trophoblast biopsy. *Pediatr Res* **18**:1032, 1984.
150. Petushkova NA: First-trimester diagnosis of an unusual case of α-mannosidosis. *Prenat Diagn* **11**:279, 1991.
151. Fukuda M, Tanaka A, Isshiki G: Variation of lysosomal enzyme activity with gestational age in chorionic villi. *J Inherit Metab Dis* **13**:862, 1990.
152. Whittem JM, Walker D: "Neuronopathy" and "pseudolipidosis" in Aberdeen Angus calves. *J Pathol Bacteriol* **74**:281, 1957.
153. Jolly RD, Slack PM, Winter PJ, Murphy CE: Mannosidosis: Patterns of storage and urinary excretion of oligosaccharides in the bovine model. *Aust J Exp Biol Med Sci* **58**:421, 1980.
154. Dorling PR: Lysosomal storage diseases in animals, in Dingle JT, Dean RT, Sly WS (eds): *Lysosomes in Biology and Pathology*. Amsterdam, Elsevier, 1984, p 347.
155. Healy PJ: Testing for undesirable traits in cattle: An Australian perspective. *J Anim Sci* **74**:917, 1996.
156. Burditt LJ, Chotai K, Hirani S, Nugent PG, Winchester BG, Blakemore WF: Biochemical studies on a case of feline mannosidosis. *Biochem J* **189**:467, 1980.
157. Walkley SU, Blakemore WF, Purpura DP: Alterations in neuronomorphology in feline mannosidosis. A Golgi study. *Acta Neuropathol* **53**:75, 1981.
158. Vandevelde M, Fankhauser R, Bichsel P, Wiesmann V, Herschkowitz N: Hereditary neurovisceral mannosidosis associated with α-mannosidase deficiency in a family of Persian cats. *Acta Neuropathol* **58**:64, 1982.
159. Abraham D, Blakemore WF, Jolly RD, Sidebotham R, Winchester B: The catabolism of mammalian glycoproteins. Comparison of the storage products in bovine, feline and human mannosidosis. *Biochem J* **215**:573, 1983.
160. Abraham D, Daniel P, Dell A, Oates J, Sidebotham R, Winchester B: Structural analysis of the major urinary oligosaccharides in feline α-mannosidosis. *Biochem J* **233**:899, 1986.
161. Warren CD, Alroy J, Bugge B, Daniel PF, Raghaven SS, Kolodny EH, Lamar JJ, Jeanloz RW: Oligosaccharides from placenta: Early diagnosis of feline mannosidosis. *FEBS Lett* **195**:247, 1986.
162. Raghavan S, Stuer G, Riviére L, Alroy J, Kolodny EH: Characterization of α-mannosidase in feline mannosidosis. *J Inherit Metab Dis* **11**:3, 1988.
163. Levade T, Graber D, Flurin V, Delisle MB, Pieraggi MT, Testut MF, Carrière JP, Salvayre R: Human β-mannosidase deficiency associated with peripheral neuropathy. *Ann Neurol* **35**:116, 1994.
164. Rodríguez-Serna M, Botella-Estrada R, Chabás A, Coll M-J, Oliver V, Febrer M-I, Aliaga A: Angiokeratoma corporis diffusum associated with β-mannosidase deficiency. *Arch Dermatol* **132**:1219, 1996.
165. Gourrier E, Thomas MP, Munnich A, Poenaru L, Asensi D, Jan D, Leraillez J: Beta mannosidosis: A new case. *Arch Pediatr* **4**:147, 1997.
166. Hu P, Wenger DA, van Diggelen OP, Kleijer WJ: Complementation studies in human and caprine β-mannosidosis. *J Inherit Metab Dis* **14**:13, 1991.
167. Tjoa S, Wenger DA, Fennessey PV: Quantitative analysis of disaccharides in the urine of β-mannosidosis patients. *J Inherit Metab Dis* **13**:187, 1990.
168. Lemonnier M, Derappe C, Poenaru L, Chester MA, Lundblad A, Svensson S, Öckerman P-A: Isolation and characterization of 4-O-β-D-mannopyranosyl-2-acetamido-2-deoxy-D-glucose from the urine of a patient with mucolipidosis II and its occurrence in normal and pathological urine. *FEBS Lett* **141**:263, 1982.
169. van Pelt J, Hokke CH, Dorland L, Duran M, Kamerling JP, Vliegenthart JFG: Accumulation of mannosyl-β(1 → 4)-N-acetylglucosamine in fibroblasts and leukocytes of patients with a deficiency of β-mannosidase. *Clin Chim Acta* **187**:55, 1990.
170. Hokke CH, Duran M, Dorland L, van Pelt J, van Sprang FJ: Novel storage products in human β-mannosidosis. *J Inherit Metab Dis* **13**:273, 1990.
171. van Pelt J, Dorland L, Duran M, Hokke CH, Kamerling JP, Vliegenthart JFG: Sialyl-α2-6-mannosyl-β1-4-N-acetylglucosamine, a novel compound occurring in urine of patients with β-mannosidosis. *J Biol Chem* **265**:19685, 1990.
172. Sopher BL, Traviss CE, Cavanagh KT, Jones MZ, Friderici KH: Purification and characterization of goat lysosomal β-mannosidase using monoclonal and polyclonal antibodies. *J Biol Chem* **267**:6178, 1992.
173. Frei JI, Cavanagh KT, Fisher RA, Hausinger RP, Dupuis M, Rathke EJS, Jones MZ: Partial purification of goat kidney β-mannosidase. *Biochem J* **249**:871, 1988.
174. Kyosaka S, Murata S, Nakamura F, Tanaka M: Purification and kinetic properties of guinea pig liver β-mannosidase. *Chem Pharm Bull* **33**:256, 1985.
175. Bernard M, Sioud M, Percheron F, Foglietti MJ: β-Mannosidase in human serum and urine. A comparative study. *Int J Biochem* **18**:1065, 1986.
176. Cooper A, Hatton C, Sardharwalla IB: Acid β-mannosidase of human plasma: Influence of age and sex on enzyme activity. *J Inherit Metab Dis* **10**:229, 1987.
177. Panday RS, van Diggelen OP, Kleijer WJ, Niermeijer MF: β-Mannosidase in human leukocytes and fibroblasts. *J Inherit Metab Dis* **7**:155, 1984.
178. Colin B, Bernard M, Foglietti MJ, Percheron F: β-D-Mannosidase in human polymorphonuclear leukocytes and lymphocytes: A comparative study. *Int J Biochem* **19**:395, 1987.

179. Iwasaki Y, Tsuji A, Omura K, Suzuki Y: Purification and characterization of β-mannosidase from human placenta. *J Biochem* **106**:331, 1989.
180. Percheron F, Foglietti MJ, Bernard M, Ricard B: Mammalian β-D-mannosidase and β-mannosidosis. *Biochimie* **74**:5, 1992.
181. McCabe NR, Biliter W, Dawson G: Preferential inhibition of lysosomal β-mannosidase by sucrose. *Enzyme* **43**:137, 1990.
182. Guadalupi R, Bernard M, Orlacchio A, Foglietti MJ, Emiliani C: Purification and properties of human urinary β-D-mannosidase. *Biochim Biophys Acta* **1293**:9, 1996.
183. Lundin L-G: A gene (Bmn) controlling β-mannosidase activity in the mouse is located in the distal part of chromosome 3. *Biochem Genet* **25**:603, 1987.
184. Schmutz SM, Moker JS, Leipprandt JR, Friderici KH: Beta-mannosidase maps to cattle chromosome 6. *Mamm Genome* **7**:474, 1996.
185. Chen H, Leipprandt JR, Traviss CE, Sopher BL, Jones MZ, Cavanagh KT, Friderici KH: Molecular cloning and characterization of bovine β-mannosidase. *J Biol Chem* **270**:3841, 1995.
186. Alkhayat AH, Draemer SA, Leipprandt JR, Macek M, Kleijer WJ, Friderici KH: Human β-mannosidase cDNA characterization and first identification of a mutation associated with human β-mannosidosis. *Hum Mol Genet* **7**:75, 1998.
187. Sopher BL, Traviss CE, Cavanagh KT, Jones MZ, Friderici KH: Bovine kidney β-mannosidase: Purification and characterization. *Biochem J* **289**:343, 1993.
188. Leipprandt JR, Kraemer SA, Haithcock BE, Chen H, Dyme JL, Cavanagh KT, Friderici KH, Jones MZ: Caprine β-mannosidase: Sequencing and characterization of the cDNA and identification of the molecular defect of caprine β-mannosidosis. *Genomics* **37**:51, 1996.
189. Blom W, Luteyn JC, Kelholt-Dijkman HH, Huijmans JGM, Loonen MCB: Thin-layer chromatography of oligosaccharides in urine as a rapid indication for the diagnosis of lysosomal acid maltase deficiency (Pompés disease). *Clin Chim Acta* **134**:221, 1983.
190. Dorland L, Wadman SK, Fabery de Jonge H, Ketting D: 1, 6-Anhydro-β-D-glucopyranose (β-glucosan), a constituent of human urine. *Clin Chim Acta* **159**:11, 1986.
191. Vietor KW, Havsteen B, Harms D, Busse H, Heyne K: Ethanolaminosis: A newly recognized, generalized storage disease with cardiomegaly, cerebral dysfunction and early death. *Eur J Pediatr* **126**:61, 1977.
192. Cooper A, Hatton C, Thornley M, Sardharwalla IB: Human β-mannosidase deficiency: Biochemical findings in plasma, fibroblasts, white cells and urine. *J Inherit Metab Dis* **11**:17, 1988.
193. Kleijer WJ, Geilen GC, van Diggelen OP, Wevers RA, Los FJ: Prenatal analyses in a pregnancy at risk for β-mannosidosis. *Prenat Diagn* **12**:841, 1992.
194. Petushkova NA, Ivleva TS, Vozniy YAM: Human chorionic β-mannosidase: Comparison with β-mannosidase from human cultured fibroblasts. *Prenat Diagn* **12**:835, 1992.
195. Jones MZ, Cunningham JG, Dade AW, Alessi DM, Mostoski UV, Vorro JR, Benítez JT, Lovell KL: Caprine β-mannosidosis: Clinical and pathological features. *J Neuropathol Exp Neurol* **421**:268, 1983.
196. Jones MZ, Kennedy FA: Caprine β-mannosidosis: Aberrant phenotype in a 5-month-old euthyroid animal. *J Inherit Metab Dis* **16**:910, 1993.
197. Abbitt B, Jones MZ, Kasari TR, Storts RW, Templeton JW, Holland PS, Castenson PE: β-Mannosidosis in twelve Salers calves. *J Am Vet Med Assoc* **198**:109, 1991.
198. Cooper A, Hatton CE, Thornley M, Sardharwalla IB: α- and β-mannosidoses. *J Inherit Metab Dis* **13**:538, 1990.
199. Jones MZ, Rathke EJS, Gage DA, Costello CE, Murakami K, Ohta M, Matsuura F: Oligosaccharides accumulated in the bovine β-mannosidosis kidney. *J Inherit Metab Dis* **15**:57, 1992.
200. Durand P, Gatti R, Borrone C, Costantino G, Cavalier S, Filocamo M, Romeo G: Detection of carriers and prenatal diagnosis for fucosidosis in Calabria. *Hum Genet* **51**:195, 1979.
201. Willems PJ, Gatti R, Darby JK, Romeo G, Durand P, Dumon JE, O'Brien JS: Fucosidosis revisited: A review of 77 patients. *Am J Med Genet* **38**:111, 1991.
202. Böck A, Fang-Kircher S, Braun F, Gerdov C, Breier F, Jurecka W, Paschke E: Another unusual case of fucosidosis. *J Inherit Metab Dis* **18**:93, 1995.
203. Fleming C, Rennie A, Fallowfield M, McHenry PM: Cutaneous manifestations of fucosidosis. *Br J Dermatol* **136**:594, 1997.
204. Durand P, Borrone CX, Della Cella G: Fucosidosis. *J Pediatr* **75**:665, 1969.
205. Loeb H, Tondeur M, Jonniaux G, Mockel-Pohl S, Vamos-Hurwitz E: Biochemical and ultrastructural studies in a case of mucopolysaccharidosis "F" (fucosidosis). *Helv Paediatr Acta* **24**:519, 1969.
206. Patel V, Watanabe I, Zeman W: Deficiency of α-L-fucosidase. *Science* **176**:426, 1972.
207. Freitag F, Kuchemann K, Blumcke S: Hepatic ultrastructure in fucosidosis. *Virchows Arch B Cell Pathol* **7**:99, 1971.
208. Zielke K, Okada S, O'Brien JS: Fucosidosis: Diagnosis by serum assay of α-L-fucosidase. *J Lab Clin Med* **79**:164, 1972.
209. Matsuda I, Arashima S, Anakura M, Ege A, Hayata I: Fucosidosis. *Tohoku J Exp Med* **109**:41, 1973.
210. Matsuda I, Arashima S, Oka Y, Mitsuyama T, Ariga S, Ikeuchi T, Ichida T: Prenatal diagnosis of fucosidosis. *Clin Chim Acta* **63**:55, 1975.
211. Borrone C, Gatti R, Trias X, Durand P: Fucosidosis: Clinical, biochemical, immunologic, and genetic studies in two new cases. *J Pediatr* **84**:727, 1974.
212. Kousseff BG, Beratis NG, Danesino C, Hirschhorn K: Genetic heterogeneity in fucosidosis. *Lancet* **2**:1387, 1973.
213. Kousseff BG, Beratis NG, Strauss L, Brill PW, Rosenfield RE, Kaplan B, Hirschhorn K: Fucosidosis type 2. *Pediatrics* **57**:205, 1976.
214. Ng WG, Donnell GN, Koch R, Bergren WR: Biochemical and genetic studies of plasma and leukocyte α-L-fucosidase. *Am J Hum Genet* **28**:42, 1976.
215. Taconis WK, Van Wiechen PJ, van Gemund JJ: Radiological findings in a case of type II fucosidosis: A case report. *Radiol Clin* (Basel) **45**:258, 1976.
216. Libert J, Van Hoof F, Tondeur M: Fucosidosis: Ultrastructural study of conjunctiva and skin and enzyme analysis of tears. *Invest Ophthalmol* **15**:626, 1976.
217. Poenaru L, Dreyfus J-C, Boue J, Nicolesco H, Ravise N, Bamberger J: Prenatal diagnosis of fucosidosis. *Clin Genet* **10**:260, 1976.
218. MacPhee GB, Logan RW: Fucosidosis in a native-born Briton. *J Clin Pathol* **30**:278, 1977.
219. Snyder RD, Carlow TJ, Ledman J, Wenger DA: Ocular findings in fucosidosis. *Birth Defects* **12**:241, 1976.
220. Troost J, Staal GEJ, Willemse J, van der Heijden MCM: Fucosidosis: I. Clinical and enzymological studies. *Neuropaediatrie* **8**:155, 1977.
221. Romeo G, Borrone C, Gatti R, Durand P: Fucosidosis in Calabria: Founder effect or high gene frequency? *Lancet* **1**:368, 1977.
222. Giovannini M, Riva E, Beluffi G, Perego O: Fucosidosis: Description of a clinical case. *Minerva Pediatr* **30**:1307, 1978.
223. Larbrisseau A, Brouchu P, Jasmin G: Fucosidose de type I: Étude anatomique. *Arch Fr Pédiatr* **36**:1013, 1979.
224. Schoondewaldt HC, Lamers KJB, Kleijnen FM, van den Berg CJMG, de Bruyn CHMM: Two patients with an unusual form of type II fucosidosis. *Clin Genet* **18**:348, 1980.
225. Alhadeff JA, Andrews-Smith GL, O'Brien JS: Biochemical studies on an unusual case of fucosidosis. *Clin Genet* **14**:235, 1978.
226. Lee FA, Donnell GN, Gwinn JL: Radiographic features of fucosidosis. *Pediatr Radiol* **5**:204, 1977.
227. Sovik O, Lie SO, Fluge G, Van Hoof F: Fucosidosis: Severe phenotype with survival to adult age. *Eur J Pediatr* **135**:211, 1980.
228. Christomanou H, Beyer D: Absence of α-fucosidase activity in two sisters showing a different phenotype. *Eur J Pediatr* **140**:27, 1983.
229. Boudet CE, Maisongrosse G, Echenne B: À propos de deux nouveaux cas de fucosidose de type II. *Bull Soc Ophthalmol Fr* **82**:91, 1982.
230. Ikeda S, Kondo K, Oguchi K, Yanagisawa N, Horigome R, Murata F: Adult fucosidosis: Histochemical and ultrastructural studies of rectal mucosa biopsy. *Neurology* **34**:561, 1984.
231. Blitzer MG, Sutton M, Miller JB, Shapira E: Brief clinical report: A thermolabile variant of α-L-fucosidase—clinical and laboratory findings. *Am J Med Genet* **20**:535, 1985.
232. Willems PJ, Garcia CA, De Smedt MCH, Martin-Jimenez R, Darby JK, Duenas DA, Granado-Villar D, O'Brien JS: Intrafamilial variability in fucosidosis. *Clin Genet* **34**:7, 1988.
233. Epinette WW, Norins AL, Drew AL: Angiokeratoma corporis diffusum with α-L-fucosidase deficiency. *Arch Dermatol* **107**:754, 1973.
234. Kornfeld M, Snyder RD, Wenger DA: Fucosidosis with angiokeratoma: Electron microscopic changes in the skin. *Arch Pathol Lab Med* **101**:478, 1977.
235. Smith EB, Graham JL, Ledman JA, Snyder RD: Fucosidosis. *Cutis* **19**:195, 1977.
236. Dvoretzky I, Fisher BK: Fucosidosis. *Int J Dermatol* **18**:213, 1979.
237. Snodgrass MB: Ocular findings in a case of fucosidosis. *Br J Ophthalmol* **60**:508, 1976.

238. Provenzale JM, Barboriak DP, Sims K: Neuroradiologic findings in fucosidosis, a rare lysosomal storage disease. *Am J Neuroradiol* **16**:809, 1995.
239. Terespolsky D, Clarke JTR, Blaser SI: Evolution of the neuroimaging changes in fucosidosis type II. *J Inherit Metab Dis* **19**:775, 1996.
240. Gordon BA, Gordon KE, Seo HC, Yang M, DiCioccio RA, O'Brien JS: Fucosidosis with dystonia. *Neuropediatrics* **26**:325, 1995.
241. Vellodi A, Cragg H, Winchester B, Young E, Young J, Downie CJC, Hoare RD, Stocks R, Banerjee GK: Allogeneic bone marrow transplantation for fucosidosis. *Bone Marrow Transp* **15**:153, 1995.
242. Dawson G, Spranger JW: Fucosidosis: A glycosphingolipidosis. *N Engl J Med* **285**:122, 1971.
243. Tsay GC, Dawson G: Oligosaccharide storage in brains from patients with fucosidosis, G_{M1}-gangliosidosis and G_{M2}-gangliosidosis (Sandhoff's disease). *J Neurochem* **27**:733, 1976.
244. Tsay GC, Dawson G, Sung S-SJ: Structure of the accumulating oligosaccharide in fucosidosis. *J Biol Chem* **251**:5852, 1976.
245. Nishigaki M, Yamashita K, Matsuda I, Arashima S, Kobata A: Urinary oligosaccharides of fucosidosis: Evidence of the occurrence of X-antgenic determinant in serum-type sugar chains of glycoproteins. *J Biochem* **84**:823, 1978.
246. Strecker G, Fournet B, Montreuil J, Dorland L, Haverkamp J, Vliegenthart JFG, Dubesset D: Structure of the three major fucosylglycoasparagines accumulating in the urine of a patient with fucosidosis. *Biochimie* **60**:725, 1978.
247. Ng Y, Kin NMK, Wolfe LS: Urinary excretion of a novel hexasaccharide and a glycopeptide analogue in fucosidosis. *Biochem Biophys Res Commun* **88**:696, 1979.
248. Lundblad A, Lundsten J, Nordén NE, Sjoblad S, Svensson S, Öckerman P-A, Gehlhoff M: Urinary abnormalities in fucosidosis: Characterization of a disaccharide and two glycoasparagines. *Eur J Biochem* **83**:513, 1978.
249. Yamashita K, Tachibana Y, Takada S, Matsuda I, Arashima S, Kobata A: Urinary glycopeptides of fucosidosis. *J Biol Chem* **254**:4820, 1979.
250. Michalski J-C, Wieruszeski J-M, Alonso C, Cache P, Montreuil J, Strecker G: Characterization and 400-MHz ^{1}H-NMR analysis of urinary fucosyl glycoasparagines in fucosidosis. *Eur J Biochem* **201**:439, 1991.
251. Ng Y, Kin NMK: Comparison of the urinary glycoconjugates excreted by patients with type I and type II fucosidosis. *Clin Chem* **33**:44, 1987.
252. Greiling H, Stuhlsatz HW, Cantz M, Gehler J: Increased urinary excretion of keratan sulfate in fucosidosis. *J Clin Chem Clin Biochem* **16**:329, 1978.
253. Staal GEJ, van der Heijden MCM, Troost J, Moes M, Borst-Eilers E: Fucosidosis and Lewis substances. *Clin Chim Acta* **76**:155, 1977.
254. Johnson SW, Alhadeff JA: Mammalian α-L-fucosidases. *Comp Biochem Physiol* [B] **99**:479, 1991.
255. Johnson SW, Piesecki S, Wang RF, Damjanov I, Alhadeff JA: Analysis of purified human liver α-L-fucosidase by western-blotting with lectins and polyclonal and monoclonal antibodies. *Biochem J* **282**:829, 1992.
256. Piesecki S, Alhadeff JA: The effect of carbohydrate removal on the properties of human liver α-L-fucosidase. *Biochim Biophys Acta* **1119**:194, 1992.
257. Roger L, Bernard M-A, Percheron F, Foglietti M-J: α-L-Fucosidase activity in normal human lymphocytes. *Clin Chim Acta* **180**:303, 1989.
258. O'Brien JS, Willems PJ, Fukushima H, de Wet JR, Darby JK, DiCioccio R, Fowler ML, Shows TB: Molecular biology of the α-L-fucosidase gene and fucosidosis. *Enzyme* **38**:45, 1987.
259. Occhiodoro T, Beckmann KR, Morris CP, Hopwood JJ: Human α-L-fucosidase: Complete coding sequence from cDNA clones. *Biochem Biophys Res Commun* **164**:439, 1989.
260. Fukushima H, Nishimoto J, Okada S: Sequencing and expression of a full-length cDNA for human α-L-fucosidase. *J Inherit Metab Dis* **13**:761, 1990.
261. White WJ, Schray KJ, Legler G, Alhadeff JA: Further studies on the catalytic mechanism of human liver α-L-fucosidase. *Biochim Biophys Acta* **912**:132, 1987.
262. Johnson K, Dawson G: Molecular defect in processing α-fucosidase in fucosidase. *Biochem Biophys Res Commun* **133**:90, 1985.
263. Johnson KF, Hancock LW, Dawson G: Synthesis and processing of lysosomal α-fucosidase in cultured human fibroblasts. *Biochim Biophys Acta* **1073**:120, 1991.
264. Wauters JG, Stuer KL, van Elsen A, Willems PJ: α-L-Fucosidase in human fibroblasts. I. The enzyme activity polymorphism. *Biochem Genet* **30**:131, 1992.
265. Andrews-Smith GL, Alhadeff JA: Radioimmunoassay determination of decreased amounts of α-L-fucosidase in fucosidosis. *Biochim Biophys Acta* **715**:90, 1982.
266. DiCioccio RA, Brown KS: Biosynthesis, processing and extracellular release of α-L-fucosidase in lymphoid cell lines of different genetic origins. *Biochem Genet* **26**:401, 1988.
267. DiCioccio RA, Darby JK, Willems PJ: Abnormal expression of α-L-fucosidase in lymphoid cell lines of fucosidosis patients. *Biochem Genet* **27**:279, 1989.
268. DiCioccio RA, Gordon BA: Defective expression of α-L-fucosidase by lymphoid cells of a fucosidosis patient. *Clin Biochem* **24**:265, 1991.
269. Turner VS, Turner BM, Kucherlapati R, Ruddle FH, Hirschhorn K: Assignment of the human α-L-fucosidase gene locus to chromosome 1 by use of a clone panel. *Birth Defects* **12**:238, 1976.
270. Turner BM, Smith M, Turner VS, Kucherlapati RS, Ruddle FH, Hirschhorn K: Assignment of the gene locus for human α-L-fucosidase to chromosome 1 by analysis of somatic cell hybrids. *Somat Cell Genet* **4**:45, 1978.
271. Corney RL, Fisher PJL, Cook J, Noades J, Robson EB: Linkage between α-fucosidase and the rhesus blood group. *Ann Hum Genet* **40**:403, 1977.
272. Carritt B, King J, Welch HM: Gene order and localization of enzyme loci on the short arm of chromosome 1. *Ann Hum Genet* **46**:329, 1982.
273. Fowler ML, Nakai H, Byers MG, Fukushima H, Eddy RL, Henry WM, Haley LL, O'Brien JS, Shows TB: Chromosome 1 localization of the human alpha-L-fucosidase structural gene with a homologous site on chromosome 2. *Cytogenet Cell Genet* **43**:103, 1986.
274. Darby JK, Willems PJ, Nakashima P, Johnsen J, Ferrell RE, Wijsman EM, Gerhard DS, Dracopoli NC, Housman D, Henke J, Fowler ML, Shows TB, O'Brien JS, Cavalli-Sforza LL: Restriction analysis of the structural α-L-fucosidase gene and its linkage to fucosidosis. *Am J Hum Genet* **43**:749, 1988.
275. Carritt B, Welch HM: An α-fucosidase pseudogene on human chromosome 2. *Hum Genet* **75**:248, 1987.
276. Kretz KA, Cripe D, Carson GS, Fukushima H, O'Brien JS: Structure and sequence of the human α-L-fucosidase gene and pseudogene. *Genomics* **12**:276, 1992.
277. Coucke P, Mangelschots K, Speleman F, Bossuyt P, Van Oostveldt P, van der Auwera B, Carritt B, Willems PJ: Assignment of the fucosidase pseudogene FUCA1P to chromosome region 2q31 → q32. *Cytogenet Cell Genet* **57**:120, 1991.
278. Eiberg H, Mohr J, Nielsen LS: Linkage of plasma α-L-fucosidase (FUCA2) and the plasminogen (PLG) system. *Clin Genet* **26**:23, 1984.
279. Murray JC, Sadler E, Eddy RL, Shows TB, Buetow KH: Evidence for assignment of plasminogen (PLG) to chromosome 6, not chromosome 4. *Cytogenet Cell Genet* **40**:709, 1985.
280. Murray JC, Buetow KH, Donovan M, Hornung S, Motulsky AG, Disteche C, Dyer K, Swisshelm K, Anderson J, Giblett E, Sadler E, Eddy R, Shows TB: Linkage disequilibrium of plasminogen polymorphisms and assignment of the gene to human chromosome 6q26–6q27. *Am J Hum Genet* **40**:338, 1987.
281. Narahara K, Tsuji K, Yokoyama Y, Namba H, Murakami M, Matsubara T, Kasai R, Fukushima Y, Seki T, Wakui K, Seino Y: Specification of small distal 6q deletions in two patients by gene dosage and *in situ* hybridization study of plasminogen and α-L-fucosidase 2. *Am J Med Genet* **40**:348, 1991.
282. Fukushima H, Dewet JR, O'Brien JS: Molecular cloning of a cDNA for human α-L-fucosidase. *Proc Natl Acad Sci USA* **82**:1262, 1985.
283. Fisher KJ, Aronson NA Jr: Isolation and sequence analysis of a cDNA encoding rat liver α-L-fucosidase. *Biochem J* **264**:695, 1989.
284. Willems PJ, Darby JK, DiCioccio RA, Nakashima P, Eng C, Kretz KA, Cavalli-Sforza LL, Shooter EM, O'Brien JS: Identification of a mutation in the structural α-L-fucosidase gene in fucosidosis. *Am J Hum Genet* **43**:756, 1988.
285. Kretz KA, Darby JK, Willems PJ, O'Brien JS: Characterization of EcoRI mutation in fucosidosis patients: A stop codon in the open reading frame. *J Mol Neurosci* **1**:177, 1989.
286. Seo H-C, Willens PJ, Kretz KA, Martin BM, O'Brien JS: Fucosidosis: Four new mutations and a new polymorphism. *Hum Mol Genet* **2**:423, 1993.
287. Yang M, Allen H, DiCioccio RA: A mutation generating a stop codon in the α-L-fucosidase gene of a fucosidosis patient. *Biochem Biophys Res Commun* **189**:1063, 1992.
288. Yang M, Allen H, DiCioccio RA: Pedigree analysis of α-L-fucosidase gene mutations in a fucosidosis family. *Biochim Biophys Acta* **1182**:245, 1993.

289. Seo H-C, Willems PJ, O'Brien JS: Six additional mutations in fucosidosis: Three nonsense mutations and three frameshift mutations. *Hum Mol Genet* **2**:1205, 1993.
290. Seo HC, Heidemann P, Lutz E, O'Brien JS: A nonsense mutation in two German patients with fucosidosis. *Hum Mutat* **6**:184, 1995.
291. Seo HC, Kunze J, Willems PJ, Kim AH, Hanfeld F, O'Brien JS: A single-base deletion mutation in a Turkish patient with fucosidosis. *Hum Mutat* **3**:407, 1994.
292. Williamson M, Cragg H, Grant J, Kretz K, O'Brien J, Willems PJ, Young E, Winchester B: A 5′ splice site mutation in fucosidosis. *J Med Genet* **30**:218, 1993.
293. Seo HC, Yang M, Tonlorenzi R, Willems PJ, Kim AH, Filocamo M, Gatti R, DiCioccio RA, O'Brien JS: A missense mutation (S63L) in α-L-fucosidase is responsible for fucosidosis in an Italian patient. *Hum Mol Genet* **3**:2065, 1994.
294. Seo HC, Meiheng Y, Kim AH, O'Brien JS, DiCioccio RA, Gordon BA: A 66-basepair insertion in exon 6 of the α-L-fucosidase gene of a fucosidosis patient. *Hum Mutat* **7**:183, 1996.
295. Cragg H, Williamson M, Young E, O'Brien J, Alhadeff J, Fang-Kircher S, Paschke E, Winchester B: Fucosidosis: Genetic and biochemical analysis of eight cases. *J Med Genet* **34**:105, 1997.
296. Cragg H, Winchester B, Seo HC, O'Brien J, Swallow D: Molecular basis of the common electrophoretic polymorphism (Fu1/Fu2) in human α-L-fucosidase. *J Med Genet* **31**:659, 1994.
297. Rowley BO, Hamilton PB: Isolation of 2-acetamido-1-β-(L-β-aspartamido)-1,2-d: deoxy-D-glucose from normal human urine. *Clin Chem* **18**:951, 1972.
298. Strecker G, Fournet B, Spik G, Montreuil J, Durand P, Tondeur M: Structure de 9 oligosaccharides et glycopeptides riches en fucose secretes dans l'urine de deux sujets atteints de fucosidose. *C R Acad Sci Paris* Ser D **284**:85, 1977.
299. McLaren J, Ng WG: Radial and linear thin layer chromatographic procedures compared for screening urines to detect oligosaccharides. *Clin Chem* **25**:1289, 1979.
300. Schindler D, Kanzaki T, Desnick RJ: A method for the rapid detection of urinary glycopeptides in α-N-acetylgalactosaminidase deficiency and other lysosomal storage diseases. *Clin Chim Acta* **190**:81, 1990.
301. Simell O, Sipila I, Autio S: Extra heating of TLC plates detects two lysosomal storage diseases, aspartylglucosaminuria and fucosidosis, during routine urinary amino acid screening. *Clin Chim Acta* **133**:227, 1983.
302. Henderson MJ, Allen JT, Holton JB, Goodall R: Extra heating of amino acids. *Clin Chim Acta* **146**:203, 1985.
303. Zielke K, Veath ML, O'Brien JS: Fucosidosis: Deficiency of α-L-fucosidase in cultured skin fibroblasts. *J Exp Med* **136**:197, 1972.
304. Wood S: A sensitive fluorometric assay for α-L-fucosidase. *Clin Chim Acta* **58**:251, 1975.
305. Wood S: Human α-L-fucosidase: A common polymorphic variant for low serum enzyme activity, studies of serum and leukocyte enzyme. *Hum Hered* **29**:226, 1979.
306. Wood S: Plasma α-L-fucosidase: Presence of a low activity in some normal individuals. *J Lab Clin Med* **88**:469, 1976.
307. DiCioccio RA, Barlow JJ, Matta KL: Specific activity of α-L-fucosidase in sera with phenotypes of either low, intermediate, or high total enzyme activity and in a fucosidosis serum. *Biochem Genet* **24**:115, 1986.
308. Butterworth J, Guy GJ: α-L-Fucosidase of human skin fibroblasts and amniotic fluid cells in tissue culture. *Clin Genet* **12**:297, 1977.
309. Kelly WR, Clague AE, Barns RJ, Bate MJ, Mackay BM: Canine α-L-fucosidosis: A storage disease of Springer Spaniels. *Acta Neuropathol* (Berlin) **60**:9, 1983.
310. Hartley WJ, Canfield PJ, Donnelly TM: A suspected new canine storage disease. *Acta Neuropathol* (Berlin) **56**:225, 1982.
311. Friend SCE, Barr SC, Embury D: Fucosidosis in an English Springer Spaniel presenting as a malabsorption syndrome. *Aust Vet J* **62**:415, 1986.
312. Healy PJ, Farrow BRH, Nicholas FW, Hedberg K, Ratcliffe R: Canine fucosidosis: A biochemical and genetic investigation. *Res Vet Sci* **36**:354, 1984.
313. Smith MO, Wenger DA, Hill SL, Matthews J: Fucosidosis in a family of American-bred English Springer Spaniels. *JAVMA*, **209**:2088, 1996.
314. Abraham D, Blakemore WF, Dell A, Herrtage ME, Jones J, Littlewood JT, Oates J, Palmer AC, Sidebotham R, Winchester B: The enzyme defect and storage products in canine fucosidosis. *Biochem J* **221**:25, 1984.
315. Barker C, Dell A, Rogers M, Alhadeff JA, Winchester B: Canine α-L-fucosidase in relation to the enzymic defect and storage products in canine fucosidosis. *Biochem J* **254**:861, 1988.
316. Taylor RM, Farrow BRH, Stewart GJ, Healy PJ: Enzyme replacement in nervous tissue after allogenic bone-marrow transplantation for fucosidosis in dogs. *Lancet* **2**:772, 1986.
317. Taylor RM, Farrow BR, Stewart GJ: Correction of enzyme deficiency by allogeneic bone-marrow transplantation following total lymphoid irradiation in dogs with lysosomal storage disease (fucosidosis). *Transplant Proc* **18**:326, 1986.
318. Taylor RM, Farrow BRH, Stewart GJ: Amelioration of clinical disease following bone marrow transplantation in fucosidase-deficient dogs. *Am J Med Genet* **42**:628, 1992.
319. Occhiodoro T, Anson DS: Isolation of the canine α-L-fucosidase cDNA and definition of the fucosidosis mutation in English Springer Spaniels. *Mammalian Genome* **7**:271, 1996.
320. Skelly BJ, Sargan DR, Herrtage ME, Winchester BG: The molecular defect underlying canine fucosidosis. *J Med Genet* **33**:284, 1996.
321. Lowden JA, O'Brien JS: Sialidosis: A review of human neuraminidase deficiency. *Am J Hum Genet* **31**:1, 1979.
322. Young ID, Young EP, Mossman J, Fielder AR, Moore JR: Neuraminidase deficiency: Case report and review of the phenotype. *J Med Genet* **24**:283, 1987.
323. Spranger J, Cantz M: Mucolipidosis I, the cherry-red spot–myoclonus syndrome and neuraminidase deficiency. *Birth Defects* **14(6B)**:105, 1978.
324. Durand P, Gatti R, Cavalieri S, Borrone C, Tondeur M, Michalski J-C, Strecker G: Sialidosis (mucolipidosis I). *Helv Paediatr Acta* **32**:391, 1977.
325. Goldstein ML, Kolodny EH, Gascon GG, Gilles FH: Macular cherry-red spot, myoclonic epilepsy, and neurovisceral storage in a 17-year-old girl. *Trans Am Neurol Assoc* **99**:110, 1974.
326. Thomas PK, Abrams JD, Swallow D, Stewart G: Sialidosis type I: Cherry-red spot–myoclonus syndrome with sialidase deficiency and altered electrophoretic mobilities of some enzymes known to be glycoproteins. *J Neurol Neurosurg Psychiatry* **42**:873, 1979.
327. Steinman L, Tharp BR, Dorfman LJ, Forno LS, Sogg RL, Kelts KA, O'Brien JS: Peripheral neuropathy in the cherry-red spot–myoclonus syndrome (sialidosis type I). *Ann Neurol* **7**:450, 1980.
328. Federico A, Cecio A, Battini GA, Michalski JC, Strecker G, Guazzi GC: Macular cherry-red spot and myoclonus syndrome. *J Neurol Sci* **48**:157, 1980.
329. Harzer K, Cantz M, Sewell AC, Dhareshwarm SS, Roggendorf W, Heckl RW, Schofer O, Thumler R, Pfeiffer J, Schlote W: Normomorphic sialidosis in two female adults with severe neurologic disease and without sialyloligosacchariduria. *Hum Genet* **74**:209, 1986.
330. Till JS, Roach ES, Burton BK: Sialidosis (neuraminidase deficiency) types I and II: Neuro-ophthalmic manifestations. *J Clin Neurol Ophthalmol* **7**:40, 1987.
331. Allegranza A, Tredici G, Marmiroli P, DiDonato S, Franceschetti S, and Mariani C: Sialidosis type I: Pathological study in an adult. *Clin Neuropathol* **8**, 266:1989.
332. Bhigjee AI, Seebaran AR, Petersen EM, Bill PLA: Sialidosis type I: First report in the Indian population. *Clin Neurol Neurosurg* **93**:115, 1991.
333. Federico A, Battistini S, Ciacci G, deStefano N, Gatti R, Durand PM, Guazzi GC: Cherry-red spot myoclonus syndrome (type I sialidosis). *Dev Neurosci* **13**:320, 1991.
334. Rapin I: Myoclonus in neuronal storage and Lafora diseases. *Adv Neurol* **43**:65, 1986.
335. Kelly TE, Graetz G: Isolated acid neuraminidase deficiency: A distinct lysosomal storage disease. *Am J Med Genet* **1**:31, 1977.
336. Bernard M, Toga M, Bernard R, Dubois D, Mariani R, Hassoun J: Pathologic findings in one case of neuronal and mesenchymal storage disease: Its relationship to lipidoses and to mucopolysaccharidoses. *Pathol Eur* **3**:172, 1968.
337. Maroteaux P, Poissonnier M, Tondeur M, Strecker G, Lemonnier M: Sialidose par déficit en alpha (2–6) neuraminidase sans atteinte neurologique. *Arch Fr Pédiatr* **35**:280, 1978.
338. Maroteaux P, Humbel R, Strecker G, Michalski J-C, Mande R: Un nouveau type de sialidose avec atteinte renale: La nephrosialidose. I Étude clinique, radiologique et nosologique. *Arch Fr Pédiatr* **35**:819, 1978.
339. Winter RM, Swallow DM, Baraitser M, Purkiss P: Sialidosis type 2 (acid neuraminidase deficiency): Clinical and biochemical features of a further case. *Clin Genet* **18**:203, 1980.

340. Oohira T, Nagata N, Akaboshi I, Matsuda I, Naito S: The infantile form of sialidosis type II associated with congenital adrenal hyperplasia: Possible linkage between HLA and the neuraminidase deficiency gene. *Hum Genet* **70**:341, 1985.
341. Laver J, Fried K, Beer SI, Iancu TC, Heyman E, Bach G, Zeigler M: Infantile lethal neuraminidase deficiency (sialidosis). *Clin Genet* **23**:97, 1983.
342. Kelly TE, Bartoshesky L, Harris DJ, McCauley RGK, Feingold M, Schott G: Mucolipidosis I (acid neuraminidase deficiency). *Am J Dis Child* **135**:703, 1981.
343. Louis JJ, Marie I, Hermier M, Nicolas A, Guibaud P: Une observation de mucolipidose de type I par déficit primaire en alpha D neuraminidase. *J Génet Hum* **31**:79, 1983.
344. Aylsworth AS, Thomas GH, Hood JL, Malouf N, Libert J: A severe infantile sialidosis: Clinical, biochemical, and microscopic features. *J Pediatr* **96**:662, 1980.
345. Johnson WG, Thomas GH, Miranda AF, Driscoll JM, Wigger JH, Yeh MN, Schwartz RC, Cohen CS, Berdon WE, Koenigsberger MR: Congenital sialidosis: Biochemical studies: Clinical spectrum in four sibs; two successful prenatal diagnoses. *Am J Hum Genet* **32**:43A, 1980.
346. Beck M, Bender SW, Reiter H-L, Otto W, Bassler R, Dancygier H, Gehler J: Neuraminidase deficiency presenting as non-immune hydrops fetalis. *Eur J Pediatr* **143**:135, 1984.
347. King M, Cockburn F, MacPhee GB, Logan RW: Infantile type 2 sialidosis in a Pakistani family — a clinical and biochemical study. *J Inherit Metab Dis* **7**:91, 1984.
348. Roth KS, Chan JC, Ghatak NR, Mamunes P, Miller WW, O'Brien JS: Acid α-neuraminidase deficiency: A nephropathic phenotype? *Clin Genet* **34**:185, 1988.
349. Rudenko G, Bonten E, Hol WGJ, d'Azzo A: The atomic model of the human protective protein/cathepsin A suggests a structural basis for galactosialidosis. *Proc Natl Acad Sci USA* **95**:621, 1998.
350. Strecker G, Peers M-C, Michalski J-C, Hondi-Assah T, Fournet B, Spik G, Montreuil J, Farriaux J-P, Marteaux P, Durand P: Structure of nine sialyl-oligosaccharides accumulated in urine of eleven patients with three different types of sialidosis. *Eur J Biochem* **75**:391, 1977.
351. Dorland L, Haverkamp J, Vliegenthart JFG, Strecker G, Michalski J-C, Fournet B, Spik G, Montreuil J: 360-MHz ^{1}H-nuclear-magnetic resonance spectroscopy of sialyloligosaccharides from patients with sialidosis (mucolipidosis I and II). *Eur J Biochem* **87**:323, 1978.
352. Strecker G, Michalski JC: Biochemical basis of six different types of sialidosis. *FEBS Lett* **85**:20, 1978.
353. Kuriyama M, Ariga T, Ando S, Suzuki M, Yamada T, Miyatake T: Four positional isomers of sialyloligosaccharides isolated from the urine of a patient with sialidosis. *J Biol Chem* **256**:12316, 1981.
354. Takahashi Y, Nakamura Y, Yamaguchi S, Orii T: Urinary oligosaccharide excretion and severity of galactosialidosis and sialidosis. *Clin Chim Acta* **203**:199, 1991.
355. van Pelt J, Kamerling JP, Bakker HD, Vliegenthart JFG: A comparative study of sialyloligosaccharides isolated from sialidosis and galactosialidosis urine. *J Inherit Metab Dis* **14**:730, 1991.
356. Nakamura Y, Takahashi Y, Hamaguchi S, Omiya S, Orii T, Yara A, Gushiken M: Severe infantile sialidosis — the characteristics of oligosaccharides isolated from the urine and the abdominal ascites. *Tohoku J Exp Med* **166**:407, 1992.
357. van Pelt J, Hard K, Kamerling JP, Vliegenthart JFG, Reuser AJJ, Galjaard H: Isolation and structural characterization of twenty-one sialyloligosaccharides from galactosialidosis urine. An intact N,N′-diacetylchitobiose unit at the reducing end of a diantennary structure. *Biol Chem Hoppe Seyler* **370**:191, 1989.
358. Scocca J, Thomas GH, Reynolds LW, Miller CS: Accumulation of [3H] sialyl-conjugates in sialidosis (sialidase deficient) fibroblasts cultured in the presence of [3H] α-N-acetyl-mannosamine. *J Inherit Metab Dis* **9**:79, 1986.
359. Thomas GH, Scocca J, Miller CS, Reynolds LW: Accumulation of N-acetylneuraminic acid (sialic acid) in human fibroblasts cultured in the presence of N-acetylmannosamine. *Biochim Biophys Acta* **37**:846, 1985.
360. Scocca JR, Thomas GH, Miller CS, Reynolds LW: Purification and characterization of sialic acid containing materials accumulated in cultured skin fibroblasts from a patient with type II sialidosis. *J Inherit Metab Dis* **10**:33, 1987.
361. Mendla K, Baumkötter J, Rosenau C, Ulrich-Bott B, Cantz M: Defective lysosomal release of glycoprotein-derived sialic acid in fibroblasts from patients with sialic acid storage disease. *Biochem J* **250**:261, 1988.
362. van Pelt J, Kamerling JP, Vliegenthart JFG, Verheijen FW, Galjaard H: Isolation and structural characterization of sialic acid–containing storage material from mucolipidosis I (sialidosis) fibroblasts. *Biochim Biophys Acta* **965**:36, 1988.
363. van Pelt J, Kamerling JP, Vliegenthart JFG, Hoogeveen AT, Galjaard H: A comparative study of the accumulated sialic acid–containing oligosaccharides from cultured human galactosialidosis and sialidosis fibroblasts. *Clin Chim Acta* **174**:325, 1988.
364. Frisch A, Neufeld EF: A rapid and sensitive assay for neuraminidase: Application to cultured fibroblasts. *Anal Biochem* **95**:222, 1979.
365. Cantz M: Sialidoses, in Schauer R (ed): *Sialic Acids*. Vienna, Springer-Verlag, 1982, p 307.
366. Cantz M, Messer H: Oligosaccharide and ganglioside neuraminidase activities of mucolipidosis I (sialidosis) and mucolipidosis II (I-cell disease) fibroblasts. *Eur J Biochem* **97**:113, 1979.
367. Lieser M, Harms E, Kern H, Bach G, Cantz M: Ganglioside G_{M3} sialidase activity in fibroblasts of normal individuals and of patients with sialidosis and mucolipidosis IV. *Biochem J* **260**:69, 1989.
368. Hiraiwa M, Nishizawa M, Uda Y, Nakajima T, Miyatake T: Human placental sialidase: Further purification and characterization. *J Biochem* **103**:86, 1988.
369. Hiraiwa M, Uda Y, Nishizawa M, Miyatake T: Human placental sialidase: Partial purification and characterization. *J Biochem* **101**:1273, 1987.
370. Ulrich-Bott B, Klem B, Kaiser R, Spranger J, Cantz M: Lysosomal sialidase deficiency: Increased ganglioside content in autopsy tissues of a sialidosis patient. *Enzyme* **38**:262, 1987.
371. Warner TG, O'Brien JS: Synthesis of 2′-(4-methylumbelliferyl)-α-D-N-acetylneuraminic acid and detection of skin fibroblast neuraminidase in normal humans and in sialidosis. *Biochemistry* **18**:2783, 1979.
372. Thomas GH, Reynolds LW, Miller CS: Characterization of neuraminidase activity of cultured human fibroblasts. *Biochim Biophys Acta* **568**:39, 1979.
373. Verheijen FW, janse HC, Van Diggelen OP, Bakker HD, Loonen MCB, Durnad P, Galjaard H: Two genetically different MU-NANA neuraminidases in human leucocytes. *Biochem Biophys Res Commun* **117**:135, 1983.
374. Verheijen FW, Palmeri S, Hoogeveen AT, Galjaard H: Human placental neuraminidase activation, stabilization and association with β-galactosidase and its protective protein. *Eur J Biochem* **149**:315, 1985.
375. Verheijen FW, Palmeri S, Galjaard H: Purification and partial characterization of lysosomal neuraminidase from human placenta. *Eur J Biochem* **162**:63, 1987.
376. van der Horst GTJ, Galjart NJ, D'Azzo A, Galjaard H, Verheijen FW: Identification and in vitro reconstitution of lysosomal neuraminidase from human placenta. *J Biol Chem* **264**:1317, 1989.
377. Potier M, Lamontagne S, Michaud L, Tranchemontagne J: Human neuraminidase is a 60 kDa-processing product of prosaposin. *Biochem Biophys Res Commun* **173**:449, 1990.
378. Hiraiwa M, Uda Y, Tsuji S, Miyatake T, Martin BM, Tayama M, O'Brien JS, Kishimoto Y: Human placental sialidase complex: Characterization of the 60 kDa protein that cross-reacts with anti-saposin antibodies. *Biochem Biophys Res Commun* **177**:1211, 1991.
379. Bonten E, van der Spoel AV, Fornerod M, Grosveld G, d'Azzo A: Characterization of human lysosomal neuraminidase defines the molecular basis of the metabolic storage disorder sialidosis. *Genes Devel* **10**:3156, 1996.
380. Galjart NJ, Gillemans N, Harris A, van der Horst GTJ, Verheijen FW, Galjaard H, D'Azzo A: Expression of cDNA encoding the human "protective protein" associated with lysosomal β-galactosidase and neuraminidase: Homology to yeast proteases. *Cell* **54**:755, 1988.
381. Jackman HL, Tan F, Tamei H, Beurling-Harbury C, Li X-Y, Skidgel RA, Erdos EG: A peptidase in human platelets that deamidates tachykinins. *J Biol Chem* **265**:11265, 1990.
382. Tranchemontagne J, Michaud L, Potier M: Deficient lysosomal carboxypeptidase activity in galactosialidosis. *Biochem Biophys Res Commun* **168**:22, 1990.
383. Potier M, Michaud L, Tranchemontagne J, Thauvette L: Structure of the lysosomal neuraminidase-β-galactosidase-carboxypeptidase multienzymic complex. *Biochem J* **267**:197, 1990.
384. Galjart NJ, Morreau H, Willemsen R, Gillemans N, Bonten EJ, d'Azzo A: Human lysosomal protective protein has cathepsin A–like activity distinct from its protective function. *J Biol Chem* **266**:14754, 1991.
385. Galjaard H, Willemsen R, Hoogeveen AT, Mancini GMS, Palmeri S, Verheijen FW, D'Azzo A: Molecular heterogeneity in human β-galactosidase and neuraminidase deficiency. *Enzyme* **38**:132, 1987.

386. D'Azzo A, Hoogeveen A, Reuser AJJ, Robinson O, Galjaard H: Molecular defect in combined β-galactosidase and neuraminidase deficiency in man. *Proc Natl Acad Sci USA* **79**:4535, 1982.
387. Mueller OT, Henry WM, Haley LL, Byers MG, Eddy RL, Shows TB: Sialidosis and galactosialidosis: Chromosomal assignment of two genes associated with neuraminidase deficiency disorders. *Proc Natl Acad Sci USA* **83**:1817, 1985.
388. Oohira T., Nagata N, Akaboshi I, Matsuda I, Naito S: The infantile form of sialidosis type II associated with congenital adrenal hyperplasia: Possible linkage between HLA and the neuraminidase deficiency gene. *Hum Genet* **70**:341, 1985.
389. Pshezhetsky AV, Richard C, Michaud L, Igdoura S, Wang S, Elsliger MA, Qu J, Leclerc D,Gravel R, Dallaire L, Potier M: Cloning, expression and chromosomal mapping of human lysosomal sialidase and characterization of mutations in sialidosis. *Nature Genet* **15**:316, 1997.
390. Halal F, Chitayat D, Parikh H, Rosenblatt B, Tranchemontagne J, Vekemans M, Potier M: Ring chromosome 20 and possible assignment of the structural gene encoding human carboxypeptidase-L to the distal segment of the long arm of chromosome 20. *Am J Med Genet* **43**:576, 1992.
391. Milner CM, Smith SV, Carrillo MB, Taylor GL, Hollinshead M, Campbell RD: Identification of a sialidase encoded in the human major histocompatibility complex. *J Biol Chem* **272**:4549, 1997.
392. Kuriyama M, Ariga T, Ando S, Suzuki M, Yamada T, Miyatake T, Igata A: Two positional isomers of sialylheptasaccharides isolated from the urine of a patient with sialidosis. *J Biochem* (Tokyo) **98**:1949, 1985.
393. Lecat D, Lemmonier M, Derappe C, Lhermitte M, Van Halbeek H, Dorland L, Vliegenthart JFG: The structure of sialyl-glyco-peptides of the O-glycosidic type, isolated from sialidosis (mucolipidosis I) urine. *Eur J Biochem* **140**:415, 1984.
394. Myers RW, Lee RT, Lee YC, Thomas GH, Reynolds LW, Uchida Y: The synthesis of 4-methylumbelliferyl α-ketoside of N-acetyl neuraminic acid and its use in a fluorometric assay for neuraminidase. *Anal Biochem* **101**:166, 1980.
395. Mueller OT, Wenger DA: Mucolipidosis I: Studies of sialidase activity and a prenatal diagnosis. *Clin Chim Acta* **109**:313, 1981.
396. Potier M, Yan LA, Womack E: Neuraminidase deficiency in the mouse. *FEBS Lett* **108**:345, 1979.
397. Igdoura SA, Gafuik C, Mertineit C, Saberi F, Pshezhetsky AV, Potier M, Trasler JM, Gravel RA: Cloning of the cDNA and gene encoding mouse lysosomal sialidase and correction of sialidase deficiency in human sialidosis and mouse **SM/J** fibroblasts. *Hum Mol Genet* **7**:115, 1998.
398. Rottier RJ, Bonten E, d'Azzo A: A point mutation in the *neu-1* locus causes the neuraminidase defect in the **SM/J** mouse. *Hum Mol Genet* **7**:313, 1998.
399. Willems PJ, Seo HC, Coucke P, Tonlorenzi R, O'Brien JS: Spectrum of mutations in fucosidosis. *Eur J Hum Genet* **7**:60, 1999.

CHAPTER 141

Aspartylglucosaminuria

Pertti Aula ■ Anu Jalanko ■ Leena Peltonen

1. **Aspartylglucosaminuria (AGU) is an autosomal recessive glycoprotein degradation defect in which glycoasparagines, mainly aspartylglucosamine, accumulate in the lysosomes of several tissues, leading to slowly progressive developmental delay. The disease has worldwide distribution, with a strong enrichment in the Finnish population due to a founder effect. The basic biochemical abnormality is the lack of activity of the lysosomal enzyme aspartylglucosaminidase (AGA), normally present at low quantities in all tissues. The corresponding cDNA and the gene on chromosome 4q have been cloned, and multiple mutations in AGU patients have been identified. Characteristically, the mutations interfere with normal folding and intracellular processing of the enzyme, resulting in a misfolded and inactive enzyme molecule. AGA has been crystallized, and its three-dimensional structure is solved. Currently it is one of the best characterized lysosomal enzymes defective in lysosomal storage diseases.**
2. **The phenotypic manifestation of aspartylglucosaminuria is characterized by global delay of psychomotor development with onset between 2 and 4 years of age. Delayed speech and motor clumsiness are often preceded by repeated upper respiratory infections. Patients reach the developmental capacities of a 5- to 6-year-old child around puberty and thereafter slowly deteriorate to the level of severe mental retardation at adulthood. Mild connective tissue changes causing coarse facial features, thick calvarium, and osteoporosis are associated with the developmental delay. A fifth of patients have epileptic seizures during the later course of the disease. Brain MRI shows abnormalities in the differentiation between gray and white matter and signs of delayed myelination.**
3. **The primary metabolic abnormality in aspartylglucosaminuria is deficient cleavage of the bond between asparagine and N-acetylglucosamine as the final step in lysosomal breakdown of glycoproteins and oligosaccharides due to defective or absent activity of the lysosomal enzyme aspartylglucosaminidase (also called glycosylasparaginase). The main abnormal degradation product is aspartylglucosamine (N-acetylglucosaminyl-asparagine), which is accumulated in large amounts in the lysosomes in neurons and glial cells in the central nervous system but also in all visceral organs and skin. Small amounts of other glycoasparagines containing additional monosaccharide units linked to the aspartylglucosamine core are also stored in the lysosomes. The same glycosasparagines and a number of other derivative structures are excreted in the urine of patients, providing an easy way to detect and screen for aspartylglucosaminuria.**
4. **Based on its three-dimensional structure, AGA was recently shown to be the only known mammalian representative so far of N-terminal hydrolases with a structure consisting of a central four-layer sandwich of α-helices and β-sheets and a catalytic N-terminal nucleophile (threonine). AGA is synthesized as a 346-amino-acid-long enzymatically inactive precursor polypeptide that during intracellular processing in endoplasmic reticulum (ER) is dimerized and cleaved into alpha- and beta-subunits of 27 kDa and 17 kDa, respectively. The structure of the catalytic center as well as the crucial amino acids for catalysis are well characterized. The heterotetrameric mature enzyme has an unusually high pH optimum of 7–9. Complete proteolytic cleavage of the N-glycosylated polypeptides precedes asparagine-N-acetylglucosamine bond hydrolysis by AGA and this activity is independent of the length of the sugar chain. AGU patients have absent or minimal activity of the AGA enzyme in cells from various sources, including brain, liver, leukocytes, and skin fibroblasts. Heterozygotes have reduced activity, to 40–60 percent of that of controls.**
5. **The gene coding for AGA is located at 4q34-35, has a total length of approximately 13 kb, and consists of nine exons. The 2.2-kb cDNA contains a 1041-bp coding region and a long 3′ untranslated region. A missense mutation (C163S) causing disruption of a disulfide bridge in the polypeptide structure is the predominant founder mutation in the Finnish population, representing 98 percent of the disease mutations. Several other "private" mutations have been detected in families with different ethnic backgrounds.**
6. **The laboratory diagnosis of AGU can be based on (a) demonstration of urinary excretion of glycoasparagines by chromatographic techniques; (b) assays of AGA activity in leukocytes, cultured fibroblasts, or, in the case of fetal diagnosis, in cultured amniotic fluid cells or in a chorionic villus sample; or (c) identification of the disease-causing mutation in the AGA gene if the mutation in the population (Finland) or in the family is known.**
7. **Two knockout mouse models of AGU have been produced, enabling new therapeutic approaches to be evaluated. No effective treatment is presently available. Bone marrow transplantation (BMT) with successful engraftment has been performed in at least three children, in whom follow-up has demonstrated biochemical normalization and disappearance of storage lysosomes. Brain MRI has shown less abnormalities post BMT, but evidence for an effect on the course of the disease will require longer follow-up.**

A list of standard abbreviations is located immediately preceding the index in each volume. Nonstandard abbreviations used in this chapter include: AGU = aspartylglucosaminuria; AGA = aspartylglucosaminidase, glycoasparaginase; MRI = magnetic resonance imaging; ER = endoplasmic reticulum; BMT = bone marrow transplantation ; AADG = aspartylglucosamine, 2-acetamido-1-L-beta-aspartamido-1,2-dideoxy-beta-D-glucose, N-acetylglucosaminyl-asparagine (GlcNAc-Asn); EEG = electroencephalogram; CT = computerized tomography; UTR = untranslated region; FISH = fluorescence *in situ* hybridization.

HISTORICAL ASPECTS

Aspartylglucosaminuria (AGU) remained undiscovered until 1968, when Pollitt, Jenner, and Merskey described the disease in a mentally retarded brother and sister in an English family.[1] Both had been developmentally slow from early years on, presented with coarse facial features and sagging skin, and excreted large amounts of aspartylglucosamine (AADG) in the urine. Seminal fluid from the brother was unable to degrade AADG, as control samples did, indicating a deficiency of the lysosomal enzyme aspartylglucosaminidase. Several cases of the disease had actually been distinguished earlier during a urinary amino acid screening of mentally retarded patients in Finland with a "peptiduria" diagnosis due to a characteristic but unidentified spot in the urinary paper chromatogram.[2] These 11 Finnish patients were soon found to have AGU,[3] and 23 new cases were subsequently identified among institutionalized mentally retarded patients in Finland. A detailed clinical investigation by Autio on 34 patients with ages ranging from 1 to 39 years delineated the phenotypic manifestations and clinical course of AGU, changing a healthy newborn to a severely retarded adult.[4] Since then it has turned out that this oligosaccharide degradation defect is the most common lysosomal storage disorder in the Finnish population, with 170 cases reported, in contrast to only approximately 60 cases known from the rest of the world.

Due to its low quantity in tissues, only small amounts of AGA, the asparagine-N-acetylglucosamine bond hydrolyzing lysosomal enzyme, could be purified at first, allowing only partial purification of the enzyme.[5,6] The human AGA enzyme was initially considered a monomeric structure[7] but was later found to be a heterotetramer consisting of two nonidentical subunits.[8,9] Crystallographic analyses finally revealed the three-dimensional structure of the protein and defined the structure of the active site and the amino acids for catalysis.[10] AGA proved to belong to a novel class of enzymes, being currently the only known mammalian representative of the N-terminal hydrolases. AGA is today one of the best-characterized lysosomal enzymes at the molecular level. The details of biosynthesis and intracellular processing are well-defined, and three-dimensional structure of AGA has shed light on lysosomal transport signals generally.[11]

Using somatic cell hybrids, the gene coding for AGA was assigned to the long arm of chromosome 4.[12] Purification of AGA protein and the production of its amino acid sequence facilitated the cloning and characterization of the corresponding cDNA and identification of disease-causing mutations.[13,14,15] As expected, a founder mutation was disclosed in the Finnish patients, one missense mutation representing 98 percent of the disease alleles. A variety of different mutations are found in patients from elsewhere.[16,17] Two transgenic mouse models of AGU have recently been produced,[18,19] allowing pathogenesis of the disease and new therapeutic possibilities to be elaborated.

CLINICAL PRESENTATION OF ASPARTYLGLUCOSAMINURIA

Two extensive clinical studies on Finnish AGU patients provide a good basis for description of the clinical findings of the disease: the original work on 34 patients by Autio[4] and a more recent study by Arvio on 121 patients.[20] Clinical data are available from other reviews as well.[21,22] Reports on AGU cases from other populations give scattered clinical data indicating a rather homogeneous phenotypic manifestation of the disease worldwide.[23]

Early Signs of AGU

Pregnancy and delivery histories of AGU cases are uneventful, and newborn babies present no signs of the disease. The diagnosis is hardly ever made or suspected before the age of 1 year unless a positive family history has provoked diagnostic studies. Retrospectively, however, unusually frequent upper respiratory tract infections with middle ear infections during the first 2 to 3 years are encountered. Enlarged pharyngeal adenoids have in some cases been removed several times. In a series of 43 children, 41 suffered from frequent respiratory infections.[24] Mild muscle hypotonia was another clinical finding noted retrospectively in several AGU infants. Hypotonia may give rise to inguinal or umbilical hernias; 20 patients out of 43 had had a hernia operation. Motor milestones and general development of these AGU children during the first year of life did not significantly differ from those of other children. The mean age at which they first walked was 14.6 months. Some infants experienced repeated unexplained gastrointestinal symptoms with diarrhea, which gradually diminished during later years (Table 141-1).

Table 141-1 Clinical Findings before Diagnosis of AGU in 43 Children, Recorded Retrospectively

Recurrent respiratory infections	39	Dental caries	5
Urinary tract infections	2	Hydrocele testis	4
Hernia Operations	20	Episodic diarrhea	3
Clubfoot or planovalgus	7	Ocular squint	2

(Modified from ref. 23)

Developmental Delay

The first sign of AGU in the majority of cases has been a delay in speech development, raising concern on the part of parents during the second and third year of life. A long time may pass, however, before any diagnostic initiatives are undertaken. In the series of 43 pediatric patients, the specific diagnosis of AGU was confirmed at a mean age of 5.5 years (range 10 months to 11 years).

Other frequent problems noted before the final diagnosis was confirmed were attention deficit, stubborn behavior, and motor clumsiness. The progressive nature of the disease is well illustrated by the developmental profile constructed on the basis of observations of 116 patients using two types of developmental testing systems by Arvio.[25] After a normal development during infancy, the developmental profile was found to consist of three sections: a period of abnormally slow but positive development up to the age of 13–16 years, a period of slow decline until 25–28 years, and a period of rapid impairment thereafter (Fig. 141-1). At the peak of development the average AGU patient is 13–16 years old with intellectual and adaptive skills comparable to those of normal children at 5–6 years old.

The severity of mental retardation in AGU thus is age related, patients under 10 years being mostly subnormal or mildly retarded, patients in the second decade being moderately to severely retarded, and adult patients all being severely retarded. The level of mental retardation on the Stanford-Binet test in two clinical series of AGU patients is presented in Table 141-2. Disorders of speech development are the cardinal features of mental retardation, with a few patients exhibiting additional signs of dysarthria. Four of 110 patients older than age 6 never learned to say a single word but could still understand simple orders. The speech of three school-age children was incomprehensible. A slow deterioration of speech takes place after puberty, and most adult patients have only a few words in their vocabulary.

Motor development is less affected than speech and intellectual capacities. A clumsy gait and poor manual motor coordination are typical of adult AGU patients. Some older patients have lost the ability to walk due to impaired balance.

Table 141-2 Level of Mental Retardation (Mean IQ) of Two Groups of Finnish AGU Patients (Stanford-Binet Test)

Age (Years)	IQ (Study 4)	IQ (Study 24)
5–9	51 (n = 7)	69 (n = 11)
10–14	32 (n = 4)	32 (n = 6)
15–20	31 (n = 3)	29 (n = 8)
>20	22 (n = 9)	22 (n = 46)

(Modified from ref. 24)

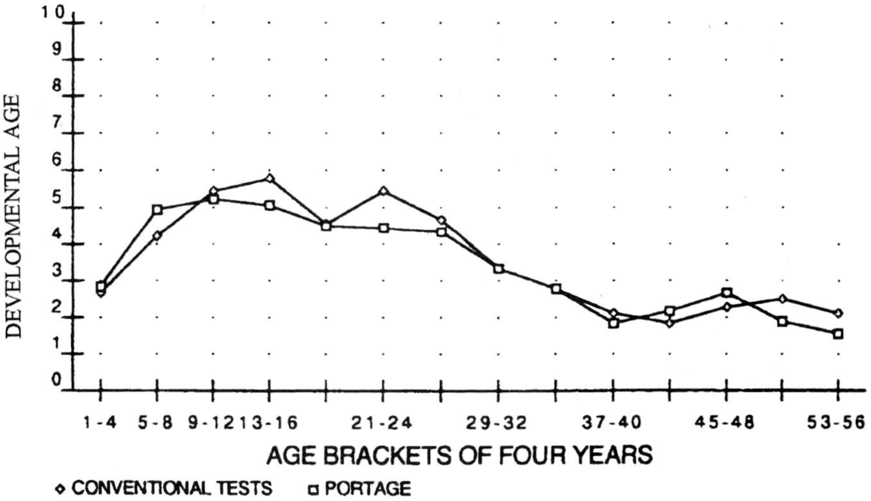

Fig. 141-1 A cross-sectional developmental profile by age of 116 AGU patients (in four-year age brackets). Developmental age (DA) was assayed with conventional psychological tests and with the Portage assessment scale. (From reference 23)

Epileptic Seizures

Approximately one fifth of AGU patients experience epileptic seizures, most of them at later stages of the disease.[26] Ten out of 23 patients over 37 years old had seizures, in contrast to only one of 35 at 7–16 years old. The major abnormality on electroencephalogram (EEG) was low amplitude. A good antiepileptic response with carbamazepine has been obtained in most cases.

Behavioral Problems

Unusually stubborn and restless behavior is typical during childhood for many patients and is sometimes also seen in older individuals. At puberty, some AGU patients, especially females, have had periods of manic excitable ("erethistic") behavior lasting for a few weeks to months.[4]

Physical Findings

The adult height of AGU patients is slightly below the height of the normal population. The mean height of 78 adult patients was at the 16th percentile for the normal Finnish population: 160 cm for females (range 143–172 cm) and 170 cm for males (range 151–186 cm).[20] Mildly abnormal facial features are present in many adults and older children with AGU, consisting of sagging skin, thick lips, low and broad nasal bridge, and coarse hair. Hypertelorism is also a frequent finding. By the time these facial features appear, developmental delay is already present; the older the patient, the more characteristic the facial features become (Fig. 141-2). The dysmorphic features may result from impaired properties of connective tissue; supporting this possibility, ultrastructural study of dermis has revealed alterations in the connective tissue matrix. The organization of collagen fiber bundles was abnormally irregular, with wide variation in the diameters of individual collagen fibrils.[27] In vitro studies in cultured fibroblasts have also shown altered collagen production in cell lines from AGU patients.[28] Hypermobility of joints, seen in several young patients, may also be associated with abnormalities of collagen fibrils. Despite abundant lysosomal storage in liver and spleen (see below), visceral enlargement is only rarely present in AGU, in contrast to several other lysosomal storage disorders.

Skeletal Changes

Thick calvarium, osteochondrotic vertebral changes, thin cortex of long bones, and generalized osteoporosis are the main radiologic findings in AGU. A thick calvarium was present in 20 out of 23 patients who were analyzed for this feature. Vertebral changes compatible with juvenile osteochondrosis were seen in 20 out of 34 patients, 13 of whom were adults. Later on, vertebral bodies are wedge-shaped with flattened intervertebral spaces. Long bones, particularly the femur and humerus, may have abnormally thin cortex, which together with generalized osteoporosis may lead to an increased tendency toward fractures.[4]

Neuroradiology

Early brain CT studies of 11 AGU patients revealed diffuse atrophy in patients more than 13 years old.[20] A recent MRI study on 12 patients ranging in age from 19 months to 32 years gave

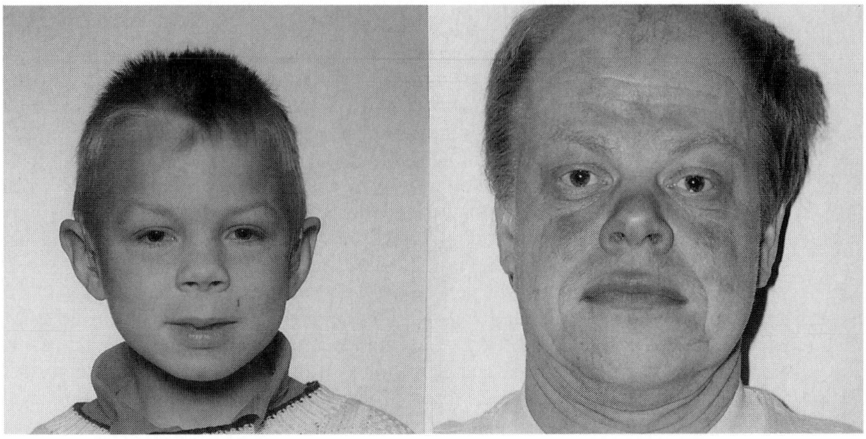

Fig. 141-2 Facial features of a 9-year-old (left) and 39-year-old patient with aspartylglucosaminuria. The older patient has rosacea-like skin changes with erythema, pustules, and telangiectasias. Facial features associated with AGU are minimal. See Color Plate 6.

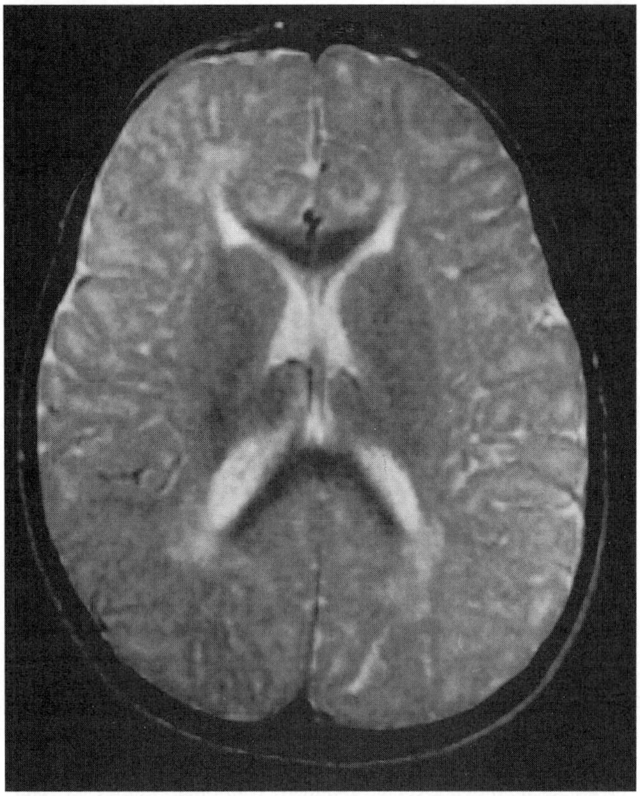

Fig. 141-3 MRI (axial slice) of a 2.6-year-old girl with AGU demonstrating several subcortical high-signal foci. Basal ganglia and thalami as well as the genu and splenium of the corpus callosum are hypointense to the adjacent white matter. Increased periventricular signal intensity is seen adjacent to the lateral ventricles. T2-weighed spin echo (Tr/te = 2500 ms/90 ms). (Courtesy of Dr. T. Autti.)

clear evidence that AGU is primarily a gray-matter disorder that also affects white matter by delaying myelination.[29] The progressive nature of the disease could be visualized. The differentiation between cortical gray matter and white matter in the cerebrum was poor in all but one young patient, becoming worse in older patients. The generally increased signal intensity on T2-weighted images of white matter was most obvious in the young patients, with many focal areas of very high signal intensity in the subcortical white matter (Fig. 141-3). The thalami showed lower signal intensity than the basal ganglia. Only the oldest patient had signs of cortical atrophy.

Clinical Findings of Non-Finnish AGU Patients

Clinical descriptions of patients from various ethnic backgrounds — known to carry different mutations in the gene encoding AGA — give the impression of a relatively homogeneous phenotype. The eight patients from three unrelated Palestinian Arab families carrying the same mutation suffer from a disease very similar to the one described above in Finnish patients. Developmental delay, physical findings, and course of the disease exhibited no mutation-specific characteristics.[23] Macroorchidism during puberty was present in three Puerto Rican brothers, who also had radiologic evidence of spondylolisthesis associated with other typical findings of AGU.[30] One Italian AGU patient had congenital methemoglobinemia due to the coincidental presence of two unrelated recessive mutations: that of the NADH-methemoglobin reductase gene at chromosome 22q and that of the AGA gene at 4q. This patient's sister had typical AGU and no methemoglobinemia.[31] Hepatosplenomegaly and hypersplenism caused by portal vein thrombosis were seen in one Canadian AGU patient, but a younger brother carrying the same two mutations had only developmental delay and facial features typical of AGU.[32] Angiokeratoma-type skin lesions were described both in the two Japanese patients[33] and in the Italian patients.[31]

General Health and Life Expectancy

The liability to infections seen during infancy and early childhood gradually disappears, and older children and adults with AGU do not suffer from respiratory infections more than other populations with mental retardation. Erythematous skin lesions with a tendency to infections on the facies are relatively common in adult patients (see Fig. 141-2). No specific changes in immunoglobulin levels or in cell-bound immunity have been recorded. Rheumatoid arthritis was recently found to be relatively frequent in AGU patients. Nine out of 164 cases (5.5 percent) showed evidence of chronic inflammatory arthritis, five with seropositive rheumatoid factors.[34]

Life expectancy is shortened in AGU. The mean age at death of 52 patients was 37.6 years (range 26–53). The immediate cause of death in several cases has been a bacterial infection such as pneumonitis or abscess.

HISTOPATHOLOGY OF AGU

Enlarged membrane-bound lysosomes, the hallmark of lysosomal storage disorders, are seen in several tissues. Cytoplasmic vacuoles can be visualized by light microscopy in cells from various tissue sources, including skin, conjunctiva, rectal mucosa, peripheral blood lymphocytes, and visceral organs.[35] The fine structure of the unit membrane-bound cytoplasmic vacuoles can have an amorphous fibrillogranular appearance, as in liver, kidney, or skin (Fig. 141-4) or contain electron-dense granular bodies, as in brain (Fig. 141-5).[36,37] Liver cells, both hepatocytes and Kupffer cells, show particularly abundant lysosomal storage, with reticular and fibrillar material, lipid droplets, and electron-dense globules. Despite the extensive vacuolization, the basic structure and function of the liver remain normal in AGU patients. Enlarged lysosomes were already seen in the liver, kidney, skin, and placenta of a 20-week fetus after termination of the pregnancy because of absence of AGA enzyme activity in cultured amniotic fluid cells.[38] The fetal central nervous system, however, had no vacuolization or any other changes.

Only one autopsy report on an AGU patient has been published, with some additional data on brain biopsy material from two adult patients.[36] The 29-year-old female patient died of bacterial pneumonitis. The brain was moderately atrophic, with generalized gyral atrophy and wide sulci. Most of the nerve cells in the cortex were distended and rounded, containing poorly defined vacuoles. The cytoplasm around the nucleus usually contained a number of coarse pigment granules with staining qualities of lipofuscin. Signs of nuclear degeneration were present. Stages of disintegration of neurons were seen, particularly in the striata. The cerebellum had a pronounced loss of Purkinje cells and hypertrophy of Bergmann glia. The basal ganglia and thalamus had signs of neuronal loss, particularly in the area of the pallidum. Slight diffuse gliosis was present in white matter. Electron microscopy (mainly of brain biopsy material) revealed electron-lucent vacuoles in neuronal cells, accompanied by large electron-dense cytosomes. The electron-dense particles consisted of membrane-bound lumps of granular material associated with opaque lipid droplets of varying sizes (Fig. 141-5). Similar findings on brain biopsy material were seen in a previous study.[37]

Brain morphology was recently investigated in four patients at autopsy in conjunction with an extensive study on magnetic resonance imaging in AGU.[29] Changes similar to those in the above-mentioned studies were seen. The basic cortical cytoarchitecture was generally preserved. Most nerve cell bodies had a distended and rounded appearance and contained poorly defined vacuoles. Cytoplasmic lipofuscin-like granules were also found. Despite the vacuolation, only a limited amount of neuronal loss was present. Vacuolation was also found in the neurons of basal ganglia and thalami. The white matter showed diffuse pallor of

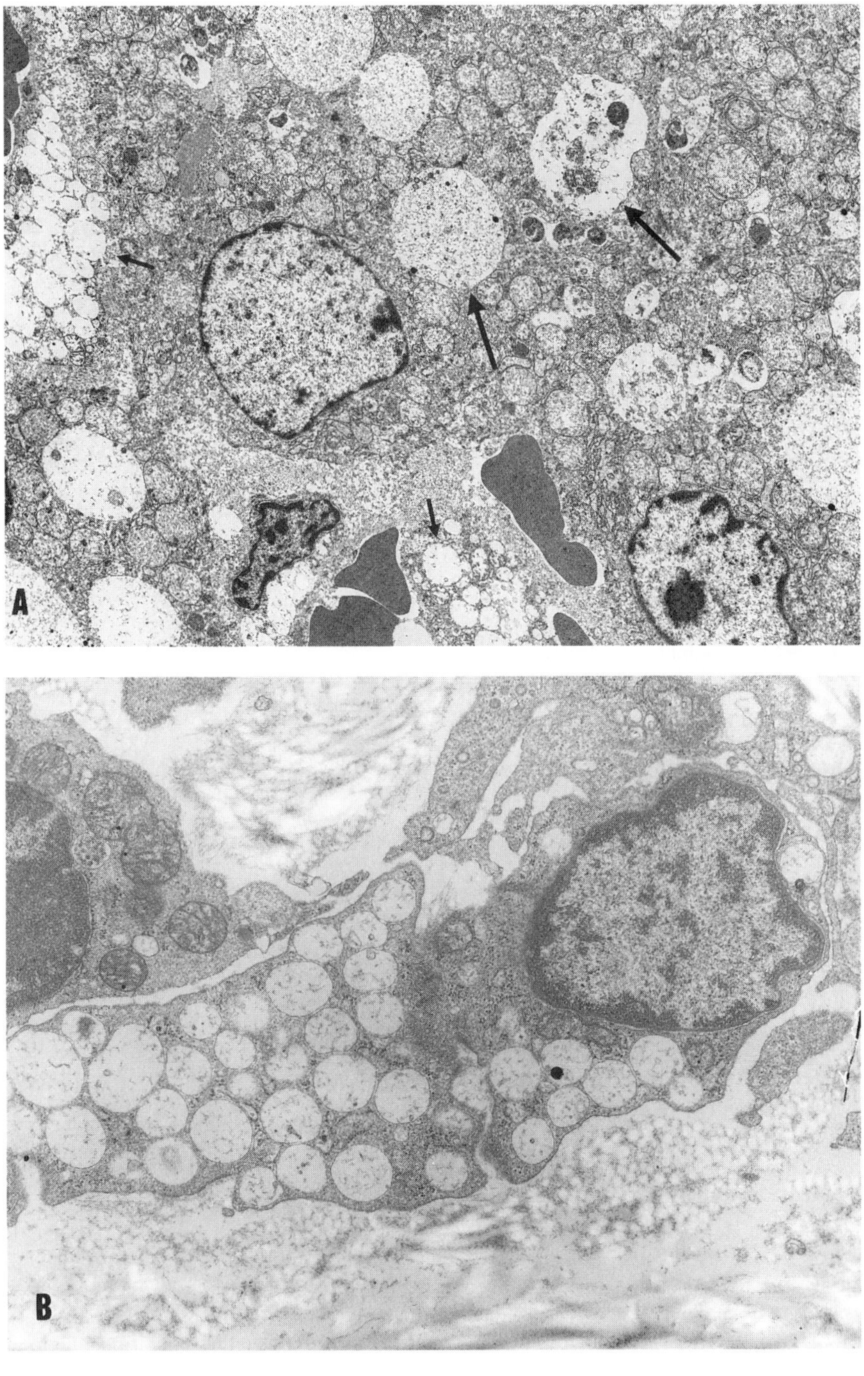

Fig. 141-4 Lysosomal storage in AGU. A) Liver tissue of an AGU patient. Large storage lysosomes in the cytoplasm of a hepatocyte (long arrows) and smaller lysosomes in the Kupffer cells (short arrows) showing amorphous material and electron-dense globules in the hepatocyte. Magnification approx. × 6000. B) Enlarged lysosomes in a fibrocyte from skin biopsy. The cytoplasm is distended by the clear storage lysosomes containing amorphous material and some membrane fragments. Magnification approx. × 18000. (*Courtesy of Dr. J. Rapola.*)

myelin staining and slight to moderate gliosis in two of the four cases.

EPIDEMIOLOGY

Since the description of the first cases of AGU in an English family, an overwhelming majority of new cases have been detected in Finland, with 170 cases in 150 families recorded today. Aspartylglucosaminuria is a prime example of the founder effect in the Finnish population, due to the small number of the founders, bottlenecks during the expansion of the population, and genetic isolation.[39] Approximately 30 autosomal recessive diseases are known to be thus enriched in the Finnish population, and a predominant founder mutation has already been identified in many of these diseases.[40] In AGU, 95 percent of patients (161) are homozygous for the Finnish founder mutation, Cys to Ser at codon 163 (C163S designated AGU_{Fin}). Five patients are compound heterozygotes with a 2-bp deletion mutation in one allele and the C163S mutation in the other allele,[41] and four patients have the founder mutation in one allele and an as yet unidentified mutation in the other allele. The founder mutation is relatively evenly distributed in the present Finnish population, with an overall carrier frequency of 1:63, well in line with the disease's incidence of 1:17,000.[42] In a series of cord blood samples from the northern (607 samples) and southwestern (553 samples) regions of Finland, carrier frequencies of 1:55 and 1:69, respectively, were obtained, a nonsignificant difference. Eleven AGU patients homozygous for the C163S mutation are known from northern Norway, an area with a large ancient Finnish emigrant population.[43] The Finnish founder mutation is also responsible for the eight AGU cases in Sweden. The C163S mutation was not found by screening a series of blood samples from Finno-Ugric populations including a total of 615 individuals (290 Estonian, 120 Finnish Saami, 90 Moksha, 75 Mari, and 40 Erza; unpublished results). The second most

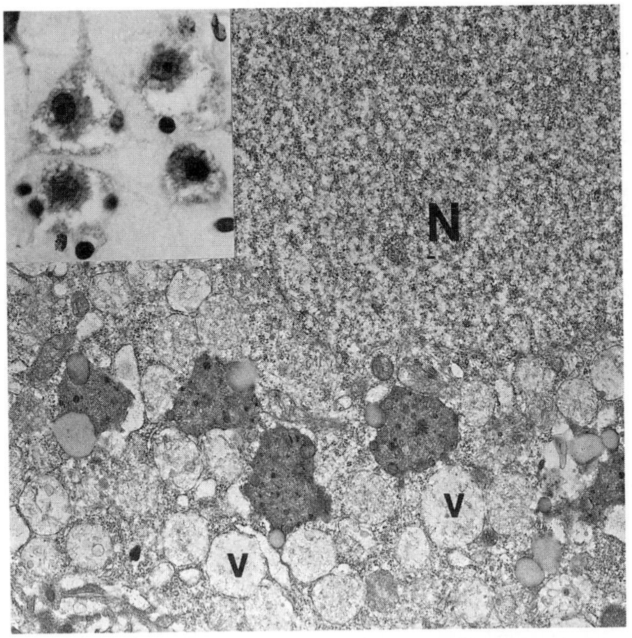

Fig. 141-5 The cytoplasm of a cerebral cortical nerve cell is studded with electron-lucent membrane-bound vacuoles (v) and dark electron-dense cytosomes. N = nucleus. Transmission electron micrograph of a brain biopsy specimen from a 26-year-old female AGU patient. Magnification approximately × 5000. Insert: The cytoplasm of cerebral cortical neurons is swollen owing to indistinct vacuolation, resembling artifactual "watery change." Paraffin section, Luxol fast blue-cresyl violet. Magnification approximately × 600. (*From Haltia M, Palo J, Autio S: Aspartlyglycosaminuria: A generalized storage disease. Morphological and histochemical studies.* Acta Neuropathol *31:243, 1975.*)

frequent AGU mutation is Ser to Pro at codon 72, a missense mutation designated S72P, found in 12 patients from four unrelated families of Palestinian Arab background.[23] Sporadic cases of AGU have been reported worldwide in people from a variety of ethnic backgrounds, including Caucasian,[1,31,32,44,45] US Hispanic[30,46] and black,[47] and Japanese.[33] A total of 44 non-Finnish patients from 27 families are known to us at the moment.

BIOCHEMISTRY AND CELL BIOLOGY OF AGU

Accumulation of Glycoasparagines

The main compound stored in the lysosomes in AGU is aspartylglucosamine (2-acetamido-1-L-β-aspartamido-1,2-dideoxy-β-D-glucose, N-acetylglucosaminyl-asparagine [AADG, GlcNAc-Asn]), due to deficient cleavage of asparagine from the residual N-acetylglucosamines as the final step in the lysosomal degradation of glycoproteins (Fig. 141-6). The enzyme responsible for the specific cleavage of the GlcNAc-Asn is lysosomal aspartylglucosaminidase (1-aspartamido-β-N-acetylglucosamine amidohydrolase, glycosylasparaginase [AGA, EC 3.5.1.26]), which on the basis of its three-dimensional structure[10] was recently proved to be the only mammalian representative of N-terminal hydrolases (see below).

Deficient hydrolysis of the GlcNAc-Asn bonds in AGU results in lysosomal accumulation of glycoasparagines and mainly of N-aspartylglucosamine. This compound, practically absent in normal tissues, has been identified in liver, spleen, kidney, thyroid, lymphocytes, and both central and peripheral neural tissue of patients with AGU.[48–51] As a minor accumulating compound, a glycoasparagine with a structure of Man-Man-GlcNAc-GlcNAc-Asn has been identified in much lower amounts. With GC-MS analysis, the amount of aspartylglucosamine in the liver of an AGU patient was on the order of 2.7 mg/g wet weight tissue and

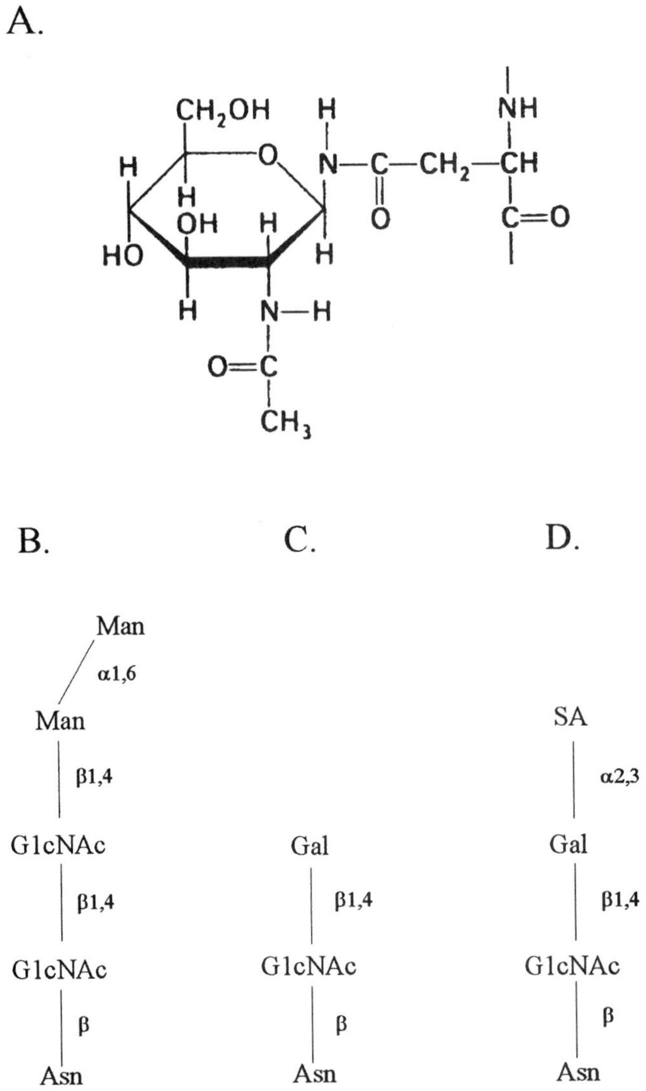

Fig. 141-6 The chemical structure of A) aspartylglucosamine (N-acetylglucosylaminyl-asparagine, AADG) and B, C, and D) some minor glycoasparagines found in the urine of AGU patients (Asn = asparagine, GlcNAc = N-acetylglucosamine, Man = mannose, Gal = galactose, SA = sialic acid).

the Man-Man-GlcNAc-GlcNAc-Asn compound was present only in a very low amount, 0.2 mg/g wet weight.[49] In peripheral blood lymphocytes only aspartylglucosamine was detected, in a concentration of 2.3 nmol/100 μg of protein.[51] The composition of the storage material is thus similar in neural and visceral tissues, but only the central nervous system cells exhibit functional disturbances leading to the clinical disease. Impaired degradation of the GlcNAc-Asn bond also results in urinary excretion of glycoasparagines, which has important clinical significance for screening and diagnosis of AGU. Like the lysosomal storage product in tissues, the major metabolite in the urine of AGU patients is aspartylglucosamine itself. Using HPLC, the mean amount of GlcNAc-Asn excreted by AGU patients (n = 15) was 1300 micromolars (range 280–3240 micromolars), equivalent to 210 μmol/mmol of creatinine (range 130–360). This was over a thousandfold more than in obligate carriers and controls, who both had barely detectable amounts of GlcNAc-Asn in urine.[52] No correlation between the severity of clinical disease and the amount of urinary excretion of GlcNAC-Asn could be demonstrated in another study, in which GC-MS was used.[53] Urinary excretion of aspartylglucosamine has also been quantitated by measuring the amount of N-acetylglucosamine liberated by chemical or enzymatic treatments.[54,55]

Small amounts of higher-order glycoasparagines are also detected in the urine of AGU patients.[56–58] As many as 14 different glycosaparagine derivatives were identified and preliminarily characterized in one study from urine of an English patient. Many of these probably represent structures formed by secondary modifications of primary abnormal degradation products. The most abundant of these is a galactosyl derivative of aspartylglucosamine, Gal-GlcNAc-Asn, a compound that probably is derived in vivo through transfer of the galactosyl moiety to aspartylglucosamine. Some of the minor glycoasparagines are sialylated, the most abundant of these having the structure α-NANA-(2→3)-β-GlcNAc-Asn (Fig. 141-6). The other minor components of urinary glycoasparagines are derivatives of aspartylglucosamine with N-acetylglucosaminyl, mannosyl, galactosyl, fucosyl, glucosyl, and N-acetylneuraminyl residues.

Synthesis, Intracellular Processing, and Tissue Distribution of AGA

AGA is synthesized as a 346-amino-acid, enzymatically inactive, precursor polypeptide with an N-terminal signal sequence of 23 amino acids that is cotranslationally removed. Upon entry into the endoplasmic reticulum (ER), two precursor molecules dimerize immediately, and this event probably triggers the cleavage of AGA into two subunits, the 27-kDa pro-α- and 17-kDa β-subunits.[59,60] The enzyme obtains its full catalytic activity during this early processing step, which presumably takes place autocatalytically.[10,61] In vitro mutagenesis studies have shown that activation requires the highly conserved sequence of Asp205-Thr206 at the active site.[62] Furthermore, His124 at the dimer interface of the two precursor molecules plays a crucial role in the initial dimerization event in the ER. The chaperon proteins of ER do not seem to be crucial for the folding of the precursor polypeptide, and the initial folding and proteolytic activation of AGA are independent of N-linked oligosaccharides.[62] After the activation cleavage step, the tetrameric AGA molecule is transported to lysosomes, where the maturation of the AGA enzyme continues by the removal of a short C-terminal peptide from the pro-α-subunit, resulting in a 24-kDa mature α-subunit.[59] The β-subunit also undergoes further maturation in lysosomes, but the processed C-terminal peptide remains linked to the so-called β'-subunit via a disulfide bridge.[60,63,64] Neither of these lysosomal trimming steps influences the enzyme activity. The intracellular processing of the AGA enzyme is depicted in Fig. 141-7.

The 24-kDa α- and 17-kDa β-subunits contain one N-glycosylation site each, both of which are utilized in vivo.[9,13] Due to heterogeneous glycosylation, the reduced subunits of the mature AGA are detected on SDS-PAGE as four polypeptide bands with molecular masses of 25, 24, 18, and 17 kDa.[9] The AGA molecule carrying mutated N-glycosylation sites in both subunits is active but totally secreted, while polypeptides carrying oligosaccharides in either of the subunits are capable of reaching the lysosomes.[63]

The amino acid sequence is known for aspartylglucosaminidases (glycoasparaginases) or asparaginases from nine species. The essential residues for the enzyme activity are conserved from bacteria to mammals, although sequence alignment reveals only 10 percent overall sequence identity. The catalytic Thr206 in the beginning of the β-subunit is absolutely conserved,[62,65,66] and the cleavage site for proteolytic activation (His204-Asp205-Thr206) is also well conserved. Other conserved residues include some amino acids on the interface between the two $\alpha\beta$ dimers, stressing the biologic importance of correct initial dimerization of the precursor polypeptides.[62]

AGA activity has been detected in a variety of species, including human, mouse, rat, bovine, porcine, and chicken,[67] as well as in prokaryotes.[68] As a "housekeeping" lysosomal enzyme, AGA is widely expressed in human tissues, including brain, liver, kidney, lung, skeletal muscle, fibroblasts, leukocytes, and placenta.

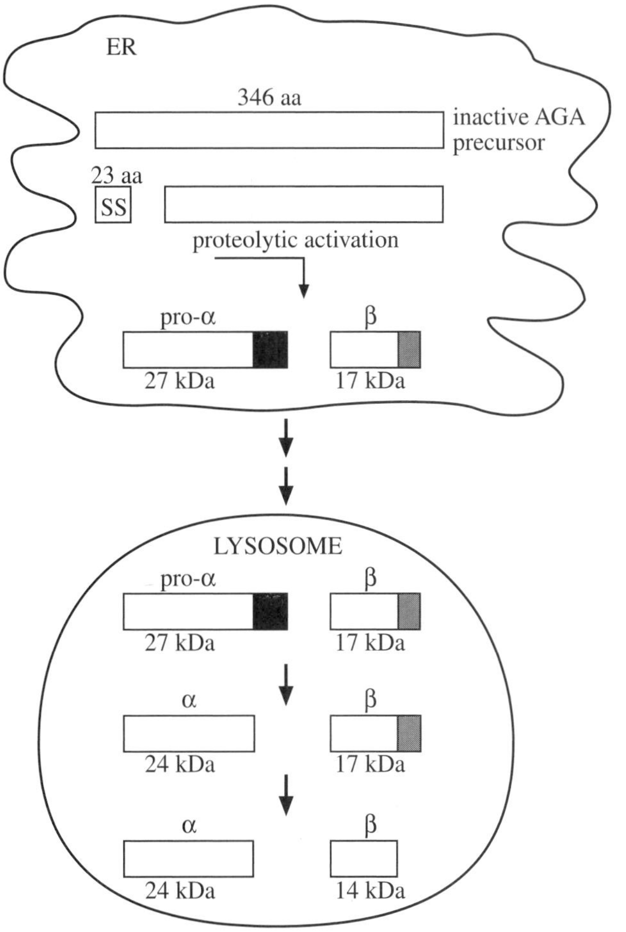

Fig. 141-7 Intracellular processing of AGA. AGA polypeptide is synthesized as a 346-amino-acid precursor polypeptide from which the signal sequence (SS) is removed by the entry into the endoplasmic reticulum (ER). The inactive precursor polypeptide is activated by a proteolytic cleavage into pro α and β subunits already in the ER. The activated enzyme matures in the lysosome where the pro α subunit is proteolytically cleaved to α. The β subunit is partially cleaved to β'.

The highest AGA activity has been measured in leukocytes, whereas fibroblasts exhibited the lowest activity.[69] Immunohistochemistry in human and mouse tissues demonstrated the strongest immunostaining in the pyramidal cells of the cerebral cortex, in hepatocytes, and in the tubule cells of the kidney.[69,70]

Structure of AGA

The recent x-ray crystallization analysis of AGA and a few other proteins revealed an entirely new enzyme family: N-terminal nucleophile (Ntn)-hydrolases, with a similar catalytic domain.[10,64] To date, other proteins of this family include glutamine 5-phosphoribosyl-1-pyrophosphate aminotransferase,[71] the proteasome β-subunit,[72] penicillin acylase,[73] and glucosamine 6-phosphate synthase.[74] All these enzymes share structural features, including a central four-layer sandwich of α-helices and β-sheets ($\alpha\beta\beta\alpha$) and a catalytic N-terminal nucleophile (cysteine, serine, or threonine) at the beginning of the β-subunit. AGA is so far the only known mammalian member of this family showing a heterotetrameric structure consisting of two α- and two β-subunits, and the characteristic Thr in the catalytic site. These characteristics of the AGA molecule would actually require reclassification of this enzyme.

The AGA polypeptide has four cysteine residues participating in a disulfide bridge formation in each subunit and one free cysteine in the N-terminal part of the α-subunit.[10,60] In vitro

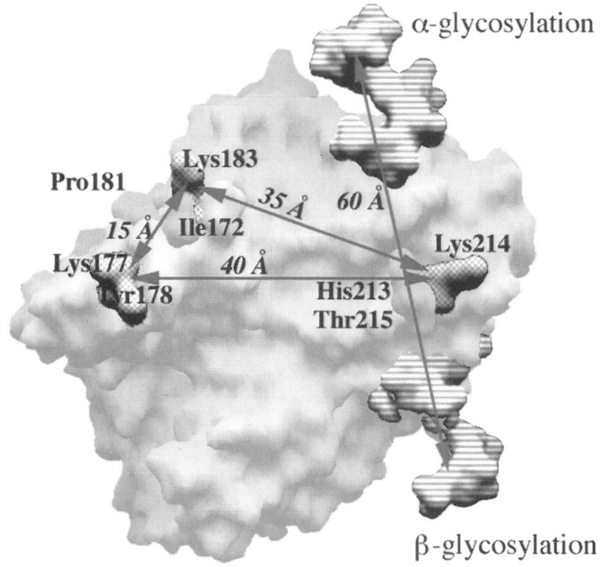

Fig. 141-8 Schematic three-dimensional representation of the surface of the AGA molecule, demonstrating the amino acids essential for phosphorylation of mannose residues and formation of the lysosomal targeting signal of AGA, one of the best-characterized lysosomal enzymes. Two modeled glycans in α- and β-subunits are shown as striped surfaces. Three dotted lysine residues and a tyrosine residue on the surface of AGA are all essential for the phosphotransferase-mediated phosphorylation of mannose residues in the oligosaccharide chains. The distances of these sites from each other are given and indicated with arrows. (*Modified from Tikkanen et al., 1997.*)

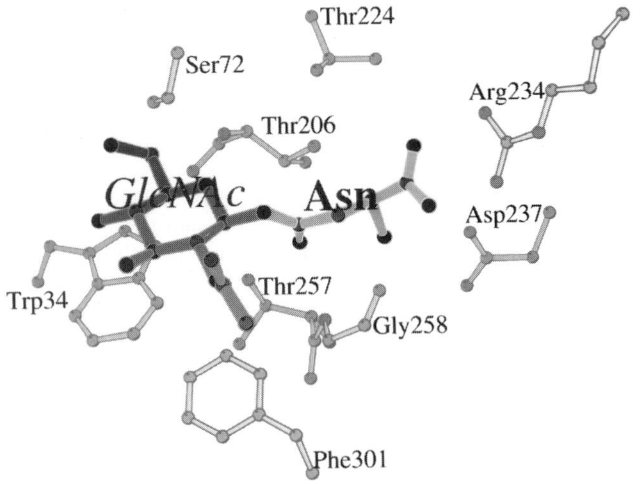

Fig. 141-9 AGA represents a novel class of lysosomal enzymes, the amidohydrolases. The figure shows the amino acid residues forming the active site of AGA based on crystal structure and functional analysis. The substrate, asparagine-linked glycosaminoglycan (in dark gray), is bound by the side chains of the amino acids of the active site (in light gray). (*Modified from Tikkanen et al., 1996.*)

mutagenesis studies have revealed that disruption of the C-terminal disulfide bond in either the α- or the β-subunit leads to a misfolded precursor molecule completely lacking activity, whereas destruction of either one of the N-terminal disulfide bonds results in decreased intracellular stability and reduced AGA activity.[60]

Recent in vitro mutagenesis studies have shed new light on the lysosomal targeting determinant in the AGA molecule. Part of this information is applicable to targeting of lysosomal enzymes generally. When all the 15 Lys-residues and several other amino acid residues were exposed on the surface of the AGA polypeptide, three lysines (Lys177, Lys183, Lys214) and one tyrosine (Tyr178) were found to be essential for the recognition of phosphotransferase, the enzyme responsible for Man-6-P labeling of lysosomal enzymes.[11] The mutants carrying substitutions in all four amino acids resulted in less than 10 percent phosphorylation and lacked lysosomal targeting of AGA. Two of the phosphotransferase binding site motifs (Lys177/Tyr178 and Lys183) were located in a loop on top of the α-subunit in the three-dimensional structure of AGA, whereas the third motif (Lys214) was located in the β-subunit (Fig. 141-8). Interestingly, the most common disease-causing mutation, C163S, interferes with the loop formation that is essential for the binding motif of the α-subunit.

The tetrameric AGA molecule thus contains two binding sites for phosphotransferase on opposite sides of the molecule, each containing parts from both αβ dimers. The N-glycosylation sites of AGA, one in each subunit, are located 20–40 Å from these crucial motifs. It has been suggested that phosphotransferase with an impressive molecular weight of 570 kDa contains two separate active sites, which actually would facilitate a single binding position on such a wide molecular surface.[75]

Catalytic Function of AGA

AGA functions as one of the final steps in the degradation pathway of glycoproteins cleaving the bond between Asn and N-acetylglucosamine. Complete proteolytic cleavage of the N-glycosylated polypeptide chain precedes hydrolysis of the asparagine-oligosaccharide bond that removes both the α-amino and α-carboxy groups of the asparagine residue. The activity of AGA is independent of the size of the sugar chain and of the lysosomal chitobiase activity that finally cleaves the bond between the two N-acetylglucosamines.[76] The reaction catalyzed by AGA primarily produces aspartic acid and 1-amino-N-acetylglucosamine, which is then nonenzymatically broken down to ammonia and N-acetylglucosamine.[77] The human enzyme which is present in all tissues has an unusually high pH optimum of 7–9.

Structural studies have shown that the active site of the heterotetrameric AGA molecule is a funnel-like cavity in which the asparagine portion of the substrate is located in the narrow tube part and the carbohydrate chain in the upper and wider part.[10] The structure of the ligand-binding pocket explains why AGA has strict requirements concerning the asparagine part of the substrate but allows variation in the oligosaccharide chain (Fig. 141-9). There are three distinct structural elements in the active site: the substrate-binding pocket, the nucleophile, and the oxyanion hole. In the substrate-binding pocket, the Asn part of the substrate is hydrogen-bonded to Arg234 (the α-carboxy group of Asn) and to Asp237 (the α-amino group of Asn), as well as to the main-chain carbonyl oxygen of Gly258. The carbohydrate part of the substrate resides in the wider cone of the active-site funnel and is probably bound by Trp34, which is essential for the enzyme activity,[66] and Phe301. The N-terminal amino acid of the β-subunit, Thr206, is the putative nucleophile in the catalysis and is hydrogen bonded to the carbonyl oxygen of the substrate. The free α-amino group of Thr206 forms a hydrogen bond with Ser72 and the Thr206 hydroxyl group with Thr224. These are not directly bound with the substrate but rather influence the properties of Thr206. The third structural element of the active site is the oxyanion hole, which is formed by Thr257 and the main-chain nitrogen of Gly258, hydrogen bonded to the carbonyl oxygen of the substrate. The pH optimum of AGA, pH 7-9, is exceptional for a lysosomal enzyme functioning in the acidic pH of lysosomes.[65] This has raised speculation as to whether AGA has an additional role outside the lysosomes.

MOLECULAR GENETICS OF AGU

The AGA Gene and Its Regulation

The gene encoding human aspartylglucosaminidase was assigned to chromosome 4q using somatic cell hybrids.[12] This was later

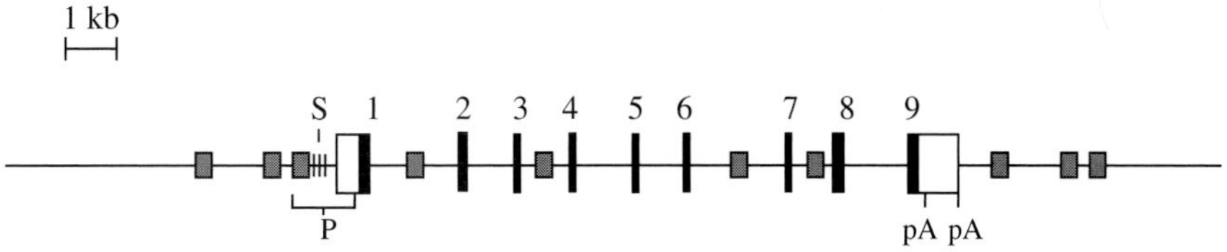

Fig. 141-10 Genomic structure of human AGA. Human AGA gene spans over 15 kb of genomic DNA and contains nine exons (black boxes). The core promoter region (P) has been defined to a 300-bp region and a silencer element (S) is located 5′ to the promoter. Two differentially utilized polyadenylation signals (pA) are located 1 kb apart from each other. The 5′ and 3′ untranslated regions are marked with white boxes. The genomic region is rich in Alu sequences (stippled boxes).

verified by linkage analysis in AGU families.[78] Fluorescence *in situ* hybridization (FISH) studies have localized the gene to 4q32-q35.[79] The mouse AGA gene has been localized to band B3 in chromosome 8, which is the mouse syntenic region of human chromosome 4q34-q35.[80] The 2.2-kb AGA cDNA, comprising a 1041-bp coding region, was cloned by two independent groups.[13,14] Human AGA cDNA contains a short, 5′ untranslated region (UTR) and a long, almost 1-kb 3′ UTR, the function of which is not known.[14,81] Due to utilization of two of the three polyadenylation signals present in human AGA cDNA, two AGA mRNA species of different sizes, 2.2 kb and 1.4 kb, have been observed in human tissues.[80] The coding regions of human and mouse AGA cDNAs are identical in length and show 84 percent homology, but the mouse AGA cDNA lacks the 3′ UTR. Only a 1.2-kb AGA transcript has been detected in mouse tissues.[80] The genomic structures of the human and mouse AGA genes have been resolved.[81,82] Both genes contain nine exons that are identical in size, and the exon-intron boundaries are also identically positioned[80] (Fig. 141-10). The human AGA gene has been reported to span approximately a 13-kb genomic region,[81] while the mouse gene covers an 11-kb region.[80]

Both human and mouse AGA genes are expressed in diverse tissues, consistent with the housekeeping role of the enzyme and suggesting stable promoter activity. In interspecies comparisons of the 5′ regions of the human and mouse AGA genes, the greatest homology was observed from nt −500 to −1000 relative to the ATG translation initiation codon. Both genes display multiple transcription start sites characteristic of housekeeping genes, but the human AGA gene contains a major transcription start site as well. Structural and functional analyses have demonstrated that the core promoter of the human AGA gene lacks a TATA element and contains two essential Sp1 binding sites, although additional contributing elements may exist. A distal silencer element at −322 to −300, reducing transcription to 22 percent, has also been identified. In northern analyses, AGA mRNA is present in a diversity of human and mouse tissues. As the main manifestations of AGU result from dysfunction of the CNS, the specific features of AGA expression in the brain have been investigated in more detail. From postnatal day 5 onward, the expression of AGA in mouse brain seems to coincide with the expression of myelin basic protein. Also, the myelinated fibers in the human infantile samples were found to be stained by anti-AGA antibodies, whereas in the adult samples they were not.[29,70] Interestingly, delayed myelination has been detected in the MRI analyses of AGU patients' brains.

AGU Mutations

The major mutation causing the AGU disease is actually a double point mutation, AGU_{FIN} ($G_{482}{\rightarrow}A + G_{488}{\rightarrow}C$), found in 98 percent of Finnish disease alleles.[14,15] Both mutations lead to amino acid substitutions in the AGA polypeptide, Arg to Gln at codon 161, designated R161Q, and C163S, respectively. These two point mutations are always found together, but the substitution of the cystine residue is solely responsible for the disease, whereas the arginine-to-glutamine change may represent a rare polymorphism.[83,84,85] Substitution of the cysteine results in the disruption of one disulfide bond in the α-subunit, leading to misfolding and retention of the precursor molecule in the ER. The other frequent mutation causing AGU in the Finnish population is a 2-bp deletion in the second exon of the AGA gene, known as AGU_{FIN} minor.[41] The AGU_{FIN} minor mutation causes a frameshift and premature translational termination codon (after 64 aa) in the AGA polypeptide. This mutation dramatically affects the transcription level of the mutant AGA allele, but a small amount of precursor polypeptide in patients' fibroblasts can be detected by metabolic labeling and immunoprecipitation. The mutation obviously leads to the creation of an early transcription termination codon, resulting in low mRNA levels but allowing readthrough on rare occasions. This polypeptide product of the readthrough remains in the precursor form and is not further processed into the mature, active form.

The search for other mutations in patients of non-Finnish origin has revealed a wide distribution of family-specific mutations throughout the coding sequence of the AGA gene[16,17] (Fig. 141-11). However, a 40-bp region in the α-subunit[41] and a 46-bp region in the C-terminal end of the β-subunit[16] seem to have an excess of disease mutations. In addition to AGU_{FIN} minor, three other mutations are known in this "hot" region for mutations, namely the Gly to Ala transition at codon 179, designated G179A, in a German patient;[16] the Thr to stop mutation at codon 192, designated T192X, in a Puerto Rican family;[30] and the Thr to Cys active site mutation at codon 214, designated T214C, in an Arab family.[61,86] This 40-bp region was found to be rich in repeats and to consist of symmetric elements previously reported in mutation hotspot regions of other genes.[87] Misalignment of short direct repeats has been suggested to be the mechanism for generation of

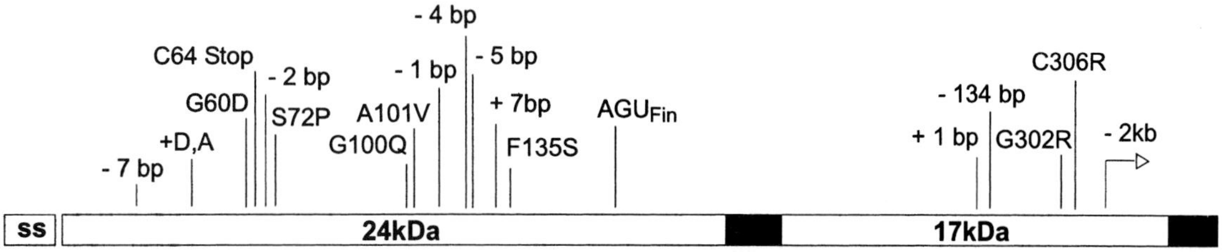

Fig. 141-11 Schematic summary of the AGU mutations. The white boxes indicate the 24-kDa α and 17-kDa β subunits. SS represents signal sequence and the black boxes indicate those areas of the polypeptide which are proteolytically cleaved off in the lysosomes.

gene deletions.[87,88] According to these models, illegitimate pairing occurs between two direct repeats during DNA replication and a repeat or part of it is deleted via secondary structure intermediates. Furthermore, DNA polymerase arrest sites (GAG) present in this particular region may be involved in the gene deletion events.[87,88]

The Effect of AGU Mutations on the AGA Molecule

Crystallographic analyses of the AGA molecule have shown that both the α- and β-subunits contain two disulfide bridges, namely Cys64–Cys69 (α), Cys163–Cys179 (α), Cys286–Cys306 (β), Cys317–Cys345 (β). Cys61, located near the N-terminus of the α-subunit, is the only cysteine residue that does not form a disulfide bond in the mature enzyme molecule.[10] The C163S mutation results in the loss of one disulfide bond in the α-subunit[14,84] and prevents the activation cleavage of the AGA precursor, leading to misfolding of the polypeptides in the ER. Thus, it seems that, in contrast to N-linked glycosylation, the formation of disulfide bonds is essential not only for the function of AGA but also for the initial folding and activation of the enzyme.

The substitution of other amino acid residues in the AGA polypeptide may also result in incorrect maturation of the enzyme. For example, substitution of His204 for serine, which is located near the precursor cleavage site (α-Asp205-Thr206-β), results in an unusual maturation of the AGA enzyme: The His204-mutated AGA precursors are not proteolytically activated in the ER but, surprisingly, are still transported into the lysosomes, where they undergo the normal maturation step of the pro-α-subunit. This results in an inactive enzyme molecule with a 24-kDa α-subunit and an abnormally long 19-kDa β-subunit.[59] Recently, a Ser to Pro mutation at codon 72, designated S72P, was found to result in processing similar to that which occurs with H204S-mutated polypeptides.[61] This indicates that the substitution of one amino acid, which may be located far from the cleavage site, may still severely affect activation of the AGA precursor.

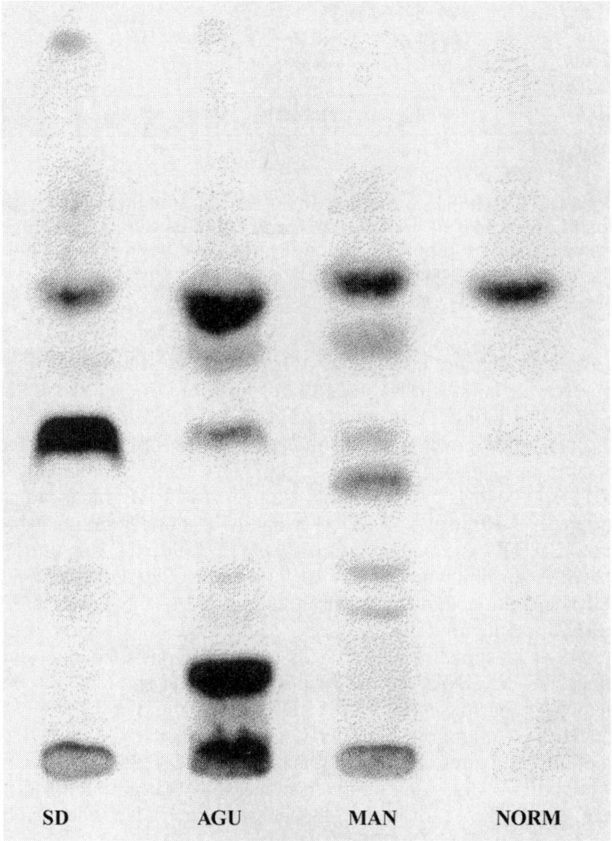

Fig. 141-12 Thin-layer chromatography of urinary oligosaccharides in aspartylglucosaminuria, mannosidosis, and Salla disease (free sialic acid storage disorder). The silica gel plate is developed in n-butanol:acetic acid:water (2:1:1 v/v), heated 10 min at 120°C, and stained with resorcinol spray.

DIAGNOSIS

Clinical Signs

The leading manifestation of AGU, the slowly progressing delay of psychomotor development, has no specific characteristics that would themselves be diagnostic. Therefore, several years may elapse after the first observations of minor changes in the child's behavior and development before the diagnosis is made. Delayed speech development and motor clumsiness in a child who has suffered from repeated upper respiratory infections warrant etiologic investigations. Analysis of urinary oligosaccharides and study of vacuolated lymphocytes are the initial screening methods, whose results can later be supplemented with assay of AGA activity in peripheral blood leukocytes. Coarse facial features in an older patient with severe mental retardation of unknown etiology are a clear indication to do diagnostic laboratory studies for AGU.

Detection of Glycoasparagines in the Urine

The constant excretion of aspartylglucosamine and other glycoasparagines in urine allows a simple and sensitive way to diagnose AGU. Several techniques based on various chromatographic or electrophoretic modifications, as recently reviewed, can be used.[89] For diagnostic and screening purposes, semi-quantitative thin-layer chromatography is convenient and widely used, with several technical modifications.[90,91] Care must be taken that, after running of the samples, the silica plates are heated up to 120°C to produce the characteristic purple color of the glycoasparagine spot with resorcinol staining (Fig. 141-12). Thin-layer chromatography of urine is widely applied as a screening test among mentally retarded patients to detect the whole group of disorders due to inherited defects in the lysosomal degradative pathways of oligosaccharides such as mannosidoses, fucosidosis, sialidoses, and free sialic acid storage diseases. A liquid chromatography-based method is also easily applicable to diagnosis and screening of AGU,[92] providing accurate quantitative results and possibilities for automation. The other techniques, such as ion-exchange chromatography,[93] GC-MS,[49] and enzymatic treatment of GlcNAc-Asn,[55] give accurate quantitative results, but they are less suitable for routine clinical laboratory diagnosis. Glycoasparagine detection in urine is a very specific test for AGU. Inadequate specimen (diluted urine) may obscure the finding, but considering the thousandfold excess of GlcNAC-Asn in patient samples, even this is unlikely to lead to a diagnostic failure. A positive urine test in a patient with clinical findings compatible with AGU confirms the diagnosis; no further diagnostic studies are necessary.

Vacuolated Lymphocytes

Examination of peripheral blood smears for vacuolated mononuclear cells has also been used as a screening test for AGU and other lysosomal disorders. The number of vacuolated cells may vary, and repeated counts (×3) of a minimum of 500 cells are recommended. In a study of 25 AGU patients, vacuolated lymphocytes were found in 19 (76 percent).[4] Cytoplasmic vacuoles, i.e., enlarged lysosomes in skin, conjunctival, or rectal biopsy in an EM study, have much more diagnostic value for this group of disorders. However, biopsies cannot be taken as freely as blood samples.

Assay of Enzyme Activity

As a household enzyme, AGA probably has activity in all tissues and cells, but for diagnostic purposes, assays of peripheral blood leukocytes or isolated lymphocytes and cultured fibroblasts are of clinical significance. A low level of AGA activity is present in plasma, but assays of cellular samples are preferable for diagnostic purposes. The method originally described by Makino, with minor modifications, works well in clinical settings.[77,94] The natural substrate aspartylglucosamine (2-acetamido-1-(β-L-aspartamido)-1,2-dideoxyglucose; 5 mM) is used at pH 7, which is the pH optimum for the enzyme. The liberated N-acetylglucosamine is measured colorimetrically with the Morgan-Elson reaction.[95] Overnight incubation is required because of the low amount of the enzyme in cells. Alternatively, the liberated AADG in permethylated form can been determined by gas liquid chromatography[95] or using direct HPLC assay.[92] These assays are more specific and sensitive than the colorimetric assay because they are devoid of the errors caused by decomposition of the glycoconjugates into hexosamines by hexosaminidases or nonspecific color formation in the Morgan-Elson reaction. Recently, fluorometric assay using a fluorylated aspartic acid derivative (L-aspartic acid-β-7-amido-4-methylcoumarin [Asp-AMC]) as substrate has been reported independently by two groups.[96,97] Fluorogenic free Asp-AMC can be measured using the same excitation and emission wavelengths commonly used when other lysosomal enzymes are assayed with umbelliferyl derivatives as substrates—355 nm and 460 nm, respectively. The fluorometric assay is more sensitive than the original colorimetric assay. Regardless of the assay system, AGU patients have shown very low (absent or less than 10 percent of normal) AGA activity both in leukocytes and in cultured fibroblasts, without any overlapping values between normal and heterozygous individuals.

Molecular Diagnosis

Direct detection of the disease-causing mutation has particular clinical significance in Finland, where 96 percent of AGU patients are homozygotes for the same founder mutation, the rest of them being compound heterozygotes with either the 2-bp deletion mutation or an unknown mutation in the other allele. The solid-phase primer extension-based minisequencing technique[98] that is visualized in Fig. 141-13 offers several advantages both in individual cases and in screening of homozygotes or heterozygous carriers. Oligonucleotide ligation assay[99] and other PCR-based mutation-specific assays[100] have also been used to detect the C163S mutation. Other AGU mutations are mainly private mutations in single families, limiting the value of molecular techniques to the index family only.

Carrier Detection and Carrier Screening

Heterozygous individuals carrying any AGU mutation in only one allele present no phenotypic manifestations, nor do they excrete glycoasparagines in urine in detectable amounts. Enzyme assay and, more recently, mutation detection are available for carrier detection. In one study using colorimetric assay, the AGA activity in peripheral blood lymphocytes among 29 obligate carriers had a mean of 34.1 U per milligram of protein (range 5–69) and the activity of 30 control individuals had a mean of 127.9 U per milligram of protein (range 91–243).[94] In another study, obligate carriers (n = 8) had a mean of 31.4 U per milligram of protein (range 17.6–42.2) and the controls (n = 6) had a mean of 74.1 U/mg (range 46.7–130.1).[96] Interestingly, the carriers of the minor Finnish AGA mutation, the 2-bp deletion leading to a premature stop codon, have AGA activity in the control range and would thus escape identification on AGA assay.[41]

Demonstration of the mutation in the AGA gene is another way to detect carriers. In the case of the Finnish founder mutation, with approximately one of every 60 individuals carrying the C163S mutation, both the individual and the population screening approach have become feasible.

The results of a series of recent studies have revealed that the prospects of large-scale AGU-carrier screening in Finland are favorable: (1) The carrier frequency of the C163S mutation was found to be on the same order of magnitude in different parts of the country, ranging from 1:55 to 1:69;[101] (2) the semiautomated solid-phase minisequencing method met the requirements of large-scale screening;[102] and (3) a pilot screening program among 2000 pregnant women at maternity health care centers indicated a high acceptance rate (95 percent) and only rare adverse reactions.[103] Nineteen carriers (1:63) were detected, but the spouses all tested negative for the founder mutation and for the other Finnish AGU mutation.

Furthermore, an earlier population survey had indicated that Finnish people mainly have a positive attitude toward gene testing in general.[104] No population-based carrier screening, however, is currently being carried out for AGU.

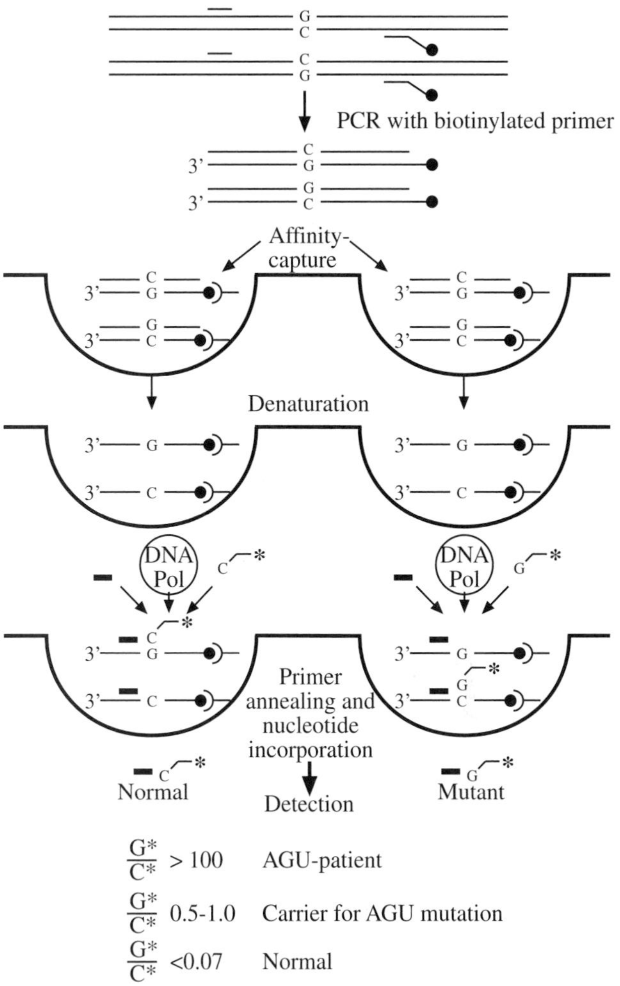

Fig. 141-13 Detection of AGU_{Fin} mutation by solid-phase minisequencing. In this technique the DNA sample is PCR-amplified with one biotinylated primer (black circle). The amplified product is attached to two streptavidin-coated microtiter wells and the normal or mutated nucleotide is detected by primer extension with a labeled nucleotide.

Prenatal Diagnosis

Amniotic fluid in pregnancies with fetuses affected with AGU does not contain aspartylglucosamine in high enough concentrations for reliable prenatal diagnosis.[105] Assay of AGA activity in cultured amniotic fluid cells,[38] or preferably in uncultured first-trimester CVS samples,[106] is a reliable way to detect fetal aspartylglucosaminuria. In the cases of affected fetuses, AGA activity has been practically absent. In recent years, molecular techniques to detect the Finnish founder mutation C163S have been the methods of choice for prenatal diagnosis in at-risk families in which both parents are carriers of the mutation. Molecular techniques can, of course, be applied in any at-risk family if the mutation has been identified.

MOUSE MODELS FOR ASPARTYLGLUCOSAMINURIA

Gene-targeted mouse models for lysosomal storage diseases offer new possibilities for studies of pathogenesis of the diseases, especially in cases with CNS manifestations.[107]

Two mouse models for AGU have recently been generated. In the first one, exon 3 was disrupted, resulting in a null-mutant phenotype without any AGA enzyme production.[18] In the other case, gene targeting disrupted exon 8, thus mimicking the human mutation, in which inactive AGA precursor polypeptide is present.[19] The mouse with exon 8 targeting produced mutant mRNA and consequently also mutant AGA precursor polypeptide, but only in brain tissue.[108] Interestingly, the wild-type animal also had severe precursor accumulation in brain,[70] which is in line with the earlier observation of slowed proteolytic processing of wild-type AGA in neurons in vitro.[109] However, active AGA in the $\alpha\beta\beta\alpha$ heterotetrameric form and all enzymatic activity were absent in the AGA −/− animals.

Typical lysosomal vacuolization was seen in the liver starting at day 14 and in the brains of day-19 embryos, extending into full-blown vacuolization of brain and visceral tissues at the age of 2 months. On EM analysis, typical storage lysosomes containing small amounts of amorphous granular material and membrane fragments on electron-clear background were seen (Fig. 141-14). The other typical finding in AGU mice was the excretion of aspartylglucosamine in the urine as shown by TLC[19] (Fig. 141-15) or by HPLC.[18]

The organs of young AGU mice appeared macroscopically normal. The first abnormal sign was observed at 6 months, as the AGA −/− mice reached 20 percent more weight than their normal littermates. A striking finding was abnormally large urinary bladders in aged AGA −/− mice, probably reflecting peripheral neuropathy affecting the autonomous nervous system innervating the bladder.[18,108] Skeletal changes were also present in the aging AGU mice. The cortices of the femur and humerus, as well as the ribs, were thicker than in wild-type animals.[108] In human disease, these changes tend to be the opposite and thickening of the bones is seen in the calvarium. From the age of 1 year on, motor coordination, mental activity, and cognitive functions were impaired. In contrast to the case in the human disease, the life span of AGU mice seems not to be shortened.

A closer analysis of the brain cytoarchitecture revealed central brain atrophy. In the central regions of the brain, the number of electron-lucent storage lysosomes in neurons increased with age and reached a plateau at the age of 2 months. Only occasional vacuoles were observed in oligodendroglia and astrocytes. Axonal dystrophy was most prominent in the basal ganglia. Neurons of the cerebral cortex were better preserved and the loss of Purkinje cells in the cerebellum was less extensive than in humans.[108]

An interesting way of monitoring brain pathology in living AGU mice is MRI, which demonstrates dilatation of the lateral ventricles from the age of 6 months on similar to that in older human patients (Fig. 141-16).

The mouse model has offered a good target for therapeutic approaches. Brain-targeted gene transfer by intraventricular injection of AGA adenovirus resulted in local disappearance of lysosomal storage granules.[110] Furthermore, as demonstrated in vitro,[109,111] AGA enzyme also migrates in vivo in neurons via mannose-6-phosphate receptor-mediated endocytosis.[110] Bone marrow transplantation of AGU mice has resulted only in the correction of peripheral tissues,[115] but enzyme replacement therapy led to partial correction of pathology in the central nervous system.[116]

THERAPY

At present there is no cure or effective treatment for AGU. Epileptic seizures have been successfully controlled with carbamazepine.

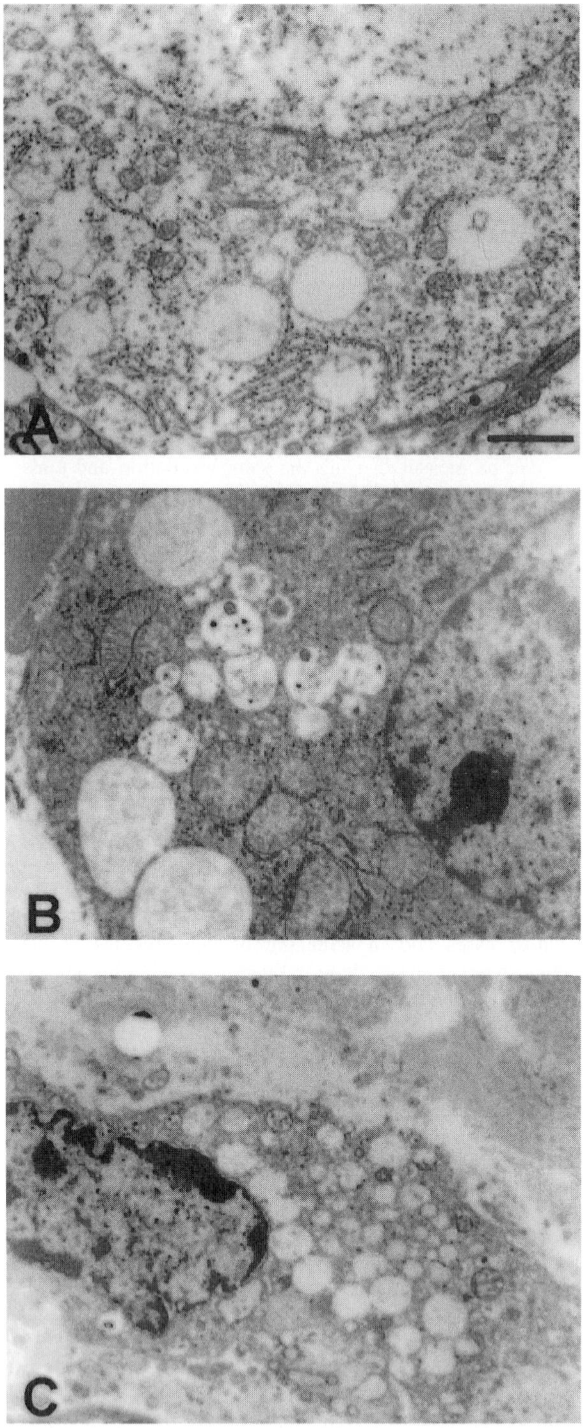

Fig. 141-14 Electron micrographs of AGU mouse brain A), liver B), and skin C) from mice of 6 weeks. Magnification bar: A) 1.25 μm.

Four AGU patients have successfully recieved allogenic bone marrow transplants. One patient, however, lost the graft during the first post-transplant year.[32,112] The ages at transplantation have ranged from 1.5 to 2.6 years, i.e., patients were at stage of absent or only mild developmental delay. The donor has been an HLA-identical relative in three cases and a matched unrelated individual in one case. Post-transplantation follow-up periods ranged from 1 to 6 years, including clinical evaluation, brain MRI, urinary glycoasparagine determinations, AGA activity assays, and EM studies of skin or rectal biopsies. Common to all cases has been

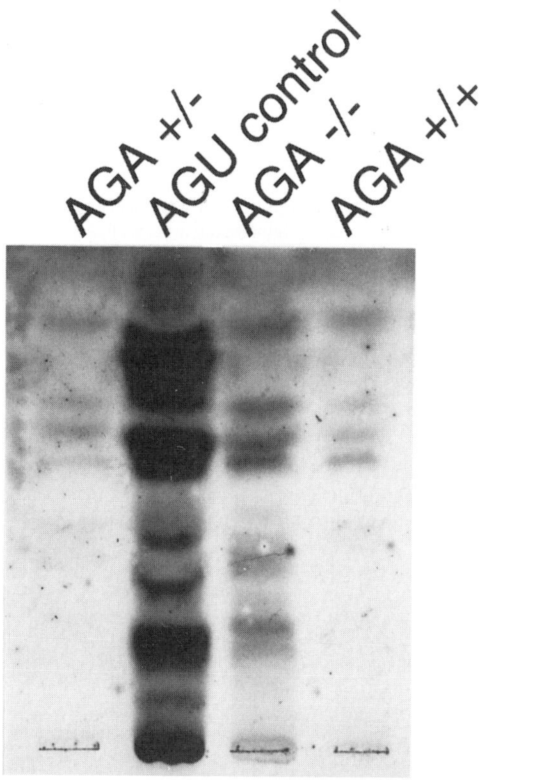

Fig. 141-15 Thin-layer chromatography of urine oligosaccharides of AGA +/+, +/− and −/− mice as well as from a human AGU patient (AGU control). (From reference 19.)

biochemical normalization, with clear reduction of urinary glycoasparagine excretion and restoration of AGA activity in peripheral blood leukocytes to levels seen in heterozygotes. Storage lysosomes in rectal biopsy specimens in two patients were undetectable three years post-transplantation. MRI studies of brain

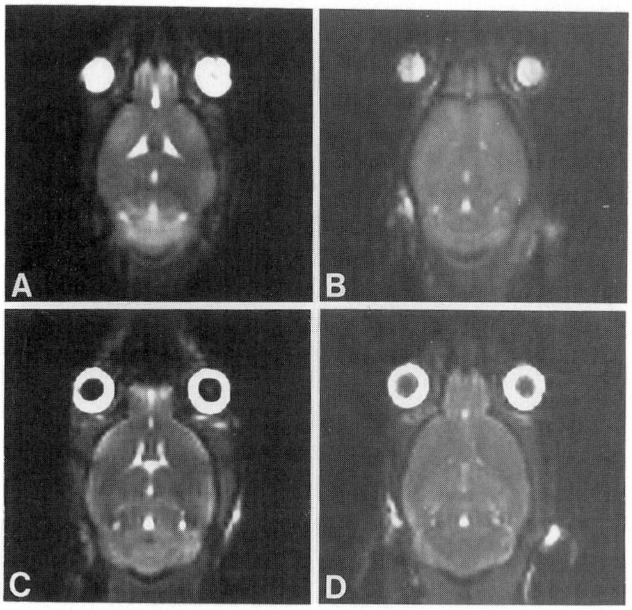

Fig. 141-16 Transversal MR images (CISS sequence) of mouse brain (A and C) AGA −/− mouse, and (B and D) AGA +/− mouse of 6 months. (From reference 19.)

before transplantation had revealed changes in cerebral myelination typical of AGU (see Neuroradiology). These abnormalities underwent changes toward normalization; fair or evident differentiation of cortical gray versus white matter was seen, and the ratios between signal intensities of deep gray matter and white matter were found to be nearly normal. The crucial criteria of a beneficial effect of BMT, intellectual improvement and/or prevention of developmental delay, cannot yet be evaluated. Since progression of the delay in AGU takes place during an extended period of approximately 10 years, much longer follow-up is needed to draw firm conclusions.

Table 141-3 AGU-Causing Mutations Reported in the Literature

Mutation	Consequence	Ethnic Origin (Reference)
POINT MUTATIONS		
488 G → C	Cys163Ser inactive precursor, no lysosomal transport	Finnish (16)
GT → TT (splice donor)	Deletion of exon 8 truncated precursor, premature stop	African-American (113)
916 T → C	Cys306Arg	American (white) (16)
179 G → A	Gly60Asp	German (16)
904 G → A	Gly302Arg	Turkish (16)
A → G in intron 3	Splicing defect, premature stop	Japanese (33)
302 G → T	Ala101Val, inactive precursor, no lysosomal transport	English (114)
192 T → A	Cys64stop, readthrough, inactive precursor	Puerto Rican (86)
214 T → C	Ser72Pro, inactive precursor, transport to lysosomes abnormal β-subunit	Arab (61)
299 G → A 404 T → C (compound heterozygote)	Gly100Gln Phe135Ser	Canadian (32)
DELETIONS		
−1 bp (− T336)	Premature stop	Dutch (16)
−5 bp (nt 367–371)	Premature stop	American (white) (114)
−7 bp (nt 101–107)	Premature stop	English (114)
−2 bp (GA between nt 193 and 200)	Premature stop	Finnish (41)
−2 kb starting from intron 8	Abnormal, inactive precursor	North American (82)
INSERTIONS		
+1 bp (800T801)	Premature stop	Spanish-American (16)
+6 bp (after 127G)	42-Asp-Ala-43	Tunisian (16)

REFERENCES

1. Pollitt RJ, Jenner FA, Merskey H: Aspartylglucosaminuria. An inborn error of metabolism associated with mental defect. *Lancet* **3**:253, 1968.
2. Palo J: Prevalence of phenylketonuria and some other metabolic disorders among mentally retarded patients in Finland. *Acta Neurol Scand* **43**:573, 1967.
3. Palo J, Mattsson K: Eleven new cases of aspartylglucosaminuria. *J Ment Defic Res* **14**:168, 1970.
4. Autio S: Aspartylglucosaminuria. Analysis of thirty-four patients. *J Ment Defic Res*, Monograph Series **1**:1, 1972.
5. Savolainen H: Isolation of the liver N-aspartyl-beta-acetylglucosaminidase in aspartylglucosaminuria. *Biochem J* **153**:749, 1976.
6. Dugal B, Strömme J: Purification and some properties of 1-aspartamido-beta-N-acetylglucosamine amidohydrolase from human liver. *Biochem J* **165**:497, 1977.
7. McGovern M, Aula P, Desnick RJ: Purification and properties of human hepatic aspartylglucosaminidase. *J Biol Chem* **258**:10743, 1983.
8. Baumann M, Peltonen L, Aula P, Kalkkinen N: Isolation of a human hepatic 60 kDa aspartylglucosaminidase consisting of three nonidentical polypeptides. *Biochem J* **262**:189, 1989.
9. Halila R, Bauman M, Ikonen E, Enomaa N, Peltonen L: Human leukocyte aspartylglucosaminidase. Evidence for two different subunits in a more complex native structure. *Biochem J* **276**:251, 1991.
10. Oinonen C, Tikkanen R, Rouvinen J, Peltonen L: Three-dimensional structure of human lysosomal aspartylglucosaminidase. *Nat Struct Biol* **2**:1102, 1995.
11. Tikkanen R, Peltola M, Oinonen C, Rouvinen J, Peltonen L: Several co-operating binding sites mediate the interaction of a lysosomal enzyme with phosphotransferase. *EMBO J* **16**:6684, 1997.
12. Aula P, Astrin KH, Francke U, Desnick RJ: Assignment of the structural gene encoding human aspartylglucosaminidase to the long arm of chromosome 4 (4q21-4qter). *Am J Hum Genet* **36**:1215, 1984.
13. Fisher KJ, Tollersrud OK, Aronson NNJ: Cloning and sequence analysis of a cDNA for human glycosylasparaginase. *FEBS Lett* **269**:440, 1990.
14. Ikonen E, Baumann M, Grön K, Syvänen A-C, Enomaa N, Halila R, Aula P, Peltonen L: Aspartylglucosaminuria: cDNA encoding human aspartylglucosaminidase and the missense mutation causing the disease. *EMBO J* **10**:51, 1991.
15. Mononen I, Heisterkamp N, Kaartinen V, Williams JC, Yates JR 3rd, Griffin PR, Hood LE, Groffen J: Aspartylglucosaminuria in the Finnish population: Identification of two point mutations in the heavy chain of glycoasparaginase. *Proc Natl Acad Sci USA* **88**:2941, 1991.
16. Ikonen E, Aula P, Grön K, Tollersrud OK, Halila R, Manninen T, Syvänen A-C, Peltonen L: Spectrum of mutations in aspartylglucosaminuria. *Proc Natl Acad Sci USA* **88**:11222, 1991.
17. Mononen I, Fisher KJ, Kaartinen V, Aronson NN Jr: Aspartylglucosaminuria: Protein chemistry and molecular biology of the most common lysosomal storage disorder of glycoprotein degradation. *FASEB J* **7**:1247, 1993.
18. Kaartinen V, Mononen I, Voncken JW, Noronkoski T, Gonzales-Gómez I, Heisterkamp N, Groffen J: A mouse model for the human lysosomal disease aspartylglucosaminuria. *Nat Med* **2**:1375, 1996.
19. Jalanko A, Tenhunen K, McKinney CE, LaMarca ME, Rapola J, Autti T, Joensuu R, et al.: Mice with aspartylglucosaminuria mutation similar to humans replicate the pathophysiology in patients. *Hum Mol Genet* **7**:265, 1998.
20. Arvio M: Life with aspartylglucosaminuria. Thesis. University of Helsinki, 1993.
21. Mononen I, Aaronson NN: Lysosomal storage diseases. *Aspartylglucosaminuria*. Berlin, Springer-Verlag, 1997.
22. Aula P, Autio S, Raivio KO, Rapola J: Aspartylglucosaminuria, in Durand P, O'Brien JS (eds): *Genetic Errors of Glycoprotein Metabolism*. Milan, Edi-Ermes, p 123 1982.
23. Zlotogora J, Ben-Neriah Z, Abu-Libdeh BY, Sury V, Zeigler M: Aspartylglucosaminuria among Palestinian Arabs. *J Inher Metab Dis* **20**:799, 1997.
24. Arvio M, Autio S, Louhiala P: Early clinical symptoms and incidence of aspartylglucosaminuria in Finland. *Acta Paediatr* **82**:587, 1993.
25. Arvio M: Follow-up in patients with aspartylglucosaminuria. Part I. The course of intellectual functions. *Acta Paediatr* **82**:469, 1993.
26. Arvio M, Oksanen V, Autio S, Gaily E, Sainio K: Epileptic seizures in aspartylglucosaminuria: a common disorder. *Acta Neurol Scand* **87**:342, 1993.
27. Näntö-Salonen K, Pelliniemi LJ, Autio S, Kivimäki T, Rapola J, Penttinen R: Abnormal collagen fibrils in aspartylglucosaminuria. Altered dermal ultrastructure in a glycogen storage disorder. *Lab Invest* **51**:464, 1984.
28. Määttä A, Järveläinen HT, Nelimarkka O, Penttinen RP: Fibroblast expression of collagens and proteoglycans is altered in aspartylglucosaminuria, a lysosomal storage disorder. *Biochim Biophys Acta* **1225**:264, 1994.
29. Autti T, Railinko R, Haltia M, Lauronen L, Vanhanen S-L, Salonen O, Aronen HJ et al.: Aspartylglucosaminuria: Radiologic course of the disease with histopathologic correlation. *J Child Neurol* **12**:369, 1997.
30. Chitayat D, Nakagawa S, Marion RW, Sachs GS, Hahm SYE, Goldman HS: Aspartylglucosaminuria in a Puerto Rican family: Additional features of a panethnic disorder. *Am J Med Genet* **31**: 527, 1988.
31. Mucumeci S, Salvati A, Schiliro G, Salvo G, Di Dio R, Caprari P: Homozygous NADH-methemoglobin reductase and aspartylglucosaminidase deficiencies in a moderately retarded Sicilian child. *Am J Med Genet* **19**:643, 1984.
32. Laitinen A, Hietala M, Haworth JC, Schroeder ML, Seargeant LE, Greenberg C, Aula P: Two novel mutations in a Canadian family and early outcome of bone marrow transplantation. *Clin Genet* **51**:174, 1997.
33. Yoshida K, Ikeda S, Yanagisawa N, Yamauchi T, Tsuji S, Hirabayshi Y: Two Japanese cases with aspartylglucosaminuria: Clinical and morphological features. *Clin Genet* **40**:318, 1991.
34. Arvio MA, Rapola JMH, Pelkonen PM: Chronic arthritis in patients with aspartylglucosaminuria. *J Rheumatol* **25**:1131, 1998.
35. Rapola J: Lysosomal storage diseases in adults. *Pathol Res Pract* **190**:759, 1994.
36. Haltia M, Palo J, Autio S: Aspartylglucosaminuria: A generalized storage disease. Morphological and histochemical studies. *Acta Neuropathol* (Berlin) **31**:243, 1975.
37. Arstila AU, Palo J, Haltia M, Riekkinen P, Autio S: Aspartylglucosaminuria. I: Fine structural studies on liver, kidney and brain. *Acta Neuropathol* (Berlin) **20**:207, 1972.
38. Aula P, Rapola J, von Koskull H, Ämmälä P: Prenatal diagnosis and fetal pathology of aspartylglucosaminuria. *Am J Med Genet* **19**:359, 1984.
39. Nevanlinna HR: The Finnish population structure. A genetic and genealogical study. *Hereditas* **71**:195, 1972.
40. De la Chapelle A: Disease gene mapping in isolated populations: The example of Finland. *J Med Genet* **30**:857, 1993.
41. Isoniemi A, Hietala M, Aula P, Jalanko A, Peltonen L: Identification of a novel mutation causing aspartylglucosaminuria reveals a mutation hotspot region in the aspartylglucosaminidase gene. *Hum Mutat* **5**:318, 1995.
42. Hietala M, Grön K, Syvänen A-C, Peltonen L, Aula P: Prospects of carrier screening of aspartylglucosaminuria in Finland. *Eur J Hum Genet* **1**:296, 1993.
43. Tollersrud OK, Nilssen O, Tranebjaerg L, Borud O: Aspartylglucosaminuria in northern Norway: A molecular and genealogical study. *J Med Genet* **31**:360, 1994.
44. Gehler J, Sewell AC, Becker C, Spranger J, Hartmann J: Aspartylglucosaminuria in an Italian family: Clinical and biochemical characteristics. *J Inherit Metab Dis* **4**:229, 1981.
45. Ziegler R, Schmidt H, Sewell AC, Weglage J, von Lengerke JH, Ullrich K: Aspartylglucosaminurie: Klinische Beschreibung von zwei deutschen Patienten. *Monatsschr Kinderheilk* **137**:454, 1989. (German)
46. Isenberg JN, Sharp HL: Aspartylglucosaminuria — psychomotor retardation masquerading as a mucopolysaccharidosis. *J Pediatr* **86**:713, 1975.
47. Hreidarsson S, Thomas GH, Valle DL, Stevenson RE, Taylor H, McCarty J, Coker SB, Green WR: Aspartylglucosaminuria in the United States. *Clin Genet* **23**:427, 1983.
48. Palo J, Savolainen H: Biochemical diagnosis of aspartylglucosaminuria. *Ann Clin Res* **5**:156, 1973.
49. Maury P: Accumulation of two glycoasparagines in the liver in aspartylglucosaminuria. *J Biol Chem* **254**:1513, 1979.
50. Maury CPJ: Accumulation of glycoprotein-derived metabolites in neural and visceral tissues in aspartylglucosaminuria. *J Lab Clin Med* **96**:838, 1980.
51. Maury P, Palo J: Characterization of the storage material of peripheral lymphocytes in aspartylglucosaminuria. *Clin Sci* **58**:165, 1980.
52. Mononen I, Kaartinen V, Mononen T: Laboratory detection of aspartylglucosaminuria. *Scand J Clin Lab Invest* suppl **191**:7, 1988.

53. Aula P, Raivio K, Maury P: Variation of urinary excretion of aspartylglucosamine and associated findings in aspartylglucosaminuria. *J Inher Metab Dis* **3**:159, 1980.
54. Borud O, Torp KH, Dahl T: Aspartylglucosaminuria. Urinary excretion of aspartylglucosamines related to mental retardation. *Monogr Hum Genet* **10**:23, 1978.
55. Sugahara K, Nishimura K, Aula P, Yamashina I: Enzymatic determination of urinary aspartylglucosamine: A rapid and sensitive method to detect aspartylglucosaminuria (AGU). *Clin Chim Acta* **72**:265, 1976.
56. Pollitt RJ, Pretty KM: The glycoasparagines in urine of a patient with aspartylglucosaminuria. *Biochem J* **141**:141, 1974.
57. Sugahara K, Akasaki M, Funakoshi I, Aula P, Yamashina I: Structural studies of glycoasparagines from urine of a patient with aspartylglucosaminuria (AGU). *FEBS Lett* **78**:284, 1979.
58. Lundblad A, Masson PK, Nordén NE, Svensson S, Öckerman P-A, Palo J: Structural determination of three glycoasparagines isolated from the urine of a patient with aspartylglucosaminuria. *Eur J Biochem* **67**:209, 1976.
59. Ikonen E, Julkunen I, Tollersrud O-K, Kalkkinen N, Peltonen L: Lysosomal aspartylglucosaminidase is processed to the active subunit complex in the endoplasmic reticulum. *EMBO J* **12**:295, 1993.
60. Riikonen A, Rouvinen J, Tikkanen R, Julkunen I, Peltonen L, Jalanko A: Primary folding of aspartylglucosaminidase: Significance of disulfide bridges and evidence of early multimerization. *J Biol Chem* **271**:21340, 1996.
61. Peltola M, Tikkanen R, Peltonen L, Jalanko A: Ser72Pro active site disease mutation in human lysosomal aspartylglucosaminidase: Abnormal intracellular processing and evidence for extracellular activation. *Hum Mol Genet* **5**:737, 1996.
62. Saarela J, Peltola M, Tikkanen R, Oinonen C, Jalanko A, Rouvinen J, Peltonen L: Activation and oligomerization of aspartylglucosaminidase. *J Biol Chem* **273**:25320, 1998.
63. Tikkanen R, Riikonen A, Ikonen E, Peltonen L: Intracellular sorting of aspartylglucosaminidase: The role of N-linked oligosaccharides and evidence of Man-6-P independent lysosomal targeting. *DNA Cell Biol* **14**:305, 1995.
64. Tikkanen R, Riikonen A, Oinonen C, Rouvinen J, Peltonen L: Functional analyses of active site residues of human lysosomal aspartylglucosaminidase: Implications for catalytic mechanism and autocatalytic activation. *EMBO J* **15**:2954, 1996.
65. Kaartinen V, Williams JC, Tomich J, Yatres JR, Hood LE, Mononen I: Glycoasparaginase from human leukocytes. Inactivation and covalent modification with diazo-oxonorvaline. *J Biol Chem* **266**:5860, 1991.
66. Riikonen A, Tikkanen R, Jalanko A, Peltonen L: Immediate interaction between the nascent subunits and two conserved amino acids trp 34 and thr 206 are needed for the catalytic activity of aspartylglucosaminidase. *J Biol Chem* **270**:4903, 1995.
67. Tollersrud O, Aronson N: Comparison of liver glycoasparaginases from six vertebrates. *Biochem J* **282**:891, 1992.
68. Tarentino AL, Quiñones G, Hauer CR, Changchien L-M, Plummer TH Jr.: Molecular cloning and sequencing analysis of *Flavobacterium meningosepticum* glycoasparaginase: A single gene encodes the alpha and beta subunits. *Arch Biochem Biophys* **316**:399, 1995.
69. Enomaa N, Lukinmaa P-L, Ikonen E, Waltimo J, Palotie A, Pateau A, Peltonen L: Expression of aspartylglucosaminidase in human tissues from normal individuals and aspartylglucosaminuria patients. *J Histochem Cytochem* **41**:981, 1993.
70. Uusitalo A, Tenhunen K, Heinonen O, Hiltunen J, Saarma M, Haltia M, Jalanko A, Peltonen L: Developmental expression of aspartylglucosaminidase in brain. *Mol Gen Metab* **67**:294, 1999.
71. Smith JL, Zaluxec EJ, Wery J, Niu L, Switzer RL, Zalkin H, Satow Y: Structure of the allosteric regulator enzyme of purine biosynthesis. *Science* **264**:1427, 1994.
72. Löwe J, Stock D, Jap B, Zwickl P, Baumeister W, Huber R: Crystal structure of the 20S proteasome from the archaeon *T. acidophilum* at 3.4 Å resolution. *Science* **268**:533, 1995.
73. Duggleby HJ, Tolley SP, Hill CP, Dodson EJ, Dodson G, Moody PCE: Penicillin acylase has a single-amino-acid catalytic centre. *Nature* **373**:264, 1995.
74. Isupov MN, Obmolova G, Butterworth S, Badet-Denisot MA, Badet B, Polikarpov I, Littlechild JA, Teplyakov A: Substrate binding is required for assembly of the active conformation of the catalytic site in Ntn amidotransferases: Evidence from the 1.8 Å crystal structure of the glutaminase domain of glucosamine-6-phosphate synthase. *Structure* **4**:801, 1996.
75. Bao M, Booth JL, Elmendorf BJ, Canfield WM: Bovine UDP-N-acetylglucosamine: lysosomal-enzyme N-acetylglucosamine-1-phosphotransferase. I. Purification and subunit structure. *J Biol Chem* **271**:31437, 1996.
76. Aronson N, Kuranda M: Lysosomal degradation of Asn-linked glycoproteins. *FASEB J* **3**:2615, 1989.
77. Makino M, Kojima T, Yamashina I: Enzymatic cleavage of glycopeptides. *Biochem Biophys Res Commun* **24**:961, 1966.
78. Grön K, Aula P, Peltonen L: Linkage of aspartylglucosaminuria (AGU) to marker loci on the long arm of chromosome 4. *Hum Genet* **85**:233, 1990.
79. Morris C, Heistercamp N, Groffen J, Williams JC, Mononen I: Chromosomal localization of the glycoasparaginase gene to 4q32-33. *Hum Genet* **88**:295, 1992.
80. Tenhunen K, Laan M, Manninen T, Palotie A, Peltonen L, Jalanko A: Molecular cloning and chromosomal assignment of the mouse aspartylglucosaminidase gene and analysis of the polypeptides by in vitro expression of cDNA. *Genomics* **30**:244, 1995.
81. Park H, Fisher KJ, Aronson NN Jr.: Genome structure of human lysosomal glycoasparaginase. *FEBS Lett* **288**:168, 1991.
82. Jalanko A, Manninen T, Peltonen L: Deletion of the C-terminal end of aspartylglucosaminidase resulting in a lysosomal accumulation disease: Evidence for a unique genomic rearrangement. *Hum Mol Genet* **4**:435, 1995.
83. Fisher KJ, Aronson NN: Characterization of the mutation responsible for aspartylglucosaminuria in three Finnish patients. *J Biol Chem* **266**:12105, 1991.
84. Ikonen E, Enomaa N, Ulmanen I, Peltonen L: In vitro mutagenesis helps to unravel the biological consequences of aspartylglucosaminuria mutation. *Genomics* **11**:206, 1991.
85. Riikonen A, Ikonen E, Sormunen R, Vehto V-P, Peltonen L, Jalanko A: Dissection of molecular consequences of a double mutation causing a lysosomal disease. *DNA and Cell Biol* **13**:257, 1994.
86. Peltola M, Chitayat D, Peltonen L, Jalanko A: Characterization of a point mutation in aspartylglucosaminidase gene: Evidence for a readthrough of a translational stop codon. *Hum Molec Genet* **3**:2237, 1994.
87. Krawczak M, Cooper DN: Gene deletions causing human genetic disease: Mechanisms of mutagenesis and the role of the local DNA sequence environment. *Hum Genet* **86**:425, 1991.
88. Kunkel TA: Misalignment-mediated DNA-synthesis errors. *Biochemistry* **29**:8003, 1990.
89. Sewell AC: Urinary oligosaccharides, in Hommes FA (ed): *Techniques in Diagnostic Human Biochemical Genetics*. New York, Wiley-Liss, 1991, p 219.
90. Humbel R, Collart M: Oligosaccharides in the urine of patients with glycoprotein storage diseases. Rapid detection by thin layer chromatography. *Clin Chim Acta* **60**:143, 1975.
91. Sewell AC: An improved thin-layer chromatographic method for urinary oligosaccharide screening. *Clin Chim Acta* **92**:411, 1979.
92. Mononen T, Parviainen M, Penttilä I, Mononen I: Liquid-chromatographic detection of aspartylglucosaminuria. *Clin Chem* **32**:501, 1986.
93. Marnela T: Automated ion-exchange chromatography in the detection of aspartylglucosaminuria. *J Chromatogr* **182**:409, 1980.
94. Aula P, Raivio K, Autio S: Enzymatic diagnosis and carrier detection of aspartylglucosaminuria using blood samples. *Pediatr Res* **10**:625, 1976.
95. Levvy GA, McAllan A: The N-acetylation and estimation of hexosamines. *Biochem J* **73**:127, 1959.
96. Mononen IT, Kaartinen VM, Williams JC: A fluorometric assay for glycosylasparaginase activity and detection of aspartylglucosaminuria. *Analyt Biochem* **208**:372, 1993.
97. Voznyi Y, Keulemans JL, Kleijer WJ, Aula P, Gray GR, van Diggelen OP: Applications of a new fluorimetric enzyme assay for the diagnosis of aspartylglucosaminuria. *J Inher Metab Dis* **16**:929, 1993.
98. Syvänen A-C, Ikonen E, Manninen T, Bergström M, Söderlund H, Aula P, Peltonen L: Convenient and quantitative determination of the frequency of a mutant allele using solid-phase minisequencing: Application to aspartylglucosaminuria. *Genomics* **12**:590, 1992.
99. Delahunty CM, Ankener W, Brainerd S, Nickerson DA, Mononen IT: Finnish-type aspartylglucosaminuria detected by oligonucleotide ligation assay. *Clin Chem* **41**:59, 1995.
100. Nilssen O, Tollersrud OK, Borud O, Tranebjaerg L: A simple and rapid PCR based method for AGU-fin determination. *Hum Molec Genet* **2**:484, 1993.

101. Hietala M, Grön K, Syvänen A-C, Peltonen L, Aula P: Prospects of carrier screening of aspartylglucosaminuria in Finland. *Eur J Hum Genet* **1**:296, 1993.
102. Hietala M, Aula P, Syvänen A-C, Isoniemi A, Peltonen L, Palotie A: DNA-based carrier screening in primary healthcare: Screening for aspartylglucosaminuria in maternity health offices. *Clin Chem* **42**:1398, 1996.
103. Hietala M, Hakonen A, Aro AR, Niemelä P, Peltonen L, Aula P: High acceptance of carrier screening among Finnish pregnant women: A pilot study using aspartylglucosaminuria gene test. *Prenat Diagn* (in press).
104. Hietala M, Hakonen A, Aro AR, Niemelä P, Peltonen L, Aula P: Attitudes toward gene testing among the general population and relatives of patients with a severe genetic disease: A survey from Finland. *Am J Hum Genet* **56**:1493, 1995.
105. Mononen I, Kaartinen V, Mononen T: Amniotic fluid glycoasparagines in fetal aspartylglucosaminuria. *J Inher Metab Dis* **11**:194, 1988.
106. Aula P, Mattila K, Piiroinen O, Ämmälä P, von Koskull H: First trimester prenatal diagnosis of aspartylglucosaminuria. *Prenat Diagn* **9**:617, 1989.
107. Suzuki K, Proia RL, Suzuki K: Mouse models of human lysosomal diseases. *Brain Path* **8**:195, 1998.
108. Tenhunen K, Uusitalo A, Autti T, Joensuu R, Kauppinen R, Haltia M, Ikonen S, Ginns EI, Jalanko A, Peltonen L: Monitoring the CNS pathology in aspartylglucosaminuria mice. *J Neuropathol Exp Neurol* **57**:1154, 1998.
109. Kyttälä A, Heinonen O, Peltonen L, Jalanko A: Expression and endocytosis of lysosomal aspartylglucosaminidase in mouse primary neurons. *J Neurosci* **57**:1154, 1998.
110. Peltola M, Kyttälä A, Heinonen O, Rapola J, Paunio T, Revah F, Peltonen L, Jalanko A: Adenovirus-mediated gene transfer results in decreased lysosomal storage in brain and total correction in liver of aspartylglucosaminuria (AGU) mouse. *Gene Ther* **5**:1314, 1998.
111. Enomaa N, Danos O, Peltonen L, Jalanko A: In vitro correction of deficient enzyme activity in a lysosomal storage disease, aspartylglucosaminuria. *Human Gene Ther* **6**:723, 1995.
112. Autti T, Santavuori P, Raininko R, Renlund M, Rapola J, Saarinen-Pihkala U: Bone-marrow transplantation in aspartylglucosaminuria. *Lancet* **349**:1366, 1998.
113. Fisher KJ, Aronson NN: Deletion of exon 8 causes glycosylasparaginase deficiency in an African American aspartylglucosaminuria (AGU) patient. *FEBS Lett* **288**:173, 1991.
114. Park H, Vettese MD, Fisher KJ, Aronson NN: Characterization of three alleles causing aspartylglucosaminuria: Two from a British family and one from an American patient. *Biochem J* **290**:735, 1993.
115. Laine M, Richter J, Fahlman C, Rapola J, Renlund M, Peltonen L, Karlsson S, Jalanko A: Correction of peripheral lysosomal accumulation in mice with aspartylglucosaminuria by bone marrow transplantation. *Exp Hematol* **27**:1467, 1999.
116. Dunder U, Kaartinen V, Valtonen P, Vaananen E, Kosma VM, Heisterkamp N, Groffen J, Mononen I: Enzyme replacement therapy in a mouse model of aspartylglucosaminuria. *FASEB J* **14**:361, 2000.

CHAPTER 142

Acid Lipase Deficiency: Wolman Disease and Cholesteryl Ester Storage Disease

Gerd Assmann ■ Udo Seedorf

1. **Deficient activity of lysosomal acid lipase results in massive accumulation of cholesteryl esters and triglycerides in most tissues of the body. Both of these lipids are substrates for the enzyme, one of the major functions of which is the hydrolysis of cholesteryl esters in various lipoproteins as they are removed from plasma by tissues in the periphery. The deficiency state is expressed in two major phenotypes: Wolman disease and cholesteryl ester storage disease.**
2. **Wolman disease occurs in infancy and is nearly always fatal before the age of 1 year. Hepatosplenomegaly, steatorrhea, abdominal distension, other gastrointestinal symptoms, adrenal calcification demonstrable on x-ray examination, and failure to thrive are observed in the first weeks of life.**
3. **Cholesteryl ester storage disease can be more benign. It may not be detected until adulthood. Lipid deposition is widespread, although hepatomegaly may be the only clinical abnormality. Hyperbetalipoproteinemia is common, and premature atherosclerosis may be severe. Adrenal calcification is rare.**
4. **Diagnosis of both disorders is based on the clinical picture combined with demonstration of acid lipase deficiency in cultured skin fibroblasts, lymphocytes, or other tissues. Both Wolman disease and cholesteryl ester storage disease are autosomal recessive disorders, involving the structural gene for acid lipase, which is located on chromosome 10q23.2-q23.3. Wolman disease is caused by a variety of different mutations, leading to complete elimination of the enzyme function. Conversely, one relatively common allele, associated with ~5 percent residual activity, is responsible for most cases of cholesteryl ester storage disease.**
5. **There is no specific therapy, but the suppression of cholesterol synthesis and apolipoprotein B production by 3-hydroxy-3-methylglutaryl coenzyme A reductase inhibitors in combination with cholestyramine treatment and a diet excluding foods rich in cholesterol and triglycerides results in a noticeable clinical improvement in at least some cases of cholesteryl ester storage disease. Prenatal diagnosis is based on the absence of acid lipase activity in cultured chorionic villus cells. In addition, genotyping of chorionic villus DNA can be used to confirm the diagnosis.**

A list of standard abbreviations is located immediately preceding the index in each volume. Nonstandard abbreviations used in this chapter include: ACAT = acyl CoA:cholesterol acyltransferase; CESD = cholesteryl ester storage disease; LAL = lysosomal acid lipase; LCAT = lecithin-cholesterol acyltransferase.

Two diseases have been independently discovered in which prodigious amounts of cholesteryl esters and often triglycerides accumulate in lysosomes. Wolman disease is the more severe form. The abnormality of lipid metabolism becomes clinically evident in the first weeks of life. The most important clinical features include hepatosplenomegaly, digestive difficulties, steatorrhea, and enlargement and calcification of the adrenal glands. The condition is usually fatal by the age of 6 months. Cholesteryl ester storage disease (CESD) is more benign, is usually compatible with survival to adulthood, and is very rarely associated with adrenal calcification.[1–4]

It is now well established that these disorders are allelic, involving mutations at the *LIPA* locus encoding a hydrolase which cleaves cholesteryl esters and triglycerides under acidic conditions (Fig. 142-1). The enzyme (EC 3.1.1.13) has been variously called lysosomal acid lipase (LAL), acid lipase, or acid esterase.

HISTORY

In 1956, Abramov, Schorr, and Wolman described an infant with abdominal distension, hepatosplenomegaly, and massive calcification of the adrenal glands.[5] In 1961, Wolman et al. reported two more affected sibs in the same family.[6] In the first report, Wolman and his colleagues[5] noted the accumulation of both cholesteryl esters and triglycerides in the liver, adrenal glands, spleen, and lymph nodes. The disorder was first called "generalized xanthomatosis with calcified adrenals" or "primary familial xanthomatosis with adrenal calcification."[5–7] Later, Crocker et al.[8] suggested the eponym Wolman disease. In retrospect, a patient described by Alexander in 1946[9] as having "Niemann-Pick disease" may have been the first with this disorder to appear in the literature.

In 1961, Wolman et al. demonstrated that most of the cholesterol was in the esterified form.[6] Later studies repeatedly confirmed these observations. In 1969, Patrick and Lake[10] demonstrated that activity of an acid hydrolase catalyzing the hydrolysis of both cholesteryl esters and triglycerides was severely deficient in the liver and spleen of patients with Wolman disease. This has been confirmed in tissues,[11,12] including cultured fibroblasts[13–16] and leukocytes,[17–19] of other patients. In 1976, Cortner et al. demonstrated that lysosomal acid lipase activity of circulating lymphocytes and cultured fibroblasts can be separated by cellogel electrophoresis into isoenzymes A and B.[13] Both Wolman disease and CESD cells showed complete absence of the A isoenzyme.[13,17]

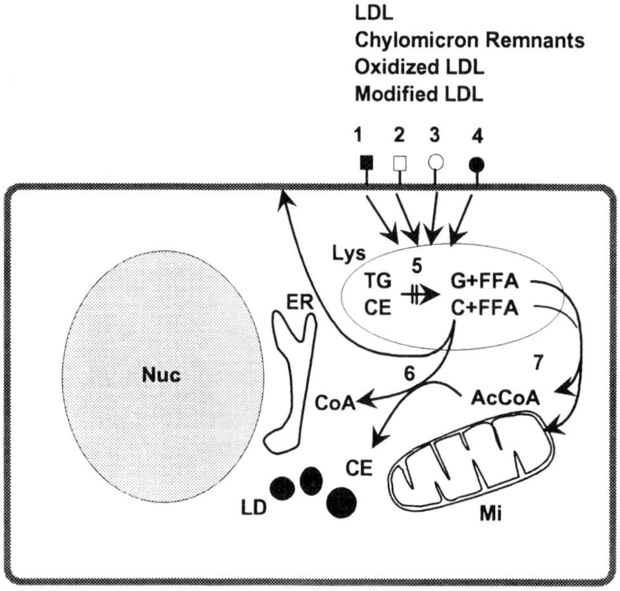

Fig. 142-1 Schematic representation of the hydrolytic site affected by the enzyme deficiency underlying acid lipase deficiency. Lipoproteins enter cells via receptor-mediated endocytosis (*1* LDL receptor; *2* chylomicron remnant receptor; *3* and *4* "scavenger receptors" for oxidized and modified LDL). Lysosomal hydrolytic degradation of lipoproteins involves acid lipase (*5*), which is defective in Wolman disease and CESD. The cellular phenotype consists of lysosomal storage of cholesteryl esters and triglycerides. Transfer- and acyl coA (ACAT; *6*)-mediated esterification of cholesterol at the lipid droplet (LD) and fatty acid transfer to mitochondrial β-oxidation via FABP (fatty acid binding protein; *7*) are absent or markedly reduced in both disorders. Nuc = nucleus; ER = endoplasmic reticulum; CE = cholesteryl esters; Mi = mitochondria; AcCoA = acyl CoA; Lys = lysosome.

Since then, more than 50 examples of Wolman disease have been described. The clinical and morphologic findings of the individual patients are presented in patient reports[5,6,8,10,11,13,17,18,20–64] and previous editions of this book.[1–4,65]

Brief published mention of CESD was first made by Fredrickson in 1963 in reference to a child with marked hyperlipidemia, whose enlarged liver was found to contain 18 percent of its wet weight as cholesteryl esters. He called the disorder "hepatic cholesterol ester storage disorder."[66] In 1967, Lageron et al.[67] and Infante el al.[68] reported a 43-year-old man with apparently the same disease under the name "polycorie cholestérolique de l'adulte." The patient had been known to have had hepatomegaly since age 14. At about the same time, Schiff et al. reported a brother and sister with similar clinical, morphologic, and biochemical abnormalities.[69] Four of their five younger sibs also had hepatomegaly. Biopsy specimens of liver from three of these sibs were interpreted as showing minimal morphologic abnormalities, suggesting a milder expression of the same inherited defect. The authors pointed out the presence of minimal cirrhosis in the liver, in addition to the fat loading of all hepatocytes seen in the other cases.

The following year, Partin and Schubert[70] described detailed studies of jejunal and duodenal biopsy specimens in the two most severely affected children of the kindred of Schiff et al.[69] The evidence they presented of cholesterol storage in the intestine was the first to indicate that the involvement of CESD extends beyond the liver. This concept has been substantiated by autopsy studies in three patients with CESD.[1,71,72] The less limited term cholesterol (or cholesteryl) ester storage disease proposed by Partin and Schubert has subsequently been used for the disorder. More than 40 reported cases of this disease have been recognized.[12,66–69,72–99] As in Wolman disease, the metabolic defect in CESD consists of severe deficiency in the activity of acid cholesteryl ester hydrolase, or acid lipase, which catalyzes the hydrolysis of both cholesteryl esters and triglycerides.

The enzymatic defect was demonstrated in several types of cells and tissues, including liver, spleen, lymph nodes, aorta, peripheral blood leukocytes, and cultured skin fibroblasts. Goldstein et al.[95] compared fibroblast extracts incubated at acid pH and intact fibroblast monolayers from normal and CESD individuals. While the cholesteryl esterase activity of mutant cell lysates was less than one-twentieth that of normal lysates, the intact mutant cells showed rates of cholesteryl ester hydrolysis that were nearly one-third that of normal cells. Subsequently, similar findings were reported with various substrates in intact fibroblasts and fibroblast lysates from Wolman disease and other CESD patients.[100] These observations led to the hypothesis that the residual activity of the mutated enzyme may be higher in CESD than in Wolman disease. More recently, this hypothesis has gained considerable support from the identification of several mutations that were detected in the *LIPA* locus from patients with either Wolman or cholesteryl ester storage disease. Anderson et al.[101] described two LAL mutations causing Wolman disease. One predicted an L179P replacement, located close to the active site at S153; the other was a frameshift mutation at nucleotide position 634 (634 insT) leading to a premature stop codon (Fs178). At about the same time, Klima et al.[102] had shown that combination of a null allele with an allele harboring a splice junction mutation in exon 8 (called $\Delta254-277_1$, or 934G → A) may cause cholesteryl ester storage disease. In their case, a G → A mutation at position −1 of the exon 8 splice donor site led to exon skipping, thereby causing deletion of codons 254–277 in the LAL mRNA. The mutated allele resulted in production of a truncated enzyme lacking 24 internal amino acids. Homozygosity for the same mutation was subsequently demonstrated in a Spanish kindred with cholesteryl ester storage disease.[103] Moreover, the mutation was found in conjunction with a T → C transition in exon 10 predicting an L336P replacement and an A → C transversion in exon 2 predicting a T(−6)P replacement in a Canadian-Norwegian kindred with cholesteryl ester storage disease.[104] The L336P replacement was identified as the second defect underlying the disease, whereas the T(−6)P replacement represented a frequent nonpathologic polymorphism. Since then, the $\Delta254-277_1$ mutation has been found either homozygous or in *trans* with other mutations in a great number of patients with CESD.[102–111] In fact, the vast majority of all patients with CESD who were studied during the past 4 years were carriers for at least one copy of this allele (Table 142-1). In contrast, the allele has so far not been found in any patient with Wolman disease. Two cases with this disorder from our laboratory resulted from the homozygous presence of alleles predicting early truncations (S112X, 454insA) of the enzyme, which would lead to absence of the catalytically active triad (located at S153). Another case was caused by homozygous presence of a TAT → TAA replacement at codon position 303, thus creating a premature stop in place of Tyr303 (Y303X). The consequence of the latter defect was a truncation of 75 amino acids from the C-terminus of the enzyme. Although the residual acid lipase activity assayed in cell extracts from three homozygous carriers of the $\Delta254-277_1$ allele and from these patients with Wolman disease was similar (2–5 percent of normal), esterification of exogenous cholesterol in the intact Wolman disease fibroblasts was almost undetectable, whereas the homozygous $\Delta254-277_1$ cell lines had residual rates of 12–24 percent. The molecular basis for the residual activity associated with the $\Delta254-277_1$ allele was elucidated by Aslanidis et al.[109] They found a small fraction of correctly spliced acid lipase mRNA (∼3–5 percent) in a compound heterozygous patient with CESD. Conversely, the truncated enzyme that is translated from abnormally spliced mRNA had no detectable cholesteryl ester hydrolyzing activity.

In view of these data, it now appears highly likely that the fact that CESD has a more benign clinical course than Wolman disease does is due to the fact that the $\Delta254-277_1$ allele leads to production of a small fraction of normal enzyme, thereby leading

Table 142-1 Genotypes of Patients with CESD or Wolman Disease

Diagnosis	Genotype*	Ethnic background	Reference
CESD	Δ254–277$_1$/G245X	Polish-German	[102,109]
CESD	Δ254–277$_1$/967del2	American	[111]
CESD	Δ254–277$_1$/Δ254–277$_1$	Spanish	[103]
CESD	Δ254–277$_1$/L336P	Canadian/Norwegian	[104]
CESD	Δ254–277$_1$/Δ254–277$_1$	Turkish	[107]
CESD	Δ254–277$_1$/L179P	American	[110]
CESD	Δ254–277$_1$/Δ254–277$_1$	Croatian	[Seedorf & Assmann, unpublished]
CESD	Δ254–277$_1$/H274Y	Italian	[105]
CESD	Δ254–277$_1$/R44X	French	[105, 275]
CESD	Δ254–277$_1$/H108P	Austrian	[106]
CESD	Δ205–253/P181L	Italian	[108]
CESD	Δ254–277$_1$/G66V	Italian	[108]
CESD	L273S/null?	Italian	[108]
CESD	H274Y/H274Y	Italian	[126]
CESD	H108R/null?	Caucasian	[127a]
Wolman	L179P/634insT	American	[101]
Wolman	438delC	Turkish	[127b]
Wolman	438delC/438delC	Turkish	[127b]
Wolman	Y303X/Y303X	Italian	[127c]
Wolman	Δ254–277$_3$/Δ254–277$_3$	African	[128]
Wolman	Δ254–277$_2$/Δ254–277$_2$	Not reported	[109]
Wolman	Y22X/Y22X	Japanese	[129]

*Nucleotides are numbered 1 to 2493 according to GenBank M74775. The signal peptide is bp 41 to 103 or amino acids (−)21 to (−)1. The mature peptide is bp 104–1237 or amino acids–334. According to recommended nomenclature, mutations with skipping of exon 8 are as follows: Δ254–277$_1$ = 934G → A; Δ254–277$_2$ = IVS8 + 1G → A; and Δ254–277$_3$ = IVS7–C → T; that skipping exon 7 is Δ295–253 = IVS6–2A → G.

to a low level of residual acid lipase activity in these patients. In contrast, Wolman disease seems to result from alleles predicting complete elimination of the enzyme function.

CLINICAL MANIFESTATIONS

Wolman Disease

Most patients with Wolman disease have had remarkably similar clinical courses. Increasing vomiting and diarrhea, hepatosplenomegaly, abdominal distension, anemia, and inanition are major clinical signs, and the child's general condition progresses rapidly downhill. Death usually occurs by age 3 to 6 months but has been protracted to as long as 14 months.[33]

The disease usually has its onset in the first weeks of life. In most cases the abnormality first noticed by the parents is persistent and forceful vomiting associated with marked abdominal distension. Several patients also had frequent and watery stools in the first few weeks of life.[30,33,37] In a few patients, jaundice[5,8,22,43] or persistent low-grade fever has been observed.[6,8]

Anemia usually appears by the sixth week and becomes more severe as the disease progresses; the hemoglobin may fall to 6 g/dl. Thrombocytopenia has not been observed. Vacuolization of lymphocytes has been noted repeatedly. The vacuoles are both intracytoplasmic and intranuclear. Lipid-laden histiocytes, or foam cells, have been observed in bone marrow aspirates as early as 40 days of age. In the later stages of the illness, the marrow almost invariably contains large numbers of foam cells. Similar cells have been observed in peripheral blood.[6] Acanthocytosis has been reported in one patient.[35] Plasma lipids are usually at the low end of the normal range.

Hepatosplenomegaly has been observed as early as the fourth day of life.[37] It is an invariable feature of the disease and may be of massive proportions. The most striking feature of Wolman disease is calcification of the adrenal glands. This abnormality has been consistently demonstrated antemortem by roentgenographic examination in all but four patients. The adrenals are markedly and symmetrically enlarged (up to 3.5 × 2.5 cm), and their normal pyramidal or semilunar shape is retained. They are extensively seeded with finely stippled or punctuate calcific deposits. The enlarged adrenals may flatten the superior poles of the kidneys,[8] but they do not deform the caliceal system or interfere with renal function. The density of the enlarged liver and the cortical calcification of the enlarged adrenals could be monitored with high sensitivity using CT (Fig. 142-2).[112]

Specific symptoms related to the central nervous system are uncommon in Wolman disease, but neurologic development is not normal. Typically alert and active at birth, the infants show progressive mental disorientation within a few weeks after the onset of the symptoms. Several case reports have noted that the optic fundi were normal and that a cherry-red spot was not present. A Babinski sign was elicited in one patient.[7] Konno et al. described a patient who had exaggerated tendon reflexes, ankle clonus, and opisthotonos.[22] Paralysis and convulsions have not been observed.

There are no specific routine laboratory observations that suggest the diagnosis. Liver function tests are frequently abnormal. Laboratory studies support the clinical observations of malabsorption and malnutrition. As determined by feeding ^{131}I-labeled triolein[35] or unlabeled fats,[37] there appears to be significant impairment of fat absorption. Histologic, biochemical, and electrophysical observations suggest that the intestinal damage in Wolman disease may be so severe as to virtually exclude the absorption of nearly any form of enteral nutrition.[64] ACTH-stimulation studies have indicated depressed adrenal responsiveness.[8,37] No gross abnormalities of the electroencephalogram have been observed in several patients.[8,22,27,35] Chromosomal analyses in two patients were normal.[22,49]

Cholesteryl Ester Storage Disease

The history and clinical course of the original patients affected with CESD are extensively discussed in previous editions of this

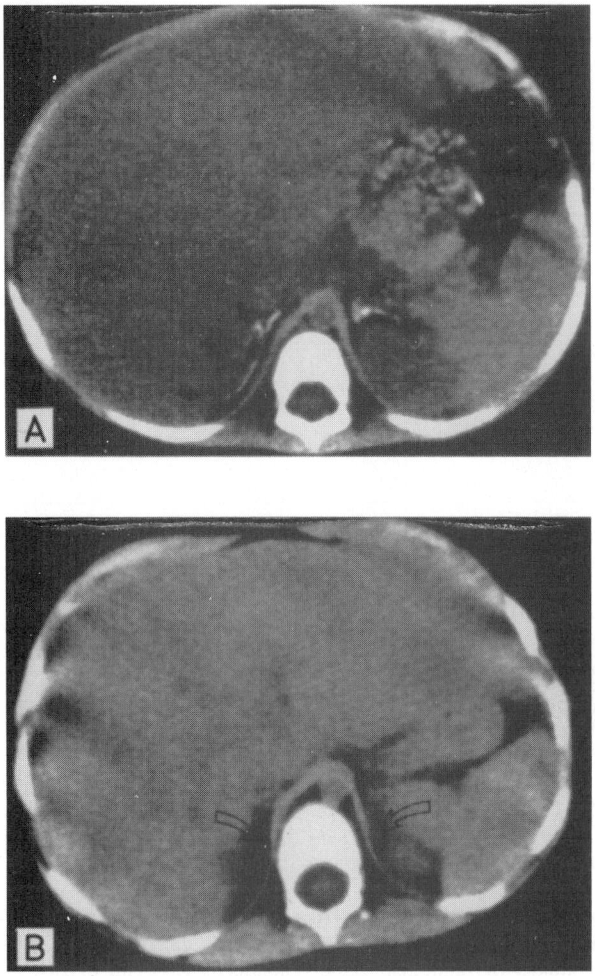

Fig. 142-2 Computed tomography. (A) Wolman disease: The liver is enlarged and has a diffuse homogeneous reduction in density. The spleen is normal in size and density. There is bilateral adrenal enlargement with linear cortical calcification (arrows). (B) CESD: There is diffuse homogenous enlargement of the liver. The spleen is normal in size and density. The adrenal glands (arrows) are normal in size, with no calcification. (*Courtesy of Dr. S.C. Hill and Dr. J.M. Hoeg and reprinted with permission.*[112])

book.[1–4,65] In contrast to Wolman disease, CESD is characterized by a relatively variable phenotype. The principal and sometimes only sign, hepatomegaly, may be evident at birth or in early childhood. Occasionally it is delayed until the second decade of life. An extremely benign variant of CESD was diagnosed in two female patients aged 43 and 56 years.[81] The clinical findings in both patients were confined to moderate, well-tolerated hepatomegaly, type IIb hyperlipoproteinemia, and xanthelasmata. Acid lipase activity was markedly deficient in peripheral leukocytes and cultured fibroblasts. In all cases of CESD, hepatomegaly apparently increases with time and eventually leads to hepatic fibrosis. The spleen has been found to be enlarged in about one-third of the patients. Massive splenomegaly and splenic abscess has been described in one patient.[79] Esophageal varices have occasionally been detected. Liver failure has developed in four patients from two families of Mexican descent. Acute liver failure developed in two patients, while chronic liver failure developed in their sib and in a patient from another family.[72,94,97,98] Jaundice has been noted in several other patients. Gallstones have not been found in any of the patients. A number of patients have had recurrent abdominal pain and occasionally some delay in puberty. A few patients had recurrent epistaxes, episodes of gastrointestinal bleeding, hypoprothrombinemia, or decreased concentration of blood clotting factor V.[90]

Malabsorption, malnutrition, or abnormalities involving the tonsils have not been described. Rarely, neurologic changes have been noticed. One patient had unexplained episodes of headache, vertigo, hypersomnia, and loss of consciousness.[68] Although adrenal calcification is rare and not prominent, finely punctuated calcific deposits may be detected on abdominal roentgenograms in some cases. One patient had roentgenographic evidence of calcification of the hepatic artery.[1,12] Exclusive of the plasma lipids, there are no distinctive abnormalities in routine laboratory tests. In some cases, bone marrow aspirates contained numerous large macrophages filled with birefringent droplets; in others, bone marrow appeared normal.[80]

PATHOLOGY

Liver

Hepatomegaly is a constant feature in Wolman disease; the liver appears to increase in size throughout the course of the illness and by age 4 months may weigh 400 g, which is about twice the normal weight.[26] The liver has a firm consistency, and the cut surface is yellow and greasy.

The normal architecture of the liver is sometimes preserved[11] but may be so distorted that the portal spaces, even though infiltrated with lymphoid cells, provide the only readily recognizable landmarks.[5,6,8,33,37] The hepatic parenchymal cells are enlarged and vacuolated, and grossly enlarged and vacuolated Kupffer cells are prominent. Large numbers of foamy histiocytes are found in the portal and periportal areas and frequently in clusters between parenchymal cells. Portal and periportal fibrosis may be marked, and there may even be frank cirrhosis. Under the electron microscope one sees that the organelles and the parenchymal cells have accumulated large osmiophilic lipid droplets. Most of these droplets are found within lysosomes[35] (Fig. 142-3). The smooth and rough endoplasmic reticulum may appear dilated and distended.[37] It is not certain from histochemical studies whether both glycerides and cholesterol accumulate in the Kupffer and parenchymal cells.[6,8,33,37] The liver in CESD also has an extraordinary orange or butter-yellow color and a smooth, soft

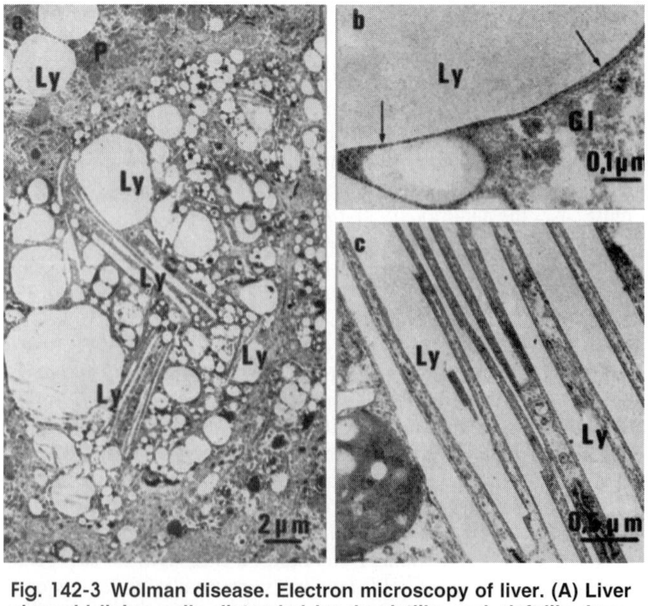

Fig. 142-3 Wolman disease. Electron microscopy of liver. (A) Liver sinusoid lining cells distended by dropletlike and cleft-like lysosomes (Ly). Dropletlike lysosomes in liver parenchymal cell (P). Magnification ×4500. (B) Membrane (arrows) of a dropletlike lysosome (Ly) in liver parenchymal cell. Glycogen granules (Gl). Magnification ×106,000. (C) High resolution microscopy of crystal cleft-like lysosomes (Ly) in liver sinusoidal cells. Magnification ×30,000. (*Courtesy of Dr. D.B. von Bassewitz.*)

texture. It is usually markedly enlarged, sometimes to twice the normal weight. Microscopic examination of the CESD liver reveals many of the same abnormalities as in Wolman disease, with some possible differences related to a disease process of much longer standing. There are (1) lipid droplets in hepatic parenchymal cells resembling those in ordinary fatty infiltration; (2) enlargement of Kupffer cells by smaller vacuoles and by periodic acid-Schiff-positive granules; (3) variable amounts of septal fibrosis, which has progressed in some patients to micronodular cirrhosis with esophageal varices; (4) focal periportal accumulations of lymphocytes, plasma cells, and foamy macrophages with little or no birefringence; and (5) vacuolization and (6) massive storage of birefringent material in hepatocytes. The Kupffer cells are greatly enlarged; have several small, indented, darkly staining nuclei; and appear more finely and uniformly vacuolated than the hepatocytes. The deposits of cholesteryl esters and triglycerides in hepatocytes appear relatively stable, while those in macrophages are transformed by peroxidation and polymerization of their fatty acids to insoluble ceroid, both in CESD and in Wolman disease.[38] The gradual formation of ceroid deposits from accumulated neutral lipid has been observed in a variety of other disease states.[113,114] In CESD, the deposits in macrophages in bone marrow, spleen, lymph nodes, and other organs tend to resemble histochemically and ultrastructurally those in hepatic macrophages, while the deposits in smooth muscle cells, perivascular cells, and endothelial cells are more similar to those in hepatocytes.

Electron microscopy of liver tissue in CESD[2,89] reveals the following: (1) There are cytoplasmic inclusions in the hepatocytes, containing material that in part seems to solubilize during the preparation and tends to form crystals after formalin fixation and storage at 4°C. (2) These inclusions are limited by trilaminar membranes 13 to 14 nm thick, consisting of a true vacuole membrane and a submembranous "halo" that is characteristic of lysosomes. There is also a thin limiting layer that has also been described in Tangier disease (Chap. 122), in which the inclusions contain cholesteryl esters but are not limited by membrane. (3) Heterogeneous storage material is found in Kupffer cells. (4) There are membrane-limited vacuoles containing partly dissolved, partly osmiophilic lipid (unsaturated fatty acids) in the epithelial cells of small bile ducts as well as in endothelial cells.

Two animal models with morphologic findings partly resembling those in hepatocytes and Kupffer cells of CESD and Wolman disease have been described. Drevon and Hovig[115] fed a semisynthetic diet containing 10 percent cottonseed oil and 1 percent cholesterol to guinea pigs and observed accumulation of multivacuolated, secondary lysosomes, membrane-bound lipid vacuoles (lipolysosomes), and myelin figures in liver. These microscopic changes were due to a marked accumulation of cholesteryl esters. Yoshida and Kuriyama[116] described Donryu rats who had inherited acid lipase deficiency in an autosomal recessive mode due to a large deletion at the 3′ end of the rat acid lipase gene.[117] Though adrenal calcification could not be found in affected animals, the spleen and liver showed massive accumulation of esterified cholesteryl oleate.[118]

Lipolysosomes (lysosomes containing large lipid droplets) can also be observed in livers of patients with various forms of hepatic injury.[115] Their numbers and sizes increase with the degree of fatty infiltration and probably represent a nonspecific finding.[119]

Adrenal Glands

The adrenal glands in Wolman disease are bright yellow and grossly and symmetrically enlarged; their configuration is, however, normal. Each gland may weigh as much as 13 g, as compared with a normal weight of 5 g. The adrenals are usually quite firm, contain flecks of gritty calcified tissue, and are difficult to cut. In cut section, the outer rim of cortex is an intense yellow and the central zone is gray or white.

Under microscopic examination it can be seen that the architecture of the outer and part of the middle zones of the cortex, that is, the zona glomerulosa and the zona fasciculata, are relatively well preserved. Many of the cells are swollen and vacuolated and contain sudanophilic lipid.[6,33] The areas corresponding to the inner fasciculata and the entire zona reticularis (the innermost portion of the cortex) are replaced by a broad zone of haphazardly arranged large cells with a vacuolated, foamy cytoplasm. Many of the cells contain anisotropic crystals or large clefts in the shape of cholesterol crystals.[37] Other foam cells seem necrotic, and their contents appear to have been released to form confluent lipid cysts. In the necrotic areas, calcification may be quite prominent. Most of the calcium occurs in fine granular deposits, but there may be areas in which it is condensed into dense lumps.[33] There is frequently extensive fibrosis in the inner half of the cortex; histochemical techniques indicate the presence of large amounts of lipid with staining properties suggestive of cholesteryl esters and triglycerides.[6,8,28,37]

Adrenal calcification is not visually observed in CESD. Extensive chemical and histopathologic examination of the adrenals in CESD has not been done.

Intestine

The small intestine of patients affected with Wolman disease is usually thickened and dilated, with a dull, opaque yellow serosa and a swollen yellow mucosa with thick, flattened, yellow villi. The changes are generally most marked in the proximal parts of the small intestine and least apparent in the terminal ileum. In the small intestine, and to some extent in the colon, the lamina propria of the mucosa is infiltrated by foamy histiocytes. Some of the mucosal cells are also foamy. The infiltration of the mucosa by foam cells converts the villi into thick club-shaped structures.[2] Some foam cells extend through the muscularis mucosa to form small clusters in the submucosa, and similar cells are present in the lymphoid tissue. Some of the cells of the muscularis mucosa also stain positively for neutral lipids with Sudan stains. Sudanophilic staining may also be present in the myenteric plexus and in foamy endothelial cells within the intestinal adventitial layer. In some cases extensive intestinal damage can be observed.[64]

Partin and Schubert originally described changes in jejunal and duodenal biopsy specimens from two patients with CESD.[70] The epithelium was normal. Beneath the epithelium in the region of the lacteals were collections of autofluorescent foam cells, which were especially densely packed in the villous tips. Large amounts of extracellular lipid were present throughout the lamina propria. This lipid appeared birefringent and stained similarly to the fat in the foam cells but was more nonpolar and showed only a weakly positive Schultz reaction. Under the electron microscope the lipid appears electron-lucent with dense rims. Ultrastructural study of the lamina propria of the small intestine of the patients revealed several interesting features.[70] The lacteal endothelium was filled with round vacuoles that distended the smooth endoplasmic reticulum and looked as if they contained lipid taken up by pinocytosis. Many macrophages surrounded the lacteals and contained numerous vacuoles that were limited by membranes and were filled with material similar to that in hepatic macrophages. Lucent lipid droplets were present in adjacent smooth muscle cells, vascular pericytes, fibroblasts, and supporting cells of nerve fibers. The ultrastructural localization of membrane-limited lipid deposits in various cell types in intestinal mucosa and submucosa was similar in other patients. In one patient, foam cells were few and small in the lamina propria of the colon and the esophagus.[1]

Other Tissues

In Wolman disease, the spleen is always grossly enlarged and by age 3 months may weigh over 200 g, as compared with the normal weight of 15 g.[6] The spleen is firm, and its cut surface is red or reddish-yellow; the surface may be mottled with yellow or brown flecks. The normal follicular architecture is replaced by a homogeneous appearance. Microscopically, only a small number of follicles are present, and they are small and compressed. Most

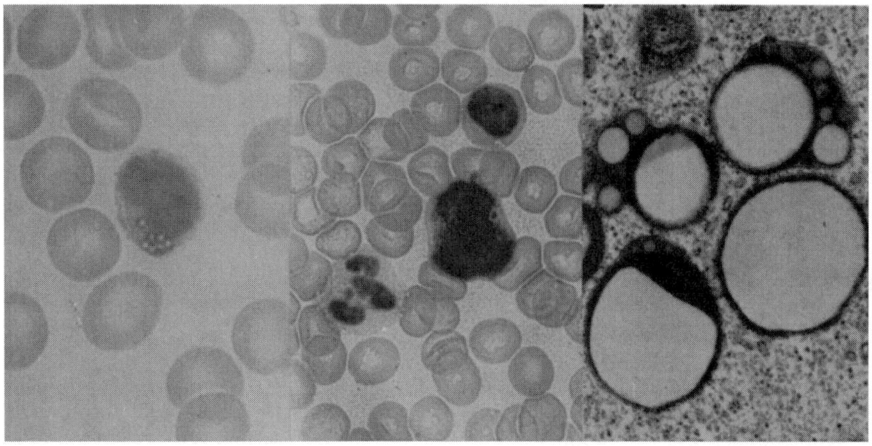

A B C

Fig. 142-4 Cholesteryl ester storage disease. Lipid storage vacuoles in lymphocytes. (A) Histochemical staining for naphthylbutyrate esterase (negative). (B) Histochemical staining for lysosomal acid phosphatase (strongly positive). (C) Electron microscopy of storage vacuoles, magnification ×60,000. (*Courtesy of Prof. H.E. Schaefer.*)

of the reticular cells are transformed into large foam cells, which make up the bulk of the organ. There is also swelling and vacuolization of endothelial cells lining the sinusoids. Lymph nodes throughout the body, particularly those in the mesentery, are enlarged, orange-yellow, firm, and elastic. Their cut surfaces are yellow and appear homogeneous. The microscopic and histochemical changes are quite similar to those found in the spleen. The bone marrow, thymus, and tonsils in Wolman disease undergo changes that are almost identical to those in the spleen and lymph nodes. Vacuolization of lymphocytes in the blood and bone marrow has often been noted in Wolman disease but is not specific to it. Excessive vacuolization of granulocytes has been reported in one case of Wolman disease.[18]

There are no gross kidney abnormalities in Wolman disease. Under the light microscope, the tubules appear normal but mesangial cells of the glomeruli may contain lipid droplets that both are sudanophilic and also stain for cholesterol.[26,33] There also may be foam cells in the interstitium. Foam cells have been observed in the thyroid,[26] testes,[8,26,33] and ovaries.[33] Wolman et al. observed sudanophilic droplets in the endothelium of capillaries of the gray matter and in swollen neurons in the medulla oblongata and the retina.[6] Crocker et al. later described the presence of foamy histiocytes in the leptomeninges.[8] They also noted a moderate decrease in the number of cortical neurons and found retarded myelination. Foam cells also occur in the interstitium of the choroid plexus.[22] Lipid storage in neurons, including Purkinje cells,[28] and sudanophilic granules within swollen microglia, periadventitial histiocytes, and possibly astrocytes have been observed in some patients.[28,32,33] One of the most extensive studies of the central nervous system in Wolman disease was made by Guazzi et al.[26,27] These investigators found an abundance of sudanophilic material and diffuse isomorphic fibrillary gliosis of the white matter, which they interpreted as sudanophilic leukodystrophy directly related to abnormal lipid storage. The autopsy was delayed for 2 days after death, however, and some of the reported changes may have been artifactual. Byrd and Powers[56] examined the peripheral and central nervous system ultrastructurally following autopsy of a 4-month-old child affected with Wolman disease. They demonstrated lipid storage in Schwann cells, perineural cells, and endoneural cells. In the central nervous system, the oligodendrocytes were the principal sites of lipid accumulation, especially in areas of active myelination.

Kamoshita and Landing[29] first made the observation that ganglion cells of the plexuses of both Auerbach and Meissner were packed with sudanophilic granules in Wolman disease. These changes were found in stomach, duodenum, and small intestine and have been repeatedly confirmed. Storage of sudanophilic lipids in sympathetic neurons has also been observed in one patient.[28]

In CESD, lipid storage in most tissues is more discrete. Foam cells were detected in the interstitium in lung and renal glomeruli.[12] Endothelial cells in numerous anatomic sites contained fine lipid droplets, as did smooth muscle cells in certain arterioles, particularly in the spleen. Electron microscopy showed that the droplets in endothelium were also limited by single, trilaminar membranes. Histologic study of the central nervous system showed no evidence of abnormal lipid storage. In contrast, abnormal lipid deposits can be detected in lymphocytes (Fig. 142-4), monocytes, and cultured skin fibroblasts of CESD patients (Fig. 142-5).[72,77,86,93,94] In lymphocytes (fresh unstained preparations), secondary lysosomes can be histochemically identified by acid phosphatase staining. The α-naphthylbutyrate esterase activity normally present in lymphocytes is completely absent from lymphocytes in CESD patients (Schaefer AE, Assmann G: unpublished data). In electron microscopy, the storage lysosomes

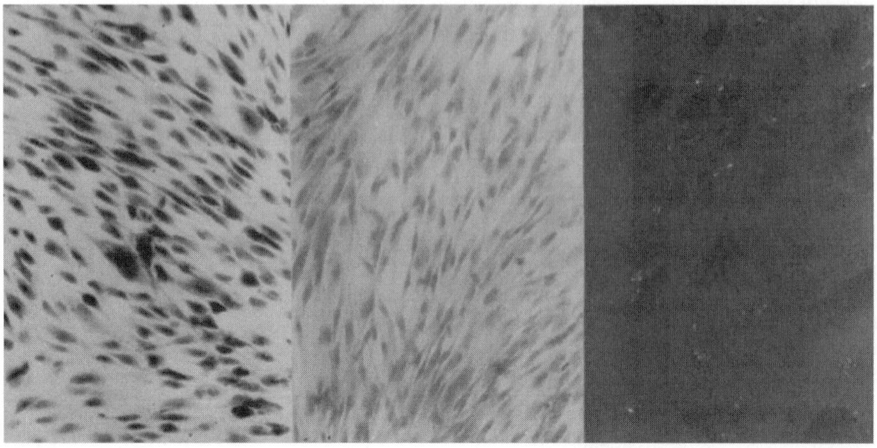

A B C

Fig. 142-5 Cholesteryl ester storage disease. (A) Normal fibroblasts stained for naphthylbutyrate esterase (strongly positive). (B) CESD fibroblasts stained for naphthylbutyrate esterase (negative). (C) CESD fibroblasts visualized in plane-polarized light birefringence (positive). (*Courtesy of Prof. H.E. Schaefer.*)

can easily be visualized through their typical trilaminar membranes. Except for lymphocytes and monocytes, blood cells are unaffected in CESD. In cultured skin fibroblasts of CESD patients, both birefringence in plane-polarized light and the absence of α-naphthylbutyrate esterase staining permit the rapid identification of acid lipase deficiency.

Atherosclerosis

On gross examination, the heart and lungs of patients with Wolman disease appear normal. Routine histologic examination of the heart also reveals no abnormalities, but in frozen sections many sudanophilic droplets may be found in the muscles[26] and vascular endothelium.[8,26] Lipid deposition in the aorta may be extensive,[38] but frank atherosclerosis has not been seen. Nevertheless, most patients affected with Wolman disease in whom postmortem examination of the arteries was made showed some degree of fat accumulation, which may be classified as fatty streaks and represent early atherosclerotic lesions.[8,11,33,38,40,44,47] The lungs contain variable numbers of foam cells in the alveoli and intestinal tissue.[8,26,33]

With the exception of one CESD patient, in whom obstructive pulmonary vascular disease developed at 15 years of age[112] and who died of liver failure at age 18,[97] none of the patients known to have CESD, including two who are in their fourth decade of life, have had clinical evidence of coronary or systemic atherosclerosis.[12] Three of the four patients who came to autopsy, however, have had anatomic evidence of a much accelerated atherosclerotic process. One patient, who died at age 21, had severe (up to 75 percent) coronary arterial luminal narrowing by atheromatous plaques, as well as striking, but functionally less severe, lesions in the circle of Willis, the abdominal aorta, and the common iliac arteries. The patient died a cardiac death, and at autopsy she also had recent cardiac necrosis, but her death appeared to be related to severe aortic valvular stenosis rather than to coronary artery disease. Another patient, who died at age 9, had a few elevated yellow plaques in the ascending aorta. Her affected sib, who died at age 8, had no abnormalities of the aorta or coronary arteries. It is not known how much of the atherosclerosis in these patients was directly related to CESD or to associated hypercholesterolemia, hyperbetalipoproteinemia, and high density lipoprotein (HDL) deficiency. Xanthomas of the type seen in familial hypercholesterolemia do not develop in patients with CESD.

The fact that most patients affected with CESD may be at risk for premature atherosclerosis is potentially of great importance. It could support the hypothesis of De Duve,[120] who suggested that a relative deficiency of LAL might lead to the accumulation of cholesteryl esters within lysosomes of arterial smooth muscle cells[121–123] and thus promote atheroma formation.

LIPID ABNORMALITIES

Wolman Disease

The principal stored lipids present in increased quantities in various tissues are cholesteryl esters and triglycerides.[1–4,65] The triglyceride concentration in the liver may be 2 to 10 times the normal value. In the spleen, the triglycerides may be elevated from eight- to a hundredfold. The triglyceride content of the adrenals has been reported in only one case,[37] in which it was half the normal value. The concentrations of monoglycerides and diglycerides were elevated five- to fifteenfold in the liver and spleen of the two patients in which they were measured[22,37] and were modestly, if at all, elevated in the adrenals of one patient.[37]

The total cholesterol concentration in liver and spleen has been elevated in every case of Wolman disease in which measurements have been reported. Although the free cholesterol concentration has frequently been greater than normal, the bulk of the increase in total cholesterol is due to the accumulation of cholesteryl esters. The cholesteryl ester content of the liver may be five to 160 times the normal value. It was shown in one case[37] that cholesteryl esters were elevated eightfold in the adrenals.[2,65] Analyses of fatty acids of triglycerides and cholesteryl esters in the liver, spleen, and other tissues of patients with Wolman disease revealed no consistent abnormality.[2,65] On examining chromatograms of published tissue analyses[33] as well as their own, Assmann and coworkers concluded that oxygenated steryl esters were also present in Wolman disease.[65] They were identified as esters of 7α- and 7β-hydroxycholesterol, 7-ketocholesterol, and 5,6β- and 5,6α-epoxycholesterol, in this order of preponderance.

An increase in the free fatty acid content of the liver and spleen has been reported in Wolman disease.[10,22] The phospholipid and glycolipid contents of the liver and the spleen have not been abnormal. Lin and coworkers[124] have reported increased quantities of alkyl and alk-1-enyl glycolipids in the liver, spleen, and adrenals of a patient with Wolman disease. No consistent abnormalities have been detected in the neutral lipids, phospholipids, or glycolipids in the nervous system.

Cholesteryl Ester Storage Disease

Chemical abnormalities in tissues in CESD are thus far known to be present in the liver, intestine, spleen, lymph node, aorta, and cultured skin fibroblasts. Lipid analyses of liver in CESD patients revealed an increase in cholesteryl esters, the concentration being 120 to 350 times normal. In one patient, 94 percent of the glyceride fraction was triglyceride, with only small amounts of diglycerides and monoglycerides as determined chromatographically.[65] The percentage distribution of hepatic phospholipids was phosphatidylcholine plus phosphatidylinositol, 49 percent; phosphatidylethanolamine, 31 percent; sphingomyelin, 11.5 percent; and lysophosphatidylcholine, 7 percent.[65] In another patient, it was concluded that sphingomyelin in liver might be increased and phosphatidylethanolamine decreased.[68] Liver glycolipids or glyceryl ethers have not been studied adequately in any patient in CESD.

In one patient, triglyceride and cholesteryl ester content was increased in the spleen and aorta, whereas in other patients, cholesterol and triglyceride analyses of spleen, kidney, lung, and cerebral gray matter were reported as normal. In cultured skin fibroblasts of several patients, the total concentration of cholesterol was close to that in controls, while the concentration of cholesteryl esters was markedly elevated. The acyl groups in the cholesteryl esters in CESD liver have been reported to be predominantly oleic and linoleic acids,[21,68,69,89] a pattern which is grossly similar to that seen in esters stored in Tangier disease, eosinophilic granuloma, and atheromas.[125] The fatty acid composition of cholesteryl esters in the intestinal mucosa of one patient did not differ markedly from that in controls or from the patient's liver.[69]

Plasma Lipids and Lipoproteins

Plasma cholesterol and triglycerides have been normal in most patients with Wolman disease in whom such measurements have been made. Elevated triglycerides and very low density lipoprotein (VLDL) cholesterol were reported in three patients.[18,33] Five patients have had unquestionable decreases in plasma HDL as determined by electrophoresis or chemical tests.[11,18,39] The severely malnourished patient described by Eto and Kitagawa had a cholesterol level of 100 mg/dl and acanthocytosis.[35]

All CESD patients for whom plasma lipid levels have been reported had hypercholesterolemia. In some this has been associated with hypertriglyceridemia. The plasma lipoprotein pattern is either II-a or II-b (see Chap. 114). The originally described patient had a persistent, marked increase in plasma low density lipoprotein (LDL) cholesterol, in concentrations of about 330 mg/dl, and variable increases in VLDL.[1] The LDL cholesterol concentrations in the patient described by Wolf et al.[74] were elevated at both 11 and 17 years of age. Her father (age 50) and sister (age 22) both had hepatomegaly and hypercholesterolemia; the mother (age 50) had no clinical or lipid abnormalities.

The cholesteryl ester:free cholesterol ratio and the pattern of cholesteryl ester fatty acid in serum is normal in CESD.[1,74] Direct investigation of the enzymatic activity of lecithin:cholesterol acyltransferase has not been done. The plasma lipoprotein abnormalities in CESD frequently include HDL abnormalities. One patient, observed over a long time, had extremely low levels of plasma HDL cholesterol, with concentrations varying from 6 to 26 mg/dl, well below the 5 percent lower limit of normal and not explained by her modest hypertriglyceridemia.[1] Another patient was also said to have low HDL (in terms of α-lipoproteins on the electrophoretic pattern).[69] One patient had an HDL cholesterol of 20 mg/dl, which was drastically increased, to 47 mg/dl, by a combined treatment including 3-hydroxy-3-methylglutaryl coenzyme A (HMG-CoA) reductase inhibition, cholestyramine administration, and low-fat diet. In one patient, who had low HDL cholesterol values on repeated determinations, an analysis of the distribution of the subfractions HDL_2 and HDL_3 by zonal centrifugation has revealed a remarkable discrepancy from normal—instead of the usual 1:10 ratio of HDL_2 to HDL_3, a 10:1 ratio was observed.[2]

GENETIC ASPECTS

Mode of Inheritance

Wolman disease is inherited as an autosomal recessive disorder involving the structural gene for acid lipase, which is located on chromosome 10q23.2-q23.3. Males and females are affected in about equal numbers. In the original family reported by Wolman and his colleagues,[5,6] three sibs died of the disease, and numerous families since have had more than one affected child. The parents of the original patients and several subsequent pairs of parents were related,[11,42,44,46] although consanguinity has been denied in the majority of the affected families.[2,65] At least six cases, possibly seven,[2,65] have been reported in Israel, and all but one of these have apparently been Jews of Iraqi or Iranian origin.[11] The other patients have been reported from North America, Western Europe, Pakistan, China, and Japan.

CESD is also inherited as an autosomal recessive disorder. A few patients had esophageal varices and a seemingly more severe disorder than the others. Some patients have not been diagnosed by enzymatic assays or tissue analyses, and the presence of hepatomegaly cannot be accepted as evidence for vertical transmission of CESD. No consanguinity in parents has yet been documented.

In general, Wolman disease and CESD can be distinguished by their very different clinical courses. In Wolman disease, there is a marked accumulation of both triglycerides and cholesteryl esters, whereas storage of cholesteryl esters is much more pronounced in CESD. Enzymatic data do not explain why tissue triglycerides are not elevated in most cases with CESD. There is, however, a certain degree of phenotypic variation among the patients with acid lipase deficiency, a phenomenon common to most inborn lysosomal diseases. Besides the acute infantile form of Wolman disease, other forms may also exist that are of later onset and follow a less severe, more prolonged course.[51] Suzuki et al. described an atypical case of Wolman disease with absence of splenomegaly and normal adrenal glands.[17] Lack of adrenal calcification was also emphasized in two further cases of Wolman disease.[18,33] On the other hand, adrenal calcification, considered pathognomonic for Wolman disease, has also been observed in CESD.[72] The time of manifestation of liver cirrhosis and the severity of related symptoms differ considerably among the reported cases of CESD. Recent genetic data indicate that patients with acid lipase deficiency represent not only homozygous expression of different alleles but frequently also genetic compounds. Thus, allelic variance may be one factor that determines the clinical expression of the disorder. On the other hand, carriers of the same mutation also revealed considerable variation in the severity of their clinical symptoms and the abnormalities of their plasma lipid values.[103,107] It thus may be assumed that the expression of CESD is strongly modulated by environmental factors and the genetic background of the patients. One example supporting this notion is a Turkish patient who was homozygous for a G → A splice junction mutation in exon 8 ($\Delta 254\text{–}277_1$, or 934G → A).[107] He developed serious liver disease soon after birth, whereas the disease progressed more slowly in all known $\Delta 277_1$ homozygotes from Western Europe. Four Mexican American children with CESD have suffered acute or chronic liver failure before adulthood, and modulating genes or a more severe allele for CESD may exist in that ethnic group.[13,72]

Acid Lipase Mutations in Patients with CESD or Wolman Disease

Cholesteryl ester storage disease. Klima et al.[102] were the first who showed that combination of a null allele with an allele harboring a splice junction mutation in exon 8 (called $\Delta 254\text{–}277_1$) may cause cholesteryl ester storage disease. In their case, a 934G → A mutation in the last coding base of exon 8 led to exon skipping, thereby causing deletion of codons 254–277 in the mRNA. The abnormal allele resulted in production of a truncated enzyme lacking 24 internal amino acids (Δ254–277). The molecular basis of the null allele was elucidated later.[109] A G → T transversion in exon 7 created a premature translation termination signal (G245X), and a second mutation that was present on the same allele led to an L179P replacement, previously also found in a compound heterozygote having Wolman disease. The genetic defects were present in a 12-year-old patient in whom (LAL) activity in cultured skin fibroblasts was reduced to approximately 9 percent of control fibroblasts. Plasma cholesterol (255 mg/dl) and LDL cholesterol (215 mg/dl) were elevated, whereas HDL cholesterol was reduced (19 mg/dl). Triglycerides were moderately elevated (141 mg/dl). There were no clinical abnormalities, with the exception of hepatosplenomegaly. Both parents had reduced LAL activity in white blood cells. The 934G → A mutation at the exon 8 splice junction has been found either homozygously or in conjunction with other mutated alleles in a great number of patients with CESD (Table 142-1).[102–111] Homozygosity for the $\Delta 254\text{–}277_1$ allele was demonstrated in several unrelated cases with cholesteryl ester storage disease.[103,107,111] The case described by Muntoni et al.[103] had relatively high acid lipase activity, which suggested that this splice defect may be associated with some residual activity. On the other hand, the patient's fasting triglyceride and cholesterol levels were higher than those of a patient in whom a null allele was combined with the $\Delta 254\text{–}277_1$ allele.[102] Another homozygote had notably more severe clinical expression of cholesteryl ester storage disease than was seen in the two originally identified patients.[107] None of these homozygotes were true homozygotes, because the mutations were present on different *LIPA* haplotypes.

Compound heterozygosity consisting of the $\Delta 254\text{–}277_1$ allele and various other mutated alleles was identified in a number of additional patients with CESD. Ameis et al.[111] found it combined with a dinucleotide deletion (1007delAG). The deletion resulted in a shifted reading frame downstream of codon 302, followed by 43 random amino acids. A premature stop at codon 345 truncated the mutant LAL protein by 34 amino acids. In a Canadian-Norwegian kindred with cholesteryl ester storage disease, the $\Delta 254\text{–}277_1$ allele was found in conjunction with a T → C transition in exon 10 predicting an L336P replacement and an A → C transversion in exon 2 encoding a T(−6)P replacement.[104] Identification of the L336P rather than the T(−6)P replacement as the second defect underlying the disease was deduced from three lines of evidence: (1) The $\Delta 254\text{–}277_1$ allele was located in *cis* with the mutation predicting T(−6)P but in *trans* with the L336P encoding allele; (2) The L336P but not the T(−6)P replacement cosegregated with low lysosomal acid lipase activity in the family; and (3) the nucleotide substitution leading to T(−6)P replacement was found in six out of 28 alleles from subjects with normal lysosomal acid lipase activity. This suggested that the T(−6)P represented a frequent nonpathologic polymorphism. A very interesting case was presented by Maslen et al.,[110] who identified compound heterozygous mutations in two siblings with cholesteryl ester storage disease. One allele was the $\Delta 254\text{–}277_1$ allele, whereas the other harbored a mutation that had previously been seen only in Wolman disease

(L179P). All other patients who were identified as compound heterozygotes for the $\Delta 254-277_1$ allele are listed in Table 142-1. Since all patients who were carriers for at least one $\Delta 254-277_1$ allele developed CESD, it may be assumed that the CESD-causing allele ameliorates the phenotype if present in *trans* with Wolman-disease-causing alleles.

As is evident from Table 142-1, the mutation at position −1 of the exon 8 splice donor site was found in every case with CESD apart from four examples. Pagani et al.[126] identified a cytosine-to-thymidine transition in position 883, predicting a missense substitution of tyrosine for histidine in codon 274. By differential oligonucleotide hybridization on an amplified white blood cell mRNA, the cytosine-to-thymidine transition was investigated in patients' family members and in the population. No normal mRNA coding for cytosine in position 883 was detectable in the propositus, and mRNA from the phenotypically normal parents coded for both cytosine and thymidine. This led to the authors' assumption that the propositus was homozygous for the mutation. Moreover, the mutation segregated in the family with decreased acid lipase activity and was not detected in mRNA from 60 normal subjects. In a second unusual case, the disease was due to a P181L mutation on one allele and an A-to-G 3′ splice site substitution (IVS6−2A → G) that caused skipping of exon 7 on the second allele (designated Δ205–253).[108] The consequence of the latter abnormality was a loss of 49 internal amino acids from the enzyme (Δ205–253). Whether the splice junction mutation affecting splicing of exon 7 permits the production of some correctly spliced transcript is currently not known. In addition, the same group found the combination of a null allele with an allele encoding an L273S replacement in another patient with CESD.[127] The L273S mutation created an additional N-glycosylation consensus (N-X-S/T) in this region. Two site-directed mutants disrupting this consensus, QMS and QML, when expressed in HeLa cells, showed not the 56-kDa form but the normal 54-kDa band, whereas deglycosylation always resulted in the major 42-kDa form, as observed with normal LAL and the L273S mutant. Thus, an additional N-glycosylation at N271 appeared responsible for the 56-kDa form of the protein produced from the L273S allele.[127] Finally, a severely affected CESD patient was heterozygous for an H108R replacement that was found in combination with a partial deletion of the *LIPA* locus.[127a] The H108R mutated enzyme had lower residual enzymatic activity than the H108P variant, suggesting that both mutations at histidine 108 may predict CESD (Table 142-2).

Wolman Disease. The $\Delta 254-277_1$ allele has so far not been found in any case with Wolman disease (Table 142-1). The first defects causing Wolman disease were described by Anderson et al.,[101] who found two mutations in a cell line from a patient with the disease. One predicted an L179P replacement, located close to the active site at S153; the second was a frameshift mutation at nucleotide position 634 (634insT) leading to a premature stop codon (Fs178). All other patients with Wolman disease in whom the underlying mutations have been studied were homozygotes. Two unrelated cases studied in our laboratory resulted from homozygous presence of alleles predicting early truncations (438delC, 454insA) of the enzyme, which would lead to absence of the catalytically active triad (located at S153). Monochorionic biamniotic twins had a homozygous TAT → TAA replacement at codon position 303, thus creating a premature stop codon in place of Tyr303 (Y303X). The consequence of this defect was a truncation of 75 amino acids from the C-terminus of the enzyme. The four patients with the truncating mutations[127b,127c] were severely affected, and all had adrenal calcification (Seedorf et al., submitted). Aslanidis et al.[109] described two children with Wolman disease who were both homozygotes for a G → A mutation at position +1 of the exon 8 splice donor site (IVS8+1G → A, or $\Delta 254-277_2$). A 3-month-old boy of African origin was homozygous for a C → T transition at position −3 of the exon 8 splice donor site (932C → T, or $\Delta 254-277_3$).[128] In a Japanese patient, the disease was caused by homozygosity for a Y22X nonsense replacement.[129]

Genotype-Phenotype Relationships

Aslanidis et al. studied two children with Wolman disease who were both homozygotes for the IVS8 + 1G → A mutation ($\Delta 254-277_2$).[109] The mutation did not permit any correct splicing. In contrast, a compound heterozygote CESD patient who had one allele with the 934G → A mutation at the exon 8 splice donor site ($\Delta 254-277_1$) revealed skipping of exon 8 in only 97 percent of the LAL hnRNA, whereas 3 percent were spliced correctly, yielding the full-length enzyme (Fig. 142-6). Expression of the Δ254–277 variant in Sf9 and H5 insect cells showed that the enzyme with the internal deletion of 24 amino acids was completely inactive. In another homozygote with Wolman disease, a 932C → T mutation ($\Delta 254-277_3$) led to exon 8 skipping and introduced a premature termination signal at amino acid 277.[128] The enzyme that was translated from the normally spliced mRNA was inactive due to presence of the nonsense codon. The shorter LAL mRNA that lacked exon 8 also lacked the nonsense codon. Therefore, protein synthesis could proceed to the natural termination codon, but the variant enzyme had an internal deletion of 24 amino acids (Δ254–277) and was therefore inactive.

The functional difference between the $\Delta 254-277_2$ Wolman disease allele and the $\Delta 254-277_1$ CESD allele was that the mutation in the first allele affected one of the invariable nucleotides of the splice consensus sequences (position +1). Conversely, the second was located in the last nucleotide of the exon. Whereas the $\Delta 254-277_2$ allele did not permit any correct splicing, the $\Delta 254-277_1$ allele allowed some correct splicing (3–5 percent of total LAL mRNA) and therefore the synthesis of functional enzyme. This showed that the level of acid lipase residual activity may distinguish the two disorders. The view that complete inactivation of lysosomal acid lipase may cause Wolman disease is also supported by three cases from our laboratory. Two resulted from homozygous presence of alleles predicting early truncations (438delC, 454insA) of the enzyme, which led to absence of the catalytically active triad (located at S153), whereas the third was caused by homozygous presence of a premature stop in place of Tyr303 (Y303X). The consequence of the latter mutation was a truncation of 75 amino acids from the C-terminus of the enzyme. Esterification of exogenous cholesterol in the intact Wolman disease fibroblasts from all three patients was almost undetectable, whereas fibroblasts from three unrelated CESD patients who were homozygotes for the $\Delta 254-277_1$ allele had residual esterification rates of 12–24 percent.[127b,127c]. Moreover, all but one of the eleven Wolman alleles, listed in Tables 142-1 and 142-2, contain either nonsense or frameshift mutations or mutations affecting the normal splicing pathway of lysosomal acid lipase mRNA. It is conceivable that all of them cause significant truncations of the enzyme and therefore are associated with complete elimination of its function. The only exception from this rule, the L179P mutation, affects a peptide segment located close to the active site at Ser153. No residual activity was found for cholesterol esters when this allele was expressed in a prokaryotic expression system.[134] In view of these data, it appears likely to us that the R44X, G245X, and 1007delAG alleles are also Wolman alleles, despite the fact that they have been detected so far only in compound heterozygotes having CESD (Table 142-2). The classification of the remaining three alleles listed in Table 142-2 (G66V, P181L, L336P) appears difficult, since they were all found in *trans* with the $\Delta 254-277_1$ CESD allele, which seems to provide protection if present in *trans* with a Wolman allele. Nonetheless, the currently available data support the concept that the comparatively benign clinical course of CESD is due to the fact that the $\Delta 254-277_1$ allele leads to production of a small fraction of normal enzyme, which is responsible for low residual acid lipase activity. Although direct proof is still lacking, residual activity may be also associated with the other alleles that have been

Table 142-2 Alleles Associated with Acid Lipase Deficiency

Clinical phenotype	Allele	Nucleotide substitution	Exon/Intron	Mechanism	Remarks/References
Wolman	Y22X	169C → A	3	Nonsense mutation	No active site [129].
Wolman*	R44X	233C → T	3	Nonsense mutation	No active site. Found in a CESD patient in *trans* with the $\Delta 254{-}277_1$ allele [275].
Not known	G66V	300G → T	4	Missense mutation	Found in a CESD patient in *trans* with the $\Delta 254{-}277_1$ allele [108].
CESD*	H108P	426A → C	4	Missense mutation	Found in a mildly affected CESD patient in *trans* with the $\Delta 254{-}277_1$ allele [106]. 4.6% residual enzymatic activity [127a].
CESD	H108R	426A → G	4	Missense mutation	Found in a CESD patient in *trans* with a partial deletion of the gene. 2.7% residual enzymatic activity [127a].
Wolman	S112X	438delC	4	Frameshift	S112X. No active site [Seedorf et al., submitted].
Wolman		454insA	4	Frameshift	No active site [Seedorf et al., submitted].
Wolman	Fs178	634insT	6	Frameshift	Insertion of one T after a stretch of 6 T. No active site [101].
Wolman	L179P	639T → C	6	Missense mutation	Nonconservative replacement close to the active site. No residual activity [101,109,110,134].
Not known	P181L	645C → T	6	Missense mutation	Found in a CESD patient in *trans* with the 934G → A allele [108].
Wolman	G245X	836G → T	7	Nonsense mutation	Found in a CESD patient in *trans* with the $\Delta 254{-}277_1$allele. Allele also contained the L179P mutation [102,109].
Not known	Δ205–253	IVS6–2A → G	7	Exon skipping	Mutation at exon 7 splice acceptor site, leading to skipping of exon 7. Encodes a Δ205–253 truncated enzyme [108].
Wolman	$\Delta 254{-}277_3$ (Q277X)	932C → T	8	Exon skipping/ nonsense	At 3rd-from-last bp of exon 8. Encodes a Δ254–277 truncated enzyme with no activity. Low levels of normally spliced mRNA containing a stop at codon 277 [128].
CESD	$\Delta 254{-}277_1$	934G → A	8	Exon skipping	At last bp of exon 8. Encodes a Δ254–277 truncated enzyme with no activity. 3–5% residual normal splicing [101–111,275].
Wolman	$\Delta 254{-}277_2$	IVS8+1G → A	8	Exon skipping	At first bp of intron 8. Encodes a Δ254–277 truncated enzyme with no activity. No residual normal splicing [109].
CESD	L273S	921T → C	8	Missense mutation	Aberrant glycosylation [108].
CESD	H274Y	923C → T	8	Missense mutation	[126].
Wolman*	Fs302	1007delAG	10	Frameshift	Found in a CESD patient in *trans* with the $\Delta 254{-}277_1$ allele [111].
Wolman	Y303X	1012T → A	10	Nonsense mutation	Y303X [127c].
Not known	L336P	1110T → C	10	Missense mutation	Found in a mildly affected CESD patient in *trans* with the $\Delta 254{-}277_1$ allele. No activity toward CE, but ~5% residual activity towards TG [104,134].

*Presumed clinical expression in the homozygous state. Nucleotide numbers refer to the cDNA and start at the ATG initiation codon. Nucleotides are numbered 1–2493 (GenBank M74775 with ATG initiation codon bp 41–43.

implicated as causing CESD (Δ205–253, L273S, H274Y). The range of the mutations that are known to cause Wolman disease implies that this disorder results from alleles predicting complete elimination of enzyme function.

Population Prevalence

Based on the relatively low numbers of verified cases that have been described in the literature since the initial descriptions of the two disorders, it has been assumed that both CESD and Wolman disease are exceedingly rare disorders. Although this is likely true for most of the known Wolman disease alleles, recent genetic data suggest that the $\Delta 254{-}277_1$ CESD allele may be among the more frequent genetic abnormalities that are present in the Caucasian population: (1) The allele has been found in various ethnic groups in several European countries, Canada, North America, and Turkey; (2) many CESD patients are $\Delta 254{-}277_1$ homozygotes despite the fact that their parents are not related and originate from geographically separated areas; and (3) the mutation is present in at least three different haplotypes (Fig. 142-7). The last fact appears interesting to us because it may suggest that the mutation

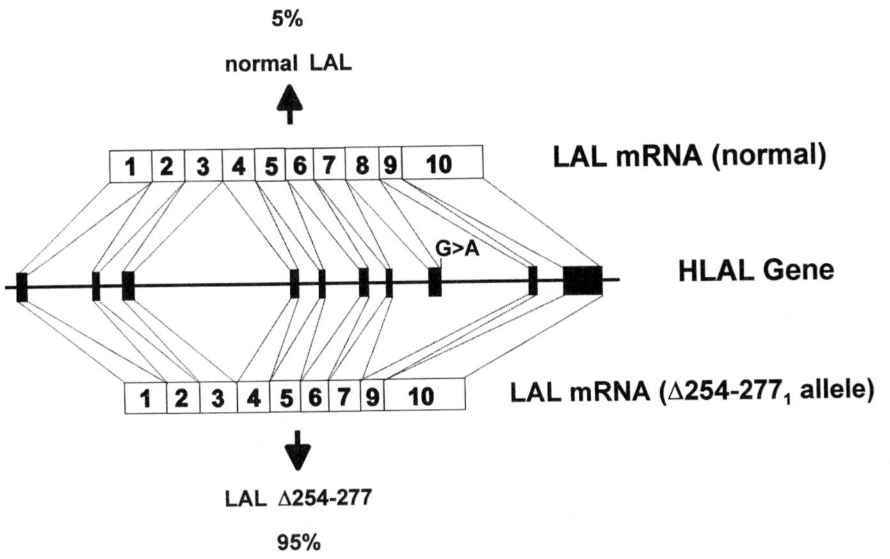

Fig. 142-6 Effect of the $\Delta 254-277_1$ allele on splicing of lysosomal acid lipase mRNA and production of normal and Δ254–277 truncated enzyme. The 10 exons are indicated by filled boxes. The mutation (934G → A) is indicated at the 3′-end of exon 8. The normal LAL mRNA accounts for ~5 percent of total mRNA; the transcript that lacks the coding information of exon 8 is ~95 percent of total mRNA produced.

occurred more than once, affecting distinct haplotypes of the locus (a mutational hot spot). Alternatively, recombination may have occurred between the respective genomic locations. Given the fact that the distance between the mutation and the polymorphic sites is small, one must assume that the mutation has already persisted in the human population for a considerable time.

Recently, we addressed the frequency of the $\Delta 254-277_1$ allele more directly by employing a mutagenically separated PCR (MS-PCR) strategy to screen for the mutation in pooled samples selected randomly from individuals who lived in Westphalia (a region in northwestern Germany). Seven heterozygotes were found in this cohort of 1887 individuals aged 20 to 70 years (0.37 percent, or 1/270). Four of them were males and three were females. The allele frequency was 0.0019, which provided an estimated homozygosity frequency of 1 in 300,000 inhabitants (~260 CESD cases in Germany) (Muntoni et al., submitted). If not due to a founder effect, this unexpectedly high frequency places the $\Delta 254-277_1$ CESD mutation among the most frequent single autosomal recessive genetic abnormalities that are currently known to exist in this population. Further studies are required in order to confirm the high prevalence of the allele in other Caucasian populations and to clarify whether the disease is underdiagnosed or whether incomplete penetrance may account for the apparent discrepancy between the estimated prevalence of $\Delta 254-277_1$ homozygosity and the low number of diagnosed CESD cases.

Heterozygote Detection

It is now well established that heterozygotes for acid lipase deficiency are detectable by enzyme assay. Young and Patrick[19] reported that leukocytes of the mother, the father, and a sib of one patient with Wolman disease contained about half the normal activity of the acid hydrolase. Lake[130] reported intermediate activity in lymphocytes on blood films prepared from obligate heterozygotes in the same family affected with Wolman disease. These authors further noted that the patient's father and mother had elevated activity of other lysosomal hydrolases in their leukocytes. A fluorometric assay of acid lipase has been described that requires only 1 ml of blood.[131] The test is sensitive enough to distinguish subnormal levels of the enzyme in obligate carriers of Wolman disease. In addition to leukocytes, cultured skin fibroblasts can be used to establish subnormal levels of acid lipase in heterozygotes.[14,131] The pedigree shown in Fig. 142-8 exemplifies the typical relationship existing between leukocyte acid lipase activities, plasma lipid anomalies, and presence of the $\Delta 254-277_1$ allele.

Thus, present data indicate that heterozygotes for both forms of acid ester hydrolase deficiency have detectable abnormalities in enzyme assays but that the two forms of the disease cannot be separated by such measurements alone. Vacuolation of peripheral lymphocytes does not allow heterozygote detection, since this has also been seen in homozygous abnormal patients and is also a common nonspecific finding in other lysosomal hydrolase deficiencies. Prenatal diagnosis of Wolman disease and CESD has been established by quantitative assays and electrophoresis of LAL in cultured amniotic fluid cells.[77,132,133] In addition, highly specific DNA diagnostic tests are available in specialized laboratories.

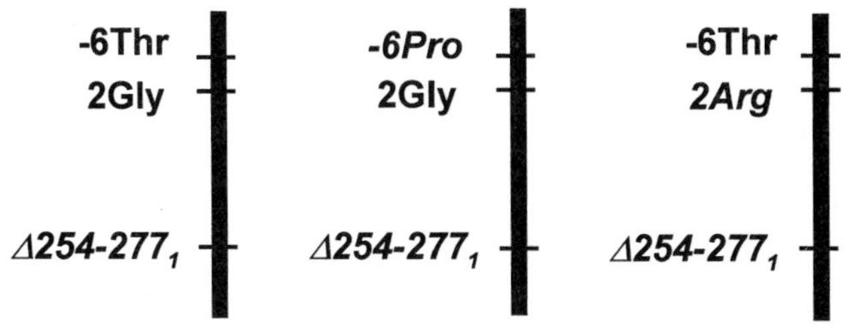

Fig. 142-7 $\Delta 254-277_1$ 934G → A haplotypes. T(−6)P and G2R are relatively frequent acid lipase gene polymorphisms that have no or only minor functional impact (allele frequencies: T(−6)P = 0.24–0.27;[276] G2R = ~0.05[107]).

PROPERTIES OF LYSOSOMAL ACID LIPASE

Intracellular Processing and Secretion

Normal concentrations of the enzyme protein and absence of lipase activity have been found in several patients with Wolman disease and CESD, suggesting that acid lipase deficiency in these patients may be the result of mutations that interfere with the catalytic activity of the enzyme.[132] Many of the mutated enzymes encoded by the alleles listed in Table 142-2 were expressed either in prokaryotic or eukaryotic expression systems, and it could be shown that all led to essentially complete inactivation of the catalytic activity.[108,109,126,127,134] On the other hand, acid lipase deficiency not only may arise from such mutations but may hypothetically be due to abnormal intracellular processing and targeting. The protein contains a 21-amino-acid-long leader sequence that belongs to a family of signal peptides directing newly synthesized proteins to the plasma membrane, secretory vesicles, and lysosomes.[135] Acid lipase is synthesized on polysomes at the rough endoplasmic reticulum (ER) and is

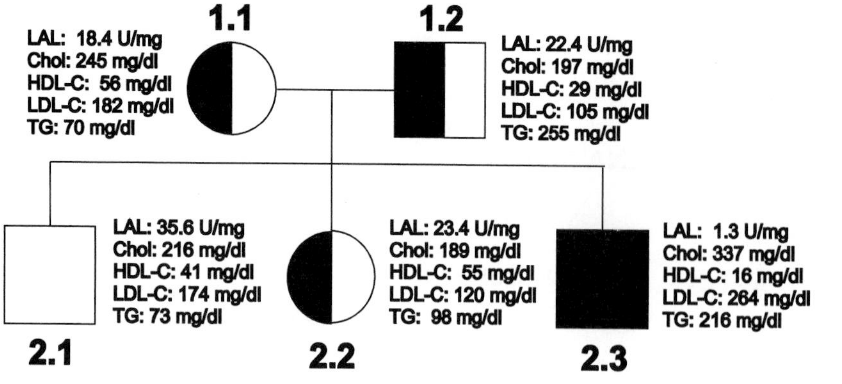

Fig. 142-8 Cosegregation of the $\Delta 254-277_1$ (934G → A) allele with reduced levels of acid lipase activity measured in peripheral blood leukocytes in a Spanish kindred with CESD, resulting from isolated presence of the $\Delta 254-277_1$ allele. 1.1 and 1.2 = heterozygous parents; 2.3 = homozygous CESD patient; 2.2 = heterozygous sister; 2.1 = normal brother.

transported to the trans-Golgi network. There, proteins with differing final locations, such as lysosomes, secretory storage vesicles, and plasma membrane proteins, are sorted to their correct destinations.[136,137] The presence of six potential N-linked glycosylation signals within the acid lipase primary structure is related to its specific targeting to the lysosomal compartment via the Man-6-P receptor pathway.[135] Deglycosylation of acid lipase by endo-β-N-acetylglucosamidase H treatment results in reduction of the molecular mass by 4 to 6 kDa. It has been shown that endoglycosidase treatment does not inhibit the catalytic activity or alter the heat stability of the enzyme but abolishes internalization by the Man-6-P receptor.[138]

It was shown with purified preparations of acid lipase secreted from fibroblasts that the glycosylated enzyme is efficiently internalized by the Man-6-P receptor system. Thus, the enzymatic defect can be corrected by addition of purified acid lipase to deficient fibroblasts.[138–140] However, coculture and cell fusion of fibroblasts from both Wolman disease and CESD subjects did not lead to correction of the enzyme deficiency, indicating that these disorders are allelic.[141]

Biochemical Assay

Though the properties of the enzyme are influenced substantially by the assay method employed, there is no standardized procedure for the assay of acid lipase/cholesteryl ester hydrolase.[142] The substrates presented to the enzyme include cholesteryl esters, glycerides, and synthetic acyl esters. Acyl moieties with great variety in chain length and extent of unsaturation and dispersions of the substrate (by detergent, solubilizing agent, application of heat and sonication, and concentration of substrates used) have been described. In addition, phospholipids and bile salts seem to stimulate the enzyme, and albumin or other proteins can serve as traps for the released fatty acids. Finally, the nature of the enzyme preparation itself (subcellular fractionations, or more or less purified enzyme) considerably affects the properties of the enzyme. Since this wide variety of assay procedures exists, it is not surprising that substantial differences in optimal pH, substrate specificity, and cofactors have been reported.

The substrates used most often are [1-^{14}C]trioleylglycerol and cholesteryl [1-^{14}C]oleate. Labeled oleic acid liberated by the enzyme's action is measured after separation by thin-layer chromatography[143] or separation from substrate by solvent extraction.[144,145] The use of synthetic substrates has the advantage of sensitivity and simplicity, but unfortunately these substrates have lower specificity. The best recommendation for dispersal of acid lipase/cholesteryl ester hydrolase substrates seems to be to use phospholipid vesicles for incorporation of radiolabeled cholesteryl esters[146] or triacylglycerols.[147] The availability of fluorescent cholesteryl esters containing fluorescent fatty acids for use in analysis of acid lipase may add a promising non-radioactive alternative that can be easily used in clinical laboratories.[148–152]

Unlike many of the lysosomal hydrolases, acid cholesteryl ester hydrolase is not very stable. It does not store well when frozen and is rapidly inactivated at elevated temperatures. For measuring acid cholesteryl esterase activity, phospholipids and bile salts are essential,[143,153,154] but there is general agreement that Ca^{2+}, Mg^{2+}, EDTA, and dithiothreitol do not significantly alter enzymatic activity.[143,154–156] However, the enzyme is inactivated by heavy metals such as copper and mercury[143,155,157–159] and by agents such as N-ethylmaleinimide, iodoacetate, and p-chloromercuribenzoate, which are reactive toward sulfhydryl groups.[153–156,159–161] Diisopropyl fluorophosphate and protamine sulfate have little inhibitory effect on acid lipase activity.[143,155] Most investigators find enzyme activity toward triacylglycerols considerably higher than that toward cholesteryl esters, which may explain the predominance of cholesteryl ester storage in most patients with CESD.

Molecular Biology of Acid Lipase

The gene encoding LAL was mapped with *in situ* hybridization techniques to chromosome 10q23.2-q23.3.[162] In addition, the entire gene structure, consisting of 10 exons dispersed over 45 kb was elucidated (GenBank X75489-X75497).[101,163] The 5′ flanking region revealed the characteristic GC-rich structure of a typical promoter for a housekeeping gene.

The amino acid sequence deduced from the nucleotide sequence of the cDNA (GenBank M74775) shows 58 and 57 percent identity with those of human gastric and rat lingual lipase, respectively, both of which are involved in the preduodenal breakdown of ingested triglycerides.[135] Conversely, the sequence lacks any significant homology with described neutral lipases. Acid lipase is distinct from hormone-sensitive lipase,[164] pancreatic lysophospholipase (bile-salt-dependent lipase/cholesterol esterase),[165–167] lecithin:cholesterol acyltransferase (LCAT),[168] and the gene family that includes lipoprotein lipase (LPL), hepatic lipase (hepatic triglyceride lipase, HTGL), and pancreatic lipase.[169–171] Nevertheless, human acid lipase shares the presence of the esterase-associated amino acid sequence motif -Gly-X-Ser-X-Gly with most other lipases, as well as with LCAT. X-ray crystallographic studies have shown that the central serines of this pentapeptide, which appears twice within the human acid lipase sequence (residues 97–101 and 151–155) are active-site catalytic residues in human pancreatic lipase,[172] hepatic lipase,[173] and pancreatic cholesterol esterase.[174] As is the case for gastric lipase, acid lipase activity is readily inhibited by sulfhydryl reagents, and thiols are required for the stability of the purified enzyme,[140,159,161,175] suggesting that cysteine residues are involved in its catalytic activity. Seven cysteine residues are present within the human acid lipase amino acid sequence, including one that is located in the proposed leader sequence. Particularly, the cysteine residue at position 240, which is also conserved in the gastric and rat lingual lipases, may be functionally related to the active site of the enzyme. Site-directed mutagenesis at two putative active centers, both with the sequence-Gly-X-Ser-X-Gly, showed that Ser153 was important to catalytic activity, whereas Ser99 was not and neither was the catalytic nucleophile.[134]

The acid lipase primary structure includes several sequence motifs that are related to its intracellular targeting to the secretory pathway and lysosomes. From the cDNA sequence, it is proposed that the protein is translated including a 21-amino-acid-long leader sequence that has the characteristics expected for a signal peptide sequence.[176] In addition, the presence of six potential N-linked glycosylation signals explains the previously described susceptibility of LAL to hydrolysis by endo-β-N-acetylglucosamidase H, resulting in a reduction of the molecular mass of the enzyme by 4 to 6 kDa. It was shown that endoglycosidase treatment does not inhibit the catalytic activity or alter the heat stability of the enzyme but abolishes internalization by the Man-6-P receptor, thereby hindering the capacity of exogeneously added enzyme to correct cholesteryl ester accumulation in cultured lipase-deficient cells.[138]

Since acid triglyceride lipase copurifies with acid cholesteryl esterase activity, it has been suggested that a single enzyme hydrolyzes both triacylglycerols and cholesteryl esters. That this assumption is correct has been demonstrated by transfection of the acid lipase cDNA into cultured cells. Transfection of the cDNA results in more than a fortyfold elevation of endogenous acid lipase activity as determined with cholesteryl oleate and triolein as the substrates.[135]

PATHOPHYSIOLOGY AT THE CELLULAR LEVEL

Lysosomal Acid Lipase in CESD and Wolman Disease

The activity of lysosomal acid lipase activity in cultured fibroblasts from patients with Wolman disease and CESD has been characterized by various methods, including enzymatic analysis and histochemical and chemical procedures. With natural substrates, the acid lipase activity in patients is less than 10 percent of that in controls and about 50 percent of that in heterozygotes in both conditions. Similar results can be obtained with a variety of artificial substrates, such as synthetic derivatives of nitrophenol or 4-methylumbelliferone. Acid lipase is distinct from phospholipase A, for there is no accumulation of phospholipids in patients affected with Wolman disease or CESD. Phospholipase A may be responsible for some of the residual activity measured with artificial substrates in some patients.

Immunologic quantification of the enzyme protein with polyclonal antibodies directed against acid lipase was performed on three patients with Wolman disease and on three CESD patients.[132] In all patients analyzed, normal concentrations of the enzyme protein and absence of lipase activity were found.

Cellogel electrophoresis of normal fibroblast extracts followed by staining for LAL using 4-methylumbelliferyl oleate demonstrates at least three acid lipase isoenzymes, labeled A, B, and C.[13] The least anodal band, A, is the most prominent one in control fibroblasts but is reduced in heterozygotes (Wolman disease) and is undetectable in both Wolman disease and CESD cells.[39] The acid lipase isoenzyme pattern observed in cultured skin fibroblasts is also present in amniotic fluid cells, lymphocytes, and several tissues (liver, spleen, lymph nodes, aorta).[13] Prenatal diagnosis of Wolman disease and CESD has been established by the combined recognition of deficiency of acid lipase and deficiency of the A band in electrophoresis of amniotic-cell extracts.[77,132,133]

The gene for the A band of acid lipase (*LIPA*) in humans has been localized initially to chromosome 10q24-q25, while B and C bands are probably controlled by one gene (*LIPB*; MIM 247980), localized to chromosome 16.[178–181] This assignment was based on electrophoretic analysis of the enzyme in hybrid cells formed from human and mouse fibroblasts. In situ hybridization led to a more precise assignment of *LIPA* at chromosome 10q23.2-q23.3.[162] Results from various inhibitors against the different bands favor the existence of a third gene (*LIPI*), independent of *LIPA* and *LIPB*.[179,181]

Studies of acid lipase with native emulsified substrates have shown that in both Wolman disease and CESD fibroblasts, acid cholesteryl ester hydrolase and triacylglycerol hydrolase activity levels are reduced proportionately,[87,182] while neutral cholesteryl ester hydrolase is preserved[183] but possibly down-regulated.[87,133] Moreover, proportional deficiencies of the two activities have also been measured in fibroblasts from patients with I-cell disease or pseudo-Hurler polydystrophy (Chap. 138).[184] The latter conditions are characterized by multiple lysosomal enzyme deficiencies due to a defect in posttranslational glycosylation as related to the Man-6-P receptor cycle.

Taken together, these findings show that cholesteryl ester hydrolase and triacylglycerol hydrolase activities in fibroblasts reside in the same enzyme molecule (A isoenzyme). It is not clear at present to what extent the B and C isoenzymes that are retained in Wolman disease and CESD fibroblasts may account for the residual enzyme activity measured in mutant cells with both artificial and radiolabeled native substrates. Wide variation in the reported residual acid lipase activity levels in Wolman disease and CESD[13,16,182,185] suggests that definitive diagnosis rests on the use of natural substrates.

Comparison of the rate of hydrolysis of cholesteryl esters with fatty acids of various chain lengths in lymphoid cell lines from normal subjects and from Wolman disease patients has shown that three cholesteryl esterases are present in normal lymphoid cell lines.[149,186–188] The first, active at pH 4.0, preferentially hydrolyzes cholesteryl esters with acyl chain lengths of more than eight carbons. This activity is severely deficient in Wolman lymphoid cell lines and corresponds to acid lipase. The second and third cholesteryl esterases, active at pH 6.0 and 8.0, respectively, hydrolyze shorter chain derivatives. The pH 6.0 and 8.0 enzymes are not deficient in Wolman lymphoid cell lines. The pH 6.0 cholesterol esterase probably corresponds to the microsomal Mn^{2+}-dependent enzyme hydrolyzing cholesteryl oleate,[189] and the pH 8.0 enzyme may correspond to a microsomal carboxyl esterase.[190]

In addition to cultured fibroblasts, leukocyte extracts can be used to establish the diagnosis of acid lipase deficiency. Acid lipase activity assayed with 4-methylumbelliferyl esters is 10 to 15 times higher in mononuclear than in polymorphonuclear leukocytes.[191] In three patients affected with Wolman disease, low leukocyte activity of β-galactosidase was reported in addition to the near absence of acid lipase activity.[18,19] The reason for this is not clear, but it might be related to a hypothetical defect in targeting of lysosomal proteins in a more general way.

Goldstein et al. compared the relative rates of hydrolysis of [^{3}H]cholesteryl linoleate-LDL in normal and mutant CESD cells. They compared fibroblast extracts incubated at acid pH and intact fibroblast monolayers.[95] While the cholesteryl esterase activity of mutant cell lysates was less than one-twentieth that of normal lysates, the intact mutant cells showed rates of cholesteryl ester hydrolysis that were nearly one-third those of the normal cells. The origin of this interesting discrepancy is not known. As the residual enzyme activity in intact CESD fibroblasts could be abolished by treatment of the cells with chloroquine, it may be concluded that the activity resides in lysosomes. Presentation of the substrate for the defective acid lipase via the lysosomal pathway in the intact cells presumably results in higher substrate availability, leading to elevated residual activity of the enzyme compared with that seen on in vitro assay.

Similar findings have been reported with various substrates in intact fibroblasts and fibroblast lysates from both Wolman disease and CESD patients.[100] Although acid lipase in cell lysates was less than 1 percent of control activity in both disorders, considerable differences were observed in intact fibroblasts from Wolman disease (10–28 percent of control) and CESD (28–49 percent of control) patients. The findings in intact cells appear to provide a biochemical explanation for the different phenotypes associated with the two disorders.

Another study[141] compared residual acid lipase activities in fibroblasts and hepatocytes from CESD and Wolman disease patients. The results of this study suggest that the enzyme activity in the fibroblasts is virtually absent in both disorders, while hepatic acid lipase was 23 percent of normal in CESD and only 4 percent of normal in Wolman disease. In addition, the activity of hepatic neutral lipase was normal in Wolman disease but increased more than twofold in CESD.

It appears from the very different clinical courses of CESD and Wolman disease that the residual acid lipase activity directed against LDL cholesteryl esters is sufficient in CESD to keep the lysosomal accumulation of cholesteryl esters and subsequent cellular damage in most extrahepatic tissues to a level compatible with a fairly normal life. In Wolman disease, the residual activity is insufficient and causes overwhelming accumulation of cholesteryl esters and destruction of cell function.

Cellular Cholesterol Metabolism in Lysosomal Acid Lipase Deficiency

Except for erythrocytes, lysosomal acid lipase is present in virtually all cells of the body. The enzyme plays an important role in the cellular processing of plasma lipoproteins and contributes to homeostatic control of lipoprotein levels in blood and to prevention of cellular lipid overloading.[12,120–123,143,192–196] In a series of elegant studies, Brown and Goldstein[197,198] and coworkers have established the obligatory role of LAL in the cellular degradation of plasma LDLs (see Chap. 120). Cultured fibroblasts take up LDL via receptor-mediated endocytosis. LDL bound to the receptor is present in coated pits on the plasma membrane and endocytosed into clathrin-coated vesicles. After removal of the clathrin coat, the endocytic vesicles fuse to form multivesicular bodies that can fuse with primary lysosomal vesicles derived from the trans-Golgi network. Subsequently, apolipoproteins, cholesteryl esters, and other lipid constituents undergo hydrolysis by lysosomal enzymes, while the LDL receptor cycles back to the cell surface.

The lysosomal degradation of LDL cholesteryl esters and triglycerides is catalyzed by the acid lipase activity (Fig. 142-1) that is deficient in Wolman disease and CESD.[95,96] Free sterol and fatty acids are liberated from the lysosomes. While fatty acids are bound by fatty acid binding protein and directed to several subcellular locations (mitochondria, peroxisomes, ER), cholesterol is partly redirected to the plasma membrane, but the bulk of the lysosomal cholesterol is transferred to the ER and initiates three important regulatory events. First, cellular synthesis of cholesterol is reduced through suppression of the activity of HMG-CoA reductase, which catalyzes the rate-limiting step in cholesterol synthesis (see Fig. 142-9). Second, transcription of the LDL receptor gene is repressed, leading gradually to a substantial reduction in the number of receptors on the cell surface and to reduced uptake of LDL. Third, cellular formation of cholesteryl esters is stimulated through activation of microsomal membrane-bound acyl-CoA:cholesterol acyltransferase (ACAT). In the reaction catalyzed by this enzyme, the bulk of incoming cholesterol, which was mainly esterified to linoleic acid in LDL, becomes reesterified predominantly with oleic (C18:1) acid or with other C14 to C18 saturated or monounsaturated fatty acids. Under certain conditions, the reesterified cholesterol may accumulate as cytoplasmic lipid droplets that resemble the droplets seen in the foam cells of atherosclerotic lesions and Tangier disease.

In fibroblasts from patients with CESD or Wolman disease, the strong regulatory effect of lysosomally metabolized lipoproteins on cholesterol metabolism is severely disturbed (Fig. 142-9). The inability to release free cholesterol from lysosomal cholesteryl esters obviously results in elevated synthesis of endogenous cholesterol, up-regulation of LDL receptor gene expression, and increased production of apo B-containing lipoproteins.[199] The combination of these effects results in a significantly elevated flux of lipoproteins into the lysosomal pathway especially of the liver, leading to even more destructive lysosomal accumulation of cholesteryl esters and triglycerides. This vicious cycle seems to be more pronounced in Wolman disease than in CESD. An attractive pathophysiological hypothesis to explain the comparatively benign clinical course of CESD compared with that of Wolman disease is

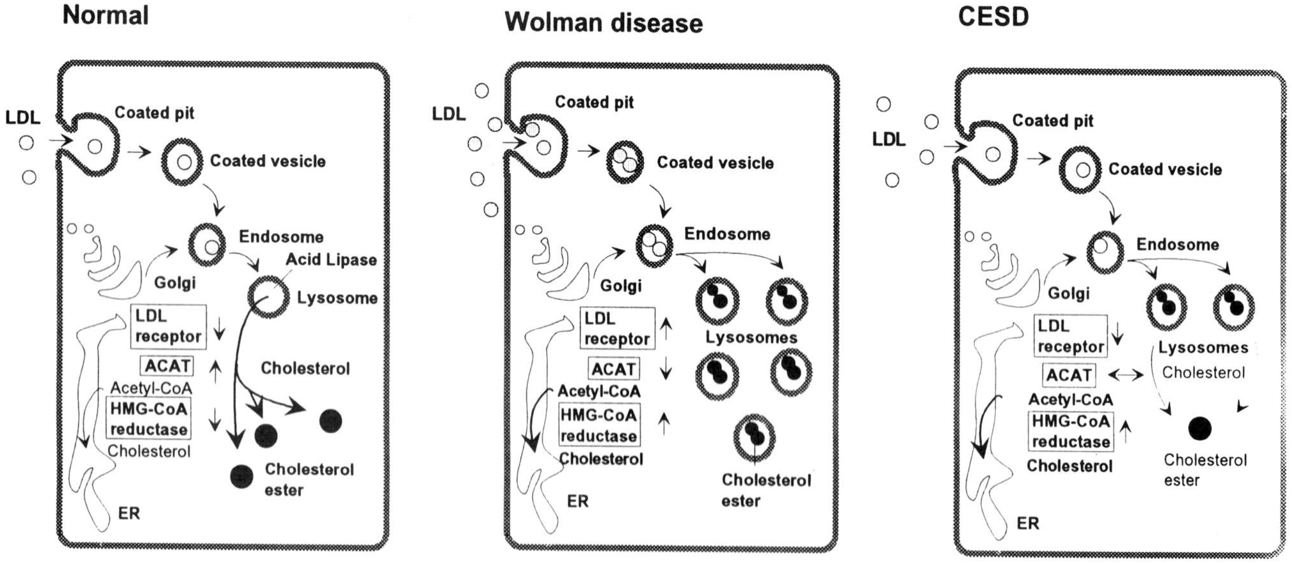

Fig. 142-9 Schematic representation of intracellular cholesterol metabolism. (A) Normal situation: Receptor-mediated endocytosis of LDL leads to cholesterol release from lysosomes, with concomitant rise in intracellular free cholesterol, which leads to activation of ACAT and cholesterol esterification of cytoplasmic lipid droplets. In addition, down-regulation of LDL receptor gene expression and HMG-CoA reductase activity results in repression of further uptake of LDL lipoproteins, as well as *de novo* synthesis of cholesterol. (B) Situation in Wolman disease: Complete deficiency of acid lipase leads to massive accumulation of lysosomal cholesteryl esters and triglycerides. Defective release of free cholesterol from lysosomes leads to up-regulation of LDL receptor gene expression and HMG-CoA reductase activity. This vicious cycle causes elevated *de novo* synthesis of cholesterol and activation of receptor-mediated endocytosis of LDL, leading to even more devastating lysosomal deposition of lipids. (C) Situation in CESD: Residual activity of acid lipase leads to reduced release of free cholesterol from lysosomes that is sufficient to down-regulate LDL receptor gene expression, thus preventing excessive accumulation of lipids in lysosomes. Elevated levels of apo B containing lipoproteins further indicate that *de novo* synthesis of cholesterol may be elevated in CESD cells.

that the relatively high residual activity of acid cholesteryl ester hydrolase is sufficient to release enough free cholesterol from the lysosomes to down-regulate expression of the LDL receptor gene and HMG-CoA reductase activity, thereby preventing excessive overload of lysosomes with lipoprotein-derived cholesteryl esters and triglycerides.

The reduced regulatory effects of LDL in acid-lipase-deficient cells can be restored when the mutant cells are cocultivated with normal fibroblasts.[96] It was shown that cholesteryl ester hydrolase is secreted by normal fibroblasts into the culture medium and can be taken up in an active form by the mutant cells via Man-6-P receptors.[138,139,200] This property of the enzyme may provide the opportunity for acid lipase replacement therapy in the future, but this has not yet been attempted.

The hydrolysis of cytoplasmic cholesteryl esters is mediated not by acid lipase but by a cytoplasmic cholesteryl ester hydrolase. This enzyme has a neutral optimal pH and therefore is called *neutral cholesteryl ester hydrolase*.[201,202] Since lysosomotrophic drugs have no effect on cholesteryl ester mobilization, it may be concluded that cytoplasmic cholesteryl esters do not reenter lysosomes for hydrolysis prior to mobilization but are quantitatively hydrolyzed in the cytoplasm. Excessive accumulation of cholesteryl ester-rich lipid droplets in the cytoplasm is characteristic of a number of pathologic conditions and might at least in part be due to reduced neutral cholesteryl esterase activity that may be reactivated by agonists of adenylate cyclase (EC 4.6.11) and cAMP-dependent protein kinase (EC 2.7.1.3.7).[145,203–208]

The liver is the principal tissue of receptor-mediated endocytosis and lysosomal degradation of LDL. In fact, it was shown that more than 70 percent of LDL is metabolized by this organ.[209,210] Thus, the hepatomegaly associated with Wolman disease and CESD is not surprising. The involvement of other tissues in both disorders is also closely correlated with their participation in receptor-mediated endocytosis and lysosomal degradation of lipoproteins. The splenomegaly associated with acid lipase deficiency is related to lysosomal storage of cholesteryl esters and triglycerides in macrophages. These cells play an important role in the removal of modified lipoproteins from the circulation. Besides the LDL receptor, macrophages express "scavenger receptors," which recognize these modified lipoproteins as ligands.[211] Unlike that of the LDL receptor, the expression of scavenger receptors is not under feedback inhibition by the intracellular cholesterol concentration.[212] Therefore, macrophages accumulate significant amounts of cholesterol by lysosomal degradation of modified LDL. In vivo, modified LDL may result from modification by malondialdehyde,[213] oxidation,[214] or LDL particle aggregation.[215,216] It was shown that malondialdehyde, which can be produced as a side product of lipid peroxidation, is a constituent of modified LDL present in atherosclerotic plaques in vivo.[213]

Adrenal calcification, which is rarely observed in CESD but always present in Wolman disease, is related to a particularly active pathway of receptor-mediated endocytosis and lysosomal degradation of LDL, which provides the sterol precursors for steroidogenesis in this tissue.[209,210] It is interesting to note that of all tissues in the body, the adrenal glands possess the highest uptake of lipoproteins on a weight basis[217,218] and that this tissue is also able to take up and utilize cholesteryl esters carried in plasma HDL.[219] Normally, the steroids secreted by the adrenals are derived in large part from lipoprotein cholesterol. However, failure of lysosomal hydrolysis of lipoprotein cholesteryl esters does not necessarily imply impairment of hormone production. Even in the complete absence of LAL activity, there are potentially at least three major sources of cholesterol available to cells to meet their metabolic needs. These include selective uptake of cholesteryl esters from HDL [via the HDL receptor pathway called scavenger receptor, class B, type I (SR-BI)], which bypass the lysosomal pathway and are hydrolyzed extralysosomally;[220–224] hydrolysis of stored cytoplasmic cholesteryl esters (involving neutral cholesteryl ester hydrolase), and cholesterol synthesized *de novo*. The distribution of abnormal lipid storage in patients with Wolman disease and CESD adds information about the quantitative importance of lysosomal degradation of lipoprotein cholesteryl esters and triglycerides in different tissues. The tissue pattern of lipid storage in Wolman disease is compatible with the observed uptake of radiolabeled LDL into various tissues of experimental animals.[209,216]

Anomalies of Plasma Lipids and Lipoproteins

Plasma cholesteryl esters are derived from two main sources: (1) esterification of cholesterol in the intestine and transport of chylomicrons containing the esters and dietary fat into plasma by way of the lymph, and (2) esterification of plasma lipoprotein-associated cholesterol by LCAT. Many details of the metabolism of chylomicrons and esterification of cholesterol via LCAT are presented in Chaps. 114–123. Once in plasma, these triglyceride-rich particles lose their triglycerides to extrahepatic tissues through the action of the capillary-bound lipase lipoprotein lipase which has an alkaline optimal pH. The particles are reduced to "core remnants" rich in cholesterol, phospholipids, and certain surface apolipoproteins. In addition to the core remnants, surface-derived discoidal cholesterol particles ("surface remnants") are formed that contain cholesterol, phospholipids, and apolipoprotein A-I.[225] These surface remnants probably bind to the HDL-binding sites on a variety of peripheral cells and are transformed to spherical HDL.[226] The core remnants are removed by the liver at a rate that appears to be directly dependent on its apoprotein composition[227,228] Present data suggest that apo E and remnant-bound LPL foster the hepatic uptake of the core remnant, while other apolipoproteins, such as apo C-III, may inhibit this function.[229,233] The uptake of chylomicron remnants is mediated by the chylomicron remnant receptor, also known as the LDL-receptor-related-protein, or α_2-macroglobulin receptor.[230–232] Binding of chylomicron remnants to this receptor directs the lipoprotein to the lysosomes, where the cholesteryl esters are hydrolyzed by the action of acid lipase,[234–238] and the liberated cholesterol is made available for further metabolism.

The hepatic uptake of lipoproteins is not confined to parenchymal cells. Also, nonparenchymal liver cells are active in binding and uptake of lipoproteins from the blood and have the capacity to degrade protein and cholesteryl ester moieties of lipoproteins.[239–242] In rat liver cells, about 50 percent of the total cholesteryl esterase activity is present in nonparenchymal cells.[242] This is compatible with the observation that cholesteryl ester storage occurs in both hepatocytes and Kupffer cells in patients affected with LAL deficiency.

While the hypercholesterolemia that has been observed in all patients with CESD may be partly explained by increased synthesis of apo B-containing lipoproteins, the precise mechanism that decreases concentrations of plasma HDL in CESD is not yet understood. Of particular interest is the abnormal ratio of HDL_2 to HDL_3 observed in one patient.[2] In this patient with elevated plasma cholesterol but normal triglycerides, lipoprotein lipase activity was found to be normal, while hepatic lipase activity was significantly reduced. Moreover, the HDL_2 fraction contained considerable amounts of apolipoprotein C-III_3, which represents the excess sialylated precursor form of apolipoprotein C-III, while C-III_2 was almost absent in this lipoprotein fraction (Fig. 142-10). In contrast, the VLDL and HDL_3 fractions did not contain detectable amounts of apolipoprotein C-III_3 but revealed a normal pattern of the other sialylated forms of apolipoprotein C-III. Thus, the regular interaction of HDL_2 with hepatocytes might be disturbed in CESD, either due to the presence of excess sialylated apolipoprotein C-III or due to down-regulation or defective function of heparin-releasable liver lipase. In a patient described by Kostner and colleagues,[243] who had elevated plasma cholesterol and triglyceride levels, lipoprotein lipase was found to be normal and hepatic lipase values increased. This patient exhibited very low levels of HDLs, which consisted almost exclusively of HDL3. The authors speculate that the low plasma HDL

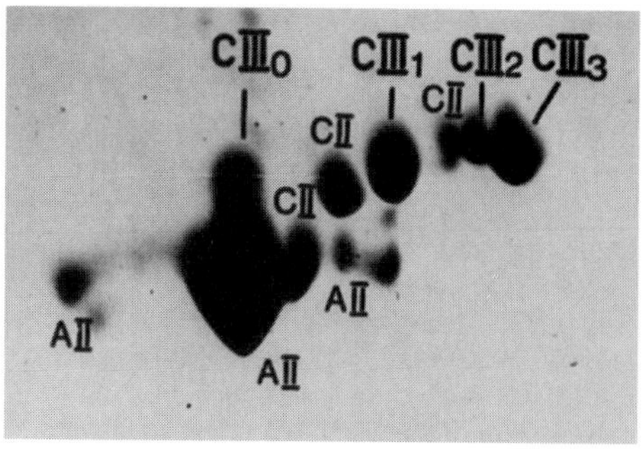

Fig. 142-10 Apolipoprotein C-III_3 in HDL_2 from a CESD patient.

levels in this patient could be a consequence of increased hepatic lipase activity.

Lysosomal Acid Lipase and Atherogenesis

Two distinct forms of lipids accumulate within various cells in arterial lesions: cytoplasmic lipid droplets and lipid-filled lysosomes.[121,122,194–196] The principal lipid found in the lysosomes of aortic cells is not cholesteryl ester but cholesterol, the product of the acid lipase reaction.[194] In addition, lipid-laden atheromatous cells reveal up to 3.5 times the acid cholesteryl esterase activity of normal aortic cells.[157] Cholesterol feeding of rabbits is associated with high aortic acid lipase activity levels, as well as other lysosomal enzyme activities, compared to control animals.[157,244,245] Under these conditions, acid lipase exhibits both cholesteryl ester-hydrolytic (optimal pH 6.6) and cholesteryl ester-synthesizing (optimal pH 6.2) activity, the latter at a rate approximately one-tenth the rate of the former.[246–248] Increased concentration of cholesterol may stimulate esterification and diminish hydrolysis, while high concentrations of lecithin produce the opposite effects.[246] Such conditions might well exist in lipid-laden lysosomes of arterial foam cells,[248] since both ACAT activity at neutral pH and cholesteryl ester synthesis at acid pH (possibly due to the reverse action of acid lipase) were found to be increased in atherogenic lesions[249–252] and in foam cells isolated from lesions.[253,254]

Further considerations suggest that low activity of acid lipase can contribute under certain conditions to cholesteryl ester accumulation and foam-cell formation in atherosclerotic lesions. In studies in which acid lipase activity was measured in mononuclear leukocytes from patients with premature coronary heart disease,[185] enzyme activity was significantly lower in the patients than in age-matched controls. However, no correlation was observed between hypercholesterolemia or hypertriglyceridemia and acid lipase activity. Analysis of acid lipase in the patients' families provided evidence for an autosomal mutation associated with (or responsible for) the reduced enzymatic activity. This genetic factor could represent an independent risk factor for premature coronary heart disease. Reductions in cholesteryl ester hydrolase activity were also measured in freshly isolated mononuclear cells from patients with primary type II hypercholesterolemia, heterozygous familial hypercholesterolemia, and familial combined hyperlipidemia.[255] Diminished acid lipase activity levels also occurred in patients with atherosclerosis of the carotid arteries.[256]

Since aortic acid lipase activity has been found to be lower in animals relatively susceptible to atherosclerosis (rabbit, swine) than in relatively resistant species (rat, dog, guinea pig),[257] a relative deficiency of aortic acid lipase may explain susceptibility to cholesterol-induced atherosclerosis. In spontaneously hypertensive rats, prolonged hypertension caused a decrease in aortic cholesteryl ester hydrolase activity.[258,259] However, in experimentally induced types of hypertension, acid cholesteryl ester hydrolase was found to be either elevated concomitantly with other lysosomal enzymes (induced with desoxycorticosterone) or unchanged, while other lysosomal enzymes were increased (induced by renal arterial constriction).[259,260] These data indicate that factors associated with some forms of hypertension may influence aortic cholesteryl ester hydrolase activity, but there are distinct differences in the response of lysosomal enzymes to etiologically different forms of hypertension.

Hajjar et al.,[261] who studied the atherogenic effect of Marek disease herpesvirus on cholesterol metabolism in cultured chicken arterial smooth muscle cells, reported that infection of these cells with Marek disease virus resulted in (1) decreased acid lipase cholesteryl esterase activity, (2) decreased excretion of cholesterol, (3) increased ACAT activity, and (4) decreased cytoplasmic neutral cholesteryl esterase activity. In addition, antigens of herpesvirus type 1, herpesvirus type 2, and cytomegalovirus have been detected in vessel walls from patients with premature coronary heart disease.[262,263] These findings suggest that infection of arterial wall cells by distinct viruses may promote the atherosclerotic process by altering cellular cholesteryl ester metabolism. In CESD, extensive premature atherosclerotic changes accompany the enzyme deficiency, whereas patients with Wolman disease usually succumb to adrenal or liver failure in infancy before vascular changes have had a chance to become manifest.

DIAGNOSIS

Wolman disease must be considered in any infant with hepatomegaly, gastrointestinal symptoms, and failure to thrive. The earliest examination should include careful attention to neurologic development. X-rays should be taken of the lungs and bones, and of the abdomen to observe the calcification of the adrenals that is almost invariably seen. Calcification of the adrenals may be observed in many other conditions, such as Addison disease,[236] adrenal teratomas,[264] hemorrhage,[5,30,33] neuroblastoma, ganglioneuroma, adrenal cysts, adrenal cortical carcinoma, and pheochromocytoma.[5,30] The presence of bilateral adrenal calcification associated with hepatosplenomegaly and gastrointestinal symptoms strongly supports the diagnosis of Wolman disease. It is noteworthy that adrenal calcification has never been seen in Niemann-Pick disease. The decreased adrenal responsiveness that has been observed in some cases of Wolman disease must be differentiated from that seen in the syndrome of X-linked adrenoleukodystrophy with adrenal insufficiency and cutaneous melanosis.[265] Adrenoleukodystrophy, having a more protracted course and definite signs of central nervous system involvement, is not easily confused with Wolman disease. Moreover, acid lipase activity is normal in fibroblasts[266] and brain tissue homogenates[267] of patients affected with adrenoleukodystrophy. Wolman disease further should be distinguished from conditions in which triglycerides instead of cholesteryl esters accumulate in tissues.[87,268] One patient with triglyceride accumulation in liver but without cholesteryl ester storage in association with acid lipase deficiency has been described.[87] Numerous metabolic diseases (galactosemia, fructose intolerance, certain disorders of amino acid metabolism) may result in secondary triglyceride accumulation. Triglyceride storage disease and neutral lipid storage disease, including the Chanarin-Dorfman syndrome, are separate biochemical and clinical entities accompanied by excessive extralysosomal triglyceride accumulation in various tissues due to number of different defects in the pathway of triglyceride mobilization.[268–270]

A severe congenital triglyceride storage disorder leading to death in the neonatal period has been reported in a unique family under the name "fatty metamorphosis of the viscera."[271] Other patients have been described with phenotypes similar to those of Wolman disease but with longer life spans.[10,36,272] Another generalized accumulation of neutral lipids, also due to a profound deficiency of acid lipase, with features of the Senior syndrome has been reported.[273,274]

CESD may be easily confused with glycogen storage disease. In both disorders, marked hepatomegaly and hyperlipidemia without splenic enlargement may appear in a child whose mental and physical development is otherwise unremarkable. Provocative tests for adequacy of glycogenolysis could be performed, but enzymatic assays of acid lipase in leukocytes and fibroblasts should be diagnostic and should preclude the need for liver biopsy to establish a diagnosis of CESD. The absence of jaundice in any patient with CESD except late in the disease suggests that the disorder need not be confused with congenital biliary cirrhosis. A normal proportion of esters in the total cholesterol in plasma should help exclude biliary obstruction. Vacuolation of hepatocytes can also be observed by light microscopy in Niemann-Pick disease type B, several forms of mucopolysaccharidoses, and G_{M1} gangliosidosis. The latter disorders can be easily distinguished from CESD by enzyme assay and have different findings on examination of cryostat sections of liver under polarized light. In CESD, liver tissue reveals birefringence, which disappears on heating the tissue to 50–60°C and reappears on cooling. Heat-sensitive birefringence of liver tissue is highly suggestive for CESD or Wolman disease and is not observed in other lysosomal deficiency state.

A child suspected to have CESD should have a biochemical study of acid lipase in leukocytes and cultured skin fibroblasts. Definitive diagnosis of acid lipase deficiency is feasible by analysis of the clinical picture and assay of acid ester hydrolase activity in freshly prepared extracts of cultured skin fibroblasts or peripheral leukocytes. Substrates for the determination of acid ester hydrolase include artificial compounds such as nitrophenyl laurate and methylumbelliferyl oleate, as well as cholesteryl oleate solubilized by detergents or incorporated into LDL. Natural substrates are more specific for acid lipase determinations and are to be preferred. Sufficient control data must be obtained; the tissue from a patient with either Wolman disease or CESD should have only 1–10 percent of normal activity. It should rarely if ever be necessary to employ open biopsy of the liver for confirmation of enzyme deficiency or abnormal storage of cholesteryl esters and triglycerides. Finally, definitive proof of the diagnosis should be obtained by elucidation of the precise molecular basis of the disease by DNA sequencing of the gene. In our laboratory, we employ a strategy of direct sequencing of all 10 exons, including the intron boundary regions and the promoter, on a solid support. The method is sensitive and specific enough to identify almost any homozygous or heterozygous mutation that is present in the relevant parts of the gene.[103,104,107]

TREATMENT

There is no specific treatment for Wolman disease or CESD. Replacement of the missing enzyme by either direct infusion or gene therapy has not been attempted. However, the suppression of cholesterol synthesis and apolipoprotein B production induced by HMG-CoA reductase inhibitors can be considered a useful therapeutic principle. It has been demonstrated in a patient with CESD that the HMG-CoA reductase inhibitor lovastatin (20 mg twice daily) resulted in significant reductions in plasma cholesterol, triglycerides, and LDL cholesterol.[199] Therapy also reduced apo B in VLDL and LDL and mevalonate levels in urine. In addition to these changes in plasma lipoproteins, this therapy might also have a beneficial effect on hepatosplenomegaly and adrenal dysfunction. Similar beneficial effects of the combined use of simvastatin (0.28 mg/kg each evening) and cholestyramine (0.22 g/kg twice daily), plus a low-cholesterol diet (37 g fat, including 168 mg/day of cholesterol), and administration of lipophilic vitamins (A, D, E, and K) were obtained with another patient. This treatment resulted in significant elevation of HDL cholesterol levels without a simultaneous rise in plasma apo A-I concentrations. One patient with CESD underwent liver transplantation for chronic liver failure and is well 2 years after the procedure,[99] but a detailed report is not available.

REFERENCES

1. Fredrickson DS, Ferrans VJ: Acid cholesteryl ester hydrolase deficiency (Wolman's disease and cholesteryl ester storage disease), in Stanbury JB, Wyngaarden JB, Fredrickson DS (eds): *The Metabolic Basis of Inherited Disease,* 4th ed. New York, McGraw-Hill, 1978, p 670.
2. Assmann G, Fredrickson DS: Acid lipase deficiency: Wolman's disease and cholesteryl ester storage disease, in Stanbury JB, Wyngaarden JB, Fredrickson DS, Goldstein JL, Brown MS (eds): *The Metabolic Basis of Inherited Disease* 5th ed. New York, McGraw-Hill, 1983, p 803.
3. Schmitz G, Assmann G: Acid lipase deficiency: Wolman disease and cholesteryl ester storage disease, in Scriver CR, Beaudet AL, Sly WS, Valle D (eds): *The Metabolic Basis of Inherited Disease,* 6th ed. New York, McGraw-Hill, 1989, p 1623.
4. Assmann G, Seedorf U: Acid lipase deficiency: Wolman disease and cholesteryl ester storage disease, in: Scriver CR, Beaudet AL, Sly WS, Valle D (eds): *The Metabolic and Molecular Bases of Inherited Disease,* 7th ed. New York, McGraw-Hill, 1995, p 2563.
5. Abramov A, Schorr S, Wolman M: Generalized xanthomatosis with calcified adrenals. *J Dis Child* **91**:282, 1956.
6. Wolman M, Sterk VV, Gatt S, Frenkel M: Primary familial xanthomatosis with involvement and calcification of the adrenals: Report of two more cases in siblings of a previously described infant. *Pediatrics* **28**:742, 1961.
7. Wolman M: Histochemistry of lipids in pathology, in Grauman W, Neumann K (eds): *Handbuch der Histochemie.* Stuttgart, Fischer-Verlag, 1964, p 228.
8. Crocker AC, Vawter GF, Neuhauser ED, Rosowsky A: Wolman's disease: Three new patients with a recently described lipidosis. *Pediatrics* **35**:627, 1965.
9. Alexander W: Niemann-Pick-disease: Report of a case showing calcification in the adrenal glands. *N Z Med J* **45**:43, 1946.
10. Patrick AD, Lake BD: Deficiency of an acid lipase in Wolman's disease. *Nature* **222**:1067, 1969.
11. Wallis K, Gross M, Kohn R, Zaidman J: A case of Wolman's disease. *Helv Paediatr Acta* **26**:98, 1971.
12. Sloan HR, Fredrickson DS: Enzyme deficiency in cholesteryl ester storage disease. *J Clin Invest* **51**:1923, 1972.
13. Cortner JA, Coates PM, Swoboda E, Schnatz JD: Genetic variation of lysosomal acid lipase. *Pediatr Res* **10**:927, 1976.
14. Kyriakides EC, Paul B, Balin JA: Lipid accumulation and acid lipase deficiency in fibroblasts from a family with Wolman's disease, and their apparent correction in vitro. *J Lab Clin Med* **80**:810, 1972.
15. Guy GJ, Butterworth J: Acid esterase activity in cultured skin fibroblasts and amniotic fluid cells using 4-methylumbelliferyl palmitate. *Clin Chim Acta* **84**:361, 1978.
16. Burton BK, Emery D, Mueller HW: Lysosomal acid lipase in cultivated fibroblasts: Characterization of enzyme activity in normal and enzymatically deficient cell lines. *Clin Chim Acta* **101**:25, 1980.
17. Suzuki Y, Kawai S, Kobayashi A, Ohbe Y, Endo H: Partial deficiency of acid lipase with storage of triglycerides and cholesterol esters in liver. *Clin Chim Acta* **69**:219, 1976.
18. Schaub J, Janka GE, Christomanou H, Sandhoff K, Permanetter W, Hubner G, Meister P: Wolman's disease: Clinical, biochemical and ultrastructural studies in an unusual case without striking adrenal calcification. *Eur J Pediatr* **135**:45, 1980.
19. Young EP, Patrick AD: Deficiency of acid esterase activity in Wolman's disease. *Arch Dis Child* **45**:664, 1970.
20. Neuhauser ED, Kirkpatrick JA, Weintraub H: Wolman's disease: A new lipidosis. *Ann Radiol* (Paris) **8**:175, 1965.
21. Rosowsky A, Crocker AC, Trites DH, Modest EJ: Gas-liquid chromatography analysis of the tissue sterol fraction in Wolman's disease and related lipidoses. *Biochim Biophys Acta* **98**:617, 1965.
22. Konno T, Fujy M, Watanuki T, Koizumi K: Wolman's disease: The first case in Japan. *Tohoku J Exp Med* **90**:375, 1966.
23. Spiegel-Adolf M, Baird HW, McCafferty M: Hematologic studies in Niemann-Pick and Wolman's disease (cytology and electrophoresis). *Cofin Neurol* **28**:399, 1966.
24. Caffey J, Silvermann FN: Pediatric x-ray diagnosis, in *Year Book Medical* 5th ed. Chicago, Year Book, 1967, p 672.
25. Sloviter HA, Janic V, Naiman JL: Lipid synthesis by red blood cell preparations in Wolman's disease (a familial lipidosis). *Clin Chim Acta* **20**:423, 1968.
26. Guazzi GC, Martin JJ, Philippart M, Roels H, Van Der Ercken H, Delbeke MJ, Vrints L: Wolman's disease. *Eur Neurol* **1**:334, 1968.

27. Guazzi GC, Martin JJ, Philippart M, Roels H, Hooft C, Van Der Ercken H, Delbeke MJ, Vrints J: Wolman's disease. Distribution and significance of the central nervous system lesions. *Pathol Eur* **3**:266, 1968.
28. Kahana D, Berant M, Wolman M: Primary familial xanthomatosis with adrenal involvement (Wolman's disease): Report of a further case with nervous system involvement and pathogenetic considerations. *Pediatrics* **42**:70, 1968.
29. Kamoshita S, Landing BH: Distribution of lesions in myenteric plexus and gastrointestinal mucosa in lipidoses and other neurological disorders of children. *Am J Clin Pathol* **49**:312, 1968.
30. Marks M, Marcus AJ: Wolman's disease. *Can Med Assoc J* **99**:232, 1968.
31. Partin JC, Mereu TR, Schubert WK: Intestinal absorptive epithelium in Wolman's cholesterol lipidoses, in Arcenaux CJ (ed): *Proceedings of the 26th Annual Meeting of the Electron Microscope Society of America*. Baton Rouge, Claitor's, 1968, p 194.
32. Wolman M: Involvement of nervous tissue in primary familial xanthomatosis with adrenal calcification. *Pathol Eur* **3**:259, 1968.
33. Marshall WC, Ockenden BC, Fosbrooke AS, Cumings JN: Wolman's disease: A rare lipidosis with adrenal calcification. *Arch Dis Child* **44**:331, 1968.
34. Werbin BZ, Wolman M: Primary familial xanthomatosis with involvement and calcification of the adrenals (Wolman's disease). *Harefuah* **74**:283, 1968.
35. Eto Y, Kitagawa T: Wolman's disease with hypolipoproteinemia and acanthocytosis: Clinical and biochemical observations. *J Pediatr* **77**:862, 1970.
36. Lake BD, Patrick AD: Wolman's disease: Deficiency of E600-resistant acid esterase activity with storage of lipids in lysosomes. *J Pediatr* **77**:862, 1970.
37. Lough J, Fawcett J, Wiegensberg B: Wolman's disease: An electron microscopic, histochemical and biochemical study. *Arch Pathol* **89**:103, 1970.
38. Lowden JA, Baron AJ, Wentworth P: Wolman's disease: A microscopic and biochemical study showing accumulation of ceroid and esterified cholesterol. *Can Med Assoc J* **102**:402, 1970.
39. Kyriakides EC, Filippone N, Paul B, Grattan W, Balint JA: Lipid studies in Wolman's disease. *Pediatrics* **46**:431, 1970.
40. Leclerc JL, Hould F, Lelievre M, Gagne F: Maladie de Wolman. Etude anatomo-clinique d'une nouvelle observation avec absence de calcifications radiologiques et macroscopiques des surrenales. *Laval Med* **42**:461, 1971.
41. Philippart M: Wolman's disease. *J Pediatr* **79**:173, 1971.
42. Raafat R, Hashemian MP, Abrishami MA: Wolman's disease: Report of two new cases with a review of the literature. *Am J Clin Pathol* **59**:490, 1973.
43. Kamalian N, Dudley AW, Beroukhim F: Wolman's disease with jaundice and subarachnoid hemorrhage. *Am J Dis Child* **126**:671, 1973.
44. Uno Y, Taniguchi A, Tanaka E: Histochemical studies in Wolman's disease: Report of an autopsy case accompanied with a large amount of milky ascites. *Acta Pathol Jpn* **23**:779, 1973.
45. Wolf H, Nolte K, Nolte R: Das neue Syndrom: Wolman-Syndrom. *Monatsschr Kinderheilkd* **121**:697, 1973.
46. Lajo A, Gracia R, Navarro M, Nistal M, Robodan B: Enfermedad de Wolman en su forma aguda infantil. *An Esp Pediatr* **7**:438, 1974.
47. Ellis JE, Patrick D: Wolman disease in a Pakistani infant. *Am J Dis Child* **130**:545, 1976.
48. Harrison RB, Francke P Jr: Radiographic findings in Wolman's disease. *Radiology* **124**:188, 1977.
49. Ozsoylu S, Gurgery A, Kocak N, Ozoran Y, Ozoran A, Kerse I, Ciliv G: Wolman's disease. A case report with lipid, chromosome and electronmicroscopic studies. *Turk J Pediatr* **19**:57, 1977.
50. von Bassewitz DB, Roggenkamp K, Strehl H, Otto H: Wolmansche Erkrankung. *Verh Dtsch Ges Pathol* **62**:530, 1978.
51. Ozoran Y, Ozoran A, Kerse I, Gurgery A, Ozsoylu S, Kocak N, Ciliv G: An ultrastructural study in a case of Wolman's disease (clinical, biochemical, light and electron microscopic study). *Turk J Pediatr* **20**:100, 1978.
52. Ho FC, Lin HJ, Chan WC: Wolman's disease: The first reported Chinese patient. *Mod Med Asia* **14**:23, 1978.
53. Schaffner T, Elner VM, Bauer M, Wissler RW: Acid lipase: A histochemical and biochemical study using triton X 100-naphtylpalmitate micelles. *J Histochem Cytochem* **26**:696, 1978.
54. Sty JR, Starshak RJ: Scintigraphy in Wolman's disease. *Clin Nucl Med* **3**:397, 1978.
55. Young LW, Sty JR, Babbitt JP: Wolman's disease. *Am J Dis Child* **133**:959, 1979.
56. Byrd JC, Powers JM: Wolman's disease: Ultrastructural evidence of lipid accumulation in central nervous system. *Acta Neuropathol* (Berlin) **45**:37, 1979.
57. Permanetter W, Muller H, Hubner G, Schaub J: Wolman's disease. *Med Welt* **30**:1783, 1979.
58. Marosvari I: Wolman disease in twins. *Acta Paediatr Hung* **26**:61, 1985.
59. Bona G, Bracco G, Gallina MR, Ivarone A, Perona A, Zaffaroni M: Wolman's disease: Clinical and biochemical findings of a new case. *J Inherit Metab Dis* **11**:423, 1988.
60. Zubov NA, Zakharova SI, Vibe AB: Wolman disease in children in the same family. *Pediatria* **5**:90, 1989.
61. Bona G, Bracco G, Gallina MR, Ivarone A, Artesani L, Perona A: A case of acid lipase deficiency: Wolman's disease. *Panminerva Med* **31**:49, 1989.
62. Wang TR, Chuang SM: A Chinese case of Wolman disease. *J Inherit Metab Dis* **12**:328, 1989.
63. Storm W, Wendel U, Sprenkamp M, Seidler A: Wolmansche Erkrankung bei einem Saugling. *Monatsschr Kinderheilkd* **138**:88, 1990.
64. Kikuchi M, Igarashii K, Noro T, Igarashi Y, Hirooka M, Tada K: Evaluation of jejunal function in Wolman's disease. *J Pediatr Gastroenterol Nutr* **12**:65, 1991.
65. Assmann G, Fredrickson DS, Sloan HR, Fales HM, Highet RI: Accumulation of oxygenated steryl esters in Wolman's disease. *J Lipid Res* **16**:28, 1975.
66. Fredrickson DS: Newly recognized disorders of cholesterol metabolism. *Ann Intern Med* **58**:718, 1963.
67. Lageron A, Caroli I, Stralin H, Barbier P: Polycorie cholesterique de l'adulte. I. Etude clinique, electronique, histochimique. *Presse Med* **75**:2785, 1967.
68. Infante R, Polonovski J, Caroli J: Polycorie cholesterique de l'adulte. II. Etude biochimique. *Presse Med* **75**:2829, 1967.
69. Schiff L, Schubert WK, McAdams AJ, Spiegel EL, O'Donnell JF: Hepatic cholesterol ester storage disease, a familial disorder. I. Clinical aspects. *Am J Med* **44**:538, 1968.
70. Partin JC, Schubert WK: Small intestinal mucosa in cholesterol ester storage disease: A light and electron microscope study. *Gastroenterology* **57**:542, 1969.
71. Fredrickson DS, Sloan HR, Ferrans VJ, Demosky SJ: Cholesteryl ester storage disease: A most unusual manifestation of deficiency of two lysosomal enzyme activities. *Trans Assoc Am Physicians* **85**:109, 1972.
72. Beaudet AL, Ferry GD, Nichols BL, Rosenberg HS: Cholesterol ester storage disease: Clinical, biochemical and pathological studies. *J Pediatr* **90**:910, 1977.
73. Orme RLE: Wolman's disease: An unusual presentation. *Proc R Soc Med* **63**:489, 1970.
74. Wolf H, Hug G, Michaelis R, Nolte K: Seltene angeborene Erkrankung mit Cholesterinester-Speicherung in der Leber. *Helv Paediatr Acta* **29**:105, 1974.
75. Alagille D, Courtecuisse V: Surcharge hepatique a esters du cholesterol (deux observations). *J Parisiennes Pediatr* **3**:465, 1970.
76. Lageron A, Gautier M, Scotto J: Particularités cliniques et histoenzymologiques de la polycorie cholestereolique chez deux enfants d'une même fratrie. *Arch Fr Pediatr* **42**:605, 1985.
77. Desai PK, Astrin KH, Thung SN, Gordon RE, Short MP, Coates PM, Desnick RJ: Cholesteryl ester storage disease: Pathologic changes in an affected fetus. *Am J Med Genet* **26**:689, 1987.
78. Tylki SA, Maciejko D, Wozniewicz B, Muszynska B: Two cases of cholesteryl ester storage disease (CESD) acid lipase deficiency. *Hepatogastroenterology* **34**:98, 1987.
79. Edelstein RA, Filling K, Pentschev P, Gal A, Chandra R, Shawker T, Guzetta P, Comly M, Kaneski C, Brady RO, Barton N: Cholesteryl ester storage disease: A patient with massive splenomegaly and splenic abscess. *Am J Gastroenterol* **83**:687, 1988.
80. D'Agostino D, Bay L, Gallo R, Chamoles N: Cholesteryl ester storage disease: Clinical, biochemical, and pathological studies of four new cases. *J Pediatr Gastroenterol Nutr* **7**:446, 1988.
81. Elleder M, Ledvinova J, Cieslar P, Kuhn R: Subclinical course of cholesterol ester storage disease diagnosed in adulthood. Report on two cases with remarks on the nature of the liver storage process. *Virchows Arch [A]* **416**:357, 1990.
82. Ekert P, Metreau JM, Zafrani ES, Fabre M, Buffet C, Etienne JP, D'humeaux D: Surcharge hépatique en esters de cholestérol. Deux nouveaux cas diagnostiques chez l'adulte. *Gastroenterol Clin Biol* **15**:441, 1991.

83. Lageron A, Lichtenstein H, Bodin F, Conte M: Polycorie cholestérolique de l'adulte: A propos d'une nouvelle observation. *Nouv Presse Med* **3**:1233, 1974
84. Lageron A, Lichtenstein H, Bodin F, Conte M: Polycorie cholestérolique de l'adulte: Aspects cliniques et histochimiques. *Med Chir Dig* **4**:9, 1975.
85. Lageron A: Histoenzymologie de la polycorie cholestérolique. *Med Chir Dig* **7**:155, 1978.
86. Gautier M, Lapons D, Raulin J: Maladie de surcharge aesters du cholésterol chez l'enfant. Etude biochimique comparative de cultures d'hepatocytes et de fibroblasts. *Arch Fr Pediatr* **35**(suppl):38, 1978.
87. Aubert-Tulkens G, van Hoof F: Acid lipase deficiency: Clinical and biochemical heterogeneity. *Acta Paediatr Belg* **32**:239, 1979.
88. Keller E, Kunnert B, Braun W: Cholesterinspeicherkrankheit der Leber im Kindesalter. *Dtsch Z Verdau Stoffwechselkr* **37**:231, 1977.
89. Kunnert B, Cossel L, Keller E: Zur Diagnostik und Morphologie der Leber bei Cholesterinester-Speicherkrankheit. *Zentralbl Allg Pathol* **123**:71, 1979.
90. Pfeiffer U, Jeschke R: Cholesterylester-Speicherkrankheit. *Virchows Arch [B]* **33**:17, 1980.
91. Kuntz HD, May B, Schejbal V, Assmann G: Cholesterinester-Speicherkrankheit der Leber. *Leber Magen Darm* **11**:258, 1981.
92. Burke JA, Schubert WK: Deficient activity of hepatic acid lipase in cholesterol ester storage disease. *Science* **176**:309, 1972.
93. Partin JC, Schubert WK: The ultrastructural and lipid composition of cultured skin fibroblasts in cholesterol ester storage disease. *Pediatr Res* **6**:393, 1972.
94. Beaudet AL, Lipson MH, Ferry GD, Nichols BLJ: Acid lipase in cultured fibroblasts: Cholesterol ester storage disease. *J Lab Clin Med* **84**:54, 1974.
95. Goldstein JL, Dana SE, Faust JR, Beaudet AL, Brown MS: Role of lysosomal acid lipase in the metabolism of plasma low density lipoprotein: Observations in cultured fibroblasts from a patient with cholesteryl ester storage disease. *J Biol Chem* **250**:8487, 1975.
96. Brown MS, Sabhani MK, Braunschede GY, Goldstein JL: Restoration of a regulatory response to low density lipoprotein in acid lipase-deficient human fibroblasts. *J Biol Chem* **251**:3277, 1976.
97. Cagle PT, Ferry GD, Beaudet AL, Hawkins EP: Clinicopathologic conference: Pulmonary hypertension in an 18-year-old girl with cholesteryl ester storage disease (CESD). *Am J Med Genet* **24**:711, 1986.
98. Ferry GD, Beaudet AL: Personal communication.
99. Kelly DR, Hoeg JM, Demosky S, Brewer HB Jr: Characterization of plasma lipids and lipoproteins in cholesteryl ester storage disease. *Biochem Med* **33**:29, 1985.
100. Burton BK, Remy WT, Raymon L: Cholesterol ester triglyceride metabolism in intact fibroblasts from patients with Wolman's disease and cholesterol ester storage disease. *Pediatr Res* **18**:1242, 1984.
101. Anderson RA, Byrum RS, Coates PM, Sando GN: Mutations at the lysosomal acid cholesteryl ester hydrolase gene locus in Wolman disease. *Proc Natl Acad Sci USA* **91**:2718, 1994.
102. Klima H, Ullrich K, Aslanidis C, Fehringer P, Lackner KJ, Schmitz G: A splice junction mutation causes deletion of a 72-base exon from the mRNA for lysosomal acid lipase in a patient with cholesteryl ester storage disease. *J Clin Invest* **92**:2713, 1993.
103. Muntoni S, Wiebusch H, Funke H, Ros E, Seedorf U, Assmann G: Homozygosity for a splice junction mutation in exon 8 of the gene encoding lysosomal acid lipase in a Spanish kindred with cholesterol ester storage disease (CESD). *Hum Genet* **95**:491, 1995.
104. Seedorf U, Wiebusch H, Muntoni S, Christensen NC, Skovby F, Nickel V, Roskos M, Funke H, Ose L, Assmann G: A novel variant of lysosomal acid lipase (Leu336 → Pro) associated with acid lipase deficiency and cholesterol ester storage disease. *Arterioscler Thromb Vasc Biol* **15**:773, 1995.
105. Redonnet-Vernhet I, Chatelut M, Basile JP, Salvayre R, Levade T: Cholesteryl ester storage disease: Relationship between molecular defects and in situ activity of lysosomal acid lipase. *Biochem Mol Med* **62**:42, 1997.
106. Gasche C, Aslanidis C, Kain R, Exner M, Helbich T, Dejaco C, Schmitz G, Ferenci P: A novel variant of lysosomal acid lipase in cholesteryl ester storage disease associated with mild phenotype and improvement on lovastatin. *J Hepatol* **27**:744, 1997.
107. Wiebusch H, Muntoni S, Funke H, Lu F, Seedorf U, Oberle S, Schwarzer U, Assmann G: A novel missense mutation (Gly2Arg) in the human lysosomal acid lipase gene is found in individuals with and without cholesterol ester storage disease (CESD). *Clin Genet* **50**:106, 1996.
108. Pagani F, Garcia R, Pariyarath R, Stuani C, Gridelli B, Paone G, Baralle FE: Expression of lysosomal acid lipase mutants detected in three patients with cholesteryl ester storage disease. *Hum Mol Genet* **5**:1611, 1996.
109. Aslanidis C, Ries S, Fehringer P, Buchler C, Klima H, Schmitz G: Genetic and biochemical evidence that CESD and Wolman disease are distinguished by residual lysosomal acid lipase activity. *Genomics* **33**:85, 1996.
110. Maslen CL, Babcock D, Illingworth DR: Occurrence of a mutation associated with Wolman disease in a family with cholesteryl ester storage disease. *J Inherit Metab Dis* **18**:620, 1995.
111. Ameis D, Brockmann G, Knoblich R, Merkel M, Ostlund RE Jr, Yang JW, Coates PM, Cortner JA, Feinman SV, Greten H: A 5′ splice-region mutation and a dinucleotide deletion in the lysosomal acid lipase gene in two patients with cholesteryl ester storage disease. *J Lipid Res* **36**:241, 1995.
112. Hill SC, Hoeg JM, Dwyer AJ, Vucich JJ, Doppman JL: CT findings in acid lipase deficiency: Wolman's disease and cholesteryl ester storage disease. *J Comput Assist Tomogr* **7**:815, 1983.
113. Ferrans VJ, Buja LM, Roberts WC, Fredrickson DS: The spleen in type I hyperlipoproteinemia: Histochemical, biochemical, microfluorimetric, and electron microscopic observations. *Am J Pathol* **64**:67, 1971.
114. Ferrans VJ, Roberts WC, Levy RI, Fredrickson DS: Chylomicrons and the formation of foam cells in type I hyperlipoproteinemia: A morphologic study. *Am J Pathol* **70**:253, 1973.
115. Drevon CA, Hovig T: The effects of cholesterol/fat feeding on lipid levels and morphological structures in liver, kidney and spleen in guinea pigs. *Acta Pathol Microbiol Scand [A]* **85**:1, 1977.
116. Yoshida H, Kuriyama M: Genetic lipid storage disease with lysosomal acid lipase deficiency in rats. *Lab Anim Sci* **40**:486, 1990.
117. Nakagawa H, Matsubara S, Kuriyama M, Yoshidome H, Fujiyama J, Yoshida H, Osame M: Cloning of rat lysosomal acid lipase cDNA and identification of the mutation in the rat model of Wolman's disease. *J Lipid Res* **36**:2212, 1995.
118. Kuriyama M, Yoshida H, Susuki M, Fujiyama J, Igata A: Lysosomal acid lipase deficiency in rats: Lipid analyses and lipase activities in liver and spleen. *J Lipid Res* **31**:1605, 1990.
119. Hayashi H, Winship DH, Sternlieb I: Lipolysosomes in human liver: Distribution in livers with fatty infiltration. *Gastroenterology* **73**:651, 1977.
120. De Duve C: Exploring cells with a centrifuge. *Science* **198**:186, 1975.
121. Goldfischer S, Schiller B, Wolinsky H: Lipid accumulation in smooth muscle cell lysosomes in primate atherosclerosis. *Am J Pathol* **78**:497, 1975.
122. Peters TJ, De Duve C: Lysosomes of the arterial wall. II. Subcellular fractionation of aortic cells from rabbits with experimental atheroma. *Exp Mol Pathol* **20**:228, 1974.
123. Peters TJ, Takano T, De Duve C: Subcellular fractionation studies on the cells isolated from normal and atherosclerotic aorta, in Porter R (ed): *Atherogenesis: Initiating Factors. CIBA Foundation Symposium, 1972*. Amsterdam, Associated Scientific, 1973, p 197.
124. Lin HJ, Lie K, Ho FC: Accumulation of glyceryl ether lipids in Wolman's disease. *J Lipid Res* **17**:53, 1976.
125. Fredrickson DS: Tangier disease, in Stanbury JB, Wyngaarden JB, Fredrickson DS (eds): *The Metabolic Basis of Inherited Disease* 2^{d} ed. New York, McGraw-Hill, 1966, p 486.
126. Pagani F, Zagato L, Merati G, Paone G, Gridelli B, Maier JA: A histidine to tyrosine replacement in lysosomal acid lipase causes cholesteryl ester storage disease. *Hum Mol Genet* **3**:1605, 1994.
127. Pariyarath R, Pagani F, Stuani C, Garcia R, Baralle FE: L273S missense substitution in human lysosomal acid lipase creates a new N-glycosylation site. *FEBS Lett* **397**:79, 1996.
127a. Ries S, Büchler C, Schindler G, Aslanidis C, Ameis D, Gasche C, Jung N, Schambach A, Fehringer P, Vanier MT, Belli DC, Greten H, Schmitz G: Different missense mutations in histidine-108 of lysosomal acid lipase cause cholesteryl ester storage disease in unrelated compound heterozygous and hemizygous individuals. *Hum Mutat* **12**:44, 1998.
127b. Mayatepek E, Seedorf U, Wiebusch H, Lenhartz H, Assmann G: Fatal genetic defect causing Wolman disease. *J Inherit Metab Dis* **22**:93, 1999.
127c. Seedorf U, Guardamagna O, Strobl W, Mayatepek E, Assmann G, Funke H: Mutation report: Wolman disease. *Hum Genet* **105**:337, 1999.

128. Ries S, Aslanidis C, Fehringer P, Carel JC, Gendrel D, Schmitz G: A new mutation in the gene for lysosomal acid lipase leads to Wolman disease in an African kindred. *J Lipid Res* **37**:1761, 1996.
129. Fujiyama J, Sakuraba H, Kuriyama M, Fujita T, Nagata K, Nakagawa H, Osame M: A new mutation (LIPA Tyr22X) of lysosomal acid lipase gene in a Japanese patient with Wolman disease. *Hum Mutat* **8**:377, 1996.
130. Lake BD: Histochemical detection of the enzyme deficiency in blood in Wolman's disease. *J Clin Pathol* **24**:617, 1971.
131. Kelly S, Bakhru-Kishore R: Fluorimetric assay of acid lipase in human leukocytes. *Clin Chim Acta* **97**:239, 1979.
132. Coates PM, Cortner J: Acid lipase in cultured amnionic fluid cells. Implications for the prenatal diagnosis of Wolman's disease. *Pediatr Res* **12**:450, 1978.
133. Christomanou H, Cap C: Prenatal monitoring of Wolman's disease in a pregnancy at risk: First case in the Federal Republic of Germany. *Hum Genet* **57**:440, 1981.
134. Sheriff S, Du H, Grabowski GA: Characterization of lysosomal acid lipase by site-directed mutagenesis and heterologous expression. *J Biol Chem* **270**:27766, 1995.
135. Anderson RA, Sando GN: Cloning and expression of cDNA encoding human lysosomal acid lipase/cholesteryl ester hydrolase. *J Biol Chem* **266**:22479, 1991.
136. Rothman ER, Orci L: Molecular dissection of the secretory pathway. *Nature* **355**:409, 1992.
137. Griffiths G, Simons K: The trans Golgi network: Sorting at the exit site of the Golgi complex. *Science* **234**:438, 1986.
138. Sando GN, Henke VL, Neufeld EF, Garvin AJ, Rowl L: Recognition and receptor-mediated endocytosis of the lysosomal acid lipase secreted by cultured human fibroblasts. *J Lipid Res* **23**:114, 1982.
139. Neufeld EF, Sando GN, Garvin AJ, Rowl L: The transport of lysosomal enzymes. *J Supramol Struct* **6**:95, 1977.
140. Sando GN, Rosenbaum LM: Human lysosomal acid lipase/cholesteryl ester hydrolase. Purification and properties of the form secreted by fibroblasts in microcarrier culture. *J Biol Chem* **260**:15186, 1985.
141. Hoeg JM, Demosky SJ Jr, Pescovitz OH, Brewer HB Jr: Cholesteryl ester storage disease and Wolman's disease: Phenotypic variants of lysosomal acid cholesteryl ester hydrolase deficiency. *Am J Hum Genet* **36**:1190, 1984.
142. Fowler SD, Brown WJ: Lysosomal acid lipase, in Borgstrom B, Brockmann HL (eds): *Lipases*. Amsterdam, Elsevier, 1984, p 329.
143. Takano T, Black WJ, Peters TJ, De Duve C: Assay, kinetics, and lysosomal localization of an acid cholesteryl esterase in rabbit aortic smooth muscle cells. *J Biol Chem* **249**:6732, 1974.
144. Belfrage P, Vaughan M: Simple liquid-liquid partition system for isolation of labeled oleic acid from mixtures with glycerides. *J Lipid Res* **10**:341, 1969.
145. Pittman RC, Khoo JC, Steinberg D: Cholesterol esterase in rat adipose tissue and its activation by cyclic adenosine 3′, 5′-monophosphate-dependent protein kinase. *J Biol Chem* **250**:4505, 1975.
146. Brecher P, Chobanian J, Small DM, Chobanian AV: The use of phospholipid residues for in vitro studies on cholesteryl-ester hydrolysis. *J Lipid Res* **17**:239, 1976.
147. Brecher P, Pynn HY, Chobanian AV: Cholesterol ester and triglyceride hydrolysis by an acid lipase from rabbit aorta. *Biochim Biophys Acta* **530**:112, 1978.
148. Salvayre R, Negre A, Maret A, Radom J, Douste-Blazy L: Maladie de Wolman et polycorie cholesterolique de l'adulte. *Ann Biol Clin (Paris)* **44**:611, 1986.
149. Negre A, Salvayre R, Rogalle P, Dang QQ, Douste-Blazy L: Acyl chain specifity and properties of cholesterol esterases from normal and Wolman lymphoid cell lines. *Biochim Biophys Acta* **918**:76, 1987.
150. Negre A, Salvayre R, Dagan A, Gatt S: New fluorometric assay of lysosomal acid lipase and its application to the diagnosis of Wolman's and cholesteryl ester storage diseases. *Clin Chim Acta* **149**:81, 1985.
151. Negre A, Salvayre R, Maret A, Vieu C, Bes JC, Borrone C, Durand P, Douste-Blazy L: Lymphoid cell lines as a model system for the study of Wolman's disease: Enzymatic, metabolic and ultrastructural investigations. *J Inherit Metab Dis* **9**:193, 1986.
152. Negre A, Dagan A, Gatt S: Pyrene-methyl lauryl ester, a new fluorescent substrate for lipases: Use for diagnosis of acid lipase deficiency in Wolman's and cholesteryl ester storage diseases. *Enzyme* **42**:110, 1989.
153. Smith AG, Brooks CW, Harland WA: Acid cholesterol ester hydrolase in pig and human aortas. *Steroid Lipids Res* **5**:150, 1974.
154. Mahadevan S, Tappel AL: Lysosomal lipases of rat liver and kidney. *J Biol Chem* **243**:2849, 1968.
155. Hayase K, Tappel AL: Specificity and other properties of lysosomal lipase of rat liver. *J Biol Chem* **245**:169, 1970.
156. Brown WJ, Sgoutas DS: Purification of rat liver lysosomal cholesteryl ester hydrolase. *Biochim Biophys Acta* **617**:305, 1980.
157. Haley NJ, Fowler S, De Duve C: Lysosomal acid cholesteryl esterase activity in normal and lipid-laden aortic cells. *J Lipid Res* **21**:961, 1980.
158. Shinomiya M, Matsuoka N, Shirai K, Saito Y, Kumagai A: Studies on cholesterol esterase in rat arterial wall. *Atherosclerosis* **33**:343, 1979.
159. Burton BK, Mueller HW: Purification and properties of human placental acid lipase. *Biochim Biophys Acta* **618**:449, 1980.
160. Hayasaka S, Hara S, Mizumo K: Partial purification and properties of acid lipase in the bovine retinal pigment epithelium. *Exp Eye Res* **25**:317, 1977.
161. Rindler-Ludwig R, Patsch W, Sailer S, Braunsteiner H: Characterization and partial purification of acid lipase from human leukocytes. *Biochim Biophys Acta* **488**:294, 1977.
162. Anderson RA, Rao N, Byrum RS, Rothshild CB, Bowden DW, Hayworth R, Pettenati M: In situ localization of the genetic locus encoding the lysosomal acid lipase/cholesteryl esterase (LIPA) deficient in Wolman disease to chromosome 10q23.2-q23.3. *Genomics* **15**:245, 1993.
163. Aslanidis C, Klima H, Lackner KJ, Schmitz G: Genomic organization of the human lysosomal acid lipase gene (LIPA). *Genomics* **20**:329, 1994.
164. Holm C, Kirchgessner TG, Svenson KL, Fredrickson G, Nilsson S, Miller CG, Schively JE, Heinzmann C, Sparkes RS, Mohandas T et al.: Hormone-sensitive lipase: Sequence, expression, and chromosomal localization to 19 cent-q13.3. *Science* **241**:1503, 1988.
165. Han JH, Stratowa C, Rutter WJ: Isolation of full-length putative rat lysophospholipase cDNA using improved methods for mRNA isolation and cDNA cloning. *Biochemistry* **26**:1617, 1987.
166. Kissel JA, Fontaine RN, Turck CW, Brockman HL, Hui DY: Molecular cloning and expression of cDNA for rat pancreatic cholesterol esterase. *Biochim Biophys Acta* **1006**:227, 1989.
167. Kyger EM, Wiegang RC, Lange RG: Cloning of the bovine pancreatic cholesterol esterase/lysophospholipase. *Biochem Biophys Res Commun* **164**:1302, 1989.
168. McLean J, Fielding C, Drayna D, Dieplinger H, Baer B, Kohr W, Henzel W, Lawn R: Cloning and expression of human lecithin-cholesterol acyltransferase cDNA. *Proc Natl Acad Sci USA* **83**:2335, 1986.
169. Wion KL, Kirchgessner TG, Lusis AJ, Schotz MC, Lawn RM: Human lipoprotein lipase complementary DNA sequence. *Science* **235**:1638, 1987.
170. Komaromy MC, Schotz MC: Cloning of rat hepatic lipase cDNA: Evidence for a lipase gene family. *Proc Natl Acad Sci USA* **84**:1526, 1987.
171. de Caro J, Boudouard M, Bonicel J, Guidoni A, Desnuelle P, Rovery M: Porcine pancreatic lipase. Completion of the primary structure. *Biochim Biophys Acta* **671**:129, 1981.
172. Winkler FK, D'Arcy A, Hunziker W: Structure of human pancreatic lipase. *Nature* **343**:771, 1990.
173. Davis RC, Stahnke G, Wong H, Doolittle MH, Ameis D, Will H, Schotz MC: Hepatic lipase: Site-directed mutagenesis of a serine residue important for catalytic activity. *J Biol Chem* **265**:6291, 1990.
174. Dispersio LP, Fontaine RN, Hui DY: Identification of the active site serine in pancreatic cholesterol esterase by chemical modification and site-specific mutagenesis. *J Biol Chem* **265**:16801, 1990.
175. Gargouri Y, Moreau H, Pieroni G, Verger R: Role of a sulfhydryl group in gastric lipases. A binding study using the monomolecular-film technique. *Eur J Biochem* **180**:367, 1989.
176. von Heijne G: A new method for predicting signal sequence cleavage sites. *Nucleic Acids Res* **14**:4683, 1986.
177. Deleted in proof.
178. van Gong N, Weil D, Hors-Cayla MC, Gross MS, Heuertz S, Foubert C, Fresal J: Assignment of the genes for human lysosomal acid lipases A and B to chromosomes 10 and 16. *Hum Genet* **55**:375, 1980.
179. Koch G, Lalley PA, Shows TB: Acid lipase 1 (LIP-I) is on mouse chromosome 19: Evidence for homologous regions of human chromosome 10 and mouse 19. *Cytogenet Cell Genet* **32**:291, 1982.
180. Koch G, Lalley PA, McAvoy M, Shows TB: Assignment of LIPA, associated with human acid lipase deficiency, to human chromosome 10 and comparative assignment to mouse chromosome 19. *Somat Cell Genet* **7**:345, 1981.

181. Gross MS, van Gong M, Hors C, Weil D, Heuertz S, Foubert C: Acid lipases and Wolman and cholesteryl ester storage diseases. *Ann Genet* **26**:10, 1983.
182. Hoeg JM, Demosky SJ, Brewer HB Jr: Characterization of neutral and acid ester hydrolase in Wolman's disease. *Biochim Biophys Acta* **711**:59, 1982.
183. Messieh S, Clarke JR, Cook HW, Spence MW: Abnormal neutral lipase activity in acid lipase deficient cultured human fibroblasts. *Pediatr Res* **17**:770, 1983.
184. Pittman RC, Williams JC, Miller A, Steinberg D: Acid acylhydrolase deficiency in I-cell disease and pseudo-Hurler polydystrophy. *Biochim Biophys Acta* **575**:399, 1979.
185. Coates PM, Langer T, Cortner JA: Genetic variations of human mononuclear leukocyte lysosomal acid lipase activity. Relationship to atherosclerosis. *Atherosclerosis* **62**:11, 1986.
186. Negre A, Salvayre R, Vuillaume M, Durant P, Douste-Blazy L: Acid lipase EC-3.1.1.3. and carboxylesterases EC-3.1.1.1. in Epstein-Barr virus transformed lymphoid cell from Wolman's disease: influence of fatty-acid structure of substrate. *Enzyme* **31**:241, 1984.
187. Negre A, Salvayre R, Durant P, Lenoir G, Douste-Blazy L: Enzyme studies on Epstein-Barr virus transformed lymphoid cell lines from Wolman's disease. Lipases, cholesterol esterase and 4-methylumbelliferyl acyl ester hydrolases. *Biochim Biophys Acta* **794**:89, 1984.
188. Salvayre R, Negre A, Maret A, Radom J, Rogalle P, Dang QQ, Gatt S, Douste-Blazy L: Lipases, cholesterylesterases and carboxylesterases in lymphoid cell lines: Substrate specificity and relation to Wolman's cholesteryl ester storage diseases and lipid storage myopathy, in Freysz L, Dreyfus H (eds): *Enzymes of Lipid Metabolism II*. New York, Plenum, 1986, p 809.
189. Coleman RA, Haynes EB: Differentiation of microsomal from lysosomal triacylglycerol lipase activities in rat liver. *Biochim Biophys Acta* **751**:230, 1983.
190. Keough DT, Zerner B: The relationship between the carboxylesterase and monoacylglycerol lipase activities of chicken liver microsomes. *Biochim Biophys Acta* **829**:164, 1985.
191. Coates PM, Cortner JA, Hoffman GM, Brown SA: Acid lipase activity of human lymphocytes. *Biochim Biophys Acta* **572**:225, 1979.
192. Sukarada T, Orimo H, Okabe H, Noma A, Murakami M: Purification and properties of cholesterol ester hydrolase from human aortic intima and media. *Biochim Biophys Acta* **424**:204, 1976.
193. Brown MS, Kovanen PT, Goldstein JL: Regulation of plasma cholesterol by lipoprotein receptors. *Science* **212**:628, 1981.
194. Shio H, Haley NJ, Fowler S: Characterization of lipid-laden aortic cells from cholesterol fed rabbits. *Lab Invest* **41**:160, 1979.
195. Shio H, Farquhar MG, De Duve C: Lysosomes of the arterial wall. IV. Cytochemical localization of acid phosphatase and catalase in smooth muscle cells and foam cells from rabbit atheromatous aorta. *Am J Pathol* **76**:1, 1974
196. Shio H, Haley NJ, Fowler S: Characterization of lipid-laden aortic cells from cholesterol-fed rabbits. II. Morphometric analysis of lipid-filled lysosomes and lipid droplets in aortic cell populations. *Lab Invest* **39**:390, 1978.
197. Brown MS, Goldstein JL: A receptor-mediated pathway for cholesterol homeostasis. *Science* **232**:34, 1986.
198. Goldstein JL, Brown MS: Regulation of the mevalonate pathway. *Nature* **343**:425, 1990.
199. Ginsberg HN, Le N, Short MP, Ramakrishnan R, Desnick RJ: Suppression of apolipoprotein B production during treatment of cholesterol ester storage disease with lovastatin. *J Clin Invest* **80**:1692, 1987.
200. Sando GN, Ma GP, Lindsley KA, Wei YP: Intercellular transport of lysosomal acid lipase mediates lipoprotein cholesteryl ester metabolism in a human vascular endothelial cell-fibroblast coculture system. *Cell Regul* **1**:661, 1990.
201. Ho YK, Brown MS, Goldstein JL: Hydrolysis and excretion of cytoplasmic cholesteryl esters by macrophages: Stimulation of high density lipoprotein and other agents. *J Lipid Res* **21**:204, 1980.
202. Brown MS, Ho YK, Goldstein JL: The cholesteryl ester cycle in macrophage foam cells. *J Biol Chem* **255**:9244, 1980.
203. Hajjar DP, Weksler BB, Falcone DJ, Hefton JM, Tack G, Minick CR: Prostacyclin modulates cholesteryl ester hydrolytic activity by its effect on cyclic adenosine monophosphate in rabbit aortic smooth muscle cell. *J Clin Invest* **70**:479, 1982.
204. Etigin OR, Hajjar DP: Nifedipine increases cholesteryl ester hydrolytic activity in lipid-laden rabbit arterial smooth muscle cells. *J Clin Invest* **75**:1554, 1985.
205. Khoo JC, Mahoney EM, Stein J: Neutral cholesterol esterase activity in macrophages and its enhancement by cAMP-dependent protein kinase. *J Biol Chem* **256**:12659, 1981.
206. Pittman RC, Steinberg D: Activatable cholesterol esterase and triacylglycerol lipase activities of rat adrenal and their relationship. *Biochim Biophys Acta* **487**:431, 1977.
207. Hajjar DP, Weksler BB: Metabolic activity of cholesterol esters in aortic smooth muscle cells is altered by prostaglandins I2 and E2. *J Lipid Res* **24**:1176, 1983.
208. Hajjar DP: Regulation of neutral cholesteryl esterase in arterial smooth muscle cells: Stimulation by agonists of adenylate cyclase and cyclic AMP-dependent protein kinase. *Arch Biochem Biophys* **247**:49, 1986.
209. Faust JR, Goldstein JL, Brown MS: Receptor-mediated uptake of low-density lipoprotein and utilization of its cholesterol for steroid synthesis in cultured mouse adrenal cells. *J Biol Chem* **252**:4861, 1977.
210. Hall PF, Nakamara M: The influence of adrenocorticotropin on transport of a cholesteryl linoleate-low-density lipoprotein complex into adrenal tumor cells. *J Biol Chem* **254**:12547, 1979.
211. Brown MS, Basu SK, Flack JR, Ho YK, Goldstein JL: The scavenger cell pathway for lipoprotein degradation: Specificity of the binding site that mediates the uptake of negatively-charged LDL by macrophages. *J Supramol Struct* **13**:67, 1980.
212. Brown MS, Goldstein JL: Lipoprotein metabolism in the macrophage: Implications for cholesterol deposition in atherosclerosis. *Annu Rev Biochem* **52**:223, 1983.
213. Haberland ME, Fong D, Cheng L: Malondialdehyde-altered protein occurs in atheroma of Watanabe heritable hyperlipidemic rabbits. *Science* **241**:215, 1988.
214. Henriksen T, Mahoney EM, Steinberg D: Enhanced macrophage degradation of biologically modified low density lipoprotein. *Atherosclerosis* **3**:149, 1983.
215. Salisbury BG, Falcone DJ, Minick CR: Insoluble low-density lipoprotein-proteoglycan complexes enhance cholesteryl ester accumulation in macrophages. *Am J Pathol* **120**:6, 1985.
216. Srinivasan SR, Vijayagopal P, Dalferes ER, Abbate B, Radhakrishnamurthy B, Berenson GS: Low-density lipoprotein retension by aortic tissue. Contribution of extracellular matrix. *Atherosclerosis* **62**:201, 1986.
217. Pittman RC, Carew TE, Attie AD, Witztum JL, Watanabe Y, Steinberg D: Receptor-dependent and receptor-independent degradation of low-density lipoprotein in normal rabbits and in receptor-deficient mutant rabbits. *J Biol Chem* **257**:7994, 1982.
218. Spady DK, Bilheimer DW, Dietschy JM: Rates of receptor-dependent and -independent low-density lipoprotein uptake in the hamster. *Proc Natl Acad Sci USA* **80**:3499, 1983.
219. Anderson JM, Dietschy JM: Relative importance of high and low-density lipoproteins in the regulation of cholesterol synthesis in the adrenal gland, ovary, and testis of the rat. *J Biol Chem* **253**:9024, 1978.
220. Varban ML, Rinninger F, Wang N, Fairchild HV, Dunmore JH, Fang Q, Gosselin ML, Dixon KL, Deeds JD, Acton SL, Tall AR, Huszar D, et al.: Targeted mutation reveals a central role for SR-BI in hepatic selective uptake of high density lipoprotein cholesterol. *Proc Natl Acad Sci USA* **95**:4619, 1998.
221. Temel RE, Trigatti B, DeMattos RB, Azhar S, Krieger M, Williams DL: Scavenger receptor class B, type I (SR-BI) is the major route for the delivery of high density lipoprotein cholesterol to the steroidogenic pathway in cultured mouse adrenocortical cells. *Proc Natl Acad Sci USA* **94**:13600, 1997.
222. Acton S, Rigotti A, Landschulz KT, Xu S, Hobbs HH, Krieger M: Identification of scavenger receptor SR-BI as a high density lipoprotein receptor. *Science* **271**:518, 1996.
223. Kozarsky KF, Donahee MH, Rigotti A, Iqbal SN, Edelman ER, Krieger M: Overexpression of the HDL receptor SR-BI alters plasma HDL and bile cholesterol levels. *Nature* **387**:414, 1997.
224. Rigotti A, Trigatti BL, Penman M, Rayburn H, Herz J, Krieger M: A targeted mutation in the murine gene encoding the high density lipoprotein (HDL) receptor scavenger receptor class B type I reveals its key role in HDL metabolism. *Proc Natl Acad Sci USA* **94**:12610, 1997.
225. Eisenberg S: High density lipoprotein metabolism. *J Lipid Res* **25**:1017, 1984.
226. Schmitz G, Robenek H, Lohmann U, Assmann G: Interaction of high-density lipoproteins with cholesteryl ester-laden macrophages: Biochemical and morphological characterization of cell surface receptor binding, endocytosis, and resecretion of high-density lipoproteins by macrophages. *EMBO J* **4**:613, 1985.

227. Faergeman O, Havel RJ: Metabolism of cholesteryl esters of rat very low-density lipoproteins. *J Clin Invest* **55**:1210, 1975.
228. Shelburne FA, Hanks J, Meyers W, Quarfordt SH: Effect of apoproteins on hepatic uptake of triglyceride emulsions in the rat. *J Clin Invest* **65**:652, 1980.
229. Hui DY, Innerarity TL, Mahley RW: Lipoprotein binding to canine hepatic membranes. Metabolically distinct apo-E and apo-B,E receptors. *J Biol Chem* **256**:5646, 1981.
230. Cooper AD, Erickson SK, Nutik R, Shrewsbury MA: Characterization of chylomicron remnant binding to rat liver membranes. *J Lipid Res* **23**:42, 1982.
231. Brown MS, Goldstein JL: Lipoprotein receptors in the liver. Control signals for plasma cholesterol traffic. *J Clin Invest* **72**:743, 1983.
232. Herz J, Hamann U, Rogne S, Myklebost O, Gausepohl H, Stanley KK: Surface location and high affinity for calcium of a 500-kd liver membrane lipoprotein receptor. *EMBO J* **7**:4119, 1988.
233. Beisiegel U, Weber W, Ihrke G, Herz J, Stanley KK: The LDL-receptor-related protein, LRP, is an apolipoprotein E-binding protein. *Nature* **341**:162, 1989.
234. Stein O, Stein Y, Goodman DS, Fidge NH: The metabolism of chylomicron cholesteryl esters in rat liver. A combined radio-autographic-electron microscopic and biochemical study. *J Cell Biol* **43**:410, 1969.
235. Floren CH, Nilsson A: Degradation of chylomicron remnant cholesteryl ester by rat hepatocyte monolayers. Inhibition by chloroquine and colchicine. *Biochem Biophys Res Commun* **74**:520, 1977.
236. Goodman ZD, Lequire VS: Transfer of esterified cholesterol from serum lipoproteins to the liver. *Biochim Biophys Acta* **398**:325, 1975.
237. Cooper AD, Yu PYS: Rates of removal and degradation of chylomicron remnants by isolated perfused rat liver. *J Lipid Res* **19**:635, 1987.
238. Floren CH, Nilsson A: Binding, interiorization and degradation of cholesteryl ester-labeled chylomicron remnant particles by rat hepatocyte monolayer. *Biochem J* **168**:483, 1977.
239. van Berkel THJC, van Tol A: In vivo uptake of human and rat low-density and high-density lipoprotein by parenchymal and nonparenchymal cells from rat liver. *Biochim Biophys Acta* **530**:299, 1978.
240. van Berkel THJC, van Tol A, Koster JF: Iodine labeled human and rat low-density and high-density lipoprotein degradation by human liver and parenchymal and nonparenchymal cells from rat liver. *Biochim Biophys Acta* **529**:138, 1978.
241. van Berkel THJC, van Tol A: Role of parenchymal and nonparenchymal rat liver cells in the uptake of cholesteryl ester-labeled serum lipoproteins. *Biochem Biophys Res Commun* **89**:1097, 1979.
242. van Berkel THJC, Vaandrager H, Kruyt JK, Koster JF: Characteristics of acid lipase and acid cholesteryl esterase in parenchymal and nonparenchymal rat liver cells. *Biochim Biophys Acta* **617**:446, 1980.
243. Kostner GM, Hadam B, Roscher A, Zechner A: Plasma lipids and lipoproteins of a patient with cholesteryl ester storage disease. *J Inherit Metab Dis* **8**:9, 1985.
244. Corey JE, Zilversmit DB: Effect of cholesterol feeding on arterial lipolytic activity in the rabbit. *Atherosclerosis* **27**:201, 1977.
245. Brecher P, Pyun HY, Chobanian AV: Effect of atherosclerosis on lysosomal cholesterol esterase activity in rabbit aorta. *J Lipid Res* **18**:154, 1977.
246. Nilsson A, Norden H, Wilhelmsson L: Hydrolysis and formation of cholesterol esters with rat liver lysosomes. *Biochim Biophys Acta* **296**:593, 1973.
247. Dousset JC, Dousset N, El Baba AM, Soula G, Douste-Blazy L: Cholesteryl ester synthetase in lysosomes of rabbit aorta. Effect of membrane bound cholesterol and physical state of substrate. *Artery* **5**:432, 1979.
248. Kritchevsky D, Kathari HV: Arterial enzymes of cholesteryl ester metabolism. *Adv Lipid Res* **16**:221, 1978.
249. Proudlock JW, Day AJ: Cholesterol esterifying enzymes of atherosclerotic rabbit intima. *Biochim Biophys Acta* **260**:716, 1972.
250. Brecher PI, Chobanian AV: Cholesterol ester synthesis in normal and atherosclerotic aortas of rabbits and rhesus monkeys. *Circ Res* **35**:692, 1974.
251. Hashimoto S, Dayton S, Alfin S, Bui PT, Baker N, Wilson L: Characteristics of the cholesterol-esterifying activity in normal and atherosclerotic rabbit aortas. *Circ Res* **34**:176, 1974.
252. Davis HR, Glagov S, Zarins CK: Role of acid lipase in cholesteryl ester accumulation during atherogenesis. *Atherosclerosis* **55**:205, 1985.
253. Schaffner T, Taylor K, Bartucci J, Fischer D, Beeson JH, Glagov S, Wissler RW: Arterial foam cells with distinctive immunomorphologic and histochemical features of macrophages. *Am J Pathol* **100**:57, 1980.
254. Proudlock JW, Day AJ, Tume RK: Cholesterol-esterifying enzymes of foam cells isolated from atherosclerotic rabbit intima. *Atherosclerosis* **18**:451, 1973.
255. Hagemenas FC, Manaugh LC, Illingworth DR, Sundberg EE, Yatsun FM: Cholesteryl ester hydrolase activity in mononuclear cells from patients with Type II hypercholesterolemia. *Atherosclerosis* **50**:335, 1984.
256. Yatsu FM, Hagemenas F, Manaugh L, Galumbos T: Cholesteryl ester hydrolase activity in human symptomatic atherosclerosis. *Lipids* **15**:1019, 1980.
257. Bonner MJ, Miller BF, Kothari HV: Lysosomal enzymes in aortas of species susceptible and resistant to atherosclerosis. *Proc Soc Exp Biol Med* **139**:1359, 1972.
258. Tomita T, Shirasaki Y, Takigucki Y, Ozalari Y, Hayashi E: Hemodynamic effects on aortic enzyme activities in spontaneously hypertensive rats. *Atherosclerosis* **37**:409, 1980.
259. Wolinsky H, Capron L, Goldfischer S, Capron F, Coltoff-Schiller B, Kasak LE: Hydrolase activities in the rat aorta: Part 2. Effect of hypertension alone and in combination with diabetes mellitus. *Circ Res* **42**:837, 1978.
260. Tomita T, Shirasaki Y, Takiguchi T, Okada T, Hayashi E: Aortic cholesterol esterase and other lysosomal enzyme activities in DOCA-salt; renal and spontaneous hypertension in the rat. *Atherosclerosis* **39**:453, 1981.
261. Hajjar DP, Falcone DJ, Fabricant CG, Fabricant J: Altered cholesteryl ester cycle is associated with lipid accumulation in herpes virus-infected arterial smooth muscle cells. *J Biol Chem* **260**:6124, 1985.
262. Melnick JL, Dressman GR, McCollum CH, Petrie BL, Burek J, Debakey ME: Cytomegalovirus antigen within human arterial smooth muscle cells. *Lancet* **2**:644, 1983.
263. Fabricant CG, Hajjar DP, Minick J: Herpesvirus infection enhances cholesterol and cholesteryl ester accumulation in cultured arterial smooth muscle cells. *Am J Pathol* **105**:176, 1983.
264. Meyers MA: Diseases of the adrenal glands, in *Radiologic Diagnosis*. Springfield, Ill., Thomas, 1963.
265. Aquilar MJ, O'Brian JS, Taber P: The syndrome of familial leukodystrophy, adrenal insufficiency, and cutaneous melanosis, in Aronson SM, Volk BW (eds): *Inborn Disorders of Sphingolipid Metabolism: Cerebral Sphingolipidoses*. New York, Pergamon, 1967, p 149.
266. Michels VV, Beaudet AL: Cholesteryl lignocerate hydrolysis in adrenoleukodystrophy. *Pediatr Res* **14**:21, 1980.
267. Ogino T, Schaumburg HH, Suzuki K, Kishimoto Y, Moser AE: Metabolic studies of adrenoleukodystrophy. *Adv Exp Med Biol* **100**:601, 1978.
268. Galton DJ, Gilbert CH, Lucey JJ, Path MRC, Walker-Smith JA: Triglyceride storage disease: A defect in activation of lipolysis in adipose tissue. *Pediatrics* **59**:442, 1977.
269. Galton DJ, Reckless JD, Gilbert CH: Triglyceride storage disease, in Collip PJ (ed): *Childhood Obesity*. Acton, Mass., Publishing Sciences, 1975, p 149.
270. Williams ML, Coleman RA, Placezk D, Grunfeld C: Neutral lipid storage disease: A possible functional defect in phospholipid-linked triacylglycerol metabolism. *Biochim Biophys Acta* **1096**:162, 1991.
271. Peremans J, De Graf PJ, Strubbe G, De Block G: Familial metabolic disorder with fatty metamorphosis of the viscera. *J Pediatr* **69**:1108, 1966.
272. Den Tandt WR, Philippart M, Nakatani S, Durand P: Triglyceride and acid lipase deficiency in triglyceride storage disease: a possible variant of Wolman's disease. *Pediatr Res* **7**:346, 1973.
273. Philippart M, Durand P, Borrone C: Neutral lipid storage with acid lipase deficiency: A new variant of Wolman's disease with features of the Senior syndrome. *Pediatr Res* **16**:954, 1983.
274. Durand P, Bugiani O, Palladini G, Barrone C, Della C, Siliato F: Nephropathie tubulo-interstitielle chronique: degenerescence tapeto retinienne et lipidose generalisée. *Arch Fr Pediatr* **28**:915, 1971.
275. Redonnet-Vernhet I, Chatelut M, Salvayre R, Levade T: A novel lysosomal acid lipase gene mutation in a patient with cholesteryl ester storage disease. *Hum Mutat* **11**:335, 1998.
276. Muntoni S, Wiebusch H, Funke H, Seedorf U, Roskos M, Schulte H, Saku K, Arakawa K, Balestrieri A, Assmann G: A missense mutation (Thr-6Pro) in the lysosomal acid lipase (LAL) gene is present with high frequency in three different ethnic populations: Impact on serum lipoprotein concentrations. *Hum Genet* **97**:265, 1996.

CHAPTER 143

Acid Ceramidase Deficiency: Farber Lipogranulomatosis

Hugo W. Moser ▪ Thomas Linke
Anthony H. Fensom ▪ Thierry Levade ▪ Konrad Sandhoff

1. **Farber disease (FD) (MIM 228000) is a genetically determined disorder of lipid metabolism associated with deficiency of lysosomal acid ceramidase and accumulation of ceramide in the lysosome.**
2. **The disease presents most commonly during the first few months after birth with a unique triad of clinical manifestations: (a) painful and progressively deformed joints; (b) subcutaneous nodules, particularly near joints and over pressure points; and (c) progressive hoarseness due to laryngeal involvement. These tissues show granulomas and lipid-laden macrophages. The liver, spleen, lung, and heart are often involved, and the nervous system may show accumulation of ceramides and gangliosides in the neurons of brain and spinal cord. The illness is progressive, and often leads to death during the first few years. Other, less frequent, phenotypes also occur, including a rapidly fatal neonatal form associated with massive hepatosplenomegaly; a form in which progressive neurologic disability associated with retinal cherry-red spots is the most prominent clinical manifestations; and somewhat milder forms with later onset and longer survival. Some patients have survived to adulthood with mild or absent neurologic involvement.**
3. **Acid ceramidase (EC 3.5.1.23) has been purified and cloned. The full-length cDNA contains a 1185-bp open-reading frame. To date, 11 different mutations have been reported in the acid ceramidase gene. The point mutations M72V and V93I were identified as polymorphisms and had no effect on the enzymatic activity. The point mutations Y36C, E138V, T222K, R254G, N320D, D331N, and P362R all significantly reduced or abolished enzymatic activity. In addition, two splice-site mutations leading to the deletion of either exon 6 or exon 13 were demonstrated in two Farber disease patients.**
4. **The ceramide that accumulates in Farber disease is confined to the lysosomal compartment, and does not appear to contribute to the multiple biomodulatory roles attributed to ceramides in other subcellular compartments. Apoptosis is apparently not increased in cultured fibroblasts of Farber disease patients.**
5. **Laboratory diagnosis is achieved by demonstration of reduced acid ceramidase activity in white blood cells, cultured skin fibroblasts, and amniocytes, or by loading studies with labeled precursors in cultured cells. Other diagnostic procedures include the demonstration of abnormally high ceramide levels in cultured cells, biopsy samples or urine, or of characteristic "Farber bodies" by electron microscope studies in biopsy samples. Prenatal diagnosis is possible.**
6. **The disease is rare. Data on 78 patients in a variety of ethnic groups have been assembled. The mode of inheritance is autosomal recessive.**
7. **There is no effective therapy. Bone marrow transplants have been performed in two patients. While there was regression of joint manifestations and subcutaneous nodules and the hoarseness improved, the overall outcome was unfavorable because of continued neurologic deterioration which led to death in both patients. Transfection with acid ceramidase cDNA corrects the biochemical defect in cultured skin fibroblasts.**
8. **Acid ceramidase activity and glucocerebrosidase activities are diminished in patients with sphingolipid activator deficiency and in a mouse model of this disorder. Clinical manifestations of this disorder resemble those of Gaucher disease.**

CLINICAL MANIFESTATIONS

Table 143-1 summarizes the clinical manifestations in 78 Farber disease patients who have been reported in the literature or are known to the authors. Diagnosis was confirmed by acid ceramidase assay or by morphologic and/or biochemical studies of biopsy or autopsy tissues.

The phenotypes have been subdivided into seven subtypes. Types 1 through 5 differ in respect to severity and sites of major tissue involvement. Type 6 is probably a fortuitous combination of type 1 Farber disease and Sandhoff disease.[1] Type 7 is represented by 1 patient and a 20-week fetal sib with combined deficiencies of glucocerebrosidase, galactocerebrosidase, and ceramidase activities[2] that were subsequently shown to be due to a complete absence of all 4 saposins (SAP-A, -B, -C, and -D) caused by a homoallelic mutation in the initiation codon of the common saposin precursor prosaposin.[3] Even though acid ceramidase activity was deficient, and ceramide accumulated in the tissues, the phenotype of this last patient resembled infantile Gaucher disease rather than Farber disease. In three patients, clinical data were insufficient to permit phenotype assignment

Type 1: Classic Farber Disease (MIM 228000)[4–23]

Thirty-five patients had the classic phenotype. The clinical presentation is so striking that diagnosis can almost be made at a glance. The characteristic features are painful swelling of joints (particularly the interphalangeal, metacarpal, ankle, wrist, knee,

Table 143-1 Farber Disease Clinical Findings

	1 (Classical)	2 (Intermediate)	3 (Mild)	4 (Neonatal)	5 (Neurologic Progression)	6 (Comb Sandhoff)	7 (SAP Deficiency)
Number of cases	35	14	11	6	7	1	1
Mean age (years)							
Onset	0.3	0.66	1.6	0	1.66	0.13	0
Death	1.45	6.25	15.8	0.16	3.6	1.1	0.3
Last follow-up	1.1	5.6	13.0	—	3.9	—	—
Nodules	100%	100%	100%	1/3	7/7	1/1	0/1
Joint involvement	100%	100%	100%	2/3	7/7	1/1	0/1
Hoarseness	100%	100%	100%	0/3	6/6	1/1	0/1
Large liver	14/20	3/7	3/7	100%	1/5	1/1	1/1
Large spleen	7/15	3/7	3/7	100%	1/5	1/1	1/1
Lung infiltrates	16/19	1/8	2/11	—	0/4	0/1	
Macular cherry-red spot	4/15	0/6	0/9	—	3/4	0/1	0/1
Lower motor neuron involvement	11/13	2/5	2/4	—	1/1	—	—
Central nervous impaired	15/22	3/10	5/9	—	7/7	1/1	1/1

and elbow), palpable nodules in relation to the affected joints and over pressure points, a hoarse cry that may progress to aphonia, feeding and respiratory difficulties, poor weight gain, and intermittent fever.

Symptoms usually first appear between ages 2 weeks and 4 months. The initial finding in most patients is painful and swollen joints or hoarseness. Attention is first drawn to the limbs and joints by diffuse swelling and hyperesthesia. Later the generalized swelling of the extremities diminishes, and nodular thickenings around the joints and tendon sheaths indicate the articular involvement. The fingers are held flexed at the interphalangeal joints, and passive motion causes pain. Joint contractures develop. The older, more mildly affected patients have shown moderate flexion contractures of the knees, wrists, and fingers. The discrete nodular subcutaneous swellings increase in size and number as the disease advances (Figs. 143-1 and 143-2). They are found most often near the interphalangeal, ankle, wrists, and elbow joints. Other frequent locations are points subject to mechanical pressure, such as the occiput and the lumbosacral region of the spine (Fig.143-1*D*). Nodules have also been observed in the conjunctiva, on the external ear, on the nostrils, and in the mouth (Fig. 143-2*B*). In a few instances, they have regressed spontaneously.

Disturbances in swallowing, vomiting, and repeated episodes of pulmonary consolidation associated with fever occur frequently in the severely involved children, and pulmonary disease is the usual cause of death. The disturbances in swallowing and respiration often are due to swelling and granuloma formation in the epiglottis and larynx. Rib and sternal retraction and asthmatic breathing attest to the obstructive element of the respiratory disease and may require tracheostomy (Fig. 143-2). Other organs are also involved relatively frequently. Seven of the severely involved patients had moderate generalized lymphadenopathy. An enlarged tongue has been reported in six patients. Six patients have had cardiac involvement, and one developed a grade 3/6 systolic murmur. The murmur was probably related to granulomatous lesions of the heart valves. Such lesions have been reported in three patients. Moderate enlargement of the liver has occurred in seven patients; a moderately enlarged spleen has been reported only once.

Evaluation of nervous system function in the severely affected young children is difficult because movement causes pain. Severe and progressive impairment of psychomotor development was reported in 15 cases; of these, 1 was complicated by probably unrelated hydrocephalus severe enough to require a shunt. Two patients had normal intelligence. Several other patients were thought to be mildly retarded or to have borderline intelligence.

Salaam-type seizures or infantile spasms were reported in two patients. Other signs of nervous system dysfunction arise mainly from the peripheral nerve involvement. Deep-tendon reflexes were diminished or absent in 11 patients. Hypotonia and muscular atrophy, which are observed frequently, may be related to the almost invariable storage of lipid in the anterior horn cells or to peripheral nerve involvement[14] and to immobility and inanition. The electromyogram may show signs of denervation. In addition, two patients showed evidence of myopathy. The cerebrospinal fluid protein level was reported in 10 patients; in 8 patients it was elevated, often markedly, and in 2 patients it was normal.

Cogan et al.[24] reported a diffuse, grayish opacification of the retina about the foveola, with a cherry-red center, but without disturbance of visual function. This abnormality, which resembles that seen in metachromatic leukodystrophy, is subtler than the cherry-red spot of Tay-Sachs disease, and was reported in six patients. A second eye abnormality is a granulomatous lesion of the conjunctiva. One patient showed corneal opacity and another lenticular opacity.

Types 2 and 3: "Intermediate" and "Mild" Forms[25–33]

Twenty-five patients were assigned to the intermediate-mild category because of longer survival and because their neurologic involvement was relatively mild. Six of the patients in these two groups had died at a mean age of 14.5 years (range 5.75 to 30 years) and 19 were alive at a mean age of 7.35 years. In 14 patients, neurologic function was thought to be normal at time of last follow-up at ages ranging from 4 to 16 years. The IQ was less than 80 in 8 patients and 3 patients showed neurologic progression and seizures beginning at 4 to 6 years of age. Eleven patients survived to age 16 or above.[28–33] We have designated these patients as representing the "mild" phenotype, but it is uncertain whether they differ significantly from the 14 patients in the "intermediate" category.

Type 4: Neonatal-Visceral

Six patients in this category are known.[9,34–36] These patients are extremely ill during the neonatal period with severe hepatosplenomegaly. The most severely involved patient presented as hydrops

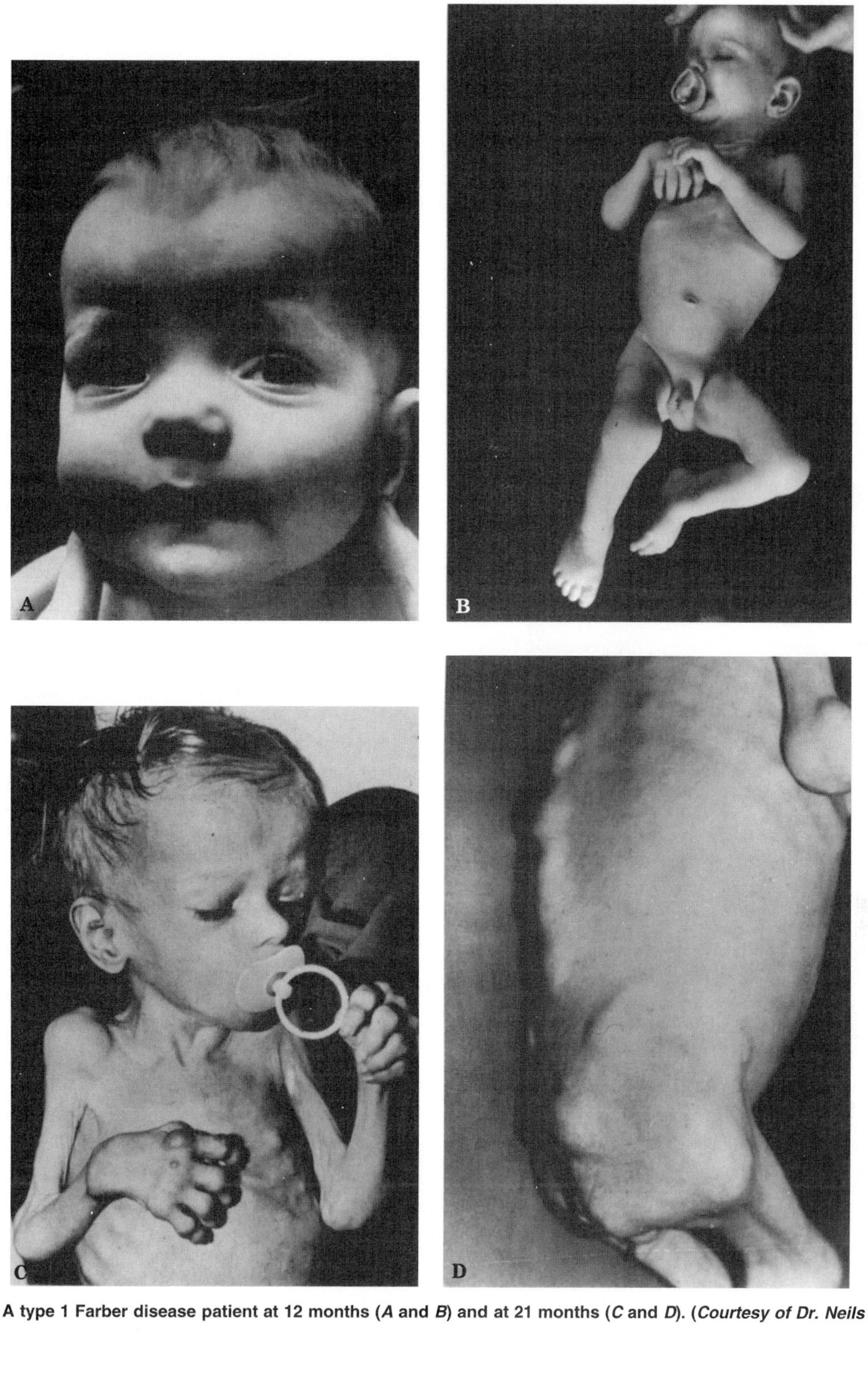

Fig. 143-1 A type 1 Farber disease patient at 12 months (*A* and *B*) and at 21 months (*C* and *D*). (*Courtesy of Dr. Neils Holboth.*)

fetalis and died on the third day. At this early age, these patients lack the characteristic clinical features of classic Farber disease, and diagnosis depends upon enzymatic and biochemical assays.

Type 5: Neurologic Progressive

Progressive neurologic deterioration and seizures were the most prominent manifestations in seven of the patients. Subcutaneous nodules and joint involvement were present but were relatively mild.[37–39] One author (HWM) followed two sisters with this phenotype. The father was Caucasian and the mother was Asian. Both children developed normally during the first year, then developed ataxia, loss of speech, and progressive paraparesis. Macular cherry-red spots were present. Subcutaneous nodules and joint involvement were present, but were mild. Postmortem study showed extensive neuronal loss and vacuolization of the cytoplasm of neurons and histiocytes with PAS-positive lipids. In contrast to classic Farber disease, the viscera were spared. Eviatar et al.[37] reported an African-American girl who, at age 2.5 years, developed progressive ataxia, tremors, rigidity, seizures, polymyoclonia, and dementia.

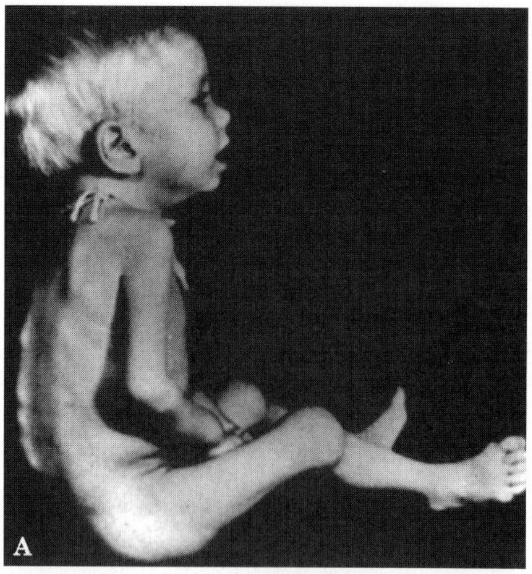

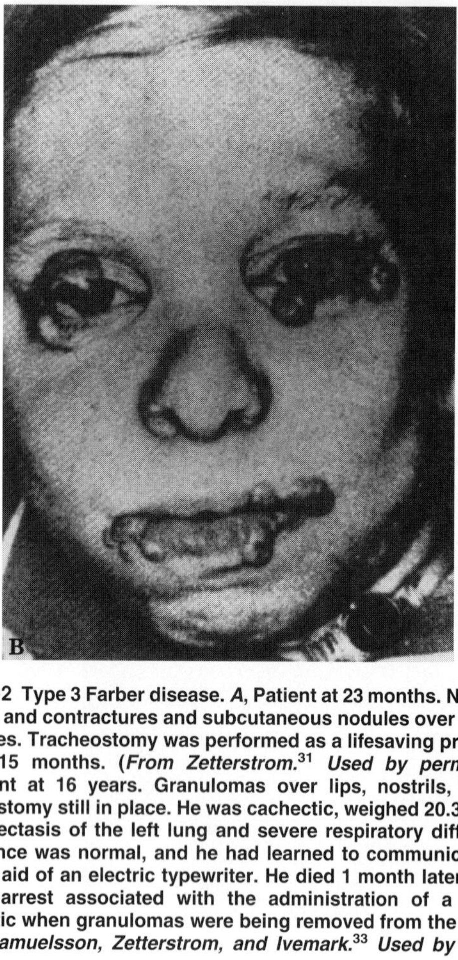

Fig. 143-2 Type 3 Farber disease. *A*, Patient at 23 months. Note joint swelling and contractures and subcutaneous nodules over spinous processes. Tracheostomy was performed as a lifesaving procedure at age 15 months. (*From Zetterstrom.*[31] *Used by permission.*) *B*, Patient at 16 years. Granulomas over lips, nostrils, eyelids. Tracheostomy still in place. He was cachectic, weighed 20.3 kg, and had atelectasis of the left lung and severe respiratory difficulties. Intelligence was normal, and he had learned to communicate well with the aid of an electric typewriter. He died 1 month later, due to cardiac arrest associated with the administration of a general anesthetic when granulomas were being removed from the eyelids. (*From Samuelsson, Zetterstrom, and Ivemark.*[33] *Used by permission.*)

Type 6: Combined Farber Disease and Sandhoff Disease

Fusch et al.[1] reported a patient who had both Farber disease and Sandhoff (MIM 268800) disease. Parents were first cousins. Studies of additional family members showed segregation of the respective genes. These data indicate that this represents a coincidental combination of two distinct genetic disorders.[40]

Type 7: Prosaposin Deficiency

This type is represented by a single patient and his 20-week fetal sib, who had a homoallelic A to T transversion in the initiation codon of the precursor protein of the sphingolipid activator proteins.[3] These proteins are now referred to as saposins or SAPs.[41] A total of four saposins have been identified. They are derived from a common precursor protein (prosaposin) through proteolytic processing,[42,43] and a review[41] recommends that they be referred to a saposins A, B, C, and D (see Chap. 134). According to this new nomenclature, saposin B is identical to SAP-1 and saposin C to SAP-2. Saposins are a group of small, nonenzymatic glycoproteins that are required for the lysosomal degradation of glycosphingolipids, including ceramide, with short, hydrophilic head-groups. Glycosphingolipids of the plasma membrane reach the lysosomal compartment of the cell after endocytosis as components of intraendosomal and intralysosomal vesicles. The interaction of the membrane-bound glycolipids with the respective water-soluble exohydrolase is mediated by saposins.[44]

Northern blotting of cultured skin fibroblasts of the patients revealed the presence of prosaposin mRNA of apparently normal size. The entire protein-coding sequence cDNA was normal except for a single nucleotide substitution in the initiation codon from the normal ATG to TTG, resulting in a lack of prosaposin. The patient's parents were fourth cousins. Both parents were heterozygous for the mutation. A subsequent pregnancy was monitored. The fetus was found to have the same defect as the proband and the pregnancy was interrupted.[3]

The phenotype of this patient resembled type 2 Gaucher disease.[2,45] Seizures were present in the neonatal period, the liver and spleen were enlarged, and storage macrophages were present in the bone marrow. The child died at 16 weeks with respiratory and circulatory failure. There was no mention of joint deformities, subcutaneous nodules, or hoarseness. However, biochemical analysis revealed significant storage of neutral glycolipids including mono-, di-, tri-, and tetrahexosylceramides in liver, kidney, and cultured skin fibroblast.[45,46] Sulfatide levels were increased in liver while ceramide storage was observed in liver and kidney. Sphingomyelin levels were normal. Ceramidase activity was 15 percent of control, glucosylceramidase was 44 percent of control, and galactosylceramidase was 13 percent of control, respectively. The biochemical findings thus show combined features of Farber disease, glucosylceramide, and galactosylceramide lipidoses.

Klein et al.[47] demonstrated through biosynthetic labeling studies that the degradation of ceramide, glucosylceramide, lactosylceramide, and ganglioside G_{M3} was impaired in cultured skin fibroblasts of these patients. Addition of purified, native SAP-D to the cell culture medium specifically reduced ceramide storage to nearly normal levels, while the addition of SAP-B had no effect on ceramide levels. These studies demonstrated for the first time that SAP-D is a required cofactor for ceramide degradation in vivo. The same study also demonstrated that the accumulation of lactosylceramide could be corrected by the addition of SAP-B. Defective lysosomal turnover of sphingomyelin-derived ceramide has also been demonstrated in SV40-transformed prosaposin-deficient fibroblasts, further emphasizing the requirement of a saposin for the degradation of ceramide in lysosomes.[48] Targeted disruption of the prosaposin gene in the mouse leads to a complex phenotype including severe leukodystrophy and widespread storage of multiple sphingolipids. The most prominent storage material in brain is lactosylceramide and neuronal storage affects perikarya, dendrites, and axons including axonal spheroids and neurofilaments.[49,50] Lactosyl-ceramide, glucosylceramide, globotriaosylceramide, sulfatide, and ceramide were all significantly increased in liver and kidney, while cholesterol, glycerophospholipids, and sphingomyelin levels were normal.[49] Apoptosis is present in cultured skin fibroblasts of this animal model.[51]

MORPHOLOGIC CHANGES

Histopathology

Studies with the light microscope show granulomatous infiltrations in the subcutaneous tissues, joints, and many other organs. The earliest lesion appears to be the accumulation of macrophages or histiocytes, and in some areas, this remains the principal pathologic feature. In other instances, there are prominent foam cells. Although in certain tissues these foamy macrophages appear to have come from elsewhere, in other tissues (such as cartilage or in the heart valve), the storage material accumulates in the chondrocytes or endocardial cells that normally exist in these locations.[4] In some instances, the lesions advance to an organized and full-blown granuloma, in which macrophages, lymphocytes, and multinucleated cells surround a core of foam cells. Older lesions show a prominent fibrotic reaction. In other lesions, the most prominent feature is the accumulation of abnormal material with the histochemical properties of a glycolipid or glycoprotein, with relatively little cellular reaction.[52]

The periarticular tissues, skin, and larynx have shown granulomatous lesions in all autopsied patients. Some of these lesions have invaded the joint capsule and on occasion the adjacent bone. The marrow in the diaphysis is much less involved.

The lungs have been involved in all the severely affected patients. They appear consolidated, and the interalveolar septums and the alveoli are infiltrated by massive numbers of macrophages. Granulomatous nodules are found on the parietal pleura. There is variability with respect to the degree of foam cell and granuloma formation. The heart has been involved in 6 of 17 autopsied patients. In three patients, there was thickening and nodule formation on the mitral and aortic valves and the chordae tendineae. Lesions are variably found in other sites, including lymph nodes, intestine, spleen, kidney, tongue, thymus, gallbladder, epithelium, and liver.

Histochemical studies of paraffin-fixed sections that had been dehydrated with lipid solvents showed material with the staining properties of mucopolysaccharides.[4] This, together with chemical assays in one patient,[12] led to the supposition that Farber disease is one of the mucopolysaccharidoses.[4,12] However, when initial sample preparation avoided lipid solvents, two types of lipid-soluble storage materials were demonstrated: one had the tinctorial properties of ceramide,[32] while the other was periodic acid-Schiff (PAS)-positive and had the staining properties of a glycolipid[6,23,52] or ganglioside.[33] These findings are consistent with biochemical assays.[6,14,61]

Except in two patients,[12,32] the nervous system was abnormal in all autopsied cases. The main change was the accumulation of storage material in neuronal cytoplasm. The accumulation was particularly prominent in the anterior horn cells in the spinal cord, but large nerve cells of the brain stem nuclei, basal ganglia, cerebellum, and retinal ganglion cells, and, to a lesser extent, the cortical neurons were also involved. Similar abnormalities occur in the peripheral nervous system, such as the autonomic ganglia, in posterior root cells, and, in some instances, in Schwann cells. The storage material is PAS-positive, and much of it is extracted with lipid solvents, which suggests that it is glycolipid.[6,52]

Ultrastructural Studies

Ultrastructural studies have been performed in 14 patients.[1,5,7,14,25,37,52–59] These have shown cytoplasmic vacuoles of irregular shape up to 2 to 3 μm in size, which probably represent lysosomes because they have a single limiting membrane and show acid phosphatase activity. While these vacuoles contain a variety of materials, the most characteristic feature is comma-shaped curvilinear tubular structures, which are referred to as Farber bodies[56] or banana bodies.[59] These consist of two dark lines separated by a clear space (Fig. 143-3). Although markedly variable, the diameter of the tubules is 14 nm on the average. It is likely that these tubular structures represent ceramide, because they can be produced in cultured fibroblasts from patients by adding ceramides containing nonhydroxy fatty acids to the growth medium.[60] Neurons and endothelial cells may also contain "zebra" bodies. These are often found in the neurons of patients with mucopolysaccharidoses or the gangliosidoses and are considered an ultrastructural expression of stored gangliosides.

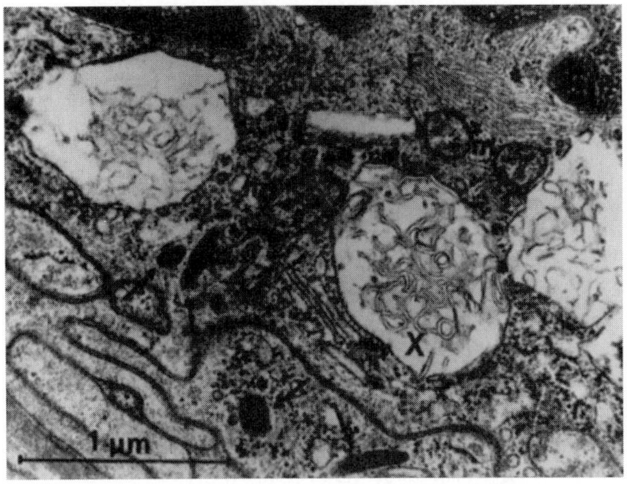

Fig. 143-3 Farber disease. Thin section of an endothelial cell with filaments (F), Wiebel-Palade bodies (arrows), mitochondria (m), and three vacuoles, one of which (x) contains "Farber bodies." Reduced from ×45,000. (*From Schmoeckel.[56] Used with permission.*)

This is consistent with the increased ganglioside level of some Farber disease tissues, as has been demonstrated biochemically[6] and histochemically.[33]

BIOCHEMICAL AND MOLECULAR STUDIES

Alterations in Chemical Composition

Accumulation of Ceramide. Accumulation of ceramide has been reported in all of the Farber disease patients in whom the tissue level of this lipid has been analyzed. High ceramide levels have been found in the subcutaneous nodules of seven patients, and ceramide may make up 20 percent of total lipids. Ceramide levels are also increased in the kidney. For the other tissues, the extent of ceramide excess appears to vary with the severity of the disease. The severely involved patients[6,14,61] showed high ceramide levels in the liver, as well as in the lungs and brain, whereas in a more mildly affected patient, liver, lung, and brain ceramide levels were normal.[32]

Unlike those of normal subjects, the ceramides of patients with Farber disease may contain significant proportions of 2-hydroxy fatty acids. In a severely involved patient, 43 percent of kidney ceramides, 39 percent of those in the cerebellum, and 10 percent of those in the liver contained 2-hydroxy fatty acids.[6,62] The 2-hydroxy acids in ceramide from the Farber disease patient consisted of cerebronic acid, which has a 24-carbon chain, and lesser amounts of C22, C20, and C28 2-hydroxy acids.[32,62] This hydroxy fatty acid pattern closely resembles that normally seen in galactocerebrosides and sulfatides. No hydroxy fatty acids were demonstrable in the ceramides isolated from the subcutaneous nodule.[32] In other respects, the composition of fatty acid and the long-chain bases in ceramide from patients with Farber disease resembled those found in control tissues. The structural differences among the ceramides that accumulate in various tissues suggest that they are produced within these tissues.[32]

Alterations in Other Tissue Components. Farber et al.[20] isolated an abnormal "lipoglycoprotein complex" from the heart, liver, and lung of their patients. This complex accounted for as much as 8 to 30 percent of total lipid but was not fully characterized. One severely involved patient had a three- to tenfold increase in G_{M3} ganglioside levels in the liver, kidney, lymph nodes, and subcutaneous nodules. Its accumulation correlated with the extent to which the tissue was infiltrated with foam cells containing PAS-positive material.[6] Sulfatide excess was documented in one patient[15] and, as already noted, the

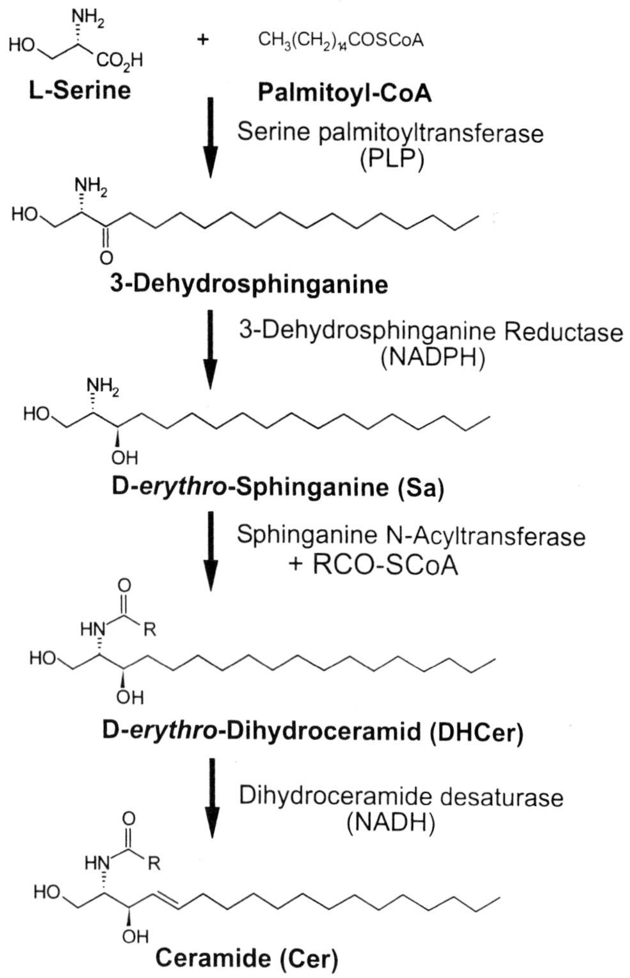

Fig. 143-4 Pathway of *de novo* ceramide biosynthesis. All enzymatic steps are located in the cytosolic leaflet of the endoplasmatic reticulum. (*Modified from van Echten-Deckert et al.*[138] *Used with permission.*)

glucocerebroside and galactocerebroside levels were increased in the type 7 patient.[2] While all these studies suggest an accumulation of glycolipid, there is variation in the extent of accumulation and type of compound. Furthermore, the chemical structure of some of these materials has not been completely defined. Nevertheless, they probably all contain ceramide, which is consistent with the defect in ceramide degradation.

Accumulation of mucopolysaccharides was reported in one patient,[12] but tissue and urinary polysaccharides were normal in three other patients.[6,10,27,32,33,52,63] As already noted, one patient with both Farber and Sandhoff Disease has been reported,[1] and this patient also shows the biochemical changes associated with the latter disorder.

Normal Ceramide Metabolism

Ceramide is an important intermediate for the synthesis and degradation of gangliosides, myelin constituents, such as galactosylceramide and sulfatide, and membrane components such as sphingomyelin and the complex glycolipids.

Ceramide Biosynthesis. *De novo* ceramide biosynthesis is initiated by the condensation of serine and palmitoyl-CoA to yield 3-dehydrosphinganine. This reaction is catalyzed by a serine palmitoyl-transferase. In a subsequent reaction, 3-dehydrosphinganine is rapidly reduced to D-erythrosphinganine by an NADH-dependent 3-ketosphinganine reductase. The acylation of sphinganine to dihydroceramide is catalyzed by a sphinganine *N*-acyltransferase.[64] The final step in the *de novo* ceramide biosynthesis, the introduction of the double bond, is catalyzed by a NAD(P)H-dependent dihydroceramide desaturase[65,66] (Fig. 143-4). Sphingosine is, therefore, not an intermediate in sphingolipid biosynthesis, and is only formed during sphingolipid degradation. All enzymatic steps of *de novo* ceramide biosynthesis are catalyzed by membrane-bound enzymes localized at the cytosolic face of the endoplasmatic reticulum (Fig. 143-5, pathway 1).

Synthesis of ceramide from sphingosine in vitro was first demonstrated by Scribney:[67]

$$\text{sphingosine} + \text{fatty acid CoA} \rightarrow \text{ceramide} + \text{CoA}$$

This reaction is catalyzed by acyl-CoA:sphingosine *N*-acyltransferase (EC 2.3.1.24). The reaction has a pH optimum of 7.5 and occurs in the microsome. Free fatty acids are not a substrate. The rates of conversion of stearoyl-, lignoceroyl-, palmitoyl-, and oleoyl-CoA were in approximate ratios of 60:12:3:1.[68] These ratios resemble the distribution of these fatty acids in brain sphingolipids, which suggests that the ceramide synthesis reaction determines the fatty acid composition of sphingolipids. There is much less specificity with respect to the long-chain base.[69]

This reaction is also used in the salvage process of catabolic products of glycosphingolipids metabolism (Fig. 143-5, pathway 2). Whereas ceramide synthesized *de novo* from sphinganine contains long chain fatty acids (C_{22}–C_{24}), recycled sphingosine is acylated with shorter-chain fatty acids (C_{16}–C_{18}) at the cytosolic face of the endoplasmatic reticulum.[69]

A pathway for ceramide biosynthesis that utilizes sphingosine, free fatty acid, and ATP has been described in rat brain.[70] The physiological role of this reaction, which occurs only in nervous tissue, has not yet been fully assessed.

Sphingomyelin as a Source of Ceramide

Ceramide can also be formed through the degradation of all sphingolipids, including the phosphosphingolipid sphingomyelin. Sphingomyelinases (EC 3.1.4.12) catalyze the reaction

$$\text{sphingomyelin} + H_2O \rightarrow \text{ceramide} + \text{phosphocholine}$$

To date, seven sphingomyelinases have been described that differ in their pH optima, cellular localization, and cation dependence. Lysosomal acid sphingomyelinase[71] is the enzyme deficient in Niemann-Pick diseases types A and B (see Chap. 144). A Zn^{2+}-dependent sphingomyelinase has been identified in bovine serum,[72] and is a product of the acid sphingomyelinase gene that occurs independent of alternative splicing. A neutral membrane-bound, Mg^{2+}-dependent sphingomyelinase[73,74] was initially reported in nervous tissues, whereas a neutral Mg^{2+}-independent sphingomyelinase[75,76] was identified in the myelin sheath and in the cytosol of leukemic cells. In addition, a Mg^{2+}- and dithiothreitol (DTT)-stimulated neutral sphingomyelinase was identified in the nuclei of rat ascites cells and different human cells.[77,78] There is also a report about a neutral sphingomyelinase localized in the chromatin and in the membrane of rat liver cell nuclei.[79,80] An alkaline sphingomyelinase has been described as being present in bile and in the digestive tract.[81,82]

Ceramide Degradation

Acid Ceramidase. Acid ceramidase (EC 3.5.1.23) catalyzes the reaction:

$$\text{ceramide} + H_2O \rightarrow \text{sphingosine} + \text{fatty acid}$$

Acid ceramidase (*N*-acylsphingosine deacylase, EC 3.5.1.23) has been purified to apparent homogeneity from human urine[83] and placenta[84] by sequential chromatography. Acid ceramidase is a heterodimeric glycoprotein with a molecular weight of approximately ~50 kDa. Under reducing conditions, acid ceramidase dissociates into two subunits designated α (molecular

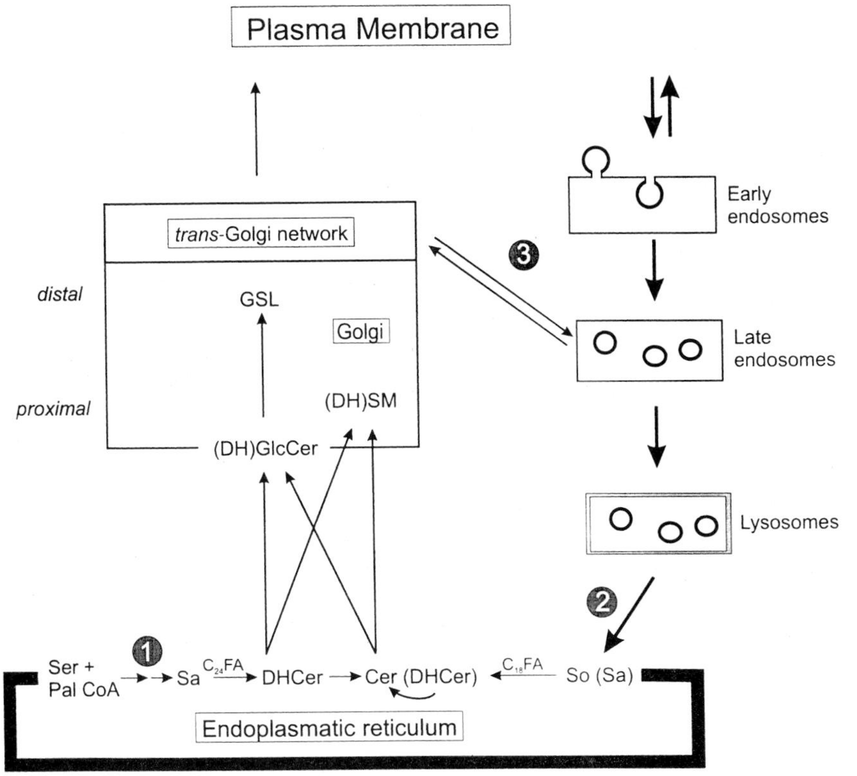

Fig. 143-5 Representation of different pathways of sphingolipid formation. Route 1 represents the *de novo* biosynthesis of glycosphingolipids (GSLs). Route 2 shows the sphingosine (So) salvage pathway. Route 3 represents recycling of native or partially hydrolyzed sphingolipids. (*Modified from van Echten-Deckert et al.*[139] *Used with permission.*) Cer = ceramide; DHCer = dihydroceramide; (DH)GlcCer = (dihydro)glucosylceramide; (DH)SM = (dihydro)sphingomyelin; GSL = glycosphingolipids; Pal CoA = palmitoyl-coenzyme A; Sa = sphinganine; Ser = serine; So = sphingosine.

weight ~13 kDa) and β (molecular weight ~40 kDa). Treatment of the purified enzyme with endoglycosidase H or peptido-*N*-glycanase F reduces the molecular mass of the β subunit to ~30 to 35 kDa and to ~27 kDa, respectively, but does not change the mass of the α subunit. This suggests that the β subunit contains five or six *N*-linked oligosaccharide chains, whereas the α subunit is not glycosylated.

Acid ceramidase, purified from human urine and placenta, is most active toward *N*-lauroylsphingosine as substrate in an in vitro, detergent-based assay system. The specific activity toward *N*-lauroylsphingosine is three to four times greater than toward *N*-oleoylsphingosine or *N*-octanoyl-sphingosine, and less toward all other substrates tested. The degradation of membrane-bound ceramide by acid ceramidase requires the presence of sphingolipid activator proteins (SAPs) and negatively charged phospholipids.[85] The importance of SAPs for ceramide hydrolysis first became evident in a patient and his fetal sib suffering from prosaposin deficiency (see Farber disease subtype 7). Biosynthetic labeling studies in fibroblasts from these patients demonstrated that supplementing the cell culture medium with purified SAP-D reduced ceramide accumulation observed in these cells.[47] The in vivo results were also confirmed by a report in which a partially purified acid ceramidase preparation was stimulated by SAP-D in an in vitro, detergent-based assay system.[86]

In an alternative assay system, the hydrolysis of membrane-bound ceramide was studied by incorporating ceramide into lipid vesicles. The conditions of the assay system and the lipid composition of the vesicles were chosen in such a way as to mimic lysosomal environment as closely as possible. In this system, acid ceramidase requires the presence of negatively charged, lysosomal lipids such as bis(monoacylglycero)phosphate (BMP) and phosphatidylinositol (PI) for ceramide hydrolysis. The most effective stimulator, however, is bis(monoacylglycero)phosphate, a lipid that was recently localized in intraendosomal structures of BHK cells[87] and in lysosomes in fibroblasts.[88] The presence of anionic lipids is also required for the stimulation of acid ceramidase activity by SAPs. In the liposomal, detergent-free assay system, both SAP-C and SAP-D are able to enhance ceramide hydrolysis by acid ceramidase. Further studies showed that ceramide hydrolysis takes place as a membrane-bound process[85] (see Fig. 143-6).

Polyclonal antibodies were raised against the purified urinary and recombinant enzyme and used to investigate the biosynthesis of the enzyme. Immunoprecipitation studies on metabolically labeled skin fibroblasts indicated that both ceramidase subunits arise from a single chain precursor of ~55 kDa. Only a minor portion of the newly synthesized acid ceramidase is secreted into the medium as a monomeric protein with a molecular weight of either ~53 to 55 kDa or ~47 to 49 kDa. Proteolytic processing of the single-chain 50-kDa precursor protein into the mature heterodimeric enzyme occurs in either the late endosomal and/or lysosomal compartments[89] (see Fig. 143-7). Preliminary studies indicated that the targeting of the enzyme to lysosomes is dependent on the mannose 6-phosphate pathway. The specific activity of the purified acid ceramidase is three to four orders of magnitude less than that of purified human acid sphingomyelinase. However, extracts of cultured human fibroblasts contain only about 10 times more acid sphingomyelinase activity (16 to 20 nmol/(mgxh) than acid ceramidase activity (0.7 to 1.2 nmol/(mgxhr), suggesting that acid ceramidase is much more abundant than acid sphingomyelinase.

Acid Ceramidase Gene and Disease-Causing Mutations. The human acid ceramidase gene spans about 30 kb and contains a total of 14 exons. The human acid ceramidase gene has been mapped to the chromosomal region 8p21.3/22.[90] The full-length cDNA that encodes human acid ceramidase has been cloned from human skin fibroblasts.[91] The full-length cDNA contains an 1185-bp open-reading frame that encodes 395 amino acids, an 1110-bp 3′-untranslated sequence, and an 18-bp poly (A) tail (see Fig. 143-8). Transient expression of the full-length cDNA in COS-1 cells led to a tenfold increase in ceramidase activity.

A total of 11 different mutations have been described in the acid ceramidase gene up to date: 2 polymorphisms (M72V and V93I) that had no affect on enzymatic activity, 7 point mutations

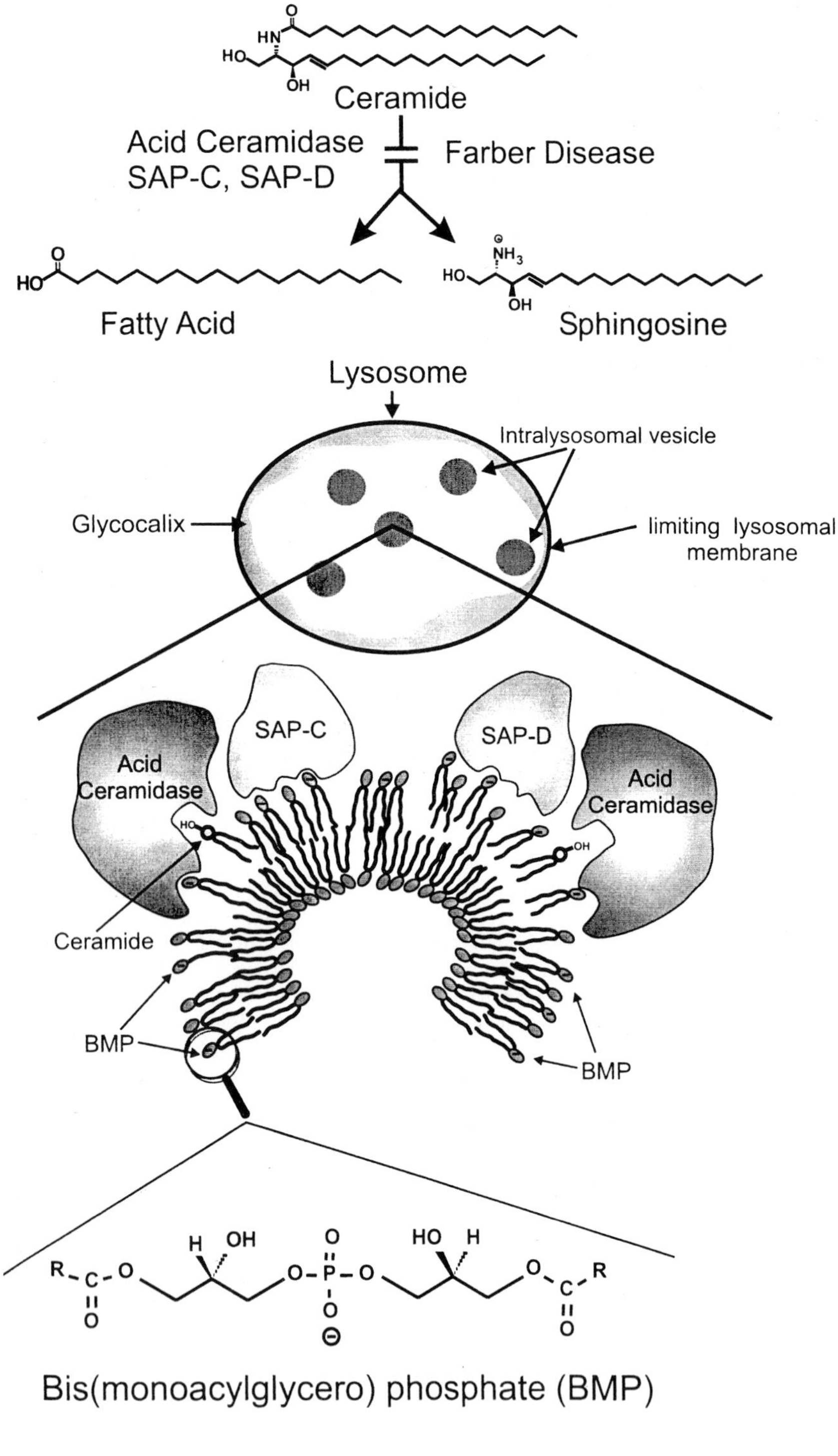

Fig. 143-6 Membrane-bound ceramide hydrolysis by acid ceramidase in the presence of sphingolipid activator proteins and bis(monoacylglycero)phosphate (BMP). According to a recent model on the topology of lysosomal digestion,[44] ceramide hydrolysis takes place on intralysosomal vesicles.

leading to various subtypes of Farber disease, and 2 additional mutations that resulted in exon deletions and also led to different subtypes of Farber disease.[91,92]

A homoallelic Y36C missense mutation was identified in a male infant of consanguineous parents. He had the typical triad of Farber disease symptoms and died at the age of 2 years (subtype 1). Expression of the mutated cDNA in COS-1 cells revealed that acid ceramidase activity was less than 5 percent of the wild-type control.[91]

A homoallelic T222K missense mutation, found in a 22-month-old girl with Farber disease whose clinical features conformed to the classic type 1 phenotype, was the first reported ceramidase mutation.[91] The acid ceramidase activity in her cultured skin fibroblasts was 5 percent of control using a detergent-based assay system. The same mutation was present in both her parents, who are consanguineous, and absent in 14 unrelated normal individuals.

A homoallelic N320D mutation was identified in a 30-month-old girl of consanguineous parents. She was diagnosed with combined Farber and Sandhoff diseases (subtype 6). In addition to the typical Farber disease symptoms, she had general motor retardation and bilateral cherry-red macular spots. Expression of mutated acid ceramidase cDNA in COS-1 cells showed that enzyme activity was reduced by as much as 90 percent in comparison to wild-type controls using a detergent-based assay system.[92]

A deletion of exon 13 in the acid ceramidase cDNA was described in a male infant, who died at the age of 3 years.[92] He

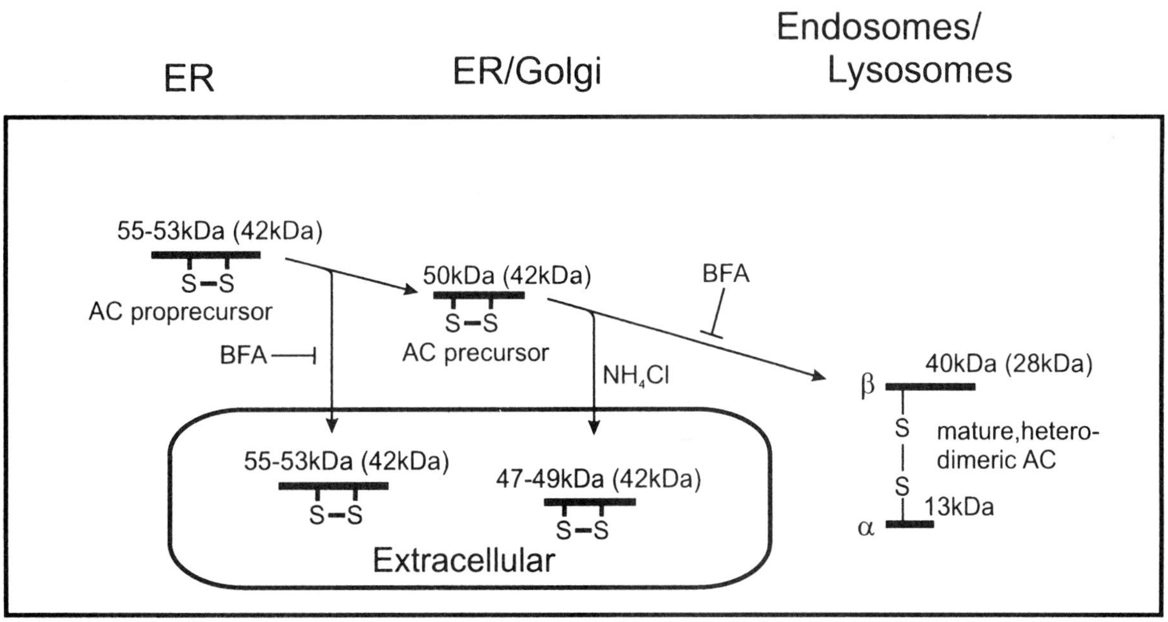

Fig. 143-7 Processing of acid ceramidase in human fibroblasts.[89] The numbers in brackets refer to the molecular weight (kDa) of the corresponding peptide. BFA = brefeldin A; ER = endoplasmatic reticulum; S-S = disulfide bridge between a and b subunit.

presented with the typical Farber disease symptoms and showed severe neurologic features (subtype 5, neurologic-progressive).

A heteroallelic N331D mutation and a deletion of exon 6 was reported in female infant suffering from the mild subtype of Farber disease (subtype 3). Her parents were nonconsanguineous; her mother transmitted the N331D allele and her father the exon 6 deletion allele.[92]

A heteroallelic E138V missense mutation[90,92] and a deletion of exon 6 were described in a female child with the mild subtype of Farber disease (subtype 3). Expression of the cDNA with the E138V mutation in COS-1 cells demonstrated that acid ceramidase activity was 5 percent of controls in a detergent-based assay, whereas expression of the cDNA with the exon deletion resulted in a mutated acid ceramidase with less than 2 percent activity as compared to controls.[92] Two further missense mutations, R254G and P362R, were identified in the genes of Farber disease patients. No data on the phenotypes of these patients were available but expression studies of these mutations indicated that while normal amounts of acid ceramidase protein was synthesized, residual enzymatic activity was less than 10 percent in comparison to wild-type controls in a detergent-based assay system.[90]

Neutral and Alkaline Ceramidases. Recently, the purification and characterization of several neutral and alkaline ceramidases were described. A membrane-bound, cation-independent nonlysosomal ceramidase was purified to apparent homogeneity from rat brain.[93] The enzyme displayed a broad pH optimum in the range from 7 to 10, and did not catalyze the reverse reaction. Two forms of a membrane-bound alkaline ceramidase were purified from guinea pig epidermis by sequential chromatography.[94] Both forms had a pH optimum for enzymatic activity in the range from 7 to 9 and were, in contrast to lysosomal acid ceramidase, most active toward *N*-linoleoylsphingosine. The alkaline ceramidase from guinea pig epidermis did not require cations for activity, and

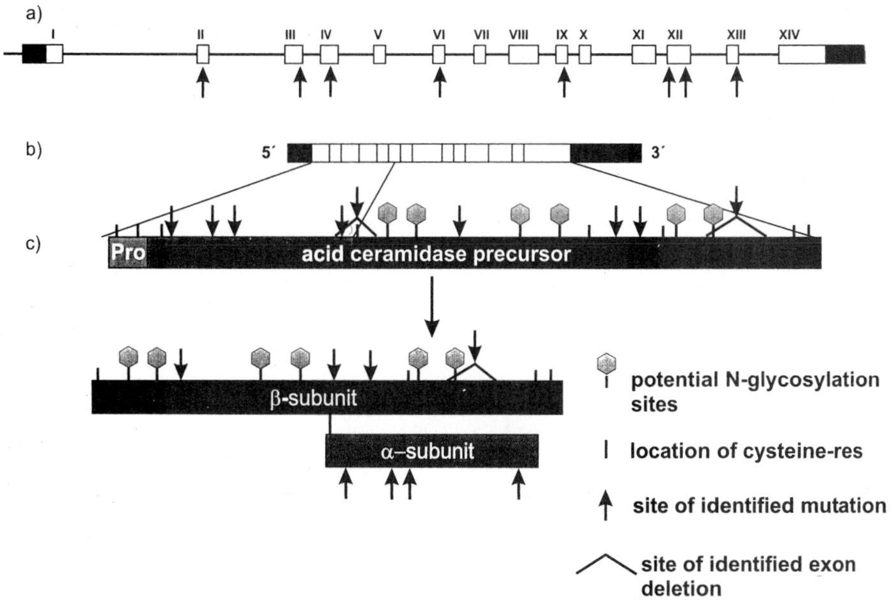

Fig. 143-8 Structure of the human acid ceramidase gene: (a) genomic structure; (b) structure of acid ceramidase cDNA; (c) illustration of acid ceramidase precursor and mature heterodimeric protein. Potential *N*-glycosylation sites, location of cysteine residues and approximate sites of point mutations are indicated. (*Modified from Kolter et al.*[140] *Used with permission.*)

did not appear to catalyze the reverse reaction, because the ceramidase reaction was strongly inhibited by sphingosine. An alkaline ceramidase was purified from a bacterial strain isolated from the skin of a patient with atopic dermatitis.[95] This bacterial alkaline ceramidase had a pH optimum in the range from 8 to 9, required the presence of Ca^{2+}, and catalyzed the reverse reaction in vitro, utilizing free fatty acids and sphingosine as substrates. These nonlysosomal ceramidases appear to have no homology to lysosomal acid ceramidase. In addition to these reports, ceramidase activity in the neutral and alkaline pH range has also been observed in a number of different tissues; for example, in the small intestine,[81] cerebellum,[96] rat kidney,[97] cultured skin fibroblasts, and white blood cells. Some of these neutral and alkaline ceramidases also appear to catalyze the reverse reaction and act upon free fatty acids rather than their CoA derivatives. The small intestine alkaline ceramidase has a pH optimum of 7.6 and may be concentrated in the brush border membrane.[81] No systematic study has yet been reported on the normal distribution of the alkaline ceramidases and/or of their substrate specificities. Of the tissues studied so far, human kidney appears to lack the alkaline ceramidase,[96] whereas this enzyme is present in rat kidney.[97] Alkaline ceramidase is clearly distinct from acid ceramidase. It is not precipitated by a monoclonal antibody against acid ceramidase,[98] and it is not deficient in Farber disease.[96,99]

PATHOGENESIS

Acid Ceramidase Deficiency and Ceramide Storage

A deficient activity of acid ceramidase was first demonstrated in postmortem tissue of two patients,[99] and in the cultured skin fibroblasts and/or white blood cells of all patients who have been studied since then.[100] The defect in this degradative enzyme accounts for the tissue accumulation of ceramide. The alkaline ceramidases appear to function normally in Farber disease.[99]

The ceramide that accumulates in Farber disease is located in the lysosome.[101–103] Turnover studies show that it results from the impaired capacity to hydrolyze the ceramide generated during the degradation of complex sphingolipids. The rate of ceramide synthesis is the same as in normal cells, and newly synthesized ceramides in Farber disease fibroblasts are directed to the synthesis of complex sphingolipids as they are in normal cells.[102]

The distribution of lesions in Farber disease and the variability of expression of the disease can only be partially explained. Neuronal storage is not unexpected because ceramide metabolism in brain is known to be active. The striking involvement of subcutaneous tissues may be accounted for by observations that ceramide has an important role in normal skin. Ceramide comprises 16 to 20 percent of the total lipids in the stratum corneum[104] and forms an essential part of the intercellular barrier that preserves the water impermeability of normal skin.[105] Some of these ceramides possess a ω-hydroxyl group on their long-chain *N*-acyl moiety, and are covalently attached to proteins on the surface of terminally differentiated keratinocytes[106] (corneocytes). This layer of protein-bound ceramide serves as the initial hydrophobic scaffold on which extracellular lipids, including cholesterol, free fatty acids, and ceramides, are deposited to form the lipid-bound envelope (LBE, see Fig. 143-9). In rare cases of complete glucocerebrosidase deficiency (see Chap. 146), the so called colloidin baby phenotype,[107,108] patients die presumably of transepidermal water loss within a few hours after birth caused by the impaired formation of the LBE. Such a severe epidermal phenotype has not been observed in Farber disease patients yet, and further studies are needed to show whether acid ceramidase plays a crucial role in the homoeostasis of the epidermal water permeability barrier.

The role of ceramide in synovial membranes has not been investigated. The relatively mild involvement of the bone marrow and reticuloendothelial system in Farber disease is surprising because these tissues are known to have a very active ceramide metabolism and are involved so strikingly in Gaucher and Niemann-Pick disease. One cannot exclude the possibility that in these tissues, ceramide is degraded by the alkaline or neutral ceramidases that are uninvolved in Farber disease, or that the ceramide that cannot be degraded is reutilized for the synthesis of glycolipids or sphingomyelin (Fig. 143-5, pathway 3). The observed variation in severity and tissue involvement in the disease is unexplained. So far, no correlation between the phenotype of Farber disease and the residual enzymatic activity, measured in detergent based assay systems, has been established.

Role of Ceramide as a "Signaling Molecule"

Ceramide appears to play a critical, but not yet fully understood, role in many aspects of cell biology (see Fig. 143-10). These are under active investigation and are described in recent reviews.[109] Although not universally accepted,[110] ceramide is thought to play a role in apoptosis.[111,112] Recent experiments demonstrate that overexpression of acid ceramidase in parental L929 cells protects from TNF-induced cell death,[113] and that ceramide mediates receptor clustering in CD95 or CD40 stimulated lymphocytes.[114] Other proposed functions include the response to stress,[111] regulation of cell growth,[115] cell senescence,[116] expression of cytokines,[117] and neuronal growth.[118] It is not certain whether these critical functions of ceramide are relevant to Farber disease because these signaling pathways appear to involve specific, nonlysosomal pools of ceramide.[112]

The Accumulated Lysosomal Ceramide in Farber Disease Does Not Cause Apoptosis, and Does Not Appear to Act as Lipid Mediator and/or Second Messenger

The demonstration that ceramide appears to modulate a large variety of cellular functions, including apoptosis, led to the inquiry whether these biomodulatory effects contribute to the pathogenesis of Farber disease. Recent studies indicate that they do not. Tohyama et al.[51] failed to demonstrate apoptosis in cultured skin fibroblasts of four Farber disease patients. Ceramide levels in these cells were 2.9 times control. Another recent study demonstrated that the ceramide present in acidic compartments is not implicated in stress-induced apoptosis. Not only was the ceramide introduced in endosomes/lysosomes unable to trigger apoptotic cell death, but also lymphoid cells and transformed fibroblasts derived from Farber patients, which accumulated ceramide in lysosomes, exhibited the same sensitivity to various apoptotic agents as normal cells. Overexpression of acid ceramidase had no effect on the apoptotic response, indicating that the lysosomal hydrolase is dispensable for this process.[118a] The lack of biomodulatory effects of ceramides in Farber disease appears to be related to the dynamics of the ceramide accumulation and the recent findings that ceramides are compartmentalized. Van Echten et al.[102] studied the turnover of ceramide in Farber disease fibroblasts with the aid of [^{14}C]serine. They showed that newly synthesized ceramide is directed toward the synthesis of complex sphingolipids at a rate similar to that in normal cells. Cellular ceramides are compartmentalized.[119] The ceramide that accumulates in Farber disease is localized to the lysosome and is the result of the impaired capacity to metabolize the ceramide derived from the degradation of the complex lipids. Biomodulatory actions appear to be exerted by those ceramides located in the inner leaflets of the plasma membrane[112] and at the cell surface in caveolae.[119] The ceramides that are in excess in Farber disease are confined to the lysosome. Chatelut et al.[120] have shown that natural ceramides, unlike their fluorescent analogues, are unable to escape from the lysosome of fibroblasts. The observation that apoptosis does not occur in Farber disease fibroblasts confirms and extends the concept that ceramide biomodulatory effects depend upon their cellular localization. Curiously, and for reasons that are not yet explained, increased apoptosis was found in cultured skin fibroblasts from the sphingolipid activator protein-deficient mouse,

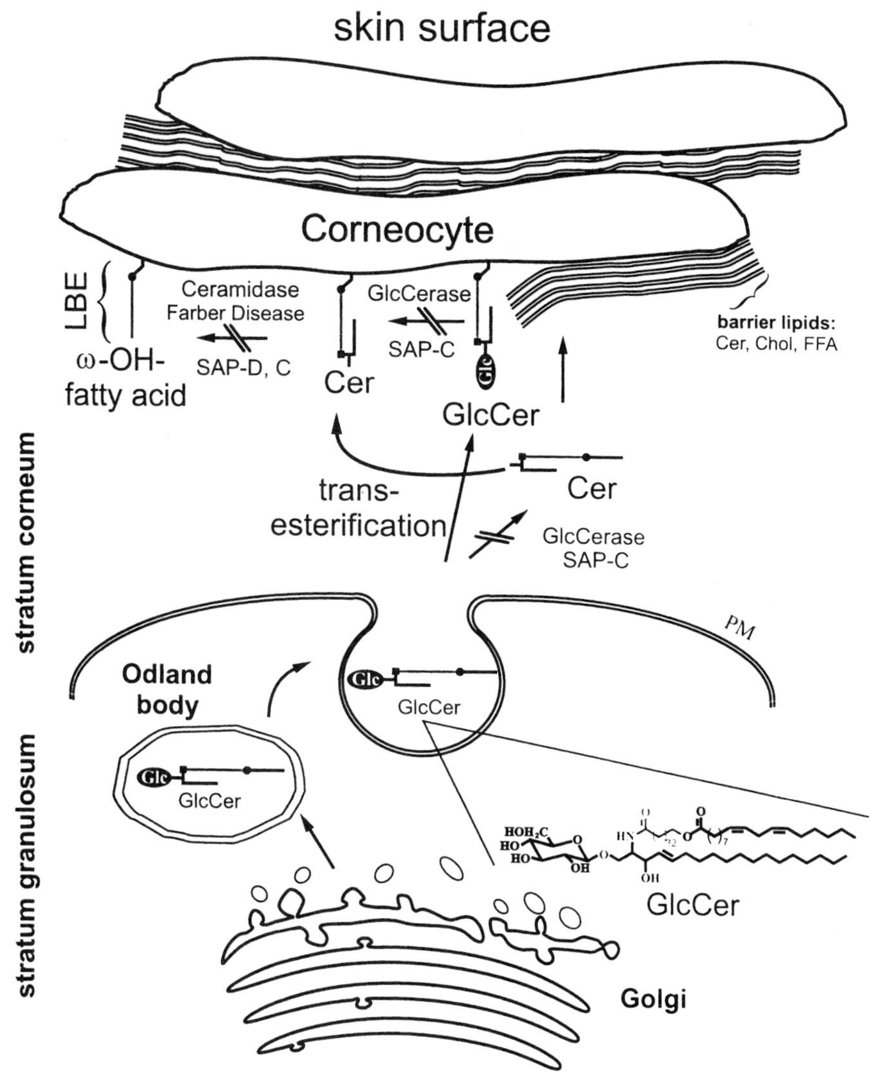

Fig. 143-9 Extracellular metabolism of GlcCer and formation of lipid-bound envelope (LBE). PM = plasma membrane; Cer = ceramide consisting of sphingosine (black) and a long-chain ω-hydroxyl fatty acid (dark grey); linoleic acid is found esterified to the ω-hydroxyl moiety. Catabolic blocks due to β-glucocerebrosidase, Sap-C, prosaposin, and possibly acid ceramidase deficiency are indicated by –//→.

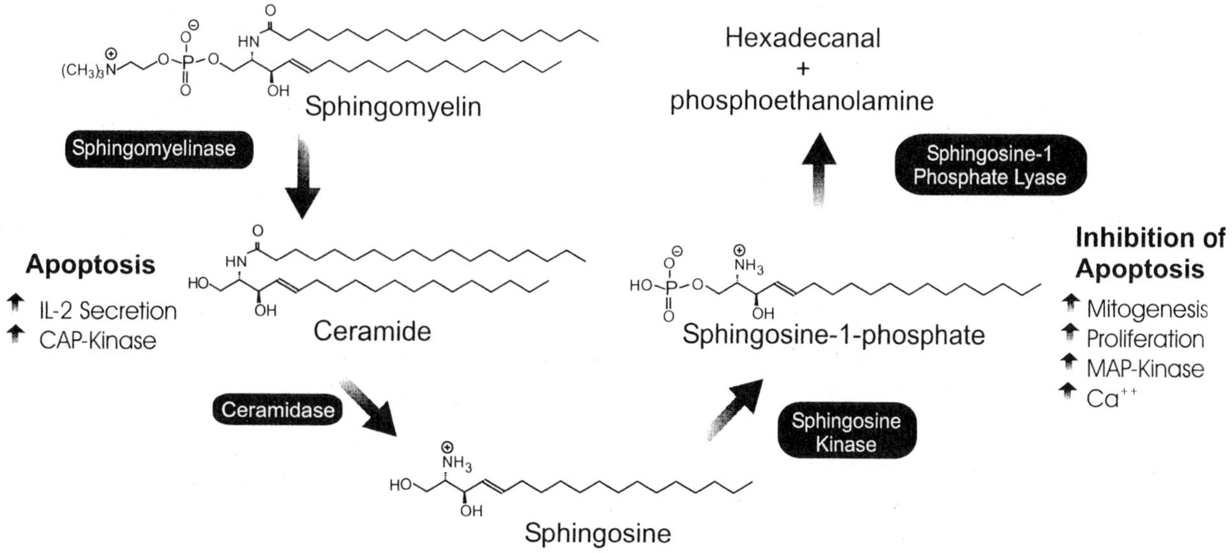

Fig. 143-10 Metabolic relationship of ceramide and sphingosine-1-phosphate. Ceramide mediates apoptotic responses whereas sphingosine-1-phosphate mediates mitogenic responses. The balance of the intracellular concentration of both sphingolipids determines the cell fate. (*Adapted from Perry et al.*[141] *Used with permission.*)

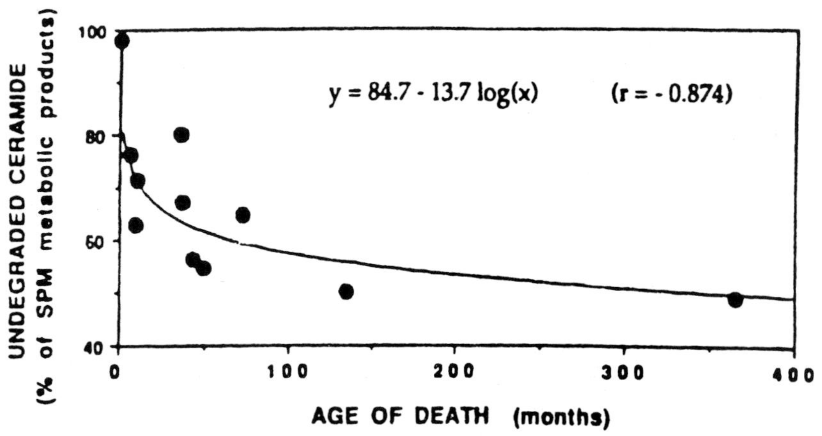

Fig. 143-11 ***In situ*** **ceramide accumulation as an antiproportional measure of residual lysosomal ceramide turnover correlates with age at death of Farber patients. Logarithmic age at death of patients correlates with ceramide accumulation: n = 11, r = 0.874 (99 percent confidence limits −0.412 to −0.979).[129]**

in which the degree of ceramide accumulation is similar to that in Farber disease fibroblasts.[51]

DIAGNOSIS

Clinical Findings

The diagnosis of classic type 1 Farber disease can be easily made clinically because the triad of subcutaneous nodules, arthritis, and laryngeal involvement is unique for this disease. Diagnostic concerns arise when one or more of these features is missing, as in juvenile rheumatoid arthritis, sarcoidosis, recurring digital fibroma of infancy, and multicentric reticulohistiocytosis,[121] or in disorders such as fibromatosis hyalina multiplex juvenilis.[122] We have found normal acid ceramidase activities in patients with these disorders and in other persons who lacked the above triad, and, conversely, all patients with the triad studied so far have shown reduced enzyme activity.

Impaired Ceramide Degradation

In vitro acid ceramidase activity in Farber disease patients is often less than 6 percent of control values. The test can be applied to postmortem tissues,[96] cultured skin fibroblasts,[123] plasma,[124] white blood cells,[9] and amniocytes.[125]

While the initial enzymatic assays used the substrate *N*-oleoyl sphingosine,[99,123,125,126] *N*-lauroylsphingosine[124,127] is the preferred substrate because it has higher sensitivity and specificity and is also most active toward the purified enzyme.[83] Impaired degradation of ceramides in Farber disease cells can also be demonstrated by loading studies with labeled precursors. These studies are of diagnostic value and permit assessment of turnover and subcellular compartmentalization. These include [^{14}C]stearic acid-labeled cerebroside sulfate. Abnormal retention of this label in the ceramide fraction has been demonstrated in Farber disease cultured skin fibroblasts,[35,128] but results in Farber disease lymphocytes do not differ from normal, presumably due to the action of an alternative degradative pathway in these cells.[35] Use of LDL-associated [^{3}H]sphingomyelin demonstrates impaired degradation of lysosomal ceramides in both Farber disease cultured fibroblasts and transformed lymphocytes, and the degree of impairment correlates to some extent with clinical disease severity (Fig. 143-11)[129]. Long-term studies with [^{14}C]serine, a substrate for a committed step in the *de novo* synthesis of ceramide and complex sphingolipids,[102] can also demonstrate the impaired degradation of ceramide in Farber disease and, as noted in the section on pathogenesis, have added valuable information on the dynamics of ceramide metabolism in Farber disease.

Ceramide Excess

Ceramide excess can easily be demonstrated qualitatively by thin-layer chromatography,[6,17] or quantitated by high-performance liquid chromatography,[130–132] or by gas-liquid chromatography combined with mass spectrometry.[32] These techniques have been applied to biopsy specimens of subcutaneous nodules[7,16,19,54,56] and liver postmortem tissues.[6,17,32] Chatelut et al.[133] validated the use of the commercially available diacylglycerol kinase kit[134,135] for the demonstration of ceramide in Farber disease cell lines. This procedure is 10 times more sensitive than the high-performance liquid chromatography methods. It is helpful to determine separately the ceramides containing α-hydroxy fatty acids. Most normal tissues contain only ceramides with nonhydroxy fatty acids, whereas both types are found in Farber disease tissue.[6,32] The level of ceramides in the subcutaneous nodule may constitute 20 percent of total lipids. Although such a finding may be diagnostic of Farber disease, this is not fully established, because there are no valid comparison samples, and it has been shown that the outer layers of normal skin contain large quantities of ceramide.[104,105] We demonstrated a two-hundredfold ceramide excess in the urine of one patient,[132] but four other patients gave normal results.

The recent demonstration that ceramide accumulation can be secondary to a mutation of the prosaposin gene[41] and that this disorder can present with an atypical severe phenotype that resembles Gaucher type 2 disease, indicates that such defects should be considered in the differential diagnosis of patients with atypical manifestations of a storage disorder.

Morphologic Studies

Other diagnostic tests include demonstration of the characteristic morphologic features on a biopsy specimen of a subcutaneous nodule or other tissue. These features include granuloma formation and the presence of macrophages with lipid cytoplasmic inclusions,[20] which are PAS-positive and are extracted by lipid solvents,[7] and which show curvilinear inclusions under the electron microscope[56] (Horowitz S, Erickson C, Struble R, personal communication). Sural nerve biopsy specimens may also show a characteristic ultrastructural abnormality.[14]

Identification of Heterozygotes

All of the obligate heterozygotes tested so far had reduced acid ceramidase activity in cultured skin fibroblasts or white blood cells.[28,54,100,123,125–127] It is likely that mutation analysis will be the most effective method for identification of heterozygotes.[90–93] The parents of the patient with the prosaponin mutation were heterozygous for this mutation.[3]

Prenatal Diagnosis

Prenatal diagnosis has been achieved by measurement of acid ceramidase activity,[125] and by loading studies[40] either on cultured amniotic cells or chorionic villus samples.

GENETICS

The reduced-acid ceramidase activity in obligate heterozygotes and pedigree data suggested an autosomal recessive mode of inheritance and this has been confirmed by mutation analysis.[90–92] Except for the Jewish population, all ethnic groups appear to be represented. Two families are Black. Among the 50 families about whom some information is available, consanguinity was present in 11. In four additional families, parents or grandparents came from the same relatively small communities. In 16 families, more than 1 sib was affected. In no instances were parents involved, and no cases were reported in previous generations.

The prevalence of Farber disease is unknown. That we have been able to document only 78 cases, coupled with the high frequency of consanguinity, suggests that it is a rare disorder. However, the recent demonstration of previously unrecognized phenotypes, coupled with the difficulty in achieving the diagnosis in such cases, raises the possibility that the incidence exceeds current estimates.

Phenotype-Genotype Correlations

The clinical severity of Farber disease correlates to some extent with the rate of degradation of sphingomyelin-derived ceramide[129] (Fig. 143-11). It does not appear to correlate with in vitro acid ceramidase activity assayed in the presence of detergents or ceramide levels in cultured skin fibroblasts of Farber disease patients.[102] Correlation with mutation analysis has not yet been assessed because only a very limited number of mutations and their corresponding phenotypes have been reported.[90–92]

THERAPY

Bone Marrow Transplant

Two patients with the classic Farber disease phenotype received bone marrow transplants (BMT) at 10 months and 18 months of age respectively.[18,136] Granulomas regressed in both patients. Joint discomfort diminished and joint mobility improved, and hoarseness diminished. Nevertheless, overall outcome was unfavorable in both patients because neurologic function continued to deteriorate and led to their death.

Although these unfavorable outcomes argue against the use of BMT in Farber disease, it may still be appropriate to consider this procedure in those Farber disease patients in whom nervous system involvement is mild or absent. The progressive joint involvement and granuloma formation cause a great deal of distress and disfigurement, and relief from this aspect of the disease would be a major benefit. In some of the less severely involved type 3 patients, nervous system involvement is mild or absent. This is documented most convincingly in the patient reported initially by Zetterstrom[31] and with later follow-up by Samuelson et al.[32,33] Although this patient had been greatly handicapped by involvement of joints and larynx and enlarging subcutaneous nodules, intellectual function was intact. At age 16 years he had an operation designed to remove a granuloma from his eyelid. He died during surgery from an anesthetic complication. Postmortem studies confirmed the diagnosis of Farber disease, but showed also that brain and lung were unaffected. BMT, which was not available at that time, might have been of great benefit to this patient. If one wishes at this time to select Farber disease patients who might benefit from BMT, the challenge is to identify relatively early those patients who are free of major nervous system involvement. Those who have seizures, psychomotor retardation, macular cherry-red spots, or impaired peripheral nerve function should be excluded. Severe pulmonary involvement also increases the risk of BMT to unacceptable levels. Serial studies should be performed because nervous system involvement may not manifest until 4 years of age or later. As noted in the section on genotype-phenotype relations, there exists some degree of correlation between biochemical alterations and disease severity, and mutation analyses may reveal other correlations in the future. It is clear at this time that the role of BMT in the therapy of Farber disease is limited, but careful evaluation may identify patients who are appropriate candidates.

Gene Therapy

Medin et al.[137] reported that the introduction of the cDNA of human acid ceramidase with a retroviral vector into Farber disease cultured skin fibroblasts restored enzyme activity completely, and normalized ceramide levels and lysosomal turnover. This study also demonstrated that transduced cells secreted normal enzyme into the medium, and that this enzyme was subsequently taken up by a process that was dependent upon the mannose-6-phosphate receptor pathway. These studies indicate that Farber disease may become a candidate for gene therapy in the future.

Currently, therapy for Farber disease is far from satisfactory. There is great need for general support for patient and family. Anti-inflammatory agents may provide relief. Laryngeal and pulmonary involvement requires close supervision and tracheostomy may be needed. One patient had hypercalcemia, possibly related to osteolytic lesions,[9] and this complication may require therapy.

REFERENCES

1. Fusch C, Huenges R, Moser HW, Sewell AC, Roggendorf W, Kusterman K, Harzer K: A case of combined Farber's and Sandhoff's disease. *Eur J Pediatr* **148**:558, 1989.
2. Harzer K, Paton B, Poulos A, Kustermann-Kuhn, Roggendorf W, Grisar T, Popp M: Sphingolipid activator protein deficiency in a 16-week-old atypical Gaucher disease patient and his fetal sibling: Biochemical signs of combined sphingolipidosis. *Eur J Pediatr* **149**:31, 1989.
3. Schnabel D, Schroder M, Furst W, Klein A, Hurwitz R, Zenk T, Weber J, Harzer K, Paton BC, Poulos A, Suzuki K, Sandhoff K: Simultaneous deficiency of sphingolipid activator proteins 1 and 2 is caused by a mutation in the initiation codon of their common gene. *J Biol Chem* **267(5)**:3312, 1992.
4. Abul-Haj SK, Martz DG, Douglas WF, Geppert LJ: Farber's disease: Report of a case with observations on its histogenesis and notes on the nature of the stored material. *J Pediatr* **61**:211, 1962.
5. Cartigny B, Libert J, Fenson AH, Martin JJ, Dhondt JL, Wyart D, Fontaine G, Farriaux JP: Clinical diagnosis of a new case of ceramidase deficiency (Farber's disease). *J Inherit Metab Dis* **8**:8, 1985.
6. Moser HW, Prensky AL, Wolfe JH, Rosman NP, Carr S, Ferreira G: Farber's lipogranulomatosis. Report of a case and demonstration of an excess of free ceramide and ganglioside. *Am J Med* **47**:869, 1969.
7. Becker H, Aubock L, Haidvogl M, Bernheimer H: Disseminated lipogranulomatosis (Farber). Case report of the 16th case of a ceramidase. *Verh Dtsch Ges Pathol* **60**:254, 1976.
8. Schonenberg H, Lindenfelser R: Farber-Syndrom. *Mschr Kinderheilk* **122**:153, 1974.
9. Antonarakis SE, Valle D, Moser HW, Kishimoto Y: Phenotypic variability in siblings with Farber disease. *J Pediatr* **104**:406, 1984.
10. Rampini S, Clausen J: Farbersche krankheit (dissemierte lipogramulomatose): Klinisches bild und zusammenfassung der chemischen befunde. *Helv Paediatr Acta* **22**:500, 1967.
11. Chanoki M, Ishii M, Fukai K, Kobayashi H, Hamada T, Murakami K, Tanaka A: Farbers lipogranulomatosis in siblings—Light and electron microscopic studies. *Br J Dermatol* **121(6)**:779, 1989.
12. Bierman SM, Edgington T, Newcomber VD, Pearson CM: Farber's disease: A disorder of mucopolysaccharide metabolism with articular, respiratory, and neurologic manifestations. *Arthritis Rheum* **9**:620, 1966.
13. Nowaczyk MJM, Feigenbaum A, Silver MM, Callahan J, Levin A, Jay V: Bone marrow involvement and obstructive jaundice in Farber lipogranulomatosis; clinical and autopsy report of a new case. *J Inherit Metab Dis* **19**:655, 1996.
14. Vital C, Battin J, Rivel J, Heheunstre JP: Aspects ultratructuraux des lesions du nerf peripherique dans un cas de maladie de Farber. *Rev Neurol* **132**:419, 1976.
15. Fujiwaki T, Hamanaka S, Koga M, Ishihara T, Nishikomori R, Kinoshita E, Furusho K: A case of Farber disease. *Acta Paediatr Jpn* **34**:72, 1992.
16. Amirhakimi GH, Haghighi P, Ghalambor A, Honari S: Familial lipogranulomatosis (Farber's disease). *Clin Genet* **9**:625, 1976.
17. Ozaki H, Mizutani M, Hayashi H, Oka E, Ohtahara S, Kimoto H, Tanaka T, Hazozaki H, Takahashi K, Suzuki Y: Farber's disease (disseminated lipogranulomatosis): The first case reported in Japan. *Acta Med Okayama* **32**:69, 1978.

18. Armfield KB, Yeager A, Krause WL, Coles C, Moser HW: Successful bone marrow transplantation in Farber disease. *Am J Hum Genet* **59**:A195, 1996.
19. Dustin P, Tondeur M, Jonniaux G, Vamos-Hurwitz E, Pelc S: La Maladie de Farber: Etude anatomo-clinique et ultrastructurale. *Bull Mem Acad R Med Belg* **128**:733, 1973.
20. Farber S, Cohen J, Uzman LL: Lipogranulomatosis. A new lipoglycoprotein storage disease. *J Mt Sinai Hosp* **24**:816, 1957.
21. Klingkowski U, Beck M, Zepp F: An 18-month-old girl with hoarseness, stiff joints, and subcutaneous nodules. *Eur J Pediatr* **157**:515, 1998.
22. Yamagata T, Yano S, Okabe I, Miyao M, Momoi MY, Yanagisawa M, Kirata H, Komatsu K: Ultrasonography and magnetic resonance imaging in Leigh disease. *Pediatr Neurol* **6(5)**:326, 1990.
23. Cvitanovic-Sojat L, Hajnzic TF, Fumic K, Pasche E, Levade T, Fensom AH, Taseski B, Mucic-Pucic B, Jurcic Z, Mataja M: Farber lipogranulomatosis type 5— Report of a new case [Abstract]. International Congress on Inborn Errors of Metabolism 245, 1997.
24. Cogan DG, Kuwabara T, Moser HW, Hazzard GW: Retinopathy in a case of Farber's lipogranulomatosis. *Arch Ophthalmol* **75**:752, 1966.
25. Burck U, Moser HW, Goebel HH, Gruttner R, Held KR: A case of lipogranulomatosis Farber: Some clinical and ultrastructural aspects. *Eur J Pediatr* **143**:203, 1985.
26. Pachman LM, Frank J, Lui M, Moser HW: Lipogranulomatosis (Farber's disease). *J Pediatr* **93**:320, 1978.
27. Barriere H, Gillot F: La lipogranulomatose de Farber. *Nouv Presse Med* **2**:767, 1973.
28. Pavone L, Moser HW, Mollica F, Reitano C, Durand P: Farber's lipogranulomatosis: Ceramidase deficiency and prolonged survival in three relatives. *Johns Hopkins Med J* **147**:193, 1980.
29. Fiumara A, Nigro F, Pavone L, Moser HW: Farber disease with prolonged survival. *J Inherit Metab Dis* **16**:915, 1993.
30. Reitano G: Acrofibrosi nodulare infantile familiare e deformante. *Rev Pediatrica Siciliana Editrice Catania* 4-Collezione Di Monografie Pediatriche. Instituto di Clinica Pediatrica dell' Universita di Catania Rivista Pediatrica Siciliana-Editroce Catania, 1959.
31. Zetterstrom R: Disseminated lipogranulomatosis (Farber's disease). *Acta Paediatr* **47**:501, 1958.
32. Samuelsson K, Zetterstrom R: Ceramides in a patient with lipogranulomatosis (Farber's disease) with chronic course. *Scand J Clin Lab Invest* **27**:393, 1971.
33. Samuelsson K, Zetterstrom R, Ivemark BI: Studies on a case of lipogranulomatosis (Farber's disease) with protracted course. Volk BW, Aronson SM (eds): *Sphingolipids, Sphingolipidoses and Allied Disorders*. New York, Plenum, 1972, p 533.
34. Pierpont ME, Wenger DA, Moser HW: Heterogeneity of clinical expression of Farber's lipogranulomatosis [Abstracts]. *Am Soc Hum Genet* **35**:111a, 1983.
35. Levade T, Tempesta MC, Moser HW, Fensom AH, Harzer K, Moser A, Salvayre R: Sulfatide and sphingomyelin loading of living cells as tools for the study of ceramide turnover by lysosomal ceramidase-implications for the diagnosis of Farber disease. *Biochem Mol Biol* **54**:117, 1995.
36. Kattner E, Schafer A, Harzer K: Hydrops fetalis: Manifestations in lysosomal storage diseases including Farber disease. *Eur J Pediatr* **156**:292, 1997.
37. Eviatar L, Sklower SL, Wisniewski K, Feldman RS, Gochoco A: Farber (lipogranulomatosis): An unusual presentation in a black child. *Pediatr Neurol* **2**:371, 1986.
38. Colamaria V, Giardina L, Simeone M, Salviati A, Fensom AH, Dalla Bernadina B: Neurologic progressive form—type 5—of Farber's lipogranulomatosis (ceraidase deficiency) in homozygotic twins [Abstract]. *European Neurological Society 3rd Meeting* 226, 1992.
39. Jameson RA, Holt PJL, Keen JH: Farber's disease (lysosomal acid ceramidase deficiency). *Ann Rheum Dis* 46:559, 1987.
40. Levade T, Enders H, Schliephacke M, Harzer K: A family with combined Farber and Sandhoff, isolated Sandhoff and isolated fetal Farber disease: Postnatal exclusion and prenatal diagnosis of Farber disease using lipid loading tests on intact cultured cells. *Eur J Pediatr* **154(8)**:643, 1995.
41. Kishimoto Y, Hiraiwa M, O'Brien JS: Saposins: Structure, function, distribution, and molecular genetics. *J Lipid Res* **33**:1255, 1992.
42. Nakano T, Sandhoff K, Stümper J, Christomanou H, Suzuki K: Structure of full-length cDNA coding for sulfatide activator, a Co-beta-glucosidase and two other homologous proteins: Two alternate forms of the sulfatide activator. *J Biochem* **105**:152, 1989.
43. O'Brien JS, Kretz KA, Dewji N, Wenger F, Fluharty AL: Coding of two sphingolipid activator proteins (SAP-1 and SAP-2) by same genetic locus. *Science* **241**:1098, 1988.
44. Kolter T, Sandhoff K: Topology of glycosphingolipid degradation. *Trends Cell Biol* **6**:98, 1996.
45. Bradova V, Smid F, Ulrich-Bott B, Roggendorf W, Paton BC, Harzer K: Prosaposin deficiency: Further characterization of the sphingolipid activator protein-deficient sibs. Multiple glycolipid elevations (including lactosylceramidosis), partial enzyme deficiencies and ultrastructure of the skin in this generalized sphingolipid storage disease. *Hum Genet* **92(2)**:143, 1993.
46. Paton BC, Schmid B, Kustermann-Kuhn B, Poulos A, Harzer K: Additional biochemical findings in a patient and fetal sibling with a genetic defect in the sphingolipid activator protein (SAP) precursor, prosaposin. Evidence for a deficiency in SAP-1 and for a normal lysosomal neuraminidase. *Biochem J* **285**:481, 1992.
47. Klein A, Henseler M, Klein C, Suzuki K, Harzer K, Sandhoff K: Sphingolipid activator protein D (sap-D) stimulates the lysosomal degradation of ceramide in vivo. *Biochem Biophys Res Commun* **200**:1440, 1994.
48. Chatelut M, Harzer K, Christomanou H, Feunteun J, Pieraggi MT, Paton BC, Kishimoto Y, O'Brien JS, Basile JP, Thiers JC, Salvayre R, Levade T: Model SV40-transformed fibroblast lines for metabolic studies of human prosaposin and acid ceramidase deficiencies. *Clin Chim Acta* **262(1-2)**:61, 1997.
49. Fujita N, Suzuki K, Vanier MT, Popko B, Maeda N, Klein A, Henseler M, Sandhoff K, Nakayasu H, Suzuki K: Targeted disruption of the mouse sphingolipid activator protein gene: A complex phenotype, including severe leukodystrophy and widespread storage of multiple sphingolipids. *Hum Mol Genet* **5**:711, 1996.
50. Oya Y, Nakayasu H, Fujita N, Suzuki K, Suzuki K: Pathological study of mice with total deficiency of sphingolipid activator proteins (SAP knockout mice). *Acta Neuropathol* **96**:29, 1998.
51. Tohyama J, Oya Y, Ezoe T, Vanier MT, Nakayasu H, Fujita N, Suzuki K: Ceramide accumulation is associated with increased apoptotic cell death in cultured fibroblasts of sphingolipid activator protein-deficient mouse but not in fibroblasts of patients with Farber disease. *J Inherit Metab Dis* **22(5)**:649, 1999.
52. Molz G: Farbersche Krankheit: Pathologisch-anatomische Befunde. *Virchows Arch* **344**:1966, 1966.
53. Rivel J, Vital C, Battin J, Heheunstre JP, Leger H: La lipogranulomatose disseminee de Farber. Etude anatomo-clinique et ultrastructurable, de deux observations. *Arch Anat Cytol Pathol* **25**:37, 1977.
54. Toppet M, Vamos-Hurwitz E, Janniaux G, Cremer N, Tondeur M, Pelc S. Farber's disease as a ceramidosis: Clinical, radiological and biochemical aspects. *Acta Paediatr Scand* **67**:113, 1978.
55. Tanaka T, Takahashi K, Hokozaki H, Kimoto H, Suzuki Y: Farber's disease (disseminated lipogranulomatosis). A pathological, histochemical and ultrastructural study. *Acta Pathol Jpn* **29**:135, 1979.
56. Schmoeckel C, Hohlfeld M: A specific ultrastructural marker for disseminated lipogranulomatosis (Farber). *Arch Dermatol Res* **266**:187, 1979.
57. Zarbin MA, Green WR, Moser HW, Morton SJ: Farber's disease: Light and electron microscopic study of the eye. *Arch Ophthalmol* **103**:73, 1985.
58. Palcoux JB, Desvignes V, Malpuech G, Charbonne F, Kantelip B, Raynaud EJ: Farber's lipogranulomatosis. *Arch Fr Pediatr* **42**:535, 1985.
59. Rauch HJ, Auboeck L: "Banana bodies" in disseminated lipogranulomatosis (Farber's disease). *Am J Dermatopathol* **5**:263, 1983.
60. Rutsaert J, Tondeur M, Vamos-Hurwitz E, Dustin P: The cellular lesions of Farber's disease and their experimental reproduction in tissue culture. *Lab Invest* **36**:474, 1977.
61. Prensky AL, Ferreira G, Carr S, Moser HW: Ceramide and ganglioside accumulation in Farber's lipogranulomatosis. *Proc Soc Exp Biol Med* **126**:725, 1967.
62. Sugita M, Connolly P, Dulaney J, Moser HW: Fatty acid composition of free ceramidase of kidney and cerebellum from a patient with Farber's disease. *Lipids* **8**:401, 1973.
63. Clausen J, Rampini S: Chemical studies of Farber's disease. *Acta Neurol Scand* **46**:313, 1970.
64. Mandon EC, Ehses I, Rother J, van Echten G, Sandhoff K: Subcellular localization and membrane topology of serine palmitoyltransferase, 3-dehydrosphinganine reductase and sphinganine N-acyltransferase in mouse liver. *J Biol Chem* **267**:11144, 1992.

65. Rother J, van Echten G, Schwarzmann G, Sandhoff K: Biosynthesis of sphingolipids. Dihydroceramide and not sphinganine is desaturated by cultured cells. *Biochem Biophys Res Commun* **189**:14, 1992.
66. Michel C, van Echten-Deckert G, Rother J, Sandhoff K, Wang E, Merrill AH: Characterization of ceramide synthesis. *J Biol Chem* **272**:22432, 1997.
67. Scribney M: Enzymatic synthesis of ceramide. *Biochim Biophys Acta* **125**:542, 1966.
68. Morell P, Radin NS: Specificity in ceramide biosynthesis from long chain bases and various fatty acyl coenzyme As by brain microsomes. *J Biol Chem* **245**:342, 1970.
69. Braun PE, Morell P, Radin NS: Synthesis of C18 and C20 dihydrosphingosines, ketodihydrosphingosines and ceramides by microsomal preparations from mouse brain. *J Biol Chem* **245**:335, 1970.
70. Singh I: Ceramide synthesis from free fatty acids in rat brain: Function of NADPH and substrate specificity. *J Neurochem* **40**:1565, 1983.
71. Quintern LE, Weitz G, Nehrkorn H, Tager JM, Schram AW, Sandhoff K: Acid sphingomyelinase from human urine: Purification and characterization. *Biochim Biophys Acta* **922**:323, 1987.
72. Schissel SL, Schuchmann EH, Williams KJ, Tabas I: Zn2+stimulated sphingo-myelinase is secreted by many cell types and is a product of the acid sphingomyelinase gene. *J Biol Chem* **271**:18431, 1996.
73. Gatt S: Magnesium-dependent sphingomylinase. *Biochim Biophys Res Commun* **68**:235, 1976.
74. Rao BG, Spence MW: Sphingomyelinase activity at pH 7.4 in human brain and a comparison to activity at pH 5.0. *J Lipid Res* **17**:506, 1976.
75. Chakraborty G, Ziemba S, Drivas A, Ledeen RW: Myelin contains neutral sphingomyelinase activity that is stimulated by tumor necrosis factor-alpha. *J Neurosci Res* **50**:466, 1997.
76. Okazaki T, Bielawska A, Domae N, Bell RM, Hannun YA: Characteristics and partial purification of a novel cytosolic, magnesium-independent, neutral sphingomyelilnase activiated in the early signal transduction of 1 alpha, 25-dihydroxyvitamin D3-induced HL-60 cell differentiation. *J Biol Chem* **269**:4070, 1994.
77. Tamiya-Koizumi T, Umekawa H, Yoshida S, Kojima K: Existence of Mg2+-dependent, neutral sphingomyelinase in nuclei of rat ascites hepatoma cells. *J Biochem* **106**:593, 1989.
78. Levade T, Vidal F, Vermeersch S, Andrieu N, Gatt S, Salvayre R: Degradation of fluorescent and radiolabelled sphingomyelins in intact cells by a non-lysosomal pathway. *Biochim Biophys Acta* **1258**:277, 1995.
79. Alessanko A, Chatterjee S: Neutral sphingomyelinase: Localization in rat liver nuclei and involvement in regeneration/proliferation. *Mol Cell Biochem* **143**:169, 1995.
80. Albi E, Viola Magni MP: Chromatin neutral sphingomyelinase and its role in hepatic regeneration. *Biochem Biophys Res Commun* **236**:29, 1997.
81. Nilsson A: The presence of sphingomyelin and ceramide cleaving enzymes in the small intestinal tract. *Biochim Biophys Acta* **176**:339, 1969.
82. Nyberg L, Duan RD, Axelsson J, Nilsson A: Identification of an alkaline sphingomyelinase activity in human bile. *Biochim Biophys Acta* **1300**:42, 1996.
83. Bernardo K, Hurwitz R, Zenk T, Desnick RJ, Ferlinz K, Schuchman EH, Sandhoff K: Purification, characterization, and biosynthesis of human acid ceramidase. *J Biol Chem* **270**:11098, 1995.
84. Linke T, Lansmann S, Sandhoff K: Purification of acid ceramidase from human placenta. *Methods Enzymol* **311**:201, 2000.
85. Linke T, Wilkening G, Sadeghlar F, Mozeall H, Bernardo K, Schuchman E, Sandhoff K: Interfacial Regulation of Acid Ceramidase Activity; Stimulation of Ceramide Degradation by Lysosomal Lipids and Sphingolipid Activator Proteins (personal publication).
86. Azuma N, O'Brien JS, Moser HW, Kishimoto Y: Stimulation of acid ceramidase by saposin D1. *Arch Biochem Biophys* **311**:354, 1994.
87. Kobayashi T, Stang E, Fang KS, de Moerloose P, Parton RG, Gruenberg J: A lipid associated with the antiphospholipid syndrome regulates endosome structure and function. *Nature* **392**:193, 1998.
88. Becker E: Magnetic isolation of lysosomes from human fibroblasts. *Characterization of lipid patterns [Dissertation]*. Bonn, University of Bonn, 1999.
89. Ferlinz K, Bernardo K, Linke T, Bär-Heine J, Lang F, Sandhoff K, Gulbins E: Processing of acid ceramidase in normal and I-cell disease fibroblasts (personal communication), 1999.
90. Li CM, Park JH, He X, Levy B, Chen F, Koji A, Adler D, Disteche CM, Koch J, Sandhoff K, Schuchmann EH: The human acid ceramidase gene: Structure, chromosomal location, mutation analysis and expression. *Genomics* **62**:223, 1999.
91. Koch J, Gartner S, Li C-M, Quintern LE, Bernardo K, Levran O, Schnabel D, Desnick RJ, Schuchman EH, Sandhoff K: Molecular cloning and characterization of a full-length complementary DNA encoding human acid ceramidase. *J Biol Chem* **271**:33110, 1996.
92. Baer-Heine J, Linke T, Ferlinz K, Sandhoff K: Identification of novel mutations in the acid ceramidase gene leading to Farber disease (personal communication), 1999.
93. El Bawab S, Bielawska A, Hannun YA: Purification and characterization of a membrane-bound nonlysosomal ceramidase from rat brain. *J Biol Chem* **274**:27948, 1999.
94. Yada Y, Higuchi K, Imokawa G: Purification and biochemical characterization of membrane-bound epidermal ceramidases from guinea pig skin. *J Biol Chem* **270**:12677, 1995.
95. Okino N, Tani M, Imayama S, Ito M: Purification and characterization of a novel ceramidase from pseudomonas aeruginosa. *J Biol Chem* **273**:14368, 1998.
96. Sugita M, Williams M, Dulaney JT, Moser HW: Ceramidase and ceramide synthesis in human kidney and cerebellum. Description of a new alkaline ceramidase. *Biochim Biophys Acta* **398**:125, 1975.
97. Spence MW, Beed S, Cook HW: Acid and alkaline ceramidase of rat tissues. *Biochem Cell Biol* **64**:400, 1986.
98. Tiffany C, Al E, Tager J, Moser HW, Kishimoto Y: The use of antibody to characterize control and Farber disease ceramidase. *J Neurochem* **48(Suppl)**:S35, 1987.
99. Sugita M, Dulaney J, Moser HW: Ceramidase deficiency in Farber's disease (lipogranulomatosis). *Science* **178**:1100, 1972.
100. Moser HW, Chen WW: Ceramidase deficiency: Farber disease, in Stanbury JB, Wyngaarden JB, Fredrickson DS, Goldstein JL, Brown MS (eds): *The Metabolic Basis of Inherited Disease*, 5th ed. New York: McGraw-Hill, 1983, p 820.
101. Sutrina SL, Chen WW: Metabolism of ceramide-containing endocytotic vesicles in human diploid fibroblasts. *J Biol Chem* **257**:3039, 1982.
102. van Echten-Deckert G, Klein A, Linke T, Heinemann T, Weisgerber J, Sandhoff K: Turnover of endogenous ceramide in cultured normal and Farber fibroblasts. *J Lipid Res* **38(12)**:2569, 1997.
103. Levade T, Leruth M, Graber D, Moisand A, Vermeersch S, Salvayre R, Courtoy PJ: In situ assay of acid sphingomyelinase and ceramidase based on LDL-mediated lysosomal targeting of ceramide-labeled sphingomyelin. *J Lipid Res* 2525, 1937.
104. Gray GM, White JR: Glycosphingolipids and ceramides in human and pig epidermis. *J Invest Dermatol* **70**:336, 1978.
105. Elias P, Brown BE, Fritsch P, Goerke G, Gray GM, White RJ: Localization and composition of lipids in neonatal mouse stratum granulosum and stratum corneum. *J Invest Dermatol* **73**:339, 1979.
106. Doering T, Holleran WM, Potratz A, Vielhaber G, Elias PM, Suzuki K, Sandhoff K: Sphingolipid activator proteins are required for epidermal permeability barrier formation. *J Biol Chem* **274**:11038, 1999.
107. Lui K, Commens C, Choong R, Jaworski R: Collodion babies with Gaucher's disease. *Arch Dis Child* **63**:854, 1988.
108. Sidransky E, Sherer DM, Ginns EI: Gaucher disease in the neonate: A distinct Gaucher phenotype is analogous to a mouse model created by targeted disruption of the glucocerebrosidase gene. *Pediatr Res* **32(4)**:494, 1992.
109. Perry DK, Hannun YA: The role of ceramide in cell signalling. *Biochim Biophys Acta* **1436**:233, 1998.
110. Hofmann K, Dixit VM: Ceramide in apoptosis — Does it really matter? *Trends Biochem Sci* **23**:374, 1998.
111. Hannun YA: Functions of ceramide in coordinating cellular responses to stress. *Science* **274**:1855, 1996.
112. Zhang P, Liu B, Jenkins GM, Hannun YA, Obeid LM: Expression of neutral sphingomyelinase identified a distinct pool of sphingomyelin involved in apoptosis. *J Biol Chem* **272(15)**:9609, 1997.
113. Strelow A, Bernardo K, Linko K, Sandhoff K, Krönke M, Adam D: Overexpression of acid ceramidase protects from tumor necrosis factor-induced cell death. *J Exp Med* (in press).
114. Grassmé H, Ferlinz K, Jekle A, Kun J, Riehle A, Mueller C, Schwarz H, Berger J, Hurwitz R, Sandhoff K, Lepple-Wienhues A, Lang F, Gulbins E: Receptor clustering is mediated by acid sphingomyelinase (personal communication).
115. Spiegel S, Merrill AH: Sphingolipid metabolism and cell growth regulation. *FASEB J* **10**:1388, 1996.

116. Venable ME, Lee JY, Smyth MJ, Bielawska A, Obeid LM: Role of ceramide in cellular senescence. *J Biol Chem* **270**:30701, 1995.
117. Pahan K, Sheikh FG, Khan M, Namboodiri A, Singh I: Sphingomyelinase and ceramide synthesis stimulate the expression of inducible nitric-oxide synthase in rat primary astrocytes. *J Biol Chem* **273**:2591, 1998.
118. Schwarz A, Futerman AH: Distinct roles for ceramide and glucosylceramide at different stages of neuronal growth. *J Neurosci* **17**:2929, 1997.
118a. Segui B, Bezombes C, Uro-Coste E, Medin JA, Andrieu-Abadle N, Auge N, Brouchet A, Laurent G, Salvayre R, Jaffrazou JP, Levade T: Stress-induced apoptosis is not mediated by endolysosomal ceramide. *FASEB J* **14**:36, 2000.
119. Liu P, Anderson RG: Compartmentalized production of ceramide at the cell surface. *J Biol Chem* **270(45)**:27179, 1995.
120. Chatelut M, Leruth M, Harzer K, Dagan A, Marchesini S, Gatt S, Salvayre R, Courtoy P, Levade T: Natural ceramide is unable to escape the lysosome, in contrast to a fluorescent analogue. *FEBS Lett* **426(1)**:102, 1998.
121. Barrow MV, Holubar K: Multicentric reticulohistiocytosis. A review of 35 patients. *Medicine (Baltimore)* **48**:287, 1969.
122. Drescher E, Woyke S, Markiewicz C, Tegi S: Juvenile fibromatosis in siblings (fibromatosis hyalina multiplex juvenilis). *J Pediatr Surg* **2**:427, 1967.
123. Dulaney JT, Milunsky A, Sidnbury J, Hobolth N, Moser HW: Diagnosis of lipogranulomatosis (Farber's disease) by use of cultured fibroblasts. *J Pediatr* **89**:59, 1976.
124. Ben-Yoseph Y, Gagne R, Parvathy MR, Mitchell DA, Momoi T: Leukocyte and plasma *N*-laurylsphingosine deacylase (ceramidase) in Farber disease. *Clin Genet* **36**:38, 1989.
125. Fensom AH, Benson PF, Neville B, Moser AB, Sulaney JT, Moser HW: The prenatal diagnosis of Farber's disease. *Lancet* **2**:990, 1979.
126. Dulaney JT, Moser HW: Farber's disease (lipogranulomatosis), in Glew RH, Peters SP (eds): *Practical Enzymology of the Sphingolipidoses*. New York, Alan R. Liss, 1977, p 283.
127. Momoi T, Ben-Yoseph Y, Nadler HL: Substrate-specificities of acid and alkaline ceramidases in fibroblasts from patients with Farber disease and control. *Biochem J* **205**:419, 1982.
128. Kudoh T, Wenger D: Diagnosis of metachromatic leukodystrophy, Krabbe disease, and Farber disease after uptake of fatty acid-labeled cerebroside sulfate into cultured skin fibroblasts. *J Clin Invest* **70**:89, 1982.
129. Levade T, Moser HW, Fensom AH, Harzer K, Moser AB, Salvayre R: Neurodegenerative course in ceramidase deficiency (Farber disease) correlates with the residual lysosomal ceramide turnover in cultured living patient cells. *J Neurol Sci* **134(1-2)**:108, 1995.
130. Iwamori M, Costello C, Moser HW: Analysis and quantitation of free ceramide containing non-hydroxy and 2-hydroxy fatty acids, and phytosphingosine by high performance liquid chromatography. *J Lipid Res* **20**:86, 1979.
131. Yahara S, Moser HW, Kolodny EH, Kishimoto Y: Reverse-phase high-performance liquid chromatography of cerebrosides, sulfatides and ceramides: Microanalysis of homolog composition without hydrolysis and application to cerebroside analysis in peripheral nerves of adrenoleukodystrophy patients. *J Neurochem* **34**:694, 1980.
132. Sugita M, Iwamori M, Evans JE, McCluer RH, Dulaney JT, Moser HW: High-performance liquid chromatography of ceramides: Application to analysis in human tissues and demonstration of ceramide excess in Farber's disease. *J Lipid Res* **15**:223, 1974.
133. Chatelut M, Feunteun J, Harzer K, Fensom AH, Basile JP, Salvayre R, Levade T: A simple method for screening for Farber disease on cultured skin fibroblasts. *Clin Chim Acta* **245(1)**:61, 1996.
134. Preiss JE, Loomis CR, Bell RM, Niedel JE: Quantitative measurement of sn-1,2-diacylglycerols. *Methods Enzymol* **141**:294, 1987.
135. van Veldhoven PP, Matthews TJ, Bolognesi DP, Bell RM: Changes in bioactive lipids, alkylacylglycerol and ceramide, occur in HIV-infected cells. *Biochem Biophys Res Commun* **187(1)**:209, 1992.
136. Souillet G, Guibaud P, Fensom AH, Maire I, Zabot MT: Outcome of displacement bone marrow transplantation in Farber's disease: A report of a case, in Hobbs JRE (ed): *Correction of Certain Genetic Diseases by Transplantation*. London, Cogent, 1989, p 137.
137. Medin JA, Takenaka T, Carpentier S, Garcia V, Basile JP, Segui B, Andrieu-Abadie N, Auge N, Salvayre R, Levade T: Retrovirus-mediated correction of the metabolic defect in cultured Farber disease cells. *Hum Gene Ther* **10(8)**:1321, 1999.
138. van Echten G, Sandhoff K: Ganglioside metabolism. Enzymology, topology, and regulation. *J Biol Chem* **268**:5341, 1993.
139. van Echten-Deckert G, Sandhoff K: Organization and topology of sphingolipid metabolism, in Pinto IM (ed): *Comprehensive Natural Products Chemistry*, vol 3. New York, Pergamon Press, 1999, p 87.
140. Kolter T, Sandhoff K: Sphingolipids-their metabolic pathways and the pathobiochemistry of neurodegenerative diseases. *Angew Chem Int Ed* **38**:1532, 1999.
141. Perry DK, Obeid LM, Hannun YA: Ceramide and regulation of apoptosis and the stress response. *Trends Cardiovasc Med* **6**:158, 1996.

CHAPTER 144

Niemann-Pick Disease Types A and B: Acid Sphingomyelinase Deficiencies

Edward H. Schuchman ▪ Robert J. Desnick

1. **Types A and B Niemann-Pick disease (NPD) are lysosomal storage disorders that result from the deficient activity of acid sphingomyelinase (ASM; EC 3.1.4.12) and the accumulation of sphingomyelin. Type A NPD is a fatal disorder of infancy characterized by failure to thrive, hepatosplenomegaly, and a rapidly progressive neurodegenerative course that leads to death by 2 to 3 years of age. In contrast, type B NPD is a phenotypically variable disorder that is usually diagnosed in childhood by the presence of hepatosplenomegaly. Most type B patients have little or no neurologic involvement and survive into adulthood. In more severely affected type B patients, progressive pulmonary infiltration causes the major disease complications.**
2. **The pathologic hallmark of types A and B NPD is the histochemically characteristic lipid-laden foam cell, often referred to as the "Niemann-Pick cell." These histiocytic cells result from the accumulation of sphingomyelin and other lipids in the monocyte-macrophage system, the primary site of pathology in this disease.**
3. **Patients with type A NPD have dramatically reduced ASM activities in their cells and tissues, generally less than 5 percent of normal depending on the enzyme source and assay system used. Type B patients, who have milder disease, have slightly higher residual ASM activities.**
4. **Types A and B NPD are both inherited as autosomal recessive traits. Somatic-cell hybridization and molecular genetic studies demonstrate that both disorders result from allelic mutations within the ASM gene. Type B NPD is panethnic, whereas Ashkenazi Jewish have a higher incidence of type A NPD; the estimated carrier frequency for type A NPD in this population is about 1:80.**
5. **The full-length cDNA and genomic sequences encoding human and murine ASM have been isolated and characterized. The human ASM gene has been mapped to the chromosomal region 11p15.1-p15.4. Although the ASM mRNA is alternatively spliced, there is only one functional transcript that encodes a 629-residue polypeptide that is cotranslationally glycosylated. Following translation/glycosylation, some of the ASM polypeptides are transported to lysosomes, while the remainder are released from cells in a form that requires Zn^{2+} cations for maximal activity.**
6. **Eighteen published mutations have been identified in the ASM gene that cause types A and B NPD. Three mutations, R496L, L302P, and fsP330, account for about 92 percent of the mutant alleles in Ashkenazi Jewish type A NPD patients. Similarly, a single lesion, ΔR608, is a common mutation in type B patients and encodes sufficient residual activity to be "neuroprotective."**
7. **The diagnosis of types A and B NPD is readily made by enzymatic determination of ASM activity in cell and/or tissue extracts. However, heterozygote detection is unreliable by enzyme assay and requires molecular studies. Prenatal diagnosis by enzymatic and/or molecular analyses of cultured amniocytes and chorionic villi has been accomplished.**
8. **Currently, there is no specific therapy for type A or B NPD. Bone marrow transplantation (BMT) studies in a "knockout" mouse model of NPD suggest that this may be a successful therapeutic approach for type B NPD, but is unlikely to alleviate the major neurologic complications of type A NPD. The ASM cDNA has been used to overexpress catalytically active enzyme in Chinese hamster ovary (CHO) cells, providing recombinant protein for the future evaluation of enzyme replacement in type B NPD. Retroviral-mediated gene transfer also corrects the metabolic defect in cultured NPD fibroblasts and hematopoietic stem cells.**

A list of standard abbreviations is located immediately preceding the index in each volume. Additional abbreviations used in this chapter include: ASM = acid sphingomyelinase; BMT = bone marrow transplant; CHO = Chinese hamster ovary; CRM = cross-reacting immunologic material; FACS = fluorescence-activated cell sorter; LTR = long terminal repeat; NPD = Niemann-Pick disease; ORF = open reading frame; SAP = sphingolipid activator protein; TK = thymidine kinase.

HISTORICAL ASPECTS

The major historical landmarks in Niemann-Pick disease (NPD) are summarized in Table 144-1. The German pediatrician Albert Niemann described the first NPD patient in 1914, an Ashkenazi Jewish infant who presented with massive hepatosplenomegaly and had a rapidly progressive neurodegenerative course that led to her death at 18 months of age.[1] At autopsy, Niemann noted that the large, lipid-laden cells in her reticuloendothelial system resembled those described in patients with nonneuronopathic type 1 Gaucher disease.[2] However, he clearly differentiated this case from Gaucher disease based on the age of onset, severe neurologic involvement, and the distinct histologic appearance of the foamy cells. Shortly after, a number of infants with similar clinical findings were described.[3,4] However, the identification of an infantile form of Gaucher disease (i.e., type 2) by Kraus in 1920[5] led many of these patients to be misclassified as having Gaucher disease variants.

In 1927, Ludwig Pick reviewed the reports of infants with rapidly progressive neurodegenerative disorders and delineated the disease described by Niemann as a unique clinical entity.[6,7] Pick's

Table 144-1 Historical Landmarks in Niemann-Pick Disease

1914	The first case of infantile (type A) NPD is described by Niemann.
1916	The stored material in NPD is identified as a phospholipid.
1927	Pick proposes that type A NPD is distinct from type 2 Gaucher disease.
1934	The accumulating phospholipid in type A NPD is identified as sphingomyelin by Klenk.
1946	NPD in adults (type B) is described by Pflander and Dusendschon.
1958	Comprehensive review of NPD is published by Crocker and Farber.
1961	Categorization of NPD into groups A to D by Crocker.
1966	The enzymatic deficiency in type A NPD is identified as ASM by Brady and colleagues.
1967	The enzymatic deficiency in type B NPD is identified as ASM by Schneider and Kennedy.
1980	Types A and B NPD are shown to be allelic and distinct from type C NPD.
1987	Highly purified preparations of human ASM are isolated.
1989	Isolation and characterization of the first cDNA encoding ASM.
1991	Identification of the first mutations causing types A and B NPD.
1991	Chromosomal localization of the ASM gene to 11p15.1-p15.4.
1992	In vitro correction of the metabolic defect in type A NPD by retroviral-mediated gene transfer.
1995	"Knock-out" mouse models of Types A and B NPD generated.

original identification of NPD as a disorder distinct from type 2 Gaucher disease was based primarily on morphologic studies; that is, he clearly identified the presence of "foam cells" that were different from those seen in Gaucher disease. Although he described this new syndrome as "lipoid cell splenomegaly," in subsequent years it became more commonly known as NPD. Twenty years later, the first adult patients with NPD (i.e., type B) were reported by Pflandler and Dusendschon;[8,9] they described two Swiss brothers with massive hepatosplenomegaly and no neurologic abnormalities who died at 29 and 33 years of age.

Wahl and Richardson performed the first comprehensive morphologic analysis of NPD in 1916.[10] Their histochemical studies indicated that the accumulating material in NPD cells was a lipid; by 1925, it was well-established that the storage material in NPD was primarily phospholipid and cholesterol.[11–14] In 1934, Klenk[15] identified the phospholipid as sphingomyelin, leading to the early suggestion that this disease was due to the lack of an enzyme that catalyzes the degradation of sphingomyelin. However, it was not until 1966 that the existence of such an enzyme was clearly demonstrated in rat liver.[16] Shortly thereafter, Brady and colleagues[17] described a deficiency of acid sphingomyelinase (ASM; EC 3.1.4.12) activity in tissue samples obtained from six infantile NPD patients. This finding was soon confirmed by Schneider and Kennedy,[18] who also reported deficient ASM activity in a 16-year-old male patient who had no neurologic involvement (i.e., type B NPD).

To date, more than 300 cases of types A and B NPD have been reported, and excellent reviews of the clinical and pathological findings are available.[19–25] In 1961, Crocker categorized the different NPD phenotypes into four clinical entities designated types A to D.[26] The type A phenotype is the infantile neurodegenerative disorder originally described by Niemann. Type B NPD is distinguished from the severe, neuronopathic type A phenotype by the absence of primary neurologic involvement, a later onset of hepatosplenomegaly, and survival into adulthood. Type C NPD patients often present with prolonged neonatal jaundice, appear normal for 1 to 2 years, and then experience a slowly progressive and variable neurodegenerative course. Their hepatosplenomegaly is less severe than in patients with type A or B NPD, and they may survive into adulthood. The underlying biochemical defect in type C patients is an abnormality in cholesterol transport, leading to the accumulation of sphingomyelin and cholesterol in their lysosomes and a secondary reduction in ASM activity[27,28] (see Chap. 145). In general, type D NPD patients develop neurologic symptoms later in childhood and have a slower neurodegenerative course than type C patients. Most individuals with type D disease share a common ancestry traceable to Acadians from Yarmouth County, Nova Scotia. Recently, the gene (*NPC1*) underlying type C NPD was identified.[29] As suggested by previous biochemical studies,[30,31] type D NPD is also caused by mutations in the *NPC1* gene.[32] In addition to these designations, Fredrickson and Sloan added type E, an indeterminate adult form,[24] and in 1978, Schneider et al.[33] described two patients with a heat-labile form of ASM and classified them as having type F NPD. All six subtypes are inherited as autosomal recessive traits.

The isolation of the cDNA and genomic sequences encoding human ASM has had a major impact on our understanding of NPD (see "The Molecular Genetics of Acid Sphingomyelinase" below). These accomplishments have provided the primary sequence of the ASM polypeptide and facilitated investigations into the nature of the molecular defects underlying the clinical heterogeneity in this disease. Importantly, identification of the mutations in the ASM gene causing types A and B NPD permits precise molecular diagnosis, reliable heterozygote detection, and phenotype/genotype correlation. In addition, the availability of the murine ASM gene sequence has led to the construction of "knock-out" mouse models of NPD that are currently used to evaluate various therapeutic approaches and to investigate the pathophysiology of this disorder.

Several different nomenclatures have been used to distinguish the different disorders classified under the eponym NPD.[25,26] In this edition, the nosology of Crocker has been retained because it has been extensively used throughout the literature. In addition, the ASM-deficient types A and B NPD and the cholesterol transport-defective type C (and type D) NPD have been delegated to separate chapters, consistent with the recognition that they are separate entities.

CLINICAL MANIFESTATIONS

Pathophysiologically, the clinical spectrum of types A and B NPD relates to the nature of the genetic defect and the resulting amount of residual ASM activity. Presumably, patients with the infantile neuronopathic type A disease have little, if any, residual ASM activity, whereas those with the milder, nonneuronopathic type B disease have sufficient residual activity to prevent the occurrence of neurologic manifestations (Table 144-2). However, this hypoth-

Table 144-2 Typical Clinical Features of Types A and B NPD

Feature	Type A	Type B
Age at onset/diagnosis	Early Infancy	Childhood/ Adolescence
Neurodegenerative course	+	−
Cherry-red macula	50%	< 10%
Hepatosplenomegaly	+	+
Marrow NPD cells	+	+
Pulmonary involvement	+/−	+
Age at death	2–3 years	Childhood/ Adulthood
Autosomal recessive inheritance	+	+
Ashkenazic Jewish predilection	+	+/−
Acid sphingomyelinase activity	< 5%	< 10%

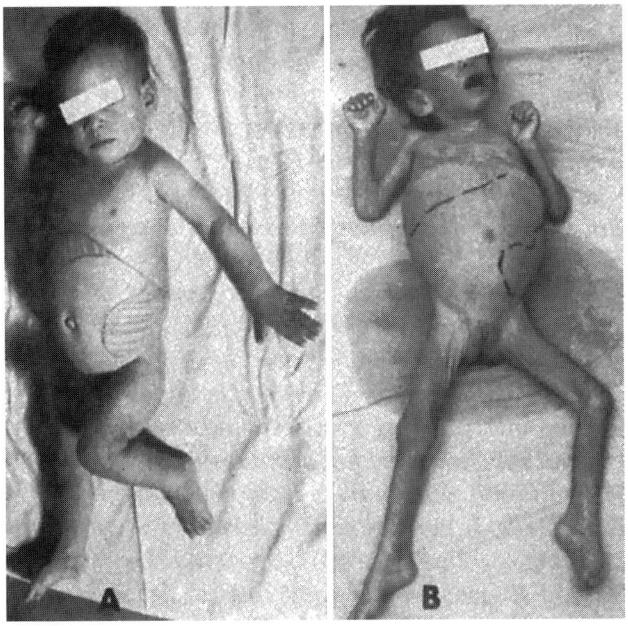

Fig. 144-1 Patient with type A NPD. *A*, Six months of age. *B*, Same patient at 22 months. (*From Fredrickson and Sloan.*[24] *Used by permission.*)

esis has been difficult to prove using in vitro assay systems and cultured cells (see "The Biochemical Defect" below). Type B patients with earlier onset and more severe disease presumably have gene lesions that result in a lesser amount of residual activity. Reviews of the clinical findings in types A and B NPD are available, and the reader should refer to these for more extensive clinical descriptions.[19–24,34] A brief clinical overview of types A and B NPD is given below.

The Type A Phenotype

The clinical presentation and course of type A NPD is relatively uniform. Pregnancy, labor, and delivery are typically unremarkable, and affected newborns appear normal at birth. Occasionally, the newborn period will be complicated by prolonged jaundice. Typically, in the first few months of life, or less frequently by 4 to 6 months, the abdomen will become protuberant and hepatosplenomegaly will be noted on physical examination (Fig. 144-1). Moderate lymphadenopathy is also present. Bone marrow examination reveals the histochemically characteristic "Niemann-Pick" foam cells. A moderate microcytic anemia, which may be responsive to iron supplementation, and a decreased platelet count occur later in the disease. Early neurologic manifestations include hypotonia and muscular weakness that are clinically manifest by feeding difficulties. Recurrent vomiting and chronic constipation are frequent complications. Due to feeding difficulties and the splenomegaly, affected infants have decreased linear growth and body weight. Cardiac function is typically normal. Most infants with type A NPD have minimal respiratory difficulties in the first year of life, with the exception of repeated bronchitis and intercurrent or aspiration pneumonias. However, chest x-ray films demonstrate infiltration of the alveoli as a uniform, diffuse reticular or finely nodular pattern in the lungs.[35]

By 6 months of age, the psychomotor retardation becomes evident. As the infant becomes progressively weaker and hypotonic, retrogression of developmental milestones is noted (e.g., the child can no longer sit). Ophthalmologic examination reveals cherry-red maculae in about half of the affected infants in the first or second year of life. Occasionally, gray granular-appearing maculae are observed (the "macular halo syndrome").[36–39] The electroretinogram is abnormal; however, impairment of vision is rare. Deep-tendon reflexes are diminished or absent, and the cerebrospinal fluid pressure and electroencephalograms are generally normal.

With advancing age, the loss of motor function and the deterioration of intellectual capabilities are progressively debilitating. In addition, affected infants exhibit striking emaciation with a protuberant abdomen and thin extremities (see Fig. 144-1). Subsequently, spasticity and rigidity are evident, and affected infants experience complete loss of contact with their environment. Seizures are rare. Hyperacusis and macrocephaly, features of Tay-Sachs disease, do not occur.

The skin of type A NPD patients may have an ochre or brownish-yellow color. Xanthomas also have been observed in some type A NPD patients, often occurring on the face and upper extremities.[21,23,40] Bony involvement is minimal considering the extensive infiltration of Niemann-Pick macrophages in the marrow. The Erlenmeyer flask deformities seen in Gaucher disease due to marrow expansion are rarely observed. However, osteoporosis is common, presumably due to infiltration and poor nutrition. Bone age, as well as serum calcium and phosphorus levels, are normal.

The Type B Phenotype

In contrast to the stereotyped type A phenotype, the clinical presentation and course of patients with type B disease are more variable (see Table 144-2). Most patients are diagnosed in infancy or childhood when enlargement of the liver and/or spleen is detected during a routine physical examination (Fig. 144-2A). At diagnosis, type B NPD patients usually have evidence of mild pulmonary involvement, usually detected as a diffuse reticular or finely nodular infiltration on the chest roentgenogram (Fig. 144-3). In most patients, hepatosplenomegaly is particularly prominent in childhood, but with increasing linear growth, the abdominal protuberance decreases and becomes less conspicuous. In mildly affected patients, the splenomegaly may not be noted until adulthood[41,42] and there may be minimal disease manifestations (Fig. 144-2B).

In most type B patients, decreased pulmonary diffusion due to alveolar infiltration becomes evident in childhood and progresses with age. Severely affected individuals may experience significant pulmonary compromise by 15 to 20 years of age. Such patients have low Po_2 values and dyspnea on exertion. Life-threatening bronchopneumonias may occur, and cor pulmonale has been described.[43] Severely affected patients also may have liver involvement leading to life-threatening cirrhosis, portal hypertension, and ascites.[44] Clinically significant pancytopenia due to secondary hypersplenism may require partial or complete splenectomy, but is rare.

In general, type B patients do not have neurologic involvement and are intellectually intact. However, there are type B NPD patients who have cherry-red maculae or a gray, granular pigmentation around the fovea;[36–38,45] notably, these patients have apparently normal intelligence and minimal to no neurologic findings (A. Crocker, personal communication). In addition, Sogawa et al.[46] reported two unrelated patients of 9 and 18 years of age who had mental retardation, and Takada et al.[47] reported two type B NPD sisters aged 9 and 13 who had vacuolated macrophages in their cerebrospinal fluid and inclusion bodies in the axons and Schwann cells of rectal biopsies, but no signs of mental retardation. Several cases of type B NPD with cerebellar ataxia also have been reported.[24,48] It is likely that these patients represent the expected clinical spectrum between the typical type A and B NPD phenotypes. Presumably, they have ASM activities that are sufficient to preclude the development of the severe type A disease, but accumulate sufficient neuronal substrate to cause mild to moderate neurologic complications. It is also possible that some of the type B patients with neurologic involvement (particularly those with cerebellar ataxia) may have been misdiagnosed and had type C NPD.

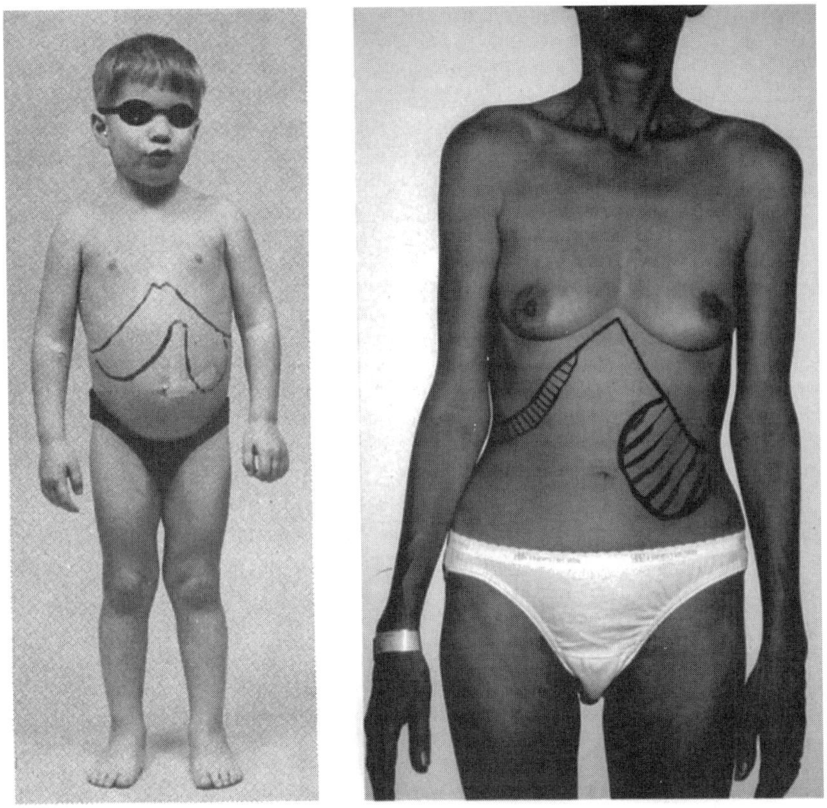

A B

Fig. 144-2 Two patients with type B NPD. ***A*, A 4.7-year-old patient with type B NPD (*From Fredrickson and Sloan.*[24] *Used by permission.*) *B*, A 44-year-old patient with type B NPD.**

PATHOLOGY

The Niemann-Pick Cell

The histologic hallmark of NPD is the pathologic "foam cell" or "Niemann-Pick cell." This histiocyte is found in clinically involved tissues and organs, primarily in the monocyte-macrophage system (Fig. 144-4). These cells should not be confused with "Gaucher cells," the histiocytic storage cell found in Gaucher disease. The two cell types can be readily distinguished by their histologic and histochemical characteristics,[49–53] as described below. The presence of NPD foam cells is not pathognomonic for NPD, because histologically similar cells are found in patients with Wolman disease, cholesterol ester storage disease, lipoprotein lipase deficiency, and in some patients with G_{M1} gangliosidosis, type 2.

The NPD foam cell is ~25 to 75 μm in diameter (smaller than the average Gaucher cell), usually has one nucleus, and the cytoplasm is generally filled with lipid droplets or particles. These droplets are usually uniform in size and give the cell its characteristic foamy appearance (Fig. 144-4). This appearance has been referred to as "mulberry-like" or "honeycomb-like."[11,12] Under polarized light, many of the droplets are birefringent, and under UV light they may appear greenish-yellow to brownish-yellow. In frozen sections, the droplets stain positive for lipid with Sudan black B and oil red O.[50] The Schultz reaction for cholesterol is positive in most NPD cells, a reaction that is negative in Gaucher cells.[51] In contrast, NPD cells stain poorly with PAS, a reaction that is positive in Gaucher cells. In bone marrow, the intracellular material may appear bluish, giving rise to the descriptive term "sea-blue histiocytes."[52] Excellent reviews

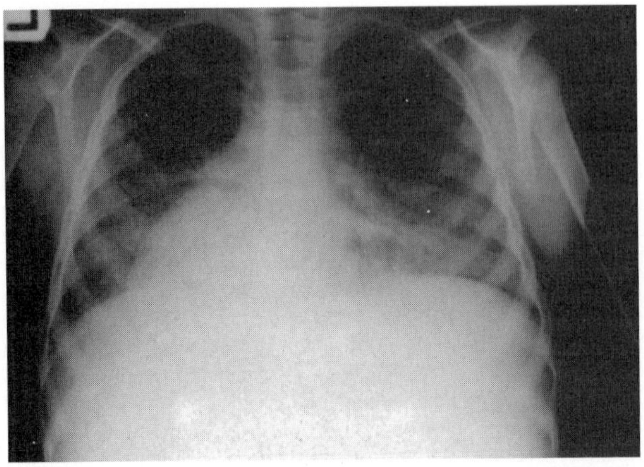

Fig. 144-3 Chest x-ray of a patient with type B NPD showing diffusely infiltrated lung fields.

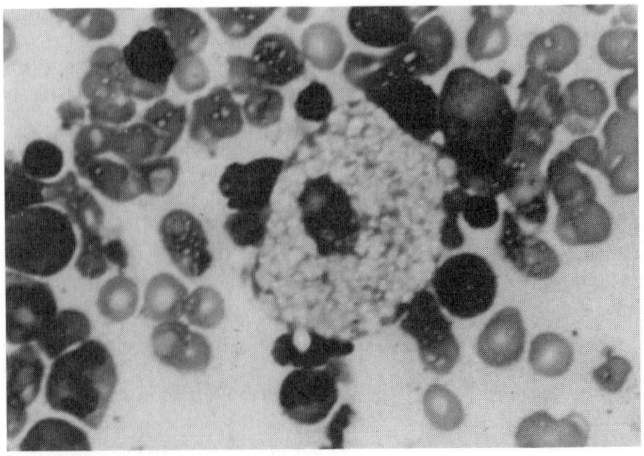

Fig. 144-4 Foam cell in a bone marrow aspirate from a patient with type A NPD.

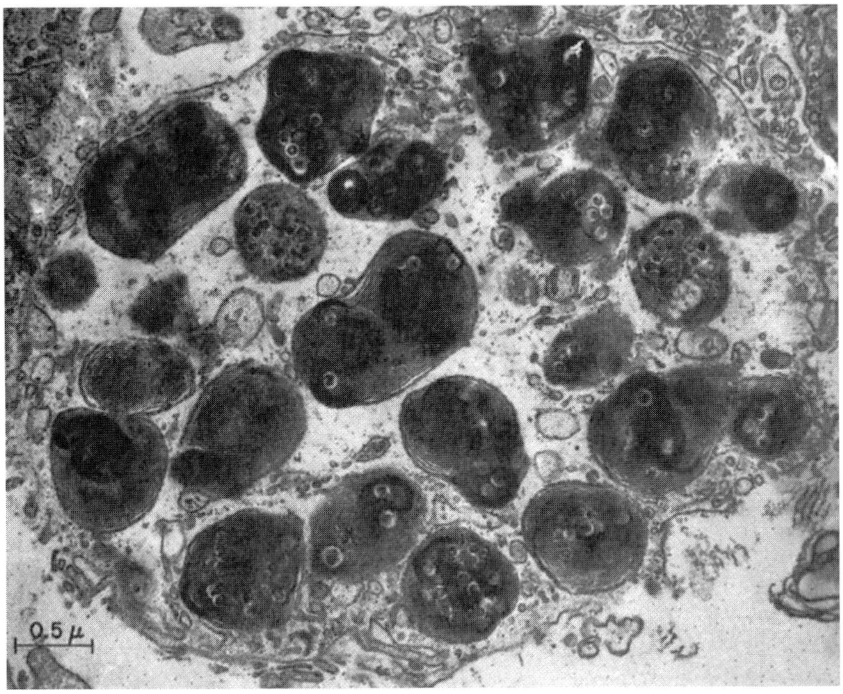

Fig. 144-5 Electron photomicrograph of a foam cell from a lymph node of a patient with type A NPD. ***(From Fredrickson and Sloan.[24] Used by permission. Photo courtesy of Dr. Robert Terry, Albert Einstein School of Medicine.)***

are available that describe the histology and histochemistry of the NPD cell.[20–22,53]

Ultrastructurally, the NPD foam cell contains numerous, granular lipid inclusions in the cytoplasm that are about 0.5 to 50 μm (Fig. 144-5). The inclusions may appear lamellar, having an average periodicity of about 50Å. They are smaller than the inclusions in Tay-Sachs disease, although there is considerable variation in their appearance. Older patients generally have the most pronounced inclusions, while in younger and mildly involved patients, the inclusion bodies are more amorphous. In contrast to Gaucher cells, in which the inclusion bodies stain strongly for acid phosphatase, the NPD cell inclusions usually stain weakly for this lysosomal marker. The inclusion bodies are often associated with ceroid granules at their surfaces.[49]

NPD cells originate from lipid-accumulating bone marrow progenitor cells.[54–56] Thus, in the NPD patient it is rare to find any tissues without some foam cells. Organs of the monocyte-macrophage system, such as the lymph nodes and spleen, often are completely infiltrated with these cells at the end stages of the disease.[57] Rarely, parenchymal cells may have a foam-cell appearance.

The foam cells found in NPD resemble those found in the sea-blue histiocyte syndrome.[58] These latter cells are macrophages that contain varying numbers of cytoplasmic granules, which impart a distinct blue color on Wright's-Giemsa stain.[59] The first reports of patients with widespread accumulation of these cells were in 1970,[60] and since then many similar patients have been described. Although the underlying defect in the sea-blue histiocyte syndrome remains unknown, some patients thought to have this syndrome based on their histopathology have, in fact, been shown to have NPD.[59,60] Thus, the diagnosis of NPD cannot be made based on histologic evidence alone. Enzymatic and/or DNA studies must be used to confirm the histologic findings.

Organ System Involvement

Central Nervous System. At autopsy, the brains of type A NPD patients appear firm and leathery.[61] The overall weight of the brain tends to be less than normal. Although the cerebellum is generally more severely affected than the cerebrum, characteristic lesions may be found in both. Histologically, the ganglion cells are swollen and pale and the cytoplasm is often filled with large vacuoles. There is frequent swelling of the dendrites, the disappearance of normal fibrillae, and a severe deficiency of myelin. Foam cells and/or lipid-laden glial cells are prominent in the brain and in the connective tissue surrounding the cerebral vessels. Similar changes occur in the spinal cord, the autonomic nuclei, and the sympathetic nerve cells in the adrenal medulla; however, the distribution of these lesions may be quite variable.

Peripheral neuropathy also has been noted in type A NPD,[62] although not as frequently or as extensively as the central nervous system involvement. Nerve conduction velocities may be severely diminished and nerve biopsies may reveal isolated fibers with demyelination and numerous dense bodies in the Schwann cells. Often, electron microscopy of nerves reveals two categories of inclusion bodies. One contains the lysosomal inclusions typical of NPD and the second is comprised mostly of myelin. Both the myelin debris and NPD inclusions have been found in axoplasm, probably originating from Schwann cell cytoplasm through axolemma lesions.

Spleen. The spleen is the most extensively involved visceral organ in both types A and B NPD. The spleen volume may be as much as 10 times normal size[63,64] and may be readily detected as early as the first month of life in type A patients. In type B NPD, the onset and severity of splenomegaly may be quite variable. At autopsy, the organ is usually firm and pale. Malpighian bodies may be seen as numerous small reddish-yellow spots. Histologically, the architecture is dramatically abnormal due to the extensive infiltration of foam cells. These cells are arranged mainly between the sinuses, but involvement of the white pulp also may be found, particularly around the arteries. In the most severe cases, the red pulp may be almost completely replaced by NPD cells. NPD cells also may appear within the numerous malpighian bodies.[21] The formation of accessory spleens in type B patients has been described.[20,21]

Lymph Nodes. The degree of lymph node involvement is variable. As the disease progresses, the lymph nodes may become extensively involved, often enlarging three to five times their normal size. Lymphadenopathy is most marked in the mesentery, the hilus of the spleen, liver, and lungs. In addition, the head of the pancreas, the thymus, and the tonsils may also be enlarged. Enlargement of peripheral nodes is not often detected. On gross examination, the nodes may appear grayish-yellow due to the infiltration of lipid-laden NPD cells in the parenchyma. As with the NPD cells of the spleen, the lymph node NPD cells may show signs of erythrocyte phagocytosis.

Bone Marrow. Because the bone marrow is the major source of cells for the monocyte-macrophage system, this organ is one of the most extensively involved in types A and B NPD. The marrow of affected individuals generally appears hyperplastic, and on histologic examination is usually infiltrated with NPD cells. In the most severely affected type A patients, NPD cells may comprise up to 3 percent of the nucleated cells of the bone marrow.[21,23] In general, the NPD cells in the bone marrow are larger than those found in other organs, and a higher percentage of multinucleated cells are observed. In contrast to the NPD cells in the spleen and lymph nodes, phagocytosis of erythrocytes is rarely seen, and the formation of other blood components in the marrow is normal in most NPD patients.

Lungs. The lungs are usually affected in both types A and B NPD, although the extent of involvement may vary considerably. In the classic studies of Crocker and Farber,[21] the weights of the lungs from type A NPD patients were found to be generally increased when compared to age-matched normal controls, the maximum being about 2.4-fold. In type B NPD patients, the lung pathology is more prominent and foam cells may be present throughout the entire organ, including in the lymphatic vessels and pulmonary arteries. Significant foam-cell infiltration of the pulmonary alveoli also may be observed.

Liver. The liver of type A NPD patients may be enlarged from 1.5- to twofold.[21,23] On gross analysis, the livers of NPD patients are firmer than normal[6] and grayish-yellow; however, histologic abnormalities may take up to 6 months to appear. The onset of hepatomegaly and histologic abnormalities may be quite variable in type B NPD. On histologic examination, large Kupffer cells and vacuolated parenchymal cells are generally visible, the former presumably becoming NPD cells during the end stages of the disease.[65] The distribution of these cells may be quite spotty, leading to a variable disruption of the liver architecture. However, the early formation of NPD cells clearly favors the sinuses, and later involves the portal areas.

Kidneys. The kidneys are only moderately involved in types A and B NPD. In fact, Crocker and Farber[21] found that at autopsy the kidneys from most type A NPD patients were slightly smaller than normal. On gross examination, the kidneys may have a fatty, light-yellow cortex. However, histologic findings have been variable. In Pick's 1927 study,[6] about 50 percent of the kidneys from type A NPD patients had visible foam cells, which originated from the tubular epithelium and glomerular endothelial cells. They may frequently be found within the glomerular capillaries and the lumen of the renal arteries. Other pathological changes in the kidneys of NPD patients have been variably noted, although kidney dysfunction has not been observed.

Eyes. Lipid-laden retinal ganglion cells, as well as vacuolated cells in the inner and outer nuclear layers and in the choroid, have been noted.[66–68] Lamellar deposits in the corneal and lens epithelium also may be found. Eye changes have been noted as early as the twenty-third week of gestation in a type A NPD fetus.[69]

Other Organs. In general, most organs of the monocyte-macrophage system contain cells with the characteristic lipid-laden appearance. In addition, large, yellow adrenal glands have been noted in a number of cases; however, adrenal insufficiency has not been found.[70] Other endocrine organs, including the gonads, thyroid, and pituitary, also may show histologic changes, but no functional abnormalities. Similar findings have been reported for the pancreas and salivary gland. In addition, the thymus of NPD patients is often strikingly yellow and massively infiltrated with foam cells. NPD cells are frequently found within the bowel wall, and vacuolated epithelial cells have been observed in the stomach and colon.[71] NPD cells also may be found between the endothelial and smooth muscle cells of the heart, and involvement of the epicardium has been noted.[23]

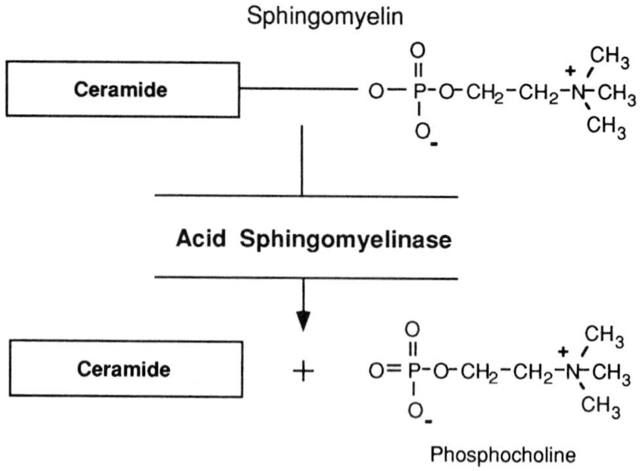

Fig. 144-6 Metabolic defect in types A and B NPD. Types A and B NPD are caused by the marked deficiency of ASM activity, leading to the accumulation of sphingomyelin in lysosomes.

THE BIOCHEMICAL DEFECT

Sphingomyelin Chemistry and Metabolism

Sphingomyelin Chemistry. The underlying biochemical defect in types A and B NPD is the deficient activity of ASM, which results in lysosomal accumulation of sphingomyelin and secondary increases in the concentrations of cholesterol and other metabolically related lipids (e.g., bis- (monoacylglycero)phosphate) (Fig. 144-6). Sphingomyelin is a phospholipid composed of a long chain base, generally sphinganine (4-amino-2-octadecene-1,3-diol), a long chain fatty acid of varying length, and a phosphocholine moiety[72–74] (Fig. 144-7). It is a common component of the plasma membrane, subcellular organelles, ER, and mitochondria, and is the major phospholipid of the myelin sheath and erythrocyte stroma.[51] Sphingomyelin comprises from 5 to 20 percent of the total phospholipid in most cell types, and is primarily localized in the plasma membrane. First discovered by Thudichum in 1884,[75] sphingomyelin can be distinguished from other phospholipids by a variety of unique chemical properties, including the fact that it contains a 2:1 ratio of nitrogen to phosphorus.

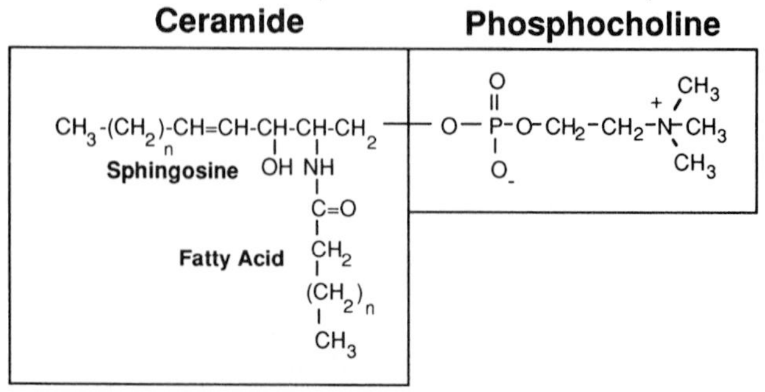

Fig. 144-7 Structure of sphingomyelin. Sphingomyelin is a phospholipid composed of a long chain base, sphingosine, a long chain fatty acid, and phosphocholine. The sphingosine and fatty acid moieties form ceramide, which is linked to the phosphocholine moiety through a phosphodiester bond.

Numerous procedures have been developed for the isolation of sphingomyelin.[76–79] Brain is the most frequent source, but lung, spleen, and liver also have been used. Purified sphingomyelin is a white powder that is only slightly soluble in cold alcohol or pyridine. It is completely insoluble in acetone and diethyl ether, but can readily form emulsions in water that exhibit birefringence.[80] Other optical properties have been noted, including a dextro-rotation in methyl alcohol/chloroform and pyridine solutions.[81] It has been suggested that sphingomyelin occurs as a zwitterion with an isoelectric point of about 6.0.[82]

The initial insights into the structure of sphingomyelin were derived from studying its hydrolysis products,[83] and it has long been recognized that a fatty acid, two nitrogenous bases, choline and sphingosine, and a phosphoric acid were essential components. The fatty acid moiety may vary, but has been most frequently identified as lignoceric acid. Palmitic and stearic acid moieties have also been found, as has the unsaturated fatty acid, nervonic acid.[84] Thannhauser and Boncoddo[85] found that brain sphingomyelin had a different fatty acid composition than sphingomyelin isolated from other tissues. Stearic, lignoceric, and nervonic acids comprised nearly all of the fatty acid moieties in brain sphingomyelins, whereas palmitic and lignoceric were the only fatty acids present in lung and spleen sphingomyelins.[79] Frankel et al.[86] proposed that brain sphingomyelin consists of salt-like complexes formed by the condensation of several adjacent molecules of choline and phosphoric acid, and that such long chain polyaminophospholipids may play a central role in producing nerve conductivity.

Sphingomyelin Synthesis. The major pathway for sphingomyelin synthesis is the enzymatic condensation of ceramide and phosphocholine[87–89] (Fig. 144-8). The enzyme catalyzing this reaction, phosphocholine ceramide transferase (i.e., sphingomyelin synthase), has been identified in various tissues, including liver, kidney, spleen, and brain. Sphingomyelin synthase transfers phosphocholine from cytidine-5′-diphosphocholine (CDP-choline) to ceramide.[87] Notably, there is a stereochemical requirement necessary for this condensation reaction to occur; that is, the sphingosine moiety of active ceramide must have the *trans* configuration of the double bond and the hydroxyl group on carbon 3 must have the threo relationship to the amino group on carbon 2. Because most of the naturally occurring sphingosine is in the erythro form, an isomerization must take place to enable the reaction to proceed. However, the nature of this isomerization has not been satisfactorily determined.

In addition to the condensation pathway, other synthetic pathways for sphingomyelin have been suggested, but not definitively proven. For example, Funjino and Negishi[90] described a pathway in brain mitochondria in which sphingosine acts as the acceptor for CDP-choline. The sphingosylphosphocholine formed serves as an acceptor for fatty acyl CoA, thus forming sphingomyelin. In addition, the direct transfer of phosphocholine from phosphatidylcholine to ceramide has been demonstrated in various cell types, and there is some evidence to suggest that phosphatidylcholine, as opposed to CDP-choline, may be the major source of phosphocholine for sphingomyelin synthesis.[90–95] The subcellular site of sphingomyelin synthesis has not been well characterized; however, there is evidence for intracellular synthesis and translocation of sphingomyelin to the plasma membrane via the *cis* cisternae of the Golgi apparatus.[91–93]

Sphingomyelin Degradation. The catabolism of sphingomyelin has been intensively studied. To date, four distinct mammalian sphingomyelinase activities have been described: (a) an intracellular, cation-independent activity with an acidic pH optimum and lysosomal localization (i.e., ASM); (b) a Mg^{2+}-dependent neutral sphingomyelinase located at the cell surface; (c) a Mg^{2+}-independent neutral sphingomyelinase; and (d) a secreted, Zn^{2+}-dependent enzyme, which also has an acidic pH optimum (see below). In addition, sphingomyelinases have been identified in various microorganisms, including *Pseudomonas aeruginosa,*[96] *Staphylococcus aureus,*[97] *Bacillus cereus,*[98,99] and *Caenorhabditis elegans.*[100] For the purpose of this review, only the human acid sphingomyelinase activities, which are deficient in types A and B NPD, are discussed in detail.

Acid Sphingomyelinase. The existence of a sphingomyelin-cleaving enzyme was demonstrated in 1940 by the pioneering work of Thannhauser and Reichel.[101] During the subsequent 25 years, similar enzymatic activities were demonstrated in various tissues, including liver,[102] brain,[103] and kidney.[104] However, it was Kanfer et al.[16] who first substantially purified a sphingomyelinase activity from rat liver in 1966 and characterized its physical and kinetic properties. Shortly thereafter, Brady and coworkers demonstrated the deficiency of this enzymatic activity in biopsied livers from patients with type A NPD.[17]

Subsequently, human ASM (EC 3.1.4.12) was purified from various sources, including placenta, brain, and urine.[105–110] Although its central role in the pathophysiology of NPD has been known for nearly 30 years, until recently the physicokinetic properties of this important hydrolytic enzyme were not well characterized. For example, the molecular weight estimates for ASM varied from about 70 to over 300 kDa. In addition, the catalytically active form of the enzyme has been described as a monomer,[108–111] dimer,[112] and tetramer,[106] and conflicting reports have appeared concerning its substrate specificity and kinetic properties. Undoubtedly, some of this variation is because different purification procedures and enzyme sources were used to isolate ASM, and that the purified enzyme aggregates readily. Furthermore, a variety of radioactive, colorimetric, and fluorescent

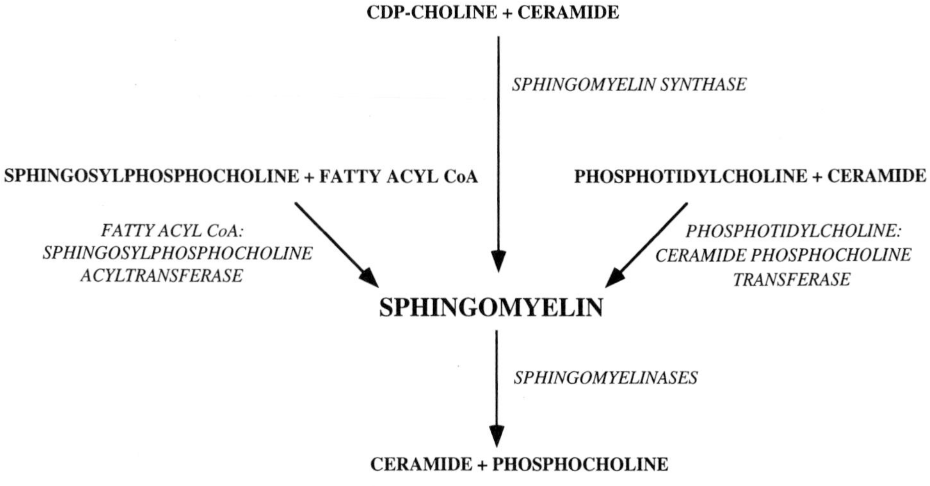

Fig. 144-8 Metabolism of sphingomyelin. Three pathways have been identified that contribute to sphingomyelin synthesis. The most common synthetic pathway involves the condensation of ceramide and CDP-choline by the enzyme sphingomyelin synthase. Sphingomyelin is degraded to ceramide and phosphocholine by the activity of sphingomyelinases.

substrates have been employed to determine the enzyme's kinetic properties, providing an additional source of variation.

The isolation of the full-length cDNA encoding human ASM has clarified some of these inconsistencies and provides further insights into the biology of ASM (see "Molecular Genetics of Acid Sphingomyelinase" below). Based on the full-length cDNA sequence, the calculated molecular weight of the ASM polypeptide is about 64 kDa, and there are 6 potential *N*-glycosylation sites. Thus, it can be predicted that the glycosylated ASM monomer is likely to be 72 to 74 kDa, consistent with the more recent molecular weight estimates.[108,109] Site-directed mutagenesis studies further revealed that five of the six glycosylation sites in human ASM are utilized, and that the two C-terminal sites are the most important for enzyme maturation and activity.[113]

Limited studies of the kinetic properties of ASM have been performed. In contrast to the neutral sphingomyelinase, it had been reported that ASM does not require divalent cations for catalytic activity because chelators such as EDTA do not inhibit the enzymatic activity.[114] However, more recent data shows that ASM is a zinc metalloprotein (see "Relationship Between Intracellular and Secretory ASM" below). In vitro ASM activity is clearly dependent on the presence of detergents, and Yedgar and Gatt[115] have shown that when the Triton X-100:sphingomyelin ratios are 4:1 or greater, the reaction displays regular Michaelis-Menten kinetics. K_m values ranging from 10 to 500 μM have been reported dependent on the substrate and assay system.[108,115,116]

There also are a number of reports that suggest that one or more sphingolipid activator proteins (SAPs) may influence the activity of ASM, thus performing a similar function in vivo that detergents such as Triton X-100 play in vitro. However, recent data obtained from knock-out mice in which the SAP precursor protein was disrupted by gene targeting, show that the ASM activity was normal or near normal in various tissues from these animals, and that no sphingomyelin was accumulated.[117] The earlier results may be explained by the fact that the ASM polypeptide contains a domain in the N-terminal portion that has high homology to the SAP proteins. Thus, it may be hypothesized that ASM does not require exogenous SAP proteins to carry out its catalytic function because it is able to do so using its own "SAP-like" sequences. This "SAP-like" domain is separated from the remainder of the protein by a proline-rich (hinge) region, perhaps linking it to a catalytic region.

Various inhibitors of ASM activity have been identified, including 5′-adenosine monophosphate (5′-AMP), tricyclic antidepressant drugs such as midalcipran,[118,119] cationic amphiphilic drugs,[120] and nephrotoxic aminoglycosides such as gentamicin.[121] The data using 5′-AMP suggested that the inhibition was noncompetitive and reversible, and that the inhibitory mechanism involved the combined effect of both the phosphate group and the purine ring. Octylglucoside is also a potent inhibitor of ASM activity and octyl-Sepharose columns have been employed in many purification schemes.[106,122] From these and other results, investigators have concluded that a carboxyl group (perhaps donated from an aspartate or a glutamate residue) and a protonated histidine are involved in sphingomyelin binding to the enzyme. Although the active site specificity involves the ceramide and diacylglycerol moieties, the presence of the phosphodiester linkage is the only absolute requirement.[107]

Apo C-III also has been shown to stimulate ASM activity in vitro.[123] This is a particularly intriguing finding in light of reports that sphingomyelinase is responsible for the aggregation and uptake of LDL particles into cultured cells.[124,125] Many of the biochemical properties of Apo C-III are similar to those of the SAP proteins (e.g., molecular weight of about 9.5 kDa; pI in the range of 4.4 to 4.6), and it has been suggested that the mechanism of ASM activation by the "SAP-like domain" and Apo C-III may be similar.[123]

Polyclonal[111,126] and monoclonal[127] antibodies have been raised against various purified ASM preparations and used to study the biosynthesis of ASM in normal and NPD fibroblasts. After labeling the cells for 16 h with [^{35}S]methionine, Jobb et al.[128] found that a single polypeptide of about 110 kDa could be immunoprecipitated from cells derived from normal individuals and that the 110-kDa polypeptide was partially processed into an 84-kDa species by 72 h. ASM also was secreted by I-cell disease fibroblasts, suggesting that the enzyme is trafficked to lysosomes by the mannose 6-phosphate receptor-mediated pathway. Recent data using recombinant ASM has suggested that the mannose 6-phosphate uptake system accounts for ~50 percent of the enzyme uptake by cultured skin fibroblasts[129] (see "Overexpression of Human ASM in Chinese Hamster Ovary Cells" below). More recent processing studies using cultured skin fibroblasts also have shown that ASM is synthesized as a 75-kDa precursor that is processed into several smaller molecular weight species (e.g., 72, 67, and 57 kDa) within lysosomes,[130] and that small amounts of the precursor form were secreted into the culture media, along with the 57-kDa form.

Other Mammalian Sphingomyelinases. In addition to the intracellular ASM, at least three other sphingomyelinases have been described in humans. Neutral sphingomyelinase is a membrane-bound enzyme with a pH optimum of about 7.5.[114,131–134] This enzyme requires Mg^{2+} for activity, is found in most mammalian tissues, and is the predominant sphingomyelinase in brain. Neutral sphingomyelinase levels are normal in types A and B NPD patients,[135] suggesting that this polypeptide is the product of a distinct gene. Recently, a cDNA clone was obtained which encodes an enzyme with many of the properties attributed to the Mg^{2+}-dependent neutral sphingomyelinase.[136] A Mg^{2+}-independent, neutral sphingomyelinase activity also has been reported,[137] as well as a Zn^{2+}-dependent acidic sphingomyelinase in human and bovine serum.[138] This latter enzyme is encoded by the same gene as the intracellular ASM, and is similarly deficient in types A and B NPD patients (see "Relationship Between Intracellular and Secreted ASM" below).

In addition to these enzymes, another acidic human sphingomyelinase was purified to apparent homogeneity from placenta.[139] Despite the molecular weight of this purified enzyme being consistent with that of ASM purified from urine,[140] none of the amino acid sequences obtained from the microsequenced proteolytic fragments were the same. Thus, this sphingomyelinase is a unique protein, distinct from ASM. The existence of another phospholipase that can cleave sphingomyelin at an acidic pH may explain some of the difficulties in developing accurate heterozygote testing for types A and B NPD by enzymatic assay. The existence of this enzyme, however, still awaits confirmation.

Relationship Between Intracellular and Secreted ASM. For many years it has been known that types A and B NPD were due to the deficient activity of lysosomal ASM. This enzyme has been studied in detail and many of its basic biochemical properties have been investigated. As noted above, it had been generally assumed that in contrast to the Mg^{2+}-dependent neutral sphingomyelinase, ASM activity was cation independent. This notion was based primarily on the fact that treatment of the enzyme with metal chelators such as EDTA did not affect enzymatic activity. In 1989, an acidic sphingomyelinase activity was reported in human and bovine serum that had the unique property of being Zn^{2+}-dependent, in contrast to intracellular ASM.[138] However, beyond this initial intriguing report, this zinc-dependent activity was not studied further until 1996, when Schissel et al.[141] reported that many different cell lines secreted a Zn^{2+}-dependent ASM with properties identical to those described for the Zn^{2+}-dependent enzyme in serum. Quite surprisingly, cells from patients with types A or B NPD were deficient in this enzymatic activity, as well as intracellular ASM. Moreover, CHO cells engineered to overexpress the human ASM cDNA (see below) overexpressed both the Zn^{2+}-dependent, secreted form of ASM, and the intracellular form that did not require zinc for catalytic activity.

Thus, the same primary ASM mRNA leads to the production of two distinct forms of ASM — one secreted from cells and requiring zinc for activity, and the other intracellular (presumably lysosomal) which does not require zinc for activation. While the biological function of the secreted ASM remains unknown, the implications for NPD are profound because mutations in the ASM gene lead to the deficiency of both enzymatic activities. Thus, it is possible that some aspects of the NPD pathology may not be due to intracellular accumulation of sphingomyelin, but instead may be related to the function of the secreted enzyme. Further clarification of the unique biologic roles of the two ASM forms and their implications for NPD is an obvious area of future research. Most recently, it was shown that the intracellular ASM, described as a cation-independent enzyme, is inactivated by the zinc-specific chelator 1,10-phenanthroline.[142] Thus, the main difference between the secreted and intracellular ASM activities is not in their zinc requirements (both require zinc cations for enzymatic activity), but rather in their intracellular trafficking and relative exposure to intracellular pools of zinc.

Overexpression of Human ASM in Chinese Hamster Ovary Cells. An important recent development that will have a major impact on the treatment of NPD is the overexpression of human ASM in CHO cells. As noted above, one difficulty encountered in the study of ASM previously was the small amounts of enzyme available from natural sources. Moreover, the enzyme obtained from tissue homogenates was prone to aggregation and difficult to purify. These limitations were overcome by overexpressing the human ASM cDNA in CHO cells using a DHFR-based amplification/expression vector system[129] similar to that used by other investigators to overexpress α-galactosidase A (see Chap. 150). Notably, ASM activity in the media of the stably transfected cells was approximately seven hundredfold greater than in the parental cells and required zinc cations for maximal activity. A rapid purification protocol was developed to isolate the recombinant human enzyme from the culture media of these overexpressing cells, permitting the purification of 5 to 10 mg of homogenous enzyme/liter of culture media. The physicokinetic properties of this enzyme have been extensively studied and appear identical to those of the native enzyme obtained from human tissues.[129] Thus, there is now an excellent source of purified human ASM available for clinical evaluation in the NPD "knock-out" mouse model (see "Animal Models" below), as well as for crystallization and other structural studies.

The Biochemical Abnormalities in Types A and B NPD

The Accumulating Lipids. ***Sphingomyelin.*** Sphingomyelin is the major lipid that accumulates in the cells and tissues of patients with types A and B NPD. In most normal tissues, sphingomyelin constitutes from 5 to 20 percent of the total cellular phospholipid content, but in tissues of types A and B NPD patients, the sphingomyelin levels may be elevated up to fiftyfold, constituting about 70 percent of the total phospholipid fraction.[118,143] The relative increases in sphingomyelin and cholesterol in various NPD tissues, including the brains of type A patients, were summarized by Spence and Callahan.[25] Presumably, the accumulation of sphingomyelin in NPD is the result of abnormal turnover of cell membranes (the major component of the intracellular sphingomyelin pool) due to the ASM deficiency. Cells of the monocyte-macrophage system, particularly in the spleen and lymph nodes, accumulate the most sphingomyelin[25] because they actively phagocytose sphingomyelin-rich membranous material. Storage in liver,[22,118,144] brain,[145] kidneys,[21] and lungs[21,22] has also been documented. Organs from types A and B NPD patients contain about the same amounts of sphingomyelin, with the notable exception that type B NPD patients have little or no lipid storage in their central nervous system.[25] Because type B NPD patients die at a much later age than those with type A NPD, the rate of sphingomyelin accumulation in type A NPD individuals is much greater than that in type B NPD patients.

Cholesterol. Tissue cholesterol levels are almost always increased in types A and B NPD. The degree of storage varies, but may be as much as 3 to 10 times normal levels. The distribution of cholesterol storage is similar to that of sphingomyelin, with cells of the monocyte-macrophage system accumulating the most. In contrast to the sphingomyelin storage, cholesterol concentrations at the time of autopsy are significantly greater in type A NPD patients than in those with type B disease.[118] Why cholesterol accumulates in the tissues of type A and B NPD patients is not clear, because the metabolic trafficking of this sterol is clearly different from that of sphingomyelin. However, increased levels of cholesterol in various phospholipid storage disease patients had been recognized in 1930,[13] leading to an erroneous hypothesis that the biochemical defect in some of these diseases was in a "phospholipid/cholesterol"-binding protein. More likely, the accumulation of cholesterol involves lipid-lipid interactions in biomembranes.[22] In support of this hypothesis, it has been demonstrated that sphingomyelin and cholesterol can form a complex with maximal van der Waals interactions between the sphingosine moiety and cholesterol carbons.[146,147] Notably, the calculated distance between the phosphate groups in this complex compares well with the periodicity of the lamellar bodies seen in NPD cells.[22] Cholesterol is a particularly good "lipid organizer,"[146] permitting strong interactions with other lipids. Thus, it is reasonable to assume that the primary storage of sphingomyelin in NPD cells leads to a secondary storage of cholesterol. Conversely, the accumulation of sphingomyelin in types C and D NPD, which results from a cholesterol transport defect (see Chap. 145), may be due to the same or a similar mechanism.

Bis(monoacylglycero)phosphate. Other than sphingomyelin and cholesterol, the major lipid that accumulates in the visceral tissues of most type A and B NPD patients is bis(monoacylglycero)phosphate. In fact, this lipid may accumulate to higher levels than sphingomyelin, perhaps as much as 85 times greater than normal levels in the livers of patients with type A NPD.[148] Normal tissues have trace amounts of bis(monoacylglycero)phosphate localized in lysosomes.[25] Although its role in the pathogenesis of NPD is not understood, the accumulation of this lipid is attributed to the increased number of lysosomes in NPD cells.[51] Notably, the storage of bis(monoacylglycero)phosphate also has been found in drug-induced lipidoses.[149]

Other Sphingolipids. There are reports of the accumulation of glycosphingolipids in NPD. These include glucocerebroside and gangliosides G_{M2} and G_{M3}.[143] In addition, lesser accumulations of lactosylceramide, globotriaosylceramide, and globotetraosylceramide also have been reported in liver and spleen[25] from NPD patients.

The Enzymatic Defect. ***Residual ASM Levels.*** Despite the fact that the enzymatic defect causing types A and B NPD has been known for almost three decades, reports on the levels of residual ASM activity have been variable due to differences in the assay procedures and enzyme sources used.[25] In general, patients with type A NPD have ASM activity levels ranging from nondetectable to less than 5 percent of normal when determined in vitro using cultured fibroblasts and/or lymphoblasts as the enzyme source.[150–153] Similar findings have been reported in tissue extracts, including liver, kidneys, and brain.[105,135,154] The ASM activities in cells and tissues obtained from type B NPD patients are more variable than those of type A. In general, the in vitro residual activities in type B NPD may range from 2 to 10 percent of normal when determined in cultured cells.[105,154,155]

Because the determination of ASM activities in vitro has proven problematic, a number of laboratories have developed *in situ* cell-loading assays to determine ASM activity. In these systems, radioactive[151,156] or fluorescent[157,158] sphingomyelin is added to the culture media of fibroblasts or lymphoblasts for uptake and transport to the lysosomes. Following a chase period, the cells are harvested, the lipids are extracted, and the amount of sphingomyelin converted to ceramide is determined. Gatt and coworkers[159] developed a modification of this technique using fluorescently labeled (pyrene) sphingomyelin and Apo E to target the substrate to lysosomes efficiently via the LDL receptor. The advantage of this technique is that it avoids hydrolysis of the exogenous substrate by contamination of the neutral sphingomyelinase activity present on the plasma membrane. Using this *in situ* assay, the residual activities in cultured cells obtained from nine type A and six type B NPD patients were determined.[159] Cells from type A NPD patients hydrolyzed only about 1 to 3 percent of the delivered sphingomyelin, whereas cells from type B patients hydrolyzed from 10 to 60 percent of the substrate, providing substantial proof that cells from type B NPD patients have higher levels of residual ASM activity than those from patients with type A NPD. Presumably, the higher levels of residual ASM activity in type B NPD prevent the development of neurologic symptoms. Notably, there are reports that the residual ASM activity in type B NPD cells can be enhanced to about normal levels by dimethyl sulfoxide (DMSO)[160,161] and cannabidiol.[162] Although these reports are intriguing, they have not been confirmed.

Immunologic Studies of the Mutant ASM. A variety of antibody preparations have been made against ASM and used to study the CRM in cultured cells from types A and B NPD patients.[128,163] However, due to difficulties in obtaining highly purified ASM, the quality of the antibodies used in these early studies remains suspect. Furthermore, because ASM is known to form aggregates and a wide range of molecular weight species have been reported, interpretation of the published immunologic studies has proven difficult. A number of NPD patients were recently analyzed for the presence of CRM using a highly specific antibody preparation raised against recombinant human ASM purified from the over-expressing CHO cells (EH Schuchman et al., unpublished results). To date, all of the type A or B patients analyzed (other than two type A patients who were homoallelic for nonsense mutations leading to truncated ASM polypeptides) have had about normal levels of ASM CRM. The availability of these high-titer, monospecific anti-ASM antibodies should facilitate further immunologic studies of the enzyme defects underlying types A and B NPD.

Sphingolipids and Signal Transduction: Implications for NPD

About 10 years ago, sphingosine was discovered to be a potent inhibitor of protein kinase C activity and of phorbol ester binding in mixed micellar assays.[164,165] Similar findings were soon reported in human platelets, neutrophils, and HL-60 cells,[166–168] raising the possibility that sphingoid bases may be important regulators of protein kinase C-mediated signal transduction. Recent reports documenting the effects of sphingolipids on protein kinase C-mediated signal transduction have been published, and it also has been suggested that some of the cellular pathology in the various sphingolipidoses may be due to sphingolipid-induced alterations in signal transduction.[169–171]

Much of the interest in the sphingolipid-mediated signal transduction field has focused on the role of ceramide (generated by sphingomyelin hydrolysis) as a second messenger in these pathways.[172,173] This so-called "sphingomyelin pathway" is a ubiquitous, evolutionarily conserved signaling system, and the Mg^{2+}-dependent and -independent neutral sphingomyelinases, as well as ASM, are implicated in the activation of this pathway. For example, activation of ASM is associated with signaling via Fas, CD28, and the interleukin-1 (IL-1) receptor.[174–176] The recent findings that ASM is actively secreted by many cell types, is stable at physiologic pH, and can be rapidly reinternalized and sequestered in endosomal compartments are supportive of a role for this enzyme in signal transduction, because it is widely assumed that the pool of ceramide that functions as a second messenger is generated at or near the cell surface, not within lysosomes.

Of particular relevance to NPD, it was recently shown that lymphoblasts from type B NPD patients failed to respond to ionizing radiation with ceramide generation and apoptosis.[177] These abnormalities were reversible on restoration of ASM activity by retroviral-mediated gene transfer of the human ASM cDNA. The ASM "knock-out" mice also expressed defects in radiation-induced ceramide generation and apoptosis in vivo.[177]

Thus, these results in the animal model system suggest that NPD patients may have subtle abnormalities in various signaling pathways, and that these abnormalities could be exacerbated by stress (e.g., radiation, infection). While there is currently no clinical evidence to support this hypothesis, future research will undoubtedly focus on the role of apoptosis in the NPD pathophysiology.

Lysosphingolipids and the NPD Pathophysiology

Lysosphingolipids, which differ from their respective parental sphingolipids by not having the amide-linked fatty acid at the 2-amino position of the sphingoid base, also are potent and reversible inhibitors of protein kinase C activity. The same hydrolytic enzymes degrade them as degrade their respective parent sphingolipids; thus, the deficiency of a particular hydrolytic enzyme leads to the accumulation of the sphingolipid and the derivative lysosphingolipid. It has been hypothesized that the accumulation of lysosphingolipids may result in cell dysfunction and cell death. In support of this hypothesis, a number of lysosphingolipids have been shown to have a role in the pathophysiology of certain sphingolipidoses, including psychosine (galactosylsphingosine) in Krabbe disease[178] and glucosylsphingosine in Gaucher disease.[179]

To date, only one lysosphingolipid, sphingosylphosphocholine (SPC), has been shown to accumulate in type A NPD.[180] Of note, SPC is a potent mitogen that, among other things, increases intracellular free Ca^{2+} uptake and induces neurite outgrowth. Moreover, it has been shown that SPC also increases the DNA-binding activity of the AP-1 transcription activator,[181] and that AP-1 binding sites are present in the ASM promoter (see "The ASM Gene," below).

GENETICS

Mode of Inheritance

The familial nature of type A NPD was noted as early as 1916, when Knox et al.[4] described the phenotype in sibs from the same family. Soon after, other investigators reported the occurrence of two or more affected sibs,[3,182,183] and by 1958, it had been clearly demonstrated that the disease was familial.[21] About equal numbers of male and female cases had been described at that time, and consanguinity had been noted in six couples with affected offspring, further supporting the autosomal recessive nature of the inheritance.

Ethnic Predilection and Incidence. Although types A and B NPD are panethnic, it is well documented that type A NPD occurs more frequently among individuals of Ashkenazi Jewish ancestry than in the general population. According to Schettler and Kahlke,[23] two-thirds of the patients reported up to 1955 were of Jewish ancestry. In the data compiled by Videbaek[184,185] and Crocker and Farber,[21] 35 of 73 patients whose ethnic history could be traced were Jewish. Indeed, Niemann's original type A patient was a Polish infant of Ashkenazi Jewish ancestry.

The carrier frequency (2pq) of type A NPD in the Ashkenazi Jewish population is estimated at about 1:80 (see "The Molecular Genetics of ASM" below), suggesting a disease incidence of about 1 in 40,000.[186] It should be noted that lipid storage has been documented in NPD fetuses,[187–190] and that type A fetuses have been reported to have a higher frequency of spontaneous abortions.[24] Therefore, the true incidence of type A NPD may be higher than what is reflected in the reported cases. Furthermore, in the early literature, type A NPD was often misdiagnosed as type 2 Gaucher disease.

The incidence of type B NPD in the Ashkenazi Jewish population is significantly less than the incidence of type A NPD. However, among non-Jewish NPD patients, the type B form is more prevalent. While accurate estimates for the frequency of type B NPD are unavailable, it occurs at a relatively high frequency within some ethnic groups.[191] Moreover, because many type B NPD patients have mild symptomology, the frequency of type B NPD is likely to be higher than what is indicated by estimates in the literature.

Allelism of Types A and B Niemann-Pick Disease

Since their original descriptions, the biochemical and genetic relationships of the clinically diverse NPD subtypes have been the subject of much speculation. In 1980, Besley et al.[192] performed a series of somatic-cell hybridization experiments with cultured cells from types A, B, and C patients. When cells from types A and B patients were fused, the ASM activities were not substantially increased (i.e., the metabolic defect could not be corrected), indicating that these two disorders were allelic and due to abnormalities in the same gene. In contrast, when cells from type C patients were fused with those from type A or B patients, the levels of ASM activity were increased to near normal levels, demonstrating that this disorder had a distinct gene defect. Biochemical and molecular studies have confirmed these findings and definitively demonstrated that types A and B NPD are due to different mutations in the ASM gene (see below). Patients with types C and D NPD have mutations in the *NPC1* gene, located on chromosome 18 (see Chap. 145).

THE MOLECULAR GENETICS OF ACID SPHINGOMYELINASE

The Human ASM cDNA

In 1989, the first cDNAs encoding human ASM were isolated.[140] Two distinct ASM cDNAs were identified (designated types 1 and 2) whose predicted amino acid sequences were colinear with peptide amino acid sequences determined from purified human urinary ASM. The type 1 cDNA contained a unique 172-bp sequence encoding 57 amino acids that was replaced in the type 2 cDNA by a 40-bp sequence encoding 13 different amino acids. From extensive library screenings, a third type of ASM cDNA also was isolated and sequenced (designated type 3).[193] Although this cDNA was colinear with the ASM amino acid sequences, it did not contain the type 1- or 2-specific sequences. In addition, the reading frame of the type 3 cDNA was altered and a premature stop codon was identified at codon 248. Northern hybridization, RNase protection, and PCR amplification analyses documented the occurrence of full-length type 1, 2, and 3 mRNAs, and suggested that the three transcripts represented about 90, 10, and 1 percent of the total cellular ASM mRNA, respectively, in fibroblasts and placenta.[193] To investigate their functional integrity, the full-length types 1, 2, and 3 cDNAs were individually subcloned into the mammalian expression vector p91023(B) and transiently expressed in COS-1 cells. Only the full-length type 1 cDNA expressed catalytically active enzyme.[193] That types 2 and 3 cDNA did not express catalytically active enzymes suggested that these mRNAs were nonfunctional and resulted from aberrant splicing of the ASM hnRNA — a hypothesis that was confirmed by analysis of the ASM genomic sequence (see "The Human ASM Gene" below).

The 2347-bp full-length type 1 cDNA had an open reading frame (ORF) of 1890 bp encoding 629 amino acids (Table 144-3). The size of the full-length type 1 cDNA was consistent with the

Table 144-3 Features of the Full-Length Type 1 Human ASM cDNA

Feature	Position
	Nucleotide
pASM-3 cDNA Insert (2385 bp)	
5′ Untranslated region (87 bp)	−87 to 1
Coding region (629 residues)	1 to 1890
3′ Untranslated region (396 bp)	1891–2286
PolyA tract (12)	2287–2298
Polyadenylation signal	
AATAAA	2253–2258
	Codon
Two in-frame ATGs	1;97
Potential *N*-Glycosylation sites	
Asn-Leu-Thr	86–88
Asn-Ile-Ser	175–177
Asn-His-Ser	335–337
Asn-Ser-Thr	395–397
Asn-Tyr-Ser	503–505
Asn-Leu-Thr	522–524

occurrence of the ~2.5-kb transcript observed in the northern hybridization experiments, the ~150-bp difference presumably due to the upstream 5′ untranslated sequences and the length of the polyA tract. Notably, two in-frame initiation codons were identified within the 5′ region.[194] Because the purified enzyme's *N*-terminus was blocked,[140] it was not known which of these potential initiation codons was utilized in vivo. However, site-directed mutagenesis and transient expression studies demonstrated that both initiation sites could function in vitro (EH Schuchman et al., unpublished results). Using the von Heijne weight-matrix method,[195] the optimal signal peptide cleavage of the ASM precursor polypeptide was predicted to occur after amino acid residue 46. The 14 amino acids preceding the signal peptide cleavage site had a particularly hydrophobic core consisting of five leucine/alanine repeats encoded by a CTGGCG hexanucleotide sequence. Six *N*-glycosylation sites were predicted in the mature ASM polypeptide (see Table 144-3), and it is now known that five of these sites are utilized.[113]

The Human ASM Gene

Genomic Structure and the Nature of Alternative Splicing. The complete ASM genomic region, including 1116 and 468 of 5′ and 3′ untranslated nucleotides, respectively, has been isolated and sequenced.[196] This housekeeping gene is about 5 kb long and is composed of 6 exons ranging in size from 77 to 773 bp and 5 introns ranging in size from 153 to 1059 bp (Fig. 144-9). Exon 2 is unusually large, encoding 258 amino acids or about 44 percent of the mature ASM polypeptide (Table 144-4). Immediately downstream from the type 2-specific sequence, within intron 2, is a single Alu 1 repeat element inserted in the reverse orientation. The Alu 1 element was placed into the "a branch" according to the classification of Jurka and Smith,[197] indicating the ancestral nature of the ASM gene. The regulatory region upstream of the ASM coding sequence was GC rich and contained putative promoter elements, including SP1, TATA, CAAT, NF-1, and AP-1 binding sites.[196]

Analysis of the genomic sequence indicated that alternative splicing of the ASM hnRNA was the molecular basis for types 1, 2, and 3 transcripts. The type 1-specific 172 bp sequence was encoded by exon 3, whereas the type 2-specific 40 bp sequence was located at the 5′ end of intron 2, followed by a cryptic donor splice site (aag gtgaat). Furthermore, there was a poor donor splice site (AAA gtgagg) at the junction of exon 3 and intron 3. Thus, the occurrence of the type 2 and 3 ASM transcripts resulted from the

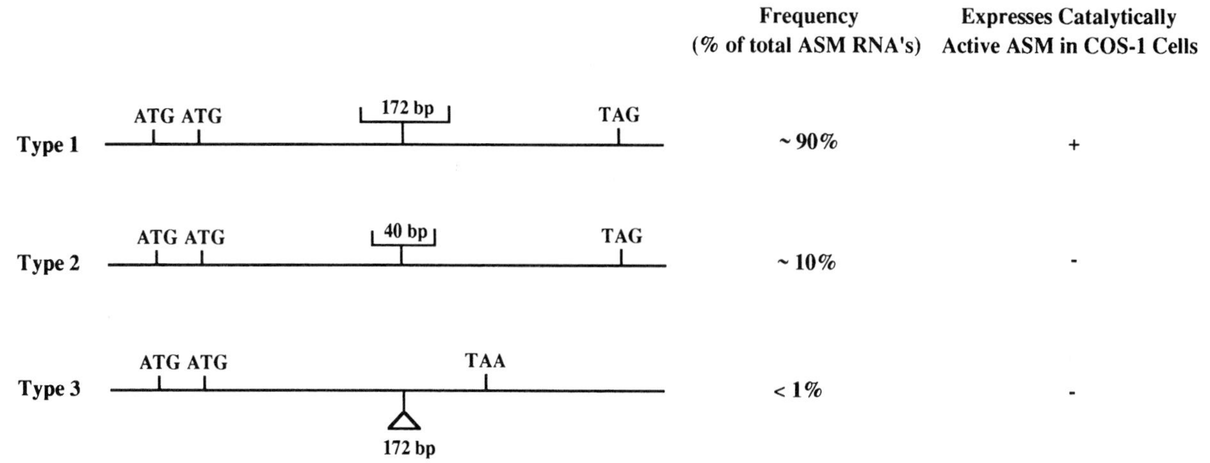

Fig. 144-9 Structure of the human ASM gene. The human ASM gene is divided into six exons (black boxes) and five introns (open boxes). The locations of the putative translation initiation and stop codons are indicated, as is the location of the Alu 1 repeat. The locations and transcriptional orientations of three other ORFs in the ASM genomic region also are shown.

fact that in about 10 percent of the hnRNAs, splicing proceeded either to the cryptic donor splice site or to the next donor site. A G-to-A transition of the nucleotide immediately adjacent to the invariant gt consensus dinucleotide in the normal donor splice site may cause these alternative splicing events, because this alteration is implicated as the cause of abnormal splicing in the proα1(I) collagen gene resulting in Ehlers-Danlos syndrome type VII.[198]

The ASM genomic region encoded three other long ORFs that predicted polypeptides of 101, 104, and 158 amino acid residues, respectively.[196] The transcriptional orientations of ORF 1 and ORF 2 were opposite those of ASM, and the predicted proteins shared no homology with ASM or any other proteins in the Swiss-Prot protein database. In contrast, ORF 3 was in the same transcriptional orientation and coding phase as the ASM gene. This ORF began within intron 2, overlapped ASM exon 3, and extended into intron 3. No known functions for these ORFs have been described.

Regional Mapping of the Human ASM Gene. Using molecular techniques, the locus for the human ASM gene was assigned to the chromosomal region 11p15.1 to p15.4 (Fig. 144-10).[199] Selective PCR amplification of a human exonic sequence and *in situ* hybridization of the radiolabeled cDNA provided independent data that assigned the gene locus (designated SMPD-1) to this narrow region on chromosome 11. Although a number of other sphingomyelinases and related phospholipases have been identified, these molecular studies identified only a single locus for human ASM, indicating the absence of homologous coding sequences and pseudogenes elsewhere in the genome. In addition, genomic Southern blotting experiments were consistent with a single ASM gene. Two other lysosomal genes have been assigned to 11p, cathepsin D to 11p15[200] and acid phosphatase 2 to 11p11.[201]

The results of these studies corrected a previous provisional assignment of the human ASM gene to chromosome 17.[202] The reason for this discrepancy is not known, although it is possible that the artificial substrate (i.e., 2-hexadecanoyl-amino-4-nitrophenol phosphorylcholine) used in the earlier study may not have been specific for ASM, particularly under the thermo-inactivation conditions used.

Polymorphisms Within the ASM Gene. Two common polymorphisms have been identified within the ASM gene leading to amino acid substitutions at codons 322 and 506. The common allele for each codon is Thr 322 (ACA) and Gly 506 (GGG).[193,203] The less common alleles are Ile 322 (ATA) and Arg 506 (AGG). Notably, the Gly 506 polymorphism created a new *MspI* restriction site, facilitating its identification by restriction enzyme analysis. In addition to these polymorphisms, the number of alanine/leucine repeats within the ASM signal peptide region are also polymorphic.[204] These common polymorphisms should be useful markers for the orientation of anonymous polymorphic sequences and/or sequence-tagged sites in the chromosomal region 11p15.

The Molecular Genetics of Murine ASM

The full-length human ASM cDNA was used to isolate the full-length cDNA encoding murine ASM.[205,206] The full-length murine ASM cDNA was 2320 bp and contained an 1884-bp ORF encoding 627 amino acids. Transient expression in COS-1 cells demonstrated the functional integrity of the murine cDNA. Overall, the nucleotide and amino acid identities between the human and murine ASM sequences were about 81 and 83 percent, respectively. Notably, five of six predicted *N*-glycosylation sites in human ASM were conserved in the mouse sequence. This was

Table 144-4 Intron-Exon Junctions in the Human ASM Gene

Exon Number	Exon Size (nt)	Codons	5′ Donor Spice Site	Intron Size (nt)	3′ Acceptor Spice Site
1	398	1–104	AG gtgagc(D1)	464	cag A (A1)
2	773	105–362	AG gtactt(D2)	1059	cag A (A2)
3	171	362–419	**AA** gtgagg(D3)	228	tag G (A3)
4	77	420–446	AG gtagga(D4)	201	cag G (A4)
5	145	446–494	TG gtgagt (D5)	153	cag G (A5)
6	778	495–630			

The underlined residues represent divergences from the 5′ donor or 3′ acceptor splice site consensus sequences; the bold AA indicates a divergence from the invariant AG dinucleotide in the 5′ donor splice site (D3) at the junction of intron 2 and exon 3.

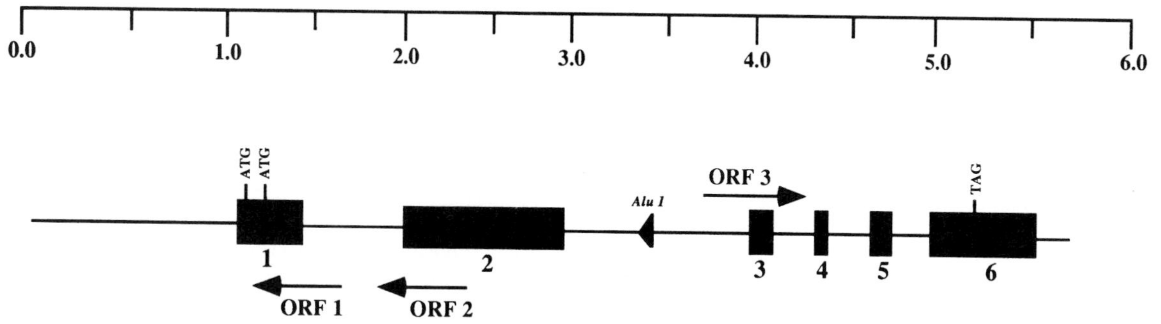

Fig. 144-10 Chromosomal localization of the human ASM gene to 11p15.1 to p15.4.

consistent with previous biochemical and molecular data, which indicated that only five of the *N*-glycosylation sites in the human polypeptide were used.[109,113]

The full-length murine ASM cDNA has been used to isolate the complete genomic region encoding murine ASM.[207] Similar to the human gene, the mouse ASM coding region was divided among six exons. The position and relative size of the ASM introns and exons were highly conserved between mice and humans, with the notable exception that intron 2 in the human gene was 1059 bp, whereas in the murine gene it was 510 bp. This was consistent with the insertion of an Alu 1 repetitive element in intron 2 of the human gene. As in the human gene, there was a poor donor splice site adjacent to exon 3 in the mouse gene. However, the cryptic donor splice site in intron 2 of the human gene was not conserved in the mouse sequence. Each of the other donor splice and acceptor sites in the murine ASM gene adhered to the consensus sequence.

To determine the chromosomal location of the murine ASM gene, a panel of nine mouse/hamster somatic-cell hybrids was analyzed using a PCR amplification detection assay.[206] Analysis of the somatic-cell hybrid panel revealed that the presence of the murine ASM gene was 100 percent concordant with the presence of mouse chromosome 7. This is consistent with the assignment of the human ASM gene to 11p15.1-p15.4, because the short arm of human chromosome 11 and mouse chromosome 7 are syntenic.

THE MOLECULAR GENETICS OF NPD

Eighteen mutations that cause types A or B NPD have been published to date. Of these, seven occurred in exon 2, three in exon 3, one each in exons 4 and 5, five in exon 6, and one in an intronic splice site (Fig. 144-11). There were 11 missense, 2 nonsense, and 3 frameshift mutations, 1 caused by an in-frame 3-base deletion that led to the removal of a single amino acid, while the other two were caused by single base alterations.

Mutations Causing Type A NPD

Ashkenazi Jewish Type A NPD Mutations. Three common mutations causing type A NPD have been identified in the Ashkenazi Jewish population[208–210] (Fig. 144-11). Two are the missense mutations R496L and L302P, and the third is a single base deletion that causes a frameshift and the introduction of a premature stop codon in the ASM coding sequence (fsP330). The R496L mutation occurred at a CpG dinucleotide, a known hotspot for mutations.[211] The R496L and L302P mutations were originally identified in unrelated Ashkenazi Jewish type A NPD patients who were homoallelic for each mutation; however, other Ashkenazi Jewish type A NPD patients have since been identified who were heteroallelic for these mutations. The fsP330 mutation has only been identified as one of the mutant ASM alleles in type A NPD patients. Fetuses homoallelic for this presumably null allele may die *in utero*. In fact, a fetus with NPD that expired *in utero* with nonimmune hydrops fetalis has been described,[212] although specific biochemical and molecular studies were not performed.

In an initial study of 27 unrelated Ashkenazi Jewish type A NPD patients (54 NPD alleles), the R496L, L302P, and fsP330 mutations were found to represent 36, 24, and 32 percent of the mutant alleles, respectively.[209,210] Thus, it was estimated that about 92 percent of the ASM alleles causing type A NPD in the

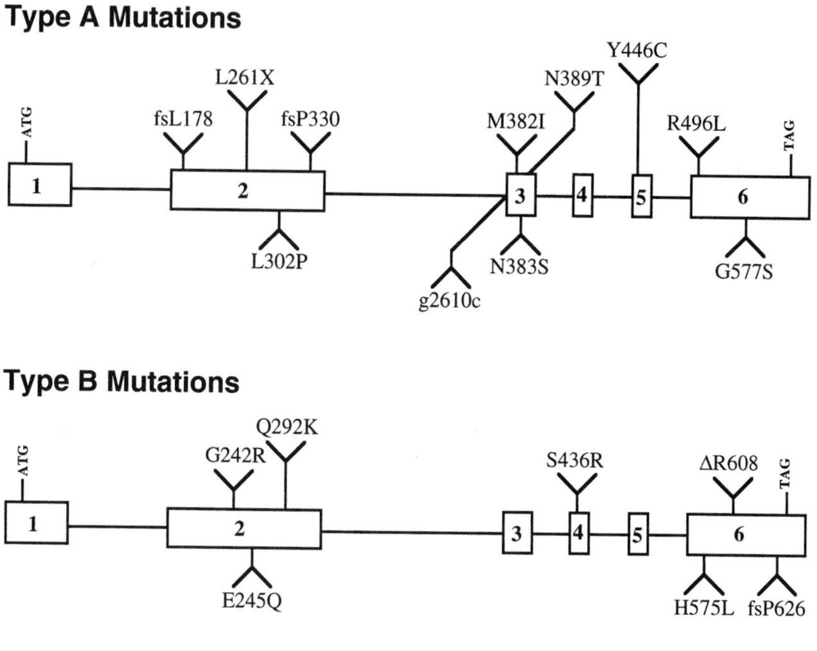

Fig. 144-11 Mutations causing types A and B NPD in the ASM gene. Mutations causing type B NPD are defined as those that express residual ASM activity and have been found as one allele in type B patients. Eleven missense, 2 nonsense, and 3 frameshift mutations are identified. In addition, there is one in-frame 3-base deletion (ΔR608) and one splice site alteration.

Ashkenazi Jewish population could be detected by testing for the presence of these three mutations. Subsequently, 1224 Ashkenazi Jewish individuals with no family history of NPD were screened for the three mutations and 14 carriers were identified (2pq = 1:80 based on 92 percent detection).[213] In contrast, the R496L mutation was found in only one of 20 non-Jewish type A NPD patients, and the L302P and fsP330 mutations have not been found in any of the 40 non-Jewish type A NPD alleles. PCR amplification and dot-blot hybridization conditions have been established and mismatched PCR primers have been constructed to detect the mutations by restriction enzyme analyses.[208–210,214]

Only one other mutation has so far been identified in the Ashkenazi Jewish type A NPD population; this mutation, designated N389T,[215] was identified as one of the mutant alleles in a single type A patient; the other allele was fsP330. Thus, N389T may be a rare cause of NPD among Ashkenazi Jewish individuals.

Non-Jewish Type A NPD Mutations. In contrast to the Ashkenazi Jewish type A NPD patients, each of the non-Jewish type A NPD patients studied has had unique, or "private," ASM mutations. To date, seven non-Jewish Type A NPD mutations have been published[216–219] (see Fig. 144-11). Of these, four are missense mutations (G242R, M382I, N383S, and G577S), one is a nonsense mutation (L261X), one is due to a single base deletion causing a frameshift mutation (fsL178), and one is due to a splice-site alteration (g2610c). It is intriguing that two of the point mutations causing type A NPD in non-Jewish individuals, M382I and M383S, occurred in adjacent codons within exon 3. As noted above, exon 3 is alternatively spliced in about 10 percent of the ASM transcripts, and transient expression studies in COS-1 cells have demonstrated that the excision of this exon leads to the loss of ASM catalytic activity. Thus, it is tempting to speculate that this region of the ASM polypeptide may encode all or part of the ASM catalytic site. Furthermore, the g2610c mutation occurred in the 3′ acceptor splice site adjacent to exon 3, consistent with this hypothesis.[219]

Mutations Causing Type B NPD

Ashkenazi Jewish Type B NPD Mutations. A mildly affected Ashkenazi Jewish type B NPD patient was identified who was heteroallelic for the type A R496L mutation and a three-base deletion that predicted the removal of an arginine residue from position 608 of the ASM polypeptide (designated ΔR608).[220] A second Ashkenazi Jewish type B patient was subsequently found to be heteroallelic for ΔR608 and a new mutation, designated H575L. Although it is intriguing that two unrelated Ashkenazi Jewish type B NPD patients carried the ΔR608 mutation, the frequency of type B NPD among Ashkenazi Jews is low, and the sample size is too small to estimate the frequency of the ΔR608 mutation in this population. No other mutations in Ashkenazi Jewish type B NPD patients have been reported to date.

Non-Jewish Type B NPD Mutations. In addition to the two unrelated patients noted above, the ΔR608 mutation is commonly found in North African type B NPD patients originating from the Maghreb region (i.e., Tunisia, Algeria, and Morocco).[191] Of 15 unrelated North African type B patients reported, 12 were homoallelic for the ΔR608 mutation and 2 were heteroallelic (i.e., 87 percent of mutant ASM alleles in this population were ΔR608). Four additional mutations causing type B NPD have been reported in non-Jewish patients.[191,216,217] Three were missense mutations (G242R, E245Q, and S436R), while the fourth was a frameshift mutation occurring at codon 626 (designated fsP626). The S436R mutation was identified as both alleles in a 19-year-old female type B patient from Japan who had moderate hepatosplenomegaly, mild pulmonary involvement, and no neuronopathic manifestations. The G242R mutation was identified as one allele in a 23-year-old American type B NPD patient of English, French, and German ancestries. The other mutant allele in this patient, N383S, did not express catalytically active ASM when transiently expressed (see below).

Expression of the ASM Mutations and Phenotype/Genotype Correlations

Eighteen mutations that cause types A and B NPD have been identified. Of these, published expression data are available for 11. As expected, the fsL178, L261X, and fsP330 mutations, each of which created premature stop codons in the ASM coding region, did not express catalytically active ASM in COS-1 cells. Thus, these mutations most likely result in truncated ASM polypeptides that are rapidly degraded. The R496L, L302P, M382I, N383S, and G577S mutations also did not express catalytically active enzyme in the transient expression system. These findings are consistent with the fact that individuals who were homoallelic for the R496L, L302P, and G577S mutations had the severe type A phenotype. In addition, a type A NPD patient has been identified who was heteroallelic for the fsL178 and M382I mutations.

In contrast, the G242R, S436R, and ΔR608 mutations expressed significant residual enzymatic activity in COS-1 cells. The ΔR608 mutation was originally identified in an Ashkenazi Jewish type B NPD patient whose other ASM allele was the type A R496L mutation.[220] Mild type B NPD patients who were homoallelic for the ΔR608 mutation also have been identified in France.[191] These observations suggest that one copy of the ΔR608 mutation is "neuroprotective," that is, it will prevent the occurrence of the neuronopathic type A phenotype. The S436R mutation was homoallelic in a mildly affected type B NPD patient from Japan who had residual activity,[47] and the G242R mutation was identified as one allele in a type B NPD patient of European ancestry. The other allele in this patient was N383S, which did not express catalytically active ASM.

These studies provide the initial basis for genotype/phenotype correlations in NPD. Within the Ashkenazi Jewish population, such genotype/phenotype correlations are useful in counseling families with newly diagnosed offspring and in decisions concerning prenatally diagnosed fetuses. In contrast, each ASM mutation in most non-Jewish families is likely to be "private" (other than ΔR608), precluding genotype/phenotype predictions unless clinical information is available from other family members or other affected individuals with the same genotype.

The Population Genetics of NPD

It is notable that two other sphingolipid storage diseases, Tay-Sachs disease and Gaucher disease, also occur more frequently among Ashkenazi Jewish individuals than in the general population (see Chaps. 146 and 153). During the past three decades, the mechanism(s) underlying the higher gene frequencies for these diseases in the Ashkenazi Jewish population has been the subject of much interest and debate. It has been suggested that higher gene frequencies for these diseases are due to a higher mutation rate, founder effect and genetic drift, and/or selection.[221–223] The molecular evidence demonstrating that two or more mutations occur in each disease argues that heterozygotes for these alleles may have had a selective advantage. Although a variety of hypotheses have been proposed to explain this selective advantage, a likely basis could be increased resistance to certain infections that were epidemic in European cities during the past two millenniums. Furthermore, the greater frequency of the three sphingolipid storage diseases among the Ashkenazim suggests a common mechanism for this selective advantage. It has been shown that certain membrane sphingolipids are involved in the recognition and binding of various bacteria and bacterial toxins, perhaps providing an explanation for the increased resistance to bacterial infections.[224] It is tempting to speculate that the slight accumulation of these membrane lipids in heterozygous individuals and the slightly higher levels of these lipids in the circulation could lead to an increased ability to bind, endocytose, and degrade these toxic agents, thereby providing a selective advantage for carriers of these mutant alleles. Although this hypothesis is intriguing, the true nature of the selective advantage for these mutations remains unknown and is an area for future investigation.

Along these lines, it was recently shown that ASM mediates entry of the bacterium *Neisseria gonorrhoeae* into epithelial cell lines and cultured skin fibroblasts.[225] Furthermore, ASM-deficient fibroblasts obtained from type A NPD patients did not internalize this bacterium, as opposed to normal fibroblasts, suggesting that NPD heterozygotes also may have some resistance to gonorrhea infection, and possibly conferring to them an increased resistance to this and perhaps other infections.

DIAGNOSIS OF TYPES A AND B NPD

Clinical Diagnosis

Patients with type A NPD present with hepatosplenomegaly, feeding problems, and failure to thrive in early infancy. The organomegaly is detectable in the first months of life. Neurologic involvement may be noted by 3 to 6 months of age. Developmental delay and/or loss of developmental milestones should signal the physician to consider NPD in the differential diagnosis. About 50 percent of the type A infants have cherry-red macular spots. In type B NPD patients, splenomegaly is usually the first manifestation detected. In most type B NPD patients, the splenic enlargement is noted in early childhood; however, in very mild cases, the enlargement may be subtle and detection may be delayed to adolescence or adulthood.

The presence of the characteristic NPD cells in the bone marrow aspirates supports the diagnosis of types A and B NPD. However, patients with types C and D NPD also have extensive infiltration of NPD cells in the bone marrow and, thus, all suspect cases should be evaluated enzymatically to confirm the clinical diagnosis.

Enzymatic Diagnosis

Types A and B NPD are readily diagnosed by the markedly deficient activity of ASM in peripheral leukocytes, cultured fibroblasts, and/or lymphoblasts. In contrast, patients with types C and D NPD have moderately decreased ASM activities (see Chap. 145), whereas patients with Gaucher disease and other storage disorders presenting with hepatosplenomegaly and/or neurologic involvement have normal or near normal levels of ASM activity. Numerous radioactive,[151,153,226–229] fluorescent[230,231] and colorimetric[226,230,232,233] substrates have been used to measure ASM activity. In general, the in vitro residual ASM activities in isolated peripheral leukocytes or in cultured fibroblasts and/or lymphoblasts from type A and B NPD patients range from less than 1 percent to a maximum of about 10 percent. Patients with type B NPD may have slightly higher levels of residual ASM activity than patients with type A disease, but this is not a reliable measure for predicting phenotypic severity. In addition to the in vitro assays, various cell-loading (i.e., *in situ*) assays have been developed to determine ASM activity.[234–240] In general, the levels of residual ASM activity determined with these *in situ* assays mimic those found with the in vitro systems.

Although the successful enzymatic identification of NPD carriers has been reported,[25] many investigators have found that heterozygote detection by in vitro or *in situ* determination of the ASM activity is problematic. The major difficulty is the significant overlap between the low-normal and high-heterozygote ranges in peripheral leukocytes and in cultured cells.

Molecular Diagnosis

The R496L, L302P, and fsP330 mutations account for about 92 percent of the mutant alleles in Ashkenazi Jewish type A NPD patients, facilitating the rapid identification of the molecular lesions in this population. PCR conditions have been developed to amplify the ASM genomic regions containing these mutations and allele-specific oligonucleotides and/or diagnostic restriction enzyme tests are available.[208–210,214] The ΔR608 mutation was identified in two of the four alleles analyzed from Ashkenazi Jewish type B NPD patients. However, because the sample size is small, the true frequency of this mutation remains unknown and additional Ashkenazi Jewish type B NPD patients must be tested. In contrast, the non-Jewish type A and B NPD patients have each had unique mutations, with the exception of ΔR608.[191]

In families in which the specific molecular lesion has been identified, family members can be accurately tested for heterozygote status by DNA analysis. Because the detectability of the type A mutations is over 90 percent among the Ashkenazi Jewish patients, molecular carrier screening can be undertaken in this population.

Prenatal Diagnosis

Prenatal diagnosis of NPD may be made reliably by measurement of ASM activities in cultured amniocytes or chorionic villi.[157,187,241,242] Although measurement of sphingomyelin turnover by cultured amniocytes has been used to diagnose type A NPD,[151,156] measurement of ASM residual activity is a more direct and reliable test. In families in which the specific ASM mutation is identified, molecular analysis of the fetal cells can provide the specific diagnosis or serve as a confirmatory test. Analyses of tissues from affected fetuses terminated in the second trimester have shown five- to tenfold increases in the level of sphingomyelin in liver and spleen.[190,243] Elevations of bis(monoacylglycero)phosphate also have been noted in the tissues of affected fetuses.

TREATMENT OF TYPES A AND B NPD

Current Status

At present, there is no specific treatment available for NPD. Orthotopic liver transplantation in an infant with type A disease[244,245] and amniotic cell transplantation[246] in several type B NPD patients have been attempted with little or no success. BMT also has been accomplished in type A NPD patients with no evidence of neurologic improvement.[247] However, BMT in one type B NPD patient was successful in reducing the spleen and liver volumes, the sphingomyelin content in the liver, the number of NPD cells in the marrow, and the radiologic infiltration of the lungs.[248]

Recently, BMT studies also were carried out in the NPD mouse model (i.e., ASMKO mice; see "Animal Models" below). An almost complete correction of the histologic and biochemical phenotype was achieved in the reticuloendothelial system organs of these animals, providing further evidence that BMT and hematopoietic stem cell-mediated gene therapy should be considered as therapeutic options for type B NPD patients. In addition, the onset of ataxia was delayed by several months in the transplanted mice, leading to an almost twofold increase in their life expectancy. This clinical result could be correlated with the recovery of the Purkinje cell layer in the transplanted animals. However, despite these positive neurologic results, the treated mice still developed ataxia (albeit at a later time point) and died prematurely.

These studies suggest that BMT may have a significant, positive effect on the clinical course of severely affected type B NPD patients if performed early in life. However, as is the case for many other genetic disorders, BMT is not a viable option for many type B NPD patients due to the lack of histocompatibly matched normal or heterozygous donors. Thus, alternative therapeutic approaches must be investigated.

Future Prospects

Enzyme Replacement Therapy. Lysosomal disorders have been important models for the development of novel therapeutic strategies since the seminal discoveries by Neufeld and others in the early 1970s that low levels of the appropriate normal enzymes could correct the metabolic defects in cultured fibroblasts from patients with storage diseases.[249,250] Among these, enzyme replacement therapy has been actively pursued for more than two decades. Until recently, this therapeutic approach was severely handicapped by the inability to produce and purify large quantities of the normal human enzymes. This limitation has been overcome by the use of mammalian expression systems to produce large amounts of recombinant proteins, and the first long-term clinical evaluations of enzyme replacement have been successfully undertaken in patients with type 1 (nonneuronopathic) Gaucher disease (see Chap. 146). Clinical trials are also underway for several other disorders. The success of enzyme therapy in Gaucher disease was due, in part, to the modification of the enzyme's oligosaccharide chains (i.e., mannose-terminated β-glucosidase) for targeting to macrophages. Because type 1 Gaucher disease and type B NPD both result from primary involvement of the monocyte-macrophage system, it is possible that infusion of a macrophage-targeted ASM glycoprotein also will be therapeutic.

Thus, type B NPD should be considered an excellent candidate for enzyme replacement therapy. The isolation of the human ASM cDNA[193] has provided the ability to stably express high levels of recombinant human ASM in mammalian expression systems (see "Overexpression of Human ASM in Chinese Hamster Ovary Cells," above), as has been accomplished for other recombinant human lysosomal enzymes.[251] The clinical efficacy of recombinant human ASM can be evaluated in the NPD mouse model. If such preclinical trials are successful, future clinical evaluation of enzyme replacement can be undertaken in type B NPD patients. For type A NPD, enzyme replacement is unlikely to be successful because the injected enzyme is not expected to cross the blood-brain barrier.

Somatic Cell Gene Therapy. The application of somatic cell gene-transfer techniques to treat selected inherited metabolic diseases, including selected lysosomal storage diseases, is currently an area of intense investigation.[252–254] To evaluate the potential of gene therapy for NPD, retroviral-mediated gene transfer was used to introduce the full-length ASM cDNA into cultured fibroblasts from unrelated type A NPD patients.[255] The ASM activities in the nontransduced cells were less than 4 percent of the mean normal levels and, consequently, these cell lines had about threefold elevated levels of sphingomyelin. Three different retroviral vectors have been evaluated: pBC140, DCTK, and MFG. pBC140 and DCTK contain the neomycin resistance gene expressed from the viral long-terminal repeat (LTR), and use heterologous promoters to express the ASM cDNA. In contrast, MFG has no selectable marker and expresses the ASM cDNA from the viral LTR. Following retroviral-mediated transduction of type A NPD fibroblasts, the ASM activities were increased up to 23 times the endogenous activity in normal fibroblasts (Table 144-5). The MFG vector consistently expressed higher levels of ASM activities than the pBC140 or DCTK vectors.

Table 144-5 In Vitro ASM Activities in Retrovirally-Transduced NPD Fibroblasts

Cell Line	Vectors	ASM Activity (nmol/h/mg protein)		Independent Infections
		Mean	Range	
Normal (n = 7)	None	76	74–106	
Type A NPD:				
Proband 1	None	0.4		
	pBC140	680	322–1221	6
	DCTK	99	76–144	4
	MFG	1097	614–1981	6
Proband 2	None	2.9		
	pBC140	703	405–889	3
	DCTK	82	66–97	3
	MFG	914	683–1095	5

Table 144-6 *In Situ* ASM Activities in Retrovirally-Transduced NPD Fibroblasts

Cell Line	Vectors	% P10-Sphingomyelin Converted to Ceramide
Normal	None	75.4 +/− 3.2
Type A NPD	None	5.9 +/− 1.4
	pBC-140	83.0 +/− 2.8
	MFG	79.5 +/− 2.1
	(Antisense)	7.5 +/− 2.8

In NPD cells transduced with either vector, the sphingomyelin content was reduced to normal levels, indicating that the vector-encoded enzyme was properly targeted to lysosomes, where it was enzymatically active and able to degrade the accumulated substrate. *In situ* cell-loading studies were also performed to evaluate the effects of retroviral-mediated gene transfer on the chemical pathology of NPD fibroblasts. When a pyrene derivative of sphingomyelin was introduced into the lysosomes of cultured fibroblasts from a type A NPD patient using Apo E-mediated endocytosis, only about 6 percent of the delivered substrate was degraded[255] (Table 144-6). In contrast, normal cells and NPD cells transduced by retroviral-mediated gene transfer were able to degrade about 80 percent of the endocytosed sphingomyelin. These results provided further evidence that retroviral-mediated gene transfer may be used to correct the metabolic defect in type A NPD cells.

Cell-loading studies also were used to develop a selection system for discrimination of untransduced and retrovirally-transduced NPD cells.[256] This selection scheme was based on the fluorescence emission of intact NPD cells, which, when loaded with pyrene- or lissamine rhodamine-labeled sphingomyelin, exceeded by three to five times those of normal or transduced cells. As a consequence, transduced cells could be efficiently sorted from nonexpressing cells by flow cytometry using a fluorescence-activated cell sorter (FACS).[255,257,258]

This selection system was originally developed using cultured skin fibroblasts from NPD patients; however, it was recently adapted to hematopoietic stem cells using a different fluorescent compound, Bodipy sphingomyelin.[259] Using bone marrow cells obtained from the NPD mouse model as an experimental system, this selection system is used to isolate a population of transduced NPD cells that are highly enriched for hematopoietic stem cells.[259] CFU-S assays carried out on the FACS-sorted cells (Table 144-7) indicate that the number of vector-positive day 14 spleen colonies is ~80 percent in animals transplanted with the sorted cells, as compared to ~30 percent in nonsorted cells. Such FACS-selected, transduced stem cells have been transplanted into NPD mice for long-term evaluation of this gene therapy procedure.

Based on these results and the encouraging BMT results obtained in the NPD mice (see above), hematopoietic stem cell-mediated gene therapy may be an effective treatment for type B NPD. The availability of a method for the selection of gene-corrected NPD stem cells also may be particularly advantageous for this disorder. Furthermore, it is now known that ASM is secreted at high levels by many cell types and is stable under

Table 144-7 PCR Analysis of CFU-S Colonies Obtained from Mice Transplanted with Retrovirally-Transduced FACS-Selected Bone Marrow

Cell Type Injected	Total Colonies Analyzed	PCR Positive Colonies
Bodipy-Selected	37	28 (76%)
Non-Selected	28	9 (32%)

physiologic conditions for long periods of time (see "Acid Sphingomyelinase," above). The secreted enzyme can be taken up readily by cells and is transported to lysosomes, facilitating in vivo cross-correction. However, many technical obstacles remain to be overcome before hematopoietic stem cell-mediated gene therapy can be accomplished successfully in human patients. This approach remains experimental and is not likely to be available to NPD families until its efficacy is proven further.

With regard to type A NPD, the results of BMT in the NPD "knock-out" mice suggest that very limited improvements in the central nervous system involvement can be achieved by hematopoietic stem-cell gene therapy. Thus, new methods, such as the use of neurotropic expression vectors or direct injection of neuronal-targeted DNA complexes, must be developed. Moreover, due to the rapid progression of the neurologic disease in type A NPD, these procedures must be accomplished in early infancy or during fetal development. Clearly, these latter studies will require extensive animal studies prior to the initiation of human clinical trials and the murine model of NPD should be particularly valuable.

ANIMAL MODELS

In the early 1980s, two naturally occurring murine models of NPD were described. In 1980, Pentchev et al.[260] described a strain of BALB/C mice with many of the characteristic NPD features, including reduced ASM activity, elevated levels of sphingomyelin and cholesterol, and clinical features such as loss of coordination, weight loss, and premature death. Shortly thereafter, Miyawaki et al.[261] described an independent strain of C57BL/6Js mice (spm/spm) with similar biochemical and clinical findings. Because reduced ASM activity leading to the accumulation of sphingomyelin and cholesterol was characteristic of NPD in humans, both strains of mice were originally described as models for the human disorder. However, it was not clear whether these mice were models for the ASM-deficient NPD subtypes (types A and B) or the cholesterol transport subtypes (types C and D). In 1984, Pentchev and colleagues[262] described the fact that the BALB/C NPD mice had an underlying defect in cholesterol transport that most resembled type C NPD in humans (see Chap. 145). Similar studies were performed on the spm/spm mice.[263] The complete ASM gene was subsequently sequenced from both strains of NPD mice, and no molecular abnormalities were identified.[206] Thus, these naturally occurring mice are models for the cholesterol transport forms of NPD, not types A or B NPD.

In 1995, two mouse models of types A and B NPD were independently constructed by gene-targeting strategies.[264,265] Although the precise targeting events differed in the two animals, the phenotypes were essentially identical. The NPD "knock-out" mice (also referred to as ASMKO mice) appeared normal at birth and developed normally until about 3 months of age, at which time mild ataxia became apparent. The ataxia progressed rapidly, leading to a severe gait abnormality by 5 months of age. Affected animals died between the sixth and eighth months of life.

Histologic analysis of the ASMKO mice revealed that the infiltration of NPD cells throughout the RES is evident by 3 months of age, and progresses rapidly until the time of death. In the central nervous system, there is an almost complete absence of Purkinje cells in the affected animals, as well as evidence of lipid-storage vacuoles in neurons. Biochemical analysis revealed that the sphingomyelin levels were elevated in various tissues from five- to fortyfold above those found in normal, age-matched littermates.

Thus, the NPD "knock-out" mice develop features of both types A and B NPD, and are an excellent model with which to evaluate various therapeutic strategies (see "Treatment of Types A and B NPD" above).

It should be noted that canine[266] and feline[267] models of NPD also have been described. However, breeding colonies were never fully established and these models were not characterized beyond their initial descriptions. It is likely that these models represent defects in cholesterol transport rather than primary ASM deficiencies.

ACKNOWLEDGMENTS

The authors acknowledge the contributions of the many individuals in our laboratories who participated in this research. In addition, we recognize the important contributions of Dr. Konrad Sandhoff's laboratory (Bonn, Germany), which collaborated on the studies of the ASM cDNA; Dr. Ira Tabas's laboratory (Columbia University, New York), which collaborated on the biology of the Zn^{2+}-activated ASM; and Dr. Richard Kolesnick's laboratory (Memorial Sloan-Kettering Cancer Center, New York), which collaborated on the role of ASM in ceramide-mediated signal transduction. These studies were supported by a research grant from the National Institutes of Health (1 R01 HD28607), the March of Dimes Birth Defects Foundation (1-1224), a grant (1 P30 HD28822) for the Mount Sinai Child Health Research Center from the National Institutes of Health, and a grant (5 M01 RR00071) for the Mount Sinai General Clinical Research Center from the National Center for Research Resources, National Institutes of Health.

REFERENCES

1. Niemann A: Ein unbekanntes Krankheitsbild. *Jahrb Kinderheilkd* **79**:1, 1914.
2. Gaucher P: De l'epithelioma primitif de la rate, hypertrophie idopathique de la rate sans leucemie. Paris, 1882.
3. Siegmund H: Lipoidzellenhyperplasie der milz und splenomegalie Gaucher. *Verh Dtsch Pathol Ges* **18**:59, 1921.
4. Knox J, Wahl W, Schmeisser A: Gaucher's disease in infants. *Bull Johns Hopkins Hosp* **27**:1, 1916.
5. Kraus E: Zur kennitnis der splenomegalie Gaucher, insbesondere der histogenese der grobzellen wucherung. *Z Angew Anat* **7**:186, 1920.
6. Pick L: Uber die lipoidzellige splenohepatomegalie typus Niemann-Pick als stoffwechselerkrankung. *Med Klin* **23**:1483, 1927.
7. Pick L: Niemann-Pick's disease and other forms of so-called xanthomases. *Am J Med Sci* **185**:601, 1933.
8. Pflander U: La maladie de Niemann-Pick dans le cadre des lipoidoses. *Schweiz Med Wochenschr* **76**, 1946.
9. Dusendschon A: Deux cas familiaux de maladie de Niemann-Pick chez adulte. Geneva, Faculte de Medicine, 1946.
10. Wahl H, Richardson M: A study of lipid content of a case of Gaucher's disease in an infant. *Arch Intern Med* **17**:238, 1916.
11. Bloom W: Splenomegaly (type Gaucher) and lipoid-histiocytosis (type Niemann). *Am J Pathol* **1**:595, 1925.
12. Bloom W: The histogenesis of essential lipoid histiocytosis (Niemann Pick disease). *Arch Pathol* **6**:827, 1928.
13. Sobotka H, Epstein E, Lichtenstein L: The distribution of lipoid in a case of Niemann-Pick's disease associated with amaurotic family idiocy. *Arch Pathol* **10**:677, 1930.
14. Sobtaka H, Gilick D, Reiner M, Tuchman L: The lipoids of spleen and liver in various types of lipidoses. *Biochemistry* **27**:2031, 1933.
15. Klenk E: Uber die natur der phosphatide der milz bei Niemann-Pickchen Krankheit. *Z Physiol Chem* **229**:151, 1934.
16. Kanfer JN, Young OM, Shapiro D, Brady RO: The metabolism of sphingomyelin. I. Purification and properties of a sphingomyelin-cleaving enzyme from rat liver tissue. *J Biol Chem* **241**:1081, 1966.
17. Brady RO, Kanfer JN, Mock MB, Fredrickson DS: The metabolism of sphingomyelin. II. Evidence of an enzymatic deficiency in Niemann-Pick disease. *Proc Natl Acad Sci U S A* **55**:366, 1966.
18. Schneider PB, Kennedy EP: Sphingomyelinase in normal human spleens and in spleens from subjects with Niemann-Pick disease. *J Lipid Res* **8**:202, 1967.
19. Baumann T, Klenk E, Scheidegger S: Die Niemann-Picksche Krankheit: eine klinische, chemische und histopathologische Studie. *Ergeb Allg Pathol U Pathol Anat* **30**:183, 1936.
20. Schettler G: . *Lipidosen Sphingomyelinoses.* Berlin, Springer, 1955.
21. Crocker A, Farber S: Niemann-Pick disease: A review of eighteen patients. *Medicine (Baltimore)* **37**:1, 1958.
22. Fredrickson D: *Sphingomyelin Lipidosis: Niemann-Pick Disease* 2nd ed. New York, McGraw-Hill, 1966.

23. Schettler G, Kahlke W: *Niemann-Pick Disease*. New York, Springer-Verlag, 1967.
24. Fredrickson D, Sloan H: *Sphingomyelin Lipidoses: Niemann-Pick Disease* 3rd ed. New York, McGraw-Hill, 1972.
25. Spence M, Callahan J: *Sphingomyelin-Cholesterol Lipidoses: The Niemann-Pick Group of Diseases*, vol. 2, 6th ed. New York, McGraw-Hill, 1989.
26. Crocker AC: The cerebral defect in Tay-Sachs disease and Niemann-Pick disease. *J Neurochem* **7**:69, 1961.
27. Pentchev PG, Comly ME, Kruth HS, Vanier MT, Wenger DA, Patel S, Brady RO: A defect in cholesterol esterification in Niemann-Pick disease (type C) patients. *Proc Natl Acad Sci U S A* **82**:8247, 1985.
28. Vanier MT, Pentchev P, Rodriguez-Lafrasse C, Rousson R: Niemann-Pick disease type C: An update. *J Inherit Metab Dis* **14**:580, 1991.
29. Carstea ED, Morris JA, Coleman KG, Loftus SK, Zhang D, Cummings C, Gu J, et al.: Niemann-Pick C1 disease gene: Homology to mediators of cholesterol homeostasis. *Science* **277**:228, 1997.
30. Butler JD, Comly ME, Kruth HS, Vanier M, Filling-Katz M, Fink J, Barton N, et al.: Niemann-Pick variant disorders: Comparison of errors of cellular cholesterol homeostasis in group D and group C fibroblasts. *Proc Natl Acad Sci U S A* **84**:556, 1987.
31. Byers DM, Rastogi SR, Cook HW, Palmer FB, Spence MW: Defective activity of acyl-CoA:cholesterol O-acyltransferase in Niemann-Pick type C and type D fibroblasts. *Biochem J* **262**:713, 1989.
32. Greer WL, Riddell DC, Gillan TL, Girouard GS, Sparrow SM, Byers DM, Dobson MJ, Neumann PE: The Nova Scotia (type D) form of Niemann-Pick disease is caused by a G3097 to T transversion in NPC1. *Am J Hum Genet* **63**:52, 1998.
33. Schneider EL, Pentchev PG, Hibbert SR, Sawitsky A, Brady RO: A new form of Niemann-Pick disease characterized by temperature-labile sphingomyelinase. *J Med Genet* **15**:370, 1978.
34. Elleder M, Jirasek A: International symposium on Niemann-Pick disease. *Eur J Pediatr* **140**:90, 1983.
35. Grunebaum M: The roentgenographic findings in the acute neuronopathic form of Niemann-Pick disease. *Br J Radiol* **49**:1018, 1976.
36. Cogan DG, Kuwabara T: The sphingolipidoses and the eye. *Arch Ophthalmol* **79**:437, 1968.
37. Cogan DG, Chu FC, Barranger JA, Gregg RE: Macula halo syndrome. Variant of Niemann-Pick disease. *Arch Ophthalmol* **101**:1698, 1983.
38. Lipson MH, O'Donnell J, Callahan JW, Wenger DA, Packman S: Ocular involvement in Niemann-Pick disease type B. *J Pediatr* **108**:582, 1986.
39. Matthews JD, Weiter JJ, Kolodny EH: Macular halos associated with Niemann-Pick type B disease. *Ophthalmology* **93**:933, 1986.
40. Maurer L: Niemann-Pick's disease, a report of four cases. *Rocky Mtn Med J* **38**:460, 1941.
41. Chan WC, Lai KS, Todd D: Adult Niemann-Pick disease—a case report. *J Pathol* **121**:177, 1977.
42. Dawson PJ, Dawson G: Adult Niemann-Pick disease with sea-blue histiocytes in the spleen. *Hum Pathol* **13**:1115, 1982.
43. Lever AM, Ryder JB: Cor pulmonale in an adult secondary to Niemann-Pick disease. *Thorax* **38**:873, 1983.
44. Tassoni JP Jr, Fawaz KA, Johnston DE: Cirrhosis and portal hypertension in a patient with adult Niemann-Pick disease. *Gastroenterology* **100**:567, 1991.
45. Hammersen G, Oppermann HC, Harms E, Blassmann K, Harzer K: Oculo-neural involvement in an enzymatically proven case of Niemann-Pick disease type B. *Eur J Pediatr* **132**:77, 1979.
46. Sogawa H, Horino K, Nakamura F, Kudoh T, Oyanagi K, Yamanouchi T, Minami R, Nakao T, Watanabe A, Matsuura Y: Chronic Niemann-Pick disease with sphingomyelinase deficiency in two brothers with mental retardation. *Eur J Pediatr* **128**:235, 1978.
47. Takada G, Satoh W, Komatsu K, Konn Y, Miura Y, Uesaka Y: Transitory type of sphingomyelinase deficient Niemann-Pick disease: clinical and morphological studies and follow-up of two sisters. *Tohoku J Exp Med* **153**:27, 1987.
48. Elleder M, Cihula J: Niemann-Pick disease (variation in the sphingomyelinase deficient group). Neurovisceral phenotype (A) with an abnormally protracted clinical course and variable expression of neurological symptomatology in three siblings. *Eur J Pediatr* **140**:323, 1983.
49. Ludatscher RM, Naveh Y, Auslaender L, Gellei B: Electron microscopic studies in lipid storage disease. *Isr J Med Sci* **17**:323, 1981.
50. Pearse A: *Histochemistry—Theoretical and Applied*. Boston, Little, Brown, 1960.
51. Brady R: *Sphingomyelin Lipidosis: Niemann-Pick Disease* 5th ed. New York, McGraw-Hill, 1983.
52. Golde DW, Schneider EL, Bainton DF, Pentchev PG, Brady RO, Epstein CJ, Cline MJ: Pathogenesis of one variant of sea-blue histiocytosis. *Lab Invest* **33**:371, 1975.
53. Brady R, King F: *Niemann-Pick's Disease*. New York, Academic, 1973.
54. Varela-Duran J, Roholt P, Ratliff NJ: Sea-blue histiocyte syndrome: A secondary degenerative process of macrophages? *Arch Pathol Lab Med* **104**:30, 1980.
55. Levade T, Salvayre R, Bes JC, Maret A, Douste-Blazy L: Biochemical and ultrastructural findings in a lymphoid cell line from Niemann-Pick disease type A. *Biol Cell* **55**:143, 1985.
56. Elleder M, Hrodek J, Cihula J: Niemann-Pick disease: Lipid storage in bone marrow macrophages. *Histochem J* **15**:1065, 1983.
57. Bes JC, Salvayre R, Levade T, Caratero C, Planel H: Ultrastructural investigations on two lymphoid cell lines from Niemann-Pick disease type B. *Biol Cell* **50**:299, 1984.
58. Long RG, Lake BD, Pettit JE, Scheuer PJ, Sherlock S: Adult Niemann-Pick disease: Its relationship to the syndrome of the sea-blue histiocyte. *Am J Med* **62**:627, 1977.
59. Landas S, Foucar K, Sando GN, Ellefson R, Hamilton HE: Adult Niemann-Pick disease masquerading as sea blue histiocyte syndrome: Report of a case confirmed by lipid analysis and enzyme assays. *Am J Hematol* **20**:391, 1985.
60. Dewhurst N, Besley GT, Finlayson ND, Parker AC: Sea-blue histiocytosis in a patient with chronic non-neuropathic Niemann-Pick disease. *J Clin Pathol* **32**:1121, 1979.
61. Hassin G: Niemann's Pick disease. *Arch Neurol Psychiatry* **24**:697, 1930.
62. Landrieu P, Said G: Peripheral neuropathy in type A Niemann-Pick disease. A morphological study. *Acta Neuropathol* **63**:66, 1984.
63. Pick L: Der Morbus Gaucher und die ihm ahnlichen Erkrankungen. *Ergeb Med Kinderheilkd* **29**:519, 1926.
64. Ivenmark B, Svennerholm L, Thoren C, Tunell R: Niemann-Pick disease in infancy: Report of two siblings with clinical, histologic and chemical studies. *Acta Paediatr* **52**:391, 1963.
65. Diezel P: Histochemical study of primary lipidoses. Oxford, Blackwell, 1957.
66. Robb RM, Kuwabara T: The ocular pathology of type A Niemann-Pick disease. A light and electron microscopic study. *Invest Ophthalmol* **12**:366, 1973.
67. Libert J, Toussaint D, Guiselings R: Ocular findings in Niemann-Pick disease. *Am J Ophthalmol* **80**:991, 1975.
68. Walton DS, Robb RM, Crocker AC: Ocular manifestations of group A Niemann-Pick disease. *Am Ophthalmol* **85**:174, 1978.
69. Howes EL Jr, Wood IS, Golbus M, Hogan ML: Ocular pathology of infantile Niemann-Pick disease. Study of fetus of 23 weeks' gestation. *Arch Ophthalmol* **93**:494, 1975.
70. Elleder M, Smid F: Adrenal changes in Niemann-Pick disease: Differences between sphingomyelinase deficiency and type C. *Acta Histochem* **76**:163, 1985.
71. Knox R, Ramsey G: Niemann-Pick's disease (essential lipoid histiocytosis). *Ann Intern Med* **6**:218, 1932.
72. Klenk E: Uber die sphingomyeline des herzmuskels. *Hoppe Seylers Z Physiol Chem* **221**:67, 1933.
73. Rouser G, Berry JF, Marinetti G, Stotz E: Studies of the structure of sphingomyelin. I. Oxidation of products of partial hydrolysis. *J Am Chem Soc* **75**:310, 1953.
74. Marinetti G, Berry JF, Rouser G, Stotz E: Studies on the structure of sphingomyelin. II. Performic and periodic acid oxidation studies. *J Am Chem Soc* **75**:313, 1953.
75. Thudichum J: A treatise on the chemical constitution of brain. Berlin, Springer, 1930.
76. Rosenheim O, Tebb M: The lipoids of the brain. Part II. A new method for the preparation of the galactosides and of sphingomyelin. *J Physiol* **41**:Proc:i, 1910.
77. Levene P: On sphingomyelin II. *J Biol Chem* **18**:453, 1914.
78. Klenk E, Rennkamp F: Uber die reindarstellung von sphingomyelin aus gehirn. *Hoppe Seyler Z Physiol Chem* **267**:145, 1941.
79. Thannhauser S, Benotti J, Boncoddo N: The preparation of pure sphingomyelin from beef lung and the identification of its component fatty acids. *J Biol Chem* **166**:677, 1946.
80. Kawamura R: *Die Cholesterinesterverfettung*. Jena, Germany, Fischer, 1911.
81. Levene P: Sphingomyelin III. *J Biol Chem* **24**:69, 1916.

82. Chain E, Kemp I: The isoelectric points of lecithin and sphingomyelin. *Biochem J* **28**:2052, 1935.
83. Deuel H: *Lipids*. New York, 1951.
84. Merz W: Untersuchungen uber das sphingomyelin. *Hoppe Seyler Z Physiol Chem* **193**:59, 1930.
85. Thannhauser S, Boncoddo N: The chemical nature of the fatty acids of brain and spleen sphingomyelin. The occurrence of saturated and unsaturated sphingosines in the sphingomyelin molecule. *J Biol Chem* **172**:141, 1948.
86. Frankel E, Bielschowsky F, Thannhauser S: Untersuchungen uber die lipoide der sangetierleber. III. Uber ein polydiaminophosphatid der Schweineleber. *Hoppe Seyler Z Physiol Chem* **218**:1, 1933.
87. Sribney M, Kennedy E: The enzymatic synthesis of sphingomyelin. *J Biol Chem* **233**:1315, 1958.
88. Brady RO, Koval GJ: The enzymatic synthesis of sphingosine. **233**:26, 1958.
89. Stoffel W, Kruger E, Melzner I: Studies on the biosynthesis of ceramide: does the reversed ceramidase reaction yield ceramides? *Hoppe-Seyler's Z Physiol Chem* **361**:773, 1980.
90. Fujino Y, Negishi T: Investigation of the enzymatic synthesis of sphingomyelin. *Biochim Biophys Acta* **152**:428, 1976.
91. Diringer H, Koch M: Biosynthesis of sphingomyelin: Transfer of phosphorylcholine from phosphatidylcholine to erythro-ceramide in a cell-free system. *Hoppe Seyler Z Physiol Chem* **354**:1661, 1973.
92. Marggraf W, Zertani R, Anderer F, Kanfer J: The role of endogenous phosphatidylcholine and ceramide in the biosynthesis of sphingomyelin in mouse fibroblasts. *Biochim Biophys Acta* **710**:314, 1982.
93. Ullman M, Radin N: The enzymatic formation of sphingomyelin from ceramide and lecithin in mouse liver. *J Biol Chem* **249**:1056, 1974.
94. Voelker D, Kennedy E: Cellular and enzymic synthesis of sphingomyelin. *Biochemistry* **21**:2753, 1982.
95. Merrill AH, Jr., Jones DD: An update of the enzymology and regulation of sphingomyelin metabolism. *Biochim Biophys Acta* **1044**:1, 1990.
96. Berka R, Vasil M: Phospholipase C (heat labile hemolysin) of *Pseudomonas aeruginosa*: Purification and preliminary characterization. *J Bacteriol* **152**:239, 1982.
97. Wadstrom T, Mollby R: Studies on extracellular proteins from *Staphylococcus aureus*: VII Studies on β-haemolysin. *Biochim Biophys Acta* **242**:308, 1971.
98. Yamada A, Tsukagoshi N, Udaka S, Sasaki T, Makino S, Nakamura S, Little C, Tomita M, Ikezawa H: Nucleotide sequence and expression in *Escherichia coli* of the gene coding for sphingomyelinase of *Bacillus cereus*. *Eur J Biochem* **175**:213, 1988.
99. Johansen T, Haugli FB, Ikezawa H, Little C: *Bacillus cereus* strain SE-1: Nucleotide sequence of the sphingomyelinase C gene. *Nucleic Acids Res* **16**:10370, 1988.
100. Lin X, Hengartner MO, Kolesnick R: *Caenorhabditis elegans* contains two distinct acid sphingomyelinases. *J Biol Chem* **273**:14374, 1998.
101. Thannhauser S, Reichel M: Studies of animal lipids. XVI. The occurrence of sphingomyelin as a mixture of sphingomyelin fatty acid ester and free sphingomyelin, demonstrated by enzymatic hydrolysis and mild saponification. *J Biol Chem* **135**:1, 1940.
102. Heller M, Shapiro B: The hydrolysis of sphingomyelin by rat liver. *Isr J Chem* **1**:204, 1963.
103. Druzhinina K, Kritzman M: Lecithinase C from animal tissue. *Biokhimiya* **17**:77, 1956.
104. Roitman A, Gatt S: Isolation of phospholipase C from rat brain. *Isr J Chem* **1**:190, 1963.
105. Callahan JW, Khalil M: Sphingomyelinases in human tissues. III. Expression of Niemann-Pick disease in cultured skin fibroblasts. *Pediatr Res* **9**:914, 1975.
106. Yamanaka T, Suzuki K: Acid sphingomyelinase of human brain: purification to homogeneity. *J Neurochem* **38**:1753, 1982.
107. Callahan JW, Jones CS, Davidson DJ, Shankaran P: The active site of lysosomal sphingomyelinase: evidence for the involvement of hydrophobic and ionic groups. *J Neurosci Res* **10**:151, 1983.
108. Quintern L, Weitz G, Nehrkorn H, Tager J, Schram A, Sandhoff K: Acid sphingomyelinase from human urine. Purification and characterization. *Biochim Biophys Acta* **922**:323, 1987.
109. Quintern LE, Zenk TS, Sandhoff K: The urine from patients with peritonitis as a rich source for purifying human acid sphingomyelinase and other lysosomal enzymes. *Biochim Biophys Acta* **1003**:121, 1989.
110. Rousson R, Vanier MT, Louisot P: Chromatofocusing of purified placental sphingomyelinase. *Biochimie* **65**:115, 1983.
111. Weitz G, Driessen M, Brouwer-Kelder EM, Sandhoff K, Barranger JA, Tager JM, Schram AW: Soluble sphingomyelinase from human urine as antigen for obtaining anti-sphingomyelinase antibodies. *Biochim Biophys Acta* **838**:92, 1985.
112. Jones C, Shankaran P, Davidson D, Poulos A, Callahan J: Studies on the structure and heterogeneity on isoelectric focusing. Studies on the structure of sphingomyelinase. *Biochem J* **209**:291, 1983.
113. Ferlinz K, Hurwitz R, Moczall H, Lansmann S, Schuchman EH, Sandhoff K: Functional characterization of the N-glycosylation sites of human acid sphingomyelinase by site-directed mutagenesis. *Eur J Biochem* **243**:511, 1997.
114. Rao B, Spence M: Sphingomyelinase activity at pH 7.4 in human brain and a comparison to activity at pH 5.0. *J Lipid Res* **17**:506, 1976.
115. Yedger S, Gatt S: Effect of Triton X-100 on the hydrolysis of sphingomyelin by sphingomyelinase of rat brain. *Biochemistry* **15**:2570, 1976.
116. Yedger S, Gatt S: Enzyme hydrolysis of sphingomyelin in the presence of bile salts. *Biochem J* **185**:749, 1980.
117. Fujita N, Suzuki K, Vanier MT, Popko B, Maeda N, Klein A, Heuseler M, Sandhoff K, Nakayasu H, Suzuki K: Targeted disruption of the mouse sphingolipid activator protein gene: A complex phenotype, including severe leukodystrophy and widespread storage of multiple sphingolipids. *Hum Mol Genet* **5**:711, 1996.
118. Vanier MT: Biochemical studies in Niemann-Pick disease. I. Major sphingolipids of liver and spleen. *Biochim Biophys Acta* **750**:178, 1983.
119. Carre JB, Boutry JM, Baumann N, Maurin Y: Acidic sphingomyelinase: relationship with anti-depressant-induced desensitization of beta-adrenoceptors. *Life Sci* **42**:769, 1988.
120. Yoshida Y, Arimoto K, Sato M, Sakuragawa N, Arima M, Satoyoshi E: Reduction of acid sphingomyelinase activity in human fibroblasts induced by AY-9944 and other cationic amphiphilic drugs. *J Biol Chem* **98**:1669, 1985.
121. Ghosh P, Chatterjee S: Effects of gentamicin on sphingomyelinase activity in cultured human renal proximal tubular cells. *J Biol Chem* **262**:12550, 1987.
122. Jones CS, Shankaran P, Callahan JW: Purification of sphingomyelinase to apparent homogeneity by using hydrophobic chromatography. *Biochem J* **195**:373, 1981.
123. Ahmad TY, Beaudet AL, Sparrow JT, Morrisett JD: Human lysosomal sphingomyelinase: Substrate efficacy of apolipoprotein/sphingomyelin complexes. *Biochemisty* **25**:4415, 1986.
124. Xu X-X, Tabas I: Sphingomyelinase enhances low-density lipoprotein uptake and ability to induce cholesteryl ester accumulation in macrophages. *J Biol Chem* **266**:24849, 1991.
125. Tabas I, Li Y, Brocia RW, Xu SW, Swenson TL, Williams KJ: Lipoprotein lipase and sphingomyelinase synergistically enhance the association of atherogenic lipoproteins with smooth muscle cells and extracellular matrix. *J Biol Chem* **268**:20419, 1993.
126. Jobb E, Callahan J: The subunit of human sphingomyelinase is not the same size in all tissues: Studies with a polyclonal rabbit serum. *J Inherit Metab Dis* **10 (Suppl 2)**:326, 1987.
127. Freeman SJ, Davidson DJ, Callahan JW: Solid-phase assay for the detection of low-abundance enzymes, and antibodies to enzymes in immune reactions, using acid sphingomyelinase as a model. *Anal Biochem* **141**:248, 1984.
128. Jobb EA, Callahan JW: Biosynthesis of sphingomyelinase in normal and Niemann-Pick fibroblasts. *Biochem Cell Biol* **67**:801, 1989.
129. He X, Miranda SRP, Dagan A, Gatt S, Schuchman EH: Overexpression of human acid sphingomyelinase in Chinese hamster ovary cells. Purification and characterization of the recombinant enzyme. *Biochem Biophys Res Comm* **1432**:251, 1999.
130. Hurwitz R, Ferlinz K, Vielhaber G, Moczall H, Sandhoff K: Processing of human acid sphingomyelinase in normal and I-cell fibroblasis. *J Biol Chem* **269**:5440, 1994.
131. Spence M, Wakkary J, Clarke J, Cook H: Localization of neutral, magnesium-stimulated sphingomyelinase in plasma membrane of cultured neuroblastoma cells. *Biochim Biophys Acta* **719**:162, 1982.
132. Noguchi E: Purification and characterization of neutral sphingomyelinase from rat brain microsomal fraction. *J Jpn Pediatr Soc* **90**:106, 1987.
133. Chatterjee S, Ghosh N: Neutral sphingomyelinase from human urine: Purification and preparation of monospecific antibodies. *J Biol Chem* **264**:12554, 1989.
134. Maruyama EN, Arima M: Purification and characterization of neutral and acid sphingomyelinases from rat brain. *J Neurochem* **52**:611, 1989.

135. Gatt S, Dinur T, Kopolovic J: Niemann-Pick disease: Presence of the magnesium-dependent sphingomyelinase in brain of the infantile form of the disease. *J Neurochem* **31**:547, 1978.
136. Tomiuk S, Hofmann K, Nix M, Zumbansen M, Stoffel W: Cloned mammalian neutral sphingomyelinase: Functions in sphingolipid signaling. *Proc Natl Acad Sci U S A* **95**:3683, 1998.
137. Okazaki T, Bielawska A, Domae N, Bell RM, Hannun YA: Characteristics and partial purification of a novel cytosolic, magnesium-independent, neutral sphingomyelinase activated in the early signal transduction of 1α,25-dihydroxyvitamin D_3-induced HL-60 cell differentiation. *J Biol Chem* **269**:4070, 1994.
138. Spence MW, Byers DM, Palmer FBSC, Cook HW: A new Zn^{2+}-stimulated sphingomyelinase in fetal bovine serum. *J Biol Chem* **264**:5358, 1989.
139. Kurth J, Stoffel W: Human placental sphingomyelinase. Purification to homogeneity, antigenic properties and partial amino-acid sequences of the enzyme. *Biol Chem Hoppe Seyler* **372**:215, 1991.
140. Quintern LE, Schuchman EH, Levran O, Suchi M, Ferlinz K, Reinke H, Sandhoff K, Desnick RJ: Isolation of cDNA clones encoding human acid-sphingomyelinase: Occurrence of alternatively processed transcripts. *EMBO J* **8**:2469, 1989.
141. Schissel SL, Schuchman EH, Williams KJ, Tabas I: Zn^{2+}-stimulated sphingomyelinase is secreted by many cell types and is a product of the acid sphingomyelinase gene. *Biol Chem* **271**:18431, 1996.
142. Schissel SL, Keesler GA, Schuchman EH, Williams KJ, Tabas I: The cellular trafficking and zinc dependence of secretory and lysosomal sphingomyelinase, two products of the acid sphingomyelinase gene. *J Biol Chem* **273**:18250, 1998.
143. Komoshita S, Aron A, Suzuki K, Suzuki K: Infantile Niemann-Pick disease. A chemical study with isolation and characterization of membranous cytoplasmic bodies and myelin. *Am J Dis Child* **117**:379, 1969.
144. Rao BG, Spence MW: Niemann-Pick disease type D: Lipid analyses and studies on sphingomyelinases. *Ann Neurol* **1**:385, 1977.
145. Besley GT, Elleder M: Enzyme activities and phospholipid storage patterns in brain and spleen samples from Niemann-Pick disease variants: A comparison of neuropathic and non-neuropathic forms. *J Inherit Metab Dis* **9**:59, 1986.
146. Vandenheuvel F: The origin, metabolism, and structure of normal human serum lipoproteins. *Can J Biochem Physiol* **40**:1299, 1962.
147. Vandenheuvel A: Study of biological structure at the molecular level with stereo model projections. I. The lipids in the myelin sheath of nerve. *J Am Oil Chem Soc* **40**:455, 1963.
148. Rouser G, Kritchevsky G, Yamamoto A, Knudson AJ, Simon G: Accumulation of a glycerolphospholipid in classical Niemann-Pick disease. *Lipids* **3**:287, 1968.
149. Yamamoto A, Adachi S, Ishikawa K, Yokomura T, Kitani T: Studies on drug-induced lipidosis. 3. Lipid composition of the liver and some other tissues in clinical cases of "Niemann-Pick-like syndrome" induced by 4,4′-diethylaminoethoxyhexestrol. *J Biochem (Tokyo)* **70**:775, 1971.
150. Gal AE, Brady RO, Hibbert SR, Pentchev PG: A practical chromogenic procedure for the detection of homozygotes and heterozygous carriers of Niemann-Pick disease. *N Engl J Med* **293**:632, 1975.
151. Vanier MT, Rousson R, Garcia I, Bailloud G, Juge MC, Revol A, Louisot P: Biochemical studies in Niemann-Pick disease. III. In vitro and in vivo assays of sphingomyelin degradation in cultured skin fibroblasts and amniotic fluid cells for the diagnosis of the various forms of the disease. *Clin Genet* **27**:20, 1985.
152. Kampine JP, Brady RO, Kanfer JN, Feld M, Shapiro D: Diagnosis of Gaucher's disease and Niemann-Pick disease with small samples of venous blood. *Science* **155**:86, 1967.
153. Poulos A, Shankaran P, Jones CS, Callahan JW: Enzymatic hydrolysis of sphingomyelin liposomes by normal tissues and tissues from patients with Niemann-Pick disease. *Biochim Biophys Acta* **751**:428, 1983.
154. Brady RO: The abnormal biochemistry of inherited disorders of lipid metabolism. *Fed Proc* **32**:1660, 1973.
155. Sloan HR, Uhlendorf BW, Kanfer JN, Brady RO, Fredrickson DS: Deficiency of sphingomyelin-cleaving enzyme activity in tissue cultures derived from patients with Niemann-Pick disease. *Biochem Biophys Res Commun* **34**:582, 1969.
156. Kudoh T, Velkoff MA, Wenger DA: Uptake and metabolism of radioactively labeled sphingomyelin in cultured skin fibroblasts from controls and patients with Niemann-Pick disease and other lysosomal storage diseases. *Biochim Biophys Acta* **754**:82, 1983.
157. Levade T, Gatt S: Uptake and intracellular degradation of fluorescent sphingomyelin by fibroblasts from normal individuals and a patient with Niemann-Pick disease. *Biochim Biophys Acta* **918**:250, 1987.
158. Levade T, Gatt S, Salvayre R: Uptake and degradation of several pyrenesphingomyelins by skin fibroblasts from control subjects and patients with Niemann-Pick disease. Effect of the structure of the fluorescent fatty acyl residue. *Biochem J* **275**:211, 1991.
159. Agmon V, Dinur T, Cherbu S, Dagan A, Gatt S: Administration of pyrene lipids by receptor-mediated endocytosis and their degradation in skin fibroblasts. *Exp Cell Res* **196**:151, 1991.
160. Sakuragawa N, Sato M, Yoshida Y, Kamo I, Arima M, Satoyoshi E: Effects of dimethyl sulfoxide on sphingomyelinase in cultured human fibroblasts and correction of sphingomyelinase deficiency in fibroblasts from Niemann-Pick patients. *Biochem Biophys Res Comm* **126**:756, 1985.
161. Sato M, Yoshida Y, Sakuragawa N, Arima M: Effects of dimethyl sulfoxide on sphingomyelinase activities in normal and Niemann-Pick type A, B and C fibroblasts. *Biochim Biophys Acta* **962**:59, 1988.
162. Burstein S, Hunter SA, Renzulli L: Stimulation of sphingomyelin hydrolysis by cannabidiol in fibroblasts from a Niemann-Pick patient. *Biochem Biophys Res Comm* **121**:168, 1984.
163. Rousson R, Bonnet J, Louisot P, Vanier MT: Presence of immunoreactive material in Niemann-Pick type A placenta using anti-sphingomyelinase rabbit gammaglobulins. *Biochim Biophys Acta* **924**:502, 1987.
164. Hannun YA, Bell RM: Lysosphingolipids inhibit protein kinase C: Implications for the sphingolipidoses. *Science* **235**:670, 1987.
165. Hannun YA, Bell RM: Functions of sphingolipids and sphingolipid breakdown products in cellular regulation. *Science* **243**:500, 1989.
166. Merrill A, Sereni A, Stevens V, Hannun Y, Bell R, Kinkade J: Inhibition of phorbol ester-dependent differentiation of human promyelocytic leukemic (HL-60) cells by sphingosine and other long-chain bases. *J Biol Chem* **261**:12610, 1986.
167. Wilson E, Olcott M, Bell R, Merrill A, Lambeth D: Inhibition of the oxidative burst in human neutrophils by sphingoid long-chain bases. Role of protein kinase C in activation of the burst. *J Biol Chem* **261**:12616, 1986.
168. Kolesnick RN: Sphingomyelinase action inhibits phorbol ester-induced differentiation of human promyelocytic leukemic (HL-60) cells. *J Biol Chem* **264**:7617, 1989.
169. Nishizuka Y: The role of protein kinase C in cell surface signal transduction and tumour promotion. *Nature* **308**:693, 1984.
170. Huterer S, Wherrett JR: Degradation of lysophosphatidylcholine by lysosomes. Stimulation of lysophospholipase C by taurocholate and deficiency in Niemann-Pick fibroblasts. *Biochim Biophys Acta* **794**:1, 1984.
171. Zhang H, Buckley NE, Gibson K, Spiegel S: Sphingosine stimulates cellular proliferation via a protein kinase C-independent pathway. *J Biol Chem* **265**:76, 1990.
172. Kolesnick RN, Kronke M: Regulation of ceramide and apoptosis. *Annu Rev Physiol* **60**:643, 1998.
173. Hannun YA: Sphingolipid second messengers: Tumor-suppressor lipids. *Adv Exp Med Biol* **400A**:305, 1997.
174. Cifone MG, De Maria R, Roncaioli P, Rippo MR, Azuma M, Lanier LL, Santoni A, Testi R: Apoptotic signaling through CD95 (Fas/Apo-1) activates an acidic sphingomyelinase. *J Exp Med* **177**:1547, 1993.
175. Boucher L-M, Wiegmann K, Futterer A, Pfeffer K, Machleidt T, Schutze S, Mak TW, Kronke M: CD28 signals through acidic sphingomyelinase. *J Exp Med* **181**:2059, 1995.
176. Liu P, Anderson RGW: Compartmentalized production of ceramide at the cell surface. *J Biol Chem* **270**:27179, 1995.
177. Santana P, Pena LA, Haimovitz-Friedman A, Martin S, Green D, McLoughlin M, Cordon-Cardo C, Schuchman EH, Fuks Z, Kolesnick R: Acid sphingomyelinase-deficient human lymphoblasts and mice are defective in radiation-induced apoptosis. *Cell* **86**:189, 1996.
178. Miyataki T, Suzuki K: Globoid cell leukodystrophy: Additional deficiency of psychosine galactosidase. *Biochem Biophys Res Commun* **48**:538, 1972.
179. Nilsson O, Svennerholm L: Accumulation of glucosylceramide and glucosylsphingosine (psychosine) in cerebrum and cerebellum in infantile and juvenile Gaucher disease. *J Neurochem* **39**:709, 1982.
180. Strasberg PM, Callahan J: Lysosphingolipid and mitochondrial function. II. Deleterious effect of sphingosylphosphorylcholine. *Biochem Cell Biol* **66**:1322, 1988.
181. Berger A, Rosenthal D, Spiegel S: Sphingosylphosphocholine, a signaling molecule which accumulates in Niemann-Pick disease type

A, stimulates DNA-binding activity of the transcription activator protein AP-1. *Proc Natl Acad Sci U S A* **92d**:5885, 1995.

182. Hamburger R: Lipoidzellige splenohepatomegalie (Type Niemann-Pick) in Verbindung mit amaurotischer Idiotie bei einem 14 Monate alten Madchen. *Jahrb Kinderheilkd* **116**:41, 1927.
183. Merksamer E, Kramer B: Niemann-Pick's disease. Report of three cases in one family. *J Pediatr* **14**:51, 1939.
184. Videbaek A: Niemann-Pick's disease, acute and chronic type. *Acta Paediatr (Upps)* **37**:95, 1949.
185. Videbaek A: Another case of Niemann-Pick's disease observed in Denmark. *Acta Paediatr (Upps)* **41**:355, 1952.
186. Goodman R: *Genetic Disorders Among the Jewish People*. Baltimore, Johns Hopkins University Press, 1979.
187. Vanier M, Boue J, Dumez Y: First-trimester prenatal diagnosis on chorionic villi and biochemical study of a foetus at 12 weeks of development. *Clin Genet* **28**:348, 1985.
188. Schoenfeld A, Ovadia J, Neri A, Abramovici A, Klibanski C: Chemical and biochemical studies in fetuses affected with Niemann-Pick disease type A. *Prenat Diagn* **2**:177, 1982.
189. Schoenfeld A, Abramovici A, Klibanski C, Ovadia J: Placental ultrasonographic biochemical and histochemical studies in human fetuses affected with Niemann-Pick disease type A. *Placenta* **6**:33, 1985.
190. Klibansky C, Chazan S, Schoenfeld A, Abramovici A: Chemical and biochemical studies in human fetuses affected with Niemann-Pick disease type A. *Clin Chim Acta* **91**:243, 1979.
191. Vanier MT, Ferlinz K, Rousson R, Duthel S, Louisot P, Sandhoff K, Suzuki K: Deletion of arginine (608) in acid sphingomyelinase is the prevalent mutation among Niemann-Pick disease type B patients from northern Africa. *Hum Genet* **92**:325, 1993.
192. Besley GT, Hoogeboom AJ, Hoogeveen A, Kleijer WJ, Galjaard H: Somatic cell hybridization studies showing different gene mutations in Niemann-Pick variants. *Hum Genet* **54**:409, 1980.
193. Schuchman EH, Suchi M, Takahashi T, Sandhoff K, Desnick RJ: Human acid sphingomyelinase: Isolation, nucleotide sequence, and expression of the full-length and alternatively spliced cDNA. *Biol Chem* **266**:8531, 1991.
194. Kozak M: An analysis of 5 noncoding sequences from 699 vertebrate messenger RNAs. *Nucleic Acids Res* **15**:8126, 1987.
195. Von Heijne G: A new method for predicting signal sequence cleavage sites. *Nucleic Acids Res* **14**:4683, 1986.
196. Schuchman EH, Levran O, Pereira LV, Desnick RJ: Structural organization and complete nucleotide sequence of the gene encoding human acid sphingomyelinase (SMPD1). *Genomics* **12**:1, 1992.
197. Jurka J, Smith T: A fundamental division in the Alu family of repeated sequences. *Proc Natl Acad Sci U S A* **85**:4775, 1988.
198. Weil D, D'Alessio M, Ramirez F, De Wet W, Cole W, Chan D, Bateman J: A base substitution in the exon of a collagen gene causes alternative splicing and generates a structurally abnormal polypeptide in a patient with Ehlers-Danlos syndrome type VII. *EMBO J* **8**:1705, 1989.
199. Pereira L, Desnick R, Adler D, Disteche C, Schuchman E: Regional assignment of the human acid sphingomyelinase gene by PCR analysis of somatic cell hybrids and in situ hybridization to 11p15.1-p15.4. *Genomics* **9**:229, 1991.
200. Henry I, Puech A, Antignac C, Couillin P, Jean-Pierre M, Ahnine L, Barichard F, et al.: Subregional mapping of BWS, CTSD, MYOD1 and T-ALL breakpoints in 11p15. *Cytogenet Cell Genet* **51**:1013, 1989.
201. Bruns G, Gerald P: Human acid phosphatase in somatic cell hybrids. *Science* **184**:480, 1974.
202. Konrad R, Wilson D: Assignment of the gene for acid lysosomal sphingomyelinase to human chromosome 17. *Cytogenet Cell Genet* **46**:641, 1987.
203. Schuchman E, Levran O, Suchi M, Desnick R: An MspI polymorphism in the human acid sphingomyelinase gene (SMPD1) at 11p15.1–p15.4. *Nucleic Acid Res* **19**:3160, 1991.
204. Wan Q, Schuchman EH: A novel polymorphism in the human acid sphingomyelinase gene due to size variation of the signal peptide region. *Biochim Biophys Acta* **1270**:207, 1995.
205. Newzella D, Stoffel W: Molecular cloning of the acid sphingomyelinase of the mouse and the organization and complete nucleotide sequence of the gene. *Biol Chem Hoppe Seyler* **373**:1233, 1992.
206. Horinouchi K, Sakiyama T, Pereira L, Lalley PA, Schuchman EH: Mouse models of Niemann-Pick disease: mutation analysis and chromosomal mapping rule out the type A and B forms. *Genomics* **18**:450, 1993.
207. Newzella D, Stoffel W: Functional analysis of the glycosylation of acid sphingomyelinase. *J Biol Chem* **271**:32089, 1996.
208. Levran O, Desnick RJ, Schuchman EH: Niemann-Pick disease: A frequent missense mutation in the acid sphingomyelinase gene of Ashkenazi Jewish type A and B patients. *Proc Natl Acad Sci U S A* **88**:3748, 1991.
209. Levran O, Desnick R, Schuchman E: A common missense mutation (L302P) in Ashkenazi Jewish type A Niemann-Pick disease patients. Transient expression studies demonstrate the causative nature of the two common Ashkenazi Jewish Niemann-Pick disease mutations. *Blood* **80**:2081, 1992.
210. Levran O, Desnick RJ, Schuchman EH: Type A Niemann-Pick disease: A frameshift mutation in the acid sphingomyelinase gene (fsP330) occurs in Ashkenazi Jewish patients. *Hum Mut* **2**:317, 1993.
211. Coulondre C, Miller J, Farabough P, Gilbert W: Molecular basis of base substitution hotspots in Escherichia coli. *Nature* **274**:775, 1978.
212. Meizner I, Levy A, Carmi R, Robinsin C: Niemann-Pick disease associated with nonimmune hydrops fetalis [see comments]. *Am J Obstet Gynecol* **163**:128, 1990.
213. Li L, Caggana M, Robinowitz J, Shabeer J, Desnick RJ, Eng CM: Prenatal screening in the Ashkenazi Jewish population: A pilot program of multiple option testing for five disorders. *Am J Hum Genet* **61 (Suppl)**:A24, 1997.
214. Schuchman EH, Miranda SRP: Niemann-Pick disease: Mutation update, genotype/phenotype correlations, and prospects for genetic testing. *Genet Test* **1**:13, 1997.
215. Schuchman EH: Two new mutations in the acid sphingomyelinase gene causing type a Niemann-Pick disease: N389T and R441X. *Hum Mutat* **6**:352, 1995.
216. Takahashi T, Suchi M, Desnick RJ, Takada G, Schuchman EH: Identification and expression of five mutations in the human acid sphingomyelinase gene causing types A and B Niemann-Pick disease. Molecular evidence for genetic heterogeneity in the neuronopathic and non-neuronopathic forms. *J Biol Chem* **267**:12552, 1992.
217. Takahashi T, Desnick RJ, Takada G, Schuchman EH: Identification of a missense mutation (S436R) in the acid sphingomyelinase gene from a Japanese patient with type B Niemann-Pick disease. *Hum Mutat* **1**:70, 1992.
218. Ferlinz K, Hurwitz R, Sandhoff K: Molecular basis of acid sphingomyelinase deficiency in a patient with Niemann-Pick disease type A. *Biochem Biophys Res Comm* **179**:1187, 1991.
219. Levran O, Desnick RJ, Schuchman EH: Identification of a 3′ acceptor splice site mutation (g2610c) in the acid sphingomyelinase gene of patients with Niemann-Pick disease. *Hum Mol Genet* **2**:205, 1993.
220. Levran O, Desnick RJ, Schuchman EH: Niemann-Pick type B disease. Identification of a single codon deletion in the acid sphingomyelinase gene and genotype/phenotype correlations in type A and B patients. *J Clin Invest* **88**:806, 1991.
221. Chase G, McKusick V: Founder effect in Tay-Sachs disease. *Am J Hum Genet* **24**:339, 1972.
222. Myrianthopoulos N, Naylor A, Aronson S: Founder effect in Tay-Sachs disease unlikely. *Am J Hum Genet* **24**:341, 1972.
223. Fraikor A: Tay-Sachs disease: Genetic drift among the Ashkenazi Jews. *Soc Biol* **24**:117, 1977.
224. Fishman P: Role of membrane gangliosides in the binding and action of bacterial toxins. *J Membr Biol* **69**:85, 1982.
225. Grassme H, Gulbins E, Brenner B, Ferlinz K, Sandhoff K, Harzer K, Lang F, Meyer TF: Acidic sphingomyelinase mediates entry of N. gonorrhoeae into nonphagocytic cells. *Cell* **91**:605, 1997.
226. Gal AE, Brady RO, Barranger JA, Pentchev PG: The diagnosis of type A and type B Niemann Pick disease and detection of carriers using leukocytes and a chromogenic analogue of sphingomyelin. *Clin Chim Acta* **104**:129, 1980.
227. Wenger DA, Kudoh T, Sattler M, Palmieri M, Yudkoff M: Niemann-Pick disease type B: prenatal diagnosis and enzymatic and chemical studies on fetal brain and liver. *Am J Hum Genet* **33**:337, 1981.
228. Chazan S, Zitman D, Klibansky C: Prenatal diagnosis of Gaucher's and Niemann-Pick diseases. Assays of glucocerebrosidase and sphingomyelinase in tissue cultures using natural substrates. *Clin Chim Acta* **86**:45, 1978.
229. Besley GT, Moss SE: Studies on sphingomyelinase and β-glucosidase activities in Niemann-Pick disease variants. Phosphodiesterase activities measured with natural and artificial substrates. *Biochim Biophys Acta* **752**:54, 1983.
230. Gatt S, Dinur T, Barenholz Y: A fluorometric determination of sphingomyelinase by use of fluorescent derivatives of sphingomyelin,

and its application to diagnosis of Niemann-Pick disease. *Clin Chem* **26**:93, 1980.
231. Klar R, Levade T, Gatt S: Synthesis of pyrenesulfonylamido-sphingomyelin and its use as substrate for determining sphingomyelinase activity and diagnosing Niemann-Pick disease. *Clin Chim Acta* **176**:259, 1988.
232. Levade T, Salvayre R, Bes J-C, Nezri M, Douste-Blazy L: New tools for the study of Niemann-Pick disease: Analogues of natural substrate and Epstein-Barr virus transformed lymphoid cell lines. *Pediatr Res* **19**:153, 1988.
233. Poulos A, Ranieri E, Shankaran P, Callahan JW: Studies on the activation of sphingomyelinase activity in Niemann-Pick type A, B, and C fibroblasts: Enzymological differentiation of types A and B. *Pediatr Res* **18**:1088, 1984.
234. Gatt S, Bierman E: Sphingomyelin suppresses the binding and utilization of low-density lipoproteins by skin fibroblasts. *J Biol Chem* **255**:3371, 1980.
235. Beaudet AL, Manschreck AA: Metabolism of sphingomyelin by intact cultured fibroblasts: Differentiation of Niemann-Pick disease type A and B. *Biochem Biophys Res Commun* **105**:14, 1982.
236. Spence MW, Clarke JT, Cook HW: Pathways of sphingomyelin metabolism in cultured fibroblasts from normal and sphingomyelin lipidosis subjects. *J Biol Chem* **258**:8595, 1983.
237. Levade T, Salvayre R, Lenoir G, Douste-Blazy L: Sphingomyelinase and nonspecific phosphodiesterase activities in Epstein-Barr virus-transformed lymphoid cell lines from Niemann-Pick disease A, B and C. *Biochim Biophys Acta* **793**:321, 1984.
238. Levade T, Salvayre R, Douste-Blazy L: Molecular forms of sphingomyelinase and non-specific phosphodiesterases in Epstein-Barr virus-transformed lymphoid cell lines from Niemann-Pick disease types A and B. *Eur J Biochem* **149**:405, 1985.
239. Levade T, Salvayre R, Maret A, Douste-Blazy L: Evidence for both endogenous and exogenous sources of the sphingomyelin storage in lymphoid cell lines from patients with Niemann-Pick disease types A and B. *J Inherit Metab Dis* **11**:151, 1985.
240. Spence MW, Cook HW, Byers DM, Palmer FB: The role of sphingomyelin in phosphatidylcholine metabolism in cultured human fibroblasts from control and sphingomyelin lipidosis patients and in Chinese hamster ovary cells. *Biochem J* **268**:719, 1990.
241. Patrick AD, Young E, Kleijer WJ, Niermeijer MF: Prenatal diagnosis of Niemann-Pick disease type A using chromogenic substrate [letter]. *Lancet* **2**:144, 1977.
242. Maziere JC, Maziere C, Hosli P: An ultramicrochemical assay for sphingomyelinase: rapid prenatal diagnosis of a fetus at risk for Niemann-Pick disease. *Monogr Hum Genet* **9**:198, 1978.
243. Epstein CJ, Brady RO, Schneider EL, Bradley RM, Shapiro D: In utero diagnosis of Niemann-Pick disease. *Am J Hum Genet* **23**:533, 1971.
244. Daloze P, Delvin EE, Glorieux FH, Corman JL, Bettez P, Toussi T: Replacement therapy for inherited enzyme deficiency: Liver orthotopic transplantation in Niemann-Pick disease type A. *Am J Med Genet* **1**:229, 1977.
245. Gartner J, Bergman I, Malatack J, Zitelli B, Jaffe R, Watkins J, Shaw B, Iwatsuki S, Starzl T: Progression of neurovisceral storage disease with supranuclear ophthalmoplegia following orthotopic liver transplantation. *Pediatrics* **77**:104, 1986.
246. Scaggiante B, Pineschi A, Sustersich M, Andolina M, Agosti E, Romeo D: Successful therapy of Niemann-Pick disease by implantation of human amniotic membrane. *Transplantation* **44**:59, 1987.
247. Bayever E, Kamani N, Ferreira P, Machin GA, Yudkoff M, Conard K, Palmieri M, Radcliffe J, Wenger DA, August CS: Bone marrow transplantation for Niemann-Pick type IA disease. *J Inherit Metab Dis* **15**:919, 1992.
248. Vellodi A, Hobbs JR, O'Donnell NM, Coulter BS, Hugh-Jones K: Treatment of Niemann-Pick disease type B by allogeneic bone marrow transplantation. *Br Med J (Clin Res Ed)* **295**:1375, 1987.
249. Sando G, Neufeld E: Recognition and receptor-mediated uptake of a lysosomal enzyme, α-l-iduronidase by cultured fibroblasts. *Cell* **12**:619, 1977.
250. Kaplan A, Achord D, Sly W: Phosphohexosyl components of a lysosomal enzyme are recognized by pinocytosis receptors of human fibroblasts. *Proc Natl Acad Sci U S A* **74**:2026, 1977.
251. Ioannou Y, Bishop D, Desnick R: Overexpression of human α-*N*-galactosidase A results in its overexpression in lysosomes and selective secretion. *J Cell Biol* **119**:1137, 1992.
252. Anderson W: Prospects for human gene therapy. *Science* **226**:401, 1984.
253. Gilboa E, Eglitis M, Kantoff P, Anderson W: Transfer and expression of cloned genes using retroviral vectors. *Biotechniques* **4**:504, 1986.
254. Desnick R, Gilboa E, Schuchman E: Human gene therapy: Strategies and prospects for inborn errors of metabolism. Advances in the Treatment of Genetic Diseases. *Proceedings of the Vth International Congress of the Inborn Errors of Metabolism Society*. New York, 1991, p 239.
255. Suchi M, Dinur T, Desnick RJ, Gatt S, Pereira L, Gilboa E, Schuchman EH: Retroviral-mediated transfer of the human acid sphingomyelinase cDNA: Correction of the metabolic defect in cultured Niemann-Pick disease cells. *Proc Natl Acad Sci U S A* **89**:3227, 1992.
256. Spence M, Cooke H, Byers D, Palmer F: The role of sphingomyelin in phosphatidylcholine metabolism in cultured human fibroblasts from control and sphingomyelin lipidosis patients and in Chinese hamster ovary cells. *Biochem J* **268**:719, 1980.
257. Hantzopoulos P, Sullenger B, Ungers G, Gilboa E: Improved gene expression upon transfer of the adenosine deaminase minigene outside the transcriptional unit of a retroviral vector. *Proc Natl Acad Sci U S A* **86**:3519, 1989.
258. Dinur T, Schuchman EH, Fibach E, Dagan A, Suchi M, Desnick RJ, Gatt S: Toward gene therapy for Niemann-Pick disease (NPD): Separation of retrovirally corrected and noncorrected NPD fibroblasts using a novel fluorescent sphingomyelin. *Hum Gene Ther* **3**:633, 1992.
259. Erlich S, Miranda SRP, Visser JWM, Dagan A, Gatt S, Schuchman EH: Fluorescence-based selection of gene-corrected hematopoietic stem and progenitor cells from acid sphingomyelinase deficient mice: Implications for Niemann-Pick disease gene therapy and the development of improved stem cell gene transfer procedures. *Blood* **93**:80, 1999.
260. Pentchev PG, Gal AE, Booth AD, Omodeo-Sale F, Fouks J, Neumeyer BA, Quirk JM, Dawson G, Brady RO: A lysosomal storage disorder in mice characterized by a dual deficiency of sphingomyelinase and glucocerebrosidase. *Biochim Biophys Acta* **619**:669, 1980.
261. Miyawaki S, Mitsuoka S, Sakiyama T, Kitagawa T: Sphingomyelinosis, a new mutation in the mouse: A model of Niemann-Pick disease in humans. *J Hered* **73**:257, 1982.
262. Pentchev P, Boothe A, Kruth H, Weintroub H, Stivers J, Brady R: A genetic storage disorder in BALB/C mice with a metabolic block in esterification of exogenous cholesterol. *J Biol Chem* **259**:5784, 1984.
263. Ohno K, Nanba E, Miyawaki S, Sakiyama T, Kitagawa T, Takeshita K: A cell line derived from sphingomyelinosis mouse shows alterations in intracellular cholesterol metabolism similar to those in type C Niemann-Pick disease. *Cell Struct Funct* **17**:229, 1992.
264. Horinouchi K, Erlich S, Perl DP, Ferlinz K, Bisgaier CL, Sandhoff K, Desnick RJ, Stewart CL, Schuchman EH: Acid sphingomyelinase deficient mice: a model of types A and B Niemann- Pick disease. *Nat Genet* **10**:288, 1995.
265. Otterbach B, Stoffel W: Acid sphingomyelinase-deficient mice mimic the neurovisceral form of human lysosomal storage disease (Niemann-Pick disease). *Cell* **81**:1053, 1995.
266. Bundza A, Lowden JA, Charlton KM: Niemann-Pick disease in a poodle dog. *Vet Pathol* **16**:530, 1979.
267. Wenger DA, Sattler M, Kudoh T, Snyder SP, Kingston RS: Niemann-Pick disease: A genetic model in Siamese cats. *Science* **208**:1471, 1980.

CHAPTER 145

Niemann-Pick Disease Type C: A Lipid Trafficking Disorder

Marc C. Patterson ▪ Marie T. Vanier ▪ Kinuko Suzuki
Jill A. Morris ▪ Eugene Carstea ▪ Edward B. Neufeld
Joan E. Blanchette-Mackie ▪ Peter G. Pentchev

1. Niemann-Pick disease type C (NP-C) is an autosomal recessive lipidosis with protean clinical manifestations, distinguished biochemically by a unique error in cellular trafficking of exogenous cholesterol that is associated with lysosomal accumulation of unesterified cholesterol. A majority of patients with this phenotype are linked genetically to chromosome 18, the locus of *NPC1*. *NPC1* is a novel gene whose predicted protein product contains between 13 and 16 transmembrane domains, and a sterol-sensing domain with homologies to Patched, HMG-CoA reductase, and SCAP. A region designated the NPC domain, conserved in yeast, nematode, and mouse, contains a leucine zipper. NP-C is distinct at clinical, biochemical, and molecular levels from the primary sphingomyelin lipidoses (Niemann-Pick disease types A and B [NP-A and NP-B, respectively]), with which it has traditionally been grouped. Niemann-Pick disease type D (NP-D) is allelic with NP-C, and should be regarded as a variant phenotype associated with a genetic isolate, rather than a distinct entity. A small group of patients belong to a second genetic complementation group that does not link to chromosome 18. These individuals are believed to have mutations in a gene provisionally designated *NPC2*.

2. The clinical manifestations of NP-C are heterogeneous. Most patients with NP-C have progressive neurologic disease, although hepatic damage is prominent in certain cases, and may be lethal in some. Variable hepatosplenomegaly, vertical supranuclear ophthalmoplegia, progressive ataxia, dystonia, and dementia characterize the "classic" phenotype. These children present in childhood, and die in the second or third decade. Other phenotypes include presentations with fetal ascites, fatal neonatal liver disease, early infantile onset with hypotonia and delayed motor development, and adult variants in which psychiatric illness and dementia predominate.

3. NP-C is panethnic. Genetic isolates have been described in Nova Scotia (formerly Niemann-Pick disease type D) and southern Colorado. Complementation studies have demonstrated two distinct groups. About 95 percent of patients link to chromosome 18q11, and thus to *NPC1*; the remainder are believed to have mutations in a second gene, provisionally designated *NPC2*.

4. NP-C has an estimated prevalence of approximately 1:150,000, making it a more common phenotype than NP-A and NP-B combined. It is likely that the true prevalence of the disease has been underestimated because of confusing terminology, the lack of a definitive diagnostic test prior to the discovery of the abnormalities of cellular cholesterol processing, and failure to recognize the clinical phenotypes.

5. Foam cells or sea-blue histiocytes are found in many tissues. Such cells are not specific for NP-C and may be absent, particularly in cases lacking visceromegaly. Characteristic inclusions (polymorphous cytoplasmic bodies) may be identified in skin and conjunctival biopsies. Neuronal storage with cytoplasmic ballooning and a variety of inclusions is present throughout the nervous system. Neurofibrillary tangles, meganeurites, and axonal spheroids are also seen.

6. In most cases of NP-C, the primary molecular defect lies in *NPC1*. Unesterified cholesterol, sphingomyelin, phospholipids, and glycolipids are stored in excess in the liver and spleen. Glycolipids are elevated in the brain, the principal target of this disease. There is no overt increase in cholesterol in the brain in human NP-C or its animal models. Partial sphingomyelinase deficiency, observed only in cultured cells (and never in leukocytes or solid tissues), represents a variable, secondary consequence of lysosomal cholesterol sequestration. Cultured fibroblasts show a unique disorder of cellular cholesterol processing, in which delayed homeostatic responses to exogenous cholesterol loading are impaired in association with cholesterol accumulation in lysosomes.

7. The diagnosis of NP-C requires both documentation of a characteristic pattern of filipin-cholesterol staining and measurement of cellular cholesterol esterification in cultured fibroblasts during LDL uptake. Candidates for such testing are identified chiefly by clinical presentation with or without supportive findings from neurophysiological tests and tissue biopsies. There is considerable variability in the

A list of standard abbreviations is located immediately preceding the index in each volume. Additional abbreviations used in this chapter include: lamp = lysosome-associated membrane proteins; LFB = Luxol fast blue; MRSI = magnetic resonance spectroscopy imaging; NP-A = Niemann-Pick disease type A; NP-B = Niemann-Pick disease type B; NP-C = Niemann-Pick disease type C; NP-D = Niemann-Pick disease type D; *NPC1* = Niemann-Pick disease type 1 gene; *NPC2* = Niemann-Pick disease type 2 gene; PCB = polymorphous cytoplasmic body; PHFs = paired helical filaments; SCAP = sterol regulatory element binding protein (SREBP) cleavage-activating protein; VSGP = vertical supranuclear gaze palsy.

degree of impairment of cholesterol trafficking in NP-C. Consequently, antenatal diagnosis has been restricted to families in which the biochemical abnormalities are pronounced. Molecular diagnosis will offer a desirable alternative in families where mutations in *NPC1* have been identified in the index case.

8. **Symptomatic treatment of seizures, dystonia, and cataplexy is effective in many patients with NP-C. Combination drug regimens have been shown to lower hepatic and plasma cholesterol levels in human NP-C. There is no evidence that such therapy alters the progression of the disease in humans or murine models.**
9. **Animal models with clinical, pathologic, and biochemical features resembling NP-C have been described in two species of mice, as well as in the cat and boxer dog. The murine ortholog of *NPC1* is mutated in the C57BLKS/J and BALB/c models.**

Major advances in our understanding of Niemann-Pick disease type C (NP-C) have occurred since the last edition of this text. Complementation studies have demonstrated that the NP-C phenotype results from mutations in two distinct genes. The gene associated with the smaller complementation group, accounting for perhaps 5 percent of NP-C patients, has not yet been identified. This gene has been provisionally designated *NPC2*.

The *NPC1* gene was cloned in 1997, conclusively demonstrating that NP-C and the sphingomyelin lipidoses (Niemann-Pick disease types A and B [NP-A and NP-B, respectively]) are distinct entities at a molecular level, confirming their earlier separation on clinical and biochemical grounds. Furthermore, it was found that NP-C is allelic with Niemann-Pick disease type D (NP-D), justifying the elimination of NP-D as an entity separate from NP-C.

As well as providing a new tool for the investigation of cellular homeostasis, the identification of *NPC1* will also provide a new means of investigating the poorly understood pathogenesis of neurodegeneration in NP-C. The latter goal is a necessary condition for the development of effective therapy for this devastating neurologic disorder.

This chapter (a) traces the historic evolution of NP-C; (b) characterizes its distinct and diverse clinical features; (c) defines its unique cellular lesions; (d) describes and evaluates various diagnostic procedures; (e) discusses potential therapeutic strategies; and (f) speculates on the role of NPC1 in cellular lipid trafficking.

HISTORY

The first recognizable description of NP-C appeared in Crocker and Farber's review of Niemann-Pick disease in 1958.[1] Until then, Niemann-Pick disease was restricted to infants conforming to Niemann's original description[2] of infantile neurodegenerative disease with hepatosplenomegaly. Crocker and Farber based their diagnosis of Niemann-Pick disease on the presence of foam cells and increased tissue sphingomyelin, thus including children with indolent or absent neurologic disease in this category. All of the classic neurologic features of NP-C were present in their patient 15, namely: vertical supranuclear gaze palsy; ataxia; dystonia; dementia; cataplexy; dysarthria; spasticity; and seizures. They also described several other presentations of NP-C, including prolonged neonatal jaundice with death in infancy (patient 2); hypotonia and delayed motor milestones (patient 9); isolated organomegaly (patient 10); seizures (patient 13); and learning and behavioral problems at school (patient 14).

Crocker later classified Niemann-Pick disease into four groups based on biochemical and clinical criteria.[3] Group A (NP-A) included the classic patients with neurodegenerative disease leading to death in infancy; group B (NP-B) patients had organomegaly without nervous system disease; group C (NP-C) patients had slowly progressive neurologic illness; and group D (NP-D) closely resembled group C, except for its restriction to a genetic isolate in Nova Scotia. Nonneural tissues in the latter two groups had relatively less sphingomyelin, and more cholesterol storage than tissue from group A and B patients.

Numerous reports in the 1960s and 1970s described a disorder now clearly recognizable as NP-C. The diagnoses included atypical cerebral lipidosis;[4] juvenile Niemann-Pick disease;[5] dystonic juvenile idiocy without amaurosis;[6] juvenile dystonic lipidosis;[7–9] giant cell hepatitis;[10] lactosylceramidosis;[11] neurovisceral storage disease with vertical supranuclear ophthalmoplegia;[12] maladie de Neville;[13] DAF (down gaze paresis, ataxia, foam cell) syndrome;[14] adult dystonic lipidosis;[15] and adult neurovisceral lipidosis.[16] The confused terminology notwithstanding, the salient clinical features of vertical supranuclear gaze palsy (VSGP),[17,18] ataxia, dystonia, and dementia were well described and clearly established NP-C as a distinct disorder.

In 1966 Brady and coworkers[19] demonstrated severe generalized sphingomyelinase deficiency in NP-A, a finding that was soon extended to type B, but not to types C and D,[20] indicating that the two latter types constituted separate entities. Hypotheses invoking the deficiency of a specific sphingomyelinase isoenzyme[21] or of a sphingomyelinase activator protein[22] were disproved[23–25] and the concept of secondary sphingomyelin lipidosis was strengthened by observations of multiple lipid storage in NP-C.[23,26] Somatic cell hybridization studies[27] supported the concept of NP-C as a separate entity. In 1982, a consensus was reached in Prague to separate the sphingomyelinase-deficient forms (NP-A and NP-B) from the other forms of Niemann-Pick disease (NP-C and NP-D).[28]

In 1984, the seminal observation by Pentchev and coworkers[29] of defective cellular esterification of exogenously derived cholesterol in the BALB/c murine model of the disease[30,31] led to the discovery of an identical lesion in NP-C and further demonstration of unique abnormalities of intracellular transport of LDL-derived cholesterol with sequestration of unesterified cholesterol in lysosomes in the disease[32–35] (see "Pathophysiology" below). From that time on, the concept of NP-C evolved from a primary sphingomyelin storage disorder to a primary cholesterol lipidosis. Strategies based on cholesterol trafficking abnormalities facilitated the early diagnosis of patients.[36,37] Mapping of the murine *spm* gene to chromosome 18[38] and subsequent correction of the metabolic lesion in mutant murine fibroblasts by human chromosome 18[39] facilitated linkage studies in the human disease. Genetic heterogeneity, with two complementation groups, was demonstrated in NP-C using combined cell hybridization and linkage studies.[40,41] The gene involved in more than 95 percent of the patients (*NPC1*) has been mapped to 18q11.[42,43] Definitive progress has been achieved with the isolation of the *NPC1* gene[43] and its murine ortholog.[44]

CLINICAL MANIFESTATIONS

NP-C is a disorder with protean manifestations that can present at any time from intrauterine life to adulthood (see Table 145-1). Manifestations may be primarily hepatic, neurologic, or psychiatric. Patients with NP-C may thus present to perinatologists, pediatricians, family practitioners, hematologists, gastroenterologists, neurologists, internists, or psychiatrists, all of whom should be familiar with this disease.

Classic Niemann-Pick Disease Type C

The "classic" NP-C patient is the product of a normal pregnancy; about half of these children have transient neonatal jaundice. Although development in early childhood is usually unremarkable, the child may be labeled as ill-behaved on entering kindergarten or school. Many years may pass before it becomes apparent that the child is slowly dementing. Meanwhile, the child is labeled as clumsy and suffers frequent falls before overt ataxia is recognized. Eye blinking or head thrusting on attempted vertical gaze may be

Table 145-1 Clinical Presentations of NP-C

Age of onset	Presentation

Perinatal period	Fetal ascites
	Neonatal jaundice
	  Benign, self-limiting
	  Rapidly fatal
	Hepatosplenomegaly
	VSGP usually absent

Early infantile	Hypotonia Delay of motor milestones Hepatosplenomegaly VSGP usually absent
Late infantile	"Clumsy," frequent falls (ataxia) Isolated organomegaly VSGP may be present
Juvenile	School failure (intellectual impairment and impaired fine movements) Behavioral problems Ataxia, dysarthria, dystonia Seizures Cataplexy VSGP present
Adolescent and adult	Progressive neurologic deterioration Dementia Psychosis VSGP may be present

noted. Gelastic cataplexy may appear at this time, with manifestations as subtle as head nodding or as dramatic as atonic collapse with injury. Dysarthria, dysphagia, and drooling contribute to educational problems by impairing communication and exposing the child to ridicule. Dystonia first manifests as posturing of a hand or foot when walking or running, and gradually becomes generalized. Partial, generalized, or mixed seizures may begin in childhood or later. Enlargement of the liver or spleen is often first detected in early childhood and usually regresses over time. In at least 10 percent of patients, hepatosplenomegaly is never detected.

The child suffers increasing physical and intellectual disability through late childhood and adolescence, eventually becoming chairbound and incapable of continuing at school. Psychiatric disturbances including psychosis may coincide with the onset of puberty. Severe dysphagia now imperils nutrition, and the upper airway is poorly protected. In many cases, spasticity or rigidity (or both) add to the burden of nursing care. Death from pulmonary complications occurs in the teenage years or early adulthood.

Variant Phenotypes

The "classic" clinical profile accounts for 50 to 60 percent of cases of NP-C in large series. Many alternative presentations have been described.

Four children with fetal ascites[45,46] have been described; only one survived the first year. Two died from hepatic failure and the other from respiratory failure.[47] Foam cells were found in the pulmonary interstitium in this patient,[47] and in another patient with progressive neonatal liver failure.[48] One child presented at 4 months with respiratory symptoms.[49] Further cases presenting with pulmonary involvement have been described.[50] A link between this aggressive pulmonary phenotype and complementation group two has been suggested.[51]

As many as half the patients with NP-C have neonatal cholestatic jaundice that is usually self-limiting;[52] in as many as 10 percent of NP-C cases, terminal hepatic failure without neurologic symptoms occurs.[10,48,49,52–55] NP-C has been reported as the second most common genetic cause of liver disease in infancy in the United Kingdom, after α_1-antitrypsin deficiency.[56] Neonatal jaundice without overt liver disease may herald a more aggressive clinical course, with neurologic abnormalities appearing in the first 4 years of life.[57] In exceptional cases, neurologic dysfunction is not apparent until adolescence.

Some children present with hypotonia and delayed motor development before 2 years of age.[52,58,59] These children invariably have hepatosplenomegaly, usually do not learn to walk, develop intention tremor and generalized spasticity, and die between 3 and 5 years of age. VSGP is not seen. This phenotype is more frequently recognized in patients from southern Europe, the Middle East, and North Africa than in those from the U.S.[60] One child was described with symptomatic peripheral neuropathy.[61] Other childhood presentations include visceromegaly discovered in the course of intercurrent illness, cataplexy with[62] or without narcolepsy,[63] or a rigid-akinetic syndrome.[64] There is considerable overlap among these early onset groups.

In contrast to these aggressive presentations, insidious onset and slow progression characterize late onset cases. Cognitive and psychiatric disturbances are prominent, and may overshadow other findings. Shulman and colleagues[65] reviewed 16 cases of NP-C with adult onset, including a new case of their own. Age of onset ranged from 18 to 59 years (mean 32 years). Signs at presentation included dysarthria (44 percent), dementia (31 percent), psychosis (25 percent), limb ataxia (25 percent), and gait ataxia (25 percent). During the course of the illness, the signs observed included dementia (81 percent), gait ataxia (75 percent), limb ataxia (69 percent), dysarthria (56 percent), VSGP (56 percent), splenomegaly (50 percent), psychosis (38 percent), extrapyramidal signs (38 percent), pyramidal signs (31 percent), dysphagia (25 percent), hepatomegaly (13 percent), and seizures (6 percent).[15,16,65–70] One patient was described with clinical and imaging findings mimicking multiple sclerosis.[71]

Two recent, biochemically well-documented observations suggest the existence of a nonneuronopathic (or, alternatively, very delayed neurologic onset) variant of NP-C. The first patient was diagnosed at the age of 46 because of an enlarged spleen that was ruptured in a traffic accident.[72] Another patient with splenomegaly and thrombocytopenia was diagnosed at age 52, following splenectomy (Massenkeil, Harzer, and Vanier, unpublished). Other similar, albeit less well documented, patients are known.[73,74] This raises the question of a possible relationship with the ill-defined patients reported as Niemann-Pick type E.[75]

Specific Symptoms and Signs

Certain manifestations of NP-C deserve separate comment. VSGP is the neurologic hallmark of this disease, and it has been present in all juvenile and adult cases examined by one author (M.C.P.). Early and late onset patients in whom this sign was not found have been reported.[65,74] Increase in saccadic latency, followed by subtle slowing of vertical saccades (upward or downward) begins in childhood, and may be accompanied by blinking or head thrusting. Older patients complain of difficulty negotiating stairs, or that their eyes become stuck at extremes of vertical gaze. Voluntary vertical gaze is completely paralyzed in the late stages of the illness, and horizontal eye movements may also be affected. Oculocephalic reflexes are preserved. The sign is easily missed if not specifically sought. Saccades should always be examined in addition to pursuit movements. For cooperative patients, an opticokinetic stimulus may be helpful. Recent studies suggest that VSGP in NP-C most likely reflects selective dysfunction of vertical burst neurons in the brain stem[76,77] (see "Pathology" below).

Cataplexy usually occurs late in the neurologic illness,[78,79] but may be the presenting feature.[62,63] Typically, the loss of postural tone is evoked by a humorous stimulus (gelastic cataplexy), and the resulting falls may lead to repeated injury.[78] This symptom also correlates with brain stem disease.[63,78–83]

EPIDEMIOLOGY AND CLINICAL GENETICS

NP-C shows autosomal recessive inheritance. Clinical heterogeneity within families is limited,[84] except when one sib has a rapidly fatal cholestatic form and another sib survives to show neurologic signs.[84,85] Few data are available on the epidemiology of NP-C, but the disease is clearly panethnic. Two genetic isolates have been described, French Acadians in Nova Scotia (formerly NP-D)[3] and Spanish-Americans in southern Colorado.[86] Their phenotypes, although variable, are indistinguishable from other patients with NP-C. A study in Yarmouth County, Nova Scotia[87] found a 1 percent incidence of NP-C and an estimated a carrier frequency between 10 and 26 percent (95 percent confidence limits). The disease is apparently much less common in the general population. A prevalence of about 1/150,000 live births has been calculated for France, West Germany, and the U.K. from the number of cases diagnosed over a 15-year period (M.T.V.). In those countries, NP-C thus appears more frequent than NP-B and NP-A combined. The prevalence of NP-C has undoubtedly been underestimated in the past, due to confusing terminology, the previous lack of specific biochemical tests, and the many variant forms of the disease.

PATHOLOGY

Human Disease

In all clinical forms of NP-C, the cardinal pathologic features are those of neurovisceral storage disease with foamy storage cells in the visceral organs and an accumulation of storage materials in neurons and glial cells in the nervous system. The severity of the pathologic manifestations varies considerably, reflecting the clinical heterogeneity of the disease.[88]

The most notable gross pathologic feature is splenomegaly with or without associated hepatomegaly. Hepatic involvement may be prominent in early life. In most juvenile or adult patients, hepatomegaly or lymphadenopathy is not seen.[60] Histopathologically, two distinct types of cells, foamy cells (macrophages) and sea-blue histiocytes are seen in bone marrow preparations.[12,15,86] Intermediate forms also occur. These cells stain variably with Luxol fast blue (LFB), periodic-acid Schiff (PAS), and Sudan black stains, and are strongly positive with the Schultz reaction for cholesterol and for acid phosphatase.[9,12,89–92] Foamy cells and sea-blue histiocytes are conspicuous in spleen (Fig. 145-1), tonsils, lymph nodes, liver, and lung. These cells tend to be clustered in the red pulp in spleen and within the sinusoids in the liver. Microvacuolation may be found in the hepatocytes.[90,91] Hepatic pathology is usually more conspicuous in the early onset cases, in which giant cell transformation of hepatocytes ("giant cell hepatitis"), cholestasis, or both have been reported.[10,48,53,55,93] In some infantile cases, severe pulmonary involvement causing death by respiratory failure has been reported.[47,50,51] Three of these early lethal pulmonary involvement cases were found to belong to the rare genetic complementation group 2 (see "Molecular Genetics" below). In adult cases, only a few foamy cells may be found in the hepatic sinusoid without significant storage in hepatocytes.[16]

Dumontel and coworkers reported the pathology of a 20-week fetus including detailed ultrastructural analysis of storage cells in the liver and spleen. They found many pleomorphic lysosomes and variously shaped crystalline structures resembling cholesterol crystals.[94] Similar crystalline structures have not been reported in postnatal NP-C cases in humans, but are seen in macrophages in the brain and liver of the murine model of NP-C[95] (see "Animal Models" below). Pathologic involvement of skin, skeletal muscle, and eye may be subtle on routine histopathologic preparation, but abnormal inclusions can be found in histiocytes at the ultrastructural level.[96–99] The cytoplasmic inclusions are polymorphic structures of various electron densities, consisting of stacked, closely packed osmiophilic membranes of varying size and thickness admixed with multiple electron-lucent vacuoles[100,101] (Figs. 145-2 and 145-3). Similar pleomorphic membranous inclusions can be also found in conjunctival epithelial cells; endothelial cells and pericytes; keratinocytes; lens epithelium; retinal ganglion cells; retinal pigment epithelium; pericytes; Schwann cells; smooth muscle cells; and fibroblasts.[96–98] Sea-blue histiocytes contain concentrically arranged, tightly packed electron-dense inclusions and lipofuscin granules.[9,89]

The brain is often atrophic, severely so in patients with a slowly progressive clinical course. Neuronal storage is the most conspicuous cerebral pathology (Fig. 145-4). Cortical neurons, in particular large pyramidal neurons in the deep cortical layers, show distended cytoplasm. In hematoxylin and eosin (H&E) preparations, pale gray-blue granular inclusions or fine vacuolation are noted in the perikarya, and axonal hillocks appear swollen (meganeurites). These granular inclusions are variably stained with PAS and/or LFB but are negative[102] or only weakly positive[89] for the histochemical stain for cholesterol. In the basal ganglia and thalamus, larger neurons tend to be more affected. The degree of neuronal cytoplasmic ballooning and distribution of such storage neurons may vary considerably in individual cases.[5,100] Golgi preparations of the cerebral cortex reveal meganeurites, ectopic neurites, and irregular focal swellings of dendrites of affected pyramidal neurons in the deep cortical layers.[103,104] These features are very similar to those of storage neurons in the

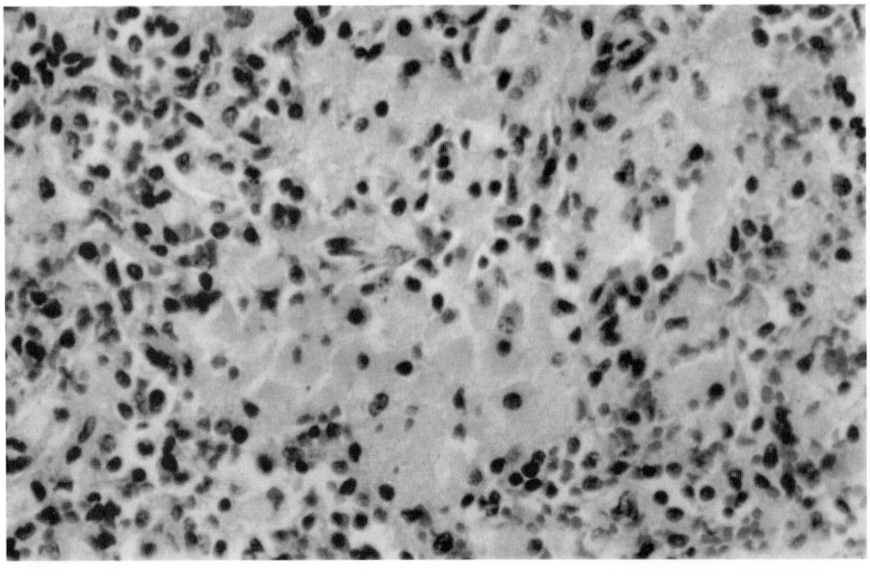

Fig. 145-1 Clusters of foamy macrophages in the spleen (H&E, ×520).

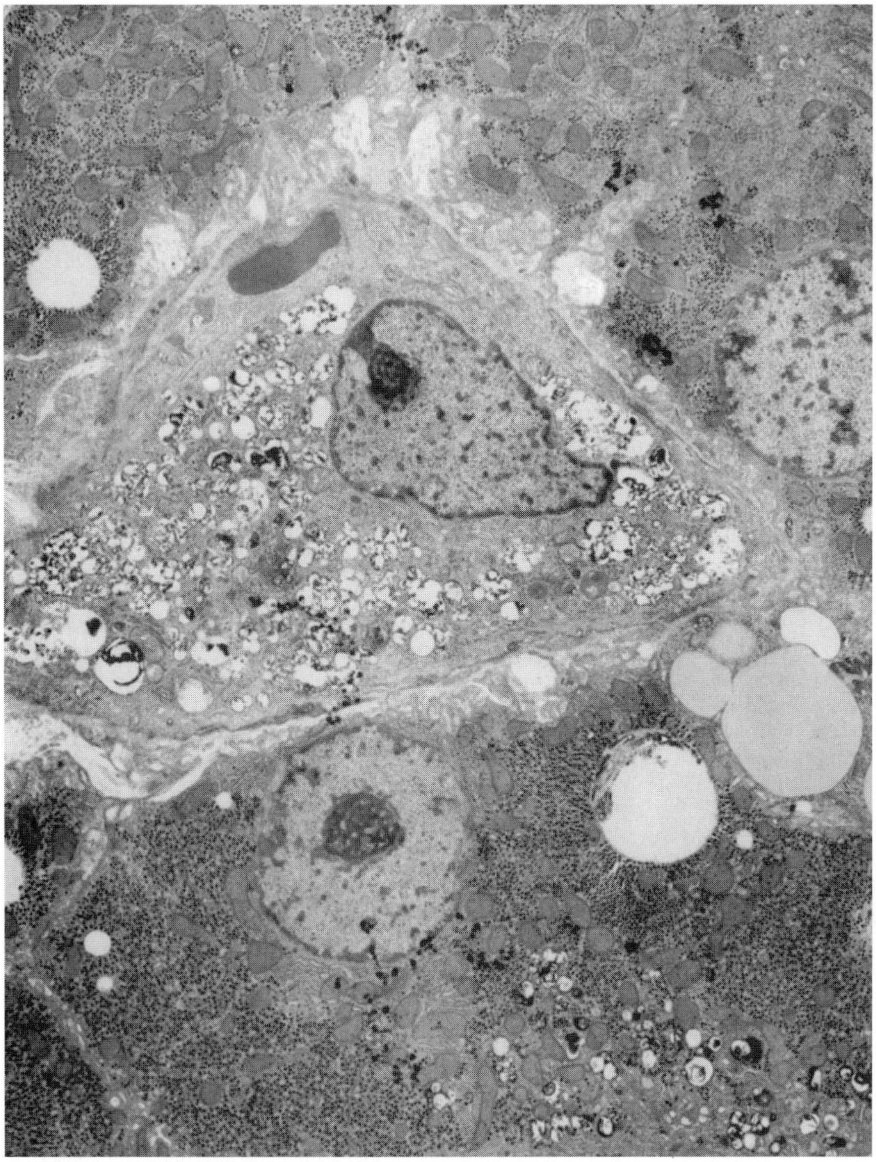

Fig. 145-2 Electron micrograph of liver showing numerous inclusions in a macrophage (Kupffer cell) in the center and surrounding hepatocytes (×8600).

gangliosidoses (see Chaps. 151 and 153). Small pyramidal neurons in the layers II, III, and IV are often devoid of storage materials.[103,104] The cerebral white matter is usually normal, although demyelination with perivascular collections of macrophages containing sudanophilic granules has been reported.[102] Neuroaxonal dystrophy in the form of axonal spheroids is found throughout the neuraxis, in particular in the thalamus (Fig. 145-5), dentate nucleus, and midbrain, including substantia nigra.[59,102] The cerebellum is variably affected by this process. In severe cases, both Purkinje and granular cells are lost and replaced with dense fibrillary gliosis.[5,59,100] Most of the surviving Purkinje cells and Golgi cells show the perikarya distended with storage materials. Antler-like swelling of Purkinje cell dendrites may be seen.[5] The perikarya of both anterior and posterior horn neurons in the spinal cord are distended with storage materials. Neuronal storage is also prominent in the myenteric plexus.[59]

Ultrastructurally, neuronal inclusions consist of heterogeneous lamellar structures, called polymorphous cytoplasmic bodies (PCBs) (Fig. 145-6). Some neurons contain cytosomes resembling the membranous cytoplasmic bodies (MCBs) of gangliosidoses, "zebra bodies," or both. Lipofuscin-like bodies or compound PCBs surrounded by a single membrane may be found in some neuronal perikarya. These complex PCBs are often associated with dilated smooth membrane profiles of Golgi apparatus. Microglia may be enlarged and often contain PCBs.[4,6,9,89,100,101] Similar inclusions are also found in hepatocytes (Fig. 145-4).

Recent studies have shown that neurofibrillary tangles (NFTs) associated with neuropil threads are consistent findings in the brains of NP-C patients with a prolonged clinical course. These NFTs consist of paired helical filaments (PHF).[67,68,105–108] Paired helical filament tau (PHFtau) in NP-C is similar to that of Alzheimer disease (AD).[109] Unlike AD, NFTs in NP-C predominantly involve the deeper layers of the cerebral cortex, thalamus, basal ganglia, hypothalamus, brain stem, and spinal cord. Entorhinal cortex, orbital gyrus, and cingulate gyrus are commonly affected. The distribution of NFTs generally parallels that of the swollen storage neurons. PHFs are found in the swollen perikarya as well as in the meganeurites. However, neurons without swollen perikarya may contain NFTs. NFTs can be found in a number of non-Alzheimer cases,[108] and thus the presence of NFTs in NP-C cases may simply represent a nonspecific neuronal response to metabolic perturbation. However, the frequent association of a prolonged clinical course and the presence of NFTs, even in patients as young as 10 years,[108] may suggest that the association is more than coincidental and reflects unique neuropathology in NP-C.

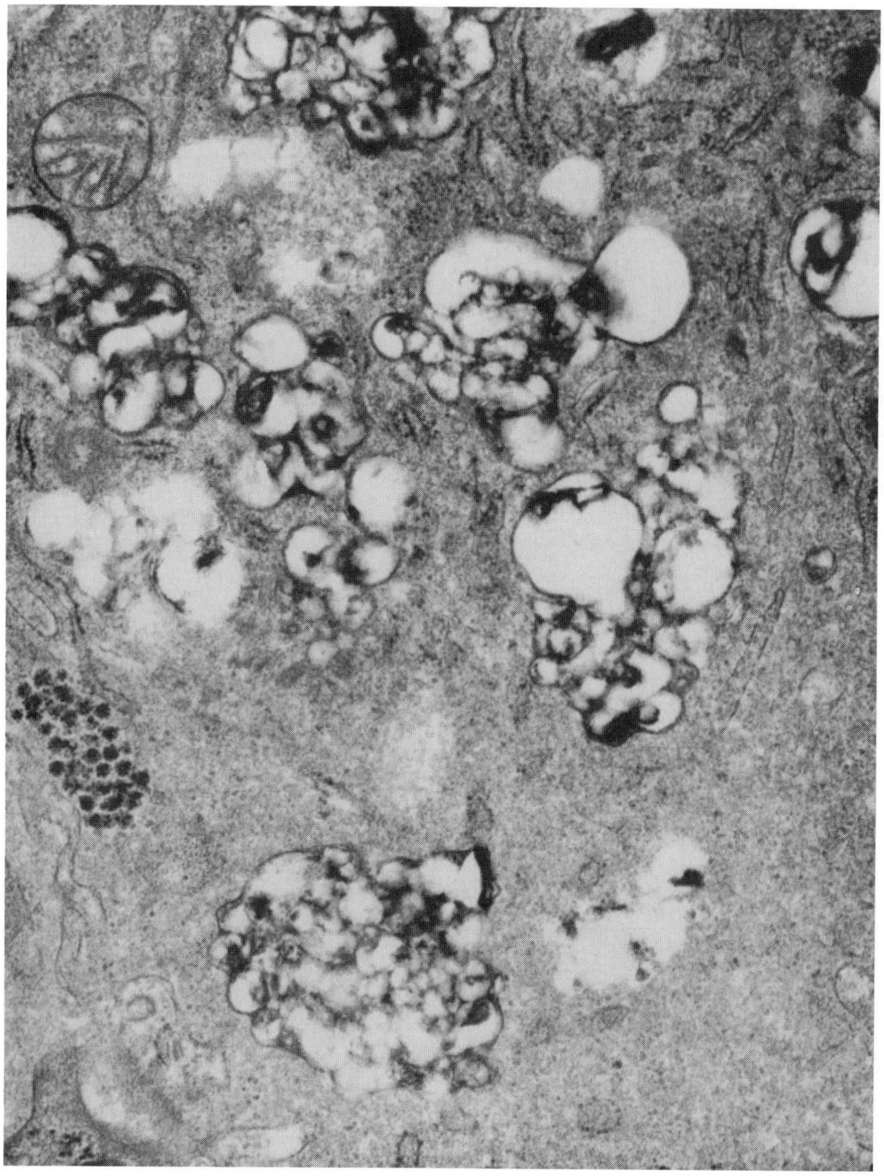

Fig. 145-3 Electron micrograph of inclusions in a hepatocyte consisting of numerous electron-lucent vacuoles and electron-dense membranes (×36,000).

Morphologic studies of the peripheral nerves are scarce. Axonal degeneration and membrane-bound lysosomal inclusions have been reported in Schwann cells, endoneurial fibroblasts, macrophages, pericytes, and endothelial cells.[61,110]

Animal Models of NP-C

A feline model,[111] canine model,[112] and two murine models (BALB/c npc^{nih} and C57BLKS/J *spm*),[95,113–115] are known. The C57BLKS/J mouse, also known as the "sphingomyelinosis" mouse, was reclassified as a model of NP-C rather than of NP-A.[116] Light and electron microscopic features of these models closely resemble human NP-C. In both canine and feline models, infiltration of foamy macrophages is extensive in the lung, liver, spleen, and lymph nodes. Hepatosplenomegaly is absent in the canine model.

Neuronal storage is prominent throughout the cerebrum. Cortical pyramidal neurons in laminae II, III, and V in the feline model exhibit meganeurite formation with or without ectopic dendritogenesis.[104] Axonal swelling or axonal spheroids is very frequent in the feline model[111] but is relatively mild in the canine model.[112] These axonal spheroids demonstrate immunoreactivity for glutamic acid decarboxylase (GAD).[104] A marked loss of Purkinje and granular cells is documented in the cerebellum of the canine model while Purkinje cells are relatively well preserved in the feline model. Segmental myelin loss is noted in the spinal roots in feline NP-C.

Two murine models have almost identical histopathology. Hepatomegaly is not apparent. Foamy macrophages can be detected in young asymptomatic mice and their numbers increase significantly with age. These foamy cells stain positively with various lectins, indicating the heterogeneous nature of the storage material.[117] Alveolar macrophages in younger mice contain osmiophilic dense granules and annulolamellar structures, but larger multilamellar concentric structures are found more frequently in the older mice.[118] The brain of the affected mice is smaller than controls, with atrophy of the cerebellum and midbrain region including colliculi.[95,114] In both murine models, neuronal storage and axonal spheroids are very conspicuous. In BALB/c npc^{nih} mice, hypomyelination and myelin degeneration have been reported,[95,115] whereas myelination is well preserved in the C57BLKS/J mice.[114] In the older mice, loss of Purkinje cells and abnormal dendritic arborization of the surviving Purkinje cells are observed.[114,119,120] Ultrastructural features of these storage neurons are closely similar to those described in feline and human NP-C and numerous concentric lamellar inclusions are found in the perikarya. Inclusions are also seen in astrocytes, oligoden-

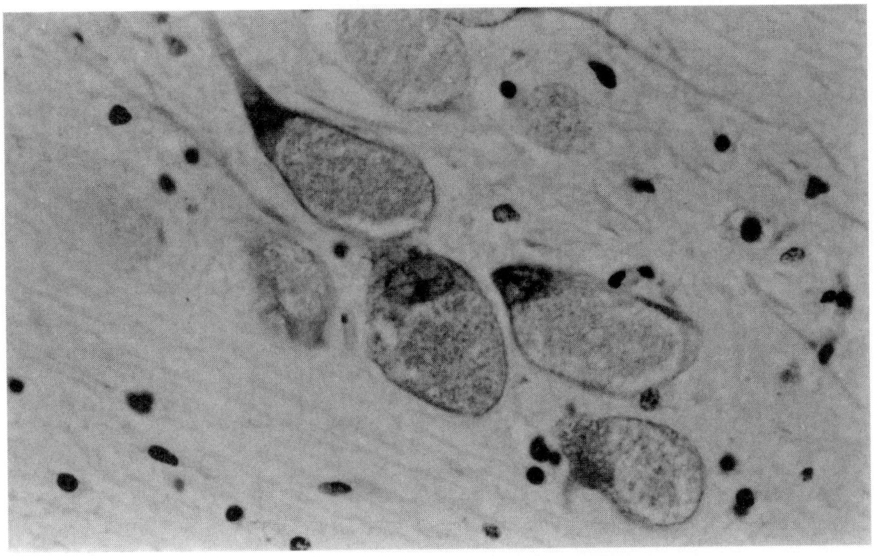

Fig. 145-4 Storage neurons with ballooned perikarya in the substantia nigra (Nissl stain, ×520).

drocytes, microglia, and vascular endothelial cells. Myelination of the spinal roots and peripheral nerves appears normal. However, teased fiber preparations of the sciatic nerve show accumulation of myelin ovoids in practically all paranodal regions of the Schwann cells in BALB/c npc^{nih} mice,[121] but myelin sheaths are reported to be preserved in C57BLKS/J mice.

Pathology in Heterozygotes

In lysosomal storage diseases, heterozygotes are usually normal. However, foamy bone marrow cells and inclusions in skin fibroblasts have been reported in the humans heterozygous for NP-C.[122,123] Furthermore, in feline obligate heterozygotes, occasional polymorphic membranous cytoplasmic inclusions have been reported in hepatocytes, biliary epithelial cells, and Kupffer cells.[124]

PATHOPHYSIOLOGY

Tissue Lipids

Liver and Spleen. A complex lipid storage pattern, with no compound predominating, is observed in liver and spleen in NP-C.[23,26] Apart from a moderate (twofold to fivefold) increase in sphingomyelin and unesterified cholesterol,[1,16,26,54,55,59,75,85,125–127] bis(monoacylglycero)phosphate,[8,23,26, 58,126,127] glucosylceramide,[26,58,59,89,128,129] and, to a lesser extent, other phospholipids and glycolipids accumulate. More lipid accumulates in spleen than in liver,[26] where alterations may be subtle.[9,130] Abnormal lipid storage is already present in the fetus and in fetal liver glucosylceramide accumulates to a greater extent in NP-C than in Gaucher disease.[37,59,94,130,131] Very similar lipid abnormalities have been reported for the murine and feline models.[30,111,132,133]

Brain. Brain lipids have been analyzed in a number of patients with NP-C, without evidence of a pathologic increase in cholesterol or sphingomyelin.[3,5,53,54,75,90,91,126,127,134–139] In cerebral cortex, the sole reported abnormalities pertain to glycolipids.[9,59,90,91,102,127,129,130,137,139–142] The most striking alterations are a many-fold increase of glucosylceramide (up to levels observed in type II Gaucher disease) and of lactosylceramide to the point that one case was initially described as lactosylceramidosis.[11,142] G_{M3} and G_{M2} gangliosides, as well as asialo-G_{M2} ganglioside, are significantly elevated. These alterations are not present in fetal brain and are discrete in the first months of postnatal life.[130,139] In white matter, these abnormalities are less marked but a varying decrease in myelin lipids has been observed.

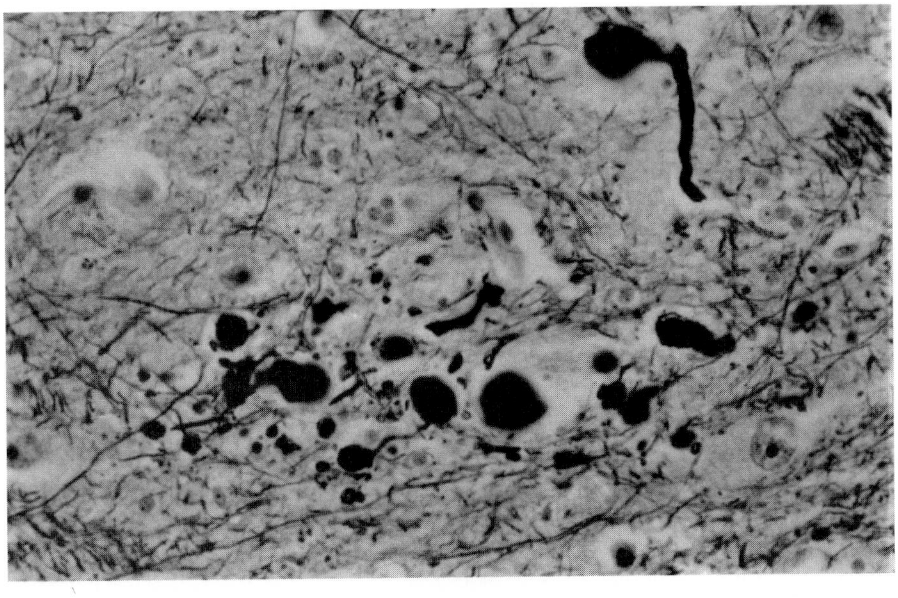

Fig. 145-5 Clustered axonal spheroids in the thalamus (Bielschowsky stain, ×520).

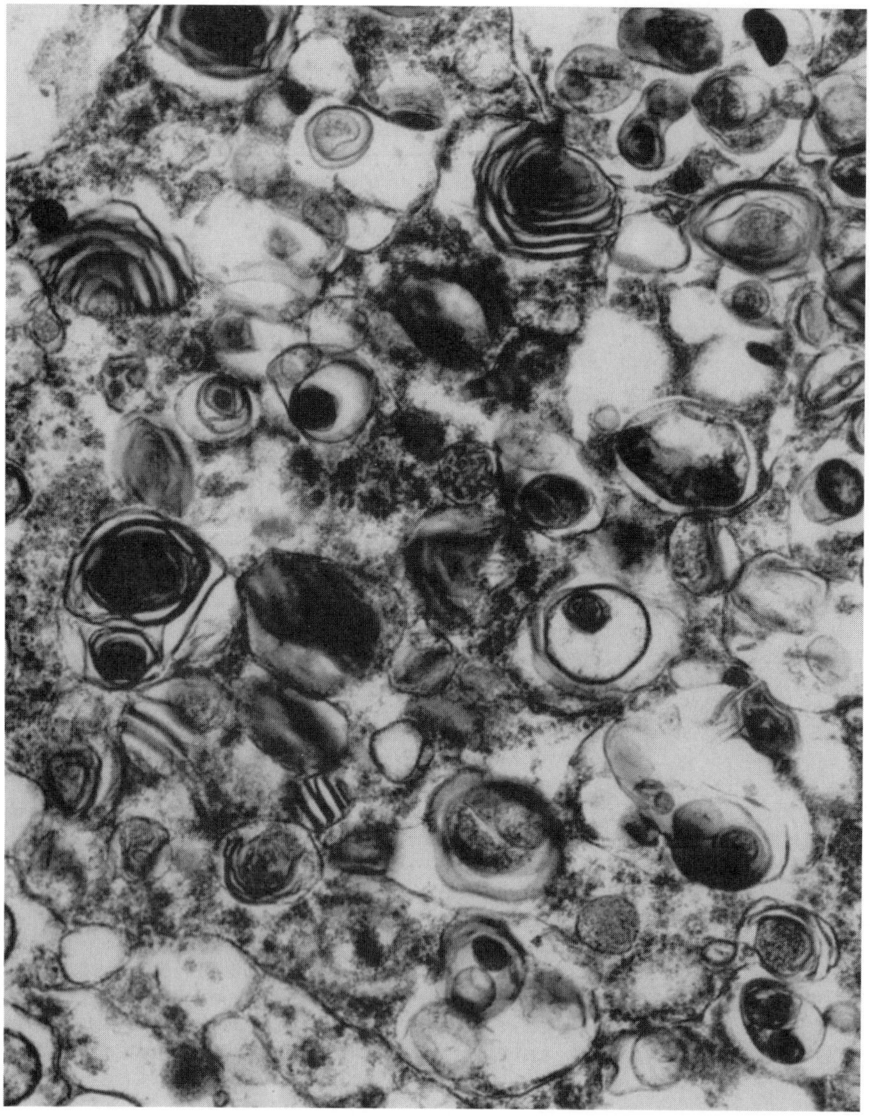

Fig. 145-6 Electron micrograph of polymorphous inclusions (PCBs) in neuronal perikarya (×66,600).

In cases with infantile onset and rapid progression of the neurologic disease, severely decreased galactosylceramide values indicate profound demyelination.[59,130,136,139] Milder changes in galactosylceramide are observed in the juvenile forms.[9,127,130] Phospholipid and cholesterol concentrations are decreased in proportion to the degree of demyelination. The biochemical findings in human NP-C brains parallel those reported for the mutant BALB/c mouse.[115]

Cellular Cholesterol Lipidosis

Elucidation of the cellular basis of NP-C occurred serendipitously in the course of the study of mutant BALB/c mice that, in retrospect, had clear biochemical and pathologic similarities to human NP-C (see "Tissue Lipids" and "Animal Models" above).[30,133] A lesion in the intracellular processing of exogenous cholesterol was demonstrated in this murine model.[29] This led to the seminal discovery that cultured NP-C fibroblasts were also deficient in their ability to synthesize cholesteryl esters during endocytic uptake of LDL[31,32] and stored abnormal amounts of unesterified cholesterol in an intravesicular compartment when cultured in a cholesterol-enriched medium.[33,143,144] Later studies from several laboratories led to more detailed understanding of the disruption in intracellular cholesterol metabolism. The subject has been reviewed by several authors.[145–150]

Internalization of LDL, its subsequent transport to lysosomes, and lysosomal hydrolysis of cholesteryl ester are not impaired in NP-C.[33,151] However, endocytosed cholesterol is sequestered in lysosomes and transport to the plasma membrane and the endoplasmic reticulum (ER) is retarded.[33–35,143,145,147,152–154] There are three principal homeostatic responses following cellular uptake of LDL cholesterol[155] (see Chap. 120): (a) attenuation of *de novo* cholesterol synthesis; (b) depression of receptor-mediated LDL uptake; and (c) activation of cellular cholesterol esterification. All of these are compromised in NP-C fibroblasts[33] (Fig. 145-7), but are normal when the same cells are treated with 25-hydroxycholesterol.[151] This indicates that the defect specifically affects the processing of endocytosed cholesterol and that the ability of the cell to respond is intact. Newly synthesized cholesterol does not appear to pass directly through the lysosome and is not affected by the sterol trafficking error.[35]

The intracellular distribution of cholesterol has been monitored with filipin, a fluorescent probe that forms specific complexes with unesterified cholesterol.[156] In cholesterol-depleted medium, little filipin-fluorescent staining is seen in either normal or NP-C fibroblasts. In normal cells, adding LDL to the medium results in enhanced filipin-cholesterol staining of the plasma membrane and some fluorescent staining of intracellular structures (Fig. 145-8*A*). In contrast, LDL uptake by NP-C cells is marked by striking filipin-cholesterol staining of perinuclear vacuoles (Fig. 145-8*B*), identified immunocytochemically as lysosomes.[34] This lysosomal sequestration of exogenous cholesterol is associated with impaired relocation to the plasma membrane.[34,35]

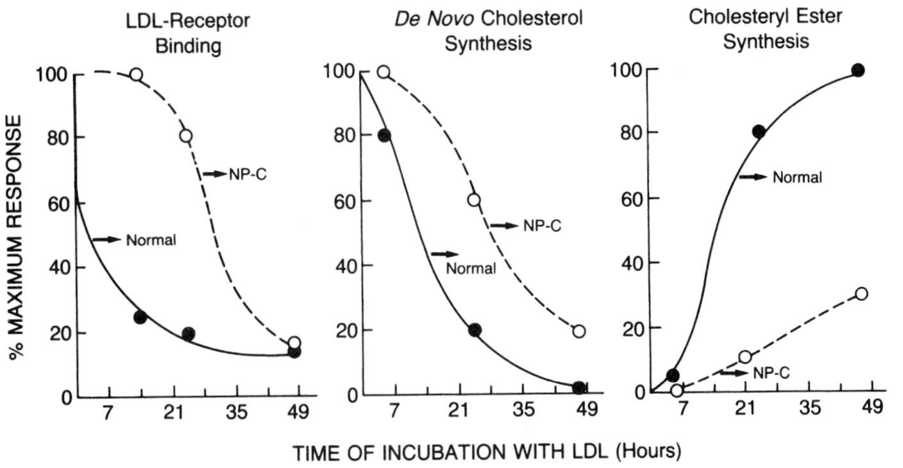

Fig. 145-7 Induction of cholesterol homeostatic responses in fibroblasts cultured with LDL. Normal and NP-C fibroblasts were cultured in lipoprotein-deficient serum to activate the LDL-receptor pathway. Cells were subsequently challenged with LDL to measure their ability to respond to the endocytic uptake and accumulation of the lipoprotein-derived cholesterol. (*Adapted from Pentchev et al.*[33] *Used by permission.*)

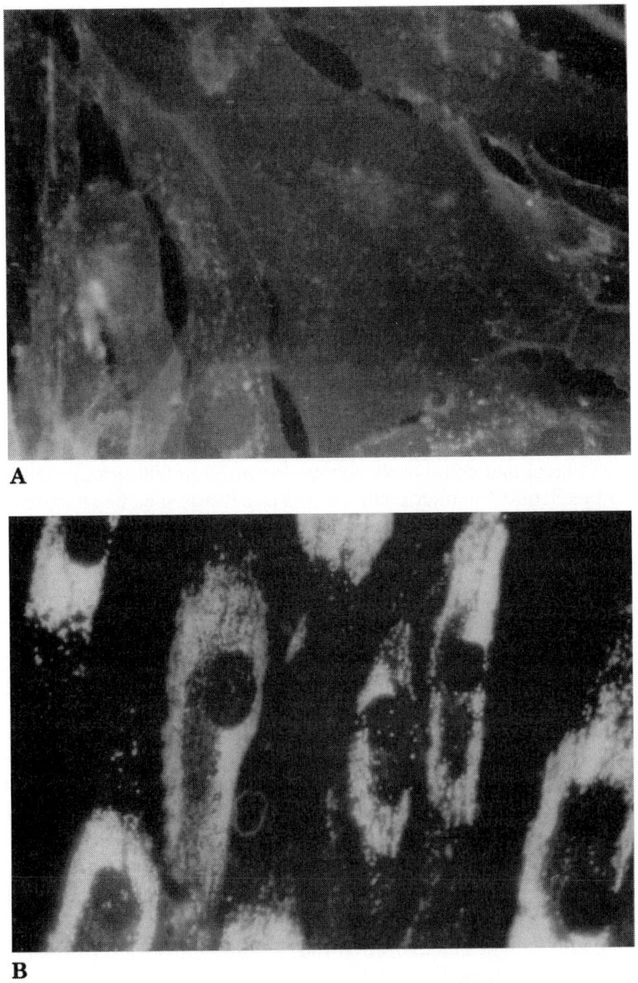

Fig. 145-8 Filipin-stained localization of unesterified cholesterol in fibroblasts cultured with LDL. Cholesterol-depleted normal (*A*) and NP-C (*B*) fibroblasts were cultured with LDL (50 mg/ml) for 24 h. Cells were subsequently fixed and stained with filipin to fluorescently label the intracellular distribution of LDL-derived cholesterol. *A*, In normal cells, cholesterol accumulation was associated with some enhanced filipin staining of the perinuclear area and the plasma membrane. *B*, In comparably treated NP-C cells, the cholesterol distribution reflected intense filipin staining of perinuclear vacuoles and reduced fluorescence of the plasma membrane. (*Courtesy of Dr. Joan Blanchette-Mackie.*)

In control fibroblasts, cholesterol egress from lysosomes may be compromised by hydrophobic amines (U-18666A, imipramine, natural sphingoid bases),[156–158] by progesterone,[159] or by inhibitors of H^+-ATPase such as bafilomycin.[160] The two first pharmacologic models have been widely used to study cellular trafficking of LDL-cholesterol.

The cellular consequences of the NP-C lesion may be traced in this order: the primary mutation leads to lysosomal sequestration of endocytosed cholesterol, to delayed induction of homeostatic regulation, and to cellular cholesterol lipidosis. The cellular distribution of cholesterol follows the descending concentration gradient: plasma membrane to endosomes to *trans*-Golgi to *cis*-Golgi to smooth endoplasmic reticulum to rough endoplasmic reticulum. The existence of this gradient implies the presence of specific trafficking mechanisms for its creation and maintenance. Exogenous cholesterol in the form of LDL enters the cell by receptor-mediated uptake,[155] and the endocytosed lipoproteins are targeted to lysosomes for hydrolysis of proteins and cholesteryl esters.[155] The mechanism of cholesterol efflux from lysosomes and transport to other sites in the cell is not well defined. Transfer of cholesterol to the plasma membrane from lysosomes appears rapid and constitutive,[161,162] but the route of trafficking is still under investigation. There is evidence for a plasma membrane-independent pathway from lysosomes to endoplasmic reticulum.[163,164] Bidirectional circulation between lysosome and plasma membrane has been suggested.[165] The NP-C mutation has provided compelling evidence that the Golgi complex plays an active role in the transport of lysosomal cholesterol to other cellular membranes.[148,150,163,166] Filipin staining of NP-C cells following LDL uptake has revealed unusually early staining of cholesterol in the Golgi apparatus in addition to lysosomal cholesterol accumulation.[153] High-resolution electron microscopy of such cells subjected to freeze-fracture cytochemistry has shown accumulation of cholesterol in the *trans*-Golgi cisternae and deficient cholesterol relocation to *cis*-medial cisternae and adjacent condensing vacuoles.[166]

It is not known if cholesterol first accumulates in the lysosome or the Golgi complex. Although the bulk of endocytosed unesterified cholesterol accumulates in lysosomes, the primary trafficking block in NP-C could affect cholesterol transport simultaneously at several organelles. Alternatively, block at an obligatory transport step at the Golgi complex could account for an upstream accumulation of cholesterol in the lysosomes. Indeed, disruption of this organelle by brefeldin-A redirects the flow of lysosomal cholesterol from the plasma membrane to the endoplasmic reticulum.[163] The abnormal distribution of cholesterol in the Golgi complex may therefore be linked to the finding that lysosomal cholesterol movement to the plasma membrane is retarded in NP-C cells.[35,163]

Notwithstanding these documented errors in cellular LDL cholesterol metabolism in cultured cells, the plasma lipoprotein profile of NP-C patients is normal. A recent study has, however, reported that intracellular trafficking of LDL-derived cholesterol is also defective in vivo in such patients.[167] Males with NP-C and same-sex controls were given [^{14}C]mevalonate intravenously, as a tracer of *de novo* synthesized cholesterol, in addition to [^{3}H]cholesteryl linoleate in LDL to monitor lipoprotein-derived sterol. The release of unesterified [^{14}C]cholesterol into the plasma and bile was normal in controls. In marked contrast, the appearance of LDL-derived [^{3}H]cholesterol in the plasma and bile was retarded in the affected individuals. The relative extent to which cholesterol transfer was delayed in the three NP-C patients correlated with the degree to which LDL cholesterol metabolism was affected in cultured fibroblasts derived from these same individuals. The kinetic data obtained in this fashion can be analyzed by compartmentalized modeling to provide a measure of both the size and turnover of the NP-C-induced cholesterol pools in vivo. This may provide a measurable endpoint for therapeutic interventions, if indeed extraneural cholesterol storage is relevant to disease progression (see "Treatment" below).

Sphingolipid Metabolism

Early studies attempted to link the NP-C mutation to a deficiency of sphingomyelin catabolism (see "History" above). Levels of sphingomyelinase activity are normal or elevated in tissues and leukocytes of NP-C patients.[20,75,126,127,131,168] In cultured fibroblasts, partial deficiency of sphingomyelinase activity[86,168,169] with decreased degradation of exogenous sphingomyelin[170–172] is found, albeit inconsistently.[52,171] It has been shown convincingly that depression of sphingomyelinase activity in NP-C-cultured fibroblasts is a secondary and reversible consequence of excessive cholesterol sequestration.[36,173] Glucosylceramidase activity is not decreased in solid tissues but often shows partial deficiency in cultured cells.[174] In contrast to human patients, solid tissues from the murine models show partial deficiencies of both sphingomyelinase and glucosylceramidase.[30,132]

G_{M2} ganglioside accumulates in lysosomes of cultured cells of patients, in spite of normal in vitro activities of hexosaminidase A.[175] There was evidence of an increased rate of biosynthesis, and accumulation occurred independently of the LDL-cholesterol uptake. Impaired cellular transport of G_{M2} ganglioside in NP-C has been suggested as a mechanism for this observation.[175–177] Nevertheless, the explanation for the storage of several glycolipids, all with a short oligosaccharide chain, in human tissues (especially brain) remains elusive, and is an area of continuing investigation.

Another intriguing observation is the many-fold elevation of free sphingoid long-chain bases, shown both in the BALB/c mouse model[178] and in human patients' tissues and cultured cells, that is apparently not modulated by LDL.[179]

Other Biochemical Abnormalities

An as yet totally unexplained observation is the deficient ferritin immunoreactivity demonstrated in liver and spleen of NP-C patients.[180,181] Some abnormal features described in the BALB/c mouse model, such as increased dolichol phosphate[182] or partial decrease of some peroxisomal β-oxidation enzymes and catalase activity in brain and liver,[183] have not been investigated in humans. One NP-C patient from a highly consanguineous family was described with additional defective peroxisomal β-oxidation of branched-chain substrates,[184] but the most likely explanation was that the patient was expressing mutations in two separate genes. Very long chain fatty acids in plasma studied in 6 NP-C patients showed normal results (Vanier, unpublished data).

Some other reported abnormalities most likely pertain to the alterations in trafficking of membrane lipids. Cystine has been shown to accumulate in lysosomes of tissues and cultured cells from both the murine BALB/c model and human NP-C, possibly as a consequence of cholesterol storage.[185] Other observations made by individual groups include high levels of caveolin-1 expression observed in liver of heterozygote mutant BALB/c mice[186] or fibroblasts of NP-C heterozygotes,[187] defective processing of apolipoprotein D found in astrocytes of the BALB/c mutant mouse,[188] and the decrease in membrane fluidity observed in cultured cells from the C57BLKS/J mouse model and from human patients.[189]

Two observations suggest some impairment of cell signaling in NP-C: the attenuated elevation of cytoplasmic calcium concentration following LDL uptake[190] and the correlation between free sphingosine levels and inhibition of phorbol dibutyrate binding in NP-C cells.[191] Alterations in neurotransmitters (serotonin, glycine, glutamate, and GABA) have also been described in the cerebellum and cortex of the BALB/c mouse model.[192]

MOLECULAR GENETICS

Genetic Heterogeneity in NP-C

The 11 patients included in the initial cell hybridization study were found to belong to the same complementation group,[69] but subsequent work[40] disclosed the existence of a minor second complementation group. A larger investigation including genetic linkage analysis definitively established that there were two separate genetic loci responsible for NP-C disease.[41] The gene defective in the large majority of NP-C families (approximately 95 percent) has been localized to chromosome 18, cloned, and designated *NPC1* (see "Identification of the *NPC1* Gene" below). The *NPC2* gene, defective in, at most, 5 percent of NP-C families (only six separate families known to date), has not yet been mapped or identified. Crossbreeding[193] and complementation[194] experiments in the C57BLKS/J and the BALB/c murine models have shown that both have allelic mutations and belong to the same complementation group as human *NPC1*.

The phenotypes of patients belonging to the two complementation groups have been thoroughly studied. Half of the patients in the *NPC2* group had suffered from the rare, rapidly fatal form with prominent lung involvement.[41] Apart from this fact, variability in the clinical and cellular phenotypes occurred in both groups, and no biochemical marker could be found that was specific to one of the groups.[41,175] This strongly suggests that the two respective gene products may function in tandem or sequentially.[41,43]

Identification of the *NPC1* Gene

The *NPC1* gene was identified through human positional cloning with the aid of the NP-C murine models. The studies of human NP-C have consistently paralleled characterization of the murine disease. In 1991, investigators linked the murine NP-C mutation in the *spm* mouse model to chromosome 18.[38] Human genomic regions that were syntenic to mouse chromosome 18 included portions of human chromosomes 5 and 18. Thirty-one stringently diagnosed NP-C families participated in a linkage study that mapped the NP-C gene to the pericentromeric region of chromosome 18.[42,43] Microcell transfer of human chromosome 18 into NP-C mouse derived 3T3 cells resulted in the restoration of cholesterol transport.[39] Linkage studies in Nova Scotia Niemann-Pick disease type D localized to 18q11, confirming that type C and type D were allelic.[195]

The NP-C critical interval on chromosome 18 was refined through genetic examination of an extended pedigree of Bedouin Arab descent, which exhibited extensive consanguinity, suggesting a homoallelic mutation. Within this family a genetic recombination narrowed the *NPC1* interval to a 1-cM region defined by markers D18S44 to D18S1388.[43] The NP-C interval was further characterized with a yeast artificial chromosome (YAC) physical map consisting of three overlapping genomic clones. These genomic clones were introduced into NP-C-like mutant CHO cells via spheroplast fusion.[196] One of the three YACs comple-

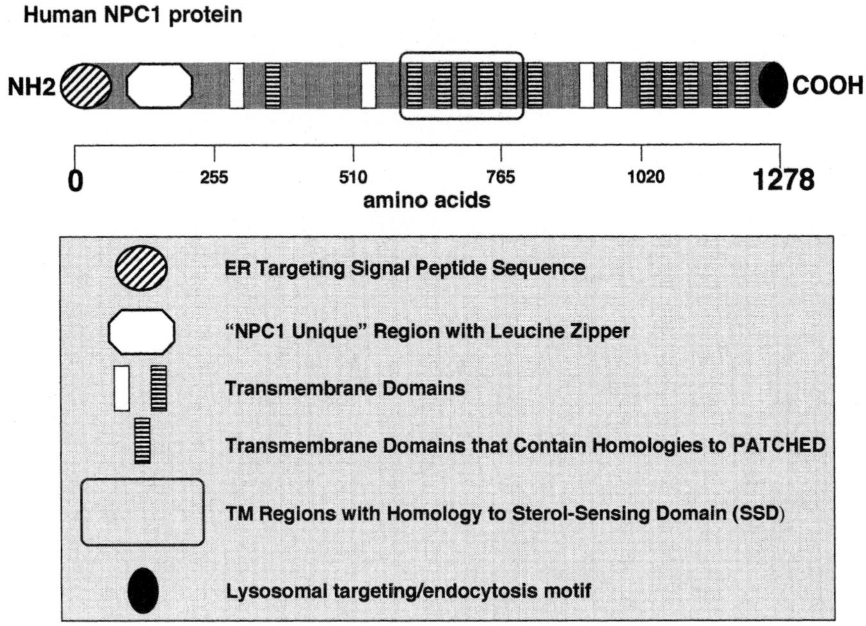

Fig. 145-9 Structure of the human NPC1 protein.

mented the NP-C phenotype. Transcripts were identified within the YAC-defined interval through sequence, exon trapping, and database analyses. The *NPC1* gene was identified based on mutation analysis of affected individuals as well as the ability to rescue the normal phenotype with the introduction of the NP-C cDNA into cultured human NP-C cells.[43] Identification of a major deletion in the murine ortholog confirmed the character of the npc^{nih} murine model.[44] The cloned human NP-C transcript was 4673 bp in length.[43]

Translation of the open-reading frame of the *NPC1* gene predicts a protein of 1278 amino acids with a molecular weight of 142 kDa. Based on amino acid sequence analysis, the NPC1 protein is predicted to be an integral membrane protein with 13 to 16 putative transmembrane domains (Fig. 145-9). The N-terminus contains a peptide sequence associated with targeting to the endoplasmic reticulum. At the C-terminus, there is a lysosomal/endocytic-targeting signal (LLNF). Amino acids 73 to 94 comprise a leucine zipper motif. This lies within a region from amino acids 55 to 165 that has high homology with other *NPC1* orthologs. A potential tyrosine phosphorylation site is located at amino acid 506. The human and mouse NPC1 proteins have 14 potential glycosylation sites. The NPC1 human protein has high homology (percent identity/percent similarity) to other NP-C orthologs: mouse (85/93), yeast *Saccharomyces cerevisiae* (34/57), and the nematode *Caenorhabditis elegans* (30/55).[43]

NPC1 has extensive homology to Patched. This homology lies within 12 of the 16 predicted transmembrane domains of NPC1.[197] Patched is the defective protein in basal cell nevus syndrome; it is also known to be involved in the Sonic hedgehog signaling pathway. The significance of this homology has yet to be defined.

The NPC1 protein also has homology to other proteins that are involved in cholesterol homeostasis. Within a five-transmembrane region of amino acids 615 to 797, there is significant homology to the sterol-sensing domains of HMG-Co A reductase, involved in cholesterol synthesis, and to the sterol regulatory element-binding protein (SREBP) cleavage-activating protein, SCAP, an activator of a transcription factor in cholesterol biosynthesis.[198,199] The sterol-sensing domains of these proteins are thought to be involved in their regulation based on the levels of sterols within the cell. It is not known whether cholesterol binds to this domain.

NP-C is a panethnic disorder with only two described founder populations, French Acadians in Nova Scotia[1,3,200] and Spanish Americans in Colorado.[86] Outside of these populations, ongoing studies in several laboratories found that a majority of patients have private mutations and are compound heterozygotes, which will complicate genotype/phenotype correlations. Eight mutations in nine unrelated individuals were defined for the identification of the *NPC1* gene, including two deletions, one insertion, and five missense mutations.[43] Mutations in the Japanese populations from 11 unrelated NP-C families have been identified, of which 2 are splicing errors.[201] The mutation in the French Acadian population of Nova Scotia has been recognized as a missense mutation.[200]

Murine Mutations

The npc^{nih} murine mutation is an insertion of an 824-bp retrotransposon-like sequence along with a 703-bp deletion of the genomic sequence consisting of 44 bp of exon sequence and 659 bp of intron sequence.[44] The resulting *NPC1* transcript has a frameshift mutation resulting in a truncated protein that is one-third the size of the NP-C protein, and that excludes 11 of the 13 transmembrane domains and the putative sterol-sensing domain. The availability of genotyping enhances the value of the npc^{nih} mouse for the study of NP-C.

CURRENT RESEARCH

The identification of the *NPC1* gene (see "Molecular Genetics" above) and its protein product promises to provide further insights into the mechanisms governing lysosomal cholesterol mobilization, and other aspects of intracellular lipid trafficking. In one study, polyclonal antiserum to a C-terminal region (amino acid residues 1256 to 1274) of the NPC1 protein has been used in immunocytochemical studies to determine its intracellular localization in cultured human fibroblasts.[202] In control cells, as well as NP-C cells whose mutations do not affect the expression of this particular epitopic region, NPC1 colocalizes with lysosome-associated membrane protein (lamp)-positive vesicles in the perinuclear region of the cell (Fig. 145-10*A*, *B*, and *C*). These vesicles are distinct and separate from the lamp-positive vesicles in which cholesterol accumulates after LDL uptake (Fig. 145-10*B*, and *C*). This segregated distribution of NPC1 and endocytosed cholesterol into separate lamp-positive vesicles is abolished when drugs are added that block lysosomal cholesterol egress.[202] The addition of the hydrophobic amine U-18666A[156] to cultured fibroblasts during the endocytic uptake of LDL causes both cholesterol and NPC1 to accumulate in the same lamp-positive vesicles (Fig. 145-10*D* and *E*). This altered relocation of NPC1 into cholesterol-engorged lysosomes suggests that NPC1 vesicles

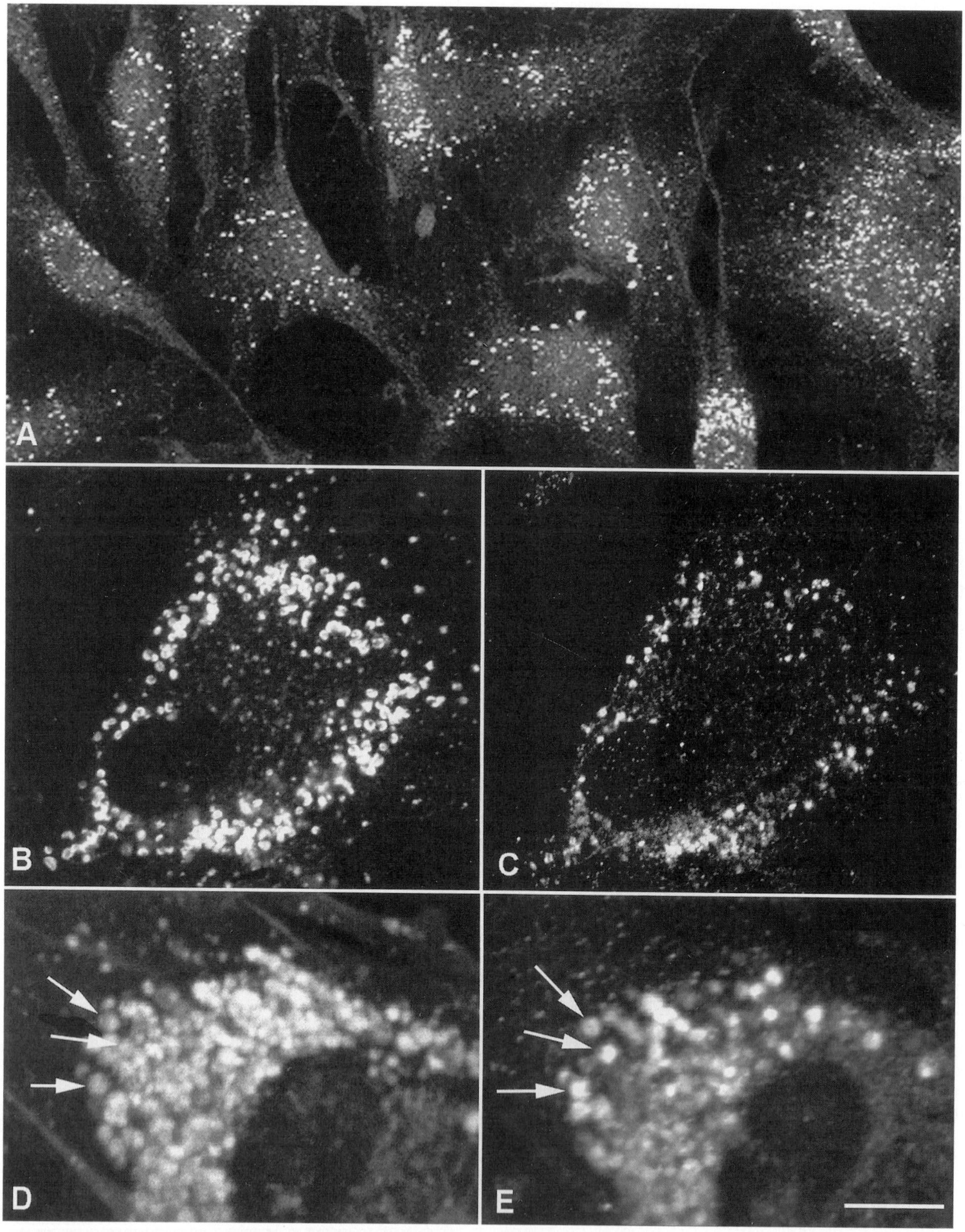

Fig. 145-10 *A*, Control human fibroblasts incubated with LDL for 24 h, immunostained with antipeptide antibodies to the C-terminus of NPC1 protein, and viewed with confocal fluorescence microscopy. NPC1 immunofluorescence is present in small granules that are distributed throughout the cytoplasm of cells.

B and *C*, Control fibroblast incubated with LDL for 24 h and immunostained with both (*B*) antibodies to a lysosomal membrane glycoprotein (lamp1) and (*C*) antipeptide antibodies to the C-terminus of NPC1 protein. The colocalization shows that NPC1 protein (*C*) is present in lamp1-positive vesicles (*B*). Note that there are many lamp1-positive lysosomes that do not contain NPC1 protein.

D and *E*, Control fibroblast incubated with LDL and U18666A for 24 h. U18666A causes an accumulation of unesterified cholesterol in lysosomes and Golgi of control cells similar to the cholesterol lipidosis in NP-C cells. Cells were stained with both filipin (*D*), to visualize unesterified cholesterol, and immunostained with (*E*) antipeptide antibodies to the C-terminus of NPC1 protein. After drug treatment NPC1 protein (*E* at arrows) is present in cholesterol-containing lysosomes (*D* at arrows). Bar = 10 μm. See Color Plate 7.

normally interact transiently with the cholesterol-enriched lysosomes to affect a relocation of this sterol pool. Further characterization of these NPC1 vesicles remains a focal point of current research.

Recent studies in NP-C cells show that the cellular defect encompasses a more global transport error than targeted disruption of cholesterol trafficking alone. Because a majority of lysosomal cholesterol relocates to the plasma membrane,[203] intracellular routing of endocytosed cholesterol can be viewed, at least in part, as tracing a retroendocytic vesicular pathway in which lysosomal components are transported to the plasma membrane.[204] This consideration encouraged a reevaluation of the trafficking defect in NP-C. Measurement of the cellular egress of an endocytosed fluid phase maker ([^{14}C]sucrose) was carried out in cultured control and NP-C fibroblasts to study trafficking through this retroendocytic vesicular pathway.[202] A discernible delay in the loss of [^{14}C]sucrose from the monolayers of NP-C fibroblasts was noted. Compartmentalized kinetic modeling of the data suggests that the difference in [^{14}C]sucrose clearance from normal and NP-C cells can be accounted for by delayed movement from a vacuolar compartment separate from, but in direct communication with, the mature lysosomes. The extent of delayed movement of sucrose through this NP-C targeted compartment (50 percent of normal)[202] closely approximates the measured delays in cholesterol relocation from lysosomes to the plasma membrane in NP-C cells.[35,163]

A model for the intracellular distribution of lysosomal cholesterol can be proposed based on these and other data. Mobilization of a majority of the lysosomal cholesterol to other membranes is likely to occur through a vesicular-mediated pathway because both specific-drug perturbations[164] and critical temperature transitions[202] known to affect vesicular trafficking markedly suppress sterol movement. Several inferences can be drawn from the [^{14}C]sucrose egress studies. The data strongly reinforce the notion of vesicular-mediated sterol trafficking because the vesicular-dependent clearance of sucrose is defective to the same extent as cholesterol in NP-C cells. That *NPC1* mutations affect the intracellular trafficking of two substances as disparate as sucrose and cholesterol suggests that the primary functional defect may target a vesicular trafficking pathway shared by these two substances. This, in turn, suggests that metabolites other than cholesterol might assume the role of offending metabolites in cells where their trafficking between the lysosomes and plasma membranes is of major physiologic significance. Solid tissues and cultured cells in NP-C contain a heterogeneous profile of accumulating material that includes several lipids in addition to cholesterol (see "Tissue Lipids" above). The possibility of alternate metabolites may explain the absence of cholesterol accumulation in the brain in humans or animals with NP-C (see "Tissue Lipids" above). Cholesterol for synthesis of myelin appears to be made locally, not imported into brain.[205] The brain in vivo has little capacity or opportunity to metabolize lipoproteins rich in cholesterol through receptor-mediated endocytosis targeted to lysosomal processing.[206] On the other hand, gray matter from NP-C brains shows extensive accumulation of glycolipids (see "Tissue Lipids" above) that are normal components of the plasma membrane[207,208] and are enriched in this organ. It might be hypothesized that the NP-C lesion leads to impaired vesicular trafficking that in turn results in cholesterol accumulation in peripheral tissues and glycolipid accumulation in the brain, where G_{M2} in particular may play an important role in pathogenesis.[209,210]

DIAGNOSIS

Accurate diagnosis of NP-C requires recognition of the many clinical phenotypes, narrowing of the differential diagnosis by the use of ancillary testing, and final confirmation by biochemical testing. The *NPC1* gene has been cloned, but to date, the majority of affected individuals are compound heterozygotes with private mutations. Thus, molecular diagnosis is not a suitable tool for

Table 145-2 Differential Diagnosis of NP-C

Clinical manifestations	Alternative diagnosis
Severe neonatal jaundice	Biliary atresia, congenital infections, α_1-antitrypsin deficiency, tyrosinemia
Isolated splenomegaly	Leukemia, lymphoma, histiocytosis, storage diseases (e.g., Gaucher, NP-A, NP-B), infections (e.g., malaria)
VSGP	G_{M2} gangliosidosis, mitochondrial diseases, glycine encephalopathy, maple syrup urine disease, dorsal midbrain syndrome
School difficulty	Attention-deficit disorder, learning disabilities, absence seizures, other dementing illnesses
Dystonia	Idiopathic torsion dystonia, doparesponsive dystonia, Wilson disease, amino and organic acidopathies (e.g., glutaric aciduria type 1), G_{M2} gangliosidosis
Dementia	Pseudodementia (depressive disorder), neuronal ceroid lipofuscinosis, subacute sclerosing panencephalitis, HIV encephalopathy
Cataplexy	Other sleep disorders, seizures, syncope, periodic paralysis

Modified with permission from Schiffmann.[247]

primary diagnosis, although it holds great promise for improvements in antenatal diagnosis and identification of heterozygotes in probands' families.

The known clinical presentations of NP-C are protean (see "Clinical Manifestations" above). The differential diagnosis is broad (see 145-2). A frequent clinical conundrum is posed by the classification of individuals with hepatosplenomegaly and foam cells in the bone marrow. Such individuals could have NP-B, but also NP-C prior to the onset of neurologic symptoms. Sphingomyelinase always shows a normal activity in leukocytes of NP-C patients, so this assay can be used to exclude sphingomyelinase-deficient types of NPD. Depression of fibroblast sphingomyelinase in NP-C is variable, but not as pronounced as in NP-B. The blood count, biochemical profile, plasma lipids, urinalysis, and cerebrospinal fluid (cells, glucose, and protein) are normal in NP-C, except in patients with hypersplenism or cholestatic jaundice.

Imaging and neurophysiologic studies are nonspecific. MRI and CT scans may be normal or show atrophy, in particular cerebellar atrophy. Changes in the periventricular white matter have been seen in some cases.[99] Proton magnetic resonance spectroscopic imaging (MRSI) in 10 patients has shown evidence of diffuse brain involvement in NP-C, beyond that apparent on routine imaging studies.[211] Patients with NP-C had significantly decreased N-acetylaspartate (NA)/creatine plus phosphocreatine (Cre) ratios in the frontal and parietal cortices, centra semiovale, and caudate, and significantly increased choline/Cre in the frontal cortex and centra semiovale, when compared to controls. The authors also noted some correlation between proton MRSI findings and clinical stage of disease as previously defined.[57] One earlier study had included a single patient who showed loss of an abnormal lipid peak on proton MRS at 13 and 19 months of cholesterol-lowering therapy.[212] Owing to differences in technique, this case cannot be readily compared to the more recent series.

The electroencephalogram may show diffuse slowing or a variety of epileptiform discharges. The latter do not always correlate with the occurrence of seizures. Central conduction times may be slowed in somatosensory and visual evoked potentials.[213] The audiologic profile, in particular the acoustic reflex, may provide evidence of brain stem dysfunction early in the course of the illness.[214] Changes in the brain stem auditory-evoked response begin with inversion of the wave V:I amplitude ratio, followed by increase in the wave I to V interpeak latency, progressing, finally, to loss of late wave forms.

Several characteristic pathologic findings have been described (see "Pathology" above). Foam cells and sea-blue histiocytes have been detected in many tissues in NP-C, but they are nonspecific.[215] Failure to demonstrate these cells in biopsies does not rule out the diagnosis of NP-C. Cases have been reported in which bone marrow biopsy was initially unrevealing,[216] only to show storage cells when the test was repeated years later.[217] Ultrastructural studies of tissue biopsies are more specific than light microscopy, and may strongly support the diagnosis of NP-C.[99,218] In early onset cases in which a liver biopsy is performed, the diagnosis of NP-C can rapidly be confirmed using as little as 5 mg of frozen tissue analyzed by thin-layer chromatography of the lipids.

Biochemical Diagnosis

The diagnosis of NP-C should no longer rely on histopathologic or tissue lipid findings alone. The discovery of abnormal LDL-cholesterol processing has established the rationale for specific biochemical testing.[32,144] The tests are usually performed on cultured fibroblasts,[32,36,88,110,219,220] although lymphocytes have been used.[221] To date, the diagnosis is best achieved by the concomitant demonstration of (a) intralysosomal accumulation of unesterified cholesterol as shown by a characteristic pattern of intense perinuclear fluorescence after challenge with LDL-enriched medium and staining with filipin (Fig. 145-8*B*), and (b) abnormal intracellular cholesterol homeostasis as defined by impaired LDL-induced cholesterol esterification.[36,60,220] A majority of NP-C cell lines (approximately 80 percent) express profound alterations of cholesterol homeostasis (classical biochemical phenotype),[32,36,52,88,110,223] but some have milder changes, especially in their esterification ability (intermediate and variant phenotypes).[36,52,130,154,219,220,224,225] The filipin test is more sensitive than cholesterol esterification assays in detecting patients with the variant phenotype.[36,60,154,220,226] Filipin staining also increases specificity because impairment of cholesterol esterification may be found in other disorders such as acid lipase deficiency, familial hypercholesterolemia, and I-cell disease. The filipin pattern in I-cell disease is abnormal, but can be differentiated from NP-C in expert hands.[36,227] In the experience of one author (M.T.V.), slight lysosomal cholesterol storage may be seen in cells from patients with sphingomyelinase-deficient types of Niemann-Pick disease.

In comprehensive investigations, no strict correlation has been observed between the severity of alteration in intracellular cholesterol homeostasis and the clinical phenotype, especially in the late infantile and juvenile onset forms.[69,74,220] A trend for adult onset patients to show a "variant" biochemical phenotype has been reported.[74] On the other hand, a consistent biochemical phenotype has been the rule within a sibship.[36,84]

More than half the obligate heterozygotes tested show a level of LDL-induced lysosomal cholesterol accumulation and possibly of cholesterol esterification intermediate between normal individuals and affected homozygotes.[36,52,74,143,220] Abnormalities in a few cases may be as pronounced as in some "variant" patients.[226] The remaining heterozygotes overlap with controls. Thus, generalized NP-C carrier screening using this strategy is not possible. Typical storage cells in bone marrow or inclusions in skin biopsies have been reported in a few parents of children with NP-C.[122,123]

Provided marked abnormalities (classical phenotype) have been demonstrated in the index case, similar tests can be used for prenatal detection of affected fetuses using cultured chorionic villus cells or amniotic fluid cells.[37,228] Because some heterozygotes may show significant alterations, prior study of both parents is advisable. By the summer of 1998, at least 150 at-risk pregnancies had been monitored in our laboratories and in those of Drs. D. Wenger, M. Ziegler, A. Fensom, and O. Van Diggelen.

Analysis of the lipids in a frozen liver biopsy (see "Tissue Lipids" above) is generally diagnostic, but occasionally may be inconclusive. Partial deficiency of sphingomyelinase activity in cultured skin fibroblasts is nonspecific and inconstant. Chitotriosidase has been found to be modestly elevated in plasma in several lysosomal diseases, although marked elevations of diagnostic value are seen only in Gaucher disease.[229] The usefulness of this enzyme as a disease marker is diminished by its relatively frequent deficiency in the general population.[230]

Molecular Diagnosis

In NP-C patients belonging to complementation group 1, at least four laboratories have initiated mutational analysis of the *NPC1* gene. In the *NPC1* cloning paper,[43] eight different mutations were reported. Most of the patients were compound heterozygotes. Subsequently, the mutation in the Nova Scotia isolate of NP-C was identified.[200] Preliminary results from the authors' laboratories and the laboratory of Dr. K. Ohno in Japan have shown that a transcript is made in most patients and that mutations occur at various locations of the gene. Most of the mutations appear to be private. A number of polymorphisms have already been observed. Consequently, with current technology, direct molecular diagnosis is not practical and may be misleading, except in specific populations such as the French Acadians in Nova Scotia and the Hispanics from southern Colorado. Nevertheless, identification of the mutation(s) in a demonstrated NP-C case is important for subsequent genetic counseling in the proband's family. Finding the mutations will make prenatal diagnosis possible for the so-called "variant" families, in which biochemical tests were not reliable. In other families, this would permit prenatal diagnosis using uncultured chorionic villi, and thus provide a result a month earlier than traditional biochemical methods. Mutational analysis would also allow accurate heterozygote testing in the proband's family.

TREATMENT

There is no specific treatment for NP-C. The identification of *NPC1* and its predicted protein product will eventually lead to new therapeutic strategies. The *NPC1* gene product appears to be an integral membrane protein, which is not likely to be readily replaced from exogenous sources including tissue transplantation. Indeed, attempts at nonspecific replacement therapy by tissue transplantation have been disappointing. In the C57BLKS/J murine model of NP-C, bone marrow transplantation[231–233] and combined liver and bone marrow transplantation[233] partially reversed tissue storage of cholesterol and sphingomyelin, but did not influence the continued neurologic deterioration.

Liver transplantation in a 7-year-old girl with NP-C and cirrhosis was similarly successful in restoring hepatic function, but failed to slow neurologic progression.[234] There has been one report of transplantation of fetal liver cells into BALB/c mutant mice, with apparent correction of the phenotype in many cells.[235,236] This study, which has not been replicated, must be interpreted cautiously, as it was performed prior to description of the murine ortholog of *NPC1*, so that genotyping of the mice prior to transplantation was not possible. Transplantation of fetal liver cells has been used in two humans.[237] The one patient for whom follow-up was available to us was engrafted twice at the ages of 8.5 and 9 years, without significant improvement of the natural history of the disease. To date, there have been no reports of bone marrow transplantation in human NP-C.

Treatment strategies to reduce intracellular cholesterol accumulation were formulated based on the hypothesis that cholesterol is an offending metabolite in NP-C. Several lines of evidence supported this assumption. Cholesterol is stored in excess in the nonneural tissues in NP-C, and the defect in cholesterol trafficking is closely associated with the primary mutation. Combinations of cholesterol-lowering agents were found to reduce hepatic stores of unesterified cholesterol in NP-C patients,[238] but there is no evidence that their outcome was improved, and several patients who elected to continue the diet long-term have subsequently succumbed to NP-C. There is a case report of a child treated with a cholesterol-lowering regimen in whom serial magnetic resonance spectroscopy studies were interpreted as showing diminution of stored cerebral lipids.[212] Follow-up data have not been published. Cholesterol-lowering drugs may be ineffective in influencing neurologic disease because cholesterol is not an offending metabolite in the brain, or, alternatively, because the agents employed do not penetrate the blood-brain barrier. Dimethyl sulfoxide, which corrects partial sphingomyelinase deficiency[239] and substantially reverses the cholesterol-trafficking abnormalities[240] in NP-C fibroblasts, has been used as a single agent in two patients. Stabilization of neurologic disease was reported in an 8-year-old girl,[241] but a 3-year-old boy showed no apparent benefit.[242]

Regardless of the availability of specific treatments for NP-C, a great deal can be offered to patients and their families in the form of symptomatic management. We found that dystonia and tremor respond to anticholinergic agents in some patients, and seizures can be controlled or diminished in frequency with antiepileptic drugs, at least early in the course of the illness. No controlled studies of the effectiveness of such treatments are available. Protriptyline,[78,79] clomipramine, and modafinil are effective in controlling cataplexy and managing accompanying sleep disturbances.

Therapy to delay or prevent puberty has been proposed as a means of ameliorating the progress of NP-C. The rationale for this approach is based on the observations (a) that progesterone can induce an NP-C like phenotype in control fibroblasts,[159] (b) that progesterone exacerbates the biochemical abnormalities in NP-C fibroblasts,[243] and (c) that symptoms of NP-C often worsen at the time of menarche. Gonadotrophin-releasing hormone analogs have been administered to some girls in an uncontrolled fashion. No data on clinical efficacy are available.

Two siblings with late onset disease, presenting with psychiatric symptoms, were treated with prednisolone with apparent improvement in symptoms, and recurrence of symptoms after steroid withdrawal.[244]

Physical therapists, speech therapists, and occupational therapists should all be involved in the care of the patient with NP-C, in order to address problems in the areas of impaired mobility, contractures, dysarthria, dysphagia, and occupation. Medical therapy notwithstanding, support of the patient and family in the course of NP-C, following long-established principles,[245] is of paramount importance. Counseling services should be available for patients and family members. Support for families with NP-C is available through umbrella organizations for children with inherited or metabolic diseases in many countries. Support groups devoted to Niemann-Pick disease have been established in the U.S. (www.nnpdf.org), the U.K. (www.nnpdf.org/npdg-uk) France (www.aafnp.org), and Germany (www.niemann-pick.de/wirveberuns.html).

Animal models will be critical for future studies of potential therapies. The genotyping of the BALB/c murine model of NP-C will facilitate its use in such experiments. Prior studies focused on reduction or removal of the accumulated offending metabolite. A new approach that has shown promise in the murine model of Tay-Sachs disease is to inhibit synthesis of a known offending metabolite, in this case G_{M2} ganglioside, prior to its accumulation.[246] Given the evidence for the role of G_{M2} ganglioside in NP-C, a trial of this agent (*N*-butyldeoxynojirimycin) in the npc^{nih} mouse may be worthwhile.

ADDENDUM

Since the manuscript for this chapter was submitted, substantial advances have occurred in our knowledge of NP-C. These are summarized in the following paragraphs.

PATHOLOGY

Falk and co-workers[248] investigated developmental expression of the *NPC1* (Npc1) mRNA with a semi-quantitative reverse transcription-polymerase chain reaction (RT-PCR). The transcript was expressed in the cerebellum in vivo and in vitro during early postnatal life, as well as in the adult cerebellum. In in vitro studies, Purkinje cells and some glial cells were immunoreactive to the antibody to anti-Npc1 antibody. They concluded that since Npc1 is expressed at similar levels throughout the development in both neurons and glia, the vulnerability of Purkinje cells in NP-C is likely to involve disruption of an interaction with other developmentally regulated proteins. In mouse brain, Prasad and co-workers[249] detected Npc1 mRNA in neurons as early as embryonic day 15. In this study, the *NPC1* gene was widely expressed in neurons, the highest levels occurring in the cerebellum and pons. The high expression in the cerebellum may account for the vulnerability of the Purkinje cells in NP-C.

Henderson et al.[250] demonstrated that embryonic striatal neurons in primary cultures from npc^{nih} mice can take up LDL-derived cholesterol but with significantly lower hydrolysis and re-esterification than in wild type neurons. Cholesterol is thought to be critical for membrane localization and function of many signaling proteins in membrane domains or "lipid rafts." These cultured NP-C neurons failed to increase neurite outgrowth in response to brain-derived neurotrophic factor (BDNF), in contrast to the response of wild type neurons. Western blotting revealed that Trk receptor expression was similar in striatal neurons from wild type and mutant mice, yet BDNF-induced tyrosine phosphorylation of Trk was essentially eliminated in neurons from npc^{nih} mice. Trk activation was also abolished in cholesterol-depleted wild type neurons. Thus, abnormal cholesterol metabolism occurs in neurons of npc^{nih} mice, even at embryonic stages, and is associated with notable lack of BDNF responsiveness. Given the importance of BDNF in neuronal survival, growth, and differentiation, the lack of BDNF responsiveness might contribute to the loss of neural function in NPC.

In contrast to the diffuse expression reported in rodents, an immunoelectron microscopic investigation of the brains of macaque monkeys found that *NPC1* was expressed predominantly in astrocytic process located in the presynaptic region, rather than in neurons.[251] These investigators also reported that the terminal fields of axons and dendrites were the earliest sites of degeneration in npc^{nih} mice, based on studies with amino-cupric-silver staining. This work remains unconfirmed to date.

Wu and co-workers[252] have found that increasing numbers of neurons were lost by apoptosis in NP-C brains with progression of the disease process in both humans and mice. Apoptosis was demonstrated in Purkinje cells in the cerebellar vermis, in cerebral cortical neurons, and in some cells in the white matter as early as 30 days of age in NP-C mice, prior to detectable neurological symptoms. The numbers of apoptotic cells increased with age.

In NP-C brains, gangliosides G_{M2} and G_{M3} accumulate. The possible role of these accumulated gangliosides in the dysfunction and eventual death of neurons in NP-C was tested by generating double knockout mice. npc^{nih} and GalNAcT -/- mice (that lack the activity of the β-1,4-GalNac transferase responsible for the synthesis of complex gangliosides) were interbred, and the clinical, pathologic, and biochemical characteristics of their double knockout offspring were studied.[253]

Positive stains for filipin and PAS best demonstrate neuronal storage in npc^{nih} mice. Neither filipin nor PAS stains were positive in the neurons of the double knockout mice, indicating absence of neuronal storage. Electron microscopic study found no neuronal inclusions typical of NP-C, and thin layer chromatography confirmed the absence of G_{M2} and complex gangliosides in the double mutant brain. The double knockout mice showed no improvement of the clinical course or neuronal degeneration compared to npc^{nih} controls. Macrophages and microglia containing cholesterol were still numerous in the brain, and visceral pathology was unchanged. Apoptotic neuronal loss appeared more pronounced and loss of Purkinje cells was clearly observed in the double knockouts by comparison with npc^{nih} controls. The absence of G_{M2} ganglioside storage from conception does not significantly influence the clinical phenotype of the NP-C in this model system.

Animal Models of NP-C

The feline model of NP-C was demonstrated to belong to the *NPC1* complementation group[254] and the generation of mutations of the homologue of *NPC1* in the nematode *C. elegans* has provided a new model system allowing studies of NP-C disease in a thoroughly characterized animal that reproduces rapidly.[255]

PATHOPHYSIOLOGY

Cell Biology

The exact function of the *NPC1* gene product is not yet elucidated and this area is under active investigation by several groups. A clear consensus has yet to emerge, but major findings may be summarized as follows.

Neufeld et al. found that the NPC1 protein was localized to late endosomes immunocytochemically and that the clearance of endocytosed ^{14}C-sucrose as well as cholesterol was defective in NP-C cells studied biochemically.[202] Both general retroendocytic trafficking and mobilization of multiple lysosomal cargo appeared defective at a late endosomal trafficking step. This mechanism would account for the accumulation of multiple lipids in NP-C cells and tissues. Site-directed mutagenesis of the NPC1 protein targeting domains of the protein responsible for its cholesterol transport function caused loss of function.[256] Confocal microscopy of living cells, using an NPC1-green fluorescent chimeric protein, documented an unusual mode of tubular membrane trafficking for the NPC1 endocytic compartment that appears linked to the NPC1 protein and cellular cholesterol content.[257] Using cytochemical techniques, it was found that cellular cholesterol levels modulate the glycolipid profile of the *NPC1* compartment. The results indicate that the *NPC1* compartment serves as a sorting station in the endocytic trafficking of both cholesterol and glycolipids. Enriching the cholesterol content of lysosomes recruits the NPC1 protein into endocytic vesicles containing glycolipids. In the presence of elevated cholesterol levels, certain glycolipids are restricted from entering the lysosomal compartment for degradation and are efficiently recycled in NPC1 sorting vesicles to the plasma membrane. Glycolipids that accumulate in NP-C cells and tissues, such as G_{M2}, are those sorted through the NPC1 compartment, while non-accumulating glycolipids such as CTH and G_{D3} are shown to traffic on to the lysosomes for probable degradation.[257] Other workers have drawn similar conclusions.[258–260]

Studies in CT60 and CT43 CHO mutants[261] disclosed that the initial movements of LDL-derived cholesterol to the plasma membrane did not require participation of the NPC1 protein. The authors concluded that the NPC1 protein cycles cholesterol from an intracellular compartment to the plasma membrane or to the endoplasmic reticulum after (and not prior to) newly hydrolyzed LDL-derived cholesterol appears in the plasma.[261] A further report concluding that cholesterol moves freely from the lysosomes to the plasma membrane in NP-C cells has appeared.[262] The latter authors considered that cholesterol accumulation in NP-C lysosomes results from an imbalance in the brisk flow of cholesterol among membrane compartments. While most authors consider that in NP-C cells, cholesterol essentially accumulates in lysosomes,[202,257,262] two reports conclude that accumulation takes place in late endosomes.[261,263]

Cholesterol balance and metabolism were quite extensively studied in mutant npc^{nih} mice. The cholesterol pool was found to expand continuously from birth in homozygous affected animals.[264] While cholesterol entering tissues through the coated-pit pathway became sequestered in the lysosomal compartment and was metabolically inactive, cholesterol that was newly synthesized or that entered cells through the SR-BI pathway was metabolized and excreted normally.[265,266]

Several reviews have addressed the subject of the role of the NPC1 protein in the broad context of intracellular cholesterol trafficking.[267–269] In general, current opinion favors a key role for the NPC1 protein in modulating vesicular trafficking of both glycolipids and cholesterol.

MOLECULAR GENETICS

NPC1 Gene Organization, NPC1 Protein Structure and Topology, Functional Domains, and *NPC1* Mutations

The genomic organization of *NPC1* is now known. The gene spans greater than 47 kb and contains 25 exons.[270] Key promoter regions have been defined.[270,271] The NPC1 protein appears to be N-glycosylated, and shows a size of 170 and 190 kDa by western blotting, in CT-60 CHO cells transfected with wild-type NPCI [256] or as native protein in human skin fibroblasts.[272] There is further evidence that the NPC1 protein resides in late endosomes and interacts transiently with lysosomes and the *trans*-Golgi network.[258] Topological analysis of NPC1 has revealed that this glycoprotein contains 13 transmembrane domains, 3 large and 4 small luminal loops, 6 small cytoplasmic loops, and a cytoplasmic tail.[273] The putative sterol-sensing domain has the same orientation as those in HMG-CoA reductase and SCAP.[273] Information regarding the functional role of different domains of the protein has been deduced from clinical studies, and by transfection of CT-60 cells with mutant NPC1. The N-terminal domain and the lysosome-targeting motif appear essential for cholesterol mobilization.[274] Mutations in the leucine-zipper motif and sterol-sensing domain inactivate the protein.[256] Homozygote missense mutations in the sterol-sensing domain correlate with a severe infantile neurological onset disease and absence of detectable NPC1 protein.[275,276] Studies in patients revealed that a cluster of mutations was located on the third large luminal, cysteine-rich loop, which is highly conserved in NPC1 orthologues, and has a sequence showing resemblance to the RING finger motif of protein kinase C.[277] This domain was shown to bind zinc[271] and also appears of particular functional interest.

Taking into account recent studies[201,272,275,277,278] and data from seven groups presented in the International Workshop "The Niemann-Pick C lesion and the role of intracellular lipid sorting in human disease" (National Institutes of Health, Bethesda, MD, October 1999), the number of *NPC1* mutations known to date exceeds 100. Mutations have been found widely distributed on the gene (leucine zipper domain excepted), with, however, about 1/3 of them located in the cysteine-rich luminal loop. With few exceptions, most mutations appear to be private. In Caucasians, only one common mutant allele, I1061T, has been identified.[278] This mutation, which in the homozygous state correlates with a juvenile neurological onset form of the disease, constitutes about 15% of alleles in patients of Western European (especially British and French) descent. The same mutation is prevalent in the Hispanic-American isolate of Colorado and New Mexico, suggesting a founder effect.[278] Mutational analysis of the *NPC1* gene is complicated by the large number of polymorphisms already recognized.[201,270]

NPC1 Gene Homologues

By EST screening, a new gene with homology to *NPC1,* named *NPC1L1*, has been isolated. It has been suggested that NPC1 and NPC1L1 form part of a new family of proteins that may have similar functions at different subcellular locations.[279]

TREATMENT

Bone marrow transplantation was performed on an NP-C patient aged 3 years and 5 months. Regression of hepatosplenomegaly and decreased infiltration of foamy macrophages in the bone marrow and lung were described 6 months after the transplant. Predictably, given the nature of the *NPC1* gene product, and the early onset of disease in this patient, neurological status continued to deteriorate, with progressive brain atrophy on serial magnetic resonance imaging (MRI). The authors concluded that bone marrow transplantation is unlikely to be an adequate treatment for NPC.[280]

Erikson et al.[281] reported that modifications of somatic cholesterol do not significantly alter the neurological course in npc^{nih} mice, confirming earlier studies.

REFERENCES

1. Crocker AC, Farber S: Niemann-Pick disease: A review of eighteen patients. *Medicine (Baltimore)* **37**:1, 1958.
2. Niemann A: Ein unbekanntes Krankheitsbild. *Jahrb Kinderheilkd* **79**:1, 1914.
3. Crocker AC: The cerebral defect in Tay-Sachs disease and Niemann-Pick disease. *J Neurochem* **7**:69, 1961.
4. Kidd M: An electron microscopical study of a case of atypical cerebral lipidosis. *Acta Neuropath (Berl)* **9**:70, 1967.
5. Norman RM, Forrester RM, Tingey AH: The juvenile form of Niemann-Pick disease. *Arch Dis Child* **42**:91, 1967.
6. Elfenbein IB: Dystonic juvenile idiocy without amaurosis, a new syndrome. Light and electron microscopic observations of cerebrum. *Johns Hopkins Med J* **123**:205, 1968.
7. De Leon GA, Kaback MM, Elfenbein IB, Percy AK, Brady RO: Juvenile dystonic lipidosis. *Johns Hopkins Med J* **125**:62, 1969.
8. Karpati G, Carpenter S, Wolfe LS, Andermann F: Juvenile dystonic lipidosis: An unusual form of neurovisceral storage disease. *Neurology* **27**:32, 1977.
9. Martin JJ, Lowenthal A, Ceuterick C, Vanier MT: Juvenile dystonic lipidosis (variant of Niemann-Pick disease type C). *J Neurol Sci* **66**:33, 1984.
10. Ashkenazi A, Yarom R, Gutman A, Abrahamov A, Russell A: Niemann-Pick disease and giant cell transformation of the liver. *Acta Paediatr Scand* **60**:285, 1971.
11. Dawson G, Matalon R, Stein RO: Lactosylceramidosis: Lactosylceramide galactosyl hydrolase deficiency and accumulation of lactosylceramide in cultured skin fibroblasts. *J Pediatr* **79**:423, 1971.
12. Neville BG, Lake BD, Stephens R, Sanders MD: A neurovisceral storage disease with vertical supranuclear ophthalmoplegia, and its relationship to Niemann-Pick disease. A report of nine patients. *Brain* **96**:97, 1973.
13. Pons G, Ponsot G, Leveque B, Lyon G: Maladie de surcharge neuroviscérale avec ophtalmoplégie supranucléaire de la verticalité et présence dans le moelle d'histiocytes bleutés ou maladie de Neville. *Ann Pediatr (Paris)* **23**:503, 1976.
14. Cogan DG, Chu FC, Bachman DM, Barranger J: The DAF syndrome. *Neuroophthalmology* **2**:7, 1981.
15. Longstreth WT Jr, Daven JR, Farrell DF, Bolen JW, Bird TD: Adult dystonic lipidosis: Clinical, histologic, and biochemical findings of a neurovisceral storage disease. *Neurology* **32**:1295, 1982.
16. Elleder M, Jirasek A, Vlk J: Adult neurovisceral lipidosis compatible with Niemann-Pick disease type C. *Virchows Arch A Pathol Anat Histopathol* **401**:35, 1983.
17. Dunn HC, Sweeney VP: Progressive supranuclear palsy in an unusual juvenile variant of Niemann-Pick disease [Abstract]. *Neurology* **21**:442, 1971.
18. Grover WD, Naiman JL: Progressive paresis of vertical gaze in lipid storage disease. *Neurology* **21**:896, 1971.
19. Brady RO, Kanfer JN, Mock MB, Fredrickson DS: The metabolism of sphingomyelin. II. Evidence of an enzymatic deficiency in Niemann-Pick disease. *Proc Natl Acad Sci U S A* **55**:366, 1966.
20. Schneider PB, Kennedy EP: Sphingomyelinase in normal human spleens and in spleens from subjects with Niemann-Pick disease. *J Lipid Res* **8**:202, 1967.
21. Callahan JW, Khalil M, Gerrie J: Isoenzymes of sphingomyelinase and the genetic defect in Niemann-Pick disease, type C. *Biochem Biophys Res Commun* **58**:385, 1974.
22. Christomanou H: Niemann-Pick disease, Type C: evidence for the deficiency of an activating factor stimulating sphingomyelin and glucocerebroside degradation. *Hoppe Seylers Z Physiol Chem* **361**:1489, 1980.
23. Harzer K, Anzil AP, Schuster I: Resolution of tissue sphingomyelinase isoelectric profile in multiple components is extraction-dependent: Evidence for a component defect in Niemann-Pick disease type C is spurious. *J Neurochem* **29**:1155, 1977.
24. Poulos A, Hudson N, Ranieri E: Sphingomyelinase in cultured skin fibroblasts from normal and Niemann-Pick type C patients. *Clin Genet* **24**:225, 1983.
25. Fujibayashi S, Wenger DA: Studies on a sphingolipid activator protein (SAP-2) in fibroblasts from patients with lysosomal storage diseases, including Niemann-Pick disease type C. *Clin Chim Acta* **146**:147, 1985.
26. Vanier MT: Biochemical studies in Niemann-Pick disease. I. Major sphingolipids of liver and spleen. *Biochim Biophys Acta* **750**:178, 1983.
27. Besley GT, Hoogeboom AJ, Hoogeveen A, Kleijer WJ, Galjaard H: Somatic cell hybridisation studies showing different gene mutations in Niemann-Pick variants. *Hum Genet* **54**:409, 1980.
28. Elleder M, Jirasek A: Niemann-Pick Disease. Report on a symposium held in Hlava's Institute of Pathology, Charles University, Prague 2nd-3rd September, 1982. *Acta Univ Carol [Med]* **29**:259, 1983.
29. Pentchev PG, Boothe AD, Kruth HS, Weintraub H, Stivers J, Brady RO: A genetic storage disorder in BALB/c mice with a metabolic block in esterification of exogenous cholesterol. *J Biol Chem* **259**:5784, 1984.
30. Pentchev PG, Gal AE, Booth AD, Omodeo-Sale F, Fouks J, Neumeyer BA, Quirk JM, et al.: A lysosomal storage disorder in mice characterized by a dual deficiency of sphingomyelinase and glucocerebrosidase. *Biochim Biophys Acta* **619**:669, 1980.
31. Pentchev PG, Comly ME, Kruth HS, Patel S, Proestel M, Weintroub H: The cholesterol storage disorder of the mutant BALB/c mouse. A primary genetic lesion closely linked to defective esterification of exogenously derived cholesterol and its relationship to human type C Niemann-Pick disease. *J Biol Chem* **261**:2772, 1986.
32. Pentchev PG, Comly ME, Kruth HS, Vanier MT, Wenger DA, Patel S, Brady RO: A defect in cholesterol esterification in Niemann-Pick disease (type C) patients. *Proc Natl Acad Sci U S A* **82**:8247, 1985.
33. Pentchev PG, Comly ME, Kruth HS, Tokoro T, Butler J, Sokol J, Filling-Katz M, et al.: Group C Niemann-Pick disease: faulty regulation of low-density lipoprotein uptake and cholesterol storage in cultured fibroblasts. *FASEB J* **1**:40, 1987.
34. Sokol J, Blanchette-Mackie J, Kruth HS, Dwyer NK, Amende LM, Butler JD, Robinson E, et al.: Type C Niemann-Pick disease. Lysosomal accumulation and defective intracellular mobilization of low density lipoprotein cholesterol. *J Biol Chem* **263**:3411, 1988.
35. Liscum L, Ruggiero RM, Faust JR: The intracellular transport of low density lipoprotein-derived cholesterol is defective in Niemann-Pick type C fibroblasts. *J Cell Biol* **108**:1625, 1989.
36. Vanier MT, Rodriguez-Lafrasse C, Rousson R, Gazzah N, Juge MC, Pentchev PG, Revol A, et al.: Type C Niemann-Pick disease: Spectrum of phenotypic variation in disruption of intracellular LDL-derived cholesterol processing. *Biochim Biophys Acta* **1096**:328, 1991.
37. Vanier MT, Rodriguez-Lafrasse C, Rousson R, Mandon G, Boue J, Choiset A, Peyrat MF, et al.: Prenatal diagnosis of Niemann-Pick type C disease: Current strategy from an experience of 37 pregnancies at risk. *Am J Hum Genet* **51**:111, 1992.
38. Sakai Y, Miyawaki S, Shimizu A, Ohno K, Watanabe T: A molecular genetic linkage map of mouse chromosome 18, including *spm*, Grl-1, Fim-2/c-fms, and Mpb. *Biochem Genet* **29**:103, 1991.
39. Kurimasa A, Ohno K, Oshimura M: Restoration of the cholesterol metabolism in 3T3 cell lines derived from the sphingomyelinosis mouse (*spm*/*spm*) by transfer of a human chromosome 18. *Hum Genet* **92**:157, 1993.
40. Steinberg SJ, Ward CP, Fensom AH: Complementation studies in Niemann-Pick disease type C indicate the existence of a second group. *J Med Genet* **31**:317, 1994.
41. Vanier MT, Duthel S, Rodriguez-Lafrasse C, Pentchev P, Carstea ED: Genetic heterogeneity in Niemann-Pick C disease: A study using somatic cell hybridization and linkage analysis. *Am J Hum Genet* **58**:118, 1996.
42. Carstea ED, Polymeropoulos MH, Parker CC, Detera-Wadleigh SD, O'Neill RR, Patterson MC, Goldin E, et al.: Linkage of Niemann-Pick disease type C to human chromosome 18. *Proc Natl Acad Sci U S A* **90**:2002, 1993.
43. Carstea ED, Morris JA, Coleman KG, Loftus SK, Zhang D, Cummings C, Gu J, et al.: Niemann-Pick C1 disease gene: Homology to mediators of cholesterol homeostasis [Comments]. *Science* **277**:228, 1997.
44. Loftus SK, Morris JA, Carstea ED, Gu JZ, Cummings C, Brown A, Ellison J, et al.: Murine model of Niemann-Pick C disease: Mutation in a cholesterol homeostasis gene [Comments]. *Science* **277**:232, 1997.

45. Maconochie IK, Chong S, Mieli-Vergani G, Lake BD, Mowat AP: Fetal ascites: An unusual presentation of Niemann-Pick disease type C [Comments]. *Arch Dis Child* **64**:1391, 1989.
46. Manning DJ, Price WI, Pearse RG: Fetal ascites: An unusual presentation of Niemann-Pick disease type C [Letter, Comment]. *Arch Dis Child* **65**:335, 1990.
47. Pin I, Pradines S, Pincemaille O, Frappat P, Brambilla E, Vanier MT, Bost M: [A fatal respiratory form of type C Niemann-Pick disease.] *Arch Fr Pediatr* **47**:373, 1990.
48. Rutledge JC: Progressive neonatal liver failure due to type C Niemann-Pick disease. *Pediatr Pathol* **9**:779, 1989.
49. Gonzalez de Dios J, Fernandez Tejada E, Diaz Fernandez MC, Ortega Paez E, Hernandez Gonzalez J, de la Vega Bueno A, Hierro Llanillo L, et al.: [The current state of Niemann-Pick disease: Evaluation of six cases.] *An Esp Pediatr* **32**:143, 1990.
50. Kovesi TA, Lee J, Shuckett B, Clarke JT, Callahon JW, Phillips MJ: Pulmonary infiltration in Niemann-Pick disease type C. *J Inherit Metab Dis* **19**:792, 1996.
51. Schofer O, Mischo B, Puschel W, Harzer K, Vanier MT: Early-lethal pulmonary form of Niemann-Pick type C disease belonging to a second, rare genetic complementation group. *Eur J Pediatr* **157**:45, 1998.
52. Vanier MT, Wenger DA, Comly ME, Rousson R, Brady RO, Pentchev PG: Niemann-Pick disease group C: Clinical variability and diagnosis based on defective cholesterol esterification. A collaborative study on 70 patients. *Clin Genet* **33**:331, 1988.
53. Ivemark BI, Svennerholm L, Thren C, Tunell R: Niemann-Pick disease in infancy. Report of two siblings with clinical histologic and chemical studies. *Acta Paediatr* **52**:391, 1963.
54. Guibaud P, Vanier MT, Malpuech G, Gaulme J, Houllemare L, Goddon R, Rousson R: [Early infantile, cholestatic, rapidly-fatal form of type C sphingomyelinosis. 2 cases.] *Pediatrie* **34**:103, 1979.
55. Jaeken J, Proesmans W, Eggermont E, Van Hoof F, Den Tandt W, Standaert L, Van Herck G, et al.: Niemann-Pick type C disease and early cholestasis in three brothers. *Acta Paediatr Belg* **33**:43, 1980.
56. Mieli-Vergani G, Howard ER, Mowat AP: Liver disease in infancy: A 20 year perspective. *Gut* **Suppl**:[FES9]S123, 1991.
57. Higgins JJ, Patterson MC, Dambrosia JM, Pikus AT, Pentchev PG, Sato S, Brady RO, et al.: A clinical staging classification for type C Niemann-Pick disease. *Neurology* **42**:2286, 1992.
58. Wiedemann HR, Debuch H, Lennert K, Caesar R, Blumcke S, Harms D, Tolksdorf M, et al.: [An infantile-juvenile, subchronically progressive lipoidosis of the sphingomyelinosis (Niemann-Pick) form—A new type? Clinical, pathohistological, electron microscopic and biochemical studies.] *Z Kinderheilkd* **112**:187, 1972.
59. Harzer K, Schlote W, Peiffer J, Benz HU, Anzil AP: Neurovisceral lipidosis compatible with Niemann-Pick disease type C: Morphological and biochemical studies of a late infantile case and enzyme and lipid assays in a prenatal case of the same family. *Acta Neuropathol (Berl)* **43**:97, 1978.
60. Vanier MT, Suzuki K: Niemann-Pick diseases, in Moser HW, Vinken PJ, Bruyn GW (eds): *Neurodystrophies and Neurolipidoses*. Vol 66, Handbook of Clinical Neurology. Amsterdam, Elsevier Science, 1996, p 133.
61. Hahn AF, Gilbert JJ, Kwarciak C, Gillett J, Bolton CF, Rupar CA, Callahan JW: Nerve biopsy findings in Niemann-Pick type II (NPC) [Comments]. *Acta Neuropathol* **87**:149, 1994.
62. Miyake S, Inoue H, Ohtahara S, Okada S, Yamano T: [A case of Niemann-Pick disease type C with narcolepsy syndrome.] *Rinsho Shinkeigaku* **23**:44, 1983.
63. Denoix C, Rodriguez-Lafrasse C, Vanier MT, Navelet Y, Landrieu P: [Cataplexy revealing an atypical form of Niemann-Pick disease type C.] *Arch Fr Pediatr* **48**:31, 1991.
64. Coleman RJ, Robb SA, Lake BD, Brett EM, Harding AE: The diverse neurological features of Niemann-Pick disease type C: A report of two cases. *Mov Disord* **3**:295, 1988.
65. Shulman LM, David NJ, Weiner WJ: Psychosis as the initial manifestation of adult-onset Niemann-Pick disease type C [Comments]. *Neurology* **45**:1739, 1995.
66. Wherrett JR, Rewcastle NB: Adult neurovisceral lipidosis. *Clin Res* **17**:665, 1969.
67. Horoupian DS, Yang SS: Paired helical filaments in neurovisceral lipidosis (juvenile dystonic lipidosis). *Ann Neurol* **4**:404, 1978.
68. Hulette CM, Earl NL, Anthony DC, Crain BJ: Adult onset Niemann-Pick disease type C presenting with dementia and absent organomegaly. *Clin Neuropathol* **11**:293, 1992.
69. Vanier MT, Rodriguez-Lafrasse C, Rousson R, Duthel S, Harzer K, Pentchev PG, Revol A, et al.: Type C Niemann-Pick disease: Biochemical aspects and phenotypic heterogeneity. *Dev Neurosci* **13**:307, 1991.
70. Lossos A, Schlesinger I, Okon E, Abramsky O, Bargal R, Vanier MT, Zeigler M: Adult-onset Niemann-Pick type C disease. Clinical, biochemical, and genetic study. *Arch Neurol* **54**:1536, 1997.
71. Grau AJ, Brandt T, Weisbrod M, Niethammer R, Forsting M, Cantz M, Vanier MT, et al.: Adult Niemann-Pick disease type C mimicking features of multiple sclerosis [Letter]. *J Neurol Neurosurg Psychiatry* **63**:552, 1997.
72. Fensom AH, Grant AR, Steinberg SJ, Ward CP, Lake BD, Logan EC, Hulman G: Case report: An adult with a non-neuronopathic form of Niemann-Pick C disease. *J Inherit Metab Dis* **22**:84, 1999.
73. Omarini LP, Frank-Burkhardt SE, Seemayer TA, Mentha G, Terrier F: Niemann-Pick disease type C: Nodular splenomegaly. *Abdom Imaging* **20**:157, 1995.
74. Vanier MT, Suzuki K: Recent advances in elucidating Niemann-Pick C disease. *Brain Pathol* **8**:163, 1998.
75. Frederickson DS, Sloan HR: Sphingomyelin lipidosis: Niemann-Pick disease, in Stanbury JB, Wyngaarden JB, Frederickson DS (eds): *The Metabolic Basis of Inherited Disease*, 3rd ed. New York, McGraw-Hill, 1972, p 783.
76. Rottach KG, von Maydell RD, Das VE, Zivotofsky AZ, Discenna AO, Gordon JL, Landis DM, et al.: Evidence for independent feedback control of horizontal and vertical saccades from Niemann-Pick type C disease. *Vision Res* **37**:3627, 1997.
77. Leigh RJ, Rottach KG, Das VE: Transforming sensory perceptions into motor commands: Evidence from programming of eye movements. *Ann N Y Acad Sci* **835**:353, 1997.
78. Kandt RS, Emerson RG, Singer HS, Valle DL, Moser HW: Cataplexy in variant forms of Niemann-Pick disease. *Ann Neurol* **12**:284, 1982.
79. Philippart M, Engel J Jr, Zimmerman EG: Gelastic cataplexy in Niemann-Pick disease group C and related variants without generalized sphingomyelinase deficiency [Letter]. *Ann Neurol* **14**:492, 1983.
80. Siegel JM: Brainstem mechanisms generating REM sleep, in Kryger MH, Roth T, Dement WC (eds): *Principles and Practice of Sleep Medicine*, Philadelphia, WB Saunders, 1989, p 115.
81. Challamel MJ, Mazzola ME, Nevsimalova S, Cannard C, Louis J, Revol M: Narcolepsy in children. *Sleep* **17**:S17, 1994.
82. Akaboshi S, Ohno K: [Niemann-Pick disease type C.] *Nippon Rinsho* **53**:3036, 1995.
83. Boor R, Reitter B: [Cataplexy in type C Niemann-Pick disease.] *Klin Padiatr* **209**:88, 1997.
84. Vanier MT, Pentchev P, Rodriguez-Lafrasse C, Rousson R: Niemann-Pick disease type C: An update. *J Inherit Metab Dis* **14**:580, 1991.
85. Yatziv S, Leibovitz-Ben Gershon Z, Ornoy A, Bach G: Clinical heterogeneity in a sibship with Niemann-Pick disease type C. *Clin Genet* **23**:125, 1983.
86. Wenger DA, Barth G, Githens JH: Nine cases of sphingomyelin lipidosis, a new variant in Spanish-American children. Juvenile variant of Niemann-Pick disease with foamy and sea-blue histiocytes. *Am J Dis Child* **131**:955, 1977.
87. Winsor EJ, Welch JP: Genetic and demographic aspects of Nova Scotia Niemann-Pick disease (type D). *Am J Hum Genet* **30**:530, 1978.
88. Fink JK, Filling-Katz MR, Sokol J, Cogan DG, Pikus A, Sonies B, Soong B, et al.: Clinical spectrum of Niemann-Pick disease type C. *Neurology* **39**:1040, 1989.
89. Gilbert EF, Callahan J, Viseskul C, Opitz JM: Niemann-Pick disease type C. Pathological, histochemical, ultrastructural and biochemical studies. *Eur J Pediatr* **136**:263, 1981.
90. Elleder M, Jirasek A, Smid F, Ledvinova J, Besley GT, Stopekova M: Niemann-Pick disease type C with enhanced glycolipid storage. Report on further case of so-called lactosylceramidosis. *Virchows Arch A Pathol Anat Histopathol* **402**:307, 1984.
91. Philippart M, Martin L, Martin JJ, Menkes JH: Niemann-Pick disease. Morphologic and biochemical studies in the visceral form with late central nervous system involvement (Crocker's group C). *Arch Neurol* **20**:227, 1969.
92. Elleder M, Jirasek A, Smid F: Niemann-Pick disease (Crocker's type C): A histological study of the distribution and qualitative differences of the storage process. *Acta Neuropathol (Berl)* **33**:191, 1975.
93. Semeraro LA, Riely CA, Kolodny EH, Dickerson GR, Gryboski JD: Niemann-Pick variant lipidosis presenting as "neonatal hepatitis." *J Pediatr Gastroenterol Nutr* **5**:492, 1986.

94. Dumontel C, Girod C, Dijoud F, Dumez Y, Vanier MT: Fetal Niemann-Pick disease type C: Ultrastructural and lipid findings in liver and spleen. *Virchows Arch A Pathol Anat Histopathol* **422**:253, 1993.
95. Higashi Y, Pentchev PG, Murayama S, Suzuki K: Pathology of Niemann-Pick type C: Studies of murine mutants, in Ikuta F (ed): *Neuropathology in Brain Research.* Amsterdam, Elsevier Science, 1991, p 85.
96. Merin S, Livni N, Yatziv S: Conjunctival ultrastructure in Niemann-Pick disease type C. *Am J Ophthalmol* **90**:708, 1980.
97. Arsenio-Nunes ML, Goutieres F: Morphological diagnosis of Niemann-Pick disease type C by skin and conjunctival biopsies. *Acta Neuropathol Suppl* **7**:204, 1981.
98. Palmer M, Green WR, Maumenee IH, Valle DL, Singer HS, Morton SJ, Moser HW: Niemann-Pick disease—Type C. Ocular histopathologic and electron microscopic studies. *Arch Ophthalmol* **103**:817, 1985.
99. Boustany RN, Kaye E, Alroy J: Ultrastructural findings in skin from patients with Niemann-Pick disease, type C. *Pediatr Neurol* **6**:177, 1990.
100. Anzil AP, Blinzinger K, Mehraein P, Dozic S: Niemann-Pick disease type C: Case report with ultrastructural findings. *Neuropädiatrie* **4**:207, 1973.
101. Pellissier JF, Hassoun J, Gambarelli D, Bryon PA, Casanova P, Toga M: [Niemann-Pick disease (Crocker's type C): Ultrastructural study of a case.] *Acta Neuropathol (Berl)* **34**:65, 1976.
102. Elleder M, Jirasek A, Smid F, Ledvinova J, Besley GT: Niemann-Pick disease type C. Study on the nature of the cerebral storage process. *Acta Neuropathol* **66**:325, 1985.
103. Braak H, Braak E, Goebel HH: Isocortical pathology in type C Niemann-Pick disease. A combined Golgi-pigmentoarchitectonic study. *J Neuropathol Exp Neurol* **42**:671, 1983.
104. March PA, Thrall MA, Brown DE, Mitchell TW, Lowenthal AC, Walkley SU: GABAergic neuroaxonal dystrophy and other cytopathological alterations in feline Niemann-Pick disease type C. *Acta Neuropathol (Berl)* **94**:164, 1997.
105. Sherriff FE, Bridges LR, De Souza DS: Non-Alzheimer neurofibrillary tangles show beta-amyloid-like immunoreactivity. *Neuroreport* **5**:1897, 1994.
106. Love S, Bridges LR, Case CP: Neurofibrillary tangles in Niemann-Pick disease type C. *Brain* **118**:119, 1995.
107. Suzuki K, Parker CC, Pentchev PG, Katz D, Ghetti B, D'Agostino AN, Carstea ED: Neurofibrillary tangles in Niemann-Pick disease type C. *Acta Neuropathol* **89**:227, 1995.
108. Suzuki K, Parker CC, Pentchev PG: Niemann-Pick disease type C: neuropathology revisited. *Dev Brain Dysf* **10**:306, 1997.
109. Auer IA, Schmidt ML, Lee VM, Curry B, Suzuki K, Shin RW, Pentchev PG, et al.: Paired helical filament tau (PHFtau) in Niemann-Pick type C disease is similar to PHFtau in Alzheimer's disease. *Acta Neuropathol* **90**:547, 1995.
110. Omura K, Suzuki Y, Norose N, Sato M, Maruyama K, Koeda T: Type C Niemann-Pick disease: Clinical and biochemical studies on 6 cases. *Brain Dev* **11**:57, 1989.
111. Lowenthal AC, Cummings JF, Wenger DA, Thrall MA, Wood PA, de Lahunta A: Feline sphingolipidosis resembling Niemann-Pick disease type C. *Acta Neuropathol* **81**:189, 1990.
112. Kuwamura M, Awakura T, Shimada A, Umemura T, Kagota K, Kawamura N, Naiki M: Type C Niemann-Pick disease in a boxer dog. *Acta Neuropathol* **85**:345, 1993.
113. Shio H, Fowler S, Bhuvaneswaran C, Morris MD: Lysosomal lipid storage disorder in NCTR-BALB/c mice. II Morphologic and cytochemical studies. *Am J Pathol* **108**:150, 1982.
114. Tanaka J, Nakamura H, Miyawaki S: Cerebellar involvement in murine sphingomyelinosis: A new model of Niemann-Pick disease. *J Neuropathol Exp Neurol* **47**:291, 1988.
115. Weintraub H, Abramovici A, Sandbank U, Pentchev PG, Brady RO, Sekine M, Suzuki A, et al.: Neurological mutation characterized by dysmyelination in NCTR-BALB/c mouse with lysosomal lipid storage disease. *J Neurochem* **45**:665, 1985.
116. Tokoro T, Yamamamoto T, Okuno A, Suzuki H, Miyawaki S, Maekawa K, Eto Y: [Impaired cholesterol esterification in Niemann-Pick disease model mouse.] *No To Hattatsu* **23**:98, 1991.
117. Weintraub H, Alroy J, DeGasperi R, Goyal V, Skutelsky E, Pentchev PG, Warren CD: Storage of glycoprotein in NCTR-Balb/C mouse. Lectin histochemistry, and biochemical studies. *Virchows Arch B Cell Pathol Incl Mol Pathol* **62**:347, 1992.
118. Manabe T, Yamane T, Higashi Y, Pentchev PG, Suzuki K: Ultrastructural changes in the lung in Niemann-Pick type C mouse. *Virchows Arch* **427**:77, 1995.
119. Tanaka J, Miyawaki S, Maeda N, Mikoshiba K: Immunohistochemical expression of P400 protein in Purkinje cells of sphingomyelinosis mouse. *Brain Dev* **13**:110, 1991.
120. Higashi Y, Murayama S, Pentchev PG, Suzuki K: Cerebellar degeneration in the Niemann-Pick type C mouse. *Acta Neuropathol* **85**:175, 1993.
121. Higashi Y, Murayama S, Pentchev PG, Suzuki K: Peripheral nerve pathology in Niemann-Pick type C mouse. *Acta Neuropathol* **90**:158, 1995.
122. Frank V, Lasson V: Ophthalmoplegic neurolipidosis, storage cells in heterozygotes. *Neuropediatrics* **16**:3, 1985.
123. Ceuterick C, Martin JJ, Foulard M: Niemann-Pick disease type C. Skin biopsies in parents. *Neuropediatrics* **17**:111, 1986.
124. Brown DE, Thrall MA, Walkley SU, Wurzelmann S, Wenger DA, Allison RW, Just CA: Metabolic abnormalities in feline Niemann-Pick type C heterozygotes. *J Inherit Metab Dis* **19**:319, 1996.
125. Spence MW, Callahan JW: Sphingomyelin-cholesterol lipidoses: The Niemann-Pick group of diseases, in Scriver CR, Beaudet AL, Sly WS, Valle D (eds): *The Metabolic Basis of Inherited Disease*, 6th ed. New York, McGraw-Hill, 1989, p 1655.
126. Besley GT, Elleder M: Enzyme activities and phospholipid storage patterns in brain and spleen samples from Niemann-Pick disease variants: A comparison of neuropathic and non-neuropathic forms. *J Inherit Metab Dis* **9**:59, 1986.
127. Rao BG, Spence MW: Niemann-Pick disease type D: Lipid analyses and studies on sphingomyelinases. *Ann Neurol* **1**:385, 1977.
128. Dacremont G, Kint JA, Carton D, Cocquyt G: Glucosylceramide in plasma of patients with Niemann-Pick disease. *Clin Chim Acta* **52**:365, 1974.
129. Dawson G: Detection of glycosphingolipids in small samples of human tissue. *Ann Clin Lab Sci* **2**:274, 1972.
130. Vanier MT, Pentchev PG, Rousson R: Pathophysiological approach of Niemann-Pick disease type C; definition of a biochemical heterogeneity and reevaluation of the lipid storage process, in Salvayre R, Douste-Blazy L, Gatt S (eds): *Lipid Storage Disorders: Biological and Medical Aspects*. New York, Plenum, 1988, p 175.
131. Vanier MT, Rousson R, Zeitouni R, Pentchev PG, Louisot P: Sphingomyelinase and Niemann-Pick disease, in Freysz L, Deyfus H, Massarelli R, Gatt S (eds): *Enzymes of Lipid Metabolism II*. New York, Plenum, 1986, p 791.
132. Miyawaki S, Mitsuoka S, Sakiyama T, Kitagawa T: Sphingomyelinosis, a new mutation in the mouse: A model of Niemann-Pick disease in humans. *J Hered* **73**:257, 1982.
133. Morris MD, Bhuvaneswaran C, Shio H, Fowler S: Lysosome storage disorder in NCTR-BALB/c mice. I Description of the disease and genetics. *Am J Pathol* **108**:140, 1982.
134. Oppenheimer DR, Norman RM, Tingey AH, Aherne WA: Histological and biochemical findings in juvenile Niemann-Pick disease. *J Neurol Sci* **5**:575, 1967.
135. Lowden JA, LaRamee MA, Wentworth P: The subacute form of Niemann-Pick disease. *Arch Neurol* **17**:230, 1967.
136. Tjiong HB, Seng PN, Debuch H, Wiedemann HR: Brain lipids of a case of juvenile Niemann-Pick disease. *J Neurochem* **21**:1475, 1973.
137. Hagberg B, Haltia M, Sourander P, Svennerholm L, Vanier MT, Ljunggren CG: Neurovisceral storage disorder simulating Niemann-Pick disease. A new form of oligosaccharidosis? *Neuropadiatrie* **9**:59, 1978.
138. Elleder M: Heterogeneity and special features of the storage process in Niemann-Pick disease, in Salvayre R, Douste-Blazy L, Gat S (eds): *Lipid Storage Disorders. Biological and Medical Aspects.* New York, Plenum Press, 1988, p 141.
139. Vanier MT: Lipid changes in Niemann-Pick disease type C brain: personal experience and review of the literature. *Neurochem Res* **24**:481, 1999.
140. Pilz H, Sandhoff K, Jatzkewitz H: Eine Gangliosidstoffwechselstörung mit Anhäufung von Ceramid-lactosid, Monosialo-Ceramid-Lactosid und Tay-Sachs-Gangliosid im Gehirn. *J Neurochem* **13**:1273, 1966.
141. Kannan R, Tjiong HB, Debuch H, Wiedemann HR: Unusual glycolipids in brain cortex of a visceral lipidosis (Niemann-Pick disease?). *Hoppe Seylers Z Physiol Chem* **355**:551, 1974.
142. Dawson G: Glycosphingolipid levels in an unusual neurovisceral storage disease characterized by lactosylceramide galactosyl hydrolase deficiency: Lactosylceramidosis. *J Lipid Res* **13**:207, 1972.
143. Kruth HS, Comly ME, Butler JD, Vanier MT, Fink JK, Wenger DA, Patel S, et al.: Type C Niemann-Pick disease. Abnormal metabolism of low-density lipoprotein in homozygous and heterozygous fibroblasts. *J Biol Chem* **261**:16769, 1986.

144. Pentchev PG, Kruth HS, Comly ME, Butler JD, Vanier MT, Wenger DA, Patel S: Type C Niemann-Pick disease. A parallel loss of regulatory responses in both the uptake and esterification of low-density lipoprotein-derived cholesterol in cultured fibroblasts. *J Biol Chem* **261**:16775, 1986.
145. Pentchev PG, Brady RO, Blanchette-Mackie EJ, Vanier MT, Carstea ED, Parker CC, Goldin E, et al.: The Niemann-Pick C lesion and its relationship to the intracellular distribution and utilization of LDL cholesterol. *Biochim Biophys Acta* **1225**:235, 1994.
146. Pentchev PG, Blanchette-Mackie EJ, Dawidowicz EA: The NP-C gene: A key to pathways of intracellular cholesterol transport. *Trends Cell Biol* **4**:365, 1994.
147. Liscum L, Underwood KW: Intracellular cholesterol transport and compartmentation. *J Biol Chem* **270**:15443, 1995.
148. Pentchev PG, Blanchette-Mackie EJ, Liscum L: Biological implications of the Niemann-Pick C mutation. *Subcell Biochem* **28**:437, 1997.
149. Liscum L, Klansek JJ: Niemann-Pick disease type C. *Curr Opin Lipidol* **9**:131, 1998.
150. Neufeld EB: What the Niemann-Pick type C gene has taught us about cholesterol transport, in Freeman DA, Chang T-Y (eds): *Intracellular Cholesterol Trafficking*. Norwell, MA, Kluwer, 1998.
151. Liscum L, Faust JR: Low-density lipoprotein (LDL)-mediated suppression of cholesterol synthesis and LDL uptake is defective in Niemann-Pick type C fibroblasts. *J Biol Chem* **262**:17002, 1987.
152. Butler JD, Comly ME, Kruth HS, Vanier M, Filling-Katz M, Fink J, Barton N, et al.: Niemann-Pick variant disorders: comparison of errors of cellular cholesterol homeostasis in group D and group C fibroblasts. *Proc Natl Acad Sci U S A* **84**:556, 1987.
153. Blanchette-Mackie EJ, Dwyer NK, Amende LM, Kruth HS, Butler JD, Sokol J, Comly ME, et al.: Type-C Niemann-Pick disease: Low-density lipoprotein uptake is associated with premature cholesterol accumulation in the Golgi complex and excessive cholesterol storage in lysosomes. *Proc Natl Acad Sci U S A* **85**:8022, 1988.
154. Argoff CE, Comly ME, Blanchette-Mackie J, Kruth HS, Pye HT, Goldin E, Kaneski C, et al.: Type C Niemann-Pick disease: Cellular uncoupling of cholesterol homeostasis is linked to the severity of disruption in the intracellular transport of exogenously derived cholesterol. *Biochim Biophys Acta* **1096**:319, 1991.
155. Brown MS, Goldstein JL: A receptor-mediated pathway of cholesterol homeostasis. *Science* **232**:34, 1986.
156. Liscum L, Faust JR: The intracellular transport of low density lipoprotein-derived cholesterol is inhibited in Chinese hamster ovary cells cultured with 3-beta-[2-(diethylamino)ethoxy]androst-5-en-17-one. *J Biol Chem* **264**:11796, 1989.
157. Rodriguez-Lafrasse C, Rousson R, Bonnet J, Pentchev PG, Louisot P, Vanier MT: Abnormal cholesterol metabolism in imipramine-treated fibroblast cultures. Similarities with Niemann-Pick type C disease. *Biochim Biophys Acta* **1043**:123, 1990.
158. Roff CF, Goldin E, Comly ME, Cooney A, Brown A, Vanier MT, Miller SP, et al.: Type C Niemann-Pick disease: Use of hydrophobic amines to study defective cholesterol transport. *Dev Neurosci* **13**:315, 1991.
159. Butler JD, Blanchette-Mackie J, Goldin E, O'Neill RR, Carstea G, Roff CF, Patterson MC, et al.: Progesterone blocks cholesterol translocation from lysosomes. *J Biol Chem* **267**:23797, 1992.
160. Furuchi T, Aikawa K, Arai H, Inoue K: Bafilomycin-A (1), a specific inhibitor of vacuolar-type H^+-ATPase, blocks lysosomal cholesterol trafficking in macrophages. *J Biol Chem* **268**:273345, 1993.
161. Brasaemle DL, Attie AD: Rapid intracellular transport of LDL-derived cholesterol to the plasma membrane in cultured fibroblasts. *J Lipid Res* **31**:103, 1990.
162. Johnson WJ, Chacko GK, Phillips MC, Rothblat GH: The efflux of lysosomal cholesterol from cells. *J Biol Chem* **265**:5546, 1990.
163. Neufeld EB, Cooney AM, Pitha J, Dawidowicz EA, Dwyer NK, Pentchev PG, Blanchette-Mackie EJ: Intracellular trafficking of cholesterol monitored with a cyclodextrin. *J Biol Chem* **271**:21604, 1996.
164. Underwood KW, Jacobs NL, Howley A, Liscum L: Evidence for a cholesterol transport pathway from lysosomes to endoplasmic reticulum that is independent of the plasma membrane. *J Biol Chem* **273**:4266, 1998.
165. Lange Y, Ye J, Steck TL: Circulation of cholesterol between lysosomes and the plasma membrane. *J Biol Chem* **273**:18915, 1998.
166. Coxey RA, Pentchev PG, Campbell G, Blanchette-Mackie EJ: Differential accumulation of cholesterol in Golgi compartments of normal and Niemann-Pick type C fibroblasts incubated with LDL: A cytochemical freeze-fracture study. *J Lipid Res* **34**:1165, 1993.
167. Shamburek RD, Pentchev PG, Zech LA, Blanchette-Mackie J, Carstea ED, VandenBroek JM, Cooper PS, et al.: Intracellular trafficking of the free cholesterol derived from LDL cholesteryl ester is defective in vivo in Niemann-Pick C disease: Insights on normal metabolism of HDL and LDL gained from the NP-C mutation. *J Lipid Res* **38**:2422, 1997.
168. Vanier MT, Revol A, Fichet M: Sphingomyelinase activities of various human tissues in control subjects and in Niemann-Pick disease—Development and evaluation of a microprocedure. *Clin Chim Acta* **106**:257, 1980.
169. Besley GT: Sphingomyelinase defect in Niemann-Pick disease, type C, fibroblasts. *FEBS Lett* **80**:71, 1977.
170. Maziere JC, Maziere C, Mora L, Routier JD, Polonovski J: *In situ* degradation of sphingomyelin by cultured normal fibroblasts and fibroblasts from patients with Niemann-Pick disease type A and C. *Biochem Biophys Res Commun* **108**:1101, 1982.
171. Kudoh T, Velkoff MA, Wenger DA: Uptake and metabolism of radioactively labeled sphingomyelin in cultured skin fibroblasts from controls and patients with Niemann-Pick disease and other lysosomal storage diseases. *Biochim Biophys Acta* **754**:82, 1983.
172. Vanier MT, Rousson R, Garcia I, Bailloud G, Juge MC, Revol A, Louisot P: Biochemical studies in Niemann-Pick disease. III. In vitro and in vivo assays of sphingomyelin degradation in cultured skin fibroblasts and amniotic fluid cells for the diagnosis of the various forms of the disease. *Clin Genet* **27**:20, 1985.
173. Thomas GH, Tuck-Muller CM, Miller CS, Reynolds LW: Correction of sphingomyelinase deficiency in Niemann-Pick type C fibroblasts by removal of lipoprotein fraction from culture media. *J Inherit Metab Dis* **12**:139, 1989.
174. Besley GT, Moss SE: Studies on sphingomyelinase and beta-glucosidase activities in Niemann-Pick disease variants. Phosphodiesterase activities measured with natural and artificial substrates. *Biochim Biophys Acta* **752**:54, 1983.
175. Yano T, Taniguchi M, Akaboshi S, Vanier MT, Tai T, Sakabura H, Ohno K: Accumulation of G_{M2} ganglioside in Niemann-Pick disease type C fibroblasts. *Proc Japan Acad Series B* **72**:214, 1996.
176. Sato M, Akaboshi S, Katsumoto T, Taniguchi M, Higaki K, Tai T, Sakuraba H, et al.: Accumulation of cholesterol and G_{M2} ganglioside in cells cultured in the presence of progesterone: An implication for the basic defect in Niemann-Pick disease type C. *Brain Dev* **20**:50, 1998.
177. Watanabe Y, Akaboshi S, Ishida G, Takeshima T, Yano T, Taniguchi M, Ohno K, et al.: Increased levels of G_{M2} ganglioside in fibroblasts from a patient with juvenile Niemann-Pick disease type C. *Brain Dev* **20**:95, 1998.
178. Goldin E, Roff CF, Miller SP, Rodriguez-Lafrasse C, Vanier MT, Brady RO, Pentchev PG: Type C Niemann-Pick disease: A murine model of the lysosomal cholesterol lipidosis accumulates sphingosine and sphinganine in liver. *Biochim Biophys Acta* **1127**:303, 1992.
179. Rodriguez-Lafrasse C, Rousson R, Pentchev PG, Louisot P, Vanier MT: Free sphingoid bases in tissues from patients with type C Niemann-Pick disease and other lysosomal storage disorders. *Biochim Biophys Acta* **1226**:138, 1994.
180. Christomanou H, Kellermann J, Linke RP, Harzer K: Deficient ferritin immunoreactivity in visceral organs from four patients with Niemann-Pick disease type C. *Biochem Mol Med* **55**:105, 1995.
181. Christomanou H, Harzer K: Ouchterlony double immunodiffusion method demonstrates absence of ferritin immunoreactivity in visceral organs from nine patients with Niemann-Pick disease type C. *Biochem Mol Med* **58**:176, 1996.
182. Schedin S, Pentchev PG, Brunk U, Dallner G: Changes in the levels of dolichol and dolichyl phosphate in a murine model of Niemann-Pick's type C disease. *J Neurochem* **65**:670, 1995.
183. Schedin S, Sindelar PJ, Pentchev P, Brunk U, Dallner G: Peroxisomal impairment in Niemann-Pick type C disease. *J Biol Chem* **272**:6245, 1997.
184. Sequeira JS, Vellodi A, Vanier MT, Clayton PT: Niemann-Pick disease type C and defective peroxisomal beta-oxidation of branched-chain substrates. *J Inherit Metab Dis* **21**:149, 1998.
185. Butler JD, Vanier MT, Pentchev PG: Niemann-Pick C disease: Cystine and lipids accumulate in the murine model of this lysosomal cholesterol lipidosis. *Biochem Biophys Res Commun* **196**:154, 1993.
186. Garver WS, Erickson RP, Wilson JM, Colton TL, Hossain GS, Kozloski MA, Heidenreich RA: Altered expression of caveolin-1 and increased cholesterol in detergent insoluble membrane fractions from liver in mice with Niemann-Pick disease type C. *Biochim Biophys Acta* **1361**:272, 1997.
187. Garver WS, Hsu SC, Erickson RP, Greer WL, Byers DM, Heidenreich RA: Increased expression of caveolin-1 in heterozygous Niemann-Pick

type II human fibroblasts. *Biochem Biophys Res Commun* **236**:189, 1997.
188. Suresh S, Yan Z, Patel RC, Patel YC, Patel SC: Cellular cholesterol storage in the Niemann-Pick disease type C mouse is associated with increased expression and defective processing of apolipoprotein D. *J Neurochem* **70**:242, 1998.
189. Koike T, Ishida G, Taniguchi M, Higaki K, Ayaki Y, Saito M, Sakakihara Y, et al.: Decreased membrane fluidity and unsaturated fatty acids in Niemann-Pick disease type C fibroblasts. *Biochim Biophys Acta* **1406**:327, 1998.
190. Yamamoto T, Tokoro T, Eto Y: The attenuated elevation of cytoplasmic calcium concentration following the uptake of low-density lipoprotein in type C Niemann-Pick fibroblasts. *Biochem Biophys Res Commun* **198**:438, 1994.
191. Rodriguez-Lafrasse C, Rousson R, Valla S, Antignac P, Louisot P, Vanier MT: Modulation of protein kinase C by endogenous sphingosine: Inhibition of phorbol dibutyrate binding in Niemann-Pick C fibroblasts. *Biochem J* **325**:787, 1997.
192. Yadid G, Sotnik-Barkai I, Tornatore C, Baker-Cairns B, Harvey-White J, Pentchev PG, Goldin E: Neurochemical alterations in the cerebellum of a murine model of Niemann-Pick type C disease. *Brain Res* **799**:250, 1998.
193. Yamamoto T, Iwasawa K, Tokoro T, Eto Y, Maekawa K: [A possible same genetic defect in two Niemann-Pick disease model mice.] *No To Hattatsu* **26**:318, 1994.
194. Akaboshi S, Yano T, Miyawaki S, Ohno K, Takeshita K: A C57BL/KsJ mouse model of Niemann-Pick disease (*spm*) belongs to the same complementation group as the major childhood type of Niemann-Pick disease type C. *Hum Genet* **99**:350, 1997.
195. Greer WL, Riddell DC, Byers DM, Welch JP, Girouard GS, Sparrow SM, Gillan TL, et al.: Linkage of Niemann-Pick disease type D to the same region of human chromosome 18 as Niemann-Pick disease type C. *Am J Hum Genet* **61**:139, 1997.
196. Gu JZ, Carstea ED, Cummings C, Morris JA, Loftus SK, Zhang D, Coleman KG, et al.: Substantial narrowing of the Niemann-Pick C candidate interval by yeast artificial chromosome complementation. *Proc Natl Acad Sci U S A* **94**:7378, 1997.
197. Johnson RL, Rothman AL, Xie J, Goodrich LV, Bare JW, Bonifas JM, Quinn AG, et al.: Human homolog of patched, a candidate gene for the basal cell nevus syndrome. *Science* **272**:1668, 1996.
198. Chin DJ, Gil G, Russell DW, Liscum L, Luskey KL, Basu SK, Okayama H, et al.: Nucleotide sequence of 3-hydroxy-3-methyl-glutaryl coenzyme A reductase, a glycoprotein of endoplasmic reticulum. *Nature* **308**:613, 1984.
199. Hua X, Nohturfft A, Goldstein JL, Brown MS: Sterol resistance in CHO cells traced to point mutation in SREBP cleavage-activating protein. *Cell* **87**:415, 1996.
200. Greer WL, Riddell DC, Gillan TL, Girouard GS, Sparrow SM, Byers DM, Dobson MJ, et al.: The Nova Scotia (type D) form of Niemann-Pick disease is caused by a G3097 $\rightarrow$ T transversion in NPC1. *Am J Hum Genet* **63**:52, 1998.
201. Yamamoto T, Nanba E, Ninomiya H, Higaki K, Taniguchi M, Zhang H, Akaboshi S, et al.: NPC1 gene mutations in Japanese patients with Niemann-Pick disease type C. *Hum Genet* **105**:10, 1999.
202. Neufeld EB, Wastney M, Patel S, Suresh S, Cooney AM, Dwyer NK, Roff CF, et al.: The Niemann-Pick C1 protein resides in a vesicular compartment linked to retrograde transport of multiple lysosomal cargo. *J Biol Chem* **274**:9627, 1999.
203. Liscum L, Dahl NK: Intracellular cholesterol transport. *J Lipid Res* **33**:1239, 1992.
204. Traub LM, Bannykh SI, Rodel JE, Aridor M, Balch WE, Kornfeld S: AP-2-containing clathrin coats assemble on mature lysosomes. *J Cell Biol* **135**:1801, 1996.
205. Jurevics H, Morell P: Cholesterol for synthesis of myelin is made locally, not imported into brain. *Neurochem* **64**:895, 1995.
206. Snipes GJ, Suter U: Cholesterol and myelin, in Bittman R (ed) *Cholesterol: Its Functions and Metabolism in Biology and Medicine*. New York, Plenum Press, 1997, p 173.
207. Yu RK, Saito M: Structure and localization of gangliosides, in Margolis RU, Margolis RK (eds): *Neurobiology of Glycoconjugates*. New York, Plenum Press, 1989, p 1.
208. Chen CS, Martin OC, Pagano RE: Changes in the spectral properties of a plasma membrane lipid analog during the first seconds of endocytosis in living cells. *Biophys J* **72**:37, 1997.
209. Walkley SU, Siegel DA, Dobrenis K, Zervas M: G_{M2} ganglioside as a regulator of pyramidal neuron dendritogenesis. *Ann N Y Acad Sci* **845**:188, 1998.
210. Walkley SU: Pyramidal neurons with ectopic dendrites in storage diseases exhibit increased G_{M2} ganglioside immunoreactivity. *Neuroscience* **68**:1027, 1995.
211. Tedeschi G, Bonavita S, Barton NW, Betolino A, Frank JA, Patronas NJ, Alger JR, et al.: Proton magnetic resonance spectroscopic imaging in the clinical evaluation of patients with Niemann-Pick type C disease. *J Neurol Neurosurg Psychiatry* **65**:72, 1998.
212. Sylvain M, Arnold DL, Scriver CR, Schreiber R, Shevell MI: Magnetic resonance spectroscopy in Niemann-Pick disease type C: Correlation with diagnosis and clinical response to cholestyramine and lovastatin. *Pediatr Neurol* **10**:228, 1994.
213. Balish M, Argoff C, Pikus A, Sato S, Grewal R, Yu K, Pentchev P, et al.: Evoked potentials in type C Niemann-Pick disease. *Ann Neurol* **28**:279, 1990 (abstr).
214. Pikus A: Audiologic profile in Niemann-Pick C. *Ann N Y Acad Sci* **630**:313, 1991.
215. Rywlin AM, Lopez-Gomez A, Tachmes P, Pardo V: Ceroid histiocytosis of the spleen in hyperlipemia: Relationship to the syndrome of the sea blue histiocyte. *Am J Clin Pathol* **56**:572, 1971.
216. Willvonseder R, Goldstein NP, McCall JT, Yoss RE, Tauxe WN: A hereditary disorder with dementia, spastic dysarthria, vertical eye movement paresis, gait disturbance, splenomegaly and abnormal copper metabolism. *Neurology* **23**:1039, 1973.
217. Yan-Go FL, Yanagihara T, Pierre RV, Goldstein NP: A progressive neurologic disorder with supranuclear vertical gaze paresis and distinctive bone marrow cells. *Mayo Clin Proc* **59**:404, 1984.
218. Libert J, Danis P: [Valve of conjunctival biopsy in the diagnosis of Niemann-Pick disease.] *Bull Soc Belge Ophtalmol* **168**:757, 1974.
219. Bowler LM, Shankaran R, Das I, Callahan JW: Cholesterol esterification and Niemann-Pick disease: An approach to identifying the defect in fibroblasts. *J Neurosci Res* **27**:505, 1990.
220. Roff CF, Goldin E, Comly ME, Blanchette-Mackie J, Cooney A, Brady RO, Pentchev PG: Niemann-Pick type-C disease: Deficient intracellular transport of exogenously derived cholesterol. *Am J Med Genet* **42**:593, 1992.
221. Argoff CE, Kaneski CR, Blanchette-Mackie EJ, Comly M, Dwyer NK, Brown A, Brady RO, et al.: Type C Niemann-Pick disease: Documentation of abnormal LDL processing in lymphocytes. *Biochem Biophys Res Commun* **171**:38, 1990.
222. Roff CF, Pastuszyn A, Strauss JF 3d, Billheimer JT, Vanier MT, Brady RO, Scallen TJ, et al.: Deficiencies in sex-regulated expression and levels of two hepatic sterol carrier proteins in a murine model of Niemann-Pick type C disease. *J Biol Chem* **267**:15902, 1992.
223. Turpin JC, Masson M, Baumann N: Clinical aspects of Niemann-Pick type C disease in the adult. *Dev Neurosci* **13**:304, 1991.
224. Byers DM, Rastogi SR, Cook HW, Palmer FB, Spence MW: Defective activity of acyl-CoA:cholesterol *O*-acyltransferase in Niemann-Pick type C and type D fibroblasts. *Biochem J* **262**:713, 1989.
225. Sidhu HS, Rastogi SA, Byers DM, Guernsey DL, Cook HW, Palmer FB, Spence MW: Regulation of low density lipoprotein receptor and 3-hydroxy-3-methyl-glutaryl-CoA reductase activities are differentially affected in Niemann-Pick type C and type D fibroblasts. *Biochem Cell Biol* **71**:467, 1993.
226. Vanier MT: Phenotypic and genetic heterogeneity in Niemann-Pick disease type C: Current knowledge and practical implications. *Wien Klin Wochenschr* **109**:68, 1997.
227. Inui K, Nishimoto J, Okada S, Yabuuchi H: Impaired cholesterol esterification in cultured skin fibroblasts from patients with I-cell disease and pseudo-Hurler polydystrophy. *Biochem Int* **18**:1129, 1989.
228. de Winter JM, Janse HC, van Diggelen OP, Los FJ, Beemer FA, Kleijer WJ: Prenatal diagnosis of Niemann-Pick disease type C. *Clin Chim Acta* **208**:173, 1992.
229. Guo Y, He W, Boer AM, Wevers RA, de Bruijn AM, Groener JE, Hollak CE, et al.: Elevated plasma chitotriosidase activity in various lysosomal storage disorders. *J Inherit Metab Dis* **18**:717, 1995.
230. Boot RG, Renkema GH, Verhoek M, Strijland A, Bliek J, de Meulemeester T, Mannens M, et al.: The human chitotriosidase gene. Nature of inherited enzyme deficiency. *J Biol Chem* **273**:25680, 1998.
231. Sakiyama T, Kitagawa T, Jhou H, Miyawaki S: Bone marrow transplantation for Niemann-Pick mice. *J Inherit Metab Dis* **6**:129, 1983.
232. Sakiyama T, Tsuda M, Owada M, Joh K, Miyawaki S, Kitagawa T: Bone marrow transplantation for Niemann-Pick mice. *Biochem Biophys Res Commun* **113**:605, 1983.
233. Yasumizu R, Miyawaki S, Sugiura K, Nakamura T, Ohnishi Y, Good RA, Hamashima Y, et al.: Allogeneic bone marrow-plus-liver trans-

plantation in the C57BL/KsJ *spm/spm* mouse, an animal model of Niemann-Pick disease. *Transplantation* **49**:759, 1990.

234. Gartner JC, Bergman I, Malatack JJ, Zitelli BJ, Jaffe R, Watkins JB, Shaw BW, et al.: Progression of neurovisceral storage disease with supranuclear ophthalmoplegia following orthotopic liver transplantation. *Pediatrics* **77**:104, 1986.
235. Veyron P, Yoshimura R, Touraine JL: Donor-derived cells in various tissues including brain of BALB/c CSD mice after fetal liver transplantation. *Transplant Proc* **28**:1778, 1996.
236. Veyron P, Mutin M, Touraine JL: Transplantation of fetal liver cells corrects accumulation of lipids in tissues and prevents fatal neuropathy in cholesterol-storage disease BALB/c mice. *Transplantation* **62**:1039, 1996.
237. Touraine JL, Laplace S, Rezzoug F, Sanhadji K, Veyron P, Royo C, Maire I, et al.: The place of fetal liver transplantation in the treatment of inborn errors of metabolism. *J Inherit Metab Dis* **14**:619, 1991.
238. Patterson MC, Di Bisceglie AM, Higgins JJ, Abel RB, Schiffmann R, Parker CC, Argoff CE, et al.: The effect of cholesterol-lowering agents on hepatic and plasma cholesterol in Niemann-Pick disease type C. *Neurology* **43**:61, 1993.
239. Sakuragawa N, Sato M, Yoshida Y, Kamo I, Arima M, Satoyoshi E: Effects of dimethylsulfoxide on sphingomyelinase in cultured human fibroblasts and correction of sphingomyelinase deficiency in fibroblasts from Niemann-Pick patients. *Biochem Biophys Res Commun* **126**:756, 1985.
240. Blanchette Mackie EJ, Dwyer NK, Vanier MT, Sokol J, Merrick HF, Comly ME, Argoff CE, et al.: Type C Niemann-Pick disease: Dimethyl sulfoxide moderates abnormal LDL-cholesterol processing in mutant fibroblasts. *Biochim Biophys Acta* **1006**:219, 1989.
241. Sakuragawa N, Ohmura K, Suzuki K, Miyazato Y: Clinical improvement with DMSO treatment in a patient with Niemann-Pick disease (type C). *Acta Paediatr Jpn* **30**:509, 1988.
242. Hashimoto K, Koeda T, Matsubara K, Ohta S, Ohno K, Ohmura K: [A case of type C Niemann-Pick disease.] *No To Hattatsu* 22:381, 1990.
243. Schiffman R: Personal communication, 1998.
244. Dreier J: Personal communication, 1998.
245. Crocker AC, Farber S: Therapeutic approaches to the lipidoses, in Aronson SM, Volk BW (eds): *Cerebral Sphingolipidoses. A Symposium on Tay-Sachs Disease and Allied Disorders.* New York, Academic, 1962, p 421.
246. Platt FM, Neises GR, Reinkensmeier G, Townsend MJ, Perry VH, Proia RL, Winchester B, et al.: Prevention of lysosomal storage in Tay-Sachs mice treated with N- butyldeoxynorjirimycin. *Science* **276**:428, 1997.
247. Schiffmann R: Niemann-Pick disease type C. From bench to bedside. *JAMA* **276**:561, 1996.
248. Falk T, Garver WS, Erickson RP, Wilson JM, Yool AJ: Expression of Niemann-Pick type C transcript in rodent cerebellum in vivo and in vitro. *Brain Res* **839**:49, 1999.
249. Prasad A, Fischer WA, Maue RA, Henderson LP: Regional and developmental expression of the Npc1 mRNA in the mouse brain. *J Neurochem* **75**:1250, 2000.
250. Henderson LP, Lin L, Prasad A, Paul CA, Chang TY, Maue RA: Embryonic striatal neurons from Niemann-Pick type C mice exhibit defects in cholesterol metabolism and neurotrophin responsiveness. *J Biol Chem* **275**:20179, 2000.
251. Patel SC, Suresh S, Kumar U, Hu CY, Cooney A, Blanchette-Mackie EJ, Neufeld EB, Patel RC, Brady RO, Patel YC, Pentchev PG, Ong WY: Localization of Niemann-Pick C1 protein in astrocytes: implications for neuronal degeneration in Niemann-Pick type C disease. *Proc Natl Acad Sci U S A* **96**:1657, 1999.
252. Wu YP, Kubota A, Suzuki K: Neuronal death and reactive glial changes in the brain of the Niemann-Pick disease type C mouse. Abstract #454.13, Society for Neuroscience, 1999.
253. Liu Y, Wu YP, Wada R, Neufeld EB, Mullin KA, Howard AC, Pentchev PG, Vanier MT, Suzuki K, Proia RL: Alleviation of neuronal ganglioside storage does not improve the clinical course of the Niemann-Pick C disease mouse. *Hum Mol Genet* **9**:1087, 2000.
254. Somers KL, Wenger DA, Royals MA, Carstea ED, Connally HE, Kelly T, Kimball R, Thrall MA: Complementation studies in human and feline Niemann-Pick type C disease. *Mol Genet Metab* **66**:117, 1999.
255. Sym M, Basson M, Johnson C: A model for Niemann-Pick type C disease in the nematode *Caenorhabditis elegans. Curr Biol* **10**:527, 2000.
256. Watari H, Blanchette-Mackie EJ, Dwyer NK, Watari M, Neufeld EB, Patel S, Pentchev PG, Strauss JF III: Mutations in the leucine zipper motif and sterol-sensing domain inactivate the Niemann-Pick C1 glycoprotein. *J Biol Chem* **274**:21861, 1999.
257. Blanchette-Mackie EJ: Intracellular cholesterol trafficking: role of the NPC1 protein. *Biochim Biophys Acta* **1486**:171, 2000.
258. Higgins ME, Davies JP, Chen FW, Ioannou YA: Niemann-Pick C1 is a late endosome-resident protein that transiently associates with lysosomes and the trans-Golgi network. *Mol Genet Metab* **68**:1, 1999.
259. Garver WS, Heidenreich RA, Erickson RP, Thomas MA, Wilson JM: Localization of the murine Niemann-Pick C1 protein to two distinct intracellular compartments. *J Lipid Res* **41**:673, 2000.
260. Hölttä-Vuori M, Määttä J, Ullrich O, Kuismanen E, Ikonen E: Mobilization of late-endosomal cholesterol is inhibited by Rab guanine nucleotide dissociation inhibitor. *Curr Biol* **10**:95, 2000.
261. Cruz JC, Sugii S, Yu C, Chang TY: Role of Niemann-Pick type C1 protein in intracellular trafficking of low density lipoprotein-derived cholesterol. *J Biol Chem* **275**:4013, 2000.
262. Lange Y, Ye J, Rigney M, Steck T: Cholesterol movement in Niemann-Pick type C cells and in cells treated with amphiphiles. *J Biol Chem* **275**:17468, 2000.
263. Kobayashi T, Beuchat MH, Lindsay M, Frias S, Palmiter RD, Sakuraba H, Parton RG, Gruenberg J: Late endosomal membranes rich in lysobisphosphatidic acid regulate cholesterol transport. *Nat Cell Biol* **1**:113, 1999.
264. Xie C, Turley SD, Pentchev PG, Dietschy JM: Cholesterol balance and metabolism in mice with loss of function of Niemann-Pick C protein. *Am J Physiol* **276**:E336, 1999.
265. Xie C, Turley SD, Dietschy JM: Cholesterol accumulation in tissues of the Niemann-Pick type C mouse is determined by the rate of lipoprotein-cholesterol uptake through the coated-pit pathway in each organ. *Proc Natl Acad Sci U S A* **96**:11992, 1999.
266. Xie C, Turley SD, Dietschy JM: Centripetal cholesterol flow from the extrahepatic organs through the liver is normal in mice with mutated Niemann-Pick type C protein (NPC1). *J Lipid Res* **41**:1278, 2000.
267. Liscum L, Munn NJ: Intracellular cholesterol transport. *Biochim Biophys Acta* **1438**:19, 1999.
268. Liscum L: Niemann-Pick type C mutations cause lipid traffic jam. *Traffic* **1**:218, 2000.
269. Incardona JP, Eaton S: Cholesterol in signal transduction. *Curr Opin Cell Biol* **12**:193, 2000.
270. Morris JA, Zhang D, Coleman KG, Nagle J, Pentchev PG, Carstea ED: The genomic organization and polymorphism analysis of the human Niemann-Pick C1 gene. *Biochem Biophys Res Commun* **261**:493, 1999.
271. Watari H, Blanchette-Mackie EJ, Dwyer NK, Watari M, Burd CG, Patel S, Pentchev PG, Strauss JF III: Determinants of NPC1 expression and action: Key promoter regions, posttranscriptional control, and the importance of a "cysteine-rich" loop. *Exp Cell Res* **259**:247, 2000.
272. Yamamoto T, Ninomiya H, Matsumoto M, Nanba E, Ohta Y, Tsutsumi Y, Yamakawa K, Millat G, Vanier MT, Pentchev PG, Ohno K: Genotype-phenotype relationship of Niemann-Pick disease type C: A possible correlation between clinical onsets and levels of Npc1 protein in isolated skin fibroblasts. *J Med Genet,* in press, 2000.
273. Davies JP, Ioannou YA: Topological analysis of Niemann-Pick C1 protein reveals that the membrane orientation of the putative sterol-sensing domain is identical to those of 3-hydroxy-3-methylglutaryl-CoA reductase and sterol regulatory element binding protein cleavage-activating protein. *J Biol Chem* **275**:24367, 2000.
274. Watari H, Blanchette-Mackie EJ, Dwyer NK, Glick JM, Patel S, Neufeld EB, Brady RO, Pentchev PG, Strauss JF III: Niemann-Pick C1 protein: Obligatory roles for N-terminal domains and lysosomal targeting in cholesterol mobilization. *Proc Natl Acad Sci U S A* **96**:805, 1999.
275. Vanier MT, Millat G, Marçais C, Rafi MA, Yamamoto T, Morris JA, Pentchev PG, Nanba E, Wenger DA: Niemann-Pick C disease: mutational spectrum in NPC1 gene and genotype/phenotype correlations. *Am J Hum Genet* **65** (suppl.):A495, 1999.
276. Vanier MT, Millat G: Niemann-Pick C disease: Insights from studies on mutated NPC1 gene and protein. *J Inherit Metab Dis* **23** (suppl. 1):232, 2000.
277. Greer WL, Dobson MJ, Girouard GS, Byers DM, Riddell DC, Neumann PE: Mutations in NPC1 highlight a conserved NPC1-specific cysteine-rich domain. *Am J Hum Genet* **65**:1252, 1999.

278. Millat G, Marçais C, Rafi MA, Yamamoto T, Morris JA, Pentchev PG, Ohno K, Wenger DA, Vanier MT: Niemann-Pick C1 disease: the I1061T substitution is a frequent mutant allele in patients of Western European descent and correlates with a classic juvenile phenotype. *Am J Hum Genet* **65**:1321, 1999.
279. Davies JP, Levy B, Ioannou YA: Evidence for a Niemann-Pick C (NPC) gene family: Identification and characterization of NPC1L1. *Genomics* **65**:137, 2000.
280. Hsu YS, Hwu WL, Huang SF, Lu MY, Chen RL, Lin DT, Peng SS, Lin KH: Niemann-Pick disease type C (a cellular cholesterol lipidosis) treated by bone marrow transplantation. *Bone Marrow Transplant* **24**:103, 1999.
281. Erickson RP, Garver WS, Camargo F, Hossain GS, Heidenreich RA: Pharmacological and genetic modifications of somatic cholesterol do not substantially alter the course of CNS disease in Niemann-Pick C mice. *J Inherit Metab Dis* **23**:54, 2000.

CHAPTER 146

Gaucher Disease

Ernest Beutler ▪ Gregory A. Grabowski

1. Gaucher disease is a lysosomal glycolipid storage disorder characterized by the accumulation of glucosylceramide (glucocerebroside), a normal intermediate in the catabolism of globoside and gangliosides.

2. Three types of Gaucher disease have been delineated. Type 1, by far the most common, is distinguished from type 2 and type 3 disease by the lack of primary central nervous system involvement. Type 2, the acute neuronopathic form of the disease, has an early onset with severe central nervous system involvement and death usually within the first 2 years of life. Patients with type 3 (subacute neuronopathic) Gaucher disease have neurologic symptoms with a later onset and a more chronic course than that observed in type 2 disease. Hepatosplenomegaly, bone lesions, and sometimes involvement of lungs and other organs occur in all forms of Gaucher disease.

3. Gaucher disease is most common in the Ashkenazi Jewish population, where the frequency of Gaucher disease-causing alleles is approximately 0.0343. The 1448C mutation exists at polymorphic levels in northern Sweden, causing type 3 disease among homozygotes.

4. The gene coding acid β-glucosidase is located on chromosome 1. A pseudogene that has maintained a high degree of homology is approximately 16 kb downstream from the active gene. A number of other active genes have been identified in the flanking regions. These include thrombospondin and metaxin. Liver/red cell pyruvate kinase is located only 71 kb downstream from the glucocerebrosidase gene.

5. Most of the disease alleles in Gaucher disease are missense mutations that lead to the synthesis of acid β-glucosidases with decreased catalytic function and/or stability. Several nonsense mutations have a moderate frequency, but occur in the heteroallelic state with a missense allele. A variety of other mutations have been found to cause Gaucher disease. Included are missense mutations, frameshift mutations, a splicing mutation, deletions, gene fusions with the pseudogene, examples of gene conversions, and total deletions. The most common mutation in the Ashkenazi Jewish population is at the cDNA nt 1226 where an A → G transition results in an N370S amino acid substitution in acid β-glucosidase. This is associated with nonneuronopathic disease only, and the clinical manifestations can be relatively mild, particularly in 1226G homozygotes. Other mutations, such as T → C at nt 1448 (L444P), are highly associated with neuronopathic disease. However, there is much diversity in phenotypic expression within all genotypes.

6. The quality of life of patients with Gaucher disease can be improved by a variety of medical and surgical procedures such as joint replacement or splenectomy. The accumulation of glucosylceramide and associated clinical manifestations can be reversed by repeated infusions of modified acid β-glucosidase (alglucerase or imiglucerase). Cure of visceral and probably skeletal manifestations of the disease can be achieved by stem cell transplantation.

7. Approximately 97 percent of mutations in Ashkenazi Jews can be detected by screening for the five most common mutations. Only about 75 percent of the mutations in non-Jewish populations can be detected in this manner. Population screening in the Ashkenazi Jewish population is feasible, but phenotypic variability makes accurate genetic counseling difficult.

INTRODUCTION AND HISTORY

The eponym Gaucher disease encompasses the heterogeneous sets of signs and symptoms in patients with defective intracellular hydrolysis of glucosylceramide (Fig. 146-1) and related glucosphingolipids. At the molecular level, these autosomal recessively inherited disorders most commonly result from mutations of the gene that encodes the lysosomal hydrolase, acid β-glucosidase [glucocerebrosidase (EC 3.2.1.45)]. Rarely, mutations at the prosaposin or "activator" locus also produce severe Gaucher disease phenotypes with glucosylceramide accumulation.

In his 1882 doctoral thesis,[1] Phillipe Charles Ernest Gaucher (1854–1918) provided the first description of the disease, which was named Gaucher disease by Brill in 1905.[2] Massive splenomegaly in a 32-year-old female was attributed to a primary splenic neoplasm. From 1895–1910 the morbid anatomy in children and adults was delineated[2–6] and the systemic nature of the disease was recognized.[7] Klaus,[8] Rusca,[9] and, later, Oberling and Woringer[10] recognized the similarities between the visceral pathologies of Gaucher disease and a rapidly progressive and fatal infantile disease involving the central nervous system, later termed the acute neuronopathic form of the disease. In 1959, Hillborg[11] described the "Norrbottnian" form of slowly progressive neuronopathic Gaucher disease in a Swedish isolate above the Arctic circle.

The familial occurrence of Gaucher disease was recognized as early as 1901,[3] but its inheritance pattern was clarified much later. Although simple autosomal dominant inheritance was suggested by Groen,[12] autosomal recessive inheritance of types 1 and 3 Gaucher disease was established by the population studies of Fried et al.[13] and Hsia et al.[14] Molecular genetic studies described later have defined the more common mutations that produce Gaucher disease. High frequencies of Gaucher disease occur in the Norrbottnian population of Sweden (type 3) and in the Ashkenazi Jewish population (type 1). However, all types are panethnic and the variants of Gaucher disease have been reported in nearly all population groups.

The metabolic nature of Gaucher disease was appreciated by Marchand in 1907[15] and the lipoidal nature of the stored material was suggested in 1916.[16] The stored material was first thought to be kerasin or galactocerebroside,[17,18] but Aghion[19] and others (see reference 20 for review) demonstrated that the major accumulated lipid was glucosylceramide. Miyatake and Suzuki suggested a pathophysiologic role for this lipid and lysosphingolipids in lysosomal storage diseases in 1973.[21] However, the storage of the minor, albeit potentially toxic, deacylated analogue glucosylsphingosine in neuronopathic variants was demonstrated only in 1984 by Svennerholm's group.[22] The enzymatic defect in Gaucher disease was shown to be due to impaired glucosylceramide

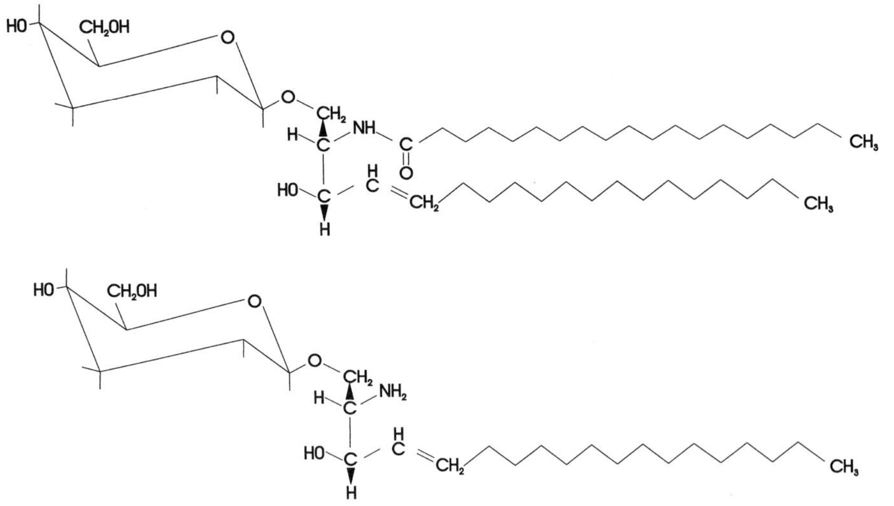

Fig. 146-1 The structure of glucosyl ceramide (glucocerebroside; above) and glucosylsphingosine (below), the major and minor glycolipids stored in Gaucher disease, respectively. Glucosylsphingosine is the deacylated analogue of glucosyl ceramide that may have a role as a toxin in the pathophysiology of Gaucher disease. Glucosylsphingosine is cleaved by acid β-glucosidase at nearly two hundredfold lesser rates than glucosyl ceramide.

hydrolysis by Brady et al.[23] and Patrick,[24] after Trams and Brady[25] demonstrated normal intracellular synthetic rates of this lipid. Because glucosylceramide (glucocerebroside), glucosylsphingosine, and, potentially, other β-glucosides are natural substrates for this enzyme, the more general terms acid β-glucosidase and lysosomal β-glucosidase are preferred to glucocerebrosidase. We use the term acid β-glucosidase in this chapter.

The specificity of acid β-glucosidase for the β-glucoside linkage was shown by Öckerman[26] and part of the enzyme's active site has been localized to the carboxy one-third of the enzyme.[27] The lysosomal localization of the enzyme was demonstrated by Weinreb et al.,[28] establishing Gaucher disease as a member of the lysosomal storage disease family. A low-molecular-weight "activator," now termed saposin C, was found by Ho and O'Brien[29] to be important for the activity of acid β-glucosidase. The gene encoding acid β-glucosidase was assigned to human chromosome 1[30,31] and mapped to 1q21.[32,33] The cDNA,[34–36] structural gene, and unprocessed pseudogene[37] were cloned and characterized between 1984 and 1988. The first missense mutation was identified in 1987 and shown to be frequent in the neuronopathic variants.[38] More recently, the cDNA[39–41] and chromosomal gene[31,42] for the unique multifunctional "activator," or prosaposin locus, have been cloned and characterized.

de Duve[43] proposed in 1964 that lysosomal enzyme deficiencies might effectively be treated by enzyme infusions, but early attempts[44,45] to treat Gaucher disease in this fashion met with only borderline success, probably largely because an adequate method for targeting infused enzyme to macrophages had not been developed. Achord et al.[46] and Stahl et al.[47] reported that macrophages possessed a glycoprotein receptor that was antagonized by mannans, and Stahl et al.[47] proposed that this might be useful in directing enzyme to macrophages in the treatment of Gaucher disease. These principles were subsequently applied in developing enzyme therapy for Gaucher disease.[48–52]

PREVALENCE

Based on the occurrence of homozygotes in the Ashkenazi Jewish population of Israel, Fried estimated a disease incidence of 1:7750[53] and 1:10,000.[13] However, because many patients with Gaucher disease do not come to medical attention, estimates based on diagnosed cases are invariably lower than the true incidence of the disorder. Although there is considerable overlap between normal and heterozygous levels of leukocyte acid β-glucosidase, efforts to predict disease incidence from such measurements have also been made. These yielded very divergent results of 1:640,[54] 1:2003,[55] and 1:3969.[56]

In contrast, it is possible to obtain quite robust estimates of gene frequencies by DNA-based screening for the more common mutations. The combined results of two studies[57,58] encompassing 2121 presumably normal Ashkenazi Jewish subjects showed that 124 were heterozygous and 6 were homozygous for the 1226G (N370S) mutation, giving a gene frequency of 0.0231. Ten of 2305 subjects were found to be heterozygous for the 84GG mutation,[58] a gene frequency of 0.00217 with a standard error of 0.00096. Thus the combined frequency of the two most common mutations is 0.0343, giving expected incidences of 1.03 per 1000 births for 1226G homozygotes and 0.14 per 1000 for 1226G/84GG heterozygotes, for a combined incidence of 1 per 855 Ashkenazi Jewish births. Homozygotes for the 84GG mutation have never been encountered and this combination may be lethal.

It is notable that the ratio of 1226G mutations to 84GG mutations is much higher in the healthy population than in the Gaucher disease population.[59] This is because numerous homozygotes for the 1226G mutation do not come to medical attention until middle age or not at all, and that they are, therefore, underrepresented in the patient population (see "Clinical Genetics and Prevention" below).

Few data are available regarding the frequency of Gaucher disease in non-Jewish populations. In Holland, a country of about 15,000,000 that is virtually without a Jewish population, between 100 and 200 cases of Gaucher disease are known, a number that is compatible with a gene frequency of about 0.005. Many of the Dutch patients have the 1226G mutation, and thus may have some Jewish ancestry. Other European countries in which a considerable number of Gaucher disease patients have been reported include Spain[60] and Portugal.[61] In both of these populations, the 1226G mutation is prevalent. A gene frequency of 0.0068 may be deduced from the Portuguese data,[62] suggesting that there may be as many as 5 cases per 100,000 population in that country. Historically, Jewish populations existed in these countries, and one may speculate that forced conversion to Christianity brought this mutation into the non-Jewish population. In non-European countries, such as Japan, the 1226G mutation has not been encountered. Without it, the overall gene frequency for Gaucher disease is probably lower still.

The high gene frequency in the Ashkenazi Jewish population has not been explained. At one time it was thought that this was simply due to the existence of a Gaucher disease mutation in a small ancestral population. But even before the molecular biology of the disease was understood, this seemed like a doubtful explanation, because Gaucher disease as well as two other lipid storage diseases, Tay-Sachs and Niemann-Pick, exhibited an extraordinarily high prevalence in the Jewish population. That there are three common mutations among Ashkenazi Jews (see

"Molecular Biology" below), makes it clear that the high gene frequency is not an accident, but rather is the result of selection; presumably heterozygotes in the Ashkenazi Jewish population enjoyed an advantage. The nature of this advantage is unknown. It has been suggested that it may be resistance to tuberculosis,[63,64] but the limited data available[65] do not support this conjecture. It is possible that the lowered blood cholesterol levels characteristic of homozygotes might in some way be related to a survival advantage of heterozygotes. In any case, it would seem that the advantage would need to be exerted at the heterozygous level, because the 84GG mutation is lethal in the homozygous form and produces very serious disease in most compound heterozygotes.

CLINICAL MANIFESTATIONS

Classification

Clinically, three major types of Gaucher disease have been delineated based on the absence (type 1) or presence and severity (types 2 and 3) of primary central nervous system involvement (Table 146-1). To avoid the nonspecific descriptors "adult," "infantile," and "juvenile," the following nosology has been adopted: type 1 = nonneuronopathic; type 2 = acute neuronopathic; type 3 = subacute neuronopathic.[66] However, within each type, even within the same ethnic and/or demographic groups, the phenotypes and genotypes can be markedly heterogeneous.

The most common form of the disease is type 1, characterized by the lack of neuronopathic involvement. This type of Gaucher disease is sometimes called the "adult" form. Although adult onset is common, onset in early childhood is the rule in those type 1 patients who have inherited more severe acid β-glucosidase mutations.

Type 2 disease, the infantile form of the disorder, is characterized by infantile onset and severe neurologic involvement, whereas type 3, the juvenile form of the disease, is characterized by neuronopathic disturbances that usually begin later in the first decade of life and progress more gradually than in the acute neuronopathic form of the disease. The distinction between severe type 1 disease and type 3 disease is often not obvious in early childhood, although certain genotypes are commonly associated with juvenile disease. Genotyping may allow provisional classification of some patients without neuronopathic disease as having a high probability of developing neurologic abnormalities.

Type 3 disease has been further subdivided. Patients with type 3a[67] disease have progressive neurologic disease dominated by myoclonus and dementia; those with 3b[67] disease have aggressive visceral and skeletal disease, but with neurologic manifestations largely limited to horizontal supranuclear gaze palsy; those with type 3c disease[68–71] have neurologic manifestations largely limited to horizontal supranuclear gaze palsy, corneal opacities, and cardiac valve calcification, but generally have little visceral disease.

Type 1 Gaucher Disease

The clinical manifestations of type 1 Gaucher disease result from engorged macrophages causing enlargement and dysfunction of the liver and spleen, displacement of normal bone marrow by storage cells, and damage to bone leading to infarctions and to fractures. Occasionally, involvement of other organs contributes to the overall clinical picture. Hypermetabolism (increased resting energy expenditure)[72] and cachexia may be present.

Severity. Type 1 Gaucher disease has a broad spectrum of severity. At one extreme, patients may be diagnosed as late as the eighth or ninth decade of life.[73–76] Some asymptomatic "patients" with the disease are ascertained only in the course of family studies or population surveys.[57,76] Such mildly affected individuals are almost invariably found to have the 1226G/1226G (N370S/N370S) genotype. The median age of appearance of the first clinical symptoms of patients with this genotype is about 30 years,[77–79] although many patients with this genotype never come to medical attention at all.

At the opposite extreme of type 1 Gaucher disease are children with massive hepatosplenomegaly associated with severe abnormalities of liver function, pancytopenias, and extensive skeletal abnormalities. Such children may die of the complications of Gaucher disease in the first or second decade of life. Almost invariably their genotypes include at least one very severely deficient allele such as the 1448C encoding the L444P mutant protein or the 84GG mutation producing a frameshift in the leader sequence.

Some patients with severe visceral (liver and spleen) enlargement have minimal skeletal involvement, while some with severe bone disease have minimal visceral disease. In other patients, visceral involvement and skeletal involvement are approximately equal in severity. The type of mutation seems to have less influence on the sites of disease involvement, than on overall visceral disease severity.

Children with moderately severe or severe Gaucher disease type 1 generally show growth retardation,[80,81] but their mental development is quite normal.

Natural History. At birth, infants with type 1 Gaucher disease are normal, and in severe cases, organomegaly becomes evident after the first year or two of life, and may progress for some years after. Bone lesions usually occur later than visceral disease. There is little progression in many or most adults with Gaucher disease. Systematic follow-up of a sizable number of patients over the age of 15 shows that changes in untreated patients, if they occur at all, are noted over decades, not over months or years.[82–85] Spleen and liver sizes do not change or only slightly so and progressive osteopenia and the occasional development of new fractures may be observed.

Table 146-1 Gaucher Disease—Clinical Types

Clinical Features	Type 1	Type 2	Type 3a	Type 3b	Type 3c
Onset	Childhood/ Adulthood	Infancy	Childhood	Childhood	Childhood
Hepatosplenomegaly	+ to +++	+	+++	+++	+
Hypersplenism	+ to +++	+	+++	+++	+
Bone crises/ fractures	+ to +++	—	++	+++	+
Neurodegenerative course	—	+++	++	+	
Survival	6–80 + years	< 2 yr	2nd to 4th decade	2nd to 4th decade	2nd to 4th decade
Ethnic predilection	Ashkenazi Jewish	Panethnic	Northern Swedish	Panethnic	Panethnic

In general, the historical data in individual patients serve as a guide to future rates of change, particularly in adults. In adults, rapid progression of previously quiescent disease is sufficiently unusual that other etiologies should be excluded before the change is attributed to Gaucher disease.

Hematologic Manifestations. Bleeding is a common presenting symptom of patients with Gaucher disease.[86] The most common cause is thrombocytopenia. Bleeding is a much less common problem in patients who have been known to have Gaucher disease for some years,[86] probably because of the ameliorating effect of splenectomy. Deficiencies of factor XI are prevalent, but may be coincidental because a deficiency of this clotting factor is common in Ashkenazi Jews,[87] the population that is most frequently affected by Gaucher disease. Abnormalities of factor IX, vWF Ag, and factor VIII have also been found, and are considered usually to be laboratory abnormalities possibly due to the presence of increased amounts of glucosylceramide in the blood.[88] However, the levels of markers for activation of coagulation thrombin-antithrombin (TAT) complex and fibrinolysis (PAP-complex fibrin-cleavage product D-dimer) have also been reported to be significantly elevated,[89] possibly due to intrasplenic activation of the coagulation cascade.[90] The possible role of hemostatic abnormalities in Gaucher disease remains unresolved.

Thrombocytopenia is the most common peripheral blood abnormality.[91] Early in the course of the disease, it is usually due to splenic sequestration of platelets and invariably responds to splenectomy.[86] Later in the course of the disease, in patients who have already undergone splenectomy, replacement of the marrow by Gaucher cells may be more important etiologically.

Anemia is usually mild, but occasionally is quite severe, with hemoglobin levels as low as 5 g/dl. Leukopenia also occurs in some patients. These changes are probably due to a combination of increased splenic sequestration, when the spleen is present, and decreased production because of replacement of the marrow by Gaucher cells.

The Spleen. Splenic enlargement is present in all but the most mildly involved. Even in those who are otherwise asymptomatic, it is commonly the presenting sign,[54,92,93] and splenomegaly is present in all symptomatic patients by physical examination or imaging.[94] In severely affected patients the spleen may be huge, filling the abdomen. The bulk of the spleen may interfere with normal food intake and it may cause dyspareunia in women. As in other states in which splenomegaly occurs, splenic infarctions occur. In rare circumstances, a large part (25 to 50 percent) of a massively enlarged spleen can infarct. Such patients present with an acute abdomen, fever, metabolic acidosis, and hyperuricemia. Selective splenic nuclide scans can be useful in delineating the presence and extent of new or old infarcts.

The Liver. Enlargement of the liver is the rule in patients with Gaucher disease.[95] When the disorder is severe, the liver may fill the entire abdomen. On physical examination, the liver is usually firm and smooth, and the right and left lobes are uniformly enlarged. Massively enlarged livers are usually hard and can have irregular surfaces. Frank hepatic failure and/or cirrhosis with portal hypertension and ascites are uncommon,[92,95] but do occur in a small percentage of patients, and bleeding from varices[96,97] may cause death. The bulk of the liver may cause distress to the patient, and episodes of pain may occur due to infarction or mechanical stress on ligaments. Minor abnormalities of liver function tests, consisting of increases in plasma transaminase and gamma-glutamyl transferase activities, are commonly present, even in mildly affected patients. Hyperbilirubinemia in Gaucher disease is usually due to infection, Gilbert syndrome, or an intercurrent illness. In patients with severe disease liver function, abnormalities may be quite serious. Jaundice attributable to Gaucher disease is a very poor prognostic sign.

Bones. The skeletal manifestations of Gaucher disease can be totally debilitating.[98] By radiographic,[98–102] scintigraphic, computed tomographic, or magnetic imaging scans,[99,103–105] nearly all affected patients have bony lesions. The Erlenmeyer flask deformity of the distal femur is a common radiographic finding, but it is not universally present. Generalized loss of bone mass has been documented and is very common, even in patients with relatively mild disease.[99,106,107]

Many patients with radiographically significant Gaucher disease of bone have few or no bony symptoms. However, episodic, excruciatingly painful "bone crises" occur in 20 to 40 percent of patients.[93] These crises are much more frequent in children and adolescents, but can occur for the first time in the third to seventh decades. The femoral head and the femoral shaft are by far the most frequently involved sites in a crisis, but these episodes occur with some frequency in the humeral heads, vertebral bodies, and ischium of the pelvis. The crisis occurs spontaneously or follows a febrile syndrome and begins with a dull, deep, aching pain in the involved bone. Over a period of about 2 to 4 days the pain may become excruciating and difficult to control with analgesics. X-ray lesions may be absent, even in the presence of severe pain. Accompanying localized tenderness, swelling, and erythema may be present. However, areas of ischemia may usually be detected on ^{99m}Tc bone scans. Within a few days the intense pain begins to subside to a dull ache that can persist for several weeks. Recurrence is often at a different location.

In children, the acute hip lesions can be misinterpreted as Legg-Calvé-Perthes disease, but this is rarely the presenting symptom of Gaucher disease. Involvement of the vertebral bodies is less common, but can lead to extensive collapse, gibbus formation, and spinal cord or nerve compression.[108] Delayed collapse of vertebrae sometimes occurs after trauma.[109] In our experience, vertebral involvement with collapse occurs most commonly during the pubertal growth spurt with rapid progression until the end of puberty. Similarly, based on observations in several hundred type 1 and 3 patients, the majority of severe bony lesions seem to appear during childhood and adolescence. This aggressive phase of bony involvement is followed in adults by a more slowly progressive process or a cessation of active bony destruction as assessed by current radiographic and MRI techniques. Although pathologic fractures of the femoral neck may occur in the third, fourth, and later decades, these usually are in areas of preexisting bony lesions. Development or redevelopment of apparent Gaucher vertebral, femoral, or other bony disease later in life is an indication to exclude malignancy, particularly multiple myeloma, or osteomyelitis. Direct erosion through the cortical bone with extravasation of Gaucher cells and formation of sinus tracts has occurred spontaneously or following surgical intervention.[110] The incidence of postmenopausal osteoporosis in women with Gaucher disease is not clearly increased (Grabowski, unpublished).

The Lungs. Although it is relatively uncommon, pulmonary failure is one of the most serious consequences of Gaucher disease. It may occur as the result of frank infiltration of lung by Gaucher cells, particularly in children,[111,112] but severe pulmonary failure also occurs in patients without demonstrable Gaucher cells in the lungs. In such patients, right-to-left intrapulmonary shunting, probably secondary to liver disease, seems to be the cause. Clubbing is generally a feature of this complication. Changes indicating both alveolar and interstitial involvement have been noted on high resolution CT scan.[113] Pulmonary hypertension also occurs in patients with type 1 Gaucher disease. This complication has been documented for at least 30 years,[114] but seems to be encountered more frequently in recent years.[112,114,115]

The Nervous System. The absence of primary central nervous system involvement defines Gaucher disease as type 1. However, central nervous symptoms can be occasionally observed as a secondary manifestation of true type 1 disease. Thus, massive systemic fat emboli involving the brain and lung[116] and compression of the spinal cord secondary to vertebral collapse[117,118] have been reported. Coagulopathies have also caused central nervous system damage.[119] Central nervous system abnormalities without other known cause have been observed in patients with adult-onset disease,[120–122] but the relationship between symptoms and putative brain involvement in these patients was unclear. Nonetheless, a high degree of concordance between Gaucher disease and neurologic disease was documented in one family.[122] An early onset of aggressive Parkinson's disease has been associated with Gaucher disease.[123] The etiologic relationships are not clear, but cannot be excluded.

Other Manifestations.

Cutaneous. Skin manifestations of Gaucher disease are infrequent and nonspecific, such as diffuse brown or yellow-brown pigmentation and easy tanning.[124] Severe neonatal ichthyosis ("collodion babies") has been described in infants with acute neuronopathic Gaucher disease.[125,126] Brownish masses of Gaucher cells have been reported to occur at the corneoscleral limbus of the eye.[127] Gaucher cells have been found in a colonic polyp[97] and the maxillary sinus.[128] Fever occurs in patients with Gaucher disease, often,[129,130] but not always,[131] in connection with bone crises.[129,130] An increased tendency toward infection has been noted in some patients, and has been attributed to a defect in neutrophil chemotaxis[132–134] or to monocyte dysfunction.[135]

Gaucher Disease and Cancer. Neoplastic disorders, particularly of the blood-forming organs, are more common in patients with Gaucher disease than in the general population.[92,136] Especially notable are lymphoproliferative diseases including chronic lymphocytic leukemia,[129,137–139] multiple myeloma,[140–144] and Hodgkin[145,146] and non-Hodgkin lymphoma.[147] The existence of monoclonal immunoglobulin spikes in the serum has also been documented in a high proportion of patients with Gaucher disease who are more than 50 years of age.[148–151] Bone tumors, including osteoblastoma[152] and malignant epithelioid hemangioendothelioma,[153] have also been diagnosed in patients with Gaucher disease, as have been chronic granulocytic leukemia[154] and breast cancer.[76,144]

Pregnancy. Patients with mild Gaucher disease appear to tolerate pregnancy well. There is little reason to believe that the course of the disease is adversely affected by the pregnancy.[155] (See reference 156 for review.) However, hematologic complications with increasing thrombocytopenia develop in more severely affected patients.[155,157] First trimester bleeding has been noted in 37 percent of a large series of pregnant patients, and only about 75 percent of the pregnancies are carried to term.[158]

Type 2 Gaucher Disease

There is a moderate degree of heterogeneity in the onset and course of even the acute neuronopathic form of the disease. Early and late onset varieties have been delineated,[54] but the overall clinical course is similar. The principal difference is in the age of onset. Indeed, Gaucher disease has been reported to manifest as hydrops fetalis[159] and we know of additional cases in which this has been the outcome.

Extensive visceral involvement with hepatosplenomegaly is the rule. Oculomotor abnormalities are often the first manifestations with the appearance of bilateral fixed strabismus[54] or of oculomotor apraxia. This may result in the appearance of rapid head thrusts as an attempt to compensate when trying to follow a moving object.[160] Hypertonia of the neck muscles with extreme arching of the neck (opisthotonus), bulbar signs, limb rigidity, seizures, and sometimes choreoathetoid movements occur, although the latter are more common in type 3 disease. A congenital ichthyosis-like cutaneous disorder may occur, and it has been suggested that the skin changes in type 2 disease may allow its early differentiation from type 3 disease and type 1.[126,161] Most infants with type 2 disease die within the first 2 years of life.[162]

Type 3 Gaucher Disease

The severity of type 3 disease is usually intermediate between that of type 1 and 2 although, as noted below, less severe forms of type 3 disease exist. Massive visceral involvement is usually present, although exceptions have been reported.[162] Neurologic symptoms similar to those observed in type 2 disease are present, but with a later onset and relatively lesser severity.

The prototype of type 3 disease is the Norrbottnian form, the clinical manifestations of which have been described in considerable detail.[163–167] The median age of onset of symptoms is at 1 year, with a range in 22 patients of 0.1 to 14.2 years. The first symptoms are usually the results of visceral involvement, with neurologic findings developing in about one-half of the children during the first decade of life. As in type 2 disease, disorders of eye movement are the usual first symptoms, with the subsequent development of other neurologic manifestations such as ataxia. Table 146-1 summarizes the distinguishing features of the three subtypes of type 3 Gaucher disease. Type 3c disease is clinically quite distinct; cardiac valve calcifications and corneal opacities are characteristic of patients homozygous for the 1342C (D409H) mutation.[69–71,168] They have not been observed with any other mutation, and the question of whether they may be the result of linkage disequilibrium with mutations in tightly linked genes in the region flanking the glucocerebrosidase gene has been raised.

CLINICOPATHOLOGIC CORRELATIONS

The Gaucher Cell

The hallmark of Gaucher disease is the presence in a variety of tissues of lipid-engorged cells with a characteristic appearance.[1] Evidence that these cells are derived from the monocyte/macrophage system includes the demonstration of pre-Gaucher monocytes and monocytoid cells with varying, but increasing, amounts of the characteristic tubular cytoplasmic inclusions in peripheral blood and bone marrow of affected patients.[169] In addition, isolated splenic Gaucher cells have macrophage surface markers.[170] The plasma membrane of Gaucher cells can be smooth or can show extensive arborization with microvilli.[171] Their surfaces can be round, ridged with the extensive folds and wrinkles that are typical of normal macrophage counterparts.[171] Intense phagocytic activity has been demonstrated in Gaucher cells in liver and spleen.[172,173] The monocyte/macrophage origin of Gaucher cells and the evolution of monocytoid cells into end-stage Gaucher macrophages have had major implications for the understanding of the pathophysiology of Gaucher disease and toward the development of targeted enzyme therapy as well as gene and cellular therapeutic strategies (see "Therapy" below).

The Gaucher cell has a distinctive appearance by light microscopy. In smears and imprints of affected tissues, Gaucher cells are about 20 to 100 μm in diameter,[169] although cells up to 200 μm can be isolated from affected bone marrows and spleens[174] (Grabowski, unpublished). These cells contain one or more nuclei and cytoplasm with a striated, fibrillary, or tubular pattern that has been likened to "wrinkled tissue paper" or "crumpled silk."[169] On Romanovsky-stained preparations these cells manifest a characteristic pale blue to gray cytoplasm. In comparison, the cells from patients with Niemann-Pick disease and other lipidoses are foam cells that contain discrete membrane-bound white or empty-appearing lipid inclusions. The Gaucher cells from a variety of tissues also stain for nonspecific esterase, and contain abundant, albeit nonuniform, iron micelles[169,173] and tartrate-resistant acid phosphatase (isozyme 5).[175,176] Erythrophagocytosis has been described[172,173] in bone marrow and spleen, and may account for some of the excess iron storage.

By electron microscopy, the cytoplasm of pre-Gaucher cells and end-stage Gaucher cells has dilated membrane-bound vesicles

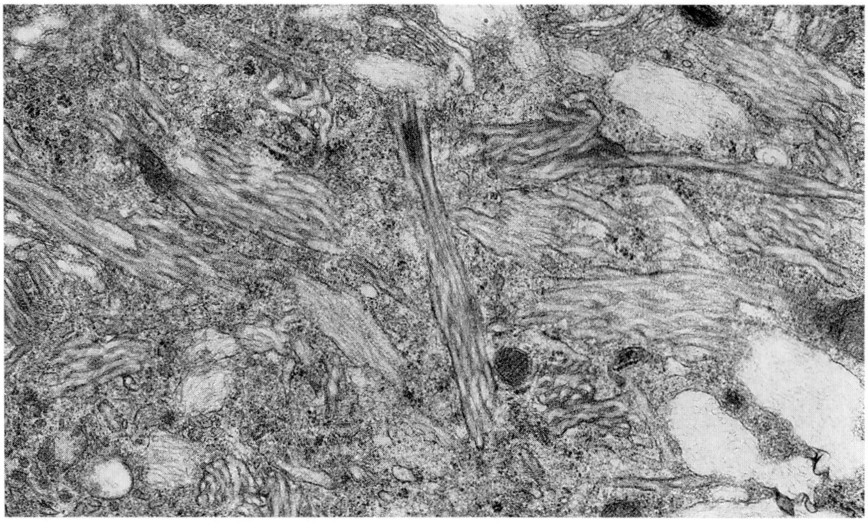

Fig. 146-2 Electron micrograph of storage material in Kupffer cells from a Gaucher disease type 3 patient (×16,000). A variety of sizes of characteristic twisted tubular appearing structures were present in elongated as well as more rounded membrane delimited organelles. (*Courtesy of Cynthia Daugherty.*)

(0.6 to 4 μm) containing characteristic twisted structures[177] (Fig. 146-2). When examined in nonembedded cells, these structures are bound by a single, limiting membrane, 250 to 500 Å wide, up to 5 μm in length, and that occur individually or in twisted pairs.[177] As viewed by x-ray diffraction, these appear as twisted bilayers.[178] Each structure contains 10 to 12 fibrils that are twisted together into a right-handed helix to form a tubule.[177] The fibrils are spaced about 80 Å apart, which is twice the length of a glucosylceramide molecule. In cross-section, each tubule has a diameter of about 350 Å.[177] These tubules are about 90 percent glucosylceramide and about 0.3 percent protein in composition.[177] Based on these observations, it has been postulated that the tubules resulted from the polymerization of glucosylceramide in a polar head-to-apolar tail manner.

Gaucher cells are distributed throughout the body, wherever macrophages reside. The largest numbers are found in spleen, sinusoids of the liver, bone marrow, and parenchyma of lymph nodes where they replace their normal counterparts, splenic, bone marrow, and lymph node macrophages, and hepatic Kupffer cells. Gaucher cells have been described in nearly every organ examined (see below). Although several theories have been suggested,[66] the evidence favors phagocytosis of the formed elements of the blood as the primary source of the accumulated intracellular lipid in the viscera. Erythrocyte fragments are present in Gaucher cells from spleen,[172,173] suggesting the erythrocyte membrane as a source of stored glycolipid. The accumulation of β-galactose, *N*-acetylglucosamine, fucose, and sialic acid-containing glycopeptides and glycans has been demonstrated in delipidated Gaucher cells from splenic red pulp, liver, and the alveolar, perivascular, and interstitial areas of the lungs.[179,180] Because these glycoconjugates are not substrates for acid β-glucosidase, their presence cannot be due to the primary enzymatic defect. They probably represent digestive remnants of phagocytosed cells or cell membranes. Because of their rapid turnover, it has been suggested that leukocyte membranes are the major source of stored glucosylceramide in visceral Gaucher cells.[181] Although this is probably the case, direct evidence of abundant phagocytosis of leukocytes is lacking. The clear demonstration that previously stored intracellular glucosylceramide is released from lysed Gaucher cells into the extracellular spaces of the spleen[172] provides a source of the elevated plasma levels of this lipid.

The Spleen

The degree of splenic enlargement is highly variable. Spleen sizes measured at autopsy,[92] surgery,[182] by computed tomography,[52] or by magnetic imaging scans[50,51] range from about 5 to over 75 times normal size when adjusted for body weight. The absolute sizes range from a few hundred grams to about 10 kg. The spleen can account for 15 to 25 percent of body weight and can have significant effects on growth and caloric requirements.[72] As determined by MRI, CT or ultrasound in 166 patients, the mean splenic volume was 21.9-fold (SD = 18.3-fold, range 1.8 to 94.9) increased over expected normal (0.2 percent of body weight) with a median of 21.5-fold.[183,184] When adjusted for body weight, the largest spleens have been found in the younger, severely affected patients with Gaucher disease types 1, 2, or 3.[92] However, some older patients (age 40 to 70 years) had spleens increased 25 to 50 times in weight.[52] Although not systematically studied, the spleen appears to increase most rapidly in size in children with type 1 or 3 disease. For individual children with these types of Gaucher disease, the rate of enlargement seems relatively constant until adolescence or early adulthood, when a clear diminution in rate occurs. Consequently, a significant acceleration in the rate of splenic enlargement in affected adults should be thoroughly evaluated to exclude malignancies or other diseases. In most cases, the amount of splenic enlargement is directly related to the degree of hypersplenism (i.e., anemia, thrombocytopenia, and, occasionally, significant leukopenia). Significant deviations from this correlation should prompt evaluations for other causes of blood dyscrasias; e.g., immune-mediated thrombocytopenia[185] and autoimmune hemolytic anemia[186] have been documented in patients with Gaucher disease.[185]

Nodules on the surface of the spleen result from regions of extramedullary hematopoiesis, collections of Gaucher cells, or resolving fibrotic infarcts.[92] These surface nodules, and their interior counterparts (0.5 to 4.5 cm in diameter), have been delineated by imaging techniques.[94] Evidence of old splenic infarcts can be found in nearly all spleens that are twentyfold larger than normal. About 20 to 40 percent of spleens have infarcts, nodules, or other structural abnormalities.[187,188] Most infarcts have been asymptomatic but subcapsular infarcts can present as localized abdominal pain. Usually point tenderness can be elicited directly over the involved area of the spleen and the pain resolves within a few days to a week. Gross examination of the Gaucher spleens reveals a hard organ that can range in color from the deep red of a normal spleen, to purple areas of extramedullary hematopoiesis, to yellow areas of resolved infarcts. The cut surface reveals extensive fibrosis, with nodular interior areas of Gaucher cell collections as well as white collections of these cells in the red pulp.[92] The fibrosis may account for the distinctly unusual occurrence of spontaneous rupture. Gaucher[1] described the microscopic appearance of these areas as resembling the alveoli of the lungs. Ultrastructural studies have demonstrated active erythrophagocytosis by Gaucher cells,[164,189] as well as the extrusion of stored glucosylceramide tubular structures into the extracellular spaces in the spleen.[173]

The Liver

Hepatic involvement by Gaucher disease is always evident on biopsy from the presence of Gaucher cells, that is, abnormal Kupffer cells, in the liver sinusoids. Importantly, even in the presence of extensive replacement of liver tissue by these Gaucher cells, the hepatocytes do not manifest grossly apparent glucosylceramide storage.[92,190] This sparing of the hepatocytes probably accounts for the low incidence of severe hepatic failure. Increases in hepatic volume from two to three times normal size are common[51,52] but massive enlargement by five- to tenfold is, in our experience, observed principally in splenectomized patients. In 254 patients, the mean hepatic volume as measured by MRI, CT, or ultrasound was 2.09-fold (SD = 0.98, range 0.73 to 7.4) increased over normal (2.5 percent of body weight) with a median of 1.83. About 20 to 35 percent of patients have abnormal signal intensities and inhomogeneities of their livers with the greater percentage of abnormalities occurring in splenectomized patients.[187,188] Grossly, the liver can be yellow-brown in the presence of nearly complete replacement by Gaucher cells, dark-red to purple in areas of extramedullary hematopoiesis, or grayish-red with white streaks from Gaucher cell infiltration. Nodules resulting from infarction or Gaucher cell infiltration can be present on the surface. As with other organs, fibrosis is the most common abnormality other than the presence of Gaucher cells. This fibrosis leads to small parenchymal nodules that contain numerous Gaucher cells. Hepatocyte regeneration does not occur in the nodules. In less involved areas, the pericellular fibrosis is most severe in the region of the central vein. Bile duct proliferation, which is typical of cirrhosis, is notably absent.[92,190] The recurrence of severe hepatic involvement followed transplantation of a liver from a normal donor into a patient with Gaucher disease.[191]

Bone

As summarized in Table 146-2, marked variation has been reported in the degree and type of bone involvement.[98,99,104,192]

The skeletal disease results from two separate processes whose interrelationships are not understood: (a) loss of bone mass and (b) complex bone marrow involvement related to the accumulation of Gaucher cells. These two processes must be separated because their pathophysiologies, documentation, and potential treatments are different. The etiology of the former is poorly understood (see "Pathophysiology" below), but accelerated bone turnover may be important.[193] The bone marrow involvement is the culmination of Gaucher cell accumulation, vascular compromise, infarction, and scarring within the marrow space. The clinical results are focal and local abnormalities leading to the majority of radiographic findings summarized in Table 146-2.

The first most general and nearly universal abnormality is the decrease in bone mass or osteoporosis.[99,100,107,194] As assessed by dual absorptiometry (DEXA), the mean bone mineral density is significantly diminished and there are good intersite correlations.[107] In comparison, the bone marrow cavity involvement is highly nonuniform and the involvement appears to progress through several stages leading to severe destruction of the bone, joints, and medullary cavity (Figs. 146-3*A* and 146-3*B*). Focal Gaucher disease includes, in approximate decreasing frequency, the femoral necks and heads; femoral shaft; humeri; vertebral bodies; tibias; ribs; pelvis; bones of the feet; calvarium; and mandible[194–196] (see reference 66 for a review). The immediate antecedents of "bone crises" are vascular compromise, infarction, and increased intramedullary pressure due to resultant edema. However, the events initiating the focal involvement are poorly understood. Microscopically, the earliest lesion appears to be increased reticulum fibers surrounding individual Gaucher cells.[92] The finding of hyperemia leading to osteopenia[98,197] and dilatation of the Haversian canals[197] suggests the presence of an inflammatory or toxic agent that initiates the pathologic process, but little correlation exists between the severity of bone disease and plasma interleukin-1 (IL-1) or IL-10 levels.[90] The lesions in bone include loss of trabeculae, fibrosis, necrosis, calcification of infarcted areas, and various stages of healing fractures.[98,99] Complete obliteration of marrow by fibrosis and osteosclerosis can occur[98–100,104] and progresses from proximal to distal with gradual replacement of bone marrow.[99] Complete loss of bone marrow perfusion has been observed.[99]

The Cardiopulmonary System

Although unusual, clinically significant cardiopulmonary disease is a very poor prognostic sign in patients with Gaucher disease. The dyspnea on exertion and tachypnea frequently observed in affected children with massive hepatosplenomegaly are usually due to limited diaphragmatic excursions. Primary involvement of the heart by Gaucher disease was reported in two adult females with Gaucher cell infiltration of the myocardium.[198,199] Amyloidosis has been observed in several cases associated with dysgammaglobulinemia.[200–202] Pericarditis[203,204] of undetermined etiology has been reported. In adults, pulmonary hypertension has been related to Gaucher cells plugging the alveolar capillaries or infiltration of lung parenchyma.[111] In a series of 13 children and adults with Gaucher disease type 1 who were evaluated by pulmonary function studies, one was hypoxemic and two others

Table 146-2 Radiologic Stages of Skeletal Lesions in Gaucher Disease Type 1

Stage	Type of lesion/site involved	Radiographic appearance
1	Diffuse osteoporosis/ tubular bones and vertebrae	Coarse trabecular pattern of osteoporosis
2	Medullary expansion/femora, long bones, ribs	Loss of normal concavity above femoral condyles; Erlenmeyer flask deformity
3	Localized destruction (osteolysis)/long bones	Small erosions (well defined or moth eaten); cortex rarefied and endosteally notched; ground-glass veiling
4	Ischemic necrosis, sclerosis, osteitis/long bones	Patch densities and erosions; serpiginous sclerotic streaks; layered periostitis; sequestra
5	Diffuse destruction; epiphyseal collapse; osteoarthrosis/hips, shoulders, vertebrae, sacroiliac joints	Flattening or irregular destruction of femoral or humeral heads; mixed lytic and sclerotic foci; larger "soap bubble" pattern

Adapted from Hermann et al.[99] and Beighten et al.[100]

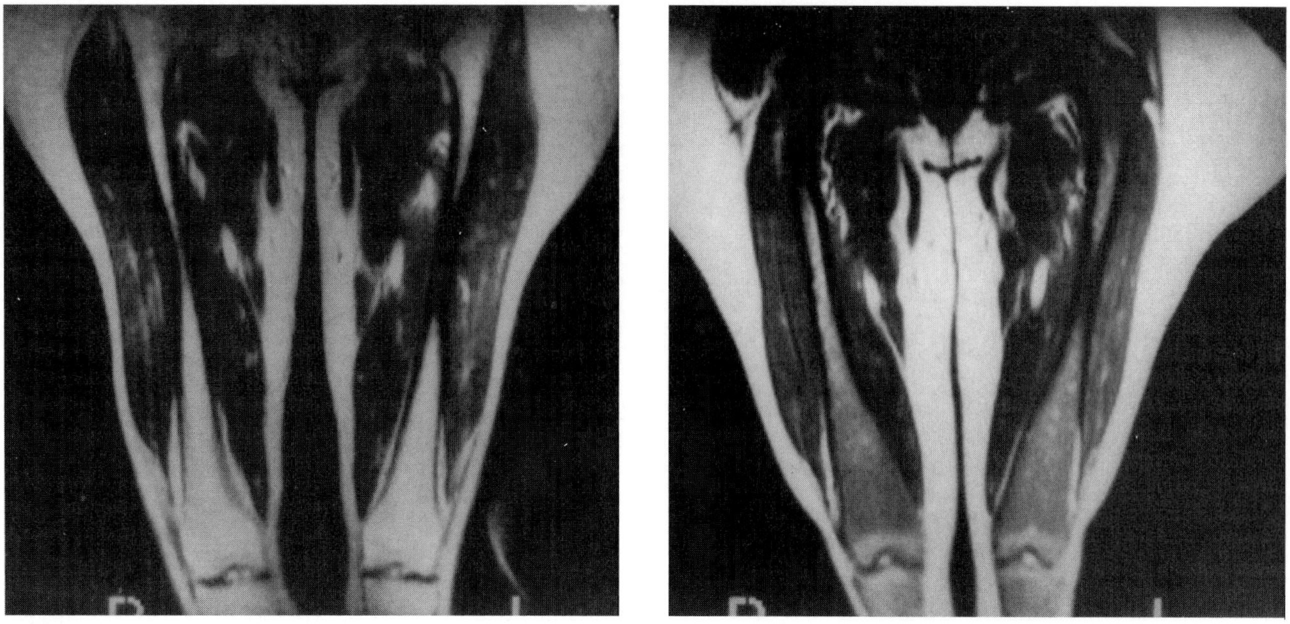

A B

Fig. 146-3 MRI T1-weighted scans of femurs in two adults with Gaucher disease type 1. In these age-matched patients, the greater whiteness of the marrow cavity and lack of major distal femoral distortion in *A* indicate lesser involvement than in *B*. The typical Erlenmeyer flask deformity and cortical bone thinning is present in *B*. The mottled, low density of the marrow cavity indicates extensive replacement of normal triglyceride with glucosyl ceramide-containing macrophages as well as other pathologic alterations (see text).

demonstrated restrictive lung disease with pulmonary infiltrates by chest x-ray.[205] The two cyanotic and hypoxemic patients ($pO_2 = 40$ to 50 mm Hg) had Gaucher cell infiltration at autopsy or the presence of Gaucher cells in bronchial lavage specimens.[206,207] In a large series, 68 percent of type 1 patients had some pulmonary function abnormalities. There was no association between the pulmonary function abnormalities, age, or genotype.[208] The clinical significance of these observations is not apparent because few patients have overt pulmonary disease. Dreborg et al.[166] have commented on the presence of reticular infiltrates on chest x-ray in several Norrbottnian patients, but they did not report clinical lung disease. In contrast, autopsy reports of nearly all patients with type 2 disease[164,180,209–211] commented on pulmonary infiltration of alveolar capillaries and frank consolidation of alveoli by Gaucher cells that could have been a contributory cause of death in these neurologically impaired children. Three patterns of pulmonary pathology have been observed in a large autopsy series:[92] (a) interstitial Gaucher cell infiltration with fibrosis; (b) alveolar consolidation and filling of alveolar spaces by Gaucher cells; and (c) capillary plugging by Gaucher cells and resultant secondary pulmonary hypertension. Pulmonary hypertension also occurs in the absence of capillary plugging by Gaucher cells[212] due to extensive thickening of the medial and intimal layers of pulmonary arterioles.[92]

Lymph Nodes

Lymph nodes in a variety of locations have been infiltrated with Gaucher cells. The lymph nodes of the neck, groin, and axilla can be enlarged and are rubbery in consistency. Very enlarged mesenteric and paraspinal nodes may be detected by computed tomography or at surgery. These can obscure the diagnosis of a malignancy and must be evaluated carefully. The thymus, Peyer's patches, adenoids, and tonsils can be involved (see reference 66 for a review).

Renal/Gastrointestinal/Endocrine

Clinically significant renal disease due to Gaucher involvement, if it exists, is rare. Gaucher cells have been found in the glomerular tufts and renal interstitium. Significant proteinuria (20 g/day) has been reported in one case, and this was associated with episodic acute glomerulonephritis.[213] Histologically, typical tubular inclusions were demonstrated in endothelial cells lining the glomerular and interstitial capillaries.[213] Only mesangial involvement was found in one other case.[214] Several other cases have been reviewed by Chander.[213]

Gastrointestinal complaints primarily relate to early satiety and a feeling of fullness due to hepatosplenomegaly. Frequent diarrhea has occurred in several patients. In the presence of massive visceromegaly with increased basal metabolic rates,[72] interference with adequate caloric intake may be a contributing cause to growth retardation and delays in skeletal maturation. A single case of colonic infiltration by Gaucher cells has been reported as the cause of lower intestinal bleeding,[97] and gastric splenosis has caused severe bleeding in one patient.[215] Nearly every autopsy on a type 2 patient has commented on the severe infiltration of the adrenal gland by Gaucher cells, but adrenal insufficiency has not been reported.

The Central Nervous System

In our experience with several autopsied cases, and in the few autopsy reports[92] on type 1 patients, periadventitial accumulation of Gaucher cells has been the only consistent abnormality in the nervous system.

Microscopic abnormalities have been found in all patients dying of type 2 Gaucher disease.[92,180,209,216–220] Neuropathologic studies of Norrbottnian[221,222] and non-Swedish type 3[92,220] patients have shown less severe involvement of the central nervous system. In contrast to other lipidoses, massive storage of material does not occur in the type 2 Gaucher disease brain. Table 146-3 summarizes the consistent light microscopic findings as condensed from the above reports.

The most striking feature is the presence of "Gaucher cells" in the perivascular Virchow-Robinow spaces in the cortex and deep white matter.[180,209,218] Not infrequently, these periadventitial cells are also found in the gray matter of the thalamus and subependymal tissues of the pons and medulla.[209] Although the exact origin of these cells is not known, they most likely are typical Gaucher cells derived from peripheral blood monocytes. These cells were excluded from the brain by the formation of a

Table 146-3 Severity and Location of Central Nervous System Abnormalities in Type 2 Gaucher Disease

Region	Neuronal loss	Gliosis	Periadventitial Gaucher cells	Neuronophagia	Free Gaucher cells
Cerebral Cortex					
Frontal	3+	2+	3+	2+	2 → 4+
Temporal	1 → 3+	2+	3+	0	3+
Parietal	4+	2+	3+	1+	2+
Occipital	1+	3+	3+	0	4+
White Matter	4+	1+	4+	0	0
Thalamus	2 → 4+	2+	1+	4+	1+
Caudate Nucleus	4+	2+	0	2 → 4+	1+
Claustrum	4+	2+	0	2+	2+
Putamen	3+	2+	0	1+	2+
Globus pallidus	4+	2+	0 → 1+	4+	0
Midbrain	2 → 4+	2+	1+	4+	0
Pons	3+	1+	1+	4+	1+
Medulla	3+	1+	1+	4+	0
Cerebellum					
Dentate nucleus	4 → 5+	0 → 1+	1 → 3+	4+	0
Purkinje layer	2+	0	0	0	0

The severity of the abnormalities range from normal (0) to very extensive changes (5+).

membrane that contained basal lamina protein collagen type IV and laminin.[222] The extraneural accumulation of these cells appears to elicit gliosis[180,209,222] and microglial proliferation[209,220] in the brain parenchyma, which approximates the perivascular Gaucher cells. The local loss of neurons was shown using antineurofilament antibody staining.[222] In some patients, immunologic studies suggested extravasation of plasma proteins into the brain parenchyma juxtaposed to the periadventitial cell accumulations.[222] Neuronal loss is widespread in the brains of type 2 patients. Large losses of neurons occur in the basal ganglia, nuclei of the midbrain, pons and medulla, and hypothalamus.[209,216,220] The dentate nucleus of the cerebellum is always severely involved. Severe neuronal loss in the cochlear nuclei and the superior olivary complex has been demonstrated by physiologic brain stem auditory-evoked responses (BAER) studies and histologic correlation in the same patients.[217] Less cell loss is observed in the cerebral cortex. When present, the cell loss is localized to the pyramidal and ganglionic layers.

Laminar necrosis of the third and fifth cortical layers has been observed in autopsy specimens[180,216,218] and in the only reported operative biopsy.[218] Cell death is also evident from crumpled, shrunken-atrophic neurons as well as those with distended cytoplasm with chromolysis and loss of Nissl substance.[209,218] Free Gaucher cells are found within brain parenchyma of the cerebral cortex, especially in the occipital lobes.[92,180,220] The numbers of these cells in cerebral cortex appear to be greater in the most severely affected patients with type 2 disease than in the type 2 patients dying later. In either case, they are few in number, and absent in type 3 patients.[92,222] Neuronophagia is prominent in involved layers of the cortex and in nuclei of the midbrain, basal ganglia, and brain stem as well as in the dentate nucleus. PAS-positive inclusions occur in neurons but the typical tubular storage structures of glucosylceramide seen in Gaucher cells are rare.[221] Light and electron microscopic studies of the brain from a 20-week-old fetus affected with a neuronopathic form of Gaucher disease were normal.[223] These pathologic findings have suggested the presence of a neurotoxic agent that leads to cellular disruption and eventual death of neurons. Direct experimental evidence for this hypothesis is lacking, but extensive chemical analyses in tissues and brains from type 2 and 3 patients[224,225] have implicated the deacylated analogue of glucosylceramide, glucosylsphingosine (Fig. 146-1), as a viable candidate toxin.

PATHOPHYSIOLOGY

The Storage Substances

The major natural substrate for acid β-glucosidase is *N*-acylsphingosyl-1-*O*-β-D-glucoside (Fig. 146-4). This compound has also been called glucosylceramide, ceramide-glucoside, and glucocerebroside. A minor, but important, substrate is glucosylsphingosine, the deacylated analogue of glucosylceramide. The enzyme that hydrolyzes the β-glucose from these substrates has been referred to as glucocerebrosidase, glucosylceramidase, ceramide β-glucosidase, and acid β-glucosidase. With some variation (see below) in chain length, the natural sphingosyl moiety is (2S,3R,4E)-2-amino-4-octadecene-1,3-diol.[226,227] Glucosylceramide is widely distributed in many mammalian tissues in small quantities as a metabolic intermediate in the synthesis and degradation of complex glycosphingolipids, such as the gangliosides or globoside. Glucosylsphingosine is not normally detected in significant amounts in tissues.

Synthesis

Glucosylceramide is synthesized from ceramide and UDP-glucose by glucosylceramide synthase.[228–231] The reaction has an optimal pH at 7.8 and K_m values of 0.12 and 0.8 mm for ceramide and UDP-glucose, respectively.[228,229] Both hydroxy and nonhydroxy fatty acylsphingosines serve as substrates.[232] This pathway is present in brain and a variety of tissues and cell types.[233–238] Although ceramide and sphingosine are synthesized in the endoplasmic reticulum, glucosylceramide is made in the *cis*-Golgi.[239] A major component of the active site of glucosylceramide synthase is on the cytoplasmic face of the *cis*-Golgi.[230,231] Glucosylceramide is the only glycosphingolipid synthesized with the polar head on the cytoplasmic surface of the Golgi. Synthesis of the higher order glycosphingolipids from glucosylceramide requires a flip-flop across the Golgi membrane during migration from *cis* to *trans*. Alternative synthetic paths occur in neuroblastoma cells via reacylation of glucosyl-sphingosine[240–242] and via dolichol-phosphate glucose in BHK-21 cells.[243] Glucosylceramide synthesized by these pathways is destined for the plasma membrane and does not contribute major amounts to the lysosomal degradative pathway. Glucosylceramide has a variety of growth and differentiation activities, particularly in neurons.[244–246] The

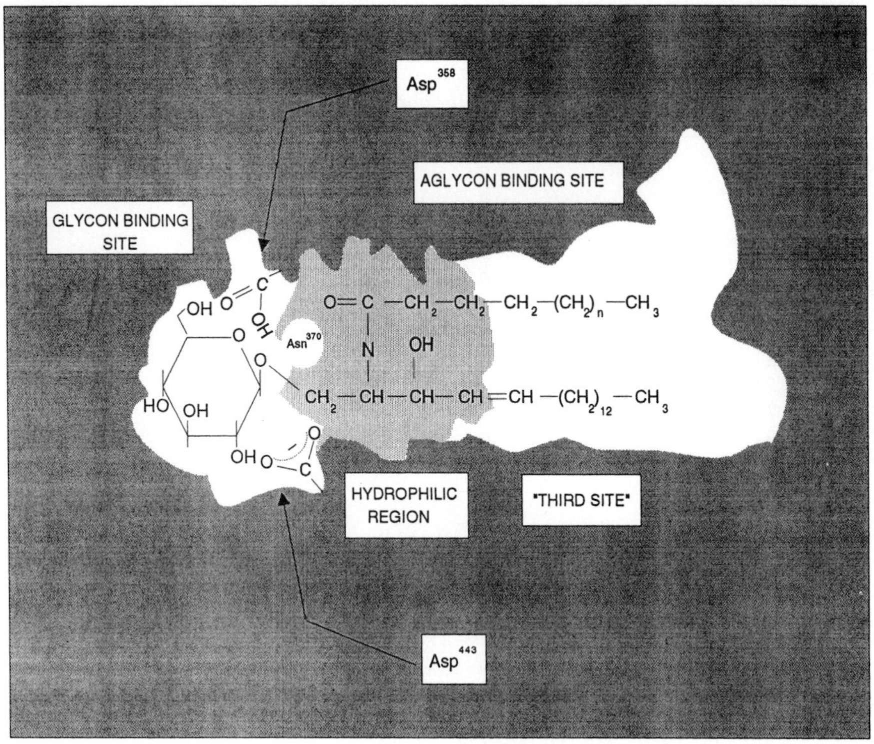

Fig. 146-4 A proposed schematic for the active site of acid β-glucosidase containing the major natural substrate, glucosyl ceramide. Glu340 and Glu235 are the nucleophile and acid/base in catalysis. Asp433 may play an assistive role in catalysis. Asn370 is important for determining the specificity of interaction at the active site and N370S is the most frequent substitution in Gaucher disease genes. The sphingosyl moiety is usually an octadecene but chain lengths vary from 16 to 22. The fatty acid acyl moiety chain length varies from 16 to 24 carbons and is dependent on the tissue source. Cleavage of the bond at the anomeric carbon releases glucose with retained configuration.

relationships of these activities to the pathogenesis of Gaucher disease remain unknown.

Catabolism

Glucosylceramide is the penultimate intermediate in the degradative pathway of most complex glycosphingolipids. Further degradation by the acid β-glucosidase produces ceramide, the latter being further degraded by acid ceramidase[247,248] to sphingosine and fatty acid. Glucosylceramide dispersions have been used to facilitate absorption of the lipid into the outer leaflet of the plasma membrane and endocytosis.[249] The fate of the internalized glucosylceramide depends on the differentiation state of the cells.[249] In differentiating cells, glucosylceramide is preferentially sorted to the Golgi apparatus following endocytosis; this does not occur in fully differentiated cells.[249,250] The method of presentation of glucosylceramide to cells also alters its subcellular location. For example, albumin solubilized glucosylceramide is found in the cytosol, and this localization may explain the very low or absent degradation of the externally added substrate in some studies of intact cells[251,252] and the fact that the rate of degradation of albumin-solubilized glucosyl ceramide in cells from Gaucher disease patients approaches normal.[253] Thus, the presentation of glucosylceramide via phagocytosis or from endogenous glycolipid degradation may significantly affect acid β-glucosidase activity and substrate flux.

Tissue and Organ Distribution and Characteristics

The properties, isolation, purification, and role of the respective glycosphingolipids in normal animals or humans as well as in patients with the lipid storage disorders have been described (see references 254 and 255 for reviews).

Plasma levels of glucosylceramide are elevated 2 to 20 times in affected patients, but such levels do not correlate with the type of Gaucher disease nor the degree of involvement within a type.[256–258] The plasma glucosylceramide is associated with lipoproteins.[256,259] Only the liver, spleen, and brains of patients with Gaucher disease have been subjected to extensive lipid analyses and characterization studies.[160,220,224,225,258,260–263] In liver and spleen there are large (twenty- to one hundredfold) increases of glucosylceramide. The fatty acid and sphingosyl base compositions of the accumulated glucosylceramides are typical of visceral organs.[225,260,261] There is a predominance of C20 to C24 fatty acids and shorter chain sphingosyl bases in all Gaucher disease variants.[225] Substantial concentrations of glucosylsphingosine are also present.[261] Increased levels of glucosylceramide are present in brains from several disease variants. However, the distribution, amount, and type of this accumulated lipid vary with the Gaucher disease variant.

Gaucher cells and glucosylceramide accumulation in type 1 disease are in the vascular periadventitial areas of the Virchow-Robinow spaces. The fatty acid and sphingosyl base compositions of the accumulated lipid in brain from one classical type 1 patient were consistent with the extraneural location and visceral origin of this lipid.[225] In comparison, composition analyses of glucosylceramide from brains of nonsplenectomized type 2 and 3 patients were consistent with a neural origin.[160,224,225] The levels of glucosylsphingosine accumulation was also increased several times over that found in the classical type 1 brain.[224,225] In splenectomized type 3 patients, much greater accumulations of glucosylceramide were found in liver and brain, when compared to their nonsplenectomized cohorts.[224,258]

PATHOGENESIS

Other than the presence of Gaucher cells, the earliest histologic abnormalities seen in a variety of tissues are the surrounding of Gaucher cells by reticulum fibers.[92] As a consequence, fibrosis in the visceral organs and gliosis in the brain appear to occur prior to or coincident with the secondary tissue events leading to advanced disease. In the visceral organs and bone, advanced disease is characterized by infarction, necrosis, and scarring. In the brain, neuronal loss is the most apparent manifestation. The regenerative capacities of visceral tissues may obscure the role of cell death as an early event in these tissues. Clearly, the extensive variation of the early and end-stage disease reflects tissue-specific characteristics: that is, the solid containment field of bone marrow, the specialized extracellular environment developed by osteoclasts, and the sinusoidal structure of the liver and spleen. Thus, only the consistent and early events in various tissues (i.e., fibrosis) can be considered if a unified pathophysiology of this disease is to be developed. In addition, unlike many other lysosomal storage diseases, most of the storage material within Gaucher cells of visceral tissues is derived from phagocytosis of cells, cell membranes, and cell debris that are external to the cell, and are not from cell-specific glycolipid synthesis. Neurons of the brain may be the only cell type in which endogenous synthesis plays an important pathogenic role. These observations suggest the presence of cytotoxic substances, that is, glucosylceramide, its lysosphingolipid derivative, glucosylsphingosine, or other glucolipids. In visceral organs from patients with type 1, 2, or 3 disease, glucosylsphingosine, if present, occurs only at exceedingly low concentrations, whereas in the central nervous system of type 2 and 3 patients significant amounts are present. The toxic role of this lysosphingolipid is consistent with the general hypothesis that the cell death and injury in glycosphingolipid storage diseases may be mediated by lysosphingolipid inhibition of protein kinase C.[264,265] However, experimental support in the lysosomal storage diseases is lacking. Glucosylceramide has been shown to have growth promoting potential in animal models.[266] In addition, macrophages release cytokines when exposed to solvent solubilized glucosylceramide.[267] Cytokine production has also been estimated by measuring mRNA levels in circulating monocytes, using RT-PCR methodology with semiquantitative analysis. Significantly increased expression of IL-1β mRNA, as well as a trend to elevated TNF-α mRNA, were found in Gaucher patients relative to healthy individuals. There were no statistically significant differences between Gaucher disease patients and controls with respect to two other tested cytokines (IL-6 and IL-8).[268] Serum levels of the macrophage-derived cytokines IL-8, IL-6, TNF-α, M-CSF, and the monocyte/macrophage activation marker sCD14, have also been investigated. Most patients showed remarkably elevated levels of M-CSF (two- to eightfold) and sCD14 (two- to fivefold) as compared to normal controls. Levels of IL-8 were elevated two- to twentyfold in all patients, whereas levels of IL-6 and TNF-α were normal.[269]

The pathogenesis of the pulmonary manifestations that occur in some patients is not clearly understood and may be multifactorial. In some patients Gaucher cells have been detected in pulmonary capillaries,[66,92,270] but direct involvement with Gaucher cells can often not be demonstrated. In patients with extensive hepatic involvement, cyanosis and clubbing can result from shunting within the lung. It has been suggested that this may be caused by an unidentified humoral factor(s) that disappears following hepatic transplantation.[191] Such right-to-left shunting has resulted in a pyogenic cerebral abscess in one adult (Grabowski, unpublished observation). Many patients with pulmonary hypertension have been treated with alglucerase, and enzyme therapy appears to have little if any effect on the course of this complication. The association between pulmonary hypertension and treatment may be fortuitous, but the cases of several patients who developed this complication only after beginning treatment have been documented.[115,271] It is possible that the closing of existing pulmonary shunts results in a rise of the pulmonary pressure.[271] Because it is well known that primary pulmonary hypertension is aggravated by pregnancy, it has also been suggested that contaminating placental proteins may play a role,[115] but there is no direct evidence for such a mechanism.

ANIMAL MODELS

A dog model of Gaucher disease[272] has, unfortunately, been lost. However, a mouse with glucocerebrosidase deficiency has been produced using the techniques of targeted disruption.[273] Homozygotes for this severe defect die within 34 h of birth and manifest extensive lysosomal glucosyl ceramide storage. A knock-in strategy has been used to create mice homozygous for the 1448C (L444P) or RecNciI (1448C [L444P], 1483C [D456P], and 1497C [V460V]) mutations.[274] Although the 1448C homozygote had more enzyme activity and less glucosylceramide storage than the homozygotes for the RecNciI mutations, both variants died within 48 h of birth, presumably from dehydration due to increased water loss through the abnormal skin.

DIAGNOSIS

Morphologic Diagnosis

Classically, the diagnosis of Gaucher disease has been most frequently suspected by detection of the specific storage cell, the Gaucher cell (see "Clinicopathology and Correlations" below). However, very similar cells (pseudo-Gaucher cells) have been described in a variety of other disorders, including chronic granulocytic leukemia,[181,275–278] thalassemia,[279,280] multiple myeloma,[281] Hodgkin disease,[282,283] lymphomas,[169,284] and acute lymphocytic leukemia,[285] and in the acquired immunodeficiency syndrome (AIDS) in a patient with *Mycobacterium avium* infections.[286] About 70 percent of patients with chronic myelogenous leukemia have pseudo-Gaucher cells in their marrow,[278] presumably due to the massively increased presentation of myeloid membranes containing glucosylceramide[181] to macrophages. These pseudo-Gaucher cells do not contain the typical tubular structures of authentic Gaucher cells.[92,169] Because biochemical and molecular techniques are less invasive and more specific, histologic diagnosis of Gaucher disease should be a means to the diagnosis only in patients in whom Gaucher disease has not been suspected previously.[287]

Although it was once believed that heterozygotes for Gaucher disease harbored a few Gaucher cells, it is now recognized that no such cells are present in carriers.

Enzymatic Diagnosis

Peripheral blood leukocytes normally contain abundant acid β-glucosidase activity and their capacity to cleave labeled glucosyl ceramide is markedly diminished in Gaucher disease.[288] However, radioactively labeled natural substrate is not generally available and, in any case, is more difficult to use than soluble artificial substrates. Under proper assay conditions synthetic, water-soluble substrates for β-glucosidase are very useful in the diagnosis of Gaucher disease. At pH 5, 4-methylumbelliferyl-β-glucoside is cleaved almost as well by intact leukocytes from Gaucher disease patients and normal controls, but at pH 4 the activity of such cells is only about 10 percent of normal.[289,290] Similar results are obtained under a variety of assay conditions using different fluorescent substrates and cell lysates with added detergent.[278,291–298] It is useful to separate lymphocytes, granulocytes, and monocytes, because the activity in these cell types differs markedly, with monocytes > lymphocytes > granulocytes.[299] Even within a given morphologic type of leukocyte, there is considerable variability in activity, and the activity is unstable, so that for optimal results to be obtained, it is necessary to process the blood within 24 h of the time that it is drawn. Cultured skin fibroblasts and amniotic fluid cells and chorionic villi are also markedly deficient in acid β-glucosidase activity[300] and can be used for diagnosis.[301–304] Demonstration of the enzyme deficiency remains the standard for establishing the diagnosis of Gaucher disease.

On average, the leukocytes and cultured skin fibroblasts of heterozygotes for Gaucher disease have about one-half normal β-glucosidase activity. However, there is considerable overlap between the lower portion of the normal range and values found in individual heterozygotes. The many methods that have been devised to increase the specificity of the assay largely represent efforts to reduce the overlap between heterozygous and normal values. Although some methods appear slightly better than other methods, considerable overlap remains. If reference values that encompass 99 percent of the normal controls are used, the assay results of at least one-third of the heterozygotes will fall within the normal range.

Enzyme-based diagnosis has not proven to be very useful in differentiating between neuronopathic disease (type 2 and type 3) and nonneuronopathic (type 1) variants. The amount of enzyme activity, measured with 4-methylumbelliferyl β-glucoside, and antigen, measured with monoclonal antibodies against acid β-glucosidase, tend to be lower in type 2 and type 3 disease, but there is considerable overlap.[305,306] It has been suggested that the use of a short acyl-chain substrate may help to differentiate the different forms of the disease.[307] In pulse-chase studies, the stability of the enzyme in type 2 disease is usually decreased while processing and stability appear to be normal in type 1 disease,[305] but there are mutations that are exceptions to this rule (see "Posttranslational Processing of Acid β-Glucosidase," below).

Diagnosis by DNA Analysis

DNA-based technology has major advantages over enzymatic diagnosis of Gaucher disease in that the results are qualitative rather than quantitative and in that the samples are extremely stable. However, although many Gaucher disease alleles have been identified, others have not. Thus, even when DNA is examined for many different known mutations, a normal result does not ensure the absence of a Gaucher disease allele. The mutations at cDNA nt 1226 (N370S) and 84 account for 80 to 90 percent of the disease-producing alleles in Ashkenazi Jewish patients with Gaucher disease. Among non-Jewish patients, mutations at nt 1448 (L444P) and 1226 (N370S) account for 70 percent of the disease-producing alleles. Thus, if Gaucher disease is suspected clinically in a Jewish patient, there is an excellent chance of being able to confirm the diagnosis by DNA analysis. Among non-Jewish patients there is also a good chance of being able to do so, but there are many more sporadic, uncommon mutations among non-Jewish patients and thus the DNA-based approach is likely to be less helpful. A variety of PCR-based techniques for facile detection of mutations have been described.[308–316]

Unlike enzyme analysis, mutation analysis has predictive value with respect to disease prognosis,[311,312,316–319] although it is not absolute[320] (see "Clinical Genetics and Prevention" below). Patients homozygous for the 1448C mutation all appear to have severe visceral disease and usually also develop neurologic disease. There have been exceptions to this in patients as old as 20 to 30 years of age.[321] On the other hand, presence of the N370S mutant enzyme appears to preclude the development of neurologic disease.[318] The 1342C (D409H) mutation manifests a characteristic phenotype including cardiac calcification, oculomotor apraxia, and corneal opacities. The relationship between the genotype and disease phenotype is described in detail below ("Relationship between genotype and phenotype").

Ancillary Studies

The activities of a number of plasma enzymes are usually increased in Gaucher disease. These include the acid phosphatase,[175,322,323] other lysosomal enzymes, such as hexosaminidase,[324] the angiotensin-converting enzyme,[325,326] and chitotriosidase.[83,327–331] Although it has been proposed that the latter enzyme, in particular, might be useful in following the course of treatment,[330,331] the relationship between disease severity and the levels of these enzymes is weak.[83] Very high plasma ferritin levels are regularly encountered in patients with Gaucher disease.[86,332] Plasma cholesterol levels tend to be lowered in unsplenectomized patients,[333] possibly due to abnormal clearance of LDL by macrophages.[334] When present, these laboratory findings support the diagnosis of Gaucher disease but they are neither required nor sufficient to make a diagnosis.

BIOCHEMISTRY

Acid β-Glucosidase

Properties. Acid β-glucosidase has been purified from a variety of species, but human tissues have been the primary source for many investigations.[335–341] Size exclusion and ion-exchange chromatography[335] or affinity chromatography using a natural activator protein[342] as the ligand provided highly purified enzyme, but in low yields (<5 percent).[343] Higher yields (≥ 20 percent) were obtained with detergent and organic solvent extraction of crude membrane preparations[336] to solubilize and delipidate this tightly membrane-associated enzyme.[344] Subsequent hydrophobic chromatography using short chain alkyl or aromatic agarose derivatives[336–338] or immobilized phosphatidylserine[345] provided additional purification. Electrophoretic and/or amino acid sequence homogeneity of preparations has been accomplished by substrate analogue affinity,[339,341,346] HPLC,[337] and immunoaffinity[340] procedures. The final specific activities of such acid β-glucosidase preparations have varied over a tenfold range (5 to 50 μmole/min/mg protein),[335–341,346] due primarily to different compositions of assay mixtures. Based on active site quantitation of homogeneous human placental acid β-glucosidase using a covalent inhibitor, bromo-[^{3}H]-conduritol B epoxide ([^{3}H]-Br-CBE), the catalytic rate constants, *k*cat, were about 2350 min^{-1} for several glucosylceramide and 4-alkyl-umbelliferyl-glucoside substrates.[347]

Human acid β-glucosidase is a homomeric glycoprotein. Partial[346] and complete[36] amino acid sequences have been determined chemically for the placental enzyme and the complete sequence deduced from the nucleotide sequences of the cDNA sequences.[35,36,348] About 13 percent of the residues are basic (lysine, arginine, or histidine) and the calculated pI value is 7.2, which is consistent with that (pI = 7.3 to 7.8) obtained experimentally for placental enzyme preparations containing only neutral mannosyloligosaccharide core.[349] The protein has about 11 percent leucine residues and 45 percent nonpolar amino acids, but transmembrane domains are not present in the mature polypeptide by computer calculations. Proteolytic digestion studies of acid β-glucosidase obtained by in vitro translation in the presence of microsomal membranes indicated the absence of a large cytoplasmic domain.[350] These and other findings[351] indicate that acid β-glucosidase is a peripheral membrane protein. No obvious basis for its tight membrane association is evident from the primary sequence. The mature human polypeptide is 497 amino acids with a calculated molecular weight of 55,575. The glycosylated enzyme from placenta has a molecular weight of about 65,000. Glucocerebrosidase II,[352] a high-molecular-weight form of acid β-glucosidase in human cells and urine, is an enzyme/saposin C aggregate. The native state of acid β-glucosidase in cells has not been resolved due to its requirement for detergent or organic solvent extraction for solubilization. Molecular weights, estimated by sedimentation and molecular exclusion chromatography, have varied from about 60,000 to 450,000.[335–339,341,346,353,354] The native molecular weight in tissues was estimated by *in situ* radioinactivation of the enzymatic activity.[353–356] Two studies[355,356] indicated that the normal enzyme may be dimeric in cells, whereas other data[353,354] were consistent with the enzyme being a monomer. The enzyme has three disulfide bonds with C126 being free (McPherson, personal communication, 1994). Compared with the human homologues, the canine and mouse cDNAs have 88 and 84 percent nucleotide identity, respectively. These cDNAs predict proteins with (a) 92 (canine)- and 87 (mouse)-amino-acid identity. A single amino acid deletion, His274, is present in the mouse sequence. (b) The cysteines were 100 percent conserved. (c) The positions of the five *N*-glycosylation sites are strictly conserved and the sequences were identical in the canine and human enzymes. Sites 1 and 2 have different amino acid contents in the mouse.[357] Additional amino acid sequence and functional studies have suggested conserved domains in the lysosomal glycosyl hydrolases.[358] These analyses identified E235 as the acid/base in catalysis that was subsequently supported by preliminary mutagenesis analysis.[359] Typical bi- and triantennery complex *N*-linked oligosaccharides are present on the human placental acid β-glucosidase.[360] Endoglycosidase F digestion analysis and site-directed mutagenesis studies suggest that the first four glycosylation sites are utilized, and that the glycosylation of the first site and/or the specific amino acid at position 19 is required to develop an active conformer.[361,362]

Enzymology

Kinetic Properties. Kinetic studies of acid β-glucosidase have been complicated by its membrane association, its requirements for detergents for solubilization, and requirements for specific amphiphiles for reconstitution of enzymatic activity. The accumulation of glucosylceramides and of small quantities of glucosylsphingosines in Gaucher disease tissues indicated that these are natural substrates for acid β-glucosidase. Glucosylceramides are insoluble in aqueous media and require a lipoidal environment for dispersion. A widely used synthetic substrate, 4MU-Glc, has greater, but limited, solubility in aqueous dispersions. Consequently, assays for acid β-glucosidase are done in heterogeneous dispersions whose physical compositions and phase states influence the physical state and activity of the enzyme as well as its interactions with effector molecules. Despite these limitations there has been a remarkable consistency in the results from various laboratories that employed (a) micellar and mixed micellar systems with combinations of polyoxyethylene ethers (e.g., Triton X-100), bile salts (e.g., sodium taurocholate[295,363]) and/or fatty acids (e.g., oleic acid), or (b) negatively charged phospholipids or glycosphingolipids dispersed by sonication. In the absence of detergents or negatively charged lipids, delipidated human,[344,364–366] bovine,[363] and murine[365] acid β-glucosidases have little hydrolytic activity. In addition, kinetic values (i.e., K_m and V_{max}) obtained in the absence of dispersants cannot be interpreted due to the aggregated state of the enzyme and glucosylceramide substrates.[364]

Effect of Negatively Charged Phospholipids and Glycosphingolipids. Because of the loss of enzyme activity early in the purification of acid β-glucosidase and the in vivo membrane association of acid β-glucosidase, specific membrane-derived lipids are needed for enzymatic activity. Dale et al.[364] found enhanced acid β-glucosidase activity toward 4MU-Glc with negatively charged phospholipids in the series, phosphatidylserine > phosphatidylinositol > phosphatidic acid. Phosphatidylethanolamine or -choline had no effect. These results have been reproduced by numerous investigators in human, bovine, and murine sources (see, e.g., references 344, 346, 363, and 366–368). In artificial membrane systems, that is, liposomes, optimal activity also required negatively charged phospholipids which bind to acid β-glucosidase.[369] Sarmientos et al.[370] found maximal activity with about 19 mole% of phosphatidylserine in liposomes, a content similar to that found in lysosomal membranes.[365] Glew and coworkers delineated some structure/activity relationships between acid β-glucosidase and negatively charged phospholipids or glycosphingolipids.[371,372] Characterization of the lipids associated with acid β-glucosidase from different tissues could provide an interesting insight into the enzyme's in vivo functional hydrophobic environment.

Activation by Saposin. Saposin C and saposin A activate acid β-glucosidase in vitro in the presence of negatively charged phospholipids. Saposin A does not appear to be a physiologic activator of acid β-glucosidase.[373] Although saposin C activated sphingomyelinase and galactosyl ceramide: β-galactosidase in vitro, storage of the substrates for these enzymes was not reported in a patient with saposin C deficiency.[374] Patients with saposin A deficiency have not yet been described. The interaction of saposin C with acid β-glucosidase has been studied extensively (see, e.g., references 29, 367, 375, and 368). Saposin C interacts directly with the enzyme[29,368] only in the presence of negatively charged phospholipids.[368,375] This effect is mediated by sequences in the COOH 50 percent of saposin C. Polyoxyethylene ether detergents or bile salts interfere with the activating effects of saposin C,[29,368] as do high concentrations of negatively charged phospholipids.[368,373,376] Berent and Radin[368] suggested that at low concentrations phosphatidylserine interacts with an enzyme anionic site, but at high concentrations it competes for the saposin C site and leads to decreasing activation effects.[373] The activating effects of saposin C require the presence of negatively charged phospholipids or glycosphingolipids.[368,375] These effects are thought to be mediated by conformational changes in acid β-glucosidase so that the interaction of phosphatidylserine conforms the enzyme into a "poised" form for the interaction with saposin C.[368] The use of inhibitory monoclonal antibodies has provided direct support for saposin C effecting a conformational change in acid β-glucosidase that enhances catalytic activity.[377]

Properties of the Active Site. The natural substrates for acid β-glucosidase are mixtures of *N*-acyl-sphingosyl-1-*O*-β-D-glucosides, glucosylceramides, with differing fatty acid acyl and sphingosyl moieties depending upon the tissue source.[260,378] 4MU-Glc also provides excellent estimates of acid β-glucosidase activity. The apparent K_m for 4MU-Glc is approximately 1.5 to 4 μM, about one hundredfold greater than that for glucosylceramides (20 to 50 μm). The enzyme activity is diprotic and has a pH optimum of about 5.5, which varies somewhat with composition of the assay mixture. A more acidic pH optimum (~4.5) is obtained in some phospholipid/saposin C-based systems. The active site is specific for D-glucose because the L-glucosyl derivative of glucosylceramide is not hydrolyzed.[379] The D-glucosyl-D-*erythro*-ceramides are better substrates than the corresponding D-glucosyl-L-*threo* derivatives.[370] Maximal in vitro hydrolytic rates are achieved with glucosylceramides containing fatty acyl acid chains of 8 to 18 carbon atoms.[380] The length of the fatty acid acyl chain had small effects on the apparent K_m values.[370,380] The absence of the C4-C5 *trans* double-bond in the sphingosyl moiety of the ceramide greatly reduces substrate affinity and the rate of hydrolysis.[370,380–382] Glucosylsphingosine and its *N*-alkylated derivatives, bearing a positive charge on the C2 nitrogen of sphingosine, are hydrolyzed at rates 25 to 100 times lower than glucosylceramides.[370,380,383,384] Such substrate analogues with C6- to C12-alkyl chains are very potent inhibitors[385] with K_i values of ~500 nM.[380,383,384] Sphingoid bases with chain lengths of 16 to 18 carbons are potent inhibitors of acid β-glucosidase, although the influence of chain length is small.[382]

Using their results[367,380,382,386–389] and previous work[385,390] of substrate specificity and inhibitor analyses, Grabowski and coworkers proposed a kinetic model of the active site of acid β-glucosidase that includes three binding sites for the glycon head group, the sphingosyl moiety, and the fatty acid acyl chain of glycosyl ceramide (Fig. 146-4). Interaction at the glycon-binding site requires a specific bonding with each hydroxyl group[388] on glucose, while the sphingosyl and fatty acid acyl binding sites are thought to accommodate hydrophobic chains up to about 16 carbon atoms in length. This model is similar to those proposed for the binding of globotriaosylceramide to saposin B[391] and phospholipids to phospholipid transfer protein.[392] Although additional supporting structural data will be required for these models, they may serve as prototypes for binding sites on lipid transfer proteins and partial or complete active sites of glycosphingolipid hydrolases.

Conduritol B epoxide (CBE), 1-D-1,2-anhydro-*myo*-inositol, derivatives are active site-directed inhibitors of many β-glucosidases and covalently bind to this site by forming an ester linkage to an enzyme nucleophile.[393] Radioactively labeled CBE derivatives were used to identify active site amino acid residues in several β-glucosidases.[27,393–395] In the human enzyme, it is Asp443.[27,396] Data obtained with CBE suggest that the catalytic mechanism of the human enzyme includes the cleavage of the β-glucosidic linkage, the release of ceramide, donation of water to a glucose-enzyme complex, and the release of β-glucose.[397] Heterologous expression of mutated enzymes has provided initial data for localization of enzyme regions that contribute to catalytic activity

Table 146-4 Common Mutations of the Glucocerebrosidase Gene that Cause Gaucher Disease

cDNA	Amino acid #	Genomic #	Base substitution	AA substitution	Phenotypic effect	Frequency	Enzymatic Effect: Catalytic	Enzymatic Effect: Stability	References
84	NA	1035	G → GG	NA	Severe	Very common	Null	Null	311
NA	IVS2 + 1	1067	G → A*	NA	Severe	Common	Null	Null	312, 457
1226	370	5841	A → G	Asn → Ser	Mild	Very common	↓Activity	Stable	577
1297	394	5912	G → T	Val → Leu	Severe	Common	↓Activity	Stable	318
1342	409	5957	G → C*	Asp → His	Severe	Common	↓↓↓Activity	Unstable	314 318
1448	444	6433	T → C*	Leu → Pro	Severe	Very common	↓↓Activity	Unstable	38
1504	463	6489	C → T	Arg → Cys	Mild	Common	↓Activity	Stable	454
1604	496	6683	G → A	Arg → His	Very Mild	Very common			312

NA = not applicable
*Pseudogene sequence.

(Fig. 146-4 and Table 146-4). These studies and the homology with the murine enzyme localize the residues involved in catalysis and possibly saposin C binding to the C-terminal 40 percent of the protein.[357,389,397,398]

Posttranslational Processing of Acid β-Glucosidase. Biosynthesis of normal acid β-glucosidase has been investigated in cultured porcine kidney cells and human skin fibroblasts.[350,399–401] Such studies were undertaken, in part, to determine the origin of three molecular weight forms of acid β-glucosidase observed by immunoelectroblotting extracts of human skin fibroblasts[402–405] and brain.[402] Total deglycosylation of acid β-glucosidase from human fibroblasts yielded only a single immunoreactive form (M_r = 56,000).[404] These results indicated that differential glycosylation produced the three steady-state enzyme forms. By metabolic labeling, the first detectable form of the human[350,399,401] and porcine[350] enzymes contained high mannosyl chains.[350,399] Over 1 to 24 h, these initial forms were transformed quantitatively into a higher molecular weight form that was partially resistant to endoglycosidase H treatment.[350,399] This transformation was due to the processing of the oligosaccharide chains to complex types within the Golgi apparatus.[350,399,401] This high-molecular-weight form was converted over about 72 h to a final glycosylated form with M_r = 59,000. Signal-sequence clipping occurs coincident with transport of the nascent polypeptide chain across the endoplasmic reticulum.[336] Unlike many other lysosomal hydrolases,[406–408] no additional proteolytic modifications occur.[350] The rate of transport of acid β-glucosidase from the endoplasmic reticulum to the Golgi apparatus was estimated at 3 h, which was longer than that for many other lysosomal enzymes.[408] The intracellular half-life was approximately 60 h, which is relatively short.[399] Lysosomal enzymes that are normally targeted to lysosomes by a mannose-6-P signal are mainly secreted from the cell in I-cell disease fibroblasts. However, acid β-glucosidase is retained under these conditions, from which observation it has been deduced that signals other than mannose-6-P are responsible for targeting acid β-glucosidase.

Saposins C and A

Definitions. A factor from Gaucher disease spleen enhanced the hydrolysis of 4MU-Glc by acid β-glucosidase.[29] This "factor" is designated heat stable factor, co-β-glucosidase, saposin C, and SAP-2 (sphingolipid activator protein 2). Saposin C is used here. The physiologic importance of saposin C was demonstrated by glucosylceramide storage and a Gaucher disease-like phenotype in two patients with a deficiency of this protein.[374,409] A second protein activator of in vitro acid β-glucosidase activity has been described and designated saposin A or protein A.[41,410] Both of these activators are derived from a single gene product by extensive proteolytic and glycosidic posttranslational processing (see "Biosynthesis and Processing" below).

Purification and Properties. The remarkable thermal stability of saposin C was exploited for its purification from normal and Gaucher disease spleens.[368,411–413] The complete amino acid sequences of the human[411] and guinea pig[41] saposin Cs have been chemically determined, and those from human[39–41,414] and rat[415] were deduced from their cDNA sequences. Saposin Cs from human, rat, and guinea pig are highly homologous. The 80-amino-acid (MW = 8950) human saposin C is an acidic glycoprotein (pI 4.2),[41] which is consistent with the presence of 20 percent acidic (Asp and Glu) amino acids. The protein also contains about 32 percent each of nonpolar and polar amino acids, as well as six cysteines and two methionines, but no tryptophans. The single *N*-linked glycosylation site is glycosylated, but only the composition of the guinea pig saposin C oligosaccharides is known.[41,416] Saposin A has been purified to homogeneity from human spleen.[410] The complete amino acid sequence has been chemically determined[410] and predicted from the cDNA sequence.[40,41,417] Similar to saposin C, saposin A is small (M_r = 9148), very acidic (calculated pI = 4.14), and has six cysteine residues that align with those in saposin C.[41] Saposin A has two *N*-glycosylation consensus sequences, both of which are occupied.[410] The human and murine saposin As are strikingly similar, with 89 percent amino acid identity.

Biosynthesis and Processing. Fujibayashi and Wenger[418,419] used rabbit antihuman saposin C antibodies in metabolic-labeling studies to demonstrate that saposin C in human skin fibroblasts had extensive proteolytic and glycosidic processing. In pulse-chase experiments, the major product following a short pulse (15 min) was a 68-kDa glycosylated species. Over 1 h, it was converted to a 73-kDa form. Subsequently, as the total amount of these two species decreased, diffuse species with M_r centered at about 12,000 and 9000 appeared. In addition, a saposin C-specific M_r = 50,000 species remained relatively constant up to 5 h of chase. The 73-kDa and 68-kDa species decreased proportionately, and were absent by about 2 to 3 h of chase. By 5 h of chase, the 12-kDa species had nearly disappeared, and the 9-kDa was predominant. Endoglycosidase F digestion studies of [^{35}S]methionine-labeled saposin C immunoprecipitates demonstrated that the 73- and 68-kDa or the 12- and 9-kDa species were glycosylated species with polypeptides of M_r = 50,000 or 7600, respectively. It is notable that very similar results were reported for the biosynthesis of saposin B,[419] which would be expected now that saposin C and saposin B have been demonstrated to be encoded by the same gene and mRNA (see Fig. 146-7). However, neither the sequence of events involved in proteolytic processing of the "prosaposin" precursor nor the potential tissue specificity have

Table 146-5 Nucleotides at 12 Positions in the Four Glucocerebrosidase Haplotypes

Glucocerebrosidase			Haplotypes											
Designation		nt Frequency	−802	−725	−614	2128	2834	3297	3747	3854	3931	4644	5135	6144
1	+	Common	a	c	c	a	c	g	g	t	g	del	c	g
2	−	Common	g	t	t	g	g	a	g	c	a	a	a	a
3	African	Common African	g	t	t	g	a	a	g	c	a	a	a	a
4	Uncommon	Rare	a	c	c	a	c	g	a	t	g	del	c	g

been elucidated. The highly homologous sulfated glycoprotein 1 (SGP-1) rat analogue of prosaposin[415] is not proteolytically processed prior to its secretion into the culture media of Sertoli cells.

Enzymatic Abnormalities in Gaucher Disease

Several investigators have suggested the existence of groups of mutant enzymes in Gaucher disease sources, based on different phenomenologic responses to various modifiers of acid β-glucosidase activity[147,346,347,365–367,380,420,421] and altered processing/stability.[305,402,404,421–423] Two groups or general classes of mutant enzymes were identified: (a) Those with decreased stability, normal interaction with inhibitors, and severely decreased catalytic rate constants. This group of mutant enzymes has been found mostly in non-Jewish type 1, 2, and 3 patients. (b) Those with essentially normal stability, decreased affinity for active site-directed inhibitors, and moderately decreased catalytic rate constants. These mutant enzymes have been found mostly in Jewish patients. Because many patients, particularly non-Jewish ones, have two different mutant acid β-glucosidase alleles, heterologous expression of mutant cDNAs was required to correlate the cellular enzyme properties with the particular mutations. The common L444P substitution (Table 146-4), as well as several other mutations, result in very unstable enzymes.[424] Several other missense mutations identified in Gaucher disease patients result in enzymes that are completely devoid of enzyme activity.[389,398,424] On the other hand, the very common N370S substitution and the rare V394L substitution produce mutant enzymes in the second group, which have residual activity, but nearly normal stability.

Saposin

Very high levels of saposin C and A have been found in Gaucher disease tissues.[425]

MOLECULAR BIOLOGY

Acid β-Glucosidase

Gene and Pseudogene Structure. The gene coding for glucocerebrosidase (GBA) has been mapped to chromosome 1 at q21.[32,33,426] The gene for acid β-glucosidase is approximately 7 kb in length and contains 11 exons. The putative TATA- and CAAT-like boxes of acid β-glucosidase promoter have been identified about 260 bp upstream from the upstream ATG start codon.[427] A 5-kb pseudogene[37] is located approximately 16 kb downstream from the acid β-glucosidase gene.[428] The pseudogene has maintained a high degree of homology with the functional gene. Although it is transcribed,[429] an unusual property for a pseudogene, it does not contain a long open-reading frame, and has a 55-bp deletion from what was once the coding region.[37] Alu sequences that have been inserted into introns[37] give the functional gene greater length than the pseudogene.

Polymorphisms in Introns and Immediate Flanking Regions. Eleven polymorphic sites are known to exist in the introns and flanking regions of the acid β-glucosidase gene.[430] Surprisingly, only four haplotypes have been found. These sites and the haplotypes that have been identified so far are summarized in Table 146-5.

Other Flanking Sequences. Flanking the functional *GBA* gene are a considerable number of other genes, some of known and some of unknown function (Fig. 146-5). Immediately upstream of *GBA* is the *cote1* gene, then further upstream is the *propin1* gene, and beyond this is the *clk2* gene. The first two genes are of unknown function, while the *clk2* gene resembles a serine/threonine kinase.[431] Immediately downstream from *GBA* is the pseudometaxin gene, and immediately downstream from the *GBA* pseudogene is the metaxin gene. Both of these genes are oriented convergently with the *GBA* genes. Unlike the *GBA* pseudogene, the metaxin pseudogene is not transcribed.[432,433] Apparently a large block of DNA containing the ancestral *GBA* gene and metaxin gene underwent duplication, and the upstream *GBA* and the downstream (with respect to *GBA*) metaxin genes were preserved as the functional genes. Further downstream from *GBA* are the polymorphic epithelial mucin gene (*MUC1*)[432] and the liver/red cell pyruvate kinase *PKLR* genes.[434,435] The latter linkage is of considerable interest because even though the 5′ ends of *GBA* and *PKLR* are 71 kb apart, polymorphic sites within these genes are in almost complete linkage disequilibrium and Gaucher disease-producing mutations are almost always in the same *PKLR* haplotype, indicating that the Gaucher disease mutations have arising recently in the human evolution probably within the past 2000 years.[436] In 50 informative meioses, no recombination was found between *GBA* and 6 markers, D1S2777, D1S2721,

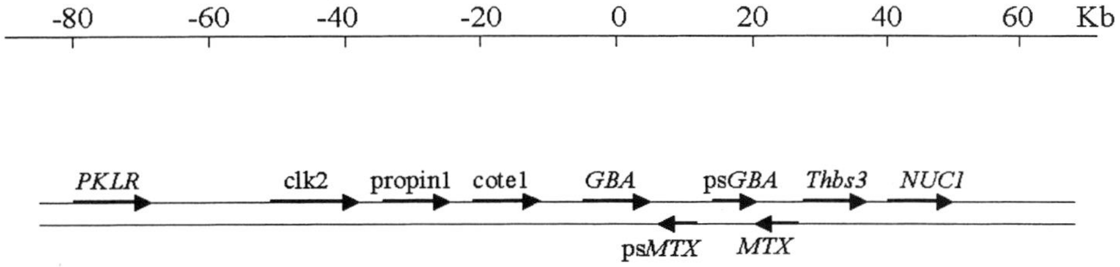

Fig. 146-5 Representation of genes surrounding the glucocerebrosidase (GBA) gene, based on several sources.[431–434,578] *PKLR* = liver/red cell pyruvate kinase; *clk2* = a gene resembling a serine/threonine kinase; *propin1* and *cote1* = two genes of unknown function; *MTX* = metaxin; *Thbs3* = thrombospondin; *MUC1* = polymorphic epithelial mucin gene; ps designates the pseudogenes.

D1S2714, D1S303, D1S1153 and D1S2140.[437] Three of these markers, D1S2777, D1S303, and D1S2140, are highly polymorphic[437] and should prove to be useful for problems in prenatal diagnosis when the mutation causing Gaucher disease has not been identified.

mRNA and cDNA. Acid β-glucosidase cDNA is about 2 kb in length.[35,36,348] Active enzyme can be produced from in vivo translation of the cDNA in a variety of eukaryotic cells, including transformed murine fibroblasts,[438,439] murine hematopoietic cells,[440] COS cells,[441] *Spodoptera frugiperda* cells infected with baculovirus,[441,442] and human hematopoietic cells.[443,444] There are two upstream ATGs that are utilized in translation.[445] The relative importance or function of these two start sites is unknown. Transfer into murine cells of human acid β-glucosidase cDNAs that were mutated so as to ablate either one or the other of the start sites, has shown that either of the two sites can produce functional enzyme in vivo.[446] The sequence between the upstream and downstream ATG is hydrophilic leader while that between the downstream ATG and the cleavage site of the leader sequence is the typical hydrophobic sequence expected in a leader sequence. It has been suggested[446] that alternatively spliced forms might create one protein product with a hydrophilic and another product with a hydrophobic leader sequence, but such spliced forms have not been identified. mRNAs of several different lengths have been detected, probably due to use of alternative polyadenylation sites,[386,447] alternative splicing,[386] or presence of pseudogene mRNA.[429]

Mutations Causing Gaucher Disease. A large number of mutations that cause Gaucher disease have been identified. Those that are encountered most commonly are summarized in Table 146-4. Comprehensive tabulations of mutations have been published periodically[448–451] and a schematic diagram is presented in Fig. 146-6.

Of the many mutations that have now been documented, only three appear to approach polymorphic frequencies in selected populations. The most common is the A → G transition at 1226G, the mutation that produces a protein with an Asn → Ser substitution at amino acid 370 of the mature protein. This mutation is present in about 6 percent of the Ashkenazi Jewish population,[59,312] and is the principal cause of the high incidence of Gaucher disease in this ethnic group. An insertion of a guanine at nt 84 of the cDNA is the second common Jewish mutation. It is found in approximately 0.6 percent of the Jewish population. Because it produces a frameshift even before the N-terminus of the mature protein, an allele bearing this drastic mutation produces no enzyme protein.[311] A T → C transition at nt 1448, producing a Leu → Pro substitution at amino acid 444 of the mature protein, is present at a relatively high frequency in the Norrbottnian population of northern Sweden.[452] The same mutation also occurs in other populations at low frequencies. It is noteworthy that the homologous position in the pseudogene is occupied by a C, just as in the Gaucher disease-producing mutation.

In some genes with the 1448C (L444P) mutation, other mutations, each corresponding to the sequence of the pseudogene, are also found. In some cases, this type of mutation, designated XOVR, represents a crossover between the functional gene and pseudogene, with loss of the genetic material between the two.[428] In other cases, the mechanism by which the abnormal gene has been formed has not been elucidated, and the alleles have merely been referred to as complex alleles,[453] pseudopattern,[454,455] or "rec" (for recombinant).[314] These may occur by mechanisms similar to that producing the XOVR mutation, or they may represent the results of gene conversion events.[456]

The relationship of mutations in the acid β-glucosidase gene to the disease itself is firmly established, not only because the mutations segregate with the disease in families, but also by the production of the mutant enzyme proteins from cloned, mutated cDNAs. Such investigations[389,398,455] have shown that the properties of the mutated enzymes approximate those that are observed in enzyme isolated from patients bearing a given mutation (see "Enzymology" above).

Relationship Between Genotype and Phenotype. Some mutations, such as the 1226G and 1297T mutations that produce the N370S and the V394L mutant enzymes, result in relatively conservative amino acid changes. At the opposite extreme, the 84GG mutation produces a frameshift close to the beginning of translation and thus cannot direct the formation of any functional enzyme. Similarly, a mutation in the first nucleotide of intron 2[59,312,457] prevents formation of any enzyme. It is to be expected, therefore, that some relationship should exist between the genotype of a patient and the severity of the clinical manifestations of the disease. In this respect, it is useful to broadly classify mutations into three categories. Mild mutations are those that are never found in patients with neuronopathic disease. The 1226G (N370S) mutation is the prototype of such a mutation. Severe mutations are those that have been associated with neuronopathic disease but that have the deduced capacity to direct the formation of some enzymes. Mutation 1448C (L444P) is the prototype of this group. Null mutations are those that are incapable of forming

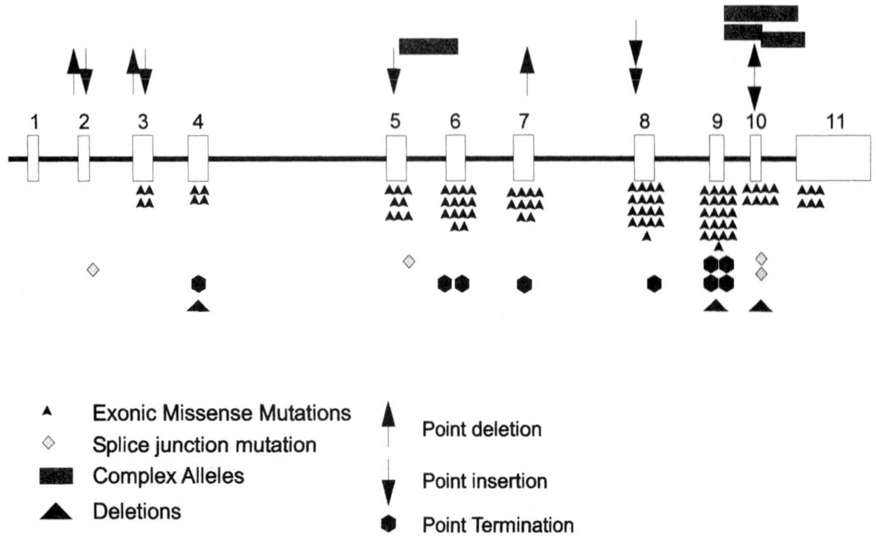

Fig. 146-6 Distribution of mutations identified in Gaucher disease. The symbols correspond to various types of mutations as indicated. The complex alleles refer to those that contain multiple missense and/or deletions that are also present in the pseudogene.

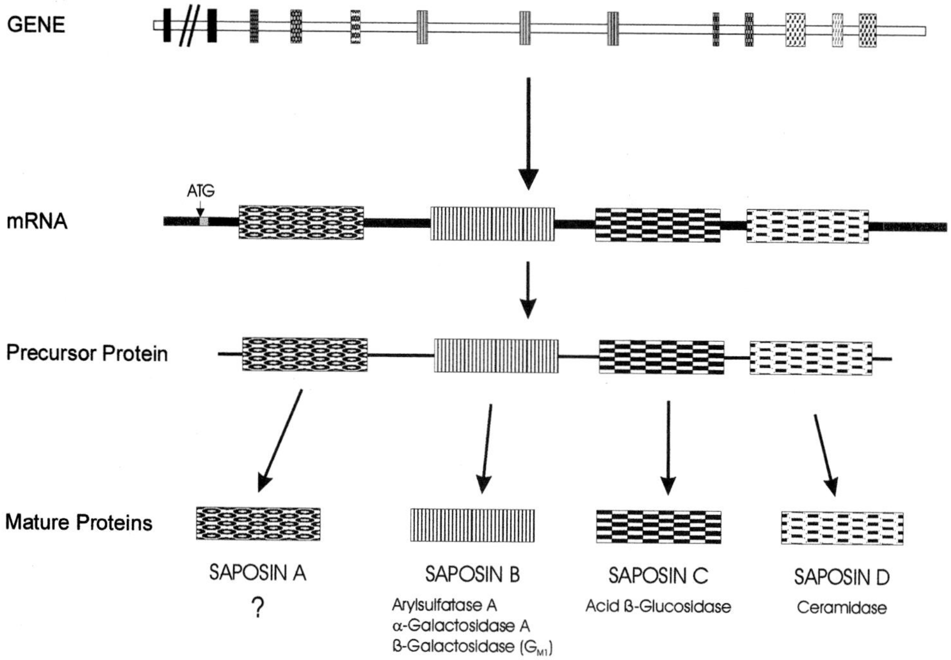

Fig. 146-7 Representations of the prosaposin genomic, RNA, and cDNA sequences. The variously shaded regions of the chromosomal gene correspond to the individual saposin regions of the gene. In the cDNA, the open reading frame includes the dark lines and the individual saposin regions. The gray shaded regions extending 5′ and 3′ correspond to untranslated sequences.

enzyme. The most common of these is the 84GG frameshift mutation. Notably such mutations have never been encountered in the homozygous state nor have there been compound heterozygotes with two different null mutations. It may be presumed that such a genotype is not compatible with life, in analogy with the glucocerebrosidase knockout mouse.[273]

Thus, a relationship exists between the type of mutation that has been inherited and the clinical phenotype. As was pointed out under "Diagnosis," homozygosity for the nt 1448C (L444P) mutation is usually associated with neuronopathic disease. In the Norrbottnian population, where the characteristic abnormality is the point mutation at nt 1448 (L444P),[318,452] the clinical phenotype is type 3 Gaucher disease. However, some patients who appear to be homozygous for the 1448C (L444P) mutation manifest type 2 disease. Additional mutations derived from the pseudogene are also present in some cases.[453] The presence of a 1226G (N370S) allele appears to preclude the development of type 2 or 3 disease. As one might expect, the disease severity is quite mild on the average in the 1226G/1226G homozygous genotype as compared with the 1226G/1448C or 1226G/84GG genotypes.[77,316–319] Particularly striking is the much later median age of first symptoms in patients homozygous for the 1226G (N370S) mutation.[59,312] Almost invariably, patients who are diagnosed in middle or old age prove to have this genotype. The mildness of this genotype is therefore underestimated when Gaucher patient populations are studied, because many with the 1226G/1226G genotype may never come to medical attention at all.[59] In one population survey,[58] 4 of 1528 apparently normal adult Ashkenazi Jewish subjects were found to have this relatively benign genotype. This genotype is uncommon in the non-Jewish population,[458] but when it occurs, the clinical phenotype is indistinguishable from that in the Jewish population.[458] In addition to these clear differences in the clinical expression of different genotypes, there is marked intragroup variation. A few patients with the 1226G/1226G genotype manifest moderately severe disease, while some patients with the 1226G/1448C and the 1226G/84GG genotypes have quite mild disease.[79,312,320] There are currently insufficient data to be certain how much of this variation is interfamily, how much is intrafamily, and how much may be due to environmental factors. It is unlikely that linked factors (such as the strength of promoters) are involved because of the marked linkage disequilibrium that exists between the 1226G mutation and even relatively distant markers.[459] However, unlinked factors (such as saposin expression or the activity of other glycohydrolases) and environmental factors (such as infections) all may play a role in disease expression.

Activator Proteins

The activator proteins for acid β-glucosidase and for other lysosomal hydrolases are discussed extensively in Chap. 134. Two species of human prosaposin mRNA arise from alternative polyadenylation[414] and the levels of mRNA expression parallel that of acid β-glucosidase; that is, the levels of prosaposin mRNA were higher in normal skin fibroblasts than in B-cells and the mRNA levels are slightly higher in the corresponding cells from Gaucher disease patients. The organization[31] and sequence[42,460] of the prosaposin gene are shown schematically in Fig. 146-7. A mutation in the saposin C region that results in a Phe or Gly for Cys substitution was reported in a patient with a Gaucher-like disease resulting from saposin C deficiency.[461,462]

THERAPY

Supportive

Even before it was possible to affect the disease process itself by enzyme replacement therapy, the morbidity associated with Gaucher disease could be mitigated somewhat by medical or surgical management of specific problems.

Bone Crises. In severe cases, hospitalization may be required for intravenous hydration and administration of narcotics for pain control. Osteomyelitis should be considered. In the absence of positive blood cultures, conservative management is generally appropriate. However, because of the high morbidity associated with bacterial osteomyelitis in Gaucher disease,[463] the involved area should be biopsied and cultured if there is a very high suspicion of infection.[197] Standard and high-dose glucocorticoid therapy has been used with some immediate effect in the treatment of severe bone crises.[464]

Splenectomy

Total Splenectomy. Splenectomy is a very effective treatment of the thrombocytopenia and, to a considerable extent, the anemia that often occurs in the course of Gaucher disease.[91,465] Splenectomy is also indicated when splenomegaly is so massive as to become symptomatic and to interfere with normal growth and development. Patients with massively enlarged spleens can respond very slowly to enzyme therapy, and splenectomy may be a more satisfactory adjunctive treatment option in those patients.[466–468] While the initial response to splenectomy is usually satisfactory, concern has been expressed about the possible effect of the removal of the spleen on progressive deposition of glycolipid in other organs.[469,470] It seems reasonable that removing an organ that serves as an important storage site would result in accelerated deposition in other organs such as the skeleton[164,470] and, in type 3 disease, the central nervous system.[222,471] The evidence that this is the case is largely anecdotal. From a review of more than 200 patients, Lee[92] concluded that the presence or absence of bony disease was unrelated to splenectomy. Other investigators have reached similar conclusions based on clinical evaluations of affected type 1 patients.[93,100,472] However, Norrbottnian patients have been found to accumulate larger amounts of glucosylceramide in the plasma and brains following splenectomy, and this correlated with a more rapid clinical deterioration.[222,224,225,258,470] The marked variability of type 1 Gaucher disease makes it difficult to resolve this controversy. We recommend conservative management, and that splenectomy be reserved for patients with moderately severe thrombocytopenia (platelet counts consistently under 40,000/μl), growth retardation, and/or mechanical cardiopulmonary compromise that are unresponsive to enzyme therapy.

Partial Splenectomy. Partial splenectomy was introduced in an attempt to obtain the therapeutic benefits of splenectomy while avoiding the possible adverse effect on the course of the disease.[473,474] The procedure was also proposed as a means of avoiding the susceptibility to sepsis that occasionally follows total splenectomy.[475] There is usually regrowth of the splenic remnant,[164,475–480] and while it is indeed possible that allowing some of the spleen to remain could prevent progression of the disease, there are no controlled studies that provide clear-cut justification for this procedure. Indeed, long-term follow-up of patients who have undergone partial splenectomy suggests little advantage for this approach, because regrowth of the spleen is associated with all of the original clinical symptoms.[480–482]

Splenic Embolization. Embolization as been advocated either as an adjunct to or a substitute for splenectomy in the treatment of Gaucher disease,[483,484] but the amount of experience with this approach is apparently quite meager.

Orthopedic Procedures. The quality of life of patients with Gaucher disease may be greatly enhanced by appropriate orthopedic surgical intervention. Hip replacement has been particularly useful in this regard,[485] and, in some cases, successful replacement of knee joints has been accomplished. Although prosthetic hip and shoulder replacement have been highly successful, care should be taken to choose the correct prosthesis length and anchoring technique for each patient depending upon the extent of the bony abnormalities in the affected limb. In patients with very extensive thinning of cortical bone, joint replacement may not be practical due to the lack of sufficient bone structure to support the prosthesis. Furthermore, joint replacement in children is not desirable because it interferes with limb growth and the prosthesis has a relatively short life.

Bisphosphonates. In 1984, aminohydroxypropylidne biphosphonate administration was reported to be effective in reversing bone disease in a patient with Gaucher disease.[486] To date, uncontrolled studies using aminohydroxypropylidene bisphosphonate (pamidronate) have been reported with encouraging results including pain relief, increase of bone density, and decrease in urinary deoxypyridinoline and hydroxyproline excretion.[487–490] However, the results of a large (> 70 patients) double-blind, randomized, controlled trial of oral alendronate in combination with enzyme therapy in adults will be complete by 2001 and will directly assess potential additive benefits of oral bisphosphonate adjunctive therapy.

Restrictions on Exercise and Sports. Once they occur, pathologic fractures often heal slowly or not at all. Collapse of vertebrae or of the femoral head has permanent sequelae. To help prevent these complications, we advise patients with Gaucher disease to avoid activities that could result in bone damage, such as competitive running, tennis, skiing, or various contact sports. Swimming is probably the safest exercise for patients with bone disease.

Enzyme Therapy

History. The history of the development of enzyme replacement therapy was recently chronicled.[491] de Duve[43] first suggested that replacement of the missing enzyme with exogenous enzyme might be a successful approach to the treatment of lysosomal storage diseases. Type 1 Gaucher disease appears to be an unusually attractive candidate for such therapy. This is because there is no primary central nervous system involvement and the target cell is the macrophage. Early attempts at replacement therapy were disappointing due to an insufficient supply of enzyme and failure to appreciate the signals needed to target enzyme efficiently to macrophages. Brady et al. administered unmodified placental acid β-glucosidase intravenously to two patients with Gaucher disease.[492–495] Liver biopsies before and after enzyme administration appeared to show clearance of glycolipid. However, in view of the heterogeneous distribution of acid β-glucosidase in liver,[45] the biopsy results were difficult to interpret. In any case, no clinical response was documented. The administration of smaller amounts of enzyme targeted to the reticuloendothelial system by encapsulation in erythrocyte ghosts that were coated with immunoglobulin was reported by Beutler et al.[45] to result in the reduction of liver size as judged by technetium scanning. However, results of the study of six additional patients using this technique[253,496–499] were disappointing. Trials of enzyme replacement were also undertaken by Belchetz and Gregoriadis[500] using liposome-entrapped enzyme. Alarming symptoms occurred after some liposome infusions, and the therapeutic results were equivocal.[501]

With the realization that the uptake of glycoproteins occurred by way of carbohydrate-specific receptors[502] and, in particular, that macrophages contained mannose-specific receptors,[503] attempts were made to target acid β-glucosidase to macrophages by modifying the oligosaccharides of the enzyme.[48,504–507] That paved the way for developing macrophage directed enzyme therapy for Gaucher disease. Industrial-scale production of human placental enzyme modified to expose covered *N*-acetylglucosamine and mannose residues (alglucerase) has made available sufficient material for prolonged clinical administration of large amounts of acid β-glucosidase. For the first time, clear-cut clinical responses were demonstrated[50,508] and readily confirmed.[51,52,77,509] In anemic patients, the hemoglobin concentration of the blood began to rise within the first few months of enzyme therapy. Similarly, rapid rises in platelet counts were observed in splenectomized patients with thrombocytopenia. The response is slower in patients whose spleen has not been removed. Regression of organomegaly was generally evident within the first 6 months of treatment, with an average decrease of excess liver volume of approximately 20 to 25 percent. Bone pain gradually decreases, but the x-ray abnormalities of bone respond very slowly. Magnetic resonance imaging shows a decrease in bone involvement. Processing of the placental extract from which the enzyme is purified is such that known viruses including the human immunodeficiency virus are destroyed. Clinical trials with recombinant enzyme (Cerezyme) indicate efficacy comparable or superior to the placenta-derived enzyme.[468]

Pharmacology. Studies of the binding of alglucerase to murine macrophages and to human monocyte-derived macrophages show that only a very small amount binds to the classical mannose receptor. Most of the mannose-terminated enzyme is bound by a low-affinity, high-copy number, mannose-dependent, but calcium-independent, receptor that is present in many cells, including endothelial cells.[510] Extensive studies in mice and rats have shown that the enzyme, given as a bolus, is rapidly cleared from the circulation $t_{\frac{1}{2}}$ ~4 to 6 min and taken up by sinusoidal cells of the liver[511–514] and spleen.[511] Immunofluorescence[511] and immunoelectron-microscopic[512,513] analyses show that the enzyme is preferentially delivered to macrophages and endothelial cells of the sinusoids of the liver and spleen, and not in significant amounts to the parenchymal cells of either organ.[511] Because of the large masses of hepatocytes, particularly, and endothelial cells in the liver, compared to Kupffer cells, quantitatively larger amounts of the enzyme were delivered to non-Kupffer cells.[514] This is consistent with the delivery of mannose-terminated ligands to endothelial cells because of their greater activity in hepatic sinusoids.[515,516] Little enzyme has been recovered from other organs including the kidneys, lungs, and brain. Studies in humans, using radiolabeled mannose-terminated acid β-glucosidase, were consistent with these findings[174] (see below). In murine bone marrow mononuclear cells, very small amounts of enzyme were recovered about 1 h after the infusion.[511] In human Gaucher disease patients, some enzyme is found in bone marrow samples, but the results are variable.[28,517] Also, the enzyme recovered from mouse liver and spleen had only about 50 to 70 percent of the catalytic capacity of the infused enzyme, indicating an inefficiency in the delivery of active enzyme to the lysosomes.[511] It is not clear if the administered enzyme attaches to the lysosomal membrane because two studies in mice and rats obtained directly opposing results.[512,518]

In a study of of ^{123}I-labeled imiglucerase and alglucerase after bolus injection into eight patients with type 1 Gaucher disease, and in one normal subject, the tracer enzyme was followed by scintigraphy and by analysis of blood, urine, and feces.[174] The tracer enzyme was cleared from blood with a $t_{\frac{1}{2}}$ ~4.7 min. Concomitantly, about 30 percent of the dose was taken up by the liver and 15 percent by the spleen. About 50 percent of the tracer was cleared rapidly from the viscera with a $t_{\frac{1}{2}}$ of 1 to 2 h and the remainder more slowly with a $t_{\frac{1}{2}}$ of 34 to 42 h. Significant enough tracer was localized to the bone marrow to determine a $t_{\frac{1}{2}}$ of 14.1 h. Infusion of alglucerase (5 U/kg bodyweight) into a Gaucher disease patient normalized the acid β-glucosidase activity within splenic Gaucher cells. At a dose of 35 U/kg over 1 h the receptor-mediated uptake in vivo was saturated, as shown by the increase in blood-clearance $t_{\frac{1}{2}}$ of tracer enzyme from 4.5 min to 12 min. These studies are concordant with the studies in normal mice and rats, but the use of a potentially partially denatured tracer enzyme may have influenced the disappearance and uptake analyses.

Because of the inefficiencies in the delivery of active enzyme to the target site of pathology, the macrophages (particularly bone marrow), the reason for the very satisfactory clinical response to aglucerase or imiglucerase at any dose remains unclear. It may be that the small amount that is taken up by macrophages is sufficient to decrease the glucosyl ceramide burden or that the enzyme removes the glycolipid from sources other than macrophages.

Adverse Events. Antibody-related and nonallergic adverse events occur in approximately 15 percent of patients receiving alglucerase or imiglucerase[519,520] (Table 146-6). Most such patients experience clusters of adverse event symptoms, not isolated reactions. Reactions can vary with each infusion, but usually patients manifest a consistent pattern of reactions during or shortly after infusions. Some patients have had recurrent adverse events one to several days following an infusion. The adverse events are similar with either enzyme preparation. Also, some patients receiving alglucerase for several years without adverse events can develop these when receiving imiglucerase. Several adverse events have been associated with (but not proven to be due to) the presence of human chorionic gonadotropin,[521–523] including menstrual disorders (spotting and irregularity), depression, weight gain, and false positive pregnancy tests. Imiglucerase does not contain chorionic gonadotropin.

Table 146-6 Hypersensitivity Reactions with Enzyme Therapy

Reaction Type (n = 105)	% of total reactions*
Pruritus	29
Urticaria	28
Rash	24
Chest discomfort/dyspnea	25
Chills	7
Nausea/vomiting	5
Abdominal cramping	5
Hypotension	4

*Several patients had more than one reaction type

Of 2462 patients who received alglucerase or imiglucerase, 11.8 percent and 13.3 percent, respectively, developed antibodies against acid β-glucosidase. Patients naive to enzyme therapy develop antibodies with a mean time of 8 months. Seroconversion after 12 months is unusual, but does occur. About half of antibody-positive patients experience adverse events. The antibodies are most frequently of the IgG1 and IgG3 subtypes, and one patient developed IgE antibody and anaphylaxis. About 90 percent of antibody-positive patients receiving alglucerase become antibody-negative (tolerized) after a mean time of approximately 28 months of continuous therapy. Among 802 patients (92 antibody-positive) who were switched from alglucerase to imiglucerase, 1.4 percent developed antibodies *de novo*, and approximately 4.5 percent, who had become antibody-negative on alglucerase, redeveloped antibodies. No patients are known to have antibodies that react only with alglucerase or imiglucerase.

Only three patients have been reported to have neutralizing antibodies.[524,525] In two cases, the antibodies inhibited the administered enzyme sufficiently to cause reappearance of progressive Gaucher disease manifestations. In one case, the antibodies appeared to interfere with the therapeutic effect of enzyme, but the disease was stable; that is, no progression was noted. Progressive disease reappeared in this adult after enzyme therapy was discontinued. Although rare (3/2462), the presence of therapeutically important neutralizing antibodies should be considered in patients who respond poorly or continue to progress when receiving sufficient amounts of enzyme for therapeutic response.

Among antibody-negative patients, less than 1 percent experience adverse events. These events are similar to those experienced by antibody-positive patients, are less specific, and can be severe. The etiology of these events is not known. Similar symptoms are experienced during imiglucerase or alglucerase infusions.

The hypersensitivity or nonallergic adverse events are treated conservatively by extending the infusion time to 3 or more hours and/or by pretreatment with antihistamines. A few patients required corticosteroids. Only a few (<10) patients had sufficiently severe adverse events to warrant discontinuation of therapy.

Selection of Patients for Treatment. The dose of alglucerase used in the early studies[50] was 60 U/kg every 2 weeks, and therapy with alglucerase or imiglucerase is still initiated at this level in most patients in the United States. Treatment of a 70-kg patient according to this schedule at the current market price of alglucerase is approximately $405,000 per year for enzyme. Additional costs are incurred for administration. Thus, enzyme therapy is extremely costly and well beyond the price range of many patients, particularly in developing countries.[526] In view of the high cost of enzyme therapy, careful consideration must be given to the question of which patients are suitable candidates. Moreover, because the preparations are relatively new, all risks of treatment may not, as yet, be appreciated. Patients with massive organomegaly and with significant cytopenias are the ones who benefit the most from therapy. Although bone disease appears to be the slowest to respond radiographically, patients with prominent bone involvement are good candidates for treatment because of the irreversibility of damage from fractures, once they occur. Patients with pulmonary shunting have a poor prognosis, and should receive enzyme replacement. The role of treatment in pulmonary hypertension secondary to Gaucher disease is not clear. Pulmonary pressures do not usually decline on treatment, and, indeed, this complication has been noted most frequently in patients already receiving enzyme replacement.[271] While young patients with active disease may benefit considerably from enzyme replacement, it is difficult to justify treatment of patients with late-onset disease who have minor degrees of organomegaly or cytopenia. As was noted under "Clinical Manifestations" above, progression does not usually occur in such adult patients. One cannot rule out the possibility that an older patient with Gaucher disease may develop a pathologic fracture, even if imaging studies of the bone do not show major abnormalities. However, the probability of such an untoward event does not seem sufficiently high to require such time- and resource-consuming intervention. Such older patients may be treated with bisphosphonate compounds prior to decisions of whether enzyme therapy is appropriate.[486–490] A gradually falling platelet count needs to be monitored, and treatment instituted if the count is persistently under 40,000 or 50,000/μL. In general, the current disease severity and progression of a constellation of signs and symptoms dictate the initiation of therapy; that is, the medical decision to institute therapy is usually not based on a single parameter.

Response to Treatment. The response of the blood counts and of the visceral organs to enzyme therapy is relatively easily documented. Liver and spleen size can be measured quite accurately by nuclear magnetic resonance (MRI) or computerized axial tomography (CAT), and somewhat surprisingly equally well with ultrasonography.[527–529] However, the transition from MRI and CT to ultrasound technologies is not straightforward and the successful use of ultrasound depends upon appropriate equipment used by experienced operators. However, under appropriate conditions the latter can provide consistent monitoring even if precision is somewhat lacking. Assessment of the response of bone disease to treatment is more difficult than assessment of visceral disease. In one comprehensive study of 12 patients utilizing noninvasive, quantitative imaging modalities (magnetic resonance score, quantitative xenon scintigraphy, and quantitative chemical shift imaging), net increases in either cortical or trabecular bone mass, as assessed by combined cortical thickness measurements and dual-energy quantitative computed tomography, respectively, occurred in 10 patients[530] after 3 to 5 years of treatment. Although the authors suggested that high doses of 130 U/Kg/month were necessary to achieve a skeletal response, the study design did not justify conclusions about dosage because only high-dose therapy was used. A subsequent double-blinded investigation of cortical bone thickness of patients treated with only 30 U/kg/month, usually given 3 times weekly, achieved similar results for cortical bone thickness changes as high-dose therapy.[531,532] All investigations show that the skeletal response to enzyme therapy is slow, if it occurs at all, and sufficiently difficult to document that great caution must be used in interpreting the data that are available. While skeletal changes occur in a period of years, increase in marrow fat as assessed by MRI occurs more rapidly, usually within the first year of enzyme therapy, and also seems to occur equally with both high- and low-dose therapy.[83,530] It is not clear, however, that such changes are relevant to the structural bone disease that Gaucher disease patients develop.

Dosage Considerations. Because of the high cost of alglucerase and imiglucerase, it is desirable to administer the preparation in as efficient a manner as possible. It is difficult to carry out clinical studies to define the most efficient mode of administration because of the great variability of both disease severity and response to treatment. However, the short intracellular half-life of exogenous acid β-glucosidase suggests that frequent administration of the enzyme would be more effective than infrequent dosing. Thus, use of one-fifth to one-ninth of the doses originally used provided results during the first 6 months of treatment, which is comparable to the results obtained with larger doses of alglucerase.[51,77,509,533–539] There are few data regarding the response after longer periods of treatment, but it is generally less robust than that observed in the initial treatment period. Anecdotal observation suggests that some patients whose response has slowed may show some acceleration if the dosage is increased.

Further studies have been recommended to establish the optimal total dose, frequency, and rate of administration,[540] but in view of the limited number of untreated patients and the marked patient-to-patient variability that is known to exist, it is unlikely that such data can ever be obtained.[541] Therefore, treatment decisions currently must be made using the available data. Analyses of these data show that no differences in response are obtained for hepatic volume or hemoglobin levels at doses between 7.5 and 60 U/Kg/2 weeks[184,542] (Fig. 146-8). The splenic response appears to be somewhat dose-dependent with smaller responses being obtained at doses less than 15 U/kg/2 weeks as compared to higher doses.[543] Recommendations that dosage be "individualized" have been made, but are difficult to implement because even within a given patient the response may vary from month to month. Analysis of the data shows that treatment "failures" are no more common at a dose of 15 U/Kg/month than at a dose of 130 U/Kg/month, which suggests that inadequate responses are not a result of inadequate dosage but rather a result of an as yet undefined characteristic of the patient that is not overcome by increase in the dose.[544]

Stem Cell Transplantation. The type 1 Gaucher disease phenotype is expressed as the result of changes in macrophages, progeny of the hematopoietic stem cell. It was, therefore, logical that allogeneic marrow transplantation be attempted. The first patient with Gaucher disease to be transplanted showed clearance of Gaucher cells from the marrow in about 6 months[545] but died of infection before 1 year. Subsequently, a number of other patients with type 1 Gaucher disease[546–548] have undergone transplantation. Although the response to transplantation has been favorable in surviving patients, there have been other deaths secondary to the transplantation procedure, which is still a high-risk form of treatment. Transplantation has also been carried out in patients with type 3 disease.[165,549–552] Although there are suggestions that the progression of neurologic disease is arrested by the procedure,[553] the long-term effects are by no means certain. In some patients, chimeras resulted from transplantation, and these patients are believed to have benefited from the chimeric state.[553,554]

The indications for stem cell transplantation are uncertain. Transplantation costs less that enzyme replacement, and may therefore be available to some patients who would not have access to enzyme therapy. Moreover, it provides a permanent cure when successful. However, it is difficult to recommend transplantation of patients with type 1 disease under most circumstances because of the 10 percent mortality incident to transplantation, even under the best circumstances, and because of adverse long-term effects on growth and development.[555–557] The risk is even higher in patients with advanced organ dysfunction, the very patients who most need

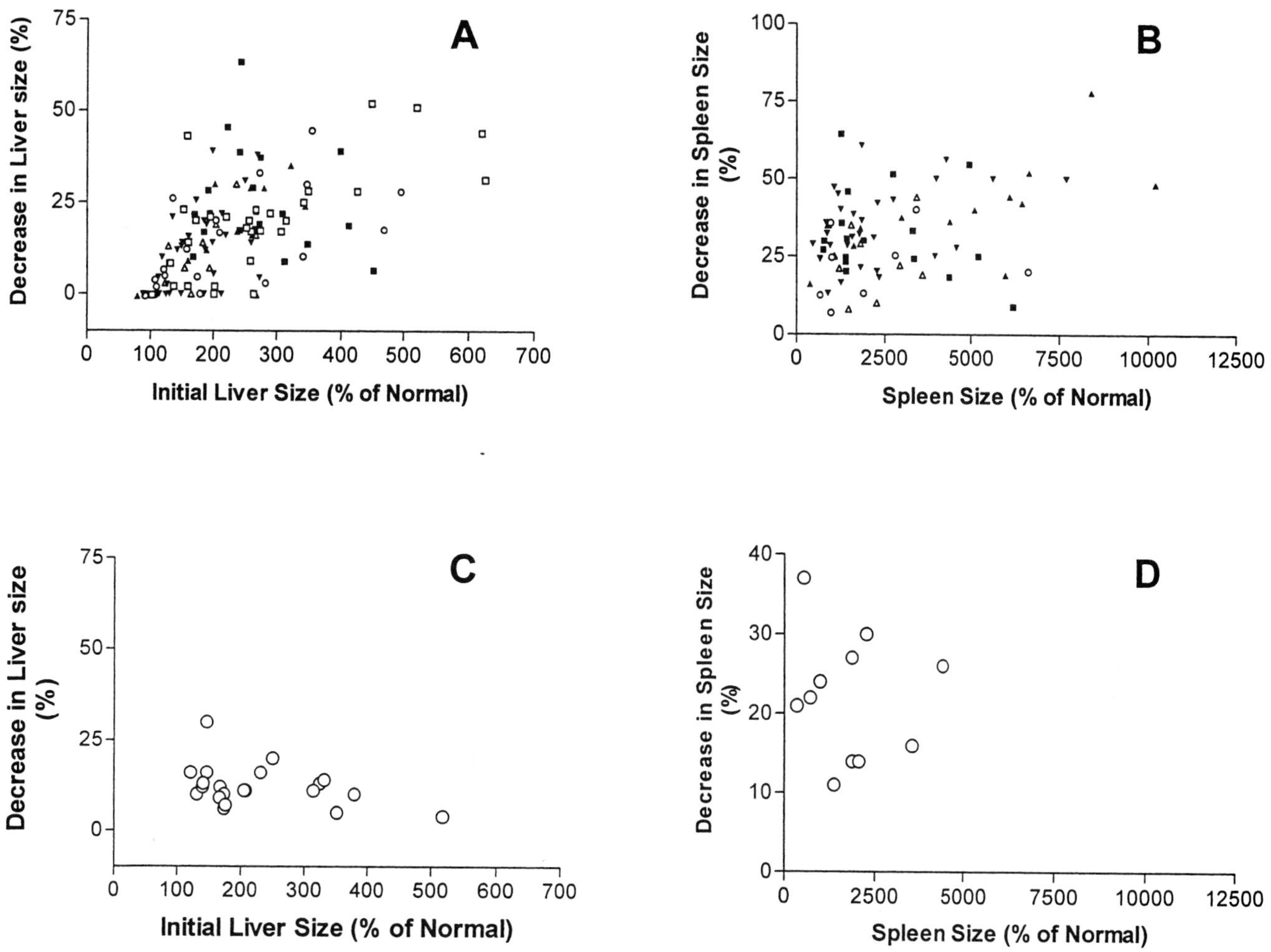

Fig. 146-8 The relationship between initial liver and spleen size and response to 6 months' therapy in doses ranging from 15 U/kg/month to 130 U/kg/month. Panels *A* (liver) and *B* (spleen) show responses to doses between 105 and 130 U/kg/month in solid symbols (130 U/Kg/month, Barton et al.[50] = ▲; 130 U/kg/mo, Grabowski et al.[579] = ▼; 105 U to 130 U/kg/month [see also Fig. 146-2], Pastores et al.[580] = ■) and doses of 30 U/Kg/month in open symbols (Beutler et al.[83] = ○; Zimran et al.[539] = □; Zimran et al.[581] = △). Panels *C* (liver) and *D* (spleen) show the response to 15 U/kg/month according to Hollak et al.[536] = ○. (*Reproduced from Beutler.[542] Used with permission.*)

treatment. Transplantation seems to be a more appropriate modality for the treatment of type 3 disease, particularly because it is unknown whether the neurologic disease could be prevented or arrested by the administration of an enzyme that does not cross the blood/brain barrier,[511] and encouraging results have been reported following stem cell transplantation.[553]

The Use of Inhibitors. Another approach to the treatment of Gaucher disease is the use of inhibitors of glucocerebrosidase synthesis. Several drugs that possess this capability are available,[558] the best known of which is 1-phenyl-2-decanoylamino-3-morpholino-1-propanol (PDMP), an inhibitor that resembles the substrate and product of the synthase.[559] PDMP decreases glucocerebroside levels in mice, rats, fish, and a variety of cultured cells. No major toxicity has been encountered, but long-term studies have not been performed. An analogous approach using *N*-butyldeoxynorjirimycin was evaluated in a Tay-Sachs mouse model with encouraging results,[560] but the lack of a suitable animal model of Gaucher disease has made it difficult to test the hypothesis that inhibitors might be therapeutically useful. In normal animal tissues, however, PDMP does rapidly lower the levels of glucosylceramide and the animals evidently do well with the lowered levels of glucosylceramide and its more complex glycolipid metabolites,[558] and a clinical study of N-butyldeoxynojirmycin has been published.[552]

Gene Transfer

Because Gaucher disease can be cured by replacing the patient's defective hematopoietic stem cell with a genetically normal stem cell from another individual, correction of the defect in the patient's own hematopoietic stem cells should be an effective way to treat this disease. However, because stem cells that produce acid β-glucosidase would not have a proliferative advantage over those that do not, cure would be expected only if the patient's untransformed cells were at least partially ablated by chemotherapy or irradiation. Thus, a rational strategy for the treatment of Gaucher disease would be marrow ablation followed by autologous transplantation with transformed hematopoietic stem cells. Considerable effort has been expended to develop the required efficient gene transfer technology.

The transfer of stable, functional acid β-glucosidase into cultured fibroblasts and transformed lymphoblasts using a retroviral vector was readily accomplished,[438,561,562] but transfer into hematopoietic stem cells is much more difficult.[446] Recently, relatively high efficiency transfer of the human acid β-glucosidase cDNA into murine and human hematopoietic stem cells or progenitors was accomplished[443,444,563] with evidence of sustained long-term expression of β-glucosidase in transplanted mice.[564–566] The use of a bicistronic vector containing, together with the glucocerebrosidase cDNA, a selectable gene has been suggested.[567] In vivo correction has been reported, but the percentage of cells transduced has been minuscule in all studies,[568] precluding the possibility of a clinical benefit.

CLINICAL GENETICS AND PREVENTION

Heterozygote Detection

As noted under "Diagnosis" above, assay of the acid β-glucosidase activity detects many, but by no means all, heterozygotes for Gaucher disease. There is considerable overlap between normal individuals and carriers, regardless of which assay procedure is used or how much care is taken in separating different white cell types from one another.

Detection of heterozygotes by DNA analysis for specific mutations is much more satisfactory. In family studies, when the specific mutation(s) in the family being examined are known, heterozygote detection is highly accurate. Barring technical errors or the existence of additional unsuspected Gaucher disease genes, every family member can be correctly classified with respect to genotype. When one or both mutations in a family are unknown, DNA analysis for specific alleles will only be accurate with respect to the known mutation. In population studies, those who have mutations for which the DNA is not examined will, of course, elude detection. In the Ashkenazi Jewish population, this problem has become a small one, because examination of DNA of Gaucher patients for just four mutations, 84GG, 1226G (N370S), IVS2(+1), and 1448C(L444P), will account for some 96.5 percent of the mutations.[312] Because the homozygous state for the 1226G (N370S) mutation frequently causes mild late onset disease, this mutation is underrepresented in the patient population, and is about twice as frequent in the general population relative to the other mutations. Examination for additional mutations that have been found in more than just a single family, that is, those at nt 1297, 1504, and 1604, brings the percentage of mutants detected in the patient population to 98 percent and that in the Ashkenazi Jewish population to 99 percent.[312] Ascertainment bias obscures genotype/phenotype correlations and complicates genetic counseling. In the Ashkenazi Jewish population, patients with the 1226G/1448C (N370S/L444P) or 1226G/null (i.e., 84GG) genotypes have earlier and more severe involvement than the 1226G (N370S) homozygotes.[183,569] However, a gross overestimate of the degree of clinical involvement of 1226G homozygotes is present because of their ascertainment by clinical presentation. The severity in 1226G/84GG or 1448C (L444P) compound heterozygous patients is sufficiently severe to allow essentially complete ascertainment. Disease gene screening of the Ashkenazi Jewish population shows gene frequencies for 1226G and 84GG of 0.0321 (1/31.2) and 0.00217 (1/460.8), respectively,[570] and predicts a 14.8:1 ratio for the 1226G/1226G to1226G/84GG genotypes. The observed ratio is 2.207, based on affected ascertainment, or a deficit of ~6.7 for the 1226G/1226G genotypes. These calculations suggest that many of the "patients" with the 1226G/1226G genotype may escape medical detection altogether or until advanced age. These findings show that the degree of "affectedness" of 1226G/1226G patients has been grossly overestimated, that the 1226G/1226G genotype is a "predisposition" to the Gaucher disease type 1 phenotype, and is insufficient to cause type 1 disease in the Ashkenazi Jewish patients.[59,570,571]

Prenatal Diagnosis

β-Glucosidase activity is readily measured in amniotic fluid cells[300] and chorionic villus samples,[572] so prenatal diagnosis is routine for all types of Gaucher disease.[55,573–575] More recently, DNA-based technology provided another quite facile means for identification of the genotype of the fetus. With the use of PCR, an ultrasensitive technique, one must be particularly concerned about contamination of fetal DNA with maternal DNA. However, because any contaminating DNA competes for the fetal DNA for the same amplifying primers, it is not anticipated that this would be a serious problem when maternal contamination is small.

Genetic Counseling

When a couple already has a child with Gaucher disease and both parents are heterozygotes, the recurrence risk, as in other autosomal recessive disorders is 1:4. Because homozygotes for the 1226G (N370S) mutation often have very mild disease, there are many instances in which one of the parents is a homozygote. Indeed, this happens with sufficient frequency that Gaucher disease was once regarded as being transmitted as an autosomal dominant disorder.[12] When one of the parents is a homozygote and the other a heterozygote, the recurrence risk is 1:2.

If the couple being counseled already has children with Gaucher disease, prediction of disease severity is easier than if there are no children with the disease. There is a considerable degree of concordance between sibs. However, sometimes there are substantial differences between sibs, particularly in disease manifestations if not severity. For example, it is not uncommon for one sib to have primarily visceral disease while another sib has mostly skeletal disease. It is less common for one sib to be severely affected while another is virtually free of disease manifestations, although this does occasionally occur.

If there are no affected children in the family, the counselor must depend on the genotype of the two parents, if it is known. In the most common circumstance, when both are 1226G (N370S) heterozygotes, they can be told that: (a) neurologic disease will not occur; (b) it is possible, but not likely, that a child homozygous for this mutation will have severe disease with early onset; and (c) it is much more likely that it will have mild disease or be essentially asymptomatic. When the fetus is at risk for the 1226G/84GG or the 1226G/1448C genotype, then the information to be given to the parents is quite different. In these genotypes, mild disease is possible, but much less probable. The median age of onset of disease in children with these genotypes is about 6 years,[77] and moderately severe disease usually develops. However, about 10 percent of the patients are exceptions, in which either of these genotypes is associated with quite mild disease. Again, neurologic disease is not expected in these genotypes. When the child is at risk for the 1448C/1448C genotype or one of its even more serious variants in which additional mutations are present (variously designated as XOVR, rec, pseudopattern, and complex allele) the prognosis is quite grave. The recombinant genotype referred to as RecTL, however, seems to result in milder manifestations than the 1448C mutation alone.[576] The likelihood of eventual, if not early, neurologic involvement is high and in any case, severe visceral and skeletal disease is to be expected. Counseling may be more difficult when one of the less common alleles is present. However, as a general rule, if such an allele has been found in a patient with neurologic disease, it may be considered to be in the same class with the 1448C(L444P) and related alleles, while if in combination with the 1448C(L444P) allele it has not resulted in neurologic disease, it may be considered to be milder in its phenotypical effect that more closely resembles the 1226G (N370S) allele.

REFERENCES

1. Gaucher PCE: De l'epithelioma primitif de la rate, hypertrophie idiopathique de la rate sans leucemie [Thesis]. Paris, 1882.
2. Brill NE, Mandelbaum FS, Libman E: Primary splenomegaly-Gaucher type. Report on one of few cases occurring in a single generation of one family. *Am J Med Sci* **129**:491, 1905.
3. Brill NE: Primary splenomegaly with a report of three cases occurring in one family. *Am J Med Sci* **121**:377, 1901.

4. Collier WA: A case of enlarged spleen in a child aged six. *Tr Path Soc London* **46**:148, 1895.
5. Picou R, Raymond F: Splenomegalic primitive epitheloma primitif de la rate. *Arch d'Med Exper et d'Anat Path* **8**:168, 1896.
6. Brill NE: A case of "splenomegalie primitif" with involvement of the haematopoietic organs. *Proc N Y Path Soc* **4**:143, 1904.
7. Schlagenhaufer F: Uber meist familiar vorkommende histologisch charakteristische splenomegalien (Typus Gaucher). *Virchows Arch Path Anat und F Klin Med* **187**:125, 1907.
8. Kraus EJ: Zur Kenntinis der Splenomegalie Gaucher, insbensondere der Histogenese der grobzellen Wucherung. *Z Angew Anat* **7**:186, 1920.
9. Rusca CL: Sul morbo del Gaucher. *Haematologica (Pavia)* **2**:441, 1921.
10. Oberling C, Woringer P: La maladie de Gaucher chez la nourrison. *Rev Franc de Pediat* **3**:475, 1927.
11. Hillborg PO: Morbus Gaucher: Norbotten. *Nord Med* **61**:303, 1959.
12. Groen JJ: Gaucher's disease: Hereditary transmission and racial distribution. *Arch Intern Med* **113**:543, 1964.
13. Fried K: Population study of chronic Gaucher's disease. *Isr J Med Sci* **9**:1396, 1973.
14. Hsia DYY, Naylor J, Bigler JA: Gaucher's disease: Report of two cases in father and son and review of the literature. *N Engl J Med* **261**:164, 1959.
15. Marchand F: Über sogenannte idiopathische splenomeglie (typus Gaucher). *MÜnch Med Wochenschr* **54**:1102, 1907.
16. Mandelbaum FS, Downey H: The histopathology and biology of Gaucher's disease (large-cell splenomegaly). *Folia Haemat* **20**:139, 1916.
17. Epstein E: Beitrag zur Chemie der Gaucherschen Krankeit. *Biochem Z* **145**:398, 1924.
18. Lieb H: Cerebrosidespeicherung bei splenomeglie Typus Gaucher. *Hoppe-Seyler's Z Physiol Chem* **140**:305, 1924.
19. Aghion H: La maladie de Gaucher dans l'enfance [Ph.D. Thesis]. Paris, 1934.
20. Schettler G, Kahlke W: Gaucher's disease, in Schettler G (ed): *Lipids and Lipidoses*. New York, Springer-Verlag, 1967, p 260.
21. Miyatake T, Suzuki K: Additional deficiency of psychosine galactosidase in globoid cell leukodystrophy: An implication to enzyme replacement therapy, in Desnick RJ, Bernlohr RW, Krivit W (eds): *Enzyme Therapy in Genetic Diseases*. Baltimore: Williams and Wilkins, 1973, p 136.
22. Conradi NG, Sourander P, Nilsson O, Svennerholm L, Erikson A: Neuropathology of the Norrbottnian type of Gaucher disease. Morphological and biochemical studies. *Acta Neuropathologica* **65**:99, 1984.
23. Brady RO, Kanfer JN, Shapiro D: Metabolism of glucocerebrosides. II. Evidence of an enzymatic deficiency in Gaucher's disease. *Biochem Biophys Res Commun* **18**:221, 1965.
24. Patrick AD: Short communications: A deficiency of glucocerebrosidase in Gaucher's disease. *Biochem J* **97**:17C, 1965.
25. Trams EG, Brady RO: Cerebroside synthesis in Gaucher's disease. *J Clin Invest* **39**:1546, 1960.
26. Öckerman PA: Identity of beta-glucosidase, beta-xylosidase, and one of the beta-galactosidase activities in human liver when assayed with 4-methylumbelliferyl-beta-d-glycoside. *Biochim Biophys Acta* **165**:59, 1968.
27. Dinur T, Osiecki Km, Legler G, Gatt S, Desnick RJ, Grabowski GA: Human acid beta-glucosidase: Isolation and amino acid sequence of a peptide containing the catalytic site. *Proc Natl Acad Sci U S A* **83**:1660, 1986.
28. Weinreb NJ, Brady RO, Tappel AL: The lysosomal localization of sphingolipid hydrolases. *Biochim Biophys Acta* **159**:141, 1968.
29. Ho MW, O'Brien JS: Gaucher's disease: Deficiency of "acid" beta-glucosidase and reconstitution of enzyme activity in vitro. *Proc Natl Acad Sci U S A* **68**:2810, 1971.
30. Devine EA, Smith M, Arredondo-Vega FX, Shafit-Zagardo B, Desnick RJ: Chromosomal localization of the gene for Gaucher disease. *Prog Clin Biol Res* **95**:511, 1982.
31. Holtschmidt H, Sandhoff K, Furst W, Kwon HY, Schnabel D, Suzuki K: The organization of the gene for the human cerebroside sulfate activator protein. *FEBS Lett* **280**:267, 1991.
32. Barneveld RA, Keijzer W, Tegelaers FPW, Ginns EI, Geurts van Kessel A, Brady RO, Barranger JA, Tager JM, Galjaard H, Westerveld A, Reuser AJJ: Assignment of the gene coding for human beta-glucocerebrosidase to the region q21-q31 of chromosome 1 using monoclonal antibodies. *Hum Genet* **64**:227, 1983.
33. Ginns EI, Choudary PV, Tsuji S, Martin B, Stubblefield B, Sawyer J, Hozier J, Barranger JA: Gene mapping and leader polypeptide sequence of human glucocerebrosidase: Implications for Gaucher disease. *Proc Natl Acad Sci U S A* **82**:7101, 1985.
34. Ginns EI, Choudary PV, Martin BM, Winfield S, Stubblefield B, Mayor J, Merkle-Lehman D, Murray GJ, Bowers LA, Barranger JA: Isolation of cDNA clones for human beta-glucocerebrosidase using the lambda gt11 expression system. *Biochem Biophys Res Commun* **123**:574, 1984.
35. Sorge J, West C, Westwood B, Beutler E: Molecular cloning and nucleotide sequence of the human glucocerebrosidase gene. *Proc Natl Acad Sci U S A* **82**:7289, 1985.
36. Tsuji S, Choudary PV, Martin BM, Winfield S, Barranger JA, Ginns EI: Nucleotide sequence of cDNA containing the complete coding sequence for human lysosomal glucocerebrosidase. *J Biol Chem* **261**:50, 1986.
37. Horowitz M, Wilder S, Horowitz Z, Reiner O, Gelbart T, Beutler E: The human glucocerebrosidase gene and pseudogene: Structure and evolution. *Genomics* **4**:87, 1989.
38. Tsuji S, Choudary PV, Martin BM, Stubblefield BK, Mayor JA, Barranger JA, Ginns EI: A mutation in the human glucocerebrosidase gene in neuronopathic Gaucher's disease. *N Engl J Med* **316**:570, 1987.
39. O'Brien JS, Kretz KA, Dewji N, Wenger DA, Esch F, Fluharty AL: Coding of two sphingolipid activator proteins (SAP-1 and SAP-2) by same genetic locus. *Science* **241**:1098, 1988.
40. Nakano T, Sandhoff K, Stumper J, Christomanou H, Suzuki K: Structure of full-length cDNA coding of sulfatide activator, a co-β-glucosidase and two other homologous proteins: Two alternate forms of the sulfatide activator. *J Biochem* **105**:152, 1989.
41. Gavrieli-Rorman E, Grabowski GA: Molecular cloning of a human co-beta-glucosidase cDNA: Evidence that four sphingolipid hydrolase activator proteins are encoded by single genes in humans and rats. *Genomics* **5**:486, 1989.
42. Gavrieli-Rorman E, Scheinker V, Grabowski GA: Structure and evolution of the human prosaposin chromosomal gene. *Genomics* **13**:312, 1992.
43. de Duve C: From cytases to lysosomes. *Fed Proc* **23**:1045, 1964.
44. Brady RO, Tallman JF, Johnson WG, Gal AE, Leahy WR, Quirk JM, Dekaban AS: Replacement therapy for inherited enzyme deficiency. Use of purified ceramide-trihexosidase in Fabry's disease. *N Engl J Med* **289**:9, 1973.
45. Beutler E, Dale GL, Guinto E, Kuhl W: Enzyme replacement therapy in Gaucher's disease: Preliminary clinical trial of a new enzyme preparation. *Proc Natl Acad Sci U S A* **74**:4620, 1977.
46. Achord DT, Brot FE, Bell CE, Sly WS: Human beta-glucuronidase: In vivo clearance and in vitro uptake by a glycoprotein recognition system on reticuloendothelial cells. *Cell* **15**:269, 1978.
47. Stahl PD, Rodman JS, Miller MJ, Schlesinger PH: Evidence for receptor-mediated binding of glycoproteins, glycoconjugates, and lysosomal glycosidases by alveolar macrophages. *Proc Natl Acad Sci U S A* **75**:1399, 1978.
48. Steer CJ, Furbish FS, Barranger JA, Brady RO, Jones EA: The uptake of agalacto-glucocerebroside by rat hepatocytes and Kupffer cells. *FEBS Lett* **91**:202, 1978.
49. Murray GJ, Doebber TW, Shen TY, Wu MS, Ponpipom MM, Bugianesi RL, Brady RO, Barranger JA: Targeting of synthetically glycosylated human placental glucocerebrosidase. *Biochem Med* **34**:241, 1985.
50. Barton NW, Brady RO, Dambrosia JM, Di Bisceglie AM, Doppelt SH, Hill SC, Mankin HJ, Murray GJ, Parker RI, Argoff CE, Grewal RP, Yu K-T: Replacement therapy for inherited enzyme deficiency — Macrophage-targeted glucocerebrosidase for Gaucher's disease. *N Engl J Med* **324**:1464, 1991.
51. Beutler E, Kay A, Saven A, Garver P, Thurston D, Dawson A, Rosenbloom B: Enzyme replacement therapy for Gaucher disease. *Blood* **78**:1183, 1991.
52. Fallet S, Sibille A, Mendelson R, Shapiro D, Hermann G, Grabowski GA: Enzyme augmentation in moderate to life-threatening Gaucher disease. *Pediatr Res* **31**:496, 1992.
53. Fried K: Gaucher's disease among the Jews of Israel. *The Bulletin of the Research Council of Israel Proceedings of the Fourth Meeting of the Israel Genetics Circle* **7B**:213, 1958.
54. Kolodny EH, Ullman MD, Mankin HJ, Raghavan SS, Topol J, Sullivan JL: Phenotypic manifestations of Gaucher disease: Clinical features in 48 biochemically verified Type I patients and comment on Type II patients, in Desnick RJ, Gatt S, Grabowski GA (eds): *Gaucher Disease: A Century of Delineation and Research*. New York, Alan R. Liss, 1982, p 33.

55. Grabowski GA, Dinur T, Gatt S, Desnick RJ: Gaucher type 1 (Ashkenazi) disease: considerations for heterozygote detection and prenatal diagnosis, in Desnick RJ, Gatt S, Grabowski GA (eds): *Gaucher Disease: A Century of Delineation and Research.* New York, Alan R. Liss, 1982, p 573.
56. Matoth Y, Chazan S, Cnaan A, Gelernter I, Klibansky C: Frequency of carriers of chronic (type I) Gaucher disease in Ashkenazi Jews. *Am J Med Genet* **27**:561, 1987.
57. Zimran A, Gelbart T, Westwood B, Grabowski GA, Beutler E: High frequency of the 1226 mutation for type I Gaucher disease among the Ashkenazi Jewish population. *Am J Hum Genet* **49**:855, 1991.
58. Beutler E, Nguyen NJ, Henneberger MW, Smolec JM, McPherson RA, West C, Gelbart T: Gaucher disease: Gene frequencies in the Ashkenazi Jewish population. *Am J Hum Genet* **52**:85, 1993.
59. Beutler E: Gaucher disease: New molecular approaches to diagnosis and treatment. *Science* **256**:794, 1992.
60. Chabas A, Cormand B, Balcells S, Gonzalez-Duarte R, Casanova C, Colomer J, Vilageliu L, Grinberg D: Neuronopathic and non-neuronopathic presentation of Gaucher disease in patients with the third most common mutation (D409H) in Spain. *J Inherit Metab Dis* **19**:798, 1996.
61. Amaral O, Pinto E, Fortuna M, Lacerda L, Sa Miranda MC: Type I Gaucher disease: Identification of N396T and prevalence of glucocerebrosidase mutations in the Portuguese. *Hum Mutat* **8**:280, 1996.
62. Lacerda L, Amaral O, Pinto R, Aerts J, Sa Miranda MC: The N370S mutation in the glucocerebrosidase gene of Portuguese type 1 Gaucher patients: Linkage to the PvuII polymorphism. *J Inherit Metab Dis* **17**:85, 1994.
63. Rotter JI, Diamond JM: What maintains the frequencies of human genetic diseases? *Nature* **329**:289, 1987.
64. Diamond JM: Jewish lysosomes. *Nature* **368**:291, 1994.
65. Kannai R, Weiler-Razell D, Elstein D, Zimran A: The selective advantage of Gaucher's disease: TB or not TB. *Isr J Med Sci* **30**:911, 1994.
66. Fredrickson DS, Sloan HR: Glucosyl ceramide lipidoses: Gaucher's disease, in Stanbury JB, Wyngaarden JB, Fredrickson DS (eds): *The Metabolic Basis of Inherited Disease.* New York, McGraw-Hill, 1972, p 730.
67. Patterson MC, Horowitz M, Abel RB, Currie JN, Yu K-T, Kaneski C, Higgins JJ, O'Neill RR, Fedio P, Pikus A, Brady RO, Barton NW: Isolated horizontal supranuclear gaze palsy as a marker of severe systemic involvement in Gaucher's disease. *Neurology* **43**:1993, 1993.
68. Uyama E, Takahashi K, Owada M, Okamura R, Naito M, Tsuji S, Kawasaki S, Araki S: Hydrocephalus, corneal opacities, deafness, valvular heart disease, deformed toes and leptomeningeal fibrous thickening in adult siblings: A new syndrome associated with beta-glucocerebrosidase deficiency and a mosaic population of storage cells. *Acta Neurol Scand* **86**:407, 1992.
69. Abrahamov A, Elstein D, Gross-Tsur V, Farber B, Glaser Y, Hada-Halpern I, Ronen S, Tafakjdi M, Horowitz M, Zimran A, Hadas-Halpern I: Gaucher's disease variant characterised by progressive calcification of heart valves and unique genotype. *Lancet* **346**:1000, 1995.
70. Chabas A, Cormand B, Grinberg D, Burguera JM, Balcells S, Merino JL, Mate I, Sobrino JA, Gonzalez-Duarte R, Vilageliu L: Unusual expression of Gaucher's disease: Cardiovascular calcifications in three sibs homozygous for the D409H mutation. *J Med Genet* **32**:740, 1995.
71. Beutler E, Kattamis C, Sipe J, Lipson M: The 1342C mutation in Gaucher's disease. *Lancet* **346**:1637, 1995.
72. Barton DJ, Ludman MD, Benkov K, Grabowski GA, LeLeiko NS: Resting energy expenditure in Gaucher's disease type 1: Effect of Gaucher's cell burden on energy requirements. *Metabolism* **38**:1238, 1989.
73. Berrebi A, Wishnitzer R, Von der Walde U: Gauchers disease: Unexpected diagnosis in three patients over seventy years old. *Nouv Rev Fr Hematol* **26**:201, 1984.
74. Brinn L, Glabman S: Gaucher's disease without splenomegaly. Oldest patient on record with review. *NY State J Med* **62**:2346, 1962.
75. Chang-Lo M, Yam LT: Gaucher's disease. Review of the literature and report of twelve new cases. *Am J Med Sci* **254**:303, 1967.
76. Beutler E: Gaucher's disease in an asymptomatic 72-year old. *JAMA* **237**:2529, 1977.
77. Beutler E: Gaucher's disease. *N Engl J Med* **325**:1354, 1991.
78. Beutler E: Modern diagnosis and treatment of Gaucher's disease. *Am J Dis Child* **147**:1175, 1993.
79. Sibille A, Eng CM, Kim S-J, Pastores G, Grabowski GA: Phenotype/genotype correlations in Gaucher disease type I: Clinical and therapeutic implications. *Am J Hum Genet* **52**:1094, 1993.
80. Kaplan P, Mazur A, Manor O, Charrow J, Esplin J, Gribble TJ, Wappner RS, Wisch JS, Weinreb NJ: Acceleration of retarded growth in children with Gaucher disease after treatment with alglucerase. *J Pediatr* **129**:149, 1996.
81. Zevin S, Abrahamov A, Hadas-Halpern I, Kannai R, Levy-Lahad E, Horowitz M, Zimran A: Adult-type Gaucher disease in children: Genetics, clinical features and enzyme replacement therapy. *QJM* **86**:565, 1993.
82. Balicki D, Beutler E: Gaucher disease. *Medicine (Baltimore)* **74**:305, 1995.
83. Beutler E, Demina A, Laubscher K, Garver P, Gelbart T, Balicki D, Vaughan L: The clinical course of treated and untreated Gaucher disease. A study of 45 patients. *Blood Cells Mol Dis* **21**:86, 1995.
84. Beutler E: Commentary: The natural history of Gaucher disease. *Blood Cells Mol Dis* **24**:82, 1998.
85. Ida H, Rennert OM, Ito T, Maekawa K, Eto Y: Type 1 Gaucher disease: Phenotypic expression and natural history in Japanese patients. *Blood Cells Mol Dis* **24**:73, 1998.
86. Zimran A, Kay AC, Gelbart T, Garver P, Saven A, Beutler E: Gaucher disease: Clinical, laboratory, radiologic and genetic features of 53 patients. *Medicine (Baltimore)* **71**:337, 1992.
87. Seligsohn U, Zitman D, Many A, Klibansky C: Coexistence of factor XI (plasma thromboplastin antecedent) deficiency and Gaucher's disease. *Isr J Med Sci* **12**:1448, 1976.
88. Billett HH, Rizvi S, Sawitsky A: Coagulation abnormalities in patients with Gaucher's disease: Effect of therapy. *Am J Hematol* **51**:234, 1996.
89. Hollak CE, Levi M, Berends F, Aerts JM, van Oers MH: Coagulation abnormalities in type 1 Gaucher disease are due to low-grade activation and can be partly restored by enzyme supplementation therapy. *Br J Haematol* **96**:470, 1997.
90. Allen MJ, Myer BJ, Khokher AM, Rushton N, Cox TM: Pro-inflammatory cytokines and the pathogenesis of Gaucher's disease: Increased release of interleukin-6 and interleukin-10. *QJM* **90**:19, 1997.
91. Medoff AS, Bayrd ED: Gauchers disease in 29 cases: Hematologic complications and effect of splenectomy. *Ann Intern Med* **40**:481, 1954.
92. Lee RE: The Pathology of Gaucher Disease, in Desnick RJ, Gatt S, Grabowski GA (eds): *Gaucher Disease: A Century of Delineation and Research.* New York, Alan R. Liss, 1982, p 177.
93. Goldblatt J, Beighton P: South African variants of Gaucher disease, in Desnick RJ, Gatt S, Grabowski GA (eds): *Gaucher Disease: A Century of Delineation and Research.* New York, Alan R. Liss, 1982, p 95.
94. Hill SC, Reinig JW, Barranger JA, Fink J, Shawker TH: Gaucher disease: Sonographic appearance of the spleen. *Radiology* **160**:631, 1986.
95. James SP, Stromeyer FW, Stowens DW, Barranger JA: Gaucher disease: Hepatic abnormalities in 25 patients, in: Desnick RJ, Gatt S, Grabowski GA (eds): *Gaucher Disease: A Century of Delineation and Research.* New York, Alan R. Liss, 1982, p 131.
96. Fellows KE, Grand RJ, Colodny AH, Orsini EN, Crocker AC: Combined portal and vena caval hypertension in Gaucher disease: The value of preoperative venography. *J Pediatr* Radiology **87**:739, 1975.
97. Henderson JM, Gilinsky NH, Lee EY, Greenwood MF: Gaucher's disease complicated by bleeding esophageal varices and colonic infiltration by Gaucher cells. *Am J Gastroenterol* **86**:346, 1991.
98. Stowens DW, Teitelbaum SL, Kahn AJ, Barranger JA: Skeletal complications in Gaucher disease. *Medicine (Baltimore)* **64**:310, 1985.
99. Hermann G, Goldblatt J, Levy RN, Goldsmith SJ, Desnick RJ, Grabowski GA: Gaucher's disease type 1: Assessment of bone involvement by CT and scintigraphy. *AJR Am J Roentgenol* **147**:943, 1986.
100. Beighton P, Goldblatt J, Sacks S: Bone involvement in Gaucher disease, in Desnick RJ, Gatt S, Grabowski GA (eds): *Gaucher Disease: A Century of Delineation and Research.* New York, Alan R. Liss, 1982, p 107.
101. Goldblatt J, Sacks S, Beighton P: The orthopedic aspects of Gaucher disease. *Clin Orthop* **137**:208, 1978.
102. Myers HS, Cremin BJ, Beighton P, Sacks S: Chronic Gaucher's disease: Radiological findings in 17 South African cases. *Br J Radiol* **48**:465, 1975.
103. Rosenthal DI, Scott JA, Barranger J, Mankin HJ, Saini S, Brady TJ, Osier LK, Doppelt S: Evaluation of Gaucher disease using magnetic resonance imaging. *J Bone Joint Surg Am* **68**:802, 1986.
104. Cremin BJ, Davey H, Goldblatt J: Skeletal complications of type I Gaucher disease: The magnetic resonance features. *Clin Radiol* **41**:244, 1990.

105. Rosenthal DI, Barton NW, McKusick KA, Rosen BR, Hill SC, Castronovo FP, Brady RO, Doppelt SH, Mankin HJ: Quantitative imaging of Gaucher disease. *Radiology* **185**:841, 1992.
106. Rosenthal DI, Mayo-Smith W, Goodsitt MM, Doppelt S, Mankin HJ: Bone and bone marrow changes in Gaucher disease: Evaluation with quantitative CT. *Radiology* **170**:143, 1989.
107. Pastores GM, Wallenstein S, Desnick RJ, Luckey MM: Bone density in Type 1 Gaucher disease. *J Bone Miner Res* **11**:1801, 1996.
108. Raynor RR: Spinal-cord compression secondary to Gaucher's disease. *J Neurosurg* **19**:902, 1962.
109. Hermann G, Goldblatt J, Desnick RJ: Kummell disease: Delayed collapse of the traumatised spine in a patient with Gaucher Type I disease. *Br J Radiol* **57**:833, 1984.
110. Gordon GL: Osseous Gaucher's disease. *Am J Med* **8**:332, 1950.
111. Schneider EL, Epstein CJ, Kaback MJ, Brandes D: Severe pulmonary involvement in adult Gaucher's disease. *Am J Med* **63**:475, 1977.
112. Kerem E, Elstein D, Abrahamov A, Ziv YB, Hadas-Halpern I, Melzer E, Cahan C, Branski D, Zimran A: Pulmonary function abnormalities in type I Gaucher disease. *Eur Respir J* **9**:340, 1996.
113. Aydin K, Karabulut N, Demirkazik F, Arat A: Pulmonary involvement in adult Gaucher's disease: High resolution CT appearance. *Br J Radiol* **70**:93, 1997.
114. Roberts WC, Fredrickson DS: Gaucher's Disease of the lung causing severe pulmonary hypertension with associated acute recurrent pericarditis. *Circulation* **35**:783, 1967.
115. Harats D, Pauzner R, Elstein D, Many A, Klutstein MW, Farfel Z, Zimran A: Pulmonary hypertension in two patients with type I Gaucher disease while on alglucerase therapy. *Acta Haematol* **98**:47, 1997.
116. Melamed E, Cohen C, Soffer D, Lavy S: Central nervous system complication in a patient with chronic Gaucher's disease. *Eur Neurol* **13**:167, 1975.
117. Hermann G, Wagner LD, Gendal ES, Ragland RL, Ulin RI: Spinal cord compression in type I Gaucher disease. *Radiology* **170**:147, 1989.
118. Markin RS, Skultety FM: Spinal cord compression secondary to Gaucher's disease. *Surg Neurol* **21**:341, 1984.
119. Grewal RP, Doppelt SH, Thompson MA, Katz D, Brady RO, Barton NW: Neurologic complications of nonneuronopathic Gaucher's disease. *Arch Neurol* **48**:1271, 1991.
120. Soffer D, Yamanaka T, Wenger DA, Suzuki K: Central nervous system involvement in adult-onset Gaucher's disease. *Acta Neuropathol (Berl)* **49**:1, 1980.
121. King JO: Progressive myoclonic epilepsy due to Gaucher's disease in an adult. *J Neurol Neurosurg Psychiatry* **38**:849, 1975.
122. Miller JD, McCluer R, Kanfer JN: Gaucher's disease: Neurologic disorder in adult siblings. *Ann Intern Med* **78**:883, 1973.
123. Neudorfer O, Giladi N, Elstein D, Abrahamov A, Turezkite T, Aghai E, Reches A, Bembi B, Zimran A: Occurrence of Parkinson's syndrome in type I Gaucher disease. *QJM* **89**:691, 1996.
124. Goldblatt J, Beighton P: Cutaneous manifestations of Gaucher disease. *Br J Dermatol* **111**:331, 1984.
125. Commens KL, Choong R, Jaworski R: Collodion babies with Gaucher's disease. *Arch Dis Child* **63**:854, 1988.
126. Sidransky E, Fartasch M, Lee RE, Metlay LA, Abella S, Zimran A, Gao W, Elias PM, Ginns EI, Holleran WM: Epidermal abnormalities may distinguish type 2 from type 1 and type 3 of Gaucher disease. *Pediatr Res* **39**:134, 1996.
127. Petrohelos M, Tricoulis D, Kotsiras I, Vouzoukos A: Ocular manifestations of Gaucher's disease. *Am J Ophthalmol* **80**:1006, 1975.
128. Schwartz MR, Weycer JS, McGavran MH: Gaucher's disease involving the maxillary sinuses. *Arch Otolaryngol Head Neck Surg* **114**:203, 1988.
129. Amstutz HC, Carey EJ: Skeletal manifestations and treatment of Gaucher's disease. *J Bone Joint Surg Am* **48**:670, 1966.
130. Draznin SZ, Singer K: Legg-Perthes' disease: A syndrome of many etiologies? With clinical and roentgenographic findings in a case of Gaucher's disease. *Am J Roentgenol* **60**:490, 1948.
131. Billings AA, Post M, Shapiro CM: Febrile reaction of Gaucher's disease. *Ill Med J* **145**:222, 1973.
132. Zimran A, Abrahamov A, Aker M, Matzner Y: Correction of neutrophil chemotaxis defect in patients with Gaucher disease by low-dose enzyme replacement therapy. *Am J Hematol* **43**:69, 1993.
133. Aker M, Zimran A, Abrahamov A, Horowitz M, Matzner Y: Abnormal neutrophil chemotaxis in Gaucher disease. *Br J Haematol* **83**:187, 1993.
134. Zimran A, Elstein D, Abrahamov A, Dale GL, Aker M, Matzner Y: Significance of abnormal neutrophil chemotaxis in Gaucher's disease. *Blood* **84**:2374, 1994.
135. Liel Y, Rudich A, Nagauker-Shriker O, Yermiyahu T, Levy R: Monocyte dysfunction in patients with Gaucher disease: Evidence for interference of glucocerebroside with superoxide generation. *Blood* **83**:2646, 1994.
136. Shiran A, Brenner B, Laor A, Tatarsky I: Increased risk of cancer in patients with Gaucher disease. *Cancer* **72**:219, 1993.
137. Chang-Lo M, Yam LT, Rubenstone AI, Schwartz SO: Gaucher's disease associated with chronic lymphocytic leukaemia, gout and carcinoma. *J Pathol* **116**:203, 1975.
138. Mark T, Dominguez C, Rywlin AM: Gaucher's disease associated with chronic lymphocytic leukemia. *South Med J* **75**:361, 1982.
139. Kaufman S, Rozenfeld V, Yona R, Varon M: Gaucher's disease associated with chronic lymphocytic leukaemia. *Clin Lab Haematol* **8**:321, 1986.
140. Garfinkel D, Sidi Y, Ben-Bassat M, Salomon F, Hazaz B, Pinkhas J: Coexistence of Gaucher's disease and multiple myeloma. *Arch Intern Med* **142**:2229, 1982.
141. Lamon J, Miller W, Tavassoli M, Longmire R, Beutler E: Specialty conference: Multiple myeloma complicating Gaucher's disease. *West J Med* **136**:122, 1982.
142. Ruestow PC, Levinson DJ, Catchatourian R, Sreekanth S, Cohen H, Rosenfeld S: Coexistence of IgA myeloma and Gaucher's disease. *Arch Intern Med* **140**:1115, 1980.
143. Benjamin D, Joshua H, Djaldetti M, Hazaz B, Pinkhas J: Nonsecretory IgD-kappa multiple myeloma in a patient with Gaucher's disease. *Scand J Haematol* **22**:179, 1979.
144. Gal R, Gukovsky-Oren S, Floru S, Djaldetti M, Kessler E: Sequential appearance of breast carcinoma, multiple myeloma and Gaucher's disease. *Haematologica (Pavia)* **73**:63, 1988.
145. Bruckstein AH, Karanas A, Dire JJ: Gaucher's disease associated with Hodgkin's disease. *Am J Med* **68**:610, 1980.
146. Cho SY, Sastre M: Coexistence of Hodgkin's disease and Gaucher's disease. *Am J Clin Pathol* **65**:103, 1976.
147. Paulson JA, Marti GE, Fink JK, Sato N, Schoen M, Karcher DS: Richter's transformation of lymphoma complicating Gaucher's disease. *Hematol Pathol* **3**:91, 1989.
148. Shoenfeld Y, Berliner S, Pinkhas J, Beutler E: The association of Gaucher's disease and dysproteinemias. *Acta Haematol* **64**:241, 1980.
149. Pratt PW, Estren F, Kochwa S: Immunoglobulin abnormalities in Gaucher's disease. Report of 16 cases. *Blood* **31**:633, 1968.
150. Turesson I, Rausing A: Gaucher's disease and benign monoclonal gammopathy. A case report with immunofluorescence study of bone marrow and spleen. *Acta Med Scand* **197**:507, 1975.
151. Liel Y, Hausmann MJ, Mozes M: Case report: Serendipitous Gaucher's disease presenting as elevated erythrocyte sedimentation rate due to monoclonal gammopathy. *Am J Med Sci* **301**:393, 1991.
152. Kenan S, Abdelwahab IF, Hermann G, Klein M, Pastores G: Osteoblastoma of the humerus associated with TYPE-I Gaucher's disease — A case report. *J Bone Joint Surg Br* **78B**:702, 1996.
153. Pins MR, Mankin HJ, Xavier RJ, Rosenthal DI, Dickersin GR, Rosenberg AE: Malignant epithelioid hemangioendothelioma of the tibia associated with a bone infarct in a patient who had Gaucher disease. *J Bone Joint Surg Am* **77-A**:777, 1995.
154. Petrides PE, le Coutre P, Müller-Höcker J, Magin E, Harzer K, Demina A, Beutler E: Coincidence of Gaucher's disease due to a private mutation and Ph' positive chronic myeloid leukemia. *Am J Hematol* **59**:87, 1998.
155. Zlotogora J, Sagi M, Zeigler M, Bach G: Gaucher disease type I and pregnancy. *Am J Med Genet* **32**:475, 1989.
156. Grabowski GA, Moskovitz J: Pregnancy in Gaucher disease: The paradigm for genetic medicine, in Platt LD, Koch R, de la Cruz F (eds): *Genetic Disorders and Pregnancy Outcome, chap 11*. London, Parthenon Publishing, 1996, p 95.
157. Menton M, Frauz M, Harzer K, Stroppel G, Franz HBG: Morbus Gaucher und Schwangerschaft. *Geburtsh u Frauenheilk* **50**:410, 1990.
158. Granovsky-Grisaru S, Aboulafia Y, Diamant YZ, Horowitz M, Abrahamov A, Zimran A: Gynecologic and obstetric aspects of Gaucher's disease: A survey of 53 patients. *Am J Obstet Gynecol* **172**:1284, 1995.
159. Sun CC, Panny S, Combs J, Gutberlett R: Hydrops fetalis associated with Gaucher disease. *Pathol Res Pract* **179**:101, 1984.
160. Conradi N, Kyllerman M, Månsson J-E, Percy AK, Svennerholm L: Late-infantile Gaucher disease in a child with myoclonus and bulbar signs: Neuropathological and neurochemical findings. *Acta Neuropathol (Berl)* **82**:152, 1991.
161. Fujimoto A, Tayebi N, Sidransky E: Congenital ichthyosis preceding neurologic symptoms in two sibs with type 2 Gaucher disease. *Am J Med Genet* **59**:356, 1995.

162. Wenger DA, Roth S, Kudoh T, Grover WD, Tucker SH, Kaye EM, Ullman MD: Biochemical studies in a patient with subacute neuropathic Gaucher disease without visceral glucosylceramide storage. *Pediatr Res* **17**:344, 1983.
163. Tibblin E, Dreborg S, Erikson A, Hakansson G, Svennerholm L: Hematological findings in the Norrbottnian type of Gaucher disease. *Eur J Pediatr* **139**:187, 1982.
164. Kyllerman M, Conradi N, Månsson J-E, Percy AK, Svennerholm L: Rapidly progressive type III Gaucher disease: Deterioration following partial splenectomy. *Acta Paediatr Scand* **79**:448, 1990.
165. Erikson A, Groth CG, Månsson J-E, Percy A, Ringdén O, Svennerholm L: Clinical and biochemical outcome of marrow transplantation for Gaucher disease of the Norrbottnian type. *Acta Paediatr Scand* **79**:680, 1990.
166. Dreborg S, Erikson A, Hagberg B: Gaucher disease — Norrbottnian type. *Eur J Pediatr* **133**:107, 1980.
167. Erikson A: Gaucher disease. Norrbottnian Type (III). Neuropaediatric and neurobiological aspects of clinical patterns and treatment. *Acta Paediatr Scand* **326**:1, 1986.
168. Uyama E, Uchino M, Ida H, Eto Y, Owada M: D409H/D409H genotype in Gaucher-like disease. *J Med Genet* **34**:175, 1997.
169. Parkin JL, Brunning RD: Pathology of the Gaucher cell, in Desnick RJ, Gatt S, Grabowski GA (eds): *Gaucher Disease: A Century of Delineation and Research.* New York, Alan R. Liss, 1982, p 151.
170. Burns GF, Cawley RJ, Flemans RJ, Higgy KE, Worman CP: Surface marker and other characteristics of Gaucher's cell. *J Clin Pathol* **30**:981, 1977.
171. Djaldetti M, Fishman P, Bessler H: The surface ultrastructure of Gaucher cells. *Am J Clin Pathol* **71**:146, 1979.
172. Pennelli N, Scaravilli F, Zacchello F: The morphogenesis of Gaucher cells investigated by electron microscopy. *Blood* **34**:331, 1969.
173. Hibbs RG, Ferrans VJ, Cipriano PR, Tardiff KJ: A histochemical and electron microscopic study of Gaucher cells. *Arch Pathol (Chicago)* **89**:137, 1970.
174. Mistry PK, Wraight EP, Cox TM: Therapeutic delivery of proteins to macrophages: implications for treatment of Gaucher's disease. *Lancet* **348**:1555, 1996.
175. Lam KW, Li CY, Yam LT, Smith RS, Hacker B: Comparison of prostatic and nonprostatic acid phosphatase. *Ann N Y Acad Sci* **390**:1, 1982.
176. Lam K-W, Desnick RJ: Biochemical properties of the tartrate-resistant acid phosphatase activity in Gaucher disease, in Desnick RJ, Gatt S, Grabowski GA (eds): *Gaucher Disease: A Century of Delineation and Research.* New York, Alan R. Liss, 1982, p 267.
177. Lee RE: The fine structure of the cerebroside occurring in Gaucher's disease. *Proc Natl Acad Sci U S A* **61**:484, 1968.
178. Lee RE, Peters SP, Glew RH: Gaucher's disease: Clinical, morphologic, and pathogenetic considerations. *Pathol Annu* **12**:309, 1977.
179. DeGasperi R, Alroy J, Richard R, Goyal V, Orgad U, Lee RE, Warren CD: Glycoprotein storage in Gaucher disease: Lectin histochemistry and biochemical studies. *Lab Invest* **63**:385, 1990.
180. Banker BQ, Miller JQ, Crocker AC: The cerebral pathology of infantile Gaucher's disease, in Aronson SM, Volk BM (eds): *Cerebral Sphingolipidoses.* New York, Academic Press, 1962, p 73.
181. Kattlove HE, Williams JC, Gaynor E, Spivack M, Bradley RM, Brady RO: Gaucher cells in chronic myelocytic leukemia: An acquired abnormality. *Blood* **33**:379, 1969.
182. Aufses AH Jr, Salky BM: The surgical management of Gaucher's Disease, in Desnick RJ, Gatt S, Grabowski GA (eds): *Gaucher Disease: A Century of Delineation and Research.* New York, Alan R. Liss, 1982, p 603.
183. Sibille A, Eng CM, Kim SJ, Pastores G, Grabowski GA: Phenotype/genotype correlations in Gaucher disease type I: Clinical and therapeutic implications. *Am J Hum Genet* **52**:1094, 1993.
184. Altman PL, Dittmer DS: *Growth*, Washington, Federation of American Societies for Experimental Biology, 1962.
185. Lester TJ, Grabowski GA, Goldblatt J, Leiderman IZ, Zaroulis CG: Immune thrombocytopenia and Gaucher's disease. *Am J Med* **77**:569, 1984.
186. Haratz D, Manny N, Raz I: Autoimmune hemolytic anemia in Gaucher's disease. *Klin Wochenschr* **68**:94, 1990.
187. Hill SC, Reinig JW, Barranger JA, Fink J, Shawker TH: Gaucher disease: Sonographic appearance of the spleen. *Radiology* **160**:631, 1986.
188. Neudorfer O, Hadas-Halpern I, Elstein D, Abrahamov A, Zimran A: Abdominal ultrasound findings mimicking hematological malignancies in a study of 218 Gaucher patients. *Am J Hematol* **55**:28, 1997.
189. Elleder M, Jirsek A: Histochemical and ultrastructural study of Gaucher cells. *Acta Neuropathol (Berl)* **7**:208, 1981.
190. James SP, Stromeyer FW, Chang C, Barranger JA: Liver abnormalities in patients with Gaucher's disease. *Gastroenterology* **80**:126, 1981.
191. Carlson DE, Busuttil RW, Giudici TA, Barranger JA: Orthotopic liver transplantation in the treatment of complications of type I Gaucher disease. *Transplantation* **49**:1192, 1990.
192. Sarnitski IP, Demidiuk PF, Guseva SA, Demidiuk SP, Monastyrskaia OS: Results of splenectomy in Gaucher's disease. *Gematol Transfuziol* **31**:39, 1986.
193. Stowens DW, Teitelbaum SL, Kahn AJ, Barranger JA: Skeletal complications of Gaucher disease. *Medicine (Baltimore)* **64**:310, 1985.
194. Katz K, Horev G, Rivlin E, Kornreich L, Cohen IJ, Gruenbaum M, Yosipovitch Z: Upper limb involvement in patients with Gaucher's disease. *J Hand Surg Am* **18**:871, 1993.
195. Bildman B, Martinez M Jr, Robinson LH: Gaucher's disease discovered by mandibular biopsy: Report of case. *J Oral Surg* **30**:510, 1972.
196. Carter LC, Fischman SL, Mann J, Elstein D, Stabholz A, Zimran A: The nature and extent of jaw involvement in Gaucher disease: Observations in a series of 28 patients. *Oral Surg Oral Med Oral Pathol Oral Radiol Endod* **85**:233, 1998.
197. Siffert RS, Platt A: Gaucher's disease: Orthopaedic considerations, in Desnick RJ, Gatt SH, Grabowski GA (eds): *Gaucher Disease: A Century of Delineation and Research.* New York, Alan R. Liss, 1982, p 617.
198. Smith RL, Hutchins GM, Sack GH Jr, Ridolfi RL: Unusual cardiac, renal and pulmonary involvement in Gaucher's disease. Interstitial glucocerebroside accumulation, pulmonary hypertension and fatal bone marrow embolization. *Am J Med* **65**:352, 1978.
199. Edwards WD, Hurdey HP, Partin JR: Cardiac involvement by Gaucher's disease documented by right ventricular endomyocardial biopsy. *Am J Cardiol* **52**:654, 1983.
200. Hrebicek M, Zeman J, Musilova J, Hodanova K, Renkema GH, Veprekova L, Ledvinova J, Hrebicek D, Sokolova J, Aerts JM, Elleder M: A case of type I Gaucher disease with cardiopulmonary amyloidosis and chitotriosidase deficiency. *Virchows Arch* **429**:305, 1996.
201. Dikman SH, Goldstein M, Kahn T, Leo MA, Weinreb N: Amyloidosis. An unusual complication of Gaucher's disease. *Arch Pathol Lab Med* **102**:460, 1978.
202. Shvidel L, Hurwitz N, Shtalrid M, Zur S, Oliver O, Berrebi A: Complex IgA gammopathy in Gaucher's disease. *Leuk Lymphoma* **20**:165, 1995.
203. Tamari I, Motro M, Neufeld HN: Unusual pericardial calcification in Gaucher's disease. *Arch Intern Med* **143**:2010, 1983.
204. Gribetz AR, Kasen L, Teirstein AS: Respiratory distress, pericarditis and inappropriate antidiuretic hormone secretion in a patient with infectious mononucleosis and Gaucher's disease. *Mt Sinai J Med* **47**:589, 1980.
205. Sloane MF, Bhuptani A, Miller A, Brown LK, Teirstein AS, Grabowski GA: Oxygen delivery defect in Gaucher's disease. *Chest* **100**:97S, 1991.
206. Carson KF, Williams CA, Rosenthal DL, Bhuta S, Kleerup E, Diaz RP, Sykes E: Bronchoalveolar lavage in a girl with Gaucher's disease. A case report. *Acta Cytol* **38**:597, 1994.
207. Tabak L, Yilmazbayhan D, Kilicaslan Z, Tascioglu C, Agan M: Value of bronchoalveolar lavage in lipidoses with pulmonary involvement. *Eur Respir J* **7**:409, 1994.
208. Kerem E, Elstein D, Abrahamov A, Bar Ziv Y, Hadas-Halpern I, Melzer E, Cahan C, Branski D, Zimran A: Pulmonary function abnormalities in type I Gaucher disease. *Eur Respir J* **9**:340, 1996.
209. Norman RM, Urich H, Lloyd OC: The neuropathology of infantile Gaucher's disease. *J Pathol Bacteriol* **72**:121, 1956.
210. Adachi M, Schneck L, Volk BW: Progress in investigations of sphingolipidoses. *Acta Neuropathol (Berl)* **43**:1, 1978.
211. Bove KE, Daugherty C, Grabowski GA: Pathological findings in Gaucher disease type 2 patients following enzyme therapy. *Hum Pathol* **26**:1040, 1995.
212. Theise ND, Ursell PC: Pulmonary hypertension and Gaucher's disease: Logical association or mere coincidence? *Am J Pediatr Hematol Oncol* **12**:74, 1990.
213. Chander PN, Nurse HM, Pirani CL: Renal involvement in adult Gaucher's disease after splenectomy. *Arch Pathol Lab Med* **103**:440, 1979.
214. Brito T, Gomes dos Reis V, Penna DO, Camargo ME: Glomerular involvement in Gaucher's disease. A light, immunofluorescent, and ultrastructural study based on kidney biopsy specimens. *Arch Pathol (Chicago)* **95**:1, 1973.

215. Chiarugi M, Martino MC, Buccianti P, Goletti O: Bleeding gastric ulcer complicating splenosis in type 1 Gaucher's disease. *Eur J Surg* **162**:63, 1996.
216. Espinas OEA, Faris AA: Acute infantile Gaucher's disease in identical twins. An account of clinical and neuropathologic observations. *Neurology* **19**:133, 1969.
217. Lacey DJ, Terplan K: Correlating auditory evoked and brainstem histologic abnormalities in infantile Gaucher's disease. *Neurology* **34**:539, 1984.
218. Adachi M, Wallace BJ, Schneck L, Volk BW: Fine structure of central nervous system in early infantile Gaucher's disease. *Arch Pathol (Chicago)* **83**:513, 1967.
219. Grafe M, Thomas C, Schneider J, Katz B, Wiley C: Infantile Gaucher's disease: A case with neuronal storage. *Ann Neurol* **23**:300, 1988.
220. Kaye EM, Ullman MD, Wilson ER, Barranger JA: Type 2 and type 3 Gaucher disease: a morphological and biochemical study. *Ann Neurol* **20**:223, 1986.
221. Conradi NG, Kalimo H, Sourander P: Reactions of vessel walls and brain parenchyma to the accumulation of Gaucher cells in the Norrbottnian type (type III) of Gaucher disease. *Acta Neuropathol (Berl)* **75**:385, 1988.
222. Conradi NG, Sourander P, Nilsson O, Svennerholm L, Erikson A: Neuropathology of the Norrbottnian type of Gaucher disease: Morphological and biochemical studies. *Acta Neuropathol (Berl)* **65**:99, 1984.
223. Kamoshita S, Odawara M, Yoshida M, Owada M, Kitagawa T: Fetal pathology and ultrastructure of neuropathic Gaucher's disease. *Adv Exp Med Biol* **68**:63, 1976.
224. Nilsson O, Svennerholm L: Accumulation of glucosylceramide and glucosylsphingosine (psychosine) in cerebrum and cerebellum in infantile and juvenile Gaucher disease. *J Neurochem* **39**:709, 1982.
225. Nilsson O, Grabowski GA, Ludman MD, Desnick RJ, Svennerholm L: Glycosphingolipid studies of visceral tissues and brain from type 1 Gaucher disease variants. *Clin Genet* **27**:443, 1985.
226. Mislow K: The geometry of sphingosine. *J Am Chem Soc* **74**:5155, 1952.
227. Carter HE, Fujino Y: Biochemistry of the sphingolipids. IX. Configuration of cerebrosides. *J Biol Chem* **221**:879, 1956.
228. Basu S, Kaufman B, Roseman S: Enzymatic synthesis of ceramide-glucose and ceramide-lactose by glycosyltransferases from embryonic chicken brain. *J Biol Chem* **243**:5802, 1968.
229. Basu S, Kaufman B, Roseman S: Enzymatic synthesis of glucocerebroside by a glucosyltransferase from embryonic chicken brain. *J Biol Chem* **248**:1388, 1973.
230. Coste H, Martel MB, Azzar G, Got R: UDP-glucoseceramide glucosyltransferase from porcine submaxillary glands is associated with the Golgi apparatus. *Biochim Biophys Acta* **814**:1, 1985.
231. Coste H, Martel MB, Got R: Topology of glucosylceramide synthesis in Golgi membranes from porcine submaxillary glands. *Biochim Biophys Acta* **858**:6, 1986.
232. Warren KR, Misra RS, Arora RC, Radin NS: Glycosyltransferases of rat brain that make cerebrosides: Substrate specificity, inhibitors, and abnormal products. *J Neurochem* **26**:1063, 1976.
233. Radin NS, Brenkert A, Arora RC, Sellinger OZ, Flangas AL: Glial and neuronal localization of cerebroside-metabolizing enzymes. *Brain Res* **39**:163, 1972.
234. Morell P, Costantino-Ceccarini EC, Radin NS: The biosynthesis by brain microsomes of cerebrosides containing non-hydroxy fatty acids. *Arch Biochem Biophys* **141**:738, 1970.
235. Shah NJ: Glycosyl transferases of microsomal fractions from brain: Synthesis of glucosylceramide and galactosylceramide during development and the distribution of glucose and galactose transferases in white and grey matter. *J Neurochem* **18**:395, 1971.
236. Brenkert A, Radin NS: Synthesis of galactosylceramide and glucosylceramide by rat brain: Assay procedures and change with age. *Brain Res* **36**:183, 1972.
237. Hammarstrom S: On the biosynthesis of cerebrosides containing nonhydroxy acids. *Biochem Biophys Res Commun* **45**:468, 1971.
238. Vunnam RR, Radin NS: Short chain ceramides as substrates for glucocerebroside synthetase. *Biochim Biophys Acta* **573**:73, 1979.
239. Sasaki T: Glycolipid transfer protein and intracellular traffic of glucosylceramide. *Experientia* **46**:611, 1990.
240. Curtino JA, Caputto R: Enzymatic synthesis of glucosylsphingosine by rat brain. *Lipids* **7**:525, 1972.
241. Curtino JA, Caputto R: Enzymatic synthesis of cerebrosides from glycosylsphingosine and stearoyl-CoA by an embryonic chicken brain preparation. *Biochem Biophys Res Commun* **56**:142, 1974.
242. Farrer RG, Dawson G: Acylation of exogenous glycosylsphingosines by intact neuroblastoma (NCB-20) cells. *J Biol Chem* **265**:22217, 1990.
243. Suzuki Y, Ecker CP, Blough HA: Enzymatic glycosylation of dolichol monophosphate and transfer of glucose from isolated dolichyl-d-glucosyl phosphate to ceramides by BHK-21 cell microsomes. *Eur J Biochem* **143**:447, 1984.
244. Schwarz A, Futerman AH: Distinct roles for ceramide and glucosylceramide at different stages of neuronal growth. *J Neurosci* **17**:2929, 1997.
245. Boldin S, Futerman AH: Glucosylceramide synthesis is required for basic fibroblast growth factor and laminin to stimulate axonal growth. *J Neurochem* **68**:882, 1997.
246. Farrer RG, Quarles RH: Extracellular matrix upregulates synthesis of glucosylceramide-based glycosphingolipids in primary Schwann cells. *J Neurosci Res* **45**:248, 1996.
247. Gatt S: Enzymatic hydrolysis of sphingolipids. I. Hydrolysis and synthesis of ceramides by an enzyme from rat brain. *J Biol Chem* **241**:3724, 1966.
248. Yavin Y, Gatt S: Further purification and properties of rat brain ceramidase. *Biochemistry* **8**:1692, 1969.
249. Kok JW, Babia T, Hoekstra D: Sorting of sphingolipids in the endocytic pathway of HT29 cells. *J Cell Biol* **114**:231, 1991.
250. Trinchera M, Ghidoni R, Sonnino S, Tettamanti G: Recycling of glucosylceramide and sphingosine for the biosynthesis of gangliosides and sphingomyelin in rat liver. *Biochem J* **270**:815, 1990.
251. Saito M, Rosenberg A: The fate of glucosylceramide (glucocerebroside) in genetically impaired (lysosomal beta-glucosidase deficient) Gaucher disease diploid human fibroblasts. *J Biol Chem* **260**:2295, 1985.
252. Barton NW, Rosenberg A: Metabolism of glucosyl (^{3}H) ceramide by human skin fibroblasts from normal and glucosyleramidotic subjects. *J Biol Chem* **250**:3966, 1975.
253. Dale GL, Beutler E: Enzyme therapy in Gaucher disease: Clinical trials and model system studies, in: Crawford MA, Gibbs DA, Watts RWE (eds): *Advances in the Treatment of Inborn Errors of Metabolism.* New York, John Wiley, 1982, p 77.
254. Kanfer IM, Hakamori S (eds): *Sphingolipid Biochemistry.* New York, Plenum Press, 1983.
255. Thompson TE: Organization of glycosphingolipids in bilayers and plasma membranes of mammalian cells. *Ann Rev Biophys Biophys Chem* **14**:361, 1985.
256. Dawson G, Oh JY: Blood glucosylceramide levels in Gaucher's disease and its distribution amongst lipoprotein fractions. *Clin Chim Acta* **75**:149, 1977.
257. Strasberg PM, Warren I, Skomorowski MA, Lowden JA: HPLC analysis of neutral glycolipids: An aid in the diagnosis of lysosomal storage disease. *Clin Chim Acta* **132**:29, 1983.
258. Nilsson O, Håkansson G, Dreborg S, Groth CG, Svennerholm L: Increased cerebroside concentration in plasma and erythrocytes in Gaucher disease: Significant differences between type I and type III. *Clin Genet* **22**:274, 1982.
259. van der Bergh FAJTM, Tager JM: Localization of neutral glycosphingolipids in human plasma. *Biochim Biophys Acta* **441**:391, 1976.
260. Nilsson O, Svennerholm L: Characterization and quantitative determination of gangliosides and neutral glycosphingolipids in human liver. *J Lipid Res* **23**:327, 1982.
261. Nilsson O, Mansson JE, Hakansson G, Svennerholm L: The occurrence of psychosine and other glycolipids in spleen and liver from the three major types of Gaucher's disease. *Biochim Biophys Acta* **712**:453, 1982.
262. Kennaway NG, Woolf LI: Splenic lipids in Gaucher's disease. *J Lipid Res* **9**:755, 1968.
263. French JH, Brotz M, Poser CM: Lipid composition of the brain in infantile Gaucher's disease. *Neurology* **19**:81, 1969.
264. Sugma S, Eto Y, Yamamoto Y, Kim SU: Psychosine cytotoxicity toward rat C6 glioma cells and the protective effects of phorbol ester and dimethylsulfoxide: Implications for therapy in Krabbe disease. *Brain Dev* **13**:104, 1991.
265. Hannun YA, Bell RM: Lysosphingolipids inhibit protein kinase C: Implications for the sphingolipidoses. *Science* **235**:670, 1987.
266. Datta SC, Radin NS: Normalization of liver glucosylceramide levels in the "Gaucher" mouse by phosphatidylserine injection. *Biochem Biophys Res Commun* **152**:155, 1988.
267. Gery I, Zigler S, Brady RO, Barranger JA: Selective effects of glucocerebroside (Gaucher's storage material) on macrophage cultures. *J Clin Invest* **68**:1182, 1981.

268. Lichtenstein M, Zimran A, Horowitz M: Cytokine mRNA in Gaucher disease. *Blood Cells Mol Dis* **23**:395, 1997.
269. Hollak CEM, Evers L, Aerts JMFG, van Oers MHJ: Elevated levels of M-CSF, sCD14 and IL8 in type 1 Gaucher disease. *Blood Cells Mol Dis* **23**:201, 1997.
270. Ross DJ, Spira S, Buchbinder NA: Gaucher cells in pulmonary-capillary blood in association with pulmonary hypertension. *N Engl J Med* **336**:379, 1997.
271. Dawson A, Elias DJ, Rubenson D, Bartz S, Garver P, Kay AC, Bloor CM, Beutler E: Development of pulmonary hypertension after alglucerase therapy in two patients with hepatopulmonary syndrome complicating type 1 Gaucher disease. *Ann Intern Med* **125**:901, 1996.
272. Van De Water NS, Jolly RD, Farrow BRH: Canine Gaucher disease-the enzymic defect. *Aust J Exp Biol Med* Sci **57**:551, 1979.
273. Tybulewicz VLJ, Tremblay ML, LaMarca ME, Willemsen R, Stubblefield BK, Winfield S, Zablocka B, Sidransky E, Martin BM, Huang SP, Mintzer KA, Westphal H, Mulligan RC, Ginns EI: Animal model of Gaucher's disease from targeted disruption of the mouse glucocerebrosidase gene. *Nature* **357**:407, 1992.
274. Liu Y, Suzuki K, Reed JD, Grinberg A, Westphal H, Hoffmann A, Döring T, Sandhoff K, Proia RL: Mice with type 2 and 3 Gaucher disease point mutations generated by a single insertion mutagenesis procedure (SIMP). *Proc Natl Acad Sci U S A* **95**:2503, 1998.
275. Albrecht M: "Gaucher-Zellen" bei chronisch myeloischer Leukaemie. *Blut* **13**:169, 1966.
276. Lee RE, Ellis LD: The storage cells of chronic myelogenous leukemia. *Lab Invest* **24**:261, 1971.
277. Rosner F, Dosik H, Kaiser SS, Lee SL, Morrison AN: Gaucher cell in leukemia. *JAMA* **209**:935, 1969.
278. Buesche G, Majewski H, Schlue J, Delventhal S, Baer-Henney S, Vykoupil KF, Georgii A: Frequency of pseudo-Gaucher cells in diagnostic bone marrow biopsies from patients with ph-positive chronic myeloid leukaemia. *Virchows Arch Int J Pathol* **430**:139, 1997.
279. Zaino EC, Rossi MB, Pham TD, Azar HA: Gaucher's cells in thalassemia. *Blood* **38**:457, 1971.
280. Bashir FY, Al-Irhayim B, Krajci D, Al-Naeb I: Thalassaemia presenting as Gaucher's disease. A case report with ultrastructural study. *Saudi Med J* **8**:407, 1987.
281. Scullin DC Jr, Shelburne JD, Cohen HJ: Pseudo-Gaucher cells in multiple myeloma. *Am J Med* **67**:347, 1979.
282. Zidar BL, Hartsock RJ, Lee RE, Glew RH, LaMarco KL, Pugh RP, Raju RN, Shackney SE: Pseudo-Gaucher cells in the bone marrow of a patient with Hodgkin's disease. *Am J Clin Pathol* **87**:533, 1987.
283. Lee KS, Chen KTK, Ahmed F, Gomez-Leon G: Acquired Gaucher's cells in Hodgkin's disease. *Am J Med* **73**:290, 1982.
284. Alterini R, Rigacci L, Stefanacci S: Pseudo-Gaucher cells in the bone marrow of a patient with centrocytic nodular non-Hodgkin's lymphoma. *Haematologica* **81**:282, 1996.
285. Knox-Macaulay H, Bhusnurmath S, Alwaily A: Pseudo-Gaucher's cells in association with common acute lymphoblastic leukemia. *South Med J* **90**:69, 1997.
286. Solis OG, Belmonte AH, Ramaswamy G, Tchertkoff V: Pseudogaucher cells in *Mycobacterium avium intracellulare* infections in acquired immune deficiency syndrome (AIDS). *Am J Clin Pathol* **85**:233, 1986.
287. Beutler E, Saven A: Misuse of marrow examination in the diagnosis of Gaucher disease. *Blood* **76**:646, 1990.
288. Kampine JP, Brady RO, Kanfer JN: Diagnosis of Gaucher's disease and Niemann-Pick disease with small samples of venous blood. *Science* **155**:86, 1967.
289. Beutler E, Kuhl W: Detection of the defect of Gaucher's disease and its carrier state in peripheral-blood leukocytes. *Lancet* **1**:612, 1970.
290. Beutler E, Kuhl W: The diagnosis of the adult type of Gaucher's disease and its carrier state by demonstration of deficiency of beta-glucosidase activity in peripheral blood leukocytes. *J Lab Clin Med* **76**:747, 1970.
291. Peters SP, Lee RE, Glew RH: A microassay for Gaucher's disease. *Clin Chim Acta* **60**:391, 1975.
292. Raghavan SS, Topol J, Kolodny EH: Leukocyte beta-glucosidase in homozygotes and heterozygotes for Gaucher disease. *Am J Hum Genet* **32**:158, 1980.
293. Daniels LB, Glew RH, Diven WF, Lee RE, Radin NS: An improved fluorometric leukocyte beta-glucosidase assay for Gaucher's disease. *Clin Chim Acta* **115**:369, 1981.
294. Klibansky C, Hoffman J, Zaizov R, Matoth Y: Gaucher's disease, chronic adult type: A comparative study of glucocerebroside and methylumbelliferyl-glucopyranoside cleaving potency in leukocytes. *Biomedicine* **20**:24, 1974.
295. Grabowski GA, Dinur T, Gatt S, Desnick RJ: Gaucher type I (Ashkenazi) disease: A new method for heterozygote detection using a novel fluorescent natural substrate. *Clin Chim Acta* **124**:123, 1982.
296. Dinur T, Grabowski GA, Desnick RJ, Gatt S: Synthesis of a fluorescent derivative of glucosyl ceramide for the sensitive determination of glucocerebrosidase activity. *Anal Biochem* **136**:223, 1984.
297. Butcher BA, Gopalan V, Lee RE, Richards TC, Waggoner AS, Glew RH: Use of 4-heptylumbelliferyl-β-D-glucoside to identify Gaucher's disease heterozygotes. *Clin Chim Acta* **184**:235, 1989.
298. Peters SP, Coyle P, Glew RH: Differentiation of beta-glucocerebrosidase from beta-glucosidase in human tissues using sodium taurocholate. *Arch Biochem Biophys* **175**:569, 1976.
299. Beutler E, Kuhl W, Matsumoto F, Pangalis G: Acid hydrolases in leukocytes and platelets of normal subjects and in patients with Gaucher's and Fabry's disease. *J Exp Med* **143**:975, 1976.
300. Beutler E, Kuhl W, Trinidad F, Teplitz R, Nadler H: Beta-glucosidase activity in fibroblasts from homozygotes and heterozygotes for Gaucher's disease. *Am J Hum Genet* **23**:62, 1971.
301. Hultberg B, Sjoblad S, Öckerman PA: 4-Methylumbelliferyl-beta-glucosidase in cultured human fibroblasts from controls and patients with Gaucher's disease. *Clin Chim Acta* **49**:93, 1973.
302. Ho MW, Seck J, Schmidt D, Veath ML, Johnson W, Brady RO, O'Brien JS: Adult Gaucher's disease: Kindred studies and demonstration of a deficiency of acid beta-glucosidase in cultured fibroblasts. *Am J Hum Genet* **24**:37, 1972.
303. Turner BM, Hirschhorn K: Properties of beta-glucosidase in cultured skin fibroblasts from controls and patients with Gaucher disease. *Am J Hum Genet* **30**:346, 1978.
304. Choy FM, Davidson RG: Gaucher's disease II. Studies on the kinetics of beta-glucosidase and the effects of sodium taurocholate in normal and Gaucher tissues. *Pediatr Res* **14**:54, 1980.
305. Beutler E, Kuhl W, Sorge J: Cross-reacting material in Gaucher disease fibroblasts. *Proc Natl Acad Sci U S A* **81**:6506, 1984.
306. Agmon V, Cherbu S, Degan A, Grace ME, Grabowski GA, Gatt S: Synthesis of novel fluorescent glycosphingolipids: Use in determining acid beta-glucosidase activity in situ and correlation with genotype in Gaucher disease. *Biochim Biophys Acta* **1170**:72, 1993.
307. Meivar-Levy I, Horowitz M, Futerman AH: Analysis of glucocerebrosidase activity using *N*-(1-[^{14}C]hexanoyl)-D-*erythro*-glucosylsphingosine demonstrates a correlation between levels of residual enzyme activity and the type of Gaucher disease. *Biochem J* **303**:377, 1994.
308. Theophilus BDM, Latham T, Grabowski GA, Smith FI: Comparison of RNase A, chemical cleavage, and GC-clamped denaturing gradient gel electrophoresis for the detection of mutations in exon 9 of the human acid β-glucosidase gene. *Nucleic Acids Res* **17**:7707, 1989.
309. Zimran A, Glass C, Thorpe VS, Beutler E: Analysis of "color PCR" by automatic DNA sequencer. *Nucleic Acids Res* **17**:7538, 1989.
310. Beutler E, Gelbart T, West C: The facile detection of the nt 1226 mutation of glucocerebrosidase by "mismatched" PCR. *Clin Chim Acta* **194**:161, 1990.
311. Beutler E, Gelbart T, Kuhl W, Sorge J, West C: Identification of the second common Jewish Gaucher disease mutation makes possible population based screening for the heterozygous state. *Proc Natl Acad Sci U S A* **88**:10544, 1991.
312. Beutler E, Gelbart T, Kuhl W, Zimran A, West C: Mutations in Jewish patients with Gaucher disease. *Blood* **79**:1662, 1992.
313. Firon N, Eyal N, Horowitz M: Genotype assignment in Gaucher disease by selective amplification of the active glucocerebrosidase gene. *Am J Hum Genet* **46**:527, 1990.
314. Eyal N, Wilder S, Horowitz M: Prevalent and rare mutations among Gaucher patients. *Gene* **96**:277, 1990.
315. Tayebi N, Cushner S, Sidransky E: Differentiation of the glucocerebrosidase gene from pseudogene by long-template PCR: Implications for Gaucher disease. *Am J Hum Genet* **59**:740, 1996.
316. Mistry PK, Smith SJ, Ali M, Hatton CSR, McIntyre N, Cox TM: Genetic diagnosis of Gaucher's disease. *Lancet* **339**:889, 1992.
317. Zimran A, Sorge J, Gross E, Kubitz M, West C, Beutler E: Prediction of severity of Gaucher's disease by identification of mutations at DNA level. *Lancet* **2**:349, 1989.
318. Theophilus B, Latham T, Grabowski GA, Smith FI: Gaucher disease: Molecular heterogeneity and phenotype-genotype correlations. *Am J Hum Genet* **45**:212, 1989.
319. Kolodny EH, Firon N, Eyal N, Horowitz M: Mutation analysis of an Ashkenazi Jewish family with Gaucher disease in three successive generations. *Am J Med Genet* **36**:467, 1990.

320. Sidransky E, Tsuji S, Martin BM, Stubblefield B, Ginns EI: DNA mutation analysis of Gaucher patients. *Am J Med Genet* **42**:331, 1992.
321. Erikson A: Gaucher disease — Norrbottnian type (III). Neuropaediatric and neurobiological aspects of clinical patterns and treatment. *Acta Paediatr Suppl* **326**:1, 1986.
322. Streifler C: Study of acid phosphatase in sera of Gaucher's disease patients, subcellular tissue fractions and platelet extracts. *Isr J Med Sci* **6**:479, 1970.
323. Robinson DB, Glew RH: Acid phosphatase in Gaucher's disease. *Clin Chem* **26**:371, 1980.
324. Öckerman PA, Köhlin P: Acid hydrolases in plasma in Gaucher's disease. *Clin Chem* **15**:61, 1969.
325. Lieberman J, Beutler E: Elevation of serum angiotensin-converting enzyme in Gaucher's disease. *N Engl J Med* **294**:1442, 1976.
326. Silverstein E, Friedland J: Elevated serum and spleen angiotensin converting enzyme and serum lysozyme in Gaucher's disease. *Clin Chim Acta* **74**:21, 1977.
327. Den Tandt WR, Van Hoof F: Marked increase of methylumbelliferyl-tetra-*N*- acetylchitotetraoside hydrolase activity in plasma from Gaucher disease patients. *J Inherit Metab Dis* **19**:344, 1996.
328. Poenaru L, Manicom J, Germain D: Chitotriosidase as a marker for diagnosis and treatment follow-up in Gaucher disease: A survey of 50 patients. *Am J Hum Genet* **59**:A205, 1996.
329. Young E, Chatterton C, Vellodi A, Winchester B: Plasma chitotriosidase activity in Gaucher disease patients who have been treated either by bone marrow transplantation or by enzyme replacement therapy with alglucerase. *J Inherit Metab Dis* **20**:595, 1997.
330. Hollak CEM, van Weely S, van Oers MHJ, Aerts JMFG: Marked elevation of plasma chitotriosidase activity. A novel hallmark of Gaucher disease. *J Clin Invest* **93**:1288, 1994.
331. Den Tandt WR, Van Hoof F: Plasma methylumbelliferyl-tetra-*N*-acetyl-β-D-chitotetraoside hydrolase as a parameter during treatment of Gaucher patients. *Biochem Mol Med* **57**:71, 1996.
332. Morgan MAM, Hoffbrand AV, Laulicht M, Luck W, Knowles S: Serum ferritin concentration in Gaucher's disease. *BMJ* **286**:1864, 1983.
333. Ginsberg H, Grabowski GA, Gibson JC, Fagerstrom R, Goldblatt J, Gilbert HS, Desnick RJ: Reduced plasma concentrations of total, low density lipoprotein and high density lipoprotein cholesterol in patients with Gaucher type I disease. *Clin Genet* **26**:109, 1984.
334. Lorberboym M, Vallabhajosula S, Lipszyc H, Pastores G: Scintigraphic evaluation of Tc-99m-low-density lipoprotein (LDL) distribution in patients with Gaucher disease. *Clin Genet* **52**:7, 1997.
335. Pentchev PG, Brady RO, Hibbert SR, Gal AE, Shapiro D: Isolation and characterization of glucocerebrosidase from human placental tissue. *J Biol Chem* **248**:5256, 1973.
336. Furbish FS, Blair HE, Shiloach J, Pentchev PG, Brady RO: Enzyme replacement therapy in Gaucher's disease: Large-scale purification of glucocerbrosidase suitable for human administration. *Proc Natl Acad Sci U S A* **74**:3560, 1977.
337. Murray GJ, Youle RJ, Gandy SE, Zirzow GC, Barranger JA: Purification of beta-glucocerebrosidase by preparative-scale high-performance liquid chromatography: The use of ethylene glycol-containing buffers for chromatography of hydrophobic glycoprotein enzymes. *Anal Biochem* **147**:301, 1985.
338. Choy FYM: Purification of human placental glucocerebrosidase using a two-step high-performance hydrophobic and gel permeation column chromatography method. *Anal Biochem* **156**:515, 1986.
339. Strasberg PM, Lowden JA, Mahuran D: Purification of glucosylceramidase by affinity chromatography. *Can J Biochem* **60**:1025, 1982.
340. Aerts JMFG, Donker-Koopman WE, Murray GJ, Barranger JA, Tager JM, Schram AW: A procedure for the rapid purification in high yield of human glucocerebrosidase using immunoaffinity chromatography with monoclonal antibodies. *Anal Biochem* **154**:655, 1986.
341. Grabowski GA, Dagan A: Human lysosomal beta-glucosidase: Purification by affinity chromatography. *Anal Biochem* **141**:267, 1984.
342. Ho MW: Specificity of low molecular weight glycoprotein effector of lipid glycosidase. *FEBS Lett* **53**:243, 1975.
343. Pentchev PG, Brady RO, Hibbert SR, Gal AE, Shapiro D: Isolation and characterization of glucocerebrosidase from human placental tissue. *J Biol Chem* **248**:5256, 1973.
344. Mueller OT, Rosenberg A: Activation of membrane-bound glucosylceramide: Beta-glucosidase in fibroblasts cultured from normal and glucosylceramidotic human skin. *J Biol Chem* **254**:3521, 1979.
345. Dale GL, Beutler E: Enzyme replacement therapy in Gaucher's disease: A rapid high-yield method for purification of glucocerebrosidase. *Proc Natl Acad Sci U S A* **73**:4672, 1976.
346. Osiecki-Newman Km, Fabbro D, Dinur T, Boas S, Gatt S, Legler G, Desnick RJ, Grabowski GA: Human acid beta-glucosidase: Affinity purification of the normal placental and Gaucher Disease splenic enzymes on *N*-alkyl-deoxynojirmycin-sepharose. *Enzyme* **35**:147, 1986.
347. Grabowski GA, Osiecki-Newman K, Dinur T, Fabbro D, Legler G, Gatt S, Desnick RJ: Human acid beta-glucosidase. Use of conduritol B epoxide derivatives to investigate the catalytically active normal and Gaucher disease enzymes. *J Biol Chem* **261**:8263, 1986.
348. Reiner O, Wilder S, Givol D, Horowitz M: Efficient in vitro and in vivo expression of human glucocerebrosidase cDNA. *DNA* **6**:101, 1987.
349. Ginns EI, Brady RO, Stowens DW, Furbish FS, Barranger JA: A new group of glucocerebrosidase isozymes found in human white blood cells. *Biochem Biophys Res Commun* **97**:1103, 1980.
350. Erickson AH, Ginns EI, Barranger JA: Biosynthesis of the lysosomal enzyme glucocerebrosidase. *J Biol Chem* **260**:14319, 1985.
351. Imai K: Characterization of beta-glucosidase as a peripheral enzyme of lysosomal membranes from mouse liver and purification. *J Biochem (Tokyo)* **98**:1405, 1985.
352. Aerts JMFG, Donker-Koopman WE, van Laar C, Brul S, Murray GJ, Wenger DA, Barranger JA, Tager JM, Schram AW: Relationship between the two immunologically distinguishable forms of glucocerebrosidase in tissue extracts. *Eur J Biochem* **163**:583, 1987.
353. Maret A, Salvayre R, Negre A, Douste-Blazy L: Properties of the molecular forms of beta-glucosidase and beta-glucocerebrosidase from normal human and Gaucher disease spleen. *Eur J Biochem* **115**:455, 1981.
354. Maret A, Potier M, Salvayre R, Douste-Blazy L: Modification of subunit interaction in membrane-bound acid beta-glucosidase from Gaucher disease. *FEBS Lett* **160**:93, 1983.
355. Choy FYM, Woo M, Potier M: In situ radiation-inactivation size of fibroblast membrane-bound acid beta-glucosidase in Gaucher type 1, type 2 and type 3 disease. *Biochim Biophys Acta* **870**:76, 1986.
356. Dawson G, Ellory JC: Functional lysosomal hydrolase size as determined by radiation inactivation analysis. *Biochem J* **226**:283, 1985.
357. O'Neill RR, Tokoro T, Kozak CA, Brady RO: Comparison of the chromosomal localization of murine and human glucocerebrosidase genes and of the deduced amino acid sequences. *Proc Natl Acad Sci U S A* **86**:5049, 1989.
358. Henrissat B, Callebaut S, Fabrega P, Lehn P, Arnon J-P, Davies G: Conserved catalytic machinery and the prediction of a common fold for several families of glycosyl hydrolases. *Proc Natl Acad Sci U S A* **92**:7090, 1995.
359. Morgenstern L, Kahn FH, Weinstein IM: Subtotal splenectomy in myelofibrosis. *Surgery* **60**:336, 1966.
360. Takasaki S, Murray GJ, Furbish FS, Brady RO, Barranger JA, Kobata A: Structure of the *N*-asparagine-linked oligosaccharide units of human placental β-glucocerebrosidase. *J Biol Chem* **259**:10112, 1984.
361. Grace ME, Grabowski GA: Human acid beta-glucosidase: Glycosylation is required for catalytic activity. *Biochem Biophys Res Commun* **168**:771, 1990.
362. Grace ME, Grabowski GA: Molecular enzymology of acid β-glucosidase, in Esen R (ed): *Glucosidases: Biochemistry and Molecular Biology.* Washington, DC, ACS Press, 1993, p 66.
363. Legler G, Liedtke H: Glucosylceramidase from calf spleen. Characterization of its active site with 4-alkylumbelliferyl-β-glucosides and *N*-alkyl derivatives of 1-deoxynojirimycin. *Biol Chem Hoppe Seyler* **366**:1113, 1985.
364. Dale GL, Villacorte D, Beutler E: Solubilization of glucocerebrosidase from human placenta and demonstration of a phospholipid requirement for its catalytic activity. *Biochem Biophys Res Commun* **71**:1048, 1976.
365. Basu A, Glew RH: Characterization of the phospholipid requirement of a rat liver β-glucosidase. *Biochem J* **224**:515, 1984.
366. Glew RH, Daniels LB, Clark LS, Hoyer SW: Enzymic differentiation of neurologic and nonneurologic forms of Gaucher's disease. *J Neuropathol Exp Neurol* **41**:630, 1982.
367. Grabowski GA, Gatt S, Kruse J, Desnick RJ: Human lysosomal beta-glucosidase: Kinetic characterization of the catalytic, aglycon, and hydrophobic binding sites. *Arch Biochem Biophys* **231**:144, 1984.
368. Berent SL, Radin NS: Beta-glucosidase activator protein from bovine spleen ("coglucosidase"). *Arch Biochem Biophys* **208**:248, 1981.
369. Vaccaro AM, Tatti M, Ciaffoni F, Salvioli R: Factors affecting the binding of glucosylceramidase to its natural substrate dispersion. *Enzyme* **42**:87, 1989.
370. Sarmientos F, Schwarzmann G, Sandhoff K: Specificity of human glucosylceramide beta-glucosidase towards synthetic glucosphingoli-

pids inserted into liposomes. Kinetic studies in a detergent-free assay system. *Eur J Biochem* **160**:527, 1986.

371. Glew RH, Basu A, LaMarco K, Prence EM: Mammalian glucocerebrosidase: Implications for Gaucher's disease. *Lab Invest* **58**:5, 1988.
372. Gonzales ML, Basu A, de Haas GH, Dijkman R, van Oort MG, Okolo AA, Glew RH: Activation of human spleen glucocerebrosidases by monoacylglycol sulfates and diacylglycerol sulfates. *Arch Biochem Biophys* **262**:345, 1988.
373. Qi X, Leonova T, Grabowski GA: Human acid β-glucosidase: Functional evaluation of human saposins expressed in E. coli. *J Biol Chem* **269**:16746, 1994.
374. Christomanou H, Aignesberger A, Linke RP: Immunochemical characterization of two activator proteins stimulating enzymic sphingomyelin degradation in vitro. Absence of one of them in a human Gaucher disease variant. *Biol Chem Hoppe Seyler* **367**:879, 1986.
375. Prence E, Chakravorti S, Basu A, Clark LS, Glew RH, Chambers JA: Further studies on the activation of glucocerebrosidase by a heat-stable factor from Gaucher spleen. *Arch Biochem Biophys* **236**:98, 1985.
376. Qi X, Qin W, Sun Y, Kondoh K, Grabowski GA: Functional organization of saposin C: Definition of the neurotrophic and acid β-glucosidase activation regions. *J Biol Chem* **271**:6874, 1996.
377. Fabbro D, Grabowski GA: Human acid beta-glucosidase: Use of inhibitory and activating monoclonal antibodies to investigate the enzyme's catalytic mechanism and saposin A and C binding sites. *J Biol Chem* **266**:15021, 1991.
378. Mansson JE, Vanier T, Svennerholm L: Changes in fatty acid and sphingosine composition of the major gangliosides of human brain with age. *J Neurochem* **30**:273, 1978.
379. Gal AE, Pentchev PG, Massey JM, Brady RO: L-glucosylceramide: synthesis, properties, and resistance to catabolism by glucocerebrosidase in vitro. *Proc Natl Acad Sci U S A* **76**:3083, 1979.
380. Osiecki-Newman K, Fabbro D, Legler G, Desnick RJ, Grabowski GA: Human acid beta-glucosidase: use of inhibitors, alternative substrates and amphiphiles to investigate the properties of the normal and Gaucher disease active sites. *Biochim Biophys Acta* **915**:87, 1987.
381. Vaccaro AM, Kobayashi T, Suzuki K: Comparison of synthetic and natural glucosylceramides as substrate for glucosylceramidase assay. *Clin Chim Acta* **118**:1, 1982.
382. Greenberg P, Merrill AH, Liotta DC, Grabowski GA: Human acid beta-glucosidase: Use of sphingosyl and *N*-alkyl-glucosylamine inhibitors to investigate the properties of the active site. *Biochim Biophys Acta* **1039**:12, 1990.
383. Vaccaro AM, Muscillo M, Suzuki K: Characterization of human glucosylsphingosine glucosyl hydrolase and comparison with glucosylceramidase. *Eur J Biochem* **146**:315, 1985.
384. Raghavan SS, Mumford RA, Kanfer JN: Isolation and characterization of glucosylsphingosine from Gaucher's spleen. *J Lipid Res* **15**:484, 1974.
385. Erickson JS, Radin NS: *N*-hexyl-*o*-glucosyl sphingosine, an inhibitor of glycosyl ceramide beta-glucosidase. *J Lipid Res* **14**:133, 1973.
386. Graves PN, Grabowski GA, Ludman MD, Palese P, Smith FI: Human acid beta-glucosidase: Northern blot and S1 nuclease analysis of mRNA from HeLa cells and normal and Gaucher disease fibroblasts. *Am J Hum Genet* **39**:763, 1986.
387. Gatt S, Dinur T, Osiecki K, Desnick RJ, Grabowski GA: Use of activators and inhibitors to define the properties of the active site of normal and Gaucher disease lysosomal beta-glucosidase. *Enzyme* **33**:109, 1985.
388. Osiecki-Newman K, Legler G, Grace M, Dinur T, Gatt S, Desnick RJ, Grabowski GA: Human acid β-glucosidase: Inhibition studies using glucose analogues and pH variation to characterize the normal and Gaucher disease glycol binding sites. *Enzyme* **40**:173, 1988.
389. Grace ME, Graves PN, Smith FI, Grabowski GA: Analyses of catalytic activity and inhibitor binding of human acid β-glucosidase by site-directed mutagenesis. Identification of residues critical to catalysis and evidence for causality of two Ashkenazi Jewish Gaucher disease Type 1 mutations. *J Biol Chem* **265**:6827, 1990.
390. Hyun JC, Misra RS, Greenblatt D, Radin NS: Synthetic inhibitors of glucocerebroside β-glucosidase. *Arch Biochem Biophys* **166**:382, 1975.
391. Wynn CH: A triple-binding-domain model explains the specificity of the interaction of a sphingolipid activator protein (SAP-1) with sulfatide, GM1-ganglioside and globotriaosylceramide. *Biochem J* **240**:921, 1986.
392. Van Paridon PA, Visser AJ, Wirtz KW: Binding of phospholipids to the phosphatidylinositol transfer protein from bovine brain as studied by steady-state and time-resolved fluorescence spectroscopy. *Biochim Biophys Acta* **898**:172, 1987.
393. Legler G: Labeling of the active center of a beta-glucosidase. *Biochim Biophys Acta* **151**:728, 1968.
394. Legler G, Harder A: Amino acid sequence at the active site of β-glucosidase A from bitter almonds. *Biochim Biophys Acta* **524**:102, 1978.
395. Bause E, Legler G: Isolation and amino acid sequence of a hexadecapeptide from the active site of β-glucosidase A_3 from *Aspergillus wentii. Hoppe-Seyler's Z Physiol Chem* **355**:438, 1974.
396. Grabowski GA, Graves PG, Grace M, Bergmann JE, Smith FI: Gaucher disease: Enzymatic and molecular studies, in Salvayre R, Douste-Blazy L, Gatt S (eds): *Lipid Storage Disorders: Biological and Medical Aspects*. New York, Plenum Press, 1988, p 793.
397. Grabowski GA, Gatt S, Horowitz M: Acid β-glucosidase: Enzymology and molecular biology of Gaucher disease. *CRC Crit Rev Biochem Mol Biol* **25**:385, 1990.
398. Grace ME, Berg A, He G, Goldberg L, Horowitz M, Grabowski GA: Gaucher disease: Heterologous expression of two alleles associated with neuronopathic phenotypes. *Am J Hum Genet* **49**:646, 1991.
399. Jonsson LMV, Murray GJ, Sorrell SH, Strijland A, Aerts JFGM, Ginns EI, Barranger JA, Tager JM, Schram AW: Biosynthesis and maturation of glucocerebrosidase in Gaucher fibroblasts. *Eur J Biochem* **164**:171, 1987.
400. Beutler E, Kuhl W: Glucocerebrosidase processing in normal fibroblasts and in fibroblasts from patients with type I, type II, and type III Gaucher disease. *Proc Natl Acad Sci U S A* **83**:7472, 1986.
401. Bergmann JE, Grabowski GA: Posttranslational processing of human lysosomal acid β-glucosidase: A continuum of defects in Gaucher disease type 1 and type 2 fibroblasts. *Am J Hum Genet* **44**:741, 1989.
402. Ginns EI, Brady RO, Pirruccello S, Moore C, Sorrell S, Furbish FS, Murray GJ, Tager J, Barranger JA: Mutations of glucocerebrosidase: Discrimination of neurologic and non-neurologic phenotypes of Gaucher disease. *Proc Natl Acad Sci U S A* **79**:5607, 1982.
403. Ginns EI, Tegelaers FPW, Barneveld R, Galjaard H, Reuser AJJ, Brady RO, Tager JM, Barranger JA: Determination of Gaucher's disease phenotypes with monoclonal antibody. *Clin Chim Acta* **131**:283, 1983.
404. Fabbro D, Desnick RJ, Grabowski GA: Gaucher disease: Genetic heterogeneity within and among the subtypes detected by immunoblotting. *Am J Hum Genet* **40**:15, 1987.
405. Beutler E, Kuhl W, Sorge J: Glucocerebrosidase "processing" and gene expression in various forms of Gaucher disease. *Am J Hum Genet* **37**:1062, 1985.
406. Hasilik A: Biosynthesis of lysosomal enzymes. *Trends Biochem Sci* **5**:237, 1980.
407. Stechel FA, Hasilik A, von Figura K: Biosynthesis, and maturation of arylsulfatase B in normal and mutant cultured human fibroblasts. *J Biol Chem* **258**:14322, 1983.
408. Hasilik A, Neufeld EF: Biosynthesis of lysosomal enzymes in fibroblasts. *J Biol Chem* **255**:4937, 1984.
409. Christomanou H, Chabás A, Pámpols T, Guardiola A: Activator protein deficient Gaucher's disease. A second patient with the newly identified lipid storage disorder. *Klin Wochenschr* **67**:999, 1989.
410. Morimoto S, Martin BM, Yamamoto Y, Kretz KA, O'Brien JS, Kishimoto Y: Saposin A: Second cerebrosidase activator protein. *Proc Natl Acad Sci U S A* **86**:3389, 1989.
411. Peters SP, Coyle P, Coffee CJ, Glew RH, Kuhlenschmidt MS, Rosenfeld L, Lee YC: Purification and properties of a heat-stable glucocerebrosidase activating factor from control and Gaucher spleen. *J Biol Chem* **252**:563, 1977.
412. Kleinschmidt T, Christomanou H, Braunitzer G: Complete amino-acid sequence of the naturally occurring A2 activator protein for enzymic sphingomyelin degradation: identity to the sulfatide activator protein (SAP-1). *Biol Chem Hoppe Seyler* **369**:1361, 1988.
413. Sano A, Radin NS, Johnson LI, Tarr GE: The activator protein for glycosylceramide β-glucosidase from guinea pig liver: Improved isolation method and complete amino acid sequence. *J Biol Chem* **263**:19597, 1988.
414. Reiner O, Dagan O, Horowitz M: Human sphingolipid activator protein-1 and sphingolipid activator protein-2 are encoded by the same gene. *J Mol Neurosci* **1**:225, 1989.
415. Collard MW, Sylvester SR, Tsuruta JK, Griswold MD: Biosynthesis and molecular cloning of sulfated glycoprotein 1 secreted by rat Sertoli cells: Sequence similarity with the 70- kilodalton precursor to sulfatide/GM1 activator. *Biochemistry* **27**:4557, 1988.
416. Sano A, Radin NS: The carbohydrate moiety of the activator protein for glucosylceramide β-glucosidase. *Biochem Biophys Res Commun* **154**:1197, 1988.

417. Morimoto S, Kishimoto Y, Tomich J, Weiler S, Ohashi T, Barranger JA, Kretz KA, O'Brien JS: Interaction of saposins, acidic lipids, and glucosylceramidase. *J Biol Chem* **265**:1933, 1990.
418. Fujibayashi S, Wenger DA: Synthesis and processing of sphingolipid activator protein-2 in cultured human fibroblasts. *J Biol Chem* **261**:15339, 1986.
419. Fujibayashi S, Wenger DA: Biosynthesis of the sulfatide/GM1 activator protein in control and mutant cultured skin fibroblasts. *Biochim Biophys Acta* **875**:554, 1986.
420. Basu A, Prence E, Garrett K, Glew RH, Ellingson JS: Comparison of N-acyl phosphatidylethanolamines with different *N*-acyl groups as activators of glucocerebrosidase in various forms of Gaucher's disease. *Arch Biochem Biophys* **243**:28, 1985.
421. Aerts JMFG, Donker-Koopman WE, Brul S, van Weely S, Sa Miranda MC, Barranger JA, Tager JM, Schram AW: Comparative study on glucocerebrosidase in spleens from patients with Gaucher disease. *Biochem J* **269**:93, 1990.
422. Tager JM, Aerts JM, Jonsson MV, Murray GJ, van Weely S, Strijland A, Ginns EI, Reuser JJ, Schram AW, Barranger JA: Molecular forms, biosynthesis and maturation of glucocerebrosidase, a membrane associated lysosomal enzyme deficient in Gaucher disease, in Freysz L, Dreyfus H, Massarelli R, Gatt S (eds): *Enzymes of Lipid Metabolism II*. New York, Plenum Press, 1986, p 735.
423. Willemsen R, van Dongen JM, Aerts JM, Schram AW, Tager JM, Goudsmit R, Reuser AJ: An immunoelectron microscopic study of glucocerebrosidase in type 1 Gaucher's disease spleen. *Ultrastruct Pathol* **12**:471, 1988.
424. Grace ME, Grabowski GA: Gaucher disease: Molecular analyses of acid β-glucosidase function. *Am J Hum Genet* **51**:169a, 1992.
425. Morimoto S, Yamamoto Y, O'Brien JS, Kishimoto Y: Distribution of saposin proteins (sphingolipid activator proteins) in lysosomal storage and other diseases. *Proc Natl Acad Sci U S A* **87**:3493, 1990.
426. Shafit-Zagardo B, Devine EA, Smith M, Arredondo GAF, Desnick RJ: Assignment of the gene for acid beta-glucosidase to human chromosome 1. *Am J Hum Genet* **33**:564, 1981.
427. Reiner O, Wigderson M, Horowitz M: Structural analysis of the human glucocerebrosidase genes. *DNA* **7**:107, 1988.
428. Zimran A, Sorge J, Gross E, Kubitz M, West C, Beutler E: A glucocerebrosidase fusion gene in Gaucher disease. Implications for the molecular anatomy, pathogenesis and diagnosis of this disorder. *J Clin Invest* **85**:219, 1990.
429. Sorge J, Gross E, West C, Beutler E: High level transcription of the glucocerebrosidase pseudogene in normal subjects and patients with Gaucher disease. *J Clin Invest* **86**:1137, 1990.
430. Beutler E, West C, Gelbart T: Polymorphisms in the human glucocerebrosidase gene. *Genomics* **12**:795, 1992.
431. Winfield SL, Tayebi N, Martin BM, Ginns EI, Sidransky E: Identification of three additional genes contiguous to the glucocerebrosidase locus on chromosome 1q21: Implications for Gaucher disease. *Genome Res* **7**:1020, 1997.
432. Long GL, Winfield S, Adolph KW, Ginns EI, Bornstein P: Structure and organization of the human metaxin gene (MTX) and pseudogene. *Genomics* **33**:177, 1996.
433. Bornstein P, McKinney CE, LaMarca ME, Winfield S, Shingu T, Devarayalu S, Vos HL, Ginns EI: Metaxin, a gene contiguous to both thrombospondin 3 and glucocerebrosidase, is required for embryonic development in the mouse: Implications for Gaucher disease. *Proc Natl Acad Sci U S A* **92**:4547, 1995.
434. Demina A, Boas E, Beutler E: Structure and linkage relationships of the region containing the human L-type pyruvate kinase (*PKLR*) and glucocerebrosidase (*GBA*) genes. *Hematopathol Mol Hematol* **11**:63, 1998.
435. Glenn D, Gelbart T, Beutler E: Tight linkage of pyruvate kinase (*PKLR*) and glucocerebrosidase (*GBA*) genes. *Hum Genet* **93**:635, 1994.
436. Beutler E: The biochemical, molecular, and population genetics of Gaucher disease, in Desnick RJ (ed): *Advances in Jewish Genetic Diseases*. New York, Oxford University Press, 1998.
437. Cormand B, Montfort M, Chabs A, Vilageliu L, Grinberg D, Chabas A: Genetic fine localization of the β-glucocerebrosidase *(GBA)* and prosaposin *(PSAP)* genes: implications for Gaucher disease genetic fine localization of the beta-glucocerebrosidase (GBA) and prosaposin (PSAP) genes: Implications for Gaucher disease. *Hum Genet* **100**:75, 1997.
438. Sorge J, Kuhl W, West C, Beutler E: Complete correction of the enzymatic defect of type I Gaucher disease fibroblasts by retroviral-mediated gene transfer. *Proc Natl Acad Sci U S A* **84**:906, 1987.
439. Sorge J, Kuhl W, West C, Beutler E: Gaucher disease: Retrovirus-mediated correction of the enzymatic defect in cultured cells. *Cold Spring Harbor Symp Quant Biol* **60**:1041, 1986.
440. Correll PH, Fink JK, Brady RO, Perry LK, Karlsson S: Production of human glucocerebrosidase in mice after retroviral gene transfer into multipotential hematopoietic progenitor cells. *Proc Natl Acad Sci U S A* **86**:8912, 1989.
441. Grabowski GA, White WR, Grace ME: Expression of functional human acid β-glucosidase in COS-1 and *Spodoptera frugiperda* cells. *Enzyme* **41**:131, 1989.
442. Martin BM, Tsuji S, LaMarca ME, Maysak K, Eliason W, Ginns EI: Glycosylation and processing of high levels of active human glucocerebrosidase in invertebrate cells using a baculovirus expression vector. *DNA* **7**:99, 1988.
443. Kohn DB, Nolta JA, Weinthal J, Bahner I, Yu XJ, Lilley J, Crooks GM: Toward gene therapy for Gaucher disease. *Hum Gene Ther* **2**:101, 1991.
444. Fink JK, Correll PH, Perry LK, Brady RO, Karlsson S: Correction of glucocerebrosidase deficiency after retroviral-mediated gene transfer into hematopoietic progenitor cells from patients with Gaucher disease. *Proc Natl Acad Sci U S A* **87**:2334, 1990.
445. Sorge JA, West C, Kuhl W, Treger L, Beutler E: The human glucocerebrosidase gene has two functional ATG initiator codons. *Am J Hum Genet* **41**:1016, 1987.
446. Beutler E, Sorge JA, Zimran A, West C, Kuhl W, Westwood B, Gelbart T: The molecular biology of Gaucher disease, in Salvayre R, Douste-Blazy L, Gatt S (eds): *Lipid Storage Disorders. Biological and Medical Aspects*. New York, Plenum, 1988, p 19.
447. Reiner O, Horowitz M: Differential expression of the human glucocerebrosidase-coding gene. *Gene* **73**:469, 1988.
448. Beutler E, Gelbart T: Mutation update: Glucocerebrosidase (Gaucher disease). *Hum Mutat* **8**:207, 1996.
449. Beutler E, Gelbart T: Hematologically important mutations: Gaucher disease. *Blood Cells Mol Dis* **23**:2, 1997.
450. Grabowski GA, Saal HM, Wenstrup RJ, Barton NW: Gaucher disease: A prototype for molecular medicine. *Crit Rev Oncol Hematol* **23**:25, 1996.
451. Mettler NE: Isolation of a microtatobiote from patients with hemolytic-uremic syndrome and thrombotic thrombocytopenic purpura and from mites in the United States. *N Engl J Med* **281**:1023, 1969.
452. Dahl N, Lagerström M, Erikson A, Pettersson U: Gaucher disease type III (Norrbottnian type) is caused by a single mutation in exon 10 of the glucocerebrosidase gene. *Am J Hum Genet* **47**:275, 1990.
453. Latham T, Grabowski GA, Theophilus BDM, Smith FI: Complex alleles of the acid β-glucosidase gene in Gaucher disease. *Am J Hum Genet* **47**:79, 1990.
454. Hong CM, Ohashi T, Yu XJ, Weiler S, Barranger JA: Sequence of two alleles responsible for Gaucher disease. *DNA Cell Biol* **9**:233, 1990.
455. Ohashi T, Hong CM, Weiler S, Tomich JM, Aerts JMFG, Tager JM, Barranger JA: Characterization of human glucocerebrosidase from different mutant alleles. *J Biol Chem* **266**:3661, 1991.
456. Baltimore D: Gene conversion: Some implications for immunoglobulin genes. *Cell* **24**:592, 1981.
457. He G-S, Grabowski GA: Gaucher disease: A $G^{+1} \rightarrow A^{+1}$ IVS2 splice donor site mutation causing exon 2 skipping in the acid β-glucosidase mRNA. *Am J Hum Genet* **51**:810, 1992.
458. Beutler E, Gelbart T: Gaucher disease mutations in non-Jewish patients. *Br J Haematol* **85**:401, 1993.
459. Beutler E: Gaucher disease phenotypes outflanked. *Genome Res* **7**:950, 1997.
460. Sun Y, Peng J, Grabowski GA: The mouse prosaposin locus: Promoter organization. *DNA Cell Biol* **16**:23, 1996.
461. Schnabel D, Schröder M, Sandhoff K: Mutation in the sphingolipid activator protein 2 in a patient with a variant of Gaucher disease. *FEBS Lett* **284**:57, 1991.
462. Rafi MA, de Gala G, Zhang XL, Wenger DA: Mutational analysis in a patient with a variant form of Gaucher disease caused by SAP-2 deficiency. *Somat Cell Mol Genet* **19**:1, 1993.
463. Bell RS, Mankin HJ, Doppelt SH: Osteomyelitis in Gaucher disease. *J Bone Joint Surg Am* **68**:1380, 1986.
464. Cohen IJ, Kornreich L, Mekhmandarov S, Katz K, Zaizov R: Effective treatment of painful bone crises in type I Gaucher's disease with high dose prednisolone. *Arch Dis Child* **75**:218, 1996.
465. Fleshner PR, Aufses AH Jr, Grabowski GA, Elias R: A 27-year experience with splenectomy for Gaucher's disease. *Am J Surg* **161**:69, 1991.

466. Krasnewich D, Dietrich K, Bauer L, Ginns EI, Sidransky E, Hill S: Splenectomy in Gaucher Disease: New management dilemmas. *Blood* **91**:3085, 1998.
467. Mistry PK, Wraight EP, Cox TM: Therapeutic delivery of proteins to macrophages: Implications for treatment of Gaucher's disease. *Lancet* **348**:1555, 1996.
468. Grabowski GA, Pastores G, Brady RO, Barton NW: Safety and efficacy of macrophage targeted recombinant glucocerebrosidase therapy. *Pediatr Res* **33**:139A, 1993.
469. Ashkenazi A, Zaizov R, Matoth Y: Effect of splenectomy on destructive bone changes in children with chronic (type I) Gaucher disease. *Eur J Pediatr* **145**:138, 1986.
470. Rose JS, Grabowski GA, Barnett SH, Desnick RJ: Accelerated skeletal deterioration after splenectomy in Gaucher type 1 disease. *Am J Roentgenol* **139**:1202, 1982.
471. Svennerholm L, Dreborg S, Erikson A, Groth CG, Hillborg PO, Håkansson G, Nilsson O, Tibblin E: Gaucher disease of the Norrbottnian type (type III). Phenotypic manifestations, in Desnick RJ, Gatt S, Grabowski GA (eds): *Gaucher Disease: A Century of Delineation and Research.* New York, Alan R. Liss, 1982, p 67.
472. Karatsis P, Rogers K: Subtotal splenectomy in Gaucher's disease: Towards a definition of critical splenic mass. *Br J Surg* **80**:399, 1993.
473. Beutler E: Newer aspects of some interesting lipid storage diseases: Tay-Sachs and Gaucher's diseases. *West J Med* **126**:46, 1977.
474. Beutler E: Gaucher disease, in Goodman RM, Motulsky AG (eds): *Genetic Diseases Among Ashkenazi Jews.* New York, Raven, 1979, p 157.
475. Guzzetta PC, Connors RH, Fink J, Barranger JA: Operative technique and results of subtotal splenectomy for Gaucher disease. *Surg Gynecol Obstet* **164**:359, 1987.
476. Rodgers BM, Tribble C, Joob A: Partial splenectomy for Gaucher's disease. *Ann Surg* **205**:693, 1987.
477. Guzzetta PC, Ruley EJ, Merrick HFW, Verderese C, Barton N: Elective subtotal splenectomy. Indications and results in 33 patients. *Ann Surg* **211**:34, 1990.
478. Bar-Maor JA: Partial splenectomy in Gaucher's disease. *Chir Gastroenterol* **2(Suppl 9)**:55, 1993.
479. Holcomb GW, III, Greene HL: Fatal hemorrhage caused by disease progression after partial splenectomy for type III Gaucher's disease. *J Pediatr Surg* **28**:1572, 1993.
480. Bar-Maor JA: Partial splenectomy in Gaucher's disease: Follow-up report. *J Pediatr Surg* **28**:686, 1993.
481. Zimran A, Elstein D, Schiffmann R, Abrahamov A, Goldberg M, Bar-Maor JA, Brady RO, Guzzetta PC, Barton NW: Outcome of partial splenectomy for type I Gaucher disease. *J Pediatr* **126**:596, 1995.
482. Freud E, Cohen IJ, Neuman M, Mor C, Zer M: Should repeated partial splenectomy be attempted in patients with hematological diseases? Technical pitfalls and causes of failure in Gaucher's disease. *J Pediatr Surg* **32**:1272, 1997.
483. Thanopoulos BD, Frimas CA, Mantagos SP, Beratis NG: Gaucher disease: Treatment of hypersplenism with splenic embolization. *Acta Paediatr Scand* **76**:1003, 1987.
484. Samama G, Brefort JL, Dolley M, Leporrier M: Huge splenomegaly in Gaucher's disease. Treatment by embolization before splenectomy. *Presse Med* **18**:1078, 1989.
485. Goldblatt J, Sacks S, Dall D, Beigton P: Total hip arthroplasty in Gaucher's disease. Long-term prognosis. *Clin Orthop* **228**:94, 1988.
486. Harinck HIJ, Bijvoet OLM, van der Meer JWH, Jones B, Onvlee GJ: Regression of bone lesions in Gaucher's disease during treatment with aminohydroxypropylidene bisphosphonate. *Lancet* **2**:513, 1984.
487. Ciana G, Cuttini M, Bembi B: Short-term effects of pamidronate in patients with Gaucher's disease and severe skeletal involvement. *N Engl J Med* **337**:712, 1997.
488. Ostlere L, Warner T, Meunier PJ, Hulme P, Hesp R, Watts RWE, Reeve J: Treatment of type 1 Gaucher's disease affecting bone with aminohydroxypropylidene bisphosphonate (pamidronate). *QJM* **79**:503, 1991.
489. Bembi B, Agosti E, Boehm P, Nassimbeni G, Zanatta M, Vidoni L: Aminohydroxypropylidene-biphosphonate in the treatment of bone lesions in a case of Gaucher's disease type 3. *Acta Paediatr* **1**:122, 1994.
490. Samuel R, Katz K, Papapoulos SE, Yosipovitch Z, Zaizov R, Liberman UA: Aminohydroxy propylidene bisphosphonate (APD) treatment improves the clinical skeletal manifestations of Gaucher's disease. *Pediatrics* **94**:385, 1994.
491. Brady RO, Barton NW: Development of effective enzyme therapy for metabolic storage disorders. *Int Pediatr* **9**:175, 1994.
492. Brady RO, Pentchev PG, Gal AE, Hibbert SR, Dekaban AS: Replacement therapy for inherited enzyme deficiency. Use of purified glucocerebrosidase in Gaucher's disease. *N Engl J Med* **291**:989, 1974.
493. Brady RO, Gal AE, Pentchev PG: Evolution of enzyme replacement therapy for lipid storage diseases. *Life Sci* **7**:1235, 1974.
494. Brady RO, Pentchev PG, Gal AE: Investigations in enzyme replacement therapy in lipid storage diseases. *Fed Proc* **34**:1310, 1975.
495. Pentchev PG, Brady RO, Gal AE, Hibbert SR: Replacement therapy for inherited enzyme deficiency. Sustained clearance of accumulated glucocerebroside in Gaucher's disease following infusion of purified glucocerebrosidase. *J Mol Med* **1**:73, 1975.
496. Beutler E: Enzyme replacement therapy. *TIBS Rev* **6**:95, 1981.
497. Beutler E, Dale GL, Kuhl W: Replacement therapy in Gaucher's disease, in Desnick RJ (ed): *Enzyme Therapy in Genetic Diseases*, 2d ed. New York, Alan R. Liss, 1980, p 369.
498. Beutler E, Dale GL: Enzyme replacement therapy, in Atkinson D, Fox CF (eds): *Covalent and Non-covalent Modulation of Protein Function.* New York, Academic Press, 1979, p 449.
499. Beutler E, Dale GL, Kuhl W: Enzyme replacement with red cells. *N Engl J Med* **296**:942, 1977.
500. Belchetz PE, Crawley JCW, Braidman IP, Gregoriadis G: Treatment of Gaucher's disease with liposome-entrapped glucocerebroside:beta-glucosidase. *Lancet* **2**:116, 1977.
501. Gregoriadis G, Weereratne H, Blair H, Bull GM: Liposomes in Gaucher Type I Disease: Use in Enzyme Therapy and the Creation of an Animal Model, in Desnick RJ, Gatt S, Grabowski GA (eds): *Gaucher Disease: A Century of Delineation and Research.* New York, Alan R. Liss, 1982, p 681.
502. Ashwell G, Morell AG: The role of surface carbohydrate in the hepatic recognition and transport of circulating glycoproteins. *Adv Enzymol* **41**:99, 1974.
503. Achord D, Brot F, Gonzalez-Noriega A, Sly W, Stahl P: Human beta-glucuronidase. II. Fate of infused human placental beta-glucuronidase in the rat. *Pediatr Res* **11**:816, 1977.
504. Furbish FS, Steer CJ, Barranger JA, Jones EA, Brady RO: The uptake of native and desialylated glucocerebrosidase by rat hepatocytes and Kupffer cells. *Biochem Biophys Res Commun* **81**:1047, 1978.
505. Pentchev PG, Kusiak JW, Barranger JA, Furbish FS, Rapoport SI, Massey JM, Brady RO: Factors that influence the uptake and turnover of glucocerebrosidase and alpha-galactosidase in mammalian liver. *Adv Exp Med Biol* **101**:745, 1978.
506. Furbish FS, Steer CJ, Krett NL, Barranger JA: Uptake and distribution of placental glucocerebrosidase in rat hepatic cells and effects of sequential deglycosylation. *Biochim Biophys Acta* **673**:425, 1981.
507. Doebber TW, Wu MS, Bugianesi RL, Ponpipom MM, Furbish FS, Barranger JA, Brady RO, Shen TY: Enhanced macrophage uptake of synthetically glycosylated human placental beta-glucocerebrosidase. *J Biol Chem* **257**:2193, 1982.
508. Barton NW, Furbish FS, Murray GJ, Garfield M, Brady RO: Therapeutic response to intravenous infusions of glucocerebrosidase in a patient with Gaucher disease. *Proc Natl Acad Sci U S A* **87**:1913, 1990.
509. Kay AC, Saven A, Garver P, Thurston DW, Rosenbloom BF, Beutler E: Enzyme replacement therapy in type I Gaucher disease. *Trans Assoc Am Phys* **104**:258, 1991.
510. Sato Y, Beutler E: Binding, internalization, and degradation of mannose-terminated glucocerebrosidase by macrophages. *J Clin Invest* **91**:1909, 1993.
511. Xu Y-H, Ponce E, Sun Y, Leonova T, Bove K, Witte DP, Grabowski GA: Tissue distribution and half-life of intravenously administered alglucerase. *Pediatr Res* **39**:313, 1996.
512. Murray GJ, Jin F-S: Immunoelectron-microscopic localization of mannose-terminal glucocerebrosidase in lysosomes of rat liver Kupffer cells. *J Histochem Cytochem* **43**:149, 1995.
513. Willemsen R, Tibbe JJ, Kroos M, Reuser A, Ginns E: A biochemical and immunocytochemical study on the targeting of alglucerase in murine liver. *Histochem J* **27**:639, 1995.
514. Bijsterbosch MK, Donker W, van de Bilt H, Van Weely S, van Berkel TJ, Aerts JM: Quantitative analysis of the targeting of mannose-terminal glucocerebrosidase. Predominant uptake by liver endothelial cells. *Eur J Biochem* **237**:344, 1996.
515. Hubbard AL, Wilson G, Ashwell G, Stukenbrok H: An electron microscope autoradiographic study of the carbohydrate recognition systems in rat liver. *J Cell Biol* **83**:47, 1979.
516. Hubbard AL, Stukenbrok H: An electron microscope autoradiographic study of the carbohydrate recognition systems in rat liver. *J Cell Biol* **83**:65, 1979.

517. Fallet S, Grace ME, Sibille A, Mendelson DS, Shapiro RS, Hermann G, Grabowski GA: Enzyme augmentation in moderate to life-threatening Gaucher disease. *Pediatric Res* **31**:496, 1992.
518. Willemsen R, Tybulewicz V, Sidransky E, Eliason WK, Martin BM, LaMarca ME, Reuser AJ, Tremblay M, Westphal H, Mulligan RC: A biochemical and ultrastructural evaluation of the type 2 Gaucher mouse. *Mol Chem Neuropathol* **24**:179, 1995.
519. Grabowski GA, Barton NW, Pastores G, Banerjee TK, McKee A, Parker C, Schiffmann R, Dambrosia JM, Hill SC, Brady RO: Enzyme therapy in Gaucher disease type 1: Comparative efficacy of mannose-terminated glucocerebrosidase from natural and recombinant sources. *Ann Intern Med* **122**:33, 1995.
520. Pastores GM, Sibille AR, Grabowski GA: Enzyme therapy in Gaucher disease type 1: Dosage efficacy and adverse effects in 33 patients treated for 6 to 24 months. *Blood* **82**:408, 1993.
521. Cohen Y, Elstein D, Abrahamov A, Hirsch H, Zimran A: HCG contamination of alglucerase: Clinical implications in low-dose regimen. *Am J Hematol* **47**:235, 1994.
522. Moscicki RA: The safety of Ceredase therapy in Gaucher disease: Adverse effects and immune response. *Clin Perspect* **2**:7, 1994.
523. Sidransky E, Dietrich Km, Ginns EI: False-positive pregnancy tests in Gaucher's disease. *Lancet* **344**:1156, 1994.
524. Ponce E, Moskovitz J, Grabowski GA: Enzyme therapy in Gaucher disease type 1: Effect of neutralizing antibodies to acid β-glucosidase. *Blood* **90**:43, 1997.
525. Brady RO, Murray GJ, Oliver KL, Leitman SF, Sneller MC, Fleisher TA, Barton NW: Management of neutralizing antibody to ceredase in a patient with type 3 Gaucher disease. *Pediatrics* **100**:E11, 1997.
526. Zimran A, Hadas-Halpern I, Abrahamov A: Enzyme replacement therapy for Gaucher's disease. *N Engl J Med* **325**:1810, 1991.
527. Cohen Y, Elstein D, Abrahamov A, Hirsch H, Zimran A: HCG contamination of alglucerase: Clinical implications in low-dose regimen. *Am J Hematol* **47**:235, 1994.
528. Elstein D, Hadas-Halpern I, Azuri Y, Abrahamov A, Bar-Ziv Y, Zimran A: Accuracy of ultrasonography in assessing spleen and liver size in patients with Gaucher disease. Comparison to computed tomographic measurements. *J Ultrasound Med* **16**:209, 1997.
529. Glenn D, Thurston D, Garver P, Beutler E: Comparison of magnetic resonance imaging and ultrasound in evaluating liver size in Gaucher patients. *Acta Haematol* **92**:187, 1994.
530. Rosenthal DI, Doppelt SH, Mankin HJ, Dambrosia JM, Xavier RJ, McKusick KA, Rosen BR, Baker J, Niklason LT, Hill SC, Miller SPF, Brady RO, Barton NW: Enzyme replacement therapy for Gaucher disease: Skeletal responses to macrophage-targeted glucocerebrosidase. *Pediatrics* **96**:629, 1995.
531. Elstein D, Hadas-Halpern I, Itzchaki M, Lahad A, Abrahamov A, Zimran A: Effect of low-dose enzyme replacement therapy on bones in Gaucher disease patients with severe skeletal involvement. *Blood Cells Mol Dis* **22**:104, 1996.
532. Beutler E: Effect of low-dose enzyme replacement therapy on bones in Gaucher disease patients with severe skeletal involvement—Commentary. *Blood Cells Mol Dis* **22**:113, 1996.
533. Figueroa ML, Rosenbloom BE, Kay AC, Garver P, Thurston DW, Koziol JA, Gelbart T, Beutler E: A less costly regimen of alglucerase to treat Gaucher's disease. *N Engl J Med* **327**:1632, 1992.
534. Hollak CEM, Aerts JMFG, van Oers MHJ: Treatment of Gaucher's disease. *N Engl J Med* **328**:1565, 1993.
535. Zimran A, Hadas-Halpern I, Zevin S, Levy-Lahd E, Abrahamov A: Low dose high frequency enzyme replacement therapy for very young children with Gaucher disease. *Br J Haematol* **85**:783, 1993.
536. Hollak CEM, Aerts JMFG, Goudsmit R, Phoa SSKS, Ek M, van Weely S, Kr von dem Borne AEG, van Oers MHJ: Individualised low-dose alglucerase therapy for type 1 Gaucher's disease. *Lancet* **345**:1474, 1995.
537. International Collaborative Gaucher Group Registry, Genzyme Therapeutics: Dosage regimens of alglucerase in Gaucher disease: A comparison of the rate and extent of clinical response. *ICGG Registry Update* 1, 1995.
538. Whittington R, Goa KL: Alglucerase. A pharmacoeconomic appraisal of its use in the treatment of Gaucher's disease. *Pharm Econ* **7**:63, 1995.
539. Zimran A, Elstein D, Levy-Lahad E, Zevin S, Hadas-Halpern I, Bar-Ziv Y, Foldes J, Schwartz AJ, Abrahamov A: Replacement therapy with imiglucerase for type 1 Gaucher's disease. *Lancet* **345**:1479, 1995.
540. McCabe ERB, Fine BA, Golbus MS, Greenhouse JB, McGrath GL, New M, O'Brien WE, Rowley PT, Sly WS, Spence MA, Stockman JA, III, Whyte M, Wilson W, Wolf B, Aerts JMFG, Barranger JA, Barton NW, Beutler E, Brady RO, Cox TM, Ekstein J, Eng CM, Erikson A, Findling DM: Gaucher disease—Current issues in diagnosis and treatment. *JAMA* **275**:548, 1996.
541. Beutler E: The cost of treating Gaucher disease. *Nat Med* **2**:523, 1996.
542. Beutler E: Enzyme replacement therapy for Gaucher disease. *Baillieres Clin Haematol* **10**:711, 1997.
543. Grabowski GA, Leslie N, Wenstrup R: Enzyme therapy for Gaucher disease: The first 5 years. *Blood Rev* **12**:215, 1998.
544. Beutler E: Treatment regimens in Gaucher's disease. *Lancet* **346**:581, 1995.
545. Rappeport JM, Ginns EI: Bone-marrow transplantation in severe Gaucher disease. *N Engl J Med* **311**:84, 1984.
546. Hobbs JR: Experience with bone marrow transplantation for inborn errors of metabolism. *Enzyme* **38**:194, 1987.
547. Hobbs JR, Shaw PJ, Jones KH, Lindsay I, Hancock M: Beneficial effect of pre-transplant splenectomy on displacement bone marrow transplantation for Gaucher's syndrome. *Lancet* **1**:1111, 1987.
548. August C, Palmieri M, Nowell P, Elkins W, D'Angelo G, Glew R, Daniels L: Bone marrow transplantation (BMT) in Gaucher's disease. *Pediatr Res* **18**:236a, 1984.
549. Ringdén O, Groth C-G, Erikson A, Bäckman L, Granqvist S, Månsson J-E, Svennerholm L: Long-term follow-up of the first successful bone marrow transplantation in Gaucher disease. *Transplantation* **46**:66, 1988.
550. Lonnqvist B, Ringden O, Wahren B, Gahrton G, Lundgren G: Cytomegalovirus infection associated with and preceding chronic graft-versus-host disease. *Transplantation* **38**:465, 1984.
551. Tsai P, Lipton JM, Sahdev I, Najfeld V, Rankin LR, Slyper AH, Ludman M, Grabowski GA: Allogenic bone marrow transplantation in severe Gaucher disease. *Pediatr Res* **31**:503, 1992.
552. Svennerholm L, Erikson A, Groth CG, Ringdén O, Månsson J-E: Norrbottnian type of Gaucher disease—Clinical, biochemical and molecular biology aspects: Successful treatment with bone marrow transplantation. *Dev Neurosci* **13**:345, 1991.
553. Ringdén O, Groth CG, Erikson A, Granqvist S, Månsson J-E, Sparrelid E: Ten years' experience of bone marrow transplantation for Gaucher disease. *Transplantation* **59**:864, 1995.
554. Chan KW, Wong LTK, Applegarth D, Davidson AGF: Bone marrow transplantation in Gaucher's disease: Effect of mixed chimeric state. *Bone Marrow Transplant* 14:327, 1994.
555. Sullivan Km, Reid CD: Introduction to a symposium on sickle cell anemia: Current results of comprehensive care and the evolving role of bone marrow transplantation. *Semin Hematol* **28**:177, 1991.
556. Storb R, Anasetti C, Appelbaum F, Bensinger W, Buckner CD, Clift R, Deeg HJ, Doney K, Hansen J, Loughran T, Martin P, Pepe M, Petersen F, Sanders J, Singer J, Stewart P, Sullivan Km, Witherspoon R, Thomas ED: Marrow transplantation for severe aplastic anemia and thalassemia major. *Semin Hematol* **28**:235, 1991.
557. Beutler E: Bone marrow transplantation for sickle cell anemia: Summarizing comments. *Semin Hematol* **28**:263, 1991.
558. Radin NS: Treatment of Gaucher disease with an enzyme inhibitor. *Glycoconj J* **13**:153, 1996.
559. Inokuchi J, Radin NS: Preparation of the active isomer of 1-phenyl-2-decanoylamino-3-morpholino-1-propanol, inhibitor of murine glucocerebroside synthetase. *J Lipid Res* **28**:565, 1987.
560. Platt FM, Neises GR, Reinkensmeier G, Townsend MJ, Perry VH, Proia RL, Winchester B, Dwek RA, Butters TD: Prevention of lysosomal storage in Tay-Sachs mice treated with *N*-butyldeoxynorjirimycin. *Science* **276**:428, 1997.
561. Choudary PV, Barranger JA, Tsuji S, Mayor J, LaMarca ME, Cepko CL, Mulligan RC, Ginns EI: Retrovirus-mediated transfer of the human glucocerebrosidase gene to Gaucher fibroblasts. *Mol Biol Med* **3**:293, 1986.
562. Choudary PV, Horowitz M, Barranger JA, Ginns EI: Gene transfer and expression of active human glucocerebrosidase in mammalian cell cultures. *DNA* **5**:78, 1986.
563. Nolta JA, Sender LS, Barranger JA, Kohn DB: Expression of human glucocerebrosidase in murine long-term bone marrow cultures after retroviral vector-mediated transfer. *Blood* **75**:787, 1990.
564. Weinthal J, Nolta JA, Yu XJ, Lilley J, Uribe L, Kohn DB: Expression of human glucocerebrosidase following retroviral vector-mediated transduction of murine hematopoietic stem cells. *Bone Marrow Transplant* **8**:403, 1991.
565. Correll PH, Colilla S, Dave HPG, Karlsson S: High levels of human glucocerebrosidase activity in macrophages of long-term reconstituted mice after retroviral infection of hematopoietic stem cells. *Blood* **80**:331, 1992.

566. Ohashi T, Boggs S, Robbins P, Bahnson A, Patrene K, Wei F-S, Wei J-F, Li J, Lucht L, Fei Y, Clark S, Kimak M, He H, Mowery-Rushton P, Barranger JA: Efficient transfer and sustained high expression of the human glucocerebrosidase gene in mice and their functional macrophages following transplantation of bone marrow transduced by a retroviral vector. *Proc Natl Acad Sci U S A* **89**:11332, 1992.
567. Ponce E, Moskovitz J, Grabowski G: Enzyme therapy in Gaucher disease type I: Effect of neutralizing antibodies to acid β-glucosidase Enzyme therapy in Gaucher disease type 1: Effect of neutralizing antibodies to acid beta-glucosidase. *Blood* **90**:43, 1997.
568. Preziosi P, Prual A, Galan P, Daouda H, Boureima H, Hercberg S: Effect of iron supplementation on the iron status of pregnant women: Consequences for newborns. *Am J Clin Nutr* **66**:1178, 1997.
569. Zimran A, Kay A, Gelbart T, Garver P, Thurston D, Saven A, Beutler E: Gaucher disease. Clinical, laboratory, radiologic, and genetic features of 53 patients. *Medicine* **71**:337, 1992.
570. Beutler E, Nguyen NJ, Henneberger MW, Smolec JM, McPherson RA, West C, Gelbart T: Gaucher disease: Gene frequencies in the Ashkenazi Jewish population. *Am J Hum Genet* **52**:85, 1993.
571. Grabowski GA: Gaucher disease: Gene frequencies and genotype/phenotype correlations. *Genet Testing* **1**:5, 1997.
572. Evans MI, Moore C, Kolodny EH, Casassa M, Schulman JD, Landsberger EJ, Karson EM, Dorfmann AD, Larsen JW Jr, Barranger JA: Lysosomal enzymes in chorionic villi, cultured amniocytes, and cultured skin fibroblasts. *Clin Chim Acta* **157**:109, 1986.
573. Schneider EL, Ellis WG, Brady RO, McCulloch JR, Epstein CJ: Infantile (type II) Gaucher's disease: In utero diagnosis and fetal pathology. *J Pediatr* **81**:1134, 1972.
574. Svennerholm L, Hakansson G, Lindsten J, Wahlstroem J, Dreborg S: Prenatal diagnosis of Gaucher disease assay of the beta-glucosidase activity in amniotic fluid cells cultivated in two laboratories with different cultivation conditions. *Clin Genet* **19**:16, 1981.
575. Heilbronner H, Wurster KG, Harzer K: Praenatale diagnose der Gaucher-krankheit. *Dtsch Med Wochenschr* **106**:652, 1981.
576. Zimran A, Horowitz M: RecTL: A complex allele of the glucocerebrosidase gene associated with a mild clinical course of Gaucher disease. *Am J Med Genet* **50**:74, 1994.
577. Tsuji S, Martin BM, Barranger JA, Stubblefield BK, LaMarca ME, Ginns EI: Genetic heterogeneity in type 1 Gaucher disease: Multiple genotypes in Ashkenazic and non-Ashkenazic individuals. *Proc Natl Acad Sci U S A* **85**:2349, 1988.
578. Adolph KW, Long GL, Winfield S, Ginns EI, Bornstein P: Structure and organization of the human thrombospondin 3 gene (THBS3). *Genomics* **27**:329, 1995.
579. Grabowski GA, Barton NW, Pastores G, Dambrosia JM, Banerjee TK, McKee MA, Parker C, Schiffmann R, Hill SC, Brady RO: Enzyme therapy in type 1 Gaucher disease: Comparative efficacy of mannose-terminated glucocerebrosidase from natural and recombinant sources. *Ann Intern Med* **122**:33, 1995.
580. Pastores GM, Sibille AR, Grabowski GA: Enzyme therapy in Gaucher disease type 1: Dosage efficacy and adverse effects in thirty-three patients treated for 6 to 24 months. *Blood* **82**:408, 1993.
581. Zimran A, Elstein D, Kannai R, Zevin S, Hadas-Halpern I, Levy-Lahad E, Cohen Y, Horowitz M, Abrahamov A: Low-dose enzyme replacement therapy for Gaucher's disease: Effects of age, sex, genotype, and clinical features on response to treatment. *Am J Med* **97**:3, 1994.
582. Cox T, Lachmann R, Hollak C, Aerts J, van Weely S, Hrebicek M, Platt F, Butters T, Dwek R, Moyses C, Gow I, Elstein D, Zimran A: Novel oral treatment of Gaucher's disease with N-butyldeoxynojirimycin (OGT 918) to decrease substrate biosynthesis. *Lancet* **355**:1481, 2000.

CHAPTER 147

Galactosylceramide Lipidosis: Globoid Cell Leukodystrophy (Krabbe Disease)

David A. Wenger ▪ Kunihiko Suzuki
Yoshiyuki Suzuki ▪ Kinuko Suzuki

1. Infantile globoid cell leukodystrophy (GLD, or Krabbe disease) is a rapidly progressive, invariably fatal disease of infants. It is transmitted as an autosomal recessive trait. The disease usually begins between ages 3 and 6 months with ambiguous symptoms, such as irritability or hypersensitivity to external stimuli, but soon progresses to severe mental and motor deterioration. Patients rarely survive the second year. Clinical manifestations are limited to the nervous system, with prominent long-tract signs. There is hypertonicity with hyperactive reflexes in the early stages, but patients later become flaccid and hypotonic. Blindness and deafness are common. Peripheral neuropathy is almost always detectable. Patients with later onset, including adult-onset, forms may present with blindness, spastic paraparesis, and dementia.

2. The presence of numerous multinucleated globoid cells, almost total loss of myelin and oligodendroglia, and astrocytic gliosis in the white matter are the morphologic basis for diagnosis. The globoid cells are hematogenous macrophages that contain undigested galactosylceramide. Segmental demyelination, axonal degeneration, fibrosis, and histiocytic infiltration are common in the peripheral nervous system.

3. Consistent with the myelin loss, the white matter is severely depleted of all lipids, particularly glycolipids. The ratio of galactosylceramide to sulfatide is abnormally high. Galactosylceramide, a sphingoglycolipid consisting of sphingosine, a fatty acid, and galactose, is normally present almost exclusively in the myelin sheath.

4. The cause of Krabbe disease is a genetic deficiency of galactosylceramidase (galactocerebroside β-galactosidase [GALC]). This lysosomal enzyme normally degrades galactosylceramide to ceramide and galactose. It is postulated that accumulation of a toxic metabolite, psychosine (galactosylsphingosine), which is also a substrate for the missing enzyme, leads to early destruction of the oligodendroglia. The total brain content of galactosylceramide is not increased. However, the extensive globoid cell reaction indicates that impaired catabolism of galactosylceramide is also an important factor in the pathogenesis.

5. Assays of GALC activity in leukocytes or cultured fibroblasts with the use of appropriate natural glycolipid substrates can readily establish a definitive diagnosis. Preventive measures are available through intrauterine diagnosis of affected fetuses by GALC assays on amniotic fluid cells or biopsied chorionic villi.

6. Treatment at this time is limited to bone marrow transplantation in patients with only minimal neurologic involvement. This seems to slow the expected course of the disease and result in improved magnetic resonance imaging findings and cerebrospinal fluid protein.

7. The human GALC gene has been mapped to chromosome 14q24.3–32.1. The human cDNA and gene have been cloned. The cDNA consists of 3795 nucleotides, including 2007 bp of coding region, 1741 bp of 3′ untranslated sequence, and 47 bp of 5′ untranslated sequence. The gene is about 56 kb, consisting of 17 exons. Analysis of the 5′ flanking region revealed GC-rich sequences, one potential SP1 binding site, and one YY1 element. Evidence for inhibitory elements were found in the 5′ flanking region and within intron 1. Over 60 disease-causing mutations have been found in patients with all types of GLD. However, a few specific mutations are found in a significant number of unrelated cases with European ancestry and within some inbred communities. In addition, a number of polymorphisms in this gene have been identified, and their role in the phenotype may be considerable.

8. GLD, also due to genetic GALC deficiency, occurs in other mammalian species, most notably in certain breeds of dogs, monkeys, and mice. Clinical and pathologic features are similar to those in the human disease. These animal models will be available for future therapy trials.

A list of standard abbreviations is located immediately preceding the index in each volume. Nonstandard abbreviations used in this chapter include: GALC = galactocerebrosidase; CSF = cerebrospinal fluid; GLD = globoid cell leukodystrophy; MLD = metachromatic leukodystrophy; CGT = UDP-gal:ceramide galactosyltransferase; FLAIR = fluid-attenuated inversion recovery.

HISTORY

In 1916, Krabbe described clinical and histologic findings in two sibs who died of an "acute infantile familial diffuse sclerosis of the brain."[1] He noted familial occurrence, early onset of spasticity, and a rapidly progressive course to death. He gave a detailed description of the globoid cells, the histologic hallmark of the disease. A retrospective search of the neuropathologic literature found two earlier descriptions of similar abnormal cells.[2,3] Collier and Greenfield[4] were the first to coin the term *globoid* to describe the numerous abnormal cells in the white matter.

An earlier suggestion[5] that globoid cells might contain kerasin (a cerebroside) was supported by subsequent chemical[6,7] and histochemical[7–10] studies. The experimental induction of the globoid cell reaction by intracerebral implantation of galactocerebroside, but not by any other lipids tested,[11–13] further supported the close relationship between globoid cells and cerebroside. Analytically, the most consistent abnormality in the white matter appeared to be a reduced ratio of sulfatide to cerebroside.[14,15] In 1970–1971, a deficiency of galactosylceramidase (galactocerebroside β-galactosidase [GALC]) was established as the underlying genetic defect of the disease.[16–19] Prenatal diagnosis of an affected fetus was first accomplished in 1971.[20] The toxic effect of a related metabolite, galactosylsphingosine (psychosine), was first proposed in 1972 as the critical biochemical pathogenetic mechanism.[21] The psychosine hypothesis has since been generally substantiated both in the human disease and in animal models.[22] In 1990, human GLD was mapped to chromosome 14.[23] The human enzyme was first purified and characterized in 1993 by Chen and Wenger.[24] The cDNA for human GALC has been cloned and sequenced, revealing the complete amino acid structure.[25,26] The gene organization and exon-intron boundaries have been determined.[27] With this information, a large number of disease-causing mutations have been identified in all types of patients. This has allowed carrier identification within families and within inbred communities. Treatment of some patients with bone marrow transplantation has been accomplished, with some degree of success.

INCIDENCE AND HEREDITY

Infantile Form

Globoid cell leukodystrophy is an autosomal recessive disorder with a wide geographic distribution. The incidence in the United States is estimated as 1 in 100,000 births. However, the incidence appears to be higher in the Scandinavian countries. Hagberg et al.[28] reported 32 Swedish cases during the period from 1953 through 1967 and calculated the incidence as 1.9 per 100,000 births. In Japan the incidence was estimated as approximately 1 in 100,000–200,000 births. Recently a report appeared on a very high incidence in a large Druze kindred in Israel.[29] The diagnosis of 12 children was confirmed by enzymatic diagnosis during the period between 1969 and 1983. There were approximately 2000 births. The calculated incidence was 6 in 1000 live births and the carrier frequency was 0.15 in this community. No Jewish patients were found in a subsequent report from the same investigators,[30] and none have been identified anywhere in the world.

Late Onset and Adult Forms

Increasing numbers of patients with the later onset forms of GLD are being diagnosed. Fifty patients with late onset Krabbe disease were summarized by Lyon et al.,[31] including 27 patients reported in response to a survey conducted by the European Federation of Child Neurology Societies in 1987 and 23 other cases reported in the literature between 1906 and 1987. These authors considered the disease to have a late onset when clinical disease started after patients had begun to walk. Of the 50 patients, 39 were of European origin, with the countries of origin as follows: Italy (9, including 8 from Sicily), France (5), Germany (4), Belgium (3), the UK (2), Norway (2), Portugal (2), Greece (1), and others. Similarly, 15 late onset cases from the United States with an age distribution between 4 and 73 were summarized recently.[32] Although distributed throughout the world, the late onset cases appear to be more common in southern Europe; seven of 10 patients reported by Fiumara et al.[33] had a late onset. In a recent report, nine of 11 patients who developed gait disturbance and vision loss were over 2 years of age.[34] The frequency of late onset cases was estimated by one of us (D.A.W.) to be approximately 10 percent of the nearly 350 of GLD diagnosed in our laboratory.

CLINICAL MANIFESTATIONS

Age of Onset and Clinical Course

The typical clinical picture of infantile GLD was described by Hagberg et al.[28] Typical infant patients develop first clinical signs and symptoms at 3 to 6 months after birth, but there are cases of very early or late onset with atypical clinical manifestations. Neurologic or nonneurologic signs were detected in some cases during the neonatal period or within several weeks after birth. Stiffness was observed during the neonatal period, with clenched fists and extended extremities.[35] Pronounced irritability and twitching may be present soon after birth.[36] Vomiting was the prominent initial sign during the first week of life in one patient.[37]

Cases of late onset have been reported with increasing frequency in recent years. Until enzymatic diagnosis became possible, the diagnosis was made on the basis of the characteristic neuropathology in late infancy,[38] childhood,[39–43] or adulthood.[44–48] There have been an increasing number of reports describing later onset forms of GLD, presenting either in childhood[49–59] or in adulthood.[60–66] Most of the recently described cases have an enzymatic diagnosis as well as a mutational analysis. Clinical manifestations in these patients are highly variable and are significantly different from those of typical infant patients.

Infantile Globoid Cell Leukodystrophy

Krabbe's original report[1] of five patients is the classic description of the clinical course and manifestations of the typical infantile disease. Hagberg[67] divided the steady and rapidly progressive clinical course into three stages. Stage I is characterized by generalized hyperirritability, hyperesthesia, episodic fever of unknown origin, and some stiffness of the limbs. The child, apparently normal for the first few months after birth, becomes hypersensitive to auditory, tactile, and visual stimuli and begins to cry frequently without apparent cause. Slight retardation or regression of psychomotor development, vomiting with feeding difficulty, and convulsive seizures may occur as initial clinical symptoms. The cerebrospinal fluid (CSF) protein level is already increased. In stage II, rapid and severe motor and mental deterioration develops. There is marked hypertonicity, with extended and crossed legs, flexed arms, and arched back. Tendon reflexes are hyperactive. Minor tonic or clonic seizures occur. Optic atrophy and sluggish pupillary reactions to light are common. Stage III is the "burnt-out" stage, sometimes reached within a few weeks or months. The infant is decerebrate and blind and has no contact with his or her surroundings. Hypertrophy of the optic nerves was observed in one patient at the late stages of the disease.[68] Deafness may occur. Patients rarely survive for more than 2 years.

Head size is often small[69–72] but may be large.[38,73] Hydrocephalus has been observed.[74] Convulsive seizures occur frequently, but infantile spasms are unusual.[75,76] In one case, a lawsuit was brought against an obstetrician on behalf of a patient who showed severe brain damage with spastic tetraplegia and infantile spasms and died at 11 months.[77] Neuropathology established the diagnosis of GLD, thus disproving the alleged intrapartum asphyxia as the cause of the condition.

The symptoms and signs are confined to the nervous system. Macular cherry-red spots have been described in one patient.[78] No visceromegaly is present. Vomiting is sometimes prominent, resulting in progressive loss of weight and emaciation. An infant was hospitalized at 8 weeks of age because of progressive feeding difficulty, generalized weakness, tachypnea, and minor motor seizures.[36] The clinical course was characterized by rapidly progressive respiratory failure and neurologic deterioration, culminating in death at age 15 weeks. The lung biopsy revealed widespread distension of alveoli and alveolar ducts by numerous large macrophage-like cells containing amorphous, electron-dense, membrane-bound cytoplasmic inclusions. However, no crystalloid or tubular inclusions typical of globoid cells were found. Bouts of hyperthermia, possibly caused by involvement of the hypothalamic system, have been reported in the absence of infection.[1,37,79] Obesity in one patient[69] was not explained by lesions in the hypothalamus. Generalized ichthyosis was present from early infancy in one patient.[80]

Involvement of the peripheral nerves was once considered uncommon in GLD. Clinical examination does not always reveal neuropathy, especially in the early stages, because symptoms and signs of central nervous system involvement are overwhelming. Krabbe, however, noted in his original five patients that knee jerks could not be elicited and that stiffness passed into a flaccid state toward the end of the disease.[1] Since the first report of the peripheral nervous system pathology by Matsuyama et al.,[81] several authors have reported absent or depressed tendon reflexes in a single examination[69,72,76,82,83] or disappearance of tendon reflexes in the course of the disease.[49,57,58,70,83,84] There are descriptions of patients with normal[38] or hyperactive[85] tendon reflexes at age 15 months.

Some patients develop slowly for the first few months after birth,[7,39,40,86] possibly because of early undetected symptoms. One patient, whose diagnosis had been established *in utero*,[87] was normal neurologically during the neonatal period, but deep tendon reflexes were already absent at 5 weeks of age, although movement and muscle tone of the extremities were apparently normal. Electromyography (EMG) revealed reduced insertional activity. At 7 weeks, peripheral nerve conduction velocity was markedly reduced. Clinically, psychomotor development was normal for the first 2 months, and weakness of neck muscles was first found at 3 months of age. These findings suggest that other patients in the literature might also have had clinical manifestations detected earlier than the reported age of onset if they had been examined more carefully.

Some patients have atypical or misleading clinical histories. Wallace et al.[88] reported a patient who developed mental deterioration, apparently after mumps, at age 5 months. Convulsions started at age 7 months. The clinical diagnosis was mumps encephalitis, and the final diagnosis was established only at autopsy. A patient with a rapid course (total 3 months) was diagnosed as having encephalitis.[89] Another patient[74] was irritable from the neonatal period, and her psychomotor development was markedly retarded by age 4 months, with intermittent opisthotonos and increasing feeding difficulties. Her head circumference increased progressively, with a bulging fontanel and a right abducens palsy 2 weeks after pneumoencephalography. The hydrocephalus persisted in spite of a ventriculoperitoneal shunt. Prominent palatal myoclonus was observed in a case at age 2 years.[33]

Late Onset Globoid Cell Leukodystrophy

Patients with late onset globoid cell leukodystrophy were often diagnosed as having "Schilder's disease" or other types of diffuse sclerosis;[90] the correct diagnosis was made only by histologic examination. The number of enzymatically confirmed cases has been increasing in recent years.[32,55–66,91–97] Most patients developed initial clinical signs and symptoms by 10 years of age, but some developed neurologic signs after 40 years of age.

Loonen et al.[55] divided 18 late onset patients into two types: late infantile (early childhood) and juvenile (late childhood). In the first group (onset at 6 months to 3 years), irritability, psychomotor regression, stiffness, ataxia, and loss of vision were the common initial symptoms. The course of most cases was progressive, resulting in death approximately 2 years after onset. In the second group (onset at 3–8 years), patients developed loss of vision, together with hemiparesis, ataxia, and psychomotor regression. The course was generally protracted, and none of the patients died during the follow-up period, which varied from 10 months to 7 years. Most patients with the late onset form showed rapid deterioration initially, followed by a more gradual progression lasting for years. Developmental delay was recorded in some cases prior to the onset of deterioration.[39,49,50,52] In three patients,[51,54,91] convulsive seizures were observed. Hemiparesis was present in two patients. Glioma was suspected in a $3\frac{1}{2}$-year-old girl with left hemiparesis and hemianopsia because of an infiltrating high-density lesion crossing the splenium of the corpus callosum.[98] A 4-year-old boy developed left paraparesis, which progressed to quadriplegia.[94] The symptoms responded to steroids and worsened on withdrawal. The case described by Goebel et al.[91] included a remission of clinical symptoms around 10 years of age. A Swedish patient was followed for 15 years from the onset of symptoms at 8 years of age.[58] At 24 years of age, the individual still can function in a sheltered environment.

The case reported by Fluharty et al.[56] may be classified as "late infantile" if the clinical signs and symptoms are considered, although the disease became manifest at $3\frac{1}{2}$ years of age. The genetic relationship among the late onset forms occurring in different age groups should be further evaluated carefully, because there are reports of cases in sibs with variable ages of onset and different clinical manifestations. A sister developed loss of vision at $5\frac{1}{2}$ years of age, while her brother became ataxic and irritable at $2\frac{3}{4}$ years.[39,50] They would be classified as juvenile and late infantile types, respectively, by the criteria of Loonen et al.[55] A recent report described two sibs in a family, one with an adult form (proband, onset 19 years) and the other with a late infantile form (brother, onset 14 months),[97] although no enzymatic confirmation was available for the brother, who died in 1972.

The number of reports on adult cases has increased recently. A female patient developed slowly progressive spastic paraparesis at 38 years of age, and MRI findings of demyelination were confined to the corticospinal tract.[99] The patient, reported as case 15 by Kolodny et al.,[32] had been shaky in childhood and walked slowly with a stiff, wide-based gait during life; progressive and generalized neurologic deterioration was observed after 40 years of age. She died of pneumonia at age 73.

Recently a senile case was reported by Takahashi et al.[100] A 64-year-old female was hospitalized for slowly progressive intention tremor and postural hand tremor lasting for 4 years. She had been healthy until 60 years of age and had worked as a nurse. Her parents were consanguineous, but there was no family history of similar diseases. On admission, mild loss of vision, opsoclonus, bilateral optic atrophy, and slightly decreased central flicker score were observed. Speech was slow and scanning. Total IQ on the Wechsler adult intelligence scale was 66. Deep tendon reflexes were hyperactive, with a positive Babinski sign. Vibration sense was mildly disturbed in the legs. Cerebellar signs and symptoms were present, and the patient could not walk without support. CSF protein was elevated, and GALC activity was low (0.29 nmol/h/mg protein, normal 2.1 ± 0.94).

The CSF protein was elevated in most cases of the late infantile type, while it was normal or only mildly elevated in the juvenile or adult patients reported.[91,93,95,98] Peripheral nerve conduction velocity is generally reduced in late infantile patients and normal in juvenile patients, with some exceptions.

CLINICAL DIAGNOSIS

In infantile cases, GLD should be strongly suspected if the following clinical features are present: onset early in infancy, irritability and muscle hypertonicity with progressive neurologic deterioration, signs of peripheral neuropathy, and elevation of CSF protein levels. In rare cases muscle hypotonia and weakness appear before CNS deterioration.[101] The disease can be differentiated from nonprogressive CNS disorders of congenital or perinatal origin on the basis of the history of normal development for the first few months after birth followed by psychomotor deterioration. Rarely, the disease may first appear to be of traumatic, inflammatory, or neoplastic origin, but careful evaluation of the clinical picture and appropriate laboratory investigation usually exclude these possibilities.

Differentiation from other degenerative diseases of infancy is often a major problem. Metachromatic leukodystrophy (MLD) usually begins in the second year of life, with slowly progressive motor disturbance as the initial symptom. Spongy degeneration of white matter begins in early infancy and is characterized by an enlarged head, initial hypotonia, and a normal CSF protein concentration. Alexander disease includes megalocephaly as a characteristic sign, but otherwise there are no specific clinical manifestations. Pelizaeus-Merzbacher disease may occur in the first year of life. The disease has a slowly progressive course, and abnormal involuntary eye movements, often described as nystagmus, are prominent and of diagnostic help. The CSF protein concentration is normal. Inheritance is X-linked recessive. The G_{M2}-gangliosidoses (Chap. 153) usually manifest themselves in the first year of life; developmental delay and macular cherry-red spots are commonly present. The initial clinical finding is sluggishness or apathy rather than hyperirritability. G_{M1}-gangliosidosis (Chap. 151) has an early onset and, both clinically and radiologically, resembles Hurler-Hunter disease more than Krabbe disease does. Patients with Gaucher disease (Chap. 146) and Niemann-Pick disease (Chaps. 144, 145) can present in the first year of life but almost always have visceromegaly.

It is practically impossible to make a clinical diagnosis of GLD in patients with atypical symptoms or courses and in patients with the late onset forms. Patients of any age with progressive deterioration of the central or peripheral nervous system should be tested for GLD. Measurement of GALC activity in leukocytes or cultured skin fibroblasts can easily make the diagnosis.

LABORATORY FINDINGS

Blood and Urine

No specific abnormalities can be found in blood chemistry tests and routine urinalysis. The CSF protein concentration is high in patients with the infantile or late infantile form. The CSF cell count is normal. The electrophoretic pattern may be of some diagnostic help; albumin and α_2-globulin levels are elevated, and β_1- and γ-globulin levels are decreased.[37,83] This pattern remains constant throughout the course of the disease and is found only in metachromatic and globoid cell leukodystrophies.[102] In one late onset patient, the protein pattern was that of blood-brain barrier damage with additional intrathecal IgG synthesis.[94]

Neuroimaging

Progressive, diffuse, and symmetric cerebral atrophy is observed on neuroimaging. Rarely is asymmetry demonstrated by computerized tomography (CT) or magnetic resonance imaging (MRI).[103,104] The CT in the early stage of the disease can be normal;[96,105] later diffuse cerebral atrophy develops involving both gray and white matter in the third stage.[103] Diffuse hypodensity of the white matter, particularly in the parieto-occipital region, may be present.[62,106] These findings are nonspecific and are observed in many white matter diseases. Localized lesions have been described in some reports: hypodensity of periventricular parieto-occipital white matter;[96] high density in the thalamus,[107] corona radiata,[108] and cerebellar cortex[108,109] (Fig. 147-1); high density in the globus pallidus changing to low density with progression of the disease;[110] and necrosis of the corpus callosum.[111] Discrete and symmetric dense areas on CT were found in the deep gray matter of the hemispheres, thalamus, posterior limb of the internal capsule, quadrigeminal plate, and cerebellum, and also in periventricular and capsular white matter.[112]

In general, MRI detects demyelination in the brainstem and cerebellum more clearly than CT at the early stage of the disease,[107] but one infant at 5 months of age had a deceptively normal MRI when CT already revealed symmetric hyperdensity involving cerebellum, thalami, caudate, corona radiata, and brainstem.[113] Another patient had a deceptively normal initial MRI at age 3 months, with progression of the white matter disease over the following 9 months.[114] The T1 value was decreased, with normal or slightly decreased T2 in white matter of the centrum semiovale.[112] In one report, a plaque-like high signal intensity in T2-weighted images and low signal intensity in T1-weighted images were characteristic of three infants in the periventricular and cerebellar white matter (Fig. 147-3).[108] On the other hand, T2-weighted and fluid-attenuated inversion recovery (FLAIR) MRI showed symmetric high intensity of the pyramidal tract and optic radiation in an adult patient who developed initial clinical manifestations at 60 years of age[100] (Fig. 147-2).

Calculation of the T2 value in the central white matter provides a basis for objective judgment for demyelinating diseases.[115] It was progressively prolonged in the occipital deep white matter and posterior part of central semiovale in late onset disease. MRI was also useful for differentiation between dysmyelination and demyelination.[116] GLD with severe demyelination showed high-intensity lesions on T2-weighted images, with a loss of diffusional anisotropy and relatively high signal intensity on diffusion-weighted images.

EEG, EMG, and Evoked Potentials

The electroencephalogram (EEG) is normal in the initial stages, but the cerebral rhythms gradually become abnormal. Background activity becomes slow and disorganized,[35,38,69,71,73,85] with changes that may be asymmetric.[73] This is often accompanied by multifocal paroxysmal or epileptic discharges.[35,38,69,75,86,117]

In accord with the clinical and pathologic observations of peripheral neuropathy, various abnormal results have been obtained by electrophysiological procedures. These include a mild increase in polyphasic motor unit potentials,[71] presence of high-amplitude neuromuscular units with a decrease in the number of units,[75] and a few fibrillations[69,71] on routine EMG. Motor nerve conduction velocity is consistently low.[49,69,71,75,79,80,117,118] Distal sensory latency of the median nerve was also prolonged in one patient.[72] EMG and nerve conduction studies were normal in an adult patient with enzymatically confirmed diagnosis,[95] but there was EMG evidence of demyelinating neuropathy in another adult.[96,97]

One study found multimodal evoked potential testing was useful for diagnostic differentiation of various types of leukodystrophies.[119] Three GLD patients had an abnormal auditory brainstem response (ABR), with a loss of rostral waves accompanied by delayed I-III interpeak latencies. Sensory evoked potentials (SEPs) were abnormal: Cortical SEP was absent and cervical SEP showed peripheral slowing. Visual evoked potentials (VEPs) were also abnormal and correlated with disease progression. In another study, prolongation of each wave component and interpeak latency was observed at early stages of the disease,[120] but later components eventually disappeared.[109,120] An adult patient showed prolonged I-III interpeak latency in ABR and prolonged N9-N19 interpeak latency in SEPs, while VEPs were normal.[97] ABR was normal in another adult patient at age 29.[95]

PATHOLOGY

Although there are some isolated reports describing pathological findings outside the nervous system,[82,121–124] the pathology of GLD is limited, for all practical purposes, to the nervous system. In a study on a muscle biopsy sample, fiber-type disproportion has been described.[125,126] Goebel et al.[127] have described typical inclusions in eccrine sweat gland epithelial cells.

Central Nervous System

Gross Pathology. The brain is usually small and atrophic, with shrunken gyri and widened sulci. The white matter is firm, reduced

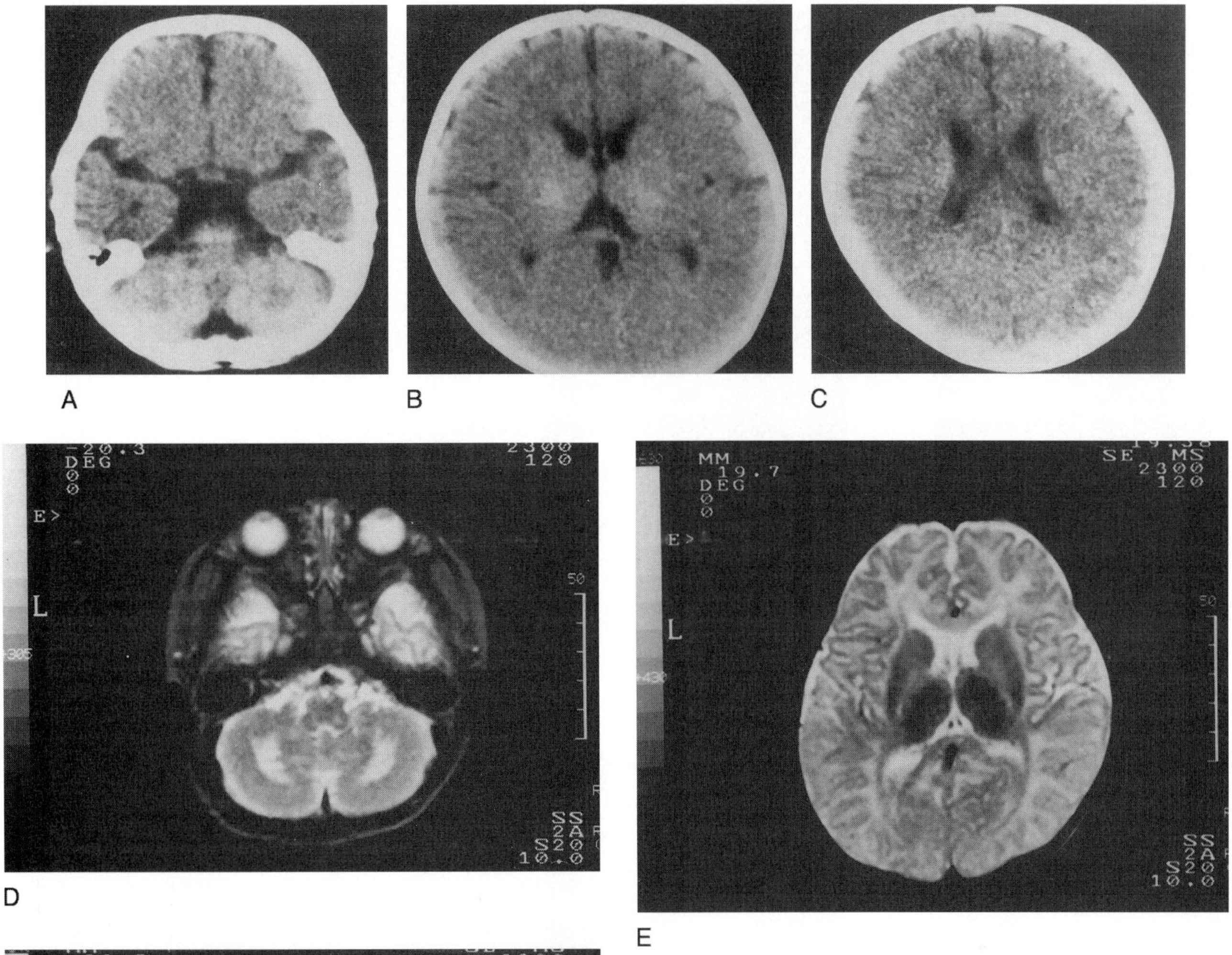

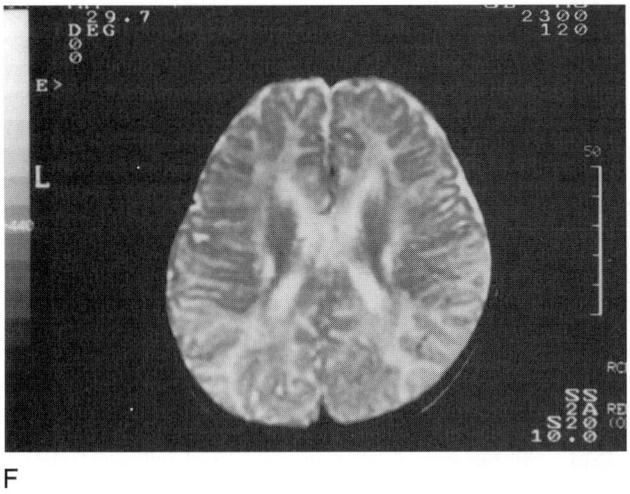

Fig. 147-1 CT and MRI images of an infant with GLD. A–C: CT at 5 months of age shows symmetrically increased density in (A) cerebellar cortex, (B) thalami, and (C) corona radiata. D–F: T2-weighted images on MRI. TR: 2,100 msec; TE 100 msec. There is an abnormally high signal intensity in cerebellar white matter (D), and slightly high signal intensity in the posterior limbs of the internal capsules (E) and periventricular cerebral white matter (F). (*From* Pediatr Neurol,[108] *by permission.*)

in volume, and of whitish-gray appearance. The ventricles are dilated. In contrast to the grossly abnormal white matter, the gray matter appears relatively normal except for a moderate reduction of cortical thickness. The junction of the gray and white matter is ill defined.

Histopathology. The major histopathologic changes are extensive demyelination, gliosis, and presence of unique macrophages, the globoid cells, in the white matter. The subcortical arcuate fibers (U-fibers) tend to be spared except in unusually severe or protracted cases, in which practically no myelin can be demonstrated within the cerebral hemispheres. Among the various white matter systems, phylogenetically newer nerve fiber tracts are usually more severely involved by the demyelinating process. Thus, the fornix, the hippocampus, the mamillothalamic tract, and the nerve fiber bundles in the basal ganglia tend to be less involved than the centrum semiovale or the cerebellar white matter.[122,128,129] In the spinal cord, the pyramidal tracts are more severely affected than the dorsal columns. In the areas of demyelination, the oligodendroglial cell population is severely diminished and globoid cells are often clustered around blood vessels (Fig. 147-3). Secondary axonal degeneration is a consistent finding. In some clinically protracted cases, the white matter may be totally gliotic, without any globoid cells.[49] If

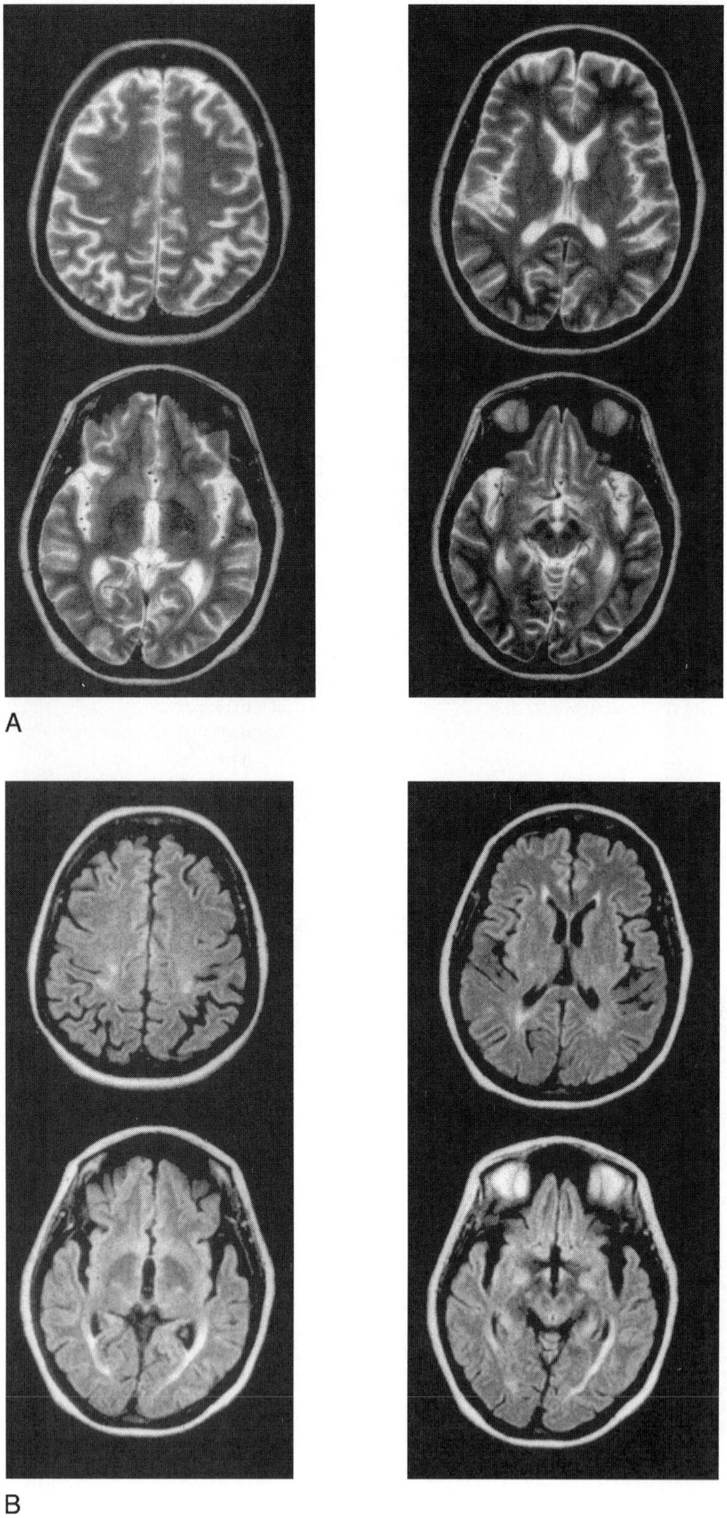

Fig. 147-2 MRI images of an adult patient with GLD. A: Axial T2-weighted images. TR 4,000 msec; TE 98 msec. B: Corresponding planes of FLAIR images. TR 10,002 msec; TE 138 msec. Bilateral pyramidal tract and optic radiation exhibits symmetrical high intensity on both images. (*Courtesy of Dr. M. Takahashi, Sumitomo Hospital, Osaka, Japan.*)

present, globoid cells have abundant cytoplasm, which stains positive with periodic acid-Schiff (PAS) stain. Characteristically, there is no sudanophilia. Intense acid phosphatase activity was demonstrated in these cells.[70,88,122,130,131] The similarities in morphologic and histochemical characteristics between the globoid cells and the glucosylceramide-containing abnormal cells in Gaucher disease were often pointed out.[5,8] There had been a long-lasting controversy as to the origin and nature of globoid cells,[4,7,132–135] but the current consensus is that these are cells of the mononuclear phagocyte lineage,[136] which have become multinucleated as the unique response to free galactosylceramide.[11–13,137] (For more details, refer to the sixth edition of this text.)

In contrast to the devastated white matter, the gray matter is generally much less affected, although neuronal degeneration in the cerebral cortex, thalamus, cerebellar nuclei, and brainstem has been reported in some cases.[7,89,132,138,139] A Golgi study indicated remarkably well-preserved dendritic processes of pyramidal neurons in the cerebral cortex.[140]

Evolution of the Histopathologic Changes. It is difficult to determine the chronologic sequence of the various histologic

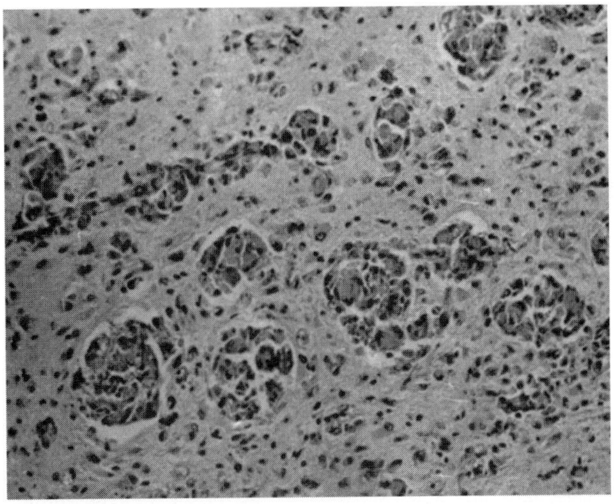

Fig. 147-3 Typical light microscopic appearance of the white matter in GLD. Conspicuous clusters of globoid cells occupy a considerable portion of whole white matter. Globoid cells are PAS-positive and often contain multiple nuclei. The remainder of the tissue is mostly occupied by reactive astrocytes. Periodic acid-Schiff (PAS) stain. Magnification × 120.

changes, because it is rarely possible to follow morphologic changes in the same patient through the course of the illness. In their classic study, D'Agostino et al.[86] attempted to reconstruct the chronologic evolution of the morphologic changes through multiple sections from three different patients. Utilizing the degree of demyelination as the criterion, they divided the course into four stages: early, advanced, late, and final. In the early lesions, mononuclear globoid cells containing PAS-positive materials are present in the white matter, with only a slight decrease in the intensity of myelin staining. In the advanced stage, myelin and axons decrease and astrocytic gliosis becomes prominent. The globoid cells are more numerous and tend to cluster around blood vessels. Many become multinucleated. In the late stage, the globoid cells become fewer in number and are mostly clumped around blood vessels. Myelin and axons are markedly diminished at this stage. The final stage is characterized by predominant astrocytic gliosis, with a few remaining globoid cells, and a total loss of myelin and axons. Later chronologic investigations using canine or murine models of GLD support accuracy of this earlier study in human patients (see "Animal Models" section).

Ultrastructure. There are many reports describing the ultrastructural pathology of GLD.[36,38,41,69,73,83,117,118,135,141–150] Mononuclear and multinucleated globoid cells are similar ultrastructurally, except for the number of nuclei. They have prominent pseudopods, moderately electron-dense granular cytoplasm containing prominent rough endoplasmic reticulum, many free ribosomes, abundant fine filaments of approximately 9–10 nm, and scattered or clustered abnormal cytoplasmic inclusions (Fig. 147-4). The inclusions have moderately electron-dense straight or curved hollow tubular profiles in longitudinal sections and appear irregularly crystalloid in cross sections (Fig. 147-5). These tubular inclusions are often scattered among the normal intracellular organelles, but sometimes they are clustered within an electron-lucent space or within an electron-dense matrix. They often have longitudinal striations of variable density, approximately 6 nm in width. Other inclusions have a structure of slender twisted tubules with rectangular or irregularly round cross sections, resembling the tubular inclusions of Gaucher disease.[73] Yunis and Lee[145] pointed out the morphologic similarities of the abnormal inclusions to negatively stained pure brain galactosylceramide. Intracerebral injection of pure galactosylceramide into rat brain produced cells that have a morphology essentially identical to that of human globoid cells, containing both types of the tubular inclusions.[151,152] Inclusions are also reported, though infrequently, in astrocytes and oligodendrocytes. Degeneration of myelin, with or without associated axonal degeneration, is widespread in the white matter, but the remaining myelin has normal multilamellar configuration with normal periodicity.

Peripheral Nervous System

The peripheral nerves are commonly affected in GLD.[69,71,81,83,143,145,153–158] The affected nerves are firm and

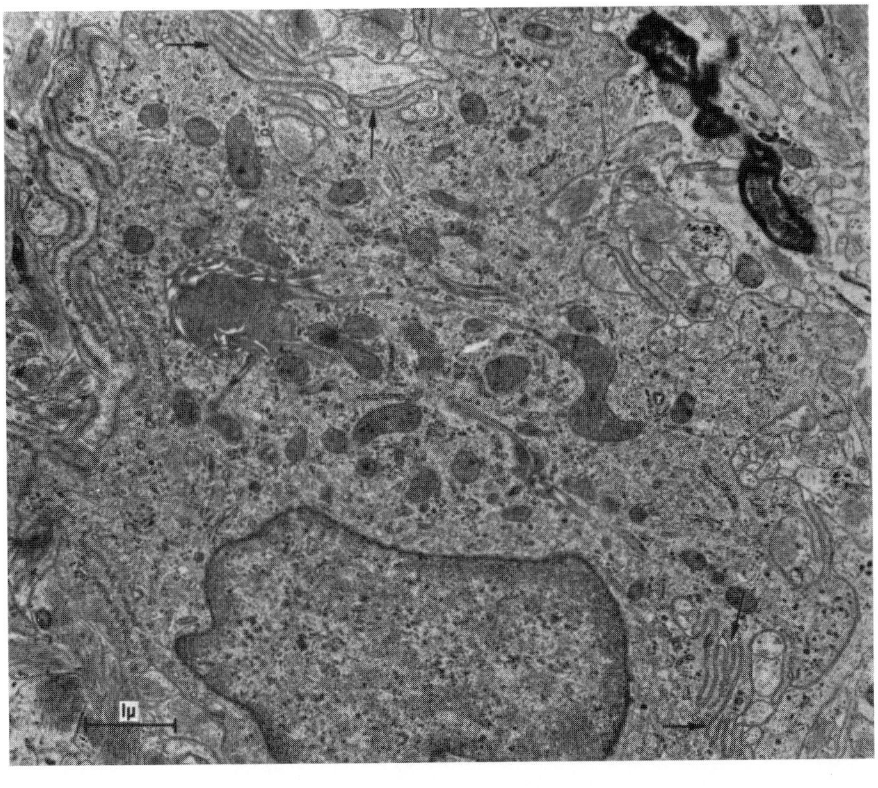

Fig. 147-4 A low-magnification electron micrograph of a globoid cell. Only one nucleus is visible. There are numerous tortuous pseudopods (arrows) which characterize this cell as a macrophage. Within the cytoplasm, near the center of the picture, there are many abnormal tubular inclusions (for details see Fig. 147-5).

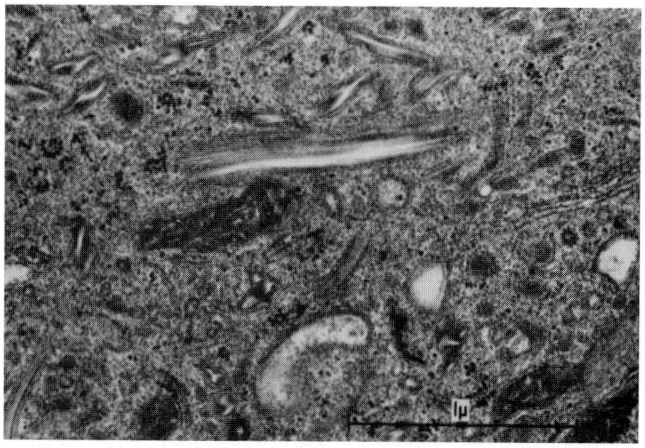

Fig. 147-5 The abnormal hollow tubules show longitudinal striations approximately 6 nm wide.

often abnormally thick and white on gross inspection. The major pathologic features are marked endoneurial fibrosis, proliferation of fibroblasts, demyelination, and infiltration or perivascular aggregation of histiocytes/macrophages containing PAS-positive materials. Teased fiber preparations clearly demonstrate segmental demyelination, increased variations in internodal length, and osmiophilic lipid droplets in paranodal Schwann cell cytoplasm.[154,158] Thinly myelinated fibers suggestive of remyelination may be present. Quantitative analysis has demonstrated a severe loss of large myelinated fibers, but the number of unmyelinated fibers was not diminished.[151] Axonal degeneration of varying degrees has been reported.[69,71,126,137,158] Ultrastructurally, inclusions similar to those in globoid cells in the brain are found in the cytoplasm of histiocytes/macrophages, as well as in the Schwann cells.[145,155,157]

Pathology of Late Onset GLD

Despite the increasing clinical reports on late onset cases in recent years, only limited information is available on their neuropathology. In late infantile and juvenile cases, neuropathologic changes are similar to those in typical infantile-onset patients. The only available description of the CNS pathology of adult-onset GLD is that by Choi et al.[159] The patients were 18-year-old identical twins. Their symptoms developed 12 and 7 months prior to death. Two months after allogeneic bone marrow transplantation, both patients died of severe graft-versus-host disease. The neuropathologic changes, almost identical in the two patients, included degeneration of the optic radiation and of the frontoparietal white matter, with secondary corticospinal tract degeneration. The frontoparietal lesions consisted of multiple necrotic foci with calcified deposits and active degeneration of the surrounding white matter with globoid cell infiltration. Small satellite foci of degeneration with globoid cells were also noted. In the peripheral nerves of patients with late onset forms, demyelination and the abnormal inclusions in Schwann cells have been described.[39,51,54,60,91,160] In a 73-year-old woman, who had the oldest reported case of GALC deficiency, loss of myelinated fibers, with disproportionately thin myelin sheaths, and Schwann cells containing needle-like inclusions were described.[160]

Pathology of Fetal Globoid Cell Leukodystrophy

Neuropathologic studies have been reported in fetuses of 20–23 weeks' gestation with GALC deficiency.[161–163] Scattered globoid cells with typical inclusions were found in the spinal cord, being more numerous in the dorsal column. Globoid cells were found in the pons in one fetus but were not found in the brainstem in other fetuses. No globoid cells were detected in the cerebrum or cerebellum. These findings are consistent with the normal sequence of myelination in the developing brain in that, at this gestational age, the telencephalon has not begun to myelinate. One report indicated a delay in myelination of both the central and peripheral nervous systems.[161] However, a comparison of an affected fetus with its unaffected fraternal twin showed no differences in degree of myelination.[163] Abnormal inclusions were found in the Schwann cells and endoneurial fibroblasts of peripheral nerves.[162]

BIOCHEMISTRY OF GALACTOSYLCERAMIDE

Chemistry of Galactosylceramide and Related Compounds

Galactosylceramide (galactocerebroside) is a sphingoglycolipid consisting of a long-chain base, sphingosine, and a galactose (Fig. 147-6). The amino group of sphingosine is acylated with long-chain fatty acid (C14–C26). N-acylsphingosine, generically called ceramide, is the basic common building block of almost all sphingolipids. Generally, the fatty acids of galactosylceramide and sulfatide in the brain are characterized by the predominance of longer-chain fatty acids (C20–C26), the lack of polyunsaturated fatty acids, and the presence of α-hydroxy acids. Approximately two-thirds of the fatty acids in cerebrosides and one-third of those in sulfatides are α-hydroxy fatty acids. These are generally absent in other lipids of the brain, including glycerophospholipids, sphingomyelin, ceramide oligohexosides, and gangliosides. In galactocerebrosides and sulfatides, particularly those in white matter, 65–80 percent of the total non-hydroxy fatty acids have chain lengths longer than 20 carbons. In the α-hydroxy fatty acids, the proportion of the longer-chain fatty acids is even greater.

Cerebroside is defined as a monohexosyl ceramide, the hexose being linked to the C-1 of ceramide by a glycosidic linkage. The hexose is either D-glucose or D-galactose. Depending on the nature of the hexose, cerebroside is named glucocerebroside (glucosylceramide) or galactocerebroside (galactosylceramide). Both the glucose and galactose are in the β anomeric configuration. Glucosylceramides occur predominantly in systemic tissues outside of the nervous system and are present only at very low concentrations in normal human brain after age 1 year. They are present in small amounts in the brains of normal human fetuses and newborns[164] and in the brains of older children with certain diseases, notably ganglioside storage disorders.[165,166] In contrast, galactosylceramide is characteristically a lipid of the nervous system, particularly of the myelin sheath. Brain sulfatides are derived from galactosylceramide, having an additional sulfate group, ester-linked to the C-3 of galactose. Sulfatides are also present at high concentrations in myelin.

There are two other metabolically related compounds that are important in the pathogenesis of GLD. Psychosine is galactosylceramide minus fatty acid ("lyso-galactosylceramide"). Although the compound is essentially absent in normal brain,[167–169] it is of potential importance when the dynamic behavior of galactosylceramide is considered in relation to the pathogenesis of the disease.

Though detailed structures of the individual moieties, such as fatty acids or sphingosines, differ among these glycosphingolipids,

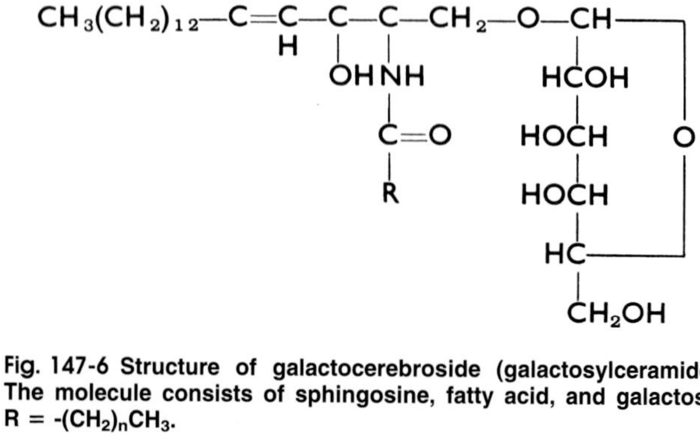

Fig. 147-6 Structure of galactocerebroside (galactosylceramide). The molecule consists of sphingosine, fatty acid, and galactose. R = $-(CH_2)_nCH_3$.

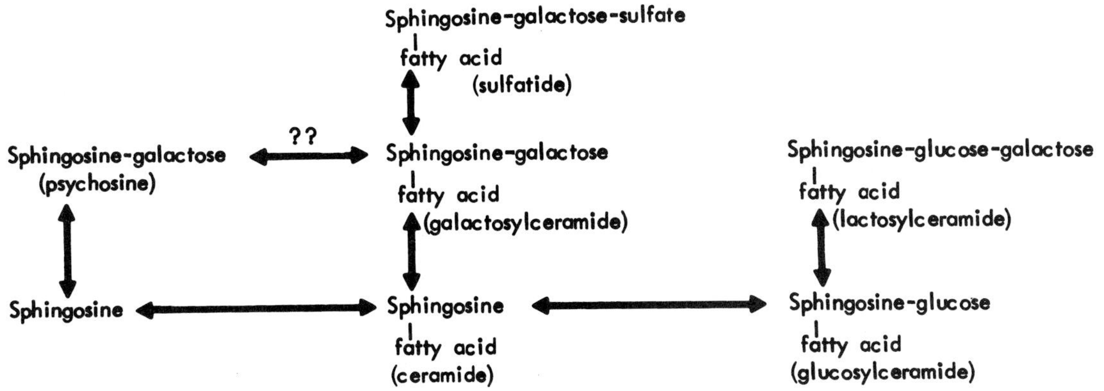

Fig. 147-7 Structural relationships between galactosylceramide and related compounds. It should be understood that the arrows between the sphingolipids do not represent reversible enzymatic reactions.

the simplified notations are convenient for purposes of most discussions in this chapter. Figure 147-7 depicts chemical and metabolic relationships among galactosylceramide and related compounds using such simplified notations.

Metabolism of Galactosylceramide and Related Compounds

Galactosylceramide is biosynthesized first by acylation of sphingosine to ceramide and then by galactosylation of ceramide by UDP-galactose:ceramide galactosyltransferase (CGT)[170,171] (Fig. 147-7). Sulfatide is then synthesized from galactosylceramide with 3′-phosphoadenosine-5′-phosphosulfate (PAPS) as the sulfate donor.[172] In addition, it has been long known that sphingosine can be directly galactosylated to form psychosine.[173] This reaction, known as the Cleland-Kennedy pathway, appears to be a dead-end pathway metabolically, because the possible alternate pathway for galactosylceramide, acylation of psychosine, has not been conclusively established. However, this dead-end pathway appears to play a crucial role in the pathogenesis of GLD.

The initial step in the lysosomal degradation of sulfatide is removal of the sulfate group to convert it to galactosylceramide. This reaction is catalyzed by cerebroside sulfate sulfatase (arylsulfatase A).[174] Deficiency of this enzyme characterizes another inherited leukodystrophy, MLD, in which abnormal accumulation of sulfatide occurs[175,176] (see Chap. 148).

Galactosylceramide is degraded to ceramide and galactose by a lysosomal hydrolytic enzyme, galactosylceramidase (galactocerebrosidase [GALC]), thus:

$$\begin{array}{c} \text{fatty acid} \\ | \\ \text{sphingosine} - \text{galactose} \\ \text{(galactosylceramide)} \end{array} \xrightarrow{\text{GALC}} \begin{array}{c} \text{fatty acid} \\ | \\ \text{sphingosine} + \text{galactose} \\ \text{(ceramide)} \end{array}$$

This enzyme, initially called cerebroside galactosidase, was first studied in detail by Radin and coworkers.[177–180] It is active on galactosylceramide with either unsubstituted or α-hydroxy fatty acids. In rat brain, GALC activity is present at 4 days of age, before myelination, when little galactosylceramide is present. The enzyme activity then rises to three to four times the 4-day level during the period of active cerebroside deposition and myelination. Activity remains high in mature animals. In humans, activity in a 72-year-old brain was the same as that in a 21-year-old brain in gray matter but was decreased to 60 percent of the activity in the young brain in white matter.[16]

Several reports described the properties of partially purified GALC.[181–186] However, in 1993 Chen and Wenger[24] succeeded in purifying GALC from human urine and brain using a series of hydrophobic affinity columns to take advantage of its extremely hydrophobic nature. As shown in Fig. 147-8, the most pure fraction from human brain consisted of bands with approximate molecular weights of 80, 50–52, and 30 based on migration on SDS-PAGE. Studies also showed that these polypeptides could aggregate into a very large complex with an estimated molecular weight greater than 800,000. The purified enzyme had very high activity toward galactosylceramide and psychosine and also had significant activity when measured using the water-soluble fluorescent substrate 4-methylumbelliferyl-β-D-galactopyrano-

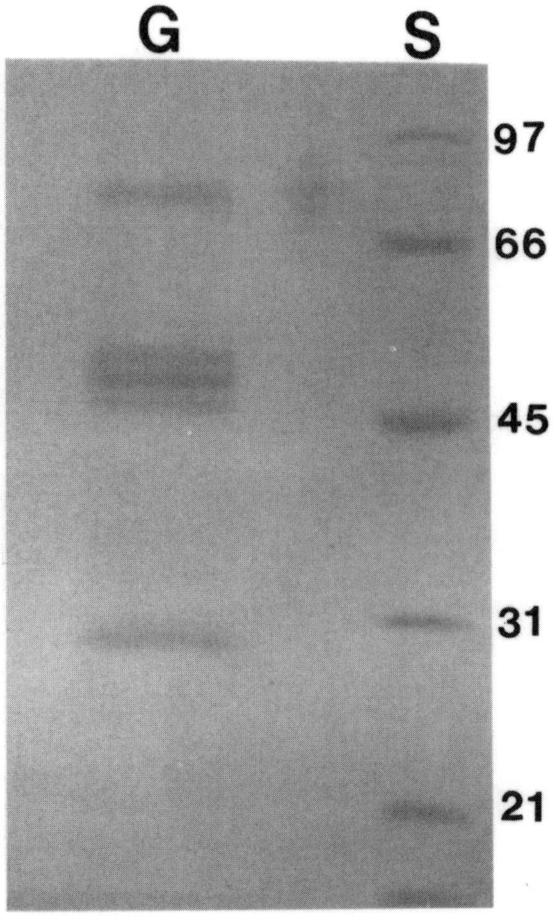

Fig. 147-8 SDS-PAGE of the most active fractions of GALC purified from human brain. G denotes the active GALC fraction, and S denotes the molecular weight standards. The gel was stained with Coomassie blue. (*From* Biochim Biophys Acta,[24] *with permission of Elsevier Science.*)

side.[24] The K_m for galactosylceramide was about 10 μM assayed in the presence of sodium taurocholate. N-terminal amino acid sequence analysis helped to confirm the relationship between the bands identified on sodium dodecylsulfate polyacrylamide gel electrophoresis. The band migrating near 80 kDa and all of the bands between 50 and 52 kDa shared the same N-terminal amino acids, while the sequence of the 30-kDa band was different. An antipeptide antibody prepared against the N-terminal amino acid sequence could detect the 80- and 50–52-kDa bands.[24] Treatment with endoglycosidase F to remove N-linked sugar chains indicated that the multiple bands near 50 kDa are not due to glycosylation differences but probably reflect proteolytic trimming during processing of the mature enzyme. Using information provided by those sequences, the cDNA for human GALC was cloned.[25] The cDNA sequence provided direct evidence that the 80-kDa band was the precursor of the 50- to 52-kDa and 30-kDa bands. As will be shown shortly, the coding region for the 50- to 52- kDa sequences is at the 5′ end of the gene and the coding region for the 30-kDa subunit is at the 3′ end of the gene. Both subunits are required for the production of active enzyme. Subsequently, Sakai and coworkers[187] purified this enzyme from human lymphocytes and reached similar conclusions, although there are some differences in the estimated molecular weights of the bands identified after gel electrophoresis of the purified fractions.

Previous studies had examined the substrate specificity of partially purified GALC. While galactosylceramide is clearly the main natural substrate, the enzyme is also active in catalyzing hydrolysis of terminal galactose from galactosylsphingosine (psychosine),[21,185–190] monogalactosyldiglyceride,[191] and, under specific assay conditions, also from lactosylceramide.[192–198] The information on the substrate specificity of the enzyme provides important information related to possible pathogenetic mechanisms, as well as to enzymatic diagnosis of the disease. It has been demonstrated that phosphatidylserine can specifically activate human brain GALC activity.[199] The hydrolysis of galactosylceramide by GALC is greatly stimulated by the presence of certain so-called sphingolipid activator proteins in the presence of acidic lipids, such as phosphatidylserine[200] (see Chap. 134).

Glycolipid Metabolism in Myelin

The distribution of galactosylceramide in mammalian organs is uniquely restricted. It is practically absent in systemic organs, except in the kidney, which normally contains appreciable amounts of galactosylceramide, although much less than the nervous system.[201,202] Brain tissue, particularly white matter, is rich in galactosylceramide and its sulfate ester, sulfatide. Galactosylceramide is mostly, if not exclusively, located in the myelin sheath and synthesized in the oligodendroglia and the Schwann cells. Thus, galactosylceramide is virtually absent in the brain before myelination and is present at abnormally low concentrations in any pathologic conditions in which severe loss of myelin occurs. The amounts of total brain galactosylceramide correlate precisely with the amounts of myelin that can be isolated from the brain, whereas amounts of other lipids do not.[203]

Myelin of adult mammalian brain generally contains galactosylceramide at a concentration of 15–18 percent of dry weight. The sum of galactosylceramide and sulfatide amounts to 20 percent of the dry weight of myelin. The content of galactosylceramide in myelin from peripheral nerves is somewhat less than that of CNS myelin.[204] In view of the unusually high concentrations of galactosylceramide and sulfatide in the myelin sheath, metabolic diseases involving these lipids (GLD and MLD) would be expected to manifest themselves primarily as disorders of white matter and peripheral nerves.

The most significant metabolic features of CNS myelin are its high rate of formation and turnover during a relatively short developmental period of active myelination and its slow turnover in the adult brain. The period of most active myelination in humans probably extends from the perinatal period to about age 18 months. Myelination does not stop after this period, and in the human brain, it may not be complete until age 20.[205] The amount of galactosylceramide in immature brain is very low compared to the concentrations of cholesterol and phospholipids. When measured by incorporation of labeled galactose administered in vivo, the rate of galactosylceramide synthesis in rat brain reaches a peak at 15–20 days, coinciding well with the most active period of myelination.[206] A similar sharp peak is observed in the activity of UDP-gal:ceramide galactosyltransferase (CGT), an enzyme that catalyzes the last step of galactosylceramide synthesis.[207] The recent cloning of rat and mouse CGT confirms that peak levels of the corresponding mRNA occur during the period of most active myelination and that relatively high mRNA levels are found in brain and kidney.[208–211] Synthesis and turnover of galactosylceramide occur at much lower rates in adult mice and rats.

Some aspects of the chemistry and metabolism of galactosylceramide are critical in considering the pathophysiology of GLD: (1) Galactosylceramide consists of sphingosine, fatty acid, and galactose. (2) Galactosylceramide is the precursor of sulfatide. (3) Both galactosylceramide and sulfatide are highly concentrated in the myelin sheath. (4) Sulfatide is normally degraded through galactosylceramide. (5) GALC degrades galactosylceramide to ceramide and galactose. (6) A few related galactolipids also serve as substrates for GALC, including psychosine, monogalactosyldiglyceride, and lactosylceramide. (7) Biosynthesis of galactosylceramide reaches a peak, coincident with the maximum period of myelination, during the first year and a half in humans. (8) GALC activity is low before myelination and increases during the active period of myelination, when myelin also turns over relatively rapidly. (9) Once formed, adult myelin is relatively stable metabolically, although there is some turnover. (10) The repair of myelin damaged by environmental insults requires a minimal level of many enzymes, including GALC, for production of stable, compact myelin.

CHEMICAL PATHOLOGY

Analytical Chemistry

Hallervorden was the first to point out the morphologic similarities of the globoid cells in GLD to the storage cells in Gaucher disease and to suggest that the globoid cells also might contain cerebroside in excess.[5] Austin[6] obtained fractions enriched in globoid cells from seven patients with GLD. He concluded that globoid cells contain unusually large amounts of galactosylceramide but little sulfatide. Such increases in galactosylceramide are confined to globoid cells. Both galactosylceramide and sulfatide levels are almost invariably much lower than normal in the white matter overall.[9,14,15,37,85,167–169,212–220]

A consistent, and perhaps the most important, analytic finding is a large increase in the amount of psychosine, primarily in the white matter but also in other organs.[167–169,221,222] It should be noted that the absolute amounts of psychosine found in the white matter of patients are still very small, approximately two orders of magnitude less than those of galactosylceramide. Even such small amounts are significant, because psychosine is essentially undetectable in normal tissues and because it is highly cytotoxic. These analytic findings provide the strongest evidence in support of the psychosine hypothesis for the pathogenetic mechanism of the disease, which will be discussed later in the "Pathophysiology" section.

Besides the abnormalities of the major glycolipids of white matter–galactosylceramides and sulfatides–lactosylceramide, glucosylceramide, digalactosylglucosyl ceramide, and globoside (N-acetylgalactosaminyl-digalactosylglucosyl ceramide) are significantly increased (refer to the sixth edition for references). These "visceral-type" sphingoglycolipids in white matter are considered intrinsic lipids of globoid cells, which are of mesodermal origin.

Unless specifically eliminated, the abnormal tubular inclusions are isolated in the conventional myelin fraction, giving erroneous analytic results. In one study,[223] the abnormal tubular inclusions were present in an even larger amount than myelin. When they were carefully eliminated, the yield of the myelin was, as expected from histologic findings, only 0.4 percent of normal. The myelin had a normal ultrastructural configuration, and its lipid composition was quite similar to that of normal myelin. In particular, the amounts of glycolipids (cerebrosides and sulfatides) were normal. Thus, in GLD the brain is capable of forming myelin with a normal morphologic appearance and normal chemical composition. However, the amount of myelin present in the white matter of the cerebral hemispheres at the terminal stage is no more than that of a 2- to 3-month-old brain.

Besides these specific chemical abnormalities, white matter in GLD typically shows increased water content and a drastic reduction of proteolipid protein and total lipid content, with a consequent relative, but not absolute, increase in protein. Cholesterol, lecithin, sphingomyelin, and ethanolamine- and serine-phospholipids are all relatively reduced to similar degrees. These findings merely reflect the devastating myelin loss. As expected from the histologic absence of sudanophilia, cholesteryl ester is not present in white matter. In contrast to that of the white matter, the chemical composition of the gray matter is relatively normal.

In keeping with the normal histologic appearance, non-neural tissues do not show conspicuous compositional changes except for the large relative increase in psychosine.[221] Suzuki[224] examined galactosylceramide levels in the kidneys of five patients and found them to be approximately 30 percent higher than normal. Since the glucosylceramide level was similarly high in patients' kidneys, it was concluded that there was no specific abnormal increase of galactosylceramide in the kidney. On the other hand, Dawson reported highly elevated levels of galactosylceramide in the livers of three patients,[225] although the actual amounts were still minute. This finding has been contradicted by a subsequent report.[169]

ENZYMATIC DEFECT

The fundamental genetic defect of GLD is a deficiency of GALC [EC 3.2.1.46] activity.[16,17] This enzyme catalyzes the lysosomal degradation of galactosylceramide to galactose plus ceramide. As expected for the fundamental genetic defect in a Mendelian autosomal recessive disorder, parents of patients with GLD, who are obligate heterozygous carriers, show GALC activity intermediate between that of normal individuals and that of patients, although there is much overlap between carriers and noncarriers due to the wide normal and carrier ranges.[64,226–228] The reasons for the wide range in values will be discussed in the "Diagnosis" section. The deficient activity of this enzyme can also be demonstrated with the other natural substrates psychosine,[21,189] monogalactosyldiglyceride,[191] or lactosylceramide.[192–198,227]

Mammalian tissues contain two genetically distinct lysosomal β-galactosidases, GALC and G_{M1}-ganglioside β-galactosidase (commonly referred to simply as "β-galactosidase"). They have different, although overlapping, substrate specificities. Deficiencies of the respective enzymes result in entirely different disorders because of the different natural substrates involved. GLD is caused by a deficiency of GALC. In the other disease, G_{M1} gangliosidosis, G_{M1} ganglioside β-galactosidase is deficient (Chap. 151). Both β-galactosidases share lactosylceramide as a substrate, and consequently lactosylceramide accumulation does not occur to any significant degree in either GLD or G_{M1} gangliosidosis. It can further be predicted that under these circumstances a specific disorder with accumulation of lactosylceramide probably does not occur in humans.[229] Kobayashi et al.[230] demonstrated that under certain assay conditions, particularly in the presence of sodium cholate, G_{M1}-ganglioside β-galactosidase could also hydrolyze galactosylceramide, but not psychosine. However, purified GALC could hydrolyze both galactosylceramide and psychosine.[24] This complex interrelationship of substrate specificity between the two β-galactosidases is important in understanding the pathogenetic mechanism of Krabbe disease.

PATHOPHYSIOLOGY

If a genetic defect of GALC is the underlying cause of GLD, we should be able to understand the morphologic and biochemical characteristics of the disease on the basis of this deficiency. These include (1) an almost total loss of myelin and oligodendroglia, (2) normal chemical composition of the remaining myelin,[223] (3) morphologic evidence of decrease in the amount of myelin during the illness,[86] (4) massive infiltration by globoid cells, and (5) absence of excess accumulation of galactosylceramide in the brain despite a block in the degradative pathway.

In 1970, Suzuki and Suzuki[16] formulated a plausible hypothesis on the evolution of the disease, based on the two unique features of galactosylceramide: (1) Galactosylceramide is almost exclusively a constituent of myelin and oligodendroglia. (2) Galactosylceramide is unique among sphingoglycolipids in its ability to elicit the globoid cell reaction when injected into normal rat brain.[11–13] According to this hypothesis, the following sequence of steps could occur in the brain of a patient with genetic GALC deficiency. Before myelination, there is practically no galactosylceramide in the brain. Therefore, lack of enzyme activity is of little consequence, although it is normally present at low activity even at the premyelination stage.[180] As soon as myelination begins, just before birth in humans, newly formed myelin begins to undergo normal turnover. This period coincides with a rapid rise of GALC activity in normal brain.[180] In the brains of patients with Krabbe disease, galactosylceramide from catabolized myelin cannot be degraded due to the lack of the enzyme. This undegraded galactosylceramide causes globoid cell infiltration. As myelination proceeds, more undegraded free galactosylceramide accumulates, stimulating more globoid cell infiltration. However, myelination cannot proceed normally, because the oligodendroglial cells disappear rapidly. When the stage of massive death of oligodendroglial cells is reached, rapid myelin breakdown occurs, because myelin is an extension of the oligodendroglial cell membrane. Myelin breakdown contributes more free cerebrosides, and these prompt a further rapid increase in globoid cells. Finally, all the oligodendroglial cells die and all the myelin is broken down. No further increase in the number of globoid cells or galactosylceramide can occur, because there is no longer any cellular source for new galactosylceramide and myelin. Therefore, the total amount of cerebroside that can accumulate in the brain during the short life span of the patient is limited by the small amount of myelin produced before the death of all the oligodendroglial cells, and such total destruction usually takes place at what would normally have been an early stage of myelination.

The unique feature of GLD is the lack of increase in the total galactosylceramide content in the brain despite the genetic defect in its catabolism. In an analogous genetic disorder, MLD, the amount of sulfatide in white matter becomes excessive as a result of defective sulfatide degradation (Chap. 148). The finding by Kobayashi et al.[230] that the other β-galactosidase, G_{M1}-ganglioside β-galactosidase, could also hydrolyze galactosylceramide under specific in vitro assay conditions raised the possibility that galactosylceramide might be catabolized in vivo by both β-galactosidases. This would be consistent with relatively rapid loss of galactosylceramide when it is loaded in cultured fibroblasts from patients with GLD.[228,229] However, the abundance of globoid cells in the white matter clearly indicates that catabolism of galactosylceramide is indeed impaired in vivo, because only free galactosylceramide is capable of inducing the globoid cell reaction.[11–13,233] The early disappearance of the oligodendroglia and the consequent early cessation of myelination therefore still appear to be the only explanation for the lack of abnormally high galactosylceramide accumulation.

Psychosine Hypothesis

In 1972, Miyatake and Suzuki formulated a hypothesis to explain the unusually rapid and complete destruction of the oligodendroglia in GLD.[21] It has become known as the psychosine hypothesis. Psychosine can be formed from UDP-galactose and sphingosine via the action of CGT (Fig. 147-7). Another potential route for psychosine formation — deacylation of galactosylceramide — could not be demonstrated in several laboratories nor by Lin and Radin's study.[234] Psychosine, with its free amino group, is known to be highly cytotoxic.[233,235,236] Psychosine is also a substrate for GALC, and patients with GLD are unable to degrade it. On the other hand, psychosine appears to be a very poor substrate for G_{M1}-ganglioside β-galactosidase.[230] Thus, it is conceivable that psychosine generated within oligodendroglia during the period of active myelination might reach a toxic level. Oligodendroglia are selectively destroyed because psychosine formation occurs primarily in these cells. This hypothesis appears to explain the early destruction of oligodendroglial cells and the resultant cessation of myelination. When analytic data on the tissue levels of psychosine[168,169,221] became available several years after it was proposed, they provided strong support for the hypothesis. In the white matter of human patients with GLD, psychosine was increased up to a hundredfold. In canine, nonhuman primate, and murine models of the disease, similar increases of psychosine were found (see "Animal Models" section).[22,237,238]

Involvement of the peripheral nervous system is expected, for here the myelin sheath also contains galactosylceramide. Histiocytes in peripheral nerves contain abnormal inclusions similar to those in the brain, but it is not clear why they are not transformed to the typical multinucleated globoid cells. The absence of discernible morphologic and functional abnormalities outside the nervous system is understandable, because normally galactosylceramide is practically absent in most non-neural tissues except for the kidney. Either a small amount of residual GALC activity or the action of acid β-galactosidase might be adequate to account for the normal turnover of renal galactosylceramide.

There is a fixed pattern of regional differences in susceptibility of the white matter to pathologic alterations. This question was approached by utilizing the canine GLD model (see "Animal Models" section).[239] In normal dogs, no consistent regional differences were found in GALC activity but in vivo turnover of galactosylceramide appeared to be more rapid in the areas of the white matter that are consistently more severely affected by the disease. Therefore, such regional differences in the metabolic activity of galactosylceramide might be at least partially responsible for the regional differences in the severity of the disease.

The fundamental metabolic defect of GLD corresponds to those in other inherited disorders of sphingolipid metabolism in which lysosomal hydrolytic enzymes involved in the degradation of particular sphingolipids are genetically defective. Of particular interest is the relationship of GLD to Gaucher disease (Chap. 146). The sphingolipid involved in Gaucher disease is glucosylceramide, and the missing enzyme is glucocerebrosidase (glucosylceramidase). Glucosylceramide and galactosylceramide differ only in the sugar moiety, and the missing enzymes are those that cleave these sugars from the respective cerebrosides. The fundamental metabolic derangements in these diseases are therefore quite similar, as are the morphologic appearances of the globoid cells and the Gaucher cells. Nevertheless, the clinical and overall pathologic features of the two diseases are entirely different. These are the consequences of the entirely different tissue distributions of galactosyl- and glucosylceramides. Galactosylceramide is located almost exclusively in the nervous system, while glucosylceramide is normally present in visceral organs and is nearly absent in the normal brain except in the early developmental stages. A massive accumulation of glucosylceramide occurs in systemic organs of Gaucher patients, while GLD is unique among the sphingolipidoses in that the total content of galactosylceramide is not elevated. It is also informative to compare GLD with MLD[240] (Chap. 148). Because galactosylceramide and sulfatide are both highly concentrated in the myelin sheath and because they are next to each other in the synthetic and catabolic pathways, both disorders manifest themselves as classic genetic disorders of myelin. On the other hand, there are several aspects for which the analogy breaks down. There is an abnormal accumulation of sulfatide in the brain, including myelin, in MLD, while, as stressed, the amount of galactosylceramide in the brain is much less than normal in GLD. Loss of the oligodendroglia occurs much earlier and is more complete in infantile GLD. Studies are lacking in adult patients who died with GLD.

MOLECULAR GENETICS

In 1990 Zlotogora et al.[23] mapped the gene for GLD to human chromosome 14 using large informative families and information localizing the gene for the twitcher mouse to chromosome 12.[241] In 1993 the human gene was further localized to region 14q24.3-q32.1 by multipoint linkage analysis.[242] *In situ* hybridization using the GALC cDNA mapped this gene to 14q31.[243] Using N-terminal amino acid sequence information, Chen et al.[25] were able to clone the human GALC cDNA. The cDNA consisted of 3795 bp, including 2007 bp of coding region, 47 bp of 5′ untranslated sequence, and 1741 bp of 3′ untranslated sequence. The coding region encodes a protein consisting of 669 amino acids with six potential glycosylation sites. It also encodes a 26-amino-acid leader sequence. The precursor protein is approximately 80–85 kDa and is processed into 50- to 52-kDa and 30-kDa subunits. The coding sequence for the 50- to 52-kDa subunit is at the 5′ end of the coding region, and the 30-kDa subunit is at the 3′ end. The initiation codon is less than optimum based on the sequences described by Kozak.[244] Sakai et al.[26] also published the cloning of the human GALC cDNA with several nucleotide changes present at polymorphic sites.

In 1995 Luzi et al.[27] described the organization of the human gene encoding GALC. It consists of 17 exons spread over about 56 kb (Fig. 147-9). Other than exons 1 and 17, they ranged in size from 39 to 181 nucleotides. The introns ranged in size from 247 nucleotides in intron 2 to about 12 kb in intron 10. The 200 nucleotides preceding the initiation codon and the 5′ end of intron 1 were very GC-rich, including 13 GGC trinucleotides. A more recent analysis of the 5′ flanking region revealed the presence of a YYI element and one potential SP1 binding site.[245] No consensus TATA box or CAAT box was detected in the 800 nucleotides preceding the initiation. A construct containing nucleotides −176 to −24 had the strongest promoter activity. However, evidence for inhibitory sequences was found just upstream of the promoter region and at the 5′ end of intron 1. Sakai and coworkers[246] also analyzed the human gene, with similar findings, although they did not note the presence of inhibitory elements in the 5′ flanking region. They noted that there was another potential initiation codon located 48 nucleotides upstream of the one previously reported.[25] However, there is no evidence that it is utilized or plays a role in tissue specific expression.

Mutation Analysis

With the nucleotide sequence available, it was possible to start analyzing the mutations in patients with GLD. Figure 147-10 shows the organization of the gene with the known mutations identified. Those on top are missense mutations, and those on the bottom involve deletions and insertions. Many of these mutations were described in a review article written by one of us (D.A.W).[247] Table 147-1 provides additional information about the known mutations. One mutation, called 502T/del, was found to be quite common in patients from northern Europe and the United States, including those with Mexican ancestry.[248,249] A rapid DNA-based test for the large deletion using genomic DNA was developed.[249] A survey conducted in patients within the Dutch population and from other parts of Europe confirmed that the 502T/del mutation makes up about 50 percent of the total mutant alleles.[250] In infant Swedish patients, this mutation makes up 75 percent of the mutant alleles (J-A Mansson and MT Vanier: personal communication).

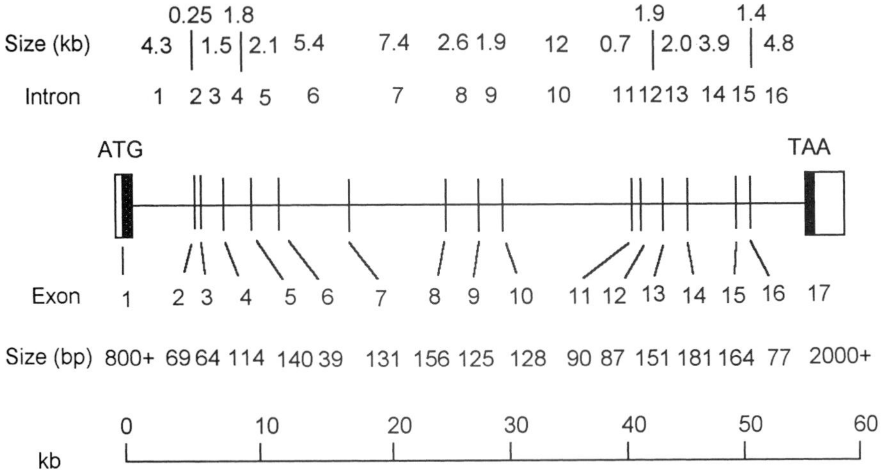

Fig. 147-9 Organization of the human GALC gene showing the 17 exons and 16 introns, and their exact or approximate sizes. The vertical bars represent the exons.

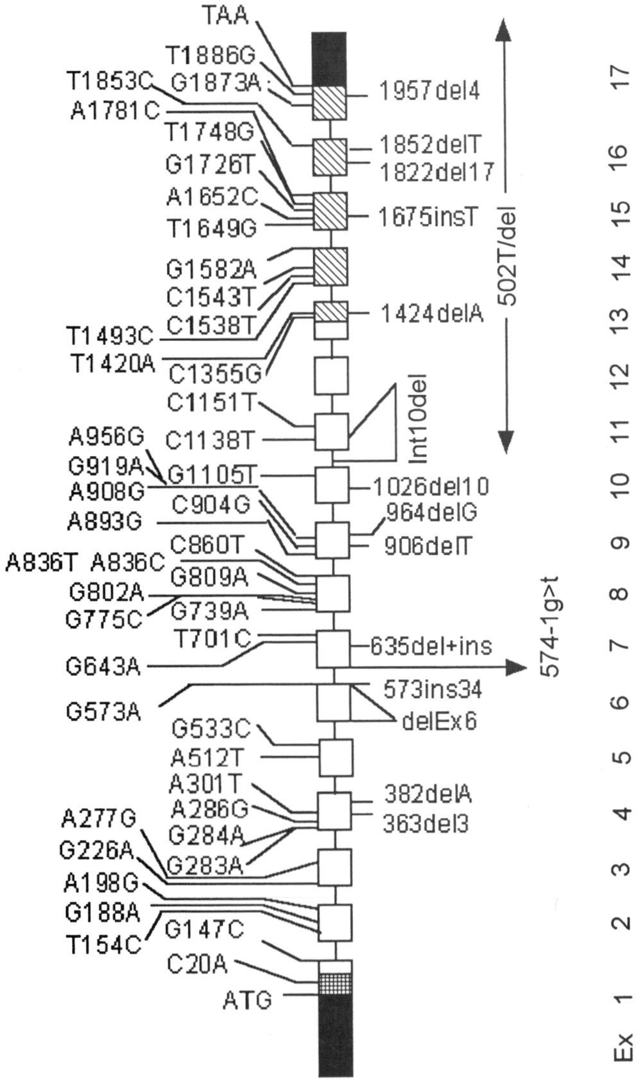

Fig. 147-10 Schematic drawing of the human GALC gene showing the location of the known mutations presented on Table (147-1). The boxes represent the 17 exons, the cross-hatched area denotes the leader peptide, the open areas show the coding region for the 50–52-kDa subunit, the lined areas show the coding region for the 30-kDa subunit, and the dark areas show the 5′ and 3′ untranslated regions. The mutations are usually numbered from the cDNA counting from the A of the initiation codon.

This mutation, consisting of a 30-kb deletion starting near the middle of intron 10 and continuing beyond the end of the gene, is always found with a known polymorphism consisting of a C-to-T transition at cDNA position 502 (counting from the A of the initiation codon), designated C502T. The 30-kb deletion eliminates all of the coding region for the 30-kDa subunit and about 15 percent of the coding region for the 50- to 52-kDa subunit. Some shortened polypeptide may be made through the use of a cryptic polyadenylation sequence located at the 5′ end of intron 10. As expected, all patients homozygous for this mutation have the infantile form of GLD. However, this mutation has been found heterozygous in a significant number of patients with late onset, including adult-onset, GLD. This mutation probably initially occurred in Sweden and traveled from there throughout Europe, Near Asia, and the United States. It has never been detected in Japanese patients.

While no other mutation is found at such high frequency among patients with GLD, a number of other mutations have been found in more than one unrelated family. Two other mutations (a C-to-T transition at nucleotide 1538, designated C1538T, and an A-to-C transversion at nucleotide 1652, designated A1652C), make up an additional 10–15 percent of the mutant alleles in infant patients with European ancestry.[247,250] Two other mutations have been found in unrelated patients and are worthy of comment. The G-to-A transition at nucleotide 809, designated G809A, is quite common among patients with late onset GLD. One of the authors (D.A.W.) has identified three infant patients of Mexican heritage who are heterozygous for one allele consisting of two changes, 1424delA plus a G-to-A transition at nucleotide 1873, designated G1873A. Kolodny et al.[251] reported only the G1873A mutation in a woman who died at age 73 with GLD. It is unknown whether the 1424delA mutation, which results in a frameshift and a premature stop codon, was present in that individual or whether the G1873A alone would cause the disease. Since the other allele in that older woman is G809A, it is probable that the presence of one copy of the G809A mutation would be enough to explain the relatively mild phenotype.

Within certain populations, some mutations have been found in more than one family. Three mutations (635del + ins; an A-to-G transition at nucleotide 198, designated A198G; and a T-to-C transition at nucleotide 1853, designated T1853C) have been found in more than one unrelated Japanese patient.[65,99,252] In Israel there are two populations with an extremely high carrier rate for Krabbe disease,[253] and they have different mutations.[254] All infant patients in the Druze population in northern Israel are homozygous for the T-to-G transversion at nucleotide 1748 (an Ile to Ser mutation at codon 583, designated I583S), and patients from a Moslem village near Jerusalem are homozygous for the G-to-A transition at nucleotide 1582 (an Asp to Asn mutation at codon

Table 147-1 Mutations[a] Found in Patients with Globoid Cell Leukodystrophy

Number	Mutation Designation	Location	cDNA Position	Base Change	Effect	Polymorphic Background[b]	Second Allele	Comments	Reference
1.	C20A	Ex1	20	TCG → TAG	S7X	502T, 1637C	#11	Adult	Luzi et al., (U)
2.	G147C	Ex1	147	GGG → GGC	G49G, missplicing	1637C	#8	Adult, Black	66, 257
3.	T154C	Ex2	154	TCC → CCC	S52P		Homo	Infantile, Arab	Rafi et al., (U)
4.	G188A	Ex2	188	CGT → CAT	R63H	1637C	#40	Adult	32, 257
5.	A198G	Ex2	198	ATA → ATG	I66M	865G	Homo	Adult, Japanese	65
6.	G226A	Ex2	226	GGT → GAT	G76D	1637C (het)[c]	#34	German	91, Rafi et al., (U)
7.	A277G	Ex3	277	ACA → GCA	T93A	1637C (het)[c]	#28	Infantile, Portuguese	Rafi et al., (U)
8.	G283A	Ex4	283	GGC → AGC	G95S	?	?		251
9.	G284A	Ex4	284	GGC → GAC	G95D	694A	#40, 45, 59	Mexican	251, Rafi et al., (U)
10.	A286G	Ex4	286	ACT → GCT	T96A	694A, 1637C	#14	Adult	62
11.	A301T	Ex4	301	ATG → TTG	M101L	1637C	#1	Adult	Luzi et al., (U)
12.	363del3	Ex4	363–365	GCTAAG → GCG	K122del	694A	#55	Greek	Rafi et al., (U)
13.	382delA	Ex4	382	ATATTA → ATTTA	FS, PS	502T, 1637C	#26	#53 on same allele, low mRNA	Rafi et al., (U)
14.	A512T	Ex5	512	GAT → GTT	D171V	502T, 1637C	#10	Adult	62
15.	G533C	Ex5	533	GGA → GCA	G178A		?	Mexican	Rafi et al., (U)
16.	535 del39	Ex6	535–573 del	del39nt	Skip Ex6	1637C	#58	Adult, Japanese	65
17.	G573A	Ex6	573	AAG → AAA	K191K, splicing error?[d]	1637C	Homo	Infantile, Portuguese	Rafi et al., (U)
18.	573ins34	Ex6	573	ins34nt from intron?[d]	FS, PS	1637C	#8	Late infantile	257
19.	574 − 1g → t	Int6	574 − 1	aagATA → aatATA	Loss of splice acceptor, del 8 bp Ex7, FS, PS	1637C	#40	Infantile, Mexican, #56 on same allele	Rafi et al., (U)
20.	635del+ins	Ex7	635	del of 12+ins 3	del 5 amino acid+ins 2	?	Homo	Infantile, Japanese	252
21.	G643A[e]	Ex7	643	GAG → AAG	E215K	1637C	#40	Juvenile, Indian	257
22.	T701C	Ex7	701	ATA → ACA	I234T		Homo	Late infantile, Greek	Rafi et al., (U)
23.	G739A	Ex8	739	GCA → ACA	A247T	1637C	#40		Rafi et al., (U)
24.	G775C	Ex8	775	GAC → CAC	D259H	694A	#40	Infantile	Rafi et al., (U)
25.	G802A	Ex8	802	GGT → AGT	G268S	?	?		251
26.	G809A	Ex8	809	GGC → GAC	G270D	1637C	Homo, #13, 40, 59		65, 251, Rafi et al., (U)
27.	A836C	Ex8	836	AAT → ACT	N279T		#40	Dutch	Rafi et al., (U)
28.	A836T	Ex8	836	AAT → ATT	N279I	1637C (het)[c]	#7	Infantile, Portugese	Rafi et al., (U)
29.	C860T	Ex8	860	TCC → TTC	S287F	1637C	Homo	Infantile, Saudi Arabian	Rafi et al., (U)
30.	A893G	Ex9	893	TAT → TGT	Y298C	1637C	#40	Infantile	257
31.	C904G	Ex9	904	CCT → GCT	P302A	?	?	Late infantile, Japanese	252
32.	906delT	Ex9	906	CTTATG → CTATG	FS, PS	1637C	?		Rafi et al., (U)
33.	A908G	Ex9	908	TAT → TGT	Y303C	694A	#40	Indian	Rafi et al., (U)
34.	G919A	Ex9	919	GGG → AGG	G307R	1637C (het)[c]	#6	German	91, Rafi et al., (U)
35.	A956G	Ex9	956	TAC → TGC	Y319C	694A	#40		Rafi et al., (U)
36.	964delG	Ex9	964	TAGAAT → TAAAT	FS, PS	1637C	#40		Rafi et al., (U)
37.	1026del10	Ex10	1026	del10nt	FS, PS		#51	Italian	Rafi et al., (U)

38.	G1105T	Ex10	1105	GAA → TAA	E369X	?	?		26
39.	Int10del	Int10/Ex11	1113+262	del in Int10 and 26 bp Ex11	?		#40		Rafi et al., (U)
40.	502T/del	Int10/end	1113+6532	del30 kb	short mRNA	502T	Homo, #4, 9, 19, 21, 23, 24, 26, 27, 30, 33, 35, 36, 39, 41, 43, 45, 47, 48, 51, 52, 56, 59	Infantile, Northern European origin, Mexican	248
41.	C1138T	Ex11	1138	CGG → TGG	R380W		Homo, #40	Infantile	Rafi et al., (U)
42.	C1151T	Ex11	1151	CCT → CTT	P384L	1637C	?		Rafi et al., (U)
43.	C1355G	Ex13	1355	ACT → AGT	T452S	694A	#40	#52 on same allele	Rafi et al., (U)
44.	T1420A	Ex13	1420	TAT → AAT	Y474N	1637C	?		Rafi et al., (U)
45.	1424delA	Ex13	1424	ATAAGG → ATAGG	FS, PS	1637C	#9, 40	Mexican, #59 on same allele	Rafi et al., (U)
46.	T1493C	Ex14	1493	TTT → TCT	F498S	694A	#47		Rafi et al., (U)
47.	C1538T	Ex14	1538	ACG → ATG	T513M	694A	Homo, #40, 46	Infantile, Northern European	Rafi et al., (U)
48.	C1543T	Ex14	1543	CGC → TGC	R515C	1637C	#40	Finnish	Rafi et al., (U)
49.	G1582A	Ex14	1582	GAT → AAT	D528N	1637C	Homo	Infantile, Israeli Arab	254
50.	T1649G	Ex15	1649	GTT → GGT	V550G	?	Homo	Non-Japanese	252
51.	A1652C	Ex15	1652	TAC → TCC	Y551S	1637C	Homo, #37, 40	Infantile, European	Rafi et al., (U)
52.	1675insT	Ex15	1675/1676	GGT → GTGT	FS, PS	694A	#40	#43 on same allele	Rafi et al., (U)
53.	G1726T	Ex15	1726	GCC → TCC	A576S	502T, 1637C	#26	#13 on same allele	Rafi et al., (U)
54.	T1748G	Ex15	1748	ATT → AGT	I583S		Homo	Infantile, Israeli Druze	254
55.	A1781C	Ex15	1781	GAT → GCT	D594A		#12	Greek	Rafi et al., (U)
56.	1822del17	Ex 16	1822	del of 17 nt	FS, PS	1637C	#40	Mexican, #19 on same allele	Rafi et al., (U)
57.	1852delT	Ex16	1852	TTAACT → TAACT	L618X		?	Mexican	Rafi et al., (U)
58.	T1853C	Ex16	1853	TTA → TCA	L618S	865G, 1637C	Homo, #16	Adult, Japanese	65, 99
59.	G1873A	Ex17	1873	GCC → ACC	A625T		#9, 26, 40	#45 on same allele[f]	251, Rafi et al., (U)
60.	T1886G	Ex17	1886	CTG → CGG	L629R		Homo	Adult	Rafi et al., (U)
61.	1957del4	Ex17	1957	del4nt	FS, PS	1637C	Homo	Infantile, Portuguese	Rafi et al., (U)

[a]In some cases more than one mutation (excluding polymorphisms) was found on the same allele.
[b]Only the least common nucleotide is shown for the following polymorphisms: C502T, G694A, A865G, and T1637C.
[c]In some cases (because only genomic DNA was available), assignment of the polymorphism to one or the other allele was not possible.
[d]It is probable that mutations #17 and #18 are the same, and that #18 results from abnormal splicing due to the nucleotide change at the 3′-end of exon 6.
[e]This may not be a disease-causing mutation, since expression studies showed significant GALC activity.[257]
[f]It is questionable whether this is a disease-causing mutation, as 1424delA (#45) is found on the same allele in all of the patients examined by one of the authors (D.A.W.). The 1424 delA mutation was not reported by De Gasperi et al.[257]
Abbreviations: Ex = exon, Int = intron, del = deletion, ins = insertion, nt = nucleotide(s), FS = frameshift, PS = premature stop codon, bp = base pair(s), homo = homozygous , U = unpublished.

528, designated D528N). Carrier testing based on the identification of the mutation in these populations has been offerred to interested individuals. Over 60 disease-causing mutations have been described (Table 147-1). It is obvious that both subunits are necessary for activity. Polymorphisms in this gene have also been found, and they play a significant role in producing the wide range of GALC values measured in the general population and the family members of affected individuals. Polymorphisms may also play a role in the development of clinical disease when inherited in multiple copies, on the same allele with another mutation, or together with a known disease-causing mutation on the other chromosome.

One mutation is worth some discussion, since it has been found to be either homozygous or heterozygous in a significant number of patients with later onset GLD.[65,247,251] In fact, one copy of this mutation, even when found together with a very severe second mutation, will result in a less severe phenotype. The G to A transition at nucleotide position 809 (D270N) has been found in later onset patients with European and Japanese ancestry. So far, all non-Japanese patients with this mutation also have a T1637C polymorphism on the same allele. This important fact was not mentioned in the paper of Furuya et al.,[65] who reported the only patient homozygous for this mutation. Their patient was from a consanguineous mating and presented with spastic gait in the second decade. Although the presence of the G809A mutation does indicate an onset of disease after the typical infantile period, it does not predict a characteristic phenotype. In fact, within families having more than one patient with the identical genotype, involving at least one copy of the G809A mutation, there can be a very wide range of clinical presentations. In two unrelated families with a total of five patients, having G809A on one allele and 502T/del on the other allele, the symptoms vary from significant neurologic impairment and mental retardation within the first decade to normal intelligence and only mild spastic paraparesis noted in the second or third decade. This clearly points to the role of other genetic and/or environmental factors in the clinical presentation of the later onset forms of GLD. A number of reports have described the onset of symptoms in older individuals within weeks after documented systemic infection or a blow to the head.[33,39,59,91]

Polymorphisms

As discussed earlier, there is a very wide range of GALC values in the "normal" population and among obligate heterozygotes.[64,226,255,256] This makes enzyme-based carrier testing in the general population almost impossible. Also, there are normal individuals, including obligate heterozygotes, who have quite low GALC activity in their leukocytes and cultured skin fibroblasts.[64,226,255,256] The polymorphic mutations that result in amino acid changes are shown in Table 147-2. While the C502T polymorphism was found in the non-Japanese population,[248] an A865G polymorphism was reported only in the Japanese population.[65,99] Expression of these mutations using COS-1 cells has demonstrated that they do result in less GALC activity than the most common genotype (Table 147-2). It has been observed by several groups that these polymorphisms occur on the same alleles as disease-causing mutations in a higher-than-expected percentage of cases.[247,250,257] In fact, some "disease-causing" mutations may be deleterious only when the polymorphism is present on the same allele. Furuya et al.[65] demonstrated by expression studies that the A198G mutation (I66M) resulted in low GALC activity only when A865G was present. The "late onset" mutation, G809A, occurs on the 1637C background, and expression studies (M.A. Rafi and D.A. Wenger, unpublished) show that there is significantly less GALC activity when the mutation is on the 1637C background. It is unclear why these polymorphisms occur together with so many disease-causing mutations.

It has also been observed by one of us (D.A.W.) that a significant number of individuals with partially low GALC activity (15–35 percent of normal) have clinical and MRI evidence of white matter disease. The age of onset, type of symptoms, and clinical course can vary greatly. PCR-based mutation analysis of the GALC gene in more than 100 such patients revealed that most have three or more polymorphic changes in the GALC gene.[247,258] In addition, all coding regions and exon-intron boundaries of six such individuals have been sequenced, with no other mutations detected. While the significance of these findings is not proven, it does raise the possibility that a certain amount of GALC activity is required for maintenance of stable myelin. However, at least two other factors must be kept in mind regarding this hypothesis. GALC activity measured in vitro, even with natural substrate, may not be indicative of in vivo activity, and other genetic or environmental factors may play a significant role in the phenotype observed. Definitive proof for this hypothesis is lacking at this time.

Table 147-2 Polymorphisms in the GALC Gene that Result in Amino Acid Changes

Nucleotide Change	Amino Acid Change	Expression[a]	Estimate of Minor Allele Frequency
C502T	R168C	80–90%	4–5%
G694A	D224N	60–70%	8–10%
A865G	I289V	80–90%[b]	?
T1637C	I546T	30–40%	40–45%
C502T/T1637C[c]	R168C/I546T	10–20%	< 2%

[a]Expression after transfection of COS-1 cells as a percentage of activity obtained with the most common allele.
[b]An estimate based on the information published by Furuya et al.[65]
[c]Both on the same allele.

As stated earlier, enzyme-based carrier testing in the general population is nearly impossible. However, carrier testing is possible in children of obligate heterozygotes, since the contribution of each allele is additive.[23,64] Also, carrier testing of individuals related to a molecularly characterized patient is relatively simple in a qualified laboratory. However, this does not help to identify carrier status in an unrelated individual who plans to have a child with a known carrier. Due to the large number of mutations already identified, mutation-based carrier testing of the general population is not feasible, except within certain inbred populations, such as the Israeli Druze and Arab populations.[254]

Gene Therapy Model Systems

With the availability of the GALC gene and cDNA, it was possible to begin preliminary studies to evaluate delivery of GALC activity to deficient cells by several methods. Two publications have described the retroviral transfer of GALC cDNA to cultured cells from human and animal models.[259,260] Transduced cultured skin fibroblasts from patients with Krabbe disease can reach very high levels of GALC activity (100 times normal), and, more important, these cells were able to secrete GALC that was rapidly and efficiently taken up by neighboring cells.[260] This could provide a mechanism for the treatment of patients through the transplantation of cells, such as hematopoietic stem cells, that can be removed from the patient and successfully transduced by a retroviral vector containing GALC cDNA. In addition to cultured skin fibroblasts, other cell types, such as rat and mouse brain astrocytes, CD34+ hematopoietic cells, twitcher mouse brain oligodendrocytes and astrocytes,[261] and mouse myoblasts, have also been transduced and produce high levels of GALC activity that can be exported and taken up by other cells. The uptake of this hydrophobic enzyme by other cells appears to be mostly by a non-mannose-6-phosphate-mediated mechanism.[260] This could be an important finding, since many neural cells are not rich in mannose-6-phosphate receptors. Very recently, human GALC cDNA was placed in several adeno-associated viral vectors and simian virus (SV40) in attempts to develop delivery systems for in vivo gene therapy. These studies are still under preliminary investigation. A transgenic mouse with the human GALC cDNA driven by the myelin basic protein promoter was developed to ensure high expression in the oligodendrocyte lineage.[262] Mice heterozygous for this mutation were mated with carriers of the twitcher mutation to develop mice heterozygous for both the twitcher mutation and the transgene. Further matings resulted in mice homozygous for the twitcher mutation and either homozygous or hemizygous for the transgene. Enzymatic expression of the GALC transgene was low, but there was evidence that the mice with two copies of the GALC gene weighed more and lived longer than mice without the transgene. There was evidence for less severe pathology and slower accumulation of psychosine in the mice with two copies of the transgene. Eventually, all the mice died with pathology similar to that of the untreated twitcher mice. While this experiment was not a great success, it does indicate that low levels of GALC activity supplied to the necessary tissues can have a positive effect. Bone marrow transplantation is the only method of treatment currently in use in human patients, but it is probable that some patients in the near future will have enzyme supplied to nervous tissues by novel approaches, including gene therapy and neural cell transplantation.

DIAGNOSIS

Brain biopsy had long been the final resort for the definitive antemortem diagnosis of GLD since Blackwood and Cumings[7] emphasized the presence of the characteristic globoid cells. The diagnostic value of peripheral nerve biopsy has not been fully explored, but in view of consistent pathologic changes, particularly on the ultrastructural level, it can be useful. Typical inclusions may be found in eccrine sweat gland epithelial cells.[127] Enzymatic diagnosis, made possible by the identification of the underlying genetic defect in 1970, superseded these invasive measures as the preferred means of diagnosis.

Assays of GALC activity in peripheral leukocytes or cultured fibroblasts offer the best and most reliable means of definitive antemortem diagnosis of GLD. Leukocytes and cultured fibroblasts are equally reliable, with the former having a clear advantage in the rapidity with which the diagnosis can be established after the specimen is obtained. The same assay is also useful for prenatal diagnosis of affected fetuses, using cultured amniotic fluid cells or biopsied chorionic villi as the enzyme source. The first prenatal detection of the disease and confirmation of the diagnosis by histologic examination and by additional enzymatic assays on the fetal specimens was accomplished in 1970, within a few months of the identification of the enzymatic defect.[20,161] Enzymatic diagnosis with the natural lipid substrate requires care, and it is advisable that the procedure be done in laboratories experienced with the assay.

Because of the broad specificity of GALC, other natural substrates can, in principle, also be used for enzymatic diagnosis of GLD. Psychosine[21,188–190] or monogalactosyl-diglyceride[191] does not provide a practical advantage, however, over the original assay for galactosylceramide hydrolysis. The enzyme is more active toward lactosylceramide,[227] but caution must attend use of this substrate for diagnosis of GLD. Since both of the lysosomal β-galactosidases can hydrolyze lactosylceramide,[194] one must use an assay system that determines exclusively the lactosylceramide-hydrolyzing activity of GALC. The procedure developed by Wenger et al.[227] is excellent for this purpose. When appropriate precautions are taken, G_{M1}-ganglioside β-galactosidase is essentially inactive toward lactosylceramide.[197,263] Conditions of assays with natural sphingolipid substrates have been carefully examined in several laboratories.[198,227,230,232,255,256,264,265–270]

With the currently available assay procedures using the natural substrates, there is no consistent difference in residual GALC activity between the classic infantile form and the late onset form. Although profound deficiency of GALC activity is almost always diagnostic for GLD, Wenger et al.[271] found very low GALC activity in several older healthy individuals. The significance of this finding in relation to the pathogenetic mechanism of the disease is unclear, but it must be kept in mind when enzymatic diagnosis is attempted. While it is a very rare occurrence, some families may require additional studies, such as a substrate-loading test in cultured skin fibroblasts.[272]

Over 1000 at-risk pregnancies have been monitored for GLD worldwide since 1970. Earlier, the prenatal diagnosis was done exclusively on cultured amniotic fluid cells. In recent years, biopsied chorionic villi have become the preferred tissue source for prenatal diagnosis. Before prenatal diagnosis is attempted, it is ideal to obtain GALC values for the parents to be sure that one of them is not low enough to cause problems with interpretation of the resulting GALC activity. Without appropriate information on the parents, there is a risk of diagnosing a carrier fetus as being affected when the normal allele has low activity due to the presence of one or more polymorphism. Of course, with the identification of mutations in many patients, prenatal diagnosis can be done by DNA analysis of a fetal sample. While this has been done in a number of pregnancies in the laboratory of one of the authors (D.A.W.), it has no real advantage over enzyme-based testing for the typical at-risk couple.

Assay of GALC activity can be useful for the identification of carriers within a family. For example, knowing the leukocyte GALC values in both heterozygous parents of a patient can make carrier testing in other offspring relatively simple in a skilled laboratory. As stated earlier, there is a large amount of overlap between the "normal" range and the carrier range. Carrier detection is inherently less reliable than diagnosis of affected patients.[226,255,256] The presence of polymorphic amino acid changes is the cause of the wide range of values measured. A large series of data has often suggested a bimodal distribution of the "normal" activity.[64,194] With the cloning of the GALC gene and identification of disease-causing and polymorphic changes, the reason for this variability is obvious.[247] While all carriers of GLD are clinically normal, there may be some evidence that subtle neurophysiological changes could be detected with careful analysis.[273,274] While studies on human heterozygotes are exceedingly difficult to control, a recent neurologic and neurobehavioral study on carriers in the murine model of the disease[275] raises a similar question.

TREATMENT

At this time the treatment options for patients with GLD are limited to hematopoietic stem cell transplantation in certain individuals who either have slowly progressive later onset forms of GLD or are diagnosed before neurologic symptoms are obvious (as occurs in some families who have prenatal testing and elect not to terminate an affected fetus or in which the diagnosis is made at birth because of family history). The recent publication of Krivit and coworkers[276] describes the successful stabilization and possible improvement in the clinical picture of four later onset patients followed for up to 9 years post transplantation. There was a lowering of the CSF protein level and an improvement in the MRI, with evidence of remyelination. One patient who had a transplant at 2 months of age is doing well and at 2 years of age is neurologically normal except for some nystagmus. An affected sib died at 13 months of age. In addition, three fetuses predicted to be affected with GLD by CVS testing at 9 weeks of age were given *in utero* bone marrow transplantation using the father as the donor.[277] The first fetus died at about 20 gestational weeks, but examination of the fetal tissues revealed significant engraftment of the donor T-cell-depleted, CD34+- selected cells. As it was postulated that too many donor cells were injected in the first case, one-thousandth the number of cells were used in the two subsequent pregnancies (Karin Blakemore, personal communication). Unfortunately, there was little, if any, engraftment detected at birth in the newborns. Both will receive postnatal transplantation of hematopoietic stem cells. Improvements in the isolation of transplantable hematopoietic stem cells from cord blood, peripheral blood, and bone marrow have improved the chances of finding a suitable donor for patients considered candidates for transplantation. Unfortunately, about 85–90 percent of patients identified with GLD are infants with significant neurologic impairment at the time of laboratory diagnosis. Only supportive care can be given to patients diagnosed too late for hematopoietic stem cell transplantation. There is mounting evidence that only a small increase in GALC activity may be needed to cause a significant improvement in clinical outcome. Future studies involving transplantation of neural cells and direct infection of the brain with viral vectors containing the GALC gene are planned with animal models.

ANIMAL MODELS

GLD caused by genetic deficiency of GALC activity also occurs in a number of animal models, including the mouse, the sheep, several breeds of dog, and the rhesus monkey.[278–286] The disease in the cat was not characterized enzymatically.[287] The clinical and pathologic features are similar to those of the human disease. At this time, twitcher mice, Cairn and West Highland White terriers, and rhesus monkeys have been studied in the most detail and are available for research.

Canine GLD

In 1963, Fankhäuser et al.[286] first reported that GLD occurs in certain strains of dogs. The disease, which has been studied extensively from the clinical, morphologic, and biochemical standpoints,[238,239,288–311] is transmitted as an autosomal recessive trait. The clinical and pathologic pictures are generally quite similar to those in the human disease. Characteristic inclusions have been documented in the kidneys of the affected dogs.[306] Consistent with the presence of inclusions, galactosylceramide levels were moderately increased in the kidney (K. Suzuki, unpublished). As in the case of human disease, the deficiency in GALC activity[307–310,312] and the progressive accumulation of psychosine in the brain[22,238] have been demonstrated in these affected dogs. In 1993, Victoria et al.[312] cloned the canine GALC cDNA and determined the mutation causing GLD in Cairn and West Highland White terriers. An A-to-C transversion at nucleotide 473 (Y158S) is the disease-causing mutation in these breeds. A rapid PCR-based test for this mutation has resulted in a North American screening program to identify carriers in these breeds. In turn, this has resulted in the establishment of a colony of carrier dogs for research at the University of Pennsylvania School of Veterinary Medicine. Affected dogs from this colony will be used to evaluate treatment options, as a step between studies in twitcher mice and in human patients. Treatment of these dogs can be followed by MRI, as is that of human patients.[313]

Recently, a number of affected Irish setters from one litter were found to have very low GALC activity (P. Carmichael and D.A. Wenger, unpublished). Sequencing has identified the disease-causing mutation as an insertion of 78 nucleotides at cDNA position 790, which results in missplicing (M.A. Rafi, P. Carmichael, D.A. Wenger, unpublished). A rapid screening test for that mutation has been developed, and more carrier dogs have been identified. A colony of these dogs will be established at the University of Georgia College of Veterinary Medicine. Other dogs have sporadically been reported to have GALC deficiency,[283,284] but these are not established as a usable colony.

Murine GLD (Twitcher)

A genetically and enzymatically authentic murine model of human GLD, known as twitcher (twi), was first detected at the Jackson Laboratory, Bar Harbor, Maine. The disease in this model is an autosomal recessive disorder, and the gene has been mapped to mouse chromosome 12.[241] Affected mice develop clinical signs at approximately 20 days, with stunted growth, twitching, and hind leg weakness. By 40 days, they reach a near-terminal stage, and even with intensive maintenance care they die before 3 months. Histopathologic findings are similar to those of human and canine GLD, both by light and electron microscopy.[314–316] Enzymatic studies with galactosylceramide and lactosylceramide as the substrates unequivocally demonstrated that GALC deficiency is the underlying lesion in this mutant.[317,318] As research tools, the canine and murine models offer complementary advantages and disadvantages. The canine model is more suitable for experiments that require relatively large amounts of tissue or dissection of different regions. On the other hand, the small size, rapid reproduction, and ease of maintenance of the mouse model make it far more convenient for experiments that require a large number of affected or heterozygous animals and for in vivo injection of isotopes. The genetic status of individual mice can be conveniently and reliably determined by GALC assays or DNA analysis using small samples of the tail tip within a day of birth.[319,320] This permits morphologic and biochemical studies of the disease process during the early critical period, well before the clinical onset of the disease.

While the pathologic findings of the brain and peripheral nerves are similar to those in human and canine disease,[314–316,321–326] one unique pathologic feature in the twitcher mouse is the abundant presence of the characteristic inclusions in the lymph nodes and kidney.[327,328] This is consistent with biochemical analyses, which demonstrated a massive accumulation of galactosylceramide in the kidneys of affected mice, in contrast to the case in human disease.[329,330] Chronologic quantitative analyses of the central and peripheral nervous systems have shown that early myelination proceeds normally but a brief period of hypomyelination and then demyelination follow.[322,323,331–335] However, the characteristic inclusions were already noted at day 5 in the Schwann cells and oligodendroglia, prior to morphologic evidence of demyelination or infiltration of macrophages.[325,332,333] As the disease progresses, the tissue level of psychosine increases dramatically in both the brain[22,333] and peripheral nerves.[331] The peripheral nerves of twitcher mice are abnormally thick, with marked endoneurial edema.[324,332,336] A role for immunologic involvement in the pathology of murine GLD has been demonstrated.[337–342] In a series of studies, Suzuki and coworkers[136,337,338] demonstrated a marked increase in Mac-1 immunopositive microglia/macrophages and major histocompatibility complex class II antigen (Ia) expressing cells at the early stages of the demyelinating process. Twitcher mice with the Ia− background (produced by mating twitcher and Ia− heterozygotes) had less severe lesions, which correlated with significantly fewer microglia/macrophages.[339] There was also less twitching in the Ia− homozygous twitcher mice. The major histocompatibility complex I antigen[340] and cytokines such as TNF-α and IL-6[341] have also been implicated in the development and progression of pathologic changes in twitcher mice. Psychosine inhibition of protein kinase C has been postulated to interfere with signal transduction and Schwann cell proliferation.[342] In addition, expression of CGT (the enzyme involved in the synthesis of galactosylceramide and psychosine) was suppressed early in the disease process.[343] The mechanism for this is not yet known.

The twitcher mouse is uniquely suited for exploration of possible routes for treatment of genetic neurologic diseases. Many reports are available on therapeutic effects of nerve grafts,[344–346] bone marrow transplantation,[347–355] and enzyme replacement with a nonmammalian β-galactosidase utilizing liposomes.[356] Increased life span, accompanied by an increase in GALC activity and a decrease in the psychosine level, has been consistently reported with bone marrow transplantation. However, all the mice died with characteristic pathologic changes. In an attempt to improve the delivery of GALC to the brain, Huppes et al.[355] transplanted hematopoietic stem cells together with intracerebral transplantation of fetal brain cells. The transplanted affected mice lived longer than untreated affected mice. The recent study utilizing a twitcher mouse with very low expression of human GALC, supplied by mating with a transgenic mouse expressing human GALC, resulted in some improvement of certain parameters but limited usefulness in the treatment of human GLD.[262] Additional references related to twitcher mice can be found in the seventh edition of this book. Two more reviews may be useful.[357,358]

Rhesus Monkey Globoid-Cell Leukodystrophy

In 1989, Baskin and coworkers[282] described pathologic findings consistent with a diagnosis of globoid cell leukodystrophy in an 11-week-old rhesus monkey. Paternity had not been determined, and a number of matings over a period of several years did not produce another affected monkey. In 1994, a more serious attempt to identify carriers by measurement of GALC activity was made, and a number of suspected male and female carriers were identified. An attempt to identify the disease-causing mutation using RNA from the obligate carrier mother was not successful. Subsequent matings produced two affected monkeys, as determined by their very low GALC activity in leukocytes and cultured skin fibroblasts. Sequencing of the GALC cDNA identified the mutation causing the low GALC activity.[359] A deletion of nucleotides A and C at positions 387 and 388 in exon 4 was found. This results in a frameshift and stop codon after 46 nucleotides. Molecular screening of 45 monkeys in the colony resulted in the identification of 22 carriers. While both affected monkeys appeared normal at birth, one rapidly lost weight and developed volitional tremors, and was euthanized. The other monkey continued to nurse but became uncoordinated and hypertonic. That monkey developed volitional tremors at 92 days of age and had severely decreased nerve conduction velocities in all motor nerves tested. The monkey was euthanized at 158 days of age;[237] pathologic evaluation revealed enlarged, firm peripheral nerves. The cerebrum, cerebellum, and spinal cord tract were heavily infiltrated with PAS-positive multinucleated globoid cells and smaller mononucleated PAS-positive macrophages. A severe lack of myelin was also noted. Changes in the peripheral nerves were also observed, including a decrease in nerve fibers and in myelin sheaths around them. While there were some inflammatory cells between nerve fibers, no globoid cells were observed. Lipid analysis of the brains revealed that there was a very large increase in the amount of pyschosine in the white matter of the affected monkeys, which increased with the age.[237] There was an overall decrease in the level of galactosylceramide and other lipids associated with myelin; however, the galactosylceramide/sulfatide ratio was normal. The lipid profile of the gray matter appeared to be normal. The kidney from the older affected monkey showed a very high amount of psychosine, compared to undetectable levels in a control monkey. These studies confirm that the rhesus monkey is an excellent model for evaluating treatment procedures. Fifteen pregnancies have occurred within this colony, including some between two carriers, and all have been monitored using molecular techniques to identify the two-nucleotide deletion using chorionic villus samples. While no affected fetuses were detected, all predictions based on the molecular tests were confirmed after birth using blood samples. This will permit the institution of treatment in affected monkeys either *in utero* or immediately after birth.

REFERENCES

1. Krabbe K: A new familial, infantile form of diffuse brain sclerosis. *Brain* **39**:74, 1916.
2. Bullard WN, Southard EE: Diffuse gliosis of the cerebral white matter in a child. *J Nerv Ment Dis* **33**:188, 1906.
3. Beneke R: Ein Fall hochgradigster ausgedehnter Sklerose des Zentralnervensystems. *Arch Kinderheilkd* **47**:420, 1908.
4. Collier J, Greenfield JG: The encephalitis periaxialis of Schilder: A clinical and pathological study with an account of two cases, one of which was diagnosed during life. *Brain* **47**:489, 1924.
5. Hallervorden J: Eine Speicherungshistiocytose des kindlichen Gehirns (Gauchersche Krankheit?). *Verh Dtsch Ges Pathol* **32**:96, 1948.
6. Austin JH: Studies in globoid (Krabbe) leukodystrophy. II. Controlled thin-layer chromatographic studies of globoid body fractions in seven patients. *J Neurochem* **10**:921, 1963.
7. Blackwood W, Cumings JN: A histochemical and chemical study of three cases of diffuse cerebral sclerosis. *J Neurol Neurosurg Psychiatry* **17**:33, 1954.
8. Diezel PB: Histochemische Untersuchungen an den Globoidzellen der familiären infantilen diffusen Sklerose vom Typus Krabbe. *Virchows Arch [Pathol Anat]* **327**:206, 1955.
9. Diezel PB: Histochemical investigation of degenerative diffuse sclerosis (leucodystrophy and diffuse sclerosis of the Krabbe type), in Cumings JN, Lowenthal A (eds): *Cerebral Lipidoses: A Symposium*. Springfield, Ill., Thomas, 1957, p 52.
10. Stammler A: Klinik, Pathologie und Histochemie der infantilen diffusen Sklerose vom Typus Krabbe. *Dtsch Z Nervenheilkd* **174**:505, 1956.
11. Austin J, Lehfeldt D, Maxwell W: Experimental "globoid bodies" in white matter and chemical analysis in Krabbe's disease. *J Neuropathol Exp Neurol* **20**:284, 1961.
12. Austin JH, Lehfeldt D: Studies in globoid (Krabbe) leucodystrophy. III. Significance of experimentally produced globoid-like elements in rat white matter and spleen. *J Neuropathol Exp Neurol* **24**:265, 1965.
13. Olsson R, Sourander P, Svennerholm L: Experimental studies on the pathogenesis of leucodystrophies. I. The effect of intracerebrally injected sphingolipids in the rat brain. *Acta Neuropathol* (Berlin) **6**:153, 1966.
14. Austin JH: Recent studies in the metachromatic and globoid body forms of diffuse sclerosis, in Folch-Pi J, Bauer H (eds): *Brain Lipids and Lipoproteins, and the Leucodystrophies*. Amsterdam, Elsevier, 1963, p 120.
15. Svennerholm L: Some aspects of biochemical changes in leucodystrophy, in Folch-Pi J, Bauer H (eds): *Brain Lipids and Lipoproteins, and the Leucodystrophies*. Amsterdam, Elsevier, 1963, p 104.
16. Suzuki K, Suzuki Y: Globoid cell leucodystrophy (Krabbe's disease): Deficiency of galactocerebroside β-galactosidase. *Proc Natl Acad Sci USA* **66**:302, 1970.
17. Suzuki K, Suzuki Y, Eto Y: Deficiency of galactocerebroside β-galactosidase in Krabbe's globoid cell leucodystrophy, in Bernsohn J, Grossman HJ (eds): *Lipid Storage Diseases: Enzymatic Defects and Clinical Implications*. New York, Academic Press, 1971, p 111.
18. Austin J, Suzuki K, Armstrong D, Brady R, Bachhawat BK, Schlenker J, Stumpf D: Studies in globoid (Krabbe) leukodystrophy (GLD). V. Controlled enzymic studies in ten human cases. *Arch Neurol* **23**:502, 1970.
19. Suzuki Y, Suzuki K: Krabbe's globoid cell leukodystrophy: Deficiency of galactocerebrosidase in serum, leukocytes, and fibroblasts. *Science* **171**:73, 1971.
20. Suzuki K, Schneider EL, Epstein CJ: In utero diagnosis of globoid cell leukodystrophy (Krabbe's disease). *Biochem Biophys Res Commun* **45**:1363, 1971.
21. Miyatake T, Suzuki K: Globoid cell leukodystrophy: Additional deficiency of psychosine galactosidase. *Biochem Biophys Res Commun* **48**:538, 1972.
22. Igisu H, Suzuki K: Progressive accumulation of toxic metabolite in a genetic leukodystrophy. *Science* **224**:753, 1984.
23. Zlotogora J, Charkraborty S, Knowleton RG, Wenger DA: Krabbe disease locus mapped to chromosome 14 by genetic linkage. *Am J Human Genet* **47**:37, 1990.
24. Chen YQ, Wenger DA: Galactocerebrosidase from human urine: Purification and partial characterization. *Biochim Biophys Acta* **1170**:53, 1993.
25. Chen YQ, Rafi MA, de Gala, G, Wenger DA: Cloning and expression of cDNA encoding human galactocerebrosidase, the enzyme deficient in globoid cell leukodystrophy. *Hum Molec Genet* **2**:184, 1993.
26. Sakai N, Inui K, Fujii N, Fukushima H, Nishimoto J, Yanagihara I, Isegawa Y, Iwamatsu A, Okada S: Krabbe disease: Isolation and characterization of a full-length cDNA for human galactocerebrosidase. *Biochem Biophys Res Commun* **198**:485, 1994.
27. Luzi P, Rafi MA, Wenger DA: Structure and organization of the human galactocerebrosidase (GALC) gene. *Genomics* **26**:407, 1995.
28. Hagberg B, Kollberg H, Sourander P, Akesson HO: Infantile globoid cell leucodystrophy (Krabbe's disease): A clinical and genetic study of 32 Swedish cases 1953–1967. *Neuropädiatrie* **1**:74, 1970.
29. Zlotogora J, Regev R, Zeigler M, Iancu TC, Bach G: Krabbe disease: Increased incidence in a highly inbred community. *Am J Med Genet* **21**:765, 1985.
30. Zlotogora J, Levy-Lahad E, Legum C, Iancu TC, Zeigler M, Bach G: Krabbe disease in Israel. *Israel J Med Sci* **27**:196, 1991.

31. Lyon G, Hagberg B, Evrard PH, Allaire C, Pavone L, Vanier M: Symptomatology of late onset Krabbe's leukodystrophy: The European experience. *Dev Neurosci* **13**:240, 1991.
32. Kolodny EH, Raghavan S, Krivit W: Late-onset Krabbe disease (globoid cell leukodystrophy): Clinical and biochemical features of 15 cases. *Dev Neurosci* **13**:322, 1991.
33. Fiumara A, Pavone L, Siciliano L, Tine A, Parano E, Innico G: Late-onset globoid cell leukodystrophy. Report on seven new patients. *Child Nerv Syst* **6**:194, 1990.
34. Barone R, Bruhl K, Stoeter P, Fiumara A, Pavone L, Beck M: Clinical and neuroradiological findings in classic infantile and late onset globoid-cell leukodystrophy (Krabbe disease). *Am J Med Genet* **63**:209, 1996.
35. Schochet SS Jr, Hardman JM, Lampert PW, Earle KM: Krabbe's disease (globoid leukodystrophy): Electron microscopic observations. *Arch Pathol* **88**:305, 1969.
36. Clarke JTR, Ozere RL, Krause VW: Early infantile variant of Krabbe globoid cell leukodystrophy with lung involvement. *Arch Dis Child* **8**:640, 1981.
37. Hagberg B, Sourander P, Svennerholm L: Diagnosis of Krabbe's infantile leukodystrophy. *J Neurol Neurosurg Psychiatry* **26**:195, 1963.
38. Nelson E, Aurebeck G, Osterberg K, Berry J, Jabbour JT, Bornhofen J: Ultrastructural and chemical studies on Krabbe's disease. *J Neuropathol Exp Neurol* **22**:414, 1963.
39. Crome L, Hanefeld F, Patrick D, Wilson J: Late onset globoid cell leukodystrophy. *Brain* **96**:84, 1973.
40. Christensen E, Melchior JC, Andersen H: Diffuse infantile familial sclerosis (Krabbe-type). *Acta Psychiatr Neurol Scand* **35**:431, 1960.
41. Liu HM: Ultrastructure of globoid leukodystrophy (Krabbe's disease) with reference to the origin of globoid cells. *J Neuropathol Exp Neurol* **29**:441, 1970.
42. Neuburger K: Zur Histopathologie der multiplen Sklerose im Kindesalter. *Z Neurol Psychiatr* **76**:384, 1972.
43. McNamara ED: Encephalitis periaxialis (Schilder). *Proc R Soc Med* **26**:297, 1933.
44. Verhaart WJC: A case of multiple sclerosis in an Indian in the Dutch East Indies. *Psychiatr Neurol Bladen* (Amsterdam) **35**:511, 1931.
45. Guillain G, Bertrand I, Gruner J: Sur un type anatomoclinique spécial de leucoencephalite à nodules morule gliogenes. *Rev Neurol* (Paris) **73**:401, 1941.
46. Ferraro A: Familial form of encephalitis periaxialis diffusa. *J Nerv Ment Dis* **66**:329, 1927.
47. Ferraro A: Familial form of encephalitis periaxialis diffusa. *J Nerv Ment Dis* **66**:479, 1927.
48. Ferraro A: Familial form of encephalitis periaxialis diffusa. *J Nerv Ment Dis* **66**:616, 1927.
49. Dunn HG, Dolman CL, Farrell DF, Tischler B, Hasinoff C, Woolf LI: Krabbe's leukodystrophy without globoid cells. *Neurology* **26**:1035, 1976.
50. Hanefeld F, Wilson J, Crome L: Die juvenile Form der Globoidzell-Leukodystrophie. *Monatsschr Kinderheilkd* **121**:293, 1973.
51. Malone MJ, Szoke MC, Looney GL: Globoid leukodystrophy. I. Clinical and enzymatic studies. *Arch Neurol* **32**:606, 1975.
52. Kolodny EH, Adams RD, Haller JS, Joseph J, Crumrine PK, Raghavan SS: Late-onset globoid cell leukodystrophy. *Ann Neurol* **8**:219, 1980.
53. Farrell DF, Swedberg K: Clinical and biochemical heterogeneity of globoid cell leukodystrophy. *Ann Neurol* **10**:364, 1981.
54. Vos AJM, Joosten EMG, Gabreëls-Festem AAWM, Gabreëls FJM: An atypical case of infantile globoid cell leukodystrophy. *Neuropediatrics* **14**:110, 1983.
55. Loonen MCB, Van Diggelen OP, Janse HC, Kleijer WJ, Aerts WFM: Late-onset globoid cell leukodystrophy (Krabbe's disease). Clinical and genetic delineation of two forms and their relation to the early infantile form. *Neuropediatrics* **16**:137, 1985.
56. Fluharty AL, Neidengard L, Holtzman D, Kihara H: Late-onset Krabbe disease initially diagnosed as cerebroside sulfatase activator deficiency. *Metab Brain Dis* **1**:187, 1986.
57. Marks HG, Scavina MT, Kolodny EH, Palmieri M, Childs J: Krabbe's disease presenting as a peripheral neuropathy. *Muscle Nerve* **20**:1024, 1997.
58. Arvidsson J, Hagberg B, Mansson J-E, Svennerholm L: Late onset globoid cell leukodystrophy (Krabbe's disease)—Swedish case with 15 years of follow-up. *Acta Paediatr* **84**:218, 1995.
59. McGuinness OE, Winrow AP, Smyth DP: Juvenile Krabbe's leukodystrophy precipitated by influenza A infection. *Dev Med Child Neurol* **38**:460, 1996.
60. Thomas PK, Halpern J-P, King RHM, Patrick D: Galactosylceramide lipidosis: Novel presentation as a slowly progressive spinocerebellar degeneration. *Ann Neurol* **16**:618, 1984.
61. Vanier M: Symptomatology of late onset Krabbe's leukodystrophy: The European experience. *Dev Neurosci* **13**:240, 1991.
62. Luzi P, Rafi MA, Wenger DA: Multiple mutations in the GALC gene in a patient with adult-onset Krabbe disease. *Ann Neurol* **40**:116, 1996.
63. Turazzini M, Beltramello A, Bassi R, Del Colle R, Silvestri M: Adult onset Krabbe's leukodystrophy: A report of 2 cases. *Acta Neurol Scand* **96**:413, 1997.
64. Wenger DA: Krabbe disease (globoid cell leukodystrophy), in Rosenberg RN, Prusiner SB, DiMauro S, Barchi RL (eds): *The Molecular and Genetic Basis of Neurological Disease.* Boston, Butterworth-Heinemann, 1997, p 485.
65. Furuya H, Kukita Y, Nagano S, Sakai Y, Yamashita Y, Fukuyama H, Inatomi Y, Saito Y, Koike R, Tsuji S, Fukumaki Y, Hayashi K, Kobayashi T: Adult onset globoid cell leukodystrophy (Krabbe disease): Analysis of galactosylceramidase cDNA from four Japanese patients. *Hum Genet* **100**:450, 1997.
66. Bernardini GL, Herrera DG, Carson D, DeGasperi R, Gama Sosa MA, Kolodny EH, Trifiletti R: Adult-onset Krabbe's disease in siblings with novel mutations in the galactocerebrosidase gene. *Ann Neurol* **41**:111, 1997.
67. Hagberg B: The clinical diagnosis of Krabbe's infantile leucodystrophy. *Acta Paediatr Scand* **52**:213, 1963.
68. Hittmair K, Wimberger D, Wiesbauer P, Zehetmayer M, Budka H: Early infantile form of Krabbe disease with optic hypertrophy: Serial MR examinations and autopsy correlation. *Am J Neuroradiol* **15**: 1454, 1994.
69. Suzuki K, Grover WD: Krabbe's leukodystrophy (globoid cell leukodystrophy): An ultrastructural study. *Arch Neurol* **22**:385, 1970.
70. Allen N, de Veyra E: Microchemical and histochemical observations in a case of Krabbe's leukodystrophy. *J Neuropathol Exp Neurol* **26**:456, 1967.
71. Hogan GR, Gutmann L, Chou SM: The peripheral neuropathy of Krabbe's (globoid) leukodystrophy. *Neurology* (Minneapolis) **19**:1093, 1969.
72. Schochet SS Jr, McCormick WF, Powell GF: Krabbe's disease: A light and electron microscopic study. *Acta Neuropath* **36**:153, 1976.
73. Yunis EJ, Lee RE: The ultrastructure of globoid (Krabbe) leukodystrophy. *Lab Invest* **21**:415, 1969.
74. Laxdal T, Hallgrimsson K: Krabbe's globoid cell leucodystrophy with hydrocephalus. *Arch Dis Child* **49**:232, 1974.
75. Yokota K, Yusa T, Mitsudome A, Takashima S, Kurokawa T, Takeshita K: An autopsy case of globoid cell leukodystrophy (Krabbe's disease). *Brain Dev* (Tokyo) **5**:296, 1973.
76. Gullotta F, Pavone L, Mollica F, Grasso S, Valenti C: Krabbe's disease with unusual clinical and morphological features. *Neuropädiatrie* **10**:395, 1979.
77. Feiden W, Bratzke H, Scharschmidt A: Geburtsschadigung oder angebörener Hirnschaden? Ein Fall eines vermeintlichen Geburtsschadens mit Globoidzell-Leukodystrophie (M Krabbe). *Geburtshilfe Frauenheilk* **51**:65, 1991.
78. Naidu S, Hofmann KJ, Moser HW, Maumenee IH, Wenger DA: Galactosylceramide β-galactosidase deficiency in association with cherry red spot. *Neuropediatrics* **19**:46, 1988.
79. Taori GM, Shalini KCM, Martin KB, Bhaktaviziam A, Bachhawat BK: Globoid leukodystrophy (Krabbe's disease). *Indian J Med Res* **58**:993, 1970.
80. Moosa A: Peripheral neuropathy and ichthyosis in Krabbe's leukodystrophy. *Arch Dis Child* **46**:112, 1971.
81. Matsuyama H, Minoshima I, Watanabe I: An autopsy case of leucodystrophy of Krabbe type. *Acta Pathol Jap* **13**:195, 1963.
82. Austin JH: Recent studies in the metachromatic and globoid forms of diffuse sclerosis. *Res Publ Assoc Res Nerv Ment Dis* **40**:189, 1962.
83. Dunn HG, Lake BD, Dolman DL, Wilson J: The neuropathy of Krabbe's infantile cerebral sclerosis (globoid cell leucodystrophy). *Brain* **92**:329, 1969.
84. Sacrez R, Levy JM, Gruner JE, Billuart J, Carlier G: La leucodystrophie de Krabbe. *Arch Fr Pediatr* **22**:641, 1965.
85. Cumings JN, Rozdilsky B: The cerebral lipid composition of the brain in six cases of Krabbe's disease. *Neurology* (Minneapolis) **15**:177, 1965.
86. D'Agostino AM, Sayre GP, Hagles AB: Krabbe's disease. *Arch Neurol* **8**:82, 1963.
87. Lieberman JS, Oshtory M, Taylor RG, Dreyfus PM: Perinatal neuropathy as an early manifestation of Krabbe's disease. *Arch Neurol* **37**:446, 1980.

88. Wallace BJ, Aronson SM, Volk BW: Histochemical and biochemical studies of globoid cell leucodystrophy (Krabbe's disease). *J Neurochem* **11**:367, 1964.
89. Osetowska E, Gail H, Lukasewicz D, Karcher D, Wisniewski H: Leucodystrophie infantile précoce (type Krabbe): (Remarques sur les proliférations gliales et les atrophies de système qui peuvent s'y observer). *Rev Neurol* (Paris) **102**:463, 1960.
90. Poser CM, van Bogaert L: Natural history and evolution of the concept of Schilder's diffuse sclerosis. *Acta Psychiatr Scand* **31**:285, 1956.
91. Goebel HH, Harzer K, Ernst JP, Bohl J, Klein H: Late-onset globoid leukodystrophy: Unusual ultrastructural pathology and subtotal β-galactocerebrosidase deficiency. *J Child Neurol* **5**:299, 1990.
92. Okada S, Kato T, Tanaka H, Takada K, Aramitsu Y: A case of late variant form of infantile Krabbe disease with a partial deficiency of galactocerebrosidase. *Brain Develop* (Tokyo) **10**:45, 1988.
93. Phelps M, Aicardi J, Vanier MT: Late-onset Krabbe's leukodystrophy. A report of four cases. *J Neurol Neurosurg Psychiatr* **54**:293, 1991.
94. Rolando S, Cremonte M, Leonardi A: Late onset globoid leukodystrophy: Unusual clinical and CSF findings. *Ital J Neurol Sci* **11**:57, 1990.
95. Grewal RP, Petronas N, Barton NW: Late-onset globoid cell leukodystrophy. *J Neurol Neurosurg Psychiatr* **54**:1011, 1991.
96. Demaerel P, Wilms G, Verdru P, Carton H, Baert AL: Findings in globoid cell leukodystrophy. *Neuroradiology* **32**:520, 1990.
97. Verdru P, Lammens M, Dom R, van Elsen A, Carton H: Globoid cell leukodystrophy: A family with both late-infantile and adult type. *Neurology* **41**:1382, 1991.
98. Epstein MA, Zimmerman RA, Rorke LB, Sladky JT: Late-onset globoid cell leukodystrophy mimicking an infiltrating glioma. *Pediatr Radiol* **21**:131, 1991.
99. Satoh J-I, Tokumoto H, Kurohara K, Yukitake M, Matsui M, Kuroda Y, Yamamoto T, Furuya H, Shinnoh N, Kobayashi T, Kukita Y, Hayashi K: Adult-onset Krabbe disease with homozygous T1853C mutation in the galactocerebrosidase gene. Unusual MRI findings of corticospinal tract demyelination. *Neurology* **49**:1392, 1997.
100. Takahashi M, Udaka F, Kameyama M, Oka N, Akagi M, Nishigaki T, Inui K: Senile-onset Krabbe's disease having a homozygous I66M mutation (abstract). *Clin Neurol*, in press.
101. Marjanovic B, Cvetkovic D, Dozic S, Todorovic S, Djuric M: Association of Krabbe leukodystrophy and congenital fiber type disproportion. *Pediatr Neurol* **15**:79, 1996.
102. Hagberg B, Svennerholm L: Metachromatic leucodystrophy—generalized lipidosis: Determination of sulfatides in urine, blood plasma and cerebrospinal fluid. *Acta Paediatr* **49**:690, 1960.
103. Lane B, Carroll BA, Pedley TA: Computerized cranial tomography in cerebral diseases of white matter. *Neurology* **28**:534, 1978.
104. Heinz ER, Drayer BP, Haenggeli CA, Painter MJ, Crumrine P: Computed tomography in white matter disease. *Radiology* **130**:371, 1979.
105. Barnes DM, Enzmann DR: The evolution of white matter disease as seen on computed tomography. *Radiology* **138**:379, 1981.
106. Ieshima A, Eda S, Matsui A, Yoshino K, Takashima S, Takeshita K: Computed tomography in Krabbe's disease: Comparison with neuropathology. *Neuroradiology* **25**:323, 1983.
107. Choi S, Enzmann DR: Infantile Krabbe disease: Complementary CT and MR findings. *Am J Neuroradiol* **14**: 1164, 1993.
108. Sasaki M, Sakuragawa N, Takashima S, Hanaoka S, Arima M: MRI and CT findings in Krabbe disease. *Pediatr Neurol* **7**:283, 1991.
109. Yamanouchi H, Kasai H, Sakuragawa N, Kurokawa T: Palatal myoclonus in Krabbe disease. *Brain Develop* (Tokyo) **13**:355,1991.
110. Yamanouchi H, Yanagisawa T, Takahashi M, Shimizu S, Hatakeyama S: Characteristic CT findings in Krabbe disease. *No to Hattatsu* (Tokyo) **22**:77, 1990.
111. Winants D, Bernard C, Galloy MA, Hoeffel JC, Vidailhet M: Scanographie et IRM de la maladie de Krabbe. *J Radiol* **69**:697, 1988.
112. Baram TZ, Goldman AM, Percy AK: Krabbe disease: Specific MRI and CT findings. *Neurology* **36**:111, 1986.
113. Finelli DA, Tarr RW, Sawyer RN, Horwitz SJ: Deceptively normal MR in early infantile Krabbe disease. *Am J Neuroradiol* **15**:167, 1994.
114. Zafeiriou DI, Anastasiou AL, Michelakaki EM, Augoustidou-Savvopoulou PA, Katzos GS, Kontopoulos EE: Early infantile Krabbe disease: Deceptively normal magnetic resonance imaging and serial neurophysiological studies. *Brain Dev* **19**:488, 1997.
115. Ono J, Kodaka R, Imai K, Itagaki Y, Tanaka J, Inui K, Nagai T, Sakurai K, Harada K, Okada S: Evaluation of myelination by means of the T2 value on magnetic resonance imaging. *Brain Dev* **15**:433, 1993.
116. Ono J, Harada K, Mano T, Sakurai K, Okada S: Differentiation of dys- and demyelination using diffusional anisotropy. *Pediatr Neurol* **16**:63, 1997.
117. Anzil AP, Blinzinger K, Mehraein P, Dorn G, Neuhauser G: Cytoplasmic inclusions in a child affected with Krabbe's disease (globoid leucodystrophy) and in the rabbit injected with galactocerebrosides. *J Neuropathol Exp Neurol* **31**:370, 1972.
118. Lyon G, Jardin L, Aicardi J: Étude au microscope éléctronique d'un nerf périphérique dans un cas de leucodystrophie de Krabbe. *J Neurol Sci* **12**:263, 1971.
119. de Meierleir LJ, Taylor MJ, Logan WJ: Multimodal evoked potential studies in leukodystrophies of children. *Can J Neurol Sci* **15**:26, 1988.
120. Yamanouchi H, Kaga M, Iwasaki Y, Sakuragawa N, Arima M: Auditory evoked responses in Krabbe disease. *Pediatr Neurol* **9**:387, 1993.
121. Austin JH: Some newer findings in Krabbe (globoid) leucodystrophy. *Trans Am Neurol Assoc* **87**:66, 1962.
122. Austin JH: Histochemical and biochemical studies in diffuse cerebral sclerosis (metachromatic and globoid-body forms), in IVth Int Congr Neuropathol vol 1. Stuttgart, Thieme, 1962, p 35.
123. Diezel PB: *Die Stoffwechselstörungen der Sphingolipoide*. Berlin, Springer-Verlag, 1957.
124. Hager H, Oehlert W: Ist die diffuse Hirnsklerose des Typ Krabbe eine entzündliche Allgemeinerkrankung? *Z Kinderheilkd* **80**:82, 1957.
125. Martin JJ, Clara R, Ceuterick C, Joris C: Is congenital fiber type disproportion a true myopathy? *Acta Neurol Belg* **76**:335, 1976.
126. Dehkharghani F, Sarnat HB, Brewster MA, Roth IS: Congenital muscle fiber-type disproportion in Krabbe's leukodystrophy. *Arch Neurol* **38**:585, 1981.
127. Goebel HH, Kimura S, Harzer K, Klein H: Ultrastructural pathology of eccrine sweat gland epithelial cells in globoid cell leukodystrophy. *J Child Neurol* **8**:171, 1993.
128. Greenfield JG, Norman RM: Demyelinating diseases, in Blackwood W, McMenemy WH, Meyer A, Norman RM, Russell DS (eds): *Greenfield's Neuropathology* 2d ed. Baltimore, Williams & Wilkins, 1963, p 475.
129. Austin JH: Globoid (Krabbe) leukodystrophy, in Minkler J (ed): *Pathology of the Nervous System*. New York, McGraw-Hill, 1968, p 843.
130. Oehmichen M, Wietholter H, Gencic M: Cytochemical markers for mononuclear phagocytes as demonstrated in reactive microglia and globoid cells. *Acta Histochem* **66**:243, 1980.
131. Oehmichen M: Enzyme-histochemical differentiation of neuroglia and microglia: A contribution to the cytogenesis of microglia and globoid cells. *Path Res Pract* **168**:244, 1980.
132. Pfeiffer J: Zur formalen Genese der Globoidzellen bei der diffusen Sklerose vom Typus Krabbe. *Arch Psychiatr Nervenkr* **195**:446, 1957.
133. Einarson L, Stromgren E: Diffuse progressive leucoencephalopathy (diffuse cerebral sclerosis) and its relationship to amaurotic idiocy: Histological and clinical aspects. *Acta Jutland* **33**:5, 1961.
134. Christensen E, Melchior JC, Negri S: A comparative study of 16 cases of diffuse sclerosis with special reference to the histopathological findings. *Acta Neurol Scand* **37**:163, 1961.
135. Oehmichen M, Gruninger H: The origin of multinucleated giant cells in experimentally induced and spontaneous Krabbe's disease (globoid cell leukodystrophy). *Beitr Pathol* **153**:111, 1974.
136. Kobayashi S, Katayama M, Bourque EA, Suzuki K, Suzuki K: The twitcher mouse: Positive immunohistochemical staining of globoid cells with monoclonal antibody against Mac-1 antigen. *Dev Brain Res* **20**:49, 1985.
137. Sourander P, Hansson HA, Olsson Y, Svennerholm L: Experimental studies on the pathogenesis of leucodystrophies. II. The effect of sphingolipids on various cell types in cultures from the nervous system. *Acta Neuropathol* (Berlin) **9**:231, 1966.
138. de Vries E: Gliomatous polio- and leucodystrophy in young child. *J Neuropathol Exp Neurol* **17**:501, 1958.
139. Schenk VW, Gluszcz A, Zelman IB: Atypical form of Krabbe-type leucodystrophy in two siblings accompanied by poliodystrophic changes. *Neuropathol Pol* **11**:117, 1973.
140. Williams RS, Ferrante RJ, Caviness VS Jr: The isolated human cortex. A Golgi analysis of Krabbe's disease. *Arch Neurol* **36**:134, 1979.
141. Andrews JM, Cancilla P: Cytoplasmic inclusions in human globoid cell leukodystrophy. *Arch Pathol* **89**:53, 1970.
142. Shaw C-M, Carlson CB: Crystalline structures in globoid-epithelioid cells: An electron microscopic study of globoid leukodystrophy (Krabbe's disease). *J Neuropathol Exp Neurol* **29**:306, 1970.

143. Lake BD: Segmental demyelination of peripheral nerves in Krabbe's disease. *Nature* **217**:171, 1968.
144. Bischoff A, Ulrich J: Peripheral neuropathy in globoid cell leukodystrophy (Krabbe's disease): Ultrastructural and histochemical findings. *Brain* **92**:861, 1969
145. Yunis EJ, Lee RE: Tubules of globoid leukodystrophy: A right-handed helix. *Science* **169**:64, 1970.
146. Blinzinger K, Anzil AP: Non-membrane bound cytoplasmic deposits in Krabbe globoid leukodystrophy. Further evidence of a revised concept of lysosomal storage diseases. *Experientia* **18**:780, 1972.
147. Yunis EJ, Lee RE: Further observations on the fine structure of globoid leukodystrophy: Peripheral neuropathy and optic nerve involvement. *Hum Pathol* **3**:371, 1972.
148. Harcourt B, Ashton N: Ultrastructure of the optic nerve in Krabbe's leukodystrophy. *Br J Ophthalmol* **57**:885, 1973.
149. Brownstein S, Meagher-Villemure K, Polomeno RC, Little JM: Optic nerve in globoid leukodystrophy (Krabbe's disease). Ultrastructural changes. *Arch Ophthalmol* **96**:864, 1978.
150. Yajima K, Fletcher TF, Suzuki K: Sub-plasmalemmal linear density: A common structure in globoid cells and mesenchymal cells. *Acta Neuropathol* **39**:195, 1977.
151. Suzuki K: Ultrastructural study of experimental globoid cells. *Lab Invest* **23**:612, 1970.
152. Andrews JM, Menkes JH: Ultrastructure of experimentally produced globoid cells in the rat. *Exp Neurol* **29**:483, 1970.
153. Sourander P, Olsson Y: Peripheral neuropathy in globoid cell leucodystrophy (Morbus Krabbe). *Acta Neuropathol* (Berlin) **11**:69, 1968.
154. Schlaepfer WW, Prensky AL: Quantitative and qualitative study of sural nerve biopsies in Krabbe's disease. *Acta Neuropathol* **20**:55, 1972.
155. Joosten EM, Krijgsman JB, Gabreëls-Festen AA, Gabreëls FJ, Baars PEC: Infantile globoid cell leukodystrophy (Krabbe's disease). Some remarks on clinical and sural nerve biopsy findings. *Dev Med Child Neurol* **16**:228, 1974.
156. Martin JJ, Ceuterick C, Martin L, Leroy JG, Nuyts JP, Joris C: Globoid cell leukodystrophy (Krabbe's disease): Peripheral nerve lesion. *Acta Neurol Belg* **74**:356, 1974.
157. Watanabe K, Hara K, Iwase K: The evolution of neurological and neurophysiological features in a case of Krabbe's globoid cell leukodystrophy. *Brain Develop* (Tokyo) **8**:432, 1976.
158. Gutmann L, Hogan G, Chou SM: The peripheral neuropathy of Krabbe's (globoid) leucodystrophy. *Electroencephalogr Clin Neurophysiol* **27**:715, 1969.
159. Choi KG, Sung JH, Brent Clark H, Krivit W: Pathology of adult-onset globoid cell leukodystrophy (GLD). *J Neuropathol Exper Neurol* **50**:336, 1991.
160. Hedley-Whyte ET, Boustany RM, Riskind P, Raghavan S, Zuñiga G, Kolodny EH: Peripheral neuropathy due to galactosylceramide-β-galactosidase deficiency (Krabbe's disease) in a 73-year-old woman. *Neuropathol Appl Neurobiol* **14**:515, 1988.
161. Ellis WG, Schneider EL, McCullough JR, Suzuki K, Epstein CJ: Fetal globoid cell leukodystrophy (Krabbe disease): Pathological and biochemical examination. *Arch Neurol* **29**:253, 1973.
162. Martin JJ, Leroy JG, Ceuterick C, Libert J, Dodinval P, Martin L: Fetal Krabbe leukodystrophy. A morphometric study of two cases. *Acta Neuropathol* **53**:87, 1981.
163. Okeda R, Suzuki Y, Horiguchi S, Fujii T: Fetal globoid cell leukodystrophy in one of twins. *Acta Neuropathol* (Berlin) **47**:151, 1979.
164. Svennerholm L: The distribution of lipids in the human nervous system. I. Analytical procedure: Lipids of foetal and newborn brain. *J Neurochem* **11**:839, 1964.
165. Suzuki K, Suzuki K, Kamoshita S: Chemical pathology of G_{M1}-gangliosidosis (generalized gangliosidosis). *J Neuropathol Exp Neurol* **28**:25, 1969.
166. Suzuki Y, Jacob JC, Suzuki K, Suzuki K: G_{M2}-gangliosidosis with total hexosaminidase deficiency. *Neurology* (Minneapolis) **21**:313, 1971.
167. Vanier M-T, Svennerholm L: Chemical pathology of Krabbe's disease. III. Ceramide hexosides and gangliosides of brain. *Acta Paediatr Scand* **64**:641, 1975.
168. Vanier M, Svennerholm L: Chemical pathology of Krabbe's disease: The occurrence of psychosine and other neutral sphingoglycolipids. *Adv Exp Med Biol* **68**:115, 1976.
169. Svennerholm L, Vanier M-T, Månsson JE: Krabbe disease: A galactosylsphingosine (psychosine) lipidosis. *J Lipid Res* **21**:53, 1980.
170. Morell P, Radin NS: Synthesis of cerebroside by brain from uridine diphosphate galactose and ceramide containing hydroxy fatty acid. *Biochemistry* **8**:506, 1969.
171. Morell P, Costantino-Ceccarini E, Radin NS: The biosynthesis by brain microsomes of cerebrosides containing nonhydroxy fatty acids. *Arch Biochem Biophys* **141**:738, 1970.
172. Balasubramanian AS, Bachhawat BK: Studies on enzymic synthesis of cerebroside sulfate from 3′-phosphoadenosine-5′-phosphosulfate. *Indian J Biochem* **2**:212, 1965.
173. Cleland WW, Kennedy EP: The enzymatic synthesis of psychosine. *J Biol Chem* **235**:45, 1960.
174. Mehl E, Jatzkewitz H: Ein Cerebrosid Sulfatase aus Schweineniere. *Z Physiol Chem* **339**:260, 1964.
175. Austin JH, Armstrong D, Shearer L: Metachromatic form of diffuse cerebral sclerosis. V. The nature and significance of low sulfatase activity: A controlled study of brain, liver and kidney in four patients with metachromatic leucodystrophy (MLD). *Arch Neurol* **13**:593, 1965.
176. Mehl E, Jatzkewitz H: Evidence for the genetic block in metachromatic leucodystrophy (ML). *Biochem Biophys Res Commun* **19**:407, 1965.
177. Hajra AK, Bowen DM, Kishimoto Y, Radin NS: Cerebroside galactosidase of brain. *J Lipid Res* **7**:379, 1966.
178. Bowen DM, Radin NS: Purification of cerebroside galactosidase from rat brain. *Biochim Biophys Acta* **152**:587, 1968.
179. Bowen DM, Radin NS: Properties of cerebroside galactosidase. *Biochim Biophys Acta* **152**:599, 1968.
180. Bowen DM, Radin NS: Cerebroside galactosidase: A method for determination and a comparison with other lysosomal enzymes in developing rat brain. *J Neurochem* **16**:501, 1969.
181. Suzuki K: Galactosylceramide galactosidase, in Ginsburg V (ed): *Methods in Enzymology,* vol 28 in *Complex Carbohydrates, Part B*. New York, Academic, 1972, p 839.
182. Suzuki Y, Suzuki K: Glycosphingolipid β-galactosidases. I. Standard assay procedures, and characterization by electrofocusing and gel filtration of the enzymes in normal human liver. *J Biol Chem* **249**:2098, 1974.
183. Suzuki Y, Suzuki K: Glycosphingolipid β-galactosidases. II. Electrofocusing characterization of the enzymes in human globoid cell leukodystrophy (Krabbe's disease). *J Biol Chem* **249**:2105, 1974.
184. Suzuki Y, Suzuki K: Glycosphingolipid β-galactosidases. IV. Electrofocusing characterization in G_{M1}-gangliosidosis. *J Biol Chem* **249**:2113, 1974.
185. Miyatake T, Suzuki K: Partial purification and the characterization of β-galactosidase from rat brain hydrolyzing glycosphingolipids. *J Biol Chem* **250**:585, 1975.
186. Awasthi YC, Lund HW, Lo JT, Srivastava SK: Sphingolipid β-galactosidases in globoid cell leukodystrophy. *Birth Defects* **14**:113, 1978.
187. Sakai N, Inui K, Midorikawa M, Okuno Y, Ueda S, Iwamatsu A, Okada S: Purification and characterization of galactocerebrosidase from human lymphocytes. *J Biochem* **116**:615, 1994.
188. Miyatake T, Suzuki K: Galactosylsphingosine galactosyl hydrolase: Partial purification and properties of the enzyme in rat brain. *J Biol Chem* **247**:5398, 1972.
189. Miyatake T, Suzuki K: Additional deficiency of psychosine galactosidase in globoid cell leukodystrophy: Implication to enzyme replacement therapy. *Birth Defects* **9**:136, 1973.
190. Miyatake T, Suzuki K: Galactosylsphingosine galactosyl hydrolase in rat brain: Probable identity with galactosylceramide galactosyl hydrolase. *J Neurochem* **22**:231, 1974.
191. Wenger DA, Sattler M, Markey SP: Deficiency of monogalactosyl diglyceride β-galactosidase activity in Krabbe's disease. *Biochem Biophys Res Commun* **53**:680, 1973.
192. Wenger DA, Sattler M, Hiatt W: Globoid cell leukodystrophy: Deficiency of lactosylceramide beta-galactosidase. *Proc Natl Acad Sci USA* **71**:584, 1974.
193. Tanaka H, Suzuki K: Lactosylceramide β-galactosidase in human sphingolipidoses: Evidence for two genetically distinct enzymes. *J Biol Chem* **250**:2324, 1975.
194. Svennerholm L, Håkansson G, Vanier MT: Chemical pathology of Krabbe's disease. IV. Studies of galactosylceramide and lactosylceramide β-galactosidases in brain, white blood cells, and amniotic fluid cells. *Acta Paediatr Scand* **64**:649, 1975.
195. Wenger DA, Sattler M, Clark C: Effect of bile salts on lactosylceramide β-galactosidase activities in human brain, liver, and cultured skin fibroblasts. *Biochim Biophys Acta* **409**:297, 1975.

196. Tanaka H, Suzuki K: Specificities of the two genetically distinct β-galactosidases in human sphingolipidoses. *Arch Biochem Biophys* **175**:332, 1976.
197. Tanaka H, Suzuki K: Substrate specificities of the two genetically distinct human brain β-galactosidases. *Brain Res* **122**:325, 1977.
198. Tanaka H, Suzuki K: Lactosylceramidase assays for diagnosis of globoid cell leukodystrophy and G_{M1}-gangliosidosis. *Clin Chim Acta* **75**:267, 1977.
199. Hanada E, Suzuki K: Specificity of galactosylceramidase activation by phosphatidylserine. *Biochim Biophys Acta* **619**:396, 1980.
200. Wenger DA, Sattler M, Roth R: A protein activator of galactosylceramide β-galactosidase. *Biochim Biophys Acta* **712**:639, 1982.
201. Makita A: Biochemistry of organ glycolipids. II. Isolation of human kidney glycolipids. *J Biochem* (Tokyo) **55**:269, 1964.
202. Martensson E: Neutral glycolipids of human kidney: Isolation, identification and fatty acid composition. *Biochim Biophys Acta* **116**:296, 1966.
203. Norton WT, Poduslo SE: Myelination in rat brain: Changes in myelin composition during brain maturation. *J Neurochem* **21**:759, 1973.
204. O'Brien JS, Sampson EL, Stern MB: Lipid composition of myelin from the peripheral nervous system. *J Neurochem* **14**:357, 1967.
205. Yakovlev P, Lecours AR: The myelogenetic cycles of regional maturation of the brain, in Minkowski A (ed): *Regional Development of the Brain in Early Life*. Oxford, Blackwell, 1967, p 3.
206. Burton RM, Sodd MA, Brady RO: The incorporation of galactose into galactolipids. *J Biol Chem* **233**:1053, 1958.
207. Costantino-Ceccarini E, Morell P: Biosynthesis of brain sphingolipids and myelin accumulation in the mouse. *Lipids* **7**:656, 1972.
208. Schulte S, Stoffel W: Ceramide UDP galactosyltransferase from myelinating rat brain: Purification, cloning, and expression. *Proc Natl Acad Sci USA* **90**:10265, 1993.
209. Stahl N, Jurevics H, Morell P, Suzuki K, Popko B: Isolation, characterization, and expression of cDNA clones that encode rat UDP-galactose:ceramide galactosyltransferase. *J Neurosci Res* **38**:234, 1994.
210. Bosio A, Binczek E, Stoffel W: Molecular cloning and characterization of the mouse CGT gene encoding UDP-galactose ceramide-galactosyltransferase (cerebroside synthetase). *Genomics* **35**:223, 1996.
211. Coetzee T, Li X, Fujita N, Marcus J, Suzuki K, Francke U, Popko B: Molecular cloning, chromosomal mapping, and characterization of the mouse UDP-galactose:ceramide galactosyltransferase gene. *Genomics* **35**:215, 1996.
212. Norman RM, Oppenheimer DR, Tingey AH: Histological and chemical findings in Krabbe's leucodystrophy. *J Neurol Neurosurg Psychiatr* **24**:223, 1961.
213. Austin J: Studies in globoid (Krabbe) leukodystrophy. I. The significance of lipid abnormalities in white matter in 8 globoid and 13 control patients. *Arch Neurol* **9**:207, 1963.
214. Tingey AH, Edgar GWF: A contribution to the chemistry of the leucodystrophies. *J Neurochem* **10**:817, 1963.
215. Jatzkewitz H: Die Leukodystrophie, Typ Scholz (metachromatische form der diffusen Sklerose) als Sphingolipoidose (Cerebrosidschwefelsäureester-Speicherkrankheit). *Z Physiol Chem* **318**:265, 1960.
216. Menkes JH, Duncan C, Moosey J: Molecular composition of the major glycolipids in globoid cell leucodystrophy. *Neurology* (Minneapolis) **16**:581, 1966.
217. Eto Y, Suzuki K: Brain sphingoglycolipids in Krabbe's globoid cell leucodystrophy. *J Neurochem* **18**:503, 1971.
218. Robinson N, Cumings JN: Biochemical and histochemical observations on Krabbe's disease (globoid body diffuse sclerosis). *Acta Neuropathol* (Berlin) **9**:280, 1967.
219. Svennerholm L, Vanier MT: Brain gangliosides in Krabbe disease, in Volk BW, Aronson SM (eds): *Sphingolipids, Sphingolipidoses and Allied Disorders*. New York, Plenum, 1972, p 499.
220. Vanier MT, Svennerholm L: Chemical pathology of Krabbe's disease. I. Lipid composition and fatty acid patterns of phosphoglycerides in brain. *Acta Paediatr Scand* **63**:494, 1974.
221. Kobayashi T, Shinoda H, Goto I, Yamanaka T, Suzuki Y: Globoid cell leukodystrophy is a generalized galactosylsphingosine (psychosine) storage disease. *Biochem Biophys Res Commun* **144**:41, 1987.
222. Kobayashi T, Goto I, Yamanaka T, Suzuki Y, Nakano T, Suzuki K: Infantile and fetal globoid cell leukodystrophy: Analysis of galactosylceramide and galactosylsphingosine. *Ann Neurol* **24**:517, 1988.
223. Eto Y, Suzuki K, Suzuki K: Globoid cell leukodystrophy (Krabbe's disease): Isolation of myelin with normal glycolipid composition. *J Lipid Res* **11**:473, 1970.
224. Suzuki K: Renal cerebroside in globoid cell leukodystrophy (Krabbe's disease). *Lipids* **6**:433, 1971.
225. Dawson G: Hepatic galactosylceramide in globoid cell leukodystrophy (Krabbe's disease). *Lipids* **8**:154, 1973.
226. Suzuki K, Suzuki Y, Fletcher TF: Further studies of galactocerebroside β-galactosidase in globoid cell leukodystrophy, in Volk BW, Aronson SM (eds): *Sphingolipids, Sphingolipidoses and Allied Disorders*. New York, Plenum, 1972, p 487.
227. Wenger DA, Sattler M, Clark C, McKelvey H: An improved method for the identification of patients and carriers of Krabbe's disease. *Clin Chim Acta* **56**:199, 1974.
228. Farrell DF, Percy AK, Kaback MM, McKhann GM: Globoid cell (Krabbe's) leukodystrophy: Heterozygote detection in cultured skin fibroblasts. *Am J Hum Genet* **25**:604, 1973.
229. Wenger DA, Sattler M, Clark C, Tanaka H, Suzuki K, Dawson G: Lactosylceramidosis: Normal activity for two lactosylceramide β-galactosidases. *Science* **188**:1310, 1975
230. Kobayashi T, Shinnoh N, Goto I, Kuroiwa Y: Hydrolysis of galactosylceramide is catalyzed by two genetically distinct acid β-galactosidases. *J Biol Chem* **260**:14982, 1985.
231. Tanaka H, Suzuki K: Globoid cell leukodystrophy (Krabbe's disease): Metabolic studies with cultured fibroblasts. *J Neurol Sci* **38**:409, 1978
232. Kobayashi T, Shinnoh N, Goto I, Kuroiwa Y, Okawauchi M, Sugihara G, Tanaka M: Galactosylceramide- and lactosylceramide-loading studies in cultured fibroblasts from normal individuals and patients with globoid cell leukodystrophy (Krabbe's disease) and G_{M1}-gangliosidosis. *Biochim Biophys Acta* **835**:456, 1985.
233. Suzuki K, Tanaka H, Suzuki K: Studies on the pathogenesis of Krabbe's leukodystrophy: Cellular reaction of the brain to exogenous galactosylsphingosine, monogalactosyl diglyceride and lactosylceramide, in Volk BW, Schneck L (eds): *Current Trends in Sphingolipidoses and Allied Disorders*. New York, Plenum, 1976, p 99.
234. Lin YN, Radin NS: Alternate pathways of cerebroside catabolism. *Lipids* **8**:732, 1973
235. Taketomi T, Nishimura K: Physiological activity of psychosine. *Jap J Exp Med* **34**:255, 1964.
236. Igisu H, Nakamura M: Inhibition of cytochrome c oxidase by psychosine (galactosylsphingosine). *Biochem Biophys Res Commun* **137**:323, 1986.
237. Baskin GB, Ratterree M, Davison BB, Falkenstein KP, Clarke MR, England JD, Vanier MT, Luzi P, Rafi MA, Wenger DA: Genetic galactocerebrosidase deficiency (globoid cell leukodystrophy, Krabbe disease) in rhesus monkeys (*Macaca mulatta*). *Lab Animal Sci* **48**:476, 1998.
238. Wenger DA, Victoria T, Rafi MA, Luzi P, Vanier MT, Vite C, Patterson DF, et al.: Globoid cell leukodystrophy in Cairn and West Highland White terriers. *J Hered* **90**:138, 1999.
239. Yamanaka T, Fletcher TF, Tiffany CW, Suzuki K: Galactosylceramide metabolism in different regions of the central nervous system: Possible correlation with regional susceptibility in genetic leukodystrophies, in Callahan JW, Lowden JA (eds): *Lysosomes and Lysosomal Storage Diseases*. New York, Raven, 1981, p 147.
240. Suzuki K: Biochemical pathogenesis of genetic leukodystrophies: Comparison of metachromatic leukodystrophy and globoid cell leukodystrophy (Krabbe disease). *Neuropediatrics* **15**(suppl):32, 1984.
241. Sweet H: Twitcher is on Ch 12. *Mouse Newslett* **75**:30, 1986.
242. Oehlmann R, Zlotogora J, Wenger DA, Knowlton RG: Localization of Krabbe disease gene (GALC) on chromosome 14 by multipoint linkage analysis. *Am J Hum Genet* **53**:1250, 1993.
243. Cannizzaro LA, Chen YQ, Rafi MA, Wenger DA: Regional mapping of human galactocerebrosidase (GALC) to 14q31 by in situ hybridization. *Cytogenet Cell Genet* **66**:244, 1994.
244. Kozak M: The scanning model for translation: An update. *J Cell Biol* **108**:229, 1989
245. Luzi P, Victoria T, Rafi M, Wenger DA: Analysis of the 5′ flanking region of the human galactocerebrosidase (GALC) gene. *Biochem Molec Med* **62**:159, 1997.
246. Sakai N, Fukushima H, Inui K, Fu L, Nishigaki T, Yanagihara I, Tatsumi N, et al.: Human galactocerebrosidase gene: Promoter analysis of the 5′-flanking region and structural organization. *Biochim Biophys Acta* **1395**:62, 1998.
247. Wenger DA, Rafi MA, Luzi P: Molecular genetics of Krabbe disease (globoid cell leukodystrophy): Diagnostic and clinical aspects. *Hum Mutat* **10**:268,1997.
248. Rafi MA, Luzi P, Chen YQ, Wenger DA: A large deletion together with a point mutation in the GALC gene is a common mutant allele in

patients with infantile Krabbe disease. *Hum Molec Genet* **4**:1285,1 995.

249. Luzi P, Rafi MA, Wenger DA: Characterization of the large deletion in the GALC gene found in patients with Krabbe disease. *Hum Molec Genet* **4**:2335, 1995.
250. Kleijer WJ, Keulemans JLM, van der Kraan M, Geilen GG, van der Helm RM, Rafi MA, Luzi P, Wenger DA, Halley DJJ, van Diggelen OP: Prevalent mutations in the GALC gene of patients with Krabbe disease of Dutch and other European origin. *J Inher Metab Dis* **20**:587, 1997.
251. Kolodny EH, Gama Sosa MA, Battistini S, Sartorato EL, Yeretsian J, MacFarlane H, Gusella J, DeGasperi R: Molecular genetics of late onset Krabbe disease. *Am J Hum Genet* **57**:A217, 1995.
252. Tatsumi N, Inui K, Sakai N, Fukushima H, Nishimoto J, Yanagihara I, Nishigaki T, Tsukamoto H, Fu L, Taniiki M, Okada S: Molecular defects in Krabbe disease. *Hum Molec Genet* **4**:1865, 1995.
253. Zlotogora J, Levy-Lahad E, Legum C, Iancu TC, Zeigler M, Bach G: Krabbe disease in Israel. *Isr J Med Sci* **27**:196, 1991.
254. Rafi MA, Luzi P, Zlotogora J, Wenger DA: Two different mutations are responsible for Krabbe disease in the Druze and Moslem Arab populations in Israel. *Hum Genet* **97**:304, 1996.
255. Svennerholm L, Vanier MT, Håkansson G, Månsson JE: Use of leukocytes in diagnosis of Krabbe disease and detection of carriers. *Clin Chim Acta* **112**:333, 1981.
256. Månsson J-E, Svennerholm L: The use of galactosylceramide with uniform fatty acids as substrates in the diagnosis and carrier detection of Krabbe disease. *Clin Chim Acta* **126**:127, 1982.
257. De Gasperi R, Gama Sosa MA, Sartorato EL, Battistini S, MacFarlane H, Gusella JF, Krivit W, Kolodny EH: Molecular heterogeneity of late onset forms of globoid-cell leukodystrophy. *Am J Hum Genet* **59**:1233, 1996.
258. Luzi P, Rafi MA, Wenger DA: Krabbe disease: Correlations between mutations in the GALC gene, GALC activity and clinical presentation. *Am J Hum Genet* **57**(Suppl):A245, 1995.
259. Gama Sosa MA, De Gasperi R, Undevia S, Yeretsian J, Rouse II SC, Lyerla TA, Kolodny EH: Correction of the galactocerebrosidase deficiency in globoid cell leukodystrophy—cultured cells by SL-3 retroviral-mediated gene transfer. *Biochem Biophys Res Commun* **218**:766, 1996.
260. Rafi MA, Fugaro J, Amini S, Luzi P, de Gala G, Victoria T, Dubell C, et al.: Retroviral vector-mediated transfer of the galactocerebrosidase (GALC) cDNA leads to overexpression and transfer of GALC activity to neighboring cells. *Biochem Molec Med* **58**:142, 1996.
261. Costantino-Ceccarini E, Luddi A, Volterrani M, Strazza M, Rafi MA, Wenger DA: Transduction of cultured oligodendrocytes from normal and twitcher mice by a retroviral vector containing human galactocerebrosidase (GALC) cDNA. *Neurochem Res* **24**:287, 1999.
262. Matsumoto A, Vanier MT, Oya Y, Kelly D, Popko B, Wenger DA, Suzuki K: Transgenic introduction of human galactosylceramidase into twitcher mouse: Significant phenotype improvement with a minimal expression. *Dev Brain Dysfunct* **19**:142, 1997.
263. Tanaka H, Meisler M, Suzuki K: Activity of human hepatic β-galactosidase toward natural glycosphingolipid substrates. *Biochim Biophys Acta* **398**:452, 1975.
264. Vanier MT, Svennerholm L, Månsson JE, Håkansson G, Bouf A, Lindsten J: Prenatal diagnosis of Krabbe disease. *Clin Genet* **20**:79, 1981.
265. Besley GT, Bain AD: Krabbe's globoid cell leukodystrophy. Studies on galactosylceramide β-galactosidase and non-specific β-galactosidase of leukocytes, cultured skin fibroblasts, and amniotic fluid cells. *J Med Genet* **13**:195, 1976.
266. Suzuki K: Globoid cell leukodystrophy (Krabbe's disease) and G_{M1}-gangliosidosis, in Glew RH, Peters SP (eds): *Practical Enzymology of Sphingolipidoses*. New York, Liss, 1977, p 101.
267. Suzuki K: Enzymatic diagnosis of sphingolipidoses. *Methods Enzymol* **50**C:456, 1978.
268. Svennerholm L: Diagnosis of the sphingolipidoses with labelled natural substrates. *Adv Exp Med Biol* **101**:689, 1978.
269. Svennerholm L, Håkansson G, Månsson JE, Vanier MT: The assay of sphingolipid hydrolases in white blood cells with labelled natural substrates. *Clin Chim Acta* **92**:53, 1979.
270. Kudoh T, Wenger DA: Diagnosis of metachromatic leukodystrophy, Krabbe disease, and Farber disease after uptake of fatty acid-labeled cerebroside sulfate into cultured skin fibroblasts. *J Clin Invest* **70**:89, 1982.
271. Wenger DA, Riccardi VM: Possible misdiagnosis of Krabbe disease. *J Pediatr* **88**:76, 1976.
272. Wenger DA, Louie E: Pseudodeficiencies of arylsulfatase A and galactocerebrosidase activities. *Develop Neurosci* **13**:216, 1991.
273. Christomanou H: Biochemical, psychometric and neurophysiological studies in heterozygotes for various lipidoses. *Hum Genet* **55**:103, 1980.
274. Christomanou H: Biochemical, genetic, psychometric and neurophysiological studies in heterozygotes of a family with globoid cell leukodystrophy (Krabbe). *Hum Genet* **58**:179, 1981.
275. Olmstead CE: Neurological and neurobehavioral development of the mutant "twitcher" mouse. *Behav Brain Res* **15**:143, 1987.
276. Krivit W, Shapiro EG, Peters C, Wagner JE, Cornu G, Kurtzberg J, Wenger DA, Kolodny EH, Vanier MT, Loes DJ, Dusenbery K, Lockman LA: Hematopoietic stem-cell transplantation in globoid-cell leukodystrophy. *N Engl J Med* **338**:1119, 1998.
277. Bambach BJ, Moser HW, Blakemore KJ, Corson VL, Griffin CA, Noga SJ, Perlman EJ, Zuckerman R, Wenger DA, Jones RJ: Engraftment following in utero bone marrow transplantation for globoid cell leukodystrophy. *Bone Marrow Transplant* **19**:399, 1997.
278. Suzuki K: "Authentic animal models" for biochemical studies of human genetic diseases, in Arima M, Suzuki Y, Yabuuchi H (eds): *Proceedings of the 4th International Symposium on Developmental Disabilities*. Tokyo, University of Tokyo Press, p 129, 1984.
279. Suzuki K, Suzuki K: Genetic galactosylceramidase deficiency (globoid cell leukodystrophy, Krabbe disease) in different mammalian species. *Neurochem Pathol* **3**:53, 1985.
280. Suzuki K, Suzuki K: Genetic animal models of Krabbe disease, in Driscoll P (ed): *Genetically-Defined Animal Models of Neurobehavioral Dysfunction*. Boston, Birkhäuser, 1992, p 24.
281. Pritchard DH, Napthine DV, Sinclair AJ: Globoid cell leukodystrophy in polled Dorset sheep. *Vet Pathol* **17**:399, 1980.
282. Baskin G, Alroy J, Li Y-T, Dayal Y, Raghavan SS, Charer L: Galactosylceramide lipidosis in Rhesus monkeys. *Lab Invest* **60**:7A, 1989.
283. Boysen GB, Tryphonas L, Harries NW: Globoid cell leukodystrophy in the blue-tick hound dog. I. Clinical manifestations. *Can Vet J* **15**:303, 1974.
284. Johnson GR, Oliver JE Jr, Selcer R: Globoid cell leukodystrophy in a beagle. *J Am Vet Med Assoc* **167**:380, 1975.
285. Fankhäuser R, Luginbühl H, Hartley WJ: Leukodystrophie vom Typus Krabbe beim Hund. *Schweiz Arch Tierheilkd* **105**:198, 1963.
286. Fletcher TF, Kurtz HJ, Low DG: Globoid cell leukodystrophy (Krabbe type) in the dog. *J Am Vet Med Assoc* **149**:165, 1966.
287. Johnson KH: Globoid leukodystrophy in the cat. *J Am Vet Med Assoc* **157**:2057, 1970
288. Jortner BS, Jonas AM: The neuropathology of globoid cell leucodystrophy in the dog: A report of two cases. *Acta Neuropathol* (Berlin) **10**:171, 1968.
289. Austin J, Armstrong D, Margolis G: Studies of globoid leukodystrophy in dogs. *Neurology* (Minneapolis) **18**:300, 1968.
290. Austin J, Armstrong D, Margolis G: Canine globoid leukodystrophy: A model demyelinating disorder. *Trans Am Neurol Assoc* **93**:181, 1968.
291. Fletcher TF: Leukodystrophy in the dog. *Minn Vet* **9**:19, 1969.
292. Austin J: Recent studies in two inborn errors of glycolipid metabolism, in Bogoch SE (ed): *The Future of the Brain Sciences*. New York, Plenum, 1969, p 397.
293. McGrath J, Schutta H, Yashen A, Steinberg A: A morphology and biochemical study of canine globoid leukodystrophy. *J Neuropathol Exp Neurol* **28**:171, 1969.
294. Hirth RS, Nielsen SW: A familial canine globoid cell leukodystrophy ("Krabbe type"). *J Small Anim Pract* **8**:569, 1967.
295. Fletcher TF, Kurtz HJ: Animal model: Globoid cell leukodystrophy in dog. *Am J Pathol* **66**:375, 1972.
296. Kurtz HJ, Fletcher TF: The peripheral neuropathy of canine globoid cell leukodystrophy (Krabbe-type). *Acta Neuropathol* (Berlin) **16**:226, 1970.
297. Fletcher TF, Kurtz HJ, Stadlan EM: Experimental Wallerian degeneration in peripheral nerves of dogs with globoid cell leukodystrophy. *J Neuropathol Exp Neurol* **30**:593, 1971.
298. Fletcher TF: Electroencephalographic features of leukodystrophic disease in the dog. *J Am Vet Med Assoc* **157**:190, 1970.
299. Fletcher TF, Lee DG, Hammer RF: Ultrastructural features of globoid cell leukodystrophy in the dog. *Am J Vet Res* **32**:177, 1971.
300. Yunis EJ, Lee RE: The morphologic similarities of human and canine globoid leukodystrophy. Thin section and freeze-fracture studies. *Am J Pathol* **85**:99, 1976.
301. Yajima K, Fletcher TF, Suzuki K: Canine globoid cell leukodystrophy. Part I. Further ultrastructural study of the typical lesion. *J Neurol Sci* **33**:179, 1977.

302. Fletcher TF, Jessen CR, Bender AP: Quantitative evaluation of spinal cord lesions in canine globoid leukodystrophy. *J Neuropathol Exp Neurol* **36**:84, 1977.
303. Yajima K: Canine globoid cell leukodystrophy: Chronological neuropathological observation in the early lesions. *Brain Dev* **12**:153, 1980.
304. Roszel JF, Steinberg SA, McGrath JT: Periodic acid-Schiff-positive cells in cerebrospinal fluid of dogs with globoid cell leukodystrophy. *Neurology* **22**:738, 1972.
305. Kurczynski TW, Kondeleon SK, MacBride RG, Dickerman LH, Fletcher TF: Studies of a synthetic substrate in canine globoid cell leukodystrophy. *Biochim Biophys Acta* **672**:297, 1981.
306. Suzuki K: Characteristic inclusions in the kidney of canine globoid cell leukodystrophy. *Acta Neuropathol* **69**:33, 1986.
307. Suzuki Y, Austin J, Suzuki K, Armstrong D, Schlenker J, Fletcher T: Studies in globoid leukodystrophy: Enzymatic and lipid findings in the canine form. *Exp Neurol* **29**:65, 1970.
308. Fletcher TF, Suzuki K, Martin F: Galactocerebrosidase activities in canine globoid leukodystrophy. *Neurology* **27**:758, 1977.
309. Suzuki Y, Miyatake T, Fletcher TF, Suzuki K: Glycosphingolipid β-galactosidases. III. Canine form of globoid cell leukodystrophy: Comparison with the human disease. *J Biol Chem* **249**:2109, 1974.
310. Kurczynski TW, Fletcher TF, Suzuki K: Lactosylceramidases in canine globoid cell leukodystrophy. *J Neurochem* **29**:37, 1977.
311. Costantino-Ceccarini E, Fletcher TF, Suzuki K: Glycolipid metabolism in the canine form of globoid cell leukodystrophy, in Volk BW, Schneck L (eds): *Current Trends in Sphingolipidoses and Allied Disorders*. New York, Plenum, 1976, p 127.
312. Victoria T, Rafi MA, Wenger DA: Cloning of the canine GALC cDNA and identification of the mutation causing globoid cell leukodystrophy in West Highland White and Cairn terriers. *Genomics* **33**:457, 1996.
313. Vite C, Cozzi F, Wenger DA, Victoria T, Haskins M: MRI and electrophysiological abnormalities in a case of canine globoid cell leukodystrophy. *J Small Anim Pract* **39**:401, 1998.
314. Duchen LW, Eicher EM, Jacobs JM, Scaravilli F, Teixeira F: A globoid cell type of leukodystrophy in the mouse: The mutant twitcher, in Baumann N (ed): *Neurological Mutations Affecting Myelination*. Amsterdam, Elsevier, 1980, p 107.
315. Duchen LW, Eicher EM, Jacobs JM, Scaravilli F, Teixeira F: Hereditary leucodystrophy in the mouse: The new mutant twitcher. *Brain* **103**:695, 1980.
316. Suzuki K, Suzuki, K: The twitcher mouse: A model of human globoid cell leukodystrophy (Krabbe's disease). *Am J Path* **111**:394, 1983.
317. Kobayashi T, Scaravilli F, Suzuki K: Biochemistry of twitcher mouse: An authentic murine model of human globoid cell leukodystrophy, in Baumann N (ed): *Neurological Mutations Affecting Myelination*. Amsterdam, Elsevier, 1980, p 253.
318. Kobayashi T, Yamamaka T, Jacobs J, Teixeira F, Suzuki K: The twitcher mouse: An enzymatically authentic model of human globoid cell leukodystrophy (Krabbe disease). *Brain Res* **202**:479, 1980.
319. Kobayashi T, Nagara H, Suzuki K, Suzuki K: The twitcher mouse: Determination of genetic status by galactosylceramidase assays on clipped tail. *Biochem Med* **27**:8, 1982.
320. Sakai N, Inui K, Tatsumi N, Fukushima H, Nishigaki T, Taniike M, Nishimoto J, Tsukamoto H, Yanagihara, Ozono K, Okada S: Molecular cloning and expression of cDNA for murine galactocerebrosidase and mutation analysis of the twitcher mouse, a model of Krabbe's disease. *J Neurochem* **66**:1118, 1996.
321. Takahashi H, Suzuki K: Globoid cell leukodystrophy: Specialized contact of globoid cell with astrocyte in the brain of twitcher mouse. *Acta Neuropath* **58**:237, 1982.
322. Nagara H, Kobayashi T, Suzuki K, Suzuki K: The twitcher mouse—normal pattern of early myelination in the spinal cord. *Brain Res* **244**:289, 1982.
323. Jacobs JM, Scaravilli F, Dearanda FT: The pathogenesis of globoid cell leukodystrophy in peripheral nerve of the mouse mutant twitcher. *J Neurol Sci* **55**:285, 1982.
324. Powell HC, Knobler RL, Myers RR: Peripheral neuropathy in the twitcher mutant—a new experimental model of endoneurial edema. *Lab Invest* **49**:19, 1983.
325. Takahashi H, Igisu H, Suzuki K, Suzuki K: The twitcher mouse: An ultrastructural study of the oligodendroglia. *Acta Neuropathol* **59**:159, 1983.
326. Takahashi H, Suzuki K: Demyelination in the spinal cord of murine globoid cell leukodystrophy (the twitcher mouse). *Acta Neuropathol* **62**:298, 1984.
327. Takahashi H, Igisu H, Suzuki, K, Suzuki K: Murine globoid cell leukodystrophy (the twitcher mouse)—the presence of characteristic inclusions in the kidney and lymph nodes. *Am J Pathol* **112**:147, 1983.
328. Takahashi H, Igisu H, Suzuki K, Suzuki K: Murine globoid cell leukodystrophy: The twitcher mouse. *Lab Invest* **50**:42, 1984.
329. Ida H, Umezawa F, Kasai E, Eto Y, Maekawa K: An accumulation of galactocerebroside in kidney from mouse globoid cell leukodystrophy (twitcher). *Biochem Biophys Res Commun* **109**:634, 1982.
330. Igisu H, Takahashi H, Suzuki K, Suzuki, K: Abnormal accumulation of galactosylceramide in the kidney of twitcher mouse. *Biochem Biophys Res Commun* **110**:940, 1983.
331. Scaravilli F, Jacobs JM, Teixeira F: Quantitative and experimental studies on the twitcher mouse, in Baumann N (ed): *Neurological Mutations Affecting Myelination*. Amsterdam, Elsevier, 1980, p 115.
332. Tanaka K, Nagara H, Kobayashi K, Goto I: The twitcher mouse: Accumulation of galactosylsphingosine and pathology of the sciatic nerve. *Brain Res* **454**:340, 1988.
333. Tanaka K, Nagara H, Kobayashi K, Goto I: The twitcher mouse: Accumulation of galactosylsphingosine and pathology of the central nervous system. *Brain Res* **482**:347, 1989.
334. Taniike M, Suzuki K: Spacio-temporal progression of demyelination in twitcher mouse: With clinico-pathological correlation. *Acta Neuropathol* **88**:228, 1994.
335. Levine SM, Wetzel DL, Eilert AJ: Neuropathology of twitcher mice: Examination by histochemistry, immunohistochemistry, lectin histochemistry and Fourier transform infrared microspectroscopy. *Int J Dev Neurosci* **12**:275, 1994.
336. Kobayashi S, Katayama M, Suzuki K, Suzuki K: The twitcher mouse: An alteration of the unmyelinated fibers in the PNS. *Am J Pathol* **131**:308, 1988.
337. Ohno M, Komiyama A, Martin PM, Suzuki K: Proliferation of microglia/macrophages in the demyelinating CNS and PNS of twitcher mouse. *Brain Res* **602**:268, 1993.
338. Ohno M, Komiyama A, Martin PM, Suzuki K: MHC class II antigen expression and T-cell infiltration in the demyelinating CNS and PNS of the twitcher mouse. *Brain Res* **652**:186, 1993.
339. Matsushima GK, Taniike M, Glimcher LH, Grusby MJ, Frelinger JA, Suzuki K, Ting JP: Absence of MHC class II molecules reduces CNS demyelination, microglial/macrophage infiltration, and twitching in murine globoid cell leukodystrophy. *Cell* **78**:645, 1994.
340. Taniike M, Marcus JR, Popko B, Suzuki K: Expression of major histocompatibility complex class I antigens in the demyelinating twitcher CNS and PNS. *J Neurosci Res* **47**:539, 1997.
341. Levine SM, Brown DC: IL-6 and TNFα expression in brains of twitcher, quaking and normal mice. *J Neuroimmunol* **73**:47, 1997.
342. Yamada H, Martin P, Suzuki K: Impairment of protein kinase C activity in twitcher Schwann cells in vitro. *Brain Res* **718**:138, 1996.
343. Taniike M, Marcus JR, Nishigaki T, Fujita N, Popko B, Suzuki K, Suzuki K: Suppressed UDP-galactose:ceramide galactosyltransferase and myelin protein mRNA in twitcher mouse brain. *J Neurosci Res* **51**:536, 1998.
344. Scaravilli F, Jacobs JM: Peripheral nerve grafting without immunological suppressive treatment in the twitcher mouse, a murine model of a human leucodystrophy. *Nature* **290**:56, 1981.
345. Scaravilli F, Jacobs JM: Improved myelination in nerve grafts from the leukodystrophic twitcher into trembler mice: Evidence for enzyme replacement. *Brain Res* **237**:163, 1982.
346. Scaravilli F, Suzuki K: Enzyme replacement in grafted nerve of twitcher mouse. *Nature* **305**:713, 1983.
347. Yeager AM, Brennan S, Tiffany C, Moser HW, Santos GW: Prolonged survival and remyelination after hematopoietic cell transplantation in the twitcher mouse. *Science* **225**:1053, 1984.
348. Seller MJ, Perkins KJ, Fensom AH: Galactosylcerebrosidase activity in tissues of twitcher mice with and without bone marrow transplantation. *J Inherit Metab Dis* **9**:234, 1986.
349. Hoogerbrugge PM, Poorthuis BJHM, Romme AE, Van de Camp JJP, Wagemaker G, van Bekkum: Bone marrow transplantation in lysosomal storage disease: Effect on enzyme levels and clinical course in the neurologically affected twitcher mouse. *J Clin Invest* **81**:1790, 1988.
350. Hoogerbrugge PM, Suzuki K, Suzuki K, Poorthuis, BJHM, Kobayashi T, Wagemaker G, van Bekkum DW: Donor-derived cells in the central nervous system of twitcher mouse after bone marrow transplantation. *Science* **239**:1035, 1988.
351. Ichioka T, Kishimoto Y, Brennan S, Santos GW, Yeager AM: Hematopoietic cell transplantation in murine globoid cell leukodystrophy (the twitcher mouse): Effects on levels of galactosylceramidase,

psychosine, and galactocerebrosides. *Proc Natl Acad Sci USA* **84**:4259, 1987.

352. Suzuki K, Hoogerbrugge PM, Poorthuis BJHM, Van Bekkum DW, Suzuki K: The twitcher mouse: CNS pathology following bone marrow transplantation (BMT). *Lab Invest* **58**:302 1988.
353. Kondo A, Hoogerbrugge PM, Suzuki K, Poorthuis BJHM, Van Bekkum DW, Suzuki K: Pathology of the peripheral nerve in the twitcher mouse following bone marrow transplantation. *Brain Res* **460**:178, 1988.
354. Yeager AM, Shinohara M, Shinn C: Hematopoietic cell transplantation after administration of high-dose Busulfan in murine globoid cell leukodystrophy (the twitcher mouse). *Pediatr Res* **29**:302, 1991.
355. Huppes W, De Groot CJ, Ostendorf RH, Bauman JG, Gossen JA, Smit V, Vijg J, et al.: Detection of migrated allogeneic oligodendrocytes throughout the central nervous system of the galactocerebrosidase-deficient twitcher mouse. *J Neurocytol* **21**:129, 1992.
356. Umezawa F, Eto Y, Tokoro T, Ito F, Maekawa K: Enzyme replacement with liposomes containing β-galactosidase from Charonia lampas in murine globoid cell leukodystrophy (twitcher). *Biochem Biophys Res Commun* **127**:663, 1985.
357. Suzuki K, Suzuki K: The twitcher mouse: A model for Krabbe disease and for experimental therapies. *Brain Pathol* **5**:249, 1995.
358. Suzuki K, Taniike M: Murine model of genetic demyelinating disease: The twitcher mouse. *Microscopy Res Tech* **32**:204, 1995.
359. Luzi P, Rafi MA, Victoria T, Baskin GB, Wenger DA: Characterization of the rhesus monkey galactocerebrosidase (GALC) cDNA and gene and identification of the mutation causing globoid cell leukodystrophy (Krabbe disease) in this primate. *Genomics* **42**:319, 1997.

CHAPTER 148

Metachromatic Leukodystrophy

Kurt von Figura ▪ Volkmar Gieselmann ▪ Jaak Jaeken

1. **Metachromatic leukodystrophy (MLD) is an autosomal recessively inherited disorder in which the desulfation of 3-0-sulfogalactosyl-containing glycolipids is defective. These sulfated glycolipids occur in the myelin sheaths in the central and peripheral nervous system and to a lesser extent in visceral organs like kidney, gallbladder, and liver. In MLD the sulfated glycolipids accumulate in lysosomes of these tissues and are responsible for their metachromatic staining. The clinical and histopathologic manifestations of MLD are dominated by the demyelination observed in the central and peripheral nervous system.**
2. **The clinical onset and severity of MLD show great variation. The late infantile form is usually recognized in the second year of life and fatal in early childhood. The juvenile form presents between age 4 and puberty; the adult form may become clinically overt at any age after puberty. In both of these variants, gait disturbance and mental regression are the earliest signs. In the childhood variants, other common signs are blindness, loss of speech, quadriparesis, peripheral neuropathy, and seizures. In the adult, behavioral disturbances and dementia are the major presenting signs, often inducing the misdiagnosis of a psychosis. The disease may progress slowly over several decades. Demonstration of demyelination by computed tomography or magnetic resonance imaging and reduced nerve conduction velocity are the major laboratory findings.**
3. **Desulfation of the 3-0-sulfogalactosyl residues in glycolipids depends on the combined action of arylsulfatase A (ASA) and saposin B, a nonenzymatic activator protein. Deficiency either of ASA or, more rarely, of saposin B causes MLD.**
4. **More than 60 different mutations have been characterized in the ASA gene. Only a few mutations occur with high frequency. Homozygosity for null alleles is the cause of the late infantile form of MLD. In the juvenile and adult forms of MLD, one or both ASA alleles are associated with at least some residual activity. There is strong evidence that the severity of the disease correlates inversely with the residual activity of ASA.**
5. **Diagnosis of MLD is based on the clinical symptoms and laboratory findings caused by the demyelination and on demonstration of the deficiency of ASA or saposin B. Prenatal diagnosis is possible by determination of ASA activity in cultured amniotic fluid cells or chorionic villi.**
6. **The diagnosis of MLD is complicated by the facts that absence of ASA activity does not prove MLD and that its presence does not exclude it. Apparent absence of ASA activity is observed in individuals homozygous for the benign ASA pseudodeficiency allele, which encodes only 5–15 percent of residual activity. Up to 2 percent of Europeans are homozygous for the pseudodeficiency allele. The apparent residual activity that is detected with the commonly used colorimetric assays for ASA in late infantile MLD, in which no functional ASA is synthesized, is in the range of that found in individuals homozygous for the pseudodeficiency allele. The latter can be identified with DNA-based assays. A further complication arises from the fact that MLD-causing mutations occur in the pseudodeficiency allele as frequently as in the wild-type ASA allele. Normal ASA activity is observed in MLD patients with a deficiency of saposin B, because the colorimetric assay for ASA does not depend on saposin B.**
7. **There is no specific treatment for MLD. Prevention of the disease is restricted to the possibility of prenatal diagnosis and carrier identification in families with known risk or in populations with a high incidence of MLD. A mouse model for MLD has been developed, which mimics most of the biochemical alterations seen in MLD but exhibits only moderate demyelination and a mild phenotype.**

HISTORICAL ASPECTS

The first description of a patient with metachromatic leukodystrophy (MLD) was published in 1910 by the German neurologist and psychiatrist Alois Alzheimer.[1] Alzheimer described the metachromatic staining of the nervous system and the clinical symptoms of a patient who would now be classified as suffering from an adult form of MLD. Alzheimer is better known for the first description of a patient with progressive senile dementia, a disease commonly designated *Alzheimer disease*. The description of this patient appeared in 1906[2] and 1907.[3] Recently it was suspected that the original Alzheimer patient in fact had an adult form of MLD.[4] If so, Alzheimer would have retained the credit for the description of the first patient with MLD but lost the credit for the description of the first patient with the disease named for him. The recent discovery of the long-lost original file of the first case of Alzheimer disease stimulated a reevaluation of Alzheimer's original diagnosis. A consensus was reached that Auguste D., whose case was reported by Alzheimer in 1907, indeed represented the first case of Alzheimer disease rather than of MLD.[5]

In 1921, Witte[6] described a patient with accumulation of metachromatic material not only in the brain but also in the liver, kidneys, and testes. Scholz,[7] in his detailed account in 1925 of three children from one family with progressive leukodystrophy, proposed that the myelin abnormality that he observed might be due to a glial cell defect. However, he failed to detect metachromatic properties in the tissues that he examined, because they had been treated with alcohol, which removed the lipid responsible for

A list of standard abbreviations is located immediately preceding the index in each volume. Nonstandard abbreviations used in this chapter include: ASA = arylsulfatase A; MLD = metachromatic leukodystrophy; ACAT = acyl CoA:cholesterol acyltransferase; CESD = cholesteryl ester storage disease; LAL = lysosomal acid lipase; LCAT = lecithin:cholesterol acyltransferase; *LIPA* = gene symbol for lysosomal acid lipase A; *LIPB* = gene symbol for lysosomal acid lipase B.

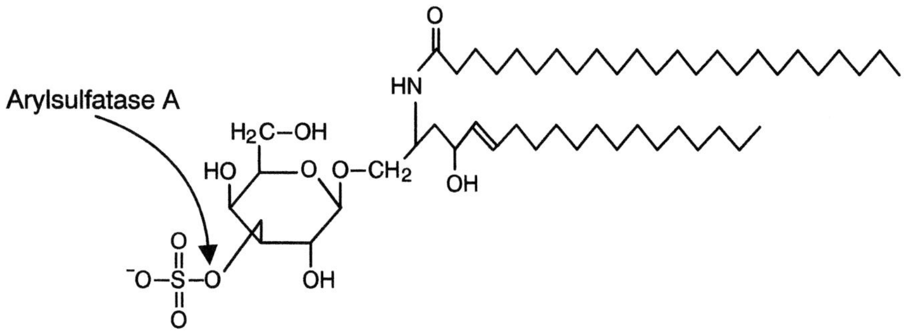

Fig. 148-1 3-0-Sulfogalactosyl ceramide (sulfatide), the major accumulating material in metachromatic leukodystrophy, and the site of action of arylsulfatase A.

the metachromasia. In 1955, von Hirsch and Peiffer[8] showed that an acetic acid-cresyl violet stain would change to brown in tissues from patients with MLD. Using this stain, Peiffer found striking metachromasia in frozen sections from the original patient of Scholz.[9] The descriptions of Scholz and Peiffer thus represent the first comprehensive report on the clinical and pathologic aspects of juvenile MLD. A third type of MLD, which begins in the late infantile period, was reported by Greenfield[10] in 1933.

Known for many years as "diffuse brain sclerosis," the disease was renamed "metachromatic leukoencephalopathy" in 1938 by Einarson and Neel.[11] Norman[12] later suggested that it be classified as a lipidosis. This was proved to be correct by the independent discoveries in 1958 and 1959, respectively, by Jatzkewitz[13] and Austin[14] of a large excess of sulfatides (3-0-sulfogalactosyl ceramides) in tissues from patients with MLD. The accumulation of this acid lipid causes the metachromasia characteristic of this disease. In 1963 Austin et al.[15] reported the deficiency of arylsulfatase A (ASA) in MLD, and 2 years later Mehl and Jatzkewitz[16] demonstrated a block in the metabolism of sulfatide (Fig. 148-1). ASA was subsequently identified as the heat-labile component of sulfatide sulfatase.[17] Mehl and Jatzkewitz[18] also described a heat-stable factor that increases the activity of sulfatide sulfatase severalfold. In rare patients with MLD, it is this factor — now known as saposin B — rather than ASA that is deficient.[19] Another disorder, which contains clinical features characteristic of MLD with signs of mucopolysaccharidosis and an ichthyosis, has been reported several times since 1965.[20] In this disorder, known as multiple sulfatase deficiency (Chap. 149), at least seven different sulfatases are deficient.[21]

Reports of apparently normal individuals with very low levels of ASA, mostly in families with MLD, began to appear in 1975.[22] This condition has been referred to as "pseudodeficiency of ASA"[23] or simply "pseudodeficiency." Subsequently, it was established that there is a relatively common allele[24] of the ASA gene that leads to low expression of the enzyme and that 1–2 percent of the European population have enzyme levels (5–15 percent of normal) that are difficult to differentiate from those of MLD patients in many assay protocols.

CLINICAL MANIFESTATIONS

The clinical entity of MLD comprises two disorders: ASA deficiency and saposin B deficiency. A related disorder, multiple sulfatase deficiency, combines the clinical features of MLD with those caused by deficiencies of other sulfatases. The frequency of ASA deficiency exceeds by far that of saposin B or multiple sulfatase deficiency.

Clinical Forms of MLD

Metachromatic leukodystrophy can be divided according to age of onset into a late infantile, a juvenile, and an adult form. The clinical features of these forms are summarized in Table 148-1.

Table 148-1 Characteristics of Late Infantile, Juvenile, and Adult Forms of MLD

Type	Age at onset (years)	Main clinical manifestations	Spinal fluid protein	Nerve conduction velocity	Urinary sulfatide excretion
Infantile	0.5–4	Gait disturbance, decreased tendon reflexes, mental regression, loss of speech, optic atrophy, ataxia, progressive spastic quadriparesis	Elevated	Slowed	Elevated
Early juvenile	4–6	Gait and postural abnormalities, emotional and behavioral disturbances, optic atrophy, progressive spastic quadriparesis	Elevated	Slowed	Elevated
Late juvenile	6–16	Behavioral abnormalities, poor school performance, language regression, gait disturbance, slowly progressive spastic tetraparesis	Elevated	Slowed	Elevated
Adult	>16	Mental regression, psychiatric symptoms, incontinence, slowly progressive spastic tetraparesis	Normal or elevated	Normal or slowed	Elevated

MLD caused by saposin B deficiency can present as any of the different forms of MLD caused by ASA deficiency. Multiple sulfatase deficiency associates the signs of MLD with those of mucopolysaccharidoses and ichthyosis. Saposin B deficiency and multiple sulfatase deficiency share with MLD elevated spinal fluid protein levels, slowed nerve conduction velocity, and increased urinary excretion of sulfatides.

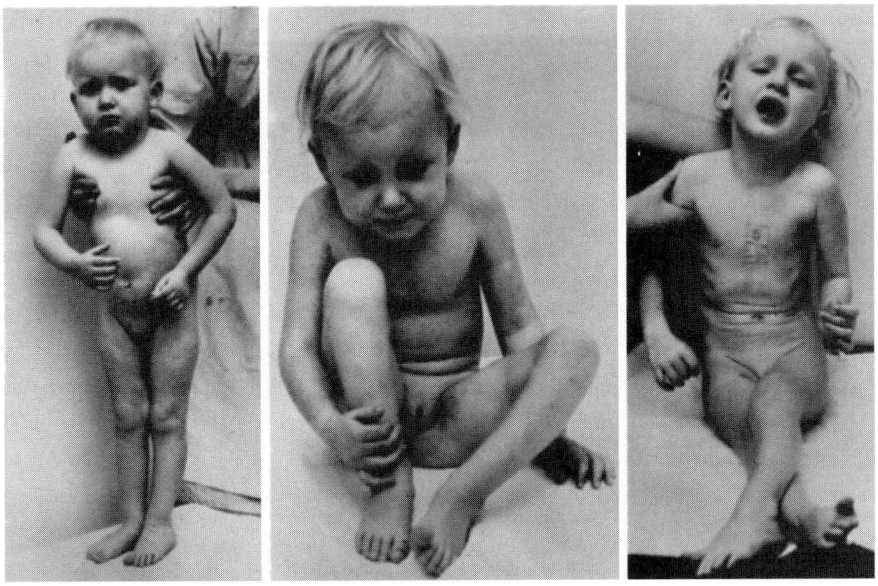

A B C

Fig. 148-2 Metachromatic leukodystrophy in late infancy. (A) The child needs to be supported when standing. (B) She can no longer stand, even with support. (C) In the late stage of the disease, the patient is no longer able to sit; note the plantar flexion of the foot and general debility. (*From Hagberg*[30] *with permission.*)

(For a review of the literature before 1993, see Kolodny and Fluharty,[25] which includes the following reviews of large series of patients[26–30]). The majority of patients are about equally divided between the late infantile and juvenile forms of MLD. The adult form of MLD accounts for some 25 percent.

Late Infantile MLD. The late infantile form of MLD (Fig. 148-2) begins between 6 months and 4 years of age. A valuable classification is that of Hagberg, who has subdivided its clinical course into four stages.[30]

Clinical stage I. Most patients have hypotonia of the legs or of all four limbs. The gait therefore becomes unsteady, and the child requires support to stand or walk. The deep tendon reflexes may be diminished or absent secondary to a progressive polyneuropathy. This stage lasts for a few months to more than 1 year.

Clinical stage II. In this stage the patient can no longer stand and shows mental regression. Speech deteriorates as a result of dysarthria and aphasia. Nystagmus is observed, as well as optic atrophy and a grayish discoloration of the macula. The neuropathy may be painful (intermittent pain in arms and legs). Ataxia and truncal titubation become obvious, and muscle tone is increased in the legs. This stage lasts only a few months.

Clinical stage III. Gradually, involvement of the pyramidal system causes the flaccid paresis to be superseded by spastic tetraplegia with pathologic reflexes such as extensor plantar reflexes, and the child becomes bedridden. Bulbar and pseudobulbar palsies occur, causing feeding difficulties and airway obstruction. Epileptic seizures occur in about 25 percent of the children.[31] Although their mental state and speech further deteriorate, these children may still be able to smile and respond.

Clinical stage IV. In this final stage, patients lose all contact with their surroundings, as they are blind and in a decerebrate state, without purposeful movements. They have to be fed through a nasogastric or gastrostomy tube. This stage may last for several years. Death usually occurs about 5 years after onset of clinical symptoms.

Juvenile MLD. The age of onset of juvenile MLD ranges from 4 to 16 years. Patients show gradual deterioration in school performance, slurred speech, gait clumsiness, and incontinence. Usually there are also emotional and behavioral disturbances. Within a year the child is no longer able to walk. Spastic paresis and cerebellar ataxia develop. Sometimes extrapyramidal features (postural abnormalities, increased muscle tone, tremor) are predominant. Contrary to the case in the infantile form, deep tendon reflexes are usually brisk. Optic atrophy develops and in about 50 percent of patients, so do seizures. Finally the child becomes bedridden with complete tetraplegia, in a decerebrate state (Fig. 148-3). There is progressive brainstem dysfunction, causing increasing difficulty in swallowing and necessitating tube feeding. The majority of patients die before the age of 20 years.

A distinction can be made between early- and late-onset forms of juvenile MLD. The early variant has its onset between 4 and 6 years and resembles the late infantile form in that gait disturbance and other motor dysfunctions are early manifestations. In the late-onset variant (onset between 6 and 16 years), behavioral abnormalities, poor school performance, and language regression appear first, followed by gait disturbance.[31] Rarely, the presenting problem is acute cholecystitis[32] or pancreatitis[33] secondary to gallbladder involvement. The latter may also manifest itself as an abdominal mass[34] or gastrointestinal bleeding from hemobilia.[35]

Adult MLD. Adult MLD has been reported at various ages beyond puberty, up to 63 years.[36,37] The patient shows a gradual decline in intellectual abilities, with poor school or job performance. He or she becomes emotionally labile and shows memory deficit, disorganized thinking, behavioral abnormalities, or psychiatric symptoms like hallucinations or delusions. Not infrequently, the initial diagnosis is schizophrenia or a psychotic depression.[38] There is also clumsiness of movements and urinary, and sometimes fecal, incontinence. Signs of peripheral neuropathy are often absent. A progressive spastic paresis of the arms and legs develops, with increased tendon reflexes and extensor plantar reflexes. Ataxia and extrapyramidal symptoms like choreiform movements and dystonia may be present, as well as optic atrophy and signs of bulbar dysfunction. Epileptic seizures are rare. During the final stages of the disease, the patient reaches a vegetative state. The duration of the disease ranges from a few years to several decades.

Saposin B Deficiency

Since the first report of saposin B deficiency by Shapiro et al. in 1979,[19] only a few patients have been described. Age of onset ranged from birth to over 30 years.[25] As might be expected, the clinical picture is indistinguishable from that of MLD caused by ASA deficiency, but the activity of ASA is normal. Deficiency of saposin B (also designated *sulfatide activator protein*) can be demonstrated in leukocytes, fibroblasts, and urine, as can sulfatide

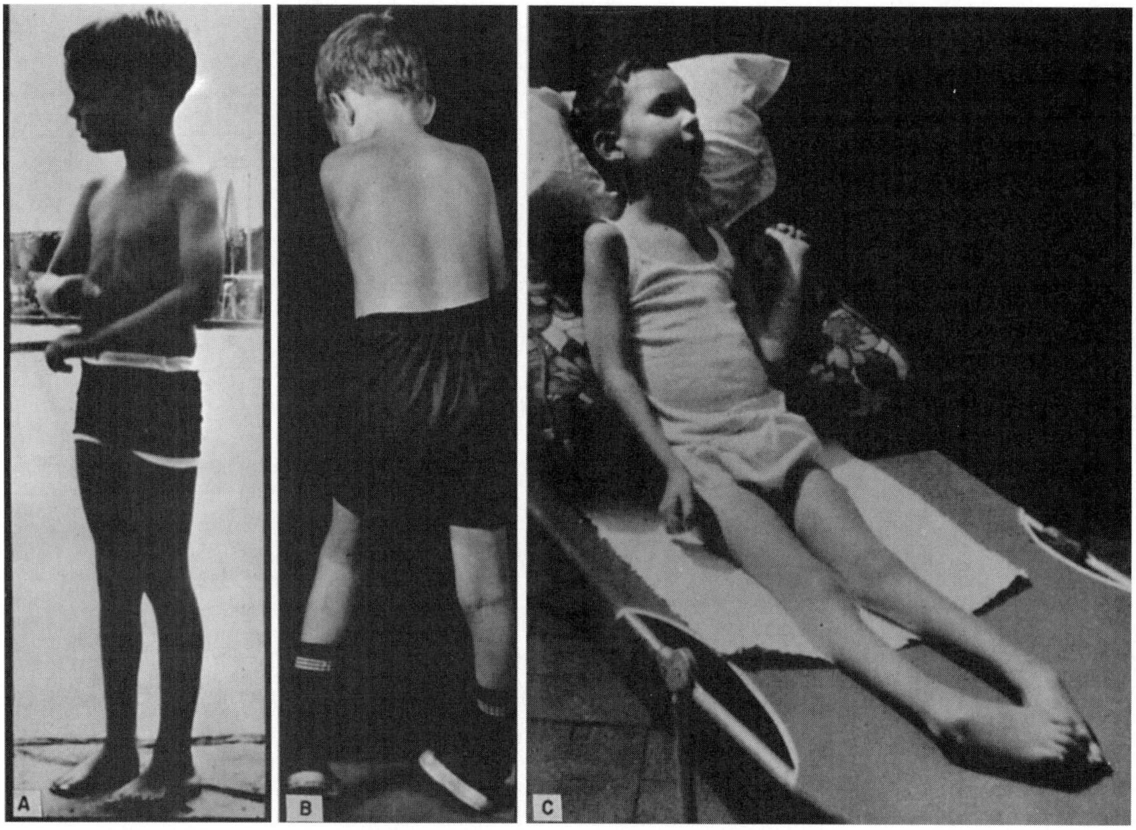

Fig. 148-3 Juvenile MLD. (A) At age $5\frac{1}{2}$ years, 1 year before onset of symptoms, the child is entirely normal. (B) At age 6 years 11 months the child has increasing gait difficulty and is unable to stand without support. (C) At the age of 8 years 10 months the patient is bedridden, has increasing difficulty in swallowing, and requires tube feeding. He is no longer able to speak but recognizes his family and displays pleasure when people pay attention to him.

storage in tissues and sulfatide excretion in urine. Saposin B deficiency is described in detail in Chap. 134.

Multiple Sulfatase Deficiency

Since multiple sulfatase deficiency was first described by Austin et al.[20] in 1965, more than 50 patients have been reported.[25,39,40] The disease, also called mucosulfatidosis or Austin disease, combines the features of MLD and several mucopolysaccharidoses. A neonatal, an early infantile ("Saudi"), an infantile, and a juvenile variant of multiple sulfatase deficiency have been described.

The infantile variant is the classic form. It associates clinical features of infantile MLD with mild features of mucopolysaccharidosis. Early development may be normal, and affected children usually acquire the ability to stand and to say a few words. During the second year of life the children lose acquired abilities and develop staring spells, spasticity, blindness, hearing loss, swallowing difficulties, convulsions, and dementia. Ichthyosis develops at 2–3 years of age. Symptoms of mucopolysaccharidosis occur at variable stages of the disease and include mild facial coarsening (may be absent), stiff joints, growth retardation, skeletal anomalies, and hepatosplenomegaly. Hydrocephalus may occur. There is usually no corneal clouding. Optic atrophy, retinal degeneration, and cherry-red macula have been reported. Age at death is usually between 10 and 18 years. A Saudi variant of multiple sulfatase deficiency has been described, with age of onset between birth and 1 year. The symptomatology comprises dwarfism, severe dysostosis multiplex, facial dysmorphism, cranial synostosis, and cervical cord compression. In rare cases, hydrocephalus develops.[39] There is no or only moderate mental retardation. Ichthyosis, deafness, and retinal degeneration are absent.

A few patients have been reported with a neonatal form of the disease and one patient with a juvenile form. The neonatal form presents at birth with severe mucopolysaccharidosis-like features; death occurs before the age of 1 year. The pathobiochemistry and the molecular defect in multiple sulfatase deficiency are the subject of Chap. 149.

LABORATORY FINDINGS

CT, MRI, and Magnetic Resonance Spectroscopy of the Brain

Computed tomography of patients with MLD reveals a symmetric decrease in the attenuation of the cerebral white matter (Fig. 148-4, upper row). This change results from gradual myelin loss and the increased water content of the remaining structures. The abnormally low density may appear first in the white matter adjacent to the lateral ventricles and is evident at a very early stage in the disease. In late infantile and juvenile cases, there is rapid progression with involvement of the entire centrum semiovale, producing ventricular enlargement. Mild cerebral atrophy may also occur. One study[41] of three children with late infantile MLD described white matter changes predominantly in the frontal lobes. However, in other patients with the late infantile form,[42,43] low attenuation in white matter was most often found in the parietal and occipital lobes.

The CT changes in adult MLD may be present before clinical signs appear and may progress more slowly. The white matter attenuation is most noticeable near the frontal and occipital horns. It may appear as large multifocal, symmetric, well-defined periventricular lucencies rather than as a uniformly diffuse leukodystrophy. As the disease progresses, significant enlargement of the ventricles and considerable cortical atrophy are observed in adult MLD.[44]

MRI (Fig. 148-4, lower row) reveals diffuse hyperintense signal in both the periventricular and subcortical white matter on T2-weighted images.[45] A bright signal may also appear in the internal capsule and corticospinal tract. The white matter lesions in

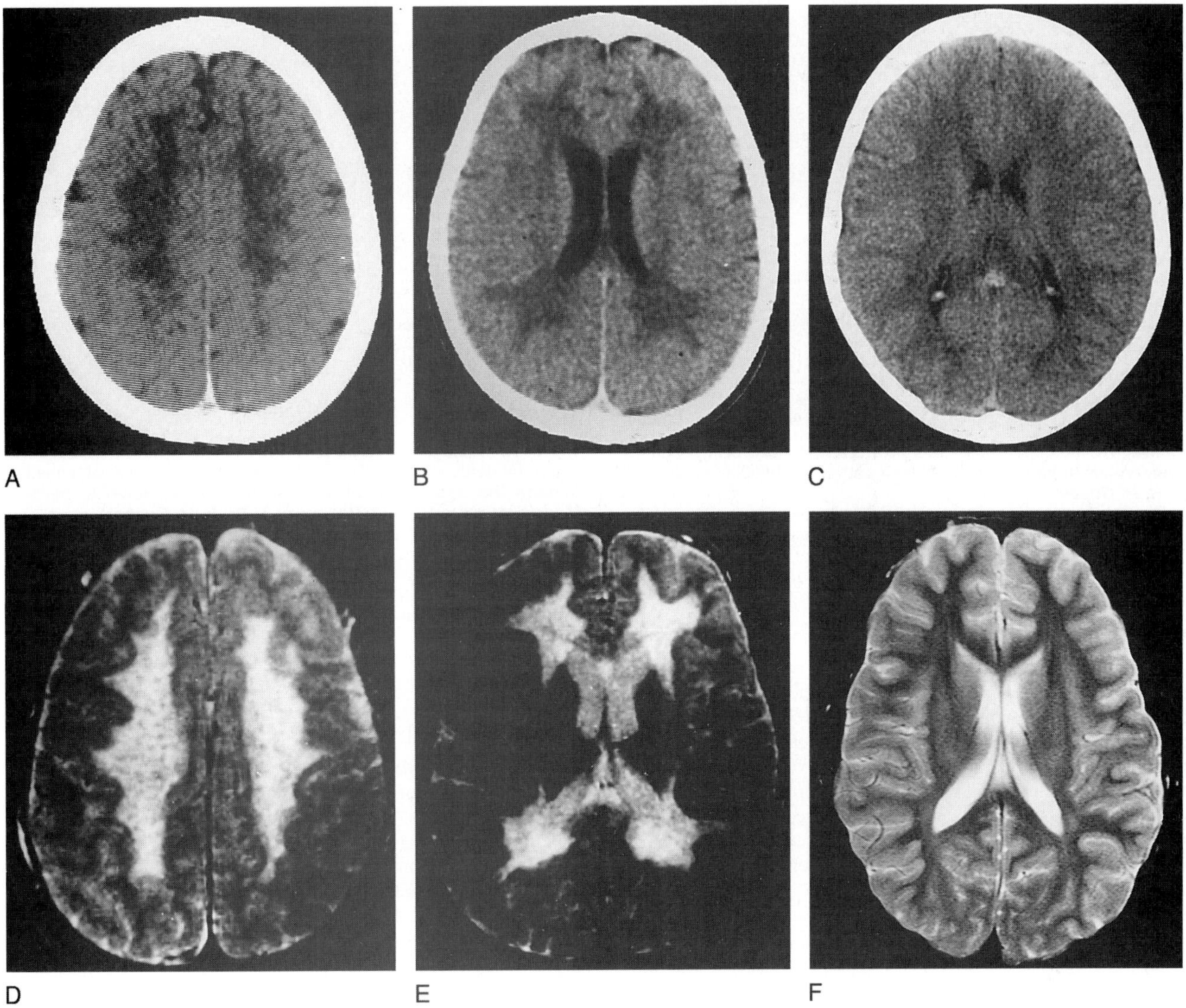

Fig. 148-4 CT and MRI of a 9-year-old patient with juvenile MLD. Upper row: Axial CT scans through the corona radiata (A) and basal ganglia plus capsula interna (B, C) of the patient (A, B) and an age-matched control (C). Extensive low-density signal (appearing dark gray) is seen throughout the deep cerebral white matter. Lower row: Axial T2-weighted MR sections at positions corresponding to those of the CT scans in the upper row. D, E: juvenile MLD; F: control. A high-density signal abnormality (appearing white) is present throughout the hemispheric white matter, sparing the U-fibers (marked by arrows in D and E) (*Courtesy of Dr. F. Hanefeld.*)

the T1-weighted images are slightly hypointense. In the early stages, the arcuate fibers are spared. The lesions do not become enhanced with contrast material. Changes on MRI in adult MLD are more impressive than those seen in CT scans.[46,47,48]

Proton magnetic resonance spectroscopy in patients with late infantile and juvenile forms of MLD revealed marked reduction of N-acetylaspartate in white and gray matter as a sign of neuroaxonal degeneration. In contrast to the case in other leukodystrophies, *myo*-inositol is increased in the white matter. *Myo*-inositol is a glial marker. Its increase in MLD may not only signify gliosis but contribute to the genesis of demyelination.[49]

Neurophysiological Studies

In the late infantile and juvenile forms of MLD, convulsions may occur late in the disease. The occurrence of partial seizures has been explained by the delay in synaptic transmission produced by demyelination. Accordingly, conduction across the corpus callosum may be insufficient to produce secondary generalization.[50]

The EEG can be normal early in the course of the disease, but sometimes it is abnormal even prior to the appearance of symptoms. As the disease advances, the EEG becomes diffusely slow and increases in amplitude, exhibiting mainly 4- to 7-Hz but also some 2- to 4-Hz activity. In a few cases, occasional bursts of spikes or of asymmetric slow-wave activity have been recorded. The discharges tend to be irregular, often with variable focal distribution. Sudden noises may stimulate a marked startle response.[50,51]

In almost all patients, motor nerve conduction velocity is decreased and sensory nerve action potentials are diminished in amplitude, with prolonged peak latency. These nerve conduction abnormalities can be present before clinical symptoms appear and thus provide evidence for the presence of peripheral neuropathy in the presymptomatic stage of MLD.[32,52–54] Different nerves are affected, each at multiple sites.[55] The delay in the afferent nerves may precede that in the efferent nerves.[56] Some patients with the late-onset variant of juvenile MLD and those with adult MLD may exhibit little or no decrease of nerve conduction velocity or any other electrophysiologic evidence of a peripheral neuropathy, even in a clinically advanced stage of their disease.[57]

Recording of brainstem auditory evoked responses in late infantile MLD shows prolongation of interpeak latencies and loss of wave components, which indicate delay or block in conduction in the eighth cranial nerve and brainstem.[58–61]These changes may occur when peripheral nerve conduction is still normal.[58] In juvenile MLD, interpeak latencies of brainstem auditory evoked responses are normal to moderately increased;[52] in adult MLD, both normal[54] and abnormal[62] responses have been reported.

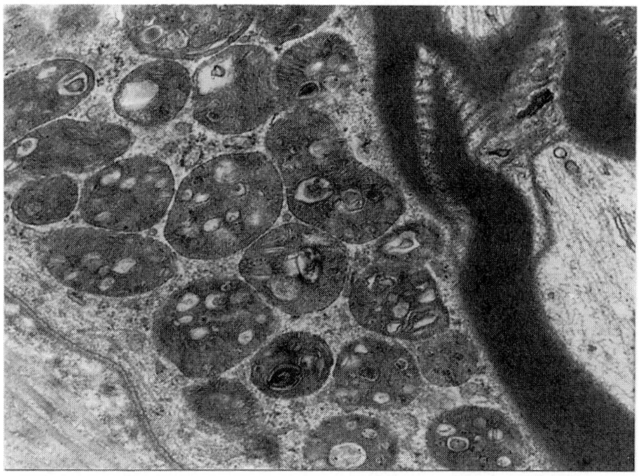

Fig. 148-5 Lysosomal inclusions in a Schwann cell of myelinated axon, typical of juvenile MLD. Magnification × 27,000. (*Courtesy of Dr. H. H. Goebel.*)

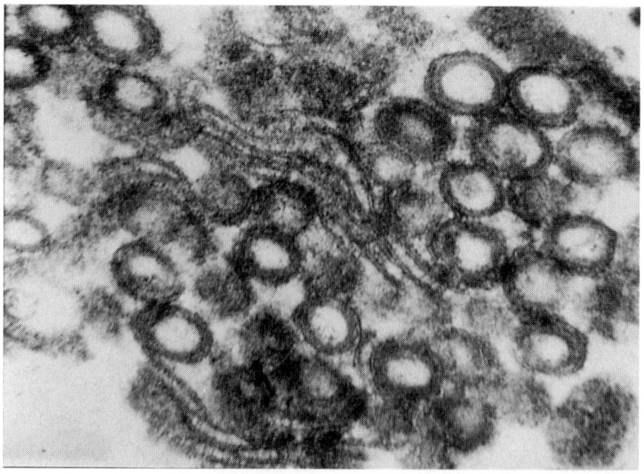

Fig. 148-7 Tuffstonelike bodies found at autopsy in the thalamus of a patient with adult MLD. The circular arrangement of lamellae imparts the impression of a tuffaceous or tuffstonelike pattern. Magnification × 153,700. (*Courtesy of Dr. H. H. Goebel.*)

Abnormalities in visual evoked responses[59–61] and in somatosensory evoked potentials[59] have also been described.[54,62–64]

Cerebrospinal Fluid

In the early stages of late infantile MLD, CSF protein may be normal, but as the disease progresses through stage II, the spinal fluid protein level may rise. Eventually, in the later stages of the disease, the level of total protein may exceed 50 mg/dl. A similar elevation in spinal fluid protein occurs in the early-onset variant of juvenile MLD. The late-onset variant of juvenile MLD may or may not exhibit an increase in spinal fluid protein. In most adult MLD patients, CSF protein is normal; raised levels have been recorded in only a few patients.[65]

The sulfatide content of CSF can be determined by HPLC.[66] Early in the course of late infantile MLD, CSF sulfatides are increased. In contrast, patients with the juvenile and adult forms studied at an intermediate or end stage of the disease have shown normal or slightly reduced levels of sulfatides in their CSF.

Gallbladder Imaging

Extensive deposition of sulfatides may occur in the epithelial layer of the gallbladder, causing papillomatous transformation and interfering with normal function. Papillomatosis of the gallbladder has been demonstrated in patients as young as 2 years of age[67] and before the first neurologic symptoms occurred.[68] Polypoid filling defects have also been seen on oral cholecystography.[69,70] Gallbladder involvement may manifest as acute cholecystitis,[32] gastrointestinal bleeding from hemobilia,[35,67] or an abdominal mass[34] or may be clinically silent.[71] Serial examination of the gallbladder with oral cholecystography[72] or radionuclide scanning may show progressive loss of function.

PATHOLOGY

Morphologic Changes

The pathology of MLD is characterized primarily by demyelination and deposits of metachromatic granules in the central and peripheral nervous system. The metachromatic deposits are spherical masses 15 to 20 μm in diameter that stain brown in frozen tissue sections when treated with a 1-percent solution of acidified cresyl violet.[8] These masses are observed not only in the nervous system but also in visceral organs. Chemical analysis of metachromatic granules has revealed a sulfatide content amounting to 39 percent of their total lipid content. The other lipid components were cholesterol and phosphatides.[73]

High-resolution electron microscopy of the storage granules revealed that the inclusions are surrounded by a membrane, supporting the idea of their lysosomal nature (Fig. 148-5).[74] The morphology of the inclusions varies, but prismatic (Fig. 148-6) and tuffstonelike (Fig. 148-7) profiles are characteristic.

In adult MLD, in addition to the characteristic prismatic and tuffstonelike profiles, composite bodies containing lipofuscin are seen. Their appearance has been attributed to accelerated formation of lipopigment in the storage lysosomes.[75]

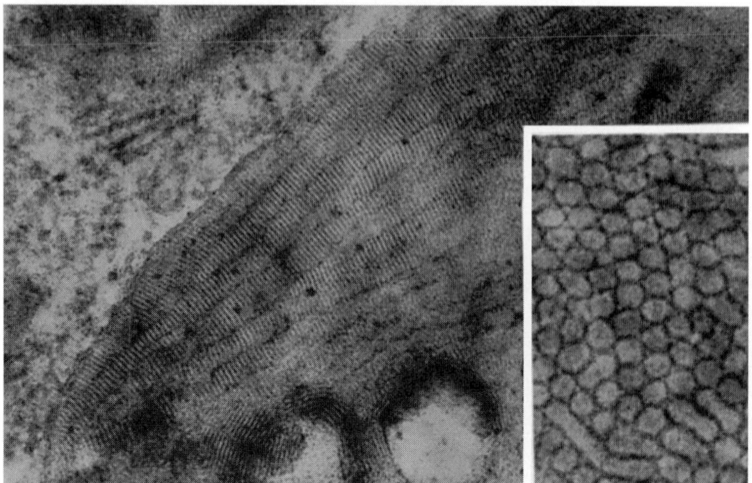

Fig. 148-6 Prismatic inclusions found at autopsy in the brain of a patient with late infantile MLD. Note the lamellar lipid leaflets with a herringbone pattern and (inset) the honeycomb pattern of the same type of structure seen in a section approximately parallel to the lamellae. Magnification × 200,000. (*From Rutsaert et al.*[327] *with permission.*)

Central Nervous System

The central white matter is reduced in amount and is firmer than normal, has a gray or sometimes brown discoloration, and in severely affected regions may show cavitation or spongy degeneration. Usually there is sparing of the U-fibers and of myelin sheaths within the central gray nuclei and optic radiation. A diminished number of intrafascicular oligodendrocytes is accompanied by a moderate to severe loss of myelin sheaths.[10] A striking accumulation of metachromatic granules is observed in macrophages that are prominent in perivascular spaces and in oligodendrocytes. They have also been observed within neurons.[76] Demyelination in the brainstem and spinal cord is prominent in late infantile MLD but much less striking in juvenile MLD.[76] A reactive gliosis is found in the areas of demyelination, and there may be partial or complete loss of axis cylinders.

The cerebellum is atrophic, with severe demyelination, prominent gliosis, and storage granules. There is a marked reduction in Purkinje cells and granule cells, and some of the surviving Purkinje cells show torpedolike swellings in the granular layer. The axon terminals of climbing fibers and mossy fibers are also missing.[77]

The retinal ganglion cells also accumulate metachromatic granules with the ultrastructural appearance of laminated bodies.[78,79] A variety of nonretinal ocular cell types (e.g., corneal epithelial and endothelial cells, keratocytes, lens fibers, and epithelial cells, as well as macrophages within the ocular meshwork and the peripheral iris) contain polymorphic lysosomal inclusions.[79]

Peripheral Nervous System

Segmental demyelination occurs in the peripheral nervous system, with metachromatic granules present in Schwann cells (Fig. 148-5) and in endoneurial macrophages.[80] These inclusions have the same ultrastructural appearance as those described above (see "Central Nervous System"). The accumulation of metachromatic material may be found in the Schwann cells at an early stage, while nerve conduction is still normal.[81] Computer-assisted morphometric analysis of sural nerves[81,82] shows reduced myelin sheath thickness for all fibers. Fibers of greater axon diameter are more severely affected than those of smaller axon diameter. The severity of demyelination of peripheral nerves correlates with the onset and duration of the disease, being milder in the early-onset and more severe in the adult-onset forms of MLD.[82]

Visceral Organs

Several visceral organs accumulate sulfatides. Tissues with excretory function are particularly affected. In the kidney, metachromatic material is present in the cells of the thin limb of the loop of Henle, the distal convoluted tubules (especially on the luminal side), the collecting tubules, and the tubule lumen and in the urine. The inclusions consist mainly of large lamellae, but some prismatic inclusions have also been observed. In the fetal period the kidney is the major site of pathology, with metachromatic granules and myelin-like membrane-bound inclusions.[83,84]

The gallbladder is small and fibrotic, and the mucosal cells and villous macrophages are distended by metachromatic material. In some cases multiple large papillomatous fronds have been noted.[34,85] Liver parenchymal cells, particularly at the periphery of the lobules, and the epithelial cells of the intrahepatic bile ducts contain abundant metachromatic material. There is similar but less striking involvement of the Kupffer cells and portal histiocytes.[86] Deposits of metachromatic lipids have been demonstrated in the islets of Langerhans,[72] the anterior pituitary,[87] the adrenal cortex,[87] and the sweat glands.[75] Accumulation of metachromatic material in the testes has been reported only in adult patients.[7] It is possible that this material was not sulfatide but seminolipid, the metabolism of which is also impaired in MLD. This sulfolipid normally is not formed in the testes before puberty and therefore would not accumulate in patients with MLD who had died before reaching puberty. The reticuloendothelial system is generally not involved.

The rectal tissue of an adult MLD patient showed histiocytes containing slightly metachromatic material stained by the Nissl technique.[62] The skeletal muscle may show fiber type disproportion, i.e., predominance and hypotrophy/atrophy of type I fibers,[88,89] as has been observed in Krabbe disease, another lysosomal leukodystrophy.[90,91]

Biochemical Changes

In late infantile MLD, there is a significant increase in the content of sulfatides in the white matter together with marked decrease in the concentration of other myelin lipids, such as cholesterol and sphingomyelin, presumably secondary to the loss of myelin. Levels of cerebroside are diminished out of proportion to those of other myelin lipids. Consequently, the cerebroside:sulfatide ratio, which in normal white matter is approximately 3, may be reduced in late infantile MLD to less than 1.[92,93] The excess of sulfatide has also been noted in isolated myelin,[94,95] including a preparation from a fetus with MLD.[96] An increased concentration of sulfatide has also been shown in the cerebellum, brainstem, and spinal cord of a 24-week fetus with MLD but was normal in the still-unmyelinated cortex.[97] The concentration of lysosulfatide, the deacylated form of sulfatide, is also increased in the cerebral white matter of patients with MLD, being 50–100 times greater than the values in control brain.[98,99] It is also much higher in MLD spinal cord and peripheral nerve than in cerebral gray matter or somatic organs. The proportion of the major gangliosides is similar in normal and MLD brain, which suggests that neuronal tissue and axons are relatively preserved.[95]

Chemical analyses of a few cases of adult MLD have disclosed differences from late infantile MLD. In adult MLD,[93] the white matter sulfatides are only moderately increased and contain more short chain and saturated fatty acid and less unsaturated fatty acid than the sulfatides from normal white matter.[100] In gray matter, the sulfatide accumulation in adult MLD is higher than that in late infantile MLD. In both types of MLD, a significant alteration also occurs in the fatty acid composition of white matter sphingomyelin[94,101] and cerebrosides.[102] The proportion of long chain fatty acids is diminished as is typical of unmyelinated or immature white matter. This probably reflects the loss of myelin, with a proportionate increase in the nonmyelinated compartment.

Sulfatide concentrations are increased in the liver, gallbladder, kidney, and urine of MLD patients, and storage in organs can already be observed in the fetus. The level in the liver is at least 10 times normal;[103] it is 10–75 times normal in the kidney,[102] and 10–100 times normal in the urine.[102,104] Both sulfatides and lactosylceramide 3-sulfates are found.[79]

BIOCHEMISTRY OF THE STORAGE MATERIAL

Sulfated Glycolipids

In MLD, the desulfation of 3-0-sulfogalactosyl-containing sphingosine- or glycerol-based glycolipids is impaired. The major sphingosine-containing sulfated glycolipids are sulfatides (3-0-sulfogalactosyl ceramides) that occur in their highest concentrations in the central and peripheral nervous system (as part of the myelin) and in the kidney.[108] They may also be found in a variety of other tissues, particularly those with a rich excretory epithelium, such as respiratory[109] and gastric mucosa,[110] gallbladder,[105] and uterine endometrium,[111] but also in body fluids, such as serum,[112] urine,[113] and CSF.[66] A lactosyl counterpart (lactosyl ceramide 3-sulfate) is also found in the kidney and is the major sulfated glycolipid in liver. The deacylated derivative of sulfatide, psychosine sulfate (also known as lysosulfatide), occurs in small amounts in the cerebral white matter, spinal cord, and kidney.[98]

Glycerol-containing sulfated glycolipids have an analogous structure, with the sulfate linked to the C-3 hydroxyl of galactose and with both acyl and alkyl ether substituents. These

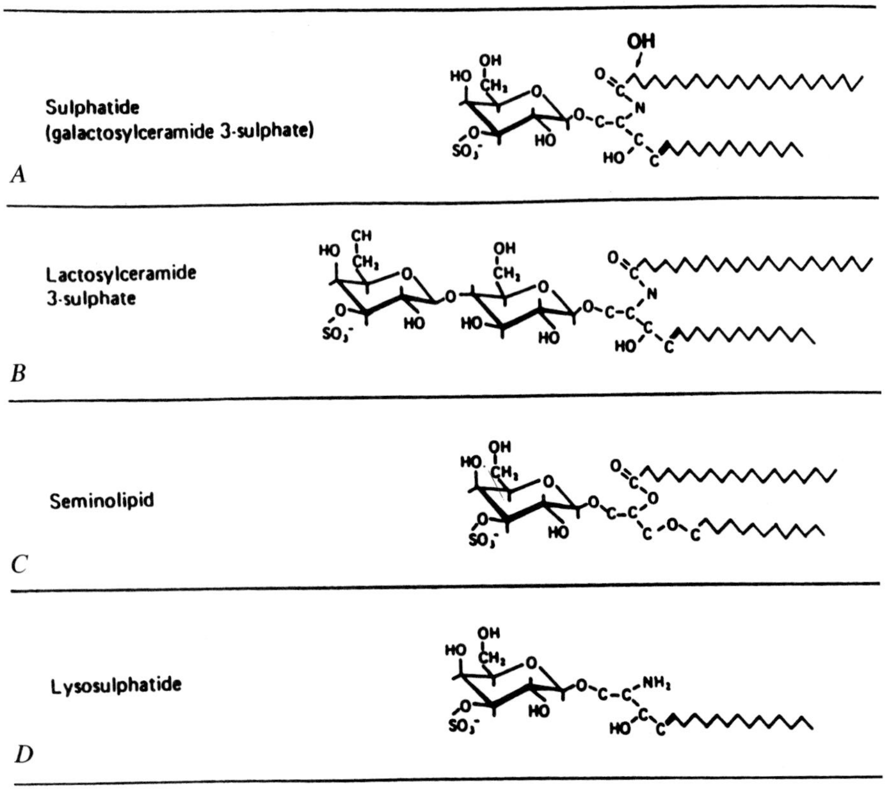

Fig. 148-8 The structure of some sulfated glycolipids. Note that a variety of fatty acyl groups and of sphingosine long chain bases are found in naturally occurring sulfatides. (A) 3-0-Sulfogalactosyl ceramide; sulfatide; 3-0-sulfogalactosyl cerebroside. (B) Lactosylceramide 3-sulfate, lactosyl sulfatide. (C) Seminolipid; 3-0-sulfogalactosyl glycerolipid. (D) 3-0-Sulfogalactosyl sphingosine; lysosulfatide; psychosine sulfate.

3-0-sulfogalactosyl glycerolipids occur in small amounts in rat brain[114] but constitute the major glycolipid constituent of mature mammalian testes and sperm;[115] hence the common name *seminolipid.*

The structures of the sulfated glycolipids of principal interest for MLD are presented in Fig. 148-8.

Sulfatides. Thudichum[116,117] first recognized the existence of a sulfur-containing lipid and named it sulfatide. In 1933, Blix[118] reported the isolation of this substance and showed it to contain equimolar amounts of cerebronic acid, sphingosine, galactose, and sulfate. It was eventually shown to be a sulfate ester of galactocerebroside with the sulfate joined by an ester linkage to the C-3 hydroxyl of galactose.[119] As is true for cerebrosides, the sphingosine base of sulfatides consists predominantly of C-18 sphingosine.[120] The structural formula of sulfatides appears in Fig. 148-8*A*.

Both sulfatides and cerebrosides contain a high proportion of long chain fatty acids and of fatty acids that contain a 2-hydroxy group. In fact, nearly all of the 2-hydroxy fatty acids found in brain lipids are constituents of these two glycolipids. In adult brain, 20–25 percent of sulfatide fatty acids contain the 2-hydroxy group, with cerebronic (C24h:0), oxynervonic (C24h:1), and the 22- and 23-carbon saturated fatty acids predominating. In fetal and immature brain, the proportion of hydroxy fatty acids is smaller. The major nonhydroxy fatty acids in sulfatides of adult brain are nervonic acid (C24n:1) and lignoceric acid (C24n:0), whereas in fetal and immature brain, medium chain fatty acids (C16n:0, C18n:0, and C18n:1) predominate. The development of the pattern characteristic of adult brain coincides with myelination.

Spinal cord sulfatides contain the same pattern of fatty acids found in cerebral white matter.[121] However, sulfatides of peripheral nerve contain significantly more saturated fatty acids, which is conducive to the formation of a tightly packed myelin membrane.[121]

The kidney is second in relative abundance of sulfatides, but its concentration is only about one-tenth that of brain. Kidney sulfatides contain more than 10 times as much behenic acid (C22n:0) as those in brain, and they also contain a higher proportion of lignoceric than nervonic acid.[102,122] Lactosylceramide 3-sulfate (Fig. 148-8*B*) is found in human kidney[122] and urine[107] and is absent from the human brain. There is also evidence for a trihexosyl sulfatide in human kidney.[123]

Sulfogalactoglycerolipids. Diacyl and alkylacyl glycerol forms of sulfogalactoglycerolipid have been characterized. Together these two lipids account for 2.1-7.2 percent of the total sulfated glycolipids in rat brain.[114] The structure of the alkylacyl form is 1-O-alkyl-2-O-acyl-3(b-3′-sulfogalactosyl) glycerol (Fig. 148-6*C*). Its common name, seminolipid, reflects the fact that it is the major sulfolipid of mammalian testes and sperm.[124] Interestingly, no sulfogalactoglycerolipid has been reported in normal human brains or in those from MLD patients.

Other Sulfated Glycolipids. A number of additional sulfated glycolipids have been recognized in recent years. Among these are a series of sulfated glycolipids found in the membrane of the intestinal epithelium.[125–127] In addition to sulfatides and lactosylceramide 3-sulfate, sulfates of glucosylceramide, trihexosylceramide, and trihexosylalkylacylglycerol have been identified. In the last, sulfation occurs at the 6-hydroxyl of the terminal sugar residue. These sulfated glycolipids are thought to play a crucial role in mucosal integrity and have been implicated in ulcer pathobiology. The kidney has also yielded a number of sulfated glycolipids of complex structure in addition to the dominant sulfatides and lactosylceramide 3-sulfate.[128–130] Sulfated gangliosides have been found in kidney[131,132] and in milk. A 3-O-sulfated glucuronic acid residue[133] has been identified as part of the antigen reacting with HNK-1, an antibody raised to membrane from a human T-cell line and reactive with a select set of cells in the developing nervous system. However, of those glycolipids tested, only sulfatides, lactosylceramide 3-sulfate, and the seminolipids have been shown to be desulfated by ASA, and there is no evidence that any of these additional sulfated glycolipids accumulate in MLD.

Biosynthesis and Degradation

Sulfatides are formed through sulfation of galactosylceramide (also designated as galactocerebroside)[134] by reaction with 3′-phosphoadenosine-5′-phosphosulfate (PAPS) as follows:

The complete absence of sulfatides in mice with disrupted galactocerebroside synthesis establishes the precursor-product relationship between galactosylceramide and sulfatide.[135,136] The reaction is catalyzed by a microsomal sulfotransferase that has been demonstrated in a variety of mammalian tissues.[137] The same enzyme can also transfer the sulfate moiety of PAPS to lactosylceramide to form lactosyl ceramide 3-sulfate. A sulfotransferase has also been described that will sulfate galactosylsphingosine and lactosylsphingosine.[137–139]

Sulfatide accounts for 3.5–4 percent of the total lipids of myelin.[94] Its synthesis is maximal during the period of myelination and proceeds more slowly in the adult. Synthesis is stimulated by cortisol[140] and reduced in neonatal hypothyroidism[141] and in the presence of psychosine.[142] Both neurons and oligodendroglial cells have sulfatide-synthesizing capability, but sulfotransferase activity is much more active in cells of glial origin.[143] Established cell lines from renal tubule epithelium have also been shown to synthesize sulfatide.[144]

Desulfation by the lysosomal enzyme ASA is the first step in the degradation of the 3-sulfogalactosyl-containing glycolipids shown in Fig. 148-8 and depends on saposin B. The latter forms complexes with the sulfated glycolipids. It is thought to facilitate the access of ASA to the sulfate groups of the membrane-integrated substrates.

Two observations point to the existence of pathways for degradation of sulfated glycolipids that bypass ASA. Recently a sulfatase was purified from mouse brain that at neutral pH hydrolyzes sulfatides but not p-nitrocatechol sulfate and is distinct from ASA.[145] The in vivo activity of this enzyme remains to be determined. The other observation refers to Epstein-Barr virus-transformed lymphoblasts, which catabolize sulfatide irrespective of the presence of ASA.[146] The desulfated glycolipids produced by ASA are further degraded by exoglycosidases (see Chap. 147 on galactosylceramidase deficiency and Chap. 151 on β-galactosidase deficiency).

Function

Sulfated glycolipids share with other membrane lipids the dual capability of hydrophilic and hydrophobic interactions. In addition, their anionic charge allows combination with inorganic cations or organic amines to maintain the electrical neutrality of the membrane. Sulfatides, an important component of the myelin sheath,[147], are located on the surface of this membrane[148] and are probably bound to myelin basic protein[149] and proteolipid protein[150] by strong ionic interactions. Together with galactosylceramides, the sulfatides maintain the insulator function of the membrane bilayer.[135,136] Sulfatides are believed to be involved in active sodium transport, serving as a cofactor for Na/K-ATPase.[151] There is evidence implicating sulfatides in binding of opiates,[152,153] GABA,[154] and serotonin[155] to their receptors. Sulfatides modulate the activity of several key enzymes. However, the physiological significance of the activation of phospholipase A_2[156] and calmodulin-dependent cyclic nucleotide phosphodiesterase[157] and of the modulation of phosphatidylinositol phosphate 3-kinase activity[158] remains to be determined.

Various cellular adhesion molecules bind specifically and with high affinity to sulfatides. These include laminin,[123,159] thrombospondin,[123,160] tenascin R,[161] and von Willebrand factor,[123,162] as well as L-selectin, the lymphocyte-homing receptor,[163] and P-selectin, the granulocyte-binding ligand.[164] Sulfatide-induced activation of L-selectin triggers tyrosine phosphorylation, activation of MAP kinase, and increase of cytosolic Ca^{2+} and potentiates the oxidative burst.[165–167] Properdin, a plasma glycoprotein;[168] cytotactin, a glial glycoprotein;[169] procollagen I N-proteinase;[170] the hepatocyte growth factor;[171] and the leech anticoagulant antistasin[172] also bind to sulfatides. The binding domain for these molecules appears to be an amino acid sequence that is common to all of them.[173] Sulfatides also induce the activation of at least three other clotting substances: prekallikrein, factor XI, and factor XII.[174–176] In this respect, it is significant that platelet sulfatide concentrations are five times those of erythrocytes.[177] Sulfatides are also believed to have anticoagulant activity in serum.[112]

Several infectious organisms have specific sulfatide-binding domains. This might account for the attraction of *Mycoplasma pneumoniae*[109,178] and *Bordetella pertussis*[179] to the respiratory epithelium and for invasion of liver cells by the malarial sporozoite.[180,181] The amino acid sequence of the binding region in the malarial proteins is similar to that found in thrombospondin, properdin, and von Willebrand factor.[180,181] Sulfatides also act as a specific ligand for binding of the gp120 envelope protein of HIV-1[182] and for binding of *Helicobacter pylori* to gastric cells.[183,184]

The sulfogalactoglycerolipids, because they are a myelin component and turn over rapidly during myelination, may have an important role in brain maturation.[114] They are also a major glycolipid of testes and spermatozoa and are thus important in spermatogenesis.[124]

ENZYME DEFECT

The primary enzyme defect in the late infantile, juvenile, and adult forms of MLD is that of ASA.[15,17,20] ASA has also been designated as sulfatidase or cerebroside 3-sulfatase, according to its major natural substrate. Other natural substrates include lactosylceramide 3-sulfate,[185] psychosine sulfate,[186] and seminolipid.[187] In MLD, ASA activity is deficient in all tissues and cells so far examined for it.

PATHOPHYSIOLOGY

The biochemical defect in all forms of MLD is a deficiency in the enzymatic hydrolysis of sulfatide. This leads to a progressive accumulation of sulfatides, mainly within lysosomes. The storage process is not uniform in all tissues and organs, and functional loss is not directly proportional to the amount of sulfatide deposited. On this basis, four categories of tissues may be defined:

1. Tissues that show little or no sulfatide accumulation and no tissue damage. These tissues include the heart, lung, spleen, skin, and bones.
2. Tissues in which there is accumulation of sulfatide but no demonstrable impairment of function. These tissues include the liver, kidney, pancreas, adrenal cortex, and sweat glands.
3. Tissues in which there is sulfatide accumulation and evidence of impaired function but in which these do not appear to contribute to the fatal outcome of the disease. This applies to the gallbladder, which, as already noted, shows sulfatide accumulation and progressive functional impairment.
4. Tissues in which sulfatide accumulation and impaired function contribute to the fatal outcome. This concerns primarily the white matter of the nervous system.

The accumulation of sulfatides probably occurs independently in each organ. It is unlikely, for example, that sulfatides from the central nervous system are deposited within the kidney. The fatty acid compositions of brain and kidney sulfatides are different,[102] and the sulfatide concentration in MLD serum is normal.[188] It is more probable that the increase in sulfatides observed in extraneural tissues reflects an *in situ* failure in the turnover of sulfatides that are normally present in plasma membranes of these tissues and serve other purposes than being structural components of myelin. The tolerance of the kidney, the gallbladder, and other extraneural tissues for sulfatides may be related to the fact that the cells most involved in the storage process fulfill an excretory function and therefore can discharge the accumulating lipid from the cell into the urine, bile, or other fluid.

The demyelination that occurs in MLD appears to be secondary to sulfatide-induced changes within the cells responsible for myelin maintenance, namely the oligodendrocytes in the central nervous system and the Schwann cells in the peripheral nervous system. Changes in the subcellular organelles of these cells are observed before any morphologic abnormalities in the myelin sheaths associated with them are detectable. In a fetus with MLD aborted in the fifth month of gestation,[189] an increase in lysosomes, some containing lamellar structured material, was found in the cerebrum and cerebellum, even though these tissues did not stain metachromatically and myelination had not yet begun. This increase in lysosomal bodies was even more marked in the oligodendroglial cells of the spinal cord. Although accumulations of metachromatic material were observed in spinal cord oligodendrocytes, the morphologic appearance of the spinal cord myelin at this stage was normal. An increase in the number of lysosomes thus appears to be the earliest pathologic change that results from the failure of sulfatide catabolism. Neuropathologic studies of two other MLD fetuses aborted in the fifth month of gestation also demonstrated cellular abnormalities at a stage at which myelin either had not yet developed or appeared morphologically normal.[96,190]

Also, in nerve biopsies from patients with MLD, a normal myelin sheath is often observed together with abundant storage material in the Schwann cell belonging to the same internodal segment of the myelin sheath.[191,192] Therefore, the abnormal accumulation of sulfatide within the lysosomes of oligodendroglial and Schwann cells and the metabolic failure of these cells precede and may trigger the events that cause demyelination. Early focal areas of demyelination would preferentially affect long tracts. This could produce delays in nerve conduction velocity and synaptic transmission and an increase in the latency period of evoked potentials. Intellectual impairment is a later event that may result from secondary damage to neurons and scrambling of information produced by slowed nerve conduction.[193]

It has been suggested that myelin breakdown in MLD results from defective resorption of sulfatides in the innermost part of the myelin sheath. Catabolism of this layer of myelin is necessary for the axon to increase its cross-sectional diameter during growth.[194] Even after maturity is reached, enzymatic failure in the resorption of myelin would prevent normal restructuring of the myelin sheath. Experiments with isotopic sulfate have confirmed the presence of two myelin compartments in adult rat myelin, one with a slow turnover rate and the other with a fast turnover rate.[195] Thus, both during growth and after the active growth phase is completed, ASA activity is needed to maintain the normal integrity of myelin.

An alternative explanation for the myelin breakdown is that the myelin formed in MLD has an abnormal composition[73,94,100,196] and is therefore unstable. This concept is supported by the findings of Ginsberg and Gershfeld,[197] who showed that lipid extracts from nervous system tissues in vitro spontaneously form a membrane bilayer at a specific, critical temperature, T^*. At any other temperature, a multilamellar state results. They found that the T^* for lipids from cerebral white matter of a normal individual and from that of a patient with multiple sclerosis was 37°C, the physiological temperature of the cell. However, myelin lipids from a patient with adult MLD yielded a T^* of less than 30°C. They concluded that the oligodendroglia in MLD white matter are initially able to counteract the imbalance caused by the excess of sulfatides and maintain myelin membrane homeostasis. They do this through changes in fatty acid composition[100] and by other adjustments in lipid metabolic pools to maintain the T^* at 37°C. However, when the cell's ability to compensate for the metabolic defect is exceeded, the difference between the body temperature and T^* widens and the myelin membrane begins to break down.[197]

Another proposed mechanism is that sulfogalactosylsphingosine (lysosulfatide), a compound closely related to galactosylsphingosine, which is known to be highly cytotoxic,[198,199] might accumulate due to its defective desulfation in MLD and cause myelin breakdown.[200] Although there is no evidence for the enzymatic deacylation of sulfatide to sulfogalactosylsphingosine,[201] Toda et al.[98,99] have shown marked accumulation of lysosulfatide in cerebral white matter, spinal cord, and sciatic nerve of six patients with MLD. They also noted substantial levels in cerebral gray matter, kidney, and liver, whereas this material was essentially undetectable in control samples. At concentrations much lower than those found even in the somatic organs of MLD patients, lysosulfatide inhibits the activity of protein kinase C[202] and cytochrome oxidase C.[99] Therefore, lysosulfatide must be considered a possible pathogenic agent in MLD.

The delay in appearance of clinical signs in the later-onset forms of MLD is difficult to explain in terms of the timetable of brain development. The period of most rapid turnover of sulfatides is presumably early in development, during the peak time of myelin formation. One would expect that the failure of enzymatic hydrolysis of sulfatides would affect brain white matter more severely at this time than at some later time. The most attractive explanation for the later-onset forms of MLD, however, is that these patients have higher residual enzyme activity[203,204] and therefore accumulate sulfatides at a slower rate.

GENETICS AND INCIDENCE OF ASA DEFICIENCY

All forms of MLD are inherited as autosomal recessive traits and are caused by allelic mutations of the ASA locus, except for the few cases of saposin B deficiency. The ASA gene has been mapped to the long arm of chromosome 22 band q13.[205,206]

The overall incidence of MLD and the frequency of the trait for MLD can only be roughly estimated. In northern Sweden, the incidence of late infantile MLD has been estimated to be 1 in 40,000.[207] This probably represents a somewhat higher figure than can be expected elsewhere, because of a clustering of 6 of the 13 cases surveyed in a single restricted geographic isolate. In France, the reported incidence of late infantile MLD is 1 in 130,000,[208] in Washington state it is 1 in 40,000,[209] and a recent survey estimates the frequency in Germany at around 1 in 170,000.[210] Several ethnic groups have a higher incidence. The Habbanite Jewish community in Israel has a particularly high frequency of late infantile MLD (1 in 75), due to a 17-percent carrier frequency and a marked tendency toward consanguineous marriages.[211] Among Arabs living in Israel, the incidence of the disease is 1 in 8,000 and most cases have been observed in a restricted area north of Nazareth.[212] Incidence rates among Eskimos and Navajo Indians are estimated to be in the ranges of 1 in 2500 and 1 in 6400, respectively.[213]

ASA

Gene and RNA

The ASA gene consists of 8 exons (103–320 nucleotides long), which encompass just 3.2 kb of genomic sequence.[214] In the promoter region, no TATA or CAAT boxes, but several GC boxes (at positions −10, −40, −50, and −60 bases) were found. These are typical positions for interaction with the transcription factor Sp1. Four transcription initiation sites were located between 367 and 387 bp upstream of the initiation codon. A polyadenylation signal follows the TGA termination codon by 95 nucleotides. The primary transcript, which is cleaved and polyadenylated at this position, yields a 2.1-kb mRNA and corresponds to the ASA cDNA that has been cloned.[215] In addition, mRNA species of 3.7 and 4.8 kb are transcribed from the ASA gene. The primary transcripts of the larger forms proceed further into the 3′ untranslated region and may be cleaved at putative polyadenylation signals further downstream.

The 2.1-kb mRNA accounts for about 90 percent and each of the longer transcripts for about 5 per cent of ASA poly $(A)^+$ RNA. The longer mRNAs are more abundant in total RNA, where they represent up to 70 percent of ASA RNA. The preferential loss of the larger transcripts in the process of purification of poly $(A)^+$ RNA suggests that they lack a poly $(A)^+$ tract.[216]

Results from a detailed analysis of a polymorphism that causes the loss of the first polyadenylation signal[216] suggest that the 2.1-kb mRNA is primarily responsible for the synthesis of ASA polypeptides and that the translational efficiency of the larger transcripts is lower. This polymorphism will be discussed in detail in "ASA Pseudodeficiency." However, the significance of the longer mRNAs remains unknown.

The 2.1-kb ASA cDNA encompasses 363 nucleotides of 5′ untranslated sequence, followed by an open reading frame of 1521 nucleotides coding sequence and 130 nucleotides of 3′ untranslated sequence. The cDNA has two ATG initiation codons separated by three nucleotides. The second codon conforms better with the optimal eukaryotic translation initiation sequence. This is followed by a 54-nucleotide sequence that predicts a typical leader peptide of 18 amino acids with a leucine-rich hydrophobic central region and an Ala-Val-Ala signal-peptidase-cleavage site. This region is followed by a 1467-bp sequence coding for 489 amino acids. A polyadenylation signal is located 95 nucleotides downstream of the termination codon. The cDNA sequence reveals three potential N-glycosylation sites. It should be noted that a small portion of the originally reported sequence between residues 359 and 401[215] was subsequently revised.[214]

ASA Protein

The ASA mRNA is translated into a 507-amino-acid precursor at the rough endoplasmic reticulum. ASA receives several post-translational modifications in the endoplasmic reticulum.

In all eukaryotic sulfatases, a formylglycine residue is found at a position where the cDNA predicts a cysteine.[217] In ASA this is cysteine 69. The formylglycine residue is generated by oxidation of the thiol group to an aldehyde. This modification is required for sulfatase activity (see below). This unique post-translational modification occurs either after or at a late stage of protein translocation, when ASA has not yet folded into its native structure. A linear sequence of 16 amino acid residues surrounding Cys69 is sufficient to direct this post-translational oxidation.[218] Deficiency of the modifying enzymes leads to the synthesis of inactive sulfatases and is causative for multiple sulfatase deficiency.[217] So far none of the components catalyzing this modification has been purified or the cDNAs cloned.

Within the lumen of the endoplasmic reticulum, the signal peptide is cleaved and the enzyme receives N-oligosaccharide side chains at each of three potential N-glycosylation sites.[219] After completion of folding, ASA is transported to the Golgi apparatus, where it is recognized as a lysosomal enzyme by the lysosomal enzyme phosphotransferase. As in other lysosomal enzymes, lysines are important for recognition of ASA by the phosphotransferase, since selective chemical modification of lysines completely abolishes the phosphorylation of the enzyme in an in vitro assay.[220] A detailed examination of the three N-linked oligosaccharide side chains of ASA revealed that mannose-6-phosphate residues are found predominantly on the first and third oligosaccharide side chains, whereas that at the second N-glycosylation site is only ineffectively phosphorylated.[219] In agreement with these data, an enzyme in which the first and third N-glycosylation sites have been abolished by in vitro mutagenesis is largely secreted.[221] Sulfation of ASA oligosaccharide side chains has also been reported, but its functional significance is unknown.[222,223]

Transport to the lysosome is accomplished via a prelysosomal acidic compartment[224] by the mannose-6-phosphate receptor pathway.[225] In contrast to other lysosomal enzymes, the majority of ASA is not proteolytically cleaved either during transport to or after arrival in the lysosome. In tissue culture, most of the enzyme is present as an unprocessed 62-kDa polypeptide.[226] Small amounts of a 57-kDa polypeptide are also found, but its precursor-product relationship to the 62-kDa form has not been established in pulse-chase experiments.[227,228] ASA purified from human placenta has been shown to consist of two different forms; again, the majority of enzyme was unprocessed and a minor fraction was found to be a product of an internal proteolytic cleavage occurring close to the C-terminus, which generated a large 51-kDa and a small 7-kDa fragment. The small fragment was postulated to be associated with the larger fragment via disulfide bridges.[229] This, however, is contradicted by the organization of disulfide bridges as determined by x-ray diffraction analysis.

ASA is a housekeeping enzyme; it is found ubiquitiously and has been purified from various sources, including liver,[230] placenta,[231] and urine.[232] Few data are available on differences in the tissue distribution of ASA activity. Except for the pig thyroid gland, in which specific activity levels twenty to sixty times higher than those in liver, kidney, and brain have been described,[233] variations occur only in a small range. In the period of myelination, ASA activity increases concomitantly with that of galactosylceramide sulfotransferase. After completion of myelination, the latter decreases, whereas ASA activity does not change.[234]

The enzyme has a low isolelectric point. Multiple molecular forms of ASA have been demonstrated in various tissues by electrophoretic separation and isoelectric focusing. These variations can be attributed to charge heterogeneity of the oligosaccharide side chains.[227,235–237] In tumor tissues, both the amount of enzyme[238] and its molecular size[222,239] are increased, the latter as a result of sialylation and phosphorylation.

ASA cleaves various sulfate-containing substrates.[240] The major physiologic substrates are sulfatides.[16,17] Other galactosyl-3-O-sulfates hydrolyzed by ASA include lactosyl ceramide 3-sulfate,[185] seminolipid,[187] and psychosine sulfate.[186] The rates of hydrolysis for several natural and artificial substrates of ASA are shown in Table 148-2. Ascorbic acid-2-sulfate is also a substrate for the enzyme. The latter compound occurs throughout the body, but it does not accumulate in MLD, apparently because it is also hydrolyzed by arylsulfatase B.[241] ASA does not hydrolyze chondroitin sulfate, 6-0-sulfogalactosyl ceramide, or galactose-6-sulfate. It only feebly attacks tyrosine-O-sulfate and is inactive toward 5-hydroxytryptamine-O-sulfate. It also has phosphodiesterase activity, because it cleaves cAMP and cGMP, although at low efficiency.[242] In vitro ASA activity is usually determined with the artificial substrate p-nitrocatecholsulfate.[243]

A time-dependent inactivation of ASA occurs during its reaction with p-nitrocatechol sulfate. Partial reactivation results on exposure to $SO_4{}^{2-}$ or certain other anions.[244] It has been proposed that the reaction between enzyme and substrate substantially modifies the enzyme, with loss of secondary structure.[245] An enzyme-antibody complex also shows anomalous kinetics but enzyme inactivation significantly lower than that for the free enzyme; presumably, this is because the antibody retards the process of structural rearrangement or covalent modification of the enzyme.[246] The anomalous kinetics of ASA make it difficult to determine initial reaction rates.

Table 148-2 Rate of Hydrolysis of Various Sulfate Esters by Arylsulfatase A

Substrate	Rate, μmol/min per mg protein
p-Nitrocatechol sulfate	160.0
4-Methylumbelliferyl sulfate	40.0
Ascorbic acid-2-sulfate	85.0
Cerebroside-3-sulfate	6.6
Seminolipid	5.0
Psychosine sulfate	3.0

SOURCE: From Farooqui and Mandel.[240]

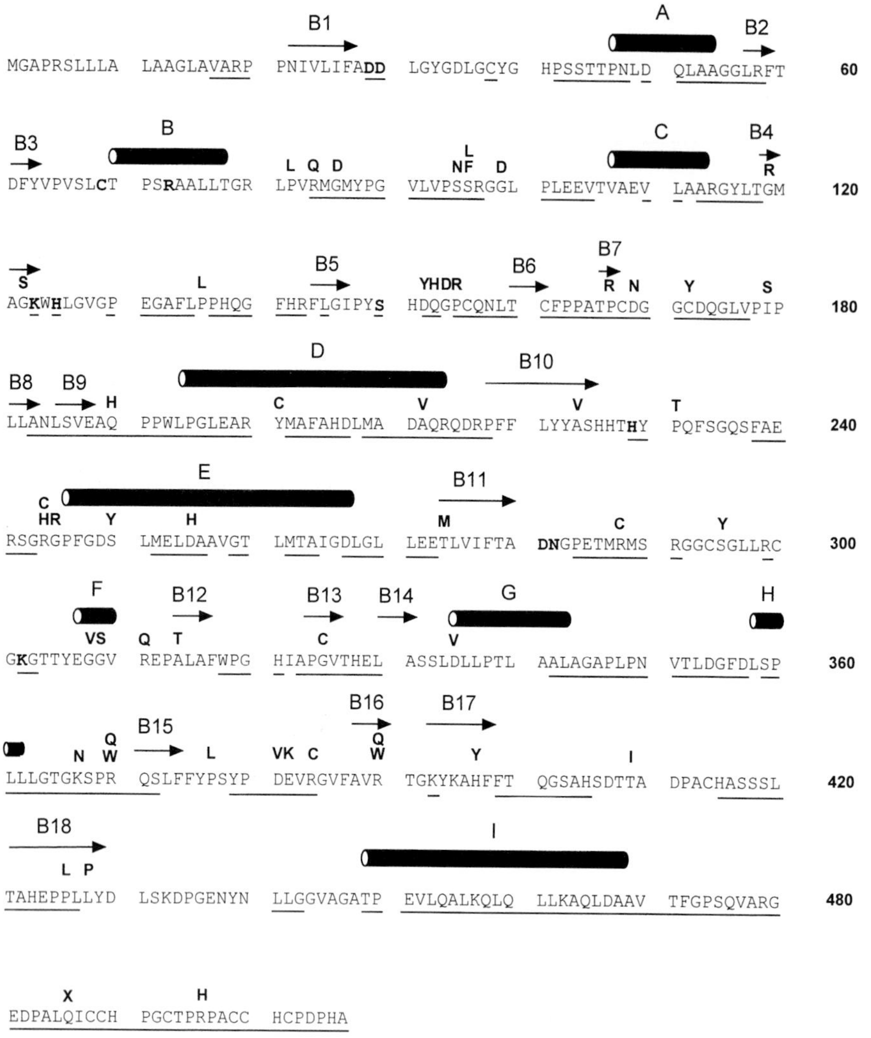

Fig. 148-9 Amino acid substitutions in the ASA polypeptide. Letters show the primary amino acid sequence of human ASA in the one-letter code. Residues located at the surface are underlined. Bold letters in the amino acid sequence indicate residues participating directly in the formation of the active center. Bold letters above the amino acid sequence indicate amino acid substitutions found in MLD patients (see Table 148-3). Tubes indicate the helices A-J and arrows the β sheets B1-B18.[247]

Recently ASA has been crystallized and its three-dimensional structure resolved.[247] At the acidic pH of lysosomes, ASA forms a homo-octamer, which is composed of dimers $(\alpha_2)_4$. The monomer structure can be described as globular and hat-like. Monomers associate to dimers through contacts between loop structures arranged on the flat part on one side of the hat-shaped monomer. At low pH values, as in lysosomes, four dimers form an octamer. Protonation/deprotonation of Glu424 regulates the tetramerization of the dimers. At pH values that induce protonation of Glu424, octamers are formed, while at higher pH values, equally charged Glu424 at the surface of dimers prevents the association.

The α/β-fold of the monomer has significant structural homology to alkaline phosphatase. Superimposition of the two structures has shown that their active centers are located at almost identical positions, which greatly facilitated the postulation of a catalytic mechanism for the sulfate ester cleavage and the assignment of residues critical for catalysis. The functionally essential formylglycine 69 is located in a positively charged pocket and acts as a ligand to an octahedrally coordinated metal ion, which is likely to be Mg^{2+}.

The critical role of the amino acids proposed to form the active site[247] (see Fig. 148-9) has been confirmed by site-directed mutagenesis and characterization of the mutant enzymes.[248] In the resting form of ASA, the aldehyde group of the formylglycine is hydrated. One of the two hydroxyl groups hydrolyzes the substrate sulfate ester via a transesterification step, resulting in a covalent intermediate. The second hydroxyl serves to eliminate sulfate through C-O cleavage and reformation of the aldehyde. Hydration of the aldehyde completes the catalytic cycle. The formation of a covalently sulfated enzyme intermediate in the first half of this catalytic cycle is analogous to the formation of the phosphorylated intermediate of alkaline phosphatase, in which a serine residue serves as acceptor for the phosphate. In the second half of the catalytic cycle, the P-O bond of the phosphorylated intermediate is hydrolyzed. An ASA mutant carrying a serine in position 69 was found to form a sulfated intermediate. Release of the sulfate was abolished by the lack of the second hydroxyl required for the elimination reaction. In contrast to alkaline phosphatase, ASA is unable to activate water and to hydrolyze the S-O bond of the sulfate intermediate.[249]

ASA Pseudodeficiency

Among Europeans, 1–2 percent of the population display a substantial deficiency of ASA activity, are clinically normal, have no signs of sulfatide storage or urinary excretion, and do not appear to have a preclinical stage of MLD.[24,250–252] These individuals have about 5–15 percent of normal ASA activity, an amount obviously sufficient to sustain normal sulfatide metabolism and phenotype. The phenomenon of ASA deficiency without clinical consequences has been termed *pseudodeficiency*.[22,23,203,253–256] It should be emphasized that this term is a misnomer, since the prefix *pseudo* suggests the deficiency to be an apparent in vitro phenomenon that does not occur in vivo. However, the deficiency is an in vivo phenomenon, since it is caused by a reduction of the amount of ASA enzyme, which will be discussed in detail below ("Molecular Genetics of ASA

Pseudodeficiency"). In spite of the fact that the term is misleading, it has been commonly accepted.

The gene encoding this low-enzyme-activity variant is allelic to the ASA gene.[257] Thus, in most cases ASA pseudodeficiency is caused by homozygosity for an ASA allele that, because of certain polymorphisms, encodes only little enzyme activity. In rare cases it may be caused by compound heterozygosity for the pseudodeficiency allele and an MLD allele.[24,252] Among Europeans, the frequency of the pseudodeficiency allele has been determined by biochemical and genetic analysis to be 10–20 percent.[250,255,258,259] To explain the high frequency of the pseudodeficiency allele, it has been speculated that heterozygotes may have some selective advantage. However, no reasonable explanation has been provided so far. ASA pseudodeficiency causes problems in diagnosis of and genetic counseling for MLD[22,23,256] (see "Diagnostic Problems"). Although it is generally accepted that homozygosity for a pseudodeficiency allele is not associated with any health risk,[203,252] there have been several reports on a higher incidence of ASA pseudodeficiency in various neurologic diseases. It therefore remains a subject of ongoing speculation whether pseudodeficiency predisposes to some neurologic disorders.[258,260–264] However, it is fair to state that in the majority of individuals pseudodeficiency has no clinical consequences.

Reports about single patients with reduced ASA activity and an otherwise unexplainable neurologic disease[265,266,267] cannot be taken as support for a causative relation between the low ASA activity and the clinical phenotype. Since 1–2 percent of the European population are ASA pseudodeficient, the association in a single patient is likely to be incidental.

Attention has also focused on individuals who are genetic compounds with an MLD allele and a pseudodeficiency allele, who have even lower ASA activity than pseudodeficiency homozygotes. Allele frequencies allow it to be calculated that this genotype should occur in about 1 in 1500 individuals.[258] Sixteen such individuals have recently been identified among relatives of MLD patients. Fourteen of these individuals were clinically normal, and two had neurologic problems.[252] However, these were minor and transient and had no resemblance to those found in MLD. This study concluded that the pseudodeficiency/MLD genotype bears no health risk and is no indication for abortion.

Molecular Genetics of ASA Pseudodeficiency

The ASA enzyme in pseudodeficient individuals consistently appeared to be 2–4 kDa smaller[268–270] than that in normal individuals. The size difference is due to a point mutation in the most C-terminal N-glycosylation site of the ASA gene, causing substitution of serine for asparagine 350. This causes the loss of one of the N-linked oligosaccharide side chains in the enzyme encoded by the pseudodeficiency allele.[216,271] Thus, whereas normal ASA has three oligosaccharide side chains, pseudodeficiency ASA bears only two. This explains the size difference of the ASA enzyme in normal individuals and those with pseudodeficiency.

Simultaneously with the detection of the N-glycosylation site polymorphism in the pseudodeficiency allele, it was noted that the major 2.1-kb mRNA species was almost completely deficient in poly $(A)^+$ RNA isolated from cells of individuals with pseudodeficiency.[216] Further investigation of the genomic sequence of such individuals revealed an additional sequence alteration — an A to G transition — in the polyadenylation signal located 95 bp downstream of the termination codon. The sequence generated by this alteration does not conform to the consensus sequence of a polyadenylation signal. Since the corresponding polyadenylation signal in the normal allele is used to generate the primary transcript from which the 2.1-kb mRNA species is derived, the second sequence alteration causes the selective loss of this mRNA species in pseudodeficiency.

Thus, the ASA pseudodeficiency allele has two polymorphisms: one leading to the loss of an N-glycosylation site and the second to the loss of a polyadenylation signal.

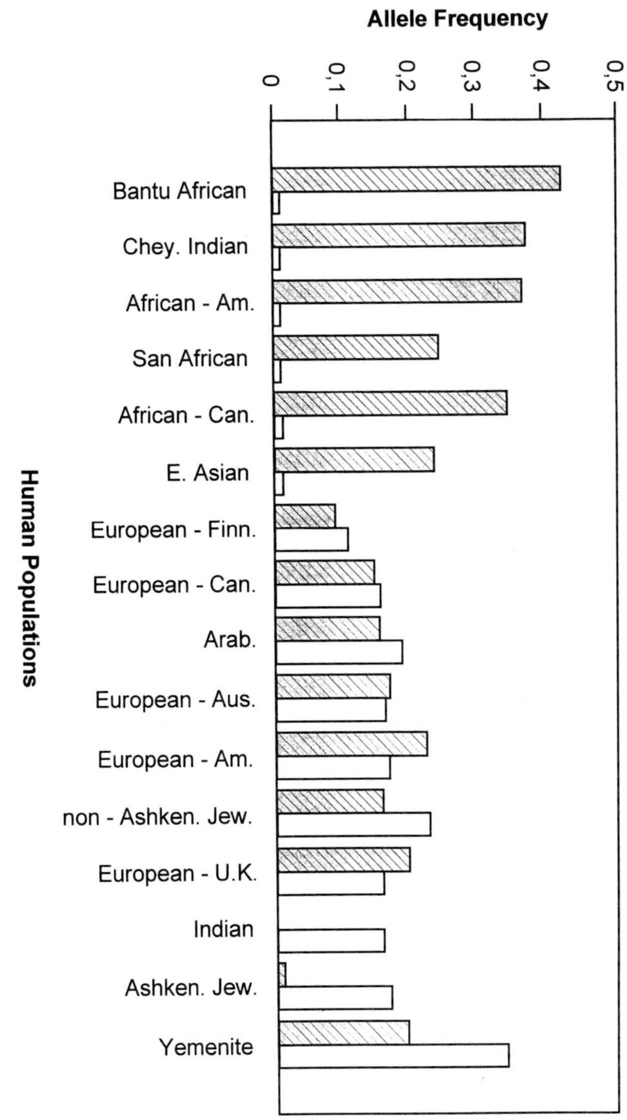

Fig. 148-10 Worldwide distribution of alleles with N-glycosylation site and polyadenylation site polymorphisms. Allele frequencies in various populations are shown. Shaded bars indicate the frequencies of an allele with the N-glycosylation site polymorphism only. White bars indicate frequencies of the allele with N-glycosylation and polyadenylation polymorphisms. (*From Ott et al.*[251] *with permission.*)

Both polymorphisms are also found independently. The N350S substitution causing loss of the N-glycosylation site seems to be a frequent allele, whereas selective loss of the polyadenylation signal seems to be rare. Two groups have determined the frequencies of the two polymorphisms in various ethnic groups (Fig. 148-10). Among Europeans the frequency of the pseudodeficiency allele was 0.075, and among Indians (from India) it was 0.125, whereas it was almost nonexistent in Africans, Asians, Cheyenne Indians, and Chinese.[251,272,273] An allele with only the N-glycosylation site polymorphism has high frequencies in East Asians and Africans — 0.21 and 0.32, respectively. Among Europeans and Indians its frequencies are lower — 0.06 and 0.01, respectively. Although the frequencies of the pseudodeficiency allele and the N-glycosylation site allele are inversely correlated in Africans/Asians and Europeans/Indians, it is interesting to note that the combined allele frequencies in both populations are almost identical. Haplotype analysis of the various alleles allowed the conclusion that the selective loss of the N-glycosylation site is the older allele and that it originated among

Africans. After the divergence of the non-African lineage, the loss of the polyadenylation signal occurred in the same allele, generating the pseudodeficiency allele. Selective loss of the polyadenylation signal has so far been reported only in three individuals. It is thus a rare allele and has also occurred on a different haplotype from that carrying the pseudodeficiency allele.[251,273]

The enzyme deficiency in pseudodeficiency can be accounted for by a decrease in enzyme protein rather than in activity.[216,270,274] The residual enzyme in pseudodeficiency appears to be enzymatically normal, since substrate affinities, pH optima, sensitivity to inhibition, and heat stability of ASA in individuals with pseudodeficiency are indistinguishable from those in controls.[255,257] Initial studies indicated that the loss of the N-glycosylation site is responsible for the decreased stability of the ASA pseudodeficiency enzyme variant. The explanation of the low enzyme activity would thus be a decreased half-life of the enzyme.[274] However, this study also noted a reduction in the synthesis of the enzyme to about 35 percent of normal. A different conclusion was reached by Gieselmann and coworkers.[216] They found no difference in expression of the enzyme activity when a cDNA with the N-glycosylation mutant was expressed in BHK cells or in human fibroblasts via retroviral gene transfer. Instead they found decreased synthesis of ASA in cultured fibroblasts of a pseudodeficient individual. This reduction in synthesis was attributed to the loss of the polyadenylation signal, which causes the deficiency of the 2.1-kb mRNA species and the reduction of poly $(A)^+$ RNA to 10 percent of control levels. This correlates well with the reduction of ASA polypeptide synthesis and enzyme activity.

The analysis of individuals carrying ASA alleles with only the N-glycosylation site or only the polyadenylation site polymorphism has indicated that the N-glycosylation site polymorphism reduces the ASA activity to about 50 percent of that of a wild-type allele,[256] while the polyadenylation site polymorphism reduces ASA activity to less than 10 percent.[256,275] This indicates that the polyadenylation site polymorphism alone can account for the reduction of activity seen with the pseudodeficiency allele. The allele with the N-glycosylation polymorphism alone can be regarded as one of presumably many alleles that encode ASA with lower or higher activity than that of the wild-type ASA.

MOLECULAR PATHOLOGY OF MLD

Mutations

Sixty-three different MLD-causing mutations have been characterized in the ASA gene (Table 148-3). Many of these mutations have been found only in single patients, demonstrating the genetic heterogeneity of the disease. Among European patients, three defective alleles occur with high frequency. One bears a splice donor site mutation of the exon 2/intron 2 border (459 + 1A → G, formerly named allele I).[276] This allele has also been found among Arabs. Haplotype analysis of three polymorphic sites in the ASA gene revealed a complete linkage disequilibrium of the haplotype and the mutation, indicating a common origin of this mutation.[277] The second most frequent allele among Europeans is characterized by an amino acid substitution at Pro426 → Leu.[276] The frequency of these two most common alleles among MLD patients has been determined by various groups and found to vary considerably among European patients. The frequency was reported to vary from 15% to 43.2% for the splice donor allele and from 16.2 to 25 percent for the Pro 426 → Leu allele.[276,278,279] Among Austrian juvenile MLD patients, the frequency of the Pro426 → Leu allele was as high as 50 percent, while in a similar selection of Polish patients it was as low as 3.5 percent.[278] The third most common allele among Europeans bears an Ile179 → Ser substitution and represents about 12 percent of mutant alleles.[278]

Various mutations have been found at higher frequencies in patients of particular ethnic groups. A Thr274 → Met substitution has been detected in several patients of Lebanese origin.[280] A single splice donor site mutation (848 + 1G → A) has been found in various patients of Alaskan Eskimo and Navajo Indian origin, suggesting a founder effect and a possible genetic link between these two populations.[281,282] An exceptionally high frequency of MLD has been noted among the small population of Habbanite Jews in Israel.[211] All patients are homozygous for a Pro377 → Leu mutation, demonstrating a founder effect in this population.[283] Indeed, the current Habbanite population originates from just a few individuals, who survived famine in the seventeenth century, when this community was still living in the Yemenite town of Habban. The pattern of alleles found in Japanese patients seems to be entirely different from that in Europeans.[284] So far the most frequent MLD allele among the Europeans has not been found among Japanese. Instead, a Gly99 → Asp mutation accounts for 30 percent of MLD alleles in Japanese patients.[284] A frequency of 1 in 8000 newborns has been noted among Arabs in Israel. Interestingly, all these patients live in a small area north of Nazareth. Because the local clustering and the tendency toward intrafamilial marriages in Arabs suggested a founder effect, it was surprising to find five different mutations, all of them occurring homozygously.[212]

The mutations analyzed so far involve seven deletions, four splice site mutations, and 53 amino acid substitutions. Deletions of 8 and 1 bp in exon 1[285] and 2,[286] respectively, cause a frameshift. An additional deletion of 12 bp occurs in exon 2.[287] A deletion of 3 bp in exon 7 causes an in-frame loss of Phe at position 398.[288] Three deletions have been found in exon 8. A 9-bp deletion causes the in-frame loss of three amino acids.[289] A deletion of an AT dinucleotide[290] and of 11 bp[291] both cause a frameshift. The latter should lead to the synthesis of a 29-amino-acid elongated protein, but no ASA cross-reacting material was detected in fibroblasts of the patient.

So far, three intronic splice donor site mutations[276,281,282,292] have been described. An exonic mutation at the exon 4/intron 4 border causes loss of the splice donor site and a concomitant substitution, Gly325 → Cys.[288] A C → T transition 22 bp downstream of the exon 8 splice acceptor site has two effects: It results in an amino acid substitution, which itself is deleterious (Thr409 → Ile), and concomitantly in the generation of a cryptic splice acceptor site 27 bp downstream of the usual site.[293] Since 75 percent of the transcripts remain correctly spliced and the amino acid substitution itself is deleterious, the latter has to be considered the major defect in the allele, which may be aggravated by the defective splicing.

Amino acid substitutions make up the largest group of mutations. Evidence that these mutations have deleterious effects on the enzyme and are not polymorphisms has in most cases been supplied by in vitro mutagenesis experiments (see Table 148-3). Occasionally, causality was assumed if amino acids that are conserved among sulfatases of different function and origin were substituted non-conservatively. Except for exon 1, amino acid substitutions have been found in all parts of the gene, with some clustering in exon 2. If the degree of amino acid conservation among different sulfatases reflects functional importance, this clustering is not surprising, since the sulfatases are particularly homologous in the N-terminal region.[294]

The effects of few amino acid substitutions on enzymatic properties, intracellular sorting, and stability have been analyzed in detail.

The second most frequent allele among European patients is characterized by a Pro 426→Leu substitution.[276] The mutant enzyme is synthesized in normal amounts and has enzymatic activity.[295,296] It is properly targeted to the lysosomes, where it is rapidly degraded.[295] Thus, the cause of deficiency is decreased intralysosomal stability. Low residual enzyme activities can be detected in cultured fibroblasts of patients. In cultured fibroblasts, the mutant enzyme can be stabilized to levels sufficient to normalize sulfatide metabolism by exposing the cells to inhibitors of cysteine proteinases.[295] This may provide a therapeutic strategy in the future.

Table 148-3 Mutations and Polymorphisms in the Human ASA Gene

Mutation	Effect	Intron/Exon	Base/codon change	Position: Gene	Position: cDNA	Phenotype	Verification by expression	Population	Restriction site alteration gain or loss	Reference
del8bp	8-bp deletion	Ex1		103–110	103–110	severe	–	-	*Bst*NI–	285
P82L	Pro82 → Leu	Ex2	CCG → CTG	394	245	severe	–	European	*Hpa*II–	372
R84Q	Arg84 → Gln	Ex2	CGG → CAG	400	251	mild	+	European	–	358,278
G86D	Gly86 → Asp	Ex2	GGC → GAC	406	257	severe	+	Muslim Arab	–	212
S95N	Ser95 → Asn	Ex2	AGC → AAC	433	284	severe	–	European	*Alu*I–	285
S96F*	Ser96 → Phe	Ex2	TCC → TTC	436	287	severe	+	European	*Sma*I–	278,299
S96L	Ser96 → Leu	Ex2	TCC → CTC	435/436	286/287	severe	+	Muslim Arab	*Sma*I–	212
G99D	Gly99 → Asp	Ex2	GGC → GAC	445	296	severe	+	Japanese	*Hae*III–	284,359
DelC446/447	1-bp deletion	Ex2	GGCCTGC → GGCTGC	446/447	297/298		–	European	*Hae*II–	286
G119R	Gly119Arg	Ex2	GGA → AGA	504	355		–	European	–	285
G122S	Gly122 → Ser	Ex2	GGC → AGC	513	364		+	Japanese/ European	*Bal*I+	360
									*Nae*I	298
del12pb	12-bp deletion	Ex2		544–555	392–403	severe	–		*Sau*I–	287
P136L	Pro136 → Leu	Ex2	CCC → CTC	559	407	severe	+	Jewish	–	371
D152Y	Asp152 → Tyr	Ex2	GAC → TAC	603	454		–		–	285
Q153H	Gln153 → His	Ex2	CAG → CAC	608	459	severe	+	Japanese	*Apa*I–	361
459+1G → A (Allele I)	Loss of splice donor site	Int2	CAGgta → CAGata	609	459+1	severe	–	European	*Mva*I	276
									*Bst*NI	369
									*Xba*I	298
G154D	Gly154 → Asp	Ex3	GGC → GAC	724	461		+	European	*Apa*I-(cDNA)	298
P155R*	Pro155 → Arg	Ex3	CCC → CGC	727	464		–	Lebanese	*Apa*I-(cDNA)	288
P167R	Pro167 → Arg	Ex3	CCT → CGT	763	500		+	European	–	298
D169N	Asp169 → Asn	Ex3	GAC → AAC	768	505		–	Polynesian	–	288
C172Y	Cys172 → Tyr	Ex3	TGT → TAT	778	515	mild	–	European	*Mae*III	372
I179S (E3P799)	Ile179 → Ser	Ex3	ATC → AGC	799	536	mild	+	European	*Pst*I	292
										278
Q190H	Gln190 → His	Ex3	CAG → CAC	833	570	severe	+	Muslim/Arab	*Fnu*4HI	212
Y201C	Tyr201 → Cys	Ex3	TAC → TGC	865	602	severe	–	South African	–	372
A212V	Ala212 → Val	Ex3	GGC → GTC	898	635	severe	+	European	*Aat*II–	278,300,363
A224V	Ala224 → Val	Ex3	GCC → GTC	934	671	mild	–	European		300
678+1G → A	Loss of splice donor site	Int3	CACgta → CACata	942	678+1	severe	–	European	*Tai*I–	372
P231T	Pro231 → Thr	Ex4	CCT → ACT	1028	691		–		–	364
R244C	Arg244 → Cys	Ex4	CGC → TGC	1067	730	severe	–	European/ Iranian	*Sst*II–	288
R244H	Arg244 → His	Ex4	CGC → CAC	1068	731	severe	–	Reunion	*Sst*II–	285
G245R	Gly245 → Arg	Ex4	GGG → AGG	1070	733	severe	+	Japanese	*Sst*II–	365
S250Y	Ser250Tyr	Ex4	TCC → TAC	1086	749	severe	–		–	285
D255H	Asp255 → His	Ex4	GAT → CAT	1100	763	severe	+	European	*Sph*I+	366
T274M	Thr274 → Met	Ex4	ACG → ATG	1158	821	severe	+	Lebanese	–	212,280,297
848+1G → A	Loss of splice donor site	Int4	TGGgta → TGGata	1186	848+1	severe	–	Navajo Indian	–	281
								Alaskan Eskimo	–	282

(Continued on next page)

Table 148-3 (Continued)

Mutation	Effect	Intron/Exon	Base/codon change	Position: Gene	Position: cDNA	Phenotype	Verification by expression	Population	Restriction site alteration gain or loss	Reference
R288C	Arg288 → Cys	Ex5	CGT → TGT	1511	862		–	European	–	288
S295Y	Ser295 → Tyr	Ex5	TCC → TAC	1533	884	severe	–	Saudi Arabian	*Msp*I–	300
G308V	Gly308 → Val	Ex5	GGC → GTC	1572	923	severe	+	Japanese	–	361
G309S	Gly309 → Ser	Ex5	GGT → AGT	1574	925	severe	+	European	–	286
R311Q	Arg311 → Gln	Ex5	CGA → CAA	1581	932		–	European	–	372
A314T	Ala314 → Thr	Ex5	GCC → ACC	1589	940	severe	–	Algerian, European	–	285
G325C*	Gly325 → Cys and loss of splice donor site	Ex5	CCGgtc → CCTgtc	1622	973		–	Indian	*Msp*I–	288
D335V	Asp355 → Val	Ex6	GAC → GTC	1743	1004	severe	+	European	–	297
K367N	Lys367 → Asn	Ex6	AAG → AAC	1840	1101	mild	–	European	–	285
R370W	Arg370 → Trp	Ex7	CGG → TGG	2093	1108	severe	+	Christian Arab	–	212
R370Q	Arg370 → Gln	Ex7	CGG → CAG	2094	1109	mild	+	Jewish	–	301
P377L*	Pro377 → Leu	Ex7	CCG → CTG	2119	1130	severe	+	Habbanite Jews	–	283
D381V	Asp381 → Val	Ex7	GAC → GCT	2131	1142	severe	+	European	–	301
E382K*	Glu382 → Lys	Ex7	GAG → AAG	2133	1144	mild	–	European	–	300
R384C	Arg384 → Cys	Ex7	CGT → TGT	2139	1150	mild	–		*Nla*IV–	285
R390W	Arg390 → Trp	Ex7	CGG → TGG	2157	1168	severe	–	Indian	–	288
								European		372
R390Q	Arg390 → Gln	Ex7	CGG → CAG	2158	1169	mild	+		–	368
H397Y	His397 → Tyr	Ex7	CAC → TAC	2178	1189	mild	+		–	368
ΔF398*	deletion Phe398/399	Ex7	TTCTTC → TTC	2181–2182	1192–1194		–	Polynesian	–	288
1204+1G → A(E7S2195)	Loss of splice donor site	Int7	AGGgta → AGGata	2194	1204+1	severe	–	European	*Bst*EII–	278,292
2320del9*	deletion Ser406–Thr408	Ex8	9-bp deletion	2320–2329	1216–1224	severe	–	European	–	289
2324delAT	2-bp deletion	Ex8	AGTGATACC → AGTGACC	2324–2325	1220–1222	severe	–		*Mae*III+	290
T409I	Thr 409 → Ile and aberrant splicing	Ex8	ACT → ATT	2330	1226	mild	+	Japanese	–	293
P426L (Allele A)	Pro426 → Leu	Ex8	CCG → CTG	2381	1277	mild	+	European	*Pst*I/*Aci*I–	276
										278
L428P	Leu429 → Pro	Ex8	CTC → CCC	2387	1283	severe	–		*Bgl*I	362
Del11bp	11-bp deletion	Ex8	11-bp deletion	2505–2515	1401–1411	severe	–	European	*Pvu*II–	278,291
Q486X	Gln486 → Stop	Ex8	CAG → TAG	2560	1456	severe	–	European	–	370
R496H	Arg496 → His	Ex8	CGC → CAC	2591	1487		–	European	–	285

Polymorphisms:										
L76P	Leu76 → Pro	Ex2	CTC → CCC	376	228				*Acc*I	302
W193C	Trp193 → Cys	Ex3	TGG → TGT	842	579				*Bgl*I	276,277
NlaIII1	–	Int4	cttg → catg	1294					*Nla*III	367
NLaIII2	–	Int4	catg → cgtg	1386					*Nla*III	367
N350S	Asn350 → Ser	Ex6	AAT → ACT	1788	1049				*Bsr*I	216
S391T	Ser391 → Thr	Ex7	AGT → ACT	2161	1072				*Bsr*I	276
*Bam*HI	–	Int7	ggatcc → ggatgc	2213					*Bam*HI	277
Poly A–	Loss of polyadenylation signal	Ex8	aataac → agtaac	2723	1620				*Mae*III	216

The mutations are listed in the first column according to their position in the gene from the 5′ to the 3′ direction. Designations given in parentheses have been used in earlier publications. Asterisks indicate mutations that have occurred on the background of the ASA pseudodeficiency allele. The S69F mutation has also been found in a non-pseudodeficiency allele in two Muslim patients (J. Zlotogora, unpublished). The next four columns give a brief description of the effect of a mutation, its exonic (Ex) or intronic (Int) location, the codon or nucleotide change, and its position in the gene or cDNA. Numbering is according to Gene/EMBL data bank submitted sequences for the cDNA J04593/J04442 and X52150 for the gene. Nucleotide number 1 is the first base of the initiation codon. The next column shows the phenotype association of the allele. "Severe" designates late infantile forms of the disease, "mild" juvenile and adult forms; ± indicates whether or not the mutation has been verified by expression studies. In the following column the association with populations is listed. If the mutation causes alteration of a restriction site it is shown in the next column, with + indicating gain and – loss of the restriction site, respectively. If a restriction site is present in neither the normal nor the mutated sequence but can be easily generated through the use of primers, it is depicted in italic letters.

A Gly309 → Ser substitution has a similar effect on the enzyme.[286] Enzymatic activity is retained, but the intralysosomal half-life is severely reduced. However, in cultured fibroblasts of the patient bearing this mutation in compound heterozygosity with a null allele, considerable residual turnover of sulfatide could be detected. This contrasts with the severe phenotype of the patient, since residual enzyme activities usually predispose to the late-onset forms of MLD. The reasons for this discrepancy are unknown. A number of amino acid substitutions (P377L, D381V, G154D, P167R, T274M, D335V) cause retention of the mutant enzyme in the endoplasmic reticulum.[277,297,298]

One patient was found to be a genetic compound of alleles, each of which has two mutations causing amino acid substitutions. Any of these amino acid substitutions is deleterious for enzyme function, as has been shown by in vitro mutagenesis experiments.[298]

To date, seven MLD-causing mutations have been described that occur on the background of the pseudodeficiency allele.[283,288,289,299,300] This fact has implications for diagnostic tests based on the detection of the polymorphisms specifying the pseudodeficiency allele (see "Diagnostic Problems" below). Five mutations on the background of the pseudodeficiency allele cause amino acid substitutions, and two cause in-frame deletions of one or two amino acids (see Table 148-3 for details).

The knowledge of the three-dimensional structure of ASA[247] will make predictions about possible effects of mutations easier. So far, none of the mutations affects any of the amino acids that are directly involved in the catalytic activity of the enzyme (Fig. 148-9). About half of the mutations affect surface residues of the enzyme; half affect interior parts. Sixty percent of all mutations occur in nonstructured loop regions of the enzyme; the remainder are found in helices and β-pleated sheets. The cysteine-rich C-terminal region, which is unique to ASA, is almost free of mutations. Several mutations affect the central β-pleated sheet (G119R, G122S, A224V, T274M, A314T, G325C), others the minor sheet (R390Q, R390W, H397W, P426L, L428P). Mutations A212V, T201Y, S250Y, D255H, G308V, and G309S occur in helices. From x-ray diffraction data it is known that residues Asp335 and Arg370 form an intramolecular salt bridge. The loss of the negative charge in allele D335V causes loss of this salt bridge and may cause incorrect folding. Indeed, it has been demonstrated that the D355V mutant is retained in the ER and has lost enzymatic activity.[297] Two mutations affect Arg370, the other partner in salt bridge formation. Substitution of tryptophan is associated with a severe type of disease,[212] substitution of Gln with a mild form.[301] Octamerization of the ASA dimers depends on hydrogen bond formation between Glu424 and Phe398. Deletion of the latter in allele ΔF398 may therefore interfere with the intralysosomal octamerization of the enzyme, but this has not been investigated. However, one should be careful in predicting effects of mutations, since, surprisingly, even non-conservative substitutions like L76P, which occurs in a helix, can be polymorphic.[302]

Genotype-Phenotype Correlations

For some of the alleles causing MLD, the effect of the mutations has been analyzed in detail. This has allowed researchers to divide the mutant alleles into two groups. The first group contains alleles in which the mutation does not allow the synthesis of any functional enzyme (null alleles). The second group contains alleles that are still associated with low amounts of residual enzyme activity (R alleles). The determination of the distribution of these alleles among patients with different forms of MLD reveals a simple genotype-phenotype correlation.

Homozygosity for null alleles always causes the severe late infantile type of disease; one copy of an R allele, with some residual enzyme activity, mitigates the course to the intermediate juvenile type of disease; and two R alleles usually produce the mild adult form of MLD.[276,278,279,303] This reveals that the amount of residual enzyme activity associated with the genotype is one determinant of the clinical course of disease. However, it is also important to note that it is not the only determinant: There is considerable overlap in the clinical courses of patients with one and those with two R alleles.[276] Similarly, intrafamilial variance in age of onset and severity of disease can also be enormous.[32] Clearly, there are other factors — genetic and/or environmental — that influence the course of disease substantially. To date none of these factors is known.

It was initially hoped that genotype-phenotype correlations would allow the precise prediction of the clinical outcome by genotype analysis. Due to the phenotypic variability determined by factors other than ASA gene mutations, this is impossible. Such an exception from the genotype-phenotype correlation is represented by patients who are heterozygous for the Pro426 → Leu (R) allele but suffer from the late infantile form of disease.[278,279] These patients may present extremes of phenotypic variation on the same ASA genotype, or the ASA allele with the Pro426 → Leu substitution may also have a second mutation that leads to a complete loss of ASA activity. Alleles with two mutations have been found in MLD.[298]

The correlation of the different clinical forms of MLD with residual enzyme activity was also established by tissue culture studies, which examined *in situ* the activity of sulfatide catabolism. These examinations revealed a correlation between the capacity of the fibroblasts to metabolize sulfatides and the age of clinical onset of the disease.[203,204,304–306] Using ^{35}S-sulfate, Porter et al.[304] found that the amount of accumulated lipid was greatest in cells from a late infantile patient; cells of juvenile patients accumulated an intermediate amount; and cells from an adult patient accumulated the least. Conversely, the amount of ^{35}S-sulfate released directly correlated with the age of onset. It should be noted that this differentiation in the range of low enzyme activities can be achieved only with sulfatide loading assay, which is the most effective way to measure the functional capacity of sulfatide catabolism (see "Diagnostic Problems" below). Determination of low enzyme activities with artificial substrates in tissue or cell homogenates of MLD patients cannot differentiate in the range of low enzyme activities. It has been estimated that enzyme activity levels in adult patients are somewhere in the range of 2–5 percent of normal enzyme activity. Individuals who are genetic compounds, with a pseudodeficiency allele and an MLD allele, have about 510 percent residual enzyme activity and are healthy.[252] Thus, the entire clinical spectrum of severely affected early-onset patients to healthy individuals occurs on the background of rather minor variations of enzyme activity, between 0 and 5 percent.

Another study has pointed out that a genotype-phenotype correlation may also exist for a clinical course in which either psychiatric or neurologic symptoms initially prevail. It seems that patients who are carriers of the I179S allele usually start with psychiatric symptoms, whereas carriers of the P426L allele show neurologic symptoms at the onset of disease.[307]

DIAGNOSIS OF MLD

Clinical Diagnosis

The initial signs of MLD may appear at any age between the first year of life and the seventh decade. Regardless of the patient's age, this diagnosis should be considered whenever progressive white matter disease is encountered. The most common ages for the disease to begin are $1\frac{1}{2}$–2 years for the late infantile variant, 4–6 years for the juvenile, and 16–26 years for the adult form. Intellectual loss, weakness, and lack of coordination are early signs. Further involvement of the long tracts eventually leads to spastic tetraparesis and incontinence. Specific signs that help to confirm the diagnosis at this stage are the presence of optic atrophy and peripheral neuropathy.

The most useful clinical laboratory tests are brain CT or MRI, measurements of nerve conduction velocity, and evoked potential

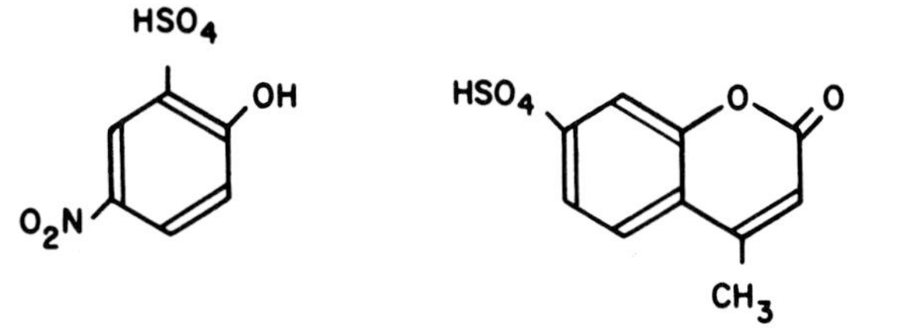

p-Nitrocatechol sulfate 4-Methylumbelliferyl sulfate

Fig. 148-11 Synthetic substrates of arylsulfatase A.

studies. All patients with significant symptomatology show changes on CT and MRI that are characteristic of brain white matter disease. In adult patients without peripheral neuropathy, nerve conduction may be normal.

Biochemical Diagnosis

Diagnosis of MLD based on clinical manifestations requires confirmation by biochemical assays. The critical diagnostic parameter for MLD is the deficiency of ASA.[15,20] Ancillary parameters comprise the catabolism of cerebroside 3-sulfate by the patient's cells and the presence of sulfatides in the urine.

ASA Determination. The most convenient and reliable sources for determination of ASA activity are peripheral blood leukocytes and cultured fibroblasts. The ubiquitous expression of ASA, however, allows the use of other tissues and body fluids for determination of its activity.[308,309,310] Although ASA is present in urine, this is a less reliable source for diagnostic purposes because of the highly variable enzyme levels in urine.[311,312]

The synthetic p-nitrocatechol sulfate and the 4-methylumbelliferyl sulfate (Fig. 148-11) are commercially available and most commonly used as substrates for colorimetric or fluorometric determination of ASA activity. The determination is complicated by the fact that both substrates are also cleaved by other arylsulfatases, most notably by arylsulfatase B, a lysosomal sulfatase codistributing with ASA. Baum et al. developed an assay for determination of ASA that is based on the inhibition of arylsulfatase B by high concentrations of NaCl.[243] Most of the published procedures represent modifications of this original assay. It should be noted that even in the absence of ASA, such assays detect an apparent residual activity 5–15 percent of that in controls. Other procedures developed to increase the specificity of the assay for ASA take advantage of the inhibition of ASA by Ag^{+}[313] or of the differential tolerance of arylsulfatases toward low temperature (Fig. 148-12A).[314] Physical separation of ASA from other arylsulfatases by ion exchange chromatography,[315] electrophoresis,[316] or isoelectric focusing[317] prior to determination of activity can also increase the specificity of the assay.

The use of the natural substrate, sulfatide, radioactively labeled in its ceramide or sulfate moiety, provides another means of selectively measuring ASA.[204,318] It should be noted that cleavage of the natural substrate requires the presence of a detergent or of

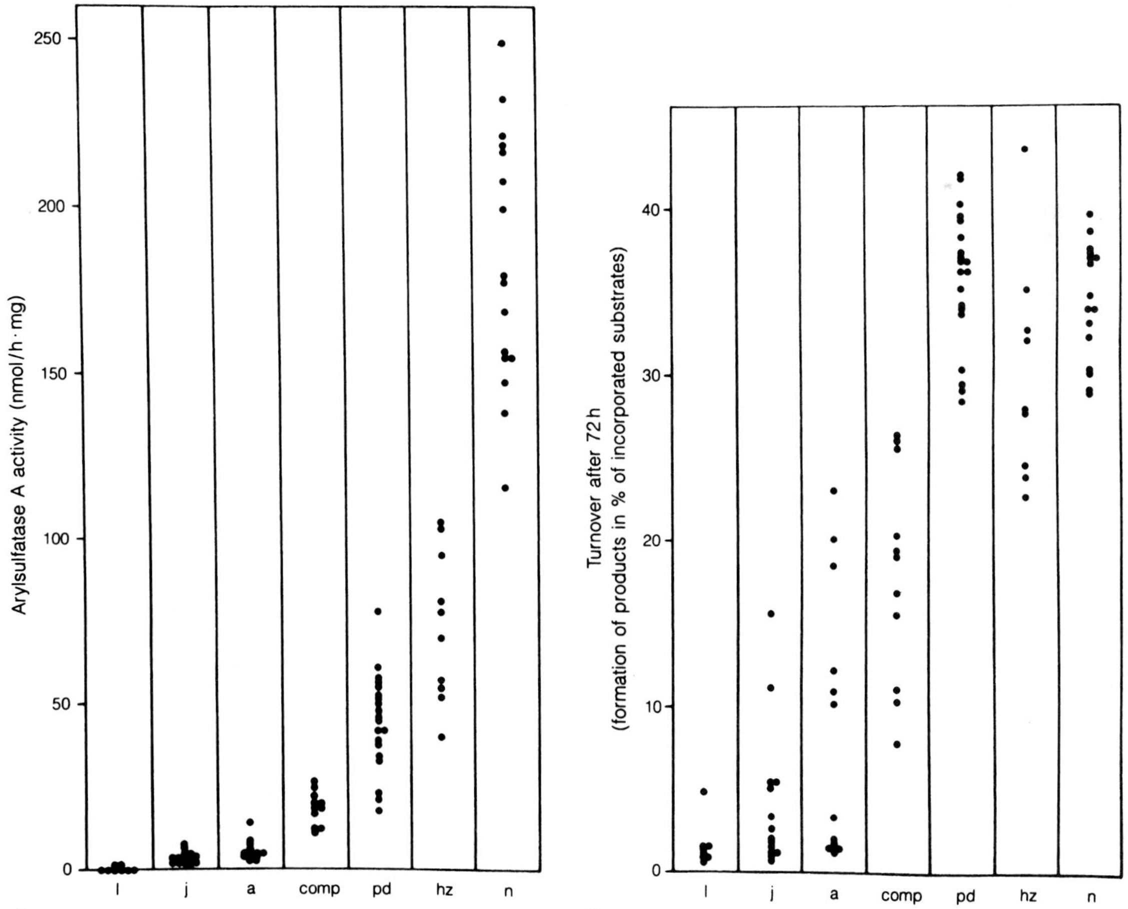

A *B*

Fig. 148-12 (A) ASA activity in homogenates of fibroblasts from MLD patients and healthy probands determined at 0°C. (B) Turnover of sulfatides in cultured skin fibroblasts (sulfatide loading test). l = late-infantile MLD; j = juvenile MLD; a = adult MLD; comp = MLD/pseudodeficiency compound heterozygotes; pd = pseudodeficiency probands; hz = obligate MLD heterozygotes; n = normal controls. (*From Leinekugel et al.*[204] *with permission.*)

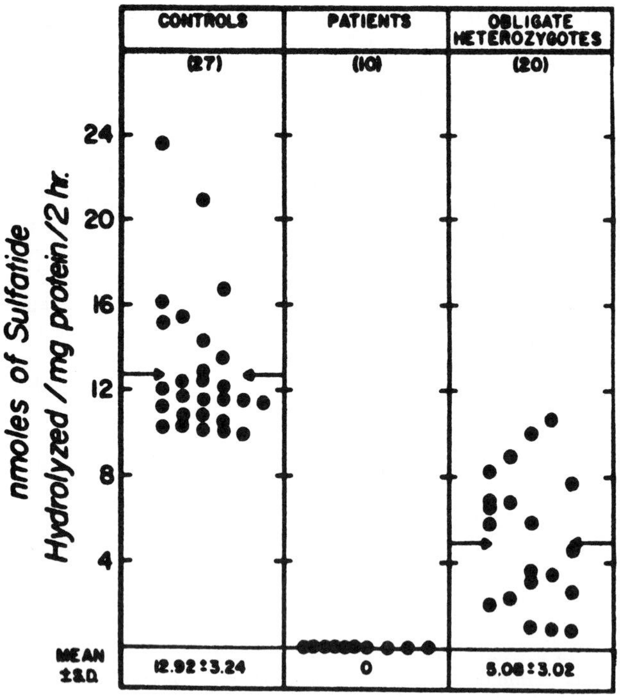

Fig. 148-13 Leukocyte ASA activity in normal controls, patients with MLD, and obligate heterozygotes. A dialyzed leukocyte sonicate was incubated for 2 h with [^{3}H] sulfatide labeled in the sphingosine portion of the molecule. The mean for each group is indicated by arrows. Note that the enzyme activity in some heterozygotes was quite low but that only in the MLD cases was it totally absent. (*Adapted from Raghavan et al.*[318])

saposin B. In the absence of ASA polypeptides, virtually no cleavage of sulfatide is observed (Fig. 148-13).

Diagnostic Problems

The major problems in enzymatic diagnosis of MLD are the frequent occurrence of the ASA pseudodeficiency allele and the rare cases of MLD that are due to the deficiency of saposin B. Individuals homozygous for the pseudodeficiency allele and compound heterozygotes carrying a pseudodeficiency allele in combination with an MLD allele have levels of residual activity that overlap with those measured in MLD patients using the conventional colorimetric or fluorometric assays for ASA. In MLD patients with a saposin B deficiency, ASA activity as determined with one of the commonly used synthetic substrates is normal. Therefore, deficiency of ASA does not necessarily prove an MLD, nor does presence of ASA activity exclude an MLD.

As discussed earlier ("Molecular Genetics of ASA Pseudodeficiency"), ASA pseudodeficiency is due to homozygosity for a frequent ASA allele that allows the expression of only about 10 percent of normal enzyme activity and is not associated with disease. However, pseudodeficiency has to be considered in genetic counseling and in diagnosis of MLD.[23,253,254,266,319] In the range of low residual enzyme activity, the conventional synthetic-substrate-based assays cannot reliably distinguish a benign pseudodeficiency from a deficiency causing MLD. ASA deficiency determined in cell homogenates with synthetic substrates does not prove MLD unless pseudodeficiency has been excluded. Individuals with pseudodeficiency who have neurologic symptoms of unknown etiology are often misdiagnosed as suffering from MLD.[266] Pseudodeficiency can be differentiated from MLD by the sulfatide loading assay.[23,320] This assay is rather laborious and expensive, but it is the only reliable procedure for differentiating pseudodeficiency from MLD. In the usual set-up, cells from a normal individual and one with pseudodeficiency metabolize comparable amounts of sulfatide in the loading assay, whereas cells from MLD patients do not.[23,286,320] Since individuals with pseudodeficiency, in contrast to MLD patients, do not excrete sulfatide in urine,[113] quantification of urinary lipid excretion may also be used to differentiate ASA deficiencies.

When genetic assays are used to differentiate between MLD and pseudodeficiency alleles[321] as the cause of ASA deficiency, it has to be kept in mind that MLD-causing mutations can occur on the background of the pseudodeficiency allele[279,283,288,289,299,300] (see Table 148-3). Thus, an individual who appears to be a carrier of a pseudodeficiency allele may well be affected with MLD. Therefore, genetic assays are to be used with caution in the differentiation of pseudodeficiency from MLD. If DNA of the index patient in the family of the person seeking genetic counseling is available, genotype analysis of the index case can help in the further differentiation. Presence of the pseudodeficiency polymorphism in the patient would constitute a clear indicator for a combined MLD/pseudodeficiency allele in the family.

If no ASA deficiency can be demonstrated in tissues of the patient but the clinical picture strongly suggests a leukodystrophy, saposin B deficiency has to be considered. The routine determination of ASA activity in leukocytes or fibroblasts is, for practical reasons, performed with an artificial, water-soluble substrate. Due to their water solubility, these substrates can be cleaved by ASA without the assistance of saposin B. Therefore, these assays do not detect a deficiency of saposin B.

The sulfatide loading test (see next paragraph) is helpful in identification of a saposin B deficiency, since cleavage of sulfatides in cells depends on the presence of both ASA and saposin B. Thus, normal enzyme activities on routine assays and lack of sulfatide cleavage in sulfatide-loading assays are indicative of MLD caused by saposin B deficiency. Determination of sulfatide in the urine of a patient provides another diagnostic parameter to substantiate the diagnosis.

Sulfatide Loading Test. This test measures the ability to degrade sulfatides in fibroblasts or other cultured cells. Sulfatides added to the culture medium are internalized and degraded by the cells. The accumulation of the sulfatides in the cells, their degradation, and the metabolic fate of the catabolic products can be followed.

The sulfatide loading test has two major applications. It is helpful if ASA activity is low but the clinical symptoms do not support the diagnosis of MLD, or if ASA activity is normal but the clinical picture is suggestive of MLD. In the former case, two pseudodeficiency alleles, or one in combination with an MLD allele, cause the low ASA activity; in the latter case, the saposin B that works in concert with ASA to degrade sulfatide in vivo is deficient.[322] In vitro tests based on the cleavage of p-nitrocatechol-sulfate, 4-methylumbelliferyl sulfate, or sulfatide plus detergent do not depend on saposin B and hence cannot detect its deficiency.

The loading test allows a clear distinction between individuals homozygous for the pseudodeficiency allele (normal catabolism of sulfatide) and MLD patients (Fig. 148-12B).[204,319] The loading test may fail to distinguish between compound heterozygotes, who carry one pseudodeficiency allele and one MLD allele, and those with the adult form of MLD.[204,323,324] It should be noted that in some loading tests semisynthetic sulfatides that carry a shortened fatty acid[204] or a fluorescent fatty acid analogue are used.[323,325,326] The structural alteration of the sulfatides may affect catabolism by ASA and saposin B. For example, sulfatides esterified with acetic acid will be degraded by ASA in vitro in the absence of saposin B, while desulfation of sulfatides with acyl chains of 6 or more carbon atoms depends on saposin B.[327] In the authors' experience, fluorescently labeled sulfatide analogues are cleaved to a considerable extent independent of saposin B. Saposin B deficiency may therefore escape detection when these semisynthetic sulfatides are used.

Sulfatide Excretion. Sulfatide excretion is highly elevated in patients with MLD. The origin of urinary sulfatides is most likely the kidney, which is second only to brain in relative abundance of sulfatides and a major site of sulfatide storage in MLD. The chemical composition of sulfatides from kidney and urine are similar and differ from that of those from brain.[102,122]

Methods for quantitative determination of urinary sulfatides involve their extraction from the urine or the urinary sediment, which contains nearly two thirds of the urinary sulfatides.[328] The sulfatides are then separated from neutral lipids and quantified by thin layer chromatography or HPLC.[113,329,330] Sulfatide excretion in individuals with low ASA (homozygotes for the pseudodeficiency allele or MLD/pseudodeficiency compound heterozygotes) is clearly distinguished from that in MLD patients.[331] Sulfatide excretion in compound heterozygotes has been reported to be normal[203,252] or slightly elevated.[331]

Heterozygote Identification and Genetic Counseling

Leukocyte and fibroblast assays for ASA using p-nitrocatechol-sulfate or sulfatides as substrates are helpful to identify carriers of MLD alleles (Fig. 148-12 and 148-13A).[204,211] Due to some overlap in enzyme values between normal individuals and carriers, the assignment of carrier status based on ASA activity determination is not unequivocal.[332] The validity of carrier assignment may be increased by inclusion of the parents and of the other members of the family. If the specific mutations causing MLD in the index case are known, carrier detection can be based on molecular techniques.

Heterozygote identification is complicated by frequent occurrence of the ASA pseudodeficiency allele.[24,250,251,273] In genetic counseling, enzyme activity levels in the heterozygous range are frequently assumed to be indicative of an MLD allele carrier status. However, in Europe, 1 out of 7 individuals is a carrier of the pseudodeficiency allele and has ASA activity in the heterozygous range. The sulfatide loading assay and sulfatide excretion are normal in individuals heterozygous for a pseudodeficiency or an MLD allele. Thus, in genetic counseling, the direct detection of pseudodeficiency allele polymorphisms is the only way to distinguish between heterozygosity for an MLD or a pseudodeficiency allele. Again, it has to be kept in mind that MLD alleles containing the pseudodeficiency polymorphisms are not distinguished from pseudodeficiency alleles by the commonly used genetic tests. Thus, there remains a low probability that an individual who is diagnosed as a carrier of a pseudodeficiency allele based on genetic assay is indeed a carrier of an MLD allele.

Determination of ASA activity in the obligate heterozygote parents of an MLD patient is most helpful in indicating whether a pseudodeficiency allele may complicate carrier assignment among the sibs of an MLD patient. If so, at least one of the parents must be an MLD/pseudodeficiency compound heterozygote with residual ASA activity in the range of that of MLD patients.

Prenatal Diagnosis

Prenatal diagnosis has been successfully accomplished for MLD by measuring activity of ASA in cultured amniotic fluid cells, chorionic villi (at 6–11 weeks of pregnancy), or cells grown from chorionic villi.[23,106,190,333,334] Direct assays of ASA activity in amniotic fluid have been used for prenatal diagnosis of MLD[84,335] but are not recommended as the only procedure to establish the diagnosis.

Activity of ASA in cultured cells depends on growth state. As is the case for many other lysosomal enzymes, activity increases significantly after the cells have grown to confluency. Therefore, careful attention must be paid to cell culture and harvesting conditions.

In any prenatal diagnosis of MLD, it is mandatory to establish whether one of the parents is a carrier of a pseudodeficiency allele (expected in 1 out of 7 parents). Otherwise, low enzyme activities in the fetus due to a benign MLD/pseudodeficiency genotype are misinterpreted as indicative of MLD. In families in which an MLD allele and a pseudodeficiency allele occur, molecular identification of the pseudodeficiency allele in the amniotic cells is required. A sulfatide loading test using cultured amniotic fluid or chorionic villi cells can also be helpful.

TREATMENT

Treatment with diets, with drugs to activate or stabilize the mutant enzyme, or with enzyme replacement by infusion of normal enzyme have been unsuccessful.[25]

Symptomatic Therapy

Physical treatment is useful to prevent contractures that would cause nursing problems. Vigabatrin, an inhibitor of GABA transaminase, has been shown to reduce spasticity and ataxia in children with MLD, and in patients who develop seizures, as it is at the same time a valuable antiepileptic drug.[336,337]

Bone Marrow Transplantation

Bone marrow transplantation has been introduced as a therapeutic option for MLD.[338–340] To understand the rationale of this therapy, some aspects of the biology of lysosomal enzymes and of microglial cells have to be explained. Newly synthesized lysosomal enzymes are not completely sorted to the lysosome, but depending on the enzyme and cell type, 10–30 percent of enzyme is secreted. The secreted enzymes can bind to mannose 6-phosphate receptors on the plasma membranes of neighboring cells. These receptors efficiently endocytose the bound lysosomal enzyme and deliver it to the lysosome. Thus, via secretion, a normal cell can donate lysosomal enzymes to a deficient recipient cell and correct the metabolic defect within this cell. In addition, various studies suggest that very low amounts of enzyme need to be endocytosed to effect metabolic correction.[204,252] Enzyme secreted by transplanted normal bone marrow cells can thus deliver enzyme to the deficient cells of the patient. In MLD the enzyme has to be delivered to the glial cells, which are not accessible to plasma enzymes due to the blood-brain barrier. It has been shown that part of the central nervous system microglia, the so-called perivascular microglia, is of monocytic lineage and thus is derived from bone marrow.[341] Thus, it is conceivable that monocytes of the donor bone marrow traverse the blood-brain barrier and become resident as perivascular microglia. These cells may secrete ASA and donate the enzyme to the deficient glial cells.

In symptomatic patients with the late infantile form of the disease, this therapy is not effective[342–344] and may even accelerate the disease.[340] Still a matter of debate is whether bone marrow transplantation in the presymptomatic stage might ameliorate the course of the disease. Several presymptomatic MLD patients have received transplants, but at the time of the reports,[342,344,345] the observation periods after transplantation were still too short to allow a final conclusion. Follow-up of these patients should inform us in the near future whether bone marrow transplantation is a valuable therapeutic option for late infantile MLD when the patients are still presymptomatic. Attempts at intrauterine bone marrow transplantation in MLD have so far failed.[346]

Bone marrow transplantation has been recommended in the juvenile and adult forms of MLD. The difficulties in evaluating the efficacy of bone marrow transplantation in the late-onset forms of MLD are illustrated by the case of a girl with the juvenile form of MLD who received a transplant at the age of 16 years. Initially the clinical course was judged as indicating considerable improvement. This was one of the index cases that led physicians to recommend transplantation in juvenile and adolescent forms of MLD.[340] However, 6 years after transplantation, the clinicians taking care of this patient concluded that her post-transplantation clinical course reflected the natural course of the disease.[347] Apart from this patient, eight patients with late-onset forms of MLD and successful engraftment have been reported.[342–344,348–351] For several of these patients, the observation period post engraftment is too short to draw conclusions about effects;[344,350] in others progression of the disease[342,343] or an arrest in progression[348,349,351] was reported. As patients with juvenile or adult forms of MLD have endogenous residual enzyme activity, less ASA has to be supplied to reach a metabolically corrective enzyme level.[204] Bone marrow transplantation is therefore more likely to be effective in late-onset than in late infantile forms of MLD. However, it has to be realized that particularly in the late-onset forms of the disease, wide variations of the clinical course have been reported, even in the same family. It is therefore difficult or even impossible to relate an arrest in the progression of the disease in an individual patient to a therapeutic effect of the transplant. To clarify whether late-onset forms of MLD will benefit from transplantation, a number of patients will have to be followed over a period of 10–20 years before conclusions can be drawn. Recommendations for or against bone marrow transplantation in presymptomatic late infantile or late-onset forms of MLD will have to take into account the mortality rate for transplantation in children with lysosomal storage disorders, which ranges from 10 to 25 percent depending on whether marrow from an HLA-identical sibling is available, and the experience that stable engraftment is obtained in about half of patients.

Gene Replacement

The cDNA for human ASA has been introduced into a recombinant retroviral vector and the virus used to infect late infantile MLD cells.[352,353] After retroviral gene transfer and selection, selected cell lines expressed ASA activities five- to tenfold higher than those expressed by normal human fibroblasts treated with the vector alone. The virally introduced gene produced mRNA, which was translated normally, and the protein precursor was postsynthetically processed and incorporated into lysosomes. Moreover, the cells could then desulfate radioactive cerebroside 3-sulfate added to the medium almost as efficiently as control cells.[352]

It can be anticipated that the beneficial effect of such gene replacement therapy will increase with the amount of enzyme secreted by the genetically modified and engrafted cells. A retroviral vector with ASA under the control of the long terminal repeat was used to transduce bone marrow of ASA-deficient mice.[354] After transduction, the bone marrow was transplanted into lethally irradiated ASA-deficient recipient mice. Serum levels of ASA were determined with a sensitive ELISA over a period of up to 9 months after transplantation. Most animals showed sustained high expression of the ASA cDNA and correspondingly high serum levels of the enzyme produced from the retroviral construct. Preliminary data point to a reduction of sulfatide storage in kidney and liver, which are the principal sites of sulfatide storage outside of the central nervous system in these mice (see "Animal Model" below).

ANIMAL MODEL

MLD has been described only in humans; there is no naturally occurring animal model. ASA-deficient mice were generated by homologous recombination in embryonic stem cells.[355] Biochemical and genetic examination of the animals demonstrated complete absence of ASA activity. Sulfatide storage was found in epithelia of the kidney, gallbladder, and lung. In the kidney, storage was confined to the loops of Henle, the distal tubules, and, to a lesser extent, the collecting ducts. Storage in nonneuronal tissues of the mice is largely identical to that in humans. In neuronal tissues, sulfatide storage was detected predominantly in the white matter and to a lesser extent in the gray matter. In the brain, sulfatide storage was found in oligodendrocytes, astrocytes, and some but not all neurons. Ultrastructural examination shows the typical lipid bilayer morphology of polar lipids and has demonstrated the intralysosomal location of the storage material. Sulfatide storage in neurons has been found in several nuclei of brainstem, spinal cord, diencephalon, and cerebellum.

Other than lipid storage, various other abnormalities were noted in the nervous systems of ASA-deficient mice. There is considerable astrogliosis in the white matter. Microglial cells appear normal in the first year of life. In the second year, microglial activation becomes apparent. Axons of the optic nerve have a reduced diameter, only 70 percent of that in controls.

In the cerebellum, the antler-like shape of the normal Purkinje cell dendritic tree was not detectable, whereas the somata of Purkinje cells were of normal morphology and number. Interestingly, no storage of sulfatide was found in Purkinje cells. In older (2-year-old) animals, Purkinje cells seem to be degenerating. The number of radial sheets extending from the Bergmann glia into the stratum moleculare is severely reduced. Since Purkinje cells and Bergmann glia extensions are in close proximity, it is tempting to speculate that glial and neuronal abnormalities are pathogenetically connected. Equivalent morphologic aberrations of Purkinje cells and Bergmann glia have not been described in humans. However, one has to realize that pathologic descriptions of human tissues are derived from gliotic final-stage brains.

Histologic examination of the inner ear revealed almost complete degeneration of glial and neural cells of the acoustic ganglion, causing deafness in the animals. This degenerative process occurs sometime between the ages of 6 and 12 months. Interestingly, alterations in brainstem auditory evoked potentials have been described as an early symptom in MLD patients.[58,59,60,61,356] However, the deafness observed in mice older than 1 year has never been documented as an early characteristic symptom in humans.

Degeneration of fibers can be seen in the peripheral nervous system of animals older than 20 months, but not to an extent comparable to that in MLD patients. In animals 20 months of age, about 30 percent of fibers of the phrenic nerve were degenerated.

The most striking difference from the human disease is the lack of demyelination in the central nervous system. This may explain the surprisingly mild phenotype of ASA deficiency in mice.

ASA-deficient mice show various neurologic and behavioral abnormalities. The gait patterns of mice were altered, with shortening of the distance between two paw prints by about 15 percent. The mice also performed significantly worse on a rotating rod. In the Morris water maze test, which is designed to evaluate spatial learning capabilities, ASA-deficient mice swam significantly more slowly than controls. The impaired swimming capabilities of the mice impeded conclusions about their learning behavior. Learning behavior in the passive avoidance test, in which the animals learn to avoid a compartment in which they receive an electric shock, was indistinguishable in normal and ASA knockout mice. Frequency of spontaneous movements as measured by the number of light beam crossings in a given time was also normal in deficient mice. The neurologic symptoms of the mice progress slowly. In the second year of life they develop a tremor of the head, and at the age of 2 years they cannot stay on a rotating rod at all and are unable to swim.

ACKNOWLEDGMENTS

The chapter on MLD was authored by Dr. Edwin H. Kolodny and Dr. Hugo W. Moser in the sixth edition and by Dr. Edwin H. Kolodny and Dr. Arvan L. Fluharty in the seventh edition. The present chapter is an updated version of the one that appeared in the seventh edition, which may be consulted for a relevant older bibliography. We gratefully acknowledge the permission to integrate large sections of the MLD chapter from the seventh edition. The authors thank Dr. Hans H. Goebel and Dr. Folker Hanefeld for assistance in preparation of this chapter and Mrs. Angelika Thiel for expert preparation of the manuscript.

REFERENCES

1. Alzheimer A: Beiträge zur Kenntnis der pathologischen Neuroglia und ihrer Beziehungen zu den Abbauvorgängen im Nervengewebe. *Nissl-Alzheimer's Histol Histopathol Arb* **3**:401, 1910.

2. Alzheimer A: Über einen eigenartigen schweren Erkrankungsprozess der Hirnrinde. *Neurologisches Zentralblatt* **23**:1129, 1906.
3. Alzheimer A: Über eine eigenartige Erkrankung der Hirnrinde. *Allgemeine Zeitschrift Psychiatrie und psychisch-gerichtliche Medizin* **64**:146, 1907.
4. Amaducci L, Sorbi S, Piacentini S, Bick KL: The first Alzheimer disease case: A metachromatic leukodystrophy? *Dev Neurosci* **13**:186, 1991.
5. Braak H: personal communication.
6. Witte F: Über pathologische Abbauvorgänge im Zentralnervensystem. *Münch Med Wochenschr* **68**:69, 1921.
7. Scholz W: Klinische, pathologisch-anatomische und erbbiologische. Untersuchungen bei familiärer, diffuser Hirnsklerose im Kindesalter. *Z Gesamte Neurol/Psychiatr* **99**:42, 1925.
8. Von Hirsch T, Peiffer J: Über histologische Methoden in der Differentialdiagnose von Leukodystrophien und Lipoidosen. *Arch Psychiatr Nervenkr* **194**:88, 1955.
9. Peiffer J: Über die metachromatischen Leukodystrophien (Typ Scholz). *Arch Psychiatr Nervenkr* **199**:386, 1959.
10. Greenfield JG: A form of progressive cerebral sclerosis in infants associated with primary degeneration of the interfascicular glia. *J Neurol Psychopathol* **13**:289, 1933.
11. Einarson L, Neel AV: Beitrag zur Kenntnis sklerosierender Entmarkungsprozesse in Gehirn mit besonderer Berücksichtigung der diffusen Sklerose. *Acta Jutlandica* **10**:1, 1938.
12. Norman RM: Diffuse progressive metachromatic leucoencephalopathy. A form of Schilder's disease related to the lipidoses. *Brain* **22**:234, 1947.
13. Jatzkewitz H: Zwei Typen von Cerebrosid-Schwefelsäureestern als sog. "Pralipoide" und Speichersubstanzen bei der Leukodystrophie, Typ Scholz (metachromatische Form der diffusen Sklerose). *Z Physiol Chem* **311**:279, 1958.
14. Austin J: Metachromatic sulfatides in cerebral white matter and kidney. *Proc Soc Exp Biol Med* **100**:361, 1959.
15. Austin JH, Balasubramanian AS, Pattabiraman TN, Saraswathi S, Basu DK, Bachhawat BK: A controlled study of enzymatic activities in three human disorders of glycolipid metabolism. *J Neurochem* **10**:805, 1963.
16. Mehl E, Jatzkewitz H: Evidence for the genetic block in metachromatic leukodystrophy (ML). *Biochem Biophys Res Commun* **19**:407, 1965.
17. Jatzkewitz H, Mehl E: Cerebroside-sulphatase and aryl sulfatase A deficiency in metachromatic leukodystrophy (ML). *J Neurochem* **16**:19, 1969.
18. Mehl E, Jatzkewitz H: Eine Cerebrosidsulfatase aus Schweineniere. *Hoppe-Seyler's Z Physiol Chem* **339**:260, 1964.
19. Shapiro LJ, Aleck KA, Kaback MM, et al: Metachromatic leukodystrophy without arylsulfatase A deficiency. *Pediatr Res* **13**:1179, 1979.
20. Austin JH, Armstrong D, Shearer L: Metachromatic forms of diffuse cerebral sclerosis. V. The nature and significance of low sulfatase activity: A controlled study of brain, liver and kidney in four patients with metachromatic leukodystrophy (MLD). *Arch Neurol* **13**:593, 1995.
21. Basner R, Von Figura K, Glössl J, Klein U, Kresse H, Mlekusch W: Multiple deficiency of mucopolysaccharide sulfatases in mucosulfatidosis. *Pediatr Res* **13**:1316, 1979.
22. Dubois G, Turpin JC, Baumann N: Absence of ASA activity in healthy father of patient with metachromatic leukodystrophy. *N Engl J Med* **293**:302, 1975.
23. Kihara H, Ho C-K, Fluharty AL, Tsay KK, Hartlage PL: Prenatal diagnosis of metachromatic leukodystrophy in a family with pseudo arylsulfatase A deficiency by the cerebroside sulfate loading test. *Pediatr Res* **14**:224, 1980.
24. Hohenschutz C, Eich P, Friedl W, Waheed A, Conzelmann E, Propping P: Pseudodeficiency of arylsulfatase A: A common genetic polymorphism with possible disease implications. *Hum Genet* **82**:45, 1989.
25. Kolodny EH, Fluharty AL: Metachromatic leukodystrophy and multiple sulfatase deficiency: sulfatide lipidosis, in Scriver CR, Beaudet AL, Sly WS, Valle D, Stanbury JD, Wyngaarden JB, Fredrickson DS (eds): *The Metabolic and Molecular Bases of Inherited Disease* 7th ed. New York, McGraw-Hill, 1995, p 2693.
26. MacFaul R, Cavanagh N, Lake BD, Stephens R, Whitfield AE: Metachromatic leucodystrophy: Review of 38 cases. *Arch Dis Child* **57**:168, 1982.
27. Hollander H: Über metachromatische Leukodystrophie. II. Relation zwischen Erkrankungsalter und Verlaufsdauer. *Arch Psychiatr Z Neurol* **205**:300, 1964.
28. Zlotogora J, Costeff H, Elian E: Early motor development in metachromatic leukodystrophy. *Arch Dis Child* **56**:309, 1981.
29. Hyde TM, Ziegler JC, Weinberger DR: Psychiatric disturbances in metachromatic leukodystrophy. Insights into the neurobiology of psychosis. *Arch Neurol* **49**:401, 1992.
30. Hagberg B: Clinical symptoms, signs and tests in metachromatic leukodystrophy, in Folch-Pi J, Bauer H (eds): *Brain Lipids and Lipoproteins and the Leukodystrophies*. Amsterdam, Elsevier, 1963, p 134.
31. Balslev T, Cortez MA, Blaser SI, Haslam RHA: Recurrent seizures in metachromatic leukodystrophy. *Pediatr Neurol* **17**:150, 1997.
32. Clarke JTR, Skomorowski MA, Chang PL: Marked clinical difference between two sibs affected with juvenile metachromatic leukodystrophy. *Am J Med Genet* **33**:10, 1989.
33. Deeg KH, Reif R, Stehr K, Hümmer KP, Harzer K: Chronisch hämorrhagische Pankreatitis bei Gallenblasenpolyposis als Erstsymptom der metachromatischen Leukodystrophie. *Monatsschr Kinderheilkd* **134**:272, 1986.
34. Tesluk H, Munn RJ, Schwartz MZ, Ruebner BH: Papillomatous transformation of the gallbladder in metachromatic leukodystrophy. *Pediatr Pathol* **9**:741, 1989.
35. Siegel EG, Lucke H, Schauer W, Creutzfeldt W: Repeated upper gastrointestinal hemorrhage caused by metachromatic leukodystrophy of the gall bladder. *Digestion* **51**:121, 1992.
36. Duyff RF, Weinstein HC: Late-presenting metachromatic leukodystrophy. *Lancet* **348**:1382, 1996.
37. Hageman ATM, Gabreëls FJM, de Jong JGN, Gabreëls-Festen AA, van den Burg CJ, van Oost BA, Wevers RA: Clinical symptoms of adult metachromatic leukodystrophy and arylsulfatase A pseudodeficiency. *Arch Neurol* **52**:408, 1995.
38. Shapiro EG, Lockman LA, Knopman D, Krivit W: Characteristics of the dementia in late-onset metachromatic leukodystrophy. *Neurology* **44**:662, 1994.
39. Al-Moutaery KR, Choudhury AR, Hassanen MO: Cervical cord compression and severe hydrocephalus in a child with Saudi variant of multiple sulfatase deficiency. *Acta Neurochir* **131**:160, 1994.
40. Suárez EC, Rodríguez AS, Tapia AG, de las Heras RS, López Rios F, Rosell MJC: Ichthyosis: The skin manifestation of multiple sulfatase deficiency. *Pediatr Dermatol* **14**:369, 1997.
41. Brismar J: CT and MRI of the brain in inherited neurometabolic disorders. *J Child Neurol* **7** (suppl):S112, 1992.
42. Jayakumar PN, Aroor SR, Jha RK, Arya BYT: Computed tomography (CT) in late infantile metachromatic leucodystrophy. *Acta Neurol Scand* **79**:23, 1989.
43. Kim TS, Kim IO, Kim WS, Choi YS, Lee JY, Kim OW, Yeon KM, et al.: MR of childhood metachromatic leukodystrophy. *Am J Neuroradiol* **18**:733, 1997.
44. Schipper HL, Seidel H: Computed tomography in late-onset metachromatic leukodystrophy. *Neuroradiology* **26**:39, 1984.
45. Demaerel P, Faubert C, Wilms G, Casaer P, Piepgras U, Baert AL: MR findings in leukodystrophy. *Neuroradiology* **33**:368, 1991.
46. Waltz G, Harik SI, Kaufmann B: Adult metachromatic leukodystrophy. Value of computed tomographic scanning and magnetic resonance imaging of the brain. *Arch Neurol* **44**:225, 1987.
47. Fisher NR, Cope SJ, Lishman WA: Metachromatic leukodystrophy: Conduct disorder progressing to dementia. *J Neurol Neurosurg Psychiatry* **50**:488, 1987.
48. Reider-Grosswasser I, Bornstein N: CT and MRI in late-onset metachromatic leukodystrophy. *Acta Neurol Scand* **75**:64, 1987.
49. Kruse B, Hanefeld F, Christen HJ, Bruhn H, Michaelis T, Hanicke T, Frahm J: Alterations of brain metabolites in metachromatic leukodystrophy as detected by localized proton magnetic resonance spectroscopy in vivo. *J Neurol* **241**:68, 1993.
50. Fukumizu M, Matsui K, Hanaoka S, Sakuragawa N, Kurokawa T: Partial seizures in two cases of metachromatic leukodystrophy: Electrophysiologic and neuroradiologic findings. *J Child Neurol* **7**:381, 1992.
51. Blom S, Hagberg B: EEG findings in late infantile metachromatic and globoid cell leukodystrophy. *Electroencephalogr Clin Neurophysiol* **22**:253, 1967.
52. Clark JR, Miller RG, Vidgoff JM: Juvenile-onset metachromatic leukodystrophy: Biochemical and electrophysiologic studies. *Neurology* **29**:346, 1979.
53. Pilz H, Hopf HC: A preclinical case of late adult metachromatic leukodystrophy? *J Neurol Neurosurg Psychiatry* **35**:360, 1972.
54. Wulff CH, Trojaborg W: Adult metachromatic leukodystrophy: Neurophysiologic findings. *Neurology* **35**:1776, 1985.
55. Miller RG, Gutmann L, Lewis RA, Sumner AJ: Acquired versus familial demyelinative neuropathies in children. *Muscle Nerve* **8**:205, 1985.

56. Cruz AM, Ferrer MT, Fueyo E, Galdós L: Peripheral neuropathy detected on an electrophysiological study as the manifestation of MLD in infancy. *J Neurol Neurosurg Psychiatry* **38**:169, 1975.
57. Brion S, Mikol J, Graveleau J: Leucodystrophie métachromatique de l'adulte jeune: étude clinique, biologique et ultra structurale. *Rev Neurol* **122**:161, 1970.
58. Brown FR, Shimizu H, McDonald JM, Moser AB, Marquis P, Chen WW, Moser HW: Auditory evoked brainstem response and high-performance liquid chromatography sulfatase assay as early indices of metachromatic leukodystrophy. *Neurology* **31**:980, 1981.
59. Markand ON, Garg BP, Demyer WE, Warren C, Worth RM: Brain stem auditory visual and somatosenosory evoked potentials in leukodystrophies. *Electroencephalogr Clin Neurophysiol* **54**:39, 1982.
60. Takakura H, Nakamo C, Kasagi S, Takashima S, Takeshita K: Multimodality evoked potentials in progression of metachromatic leukodystrophy. *Brain Dev* **7**:424, 1985.
61. De Meirleir LJ, Taylor MJ, Logan WJ: Multimodal evoked potential studies in leukodystrophy of children. *Can J Neurol Sci* **15**:26, 1988.
62. Klemm E, Conzelmann E: Adult-onset metachromatic leucodystrophy presenting without psychiatric symptoms. *J Neurol* **236**:427, 1989.
63. Carlin L, Roach ES, Riela A, Spudis E, McLean WT Jr: Juvenile metachromatic leukodystrophy: Evoked potentials and computed tomography. *Ann Neurol* **13**:105, 1983.
64. Philippart M, Nuwer MR, Packwood J: Presymptomatic adult-onset metachromatic leukodystrophy (MLD): Electrophysiological and clinical correlations. *Neurology* **40**(suppl 1):128, 1990.
65. Markiewicz D, Adamczewska-Goncerzewicz Z, Zelman IB, Dynecki J, Bieniasz J: A case of metachromatic leukodystrophy with a chronic course (clinical-morphological-biochemical study). *Neuropathol Pol* **16**:233, 1978.
66. Kaye EM, Ullman MD, Kolodny EH, Krivit W, Rischert JC: Possible use of CSF glycosphingolipids for the diagnosis and therapeutic monitoring of lysosomal storage diseases. *Neurology* **42**:2290, 1992.
67. Oak S, Rao S, Karmakow S, Kulkarni B, Kaltgutkar A, Malde A, Naik L: Papillomatosis of the gallbladder in metachromatic leukodystrophy. *Pediatr Surg Int* **12**:424, 1997.
68. Ries M, Deeg KH: Polyposis of the gallbladder associated with metachromatic leukodystrophy. *Eur J Pediatr* **152**:450, 1993.
69. Kleinman P, Winchester P, Volbert F: Sulfatide cholecystosis. *Gastrointest Radiol* **1**:99, 1976.
70. Burgess JH, Kaffayan B, Slungaard RK, Gilbert E: Papillomatosis of the gallbladder associated with metachromatic leukodystrophy. *Arch Pathol Lab Med* **109**:79.
71. Fock JM, Begeer JH, Prins TR: Metachromatic leukodystrophy and coincidental finding of papillomatosis of the gallbladder. A case report. *Neuropediatrics* **26**:55, 1996.
72. Hagberg B, Sourander P, Svennerholm L: Sulfatide lipidosis in childhood: Report of a case investigated during life and at autopsy. *Am J Dis Child* **104**:644, 1962.
73. Suzuki K, Suzuki K, Chen GC: Isolation and chemical characterization of metachromatic granules from a brain with metachromatic leukodystrophy. *J Neuropathol Exp Neurol* **26**:537, 1967.
74. Takahashi K, Naito M: Lipid storage disease: Part II. Ultrastructural pathology of lipid storage cells in sphingolipidoses. *Acta Pathol Jpn* **35**:385, 1985.
75. Goebel HH, Busch H: Abnormal lipopigments and lysosomal residual bodies in metachromatic leukodystrophy. *Adv Exp Med Biol* **266**:299, 1990.
76. Takashima S, Matusui A, Fujii Y, Nakamura H: Clinico-pathological differences between juvenile and late infantile metachromatic leukodystrophy. *Brain Dev* **3**:365, 1981.
77. Yamano T, Ohta S, Shimada M, Okada S, Yutaka T, Yabuuchi H: Neuronal depletion of cerebellum in late infantile metachromatic leukodystrophy. *Brain Dev* **2**:359, 1980.
78. Goebel HH, Busch-Hettwer H, Bohl J: Ultrastructural study of the retina in late infantile metachromatic leukodystrophy. *Ophthalmic Res* **24**:103, 1992.
79. Scott IU, Green WR, Goyal AK, de la Cruz Z, Naidu S, Moser H: New sites of ocular involvement in late-infantile metachromatic leukodystrophy revealed by histopathologic studies. *Graefes Arch Clin Exp Ophthalmol* **231**:189, 1993.
80. Martin JJ, Ceuterick C, Mercelis R, Joris C: Pathology of peripheral nerves in metachromatic leukodystrophy. A comparative study of ten cases. *J Neurol Sci* **53**:95, 1985.
81. Alves D, Pires MM, Guimarães A, Miranda MC: Four cases of late onset metachromatic leucodystrophy in a family: Clinical, biochemical and neuropathological studies. *J Neurol Neurosurg Psychiatry* **49**:1423, 1986.
82. Bardosi A, Friede R, Ropte S, Goebel HH: A morphometric study on sural nerves in metachromatic leukodystrophy. *Brain* **110**:683, 1987.
83. LeRoy JG, Van Elsen A, Martin JJ, Dumaon JE, Hulet AE, Okada S, Navarro C: Infantile metachromatic leukodystrophy: Confirmation of a prenatal diagnosis. *N Engl J Med* **288**:1365, 1973.
84. Eto Y, Tahara T, Koda N, Yamaguchi S, Ito F, Okuno A: Prenatal diagnosis of metachromatic leukodystrophy. A diagnosis by amniotic fluid and its confirmation. *Arch Neurol* **39**:29, 1982.
85. Malde AD, Naik LD, Pantvaidya SH, Oak SN: An unusual presentation in a patient with metachromatic leukodystrophy. *Anaesthesia* **52**:690, 1997.
86. Resibois A: Electron microscopic studies of metachromatic leukodystrophy. IV. Liver and kidney alterations. *Pathol Eur* **6**:278, 1971.
87. Wolfe HJ, Peitra GG: The visceral lesions of metachromatic leukodystrophy. *Am J Pathol* **44**:921, 1964.
88. Werneck LC, Pereira JL, Bruck I: Metachromatic leukodystrophy: Report of two cases with histochemistry of nerves and muscles. *Arquivos de Neuropsiquiatría* **38**:237, 1980.
89. Krendel DA, Shutter LA, Holt PJ: Fiber type disproportion in metachromatic leukodystrophy. [Letter] *Muscle Nerve* **17**:1352, 1994.
90. Martin JJ, Clara R, Ceuterick CL, Joris CL: Is congenital fiber type disproportion a true myopathy? *Acta Neurol Belg* **76**:335, 1976.
91. Dehkharghani F, Saraut HB, Brewster MA, Roth SI: Congenital muscle fiber type disproportion in Krabbe's leukodystrophy. *Arch Neurol* **38**:585, 1981.
92. Svennerholm L: Some aspects of the biochemical changes in leucodystrophy, in Folch-Pi J, Bauer H (eds): *Brain Lipids and Lipoproteins, and the Leucodystrophies*. Amsterdam, Elsevier, 1963, p 104.
93. Harzer K, Kustermann-Kuhn B: Brain glycolipid content in a patient with pseudoarylsulfatase A deficiency and coincidental diffuse disseminated sclerosis, and in patients with metachromatic, adreno-, and other leukodystrophies. *J Neurochem* **48**:62, 1987.
94. Norton WR, Poduslo SE: Biochemical studies of metachromatic leukodystrophy in three siblings. *Acta Neuropathol* (Berlin) **57**:188, 1982.
95. Rosengren B, Fredman P, Månsson J-E, Svennerholm L: Lysosulfatide (galactosylsphingosine-3-O-sulfate) from metachromatic leukodystrophy and normal human brain. *J Neurochem* **52**:1035, 1989.
96. Poduslo SE, Tennekoon G, Price D, Miller K, McKhann GM: Fetal metachromatic leukodystrophy: Pathology, biochemistry and a study of in vitro enzyme replacement in CNS tissue. *J Neuropathol Exp Neurol* **35**:622, 1976.
97. Baier W, Harzer K: Sulfatides in prenatal metachromatic leukodystrophy. *J Neurochem* **41**:1766, 1983.
98. Toda K-I, Kobavashi T, Goto I, Ohno K, Eto Y, Inui K, Okada S: Lysosulfatide (sulfogalactosylsphingosine) accumulation in tissues from patients with metachromatic leukodystrophy. *J Neurochem* **55**:1585, 1990.
99. Toda K, Kobayashi, T, Goto I, Kurokawa T, Ogomori K: Accumulation of lysosulfatide (sulfogalactosylsphingosine) in tissues of a boy with metachromatic leukodystrophy. *Biochem Biophys Res Commun* **159**:605, 1989.
100. Pilz H, Heipertz R: The fatty acid composition of cerebrosides and sulfatides in a case of adult metachromatic leukodystrophy. *Z Neurol* **206**:203, 1974.
101. Stallberg-Stenhagen S, Svennerholm L: Fatty acid composition of human brain sphingomyelin: Normal variation with age and changes during myelin disorders. *J Lipid Res* **6**:46, 1965.
102. Malone MJ, Stoffyn P: A comparative study of brain and kidney glycolipids in metachromatic leukodystrophy. *J Neurochem* **13**:1037, 1966.
103. Moser HW, Sugita M, Snag MD, Williams M: Liver glycolipids, steroid sulfates and steroid sulfatase in a form of metachromatic leukodystrophy associated with multiple sulfatase deficiencies, in Volk BW, Aronson SM (eds): *Sphingolipids, Sphingolipidoses and Allied Disorders (Advances in Experimental Medicine and Biology vol 19)*. New York, Plenum, 1972, p 429.
104. Nishio H, Kodama S, Matsuo T: Analysis of fatty acids and sphingosines from urinary sulfatides in a patient with metachromatic leukodystrophy by gas chromatography-mass spectrometry. *Brain Dev* **7**:614, 1985.

108. Kikkawa Y, Mimura A, Inage Z: Regional distribution of sulfatide in human kidney, and anti-sulfatide antibodies in sera from patients with nephritis detected by TLC immunostaining. *Nippon Jinzo Gakkai Shi* 33:635, 1991.
109. Krivan HC, Olson LD, Barile MF, Ginsburg V, Roberts DD: Adhesion of *Mycoplasma pneumoniae* to sulfated glycolipids and inhibition by dextran sulfate. *J Biol Chem* **264**:9283, 1989.
110. Natomi H, Sugano K, Takaku F, Iwamori M: Glycosphingolipid composition of the gastric mucosa. A role of sulfatides in gastrointestinal mucosal defense? *J Clin Gastroenterol* **12**(suppl 1):552, 1990.
111. Takamatsu K: Phytosphingosine-containing neutral glycosphingolipids and sulfatides in the human female genital tract: Their association in the cervical epithelium and the uterine endometrium and their dissociation in the mucosa of fallopian tube with the menstrual cycle. *Keio J Med* **41**:161, 1992.
112. Zhu XH, Hara A, Taketomi T: The existence of galactosyl ceramide 3-sulfate in serums of various mammals and its anticoagulant activity. *J Biochem* 110:241, 1991.
113. Molzer B, Sundt-Heller R, Kainz-Korschinsky M, Zobel M: Elevated sulfatide excretion in heterozygotes of metachromatic leukodystrophy: Dependence on reduction of arylsulfatase A activity. *Am J Med Genet* **44**:523, 1992.
114. Ishizuka I, Inomata M, Ueno K, Yamakawa T: Sulphated glyceroglycolipid in rat brain. Structure, sulphation in vivo, and accumulation in whole brain during development. *J Biol Chem* **253**:898, 1978.
115. Ishizuka I, Suzuki M, Yamakawa T: Isolation and characterization of a novel sulfoglycolipid, 'seminolipid,' from boar testis and spermatozoa. *J Biochem* **73**:77, 1973.
116. Thudichum JLW: *A Treatise on the Chemical Constitution of Brain*. London, Balliere, 1884.
117. Thudichum JLW: Die chemische Konstitution des Gehirns des Menschen und der Tiere. Tübingen, Franz Pietzeker, 1901.
118. Blix G: Zur Kenntnis der schwefelhaltigen Lipidstoffe des Gehirns: Über Cerebronschwefelsäure. *Hoppe-Seyler's Z Physiol Chem* **219**:82, 1933.
119. Stoffyn P, Stoffyn A: Structure of sulfatides. *Biochim Biophys Acta* **70**:218, 1963.
120. Stoffyn PJ: The structure and chemistry of sulfatides. *J Am Oil Chem Soc* **43**:69, 1966.
121. Svennerholm L, Bostrom K, Fredman P, Jungbjer B, Månsson JE, Rynmark BM: Membrane lipids of human peripheral nerve and spinal cord. *Biochim Biophys Acta* **1128**:1, 1992.
122. Martensson E: Sulfatides of human kidney: Isolation, identification, and fatty acid composition. *Biochim Biophys Acta* **116**:521, 1966.
123. Roberts DD, Rao CN, Liotta LA, Gralnick HR, Ginsburg V: Comparison of the specificities of laminin, thrombospondin, and von Willebrand factor for binding to sulfated glycolipids. *J Biol Chem* **261**:6872, 1986.
124. Kornblatt MJ, Knapp A, Levine M, Schachter H, Murray RK: Studies on the structure and formation during spermatogenesis of sulphoglycerogalactolipid of rat testis. *Can J Biochem* **52**:689, 1974.
125. Leffler H, Hansson C, Stromberg N: A novel sulfoglycosphingolipid of mouse small intestine, IV^3-sulfogangliotetraosylceramide, demonstrated by negative ion fast atom bombardment mass spectrometry. *J Biol Chem* **261**:1440, 1986.
126. Slomiany BL, Piotrowski J, Nishikawa N, Slomiany A: Enzymatic sulfation of salivary mucins: Structural features of 35S-labeled oligosaccharides. *Biochem Biophys Res Commun* **157**:61, 1988.
127. Liau YH, Lopez RA, Slomiany A, Slomiany BL: Helicobacter pylori lipopolysaccharide effect on the synthesis and secretion of gastric sulfomucin. *Biochem Biophys Res Commun* **184**:1411, 1992.
128. Nagai KI, Roberts DD, Toida T, Matsumoto H, Kushi Y, Handa S, Ishizuka I: Mono-sulfated globotetraosylceramide from human kidney. *J Biochem* **106**:878, 1989.
129. Tadano K, Ishizuka I: Bi-sulfoglycosphingolipid containing a unique 3-*O*-sulfated N-acetylgalactosamine from rat kidney. *J Biol Chem* **257**:9294, 1982.
130. Iida N, Toida T, Kushi Y, Handa S, Fredman P, Svennerholm L, Ishizuka I: A sulfated glucosylceramide from rat kidney. *J Biol Chem* **264**:5974, 1989.
131. Tadano K, Ishizuka I, Matsuo M, Matsumoto S: Bi-sulfated gangliotetraosylceramide from rat kidney. *J Biol Chem* **257**:13413, 1982.
132. Ishizuka I, Nagai KI, Kawaguchi K, Tadano-Aritomi K, Toida T, Hirabayashi Y, Li YT, et al.: Preparation and enzymatic degradation of monosulfogangliotriaosylceramide. *J Biol Chem* **260**:11256, 1985.
133. Chou DKH, Ilyas AA, Evans JE, Costello C, Quarles RH, Jungalwala FB: Structure of sulfated glucuronyl glycolipids in the nervous system reacting with HNK-1 antibody and some IgM paraproteins in neuropathy. *J Biol Chem* **261**:11717, 1986.
134. Hauser G: Labeling of cerebrosides and sulfatides in rat brain. *Biochim Biophys Acta* **84**:212, 1964.
135. Bosio A, Binzek E, Stoffel W: Functional breakdown of the lipid bilayer of the myelin membrane in central and peripheral nervous system by disrupted galactocerebroside synthesis. *Proc Natl Acad Sci USA* **93**:13280, 1996.
136. Coetzee T, Fujita N, Dupree J, Shi R, Blight A, Suzuki K, Suzuki D, et al.: Myelination in the absence of galactocerebroside and sulfatide: Normal structure with abnormal function and regional instability. *Cell* **86**:209, 1996.
137. Farrell DF, McKhann GM: Characterization of cerebroside sulfotransferase from rat brain. *J Biol Chem* **246**: 4694, 1971.
138. Farrell DF: Enzymatic sulphation of some galactose-containing sphingolipids in developing rat brain. *J Neurochem* **23**:219, 1974.
139. Honke K, Tsuda M, Hirahara Y, Ishii A, Makita A, Wada Y: Molecular cloning and expression of cDNA encoding human 3′-phosphoadenylsulfate: Galactosylceramide 3′-sulfotransferase. *J Biol Chem* **272**:4864, 1997.
140. Marcelo AJ, Pieringer RA: Hydrocortisone regulates arylsulfatase A (cerebroside-3-sulfate-3-sulfohydrolase) by decreasing the quantity of the enzyme in cultures of cells dissociated from embryonic mouse cerebra. *Neurochem Res* **15**:937, 1990.
141. Harris RA, Loh HH: Brain sulfatide and non-lipid sulfate metabolism in hypothyroid rats. *Res Commun Chem Pathol Pharmacol* **24**:169, 1979.
142. Ida H, Eto Y, Maekawa K: Biochemical pathogenesis of demyelination in globoid cell leukodystrophy (Krabbe's disease): The effects of psychosine upon oligodendroglial cell culture. *Acta Paediatr Jpn* (Overseas Ed) **32**:20, 1990.
143. Benjamins JA, Guarnieri M, Miller K, Sonneborn CM, McKhann GM: Sulfatide synthesis in isolated oligodendroglial and neuronal cells. *J Neurochem* **23**:751, 1974.
144. Ishizuka I, Tadano K, Nagata N, Niimura Y, Nagai Y: Hormone-specific responses and biosynthesis of sulfolipids in cell lines derived from mammalian kidney. *Biochim Biophys Acta* **541**:467, 1978.
145. Sundaram SK, Tan JH, Lev M: A neutral galactocerebroside sulfate sulfatidase from mouse brain. *J Biol Chem* **270**:10187, 1995.
146. Tempesta MC, Salvayre R, Levade T: Functional compartments of sulphatide metabolism in cultured living cells: Evidence for the involvement of a novel sulphatide-degrading pathway. *Biochem J* **297**:479, 1994.
147. Norton WT, Poduslo SE: Myelination in rat brain: Changes in myelin composition during brain maturation. *J Neurochem* **21**:759, 1973.
148. Arvanitis D, Dumas M, Szuchet S: Myelin palingenesis. 2. Immunocytochemical localization of myelin/oligodendrocyte glycolipids in multilamellar structures. *Dev Neurosci* **14**:328, 1992.
149. London Y, Vossenberg FGA: Specific interaction of central nervous system myelin basic protein with lipid. *Biochim Biophys Acta* **478**:478, 1973.
150. Vacher M, Waks M, Nicot C: Myelin proteins in reverse micelles: Tight lipid association required for insertion of the Folch-Pi proteolipid into a membrane-mimetic system. *J Neurochem* **52**:117, 1989.
151. Rintoul DA, Welti R: Thermotropic behavior of mixtures of glycosphingolipids and phosphatidylcholine: Effect of monovalent cations on sulfatide and galactosylceramide. *Biochemistry* **28**:26, 1989.
152. Loh HH, Lay PY, Ostwald T, Cho TM, Way EL: Possible involvement of cerebroside sulfate in opiate receptor binding. *Fed Proc* **37**:147, 1978.
153. Craves FB, Zalc B, Leybin L, Baumann N, Loh HH: Antibodies to cerebroside sulfate inhibit the effects of morphine and β-endorphin. *Science* **207**:75, 1980.
154. Ebadi M, Chweh A: Inhibition by arylsulfatase A of Na-independent $[^3H]$-GABA and $[^3H]$-muscinol binding to bovine cerebellar synaptic membranes. *Neuropharmacology* **19**:105, 1980.
155. Miyakawa A, Ishitani R: Butanol extracts from myelin fragments: Identification of 5-hydroxytryptamine binding components. *Life Sci* **31**:1427, 1982.
156. Maggio B, Bianco ID, Montich GG, Fidelio GD, Yu RK: Regulation by gangliosides and sulfatides of phospholipase A_2 activity against dipalmitoyl and dilauroylphosphatidylcholine in small unilamellar bilayer vesicles and mixed monolayers. *Biochem Biophys Acta* **1190**:137, 1994.
157. Higashi H, Yamagata T: Full activation without calmodulin of calmodulin-dependent cyclic nucleotide phosphodiesterase by acidic

glycosphingogolipids: G_{M3}, sialosylneolactotetraosyl ceramide and sulfatide. *FEBS Lett* **314**:53, 1992.
158. Woscholski R, Kodaki T, Palmer RH, Waterfield MD, Parker PJ: Modulation of the substrate specificity of the mammalian phosphatidylinositol-3-kinase by cholesterolsulfate and sulfatide. *Biochemistry* **34**:11489, 1995.
159. Taraboletti G, Rao CN, Krutzsch HK, Liotta LA, Roberts DD: Sulfatide-binding domain of the laminin A chain. *J Biol Chem* **265**:12253, 1990.
160. Guo NH, Krutzsch HC, Negre E, Vogel T, Blake DA, Roberts DD: Heparin- and sulfatide-binding peptides from the type I repeats of human thrombospondin promote melanoma cell adhesion. *Proc Natl Acad Sci USA* **89**:3040, 1992.
161. Pesheva P, Gloor S, Schachner M, Probstmeier R: Tenascin R is an intrinsic autocrine factor for oligodendrocyte differentiation and promotes cell adhesion by a sulfatide mechanism. *J Neurosci* **17**:4642, 1997.
162. Christophe O, Obert B, Meyer D, Girma JP: The binding domain of von Willebrand factor to sulfatides is distinct from those interacting with glycoprotein Ib, heparin, and collagen and residues between amino acid residues Lev 512 and Lys 673. *Blood* **78**:2310, 1991.
163. Suzuki Y, Toda Y, Tamatani T, Watanabe T, Suzuki T, Nakao T, Murase K, et al.: Sulfated glycolipids are ligands for a lymphocyte homing receptor, L-selectin (LECAM-1), binding epitope in sulfated sugar chain. *Biochem Biophys Res Commun* **190**:426, 1993.
164. Todderud G, Alford J, Millsap KA, Aruffo A, Tramposch KM: PMN binding to P-selectin is inhibited by sulfatide. *J Leukocyte Biol* **52**:85, 1992.
165. Waddell TK, Fialkow L, Chan CK, Kishimoto TK, Downey GP: Signaling function of L-selectin. Enhancement of tyrosine phosphorylation and activation of MAP kinase. *J Biol Chem* **270**:15403, 1995.
166. Bengtsson T, Grenegård M, Olsson A, Sjögren F, Stendahl O, Zalavary S: Sulfatide induced L-selectin activation generates intracellular oxygen radicals in human neutrophils: Modulation by extracellular adenosine. *Biochim Biophys Acta* **1313**:119, 1996.
167. Laudanna C, Constantin G, Baron P, Scarpini E, Scarlato G, Cabrini G, Dechecchi C, et al.: Sulfatides trigger increase of cytosolic free calcium and enhanced expression of tumor necrosis factor-alpha and interleukin-8 mRNA in human neutrophils. Evidence for a role of L-selectin as a signaling molecule. *J Biol Chem* **269**:4021, 1994.
168. Holt GD, Pangburn MK, Ginsburg V: Properdin binds to sulfatide [Gal(3-SO_4)β1-1Cer] and has a sequence homology with other proteins that bind sulfated glycoconjugates. *J Biol Chem* **265**:2852, 1990.
169. Crossin KL, Edelman GM: Specific binding of cytotactin to sulfated glycolipids. *J Neurosci Res* **33**:631, 1992.
170. Colige A, Li SW, Sieron AL, Nusgens BV, Prockop DJ, Lapiere CM: cDNA cloning and expression of bovine procollagen I N-proteinase: A new member of the superfamily of zinc-metalloproteinases with binding sites for cells and other matrix components. *Proc Natl Acad Sci USA* **94**:2374, 1997.
171. Kobayashi T, Honke K, Miyazaki I, Matsumoto K, Nakamura T, Ishizuka I, Makita A: Hepatocyte growth factor specifically binds to sulfoglycolipids. *J Biol Chem* **269**:9817, 1994.
172. Brankamp RG, Manley GD, Owen TJ, Krstenansky JL, Smith PL, Cardin AD: Demonstration that [$A^{103,106,108}$] antistasin 93-119 inhibits the specific binding of antistasin to sulfatide [Gal(3-SO_4)β1-1Cer]. *Biochem Biophys Res Commun* **181**:246, 1991.
173. Guo NH, Krutzsch HC, Negre E, Zabrenetzky VS, Roberts DD: Heparin-binding peptides from the type I repeats of thrombospondin. Structural requirements for heparin binding and promotion of melanoma cell adhesion and chemotaxis. *J Biol Chem* **267**:19349, 1992.
174. Weerasinghe KM, Scully MF, Kakkar VV: Inhibition of the cerebroside sulphate (sulphatide)-induced contact activation reactions by platelet factor four. *Thromb Res* **33**:625, 1984.
175. Schiffman S, Rosenfeld R, Retzios AD: Interaction of factor XI and sulfatide. *Thromb Res* **41**:575, 1986.
176. Ratnoff OD, Everson B, Embury PM, Zaits NP, Anderson JM, Emanuelson MM, Malemud CJ: Inhibition of the activation of Hageman factor (factor XII) by human vascular endothelial cell culture supernates. *Proc Natl Acad Sci USA* **88**:10740, 1991.
177. Hånsson CG, Karlsson KA, Samuelsson BE: The identification of sulphatides in human erythrocyte membrane and their relation to sodium-potassium dependent adenosine triphosphatase. *J Biochem* **83**:813, 1978.
178. Olson LD, Gilbert AA: Characteristics of *Mycoplasma hominis* adhesion. *J Bacteriol* **175**:3224, 1993.
179. Brennan MJ, Hannah JH, Leininger E: Adhesion of *Bordetella pertussis* to sulfatides and to the GalNAc b4 Gal sequence found in glycosphingolipids. *J Biol Chem* **266**:18827, 1991.
180. Cerami C, Kwakye-Berko F, Nussenzweig V: Binding of malarial circumsporozoite protein to sulfatides [Gal(3-SO_4)β1-Cer] and cholesterol-3-sulfate and its dependence on disulfide bond formation between cysteines in region II. *Mol Biochem Parasitol* **54**:1, 1992.
181. Muller HM, Reckmann I, Hollingdale MR, Bujard H, Robson KJ, Crisanti A: Thrombospondin related anonymous protein (TRAP) of *Plasmodium falciparum* binds specifically to sulfated glycoconjugates and to HepG2 hepatoma cells suggesting a role for this molecule in sporozoite invasion of hepatocytes. *EMBO J* **12**:2881, 1993.
182. Van Den Berg LH, Sadiq SA, Lederman S, Latov N: The gp120 glycoprotein of HIV-1 binds to sulfatide and to the myelin associated glycoprotein. *J Neurosci Res* **33**:513, 1992.
183. Kamisago S, Iwamori M, Tai T, Mitamura K, Yazaki Y, Sugano K: Role of sulfatides in adhesion of *Helicobacter pylori* to gastric cancer cells. *Infect Immun* **64**:624, 1996.
184. Huesca M, Borgia S, Hoffman P, Lingwood CA: Acidic pH changes receptor binding specificity of *Helicobacter pylori*: A binary adhesion model in which surface heat shock (stress) proteins mediate sulfatide recognition in gastric colonization. *Infect Immun* **64**:2643, 1996.
185. Harzer K, Benz HU: Deficiency of lactosyl sulfatide sulfatase in metachromatic leukodystrophy (sulfatidosis). *Hoppe-Seyler's Z Physiol Chem* **355**:744, 1974.
186. Fisher G, Reiter S, Jatzkewitz H: Enzymic hydrolysis of sulphosphingolipids and sulphoglycerolipids by sulphatase A in the presence and absence of activator protein. *Hoppe-Seyler's Z Physiol Chem* **359**:863, 1978.
187. Yamaguchi S, Aoki K, Handa S, Yamakawa T: Deficiency of seminolipid sulphatase activity in brain tissue of metachromatic leukodystrophy. *J Neurochem* **24**:1087, 1975.
188. Svennerholm E, Svennerholm L: Isolation of blood serum glycolipids. *Acta Chem Scand* **16**:1282, 1962.
189. Meier C, Bischoff A: Sequence of morphological alterations in the nervous system of metachromatic leukodystrophy: Light- and electron-microscopic observations in the central and peripheral nervous system in a prenatally diagnosed foetus of 22 weeks. *Acta Neuropathol* (Berlin) **36**:369, 1976.
190. LeRoy JG, Van Elsen A, Martin JJ, Dumaon JE, Hulet AE, Okada S, Navarro C: Infantile metachromatic leukodystrophy: Confirmation of a prenatal diagnosis. *N Engl J Med* **288**:1365, 1973.
191. Argyrakis A, Pilz H, Goebel HH, Muller D: Ultrastructural findings of peripheral nerve in a preclinical case of adult metachromatic leukodystrophy. *J Neuropathol Exp Neurol* **36**:693, 1977.
192. Grégoire A, Périer O, Dustin P: Metachromatic leukodystrophy, an electron microscopic study. *J Neuropathol Exp Neurol* **25**:617, 1966.
193. Morell P: A correlative synopsis of the leukodystrophies. *Neuropediatrics* **15**:62, 1984.
194. Austin J: Metachromatic leukodystrophy (sulfatide lipidosis), in Hers HG, Van Hoof F (eds): *Lysosomes and Lysosomal Storage Diseases*. New York, Academic, 1973, p 411.
195. Davison AN, Gregson NA: Metabolism of cellular membrane sulpholipids in the rat brain. *Biochem J* **98**:915, 1966.
196. O'Brien JS, Sampson EL: Myelin membrane: A molecular abnormality. *Science* **150**:1613, 1965.
197. Ginsberg L, Gershfeld NL: Membrane bilayer instability and the pathogenesis of disorders of myelin. *Neurosci Lett* **130**:133, 1991.
198. Tanaka K, Nagara H, Kobayashi T, Goto I: The twitcher mouse: Accumulation of galactosylsphingosine and pathology of the sciatic nerve. *Brain Res* **454**:340, 1988.
199. Tanaka K, Nagara H, Kobayashi T, Goto I: The twitcher mouse: Accumulation of galactosylsphingosine and pathology of the central nervous system. *Brain Res* **482**:347, 1989.
200. Eto Y, Wiesmann U, Herschkowitz NN: Sulfogalactosyl sphingosine sulfatase: Characteristic of the enzyme and its deficiency in metachromatic leukodystrophy in human cultured skin fibroblasts. *J Biol Chem* **249**:4955, 1974.
201. Suzuki K: Biochemical pathogenesis of genetic leukodystrophies: Comparison of metachromatic leukodystrophy and globoid cell leukodystrophy (Krabbe's disease). *Neuropediatrics* **15**:32, 1984.
202. Hannun YA, Bell RM: Lysosphingolipids inhibit protein kinase C: Implications for the sphingolipidoses. *Science* **235**:670, 1987.
203. Kappler J, Leinekugel P, Conzelmann E, Kleijer WJ, Kohlschutter A, Tonnesen T, Rochel M, et al.: Genotype-phenotype relationship in various degrees of arylsulfatase A deficiency. *Hum Genet* **86**:463, 1991.

204. Leinekugel P, Michel S, Conzelmann E, Sandhoff K: Quantitative correlation between the residual activity of β-hexosaminidase A and arylsulfatase A and the severity of the resulting lysosomal storage diseases. *Hum Genet* **88**:513, 1992.
205. Bruns GAP, Mintz BJ, Leary AC, Regina VM, Gerald PS: Expression of human arylsulfatase-A in man-hamster somatic cell hybrids. *Cytogenet Cell Genet* **22**:182, 1978.
206. Phelan MC, Thomas GR, Saul RA, Rogers RC, Taylor HA, Wenger DA, McDermid HE: Cytogenetic, biochemical and molecular analyses of a 22q13 deletion. *Am J Med Genet* **43**:872, 1992.
207. Gustavson K-H, Hagberg B: The incidence and genetics of metachromatic leucodystrophy in northern Sweden. *Acta Paediatr Scand* **60**:585, 1971.
208. Guibaud P, Garcia I, Guyonnet CL: La detection de l'heterozygotisme pour la sulfatidase. *Lyon Med* **229**:1215, 1973.
209. Farrell DF: Heterozygote detection in MLD. Allelic mutations at the ARA locus. *Hum Genet* **59**:129, 1981.
210. Heim P, Claussen M, Hoffmann B, Conzelmann E, Gartner J, Harzer K, Hunnerian DH, et al.: Leukodystrophy incidence in Germany. *Am J Med Genet* **71**:475, 1997.
211. Zlotogora J, Bach G, Varak V, Elian E: Metachromatic leukodystrophy in the Habbanite Jews: High frequency in a genetic isolate and screening for heterozygotes. *Am J Hum Genet* **32**:663, 1980.
212. Heinisch U, Zlotogora J, Kafert S, Gieselmann V: Multiple mutations are responsible for the high frequency of metachromatic leukodystrophy in a small geographic area. *Am J Hum Genet* **56**:51, 1995.
213. Wenger D, personal communication.
214. Kreysing J, von Figura K, Gieselmann V: Structure of the arylsulfatase A gene. *Eur J Biochem* **191**:627, 1990.
215. Stein C, Gieselmann V, Kreysing J, Schmidt B, Pohlmann R, Waheed A, Meyer HE, et al.: Cloning and expression of human arylsulfatase A. *J Biol Chem* **264**:1252, 1989.
216. Gieselmann V, Polten A, Kreysing J, von Figura K: Arylsulfatase A pseudodeficiency: Loss of a polyadenylation signal and N-glycosylation site. *Proc Natl Acad Sci USA* **86**:9436, 1989.
217. Schmidt B, Selmer T, Ingendoh A, von Figura K: A novel amino acid modification in sulfatases that is defective in multiple sulfatase deficiency. *Cell* **82**:271, 1995.
218. Dierks T, Schmidt B, von Figura K: Conversion of cysteine to formylglycine: A protein modification in the endoplasmic reticulum. *Proc Natl Acad Sci USA* **94**:11963, 1997.
219. Sommerlade H J, Selmer T, Ingendoh A, Gieselmann V, von Figura K, Neifer K, Schmidt B: Glycosylation and phosphorylation of arylsulfatase A. *J Biol Chem* **269**:20977, 1994.
220. Polten A, unpublished.
221. Gieselmann V, Schmidt B, von Figura K: In vitro mutagenesis of potential N-glycosylation sites of arylsulfatase A. Effects on glycosylation, phosphorylation and intracellular sorting. *J Biol Chem* **267**:13262, 1992.
222. Waheed A, Van Etten RL: Phosphorylation and sulfation of arylsulfatase A accompanies biosynthesis of the enzyme in normal and carcinoma cell lines. *Biochim Biophys Acta* **847**:53, 1985.
223. Braulke T, Hille A, Huttner HB, Hasilik A, von Figura K: Sulfated oligosaccharides in human lysosomal enzymes. *Biochem Biophys Res Commun* **143**:178, 1987.
224. Kelly BM, Yu CZ, Chang PL: Presence of a lysosomal enzyme, arylsulfatase-A, in the prelysosome-endosome compartments of human cultured fibroblasts. *Eur J Cell Biol* **48**:71, 1989.
225. Braulke T, Tippmer S, Chao HJ, von Figura K: Insulin-like growth factors I and II stimulate endocytosis but do not affect sorting of lysosomal enzymes in human fibroblasts. *J Biol Chem* **265**:6650, 1990.
226. Gieselmann V, unpublished.
227. Waheed A, Hasilik A, von Figura K: Synthesis and processing of arylsulfatase A in human skin fibroblasts. *Hoppe-Seyler's Z Physiol Chem* **363**:425, 1982.
228. Steckel F, Hasilik A, von Figura K: Synthesis and stability of arylsulfatase A and B in fibroblasts from multiple sulfatase deficiency. *Eur J Biochem* **151**:141, 1985.
229. Fujii T, Kobayashi T, Honke K, Gasa S, Ishikawa M, Shimizu T, Makita A: Proteolytic processing of human lysosomal arylsulfatase A. *Biochim Biophys Acta* **1122**:93, 1992.
230. James GT, Thach AB, Klassen L, Austin JH: Studies in metachromatic leukodystrophy: XV. Purification of normal and mutant arylsulfatase A from human liver. *Life Sci* **37**:2365, 1985.
231. Farooqui AA: Purification and properties of arylsulfatase A from human placenta. *Arch Int Physiol Biochim* **84**:479, 1976.
232. Laidler PM, Waheed A, Van Etten RL: Structural and immunochemical characterization of human urine arylsulfatase A purified by affinity chromatography. *Biochim Biophys Acta* **827**:73, 1985.
233. Selmi S, Maire I, Rousset B: Evidence for the presence of a very high concentration of arylsulfatase A in the pig thyroid: Identification of arylsulfatase A subunits as the two major glycoproteins in purified thyroid lysosomes. *Arch Biochem Biophys* **273**:170, 1989.
234. Van Der Pal RH, Klein W, Van Golde LM, Lopes-Cardozo M: Galactosylceramide sulfotransferase, arylsulfatase A and cerebroside sulfatase activity in different regions of developing rat brain. *Biochim Biophys Acta* **1043**:91, 1990.
235. Manowitz P, Fine LV, Nora R, Chokroverty S, Nathan PE, Fazzaro JM: A new electrophoretic variant of arylsulfatase A. *Biochem Med Metab Biol* **39**:117, 1988.
236. Poretz RD, Yang RS, Canas B, Lackland H, Stein S, Manowitz P: The structural basis for the electrophoretic isoforms of normal and variant human platelet arylsulphatase A. *Biochem J* **287**:979, 1992.
237. Sarafian TA, Tsay KK, Jackson WE, Fluharty AL, Kihara H: Studies on the charge isomers of arylsulfatase A. *Biochem Med* **33**:372, 1985.
238. Mituhashi K, Maru A, Koyanagi T, Ishibashi T, Imai Y, Gasa S, Taniguchi N, et al.: Arylsulfatase A activities in urine and tissues taken from bladder cancer patients. *Jpn J Exp Med* **54**:211, 1984.
239. Nakamura M, Gasa S, Makita A: Arylsulfatase A form normal human lung and lung tumors showed different patterns of microheterogeneity. *J Biochem* **96**: 207, 1984.
240. Farooqui AA, Mandel P: Recent developments in the biochemistry of globoid and metachromatic leucodystrophies. *Biomedicine* **26**:232, 1977.
241. Roy AB: L-ascorbic acid 2-sulphate. A substrate for mammalian arylsulphatases. *Biochim Biophys Acta* **377**:356, 1975.
242. Uchida T, Egami F, Roy AB: 3′,5′-Cyclic nucleotide phosphodiesterase activity of the sulphatase A of ox liver. *Biochim Biophys Acta* **657**: 356, 1981.
243. Baum H, Dodgson KS, Spencer B: The assay of arylsulphatases A and B in human urine. *Clin Chim Acta* **4**:453, 1950.
244. Roy AB, Mantle TJ: The anomalous kinetics of sulphatase A. *Biochem J* **261**:689, 1989.
245. Waheed A, Van Etten RL: The structural basis of the anomalous kinetics of rabbit liver arylsulfatase A. *Arch Biochem Biophys* **203**:11, 1980.
246. Rybarska-Stylinska J, Van Etten RL: Antigen-antibody interactions and the anomalous kinetics of arylsulfatase A. *Biochim Biophys Acta* **570**:107, 1979.
247. Lukatela G, Krauss N, Theis K, Selmer T, Gieselmann V, von Figura K, Saenger W: Crystal structure of human arylsulfatase A: The aldehyde function and the metal ion at the active site suggest a novel mechanism for sulfate ester hydrolysis. *Biochemistry* **37**: 3654, 1998.
248. Waldow A, Schmidt B, Dierks T, von Bülow R, von Figura K: Amino acid residues forming the active site of arylsulfatase A. Role in catalytic activity and substrate binding. *J Biol Chem* **274**: 12284, 1999.
249. Recksiek M, Selmer T, Dierks T, Schmidt B, von Figura K: Sulfatases: Trapping of the sulfated enzyme intermediate by substituting the active site formylglycine. *J Biol Chem* **273**:6069, 1998.
250. Nelson PV, Carey WF, Morris CP: Population frequency of the arylsulfatase A pseudo-deficiency allele. *Hum Genet* **87**:87, 1991.
251. Ott R, Waye JS, Chang PL: Evolutionary origins of two tightly linked mutations in arylsulfatase-A pseudodeficiency. *Hum Genet* **101**:135, 1997.
252. Penzien JM, Kappler J, Herschkowitz N, Schuknecht B, Leinekugel P, Propping P, Tonnesen T, et al.: Compound heterozygosity for metachromatic leukodystrophy and arylsulfatase A pseudodeficiency alleles is not associated with progressive neurological disease. *Am J Hum Genet* **52**:557, 1993.
253. Lott IT, Dulaney JT, Milunsky A, Hoefnagel D, Moser HW: Apparent biochemical homozygosity in two obligatory heterozygotes for metachromatic leukodystrophy. *J Pediatr* **89**:438, 1976.
254. DuBois G, Harzer K, Baumann N: Very low arylsulfatase A and cerebroside sulfatase activities in leukocytes of healthy members of metachromatic leukodystrophy family. *Am J Hum Genet* **29**:191, 1977.
255. Herz B, Bach G: Arylsulfatase A in pseudo deficiency. *Hum Genet* **66**:147, 1984.
256. Shen N, Zhen-Guo L, Waye JS, Francis G, Chang PL: Complications in the genotypic molecular diagnosis of pseudo arylsulfatase A deficiency. *Am J Med Genet* **45**:631, 1993.
257. Chang PL, Davidson RG: Pseudo arylsulfatase A deficiency in healthy individuals: Genetic and biochemical relationship to metachromatic leukodystrophy. *Proc Natl Acad Sci USA* **80**:7323, 1983.

258. Propping P, Friedl W, Huschka M, Schlor KH, Reimer F, Lee-Vaupel M, Conzelmann E, et al.: The influence of low arylsulfatase A on neuropsychiatric morbidity: A large-scale screening in patients. *Hum Genet* **74**:244, 1986.
259. Schaap T, Zlotogora J, Elian E, Barak Y, Bach G: The genetics of the arylsulfatase A locus. *Am J Hum Genet* **33**:531, 1981.
260. Kappler J, Potter W, Gieselmann V, Kiessling W, Friedl W, Propping P: Phenotypic consequences of low arylsulfatase A genotypes, ASAp/ASAp and ASA−/ASAp: Does there exist an association with multiple sclerosis? *Dev Neurosci* **13**:228, 1991.
261. Mahon-Haft H, Stone RK, Johnson R, Shah S: Biochemical abnormalities of metachromatic leukodystrophy in an adult psychiatric population. *Am J Psychiatry* **138**:1372, 1981.
262. Shah SN, Johnson RC, Stone RK, Mahon-Haff H: Prevalence of partial cerebroside sulfate sulfatase (arylsulfatase A) defect in adult psychiatric patients. *Biol Psychiatry* **20**:50, 1985.
263. Heavey AM, Philpot MP, Fensom AH, Jackson M, Crammer JL: Leucocyte arylsulphatase A activity and subtypes of chronic schizophrenia. *Acta Psychiatr Scand* **82**:55, 1990.
264. Sangiorgi S, Ferlini A, Zanetti A, Mochi M: Reduced activity of arylsulfatase A and predisposition to neurological disorders: Analysis of 140 pediatric patients. *Am J Med Genet* **40**:365, 1991.
265. Naylor MW, Alessi NE: Pseudoarylsulfatase A deficiency in a psychiatrically disturbed adolescent. *J Am Acad Child Adolesc Psychiatry* **28**:444, 1989.
266. Kappler J, Watts RWE, Conzelmann E, Gibbs DA, Propping P, Gieselmann V: Low arylsulphatase A activity and choreoathetotic syndrome in three siblings: Differentiation of pseudodeficiency from metachromatic leukodystrophy. *Eur J Pediatr* **150**:287, 1991.
267. Sangiorgi S, Mochi M, Capellari S, Pietrobello MV, Marchello L, Montagna P: Movement disorders in arylsulfatase A pseudodeficiency, ASAPD. *Neurology* **42**(suppl 3):155, 1992.
268. Bach G, Neufeld EF: Synthesis and maturation of cross-reactive glycoprotein in fibroblasts deficient in arylsulfatase A activity. *Biochem Biophys Res Commun* **112**:198, 1983.
269. Fluharty AL, Meek WE, Kihara H: Pseudo arylsulfatase A deficiency: Evidence for a structurally altered enzyme. *Biochem Biophys Res Commun* **112**:191, 1983.
270. Kihara H, Meek WE, Fluharty AL: Attenuated activities and structural alterations of arylsulfatase A in tissues from subjects with pseudo arylsulfatase A deficiency. *Hum Genet* **74**:59, 1986.
271. Waheed A, Steckel F, Hasilik A, von Figura K: Two allelic forms of human arylsulfatase A with different numbers of asparagine-linked oligosaccharides. *Am J Hum Genet* **35**:228, 1983.
272. Hwu WL, Tsai LP, Wang WC, Chuang SC, Wang PJ, Wang TR: Arylsulfatase A pseudodeficiency in Chinese. *Hum Genet* **97**:148, 1996.
273. Ricketts MH, Goldman D, Long JC, Manowitz P: Arylsulfatase A pseudodeficiency-associated mutations: Population studies and identification of a novel haplotype. *Am J Med Genet* **67**:387, 1996.
274. Ameen M, Chang PL: Pseudo arylsulfatase A deficiency. Biosynthesis of an abnormal arylsulfatase A. *FEBS Lett* **219**:130, 1987.
275. Leistner S, Young E, Meancy C, Winchester B: Pseudodeficiency of arylsulfatase A: Strategy for clarification of genotype in families of subjects with low ASA activity and neurological symptoms. *J Inherit Metab Dis* **18**:710, 1995.
276. Polten A, Fluharty AL, Fluharty CB, Kappler J, von Figura K, Gieselmann V: Molecular basis of different forms of metachromatic leukodystrophy. *N Engl J Med* **324**:18, 1991.
277. Zlotogora J, Furman-Shaharabani Y, Harris A, Barth M L, von Figura K, Gieselmann V: A single origin for the most frequent mutation causing late infantile metachromatic leucodystrophy. *J Med Genet* **31**:672, 1994.
278. Berger J, Loschl B, Bernheimer H, Lugowska A, Tylki-Szymanska A, Gieselmann V, Molzer B: Occurrence, distribution, and phenotype of arylsulfatase A mutations in patients with metachromatic leukodystrophy. *Am J Med Genet* **69**:335, 1997.
279. Barth ML, Fensom A, Harris A: Prevalence of common mutations in the arylsulphatase A gene in metachromatic leukodystrophy patients diagnosed in Britain. *Hum Genet* **91**:73, 1993.
280. Harvey JS, Nelson PV, Carey WF, Robertson EF, Morris CP: An arylsulfatase A (ARSA) missense mutation (T274M) causing late-infantile metachromatic leukodystrophy. *Hum Mutat* **2**:261, 1993.
281. Pastor-Soler NM, Rafi MA, Hoffman JD, Hu D, Wenger DA: Metachromatic leukodystrophy in the Navajo Indian population: A splice site mutation in intron 4 of the arylsulfatase A gene. *Hum Mutat* **4**:199, 1994.
282. Pastor-Soler NM, Schertz EM, Rafi MA, de Gala G, Wenger DA: Metachromatic leukodystrophy among southern Alaskan Eskimos: Molecular and genetic studies. *J Inherit Metab Dis* **18**:326, 1995.
283. Zlotogora J, Bach G, Bösenberg C, Barak Y, von Figura K, Gieselmann V: Molecular basis of late infantile metachromatic leukodystrophy in the Habbanite Jews. *Hum Mutat* **5**:137, 1995.
284. Eto Y, Kawame H, Hasegawa Y, Ohashi T, Ida H, Tohoro T: Molecular characteristics in Japanese patients with lipidosis: Novel mutations in metachromatic leukodystrophy and Gaucher disease. *Mol Cell Biochem* **119**:179, 1993.
285. Draghia R, Letourner F, Drugan C, Manicom J, Blanchot C, Kahn A, Poenaru L, Caillaud C: Metachromatic leukodystrophy: Identification of the first deletion in exon 1 and of nine novel point mutations in the arylsulfatase A gene. *Hum Mutat* **9**:234, 1997.
286. Kreysing J, Bohne W, Bösenberg C, Marchesini S, Turpin JC, Baumann N, von Figura K, Gieselmann V: High residual arylsulfatase A (ARSA) activity in a patient with late-infantile metachromatic leukodystrophy. *Am J Hum Genet* **53**:339, 1993.
287. Luyten JA, Wenink PW, Steenbergen-Spanjers GC, Wevers RA, Ploos van Amstel HK, de Jong JG, van den Heuvel LP: Metachromatic leukodystrophy: A 12-bp deletion in exon 2 of the arylsulfatase A gene in a late infantile variant. *Hum Genet* **96**:357, 1995.
288. Harvey JS, unpublished.
289. Regis S, Filocamo M, Stroppiano M, Corsolini F, Caroli F, Gatti R: A 9-bp deletion (2320del9) on the background of the arylsulfatase A pseudodeficiency allele in a metachromatic leukodystrophy patient and in a patient with nonprogressive neurological symptoms. *Hum Genet* **102**:50, 1998.
290. Regis S, Carrozzo R, Filocamo M, Serra G, Mastropaolo C, Gatti R: An AT-deletion causing a frameshift in the arylsulfatase A gene of a late infantile metachromatic leukodystrophy patient. *Hum Genet* **96**:233, 1995.
291. Bohne W, von Figura K, Gieselmann V: An 11 bp deletion in the arylsulfatase A gene of a patient with late infantile metachromatic leukodystrophy. *Hum Genet* **87**:155, 1990.
292. Fluharty AL, Fluharty CB, Bohne W, von Figura K, Gieselmann V: Two new arylsulfatase A (ARSA) mutations in a juvenile metachromatic leukodystrophy (MLD) patient. *Am J Hum Genet* **49**:1340, 1991.
293. Hasegawa Y, Kawame H, Ida H, Ohashi T, Eto Y: Single exon mutation in arylsulfatase A gene has two effects: Loss of enzyme activity and aberrant splicing. *Hum Genet* **93**:415, 1994.
294. Tomatsu S, Fukuda S, Masue M, Sukegawa K, Fukao T, Yamagishi A, Hori T, et al.: Morquio disease: Isolation, characterization and expression of full-length cDNA for human N-acetylgalactosamine-6-sulfate sulfatase. *Biochem Biophys Res Commun* **181**:677, 1991.
295. von Figura K, Steckel F, Hasilik A: Juvenile and adult metachromatic leukodystrophy: Partial restoration of arylsulfatase A (cerebroside sulfatase) activity by inhibitors of thiol proteinases. *Proc Natl Acad Sci USA* **80**:6066, 1983.
296. von Figura K, Steckel F, Conary J, Hasilik A, Shaw E: Heterogeneity in late-onset metachromatic leukodystrophy. Effect of inhibitors of cysteine proteinases. *Am J Hum Genet* **39**:371, 1986.
297. Hess B, Kafert S, Heinisch U, Wenger DA, Zlotogora J, Gieselmann V: Characterization of two arylsulfatase A missense mutations D335V and T274M causing late infantile metachromatic leukodystrophy. *Hum Mutat* **7**:311, 1994.
298. Kappler J, Sommerlade HJ, von Figura K, Gieselmann V: Complex arylsulfatase A alleles causing metachromatic leukodystrophy. *Hum Mutat* **4**:119, 1994.
299. Gieselmann V, Fluharty A, Tonnesen T, von Figura K: Mutations in the arylsulfatase A pseudodeficiency allele causing metachromatic leukodystrophy. *Am J Hum Genet* **49**:407, 1991.
300. Barth ML, Fensom A, Harris A: Missense mutations in the arylsulphatase A genes of metachromatic leukodystrophy patients. *Hum Mol Genet* **2**:2117, 1993.
301. Kafert S, unpublished.
302. Berger J, Gmach M, Fae I, Molzer B, Bernheimer H: A new polymorphism of arylsulfatase A within the coding region. *Hum Genet* **98**:348, 1996.
303. Gieselmann V, Zlotogora J, Harris A, Wenger DA, Morris CP: Molecular genetics of metachromatic leukodystrophy. *Hum Mutat* **4**:233, 1994.
304. Porter MT, Fluharty A, Trammell J, Kihara H: A correlation of intracellular cerebroside sulfatase activity in fibroblasts with latency in metachromatic leukodystrophy. *Biochem Biophys Res Commun* **44**:660, 1971.

305. Porter MT, Fluharty AL, Harris SE, Kihara H: The accumulation of cerebroside sulfates by fibroblasts in culture from patients with late infantile metachromatic leukodystrophy. *Arch Biochem Biophys* **138**:646, 1970.
306. Conzelmann E, Sandhoff K: Partial enzyme deficiencies: Residual activities and the development of neurologic disorders. *Dev Neurosci* **6**:58, 1983/84.
307. Tylki-Szymanska A, Berger J, Loschl B, Lugowska A, Molzer B: Late juvenile metachromatic leukodystrophy (MLD) in three patients with a similar clinical course and identical mutation on one allele. *Clin Genet* **50**:287, 1996.
308. DuBois G, Turpin JC, Georges MC, Baumann N: Arylsulfatase A and B in leukocytes: A comparative statistical study of late infantile and juvenile forms of metachromatic leukodystrophy and controls. *Biomedicine* **33**:2, 1980.
309. Porter MT, Fluharty AL, Kihara H: Metachromatic leukodystrophy: Arylsulfatase-A deficiency in skin fibroblast cultures. *Proc Natl Acad Sci USA* **62**:887, 1969.
310. Beratis NG, Aron AM, Hirschhorn K: Metachromatic leukodystrophy: Detection in serum. *J Pediatr* **83**:824, 1973.
311. Thomas GH, Howell RR: Arylsulfatase A activity in human urine: Quantitative studies on patients with lysosomal disorders including metachromatic leukodystrophy. *Clin Chim Acta* **36**:99, 1972.
312. Hultberg B: Fluorometric assay of the arylsulphatases in human urine. *J Clin Chem Clin Biochem* **17**:795, 1979.
313. Christomanou H, Sandhoff K: A sensitive fluorescence assay for the simultaneous and separate determination of arylsulphatases A and B. *Clin Chim Acta* **79**:527, 1977.
314. Lee-Vaupel M, Conzelmann E: A simple chromogenic assay for arylsulfatase A. *Clin Chim Acta* **164**:171, 1987.
315. Humbel R: Rapid method for measuring arylsulfatase A and B in leucocytes as a diagnosis for sulfatidosis, mucosulfatidosis and mucopolysaccharidosis VI. *Clin Chim Acta* **68**:339, 1976.
316. Li ZG, Waye JS, Chang PL: Diagnosis of arylsulfatase A deficiency. *Am J Med Genet* **43**:976, 1992.
317. Chang PL, Rosa NE, Varey PA, Kihara H, Kolodny EH, Davidson RG: Diagnosis of pseudo-arylsulfatase A deficiency with electrophoretic techniques. *Pediatr Res* **18**:1042, 1984.
318. Raghavan SS, Gajewski A, Kolodny EH: Leukocyte sulfatidase for the reliable diagnosis of metachromatic leukodystrophy. *J Neurochem* **36**:724, 1981.
319. Baldinger S, Pierpont ME, Wenger DA: Pseudodeficiency of arylsulfatase A: A counseling dilemma. *Clin Genet* **31**:70, 1987.
320. Fluharty AL, Stevens RL, Kihara H: Cerebroside sulfate hydrolysis by fibroblasts from a metachromatic leukodystrophy parent with deficient arylsulfatase. *J Pediatr* **92**:782, 1978.
321. Gieselmann V: An assay for the rapid detection of the arylsulfatase A pseudodeficiency allele facilitates diagnosis and genetic counseling for metachromatic leukodystrophy. *Hum Genet* **86**:251, 1991.
322. Stevens RL, Fluharty AL, Kihara H, Kaback MM, Shapiro LJ, Marsh B, Sandhoff K, et al.: Cerebroside sulfatase activator deficiency induced metachromatic leukodystrophy. *Am J Hum Genet* **33**:900, 1981.
323. Bach G, Dagen A, Herz B, Gatt S: Diagnosis of arylsulfatase A deficiency in intact cultured cells using a fluorescent derivative of cerebroside sulfate. *Clin Genet* **31**:211, 1987.
324. Hreidarsson SJ, Thomas GH, Kihara H, Fluharty AL, Kolodny EH, Moser HW, Reynolds LW: Impaired cerebroside sulfate hydrolysis in fibroblasts of sibs with "pseudo" arylsulfatase A deficiency without metachromatic leukodystrophy. *Pediatr Res* **17**:701, 1983.
325. Marchesini S, Preti A, Aleo MF, Casella A, Dagan A, Gatt S: Synthesis, spectral properties and enzymatic hydrolysis of fluorescent derivatives of cerebroside sulfate containing long-wavelength-emission probes. *Chem Phys Lipids* **53**:165, 1990.
326. Viani P, Marchesini S, Cestaro B, Gatt S: Correlation of the dispersion state of pyrene cerebroside sulfate and its uptake and degradation by cultured cells. *Biochim Biophys Acta* **1002**:20, 1989.
327. Vogel A, Schwarzmann G, Sandhoff K: Glycosphingolipid specificity of the human sulfatide activator protein. *Eur J Biochem* **200**:591, 1991.
328. Natowicz MR, Prence EM, Chaturvedi P, Newburg DS: Urine sulfatides and the diagnosis of metachromatic leukodystrophy. *Clin Chem* **42**:232, 1996.
329. Philippart M, Sarlieve L, Meurant C, Mechler L: Human urinary sulfatides in patients with sulfatidosis (metachromatic leukodystrophy). *J Lipid Res* **12**:434, 1971.
330. Strasberg PMA, Warren I, Skomorowski M-A, Lowden JA: HPLC analysis of urinary sulfatide: An aid in the diagnosis of metachromatic leukodystrophy. *Clin Biochem* **18**:92, 1985.
331. Lugowska A, Tylki-Szymanska A, Berger J, Molzer B: Elevated sulfatide excretion in compound heterozygotes of metachromatic leukodystrophy and ASA-pseudodeficiency allele. *Clin Biochem* **30**:325, 1997.
332. Kihara H, Porter MT, Fluharty AL, Scott ML, De La Flor SD, Trammell JL, Nakamura RN: Metachromatic leukodystrophy: Ambiguity of heterozygote identification. *Am J Ment Defic* **77**:389, 1973.
333. Kihara H, Fluharty AL, Tsay KK, Bachman RP, Stephens JD, Won NG: Prenatal diagnosis of pseudo arylsulfatase A deficiency. *Prenat Diagn* **3**:29, 1983.
334. Desnick RJ, Schuette JL, Golbus MS, Jackson L, Lubs HA, Ledbetter DH, Mahoney MJ, et al.: First-trimester biochemical and molecular diagnoses using chorionic villi: High accuracy in the US collaborative study. *Prenat Diagn* **12**:357, 1992.
335. Borrensen A-L, Van Derhagen CB: Metachromatic leukodystrophy. II. Direct determination of arylsulphatase A activity in amniotic fluid. *Clin Genet* **4**:442.
336. Jaeken J, Casaer P, De Cock P, Francois B: Vigabatrin in GABA metabolism disorders. *Lancet* **1**:1074, 1989.
337. Kurlemann G, Palm DG: Vigabatrin in metachromatic leucodystrophy: Positive influence on spasticity. *Dev Med Child Neurol* **33**:182, 1991.
338. Krivit W, Shapiro EG: Bone marrow transplantation for storage diseases, in Desnick RJ (ed): *Treatment of Genetic Disease*. New York, Churchill Livingstone, p 203, 1991.
339. Krivit W, Shapiro E, Lockman L, Kennedy W, Dhuna A, Ringden O, Henslee-Downey J, Yeager A, Wenger D, Bayever E: Recommendations for treatment of metachromatic leukodystrophy by bone marrow transplantation based on a review of seven patients who have been engrafted for at least 1 year. COGENT II, in Hobbs JR (ed): *Correction of Certain Genetic Diseases by Transplantation*. London, Westminster Medical School Press, p 57, 1992.
340. Krivit W, Lockman LA, Watkins PA, Hirsch J, Shapiro EG: The future for treatment by bone marrow transplantation for adrenoleukodystrophy, metachromatic leukodystrophy, globoid cell leukodystrophy and Hurler syndrome. *J Inher Metabol Dis* **18**:398, 1995.
341. Krall WJ, Challita PM, Perlmutter LS, Skelton DC, Kohn DB: Cells expressing human glucocerebrosidase from a retroviral vector repopulate macrophages and central nervous system microglia after murine bone marrow transplantation. *Blood* **83**:2737, 1994.
342. Malm G, Ringden O, Winiarski J, Grondahl E, Uyebrant P, Eriksson J, Hakansson H, et al.: Clinical outcome in four children with metachromatic leukodystrophy treated by bone marrow transplantation. *Bone Marrow Transplant* **17**:1003, 1996.
343. Hoogerbrugge PM, Brouwer OF, Bordigoni P, Ringden O, Kapaun P, Ortega JJ, O'Meara A, et al.: Allogeneic bone marrow transplantation for lysosomal storage diseases. *Lancet* **345**:1398, 1995.
344. Shapiro EG, Lockman LA, Balthazor M, Krivit W: Neuropsychological outcomes of several storage diseases with and without bone marrow transplantation. *J Inher Metab Dis* **18**:413, 1995.
345. Pridjian G, Humbert J, Willis J, Shapira E: Presymptomatic late infantile metachromatic leukodystrophy treated with bone marrow transplantation. *J Pediatr* **125**:755, 1994.
346. Slavin S, Naparstek E, Ziegler M, Lewin A: Clinical application of intrauterine bone marrow transplantation for treatment of genetic diseases—feasibility studies. *Bone Marrow Transplant* **9**(suppl 1):189, 1992.
347. Kapaun P, Dittmann RW, Granitzny B, Eickhoff W, Wulbrand H, Neumaier-Probst E, Zander A, et al.: Slow progression of juvenile metachromatic leukodystrophy six years after bone marrow transplantation. *J Child Neurol* **14**:222, 1999.
348. Navarro C, Domínguez C, Fernández JM, Fachal C, Alvárez M: Case report: Four-year follow-up of bone-marrow transplantation in late juvenile metachromatic leukodystrophy. *J Inher Metab Dis* **18**:157, 1995.
349. Stillman AE, Krivit W, Shapiro E, Lockman L, Latchaw RE: Serial MR after bone marrow transplantation in two patients with metachromatic leukodystrophy. *Am J Neuroradiol* **15**:1929, 1994.
350. Guffon N, Souillet G, Maire I, Dorche C, Mathieu M, Guibaud P: Juvenile metachromatic leukodystrophy: Neurological outcome two years after bone marrow transplatation. *J Inher Metab Dis* **18**: 159, 1995.
351. Kidd D, Nelson J, Jones F, Dusoir H, Wallace I, McKinstry S, Patterson V: Long-term stabilization after bone marrow transplantation in juvenile metachromatic leukodystrophy. *Arch Neurol* **55**:98, 1998.

352. Rommerskirch W, Fluharty AL, Peters C, Von Figura K, Gieselmann V: Restoration of arylsulfatase A activity in human metachromatic leukodystrophy fibroblasts via retroviral-vector-mediated gene transfer. *Biochem J* **280**:459, 1991.
353. Rommerskirch W, von Figura K: Multiple sulfatase deficiency: Catalytically inactive sulfatases are expressed from retrovirally introduced sulfatase cDNAs. *Proc Natl Acad Sci USA* **89**:2561, 1992.
354. Matzner U, personal communication.
355. Hess B, Saftig, P, Hartmann D, Coenen R, Lüllmann-Rauch R, Goebel HH, Evers M, von Figura K, D'Hooge R, Nagels G, De Deyn P, Peters C, Gieselmann V: Phenotype of arylsulfatase A-deficient mice: Relationship to human metachromatic leukodystrophy. *Proc Natl Acad Sci USA* **93**:14821, 1996.
356. Lutschg J: Pathophysiological aspects of central and peripheral myelin lesions. *Neuropediatrics* **15**(suppl):24, 1984.
357. Rutsaert J, Menu R, Resibois A: Ultrastructure of sulfatide storage in normal and sulfatase-deficient fibroblasts in vitro. *Lab Invest* **29**:527, 1973.
358. Kappler J, von Figura K, Gieselmann V: Late onset metachromatic leukodystrophy: Molecular pathology in two siblings. *Ann Neurol* **31**:256, 1992.
359. Kondo R, Wakamatsu N, Yoshino H, Fukuhara N, Miyatake T, Tsuji S: Identification of a mutation in the arylsulfatase A gene of a patient with adult type metachromatic leukodystrophy. *Am J Hum Genet* **48**:971, 1991.
360. Honke K, Kobayashi T, Fujii T, Gasa S, Xu M, Takamaru Y, Kondo R, Tsuji S, Makita A: An adult-type metachromatic leukodystrophy caused by substitution of serine for glycine-122 in arylsulfatase A. *Hum Genet* **92**:451, 1993.
361. Tsuda T, Hasegawa Y, Eto Y: Two novel mutations in a Japanese patient with the late infantile form of metachromatic leukodystrophy. *Brain Dev* **18**:400, 1996.
362. Regis S, Filocoma M, Stroppiano M, Corsolini F, Gatti R: A T → C transition causing a Leu → Pro substitutions in a conserved region of the arylsulfatase A gene in a late infanite metachromatic leukodystrophy patient. *Clin Genet* **52**:65, 1997.
363. Coulter-Mackie MB, Gagnier L, Beis MJ, Applegarth DA, Cole DE, Gordon K, Ludman MD: Metachromatic leucodystrophy in three families from Nova Scotia, Canada: A recurring mutation in the arylsufatase A gene. *J Med Genet* **34**:493, 1997.
364. Cailaud C, Blanchot C, Akli S, Crosnier JM, Puech JP, Kahn A, Poenaru L: Molecular basis of late infantile metachromatic leukodystrophy in France. *ESGLD Workshop*, Delphi, Greece, Abstract, 1993.
365. Hasegawa Y, Kawame H, Eto Y: Mutations in the arylsulfatase A gene of Japanese patients with metachromatic leukodystrophy. *DNA Cell Biol* **12**:493, 1993.
366. Lissens W, Vervoort R, van Regemorter N, van Bogaert P, Freund M, Verellen-Dumoulin C, Seneca S, Liebers I: A D255*T substitution in the arylsulfatase A gene of two unrelated Belgian patients with late infantile metachromatic leukodystrophy. *J Inherit. Metab Dis* **19**: 782, 1996.
367. Coulter-Mackie M, Gagnier L: Two new polymorphisms in the arylsulfatase A gene and their haplotype associations with normal, metachromatic leukodystrophy and pseudodeficiency alleles. *Am J Med Genet* **73**:32, 1997.
368. Coulter-Mackie M, Gagnier L: Two novel mutations in the arylsulfatase A gene associated with juvenile (R390Q) and adult onset (H397Y) metachromatic leukodystrophy. *Hum Mutat* **1**:254, 1998.
369. Berger J, Molzer B, Gieselmann V, Bernheimer H: Simultaneous detection of the two most frequent metachromatic leukodystrophy mutations. *Hum Genet* **92**:421 (1993).
370. Harvey JD, Carey WF, Nelson PV, Morris CP: Metachromatic leukodystrophy: A nonsense mutation (Q486X) in the arylsulfatase A gene. *Hum Mol Genet* **3**:207, 1994.
371. Kafert S, Heinisch U, Zlotogora J, Gieselmann V: A missense mutation P136L in the arylsulfatase A gene causes instability and loss of activity of the mutant enzyme. *Hum Genet* **95**:201, 1995.
372. Barth ML, Fensom A, Harris A: Identification of seven novel mutations associated with metachromatic leukodystrophy. *Hum Mutat* **6**: 170, 1995.

CHAPTER 149

Multiple Sulfatase Deficiency and the Nature of the Sulfatase Family

John J. Hopwood ▪ Andrea Ballabio

1. **Multiple sulfatase deficiency (MSD) is a rare autosomal recessive disorder with a prevalence of about 1 in 1.4 million births, characterized by deficiencies in all 12 known sulfatases and leading to a clinical presentation that generally resembles late infantile metachromatic leukodystrophy. However, like those of all lysosomal storage disorders, the clinical presentation and progression of MSD are clinically heterogeneous.**
2. **In MSD all sulfatase polypeptides have reduced catalytic activities toward their natural substrates. This reduced activity is caused by a deficiency in a modification system that generates an α-formylglycine residue by the oxidation of the thiol group of an active site cysteine conserved in all members of the mammalian sulfatase family.**
3. **This novel protein modification occurs before the sulfatase polypeptide is folded to a native structure and at a late stage of or after cotranslational protein translocation into the endoplasmic reticulum.**
4. **The aldehyde group of the α-formylglycine residue may accept sulfate during sulfate ester cleavage, leading to formation of a covalently sulfated enzyme complex.**
5. **The active sites of all sulfatases probably have four conserved amino acid residues involved in metal ion coordination and at least five residues involved in the catalytic mechanism.**
6. **The active sites of sulfatases and of alkaline phosphatase share remarkable structural homology.**
7. **Diagnosis of MSD can be made biochemically from the characteristic pattern of sulfatase deficiencies observed in various cell types. Affected individuals have abnormal urinary oligosaccharide, mucopolysaccharide, and glycopeptide profiles. Prenatal diagnosis is reliable, and carrier detection may be possible.**
8. **There is no definitive treatment for patients with MSD.**

A list of standard abbreviations is located immediately preceding the index in each volume. Additional abbreviations used in this chapter include: ASA = arylsulfatase A, galactose-3-sulfatase, sulfatidase; ASB = arylsulfatase B, N-acetylgalactosamine-4-sulfatase; ASC = arylsulfatase C, steroid sulfatase; ASD = arylsulfatase D; ASE = arylsulfatase E; ASF = arylsulfatase F; GlN6S = glucosamine-6-sulfatase; MLD = metachromatic leukodystrophy; MPS = mucopolysaccharidosis; MSD = multiple sulfatase deficiency.

INTRODUCTION

The existence of sulfatases has been known for almost 90 years. The sulfatases catalyze the hydrolysis of sulfate esters such as O-sulfates and N-sulfates.

$$\text{R-OSO}_3^- + \text{H}_2\text{O} \rightarrow \text{R-OH} + \text{H}^+ + \text{SO}_4^{2-}$$
$$\text{R-NHSO}_3^- + \text{H}_2\text{O} \rightarrow \text{R-NH}_3^+ + \text{SO}_4^{2-}$$

Their importance in modern medicine and biochemistry has been appreciated over the past 40 years, when the association of deficiencies in many of the sulfatases with a number of clinical syndromes was discovered.

It is now recognized that the hydrolysis of sulfate esters requires the action of a family of sulfatase enzymes. These sulfatases share structure and function characteristics to achieve cleavage of O- and N-linked sulfate esters.[1] In fact, sulfatases also share structural and functional characteristics with phosphatases.[2] Sulfate ester substrates include complex molecules such as sulfated glycosaminoglycans, glycolipids, glycopeptides, and hydroxysteroids. At least 12 different sulfatases are needed for the hydrolysis of these complex substrates. Sulfatases appear to act on small molecules or at the nonreducing, or polar, end of the sulfated macromolecular compounds. A number of different cellular locations are involved in the hydrolysis of these substrates. Eight different sulfatases act in the lysosome to desulfate glycosaminoglycans, glycolipids, and glycopeptides, whereas four different sulfatases act on sulfated hydroxysteroids and other, as yet unknown, substrates in neutral cellular compartments, including microsomes, endoplasmic reticulum, and the Golgi network.

Recent reports have identified the likely locations and natures of the active sites of all sulfatases. A rare inherited disorder in which activity of all sulfatases is deficient has been shown to result from a failure to post-translationally convert a specific cysteine residue to an alpha-formylglycine residue (reviewed by von Figura et al.;[3] also see Chap. 148).

A complex mixture of sulfate ester substrates is found to accumulate in this disorder. A number of genetic disorders also result from deficiency of the activity of a specific sulfatase and accumulate sulfate ester substrates specific to that sulfatase. One of these, metachromatic leukodystrophy (MLD) (see Chap. 148), results from a deficiency of galactose-3-sulfatase (arylsulfatase A [ASA]) and the accumulation of cerebroside-3-sulfate (sulfatide, a glycolipid containing a polar head galactose-3-sulfate residue).

Maroteaux-Lamy syndrome (mucopolysaccharidosis type VI [MPS VI]) (see Chap. 136) results from a deficiency of N-acetylgalactosamine-4-sulfatase (arylsulfatase B [ASB]) and the accumulation of the glycosaminoglycans dermatan sulfate and chondroitin sulfate. In their catalytic reactions, both ASA and ASB are relatively nonspecific and cleave a wide range of synthetic substrates. However, in vivo, both of these enzymes are highly specific for their natural substrates. The physiological substrate for ASA is the "activator (saposin B) solubilized" cerebroside-3-sulfate; those for ASB are the 4-sulfated nonreducing terminals of dermatan sulfate and chondroitin-4-sulfate glycosaminoglycan chains.

A deficiency in hydrolytic function or cellular location of these sulfatases may lead to a clinical phenotype ranging from extremely severe and life threatening with an early death to reduced quality of life and life expectancy. All of these disorders result from the primary storage of the complex sulfate ester substrate, often causing secondary storage of other compounds that may also have toxic effects on cellular function.

In this chapter, the condition known as multiple sulfatase deficiency (MSD) and the general properties of the family of sulfatases will be reviewed.

MULTIPLE SULFATASE DEFICIENCY CLINICAL PHENOTYPE AND DIAGNOSIS

Clinical

Austin described the first case of MSD in two siblings in 1963 and 1965.[4,5] Since then a number of MSD patients have been described by many different investigators.[6] A complex clinical phenotype is often observed in MSD patients. The clinical phenotype may include features characteristic of single sulfatase deficiencies, such as rapid neurologic deterioration and developmental delay. The clinical phenotype of MSD generally resembles late infantile MLD. Deficiencies of other sulfatases besides ASA lead to storage of other substrates and other clinical phenotypes, such as those consistent with attenuated mucopolysaccharidoses, for example: low-level dysostosis multiplex, coarse facies, stiff joints, and deafness. Reduced arylsulfatase C (ASC) levels may lead to ichthyosis. Two boys presented at 1 year of age with developmental delay from birth, mildly coarse facial features, and hepatomegaly suggestive of a mucopolysaccharidosis (MPS), particularly MPS type II (MPS II), but were shown to have MSD. These findings suggest that MSD should be considered as a possible diagnosis in young patients with MPS symptoms.[7] One patient presented at birth with dysmorphic features, hydrocephalus, chondrocalcificans congenita, heart abnormalities, excessive mucopolysacchariduria, and a profound deficiency in a number of sulfatases in plasma, leukocytes, and cultured skin fibroblasts.[8]

Early development may be normal following an often rapid clinical progression, with neurodegeneration leading to early death within a few years of clinical onset.

The prevalence of MSD in Australia is 1 in 1.4 million births, compared to 1 in 92,000 and 1 in 235,000 for MLD and MPS VI, respectively.[9]

Biochemical Diagnosis

Biochemical confirmation of a diagnosis of MSD is made by measuring the pattern of sulfatase activities in leukocytes, plasma, and cultured fibroblasts from individual patients. In general there is reduced arylsulfatase A, B, and C activity together with reduced sulfamidase and iduronate-2-sulfatase levels. Leukocytes display granulation abnormalities. Patients may be classified according to the relative levels of residual sulfatase activity in cultured skin fibroblasts. Generally, the lower these levels, the more severe the clinical phenotype.

Heterozygotes have been reported to have intermediate sulfatase levels in cultured skin fibroblasts compared with affected and unaffected controls.[10]

Prenatal diagnosis of MSD has been made following amniocentesis, using the pattern of reduced sulfatase activities in cultured amniotic cells as a criterion for diagnosis. This method is reliable but can give only a late second-trimester diagnosis. A prenatal diagnosis in the first trimester was achieved by demonstrating markedly reduced activities of arylsulfatases and sulfamidase in direct assay of chorionic villi. The diagnosis was confirmed by assay of cultured cells derived from villi and fetal skin.[11]

Treatment

There is no known treatment for MSD, but a number of clinical trials are planned to evaluate the efficacy of enzyme replacement therapy in patients with deficient activity of individual sulfatases. There has been considerable success with the application of enzyme replacement therapy for MPS VI cats treated from birth with weekly infusions of recombinant human N-acetylgalactosamine-4-sulfatase.[12,13,14] A number of sulfatases have been expressed and the resultant recombinant enzyme purified and characterized. These include:

Iduronate-2-sulfatase,[15] involved in MPS II
Sulfamidase,[16] involved in MPS IIIA
Glucosamine-6-sulfatase,[17] involved in MPS IIID
N-acetylgalactosamine-6-sulfatase,[18] involved in MPS IVA
N-acetylgalactosamine-4-sulfatase,[19] involved in MPS VI

These studies have encouraged activities to evaluate the efficacy of enzyme replacement therapies, particularly in patients in whom clinical signs from central nervous system pathology are not present. These conditions include all MPS IVA and VI patients, and attenuated MPS II patients. All MPS IIIA and IIID patients have or will develop clinical signs generated from storage pathology present in the central nervous system and would therefore be unlikely to respond to therapy relying on the passage of the therapeutic enzyme through the blood-brain barrier into the brain.

THE SULFATASE FAMILY

Twelve sulfatases, with exquisite substrate structure specificities, have been characterized in recent times. Most of these individual sulfatases have been characterized as a result of the linking of a clinical condition to a deficiency of function of one of these enzymes. These are listed in Table 149-1. Ten sulfatases have had their genes isolated and characterized. Many mutations causing sulfatase dysfunction and leading to clinical problems have been defined. The clinical nature and molecular genetic detail for each sulfatase deficiency have been described (see Chaps. 136, 148, 166).

Except for the membrane-spanning region present in ASC, ASD, ASE, and ASF, sulfatases generally have similar polypeptide lengths but different sizes as a result of different levels of glycosylation.

Research into the biochemical cause of MSD has identified a novel modification that appears to be common to all sulfatases.[3] This modification causes the conversion of a conservative cysteine to an α-formylglycine residue (Fig. 149-1).

STRUCTURE AND FUNCTION OF SULFATASES

Molecular Structure

The crystal structures of ASB and ASA were determined independently in x-ray diffraction studies of crystals of each enzyme at resolutions of 2.5 and 2.1 Å, respectively.[2,20] A comparison of the overall shapes of ASA and ASB shows that they are similar and consist of two domains. One domain has a larger N-terminal region, containing a large central β-sheet flanked by α-helices, and a smaller second C-terminal domain, consisting of a small antiparallel β-sheet with a tightly packed associated

Table 149-1 **The Sulfatase Gene Family**

Enzyme	Subcellular Localization	Natural Substrate	Chromosomal Localization	Disease
I2S	Lysosome	DS/HS	Xq27–28	MPS II
GINS	Lysosome	HS	17q25.3	MPS IIIA
GIN6S	Lysosome	HS	12q14	MPS IIID
GalN6S	Lysosome	CS/KS	16q24	MPS IVA
ASB	Lysosome	DS	5q13–q14	MPS VI
GAS	Lysosome?	HS?	unknown	unknown
GIN3S	Lysosome?	HS?	unknown	unknown
ASA	Lysosome	sulfatide	22q13	MLD
ASC	Microsomes	sulfated steroids	Xp22.3	XLI
ASD	ER	unknown	Xp22.3	unknown
ASE	Golgi network	unknown	Xp22.3	CP
ASF	ER	unknown	Xp22.3	unknown

Abbreviations: I2S = iduronate-2-sulfatase; GINS = sulfamidase; GIN6S = glucosamine-6-sulfatase; Gal6S = N-acetylgalactosamine-6-sulfatase; ASB = arylsulfatase B, N-acetylgalactosamine-4-sulfatase; GAS = glucuronate-2-sulfatase; GIN3S = glucosamine-3-sulfatase; ASA = arylsulfatase A, galactose-3-sulfatase, sulfatidase; ASC = arylsulfatase C, steroid sulfatase; ASD = arylsulfatase D; ASE = arylsulfatase E; ASF = arylsulfatase F; DS = dermatan sulfate; HS = heparan sulfate; CS = chondroitin sulfate; KS = keratan sulfate; MPS = mucopolysaccharidosis; MLD = metachromatic leukodystrophy; XLI = X-linked ichthyosis; CP = chondrodysplasia punctata.

long C-terminal α-helix. The smaller domain ends in a long loop that wraps around the length of the entire molecule. Residues involved in the octamerization of ASA are all located in the C-terminal domain. ASA and ASB share amino acid sequence homology, with nearly one-third showing sequence identity and nearly half differing only by conservative changes. The N-terminal domains show a significantly higher degree of homology than the C-terminal domains. Most secondary structural elements occupy identical positions in ASA and ASB, with superimposable protein core regions and with some variation in the flexible loop regions.

Active Site

Purification of the active and inactive sulfatases expressed in normal control and multiple sulfatase deficiency cells suggests that the latter are deficient in a factor required for the post-translational modification of all sulfatases to convert them to catalytically active enzymes (Fig. 149-1). In a most elegant study, Schmidt et al.[21] were able to show that purified ASA, when digested with trypsin, produced a peptide mixture containing a peptide fragment that included residues 59 to 73 with a 2-amino-3-oxopropanoic acid (α-formylglycine) at position 69, where a cysteine residue was predicted from the ASA genetic code. The presence of this aldehyde group in place of a cysteine blocked the sequencing from proceeding through this tryptic fragment. Reduction of this tryptic fragment with sodium borohydride produced a serine at position 69 and allowed Edman sequencing to proceed. The aldehyde at residue 69 of the intact polypeptide was also reactive with a variety of compounds, such as p-nitroaniline, dinitrophenylhydrazide, and glycerol, to form a Schiff base, a hydrazone, and semiacetal products, respectively.

The active sites of sulfatases have been characterized within the crystal structures of the two sulfatases so far crystallized.[2,20] A number of structural similarities have been observed between ASA and ASB. These include a divalent metal ion located at the base of a substrate-binding pocket and a modified active site cysteine stabilized through a number of hydrogen bonds from highly conserved residues (Table 149-2). The conserved residues in the substrate-binding pocket appear to have identical functions in the catalytic mechanisms involving the generation of intermediate enzyme-sulfate ester and substrate complex reactions.

The critical residues involved in hydrogen-bonding reactions in the active site (Fig. 149-2) are conserved in most sulfatases (Tables 149-2, 149-3). This supports the common role of these residues to form a structurally similar active site pocket in all of the sulfatases, despite the different substrate structures they hydrolyze. This also means that all of these sulfatases use a common catalytic mechanism to hydrolyze their structurally different substrates.

However, there are some differences in these active site residues that may be informative regarding the evolution of the sulfatase family of proteins. For example, all of the sulfatases, including bacterial sulfatases, have conserved the double aspartic acid residues (e.g., Asp53 and Asp54 in ASB, Fig. 149-2) that are involved in the coordination of the metal ion. The other residues involved in metal ion coordination, the aspartic acid and asparagine doublet (e.g. Asp300 and Asn301 in ASB, Fig. 149-2), show differences between sulfatases. Whereas the aspartic acid

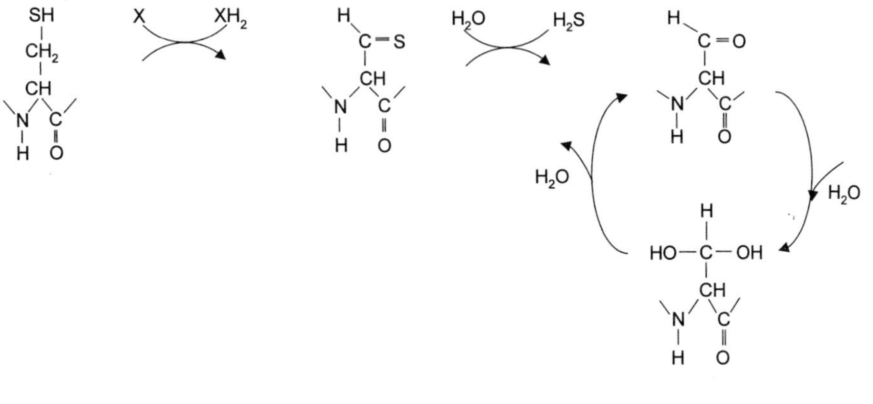

Fig. 149-1 Proposed scheme for the conversion of the active site cysteine to α-formylglycine. In the first step, the thiol group of cysteine is oxidized to a thioaldehyde using an acceptor molecule to remove hydrogen. The next step has the thioaldehyde releasing hydrogen sulfide; the third step is the hydration of the aldehyde.

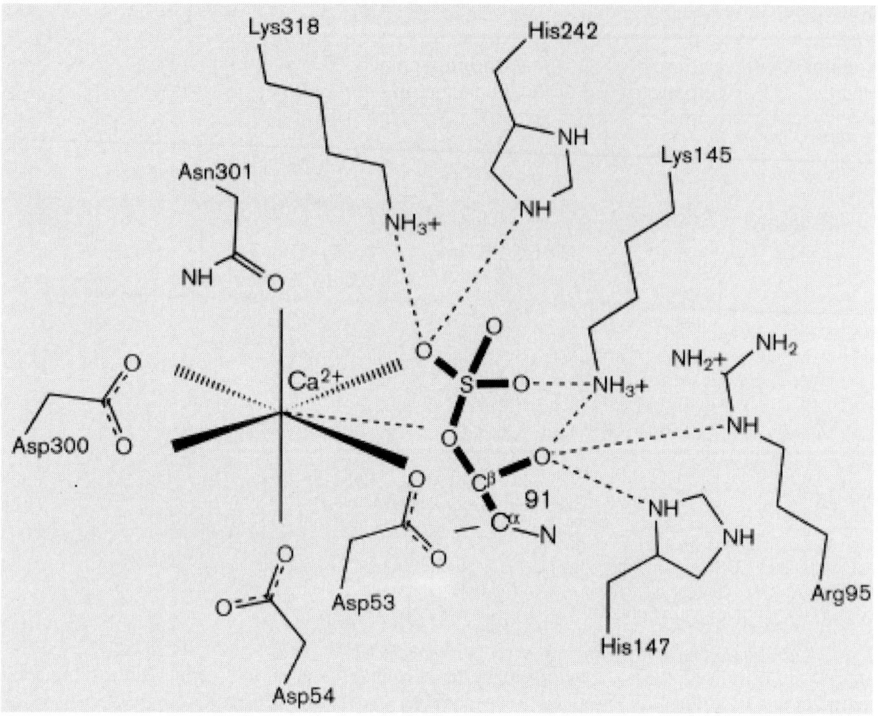

Fig. 149-2 Sketch view of catalytic site of ASB (adapted from Bond et al.[2]) showing hydrogen-bonded interactions (dashed lines) that stabilize the sulfate ester. The seven-coordinate-metal ion is on the left. A salt-bridge interaction between Lys145 and the O (carboxyl) atom of Asp53, which is not coordinated to the metal ion, and a number of charges and double bonds are omitted from the figure for clarity.

(Asp300 in ASB) is conserved in all mammalian sulfatases and alkaline phosphatase, the asparagine (Asn301 in ASB) is present in all lysosomal sulfatases except iduronate-2-sulfatase, in which this residue is a histidine (Table 149-3, H335). ASC has a glutamine in place of the asparagine, suggesting that this residue in this neutral sulfatase is probably also involved in metal ion coordination.

Variation of the amino acid in the metal ligand coordination pocket may reflect ability of a specific sulfatase to bind different metal ions, for example, calcium or magnesium. Like iduronate-2-sulfatase, ASD, ASE, and alkaline phosphatase have a histidine residue in place of the asparagine residue 301 (see Fig. 149-2). This suggests that some drift has been possible during evolution of these sulfatases that has maintained the general catalytic mechanism. However, major differences amongst present day mammalian sulfatases, such as substrate specificity, are likely to have arisen during evolution by a process of mutation and selection. The arginine residue that is always 4 residues toward the C-terminus of all sulfatases is similarly placed in relation to the essential serine residue in alkaline phosphatase and *Klebsiella pneumoniae* sulfatase. The other doublet of residues, lysine 145 and histidine 147 (Fig. 149-2), appears to have a role in the catalytic mechanism, possibly that of stabilizing the α-formylglycine residue. The histidine-histidine pair (ASB, residues 147 and 242) may be involved in the nucleophile and proton donor in the catalytic mechanism, whereas the two lysines (ASB, residues 145 and 318) are probably involved as proton-tunneling or hydrogen-bonded bases assisting the protonation and deprotonation of the histidine residues (ASB, residues 147 and 242) in the active site. The lysine-histidine doublet (ASB, residues 145 and 147) is conserved in all of the sulfatases listed in Table 149-3 except where the histidine residue (ASB, residue 125) is replaced with a leucine in GlN6S or the histidine is three (ASB, asparagine 301 replaced with histidine), instead of the usual two, amino acid residues from the lysine in iduronate-2-sulfatase.

Table 149-2 Active Site Residues Conserved Between ASA and ASB

Residue	Position: ASA	Position: ASB	Proposed Function
Aspartic acid	29	53	metal coordination
Aspartic acid	30	54	metal coordination
Aspartic acid	281	300	metal coordination
Asparagine	282	301	metal coordination
Cysteine	69	91	α-formylglycine
Arginine	73	95	catalytic mechanism
Lysine	123	145	catalytic mechanism
Histidine	125	147	catalytic mechanism
Histidine	229	242	catalytic mechanism
Lysine	302	318	catalytic mechanism

The functions of the conserved active site amino acid residues in ASA and listed in Tables 149-2 and 149-3 were systematically analyzed.[22] In this study, each residue was conservatively substituted and the K_m, V_{max}, and pH optimum of the mutant polypeptide toward an artificial substrate determined. Results indicated that each of the eight residues listed (Tables 149-2, 149-3) has a critical function for catalytic activity. Lysine 123 and 302 in ASA may be involved in substrate binding, since substitution of alanine for these residues leads to more than a tenfold increase in the K_m.[22] These two lysine residues may bind the sulfate group of the sulfatide substrate. It is likely that substitutions for the equivalent residues in other sulfatases will similarly influence their catalytic properties.

Multiple Sulfatase Factor

Thus far, as all sulfatases function in the secretory pathway of eukaryotic cells (Table 149-1), it is likely that the activation step occurs early in the polypeptide transcription and before complete folding to a native structure has been completed. Dierks et al. reported that an in vitro translation system supplemented with import-competent microsomes and a transcript coding for residues 19 to 200 of ASA and the signal peptide of preprolactin was able to convert a significant proportion of cysteine 69 into 2-amino-3-oxopropanoic acid (α-formylglycine).[23] In the absence of microsomes, cysteine 69 was not converted to the aldehyde. They were able to show that a linear sequence of 16 amino acids, from residues 65 to 80, was all that was needed for the direct oxidation of cysteine 69 in the microsome system, suggesting that this

Table 149-3 Comparison of Active Site Residues Between Sulfatases/Alkaline Phosphatase

	Amino Acid Position in Various Sulfatases										
Residue	**ASA**	**ASB**	**GIN6S**	**ASC**	**Gal6S**	**I2S**	**GINS**	**ASD**	**ASE**	**Kleb**	**ALK**
D	29	53	55	35	39	45	31	49	46	55	D
D	30	54	56	36	40	46	32	50	47	56	G
D	281	300	326	342	288	334	273	356	353		D
N	282	301	327	343Q	289	335H	274	357H	354H		H
C	69	91	91	75	79	84	70	89	86	72S	S
R	73	95	95	79	83	88	74	93	90	76	A
K	123	145	149	134	140	135	123	148	145		
H	125	147	151L	136	142	138	125	150	147		
H	229	242	H	H	236	P/A	P/A	305	301		D
K	302	318	305	K	267	P/A	303	335	332		

Abbreviations: P/A = poor alignment; Kleb = *Klebsiella pneumoniae* sulfatase; ALK = alkaline phosphatase; I2S = iduronate-2-sulfatase; GINS = sulfamidase; GIN6S = glucosamine-6-sulfatase; Gal6S = N-acetylgalactosamine-6-sulfatase; ASB = arylsulfatase B, N-acetylgalactosamine-4-sulfatase; ASA = arylsulfatase A, galactose-3-sulfatase, sulfatidase; ASC = arylsulfatase C, steroid sulfatase; ASD = arylsulfatase D; ASE = arylsulfatase E.

modification occurs in the endoplasmic reticulum before protein folding is complete.

Dierks et al. investigated translation steps that may influence the oxidation of cysteine 69 in ASA.[23,24] In translation intermediates produced in translocation-arrested systems, N-glycosylation at position 87 was able to proceed without modification of the cysteine 69 residue. Oxidation of cysteine 69 occurred only after the nascent polypeptide was released and chased through the microsomal system following the addition of puromycin to the incubation mixture. This finding supports a mechanism of translation in which the ASA polypeptide needs to be released from the ribosome before cysteine 69 is oxidized.

A number of amino acid residues within this ASA fragment are conserved between eukaryotic sulfatases. Although some of these conserved residues are candidates for recognition by the enzyme(s) involved in the oxidation of sulfatases, it is also likely that they are involved in overall function of the active site of sulfatases (see above). Substitution of several conserved residues in this ASA peptide region impaired (but did not completely eliminate) the oxidation of the cysteine 69 residue or reduced sulfatase activity without influencing the level of cysteine 69 modification. The amino acid sequence in residues adjacent to cysteine 69 is reported not to be essential in the oxidation reaction catalyzed by the multiple sulfatase factor.[25] In this study it was shown that within residues 68 to 86 of ASA, flanking the cysteine residue 69, there were no essential residues other than the cysteine required for the important active site post-translation oxidation reaction. In fact, substitution of the highly conserved leucine 68, proline 71, and alanine 74 within the heptapeptide LCTPSRA reduced the α-formylglycine production only to about 30–50 percent of that of the wild-type sequence.

The modification of cysteine to α-formylglycine in ASA is directed by the short linear sequence CTPSR motif containing the cysteine residue to be modified.[26] Systematic substitution of these residues demonstrated that cysteine, proline, and arginine are key residues within the motif. The serine and threonine residues could be individually but not simultaneously substituted without interfering with the conversion of cysteine to α-formylglycine. They further demonstrated that seven additional residues, AALLTGR, directly following the CTPSR motif in ASA, may have an auxiliary function in presenting the cysteine residue to the multiple sulfatase factor. An important point is that the LTGR sequence is conserved in most mammalian sulfatases.

A sequence very similar to the CTPSA motif is also present in bacterial sulfatases, e.g., *Klebsiella pneumoniae* (Table 149-3). However, there is a serine in place of the essential cysteine that is modified to α-formylglycine in human arylsulfatases. Miech et al. have reported that the α-formylglycine residue is formed from this serine residue in the *Klebsiella pneumoniae* sulfatase.[27] Interestingly, when the human sulfatase essential cysteine is replaced with a serine residue, these sulfatases are inactive,[23,28] suggesting the existence of both cysteine-specific and serine-specific sulfatase-modifying enzymes.

Metal-Binding Site

The metal coordination sites are conserved between ASA and ASB (Table 149-2). However, the metal ion reported in ASA is Mg^{2+} and that in ASB Ca^{2+}. In ASA the Mg^{2+} ion is reported to be coordinated through six ligands, whereas ASB has a Ca^{2+} coordinated through seven ligands. The metal ions in both structures were chosen based on refinement of crystallographic data, and there is some uncertainty about whether the modeled metal ion has been introduced or exchanged for the naturally occurring metal ion during the purification of the sulfatase. The ASA used in the crystallographic studies was subjected to an immune purification step that used molar concentrations of Mg^{2+}. Similarly, it cannot be assumed for ASB that the ion is Ca^{2+} in vivo, as the purification and crystallization of the enzyme may have caused the endogenous ion to be replaced.

Four amino acid residues that are conserved between sulfatases are involved in the coordination of the metal ion in the active site. The three aspartic acid residues (53, 54, and 300; see Fig. 149-2) in this group are present in all sulfatases. The other residue, an asparagine in Fig. 149-2, can be replaced with a glutamine in ASC and with a histidine in iduronate-2-sulfatase, ASD, ASE, and alkaline phosphatase (Table 149-3). Aspartic acid residues are typically found in the setting of chelation with calcium ions, whereas amino groups are more likely to favor chelation with magnesium ions. The metal ion probably acts as a Lewis acid in the catalytic mechanism, helping to stabilize the negative charge on the coordinated oxygen atom from the sulfate ion (Fig. 149-2).

Enzyme Mechanism

Based on the high degree of structural similarity of their active sites, the reaction mechanisms of ASA and ASB appear to share some properties with each other and with alkaline phosphatase.[2,20] The reaction mechanism of ASB as described has the covalently linked sulfate being released by hydrolysis involving a nucleophilic attack, possibly by water, as has been proposed for alkaline phosphatase,[2,29] or released as part of an equilibrium reaction with the free aldehyde form. The nonreducing end 4-sulfate ester of the glycosaminoglycan substrate binds to the enzyme to form a covalent ester with the α-formylglycine residue at position 91 (Fig. 149-3*A*). This intermediate may then undergo hydrolysis following a nucleophilic attack to release the glycosaminoglycan and leaving the sulfate bound to the enzyme (Fig. 149-3*A*).

The precise order of addition and removal of reactants and products operating between the α-formylglycine residue in the

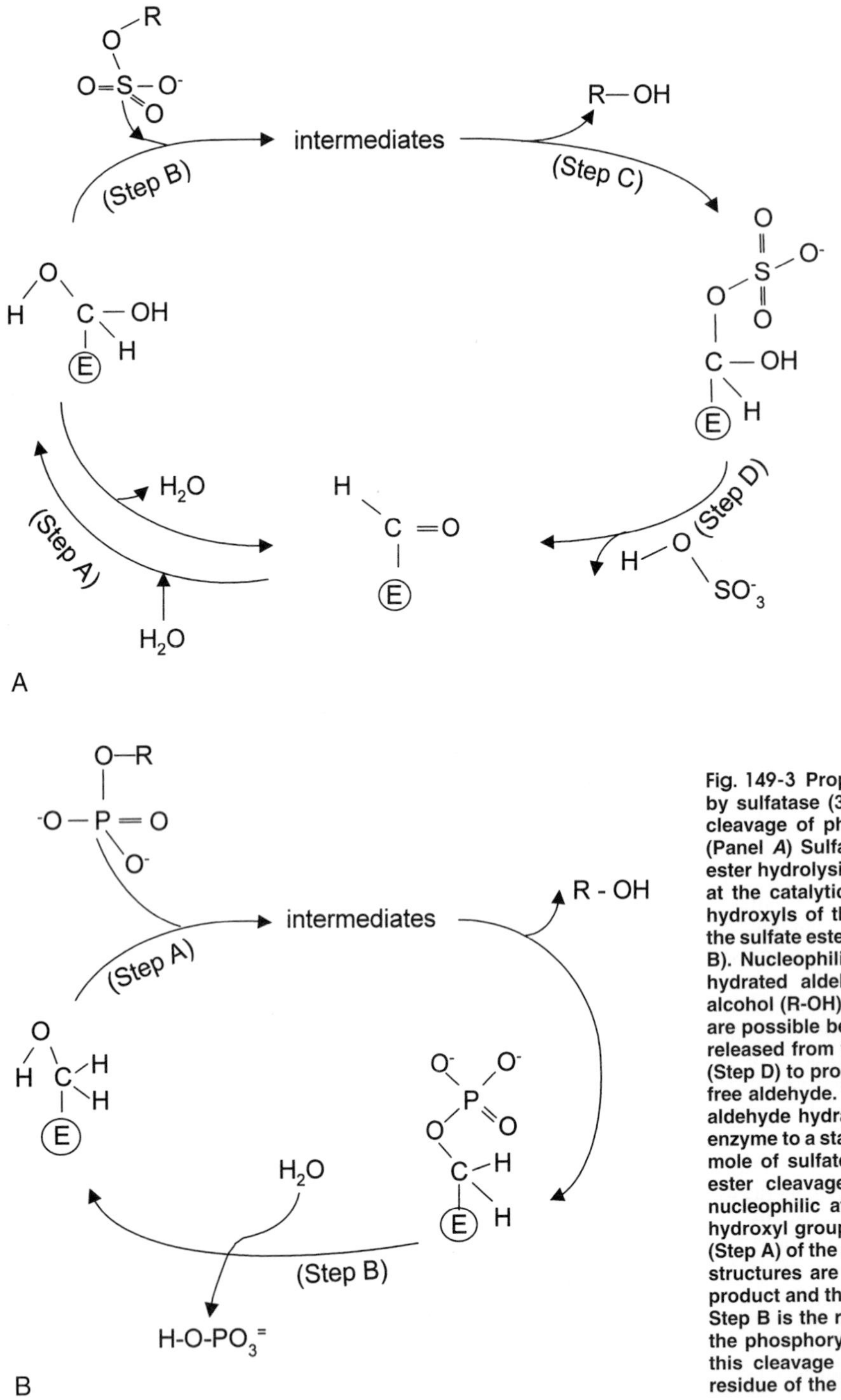

Fig. 149-3 **Proposed scheme for the cleavage of sulfate esters by sulfatase (3*A*) compared with a scheme proposed for the cleavage of phosphate esters by alkaline phosphatase (3*B*). (Panel *A*) Sulfate ester cleavage. In the cycle shown, sulfate ester hydrolysis begins with formation of an aldehyde hydrate at the catalytic α-formylglycine residue (Step A). One of the hydroxyls of the aldehyde hydrate then attacks the sulfur of the sulfate ester to form an enzyme-sulfate ester complex (Step B). Nucleophilic attack of one of the hydroxyl groups of the hydrated aldehyde eventually leads to the release of the alcohol (R-OH) in Step C. A number of intermediate structures are possible between Steps B and C. The sulfate ester is then released from the sulfated enzyme by an elimination reaction (Step D) to produce an inorganic sulfate and an enzyme with a free aldehyde. The free aldehyde is then hydrated to yield the aldehyde hydrate form of the sulfatase (Step A) to return the enzyme to a state in which it is ready to interact in Step B with a mole of sulfate ester to be hydrolyzed. (Panel *B*) Phosphate ester cleavage. Phosphate ester hydrolysis begins with a nucleophilic attack of the phosphate ester substrate by the hydroxyl group of the catalytic serine residue and the release (Step A) of the alcohol (R-OH). Again, a number of intermediate structures are possible to achieve the release of the alcohol product and the phosphate intermediate bound to the enzyme. Step B is the release of inorganic phosphate by hydrolysis of the phosphorylated enzyme with water. The other product of this cleavage reaction is the regenerated active site serine residue of the phosphatase.**

sulfatase, the sulfate ester substrate, and water has not been established.

Figure 149-3*B* shows the proposed scheme for hydrolysis of phosphate esters by alkaline phosphatase. Phosphate ester cleavage with nucleophilic attack of the phosphate by the hydroxyl group of the essential serine leads to the replacement of the substrate alcohol and the release of phosphate from the phosphorylated enzyme by hydrolysis to cleave the phosphate ester bond and regenerate the essential serine hydroxyl group on the enzyme.

SULFATASE GENES AND EVOLUTION OF A FAMILY OF GENES

Some amino acid sequence homology has been found for sulfatases from all eukaryotes. This homology is over the full length of the sequence but is highest in the N-terminal third. Amino acid sequence conservation suggests that sulfatases are members of an evolutionarily conserved gene family sharing a common ancestor. This ancestral gene, which has probably undergone duplication events during evolution, may be related to those currently present in lower eukaryotes. As sulfatase genes share a relatively low degree of identity at the DNA level and generally have different chromosomal locations, it is likely that some duplication events occurred quite early in evolution. The exception to the spread of chromosomal locations observed for most sulfatase genes is a cluster of sulfatase genes on the distal short arm of the human X chromosome (Xp22.3). These genes include ASC, ASD, ASE, and ASF, which cluster in a 200-kb region of DNA.[30,31] This cluster is 150 kb proximal to the pseudo-autosomal boundary. These genes escape X inactivation and share a pseudoautosomal region between X and Y chromosomes.

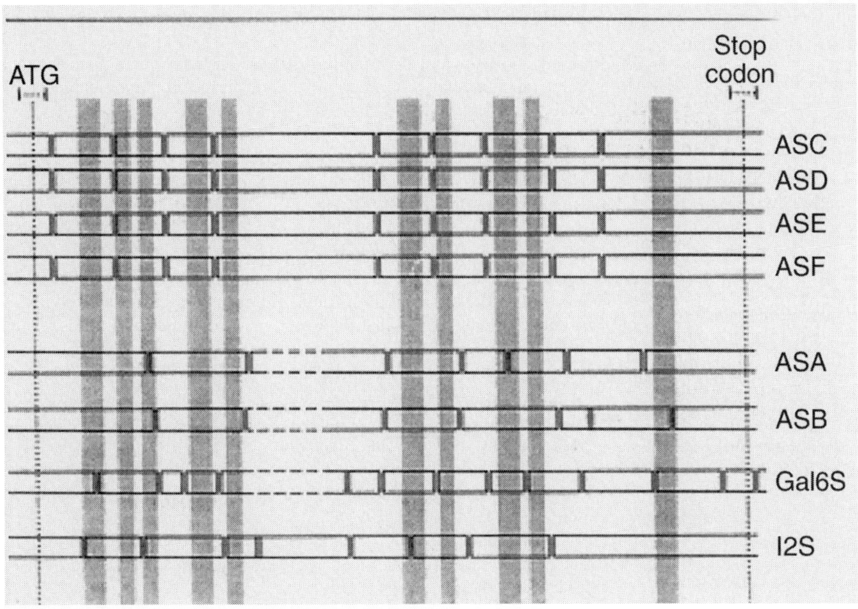

Fig. 149-4 Comparison of the genomic organization of human sulfatase genes (adapted from Parenti et al.[1]). Open rectangles indicate exons; horizontal dashed lines indicate sequences absent from the protein alignment; shaded bars indicate regions of high homology among all sulfatases. Abbreviations: I2S = iduronate-2-sulfatase; ASA = arylsulfatase A, galactose-3-sulfatase, sulfatidase; ASB = arylsulfatase B, N-acetylgalactosamine-4-sulfatase, ASC = arylsulfatase C, ASD = arylsulfatase D, ASE = arylsulfatase E, ASF = arylsulfatase F.

The four X-linked arylsulfatase genes have very similar genomic structures, with intron/exon boundaries at the same positions (Fig. 149-4). A common genomic organization and a high degree of DNA sequence homology support an evolutionary process of gene duplication of a common ancestral sulfatase gene present in the pseudoautosomal region of the X chromosome. Parenti et al.[1] have speculated that the duplication events that formed the cluster of sulfatase genes occurred before the X and Y copies of these genes diverged. Repositioning of the sulfatase cluster on the Y chromosome then occurred by a series of complex rearrangements, which were confirmed using mapping studies of the X-linked sulfatases.

Another sulfatase on the X chromosome that has been shown to have undergone a recent duplication is iduronate-2-sulfatase.[32–34] The presence of repeat sequences within 20 kb of the iduronate-2-sulfatase gene may indicate a pseudogene or possibly a functionally related gene. Other repeat sequences have been identified between these two regions that may have been involved in the duplication event.

SUBSTRATE BINDING POCKET IN THE ACTIVE SITE OF SULFATASES

Arylsulfates are hydrolyzed by all sulfatases. However, some sulfatases, known as arylsulfatases, are able to hydrolyze arylsulfates several thousand times more efficiently than others (Table 149-4), whereas the catalytic action of these sulfatases toward their natural substrates shows they have much higher affinities and turnover rates (Table 149-5). There are five (or maybe six) arylsulfatases (A, B, C, D, E, and F; Table 149-2). It is expected that these sulfatases will also specifically hydrolyze their natural substrate sulfate esters with higher affinities and turnover characteristics.

Nothing is known about the structure of the active site that influences the binding of a specific substrate to each sulfatase and then directs the extremely specific and efficient hydrolysis of this bound sulfate ester. Cocrystallization of specific substrate inhibitors and of each specific sulfatase, followed by analysis of the intramolecular interactions between substrate and enzyme, will help to determine the specific amino acid residues involved in determining substrate specificity for each sulfatase.

MUTATIONS IN CONSERVED REGIONS OF STRUCTURE

Sulfatases and Human Disease

Not surprisingly, a number of mutations have been identified in the critical regions of the active site (Fig. 149-2; Tables 149-2, 149-3). A natural mutation that replaces the active site cysteine residue 84 in iduronate-2-sulfatase with an alanine was reported to abolish enzyme activity, confirming that this residue is required for sulfatase activity.[35]

SULFATASE AND PHOSPHATASE STRUCTURAL HOMOLOGY

Active Site Homologies

The active sites of sulfatases and alkaline phosphatase share remarkable structural homology.[2,20] The active site of ASB carries

Table 149-4 Catalytic Properties of a Number of Specific Sulfatases Toward the Artificial Substrate 4-Methylumbelliferylsulfate (MUS)

	K_m mM	V_{max} (nmol/min/mg)	pH optimum
GINS	4.8	114	5.4
GIN6S	5.8	10	5.2
I2S	12.4	300	5.6
Gal6S	4.4	120	4.7
ASB	1.2	48485	5.6

Abbreviations: 12S = iduronate-2-sulfatase; GINS = sulfamidase; GIN6S = glucosamine-6-sulfatase; Gal6S = N-acetylgalactosamine-6-sulfatase; ASB = arylsulfatase B, N-acetylgalactosamine-4-sulfatase.

Table 149-5 Catalytic Properties of Sulfatases Toward Their Native Substrates

	K_m (μ/M)	V_{max} (μmol/min/mg)	pH optimum
GINS	10.7	0.80	5.2
GIN6S	48.2	0.049	6.0
I2S	3.0	3.4	4.5
Gal6S	12.5	1.5	4.7
ASB	60	20	5.6
GAS	0.3	12.8	3.2

Abbreviations: I2S = iduronate-2-sulfatase; GINS = sulfamidase; GIN6S = glucosamine-6-sulfatase; Gal6S = N-acetylgalactosamine-6-sulfatase; ASB = arylsulfatase B, N-acetylgalactosamine-4-sulfatase; GAS = glucuronate-2-sulfatase.

a Ca^{2+} ion and a sulfate ester at modified cysteine 91, whereas for alkaline phosphatase, a Zn^{2+} and a hydroxyl of serine 102 are involved in the hydrolysis of sulfate and of phosphate esters, respectively. The ASA active site has an Mg^{2+} ion and an aldehyde modified at cysteine 69. Recksiek et al. have demonstrated the similarity of the catalytic mechanisms of sulfatases and of alkaline phosphatase by studying ASA and ASB with their active site cysteine (residue 69 and 91) replaced with serine residues.[36] When these mutant sulfatases were incubated with sulfate ester substrates, the hydrolyzed sulfate was covalently linked to the active site serine. Each sulfated sulfatase remained sulfated at pH 5 but lost its sulfate ester at an alkaline pH. The active site serine of alkaline phosphatase is transesterified with phosphate from the phosphate ester substrate during the first half of the catalytic mechanism (Fig. 149-3*B*). In the second part of the reaction, the active site serine phosphate ester is hydrolyzed. Thus, sulfatases and phosphatases have in common the formation of a covalent ester intermediate. A very low level of phosphatase activity was detected in ASB.[2]

ACKNOWLEDGMENTS

We thank Dr. Peter Clements for discussions about ASB structure and catalytic mechanisms.

REFERENCES

1. Parenti G, Meroni G, Ballabio A: The sulfatase gene family. *Curr Opin Genet Dev* **7**:386, 1997.
2. Bond CS, Clements PR, Ashby SJ, Collyer CA, Harrop SJ, Hopwood JJ, Guss JM: Structure of a human lysosomal sulfatase. *Structure* **5**:277, 1997.
3. von Figura K, Schmidt B, Selmer T, Dierks T: A novel protein modification generating an aldehyde group in sulfatases—its role in catalysis and disease. *Bioessays* **20**:505, 1998.
4. Austin JH: Recent studies in the metachromatic and globoid body forms of diffuse sclerosis, in Folch-Pi, Bauer H (eds): *Brain Lipids and Lipoproteins, and Leucodystrophies*. Amsterdam, Elsevier, 1963, p 120.
5. Austin JH: Mental retardation, metachromatic leucodystrophy (sulfatide lipidosis, metachromatic leucoencephalopathy), in Carter CH (ed): *Medical Aspects of Mental Retardation*. Springfield, Thomas, 1965, p 768.
6. Kolodny EH, Fluharty AL: Metachromatic leukodystrophy and multiple sulfatase deficiency: Sulfatide lipidosis, in Scriver CR, Beaudet AL, Sly WS, Valle D (eds): *The Metabolic and Molecular Bases of Inherited Disease*, 7th ed. New York, McGraw-Hill, 1995, p 2693.
7. Burk RD, Valle D, Thomas GH, Miller C, Moser A, Moser H, Rosenbaum KN: Early manifestations of multiple sulfatase deficiency. *J Pediatr* **104**:574, 1984.
8. Burch M, Fensom AH, Jackson M, Pitts-Tucker T, Congdon PJ: Multiple sulphatase deficiency presenting at birth. *Clin Genet* **30**:409, 1986.
9. Meikle PJ, Hopwood JJ, Clague AE, Carey WF: Prevalence of lysosomal storage disorders. *JAMA* **281**:249, 1999.
10. Eto Y, Tokoro T, Ito F: Chemical compositions of acid mucopolysaccharides in urine and tissues of patients with multiple sulphatase deficiency. *J Inherit Metab Dis* **4**:161, 1981.
11. Patrick AD, Young E, Ellis C, Rodeck CH: Multiple sulphatase deficiency: Prenatal diagnosis using chorionic villi. *Prenat Diagn* **8**:303, 1988.
12. Crawley AC, Brooks DA, Muller VJ, Peterson BA, Isaac EL, Bielicki J, King BM, Boulter CD, Moore AJ, Fazzalari NL, Anson DS, Byers S, Hopwood JJ: Enzyme replacement therapy in a feline model of Maroteaux-Lamy syndrome. *J Clin Invest* **97**:1864, 1996.
13. Crawley AC, Niedzielski KH, Isaac EL, Davey RC, Byers S, Hopwood JJ: Enzyme replacement therapy from birth in a feline model of mucopolysaccharidosis type VI. *J Clin Invest* **99**:651, 1997.
14. Byers S, Nuttall JD, Crawley AC, Hopwood JJ, Smith K, Fazzalari NL: Effect of enzyme replacement on bone formation in a feline model of mucopolysaccharidosis type VI. *Bone* **21**:425, 1997.
15. Bielicki J, Hopwood JJ, Wilson PJ, Anson DS: Recombinant human iduronate-2-sulphatase: Correction of mucopolysaccharidosis-type II fibroblasts and characterization of the purified enzyme. *Biochem J* **289**:241, 1993.
16. Bielicki J, Hopwood JJ, Melville EL, Anson DS: Recombinant human sulphamidase: expression, amplification, purification and characterization. *Biochem J* **329**:145, 1998.
17. Litjens T, Bielicki J, Anson DS, Friderici K, Jones MZ, Hopwood JJ: Expression, purification and characterization of recombinant caprine N-acetylglucosamine-6-sulphatase. *Biochem J* **327**:89, 1997
18. Bielicki J, Fuller M, Guo X-H, Morris CP, Hopwood JJ, Anson DS: Expression, purification and characterization of recombinant human N-acetylgalactosamine-6-sulphatase. *Biochem J* **311**:333, 1995.
19. Anson DS, Taylor JA, Bielicki J, Harper GS, Peters C, Gibson GJ, Hopwood JJ: Correction of human mucopolysaccharidosis type-VI fibroblasts with recombinant N-acetylgalactosamine-4-sulphatase. *Biochemical Journal* **284**:789, 1992.
20. Lukatela G, Krauss N, Theis K, Selmer T, Gieselmann V, von Figura K, Saenger W: Crystal structure of human arylsulfatase A: The aldehyde function and the metal ion at the active site suggest a novel mechanism for sulfate ester hydrolysis. *Biochemistry* **37**:3654, 1998.
21. Schmidt B, Selmer T, Ingendoh A, von Figura K: A novel amino acid modification in sulfatases that is defective in multiple sulfatase deficiency. *Cell* **82**:271, 1995.
22. Waldow A, Schmidt B, Dierks T, von Bulow R, von Figura K: Amino acid residues forming the active site of arylsulfatase A. *J Biol Chem* **274**:12284, 1999.
23. Dierks T, Schmidt B, von Figura K: Conversion of cysteine to formylglycine—a protein modification in the endoplasmic reticulum. *Proc Natl Acad Sci USA* **94**:11963, 1997
24. Dierks T, Miech C, Hummerjohann J, Schmidt B, Kertesz MA, von Figura K: Post-translational formation of formylglycine in prokaryotic sulfatases by modification of either cysteine or serine. *J Biol Chem* **273**:25560, 1998.
25. Knaust A, Schmidt B, Dierks T, von Bulow R, von Figura K: Residues critical for formylglycine formation and/or catalytic activity of arylsulfatase A. *Biochemistry* **37**:13941, 1998.
26. Dierks T, Lecca MR, Schlotterhose P, Schmidt B, von Figura K: Sequence determinants directing conversion of cysteine to formylglycine in eukaryotic sulfatases. *EMBO J* **18**:2084, 1999.
27. Miech C, Dierks T, Selmer T, von Figura K, Schmidt B: Arylsulfatase from *Klebsiella pneumoniae* carries a formylglycine generated from a serine. *J Biol Chem* **273**:4835, 1998.
28. Brooks DA, Robertson DA, Bindloss C, Litjens T, Anson DS, Peters C, Morris CP, Hopwood JJ: Two site-directed mutations abrogate enzyme activity but have different effects on the conformation and cellular content of the N-acetylgalactosamine 4-sulphatase protein. *Biochem J* **307**:457, 1995.
29. Sowadski JM, Handschumacher MD, Krishna Murthy HM, Foster BA, Wyckoff HW: Refined structure of alkaline phosphatase from *Eschericha coli* at 2.8 Å resolution. *J Molec Biol* **186**:417, 1985.
30. Franco B, Meroni G, Parenti G, Levilliers J, Bernard L, Gebbia M, Cox L, Maroteaux P, Sheffield L, Rappola GA, Andria G, Petit C, Ballabio A: A cluster of sulfatase genes on Xp22.3. *Cell* **81**:15, 1995.
31. Puca A, Zollo M, Repetto M, Andolfi G, Guffanti A, Simon G, Ballabio A, Franco B: Identification by shotgun sequencing, genomic organisation and functional analysis of a fourth arylsulphatase gene (ARSF) from the Xp22.3 region. *Genomics* **42**:192, 1997.
32. Wilson PJ, Meaney CA, Hopwood JJ, Morris CP: Sequence of the human iduronate-2-sulfatase (IDS) gene. *Genomics* **17**:773, 1993.
33. Timms KM, Lu F, Shen Y, Pierson CA, Muzny DM, Gu Y, Nelson DL, Gibbs RA: 130 kb of DNA sequence reveals two new genes and a regional duplication distal to the human iduronate-2-sulfate sulfatase locus. *Genome Res* **5**:71, 1995.
34. Bondeson M-L, Malmgren H, Dahl N, Carlberg BM, Pettersson U: Presence of an IDS-related locus (IDS2) in Xq28 complicates the mutational analysis of Hunter syndrome. *Eur J Hum Genet* **3**:219, 1995.
35. Millat G, Froissart R, Maire I, Bozon D: Characterization of iduronate sulphatase mutants affecting N-glycosylation sites and the cysteine-84 residue. *Biochem J* **326**:243, 1997.
36. Recksiek M, Selmer T, Dierks T, Schmidt B, von Figura K: Sulfatases, trapping of the sulfated enzyme intermediate b substituting the active site formylglycine. *J Biol Chem* **273**:6096, 1998.

CHAPTER 150

α-Galactosidase A Deficiency: Fabry Disease

Robert J. Desnick ▪ Yiannis A. Ioannou ▪ Christine M. Eng

1. Fabry disease is an X-linked recessive inborn error of glycosphingolipid catabolism resulting from the deficient activity of the lysosomal hydrolase α-galactosidase A in tissues and fluids of affected hemizygous males. Most heterozygous female carriers of the gene have an intermediate level of enzymatic activity.

2. The enzymatic defect leads to the systemic deposition of glycosphingolipids with terminal α-galactosyl moieties, predominantly globotriaosylceramide and, to a lesser extent, galabiosylceramide and blood group B substances. Hemizygous males have extensive deposition of these glycosphingolipid substrates in body fluids and in the lysosomes of endothelial, perithelial, and smooth-muscle cells of blood vessels. Deposition also occurs in ganglion cells, and in many cell types in the heart, kidneys, eyes, and most other tissues.

3. Clinical manifestations in classically affected hemizygotes who have no detectable α-galactosidase A activity include the onset during childhood or adolescence of pain and paresthesias in the extremities, vessel ectasia (angiokeratoma) in skin and mucous membranes, and hypohidrosis. Corneal and lenticular opacities also are early findings. With increasing age, proteinuria, hyposthenuria, and lymphedema appear. Severe renal impairment leads to hypertension and uremia. Death usually occurs from renal failure or from cardiac or cerebrovascular disease. Atypical hemizygotes with residual α-galactosidase A activity may be asymptomatic or have late-onset, mild disease manifestations primarily limited to the heart (the "cardiac variant").

4. Heterozygous females may have an attenuated form of the disease. They usually are asymptomatic, although rarely can be as severely affected as hemizygous males. The most frequent clinical finding in females is the characteristic whorl-like corneal epithelial dystrophy observed by slit-lamp microscopy.

5. Confirmation of the clinical diagnosis in affected hemizygotes requires the demonstration of deficient α-galactosidase A activity in plasma, leukocytes, or tears, or increased levels of globotriaosylceramide in plasma or urinary sediment. Heterozygous females may have intermediate levels of enzymatic activity and accumulated substrate. More accurate diagnosis of heterozygous females can be accomplished by detection of a molecular lesion in the α-galactosidase A gene or by linkage analysis in families with an affected male.

6. The disorder is transmitted by the X-linked gene encoding α-galactosidase A, which has been localized to the X-chromosomal region, Xq22.1. The human α-galactosidase A cDNA and genomic sequences have been isolated, characterized, and over 150 mutations have been identified including partial gene rearrangements, splice-junction defects, and point mutations, which emphasize the heterogeneity of the molecular lesions causing this disease.

7. Prenatal diagnosis can be accomplished by demonstration of deficient α-galactosidase A activity and an XY karyotype, by haplotype linkage analysis, and/or most accurately by demonstration of the specific α-galactosidase A mutation in chorionic villi or cultured amniotic cells.

8. Low maintenance dosages of diphenylhydantoin or carbamazepine may provide relief of the excruciating pain and constant discomfort. Oral anticoagulants are recommended for stroke-prone patients. Renal dialysis and transplantation are effective in the treatment of end-stage renal disease. Clinical trials of direct enzyme replacement indicate the potential value of this therapeutic approach.

Fabry disease, an inborn error of glycosphingolipid catabolism, results from the defective activity of the lysosomal enzyme, α-galactosidase A. The enzymatic defect, transmitted by an X-linked recessive gene, leads to the progressive deposition of neutral glycosphingolipids with terminal α-galactosyl moieties in the lysosomes of most visceral tissues and in body fluids. The predominant glycosphingolipid accumulated is globotriaosylceramide, or galactosyl($\alpha 1 \rightarrow 4$)-galactosyl-($\beta 1 \rightarrow 4$)-glucosyl-($\beta 1 \rightarrow 1'$)-ceramide (Fig. 150-1). The birefringent deposits are primarily found in the lysosomes of the vascular endothelium. Progressive endothelial glycosphingolipid accumulation results in ischemia and infarction, and leads to the major clinical manifestations of the disease. The glycosphingolipids also accumulate in perithelial and smooth-muscle cells of the cardiovascular-renal system. To a lesser extent, they accumulate in reticuloendothelial, myocardial, and connective tissue cells; in epithelial cells of the cornea, kidney, and other tissues; and in ganglion and perineural cells of the autonomic nervous system. Clinically, hemizygous males have a characteristic skin lesion, which led to the descriptive name of angiokeratoma corporis diffusum universale. They also have acroparesthesias, episodic crises of excruciating pain, corneal and lenticular opacities, hypohidrosis, and cardiac and renal dysfunction. Death usually occurs in adult life from renal, cardiac, and/or cerebral complications of the vascular disease. Heterozygous females are usually asymptomatic and are most likely to show the corneal opacities, but may develop cardiac involvement in late adulthood.

A list of standard abbreviations is located immediately preceding the index in each volume. Additional abbreviations used in this chapter include: ATK = agammaglobulinemia tyrosine kinase; EMG = electromyogram; Gal T-6 = UDPGal:LacCer($\alpha 1 \rightarrow 4$) galactosyltransferase; M6P = mannose-6-phosphate; M6PR = mannose-6-phosphate receptor; pI = isoelectric point; SAP = sphingolipid activator protein; TGN = *trans*-Golgi network.

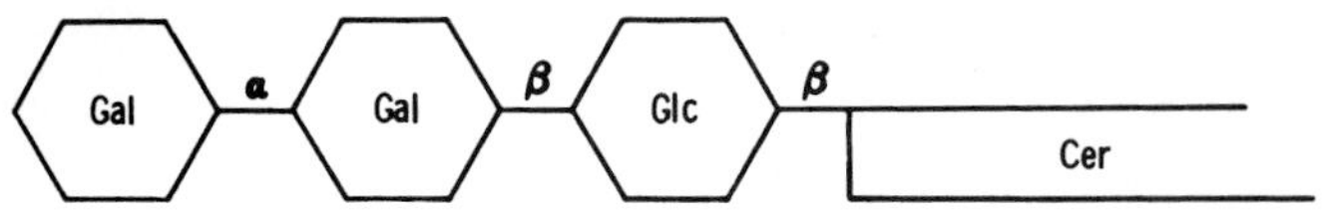

Fig. 150-1 Globotriaosylceramide (galactosyl(α1 → 4)galactosyl(β1 → 4)glucosyl(β1 → 1′) ceramide).

HISTORICAL ASPECTS

In 1898, two dermatologists, Anderson[1] in England and Fabry[2] in Germany, independently described the first patients with angiokeratoma corporis diffusum. Anderson designated his case as one of angiokeratoma. His original patient was a 39-year-old male who had proteinuria, finger deformities, varicose veins, and lymphedema. Because of the proteinuria, Anderson suspected that the disease was a generalized disorder and astutely suggested that abnormal vessels might be present in the kidneys as well as in the skin. He also correctly noted that "the vascular lesion was not a new formation, as implied by the suffix "oma," but an ectasia of cutaneous capillaries."[1] Fabry originally made the diagnosis of purpura nodularis in a 13-year-old male whom he followed over the next 30 years. He documented the presence of albuminuria, further described the cutaneous lesions, noting the presence of small vessel aneurysms,[3] and subsequently classified his case as one of angiokeratoma corporis diffusum, a designation that has persisted, particularly among dermatologists.

Several individuals made early contributions to the clinical description of the disease. Steiner and Voerner[4] and Gunther[5] described a hemizygous male with anhidrosis and intermittent acroparesthesias that were aggravated by hot or cold weather. Examination of a skin biopsy showed atrophy of the sweat glands and aneurysmal dilatation of the capillaries. Weicksel[6] first described the characteristic corneal opacities and the vascular abnormalities in the conjunctiva and retina. In 1947, Pompen and coworkers[7] reported the first postmortem findings in two affected brothers who died from renal failure. The most significant observation was the presence of abnormal vacuoles in blood vessels throughout their bodies. On the basis of these findings, they suggested that the disease was a generalized storage disorder. Subsequently, Scriba definitively established the lipid nature of the storage material,[8] and Hornbostel and Scriba were the first to confirm the diagnosis histologically in a living patient by demonstrating the refractile lipid deposits in vessels of a skin biopsy specimen.[9] Although the familial occurrence of the disease was recognized earlier,[10] it was not until 1965 that Opitz et al.[11] documented the X-linked recessive inheritance of the disorder by pedigree analysis.

In 1963, Sweeley and Klionsky[12] isolated and characterized two neutral glycosphingolipids—globotriaosylceramide (Gal-Gal-Glc-Cer) and galabiosylceramide (Gal-Gal-Cer)—from the kidney of a Fabry hemizygote obtained at autopsy. On the basis of these findings, they classified Fabry disease as a sphingolipidosis. Subsequent chemical analyses of various Fabry tissues and fluids[13–16] have demonstrated the marked accumulation of globotriaosylceramide, and to a lesser extent, galabiosylceramide.[12,14,16] In addition, the abnormal accumulation of blood group B substances, glycosphingolipids with terminal α-galactosyl moieties, has been reported in affected individuals with B or AB blood types.[17] In 1967, Brady et al.[18] demonstrated that the enzymatic defect was in ceramide trihexosidase, a lysosomal galactosyl hydrolase required for the catabolism of globotriaosylceramide (see Fig. 150-1). Kint,[19] using synthetic substrates, characterized the defective enzymatic activity as an α-galactosyl hydrolase. Shortly thereafter, it was recognized that there were two enzymes (designated α-galactosidases A and B) that hydrolyzed synthetic substrates with α-galactosyl moieties, α-galactosidase A being deficient in Fabry disease. It was shown subsequently that α-galactosidase B was an α-*N*-acetylgalactosaminidase,[20,21] the lysosomal hydrolase shown to be deficient in the infantile and later-onset forms of Schindler disease[22] and its adult-onset form, which presents with angiokeratoma and glycopeptiduria.[23] Thus, there appears to be only one lysosomal α-galactosidase (designated α-galactosidase A), the enzyme defective in Fabry disease.

The elucidation of the specific enzymatic defect in Fabry disease permitted the enzymatic diagnosis of affected hemizygous males, presumptive identification of heterozygous carrier females,[24,25] and the prenatal diagnosis of affected male fetuses.[26,27] In addition, pilot trials of α-galactosidase A replacement with the purified human enzyme were reported.[28–30] The subsequent isolation of the full-length cDNA[31–33] and the entire genomic sequence[33] for human α-galactosidase A permitted characterization of disease mutations, improved carrier identification and prenatal diagnosis, and stimulated efforts to treat the disease with purified recombinant enzyme or by gene therapy. Clinical trials of enzyme replacement therapy using recombinant human α-galactosidase A are currently under active investigation. Various designations have been used to identify this disorder. In keeping with the terminology applied to other lipidoses and for the benefit of information retrieval, it seems advisable to refer to the disease by its specific enzymatic defect and to retain the commonly used eponym. Thus, an appropriate designation is α-galactosidase A deficiency: Fabry disease.

CLINICAL MANIFESTATIONS

The Classically Affected Hemizygote

The clinical manifestations of Fabry disease result predominantly from the progressive deposition of globotriaosylceramide in the vascular endothelium (Table 150-1). Clinical onset usually occurs during childhood or adolescence, but it may be delayed until the second or third decade. Early manifestations include periodic crises of severe pain in the extremities (acroparesthesias), the appearance of vascular cutaneous lesions (angiokeratoma), hypohidrosis, and the characteristic corneal and lenticular opacities.

The frequency of Fabry disease has not been determined; the disease is rare, and it is estimated that the incidence is about 1 in 40,000 males. The disorder is panethnic and patients representing all ethnic groups, including Caucasian, African, Hispanic, American Indian, and Asian, have been observed.[34]

Pain. The most debilitating symptom of Fabry disease is pain. Two types have been described: episodic crises and constant discomfort.[10,35] The painful crises most often begin in childhood or early adolescence and signal clinical onset of the disease. Lasting from minutes to several days, these "Fabry crises" consist

Table 150-1 Major Clinical Manifestations in Hemizygotes with Fabry Disease

Vascular Glycolipid Deposition	Manifestations
Skin	Angiokeratoma
Peripheral nerves (autonomic system)	Excruciating pain, acroparesthesias, hypohidrosis
Heart	Ischemia and infarctions
Brain	Transient ischemic attacks, strokes
Kidney	Renal failure

NOTE: Average age at death, 41 years.[82]

of agonizing, burning pain felt initially in the palms and soles. Often the pain radiates to the proximal extremities and other parts of the body. Attacks of abdominal or flank pain may simulate appendicitis or renal colic.[36] The painful crises are usually triggered by fever, exercise, fatigue, emotional stress, or rapid changes in temperature and humidity. With increasing age, the periodic crises usually decrease in frequency and severity; however, in some patients, they may occur more frequently, and the pain can be so excruciating that the patient may contemplate suicide.[37,38] Because the pain usually is associated with a low-grade fever and an elevated erythrocyte sedimentation rate, these symptoms frequently have led to the misdiagnosis of rheumatic fever, neurosis, or erythromelalgia.[35,38–41]

In addition to these intermittent crises, most patients complain of a nagging, constant discomfort in their hands and feet characterized by burning, tingling paresthesias.[35] These acroparesthesias may occur daily, usually during late afternoon, and may represent an attenuated form of the excruciating episodic crises. Although pain is a hallmark of the disease, about 10 to 20 percent of older patients deny any history of Fabry crises or acroparesthesias. In many instances, patients learn to adapt to the pain by changing their lifestyles in an effort to avoid precipitating factors.

Skin Lesions. Angiectases may be one of the earliest manifestations and may lead to diagnosis in childhood. There is a progressive increase in the number and size of these cutaneous vascular lesions with age. Classically, the angiokeratomas develop slowly as individual punctate, dark red to blue-black angiectases in the superficial layers of the skin (Fig. 150-2). The lesions may be flat or slightly raised and do not blanch with pressure. There is a slight hyperkeratosis notable in larger lesions. Clusters of lesions are most dense between the umbilicus and the knees and have a tendency toward bilateral symmetry. The hips, back, thighs, buttocks, penis, and scrotum are most commonly involved, but there is a wide variation in the pattern of distribution and density of the lesions. Involvement of the oral mucosa and conjunctiva is common, and other mucosal areas may also be involved. Variants without the characteristic skin lesions have been reported[42–45] (see "Atypical Hemizygotes; Cardiac Variants" below).

Although the angiectases may not be readily apparent in some patients, careful examination of the skin, especially the scrotum and umbilicus, may reveal isolated lesions. In addition to these vascular lesions, anhidrosis, or more commonly hypohidrosis, is an early and almost constant finding.

Cardiac, Cerebral, and Renal Vascular Manifestations. With increasing age, the major morbid symptoms of the disease result from the progressive deposition of glycosphingolipid in the cardiovascular-renal system. Cardiac disease occurs in most hemizygous males. Early findings include left ventricular enlargement, valvular involvement, and conduction abnormalities.[46,47] Mitral insufficiency is the most frequent valvular lesion and is typically present in childhood or adolescence. Involvement of the myocardium and possibly the conduction system results in electrocardiographic abnormalities that may show left-ventricular hypertrophy, ST segment changes, and T-wave inversion. Other abnormalities including arrhythmias, intermittent supraventricular tachycardias, and a short PR interval have been described.[48–50] Intracardiac pacing has shown rapid conduction through the AV node.[51] The PR interval decreased over a 10-year period in two hemizygotes, indicating an accelerated atrioventricular conduction with progressive lipid deposition in the bundle of His.[52] Patients with complete atrioventricular block and/or sinus node dysfunction have been reported.[10,48,53] Several patients with electrocardiographic changes indicating infarction had no evidence of myocardial necrosis at postmortem examination; the EKG changes were probably related to glycosphingolipid deposition in the myocardium.[47] Echocardiographic studies demonstrate an increased incidence of mitral valve prolapse and an increased thickness of the interventricular septum and the left ventricular posterior wall.[54–56] The two-dimensional and M-mode echocardiographic findings in Fabry hemizygotes are similar to those in cardiac amyloidosis patients.[57] MRI reveals marked concentric hypertrophy and increased signal intensity of the left ventricular wall.[58] The T2 relaxation time is markedly prolonged throughout the left ventricular myocardium; values are greater than those seen in patients with hypertension or hypertrophic cardiomyopathy, presumably because of myocardial glycolipid deposition.[58] In addition, hypertrophic obstructive cardiomyopathy secondary to glycosphingolipid infiltration in the interventricular septum has been reported.[59] Typical severe angina in a 27-year-old hemizygote due to glycolipid deposition in the coronary arteries was successfully treated by coronary bypass.[60] Late manifestations may include angina pectoris, myocardial ischemia and infarction, congestive heart failure, and severe mitral regurgitation.[46,47] These findings may be accentuated by systemic hypertension related to vascular involvement of renal parenchymal vessels. Cerebrovascular manifestations result primarily from multifocal small-vessel involvement and may include thromboses, transient ischemic attacks, basilar artery ischemia and aneurysm, seizures, hemiplegia, hemianesthesia, aphasia, labyrinthine disorders, or frank cerebral hemorrhage.[10,61–69] A review of 43 reported cases revealed an average age at onset of 33.8 years. The most frequent symptoms in descending order were hemiparesis, vertigo/dizziness, diplopia, dysarthria, nystagmus, nausea/vomiting, head pain, hemiataxia, and gait ataxia. The recurrence rate was 76 percent. These manifestations are predominantly due to dilative arteriopathy of the vertebrobasilar circulation.[70] MRI and proton MRS imaging have proved useful in the evaluation of cerebrovascular involvement;[69,71,72] in fact, MRI was more effective in detecting lacunar infarcts than was CT.[73] Personality changes and psychotic behavior may become manifest with increasing age.[73–76] A transient state of disorientation and confusion may occur in association with electrolyte imbalance, usually secondary to renal

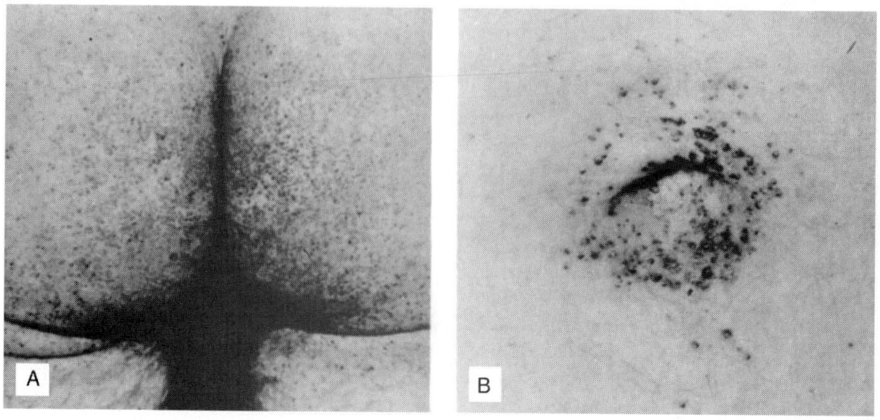

Fig. 150-2 Clusters of dark-red to blue angiokeratomas (telangiectases) on the buttocks (*A*) and in the umbilical area (*B*) of a hemizygote with Fabry disease.

disease.[77] Severe neurologic signs may be present without evidence of major thrombosis or hypertension and are presumably due to multifocal small-vessel occlusive disease.[77,78]

Progressive glycosphingolipid deposition in the kidney results in proteinuria and other signs of renal impairment, with gradual deterioration of renal function and development of azotemia in middle age. During childhood and adolescence, protein, casts, red cells, and desquamated kidney and urinary tract cells may appear in the urine. Birefringent lipid globules with characteristic "Maltese crosses" can be observed free in the urine and within desquamated urinary sediment cells by polarization microscopy. With age, progressive renal impairment is evidenced by significant proteinuria, isosthenuria (specific gravities of 1.008 to 1.012), and alterations of other renal tubular functions including tubular reabsorption, secretion, and excretion.[79] Polyuria and a syndrome similar to vasopressin-resistant diabetes insipidus occasionally develop. On MRI examination, there is gradual loss of cortico-medullary differentiation. In addition, there may also be an increase in the incidence of simple renal cysts.[80] Gradual deterioration of renal function and the development of azotemia usually occur in the third to fifth decades of life, although renal failure has been reported in the second decade.[81] Death most often results from uremia, unless chronic hemodialysis or renal transplantation is undertaken. The mean age at death of 94 affected males who were not treated for uremia was 41 years,[82] but occasionally an affected male has survived into his sixties.

Ocular Features. Ocular involvement is most prominent in the cornea, lens, conjunctiva, and retina.[40,83,84] A characteristic corneal opacity, observed only by slit-lamp microscopy, is found in affected males and in most heterozygous females (Fig. 150-3). The earliest lesion is a diffuse haziness in the subepithelial layer. In more advanced cases, the opacities appear as whorled streaks extending from a central vortex to the periphery of the cornea. Typically, the whorl-like opacities are inferior and cream-colored; however, they range from white to golden-brown and may be very faint.[84] An identical, familial corneal dystrophy, termed cornea verticillata, was described by Gruber in 1946;[85] subsequent investigation of these patients revealed that they were hemizygous and heterozygous for Fabry disease.[86] An indistinguishable, drug-induced phenocopy of the Fabry corneal dystrophy occurs in patients on long-term chloroquine or amiodarone therapy (see "Diagnosis" below).

Two specific types of lenticular changes have been described (Fig. 150-4). A granular anterior capsular or subcapsular deposit has been observed in about one-third of hemizygous males, but rarely in heterozygous females. Typically, these lenticular opacities are bilateral and inferior in position. They frequently appear in a "propeller-like" distribution, that is, wedge-shaped with their bases near the lenticular equator and aligned radially with the apexes toward the center of the anterior capsule. A second, and possibly pathognomonic, lenticular opacity has been observed in both hemizygous and heterozygous individuals.[40,83] It may be the first ocular manifestation to appear. The opacity is posterior and linear, and appears as a whitish, almost translucent, spoke-like deposit of fine granular material on or near the posterior lens capsule. These lines usually radiate from the central part of the posterior cortex. This unusual opacity has been termed the Fabry cataract[40] and is best seen by retroillumination.

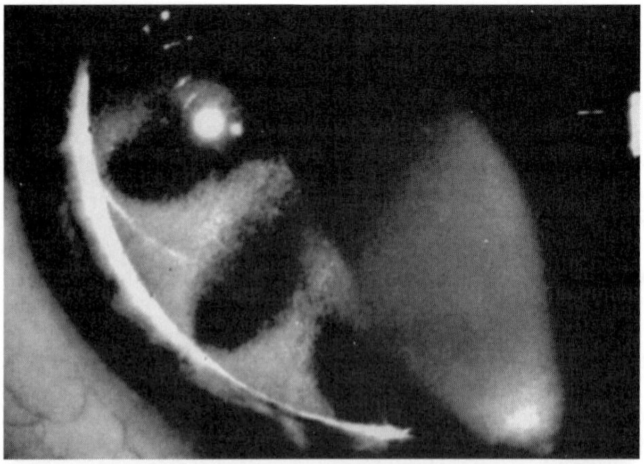

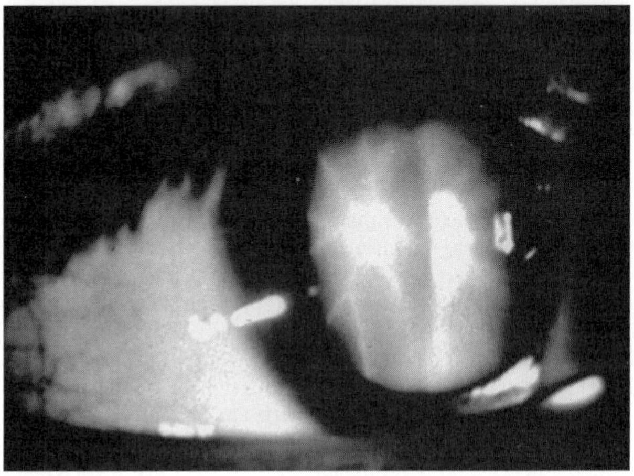

Fig. 150-4 Lenticular changes include the anterior capsular opacity shown with a "propeller-like" distribution (above) and the posterior opacity or "Fabry cataract" (below), which is best seen by retroillumination and may be unique to Fabry hemizygotes and heterozygotes. (*Reproduced from Sher et al.*[40] *Used by permission.*)

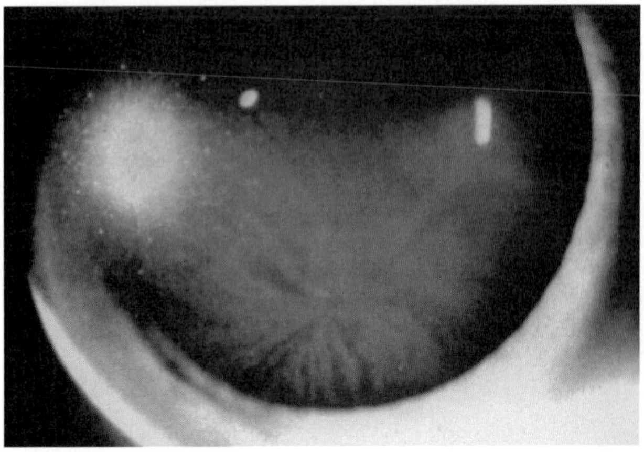

Fig. 150-3 Corneal opacity in a heterozygote observed by slit-lamp microscopy. The corneal involvement results from subepithelial glycosphingolipid deposition. (*Reproduced from Sher et al.*[40] *Used by permission.*)

Conjunctival and retinal vascular lesions are common and represent part of the diffuse systemic vascular involvement. These vascular lesions occur early in life in normotensive individuals and are characterized by mild to marked tortuosity of the conjunctival and retinal vessels. There is an aneurysmal dilatation of thin-walled venules as well as angulation and segmental, sausage-like dilatation of veins typically seen on the inferior bulbar conjunctiva. As the disease progresses, retinal changes associated with the development of hypertension and uremia may be superimposed. Vision is not impaired by the vascular lesions in the conjunctiva and retina or by the corneal dystrophy. However, acute visual loss has occurred in males as a result of unilateral total central retinal artery occlusion.[40,87]

Other ocular findings have included lid edema in the absence of renal insufficiency, myelinated nerve fibers radiating from the optic disk, mild optic atrophy, papilledema, peripapillary edema, nystagmus, internuclear ophthalmoplegia, and retinal vein occlusion.[34,40,83,84,88]

Gastrointestinal Manifestations. Episodic diarrhea, abdominal pain, and, to a lesser extent, nausea, vomiting, and flank pain are the most common gastrointestinal complaints.[89,90] These symptoms may be related to the deposition of glycosphingolipid in intestinal small vessels and in the autonomic ganglia of the bowel.[91] Achalasia and jejunal diverticulosis, which may lead to perforation of the small bowel, have been described.[92,93] Although intestinal malabsorption has been reported, it is not a recognized feature of the disease. Radiologic studies may reveal thickened, edematous folds and mild dilatation of the small bowel; a granular-appearing ileum; and the loss of haustral markings throughout the colon, particularly in the distal segments.[89] While a significant proportion of affected males manifest gastrointestinal symptoms, approximately 33 percent, these are not universal findings. The symptomatology and pathophysiology of the gastrointestinal involvement have been reviewed.[89,91,94]

Other Clinical Features. Because of the widespread visceral distribution of the glycosphingolipid deposits, signs and symptoms of this disorder arise in many other organ systems. Minor changes in electroencephalogram (EEG) and electromyelogram (EMG) findings as well as slowed and latent peripheral nerve conduction abnormalities may be observed.[95] Auditory and vestibular abnormalities have been described[69] and high frequency hearing loss is a nearly universal finding in affected males. Several patients have had chronic bronchitis, wheezing respiration,[10] or dyspnea with alveolar capillary block.[96] In many hemizygotes, pulmonary function studies indicate a mild obstructive component, and primary pulmonary involvement has been reported in the absence of cardiac or renal disease.[97,98] In older hemizygotes, pulmonary function studies may show significant airflow obstruction, reduced diffusing capacity, and a reduction in the V_{max25} values; smokers had greater airflow obstruction than expected from smoking alone.[99] In a study of 25 unselected, consecutive classically affected males, 36 percent had airway obstruction on spirometry, a finding that was associated with age (>26 years), but only weakly associated with smoking.[98] Roentgenographic studies may reveal hyperinflation and/or bullous disease. Lymphedema of the legs may be present in adulthood without hypoproteinemia, varices, or any clinically manifest vascular disease.[100,101] This manifestation presumably reflects the progressive glycosphingolipid deposition in the lymphatic vessels and lymph nodes. Patients have presented with prominent lymphadenopathy as their only finding[102] and enlarged lymph nodes secondary to deposition of GL-3 have been seen at biopsy. Many patients have varicosities and hemorrhoids. Priapism also has been reported.[103–106]

Anemia is probably due to decreased erythrocyte survival.[107] A decreased serum iron concentration, normal erythrocyte fragility, and an elevated reticulocyte count have been reported.[34] Increased platelet aggregation and a high concentration of β-thromboglobulin have been described.[108] Lipid-laden, foamy-appearing macrophages are present in the bone marrow.[109] The spleen is not enlarged.

Many patients have evidence of musculoskeletal involvement. A characteristic permanent deformity arises from changes in the distal interphalangeal joint of the fingers, causing limited extension of the terminal joints.[10] The bony changes are characterized by multiple enthesopathic ossifications at the insertions of fibrous structures and by intra- and extraarticular erosions.[110] The following have been described: avascular necrosis of the head of the femur or talus; multiple, small infarct-like opacities in the femoral heads; and involvement of the metacarpals, metatarsals, and temporomandibular joint.[34]

Many affected males appear to have retarded growth or delayed puberty and sparse, fine facial and body hair. In some kindreds, affected males have a characteristic acromegaly-like facies.[34] Affected individuals may complain of fatigue and weakness and may be incapacitated for prolonged periods.

Atypical Hemizygotes

The Cardiac Variant. Fabry hemizygotes have been described who were essentially asymptomatic at ages when classic hemizygotes would be severely affected or would have died from the disease[44,111–120] (Table 150-2). Many of these variants were identified serendipitously during evaluation of other unrelated medical problems or of their family members. In contrast to patients with the classic phenotype who have no detectable α-galactosidase A activity, atypical variants have residual activity compatible with their milder phenotypes (see "Residual Activity in Atypical Hemizygotes" below). Recent reports have described several patients with late-onset cardiac or cardiopulmonary disease.[44,111,115–120] These individuals were essentially asymptomatic during most of their lives and did not experience the early classic manifestations including acroparesthesias, angiokeratoma, corneal and lenticular opacities, and anhidrosis. Most were diagnosed after the onset of cardiac manifestations and most were found to have mild proteinuria. These "cardiac variants" had cardiomegaly, typically involving the left ventricular wall and interventricular septum, and electrocardiographic abnormalities consistent with a cardiomyopathy. Others had nonobstructive hypertrophic cardiomyopathy and/or myocardial infarctions.

Among early descriptions of the atypical cardiac variants were two independent reports of males of Italian descent who were identified at ages 38 and 42 years during evaluations for hypercholesterolemia[44,114] and rheumatoid arthritis,[111] respectively. The finding of proteinuria in each led to renal biopsies that revealed ultrastructural findings consistent with Fabry disease. Low levels of α-galactosidase A activity confirmed their diagnoses. Neither had acroparesthesias, angiokeratoma, anhidrosis, or corneal opacities. The atypical hemizygote with poorly controlled hypercholesterolemia had normal renal function until his death at age 49 from a second myocardial infarction.[44] The hemizygote with rheumatoid arthritis remained asymptomatic at 55 years of age with normal creatinine clearance and renal concentrating values, and with mild left-ventricular hypertrophy on echocardiography.[77,111] Another well-characterized cardiac variant was a 54-year-old male of German descent with isolated myocardial involvement identified following a diagnostic endocardial biopsy that revealed ultrastructural findings in the myocardium that were suggestive of Fabry disease.[120] However, careful ultrastructural examination of endothelial cells in the endomyocardium, liver, skeletal muscle, rectum, and skin failed to demonstrate the expected glycolipid deposition. The patient denied a history of acroparesthesias and did not have the other classical disease manifestations of Fabry disease. An Italian patient with a long history of atrial fibrillation was found on endomyocardial biopsy to have severely hypertrophied myocardiocytes filled with the typical concentric lamellar inclusions and low α-galactosidase A activity.

Two cardiac variants of Czech and Japanese descent were diagnosed at postmortem examination.[115,119] The Czech patient had hypertension, dyspnea, marked left-ventricular hypertrophy with ischemic changes, and atrial enlargement; he died at age 63 from a pulmonary embolism and cardiac failure. Autopsy findings revealed marked cardiomegaly and concentric left-ventricular hypertrophy with no evidence of left-ventricular obstruction. Storage of globotriaosylceramide was confined to the myocardium. Histochemical and/or ultrastructural examination revealed no evidence of glycolipid deposition in coronary or pulmonary arteries, aorta, brain, kidney, liver, or pancreas. The Japanese patient had a history of dyspnea, proteinuria, and nonspecific EKG abnormalities including abnormal Q waves and interventricular conduction disturbances. He died at age 71. At autopsy, significant deposition of globotriaosylceramide in the myocardium was detected immunohistochemically with a mouse monoclonal

Table 150-2 Findings in Atypical Hemizygotes*

Reference number	Ancestry	Age at diagnosis	Angiokeratoma	Acroparesthesias	Corneal opacity	Anhidrosis	Proteinuria	Cardiomegaly/ cardiomyopathy	Glycolipid deposition	Residual enzymatic activity	Mutation
44	Italian	31	–	–	–	–	+	+	+	+	
111	Italian	42	–	–	–	–	+	+		+	N215S
112	Arab	51	–		–	–	–	–		+	
113	Japanese	26	–	+	–	–	–	–	+	+	
115	Japanese	71†				–		+			
116, 117	Japanese	63	–	–	–	–	–	+		+	S279E
116, 118	Japanese	52	–	–		–	–	+		+	R301Q
119	Czech	63†	–	–	–	–		+	+	+	N215S
120	German	54	–	–	–	–	+	+	+	+	M296V
121	Japanese	62	–	–	–	–		+		+	M296I
121	Japanese	55	–	–	–	–		+		+	A20P

*Plus (+) or minus (–) indicates presence or absence of the clinical or biochemical finding.
†Diagnosis made at autopsy.

antibody to the pathogenic glycosphingolipid, but no accumulation occurred in the kidney or liver. The incidence of the cardiac variant is unknown. However, in a study of 230 Japanese males with left ventricular hypertrophy, seven (3 percent) were found to have low plasma α-galactosidase A activity and/or α-galactosidase A mutations, suggesting that the variant form of Fabry disease may be underdiagnosed.[121] These variants emphasize the need to include Fabry disease in the differential diagnosis of patients with hypertrophic cardiomyopathy and cardiac disease of unknown etiology.

Other Variants. In addition to the cardiac variants, several other atypical hemizygotes have been reported. For example, Kobayashi et al. described a 26-year-old Japanese male who experienced acroparesthesias but who did not have angiokeratoma, hypohidrosis, or keratopathy.[113] Bach et al. reported an asymptomatic 51-year-old male of Arab descent[112] who was identified after his daughter was found to have lupus nephritis and lesions characteristic of Fabry disease in a renal biopsy sample.[122] There are several reports of males who have disease manifestations confined to the kidney.[123,124] Several such patients were identified among renal dialysis patients in Japan who lacked the classical manifestations of Fabry disease, that is, angiokeratoma, corneal opacities, and acroparesthesias.[125] It is likely that additional, mildly affected or asymptomatic variants will continue to be detected in the future. Astute recognition of subtle clinical manifestations or the observation of abnormal ultrastructural findings suggest the diagnosis of Fabry disease. Subsequent biochemical and molecular studies can definitively establish the diagnosis (see "Diagnosis" below). Clearly, there is a spectrum of disease ranging from the classic full phenotype to mildly affected individuals with significant residual α-galactosidase A activity and markedly lower substrate accumulation in certain tissues, especially the vascular endothelium. It is notable that certain α-galactosidase A mutations occurring in patients described as cardiac variants (i.e., R112H, R301Q, and G328R) also have been reported in patients with classical disease.[126] The finding of patients with the same α-galactosidase A mutations, but different phenotypes, suggests that other modifying factors may contribute to differences in phenotype (see below "Genotype/Phenotype Correlations").

The Heterozygote. The clinical course and prognosis of heterozygotes differ significantly from those of hemizygotes.[34] Heterozygotes experience little difficulty in adult life at ages when hemizygous males already have severe renal and/or cardiac involvement. Although most biochemically documented heterozygotes are asymptomatic throughout a normal life span, with increasing age some manifest minor symptoms of the disease (Table 150-3). Approximately 30 percent of heterozygotes have a few isolated skin lesions, less than 10 percent have acroparesthesias, and about 70 percent have the whorl-like corneal dystrophy.[127] Some heterozygotes develop cardiac involvement with advanced age.[128] However, a few heterozygotes have been described with disease as severe as that observed in classically affected hemizygous males.[46,129–131] In contrast, obligate heterozygotes (daughters of affected hemizygous males) without any clinical manifestations and with normal levels of leukocyte α-galactosidase A and urinary sediment glycosphingolipids have been reported.[130,132] Indeed, asymptomatic and symptomatic monozygotic female twins have been described.[133–135] Such markedly variable expression is expected in females heterozygous for X-linked diseases as a result of random X inactivation.[136] At the cellular level, heterozygotes for most X-linked enzymatic defects have two populations of cells, one with mutant and the other with normal enzymatic activity resulting from the random inactivation of one X chromosome in each cell early in embryogenesis. Representatives of two such populations have been cloned from cultured skin fibroblasts from obligate heterozygotes, one with normal and the other with defective

Table 150-3 Clinical Manifestations in Heterozygotes for Fabry Disease

Manifestation	Estimated Incidence (by percentage)*	Remarks
Corneal dystrophy	∼70	Useful for heteozygote detection
Angiokeratoma	∼30	Single or isolated lesions
Acroparesthesias	<10	Infrequent; hands, feet, and lower abdomen
Hypohidrosis	<1	Rare variants†
Cardiac involvement	<1	Rare variants†
Central nervous system involvement	<1	Rare variants†
Renal failure	<1	Rare variants†

*Based on review of over 122 heterozygous females, 1 to 85 years of age, evaluated by the authors.
†Rare female variants with 0 to 5% α-galactosidase A activity.

α-galactosidase A activity.[137] Preferential inactivation of either the affected or unaffected X-chromosome has been shown to be the mechanism of discordant expression of Fabry disease in one set of monozygotic twins with a *de novo* mutation in the α-galactosidase A gene.[135] Ultrastructural examination of renal tissue from heterozygotes also demonstrated two populations of glomerular, interstitial, and vascular cells: one normal, the other with observed glycosphingolipid deposition.[138,139] Similar findings were observed in cardiac tissues from a heterozygote.[139]

Of more than 150 heterozygotes reported in the literature, corneal involvement is the most frequent and often the only manifestation.[40] Frequently, the corneal dystrophy is more prominent than in affected males in the same family. However, about 30 percent of biochemically documented and/or obligate heterozygous females do not have corneal opacities.[10,83,132,140] The skin lesions are absent or much less prominent in carrier females than in affected males. Isolated lesions may occasionally be observed on the breasts, lips, and trunk. The cutaneous involvement may be more prominent in heterozygotes who also accumulate blood group B substances. The lesions have been detected in heterozygotes during childhood. Skin biopsies of clinically uninvolved skin from obligate heterozygotes obtained in the first decade of life contain glycosphingolipid deposits in the vascular endothelial and muscularis cells. Other manifestations may include intermittent pain in the extremities, edema (particularly of the ankles), vascular lesions in the conjunctiva and retina, and cardiovascular changes such as hypertension, electrocardiographic abnormalities, and left-ventricular hypertrophy.[10,43,82] Cerebrovascular complications are rare and have included memory loss, dizziness, ataxia, hemiparesis, and hemisensory symptoms.[70] Basilar artery aneurysms also have been reported. Renal findings in heterozygotes include hyposthenuria; erythrocytes, leukocytes, and granular and hyaline casts in the urinary sediment; proteinuria; and other signs of renal impairment. Mucosal lesions, hypohidrosis, and diarrhea have been recorded less frequently. Heterozygotes may develop arthritis in the distal interphalangeal joints of the fingers.

PATHOLOGY

Morphologically, Fabry disease is characterized by widespread tissue deposits of crystalline glycosphingolipids, which show birefringence with characteristic "Maltese crosses" under polarization microscopy. The glycosphingolipid is deposited in all areas of the body and occurs predominantly in the lysosomes of endothelial, perithelial, and smooth-muscle cells of blood vessels

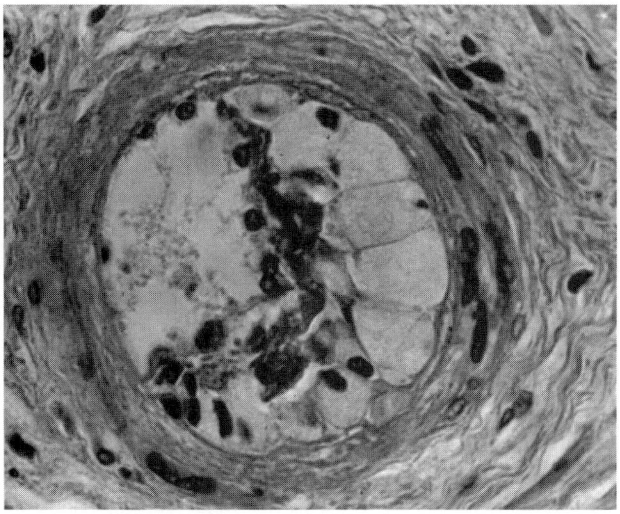

Fig. 150-5 Photomicrograph of a prostatic arteriole showing the hypertrophied, lipid-laden endothelial cells encroaching on the vascular lumen. H&E, × 600.

(Fig. 150-5) and, to a lesser degree, in histiocytic and reticular cells of connective tissue. Lipid deposits are also prominent in epithelial cells of the cornea and glomeruli and tubules of the kidney, in muscle fibers of the heart, and in ganglion cells of the autonomic system. Glycosphingolipid deposition does not occur in hepatocytes but is present in the liver sinus endothelial and Kupffer cells.[141]

Skin

The skin lesions are telangiectases or small superficial angiomas. After a silent period, cumulative vascular damage eventually leads to clinically apparent and progressive angiectases. This sequence is suggested by the biopsy finding of lipid deposits in areas of clinically normal skin[142,143] or in patients with no skin lesions[144] and by recognition of patients who have visceral lesions but whose skin lesions were either of minimal consequence or delayed. The early pathologic involvement has been observed in the vascular endothelium and perithelium of clinically normal skin from a 1-year-old affected male.[143]

Capillaries, venules, and arterioles contain pathologic lipid storage in the endothelium, perithelium, and smooth muscle (Fig. 150-6). There is marked dilatation of the capillaries of the dermal papillae. Deeper vessels show less dilatation and aneurysm formation. Lipid stores have been noted in arrectores pilorum muscles, sweat gland epithelium, and perineural cells.[142–146] Similar findings have been observed in gingival tissues. Atrophic or scarce sweat and sebaceous glands have been reported.[96] Ultrastructural examination of eccrine sweat glands revealed numerous cytoplasmic inclusions in the clear cells of the secretory coil, coiled duct, and basal cells of the straight duct. Inclusions were also observed in unmyelinated axons innervating the sweat gland and the small blood vessels around the gland, which had marked involvement of the vascular endothelium.[147]

The fully developed classic lesions are usually located in the upper dermis, where they may produce elevation, flattening, or hypertrophy of the epithelium. The larger lesions may have a slight to moderate hyperkeratosis; hence the term angiokeratoma. As in all forms of angiokeratomas, the hypertrophy and hyperkeratosis may be secondary to pressure on the epithelium by the underlying dilated vessel.

Kidney

The lesions are due to the accumulation of glycosphingolipids primarily in epithelial cells of the glomerulus (Fig. 150-7) and of the distal tubules (Fig. 150-8). In later stages, and to a lesser degree, proximal tubules, interstitial histiocytes, and interstitial cells may show lipid accumulation. Lipid-laden distal tubular epithelial cells desquamate and may be detected in the urinary sediment.[14] These cells have been shown to account for about 75 percent of the urinary cells shed by an affected hemizygote.[148]

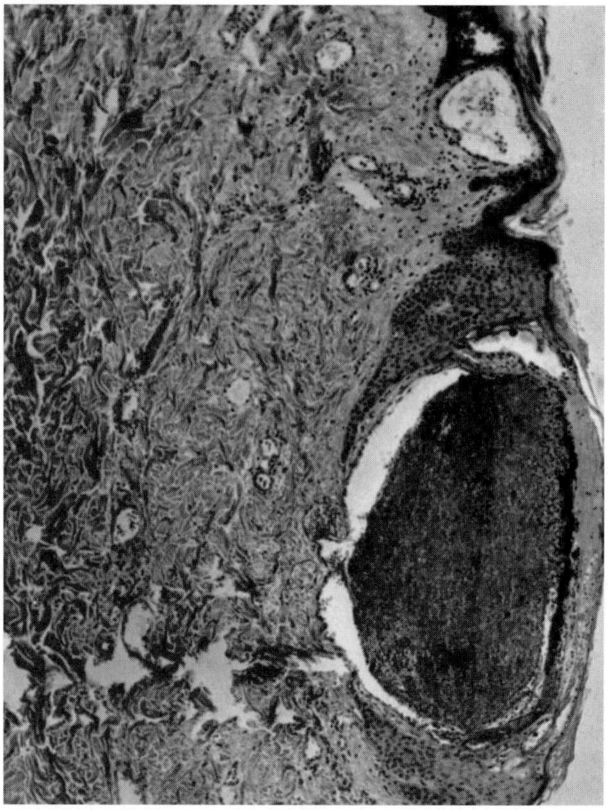

Fig. 150-6 Photomicrograph of the skin lesion reveals dilated vascular channels of varying size in the upper dermis. The vessels may contain thrombi, and the overlaying epithelium may be thinned, ulcerated, and/or keratotic. H&E, × 65.

Concurrently, renal blood vessels are involved progressively and often extensively. A late finding is arterial fibrinoid deposits, which may result from the necrosis of severely involved muscular cells.[7,138] Other histologic changes in the kidney are the sequelae of nonspecific, end-stage renal disease with evidence of severe arteriolar sclerosis, glomerular atrophy and fibrosis, tubular atrophy, diffuse interstitial fibrosis, and other secondary changes. Renal size increases during the third decade of life, followed by a decrease in the fourth and fifth decades. The renal involvement has been the subject of a recent report[80] and older comprehensive reviews.[79,145,149,150]

Nervous System

Vascular involvement also is prominent in the nervous system[151–158] and presumably accounts for the observation of minor EEG and EMG abnormalities in these patients. In addition, vascular ischemia and lipid deposition in the perineurium may cause the peripheral nerve conduction abnormalities of slowed conduction velocities and distal latency, respectively.[95] In both heterozygotes and affected hemizygotes, glycosphingolipid deposition in nervous tissue appears to be limited to perineural sheath cells of peripheral nerves, neurons of the peripheral and central autonomic nervous system, and certain primary neurons of somatic afferent pathways.[8,153–157,159] Lipid deposition has been observed in Schwann cells by some but not all investigators.[156,157] Qualitative[153–156] and quantitative[155] studies of peripheral sensory neurons in sural nerves and spinal ganglia have shown preferential loss of small myelinated and unmyelinated fibers as well as small

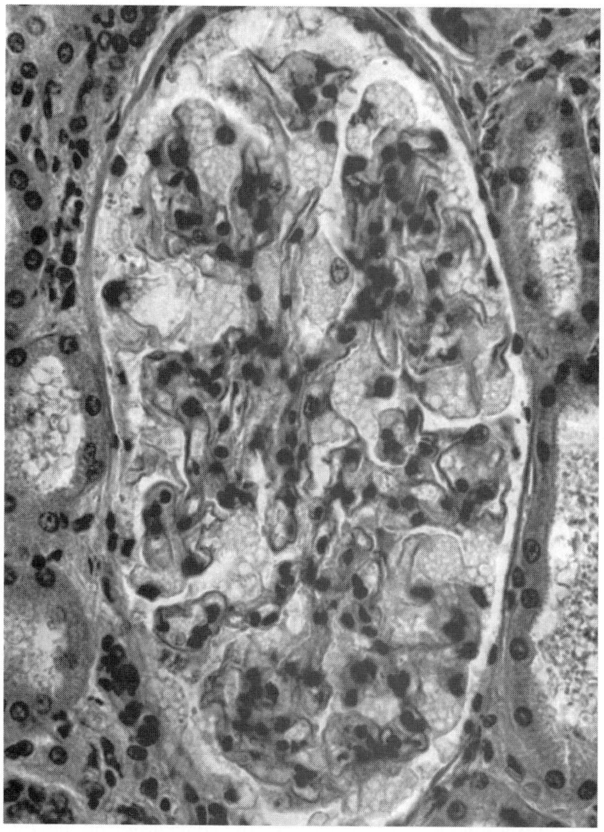

Fig. 150-7 Photomicrograph of a glomerulus from a 35-year-old classically affected male. The epithelial cells of the parietal and visceral layers of Bowman's capsule show multiple vacuoles from which the stored glycosphingolipids were extracted. Zenker's fixation, paraffin embedding. H&E, × 225.

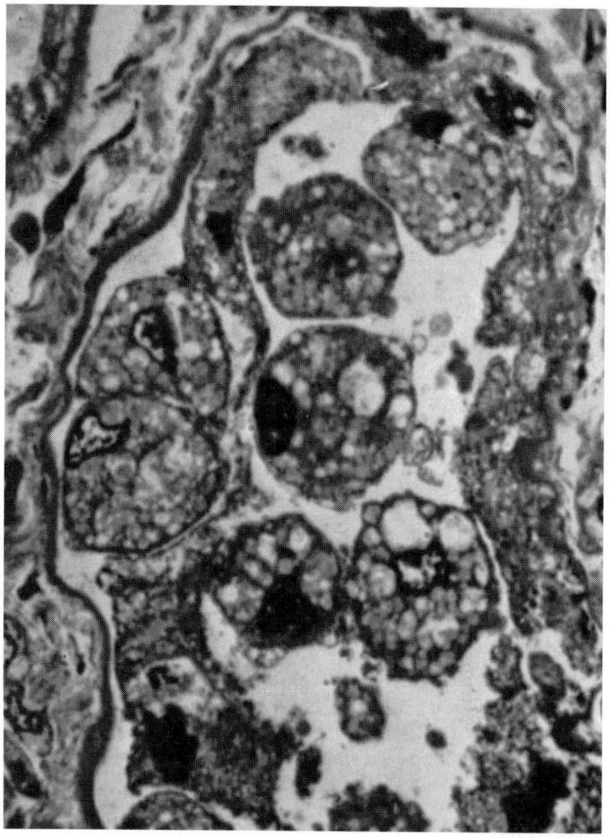

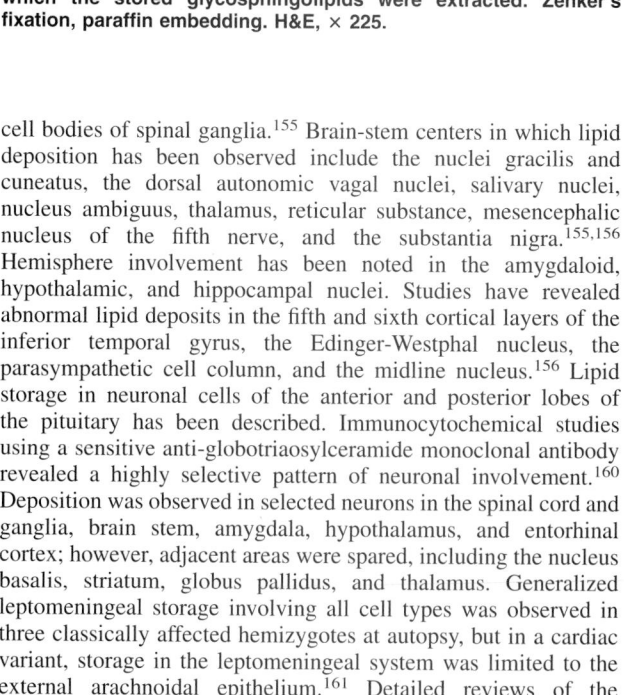

Fig. 150-8 Photomicrograph of the lipid-laden cells in the lining and in the lumen of a renal tubule. Formalin fixation, post fixation in osmium tetroxide, and embedding in Vestopal; 1-mm-thick section; × 1000.

cell bodies of spinal ganglia.[155] Brain-stem centers in which lipid deposition has been observed include the nuclei gracilis and cuneatus, the dorsal autonomic vagal nuclei, salivary nuclei, nucleus ambiguus, thalamus, reticular substance, mesencephalic nucleus of the fifth nerve, and the substantia nigra.[155,156] Hemisphere involvement has been noted in the amygdaloid, hypothalamic, and hippocampal nuclei. Studies have revealed abnormal lipid deposits in the fifth and sixth cortical layers of the inferior temporal gyrus, the Edinger-Westphal nucleus, the parasympathetic cell column, and the midline nucleus.[156] Lipid storage in neuronal cells of the anterior and posterior lobes of the pituitary has been described. Immunocytochemical studies using a sensitive anti-globotriaosylceramide monoclonal antibody revealed a highly selective pattern of neuronal involvement.[160] Deposition was observed in selected neurons in the spinal cord and ganglia, brain stem, amygdala, hypothalamus, and entorhinal cortex; however, adjacent areas were spared, including the nucleus basalis, striatum, globus pallidus, and thalamus. Generalized leptomeningeal storage involving all cell types was observed in three classically affected hemizygotes at autopsy, but in a cardiac variant, storage in the leptomeningeal system was limited to the external arachnoidal epithelium.[161] Detailed reviews of the neurologic findings are available.[156,159,160]

Eye

Histologically, abnormal glycosphingolipid deposits are found in endothelial, perivascular, and smooth-muscle cells of all ocular and orbital vessels, in smooth muscle of the iris and ciliary body, in perineural cells, and in connective tissue of the lens and cornea.[162,163] Inclusions have been found in the epithelium of the conjunctiva, cornea, and lens, and, by electron microscopy, in the basal layer of conjunctival epithelial cells, in the surface epithelium, and in the conjunctival goblet cells.[164] There may be hyperplasia and edema of corneal epithelial cells. Bowman's membrane appears normal, and no deposits are observed in the stroma or endothelium by light or electron microscopy. It has been suggested that the whorl-like corneal dystrophic pattern may result from the formation of a series of subepithelial ridges or from the reduplication of the basement membrane.[162,163]

Heart

The progressive deposition of glycosphingolipid in myocardial cells and valvular fibrocytes appears to be a primary cause of cardiac disease in affected hemizygotes and some heterozygotes.[16,46,47] Gross cardiomegaly involving all chambers has been observed. Most commonly, the left atrium and ventricle are enlarged, and the ventricular walls and septum are markedly thickened; right atrial and ventricular dilatation and enlargement are variable findings. Within the myocardial cells, there is extensive glycosphingolipid deposition around the nucleus and between myofibrils. The vessels show marked hypertrophy of the endothelial cells and smooth-muscle cells secondary to lipid deposition.

Mitral and tricuspid valves have numerous lipid-laden cells embedded in fibrous tissue.[16] The most common valvular defect is thickening and interchordal hooding of the leaflets of the mitral valve, with normal chordae tendineae and either normal or thickened and shortened papillary muscles. This defect may lead to the high incidence of mitral valve prolapse. The tricuspid valve may be similarly involved; the aortic and pulmonary valves are usually normal. Clinical and pathologic features of cardiac involvement in both affected hemizygotes and heterozygotes have been reviewed.[16,46,47]

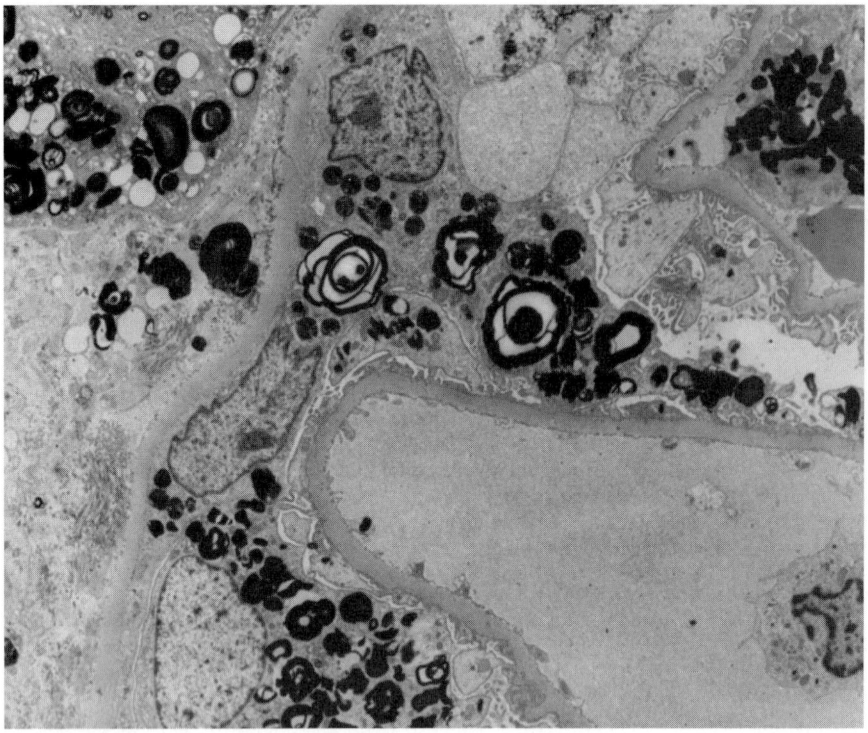

Fig. 150-9 Electron photomicrograph of a portion of a glomerulus, adjacent tubule, and an interstitial cell from a 32-year-old classically affected hemizygote. Note the numerous concentric lamellar inclusions in the lysosomes of the podocytes, Bowman's capsular epithelium, interstitial cells, and tubular epithelium. × 6200. *(Courtesy Dr. S.K. Lee and Ms. C.E. Sheehan, Albany Medical College.)*

Other Tissues

Many other organs, including the adrenal glands, gastrointestinal tract, liver, placenta, pancreas, prostate, testis, thyroid, and urinary bladder, show involvement of the blood vessels, smooth muscle, ganglia, and nerves. In addition, vacuoles or lipid stores have been demonstrated in epithelial cells, mucous glands, synovial membrane, smooth muscle of the bronchus, alveolar ciliated epithelial cells and goblet cells, type II alveolar epithelial pneumocytes, and skeletal muscle.[165] No inclusions have been found in alveolar macrophages. Involvement of reticuloendothelial cells has been noted in the bone marrow, liver, spleen, and lymph nodes.[34] Histologic examination of temporal bones from affected hemizygotes revealed strial and spiral ligament atrophy in all turns, hair cell loss mainly in the basal turns, and a decreased number of spiral ganglia.[166]

Histochemistry and Ultrastructure

The accumulated glycosphingolipids are birefringent and show a Maltese cross configuration in polarized light. They can be stained in frozen sections with lipid-soluble dyes, and may be removed from tissues by the process of dehydration and embedding in paraffin. If lipid-solubilizing procedures are used, empty vacuoles are observed by light microscopy. Most of the lipid crystals are retained through alcohol dehydration but are lost on exposure to xylene or pyridine. Exposure of formalin-fixed tissue to 3 percent potassium chromate for 1 week helps to preserve the lipid; improved fixation of the lipid deposits can be achieved with 1 percent calcium formol. A comparison of various fixation and embedding techniques to preserve the storage material has been reported.[167] A modified periodic acid-Schiff (PAS) stain specific for neutral glycosphingolipids[168] and a positive test for sphingosine[169] have served to confirm the chemical identification of the accumulated glycosphingolipids. Peroxidase-conjugated or fluorescent-labeled *Bandeiraea simplicifolia* lectin, which is specific for α-*D*-galactosyl residues, and antiglobotriaosylceramide antibodies also have been used to stain the glycosphingolipid substrates selectively.[148,167,170] The ultrastructural characteristics of the lesions and of the lipid inclusions in various tissues from affected hemizygotes have been described extensively.[171–173] At high resolution, a typical pattern of concentric or lamellar inclusions with alternating light- and dark-staining bands is observed (Fig. 150-9). The periodicity of these bands has been reported variably as 40 to 50 Å, 50 to 60 Å, 60 to 65 Å, or as great as 98 Å. The electron-dense component is 20 to 30 Å in thickness with coarser periods of 150 to 200 Å.

THE METABOLIC DEFECT IN FABRY DISEASE

Nature of the Accumulated Glycosphingolipids

The deficient activity of α-galactosidase A in patients with Fabry disease leads to the progressive accumulation of glycosphingolipids with terminal α-*D*-galactosyl residues in the lysosomes of most nonneural tissues and in body fluids. These substances are members of a family of structurally and metabolically related glycosphingolipids that are widely distributed in human tissues as normal surface constituents of plasma membranes[174,175] and of some intracellular membranes, including those of the Golgi and lysosomes.[176] In the plasma, they are associated with lipoproteins, with the highest concentration found in the low density lipoprotein fraction.[177–180] The concentrations of the individual neutral glycosphingolipids in the various lipoprotein fractions are presented in a previous edition of this text.[34]

Glycosphingolipid Structure. The lipoidal moiety of the amphipathic glycosphingolipids is a hydrophobic structure called ceramide, which consists of a mixture of 4-sphingenine (sphingosine) and related long chain aliphatic amines joined by amide linkages to various fatty acids. In neutral glycosphingolipids, the fatty acid moieties are primarily saturated and monounsaturated compounds with chain lengths from C16 to C26. Carbohydrate groups are covalently attached by a glycosidic linkage between the reducing end of the carbohydrate and the terminal hydroxyl group of the ceramide. The carbohydrate moiety may vary from a simple monosaccharide (cerebrosides) to large branched-chain oligosaccharides with 20 or more sugar residues.

The glycosphingolipids that accumulate in Fabry disease are neutral glycosphingolipids, as contrasted with the negatively

Table 150-4 Neutral Glycosphingolipids with Terminal α-Galactosyl Moieties of Human Origin

Chemical Structure	Trivial Name	Approved Nomenclature	Suggested Abbreviation
Gal (α1 → 4)Gal (β1 → 4)Glc(β1 → 1′)Cer	Ceramide trihexoside (trihexosylceramide)	Globotriaosylceramide	$GbOse_3Cer$
Gal (α1 → 4)Gal(β1 → 1′)Cer	Digalactosylceramide	Galabiosylceramide	$GaOse_3Cer$
Gal(α → 3)Gal (2 ← 1αFuc) (β1 → 3)GlcNAc-(β1 → 3) Gal(β1 → 4)Glc(β1 → 1′)Cer	Blood group B glycolipid	IV^2-α-Fucosyl-IV^3-α-galactosyl-lactotetraosylceramide	IV^2-α-Fucosyl-IV^3-α-Gal-$LcOse_4Cer$
Gal (α1 → 3)Gal (2 ← 1αFuc) (β1 → 4)GlcNAc-(β1 → 3) Gal(β1 → 4)Glc(β1 → 1′)Cer	Blood group B_1 glycolipid	IV^2-α-Fucosyl-IV^3-α-galactosyl-neolactotetraosylceramide	IV^2-α-Fucosyl-IV^3-α-Gal-$LcnOse_4Cer$
Gal(α1 → 4)Gal(β1 → 4)GlcNAc-(β1 → 3)Gal(β1 → 4)Glc(β1 → 1′)Cer	Blood group B_1 glycolipid	IV^2-α-Galactosyl-neolacto-tetraosylceramide	IV^2-α-Gal-$LcnOse_4Cer$

For more complete information on glycosphingolipid structure, see Macher and Sweeley.[182]

charged gangliosides and sulfoglycosphingolipids (sulfatides). The neutral glycosphingolipids have been grouped into families based on their structural or biosynthetic relationships, and these groups have provided the basis for their nomenclature.[181,182] The complete structural determination of individual neutral glycosphingolipids can be accomplished by proton resonance spectroscopy. Application of two-dimensional spin-echo J-correlated spectroscopy, nuclear Overhauser-effect spectroscopy, and J-relayed coherence transfer spectroscopy has permitted the complete delineation of the molecular structure, anomeric linkage, and linkage position of these glycosphingolipids.[183] Enzymes that specifically cleave the oligosaccharide moiety from ceramide[184,185] allow separate analyses of the carbohydrate and ceramide portions of various neutral and acidic glycosphingolipids. The structures and nomenclature for the neutral glycosphingolipids of human origin that have terminal α-*D*-galactosyl moieties are indicated in Table 150-4. More detailed information on glycosphingolipid structure, isolation, quantitation methods, and tissue distribution is available in several reviews.[175,186–188]

Globotriaosylceramide. In Fabry disease, there is widespread accumulation of the glycosphingolipid, globotriaosylceramide [Gal(α1 → 4)Gal(β1 → 4)-Glc(β1 → 1′)Cer], particularly in the lysosomes of vascular endothelial and smooth-muscle cells as well as in epithelial and perithelial cells of most organs. The positions of the glycosidic linkages, the anomeric configurations of these linkages, and the fatty acid compositions of globotriaosylceramides from normal and Fabry tissues have been rigorously established.[189] Such analyses have demonstrated that the accumulated glycosphingolipids isolated from tissues of patients with Fabry disease are identical to those of normal tissues.[190] Globotriaosylceramide is identical to the rare p^k blood group antigen on human erythrocytes[191–193] and has been used as a cell-specific marker for Burkitt lymphoma.[194–197] The complete structure of this glycosphingolipid is shown in Fig. 150-10*A*. Its stereoselective, total chemical synthesis has been accomplished.[198,199]

In normal individuals, the highest concentrations of globotriaosylceramide were found in the kidney, followed by aorta, spleen, and liver.[15,190,200–203] As a function of body mass, however, kidney, liver, lung, and erythrocytes contribute much of the normal glycolipid load. In classic hemizygotes with Fabry disease, increased concentrations of globotriaosylceramide were found in all analyzed sources except erythrocytes,[13,15,200,201,203] which indicates that most tissues are involved in the catabolism of these glycosphingolipids. The magnitude of accumulation of globotriaosylceramide in Fabry hemizygotes was thirty- to more than three hundredfold higher than normal levels.[15,200,201] The highest concentrations were found in kidney, lymph nodes, heart, prostate, striated muscle, and autonomic ganglia.[12,15,200,201] In contrast, a symptomatic 55-year-old heterozygote had globotriaosylceramide levels in the heart, liver, and kidney that were 3.2, 3.7, and 6.8 times greater than those in normal controls.[204]

Galabiosylceramide. A second neutral glycosphingolipid, galabiosylceramide [Gal(α1 → 4)Gal(β1 → 1′)Cer], also accumulates to abnormally high concentrations in Fabry hemizygotes and to a lesser extent in heterozygotes. The deposition of galabiosylceramide is tissue-specific, because this substrate has been detected only in the kidney, pancreas, right heart, lung, urinary sediment, and spinal and sympathetic ganglia.[12,14–16,200,205] The complete chemical structure of galabiosylceramide obtained from normal and Fabry kidney has been established[189] and is shown in Fig. 150-10*B*.

Blood Group B and P Glycosphingolipids. Two additional accumulated glycosphingolipids were identified in the pancreas of a Fabry hemizygote who had the blood group B and B1 antigens.[17] In human erythrocytes, there are two neutral glycosphingolipids with terminal α-galactosyl residues that inhibit blood group B-specific hemagglutination, the blood group B glycosphingolipid [Gal(α1 → 3)Gal(2←1αFuc)(β1 → 3)GlcNAc(β1 → 3)Gal(β1 → 4) Glc (β1 → 1′)Cer] and the blood group B1 glycosphingolipid [Gal(α1 → 3)Gal(2←1αFuc)(β1 → 4)GlcNAc(β1 → 3)Gal(β1 → 4) Glc(β1 → 1′)Cer].[17,189,206] The structures of the blood group B and B1 glycosphingolipids isolated from Fabry pancreas were established by biochemical, enzymatic, and immunologic methods and were identical to those of the B and B1 glycosphingolipids of normal human erythrocytes.[17,189] Their complete structures are shown in Fig. 150-10*C* and *D*. In general, glandular epithelial tissues such as stomach, pancreas, and intestine are rich sources of these fucose-containing neutral glycosphingolipids, whereas parenchymatous organs and erythrocytes contain lower quantities. The concentrations of the B and B1 antigens in the Fabry pancreas analyzed were approximately 50 percent of the level of the accumulated globotriaosylceramide.[17] Thus, Fabry hemizygotes and heterozygotes who have blood group B and AB accumulate four glycosphingolipid substrates, whereas patients with A or O blood groups accumulate only globotriaosylceramide and galabiosylceramide.

A fifth neutral glycosphingolipid that can accumulate in Fabry disease is the P1 blood group antigen. In the P blood group system, the p^k and p antigens have been shown to be globotriaosylceramide and globotetraosylceramide [GalNAc(β1 → 3)Gal(α1 → 4)Gal(β1 → 3)Glc(β1 → 1′)Cer].[191–193] Although blood group p^k and p are rare, the P1 antigen [Gal(α1 → 4)Gal(β1 → 4)GlcNAc(β1 → 3) Gal(β1 → 4)-Glc(β1 → 1′)Cer] is present in about 75 percent of the population.[193] To date, the accumulation of the P1 substance in Fabry disease has not been documented, nor has the possibility of increased disease severity due to the accumulation of this blood group substance been assessed.

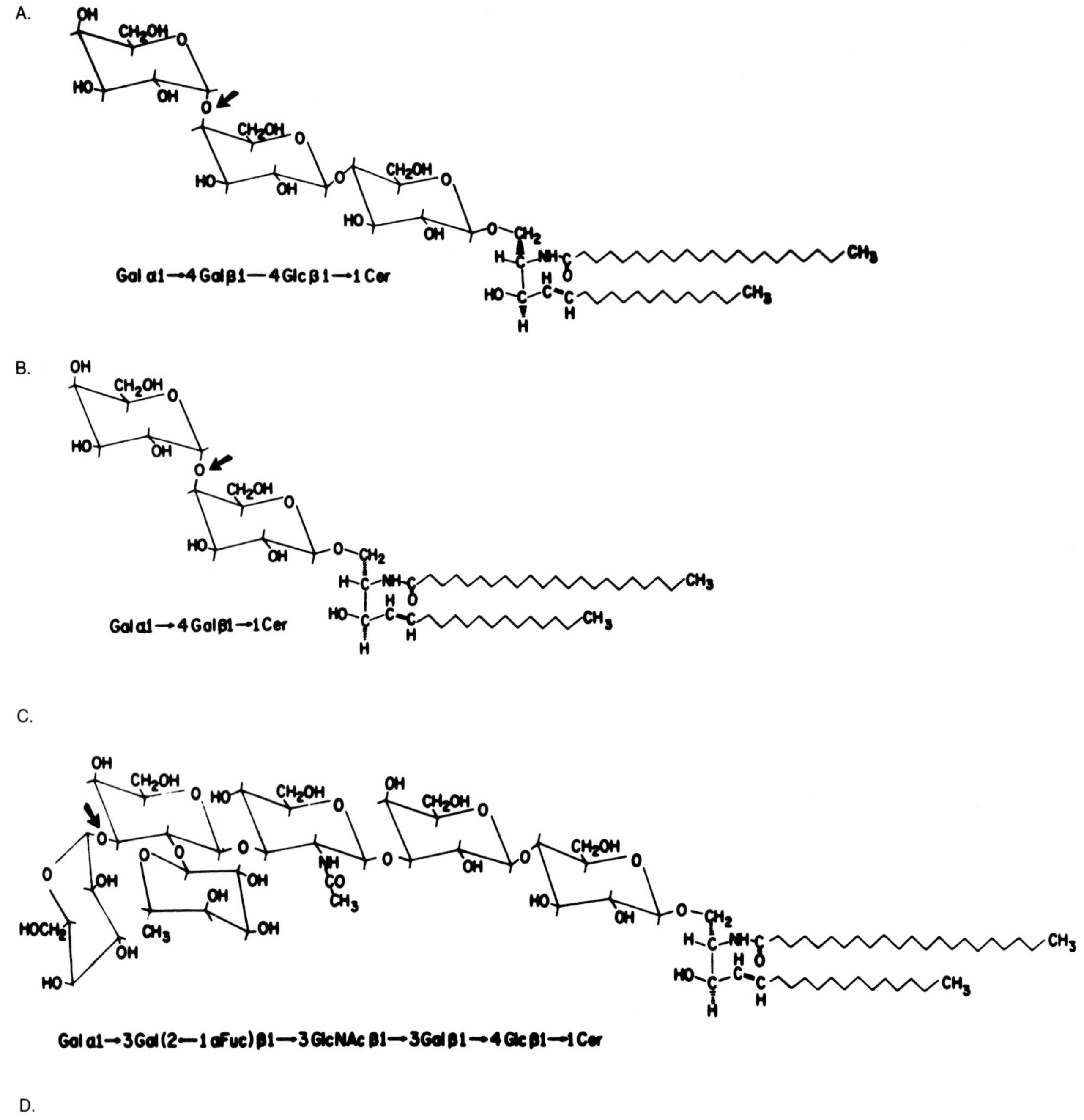

Fig. 150-10 Complete chemical structures of the neutral glycosphingolipids that accumulate in Fabry disease. *A*, Globotriaosylceramide, the major accumulated substrate. *B*, Galabiosylceramide. *C* and *D*, The blood group B and B1 antigenic glycosphingolipids, respectively, which accumulate in blood group B and AB patients. The arrows indicate the α-galactosyl bonds, which are normally cleaved by α-galactosidase A.

Glycosphingolipid Biosynthesis. Neutral glycosphingolipids are synthesized by sequential enzymatic reactions involving the stepwise addition of monosaccharide units to acceptors, which then become the appropriate substrates for subsequent enzymes in the pathway. This process, in which sugar nucleotides serve as donors of the carbohydrate residues, requires the concerted action of a group of glycosyltransferases that may be closely associated in a subcellular membrane as a multienzyme complex. A more extensive treatment of glycosphingolipid biosynthesis can be found in a previous edition of this chapter[189] and in reviews.[207–210]

In the following section, discussion is limited to the biosynthetic steps involved in the addition of the terminal α-galactosyl residues to the glycosphingolipids that accumulate in Fabry disease. These biosynthetic reactions are mediated by different α-galactosyltransferases that attach the galactose moiety from the sugar nucleotide, UDP-galactose (UDP-Gal), to the glycosphingolipid acceptor by an α-anomeric linkage. The α-galactosyltransferases involved in glycosphingolipid biosynthesis are important, because their specific activity and tissue-specific and/or regulated expression determine the cell and tissue distribution and the amount of the individual glycosphingolipids that accumulate in this disease. For example, lactosylceramide [Gal(β1 → 4)Glc(β1 → 1)Cer; LacCer] is found in all tissues and is the common precursor for the biosynthesis of certain neutral glycosphingolipids and gangliosides, whereas galactosylcerebroside [Gal(β1 → 1′)Cer], the precursor of galabiosylceramide, occurs primarily in the brain and kidney. Because the α-galactosyltransferase that recognizes galactosylcerebroside as an acceptor is present in kidney and not brain (see below), galabiosylceramide is not synthesized in the brain, consistent with the limited neuronopathic involvement in Fabry disease.

UDPGal:LacCer(α1 → 4)galactosyltransferase (GalT-6)[207] catalyzes the synthesis of globotriaosylceramide by addition of an α-galactosyl moiety to LacCer. The transferase has been highly purified from rat liver and is composed of two nonidentical subunits with molecular weights of about 65 and 22 kDa.[211] This enzyme is highly specific for LacCer and does not transfer α-galactosyl residues for the formation of galabiosylceramide or the blood group B or P1 antigens. The GalT-6 gene has been isolated from a cosmid library constructed from a human Burkitt lymphoma cell line, and the active enzyme has been expressed in mouse L5178 cells transfected with this gene.[212]

UDPGal:Gal(β1 → 1′)Cer(α1 → 4)galactosyltransferase catalyzes the synthesis of galabiosylceramide and has been characterized in crude particulate fractions of rat kidney.[213] The activity was differentiated from GalT-6 by its greater sensitivity to heat denaturation. Notably, the activity was present in kidney but not in brain, spleen, liver, or lung, consistent with the observed tissue distribution of galabiosylceramide in Fabry patients.

UDPGal:Gal(β1 → 4)GlcNAc[(β1 → 3) or (β1 → 4)Gal(β1 → 4)Glc(β1 → 1′)Cer(α1 → 3) galactosyltransferase catalyzes the synthesis of the B and B1 blood group glycosphingolipids.[214] Interestingly, there are two alleles for this transferase, designated B1 and B2.[215] The B1 allele produces the normal galactosyltransferase (B1) found in Caucasians, whereas the B2 allele, which is found primarily in blacks and Asians, encodes the B2 enzyme, which has a higher activity and a lower K_m for H substance. In fact, in AB blood type individuals, the B2 enzyme converts H substance to blood group B and B1 glycosphingolipids so efficiently that little blood group A glycosphingolipid is synthesized.[193] In black and Asian populations, the frequency of the B2 allele in B blood group individuals is about 30 to 40 percent and 10 percent, respectively. The occurrence of the B2 allele in affected hemizygotes with Fabry disease who are blood group type AB will result in the synthesis and subsequent accumulation of blood group B glycosphingolipids, at levels near those observed in blood group B homozygotes.[17] UDPGal:Gal(β1 → 4)GlcNAc(β1 → 3)Gal(β1 → 4)Glc(β1 → 1′)Cer(α1 → 4)galactosyltransferase (GalT-5) catalyzes the synthesis of the P1 blood group glycosphingolipid. The enzyme has been studied in crude preparations from rabbit bone marrow, bovine spleen, and human cultured lymphoblasts.[216–218] It is notable that the terminal α-anomeric linkage in the P1 substance is α1 → 4, whereas the terminal galactosyl linkages in the B and B1 glycosphingolipids are α1 → 3. The α1 → 4 linkage on the P1 glycosphingolipid apparently prevents the addition of fucose to the penultimate galactose in the P1 glycosphingolipids.

Plasma-neutral glycosphingolipids are synthesized primarily in the liver, where they are incorporated into lipoprotein particles.[219] This concept is supported by the kinetics of their turnover in plasma after incorporation in vivo of [^{14}C]glucose in pig[220] or [6,6-$^{2}H_2$]glucose in humans;[221] these kinetics are comparable to those observed with triacyl-sn-glycerols and phospholipids after pulse-labeling with fatty acids or inorganic phosphate.[222] The studies suggested that about 25 percent of the plasma glycosphingolipid pool was newly synthesized each day.[220] The reappearance of ^{14}C-glycosphingolipids in porcine plasma at 60 days after labeling indicated that a portion of the plasma glycosphingolipid pool is derived from senescent erythrocytes.[220] Thus, it appears that the liver and bone marrow are the primary synthetic sources of plasma glycosphingolipids. Because convincing evidence has been provided that erythrocyte glycosphingolipids, with carbohydrate moieties longer than those of glucosylceramide, do not exchange with lipoprotein glycosphingolipids in the circulation,[159,198] transfer must occur in tissues—presumably via specific transport proteins for glycosphingolipids that have been identified in spleen and liver.[223,224] The rate of exchange of plasma glycosphingolipids with those in plasma membranes has not been determined.

Catabolism. Glycosphingolipids are degraded in a stepwise fashion by a family of specific exoglycosidases, as illustrated by the pathway shown in Fig. 150-11 for the catabolism of globotetraosylceramide, galabiosylceramide, and the blood group B and P1 active hexa- and pentaglycosylceramides. Reactions catalyzed by individual glycosidases involved in these pathways have been extensively studied in cell-free extracts. Most of the enzymes have been obtained in relatively pure form, and their kinetic properties and substrate specificities determined. Virtually all of these exoglycosidases are glycoproteins with optimal catalytic activity at acidic pH. They occur predominantly, but not exclusively, in lysosomes. The existence of multiple forms of many of these enzymes may be related to their subcellular distribution, differences in their substrate specificities, and chemical heterogeneity due to structurally different carbohydrate moieties or subunit peptides, or both. In vivo, certain hydrophobic glycosphingolipid substrates are made available for hydrolysis by specific noncatalytic "activator" proteins that act as biologic detergents.[225,226] The resulting glycosphingolipid-glycoprotein complexes appear to be the true substrates for these glycosidases (with the notable exception of the glucocerebrosidase activator, which is an enzyme cofactor).[225,226] The lysosomal glycosidases involved in glycosphingolipid metabolism have been the subject of several reviews.[176,225–231]

α-Galactosidase A: The Enzymatic Defect in Fabry Disease

The enzymatic defect in Fabry disease is the deficient activity of the lysosomal enzyme, α-galactosidase A. Following the identification of globotriaosylceramide and galabiosylceramide as the accumulated substrates in Fabry disease,[12] Brady and coworkers synthesized globotriaosylceramide with a radiolabeled terminal galactosyl moiety and used the radiolabeled glycosphingolipid to demonstrate the presence of a galactosidase in normal intestinal tissue and its deficient activity in intestinal biopsy specimens from hemizygotes with Fabry disease.[18] The anomeric specificity of the deficient galactosidase activity was determined in 1970 by Kint, who demonstrated that leukocytes from hemizygotes with Fabry disease were deficient in an α-galactosidase assayed with either synthetic substrate, p-nitrophenyl-α-*D*-galactoside or

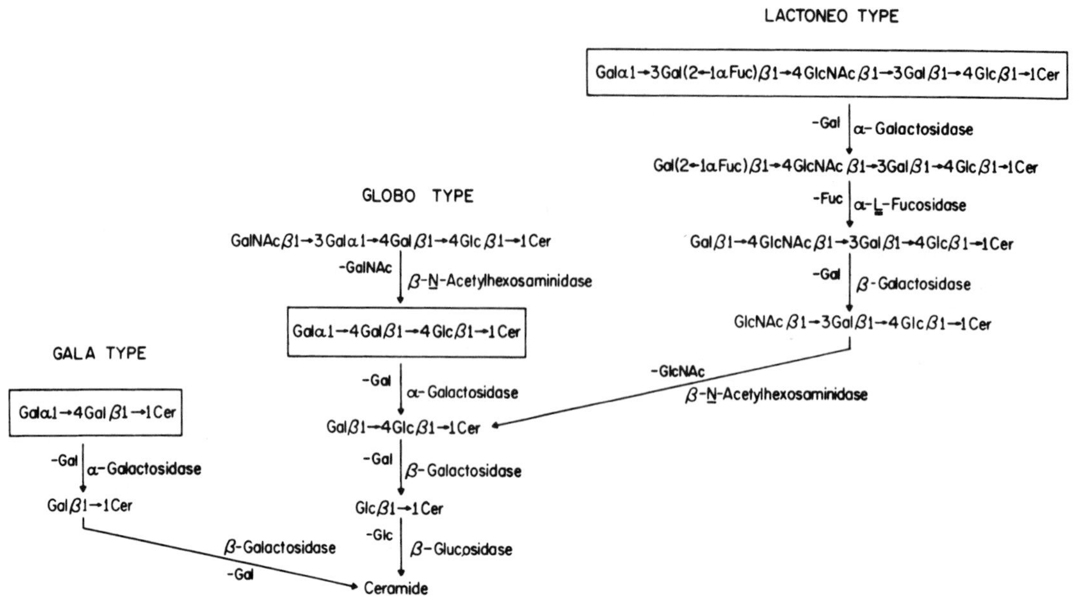

Fig. 150-11 Pathway for the catabolism of neutral glycosphingolipids involving the stepwise hydrolysis of individual sugar residues by specific glycosyl hydrolases. The accumulated substrates in Fabry disease—galabiosylceramide, globotriaosylceramide, and the blood group B glycosphingolipids—are indicated.

4-methylumbelliferyl-α-*D*-galactoside.[19] The identification of the anomeric linkage was confirmed in subsequent spectroscopic and enzymatic studies, which demonstrated that globotriaosylceramide from Fabry kidney has an $\alpha 1 \rightarrow 4$ linkage in the terminal galactosyl moiety.[232–236] Investigators documented the deficient activity of an α-galactosidase in affected hemizygotes and obligate heterozygotes using the radiolabeled natural substrate, globotriaosylceramide,[18] and/or synthetic chromogenic or fluorogenic substrates.[19,25,237]

α-Galactosidases A and B. Early studies with synthetic substrates revealed that classically affected hemizygotes had a level of α-galactosidase activity that was approximately 10 to 25 percent of that observed in the respective source from normal individuals.[25,237–239] The residual α-galactosidase activity in Fabry hemizygotes was thermostable and was not inhibited by myoinositol, whereas 80 to 90 percent of the total α-galactosidase activity in normal individuals was thermolabile and myoinositol-inhibitable.[25,237,238,240–242] Based on these studies with synthetic substrates, the two activities initially were thought to represent α-galactosidase isozymes and were designated α-galactosidases A and B.[217] The two "isozymes" were separable by electrophoresis, isoelectric focusing, and ion-exchange chromatography. After neuraminidase treatment, the electrophoretic migrations and pI values of α-galactosidases A and B were very similar,[19,243] suggesting that the two enzymes were the differentially glycosylated products of the same gene. The finding that the purified glycoprotein enzymes had similar physical properties, including subunit molecular mass (~46 kDa), homodimeric structures, and amino acid compositions, also indicated their structural relatedness.[20,21,239,244] However, the subsequent demonstration that polyclonal antibodies against α-galactosidase A or B did not cross-react with the other enzyme,[21,244] that only α-galactosidase A activity was deficient in hemizygotes with Fabry disease, and that the genes for α-galactosidases A and B mapped to different chromosomes,[34] clearly established that these enzymes were genetically distinct. Thus, it was not surprising when α-galactosidase B was shown in 1977 to be an α-*N*-acetylgalactosaminidase, a homodimeric glycoprotein that hydrolyzed artificial and natural substrates with terminal α-acetylgalactosaminyl moieties[20,21] including various *O*- and *N*-linked glycopeptides and glycoproteins, glycosphingolipids, and the proteoglycan, cartilage keratan sulfate II.[34] Further molecular studies demonstrated that the two enzymes were encoded by separate but evolutionarily related genes.[245,246] The deficient activity of α-galactosidase B is the specific enzymatic defect in a recently described neuroaxonal dystrophy known as Schindler disease[22] and its adult variant, which presents with angiokeratoma and glycopeptiduria (see Chap. 139).[23,247,248]

Purification. Human α-galactosidase A has been purified to homogeneity from various tissues and plasma. Most purification procedures employ a series of chromatographic steps, typically including chromatography on concanavalin A Sepharose, diethylaminoethyl (DEAE)-cellulose, hydroxyapatite and the α-galactosidase affinity resin, *N*-6-aminohexanoyl-α-*D*-galactosylamine coupled to Sepharose.[249–251] Although α-galactosidase B also binds to the affinity resin, it can be preferentially eluted, or prevented from binding, with *N*-acetylgalactosamine. By such procedures, human α-galactosidase A has been highly purified from liver,[252] spleen,[250] placenta,[250,253] and plasma.[250] The most highly purified material has been isolated from human lung by using high-performance liquid chromatography (HPLC) gel filtration to remove minor (<5 percent) contaminants.[34,250] Modifications of these procedures have been used to purify to homogeneity the recombinant human α-galactosidase A secreted by stably expressing Chinese hamster ovary (CHO) cells.[254]

Physical Properties. The native α-galactosidase A from human sources is a protein of approximately 101 kDa.[250,252,255,256] Polyacrylamide gel electrophoresis in the presence of sodium dodecylsulfate has consistently shown a single diffuse subunit band of about 49 kDa,[31,250,255,257] indicating that the enzyme has a homodimeric structure. The enzyme is a glycoprotein containing 5 to 15 percent asparagine-linked complex and high-mannose oligosaccharide chains.[249,250,256–258] Multiple forms are observed on isoelectric focusing of purified preparations from plasma and various tissues (Fig. 150-12). The isoelectric points of the tissue forms of α-galactosidase A ranged from 4.3 to as high as 5.1,[244,250,252,256] whereas the plasma form had a pI of 4.2.[250,255] The plasma and tissue forms of the enzyme were converted by neuraminidase to a single form with a sharp isoelectric focusing band of higher pI (5.1), which suggested that the heterogeneity resulted from variations in the amount of sialic acid on the

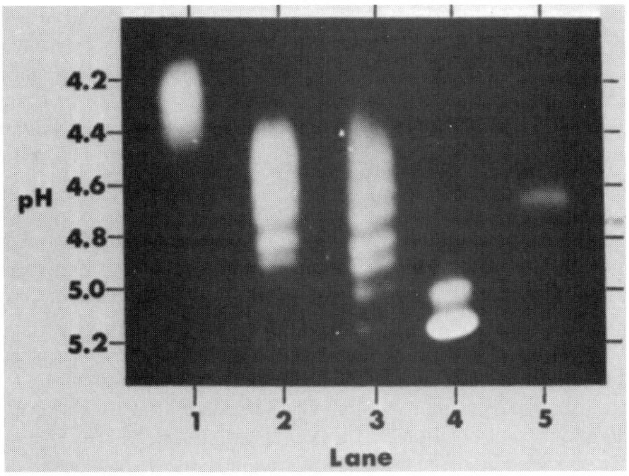

Fig. 150-12 Isoelectric focusing of purified α-galactosidase A. Lane 1, plasma form; lanes 2 and 3, splenic forms (different preparations); lane 4, placental form; lane 5, placental α-galactosidase B (α-*N*-acetylgalactosaminidase). (*Reproduced from Bishop and Desnick.*[250] *Used by permission.*)

carbohydrate chains. Such studies indicated that the plasma form contained 10 to 12 sialic acid residues, whereas the placental form of α-galactosidase A had only one or two residues.[250] The negatively-charged sialic acid residues were presumably responsible for the prolonged circulatory half-life of enzyme administered intravenously to patients with Fabry disease,[249] and may also determine which organs acquire enzyme activity after infusion (see below, "Structure-Function Studies of α-Galactosidase A").

Kinetic Properties. α-Galactosidase A isolated from normal tissues and fluids is a relatively heat-labile glycoprotein that catalyzes the hydrolysis of substrates possessing terminal α-galactosidic residues, including various synthetic water-soluble substrates and naturally occurring glycosphingolipids and glycoproteins. Maximal activity of α-galactosidase A with the artificial substrate 4-methylumbelliferyl-α-*D*-galactopyranoside is obtained at pH 4.6. The K_m of the reaction with this substrate is approximately 2 mM.[20,237,244,250,252,255,259] With the detergent-solubilized glycosphingolipid substrate globotriaosylceramide, the pH optimum is 3.8 to 4.0, and the K_m is 0.1 to 0.2 mM.[250,252,255,259] The turnover number[260] of the most highly purified human α-galactosidase A is approximately $6 \times$: 10^3 min^{-1}.[34,250]

Several substrate analogues of globotriaosylceramide have been described that could serve as useful tools for the study of α-galactosidase A structure and function. Conduritol C trans-epoxide is a moderately effective inactivator and presumably forms a covalent bond with an active carboxyl group in the catalytic site.[261] The glucose analogue of this compound has been used to identify active site peptides in yeast[262] and almond[263] glucosidases as well as in human glucocerebrosidase.[264] In addition, potent competitive inhibitors of coffee bean α-galactosidase A have been described; 1,4-dideoxy-1,4-imino-*D*-lyxitol and 1,5-dideoxy-1,5-imino-*D*-galactitol had reported K_i values of 0.2 and 0.4 μM, respectively.[265,266] Other inhibitors are described below (see "Chemical Chaperons"). Recently, 16 imino sugars were evaluated as potential α-galactosidase A potent competitive inhibitors.[267] Among them, 1-deoxy-galactonojirimycin was the most potent inhibitor of α-galactosidase A with an IC_{50} value of 0.04 μM. α-*Galacto*-homonojirimycin, α-*allo*-homonojirimycin and β-1-*C*-butyl-deoxygalactonojirimycin were effective inhibitors with IC_{50} values of 0.21 μM, 4.3 μM, and 16 μM, respectively. The K_m values were determined to be 0.04 μM (1-deoxy-galactonojirimycin), 0.25 μM (α-*galacto*-homonojirimycin), 2.6 μM (α-*allo*-homonojirimycin) and 16 μM (β-1-*C*-butyl-deoxy-galactonojirimycin), respectively. *N*-Alkylation, deoxygenation at C-2, and epimerization at C-3 of 1-deoxy-galactonojirimycin markedly lowered or abolished its inhibition toward α-galactosidase A. The in vitro cleavage of globotriaosylceramide by α-galactosidase A requires the addition of an appropriate detergent, such as sodium taurocholate, to make the substrate available through the formation of mixed micelles. In vivo hydrolysis of globotriaosylceramide, as well as certain other glycosphingolipids and gangliosides, is mediated by "activator" proteins (designated sphingolipid activator proteins [SAPs]) that form complexes with specific glycosphingolipids.[231,268,269] SAP-B (also called SAP-1 or saposin B) is a 22-kDa glycoprotein,[270–273] encoded by a gene localized to chromosome 10q22.1,[274–276] which binds to sulfatide, G_{M1} ganglioside, and globotriaosylceramide and renders these glycosphingolipids available (i.e., soluble) for hydrolysis by their respective lysosomal enzymes. Studies with insect-cell derived recombinant human α-galactosidase A in a detergent-free liposomal system demonstrated that degradation of globotriaosylceramide was dependent on the presence of both α-galactosidase A and SAP-B.[277] The presence of SAP-A, SAP-C, or SAP-D had no affect on degradation. Human hepatic SAP-B has been purified to homogeneity by several investigators,[270,278,279] and its cDNA and genomic sequences have been isolated and characterized.[280,281] Of note, the SAP-B concentration was normal in various tissues from a classically affected male with Fabry disease.[282] The inherited deficiency of SAP-B activity results in a recessive disorder that is phenotypically similar to metachromatic leukodystrophy,[283–286] a severe neurodegenerative disease (see Chap. 148). In patients with SAP-B deficiency, the α-galactosidase A, β-galactosidase, and cerebroside sulfatase activities were not detectable in urine.[271] Kinetic and immunologic analyses in these patients have documented the absence of the SAP-B protein.[271,284–286] Notably, the concentrations of globotriaosylceramide and galabiosylceramide in the urinary sediment of the SAP-B-deficient patients were markedly elevated,[271] similar to the pattern seen in urinary sediment from Fabry hemizygotes.[14] Thus, SAP-B-deficient homozygotes have at least three enzyme deficiencies, and the disease phenotype results from the accumulation of their respective substrates. Comprehensive reviews concerning the activator proteins are available.[269,287–289]

Enzyme Biosynthesis and Processing. Biosynthetic studies in cultured human cells have shown that the α-galactosidase A glycoprotein subunit is synthesized as a precursor peptide that is processed to the mature lysosomal subunit.[257,290] Metabolic labeling studies in cultured human fibroblasts[290] have identified a 50-kDa precursor that was processed via 47- to 50-kDa intermediates over several days to a mature lysosomal form of 46 kDa (Fig. 150-13). The transport to lysosomes is dependent on mannose-6-phosphate receptors, because the enzyme was secreted as a 52-kDa glycosylated precursor in mucolipidosis II cells or in the presence of NH_4Cl.[290] Studies of the *N*-linked oligosaccharide carbohydrate chains of the secreted precursor and intracellular lysosomal forms of the recombinant human enzyme are described above (see "Analysis of *N*-Linked Oligosaccharide Structures of Recombinant α-Galactosidase A").

Defective α-Galactosidase A in Fabry Disease

Several classes of mutations in the α-galactosidase A gene have been identified by biochemical and immunologic analyses. These include classic hemizygotes with no detectable α-galactosidase A activity or enzyme protein, classic hemizygotes with no enzymatic activity but detectable levels of enzyme protein, and atypical hemizygotes with residual α-galactosidase A activity and protein (see below). Immunologic techniques have been employed to determine the presence or absence of nonfunctional enzyme protein in classically affected males with essentially no detectable α-galactosidase A activity. Using rabbit anti-human α-galactosidase A antibodies, Beutler and Kuhl,[244,291] Rietra et al.,[292] and Hamers et al.[293] were unable to detect cross-reacting immunologic material (CRIM) in fibroblasts, leukocytes, urine, or renal tissue

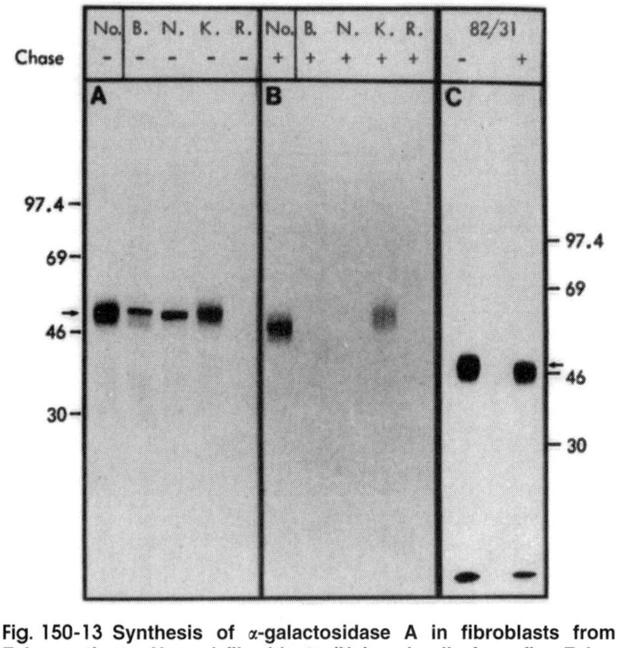

Fig. 150-13 Synthesis of α-galactosidase A in fibroblasts from Fabry patients. Normal fibroblasts (No) and cells from five Fabry hemizygotes (B, N, K, R, and 82/31) were labeled with [^{35}S] methionine for 4 h and harvested after labeling or after a chase for 2 days. α-Galactosidase A (arrows) was immunoprecipitated from cell extracts. See text for details. (*Reproduced from Lemansky et al.*[290] *Used by permission.*)

from eight classically affected hemizygotes from seven unrelated Fabry families. On the basis of these findings, they independently concluded that the mutations in these families were CRIM-negative. Thus, the inability to detect any residual α-galactosidase A activity in these Fabry sources was consistent with the absence of the enzyme protein.

Our laboratory also has evaluated the α-galactosidase A CRIM status in hemizygotes with Fabry disease. Using a monospecific rabbit antibody to homogeneous placental α-galactosidase A (which does not cross-react with α-galactosidase B), the presence of CRIM was evaluated by rocket immunoelectrophoresis in tissues from six unrelated, classically affected hemizygotes who had no detectable α-galactosidase A activity by assay of the immunoprecipitated protein. Renal or splenic tissues from four hemizygotes were CRIM-negative, but CRIM corresponding to about 1 to 5 percent of normal enzyme protein levels was detected in the tissues of two other hemizygotes.

Recently, we evaluated the α-galactosidase A CRIM status of an additional 26 classically affected hemizygotes with no detectable α-galactosidase activity who had specific missense or nonsense mutations (Ashton-Prolla et al., personal communication). CRIM status was assessed using an affinity-purified monospecific rabbit polyclonal antibody against purified recombinant human α-galactosidase A in an ELISA assay. All 26 unrelated males were CRIM-negative. Thus, the presence or absence of enzyme protein in classically affected males demonstrates the biochemical heterogeneity of the mutations causing this disease.

Affected males with classic disease manifestations have been observed who have plasma α-galactosidase A activities that were in the normal range (12 to 18 nmol/hr/ml, respectively; normal range 7.8 to 14.6 nmol/hr/ml), but deficient activity in peripheral leukocytes (0.7 to 2.1 U/mg protein, respectively; normal range 21.5 to 50 U/mg protein). In one patient the diagnosis of Fabry disease was made following a renal biopsy for proteinuria and deteriorating renal function. He had classic symptoms including angiokeratoma, hypohidrosis, and acroparesthesias. An affected nephew had the same biochemical and clinical phenotype. Molecular analysis revealed a missense mutation in which aspartic acid was substituted for the normal asparagine at position 244 (D244N). This lesion created a new glycosylation consensus sequence. The additional oligosaccharide chain apparently stabilized the enzyme at neutral pH, but the enzyme was nonfunctional and/or unstable at lysosomal pH. In vitro expression of the mutant enzyme protein in COS-1 cells showed high levels of activity in media and decreased hydrolysis of the natural substrate (Ashton-Prolla et al., personal communication).

A second unrelated male with a similar biochemical phenotype was diagnosed with Fabry disease prior to renal transplantation. He had a history of non-insulin-dependent diabetes and coronary artery disease requiring angioplasty. While he denied acroparesthesias, hypohidrosis, or angiokeratoma, he did have conjunctival changes consistent with Fabry disease. This patient had a missense mutation that resulted in the substitution of lysine for glutamic acid at position 59 (E59K). The expressed E59K protein had normal stability at pH 7.4, but was unstable at pH 4.6. Using the fluorescent substrate, a significant decrease in hydrolysis was observed. Fluorescence microscopy revealed a normal subcellular targeting pattern. Thus, these patients had mutant enzymes that were stable at neutral pH, but were unstable at lysosomal pH, thereby resulting in Fabry disease. Such findings emphasize the need to assay α-galactosidase A activity in cells for accurate diagnosis of symptomatic patients with normal plasma enzymatic activity.

The biosynthesis of α-galactosidase A in normal individuals and several Fabry hemizygotes has been studied.[290] As shown in Fig. 150-13, four different patterns were observed in classically affected hemizygotes. One hemizygote synthesized no enzyme precursor (R, Fig. 150-13*A*); two synthesized the precursor, but no enzyme protein was detected after a 4-day chase (B and N, Fig. 150-13*B*), indicating the instability of the mutant protein; and a fourth hemizygote synthesized an apparently normal enzyme precursor and mature lysosomal protein, but the protein was unable to hydrolyze the natural substrate (82/31, Fig. 150-13*C*). In a fifth hemizygote, who was an atypical variant with about 20 percent residual activity in cultured fibroblasts, the biosynthetic processing was delayed (K, Fig. 150-13*D*). The precursor was cleaved to an intermediate and then to the mature lysosomal subunit at a slower rate, suggesting a structural mutation that retarded the normal transport from the endoplasmic reticulum through the Golgi and endosomes to the lysosome. These findings further emphasize the heterogeneity in the mutations responsible for this disease and suggest that correlation with the specific molecular lesions in these and other patients may provide a relationship between structure-function of α-galactosidase A correlations (see "Molecular Pathology of Fabry Disease").

Residual Activity in Atypical Variants

Among lysosomal storage disorders, the rate of clinical progression in Fabry disease is among the slowest, reflecting the normally low rate of substrate metabolism. Therefore, variants with residual activity who are asymptomatic or express subtle renal and/or cardiac manifestations of the disease would be expected to present at advanced age. Patients with such rare variants have been described with milder manifestations of disease, including the "cardiac variants" (see "Atypical Hemizygotes; Cardiac Variants" above and Table 150-2).[44,111–120] In contrast to the classically affected hemizygotes, who have essentially no detectable α-galactosidase A activity, biochemical investigation of the atypical variants has revealed the presence of residual α-galactosidase A activity and cross-reactive immunologically detectable enzyme protein (CRIM) (see above "Defective α-Galactosidase A in Fabry Disease"), consistent with the attenuation or absence of the classical clinical manifestations. Several of the reported cardiac variants have been the subjects of biochemical studies. The 38-year-old Italian cardiac variant described by Clarke et al.[44] had ~20 percent of normal α-galactosidase A activity in his fibroblasts, and urinary sediment globotriaosylceramide levels in the heterozygote range. His residual α-galactosidase A activity in cultured fibroblasts was partially purified and shown to have kinetic and thermostability properties similar to those of α-galactosidase A from normal fibroblasts.[114]

The 42-year-old Italian cardiac variant who presented with severe rheumatoid arthritis[111] had residual α-galactosidase A activity that was about 1 percent of normal in plasma and urine and was subsequently shown to have the common N215S α-galactosidase A mutation.[294] Immunoprecipitation with monospecific anti-α-galactosidase A antibodies demonstrated residual activity in granulocytes, lymphocytes, platelets, liver, and cultured fibroblasts ranging from 9 to 37 percent of the respective normal levels. The immunoprecipitated residual α-galactosidase A activity from fibroblasts had the same kinetic and physical properties as the immunoprecipitated enzyme from normal fibroblasts. Rocket immunoelectrophoresis studies demonstrated that the level of α-galactosidase A activity corresponded to the amount of enzyme protein. However, compared with the normal enzyme, the residual fibroblast α-galactosidase A was more thermolabile at pH 4.6 and 50°C, and significantly less stable at pH 7.4 and 37°C. This finding was consistent with the extremely low enzyme levels in plasma and urine. Interestingly, the levels of globotriaosylceramide in plasma and urinary sediment were both in the low heterozygote range. No lysosomal inclusions were observed in hepatocytes or Kupffer cells in percutaneously biopsied liver, although ultrastructural evidence of glycosphingolipid was observed in a kidney biopsy. These findings were consistent with the N215S mutation resulting in an unstable enzyme with normal kinetics. In this variant, it appeared that 10 to 40 percent of normal intracellular activity was sufficient to prevent the major clinical manifestations of the disease. In addition, the finding of only 1 percent of enzymatic activity in the plasma and low levels of plasma globotriaosylceramide suggested that circulating enzyme was not required to catabolize the plasma substrate.

Of the cardiac variants, the 54-year-old German cardiac variant described by von Scheidt et al.[120] has been extensively studied (see above, "Atypical Hemizygotes: The "Cardiac Variant"). This variant who had the M296V α-galactosidase A mutation had the typical lysosomal inclusions in myocytes from an endocardial biopsy, but no histologic or ultrastructural evidence of lysosomal substrate deposition in myocardial capillaries or in other biopsied tissues. The patient's plasma globotriaosylceramide concentration (4.2 nmol/ml) was only slightly higher than the levels in his normal brothers (3.6 and 4.0 nmol/ml), whereas his urinary sediment concentration was at the low end of the heterozygote range. His α-galactosidase A activities ranged from 2 to 22 percent of the respective normal mean values in granulocytes (lowest), urine, lymphocytes, cultured lymphoblasts and fibroblasts, and plasma (highest). The disease manifestations in this 54-year-old variant were limited to the myocardium; there was no histologic evidence of small-vessel involvement or clinically manifest renal disease. Apparently the mutant enzyme in this variant with the M296V mutation was sufficiently active in vivo to markedly limit substrate deposition. Similar biochemical findings have been observed in the other cardiac variants (see Table 150-2).

Of interest is the 26-year-old Japanese variant described by Kobayashi et al.[113] who had no detectable α-galactosidase A activity in cultured fibroblasts when assayed with synthetic substrates. However, loading studies conducted in cultured fibroblasts demonstrated hydrolysis of some of the exogenously supplied substrate, which suggested the presence of residual activity toward the natural substrate.

Finally, a 51-year-old asymptomatic Arab male described by Bach and colleagues[112] had 10 percent of normal α-galactosidase A activity in cultured skin fibroblasts and normal levels of globotriaosylceramide in his urinary sediment. Further enzymatic studies revealed that the residual enzymatic activity had a K_m value that was fourfold higher than normal and an increased stability.

Recently, we evaluated the α-galactosidase A CRIM status of six unrelated cardiac variants who had residual α-galactosidase activity and whose mutations were known (E59K, R112H, F113L, D244N, M296V, and R356W). Using an affinity-purified monospecific rabbit polyclonal antibody against purified recombinant human α-galactosidase A in an ELISA assay, all six variant males were CRIM-positive with CRIM levels of 1.1 to 7.8 percent of normal (Ashton-Prolla et al., personal communication).

THE MOLECULAR GENETICS OF α-GALACTOSIDASE A

Our understanding of human α-galactosidase A and Fabry disease has been advanced dramatically by the isolation of the full-length cDNA and entire genomic sequence encoding this lysosomal enzyme.[31–33] The full-length cDNA sequence provided the primary structure of the enzyme precursor, including the signal peptide. The subsequent isolation and sequencing of the entire chromosomal gene for α-galactosidase A allowed characterization of the structural organization and regulatory elements of this housekeeping gene.[32,33] *In situ* hybridization, restriction fragment length polymorphism (RFLP) studies, and the recent isolation and analyses of yeast artificial chromosomes (YACs) containing the α-galactosidase A gene and flanking markers[295–298] provided both genetic and physical mapping of the α-galactosidase A gene to the Xq22.1 region of the X chromosome. Initial studies of the mutations in unrelated Fabry families have identified a variety of lesions underlying the molecular genetic heterogeneity of this disease (see "Molecular Pathology of Fabry Disease" below). More accurate carrier diagnosis has become possible by identification of the specific lesions in families or by analysis of closely linked polymorphisms (see "Diagnosis" below). Eukaryotic expression of the full-length cDNA has resulted in the production of large amounts of active enzyme for characterization, crystallization, and trials of enzyme replacement therapy (see "Treatment" below). In addition, site-specific mutagenesis has been employed to provide information on the structure and function of the enzyme.

Gene Assignment

The locus for human α-galactosidase A was assigned to the X chromosome in 1970 when Kint convincingly demonstrated that the defective globotriaosylceramide hydrolysis in Fabry disease was due to the deficient activity of α-galactosidase A.[19] Gene-mapping studies of human-hamster somatic cell hybrids localized the α-galactosidase A gene to a region on the long arm of the X chromosome, Xq21 → q24.[299,300] Subsequently, the regional assignment was narrowed to Xq21 → q22 by using a series of somatic cell hybrids made from a human cell line with an X,2,15 translocation, 46X,t(X;2;15)(q22;p12;p12).[301] This localization was further refined to the region Xq22 by *in situ* hybridization using the radiolabeled cDNA as a probe.[34,302] In addition, the restriction fragments detected in genomic DNA by Southern hybridization, using the full-length cDNA as a probe, exactly matched those identified by restriction mapping of genomic clones for α-galactosidase A, which indicated the absence of closely related sequences or pseudogenes.[303] Thus, the *in situ* and Southern hybridization studies established the occurrence of a single X-chromosomal gene for human α-galactosidase A.

The gene assignment was localized to Xq22 by RFLP studies that indicated that the α-galactosidase A locus was closely linked to the anonymous X-chromosome probes DXS17 and DXS87, but not to DXS11 or DXYS1.[304–307] The Xq22 region spans approximately 10 to 12 megabases (Mb) of genomic DNA in the proximal long arm of the X chromosome. Detailed physical maps of this region have been constructed by pulsed-field gel electrophoresis and radiation hybrid mapping.[308] Recently, YACs containing the α-galactosidase A gene were isolated, and the order and distances of the flanking markers were defined.[295,296] These studies identified several CpG islands in the Xq22 region that predicted the presence of a high density of functional genes in this area.[295,297] More recently, an integrated STS/YAC physical, genetic, and transcript map of human X-chromosomal region

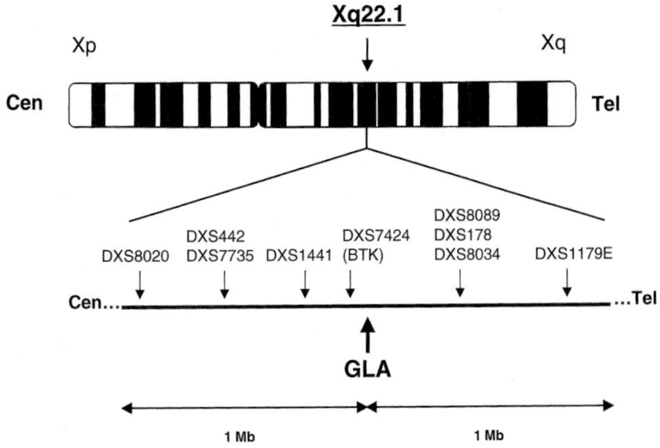

Fig. 150-14 Idiogram of the human G-banded X chromosome illustrating the position of band Xq22.1 (below) and the genomic map of the α-galactosidase A (GLA) gene and selected flanking markers with distances centromeric (−1 Mb) and telomeric (+1 Mb) from the α-galactosidase A locus indicated above. (After[296,298])

containing the α-galactosidase A gene has further defined its position and relevant flanking genes and polymorphic markers (Fig. 150-14).[298] Several other genes involved in genetic disorders were found in the vicinity of α-galactosidase A. These include the α5(IV) collagen gene COL4A5[309] that is defective in Alport syndrome,[310] PLP in Pelizaeus-Merzbacher disease and spastic paraplegia,[311,312] and the agammaglobulinemia tyrosine kinase (BTK) gene that is defective in Bruton agammaglobulinemia.[313] To date, over 30 genes as well as 56 unique expressed sequences have been identified in the region of Xq21.3-q23/24.[298]

The 1999 combined map covers the region Xq21.3 to Xq23/24 and provides 100 kb inter-STS resolution in 291 YACs formatted with 201 STS.[298] Thirty dinucleotide repeat markers and 51 unique expressed sequence tags (ESTs) have been placed on this map. The order of some of the polymorphic markers and genes within 5 Mb of α-galactosidase A include cen···DXS8077-DXS454-DXS1231-DXS8034-DXS8020-BTK-GLA-DXS8089-PRKC1-DXS101-DXS1106-DXS8096-PLP-DXS1191-DXS8075-DXS95-DXS17···tel. Useful flanking markers for haplotyping patients include DXS8020, DXS442, DXS7424, DXS8089, DXS178, and DXS8034, all within 1 Mb of the α-galactosidase A gene (Fig. 150-14). The closest centromeric gene, *BTK*, was determined by sequencing to be ~9 kb from α-galactosidase A.[314] The availability of this X21.3-Xq23 contig facilitated the identification of useful polymorphic simple sequence repeats for rapid heterozygote detection and prenatal diagnosis in families whose specific mutations have not been identified (see "Molecular Diagnosis of Heterozygotes" below). This region and the entire sequence of the X chromosome is being determined as part of the Human Genome Project and should become available shortly.

The α-Galactosidase A cDNA

Isolation and Characterization of the Full-Length cDNA. The full-length cDNA encoding human α-galactosidase A was isolated, sequenced, and expressed in COS-1 cells.[31,32,315,316] The pcDAG126 full-length cDNA contained 60 bp of 5′ untranslated sequence, the initiation codon, and the entire open reading frame, which encoded a 31-amino-acid signal peptide and the 398 residues of the mature enzyme subunit. The 1290-bp coding sequence predicted unglycosylated precursor and mature enzyme subunits of $M_r = 48{,}772$ and 45,356, respectively. The signal peptide predicted for the precursor subunit was consistent in size with that predicted from maturation studies in which human α-galactosidase A was synthesized as an ~55-kDa precursor glycoprotein and then was proteolytically cleaved to the mature ~51-kDa lysosomal glycoprotein.[290] The weight-matrix method of von Heijne[317] predicted cleavage at the signal peptide after Ala-31 (score = 7.36). This site was consistent with Leu-32 being the amino-terminal residue, as established by microsequencing of the purified enzyme.[31,316] The predicted signal peptide had typical features,[317,318] including a basic amino acid in the first five residues followed by a central hydrophobic core of 15 residues, two α-helix breakers (proline or glycine) −4 to −8 residues from the cleavage site, a more polar C-terminal region, and the most frequently observed C-terminal sequence, Ala-X-Ala. The microsomal cleavage of the signal peptide appears to be the only amino-terminal processing step in the biosynthesis of α-galactosidase A as is the case with several other human lysosomal enzymes,[319] although some enzymes contain pre and pro segments, which require a second cleavage to form the mature polypeptide.[320,321]

Analysis of the predicted amino acid sequence revealed four possible *N*-glycosylation sites. The four sites were located in β-turns within hydrophilic regions of the enzyme[322] consistent with their probable surface localization. Of the four, only three sites were occupied[323] (see "Structure-Function Studies of Human α-Galactosidase A" below). The most C-terminal site, Asn-Pro-Thr, which is rarely glycosylated,[319] was not used. Consistent with these findings, three oligosaccharide chains per subunit were suggested by previous studies of purified α-galactosidase A from human plasma and spleen[250] and immunoprecipitated enzyme from cultured cells.[257]

An unusual feature of most α-galactosidase A cDNAs isolated from different libraries was the absence of a 3′ untranslated sequence.[31–34] The polyadenylation signal sequence was in the coding region 12 bp from the termination codon, which was followed by the poly(A) tract. This finding is very rare among human nuclear-encoded mRNAs.[324] In two other α-galactosidase A cDNAs, pcDAG7 and pcDAG41, the TAA termination codons were followed by the short 3′ untranslated sequences, AATGTTT and AATGTC,[33] respectively, whereas a previously reported cDNA279 had the sequence AATGTT. Thus, although the majority of the isolated α-galactosidase A cDNAs lack a 3′ untranslated sequence, alternative cleavage and polyadenylation can result in a short 6- or 7-bp untranslated sequence following the termination codon. These alternative, short 3′ regions may indicate microheterogeneity of mRNAs due to alternative sites for the primary α-galactosidase A cleavage reaction.[325] Additionally, a second upstream (−28 bp from the termination codon) polyadenylation signal, AATACA, may be involved in the variant cleavages. Whatever the mechanism responsible for these alternative 3′ sequences, it is notable that the α-galactosidase A transcript does not require a 3′ untranslated region for expression in human cells.

Searches of amino acid and nucleotide sequence databases identified a few sequences with very limited similarity to human α-galactosidase A.[32] The notable exception was human α-galactosidase B (α-*N*-acetylgalactosaminidase; see Schindler disease in Chap. 139), which had remarkable nucleotide and amino acid homology with α-galactosidase A, suggesting an evolutionary relationship.[245,246] Alignment of their cDNA sequences required only four gaps and two insertions of three nucleotides each (see "The α-Galactosidase Gene Family" below).

The α-Galactosidase A Gene

Structural Organization. The entire 12-kb α-galactosidase A gene, which contains seven exons, has been completely sequenced.[33] The exons range in length from 92 to 291 bp, whereas the introns vary from 200 bp to 3.7 kb (Fig. 150-15). All intron-exon splice junctions follow the "GT/AG" rule[326] and are consistent with the consensus sequences for splice junctions of RNA polymerase II-transcribed genes.[327] Exon 1 contains the entire 5′ untranslated region, the sequence encoding the signal peptide, and the first 33 residues of the mature enzyme subunit. Intron 1 contained an 84-bp CT repeat that was not polymorphic. There were 12 *Alu* repetitive elements distributed throughout the intervening sequences and in the 3′ flanking region (see Fig. 150-15). These 300-nucleotide middle repetitive elements constituted about 30 percent of the gene. Thus, the α-galactosidase

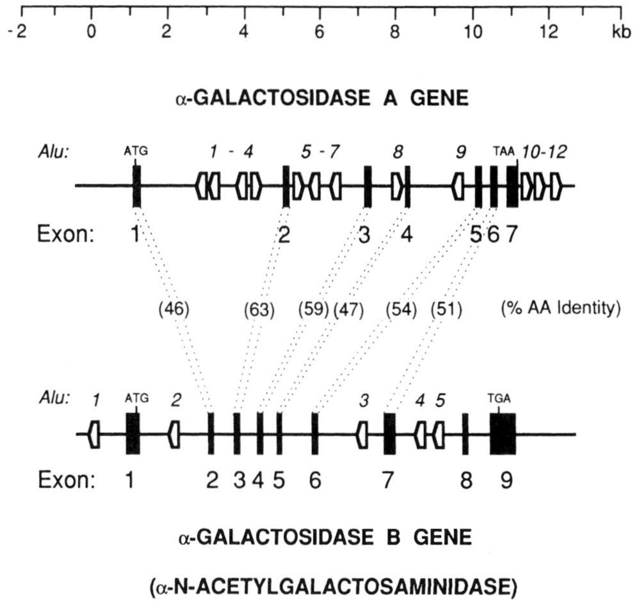

Fig. 150-15 Structures of the α-galactosidase A and B genes. Exons are denoted by solid rectangles. The positions and orientations of the *Alu* repeats are indicated. Homologous exons are denoted by dashed lines, and the percentage amino acid identity is indicated in parentheses.

A gene is one of the most *Alu*-rich genes with ~1 *Alu*/kb. When categorized into the *Alu* "subfamilies" according to the classification of Jurka and Smith,[328] all 12 *Alu* elements had sequences homologous to the more modern "S subfamily"; 9 were further subdivided into the older "a branch," 2 were assigned to the more recent "b branch," and 1 to the intermediate "c branch."[328] When each of these repeats was aligned with the consensus sequence, the percent divergence (based on the number of mismatches due to base substitutions, insertions, and/or deletions) ranged from 9 to 15. Analogously, comparison of the *Alu* sequences to each other revealed a divergence of 12 to 21 percent, which suggested that each *Alu* resulted from a separate retroposition event. Of the 24 CpG dinucleotides in the *Alu* consensus sequence, the number in each of the 12 *Alu* repeats in the α-galactosidase A gene that presumably had undergone spontaneous deamination of 5-methylcytosine to thymidine ranged from 8 to 20.[33,329]

Regulatory Elements. ">The α-galactosidase A gene contains several putative regulatory elements in the 5′ flanking region, including a TAATAA sequence, five CCAAT box sequences, and two GC box consensus sequences for the promoter-binding transcription factor Sp1.[33] Several potential enhancer-binding sites are present, including the conserved recognition motif (TGACTCA) of the AP1 enhancer-binding protein,[330] the immunoglobin "OCTA" enhancer element,[331] a reverse complement of the c-fos enhancer element GATGTCC,[332] and four direct repeats of the "chorion box" enhancer.[333] As yet, the functional significance of these putative promoter-enhancer elements in the regulation of α-galactosidase A gene expression has not been defined. Of interest, a −30G to −30A substitution in a putative NF-kB/Ets consensus binding site was detected in normal individuals who expressed two to threefold elevations in their plasma α-galactosidase A levels. In vitro translation studies of normal and −30A transcripts revealed similar levels of enzyme protein, suggesting that the point mutation enhanced transcription.[334]

The α-galactosidase A gene contains a methylation-free island, or "HTF island," in the region upstream from the initiation ATG (bp −660 to +1) that includes the indicative *Sac*II site.[335] These DNA islands are sequences of 500 to 2000 bp that are enriched in CpG dinucleotides (CpG/GpC > 1.0) in GC-rich regions (>50 percent) and are typically found in "housekeeping" genes.[336] The G + C content of this region in the α-galactosidase A gene is 54 percent, and the CpG/GpC dinucleotide ratio is 1.4. HTF islands have been implicated in maintaining the inactivation of X-linked genes.[337,338] Analysis of the methylation patterns in this region in active versus inactive X chromosomes should be of interest.[339]

The 3′-Flanking Region. As noted above, the 3′-untranslated region in α-galactosidase A cDNAs was absent or extremely short (i.e., 5 to 7 bp). Sequencing of the 3′-flanking region of the genomic clone indicated that this was not an artifact of cDNA library construction.[32,33] The 3′-flanking region also contained sequences with similarities to the consensus downstream elements, YGTGTTYY ("GT-box") and Tn ("T-rich") that are involved in polyadenylation.[340–342] Because two pairs of these downstream elements occur in the α-galactosidase A gene, it is possible that the alternative cleavage sites may be due to the presence of these additional, more 3′ elements.

The α-Galactosidase Gene Family. As noted above, human α-galactosidases A and B had similar biochemical properties, and the subsequent isolation of their respective full-length cDNAs revealed remarkable overall identity of their predicted amino acid sequences (46.9 percent).[245] Subsequent isolation and sequencing of the entire 14-kb gene encoding human α-galactosidase B (located at chromosome 22q11) permitted comparison of its genomic organization with that of α-galactosidase A.[246] Six of the eight α-galactosidase B introns (2 through 7) interrupted the gene at positions identical to those of all six introns in the α-galactosidase A genomic sequence (see Fig. 150-15). The percentage amino acid identity between the homologous α-galactosidase A exons 1 through 6 and α-galactosidase B exons 2 through 7 ranged from 46.2 to 62.7 (49.2 to 66.1 percent isofunctional similarity), with only a few single amino acid gaps (see Fig. 150-15). In contrast, the homology between α-galactosidase A exon 7 and α-galactosidase B exons 8 and 9 dropped significantly to 15.8 percent, with multiple gaps. The divergence between the two coding regions occurred at nt 957 of the α-galactosidase B cDNA, which is the last nucleotide in α-galactosidase B exon 7. The homologous intron placement and remarkable amino acid identity of the six exonic sequences suggest that the α-galactosidase B and α-galactosidase A genes had a common origin. Presumably, they were duplicated from a common ancestral gene and underwent subsequent divergence to acquire their specific functions.[343] A similar mechanism has been proposed for the evolution of the β-hexosaminidase α- and β- chains[344] and the functional β-glucosidase gene and adjacent pseudogene.[345] Lack of homology between α-galactosidase B and α-galactosidase A after α-galactosidase B exon 7 suggests that this position may represent the 3′ boundary of the common ancestral gene. Additional support for this concept is derived from the finding of predicted amino acid homology in human α-galactosidase B cDNA with the human, yeast, and *E. coli* α-galactosidase cDNAs,[32,346,347] which suggests that α-galactosidase B exons 2 through 7 were conserved functional domains common to these enzymes. Thus, there is an α-galactosidase family of genes that share functional domains. Subsequent structure-function and crystallographic studies should permit further assessment of the "α-galactosidase-specific" domains that have been conserved in evolution.

The Murine α-Galactosidase A Gene. The murine α-galactosidase A cDNA and genomic sequences have been isolated and characterized.[348,349] The cDNA predicts a subunit of 419 residues that are highly homologous (79 percent) with its human counterpart, including the 31-residue leader sequence. The murine cDNA has two polyadenylation sites that generate ~1.4 and ~3.6 kb transcripts. All intron/exon junctions are in the same positions as in the human ortholog. The murine promoter was TATA-less and had Sp1 and AP1 elements, like its human counterpart.

Expression of Recombinant α-Galactosidase A

Prokaryotic Expression. To evaluate expression of the unglycosylated protein in *E. coli*, the λAG18 cDNA, which encodes the mature form of α-galactosidase A, and a derivative cDNA construct containing the signal peptide sequence were inserted into the ptrpL1 plasmid containing the regulatable Trp promoter.[350] Low-level expression of the human enzyme was detected immunologically in maxicell experiments, but detection of activity using synthetic substrates was not possible. Subsequently, Ioannou et al.[351] inserted the full-length pcDAG126 cDNA into the prokaryotic secretion expression vector PIN-III-omp A[352] and detected significant levels of active human α-galactosidase A in *E. coli* K12 strain M2701[353] in which the bacterial α-galactosidase A gene, *melA*, is defective. However, the unglycosylated form of human α-galactosidase A produced in *E. coli* was unstable, indicating the importance of glycosylation (see "Structure-Function Studies of Human α-Galactosidase A" below) and precluding the large-scale microbial production of the human enzyme.

Mammalian Expression. Human α-galactosidase A has been transiently expressed in COS-1 and other cultured cells.[254] Active enzyme is detected primarily in cellular lysosomes, but also in the media. *N*-terminal purification or expression tags impair enzymatic activity, indicating the importance of the *N*-terminal structure in enzyme function. In contrast, *C*-terminal tags have had little, if any, effect on enzyme stability or function.[354,355] Consistent with this finding, deletion of 2 to 10 *C*-terminal amino acids enhanced enzymatic activity up to sixfold, while deletion of 12 or more *C*-terminal residues resulted in the complete loss of activity.[356] Of note, the highly homologous murine ortholog encodes 419 residues, lacking the last 10 *C*-terminal residues in the human enzyme.[349,357]

Human α-galactosidase A has been successfully overexpressed in CHO cells by a stable amplification strategy, and its biosynthesis and targeting have been investigated.[254] Clone AGA5.3, which was the highest enzyme overexpressor, produced intracellular α-galactosidase A levels of 20,900 U/mg (100 μg of enzyme/10^7 cells) and secreted ~13,000 U (75 μg/10^7 cells) per day. Ultrastructural examination of these cells revealed numerous 0.25 to 15 μM crystalline structures in the dilated *trans*-Golgi network (TGN) and in lysosomes (Fig. 150-16*A* and *B*). These crystalline structures were stained with immunogold particles using affinity-purified anti-human α-galactosidase A antibodies (Fig. 150-16*C*). Pulse-chase studies revealed that ~65 percent of the recombinant α-galactosidase A synthesized by these cells was secreted, while endogenous CHO lysosomal enzymes were not, which indicated that the α-galactosidase A secretion was specific. The intracellular and secreted forms of human α-galactosidase A were normally glycosylated, processed, and phosphorylated. The secreted enzyme had mannose-6-phosphate (M6P) moieties, and bound the immobilized 215-kDa mannose-6-phosphate receptor (M6PR). The uptake of the secreted enzyme by Fabry fibroblasts was inhibited by 2 mM M6P. These studies demonstrated that the overexpressed enzyme's selective secretion did not result from oversaturation of the M6PR-mediated pathway or abnormal binding to the M6PR. In fact, the overexpression of acid sphingomyelinase and α-galactosidase B in these amplifiable expression vectors resulted in their respective selective secretion.[254] These findings led other investigators to overexpress lysosomal cDNAs in this or related systems, resulting in their high level expression, selective secretion, and easier purification.[358–363] The mechanism of the enzyme's selective secretion has not been investigated, but several explanations have been advanced including an aggregation-secretion model and the possibility of specific, but rate-limiting chaperons for transport to the lysosome.[254]

The stable overexpression of human α-galactosidase A permitted the large-scale production of both lysosomal and secreted forms of this enzyme for characterization, crystallization, and for clinical trials of enzyme replacement.[254] Characterization of the purified cellular and secreted forms revealed that both were homodimeric glycoproteins with subunit molecular weights of 53 and 57 kDa, respectively. Microsequencing of each form demonstrated the same 15 *N*-terminal amino acids. The pH optimum of both forms was 4.6, but the cellular form had a higher pI than the secreted enzyme (4.6 versus 3.7). The K_m values of the cellular and secreted forms toward the synthetic substrate, 4-methylumbelliferyl-α-*D*-galactopyranoside, were similar (1.3 and 1.9 mM, respectively), and both forms hydrolyzed the natural glycolipid substrate, globotriaosylceramide. Both the cellular and secreted forms contained high-mannose-type and complex-type oligosaccharides with terminal Manα and Galβ(1,4)GlcNAc residues (see below "Analysis of *N*-Linked Oligosaccharide Structures of Recombinant α-Galactosidase A"). Both forms were phosphorylated, had M6P moieties, and were efficiently internalized by Fabry fibroblasts via the M6PR system. The properties of the recombinant secreted and cellular forms were essentially the same as those of the forms purified from human plasma and tissues, respectively (Ioannou et al., personal communication).

Structure-Function Studies of Human α-Galactosidase A

***N*-Glycosylation Site Occupancy and Structure of the Oligosaccharides.** To determine the role of the four consensus *N*-glycosylation sites in the α-galactosidase A cDNA, site-directed mutagenesis and transient expression in COS-1 cells were performed. Each site was individually eliminated by engineering an asparagine (N) to glutamine (Q) substitution (Fig. 150-17). Transient expression in COS-1 cells of each construct (N139Q, N192Q, N215Q, and N408Q) and analysis of the subunit

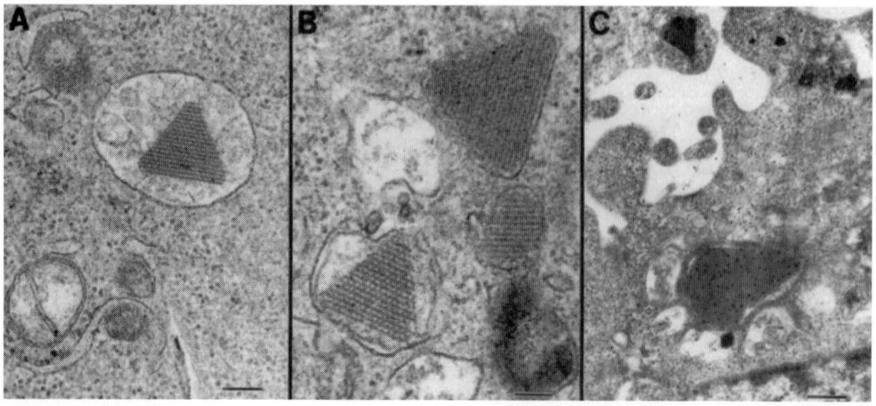

Fig. 150-16 Electron photomicrographs of AGA5.3-1000Mx cells showing crystalline structures of overexpressed human α-galactosidase A in single membrane-limited vacuoles (*A*) and in vesicles, presumably in the dilated *trans*-Golgi (*B*). *C*, Immunoelectron microscopic localization of human α-galactosidase A with 10-nm colloidal gold particles. Bars: *A*, 0.15 μm; *B*, 0.10 μm; *C*, 0.31 μM. (*Reproduced from Ioannou et al.[254] Used with permission.*)

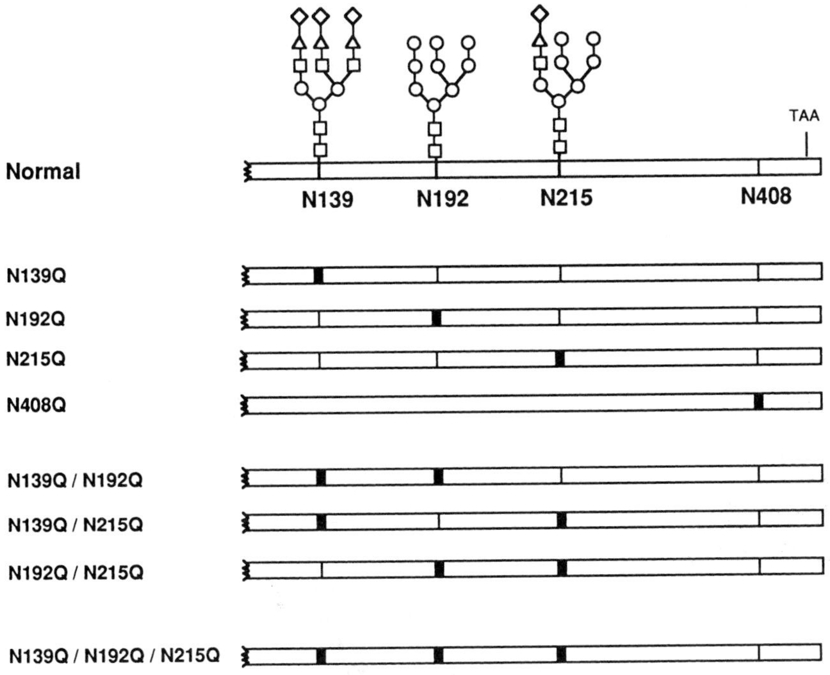

Fig. 150-17 Expression constructs for α-galactosidase A mutated at each glycosylation consensus sequence by an asparagine (N) to glutamine (Q) substitution. Transient expression of single-site constructs, N139Q, N192Q, N215Q, and N408Q, in COS-1 cells demonstrated that site N408 is not occupied. Double- and triple-site mutant constructs, N139Q/N192Q, N139Q/N215Q, N192Q/N215Q, and N139Q/N192Q/N215Q, expressed highly unstable proteins that were trapped in the endoplasmic reticulum.

molecular weights of the expressed enzymes revealed that the first three sites were occupied, but that site 4 (N408) was not. Further, transient expression of the N139Q, N192Q, and N408Q constructs resulted in near-normal levels of enzyme activity in COS-1 cells, whereas the N215Q construct expressed about 50 percent of normal intracellular levels (Table 150-5). All of the glycosylation mutant constructs expressed enzymes that were relatively unstable (N215Q < N139Q < N192Q) in the culture media at pH 7.2. Elimination of any two glycosylation sites, or of all three, resulted in unstable enzyme proteins that were degraded in the endoplasmic reticulum. Interestingly, the N139Q/N192Q double mutant, which had a functional N215 site, had ~30 to 40 percent of the activity expressed by the normal construct.[323] Thus, glycosylation at site 3 was critical for the formation of soluble, active enzyme, as well as transport to the lysosome. Absence of the site 3 hybrid-type oligosaccharide exposed an adjacent, normally protected, hydrophobic region, resulting in aggregation of the enzyme polypeptide in the endoplasmic reticulum. In support of this concept, Endo H-treated enzyme or mannose-terminated enzyme expressed in *Autographa californica* cells using the baculovirus system also aggregated when concentrated, emphasizing that site 3 occupancy by a hybrid-type oligosaccharide was required for enzyme solubility.[323] Of interest, and consistent with these site-specific mutagenesis experiments, the affected hemizygotes with the N215S mutation have residual enzymatic activity and the atypical cardiac variant phenotype (see "Atypical Hemizygotes: Cardiac Variants" and "Residual Activity in Atypical Variants" above).

Table 150-5 **Transient Expression of α-Galactosidase A Glycosylation Mutants in COS-1 Cells**

Glycosylation mutant construct	% Normal expressed activity* Intracellular	Media
Normal	100	100
N139Q	90	26
N192Q	95	42
N215Q	47	3.4
N408Q	100	100
N139Q + N192Q	35	35
N139Q + N215Q	15	4.5
N192Q + N215Q	15	2.2
N139Q + N192Q + N215Q	18	3.0

*Following electroporation of 20 μg of each construct into 2 × 10^6 COS-1 cells, transfected cells were grown and harvested at 48 h and the total α-galactosidase A activity was determined. Values are the mean of three independent experiments and the percentage of the activity expressed by the normal construct (~2,500 U/mg) minus the COS-1 background (~120 U/mg).[254]

Analysis of *N*-Linked Oligosaccharide Structures of Recombinant α-Galactosidase A. Recently, the complete carbohydrate structures of the *N*-linked oligosaccharides of the intracellular (i.e., lysosomal) and secreted forms of human recombinant α-galactosidase A were determined.[258] The secreted enzyme's oligosaccharides were remarkably heterogeneous, having high mannose (63 percent), complex (30 percent), and hybrid (5 percent) structures. The major high mannose oligosaccharides were $Man_{5\text{-}7}GlcNAc_2$ species. Approximately 40 percent of the high mannose and 30 percent of the hybrid oligosaccharides had phosphate monoester groups. The complex oligosaccharides were mono-, bi-, 2,4-tri-, 2,6-tri-, and tetra-antennary with or without core-region fucose, many of which had incomplete outer chains. Approximately 30 percent of the complex oligosaccharides were mono- or disialylated. Sialic acids were mostly *N*-acetylneuraminic acid and occurred in exclusively in α2,3-linkage. In contrast, the intracellular enzyme had only small amounts of complex chains (7.7 percent) and had predominantly high mannose oligosaccharides (92 percent), mostly $Man_{5\text{-}7}GlcNAc_2$ and smaller species, of which only 3 percent were phosphorylated. The complex oligosaccharides were fucosylated and had the same antennary structures as the secreted enzyme. The highly heterogeneous secreted forms presumably were due to the high level expression and impaired glycosylation in the *trans*-Golgi network, and the predominantly $Man_{5\text{-}7}GlcNAc_2$ cellular glycoforms resulted from carbohydrate trimming in the lysosome.[254,258]

Determination of the Active Site Aspartate. Studies of various bacterial glycosidases have identified specific aspartate (D) or glutamate residues that are the nucleophiles in their respective active sites.[364] On the basis of an analysis of the conserved aspartate residues in α-galactosidase A sequences from humans and other species, six highly conserved aspartate residues (D92, D93, D109, D165, D264, and D322) were identified. Expression constructs were synthesized in which each of the conserved aspartates was mutagenized to an asparagine. Each of these constructs transiently expressed normal or near-normal amounts of activity, and the expressed enzymes had the same K_m toward the artificial substrate, 4-methylumbelliferyl-α-*D*-galactopyranoside, with the notable exception of D93N, which exhibited no activity.[365] All of the transiently expressed mutant enzymes, including D93N, bound an immobilized substrate analogue and were competitively eluted with galactose. Further studies with the D93E construct, designed with the more conservative D-to-E substitution, resulted in an expressed enzyme with very low activity, indicating that residue D93 is a strong candidate for the nucleophile involved in the hydrolysis of α-galactosyl moieties by human α-galactosidase A.

Crystallography and X-Ray Diffraction. The stable expression of high levels of recombinant human α-galactosidase A (see above) permitted purification of large amounts of the enzyme for crystallization and preliminary diffraction analysis.[366] Diffractable crystals were grown by the "hanging drop" method of vapor diffusion. X-ray diffraction data collected from these crystals indicated that the crystals belong to the orthorhombic space group C2221 with cell dimensions of a = 93.8 Å, b = 141.1 Å, and c = 184.4 Å. The crystals diffracted to a resolution of 3 Å, and native data were collected to 3.5-Å resolution. Assuming a dimer per asymmetric unit of total molecular mass 110 kDa (with oligosaccharide structures), the Matthews coefficient was $V_m = 2.77$ Å/dalton, corresponding to a solvent content of 55 percent. The self-rotation function indicated the presence of a noncrystallographic twofold axis relating the dimeric subunits.

MOLECULAR PATHOLOGY OF FABRY DISEASE

The availability of the full-length cDNA[31,32] and genomic sequences[33] for human α-galactosidase A has permitted the investigation of the nature and frequency of the mutations causing Fabry disease. Techniques employed to analyze the molecular lesions include Southern and northern hybridization analyses, RNase A studies, PCR amplification of genomic DNA or reverse-transcribed mRNA for subsequent DNA sequencing by dideoxy nucleotide sequencing, cycle sequencing or automated sequencing, fluorescent chemical cleavage, fluorescence-assisted mismatch analysis, and single-strand conformational polymorphism analysis, among others. Such studies have demonstrated the variety of molecular lesions that cause Fabry disease, examples of which are discussed below. To date, over 150 mutations have been identified in the Human Gene Mutation Database (HGMD) (www.uwcm.ac.uk/uwcm/mg/hgmd0.html), in a gene which encodes a 421-residue subunit. Most of the mutations were "private," confined to individual pedigrees. Mutations that have been identified in more than one family mostly occurred at CpG dinucleotides. Alternatively, the families that share the same mutation are frequently found by haplotype analysis to be distant members of the same pedigree.[126,367] Characterization of these lesions has provided information on the nature and frequency of the mutations causing this disease as well as insights into the structure-function relationships of this lysosomal hydrolase. Moreover, the identification of the mutation in a given Fabry family permits the precise diagnosis of other family members by the use of mutation-specific detection methods, such as targeted DNA sequencing or allele-specific oligonucleotide hybridization. With the prospect of enzyme replacement therapy for Fabry disease, it is possible that knowledge of a patient's mutation may be important in devising genotype-specific treatment regimens. The major types of mutations causing Fabry disease are discussed below. Of the over 150 mutations recorded in the HGMD (Fig. 150-18), 71.6 percent were coding region missense or nonsense mutations, 6.5 percent were RNA processing defects, and 21.9 percent were large or small gene rearrangements. In addition, four complex mutations have been described.

The location of the reported mutations provides some insights into structure/function relationships of this enzyme. Mutations appear to occur randomly throughout the gene with some notable exceptions: there is only one reported mutation between the initiation codon and codon 31 (the region containing the signal peptide that controls targeting to the endoplasmic reticulum), and the 3′ end of exons 3 and 4 and the 5′ ends of exon 4 and 5 have no reported mutations. Interestingly, 23 percent of the nonsense mutations and 29 percent of the small insertions and deletions occurred in exon 7, thus indicating that the carboxy-terminal residues are critical for enzyme function, even though some of the nonsense mutations occurred at residues with a low degree of conservation, for example, Q386X and W399X. These observations may indicate that specific regions are either crucial to the function of this gene or that mutations in other regions may not generate a phenotype.

Coding Region Mutations. Approximately 70 percent of the mutations causing Fabry disease are missense or nonsense mutations. Of the coding region single-base alterations listed in the HGMD, 84 percent were missense mutations and 16 percent were nonsense mutations.[120,294,303,368–374] Point mutations have been described in all exons. However, exons 4 and 7 were relatively underrepresented with only 3 and 12 mutations respectively, while the remaining mutations were equally distributed among the other exons. Although most of the missense and nonsense mutations were detected in classically affected hemizygotes, several missense mutations (I91T,[372] R112H,[371] F113L,[372] P146S,[369] N215S,[294,368] M296V,[303] Q279E,[117,294] and R301Q[118,120]) were identified in asymptomatic or cardiac variants of Fabry disease.

RNA Processing Defects. Ten mutations altering the processing of the α-galactosidase A transcript have been described in classically affected hemizygotes.[294,372,374–380] Most occur at the 5′-splice donor sites, though four 3′-splice acceptor site alterations have been described. Many of these mutations have undergone further molecular characterization to demonstrate the RNA processing defect. For example, The IVS6^{+1} mutation was shown to result in exon skipping.[376] Northern hybridization analysis of affected males initially detected a shortened 1.25-kb α-galactosidase A mRNA, which was present at 50 to 60 percent of normal abundance. Heterozygotes had both the normal 1.45-kb and the shorter 1.25-kb transcript. RNase A protection analysis identified a deletion of about 200 bp that included all of exon 6. The exon 6 deletion resulted from a gt → tt substitution of the invariant 5′-donor splice consensus site of intron 6, causing abnormal splicing of the α-galactosidase A pre-mRNA. Similar studies have been carried out with the IVS3^{-1} mutation.[374]

Gene Rearrangements. The frequency of gene rearrangements in the α-galactosidase A gene causing Fabry disease was assessed in 165 unrelated patients by Southern hybridization analysis using the full-length α-galactosidase A cDNA as a probe[303] or by multiplex PCR amplification of the entire α-galactosidase A coding region.[381] The latter method determines the size of each of the seven exons in four PCR products that are simultaneously amplified and provides rapid screening for large (> 50 to 100 bp) insertions or deletions. By these two methods, one partial gene duplication and five partial gene deletions were identified,[303] a frequency of ~5 percent, which is similar to that reported for other X-linked diseases.[382] To date, no total gene deletions have been identified. Interestingly, a patient has been described with both Fabry disease and Duchenne muscular dystrophy, indicating that he had concurrent deletions in both Xp21 and Xq22.[383]

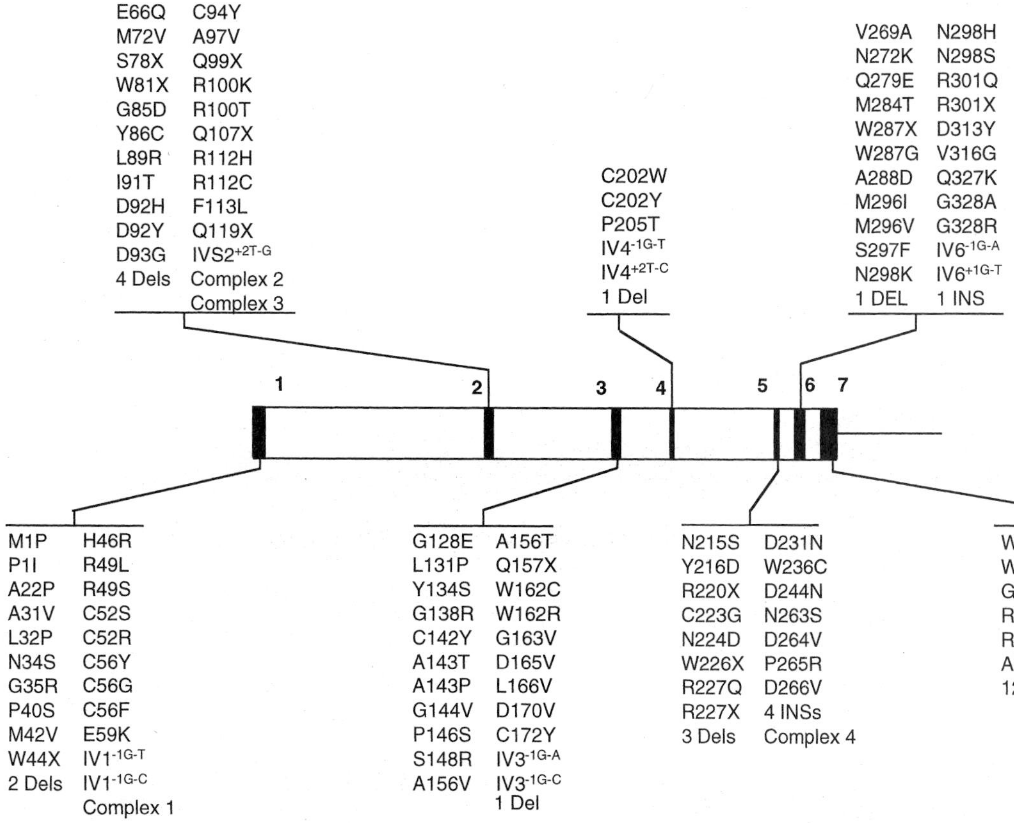

Fig. 150-18 Schematic of the α-galactosidase A gene indicating the relative position of the seven exons and listing the mutations identified in each. Numbers for deletions or insertions refer to nucleotide position in the α-galactosidase A cDNA sequence. ins = insertion; Δ = deletion; IVS = intervening sequence; see the Human Gene Mutation Database (www.uwcm.ac.uk/uwcm/mg/hgmd0.html) listing for GLA for additional information about the mutations.

α-Galactosidase A Small Insertions and Deletions. In contrast to the rarity of large deletions or duplications, a number of small insertions and deletions have been described in the α-galactosidase A coding sequence in unrelated Fabry patients (see HGMD for list and references). These rearrangements result in either frameshift mutations that lead to premature chain termination or insertion or deletion of one or more amino acids (e.g., 257del18). Of the 30 small insertions and deletions reported to date, 43 percent occurred in exon 7. That a large proportion of the small gene rearrangements occurred in this exon indicates that it is highly susceptible to gene rearrangements and that a mutational "hot spot" may exist in the region of codons 353 to 365.[372] An additional "hot spot" for deletions also was identified in exon 2 from codons 111 to 122.[294]

Complex Mutations. Four complex mutations, which are defined as mutations involving at least two presumably simultaneous mutational events, have been identified in patients with Fabry disease. These occur in exons 1, 2, and 5 of the α-galactosidase A gene.[372,384] In part, these mutations are termed complex because they cannot be readily explained by the usual mutational mechanisms. These mutations are g1312TGCAC → GCTCG in exon 1, g5115GGCAGAGCTCATG → GCAGAGCCA and c356AGCTAGCT → AGCCAACT in exon 2, and c654ATCCGA → AATCGA in exon 5. Complex mutations have been identified in several genes, including the LDL receptor gene,[385] the HPRT gene,[386] and the serum cholinesterase gene.[387] The exon 1 rearrangement resulted from a series of sequence alterations occurring between the tetranucleotide short direct repeat CTGG (normal sequence = CTGG CTGCA CTGG; mutant sequence = CTGG CGCTC GTGG). The α-galactosidase A exon 2 complex rearrangement g5115GGCAGAGCTCATG → GCAGAGCCA involved a series of three small deletions in a 13-bp region (G GCA GAG CTC ATG) from nucleotide 216 to 218. There were a total of four bases deleted and therefore a frameshift was predicted at codon 72.[372] The other exon 2 complex mutation, c356AGCTAGCT → AGCCAACT, resulted from a mutation(s) that altered the underlined two bases in the sequence AGC<u>T</u>A<u>G</u>CT to AGCCAACT. The mutant sequence predicted the in-frame substitution of L120 and A121 to P120 and T121 (L120P and A121T).[384] The complex mutation in exon 5 involved the insertion of an adenosine residue after nucleotide 654 (duplication of the A at position 654) and the deletion of the cytosine at position 656 (ATC CGA to AAT CGA). These base changes predicted an isoleucine to asparagine substitution at position 219 (I219N).[384] Interestingly, the adenosine duplication was preceded by three other adenosine residues (nucleotides 651 to 653). Various mechanisms have been proposed for the generation of these mutations: these include gene conversion between evolutionarily-related sequences[388] or misalignment of "quasi-palindromic" sequences during DNA replication and the subsequent deletion or insertion of bases that might serve to stabilize a hairpin loop.[389] Analysis of the α-galactosidase A sequences in exons 1 and 5 does not support gene conversion as the mutational mechanism for generation of these complex mutations. The existence of several alterations involving multiple insertion and deletion events is unique to the α-galactosidase A gene.

Common Molecular Lesions in Fabry Disease. As noted above, most of the reported mutations have been private (i.e., confined to a single Fabry pedigree). In fact, the discovery that two presumably unrelated families had identical mutations has frequently led to linking of two distant arms of the same pedigree. In contrast, mutations occurring at CpG dinucleotides have been found in unrelated families of different ethnic or geographic backgrounds. Of the 14 CpG dinucleotides in the α-galactosidase A coding sequence, point mutations have been described in eight (in codons 49, 112, 142/143, 220, 227, 301, 342, and 356); codons 49, 112, 227, 301, and 342 had mutations at both the C and G of their respective CpG dinucleotides. These include R49L, R49S, R112C, R112H, R227Q, R227X, R301Q, R301X, R342Q, and R342X mutations. R227Q and R227X, which occurred at a CpG nucleotide, were the most common mutations causing the classic phenotype. Taken together, they were found in 5 percent (8 of 148) of unrelated Fabry families studied,[294] including families whose mutant alleles could be traced to Danish, English, German, Indian, Irish, Italian, and Polish ancestries. Two families with the R227Q mutation were of German descent, but a common ancestor or demographic region could not be identified. Several apparently unrelated families have had either the R112C or R112H or the R342Q or R342X mutations.[368,369] Therefore, these CpG associated mutations account for the vast majority of recurrent molecular lesions seen in Fabry disease families. The high frequency of mutations at CpG dinucleotides is consistent with their recognition as mutational hot spots due to the deamination of methylcytosine to thymidine.[390] However, N215S, a common mutation among atypical hemizygotes who were asymptomatic or had mild disease manifestations (i.e., cardiac variants), did not occur at a CpG dinucleotide.[119,294,368]

Genotype/Phenotype Correlations

Affected hemizygotes with the classic disease manifestations and no detectable α-galactosidase A activity had a variety of α-galactosidase A lesions, including large and small gene rearrangements, splicing defects, and missense or nonsense mutations. In contrast, all of the asymptomatic or mildly affected atypical hemizygotes (see Table 150-2) had missense mutations that expressed residual α-galactosidase A activity (see "Residual Activity in Atypical Hemizygotes" above). However, efforts to establish genotype/phenotype correlations have been limited, because most Fabry patients had private mutations, and attempts to predict the phenotype require more extensive clinical information from unrelated patients with the same genotype. In addition, attempts to predict the clinical phenotype on the basis of the type or location of a molecular lesion are premature. For example, several atypical mild mutations, N215S, Q279E, M296V, and R301Q, are located in exons 5 and 6. However, other nearby missense mutations, such as S297F, which is adjacent to M296V, result in severe disease. The type of amino acid change (i.e., isofunctional versus altered charge) also fails to predict a classic or mild phenotype. Thus, the clinical severity of private missense mutations detected in Fabry families with few or only young patients is difficult to predict. However, it is anticipated that future crystallographic studies may provide useful structure-function information for genotype/phenotype correlations. Moreover, the influence of modifier genes or other genetic factors on the severity of the disease phenotype may be important since individuals from different pedigrees who share the same mutation and even members of the same family, can have markedly variable phenotypes. In fact, patients from unrelated families with the R112H, R301Q, and G328R mutations have had the classic disease phenotype in one family whereas affected hemizygotes in the other family had mild disease manifestations.[117,126] These occurrences, although rare at present, may become more frequent as more Fabry families are genotyped.

Insights into the structure-function relationships of specific α-galactosidase A amino acids and domains can be gained by noting the position of the point mutations causing classic or variant Fabry disease and their relative conservation in the over 20 homologues encoding α-galactosidase A or the evolutionarily related enzyme α-*N*-acetylgalactosaminidase (α-galactosidase B)[245] currently recorded in the GenBank database. For example, two mutations involving cysteine residues (C94Y and C202Y) were highly conserved in 85 percent and 90 percent of the sequences analyzed, respectively, indicating their probable importance in the formation of intramolecular disulfide bridges in the enzyme polypeptide. In a study of 35 novel α-galactosidase A mutations, several observations were made regarding the location of mutations in conserved regions.[372] In this study, seven missense mutations (Y86C, L89P, I91T, D92Y, C94Y, R100T, and F113L) occurred in exon 2, in a highly conserved region presumed to contain residues in the active site.[365] Six of the seven exon 2 missense mutations were highly conserved in the 20 α-galactosidase A and α-galactosidase B sequences examined (ranging from 80 percent to 95 percent conserved), with the divergence occurring in the bacterial sequences. Moreover, the mutations in two cardiac variants were also located in exon 2 and occurred at moderately to highly conserved residues (I91T, 80 percent; F113L, 85 percent), further demonstrating the functional importance of this region. Other mutations that occurred at highly conserved (> 75 percent) residues were Y134S, S148R, D170V, N263S, and W287C, indicating their importance in the activity and/or stability of the enzyme. Certain mutations occurred in positions that were conserved residues only in mammalian α-galactosidase A sequences (e.g., A31V, H46R, A97V, and L89P). Presumably, substitutions occurring at less essential residues would be neutral or may retain sufficient enzymatic function to be clinically insignificant.

PATHOPHYSIOLOGY

The pattern of glycosphingolipid deposition in Fabry disease, particularly its predilection for vascular endothelial and smooth-muscle cells, is uniquely different from that seen in other glycosphingolipidoses.[391] However, the origin of the accumulated glycosphingolipid substrates has not been fully clarified. A significant contribution comes from endogenous synthesis and subsequent lysosomal accumulation of terminal α-galactosyl containing glycosphingolipids following autophagy of cellular membranous material containing these lipid substrates. Endogenous metabolism is a major source of substrate accumulation in avascular sites such as cornea and in neural cells, which presumably are protected from the increased circulating levels of globotriaosylceramide by the blood-brain barrier. In addition, the turnover of globotriaosylceramide, and particularly its precursor, globotetraosylceramide (globoside), which are present in high concentrations in normal renal tissue, are presumably responsible for the endogenous renal deposition of the Fabry substrates.

The unique cellular and tissue distribution of accumulated globotriaosylceramide, particularly in the vascular endothelium (Fig. 150-19) and smooth muscle, suggests that a significant intracellular contribution may be derived by the endocytosis or diffusion of globotriaosylceramide from the circulation, where the concentration is three- to tenfold higher than in normal individuals. The circulating globotriaosylceramide is primarily transported in the LDL and HDL lipoproteins.[177–179,189,392] In plasma from affected hemizygotes, the accumulated globotriaosylceramide is distributed in the LDL and HDL fractions in proportions similar to those in normal plasma, approximately 60 and 30 percent, respectively. The finding that little, if any, substrate deposition occurs in Fabry hepatocytes (in contrast to the accumulation in Kupffer cells)[141,167,393] supports the contention that globotriaosylceramide synthesized in hepatocytes is associated with the lipoproteins and secreted as a complex.[394] In support of this concept is the fact that patients with hypercholesterolemia have proportional plasma elevations of both LDL and neutral glycosphingolipids, including globotriaosylceramide.[177] The circulating globotriaosylceramide then presumably gains access to vascular endothelial and smooth-muscle cells throughout the body by the high-affinity lipoprotein receptor-mediated uptake pathway.[395–397] Deposits in other tissues may also be derived to a lesser extent from receptor-independent diffusion or by non-absorptive endocytosis of globoside- or globotriaosylceramide-lipoprotein complexes from the plasma. Because lysosomes in all cells are deficient in the α-galactosidase A activity needed to degrade the deposited glycosphingolipids, the glycosphingolipids accumulate within extended multivesicular bodies or, in more

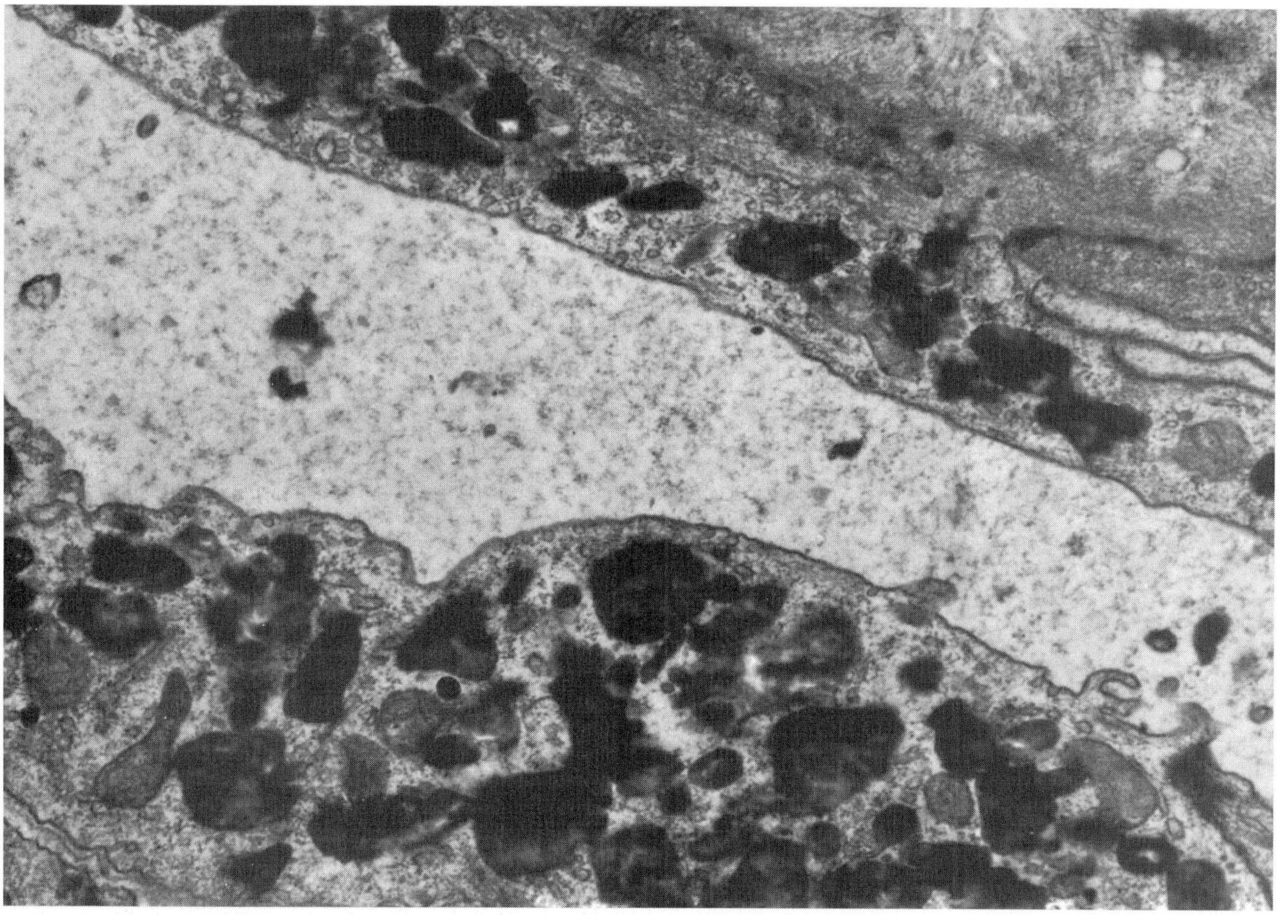

Fig. 150-19 Electron micrograph of a section of an arteriole from a classically affected hemizygote, showing the marked accumulation of concentric lamellar inclusions in the lysosomes of the vascular endothelium. The progressive lysosomal deposition of the glycosphingolipid substrate leads to the narrowing and eventual occlusion of the vascular lumen. ×25,000. (*Courtesy of Dr. J.G. White, University of Minnesota.*)

advanced stages, as free intracytoplasmic masses, which may lead to cellular dysfunction or degeneration.

In addition to their biosynthesis in hepatocytes, glycosphingolipids are synthesized in the bone marrow, where they become incorporated into the membranes of the formed blood elements.[13,220,398] It has been postulated that erythrocyte globoside, the predominant glycosphingolipid of erythrocytes and the catabolic precursor of globotriaosylceramide (see Fig. 150-11), may be another major metabolic source of the circulating pathogenic lipid. Globoside is presumably released into the circulation from senescent erythrocytes[220] and is subsequently catabolized (presumably in the spleen) to globotriaosylceramide. In Fabry disease, the globotriaosylceramide cannot be metabolized and may be partly released into the circulation, where it can be incorporated into both HDL and LDL fractions,[394] and/or rapidly cleared by the liver as has been shown for intravenously administered neutral glycosphingolipids.[399] Thus, the turnover of erythrocyte and other membrane glycosphingolipids may contribute significantly to the substrate load in Fabry disease. In addition, a minor amount of globotriaosylceramide may be "excreted" into the circulation from the secondary lysosomes of various cell types throughout the body. Because the glycosphingolipid cannot be catabolized in the circulation, it would slowly accumulate at a rate reflecting the turnover of various cells, the contribution from exocytosis, and lipoprotein uptake and/or diffusion. The progressive accumulation of the glycosphingolipid substrates as a function of age in the α-galactosidase A-deficient mice supports this notion.[357]

The metabolism of at least two other glycosphingolipids is also abnormal, as demonstrated by the accumulation of galabiosylceramide and the blood group B substances. Hemizygous and heterozygous individuals who are blood group B or AB appear to be more severely affected, presumably because of the additional accumulation of B-specific glycosphingolipids.[400,401] Thus, the total amount of glycosphingolipid stored in a given tissue depends on time, the rate of accumulation from intracellular and circulatory sources, the possibilities for excretion, the individual's ABO blood type, and the presence or absence of residual α-galactosidase A activity (see "Residual Activity in Atypical Hemizygotes" above).

The pattern of glycosphingolipid accumulation, predominantly in the cardiovascular-renal system, best correlates pathophysiologically with the major clinical manifestations of the disease as selectively described below.

Vasculature

Narrowing, dilatation, motor unresponsiveness, and instability of blood vessels are major features of the altered physiology in Fabry disease. The swollen vascular endothelial cells, often accompanied by endothelial proliferation, encroach on the lumen (see Figs. 150-5 and 150-19), causing a focal increase of intraluminal pressure, dilatation, and angiectases as well as peripheral ischemia or frank infarction.[173] Such changes are frequently the precursors of thromboses and infarcts of the brain and other tissues. Muscle and peripheral nerve ischemia may contribute to the pain or fatigue.[157,402]

There may be progressive aneurysmal dilatation of the weakened vascular wall. This process is apparent in the progressive dilatation and microaneurysm formation of the retinal and conjunctival vessels and in the transition from normality to telangiectasia and frank angiokeratoma in the skin. Observed alterations of vasomotor control may reflect either the vascular lesions themselves or the extensive glycosphingolipid deposits in autonomic ganglia and perineural sheath cells.[158,402,403] Hemizygotes and heterozygotes with Fabry disease demonstrate an impaired ability for vasoconstriction, and the more severely involved hemizygotes also show an inability to vasodilate. Such a combined vascular and neural lesion may also explain the clinically observed temperature intolerance.

Nervous System

The involvement of peripheral and central autonomic nerve cells may be responsible for the paresthesias, pain, hypohidrosis, gastrointestinal symptoms like nausea and diarrhea, and a variety of vague neurologic signs and symptoms. Fukuhara et al.[402] found marked degeneration of the secretory cells and myoepithelial cells of sweat glands by electron microscopy, and proposed that the hypohidrosis was due to local lipid deposition rather than to autonomic nervous system involvement. Yamamoto et al. found slightly decreased skin sympathetic nerve activity in a heterozygote with anhidrosis and concluded that the lack of sweating was due to sweat gland dysfunction as well as abnormal skin sympathetic nerve activity.[404] The episodic fevers may be related to lesions of the hypothalamus.[82] The observation of a selective decrease in the number of unmyelinated and small myelinated fibers in peripheral nerves[17,95,148,152–156,405–409] has led to the suggestion that the selective damage to these fibers may account for the pain production and hypohidrosis in this disorder. Studies of autonomic function revealed sympathetic and parasympathetic dysfunction, particularly in distal cutaneous responses.[133,406] Abnormalities of cutaneous thermal sensation suggest involvement of small myelinated fibers.[69] The diminished cutaneous flare responses are presumably due to the involvement and loss of peripheral unmyelinated fibers.[410] The exclusive glycolipid deposition in dorsal root ganglia observed at autopsy of one hemizygote led to the suggestion that the pain resulted from sensory root ganglia involvement.[411] Alternatively, it has been suggested that the lipid deposition in the vasa nervorum may lead to the acroparesthesias rather than involvement of the autonomic nervous system.[402,406,407]

Kidney

The observed abnormalities in renal function have their basis in lesions of the nephron and of the renal vasculature, and possibly in disorders of the posterior pituitary and hypothalamus. Glycosphingolipid deposits antedate clinical signs and symptoms. During this early period, the lesions of the renal vasculature are less prominent than those of the nephron, and renal architecture is maintained. The observed mild proteinuria may be explained by alteration of the glomerular epithelial cells and their foot processes[149] and/or by increased desquamation of lipid-laden tubular epithelial cells.[148] Loss of renal concentrating ability with polyuria and polydipsia may occur well in advance of a significant decrease in glomerular filtration or evidence of renal failure.[79] The defect in concentrating ability may be due to decreased water permeability of the distal tubules and collecting ducts secondary to lipid deposition. The diabetes insipidus-like syndrome, which is not related to faulty electrolyte transfer in distal tubules, may result from tubular insensitivity to antidiuretic hormone or to combined dysfunction of the renal tubular cells and lesions of the glycosphingolipid-laden supraoptic nucleus and antidiuretic center of the hypothalamus. The later and more severe renal changes are the result of vascular lesions and of systemic hypertension.

Heart

The progressive deposition of glycosphingolipids in the myocardial cells, the valvular fibroblasts, and the coronary vessels is the primary cause of cardiac disease in affected hemizygotes and some heterozygotes.[16,46,47] The frequent findings of left ventricular hypertrophy and mitral insufficiency are presumably related to the fact that the left ventricular myocardium and the mitral valve are the sites of the most marked lipid deposition in the heart.[16] The abnormally short PR interval, the Wenckebach phenomenon, Wolff-Parkinson-White syndrome, complete atrioventricular block, and the finding of cardiomyopathy on EKG may be related to lipid deposition in the myocardium and/or conduction system.[48,55,412] The marked deposition of globotriaosylceramide in the coronary arteries leads to myocardial ischemia and frank infarction.[16,46,47,60]

The findings in atypical variants indicate that manifestations of Fabry disease can be limited to the heart. The specific cardiac involvement in these patients is presumably due to "mild" α-galactosidase A mutations. The mechanism of this limited involvement may be related to the observation that the myocardium is an early site of glycosphingolipid deposition, as demonstrated by the accumulation of this lipid in the heart and kidneys of affected fetuses.[77] With age, the progressive myocardial deposition is manifested first by hypertrophy and then by dilatation, both being aggravated by additional valvular abnormalities. However, most patients with the classic phenotype die of complications of the renal and vascular involvement before the myocardial manifestations become debilitating. In contrast, patients with atypical form may have sufficient residual α-galactosidase A activity to protect the kidneys and vascular endothelium, but the level of enzyme activity in the heart may be inadequate to prevent the progressive deposition of glycosphingolipid in myocardial cells. In later adulthood, myocardial disease develops in these patients and leads to a clinical phenotype of Fabry disease confined to the myocardium. The very late development of myocardial symptoms in heterozygous females who have low levels of α-galactosidase A activity (due to random X-inactivation) presumably also results from this pathologic process.

Other Involvement

Pulmonary symptoms have been attributed to involvement of lung vasculature or bronchial and mucous gland epithelium.[99] The airflow obstruction may be due to the loss of elastic recoil secondary to lipid deposition in lung parenchyma. The lymphedema presumably results from lymphatic obstruction or venous insufficiency secondary to lipid-laden endothelial cells. Histochemical evidence of glycosphingolipid accumulation in neurons and nerve fibers of intestinal nerve plexuses and smooth muscle[92] may account for the uncoordinated intestinal smooth-muscle activity in Fabry hemizygotes, which may lead to complaints of chronic diarrhea or constipation. Glycolipid deposition in the myenteric and submucosal plexuses and a marked decrease in argyrophilic neurons were observed in an involved segment of bowel from a Fabry hemizygote who had jejunal diverticulosis and perforation. The abdominal pain may be due to deposits in the vessels and nerves supplying the bowel, but large vessel disease of the superior mesenteric artery has also been described.[413]

Reports of growth retardation, delayed puberty, slow beard growth, or impaired fertility associated with a decrease of gonadotropins may correlate with observations of testicular atrophy[414] or with glycosphingolipid storage in the interstitial cells of the testis or in anterior and posterior lobes of the pituitary gland.[167] Reports of priapism may be related to autonomic nervous system and vascular glycosphingolipid deposition.[105] No explanations have been offered for the frequently observed acromegalic appearance.

DIAGNOSIS

Genetic counseling should be offered to all families in which the diagnosis of Fabry disease is made (see "Genetic and Family Counseling" below).[415] Inheritance of the Fabry gene from affected hemizygotes or heterozygotes should be considered, because both genotypes transmit the gene. In each extended family, all at-risk males should be diagnostically evaluated. All at-risk females in a pedigree should be examined clinically and biochemically for heterozygote identification. In addition, it may be necessary to carry out molecular studies in order to determine more accurately the genotype of women at risk for inheriting the disease gene (see "Molecular Diagnosis of Fabry Heterozygotes" below). Fabry disease has been detected antenatally from cultured fetal cells and amniotic fluid obtained by amniocentesis as well as from chorionic villi (see "Prenatal Diagnosis" below).

Clinical Evaluation

The clinical diagnosis in affected males is most readily made from the history and by observation of the characteristic skin lesions and corneal dystrophy. The most common childhood symptom before the appearance of the cutaneous lesions is recurrent fever in association with pain of the hands and feet. The disorder has often been misdiagnosed as rheumatic fever, neurosis, erythromelalgia, or collagen vascular disease. Differential diagnosis of the cutaneous lesions must exclude the angiokeratoma of Fordyce,[416,417] angiokeratoma of Mibelli,[177,418] and angiokeratoma circumscriptum,[419,420] none of which has the typical histologic or ultrastructural pathology of the Fabry lesion (see Fig. 150-6). The angiokeratomas of Fordyce are similar in appearance to those of Fabry disease, but are limited to the scrotum, and usually appear after age 30. The angiokeratomas of Mibelli are warty lesions on the extensor surfaces of extremities in young adults and are associated with chilblains. Angiokeratoma circumscriptum or naeviformus can occur anywhere on the body, is clinically and histologically similar to those of Fordyce, and is not associated with chilblains.

Angiokeratoma, reportedly similar to or indistinguishable from the clinical appearance and distribution of the cutaneous lesions in Fabry disease, have been described in patients with other lysosomal storage diseases, including fucosidosis,[421,422] sialidosis (α-neuraminidase deficiency with or without β-galactosidase deficiency),[423,424] adult-type β-galactosidase deficiency,[425] aspartylglucosaminuria,[426] adult-onset α-galactosidase B deficiency,[23,247,248] β-mannosidase deficiency,[427] and a lysosomal disorder that presents with mental retardation and some features of the mucopolysaccharidoses.[428] Ultrastructural examination of these lesions reveals lysosomal substrate deposition that differs in the fine structural appearance of the respective storage material. In addition, patients with classic-appearing angiokeratoma but no other clinical symptoms or morphologic evidence of lysosomal storage have been described;[429,430] these patients have had normal levels of α-galactosidase A and other lysosomal enzymes. Clinical and pathologic details of the differential diagnosis of the skin lesions are available in reviews.[142,431–433]

Presumptive diagnosis of affected males can be made by observation of the characteristic corneal dystrophy on slit-lamp examination and by demonstration of the birefringent inclusions in the urinary sediment. Women suspected of being heterozygous carriers of the Fabry gene should be carefully examined for evidence of the corneal opacity and for isolated skin lesions, particularly on the breasts, back, trunk, and posterolateral thighs. Heterozygote detection also may be accomplished by the histologic or immunologic finding of lipid-laden cells in biopsied skin and tissues or in the urinary sediment.[434]

Phenocopies

A phenocopy is a phenotypic mimic or simulation of a specific genetic trait. Because a phenocopy is usually the result of environmental factors, it is not inherited. There are two such phenocopies for Fabry disease, one that mimics the characteristic corneal opacity and another that causes functional and ultrastructural renal changes resembling those in hemizygotes. Because the diagnosis of Fabry disease is often suspected on the basis of an eye examination or renal evaluation for proteinuria, these phenocopies have significant diagnostic import.

The whorl-like keratopathy of Fabry disease is readily distinguished from the corneal opacities of other lysosomal storage disorders, but is clinically and ultrastructurally identical to the corneal dystrophy associated with long-term chloroquine therapy.[435,436] Chloroquine has been shown to concentrate rapidly in lysosomes, increase the intralysosomal pH, decrease the activity of specific lysosomal hydrolases, alter the rate of proteolysis, and cause the formation of lysosomal inclusions. On the basis of these findings, it has been proposed that the chloroquine-induced keratopathy results from the pH inactivation of lysosomal α-galactosidase A and the subsequent accumulation of globotriaosylceramide.[436] In support of this concept is the finding that corneal α-galactosidase A is more sensitive to increasing pH in vitro than other lysosomal hydrolases.[33,437] Similar studies have shown that chloroquine inactivated the α-galactosidase A activity in cultured human skin fibroblasts.[438] These findings demonstrate the likely mechanism responsible for the phenocopy and represent the first biochemical elucidation of a human phenocopy. More recently, amiodarone has been shown to cause a phenocopy of the Fabry keratopathy. The mechanism underlying the amiodarone-induced pathology has not been characterized,[439] although it is presumed to act like chloroquine. Lipid-laden lysosomes have been observed in nerve and muscle biopsy specimens of amiodarone-treated patients who developed a neuromyopathy.[440]

Another tissue-specific phenocopy of Fabry disease occurs in individuals who are environmentally exposed to silica dust. The pulmonary complications of silicolipoproteinosis have been described, but the renal manifestations of proteinuria and lipiduria have received little attention. Ultrastructural examination of renal tissue from these individuals has revealed the typical electron-dense lamellar inclusions in the lysosomes of glomerular epithelial and endothelial cells and proximal and distal tubular cells observed in Fabry disease.[34,441] The levels of α-galactosidase A and urinary sediment glycosphingolipids were normal in one such patient.[441] Although the mechanism responsible for the silica-induced phenocopy is unknown, the finding of such lesions in biopsied renal tissue should include silicosis as well as Fabry disease in the differential diagnosis.

Biochemical Diagnosis of Affected Hemizygotes

All suspect hemizygotes should be confirmed biochemically by the demonstration of deficient α-galactosidase A activities in plasma or serum, leukocytes, tears, biopsied tissues, or cultured skin fibroblasts or lymphoblasts.[25,237,238,240,442,443] Classically affected hemizygotes usually have no detectable α-galactosidase A activity when the assay is performed with synthetic substrates for α-galactosidase A with the addition of *N*-acetylgalactosamine in the reaction mixture to inhibit the α-galactosidase B activity.[443] This assay modification permits the reliable diagnosis of classically affected hemizygotes (Fig. 150-20).

Atypical hemizygotes may be detected by the presence of residual α-galactosidase A activity ranging from less than 5 to 35 percent of normal. Variants have been detected with high levels of activity in plasma (~30 percent) and low levels (2 to 10 percent) in cellular sources, with absent or low levels in plasma and higher levels (5 to 25 percent) in cultured cells and tissues, and with low but detectable residual activity in both plasma and cellular sources.[111,112,114,120] In most variants studied, the levels of residual activity have been highest (20 to 30 percent of normal) in cultured skin fibroblasts.[111–114,120] The kinetic and stability properties of the residual α-galactosidase A should be determined, as should the levels of globotriaosylceramide in various fluid and cellular sources. Such studies are required in order to establish the biochemical diagnosis of atypical variants and to gain information on the structural and functional properties of these mutant enzymes.

Molecular Diagnosis of Fabry Heterozygotes

The biochemical identification of female carriers of the Fabry gene is less reliable because of random X-chromosomal inactivation.[136] Many heterozygous females can be detected by intermediate levels of α-galactosidase A activity in various sources. However, because

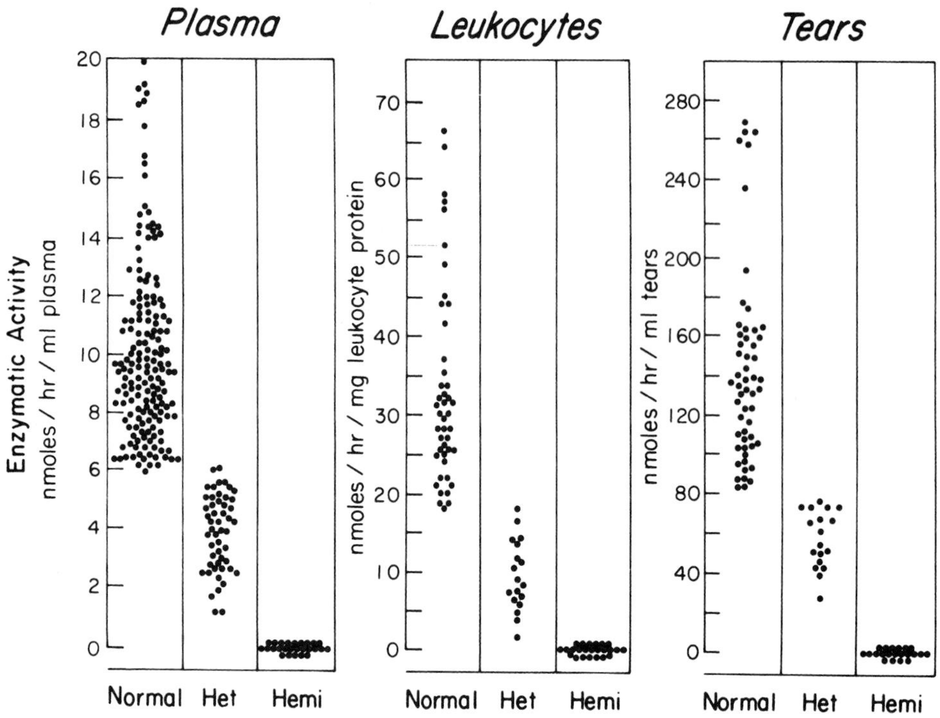

Fig. 150-20 Levels of α-galactosidase A activity in plasma (or serum),[237] isolated leukocytes,[237] and tears[25] from normal individuals (N) and heterozygotes (Het) and hemizygotes (Hemi) with Fabry disease.

of random X-chromosomal inactivation, heterozygotes can express levels of enzymatic activity ranging from essentially zero to normal. Thus, reports of obligate heterozygotes with normal α-galactosidase A activity and no keratopathy[1,20,83,444] are not unexpected and emphasize the need for precise carrier detection. In addition, recent evidence suggests that inactivated X-chromosomal genes may become reactivated as a result of aging and decreased levels of 5-methyldeoxycytidine.[445–447] Thus, the demethylation of X-chromosomal genes may explain the not-infrequent observation that older obligate heterozygotes have levels of α-galactosidase A activity at the high end of the heterozygote range or within the normal range.[77] Clearly, this aging phenomenon may further obscure precise enzymatic diagnosis of heterozygotes.

In the past, attempts to accurately establish heterozygosity required the demonstration of both normal and mutant cell populations by α-galactosidase A assays of single hair roots[62,448–450] or by the laborious and procedurally difficult cloning,[137] cell sorting of individual fibroblasts,[451] or immunofluorescence imaging using confocal laser scanning microscopy of individual fibroblasts.[434] These studies are extremely time-consuming, require special expertise to perform, and may be difficult to interpret.[130] More recent molecular analyses of the specific gene defect in each family or the use of α-galactosidase A-specific polymorphisms[306] or closely linked X-chromosomal anonymous DNA sequences[452–455] have provided more accurate heterozygote detection. The identification of a gene rearrangement, a restriction endonuclease cleavage site alteration, or a specific point mutation detectable by use of a specific restriction enzyme or synthetic oligonucleotide probe permits the precise diagnosis of heterozygotes in families with specific alterations. Advances in rapid DNA sequencing make more feasible the identification of mutations in all Fabry patients. Certainly, for all families in which the molecular lesion has been identified, precise molecular carrier detection should be offered. Alternatively, molecular diagnoses may be accomplished using indirect methods. These include the analysis of α-galactosidase-A-specific polymorphisms[306] as well as for anonymous X-chromosomal polymorphic sequences that are closely linked to the α-galactosidase A locus as shown in Fig. 150-14.[455,456]

Locus-Specific Polymorphisms. Variants for the CT repeat in intron 1 or for the *Alu* elements in the α-galactosidase A gene have not been detected in normal individuals or members of unrelated Fabry families. Six α-galactosidase A-specific polymorphisms have been identified in various ethnic and racial groups. Using over 40 different restriction endonucleases, only two single nucleotide polymorphisms (SNPs) in and adjacent to the α-galactosidase A gene were detected,[34,306] a frequency consistent with that found in other X-linked sequences.[452,457] The *Sac*I and *Nco*I RFLPs are in intron 4 and about 10 kb downstream from the stop codon of the α-galactosidase A gene, respectively. The rare form of the *Sac*I polymorphism was observed in 8 percent of normal alleles and in only 2 percent of unrelated Fabry families studied.[34] The rare form of the *Nco*I polymorphism was observed in 13 to 20 percent of normal alleles[458] and in 12 percent of the 75 Fabry families analyzed.[34,306] The power of these locus-specific RFLPs for precise carrier detection has been demonstrated in a large Fabry family.[459] A multiallelic polymorphic system of three sequence alterations at −10, −12, and −30 in the 5′ untranslated region of the α-galactosidase A gene has been identified.[458] The combined frequency of the three polymorphisms in a normal population was ~10 percent. In addition, a 7-bp deletion polymorphism in intron 2, detected by single-strand conformational polymorphism analysis, was found to occur with an allele frequency of 0.12.[458]

Linked Polymorphic Anonymous DNA Sequences. Another approach for heterozygote detection in Fabry families in which the specific molecular lesions have not been identified is the use of anonymous polymorphic DNA sequences that are closely linked to the Fabry locus at Xq22.1. Previously, several such RFLPs had been identified, including DXS17, DXS72, DXS87, DXS88, DXS94, DXS106, DXS287, and PLP.[304–306,460–463] Studies of the segregation of DXS17 and DXS87 in five informative Fabry families proved the usefulness of these probes;[304,305] however, they were found to be informative in only 70 percent of 42 families.[34,77,306] More recent genetic and physical mapping studies of the Xq21.3-q23/24 region[295–298,308] have identified several dinucleotide repeats that closely flank α-galactosidase A. By the evaluation of these highly informative short tandem repeats

(DXS458, DXS454, DXS178, DXS101, DXS94, DXS17, and DXS7424), and the two RFLPs that are closely linked to the α-galactosidase A gene, rapid, accurate molecular carrier detection or prenatal diagnoses have been achieved.[455,456] Three of these markers, DXS7424, DXS178, and DXS101, flank α-galactosidase A and lie within 1 cM of the gene; their proximity to the α-galactosidase A gene significantly limits the risk of misdiagnosis due to recombinational events. These loci are all highly polymorphic, thereby increasing the likelihood that individuals will be informative and their genotypes can be assigned. In addition, these polymorphic flanking markers can be used to determine the haplotype of patients who have the same α-galactosidase A mutation in order to assess if the same mutation arose independently on different chromosomes or if the patients have a common haplotype suggesting that they share a common ancestor.[126]

Generation of a Mouse Knock-Out with α-Galactosidase A Deficiency. In order to characterize the pathophysiology of Fabry disease and to evaluate potential treatment modalities such as enzyme and gene replacement therapies, a mouse model of α-galactosidase A deficiency was generated by targeted disruption of the α-galactosidase A gene in mouse embryonic stem (ES) cells. Tissues from adult hemizygous males and homozygous females for the null allele had no detectable α-galactosidase A activity.[357,464] Adult α-galactosidase A-deficient mice had elevated levels of globotriaosylceramide in all tissues analyzed, including liver, spleen, heart, kidney, skin, and plasma. Globotriaosylceramide levels increased with age; however, the mice did not have a clinical phenotype. Thus, they provide a biochemical model of Fabry disease but only permit limited studies of the disease pathogenesis. However, the α-galactosidase A-deficient animals provide an excellent model for evaluation of enzyme or gene replacement therapy for Fabry disease by allowing the determination of the effects of recombinant enzyme administration or gene delivery strategies on globotriaosylceramide storage and reaccumulation (see below, "Treatment").

TREATMENT

Medical Management

In Fabry disease, the chronicity of the clinical events causes severe debilitation and incapacity that extends over years. The single most debilitating and morbid aspect of Fabry disease is the excruciating pain. The pathophysiological events that cause the incapacitating episodes of pain or the chronic burning acroparesthesias have not been clarified. Numerous drugs have been tried for the relief of these agonizing pains.[10] The α-adrenergic blocking agent, phenoxybenzamine, which increases peripheral vascular flow has been administered for pain relief, although this drug provided relief in a hemizygote on several occasions, priapism and epistaxis were early complications in two other hemizygotes.[104] With the exception of centrally acting narcotic analgesics, such as morphine,[465,466] conventional analgesic agents have not been helpful. However, prophylactic administration of low-maintenance dosages of diphenylhydantoin have been found to provide relief from the periodic crises of excruciating pain and constant discomfort in hemizygotes and heterozygotes.[35] Lenoir et al.[467] noted that carbamazepine also provided pain relief. The combination of diphenylhydantoin and carbamazepine may significantly reduce the frequency and severity of the pain.[468] Subsequent reports have further documented the effectiveness of diphenylhydantoin and/or carbamazepine in the prevention and amelioration of these debilitating episodes.[469] The potential side effects of gingival hypertrophy with diphenylhydantoin and dose-related autonomic complications with carbamazepine, including urinary retention, nausea, vomiting, and ileus, have been recorded.[470] A report describing the use of neurotrophin, an extract from the inflamed skin of vaccinia virus-inoculated rabbits that has been used as an analgesic in Japan, was reported to provide pain relief in a Fabry patient when used in combination with carbamazepine.[470,471] Gabapentin (neurontin) and amitriptyline also have had anecdotal success in managing Fabry crises. Some patients report relief from the use of nonsteroidal anti-inflammatory drugs, but these agents should be used conservatively, if at all, due to potential renal toxicity.

Care of patients with regard to cardiac, pulmonary, gastrointestinal, and central nervous system manifestations remains nonspecific and symptomatic. Successful cardiac transplantation of a heterozygote with end-stage cardiomyopathy has been reported.[472] Obstructive lung disease has been documented in older hemizygotes and heterozygotes, with more severe impairment in smokers. Therefore, patients should be discouraged from smoking.[98] Patients with reversible obstructive airway disease may benefit from bronchodilation therapy. Patients with gastrointestinal manifestations due to delayed gastric emptying have experienced clinical improvement with the oral prokinetic drug, metoclopramide.[473] Prophylactic oral anticoagulants are recommended for stroke-prone patients. Angiokeratoma can be removed for cosmetic appearance or other indications by argon laser treatment with little, if any, scarring.[474–476] Since few patients have requested such cosmetic therapy, experience is limited.

Dialysis and Renal Transplantation

Because renal insufficiency is the most frequent late complication in patients with this disease, chronic hemodialysis and/or renal transplantation have become lifesaving procedures.[477,478] Contrary to an unfavorable early report,[479] more recent experience has indicated the clear benefit of transplantation for this disease.[477,480,481] Successful transplantation will correct renal function, and the engrafted kidney will remain histologically free of endogenous glycolipid deposition,[482,483] because the normal α-galactosidase A in the allograft will catabolize endogenous renal glycosphingolipid substrates. Reports of substrate accumulation in transplanted cadaveric kidneys have identified rare, isolated deposits, observable only by electron microscopy in infiltrating mononuclear cells[482,484] or nonglomerular capillary endothelial cells.[167,485,486] Presumably these endothelial cells are derived from the recipient and are α-galactosidase A-deficient.[487] Thus, renal transplantation for Fabry patients with end-stage renal disease is an efficacious procedure. However, living-related transplantation of kidneys donated from Fabry heterozygotes, which may already contain significant substrate deposition, should be avoided. In one reported patient, transplantation of a heterozygous allograft resulted in renal dysfunction five years later.[488] Therefore, all potential related donors must be carefully evaluated so that affected hemizygotes and heterozygotes for the Fabry gene are excluded. Since enzyme analysis does not reliably diagnose heterozygotes, it is necessary to demonstrate the specific α-galactosidase A mutation or disease haplotype in relatives who are potential donors. Also, the immune function in Fabry hemizygotes has been shown to be similar to that in other uremic patients, indicating that there is no immunologic contraindication to transplantation in this disease.[489] However, the formation of anti-α-galactosidase A antibodies has been demonstrated following acute rejection[490] in a recipient who was later shown to be CRIM-negative.[77]

For those patients who are unable or unwilling to undergo renal transplantation, chronic hemodialysis is an effective measure. In addition, the experience with peritoneal dialysis has been both long term and successful.[478] Use of angiotensin converting enzyme (ACE) inhibitors should be considered to prolong renal function in affected patients.

Genetic and Family Counseling

Fabry disease is inherited as an X-linked recessive trait.[11] All sons of affected males are unaffected, but all daughters are obligate carriers for the mutant gene. For each pregnancy of a female carrier, there is a 50 percent chance of passing the mutant gene to a male who would be affected, and a 50 percent chance of passing the mutant gene to a female, who would be a carrier. Biochemical and molecular testing of all suspect heterozygotes, genetic counseling, and prenatal diagnostic studies should be made available to all at-risk families (see "Diagnosis" above). Family and vocational counseling should be provided, especially to families with affected children. Often, parents, teachers, and/or physicians misinterpret the excruciating pain experienced during childhood as malingering, especially in the absence of any objective physical or laboratory findings. Because physical exertion, emotional stress, fatigue, and rapid changes in the environmental temperature and humidity can trigger these painful episodes, appropriate arrangements must be made with physical education teachers, employers, and other individuals to minimize or eliminate activities that may precipitate the painful crises. In addition, affected males should be allowed to participate in selected activities and be permitted to stop these activities at their own discretion. Within these limitations, reasonable occupational and vocational objectives should be pursued. Vocational counseling should discourage occupations that require significant manual dexterity, physical exertion, emotional stress, or exposure to extremes in temperature or rapid changes in temperature or humidity.

Prenatal Diagnosis

Prenatal diagnosis of Fabry disease can be accomplished by the assay of α-galactosidase A activity in chorionic villi obtained at 9 to 10 weeks of pregnancy or in cultured amniotic cells obtained by amniocentesis at approximately 15 weeks of pregnancy.[26,27,491–493] The prenatal diagnosis of an affected male fetus minimally requires the demonstration of deficient α-galactosidase A activity and an XY karyotype. It should be noted that the demonstration of the specific molecular lesion in the α-galactosidase A gene, if known in the family, is an important and often diagnostic adjunct to the enzyme assay.

Biochemical and ultrastructural studies of tissues from fetuses with Fabry disease have been reported.[26,491–494] Consistent with the prenatal diagnosis, the α-galactosidase A activity was deficient in all tissues studied; slightly increased concentrations of globotriaosylceramide were found in all tissues analyzed, with the exception of neural tissues.[491] Histologic and light-microscopic examination of various tissues were unremarkable, but ultrastructural examination revealed electron-dense concentric lamellar inclusions in the lysosomes of vascular endothelium, myocardium, renal tubules, epithelial and endothelial cells of renal glomeruli, and epithelial cells of the cornea.[493]

Enzyme Replacement

Attempts to replace the defective α-galactosidase A activity with normal enzyme have been undertaken. Early studies using partially purified α-galactosidase A from fig,[495] coffee bean,[496] and human sources[497–500] added to the media of cultured skin fibroblasts from Fabry hemizygotes demonstrated the ability of the exogenous enzyme to gain access to and catabolize the accumulated substrate, globotriaosylceramide. These in vitro studies indicated the feasibility of enzyme replacement and demonstrated that low levels (< 5 percent) of exogenous enzyme, particularly the high-uptake form,[498,499] were capable of normalizing substrate metabolism.

Several in vivo exploratory studies of enzyme replacement were undertaken in the 1970s to determine whether such endeavors can decrease the circulating accumulated substrate concentration. Normal plasma containing active enzyme was administered to affected males with Fabry disease.[28] Although active enzyme and decreased levels of globotriaosylceramide were demonstrated in the recipients' plasmas, the major limitation was the short half-life (~95 min) of the infused enzymatic activity. Subsequently in 1973, Brady and coworkers[29] intravenously administered single doses to two patients (6000 and 11,000 units, respectively) of a partially purified tissue form of α-galactosidase A from human placenta. The exogenous activity was rapidly cleared from the recipients' circulation with half-lives of 10 and 12 min, respectively. The plasma substrate was decreased about 50 percent at 45 min with a return to the preinfusion level by 48 h. In addition, the administered activity was detected in percutaneously biopsied liver at 1 h.[501]

In 1979, a clinical trial of enzyme replacement was performed involving multiple injections of purified splenic and plasma forms of α-galactosidase A into two brothers with Fabry disease.[249] This trial confirmed the previously observed differences in clearance rates of enzyme from the circulation and demonstrated for the first time the differential substrate depletion and reaccumulation kinetics for enzyme purified from tissue versus plasma sources.[30] The differential plasma clearance of these enzyme forms was presumably related to differences in the posttranslational modifications of these glycoproteins. The splenic form, which was rapidly cleared from the circulation ($t_{1/2}$ ~10 min), contained few charged sialic acid and/or phosphate residues. The plasma form, however, was highly sialylated and phosphorylated and was retained in the circulation ($t_{1/2}$ ~70 min).[249] These results are in accordance with the Ashwell model for the prolonged retention of sialylated glycoproteins in the circulation and the rapid clearance of desialylated glycoproteins.[502]

A marked difference in the clearance of circulating substrate was observed after these isozymes were administered.[30,249,503] Administration of α-galactosidase A isolated from human spleen effected a rapid decrease in the plasma concentration of accumulated substrate. The level of the circulating substrate decreased to approximately 50 percent of the preinfusion values 15 min after injection, followed by a rapid return to preinfusion levels by 2 to 3 h. In contrast, the administration of α-galactosidase A from human plasma resulted in a prolonged depletion of the circulating substrate. At 2 h after injection, the levels of globotriaosylceramide were decreased by 50 to 70 percent of the preinfusion values. Significantly, low levels were retained up to 12 to 24 h, and the substrate levels slowly returned to preinfusion levels after 36 to 72 h. When the total amount of substrate cleared with time was calculated by integrating the mean concentrations of globotriaosylceramide, the plasma enzyme appeared to have cleared about 25 times more substrate over time than did the splenic form. When two doses were administered on subsequent days, the plasma substrate level was reduced to the normal range.[30] In addition, these clinical trials demonstrated that multiple doses of either partially purified enzyme, administered over a 117-day period, did not elicit an immune response in the recipients. Although the amounts of enzyme administered were small, these studies demonstrated the feasibility of enzyme therapy for Fabry disease.

Recently, preclinical and clinical trials of human recombinant α-galactosidase A have been undertaken. Initial preclinical studies involved the administration of recombinant α-galactosidase A produced in CHO cells[254] into α-galactosidase A-deficient knockout mice (see above). Initial studies evaluated four different recombinant α-galactosidase A glycoforms, each differing in their glycosylation and/or phosphorylation (Ioannnou and Desnick, personal communication). The biodistribution, pharmacokinetics, and stability of these glycoforms were analyzed in vivo. At doses of 1 to 10 mg/kg body weight, over 90 percent of recovered enzyme activity of all four glycoforms was found in the liver and spleen, with 1 to 3 percent recovered in the heart and kidney, and no detectable enzyme in the brain. The half-life in plasma was less than 5 min for each glycoform. An α-galactosidase A glycoform with the highest degree of sialylation, was further analyzed for its ability to correct the enzyme deficiency in various tissues. Following administration of this lysosomal glycoform, the activity of α-galactosidase A reached wild type levels or higher in most tissues analyzed. The enzyme's half-life in liver lysosomes was ~40 hr, and was ~20 hr in the spleen and kidney. Multiple doses of α-galactosidase A resulted in the hydrolysis of the accumulated globotriaosylceramide in the liver, heart, kidney, and plasma.

Single doses of administered α-galactosidase A (0.3 to 10 mg enzyme/kg body weight) demonstrated that the metabolism of globotriaosylceramide in liver, spleen, heart, and kidney was dose-dependent, as demonstrated by a quantitative ELISA assay.[504] These preclinical studies provided the rationale for clinical trials of enzyme replacement therapy.

Independent Phase 1/2 and Phase 1 clinical trials recently have been undertaken using human α-galactosidase A produced in CHO cells and in human fibroblasts, respectively. Subsequently, independent Phase 3 and Phase 2 clinical trials were undertaken. At the time of this writing, the latter trials are being analyzed and no results are available.

Other Therapeutic Endeavors

Fetal Liver Transplantation. Fetal liver has been transplanted in three hemizygotes with Fabry disease in an attempt to replace the deficient enzyme.[505] The rise and subsequent fall in the levels of serum α-fetoprotein evidenced the initial survival and subsequent maturation (or possible loss) of the fetal cells.[506] Following transplantation, the α-galactosidase A levels in serum and leukocytes were unchanged, and the substrate levels in urine and serum were slightly decreased. However, the recipients noted subjective clinical improvement (e.g., increased sweating, no acroparesthesias, slightly decreased angiokeratoma). No further documentation of the effectiveness of fetal liver transplantation has been reported.

Experimental Bone Marrow Transplantation. To date, bone marrow transplantation has not been reported in patients with Fabry disease. However, normal murine bone marrow has been transplanted into α-galactosidase A-deficient mice.[507,508] In recipient mice with significant engraftment, decreased concentrations of globotriaosylceramide were noted in liver, spleen, and heart, but not in the kidney. Thus, extrapolation to patients with Fabry disease would have to evaluate the risk of the procedure and the possibility that successful transplantation may not alter the course of the renal disease.

Substrate Depletion. Another approach to deplete the accumulated circulating substrate has been chronic plasmapheresis.[509] This strategy was designed to deplete the accumulated substrate from the circulation before its deposition in the vascular wall and other cellular sites. Three plasmaphereses, performed at 2-day intervals, resulted in the removal of 23 mg and a 70 percent reduction of the level of circulating globotriaosylceramide to a value within the normal range. The plasma substrate levels slowly returned to preplasmapheresis levels in 5 days. Similar results were observed with chronic plasmapheresis performed over a 6-month period.[510,511] The major question with this approach is whether intervention by chronic plasmapheresis can deplete more substrate than that newly synthesized, so that the net result will be to decrease substrate deposition in the target sites of pathology, particularly the vascular endothelium. Another therapeutic attempt to decrease the plasma substrate levels involved chronic phlebotomies, which were performed in an attempt to remove senescent erythrocytes, a source of the accumulated glycosphingolipid.[512] However, following chronic blood depletion for almost 6 months, the levels of plasma globotriaosylceramide unexpectedly increased, which indicated that this approach was not therapeutic. Reviews of the various approaches for the treatment of enzyme deficiency diseases are available.[510,513]

Substrate Deprivation. Another approach to deplete the accumulated globotriaosylceramide and related glycolipids is "substrate deprivation." In this strategy, potent inhibitors of glycosylceramide synthase are used to decrease the synthesis of glucosylceramide (Glc-Cer), the precursor of globotriaosylceramide. A variety of inhibitors have been evaluated including *N*-butyldeoxnojirimycin and 1-phenyl-2-palmitoylamino-3-pyrrolidino-1-propanol-based compounds.[514] These inhibitors have reduced the globotriaosylceramide concentrations in lymphoblasts from Fabry patients; however, their in vivo safety and effects on the accumulated substrate have not been clinically evaluated.

Chemical Chaperons. Okumiya and colleagues reported that certain missense mutations produced catalytically active mutant enzymes that apparently were unstable and degraded in the endoplasmic reticulum under normal physiologic conditions, but could be stabilized by galactose or melibiose under in vitro conditions.[515,516] This approach was evaluated in an Italian cardiac variant with the G328R mutation.[517] Every other day intravenous infusion of 1 gm/kg of galactose resulted in marked improvement in cardiac function. Thus, for missense mutations that produce residual, but unstable, enzymatic activity, the use of small molecular inhibitors that bind to the active site and stabilize the enzyme for transport to the lysosome may prove therapeutic. However, this approach may be limited to cardiac variant patients who have residual activity and later-onset milder disease.

Recently, it was shown that 1-deoxy-galactonojirimycin (DGJ), a potent competitive inhibitor of α-galactosidase A, effectively enhanced the residual α-galactosidase A activity in Fabry lymphoblasts from cardiac variant patients, when administrated at concentrations lower than that usually required for intracellular inhibition of the enzyme.[518] The inhibitor appeared to accelerate transport and maturation of the mutant enzyme. Oral administration of DGJ to transgenic mice overexpressing the mutant R301Y α-galactosidase A allele substantially elevated the enzyme activity in some organs. These findings suggested that the administration of competitive inhibitors as "chemical chaperons" at subinhibitory intracellular concentrations for the treatment of the cardiac variant patients with residual α-galactosidase A activity may be efficacious.

Experimental Gene Therapy. The results of enzyme replacement studies and the lack of neuropathology make Fabry disease an ideal candidate disease for gene replacement. Early attempts focused on the construction of retroviral vectors that expressed the α-galactosidase A cDNA. These vectors were driven by the Harvey murine sarcoma virus and contained a bicistronic expression cassette composed of MDR1 (P-glycoprotein) for selection, an internal ribosome entry sequence (IRES) followed by the α-galactosidase A cDNA.[519,520] Expression of the α-galactosidase A activity using these vectors was obtained in vitro.[519] In addition, it was shown that the α-galactosidase A protein was secreted by positively transduced cells and that the enzyme was taken up by neighboring cells,[520] suggesting that this bystander effect could be advantageous for the treatment of Fabry disease by gene therapy. However, the major limitations of these vectors were the low expression of the second gene (the α-galactosidase A) in this bicistronic arrangement. Attempts to circumvent this limitation included the selection of transduced cells with vincristine, a drug that amplifies the MDR1 protein and thus, the full cistron including the α-galactosidase A.[521] However, the applicability of this selection procedure in vivo may not be practical. Subsequently, a different retroviral vector was used to transduce CD34(+) hematopoietic progenitor cells in vitro.[522] In addition, an adenoviral vector was used to correct the enzyme deficiency in Fabry fibroblasts.[523]

The first in vivo gene therapy was recently reported.[524] Recombinant adenoviral vectors expressing the the α-galactosidase A cDNA were constructed and injected intravenously into Fabry knockout mice.[357] This treatment caused an increase of the α-galactosidase A activity in all tissues analyzed including the liver, lung, spleen, muscle, heart, and kidney.[524] The activities observed were higher that those in normal mouse tissues, however, expression of the α-galactosidase A did not persist. By 12 weeks post-injection of the adenoviral vector, only 10 percent of the activity observed on day 3 remained. Most importantly however, the increase of the α-galactosidase A in treated mice coincided with a concomitant decrease of accumulated globotriaosylceramide to near normal levels for up to 6 months post treatment in the tissues studied. In another study, murine bone marrow cells were transduced with a retroviral vector and then transplanted into irradiated recipients.[355,525] The transplanted cells were detected in the peripheral blood nine weeks later and the activity of the engineered fusion protein was demonstrated. These results suggest that gene replacement represents a viable future approach for the treatment of Fabry disease provided that the obstacles of persistent expression and potential immunologic inactivation are overcome.

Future Prospects. The prospects for effective treatment of Fabry disease are promising. Enzyme replacement therapy using recombinant human α-galactosidase A is currently being evaluated in clinical trials. Other modes of therapy such as biochemical stabilization and enhancement of enzymatic activity using α-galactosidase inhibitors as "chemical chaperons"[518] and gene therapy[524] are being investigated. It is likely that in the near future, the outlook for Fabry patients will improve markedly and the emphasis will be on recognition of the often subtle early clinical features of the disease and on the diagnosis of at-risk family members so that treatment can be instituted early.

ACKNOWLEDGMENTS

The authors express their sincerest appreciation to the many Fabry patients and their families who have been the primary contributors to this review. In addition, we thank the nursing staff of the Mount Sinai General Clinical Research Center for their superb care of these patients. We thank Dr. Kenneth H. Astrin for critical review and assistance in the preparation of this manuscript. This work was supported in part by a grant (MERIT Award 5 R01 DK4045) from the National Institutes of Health, a grant (5 M01 RR00071) for the Mount Sinai General Clinical Research Center Program from the National Center of Research Resources, National Institutes of Health, and a grant (5P30 HD28822) for the Mount Sinai Child Health Research Center from the National Institutes of Health.

REFERENCES

1. Anderson W: A case of angiokeratoma. *Br J Dermatol* **10**:113, 1898.
2. Fabry J: Ein Beitrag Zur Kenntnis der Purpura haemorrhagica nodularis (Purpura papulosa hemorrhagica Habrae). *Arch Dermatol Syph* **43**:187, 1898.
3. Fabry J: Weiterer Beitrag zur klinik des Angiokeratoma naeviforme (Naevus angiokeratosus). *Dermatol Wochenschr* **90**:339, 1930.
4. Steiner L, Voerner H: Angiomatosis miliaris: Eine ideiopathische Gefasserkrankung. *Dtsch Arch Klin Med* **96**:105, 1909.
5. Gunther H: Anhidrosis and Diabetes insipidus. *Z Klin Med* **78**:53, 1913.
6. Weicksel J: Angiomatosis, bzw. Angiokeratosis universalis (eine sehr seltene Haut-und Gafasskrankheit). *Dtsch Med Wochenschr* **51**:898, 1925.
7. Pompen AWM, Ruiter M, Wyers JJG: Angiokeratoma corporis diffusum (universale) Fabry, as a sign of internal disease: Two autopsy reports. *Acta Med Scand* **128**:234, 1947.
8. Scriba K: Zur Pathogenese des Angiokeratoma corporis diffusum Fabry mit cardio-vasorenalem Symptomenkomplex. *Verh Dtsch Ges Pathol* **34**:221, 1950.
9. Hornbostel H, Scriba K: Zur Diagnostik des Angiokeratoma Fabry mit kardiovasorenalem Symptomenkomplex als posphatidspeicherungs-krankheit durch Probeexcision der Haut. *Klin Wochenschr* **31**:68, 1953.
10. Wise D, Wallace H, Jellinck E: Angiokeratoma corporis diffusum: A clinical study of eight affected families. *Q J Med* **31**:177, 1962.
11. Opitz JM, Stiles FC, Wise D, von Gemmingen G, Race RR, Sander R, Cross EG, de Groot WP: The genetics of angiokeratoma corporis diffusum (Fabry's disease), and its linkage with Xg(a) locus. *Am J Hum Genet* **17**:325, 1965.
12. Sweeley CC, Klionsky B: Fabry's disease: Classification as a sphingolipidosis and partial characterization of a novel glycolipid. *J Biol Chem* **238**:3148, 1963.
13. Vance DE, Krivit W, Sweeley CC: Concentrations of glycosyl ceramides in plasma and red cells in Fabry's disease, a glycolipid lipidosis. *J Lipid Res* **10**:188, 1969.
14. Desnick RJ, Dawson G, Desnick SJ, Sweeley CC, Krivit W: Diagnosis of glycosphingolipidoses by urinary-sediment analysis. *N Engl J Med* **284**:739, 1971.
15. Schibanoff JM, Kamoshita S, O'Brien JS: Tissue distribution of glyco-sphingolipids in a case of Fabry's disease. *J Lipid Res* **10**:515, 1969.
16. Desnick RJ, Blieden LC, Sharp HL, Hofschire PJ, Moller JH: Cardiac valvular anomalies in Fabry disease. Clinical, morphologic, and biochemical studies. *Circulation* **54**:818, 1976.
17. Wherrett JR, Hakomori SI: Characterization of a blood group B glycolipid accumulating in the pancreas of a patient with Fabry's disease. *J Biol Chem* **248**:3046, 1973.
18. Brady RO, Gal AE, Bradley RM, Martensson E, Warshaw AL, Laster L: Enzymatic defect in Fabry's disease. Ceramidetrihexosidase deficiency. *N Engl J Med* **276**:1163, 1967.
19. Kint JA: Fabry's disease: α-Galactosidase deficiency. *Science* **167**:1268, 1970.
20. Dean KJ, Sung SS, Sweeley CC: The identification of α-galactosidase B from human liver as an α-*N*-acetylgalactosaminidase. *Biochem Biophys Res Commun* **77**:1411, 1977.
21. Schram AW, Hamers MN, Tager JM: The identity of alpha-galactosidase B from human liver. *Biochim Biophys Acta* **482**:138, 1977.
22. Schindler D, Bishop DF, Wolfe DE, Wang AM, Egge H, Lemieux RU, Desnick RJ: Neuroaxonal dystrophy due to lysosomal α-*N*-acetylga-lactosaminidase deficiency. *N Engl J Med* **320**:1735, 1989.
23. Kanzaki T, Wang AM, Desnick RJ: Lysosomal alpha-*N*-acetylgalacto-saminidase deficiency, the enzymatic defect in angiokeratoma corporis diffusum with glycopeptiduria. *J Clin Invest* **88**:707, 1991.
24. Desnick RJ, Allen KY, Desnick SJ, Raman MK, Bernlohr RW, Krivit W: Fabry disease: Enzymatic diagnosis of hemizygotes and hetero-zygotes. α-Galactosidase activities in plasma, serum, urine and leukocytes. *J Lab Clin Med* **81**:157, 1973.
25. Johnson DL, Del Monte MA, Cotlier E, Desnick RJ: Fabry disease: Diagnosis of hemizygotes and heterozygotes by α-galactosidase A activity in tears. *Clin Chim Acta* **63**:81, 1975.
26. Brady RO, Uhlendorf BW, Jacobson CB: Fabry's disease: Antenatal detection. *Science* **172**:174, 1971.
27. Desnick R, Sweeley C: Prenatal detection of Fabry's disease (1971), in Dorfman A (ed): *Antenatal Diagnosis*. Chicago, University of Chicago Press, 1971, p 185.
28. Mapes CA, Anderson RL, Sweeley CC, Desnick RJ, Krivit W: Enzyme replacement in Fabry's disease, an inborn error of metabolism. *Science* **169**:987, 1970.
29. Brady RO, Tallman JF, Johnson WG, Gal AE, Leahy WR, Quirk JM, Dekaban AS: Replacement therapy for inherited enzyme deficiency. Use of purified ceramidetrihexosidase in Fabry's disease. *N Engl J Med* **289**:9, 1973.
30. Desnick RJ, Dean KJ, Grabowski GA, Bishop DF, Sweeley CC: Enzyme therapy XVII: Metabolic and immunologic evaluation of α-galactosidase A replacement in Fabry disease. *Birth Defects Orig Artic Ser* **16**:393, 1980.
31. Bishop DF, Calhoun DH, Bernstein HS, Hantzopoulos P, Quinn M, Desnick RJ: Human α-galactosidase A: Nucleotide sequence of a cDNA clone encoding the mature enzyme. *Proc Natl Acad Sci U S A* **83**:4859, 1986.
32. Bishop DF, Kornreich R, Desnick RJ: Structural organization of the human alpha-galactosidase A gene: Further evidence for the absence of a 3′ untranslated region. *Proc Natl Acad Sci U S A* **85**:3903, 1988.
33. Kornreich R, Desnick RJ, Bishop DF: Nucleotide sequence of the human α-galactosidase A gene. *Nucl Acids Res* **17**:3301, 1989.
34. Desnick RJ, Bishop DF; Fabry disease: α-Galactosidase A deficiency and Schindler disease: α-*N*-acetylgalactosaminidase deficiency, in Stanbury, JB, Wyngaarden JB, Fredrickson DS, Goldstein JL, Brown MS (eds): *The Metabolic Basis of Inherited Disease*, 6th ed. New York, McGraw-Hill, 1989, p 1751.
35. Lockman LA, Hunninghake DB, Krivit W, Desnick RJ: Relief of pain of Fabry's disease by diphenylhydantoin. *Neurology* **23**:871, 1973.
36. Rahman A, Simcone F, Hackel D, Hall PI, Hirsch E, Harris J: Angiokeratoma corporis diffusum universale (hereditary dystopic lipidosis). *Trans Assoc Am Physicians* **74**:366, 1961.
37. Burda CD, Winder PR: Angiokeratoma corporis diffusum universale (Fabry's disease) in female subjects. *Am J Med* **42**:293, 1967.
38. Bagdale JD, Parker F, Ways PO, Morgan TE, Lagunoff D, Eidelman S: Fabry's disease. A correlative clinical, morphologic, and biochemical study. *Lab Invest* **18**:681, 1968.
39. Johnston A, Weller S, Warland B: Angiokeratoma corporis diffusum. Some clinical aspects. *Arch Dis Child* **43**:73, 1968.

40. Sher NA, Letson RD, Desnick RJ: The ocular manifestations in Fabry's disease. *Arch Ophthalmol* **97**:671, 1979.
41. Lazareth I: [False erythermalgia]. *J Mal Vasc* **21**:84, 1996.
42. Urbain G, Peremans J, Philippart M: Fabry's disease without skin lesions. *Lancet* **1**:1111, 1967.
43. Wallace RD, Cooper WJ: Angiokeratoma corporis diffusum universale (Fabry). *Am J Med* **39**:656, 1965.
44. Clarke JT, Knaack J, Crawhall JC, Wolfe LS: Ceramide trihexosidosis (Fabry's disease) without skin lesions. *N Engl J Med* **284**:233, 1971.
45. Ainsworth S, Smith R: A case study of Fabry's disease occurring in a Black kindred without peripheral neuropathy or skin lesions. *Lab Invest* **38**:373, 1978.
46. Ferrans VJ, Hibbs RG, Burda CD: The heart in Fabry's disease. A histochemical and electron microscopic study. *Am J Cardiol* **24**:95, 1969.
47. Becker AE, Schoorl R, Balk AG, van der Heide RM: Cardiac manifestations of Fabry's disease. Report of a case with mitral insufficiency and electrocardiographic evidence of myocardial infarction. *Am J Cardiol* **36**:829, 1975.
48. Mehta J, Tuna N, Moller JH, Desnick RJ: Electrocardiographic and vectorcardiographic abnormalities in Fabry's disease. *Am Heart J* **93**:699, 1977.
49. Efthimiou J, McLelland J, Betteridge DJ: Short PR intervals and tachyarrhythmias in Fabry's disease. *Postgrad Med J* **62**:285, 1986.
50. Pochis WT, Litzow JT, King BG, Kenny D: Electrophysiologic findings in Fabry's disease with a short PR interval. *Am J Cardiol* **74**:203, 1994.
51. Matsui S, Murakami E, Takekoshi N, Hiramaru Y, Kin T: Cardiac manifestations of Fabry's disease. Report of a case with pulmonary regurgitation diagnosed on the basis of endomyocardial biopsy findings. *Jpn Circ J* **41**:1023, 1977.
52. Rowe JW, Caralis DG: Accelerated atrioventricular conduction in Fabry's disease: A case report. *Angiology* **29**:562, 1978.
53. Suzuki M, Goto T, Kato R, Yamauchi K, Hayashi H: Combined atrioventricular block and sinus node dysfunction in Fabry's disease. *Am Heart J* **120**:438, 1990.
54. Bass JL, Shrivastava S, Grabowski GA, Desnick RJ, Moller JH: The M-mode echocardiogram in Fabry's disease. *Am Heart J* **100**:807, 1980.
55. Goldman ME, Cantor R, Schwartz MF, Baker M, Desnick RJ: Echocardiographic abnormalities and disease severity in Fabry's disease. *J Am Coll Cardiol* **7**:1157, 1986.
56. Sakuraba H, Yanagawa Y, Igarashi T, Suzuki Y, Suzuki T, Watanabe K, Ieki K, Shimoda K, Yamanaka T: Cardiovascular manifestations in Fabry's disease. A high incidence of mitral valve prolapse in hemizygotes and heterozygotes. *Clin Genet* **29**:276, 1986.
57. Cohen IS, Fluri-Lundeen J, Wharton TP: Two dimensional echocardiographic similarity of Fabry's disease to cardiac amyloidosis: A function of ultrastructural analogy? *J Clin Ultrasound* **11**:437, 1983.
58. Matsui S, Murakami E, Takekoshi N, Nakatou H, Enyama H, Takeda F: Myocardial tissue characterization by magnetic resonance imaging in Fabry's disease. *Am Heart J* **117**:472, 1989.
59. Colucci WS, Lorell BH, Schoen FJ, Warhol MJ, Grossman W: Hypertrophic obstructive cardiomyopathy due to Fabry's disease. *N Engl J Med* **307**:926, 1982.
60. Fisher EA, Desnick RJ, Gordon RE, Eng CM, Griepp R, Goldman ME: Fabry disease: An unusual cause of severe coronary disease in a young man. *Ann Intern Med* **117**:221, 1992.
61. Bethune J, Landrigan P, Chipman C: Angiokeratoma corporis diffusum (Fabry's disease in two brothers). *N Engl J Med* **264**:1280, 1961.
62. Beaudet AL, Caskey CT: Detection of Fabry's disease heterozygotes by hair root analysis. *Clin Genet* **13**:251, 1978.
63. Maisey DN, Cosh JA: Basilar artery aneurysm and Anderson-Fabry disease. *J Neurol Neurosurg Psychiatry* **43**:85, 1980.
64. van Roey A, Wellens W: Angiokeratoma corporis diffusum van Fabry. *Arch Belg Dermatol Syph* **17**:325, 1961.
65. Duperrat B: L'Angiokeratome diffus de Fabry (angiokeratoma corporis diffusum). *Presse Med* **67**:1814, 1959.
66. Curry H, Fleisher T: Angiokeratoma corporis diffusum: A case report. *JAMA* **175**:864, 1961.
67. Stoughton R, Clendenning W: Angiokeratoma corporis diffusum (Fabry). *Arch Dermatol* **79**:601, 1959.
68. Guin GH, Burns WA, Saini N, Jones WP: Diffuse angiokeratoma (Fabry's disease): Case report. *Mil Med* **141**:259, 1976.
69. Morgan SH, Rudge P, Smith SJ, Bronstein AM, Kendall BE, Holly E, Young EP, Crawfurd MD, Bannister R: The neurological complications of Anderson-Fabry disease (alpha-galactosidase A deficiency)—Investigation of symptomatic and presymptomatic patients. *Q J Med* **75**:491, 1990.
70. Mitsias P, Levine SR: Cerebrovascular complications of Fabry's disease. *Ann Neurol* **40**:8, 1996.
71. Crutchfield KE, Patronas NJ, Dambrosia JM, Frei KP, Banerjee TK, Barton NW, Schiffmann R: Quantitative analysis of cerebral vasculopathy in patients with Fabry disease. *Neurology* **50**:1746, 1998.
72. Tedeschi G, Bonavita S, Banerjee TK, Virta A, Schiffmann R: Diffuse central neuronal involvement in Fabry disease: A proton MRS imaging study. *Neurology* **52**:1663, 1999.
73. Moumdjian R, Tampieri D, Melanson D, Ethier R: Anderson-Fabry disease: A case report with MR, CT, and cerebral angiography. *Am J Neuroradiol* **10**:S69, 1989.
74. Liston EH, Levine MD, Philippart M: Psychosis in Fabry disease and treatment with phenoxybenzamine. *Arch Gen Psychiatry* **29**:402, 1973.
75. Steward VW, Hitchcock C: Fabry's disease (angiokeratoma corporis diffusum). A report of 5 cases with pain in the extremities as the chief symptom. *Pathol Eur* **3**:377, 1968.
76. Mendez MF, Stanley TM, Medel NM, Li Z, Tedesco DT: The vascular dementia of Fabry's disease. *Dement Geriatr Cogn Disord* **8**:252, 1997.
77. Desnick R: Unpublished results.
78. Brown A, Milne J: Diffuse angiokeratoma: Report of two cases with diffuse skin changes, one with neurological symptoms and splenomegaly. *Glasgow J Med* **33**:361, 1952.
79. Pabico RC, Atancio BC, McKenna BA, Pamukcoglu T, Yodaiken R: Renal pathologic lesions and functional alterations in a man with Fabry's disease. *Am J Med* **55**:415, 1973.
80. Glass RBJ, Norton KI, Parsons R, Eng CM, Desnick RJ: Renal changes in Fabry disease: MRI and sonographic correlation with renal function in affected males and carrier females. (in review)
81. Sheth KJ, Roth DA, Adams MB: Early renal failure in Fabry's disease. *Am J Kidney Dis* **2**:651, 1983.
82. Colombi A, Kostyal A, Bracher R, Gloor F, Mazzi R, Tholen H: Angiokeratoma corporis diffusum—Fabry's disease. *Helv Med Acta* **34**:67, 1967.
83. Spaeth GL, Frost P: Fabry's disease. Its ocular manifestations. *Arch Ophthalmol* **74**:760, 1965.
84. Franceschetti AT: [Cornea verticillata (Gruber) and its relation to Fabry's disease (angiokeratoma corporis diffusum)]. *Ophthalmologica* **156**:232, 1968.
85. Gruber H: Cornea verticillata. *Ophthalmologica* **111**:120, 1946.
86. Terlinde R, Richard G, Lisch W, Ulrich K: Ruckbildung der Cornea verticillata bei Morbus-Fabry durch Kontaktlinsen. Erste beobachtungen. *Contactologia* **4**:20, 1982.
87. Andersen MV, Dahl H, Fledelius H, Nielsen NV: Central retinal artery occlusion in a patient with Fabry's disease documented by scanning laser ophthalmoscopy. *Acta Ophthalmol (Copenh)* **72**:635, 1994.
88. Oto S, Kart H, Kadayifcilar S, Ozdemir N, Aydin P: Retinal vein occlusion in a woman with heterozygous Fabry's disease. *Eur J Ophthalmol* **8**:265, 1998.
89. Rowe JW, Gilliam JI, Warthin TA: Intestinal manifestations of Fabry's disease. *Ann Intern Med* **81**:628, 1974.
90. Nelis GF, Jacobs GJ: Anorexia, weight loss, and diarrhea as presenting symptoms of angiokeratoma corporis diffusum (Fabry-Anderson's disease). *Dig Dis Sci* **34**:1798, 1989.
91. Sheth KJ, Werlin SL, Freeman ME, Hodach AE: Gastrointestinal structure and function in Fabry's disease. *Am J Gastroenterol* **76**:246, 1981.
92. Friedman LS, Kirkham SE, Thistlethwaite JR, Platika D, Kolodny EH, Schuffler MD: Jejunal diverticulosis with perforation as a complication of Fabry's disease. *Gastroenterology* **86**:558, 1984.
93. Roberts DH, Gilmore IT: Achalasia in Anderson-Fabry's disease. *J R Soc Med* **77**:430, 1984.
94. O'Brien BD, Shnitka TK, McDougall R, Walker K, Costopoulos L, Lentle B, Anholt L, Freeman H, Thomson AB: Pathophysiologic and ultrastructural basis for intestinal symptoms in Fabry's disease. *Gastroenterology* **82**:957, 1982.
95. Sheth KJ, Swick HM: Peripheral nerve conduction in Fabry disease. *Ann Neurol* **7**:319, 1980.
96. Parkinson J, Sunshine A: Angiokeratoma corporis diffusum universale (Fabry) presenting as suspected myocardial infarction and pulmonary infarcts. *Am J Med* **31**:951, 1961.
97. Kariman K, Singletary WV Jr., Sieker HO: Pulmonary involvement in Fabry's disease [Letter]. *Am J Med* **64**:911, 1978.
98. Brown LK, Miller A, Bhuptani A, Sloane MF, Zimmerman MI, Schilero G, Eng CM, Desnick RJ: Pulmonary involvement in Fabry disease. *Am J Respir Crit Care Med* **155**:1004, 1997.

99. Rosenberg DM, Ferrans VJ, Fulmer JD, Line BR, Barranger JA, Brady RO, Crystal RG: Chronic airflow obstruction in Fabry's disease. *Am J Med* **68**:898, 1980.
100. Gemignani F, Pietrini V, Tagliavini F, Lechi A, Neri TM, Asinari A, Savi M: Fabry's disease with familial lymphedema of the lower limbs. Case report and family study. *Eur Neurol* **18**:84, 1979.
101. Lozano F, Garcia-Talavera R, Gomez-Alonso A: An unusual cause of lymphoedema—Confirmed by isotopic lymphangiography. *Eur J Vasc Surg* **2**:129, 1988.
102. Mayou SC, Kirby JD, Morgan SH: Anderson-Fabry disease: An unusual presentation with lymphadenopathy. *J R Soc Med* **82**:555, 1989.
103. Wilson SK, Klionsky BL, Rhamy RK: A new etiology of priapism: Fabry's disease. *J Urol* **109**:646, 1973.
104. Funderburk SJ, Philippart M, Dale G, Cederbaum SD, Vyden JK: Letter: Priapism after phenoxybenzamine in a patient with Fabry's disease. *N Engl J Med* **290**:630, 1974.
105. Garcia-Consuegra J, Padron M, Jaureguizar E, Carrascosa C, Ramos J: Priapism and Fabry disease: A case report. *Eur J Pediatr* **149**:500, 1990.
106. Foda MM, Mahmood K, Rasuli P, Dunlap H, Kiruluta G, Schillinger JF: High-flow priapism associated with Fabry's disease in a child: A case report and review of the literature. *Urology* **48**:949, 1996.
107. Krivit W, Vance D, Desnick R, Whitecar J, Sweeley C: Red cell physiology in Fabry's disease. *J Lab Clin Med* **12**:906, 1968.
108. Igarashi T, Sakuraba H, Suzuki Y: Activation of platelet function in Fabry's disease. *Am J Hematol* **22**:63, 1986.
109. Fessas P, Wintrobe M, Cartwright G: Angiokeratoma corporis diffusum universale (Fabry): First American report of a rare disorder. *Arch Intern Med* **95**:469, 1955.
110. Fischer E: Fabry disease, a disease with rheumatic aspects: Radiology of soft tissue and bone changes in the hand. *Z Rheumatol* **45**:36, 1986.
111. Bishop DF, Grabowski GA, Desnick RJ: Fabry disease: An asymptomatic hemizygote with significant residual α-galactosidase A activity. *Am J Hum Genet* **33**:71A, 1981.
112. Bach G, Rosenmann E, Karni A, Cohen T: Pseudodeficiency of alpha-galactosidase A. *Clin Genet* **21**:59, 1982.
113. Kobayashi T, Kira J, Shinnoh N, Goto I, Kuroiwa Y: Fabry's disease with partially deficient hydrolysis of ceramide trihexoside. *J Neurol Sci* **67**:179, 1985.
114. Romeo G, D'Urso M, Pisacane A, Blum E, De Falco A, Ruffilli A: Residual activity of alpha-galactosidase A in Fabry's disease. *Biochem Genet* **13**:615, 1975.
115. Ogawa K, Sugamata K, Funamoto N, Abe T, Sato T, Nagashima K, Ohkawa S: Restricted accumulation of globotriaosylceramide in the hearts of atypical cases of Fabry's disease. *Hum Pathol* **21**:1067, 1990.
116. Nagao Y, Nakashima H, Fukuhara Y, Shimmoto M, Oshima A, Ikari Y, Mori Y, Sakuraba H, Suzuki Y: Hypertrophic cardiomyopathy in late-onset variant of Fabry disease with high residual activity of alpha-galactosidase A. *Clin Genet* **39**:233, 1991.
117. Ishii S, Sakuraba H, Suzuki Y: Point mutations in the upstream region of the alpha-galactosidase A gene exon 6 in an atypical variant of Fabry disease. *Hum Genet* **89**:29, 1992.
118. Sakuraba H, Oshima A, Fukuhara Y, Shimmoto M, Nagao Y, Bishop DF, Desnick RJ, Suzuki Y: Identification of point mutations in the α-galactosidase A gene in classical and atypical hemizygotes with Fabry disease. *Am J Hum Genet* **47**:784, 1990.
119. Elleder M, Bradova V, Smid F, Budesinsky M, Harzer K, Kustermann-Kuhn B, Ledvinova J, Belohlavek, Kral V, Dorazilova V: Cardiocyte storage and hypertrophy as a sole manifestation of Fabry's disease. Report on a case simulating hypertrophic non-obstructive cardiomyopathy. *Virchows Arch A Pathol Anat Histopathol* **417**:449, 1990.
120. von Scheidt W, Eng CM, Fitzmaurice TF, Erdmann E, Hubner G, Olsen EG, Christomanou H, Kandolf R, Bishop DF, Desnick RJ: An atypical variant of Fabry's disease with manifestations confined to the myocardium. *N Engl J Med* **324**:395, 1991.
121. Nakao S, Takenaka T, Maeda M, Kodama C, Tanaka A, Tahara M, Yoshida A, Kuriyama M, Hayashibe H, Sakuraba H, et al.: An atypical variant of Fabry's disease in men with left ventricular hypertrophy. *N Engl J Med* **333**:288, 1995.
122. Rosenmann E, Kobrin I, Cohen T: Kidney involvement in systemic lupus erythematosus and Fabry's disease. *Nephron* **34**:180, 1983.
123. Ko YH, Kim HJ, Roh YS, Park CK, Kwon CK, Park MH: Atypical Fabry's disease. An oligosymptomatic variant. *Arch Pathol Lab Med* **120**:86, 1996.
124. Meroni M, Spisni C, Tazzari S, Di Vito R, Stingone A, Bovan I, Torri Tarelli L, Sessa A: Isolated glomerular proteinuria as the only clinical manifestation of Fabry's disease in an adult male. *Nephrol Dial Transplant* **12**:221, 1997.
125. Nakao S, Kodama C, Takenake T, Tanaka A, Yuichiro Y, Yoshida A, Kanzaki T, Enriquez ALD, Eng CE, Tanaka H, Desnick RJ: Fabry disease: Detection of undiagnosed patients undergoing chronic hemodialysis. In review.
126. Ashton-Prolla P, Tong B, Shabbeer J, Eng CM, Desnick RJ: 22 novel mutations in the α-galactosidase A gene and genotype/phenotype correlations including mild hemizygotes and severely affected heterozygotes. *J Invest Med* **48**:227, 2000.
127. Franceschetti AT: Fabry disease: Ocular manifestations. *Birth Defects Orig Artic Ser* **12**:195, 1976.
128. Broadbent JC, Edwards WD, Gordon H, Hartzler GO, Krawisz JE: Fabry cardiomyopathy in the female confirmed by endomyocardial biopsy. *Mayo Clin Proc* **56**:623, 1981.
129. Desnick RJ, Simmons RL, Allen KY, Woods JE, Anderson CF, Najarian JS, Krivit W: Correction of enzymatic deficiencies by renal transplantation: Fabry's disease. *Surgery* **72**:203, 1972.
130. Rietra P, Brouwer-Kelder E, de Groot W, Tager J: The use of biochemical parameters for the detection of carriers of Fabry's disease. *J Mol Med* **1**:237, 1976.
131. Van Loo A, Vanholder R, Madsen K, Praet M, Kint J, De Paepe A, Messiaen L, Lameire N, Hasholt L, Sorensen SA, Ringoir S: Novel frameshift mutation in a heterozygous woman with Fabry disease and end-stage renal failure. *Am J Nephrol* **16**:352, 1996.
132. Avila JL, Convit J, Velazquez-Avila G: Fabry's disease: normal alpha-galactosidase activity and urinary-sediment glycosphingolipid levels in two obligate heterozygotes. *Br J Dermatol* **89**:149, 1973.
133. Levade T, Giordano F, Maret A, Marguery MC, Bazex J, Salvayre R: Different phenotypic expression of Fabry disease in female monozygotic twins. *J Inherit Metab Dis* **14**:105, 1991.
134. Marguery MC, Giordano F, Parant M, Samalens G, Levade T, Salvayre R, Maret A, Calvas P, Bourrouillou G, Cantala P, et al.: Fabry's disease: Heterozygous form of different expression in two monozygous twin sisters. *Dermatology* **187**:9, 1993.
135. Redonnet-Vernhet I, Ploos van Amstel JK, Jansen RP, Wevers RA, Salvayre R, Levade T: Uneven X inactivation in a female monozygotic twin pair with Fabry disease and discordant expression of a novel mutation in the alpha-galactosidase A gene. *J Med Genet* **33**:682, 1996.
136. Lyon M: Gene action in the X-chromosome of the mouse (Mus musculus L.). *Nature* **190**:372, 1961.
137. Romeo G, Migeon BR: Genetic inactivation of the alpha-galactosidase locus in carriers of Fabry's disease. *Science* **170**:180, 1970.
138. Gubler MC, Lenoir G, Grunfeld JP, Ulmann A, Droz D, Habib R: Early renal changes in hemizygous and heterozygous patients with Fabry's disease. *Kidney Int* **13**:223, 1978.
139. Itoh K, Takenaka T, Nakao S, Setoguchi M, Tanaka H, Suzuki T, Sakuraba H: Immunofluorescence analysis of trihexosylceramide accumulated in the hearts of variant hemizygotes and heterozygotes with Fabry disease. *Am J Cardiol* **78**:116, 1996.
140. Desnick RJ, Ioannou YA, Eng CM: α-Galactosidase A deficiency: Fabry disease in Scriver CR, Beaudet AL, Sly WS, Valle D (eds): *The Metabolic Basis of Inherited Disease*, 7th ed. New York, McGraw-Hill, 1995, p 2741.
141. Elleder M: Fabry's disease: Absence of storage as a feature of liver sinus endothelium. *Acta Histochem* **77**:33, 1985.
142. Sagebiel RW, Parker F: Cutaneous lesions of Fabry's disease: Glycolipid lipidosis; light and electron microscopic findings. *J Invest Dermatol* **50**:208, 1968.
143. Breathnach SM, Black MM, Wallace HJ: Anderson-Fabry disease. Characteristic ultrastructural features in cutaneous blood vessels in a 1-year-old boy. *Br J Dermatol* **103**:81, 1980.
144. Tarnowski WM, Hashimoto K: New light microscopic skin findings in Fabry's disease. Study of four patients using plastic-embedded tissue. *Acta Derm Venereol* **49**:386, 1969.
145. Morel-Maroger L, Ganter P, Ardaillou R, Cathelineau G, Richet G: Histochemical study of a lipid thesaurismosis with renal, cutaneous and neurologic involvement. Its relation to Fabry's angiokeratosis and familial renal cytodystrophy. *Bull Mem Soc Med Hop Paris* **117**:49, 1966.
146. Hashimoto K, Gross B, Lever W: Angiokeratoma corporis diffusum (Fabry): Histochemical and electron microscopic studies of the skin. *J Invest Dermatol* **44**:119, 1965.
147. Lao LM, Kumakiri M, Mima H, Kuwahara H, Ishida H, Ishiguro K, Fujita T, Ueda K: The ultrastructural characteristics of eccrine sweat glands in a Fabry disease patient with hypohidrosis. *J Dermatol Sci* **18**:109, 1998.

148. Chatterjee S, Gupta P, Pyeritz RE, Kwiterovich POJ: Immunohistochemical localization of glycosphingolipid in urinary renal tubular cells in Fabry's disease. *Am J Clin Pathol* **82**:24, 1984.
149. McNary W, Lowenstein L: A morphological study of the renal lesion in angiokeratoma corporis diffusum universale (Fabry's disease). *J Urol* **93**:641, 1965.
150. Burkholder PM, Updike SJ, Ware RA, Reese OG: Clinicopathologic, enzymatic, and genetic features in a case of Fabry's disease. *Arch Pathol Lab Med* **104**:17, 1980.
151. Grunnet ML, Spilsbury PR: The central nervous system in Fabry's disease. An ultrastructural study. *Arch Neurol* **28**:231, 1973.
152. Cable WJ, Kolodny EH, Adams RD: Fabry disease: Impaired autonomic function. *Neurology* **32**:498, 1982.
153. Kocen RS, Thomas PK: Peripheral nerve involvement in Fabry's disease. *Arch Neurol* **22**:81, 1970.
154. Kahn P: Anderson-Fabry disease: A histopathological study of three cases with observations on the mechanism of production of pain. *J Neurol Neurosurg Psychiatry* **36**:1053, 1973.
155. Ohnishi A, Dyck P: Loss of small peripheral sensory neurons in Fabry disease. Histologic and morphometric evaluation of cutaneous nerves, spinal ganglia, and posterior columns. *Arch Neurol* **31**:120, 1974.
156. Sung J, Hayano M, Mastri A, Desnick R: Neuropathology and neural glycosphingolipid deposition in Fabry's disease. *Excerpta Med Cong Ser* **1**:267, 1975.
157. Sung JH: Autonomic neurons affected by lipid storage in the spinal cord in Fabry's disease: Distribution of autonomic neurons in the sacral cord. *J Neuropathol Exp Neurol* **38**:87, 1979.
158. Cable WJ, Dvorak AM, Osage JE, Kolodny EH: Fabry disease: Significance of ultrastructural localization of lipid inclusions in dermal nerves. *Neurology* **32**:347, 1982.
159. Rahman A, Lindenberg R: The neuropathology of hereditary dystopic lipidosis. *Arch Neurol* **9**:373, 1963.
160. de Veber GA, Schwarting GA, Kolodny EH, Kowall NW: Fabry disease: Immunocytochemical characterization of neuronal involvement. *Ann Neurol* **31**:409, 1992.
161. Elleder M, Christomanou H, Kustermann-Kuhn B, Harzer K: Leptomeningeal lipid storage patterns in Fabry disease. *Acta Neuropathol* **88**:579, 1994.
162. Witschel H, Mathyl J: Morphological bases of the specific ocular changes in Fabry's disease. *Klin Monatsbl Augenheilkd* **154**:599, 1969.
163. Font RL, Fine BS: Ocular pathology in Fabry's disease. Histochemical and electron microscopic observations. *Am J Ophthalmol* **73**:419, 1972.
164. Macrae WG, Ghosh M, McCulloch C: Corneal changes in Fabry's disease: A clinico-pathologic case report of a heterozygote. *Ophthalmic Paediatr Genet* **5**:185, 1985.
165. Uchino M, Uyama E, Kawano H, Hokamaki J, Kugiyama K, Murakami Y, Yasue H, Ando M: A histochemical and electron microscopic study of skeletal and cardiac muscle from a Fabry disease patient and carrier. *Acta Neuropathol* **90**:334, 1995.
166. Schachern PA, Shea DA, Paparella MM, Yoon TH: Otologic histopathology of Fabry's disease. *Ann Otol Rhinol Laryngol* **98**:359, 1989.
167. Faraggiana T, Churg J, Grishman E, Strauss L, Prado A, Bishop DF, Schuchman E, Desnick RJ: Light- and electron-microscopic histochemistry of Fabry's disease. *Am J Pathol* **103**:247, 1981.
168. Lehner T, Adams CW: Lipid histochemistry of Fabry's disease. *J Pathol Bacteriol* **95**:411, 1968.
169. van Mullem P, Ruiter M: Histochemical studies on lipid metabolism in so-called Fabry's disease (angiokeratoma corporis diffusum). *Arch Klin Exp Derm* **232**:148, 1968.
170. Robinson D, Khalfan H: Fabry's disease. Identification of carrier status by fluorescent/electron binding. *Biochem Soc Trans* **12**:1063, 1984.
171. van Mullem P, Ruiter M: Fine structure of the skin in angiokeratoma corporis diffusum (Fabry's disease). *J Pathol* **101**:221, 1970.
172. Hashimoto K, Lieberman P, Lamkin NJ: Angiokeratoma corporis diffusum (Fabry disease). A lysosomal disease. *Arch Dermatol* **112**:1416, 1976.
173. Nakamura T, Kaneko H, Nishino I: Angiokeratoma corporis diffusum (Fabry disease): Ultrastructural studies of the skin. *Acta Derm Venereol* **61**:37, 1981.
174. Steck T, Dawson G: Topographical distribution of complex carbohydrates in the erythrocyte membrane. *J Biol Chem* **239**:2135, 1974.
175. Thompson T, Tillack T: Organization of glycosphingolipids in bilayers and plasma membranes of mammalian cells. *Ann Rev Biophys Chem* **14**:361, 1985.
176. Dawson G: Glycolipid catabolism, in Horowitz M, Pigman W (eds): *The Glycoconjugate II*. New York, Academic Press, 1978, p 225.
177. Dawson G, Kruski AW, Scanu AM: Distribution of glycosphingolipids in the serum lipoproteins of normal human subjects and patients with hypo- and hyper-lipidemias. *J Lipid Res* **17**:125, 1976.
178. Clarke JT, Stoltz JM, Mulcahey MR: Neutral glycosphingolipids of serum lipoproteins in Fabry's disease. *Biochim Biophys Acta* **431**:317, 1976.
179. Chatterjee S, Kwiterovich POJ: Glycosphingolipids and plasma lipoproteins: A review. *Can J Biochem Cell Biol* **62**:385, 1984.
180. Kundu S, Diego I, Osovitz S, Marcus D: Glycosphingolipids of human plasma. *Arch Biochem Biophys* **238**:388, 1985.
181. Yang H, Lund T, Niebuhr E, Norby S, Schwartz M, Shen L: A deletion panel of the long arm of the X chromosome: Subregional localization of 22 DNA probes. *Hum Genet* **85**:25, 1990.
182. Macher B, Sweeley C: Glycosphingolipids: Structure, biological source and nomenclature. *Methods Enzymol* **50C**:236, 1978.
183. Gasa S, Nakamura M, Makita A, Ikura M, Hikichi K: Complete structural analysis of globoseries glycolipids by two-dimensional nuclear magnetic resonance. *Eur J Biochem* **155**:603, 1986.
184. Ito M, Yamagata T: A novel glycosphingolipid-degrading enzyme cleaves the linkage between the oligosaccharide and ceramide of neutral and acidic glycosphingolipids. *J Biol Chem* **261**:14278, 1986.
185. Li S-C, Degasperi R, Muldrey J, Li Y-T: A unique glycosphingolipid-splitting enzyme (ceramide-glycanase from leech) cleaves the linkage between the oligosaccharide and the ceramide. *Biochem Biophys Res Commun* **141**:346, 1986.
186. Kannagi R, Watanabe K, Hakomori S-I: Isolation and purification of glycosphingolipids by high-performance liquid chromatography. *Methods Enzymol* **138**:3, 1987.
187. Ulman M, McCluer R: High-pressure chromatography analysis of neutral glycosphingolipids: Perbenzoylated mono-, di-, tri- and tetraglycosylceramides. *Methods Enzymol* **138**:117, 1987.
188. Karlsson KA: On the character and functions of sphingolipids. *Acta Biochem Pol* **45**:429, 1998.
189. Desnick RJ, Sweeley CC: Fabry disease: α-Galactosidase A deficiency, in Stanbury JB, Fredrickson DS, Goldstein JL, Brown MS (eds): *The Metabolic Basis of Inherited Disease*. New York, McGraw Hill, 1983, p 906.
190. Martensson E: Neutral glycolipids of human kidney. Isolation, identification and fatty acid composition. *Biochim Biophys Acta* **116**:296, 1966.
191. Naiki M, Marcus DM: Human erythrocyte P and Pk blood group antigens: Identification as glycosphingolipids. *Biochem Biophys Res Commun* **60**:1105, 1974.
192. Naiki M, Marcus D: An immunochemical study of the human blood group P1, P, and Pk glycosphingolipid antigens. *Biochemistry* **14**:4837, 1975.
193. Marcus D, Naiki M, Kundu S: Abnormalities in the glycosphingolipid content of human Pk and P erythrocytes. *Proc Natl Acad Sci U S A* **73**:3263, 1976.
194. Wiels J, Holmes EH, Cochran N, Tursz T, Hakomori S: Enzymatic and organizational difference in expression of a Burkitt lymphoma-associated antigen (globotriaosylceramide) in Burkitt lymphoma and lymphoblastoid cell lines. *J Biol Chem* **259**:14783, 1984.
195. Nudelman E, Kannagi R, Hakomori S, Parsons M: A glycolipid antigen associated with Burkitt lymphoma defined by a monoclonal antibody. *Science* **220**:509, 1983.
196. Wils P, Junqua S, Le Pecq JB: Determination of antibody-complement mediated cytotoxicity using ATP release induced by a monoclonal antibody against the Burkitt lymphoma associated globotriaosylceramide antigen. *J Immunol Methods* **87**:217, 1986.
197. Cohen A, Hannigan GE, Williams BR, Lingwood CA: Roles of globotriaosyl and galabiosylceramide in verotoxin binding and high affinity interferon receptor. *J Biol Chem* **262**:17088, 1987.
198. Shapiro D, Acher AJ: Total synthesis of ceramide trihexoside accumulating with Fabry's disease. *Chem Phys Lipids* **22**:197, 1978.
199. Koike K, Sugimoto M, Sato S, Ito Y, Nakahara Y, Ogawa T: Total synthesis of globotriaosyl-E and Z-ceramides and isoglobotriaosyl-E-ceramide. *Carbohydr Res* **163**:189, 1987.
200. Miyatake T: A study on glycolipids in Fabry's disease. *Jpn J Exp Med* **39**:35, 1969.
201. Lou H: A biochemical investigation of angiokeratoma corporis diffusum. *Acta Pathol Microbiol Scand* **68**:332, 1966.
202. Snyder PJ, Krivit W, Sweeley C: Generalized accumulation of neutral glycosphingolipids with G_{m2} ganglioside accumulation in the brain. *J Lipid Res* **13**:128, 1972.

203. Vance DE, Sweeley CC: Quantitative determination of the neutral glycosyl ceramides in human blood. *J Lipid Res* **8**:621, 1967.
204. Hozumi I, Nishizawa M, Ariga T, Miyatake T: Biochemical and clinical analysis of accumulated glycolipids in symptomatic heterozygotes of angiokeratoma corporis diffusum (Fabry's disease) in comparison with hemizygotes. *J Lipid Res* **31**:335, 1990.
205. Hozumi I, Nishizawa M, Ariga T, Inoue Y, Ohnishi Y, Yokoyama A, Shibata A, Miyatake T: Accumulation of glycosphingolipids in spinal and sympathetic ganglia of a symptomatic heterozygote of Fabry's disease. *J Neurol Sci* **90**:273, 1989.
206. Koskielak J, Piasek A, Gorniak H, Gardas A, Gregor A: Structures of fucose-containing glycolipids with H and B blood group activity and of sialic acid and glucosamine-containing glycolipid of human erythrocyte membrane. *Eur J Biochem* **37**:214, 1973.
207. Basu M, De T, Das K, Kyle J, Chon H-C, Schaeper R, Basu S: Glycolipids. *Methods Enzymol* **138**:575, 1987.
208. Stults CL, Sweeley CC, Macher BA: Glycosphingolipids: Structure, biological source, and properties. *Methods Enzymol* **179**:167, 1989.
209. Shayman JA, Radin NS: Structure and function of renal glycosphingolipids [Editorial]. *Am J Physiol* **260**:F291, 1991.
210. Ichikawa S, Hirabayashi Y: Glucosylceramide synthase and glycosphingolipid synthesis. *Trends Cell Biol* **8**:198, 1998.
211. Taniguchi N, Yanagisawa K, Makita A, Naiki M: Purification and properties of rat liver globotriaosylceramide synthase, UDP-galactose: lactosylceramide α1,4-galactosyltransferase. *J Biol Chem* **260**:4908, 1985.
212. Kojima H, Tsuchiya S, Sekiguchi K, Gelinas R, Hakomori S: Predefined gene transfer for expression of a glycosphingolipid antigen by transfection with a cosmid genomic library prepared from a cell line in which the specific glycosphingolipid is highly expressed. *Biochem Biophys Res Commun* **143**:716, 1987.
213. Martensson E, Ohman R, Graves M, Svennerholm L: Galactosyltransferases catalyzing the formation of the galactosyl-galactosyl linkage in glycosphingolipids. *J Biol Chem* **249**:4132, 1974.
214. Nagai M, Dave V, Muensch H, Yoshida A: Human blood group glycosyltransferase II. Purification of galactosyltransferase. *J Biol Chem* **253**:380, 1978.
215. Yoshida A: The existence of atypical blood group galactosyltransferase which causes an expression of A2 character in A1B red blood cells. *Am J Hum Genet* **35**:1117, 1983.
216. Basu M, Basu S: Enzymatic synthesis of a blood group B-related pentaglycosylceramide by an α-galactosyltransferase from rabbit bone marrow. *J Biol Chem* **248**:1700, 1973.
217. Basu S, Basu M, Kyle J, De T, Das K, Schaeper R in Freysz Z, Gatt S (eds): *Enzymes of Lipid Metabolism*. New York, Plenum, 1986.
218. Iizuka S, Chen SH, Yoshida A: Studies on the human blood group P system: An existence of UDP-Gal:lactosylceramide alpha 1–4 galactosyltransferase in the small p type cells. *Biochem Biophys Res Commun* **137**:1187, 1986.
219. Brown M, Kovanen P, Goldstein J: Regulation of plasma cholesterol by lipoprotein receptors. *Science* **212**:628, 1981.
220. Dawson G, Sweeley CC: In vivo studies on glycosphingolipid metabolism in porcine blood. *J Biol Chem* **245**:410, 1970.
221. Vance DE, Krivit W, Sweeley CC: Metabolism of neutral glycosphingolipids in plasma of a normal human and a patient with Fabry's disease. *J Biol Chem* **250**:8119, 1975.
222. Entenman C, Chaikoff I, Zilversmit D: Removal of plasma phospholipids as a function of the liver: The effect of exclusion of the liver on the turnover rate of plasma phospholipids as measured with radioactive phosphorus. *J Biol Chem* **166**:15, 1946.
223. Metz R, Radin N: Glucosylceramide uptake protein from spleen cytosol. *J Biol Chem* **255**:4463, 1980.
224. Bloj B, Zilversmit D: Accelerated transfer of neutral glycosphingolipids and ganglioside GM1 by a purified lipid transfer protein. *J Biol Chem* **256**:5988, 1981.
225. Furst W, Sandhoff K: Activator proteins and topology of lysosomal sphingolipid catabolism. *Biochim Biophys Acta* **1126**:1, 1992.
226. Sandhoff K, van Echten G, Schroder M, Schnabel D, K: S: Metabolism of glycolipids: The role of glycolipid-binding proteins in the function and pathobiochemistry of lysosomes. *Biochem Soc Trans* **20**:1992.
227. Salvayre R, Negre A, Maret A, Douste-Blazy L: Alpha-galactosidases and alpha-*N*-acetylgalactosaminidase. Biochemical bases of Fabry's disease. *Pathol Biol (Paris)* **32**:269, 1984.
228. Glew R, Peters S: *Practical Enzymology of the Sphingolipidoses*. New York, A. R. Liss, 1977.
229. Kusiak J, Quirk J, Brady R: Ceramide trihexoside from human placenta. *Methods Enzymol* **50**:529, 1978.
230. Desnick R: Enzyme Therapy in Genetic Diseases, R J Desnick, ed., p544, vol. 2. New York, Alan R. Liss, 1980.
231. Conzelmann E, Sandhoff K: Glycoplipid and glycoprotein degradation. *Adv Enzymol* **60**:90, 1987.
232. Bensaude I, Callahan J, Philippart M: Fabry's disease as an α-galactosidosis: Evidence for an α-configuration in trihexosyl ceramide. *Biochem Biophys Res Commun* **43**:913, 1971.
233. Clarke JTR, Wolfe LS, Perlin AS: Evidence for an a terminal α-D-galactopyranosyl residue in galactosyl-galactosyl-glucosyl ceramide from human kidney. *J Biol Chem* **246**:5563, 1971.
234. Hakomori SI, Siddiqui B, Li YT, Li SC, Hellerqvist CB: Anomeric structures of globoside and ceramide trihexoside of human erythrocytes and hamster fibroblasts. *J Biol Chem* **246**:2271, 1971.
235. Handa S, Ariga T, Miyatake T, Yamakawa T: Presence of alpha-anomeric glycosidic configuration in the glycolipids accumulated in kidney with Fabry's disease. *J Biochem (Tokyo)* **69**:625, 1971.
236. Li YT, C. LS: Anomeric configuration of galactose residues in ceramide trihexosides. *J Biol Chem* **246**:3769, 1971.
237. Desnick RJ, Allen KY, Desnick SJ, Raman MK, Bernlohr RW, Krivit W: Fabry's disease: Enzymatic diagnosis of hemizygotes and heterozygotes. Alpha-galactosidase activities in plasma, serum, urine, and leukocytes. *J Lab Clin Med* **81**:157, 1973.
238. Beutler E, Kuhl W: Biochemical and electrophoretic studies of α-galactosidase in normal man, in patients with Fabry's disease, and in Equidae. *Am J Hum Genet* **24**:237, 1972.
239. Rietra PJ, Van den Bergh FA, Tager JM: Properties of the residual alpha-galactosidase activity in the tissues of a Fabry hemizygote. *Clin Chim Acta* **62**:401, 1975.
240. Wood S, Nadler HL: Fabry's disease: Absence of an α-galactosidase isozyme. *Am J Hum Genet* **24**:250, 1972.
241. Beutler E, Kuhl W: Relationship between human α-galactosidase isozymes. *Nature New Biol* **239**:207, 1972.
242. Crawhall JC, Banfalvi M: Fabry's disease: Differentiation between two forms of α-galactosidase by myoinositol. *Science* **177**:527, 1972.
243. Kint J, Carton D in Van Hoof F, (ed) Fabry's disease: *Lysosomes and Storage Diseases*. New York, Academic Press, 1973, p 347.
244. Beutler E, Kuhl W: Purification and properties of human α-galactosidases. *J Biol Chem* **247**:7195, 1972.
245. Wang A, Bishop D, Desnick R: Human α-*N*-acetylgalactosaminidase: Molecular cloning, nucleotide sequence, and expression of a full-length cDNA. *J Biol Chem* **265**:21859, 1990.
246. Wang A, Desnick R: Structural organization and complete sequence of the human α-*N*-acetylgalactosaminidase gene: Homology with the α-galactosidase A gene provides evidence for evolution from a common ancestral gene. *Genomics* **10**:133, 1991.
247. Kanzaki T, Yokota M, Mizuno N, Matsumoto Y, Hirabayashi Y: Novel lysosomal glycoamino acid storage disease with angiokeratoma corporis diffusum. *Lancet* **1**:875, 1989.
248. Kanzaki T, Yokota M, Irie F, Hirabayashi Y, Wang AM, Desnick RJ: Angiokeratoma corporis diffusum with glycopeptiduria due to deficient lysosomal α-*N*-acetylgalactosaminidase activity. *Arch Dermatol* **129**:460, 1993.
249. Desnick RJ, Dean KJ, Grabowski G, Bishop DF, Sweeley CC: Enzyme therapy in Fabry disease: Differential in vivo plasma clearance and metabolic effectiveness of plasma and splenic α-galactosidase A isozymes. *Proc Natl Acad Sci U S A* **76**:5326, 1979.
250. Bishop DF, Desnick RJ: Affinity purification of α-galactosidase A from human spleen, placenta, and plasma with elimination of pyrogen contamination. Properties of the purified splenic enzyme compared to other forms. *J Biol Chem* **256**:1307, 1981.
251. Harpaz N, Flowers HM, Sharon N: Purification of coffee bean α-galactosidase by affinity chromatography. *Biochim Biophys Acta* **391**:213, 1974.
252. Dean KJ, Sweeley CC: Studies on human liver α-galactosidases. I. Purification of α-galactosidase A and its enzymatic properties with glycolipid and oligosaccharide substrates. *J Biol Chem* **254**:9994, 1979.
253. Mayes JS, Beutler E: Alpha-galactosidase A from human placenta. Stability and subunit size. *Biochim Biophys Acta* **484**:408, 1977.
254. Ioannou YA, Bishop DF, Desnick RJ: Overexpression of human α-galactosidase A results in its intracellular aggregation, crystallization in lysosomes and selective secretion. *J Cell Biol* **119**:1137, 1992.
255. Bishop DF, Sweeley CC: Plasma α-galactosidase A: Properties and comparisons with tissue α-galactosidases. *Biochim Biophys Acta* **525**:399, 1978.
256. Kusiak JW, Quirk JM, Brady RO: Purification and properties of the two major isozymes of α-galactosidase from human placenta. *J Biol Chem* **253**:184, 1978.

257. LeDonne J, N. C., Fairley JL, Sweeley CC: Biosynthesis of α-galactosidase A in cultured Chang liver cells. *Arch Biochem Biophys* **224**:186, 1983.
258. Matsuura F, Ohta M, Ioannou YA, Desnick RJ: Human α-galactosidase A: Characterization of the *N*-linked oligosaccharides on the intracellular and secreted glycoforms overexpressed by Chinese hamster ovary cells. *Glycobiology* **8**:329, 1998.
259. Ho M: Hydrolysis of ceramide trihexoside by a specific α-galactosidase from human liver. *Biochem J* **133**:1, 1973.
260. Segal I: *Enzyme Kinetics: Behavior and Analysis of Rapid Equilibrium and Steady-State Enzyme Systems*. New York, John Wiley, 1975.
261. Legler G, Herrchen M: Active site-directed inhibition of galactosidases by conduritol C epoxides (1, 2 anhydro-epi- and neo-inositol). *FEBS Lett* **135**:139, 1981.
262. Bause E, Legler G: Isolation and structure of a tryptic glycopeptide from the active site of β-glucosidase A3 from *Aspergillus wentii*. *Biochim Biophys Acta* **626**:459, 1980.
263. Legler G, Harder A: Amino acid sequence at the active site of β-glucosidase A from bitter almonds. *Biochim Biophys Acta* **524**:102, 1978.
264. Grabowski G, Osiecki-Newman K, Dinur T, Fabbro D, Legler G, Gatt S, Desnick R: Human acid β-glucosidase. Use of conduritol B epoxide derivatives to investigate the catalytically active normal and Gaucher disease enzymes. *J Biol Chem* **261**:8263, 1986.
265. Fleet G, Nicholas S, Smith P, Evans S, Fellows L, Nash R: Potent competitive inhibition of α-galactosidase and α-glucosidase activity by 1,4-dideoxy-1,4-iminopentitols: Synthesis of 1,4-dideoxy-1,4-imino-D-lyxitol and of both enantiomers of 1,4-dideoxy-1,4-iminoarabinitol. *Tet Lett* **26**:3127, 1985.
266. Bermotas R, Pezzone M, Ganem B: Synthesis of (+) = 1,5-dideoxy-1,5-imino-D-galactitol, a potent α-D-galactosidase inhibitor. *Carbohydr Res* **167**:305, 1987.
267. Asano N, Ishii S, Kizu H, Ikeda K, Yasuda K, Kato A, Martin OR, Fan J-Q: Correlations between in vitro inhibition and intracellular enhancement of lysosomal α-galactosidase A activity in Fabry lymphoblasts by 1-deoxygalactonojirimycin and its derivatives. *Euro J Biochem* **267**:4179, 2000.
268. Mehl E, Jatzkewitz H: Eine cerebrosidsulfatase aus schweineniere. *Hoppe-Seyler's Z Physiol Chem* **339**:260, 1964.
269. Bierfreund U, Kolter T, Sandhoff K: Sphingolipid hydrolases and activator proteins. *Methods Enzymol* **311**:255, 2000.
270. Gartner S, Conzelmann E, K S: Activator protein for the degradation of globotriaosylceramide by human α-galactosidase. *J Biol Chem* **258**:12378, 1983.
271. Li SC, Kihara H, Serizawa S, Li YT, Fluharty AL, Mayes JS, Shapiro LJ: Activator protein required for the enzymatic hydrolysis of cerebroside sulfate. Deficiency in urine of patients affected with cerebroside sulfatase activator deficiency and identity with activators for the enzymatic hydrolysis of GM1 ganglioside and globotriaosylceramide. *J Biol Chem* **260**:1867, 1985.
272. Vogel A, Furst W, Abo-Hashish MA, Lee-Vaupel M, Conzelmann E, Sandhoff K: Identity of the activator proteins for the enzymatic hydrolysis of sulfatide, ganglioside GM1, and globotriaosylceramide. *Arch Biochem Biophys* **259**:627, 1987.
273. Dewji N, Wenger D, O'Brien J: Nucleotide sequence of cloned cDNA for human sphingolipid activator protein 1 precursor. *Proc Natl Acad Sci U S A* **84**:8652, 1987.
274. Kao F, Law M, Hartz J, Jones C, Zhang X-L, Dewji N, O'Brien J, Wenger D: Regional localization of the gene coding for sphingolipid activator protein SAP-1 on human chromosome 10. *Somat Cell Mol Genet* **13**:685, 1987.
275. Bar-Am I, Avivi L, Horowitz M: Assignment of the human prosaposin gene (PSAP) to 10q22.1 by fluorescence in situ hybridization. *Giraffidae*, okapi (*Okapiajohnstoni*), and giraffe (*Giraffa camelopardalis*): Evidence for ancestral telomeres at the okapi polymorphic rob (4;26) fusion site. *Cytogenet Cell Genet* **72**:316, 1996.
276. Cormand B, Montfort M, Chabas A, Vilageliu L, Grinberg D: Genetic fine localization of the beta-glucocerebrosidase (GBA) and prosaposin (PSAP) genes: Implications for Gaucher disease. *Hum Genet* **100**:75, 1997.
277. Kase R, Bierfreund U, Klein A, Kolter T, Itoh K, Suzuki M, Hashimoto Y, Sandhoff K, Sakuraba H: Only sphingolipid activator protein B (SAP-B or saposin B) stimulates the degradation of globotriaosylceramide by recombinant human lysosomal α-galactosidase in a detergent-free liposomal system. *FEBS Lett* **393**:74, 1996.
278. Fischer G, Jatzkewitz H: The activator of cerebroside-sulphatase. A model of the activation. *Biochim Biophys Acta* **528**:69, 1978.
279. Li S-C, Li Y-T: An activator stimulating the enzymic hydrolysis of sphingoglycolipids. *J Biol Chem* **251**:1159, 1976.
280. Rorman EG, Grabowski GA: Molecular cloning of a human co-beta-glucosidase cDNA: Evidence that four sphingolipid hydrolase activator proteins are encoded by single genes in humans and rats. *Genomics* **5**:486, 1989.
281. Rorman EG, Scheinker V, Grabowski GA: Structure and evolution of the human prosaposin chromosomal gene. *Genomics* **13**:312, 1992.
282. Morimoto S, Yamamoto Y, O'Brien JS, Kishimoto Y: Distribution of saposin proteins (sphingolipid activator proteins) in lysosomal storage and other diseases. *Proc Natl Acad Sci U S A* **87**:3493, 1990.
283. Shapiro L, Aleck K, Kaback M, Itabashi H, Desnick R, Brand N, Stevens R, Fluharty A, Kihara H: Metachromatic leukodystrophy without arylsulfatase A deficiency. *Pediatr Res* **13**:1179, 1979.
284. Stevens R, Fluharty A, Kihara H, Kaback M, Shapiro L, Marsh B, Sandhoff K, Fischer G: Cerebroside sulfatase activator deficiency induced metachromatic leukodystrophy. *Am J Hum Genet* **33**:900, 1981.
285. Hahn A, Gordon B, Feleki V, Hinton G, Gilbert J: A variant form of metachromatic leukodystrophy without arylsulfatase deficiency. *Ann Neurol* **12**:33, 1982.
286. Inui K, Emmett M, Wenger D: Immunological evidence for deficiency of an activator protein for sulfatide sulfatase in a variant form of metachromatic leukodystrophy. *Proc Natl Acad Sci U S A* **80**:3074, 1983.
287. Sandhoff K, Kolter T: Processing of sphingolipid activator proteins and the topology of lysosomal digestion. *Acta Biochim Pol* **45**:373, 1998.
288. Sandhoff K, Kolter T, Van Echten-Deckert G: Sphingolipid metabolism. Sphingoid analogs, sphingolipid activator proteins, and the pathology of the cell. *Ann N Y Acad Sci* **845**:139, 1998.
289. Kolter T, Sandhoff K: Recent advances in the biochemistry of sphingolipidoses. *Brain Pathol* **8**:79, 1998.
290. Lemansky P, Bishop DF, Desnick RJ, Hasilik A, von Figura K: Synthesis and processing of alpha-galactosidase A in human fibroblasts. Evidence for different mutations in Fabry disease. *J Biol Chem* **262**:2062, 1987.
291. Beutler E, Kuhl W: Absence of cross-reactive antigen in Fabry's disease. *N Engl J Med* **289**:694, 1973.
292. Rietra PJ, Molenaar JL, Hamers MN, Tager JM, Borst P: Investigation of the alpha-galactosidase deficiency in Fabry's disease using antibodies against the purified enzyme. *Eur J Biochem* **46**:89, 1974.
293. Hamers MN, Wise D, Ejiofor A, Strijland A, Robinson D, Tager JM: Relationship between biochemical and clinical features in an English Anderson-Fabry family. *Acta Med Scand* **206**:5, 1979.
294. Eng CM, Resnick-Silverman LA, Niehaus DJ, Astrin KH, Desnick RJ: Nature and frequency of mutations in the α-galactosidase A gene that cause Fabry disease. *Am J Hum Genet* **53**:1186, 1993.
295. Vetrie D, Bobrow M, Harris A: Construction of a 5.2-megabase physical map of the human X chromosome at Xq22 using pulsed-field gel electrophoresis and yeast artificial chromosomes. *Genomics* **19**:42, 1994.
296. Vetrie D, Kendall E, Coffey A, Hassock S, Collins J, Todd C, Lehrach H, Bobrow M, Bentley DR, Harris A: A 6.5-Mb yeast artificial chromosome contig incorporating 33 DNA markers on the human X chromosome at Xq22. *Genomics* **19**:42, 1994.
297. Kendall E, Evans W, Jin H, Holland J, Vetrie D: A complete YAC contig and cosmid interval map covering the entirety of human Xq21.33 to Xq22.3 from DXS3 to DXS287. *Genomics* **43**:171, 1997.
298. Srivastava AK, McMillan S, Jermak C, Shomaker M, Copeland-Yates SA, Sossey-Alaoui K, Mumm S, Schlessinger D, Nagaraja R: Integrated STS/YAC physical, genetic, and transcript map of human Xq21.3 to q23/q24 (DXS1203-DXS1059). *Genomics* **58**:188, 1999.
299. Grzeschik K, Grzeschik A, Banhof S, Romeo G, Siniscalco M, van Som Eren H, Meera Khan P, Westerveld A, Bootsma D: X-Linkage of human α-galactosidase. *Nature New Biol* **204**:48, 1972.
300. Miller O, Siniscalco M: Report of the committee on the genetic constitution of the X and Y chromosomes. *Cytogenet Cell Genet* **32**:121, 1982.
301. Fox M, Dutoit D, Warnich L, Retief A: Regional localization of α-galactosidase (GLA) to Xpter-q22, hexosaminidase B (HEXB) to 5q13-qter, and arylsulfatase B (ARSB) to 5pter-q13. *Cytogenet Cell Genet* **38**:45, 1984.
302. Bishop D, Calhoun D, Bernstein H, Quinn M, Hantzopoulos P, Desnick R: Molecular cloning and nucleotide sequencing of a cDNA encoding human α-galactosidase A. *Am J Hum Genet* **37**:A144, 1985.
303. Bernstein HS, Bishop DF, Astrin KH, Kornreich R, Eng CM, Sakuraba H, Desnick RJ: Fabry disease: Six gene rearrangements and an exonic

point mutation in the alpha-galactosidase gene. *J Clin Invest* **83**:1390, 1989.

304. Morgan SH, Cheshire JK, Wilson TM, MacDermot K, Crawfurd MA: Anderson-Fabry disease—Family linkage studies using two polymorphic X-linked DNA probes. *Pediatr Nephrol* **1**:536, 1987.
305. MacDermot KD, Morgan SH, Cheshire JK, Wilson TM: Anderson Fabry disease, a close linkage with highly polymorphic DNA markers DXS17, DXS87 and DXS88. *Hum Genet* **77**:263, 1987.
306. Desnick RJ, Bernstein HS, Astrin KH, Bishop DF: Fabry disease: Molecular diagnosis of hemizygotes and heterozygotes. *Enzyme* **38**:54, 1987.
307. Yang H, Niebuhr E, Norby S, Lund T, Schwartz M: Subregional localization of myelin proteolipid protein to Xq21.33-Xq22 by deletion mapping. *Cytogenet Cell Genet* **46**:722, 1987.
308. O'Reilly M-A, Alterman L, Zijlstra J, Malcolm S, Levinsky R, Kinnon C: Pulsed-field gel electrophoresis and radiation hybrid mapping analyses enable the ordering of eleven DNA loci in Xq22. *Genomics* **15**:275, 1993.
309. Hostikka S, Eddy R, Byers M, Hoyhtya M, Shows T, Tryggvason K: Identification of a distinct type IV collagen α-chain with restricted kidney distribution and assignment of its gene to the locus of X-linked Alport syndrome. *Proc Natl Acad Sci U S A* **87**:1606, 1990.
310. Barker D, Hostikka S, Zhou J, Chow L, Oliphant A, Gerken S, Gregory M, Skolnick M, Atkin C, Tryggvason K: Identification of mutations in the COL4A5 collagen gene in Alport syndrome. *Science* **248**:1224, 1990.
311. Willard HF, Riordan JR: Assignment of the gene for myelin proteolipid protein to the X chromosome: Implications for X-linked myelin disorders. *Science* **230**:940, 1985.
312. Saugier-Veber P, Munnich A, Bonneau D, Rozet JM, Le Merrer M, Gil R, Boespflug-Tanguy O: X-linked spastic paraplegia and Pelizaeus-Merzbacher disease are allelic disorders at the proteolipid protein locus. *Nat Genet* **6**:257, 1994.
313. Vetrie D, Vorechovsky I, Sideras P, Holland J, Davies A, Flinter F, Hammarstrom L, Kinnon C, Levinsky R, Bobrow M, Smith C, Bentley D: The gene involved in X-linked agammaglobulinaemia is a member of the src family of protein-tyrosine kinases. *Nature* **361**:226, 1993.
314. Oeltjen JC, Liu X, Lu J, Allen RC, Muzny D, Belmont JW, Gibbs RA: Sixty-nine kilobases of contiguous human genomic sequence containing the alpha-galactosidase A and Bruton's tyrosine kinase loci. *Mamm Genome* **6**:334, 1995.
315. Tsuji S, Martin B, Kaslow D, Migeon B, Choudary P, Stubblefield B, Mayor J, Murray G, Barranger J, Ginns E: Signal sequence and DNA-mediated expression of human lysosomal α-galactosidase A. *Eur J Biochem* **165**:275, 1987.
316. Bishop DF, Kornreich R, Eng CM, Ioannou YA, Fitzmaurice TF, Desnick RJ: Human α-galactosidase: Characterization and eukaryotic expression of the full-length cDNA and structural organization of the gene, in Salvayre R, Douste-Blazy L, Gatt S (eds): *Lipid Storage Disorders*. New York, Plenum, 1988, p 809.
317. von Heijne G: A new method for predicting signal sequence cleavage sites. *Nucleic Acids Res* **14**:4683, 1986.
318. Watson M: Compilation of published signal sequences. *Nucleic Acids Res* **12**:5145, 1984.
319. Aubert J-P, Biserte G, Loucheux-Lefebvre M-H: Carbohydrate-peptide linkage in glycoproteins. *Arch Biochem Biophys* **175**:410, 1976.
320. Sorge J, West C, Westwood B, Beutler E: Molecular cloning and nucleotide sequence of human glucocerebrosidase cDNA. *Proc Natl Acad Sci U S A* **82**:7289, 1985.
321. Faust P, Kornfeld S, Chirgwin J: Cloning and sequence analysis of cDNA for human cathepsin D. *Proc Natl Acad Sci U S A* **82**:4910, 1985.
322. Myerowitz R, Piekarz R, Neufeld E, Shows T, Suzuki K: Human β-hexosaminidase α-chain: Coding sequence and homology with the β chain. *Proc Natl Acad Sci U S A* **82**:7830, 1985.
323. Ioannou Y, Zeidner K, Grace M, Desnick R: Human α-galactosidase A: Glycosylation site 3 is essential for enzyme solubility. *Biochem J* **332**:789, 1998.
324. Jenh C-H, Deng T, Li D, Dewille J, Johnson L: Mouse thymidylate synthase messenger RNA lacks a 3′ untranslated region. *Proc Natl Acad Sci U S A* **83**:8482, 1986.
325. Birnstiel M, Busslinger MKS: Transcription termination and 3′ processing: The end is in site! *Cell* **41**:349, 1985.
326. Breathnach R, Chambon P: Organization and expression of eucaryotic split genes coding for proteins. *Ann Rev Biochem* **50**:349, 1981.
327. Mount SM: A catalog of splice junction sequences. *Nucl Acids Res* **10**:459, 1982.
328. Jurka J, Smith T: A fundamental division in the Alu family of repeated sequences. *Proc Natl Acad Sci U S A* **85**:4775, 1988.
329. Kornreich R, Bishop DF, Desnick RJ: The gene encoding alpha-galactosidase A and gene rearrangements causing Fabry disease. *Trans Assoc Am Physicians* **102**:30, 1989.
330. Lee W, Mitchell P, Tjian R: Purified transcription factor AP-1 interacts with TPA-inducible enhancer elements. *Cell* **49**:741, 1987.
331. Lenardo M, Pierce J, Baltimore D: Protein-binding sites in Ig gene enhancers determine transcriptional activity and inducibility. *Science* **236**:1573, 1987.
332. Prywes R, Roeder R: Inducible binding of a factor to the c-fos enhancer. *Cell* **47**:777, 1986.
333. Spoerel N, Nguyen HT, Kafatos FC: Gene regulation and evolution in the chorion locus of *Bombyx mori*. Structural and developmental characterization of four eggshell genes and their flanking DNA regions. *J Mol Biol* **190**:23, 1986.
334. Fitzmaurice TF, Desnick RJ, Bishop DF: Human alpha-galactosidase A: high plasma activity expressed by the −30G → A allele. *J Inherit Metab Dis* **20**:643, 1997.
335. Lindsay S, Bird A: Use of restriction enzymes to detect potential gene sequences in mammalian DNA. *Nature* **327**:336, 1987.
336. Bird A: CpG-rich islands and the function of DNA methylation. *Nature* **321**:209, 1986.
337. Yang T, Caskey T: Nuclease sensitivity of the mouse HPRT gene promoter region: Differential sensitivity on the active and inactive X-chromosomes. *Mol Cell Biol* **7**:2994, 1987.
338. Keith D, Singer-Sam J, Riggs A: Active X chromosome DNA is unmethylated at eight CCGG sites clustered in a guanine-plus-cytosine-rich island at the 5′ end of the gene for phosphoglycerate kinase. *Mol Cell Biol* **6**:4122, 1986.
339. Mohandas T, Sparkes R, Bishop D, Desnick R, Shapiro L: Frequency of reactivation and variability in expression of X-linked enzyme loci. *Am J Hum Genet* **36**:916, 1984.
340. McDevitt M, Hart R, Wong W, Nevins J: Sequences capable of restoring poly (A) site function define two distinct downstream elements. *EMBO J* **5**:2907, 1986.
341. Gil A, Proudfoot N: Position-dependent sequence elements downstream of AAUAAA are required for efficient rabbit β-globin mRNA 3′ end formation. *Cell* **49**:399, 1987.
342. McLauchlan J, Gaffney D, Whitton J, Clements J: The consensus sequence YGTGTTYY located downstream from the AATAAA signal is required for efficient formation of mRNA 3′ termini. *Nucleic Acids Res* **13**:1347, 1985.
343. Maeda N, Smithies O: The evolution of multi-gene families: Human haptoglobin genes. *Ann Rev Genet* **20**:81, 1986.
344. Proia R: Gene encoding the human β-hexosaminidase chain: Extensive homology of intron placement in the α- and β-chain genes. *Proc Natl Acad Sci U S A* **85**:1883, 1988.
345. Horowitz M, Wilde S, Horowitz Z, Reiner O, Gelbart T, Beutler E: The human glucocerebrosidase gene and pseudogene: Structure and evolution. *Genomics* **4**:87, 1989.
346. Liljestrom PL, Liljestrom P: Nucleotide sequence of the *mel*A gene, coding for α-galactosidase in *Escherichia coli* K-12. *Nucleic Acids Res* **15**:2213, 1987.
347. Liljestrom PL: The nucleotide sequence of the yeast MEL1 gene. *Nucleic Acids Res* **13**:7257, 1985.
348. Ohshima T, Murray GJ, Nagle JW, Quirk JM, Kraus MH, Barton NW, Brady RO, Kulkarni AB: Structural organization and expression of the mouse gene encoding alpha-galactosidase A. *Gene* **166**:277, 1995.
349. Gotlib RW, Bishop DF, Wang AM, Zeidner KM, Ioannou YA, Adler DA, Disteche CM, Desnick RJ: The entire genomic sequence and cDNA expression of mouse α-galactosidase A. *Biochem Mol Med* **57**:139, 1996.
350. Hantzopoulos PA, Calhoun DH: Expression of the human alpha-galactosidase A in Escherichia coli K-12. *Gene* **57**:159, 1987.
351. Ioannou Y, Desnick R, Bishop D: unpublished results.
352. Ghrayeb J, Kimura H, Takahara M, Hsiung H, Masui Y, Inouye M: Secretion cloning vectors in *Escherichia coli*. *EMBO J* **3**:2437, 1984.
353. Schmitt R: Analysis of melibiose mutants deficient in α-galactosidase and thiomethylgalactoside permease II in *Escherichia coli* K-12. *J Bacteriol* **96**:462, 1968.
354. Ioannou YA: *Human Genetics*. New York, City University of New York, 1992, p 1.
355. Takenaka T, Qin G, Brady RO, Medin JA: Circulating alpha-galactosidase A derived from transduced bone marrow cells: Relevance for corrective gene transfer for Fabry disease. *Hum Gene Ther* **10**:1931, 1999.

356. Miyamura N, Araki E, Matsuda K, Yoshimura R, Furukawa N, Tsuruzoe K, Shirotani T, Kishikawa H, Yamaguchi K, Shichiri M: A carboxy-terminal truncation of human alpha-galactosidase A in a heterozygous female with Fabry disease and modification of the enzymatic activity by the carboxy-terminal domain. Increased, reduced, or absent enzyme activity depending on number of amino acid residues deleted. *J Clin Invest* **98**:1809, 1996.
357. Wang AM, Ioannou YA, Zeidner KM, Gotleb RW, Dikman S, Stewart CL, Desnick RJ: Generation of a mouse model with α-galactosidase A. *Am J Hum Genet* **59**:A208, 1996.
358. Kakkis ED, Matynia A, Jonas AJ, Neufeld EF: Overexpression of the human lysosomal enzyme alpha-l-iduronidase in Chinese hamster ovary cells. *Protein Expr Purif* **5**:225, 1994.
359. Van Hove JLK, Yang HW, Wu J-Y, Brady RO, Chen Y-T: High-level production of recombinant human lysosomal acid α-glucosidase in Chinese hamster ovary cells which targets to heart muscle and corrects glycogen accumulation in fibroblasts from patients with Pompe disease. *Proc Natl Acad Sci U S A* **93**:65, 1996.
360. Zhao KW, Faull KF, Kakkis ED, Neufeld EF: Carbohydrate structures of recombinant human alpha-l-iduronidase secreted by Chinese hamster ovary cells. *J Biol Chem* **272**:22758, 1997.
361. Litjens T, Bielicki J, Anson DS, Friderici K, Jones MZ, Hopwood JJ: Expression, purification and characterization of recombinant caprine *N*-acetylglucosamine-6-sulphatase. *Biochem J* **327**:89, 1997.
362. Bielicki J, Hopwood JJ, Melville EL, Anson DS: Recombinant human sulphamidase: Expression, amplification, purification and characterization. *Biochem J* **329**:145, 1998.
363. He X, Miranda SR, Xiong X, Dagan A, Gatt S, Schuchman EH: Characterization of human acid sphingomyelinase purified from the media of overexpressing Chinese hamster ovary cells. *Biochim Biophys Acta* **1432**:251, 1999.
364. Legler G: Glycoside hydrolases: Mechanistic information from studies with reversible and irreversible inhibitors. *Adv Carbohydr Chem Biochem* **48**:319, 1990.
365. Zeidner K, Ioannou Y, Desnick R: Human α-galactosidase A active site residue: Determination by homology, mutagenesis and transient expression [Abstract]. *Am J Hum Genet* **53**:168A, 1993.
366. Murali R, Ioannou YA, Desnick RJ, Burnett RM: Crystallization and preliminary x-ray analysis of human alpha-galactosidase A complex. *J Mol Biol* **239**:578, 1994.
367. Topaloglu AK, Ashley GA, Tong B, Shabbeer J, Astrin KH, Eng CM, Desnick RJ: Twenty novel mutations in the α-galactosidase A gene causing Fabry disease. *Mol Med* **5**:806, 1999.
368. Davies JP, Winchester BG, Malcolm S: Mutation analysis in patients with the typical form of Anderson-Fabry disease. *Hum Mol Genet* **2**:1051, 1993.
369. Ploos van Amstel JK, Jansen RP, de Jong JG, Hamel BC, Wevers RA: Six novel mutations in the α-galactosidase A gene in families with Fabry disease. *Hum Mol Genet* **3**:503, 1994.
370. Koide T, Ishiura M, Iwai K, Inoue M, Kaneda Y, Okada Y, Uchida T: A case of Fabry's disease in a patient with no alpha-galactosidase A activity caused by a single amino acid substitution of Pro-40 by Ser. *FEBS Lett* **259**:353, 1990.
371. Eng CM, Desnick RJ: Molecular basis of Fabry disease: Mutations and polymorphisms in the human α-galactosidase A gene. *Hum Mutat* **3**:103, 1994.
372. Eng CM, Ashley GA, Burgert TS, Enriquez AL, D'Souza M, Desnick RJ: Fabry disease: Thirty-five mutations in the α-galactosidase A gene in patients with classic and variant phenotypes. *Mol Med* **3**:174, 1997.
373. Davies JP, Eng CM, Malcolm S, MacDermot K, Winchester B, Desnick RJ: Fabry disease: Fourteen α-galactosidase A mutations in unrelated families from the United Kingdom and other European countries. *Eur J Hum Genet* **4**:219, 1996.
374. Germain DP, Poenaru L: Fabry disease: Identification of novel alpha-galactosidase A mutations and molecular carrier detection by use of fluorescent chemical cleavage of mismatches. *Biochem Biophys Res Commun* **257**:708, 1999.
375. Yokoi T, Shinoda K, Ohno I, Kato K, Miyawaki T, Taniguchi N: A 3′ splice site consensus sequence mutation in the intron 3 of the alpha-galactosidase A gene in a patient with Fabry disease. *Jinrui Idengaku Zasshi* **36**:245, 1991.
376. Sakuraba H, Eng CM, Desnick RJ, Bishop DF: Invariant exon skipping in the human alpha-galactosidase A pre-mRNA: A g^{+1} to t substitution in a 5′-splice site causing Fabry disease. *Genomics* **12**:643, 1992.
377. Davies J, Christomanou H, Winchester B, Malcolm S: Detection of 8 new mutations in the alpha-galactosidase A gene in Fabry disease. *Hum Mol Genet* **3**:667, 1994.
378. Okumiya T, Ishii S, Kase R, Kamei S, Sakuraba H, Suzuki Y: Alpha-galactosidase gene mutations in Fabry disease: Heterogeneous expressions of mutant enzyme proteins. *Hum Genet* **95**:557, 1995.
379. Okumiya T, Takenaka T, Ishii S, Kase R, Kamei S, Sakuraba H: Two novel mutations in the alpha-galactosidase gene in Japanese classical hemizygotes with Fabry disease. *Jpn J Hum Genet* **41**:313, 1996.
380. Chen CH, Shyu PW, Wu SJ, Sheu SS, Desnick RJ, Hsiao KJ: Identification of a novel point mutation (S65T) in alpha-galactosidase A gene in Chinese patients with Fabry disease. *Hum Mutat* **11**:328, 1998.
381. Kornreich R, Desnick RJ: Fabry disease: Detection of gene rearrangements in the human alpha-galactosidase A gene by multiplex PCR amplification. *Hum Mutat* **2**:108, 1993.
382. Kornreich R, Bishop DF, Desnick RJ: α-galactosidase A gene rearrangements causing Fabry disease: Identification of short direct repeats at breakpoints in an Alu-rich gene. *J Biol Chem* **265**:9319, 1990.
383. Takenaka T, Sakuraba H, Hashimoto K, Fujino O, Fujita T, Tanaka H, Suzuki Y: Coexistence of gene mutations causing Fabry disease and Duchenne muscular dystrophy in a Japanese boy. *Clin Genet* **49**:255, 1996.
384. Eng CM, Niehaus DJ, Enriquez AL, Burgert TS, Ludman MD, Desnick RJ: Fabry disease: Twenty-three mutations including sense and antisense CpG alterations and identification of a deletional hot-spot in the alpha-galactosidase A gene. *Hum Mol Genet* **3**:1795, 1994.
385. Yamakawa-Kobayashi K, Kobayashi T, Yanagi H, Shimakura Y, Satoh J, Hamaguchi H: A novel complex mutation in the LDL receptor gene probably caused by the simultaneous occurrence of deletion and insertion in the same region. *Hum Genet* **93**:625, 1994.
386. Gibbs RA, Nguyen P-N, McBride LJ, Koepf SM, Caskey CT: Identification of mutations leading to the Lesch-Nyhan syndrome by automated direct DNA sequencing of in vitro amplified cDNA. *Proc Natl Aca Sci U S A* **86**:1919, 1987.
387. Nogueira CP, McGuire MC, Graeser C, Bartels CF, Arpagaus M, Van der Spek AF, Lightstone H, Lockridge O: Identification of a frameshift mutation responsible for the silent phenotype of human serum cholinesterase, Gly 117 (GGT → GGAG). *Am J Hum Genet* **46**:934, 1990.
388. Pease LR, Horton RM, Pullen JK, Yun TJ: Unusual mutation clusters provide insight into class I gene conversion mechanisms. *Mol Cell Biol* **13**:4374, 1993.
389. Cooper A, Sardharwalla I, Roberts M: Human β-mannosidase deficiency. *N Engl J Med* **315**:1231, 1986.
390. Cooper C, Youssoufian H: The CpG dinucleotide and human genetic disease. *Hum Genet* **78**:151, 1988.
391. Johnson DL, Desnick RJ: Molecular pathology of Fabry's disease. Physical and kinetic properties of alpha-galactosidase A in cultured human endothelial cells. *Biochim Biophys Acta* **538**:195, 1978.
392. van den Bergh F, Tager J: Localization of neutral glycosphingolipids in human plasma. *Biochim Biophys Acta* **441**:391, 1976.
393. Meuwissen SG, Dingemans KP, Strijland A, Tager JM, Ooms BC: Ultrastructural and biochemical liver analyses in Fabry's disease. *Hepatology* **2**:263, 1982.
394. Clarke JTR, Stoltz JM: Uptake of radiolabeled galactosyl-(α1–4)-galactosyl-(β1–4)-glucosylceramide by human serum lipoproteins in vitro. *Biochim Biophys Acta* **441**:165, 1976.
395. Stein O, Stein Y: High-density lipoproteins reduce the uptake of low-density lipoproteins by human endothelial cells in culture. *Biochem Biophys Acta* **431**:363, 1976.
396. Goldstein J, Brown M: The low-density lipoprotein pathway and its relation to atherosclerosis. *Ann Rev Biochem* **46**:897, 1977.
397. Vlodavsky I, Fielding P, Fielding C, Gospodarowicz D: Role of contact inhibition in the regulation of receptor-mediated uptake of low-density lipoprotein in cultured vascular endothelial cells. *Proc Natl Acad Sci U S A* **75**:356, 1979.
398. Tao R: *Biochemistry and Metabolism of Mammalian Blood Glycosphingolipids*. Lansing, MI, Michigan State University. Ph.D. thesis, 1973.
399. Barkai A, Di Cesare JL: Influence of sialic acid groups on the retention of glycosphingolipids in blood plasma. *Biochim Biophys Acta* **398**:287, 1975.
400. Kahlke W: Angiokeratoma corporis diffusum (Fabry's disease), in Schettler G (ed): *Lipids and Lipidoses*. Berlin, Springer, 1967, p 332.
401. Ledvinova J, Poupetova H, Hanackova A, Pisacka M, Elleder M: Blood group B glycosphingolipids in alpha-galactosidase deficiency (Fabry disease): Influence of secretor status. *Biochim Biophys Acta* **1345**:180, 1997.

402. Fukuhara N, Suzuki M, Fujita N, Tsubaki T: Fabry's disease on the mechanism of the peripheral nerve involvement. *Acta Neuropathol (Berl)* **33**:9, 1975.
403. Seino Y, Vyden JK, Philippart M, Rose HB, Nagasawa K: Peripheral hemodynamics in patients with Fabry's disease. *Am Heart J* **105**:783, 1983.
404. Yamamoto K, Sobue G, Iwase S, Kumazawa K, Mitsuma T, Mano T: Possible mechanism of anhidrosis in a symptomatic female carrier of Fabry's disease: An assessment by skin sympathetic nerve activity and sympathetic skin response. *Clin Auton Res* **6**:107, 1996.
405. Gemignani F, Marbini A, Bragaglia MM, Govoni E: Pathological study of the sural nerve in Fabry's disease. *Eur Neurol* **23**:173, 1984.
406. Dvorak AM, Cable WJ, Osage JE, Kolodny EH: Diagnostic electron microscopy. II. Fabry's disease: Use of biopsies from uninvolved skin. Acute and chronic changes involving the microvasculature and small unmyelinated nerves. *Pathol Annu* **16**:139, 1981.
407. Tome FM, Fardeau M, Lenoir G: Ultrastructure of muscle and sensory nerve in Fabry's disease. *Acta Neuropathol (Berl)* **38**:187, 1977.
408. Pellissier JF, Van Hoof F, Bourdet-Bonerandi D, Monier-Faugere MC, Toga M: Morphological and biochemical changes in muscle and peripheral nerve in Fabry's disease. *Muscle Nerve* **4**:381, 1981.
409. Scott LJ, Griffin JW, Luciano C, Barton NW, Banerjee T, Crawford T, McArthur JC, Tournay A, Schiffmann R: Quantitative analysis of epidermal innervation in Fabry disease. *Neurology* **52**:1249, 1999.
410. Walker F: Histamine flare in Fabry's disease [Letter]. *Neurology* **33**:387, 1983.
411. Gadoth N, Sandbank U: Involvement of dorsal root ganglia in Fabry's disease. *J Med Genet* **20**:309, 1983.
412. Ikari Y, Kuwako K, Yamaguchi T: Fabry's disease with complete atrioventricular block: Histological evidence of involvement of the conduction system. *Br Heart J* **68**:323, 1992.
413. Jardine DL, Fitzpatrick MA, Troughton WD, Tie AB: Small bowel ischaemia in Fabry's disease. *J Gastroenterol Hepatol* **9**:201, 1994.
414. Vogelberg K, Solbach H, Gries F: Lipoidchemische Untersuchun gen beim Angiokeratoma corporis diffusum (Fabry syndrome). *Klin Wochenschr* **47**:916, 1969.
415. Sorensen SA, Hasholt L: Attitudes of persons at risk for Fabry's disease towards predictive tests and genetic counselling. *J Biosoc Sci* **15**:89, 1983.
416. Fordyce J: Angiokeratoma of the scrotum. *J Cutan Genitourin Dis* **14**:81, 1896.
417. Imperial R, Heliwig E: Angiokeratoma of the scrotum (Fordyce type). *J Urol* **98**:397, 1967.
418. Traub E, Tolmach J: Angiokeratoma. Comprehensive study of the literature and report of a case. *Arch Derm Syph* **24**:39, 1931.
419. Dammert K: Angiokeratosis naeviformis — A form of naevus telangiectateus lateralis (naevus flammeus). *Dermatologica* **130**:17, 1965.
420. Goldman L, Gibson SH, Richfield DF: Thrombotic angiokeratoma circumscriptum simulating melanoma. *Arch Dermatol* **117**:138, 1981.
421. Epinette WW, Norins AL, Drew AL, Zeman W, Patel V: Angiokeratoma corporis diffusum with α-L-fucosidase deficiency. *Arch Dermatol* **107**:754, 1973.
422. Fleming C, Rennie A, Fallowfield M, McHenry PM: Cutaneous manifestations of fucosidosis. *Br J Dermatol* **136**:594, 1997.
423. Miyatake T, Atsumi T, Obayaski T, Mizuno Y, Ando S, Ariga T, Matsui-Nakamura K: Adult type neuronal storage disease with neuraminidase deficiency. *Ann Neurol* **6**:232, 1978.
424. Ishibashi A, Tsuboi R, Shinmei M: β-Galactosidase and neuraminidase deficiency associated with angiokeratoma corporis diffusum. *Arch Dermatol* **120**:1344, 1984.
425. Wenger D, Sattler M, Mueller O, Myers G, Schneider R, Nixon G: Adult GM1 gangliosidosis: Clinical and biochemical studies on two patients and comparison to other patients called variant or adult GM1 gangliosidosis. *Clin Genet* **17**:323, 1980.
426. Gehler J, Sewell AC, Becker C, Hartmann J, Spranger J: Clinical and biochemical delineation of aspartyl glycosaminuria as observed in two members of an Italian family. *Helv Paediatr Acta* **36**:179, 1981.
427. Rodriguez-Serna M, Botella-Estrada R, Chabas A, Coll MJ, Oliver V, Febrer MI, Aliaga A: Angiokeratoma corporis diffusum associated with beta-mannosidase deficiency. *Arch Dermatol* **132**:1219, 1996.
428. McCallum DI, Macadam RF, Johnston AW: Angiokeratoma corporis diffusum with features of a mucopolysaccharidosis. *J Med Genet* **17**:21, 1980.
429. Holmes RC, Fensom AH, McKee P, Cairns RJ, Black MM: Angiokeratoma corporis diffusum in a patient with normal enzyme activities. *J Am Acad Dermatol* **10**:384, 1984.
430. Crovato F, Rebora A: Angiokeratoma corporis diffusum and normal enzyme activities [Letter]. *J Am Acad Dermatol* **12**:885, 1985.
431. Frost P, Tamala Y, Spaeth GL: Fabry's disease — Glycolipid lipidosis. Histochemical and electron microscopic studies of two cases. *Am J Med* **40**:618, 1966.
432. Imperial R, Heliwig E: Angiokeratoma: A clinicopathological study. *Arch Dermatol* **95**:166, 1967.
433. Van Mullem P, Ruiter M: Electron microscopic study of the skin in angiokeratoma corporis diffusum. *Arch Klin Exp Dermatol* **226**:453, 1966.
434. Itoh K, Kotani M, Tai T, Suzuki H, Utsunomiya T, Inoue H, Yamada H, Sakuraba H, Suzuki Y: Immunofluorescence imaging diagnosis of Fabry heterozygotes using confocal laser scanning microscopy. *Clin Genet* **44**:302, 1993.
435. Francois J, de Becke L: Les manifestations oculaires de l'intoxication chloroquine. *Ann Oculist* **198**:513, 1965.
436. Desnick R, Doughman D, Riley F, Whitley C: Fabry keratopathy: Molecular pathology of the chloroquine-induced phenocopy. *Am J Hum Genet* **26**:A26, 1974.
437. Whitley C: *Studies of Heritable and Induced Lysosomopathies*. Mnneapolis, University of Minnesota. Ph.D. Thesis, 1977.
438. de Groot P, Elferink R, Hollemans M, Strijland A, Westerveld A, Meera Khan P, Tager J: Inactivation by chloroquine of α-galactosidase in cultured human skin fibroblasts. *Exp Cell Res* **136**:327, 1981.
439. Whitley CB, Tsai MY, Heger JJ, Prystowsky EN, Zipes DP: Amiodarone phenocopy of Fabry's keratopathy [Letter]. *JAMA* **249**:2177, 1983.
440. Dudognon P, Hauw J, de Baecque C, et al.: Amiodarone neuropathy: Clinical and pathological study of a new drug induced lipidosis. *Rev Neurol* **135**:527, 1979.
441. Banks DE, Milutinovic J, Desnick RJ, Grabowski GA, Lapp NL, Boehlecke BA: Silicon nephropathy mimicking Fabry's disease. *Am J Nephrol* **3**:279, 1983.
442. Ho MW, Beutler S, Tennant L, O'Brien JS: Fabry's disease: Evidence for a physically altered α-galactosidase. *Am J Hum Genet* **24**:256, 1972.
443. Mayes JS, Scheerer JB, Sifers RN, Donaldson ML: Differential assay for lysosomal alpha-galactosidases in human tissues and its application to Fabry's disease. *Clin Chim Acta* **112**:247, 1981.
444. Francois J: Heterozygotes for sex-linked traits and Mary Lyon's inactivation theory. XIV Fabry's dystopic lipidosis, in Proceedings of the III International Congress of Human Genetics. Baltimore, MD, Johns Hopkins University Press, 1967, p 423.
445. Holliday R: Strong effects of 5-azacytidine on the in vitro life span of human diploid fibroblasts. *Exp Cell Res* **166**:543, 1986.
446. Wareham KA, Lyon MF, Glenisler PH, Williams ED: Age-related reactivation of an X-linked gene. *Nature* **327**:725, 1987.
447. Wilson V, Smith R, Ma S, RG C: Genomic 5-methyldeoxycytidine decreases with age. *J Biol Chem* **262**:9948, 1987.
448. Grimm T, Wienker TF, Ropers HH: Fabry's disease: Heterozygote detection by hair root analysis. *Hum Genet* **32**:329, 1976.
449. Spence MW, Goldbloom AL, Burgess JK, D'Entremont D, Ripley BA, Weldon KL: Heterozygote detection in angiokeratoma corporis diffusum (Anderson-Fabry disease). Studies on plasma, leucocytes, and hair follicles. *J Med Genet* **14**:91, 1977.
450. Vermorken AJ, Weterings PJ, Spierenburg GT, van Bennekom CA, Wirtz P, deBruyn CH, Oei TL: Fabry's disease: Biochemical and histochemical studies on hair roots for carrier detection. *Br J Dermatol* **98**:191, 1978.
451. Jongkind JF, Verkerk A, Niermeijer MF: Detection of Fabry's disease heterozygotes by enzyme analysis in single fibroblasts after cell sorting. *Clin Genet* **23**:261, 1983.
452. Williard H, Skolnick M, Pearson P, Mandel J-L: Report of the committee on human gene mapping by recombinant DNA techniques, in human gene mapping 11. *Cytogenet Cell Genet* **58**:853, 1991.
453. Kornreich R, Astrin KH, Desnick RJ: Amplification of human polymorphic sites in the X-chromosomal region q21.33 to q24: DXS17, DXS87, DXS287, and alpha-galactosidase A. *Genomics* **13**:70, 1992.
454. Caggana M, Ashley CA, Desnick RJ, Eng CM: Fabry disease: Molecular carrier detection and prenatal diagnosis by analysis of closely linked polymorphisms at Xq22.1. *Am J Med Genet* **71**:329, 1997.
455. Ashton-Prolla P, Ashley GA, Giuglianai R, Pires RF, Desnick RJ, Eng CM: Fabry disease: Comparison of enzymatic, linkage and mutation analysis in a family with a novel mutation (30delG). *Am J Med Genet* **84**:420, 1999.

456. Caggana M, Ashley GA, Desnick RJ, Eng CM: Fabry disease: Molecular carrier detection and prenatal diagnosis by analysis of closely linked polymorphisms at Xq22.1. *Am J Med Genet* **71**:329, 1997.
457. Hofker M, Skraastad M, Bergen A, Wapenaar M, Bakker E, Millington-Ward A, van Ommen G, Pearson P: The X chromosome shows less genetic variation at restriction sites than the autosomes. *Am J Hum Genet* **39**:438, 1986.
458. Davies JP, Winchester BG, Malcolm S: Sequence variations in the first exon of alpha-galactosidase A. *J Med Genet* **30**:658, 1993.
459. Kirkilionis AJ, Riddell DC, Spence MW, Fenwick RG: Fabry disease in a large Nova Scotia kindred: Carrier detection using leucocyte alpha-galactosidase activity and a *Nco*I polymorphism detected by an alpha-galactosidase cDNA clone. *J Med Genet* **28**:232, 1991.
460. Davatelis G, Siniscalco M, Szabo P: An anonymous single copy X-chromosome clone DXS94 from Xq11-Xq21 identifies a common RFLP. *Nucleic Acids Res* **15**:4694, 1987.
461. Schmeckpeper B, Davis J, Willard H, Smith K: An anonymous single-copy X-chromosome RFLP for DXS72 from Xq13-Xq22. *Nucleic Acids Res* **13**:5724, 1985.
462. Keppen L, Leppert M, O'Connell P, Yusuke N, Stauffer D, Lathrop M, Lalouel J-M, White R: Etiological heterogeneity in X-linked spastic paraplegia. *Am J Hum Genet* **41**:933, 1987.
463. Wu J-S, Riordan J, Willard H, Milner R, Kidd K: Msp RFLP for X-linked proteolipid protein gene (PLP) identified with either rat or human PLP cDNA clone. *Nucleic Acids Res* **15**:1882, 1987.
464. Ohshima T, Murray GJ, Swaim WD, Longenecker G, Quirk JM, Cardarelli CO, Sugimoto Y, Pastan I, Gottesman MM, Brady RO, Kulkarni AB: alpha-Galactosidase A-deficient mice: A model of Fabry disease. *Proc Natl Acad Sci U S A* **94**:2540, 1997.
465. Gordon KE, Ludman MD, Finley GA: Successful treatment of painful crises of Fabry disease with low-dose morphine [see comments]. *Pediatr Neurol* **12**:250, 1995.
466. Philippart M: Treatment of painful crises of Fabry disease with morphine [Letter; Comment]. *Pediatr Neurol* **13**:268, 1995.
467. Lenoir G, Rivron M, Gubler MC, Dufier JL, Tome FS, Guivarch M: [Fabry's disease. Carbamazepine therapy in acrodyniform syndrome]. *Arch Fr Pediatr* **34**:704, 1977.
468. Atzpodien W, Kremer GJ, Schnellbacher E, Denk R, Haferkamp G, Bierbach H: [Angiokeratoma corporis diffusum (Fabry's disease). Biochemical diagnosis in plasma]. *Dtsch Med Wochenschr* **100**:423, 1975.
469. Duperrat B, Puissant A, Saurat JH, Delanoe MJ, Doyard PA, Grunfeld JP: [Proceedings: Fabry's disease, angiokeratomas present at birth. Effect of diphenylhydantoin on painful attacks]. *Ann Dermatol Syphiligr* **102**:392, 1975.
470. Filling-Katz MR, Merrick HF, Fink JK, Miles RB, Sokol J, Barton NW: Carbamazepine in Fabry's disease: Effective analgesia with dose-dependent exacerbation of autonomic dysfunction. *Neurology* **39**:598, 1989.
471. Inagaki M, Ohno K, Ohta S, Sakuraba H, Takeshita K: Relief of chronic burning pain in Fabry disease with neurotrophin. *Pediatr Neurol* **6**:211, 1990.
472. Cantor WJ, Daly P, Iwanochko M, Clarke JT, Cusimano RJ, Butany J: Cardiac transplantation for Fabry's disease. *Can J Cardiol* **14**:81, 1998.
473. Argoff CE, Barton NW, Brady RO, Ziessman HA: Gastrointestinal symptoms and delayed gastric emptying in Fabry's disease: Response to metoclopramide. *Nucl Med Commun* **19**:887, 1998.
474. Newton JA, McGibbon DH: The treatment of multiple angiokeratomata with the argon laser. *Clin Exp Dermatol* **12**:23, 1987.
475. Hobbs ER, Ratz JL: Argon laser treatment of angiokeratomas. *J Dermatol Surg Oncol* **13**:1319, 1987.
476. Lapins J, Emtestam L, Marcusson JA: Angiokeratomas in Fabry's disease and Fordyce's disease: Successful treatment with copper vapour laser. *Acta Derm Venereol* **73**:133, 1993.
477. Donati D, Novario R, Gastaldi L: Natural history and treatment of uremia secondary to Fabry's disease: An European experience. *Nephron* **46**:353, 1987.
478. Tsakiris D, Simpson HK, Jones EH, Briggs JD, Elinder CG, Mendel S, Piccoli G, dos Santos JP, Tognoni G, Vanrenterghem Y, Valderrabano F: Report on management of renal failure in Europe, XXVI, 1995. Rare diseases in renal replacement therapy in the ERA-EDTA Registry. *Nephrol Dial Transplant* **11**:4, 1996.
479. Maizel SE, Simmons RL, Kjellstrand C, Fryd DS: Ten-year experience in renal transplantation for Fabry's disease. *Transplant Proc* **13**:57, 1981.
480. Erten Y, Ozdemir FN, Demirhan B, Karakayali H, Demirag A, Akkoc H: A case of Fabry's disease with normal kidney function at 10 years after successful renal transplantation. *Transplant Proc* **30**:842, 1998.
481. Ramos EL, Tisher CC: Recurrent diseases in the kidney transplant. *Am J Kidney Dis* **24**:142, 1994.
482. Mosnier JF, Degott C, Bedrossian J, Molas G, Degos F, Pruna A, Potet F: Recurrence of Fabry's disease in a renal allograft eleven years after successful renal transplantation. *Transplantation* **51**:759, 1991.
483. Peces R: Is there true recurrence of Fabry's disease in the transplanted kidney *Nouv Presse Med* **8**:1499, 1979.
484. Clarke JT, Guttmann RD, Wolfe LS, Beaudoin JG, Morehouse DD: Enzyme replacement therapy by renal allotransplantation in Fabry's disease. *N Engl J Med* **287**:1215, 1972.
485. Friedlaender MM, Kopolovic J, Rubinger D, Silver J, Drukker A, Ben-Gershon Z, Durst AL, Popovtzer MM: Renal biopsy in Fabry's disease eight years after successful renal transplantation. *Clin Nephrol* **27**:206, 1987.
486. MacMahon J, Tubbs R, Gephardt G, Steinmuller D: Pseudorecurrence of Fabry's disease in renal allograft. *Lab Invest* **54**:42A, 1986.
487. Sinclair R: Origin of endothelium in human renal allograft. *Br Med J* **11**:15, 1972.
488. Popli S, Molnar ZV, Leehey DJ, Daugirdas JT, Roth DA, Adams MB, Cheng JC, Ing TS: Involvement of renal allograft by Fabry's disease. *Am J Nephrol* **7**:316, 1987.
489. Donati D, Sabbadini M, Capsoni F, Baratelli L, Cassani D, de Maio A, Frattini G, Martegani M, Gastaldi L: Immune function and renal transplantation in Fabry's disease. *Proc Eur Dialysis Transplant Assoc* **21**:686, 1984.
490. Voglino A, Paradisi M, Dompe G, Onetti Muda A, Faraggiana T: Angiokeratoma corporis diffusum (Fabry's disease) with unusual features in a female patient. Light- and electron-microscopic investigatioin. *Am J Dermatopathol* **10**:343, 1988.
491. Desnick R, Raman M, Bendel R, Kersey J, Lee J, Krivit W: Prenatal diagnosis of glycosphingolipidoses: Sandhoff's (SD) and Fabry's diseases (FD). *J Pediatr* **83**:149, 1973.
492. Malouf M, Kirkman H, Buchanan P: Ultrastructural changes in antenatal Fabry's disease. *Am J Pathol* **82**:132, 1976.
493. Kleijer WJ, Hussaarts-Odijk LM, Sachs ES, Jahoda MG, Niermeijer MF: Prenatal diagnosis of Fabry's disease by direct analysis of chorionic villi. *Prenat Diagn* **7**:283, 1987.
494. Elleder M, Poupetova H, Kozich V: Fetal pathology in Fabry's disease and mucopolysaccharidosis type I. *Cesk Patol* **34**:7, 1998.
495. Dawson G, Matalon R, Li YT: Correlation of the enzymic defect in cultured fibroblasts from patients with Fabry's disease: treatment with purified alpha-galactosidase from ficin. *Pediatr Res* **7**:684, 1973.
496. Osada T, Kuroda Y, Ikai A: Endocytotic internalization of alpha-2-macroglobulin: alpha-galactosidase conjugate by cultured fibroblasts derived from Fabry hemizygote. *Biochem Biophys Res Commun* **142**:100, 1987.
497. Johnson D, Desnick R: Unpublished results.
498. Mayes JS, Cray EL, Dell VA, Scheerer JB, Sifers RN: Endocytosis of lysosomal alpha-galactosidase A by cultured fibroblasts from patients with Fabry disease. *Am J Hum Genet* **34**:602, 1982.
499. Hasholt L, Sorensen SA: ConA-mediated binding and uptake of purified alpha-galactosidase A in Fabry fibroblasts. *Exp Cell Res* **148**:405, 1983.
500. Hasholt L, Sorensen SA: A microtechnique for quantitative measurements of acid hydrolases in fibroblasts. Its application in diagnosis of Fabry disease and enzyme replacement studies. *Clin Chim Acta* **142**:257, 1984.
501. Brady RO, Pentchev PG, Gal AE, Hibbert SR, Dekaban AS: Replacement therapy for inherited enzyme deficiency. Use of purified glucocerebrosidase in Gaucher's disease. *N Engl J Med* **291**::989, 1974.
502. Ashwell G, Morell AG: The role of surface carbohydrates in the hepatic recognition and transport of circulating glycoproteins. *Adv Enzymol* **41**:99, 1974.
503. Bishop DF, Kovac CR, Desnick RJ: Enzyme therapy XX: Further evidence for the differential *in vivo* fate of human splenic and plasma forms of α-galactosidase A in Fabry disease. Recovery of exogenous activity from hepatic tissue, J. W. Callahan JW, Lowden, JA (eds): *Lysosomes and Lysosomal Storage Diseases*. New York, Raven Press, 1981, p. 381.
504. Zeidner K, Desnick R, and Ioannou Y: Quantitative determination of globotriaosylceramide by immunodetection of glycolipid-bound recombinant verotoxin B subunit. *Anal Biochem* **267**:104, 1999.

505. Touraine JL, Malik MC, Perrot H, Maire I, Revillard JP, Grosshans E, Traeger J: Fabry's disease: Two patients improved by fetal liver cells. *Nouv Presse Med* **8**:1499, 1979.
506. Grosshans E: The general review on Fabry's disease [Letter]. *Ann Dermatol Venereol* **113**:277, 1986.
507. Simonaro CM, Gordon RE, Ioannou YA, Desnick RJ: Fabry disease: Bone marrow transplantation in α-galactosidase A deficient mice reverses substrate accumulation, except in the kidney. *Am J Hum Genet* **65**:A503, 1999.
508. Ohshima T, Schiffmann R, Murray GJ, Kopp J, Quirk JM, Stahl S, Chan CC, Zerfas P, Tao-Cheng JH, Ward JM, Brady RO, Kulkarni AB: Aging accentuates and bone marrow transplantation ameliorates metabolic defects in Fabry disease mice. *Proc Natl Acad Sci U S A* **96**:6423, 1999.
509. Pyeritz RE, Ullman MD, Moser AB, Braine HG, Moser HW: Plasma exchange removes glycosphingolipid in Fabry disease. *Am J Med Genet* **7**:301, 1980.
510. Desnick RJ, Grabowski GA: Advances in the treatment of inherited metabolic diseases. *Adv Hum Genet* **11**:281, 1981.
511. Moser HW, Braine H, Pyeritz RE, Ullman D, Murray C, Asbury AK: Therapeutic trial of plasmapheresis in Refsum disease and in Fabry disease. *Birth Defects Orig Artic Ser* **16**:491, 1980.
512. Beutler E, Westwood B, Dale GL: The effect of phlebotomy as a treatment of Fabry disease. *Biochem Med* **30**:363, 1983.
513. Desnick R: RJ Desnick, ed *Treatment of Genetic Diseases*. New York, Churchill Livingstone, pp 331, 1991.
514. Abe A, Arend LJ, Lingwood C, Brady RO, Shayman JA: Glycosphingolipid depletion in Fabry disease lymphoblasts with potent inhibitors of glucosylceramide synthase. *Kidney Int* **16**:446, 2000.
515. Okumiya T, Ishii S, Takenaka T, Kase R, Kamei S, Sakuraba H, Suzuki Y: Galactose stabilizes various missense mutants of alpha-galactosidase in Fabry disease. *Biochem Biophys Res Commun* **214**:1219, 1995.
516. Okumiya T, Takata T, Sasaki M, Sakuraba H: Alpha-galactosidase gene mutation and its expression product in Fabry disease (alpha-galactosidase deficiency). *Rinsho Byori* **45**:127, 1997.
517. Frustaci A, Chimenti C, Ricci R, Natale L, Russo MA, Maseri A, Eng CE, Desnick RJ: Galactose infusion therapy improves cardiac function in the cardiac variant of Fabry disease. Two-year experience of galactose-mediated enzyme enhancement. (In review)
518. Fan JQ, Ishii S, Asano N, Suzuki Y: Accelerated transport and maturation of lysosomal alpha-galactosidase A in Fabry lymphoblasts by an enzyme inhibitor. *Nat Med* **5**:112, 1999.
519. Sugimoto Y, Aksentijevich I, Murray GJ, Brady RO, Pastan I, Gottesman MM: Retroviral coexpression of a multidrug resistance gene (MDR1) and human alpha-galactosidase A for gene therapy of Fabry disease. *Hum Gene Ther* **6**:905, 1995.
520. Medin JA, Tudor M, Simovitch R, Quirk JM, Jacobson S, Murray GJ, Brady RO: Correction in *trans* for Fabry disease: Expression, secretion and uptake of alpha-galactosidase A in patient-derived cells driven by a high-titer recombinant retroviral vector. *Proc Natl Acad Sci U S A* **93**:7917, 1996.
521. Sugimoto Y, Tsuruo T: In vivo drug-selectable markers in gene therapy. *Leukemia* **11(Suppl 3)**:552, 1997.
522. Takiyama N, Dunigan JT, Vallor MJ, Kase R, Sakuraba H, Barranger JA: Retrovirus-mediated transfer of human alpha-galactosidase A gene to human CD34+ hematopoietic progenitor cells. *Hum Gene Ther* **10**:2881, 1999.
523. Ohsugi K, Kobayashi K, Sakuraba H, Sakuragawa N: Enzymatic corrections for cells derived from Fabry disease patients by a recombinant adenovirus vector. *J Hum Genet* **45**:1, 2000.
524. Ziegler RJ, Yew NS, Li C, Cherry M, Berthelette P, Romanczuk H, Ioannou YA, Zeidner KM, Desnick RJ, Cheng SH: Correction of enzymatic and lysosomal storage defects in Fabry mice by adenovirus-mediated gene transfer. *Hum Gene Ther* **10**:1667, 1999.
525. Takenaka T, Hendrickson CS, Tworek DM, Tudor M, Schiffmann R, Brady RO, Medin JA: Enzymatic and functional correction along with long-term enzyme secretion from transduced bone marrow hematopoietic stem/progenitor and stromal cells derived from patients with Fabry disease. *Exp Hematol* **27**:1149, 1999.

CHAPTER 151

β-Galactosidase Deficiency (β-Galactosidosis): G_{M1} Gangliosidosis and Morquio B Disease

Yoshiyuki Suzuki ▪ Akihiro Oshima ▪ Eiji Nanba

1. Hereditary deficiency of lysosomal acid β-galactosidase (β-galactosidosis) is expressed clinically as two different diseases, G_{M1} gangliosidosis and Morquio B disease. The mode of inheritance is autosomal recessive. G_{M1} gangliosidosis is a neurosomatic disease occurring mainly in early infancy (infantile form; type 1). Developmental arrest is observed a few months after birth, followed by progressive neurologic deterioration and generalized rigospasticity with sensorimotor and psychointellectual dysfunctions. Macular cherry-red spots, facial dysmorphism, hepatosplenomegaly, and generalized skeletal dysplasia are usually present in infantile cases. Cases of later onset have been described as late infantile/juvenile form (type 2) or adult/chronic form (type 3). They are observed as progressive neurologic diseases in childhood or in young adults. Dysmorphic changes are less prominent or absent in these clinical forms, although vertebral dysplasia is often detected by radiographic studies. No specific neurologic manifestations are known for late infantile/juvenile patients with G_{M1} gangliosidosis. Extrapyramidal signs of protracted course, mainly presenting as dystonia, are the major neurologic manifestation in adults with G_{M1} gangliosidosis.

2. Morquio B disease is clinically a mild phenotype of Morquio A disease. It is expressed as generalized skeletal dysplasia with corneal clouding, resulting in short stature, pectus carinatum (sternal protrusion), platyspondylia, odontoid hypoplasia, kyphoscoliosis, and genu valgum. There is no central nervous system involvement, although spinal cord compression may occur at the late stage of the disease. Intelligence is normal, and hepatosplenomegaly is not present. X-ray changes are of pathognomonic significance.

3. There is diffuse atrophy of the brain in patients with early onset G_{M1} gangliosidosis. Neurons are filled with numerous membranous cytoplasmic bodies (MCB), and inclusions of other types are observed in glial cells: pleomorphic lipid bodies, membranovesicular bodies, or large compact oval deposits. There are histiocytes with distended cytoplasm in visceral organs. Cytoplasmic inclusions observed under electron microscopy are different from MCB in neurons. They are vacuoles filled with fine granular, tubular, or amorphous osmiophilic material. These changes are less prominent in cases of mild phenotypic expression.

4. Glycoconjugates with terminal β-galactose are increased in tissues and urine from patients with G_{M1} gangliosidosis and Morquio B disease. Ganglioside G_{M1} and its asialo derivative G_{A1}, accumulate in the G_{M1} gangliosidosis brain. High amounts of oligosaccharides derived from keratan sulfate or glycoproteins have been reported in visceral organs and urine from G_{M1} gangliosidosis or Morquio B disease patients. Undersulfated keratan sulfate has also been described.

5. Two lysosomal enzymes are known for hydrolysis of terminal β-linked galactose at acidic pH in various glycoconjugates. One is an enzyme usually called β-galactosidase (EC 3.2.1.23), catabolizing ganglioside G_{M1}, galactose-containing oligosaccharides, keratan sulfate, and other β-galactose-containing glycoconjugates (G_{M1} β-galactosidase). The enzyme activity is markedly reduced or almost completely deficient in cells and body fluids from patients with β-galactosidosis. Heterogeneous kinetic or physicochemical properties have been found in the mutant enzymes. The degree of substrate storage and residual enzyme activity is correlated with the severity of each clinical phenotype; infantile G_{M1} gangliosidosis shows the highest substrate storage and the lowest residual enzyme activity as compared with other milder phenotypes. The second genetically different β-galactosidase is galactosylceramidase (galactocerebrosidase; EC 3.2.1.46), catabolizing galactosylceramide, galactosylsphingosine, and other lipid compounds. Genetic deficiency of this enzyme results in globoid cell leukodystrophy, which is another neurometabolic disease.

6. The human β-galactosidase gene has been mapped on chromosome 3 (3p21.33). The cDNA codes for a protein of 677 amino acids, including a putative signal sequence of 23 amino acids and 7 potential asparagine-linked glycosylation sites. The gene spans more than 60 kb, and contains 16 exons. The promoter has the characteristics of a housekeeping gene, with GC-rich stretches and five SP1 transcription elements on the two strands. Molecular genetic analysis revealed heterogeneous gene mutations in all clinical forms of β-galactosidosis, such as missense/nonsense mutation, insertion/duplication, and insertion causing splicing defect. Neither the type nor location of mutation in the gene is correlated to the clinical phenotype. Five common mutations have been known: R482H in Italian patients with infantile G_{M1} gangliosidosis; R208C in American patients with infantile G_{M1} gangliosidosis, R201C in Japanese patients with juvenile G_{M1} gangliosidosis; I51T

in Japanese patients with adult G_{M1} gangliosidosis; and W273L in Caucasian patients with Morquio B disease. Restriction analysis has been successfully performed for the diagnosis of the common mutations in new patients.

7. **G_{M1} gangliosidosis has been recorded in cats, dogs, sheep, and calves. These animals showed various central nervous system manifestations. β-Galactosidase is deficient, and storage of G_{M1} and oligosaccharides has been confirmed. Furthermore, mouse models have been generated by disruption of the β-galactosidase gene. The β-galactosidase-deficient knockout mouse presented with progressive neurologic manifestations a few months after birth. Clinical, pathologic, and biochemical analysis indicated that this also is an authentic model of human G_{M1} gangliosidosis.**
8. **Morphologic, pharmacologic, and biochemical aberrations have been found in the brain of G_{M1} gangliosidosis patients and animals. Meganeurites and ectopic dendrogenesis are observed in G_{M1} gangliosidosis, and the extent of meganeurite development is related to the onset, severity, and clinical course of the disease. Various pharmacologic abnormalities have been observed in feline G_{M1} gangliosidosis, such as cholinergic dysfunction, neuroaxonal dystrophy in GABAergic neurons, and alteration of phospholipase C and adenyl cyclase activities. These data suggest that morphologic and metabolic effects occur in the presence of excessive storage of ganglioside G_{M1}.**

HISTORY

In 1959, Norman et al.[1] reported a patient with a specific form of amaurotic idiocy—"Tay-Sachs disease with visceral involvement." Clinical and pathologic findings resembled those of Tay-Sachs disease, but lipid-laden histiocytes were observed in extraneural tissues. The stored material was ganglioside, and not sphingomyelin. Craig et al.[2] also described an infant with clinical and radiologic features suggestive of Hurler disease—"an unusual storage disease resembling the Hurler-Hunter disease." The "foam-cell" histiocytes that were found in viscera did not contain mucopolysaccharides.

Subsequently, after a preliminary study of four patients with "pseudo-Hurler disease,"[3] Landing et al.[4] established a new disease, called "familial neurovisceral lipidosis," as a clinicopathological entity. Their eight patients showed (a) clinical and radiologic findings suggesting those of Hurler disease (psychomotor deterioration with dysmorphism); (b) pathologic features resembling those of Niemann-Pick disease, but with certain distinctive features, including involvement of glomerular epithelium; and (c) histochemical properties of the stored material differing from those seen with previously defined lipidoses. Biochemical analysis revealed generalized accumulation of ganglioside G_{M1} in brain and viscera,[5] and the term *generalized gangliosidosis* was proposed as a new inborn error of metabolism.[5] Clinical signs and symptoms developed in early infancy in all patients in these reports. The same disease was described as a biochemically special form of infantile amaurotic idiocy,[6] Tay-Sachs disease with visceral involvement,[7] familial infantile amaurotic idiocy with visceral involvement,[8] Landing disease,[9] generalized gangliosidosis of Norman-Landing type,[10] and G_{M1} gangliosidosis.[11]

Later, cases were recognized of later onset ("late infantile systemic lipidosis") without distinctive clinical or radiologic features.[12,13] Storage of G_{M1} was remarkable in brain but not in viscera. The patients with this G_{M1} storage disease were subsequently divided into two clinical forms on the basis of clinical and biochemical data.[14] Type 1 is characterized by the onset of neurologic deterioration and visceromegaly before 6 months of age, associated with dysmorphism and skeletal deformities, and type 2 by later onset (7 to 14 months) without specific physical findings.

β-Galactosidase deficiency was demonstrated first by Okada and O'Brien,[15] and then a widespread biochemical screening started. As a result, patients with later onset[16,17] and atypical cases in adults with more protracted clinical courses[18] were found. Extrapyramidal signs and symptoms were the major manifestations in adults, starting around 10 years of age and progressing very slowly over 20 years.[18] Otherwise, there were no specific neurologic or somatic abnormalities except for slight vertebral deformities (flattening). Biochemical screening detected a specific deficiency of β-galactosidase in leukocytes and serum. This disease was classified as the adult form of G_{M1} gangliosidosis.[18]

On the other hand, spondyloepiphyseal dysplasia and somatic dysmorphism were found in a patient with β-galactosidase deficiency.[19] Intelligence was normal, and no signs of central nervous system involvement were detected. It was described as a Morquio-like syndrome in another report,[20] and a conclusion was drawn for β-galactosidase deficiency in Morquio B disease as a primary genetic defect due to allelic mutation of the enzyme gene.[21]

The molecular basis of these phenotypic variations became evident when a cDNA clone for human β-galactosidase was cloned and sequenced.[22] Various mutations of the β-galactosidase gene were found in both G_{M1} gangliosidosis and Morquio B disease,[23,24] with some overlap between them,[25] and the term *β-galactosidosis* was proposed on the basis of these molecular genetic observations.[25]

CLINICAL AND GENETIC ASPECTS

As described above, two diseases have been recognized for human β-galactosidase deficiency—a neurodegenerative disease with visceral involvement (G_{M1} gangliosidosis), and a generalized bone disease without central nervous system involvement (Morquio B disease). Originally, they were reported separately as different diseases, but molecular analysis has confirmed allelic mutations of the same gene in these diseases with diverse phenotypic expressions. In this chapter, however, they are described individually because of distinct clinical manifestations.

G_{M1} Gangliosidosis

Incidence and Heredity. G_{M1} gangliosidosis is a rare disease with heterogeneous clinical manifestations. The mode of inheritance is autosomal recessive in all clinical types. Both sexes are affected equally. The incidence of the disease is not known. The infantile form of the disease is described more often than the others. Patients of various ethnic origins have been reported, including Algerian, Belgian, Dutch, English, French, German, Indian, Italian, Japanese, Jewish, Mexican, Polish, Puerto Rican, Saudi Arabian, Swedish, Swiss, and others. Among them, a high incidence has been reported in the population of Malta.[26] Between 1970 and 1993, 149,750 live birth were recorded, and G_{M1} gangliosidosis was confirmed in 23 males and 17 females from 33 families without consanguinity. The incidence was calculated at 1/3700 live births. Adult patients have been reported most often in Japan, but the incidence is not known.

Age of Onset and Clinical Course. In typical cases, the disease is recognized early in infancy. Psychomotor development is retarded from birth in some patients, but the age of onset is variable among the patients with the infantile form (type 1). Cases of later onset have been reported less frequently, and classified clinically as late infantile or juvenile (type 2), adult or chronic (type 3), and other variant types, mainly on the basis of the age of onset and clinical course.[27] Further subclassification was proposed in some reports,[28–31] but clinical classification is not always easy for individual cases. Phenotypic variation has been observed in a family.[31] Early development is normal in the late onset forms, and signs of the central nervous system involvement gradually appear

Table 151-1 Major Clinical Types of Hereditary β-Galactosidase Deficiency (β-Galactosidosis)

	G_{M1} Gangliosidosis			Morquio B disease
Clinical type	Infantile (Type 1)	Late infantile/ juvenile (Type 2)	Chronic/adult (Type 3)	
Major phenotypic expression	Generalized neurosomatic	Generalized neurovertebral	Localized neurovertebral	Generalized skeletal
Onset	0–6 mo	7 m–3 yr	3–30 yr	5–10 yr
Course	<2 y	1–5 y	10–30 y	>30 y
Central nervous system	Generalized	Generalized	Localized	–
Mental	+++	++	+ or –	–
Major motor	Pyramidal	Pyramidal	Extrapyramidal	–
Peripheral nervous system	–	–	–	–
Muscle	–	–	+ or –	–
Cherry-red spots	+	+ or –	–	–
Hepatosplenomegaly	+	+ or –	–	–
Dysmorphism	+ or –	+ or –	–	–
Skeletal system	Generalized	Localized	Localized	Generalized
Storage				
Ganglioside G_{M1}	+++	++	+	–
Oligosaccharides	+++	++	+	+
Keratan sulfate	+	+	ND	+++
β-Galactosidase	Deficient	Deficient	Deficient	Deficient
Common gene mutation	R482H (Italian) R208C (American)	R201C (Japanese)	I51T (Japanese)	W273L (Caucasian)

ND = not described.

at various ages between late infancy and young adulthood. In general, the clinical course is related to the age of onset.

Signs and symptoms of the central nervous system progress rapidly in the cases of early onset, and the infant becomes vegetative with generalized rigospasticity within a year after birth. The clinical course is protracted in the cases of later onset. In exceptional cases, it takes 10 to 30 years before the patient is completely disabled and bedridden. Patients with type 1 or type 3 disease show relatively conspicuous clinical manifestations. Nonspecific signs and symptoms appear in childhood in cases grossly designated as type 2. Clinical, biochemical, and genetic findings of these three types are summarized in Table 151-1.

Infantile (Type 1) G_{M1} Gangliosidosis. Clinical signs and symptoms appear in early infancy after normal development, but some patients show physical or neurologic abnormalities immediately after birth.[10,32–36] In severe cases, appetite is poor, sucking is weak, and weight gain is subnormal in the neonatal period. Ascites and/or edema of the extremities are sometimes observed.

In most cases, developmental arrest or delay in developmental milestones is observed at 3 to 6 months of age. Then the signs of severe brain damage become obvious. Definite functional deterioration of the nervous system follows within several months. The patient may show an exaggerated startle response to sounds.[33,37,38] Deep tendon reflexes are hyperactive, and pyramidal signs are positive. Generalized muscle hypotonia at the initial stage of the disease is gradually changed to rigospasticity later, associated with frequent convulsive seizures.

Macular cherry-red spots are of pathognomonic significance. Corneal clouding is often observed. Optic atrophy is present at the late stage of the disease, and the retina becomes edematous.[39] Hepatosplenomegaly is almost always present. Clinical signs of peripheral nerve involvement have not been described.

In typical cases, dysmorphism and generalized skeletal dysplasia are evident and progressive. The following dysmorphic changes have been described: coarse and thick skin; frontal bossing; depressed nasal bridge; large, low-set ears; increased distance between nose and upper lip; hirsutism on the forehead and neck; gingival hypertrophy; and macroglossia.[27,33] Dorsolumbar kyphoscoliosis is present. Hands are broad, and fingers are short and stubby. Interosseous muscles are atrophic. Joints are stiff, with generalized contractures.

However, these typical dysmorphic expressions are not always obvious in infantile patients.[36] In fact, many patients have presented with neurodegenerative disease without remarkable physical changes. A number of G_{M1} gangliosidosis cases have been known in Japan, but only a few of them presented with the well-known physical changes described above (Fig. 151-1*A* to *C*). It is therefore not always easy to determine the clinical type of a patient on the basis of the specific physical changes.

The patient becomes vegetative with generalized rigospasticity and joint contractures at the late stage of the disease. Death ensues within a few years after the onset of the disease.

Late Infantile/Juvenile (Type 2) G_{M1} Gangliosidosis. G_{M1} gangliosidosis of late onset has been roughly grouped into two subtypes—the late infantile/juvenile and adult/chronic forms. Clinical manifestations in adult patients are uniform, but the patients with relatively early onset (late infancy and childhood) present with heterogeneous phenotypic expressions.

The report by Gonatas and Gonatas[12] described a case of "late infantile lipidosis," but the patient's psychomotor development had been retarded in early infancy, and he smiled and watched his mother only at 8 to 10 months of age. He could never sit without support. Definite deterioration started by 14 months, and myoclonic seizures and generalized convulsions occurred for 2 months before his death at 25 months.

Two sibs in the report of Derry et al.[14] had almost the same clinical course after the deterioration started. However, their early development was normal up to age 1. They started walking without support at 10 to 11 months, but became less responsive and had difficulty feeding at 13 months and stopped walking at 14 months, and progressive stiffness developed thereafter. By 2 years of age, they were in a state of spastic quadriplegia. Babinski reflex

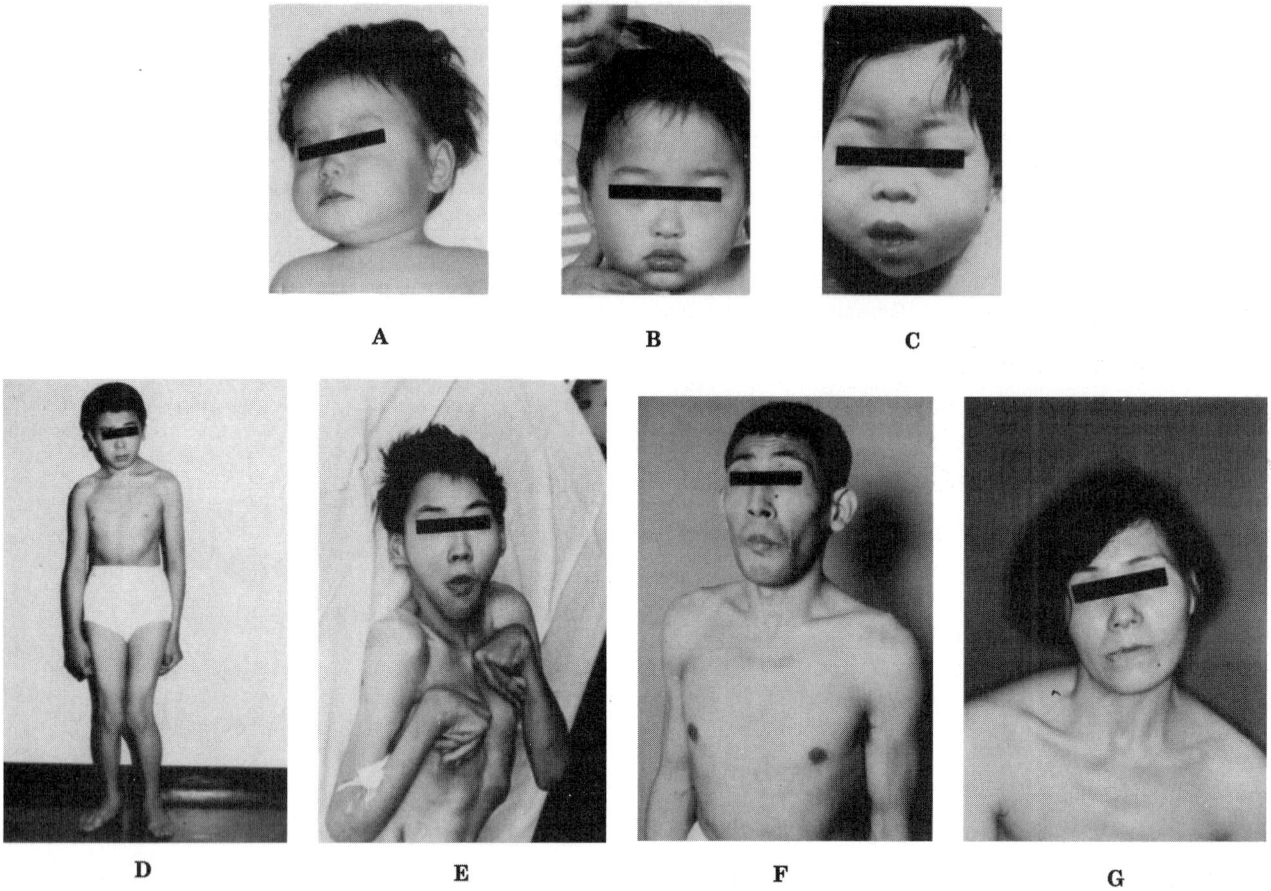

Fig. 151-1 Patients with G_{M1} gangliosidosis. ***A,*** **Infantile form, 1 year, 4 months, female; not dysmorphic. (*Courtesy of Dr. Y. Tanabe, Chiba Children's Hospital, Chiba, Japan.*)** ***B,*** **Infantile form, 1 year, male; not dysmorphic. (*Courtesy of Dr. M. Segawa, Segawa Children's Neurological Clinic, Tokyo, Japan.*)** ***C,*** **Infantile form, 8 months, female; dysmorphic. (*Courtesy of Dr. K. Inui, Osaka University, Osaka, Japan.*)** ***D,*** **Juvenile form, 13 years, male. (*Reproduced from Takamoto et al.*[43] *Used by permission.*)** ***E,*** **Chronic form, 25 years, female. (*Courtesy of Dr. A. Ishizaki, Fuchu Medical Center for the Handicapped, Tokyo, Japan.*)** ***F,*** **Adult form, 29 years, male.[18]** ***G,*** **Adult form, 38 years, female.[54] (*Courtesy of Dr. T. Nakano, Shinshu University, Matsumoto, Japan.*)**

and tonic neck reflex were positive. Optic disks were pale, but cherry-red spots were not observed. There was neither visceromegaly nor dysmorphism described for infantile G_{M1} gangliosidosis. Bone x-ray was normal; no deformities or dysplasias were found. On the basis of the findings in these cases, Derry et al.[14] divided G_{M1} gangliosidosis into types 1 (infantile) and 2 (late infantile). An almost identical clinical picture was reported by Hooft et al.[40] Progressive deterioration started at 13 months, without cherry-red spots, visceromegaly, dysmorphism, or x-ray skeletal changes, although the patient's hands were short and broad.

Five patients from two families showed similar clinical courses, and were reported to have "juvenile G_{M1} gangliosidosis."[16] Gait disturbance was observed at 12 to 18 months, and then psychomotor deterioration became evident. No specific general somatic abnormalities were found. Convulsive seizures occurred frequently after 2 years and were not controlled by anticonvulsants at 3 to 5 years. One of them died after aspiration at 57 months.

Cases of later onset and protracted course have been reported — an 11-year-old boy (onset, 2 years),[41] a 10-year-old girl (onset, 6 years),[42] and a 12-year-old girl (onset, 6 years).[17] Cherry-red spots, visceromegaly, and dysmorphism are absent in most cases (Fig. 151-1*D* and *E*). Atypical cherry-red spots were described in one case.[43] Skeletal dysplasia may not be present,[40,42,44] but has been reported in many patients.

G_{M1} Gangliosidosis in Adults (Adult/Chronic Form; Type 3). In 1977, we reported six Japanese patients with hereditary β-galactosidase deficiency.[18] Three young adults (15 to 22 years) showed progressive cerebellar ataxia, action myoclonus, cherry-red spots, and dysmorphism. Intracellular β-galactosidase activity was low (10 percent of normal), but plasma enzyme activity was normal. Similar cases had been reported previously as a variant of G_{M1} gangliosidosis or a "mucolipidosis."[45–49] After a careful clinical and enzymatic study, we concluded that (a) this group had a new disease different from G_{M1} gangliosidosis or mucopolysaccharidosis, and (b) β-galactosidase deficiency is a secondary biochemical abnormality caused by another basic molecular defect.

The other two sibs, ages 34 and 30, showed different phenotypic expressions, with progressive pyramidal and extrapyramidal disease and muscle atrophy, but without dysmorphism or cherry-red spots. β-Galactosidase activity was extremely low in their leukocytes, fibroblasts, and plasma. Their parents showed half-normal enzyme activity, and we concluded that they represent a new clinical type (adult type) of G_{M1} gangliosidosis caused by a genetic defect of β-galactosidase.[18] This conclusion was subsequently supported by demonstration of an increase of ganglioside G_{M1} in fibroblasts,[50] and genetic complementation analysis.[51] This is a rare clinical form; about 20 families have been reported, mainly in Japan,[52–62] and a few in other areas.[63–67]

Dystonia is the major neurologic manifestation (Fig. 151-1*E* to *G*). Early development is normal. A study of 16 Japanese patients with adult/chronic G_{M1} gangliosidosis revealed that the disease started at 3 years in two sibs, at 4 years in one case, and at 6 to 8 years in four cases.[60] The age of onset was variable in some sibs; it was 19, 30, and 30 years in one family, 4 and 27 years in the second family,[60] 17 and 19 years in the third family, and 3, 3, and 11 to 12 years in the fourth family. The onset was probably 4 to 7 years in the case of Wenger et al.,[65] 2.5 to 3 years in the case of Goldman et al.,[66] and 3 years in the case of Nardocci et al.[68] The severity of phenotypic expressions was remarkably different in two sibling cases of chronic G_{M1} gangliosidosis.[69] The elder sister developed left hip joint pain and gait disturbance at age 27. Early development of the younger brother was retarded in infancy, and progressive psychomotor deterioration became manifest in childhood. Both patients were homozygous for the I51T mutation. The pathogenesis of this discordant phenotypic expression is not known.

Gait or speech disturbance is the first sign in most cases. Dystonic posture develops gradually. Severe dystonia caused masticatory impairment in one patient.[61] Pyramidal signs are present. Deterioration of intellectual activity is not remarkable. Cherry-red spots are not observed, but corneal clouding has been recorded in some cases. Dysmorphism is not obvious. Slight vertebral changes are usually described. Clinical data on the Japanese patients are summarized in Table 151-2.

In some "chronic" cases, progressive neurologic signs and symptoms appeared at age 2 to 3, but the course was protracted with long survival. Postmortem examinations confirmed the diagnosis in two cases neuropathologically and biochemically.[66,70,71] One patient[70] was spastic, decerebrate, and underweight by age 7, and died at 17 years. Ocular signs (cherry-red spots, corneal clouding) and visceromegaly were never observed, but there was mild spondylodysplasia. Her features became coarse, her nasal bridge was slightly depressed, and her forehead developed bossing in the last few years of her life. Autofluorescent material accumulated strikingly in cerebral neurons as seen in neuronal ceroid lipofuscinosis, in addition to storage of ganglioside G_{M1}. The phenotype of this case was originally classified as the late infantile/juvenile form with protracted clinical course.

The case reported by Takamoto et al.[43] is phenotypically similar to adult patients, presenting mainly with dystonia and dysostosis, but atypical cherry-red spots were present. Subsequent clinical follow-up was not possible.

Atypical Clinical Manifestations. Numerous telangiectasias, isolated or in groups, were recorded on the abdomen, pubis, thighs, and face of an infantile patient;[37] a small dilated vessel was surrounded by stellar-ranged distended capillaries, which faded easily under pressure. Angiokeratoma was one of the prominent clinical signs in a few infants with G_{M1} gangliosidosis.[72,73] β-Galactosidase was deficient, but neuraminidase was normal. The clinical course and manifestations were typical of infantile G_{M1} gangliosidosis with dysmorphism, visceromegaly, and neurologic signs and symptoms in early infancy. The lesions were pinhead-sized, purplish, slightly raised, and scattered on the chest, abdomen, thighs, and forearm. They did not blanch with pressure. Foamy endothelial cells were observed in the cutaneous blood vessels in one patient.[74] Extensive Mongolian spots have been described in some cases of infantile G_{M1} gangliosidosis.[73–77]

Cardiac involvement has been another striking manifestation in some patients.[78–82] Cardiomyopathy was observed in an infant with dysmorphism, skeletal dysplasia, and visceromegaly.[78] Corneal opacities or cherry-red spots were not present. A grade 2/6 systolic murmur was heard along the left sternal border. An EKG showed incomplete bundle branch block. At autopsy, the myocardium was pale brown and waxy. Microscopically, myofibers were vacuolated and hypertrophied. The mitral valve leaflets were thick and nodular with vacuolated histiocytes and fibrous tissue. The right coronary artery was partially occluded by a large intimal atherosclerotic plaque containing ballooned cells.

Congenital cardiomyopathy, muscular weakness, and hypotonia were the major symptoms in a male infant, who subsequently developed hepatosplenomegaly and died from heart failure at 8 months of age.[80] His clinical condition resembled that of Pompe disease (infantile glycogenosis II); lymphocytes were vacuolated, and vacuolar inclusions were finely granular and membranous. Axons of intradermal nerve fascicles were often tightly packed with mitochondria and dense bodies, and Schwann cells contained

Table 151-2 Clinical Summary of Japanese Patients with Adult/Chronic G_{M1} Gangliosidosis

Family	1	2	3	4			5	6	7	8		9		10		
Case				1	2	3				1	2	1	2	1	2	3
Sex	F	F	M	F	M	M	M	M	M	F	M	M	F	M	M	M
Age (yr) at onset	7	13	10	19	30	30	8	6	7	27	4	17	19	11	3	3
Age (yr) at diagnosis	25	22	37	38	45	43	46	53	32	29	27	40	34	33	31	28
Clinical manifestations*																
Initial sign	G/S	S	S	G/S	G	G	G/S	S	S	G	S	S	H	S	G/S	G/S
MR/MD	+	−	−	−	−	−	−	−	−	−	−	−	−	+	+	+
Speech	+	+	+	+	+	+	+	+	+	+	+	+	+	+	+	+
Gait	9	+	+	+	+	+	+	49	29	+	+	+	+	+	22	26
Pyr/ExPyr	−/+	−/+	−/+	−/+	−/+	−/+	−/+	−/+	−/+	+/+	−/+	−/+	−/+	+/+	−/+	+/+
Muscle	+	−	−	−	−	−	−	−	+	−	−	−	−	−	−	+
Cornea	−	+	−	−	−	−	−	−	+	−	−	−	−	−	+	−
Bone	+	+	+	+	−	−	+	+	+	+	+	−	−	+	+	+
Laboratory data†																
CT/MRI	Ab	N	Ab	Ab	N		Ab	Ab	Ab	N		Ab	Ab	Ab	Ab	Ab
Bone marrow		−		−					+							+
β-Galactosidase	4.2	7.0	5.7	7.3	8.5	4.4	5.3	7.0	7.9	8.9	5.4	4.7	2.7	5.0	5.0	5.0

*Initial signs and symptoms: G = gait disturbance; S = speech disturbance; H = disturbance of hand movements; MR/MD = mental retardation/deterioration; Speech = speech disturbance; Gait = gait disturbance (numbers denote age at onset of gait disturbance); Pyr/ExPyr = pyramidal and extrapyramidal signs; Muscle = muscle atrophy; Cornea = corneal opacity; Bone = vertebral dysplasia (mainly flattening of vertebral bodies).

†CT/MRI: neuroimaging (computed tomography and/or magnetic resonance imaging [N = normal; Ab = abnormal]); Bone marrow = foam cells in bone marrow; β-Galactosidase = enzyme activity expressed as percent of normal in fibroblasts (substrate: 4-methylumbelliferyl β-galactoside).

SOURCE: Data from reference 60.

membrane-bound lamellar bodies. β-Galactosidase deficiency was found in plasma, leukocytes, and fibroblasts from the patient.

In another female patient, progressive cardiomyopathy (congestive heart failure) and skeletal myopathy (hypotonia and weakness) developed at 4 months of age.[82] α-Glucosidase was normal, but β-galactosidase was found to be deficient. Progressive neurologic manifestations appeared at 9 months, and the patient died at 12 months. Bone dysplasia was not found in this case.

Involvement of the respiratory tract was remarkable in two infants.[83,84] Repeated respiratory infections occurred in one case, and the patient died at 10.5 months from respiratory failure.[83] Alveolar lumina were often completely filled with phagocytic cells.

Hydrops fetalis or ascites in the neonatal period has been reported.[85–87] Venoportography and portal vein pressure were normal.[85] Heavy infiltration of the capillary endothelial cells may have been the cause of the ascites. Administration of salt-free albumin, resulting in better colloid osmotic pressure, temporarily improved the ascites in the patients. In a normal-appearing infant born to a previously unaffected family, progressive, third-trimester oligohydramnios and fetal growth retardation had been documented by ultrasonography. Routine placental examination revealed vacuolization of syncytiotrophoblasts, intermediate trophoblasts, and stromal Hofbauer cells.[88] Subsequent enzyme assays confirmed the diagnosis of G_{M1} gangliosidosis.

Laboratory Findings

Peripheral Blood. Blood counts are normal. Vacuolation of lymphocytes (up to 80 percent) has been recorded in many cases,[10,33,37–39] but is less frequent in late onset cases, particularly in adults. Vacuoles appear empty on electron microscopy. Lymphocytes and neutrophils show basophilic cytoplasmic granules that are slightly positive for toluidine blue stain.[37] Routine blood chemistry is normal. Type IV hyperlipidemia was recorded in two unrelated families; triglycerides and pro-β-lipoprotein were increased.[89] Serum alkaline phosphatase activity was increased in five patients in three reports.[87,90,91] Scattered accumulation of osteoblasts and osteoclasts was found in bone marrow aspirates from one patient.[90] However, the osteoblastosis as a source of hyperphosphatasemia was not supported in the second report.[91] This biochemical abnormality could be an early biologic marker of the disease.

Bone Marrow. Large foam cells or ballooned cells (Fig. 151-2) are present in the bone marrow,[37] but in fewer numbers than in Gaucher disease or Niemann-Pick disease. The cytoplasm is finely vacuolated but does not stain with Sudan III. Lymphocytes are highly vacuolated as in the peripheral blood. Vacuolation is less frequently found in adult cases,[59] and may not be observed in late infantile/juvenile[40] or adult cases.[66] Sea-blue histiocytes

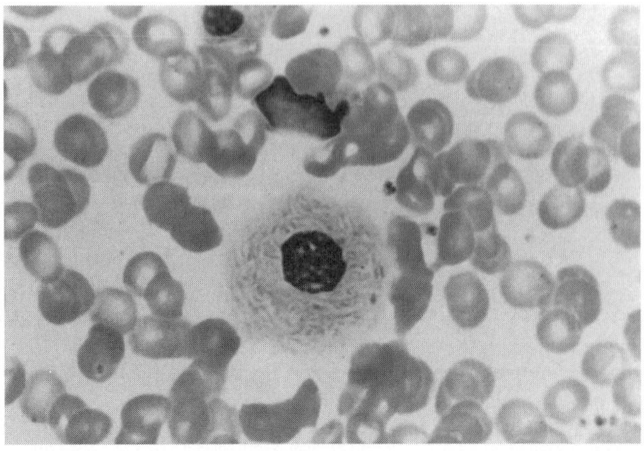

Fig. 151-2 Ballooned histiocyte in the bone marrow of a patient with chronic form of G_{M1} gangliosidosis (17 years, male). (*Courtesy of Dr. M. Yanagisawa, Jichi Medical School, Tochigi, Japan.*)

were present in two sibs with juvenile G_{M1} gangliosidosis.[92] Osteoblastosis was observed in one patient as described above.[90]

Urinalysis. Routine urinalysis is normal. Foamy mononuclear cells may be found in the urinary sediment.[33] Cetylpyridinium chloride (CPC)-precipitable urinary mucopolysaccharides are normal or only slightly elevated.

Cerebrospinal Fluid (CSF). Cell counts and protein are normal. G_{M1} was increased in cerebrospinal fluid by radioassay in adult patients as well as in earlier onset patients.[66] On the other hand, G_{M1} was not detected in plasma or cerebrospinal fluid from an adult patient by an immunostaining method, but an increase was found in infantile and juvenile cases.[59,93] An increase of G_{M1} was confirmed in patients with G_{M1} gangliosidosis using HPLC.[94] G_{M1} in CSF may be helpful in the diagnosis and monitoring of G_{M1} gangliosidosis.

Electrocardiography and Echocardiography. Signs of ventricular hypertrophy were found in the patients with cardiomyopathy.[78–82] Prominent left ventricular forces, with a normal PR interval and tall QRS complexes, were present in one case,[82] and left-axis deviation in the frontal plane was present in another case.[80] Echocardiography showed dilatation of the left ventricle with poor contractility.[80,82] A negative T wave was observed by EKG at precordial leads in one case,[43] and myocardial damage was suspected.

Electromyography. No detectable signs of denervation have been recorded. The number, duration, or amplitude of muscle excitability potentials is normal. H-reflex was demonstrable, but weak and inconsistent, in one patient.[38] Nerve conduction velocities are normal.

Electroencephalography and Electroretinography. EEG may be normal at the initial stage of disease.[13,37] Generalized dysrhythmia with irregular slow activity at the initial stages[38,39] becomes increasingly pronounced around 2 to 3 years of age in infantile form patients.[95] Fluctuating 4 to 5 cycles per second, rhythmic activity was often prominent in the temporal region in type 2 patients.[95] Paroxysmal activity was not a conspicuous feature,[96] but epileptogenic foci are observed in many patients.[39] A normal EEG has been recorded for a case of chronic G_{M1} gangliosidosis.[63]

Electroretinogram was normal in all patients studied, but visual-evoked potential was variably altered.[95]

Bone X-ray Imaging. Bone changes are generally prominent in patients with clinically severe patients, but there are cases of rapid psychomotor deterioration in early infancy with minimal bone dysplasia.[36] No detectable bone changes were reported in a case of late infantile G_{M1} gangliosidosis.[40] Bones are generally rarefied with coarse trabeculation. Vertebral deformities are remarkable; hypoplasia and anterior beaking at the thoracolumbar region[10,17,33,37] and anterior notch deformity occur (Fig. 151-3*A* and *B*).[97] The pathogenesis of the thoracolumbar junction deformity has been explained to be the result of an anteriorly herniated intervertebral disk following prolonged kyphosis,[98] or as the effect of longstanding gravitational pressure and stress on the growth and development of the vertebral body.[99]

Bone age is retarded.[13] Long bones are short, and the midshaft region is wider, tapering both proximally and distally. Metacarpal bones become wedge-shaped with a constriction proximally;[10,33] the fifth metacarpal is frequently the most expanded and deformed. Cloaking of the humerus occurs due to subperiosteal new bone formation. With increasing age, the externally thickened cortical wall is removed (“reamed out”) by expansion of the medullary cavity, resulting in a synchronous thinning of the cortical wall.[33]

Other bones are also involved: thick skull;[17] shallow and elongated pituitary fossa (shoe-shaped sella);[10] widened spatulate ribs;[10] flared ilia;[4] acetabular dysplasia and flattened femoral heads with irregular ossification;[17,43,100] and dislocation of bilateral hip joints.[10]

Bone changes in adult/chronic patients are characterized by mild anterior beaking of lumbar vertebral bodies (Fig. 151-3*D*), platyspondylia (Fig. 151-3*C* and *G*),[54,58] diminished intervertebral spaces, scoliosis (Fig. 151-3*F*),[54] acetabular hypoplasia, and flattened femoral heads[53,54,58,59,65] (Fig. 151-3*E*).

Neuroimaging. Cranial CT and MRI show diffuse atrophy of the central nervous system (generalized cortical atrophy and enlargement of the ventricular system) and features of myelin loss in the cerebral white matter in early onset patients (Fig. 151-4*A*). CT scan revealed an increasing white matter involvement in one case,[101] with generalized areas of reduced density early in the course of the disease.

In adult cases, CT shows diffuse but mild cerebral atrophy,[58,59] or localized atrophy of the head of the caudate nucleus.[66] In some other cases, CT was normal,[54,55] or the frontal horns of the lateral ventricles were only slightly dilated,[52,54] suggesting a slight atrophy of the head of the caudate nucleus (Fig. 151-4*B*).

A patient with infantile G_{M1} gangliosidosis showed at age 34 months high signal intensity in the basal ganglia and low signal intensity in the white matter on T_1-weighted MRI, and low signal intensity in the basal ganglia and high signal intensity in the white matter on T_2-weighted MRI (Fig. 151-5*A*).[102] Similar changes were observed in an 11-year-old patient with chronic G_{M1} gangliosidosis,[103] with bilaterally symmetric low intensity in the putamen and globus pallidus on T_2-weighted images. In this case, single-photon-emission computed tomography using ^{99}Tc-HMPAO showed bilateral hyperperfusion in the basal ganglia that decreased gradually during 1 year of observation. In contrast, proton-density and T_2-weighted MRI showed symmetric hyperintense lesions of both putamina in adult patients (Fig. 151-5*B*).[58,59] Symmetric hyperintensity was seen in both putamina.

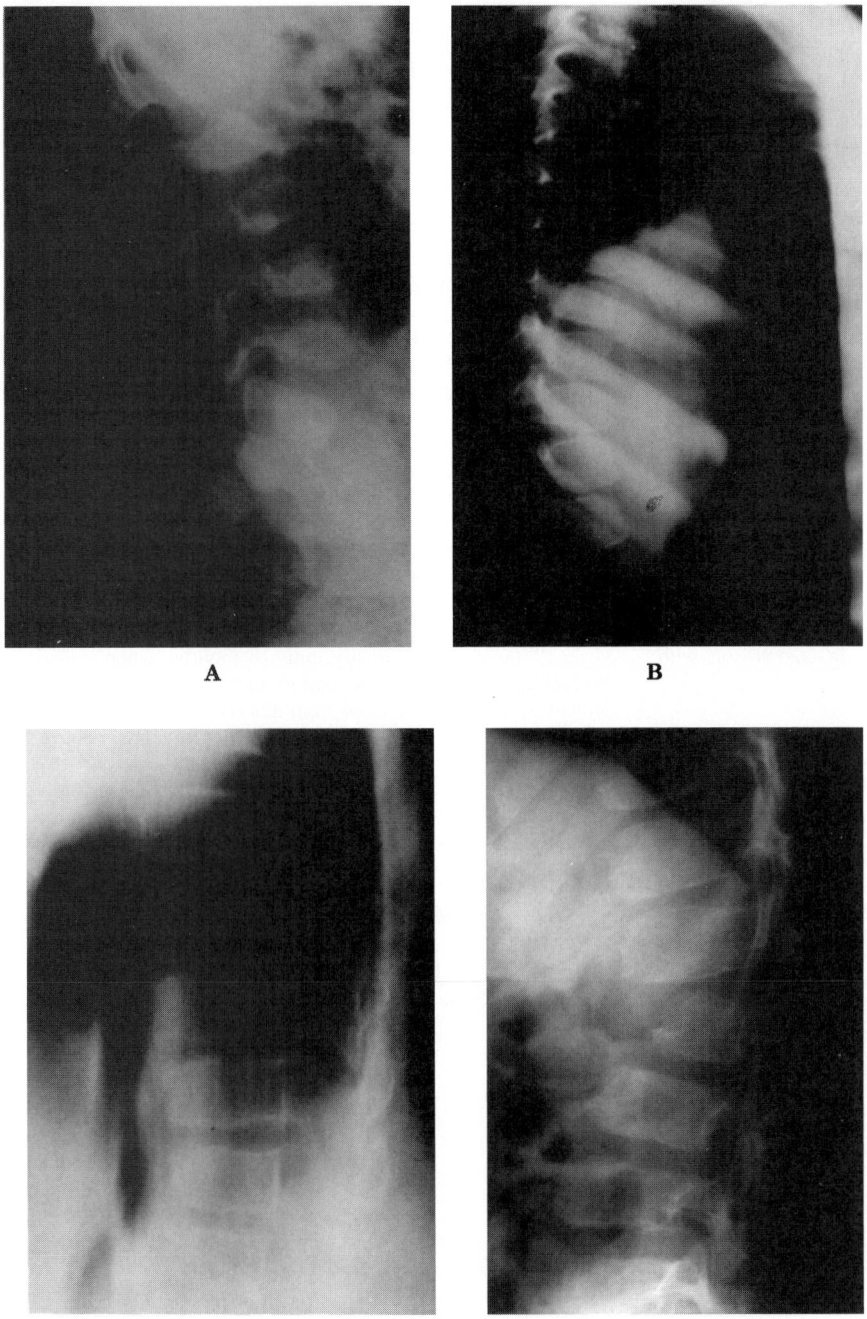

A B C D

Fig. 151-3 Bone x-ray film of G_{M1} gangliosidosis patients. *A*, Infantile form, 2 years, 5 months. (*Courtesy of Dr. Y. Kubota, Mito Saiseikai Hospital, Mito, Japan.*) *B*, Juvenile form, 7 years, male (*Courtesy of Dr. Y. Koizumi, Hitachi General Hospital, Hitachi, Japan.*) *C*, Juvenile form, 13 years, male.[43] (*Courtesy of K. Takamoto, Tokyo Metropolitan Neurological Hospital, Tokyo, Japan.*) *D and E*, Chronic form, 17 years, male. (*Courtesy of Dr. M. Yanagisawa, Jichi Medical School, Tochigi, Japan.*) *F*, Adult form, 22 years, female. (*Courtesy of Dr. M. Ushiyama, Shinshu University, Matsumoto, Japan.*) *G*, Chronic form, 38 years, female.[54] (*Courtesy of Dr. T. Nakano, Shinshu University, Matsumoto, Japan.*)

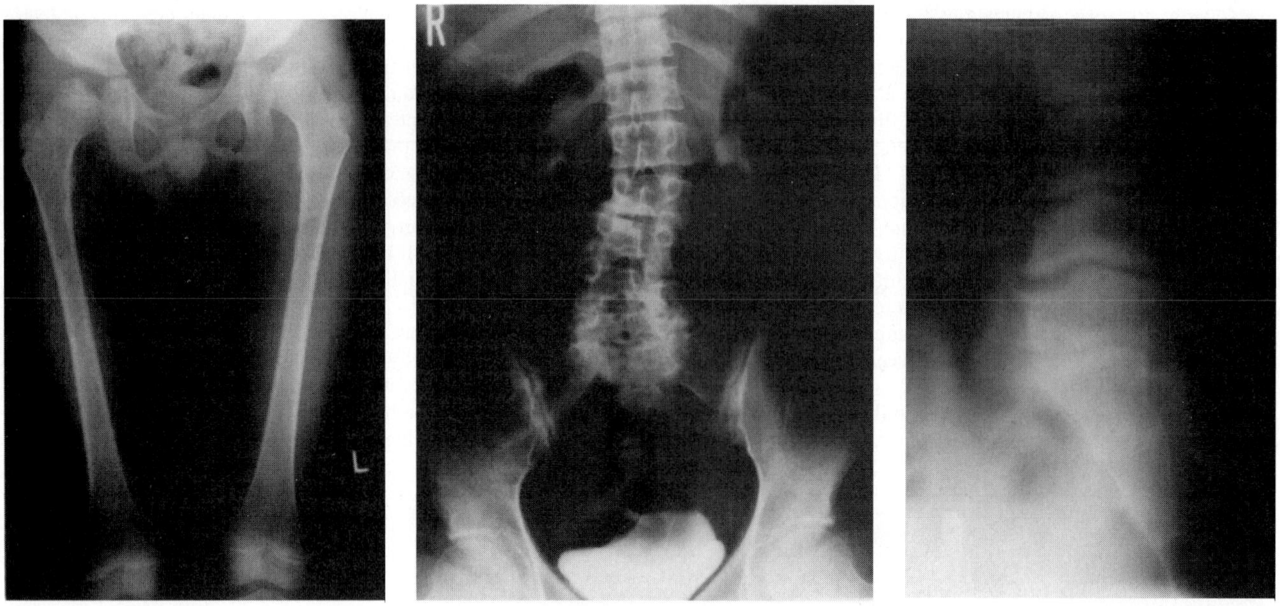

E F G

Fig. 151-3 (Continued)

Calcification in the basal ganglia was demonstrated by cranial plain x-ray imaging in a case of juvenile G_{M1} gangliosidosis.[17]

Morquio B Disease

Morquio disease has been defined clinically as a hereditary generalized skeletal dysplasia with corneal clouding.[104] There is no central nervous system involvement, and intelligence is normal. Excessive excretion of keratan sulfate in urine is the hallmark of this disease, and deficiency of *N*-acetylgalactosamine-6-sulfate sulfatase was found in patients with typical clinical manifestations (Morquio A disease).[105] A mild phenotype with β-galactosidase deficiency was recognized later,[19] and designated Morquio B disease.[20] Allelic mutation of the β-galactosidase gene was suggested by cell hybridization studies,[21] and direct gene analysis confirmed gene mutations different from those for G_{M1} gangliosidosis.[24] Table 151-1 summarizes the major findings in this clinical form of β-galactosidase deficiency in comparison with G_{M1} gangliosidosis.

Incidence and Heredity. Morquio B disease is a rare autosomal recessive disease. Sixteen cases from 10 families were known to the authors by the end of 1997[19,20,106–112] (Table 151-3). The incidence of this disease has not been calculated. Nine males and seven females were affected. The patients from eight families were of Arab, Austrian, Dutch, Greek, Italian, Japanese, Polish, or South African descents; no ethnic ancestry has been recorded for the other two families.

Clinical Manifestations. Morquio disease is a systemic bone disease. Type B disease is considered a mild phenotype, but clinical manifestations are variable. There is an overlap in severity between severe type B and mild type A diseases.[110]

Developmental milestones are normal in infancy and early childhood. The first sign of this disease is growth retardation; the patient is noted to have short stature in childhood. The first patient reported by O'Brien et al.[19] was normal in stature. However, as shown in Table 151-3, the patients visited physicians with other complaints. The proband in three sib cases[109] was referred to a physician at 4.5 years because of "stiffness" of motor performance, such as running and hopping. Two sibs, a brother and a sister,[110] developed normally until 18 months, when at least the brother could walk without support and could speak in sentences. However, he slowly declined from this stage on, with deterioration of speech, understanding, and intellect.

Physical deformities progress with age, and characteristic changes have been observed, including short-trunk dwarfism, sternal protrusion (pectus carinatum), kyphoscoliosis with platyspondylia, genu valgum, swelling of distal ends of long bones, and

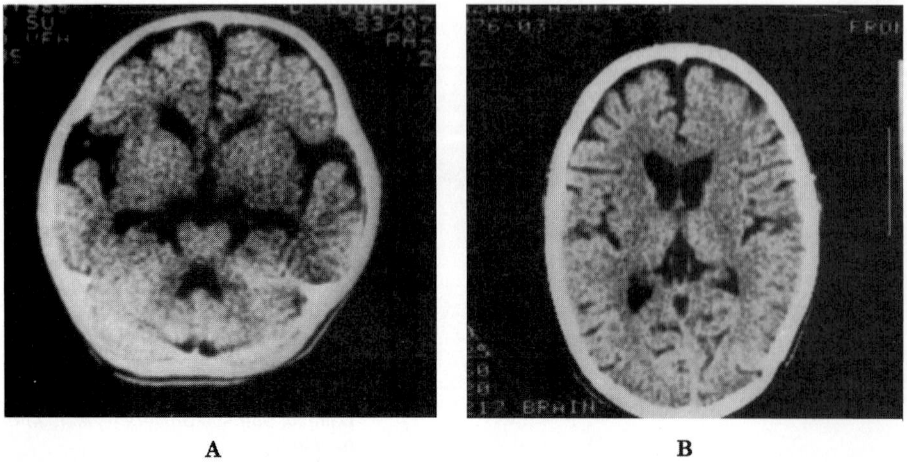

A B

Fig. 151-4 Cranial CT of G_{M1} gangliosidosis. *A*, Infantile form, 1 year, male. (*Courtesy of Dr. M. Segawa, Segawa Children's Neurological Clinic, Tokyo, Japan.*) *B*, Adult form, 38 years, female. (*Reproduced from Nakano et al.*[54] *Used by permission.*)

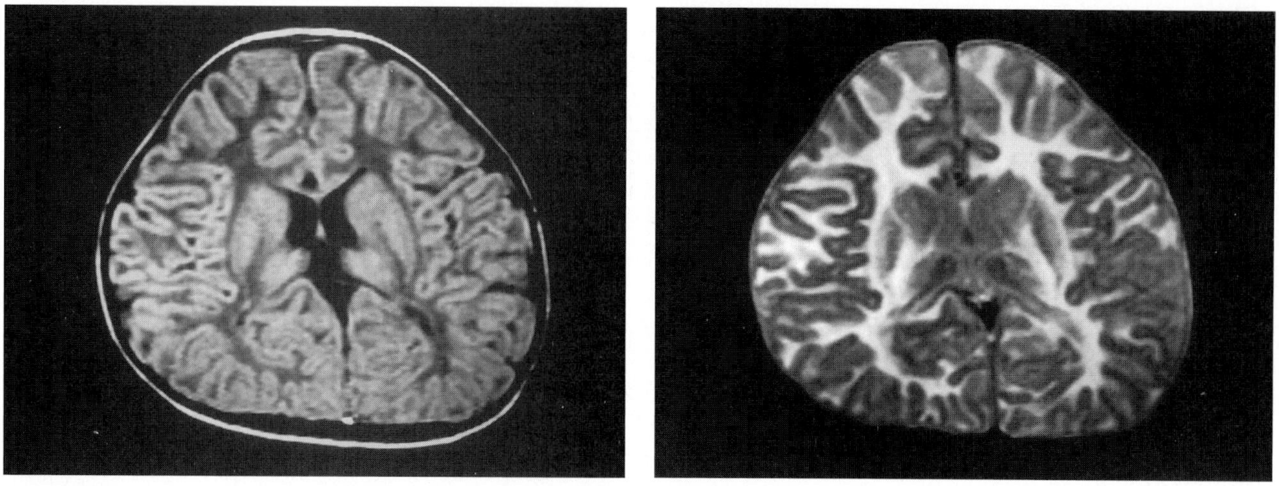

A B

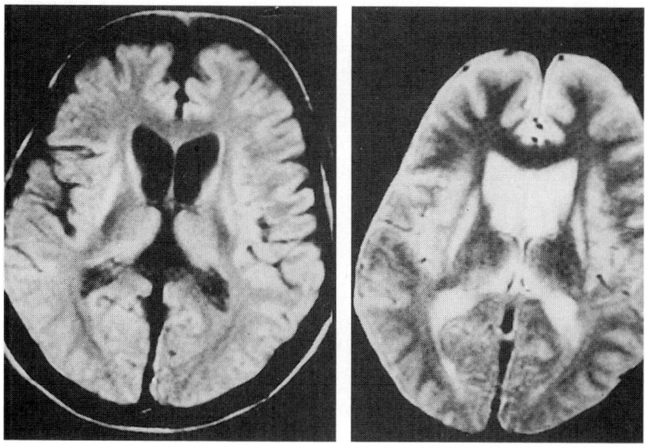

C D

Fig. 151-5 MRI of patients with G_{M1} gangliosidosis. *A*, Infantile form, 34 months, male. Left panel: T_1-weighted image (TR/RE: 560/26). Symmetric hyperintensity in the thalami, caudate nuclei, and lenticular nuclei, with wave-shaped hyperintensity in the cerebral cortex (particularly in the temporal lobe), and decreased signal intensity in the entire white matter. Right panel: T_2-weighted image (2000/100). High signal intensity in the white matter and low intensity in the basal ganglia and thalami (particularly in the medial regions). (*Reproduced from Kobayashi and Takashima.*[102] *Used by permission.*) *B*. Adult form, 32 years, male. Left panel: Proton density image (TR/TE: 2000/25. Right panel: T_2-weighted image (TR/TE: 2000/100). Symmetric hyperintensity in both putamina. (*Reproduced from Inui et al.*[59] *Used by permission.*)

odontoid hypoplasia (Fig. 151-6). The patient of O'Brien et al.,[19] who had been normal in height, had lower back and lower extremity pain at age 10, and then pain and limited movements of hip joints. Overt corneal clouding has been described in several cases.[19,20,107,108] Slit-lamp examination revealed minimal clouding in almost all cases examined.[106,110]

Joints are bulged and deformed. The carrying angle of elbows is increased, and slight ulnar deviation of hands is present. Wrist and interphalangeal joints are thickened. Genu valgum is prominent. A marked varus deformity of thighs is present. Range of motion is not much restricted except for hip joints. The neck and trunk are relatively short as compared with the extremities. Pectus carinatum, barrel-shaped chest, and thoracolumbar kyphosis with gibbus formation are common.

Patients do not have facial dysmorphism, enamel hypoplasia, cardiac murmurs, or visceromegaly. Cherry-red spots have not been recorded. Neurologic examination is negative; there are no pyramidal, extrapyramidal, or cerebellar signs. However, increased muscle tone and pathologically brisk tendon reflexes may appear due to cervical myelopathy. Intelligence is normal in all cases reported, except for two sibs with progressive mental regression.[110]

The clinical course is generally more prolonged than that for Morquio A disease patients, although there is a wide variation in severity and course of the disease. Surgical intervention was necessary in two cases: posterior cervical fusion was performed for anterior subluxation of C-1 on C-2 due to odontoid hypoplasia,[20] and arthrotomy of knee joint due to interposition of a discoid lateral meniscus in one case.[109]

The sibs reported by Giugliani et al.[110] showed progressive deterioration of the central nervous system manifestations. After 18 months of normal development, they slowly declined and could not walk at 11 years and 8 years, respectively. The pathogenesis of this unique clinical manifestation is not known.

Laboratory Findings

Blood. Blood counts are normal. Vacuolation was observed in 1 percent of lymphocytes in peripheral blood from a patient (normal).[19] Lymphocyte vacuoles were not found in Pappenheim or Alcian blue-stained blood smears in another case.[106] No specific abnormality has been described for clinical blood chemistry.

Urine. Routine urinalysis is negative. For metabolic screening, a 5 to 10 percent solution of CPC or cetyltrimethyl ammonium bromide is added to precipitate mucopolysaccharides, but keratan sulfate is not easily precipitated by this procedure. Uronic acid-containing mucopolysaccharides are normal in amount by quantitation with Alcian blue.[110] Accordingly, diagnosis of keratan sulfaturia has been overlooked in some patients. Qualitative analysis of mucopolysaccharides showed an increase of keratan sulfate by thin-layer chromatography[107,110] or by two-dimensional electrophoresis.[110] However, the pattern was indistinguishable from that for G_{M1} gangliosidosis.[110] An oligosaccharide pattern similar to that in G_{M1} gangliosidosis was observed by thin-layer chromatography.[107,111]

Bone X-ray Imaging. Platyspondylia is the most remarkable hallmark of Morquio disease. The following changes have been

Table 151-3 Clinical Summary of Reported Cases of Morquio B Disease

Family	1	2	3	4	5		6	7			8		9			10	11	
Case					1	2		1	2	3	1	2	1	2	3		1	2
Reference	19	20	106		07		108		109		110			111		112	302	
Ethnic origin*	Ital	Wh	Gr	Aus	Wh		Pol		Dut		Arab			SA		Jpn	Ital	
Consanguinity	–	–	–		–		–		–		+			–			–	
Sex	F	F	M	M	M	F	M	F	M	F	M	F	M	M	F	M	F	F
Age (yr) at diagnosis	14	23	6	25	7	5	7	17	15	11	11	8	15	12	13	15	25	20
Age (yr) at onset	10	9	4	2–3	1		Inf	4	11	7	1.5	1.5				7	6	6
Initial sign†	HP	HP BD GD	GR	GR	GD		BD	GD	GD	GD	PMD	PMD				BD	BD	BD
Short stature	–	+	+	+	+		+	+	+	+	+	+	+	+	+	+	+	+
Intelligence‡	N	N	N	N	N	N	N	N	N	N	L	L	N	N	N	LN	N	N
Corneal opacity	+	+	+	+	+	+	+	+	+	+	+	–				–	–	–
Systolic heart murmur		–	–	–	1/6	–	–	–	–		2/6					–		
Liver/spleen (cm/cm palpable)	–/–	–/–	1/–	4/–	–/–	–/–	–/–	–/–	–/–							–/–		
Joint limitation#	H	F	–	–	–		–	+					–	–	–	–		
Ligamentous laxity	–	–	–	–	±	–	–	–	–				+	+	+	–		
Kyphoscoliosis	+	+	+	+	+	+	+	+	+	+	+	+	+	+	+	+	+	+
Platyspondylia	+	+	+	+	+	+	+	+	+	+	+	+	+	+	+	+	+	+
Pectus carinatum		±	–	+	+		+		+		+		+	+	+	–		
Hip joint§	+	+	+	+	+		+	+		+	+	+	+	+	+	+		
Genu valgum		±	±	+	+	+	+	+	+	+			+	+	+	+		
Urinary MPS/OS¶		KS	KS	KS	KS		HN	KS	KS	KS	KS OS	KS OS	OS	OS	KS OS	KS OS		
MUβ-Gal**	3.5 2.4	3.9				6.2		8.3 6	6		2.4 3.4	2.7 3.2	<5	<5	<5	3.5		2.7
PNB β-Gal**		17.3	7.4	6	17.0	2.9	3.5											
Gene mutation				W273L ?		W273L W509C	W273L W273L							Spl2 Spl2		Y83H R482C	W273L R482H	W273L R482H

*Ital = Italian; Wh = Caucasian; Gr = Greek; Aus = Australian; Pol = Polish; Dut = Dutch; SA = South African; Jpn = Japanese.
†Initial signs and symptoms: HP = hip pain; GD = gait disturbance (waddling gait); BD = bone deformity; PWD = psychomotor deterioration.
‡N = Normal; L = Low; LN = Low normal.
#H = hip joints; F = finger joints.
§Dysplasia of acetabulum and/or femoral head.
¶MPS = mucopolysaccharides; OS = oligosaccharides; KS = keratan sulfate; HN = high normal.
**MU β-gal = 4-methylumbelliferyl β-galactosidase; PNP β-gal = p-nitrophenyl β-galactosidase. Enzyme activity is expressed as percent of normal in fibroblasts (or in leukocytes [underlined]).

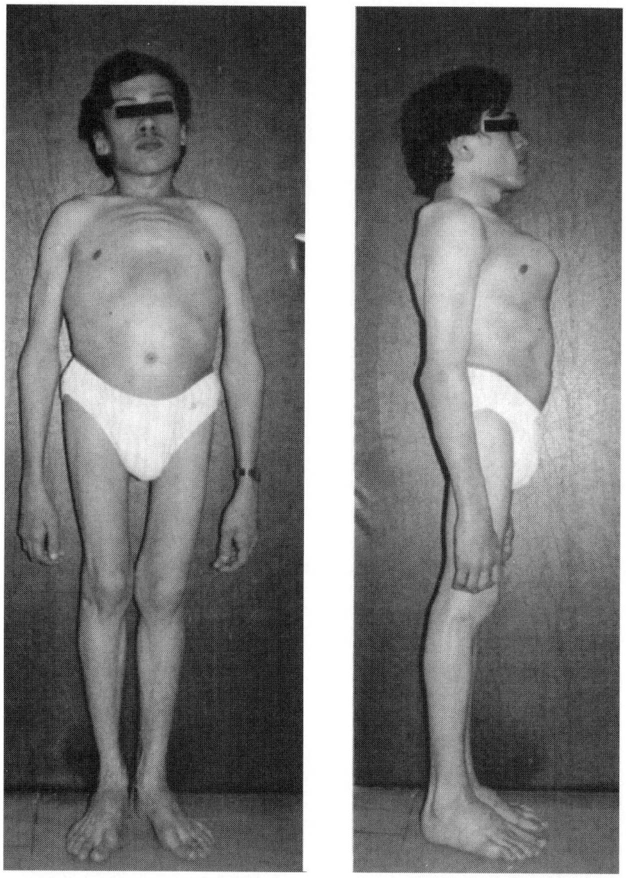

Fig. 151-6 Patient with Morquio B disease.[108] *(Courtesy of Dr. J. Zaremba, Institute of Psychiatry and Neurology, Warsaw, Poland.)*

observed in vertebral bones: loss of normal cervical and lumbar lordosis, with some accentuation of the lumbosacral angle; thoracolumbar kyphosis; mild to moderate flattening of the vertebral bodies (platyspondylia); narrowing of interpediculate spaces; protrusion of anterior borders like a tongue and a humplike plate leading up to a markedly narrowed disk space; narrowing of the sagittal diameter of the spinal canal; and hypoplastic odontoid process. Large maxillary sinuses are also described.[20]

Bones of the hand show abnormally angular metacarpal epiphyses, moderate brachymetacarpia, tongue-shaped narrowing of the distal ends of proximal phalanges, angular carpal bones, and round navicular bones.[19] Bone age was retarded in one case.[109] The following deformities have been described for the bones of lower extremities: coxa vara deformity with extreme flattening of the femoral heads; irregular sclerosis of the acetabular roof;[19] mild valgus deformity of both knees; knock-knee;[107] flattened medial condyles, with mild concavity of contour and some sclerotic margins;[107] outfolded pelvis;[107] narrow pelvis;[110] and dysplastic hip joints.

NOSOLOGY AND NOMENCLATURE

A human disease caused by β-galactosidase deficiency occurring mainly in infants was first designated as G_{M1} gangliosidosis. However, further diagnostic screening of β-galactosidase deficiency revealed atypical variants and late-onset variants in older children and adults with various clinical manifestations, mainly those of the central nervous system or the skeletal system. They have been classified as G_{M1} gangliosidosis or a mucopolysaccharidosis (Morquio-like disease) on the basis of the clinical characteristics and the storage compound initially detected in each laboratory. However, after detailed biochemical analysis, the spectrum of substrate storage was found to overlap between these two disease categories (G_{M1} gangliosidosis and Morquio B disease) that had originally been thought to be completely different from each other.

The distinction between them is becoming less clear, and a new framework for understanding the β-galactosidase deficiency disorders is necessary. The major phenotypic manifestations of β-galactosidase deficiency are grossly grouped into those for the central nervous system, those for the skeletal system, and those for other organs mainly described as "dysmorphism" (see Table 151-1). Early onset G_{M1} gangliosidosis is characterized as generalized encephalopathy with generalized or localized dysostosis; the infantile form as generalized encephalopathy with generalized dysostosis; and the late infantile/juvenile form as generalized encephalopathy with localized (vertebral) dysostosis. Adult or chronic form G_{M1} gangliosidosis manifests itself as an extrapyramidal system disorder (localized encephalopathy) with vertebral dysplasia. On the other hand, Morquio B disease is understood as a generalized dysostosis of another type without central nervous system involvement.

The genetic basis of each subtype has been partly clarified. Gene mutations are heterogeneous for Japanese patients with infantile G_{M1} gangliosidosis, while the other three subtypes were each found to have common mutations among the patients studied until 1992. The whole spectrum of these different manifestations may be compiled in a group of diseases "β-galactosidosis."[25]

At present there is no clear border between G_{M1} gangliosidosis and Morquio B disease. Biochemical analysis suggests that there is considerable overlap for stored material and enzyme activity. In fact, a few cases are known to the authors with expressions of both G_{M1} gangliosidosis and Morquio B disease combined in single patients, such as the sib cases in family 8 in Table 151-3.[110] They had skeletal dysplasia clinically compatible with that for Morquio B disease, with additional manifestations of progressive neurologic disease.

PATHOLOGY

Infantile and Late Infantile/Juvenile G_{M1} Gangliosidosis

Central Nervous System

Gross Morphology. Morphologic aspects of infantile and late infantile form patients were well documented in early reports by Landing et al.,[4] Gonatas and Gonatas,[12] and Suzuki et al.[13,113] Grossly, the brain is atrophic in the gray matter of cerebrum and cerebellum. Atrophy is more prominent in infantile than in late onset cases.

Light Microscopy. Cortical architecture is distorted, and the number of neurons is reduced.[16] Cytoplasm is distended in neurons and glial cells in all layers of the cerebral and cerebellar cortex, basal ganglia, brain stem, and spinal cord (Fig. 151-7*A*). The nuclei are eccentrically placed and pyknotic. The cytoplasm contains finely granular material which stains pale pink with hematoxylin & eosin (HE) and PAS, and occasionally stains with Luxol fast blue.[16] Many acid phosphatase positive granules are seen in the distended neuronal perikarya, axons, and dendrites.[13] They are uniform in size and appear slightly larger than normal neuronal lysosomes. Frozen sections stained strongly PAS-positive in the cytoplasm of neurons in one patient,[12] but did not stain with Sudan black B, Sudan IV, or PAS in another patient.[4] Acid mucopolysaccharide stains were positive in the original patient of Landing et al.[4] Metachromatic material is not present. No cellular infiltrates or any significant gliosis is observed in the cortex. Astroglial infiltration and scant myelin were observed in the central white matter from an infantile case.[4] Myelin stain suggests mild demyelination.[12]

Lipofuscin has been described in G_{M1} gangliosidosis neurons.[13,71,114] Accumulation was remarkable in the case with prolonged survival (onset, 2 years; autopsy, 17 years) reported by

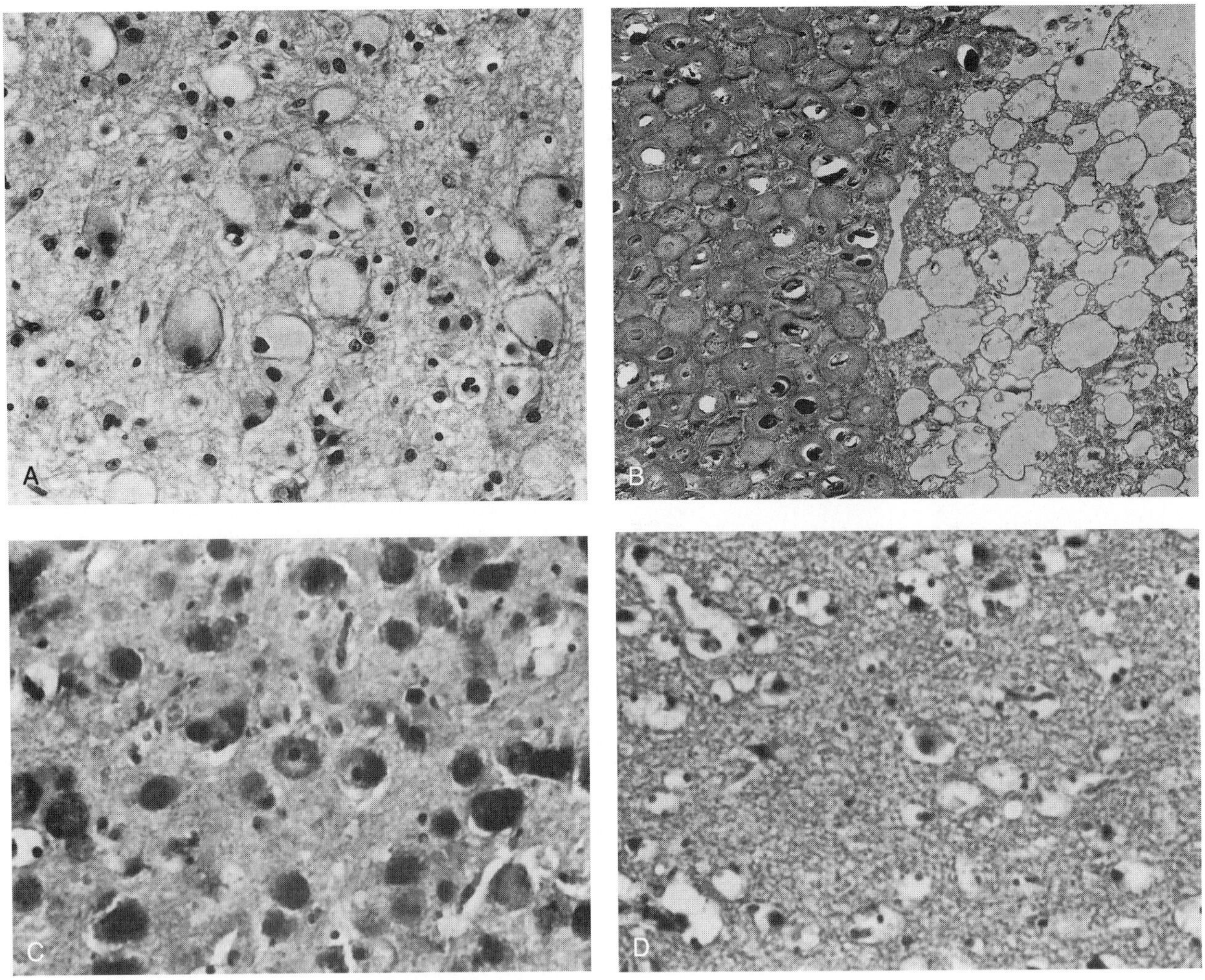

Fig. 151-7 Neuronal changes in G_{M1} gangliosidosis. *A*, Late infantile form, 5 years, male. Ballooning of neurons in the frontal cortex. HE stain, × 180. (*Courtesy of Dr. Yoshio Morimatsu, Tokyo Metropolitan Institute of Neuroscience, Fuchu, Japan.*) *B*, Infantile form, 5 years, male. Numerous MCB in the cytoplasm of a Purkinje cell in the cerebellum. × 6300. (*Courtesy of Dr. Yoshio Morimatsu, Tokyo Metropolitan Institute of Neuroscience, Fuchu, Japan.*) *C*, Adult form. Head of caudate nucleus. Almost all neurons are markedly distended with Luxol fast blue (LFB)-stained material within the cytoplasm. LFB-HE stain, ×1000. (*Courtesy of Dr. Junichi Tanaka, Tokyo Jikei University School of Medicine, Tokyo, Japan.*) *D*, Adult form. Cerebral cortex. Neurons are fairly well preserved in size, shape, number, and distribution. An occasional distended neuron is visible in the central field. LFB-HE stain, ×500. (*Courtesy of Dr. Junichi Tanaka, Tokyo Jikei University School of Medicine, Tokyo, Japan.*)

Lowden et al.[71] This unusual longevity may have led to an increased amount of lipofuscin. Gaucher-like cells with numerous intracytoplasmic striations were found in a case of juvenile G_{M1} gangliosidosis.[41] They were intensely positive for PAS stain and negative for various lipid stains.

Storage was also found in peripheral nerves[115] and astroglia.[114] Retinal neurons were investigated in one case.[116] The ganglion-cell layer is almost completely degenerated. Remaining neurons are strongly ballooned. Infiltration of glial cells with Luxol fast blue-positive material in the cytoplasm is remarkable. Optic atrophy corresponds to strong glial infiltration.

These histologic changes may be less severe in late infantile or juvenile patients, although the lesions are essentially the same as in infantile patients;[42,117] not all neurons are uniformly affected.

Electron Microscopy. The cytoplasm of neurons is filled with numerous concentrically arranged inclusion bodies, such as those in Tay-Sachs disease MCB (Fig. 151-7*B*).[118] They are 0.5 to 3 μm in diameter,[12,13] consist of parallel arrays of membranes usually arranged in a circumferential fashion, and replace largely normal cytoplasmic constituents. The membranes in the center often have an orientation roughly perpendicular to the outer membranes that are circumferentially arranged. The periodicity is 50 to 60 Å,[12,13] and the dimensions of the dense line and light band are 30 Å and 20 Å, respectively.[12] Splitting of the dense line is often seen. The core of the MCB is amorphous or polymorphic, with variable collections of vesicles, granules, and highly electron-opaque material. There is no distinct outer membrane enclosing it, but concentric layers of membranes limit each body.

These inclusion bodies are densely packed in the cell, and the small space between them is filled with mitochondria, smooth vesicles or membranous profiles, and ribosomes. They are also seen in axons and dendrites.[13] MCB is an ordinary molecular complex, and, in fact, was induced by a combination of gangliosides, cholesterol, phospholipids, cerebrosides, and casein hydrolysates.[119] MCB is observed in the brain stem of affected fetuses.

Inclusion bodies with other structures are also observed in glial cells from late infantile cases.[12,13] They are polymorphic, pleomorphic lipid bodies (PLB), membranovesicular bodies (MVB),[12,120] or large compact oval deposits.[16] MVB may be a precursor of lipofuscin,[12] but they may not be the result of intracellular synthesis, as their presence is related to phagocytic activity of these cells.[12,13,120] PLB are surrounded by a limiting membrane and are composed of stacked or circularly layered lamellae with a granular substance of moderate electron opacity.

MVB are composed of stacks of circular arrangements of membranes. Large compact oval deposits are bounded by broken single membranes, and consist of irregularly accumulated curvilinear lamellae that blend into an amorphous matrix of moderate electron opacity.

In the white matter, many degenerated axons are distended with abnormal mitochondria, lamellated dense bodies, and amorphous granular debris.[13,120] Degeneration of myelin is also observed with or without accompanying axonal degeneration.[13]

MCB in the retina are exclusively confined to the ganglion cells.[120] Their appearance is different from those in the brain; membranes are irregularly arranged, forming a water-silk pattern surrounded by amorphous material.

General Pathology

Gross Morphology. Marked hepatosplenomegaly is observed in infantile onset cases, but later onset cases show visceral organs of normal size. Generalized skeletal dysplasia is grossly observed in infantile patients.

Light Microscopy. Histiocytes with distended cytoplasm filled with a finely granular material are observed in liver, spleen, lymph nodes, thymus, lung, intestine, interlobular septa of pancreas, and bone marrow.[4,12,13] Vacuolation has also been observed in the pituitary gland, thyroid glands, salivary glands, sweat glands, and vascular endothelial cells.[115,120] They stain intensely with PAS in paraffin-embedded tissue. Alcian blue and toluidine blue stains are positive.[121] The nuclei are small and pyknotic, and eccentric in location. Vacuolation has not been found in the islets of Langerhans, adrenal cortex, or skeletal muscle.[115]

Renal glomerular epithelium is usually swollen,[4,13] and this characteristic lesion is not found in any other lipid storage disease except Fabry disease.[33] The glomerular epithelial cells store large quantities of cytoplasmic material, giving the glomerulus a swollen appearance.[4] The storage material is very soluble in aqueous fixatives, and empty vacuoles remain after fixation for electron microscopy.[9,32] Vacuoles were also found in renal tubules.[115] In the frozen-dried tissue fixed with formaldehyde gas, the material in the vacuoles is retained and stains with hematoxylin, Alcian blue, PAS, and aldehyde fuchsin. This material also shows metachromasia with toluidine blue.[32]

Cardiac lesions are often reported. Mitral and tricuspid valves show a sparsely cellular connective tissue.[12,78] Vacuolation of cardiac muscles has been observed.[35,78,115,122] Foam cells were seen in the interstitial tissue, heart valves, subendocardial tissues, and adventitia of coronary arteries and large arteries including aorta.[115] Hepatic parenchymal cells are enlarged,[16] and foam cells are present in the portal triads and gallbladder mucosa.[115]

Tissues of a patient at autopsy revealed accumulation of a lipid with histochemical characteristics of gangliosides in the brain; this lipid was positive for Sudan black B and Bial stains, and soluble in alcohol, hot water, chloroform-methanol, and pyridine. On the other hand, the storage material in liver was PAS- and Alcian blue-positive, Sudan black-negative, and could not be extracted by lipid solvents. This material was considered to be an acid polysaccharide different from ganglioside.[123]

Ocular pathology demonstrated two different lesions.[124] Foamy changes were present in the epithelial cells, histiocytes, and keratocytes of cornea. Colloidal iron and Alcian blue stains are positive for mucopolysaccharides, and become negative after treatment with β-galactosidase. Descemet membrane is normal. The retinal ganglion cells were markedly distended, especially in the macular region. They did not stain with HE or PAS. Electron microscopy revealed numerous MCB in the cytoplasm. These findings, together with electron microscopic observations, suggest mucopolysaccharide storage in the cornea and ganglioside storage in retinal ganglion cells.[124]

Cultured skin fibroblasts contain vacuoles with fine granular material that shows metachromatic stain with toluidine blue O when fixed in acetic acid.[44,116,125] Gaucher-like cells in the bone marrow from one patient were clearly distinguished from Gaucher cells;[41] in another case, membrane-bound inclusions of various sizes were arranged in a mosaic pattern and filled with fibrillar material with a "crinkled paper" appearance.[17] Intermingled tubular structures are usually narrow compared with those in Gaucher cells.[41]

In late onset cases, the histologic changes are generally less prominent, or patients may exhibit no evidence of visceral involvement.[117]

Electron Microscopy. Endothelial and mesangial cells in glomeruli, visceral and parietal epithelial cells of Bowman's capsule, and proximal tubule cells contain vacuoles that are filled with fine granular material or that are, on occasion, filled with amorphous osmiophilic material.[115] The cytoplasm of the macrophages in the liver and spleen appears to be divided into many small compartments. Each compartment is filled with interwoven bundles of many fine tubular structures, which are different in size and shape from MCB in the brain.[13,17] Roels et al.[120] did not observe this tubular material in their case.

Two types of inclusions are present in hepatocytes—polymorphic, dense membrane-limited bodies, and cytoplasmic, multivacuolated, lysosome-like bodies (mainly in peribiliary canalicular regions).[16] The vacuoles contain thin filaments of low electron density that are arranged irregularly.[35,110] Rarely, round lamellated bodies of various sizes are found.

Muscle fibers show vacuoles of various sizes containing fine granular material.[115] On the other hand, two types of inclusions have been observed in extramuscular cells, with nonspecific changes in muscle fibers.[126] These are moderately electron-dense and polymorphic material, probably corresponding to ganglioside accumulation, in Schwann cells of intramuscular nerves, and vacuolar inclusions, probably containing polysaccharides in perineurial cells, endothelium, pericytes of blood vessels, and muscle satellite cells. Electron-dense granules are seen in the heart muscle, and amorphous, electron-dense bodies without clear substructure are present in endothelial cells and interstitial cells in the heart.[122]

The vesicles in the cells of cornea consist of a single membrane, and contain small amounts of finely granular material. Retinal ganglion cells show numerous MCB composed of concentric and/or parallel lamellae bounded by a single membrane.[124]

Adult/Chronic G_{M1} Gangliosidosis

Central Nervous System

Gross Morphology. The brain of the patient reported by Goldman et al.[66] was small, but displayed only a slight degree of frontal cortical atrophy. The ventricular system was not dilated. Midbrain, pons, medulla, cerebellum, and spinal cord were grossly unremarkable. Gross abnormality was localized in the basal ganglia with firm consistency; caudate nucleus, putamen, and globus pallidus were shrunken and somewhat yellow. In an autopsy case of adult G_{M1} gangliosidosis,[127] pathologic lesions were most prominent in the caudate nucleus and putamen, and, to a lesser degree, in the amygdala, globus pallidus, and Purkinje cells. The other areas of the central nervous system were relatively spared. It was concluded that this selective neuronal involvement reflected a more active turnover of ganglioside G_{M1} in the affected areas than elsewhere in the central nervous system.

Light Microscopy. Neurons of basal ganglia show markedly swollen perikarya, the cytoplasm displaying an eosinophilic, slightly granular appearance with HE stain.[66] These changes are marked in the anterior putamen and head of the caudate nucleus (Fig. 151-7*C*). Neuronal loss and gliosis were observed in their superior part. The cell loss was greater in the more posterior parts of the nuclei. The cytoplasm of the enlarged neurons stains brightly with PAS with or without diastase, but somewhat less well with Sudan black or oil red O. There is no intraneuronal storage in the cerebral cortex or other deep cerebral nuclei (thalamus, subthalamic nucleus, amygdala, hypothalamus, and mammillary body) (Fig. 151-7*D*). Cytoarchitecture is normal in several areas of cerebral or cerebellar cortex. Neurons of midbrain, pons, medulla, spinal cord, and dorsal root ganglia are all normal.

Dilated proximal processes of medium-sized spiny neurons (meganeurites) were demonstrated on Golgi preparations of basal ganglia.[66] Axons arose from the distal part of the meganeurite. Dendrites were irregular in shape, with focal thickening and loss of spines. Purkinje cells showed focal swellings within their dendritic trees (megadendrites).

Electron Microscopy. Goldman et al.[66] described in detail the structure of inclusion bodies from a patient with adult form G_{M1} gangliosidosis. Various intracytoplasmic inclusions were observed in neurons of basal ganglia: (a) membranous cytoplasmic bodies with concentrically arranged lamellae surrounding a granular or lucent core; (b) pleomorphic inclusions, irregular in shape, containing elements of MCB intermixed with granular material and short, curvilinear profiles; (c) large membrane-bound aggregates; and (d) membrane-bound collections of vesicular profiles or large, dense aggregates in astrocytes of the basal ganglia. Membranous inclusions were rare in Purkinje cells. The neuronal inclusions of cerebellar cortex were small and membrane-bound, containing various membranous and vesicular profiles and granular material.

General Pathology

Light Microscopy. In the case of Goldman et al.,[66] intracellular storage was observed in the reticuloendothelial system; vacuolated Kupffer cells or histiocytes in liver, spleen, bone marrow, lamina propria of the gastrointestinal tract, and glomerular epithelium of the kidney. The cytoplasm of these cells showed PAS-positive, diastase-resistant staining in a granular pattern. Lipofuscin was slightly increased in hepatic cells.

Rectal biopsy shows cytoplasmic granules in the rectal histiocytes. They are strongly or moderately positive for PAS, and faintly positive for Sudan black B.[54,55] Various lectin stains indicated the presence of acidic glycoconjugates, containing abundant terminal β-galactose residues in histiocytes.[55]

Microscopic examination of the vertebral body in an infantile case[97] demonstrated an excessive accumulation of hyaline cartilage in the region of anterior notch deformity at the thoracolumbar junction. Columnar and palisading cartilaginous cells were detected along the posterior superior portion of the body. This finding suggested an asymmetric growth process, rather than a localized dysplasia.

Electron Microscopy. Kupffer cells contained numerous vacuoles of varying sizes bounded by a single membrane.[66] Some were empty, but others contained fibrillar material. In one patient, rectal biopsy showed abundant cytoplasmic inclusion bodies in autonomic neurons.[54]

Morquio B Disease

Dermis and epidermis were normal except for occasional extralysosomal U-shaped, round, or irregular lamellar inclusions in cutaneous nerves.[19] They were not enclosed by a limiting membrane, and were comprised of lamellae with alternating light and dense lines. In another case,[20] biopsy of bulbar conjunctiva revealed intracytoplasmic vacuoles limited by single unit membranes containing fine fibrinogranular material typically seen in mucopolysaccharidoses.

STORAGE COMPOUNDS

The enzyme β-galactosidase has catalytic activities toward glycoconjugates containing a terminal β-galactosidic linkage. Three major groups of compounds have been identified in the cells from patients with β-galactosidase deficiency: ganglioside G_{M1} and its asialo derivative G_{A1}, glycoprotein-derived oligosaccharides, and keratan sulfate.

Glycosphingolipids

Gangliosides were discovered as a new group of glycolipids stored in Tay-Sachs disease,[128] and the monosialoganglioside G_{M1} was the first ganglioside to be analyzed for its structure. G_{M1}'s structure consisted of oligosaccharides and hydrophobic ceramide moiety that were linked together by a glycosidic linkage:[129]

$$\begin{array}{c}\text{Gal}\beta1\text{–}3\text{GalNAc}\beta1\text{–}4\text{Gal}\beta1\text{–}4\text{Glc}\beta1\text{–}1\text{Cer}\\ 3\\ |\\ \text{NeuAc}\alpha2\end{array}$$

Gangliosides are normal components of cell plasma membranes, concentrated in neuronal membranes, especially in the regions of nerve endings and dendrites. The hydrophilic oligosaccharide chain extends into the extracellular space. G_{M1} is the major ganglioside in brains of vertebrates.

At the membrane level, gangliosides display a broad capability of interactions.[130] They act as binding molecules for toxins and hormones, and are also involved in cell differentiation and cell-cell interaction. G_{M1} is well known as a specific receptor of subunit B of cholera toxin. Long-term injection of G_{M1} selectively modulates serotonin receptors.[131,132] Among various gangliosides, only G_{M1} was shown to be necessary to support synaptic transmission in Schaffer collateral-pyramidal cell synapses.[131]

Biosynthesis of gangliosides is catalyzed by a group of membrane-bound transferases. They are transported from the membranes to lysosomes, where they are degraded in a stepwise manner by acid hydrolases starting at the hydrophilic end of the molecules. In fact, the catabolic pathways were mostly studied on the basis of sphingolipid storage diseases. Sphingolipid hydrolases are bond-specific, and degrade different glycoconjugates. Mutation of a gene coding for a lysosomal hydrolase results in its deficiency, and causes intralysosomal accumulation of substrates. The water-insoluble lipid substrates form a complex with proteins, appearing as pathologic storage bodies in somatic cells.

The desialylated derivative of ganglioside G_{M1} (G_{A1}) is not the major component of cell membranes, and its function has not been fully determined. However, this compound also accumulates excessively in neuronal cells.[133]

Glycoproteins and Oligosaccharides

Glycoproteins are widely distributed macromolecules with a variety of functional implications. They are found in serum, urine, various secretions, intracellular and plasma membranes, and extracellular spaces of connective tissue. Many enzymes and hormones are also glycoproteins. The protein portion is variable, and the carbohydrate portion consists mainly of sialic acid, galactose, mannose, *N*-acetylglucosamine, fucose, and *N*-acetylgalactosamine. Glucose, arabinose, and xylose are rarely found in glycoproteins.

Two major types of sugar-amino acid linkage are present: (a) *N*-acetylglucosamine linked to the amide nitrogen of asparagine (*N*-glycosidic linkage) and (b) *N*-acetylgalactosamine linked to the hydroxy group of serine or threonine (*O*-glycosidic linkage). β-Galactoside linkage is present in both molecular species. The structure and function of glycoproteins have been extensively reviewed.[134–137]

The *N*-linked oligosaccharide is first synthesized as a unique lipid intermediate, dolichol-oligosaccharide, by sequential addition of individual sugar residues to dolichol phosphate linkage, consisting of dolichol (Dol), phosphate (P), *N*-acetylglucosamine (GlcNAc), mannose (Man), and glucose (Glc):

$$\text{Glc}_3\text{Man}_9\text{GlcNAc}_2\text{–P–P–Dol}$$

This dolichol-linked oligosaccharide is then transferred cotranslationally to asparagine of the Asn-X-Ser/Thr sequence in nascent polypeptides within the lumen of RER, and the biosynthesis continues and terminates in the smooth SER/Golgi apparatus, where the oligosaccharide moiety is subjected to trimming and addition of other sugars, to form complex-type oligosaccharides. For the biosynthesis of *O*-lin ked oligosaccharides, *N*-acetylgalactosamine is linked posttranslationally, first to serine or threonine in the peptide, and then other sugars are added sequentially.

The degradation of glycoproteins occurs predominantly in lysosomes. Almost all lysosomal enzymes that catalyze the catabolism of glycoconjugates are glycoproteins themselves. Proteolytic enzymes first degrade the protein core of glycoprotein. The aspartylglucosamine linkage in the partial breakdown product (glycopeptide) is then hydrolyzed by an enzyme aspartylglucosaminidase. The free oligosaccharides are subjected to stepwise cleavage of monosaccharides by exoglycosidases from the nonreducing end of the carbohydrate chain. Hereditary β-galactosidase deficiency results in a defect of cleavage at the galactose moiety, and storage of galactose-containing oligosaccharides ensues.

Keratan Sulfate

Mucopolysaccharides are generally high-molecular-weight compounds with the repeating structure of disaccharides consisting of hexosamine and uronic acid. However, unlike other mucopolysaccharides, keratan sulfate does not contain uronic acid and consists of β-linked galactose (Gal) residues alternating with β-linked *N*-acetylglucosamine residues:

$$\text{Gal(6S)}\beta\text{1–4GlcNAc(6S)}\beta\text{1–3Gal(6S)}\beta\text{1–4GlcNAc(6S)}$$

Both monosaccharides may be sulfated at their C-6 positions. Keratan sulfate exists in a proteoglycan linked with chondroitin sulfate. After proteolysis, free keratan sulfate chains are hydrolyzed stepwise by a series of exoenzymes, including galactose 6-sulfatase, β-galactosidase, glucosamine 6-sulfatase, and β-hexosaminidase A and B. Endoglycosidase activity toward keratan sulfate has not been described.

Removal of 6-sulfate on the galactose moiety is necessary for β-galactosidic hydrolysis by β-galactosidase. Specific diseases are known to result from deficiency of one of these four enzymes: galactose 6-sulfatase for Morquio A disease, β-galactosidase for Morquio B disease, glucosamine 6-sulfatase for Sanfilippo D disease, and β-hexosaminidase for G_{M2} gangliosidosis. However, keratan sulfate does not accumulate in G_{M2} gangliosidosis, as hexosaminidase S is not deficient and is able to hydrolyze both β-GlcNAc and β-GlcNAc-6S in this disease.[138]

Keratan sulfate is one of the natural substrates for acid β-galactosidase, and is a part of proteoglycan. Two types of keratan sulfate, I and II, have been distinguished.[139] The former is linked to protein via the *N*-glycosidic linkage between *N*-acetylglucosamine and the amide group of an asparagine residue;[140] it is a major component of cornea. The latter is linked to protein via *O*-glycosidic linkages between *N*-acetylgalactosamine (a minor component) and the hydroxyl group of threonine/serine residue;[141] it is a component of skeletal tissues.

Storage Material in β-Galactosidosis

Ganglioside G_{M1} and Asialo G_{M1} (G_{A1}). Storage of ganglioside G_{M1} has been the most prominent observation for G_{M1} gangliosidosis since the first reports by Jatzkewitz and Sandhoff,[6] Jatzkewitz et al.,[142] O'Brien et al.,[5] and Ledeen et al.[143] Extensive analytical studies were subsequently performed by Suzuki et al.[13,133] The stored G_{M1} has the same fatty acid composition, sugar composition and sequence, and glycosidic linkages as normal G_{M1}. An enormous increase of G_{M1} and, to a lesser extent, of G_{A1}, has been found in brain from G_{M1} gangliosidosis patients; the total amount of ganglioside sialic acid is increased threefold to fivefold in the cerebral gray matter, and G_{M1} is the major component in distribution (75 to 80 percent of total ganglioside sialic acid; control values, 15 to 20 percent). The total increase of G_{A1} is fourfold to twentyfold in the gray matter, but no definite increase is observed in the white matter. G_{M1} constitutes about one third of the dry weight of pure isolated MCB. Storage of G_{M1} was detected by specific binding of cholera toxin B subunit,[144] immunoassay,[59,93] and radioassay,[66] as well as by conventional biochemical analysis. Lysocompounds of G_{M1} and asialo G_{M1} were reported to be increased in the brain of patients with infantile, late infantile, and adult G_{M1} gangliosidosis.[145] These cytotoxic lysosphingolipids may be of pathogenetic significance in G_{M1} gangliosidosis.

Visceral organs also show an abnormal increase of G_{M1}.[34,133] A normal ganglioside pattern was reported in the liver of a patient with late infantile G_{M1} gangliosidosis.[40] An increase of G_{M1} was observed in erythrocytes from a patient with G_{M1} gangliosidosis,[146] but lipid-bound sialic acid was normal in erythrocytes and highly increased in another late infantile patient.[40] G_{M1} was apparently normal in fibroblasts from one patient.[37] No definite conclusion was made for the ganglioside pattern in fibroblasts from G_{M1} gangliosidosis patients.[125]

The extent of G_{M1} storage in the brain is not significantly different between infantile and late infantile/juvenile cases.[33,34,133,147] Accumulation of G_{M1} is detected only in caudate nucleus and putamen in adult or chronic cases.[70]

Abnormalities of Other Lipids. Glucosylceramide and lactosylceramide are increased in the brain in G_{M1} gangliosidosis as well as in G_{M2} gangliosidosis. White matter shows chemical manifestations of myelin breakdown, including low proteolipid protein, low total lipid, and presence of esterified cholesterol.[40,133] Decrease of major cerebral lipids (cholesterol, phospholipids, cerebroside, sulfatide) was more remarkable in an infantile form patient than in a juvenile form patient.[147] In addition, other unusual neutral sphingolipids were found only in the infantile patient. They are tentatively identified as fucolipids consisting of glucose, galactose, *N*-acetylglucosamine, and fucose (1:2:1:1, and 1:3:2:2); lacto-*N*-fucopentaose II (lacto-*N*-difucooctanose), and lacto-*N*-fucopentaose III.[148]

Glycolipids are normal in visceral organs, but a large amount of cholesterol glucuronide was found in a juvenile patient.[149]

Oligosaccharides and Keratan Sulfate. Galactose-containing oligosaccharides and undersulfated keratan sulfate and its partial degradation derivatives have been demonstrated in urine and liver from β-galactosidase-deficient patients.[133,150,151]

Keratan Sulfate and Keratan Sulfate-Derived Oligosaccharides. Vacuoles in visceral organs of G_{M1} gangliosidosis patients contain highly water-soluble compounds, suggesting the presence of compounds other than lipids. A mucopolysaccharide was detected in large amounts in liver and spleen of G_{M1} gangliosidosis patients.[133,152] It was tentatively identified as keratan sulfate on the basis of its behavior in the preparative procedure, composition (almost equimolar galactose and hexosamine), and electrophoretic and thin-layer chromatographic mobilities. The presence of very soluble sialomucopolysaccharide, which contained small amounts of galactosamine, mannose, and fucose, in addition to galactose and glucosamine, was also reported.[133,152] Results of further characterization of this compound have not been reported.

Wolfe et al.[44] detected two types of undersulfated keratan sulfate-like mucopolysaccharides in the urine of a late infantile case. One type was precipitated by CPC, and migrated on Sepharose electrophoresis like standard cartilage keratan sulfate. The other was not precipitated by CPC, and was free of uronic acid. The sugar composition closely resembled the material from the liver of another autopsy patient. Urinary mucopolysaccharides were markedly increased in an infantile case,[88] but the preparation contained significant amounts of uronic acid and galactosamine, major constituents of chondroitin sulfate.

The mucopolysaccharides accumulating in the liver of a patient with infantile G_{M1} gangliosidosis contained galactose and glucosamine as the major carbohydrate constituents, with small amounts of sulfate, sialic acid, and galactosamine.[150] Threonine was found in the keratan sulfate fraction.[153] Mucopolysaccharides were not precipitated by CPC. The structure was similar to the skeletal form of keratan sulfate. However, sulfate was extremely low in content in the mucopolysaccharide from the G_{M1} gangliosidosis liver as compared with normal human skeletal keratan sulfate.

Tsay et al.[154,155] determined the structure of "keratosulfate-like" oligosaccharide from the liver of a patient with infantile G_{M1} gangliosidosis. It was identified as an octahexosyl glycopeptide, probably representing the desulfated linkage region of skeletal keratan sulfate with the structure as follows.

```
                                              Thr
                                               |
Galβ1-4[GlcNAcβ1-3Gal]2β1-4GlcNAcβ1-6GalNAc
                                               3
                                               |
                                             Galβ1
```

The amount of urinary keratan sulfate in G_{M1} gangliosidosis is less than that for Morquio B disease patients.[21]

Keratan sulfate excretion is markedly increased in the patients with Morquio B disease;[19] it constituted 31 percent and 26 percent of total mucopolysaccharides in two cases.[106,109,110] Chondroitin sulfate, which is often observed in Morquio A disease, is not increased.[106,110] Undersulfated keratan sulfate was detected in the CPC-nonprecipitable fraction of one patient.[20]

Glycoprotein-Derived Oligosaccharides. A large number of galactose-containing oligosaccharides have been found in the liver[155,156] and urine[157–165] of G_{M1} gangliosidosis patients, and urine of a Morquio B disease patient.[166] They are heterogeneous, consisting of widely ranging molecular weights (see reference 408 for details).[167] Abnormal oligosaccharide bands were visualized on thin-layer chromatography in an infantile G_{M1} gangliosidosis patient.[21] The most abundant material is an octasaccharide.[156,168,169] The octasaccharide band structure indicates a block in glycoprotein catabolism, not related to keratan sulfate, at the step of β-galactosidic cleavage, subsequent to hydrolysis by endo-*N*-acetylglucosaminidase (sugar-peptide linkage), neuraminidase (sialic acid), and α-fucosidase (fucose). Some of the bands are detected in both liver and urine. They appear to have derived from incomplete degradation of erythrocyte stromal glycoproteins[156] or immunoglobulins.[157]

Neutral oligosaccharides were increased in the urine from adult patients;[170] the pattern was identical to that reported in type 2 G_{M1} gangliosidosis.[52–54] However, the pattern was indistinguishable from that in normal control urine.[21] Two major oligosaccharides were isolated from the urine of a patient with adult G_{M1} gangliosidosis.[165] The first was one of the most common urinary oligosaccharides found in type 1 and type 2 patients, but the amount was much less than that of a type 2 patient. The second oligosaccharide had not been described previously in G_{M1} gangliosidosis. Hepatic glycoproteins were normal in the liver of an autopsied patient.[70]

Four types of oligosaccharides have been identified in the tissues and urine of cats affected with G_{M1} gangliosidosis.[171–173] Oligosaccharide analysis of the liver from Beagle dogs with G_{M1} gangliosidosis revealed carbohydrate sequences nearly identical to those in oligosaccharides stored in the human disease.[172] However, the Beagle carbohydrate sequences differ from the human compounds in that they contain two glucosamine residues at the reducing terminus instead of one.[171] There also may be differences between humans and dogs in glycoprotein metabolism or structure.

Asparagine-linked sugar chains of sphingolipid activator protein 1 were identified in normal and G_{M1} gangliosidosis livers.[174] Eight degradation products from complex-type sugar chains were present in the normal liver; the sugar chains were of sialylated or nonsialylated monoantennary to tetra-antennary complex-type in G_{M1} gangliosidosis, different from those in normal liver.

Oligosaccharide excretion is increased in Morquio B disease.[108] The oligosaccharide pattern is similar to that in G_{M1} gangliosidosis,[106,109,110] but the intensity of all bands is considerably less for Morquio B patients.[110] In another report,[21] the patterns were different from that for G_{M1} gangliosidosis. Six different oligosaccharides have been identified from the urine of a patient with Morquio B disease.[166] Three oligosaccharides were identical to those reported for G_{M1} gangliosidosis, and the other three were novel oligosaccharides in this patient.

Correlation of Phenotype and Substrate Storage. The degree of storage of G_{M1} does not correlate with the age of onset or severity of phenotypic expression, at least for infantile and late infantile cases.[13,34,133] In an experiment using cultured human fibroblasts, a relative increase of G_{M1} was demonstrated in three different forms of G_{M1} gangliosidosis[50] (Fig. 151-8). Gangliosides in the cells were radiolabeled with ^{14}C-galactose in the culture medium. G_{M3} was the major ganglioside in control cells, and a relative increase of G_{M1} was observed in cells from the patients. The degree of increase was inversely correlated to the age of onset.

The amounts of total urinary oligosaccharides are the highest in type 1 (infantile) G_{M1} gangliosidosis; the amounts for type 2 patients were approximately one-tenth of those for type 1 patients.[160] Oligosaccharides with long outer chains (Galβ1–

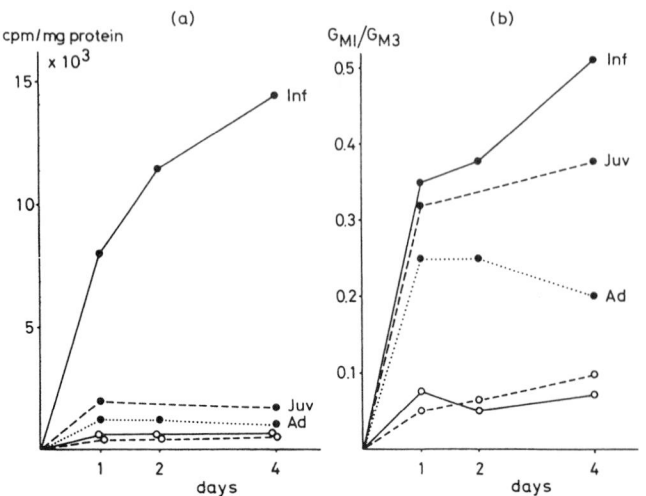

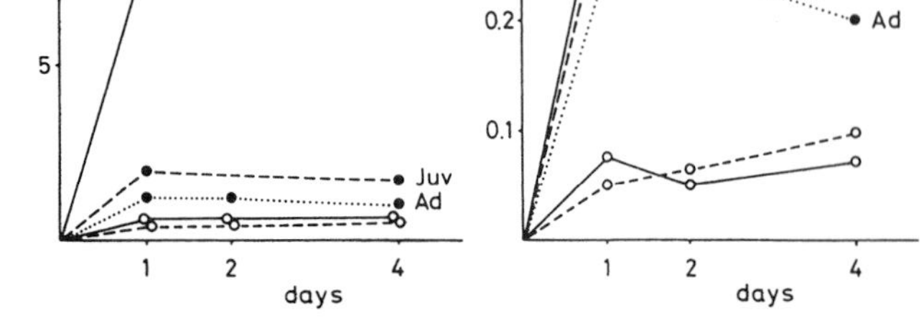

Fig. 151-8 Storage of G_{M1} in fibroblasts with G_{M1} gangliosidosis. Gangliosides were labeled with ^{14}C-galactose, and the radioactivity in the G_{M1} and G_{M3} fractions was determined. Values are expressed as (a) G_{M1}/protein, and (b) G_{M1}/G_{M3} ratio. ○, controls; ●, patients. Inf = infantile form; Juv = juvenile form; Ad = adult form. (*Reproduced from Suzuki et al.*[50] *Used by permission.*)

4GlcNAcβ1–3Galβ1–4GlcNAcβ1–or longer) were reported not to be detectable in the urine from type 2 patients,[160] but most of the oligosaccharides were later found to be present in the latter.[162] Results of comparative quantitative analysis of urinary oligosaccharides have not been reported between G_{M1} gangliosidosis and Morquio B disease patients, although some oligosaccharides are present in both phenotypes.[158,160,162,166]

ENZYME DEFECT

Lysosomal Acid β-Galactosidase

Two lysosomal enzymes are known for hydrolysis of terminal β-linked galactose at acidic pH in various glycoconjugates. One is G_{M1} β-galactosidase (EC 3.2.1.23), catabolizing ganglioside G_{M1}, G_{A1}, lactosylceramide, asialofetuin, galactose-containing oligosaccharides, and keratan sulfate (G_{M1} β-galactosidase). The other genetically different enzyme is galactosylceramidase (galactocerebrosidase; EC 3.2.1.46), catabolizing galactosylceramide, galactosylsphingosine, lactosylceramide, and monogalactosyl diglyceride. Hereditary deficiency of the latter results in a neurometabolic disease, globoid cell leukodystrophy (see Chap. 147).

G_{M1} β-galactosidase is often designated simply as β-galactosidase, and we follow this nomenclature in this chapter. Artificial substrates are currently used for simple and sensitive assays of this enzyme. These include 4-methylumbelliferyl-β-D-galactopyranoside (fluorogenic) and *p*-nitrophenyl-β-D-galactopyranoside (chromogenic). However, more sensitivity is often required for the diagnostic purpose, using small amounts of clinically available samples. Some techniques have been reported for single cell assays[175] and for microassays using microtiter plates,[176,177] high-performance liquid chromatography,[178] or chemiluminescence.[179]

β-Galactosidase is present in a variety of human tissues and body fluids. The enzyme activity is higher in systemic organs, including fibroblasts and lymphocytes, than in the central nervous system. The enzyme has been studied in human liver,[180–187] brain,[188,189] skin fibroblasts,[176,190–194] kidney,[195] urine,[196] placenta,[197] and leukocytes.[198,199]

The optimal pH of β-galactosidase is approximately 4.5. It is thermolabile and activated by chloride ions;[200,201] its activity is inhibited in the presence of mucopolysaccharides,[202,203] and partially restored by the addition of CPC[202,203] or chloride ions.[204] Specific inhibitors of β-galactosidase have been developed, including *N*-bromoacetyl-β-galactosylamine,[205] β-D-galactopyranosylmethyl-*p*-nitrophenyltriazene,[206] *N*-substituted (β-D-galactopyranosylmethyl)amines,[207] and diazomethyl-β-D-galactopyranosyl ketone.[208] β-D-Galactopyranosylmethyl-*p*-nitrophenyltriazene was used to establish an in vitro model of G_{M1} gangliosidosis.[209]

Multiple forms of β-galactosidase have been separated on the basis of molecular weight or electrophoretic mobility. Molecular weights of β-galactosidases purified from human liver are 65, 150, and 700 kDa, probably representing monomeric, dimeric, and multimeric forms, respectively.[183,185,188] Immunologic studies suggested that the high-molecular-weight form is a multimeric aggregate of the monomer.[182]

In human fibroblasts, β-galactosidase is synthesized as a high-molecular-weight precursor of 84 to 85 kDa, which is processed via an intermediate form to the 64-kDa mature enzyme.[210,211] After processing, the monomeric-form protein aggregates to a homomultimer of approximately 700 kDa. A multifunctional glycoprotein (protective protein/cathepsin A) is necessary for aggregation of β-galactosidase in vivo.[192,210] The half-life of aggregated β-galactosidase is approximately 10 days.[212] In the absence of protective protein/cathepsin A, the β-galactosidase precursor is subjected to an abnormal trimming, which precludes its normal processing and expression of catalytic activity.[213]

β-Galactosidase is a glycoprotein containing 7.5 to 9 percent carbohydrate.[181,184,186] Frost et al.[184] isolated a dimeric form of β-galactosidase from human liver; it contained high amounts of acid and neutral amino acids, and low amounts of basic and sulfur-containing amino acids. β-Galactosidase is a soluble lysosomal enzyme with a high content of complex-type oligosaccharides and a low content of oligomannoside-type oligosaccharides.[186] A calculation indicated three carbohydrate chains per enzyme molecule on average.[186]

Natural Substrates for β-Galactosidase

Sphingolipids. Hydrolysis of G_{M1} has been studied for various tissues and cells, including human leukocytes,[214,215] human fibroblasts,[215] human liver,[181,188,214,216] human placenta,[217] rabbit brain,[217] and rat brain.[218] Some reports have discussed the spectrum of substrate specificity.[219–222] In vitro enzyme studies demonstrated that the only substrate common to the two β-galactosidases, G_{M1}-cleaving enzyme and galactosylceramide-cleaving enzyme, is lactosylceramide.[221,222] The terminal galactose in most sphingolipids is cleaved by G_{M1} β-galactosidase, except for galactosylceramide and galactosylsphingosine. Lactosylceramide is hydrolyzed by both enzymes.[190,220,222] The enzymic hydrolysis of liposome-integrated lactosylceramide is significantly dependent on the structure of its lipophilic aglycon moiety, with increasing length of its fatty acyl chain.[223] However, in the presence of detergents, the degradation rate is independent of the acyl chain length.

Bile salts have been added into the enzyme assay mixture for stimulation of hydrolysis of G_{M1} in vitro; this stimulation occurs probably by a detergent effect on the substrate and an interaction between bile salts and the enzyme molecule.[224] Shiraishi et al.[224] reported that the hydrolysis of G_{M1} by β-galactosidase was greatly enhanced by the addition of heptakis(2,6-di-*O*-methyl)-β-cyclodextrin or α-cyclodextrin in the assay mixture. They concluded that these compounds stimulated the hydrolysis by formation of an inclusion complex between G_{M1} and cyclodextrin without enzyme-protein interaction.

Carbohydrates. β-Galactosidase is also involved in the degradation of keratan sulfate and glycoprotein-derived oligosaccharides. A few enzymatic studies have been reported.[21,225] More evidence for β-galactosidase's role in carbohydrate degradation has accumulated from analysis of the storage material in urine or liver from β-galactosidase-deficient patients as described above.

Protective Protein/Cathepsin A

Protective protein is a glycoprotein associated with β-galactosidase and neuraminidase in the lysosome, stabilizing the former and activating the latter.[192,210,226,227] It is synthesized in human fibroblasts as a 54-kDa precursor, which is processed to a mature form, a heterodimer of 32- and 20-kDa subunits held together by a disulfide bond, and aggregates with monomeric β-galactosidase to form a high-molecular-weight complex involving neuraminidase.[192,210,211,228–230]

Some recent studies reveal that this is a multifunctional enzyme protein with serine esterase activities — acid carboxypeptidase at pH 5.6, esterase at pH 7.0, and C-terminal deamidase at pH 7.0.[231,232] It also has cathepsin A-like activity.[233] Genetic defect of protective protein results in combined deficiency of β-galactosidase and neuraminidase (galactosialidosis)[234,235] (see Chap. 152). A defect in multimerization of β-galactosidase has been reported in fibroblasts from galactosialidosis patients; the monomeric enzyme is rapidly degraded by thiol proteases, and the enzyme activity is restored by their inhibitors.[192,212,236,237] Protease inhibitors are effective also for preventing rapid degradation of exogenous *Aspergillus oryzae* β-galactosidase in human fibroblasts.[238]

Activator Protein

Some water-soluble hydrolases need nonenzymic, low-molecular-weight factors (activator proteins) for degradation of sphingolipids in the lysosome (see Chap. 134). They act as physiological detergents that facilitate enzyme-substrate interactions. Sphingolipid activator protein 1 (SAP-1), or saposin B, is required for in vivo cleavage of ganglioside G_{M1} by β-galactosidase.[239,240]

Saposin B is a 9-kDa glycoprotein that stimulates degradation of sulfatides[241–243] and trihexosylceramide[244] by arylsulfatase A and α-galactosidase, respectively. Saposin B and three other thermostable proteins (saposins A, C, and D) are derived from a single high-molecular-weight precursor (prosaposin) by proteolytic processing.[245–247] Saposin B forms water-soluble complexes with both lactosylceramide and G_{M1}, and these complexes are recognized by β-galactosidase as optimal substrates in the same mode.[223] A synthetic peptide corresponding to a predicted α-helix of saposin B, spanning the amino acid residues 52 to 69, has been suggested to play a major role in the recognition and binding to G_{M1} by this activator protein.[248]

Mutant β-Galactosidase

Residual Enzyme Activity. A genetic defect of β-galactosidase in man is responsible for G_{M1} gangliosidosis and Morquio B disease. A profound loss of enzyme activity against natural substrates (G_{M1} and G_{A1}) and artificial substrates has been found in infantile and juvenile G_{M1} gangliosidosis patients (Table 151-4). Less than 5 percent of the control values is found in liver and brain,[188] and almost total loss of activity in leukocytes and fibroblasts.[23,215,249,250] Patients with adult form G_{M1} gangliosidosis have higher residual β-galactosidase activity (5 to 10 percent of control values).[23,51,60] β-Galactosidase activity toward a radiolabeled trisaccharide derived from shark cartilage keratan sulfate was low in fibroblasts from G_{M1} gangliosidosis patients.[251]

Morquio B disease patients show β-galactosidase activity (Table 151-4) that is 5 to 10 percent of control values[106] or less than 5 percent.[111] Residual enzyme activity in fibroblasts was variable toward three different substrates.[19] It was 7 percent for G_{M1}, 1.4 percent for asialofetuin, and 3.5 percent for 4-methylumbelliferyl β-galactoside. It exhibited normal thermostability, and had a normal optimal pH. The K_m for *p*-nitrophenyl β-D-galactoside was fivefold higher than normal.[106,110,252] Mutant β-galactosidase in Morquio B disease had no detectable affinity toward either keratan sulfate or oligosaccharides isolated from patient urine,[21] but a high residual activity of the mutant enzyme was found toward G_{M1} in the presence of partially purified G_{M1}-activator protein.[253] G_{M1} activator thus stimulated G_{M1} hydrolysis by the Morquio B mutant enzyme, but did not stimulate keratan sulfate hydrolysis.[253]

In general, serum β-galactosidase activity is low in G_{M1} gangliosidosis, particularly after long-term clotting of the whole blood.[254] In the cases of juvenile G_{M1} gangliosidosis with homozygous R201C mutation, however, serum enzyme activity was normal and only relatively low, even after long-term clotting,[255] showing a pattern similar to that in galactosialidosis. The R201C mutation is known to produce a mutant enzyme protein with a defect in molecular interaction with protective protein/carboxypeptidase,[256] which is probably a common molecular mechanism for the β-galactosidosis caused by this mutation and for galactosialidosis.

The activities of lysosomal enzymes other than β-galactosidase are usually normal or increased at most threefold to fourfold in plasma from patients with β-galactosidase deficiency. However, markedly increased activities of plasma lysosomal enzymes that were comparable to those seen in I-cell disease, were found in fibroblasts from a patient with a single deficiency of β-galactosidase, thus excluding the diagnosis of I-cell disease.[256] The reason for this unusual observation is not known.

Substrate Loading in Culture Cells. Uptake and degradation of G_{M1} and G_{A1} in cultured fibroblasts were studied in patients with β-galactosidase deficiency after lipid loading in the culture medium.[257–260] In infantile G_{M1} gangliosidosis, the loaded substrates were hardly hydrolyzed and remained in the cells on any day of culture. However, fibroblasts from adult G_{M1} gangliosidosis and Morquio B disease patients hydrolyzed the substrates at nearly normal rates. The *in situ* metabolism of G_{M1} and G_{A1} may be normal, even though in vitro β-galactosidase activities are very low. This result seems compatible with the findings that G_{M1} and G_{A1} do not accumulate in somatic cells of patients with these clinical types of β-galactosidosis, except in basal ganglia.

Mutant Enzyme. Somatic cell hybridization studies showed that the different forms of G_{M1} gangliosidosis and Morquio B disease are based on different mutations in the same gene on chromosome 3.[21,51,261–263] Previous immunologic studies using antiserums against purified human β-galactosidase demonstrated the presence of normal amounts of CRM in liver and fibroblasts from infantile and adult form G_{M1} gangliosidosis patients.[120,264] Normal amounts of CRM were found in cells from juvenile G_{M1} gangliosidosis patients,[182] but a reduction or increase was reported when compared with controls.[265,266] Abnormal electrophoretic migration, a high K_m, and a high antigenic activity per unit of catalytic activity were found in one case.[234]

In one study, the enzyme protein was labeled in vivo in fibroblasts, immunoprecipitated, and fractionated by sucrose-density gradient centrifugation.[193] An 85-kDa precursor was normally synthesized in infantile and adult G_{M1} gangliosidosis cells, but more than 90 percent of the enzyme was degraded at one of the early steps in the posttranslational processing. The residual enzyme was a 64-kDa mature form in adult G_{M1} gangliosidosis, with normal catalytic properties and reduced aggregation to multimers. A contradictory result was obtained in another study using a precursor-specific antibody.[267] An immunoprecipitation analysis revealed that the precursor protein primarily accounted for the residual enzyme activity in fibroblasts from an adult G_{M1} gangliosidosis patient, and that the mature protein accounted for the activity in fibroblasts from a juvenile G_{M1} gangliosidosis patient. In Morquio B disease, the mutation of the enzyme did not

Table 151-4 Residual β-Galactosidase Activity in Fibroblasts from Patients with β-Galactosidosis

		G_{M1} Gangliosidosis*				
Substrate		Infantile	Juvenile	Adult	Morquio B disease*	Reference
4MU*		0.07–1.3	0.3–4.8	0.6–8.9	1.5–12.3	19, 23, 51, 106, 110, 111, 250, 251, 265
G_{M1}	(A)#		4.6–9.4		2.9–25	17, 19, 106, 265
	(B)§	0.1–0.6	0.6–2.0	1.1–4.4		265

4MU = 4-methylumbelliferyl β-galactopyranoside; G_{M1} = ganglioside G_{M1}.
*Enzyme activity = percent of control mean activity per protein (min-max).
#Enzyme activity = percent of control mean activity per protein (min-max).
§Enzyme activity = percent of control mean activity per amount of CRM (min-max).

interfere with posttranslational processing or intralysosomal aggregation.[193] The mature mutant W273L gene product showed a total loss of affinity toward a synthetic substrate, although its precursor protein was measurable, with relatively high K_m as compared with the wild-type enzyme.[268]

Phosphorylation of precursor β-galactosidase was reported to be defective in both infantile and adult form G_{M1}-gangliosidosis fibroblasts.[193] The impairment of phosphorylation could be due to conformational changes of the precursor, resulting in secretion into culture medium, instead of compartmentalization into lysosomes. An immunoelectron microscopic study demonstrated the precursor form of the enzyme in RER and Golgi apparatus, but the enzyme molecule was not detected in lysosomes.[269]

Characterization of Mutant Gene Products. The following results have been observed by expression of mutant genes in G_{M1} gangliosidosis fibroblasts, followed by intracellular turnover analysis of the mutant enzyme protein.[270]

The expression product of the mutant gene W273L (Table 151-5), commonly found in Morquio B disease, is sorted to lysosomes, aggregated with protective protein, and stabilized. A stable mature enzyme has been detected in previous biologic and immunologic studies on Morquio B disease patients, although their genotypes were not known.[21,193,225] This observation was further confirmed by another experiment, using three different forms of human β-galactosidase antibody: a high-molecular-weight multienzyme complex, a recombinant 84-kDa precursor, and a 64-kDa tryptic product of the precursor (an analog of the mature form enzyme).[271] Immunoprecipitation and immunostaining studies demonstrated normal patterns in Morquio B disease, except that the residual enzyme activity was markedly reduced. Formation of a complex in the lysosome (β-galactosidase, neuraminidase, and protective protein) may be related to catabolism of G_{M1}; this substrate is almost normally hydrolyzed in fibroblasts derived from Morquio B patients.[258]

The product of R201C (Table 151-5), a common mutation in late infantile/juvenile G_{M1} gangliosidosis, is sorted to the lysosome but not aggregated with protective protein. The mature enzyme is rapidly degraded in the lysosome as in galactosialidosis with protective protein/cathepsin A gene mutations.

The product of I51T (Table 151-5), a common mutation in adult/chronic G_{M1} gangliosidosis among Japanese patients, was not phosphorylated. Sorting of the mutant enzyme to lysosomes was disturbed at the Golgi apparatus, and only a small amount of the mutant enzyme reached the lysosome. Endogenous protective protein/cathepsin A may stabilize the mutant enzyme. The phosphorylation defect was present at the Golgi apparatus in a mutant cell strain of adult G_{M1} gangliosidosis,[194] and the inactive precursor was secreted in the culture medium. The amount of the mutant enzyme molecule is reduced,[164,193,269] but most of the enzyme activity is in the lysosome. The mutant enzyme is as stable as wild-type β-galactosidase.[272] Further details of the molecular defect are not known.

Table 151-5 Mutant β-Galactosidase of Intracellular Turnover in β-Galactosidosis

Phenotype	Mutation	Ethnic origin	Molecular defect
G_{M1} Gangliosidosis			
Infantile	R482H	Italian	Biosynthesis*
	R208C	American	
Juvenile/Adult	R201C	Japanese	Complex formation¶
	R201H	Caucasian	
Adult	I51T	Japanese	Transport#
	T82M	Caucasian	
Morquio B	W273L	Caucasian	Substrate specificity§
	Y83H	Japanese	

Expression products of common mutation genes for each clinical phenotype are listed for correlative comparison.
*Defect in protein biosynthesis.
¶Molecular interaction between β-galactosidase and protective protein/cathepsin A.
#Intracellular transport of the β-galactosidase protein to the lysosome.
§Altered substrate specificity of the mutant enzyme.

Correlation of Phenotype and Enzyme Defect. Quantitative and qualitative studies have been performed in each clinical subtype of β-galactosidosis. Residual enzyme activities toward synthetic substrates or ganglioside G_{M1} were not clearly correlated to severity of clinical manifestations in infantile, late infantile, or juvenile form patients.[17,34,198] On the other hand, more residual enzyme activity was found in type 2 patients than in type 1 patients.[50,191] Adults with G_{M1} gangliosidosis show higher residual enzyme activities than the patients with other clinical forms.[23,50,51] Residual β-galactosidase activity is also relatively high in Morquio B patients. Direct comparison of the data from different laboratories with different enzyme sources and different substrates is difficult, but the amount of residual enzyme activity seems to have an inverse correlation with the age of onset or clinical severity. No data have been demonstrated for further comparative characterization of mutant enzymes between adult G_{M1} gangliosidosis and Morquio B disease.

Differences in optimal pH, thermostability, and electrophoretic mobility have also been reported.[191,250,273,274] Two clinical forms (infantile and juvenile) occurred in a single family, and different isoelectric focusing patterns were elicited,[275] but further molecular analysis was not performed.

Neutral β-Galactosidase

An enzyme was found in human liver with β-galactosidase activity at neutral pH. It is different from the acid enzyme, and cleaves synthetic substrates with both aryl β-galactoside and β-glucoside linkages, but not G_{M1} or asialofetuin.[180] Antibodies against acid and neutral β-galactosidases do not cross-react with each other.[265,276] In G_{M1} gangliosidosis liver, the neutral β-galactosidase activity is normal[265] or high.[277] This enzyme activity shows a bimodal distribution in human liver, with a high-activity group and a low-activity group (10 percent of the high-activity group).[278] No clinical symptoms have been described even in individuals with extremely low enzyme activity.

MOLECULAR GENETICS OF β-GALACTOSIDASE DEFICIENCY

Molecular Genetics of β-Galactosidase

Gene Assignment. The structural gene coding for human acid β-galactosidase was initially assigned to chromosome 22,[279] and subsequently to chromosome 3.[262,263,280,281] Actually, two loci, one on chromosome 3 and one on 22, were required for the full gene expression.[282] Using human-mouse or human-hamster hybrids and anti-β-galactosidase antibody, the structural gene for β-galactosidase was assigned to chromosome 3p21-3q21[283] and 3cen-3pter.[284] Hybridization of the β-galactosidase cDNA probe to human-mouse somatic cell hybrids revealed the β-galactosidase gene is located in the 3p21-3pter region.[285] Finally, fluorescence *in situ* hybridization recently confirmed the localization at 3p21.33.[286] Several data indicate that the second locus is actually on chromosome 20 and that it codes for protective protein/cathepsin A (see Chap. 152).

β-Galactosidase cDNA. A 2.4-kb full-length cDNA for human placental β-galactosidase was isolated and designated GP8.[22] Expression of the functional molecule in transfected COS (CV-1 transformed by an origin-defective SV40) cells confirmed that the clone GP8 encoded a functional sequence, a protein of 677 amino acids, including a putative signal sequence of 23 amino acids and 7 potential asparagine-linked glycosylation sites.

Two additional 2.4- and 2.0-kb clones were isolated independently.[285,287] The amino acid sequence of the 2.4-kb clone was corrected at position 10 [Pro(CCT) → Leu(CTT)] and position 200 to 201 [Leu(CTC)Ala(GCG) → Leu(CTG)Arg(CGC)]. Sequence analysis of apparently normal subjects and patients with G_{M1} gangliosidosis or Morquio B disease revealed that Leu10 is most common, but Pro10 is also found in less than 10 percent of the subjects analyzed. The expression products of the cDNAs GP8 (with Pro10) and GPN (with Leu10) exhibited almost the same catalytic activity.[23] Pro10 is probably a neutral polymorphism.

The other shorter clone of 2.0 kb is a product of alternative splicing.[287] Exons 2, 3, and 5 are skipped. The band corresponding to the 2.0-kb cDNA was hardly visualized by northern blot analysis. Its expression product was not active toward a fluorogenic substrate, 4-methylumbelliferyl β-galactoside, and failed to be sorted to lysosomes. Alternative splicing has been observed also for other lysosomal enzymes, but its physiological significance is unknown.[288]

A full-length cDNA clone for mouse β-galactosidase was isolated on the basis of homology with the human gene.[289] The degree of similarity between the human and mouse enzymes was nearly 80 percent in the amino acid sequence, and five of seven putative glycosylation sites in the human sequence are conserved.

cDNA Expression. Full-length cDNAs were expressed in COS-1 cells to characterize the gene products.[22,287,289,290] Transient expression led to an increase in β-galactosidase activity up to fivefold 3 days after transfection, and precursors of 84 and 88 kDa were detected by immunoprecipitation from the extract of the transfected cells. The 88-kDa precursor, secreted from transiently transfected[287] or stably transformed[290] COS cells, was efficiently taken up and processed to the 64-kDa mature form by fibroblasts derived from patients with G_{M1} gangliosidosis.[290]

The cDNA was also expressed in fibroblasts derived from a patient with infantile G_{M1} gangliosidosis and transformed by adenovirus-SV40 recombinant virus.[23] It was first subcloned into the pCAGGS expression vector,[291] and then transfected to the transformed mutant fibroblasts that do not express β-galactosidase activity. Detection of the residual enzyme activity expressed by the mutant β-galactosidase gene is possible in this system. No increase of the enzyme activity was detected in COS cells transfected with mutant genes; the endogenous β-galactosidase activity in the host cells was much higher than the residual mutant enzyme activity. In this system, newly synthesized gene products are overexpressed, the endogenous protective protein is relatively deficient, and the enzyme molecule is rapidly degraded.

Overexpression of β-galactosidase has been achieved in the baculovirus-Sf9 (*Spodoptera frugiperda*) system[292–294] and the baculovirus-TN 368 (*Trichoplusia ni*) system.[294] TN 368 cells produced β-galactosidase more efficiently than Sf9 cells on a per-cell basis. However, the Sf9 cell-density varied markedly, and more enzyme activity was recovered at the highest density.

Organization of β-Galactosidase Gene. The human β-galactosidase gene spans more than 60 kb, and contains 16 exons.[295] The ATG translation initiation was numbered as position 1. The promoter activity is located on the 236-bp *Pst* fragment (−261 to −26). The 851-bp *Pst* fragment (−1112 to −262) negatively regulates the initiation of transcription. The promoter has the characteristics of a housekeeping gene, with GC-rich stretches and five SP1 transcription elements on the two strands. The major multiple cap site of mRNA is −53. The mouse β-galactosidase gene spans more than 80 kb, but intron-exon organization is well conserved.[296]

Molecular Pathology of β-Galactosidase Deficiency

Analysis of Mutant Genes. Mutant genes in various clinical forms of human β-galactosidase deficiency have been analyzed. Southern blot analysis did not detect gross gene rearrangements. mRNA was not detected or reduced by northern blotting,[287,297] or abnormally large in size[20] in patients with infantile G_{M1} gangliosidosis, but no abnormality was observed in patients with other clinical subtypes. For patients with normal amounts of mRNA, mutant genes were identified by reverse transcriptase treatment of mRNA, PCR amplification of cDNA, cloning into m13 bacteriophage, and sequencing. The mutation was confirmed, in some cases, by restriction analysis of the PCR-amplified exon comprising the mutation site.

Gene mutations identified in G_{M1} gangliosidosis and Morquio B disease are summarized in Table 151-6. They include missense/nonsense mutation,[23,24,60,297–304] duplication/insertion,[304,305] and insertion causing splicing defect.[112,298,306] Deletion has not been found. Neither the type nor location of mutation in the gene was correlated to the phenotype of the patients with β-galactosidosis. However, five common mutations have been found in different clinical phenotypes: R482H in Italian patients with infantile G_{M1} gangliosidosis,[299] R208C in American patients with infantile G_{M1} gangliosidosis,[300] R201C in Japanese patients with juvenile G_{M1} gangliosidosis,[23,297] I51T in Japanese patients with adult G_{M1} gangliosidosis,[23] and W273L in Caucasian patients with Morquio B disease.[24] The R208C mutation has been suggested to have originated from Puerto Rican ancestry.[300] The R482H mutation had also been identified in Morquio B disease as well as in infantile G_{M1} gangliosidosis.[24,299] There is no clear genetic distinction between the two clinical phenotypes; one with generalized neurosomatic manifestations and the other with generalized skeletal dysplasia without central nervous system involvement. This observation supports our nomenclature of β-galactosidosis.[25]

The mutant gene products had almost normal enzyme activity (L10P polymorphism; 10Leu → Pro/CTT → CCT), about 10 percent normal activity (I51T, R201C, W273L), or less than 1 percent (others).

Figure 151-9 presents the results of restriction analysis on families with adult G_{M1} gangliosidosis. The combination of exon 2 amplification and restriction analysis is useful for the diagnosis of the I51T mutation, expressing adult G_{M1} gangliosidosis, which is common among the Japanese population; 16 patients were homozygotes and 1 was a compound heterozygote for this mutation.[60]

Phenotype-Genotype Correlation. Gene mutations are heterogeneous among Japanese patients with infantile G_{M1} gangliosidosis, mostly compound heterozygotes without consanguinity. The mRNA amount is reduced in most patients, and the mutant genes expressed no detectable enzyme activity. Infantile G_{M1} gangliosidosis has been the most common phenotype among the human β-galactosidase deficiencies. It is expected that most β-galactosidase gene mutations express no or extremely low residual enzyme activity.

For other phenotypes with milder clinical manifestations, these characteristics were observed in our studies:[23,24,60] (a) three gene mutations, R201C, I51T, and W273L, were always found for late infantile/juvenile G_{M1} gangliosidosis, adult/chronic G_{M1} gangliosidosis, and Morquio B disease, respectively, in specific ethnic populations; and (b) patients are either homozygotes or compound heterozygotes, but the expression products of counterpart mutant genes (R457Q, R482H, W509C) showed no enzyme activity; any combination of these second mutant genes results in infantile G_{M1} gangliosidosis.

The three common mutant genes produce reduced but active enzymes. Partial breakdown of natural substrates, ganglioside G_{M1}, oligosaccharide, and keratan sulfate, probably results in mild phenotypic expression in different ways. For late infantile/juvenile G_{M1} gangliosidosis, no obvious difference was observed in clinical manifestations between homozygotes and compound heterozygotes. For adult/chronic G_{M1} gangliosidosis, the age of onset and clinical signs were similar, but a compound heterozygote

Table 151-6 **β-Galactosidase Gene Mutations in β-Galactosidosis**

Mutation	Exon	Amino acid	Base	Phenotype*	Ethnic origin	Ref
Spl1	Int 1	Ins 20 bp; ex1/2	GC/gta → GCGTTA	Adult G_{M1}	Caucasian	298
R49C	2	49Arg → Cys	145C → T	Inf G_{M1}	Japanese	297
I51T	2	51Ile → Thr	152T → C	Adult G_{M1}	Japanese	23, 60
Spl2	Int 2	Ins 32 bp; ex2/3	ag/GT → AAGT	MB	Caucasian	112
T82M	2–3	82Thr → Met	245C → T	Adult G_{M1}	Caucasian	298, 301
Y83H	3	83Tyr → His	247T → C	MB	Japanese	302
Dup254	3	Duplication	#254–276	Inf G_{M1}	Japanese	305
G123R	3	123Gly → Arg	367G → A	Inf G_{M1}	Japanese	23
R201C	6	201Arg → Cys	601C → T	Juv G_{M1}	Japanese	23, 297
R201H	6	201Arg → His	602G → A	Adult G_{M1}	Caucasian	302
R208C	6	208Arg → Cys	622C → T	Inf G_{M1}	American¶	303, 303
Ins9bp:ex6	6	Ins GluAsnPhe	CAGAATTTT	Adult G_{M1}	American¶	304
Spl6	Int 6	Ins 9 bp; ex6/7	acaa → ag/AA	Juv G_{M1}	Japanese	306
P263S	7	263Pro → Ser	787C → T	Adult G_{M1}	Unknown	302
N266S	8	266Asn → Ser	797A → G	Adult G_{M1}	American¶	304
W273L	8	273Trp → Leu	818G → T	MB	Caucasian	24
Y316C	9	316Tyr → Cys	947A → G	Inf G_{M1}	Japanese	23
N318H	9	318Asn → His	952A → C	Juv G_{M1}–MB	Greek	302
Dup1069	11–12	Duplication	#1069–1233	Inf G_{M1}	Japanese	23
S434L	13	434Ser → Leu	1301C → T	Inf G_{M1}	English¶	#
R457X	14	457Arg → Ter	1369C → T	Inf G_{M1}	Japanese	297
R457Q	14	457Arg → Gln	1370G → A	Adult G_{M1}	Japanese	23
R482H	14	482Arg → His	1445G → A	MB Inf G_{M1}	Caucasian/Italian	24, 299, 302
R482C	14	482Arg → Cys	1444C → T	MB	Japanese	302
G494C	15	494Gly → Cys	1480G → T	Inf G_{M1}	Japanese	23
W509C	15	509Trp → Cys	1527G → T	MB	Caucasian	24, 302
K578R	15	578Lys → Arg	1733A → G	Inf G_{M1}	Caucasian	300
R590H	16	590Arg → His	1769G → A	Juv G_{M1}	Caucasian	300
E632G	16	632Glu → Gly	1895A → G	Juv G_{M1}	Caucasian	300

*Inf G_{M1} = infantile G_{M1}-gangliosidosis; Juv G_{M1} = juvenile G_{M1}-gangliosidosis; Adult G_{M1} = adult G_{M1}-gangliosidosis; MB = Morquio B disease

#Nanba E: Unpublished data.
¶Ethnic origin not specified.

I51T/R457Q had a relatively rapid clinical course as compared to homozygotes I51T/I51T.[60]

PATHOGENESIS

G_{M1} has been suggested to have antineurotoxic, neuroprotective, and neurorestorative effects on various central transmitter systems.[307] It may be used for treating neuroinjury and a variety of degenerative conditions, including aging. On the other hand, as already described in this chapter, morphologic, pharmacologic, and biochemical changes have been demonstrated in human and animal diseases involving catabolism of ganglioside G_{M1} and related complex carbohydrates, resulting in excessive storage of these compounds.

Ganglioside G_{M1} stimulates neurite outgrowth as a morphologic expression of neuronal differentiation, and enhances the action of nerve growth factor. Golgi and electron microscopic studies of cortical neurons demonstrated large neural processes (meganeurites) in several lysosomal storage diseases (G_{M2} gangliosidosis, Hurler disease, and neuronal ceroid lipofuscinosis).[308] Meganeurites develop between the base of the perikaryon and the initial portion of the axon, particularly in pyramidal neurons. Dendritic growth also occurs at aberrant sites (ectopic dendrogenesis).[309] The extent of meganeurite development is related to the onset, severity, and clinical course of the disease. Inhibition of neurite initiation occurred in Neuro-2a neuroblastoma cells, when the cell-surface G_{M1} was blocked by the B subunit of cholera toxin or anti-G_{M1} antibody, but no effect was observed on preformed neurites.[310]

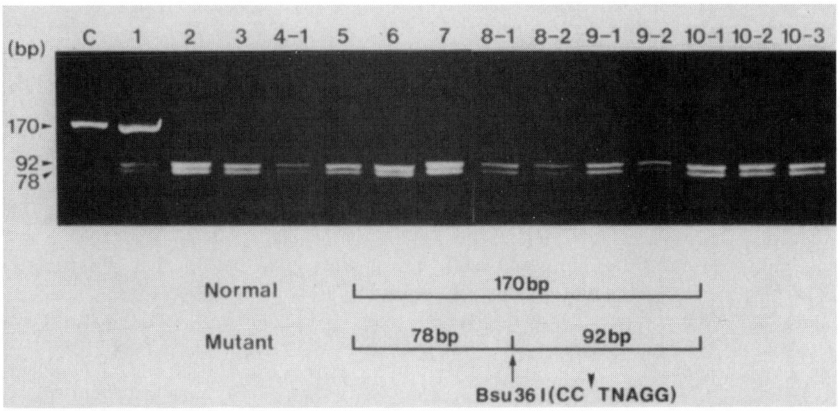

Fig. 151-9 **Restriction analysis of genomic DNA from 14 patients with adult/chronic G_{M1} gangliosidosis. A 170-bp fragment was PCR-amplified, digested with *Bsu*36I, electrophoresed, and stained with ethidium bromide. The lane number corresponds to the family number in Table 151-2. The I51T mutant allele is digested to produce two smaller fragments, 92 and 78 bp. All patients in this study were homozygous for the I51T mutation (genotype: I51T/I51T), except patient 1 (compound heterozygote: I51T/R457Q). (*Reproduced from Yoshida et al.*[60] *Used by permission.*)**

Similar morphologic changes were subsequently observed for feline G_{M1} gangliosidosis.[311,312] MCB were densely packed in meganeurites except near their peripheral area. Meganeurites were present on pyramidal neurons, granule cells of the fascia dentata, and spiny neurons of the caudate nucleus. Neurite outgrowth from meganeurites is particularly prominent in this feline mutant. The onset of ectopic neurite growth occurred after the elaboration of dendrites on cortical pyramidal neurons.[313] There was a greater tendency toward formation of meganeurites in sheep with G_{M1} gangliosidosis, whereas the growth of ectopic axon hillock neurites without meganeurites predominated in cats with G_{M2} gangliosidosis.[313] There are probably two separate driving forces behind somadendritic abnormalities of pyramidal neurons in the two types of gangliosidoses.

In another study, significant changes in neuronal connectivity were found in the cerebral cortex, such as degenerative changes in axons and synapses of inhibitory neurons, and regrowth of dendrites and new synapse formation ("rewiring") involving pyramidal neurons.[314] In addition, G_{M1} was found in the nuclear membrane of neuroblastoma cells and cerebellar granule cells in association with neurite outgrowth.[315] The total ganglioside and G_{M1} concentrations correspond to the extent of the meganeurite formation in the feline disease,[316] and a reduced fluidity of synaptosomal membranes was found.[317] These data suggest that storage of G_{M1} is closely related to abnormal synaptogenesis in this disease.

G_{M1} also associated tightly with Trk, the high-affinity tyrosine kinase-type receptor for the nerve growth factor (NGF), enhancing neurite outgrowth and neurofilament expression in rat PC12 cells[318] and C6trk$^+$ cells, a derivative of C6-2B glioma cells.[319] In the latter, tyrosine phosphorylation of trkA target proteins, such as extracellular signal-regulated kinases and *suc*-associated neurotrophic factor-induced tyrosine-phosphorylated target, also were activated. However, administration of G_{M1} had no effect on the Trk protein, although it partially restored NGF and NGF mRNA in frontal cortex and hippocampus in the brain of aged rats, which showed moderate decreases of both Trk and NGF as compared with those in the brain of young rats.[318,320]

Cholinergic function was altered in the brain of cats with G_{M1} gangliosidosis.[321,322] Acetylcholine synthesis and its K^+-stimulated release were increased in cerebral cortex and hippocampal slices. Choline acetyltransferase activity was not significantly different from that in controls. However, the decreased activity of choline acetyltransferase in aged rats was enhanced by treatment with G_{M1} in the striatum and frontal cortex, but not in the hippocampus.[323] In another experiment, a decrease in high-affinity uptake of glutamate, γ-aminobutyrate, and norepinephrine was observed in synaptosomes in feline G_{M1} gangliosidosis.[324] Neuroaxonal dystrophy was observed in GABAergic neurons in feline models of lysosomal storage disorders (G_{M1} gangliosidosis, G_{M2} gangliosidosis, α-mannosidosis, mucopolysaccharidosis I).[325] A resulting defect in neurotransmission in inhibitory circuits may be an important factor underlying brain dysfunction in them.

Phosphoinositol-specific phospholipase C and adenyl cyclase activities were altered in the membranes of cerebral cortex from cats with G_{M1} gangliosidosis.[326] Phospholipase C did not respond to stimulation by GTPγS, carbachol, or fluoroaluminate, but was normally activated by calcium. Basal adenyl cyclase activity was increased threefold in the brains of affected cats. Plasma membrane-localized G_{M1} modulates prostaglandin E1-induced cAMP in Neuro-2a neuroblastoma cells;[327] treatment with neuraminidase, an enzyme that increases cell surface G_{M1}, or with nM concentrations of G_{M1} elevated cAMP in these cells. However, higher concentrations of exogenous G_{M1} progressively inhibited adenyl cyclase, and induced a dose-responsive fall off in cAMP elevation.

The B subunit of cholera toxin, which binds specifically to ganglioside G_{M1} in the outer leaflet of the cell membrane, was found to induce an increase of calcium and manganese influx in N18 cells.[328] Activation of an L-type voltage-dependent calcium channel has been suggested. This channel modulation by G_{M1} has important implications for its role in neural development, differentiation, and regeneration, and electrical excitability of neurons, possibly under pathologic conditions due to an abnormal storage of G_{M1}. On the other hand, G_{M1} reduced the ethanol-induced activation of phospholipase A2 in synaptosomal preparations from rat brain.[329] This neuroprotective effect against ethanol on the nervous system is probably induced by influencing deacylation/reacylation of membrane phospholipids.

These data suggest that various morphologic and metabolic aberrations occur in the brains of G_{M1} gangliosidosis patients and animals. However, the pathogenesis of localized encephalopathy is not known in adults with G_{M1} gangliosidosis. Furthermore, the pathogenetic role of oligosaccharides or keratan sulfate has not been investigated for the development of morphologic abnormalities occurring mainly in the mesodermal tissues. Understanding the information-processing system induced by ganglioside G_{M1} and possibly other galactose-containing glycoconjugates may provide further insight into the precise mechanisms of brain dysfunction in β-galactosidase-deficient disorders and also of dendritic elaboration and synapse formation in the developing nervous system.

DIAGNOSIS

Clinical Diagnosis

The diagnostic procedure starts with careful clinical evaluation of a patient with neurosomatic manifestations of unknown origin. The possibility of G_{M1} gangliosidosis should always be considered for patients with progressive neurologic deterioration, or developmental retardation with signs of general somatic changes, particularly of the skeletal system and connective tissue, with or without visceromegaly, in infancy. It should be remembered, however, that many cases of G_{M1} gangliosidosis do not present with specific somatic manifestations like facial dysmorphism, visceromegaly, or remarkable bone changes. Clinical diagnosis of patients with the onset after infancy is more difficult, as no specific signs or symptoms have been described, except for deteriorating clinical course and slight vertebral deformities common to disorders of complex carbohydrates (mucopolysaccharides and glycoprotein-derived oligosaccharides).

Dysmorphism and skeletal dysplasias are important clinical signs for differential diagnosis in infancy, late infancy, and childhood. Biochemical screening of urinary mucopolysaccharides and oligosaccharides, as well as enzyme studies, should be performed for excluding mucopolysaccharidoses, multiple sulfatase deficiency, α-mannosidosis, β-mannosidosis, fucosidosis, aspartylglucosaminuria, I-cell disease, sialidosis, galactosialidosis, and other related diseases.

Macular cherry-red spots, if present, are important for consideration of lysosomal storage diseases. Several diseases have been recognized with this unique finding in the optic fundi: G_{M2} gangliosidosis (Tay-Sachs disease, Sandhoff disease, AB variant), G_{M1} gangliosidosis, Niemann-Pick disease, sialidosis, and galactosialidosis show typical macular changes. Similar but not typical changes have been described in cases of other lysosomal diseases such as metachromatic leukodystrophy, globoid-cell leukodystrophy, and Gaucher disease.

G_{M1} gangliosidosis in adults is considered a discrete clinical entity. Progressive extrapyramidal disease, mainly presenting as dystonia, associated with vertebral dysplasia, is an important diagnostic point. Any adult patient with this combination of neuroskeletal signs, unless associated with other specific manifestations indicating diagnosis, should be considered for enzymatic screening of β-galactosidase deficiency.

Rectal biopsy can be of diagnostic help; the neuronal cytoplasm is ballooned with storage material.[55,330] Skin biopsy may afford a clue to diagnosis, if sweat glands are studied carefully; the cells of secretory coils are swollen and vacuolated with faintly visible small granules.[331] Cytoplasmic vesicles were observed in the endothelial cells of conjunctiva, producing a mechanical narrowing of the lumen.[332] The storage material was similar to that seen in fibroblasts from skin or of visceral organs in G_{M1} gangliosidosis. The conjunctiva provides a ready source for biopsy and diagnostic evaluation. Various lectin stains indicate the presence of acidic glycoconjugates in histiocytes containing abundant terminal β-galactose residues.[55]

Clinical diagnosis of Morquio disease is not difficult. Skeletal deformities are unique, and enzyme assays will confirm the diagnosis of type B disease. However, bone changes on x-ray films are not specific to G_{M1} gangliosidosis; mucopolysaccharidoses and glycoprotein disorders can show almost the same pictures. Further biochemical analysis is necessary for the final diagnosis.

Biochemical Diagnosis

Analysis of Storage Compounds. The analytical hallmark of G_{M1} gangliosidosis is the abnormal accumulation of ganglioside G_{M1} in tissues. Because the levels of gangliosides in extraneural tissues are very low, lipid analyses for diagnostic purposes are usually limited to the brain. The total concentration of brain gangliosides may be 3 to 5 times normal in the gray matter and may be as high as 10 times in the white matter.[133] About 90 to 95 molar percent of the total ganglioside is G_{M1} in contrast to 22 to 25 molar percent in normal brain; the actual increase of G_{M1} in the gray matter is up to twentyfold normal.

The determination of G_{M1} accumulation in the brain by means of thin-layer chromatography[333] is convenient, but its applicability is usually restricted to postmortem examination. An immunologic method for determination of gangliosides in cerebrospinal fluid using enzyme-immunostaining and densitometry has been reported,[334] and an increase of G_{M1} was confirmed in the cerebrospinal fluid from infantile patients.[59,93,94] G_{M1} was not detected in adult patients.

Galactose-containing oligosaccharides are excreted in the urine of patients with G_{M1} gangliosidosis and Morquio B disease.[158–160,163,166,335,336] Thin-layer chromatographic or HPLC analysis of the urinary oligosaccharides is employed as an ancillary diagnostic test. The concentration of the urinary oligosaccharides correlates with the severity of the disease.[160,336] Analysis of urinary mucopolysaccharides and the demonstration of the excessive excretion of keratan sulfate are the earliest biochemical procedures available for diagnosis of Morquio B disease.

Enzyme Diagnosis. The most common biochemical parameter is the activity of β-galactosidase. For enzyme diagnosis of G_{M1} gangliosidosis and Morquio B disease, leukocytes, fibroblasts, and solid tissues can usually be used as enzyme sources (Fig. 151-10*A* and *B*). Serum might potentially be useful, but it is known that β-galactosidase activity in serum changes contingent on the preparation conditions such as the time allowed for clotting.[254] In fact, the data using serum have not been reliable or reproducible, when serum was used as the sole enzyme source for diagnostic assay for G_{M1} gangliosidosis. Plasma gives more reliable enzymatic results for the diagnosis of G_{M1} gangliosidosis.

β-Galactosidase activity is also present in urine, but there is an enormous range of variation in this enzyme activity in normal urine. The ratio of β-hexosaminidase to β-galactosidase should be used for diagnosis. In view of the ready availability of other enzyme sources, the use of urine is not recommended. Tears may be used for diagnostic enzyme assays.[337]

Artificial substrates such as *p*-nitrophenyl β-galactopyranoside or 4-methylumbelliferyl β-galactopyranoside are readily available; the latter is fluorogenic, sensitive, and widely used. In infantile and juvenile G_{M1} gangliosidosis, β-galactosidase activity is almost completely deficient, but a considerable residual enzyme activity is detected in adult G_{M1} gangliosidosis and Morquio B disease by enzyme assays in leukocytes or fibroblasts using artificial substrates. In addition, a recent report suggested that new fluorogenic substrates, 4-fluoromethylumbelliferyl derivatives, were convenient for revealing glycosidase activities directly in tissue samples,[338] as 4-fluoromethylumbelliferone exhibits more contrast yellow fluorescence under the UV light than the blue light

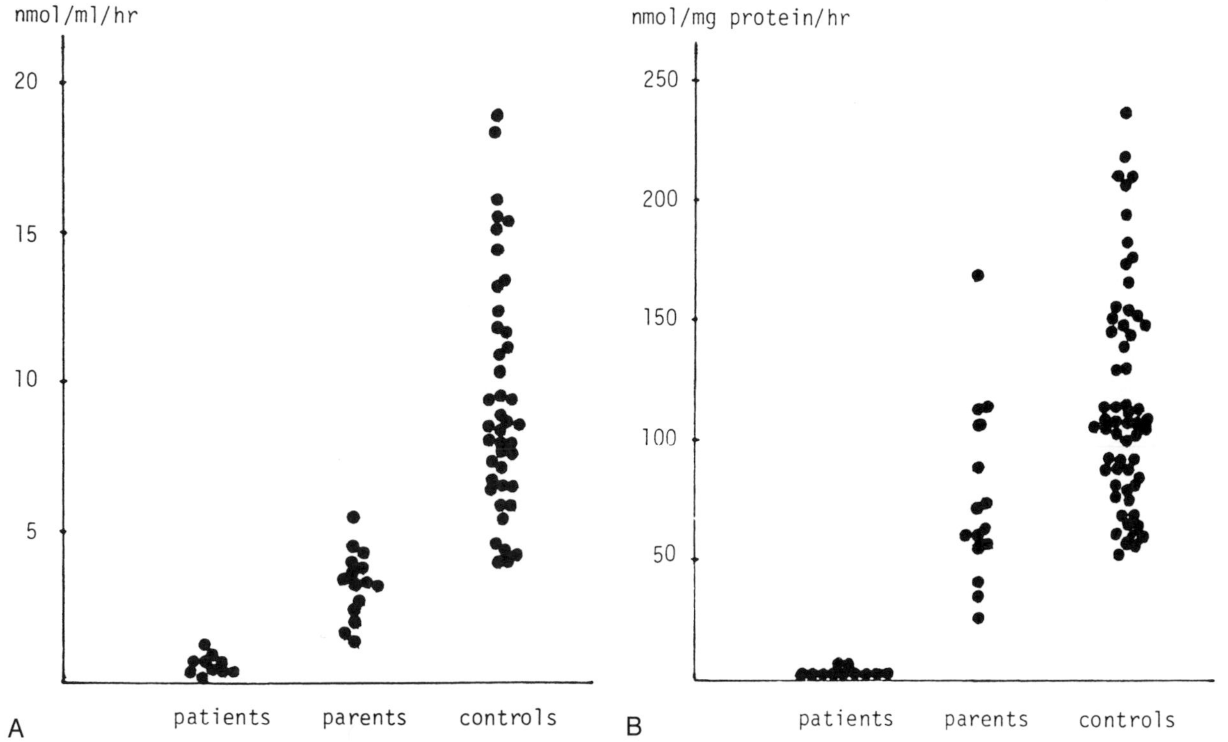

Fig. 151-10 **β-Galactosidase activity in plasma and leukocytes from patients with infantile G_{M1} gangliosidosis. *A*, Plasma. *B*, Leukocytes. Enzyme assays give a clear diagnosis of the patients. However, there is more overlap between the normal individual group and obligate heterozygotes when leukocytes (a mixture of granulocytes and lymphocytes) are used for enzyme assay. (*Y. Suzuki, personal data.*)**

of 4-methylumbelliferone upon exposure of the enzyme activity on solid supports.

However, these substrates can also be degraded by galactosylceramidase, which is commonly increased in G_{M1} gangliosidosis, and ambiguous results are sometimes obtained with the white matter, which is normally rich in galactosylceramidase. Hydrolysis of 4-methylumbelliferyl β-galactopyranoside by the white matter from G_{M1} gangliosidosis patients ranged from 20 to 25 percent of normal values.[221,225] The use of the natural substrate—radiolabeled G_{M1} or G_{A1}—is recommended when the results with the artificial substrates are equivocal.[215]

A newly developed fluorophor may overcome this problem. *O*-[4-(1-imidazolyl)butyl]2,3-dicyano-1,4-hydroquinonyl β-D-galactopyranoside (Im-DCH-β-Gal)[339] was shown to be a specific substrate for human lysosomal β-galactosidase in cell homogenates. Furthermore, its tetraacetate derivative, Im-DCH-β-Gal$(OAc)_4$, was taken up and hydrolyzed by normal fibroblasts but not hydrolyzed in the enzyme-deficient cells. The rates of uptake and deacetylation were similar for normal and mutant cells. Another fluorogenic substrate, 5-chloromethylfluorescein di-α-D-galactopyranoside, was used for monitoring *lacZ* gene expression in cultured cells.[340] It is far more sensitive than the conventional X-gal cytochemistry, and may be useful for monitoring gene expression of human α-galactosidase after gene therapy or protein therapy in future. Another staining method based on TNBT (tetranitroblue tetrazolium) reduction and precipitation has been proposed as a sensitive procedure for immunohistochemistry and *in situ* hybridization of β-galactosidase and its mRNA.[341] These compounds will be useful as a fluorescent marker for detecting genetic β-galactosidase mutants.

It is also important to determine other enzyme activities, including neuraminidase for differential diagnosis of secondary β-galactosidase deficiency, such as galactosialidosis, I-cell disease, mucolipidosis III, and mucopolysaccharidoses other than Morquio B disease.

Table 151-7 Restriction Analysis and Screening of the Mutant β-Galactosidase Gene

	Restriction enzyme			Screening	
Mutation	**Site***	**Enzyme**	**Ref**	**Method**	**Ref**
R49C	−	*Bbv*I/*Bso*Fi		ASO	297
I51T	+	*Bsu*36I/*Sau*I	23, 58		
T82M	+	*Msl*I		ASO	298
Y83H	+	*Nla*III			
G123R	−	*Sma*I/*Apa*I			
R201C	−	*Bsp*MI	23, 264		
R201H	−	*Hha*I		SSCP	304
R208C	N			ASO	300, 303
P263S	+	*Bam*HI			
N266S	+	*Cla*I		SSCP	304
W273L	+	*Stu*I†	24		
Y316C	N				
N318H	+	*Nla*III			
S434L	−	*Mbo*II			
R457X	N				
R457Q	N				
R482H	+	*Nsp*I	24		
R482C	−	*Afl*III		ASO	299
G494C	N				
W509C	+	*Rsa*I	24		
K577R	N			ASO	303
R590H	N			ASO	300
E632G	N			ASO	303

*+ = restriction site generated; − = restriction site eliminated; N = neither generated nor eliminated.
†Restriction site produced by adding a second mutation by PCR.
ASO = allele-specific oligonucleotide hybridization (= dot blot analysis).
SSCP = single-strand conformation polymorphism.

Gene Diagnosis

In principle, direct sequencing is possible for the diagnosis of a new gene mutation in a patient. It requires time and labor, and its clinical application is not practical at present. However, once a mutation is established for a family with β-galactosidase deficiency, rather simple procedures can be taken for rapid genetic diagnosis. The mutation is easily detected by restriction digestion, allele-specific oligonucleotide hybridization, single-strand conformation polymorphism, or amplification refractory mutation system, in combination with PCR amplification.

In fact, restriction analysis methods have been developed for several mutations, including the common mutations described above. The *Bsu*36I restriction analysis has been performed for gene diagnosis of 14 adult/chronic form G_{M1} gangliosidosis patients from 10 different Japanese families.[60] The result showed that all 14 patients examined had a common single-base substitution of I51T. Thirteen were homozygotes, and one was a compound heterozygote of this common mutation associated with another base substitution.

Restriction analysis is possible for many β-galactosidase gene mutations, and other simple screening methods also are available (Table 151-7). They can be applied for detecting heterozygous carriers as well as affected patients.

Heterozygous Carrier Diagnosis

Carrier detection is important for genetic counseling and prenatal diagnosis. Reliability of enzymatic heterozygote detection depends on two factors: (a) accuracy of assays, and (b) variation of enzymatic activity among a general population and a variation in a single individual under the influence of age and physical conditions. Appropriate precautions and careful standardization of the enzyme assay are necessary.

When a sufficiently large number of specimens are examined, the average of β-galactosidase activities of known heterozygotes gives an intermediate value between normal subjects and affected patients, with a high statistical significance (Fig. 151-10*A* and *B*). However, varying degrees of overlap occur between normal homozygotes and heterozygous carriers. It is well known that the enzyme diagnosis for heterozygous carriers is not always reliable.

Gene diagnosis will provide a more reliable method for the detection of heterozygous carriers, if an appropriate method is available for a certain mutant gene. The diagnosis of I51T mutation heterozygotes was established in eight parents and two sibs from four different Japanese families with adult/chromic G_{M1} gangliosidosis[60] (Fig. 151-11). Heterozygous carriers are diagnosed by restriction analysis or allele-specific oligonucleotide hybridization for known gene mutations. Single-strand conformation polymorphism also is useful for screening of an unknown mutation, although it does not provide information about the mutant gene structure (Table 151-7).

Prenatal Diagnosis

Assays of β-galactosidase activity in cultured amniotic fluid cells or chorionic villi are used for prenatal diagnosis, and it has been successfully performed for G_{M1} gangliosidosis.[342–347] A rapid diagnosis was made possible by microchemical assays;[345] the use of 10 to 30 freeze-dried cells for single enzyme assays requires only a few hundred cells growing within 9 to 12 days after amniocentesis. However, special microassay methods have become unnecessary since the development of chorionic villi sampling for rapid prenatal diagnosis with sufficient amounts of cell samples from fetuses. A survey was made on the first trimester prenatal diagnosis of metabolic diseases using chorionic villi in countries from the European Community.[348] As of December 1985, 258 diagnoses were made for 38 different metabolic diseases; 56 affected fetuses (22 percent) were detected. Among them, 11 fetuses were subjected to prenatal diagnosis of G_{M1}

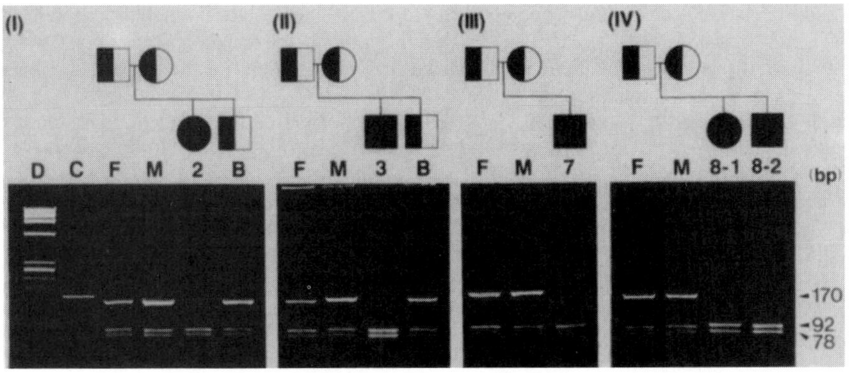

Fig. 151-11 Restriction analysis of the family members of adult G_{M1} gangliosidosis patients. The lane number corresponds to the family number in Fig. 151-9. F = father; M = mother; B = brother; C = normal control; D = DNA markers (øx174 phage DNA/*Hae*II digest). (*Reproduced from Yoshida et al.*[60] *Used by permission.*)

gangliosidosis — 1 in Denmark, 6 in France, 1 in Italy, and 3 in United Kingdom. One affected patient was found in France.

An early prenatal diagnosis was accomplished by analyzing galactosyl-oligosaccharides accumulating in amniotic fluid at 14 weeks' gestation, with HPLC.[336] The pattern of amniotic oligosaccharides was almost identical to that in the urine from postnatal G_{M1} gangliosidosis patients, but the concentration was about one-fifth that in urine. Accordingly, a highly sensitive assay method is necessary for prenatal diagnosis.

The diagnosis of affected fetuses was confirmed by histologic demonstration of MCB in spinal cord motor neurons[344,349] or basal ganglia,[346] zebra bodies in dorsal-root ganglion cells,[342] pleomorphic electron-dense bodies in axons,[350] or membrane-limited vacuoles in Schwann cells.[350] Vacuolation of hepatocytes, and renal glomerular and tubular epithelial cells were recorded in a fetus affected with infantile G_{M1} gangliosidosis.[350] MCB were abundant in retinal ganglion cells.[351] Marked retinal lesions were reported in two other cases.[352,353]

Biochemical analysis revealed an increase of G_{M1} in the fetal brain,[344,347,353] and β-galactosidase deficiency in liver or brain.[342,344] An affected fetus was aborted with intrauterine hypertonic-saline instillation.[344] Fetal tissues were adequate for subsequent biochemical diagnosis.

TREATMENT

Therapeutic experiments using cultured cells have been reported to enhance the uptake of the exogenous enzyme and to prolong its intracellular half-life. Enzyme replacement of cultured cells from cats with G_{M1} gangliosidosis was tried with the liposome-entrapped enzyme, and the storage of glycopeptides decreased.[354] A thiol protease inhibitor prolonged the effect of exogenous β-galactosidase in human G_{M1} gangliosidosis fibroblasts.[238]

Allogeneic bone marrow transplantation was performed in an 81-day-old Portuguese water dog affected with G_{M1} gangliosidosis, using a dog leukocyte antigen-identical sibling as donor.[354] Complete engraftment was achieved, and β-galactosidase activity in leukocytes of the transplanted dog was similar to that in the donor. However, neither subsequent clinical course nor the enzyme activity was modified. It was concluded that bone marrow transplantation early in life is ineffective in canine G_{M1} gangliosidosis.

Amniotic tissue transplantation was tried on a patient with Morquio B disease.[355] No clinical improvement was observed. Only conservative therapy has been performed for human G_{M1} gangliosidosis patients. Dystonia was markedly improved dose-dependently by oral administration of trihexyphenidyl in an adult G_{M1} gangliosidosis patient.[356] No side effects were observed. The extrapyramidal signs in adults with G_{M1} gangliosidosis are probably caused by hypofunction of dopaminergic neurons or relative hyperactivity of cholinergic neurons in the basal ganglia.

Recently, we tried adenovirus-mediated gene transfer into tissues of G_{M1}-gangliosidosis knockout mice. The recombinant virus expressing human β-galactosidase under the control of the CAG promoter was injected intravenously. β-Galactosidase activity was expressed in liver and spleen in 4-month-old affected mice, with a correction of abnormal urinary oligosaccharide pattern. This effect lasted for at least 1 month. However, no activity was detected in the brain. On the contrary, a high β-galactosidase activity was observed in most of the organs examined, including the brain, in newborn affected mice. Storage of ganglioside G_{M1} was less pronounced as compared with untreated mice at 10 days after administration (Oshima A et al., unpublished data).

ANIMAL MODELS

Animal models of G_{M1} gangliosidosis have been recorded in cats,[357–360] dogs,[361–364] sheep,[365–368] and calves.[369–371] They are domestic animals with spontaneously occurring storage diseases. Although inbred strains of laboratory rodents had not been reported, mouse models of G_{M1} gangliosidosis were recently created through targeted disruption of the β-galactosidase gene.[372–374] All the model animals show central nervous system manifestations with a specific deficiency of β-galactosidase.

Feline G_{M1} Gangliosidosis

A neurologic disorder with clinical, morphologic, biochemical, and genetic similarities to human G_{M1} gangliosidosis has been described in two families of Siamese cats[322,357,358,375,376] and in two families of short-haired domestic cats.[172,359,360,377] Affected kittens appear normal at birth, and tremors of the head and hind limbs are first noted at 2 to 3 months of age, followed by generalized dysmetria and spastic quadriplegia. Affected cats show exaggerated acousticomotor response, impaired vision, and generalized convulsive seizures by 1 year of age. This disease is transmitted as an autosomal recessive trait.

A widespread neuronal vacuolation is observed microscopically in brain, retina, spinal cord, and peripheral ganglia. Numerous MCB are observed electron microscopically, with multiple concentric lamellae simulating those in the human disease. Lesions outside the nervous system are limited to hepatocellular vacuolation and aspermatogenesis.

Neutral oligosaccharides are markedly increased in the tissues and urine of affected cats.[172] The core structure of a hexasaccharide has been identified as Galβ–GlcNAc–Man–Man–GlcNAc with an additional *N*-acetylglucosamine.[171,173] Four major types of oligosaccharides were proposed by Barker et al.[172] Their structures suggest that they arise from incomplete catabolism of *N*-glycans of glycoproteins.

A family of Siamese cats,[322,357,375,376] which was extensively investigated clinically and biochemically, is linked to late infantile/juvenile G_{M1} gangliosidosis in humans.[173,360,378] The cats developed normally until the age of 4 months, and then neurologic manifestations followed. Physical appearance was normal, and no hepatosplenomegaly was observed. Electrodiagnostic tests revealed that motor and sensory nerve conduction velocities remained within normal limits, but spinal-evoked potentials indicated slowing in conduction velocity and brain stem auditory-evoked responses indicated prolonged latencies.[379] Some residual enzyme activity of β-galactosidase was detected in brain (15 percent of normal).[357] β-Galactosidase deficiency has been demonstrated in brain, kidney, liver, spleen, skin, cultured fibroblasts, and cultured conjunctival cells,[380] associated with remarkable accumulation of ganglioside G_{M1}. The mutant enzyme has a reduced K_m for 4-methylumbelliferyl β-galactoside, high K_m for G_{M1} and asialofetuin, increased thermostability, and a shift of isoelectric point.[378]

Several investigations into the pathogenesis of neuronal dysfunction have been performed using this feline model of human disease. These showed: (a) increased gangliosides, cholesterol, and phospholipids in synaptosomal membranes;[317] (b) reduced fluidity of synaptosomal membranes;[317] (c) meganeurites between the soma and initial axon segment, and aberrant secondary neurites,[311,312] suggesting a possible role for gangliosides in neuronal differentiation and synaptogenesis;[309,311] (d) a gradient in total ganglioside and G_{M1} concentration and the proportion of docosanoate (22:0) in G_{M1}, corresponding to the morphologic gradient of meganeurite formation (cerebral cortex > caudate = thalamus > cerebellum);[316] (e) increased acetylcholine synthesis and release in cerebral cortex and hippocampal slices;[321,322] (f) decrease of high-affinity uptake of glutamate, γ-aminobutyrate, and norepinephrine in synaptosomes;[324] (g) alteration of phospholipase C and adenyl cyclase activities;[326] (h) alteration of evoked synaptic activity patterns in cortical pyramidal neurons;[381] (i) reduced calcium flux in synaptosomes;[382] (j) quantitatively and qualitatively normal phorbol ester receptors in the brain;[383] and (k) common occurrence of glutamic acid decarboxylase-immunoreactive spheroids in many brain regions, whereas limited in distribution in other diseases.[325] These data suggest that various morphologic and metabolic aberrations occur in the presence of excessive storage of ganglioside G_{M1}.

Canine G_{M1} Gangliosidosis

The canine disease has been described in mixed-breed beagle dogs,[361] English springer spaniels,[363,384] and Portuguese water dogs.[364,385] Two canine models, English springer spaniel and Portuguese water dog, have been compared.[384] The clinical course and severity of skeletal dysplasia and progressive neurologic impairment were similar in both models. The skeletal lesions in both canine models were similar to those in a child with G_{M1} gangliosidosis.[386] However, dwarfism and coarse facial features were seen only in English springer spaniels; glycoproteins containing polylactosaminoglycans were found in visceral organs. Portuguese water dogs did not show these clinical or biochemical changes. They may represent different mutations of the β-galactosidase gene. It seems difficult and inappropriate to apply clinical classification of G_{M1} gangliosidosis in humans to these model animals.[384] Dysostosis multiplex, dwarfism, and orbital hypertelorism with coarse facial features were found in the cases reported by Alroy et al.,[363] probably representing a model of infantile G_{M1} gangliosidosis.

Pathologic and biochemical changes are similar to those in the feline cases described above.[387] The ultrastructural and biochemical features suggested that the disease in the first reported dog had features similar to both the infantile and juvenile form of human G_{M1} gangliosidosis (Table 151-1).[362] Serial MRI studies revealed an abnormal signal intensity of cerebral and cerebellar white matter observed on T_2-weighted images.[387]

Analysis of the major oligosaccharides accumulating in the dog revealed that compounds are nearly identical to the oligosaccharides stored in human G_{M1} gangliosidosis liver, but they differ from the human compounds uniquely, because they contain two GlcNAc residues at the reducing terminus instead of one, suggesting that there may be significant differences in glycoprotein metabolism or structure between mammalian species.[171] Kinetic properties of the mutant enzyme in affected dogs were identical to those from normal dogs, but the amount of CRM was markedly reduced.[388]

Antiserum raised against purified human liver β-galactosidase cross-reacted with the enzyme from dog liver, but not with those from cat liver or *Escherichia coli*.[389] Furthermore, 21 of the 24 tryptic peptides of the dog β-galactosidase were homologous with those of the human enzyme. A partial canine β-galactosidase cDNA was 86 percent homologous to the human counterpart, and preliminary analysis of a genomic library indicated conservation of exon number and size.[390] Based on these observations, it was concluded that dog and human β-galactosidases are structurally similar, and that canine G_{M1} gangliosidosis is an excellent model for the human disease.

Retarded endochondral ossification and osteoporosis were observed at 2 months of age in canine G_{M1} gangliosidosis, and focal cartilage necrosis within lumbar vertebral epiphyses in older puppies.[386] The lesions were characterized histologically by chondrocytic hypertrophy and lysosomal accumulation of storage materials. These changes were similar to those in a human child with G_{M1} gangliosidosis. Chondrocytes from affected dogs cultured in agarose contained numerous large vacuoles, and had a reduction in mitosis and Alcian blue staining proteoglycans.[391] This culture system may be a useful method for studying the biology of cartilage leading to skeletal abnormalities in lysosomal storage diseases.

Ovine G_{M1} Gangliosidosis

An inherited disease associated with deficiencies of β-galactosidase (5 percent normal) and α-neuraminidase (20 percent normal) has been observed in sheep.[368,392] The neuraminidase activity was not restored after addition of leupeptin in the culture medium of fibroblasts.[365,366] Neuronal storage was much more extensive than visceral storage. Kupffer cells and macrophages from bone marrow were affected similarly to but less severely than hepatocytes and renal epithelial cells, whereas hematopoietic cells and chondrocytes were unaffected.[392] Results of lectin histochemistry suggested that the stored material in this disease has terminal saccharide moieties consisting of β-galactose, *N*-acetylneuraminic acid, and *N*-acetylgalactosamine.[393] An interspecific genetic complementation analysis indicated that the ovine β-galactosidase deficiency is due to a mutation at the genetic locus homologous with that of human G_{M1} gangliosidosis and Morquio B disease in humans.[394] A genetic defect in lysosomal β-galactosidase may cause the deficiency of lysosomal α-neuraminidase in sheep.[365,395]

The initial clinical sign of ovine G_{M1} gangliosidosis is ataxia around 5 months of age, and neurologic deterioration follows:[365,366] ataxia, conscious proprioceptive deficit most severe in the hind limbs, blindness, and recumbency.[396] An ovine fetus affected with G_{M1} gangliosidosis at 4 months of gestation (normal gestation 5 months) showed marked cytoplasmic enlargement and vacuolation of central and peripheral nervous system neuronal soma and of hepatocytes and renal epithelial cells.[397] This case indicates the need for prenatal initiation of therapy. Vacuolization seems to be not the single cause of clinical signs in the ovine disease, as the clinical signs do not commence until at least 5 months after vacuolization is histologically apparent.

Another form of ovine G_{M1} gangliosidosis was recently reported.[367] Neurologic signs were observed at approximately 1 month of age. A specific deficiency of β-galactosidase was found, with relatively high residual activity (10 percent), as compared with that described above. Neuraminidase activity was normal. Storage of G_{M1} and asialo G_{M1} was not reported for this case. In both ovine cases, molecular genetic analysis has not been performed.

Bovine G_{M1} Gangliosidosis

Pathologic, biochemical, and enzymatic studies were performed in Friesian calves with G_{M1} gangliosidosis. G_{M1} accumulated in

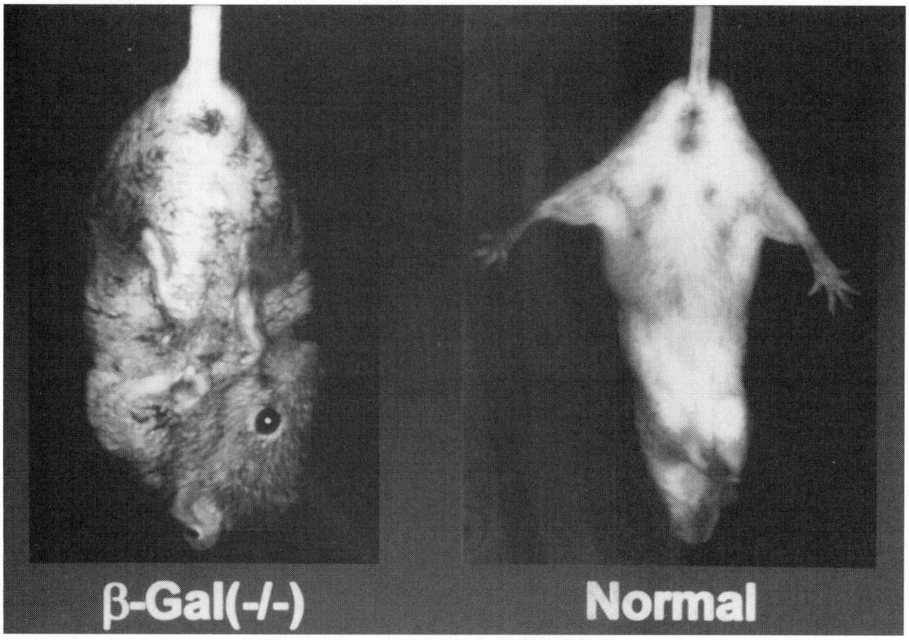

Fig. 151-12 Abnormal posture of a β-galactosidase-deficient mouse in the downward vertical position. *A,* An affected α-Gal (−/−) mouse (8 months old) huddles himself with all limbs flexed and paws clenched. *B,* A normal α-Gal (+/+) littermate with normal reaction. (*Reproduced from Matsuda et al.*[373] *Used by permission.*)

neurons, and β-galactosidase deficiency was confirmed.[367,371,399–401] However, morphologic hepatic changes were minimal or absent, without significant elevation of mucopolysaccharides.[398] Vision is impaired at the late stage of the disease. The ocular lesions were confined to retina and optic nerves.[399] Retinal ganglion cells and amacrine cells in the inner nuclear layer are distended with dense aggregates of MCB. Wallerian degeneration is present in the optic nerves.

Murine G_{M1} Gangliosidosis Generated by Gene Targeting (Knockout Mouse)

Gene targeting in embryonic stem cells generated mouse models[372–374] for conventional laboratory use. Homozygous mutants were born normally and apparently healthy until 4 months of age, although poor achievement on the water maze test was observed in some mutant mice after 2 months. Then, horizontal movement became slow, and rearing or vertical climbing became less frequent. By 6 to 8 months, definite gait disturbance with mild shaking was observed and spastic diplegia progressed. When hung vertically with the tail held upward, they huddled themselves with all four limbs flexed (Fig. 151-12). Normal mice always extended their limbs in the downward vertical direction. At the terminal stage, generalized and progressive paralysis appeared, and the affected mice died of extreme emaciation at 7 to 10 months of age. Hepatosplenomegaly or skeletal dysplasia is not detected. About half of homozygote pairs could produce at least one litter; thus, the knockout mice could be maintained as homozygous mutants.[373]

Three biochemical markers confirmed that the affected mice are authentic model of human G_{M1} gangliosidosis: generalized β-galactosidase deficiency, abnormal storage of G_{M1} in brain and other tissues (Fig. 151-13), and hyperexcretion of urinary oligosaccharides.

Although some neuronal cells with distended cytoplasm were observed in spinal cord and brain stem at 3 days after birth, no pathologic changes in other areas of the brain are observed in newborn affected mice. The number of degenerated neurons with distended cytoplasm increases after 2 weeks of age, and then the central nervous system becomes diffusely and severely affected within 4 to 8 weeks. These pathologic changes are correlated with accumulation of G_{M1} and asialo G_{M1} in the brain. HPTLC analysis showed that the G_{M1} content of the mutant mouse brain was not pathologically increased at birth. An increase of G_{M1} and asialo G_{M1} occurred rapidly to the same degree of storage. This remarkable accumulation of asialo G_{M1} may be explained by a metabolic turnover of G_{M1} to asialo G_{M1} catalyzed by a specific neuraminidase in mice. A recent report has confirmed that intact and living cells of neurotumoral nature express a neuraminidase that hydrolyzes ganglioside G_{M1} and G_{M2}.[400] This degradative process seems to occur in lysosomes, as it is blocked by the conditions preventing endocytosis or inhibiting lysosomal enzyme activities.

Skeletal dysplasia is observed in human patients with infantile G_{M1} gangliosidosis and Morquio B disease, but not in mutant mice. Urinary mucopolysaccharides were normal in amount and pattern in mutant mice. The mouse does not synthesize keratan sulfate in the skeletal system.[401] In another report, the mouse rib

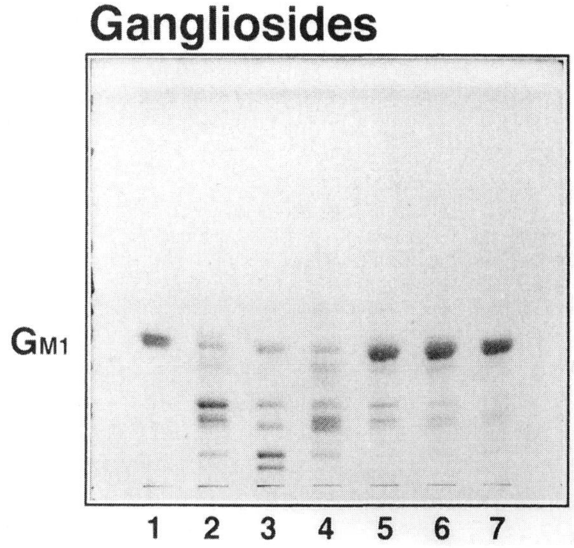

Fig. 151-13 Thin-layer chromatographic pattern of mouse brain gangliosides. Resorcinol stain. −/− = affected knockout mouse; +/+ = normal mouse. Age, 7 months. A remarkable increase in ganglioside G_{M1} is observed in three different areas of the brain. A = cerebral hemisphere; B = brain stem; C = cerebellum. (*Courtesy of Dr. Junichiro Matsuda, National Institute of Infectious Diseases, Tokyo, Japan.*)

cartilage contained only small amounts of keratan sulfate of extremely small size.[402] It may explain an apparent lack of skeletal dysplasia in mutant mice, although more time may be necessary for development of generalized skeletal dysplasias.[373]

REFERENCES

1. Norman RM, Urich H, Tingey AH, Goodbody RA: Tay-Sachs' disease with visceral involvement and its relationship to Niemann-Pick disease. *J Pathol Bacteriol* **78**:409, 1959.
2. Craig JM, Clarke JT, Banker BQ: A metabolic neurovisceral disorder with the accumulation of an unidentified substance: A variant of Hurler's syndrome? *Am J Dis Child* **98**:577, 1959.
3. Landing BH, Rubinstein JH: Biopsy diagnosis of neurologic diseases in children with emphasis on the lipidoses, in Aronson SM, Volk BW (eds): *Cerebral Sphingolipidoses*, New York, Academic Press, 1962, p 1.
4. Landing BH, Silverman FN, Craig JM, Jacoby MD, Lahey ME, Chadwick DL: Familial neurovisceral lipidosis. *Am J Dis Child* **108**:503, 1964.
5. O'Brien JS, Stern MB, Landing BH, O'Brien JK, Donnell GN: Generalized gangliosidosis. Another inborn error of metabolism? *Am J Dis Child* **109**:338, 1965.
6. Jatzkewitz H, Sandhoff K: On a biochemically special form of infantile amaurotic idiocy. *Biochim Biophys Acta* **70**:354, 1963.
7. Norman RM, Tingey AH, Newman CGH, Ward SP: Tay-Sachs disease with visceral involvement and its relation to gargoylism. *Arch Dis Child* **39**:634, 1964.
8. Attal C, Farkas-Bargeton E, Edgar GWF, Pham-Huu-Trung GF, Girard F, Moziconacci P: Idiotie amaurotique infantile familiale avec surcharge viscerale. *Ann Pédiatr* **14**:1725, 1967.
9. Sacrez R, Juif JG, Gigonet JM, Gruner JE: La maladie de Landing, ou idiotie amaurotique infantile précoce avec gangliosidoes généralisée. *Pédiatrie* **22**:143, 1967.
10. Seringe P, Plainfosse B, Lautmann F, Lorilloux J, Galamy G, Berry JP, Watchi J-M: Gangliosidose généralisée, du type Norman-Landing, á G_{M1}. *Ann Pédiatr* **15**:685, 1968.
11. Suzuki K, Chen GC: Brain ceramide hexosides in Tay-Sachs' disease and generalized gangliosidosis (G_{M1}-gangliosidosis). *J Lipid Res* **8**:105, 1967.
12. Gonatas NK, Gonatas J: Ultrastructural and biochemical observations on a case of systemic late infantile lipidosis and its relationship to Tay-Sachs disease and gargoylism. *J Neuropathol Exp Neurol* **24**:318, 1965.
13. Suzuki K, Suzuki K, Chen GC: Morphological, histochemical and biochemical studies on a case of systemic late infantile lipidosis (generalized gangliosidosis). *J Neuropathol Exp Neurol* **27**:15, 1968.
14. Derry DM, Fawcett JS, Andermann F, Wolfe LS: Late infantile systemic lipidosis. Major monosialogangliosidosis. Delineation of two types. *Neurology* **18**:340, 1968.
15. Okada S, O'Brien JS: Generalized gangliosidosis: β-Galactosidase deficiency. *Science* **160**:1002, 1968.
16. O'Brien JS, Ho MW, Veath ML, Wilson JF, Myers G, Opitz JM, ZuRhein GM, Spranger JW, Hartmann HA, Haneberg B, Grosse FR: Juvenile G_{M1}-gangliosidosis: clinical, pathological, chemical and enzymatic studies. *Clin Genet* **3**:411, 1972.
17. Lowden JA, Callahan JW, Norman MG: Juvenile G_{M1}-gangliosidosis. Occurrence with absence of two β-galactosidase components. *Arch Neurol* **31**:200, 1974.
18. Suzuki Y, Nakamura N, Fukuoka K, Shimada Y, Uono M: β-Galactosidase deficiency in juvenile and adult patients. Report of six Japanese cases and review of literature. *Hum Genet* **36**:219, 1977.
19. O'Brien JS, Gugler E, Giedion A, Wiesmann U, Herschkowitz N, Meier C, Leroy J: Spondyloepiphyseal dysplasia, corneal clouding, normal intelligence and acid β-galactosidase deficiency. *Clin Genet* **9**:495, 1976.
20. Arbisser AI, Donnelly KA, Scott CI, Di Ferrante N, Singh J, Stevenson RE, Aylesworth AS, Howell RR: Morquio-like syndrome with β-galactosidase deficiency and normal hexosamine sulfatase activity: mucopolysaccharidosis IVB. *Am J Med Genet* **1**:195, 1977.
21. van der Horst GTJ, Kleijer WJ, Hoogeveen AT, Huijmans JGM, Blom W, van Diggelen OP: Morquio B syndrome: A primary defect in β-galactosidase. *Am J Med Genet* **16**:261, 1983.
22. Oshima A, Tsuji A, Nagao Y, Sakuraba H, Suzuki Y: Cloning, sequencing, and expression of cDNA for human β-galactosidase. *Biochem Biophys Res Commun* **157**:238, 1988.
23. Yoshida K, Oshima A, Shimmoto M, Fukuhara Y, Sakuraba H, Yanagisawa N, Suzuki Y: Human β-galactosidase gene mutations in G_{M1}-gangliosidosis: A common mutation among Japanese adult/chronic cases. *Am J Hum Genet* **49**:435, 1991.
24. Oshima A, Yoshida K, Shimmoto M, Fukuhara Y, Sakuraba H, Suzuki Y: Human β-galactosidase gene mutations in Morquio B disease. *Am J Hum Genet* **49**:1091, 1991.
25. Suzuki Y, Oshima A: A β-galactosidase gene mutation identified in both Morquio B disease and infantile G_{M1}-gangliosidosis. *Hum Genet* **91**:407, 1993.
26. Lenicker HM, Vassallo AP, Young EP, Attard MS: Infantile generalized G_{M1} gangliosidosis: high incidence in the Maltese Islands. *J Inherit Metab Dis* **20**:723, 1997.
27. O'Brien JS: β-Galactosidase deficiency (G_{M1}-gangliosidosis, galactosialidosis, and Morquio syndrome type B); ganglioside sialidase deficiency (mucolipidosis IV), in Scriver CR, Beaudet AL, Sly WS, Valle D (eds): *The Metabolic Basis of Inherited Disease*, 6th ed. New York, McGraw-Hill, 1989, p 1797.
28. Orii T, Sukegawa K, Kudoh T, Horino K, Nakao T: Three G_{M1}-gangliosidoses and a variant of β-galactosidase deficiency. *Tohoku J Exp Med* **117**:197, 1975.
29. Orii T, Sukegawa K, Nakao T: A variant of G_{M1}-gangliosidosis type 2 and enzymic differences between G_{M1}-gangliosidosis types 1 and 2. *Tohoku J Exp Med* **117**:99, 1975.
30. Kudoh T, Orii T, Nakao T, Sakagami T: Three cases of G_{M1}-gangliosidosis. *Clin Chim Acta* **70**:277, 1976.
31. Farrell DF, Ochs U: G_{M1} gangliosidosis: Phenotypic variation in a single family. *Ann Neurol* **9**:225, 1981.
32. Scott RC, Lagunoff D, Trump BF: Familial neurovisceral lipidosis. *J Pediatr* **71**:357, 1967.
33. O'Brien JS: Generalized gangliosidosis. *J Pediatr* **75**:167, 1969.
34. Suzuki Y, Crocker AC, Suzuki K: G_{M1}-gangliosidosis. Correlation of clinical and biochemical data. *Arch Neurol* **24**:58, 1971.
35. Nihei K, Abe T, Kamoshita S: An autopsy case of generalized gangliosidosis. *Clin Neurol* **12**:329, 1972.
36. Fricker H, O'Brien JS, Vassella F, Gugler E, Muhlethaler JP, Spycher M, Wiesmann UN, Herschkowitz N: Generalized gangliosidosis: Acid β-galactosidase deficiency with early onset, rapid mental deterioration and minimal bone dysplasia. *J Neurol* **213**:273, 1976.
37. Hooft C, Senesael L, Delbeke MJ, Kint J, Dacremont G: The G_{M1}-gangliosidosis (Landing disease). *Eur Neurol* **2**:225, 1969.
38. Feldges A, Muller HJ, Buhler E, Stalder G: G_{M1}-gangliosidosis. I. Clinical aspects and biochemistry. *Helv Paediatr Acta* **28**:511, 1973.
39. Hubain P, Adam E, Dewelle A, Druez G, Farriaux JP, Dupont A: Étude d'une observation de gangliosidose á G_{M1}. *Helv Paediatr Acta* **24**:337, 1969.
40. Hooft C, Vlietinck RF, Dacremont G, Kint JA: G_{M1} gangliosidosis type II. *Eur Neurol* **4**:1, 1970.
41. Hakozaki H, Takahashi K, Naito M, Kojima M, Koizumi Y, Nonomiya N: Gaucher-like cells in juvenile G_{M1}-gangliosidosis and in β-thalassemia — A histochemical and ultrastructural observation. *Acta Pathol Jpn* **29**:303, 1979.
42. Patton VM, Dekaban AS: G_{M1}-gangliosidosis and juvenile cerebral lipidosis. Clinical, histochemical, and chemical study. *Arch Neurol* **24**:529, 1971.
43. Takamoto K, Beppu H, Hirose K, Uono M: Juvenile β-galactosidase deficiency with mental deterioration, dystonic movement, pyramidal symptoms, dysostosis and cherry red spot. *Clin Neurol* **20**:339, 1980.
44. Wolfe LS, Callahan J, Fawcett JS, Andermann F, Scriver CR: G_{M1}-gangliosidosis without chondrodystrophy or visceromegaly. β-Galactosidase deficiency with gangliosidosis and the excessive excretion of a keratan sulfate. *Neurology* **20**:23, 1970.
45. Goldberg MF, Cotlier E, Fichenscher LG, Kenyon K, Enat R, Borowsky SA: Macular cherry-red spot, corneal clouding, and β-galactosidase deficiency. Clinical, biochemical, and electron microscopic study of a new autosomal recessive storage disease. *Arch Intern Med* **128**:387, 1971.
46. Orii T, Minami R, Sukegawa K, Sato S, Tsugawa S, Horino K, Miura R, Nakao T: A new type of mucolipidosis with β-galactosidase deficiency and glycopeptiduria. *Tohoku J Exp Med* **107**:303, 1972.
47. Guazzi G, Ghetti B, Barbieri F, Cecio A: Myoclonus-epilepsy with cherry-red spot in adult: a peculiar form of mucopolysaccharidosis (a clinical, genetical, chemical and ultrastructural study). *Acta Neurol* **28**:542, 1973.
48. Koster JF, Niermeijer MF, Loonen MCB, Galjaard H: β-Galactosidase deficiency in an adult: A biochemical and somatic cell genetic study on a variant of G_{M1}-gangliosidosis. *Clin Genet* **9**:427, 1976.

49. Yamamoto A, Adachi S, Kawamura S, Takahashi M, Kitani T, Ohtori T, Shiji Y, Nishikawa M: Localized β-galactosidase deficiency. Occurrence in cerebellar ataxia with myoclonus epilepsy and macular cherry-red spot—A new variant of G_{M1}-gangliosidosis? *Arch Intern Med* **134**:627, 1974.
50. Suzuki Y, Nakamura N, Fukuoka K: G_{M1}-gangliosidosis: accumulation of ganglioside G_{M1} in cultured skin fibroblasts and correlation with clinical types. *Hum Genet* **43**:127, 1978.
51. Suzuki Y, Furukawa T, Hoogeveen AT, Verheijen F, Galjaard H: Adult type G_{M1}-gangliosidosis: A complementation study on somatic cell hybrids. *Brain Dev* **1**:83, 1979.
52. Ohta K, Tsuji S, Atsumi T, Mizuno Y, Miyatake T, Yahagi T: Biochemical and clinical studies on type 3 (adult type) G_{M1} gangliosidosis. *Clin Neurol* **23**:191, 1983.
53. Ohta K, Tsuji S, Mizuno Y, Atsumi T, Yahagi T, Miyatake T: Type 3 (adult) G_{M1}-gangliosidosis: Case report. *Neurology* **35**:1490, 1985.
54. Nakano T, Ikeda S, Kondo K, Yanagisawa N, Tsuji S: Adult G_{M1}-gangliosidosis: Clinical patterns and rectal biopsy. *Neurology* **35**:875, 1985.
55. Ushiyama M, Ikeda S, Nakayama J, Yanagisawa N, Hanyu N, Katsuyama T: Type III (chronic) G_{M1}-gangliosidosis. Histochemical and ultrastructural studies of rectal biopsy. *J Neurol Sci* **71**:209, 1985.
56. Mutoh T, Naoi M, Takahashi A, Hoshino M, Nagai Y, Nagatsu T: Atypical adult G_{M1} gangliosidosis: Biochemical comparison with other forms of primary β-galactosidase deficiency. *Neurology* **36**:1237, 1986.
57. Mutoh T, Sobue I, Naoi M, Matsuoka Y, Kiuchi K, Sugimura K: A family with β-galactosidase deficiency: Three adults with atypical clinical patterns. *Neurology* **35**:54, 1986.
58. Uyama E, Terasaki T, Owada M, Naito M, Araki S: Three siblings with type 3 G_{M1}-gangliosidosis—Pathophysiology of dystonia and MRI findings. *Clin Neurol* **30**:819, 1990.
59. Inui K, Namba R, Ihara Y, Nobukuni K, Taniike M, Midorikawa M, Tsukamoto H, Okada S: A case of chronic G_{M1} gangliosidosis presenting as dystonia: Clinical and biochemical studies. *J Neurol Sci* **237**:491, 1990.
60. Yoshida K, Oshima A, Sakuraba H, Nakano T, Yanagisawa N, Inui K, Okada S, Uyama E, Namba R, Kondo K, Iwasaki S, Takamiya K, Suzuki Y: G_{M1}-gangliosidosis in adults: Clinical and molecular analysis of 16 Japanese patients. *Ann Neurol* **31**:328, 1992.
61. Hirayama M, Kitagawa Y, Yamamoto S, Tokuda A, Mutoh T, Hamano T, Aita T, Kuriyama M: G_{M1} gangliosidosis type 3 with severe jaw-closing impairment. *J Neurol Sci* **152**:99, 1997.
62. Uyama E, Terasaki T, Watanabe S, Naito M, Owada M, Araki S, Ando M: Type 3 G_{M1} gangliosidosis: Characteristic MRI findings correlated with dystonia. *Acta Neurol Scand* **86**:609, 1992.
63. Stevenson RE, Taylor HA, Parks SE: β-Galactosidase deficiency: Prolonged survival in three patients following early central nervous system deterioration. *Clin Genet* **13**:305, 1978.
64. Wenger DA, Goodman SI, Myers GG: β-Galactosidase deficiency: Prolonged survival in three patients following early central nervous system deterioration. *Lancet* **2**:1319, 1974.
65. Wenger DA, Sattler M, Mueller T, Myers GG, Schneiman RS, Nixon GW: Adult G_{M1}-gangliosidosis: Clinical and biochemical studies on two patients and comparison to other patients called variant or adult G_{M1} gangliosidosis. *Clin Genet* **17**:323, 1980.
66. Goldman JE, Katz D, Rapin I, Purpura DP, Suzuki K: G_{M1}-gangliosidosis presenting as dystonia: I. Clinical and pathological features. *Ann Neurol* **9**:465, 1981.
67. Guazzi GC, D'Amore I, Van Hoof F, Fruschelli C, Alessandrini C, Palmeri S, Federico A: Type 3 (chronic) G_{M1} gangliosidosis presenting as infanto-choreo-athetotic dementia, without epilepsy, in three sisters. *Neurology* **38**:1124, 1988.
68. Nardocci N, Bertagnolio B, Rumi V, Combi M, Bardelli P, Angelini L: Chronic G_{M1} gangliosidosis presenting as dystonia: Clinical and biochemical studies in a new case. *Neuropediatrics* **24**:164, 1993.
69. Yamashita M, Yamasaki M, Kusaka H, Imai T, Inui K: Two siblings of type 3 G_{M1} gangliosidosis with different clinical features and different ages of onset. *Clin Neurol* **33**:631, 1993.
70. Kobayashi T, Suzuki K: Chronic G_{M1} gangliosidosis presenting as dystonia: II. Biochemical studies. *Ann Neurol* **9**:476, 1981.
71. Lowden JA, Callahan JW, Gravel RA, Skomorowski MA, Becker L, Groves J: Type 2 G_{M1}-gangliosidosis with long survival and neuronal ceroid lipofuscinosis. *Neurology* **31**:719, 1981.
72. Goetting MG, Dasouki MJ: Cerebral atrophy, macrosomia, and cutaneous telangiectasia in G_{M1} gangliosidosis. *J Pediatr* **107**:644, 1985.
73. Beratis NG, Varvarigou Frimas A, Beratis S, Sklower SL: Angiokeratoma corporis diffusum in G_{M1} gangliosidosis, type 1. *Clin Genet* **36**:59, 1989.
74. Tang TT, Esterly NB, Lubinsky MS, Oechler HW, Harb JM, Franciosi RA: G_{M1}-gangliosidosis type 1 involving the cutaneous vascular endothelial cells in a black infant with multiple ectopic Mongolian spots. *Acta Derm Venereol* **73**:412, 1993.
75. Weissbluth M, Esterly NB, Caro WA: Report of an infant with G_{M1}-gangliosidosis type I and extensive and unusual mongolian spots. *Br J Dermatol* **104**:195, 1981.
76. Selsor LC, Lesher JLJ: Hyperpigmented macules and patches in a patient with G_{M1} type 1 gangliosidosis. *J Am Acad Dermatol* **20**:878, 1989.
77. Esterly NB, Weissbluth M, Caro WA: Mongolian spots and G_{M1} type 1 gangliosidosis. *J Am Acad Dermatol* **22**:320, 1990.
78. Hadley RN, Hagstrom JWC: Cardiac lesions in a patient with familial neurovisceral lipidosis (generalized gangliosidosis). *Am J Clin Pathol* **55**:237, 1971.
79. Benson PF, Barbarik A, Brown SP, Mann TP: G_{M1}-generalized gangliosidosis variant with cardiomegaly. *Postgrad Med J* **52**:159, 1976.
80. Kohlschütter A, Sieg K, Schulte FJ, Hayek HW, Goebel HH: Infantile cardiomyopathy and neuromyopathy with β-galactosidase deficiency. *Eur J Pediatr* 139:75, 1982.
81. Rosenberg H, Frewen TC, Li MD, Gordon BL, Jung JH, Finlay JP, Roy PL, Grover D, Spence M: Cardiac involvement in diseases characterized by β-galactosidase deficiency. *J Pediatr* **106**:78, 1985.
82. Charrow J, Hvizd MG: Cardiomyopathy and skeletal myopathy in an unusual variant of G_{M1} gangliosidosis. *J Pediatr* **108**:729, 1986.
83. Heyne K, von der Linde J, Trübsbach A: Die Lungenerkrankung bei generalisierter G_{M1}-Gangliosidose. *Helv Paediatr Acta* **27**:591, 1972.
84. Matsumoto T, Matsumoto H, Taki T, Takagi T, Fukuda Y: Infantile G_{M1}-gangliosidosis with marked manifestation of lungs. *Acta Pathol Jpn* **29**:269, 1979.
85. Abu-Dalu KI, Tamary H, Livni N, Rivkind AI, Yatziv S: G_{M1}-gangliosidosis presenting as neonatal ascites. *J Pediatr* **100**:940, 1982.
86. Bonduelle M, Lissens W, Goossens A, De Catte L, Foulon W, Denis R, Jauniaux E, Liebaers I: Lysosomal storage diseases presenting as transient or persistent hydrops fetalis. *Genet Counsel* **2**:227, 1991.
87. Denis R, Wayenberg JL, Vermeulen M, Gorus F, Gerlo E, Lissens W, Liebaers I, Jauniaux E, Vamos E: Hyperphosphatasemia in early diagnosed infantile G_{M1} gangliosidosis presenting as transient hydrops fetalis. *Acta Clin Belg* **51**:320, 1996.
88. Roberts DJ, Ampola MG, Lage JM: Diagnosis of unsuspected fetal metabolic storage disease by routine placental examination. *Pediatr Pathol* **11**:647, 1991.
89. Knight JA, Myers GG: Type IV hyperlipidemia in the G_{M1}-gangliosidoses. *Am J Clin Pathol* **59**:124, 1973.
90. Mogilner BM, Barak Y, Amitay M, Zlotogora J: Hyperphosphatasemia in infantile G_{M1} gangliosidosis: Possible association with microscopic bone marrow osteoblastosis. *J Pediatr* **117**:758, 1990.
91. Denis R, Wayemberg JL, Vermeulen M, Gorus F, Liebaers I, Vamos E: Hyperphosphatasemia in G_{M1} gangliosidosis. *J Pediatr* **120**:164, 1992.
92. Gascon GG, Ozand PT, Erwin RE: GM1 gangliosidosis type 2 in two siblings. *J Child Neurol* **7(Suppl)**:S41, 1992.
93. Yamanaka T, Hirabayashi Y, Koketsu K, Higashi H, Matsumoto M: Highly sensitive analysis of gangliosides in human cerebrospinal fluid with neurological diseases. *Jpn J Exp Med* **37**:131, 1987.
94. Kaye EM, Ullman MD, Kolodny EH, Krivit W, Rischert JC: Possible use of CSF glycosphingolipids for the diagnosis and therapeutic monitoring of lysosomal storage diseases. *Neurology* **42**:2290, 1992.
95. Harden A, Martinovic Z, Pampiglione G: Neurophysiological studies in G_{M1}-gangliosidosis. *Ital J Neurol Sci* **3**:201, 1982.
96. Pampiglione G, Harden A: Neurophysiological investigations in G_{M1} and G_{M2} gangliosidoses. *Neuropediatrics* **15(Suppl)**:74, 1984.
97. Rabinowitz JG, Sacher M: Gangliosidosis (G_{M1}). A re-evaluation of the vertebral deformity. *AJR Am J Roentgenol* **121**:155, 1974.
98. Swischuk LE: Beaked, notched or hooked vertebrae. *Radiology* **95**:661, 1970.
99. Gooding CA, Neuhauser EBD: Growth and development of vertebral body in presence or absence of normal stress. *AJR Am J Roentgenol* **93**:388, 1965.
100. Severi F, Magrini U, Tettamanti G, Bianchi E, Lanzi G: Infantile G_{M1} gangliosidosis. Histochemical, ultrastructural and biochemical studies. *Helv Paediatr Acta* **26**:192, 1971.
101. Curless RG: Computed tomography of G_{M1} gangliosidosis. *J Pediatr* **105**:964, 1984.

102. Kobayashi O, Takashima S: Thalamic hyperdensity on CT in infantile G_{M1}-gangliosidosis. *Brain Dev* **16**:472, 1994.
103. Tanaka R, Momoi T, Yoshida A, Okumura M, Yamakura S, Takasaki Y, Kiyomasu T, Yamanaka C: Type 3 G_{M1} gangliosidosis: Clinical and neuroradiological findings in an 11-year-old girl. *J Neurol* **242**:299, 1995.
104. McKusick VA: *Heritable Disorders of Connective Tissue*, 4th ed. St. Louis, Mosby, 1972.
105. Matalon R, Arbogast B, Justice P, Brandt EK, Dorfman A: Morquio's syndrome. Deficiency of a chondroitin sulfate *N*-acetylhexosamine sulfate sulfatase. *Biochem Biophys Res Commun* **61**:759, 1974.
106. Groebe H, Krins M, Schmidberger H, von Figura K, Harzer K, Kresse H, Paschke E, Sewell A, Ullrich K: Morquio syndrome (mucopolysaccharidosis IV B) associated with β-galactosidase deficiency. Report of two cases. *Am J Hum Genet* **32**:258, 1980.
107. Trojak JE, Ho CK, Roesel RA, Levin LS, Kopits SE, Thomas GH, Toma S: Morquio-like syndrome (MPS IVB) associated with deficiency of a β-galactosidase. *Johns Hopkins Med J* **146**:75, 1980.
108. Pronicka E, Tylki A, Czartoryska B, Gorska D: Three cases of β-galactosidase deficiency. *Klin Pädiatr* **193**:343, 1981.
109. van Gemund JJ, Giesberts MA, Eerdmans RF, Blom W, Kleijer WJ: Morquio-B disease, spondyloepiphyseal dysplasia associated with acid β-galactosidase deficiency. Report of three cases in one family. *Hum Genet* **64**:50, 1983.
110. Giugliani R, Jackson M, Skinner SJ, Vimal CM, Fensom AH, Fahmy N, Sjovall A, Benson PF: Progressive mental regression in siblings with Morquio disease type B (mucopolysaccharidosis IV B). *Clin Genet* **32**:313, 1987.
111. Beck M, Petersen EM, Spranger J, Beighton P: Morquio's disease type B (β-galactosidase deficiency) in three siblings. *S Afr Med J* **72**:704, 1987.
112. Ishii N, Oohira T, Oshima A, Sakuraba H, Endo F, Matsuda I, Sukegawa K, Orii T, Suzuki Y: Clinical and molecular analysis of a Japanese boy with Morquio B disease. *Clin Genet* **48**:103, 1995.
113. Suzuki K, Suzuki Ki, Chen GC: G_{M1}-gangliosidosis (generalized gangliosidosis). Morphology and chemical pathology. *Pathol Eur* **3**:389, 1968.
114. Roels H: Generalized G_{M1} gangliosidosis: An electron-microscopic study of the brain. *Arch Dis Child* **45**:150, 1970.
115. Mihatsch MJ, Ohnacker H, Riede UN, Remagen W, von Bassewitz DB, Schuppler J, Meier-Ruge W: G_{M1}-gangliosidosis. II. Morphological aspects and review of the literature. *Helv Paediatr Acta* **28**:521, 1973.
116. Pfeiffer RA, Diekmann L, Wierich W, von Bassewitz DB, Jünemann G, Damaske E, Werries E, Wässle K: Klinische, pathologische und biochemische Untersuchungen in einem Fall von infantiler generalisierter Gangliosidose (G_{M1}-Mucolipidose). *Z Kinderheilkd* **112**:23, 1972.
117. Patel V, Goebel HH, Watanabe I, Zeman W: Studies on G_{M1}-gangliosidosis, type II. *Acta Neuropathol* **30**:155, 1974.
118. Terry RD, Weiss M: Studies in Tay-Sachs disease. II. Ultrastructure of the cerebrum. *J Neuropathol Exp Neurol* **22**:18, 1963.
119. Samuels S, Gonatas NK, Weiss M: Formation of the membranous cytoplasmic bodies in Tay-Sachs disease. An in vitro study. *J Neuropathol Exp Neurol* **24**:256, 1965.
120. Roels H, Quatacker J, Kint A, Van der Eecken H, Vrints L: Generalized gangliosidosis-G_{M1} (Landing disease). II. Morphological study. *Eur Neurol* **3**:129, 1970.
121. Joshua GE, Bhaktaviziam A, Sudarazanam D, Basu DK: G_{M1}-gangliosidosis in a South Indian child—A clinicopathological and biochemical study. *Indian J Med Res* **62**:788, 1974.
122. Backwinkel K-P, von Bassewitz DB, Diekmann L, Themann H: Ultrastructure of heart muscle in generalized gangliosidosis G_{M1}. *Z Kinderheilkd* **110**:104, 1971.
123. Farkas-Bargeton E: Idiotie amautorique infantile avec surcharge viscerale. *Excerpta Medica Int Congr Ser* **100**:135, 1965.
124. Emery JM, Green WR, Wyllie RG, Howell RR: G_{M1}-gangliosidosis. Ocular and pathological manifestations. *Arch Ophthalmol* **85**:177, 1971.
125. Callahan JW, Pinsky L, Wolfe LS: G_{M1}-gangliosidosis (type II): Studies on a fibroblast cell strain. *Biochem Med* **4**:295, 1970.
126. Tomé FMS, Fardeau M: Ultrastructural study of a muscle biopsy in a case of G_{M1} gangliosidosis type I. *Pathol Eur* **11**:15, 1976.
127. Yoshida K, Ikeda S, Kawaguchi K, Yanagisawa N: Adult G_{M1}-gangliosidosis: Immunohistochemical and ultrastructural findings in an autopsy case. *Neurology* **44**:2376, 1994.
128. Klenk E: Beiträge zur Chemie der Lipidosen. I. Niemann-Pick'sche Krankheit und amaurotische Idiotie. *Hoppe-Seylers Z Physiol Chem* **262**:128, 1939/40.
129. Kuhn R, Wiegandt H: Die Konstitution der Ganglio-N-tetraose und des Gangliosids G_1. *Chem Ber* **96**:866, 1978.
130. Sonnino S, Acquotti D, Riboni L, Giuliani A, Kirschner G, Tettamanti G: New chemical trend in ganglioside research. *Chem Phys Lipids* **42**:3, 1986.
131. Wieraszko A, Seifert W: Evidence of the functional role of monosialoganglioside G_{M1} in synaptic transmission in the rat hippocampus. *Brain Res* **371**:305, 1986.
132. Agnati LF, Benfenati F, Cavichilolo L, Fuxe K, Toffano G: Selective modulation of [^{3}H]-spiperone labeled 5-HT receptors by subchronic treatment with the ganglioside G_{M1} in the rat. *Acta Physiol Scand* **117**:311, 1983.
133. Suzuki K, Suzuki Ki, Kamoshita S: Chemical pathology of G_{M1}-gangliosidosis (generalized gangliosidosis). *J Neuropathol Exp Neurol* **28**:25, 1969.
134. Lennarz WJ: *The Biochemistry of Glycoproteins and Proteoglycans*. New York, Plenum Press, 1980.
135. Kornfeld R, Kornfeld S: Assembly of asparagine-linked oligosaccharides. *Annu Rev Biochem* **54**:631, 1985.
136. Rademacher TW, Prekh RB, Dwek RA: Glycobiology. *Annu Rev Biochem* **57**:785, 1988.
137. Schachter H, Brockhausen I: The biosynthesis of branched *O*-glycans. *Symp Soc Exp Biol* **43**:1, 1989.
138. Hopwood JJ, Morris CP: The mucopolysaccharidoses. Diagnosis, molecular genetics and treatment. *Mol Biol Med* **7**:381, 1990.
139. Meyer K: Biochemistry and biology of mucopolysaccharides. *Am J Med* **47**:664, 1969.
140. Baker JR, Cifonelli JA, Roden L: The linkage of corneal keratan sulfate to protein. *Connect Tissue Res* **3**:149, 1975.
141. Bray RA, Lickerman R, Meyer K: Structure of human skeletal keratosulfate. *J Biol Chem* **242**:3373, 1967.
142. Jatzkewitz H, Pilz H, Sandhoff K: Quantitative Bestimmungen von Gangliosiden und ihre neuraminäurefreien Derivaten bei infantilen, juvenilen und adulten Formen der amaurotischen Idiotie und einer spätinfantilen biochemischen Sonderform. *J Neurochem* **12**:135, 1965.
143. Ledeen R, Salsman K, Gonatas J, Taghavy A: Structure comparison of the major monosialogangliosides from brains of normal human, gargoylism, and late infantile systemic lipidosis. Part I. *J Neuropathol Exp Neurol* **24**:341, 1965.
144. Iwamasa T, Ohshita T, Nashiro K, Iwanaga M: Demonstration of G_{M1}-ganglioside in nervous system in generalized G_{M1} gangliosidosis using cholera toxin B subunit. *Acta Neuropathol* **73**:357, 1987.
145. Kobayashi T, Goto I, Okada S, Orii T, Ohno K, Nakano T: Accumulation of lysosphingolipids in tissues from patients with G_{M1} and G_{M2} gangliosidoses. *J Neurochem* **59**:1452, 1992.
146. Weiss MJ, Krill AE, Dawson G, Hindman J, Cotlier E: G_{M1}-gangliosidosis type I. *Am J Ophthalmol* **76**:999, 1973.
147. Kasama T, Taketomi T: Abnormalities of cerebral lipids in G_{M1}-gangliosidoses, infantile, juvenile, and chronic type. *Jpn J Exp Med* **56**:1, 1986.
148. Taketomi T, Hara A, Kasama T: Cerebral and visceral organ gangliosides and related glycolipids in G_{M1}-gangliosidosis type 1, type 2 and chronic type. *Adv Exp Med Biol* **174**:419, 1984.
149. Taketomi T, Hara A, Kasama T: Abnormalities in cerebral lipids and hepatic cholesterol glucuronide of a patients with G_{M1}-gangliosidosis type 2, in Makita A, Handa S, Taketomi T, Nagai Y (eds): *New Vistas in Glycolipid Research*. New York, Plenum, 1982, p 291.
150. Callahan JW, Wolfe LS: Isolation and characterization of keratan sulfates from the liver of a patient with G_{M1}-gangliosidosis type I. *Biochim Biophys Acta* **215**:527, 1970.
151. Howell R: Mild Morquio syndrome (MPS-IVB) with keratan sulfaturia but normal 6-sulfatase activity. *Am J Med Genet* **1**:195, 1977.
152. Suzuki K: Cerebral G_{M1}-gangliosidosis: chemical pathology of visceral organs. *Science* **159**:1471, 1968.
153. Calatroni A: Fractionation and characterization of glycopeptides and oligosaccharides from the liver of a patient with G_{M1}-gangliosidosis type I. *Ital J Biochem* **23**:329, 1974.
154. Tsay GC, Dawson G: Structure of the "keratosulfate-like" material in liver from a patient with G_{M1}-gangliosidosis (β-D-galactosidase deficiency). *Biochem Biophys Res Commun* **52**:759, 1973.
155. Tsay GC, Dawson G, Li Y-T: Structure of the glycopeptide storage material in G_{M1} gangliosidosis. Sequence determination with specific endo- and exoglycosidases. *Biochim Biophys Acta* **385**:305, 1975.

156. Wolfe LS, Senior RG, Ng Ying Kin NMK: The structure of oligosaccharides accumulating in the liver of G_{M1}-gangliosidosis, type I. *J Biol Chem* **249**:1828, 1974.
157. Ng Ying Kin NMK, Wolfe LS: Characterization of oligosaccharides and glycopeptides excreted in the urine of G_{M1}-gangliosidosis patients. *Biochem Biophys Res Commun* **66**:123, 1975.
158. Lundblad A, Sjoblad S, Svensson S: Characterization of a penta- and an octasaccharide from urine of a patient with juvenile G_{M1}-gangliosidosis. *Arch Biochem Biophys* **188**:130, 1978.
159. Ohkura T, Yamashita K, Kobata A: Urinary oligosaccharides of G_{M1}-gangliosidosis. Structures of oligosaccharides excreted in the urine of type 1 but not in the urine of type 2 patients. *J Biol Chem* **256**:8485, 1981.
160. Yamashita K, Ohkura T, Okada S, Yabuuchi H, Kobata A: Urinary oligosaccharides of G_{M1}-gangliosidosis. Different excretion patterns of oligosaccharides in the urine of type 1 and type 2 subgroups. *J Biol Chem* **256**:4789, 1981.
161. Warner TG, Robertson AD, O'Brien JS: Diagnosis of G_{M1}-gangliosidosis based on detection of urinary oligosaccharides with high performance liquid chromatography. *Clin Chim Acta* **127**:313, 1983.
162. Takahashi Y, Orii T: Severity of G_{M1} gangliosidosis and urinary oligosaccharide excretion. *Clin Chim Acta* **179**:153, 1989.
163. Takahashi Y, Orii T: Diagnosis of subtypes of G_{M1} gangliosidosis in vitro and in vivo using urinary oligosaccharides as substrates. *Clin Chim Acta* **179**:219, 1989.
164. Michalski JC, Lemoine J, Wieruszeski JM, Fournet B, Montreuil J, Strecker G: Characterization of a novel type of chain terminator Galβ1-6Galβ1-4GlcNAc in an oligosaccharide related to *N*-glycosylated protein glycans isolated from G_{M1} the urine of patients with gangliosidosis. *Eur J Biochem* **198**:521, 1991.
165. Tsuji S, Ariga T, Ando S, Tanaka Y, Kon K, Yahagi T, Ohta K, Miyatake T: Isolation and characterization of major urinary oligosaccharides excreted by a patient with type 3 G_{M1} gangliosidosis. *J Biochem* **109**:722, 1991.
166. Michalski JC, Strecker G, van Halbeek H, Dorland L, Vliegenthart JF: The structures of six urinary oligosaccharides that are characteristic for a patient with Morquio syndrome type B. *Carbohydr Res* **100**:351, 1982.
167. Suzuki Y, Sakuraba H, Oshima A: β-Galactosidase deficiency (β-galactosidosis): G_{M1} gangliosidosis and Morquio B disease, in Scriver CR, Beaudet AL, Sly WS, Valle D (eds): *The Metabolic and Molecular Bases of Inherited Disease*, 7th ed. New York, McGraw-Hill, 1995, p 2785.
168. Strecker G, Montreuil J: Glycoproteins and glycoproteinases. *Biochimie* **61**:1199, 1979.
169. Strecker, G. Oligosaccharides in lysosomal storage diseases, in Callahan JW, Lowden JA (eds): *Lysosomes and Lysosomal Storage Diseases*. New York, Raven Press, 1981, p 95.
170. Taylor HA, Stevenson RE, Parker SE: β-Galactosidase deficiency: Studies of two patients with prolonged survival. *Am J Med Genet* **5**:235, 1980.
171. Warner TG, O'Brien JS: Structure analysis of the major oligosaccharides accumulating in canine G_{M1} gangliosidosis liver. *J Biol Chem* **257**:224, 1982.
172. Barker CG, Blakemore WF, Dell A, Palmer AC, Tiller PR, Winchester BG: G_{M1} gangliosidosis (type 1) in a cat. *Biochem J* **235**:151, 1986.
173. Holmes EW, O'Brien JS: Hepatic storage of oligosaccharides and glycolipids in a cat affected with G_{M1} gangliosidosis. *Biochem J* **175**:945, 1978.
174. Yamashita K, Inui K, Totani K, Kochibe N, Furukawa M, Okada S: Characteristics of asparagine-linked sugar chains of sphingolipid activator protein 1 purified from normal human liver and G_{M1}-gangliosidosis (type 1) liver. *Biochemistry* **29**:3030, 1990.
175. Suzuki Y, Yokota S, Kobayashi N, Kato T: Application of ultramicrotechnique for the diagnosis of hereditary metabolic diseases. *Acta Paediatr Jpn* **23**:44, 1981.
176. Furuya T, Suzuki Y, Momoi T: Acid β-galactosidase from human fibroblasts. A microscale purification method monitored by a highly sensitive enzyme assay. *J Biochem* **99**:437, 1986.
177. Arvisdon DN, Schneider TD, Stormo GD: Automated kinetic assay of β-galactosidase activity. *Biotechniques* **11**:733, 1991.
178. Naoi M, Kondoh M, Mutoh T, Takahashi T, Kojima T, Hirooka T, Nagatsu T: Microassay for G_{M1} ganglioside β-galactosidase activity using high-performance liquid chromatography. *J Chromatogr* **426**:75, 1988.
179. Jain VK, Magrath IT: A chemiluminescent assay for quantitation of β-galactosidase in the femtogram range: Application to quantitation of β-galactosidase in *lac*Z-transfected cells. *Anal Biochem* **199**:119, 1991.
180. Ho MW, Cheetham P, Robinson D: Hydrolysis of G_{M1}-ganglioside by human liver β-galactosidase isoenzymes. *Biochem J* **136**:351, 1973.
181. Norden AGW, Tennant LL, O'Brien JS: G_{M1} ganglioside β-galactosidase A. Purification and studies of the enzyme from human liver. *J Biol Chem* **249**:7969, 1974.
182. O'Brien JS: Molecular genetics of G_{M1} β-galactosidase. *Clin Genet* **8**:303, 1975.
183. Cheetham PSJ, Dance NE: The separation and characterization of the methylumbelliferyl β-galactosidase of human liver. *Biochem J* **157**:189, 1976.
184. Frost RG, Holmes EW, Norden AGW, O'Brien JS: Characterization of purified human liver acid β-D-galactosidase A_2 and A_3. *Biochem J* **175**:181, 1978.
185. Heyworth CM, Neumann EF, Wynn CH: The stability and aggregation properties of human liver acid β-galactosidase. *Biochem J* **193**:773, 1981.
186. Overdijk B, Hiensch-Goormachtig EFJ, Beem EP, van Steijn GJ, Trippelvitz LAW, Lisman JJW, van Halbeek H, Mutsaers JHGM, Vliegenthart JFG: The carbohydrate structures of β-galactosidase from human liver. *Glycoconjugate J* **3**:339, 1986.
187. Mutoh T, Naoi M, Nagatsu T, Takahashi A, Matsuoka Y, Hashizume Y, Fujiki N: Purification and characterization of human liver β-galactosidase from a patient with the adult form of G_{M1} gangliosidosis and a normal control. *Biochim Biophys Acta* **964**:244, 1988.
188. Norden AGW, O'Brien JS: Ganglioside G_{M1} β-galactosidase: Studies in human liver and brain. *Arch Biochem Biophys* **159**:383, 1973.
189. Lisman JJW, Hoogewinkel GJM: Kinetic properties of β-galactosidase of human tissue. *Neurobiology* **4**:167, 1974.
190. Tanaka H, Suzuki K: Substrate specificities of the two genetically distinct human brain β-galactosidases. *Brain Res* **122**:325, 1977.
191. Pinsky L, Miller J, Shanfield B, Watters G, Wolfe LS: G_{M1} gangliosidosis in skin fibroblast culture: Enzymatic differences between types 1 and 2 and observations on a third variant. *Am J Hum Genet* **26**:563, 1974.
192. Hoogeveen AT, Verheijen FW, Galjaard H: The relation between human lysosomal β-galactosidase and its protective protein. *J Biol Chem* **258**:12143, 1983.
193. Hoogeveen AT, Graham-Kawashima H, D'Azzo A, Galjaard H: Processing of human β-galactosidase in G_{M1}-gangliosidosis and Morquio B syndrome. *J Biol Chem* **259**:1974, 1984.
194. Hoogeveen AT, Reuser AJ, Kroos M, Galjaard H: G_{M1}-gangliosidosis. Defective recognition site on β-galactosidase precursor. *J Biol Chem* **261**:5702, 1986.
195. Dance N, Price RG, Robinson D, Stirling JL: β-Galactosidase, β-glucuronidase and *N*-acetyl-β-glucosaminidase in human kidney. *Clin Chim Acta* **24**:189, 1969.
196. Kress BC, Miller AL: Characterization of the acid β-D-galactosidases from human urine. *Clin Chim Acta* **85**:23, 1978.
197. Lo J, Mukerji K, Awasthi YC, Hanada E, Suzuki K, Srivastava SK: Purification and properties of sphingolipid β-galactosidases from human placenta. *J Biol Chem* **254**:6710, 1979.
198. Singer HS, Schafer IA: Clinical and enzymatic variations in G_{M1} generalized gangliosidosis. *Am J Hum Genet* **24**:454, 1972.
199. Kolodny EH, Mumford RA: Human leukocyte acid hydrolyses: Characterization of eleven lysosomal enzymes and study of reaction conditions for their automated analysis. *Clin Chim Acta* **70**:247, 1976.
200. Ho MW, O'Brien JS: Stimulation of acid β-galactosidase activity by chloride ions. *Clin Chim Acta* **30**:531, 1970.
201. Ho MW, O'Brien JS: Differential effect of chloride ions on β-galactosidase isoenzymes: A method for differential assay. *Clin Chim Acta* **32**:443, 1971.
202. Kint JA: Antagonistic action of chondroitin sulphate and cetylpyridinium chloride on human liver β-galactosidase. *FEBS Lett* **36**:53, 1973.
203. Kint JA, Dacremont G, Carton D, Orye E, Hooft C: Mucopolysaccharidosis: Secondarily induced abnormal distribution of lysosomal isoenzymes. *Science* **181**:352, 1973.
204. Ho MW, Fluharty A: Chloride ions cancel out inhibition of β-galactosidase activity by acid mucopolysaccharides. *Nature* **253**:660, 1975.
205. Meisler M: Inhibition of human liver β-galactosidases and β-glucosidase by *N*-bromoacetyl-β-galactosylamine. *Biochim Biophys Acta* **410**:347, 1975.

206. van Diggelen OP, Galjaard H, Sinnott ML, Smith PJ: Specific inactivation of lysosomal glycosidases in living fibroblasts by the corresponding glycosylmethyl-*p*-nitrophenyltriazenes. *Biochem J* **188**:337, 1980.
207. BeMiller JN, Gilson RJ, Myers RW, Santoro MM, Yadav MP: *N*-substituted (β-D-galactopyranosylmethyl)amines as reversible inhibitors of β-D-galactosidase. *Carbohydr Res* **250**:93, 1993.
208. BeMiller JN, Gilson RJ, Myers RW, Santoro MM: Suicide-substrate inactivation of β-galactosidase by diazomethyl β-D-galactopyranosyl ketone. *Carbohydr Res* **250**:101, 1993.
209. Singer HS, Tiemeyer M, Slesinger PA, Sinnott ML: Inactivation of G_{M1}-ganglioside β-galactosidase by a specific inhibitor: A model for ganglioside storage disease. *Ann Neurol* **21**:497, 1987.
210. D'Azzo A, Hoogeveen A, Reuser AJ, Robinson D, Galjaard H: Molecular defect in combined β-galactosidase and neuraminidase deficiency in man. *Proc Natl Acad Sci U S A* **79**:4535, 1982.
211. Nanba E, Tsuji A, Omura K, Suzuki Y: G_{M1}-gangliosidosis: Abnormalities in biosynthesis and early processing of β-galactosidase in fibroblasts. *Biochem Biophys Res Commun* **152**:794, 1988.
212. van Diggelen OP, Hoogeveen AT, Smith PJ, Reuser AJ, Galjaard H: Enhanced proteolytic degradation of normal β-galactosidase in the lysosomal storage disease with combined β-galactosidase and neuraminidase deficiency. *Biochim Biophys Acta* **703**:69, 1982.
213. Okamura-Oho Y, Zhang S, Hilson W, Hinek A, Callahan JW: Early proteolytic cleavage with loss of a C-terminal fragment underlies altered processing of the beta-galactosidase precursor in galactosialidosis. *Biochem J* **313**:787, 1996.
214. Suzuki Y, Fukuoka K, Wey JJ, Handa S: β-Galactosidase in mucopolysaccharidoses and mucolipidoses. Deficiency of G_{M1} β-galactosidase in liver and leukocytes. *Clin Chim Acta* **75**:91, 1977.
215. Raghavan SA, Gajewski A, Kolodny EH: G_{M1}-ganglioside β-galactosidase in leukocytes and cultured fibroblasts. *Clin Chim Acta* **81**:47, 1977.
216. Miller AL, Frost RG, O'Brien JS: Purified human liver acid β-galactosidase possessing activity towards G_{M1}-ganglioside and lactosylceramide. *Biochem J* **165**:591, 1977.
217. Callahan JW, Gerrie J: Purification of G_{M1}-ganglioside and ceramide lactoside β-galactosidase from rabbit brain. *Biochim Biophys Acta* **391**:141, 1975.
218. Gatt S: Enzymatic hydrolysis of sphingolipids. V. Hydrolysis of monosialoganglioside and hexosylceramides by rat brain β-galactosidase. *Biochim Biophys Acta* **137**:192, 1967.
219. Suzuki Y, Suzuki K: Glycosphingolipid β-galactosidases I. Standard assay procedures and characterization by electrofocusing and gel filtration of the enzymes in normal human liver. *J Biol Chem* **249**:2098, 1974.
220. Tanaka H, Suzuki K: Lactosylceramide β-galactosidase in human sphingolipidoses. Evidence for two genetically distinct enzymes. *J Biol Chem* **250**:2324, 1975.
221. Tanaka H, Meisler M, Suzuki K: Activity of human hepatic β-galactosidase toward natural glycosphingolipid substrates. *Biochim Biophys Acta* **398**:452, 1975.
222. Tanaka H, Suzuki K: Specificities of the two genetically distinct β-galactosidases in human sphingolipidoses. *Arch Biochem Biophys* **175**:332, 1976.
223. Zschoche A, Furst W, Schwarzmann G, Sandhoff K: Hydrolysis of lactosylceramide by human galactosylceramidase and G_{M1}-β-galactosidase in a detergent-free system and its stimulation by sphingolipid activator proteins, *sap*-B and *sap*-C. *Eur J Biochem* **222**:83, 1994.
224. Shiraishi T, Hiraiwa M, Uda Y: Effects of cyclodextrins on the hydrolysis of ganglioside G_{M1} by acid β-galactosidases. *Glycoconjugate J* **10**:170, 1993.
225. Paschke E, Niemann R, Strecker G, Kresse H: Aggregation properties of β-galactosidase of human urine and degradation of its natural substrates by a purified preparation of the enzyme. *Biochim Biophys Acta* **704**:134, 1982.
226. Verheijen F, Palmeri S, Hoogeveen AT, Galjaard H: Human placental neuraminidase. *Eur J Biochem* **149**:315, 1985.
227. Verheijen F, Palmeri S, Galjaard H: Purification and partial characterization of lysosomal neuraminidase from human placenta. *Eur J Biochem* **162**:63, 1987.
228. Galjart NJ, Gillemans N, Harris A, van der Horst GTT, Verheijen FW, Galjaard H, D'Azzo A: Expression of cDNA encoding the human protective protein associated with lysosomal β-galactosidase and neuraminidase: homology to yeast proteases. *Cell* **53**:755, 1988.
229. van der Horst GTJ, Galjart NJ, D'Azzo A, Galjaard H, Verheijen FW: Identification and *in vitro* reconstitution of lysosomal neuraminidase from human placenta. *J Biol Chem* **264**:1317, 1989.
230. Potier M, Michaud L, Tranchemontagne J, Thauvette L: Structure of the lysosomal neuraminidase-β-galactosidase-carboxypeptidase multienzymic complex. *Biochem J* **267**:197, 1990.
231. Jackman HL, Tan F, Tamei H, Beurling-Harbury C, Li X-Y, Skidgel RA, Erdos EG: A peptidase in human platelets that deamidates tachykinins. *J Biol Chem* **256**:11265, 1990.
232. Kase R, Itoh K, Takiyama N, Oshima A, Sakuraba H, Suzuki Y: Galactosialidosis: simultaneous deficiency of esterase, carboxy-terminal deamidase and acid carboxypeptidase activities. *Biochem Biophys Res Commun* **172**:1175, 1990.
233. Galjart NJ, Morreau H, Willemsen R, Gillemans N, Bonten EJ, D'Azzo A: Human lysosomal protective protein has cathepsin A-like activity distinct from its protective function. *J Biol Chem* **266**:14754, 1991.
234. Suzuki Y, Sakuraba H, Yamanaka T, Ko Y-M, Iimori Y, Okamura Y, Hoogeveen AT: Galactosialidosis: a comparative study of clinical and biochemical data on 22 patients, in Arima M, Suzuki Y, Yabuuchi H: *The Developing Brain and Its Disorders*. Basel, Karger, 1985, p 161.
235. Galjaard H, Willemsen R, Hoogeveen AT, Mancini GM, Palmeri S, Verheijen FW, D'Azzo A: Molecular heterogeneity in human β-galactosidase and neuraminidase deficiency. *Enzyme* **38**:132, 1987.
236. Suzuki Y, Sakuraba H, Hayashi K, Suzuki K, Imahori K: β-Galactosidase-neuraminidase deficiency: Restoration of β-galactosidase activity by protease inhibitors. *J Biochem* **90**:271, 1981.
237. Sakuraba H, Suzuki Y, Akagi M, Sakai M, Amano N: β-Galactosidase-neuraminidase deficiency (galactosialidosis): Clinical, pathological, and enzymatic studies in a postmortem case. *Ann Neurol* **13**:497, 1983.
238. Ko Y-M, Yamanaka T, Umeda M, Suzuki Y: Effects of thiol protease inhibitors on intracellular degradation of exogenous β-galactosidase in cultured human skin fibroblasts. *Exp Cell Res* **148**:525, 1983.
239. Li SC, Li YT: An activator stimulating the enzymic hydrolysis of sphingoglycolipids. *J Biol Chem* **251**:1159, 1976.
240. Wenger DA, Inui K: Studies on the sphingolipid activator protein for the enzymatic hydrolysis of G_{M1} ganglioside and sulfatide, in Barranger JA, Brady RO: *Molecular Basis of Lysosomal Storage Disorders*. New York, Academic Press, 1984, p 61.
241. Mehl E, Jatzkewitz H: Eine Cerebrosidsulfatase aus Schweineniere. *Hoppe-Seylers Z Physiol Chem* **339**:260, 1964.
242. Mehl E, Jatzkewitz H: Cerebroside-3-sulfate as a physiological substrate of arylsulfatase A. *Biochim Biophys Acta* **151**:619, 1968.
243. Jatzkewitz H, Stinshoff K: An activator of cerebroside sulfatase in human normal liver and in cases of congenital metachromatic leukodystrophy. *FEBS Lett* **32**:129, 1973.
244. Gartner S, Conzelmann E, Sandhoff K: Activator protein for the degradation of globotriaosylceramide by human α-galactosidase. *J Biol Chem* **258**:12378, 1983.
245. O'Brien JS, Kretz KA, Dewji N, Wenger DA, Esch F, Fluharty AL: Coding of two sphingolipid activator proteins (SAP-1 and SAP-2) by same genetic locus. *Science* **241**:1098, 1988.
246. Sano A, Radin NS, Johnson LL, Tarr GE: The activator protein for glucosylceramide β-glucosidase from guinea pig liver. *J Biol Chem* **263**:19579, 1988.
247. Nakano T, Sandhoff K, Stümper J, Christomanou H, Suzuki K: Structure of full-length cDNA coding for sulfatide activator, a co-β-glucosidase and two other homologous proteins: two alternate forms of the sulfatide activator. *J Biochem* **105**:152, 1989.
248. Champagne M-J, Lamontagne S, Potier M: Binding of G_{M1} ganglioside to a synthetic peptide derived from the lysosomal sphingolipid activator protein saposin B. *FEBS Lett* **349**:439, 1994.
249. Galjaard H, Reuser A JJ: Clinical, biochemical and genetic heterogeneity in gangliosidoses, in Harkness RA, Cockburn F (eds): *Inborn Errors of Metabolism: The Cultured Cell*. St. Leonardgate, MTP Press, 1977, p 139.
250. Pinsky L, Powell E, Callahan J: G_{M1}-gangliosidosis types 1 and 2: Enzymatic differences in cultured fibroblasts. *Nature* **228**:1093, 1970.
251. Yutaka T, Okada S, Kato T, Yabuuchi H: Impaired degradation of keratan sulfate in G_{M1}-gangliosidosis. *Clin Chim Acta* **125**:233, 1982.
252. Czartoryaka B, Gorska D, Abramowicz T: Kinetic properties of β-galactosidase in Morquio B disease. *Acta Anthropogenet* **7**:301, 1983.
253. Paschke E, Kresse H: Morquio disease, type B: Activation of G_{M1}-β-galactosidase by G_{M1}-activator protein. *Biochem Biophys Res Commun* **30**:568, 1982.
254. Sakuraba H, Iimori Y, Suzuki Y, Kint JA, Akagi A: Galactosialidosis: Low β-galactosidase activity in serum after long-term clotting. *Ann Neurol* **18**:261, 1985.

255. Ishii N, Oshima A, Sakuraba H, Fukuyama Y, Suzuki Y: Normal serum β-galactosidase in juvenile G_{M1}-gangliosidosis. *Pediatr Neurol* **10**:317, 1994.
256. Prence EM, Natowicz MR: Unusual biochemical presentation of G_{M1} gangliosidosis: Markedly elevated levels of multiple plasma lysosomal enzyme activities. *J Inherit Metab Dis* **16**:897, 1993.
257. Kobayashi T, Shinnoh N, Goto I, Kuroiwa Y, Okawauch M, Sugihara G, Tanaka M: Galactosylceramide- and lactosylceramide-loading studies in cultured fibroblasts from normal individuals and patients with globoid cell leukodystrophy (Krabbe's disease) and G_{M1}-gangliosidosis. *Biochim Biophys Acta* **835**:456, 1985.
258. Kobayashi T, Shinnoh N, Kuroiwa Y: Incorporation and degradation of G_{M1} ganglioside and asialo G_{M1} ganglioside in cultured fibroblasts from normal individuals and patients with β-galactosidase deficiency. *Biochim Biophys Acta* **875**:115, 1986.
259. Midorikawa M, Inui K, Okada S, Yabuuchi H, Ogura K, Handa S: Uptake and metabolism of radiolabelled G_{M1}-ganglioside in skin fibroblasts from controls and patients with G_{M1}-gangliosidosis. *J Inherit Metab Dis* **14**:721, 1991.
260. Schmid B, Paton BC, Sandhoff K, Harzer K: Metabolism of G_{M1} ganglioside in cultured skin fibroblasts: anomalies in gangliosidoses, sialidoses, and sphingolipid activator protein (SAP, saposin) 1 and prosaposin deficient disorders. *Hum Genet* **89**:513, 1992.
261. Galjaard H, Hoogeveen A, de Wit Verbeek HA, Reuser AJ, Ho MW, Robinson D: Genetic heterogeneity in G_{M1}-gangliosidosis. *Nature* **257**:60, 1975.
262. Bruns GAP, Leary AC, Regina VM, Gerald PS: Lysosomal β-D-galactosidase in man-hamster somatic cell hybrids. *Cytogenet Cell Genet* **22**:177, 1978.
263. Shows TB, Scrafford-Wolff L, Brown JA, Meisler M: Assignment of a β-galactosidase gene (β-Gal A) to chromosome 3 in man. *Cytogenet Cell Genet* **22**:219, 1978.
264. Ben-Yoseph Y, Burton BK, Nadler HL: Quantitation of the enzymically deficient cross-reacting material in G_{M1} gangliosidoses. *Am J Hum Genet* **29**:575, 1977.
265. Meisler M, Rattazzi MC: Immunological studies of β-galactosidase in normal human liver and in G_{M1} gangliosidosis. *Am J Hum Genet* **26**:683, 1974.
266. Norden AG, O'Brien JS: An electrophoretic variant of β-galactosidase with altered catalytic properties in a patient with G_{M1} gangliosidosis. *Proc Natl Acad Sci U S A* **72**:240, 1975.
267. Takiyama N, Itoh K, Oshima A, Sakuraba H, Suzuki Y: Characterization of an anti-β-galactosidase antibody recognizing a precursor but not a mature enzyme in solution. *Biochem Biophys Res Commun* 193:526, 1993.
268. Fukuhara Y, Oshima A, Suzuki Y: Altered substrate affinity of a mutant β-galactosidase causing Morquio B disease. *Dev Brain Dysfunct* **10**:119, 1997.
269. Willemsen R, Hoogeveen AT, Sips HJ, van Dongen JM, Galjaard H: Immunoelectron microscopical localization of lysosomal β-galactosidase and its precursor forms in normal and mutant human fibroblasts. *Eur J Cell Biol* **40**:9, 1986.
270. Oshima A, Yoshida K, Itoh K, Kase R, Sakuraba H, Suzuki Y: Intracellular processing and maturation of mutant gene products in hereditary β-galactosidase deficiency (β-galactosidosis). *Hum Genet* **93**:109, 1994.
271. Takiyama N, Itoh K, Shimmoto M, Nishimoto J, Inui K, Sakuraba H, Suzuki Y: Molecular form and subcellular distribution of acid β-galactosidase in fibroblasts from patients with G_{M1} gangliosidosis, Morquio B disease and galactosialidosis. *Brain Dev* **19**:126, 1997.
272. van Diggelen OP, Schram AW, Sinnott ML, Smith PJ, Robinson D, Galjaard H: Turnover of β-galactosidase in fibroblasts from patients with genetically different types of β-galactosidase deficiency. *Biochem J* **200**:143, 1981.
273. Chou L, Kaye CI, Nadler HL: Brain β-galactosidase and G_{M1}-gangliosidosis. *Pediatr Res* **8**:120, 1974.
274. Yutaka T, Okada S, Mimaki K, Sugita T, Yabuuchi H: Enzymatic study of G_{M1}-gangliosidosis. *Clin Chim Acta* **59**:283, 1975.
275. Farrell DF, MacMartin MP: G_{M1} gangliosidosis: enzymatic variation in a single family. *Ann Neurol* **9**:232, 1981.
276. Ben-Yoseph Y, Shapira E, Edelman D, Burton BK, Nadler HL: Purification and properties of neutral β-galactosidases from human liver. *Arch Biochem Biophys* **184**:373, 1977.
277. Suzuki Y, Hayakawa T, Yazaki M, Hiratani Y: G_{M1}-gangliosidosis. A variant with high activity of hepatic neutral β-galactosidase. *Eur J Pediatr* **122**:177, 1976.
278. Cheetham PSJ, Dance NE, Robinson D: A benign deficiency of type B β-galactosidase in human liver. *Clin Chim Acta* **83**:67, 1978.
279. de Wit J, Hoeksema HL, Hally D, Hagemeijer A, Bootsma D, Westerveld A: Regional localization of a β-galactosidase locus on human chromosome 22. *Somat Cell Genet* **3**:351, 1977.
280. Shows TB, Scrafford Wolff LR, Brown JA, Meisler MH: G_{M1}-gangliosidosis: Chromosome 3 assignment of the β-galactosidaseA gene (βGAL_A). *Somat Cell Genet* **5**:147, 1979.
281. Sips HJ, de Wit-Verbeek HA, de Wit J, Westerveld A, Galjaard H: The chromosomal localization of human β-galactosidase revisited: a locus for β-galactosidase on human chromosome 3 and for its protective protein on human chromosome 22. *Hum Genet* **69**:340, 1985.
282. de Wit J, Hoeksema HL, Bootsma D, Westerveld A: Assignment of structural β-galactosidase loci to human chromosomes 2 and 22. *Hum Genet* **51**:259, 1979.
283. Naylor SL, Elliott RW, Brown JA, Shows TB: Mapping of aminoacylase-1 and β-galactosidase-A to homologous regions of human chromosome 3 and mouse chromosome 9 suggests location of additional genes. *Am J Hum Genet* **34**:235, 1982.
284. Jones C, Miller YE, Palmer D, Morse H, Kiry M, Patterson D: Regional mapping of human chromosome 3. *Cytogenet Cell Genet* **37**:500, 1984.
285. Yamamoto Y, Hake CA, Martin BM, Kretz KA, Ahern-Rindall AJ, Naylor SL, Mudd M, O'Brien JS: Isolation, characterization, and mapping of a human acid β-galactosidase cDNA. *DNA Cell Biol* **9**:119, 1990.
286. Takano T, Yamanouchi Y: Assignment of human β-galactosidase-A gene to 3p21.33 by fluorescence in situ hybridization. *Hum Genet* **92**:403, 1993.
287. Morreau H, Galjart NJ, Gillemans N, Willemsen R, van der Horst GT, D'Azzo A: Alternative splicing of β-galactosidase mRNA generates the classic lysosomal enzyme and a β-galactosidase-related protein. *J Biol Chem* **264**:20655, 1989.
288. Oshima A, Kyle LW, Miller RD, Hoffman JW, Powell PP, Grubb JH, Sly WS, Tropak M, Guise KS, Gravel RA: Cloning, sequencing, and expression of cDNA for human β-glucuronidase. *Proc Natl Acad Sci U S A* **84**:685, 1987.
289. Nanba E, Suzuki K: Molecular cloning of mouse acid β-galactosidase cDNA: Sequence, expression of catalytic activity and comparison with the human enzyme. *Biochem Biophys Res Commun* **173**:141, 1990.
290. Oshima A, Itoh K, Nagao Y, Sakuraba H, Suzuki Y: β-Galactosidase-deficient human fibroblasts: uptake and processing of the exogenous precursor enzyme expressed by stable transformant COS cells. *Hum Genet* **85**:505, 1990.
291. Niwa H, Yamamura K, Miyazaki J: Efficient selection for high-expression transfectants with a novel eukaryotic vector. *Gene* **108**:193, 1991.
292. Itoh K, Oshima A, Sakuraba H, Suzuki Y: Expression, glycosylation, and intracellular distribution of human β-galactosidase in recombinant baculovirus-infected *Spodoptera frugiperda* cells. *Biochem Biophys Res Commun* **167**:746, 1990.
293. Itoh K, Oshima A, Sakuraba H, Suzuki Y: Characterization and purification of human β-galactosidase overexpressed in recombinant baculovirus-infected *Spodoptera frugiperda* cells. *J Inherit Metab Dis* **14**:813, 1991.
294. Ogonah O, Shuler ML, Granados RR: Protein production (β-galactosidase) from a baculovirus vector in *Spodoptera frugiperda* and *Trichpolusia ni* cells in suspension culture. *Biotechnol Lett* **13**:265, 1991.
295. Morreau H, Bonten E, Zhou XY, D'Azzo A: Organization of the gene encoding human lysosomal β-galactosidase. *DNA Cell Biol* **10**:495, 1991.
296. Nanba E, Suzuki K: Organization of the mouse acid β-galactosidase. *Biochem Biophys Res Commun* **178**:158, 1991.
297. Nishimoto J, Nanba E, Inui K, Okada S, Suzuki K: G_{M1}-gangliosidosis (genetic β-galactosidase deficiency): Identification of four mutations in different clinical phenotypes among Japanese patients. *Am J Hum Genet* **49**:566, 1991.
298. Chakraborty S, Rafi MA, Wenger DA: Mutations in the lysosomal β-galactosidase gene that cause the adult form of G_{M1} gangliosidosis. *Am J Hum Genet* **54**:1004, 1994.
299. Mosna G, Fattore S, Tubiello G, Brocca S, Trubia M, Gianazza E, Gatti R, Danesino C, Minelli A, Piantanida M: A homozygous missense arginine to histidine substitution at position 482 of the β-galactosidase in an Italian infantile G_{M1}-gangliosidosis patient. *Hum Genet* **90**:247, 1992.

300. Boustany R-M, Qian W-H, Suzuki K: Mutations in acid β-galactosidase cause G_{M1}-gangliosidosis in American patients. *Am J Hum Genet* **53**:881, 1993.
301. Morrone A, Morreau H, Zhou XY, Zammarchi E, Kleijer WJ, Galjaard H, D'Azzo A: Insertion of a T next to the donor splice site of intron 1 causes aberrantly spliced mRNA in a case of infantile G_{M1}-gangliosidosis. *Hum Mutat* **3**:112, 1994.
302. Ishii N, Oshima A, Sakuraba H, Osawa M, Suzuki Y: β-Galactosidosis (genetic β-galactosidase deficiency): Clinical and genetic heterogeneity of the skeletal form. *Dev Brain Dysfunct* **8**:40, 1995.
303. Chiu NC, Qian WH, Shanske AL, Brooks SS, Boustany RM: A common mutation site in the β-galactosidase gene originates in Puerto Rico. *Pediatr Neurol* **14**:53, 1996.
304. Kaye EM, Shalish C, Livermore J, Taylor HA, Stevenson RE, Breakefield XO: β-Galactosidase gene mutations in patients with slowly progressive G_{M1} gangliosidosis. *J Child Neurol* **12**:242, 1997.
305. Oshima A, Yoshida K, Ishizaki A, Shimmoto M, Fukuhara Y, Sakuraba H, Suzuki Y: G_{M1}-gangliosidosis: Tandem duplication within exon 3 of β-galactosidase gene in an infantile patient. *Clin Genet* **41**:235, 1992.
306. Fukushima H, Tsukamoto H, Nishimoto J, Inui K, Minami R, Ishikawa Y, Okada S: A new gene mutation in juvenile G_{M1}-gangliosidosis. *J Inherit Metab Dis* **9**:112, 1993.
307. Hadjiconstantinou M, Neff NH: G_{M1} ganglioside: In vivo and in vitro trophic actions on central neurotransmitter systems. *J Neurochem* **70**:1335, 1998.
308. Purpura DP, Suzuki K: Distortion of neuronal geometry and formation of aberrant synapses in neuronal storage disease. *Brain Res* **116**:1, 1976.
309. Purpura DP: Ectopic dendritic growth in mature pyramidal neurones in human ganglioside storage disease. *Nature* **276**:520, 1978.
310. Wu G, Nakamura K, Ledeen RW: Inhibition of neurite outgrowth of neuroblastoma Neuro-2A cells by cholera toxin B-subunit and anti-G_{M1} antibody. *Mol Chem Neuropathol* **21**:259, 1994.
311. Purpura DP, Baker HJ: Meganeurites and other aberrant processes of neurons in feline G_{M1}-gangliosidosis: A Golgi study. *Brain Res* **143**:13, 1978.
312. Purpura DP, Pappas GD, Baker HJ: Fine structure of meganeurites and secondary growth processes in feline G_{M1}-gangliosidosis. *Brain Res* **143**:1, 1978.
313. Walkley SU, Baker HJ, Rattazzi MC: Initiation and growth of ectopic neurites and meganeurites during postnatal cortical development in ganglioside storage disease. *Brain Res Dev Brain Res* **51**:167, 1990.
314. Walkley SU, Wurzelmann S: Alterations in synaptic connectivity in cerebral cortex in neuronal storage disorders. *Ment Retard Dev Disabil Res Rev* **1**:183, 1995.
315. Wu G, Lu Z-H, Ledeen RW: Induced and spontaneous neurogenesis are associated with enhanced expression of ganglioside G_{M1} in the nuclear membrane. *J Neurosci* **15**:3739, 1995.
316. Byrne MC, Ledeen RW: Regional variation of brain gangliosides in feline G_{M1} gangliosidosis. *Exp Neurol* **81**:210, 1983.
317. Wood PA, McBride MR, Baker HJ, Christian ST: Fluorescence polarization analysis, lipid composition and Na^+,K^+-ATPase kinetics of synaptosomal membranes in feline G_{M1} and G_{M2}-gangliosidosis. *J Neurochem* **44**:947, 1985.
318. Mutoh T, Tokuda A, Miyadai T, Hamaguchi M, Fujiki N: Ganglioside G_{M1} binds to the Trk protein and regulates receptor function. *Proc Natl Acad Sci U S A* **92**:5087, 1995.
319. Rabin SJ, Mocchetti I: G_{M1} ganglioside activates the high-affinity nerve growth factor receptor *trkA*. *J Neurochem* **65**:347, 1995.
320. Duchemin AM, Neff NH, Hadjiconstantinou M: G_{M1} increases the content and mRNA of NGF in the brain of aged rats. *NeuroReport* **8**:3823, 1997.
321. Baker HJ, Jope RS: Increased metabolism of acetylcholine in brain of cats with G_{M1} gangliosidosis. *Brain Res* **343**:363, 1985.
322. Jope RS, Baker HJ, Conner DJ: Increased acetylcholine synthesis and release in brains of cats with G_{M1} gangliosidosis. *J Neurochem* **46**:1567, 1986.
323. Gugliotta P, Pacchioni D, Bussolati G: Staining reaction for β-galactosidase in immunocytochemistry and *in situ* hybridization. *Eur J Histochem* **36**:143, 1992.
324. Singer HS, Coyle JT, Weaver DL, Kawamura N, Baker HJ: Neurotransmitter chemistry in feline G_{M1} gangliosidosis: A model for human ganglioside storage disease. *Ann Neurol* **12**:37, 1982.
325. Walkley SU, Baker HJ, Rattazzi MC, Haskins ME, Wu JY: Neuroaxonal dystrophy in neuronal storage disorders: Evidence for major GABAergic neuron involvement. *J Neurol Sci* **104**:1, 1991.
326. Claro E, Wallace MA, Fain JN, Nair BG, Patel TB, Shanker G, Baker HJ: Altered phosphoinositide-specific phospholipase C and adenyl cyclase in brain cortical membranes of cats with G_{M1} and G_{M2} gangliosidosis. *Brain Res Mol Brain Res* **11**:265, 1991.
327. Wu G, Lu Z-H, Ledeen RW: G_{M1} ganglioside modulates prostaglandin E1 stimulated adenylyl cyclase in neuro-2A cells. *Glycoconjugate J* **13**:235, 1996.
328. Carlson RO, Masco D, Brooker G, Spiegel S: Endogenous ganglioside G_{M1} modulates L-type calcium channel activity in N18 neuroblastoma cells. *J Neurosci* **14**:2272, 1994.
329. Hungund BL, Zheng Z, Lin L, Barkai AI: Ganglioside G_{M1} reduces ethanol induced phospholipase A2 activity in synaptosomal preparations from mice. *Neurochem Int* **25**:321, 1994.
330. Ikeda S, Ushiyama M, Nakano T, Kikkawa T, Kondo K, Yanagisawa N: Ultrastructural findings of rectal and skin biopsies in adult G_{M1}-gangliosidosis. *Acta Pathol Jpn* **36**:1823, 1986.
331. Drut R: Eccrine sweat gland involvement in G_{M1} gangliosidosis. *J Cutan Pathol* **5**:35, 1978.
332. Boniuk V, Ghosh M, Galin MA: Conjunctival eye signs in G_{M1} type 1 gangliosidosis. *Birth Defects* **12**:543, 1976.
333. Berra B, di Palma S, Primi DA: High performance thin layer chromatography of neutral and acidic glycolipids: Application to the chemical diagnosis of lipid storage diseases. *Biochem Exp Biol* **13**:79, 1977.
334. Hirabayashi Y, Koketsu K, Higashi H, Suzuki Y, Matsumoto M, Sugimoto M, Ogawa T: Sensitive enzyme-immunostaining and densitometric determination of ganglio-series gangliosides on thin-layer plate: pmol detection of gangliosides in cerebrospinal fluid. *Biochim Biophys Acta* **876**:178, 1986.
335. Sewell AC, Gehler J, Spranger J: Urinary oligosaccharide screening in patients with β-galactosidase deficiency. *Eur J Pediatr* **133**:269, 1980.
336. Warner TG, Robertson AD, Mock AK, Johnson WG, O'Brien JS: Prenatal diagnosis of G_{M1} gangliosidosis by detection of galactosyl-oligosaccharides in amniotic fluid with high-performance liquid chromatography. *Am J Hum Genet* **35**:1034, 1983.
337. Tsuboyama A, Miki F, Yoshida M, Ogura Y, Miyatake T: The use of tears for diagnosis of G_{M1} gangliosidosis. *Clin Chim Acta* **80**:237, 1977.
338. Karpova EA, Voznyi Y, Dudukina TV, Tsvetkova IV: 4-Trifluoromethylumbelliferyl glycosides as new substrates for revealing diseases connected with hereditary deficiency of lysosome glycosidases. *Biochem Int* **24**:1135, 1991.
339. Kaneski CR, French SA, Brescia M-R, Harbour MJ, Miller SFP: Hydrolysis of a novel lysosomotropic enzyme substrate for β-galactosidase within intact cells. *J Lipid Res* **35**:1441, 1994.
340. Brustugun OT, Mellgren G, Gjertsen BT, Bjerkvig R, Doskeland SO: Sensitive and rapid detection of β-galactosidase expression in intact cells by microinjection of fluorescent substrate. *Exp Cell Res* **219**:372, 1995.
341. Fong TG, Neff NH, Hadjiconstantinou M: Systemic administration of G_{M1} ganglioside increases choline acetyltransferase activity in the brain of aged rats. *Exp Neurol* **132**:157, 1995.
342. Lowden JA, Cutz E, Conen PE, Rudd N, Doran TA: Prenatal diagnosis of G_{M1}-gangliosidosis. *N Engl J Med* **288**:225, 1973.
343. Booth CW, Gerbie AB, Nadler HL: Intrauterine detection of G_{M1}-gangliosidosis, type 2. *Pediatrics* **52**:521, 1973.
344. Kaback MM, Sloan HR, Sonneborn M, Herndon RM: G_{M1}-gangliosidosis type I: in utero detection and fetal manifestations. *J Pediatr* **82**:1037, 1973.
345. Kleijer WJ, Van der Veer E, Niermeijer MF: Rapid prenatal diagnosis of G_{M1}-gangliosidosis using microchemical methods. *Hum Genet* **33**:299, 1976.
346. Kudoh T, Kikuchi K, Nakamura F, Yokoyama S, Karube K, Tsugawa S, Minami R, Nakao T: Prenatal diagnosis of G_{M1}-gangliosidosis: Biochemical manifestations in fetal tissues. *Hum Genet* **44**:287, 1978.
347. Ida H, Eto Y, Maekawa K: G_{M1}-gangliosidosis: Morphological and biochemical studies. *Brain Dev* **11**:394, 1989.
348. Poenaru L: First trimester prenatal diagnosis of metabolic diseases: A survey in countries from the European Community. *Prenat Diag* **7**:333, 1987.
349. Percy AK, McCormick UM, Kaback MM, Herndon RM: Ultrastructure manifestations of G_{M1} and G_{M2} gangliosidosis in fetal tissues. *Arch Neurol* **28**:417, 1973.
350. Yamano T, Shimada M, Okada S, Yutaka T, Kato T, Inui K, Yabuuchi H: Ultrastructural study on nervous system of fetus with G_{M1}-gangliosidosis type 1. *Acta Neuropathol* **61**:15, 1983.

351. Cogan DG, Kuwabara T, Kolodny E, Driscoll S: Gangliosidoses and the fetal retina. *Ophthalmology* **91**:508, 1984.
352. Bieber FR, Mortimer G, Kolodny EH, Driscoll SG: Pathologic findings in fetal G_{M1} gangliosidosis. *Arch Neurol* **43**:736, 1986.
353. Schmitt Graff A: Manifestation of infantile G_{M1} gangliosidosis in the fetal eye. An electron microscopic study. *Graefes Arch Clin Exp Ophthalmol* **226**:84, 1988.
354. O'Brien JS, Storb R, Raff RF, Harding J, Appelbaum F, Morimoto S, Kishimoto Y, Graham T, Ahern Rindell A, O'Brien SL: Bone marrow transplantation in canine G_{M1} gangliosidosis. *Clin Genet* **38**:274, 1990.
355. Tylki Szymanska A, Maciejko D, Kidawa M, Jablonska Budaj U, Czartoryska B: Amniotic tissue transplantation as a trial of treatment in some lysosomal storage diseases. *J Inherit Metab Dis* **8**:101, 1985.
356. Ushiyama M, Hanyu N, Ikeda S, Yanagisawa N: A case of type III (adult) G_{M1}-gangliosidosis that improved markedly with trihexyphenidyl. *Clin Neurol* **26**:221, 1986.
357. Baker HJJ, Lindsey JR, McKhann GM, Farrell DF: Neuronal G_{M1}-gangliosidosis in a Siamese cat with β-galactosidase deficiency. *Science* **174**:838, 1971.
358. Handa S, Yamakawa T: Biochemical studies in cat and human gangliosidosis. *J Neurochem* **18**:1275, 1971.
359. Blakemore WF: G_{M1}-Gangliosidosis in a cat. *J Comp Pathol* **82**:179, 1972.
360. Barnes IC, Kelly DF, Pennock CA, Randall JA: Hepatic β-galactosidase and feline G_{M1}-gangliosidosis. *Neuropathol Appl Neurobiol* **7**:463, 1981.
361. Read DH, Harrington DD, Keenana TW, Hinsman EJ: Neuronal-visceral G_{M1} gangliosidosis in a dog with β-galactosidase deficiency. *Science* **194**:442, 1976.
362. Rodriguez M, O'Brien JS, Garrett RS, Powell HC: Canine G_{M1}-gangliosidosis. An ultrastructural and biochemical study. *J Neuropathol Exp Neurol* **41**:618, 1982.
363. Alroy J, Orgad U, Ucci AA, Schelling SH, Schunk KL, Warren CD, Raghavan SS, Kolodny EH: Neurovisceral and skeletal G_{M1}-gangliosidosis in dogs with β-galactosidase deficiency. *Science* **229**:470, 1985.
364. Saunders GK, Wood PA, Myers RK, Shell LG, Carithers R: G_{M1}-gangliosidosis in Portuguese water dogs: Pathologic and biochemical findings. *Vet Pathol* **25**:265, 1988.
365. Ahern-Rindell AJ, Murnane RD, Prieur DJ: β-Galactosidase activity in fibroblasts and tissues from sheep with a lysosomal storage disease. *Biochem Genet* **26**:733, 1988.
366. Prieur DJ, Ahern Rindell AJ, Murnane RD: Ovine G_{M1}-gangliosidosis. *Am J Pathol* **139**:1511, 1991.
367. Skelly BJ, Jeffrey M, Franklin RJM, Winchester BG: A new form of ovine G_{M1}-gangliosidosis. *Acta Neuropathol* **89**:374, 1995.
368. Murnane RD, Prieur DJ, Ahern-Rindell AJ, Parish SM, Collier LL: The lesions of an ovine lysosomal storage disease. Initial characterization. *Am J Pathol* **134**:263, 1989.
369. Donnelly WJ, Sheahan BJ, Kelly M: β-Galactosidase deficiency in G_{M1}-gangliosidosis of Friesian calves. *Res Vet Sci* **15**:139, 1973.
370. Donnelly WJ, Sheahan BJ, Rogers TA: G_{M1} gangliosidosis in Friesian calves. *J Pathol* **111**:173, 1973.
371. Donnelly WJ, Kelly M: Leukocyte β-galactosidase activity in the diagnosis of bovine G_{M1} gangliosidosis. *Vet Rec* **100**:318, 1977.
372. Matsuda J, Suzuki O, Oshima A, Ogura A, Naiki M, Suzuki Y: Neurological manifestations of knockout mice with β-galactosidase deficiency. *Brain Dev* **19**:19, 1997.
373. Matsuda J, Suzuki O, Oshima A, Ogura A, Noguchi Y, Yamamoto Y, Asano T, Takimoto K, Sukegawa K, Suzuki Y, Naiki M: β-Galactosidase-deficient mouse as an animal model for G_{M1}-gangliosidosis. *Glycoconjugate J* **14**:729, 1997.
374. Hahn CN, del Pilar M, Schroder M, Vanier MT, Hara Y, Suzuki K, D'Azzo A: Generalized CNS disease and massive G_{M1}-ganglioside accumulation in mice defective in lysosomal acid β-galactosidase. *Hum Mol Genet* **6**:205, 1997.
375. Farrell DF, Baker HJ, Herndon RM, Lindsey JR, McKhann GM: Feline G_{M1}-gangliosidosis: Biochemical and ultrastructural comparisons with the disease in man. *J Neuropathol Exp Neurol* **32**:1, 1973.
376. Baker HJ, Lindsey JR: Animal model: Feline G_{M1} gangliosidosis. *Am J Pathol* **74**:649, 1974.
377. Murray JA, Blakemore WF, Barnett KC: Ocular lesions in cats with G_{M1}-gangliosidosis with visceral involvement. *J Small Anim Prac* **18**:1, 1977.
378. Holmes EW, O'Brien JS: Feline G_{M1} gangliosidosis: Characterization of the residual liver acid β-galactosidase. *Am J Hum Genet* **30**:505, 1978.
379. Steiss JE, Baker HJ, Braund KG, Cox NR, Wright JC: Profile of electrodiagnostic abnormalities in cats with G_{M1} gangliosidosis. *Am J Vet Res* **58**:706, 1997.
380. Nowakowski RW, Thompson JN, Baker HJ: Diagnosis of feline G_{M1}-gangliosidosis by enzyme assay of cultured conjunctival cells. *Invest Ophthalmol Vis Sci* **29**:487, 1988.
381. Karabelas AB, Walkley SU: Altered patterns of evoked synaptic activity in cortical pyramidal neurons in feline ganglioside storage disease. *Brain Res* **339**:329, 1985.
382. Koenig ML, Jope RS, Baker HJ, Lally KM: Reduced Ca^{2+} flux in synaptosomes from cats with G_{M1} gangliosidosis. *Brain Res* **424**:169, 1987.
383. Shanker G, Baker HJ: Phorbol ester receptors in cerebral cortex of cats with G_{M1} gangliosidosis. *Neurochem Res* **16**:11, 1991.
384. Alroy J, Orgad U, De Gasperi R, Richard R, Warren CD, Knowles K, Thalhammer JG, Raghavan SS: Canine G_{M1}-gangliosidosis. A clinical, morphologic, histochemical, and biochemical comparison of two different models. *Am J Pathol* **140**:675, 1992.
385. Shell LG, Potthoff AI, Carithers R, Katherman A, Saunders GK, Wood PA, Giger U: Neuronal-visceral G_{M1} gangliosidosis in Portuguese water dogs. *J Vet Intern Med* **3**:1, 1989.
386. Alroy J, Knowles K, Schelling SH, Kaye EM, Rosenberg AE: Retarded bone formation in G_{M1}-gangliosidosis: A study of the infantile form and comparison with two canine models. *Virchows Archiv* **426**:141, 1995.
387. Kaye EM, Alroy J, Raghavan SS, Schwarting GA, Adelman LS, Runge V, Gelblum D, Thalhammer JG, Zuniga G: Dysmyelinogenesis in animal model of G_{M1} gangliosidosis. *Pediatr Neurol* **8**:255, 1992.
388. Rittmann LS, Tennant LL, O'Brien JS: Dog G_{M1} gangliosidosis: Characterization of the residual liver acid β-galactosidase. *Am J Hum Genet* **32**:880, 1980.
389. Hubert JJ, O'Brien JS: Dog and human acid β-D-galactosidases are structurally similar. *Biochem J* **213**:473, 1983.
390. Ahern-Rindell AJ, Kretz KA, O'Brien JS: Comparison of the canine and human acid β-galactosidase gene. *Am J Med Genet* **63**:340, 1996.
391. Alroy J, De Gasperi R, Warren CD: Application of lectin histochemistry and carbohydrate analysis to the characterization of lysosomal storage diseases. *Carbohydr Res* **213**:229, 1991.
392. Murnane RD, Ahern-Rindell AJ, Prieur DJ: Ultrastructural lesions of ovine G_{M1} gangliosidosis. *Modern Pathol* **4**:755, 1991.
393. Murnane RD, Ahern-Rindell AJ, Prieur DJ: Lectin histochemistry of an ovine lysosomal storage disease with deficiency of β-galactosidase and α-neuraminidase. *Am J Pathol* **135**:623, 1989.
394. Ahern-Rindell AJ, Murnane RD, Prieur DJ: Interspecific genetic complementation analysis of human and sheep fibroblasts with β-galactosidase deficiency. *Somat Cell Mol Genet* **15**:525, 1989.
395. Ahern-Rindell AJ, Prieur DJ, Murnane RD, Raghavan SS, Daniel PF, McCluer RH, Walkley SU, Parish SM: Inherited lysosomal storage disease associated with deficiencies of β-galactosidase and α-neuraminidase in sheep. *Am J Med Genet* **31**:39, 1988.
396. Murnane RD, Prieur DJ, Ahern-Rindell AJ, Holler LD, Parish SM: Clinical and clinicopathologic characteristics of ovine G_{M1} gangliosidosis. *J Vet Intern Med* **8**:221, 1994.
397. Murnane RD, Wright RWJ, Ahern Rindell AJ, Prieur DJ: Prenatal lesions in an ovine fetus with G_{M1} gangliosidosis. *Am J Med Genet* **39**:106, 1991.
398. Johnson AH, Donnelly WJ, Sheahan BJ: The glycosaminoglycan content of the liver in bovine G_{M1} gangliosidosis. *Res Vet Sci* **22**:256, 1977.
399. Sheahan BJ, Donnelly WJ, Grimes TD: Ocular pathology of bovine G_{M1}-gangliosidosis. *Acta Neuropathol* **41**:91, 1978.
400. Riboni L, Caminiti A, Bassi R, Tettamanti G: The degradative pathway of gangliosides G_{M1} and G_{M2} in neuro-2a cells by sialidase. *J Neurochem* **64**:451, 1995.
401. Venn G, Mason RM: Absence of keratan sulphate from skeletal tissues of mouse and rat. *Biochem J* **228**:443, 1985.
402. Wikstrom B, Engfeldt B, Heinegard D, Hjerpe A: Proteoglycans and glycosaminoglycans in cartilage from the brachymorphic (*bm/bm*) mouse. *Collagen Related Res* **5**:193, 1985.

CHAPTER 152

Galactosialidosis

Alessandra d'Azzo ▪ Generoso Andria
Pietro Strisciuglio ▪ Hans Galjaard

1. **Galactosialidosis is a lysosomal storage disease associated with a combined deficiency of β-galactosidase and neuraminidase, secondary to a defect of another lysosomal protein, the protective protein/cathepsin A (PPCA).**
2. **All patients have clinical manifestations typical of a lysosomal disorder, such as coarse facies, cherry-red spots, vertebral changes, foam cells in the bone marrow, and vacuolated lymphocytes. Three phenotypic subtypes are recognized. The early infantile form is associated with fetal hydrops, edema, ascites, visceromegaly, skeletal dysplasia, and early death. Hepatosplenomegaly, growth retardation, cardiac involvement, and rare occurrence of important neurologic signs characterize the late infantile type. The majority of reported patients belong to the juvenile/adult group and are mainly of Japanese origin. Myoclonus, ataxia, angiokeratoma, mental retardation, neurologic deterioration, absence of visceromegaly, and long survival are quite characteristic of this subtype.**
3. **Sialyloligosaccharides accumulate in lysosomes and are excreted in body fluids. Ultrastructural analysis of central, peripheral, and autonomic nervous systems, retina, liver, kidney, skin, and lymphocytes shows numerous membrane-bound vacuoles and, in some tissues, many membranous cytoplasmic bodies.**
4. **The autosomal gene encoding human PPCA that has been localized on chromosome 20q13.1 transmits the disorder. The PPCA cDNA and genomic sequences have been used to analyze the mutations causing galactosialidosis. Mainly single-base substitutions or splice-junction defects have been identified in patients with different clinical phenotypes. Correlation of genotype with disease severity has emerged from structure/function studies of the mutant enzyme.**
5. **PPCA associates with β-galactosidase and neuraminidase in an early biosynthetic compartment. By virtue of this association the two glycosidases are correctly routed to the lysosome and are protected against rapid intralysosomal proteolysis. Mammalian PPCA is a multifunctional enzyme with distinct protective and catalytic activities. It is synthesized as a 54-kDa precursor that is processed into two disulfide-linked chains of 32 and 20 kDa by endoproteolytic removal of a 2-kDa peptide. The enzyme is active at both acidic and neutral pH and functions as cathepsin A/deamidase/esterase on a subset of neuropeptides, including substance P, oxytocin, and endothelin I. This activity was found to be deficient in all patients with galactosialidosis so far tested.**
6. **The three-dimensional structure of the PPCA precursor has been solved by a combination of molecular replacement and twofold density averaging. The structure revealed an unusual inactivation mechanism of the zymogen that explains how removal of the 2-kDa peptide triggers activation. A number of amino acid substitutions found in defective PPCA from different galactosialidosis patients have been localized in the three-dimensional structure. There appears to be a significant correlation between the effect of each mutation on the integrity of protein structure and the general severity of the clinical phenotype.**
7. **The disease can be suspected in patients with clinical features of a lysosomal storage disease showing sialyloligosacchariduria on thin-layer chromatography. The demonstration of a combined deficiency of β-galactosidase and neuraminidase in lymphocytes and/or cultured skin fibroblasts is the preferred method of biochemical diagnosis. Assaying only the cathepsin A activity of PPCA might give a false negative result because, in principle, a mutation could affect the protective function but not the catalytic activity. However, carrier detection should be based on assays involving the primary defect.**
8. **Prenatal diagnosis has been established by demonstrating a combined β-galactosidase/neuraminidase deficiency in cultured amniotic fluid cells. Furthermore, sialyloligosaccharides in deproteinized amniotic fluid supernatant were detected in the case of an affected fetus.**
9. **Mice homozygous for a null mutation at the PPCA locus develop a phenotype closely resembling human patients with the severe form of galactosialidosis. Excessive excretion of sialyloligosaccharides in urine is diagnostic of the disease. Systemic organ pathology can be fully corrected by transplanting null mutants with bone marrow from transgenic mice overexpressing human PPCA in specific hemopoietic lineages.**

HISTORICAL ASPECTS

In the years after Okada and O'Brien's[1] discovery that β-galactosidase deficiency was the primary defect in generalized gangliosidosis, a dozen or so patients with different clinical features and time of onset of symptoms were reported. Some were presented as having a new variant of G_{M1} gangliosidosis, distinct from the infantile and juvenile forms of the disease but with similar residual activity for the enzyme.[2–11]

Complementation studies after somatic cell hybridization[12] revealed that the 3-year-old patient described by Pinsky et al.[8] and the adult patient reported by Loonen et al.[9] had different gene mutations from those present in patients with the infantile or juvenile form of G_{M1} gangliosidosis. These results were difficult to explain by the sole involvement of β-galactosidase[12–14] because this enzyme was known to exist in different aggregated forms of one polypeptide[15] and intragenic complementation had never been described in mammalian cells.

In 1978, Wenger et al.[16] discovered a coexistent deficiency of neuraminidase and β-galactosidase in leukocytes and cultured

A list of standard abbreviations is located immediately preceding the index in each volume. Additional abbreviations used in this chapter include: PPCA = protective protein/cathepsin A; CPY = carboxypeptidase Y; CPW = wheat serine carboxypeptide; DFP = diisopropylfluorophosphate.

fibroblasts from a 12-year-old patient, previously considered a variant form of G_{M1} gangliosidosis.[17] A similar combined deficiency was subsequently detected in patients belonging to one of the complementation groups mentioned above and in other patients with atypical symptoms of single β-galactosidase and/or neuraminidase deficiency.[18–24] At that time, most investigators believed that the neuraminidase deficiency was the primary cause of the disease in these patients. However, complementation studies[25] demonstrated that neuraminidase activity was corrected in heterokaryons obtained by fusion of fibroblasts from patients with a combined β-galactosidase/neuraminidase deficiency with fibroblasts from sialidosis patients with an isolated neuraminidase deficiency. In the same study, cocultivation of the two cell types led to a partial restoration of neuraminidase activity in the β-galactosidase/neuraminidase-deficient cells. It was postulated that a third glycoprotein could be responsible for correcting an essential posttranslational processing step of the two glycosidases. Subsequently, this "corrective factor" was shown to restore both β-galactosidase and neuraminidase activities in cells with a combined deficiency.[26]

Using a suicide substrate for β-galactosidase, van Diggelen et al.[27] demonstrated that in β-galactosidase/neuraminidase-deficient cells this enzyme had normal hydrolytic properties but its half-life was reduced to less than 1 day, as compared to 10 days in normal cells. Uptake experiments with purified placental β-galactosidase further established that the enhanced turnover of β-galactosidase in mutant cells was caused by rapid degradation of the enzyme molecules,[28] which could partly be prevented by inhibitors of lysosomal proteases.[29–31]

The elucidation of the specific defect[31] identified the disorder associated with a combined β-galactosidase/neuraminidase deficiency as a new clinical and biochemical condition that was designated galactosialidosis.[32]

CLINICAL MANIFESTATIONS

The number of patients with a clear-cut diagnosis of galactosialidosis, reported in the literature or known to us, is approximately 80 (Table 152-1). They have been classified in the three following categories,[32,33] based on age of onset and severity of clinical manifestations: early (severe) infantile type, late (mild) infantile type, and juvenile/adult type.

Early Infantile Type

The early (severe) infantile form of galactosialidosis has been observed in 19 patients[20,34–48] who presented between birth and 3 months of age with fetal hydrops, neonatal edema, kidney involvement (proteinuria), coarse facies, inguinal hernias, and telangiectasias. Telangiectasias have been rarely reported in the other two phenotypes. The patients also developed visceromegaly, psychomotor delay, and skeletal changes, particularly in the spine. Skeletal changes were less prominent in patients with the early

Table 152-1 Clinical Features of Galactosialidosis

	Early Infantile	Late Infantile	Juvenile/Adult
Number of patients (families)	20 (19)	13 (12)	49 (38)
Sex (male/female)	7M/10F	7M/6F	30M/19F
Ethnic origin (Japanese/Caucasian)	5J/12C	10C	42J/4C
Families with parental consanguinity	5/19	3/10	18/36
Age at onset of symptoms (mean)	0–90 (12) days	0–48 (11)	1–40 (16) years
Coarse facies	17/18	10/10	48/49
Macrocephaly	1/4	7/10	3/8
Growth disturbance	6/6	7/11	15/24
Hepatosplenomegaly	18/18	13/13	5/41
Fetal hydrops, ascites	14/14	2/6	0/23
Kidney involvement	6/8	4/8	0/10
Heart involvement	7/9	8/9	16/16
Hernias	7/10	7/7	8/11
Angiokeratoma	2/8	2/7	21/41
Telangiectasias	7/8	1/5	2/6
Seizures	1/5	2/5	13/30
Myoclonus	0/4	1/7	35/47
Ataxia		0/6	32/41
Pyramidal tract signs	1/4	3/7	8/30
Progressive neurologic course	5/5	1/6	18/23
Mental retardation	11/11	7/11	20/45
Cherry-red spots	3/12	5/11	30/41
Lens opacity	1/4	2/7	11/18
Corneal clouding	5/8	5/8	32/40
Loss of visual acuity	2/3	1/5	32/35
Hearing loss	1/2	5/7	18/31
Joint stiffness	6/10	2/6	9/13
Dysostosis multiplex	7/7	6/8	10/15
Vertebral changes	8/9	6/9	34/35
Foam cells (lymphocytes/bone marrow)	12/12	8/8	24/24
Course: alive	0/19	12/13	45/48
Course: age at last exam (range/mean)		1–26/13 years	3–59/28 years
Course: dead	18/18	1/13	3/45
Course: age at death (range/mean)	0–20/7 months	15	13–45/27 years

The table is based on the case reports quoted in the section "Clinical Manifestations." Updates of reported patients and data on unpublished cases were kindly provided by Drs. G. Berry, N.U. Bosshard, R. Giugliani, A. Groener, G. Hoganson, A. Nivelon-Chevalier, S. Savasta, K. Ullrich, and G. Watters.

infantile form than in those with the late infantile or juvenile/adult forms, possibly because of their short life span. Ocular abnormalities, such as corneal clouding and fundal changes, ranging from a grayish disk to a cherry-red spot, have been described in five infants.[34,35,41,42] Heart involvement consisting of cardiomegaly, thickened septum, and cardiac failure has often been documented.[34–36,40,43,44] Death occurred at an average age of 7 months, probably as a result of renal and cardiac failure.[37,40] The early infantile type of galactosialidosis may be associated with fetal loss. Two families with a history of recurrent fetal hydrops were reported by Kleijer et al.[20] and Landau et al.[46] A further case with severe infantile presentation, characterized by an unusual association of congenital malformations, is not included in Table 152-1, because biochemical findings, including a high residual activity of neuraminidase, are not typical of galactosialidosis.[49]

Late Infantile Type

A distinct phenotype, defined as late (mild) infantile, has been observed in 13 patients.[8,32,43,50–57] They presented symptoms in the first months of life. One patient showed a severe neonatal presentation typical of the early infantile phenotype, with ascites and edema, and a mild course later on.[55] The clinical picture at onset was generally characterized by coarse facies (Fig. 152-1), hepatosplenomegaly, and dysostosis multiplex, affecting especially the spine. Cherry-red spots and/or corneal clouding were observed in six patients,[32,43,52,53,56,57] whereas no ocular abnormalities were detected in two others at the end of their second decade of life.[50,51] A Kayser-Fleischer ring was described in a 4-year-old patient.[54] In all patients but one, severe neurologic manifestations, such as myoclonus or ataxia, were absent. Seizures (generalized convulsions, petit mal) have been transiently observed in two patients.[8,32] Progressive neurologic course was reported in one case. Mental retardation, generally mild or very mild, was observed in seven patients.[8,32,53–56] Okamuro-Ono et al.[58] proposed a neurologic subgroup of late infantile galactosialidosis, mainly on the basis of four patients reported by Ozand et al.[43] However, these patients, not included in Table 152-1, showed normal activity of cathepsin A and a very low β-galactosidase residual activity. A common feature in late infantile patients seems to be the heart involvement, characterized by valvular disease. Echocardiography revealed thickened mitral and aortic valves with hemodynamic evidence of valvular insufficiency. Hearing loss of conductive or mixed type is frequently noted. All patients but one are alive. A growth disturbance, partly due to the spine involvement and often associated with muscular atrophy, is apparent in the majority of these patients.

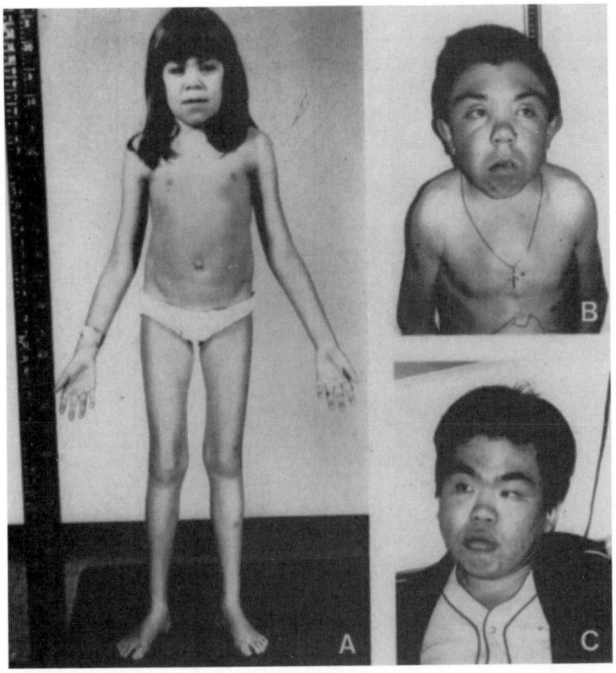

Fig. 152-1 Clinical features of galactosialidosis. ***A,*** **An 8.5-year-old girl with the late infantile form of the disease. (*Courtesy of Dr. William S. Sly.*)** ***B,*** **An 18-year-old patient with late infantile galactosialidosis.** ***C,*** **A 17-year-old juvenile patient. (*Courtesy of Dr. Yoshiyuki Suzuki.*)**

Juvenile/Adult Type

Approximately 60 percent of the reported patients can be classified in the group of juvenile/adult galactosialidosis.[6,10,16,21,22,36,37,59–68] The reason for this dual designation is that the clinical course is variable and characterized by a broad and continuous spectrum of severity and age of onset. The mean age of presentation is 16 years, but in one patient, the first symptoms appeared as late as 40 years of age,[37] and in another patient, the first symptoms appeared as early as 1 year of age.[62] Patients with juvenile/adult galactosialidosis are mostly of Japanese origin. Parental consanguinity has been reported in half of the families. Coarse facies is a recurrent finding, although it is less marked than in other lysosomal storage diseases (see Fig. 152-1). Spinal changes, like platyspondylia of thoracic and lumbar vertebrae, are commonly diagnosed, whereas more general dysostosis multiplex seems rare. Major neurologic manifestations include myoclonus, cerebellar ataxia, generalized seizures, and mental retardation with deterioration. Hyperactive deep tendon reflexes are more frequently observed than clear-cut pyramidal tract signs.[36] Typical eye abnormalities consist of bilateral cherry-red spots and corneal clouding with loss of visual acuity, which presents in the second decade of life. Punctate lens opacity was reported in a few patients. Color blindness has been diagnosed in 5 of 29 male patients.[59,62] Angiokeratoma, similar to that observed in Fabry disease and fucosidosis, is present in about half of the juvenile/adult patients and observed almost exclusively in this category of galactosialidosis. This skin lesion has been noticed as early as 3 years of age[37,62] and as late as the fourth decade of life.[21] Nearly all patients have a normal-size liver and spleen, in striking contrast with the patients having the infantile forms.

In summary, all galactosialidosis patients present with clinical features suggestive of a lysosomal storage disease, including coarse facies, cherry-red spots, vertebral changes, foam cells in the bone marrow, and vacuolated lymphocytes in blood smears. Fetal hydrops, ascites, and kidney failure are specific for the early infantile form. The late infantile type seems to be characterized by hepatosplenomegaly, growth retardation, cardiac involvement, and rare occurrence of important neurologic signs. The presence of myoclonus, ataxia, and angiokeratoma in patients who have no visceromegaly is typical of the juvenile/adult form.

The clinical phenotypes of galactosialidosis resemble those described in sialidosis, due to the isolated deficiency of neuraminidase (the reader is referred to Chap. 140 for details on the clinical, biochemical, and genetic aspects of this disorder). The most striking similarity is between the early infantile form of galactosialidosis and the so-called congenital form of sialidosis: visceromegaly, hydrops, ascites, and early death characterize both phenotypes. At the other end of the spectrum, a comparison might be attempted between the forms with a later onset (juvenile/adult). Both groups share the absence of visceromegaly and most neurologic and ocular manifestations, namely myoclonus, ataxia, seizures, cherry-red spots, and loss of visual acuity. However, adult-onset sialidosis patients lack any dysmorphic features. The late infantile/childhood forms of galactosialidosis and sialidosis are also similar except for the milder neurologic involvement in the galactosialidosis patients. These observations point to a major role for neuraminidase deficiency in the pathogenesis of galactosialidosis. A clear understanding of the contribution of the cathepsin A deficiency and partial β-galactosidase deficiency to the phenotypic abnormalities present in galactosialidosis awaits further biochemical and clinical assessments.

PATHOLOGY

Morphologic Studies

Pathologic studies of brain, peripheral and autonomic nervous systems, retina and optic nerve, liver, kidney, skin, rectal mucosa, and small intestine have been reported in a few patients.

Postmortem examination of a 14-month-old girl with the early infantile form of the disease showed multiple cortical-subcortical infarctions in the brain due to a compromised circulation as a consequence of endothelial luminal encroachment.[45] Extensive vacuolation was detected by electron microscopy in the endothelial cells lining the cerebral blood vessels, in neurons and glial cells of the brain and the spinal cord, and in liver and kidney specimens.[45] Because endothelial vacuolation and focal cerebrovascular lesions had not been previously described, these authors suggested that these features could be specific for the severe early infantile form of the disease. Other ultrastructural neuronal findings were similar to those reported in other juvenile/adult cases, as described below.

Macroscopic examination of the brain during autopsy of a 13-year-old boy with the juvenile form showed marked atrophy of the globus pallidus, thalamus, dentate nucleus, and optic nerves.[69] Light microscopy indicated a severe neuronal loss with fibrillary gliosis in the globus pallidus, thalamus, and cerebellum. Abundant storage materials were seen in the basal forebrain and motor nuclei of the spinal cord and brain stem.[69] Histochemical analysis revealed that the storage material was heterogeneous and differed in the neurons from various anatomic regions. In the basal ganglia, thalamus, and dentate nucleus, the storage material was autofluorescent and strongly positive for Sudan black B and periodic acid-Schiff (PAS) staining. In the motor nuclei of spinal cord and brain stem, the storage material was not autofluorescent and was negative for Sudan black B, but it was weakly positive for PAS staining. Ultrastructural investigation showed a variety of inclusions, such as membranous cytoplasmic bodies, parallel or wavy-lamellar structures, tortuous tubular inclusions, lipofuscin-like pleomorphic bodies, and cytoplasmic vacuoles with fine granules and lamellar material.[69] Similar neuropathologic findings were described in an adult patient with galactosialidosis,[70] as well as in the early infantile case.[45]

Ultrastructural examination of sural nerve biopsy or peripheral nerve bundles of the dermis revealed membrane-bound vacuoles containing fine granular material in the Schwann cells and perineurial and endoneurial epithelium.[19,67,71] The neurons in the paravertebral sympathetic ganglia and myenteric plexus of the rectum contained concentric lamellar inclusions.[19,67]

Gross examination of the retina and optic nerve in another Japanese patient[72] showed marked loss of ganglion cells in the retina as well as myelinated nerve fibers in the optic nerve. Histochemical staining revealed abnormal storage of phospholipids, proteinaceous material, and a lipofuscin-like substance in the residual swollen ganglion cells of the retina. Ultrastructural analysis showed two types of intracytoplasmic inclusion bodies in the retinal ganglion cells and amacrine cells. Some inclusion bodies showed an almost concentric, wavy, or partially parallel structure. Others were membrane-bound, with partially crossing and parallel lamellar structures, and tiny lipid droplets. The optic nerve showed no inclusion bodies.

Hepatocytes and Kupffer cells in the liver, as well as glomerular and tubular epithelial cells in the kidney, were filled with numerous membrane-bound vacuoles.[39,45,73] Vacuolar inclusions and concentric lamellar inclusions were seen in cultured skin fibroblasts.[74] Cytoplasmic vacuoles were also found in the endothelial cells of renal vessels or of biopsied angiokeratoma specimens.[39,45,71] Peripheral lymphocytes had several cytoplasmic vacuoles, which showed negative results when stained with Giemsa, PAS, toluidine blue, and Sudan black B and III. At electron microscopy examination, the vacuoles were membrane-bound and 0.5 to 1 μM in diameter.[19,39]

These pathologic findings are similar to those seen in G_{M1} gangliosidosis and sialidosis.[75,76] (for details see Chaps. 140 and 151).

THE METABOLIC DEFECT IN GALACTOSIALIDOSIS

Chemical Analysis of Storage Compounds

Glycoproteins have a polypeptide backbone with covalently linked carbohydrate chains that present a great structural heterogeneity. One of the major classes of carbohydrate chains in glycoproteins consists of the *N*-glycosidic chains, characterized by the linkage of *N*-acetylglucosamine to asparagine.[77] The other group of carbohydrate chains commonly present in glycoproteins involves an *O*-glycosidic linkage of *N*-acetylgalactosamine to threonine or serine. Sialic acid residues are usually present at the nonreducing terminus of both types of carbohydrate chains, linked by either α2-3 or α2-6 bonds.

A primary or secondary neuraminidase defect affects the cleavage of both α2-3- and α2-6-linked sialic acid residues,[78] leading to accumulation of *N*-acetyllactosamine type of sialyloligosaccharides, with the mannose β1-4 *N*-acetylglucosamine sequence at the reducing terminus in common.[79–84]

Sialyloligosaccharides. Isolation and structural characterization of sialic acid-bound storage compounds has been performed in fibroblasts and urine (Fig. 152-2) of sialidosis and galactosialidosis patients.[85,86] In addition, sialyloligosaccharides have been analyzed from the placenta of a fetus with galactosialidosis.[87] In both sialidosis and galactosialidosis fibroblasts, the same fully sialylated di- and triantennary oligosaccharides of the *N*-glycosidic type were detected.[85] The only difference was the presence of more α2-6-linked sialic acid in accumulated oligosaccharides of sialidosis fibroblasts. A comparative study of storage compounds from urine of galactosialidosis and sialidosis patients also showed that the same sialyloligosaccharides are present in both diseases.[86] Again the sialylated compounds in the urine of sialidosis patients had predominantly α2-6-linked sialic acid residues. Some partially sialylated carbohydrate chains were also isolated from urine of sialidosis and galactosialidosis patients. These compounds are probably formed in body fluids, because they are not detected in cultured fibroblasts from these patients (Fig. 152-2). The structural characterization of storage compounds from the placenta of a human galactosialidosis fetus revealed 16 fully sialylated oligosaccharides of the *N*-glycosidic type.[87] None of them presented terminal galactose residues.

These results indicate that there are no significant differences in the sialyloligosaccharides isolated from urine and fibroblasts of patients affected with either sialidosis or galactosialidosis. The additional β-galactosidase deficiency in the disease does not seem to play a role in the pathogenesis. Alternatively, the residual β-galactosidase activity might be sufficient to remove terminal galactose residues. Finally, the difference in the relative amounts of α2-6- versus α2-3-bound sialic acid residues in stored oligosaccharides isolated from patients' materials could be due to a different residual activity and/or specificity of neuraminidase toward sialic acid α2-3 and α2-6 linkages. Another explanation might be that there is a variation in the activity of sialyltransferases.[86] No studies are available on products of O-linked glycosidic chains that are also expected to accumulate in disorders associated with neuraminidase deficiency.

Other Compounds. Accumulation of G_{M3}, G_{M2}, G_{M1}, and G_{D1a} gangliosides has been described in sympathetic and spinal ganglia and in gray matter of the spinal cord of juvenile/adult galactosialidosis patients.[60,67] Lactose ceramide G_{A2} and G_{A1} gangliosides were also accumulated in sympathetic and spinal

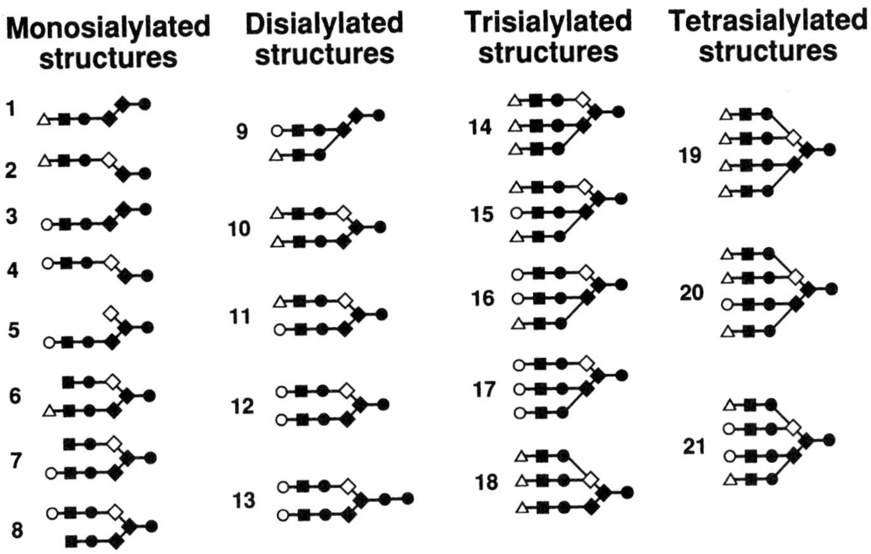

Fig. 152-2 Structures of sialyloligosaccharides isolated from galactosialidosis urine. The structures are represented by shorthand symbolic notation: ■ = Gal; ● = GlcNAc; ◆ = Man α1-3; ◇ = Man α1-6; ○ = NeuAc α2-6; △ = NeuAc α2-3. (*Adapted from J. van Pelt et al.*[173])

ganglia. The defect of lysosomal neuraminidase might play a role in the degradation of G_{M3} and G_{D1a} gangliosides, as suggested by in vivo studies.[88] In vitro experiments have confirmed this hypothesis and have also shown that ganglioside catabolism by lysosomal neuraminidase might require the sphingomyelin activator.[70,89]

The accumulation of G_{M1} ganglioside has been suggested to be a consequence of the decreased β-galactosidase activity.[60] Storage of an amylopectin-like polysaccharide was demonstrated in the liver of a patient with juvenile galactosialidosis.[73]

The Elucidation of the Primary Defect

Evidence for the existence of PPCA as a distinct biochemical entity came from studies on human β-galactosidase and neuraminidase in normal and deficient fibroblasts and tissues. Initial immunoprecipitation experiments using antihuman-β-galactosidase polyclonal antibodies demonstrated that the enzyme was synthesized in normal fibroblasts as an 85-kDa glycosylated precursor, and posttranslationally converted through a number of steps into a mature 64-kDa form.[31] In contrast, in galactosialidosis fibroblasts, a normally synthesized β-galactosidase precursor was only partially processed into a 66-kDa intermediate that was degraded within 12 to 24 h. Addition of the protease inhibitor leupeptin to the culture medium of deficient cells partly prevented this degradation.[29–31] In the same immunoprecipitates, hitherto unknown polypeptides of 54, 32, and 20 kDa were coprecipitated with anti-β-galactosidase antibodies from normal fibroblasts, but not from fibroblasts of a patient with the early infantile form of galactosialidosis.[31] The 54-kDa protein appeared to be the precursor of the 32-and 20-kDa polypeptides, that was also released extracellularly after treatment of cells with ammonium chloride.[31,90] The identity between this protein and the "corrective factor" described earlier[26] was established by the normalization of the β-galactosidase maturation pattern in galactosialidosis cells after uptake of the secreted 54-kDa precursor.[31,90] On the basis of these studies, it was concluded that the primary defect in galactosialidosis was the absence or deficiency of the 32/20-kDa "protective protein" and its 54-kDa precursor. It was postulated that this protein was needed to protect β-galactosidase against rapid proteolytic degradation in the lysosomal environment, and was required to unite β-galactosidase monomers and neuraminidase in a complex.[31]

After the isolation of the protective protein cDNA, Galjart et al.[91] demonstrated that fibroblasts from an early infantile galactosialidosis patient were devoid of protective protein mRNA. Transient expression of the cDNA in COS-1 cells resulted in the synthesis of a 54-kDa precursor that was converted into a 32/20-kDa two-chain product, and was also secreted in large amounts. When this secreted precursor was taken up by galactosialidosis fibroblasts via a mannose-6-phosphate receptor-mediated endocytosis, it was routed to lysosomes, where it was correctly processed and where it restored β-galactosidase and neuraminidase activities.[91] These findings established that the cDNA-encoded precursor yielded a biologically functional protein, and proved unequivocally the nature of the primary defect in galactosialidosis.

PPCA/β-Galactosidase/Neuraminidase Complex

The triple enzyme deficiency in galactosialidosis provided genetic evidence that both neuraminidase and β-galactosidase are dependent on PPCA for their correct lysosomal function. Biochemical evidence for the existence of the three enzymes in a complex came from copurification studies. It was first observed that 85 percent of the active β-galactosidase in normal cells was resolved by gel filtration in a high-molecular-weight aggregate containing small amounts of the 32- and 20-kDa polypeptides. In galactosialidosis cells, instead, the residual β-galactosidase activity was detected only as a low molecular weight form that could be converted into the high molecular weight aggregate by addition of the 54-kDa precursor to the culture medium.[90] Based on this observation, it was proposed that one of the functions of the protective protein was to promote the aggregation of β-galactosidase molecules, thereby preventing their rapid proteolytic degradation.[90] Other investigators also found a correlation between aggregation and stability of β-galactosidase in human liver[92] and porcine spleen.[93]

Experiments aimed at purifying lysosomal neuraminidase showed that this enzyme could be isolated together with the protective protein and β-galactosidase from mammalian tissues and cultured cells.[94–98] When dissociated from the complex, neuraminidase was inactive.[95] Furthermore, monospecific antibodies against the 32-kDa protein coprecipitated both β-galactosidase and neuraminidase activities from purified placental preparations, indicating that the three proteins were able to associate.[95] In vitro reconstitution assays contributed the first biochemical proof that an inactive 66-kDa neuraminidase required the presence of the protective protein to become active, although in this study the identity of the neuraminidase polypeptide turned out to be incorrect.[99] It was also postulated that additional interaction of this enzyme with β-galactosidase increased its stability.[99] This was in agreement with the early observation that neuraminidase was apparently less stable in G_{M1} gangliosidosis cells with an isolated β-galactosidase deficiency.[100]

Following the identification of the catalytic activity of PPCA,[91] all three enzyme activities were shown to copurify, using either β-galactosidase or PPCA affinity matrices.[101–105] In mammalian tissues, however, only a small percentage of mature β-galactosidase and PPCA are consistently found in the complex (as low as 1 to 2 percent), which nevertheless contains all of the neuraminidase activity.[102–105] These studies support the notion that lysosomal neuraminidase activity cannot be isolated individually apart from the complex, whereas PPCA and β-galactosidase can exist independently in alternative forms[90,106] (see also references above). Estimates of the molecular weight of the multienzyme complex range from ~680 kDa[101] to ~1300 kDa.[102,103] In a few instances, the calculation of the relative number of PPCA versus β-galactosidase molecules present in the complex has been attempted,[107,108] but the determination of its stoichiometry awaits a clear understanding of the interrelationship between all components. Furthermore, recent studies indicated that *N*-acetylgalactosamine-6-sulfate sulfatase (GALNS) is also a component of the large multienzyme complex containing neuraminidase activity.[103] GALNS is required for the first step of keratan sulfate degradation, prior to the β-galactosidase-catalyzed second step (see Chap. 136). GALNS activity was found to be 6 to 40 percent of its normal value in fibroblasts from galactosialidosis patients, whose urinary secretion of keratan sulfate is comparable to that of patients with a primary GALNS deficiency.[103] These data suggest that this enzyme may also depend on PPCA for its lysosomal function.

The recent isolation of the cDNA for lysosomal neuraminidase[109–111] has allowed the definition of the molecular basis of sialidosis and the initiation of molecular and biochemical studies addressing the influence of PPCA in the generation and maintenance of neuraminidase and β-galactosidase activities. Transient expression of the neuraminidase cDNA in deficient galactosialidosis fibroblasts unequivocally showed that the enzyme is not activated in these cells unless it is coexpressed with PPCA.[109] Furthermore, neuraminidase activity increases in cDNA-transfected sialidosis and galactosialidosis cells in a PPCA-dependent manner.[109] It is now understood that neuraminidase and β-galactosidase interact with PPCA in an early biosynthetic compartment and require this association to be correctly compartmentalized in lysosomes.[112,113] Because active neuraminidase remains associated with mature PPCA, this interaction apparently is needed to maintain catalytic activity,[113] in agreement with the purification studies mentioned earlier. The relatively short half-life of lysosomal neuraminidase, on the other hand, may be important to control neuraminidase activity in the endosomal/lysosomal pathway.[113] In the absence of PPCA, neuraminidase is eventually subjected to rapid proteolysis.[114] Taken together, these findings provide strong evidence for a new role of PPCA as an intracellular transport protein.[113]

Primary Structure and Biosynthesis

Human PPCA is synthesized as a 480-amino acid precursor[91] containing a conventional hydrophobic signal peptide of 28 residues, two *N*-linked glycosylation sites (Asn117 and Asn305) and nine cysteines (Fig. 152-3). The glycosylated precursor of 54 kDa dimerizes soon after synthesis in the endoplasmic reticulum[115] and acquires the mannose-6-phosphate recognition marker only on the oligosaccharide chain linked to Asn117.[112] Both events are essential for the proper intracellular transport and lysosomal localization of the precursor molecule.[112,115] In the endosomal/lysosomal compartment, the precursor undergoes a protease-mediated maturation process that occurs in two steps (Fig. 152-3): an initial endoproteolytic cleavage, leading to a 34-kDa and a 20-kDa inactive intermediate, is followed by the removal of a 2-kDa "linker" or "excision" peptide from the

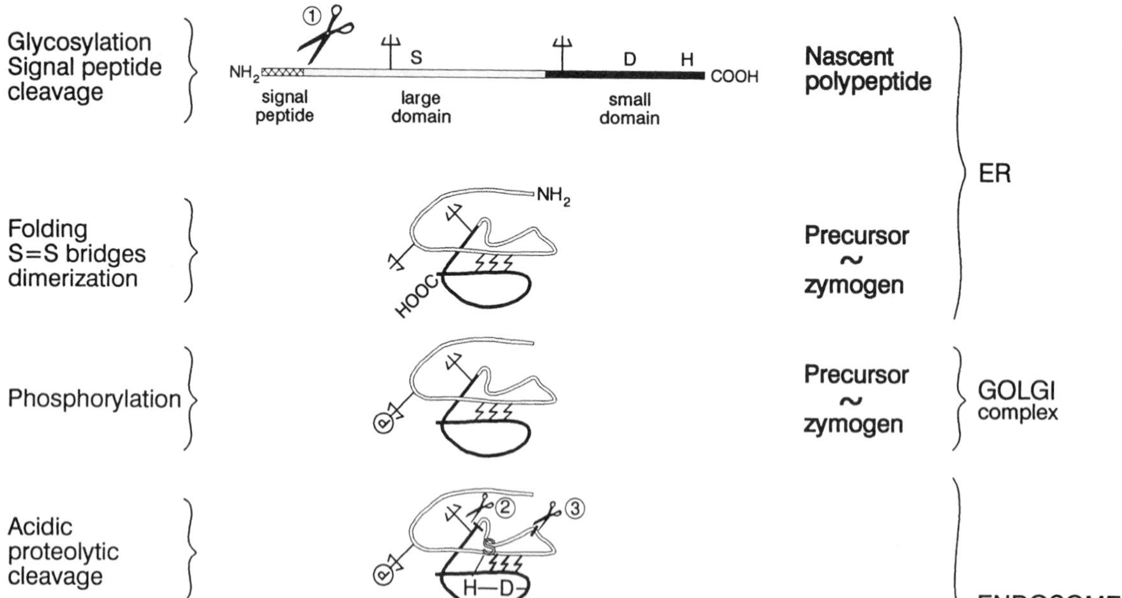

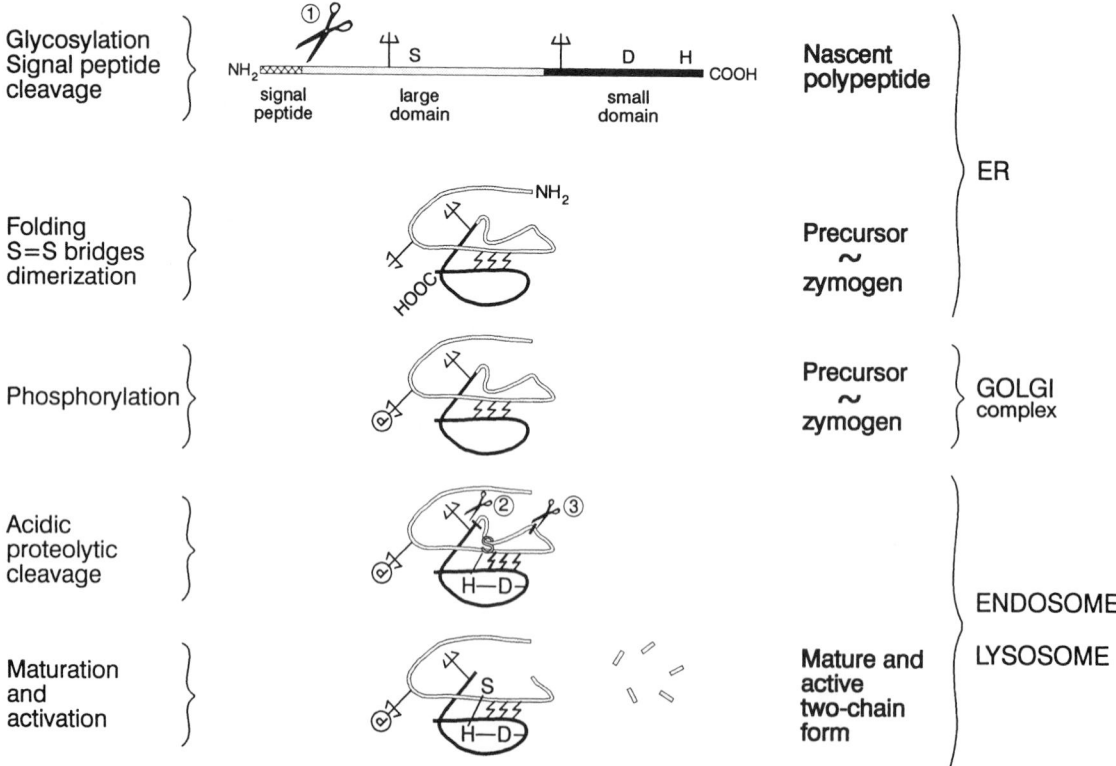

Fig. 152-3 Model for the biosynthesis and processing of human protective protein. Three proteolytic processing steps are thought to occur during the life cycle of the protective protein: (1) signal peptide cleavage; (2) the first endosomal/lysosomal endoprotease cleavage; and (3) C-terminal trimming of the 32-kDa polypeptide. Oligosaccharide side chains on the two subunits can be distinguished by the fact that only the one on the 32-kDa subunit carries the mannose-6-phosphate recognition marker. The intermediate stretch of amino acids between the 32- and 20-kDa chains is placed in front of the serine active site residue in the precursor/zymogen. The serine (S), histidine (H), and aspartic acid (D) make up the "catalytic triad" in the active, fully processed, mature protective protein.

C-terminus of the large domain.[116–118] The mature and functional protein present in lysosomes consists of two subunits of 32 and 20 kDa, held together by disulfide bridges. Amino acid sequencing of tryptic peptides from mature PPCA isolated from placenta has shown that residue Arg284 is still present in the 32-kDa chain after maturation,[91] while Met299 is the first residue in the 20-kDa chain.[91,119] The excision peptide thus comprises, at most, residues Met285–Arg298. The PPCA maturation process can be mimicked in vitro by limited proteolysis of the precursor with trypsin, probably cleaving at sites Arg284, Arg298, and Arg292.[115,117] The structural basis of catalytic activation has become apparent after the determination of the three-dimensional structure of the PPCA precursor.[118]

Homology of the Protective Protein to Serine Carboxypeptidases

In addition to that of human protective protein, the amino acid sequences of the mouse and chicken homologues have also been determined from their cloned cDNAs.[115,120] The three proteins are extremely conserved, with homology scores ranging from 67 percent (chicken/human) and 66 percent (chicken/mouse) to 87 percent (mouse/human).

Analysis of the primary structure of the cDNA-encoded human protein[116] revealed its similarity to serine carboxypeptidases.[121] PPCA has approximately 30 percent sequence identity to two yeast carboxypeptidases, carboxypeptidase Y (CPY) and the KEX1 gene products,[91,122,123] as well as to the wheat serine carboxypeptidase CPW.[124] The active site serine has been determined for both CPY and the KEX1 gene products.[123,125] This residue, at position 150 in the human PPCA, resides in a stretch of six amino acids (GESYA(G)G) found in all serine carboxypeptidases.[126] This domain is present in the 32-kDa subunit of the mature enzyme. A second highly conserved region of four amino acids (HXMP) is located in the 20-kDa chain and includes histidine residue 429. It has been suggested that, as in endopeptidases, the essential serine residue in carboxypeptidases is activated by the concerted action of two other residues, a histidine and an aspartic acid.[121] These three amino acids form the "catalytic triad." Based on sequence alignment with serine carboxypeptidases the catalytic triad in the protective protein was proposed to be formed by the residues Ser150, His429, and Asp372.[91]

The serine carboxypeptidase activity of the protective protein was first predicted by its capacity to bind to the serine protease inhibitor diisopropylfluorophosphate (DFP).[91,120] This compound specifically modifies the seryl residue in the active site of serine proteases and inactivates these enzymes. Both human and mouse proteins, overexpressed in COS-1 cells, bound radiolabeled DFP, but only in their processed two-chain state. The liberation of the catalytic activity entailed maturation of the precursor that behaved as a zymogen.[116,120] Following this initial observation, Tranchemontagne et al. demonstrated that in a purified preparation of the complex, the protective protein was catalytically active toward the *N*-blocked dipeptide Z-Phe-Leu, commonly used to assay CPY. These authors named this carboxypeptidase "carb L" and reported its deficiency in three galactosialidosis patients.[127]

Some of the biochemical characteristics of the protective protein, however, correlated well with those of a previously identified lysosomal carboxypeptidase, cathepsin A.[116] This enzyme was partially purified from different tissues and species, and shown to exist in small and large aggregates.[128,129] An accurate assessment of the quaternary structure and inhibitor profile of cathepsin A purified from pig kidney were reported by Miller et al.[130] Besides its carboxypeptidase activity, cathepsin A can also function as a peptidyl aminoacylamidase.[128] Several lines of evidence have led to the identification of the protective protein as cathepsin A: (a) Jackman et al.[119] reported the purification of a deamidase/carboxypeptidase, released from human platelets, consisting of disulfide-linked 32/20-kDa chains with N-terminal sequences identical to those of the protective protein. The purified enzyme was shown to homodimerize at acidic pH and to catalyze

Table 152-2 Cathepsin A-like Activity in Normal and Mutant Fibroblasts*

Cell Strain	Cathepsin A-like activity (milliunits† mg protein)
Normal fibroblasts ($n = 50$)	$x = 264$ (SD = 60)
Early infantile galactosialidosis	
Patient 1 (ref. 20)	0.8
Patient 2 (unpublished)	0.1
Late infantile galactosialidosis	
Patient 1 (ref. 32)	2.3
Patient 2 (ref. 32)	10.9
Juvenile/adult galactosialidosis (ref. 53)	5.6
Parents late infantile patient 1 (ref. 32)	
Mother	120
Father	117
G_{M1} gangliosidosis	355

*Cell homogenates of cultured fibroblasts were incubated for 30 min at 37°C in 50 m*M* 2-[*N*-Morpholino]ethanesulfonic acid (MES) pH 5.5, containing 1.5 m*M* Z-Phe-Ala. Cathepsin A-like activity was determined by indirect fluorimetric quantitation of liberated alanine.

†One milliunit is defined as the enzyme activity that releases 1 n*M* alanine per minute.

SOURCE: Adapted from Galjart et al.[88] Used with permission.

the hydrolysis of a selected number of bioactive peptides in vitro, including substance P, oxytocin, angiotensin I, and endothelin I.[119,131] (b) Overexpression of the protective protein in COS-1 cells and galactosialidosis fibroblasts resulted in an increase in cathepsin A activity.[109,116] (c) Monospecific polyclonal antibodies raised against native human protective protein precursor precipitated virtually all carboxypeptidase activity towards the acylated dipeptide Z-Phe-Ala,[116] known to be a specific substrate for cathepsin A.[132] (d) Using this artificial substrate, less than 1 percent cathepsin A activity was detected in fibroblasts from patients with different forms of galactosialidosis.[116,133] Heterozygotes had approximately 50 percent of control activity (Table 152-2). (e) The protective protein has been directly purified using cathepsin A-specific affinity matrices.[102,134]

PPCA — A Multifunctional Enzyme

A genetic approach was initially chosen to address the question of whether the cathepsin A activity of the protein was linked to its protective function towards β-galactosidase and neuraminidase. Genetically engineered active site mutants were generated with a single amino acid substitution at the serine or histidine residues of the catalytic triad.[116] These catalytically inactive proteins displayed a normal pattern of biosynthesis, processing, and secretion when expressed in COS-1 cells.[116] However, both secreted mutant precursors, endocytosed by galactosialidosis fibroblasts, were still able to correct β-galactosidase and neuraminidase activities as efficiently as the wild-type precursor.[116] These data clearly indicated that the catalytic and protective functions of PPCA are separable, which is why the enzyme is now termed PPCA.

It was further demonstrated that aside from its cathepsin A activity at acidic pH, PPCA maintains deamidase, and esterase activities at neutral pH.[119,131,135] In vitro the enzyme can deamidate neuropeptides, such as substance P and neurokinin, and act as carboxypeptidase on oxytocin-free acid, bradykinin, and endothelin I.[119,131] Mature PPCA is released from thrombin-stimulated human platelets and from ionophore B-stimulated natural killer cells,[119,135] and is detected in granules of human IL-2-activated killer cells.[135] The carboxypeptidase, deamidase, and esterase activities of the enzyme were found to be deficient in

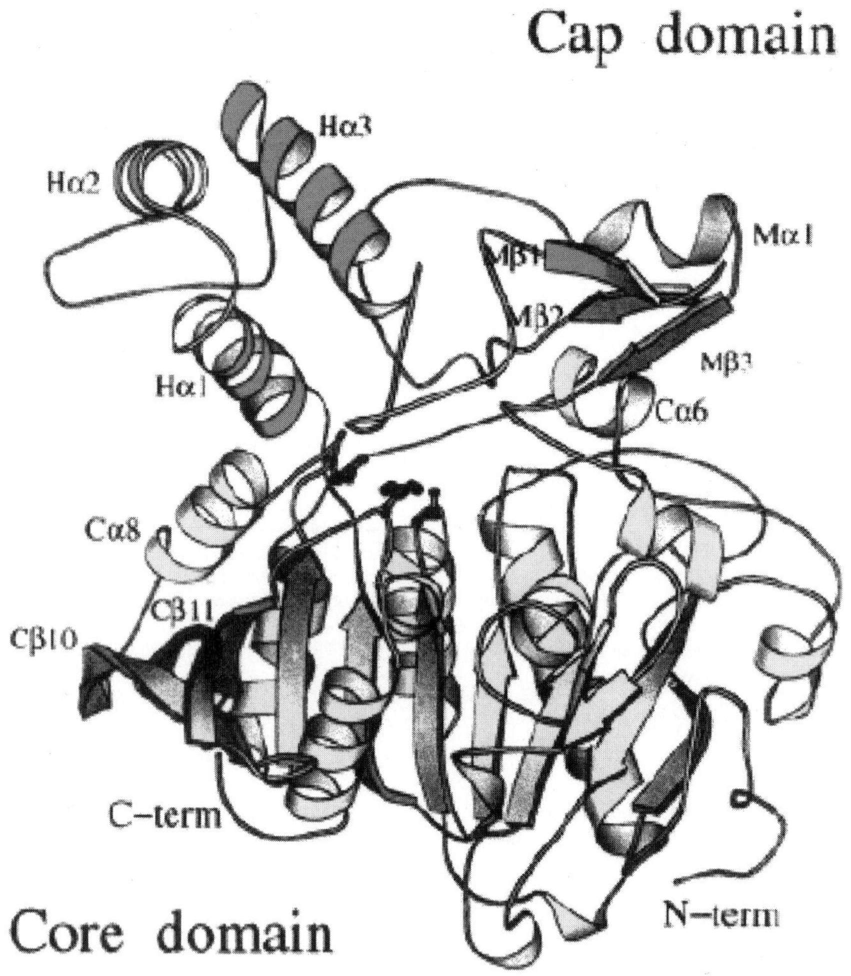

Fig. 152-4 Ribbon diagram of the PPCA monomer (monomer 1), showing the positions of the "core" and "cup" domains. The cup domain includes a three helical subdomain (left) and a maturation subdomain (right) which consist of a small mixed β-sheet containing the excision peptide involved in enzyme inactivation. The side chains of the catalytic triad Ser150, His 429, and Asp372 (from right to left) in the active site of PPCA housed by the core domain are indicated. Some secondary structure elements are labeled. (*Derived from Rudenko et al.*[118])

lymphoblastoid cells and fibroblasts from 16 galactosialidosis patients of Japanese origin.[136] In addition, Itoh et al.[137] demonstrated that an enzyme hydrolyzing the C-terminus of endothelin I was deficient in tissues from a galactosialidosis patient, and implicated PPCA as a major endothelin-degrading enzyme present in human tissues. Together these findings implied that PPCA may also be involved in extralysosomal processes, such as the inactivation of bioactive peptides or granzyme-mediated cellular toxicity.[138] The separable functions of PPCA could relate to the existence of different pools of free and associated forms of the enzyme in human tissues.[95] These pools might vary among distinct cell types and organs, and differentially catabolize a broad spectrum of substrates. Thus, although the pathology of galactosialidosis patients is primarily caused by lysosomal dysfunction, the possibility still remains that some of their symptoms are related to extracellular activities of PPCA.

A better understanding of the functions of PPCA requires the identification of substrates that are targets of the enzyme in vivo.

Three-Dimensional Structure of the Human PPCA Precursor. The crystal structure of the 108-kDa dimer of PPCA precursor has been solved to 2.2 Å resolution by a combination of molecular replacement and twofold density averaging.[118] As Fig. 152-4 shows, the protein fold is divisible into two domains. The first "core" domain, housing the catalytic triad, is very similar to a domain found in CPW and CPY and other proteases and lipases with different catalytic properties.[118] These enzymes, including human PPCA, are member of the hydrolase fold family.[139–141] The second is the "cap" domain, which consists of a helical subdomain and a maturation subdomain comprising the excision peptide. Both the core domain and helical subdomain in the PPCA dimer contribute to formation of the dimer interface; the maturation subdomain is not involved. Although PPCA and CPW both form dimers, comparing the configuration of the subunits in each enzyme reveals a significant 15° rotational difference, which has been impossible to predict by homology modeling.[142] The structure determination also revealed that the maturation subdomain, consisting of 49 amino acids including the 14 residues of the excision peptide, plays a critical role in enzyme activation.[118] The active site is filled by a peptide from this subdomain, shielding the catalytic triad and substrate binding sites from the solvent. Unexpectedly, these residues blocking the active site do not coincide with the excision peptide, which is found at the protein surface where it is solvent and protease-accessible. Hence, mere removal of the excision peptide is not sufficient to activate the enzyme. This mode of activation of PPCA is unique among proteases with known structures. While the catalytic triad is already correctly poised for catalysis in the zymogen, the peptide physically blocking the active site is not removed during enzyme activation, but refolds after cleavage of the excision peptide to render the catalytic cleft substrate accessible.

MOLECULAR GENETICS

Gene Assignment

The chromosomal localization of the human PPCA locus was controversial at first. Sips et al.[143] assigned the gene to chromosome 22 by using an antibody that recognized both human β-galactosidase and protective protein to screen human/mouse and human/Chinese hamster somatic cell hybrids. Mueller et al.[144] instead localized the gene involved in galactosialidosis to chromosome 20 by scoring for an increase of neuraminidase activity over the mouse background in human/mouse somatic cell hybrids. Using the PPCA cDNA as a probe for *in situ* hybridization of human metaphase spreads, the locus for human PPCA was unequivocally assigned to chromosome 20q13.1.[145]

The PPCA Gene

YAC and cosmid clones containing the entire PPCA gene and flanking sequences have been isolated and characterized.[146] The gene spans 7.5 kb of genomic DNA and comprises 15 exons. Their sizes range from ~27 bp to 450 bp, whereas the introns vary from 0.07 kb to 1.85 kb.[146] All intron-exon splice junctions follow the GT/AG rule.[147] Exon I of the human gene contains the short 5′ untranslated region, and exons 2 to 15 comprise the coding region, 3′ untranslated region, and the polyadenylation signal. An unusual feature was discovered through the analysis of the PPCA gene structure.[146] The last 58 nucleotides of exon 15 that are part of the 3′ untranslated region overlap with the 3′ end of the gene encoding the phospholipid transfer protein (PLTP).[148,149] At the moment it is not clear whether the two genes influence each other's expression and regulation.

Comparative studies of the human and mouse PPCA genes were used to identify promoter elements that regulate their expression.[150] The 5′ genomic regions of the two genes are strikingly similar in both organization and nucleotide sequence. The human gene is transcribed into a single PPCA transcript of 1.8 kb, which is expressed ubiquitously, but at different levels in human tissues. In contrast, mouse tissues have a major 1.8-kb transcript, similar to the human, and a minor 2.0-kb transcript, unique to the mouse. Both murine mRNAs are differentially expressed and vary in their 5′ untranslated regions. Thus, the human gene contains only one 5′ untranslated exon (exon 1), whereas the mouse gene has two exons, 1a and 1b, found in the large and the small mRNAs, respectively.

The mouse 2.0-kb mRNA is transcribed from an upstream TATA-box-containing promoter, which is absent in the human gene. A downstream promoter, found in both human and mouse genes, gives rise to the 1.8-kb mRNA common to the two species. This promoter bears some features of housekeeping gene promoters, including putative Sp1 binding sites. In addition, it carries three highly conserved USF/MLTF sequence motifs,[151] also known as E boxes.[152,153] Transcription factors such as MyoD, kE2-binding protein, and c-Myc are known to bind to these elements,[152–154] but functional studies are required to ascertain the importance of these motifs in the regulation of the PPCA gene. It is noteworthy that an exon 1a-specific mouse probe and the corresponding homologous region of the human gene detect on multitissue northern blots an extra mRNA of ~1.0 kb, which is well expressed in heart and skeletal muscle.[150] However, the nature of this transcript is still unknown.

Molecular Pathology

Few biochemical and molecular studies have been performed in galactosialidosis patients with distinct clinical phenotypes. Immunoprecipitation analyses have shown that fibroblasts from a patient with the early infantile type of the disease were devoid of immunoprecipitable PPCA protein.[31,155] This finding was consistent with the observation that the same patient completely lacked PPCA mRNA.[91] Therefore, the 43-kDa precursor detected in the same patient in another immunoprecipitation study[156] must have been a contaminant protein nonspecificically brought by the antibodies. In fibroblasts from two late infantile patients, a higher-than-normal amount of the 54-kDa PPCA precursor was immunoprecipitated[155,157] together with trace amounts of the 32-kDa subunit of mature PPCA. It was suggested that this feature was distinctive for late infantile patients and could account for their milder clinical phenotype. A small amount of a normally sized precursor was also detected in another patient with the juvenile/adult form.[9,155] However, a number of juvenile/adult Japanese patients were shown to synthesize precursor polypeptides of heterogeneous molecular masses ranging from 45 to 63 kDa.[156]

A better understanding of the genotype-phenotype correlation in galactosialidosis has emerged from the identification of various mutations, especially when expression and structural studies are performed. Most of the mutations reported to date have been identified in Japanese patients. Based on their clinical manifestations and distribution of mutant alleles, these patients are classified in two groups: type I and type II.[158] Type I patients have the severe phenotype with a neonatal or early infantile onset; only three patients of this type have been analyzed at the molecular level and they were genotypically different.[37,48,158] A substitution of Ser-90 with Leu was found in one severe neonatal case in compound heterozygosity with a Tyr395Cys substitution,[159] which is apparently quite common in Japanese patients. The latter mutation was also present in the other two early infantile patients, one of whom carried it in the homozygous state.[48] Type II patients include the juvenile/adult group and share a single base substitution at the donor splice site of intron 7, causing aberrant splicing of the precursor mRNA and the skipping of exon 7 (SpDEx7).[37,158,160] These patients were further divided into subtypes IIA (more severe, juvenile onset) and IIB (less severe, adult onset).[37,158] Juvenile patients of the IIA subtype carry the SpDEx7 mutation in compound heterozygosity with three different missense mutations, resulting in the amino acid substitutions Gln49Arg and Trp65Arg, as well as the Tyr395Cys found also in neonatal cases.[37,158,159] Transient expression in a galactosialidosis cell line of mutant cDNAs with either of these point mutations did not correct their combined β-galactosidase and neuraminidase deficiency and resulted in low levels of cathepsin A activity.[158] Adult patients, belonging to the IIB subtype, are normally homozygous for the SpDEx7 lesion.[37] It was postulated that this is a leaky mutation, allowing a small amount of correctly spliced transcript to occur in homozygous patients with a mild presentation. The exception of two severe juvenile patients, homozygous for the SpDEx7 mutation, has to be considered, however, if a correct genotype-phenotype correlation is to be made for this group of patients.

To date, eight Caucasian galactosialidosis patients with the early or late infantile phenotype and one juvenile/adult patient of Japanese/Dutch origin have been analyzed at the molecular level.[55,56,115,158] All patients included in the study by Zhou et al.[55] had detectable PPCA mRNA. These authors have identified three new single amino acid substitutions in two early infantile patients, Val104Met, Leu208Pro, and Gly411Ser. The former two were present in compound heterozygosity in one patient; the third was detected in the only transcribed allele of the other patient. Another amino acid change, Ser23Tyr, was found in the juvenile/adult case in combination with the SpDEx7 mutation. This patient clearly belonged to the Japanese subtype IIA, according to the classification of Shimmoto et al.[158] These amino acid substitutions were shown to hamper phosphorylation and, hence, lysosomal localization and maturation of the mutant PPCA precursors.[55] Coexpression studies with the neuraminidase cDNA in COS-1 cells[113] have further demonstrated that Val104Met and Leu208Pro mutants are still able to associate with neuraminidase but retain the enzyme in a prelysosomal compartment and prevent its activation. These findings explain why neuraminidase is so profoundly affected in patients that synthesize transport-incompetent PPCA.

The small group of patients with either the intermediate early infantile/late infantile or the late infantile form comprises two Americans, one of whom is of French/German origin,[51] two Canadians,[8,52] and one Italian.[32] Two amino acid substitutions, Phe412Val[115] and Tyr221Asn,[55,158] are shared by all five late infantile cases. These mutations appear to be pathognomonic for this phenotype, and determine the clinical outcome depending on whether they are present together or in combination with other mutations. The latter include a single base deletion and yet another amino acid change (Met378Thr), which generates an additional

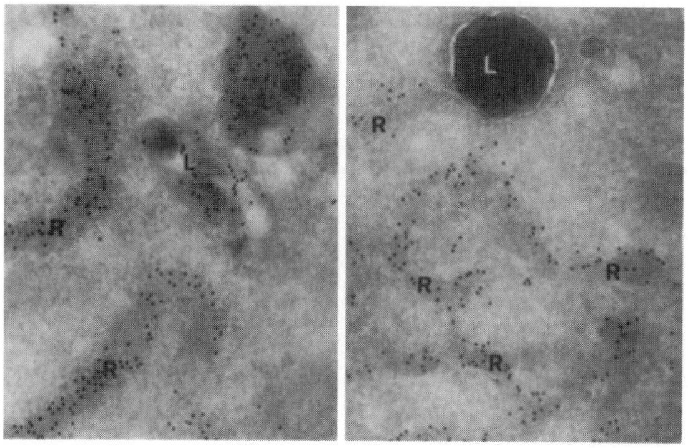

A B

Fig. 152-5 Subcellular localization of overexpressed normal and mutant proteins. Cryosections of COS-1 cells, transfected with wild-type (*A*) or the Phe-412 → Val (*B*) constructs, were incubated with anti–PPCA antibodies followed by goat anti-(rabbit IgG)-gold labeling. In *A*, extensive labeling of rough endoplasmic reticulum structures (R) and lysosomes (L) is detected. In contrast, *B* shows strong labeling of the rough endoplasmic reticulum (R) but only a few gold particles in a lysosome (L). Magnification: ×65,000. (*Courtesy of Rob Willemsen, Erasmus University, Rotterdam.*)

glycosylation site.[55] Within the late infantile group, patients with the Phe412Val mutation are clinically more severe than those with the Tyr221Asn substitution. For example, the patient homozygous for the Phe412Val mutation[23] has prominent ocular and skeletal involvement, whereas the patient who carries both amino acid changes is free of symptoms in both eyes and bones.[8]

Expression studies in COS-1 cells[113,115] have shown that Phe412Val impairs dimerization of the mutant PPCA precursor, causing its partial retention in the endoplasmic reticulum and its rapid degradation following proteolytic processing in lysosomes (Fig. 152-5). The Asn221-mutant protein behaves similarly, but its intralysosomal stability is intermediate between that of wild-type and Val412-PPCA.[55] In agreement with early immunoprecipitation studies,[157] detectable amounts of mature Asn221-PPCA accumulate in lysosomes and have residual cathepsin A activity. Moreover, when coexpressed with neuraminidase, this mutant PPCA has the capacity to transport a small portion of the enzyme to the lysosomes, resulting in low levels of neuraminidase activity.[113] Recently, a patient of Polish/Italian/Canadian origin with an unusual late infantile phenotype was reported by Richard et al.[56] The authors identified two new frameshift mutations in the PPCA gene of this patient that were caused by a two-nucleotide deletion, C517delTT, and an intronic mutation, IVS8+9C → G, resulting in abnormal splicing and a five-nucleotide insertion in the mRNA. Although both mutations give rise to the synthesis of truncated and inactive proteins, low amounts of a catalytically active PPCA were detected in fibroblasts from the patients, suggesting that a small pool of mRNA molecules is spliced normally.

Eleven amino acid substitutions (Fig. 152-6) identified in mutant PPCAs from clinically different galactosialidosis patients have been modeled in the three-dimensional structure of the wild-type enzyme precursor.[118,161] Of these mutations, nine are located in positions that drastically alter the folding and stability of the variant protein. In contrast, the remaining two, Phe412Val and Tyr221Asn, have a milder effect on protein structure. Remarkably, none of the mutations occurred at the active site of PPCA or at the protein surface, which would have disrupted the catalytic activity or protective function of the protein. Instead, there appears to be a remarkable correlation between the effect of the amino acid change on the integrity of protein structure and the general severity of the clinical phenotype.[161] The high number of folding defects in galactosialidosis may reflect the fact that a single point mutation is unlikely to affect both the β-galactosidase and neuraminidase binding sites of PPCA at the same time to produce the double glycosidase deficiency. Mutations that affect folding of the protein, however, disrupt every function of PPCA simultaneously. These studies provide the first structural explanation for the failure of a lysosomal mutant protein to reach its final destination, and further substantiate the correlation between the clinical severity of galactosialidosis and the amount of residual protein found in lysosomes.

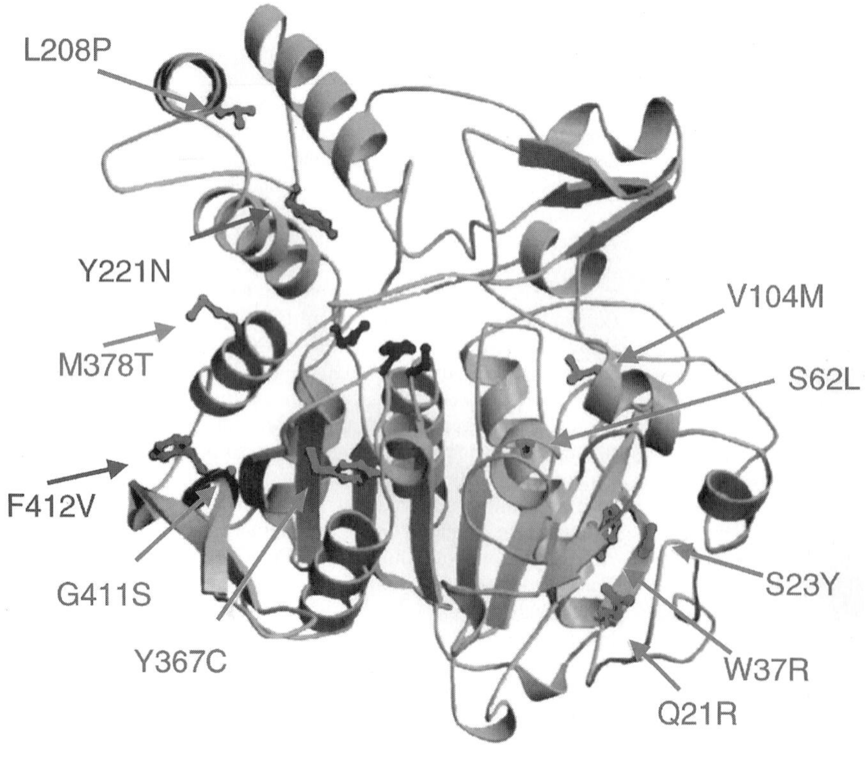

Fig. 152-6 Diagram of the PPCA monomer, which is present as a dimer in the crystal structure. The PPCA mutations found in galactosialidosis patients that have been modeled in the crystal structure are indicated. (*Adapted from Rudenko et al.*[161] *Used with permission.*)

GENETICS

Galactosialidosis is transmitted as an autosomal recessive trait. This mode of inheritance is supported by the high rate of consanguinity among parents of affected individuals and by molecular and biochemical analyses of obligate heterozygotes. The first evidence for PPCA heterozygosity came from the finding that fibroblasts from the parents of an early infantile patient had markedly reduced amounts of PPCA mRNA.[91] Currently, the enzymatic assay of cathepsin A activity is the first-choice method to demonstrate values intermediate between controls and patients in fibroblasts from obligate heterozygotes.[116,133,162]

DIAGNOSIS

The combination of clinical and pathologic manifestations of a lysosomal storage disease with sialyloligosacchariduria is the first clue to the diagnosis. Enzyme studies on white blood cells or cultured skin fibroblasts should confirm the triple enzyme deficiency. It is still advisable for clinical diagnostic purposes to demonstrate the combined β-galactosidase and neuraminidase deficiency, in addition to measuring the cathepsin A activity,[116,127,133,136] because there may be galactosialidosis patients who have a mutation interfering with the protective, but not the catalytic, function of PPCA.

As a result of the severe neuraminidase deficiency, galactosialidosis patients excrete an excessive amount of sialyloligosaccharides in their urine. Sialyloligosacchariduria can be easily ascertained by thin-layer chromatography,[35,38,66,116,163,164] although this assay does not discriminate between patients with galactosialidosis and sialidosis, or patients with different forms of galactosialidosis.[51,68] Thus, the identification of sialyloligosacchariduria in a patient with a typical lysosomal storage disease must be followed by additional enzyme assays to establish an exact diagnosis.

Enzyme Assays

β-Galactosidase and neuraminidase activities are usually measured in white blood cells and/or cultured fibroblasts by using the respective fluorogenic 4-methylumbelliferyl substrates.[165] Irrespective of the clinical severity, the residual β-galactosidase activity, assayed with an artificial substrate, is usually 5 to 15 percent of control values. Neuraminidase activity is reduced to less than 1 percent of normal levels. A higher residual neuraminidase activity can be detected in total white blood cell homogenates, because leukocytes contain two different enzymes active toward 4-methylumbelliferyl-α-D-*N*-acetylneuraminate. Only one type, predominant in lymphocytes (more than 80 percent), is deficient in galactosialidosis.[166,167] Thus, the use of isolated lymphocytes is to be preferred for diagnostic purposes. Tsuji et al.[61] used lymphocytes for the diagnosis of four patients with the adult form of galactosialidosis and discriminated between neuraminidase activity in a lysosomal fraction and that in the plasma membrane. Only the former reliably distinguished patients from carriers and from controls.

The occurrence of different types of neuraminidases should also be considered when interpreting enzyme activities in organ material from patients with galactosialidosis. Using 4-methylumbelliferyl-α-D-*N*-acetylneuraminate as a substrate, Suzuki et al.[62] reported 27 percent residual neuraminidase activity in liver and 76 percent in brain in a study of 22 patients with the juvenile/adult form of the disease. An explanation for this high residual activity could be that a relatively high amount of ganglioside neuraminidase is present in the plasma membrane that is not affected by the mutation(s) of PPCA.[168]

Natural substrates like fetuin, sialyllactitol, and [^{3}H]sialyllactose have also been used to assay the neuraminidase activity in galactosialidosis patients.[16,168] Less than 1 percent residual activities were measured in cultured fibroblasts using these substrates, whereas the activities toward G_{M3} and G_{D1a} gangliosides were normal.

As discussed earlier in this chapter, the discovery of the homology of the protective protein with serine carboxypeptidases[91] stimulated the search for assays of the primary protein defect in galactosialidosis. Initially, Tranchemontagne et al.[127] measured the carboxypeptidase activity with 0.75 mM Z-L-phenylalanine-L-leucine as a substrate at pH 5.5 and found 1 to 2 percent residual activity in fibroblasts from three patients with the late infantile or juvenile form of galactosialidosis. Using the same substrate, Kase et al.[136] also found a carboxypeptidase deficiency in fibroblasts from seven patients with the adult form of galactosialidosis. Galjart et al.[116] introduced the use of the *N*-blocked dipeptide Z-L-phenylalanine-L-alanine for the assay of cathepsin A and demonstrated its deficiency in various forms of galactosialidosis. Cells from parents of a patient with the late infantile form of the disease had cathepsin A values intermediate between homozygotes and controls (see Table 152-2).

PPCA has a substrate preference for hydrophobic residues in the P1 and/or P1′ binding pocket.[118,131] In turn, *N*-blocked acylated dipeptides, like Z-Phe-Ala or Z-Phe-Leu, are currently being used to accurately assay cathepsin A activity in normal cultured fibroblasts and tissues, as well as in galactosialidosis material (see above). In addition, a colorimetric assay for cathepsin A has been developed[108] that makes use of furylacryloyl (FA)-Phe-X dipeptides as substrates. Using this method, these authors confirmed that the enzyme has the highest affinity for substrates with hydrophobic (Phe, Leu) or positively charged (Arg) residues in P1′ position. Substrates like FA-Phe-Phe, FA-Phe-Leu, and FA-Phe-Ala have the highest specificity.

Using Z-Phe-Ala as substrate, a comprehensive analysis was recently carried out on 20 galactosialidosis patients of different ethnic origins and 9 of their heterozygous parents.[133] Interestingly, a clear correlation is observed between levels of residual cathepsin A activity and severity of the clinical phenotypes. These authors have also shown that cathepsin A has considerable activity in chorionic villi and amniocytes, but is deficient in these samples from a pregnancy with an affected fetus. These results emphasize the importance of including the cathepsin A assay for prenatal diagnosis of galactosialidosis.

Prenatal Diagnosis

The first prenatal diagnosis of galactosialidosis was established by measuring β-galactosidase and neuraminidase activities in cultured amniotic fluid cells.[20] The β-galactosidase activity was reduced to about 10 percent of control values, whereas neuraminidase activity was barely detectable. After termination of the pregnancy, the prenatal diagnosis was confirmed by measuring a combined β-galactosidase and neuraminidase deficiency in fetal liver, and an increased sialic acid content in liver and brain.

A second prenatal diagnosis has been performed by enzyme analysis in amniotic fluid cells.[169] In addition, thin-layer chromatography of deproteinized amniotic fluid supernatant revealed sialyloligosaccharides that were not present in control samples. After termination of the pregnancy, the prenatal diagnosis was confirmed by enzyme analysis of fetal skin fibroblasts and placental cell cultures.

ANIMAL MODELS

Inbred sheep have been shown to have deficiencies of β-galactosidase and neuraminidase in several tissues.[170] The sheep initially presented with mild neurologic signs at 4 to 6 months, which culminated rapidly, over a period of 2 weeks to 2 months, in severe ataxia and coma. Biochemical and enzymatic evaluations disclosed a combined deficiency of β-galactosidase and neuraminidase storage of G_{M1} ganglioside, asialo-G_{M1} ganglioside, and neutral long chain oligosaccharides in brain, as well as urinary excretion of neutral long chain oligosaccharides. Histopathologic studies showed marked vacuolation of neurons, hepatocytes, and renal epithelial cells. Clinical signs appeared to be associated

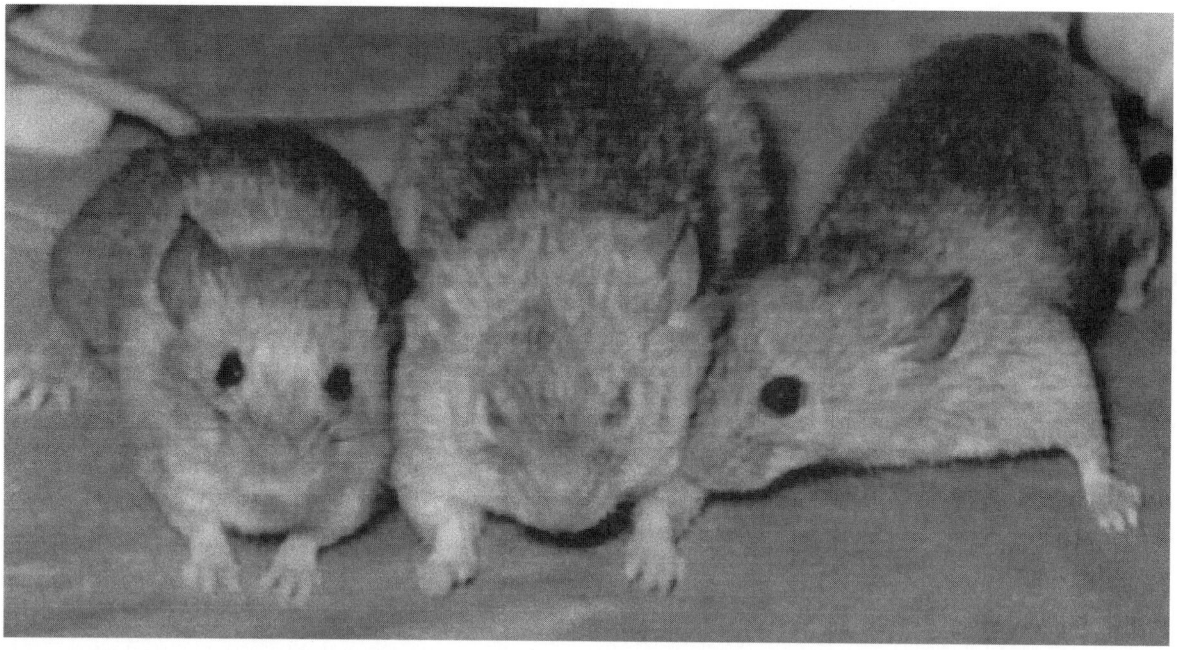

Fig. 152-7 Gross phenotypic appearance of a PPCA −/− mouse (middle) at 10 months of age, compared to a wild type +/+ littermate (right), and a −/− littermate (left) transplanted 5 months earlier with transgenic BM. The affected mouse has a broad face, disheveled coat, and swollen limbs and eyelids. In contrast, the BMT mouse clearly has improved in appearance. Evidence of edema has disappeared, and the coat is shiny and full. (Derived from Zhou et al.[172])

mainly with neuronal storage. However, there are several important differences between this condition in the sheep and human galactosialidosis, which suggest that they are distinct entities. The ratio of the residual activity of β-galactosidase and neuraminidase present in the sheep (5 percent and 20 percent, respectively) is the reverse of that in the human galactosialidosis (5 to 15 percent and 1 to 2 percent, respectively). The gene dosage effect underlined by intermediate levels of β-galactosidase activity in heterozygous sheep has not been observed in parents of human patients.[23] Finally, the increase of β-galactosidase activity observed in human galactosialidosis fibroblasts after treatment with leupeptin[171] was absent in fibroblasts from affected sheep.

Mouse Model of Galactosialidosis and Therapy

Using homologous recombination in murine embryonic stem cells, a mouse line was recently generated that carries a targeted null mutation in the PPCA gene.[172] Molecular and biochemical characteristics of PPCA −/− mice correlate closely with those in humans with the most severe form of galactosialidosis. The engineered mutation renders homozygous −/− mice unable to encode the protein, as established by assaying cathepsin A activity in fibroblasts and tissues from mutant animals. The deficiency of cathepsin A is directly paralleled by a severely reduced activity of lysosomal neuraminidase in all tissues. However, contrary to what would be predicted from the human disease, β-galactosidase levels vary considerably, being ~20 percent of normal levels in fibroblasts, as found in galactosialidosis patients, but higher than normal in liver. The apparent discrepancy with the human condition is difficult to explain on the basis of what has been reported for human material, which is limited to a few autopsy cases from adult Japanese patients.[62,70] Thus, it is quite possible that the findings in PPCA −/− mice actually reflect the situation in patients. Alternatively, the difference may be caused by species-specific variation in substrate metabolism. It is, however, clear that murine β-galactosidase seems to be less dependent for its stability and activity on complex formation with PPCA than is murine neuraminidase. The consequences of the severe neuraminidase, rather than β-galactosidase, deficiency are seen in the storage products present in urine of −/− mice; these are mainly sialylated oligosaccharides, as is the case in human patients.[70,173]

Although viable and fertile, mutant mice have a shorter lifespan (10 to 12 months) and present with signs of the disease soon after birth. Most of their tissues, including the central nervous system, show characteristic vacuolation of specific cells attributable to lysosomal storage. Regional distribution of accumulating neurons and glial cells is particularly evident in the brain, with consistent loss of Purkinje cells in the cerebellum. This distribution of affected cells in PPCA −/− tissues coincides closely, but not entirely, with the expression pattern of PPCA mRNA and protein in specific cell types.[174] This apparent discrepancy may relate to a distinct requirement of PPCA function in different cells and/or physiological conditions. As seen in Fig. 152-7, the gross appearance of affected mice overall worsens with age. Ataxic movements and tremor accompany progressive and diffuse edema. Nephropathy, which is a major complication and cause of death in early infantile patients, is also the most apparent cause of physical deterioration in affected mice. Thus, this mouse model provides an attractive opportunity to study the pathogenesis and pathophysiology of the disease and to evaluate therapies that could be eventually useful for treating patients.

The first therapeutic trial on the galactosialidosis mice has been attempted.[172] Affected mice were treated by bone marrow transplantation (BMT), using an approach that is based on the hypothesis that substantial secretion of PPCA by genetically modified BM cells could translate into a more timely and effective correction of the lesions in cells that internalize the corrective protein. For this purpose, transgenic mice were generated in which expression of a human PPCA transgene is driven by the β-globin promoter and locus control region of the β-globin.[175] The transgenic mice overproduce the heterologous human protein in erythroid precursor cells, and differentially secrete it at high levels.[172] BM from these transgenic mice, as well as from normal mice, was transplanted into lethally irradiated PPCA −/− mice ranging in age from 2.5 to 5 months. Functional PPCA, provided by both transgenic and normal BM cells, was found to be sufficient to correct the accumulation of sialyloligosaccharides in urine. Furthermore, transplanted animals outlive the affected mice and show complete reversal of their gross phenotype (Fig. 152-7, *left*). Histopathologic examination of their tissues demonstrates that transplantation of the overexpressing BM is more effective than normal BM for clearing storage in cells of visceral organs that undergo complete reversal of the lesions. Correction in the central nervous system is only partial, although detailed evaluation of its extent awaits fine mapping of the affected cells in different regions of the brain and the analysis of a larger number of treated mice. These findings give the first indication of the potential of overproducing and secreting hematopoietic cells for the treatment of galactosialidosis.

REFERENCES

1. Okada S, O'Brien J: Generalized gangliosidosis. Beta-galactosidase deficiency. *Science* **160**: 1002, 1968.
2. Derry D, Fawcett J, Andermann F, Wolfe L: Late infantile systemic lipidosis. *Neurology* **18**:340, 1968.
3. Wolfe L, Callahan J, Fawcett J, Andermann F, Scriver C: G_{M1} gangliosidosis without chondrodystrophy or visceromegaly. *Neurology* **20**:23, 1970.
4. Goldberg M, Cotlier E, Fichenser L, Kenyon K, Ernst R, Borowsky S: Macular cherry-red spot, corneal clouding and β-galactosidase deficiency. *Arch Intern Med* **128**:387, 1971.
5. O'Brien J, Ho M, Veath M, Wilson J, Myers G, Opitz J, ZuRhein G, et al.: Juvenile G_{M1}-gangliosidosis, clinical, pathological, chemical and enzymatic studies. *Clin Genet* **3**:411, 1972.
6. Orii T, Minami R, Sukegawa K, Sato S, Tsugawa S, Horino K, Miura R, et al.: A new type of mucolipidosis with β-galactosidase deficiency and glycopeptiduria. *Tohoku J Exp Med* **107**:303, 1972.
7. Lowden J, Callahan J, Norman M, Thain M, Prichard J: Juvenile G_{M1}-gangliosidosis: Occurrence with absence of two β-galactosidase components. *Arch Neurol* **31**:200, 1974.
8. Pinsky L, Miller J, Shanfield B, Watters G, Wolfe LS: G_{M1} gangliosidosis in skin fibroblast culture: Enzymatic difference between types 1 and 2 and observations on a third variant. *Am J Hum Genet* **26**:563, 1974.
9. Loonen M, Lugt Lvd, Francke C: Angiokeratoma corporis diffusum and lysosomal enzyme deficiency. *Lancet* **ii**:785, 1974.
10. Yamamoto A, Adachi S, Kawamura S, Takahashi M, Kitani T, Ohtori T, Shinji Y, et al.: Localized β-galactosidase deficiency. Occurrence in cerebellar ataxia with myoclonus epilepsy and macular cherry-red spot. A new variant of G_{M1}-gangliosidosis. *Arch Inter Med* **134**:627, 1974.
11. Wenger D, Goodman S, Meijers G: β-galactosidase deficiency in young adults. *Lancet* **ii**:1319, 1974.
12. Galjaard H, Hoogeveen AT, Keijzer W, de Wit-Verbeek HA, Reuser AJJ, Ho MW, Robinson D: Genetic heterogeneity in G_{M1}-gangliosidosis. *Nature* **257**:60, 1975.
13. Galjaard H, Reuser A: Clinical, biochemical and genetic heterogeneity in gangliosidosis, in Harkness R, Cockburn F (eds): *The Cultured Cell and Inherited Metabolic Disease*. St. Leonardgate Lancashire, UK, MTP Press, 1977, p. 139.
14. O'Brien J: Molecular genetics of G_{M1}-β-galactosidase. *Clin Genet* **3**:303, 1975.
15. Norden AGW, Tennant L, O'Brien JS: Ganglioside G_{M1} β-galactosidase A: Purification and studies of the enzyme from human liver. *J Biol Chem* **249**:7969, 1974.
16. Wenger DA, Tarby TJ, Wharton C: Macular cherry-red spots and myoclonus with dementia: Coexistent neuraminidase and β-galactosidase deficiencies. *Biochem Biophys Res Commun* **82**:589, 1978.
17. Justice P, Wenger D, Naidu S, Rosenthal I: Enzymatic studies in a new variant of G_{M1}-gangliosidosis in an older child. *Pediatr Res* **11**:407, 1977.
18. Miyatake T, Yamada T, Suzuki M, Pallmann B, Sandhoff K, Ariga T, Atsumi T: Sialidase deficiency in adult-type neuronal storage disease. *FEBS Lett* **97**:257, 1979.
19. Kobayashi T, Ohta M, Goto I, Tanaka Y, Kuroiwa Y: Adult type mucolipidosis with β-galactosidase and sialidase deficiency. *J Neurol* **221**:137, 1979.
20. Kleijer WJ, Hoogeveen A, Verheijen FW, Niermeijer MF, Haljaard H, O'Brien JS, Warner TG: Prenatal diagnosis of sialidosis with combined neuraminidase and β-galactosidase deficiency. *Clin Genet* **16**:60, 1979.
21. Suzuki Y, Fukuoka K, Sakuraba H: β-galactosidase-neuraminidase deficiency with cerebellar ataxia and myoclonus, in Sobue I (ed): *Spinocerebellar Degenerations*. Tokyo, University of Tokyo, 1980, p 339.
22. Okada S, Yutaka T, Kato T, Ikehara C, Yabuuchi H, Okawa M, Inui M, et al.: A case of neuraminidase deficiency associated with a partial β-galactosidase defect. Clinical, biochemical, and radiological studies. *Eur J Pediatr* **130**:239, 1979.
23. Andria G, Giudice ED, Reuser A: Atypical expression of β-galactosidase deficiency in a child with Hurler-like features but without neurological abnormalities. *Clin Genet* **14**:16, 1978.
24. Reuser A, Andria G, Wit-Verbeek Ed, Hoogeven A, Giudice Ed, Halley D: A two-year-old patient with an atypical expression of G_{M1}-β-galactosidase deficiency: Biochemical, immunological and cell genetic studies. *Hum Genet* **46**:11, 1979.
25. Hoogeveen AT, Verheijen FW, d'Azzo A, Galjaard H: Genetic heterogeneity in human neuraminidase deficiency. *Nature* **285**:500, 1980.
26. Hoogeveen A, d'Azzo A, Brossmer R, Galjaard H: Correction of combined beta-galactosidase/neuraminidase deficiency in human fibroblasts. *Biochem Biophys Res Commun* **103**:292, 1981.
27. van Diggelen OP, Schram AW, Sinnott ML, Smith PJ, Robinson D, Galjaard H: Turnover of beta-galactosidase in fibroblasts from patients with genetically different types of beta-galactosidase deficiency. *J Biol Chem* **200**:143, 1981.
28. van Diggelen O, Hoogeveen A, Smith P, Reuser A, Galjaard H: Enhanced proteolytic degradation of normal β-galactosidase in the lysosomal storage disease with combined β-galactosidase and neuraminidase deficiency. *Biochim Biophys Acta* **703**:69, 1982.
29. Galjaard H, Hoogeveen A, Verheijen F, van Diggelen O, Konings A, d'Azzo A, Reuser A: Relationship between clinical, biochemical and genetic heterogeneity in sialidase deficiency, in Tettamanti G, Durant P, Donato SD (eds): *Sialidases and Sialidoses*. Milan, Italy, Edi Ermes, 1981, p 317.
30. Suzuki Y, Sakuraba H, Hayashi K, Suzuki K, Imahori K: β-galactosidase-neuraminidase deficiency: Restoration of β-galactosidase activity by protease inhibitors. *J Biochem* **90**:271, 1981.
31. d'Azzo A, Hoogeveen A, Reuser AJ, Robinson D, Galjaard H: Molecular defect in combined beta-galactosidase and neuraminidase deficiency in man. *Proc Natl Acad Sci U S A* **79**:4535, 1982.
32. Andria G, Strisciuglio P, Pontarelli G, Sly WS, Dodson WE: Infantile neuraminidase and β-galactosidase deficiencies (galactosialidosis) with mild clinical courses, in Tettamanti G, Durand P, DiDonato SD (eds): *Sialidases and Sialidoses*. Milan, Italy, Edi Ermes, 1981, p 379.
33. Spranger J, Mucolipidosis I: Phenotype and nosology, in Tettamanti G, Durand P, Di Donato SD (eds): *Sialidases and Sialidoses*. Milan, Italy, Edi Ermes, 1981, p 303.
34. Gravel R, Lowden J, Callahan J, Wolfe L, Kin NNY: Infantile sialidosis: A phenocopy of type 1 G_{M1} gangliosidosis distinguished by genetic complementation and urinary oligosaccharides. *Am J Hum Genet* **31**:669, 1979.
35. Lowden J, Cutz E, Skomorowski M: Infantile type 2 sialidosis with β-galactosidase deficiency, in Tettamanti G, Durand P, Donato SD (eds): *Sialidases and Sialidoses*. Milan, Italy, Edi Ermes, 1981, p 261.
36. Suzuki Y, Nanba E, Tsuji A, Yang R-C, Okamura-Oho Y, Yamanaka T: Clinical and genetic heterogeneity in galactosialidosis. *Brain Dysfunct* **1**:285, 1988.
37. Takano T, Shimmoto M, Fukuhara Y, Itoh K, Kase R, Takiyama N, Kobayashi T, et al.: Galactosialidosis: Clinical and molecular analysis of 19 Japanese patients. *Brain Dysfunct* **4**:271, 1991.
38. Okada S, Sugino H, Kato T, Yutaka T, Koike M, Dezawa T, Yabuuchi H, et al.: A severe infantile sialidosis (β-galactosidase-β-neuraminidase deficiency) mimicking G_{M1}-gangliosidosis type 1. *Eur J Pediatr* **140**:295, 1983.
39. Yamano T, Dezawa T, Koike M, Okada S, Shimada M, Sugino H, Yauuchi H: Ultrastructural study on a severe infantile sialidosis (β-galactosidase-β-neuraminidase deficiency). *Neuropediatrics* **16**:109, 1985.
40. Sewell AC, Pontz BF, Weitzel D, Humberg C: Clinical heterogeneity in infantile galactosialidosis. *Eur J Pediatr* **146**:528, 1987.
41. Zammarchi E, Donati MA, Marrone A, Donzelli G, Zhou XY, d'Azzo A: Early infantile galactosialidosis: Clinical, biochemical, and molecular observations in a new patient. *Am J Med Genet* **64**:453, 1996.
42. Carton D, Leroy J, Dacremont G, Elsen A, Vanhaesebrouck P, van Hille J, Kint J: A neonate with galactosialidosis [Abstract], in *International Symposium on Lysosomal Diseases*. Münster, Germany, 1989.
43. Ozand P, Gascon G: Heterogeneity of carboxypeptidase activity in infantile-onset galactosialidosis. *J Child Neurol* **7**:S31, 1992.
44. Kyllerman M, Månsson L, Westphal O, Conradi N, Nellström H: Infantile galactosialidosis with congenital adrenal hyperplasia and renal hypertension. *Pediatr Neurol* **9**:318, 1993.
45. Nordborg C, Kyllerman M, Conradi N, Månsson J: Early infantile galactosialidosis with multiple brain infarctions: morphological, neuropathological and neurochemical findings. *Acta Neuropathol* **93**:24, 1997.

46. Landau D, Zeigler M, Shinwell E, Meisner I, Bargal R: Hydrops fetalis in four siblings caused by galactosialidosis. *Isr J Med Sci* **31**:321, 1995.
47. Itoh K, Miharu N, Ohama K, Mizoguchi N, Sakura N, Sakuraba H: Fetal diagnosis of galactosialidosis (protective protein/cathepsin A deficiency). *Clin Chim Acta* **266**:75, 1997.
48. Itoh K, Shimmoto M, Utsumi K, Mizoguchi N, Miharu N, Ohama K, Sakuraba H: Protective protein/cathepsin A loss in cultured cells derived from an early infantile form of galactosialidosis patients homozygous for the A 1184-G transition (Y395C mutation). *Biochem Biophys Res Commun* **247**:12, 1998.
49. Say B, Hommes F, Malik S, Carpenter N: An infant with multiple congenital abnormalities and biochemical findings suggesting a variant of galactosialidosis. *J Med Genet* **29**:423, 1992.
50. Andria G, del Giudice E, Reuser AJJ: Atypical expression of β-galactosidase deficiency in a child with Hurler-like features but without neurological abnormalities. *Clin Genet* **14**:16, 1978.
51. Strisciuglio P, Sly WS, Dodson WE, McAlister WH, Martin TC: Combined deficiency of β-galactosidase and neuraminidase: Natural history of the disease in the first 18 years of an American patient with late infantile onset form. *Am J Med Genet* **37**:573, 1990.
52. Chitayat D, Applegarth DA, Lewis J, Dimmick JE, McCormick AQ, Hall JG: Juvenile galactosialidosis in a white male: A new variant. *Am J Med Genet* **31**:887, 1988.
53. Yuce A, Kocak N, Besley G: Galactosialidosis in two siblings. *Turk J Pediatr* **38**:85, 1996.
54. Mongalgi M, Toumi N, Cheour M, Vanier M, Debbabi A: La galactosialidose avec anneau de Kayser-Fleischer. *Arch Fr Pediatr* **19**:193, 1992.
55. Zhou X-Y, van der Spoel A, Rottier R, Hale G, Willemsen R, Berry GT, Strisciuglio P, et al.: Molecular and biochemical analysis of protective protein/cathepsin A mutations: Correlation with clinical severity in galactosialidosis. *Hum Mol Genet* 5:1977, 1996.
56. Richard C, Tranchemontagne J, Elsliger M, Mitchell G, Potier M, Pshezhetsky A: Molecular pathology of galactosialidosis in a patient affected with two new frameshift mutations in the cathepsin A/ protective protein gene. *Hum Mutat* **11**:461, 1998.
57. Sugayama S, Utagawa C, Bertola D, Giugliana R, Burin M, Coelho J, d'Azzo A, et al.: Galactosialidosis in a 18-year-old Brazilian boy [Abstract], in *Ninth International Congress of Human Genetics*. Rio de Janeiro, Brazil, 1996.
58. Okamura-Oho Y, Zhang S, Callahan J: The biochemistry and clinical features of galactosialidosis. *Biochim Biophys Acta* **1225**:244, 1994.
59. Matsuo T, Egawa I, Okada S, Suetsugu M, Yamamoto K, Watanabe M: Sialidosis type 2 in Japan. Clinical study in two siblings cases and review of literature. *J Neurol Sci* **58**:45, 1983.
60. Yoshino H, Miyashita K, Miyatani N, Ariga T, Hashimoto Y, Tsuji S, Oyanagi K, et al.: Abnormal glycosphingolipid metabolism in the nervous system of galactosialidosis. *J Neurol Sci* **97**:53, 1990.
61. Tsuji S, Yamada T, Ariga T, Toyoshima I, Yamaguchi H, Kitahara Y, Miyatake T, et al.: Carrier detection of sialidosis with partial β-galactosidase deficiency by the assay of lysosomal sialidase in lymphocytes. *Ann Neurol* **15**:181, 1984.
62. Suzuki Y, Sakuraba H, Yamanaka T, Ko YM, Limori Y, Okamura Y, Hoogeveen AT: Galactosialidosis: A comparative study of clinical and biochemical data on 22 patients, in Arima M, Suzuki Y, Yabuuchi H (eds): *The Developing Brain and Its Disorders XX*. Tokyo, University of Tokyo Press, 1984, p 161.
63. Suzuki Y, Nakamura N, Fukuoka K, Shimada F, Uono M: β-Galactosidase deficiency in juvenile and adult patients. *Hum Genet* **36**:219, 1977.
64. Tsuji S, Yamada T, Tsutsumi A, Miyatake T: Neuraminidase deficiency and accumulation of sialic acid in lymphocytes in adult type sialidosis with partial β-galactosidase deficiency. *Ann Neurol* **11**:541, 1982.
65. Maire I, Nivelon-Chevallier A: Combined deficiency of β-galactosidase and neuraminidase: Three affected siblings in a french family. *J Inherit Metab Dis* **4**:221, 1981.
66. Loonen MCB, Reuser AJJ, Visser P, Arts WFM: Combined sialidase and β-galactosidase deficiency. Clinical, morphological and enzymological observations in a patient. *Clin Genet* **26**:139, 1984.
67. Miyatake T, Atsumi T, Obayashi T, Mizuno Y, Ando S, Ariga T, Matsui-Nakamura K, et al.: Adult type neuronal storage disease with neuraminidase deficiency. *Ann Neurol* **6**:232, 1979.
68. Kuriyama M, Miyatake T, Owada M, Kitagawa T: Neuraminidase activities in sialidosis and mucolipidosis. *J Neurol Sci* **54**:181, 1982.
69. Oyanagi K, Ohama E, Miyashita K, Yoshino H, Miyatake T, Yamazaki M, Ikuta F: Galactosialidosis: Neuropathological findings in a case of the late-infantile type. *Acta Neuropathol* **82**:331, 1991.
70. Amano N, Yokoi S, Akagi M, Sakai M, Yagishita S, Nakata K: Neuropathological findings of an autopsy case of adult β-galactosidase and neuraminidase deficiency. *Acta Neuropathol* **61**:283, 1983.
71. Ishibashi A, Tsuboi R, Shinmei M: β-galactosidase and neuraminidase deficiency associated with angio keratoma corporis diffusum. *Arch Dermatol* **120**:1344, 1984.
72. Usui T, Sawaguchi S, Abe H, Iwata K, Oyanagi K: Late-infantile type galactosialidosis—Histopathology of the retina and optic nerve. *Arch Ophthalmol* **109**:542, 1991.
73. Suzuki Y, Nakamura N, Shimada Y, Yotsumoto H, Endo H, Nagashima K: Macular cherry-red spots and β-galactosidase deficiency in an adult patient. An autopsy case with progressive cerebellar ataxia, myoclonus, thrombocytopathy, and accumulation of polysaccharide in liver. *Arch Neurol* **34**:157, 1977.
74. Takahashi K, Naito M, Suzuki Y: Genetic mucopolysaccharidoses, mannosidosis, sialidosis, galactosialidosis, and I-cell disease. *Acta Pathol Jpn* **37**:385, 1987.
75. Ikeda S, Ushiyama M, Nakano T, Kikkawa T, Kondo K, Yanagisawa N: Ultrastructural findings of rectal and skin biopsies in adult G_{M1} gangliosidosis. *Acta Pathol Jpn* **36**:1823, 1986.
76. Aylsworth A, Thomas G, Hood J, Malouf N, Libert J: A severe infantile sialidosis: Clinical biochemical and microscopic features. *J Pediatr* **96**:662, 1980.
77. Kornfeld S, Kornfeld R: Comparative aspects of glycoprotein structure. *Ann Rev Biochem* **45**:217, 1976.
78. Lowden J, O'Brien J: Sialidosis: A review of human neuraminidase deficiency. *Am J Hum Genet* **31**:1, 1979.
79. Dorland L, Haverkamp J, Vliegenthart J, Strecker G, Michalski J, Fournet B, Spik G, et al.: 360 MHz nuclear-magnetic-resonance spectroscopy of sialyloligosaccharides from patients with sialidosis (mucolipidosis I and II). *Eur J Biochem* **87**:323, 1978.
80. Koseki M, Tsurumi K: Structure of a novel sialyloligosaccharide from the urine of a patient with mucolipidosis. *Tohoku J Exp Med* **124**:361, 1978.
81. Koseki M, Tsurumi K: The structure of a new sialic acid-containing decasaccharide from the urine of a patient with mucolipidosis. *Tohoku J Exp Med* **128**:39, 1979.
82. Kuriyama M, Ariga T, Ando S, Suzuki M, Yamada T, Miyatake T: Four positional isomers of sialyloligosaccharides isolated from the urine of a patient with sialidosis. *J Biol Chem* **256**:12316, 1981.
83. Kuriyama M, Ariga T, Ando S, Suzuki M, Yamada T, Miyatake T, Igata A: Two positional isomers of sialylheptasaccharides isolated from the urine of a patient with sialidosis. *J Biochem* **98**:1049, 1985.
84. Strecker G, Peers M, Michalski J, Hondi-Assah T, Fournet B, Spik G, Montreuil J, et al.: Structures of nine sialyloligosaccharides accumulated in urine of eleven patients with three different types of sialidosis. Mucolipidosis II and two new types of mucolipidosis. *Eur J Biochem* **75**:391, 1977.
85. van Pelt J, Kamerling JP, Vliegenthart JF, Hoogeveen AT, Galjaard H: A comparative study of the accumulated sialic acid-containing oligosaccharides from cultured human galactosialidosis and sialidosis fibroblasts. *Clin Chim Acta* **174**:325, 1988.
86. van Pelt J, Bakker H, Kamerling J, Vliegenthart J: A comparative study of sialyloligosaccharides isolated from sialidosis and galactosialidosis urine. *J Inherit Metab Dis* **14**:730, 1991.
87. van Pelt J, van Kuik JA, Kamerling JP, Vliegenthart JF, van Diggelen OP, Galjaard H: Storage of sialic acid-containing carbohydrates in the placenta of a human galactosialidosis fetus. Isolation and structural characterization of 16 sialyloligosaccharides. *Eur J Biol Chem* **177**:327, 1988.
88. Mancini GM, Hoogeveen AT, Galjaard H, Mansson JE, Svennerholm L: Ganglioside G_{M1} metabolism in living human fibroblasts with β-galactosidase deficiency. *Hum Genet* **73**:35, 1986.
89. Fingerhut R, van der Horst GTJ, Verheijen FW, Conzelmann E: Degradation of gangliosides by the lysosomal sialidase requires an activator protein. *Eur J Biochem* **208**:623, 1992.
90. Hoogeveen AT, Verheijen FW, Galjaard H: The relation between human lysosomal beta-galactosidase and its protective protein. *J Biol Chem* **258**:12143, 1983.
91. Galjart NJ, Gillemans N, Harris A, van der Horst GTJ, Verheijen FW, Galjaard H, d'Azzo A: Expression of cDNA encoding the human "protective protein" associated with lysosomal beta-galactosidase and neuraminidase: Homology to yeast proteases. *Cell* **54**:755, 1988.
92. Heyworth C, Neumann E, Wynn C: The stability and aggregation properties of human liver acid β-D-galactosidase. *Biochem J* **193**:773, 1981.

93. Yamamoto Y, Nishimura K: Aggregation-dissociation and stability of acid β-galactosidase purified from porcine spleen. *Int Biochem* **4**:327, 1986.
94. Verheijen F, Brossmer R, Galjaard H: Purification of acid beta-galactosidase and acid neuraminidase from bovine testis: Evidence for an enzyme complex. *Biochem Biophys Res Commun* **108**:868, 1982.
95. Verheijen FW, Palmeri S, Hoogeveen AT, Galjaard H: Human placental neuraminidase. Activation, stabilization and association with beta-galactosidase and its protective protein. *Eur J Biochem* **149**:315, 1985.
96. Yamamoto Y, Fujie M, Nishimura K: The interrelation between high- and low-molecular-weight forms of G_{M1}-β-galactosidase purified from porcine spleen. *J Biol Chem (Tokyo)* **92**:13, 1982.
97. Yamamoto Y, Nishimura K: Copurification and separation of β-galactosidase and sialidase from porcine testis. *J Biol Chem (Tokyo)* **19**:435, 1987.
98. Hiraiwa M, Nishizawa M, Uda Y, Nakajima T, Miyatake T: Human placental sialidase: Further purification and characterization. *J Biochem* **103**:86, 1988.
99. van der Horst G, Galjart NJ, d'Azzo A, Galjaard H, Verheijen FW: Identification and in vitro reconstitution of lysosomal neuraminidase from human placenta. *J Biol Chem* **264**:1317, 1989.
100. Cantz M, Gehler J, Spranger J: Mucolipidosis I: Increased sialic acid content and deficiency of an α-*N*-acetylneuraminidase in cultured fibroblasts. *Biochem Biophys Commun* **74**:732, 1977.
101. Potier M, Michaud L, Tranchemontagne J, Thauvette L: Structure of the lysosomal neuraminidase-beta-galactosidase-carboxypeptidase multienzymic complex. *Biochem J* **267**:197, 1990.
102. Pshezhetsky AV, Potier M: Direct affinity purification and supramolecular organization of human lysosomal cathepsin A. *Ach Biochem Biophys* **313**:64, 1994.
103. Pshezhetsky A, Potier M: Association on *N*-acetylgalactosamine-6-sulfate sulfatase with the multienzyme lysosomal complex of β-galactosidase, cathepsin A, and neuraminidase. *J Biol Chem* **271**:28359, 1996.
104. Hiraiwa M, Kishimoto Y: Saposins and sphingolipid metabolisms. *Seikagaku* **68**:464, 1996.
105. Hiraiwa M, Saitoh M, Arai N, Shiraishi T, Odani S, Uda Y, Ono T, et al.: Protective protein in the bovine lysosomal beta-galactosidase complex. *Biochim Biophys Acta* **1341**:189, 1997.
106. Hubbes M, d'Agrosa RM, Callahan JW: Human placental β-galactosidase. Characterization of the dimer and complex forms of the enzyme. *Biochem J* **285**:827, 1992.
107. Pshezhetsky A, Potier M: Stoichiometry of human lysosomal carboxypeptidase-beta-galactosidase complex. *Biochem Biophys Res Commun* **195**:354, 1993.
108. Pshezhetsky AV, Vinogradova MV, Elsliger MA, el-Zein F, Svedas VK, Potier M: Continuous spectrophotometric assay of human lysosomal cathepsin A/protective protein in normal and galactosialidosis cells. *Anal Biochem* **230**:303, 1995.
109. Bonten E, van der Spoel A, Fornerod M, Grosveld G, d'Azzo A: Characterization of human lysosomal neuraminidase defines the molecular basis of the metabolic storage disorder sialidosis. *Genes Dev* **10**:3156, 1996.
110. Milner C, Smith S, Carrillo M, Taylor G, Hollinshead M, Campbell R: Identification of a sialidase encoded in the human major histocompatibility complex. *J Biol Chem* **272**:4549, 1997.
111. Pshezhetsky A, Richard C, Michaud L, Igdoura S, Wang S, Elsliger M, Qu J, et al.: Cloning, expression and chromosomal mapping of human lysosomal sialidase and characterization of mutations in sialidosis. *Nat Genet* **15**:316, 1997.
112. Morreau H, Galjart NJ, Willemsen R, Gillemans N, Zhou XY, d'Azzo A: Human lysosomal protective protein. Glycosylation, intracellular transport, and association with β-galactosidase in the endoplasmic reticulum. *J Biol Chem* **267**:17949, 1992.
113. van der Spoel A, Bonten E, d'Azzo A: Transport of human lysosomal neuraminidase to mature lysosomes requires protective protein/cathepsin A. *EMBO J* **17**:1588, 1998.
114. Vinogradova M, Michaud L, Mezentsev A, Lukong K, El-Alfy M, Morales C, Potier M, et al.: Molecular mechanism of lysosomal sialidase deficiency in galactosialidosis involves its rapid degradation. *Biochem J* **330**:641, 1998.
115. Zhou XY, Galjart NJ, Willemsen R, Gillemans N, Galjaard H, d'Azzo A: A mutation in a mild form of galactosialidosis impairs dimerization of the protective protein and renders it unstable. *EMBO J* **10**:4041, 1991.
116. Galjart NJ, Morreau H, Willemsen R, Gillemans N, Bonten EJ, d'Azzo A: Human lysosomal protective protein has cathepsin A-like activity distinct from its protective function. *J Biol Chem* **266**:14754, 1991.
117. Bonten EJ, Galjart NJ, Willemsen R, Usmany M, Vlak JM, d'Azzo A: Lysosomal protective protein/cathepsin A: Role of the "linker" domain in catalytic activation. *J Biol Chem* **270**:26441, 1995.
118. Rudenko G, Bonten E, d'Azzo A, Hol WGJ: Three-dimensional structure of the human "protective protein": Structure of the precursor form suggests a complex activation mechanism. *Structure* **3**:1249, 1995.
119. Jackman HL, Tan FL, Tamei H, Buerling-Harbury C, Li XY, Skidgel RA, Erdos EG: A peptidase in human platelets that deamidates tachykinins. Probable identity with the lysosomal "protective protein." *J Biol Chem* **265**:11265, 1990.
120. Galjart NJ, Gillemans N, Meijer D, d'Azzo A: Mouse "protective protein." cDNA cloning, sequence comparison, and expression. *J Biol Chem* **265**:4678, 1990.
121. Breddam K: Serine carboxypeptidases. A review. *Carlsberg Res Commun* **51**:83, 1986.
122. Valls L, Hunter C, Rothman J, Stevens T: Protein sorting in yeast: The localization determinant of yeast vacuolar carboxypeptidase. *Cell* **48**:887, 1987.
123. Dmochowska A, Dignard D, Henning D, Thomas DY, Bussey H: Yeast KEX1 gene encodes a putative protease with a carboxypeptidase B-like function involved in killer toxin and alpha-factor precursor processing. *Cell* **50**:573, 1987.
124. Breddam K, Sorensen S, Svendsen I: Primary structure and enzymatic properties of carboxypeptidase II from wheat bran. *Carlsberg Res Commun* **52**:297, 1987.
125. Hayashi R, Moore S, Stein W: Serine at the active center of yeast carboxypeptidase. *J Biol Chem* **248**:8366, 1973.
126. Brenner S: The molecular evolution of genes and proteins: a tale of two serines. *Nature* **334**:528, 1988.
127. Tranchemontagne J, Michaud L, Potier M: Deficient lysosomal carboxypeptidase activity in galactosialidosis. *Biochem Biophys Res Commun* **168**:22, 1990.
128. McDonald J, Barrett A (eds): Lysosomal carboxypeptidase A, *in Mammalian Proteases: A Glossary and Bibliography.* New York, Academic Press, 1986, p 186.
129. Doi E, Kawamura Y, Matoba T, Hata T: Cathepsin A of two different molecular sizes in pig kidney. *J Biochem* **75**:889, 1974.
130. Miller J, Changaris D, Levy R: Purification, subunit structure and inhibitor profile of cathepsin A. *J Chromatogr* **627**:153, 1992.
131. Jackman HL, Morris PW, Deddish PA, Skidgel RA, Erdos EG: Inactivation of endothelin I by deamidase (lysosomal protective protein). *J Biol Chem* **267**:2872, 1992.
132. Kawamura Y, Matoba T, Hata T, Doi E: Substrate specificities of cathepsin A, L and A, S from pig kidney. *J Biochem* **81**:435, 1977.
133. Kleijer WJ, Geilen GC, Janse HC, van Diggelen OP, Zhou X-Y, Galjart NJ, Galjaard H, et al.: Cathepsin A deficiency in galactosialidosis: Studies of patients and carriers in 16 families. *Pediatr Res* **39**:1067, 1996.
134. Matsuzaki H, Ueno H, Hayashi R, Liao T: Bovine spleen cathepsin A: Characterization and comparison with the protective protein. *J Biochem (Tokyo)* **123**:701, 1998.
135. Hanna WL, Turbov JM, Jackman HL, Tan F, Froelich CJ: Dominant chymotrypsin-like esterase activity in human lymphocyte granules is mediated by the serine carboxypeptidase called cathepsin A-like protective protein. *J Immunol* **153**:4663, 1994.
136. Kase R, Itoh K, Takiyama N, Oshima A, Sakuraba H, Suzuki Y: Galactosialidosis: Simultaneous deficiency of esterase, carboxy-terminal deamidase and acid carboxypeptidase activities. *Biochem Biophys Res Commun* **172**:1175, 1990.
137. Itoh K, Kase R, Shimmoto M, Satake A, Sakuraba H, Suzuki Y: Protective protein as an endogenous endothelin degradation enzyme in human tissues. *J Biol Chem* **270**:515, 1995.
138. Skidgel R, Erdos E: Cellular carboxypeptidases. *Immunol Rev* **161**:129, 1998.
139. Liao D, Breddam K, Sweet B, Bullock T, Remington S: Refined atomic model of wheat serine carboxypeptidase II at 2.2 Å resolution. *Biochemistry* **31**:9796, 1992.
140. Endrizzi J, Breddam K, Remington S: 2.8-Å structure of yeast serine carboxypeptidase. *Biochemistry* **33**:11106, 1996.
141. Ollis D, Goldman A: The α/β hydrolase fold. *Protein Eng* **5**:197, 1992.
142. Elsliger MA, Potier M: Homologous modeling of the lysosomal protective protein/carboxypeptidase L: Structural and functional implications of mutations identified in galactosialidosis patients. *Proteins* **18**:81, 1994.
143. Sips HJ, de Wit-Verbeek HA, de Wit J, Westerveld A, Galjaard H: The chromosomal localization of human β-galactosidase revisited: A locus for β-galactosidase on human chromosome 3 and for its protective protein on human chromosome 22. *Hum Genet* **69**:340, 1985.

144. Mueller OT, Henry WM, Haley LL, Byers MG, Eddy RL, Shows TB: Sialidosis and galactosialidosis: Chromosomal assignment of two genes associated with neuraminidase-deficiency disorders. *Proc Natl Acad Sci U S A* **83**:1817, 1986.
145. Wiegant J, Galjart NJ, Raap AK, Dazzo A: The gene encoding human protective protein (PPGB) is on chromosome-20. *Genomics* **10**:345, 1991.
146. Shimmoto M, Nakahori Y, Matsushita I, Shinka T, Kuroki Y, Itoh K, Sakuraba H: A human protective protein gene partially overlaps the gene encoding phospholipid transfer protein on the complementary strand of DNA. *Biochem Biophys Res Comm* **220**:802, 1996.
147. Mount S: A catalogue of splice junction sequences. *Nucleic Acids Res* **10**:459, 1982.
148. Day J, Albers J, Lofton-Day C, Ching A, Grant F, O'Hara P, Marcovina S, et al.: Complete cDNA encoding human phospholipid transfer protein from human endothelial cells. *J Biol Chem* **269**:9388, 1994.
149. Whitmore T, Day J, Albers J: Localization of the human phospholipid transfer protein gene to chromosome 20q12-q13.1. *Genomics* **28**:599, 1995.
150. Rottier R, d'Azzo A: Identification of the promoters for the human and murine protective protein/cathepsin A genes. *DNA Cell Biol* **16**:599, 1997.
151. Sawadogo M, Roeder RG: Interaction of a gene-specific transcription factor with the adenovirus major late promoter upstream of the TATA box region. *Cell* **43**:165, 1985.
152. Murre C, McCaw PS, Baltimore D: A new DNA binding and dimerization motif in immunoglobulin enhancer binding, daughterless, MyoD, and myc proteins. *Cell* **56**:777, 1989.
153. Blackwell TK, Kretzner L, Blackwood EM, Eisenman RN, Weintraub H: Sequence-specific DNA binding by the c-myc protein. *Science* **250**:1149, 1990.
154. Blackwell TK, Weintraub H: Differences and similarities in DNA-binding preferences of MyoD and E2A protein complexes revealed by binding site selection. *Science* **250**:1104, 1990.
155. Palmeri S, Hoogeveen AT, Verheijen FW, Galjaard H: Galactosialidosis: Molecular heterogeneity among distinct clinical phenotypes. *Am J Hum Genet* **38**:137, 1986.
156. Nanba E, Tsuji A, Omura K, Suzuki Y: Galactosialidosis: Molecular heterogeneity in biosynthesis and processing of protective protein for β-galactosidase. *Hum Genet* **80**:329, 1988.
157. Strisciuglio P, Parenti G, Giudice C, Lijoi S, Hoogeveen AT, d'Azzo A: The presence of a reduced amount of 32-kd "protective" protein is a distinct biochemical finding in late infantile galactosialidosis. *Hum Genet* **80**:304, 1988.
158. Shimmoto M, Fukuhara Y, Itoh K, Oshima A, Sakuraba H, Suzuki Y: Protective protein gene mutations in galactosialidosis. *J Clin Invest* **91**:2393, 1993.
159. Fukuhara Y, Takano T, Shimmoto M, Oshima A, Takeda E, Kuroda Y, Sakuraba H, et al.: A new point protection of protective protein gene in two Japanese siblings with juvenile galactosialidosis. *Brain Dysfunct* **5**:319, 1992.
160. Shimmoto M, Takano T, Fukuhara Y, Oshima A, Sakuraba H, Suzuki Y: Japanese-type adult galactosialidosis—A unique and common splice junction mutation causing exon skipping in the protective protein/carboxypeptidase gene. *Proc Japan Acad Series B Phys Biol Sci* **66**:217, 1990.
161. Rudenko G, Bonten E, Hol W, d'Azzo A: The atomic model of the human protective protein/cathepsin A suggests a structural basis for galactosialidosis. *Proc Natl Acad Sci U S A* **95**:621, 1998.
162. Itoh K, Takiyama N, Nagao Y, Oshima A, Sakuraba H, Potier M, Suzuki Y: Acid carboxypeptidase deficiency in galactosialidosis. *Jpn J Human Genet* **36**:171, 1991.
163. Sewell A: An improved thin layer chromatographic method for urinary oligosaccharide screening. *Clin Chim Acta* **92**:411, 1979.
164. Kuriyama M, Okada S, Tanaka Y, Umezaki H: Adult mucolipidosis with β-galactosidase and neuraminidase deficiencies. *J Neurol Sci* **46**:245, 1980.
165. Galjaard H (ed): *Genetic Metabolic Diseases, Early Signs and Prenatal Analysis.* New York, Elsevier/North Holland Biomedical, 1980.
166. Suzuki Y, Sakuraba H, Potier M, Akagi M, Sakai M, Beppu H: β-Galactosidase-neuraminidase deficiency and accumulation of sialic acid in lymphocytes in adult type sialidosis with partial β-galactosidase deficiency. *Ann Neurol* **11**:543, 1982.
167. Verheijen FW, Janse HC, van Diggelen OP, Bakker HD, Loonen MC, Durand P, Galjaard H: Two genetically different MU-NANA neuraminidases in human leucocytes. *Biochem Biophys Res Commun* **117**:470, 1983.
168. Tettamanti G, Durant P, Donato SD (eds): *Sialidases and Sialidoses.* Milan, Italy, Edi Ermes, 1981.
169. Sewell AC, Pontz BF: Prenatal diagnosis of galactosialidosis. *Prenat Diagn* **8**:151, 1988.
170. Ahern-Rindell AJ, Prieur DJ, Murnane RD, Raghavan SS, Daniel PF, McCluer RH, Walkley SU, et al.: Inherited lysosomal storage disease associated with deficiencies of α-galactosidase and β-neuraminidase in sheep. *Am J Med Genet* **31**:39, 1988.
171. Strisciuglio P, Creek K, Sly W: Complementation, cross reaction and drug correction studies of combined β-galactosidase and neuraminidase deficiency in human fibroblasts. *Pediatr Res* **18**:167, 1984.
172. Zhou XY, Morreau H, Rottier R, Davis D, Bonten E, Gillemans N, Wenger D, et al.: Mouse model for the lysosomal disorder galactosialidosis and correction of the phenotype with over-expressing erythroid precursor cells. *Genes Dev* **9**:2623, 1995.
173. van Pelt J, Hard K, Kamerling JP, Vliegenthart JF, Reuser AJ, Galjaard H: Isolation and structural characterization of twenty-one sialyloligosaccharides from galactosialidosis urine. An intact *N, N'*-diacetylchitobiose unit at the reducing end of a diantennary structure. *Biol Chem Hoppe Seyler* **370**:191, 1989.
174. Rottier R, Hahn C, Mann L, Martin M, Smeyne R, Suzuki K, d'Azzo A: Lack of PPCA expression only partially coincides with lysosomal storage in galactosialidosis mice: Indirect evidence for spatial requirement of the catalytic rather than the protective function of PPCA. *Hum Mol Gen* **7**:1787, 1998.
175. Grosveld F, Blom van Assendelft G, Greaves DR, Kollias G: Position-independent, high-level expression of the human β-globin gene in transgenic mice. *Cell* **51**:975, 1987.

CHAPTER 153

The G_{M2} Gangliosidoses

Roy A. Gravel ■ Michael M. Kaback ■ Richard L. Proia
Konrad Sandhoff ■ Kinuko Suzuki ■ Kunihiko Suzuki

1. **The G_{M2} gangliosidoses are a group of inherited disorders caused by excessive accumulation of ganglioside G_{M2} and related glycolipids in the lysosomes, mainly of neuronal cells. The enzymatic hydrolysis of ganglioside G_{M2} requires that it be complexed with a substrate-specific cofactor, the G_{M2} activator. There are two isoenzymes of β-hexosaminidase, Hex A, structure $\alpha\beta$, and Hex B, structure $\beta\beta$ where only Hex A can act on the ganglioside G_{M2}/G_{M2} activator complex. Defects in any of three genes may lead to G_{M2} gangliosidosis: *HEXA*, which encodes the α-subunit of Hex A; *HEXB*, which encodes the β-subunit of Hex A and Hex B; or *GM2A*, which encodes the monomeric G_{M2} activator. There are three forms of G_{M2} gangliosidosis: (a) Tay-Sachs disease and variants, resulting from mutations of the *HEXA* gene, are associated with deficient activity of Hex A but normal Hex B; (b) Sandhoff disease and variants, resulting from mutations of the *HEXB* gene, are associated with deficient activity of both Hex A and Hex B; and (c) G_{M2} activator deficiency, due to mutation of the *GM2A* gene, is characterized by normal Hex A and Hex B but the inability to form a functional ganglioside G_{M2}/G_{M2} activator complex. There are also pseudodeficient or clinically benign "disorders" characterized by biochemical defects of Hex A but functional activity toward ganglioside G_{M2}. The gross pathology is very similar in Tay-Sachs disease, Sandhoff disease and G_{M2} activator deficiency, except that there is also involvement of the visceral organs in Sandhoff disease. The most pronounced cellular change is the presence of swollen neurons with storage material in lysosomes throughout the nervous system. Characteristic inclusions are the so-called membranous cytoplasmic bodies.**
2. **The hexosaminidases and G_{M2} activator are glycoproteins that are synthesized in the lumen of the ER and processed through the Golgi. They are transported to the lysosome via the mannose-6-phosphate receptor where they are processed further to their final "mature" forms. Hex A and Hex B hydrolyze a broad spectrum of substrates that are specific for terminal GlcNAc or GalNAc residues in β-linkage. Active site residues and the mechanism of catalysis are being revealed through mutagenesis, photoaffinity labeling with substrate analogs, and studies of chimeric α-β enzyme. In addition to the hydrolysis of ganglioside G_{M2} by only Hex A, both isoenzymes will catabolize glycoproteins, glycosaminoglycans, and glycolipids. They will also hydrolyze synthetic substrates of which the most sensitive and commonly used is β-GlcNAc derivative of 4-methylumbelliferone (4MUG). It is recognized by both Hex A and Hex B and does not require the G_{M2} activator. Using 4MUG, Hex A and Hex B can be distinguished by taking advantage of different thermal or other characteristics of the isoenzymes. A related compound cleaved by Hex A (and Hex S), but not Hex B, is 4-methylumbelliferyl-GlcNAc-6-sulfate (4MUGS). Substrate such as 4MUG or 4MUGS are used for routine diagnostic testing and for screening of carriers of *HEXA* or *HEXB* alleles.**
3. **The clinical phenotypes associated with each of the different biochemical variants vary widely from infantile-onset, rapidly progressive neurodegenerative disease culminating in death before age 4 years (classical Tay-Sachs disease and Sandhoff disease, as well as G_{M2} activator deficiency) to later-onset, subacute or chronic, progressive neurologic conditions compatible with survival into childhood or teens (subacute form) or long survival (chronic form). Chronic forms include several different clinical phenotypes in which symptoms referable to one or another part of the central nervous system dominate, including progressive dystonia, spinocerebellar degeneration, motor neuron disease, or psychosis.**
4. **At least 92 specific *HEXA*, 26 *HEXB*, and 4 *GM2A* mutations have been characterized to date. The majority of mutations cause the severe, infantile-onset disease. Mutations causing subacute or chronic forms show correlation between the level of residual activity toward G_{M2} ganglioside and a combination of the level of ganglioside G_{M2} normally present in the cells in question. Several mutations are responsible for special subtypes of Hex A deficiency. The B1 subtype includes *HEXA* mutations in the putative catalytic domain of the α-subunit. They do not interfere with the synthesis of the Hex A heterodimer and leave intact Hex A activity toward 4MUG due to the functional β-subunit, but are inactive toward 4MUGS or G_{M2} ganglioside. Other mutations, causing the chronic disease phenotype, result in an unstable protein that may fail to associate with the β-subunit or are otherwise incompletely processed. Hex A pseudodeficiency is caused by point mutations that leave the Hex A with reduced but variable activity with synthetic substrates, but with sufficient ganglioside G_{M2} hydrolyzing activity to escape disease.**
5. **Heterozygotes for any one of the defects are asymptomatic; thus all G_{M2} gangliosidosis variants are inherited in an autosomal recessive fashion (*HEXA* maps to chromosome**

A list of standard abbreviations is located immediately preceding the index in each volume. The nomenclature and abbreviations of gangliosides, sphingolipids, and oligosaccharide or constituent sugars not in the standard list are given in Fig. 153-2. Additional abbreviations used in this chapter include: Hex A, Hex B, Hex S = β-hexosaminidase A, B, S, respectively; *HEXA* and *Hexa*, genes encoding α-subunit of Hex A isoenzyme in humans and mice, respectively; *HEXB* and *Hexb*, genes encoding β-subunit of Hex A and Hex B isoenzymes in humans and mice, respectively; *GM2A* and *Gm2a*, genes encoding G_{M2} activator in humans and mice, respectively; *GM2AP* = pseudogene related to *GM2A*; ER = endoplasmic reticulum; MUG = 4-methylumbelliferone; MCB = membranous cytoplasmic body.

GenBank accession numbers for human sequences are: *HEXA* mRNA, NM 00520; *HEXB* mRNA, NM 00521; and *GM2A* mRNA, X61095.

15 and *HEXB* and *GM2A* to chromosome 5). The availability of rapid and inexpensive methods for the identification of heterozygotes for Hex A deficiency has made possible large programs for family and population screening. Furthermore, when coupled with DNA-based diagnostics, mutations leading to infantile, subacute, or chronic disease can be distinguished. This has importance in recognizing the presence of pseudodeficiency alleles that are not easily distinguished biochemically. In the general population, heterozygote frequencies are estimated at 0.006 for *HEXA* mutations and 0.0036 for *HEXB* mutations. About 35 percent of alleles are accounted for by two mutations associated with the infantile phenotype and a further 5 percent by a prevalent chronic mutation. Of particular importance is that ~35 percent of non-Jewish individuals are heterozygous for one of the two pseudodeficiency mutations. In some ethnic groups, much higher carrier frequencies are observed. Among the Ashkenazi Jewish people in North America and in Israel, the heterozygote frequency for *HEXA* mutations is 0.033. This includes two "infantile" mutations that account for 90 to 95 percent of the total, the chronic mutation that accounts for 3 percent, and the pseudodeficiency mutations that account for 2 percent of the alleles. Extensive genetic counseling and monitoring of fetuses at risk has reduced the incidence of Tay-Sachs disease in the Ashkenazi Jewish population by almost 90 percent.

6. **Murine models for the three G_{M2} gangliosidoses have been generated by targeted gene disruption. Sandhoff mice, lacking Hex A and Hex B, accumulate ganglioside G_{M2} and glycolipid G_{A2} in nervous tissue, show a characteristic neuropathology and a progressive, severe neurodegenerative disease culminating in death at 4 to 4.5 months of age. Tay-Sachs mice, lacking only Hex A, accumulate G_{M2} to a lesser extent with negligible G_{A2}, have a less extensive and more restricted neuropathology, and escape disease to at least 1 year of age. These mice bypass the Hex A defect by catabolizing accumulating G_{M2} via G_{A2} and lactosylceramide by the action of sialidase and Hex B. The mouse model of G_{M2} activator deficiency results in a functional deficiency of Hex A and Hex B activities. These mice accumulate G_{M2} and a low amount of G_{A2} and have a motor deficit, but with a normal life span. The double-mutant mice, derived by crossbreeding, have deficient α and β subunits of Hex A. They lack Hex A, Hex B, and the Hex S α dimer characteristic of Sandhoff disease. In addition to their ganglioside storage disease, these mice show features of severe mucopolysaccharidosis and accumulate and excrete glycosaminoglycans, findings that underscore the importance of the Hex S residual activity in Sandhoff disease.**
7. **Specific therapy for G_{M2} gangliosidosis is not available to date, although all Hex A-deficiency variants can be diagnosed prenatally from amniotic fluid, cultured amniotic fluid cells, or chorionic villus biopsies. Several approaches to therapy are being investigated in animal or cell-culture models of the G_{M2} gangliosidoses. These approaches include enzyme replacement therapy, bone marrow and neural progenitor cell transplantation, gene therapy, and substrate deprivation therapy, the last by drug-mediated restriction of ganglioside biosynthesis in mutant mice.**

HISTORICAL INTRODUCTION

Warren Tay,[1] a British ophthalmologist, was the first to draw attention to the clinical characteristics of "infantile amaurotic idiocy" when, in 1881, he observed a cherry-red spot in the retina of a 1-year-old child with mental and physical retardation. The American neurologist Bernard Sachs noted the distended cytoplasm of neurons that is characteristic of the disease.[2] He coined the term *amaurotic family idiocy* in 1896,[3] and recognized the prevalence of the disease in Jews. Further progress in understanding Tay-Sachs disease, as it became known, had to await developments in chemical, biochemical, and histochemical analysis. It was not until the 1930s that the German biochemist Ernst Klenk[4,5] identified the storage material in the brains of patients with amaurotic idiocy as a new group of acidic glycosphingolipids. He named these sialic acid-containing glycolipids *gangliosides* because of their high concentration in normal ganglion cells.[6] The main neuronal storage compound in Tay-Sachs disease, ganglioside G_{M2} (Fig. 153-1), was identified by Svennerholm in 1962,[7] and its structure was elucidated by Makita and Yamakawa.[8]

This set the stage for the identification of the underlying defect in Tay-Sachs disease. The presence of a terminal, β-linked *N*-acetylgalactosamine residue in ganglioside G_{M2} implicated a defect in the glycohydrolase, hexosaminidase, as the offending lesion. Yet, hexosaminidase levels in Tay-Sachs patients were nearly always normal or slightly elevated. In 1968, Robinson and Stirling[9] showed by electrophoresis that the hexosaminidase of human spleen could be separated into two forms, an acidic, heat-labile form, hexosaminidase A, and a basic, heat-stable form, hexosaminidase B. This proved to be the key as Okada and

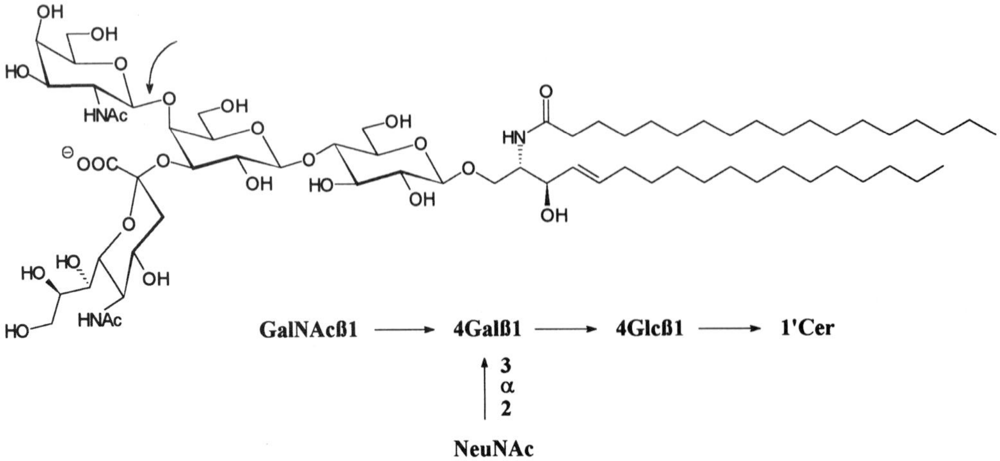

Fig. 153-1 Structure of ganglioside G_{M2}. The arrow indicates the bond to be cleaved by hexosaminidase A.

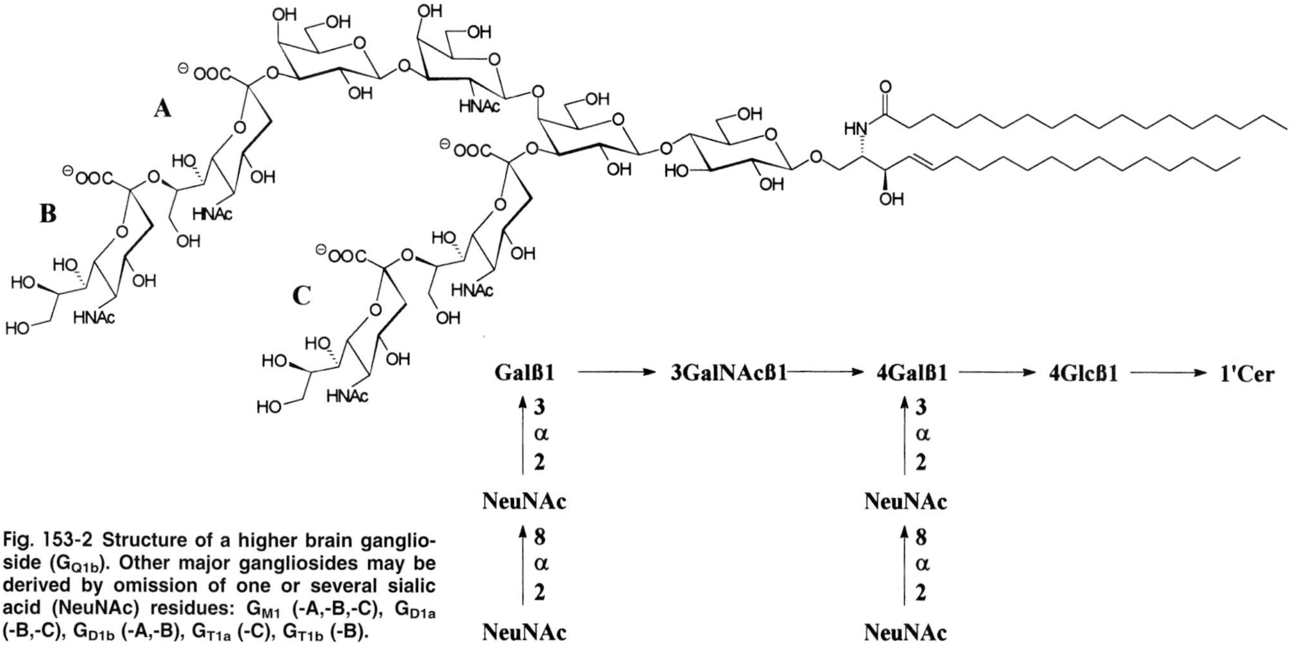

Fig. 153-2 Structure of a higher brain ganglioside (G_{Q1b}). Other major gangliosides may be derived by omission of one or several sialic acid (NeuNAc) residues: G_{M1} (-A,-B,-C), G_{D1a} (-B,-C), G_{D1b} (-A,-B), G_{T1a} (-C), G_{T1b} (-B).

O'Brien[10] showed in 1969 that the activity of the hexosaminidase A component was missing in Jewish patients with Tay-Sachs disease. These findings soon led to biochemical diagnosis of the disease and to carrier screening and prenatal diagnosis in at-risk pregnancies.[11,11A] Significantly, Sandhoff[12,13] showed that some patients who were non-Jewish were missing both hexosaminidase A and B or, paradoxically, neither isoenzyme. These results were not fully understood until the structure of the hexosaminidase isoenzymes, their substrate specificities, and the role of the G_{M2} activator, a substrate-specific cofactor of hexosaminidase A, were worked out in the ensuing years. These patients are now recognized as having Sandhoff disease or the AB-variant of the disease, respectively. A useful and comprehensive term, *G_{M2} gangliosidosis* was introduced by Suzuki and Chen[14] for disorders characterized by a primary accumulation of ganglioside G_{M2} resulting from a block in its catabolism. The cloning of the cDNAs and genes coding for the α and β subunits of hexosaminidase and for the G_{M2} activator protein has led to a molecular definition of all three disorders making up the G_{M2} gangliosidoses.

GANGLIOSIDES

The G_{M2} gangliosidoses produce disease because the inability to catabolize ganglioside G_{M2} to its constituent metabolites results in its accumulation to massive levels in the lysosomes of cells of the nervous system, causing a biochemical and clinical pathology that may ultimately be fatal. To understand disease mechanisms resulting from excessive ganglioside storage in the nervous system requires an understanding of their complex biosynthesis and degradation. This section summarizes the biologic role of gangliosides in neurons, their biosynthesis through the ER and Golgi, their distribution in the plasma membrane, and their degradation in the lysosome.

Structure and Function

Gangliosides[15–17] are glycosphingolipids consisting of a hydrophobic ceramide (*N*-acylsphingosine) and a hydrophilic oligosaccharide chain bearing one or more *N*-acetylneuraminic acid (sialic acid, NeuAc) residues. Kuhn and Wiegandt[18] established the first ganglioside structure in 1963 for the monosialoganglioside G_{M1}. The ganglioside nomenclature used in this article is that of Svennerholm.[19] The relevant structures are summarized in Fig. 153-2. In adult human brain, at least 12 different gangliosides have been identified, 4 of which, gangliosides G_{M1}, G_{D1a}, G_{D1b}, and G_{T1b}, make up more than 90 percent of the total. They all contain the same tetrasaccharide chain to which one (G_{M1}), two (G_{D1a} and G_{D1b}), or three (G_{T1b}) sialic acid residues are attached (Fig. 153-2). In gangliosides G_{M2} and G_{M3}, the oligosaccharide chain is incomplete and consists of a trisaccharide (gangliotriaose) or disaccharide (lactose), respectively, to which a sialic acid is bound.

Gangliosides are typical components of the outer leaflet of plasma membranes of animal cells. They are anchored by their hydrophobic ceramide moiety so that their hydrophilic oligosaccharide chains extend into the extracellular space.[20] They form cell-type-specific patterns that change with cell differentiation and cell transformation[21] and, as cell surface markers, are likely to be involved in cell differentiation and cell-cell interaction.[22,23] Although their physiological functions are still obscure, specific gangliosides are implicated as binding sites on cell surfaces for viruses and bacterial toxins, and as coreceptors for hormones, for example, thyroid-stimulating hormone, growth factors, interferons, and in cell mobility (for reviews see references 15 and 24 to 28).

The highest ganglioside content is found in the gray matter of the brain,[29] although the ganglioside content and pattern differ widely between different portions of the brain[30] and change significantly during ontogenesis.[31–35] Whereas the gangliosides of the central nervous system belong almost exclusively to the ganglio series (Fig. 153-2), those of peripheral nerves (approximately 0.1 μM NeuAc per gram wet weight[36]) and extraneural tissues (0.1 to 0.4 μM NeuAc per gram wet weight[18]) contain high proportions of gangliosides of the lacto series, for example, (Gal(β1 → 3)GlcNAc(β1 → 3)Gal(β1 → 4)Glc,[37–40] or globo series, for example, GalNAc(β1 → 3)Gal(α1 → 4) Galβ(1 → 4)Glc.[41,42] Major gangliosides of peripheral nerves are G_{M3} and G_{D3}; a major ganglioside of peripheral nerve myelin is NeuAc(α2 → 3)Gal(β1 → 4)GlcNAc(β1 → 3)Gal(β1 → 4) Glc(β1-1′)Cer.[43]

Gangliosides are highly concentrated in neuronal plasma membranes,[29,44] especially in regions of nerve endings and dendrites.[45] The bulk of brain ganglioside is localized in neurons, but glial cells, such as oligodendrocytes and astrocytes, and other cell types also have their unique ganglioside composition.[46–48]

The function of gangliosides in neuronal plasma membranes is unknown. Knockout mice with disrupted biosynthesis of complex gangliosides (G_{M2}/G_{D2} synthase deficiency) develop a histologically normal nervous system but show minor neurologic deficits, such as in neuronal conduction velocity and behavioral tests.[49] As Ca^{2+}-binding sites, gangliosides have been implicated indirectly in neuronal transmission.[29,50] They have also been shown to have neurotigenic and neurotrophic effects, in that they can induce differentiation in some primary neuronal cultures and neuroblastoma cell lines. Exogenously added gangliosides also facilitate *in vivo* survival and repair of damaged neurons in both the central and peripheral nervous systems.[17,51–56] Neuronal, tri-, and tetrasialogangliosides are ligands of myelin-associated glycoprotein and have been implicated in the interactions of myelinating glial cells with neuronal axons.[57]

Biosynthesis and Intracellular Transport

Ganglioside biosynthesis starts from ceramide, which is formed at the cytosolic leaflet of the endoplasmic reticulum.[58] The glycosyl chain is assembled in a stepwise manner by sequential addition of the individual sugar and sialyl residues to the growing glycolipid. The glycosyl residues are donated by the respective uridine-5′-diphosphate (UDP) derivatives, while the active species for the sialyl residue is the cytosine-5′-monophosphate derivative (CMP-NeuAc). Glucosylceramide is formed at the cytosolic leaflet of the Golgi membranes,[59] whereas the remaining steps are catalyzed by membrane-bound glycosyltransferases at the luminal surface of the Golgi stacks.[60,61] The precursor of the major ganglioside series, G_{M3} and G_{D3}, are formed by specific glycosyltransferases in early Golgi compartments.[62–64] These precursors are converted to the complex gangliosides of the a and b series by an identical set of quite nonspecific glycosyltransferases[65] in later Golgi compartments.[64,66] The cDNAs for many of the glycosyltransferases involved in glycosphingolipid biosynthesis have been cloned.[67]

It is now believed that, after synthesis in the Golgi apparatus, gangliosides are transported to the plasma membrane by vesicle flow.[64,68] Studies *in vitro* suggest that oligosialogangliosides can be partially degraded there to ganglioside G_{M1} by a membrane-based sialidase that is regulated by the organization and physical properties of the membranes.[69]

In neurons, synthesis and degradation of gangliosides apparently occur in the cell body but not in the axons or nerve terminals. The latter structures receive gangliosides by fast anterograde axonal transport and discharge them by retrograde axonal transport.[70,71]

Ganglioside Degradation

The catabolism of gangliosides and other sphingolipids has been studied intensively in many laboratories during the past 30 years, primarily to understand the molecular basis of the inherited lipidoses and their steadily increasing heterogeneity. The degradation of gangliosides occurs in the lysosome where exohydrolases remove the sugars from the hydrophilic end sequentially to the ceramide core. It is here, in the lysosomes, that the collection of disorders comprising the ganglioside storage diseases has its enzyme defects. Indeed, for virtually every enzyme taking part in the catabolism of gangliosides, there is a corresponding genetic disease (reviewed in other chapters of this book as well as in references 72 to 74). These diseases are highly heterogeneous both biochemically and clinically, partly because defects giving partial enzyme activity can show a reduced accumulation of substrates and partly because the level of enzyme or the propensity to accumulate substrate varies from tissue to tissue. The lysosomal hydrolases, and consequently their inherited deficiencies, are found in all organs, body fluids, and cells (with the exception of erythrocytes), but the lipid substrates accumulate predominantly in the organs in which they are synthesized. Therefore defects in ganglioside catabolism will lead mainly to neuronal storage. The lysosomal storage characteristic of these disorders results from the accumulation of the partially degraded gangliosides that are not recycled and that cannot easily escape the organelle.[60] Only small amounts of the accumulating lipids leave the cells in which they were synthesized; they may be detected in cerebrospinal fluid and in urine.

The degradation of glycosphingolipids occurs in the acidic compartments of the cell, the endosomes and the lysosomes. Components of the plasma membrane containing glycosphingolipids destined for degradation are endocytosed and passed through the endosomal compartments to reach the lysosome.[75] The observation of multivesicular bodies in the early and late endosomal reticulum[75,76] suggests that parts of the endosomal membrane, presumably enriched in components derived from the plasma membrane, bud off into the endosomal lumen to form intraendosomal vesicles. Through successive steps of membrane fusion and fission, these vesicles find their way into the lysosome, in part as intralysosomal vesicles with their component glycoconjugates facing into the lysosomal milieu for degradation.[77]

In human tissues, ganglioside G_{M2} is degraded in the lysosomal milieu by β-hexosaminidase A, which removes the terminal *N*-acetylgalactosaminyl residue. However, the water-soluble enzyme cannot alone degrade membrane-bound ganglioside G_{M2} due to steric hindrance by the membrane surface. This is accomplished by the enzyme acting on a ganglioside G_{M2}/G_{M2} activator complex as substrate (Fig. 153-3). The G_{M2} activator acts to lift the ganglioside from the membrane surface and presents it to the water-soluble enzyme for hydrolysis of the terminal sugar.[76,78] In human tissues, sialidase has little activity toward ganglioside G_{M2}, even though sialic acid is also in a terminal position. Eventually, ganglioside G_{M2} is broken down in the lysosomes to individual hexoses, fatty acid and D-E-sphingosine. The latter down-regulates serine-palmitoyl transferase, catalyzing the first committed step in sphingolipid biosynthesis.[79] This down-regulation is presumably reduced in sphingolipid storage diseases.

THE HEXOSAMINIDASES AND G_{M2} ACTIVATOR

The presence of an *N*-acetyl-β-D-glucosaminidase in mammalian tissue was first reported in 1936.[80] It was later shown that the same enzyme hydrolyzes the β-glycosidic bond of the two amino sugars, *N*-acetyl-D-glucosamine and *N*-acetyl-D-galactosamine.[9,81–87] The enzyme was therefore called *β-hexosaminidase* or simply *hexosaminidase* (EC 3.2.1.52). It has also been listed as *β-N*-acetylglucosaminidase (NAG, EC 3.2.1.30) in *Enzyme Nomenclature*, although this term is inappropriate for the mammalian enzyme. Nevertheless, it is still commonly used to describe the serum and urine forms of hexosaminidase. It was found to be localized to the lysosome by subcellular fractionation,[9,88,89] consistent with its acidic pH optimum. Through the remainder of this chapter, the isoenzymes of hexosaminidase, such as β-hexosaminidase A and β-hexosaminidase B, will be written as Hex A and Hex B, respectively.

Protein Structure

Our understanding of the structural relationship between Hex A and Hex B came initially from an immunological characterization by Srivastava and Beutler[90] who showed that Hex A was composed of at least two nonidentical subunits, one an acidic α subunit and the other a basic β subunit, and that Hex B was composed only of β subunits. Thus, the absence of Hex A activity in Tay-Sachs disease and of both enzyme activities in Sandhoff disease was explainable. Mutations of the α subunit in Tay-Sachs disease would lead to Hex A deficiency without affecting Hex B activity. Mutations of the common β subunit in Sandhoff disease would result in a deficiency of both Hex A and Hex B activities. Subsequently, the small amount of residual Hex activity in tissues of patients with Sandhoff disease was found to be due to a third, unstable isoenzyme with a very acidic pI.[13,91,92] This isoenzyme, Hex S, contained only α subunits.[92–94] The involvement of two genes was also demonstrated in somatic cell hybrids. It was shown

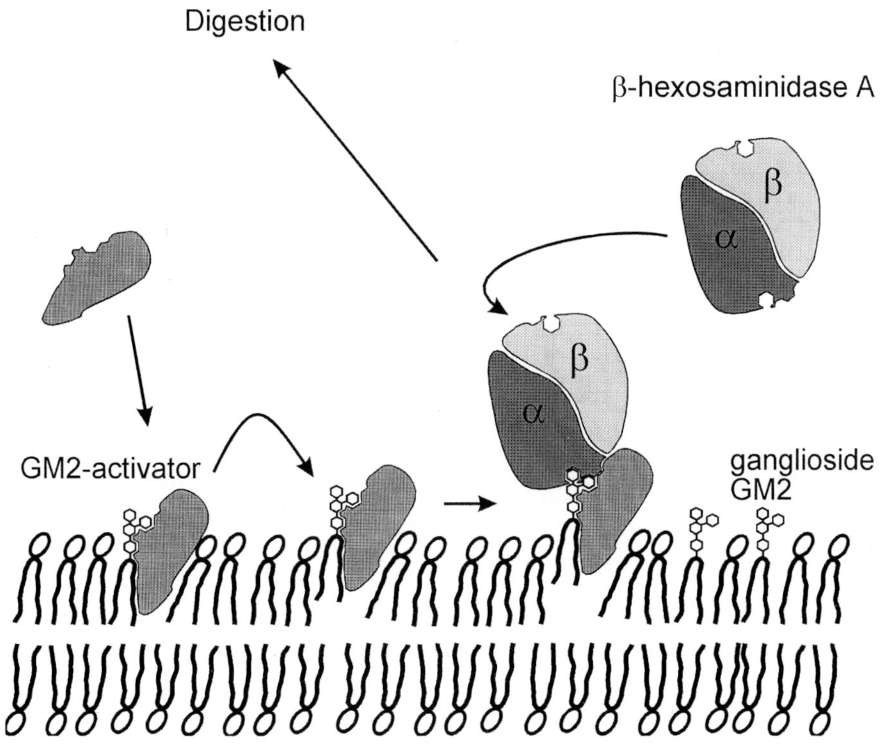

Fig. 153-3 Model for the G_{M2} activator-stimulated degradation of ganglioside G_{M2} by Hex A. The G_{M2} activator binds one molecule of membrane-bound ganglioside G_{M2} and lifts it out of the membrane. The activator-lipid complex is recognized by the water soluble Hex A, which cleaves the lipid substrate.[77]

by several laboratories that expression of human Hex B required only the presence of chromosome 5, whereas Hex A required chromosomes 5 and 15 simultaneously.[95–97] This confirmed the two-polypeptide model and showed that the α and β subunits were encoded by distinct genes (Fig. 153-4).

Subsequent research addressed the polypeptide composition of Hex A and Hex B. It was not until 1980 that structures approximating the current view were proposed (Fig. 153-5; reviewed in reference [98]). Mahuran and colleagues,[99,100] who purified the enzyme from human placenta, and Hasilik and Neufeld,[101] who studied the enzyme immunoprecipitated from radiolabeled fibroblasts, concluded that the α subunit of Hex A contained a single polypeptide, M_r ~55,000, while the β subunit in either Hex A or Hex B was comprised of at least two smaller polypeptides, M_r ~20,000 to 30,000. These were designated β_a and β_b.[100] Importantly, pulse-chase experiments showed that the α and β polypeptides were synthesized as larger precursors, the propolypeptides, which were glycosylated at multiple sites and proteolytically processed to their mature forms.[101,102] A more precise definition of the peptide components of the α and β subunits was derived later by aligning N-terminal sequences with the deduced amino acid sequences of corresponding cDNA clones (see "Structure of the *HEXA*, *HEXB*, and *GM2A* cDNAs and Genes" below).

The G_{M2} activator was purified in 1979[103] and sequenced in its entirety in 1990.[104] It is a small, M_r ~22,000, acidic (pI ~4.8), heat-stable monomer of 160 amino acids. Like the subunits of Hex A, it is a glycoprotein that is derived from the N-terminal proteolytic cleavage in the lysosome of a larger precursor, M_r

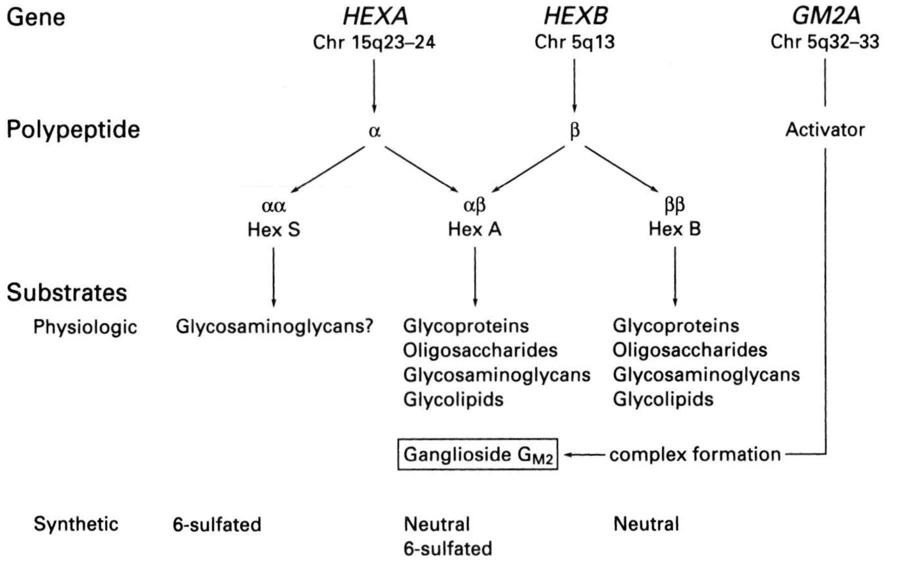

Fig. 153-4 The β-hexosaminidase gene system. Three polypeptides, each encoded by a different gene, are needed for the degradation of ganglioside G_{M2}: the α- and β-subunits of the Hex A isoenzyme and the G_{M2} activator protein that binds the ganglioside and presents it to the enzyme. (For explanation of the various substrates, see text.)

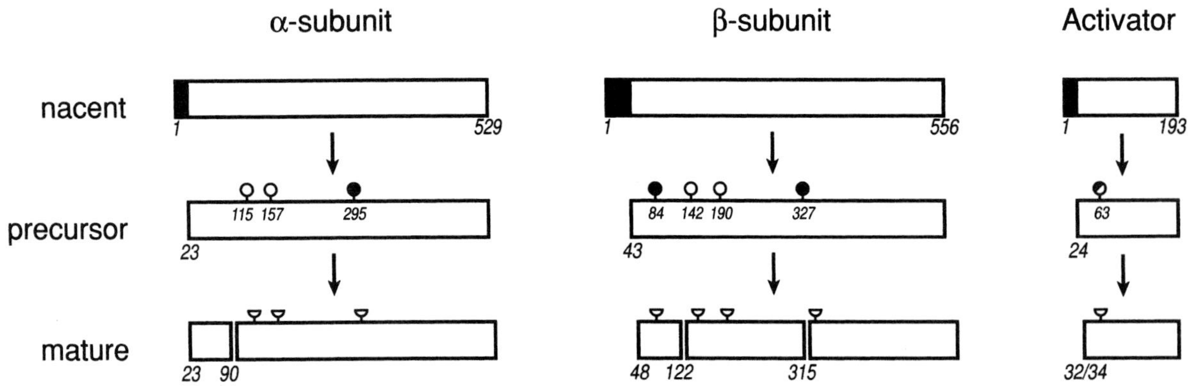

Fig. 153-5 Posttranslational modifications of the β-hexosaminidase subunits and the activator protein. Bars represent the polypeptides. The numbers below the bars represent the amino acids of the termini. The filled bars represent the signal peptides. The numbers in the bars represent the asparagine residues modified by oligosaccharides. Asparagine residue 142 on the β-subunit is incompletely glycosylated. The circles represent oligosaccharides. Filled circles indicate preferred phosphorylation sites. The activator oligosaccharide is incompletely phosphorylated and is represented by the partially filled circle. Half circles indicate degraded oligosaccharide structures. The fragments of the mature hexosaminidase subunits are held together by disulfide bonds (not shown).

~24,000.[105] A truncated form of the G_{M2} activator, referred to as the G_{M2A} protein, has also been identified through cDNA cloning.[106,107] The G_{M2} activator is not related to other sphingolipid activator proteins, such as the saposins A-D, which are proteolytically derived from a single multiactivator protein (reviewed in references 76 and 108). Instead, the G_{M2} activator is encoded uniquely by its own gene, *GM2A*, and the two forms of the protein appear to be derived by alternate splicing.[107] A deficiency of the G_{M2} activator is responsible for the final class of patients, the AB variant, who have neither Hex A nor Hex B activity, but who, nonetheless, store ganglioside G_{M2}[109] (reviewed in reference 76).

Biosynthesis and Posttranslational Modifications

The expression of Hex A, Hex B, and the G_{M2} activator in lysosomes requires biosynthetic processing by components of the secretory and lysosomal pathways. The posttranslational modifications acquired by the polypeptides during their biosynthesis are characteristic features of the cellular organelles, the ER, Golgi, *trans*-Golgi network and lysosome, through which they transit and ultimately reside.

Endoplasmic Reticulum. The ER contains the cellular machinery for translation, *N*-linked glycosylation, disulfide-bond formation, and folding and assembly of polypeptides.[110–112] Also present is a quality control apparatus that can retain incompletely or improperly folded polypeptides and remove them by degradation.[113]

The α- and β-subunits of hexosaminidase[114–117] and the G_{M2} activator[118] are each initially synthesized with aminoterminal, hydrophobic signal sequences. These sequences are removed by the signal peptidase during cotranslational targeting into the lumen of the ER. Here the oligosaccharyltransferase transfers preassembled high-mannose oligosaccharides from a dolichol-linked oligosaccharide donor onto asparagine acceptor sites in the nascent polypeptides—three onto the α-subunit,[119] four onto the β-subunit,[120,121] and a single glycan onto the G_{M2} activator protein.[104] The elimination of individual oligosaccharides acceptor sites on the α or β-subunits does not greatly alter hexosaminidase activity.[119,121] However, the loss of all three oligosaccharides on the α-subunit impairs proper protein folding and causes the misfolded subunit to become entrapped in the ER.[119] The single oligosaccharide on the G_{M2} activator is dispensable for both functional activity and cellular transport to lysosomes.[122,123]

With the exception of one linkage,[124] the arrangement of the disulfide bonds is not known for the subunits of hexosaminidase. For the G_{M2} activator protein, the location of each of its four disulfide bonds has been determined.[118]

The assembly of the precursor subunits is a critical event in the natural history of hexosaminidase. Dimerization is required for catalytic activity[125,126] and results in the three forms of the enzyme—Hex A (αβ), Hex B (ββ) and Hex S (αα)—each with different substrate specificity. Significantly, subunit assembly is a process that is sensitive to disruption by mutation in the G_{M2} gangliosidoses.[127] Dimerization of β-subunits to form Hex B occurs in the ER rapidly after entry.[125] In contrast, the assembly of α and β-subunits to form Hex A is a much slower process. Newly synthesized, unassembled α-subunits enter a pool that is retained prelysosomally prior to assembly with β-subunits.[126] The assembly of α-subunits with newly synthesized β-subunits takes place over several hours after the synthesis of the α-subunits. After assembly, the heterodimers are rapidly delivered to lysosomes. The precise location of αβ assembly has not been established. However, an endoplasmic reticulum site is probable because retention of unassembled polypeptides is a general property of this organelle.[113]

Golgi. In the Golgi, and in pre-Golgi compartments, proteins destined for lysosomes are recognized by UDP-*N*-acetylglucosamine 1-phosphotransferase, which transfers GlcNAc-phosphate onto mannose residues of the oligosaccharide side chains.[128,129] The recognition of the attachment sites by the phosphotransferase is determined by the position of key contact points, dominated by lysine residues, on the surface of the lysosomal protein.[130–136] The terminal Glc-Nac residue is next removed by a second Golgi-resident enzyme that exposes the mannose-6-phosphate structure essential to lysosomal targeting. Finally, the mannose-6-phosphate residues are recognized by receptors that sort the glycoproteins to lysosomes. Although the majority of lysosomal proteins utilize this pathway, some proteins are sorted to lysosomes by a pathway independent of mannose-6-phosphate.[137–139]

For the α and β-subunits, there is some specificity with which particular oligosaccharides are phosphorylated. On the α-subunit, the first and fourth oligosaccharide are preferentially phosphorylated.[121] On the β-subunit, the third, corresponding to the fourth on the α-subunit, is the site of preferential phosphorylation.[119] This specificity of phosphorylation may reflect the relative distances between the phosphotransferase recognition determinants and the oligosaccharide chains.[140] At present, the recognition determinant on hexosaminidase subunits has not been identified. The lysosomal targeting of hexosaminidase is heavily dependent on the mannose-6-phosphate recognition marker as illustrated by the nearly complete secretion of precursor enzyme in I-cell fibroblasts.[141]

The single glycan on the activator protein is predominantly a nonphosphorylated, complex-type oligosaccharide.[123,142] Less than 10 percent of the activator glycans synthesized in human keratinocytes contain phosphate. Interestingly, completely nonglycosylated activator protein is delivered to lysosomes, both through a biosynthetic route and by endocytosis of endogenous protein.[123,142] Thus, unlike hexosaminidase, the G_{M2} activator can be targeted to lysosomes independent of the mannose-6-phosphate pathway.

A substantial fraction of newly synthesized proteins escapes the lysosomal pathway and is secreted.[143] These precursors generally differ from their intracellular counterparts by an increase in the complexity of their oligosaccharides. They are subject to uptake by cell-surface receptors and delivery to lysosomes.

Lysosomes. The major modifications that occur in lysosomes are proteolytic and glycosidic processing.[143] Although required in some cases for enzymatic activity to be expressed, for most resident lysosomal proteins the processing appears to be adventitious. The hexosaminidase subunits are proteolytically cleaved in lysosomes.[141] Internal cleavages, with trimming of termini, yield a mature α-subunit consisting of two peptides[116,144,145] and a mature β-subunit containing three peptides.[115,121,145] In each case, the peptide fragments are covalently linked by disulfide bonds. The mature activator protein is formed in lysosomes after loss of either eight or nine amino acids from its amino terminus.[104] None of the polypeptide cleavages is prerequisite for acquisition of catalytic activity because the precursor enzyme[101] and activator[105] are fully active. The oligosaccharides of the hexosaminidase subunits[120] and activator protein[123] is extensively degraded in lysosomes without noticeable effects on activity.

Substrate Specificity

Like most lysosomal glycosidases, hexosaminidases hydrolyze a broad spectrum of substrates (Fig. 153-4). They are specific for only the terminal nonreducing sugar (GlcNAc or GalNAc) in β linkage.[146] The nature of the aglycone component is of little importance, and this has made it possible to develop numerous synthetic substrates (reviewed in reference 87). The most sensitive and commonly used synthetic substrate is the β-GlcNAc derivative of the fluorogenic compound, 4-methylumbelliferone (MUG).[147] It is recognized by both Hex A and Hex B and does not require the G_{M2} activator protein for activity. 4-Methylumbelliferyl-GlcNAc-6-SO_4 in β linkage (MUGS),[148] a related compound with specificity for the α catalytic sites of Hex A and Hex S, was developed based on the substrate specificity studies by Kresse[149,150] (see "Enzyme Assays" below).

Both the α and β subunits of hexosaminidase possess an active site,[151] although dimer formation, as Hex S ($\alpha\alpha$), Hex B ($\beta\beta$), or Hex A ($\alpha\beta$), is required for catalytic activity.[126] Furthermore, the α and β subunits have somewhat different substrate specificities.[151] The β subunit preferentially hydrolyzes neutral water-soluble substrates, including the MUG synthetic substrate. The α subunit, however, also hydrolyzes negatively charged substrates such as ganglioside G_{M2} or polysaccharides with a penultimate charged (uronic acid) residue, as in dermatan sulfate or chondroitin sulfate.[151,152] Substrates with a negative charge on the terminal *N*-acetylglucosamine, as in the GlcNAc-6-SO_4 residue in keratan sulfate[149,153] or the MUGS artificial substrate, are also hydrolyzed by the α subunit.

The kinetic constants of Hex A and Hex B toward the neutral MUG have been found to be very similar, with K_m/V_{max} values of 0.91 mM/1.8 $\times$ 10^{-4} mol/min/mg and 0.90 mM/4.4 $\times$ 10^{-4} mol/min/mg, respectively.[151] They also have an identical pH optimum of 4.4 for MUG.[154–157] They differ with respect to the hydrolysis of MUGS. The K_m for Hex B is 3.4 mM, 10 times higher than the values determined for Hex A and Hex S, reflecting the specificity of the α subunit for negatively charged substrates.[151] However, the specific activity of Hex S towards the MUGS substrate was reported to be only one-fifth that of Hex A, perhaps reflecting the inherent instability of this isoenzyme during purification.[151] Recent studies with recombinant Hex S produced in insect cells resulted in a twofold higher specific activity (6.8 $\times$ 10^{-5} mol/min/mg) than that for Hex A.[158] Mouse Hex S presumably also exhibits some minor hydrolyzing activities toward ganglioside G_{M2} and G_{A2} *in vivo*—so far not detected *in vitro*—as indicated by the increased neuronal glycolipid storage in double-knockout mice (*Hexa* −/−;*Hexb* −/−) with a defect of all three hexosaminidases, Hex A, Hex B, and Hex S (G_{M2} = 1.15 and G_{A2} = 2.4 μmol/g wet weight) compared to *Hexb* −/− knockout mice still expressing Hex S (G_{M2} = 0.76 and G_{A2} = 1.9 μmol/g wet weight).[159]

Whereas in human cells ganglioside G_{M2} is hydrolyzed almost exclusively by Hex A in the presence of the G_{M2} activator, in mice, ganglioside G_{M2} is also degraded by a lysosomal sialidase. Therefore, the catabolic block in *Hexa* −/− knockout mice is partially bypassed by mouse sialidase converting G_{M2} to G_{A2}, which is then slowly degraded by Hex B, presumably with the help of the G_{M2} activator.[159–161]

Active Sites of Hexosaminidases and Catalysis

Lysosomal hexosaminidases catalyze the hydrolysis of their glycoside substrates by a "retaining" mechanism[162] in which the anomeric configuration at C1 of the substrate is retained in the product.[163,164] Most glycosidases employ an acid catalysis mechanism of substrate hydrolysis (Fig. 153-6). One amino acid residue of the enzyme functions as a proton donor that protonates the glycosidic oxygen, while another residue functions as an anion that stabilizes the cationic transition state or acts as a nucleophile.[163,165] By analogy with the widely cited mechanism for retaining β-glucosidases,[163] *N*-acetyl-β-D-hexosaminidases may operate by stabilizing the transition state, leading to a covalent enzyme-substrate complex (Fig. 153-6, upper path).[166] Alternatively, the configuration-retaining aspect of some *N*-acetyl-β-D-hexosaminidases, probably also including the human enzymes, may be attributed to the participation of the neighboring C-2 acetamido group, leading initially to a cyclized oxazolone intermediate (Fig. 153-6, lower path).[167,168]

Recently, some progress was made in the identification of the active site residues of the hexosaminidases. Photoaffinity labeling of purified Hex B with a substrate analogue carrying a carbene precursor identified Glu355 at the substrate binding site.[169] Changing Glu355 to other amino acids by site-directed mutagenesis results in loss of enzymatic activity without impairing substrate binding, thus indicating that Glu355 is involved in the catalytic cation of Hex B.[170] This is supported by the position of Glu355 modeled against the the x-ray crystallographic structure analysis of a bacterial chitobiase (*Serratia marcescens*). The bacterial enzyme and Hex A and Hex B belong to family 20 of glycosyl hydrolases, in which the members of any one family share sequence and folding characteristics and mechanistic stereochemistry. This analysis identified Glu-540 of bacterial chitobiase as the catalytic residue.[171] By sequence alignment, Glu-540 corresponds to Glu355 of the β subunit and Glu323 of the α subunit of human hexosaminidase. Recent studies employing site-directed mutagenesis and expression confirmed α:Glu323 as the putative active site residue in Hex A.[172]

According to the crystal structure of bacterial chitobiase, the catalytic domain, conserved in family 20 of glycosyl hydrolases, is defined by a central region forming a $(\beta\alpha)_8$ barrel fold.[171] Modeling of the catalytic domain of Hex A against the structure of chitobiase brings α:Glu323 in proximity to the substrate-binding cleft and leaves it spatially arranged so as to facilitate catalysis.[172] In contrast, α:Asp163, which corresponds to β:Asp196 and which was also investigated as a candidate active-site residue in the β subunit,[173] appears to be remote from the catalytic domain. Also of note are mutations in the *HEXA* gene that inactivate the active site of the α subunit of Hex A while leaving the β site active. Such

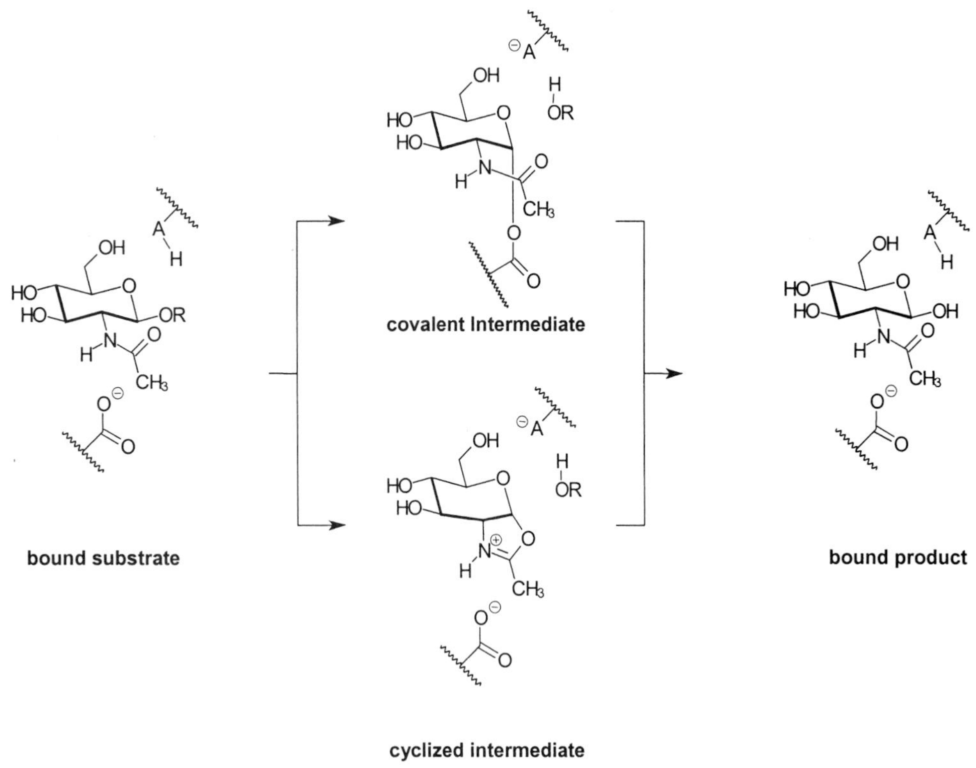

Fig. 153-6 Proposed mechanisms for the hydrolysis of the glycosidic bond by *N*-acetyl-β-hexosaminidase (i.e., Hex A or Hex B) via a covalent enzyme-substrate complex (upper path) or via participation of the neighboring C-2 acetamido group and a cyclized oxazolone intermediate (lower path). (*Reproduced from Knapp et al.*[165] *Used by permission.*)

mutations, causing the B1 phenotype of G_{M2} gangliosidosis, include the basic residue α:Arg178[151,174–176] and the acidic residue α:Asp258.[176,177] They appear to be essential for proper formation and stabilization of the active site domain but apparently are not directly involved in catalysis[171] (Fig. 153-7; see "Mutations Associated with Subacute Variant of Tay-Sachs Disease" below).

Hydrolysis of ganglioside G_{M2} by Hex A requires interaction with the G_{M2} activator protein.[103] To identify domains needed for the activator-stimulated hydrolysis of ganglioside G_{M2}, chimeric Hex enzymes were generated by fusion of different segments of the α and β subunits.[178,179] The results indicate that the ability of the α subunit to bind negatively charged substrates is located in residues α 132 to 283,[178] whereas β subunit amino acids 225 to 556 contribute an essential function in the G_{M2}-hydrolyzing activity of Hex A.[179]

Role of the G_{M2} Activator Protein

It is evident from the occurrence of the three forms of G_{M2} gangliosidosis that only Hex A can hydrolyze ganglioside G_{M2} *in vivo* and that it requires the presence of the G_{M2} activator to do so. Mechanistically, the activator forms a 1:1 complex with gangliosides, and it is the complex that is presented to the enzyme for hydrolysis. It can also form a complex with G_{A2} because Hex B has ~3 percent residual activity toward G_{A2} in the presence of the activator.[103] Although the activator binds to a wide variety of negatively charged glycosphingolipids,[180] the binding affinity decreases in the order $G_{M2} \gg G_{T1b} \gg G_{M1} > G_{b4} > G_{M3} > G_{A2}$.[181,182] These data indicate that the activator contains a specific carbohydrate binding site that recognizes the sialic acid,[183] as well as another for the GalNAc residue, recently confirmed using recombinant activator.[107] The activator must also bind to the ceramide moiety in order to extract the ganglioside from the membrane. *In vitro*, the G_{M2} activator can remove labeled gangliosides from one liposome and insert them into another liposome.[182] Thus, the G_{M2} activator does not activate Hex A, but rather may function both to transport ganglioside G_{M2} from the lysosomal membrane and, as a complex with the glycolipid, present it to Hex A for hydrolysis (Fig. 153-3).

Certain detergents, for example, taurodeoxycholate (2 mM), can be used to replace the G_{M2} activator *in vitro*. Hex S can also hydrolyze ganglioside G_{M2} in the presence of detergents, whereas the Hex B residual activity remains low (~17 percent of Hex A levels); however, G_{A2} ganglioside becomes a better substrate for Hex B than Hex A.[103] These data are consistent with a role for negative charges in determining the substrate specificity of Hex isoenzymes (above). They also indicate that the activator behaves like a mild detergent, but with specificity for Hex A. Thus, the α subunit supplies the active site for ganglioside G_{M2} hydrolysis, but the presence of the β subunit in the Hex A dimer is necessary for the correct binding of the ganglioside G_{M2}/G_{M2} activator complex (Fig. 153-3).

Interestingly, when either the oligosaccharide chain of the ganglioside is elongated, as in GalNAc-G_{D1a} ganglioside, or the fatty acid is shortened, the resulting molecule can become a substrate for Hex A alone.[78] The effect of the former modification is to extend the target β-GalNAc residue far enough into the aqueous environment to make it accessible to Hex A for hydrolysis. The effect of the latter is to make the potential substrate more water soluble, allowing Hex A to hydrolyze each molecule as it is dissolved. Thus, the function of the G_{M2} activator is to overcome the inability of water-soluble Hex A to bind, due to steric hindrance, and hydrolyze the target β-GalNAc residue on the terminus of the membrane-bound ganglioside G_{M2}.[78] It follows that Hex A does not recognize or bind to any other portions of the ganglioside molecule. These data demonstrate the validity of using small water-soluble synthetic substrates, such as MUGS, to measure the competence of the α-catalytic site in Hex A to hydrolyze ganglioside G_{M2}. What MUGS cannot measure is any change in the ability of Hex A (requiring portions of both subunits) to bind the G_{M2} activator. Thus, it is possible, and it was suggested in one case,[184,185] that a *HEXA* or *HEXB* mutation could adversely affect activator binding without affecting the catalytic site, that is, activity towards the 4-MUGS substrate.

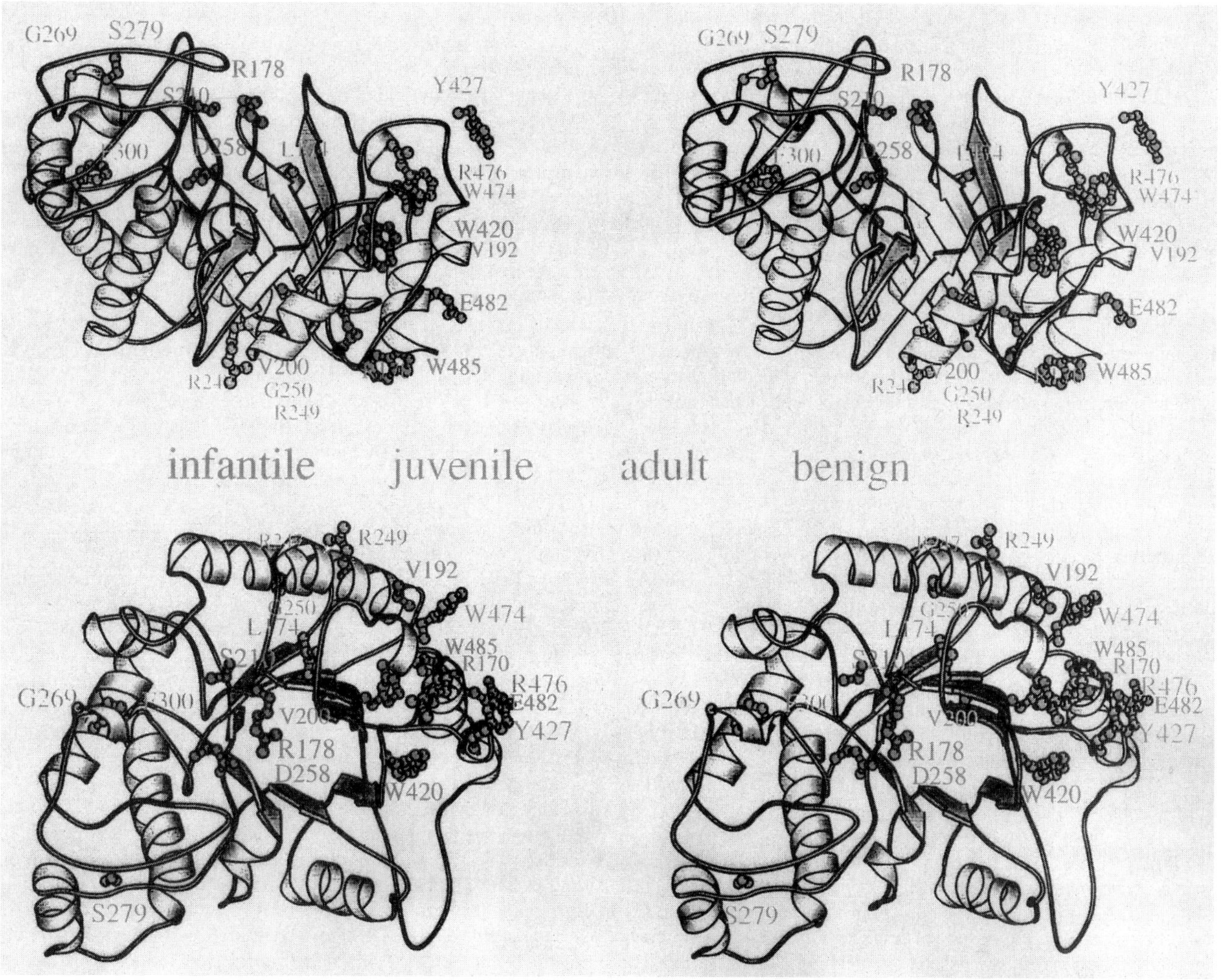

Fig. 153-7 Stereoviews of predicted structure of Hex active site region showing sites of selected mutations coded by phenotypic classification (mutations referenced in original publication), infantile, juvenile (subacute), adult (chronic), and benign (pseudo-deficiency) mutations. The online version of MMBID presents these mutant residues in color: red for infantile, orange for juvenile, green for adult, blue for benign. The lower view shows the predicted $(\beta\alpha)_8$-barrel motif from the top, the upper view is turned 90° on its axis. (*Reproduced from Tews et al.*[171] *Used by permission.*)

STRUCTURE OF THE *HEXA*, *HEXB*, AND *GM2A* cDNAs AND GENES

In the mid-1980s, the structural characterization of Hex A and Hex B was given a major boost with the isolation of cDNA clones coding for the α[186–188] and β subunits.[189] These efforts revealed the amino acid sequences as deduced from the cDNAs and positioned proteolytic cleavage and oligosaccharide binding sites determined from protein or peptide sequences (see "Protein Structure" above).

As the primary amino acid sequences of the α and β chains were determined, it became obvious, even from a small amount of sequence data, that they shared a large degree of primary structure homology.[187] When the nearly complete sequences were compared, there was an overall 57 percent sequence identity.[188] As well, the structures of the *HEXA* and *HEXB* genes showed a striking degree of homology, both in the number and placement of exon/intron junctions.[190] Twelve of the 13 introns interrupt the genes at corresponding positions. Despite their location on different chromosomes, these data suggested that the *HEXA* and *HEXB* genes arose from a common ancestor.

With the isolation of the cDNAs, the cloning of the *HEXA* and *HEXB* genes followed. The *HEXA* gene is 35 kb in length and contains 14 exons.[191] It was mapped to chromosome 15q23 → q24.[192] The *HEXB* gene is approximately 45 kb long and also contains 14 exons.[190,193] It was mapped to chromosome 5q13.[194] In both genes, most of the promoter activity resides within 100 or 150 bp, respectively, of the ATG initiation codon.[195] Both promoters are GC rich and have the appearance of housekeeping genes. The corresponding mouse genes are more compact but share identical positioning of the splice sites and essential structure of the promoters.[195–198] The tissue distribution of mRNAs, investigated in the mouse, is very different between the two genes, with testis and adrenal the major sites of expression of the *Hexa* gene, and kidney and epididymis the major sites for the *Hexb* gene. In the mouse *Hexa* gene, transcription is initiated from a cluster of sites centered approximately 32 bp from the ATG initiation codon.[197]

Finally, cDNA clones encoding the G_{M2} activator were isolated.[106,199–201] As well, its amino acid sequence was independently determined by Edman degradation.[104] The *GM2A* gene is ~16 kb long and contains four exons.[107,200] *GM2A* was mapped to chromosome 5q31.1-31.3[202–204] and a pseudogene, *GM2AP*, was mapped to chromosome 3.[204] Alternate splicing involving intron 3 and exon 4 is responsible for the two forms of activator protein predicted in cells. The predominant 160-amino-acid-long form is encoded by exons 1 to 4. The smaller truncated form, deduced from cDNA sequences, shares the first 109 amino acids translated from exons 1 to 3, but terminates in the tripeptide VST translated from a subset of mRNA that does not undergo splicing of intron

3.[106,107] Studies by Li and colleagues[107] have shown that while the G_{M2} activator supports the hydrolysis of GalNac or NeuAc from ganglioside G_{M2} and GalNac-G_{D1a}, recombinant G_{M2A} protein supports only NeuAc release. These data indicate that the N-terminal region of the G_{M2} activator recognizes the NeuAc moiety, while the C-terminal region contributes in an essential way to GalNac binding. The mouse *GM2A* gene has a similar structure to the human gene and contains a GC-rich promoter with CCAAT and Sp1 sites.[205,206] Expression is strongest in kidney and testis.

THE G_{M2} GANGLIOSIDOSIS VARIANTS

The genetic basis of G_{M2} gangliosidosis is complex, because, as described above, three lysosomal polypeptides, encoded by three distinct genes, are essential for normal catabolism of ganglioside G_{M2} *in vivo* — the α and β subunits of Hex A and the G_{M2} activator protein (Fig. 153-4). Mutations in any of the three genes encoding these proteins may give rise to G_{M2} gangliosidosis. Tay-Sachs disease and its variants are due to deficiency of Hex A activity. They are caused by mutations of the *HEXA* gene encoding the α subunit; Hex B activity is normal or increased. Sandhoff disease and its variants are characterized by combined deficiency of Hex A and Hex B activities. Their genetic lesions are in the *HEXB* gene encoding the β subunit common to Hex A and Hex B. The AB variant of G_{M2} gangliosidosis is caused by mutations of the *GM2A* gene encoding the G_{M2} activator protein. In this variant, Hex A and Hex B are structurally and functionally normal, and activities of the enzymes are normal when measured with the use of synthetic, nonlipid substrates. However, hydrolysis of ganglioside G_{M2} by Hex A *in vivo* is impaired by absent or defective formation of the ganglioside G_{M2}/G_{M2} activator complex.

Classification and Nomenclature

Various nomenclatures have been proposed to describe the different forms of G_{M2} gangliosidosis. In 1971, Sandhoff et al.[13] proposed a classification based on the hexosaminidase isoenzyme remaining functional in the tissues of affected patients: variant B due to presence of Hex B and absence of Hex A; variant 0 due to absence of both Hex A and Hex B; and variant AB corresponding to G_{M2} activator defects. In the previous edition of this chapter[207] and continued here, we made use of a nomenclature that employs clinical designations for the various forms of the disease and gene designations to describe the relevant mutations. Accordingly, Tay-Sachs disease and variants refer to G_{M2} gangliosidosis due to *HEXA* mutations; Sandhoff disease and variants refer to G_{M2} gangliosidosis due to *HEXB* mutations; and G_{M2} activator deficiency refers to G_{M2} gangliosidosis due to *GM2A* mutations.

The large spectrum of clinical and enzymologic variants of Tay-Sachs and Sandhoff diseases has made a simplistic nomenclature an elusive goal. Descriptive terms referring to the age of onset and/or the clinical course, such as late-onset, juvenile, adult, subacute, or chronic, are often used to designate variants. These terms are pragmatically convenient, but are often arbitrary and imprecise. Generally, the later the clinical onset the slower the disease progression, although patients are known with the onset in their infancy and a clinical course lasting decades.[208]

Tay-Sachs Disease and Variants. Deficiency or defects of the α subunit of Hex A[209–212] may block the formation of intact Hex A and the minor isoenzyme, Hex S (the $\alpha\alpha$ dimer); however, the nonmutant β subunits still associate to form Hex B. Biochemically, this disorder is characterized by normal or elevated levels of Hex B[10,13,91] and has therefore been referred to as *variant B* of G_{M2} gangliosidosis.[13] The eponym *Tay-Sachs disease* usually refers to the infantile form of the disease.

A few patients with G_{M2} gangliosidosis synthesize an α subunit that associates almost normally with the β subunit, but is devoid of catalytic activity toward ganglioside G_{M2}.[213] The resulting dimer, $\alpha\beta$, behaves like normal Hex A in some respects, such as isoelectric point, heat stability and activity toward commonly used synthetic substrates, but it is inactive toward the physiological substrate, ganglioside G_{M2} and also toward the sulfated synthetic substrate, 4-methylumbelliferyl *N*-acetylglucosamine 6-sulfate (MUGS; see "Substrate Specificity" above).[214,215] This variant, called the *B1 variant*, was first thought to be a form of G_{M2} activator deficiency,[216,217] but was later shown to be allelic with other α subunit deficiencies.[218]

Numerous other variants of Hex α subunit deficiencies have been described since the late 1960s, many with genetic and/or enzymologic characterizations. They encompass a clinical spectrum ranging from *subacute* to *chronic* forms of the disease in which the onset of symptoms of disease may be delayed from a few years to decades. By and large the clinical phenotype correlates well with the enzymatic outcome of the genetic lesion, where the higher the residual activity of Hex A in the lysosome, the later the onset and milder the disease manifestations (see "Degree of Enzyme Deficiency and Development of Different Clinical Diseases" below).

Sandhoff Disease and Variants. Patients with defects of the β subunit have deficiencies of both Hex A and Hex B.[12,13] This variant has been designated *variant 0*, indicating zero hexosaminidase activity. The eponym *Sandhoff disease* is a reference to the first reported differentiation of this variant from classical Tay-Sachs disease by Sandhoff and his colleagues.[12] The small residual hexosaminidase activity in the tissues of patients with infantile Sandhoff disease is due to the presence of α subunit dimers, called Hex S.[93] Hex S had been considered physiologically irrelevant until recent studies of a mouse model doubly deficient in both subunits of hexosaminidase.[219]

Patients with infantile Sandhoff disease are essentially indistinguishable clinically from patients with infantile Tay-Sachs disease. The disease was discovered purely based on enzymology.[220] The clinical features of patients with late-onset/chronic forms are also similar to those of Tay-Sachs disease variants of corresponding ages. Despite accumulation of additional substances, such as globoside and fragments of oligosaccharides in the liver, spleen, kidney, and other systemic organs, clinically detectable organomegaly, skeletal abnormalities or abnormal bone marrow cells are not common in patients with Hex β subunit defects. The presence of such signs is more indicative of G_{M1}-gangliosidosis. Patients excrete abnormal amounts of hexosamine-containing glycoprotein fragments that can be of some diagnostic value.[221,222] Late-onset variants of Sandhoff disease have also been described in which the onset of symptoms is delayed for 2 to 10 years (subacute variants), or even into late adult life (chronic variants).

G_{M2} Activator Deficiency (AB Variant). In 1969, Sandhoff described a patient with infantile "Tay-Sachs disease" who showed normal activities of Hex A and Hex B.[220,223] Both the α and β subunits are genetically intact in this disorder, and thus the major hexosaminidase isozymes, A and B, are functionally normal.[224] It was termed "AB variant" to denote that the hexosaminidase isozymes were normal. G_{M2} activator deficiency is exceedingly rare. The number of known cases is too small to assess geographic and ethnic distribution, but there is no obvious concentration in any groups. An African-American patient was among the early reported cases.[225] The clinical and biochemical phenotype is very similar to those of the classical infantile Tay-Sachs disease. One late infantile patient originally reported to have an "atypical" AB-variant disease later turned out to have the B1 variant form of the disease (hexosaminidase α subunit defect).[214,216] All AB-variant patients so far known are of the infantile phenotype. The patient described in the literature as adult G_{M2} activator-deficient is most likely not a case of G_{M2} activator deficiency because the brain gangliosides showed only minor relative increases of monosialogangliosides, a highly nonspecific finding seen in many neurodegenerative disorders, and because no evidence of impaired G_{M2} ganglioside degradation was provided.[226]

Clinical Phenotypes

Classical infantile Tay-Sachs disease was the only known genetic gangliosidosis until enzymatic identification became possible. On a clinicopathologic basis, the group of neurogenetic disorders now known as neuronal ceroid-lipofuscinosis (Batten, Bielschowski-Jansky, Spielmeyer-Vogt-Sjøgren, Kuf, etc.) were erroneously considered late-onset forms of Tay-Sachs disease ("familial amaurotic idiocies"). Clarification of the enzymatic basis of G_{M2} gangliosidosis brought not only the delineation of the three genetically distinct forms of the disease, but also the recognition that they exist in many clinical and enzymologic variant forms.

The clinical phenotypes associated with G_{M2} gangliosidosis variants vary widely. They range from infantile-onset, rapidly progressive neurodegenerative disease culminating in death before age 4 years (classical Tay-Sachs and Sandhoff diseases and G_{M2} activator deficiency) to late, adult-onset, slowly progressive neurologic conditions compatible with long survival with little or no effect on intellect.[227–231] The different variants of G_{M2} gangliosidosis have been subclassified clinically according to the age of the onset of symptoms into infantile, juvenile, and adult variants. These classifications are often arbitrary, as many patients fall between the categories and some patients who survive into adulthood can have clinical onset in their infantile period.[208] Marked clinical variability is seen even within the same family; complete dementia by age 20 years in one individual has been reported occurring along with very slowly progressive disease in other affected members of the same family, who functioned well into their sixth or seventh decades of life.[232]

A classification of the late-onset variants of the disease based more broadly on the different clinical phenotypes that have been described would be more useful to the clinician and was introduced in the previous edition.[207] The clinical designations recognize the dominance of the encephalopathy rather than age of onset as the primary clinical delineator: *infantile acute encephalopathic G_{M2} gangliosidosis*, which corresponds to the classical infantile form with which the term should remain interchangeable; *subacute encephalopathic G_{M2} gangliosidosis*, which includes late infantile and juvenile onset forms showing a pervasive clinical course usually fatal in childhood or early adulthood; and *chronic encephalopathic G_{M2} gangliosidosis*, which includes some juvenile and adult onset forms comprising a diversity of phenotypes generally compatible with long survival. These are abbreviated the "infantile," "subacute," and "chronic" forms in the text.

Infantile Acute G_{M2} Gangliosidosis

The clinical phenotypes of the acute infantile form of any of the three genetic G_{M2} gangliosidoses, Tay-Sachs disease, Sandhoff disease and G_{M2} activator deficiency, are essentially indistinguishable. Affected infants generally appear completely normal at birth. The clinical manifestations are almost exclusively neurologic with primary involvement of gray matter. The earliest sign of the disease, often only appreciated in retrospect, is mild motor weakness beginning at 3 to 5 months of age. Parents first notice nonspecific and subtle slowdown of growth and dullness of responses to outside stimuli; they sense "something is not quite right." An exaggerated startle response to sharp, though not necessarily loud, sounds is commonly observed at an early stage. This is characterized by sudden extension of both upper and lower extremities, resembling the early components of the normal Moro reflex, but often associated with myoclonic jerks.

Soon regression and loss of already acquired mental and motor skills become obvious. A fundamental aspect of the clinical course of all genetic gangliosidoses is their progressive nature. It is therefore critically important to evaluate patients carefully not only against the standard of normal development at any particular time point but longitudinally to ascertain *regression* of clinical parameters. A static clinical status can be mistakenly perceived as regression because of the relative advances of the normal developmental curve. Progressive weakness and hypotonia, associated with poor head control and with either failure to achieve or loss of gross motor skills, such as crawling and sitting unsupported by 6 to 10 months of age, are often the features that prompt parents to seek medical attention. Seizures of various forms are rare as the presenting symptom but occur often after several months of other neurologic manifestations. Progressive visual difficulty with delayed visual-evoked potential is common. In some cases, decreasing visual attentiveness, associated with unusual eye movements, raises parental concerns about the child's vision, leading to ophthalmologic consultation. Ophthalmoscopic examination often reveals macular pallor with marked prominence of the fovea centralis, the so-called cherry-red spot (Fig. 153-8), immediately raising the possibility of Tay-Sachs disease or one of a small number of other neurodegenerative storage diseases. Although not pathognomonic of infantile G_{M2} gangliosidosis, this finding is seen in virtually all patients with infantile Tay-Sachs or Sandhoff disease. One author observed a faint cherry-red spot by indirect ophthalmoscopy as early as 2 days of age in an affected infant born to a family with a previous child with Tay-Sachs disease (M.M. Kaback, unpublished).

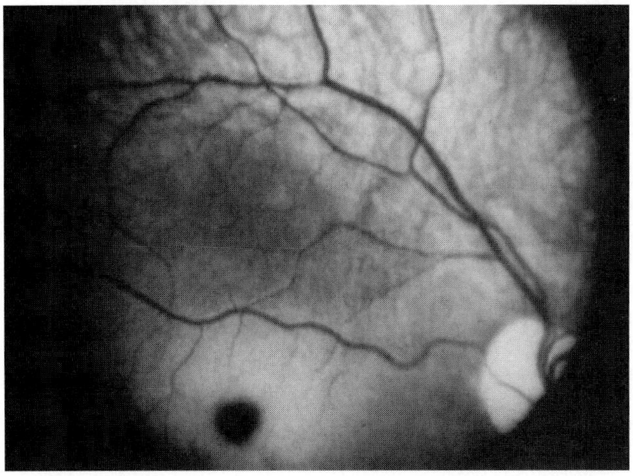

Fig. 153-8 "Cherry red" spot in the fundus of an infantile Tay-Sachs patient (at bottom left).

After 8 to 10 months of age, progression of the disease is rapid. This period is marked by increasing paucity of spontaneous or purposeful voluntary movement and the infant becomes progressively less responsive to parents and surroundings. Hyperacusis and the resulting startle reaction become prominent. Vision deteriorates rapidly, although the ability to distinguish light and darkness may be preserved. Seizures are common by the end of the first year of life. They are highly variable in type; subtle partial-complex seizures or absence attacks typically become more frequent and more severe with time. Partial, though rarely complete, seizure control can usually be achieved using conventional anticonvulsant medications, such as benzodiazepines. The electroencephalographic changes in the disease are relatively mild for much of the first year of life but then show rapidly progressive deterioration until death.[233] The electroretinogram is consistently normal; however, visual-evoked potentials are abnormal from the early stages of the disease, and the cortical response is generally abolished by 12 to 16 months of age. Progressive enlargement of the head (macrocephaly) typically begins by 18 months of age; it results from reactive cerebral gliosis and is not due to hydrocephaly.

Further deterioration in the second year of life invariably leads to decerebrate posturing, difficulties in swallowing, increasing seizure activity, and eventually to a completely unresponsive, vegetative state. Death is usually caused by bronchopneumonia resulting from stasis or aspiration coupled with depressed cough. Although children with infantile G_{M2} gangliosidosis usually do not live beyond 2 to 4 years of age, one child with Tay-Sachs disease is known to have survived to age 6.

Four patients with infantile Tay-Sachs disease were followed with neuroimaging through different clinical phases of the disease.[234] At the initial phase, the basal ganglia and cerebral white matter showed low density on CT and high signal intensity on T2-weighted MRI. Enlargement of the caudate nucleus was observed during the first and second stage, and the low density of the white matter on CT continued throughout the course. In the last phase, the whole brain appeared atrophic despite the enlarged head.

The occurrence of this clinical phenotype in a child of Ashkenazi Jewish parents strongly suggests a diagnosis of Tay-Sachs disease. Sandhoff disease and G_{M2} activator deficiency are panethnic, although small pockets of high incidence populations are recorded. Enzymatic diagnosis can readily distinguish Tay-Sachs and Sandhoff disease. However, the clinical phenotype and normal Hex A and Hex B are insufficient for the diagnosis of G_{M2} activator deficiency because most people in the general population have the normal hexosaminidase complement. Positive evidence of defective G_{M2} activator, either on the gene or protein level, or evidence of defective G_{M2} ganglioside degradation, either as a massive accumulation in the brain or metabolically in cultured cells, is required for definitive diagnosis.

Late-Onset Forms

No patients are known with a late-onset or adult form of G_{M2} activator deficiency. The clinical phenotype varies widely among the late-onset, variant forms of Tay-Sachs and Sandhoff diseases. Onset can be at any time from the late infantile period to adult age. Macular cherry red spots are less frequent, particularly in the adult patients. If a somewhat simplistic generalization can be made regarding the clinical manifestations of later-onset forms, involvement of the deeper brain structures are more prominent compared to the overwhelming generalized gray matter involvement in the infantile form. Manifestations include dystonia, other extrapyramidal signs, such as ataxia, choreoathetoid movements, the signs of spinocerebellar degeneration and ALS-like motor neuron involvement. Psychotic manifestations are not uncommon among patients with late-onset forms. On the other hand, in some older patients, mental capacity can be well preserved, although severe dysarthria often masks the preserved intelligence. Most of the older variants were recognized when the enzymatic diagnosis of the disease became feasible.

Subacute G_{M2} Gangliosidosis. Generally, the onset of the subacute disease is heralded by the development of ataxia and incoordination between 2 and 10 years of age. Developmental regression and dementia, particularly involving speech and life skills, are prominent features of this variant. In addition to progressive psychomotor deterioration, the course of the disease is characterized by increasing spasticity and the development of seizures by the end of the first decade of life.[235–238] Loss of vision occurs much later than in the infantile disease, and macular degeneration is variable. Instead, optic atrophy and retinitis pigmentosa may be seen late in the course of this condition. A vegetative state with decerebrate rigidity develops by 10 to 15 years of age, followed within a few years by death, usually due to intercurrent infection.

In some cases, described by some as late-infantile G_{M2} gangliosidosis, the disease takes a particularly aggressive course, culminating in death in 2 to 4 years.[239] This subacute phenotype has been described in patients with *HEXA* or *HEXB* mutations. Many of the patients who were reported as having late-infantile or juvenile forms of the disease had *HEXA* mutations associated with the B1 variant biochemical phenotype.[240–243] A patient described as having a juvenile form of Hex A deficiency, later recognized as most likely having the enzymologically unique B1 variant form, presented the typical clinical course of the subacute disease occurring in the juvenile age group.[238] The patient, a Puerto Rican girl, developed normally. Soon after she started elementary school, she developed clumsiness and fell readily. She started losing her mental capacity slowly beginning at about 6 years, and developed seizures at 8 years and cerebellar signs at 9 years. Pyramidal signs and dystonia became prominent between 9.5 to 11 years, and dysphagia was difficult to manage by 14 years. She became areflexic at 14 years and died at 14.5 years.

Chronic G_{M2} Gangliosidosis. Patients with the chronic form of the disease have their clinical onset anywhere from childhood to well into adulthood.[227,229,231,244,245] Variations in the clinical manifestations and courses are extreme. For example, in an Ashkenazi Jewish family with three sibs affected by Hex A deficiency,[208] all developed clear clinical symptoms around 2 years of age. Yet, despite the relatively early onset, the disease progressed very slowly with primarily pyramidal and extrapyramidal signs. One affected sib died of phenothiazine intoxication at 16 years, but the others survived into their forties. Mental capacity remained intact throughout the course of the disease, although communication was difficult because of the motor disturbance.

As in the case of infantile acute and subacute subtypes of G_{M2}-gangliosidosis, the clinical differentiation of chronic variants due to hexosaminidase α subunit deficiency (Tay-Sachs disease variants) from those due to β subunit deficiency (Sandhoff disease variants) is generally not possible. However, the former are much more common than the latter, and, as stated already, late-onset chronic forms of G_{M2} activator deficiency are not known.

Neurologic and Psychiatric Manifestations Commonly Associated with Chronic G_{M2} Gangliosidosis

In contrast to the stereotypical clinical manifestations of the infantile forms of G_{M2} gangliosidosis, the spectrum of the clinical phenotypes of late-onset forms is wide and complex. There is no single "Gestalt" that gives away the underlying nature of the disease. It is important to remember that many neurologic manifestations of the late-onset forms are also shared by some unrelated neurodegenerative disorders, such as Friedreich ataxia or amyotrophic lateral sclerosis, as well as by late-onset variants of other genetic lysosomal sphingolipidoses. As already indicated, preponderance of symptoms due to lower central nervous system structures is common among the late-onset forms of these disorders. Some of the common neurologic features seen in late-onset forms are summarized from the literature in the following paragraphs.

Dystonia. Dystonia and other extrapyramidal signs, such as choreic movements, athetosis, and ataxia, are common in many of the late-onset variants of G_{M2} gangliosidosis. However, in some patients, slowly progressive dystonia dominates the clinical course of the disease, and psychomotor regression is less prominent or absent. Two patients, classified as having juvenile variants of Tay-Sachs disease, are reported to have shown evidence of dystonic posturing and other extrapyramidal signs from early childhood and were severely affected by 10 years of age;[246,247] another presented as a young adult.[248] The disease was due to Hex A deficiency, and the dystonia was associated with other extrapyramidal signs (choreoathetosis, ataxia), muscle wasting, and dementia.

Spinocerebellar Degeneration. The clinical phenotype reminiscent of Friedreich spinocerebellar degeneration is common among patients with subacute or chronic forms of G_{M2} gangliosidosis. In one clinical variant, cerebellar signs were dominant in the clinical phenotype.[208,249,250] Dysarthria, ataxia, incoordination, and abnormalities of posture develop between 2 and 10 years of age.

Mentation and verbal intelligence remain intact, although these are often difficult to test due to the severe motor involvement. In some cases, the prominence of cerebellar symptoms (ataxia, dysmetria, intention tremor, and dysdiadochokinesia), along with spasticity, muscle wasting, weakness, and pes cavus deformities, suggests an atypical form of spinocerebellar degeneration with normal or increased deep tendon reflexes (atypical Friedreich ataxia).[208,250–252] Results of sensory examination are usually normal. However, an early and severe sensory loss was reported in siblings with hexosaminidase β subunit defects in their sixth and seventh decades with motor neuron disease and cerebellar ataxia.[253,254]

Motor Neuron Disease. A number of patients have been reported who showed a pattern of progressive muscle wasting and weakness, fasciculations, and secondary skeletal abnormalities indistinguishable from progressive adolescent-onset spinal muscular atrophy (Kugelberg-Welander disease).[255,256] In still others, the condition resembles late-onset spinal muscular atrophy with onset in early adulthood.[244,257] Muscle weakness is the most prominent clinical abnormality. Upper motor neuron signs are absent. Most of these patients had a late onset form of hexosaminidase α subunit defects.

Many patients with late-onset G_{M2} gangliosidosis due to either hexosaminidase α or β subunit defects have been reported to have muscle wasting and weakness associated with upper, rather than lower, motor neuron abnormalities.[245,258–260] Although this type is often referred to as "amyotrophic lateral sclerosis phenotype," it is a misnomer because both upper and lower motor neurons are consistently affected in amyotrophic lateral sclerosis.

Electrophysiology. Electromyographic findings in these late-onset variations of G_{M2}-gangliosidosis are generally consistent with chronic active denervation with reinnervation, showing spontaneous activity (fasciculations, fibrillation potentials), decreased recruitment, and high-amplitude, polyphasic motor-unit potentials consistent with anterior horn cell disease.[229,230,244,245,261] Nerve conduction velocities are usually normal.[244] Muscle biopsy shows denervation atrophy.[244,258,262]

EEG and Rectal Biopsy. The electroencephalograph in all the late-onset variants of the disease is generally unremarkable.[262] Rectal biopsy with electron microscopic examination of neurons of the myenteric plexus shows presence of ganglion cells distended with concentrically arranged, membranous cytoplasmic bodies (MCB), as are seen in the brain in the more severe clinical variants of G_{M2} gangliosidosis.[229,231,244]

Neuroimaging Studies. CT scans and MR imaging of the brain generally show severe cerebellar atrophy, often with some cerebral atrophy.[248,258,263,264] Apparent discrepancies between the clinical phenotype and neuroimaging findings were reported in 10 Ashkenazi Jewish patients with late-onset G_{M2} gangliosidosis due to Hex A deficiency.[265] All patients showed prominent cerebellar atrophy, particularly of vermis, and normal cerebral hemispheres. No correlation was found with the clinical onset, course, and severity of the neurologic impairment. The cerebral hemispheres appeared normal in seven patients with intellectual deterioration, and in six patients with psychotic episodes. The most prominent cerebellar atrophy was present in the only patient in this group who showed no cerebellar signs.

Psychosis. Psychiatric abnormalities are relatively common in late-onset G_{M2} gangliosidosis, affecting as much as 40 percent of patients with the disease. They may occur as the presenting or most prominent feature of the condition, or more often on a background of the other neurodegenerative clinical phenotypes.[230,262,266,267] The psychiatric manifestations of disease include acute hebephrenic schizophrenia associated with marked disorganization of thought, agitation, delusions and hallucinations, and paranoia, as well as recurrent psychotic depression. The clinical response to conventional antipsychotic or antidepressant therapy is unpredictable and generally poor. The poor response to tricyclic antidepressants and phenothiazines has been attributed to the observation that these drugs inhibit Hex A activity *in vitro* and induce lysosomal lipidosis in fibroblasts and accumulation of lipids in experimental animals *in vivo*.[268–270] Treatment with lithium salts and electroconvulsive therapy has been reported to be beneficial, at least in ameliorating the episodes of psychotic depression.[271]

Other Neurologic Abnormalities. A variety of other neurologic abnormalities have been described in association with the major clinical phenotypes described above. Except for patients with a subacute phenotype, dementia is generally not a prominent feature of the late-onset variants of G_{M2} gangliosidosis presenting in adolescence or adulthood, although many patients show some evidence of organic brain syndrome.[244] On the other hand, Mitsumoto et al.[258] reported severe chronic organic brain syndrome in a 28-year-old patient with a motor neuron disease phenotype due to Hex A deficiency. Federico et al.[263] reported various neurovegetative abnormalities, including bradycardia, postural hypotension, and impaired esophageal motility, in their patients with *HEXB* mutations, and a phenotype of amyotrophic lateral sclerosis. Supranuclear gaze palsies and nystagmus have been described in patients with late-onset G_{M2} gangliosidosis.[272] In the slowly progressive, chronic forms of G_{M2} gangliosidosis, vision is rarely affected, and results of funduscopic examination are generally unremarkable.

PATHOLOGY

A detailed discussion of the pathology of G_{M2} gangliosidosis is presented in the previous editions of this volume[207,273] and is only briefly summarized here.

Tay-Sachs Disease and Variants

Reflecting the clinical picture, the pathology is confined to the nervous system. Three clinical phenotypes — corresponding to the acute infantile form or classical Tay-Sachs disease, the subacute juvenile form, and the chronic adult form — are known. The pathology of infantile Tay-Sachs disease was described in detail in earlier publications.[274] The brain is atrophic during the early stage, but brain weight and size gradually increase. In children who live past the twenty-fourth month, the brain weight is reported to be markedly increased. Histopathology is that of classical neuronal storage disease and essentially all neurons throughout the central nervous system and peripheral nervous system (PNS), including retinal ganglion cells, are swollen with storage material. The nuclei, Nissl substance and other normal subcellular organelles are displaced to the periphery of the neuronal perikarya (Fig. 72-5 in the sixth edition of this volume[273]). The storage material is strongly stained with periodic acid Schiff (PAS) stain on frozen section but not on paraffin section. The classic work of Terry and colleagues[275,276] established the most essential aspect of the ultrastructural pathology of infantile Tay-Sachs disease. The neuronal perikarya are filled with discrete concentrically arranged multilamellar membranous bodies (membranous cytoplasmic bodies (MCBs); Fig. 153-9), which are composed of cholesterol, phospholipid, and G_{M2} ganglioside. Acid phosphatase activity is demonstrated on MCBs histochemically,[274] identifying them as altered secondary lysosomes. The MCBs also accumulate in the "meganeurites" occurring proximal to axonal initial segments in pyramidal neurons that frequently give rise to secondary neurites and form aberrant synaptic contacts[277] (Fig. 72-6 in the sixth edition of this volume[273]). The abnormal wiring of the neuronal circuits by the formation of aberrant synaptic contacts has been suggested to play a significant role in neuronal dysfunction in patients with gangliosidosis and other neuronal storage diseases.[278] Increased numbers of apoptotic cells have been

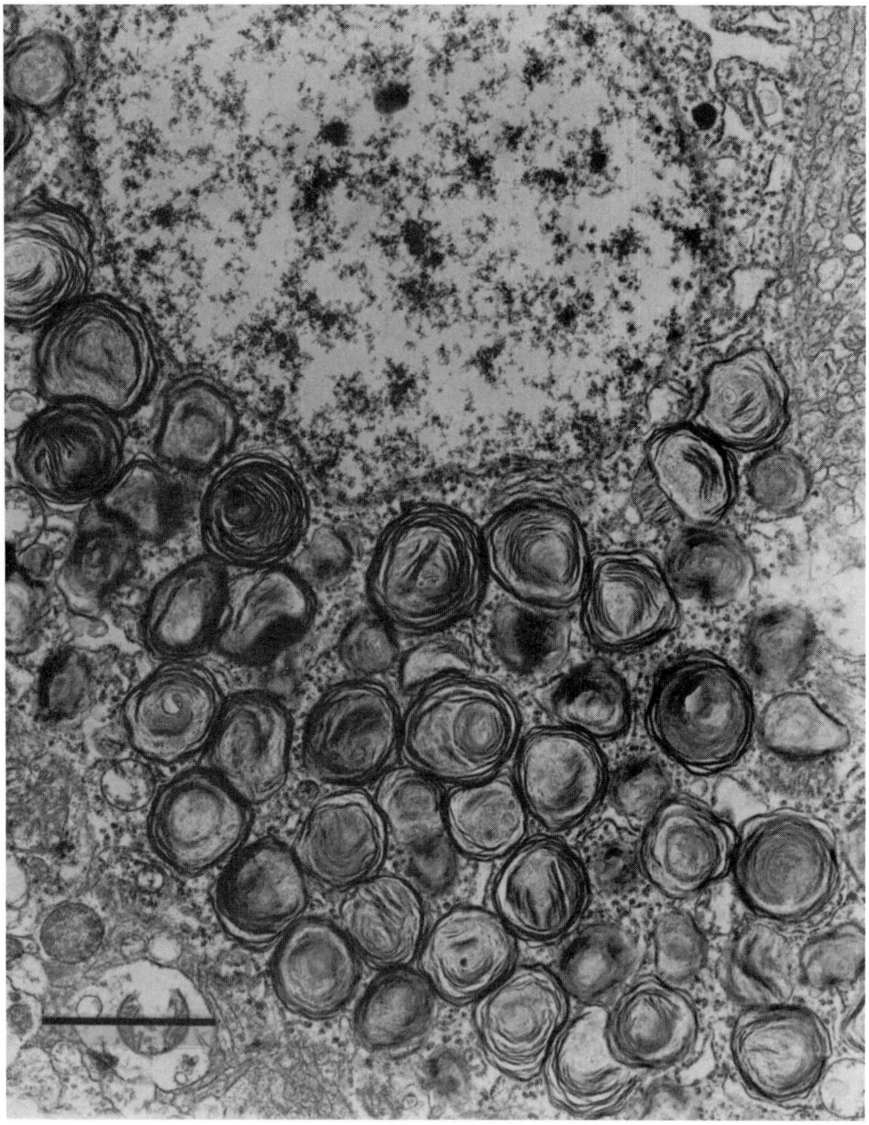

Fig. 153-9 Membranous cytoplasmic bodies (MCBs) occupy neuronal perikarya. Line indicates 1 μm.

demonstrated in the brain of the infantile type of Tay-Sachs and Sandhoff diseases, as well as in the murine model.[279]

The neuronal pathology in the central nervous system in subacute or chronic forms is generally less severe than that in the infantile form, and tends to be more conspicuous in the hypothalamus, cerebellum, brain stem, and spinal cord than in the cerebral cortex.[280] Also neuronal storage material in late-onset cases tends to be more heterogenous and often has stain characteristics similar to lipofuscin pigments. The neurons in the myenteric plexus or other visceral autonomic ganglia, however, show marked cytoplasmic swelling similar to that seen in the infantile form and contain MCBs. Several well-defined clinical phenotypes are identified in these late-onset forms. However, due to limited numbers of postmortem examinations of these cases, clinicopathologic correlations are incomplete.[252] Abnormal storage material can be detected in the fetus upon ultrastructural examination of the spinal cord, dorsal root ganglion, and so on.[281,282]

In the B1 variant of Tay-Sachs disease, the neuropathology is similar to other types of G_{M2} gangliosidosis, but neuronal storage is milder than in infantile Tay-Sachs disease.[216,283,284] The cerebrum and cerebellum are atrophic. Neuronal storage shows some regional variability. Ultrastructural features of neuronal storage material are more heterogeneous, and storage in glial cells is noted as well. Meganeurite formation is conspicuous. There is no storage in visceral organs.

Sandhoff Disease and Variants

Neuropathology is generally similar to Tay-Sachs disease. However, yellowing of the cerebral cortex and deeper structures has been documented in Sandhoff disease possibly owing to accumulated asialoganglioside.[285,286] Also, additional accumulation of sphingoglycolipids with a terminal hexosamine residue and of fragments of undigested glycoprotein in systemic organs, and strongly PAS-positive materials, can be demonstrated in Kupffer cells in the liver, histiocytes in the spleen, lymph nodes and lung, and renal tubular epithelium on frozen section. These storage cells, however, appear vacuolated on routine hematoxylin and eosin-stained paraffin sections. The storage material in these visceral organs are composed of heterogeneous lamellar structures, some of which resemble MCBs.[285–287] The PAS-positive materials in systemic tissues are not seen in patients with Tay-Sachs disease and its variants or with G_{M2} activator deficiency and serve as a diagnostic criterion to distinguish Sandhoff disease and variants from the other two genetic forms of G_{M2} gangliosidosis. In late-onset cases, other than a report describing neurons containing typical MCBs in the myenteric plexus,[288] studies on the pathology of systemic organs is limited.

Table 153-1 Lipids Accumulating in the G_{M2} Gangliosidoses

Substance	Structure	References
G_{A2}	GalNAc(β1 → 4)Gal(β1 → 4) Glc(β1 → 1′)Cer	13, 496
G_{D2}	GalNAc(β1 → 4)[NeuAc(α2 → 8) NeuAc(a2 → 3)]Gal(β1 → 4) Glc(β1 → 1′)Cer	497
Globoside	GalNAc(β1 → 3)Gal(α1 → 4) Gal(β1 → 4)Glc(β1 → 1′)Cer	13, 496, 498
Lyso-G_{M2}	GalNAc(β1 → 4)[NeuAc(α2 → 3)] Gal(β1 → 4)Glc(β1 → 1′) Sphingosine	453, 454
G_{D1a}-GalNAc	GalNAc(β1 → 4)[NeuAc(α2 → 3)] Gal(β1 → 3)GalNAc(β1 → 4) [NeuAc(a2 → 3)]Gal(β1 → 4) Glc(β1 → 1′)Cer	497
G_{M1b}-GalNAc	GalNAc(β1 → 4)[NeuAc(α2 → 3)] Gal(β1 → 3)GalNAc(β1 → 4) Gal(β1 → 4)Glc(β1 → 1′)Cer	499
G_{M1a}-GalNAc	GalNAc(β1 → 4)Gal(β1 → 3) GalNAc(β1 → 4)[NeuAc(α2 → 3)] Gal(β1 → 4)Glc(β1 → 1′)Cer	500
G_{M3}*	NeuAc(α2 → 3)Gal(β1 → 4) Glc(β1 → 1′)Cer	501
G_{D3}*	NeuAc(α2 → 8)NeuAc(α2 → 3) Gal(β1 → 4)Glc(β1 → 1′)Cer	501

*Gangliosides G_{M3} and G_{D3} are not substrates for hexosaminidases. Thus, their storage is probably secondary.

G_{M2} Activator Deficiency

The neuropathology is essentially indistinguishable from that of Tay-Sachs disease or Sandhoff disease at the light microscope level. However, at the ultrastructural level, cerebral cortical neurons reveal Zebra bodies in addition to MCBs, and heterogeneous inclusions are found in astrocytes, oligodendrocytes, and microglia, features that are somewhat different from classical Tay-Sachs disease[216,225] (case 2). Visceral organs are not involved.

STORAGE COMPOUNDS

Almost all storage compounds are either substrates of Hex A or of both Hex A and Hex B. They contain, as the terminal nonreducing sugar moiety, either *β-N*-acetylgalactosamine (on most of the accumulating glycolipids) or *β-N*-acetylglucosamine (on most of the accumulating oligosaccharides).

Glycolipids

The major neuronal storage compound of all variants of G_{M2} gangliosidosis is ganglioside G_{M2} (Fig. 153-1). Its accumulation starts at an early embryonic age and has been observed in the brain of 18 to 20-week-old Tay-Sachs fetuses (100 to 150 nmol ganglioside G_{M2} per gram wet weight).[289,290] Other accumulating lipids are listed in Table 153-1.

The extent of accumulation of the major lipids in G_{M2} gangliosidosis brain was summarized in the previous edition of this volume.[207] All accumulating lipids are amphiphilic membrane components that precipitate together with other membrane components, such as phospholipids, cholesterol, and proteins, mostly in multilamellar cytoplasmic bodies in the cells in which they have been synthesized.

At the storage level, infantile Sandhoff disease is distinguished from both Tay-Sachs disease and G_{M2} activator deficiency by a pronounced accumulation of globoside in visceral organs, and from Tay-Sachs disease by an increased storage of G_{A2} in the brain. The process of lipid accumulation affects primarily the gray matter (Table 72-4 in the sixth edition of this volume[273]) and is accompanied by a decrease of major gangliosides (G_{M1}, G_{D1a}, G_{D1b}, and G_{T1b}). In infantile Tay-Sachs disease, these gangliosides are decreased to 20 to 50 percent of control levels.[13,291] This process is less pronounced in infantile Sandhoff disease and in infantile G_{M2} activator deficiency. A demyelination observed in all infantile variants seems to be secondary to nerve cell degeneration and is reflected at the biochemical level in a sharp decrease in the amount of lipids characteristic of myelin. Cerebrosides and sulfatides are usually decreased in infantile Tay-Sachs disease and Sandhoff disease to levels less than 30 percent of control values; in one case of infantile G_{M2} activator deficiency, the cerebroside level was 10 percent and sulfatide level 40 percent of control.[13]

The extent of lipid accumulation in the late-onset subacute or chronic forms of G_{M2} gangliosidosis is much less pronounced than in infantile forms (Table 72-4 in the sixth edition of this volume[273] and references 238 and 291). Lipid accumulation in infantile acute forms is excessive and ubiquitous throughout the nervous system. In the subacute and chronic forms, the cortex is almost uninvolved. The hippocampus and the nuclei of the brain stem, the spinal cord, and the granular cells in the cerebellum and the retina are mostly affected.[276,291,292]

Oligosaccharides

Oligosaccharides that are derived from glycoproteins and contain terminal *β*-glycosidically linked *N*-acetylglucosaminyl residues are ubiquitous storage compounds in Sandhoff disease. In contrast to glycolipids, accumulating oligosaccharides are water-soluble and can be excreted in the urine. Oligosaccharides identified so far are degradation products of asparagine-linked glycoproteins. They originate by the combined action of proteases, *β*-endo-*N*-acetylglucosaminidase, sialidase, and *β*-galactosidase. The amount of stored and excreted oligosaccharides is given in Tables 72-6 and 72-7 in the sixth edition of this volume.[273] In contrast to the storage of oligosaccharides derived from glycoproteins, accumulation of glycosaminoglycans has never been clearly documented.

Physiologic Significance of the Enzymatic Components Deduced from Storage Products

The roles played by the various hexosaminidase isoenzymes and by the G_{M2} activator in the catabolism of various classes of glycoconjugates is deducible from the substances that accumulate in the different enzymatic variants of infantile G_{M2} gangliosidosis (see Tables 72-3 to 72-7 in the sixth edition of this volume[273]).

Glycolipids. Patients who lack Hex A and the minor Hex S isoenzyme but who have Hex B in normal or elevated amounts, accumulate glycolipids G_{M2} and G_{A2} (and a few minor gangliosides; for review see reference [273]) in neurons. This indicates that these two lipids cannot be degraded by Hex B. As outlined above, the glycolipids are not attacked directly by Hex A but are first solubilized by the G_{M2} activator protein, and the resulting glycolipid-activator complex is the substrate of the enzymatic reaction. Studies *in vitro* showed that human Hex B does not interact with this complex.[103,109] In accordance with these results, patients with the rare deficiency of the G_{M2} activator protein also accumulate ganglioside G_{M2} and glycolipid G_{A2}.[13,109] The structural basis of this substrate specificity is discussed in the section on activator proteins (see "Role of the G_{M2} Activation Protein" above). The lower accumulation of glycolipid G_{A2} in α-subunit deficiency as compared to *β*-subunit deficiency may be explained by a small but significant activity of Hex B (approximately 3 percent that of Hex A as measured *in vitro*) with this substrate in the presence of the G_{M2} activator.[103] The degradation of kidney globoside is still an open question. This glycolipid accumulates in Sandhoff disease but not in the other variants,[13] indicating that it also can be degraded by Hex B.

Glycoproteins and Oligosaccharides. Significant tissue accumulation and urinary excretion of glycoprotein-derived oligosaccharides have so far been found only when both hexosaminidases are deficient,[273,293] making it evident that these water-soluble substrates can also be hydrolyzed by Hex B.

THE MOLECULAR DEFECTS

As typical of other genetic diseases, several classes of mutations have been identified, including partial gene deletions, small insertions or deletions, and base substitutions. In general, mutations causing the production of no mRNA or highly unstable mRNA, which results in complete absence of enzyme activity, are associated with early onset of symptoms and a fulminant clinical course. Less-severe point mutations, compatible with the production of stable mRNA and some detectable mutant enzyme protein and residual enzyme activity, are associated with late onset and slow progression of the disease. Appendices 153-A to C, and an active mutation database (http://data.mch.mcgill.ca/), contain lists of the mutations identified to date in the G_{M2} gangliosidoses with a brief comment on the associated biochemical and clinical phenotype where available. A clear statement of phenotype requires the occurrence of homozygotes and this is indicated in the table. However, homozygotes for many of the rare mutations have not been described. In these instances, it is anticipated that the clinical phenotype correlates more closely with the genetically less severe of the two alleles. Many of the mutations have been associated with particular ethnic groups or geographic isolates. This is also indicated in the table and is discussed more fully in "Incidence and Heredity" below.

Mutations in the *HEXA* Gene

The following sections described *HEXA* gene mutations according to clinical phenotype. Note the positions of mutations causing amino acid substitutions on the structure of the active site of Hex A (α subunit), which positions were derived by modeling against the structure of bacterial chitobiase (Fig. 153-7; see "Active Sites of Hexosaminidases and Catalysis" above). The figure illustrates the distribution of mutations against the clinical phenotypes of affected patients.

Mutations Associated with Infantile Tay-Sachs Disease. Of the approximately 92 mutations identified to date, most are associated with the infantile phenotype. All of the small insertions or deletions that produce frameshifts and the nucleotide substitutions that produce stop codons result in this clinical phenotype. All of these mutations are biochemically CRM-negative. Most splice mutations fall into this category, but there are important exceptions (see following section).

The most frequent, best known, and most studied of the G_{M2} gangliosidoses is classical infantile Tay-Sachs disease. The first mutation identified was a 7.6-kb deletion at the 5′ end of the *HEXA* gene in a French Canadian patient.[294,295] The deletion extends from about 2 kb upstream of the 5′ end of the gene into intron 1. It appears to have arisen from recombination between two Alu sequences. The result is an mRNA-negative, CRM-negative biochemical phenotype.

This was followed by the identification of two mutations accounting for most of the infantile Tay-Sachs disease occurring in Ashkenazi Jews (see "Incidence and Heredity" below). These mutations also result in CRM-negative biochemical phenotypes, although the gene is transcriptionally active in both cases. The most frequent allele is a 4-bp insertion in exon 11, 1278ins4, which creates a frameshift and downstream stop codon in the coding sequence.[296] While the *HEXA* gene is transcribed normally, the mRNA is undetectable by northern blotting.[297] This is not unusual for mRNAs containing stop codons, but it is unexpected in this case, considering that the mutation is so close to the 3′ end of the gene.[298] Interestingly, transient expression of the mutant cDNA resulted in the production of a full-size, stable mRNA, and the synthesis of a truncated α polypeptide.[299] In contrast, stable expression of a mutant sequence, as a minigene, was associated with an unstable mRNA.[300] The matter was resolved by Boles et al.[300] who showed that deletion of one nucleotide to restore the reading frame also restored mRNA stability, confirming that the frameshift is solely responsible for the mRNA instability in patients. The second major Ashkenazi allele is a donor splice junction mutation in intron 11.[301–303] It results in the production of several aberrantly spliced mRNAs (see below).

The different mutations predominating in infantile Tay-Sachs disease in Ashkenazi Jews and French Canadians set the stage for the discovery of extensive allelic heterogeneity which, as in many genetic diseases, is proving to be the rule in the general population, and, perhaps less expected, in population clusters as well (see "Incidence and Heredity" below).

Many mutations that cause infantile Tay-Sachs disease are CRM-positive. Several multibase mutations that fall into this category are in-frame deletions. Three mutations result in deletion of a single amino acid, 304delF (or 305)[304,305] and 320delG (or 321)[306] and 402delK,[307] and one other shows loss of six amino acids, 347delDFKQLE.[308] The first two are deletions of one of two adjacent, identical amino acids, perhaps due to strand slippage during replication or crossing over between tandemly repeated short sequences. Only 304delF has been described biochemically. It results in the expression of a stable α polypeptide that is defective in subunit association so that no Hex A is formed. Among the point mutations resulting in amino acid substitutions, all would be expected to result in the translation of an α polypeptide. Significantly, of the 48 amino acid substitutions described, fully half are associated with an infantile phenotype. The mutations have a variety of effects from defective processing or subunit assembly to defective catalytic activity (Appendix 153A and Fig. 153-7).

Mutations Affecting Protein Processing. Several mutations have been described that affect subunit assembly or processing of the newly synthesized α precursor polypeptide. Most were detected at the 3′ end of the protein, although there is no direct evidence for a sequence or structure near the C-terminus that is specifically involved in subcellular transport. The mutant proteins appear to fall into two groups. In one group, the α precursor is retained in an early compartment, probably the ER. The protein fails to be phosphorylated, does not combine with the β subunit to form Hex A, is not processed to mature form (i.e., it does not reach the lysosome), and is not secreted. In the case of E482K,[309,310] the mutant protein could only be extracted with the use of strong detergents.[114] Other mutations showing this behavior include R499H[311] and 1510delC (at R504).[312,313] The latter results in a protein truncated by 22 amino acids. Interestingly, R499H was discovered in a patient with the subacute encephalopathic disease who was a compound heterozygote with a functionally null second allele. This patient had 3 percent residual enzyme activity with G_{M2} ganglioside as substrate.

In the second class of protein-processing mutations, the α precursor is phosphorylated but fails to associate with β subunits. It is not processed to mature form. It is secreted after treatment of the cells with ammonium chloride, but as unprocessed monomers rather than $\alpha\alpha$ or $\alpha\beta$ dimers. R504C[314] and R504H[311] show this biochemical phenotype as does G269S,[127] a mutation that is found in patients with late-onset disease (see below). Patients homozygous for R504 mutations vary in severity of clinical expression according to the amino acid substitution. One patient homozygous for R504C and another patient with the mutation occurring along with a functionally null donor splice mutation presented with an infantile acute encephalopathic clinical phenotype. In contrast, a patient homozygous for R504H and another with the mutation occurring along with the common and functionally null 1278ins4 insertion mutation had a subacute (juvenile) disease.

Mutations Affecting mRNA Processing. Most splicing mutations produce a functionally null biochemical phenotype and, as such, are associated with infantile Tay-Sachs disease (exceptions are noted in the next section). Investigations into the nature of the mRNA species resulting from splice mutations often reveal the presence of transcribed RNA, but detailed analysis has shown them to be abnormal in structure and coding for partially deleted or otherwise truncated proteins. Indeed, in most cases, the level of mRNA in cells is so low that the RNA transcripts must be either highly unstable or they do not reach the cytoplasm. Fourteen splice mutations have been described, 10 of which affect the donor site. Two donor splice mutations have been examined in detail. The first, IVS12+1G → C,[301–303] one of the major alleles in Ashkenazi Jewish Tay-Sachs disease, was shown to result in the production of a diverse array of splice products.[303,315] Most read through into intron 12 or skip exon 12. Some of these species also lack one or more upstream exons. In another donor splice mutation, IVS9+1G → A,[305,316,317] the low level of mRNAs detected were made up mainly of species utilizing cryptic donor sites in exon 9 or intron 10 or that skipped exon 9. In both examples, normal sequences expressed at these alleles were not detected.

Most splice mutations produce an infantile acute phenotype when homozygous or present in combination with a second infantile mutation. However, exceptions would be expected if some measure of normal splicing occurs, with consequent detectable level of Hex A activity. An example is IVS7−7G → A observed in a patient with the chronic disease.[318] The second allele was a frameshift, confirming that the mild disease was due to the splice mutation. The estimated 3 percent normal mRNA level was correlated with about 5 percent Hex A-specific enzyme activity. Other examples have either had a second allele known to be associated with a milder than infantile disease or the second allele was not identified so that no conclusion could be drawn.

Mutations Associated with Subacute Variants of Tay-Sachs Disease. Several mutations have been associated with the subacute encephalopathic clinical phenotype (Appendix 153A and "juvenile" mutations in Fig. 153-7). The later onset and slower course of the disease in these patients is due to the presence of some residual level of ganglioside G_{M2}-hydrolyzing activity. For example, Akli et al.[319] reported a patient with an exon mutation affecting splicing who had a late-infantile form of the disease. The patient was homozygous for a silent mutation, 570G → A (L190L), occurring in the last nucleotide of exon 5. The result was a reduced level of mRNA, most of which was deleted for exon 5. However, a small amount of normal mRNA was detected that was compatible with enzymatic data showing 2.5 percent residual Hex A activity in fibroblasts (MUG assay). Further, the enzyme showed normal biochemical properties compatible with the correct splicing in the minor mRNA. Therefore, this patient's milder course can be ascribed to the low level of correct splicing permitted by this type of mutation.

Other mutations resulting in a milder disease include certain amino acid substitutions. One of these occurred in a patient homozygous for G250D in exon 7.[320] Expression of the mutant cDNA in COS cells cotransfected with a normal β cDNA gave about 12 percent of the Hex A activity observed in cells doubly transfected with normal α and β cDNAs. Interestingly, transfection with α cDNA alone gave no Hex S activity over background, indicating the importance of the α/β transfection for the analysis of this type of mutation. The processing of the mutant α chain has not been examined. Two mutations—R499H and R504H—that affect α-chain processing are also associated with a subacute clinical phenotype in patients. The implication is that the more conservative His substitution (compared to Cys, which generated an infantile phenotype) must allow some mutant α chain to become phosphorylated, associate with β chains, and be delivered to the lysosome.

B1 Mutation. An important class of mutation is represented by the B1 variant of Tay-Sachs disease, largely worked out by Suzuki and colleagues (reviewed in reference 240). Affected individuals produce Hex A that is active toward the commonly used MUG substrate, but not active toward MUGS or ganglioside G_{M2}. The MUG activity is within carrier range in compound heterozygotes with a functionally null second allele, and can be near normal in homozygotes.[240,259] The explanation is that an α mutation inactivates the polypeptide but does not interfere with subunit association and processing to the lysosome. The result is that the Hex A activity is derived from the activity of the β subunit.[214] The mutant enzyme can hydrolyze MUG but not MUGS or G_{M2} ganglioside. The paradigm mutation is R178H,[175,241,321,322] which is common in Portuguese and responsible for most cases of the B1 variant (see "Incidence and Heredity" below). These mutations are associated with a severe subacute phenotype (late infantile) when present along with a null allele; however, the phenotype is considerably ameliorated when in homozygous form, showing a later onset during early childhood and slower progression (juvenile onset). The implication is that the defective Hex A produced, that is, the α chain, has some minimal activity toward G_{M2} ganglioside, so that a homozygote would effectively have twice the activity of a compound heterozygote that has a nonexpressing second allele.

Other mutations at the same R178 codon have been identified. One is R178C, which is biochemically and clinically similar to R178H and so can also be classified as of the B1 biochemical phenotype.[321] Another is R178L.[323] However, in this case, the activity toward MUG is only 19 percent of normal and the phenotype is clinically more severe (infantile acute form; second allele is a nonsense mutation). The implication is that the α chain mutation disrupts not only α chain function but also the conformation or stability of the $\alpha\beta$ dimer. Although G_{M2} gangliosidase was not assayed, the clinical phenotype suggests that it must be very low.

Mahuran and colleagues[174] reproduced the R178H mutation in the homologous site in the β subunit (β:R211H) by site-directed mutagenesis and showed that the resulting Hex B, produced by expression in COS cells, was now catalytically inactive although biosynthetic processing and stability were also affected. The less disruptive β:R211K mutation produced a Hex B that was structurally indistinguishable from normal but with markedly reduced catalytic activity.[176] These data suggest that the β:R211 and, by extrapolation α:R178, participate in the active site of the enzyme (see "Active Sites of Hexosaminidases and Catalysis" above and Fig. 153-7).

Other patients, described as having a B1 phenotype, had the relevant mutation at yet another site. Bayleran et al.[177] described two patients with infantile Tay-Sachs disease who had ~16 percent Hex A activity with MUG (30 percent using chromatographic determination of Hex A) but <1 percent with MUGS.[177] Using inhibitors to distinguish the α and β subunit activities in Hex A, they showed that the MUG activity was confined to the β subunit. Further, they showed that the α subunit mutation affected the catalytic rate without affecting substrate binding. Subsequently, they identified a mutation, D258H, that was common to both patients (the second allele was a frameshift in one case and R170W in the other)[324] and suggested that D258 may participate catalytically in the cleavage of the glycoside bond (see "Active Sites of Hexosaminidases and Catalysis" above and Fig. 153-7).

Thus, at least two α subunit sites, R178 and D258, appear to inactivate the α subunit while retaining full or partial $\alpha\beta$ integrity. Both may be candidates for participation in or near the catalytic site of the enzyme and occur at sites conserved among Hex A, Hex B and the hexosaminidase from *D. discoideum.*

Mutations Associated with the Chronic Form of Tay-Sachs Disease. Several α subunit mutations are associated with late-onset chronic G_{M2} gangliosidosis. Mechanistically, this is invariably due to the retention of partial Hex A activity. One major mutation is G269S,[325,326] which occurs with significant frequency in the Ashkenazi Jewish population (see "Incidence and Heredity" below). Patients with the G269S mutation synthesize the α chain precursor, but the mutant polypeptide is unstable and fails to associate with β subunits.[127,327] The small amount of polypeptide that does associate would account for the residual Hex A activity expressed in these patients. However, the amount of Hex A activity produced is variable and is likely a reflection of the size and turnover rate of the α precursor pool in the ER, where the association with β subunits occurs.[327] This may explain the marked clinical heterogeneity associated with the chronic encephalopathic disease, even within families. Subtle changes in the rate of early processing steps may have profound influence on the residual Hex A activity. Indeed, these fluctuations may vary from tissue to tissue. As described earlier for other mutations yielding partial enzyme activity, homozygotes would be expected to have higher enzyme activities and a correspondingly milder clinical phenotype.[328] A second mutation at G269, G269D, was identified in an infant with the infantile acute phenotype.[307] This outcome suggests that it is not the position of the mutated amino acid that is responsible for the mild disease in G269S but the conservative change to Ser.

Several other mutations have been associated with the chronic encephalopathic phenotype. One mutation is Y180H, which, like G269S, is associated with an unstable protein and impaired Hex A biosynthesis.[329] Other mutations causing the chronic disease that have not been studied in detail include K197T, R252H, and V391M.[330–332] In the latter two examples, the second allele was the major B1 mutation, R178H, so that the affected patients showed an overriding B1 biochemical phenotype as well.

Hex A-Minus Pseudodeficiency. A complication of the use of artificial substrates for the assay of Hex has been the identification of individuals who have an apparent deficiency of Hex A activity but who are nonetheless healthy. They have been called "pseudodeficient" or "Hex A minus" normal.[230,333–336] Most pseudodeficient individuals have been identified through carrier screening or during prenatal diagnosis. Importantly, one such subject was also the mother of a child with infantile Tay-Sachs disease,[333] suggesting the involvement of disease alleles in their genotype. Triggs-Raine et al.[337] screened several pseudodeficient subjects for *HEXA* mutations and identified the amino acid substitution, R247W, present in each case. All were compound heterozygotes coupled with a true Tay-Sachs mutation. Most of the subjects were Ashkenazi Jews and the second mutation was either the 1278ins4 insertion or the intron 12-splice mutation common in the population. The enzymatic defect is due to an α subunit that is defective toward MUG or MUGS, but which is normal toward ganglioside G_{M2}.[335,337,338] Recently, Triggs-Raine[339] identified a second pseudodeficiency allele, R249W, near the first. Both mutations reduce net enzymatic activity, not by affecting the processing of the α-subunit, that is, phosphorylation, targeting, or secretion, or by affecting its catalytic function, but by reducing its stability *in vivo*.[340] A third mutation in this region, D250G, is associated with a subacute (juvenile onset) phenotype and different biochemistry (Appendix 153A).

Mutations in the *HEXB* Gene

Sandhoff disease and its variants are also caused by a heterogeneous group of mutations. Mutation studies are not as far advanced as in the case of the *HEXA* gene, but both CRM-positive and CRM-negative mutations have been encountered and clinical severity correlates with the residual activity of the Hex A isoenzyme. Some two dozen mutations have been described, the vast majority of which are associated with infantile Sandhoff disease. At this point, it is important to note that the literature contains an ambiguity of the position of the initiation codon and consequent confusion in the numbering of coding sequence mutations. There are three in-frame ATG codons at the 5′ end of the gene.[189,193] While all three ATG codons are capable of translation initiation *in vitro*,[125] only the first is functional *in vivo*.[341] However, when first reported, only the second and third ATG were noted in one report,[190] with the result that some mutation reports have counted from the second ATG in assigning amino acid positions. Where this occurs, the addition of 36 nucleotide or 12 amino acid positions restores the correct count. Appendix 153B indicates some of these corrections.

Mutations Associated with Infantile Sandhoff Disease. The most common disease mutation thus far identified is a 16-kb deletion spanning the promoter, exons 1 to 5 and part of intron 5.[342] It appears to be derived from recombination between two Alu sequences, with the breakpoints occurring at the midpoint in each case. The result is the regeneration of an intact Alu element in the deletion sequence. In homozygous form, it is associated with the infantile Sandhoff disease. A second deletion, originally described as covering about 50 kb of DNA by pulse-field electrophoresis,[343] is the same mutation.[344]

An independent 50-kb deletion mutation has been identified that is not related to the 16-kb deletion.[345] This mutation was observed in a single family. It begins upstream of the promoter region and includes exons 1 to 6 and part of intron 6. The distinct termination sites of del16kb in intron 5 and del50kb in intron 6 confirm them as independent mutations.

Other deletions involve single or small numbers of nucleotides and most, with two exceptions (below), are associated with an infantile presentation. Other mutations causing infantile disease include several amino acid substitutions, one nonsense mutation, and several splice mutations. Among the amino acid substitutions, only 3 of the 10 described mutations can be reliably linked to the infantile disease (S62L, S255R, and C534Y). One exon mutation affecting splicing is 1242G → A. This is a silent mutation at K414, with the mutation occurring at the last nucleotide of exon 10. It results in a severely reduced amount of mRNA, comprised mainly of abnormal species and a net presence of about 1 percent normal mRNA.

Mutations Associated with Subacute or Chronic Forms of Sandhoff Disease. One patient, who presented with clinical motor neuron disease, juvenile spinomuscular atrophy phenotype, was a compound heterozygote for two point mutations of I207V and Y456S.[184] Neither mutation has been seen in a homozygote or coupled with a null allele, so it is not possible to assess their individual impact on Hex A activity. Presumably, at least one of the mutations is associated with a late-onset clinical course, while the second may be more severe or similar to the first.

Another amino acid substitution identified is P417L. This mutation is unusual in that it affects splicing rather than β chain processing or activity, although it is located at nucleotide position 8 (1252C → T) of exon 11. Wakamatsu et al.[346] identified the mutation in homozygous form in a Japanese patient presenting with the subacute encephalopathic disease (juvenile Sandhoff disease). In COS expression experiments, the mutation inhibited correct splicing at the 3′ acceptor site of intron 10, as was found for the patient's cells. Instead, it promoted the selection of a cryptic acceptor site within exon 11 or skipping of exon 11 altogether. Significantly, the normal mRNA (called P1) and the mRNA with the cryptic acceptor site (P2) were both found to be present in normal cells (99.4 percent and 0.6 percent, respectively). Except for the production of trace amounts of mRNA lacking exon 11 (P3), the effect of the mutation seemed to be more a shift in the ratio rather than the creation of new species of mRNA. The result was a reduction in the level of β mRNA to 8 percent of normal and a P1:P2:P3 ratio of 11:2:1. These data illustrate the possibility that abnormal mRNA species that are detected in mutant cells may sometimes be rare species found in normal cells, but not seen because of the presence of overwhelming amounts of the normal transcript.

Curiously, a Caucasian family has been reported in which five patients, who were compound heterozygotes for the same P417L mutation along with a null allele, presented very late with mild disease or were asymptomatic.[347] The proband had the mutation coupled with the 16 kb deletion. The implication from the foregoing is that half the normal amount of mRNA might be produced and the result should therefore be a clinical presentation more severe than in the homozygote. Instead, the patient presented at age 51 with a 9-year history of chronic diarrhea and findings suggestive of impairment of the autonomic nervous system; like most patients with late-onset disease, the patient had MCBs in intestinal neurons. The four affected siblings, ages 51 to 61 years, were asymptomatic. These data illustrate the highly variable expression of the mutation between different patients and among different tissues in the same patient.

Two other mutations resulting in the insertion of several amino acids near the 3′ end of the gene affect β subunit processing. One was caused by a nucleotide substitution in intron 12, IVS12−26G → A, which generated a cryptic acceptor site.[264,348,349] The result is the in-frame insertion of eight amino acids between exon 12 and 13. The second, involving duplication of 18 bp from −16 to +2 at the IVS-13/exon 14 junction, resulted in the insertion of six amino acids at the beginning of exon 14.[349] In both cases, the resulting elongated β chain appears to fail to fold properly and is not processed. However, in both cases a small amount of correct splicing appears to be responsible for the formation of a small but highly variable amount of normal Hex A. This has resulted in a variable clinical phenotype, including patients with a subacute (juvenile) disease or an asymptomatic individual in the case of the IVS-12 splice mutation[264,349] and an asymptomatic individual in a case of the IVS-13 insertion.[349] An important caveat is that the second allele has not been identified in any of these individuals. In all of these individuals, Hex B was virtually absent. This biochemical phenotype, Hex A-plus/Hex B-minus, was originally called "Hexosaminidase Paris" by Dreyfus and colleagues.[350] These results suggest that the C-terminal sequence of the β subunit, like the α subunit, appears to be important in its proper folding or initial processing.

Several mutations have been identified that are responsible for the generation of a thermolabile β subunit and a chronic disease or asymptomatic presentation. They include P504S, R505Q, and A543T, all clustered at the C-terminus of the protein.[185,351–353] In the case of P504S, it was shown that the mutant β chain showed increased retention in the ER and the mutant Hex A showed a reduced activity toward ganglioside G_{M2}/G_{M2} activator complex relative to MUGS.[185]

A frequent mutation, 1751delTG, has been described in the 3′ UTR of the *HEXB* gene seven nucleotides 5′ of the first polyadenylation site that reduces the level of enzyme activity.[354] Leukocyte total hexosaminidase and Hex B activities were shown to be about 70 percent of normal while serum hexosaminidase was not affected appreciably. Adult individuals with the TG deletion on one allele and a null mutation on the other were asymptomatic. The mutation appears to result in reduction in the level of mRNA containing it. The mechanism remains unknown but possibilities included impact on secondary structure in the UTR and disruption of a nuclear matrix attachment region.

Mutations in the *GM2A* Gene

Only four mutations have been documented in the *GM2A* gene encoding the G_{M2} activator (Appendix 153C). All have been homozygous in patients who have had an infantile acute encephalopathic disease and absent Hex A activity toward ganglioside G_{M2}. The first reported mutation, C138R,[355,356] proved to have defective Hex A binding but normal interaction with G_{M2} ganglioside.[357] A second point mutation, R169P, was negative by western blot, suggesting instability of the mutant protein.[358] The other mutations include a single amino acid deletion, delK88, and a frameshift, 410delA, which were associated with unstable proteins that appeared to be degraded in the ER or Golgi.[359] An additional Japanese patient with infantile acute disease and absent G_{M2} activator by western blot has been described, but the mutation(s) has yet to be identified.[360]

DIAGNOSIS AND CARRIER DETECTION

Biochemical Methods

Metabolite Assays. Historically, diagnosis in this group of disorders depended on clinical history and physical findings, as well as on histopathologic/or biochemical determinations derived from biopsied material (e.g., myenteric plexus or brain) or postmortem specimens. Because extraneural tissues possess very low levels of gangliosides, lipid analyses for diagnostic purposes were usually limited to nervous tissue, and their applicability restricted to postmortem examinations or to verification of a prenatal diagnosis after abortion. A four- to fivefold ganglioside G_{M2} accumulation has been observed in G_{M2} gangliosidosis fetuses as early as 18 to 20 weeks gestation,[289,361] although MCBs have been detected earlier by electron microscopy (see "Pathology" above).

In contrast, the *N*-acetylglucosaminyl oligosaccharides that accumulate in almost all tissues of patients with Sandhoff disease are also excreted in the urine in considerable amount (see Table 72-7 in the sixth edition of this volume[273]). Analysis of urinary oligosaccharides may, therefore, be used for the diagnosis of this G_{M2} gangliosidosis variant.[362] A much lower, but still significant, level of such oligosaccharides was also found in the amniotic fluid of fetuses affected with Sandhoff disease, providing an adjunct to enzymatic studies for prenatal diagnosis.[293]

With the development of specific enzymatic and/or molecular diagnostic methods, specific delineation of the heterozygous, homozygous, and (in most instances) even the compound heterozygous states, can be achieved with readily available tissues or body fluids such as serum, leukocytes, mouthwashing-derived buccal cells, tears, skin fibroblasts, amniocytes, and chorionic villi. These approaches are discussed below.

Enzyme Assays. The discovery of the enzymatic defects underlying Sandhoff disease and Tay-Sachs disease in 1968 and 1969, respectively, greatly simplified the approach to diagnosis of these ganglioside G_{M2}-storage disorders and their variants. In particular, the utilization of synthetic substrates (fluorogenic or colorimetric) for the quantification of the lysosomal hexosaminidases made diagnosis of these conditions relatively straightforward and rapid. The nature of the aglycone portion of the substrate is usually of little importance for the action of hexosaminidase A and B. Although, as the name hexosaminidase implies, the enzymes accept both *N*-acetylglucosaminides and *N*-acetylgalactosaminides, the glucosaminides are usually preferred because they are more sensitive (hydrolyzed faster) and less expensive.

With the few exceptions stated below, the enzymes can be assayed in any tissue sample or body fluid that can be obtained from the patient. Most convenient specimens are serum and leukocytes.

Hex A Deficiency (Tay-Sachs Disease and Variants). The diagnosis of α subunit defects due to mutations of the *HEXA* gene requires the specific demonstration of deficient activity of Hex A in the presence of a normal or even elevated activity of the Hex B isoenzyme. This can be done after separation of Hex A and Hex B and assay by synthetic chromogenic or fluorogenic substrates that are hydrolyzed by both isoenzymes; or, without the need for separation, the assay can be done with a substrate that is specifically hydrolyzed by Hex A. Separation of the isoenzymes is usually achieved with ion-exchange chromatography,[363–367] isoelectric focusing,[368–371] or electrophoresis in starch gels[9,10,372] or on cellulose acetate.[373–375] While electrophoretic separation allows only a qualitative assay, the other techniques permit the quantitative determination of each of the two isoenzymes.

Table 153-2 Degradation of Ganglioside G_{M2} by Extracts of Fibroblasts from Patients with G_{M2} Gangliosidosis

Probands	Ganglioside G_{M2} Degradation pmol/(h·mg·AU)* Mean	Range
Controls, $n = 9$	535	296–762
Heterozygotes, $n = 4$ (different genotypes)	285	121–395
Tay-Sachs disease and Variants (*HEXA* gene defects):		
Infantile, $n = 5$	2.40	0.8–3.8
Subacute, $n = 5$	15.8	13.6–18.0
Chronic, $n = 9$	19.1	13.1–32.8
Sandhoff disease and Variants (*HEXB* gene defects)		
Infantile, $n = 2$	6.6	3.6–9.5
Subacute, $n = 3$	23.3	9.5–39.4
Healthy adult, $n = 2$	105	75–143

*AU = activator unit as defined in reference[502]

More rapid, and still highly accurate, methods frequently used for large-scale screening purposes are based on the lower thermal[11,364,376] or pH stability[377] of Hex A. At pH 4.4, Hex B is comparatively stable up to 55°C, whereas Hex A is inactivated with a half-life of some 10 min at 50°C[94,157] and 3 min at 55°C.[157] (At pH 6.0, 50°C, Hex A, especially in purified form, is largely converted to Hex B[155,378] due to rearrangement of subunits.) Total activity is measured before and after selective denaturation of Hex A and the activity of this isoenzyme is calculated from the difference. Problems may arise with these methods in some extremely unusual cases, such as in families that harbor an allele coding for a heat-labile, but functionally active, β subunit.[379,380]

The discovery of Kresse and coworkers[149,150] that the Hex A but not the Hex B isoenzyme releases intact *N*-acetylglucosamine-6-sulfate from keratan sulfate led to the development of the corresponding synthetic substrates, *p*-nitrophenyl- and 4-methylumbelliferyl-6-sulfo-*N*-acetyl-β-D-glucosaminide,[148,149,151,381] which are hydrolyzed almost exclusively by Hex A (and probably also by the minor Hex S isoenzyme[153]) but only very poorly by Hex B. These sulfated substrates have proven useful in the diagnosis of Tay-Sachs disease, and particularly the B1 variant.[290,382,383] Unfortunately, assays with this substrate do not distinguish heterozygotes for the pseudodeficiency alleles[337] nor are they as sensitive as the standard substrates in the detection of carriers for other α-subunit mutations (M.M. Kaback, unpublished). It should also be noted that for assaying Hex activity with these sensitive 4-MU derivatives, dilutions should be made with citrate-phosphate buffer (acetate buffer is inhibitory) containing 0.1 to 0.3 percent hexosaminidase-free albumin.

The most specific method for the determination of Hex A activity employs the natural substrate, ganglioside G_{M2}, in the presence of the activator protein. The use of detergents for this purpose[384,385] should be discouraged because they are likely to change the substrate specificities of the isoenzymes and also to denature them,[386] and may thus lead to incorrect results. With an improved assay system,[387] it has been possible to determine the residual ganglioside G_{M2} hydrolase activity in crude extracts of fibroblasts and to discriminate between different clinical variants of G_{M2} gangliosidosis (Table 153-2; see also section on "Degree of Enzyme Deficiency and Development of Different Clinical Diseases" below). The requirements, however, for appropriately labeled ganglioside G_{M2}, its limited stability, and the need for fresh G_{M2} activator in this natural substrate assay make this method difficult, time-consuming, and expensive. It also requires a certain minimal enzyme concentration so that it cannot be applied to serum or urine. Still, it may be valuable for certain diagnostic applications. For example, it is useful for prenatal diagnosis of the B1 variant, which has high residual Hex A activity toward the usual synthetic substrates,[290] or for the discrimination between infantile and chronic variants, which may occur in the same family.[232] In those instances where specific mutations are known to segregate in each parent, molecular diagnosis can replace the need for this difficult assay (see "Molecular Diagnosis" below.

Prenatal diagnosis may be performed with cultured amniotic fluid cells, which are similar to fibroblasts in their hexosaminidase content and pattern. Caution should be exercised in using amniotic fluid as the sole enzyme source because the presence of an acidic heat-stable enzyme, presumably Hex B complexed with acidic mucopolysaccharides, may mimic Hex A.[388] Chorionic villus tissue, either directly and/or after cultivation *in vitro* also can be employed for the prenatal diagnosis of the G_{M2} gangliosidoses (see below).

Hex A and Hex B Deficiency (Sandhoff Disease and Variants). The absence or near-absence of total β-hexosaminidase activity can, in principle, be demonstrated with any one of the substrates used for Tay-Sachs diagnosis, provided that the preservation of the specimen to be assayed is checked to rule out artifacts due to deterioration of the sample. In our experience, the ratio of total hexosaminidase to β-galactosidase is a reliable indicator. If diagnostic material is to be stored for any period of time or to be sent to other laboratories, it should be kept frozen.

Where both an infantile Sandhoff disease mutation and a β-subunit pseudodeficiency mutation occur within the same family,[350,389] prenatal diagnosis may be particularly problematic. Here, the use of molecular methods (DNA-based diagnosis) is particularly critical to identify the mutations involved and to resolve any diagnostic dilemma.

G_{M2} Activator Deficiency (Variant AB). G_{M2} activator deficiency gangliosidosis is the most difficult form of G_{M2} gangliosidosis to diagnose. To date, biochemical diagnosis has only been made from cultured skin fibroblasts and postmortem analysis of autopsy tissues. Three different methods have been used: (a) An assay system was developed to determine the G_{M2} activator activity in fibroblast extracts on the basis of their ability to stimulate hydrolysis of ganglioside G_{M2} by purified Hex A *in vitro*.[214] Although values are generally low, an accurate distinction can be made between G_{M2} activator-deficient cells and others (Table 72-9 in the sixth edition of this volume[273]). (b) The G_{M2} activator protein was assayed immunochemically in fibroblast extracts with an ELISA.[390] (c) Radiolabeled ganglioside G_{M2} was fed to skin fibroblasts in cell culture (see below). The deficit of variant AB cells in the degradation of this substrate could be corrected by the addition of purified G_{M2} activator to the culture medium (Fig. 153-10).

Metabolic Studies in Cultured Cells. Studies of the metabolism of exogenously added radiolabeled ganglioside G_{M2} in cultured skin fibroblasts may provide a useful alternative for diagnosis of unusual G_{M2} gangliosidosis variants,[228,391] particularly when enzyme assays are inconclusive, as in G_{M2} activator deficiency, or where specific mutations in a given family are unidentified. Gangliosides dissolved in culture medium (preferably with low content of fetal calf serum)[392] insert into the cell membrane[393] and are internalized and metabolized like endogenous glycolipids. If the radiolabel is in the sphingosine base, almost all labeled products are neutral lipids.[391,392] When, after a few days of feeding, the lipids are extracted from the cells and separated by ion-exchange chromatography, the percentage of radioactivity in the neutral lipids fraction is a reliable measure of the degradative capability of the cells.[392] Alternatively, the less polar products may

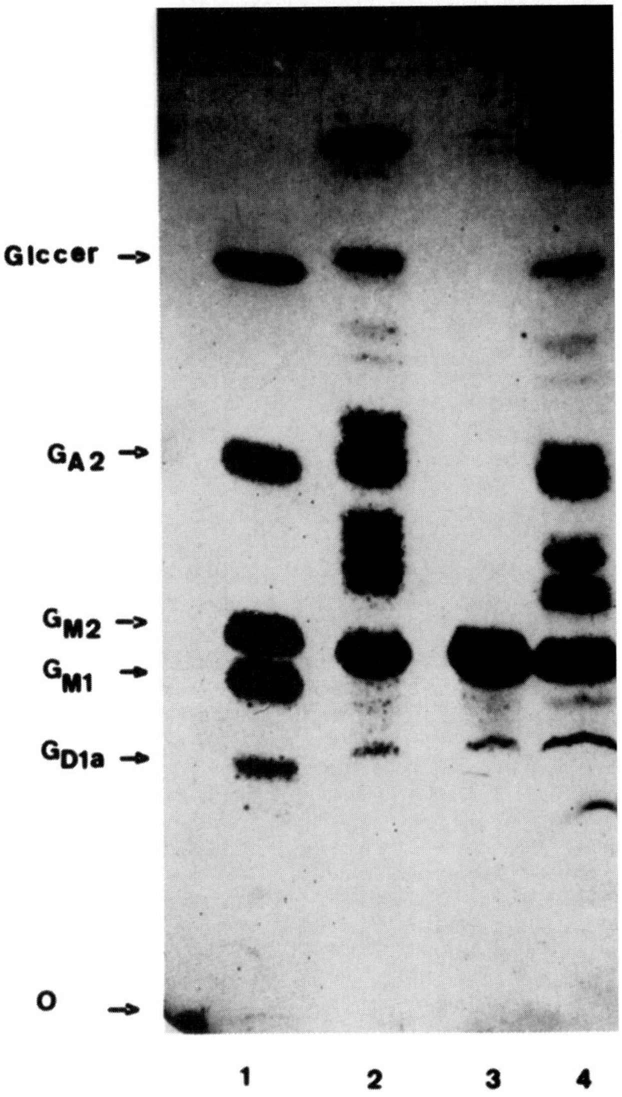

Fig. 153-10 Metabolism of ganglioside G_{M2} in G_{M2} activator-deficient fibroblasts. [^{3}H]Ganglioside G_{M2} was added to the culture medium of skin fibroblasts. After 70 h, the lipids were extracted, separated on thin-layer chromatography plates and the radioactive spots visualized with fluorography. Lane 1 = standards; lane 2 = normal control cells; lane 3 = G_{M2} activator-deficient cells, 30 μg of purified G_{M2} activator protein added with the ganglioside substrate.

be separated from unreacted ganglioside substrate by partitioning in a water-chloroform-methanol two-phase system.[391]

Molecular Diagnosis

As discussed in "The Molecular Defects" section above, at least 92 specific α-chain mutations have been characterized to date. Large and small deletions, missense, nonsense, frameshift, and splice site alterations have been delineated, spanning this 14-exon, 40-kb gene. Some 40 percent of the listed mutations occur at CpG dinucleotide sites. Specific mutations associated with B_1, and subacute and chronic variants, have been characterized in patients with these disorders, usually in compound heterozygosity with one of the more common infantile alleles. Two alleles, R247W and R249W (both at CpG sites) are associated with pseudodeficiency (resulting in *reduced synthetic* substrate hydrolysis but *unimpaired natural* substrate cleavage)[337,339,340] (see section on "Hex A-minus Pseudodeficiency" above).

In a given family where known mutation(s) are segregating, specific diagnosis of the heterozygous, homozygous, or compound heterozygous states can be made (either pre- or postnatally) by direct DNA-based mutation analysis techniques. Where specific mutations have not been assessed in a family, but initial enzymatic tests indicate either homozygosity or heterozygosity for an α-chain mutation, specific mutation analyses should be done for more accurate genetic counseling and to ensure *the absence* of a biologically benign pseudodeficiency allele.

With regard to β-chain defects, 26 mutations (including 3 asymptomatic alleles) have been delineated thus far. Again, where specific β-subunit mutations have been identified in a family, the highest level of specificity and genetic counseling accuracy is achieved through DNA-based mutation analysis in relatives (for heterozygote testing) or for prenatal diagnostic purposes. Where such mutations are undetermined, a strategy similar to that described with α-chain defects should be employed (mutation analysis to rule out pseudodeficiency alteration(s) or other known genetic variants). Here, also, the *sequential use* of "gene product" testing first (Hex A and Hex B isoenzyme activities), followed by molecular analyses is optimal.

Population Screening for G_{M2} Gangliosidosis Heterozygotes

Screening for *HEXA* Mutations. Reduced Hex A has been demonstrated (using synthetic Hex substrates) in serum,[376] leukocytes,[394] fibroblasts,[395] and tears[396] of obligate heterozygotes for essentially all known Tay-Sachs disease (α-subunit) mutations. This capability provided the basis for the development of simple, inexpensive, and highly accurate methods for heterozygote identification.[11,11A] Furthermore, because of the ethnic predilection for this disorder and the availability of genetic counseling and prenatal diagnosis, a rationale was established for population screening among reproductive-age Jewish individuals.[397] In this way, individuals identified as heterozygotes and, even more critically, couples in which both members were carriers, could be made aware of their risk status prior to the birth of any affected offspring. With comprehensive genetic counseling, such families could choose, if they desired, to monitor all subsequent pregnancies by prenatal diagnosis and to carry to term only those pregnancies in which the fetus was found not to be affected with the deficiency disorder. If a fetus was found affected, a family could choose to terminate the pregnancy. Albeit an imperfect solution, such an interim approach could provide at-risk families, if they chose, a selective means to have only unaffected offspring, while preventing the birth of children destined to deteriorate and die with an untreatable disease.

Large-scale population screening for Tay-Sachs disease heterozygotes began in the early 1970s in Jewish communities throughout North America.[398,399] Subsequently, such programs

Table 153-3 **Tay-Sachs Disease Heterozygote Screening 1971–1998**

Country	No. tested	Carriers	At-risk couples
United States	925,876	35,372	795
Israel	302,395	7,277	380
Canada	65,813	3,301	62
South Africa	15,138	1,582	52
Europe	17,725	1,127	37
Brazil	1,027	72	20
Mexico	655	26	0
Argentina	84	5	0
Australia	3,334	102	4
TOTALS	1,332,047	48,864	1,350

were initiated in countries throughout the world.[400] As of mid-1998, more than 1,332,000 young adults were screened voluntarily to determine their Tay-Sachs disease carrier status. Over 48,000 heterozygotes were detected and, most critically, 1350 at-risk couples identified (both partners were carriers). None of these couples previously had children with Tay-Sachs disease or any other G_{M2} gangliosidosis. These results are summarized in Table 153-3.

Such screening efforts generally have employed automated thermal or pH fractionation of serum hexosaminidases,[377,378] which measures total Hex activity as well as the specific quantification of the Hex A fraction (that fraction inactivated either by defined exposure to heat or low pH). Follow-up leukocyte Hex profiles are then employed for confirmation of carrier status or for clarification of status in individuals with inconclusive or "unusual" serum profiles, or where confounding factors may be present, such as pregnancy, birth-control medication, unusual drugs, and selected current illnesses. Heterozygotes for nearly all the α-subunit mutations are identifiable by a significant reduction in serum and leukocyte Hex A activity (including carriers of the pseudodeficiency alleles). The one exception is seen in B_1 variant heterozygotes whose Hex A levels, with the usual substrates, are generally in the "indeterminate" or low noncarrier ranges. Fortunately, the frequency of the B_1 variant disorder is quite low even in the general population, and not yet described in Jewish patients, making "missed" carriers in enzyme-based screening programs exceedingly unlikely. For this variant, carrier detection, like homozygote diagnosis, requires the use of specific Hex A substrates or specific DNA-based mutation testing.

These routine screening methods (enzymatic) do not permit a distinction to be made, however, between the different *HEXA* mutations. Carriers of *HEXA* mutations for the variant α-subunit conditions (e.g., subacute or chronic G_{M2} gangliosidosis) are indistinguishable enzymatically from heterozygotes for classic Tay-Sachs disease. These distinctions can be made only by the adjunct use of DNA-based mutation analysis in enzyme-defined carriers. For initial population screening, enzyme-based testing is regarded as optimal because the Hex A test identifies the vast majority of mutant genotypes, whereas DNA tests are limited by their unique specificity for each particular mutation.[401] Once defined by enzymatic testing, however, mutational analysis has an essential and critical role, in all carrier/carrier couples, in order to define the nature of the ganglioside G_{M2} disorder for which the couple is at-risk—infantile, subacute, or chronic. Most particularly, a pseudodeficiency allele in either of the apparently heterozygous parents obviates the risk for any neurologically significant condition in their offspring. The compound heterozygous fetus would be enzymatically deficient, that is, Hex A-minus with synthetic substrates, but would be expected to never develop neurologic impairment. Accordingly, invasive prenatal diagnostic procedures with their contingent risks are not indicated.

Approximately *35 percent of non-Jewish* individuals identified to be "TSD-heterozygotes" by Hex A determination are actually carriers of a pseudodeficiency mutation.[337] Follow-up DNA analysis is essential in all enzymatically-defined carriers to evaluate this possibility. In Jewish carriers identified by Hex A screening, only approximately 2 percent are found to have such pseudodeficient alterations.[316] Again, specific mutation analysis can be employed to resolve this issue.

Screening for *HEXB* Mutations. Serum and leukocyte Hex profiles employed for Tay-Sachs disease carrier identification can also be utilized for the delineation of heterozygotes for β-subunit mutations.[402] Such heterozygotes are characterized by significantly low total hexosaminidase-specific activities with a *relatively increased* fraction of Hex A (thermal or acid-labile). In this way, heterozygotes for Sandhoff disease and most other variant β-subunit mutations can be distinguished. Again, follow-up mutation analysis of enzymatic-defined carriers should be utilized to rule out pseudodeficiency and for enhanced genetic counseling purposes.

Table 153-4 Prenatal Diagnosis of Tay-Sachs Disease Worldwide Experience, 1969–1998

	Couples Identified At-Risk By:		
	Prior Offspring	Carrier Screening	Total
Pregnancies monitored	1399	1747	3146
Affected fetuses	336	268	604
Elective abortions	318	267	585*
Tay-Sachs disease fetuses missed	2	1	3
Unaffected offspring born	1038	1428	2466

*Eighteen infants affected with infantile Tay-Sachs disease, 1 with adult-onset disorder as predicted.

Prenatal Diagnosis

As described above, both Hex A and Hex B are readily quantitated in normal fetal tissues obtained in early to mid gestation, including amniotic fluid, uncultured or cultured amniocytes, and direct or cultured material derived from chorionic villus samples. Such normative data provide the basis for the intrauterine detection of Tay-Sachs disease, Sandhoff disease, and most of the other G_{M2} gangliosidoses. For G_{M2} activator deficiency, prenatal diagnosis should be possible through direct assessment of cellular ganglioside G_{M2} degradation or quantitative (functional or immunologic) studies of the G_{M2} activator itself.

The prenatal diagnosis of Tay-Sachs disease was first accomplished in 1970.[372,403,404] This capability, as stated previously, provided a rationale for prospective population heterozygote screening. At first, prenatal testing was employed only in pregnancies in couples in which prior affected offspring had been born. More recently, the majority of pregnancies monitored for fetal Tay-Sachs disease, either by amniocentesis at 16 to 18 weeks or by chorionic villus sampling at 9 to 12 weeks,[405,406] has been in couples identified to be at risk through heterozygote testing. Table 153-4 reflects the worldwide experience with prenatal diagnosis through mid-1998.

The frequency of fetuses affected with Tay-Sachs disease is significantly less than the 25 percent expected (Table 153-4) because the data include a significant number of monitored pregnancies in which the actual risk was substantially less than 25 percent or was even negligible (e.g., remarried parent of a prior child with Tay-Sachs disease requesting the procedure for reassurance; one parent identified as a carrier and the other unavailable or inconclusive through screening; etc.). In the 19 instances in which a prenatal diagnosis of Tay-Sachs disease was made but the pregnancies went to term, the diagnosis was made too late in pregnancy for legal termination to be performed, or there were parental moral or religious proscriptions against abortion. Eighteen children manifested classic Tay-Sachs disease in infancy, and one (a twin) has a late-onset form, as predicted.

With molecular DNA-based diagnostic techniques, an enhanced level of specificity is gained in the prenatal detection of G_{M2} gangliosidoses. Where specific mutations are identified in each parent, the identification of homozygosity or compound heterozygosity in the fetus is straightforward.[407] Where such mutations are not known or have not been identified, then enzymatic tests in combination with selected specific mutation tests (to rule out compound heterozygosity with a pseudodeficiency allele) are critical. In this way, an unaffected Hex A minus normal fetus would not be confused with one affected by a neurologically significant G_{M2} storage disorder.

INCIDENCE AND HEREDITY

Gene Frequencies and Disease Incidence

Earlier estimates of the gene frequencies for the Tay-Sachs disease allele in Jewish and non-Jewish North American populations were based on disease incidence figures developed from death certificate information.[408,409] By Hardy-Weinberg analysis, a disease incidence of about 1 in 4000 Ashkenazi Jewish births predicted a carrier rate for Tay-Sachs disease of between 1 in 30 and 1 in 40 among Jewish Americans of central and eastern European extraction. Among non-Jews and Sephardic Jews, the disease incidence was observed to be 100 times less frequent, corresponding to one-tenth the carrier frequency (about 1 in 300). Such figures can only be viewed as estimates because of ascertainment bias and possible misdiagnosis. Clearly, misdiagnosis of Sandhoff disease as Tay-Sachs disease (particularly prior to the introduction of biochemical methods for their differentiation) would result in an inflated Tay-Sachs disease carrier estimate, or, conversely, missed diagnoses of Tay-Sachs disease would cause underestimates of the heterozygote frequency in either population.

More recently, carrier frequency estimates for Tay-Sachs disease were made directly from data obtained in large-scale population-screening programs in the United States and Canada.[410] Importantly, however, enzymologic identification of Tay-Sachs or Sandhoff disease heterozygotes does not distinguish between the large number of *HEXA* or *HEXB* mutations causing these disorders and their variants. Also, the pseudodeficiency mutations in each gene are similarly not distinguished by enzymatic testing. Accordingly, if enzymologic data alone are used to calculate gene frequencies and disease incidence, considerable overestimates would be expected. Several studies have been done using mutation analysis in DNA from enzyme-defined carriers to resolve this issue. The findings are in close agreement.[401,411–414]

In the Ashkenazi Jewish population, three distinct *HEXA* mutations — two associated with infantile Tay-Sachs disease and a third found in essentially all patients identified to date with late-onset (adult or chronic) G_{M2} gangliosidosis — account for 95 to 98 percent of all Jewish heterozygotes.[401,411–414] About 1 in 50 Jewish carriers are found to have a pseudodeficiency mutation and another 2 percent (approximately) remain unidentified after testing for the 6 most common mutant alleles (including the 2 pseudodeficiency mutations).[415] The most common mutation among Jewish carriers is the four-base insertion in exon 11 (1278ins4). This alteration accounts for 75 to 80 percent of all *HEXA* mutations in this population. The mutation in intron 12 (IVS12+1G → C) is found in approximately 15 percent of Jewish carriers and the late-onset alteration in exon 7 (G269S) in approximately 3 percent of Jewish carriers.

Among non-Jewish heterozygotes, including both obligate and screening program-identified carriers, the mutation pattern is vastly different.[316] Approximately 20 percent of non-Jewish carriers have the same 1278ins4 insertion as seen in Jewish carriers; *none* have been identified with the IVS12+1G → C mutation; and approximately 5 percent carry the exon 7 (G269S) mutation associated with the chronic phenotype. An abnormal splice site mutation at IVS9+1G → A is found in about 15 percent of non-Jewish carriers in the U.S.[316] This alteration has not been seen in more than 200 Jewish carriers examined for it. Of particular importance is that approximately 35 percent of non-Jewish enzyme-defined carriers are found to be heterozygous for one of the two pseudodeficiency mutations — R247W or R249W.[337,339]

Overall, approximately 40 to 50 percent of non-Jewish enzymatically confirmed carriers (both obligate and through screening) are "negative" after mutation analysis for the six most frequent alterations.[416] As most of the remaining mutations described to date occur in diverse populations with low overall frequencies, or in isolated population groups, or as "private" mutations in single or very few families, it would be prohibitive to test every carrier identified for all mutations. Rather, selected mutational testing for specific alterations found in the particular ethnic group of an individual with heterozygous enzymatic levels is appropriate, for example, testing for the 7.6-kb deletion in non-Jewish French Canadians or the IVS9+1 mutation in enzymatic carriers of French or Celtic backgrounds.

With appropriate adjustments made for pseudodeficiency alleles in both Jewish and non-Jewish North American populations, it is possible to calculate *HEXA* mutation frequencies and disease incidence figures for these two populations. In a cohort of 46,304 Jewish individuals tested through the California Tay-Sachs Disease Prevention program, enzyme-defined heterozygotes were identified with a frequency of 0.033 (1 in 30). Pseudodeficiency mutations account for approximately 2 percent of these "carriers," reducing the disease-related carrier rate to 0.032 (1 in 31). If these were solely infantile mutations, this would predict a Tay-Sachs disease phenotype in 1 of 3900 Jewish infants born. Because 3 percent of Jewish carriers have the late-onset G269S mutation, and perhaps another 2 percent (estimated) carry other noninfantile phenotype-associated mutations, the infantile disease frequency in Jews would be reduced to approximately 1 in 4100 births.

The result of testing 34,532 "non-Jewish" individuals in the same program was an enzyme-based carrier rate of 0.006 or 1 in 167 persons tested. This would predict a Tay- Sachs disease incidence among non-Jewish infants of about 1 in 112,000 births, or as many as 40 non-Jewish cases each year in the U.S. Clearly, this is an overestimate. However, consideration of the current findings — that 35 percent of non-Jewish "carriers" actually are heterozygotes for a pseudodeficiency allele — resolves this dilemma. The disease-related α-subunit mutation carrier rate now becomes 0.0039 (1 in 256 non-Jewish individuals). With 5 percent of non-Jewish heterozygotes found to carry the late-onset mutation (G269S), and estimating about the same fraction of enzyme-defined carriers to have other *noninfantile* mutations, the predicted incidence of Tay-Sachs disease in non-Jewish American infants is about 1 in 320,000 births, almost exactly that observed.

Although enzyme-based estimates of the frequencies of *HEXB* alleles in both Jewish and non-Jewish populations are available, no systematic DNA-based mutation frequencies are available at present. Also, no frequency estimates can yet be made about the pseudodeficiency allele(s) in either population. Accordingly, only rough estimates can be made about heterozygote frequencies for *HEXB* mutations. Of 22,043 Jewish individuals enzymatically tested for β-subunit deficiencies, a total of 44 (0.0020) were identified as heterozygotes, or 1 in 500 Jewish persons. This predicts a birth rate frequency of Sandhoff disease (or later-onset variant) of about 1 in 1,000,000 Jewish births. By contrast, 1 in 278 (0.0036) non-Jewish individuals tested (in a cohort of 32,342 persons) were found to be β-subunit-deficient carriers. This indicates a birth rate of β-subunit-deficient individuals (either homozygotes or compound heterozygotes) of 1 in 309,000 births.

These projections are consistent with the annual worldwide surveillance data for newly diagnosed ganglioside G_{M2} disorders, initiated for Tay-Sachs disease in 1980 and for other ganglioside G_{M2} storage disorders in 1982. One expects a Jewish infant to be born with Sandhoff disease in North America once every 10 to 15 years. One has been reported since data collection was initiated. Similarly, about 15 to 20 births of non-Jewish infants with Sandhoff disease is expected each year in North America. From 1982 to 1992, the diagnosis of classic Sandhoff disease was made in 148 non-Jewish infants, consistent with the rate predicted.

Heredity and Population Genetics

A pattern of autosomal recessive inheritance is evident with all of the G_{M2} ganglioside storage disorders. *HEXA*, *HEXB* and *GM2A* mutations all show allelic heterogeneity. As tabulated (Appendices 153A to C and database at http://data.mch.mcgill.ca/), 92 *HEXA*,

26 *HEXB*, and 4 *GM2A* mutations have been identified to date. Most of these alterations represent "private" mutations and have been delineated in single (or very few) families. Others appear in small isolated populations (or highly inbred groups); only a few have been found in multiple cases in diverse populations.

***HEXA* Mutations.** Infantile G_{M2} gangliosidosis due to *HEXA* mutations (Tay-Sachs disease) has been reported throughout the world in "non-Jewish" infants of diverse ethnic groups.[417] An increased incidence of this ganglioside G_{M2} disorder has been reported in at least five geographic isolates—in Switzerland,[418] in Japan,[419] in a Pennsylvania Dutch group in Pennsylvania,[420] in a French-Canadian deme in Eastern Quebec,[421] and among Cajuns in southern Louisiana.[422] Where determined, the underlying mutation(s) differ in each group. At least two novel mutations are observed in non-Jewish French Canadians, the 7.6-kb deletion at the 5′ end of the *HEXA* gene and a G to A alteration at IVS7+1.[295,423] These occur in different subisolates among the Quebecois, one of which, the deletion mutation, has been traced to probable founders.[424] The four-base insertion, 1278ins4, seen most commonly in Ashkenazi Jews, has also been detected.[425]

At least two mutations also are described among the Cajuns: the IVS9+1G → A transition and 1278ins4.[426] In the Pennsylvania Dutch isolate, the IVS9+1 allele accounts for most of the heterozygotes and a pseudodeficiency mutation, R247W, is also frequent in this group.[427] The IVS9+1 mutation also has been identified in non-Jewish patients and obligate heterozygotes of Celtic and French origins.[305,316,317] This may account for the presence of this mutation in the Cajun population and its relatively high frequency in non-Jewish Americans of English, Irish, and Scottish ancestry.

Among Moroccan Jewish patients with Tay-Sachs disease (and family members), a different mutation predominates. Here the two infantile mutations seen in Ashkenazi Jews, 1278ins4 and IVS12+1G → C, are not commonly found. Rather, a three-base deletion, 910delTTC in exon 8, resulting in the loss of F304 or 305, is most often observed.[304,428]

The major *HEXA* allele among the Japanese is a nucleotide transversion at an acceptor splice site, IVS5−1G → T.[429] It accounted for 80 percent (38/48) of the mutant alleles examined. In African Americans, several unrelated patients (one homozygous) were found to have an analogous mutation in a different intron, IVS4−1G → T.[430] Many other mutations (Appendix 153A) have been reported to date in individual families with infantile Tay-Sachs disease probands from widely diverse population groups. In most instances, these patients are found to be either compound heterozygotes with a more common null allele or, where consanguinity is evident or suspected, homozygotes for the rare mutation.

With regard to *HEXA* mutations associated with later-onset forms (B_1 variant, subacute, chronic) a similar pattern to the infantile mutations is observed. The B_1 variant is associated with several different mutations. The most common B1 mutation, the 533G → A transition in exon 5 (R178H), was first identified in a Puerto Rican patient, and subsequently in several patients from a defined region of Portugal. Most recently, the same alteration was detected in individuals with diverse European backgrounds.[241,321] A cystine substitution in the same site (codon 178) is described in Czechoslovakian patients with this variant.[321]

Different mutations are associated with Hex A-deficient subacute forms of G_{M2} gangliosidosis. Two similar alterations, R499H and R504H, have been identified (the latter in homozygous form) in Scotch-Irish, Assyrian, and Armenian patients.[311] A third mutation, G250D, was found in a Lebanese child (homozygous) whose parents were first cousins.[320,431]

***HEXB* Mutations.** Several isolated populations in different areas of the world have been shown to have an increased incidence of Sandhoff disease. Of significance is a sizable geographic isolate of the Creole population in the northern part of Argentina,[432–434] where 65 cases of Sandhoff disease have been diagnosed since 1975. The carrier frequency in the region is estimated at 1 in 26.[433] An increased frequency of the disorder has also been found in an inbred community of Metis Indians in northern Saskatchewan,[435] among Lebanese-Canadians,[421] as well as in Lebanon.[436] Recent population screening data from California suggest a relatively increased Sandhoff disease gene frequency among Hispanics of Mexican or Central American origins as well.[437]

Although only limited, mutation-based population surveys have been reported to date for the 26 *HEXB* mutations, several findings are of interest. The most common mutation described to date is a 16-kb deletion in the 5′ region of the *HEXB* gene extending from the promoter region into intron 5.[342] This is seen predominantly in French and French-Canadian patients, and may account for as much as one-third of *HEXB* mutations. When homozygous, this is associated with infantile disease. In compound heterozygosity with several reported missense mutations, phenotypes have been milder, that is, subacute or chronic.[342] Two distinct null mutations have been described in Sandhoff patients of Argentinian origin, a G to A transition (IVS2+1) and a four-base deletion (784del4) in exon 7.[438] The former was identified in 26 and the latter in 1 of 27 independent disease or obligate alleles examined.[439]

Mutation Origins. For Tay-Sachs disease in the Ashkenazi Jewish population, it has been suggested that the initial mutation for this disorder occurred sometime after 70 A.D. (the second Diaspora of the Jews from Palestine) and before the year 1100 A.D. in areas of central-eastern Europe that now correspond to Austria, the Czech and Slovak republics, and Hungary.[410] Previously, the mutation was believed to have originated farther north in regions that are now northeastern Poland and northwestern Russia.[440] As Sephardic Jews and other non-Ashkenazi groups do not appear to carry this gene(s) in increased frequency (with the exception of Moroccan Jews who harbor a different mutation), such historic dating seems appropriate.

The relatively high frequencies of three *HEXA* mutations in the Ashkenazi Jewish population, and the persistence of the same and additional *HEXA* mutations in other diverse non-Jewish populations, have led to considerable discussion as to the genetic rationale for the retention of these deleterious or lethal alleles (in homozygous or compound heterozygous forms) in these populations. Two major arguments have been posed (which, in fact, may not be mutually exclusive). On the one hand, founder effects with genetic drift could account for this observation.[441,442] Alternatively, others argue that some selective environmental factor may have conferred a biologic advantage (increased fitness) in heterozygotes as a more likely explanation.[440] A suggestion has been made that relative resistance to pulmonary disease, particularly tuberculosis, might have been operative for many centuries in eastern and central Europe where the Ashkenazim lived, often under extremely demanding environmental conditions.[443]

The observed increase in incidence of three other genetically distinct lysosomal lipid storage disorders, Gaucher disease, Niemann-Pick disease, and mucolipidosis IV, in this same population (possibly resulting in similar benefits to heterozygotes for these autosomal recessive mutations) lends weight to this hypothesis.[444] It is intriguing to speculate that some subtle (as yet undetermined) alteration in cell membrane sphingolipid composition or distribution—the result of reduced lysosomal hydrolase activity in the heterozygote—could affect cellular responses (host defense mechanisms) that contribute to susceptibility to pathogens such as *M. tuberculosis*.

The impact of carrier detection programs and the provision of a mechanism for selective reproduction in at-risk couples (through the monitoring of all at-risk pregnancies and the termination of those in which the fetus is found to be affected) has raised questions as to the impact such efforts might have on the gene

Table 153-5 Incidence of Tay-Sachs Disease in the United States and Canada, 1970–1997

	Jewish	Non-Jewish	Total
1970	30–40*	6–10*	40–50*
1980	13	11	24
1982	9	7	16
1983	2	9	11
1985	6	5	11
1987	6	11	17
1989	4	11	15
1991	3	7	10
1993	4	13	17
1995	3	15	18
1997	5	13	18

*Estimates based on Myrianthropoulous,[408] Aronson,[409] Aronson et al.,[417] and O'Brien.[503]

frequency for the Tay-Sachs disease allele in the Jewish and general populations. Because the vast majority of autosomal recessive genes are passed from one generation to the next through heterozygote-nonheterozygote matings, it is clear that the impact on overall gene frequency is minimal. In fact, such a program does not increase the gene frequency at all. Rather, it reduces slightly the rate at which the mutant gene(s) would be expected to be lost from the population.

While the influence of applied technology on gene frequency is trivial, the overall impact on disease incidence can be profound. Unquestionably, the advent of prenatal diagnosis for Tay-Sachs disease and the concomitant development of wide-scale community education, carrier screening, and genetic counseling programs throughout North America have contributed greatly to the reduced incidence of Tay-Sachs disease observed in Jewish infants in the United States and Canada since 1970. These data are presented in Table 153-5. Note that as such programs have been targeted primarily (but not exclusively) to the higher risk Jewish population, the reduction in disease incidence in that group (approaching 90 percent) is not matched by a comparable reduction in incidence in the non-Jewish population. In fact, since the mid- to late-1980s, more cases of classic Tay-Sachs disease have been identified annually in non-Jewish infants than in Jewish ones. This, of course, represents a relative increase only, because the number of new cases diagnosed annually in non-Jewish children has remained unchanged or only slightly increased (perhaps the result of increased intermarriage), while the number of cases in Jewish infants has dropped precipitously.

PATHOGENESIS

Possible Pathogenic Factors Involved in the Development of the Gangliosidoses

The pathogenic mechanisms that lead to the malfunctioning of neuronal circuitry in ganglioside storage diseases are not yet understood. Some factors seem quite obviously to be involved (although their exact contribution remains unclear), while the involvement of others is more speculative.

Monosialogangliosides are amphiphiles that aggregate in aqueous solutions having a critical micellar concentration around 10^{-8} to 10^{-10} M.[445] *In vivo* they occur as components of cellular membranes and are degraded in the lysosomes. In case of blocked catabolism they accumulate and precipitate in the lysosomal compartments of cells in which they are synthesized together with other lipophilic membrane components, phospholipids, cholesterol, and amphiphilic proteins and peptides. In the severe infantile cases, the accumulation of ganglioside G_{M2} alone may amount to 12 percent of dry brain weight (see "Storage Compounds" above) and the resulting storage granules (MCB) may fill the entire cytoplasm of a neuronal cell body (see "Pathology" above). Although the storage compounds themselves are normal, nontoxic membrane components, this excessive accumulation is likely to interfere with intracellular transport and other activities.

In late-onset forms of the disease, glycolipid accumulation is much less pronounced than in infantile forms, suggesting that other mechanisms should also be considered for the pathogenesis of gangliosidoses. Purpura and Suzuki[277] demonstrated formation of meganeurites and tremendous increase of synaptic spines on neurons in patients with ganglioside storage diseases. Similar findings have been reported for some animal models of other neuronal storage diseases[446–449] and suggest formation of misconnections in the nervous tissue.

Preliminary evidence suggests the possibility that in G_{M2} gangliosidosis cells, the undegraded storage material is not confined to secondary lysosomes, but can, to some extent, be recycled and reach other compartments, such as Golgi and plasma membrane, by normal membrane flow.[445] Such an effect might lead to changes in the content and pattern of gangliosides in the plasma membrane. Although convincing proof is still lacking, gangliosides are implicated in cell-cell recognition phenomena,[57] including synaptogenesis. An altered ganglioside pattern on neuronal surfaces might thus interfere with the establishment of proper connections.

Another possible mechanism in pathogenesis might be the formation of toxic compounds, by analogy with the occurrence of glycosylsphingosine and galactosylsphingosine in Gaucher and Krabbe diseases, respectively.[450–452] Indeed, lysoganglioside G_{M2} (II3-sialylgangliotriaosylsphingosine) was found in the brain of patients with Tay-Sachs disease (~15 nmol per gram wet weight[453–455]) and in the brain of patients with Sandhoff disease (~45 nmol per gram wet weight in one study[454] and 6 to 12 nmol per gram wet weight in another[455,456]), but not in normal human brain. Like other psychosine derivatives and lysolecithin, lysoganglioside G_{M2} has lytic properties and is toxic in cell culture.[453] However, the concentration of lysoganglioside is some 300 to 600 times lower than that of the main storage compound, ganglioside G_{M2}. In view of this ratio and of the different lysoganglioside G_{M2} levels reported so far for brains of patients with Tay-Sachs and Sandhoff diseases, it appears unlikely that the toxicity of this compound is the immediate cause of cell death. Hannun and Bell[457] reported that lysosphingolipids are potent inhibitors of protein kinase C and thus may interfere with signal transduction in nerve cells.

An involvement of other factors besides the neuronal storage of glycolipids G_{M2} and G_{A2} in the pathogenesis of G_{M2} gangliosidosis is suggested by bone marrow transplantation (BMT) experiments in *Hexb−/−* (Sandhoff disease) mice[458] (see "Animal Models" below). BMT extended the life span of these knockout mice from ~4.5 months to 8 months and slowed their neurologic deterioration. It also corrected glycolipid storage in the visceral organs, however, without a clear reduction of brain glycolipid storage. These observations suggest a complex pathogenetic mechanism that may well involve lytic compounds, for example, in the blood circulation and/or cytokines generated by colloidal iron-positive macrophages in the brain, which were heavily reduced in BMT Sandhoff mice. BMT may also selectively reduce levels of minor, more water-soluble, toxic metabolites, such as lyso-G_{M2}, that may mediate neuropathogenesis in this disorder.[458]

Degree of Enzyme Deficiency and Development of Different Clinical Diseases

Although all cases of Tay-Sachs disease and variants are caused by allelic mutations of the *HEXA* gene, the discussion in this review underscores the tremendous clinical heterogeneity derived from the expression of different mutations. Although fewer mutations are known, the same is evident for Sandhoff disease and its variants.

At the biochemical level, this heterogeneity is paralleled by a corresponding variation in the extent and pattern of glycolipid accumulation in different regions of the brain. Infantile forms have an excessive and ubiquitous neuronal glycolipid storage (up to 12 percent of the brain dry weight). Late onset forms show much-less pronounced accumulation, which is restricted to specific brain regions, the cortex being almost unimpaired, whereas the hippocampus, the nuclei of the brain stem, and spinal cord, as well as the granular cells in the cerebellum and retina, are markedly affected.[276,291,292] Thus, different allelic mutations in one gene locus lead to variable clinical and neuropathologic expression. A crucial difference between the various clinical manifestations (e.g., the infantile and adult forms) is different residual activity against the natural ganglioside G_{M2} substrate of Hex A.

Unfortunately, the *in vivo* activity of mutant enzymes against their natural substrates cannot be determined directly. The experimental approaches that are so far considered to yield the best approximations are (a) feeding of ganglioside G_{M2} to cultivated fibroblast and (b) *in vitro* determination of enzyme activity in fibroblasts homogenates, using the natural substrate in the presence of the G_{M2} activator protein. Data obtained with the latter method indicate that chronic and subacute patients with α-subunit defects have some residual activity, i.e., significantly higher that of infantile forms of G_{M2} gangliosidosis (Table 153-2).[387] Residual activities in the range of 10 to 20 percent of the mean control value appear to be compatible with normal life. These findings stress the importance of small variations of the low residual enzyme activity for the development of a different clinical course of the disease.

Sandhoff and colleagues developed a kinetic model relating enzyme activity to substrate turnover that can account for the observation that as little as 10 to 15 percent Hex A activity may be sufficient to sustain normal catabolism of ganglioside G_{M2}, and that small variations in Hex A activity below this value (i.e., below 5 percent activity) can greatly influence the clinical course of the disease.[459,460] According to the model, the catabolism of the substrate would increase steeply with small increases in residual Hex A activity resulting from different mutation types. Indeed, this was born out experimentally in ganglioside G_{M2} loading experiments using fibroblasts cultures from patients with infantile, subacute or chronic forms of G_{M2} gangliosidosis due to α, β, or G_{M2} activator deficiency.[460]

This explains why heterozygotes, with 30 to 70 percent reduction in enzyme activity, show normal ganglioside G_{M2} catabolism. Only when the residual activity falls below a critical threshold would the overall turnover rate be reduced. In this case, the substrate accumulation would be proportional to the difference between threshold activity and the smaller actual residual activity in the lysosome. Because influx of the substrate as well as enzyme activity differ in different organs or cell types and may even vary between individual cells (e.g., neurons), the consequence of a mutation on different organs or cell types may be quite variable. For instance, in late-onset chronic forms of the disease having residual ganglioside G_{M2}-cleaving activity, neurons with a low rate of ganglioside biosynthesis might easily tolerate the enzyme defect. Conversely, in cells with a high rate of ganglioside biosynthesis, the influx rate would exceed the maximal capacity of the enzyme and the cells would suffer from irreversible glycolipid accumulation. Thus, in contrast to infantile forms in which all neurons are affected and the relative metabolic rates merely determine the temporal sequence of symptoms, in late-onset forms the function and viability of some neurons are affected preferentially, while others may remain unimpaired.

ANIMAL MODELS

Naturally Occurring Animal Model of G_{M2} Gangliosidosis

G_{M2} gangliosidosis has been reported in dogs,[461–464] cats,[465–467] and pig.[468,469] In all species, abundant neuronal storage is a conspicuous feature, but visceral storage is noted only in feline G_{M2} gangliosidosis. The feline model is homologous with human Sandhoff disease. Meganeurites as seen in human G_{M2} gangliosidosis have been reported in canine[464] and feline[470] models. Using Golgi and combined Golgi-electron microscopic studies, Walkley and collaborators described ectopic neurite growth on pyramidal neurons of cerebral cortex and multipolar cells of amygdala and claustrum in the feline model. These neurites commonly possess asymmetric synapses. They have shown that a strong correlation exists between ectopic neurite growth and accumulation of G_{M2} ganglioside.[278,448,471,472]

Murine Models of G_{M2} Gangliosidosis Generated by Targeted Gene Disruption

Three groups have independently generated murine models of Tay-Sachs disease, Sandhoff disease, and G_{M2} activator deficiency using gene-targeting techniques.[159,160,473–476] Unlike human G_{M2} gangliosidosis, phenotypic differences among these murine models are notable.

Tay-Sachs Disease Models. Three mouse models of Tay-Sachs disease have been derived independently by interruption of exon 8[474–476] or exon 11[160] of the *Hexa* gene with the neomycin cassette. In each case, a near total deficiency of Hex A and normal levels of Hex B were found. Most strikingly, the Tay-Sachs mice showed no clinical phenotype or behavior abnormalities to at least 1 year of age in stark contrast to the human disorder. Progressive accumulation of ganglioside G_{M2} in the form of MCBs identical to those found in patients were detected in restricted regions of the brains of the mice. Areas of prominent G_{M2} storage are noted primarily in neurons in the cerebral cortex, amygdala, piriform cortex, hippocampus, hypothalamus, and so on, with relatively little storage in the basal ganglia and thalamus (Figs. 153-11 and 153-12). In the cerebral cortex, large pyramidal neurons show more storage than other cortical neurons. The storage material stains strongly with PAS stain on frozen section, is immunoreactive with antibody to G_{M2} ganglioside,[160] and consists of MCBs at the ultrastructural level. Most notably, storage neurons are very rare in the cerebellum or spinal cord.[160,475] No storage is reported in visceral organs at the light microscopic level, but moderate lysosomal storage is reported at the ultrastructural level.[474]

Sandhoff Disease Models. Two Sandhoff disease model mouse lines have been produced by targeted gene disruption of the *Hexb* gene through insertion of the neomycin cassette into exon 13[159] or exon 2.[160] The Sandhoff-disease mice were deficient in both the Hex A and Hex B isozymes, and produced only small quantities of Hex S. Beginning about 3 months after birth, the Sandhoff mice underwent a progressive and severe neurodegenerative course. The most prominent phenotypic features of the mice were abnormalities in motor function, initially presenting as defects in balance and coordination, and evolving by 4 months to almost complete absence of limb movement with significant muscle wasting and hind limb rigidity. The animals died by 4 to 4.5 months of age. Histopathologically, neuronal storage was far more extensive than in the Tay-Sachs mice (Figs. 153-11 and 153-12).

In *Hexb*−/− mice, neuronal storage is diffusely observed throughout neuraxes. Extensive storage is noted in neurons in the cerebellum, brain stem, spinal cord, retina, and myenteric plexus. Storage is noted in small round cells that stain positive with the lectin RCA-1, indicating microglia/macrophages. These cells tend to be localized to perivascular regions. They stain with PAS, Alcian blue, and also colloidal iron. Similar storage macrophages are observed in the visceral organs and of the renal tubular epithelium. On the other hand, neuronal storage material does not stain with any of these stains on paraffin sections, although it stains strongly with PAS on frozen section. G_{M2} ganglioside immunostaining is detected only in frozen sections. Cerebral white matter is hypomyelinated and myelin/axonal degeneration is recognized in the spinal white matter[159,160] (Fig. 153-11).

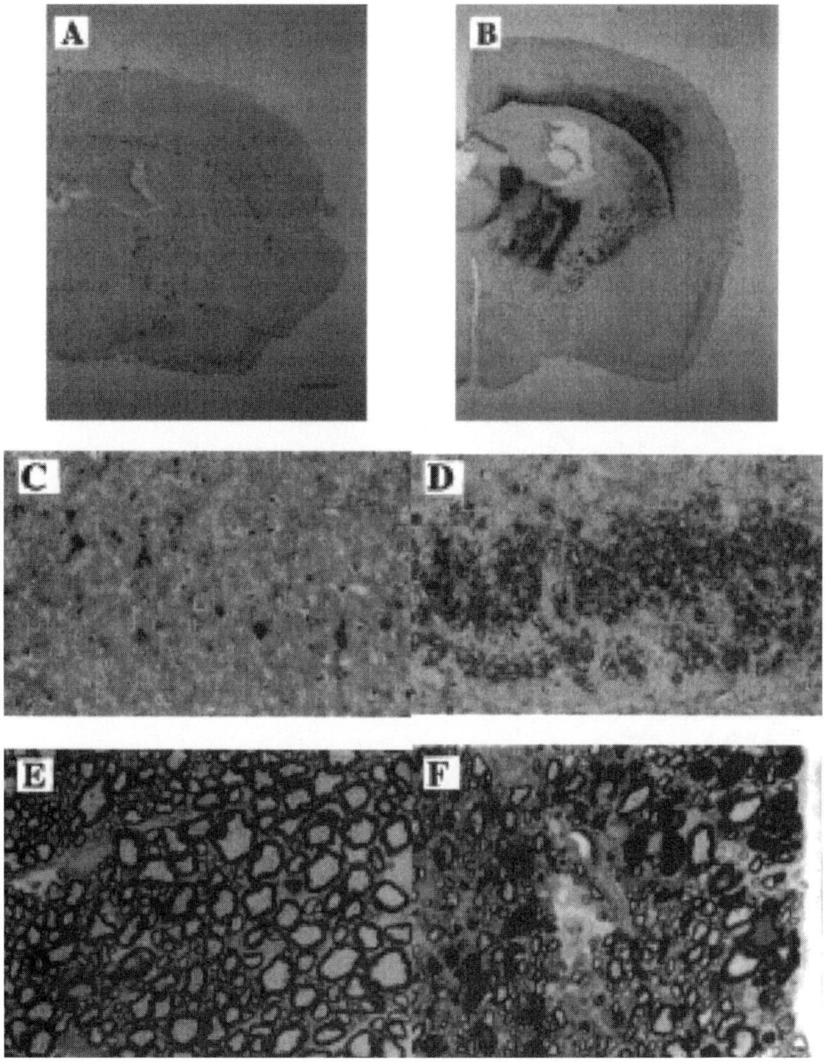

Fig. 153-11 Neuropathology of *Hexa–/–* (A,C) and *Hexb–/–* (B,D,F) mice (3 to 4.5 months of age). E is from a wild-type mouse. *A, B,* Coronal sections of forebrain immunostained with mouse-human chimeric monoclonal antibody recognizing G_{M2} (brown stain); bar = 667 μm. *C, D,* CA3 region of hippocampus showing PAS-positive storage material; ×325. *E, F,* Ventrolateral field of the spinal cord showing myelin profiles; bar = 17 μm. (*Panels A and B from Phaneuf et al.*[160] *Used by permission.*)

Apoptotic death of neurons was observed in the Sandhoff, but not in the Tay-Sachs, disease model.[279] Bulk G_{M2} ganglioside storage in the brains of the Sandhoff mice was two to four times higher than in the Tay-Sachs mice. G_{A2} glycolipid (asialo-G_{M2}) was also highly elevated in Sandhoff mice. The Tay-Sachs mice did not accumulate G_{A2}. The Sandhoff-disease mice also accumulated glycolipid in visceral organs and excreted oligosaccharides in their urine.[160,458]

G_{M2} Activator Deficiency Model. The gene-targeting procedure deleted the protein coding regions of exons 3 and 4 of the *Gm2a* gene and produced a null allele.[473] These mice had defects in motor function; however, the mice had a normal life span and were fertile. The G_{M2} activator-deficient mice demonstrated neuronal storage but only in restricted regions of the brain (piriform, entorhinal cortex, amygdala, and hypothalamic nuclei) reminiscent of the Tay-Sachs model mice (Fig. 153-12). Unlike the Tay-Sachs model, they displayed significant storage in the cerebellar Purkinje and granular cells. Also, like the Tay-Sachs mice, little storage was observed in the spinal cord or visceral organs. The abnormal ganglioside storage in the activator-deficient mice consisted of G_{M2} with a low amount of G_{A2}.

Phenotypic Variation Among the Mouse Models. It is striking that unlike the nearly identical clinical course of Tay-Sachs disease, Sandhoff disease and the G_{M2} activator deficiency in humans, the corresponding mutant mouse models vary greatly in phenotype. The great phenotypic differences among the models are the result of distinctive ganglioside degradation pathways in mice and humans (Fig. 153-13). In humans, G_{M2} ganglioside is degraded nearly exclusively by Hex A in collaboration with the activator protein to yield G_{M3}. The absence of either Hex A in Tay-Sachs and Sandhoff disease patients, or the G_{M2} activator protein in G_{M2} activator deficiency patients, causes a nearly total block of this pathway and results in massive accumulation of ganglioside G_{M2} in neurons with attendant neurodegeneration. In mice, ganglioside G_{M2} can be degraded by two pathways (Fig. 153-13). One is identical to the human pathway. The second is essentially unique to the mouse and is initiated by sialidase acting on G_{M2} to yield G_{A2}. The G_{A2} is then degraded by either Hex A with activator protein or, to a lesser extent, by Hex B with the G_{M2} activator protein. In Tay-Sachs mice, the absence of Hex A blocks the G_{M2} to G_{M3} pathway. However, Hex B, likely with G_{M2} activator, can slowly degrade G_{A2} generated by the mouse sialidase, explaining the modest storage and the absence of a clinical phenotype. In contrast, when both Hex A and Hex B are absent in the Sandhoff-disease mice both pathways are blocked producing high levels of G_{M2} and G_{A2} storage, and a severe clinical phenotype. In the G_{M2} activator-deficiency model, the G_{M2} to G_{M3} pathway is blocked by the absence of the activator protein

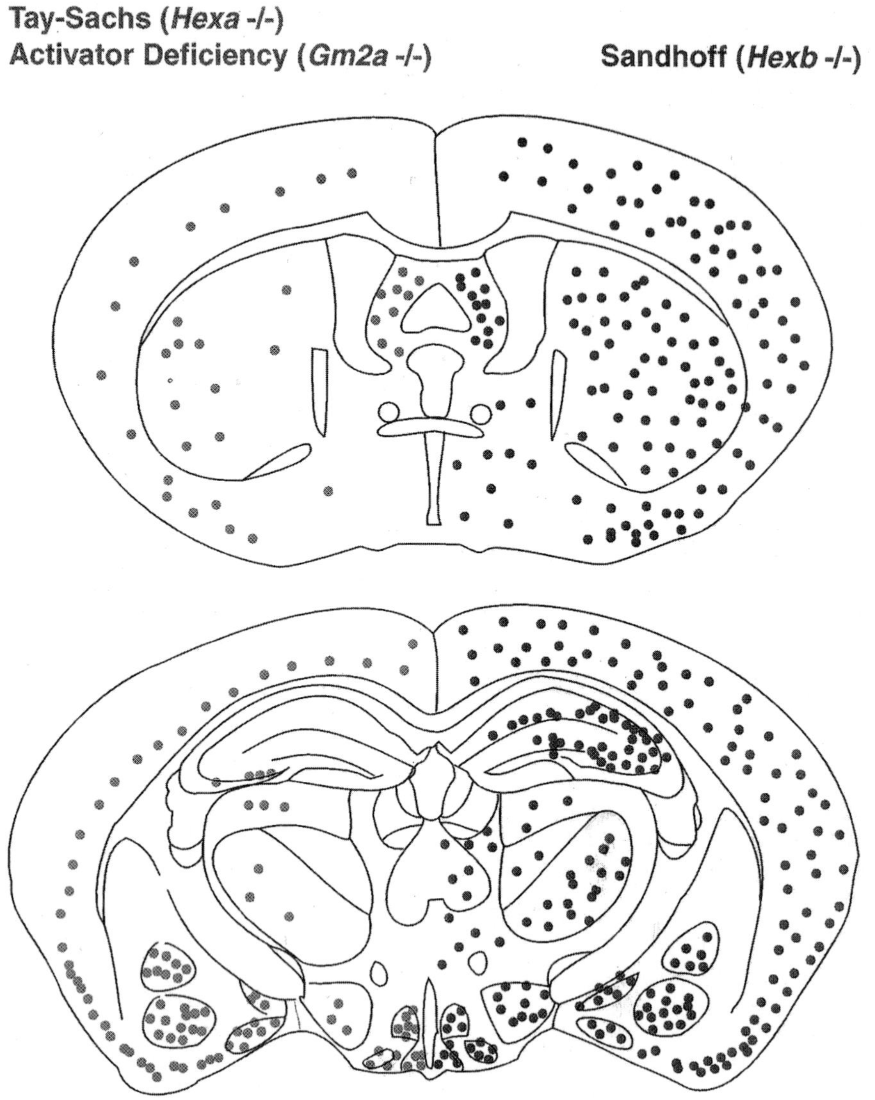

Fig. 153-12 Diagrams showing the distribution of storage material in the brain of mouse models of Tay-Sachs disease and G_{M2} activator deficiency (left half) and Sandhoff disease (right half).

resulting in a regional distribution of storage similar to the Tay-Sachs model (Fig. 153-12). Without the G_{M2} activator, the degradation of G_{A2} by β-hexosaminidase proceeds, but at a suboptimal rate, resulting in higher levels of glycolipid G_{A2} with increased storage in the cerebellum and defects in motor function. The model of ganglioside degradation in the mouse is based on the glycolipids accumulated in the mutant mice,[159,160,473,476] degradation of labeled ganglioside in fibroblast cultures,[159,473] and the enzymatic specificity of mouse β-hexosaminidase and G_{M2} activator protein.[161]

Double-Mutant Mice Totally Deficient in β-Hexosaminidase. Through cross-breeding of mice carrying disrupted *Hexa* and *Hexb* genes, mice totally deficient in β-hexosaminidase have been generated.[219,477] Without functional *Hexa* or *Hexb* genes all three hexosaminidase isozymes, Hex A, Hex B, and Hex S, are absent. Humans with such deficiency have not been described. In addition to gangliosidosis, these mice showed many features of severe mucopolysaccharidosis. The mice exhibited dysmorphic features, dysostosis multiplex, excreted glycosaminoglycans (GAGs) in the urine and accumulated GAGs in cells and tissues. The pathology of these mice was also similar to that found in mucopolysaccharidosis patients. Macrophages storing GAGs were abundant and found in many tissues. Storage was also apparent in other tissue elements such as chondrocytes, osteocytes, splenic sinusoidal cells, and smooth muscle cells in the media of the aorta and arteries. Other than hexosaminidase, no deficiency of other lysosomal enzymes involved in GAG degradation was found.[478] These striking features of mucopolysaccharidosis were not seen in either the Tay-Sachs or the Sandhoff model. The mucopolysaccharidosis phenotype of the total hexosaminidase-deficient mice proves that hexosaminidase is essential for the degradation of GAGs (Chap. 136) and that there is redundancy among the hexosaminidase isozymes for this function. The lack of a strong mucopolysaccharidosis phenotype in the Sandhoff disease model suggests that Hex S, the only hexosaminidase isozyme present in these animals, may play a physiologic role in the degradation of GAGs.

THERAPY

For the most part, treatment for any of the G_{M2} gangliosidoses is restricted to supportive care and appropriate management of intervening problems, such as maintenance of adequate nutrition and hydration, management of infectious disease, and control of seizures when and where they occur (see "Psychosis" above). In

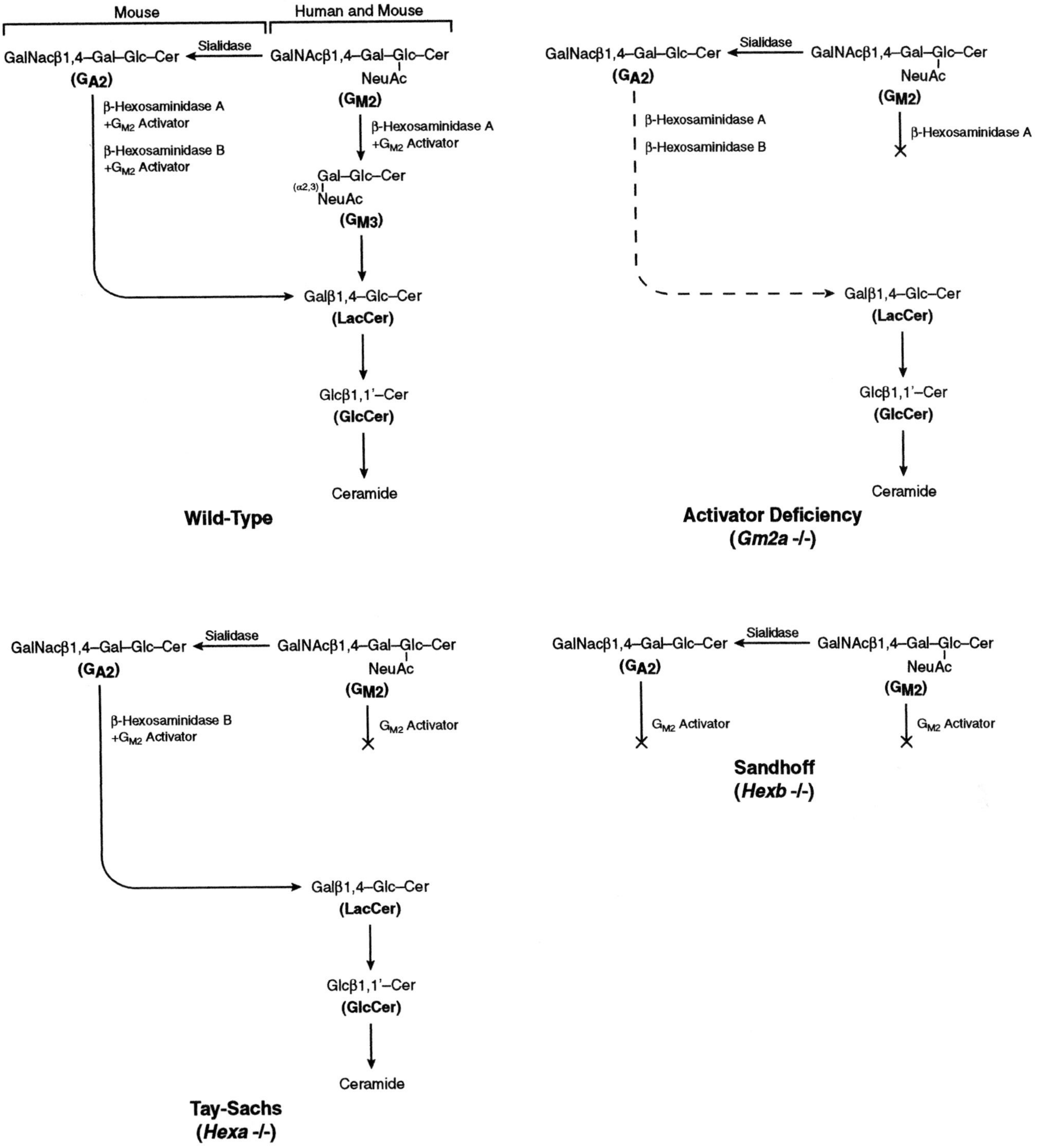

Fig. 153-13 The ganglioside degradation pathways in G_{M2} gangliosidosis mice. The scheme illustrates the alternative catabolism of G_{M2} via G_{M3} (action of Hex A) or G_{A2} (action of sialidase and Hex B) in the mouse. In humans, the predominant route of catabolism is via G_{M3}. The dotted line indicates a reduced extent of catabolism of G_{A2} by Hex A or Hex B in mice with G_{M2} activator deficiency. The scheme does not account for a minor contribution of Hex S on ganglioside degradation.

the most disabling conditions, bowel management is frequently a continuing problem. At present, there is no specific therapy that will halt the progression or reverse the clinical manifestations of the G_{M2} gangliosidoses. However, a number of different therapeutic approaches are being evaluated.

Enzyme Replacement Therapy

The success of enzyme replacement therapy for the treatment of nonneuronopathic (type I) Gaucher disease (Chap. 146) suggests that a similar approach might be beneficial for the G_{M2} gangliosidoses. Unfortunately, early attempts at enzyme replacement in the G_{M2} gangliosidoses were unsuccessful[479,480] and pointed out two major obstacles that must be overcome before enzyme therapy can be successfully applied. Of paramount importance is a means of introducing of enzyme into the central nervous system. In contrast to type I Gaucher disease, the principal clinical manifestations of the G_{M2} gangliosidoses occur within the central nervous system. Unfortunately, delivery of enzyme to the central nervous system is severely retarded by the blood-brain barrier (BBB). Methods to circumvent the BBB include intrathecal administration of enzyme[480] and osmotic disruption of the BBB prior to the intra-arterial administration of enzyme.[481]

A second challenge for successful enzyme replacement is efficient targeting of enzyme to neuronal lysosomes. Enzyme isolated from body tissues lacks the mannose-6-phosphate recognition marker that could permit neuronal uptake.[120] Recombinant Hex A, synthesized in expression systems that introduce the mannose-6-phosphate modification, has not yet been produced in sufficient quantities for therapeutic trials. An alternative approach for targeting enzyme to neurons was taken with the covalent attachment of the polysialylganglioside-binding domain of tetanus toxin (fragment C) to placental Hex A.[482] *In vitro* experiments have demonstrated enhanced binding and uptake of the Hex A-fragment C conjugate by neurons and the elimination of G_{M2} storage from neuronal cultures derived from Sandhoff-disease cats.[482]

Recombinant activator protein has been produced in large quantities and is efficiently endocytosed by cells through a carbohydrate-independent mechanism.[118,122,483] If the recombinant activator protein is also endocytosed by neurons, it may be useful for replacement therapy in the AB variant.

Cell Therapy

Cell therapy for the G_{M2} gangliosidoses involves the transplantation of cells to provide a long-term source of Hex A or the activator protein to affected tissues. BMT has emerged as a potentially effective cell therapy for some types of lysosomal storage disorders. After engraftment, donor-derived monocytes, macrophages, and microglia repopulate target organs and deliver the missing lysosomal enzyme.[484] In some lysosomal disease patients, BMT has produced dramatic improvement in many of the somatic manifestations of the diseases.[485,486] Less clear-cut has been the effectiveness of BMT in preventing or reversing central nervous system manifestations. The experience of treating G_{M2} gangliosidosis patients with BMT is very limited. BMT treatment of a Tay-Sachs patient and a Sandhoff patient, both at about 1 year of age and after onset of significant neurologic symptoms, yielded little or no benefit.[485]

Recent experiments using the mouse model of Sandhoff disease[159] show that syngeneic bone marrow transplantation prior to the onset of neurologic symptoms, at about 2 weeks of age, increased life span from about 4 to 4.5 months to 6 to 8 months.[458] BMT was highly effective in eliminating or reversing the pathology and glycolipid storage in somatic tissues. The somatic improvement was consistent with a substantial increase of hexosaminidase activity in visceral organs. In the brain and spinal cord, a much smaller increase of hexosaminidase activity was found and appeared to be due to donor-derived microglia or macrophages infiltrating the central nervous system. Significantly, BMT ameliorated some neurologic manifestations associated with disease. In light of the lengthened life span and the neurologic improvement after BMT, it was surprising that neither a reduction in neuronal pathology nor glycolipid storage in the brain was detected. Possible explanations for the neurologic improvement after BMT are: (a) very localized correction of neuronal storage; (b) reduction of neurotoxic lysogangliosides such as lyso-G_{M2} that may be present in brain or released by visceral organs; or (c) replacement of the enzyme-deficient microglia population with normal microglia, which may delay their possible activation and mediation of central nervous system pathology.

The small amount of enzyme introduced into the central nervous system and inability to significantly impact neuronal storage would suggest that, without a significant increase in the capacity of microglia to secrete hexosaminidase, BMT may not be effective for infantile forms of the G_{M2} gangliosidoses. However, a small increase in central nervous system enzyme activity by BMT could potentially improve the clinical course of the later-onset forms of the disorder.

A second form of cell therapy uses neural progenitor cells for implantation into the central nervous system.[487] These cells, when implanted into the central nervous system, can differentiate into neurons, astrocytes, and oligodendrocytes, and have the ability to integrate throughout the neuraxis and supply the missing enzyme. The neural progenitor cell strategy has been tested in the MPS VII mouse, a model with central nervous system involvement.[488] β-Glucuronidase-secreting neural progenitors, transplanted into the brains of newborn mice, produced diffuse expression of the enzyme and eliminated storage in the neurons and glia of the disease model mice. The same neural progenitors were transduced with a *HEXA* cDNA containing retrovirus to produce cell lines overproducing the α-subunit.[489] When implanted into the cerebral ventricles of newborn wild-type mice, these cells produced high levels of hexosaminidase activity for extended periods of time. This approach has not yet been tested in animal models of the G_{M2} gangliosidoses.

Gene Therapy

Gene therapy strategies for the G_{M2} gangliosidoses could involve either an ex vivo approach in which cells are first transduced with recombinant vector containing *HEXA*, *HEXB*, or *GM2A* cDNA, and then transplanted, or an *in situ* approach in which the recombinant vector is introduced directly into the central nervous system. Possible cellular vehicles for ex vivo applications include hematopoietic stem cells, neural progenitor cells (discussed above), or fibroblasts.[490] At present, most gene therapy experiments related to the G_{M2} gangliosidoses have involved the production of recombinant virus, either retrovirus[491] or adenovirus,[492] containing the *HEXA* cDNA and transduction of cells *in vitro*.

Substrate Deprivation Therapy

A novel approach to the treatment of the G_{M2} gangliosidoses and other sphingolipidoses is substrate deprivation therapy. According the threshold model for lysosomal storage,[460] accumulation of glycolipid will be prevented if the rate of degradation conferred by the residual lysosomal enzyme activity in the patients exceeds the rate of substrate influx into lysosomes. Substrate deprivation therapy employs an inhibitor to lower glycosphingolipid synthesis and the corresponding rate of substrate influx into lysosomes. If synthesis is lowered sufficiently, the patient's residual enzyme activity will be able to completely degrade the substrate and prevent or eliminate lysosomal storage. Recent investigations have focused on *N*-butyldeoxynojirimycin (NB-DNJ), an inhibitor of glucosylceramide synthase, the enzyme catalyzing the first step of glucosylceramide-based glycosphingolipids.[493] Platt and colleagues tested the effectiveness of NB-DNJ by oral administration to the Tay-Sachs mouse model.[494] Treatment resulted in an approximately 50 percent reduction of G_{M2} ganglioside accumulation in the brains of the treated, as compared to untreated, Tay-Sachs mice. A corresponding diminution in the severity of neuropathology was also observed. The only other effect of the drug treatment was a reduction in the size of spleen and thymus. The drug treatment was also recently evaluated in the symptomatic Sandhoff-disease model.[495] The drug treatment improved neurologic function of the mice and lengthened their life span by 40 percent. G_{M2} and G_{A2} storage was reduced by 30 to 40 percent in the brain. Because the effectiveness of this approach is dependent on the level of residual lysosomal enzyme activity, the later-onset forms of the disease would be expected to respond better to NB-DNJ therapy than the infantile forms. Finally, because NB-DNJ lowers synthesis of all glucosylceramide-based glycolipids, it is a potentially suitable therapeutic for all three forms of G_{M2} gangliosidosis as well as for other glycosphingolipidoses including Gaucher disease (Chap. 146), Fabry disease (Chap. 150) and G_{M1} gangliosidosis (Chap. 151).

Appendix 153A **Mutations in Tay-Sachs Disease and Variants**

Mutation	Location	Expected Result	Biochemical Phenotype	Clinical Phenotype*	Origin	References
Del7.6 kb	5′ to IVS-1	no mRNA	Abnormal Southern blot, mRNA undetectable in homozygotes	Infantile acute (patient homozygous)	French Canadian	294, 295, 424
1A → G	Exon 1	Met1Val		Infantile acute	Black American	306
1A → T	Exon 1	Met1Leu	mRNA at 1/3 level of wild type allele; absence of enzyme activity with MUGS after transfection in HeLa cells	Chronic (second allele Gly269Ser)	Ukrainian	504
2T → C	Exon 1	Met1Thr		Severe subacute (second allele Pro25Ser)	English	505
73C → T	Exon 1	Pro25Ser	Patient fibroblasts contain pro-α but no mature α	Severe subacute (second allele Met1Thr)	English	505
78G → A	Exon 1	Trp26Stop		Infantile acute (second allele Arg178Leu)	English	323
116T → G	Exon 1	Leu39Arg	Decreased amount of α precursor and absent mature α subunit	Infantile acute (second allele 1278insTATC)	Polish	330
316C → T	Exon 2	Gln106 → Stop		Infantile acute	Mixed European	307
G → C	+1 IVS-2	Abnormal splicing		Infantile acute	German/ Irish/English	323
G → A	+1 IVS-2	Abnormal splicing	Low level of mRNA lacking exon 2	Infantile acute	French	305
379C → T	Exon 3	Leu127Phe		Infantile acute	Mixed European	307
380T → G	Exon 3	Leu127Arg		Infantile acute	Italian	330
409C → T	Exon 3	Arg137Stop	mRNA undetectable (second allele 1278insTATC)	Infantile acute	French	305, 306
G → T	+1 IVS-3	Abnormal splicing	mRNA lacking exon 3	Infantile acute	Japanese	506
423delTT	Exon 4	Frameshift	Absent mRNA on Northern blot	Infantile acute (patient homozygous)	French	330
436delG	Exon 4	Frameshift		Infantile acute (patient homozygous)	Black American	306
InsT	+3 IVS-4	Abnormal splicing	Severely reduced mRNA lacking exon 4	Infantile acute (patient homozygous)	Israeli Bedouin	507
G → A	+5 IVS-4	Abnormal splicing	3% mRNA lacking exon 4 (second allele 1278insTATC)	Infantile acute	French	305
G → T	−IVS-4	Abnormal splicing		Infantile acute (patient homozygous)	Black American	430
477delTG	Exon 5	Frameshift		Infantile acute	English	323
496C → G	Exon 5	Arg166Gly	Reduced activity with MUG, MUGS; altered Km with MUG; increased heat stability of Hex A	Severe subacute (second allele is 498delC)	Syrian	508
496delC	Exon5	Frameshift	mRNA at 5% of normal level for this allele	Severe subacute (second allele Ser279Pro)	Israeli Druze	509
498delC	Exon5	Frameshift		Severe subacute (second allele Arg166Gly)	Syrian	508

(Continued on next page)

Appendix 153A (Continued)

Mutation	Location	Expected Result	Biochemical Phenotype	Clinical Phenotype*	Origin	References
508C → T	Exon 5	Arg170Trp	Not established; second allele (Asp258His) is B1-type	Infantile acute	French Canadian	324
509G → A	Exon 5	Arg170Gln	Mutation generates cryptic acceptor site in exon 5 giving in frame deletion of 17 amino acids; processed to mature enzyme of reduced size and in reduced amount; in COS transfection presumptive α dimer formed in reduced size and amount	Infantile acute	Japanese; Moroccan Jews (17/44 enzyme defined carriers); Scottish	330, 428, 510, 511
532C → T	Exon 5	Arg178Cys	"B1"-type catalytic defect; in COS transfection, Hex S is inactive	Infantile acute	Czechoslovakian	321
533G → A	Exon 5	Arg178His	Near normal Hex A activity with MUG substrate; absent MUGS/G_{M2} hydrolysis = B1 biochemical phenotype; in COS transfection, Hex S is inactive	Subacute in homozygotes (more severe in compound heterozygotes with null allele)	Common in Portuguese; other European	175, 214, 241, 321, 322
533G → T	Exon 5	Arg178Leu	19% serum Hex A activity with MUG substrate; second allele (Trp26Stop) is null	Infantile acute	English	323
538T → C	Exon 5	Tyr180His	Unstable, thermolabile α chain when expressed in COS cells, impaired Hex A formation	Chronic (second mutation 1278insTATC)	Ashkenazi Jewish	329
540C → G	Exon 5	Tyr180Stop		Infantile acute	Moroccan Jew	428, 511
547insA	Exon 5	Frameshift	CRM negative in fibroblasts	Infantile acute (patient homozygote)	Chinese	310
570G → A	Exon 5 (also described as −1 position of exon 5)	Silent change in last amino acid (190Leu) of exon	7% mRNA lacking exon 5 and 3% normal-size mRNA containing silent mutation; suggest residual Hex A (2.5%) due to normal enzyme	Severe subacute (patient homozygous)	Tunisian	319
G → A	+1 IVS-5	Abnormal splicing		Infantile acute (patient homozygous)	Turkish	512
A → G	−2 IVS-5	Abnormal splicing	mRNA lacking exon 6	Enzyme defined carrier	Moroccan Jews (6/44 samples)	511
G → T	−1 IVS-5	Abnormal splicing	mRNA lacking exon 6	Infantile acute (patient homozygous)	Japanese (present in 38/48 mutant alleles)	429
574G → C, 598G → A	Exon 6	Val192Leu, Val200Met	Not a B1-type mutation as previously proposed; absent Hex A activity and degraded α subunit in patient fibroblasts; Val192Leu α chain expressed in COS cells fails to form αβ dimer or mature α subunit; Val200Met α chain gives active Hex A (second allele G → A +1 IVS-9)	Infantile acute		513–515
587A → G	Exon 6	Asn196Ser		Identified in enzyme defined carrier	US French Canadian	516

Appendix 153A (Continued)

Mutation	Location	Expected Result	Biochemical Phenotype	Clinical Phenotype*	Origin	References
590A → C	Exon 6	Lys197Thr	No biochemical analysis; second mutation observed in subacute patient suggesting Lys197Thr may be milder allele	Chronic (second mutation Arg499His)	Dutch	330
611A → G	Exon 6	His204Arg		Infantile acute	German	330
629C → T	Exon 6	Ser210Phe		Infantile acute (patient homozygous)	Algerian	305
632T → C	Exon 6	Phe211Ser		Infantile acute	Italian	330
G → A	+1 IVS-6	Abnormal splicing	mRNA lacking exon 6 with in frame loss of 34 amino acids (compatible with subacute phenotype?)	Subacute, chronic patients (second allele not identified)	American	330
677C → T	Exon 7	Ser226Phe			Azore	307
739C → T	Exon 7	Arg247Trp	Reduced activity toward MUG, MUGS, low normal ganglioside G_{M2} hydrolysis; catalytically normal enzyme in fibroblasts and when expressed in COS cells; normal synthesis of pro-α and reduced stability of the mature α subunit in fibroblasts and when expressed in COS cells; slower maturation of α subunit in COS cells = "Hex A pseudodeficiency"	Asymptomatic in compound heterozygotes with null alleles	Diverse (accounts for 32% of non-Jewish enzyme-defined carriers; not detected in Ashkenazi Jews)	337, 340
745C → T	Exon 7	Arg249Trp	Reduced activity toward MUG, MUGS, low normal ganglioside G_{M2} hydrolysis; catalytically normal enzyme in fibroblasts and when expressed in COS cells; normal synthesis of pro-α and reduced stability of the mature α subunit in fibroblasts and when expressed in COS cells; slower maturation of α subunit in COS cells = "Hex A pseudodeficiency"	Asymptomatic in compound heterozygotes with null alleles	Diverse (accounts for 6% of non-Jewish enzyme-defined carriers; not detected in Ashkenazi Jews)	340, 517
748G → A	Exon 7	Gly250Ser	Possibly benign; unpublished reference to reduced enzyme activity,	Detected in enzyme defined carriers	US French Canadians (in 4/36 samples)	516
749G → A	Exon 7	Gly250Asp	α Unstable, unphosphorylated; COS transfection shows absent Hex S activity but intermediate activity (as Hex A) if co-transfected with β	Subacute (patient homozygous)	Lebanese	320, 518
755G → A	Exon 7	Arg252His	B1 biochemical phenotype due to Arg178His allele	Chronic (second allele Arg178His)	Portuguese	331

(Continued on next page)

Appendix 153A (Continued)

Mutation	Location	Expected Result	Biochemical Phenotype	Clinical Phenotype*	Origin	References
772G → C	Exon 7	Asp258His	16% MUG, <1% MUGS Hex A activity; mutant Hex A more heat stable than normal (second allele 927delCT) = B1 biochemical phenotype	Infantile acute	Scottish-Irish	177, 324
805G → A	Exon 7	Gly269Ser	Reduction in mRNA level due to presumptive defect in splicing; reduced level of α subunit and defective subunit association; in COS transfection α unstable, soluble, phosphorylated	Chronic (homozygotes at mild end of spectrum)	Diverse; Ashkenazi Jews, 3% of alleles	127, 325, 326, 328; screening in 401, 411, 412, 414
G → A	+1 IVS-7	Abnormal splicing	mRNA undetectable (second allele del7.6 kb)	Infantile acute	French Canadian	519
G → C	+1 IVS-7	Abnormal splicing	Trace mRNA lacking exon 7	Infantile acute (patient homozygous)	Portuguese	520
G → A	−7 IVS-7	Abnormal splicing	mRNA level 20% of normal made up of 10% normal sequence mRNA and 6% mRNA lacking exon 8, as well as 3% mRNA due to second allele; normal mRNA fraction accounts for reduced level of functional enzyme (MUGS activity 5% of normal)	Chronic (second allele 1278insTATC)	English	318
806G → A	Exon 8	Gly269Asp		Infantile acute		307
835T → C	Exon 8	Ser279Pro	Deficient enzyme activity when expressed in COS cells	Severe subacute (second allele 496delC)	Israeli Druze	509
902T → G	Exon 8	Met301Arg		Infantile acute	Yugoslavian	521
910delTTC	Exon 8	304delPhe	Defective subunit assembly and secretion; in COS transfection, precursor stable, no Hex S activity	Infantile acute	Moroccan Jews (17/44 enzyme defined carriers), French, Irish	304, 305, 428,511
927delCT	Exon 8	Frameshift		Infantile acute	French Canadian	324
941A → T	Exon 8	Asp314Val			Ashkenazi Jewish/Irish-English	307
958delGGA	Exon 8	320delGly		Severe subacute	Irish	306
A → G	+3 IVS-8	Abnormal splicing	mRNA lacking exon 8	Severe subacute (second allele Arg178His)	German/Hungarian/Irish	522
987G → A	Exon 9	Trp329Stop		Infantile acute	German/English	306
1003A → T	Exon 9	Ile335Phe		Obligate carrier (four affected pregnancies)	Non-Jewish	308
1039del18	Exon 9	347delDFKQLE		Obligate carrier (affected pregnancy)	Ashkenazi Jewish	308
G → A	+1 IVS-9	Abnormal splicing	Low level of mRNA with cryptic splices in exon 9, IVS-9; no normal mRNA	Infantile acute	diverse; probable Celtic origin	305, 316, 317
DelTCTCC	−12 to −8 IVS-9	Abnormal splicing	Low mRNA, most missing exon 10 (second allele +$TATC_{1278}$)	Infantile acute	Polish	323
G → T	−1 IVS-9	Abnormal splicing		Infantile acute	Irish/French	523

Appendix 153A (Continued)

Mutation	Location	Expected Result	Biochemical Phenotype	Clinical Phenotype*	Origin	References
1164C → G	Exon 11	Ile388Met		Enzyme defined carrier	US French Canadians	516
1168C → T	Exon 11	Gln390Stop		Obligate carrier		307
1171G → A	Exon 11	Val391Met	52% MUG, <3% MUGS Hex A activity = B1 biochemical phenotype (due to Arg178His allele); allele shows high (60% of normal) Hex A activity in carrier father suggestive of mild impact of mutation on enzyme function	Chronic (second allele) Arg178His	Greek	332
1176G → A	Exon 11	Trp392Stop	Trace mRNA on Northern blot	Infantile acute (second mutation 1278insTATC)	Ashkenazi Jewish	524
C_{1177} → T	Exon 11	Arg393Stop	undetectable mRNA	Infantile acute (patient homozygous)	French, Turkish	305, 512
1182delG	Exon 11	Frameshift		Infantile acute	Non-Jewish	308
1204delAAG	Exon 11	delLys402	Unknown	Enzyme defined allele		307
1260G → C	Exon 11	Trp420Cys	In COS transfection, presumptive Hex S is inactive	Infantile acute	German	525
1278insTATC	Exon 11	Frameshift	Absent mRNA in patient cells, normal transcription; stable mRNA with truncated, unprocessed α after expression in COS cells	Infantile acute	major allele in Ashkenazi Jews (75–80% of alleles); diverse	296, 297, 299; screening in 401, 411–414,511
1334delC	Exon 12	Frameshift	Absent Hex A activity	Infantile acute (patient homozygous)	Portuguese	526
1360G → A	Exon 12	Gly454Ser		Infantile acute	Italian	330
1363G → A	Exon 12	Gly455Arg	24% MUG, <2% MUGS Hex A activity = B1 biochemical phenotype due to Arg178His allele; Gly455Arg not evaluated but severity of phenotype and absent MUGS activity suggests major impact on Hex A	Severe subacute (second allele Arg178His)	Portuguese	526
1373G → A	Exon 12	Cys458Tyr	Normal-sized mRNA; expressed allele has no enzyme activity	Infantile acute	Japanese	506
G → C	+1 IVS-12	Abnormal splicing	Trace level of abnormal mRNA with retention of intron 12 or exclusion of exon 12	Infantile acute	Ashkenazi Jewish (15% of alleles), Moroccan Jew	301–303, 315, 527; screening in 401, 411–414, 511
1422G → C	Exon 13	Trp474Cys	Absent α subunit in fibroblasts; pro-α precursor and small amount of mature α synthesized in COS cells when coexpressed with β subunit	Subacute (second allele 1278insTATC)	German-Dutch	340
1444G → A	Exon 13	Glu482Lys	Level of mRNA normal; early defect in processing or retained in ER	Infantile acute (patient homozygous)	Italian, Chinese, Moroccan Jew	114, 309, 310, 511
1451T → C	Exon 13	Leu484Gln		Infantile acute	Japanese	506

(Continued on next page)

Appendix 153A (Continued)

Mutation	Location	Expected Result	Biochemical Phenotype	Clinical Phenotype*	Origin	References
1453T → C	Exon 13	Trp485Arg	COS cell transfection gives no Hex S activity or detectable mature α	Infantile acute	Chinese	310
1495C → T	Exon 13	Arg499Cys		Chronic (second allele Gly269Ser)	Slavic/Irish/ English/ Polish	306
1496G → A	Exon 13	Arg499His	Early processing defect; retained in the ER and degraded	Subacute (second allele is 1278insTATC)	Scottish-Irish	311
1510delC	Exon 13	Frameshift	Apparent normal level of mRNA; truncated α defective in early processing and degraded	Infantile acute (patient homozygous)	Italian	312, 313
C1510 → T	Exon 13	Arg504Cys	In COS transfection fails to form α dimer, no enzyme activity	Infantile acute (patient homozygous)	French, Algerian, German?	305, 314
1511G → A	Exon 13	Arg504 His	α does not associate with β, is phosphorylated, does not reach lysosome but is secreted after NH_4Cl treatment primarily as α monomer; in COS transfection fails to form α dimer	Subacute (patient homozygous)	Assyrian, Lebanese, East European	311, 330, 528
1549insC	Exon 14	Frameshift		Infantile acute	Ecuadorean	307

*Clinical phenotypes as desribed in text:
Infantile acute = Infantile acute encephalopathic phenotype; formerly "infantile onset"
Subacute = Subacute encephalopathic phenotype; formerly "juvenile onset;" note that "late infantile" is more severe form of subacute phenotype
Chronic = Chronic encephalopathic phenotype; formerly "chronic" or "adult onset"

Appendix 153B Mutation in Sandhoff Disease and its Variants

Mutation	Location	Expected Result	Biochemical Phenotype	Clinical Phenotype*	Origin	References
del16 kb	5′ end to IVS-5 (reported as a "del50 kb" in[343,344,529])	absent mRNA	Abnormal Southern blot, mRNA undetectable due to deletion of 16 kb between two Alu sequences	Infantile acute	diverse; ~30% of Sandhoff alleles	342–344, 529
del50kb	5′ end to IVS-6	Absent mRNA	Abnormal Southern blot, mRNA undetectable ikely due to deletion of 50 kb between two L1 sequences (only 3' side characterized)	Infantile acute		345
delA76	Exon 1	Frameshift	Reduced mRNA of normal size	Infantile acute (patient homozygous)	Greek-Cypriot Maronite	530
185C → T	Exon 1	Ser62Leu		Infantile acute (second allele del50kb)		345
G → A	+1 IVS-2	Abnormal splicing	Absent mRNA	Infantile acute (patient homozygous)	Argentinean (30/31 alleles)	434, 438, 439
A_{619} → G	Exon 5	Ile207Val	30% (MUG), 21% (MUGS) Hex A; absent Hex B; β chain only in Hex A; suggested defect in G_{M2} activator association for this allele (see Tyr456Ser)	Subacute (second allele Tyr456Ser)		184, 259

Appendix 153B (Continued)

Mutation	Location	Expected Result	Biochemical Phenotype	Clinical Phenotype*	Origin	References
765C → G	Exon 6	Ser255Arg	Observed in cis with Pro417Leu (see Pro417Leu entry)	Infantile acute, in cis with P417L (patient homozygous)	Japanese	531
772delG	Exon 7	Frameshift	Absent mRNA by Northern (total Hex β mRNA 1.6% of normal, with second allele 1305delAG)	Infantile acute	Caucasian; Indian	532–534
782delCTTT	Exon 7	Frameshift	Absent mRNA	Infantile acute (second allele +1 IVS-2 G → A)	Argentinean	439
850C → T	Exon 7	Arg284Stop	Absent mRNA by Northern blotting (total Hex β mRNA 0.3% with second allele null)	Infantile acute (second allele del16 kb deletion)		534
926G → A (reported at 890)	Exon 8	Cys309Tyr (reported at 297)		Chronic (second allele is Pro417Leu which is likely responsible for chronic phenotype)	Italian	535
+5G → C	IVS-8	Abnormal splicing	MRNA lacks last four nucleotides of exon 8 causing frameshift; confirmed in by expression in CHO cells	Infantile acute	Greek-Cypriot	536
1242G → A (reported as 1206)	Exon 10	Lys414Lys (last nucleotide of exon; amino acid position reported as 402)	Overall 4% β mRNA in fibroblasts comprised of 82% lacking exon 10, 11% normal structure, 7% lacking exon 10+5' insertion flanking exon 11 due to cryptic acceptor site	Infantile acute (patient homozygous)	Italian	537
−17A → G	IVS-10	Abnormal splicing	Absence of normal mRNA; cryptic acceptor splice at −37 of IVS-10	Infantile acute (patient homozygous)	Japanese	531
C_{1250} → T (±362A → G±765C → G); reported as 1214C → T in[535]	Exon 11	Pro417 → Leu (±Lys121Arg ±Ser255Arg); Lys121Arg is benign polymorphism (reported as Pro405Leu in 35059)	MRNA 30% normal structure, 70% with cryptic acceptor in exon 11; mutant Hex B expressed in COS cells shows 70% activity of normal enzyme; when coupled with Ser255Arg in cis, Hex B activity reduced to 30% of normal	Subacute or mild chronic phenotype; infantile phenotype when P417L is in cis with S255R in homozygote	Japanese, French Canadian, Italian	346, 531, 535, 538
delAG1305	Exon 11	Frameshift	Absent mRNA by Northern (total mRNA Hex β 1.6%, with second allele also frameshift)	Infantile acute (second allele ÄG_{772})	Caucasian, Indian	532–534
delT1344	Exon 11	Frameshift	MRNA detectable by Northern blotting; total mRNA is 18% (36% of single gene dose as second allele null)	Infantile acute (second allele is del16 kb deletion)		534
A_{1367} → C	Exon 11	Tyr456 → Ser	30% (MUG) 21% (MUGS) Hex A, absent Hex B; β chains only in Hex A; suggested defect in β·β association for this allele (see Ile207Ser)	Subacute (second alelle Ile207Val)		184, 259

(Continued on next page)

Appendix 153B (Continued)

Mutation	Location	Expected Result	Biochemical Phenotype	Clinical Phenotype*	Origin	References
G → A	−26 IVS-12	8 amino acid insertion before exon 13 due to cryptic slice acceptor	"Hexosaminidase Paris" = (Hex A^+/B^-); early defect in β subunit processing; fails to fold properly; does not associate with α is not phosphorylated; residual Hex A activity likely due to small amount of normal β to give 3–6% Hex A activity in subacute patients to 9–10% Hex A activity in asymptomatic subjects; Hex B activity absent	Subacute or Asymptomatic	French, Japanese, Canadian,	264, 348–350
1510C → T	Exon 13	Pro504Ser	~20% MUG, MUGS activity mainly in pro-enzyme form in fibroblasts; predominant accumulation of pro-β in ER in transfected CHO cells; mutant Hex A shows 1/3 activity toward G_{M2} compared to MUGS	Chronic (second allele del16kb)		185
1514G → A	Exon 13	Arg505Gln	β transfection of COS cells produces thermolabile Hex	Chronic (second allele null)		351
1601G → A (reported at 1565)	Exon 13	Cys534Tyr (reported at 522)		Infantile acute (patient homozygous)	Japanese	539
dupl 18 bp I13E14–16	−16 to +2 IVS-13/ Exon 14	6 amino acid insertion at beginning of exon 14	"Hexosaminidase Paris" = (Hex A^+/B^-); early defect in β subunit processing; fails to fold properly; does not associate with á is not phosphorylated; residual Hex A activity likely due to small amount of normal β	Asymptomatic (second allele null)		349, 350
T → G	+2 IVS-13	Abnormal splicing	8% of normal total Hex activity represented by Hex S; mRNA containing 48 bp insertion at junction between exons 13 and 14 as a result of using cryptic donor splice site due to mutation of natural site (second allele unidentified null)	Infantile acute	Italian	540
1627G → A	Exon 14		Heat labile Hex B		Jews, Arabs	353
1751delTG	Exon 14	Deletion at 7 nc 5' of first polyadenylation site (published sequence[193] contains deletion)	30% reduction in leukocyte total Hex and Hex B due to mutation in 3' UTR, plasma Hex unchanged; reduction in level of mRNA containing the mutation	Benign	Argentinean (10% allele frequency; also frequent in other populations, % unknown)	354

*See Appendix A for explanation of clinical phenotypes

Appendix 153C Mutation in the AB Variant (G_{M2} Activator Deficiency)

Mutation	Location	Expected Result	Biochemical Phenotype	Clinical Phenotype*	Origin	References
262delAAG	Exon	Deletion of Lys88	Normal level of mRNA; premature degradation of protein in ER or Golgi	Infantile acute (patient homozygous)		359
410delA	Exon	Frameshift	Normal level of mRNA; premature degradation of truncated protein in ER or Golgi	Infantile acute (patient homozygous)		359
412T → C	Exon	Cys137Arg	Protein expressed in E. coli shows normal G_{M2} activator binding; absent Hex A binding.	Infantile acute (patient homozygous)		356
506G → C	Exon	Arg169Pro	Transfected BHK cells are negative by Western blot	Infantile acute (patient homozygous)		358

*See Appendix A for explanation of clinical phenotypes

REFERENCES

1. Tay W: Symmetrical changes in the region of the yellow spot in each eye of an infant. *Trans Ophthalmol Soc UK* **1**:155, 1881.
2. Sachs B: On arrested cerebral development with special reference to its cortical pathology. *J Nerv Ment Dis* **14**:541, 1887.
3. Sachs B: A family form of idiocy, generally fatal associated with early blindness. *J Nerv Ment Dis* **21**:475, 1896.
4. Klenk E: Über die Natur der Phosphatide und anderer Lipoide des Gehirns und der Leber bei der Niemann-Pick'schen Krankheit. *Hoppe Seyler's Z Physiol Chem* **235**:24, 1935.
5. Klenk E: Beitrage zur Chemie der Lipidosen. I. Niemann-Pick'schen Krankheit und amaurotische Idiotie. *Hoppe Seyler's Z Physiol Chem* **262**:128, 1939.
6. Klenk E: Über die ganglioside, eine neue Gruppe von zuckerhaltigen Gehirnlipoiden. *Z Physiol Chem* **273**:76, 1942.
7. Svennerholm L: The chemical structure of normal human brain and Tay-Sachs gangliosides. *Biochem Biophys Res Commun* **9**:436, 1962.
8. Makita A, Yamakawa T: The glycolipids of the brain of Tay-Sachs disease. The chemical structure of globoside and main ganglioside. *Jpn J Exp Med* **33**:361, 1963.
9. Robinson D, Stirling J: N-acetyl-beta-glucosaminidases in human spleen. *Biochem J* **107**:321, 1968.
10. Okada S, O'Brien J: Tay-Sachs disease: Generalized absence of a beta-d-*N*-acetylhexosaminidase component. *Science* **165**:698, 1969.
11. Kaback M: Thermal fractionation of serum hexosaminidases: Heterozygote detection and diagnosis of Tay-Sachs disease. *Methods Enzymol* **28**:862, 1972.
11a. Kaplan F: Tay-Sachs disease carrier screening: A model for prevention of genetic disease, in Genetic Testing **2**(4):271, 1998.
12. Sandhoff K, Andreae U, Jatzkewitz H: Deficient hexosaminidase activity in an exceptional case of Tay-Sachs disease with additional storage of kidney globoside in visceral organs. *Pathol Eur* **3**:278, 1968.
13. Sandhoff K, Harzer K, Wassle W, Jatzkewitz H: Enzyme alterations and lipid storage in three variants of Tay-Sachs disease. *J Neurochem* **18**:2469, 1971.
14. Suzuki K, Chen GC: Brain ceramide hexosides in Tay-Sachs disease and generalized gangliosidosis. *J Lipid Res* **8**:105, 1967.
15. Wiegandt H: The gangliosides, in Agranoff B, Aprison M (eds): *Advances in Neurochemistry.* New York, Plenum, 1982, p 149.
16. Svennerholm L: Gangliosides and synaptic transmission, in Svennerholm L, Mandel P, Dreyfus H, Urban P-F (eds): *Structure and Function of Gangliosides*. New York, Plenum, 1980, p 533.
17. Ledee RW, RK, Rappor, MM, Suzuki K: *Ganglioside Structure, Function and Biomedical Potential*. New York, Plenum Publishing, 1984.
18. Kuhn R, Wiegandt H: Die konstitution der gangliotetraose und des gangliosids GI. *Chem Berl* **96**:866, 1963.
19. Svennerholm L: Chromatographic separation of human brain gangliosides. *J Neurochem* **10**:613, 1963.
20. Thompson T, Tillack T: Organization of glycosphingolipids in bilayers and plasma membranes of mammalian cells. *Ann Rev Biophys Chem* **14**:361, 1985.
21. Hakomori S-I: Glycosphingolipids as differentiation-dependent, tumor-associated markers and as regulators of cell proliferation. *Trends Biochem Sci* **9**:453, 1984.
22. Roseman S: Studies on specific intercellular adhesion. *J Biochem* **97**:709, 1985.
23. Varki A, Hooshmand F, Diaz S, Varki N, Hedrick S: Developmental abnormalities in transgenic mice expressing a sialic acid-specific 9-0-acetylesterase. *Cell* **65**:65, 1991.
24. Akawa T, Nagai Y: Glycolipids at the cell surface and their biological functions. *Trends Biochem Sci* **3**:128, 1978.
25. Svennerholm L: Biological significance of gangliosides. *Colloque INSERM/CNRS* **126**:21, 1984.
26. Thompson L, Horowitz P, Bently K, Thomas D, Alderete J, Klebe R: Localization of the ganglioside-binding site of fibronectin. *J Biol Chem* **261**:5209, 1986.
27. Kielczynski W, Bartolomeusz R, Eckardt G, Harrison L: The thyrotropin receptor ganglioside in a rat thyroid cell line (FRTL-5) is a GD1a lactone. *Clycoconjugate J* **8**:164, 1991.
28. Kojima N, Hakomori S: Molecular mechanisms of cell motility 3. Cell adhesion, spreading and motility of GM3-expressing cell based on glycolipid-glycolipid interaction. *J Biol Chem* **266**:17552, 1991.
29. Ando S: Gangliosides in the nervous system. *Neurochem Int* **5**:507, 1983.
30. Kracun I, Rosner H, Cosovic C, Stavljenic A: Topographical atlas of the gangliosides of the adult human brain. *J Neurochem* **43**:979, 1984.
31. Vanier MT, Holm M, Ohman R, Svennerholm L: Developmental profiles of gangliosides in human and rat brain. *J Neurochem* **18**:581, 1971.
32. Suzuki K: The patterns of mammalian brain gangliosides. III regional and developmental differences. *J Neurochem* **12**:969, 1965.
33. Yusuf HK, Merat A, Dickerson JWT: Effect of development of the gangliosides of human brain. *J Neurochem* **28**:1299, 1977.
34. Martinez M, Ballabriga A: A chemical study on the development of the human forebrain and cerebellum during the growth spurt period. I. Gangliosides and plasmalogens. *Brain Res* **159**:351, 1981.
35. Seyfried T, Miyazawa N, Yu R: Cellular localization of gangliosides in the developing mouse cerebellum: analysis using the weaver mutant. *J Neurochem* **41**:491, 1983.
36. Svennerholm L, Bruce A, Mansson J, Raysnark B, Vanier M: Sphingolipids of human skeletal muscle. *Biochim Biophys Acta* **280**:626, 1972.
37. Wiegandt H, Bücking W: Carbohydrate components of extraneural gangliosides from bovine and human spleen, and bovine kidney. *Eur J Biochem* **15**:287, 1970.
38. Chien J, Hogan E: Characterization of two gangliosides of the paragloboside series from chicken skeletal muscle. *Biochim Biophys Acta* **620**:454, 1980.
39. Ghidoni R, Sonnino S, Masserini M, Orlando P, Tettamanti G: Specific tritium labeling of gangliosides at the 3-position of sphingosines. *J Lipid Res* **22**:1286, 1981.
40. Rosner H: Isolation and preliminary characterization of novel polysialogangliosides from embryonic chick brain. *J Neurochem* **37**:993, 1981.

41. Chien J-L, Hogan E: Glycosphingolipids of chicken skeletal muscle, in Yamakawa T, Osawa T, Handa S (eds): *Glycoconjugates*. Tokyo, Japan Scientific Societies Press, 1981, p 74.
42. Breimer M, Hansson G, Karlsson K, Leffler H: Glycosphingolipids of rat tissues. Different composition of epithelial and nonepithelial cells of small intestine. *J Biol Chem* **257**:557, 1982.
43. Chou K, Nolan C, Jungalwala F: Composition and metabolism of gangliosides in rat peripheral nervous system during development. *J Neurochem* **39**:1547, 1982.
44. Ledeen RW: Ganglioside structures and distribution: Are they localized at the nerve ending? *J Supramol Struct* **8**:1, 1978.
45. Hansson HA, Holmgren J, Svennerholm L: Ultrastructural localization of cell membrane GM1 ganglioside by cholera toxin. *Proc Natl Acad Sci U S A* **74**:3782, 1977.
46. Byrne MC, Farooq M, Sbaschnig Agler M, Norton WT, Ledeen RW: Ganglioside content of astroglia and neurons isolated from maturing rat brain: Consideration of the source of astroglial gangliosides. *Brain Res* **461**:87, 1988.
47. Sbaschnig Agler M, Dreyfus H, Norton WT, Sensenbrenner M, Farooq M, Byrne MC, Ledeen RW: Gangliosides of cultured astroglia. *Brain Res* **461**:98, 1988.
48. van Echten G, Sandhoff K: Modulation of ganglioside biosynthesis in primary cultured neurons. *J Neurochem* **52**:207, 1989.
49. Takamiya K, Yamamoto A, Furukawa K, Yamashiro S, Shin M, Okada M, Fukumoto S, et al: Mice with disrupted GM2/GD2 synthase gene lack complex gangliosides but exhibit only subtle defects in their nervous system. *Proc Natl Acad Sci U S A* **93**:10662, 1996.
50. Rahmann H, Rosner H, Breer H: A functional model of sialoglycomacromolecules in synaptic transmission and memory formation. *J Theor Biol* **57**:231, 1976.
51. Hanai N, Nores GA, MacLeod C, Torres Mendez CR, Hakomori S: Ganglioside-mediated modulation of cell growth. Specific effects of GM3 and lyso-GM3 in tyrosine phosphorylation of the epidermal growth factor receptor. *J Biol Chem* **263**:10915, 1988.
52. Ledeen R: Gangliosides of the neuron. *TINS* **8**:169, 1985.
53. Schengrund CL: The role(s) of gangliosides in neural differentiation and repair: A perspective. *Brain Res Bull* **24**:131, 1990.
54. Faron H, Alho H, Bertolino M, Ferret B, Guidotti A, Costa E: Gangliosides prevent glutamate and kainate neurotoxicity in primary neuronal cultures of neonatal rat cerebellum and cortex. *Proc Natl Acad Sci U S A* **85**:7351, 1988.
55. Manev H, Favaron M, Vicini S, Guidotti A, Costa E: Glutamate-induced neuronal death in primary cultures of cerebellar granule cells: Protection by synthetic derivatives of endogenous sphingolipids. *J Pharmacol Exp Ther* **252**:419, 1990.
56. Geisler FH, Dorsey FC, Coleman WP: Recovery of motor function after spinal-cord injury — A randomized, placebo-controlled trial with GM-1 ganglioside. *N Engl J Med* **324**:1829, 1991.
57. Yang LJ, Zeller CB, Shaper NL, Kiso M, Hasegawa A, Shapiro RE, Schnaar RL: Gangliosides are neuronal ligands for myelin-associated glycoprotein. *Proc Natl Acad Sci U S A* **93**:814, 1996.
58. Mandon E, Ehses I, Rother J, van Echten G, Sandhoff K: Subcellular localization and membrane topology of serine palmitoyltransferase, 3-oxo-sphinganine reductase and sphinganine *N*-acyltransferase in mouse liver. *J Biol Chem* **267**:11144, 1992.
59. Hakomori S: Bifunctional role of glycosphingolipids. Modulators for transmembrane signaling and mediators for cellular interactions. *J Biol Chem* **265**:18713, 1990.
60. Schwarzmann G, Sandhoff K: Metabolism and intracellular transport of glycosphingolipids. *Biochemistry* **29**:10865, 1990.
61. Van Echten G, Iber H, Stotz H, Takatsuki A, Sandhoff K: Uncoupling of ganglioside biosynthesis by Brefeldin A. *Eur J Cell Biol* **51**:135, 1990.
62. Trinchera M, Ghidoni R: Two glycosphingolipid sialyltransferases are localized in different sub-Golgi compartments in rat liver. *J Biol Chem* **264**:15766, 1989.
63. Trinchera M, Pirovano B, Ghidoni R: Sub-Golgi distribution in rat liver of CMP-NeuAc GM3- and CMP-NeuAc:GT1b alpha $2 \rightarrow 8$ sialyltransferases and comparison with the distribution of the other glycosyltransferase activities involved in ganglioside biosynthesis. *J Biol Chem* **265**:18242, 1990.
64. Iber H, van Echten G, Sandhoff K: Fractionation of primary cultured neurons: Distribution of sialyltransferases involved in ganglioside biosynthesis. *J Neurochem* **58**:1533, 1992.
65. Sandhoff K, Yusuf H: Glycosphingolipid biosynthesis [Minireview]. *TIGG* **3**:152, 1991.
66. van Echten G, Sandhoff K: Ganglioside Metabolism: Enzymology, topology, and regulation. *J Biol Chem* **268**:5341, 1993.
67. Takahashi K, Ogura Y, Kawarada Y: Pathophysiological changes caused by occlusion of blood flow into the liver during hepatectomy in dogs with obstructive jaundice: Effects of intestinal congestion. *J Gastroenterol Hepatol* **11**:963, 1996.
68. Miller-Prodraza H, Fishman PH: Effect of drugs and temperature on biosynthesis and transport of glycosphingolipids in cultured neurotumor cells. *Biochim Biophys Acta* **804**:44, 1984.
69. Scheel G, Acevedo E, Conzelmann E, Nehrkorn H, Sandhoff K: Model for the interaction of membrane-bound substrates and enzymes. Hydrolysis of ganglioside GD1a by sialidase of neuronal membranes isolated from calf brain. *Eur J Biochem* **127**:245, 1982.
70. Landa C, Maccioni H, Caputto R: The site of synthesis of gangliosides in the chick optic system. *J Neurochem* **33**:825, 1979.
71. Ledeen R, Skrivanek J, Nunez J, Sclafani J, Norton W, Farooq M: Implications of the distribution and transport of gangliosides in the nervous system, in Rappaport M, Gorio A (eds): *Gangliosides in Neurological and Neuromuscular Function*. New York, Raven Press, 1981, p 211.
72. Neufeld E, Lim T, Shapiro L: Inherited disorders of lysosomal metabolism. *Annu Rev Biochem* **44**:357, 1975.
73. Sandhoff K: The biochemistry of sphingolipid storage diseases. *Angew Chem Int Ed* **16**:273, 1977.
74. Neufeld E: Lysosomal storage disorders. *Annu Rev Biochem* **60**:257, 1991.
75. Sandhoff K, Kolter T: Topology of glycosphingolipid degradation. *Trends Cell Biol* **6**:98, 1996.
76. Furst W, Sandhoff K: Activator proteins and topology of lysosomal sphingolipid catabolism. *Biochim Biophys Acta* **1126**:1, 1992.
77. Kolter T, Sandhoff K: Recent advances in the biochemistry of sphingolipidoses. *Brain Pathol* **8**:79, 1998.
78. Meier EM, Schwarzmann G, Fürst W, Sandhoff K: The human GM2 activator protein. A substrate specific cofactor of beta-hexosaminidase A. *J Biol Chem* **26**:1879, 1991.
79. Mandon E, van Echten G, Birk R, Schmidt RR, Sandhoff K: Sphingolipid biosynthesis in cultured neurons — Down-regulation of serine palmitoyltransferase by sphingoid bases. *Eur J Biochem* **198**:667, 1991.
80. Watanabe K: Biochemical studies on carbohydrates. XXII. Animal *β-N*-monoacetylglucosaminidase. *J Biochem (Tokyo)* **24**:297, 1936.
81. Woolen J, Heyworth R, Walker P: Studies on glucosaminidase 3. Testicular *N*-acetyl-*β*-glucosaminidase and *N*-acetyl-*β*-galactosaminidase. *Biochem J* **78**:111, 1961.
82. Walker P, Woollen J, Heyworth R: Studies on glucosaminidase 5. Kidney *N*-acetyl-*β*-glucosaminidase and *N*-acetyl-*β*-galactosaminidase. *Biochem J* **79**:288, 1961.
83. Woollen J, Walker P, Heyworth R: Studies on glucosaminidase 6. *N*-Acetyl-*β*-glucosaminidase and *N*-acetyl-*β*-galactosaminidase activities of a variety of enzyme preparations. *Biochem J* **79**:294, 1961.
84. Weissmann B, Hadjiioannou S, Tornheim J: Oligosaccharase activity of *β-N*-acetyl-D-glucosaminidase of beef liver. *J Biol Chem* **239**:59, 1964.
85. Frohwein YZ, Gatt S: Isolation of *β-N*-acetylglucosaminidase and *β-N*-acetylgalactosaminidase from calf brain. *Biochemistry* **6**:2775, 1967.
86. Sandhoff K, Wassle W: Anreicherung und charakterisierung zweir formen der menschlichen *N*-acetyl-*β*-d-hexosaminidase. *Hoppe Seyler's Z Physiol Chem* **352**:1119, 1971.
87. Robinson D, Jordan TW, Horsburgh T: The *N*-acetyl-*β*-d-hexosaminidase of calf and human brain. *J Neurochem* **19**:1975, 1972.
88. Sellinger OZ, Beaufay H, Jacques P, Doyen A, De Duve C: Tissue fractionation studies. 15. Intracellular distribution and properties of *β-N*-acetylglucosaminidase and *β*-galactosidase in rat liver. *Biochem J* **74**:450, 1960.
89. Conchie J, Hay A: Mammalian glycosidases. 4. The intracellular localization of *β*-galactosidase, *α*-mannosidase, *β-N*-acetylglucosaminidase and *α*-L-fucosidase in mammalian tissues. *Biochem J* **87**:354, 1963.
90. Srivastava S, Beutler E: Hexosaminidase A and hexosaminidase B: Studies in Tay-Sachs disease and Sandhoff's disease. *Nature* **241**:463, 1973.
91. Sandhoff K: Variation of beta-*N*-acetylhexosaminidase pattern in Tay-Sachs disease. *FEBS Lett* **4**:351, 1969.
92. Ikonne JU, Rattazzi MC, Desnick RJ: Characterization of hex-S, the major residual *β*-hexosaminidase activity in type O GM2-gangliosidosis. *Am J Hum Genet* **27**:639, 1975.

93. Beutler E, Kuhl W, Comings D: Hexosaminidase isoenzyme in type 0 GM2 gangliosidosis (Sandhoff-Jatzkewitz disease). *Am J Hum Genet* **27**:628, 1975.
94. Geiger B, Arnon R, Sandhoff K: Immunochemical and biochemical investigation of hexosaminidase S. *Am J Hum Genet* **29**:508, 1977.
95. Lalley PA, Rattazzi MC, Shows TB: Human β-d-*N*-acetylhexosaminidases A and B: Expression and linkage relationships in somatic cell hybrids. *Proc Natl Acad Sci U S A* **71**:1569, 1974.
96. Boedecker HJ, Mellman WJ, Tedesco TA, Croce CM: Assignment of the human gene for hex B to chromosome 5. *Exp Cell Res* **93**:468, 1975.
97. Chern J, Beutler E, Kuhl W, Gilbert F, Mellman WJ, Croce CM: Characterization of heteropolymeric hexosaminidase A in human X mouse hybrid cells. *Proc Natl Acad Sci U S A* **73**:3637, 1976.
98. Mahuran D, Novak A, Lowden JA: The lysosomal hexosaminidase isozymes. *Isozymes Curr Top Biol Med Res* **12**:229, 1985.
99. Mahuran DJ, Lowden JA: The subunit and polypeptide structure of hexosaminidase from human placenta. *Can J Biochem* **58**:287, 1980.
100. Mahuran DJ, Tsui F, Gravel RA, Lowden JA: Evidence for two dissimilar polypeptide chains in the beta 2 subunit of hexosaminidase. *Proc Natl Acad Sci U S A* **79**:1602, 1982.
101. Hasilik A, Neufeld EF: Biosynthesis of lysosomal enzymes in fibroblasts: Synthesis as precursors of higher molecular weight. *J Biol Chem* **255**:4937, 1980.
102. Hasilik A, Neufeld E: Biosynthesis of lysosomal enzymes in fibroblasts: Phosphorylation of mannose residues. *J Biol Chem* **255**:4946, 1980.
103. Conzelmann E, Sandhoff K: Purification and characterization of an activator protein for the degradation of glycolipids GM2 and GA2 by hexosaminidase A. *Physiol Chem* **360**:1837, 1979.
104. Fürst W, Schubert J, Machleidt W, Meyer HE, Sandhoff K: The complete amino-acid sequences of human ganglioside GM2 activator protein and cerebroside sulfate activator protein. *Eur J Biochem* **192**:709, 1990.
105. Burg J, Banerjee A, Sandhoff K: Molecular forms of GM2-activator protein. A study on its biosynthesis in human skin fibroblasts. *Biol Chem Hoppe Seyler* **366**:887, 1985.
106. Nagarajan S, Chen H, Li S, Li Y, Lockyer JM: Evidence for two cDNA clones encoding human GM2-activator protein. *Biochem J* **282**:807, 1992.
107. Wu YY, Sonnino S, Li YT, Li SC: Characterization of an alternatively spliced GM2 activator protein, GM2A protein. An activator protein which stimulates the enzymatic hydrolysis of *N*-acetylneuraminic acid, but not *N*-acetylgalactosamine, from GM2. *J Biol Chem* **271**:10611, 1996.
108. O'Brien J, Kishimoto Y: Saposin proteins: Structure, function and role in human lysosomal storage disorders. *FASEB J* **5**:301, 1991.
109. Conzelmann E, Sandhoff K: AB variant of infantile G_{M2} gangliosidosis: Deficiency of a factor necessary for stimulation of hexosaminidase A-catalyzed degradation of ganglioside G_{M2} and glycolipid G_{A2}. *Proc Natl Acad Sci U S A* **75**:3979, 1978.
110. Gaut JR, Hendershot LM: The modification and assembly of proteins in the endoplasmic reticulum. *Curr Opin Cell Biol* **5**:589, 1993.
111. Rapoport TA, Rolls MM, Jungnickel B: Approaching the mechanism of protein transport across the ER membrane. *Curr Opin Cell Biol* **8**:499, 1996.
112. Suzuki T, Yan Q, Lennarz WJ: Complex, two-way traffic of molecules across the membrane of the endoplasmic reticulum. *J Biol Chem* **273**:10083, 1998.
113. Hammond C, Helenius A: Quality control in the secretory pathway. *Curr Opin Cell Biol* **7**:523, 1995.
114. Proia RL, Neufeld EF: Synthesis of beta-hexosaminidase in cell-free translation and in intact fibroblasts: An insoluble precursor alpha chain in a rare form of Tay-Sachs disease. *Proc Natl Acad Sci U S A* **79**:6360, 1982.
115. Quon DV, Proia RL, Fowler AV, Bleibaum J, Neufeld EF: Proteolytic processing of the beta-subunit of the lysosomal enzyme, beta-hexosaminidase, in normal human fibroblasts. *J Biol Chem* **264**:3380, 1989.
116. Little LE, Lau MM, Quon DV, Fowler AV, Neufeld EF: Proteolytic processing of the alpha-chain of the lysosomal enzyme, beta-hexosaminidase, in normal human fibroblasts. *J Biol Chem* **263**:4288, 1988.
117. Stirling J, Leung A, Gravel RA, Mahuran D: Localization of the pro-sequence within the total deduced primary structure of human beta-hexosaminidase B. *FEBS Lett* **231**:47, 1988.
118. Schutte CG, Lemm T, Glombitza GJ, Sandhoff K: Complete localization of disulfide bonds in GM2 activator protein. *Protein Sci* **7**:1039, 1998.
119. Weitz G, Proia RL: Analysis of the glycosylation and phosphorylation of the alpha- subunit of the lysosomal enzyme, beta-hexosaminidase A, by site-directed mutagenesis. *J Biol Chem* **267**:10039, 1992.
120. O'Dowd BF, Cumming DA, Gravel RA, Mahuran D: Oligosaccharide structure and amino acid sequence of the major glycopeptides of mature human beta-hexosaminidase. *Biochemistry* **27**:5216, 1988.
121. Sonderfeld-Fresko S, Proia RL: Analysis of the glycosylation and phosphorylation of the lysosomal enzyme, beta-hexosaminidase B, by site-directed mutagenesis. *J Biol Chem* **264**:7692, 1989.
122. Klima H, Klein A, van Echten G, Schwarzmann G, Suzuki K, Sandhoff K: Over-expression of a functionally active human GM2-activator protein in *Escherichia coli*. *Biochem J* **292**:571, 1993.
123. Glombitza GJ, Becker E, Kaiser HW, Sandhoff K: Biosynthesis, processing, and intracellular transport of GM2 activator protein in human epidermal keratinocytes. The lysosomal targeting of the GM2 activator is independent of a mannose-6-phosphate signal. *J Biol Chem* **272**:5199, 1997.
124. Sagherian C, Poroszlay S, Vavougios G, Mahuran D: Proteolytic processing of the pro beta chain of beta-hexosaminidase occurs at basic residues contained within an exposed disulfide loop structure. *Biochem Cell Biol* **71**:340, 1993.
125. Sonderfeld-Fresko S, Proia RL: Synthesis and assembly of a catalytically active lysosomal enzyme, beta-hexosaminidase B, in a cell-free system. *J Biol Chem* **263**:13463, 1988.
126. Proia RL, d'Azzo A, Neufeld EF: Association of alpha- and beta-subunits during the biosynthesis of beta-hexosaminidase in cultured human fibroblasts. *J Biol Chem* **259**:3350, 1984.
127. d'Azzo A, Proia RL, Kolodny EH, Kaback MM, Neufeld EF: Faulty association of alpha- and beta-subunits in some forms of beta-hexosaminidase A deficiency. *J Biol Chem* **259**:11070, 1984.
128. Kornfeld S, Mellman I: The biogenesis of lysosomes. *Ann Rev Cell Biol* **5**:483, 1989.
129. von Figura K, Hasilik A: Lysosomal enzymes and their receptors. *Ann Rev Biochem* **55**:167, 1986.
130. Dustin ML, Baranski TJ, Sampath D, Kornfeld S: A novel mutagenesis strategy identifies distantly spaced amino acid sequences that are required for the phosphorylation of both the oligosaccharides of procathepsin D by *N*-acetylglucosamine 1-phosphotransferase. *J Biol Chem* **270**:170, 1995.
131. Yoshida H, Kuriyama M: Genetic lipid storage disease with lysosomal acid lipase deficiency in rats. *Lab Anim Sci* **40**:486, 1990.
132. Baranski TJ, Koelsch G, Hartsuck JA, Kornfeld S: Mapping and molecular modeling of a recognition domain for lysosomal enzyme targeting. *J Biol Chem* **266**:23365, 1991.
133. Baranski TJ, Cantor AB, Kornfeld S: Lysosomal enzyme phosphorylation. I. Protein recognition determinants in both lobes of procathepsin D mediate its interaction with UDP-GlcNAc:lysosomal enzyme *N*-acetylglucosamine-1-phosphotransferase. *J Biol Chem* **267**:23342, 1992.
134. Cuozzo JW, Tao K, Wu QL, Young W, Sahagian GG: Lysine-based structure in the proregion of procathepsin L is the recognition site for mannose phosphorylation. *J Biol Chem* **270**:15611, 1995.
135. Cuozzo JW, Sahagian GG: Lysine is a common determinant for mannose phosphorylation of lysosomal proteins. *J Biol Chem* **269**:14490, 1994.
136. Tikkanen R, Peltola M, Oinonen C, Rouvinen J, Peltonen L: Several cooperating binding sites mediate the interaction of a lysosomal enzyme with phosphotransferase. *EMBO J* **16**:6684, 1997.
137. Glickman JN, Kornfeld S: Mannose 6-phosphate-independent targeting of lysosomal enzymes in I-cell disease B lymphoblasts. *J Cell Biol* **123**:99, 1993.
138. McIntyre GF, Erickson AH: Procathepsins L and D are membrane-bound in acidic microsomal vesicles. *J Biol Chem* **266**:15438, 1991.
139. Tikkanen R, Enomaa N, Riikonen A, Ikonen E, Peltonen L: Intracellular sorting of aspartylglucosaminidase: The role of *N*-linked oligosaccharides and evidence of Man-6-P-independent lysosomal targeting. *DNA Cell Biol* **14**:305, 1995.
140. Cantor AB, Kornfeld S: Phosphorylation of Asn-linked oligosaccharides located a novel sites on the lysosomal enzyme cathepsin D. *J Biol Chem* **267**:23357, 1992.
141. Hasilik A, Neufeld EF: Biosynthesis of lysosomal enzymes in fibroblasts. Phosphorylation of mannose residues. *J Biol Chem* **255**:4946, 1980.

142. Rigat B, Wang W, Leung A, Mahuran DJ: Two mechanisms for the recapture of extracellular GM2 activator protein: Evidence for a major secretory form of the protein. *Biochemistry* **36**:8325, 1997.
143. Hasilik A: The early and late processing of lysosomal enzymes: Proteolysis and compartmentation. *Experientia* **48**:130, 1992.
144. Mahuran DJ, Neote K, Klavins MH, Leung A, Gravel RA: Proteolytic processing of pro-alpha and pro-beta precursors from human beta-hexosaminidase. Generation of the mature alpha and beta a beta b subunits. *J Biol Chem* **263**:4612, 1988.
145. Hubbes M, Callahan J, Gravel R, Mahuran D: The amino-terminal sequences in the pro-alpha and -beta polypeptides of human lysosomal beta-hexosaminidase A and B are retained in the mature isozymes. *FEBS Lett* **249**:316, 1989.
146. Ledeen R, Salsman K: Structure of the Tay-Sachs ganglioside. *Biochemistry* **4**:2225, 1965.
147. Kaback M, Bailin G, Hirsch P, Roy C: Automated thermal fractionation of serum hexosaminidase: Effects of alteration in reaction variables and implications for Tay-Sachs disease heterozygote screening and prevention, in Kaback M, Rimoin D, O'Brien J (eds): *Tay-Sachs Disease: Screening and Prevention*. New York, Alan R. Liss, 1977, p 197.
148. Bayleran J, Hechtman P, Saray W: Synthesis of 4-methylumbelliferyl-beta-D-*N*-acetylglucosamine-6-sulfate and its use in classification of GM2 gangliosidosis genotypes. *Clin Chim Acta* **143**:73, 1984.
149. Kresse H, Fuchs W, Glossl J, Holtfrerich D, Gilberg W: Liberation of *N*-acetylglucosamine-6-sulfate by human beta-*N*-acetylhexosaminidase. *J Biol Chem* **256**:12926, 1981.
150. Ludolph T, Paschke E, Glossl J, Kresse H: Degradation of keratan sulphate by beta-*N*-acetylhexosaminidases A and B. *Biochem J* **193**:811, 1981.
151. Kytzia HJ, Sandhoff K: Evidence for two different active sites on human beta- hexosaminidase A. Interaction of GM2 activator protein with beta-hexosaminidase A. *J Biol Chem* **260**:7568, 1985.
152. Bearpark TM, Stirling JL: A difference in the specificities of human liver *N*-acetyl-beta-hexosaminidases A and B detected by their activities towards glycosaminoglycan oligosaccharides. *Biochem J* **173**:997, 1978.
153. Kytzia HJ, Hinrichs U, Sandhoff K: Diagnosis of infantile and juvenile forms of GM2 gangliosidosis variant 0. Residual activities toward natural and different synthetic substrates. *Hum Genet* **67**:414, 1984.
154. Wenger D, Okada S, O'Brien J: Studies on the substrate specificity of hexosaminidase A and B from liver. *Arch Bioch Biophys* **153**:116, 1972.
155. Tallman J, Brady R, Quirk J, Villalba M, Gal A: Isolation and relationship of human hexosaminidases. *J Biol Chem* **249**:3489, 1974.
156. Wiktorowicz JE, Awasthi YC, Kurosky A, Srivastava SK: Purification and properties of human kidney-cortex hexosaminidases A and B. *Biochem J* **165**:49, 1977.
157. Conzelmann E, Sandhoff K, Nehrkorn H, Geiger B, Arnon R: Purification, biochemical and immunological characterization of hexosaminidase A from variant AB of infantile GM2 gangliosidosis. *Eur J Biochem* **84**:27, 1978.
158. Ließem B: *Dissertation*. Bonn, Universität Bonn, 1996.
159. Sango K, Yamanaka S, Hoffmann A, Okuda Y, Grinberg A, Westphal H, McDonald MP, et al: Mouse models of Tay-Sachs and Sandhoff diseases differ in neurologic phenotype and ganglioside metabolism. *Nat Genet* **11**:170, 1995.
160. Phaneuf D, Wakamatsu N, Huang JQ, Borowski A, Peterson AC, Fortunato SR, Ritter G, et al: Dramatically different phenotypes in mouse models of human Tay-Sachs and Sandhoff diseases. *Hum Mol Genet* **5**:1, 1996.
161. Yuziuki JA, Bertoni C, Beccari T, Orlacchio A, Wu YY, Li SC, Li YT: Specificity of mouse GM2 activator protein and beta-*N*-acetylhexosaminidases A and B. Similarities and differences with their human counterparts in the catabolism of GM2. *J Biol Chem* **273**:66, 1998.
162. Lai EC, Withers SG: Stereochemistry and kinetics of the hydration of 2-acetamido-D-glucal by beta-*N*-acetylhexosaminidases. *Biochemistry* **33**:14743, 1994.
163. Sinnott ML: Catalytic mechanism of enzymic glycosyl transfer. *Chem Rev* **90**:1171, 1990.
164. Tomme P, Claeyssens M: Identification of a functionally important carboxyl group in cell biohydrolase 1 from *Trichoderma reesi*—A chemical modification study. *FEBS Lett* **243**:239, 1989.
165. Knapp S, Vocadlo D, Gao ZN, Kirk B, Lou JP, Withers SG: NAG-thiazoline, an *N*-acetyl-beta-hexosaminidase inhibitor that implicates acetamido participation. *J Am Chem Soc* **118**:6804, 1996.
166. Koshland DE: Stereochemistry and the mechanism of enzymatic reactions. *Biol Rev* **28**:416, 1953.
167. Lowe G, Sheppard G, Sinnott ML, Williams A: Lysozyme-catalysed hydrolysis of some beta-aryl di-*N*-acetylchitobiosides. *Biochem J* **104**:893, 1967.
168. Jones CS, Kosman DJ: Purification, properties, kinetics, and mechanism of beta-*N*-acetylglucosamidase from *Aspergillus niger*. *J Biol Chem* **255**:11861, 1980.
169. Liessem B, Glombitza GJ, Knoll F, Lehmann J, Kellermann J, Lottspeich F, Sandhoff K: Photoaffinity labeling of human lysosomal beta-hexosaminidase B. Identification of Glu-355 at the substrate binding site. *J Biol Chem* **270**:23693, 1995.
170. Pennybacker M, Schuette CG, Liessem B, Hepbildikler ST, Kopetka JA, Ellis MR, Myerowitz R, et al: Evidence for the involvement of Glu-355 in the catalytic action of human beta-hexosaminidase B. *J Biol Chem* **272**:8002, 1997.
171. Tews I, Perrakis A, Oppenheim A, Dauter Z, Wilson KS, Vorgias CE: Bacterial chitobiase structure provides insight into catalytic mechanism and the basis of Tay-Sachs disease. *Nat Struct Biol* **3**:638, 1996.
172. Fernandes MJ, Yew S, Leclerc D, Henrissat B, Vorgias CE, Gravel RA, Hechtman P, et al: Identification of candidate active site residues in lysosomal beta-hexosaminidase A. *J Biol Chem* **272**:814, 1997.
173. Tse R, Vavougios G, Hou Y, Mahuran DJ: Identification of an active acidic residue in the catalytic site of beta-hexosaminidase. *Biochemistry* **35**:7599, 1996.
174. Brown CA, Neote K, Leung A, Gravel RA, Mahuran DJ: Introduction of the alpha subunit mutation associated with the B1 variant of Tay-Sachs disease into the beta subunit produces a beta-hexosaminidase B without catalytic activity. *J Biol Chem* **264**:21705, 1989.
175. Ohno K, Suzuki K: Mutation in GM2-gangliosidosis B1 variant. *J Neurochem* **50**:316, 1988.
176. Brown CA, Mahuran DJ: Active arginine residues in beta-hexosaminidase. Identification through studies of the B1 variant of Tay-Sachs disease. *J Biol Chem* **266**:15855, 1991.
177. Bayleran J, Hechtman P, Kolodny E, Kaback M: Tay-Sachs disease with hexosaminidase A: Characterization of the defective enzyme in two patients. *Am J Hum Genet* **41**:532, 1987.
178. Tse R, Wu YJ, Vavougios G, Hou Y, Hinek A, Mahuran DJ: Identification of functional domains within the α and β subunits of β-hexosaminidase A through the expression of α-β fusion proteins. *Biochemistry* **35**:7599, 1996.
179. Pennybacker M, Liessem B, Moczall H, Tifft CJ, Sandhoff K, Proia RL: Identification of domains in human beta-hexosaminidase that determine substrate specificity. *J Biol Chem* **271**:17377, 1996.
180. Hama Y, Li YT, Li SC: Interaction of GM2 activator protein with glycosphingolipids. *J Biol Chem* **272**:2828, 1997.
181. Smiljanic-Georgijev N, Rigat B, Xie B, Wang W, Mahuran DJ: Characterization of the affinity of the G(M2) activator protein for glycolipids by a fluorescence dequenching assay. *Biochim Biophys Acta* **1339**:192, 1997.
182. Conzelmann E, Burg J, Stephan G, Sandhoff K: Complexing of glycolipids and their transfer between membranes by the activator protein for degradation of lysosomal ganglioside GM2. *Eur J Biochem* **123**:455, 1982.
183. Li SC, Serizawa S, Li YT, Nakamura K, Handa S: Effect of modification of sialic acid on enzymic hydrolysis of gangliosides GM1 and GM2. *J Biol Chem* **259**:5409, 1984.
184. Banerjee P, Siciliano L, Oliveri D, McCabe NR, Boyers MJ, Horwitz AL, Li SC, et al: Molecular basis of an adult form of beta-hexosaminidase B deficiency with motor neuron disease. *Biochem Biophys Res Commun* **181**:108, 1991.
185. Hou Y, McInnes B, Hinek A, Karpati G, Mahuran D: A Pro504 → Ser substitution in the beta-subunit of beta-hexosaminidase A inhibits alpha-subunit hydrolysis of GM2 ganglioside, resulting in chronic Sandhoff disease. *J Biol Chem* **273**:21386, 1998.
186. Myerowitz R, Proia RL: cDNA clone for the alpha-chain of human beta-hexosaminidase: Deficiency of alpha-chain mRNA in Ashkenazi Tay-Sachs fibroblasts. *Proc Natl Acad Sci U S A* **81**:5394, 1984.
187. Myerowitz R, Piekarz R, Neufeld EF, Shows TB, Suzuki K: Human beta-hexosaminidase alpha chain: Coding sequence and homology with the beta chain. *Proc Natl Acad Sci U S A* **82**:7830, 1985.
188. Korneluk RG, Mahuran DJ, Neote K, Klavins MH, O'Dowd BF, Tropak M, Willard HF, et al: Isolation of cDNA clones coding for the alpha-subunit of human beta-hexosaminidase. Extensive homology between the alpha- and beta-subunits and studies on Tay-Sachs disease. *J Biol Chem* **261**:8407, 1986.

189. O'Dowd BF, Quan F, Willard HF, Lamhonwah AM, Korneluk RG, Lowden JA, Gravel RA, et al: Isolation of cDNA clones coding for the beta subunit of human beta-hexosaminidase. *Proc Natl Acad Sci U S A* **82**:1184, 1985.
190. Proia RL: Gene encoding the human beta-hexosaminidase beta chain: Extensive homology of intron placement in the alpha- and beta-chain genes. *Proc Natl Acad Sci U S A* **85**:1883, 1988.
191. Proia RL, Soravia E: Organization of the gene encoding the human beta-hexosaminidase alpha-chain. *J Biol Chem* **262**:5677, 1987.
192. Takeda K, Nakai H, Hagiwara H, Tada K, Shows TB, Byers MG, Myerowitz R: Fine assignment of beta-hexosaminidase A alpha-subunit on 15q23-q24 by high resolution in situ hybridization. *Tohoku J Exp Med* **160**:203, 1990.
193. Neote K, Bapat B, Dumbrille Ross A, Troxel C, Schuster SM, Mahuran DJ, Gravel RA: Characterization of the human HEXB gene encoding lysosomal beta- hexosaminidase. *Genomics* **3**:279, 1988.
194. Fox MF, DuToit DL, Warnich L, Retief AE: Regional localization of alpha-galactosidase (GLA) to Xpter → q22, hexosaminidase B (HEXB) to 5q13 → qter, and arylsulfatase B (ARSB) to 5pter → q13. *Cytogenet Cell Genet* **38**:45, 1984.
195. Norflus F, Yamanaka S, Proia RL: Promoters for the human beta-hexosaminidase genes, HEXA and HEXB. *DNA Cell Biol* **15**:89, 1996.
196. Yamanaka S, Johnson ON, Norflus F, Boles DJ, Proia RL: Structure and expression of the mouse beta-hexosaminidase genes, Hexa and Hexb. *Genomics* **21**:588, 1994.
197. Wakamatsu N, Benoit G, Lamhonwah AM, Zhang ZX, Trasler JM, Triggs-Raine BL, Gravel RA: Structural organization, sequence, and expression of the mouse HEXA gene encoding the alpha subunit of hexosaminidase A. *Genomics* **24**:110, 1994.
198. Triggs-Raine BL, Benoit G, Salo TJ, Trasler JM, Gravel RA: Characterization of the murine beta-hexosaminidase (HEXB) gene. *Biochim Biophys Acta* **1227**:79, 1994.
199. Schroder M, Klima H, Nakano T, Kwon H, Quintern LE, Gartner S, Suzuki K, et al: Isolation of a cDNA encoding the human GM2 activator protein. *FEBS Lett* **251**:197, 1989.
200. Klima H, Tanaka A, Schnabel D, Nakano T, Schroder M, Suzuki K, Sandhoff K: Characterization of full-length cDNAs and the gene coding for the human GM2 activator protein. *FEBS Lett* **289**:260, 1991.
201. Xie B, McInnes B, Neote K, Lamhonwah AM, Mahuran D: Isolation and expression of a full-length cDNA encoding the human GM2 activator protein. *Biochem Biophys Res Commun* **177**:1217, 1991.
202. Burg J, Conzelmann E, Sandhoff K, Solomon E, Swallow DM: Mapping of the gene coding for the human GM2 activator protein to chromosome 5. *Ann Hum Genet* **49**:41, 1985.
203. Heng HHQ, Xie B, Shi X-M, Tsui L-C, Mahuran DJ: Refined mapping of the GM2 activator protein (GM2A) locus to 5q31.3-33.1, distal to the spinal muscular atrophy locus. *Genomics* **18**:429, 1993.
204. Xei B, Kennedy J, McInnes B, Auger D, Mahuran D: Identification of a processed pseudogene related to the functional gene encoding the GM2 activator protein: Localization of the pseudogene to human chromosome 3 and the functional gene to human chromosome 5. *Genomics* **14**:796, 1992.
205. Yamanaka S, Johnson ON, Lyu MS, Kozak CA, Proia RL: The mouse gene encoding the GM2 activator protein (Gm2a): cDNA sequence, expression, and chromosome mapping. *Genomics* **24**:601, 1994.
206. Bertoni C, Appolloni MG, Stirling JL, Li SC, Li YT, Orlacchio A, Beccari T: Structural organization and expression of the gene for the mouse GM2 activator protein. *Mamm Genome* **8**:90, 1997.
207. Gravel RA, Clarke JTR, Kaback MM, Mahuran D, Sandhoff K, Suzuki K: The GM2 gangliosidoses, in Scriver CR, Beaudet AL, Sly WS, Valle D (eds): *The Metabolic and Molecular Bases of Inherited Disease*. New York, McGraw-Hill, 1995, p 2839.
208. Rapin I, Suzuki K, Suzuki K, Valsamis MP: Adult (chronic) GM2-gangliosidosis. Atypical spinocerebellar degeneration in a Jewish sibship. *Arch Neurol* **33**:120, 1976.
209. Bartholomew W, Rattazzi M: Immunochemical characterization of human β-D-*N*-acetylhexosaminidase from normal individuals and patients with Tay-Sachs disease. *Int Arch Allergy Appl Immunol* **46**:512, 1974.
210. Carroll M, Robinson D: Immunological properties of *N*-acetyl-β-D-glucosaminidase of normal human liver and of GM2 gangliosidosis liver. *Biochem J* **131**:91, 1973.
211. Geiger B, Navon R, Ben-Yoseph Y, Arnon R: Specific determination of *N*-acetyl-β-D-hexoaminidase isoenzymes A and B by radio-immunoassay and radial immunodiffusion. *J Biochem* **56**:311, 1975.
212. Srivastava S, Beutler E: Studies on human β-D-*N*-acetylhexosaminidases III. Biochemical genetics of Tay-Sachs and Sandhoff's diseases. *J Bio Chem* **249**:2054, 1974.
213. Kytzia H-J, Sandhoff K: Evidence for two different active sites on human beta- hexosaminidase A. Interaction of GM2 activator protein with beta-hexosaminidase A. *J Biol Chem* **260**:7568, 1985.
214. Kytzia HJ, Hinrichs U, Maire I, Suzuki K, Sandhoff K: Variant of GM2-gangliosidosis with hexosaminidase A having a severely changed substrate specificity. *EMBO J* **2**:1201, 1983.
215. Li YT, Hirabayashi Y, Li SC: Differentiation of two variants of type-AB GM2-gangliosidosis using chromogenic substrates. *Am J Hum Genet* **35**:520, 1983.
216. Goldman JE, Yamanaka T, Rapin I, Adachi M, Suzuki K: The AB-variant of GM2-gangliosidosis. Clinical, biochemical, and pathological studies of two patients. *Acta Neuropathol (Berl)* **52**:189, 1980.
217. Li S-C, Hirabayashi Y, Li Y-T: A protein activator for the enzymic hydrolysis of GM2 ganglioside. *J Biol Chem* **256**:6234, 1981.
218. Sonderfeld S, Brendler S, Sandhoff K, Galjaard H, Hoogeveen AT: Genetic complementation in somatic cell hybrids of four variants of infantile GM2 gangliosidosis. *Hum Genet* **71**:196, 1985.
219. Sango K, Mcdonald MP, Crawley JN, Mack ML, Tifft CJ, Skop E, Starr CM, et al: Mice lacking both subunits of lysosomal beta-hexosaminidase display gangliosidosis and mucopolysaccharidosis. *Nat Genet* **14**:348, 1996.
220. Sandhoff K: Variation of β-hexosaminidase pattern in Tay-Sach disease. *FEBS Lett* **4**:351, 1969.
221. Suzuki Y, Jacob K, Suzuki K, Kutty KM, Suzuki K: GM2-gangliosidosis with total hexosaminidase deficiency. *Neurology* **21**:313, 1971.
222. Strecker G, Herlant-Peers M-C, Fournet B, Montreuil J: Structure of seven oligosaccharides excreted in the urine of a patient with Sandhoff's Disease (GM2 gangliosidosis-Variant 0). *Europ J Biochem* **81**:165, 1977.
223. Conzelmann E, Sandhoff K: AB variant of infantile GM2 gangliosidosis: Deficiency of a factor necessary for stimulation of hexosaminidase A-catalyzed degradation of ganglioside GM2 and glycolipid GA2. *Proc Natl Acad Sci U S A* **75**:3979, 1978.
224. Conzelmann E, Sandhoff K, Nehrkorn H, Geiger B, Arnon R: Purification, biochemical and immunological characterisation of hexosaminidase A from variant AB of infantile GM2 gangliosidosis. *Eur J Biochem* **84**:27, 1978.
225. de Baecque CM, Suzuki K, Rapin I, Johnson AB, Wethers DL, Suzuki K: GM2-gangliosidosis, AB variant. Clinicopathological study of a case. *Acta Neuropathol* **33**:207, 1975.
226. O'Neil B, Butler AB, Young E, Falk PM, Bass NH: Adult-onset GM2 gangliosidosis. Seizures, dementia, and normal pressure hydrocephalus associated with glycolipid storage in the brain and arachnoid granulation. *Neurology* **28**:1117, 1978.
227. Johnson WG: The clinical spectrum of hexosaminidase deficiency disease. *Neurology* **31**:1453, 1981.
228. Kolodny E, Raghavan S: GM2-gangliosidosis. Hexosaminidase mutations not of the Tay-Sachs type produce unusual clinical variants. *Trends Neurosci* **6**:16, 1983.
229. Navon R: Molecular and clinical heterogeneity of adult GM2 gangliosidosis. *Dev Neurosci* **13**:295, 1991.
230. Navon R, Argov Z, Frisch A: Hexosaminidase A deficiency in adults. *Am J Med Genet* **24**:179, 1986.
231. Federico A, Palmeri S, Malandrini A, Fabrizi G, Mondelli M, Guazzi GC: The clinical aspects of adult hexosaminidase deficiencies. *Develop Neurosci* **13**:280, 1991.
232. Navon R, Argov Z, Brand N, Sandbank U: Adult GM2 gangliosidosis in association with Tay-Sachs disease: A new phenotype. *Neurol* **31**:1397, 1981.
233. Pampiglione G, Privett G, Harden A: Tay-Sachs disease: Neurophysiological studies in 20 children. *Develop Med Child Neurol* **16**:201, 1974.
234. Fukumizu M, Yoshikawa H, Takashima S, Sakuragawa N, Kurokawa T: Tay-Sachs disease: Progression of changes on neuroimaging in four cases. *Neuroradiology* **34**:483, 1992.
235. Brett EM, Ellis RB, Haas L, Ikonne JU, Lake BD, Patrick AD, Stephen R: Late onset GM2 gangliosidosis: Clinical, pathological and biochemical studies in eight patients. *Arch Dis Child* **48**:775, 1973.
236. MacLeod PM, Wood S, Jan JE, Applegarth DA, Doman CL: Progressive cerebellar ataxia, spasticity, psychomotor retardation, and hexosaminidase deficiency in a 10-year old child: Juvenile Sandhoff disease. *Neurology* **27**:571, 1977.

237. Menkes JH, O'Brien JS, Okada S, Grippo J, Andrews JM, Cancilla PA: Juvenile GM2 gangliosidosis: Biochemical and ultrastructural studies on a new variant of Tay-Sachs disease. *Arch Neurol* **25**:14, 1971.
238. Suzuki K, Rapin I, Suzuki Y, Ishii N: Juvenile GM2-gangliosidosis: Clinical variant of Tay-Sachs disease or a new disease. *Neurology* **20**:190, 1970.
239. Harmon DL, Gardner-Medwin D, Stirling JL: Two new mutations in a late infantile Tay-Sachs patient are both in exon 1 of the β-hexosaminidase α subunit gene. *J Med Genet* **30**:123, 1993.
240. Suzuki K, Vanier MT: Biochemical and molecular aspects of late-onset GM2- gangliosidosis: B1 variant as a prototype. *Dev Neurosci* **13**:288, 1991.
241. Dos Santos MR, Tanaka A, Sa Miranda MC, Ribeiro MG, Maia M, Suzuki K: GM2-gangliosidosis B1 variant: analysis of beta-hexosaminidase alpha gene mutations in 11 patients from a defined region in Portugal. *Am J Hum Genet* **49**:886, 1991.
242. Ribeiro MG, Pinto RA, Dos Santos MR, Maia M, Sá Miranda MC: Biochemical characterization of β-hexosaminidase in different biological specimens from eleven patients with GM2-gangliosidosis B1 variant. *J Inherit Metab Dis* **14**:715, 1991.
243. Maia M, Alves D, Ribeiro G, Pinto R, Sá Miranda MC: Juvenile GM2 gangliosidosis variant B1: Clinical and biochemical study in seven patients. *Neuropediatrics* **21**:18, 1990.
244. Navon R, Argov AZ, Brand N, Sandbank U: Adult GM2 gangliosidosis in association with Tay-Sachs disease: A new phenotype. *Neurology* **31**:1397, 1981.
245. Yaffe M, Kaback M, Goldberg M, Miles G, Itabashi H, McIntyre H, Mohandas T: An amyotrophic lateral sclerosis-like syndrome with hexosaminidase A deficiency: A new type of GM2 gangliosidosis. *Neurology* **29**:611, 1979.
246. Meek D, Wolfe LS, Andermann E, Andermann F: Juvenile progressive dystonia: A new phenotype of GM2 gangliosidosis. *Ann Neurol* **15**:348, 1984.
247. Nardocci N, Bertagnolio B, Rumi V, Angelini L: Progressive dystonia symptomatic of juvenile GM2-gangliosidosis. *Mov Disorders* **7**:64, 1992.
248. Oates CE, Bosch EP, Hart MN: Movement disorders associated with chronic GM2 gangliosidosis. Case report and review of the literature. *Eur Neurol* **25**:154, 1986.
249. Johnson WG, Chutorian A, Miranda A: A new juvenile hexosaminidase deficiency disease presenting as cerebellar ataxia. Clinical and biochemical studies. *Neurology* **27**:1012, 1977.
250. Willner JP, Grabowski GA, Gordon RE, Bender AN, Desnick RJ: Chronic GM2 gangliosidosis masquerading as atypical Friedreich ataxia: Clinical, morphologic and biochemical studies of nine cases. *Neurology* **31**:787, 1981.
251. Oonk JGW, van der Helm HJ, and Martin JJ: Spinocerebellar degeneration: Hexosaminidase A and B deficiency in two adult sisters. *Neurology* **29**:380, 1979.
252. Hund E, Grau A, Fogel W, Forsting M, Cantz M, Kustermann-Kuhn B, Harzer, et al: Progressive cerebellar ataxia, proximal neurogenic weakness and ocular motor disturbances: Hexosaminidase A deficiency with late clinical onset in four siblings. *J Neurol Sci* **145**:25, 1997.
253. Schnorf H, Bosshard NU, Gitzelmann R, Spycher MA, Isler P, Waespe W: Adult form of G_{M2} gangliosidosis: Three siblings with hexosaminidase A and B deficiency (Sandhoff disease) and review of the literature. *Schweiz Med Wochenschr* **126**:757, 1996.
254. Schnorf H, Gitzelmann R, Bosshard NU, Spycher M, Waespe W: Early and severe sensory loss in three adult siblings with hexosaminidase A and B deficiency (Sandhoff disease). *J Neurol Neurosurg Psychiatry* **59**:520, 1995.
255. Johnson WG, Wigger HJ, Karp HR, Glaubiger LM, Rowland LP: Juvenile spinal muscular atrophy: A new hexosaminidase deficiency phenotype. *Ann Neurol* **11**:11, 1982.
256. Parnes S, Karpati G, Carpenter S, Ng Ying Kin NMJ, Wolfe LS, Suranyi L: Hexosaminidase A deficiency presenting as atypical juvenile onset muscular dystrophy. *Arch Neurol* **42**:1176, 1985.
257. Karni A, Navon R, Sadeh M: Hexosaminidase A deficiency manifesting as spinal muscular atrophy of late onset. *Ann Neurol* **24**:451, 1988.
258. Mitsumoto H, Sliman RJ, Schafer IA, Sternick CS, Kaufman B, Wilbourn A, Horwitz SJ: Motor neuron disease and adult hexosaminidase A deficiency in two families: Evidence for multisystem degeneration. *Ann Neurol* **17**:378, 1985.
259. Cashman NR, Antel JP, Hancock LW, Dawson G, Horowitz AL, Johnson WG, Huttenlocher PR, et al: *N*-Acetyl-β-hexosaminidase β locus defect and juvenile motor neuron disease. A case study. *Ann Neurol* **19**:568, 1986.
260. Oyanagi K, Ohama E, Miyashita K, Yoshino H, Miyatake T, Yamazaki M, Ikuta F: Galactosialidosis: Neuropathological findings in a case of the late infantile type. *Acta Neuropathol (Berl)* **82**:331, 1991.
261. Mondelli M, Rossi A, Palmeri S, Rizzuto N, Federico A: A neurophysiological study in chronic GM2 gangliosidosis (hexosaminidase A and B deficiency), with motor neuron disease phenotype. *Ital J Neurol Sci* **10**:433, 1989.
262. Argov Z, Navon R: Clinical and genetic variations in the syndrome of adult GM2 gangliosidosis resulting from hexosaminidase A deficiency. *Ann Neurol* **16**:14, 1984.
263. Federico A, Ciacci G, D'Amore I, Pallini R, Palmeri S, Rossi A, Rizzuto N, et al: GM2 gangliosidosis with hexosaminidase A and B defect: Report of a family with motor neuron disease-like phenotype. *J Inherit Metab Dis* **9**:307, 1986.
264. Mitsuo K, Nakano T, Kobayashi T, Goto I, Taniike M, Suzuki K: Juvenile Sandhoff disease: A Japanese patient carrying a mutation identical to that found earlier in a Canadian patient. *J Neurol Sci* **98**:277, 1990.
265. Streifler JY, Gornish M, Hadar H, Gadoth N: Brain imaging in late-onset GM2 gangliosidosis. *Neurology* **43**:2055, 1993.
266. Lichtenberg P, Navon R, Wertman E, Dasberg H, Lerer B: Post-partum psychosis in adult GM2-gangliosidosis: A case report. *Brit J Psychiat* **153**:387, 1988.
267. Streifler J, Golomb M, Gadoth N: Psychiatric Features of Adult GM2-Gangliosidosis. *Br J Psychiatry* **155**:410, 1989.
268. Albouz S, Le Saux F, Wenger D, Hauw JJ, Baumann N: Modifications of sphingomyelin and phosphatidylcholine metabolism by tricyclic antidepressants and phenothiazine. *Life Sci* **38**:357, 1986.
269. Navon R Baram D: Depletion of cellular beta-hexosaminidase by imipramine is prevented by dexamethasone: Implications for treating psychotic hexosaminidase A deficient patients. *Biochem Biophys Res Commun* **148**:1098, 1987.
270. Palmeri S, Mangano L, Battisti C, Malandrini A, Federico A: Imipramine induced lipidosis and dexamethasone effect: Morphological and biochemical study in normal and chronic GM2 gangliosidosis fibroblasts. *J Neurol Sci* **110**:215, 1992.
271. Renshaw PF, Stern TA, Welch C, Schouten R, Kolodny EH: Electroconvulsive therapy treatment of depression in a patient with adult GM2-gangliosidosis. *Ann Neurol* **31**:342, 1992.
272. Harding AE, Young EP, Schon F: Adult onset supranuclear ophthalmoplegia, cerebellar ataxia, and neurogenic proximal muscle weakness in a brother and sister: Another hexosaminidase A deficiency syndrome. *J Neurol Neurosurg Psychiat* **50**:687, 1987.
273. Sandhoff K, Conzelmann E, Neufeld EF, Kaback MM, Suzuki K: The G_{M2} gangliosidoses, in Scriver CR, Beaudet AL, Sly WS, Valle D (eds): *The Metabolic Basis of Inherited Disease*. New York, McGraw-Hill, 1989, p 1807.
274. Volk B, Schneck L, Adachi M: Clinic, pathology and biochemistry of Tay-Sachs disease, in Vinken P, Bruyn G (eds): *Textbook of Neurology*. Amsterdam, North-Holland Publishing, 1970, p 385.
275. Terry RD, Korey: Membranous cytoplasmic granules in infantile amaurotic idiocy. *Nature* 100, 1960.
276. Terry R, Weiss M: Studies on Tay-Sachs disease: II. Ultrastructure of the cerebrum. *J Neuropathol Exp Neurol* **22**:18, 1963.
277. Purpura DP, Suzuki K: Distortion of neuronal geometry and formation of aberrant synapses in neuronal storage disease. *Brain Res* **116**:1, 1976.
278. Walkley SU: Pyramidal neurons with ectopic dendrites in storage diseases exhibit increased GM2 ganglioside immunoreactivity. *Neuroscience* **68**:1027, 1995.
279. Huang JQ, Trasler JM, Igdoura S, Michaud J, Hanal N, Gravel RA: Apoptotic cell death in mouse models of GM2 gangliosidosis and observations on human Tay-Sachs and Sandhoff diseases. *Hum Mol Genet* **6**:1879, 1997.
280. Suzuki K: Neuropathology of late onset gangliosidoses. A review. *Dev Neurosci* **13**:205, 1991.
281. Navon R, Sandbank U, Frisch A, Baram D, Adam A: Adult-onset GM2 gangliosidosis diagnosed in a fetus. *Prenat Diagn* **6**:169, 1986.
282. Adachi M, Schneck L, Volk BW: Ultrastructural studies of eight cases of fetal Tay-Sachs disease. *Lab Invest* **30**:102, 1974.
283. Goebel HH, Stolte G, Kustermann Kuhn B, Harzer K: B1 variant of GM2 gangliosidosis in a 12-year-old patient. *Pediatr Res* **25**:89, 1989.

284. Benninger C, Ullrich-BotT B, Zhan SS, Schmitt HP: GM2D gangliosidosis B1 variant in a boy of German/Hungarian descent. *Clin Neuropath* **12**:196, 1993.
285. Dolman CL, Chang E, Duke RJ: Pathologic findings in Sandhoff disease. *Arch Pathol* **96**:272, 1973.
286. Hadfield MG, Mamunes P, David RB: The pathology of Sandhoff's disease. *J Path* **123**:137, 1977.
287. Suzuki K: Neuronal storage disease: A review, in Zimmerman HM (ed): *Progress in Neuropathology*. New York, Grune & Stratton, 1976, p 173.
288. Rubin M, Karpati G, Wolfe LS, Carpenter S, Klavins MH, Mahuran DJ: Adult onset motor neuronopathy in the juvenile type of hexosaminidase A and B deficiency. *J Neurol Sci* **87**:103, 1988.
289. Hoffman LM, Amsterdam D, Brooks SE, Schneck L: Glycosphingolipids in fetal Tay-Sachs disease brain and lung cultures. *J Neurochem* **29**:551, 1977.
290. Conzelmann E, Nehrkorn H, Kytzia HJ, Sandhoff K, Macek M, Lehovsky M, Elleder M, et al: Prenatal diagnosis of GM2 gangliosidosis with high residual hexosaminidase A activity (variant B1; pseudo AB variant). *Pediatr Res* **19**:1220, 1985.
291. Jatzkewitz H, Pilz H, Sandhoff K: The quantitative determination of gangliosides and their derivatives in different forms of amaurotic idiocy. *J Neurochem* **12**:135, 1965.
292. Escola J: Uber die Prozebausbreitung der amaurotischen idiotie im zentralnervensystem in verschiedenen lebensaltern und besonderheiten der spatform gegenuber der pigmentatrophie. *Arch Psychiat Nervenkr* **202**:95, 1961.
293. Warner TG, Turner MW, Toone JR, Applegarth D: Prenatal diagnosis of infantile GM2 gangliosidosis type II (Sandhoff disease) by detection of *N*-acetylglucosaminyl-oligosaccharides in amniotic fluid with high-performance liquid chromatography. *Prenat Diagn* **6**:393, 1986.
294. Myerowitz R, Hogikyan ND: Different mutations in Ashkenazi Jewish and non-Jewish French Canadians with Tay-Sachs disease. *Science* **232**:1646, 1986.
295. Myerowitz R, Hogikyan ND: A deletion involving Alu sequences in the beta-hexosaminidase alpha-chain gene of French Canadians with Tay-Sachs disease. *J Biol Chem* **262**:15396, 1987.
296. Myerowitz R, Costigan FC: The major defect in Ashkenazi Jews with Tay-Sachs disease is an insertion in the gene for the alpha-chain of beta-hexosaminidase. *J Biol Chem* **263**:18587, 1988.
297. Paw BH, Neufeld EF: Normal transcription of the beta-hexosaminidase alpha-chain gene in the Ashkenazi Tay-Sachs mutation. *J Biol Chem* **263**:3012, 1988.
298. Mashima Y, Murakami A, Weleber RG, Kennaway NG, Clarke L, Shiono T, Inana G: Nonsense-codon mutations of the ornithine aminotransferase gene with decreased levels of mutant mRNA in gyrate atrophy. *Am J Hum Genet* **51**:81, 1992.
299. Nishimoto J, Tanaka A, Nanba E, Suzuki K: Expression of the beta-hexosaminidase alpha subunit gene with the four-base insertion of infantile Jewish Tay-Sachs disease. *J Biol Chem* **266**:14306, 1991.
300. Boles DJ, Proia RL: The molecular basis of HEXA mRNA deficiency caused by the most common Tay-Sachs disease mutation. *Am J Hum Genet* **56**:716, 1995.
301. Arpaia E, Dumbrille Ross A, Maler T, Neote K, Tropak M, Troxel C, Stirling JL, et al: Identification of an altered splice site in Ashkenazi Tay-Sachs disease. *Nature* **333**:85, 1988.
302. Myerowitz R: Splice junction mutation in some Ashkenazi Jews with Tay-Sachs disease: Evidence against a single defect within this ethnic group. *Proc Natl Acad Sci U S A* **85**:3955, 1988.
303. Ohno K, Suzuki K: A splicing defect due to an exon-intron junctional mutation results in abnormal beta-hexosaminidase alpha chain mRNAs in Ashkenazi Jewish patients with Tay-Sachs disease. *Biochem Biophys Res Commun* **153**:463, 1988.
304. Navon R, Proia RL: Tay-Sachs disease in Moroccan Jews: Deletion of a phenylalanine in the alpha-subunit of beta-hexosaminidase. *Am J Hum Genet* **48**:412, 1991.
305. Akli S, Chelly J, Lacorte JM, Poenaru L, Kahn A: Seven novel Tay-Sachs mutations detected by chemical mismatch cleavage of PCR-amplified cDNA fragments. *Genomics* **11**:124, 1991.
306. Mules EH, Hayflick S, Miller CS, Reynolds LW, Thomas GH: Six novel deleterious and three neutral mutations in the gene encoding the alpha-subunit of hexosaminidase A in non-Jewish individuals. *Am J Hum Genet* **50**:834, 1992.
307. Akerman BR, Natowicz MR, Kaback MM, Loyer M, Campeau E, Gravel RA: Novel mutations and DNA-based screening in non-Jewish carriers of Tay-Sachs disease. *Am J Hum Genet* **60**:1099, 1997.
308. Tomczak J, Grebner EE: Three novel beta-hexosaminidase A mutations in obligate carriers of Tay-Sachs disease. *Hum Mutat* **4**:71, 1994.
309. Nakano T, Muscillo M, Ohno K, Hoffman AJ, Suzuki K: A point mutation in the coding sequence of the beta- hexosaminidase alpha gene results in defective processing of the enzyme protein in an unusual GM2-gangliosidosis variant. *J Neurochem* **51**:984, 1988.
310. Akalin N, Shi H-P, Vavougios G, Hechtman P, Lo W, Scriver CR, Mahuran D, et al: Novel Tay-Sachs disease mutations from China. *Hum Mutat* **1**:40, 1992.
311. Paw BH, Moskowitz SM, Uhrhammer N, Wright N, Kaback MM, Neufeld EF: Juvenile GM2 gangliosidosis caused by substitution of histidine for arginine at position 499 or 504 of the alpha-subunit of beta- hexosaminidase. *J Biol Chem* **265**:9452, 1990.
312. Zokaeem G, Bayleran J, Kaplan P, Hechtman P, Neufeld EF: A shortened beta-hexosaminidase alpha-chain in an Italian patient with infantile Tay-Sachs disease. *Am J Hum Genet* **40**:537, 1987.
313. Lau MM, Neufeld EF: A frameshift mutation in a patient with Tay-Sachs disease causes premature termination and defective intracellular transport of the alpha-subunit of beta-hexosaminidase. *J Biol Chem* **264**:21376, 1989.
314. Paw BH, Wood LC, Neufeld EF: A third mutation at the CpG dinucleotide of codon 504 and a silent mutation at codon 506 of the HEX A gene. *Am J Hum Genet* **48**:1139, 1991.
315. Ohno K, Suzuki K: Multiple abnormal beta-hexosaminidase alpha chain mRNAs in a compound-heterozygous Ashkenazi Jewish patient with Tay-Sachs disease. *J Biol Chem* **263**:18563, 1988.
316. Akerman BR, Zielenski J, Triggs Raine BL, Prence EM, Natowicz M, Lim-Steele JST, Kaback MM, et al: A mutation common in non-Jewish Tay-Sachs disease: Frequency and RNA studies. *Hum Mutat* **1**:303, 1992.
317. Landels EC, Green PM, Ellis IH, Fensom AH, Bobrow M: Beta-hexosaminidase splice site mutation has a high frequency among non-Jewish Tay-Sachs disease carriers from the British Isles. *J Med Genet* **29**:563, 1992.
318. Fernandes MJ, Hechtman P, Boulay B, Kaplan F: A chronic GM2 gangliosidosis variant with a HEXA splicing defect: Quantitation of HEXA mRNAs in normal and mutant fibroblasts. *Eur J Hum Genet* **5**:129, 1997.
319. Akli S, Chelly J, Mezard C, Gandy S, Kahn A, Poenaru L: A "G" to "A" mutation at position -1 of a $5'$ splice site in a late infantile form of Tay-Sachs disease. *J Biol Chem* **265**:7324, 1990.
320. Trop I, Kaplan F, Brown C, Mahuran D, Hechtman P: A glycine250 $\rightarrow$ aspartate substitution in the alpha-subunit of hexosaminidase A causes juvenile-onset Tay-Sachs disease in a Lebanese-Canadian family. *Hum Mutat* **1**:35, 1992.
321. Tanaka A, Ohno K, Sandhoff K, Maire I, Kolodny EH, Brown A, Suzuki K: GM2-gangliosidosis B1 variant: Analysis of beta-hexosaminidase alpha gene abnormalities in seven patients. *Am J Hum Genet* **46**:329, 1990.
322. Tanaka A, Ohno K, Suzuki K: GM2-gangliosidosis B1 variant: A wide geographic and ethnic distribution of the specific beta-hexosaminidase alpha chain mutation originally identified in a Puerto Rican patient. *Biochem Biophys Res Commun* **156**:1015, 1988.
323. Triggs Raine BL, Akerman BR, Clarke JT, Gravel RA: Sequence of DNA flanking the exons of the HEXA gene, and identification of mutations in Tay-Sachs disease. *Am J Hum Genet* **49**:1041, 1991.
324. Fernandes M, Kaplan F, Natowicz M, Prence E, Kolodny E, Kaback M, Hechtman P: A new Tay-Sachs disease B1 allele in exon 7 in two compound heterozygotes each with a second novel mutation. *Hum Mol Genet* **1**:759, 1992.
325. Navon R, Proia RL: The mutations in Ashkenazi Jews with adult GM2 gangliosidosis, the adult form of Tay-Sachs disease. *Science* **243**:1471, 1989.
326. Paw BH, Kaback MM, Neufeld EF: Molecular basis of adult-onset and chronic GM2 gangliosidoses in patients of Ashkenazi Jewish origin: Substitution of serine for glycine at position 269 of the alpha-subunit of beta-hexosaminidase. *Proc Natl Acad Sci U S A* **86**:2413, 1989.
327. Brown CA, Mahuran DJ: β-Hexosaminidase isozymes from cells cotransfected with α and β cDNA constructs: Analysis of the α subunit missense mutation associated with the adult form of Tay-Sachs disease. *Am J Hum Genet* **53**:497, 1993.
328. Navon R, Kolodny EH, Mitsumoto H, Thomas GH, Proia RL: Ashkenazi-Jewish and non-Jewish adult GM2 gangliosidosis patients share a common genetic defect. *Am J Hum Genet* **46**:817, 1990.

329. De Gasperi R, Gama SM, Battistini S, Yeretsian J, Raghavan S, Zelnik N, Leshinsky E, et al: Late-onset GM2 gangliosidosis: Ashkenazi Jewish family with an exon 5 mutation (Tyr180 → His) in the Hex A alpha-chain gene. *Neurology* **47**:547, 1996.
330. Akli S, Chomel JC, Lacorte JM, Bachner L, Poenaru A, Poenaru L: Ten novel mutations in the HEXA gene in non-Jewish Tay-Sachs patients. *Hum Mol Genet* **2**:61, 1993.
331. Ribeiro MG, Sonin T, Pinto RA, Fontes A, Ribeiro H, Pinto E, Palmeira MM, et al: Clinical, enzymatic, and molecular characterisation of a Portuguese family with a chronic form of GM2-gangliosidosis B1 variant. *J Med Genet* **33**:341, 1996.
332. Navon R, Khosravi R, Korczyn T, Masson M, Sonnino S, Fardeau M, Eymard B, et al: A new mutation in the HEXA gene associated with a spinal muscular atrophy phenotype. *Neurology* **45**:539, 1995.
333. Vidgoff J, Buist N, O'Brien J: Absence of β-*N*-acetyl-d-hexosaminidase A activity in a healthy women. *Am J Hum Genet* **25**:372, 1973.
334. Kelly TE, Reynolds LW, O'Brien JS: Segregation within a family of two mutant alleles for hexosaminidase A. *Clin Genet* **9**:540, 1976.
335. Grebner EE, Mansfield DA, Raghavan SS, Kolodny EH, d'Azzo A, Neufeld EF, Jackson LG: Two abnormalities of hexosaminidase A in clinically normal individuals. *Am J Hum Genet* **38**:505, 1986.
336. O'Brien JS, Tennant L, Veath ML, Scott CR, Bucknall WE: Characterization of unusual hexosaminidase A (HEX A) deficient human mutants. *Am J Hum Genet* **30**:602, 1978.
337. Triggs Raine BL, Mules EH, Kaback MM, Lim Steele JST, Dowling CE, Akerman BR, Natowicz MR, et al: A pseudodeficiency allele common in non-Jewish Tay-Sachs carriers: Implications for carrier screening. *Am J Hum Genet* **51**:793, 1992.
338. Thomas GH, Raghavan S, Kolodny EH, Frisch A, Neufeld EF, O'Brien JS, Reynolds LW, et al: Nonuniform deficiency of hexosaminidase A in tissues and fluids of two unrelated individuals. *Pediat Res* **16**:232, 1982.
339. Cao Z, Natowicz MR, atowicz MR, aback MM, im-Steele JS, Prence EM, Brown D, et al: A second mutation associated with apparent beta-hexosaminidase A pseudodeficiency: Identification and frequency estimation. *Am J Hum Genet* **53**:1198, 1992.
340. Cao Z, Petroulakis E, Salo T, Triggs-Raine B: Benign HEXA mutations, C739T(R247W) and C745T(R249W), cause beta-hexosaminidase A pseudodeficiency by reducing the alpha-subunit protein levels. *J Biol Chem* **272**:14975, 1997.
341. Neote K, Brown CA, Mahuran DJ, Gravel RA: Translation initiation in the HEXB gene encoding the beta-subunit of human beta-hexosaminidase. *J Biol Chem* **265**:20799, 1990.
342. Neote K, McInnes B, Mahuran DJ, Gravel RA: Structure and distribution of an Alu-type deletion mutation in Sandhoff disease. *J Clin Invest* **86**:1524, 1990.
343. Bikker H, van den Berg FM, Wolterman RA, de Vijlder JJ, Bolhuis PA: Demonstration of a Sandhoff disease-associated autosomal 50-kb deletion by field inversion gel electrophoresis. *Hum Genet* **81**:287, 1989.
344. Bolhuis PA, Bikker H: Deletion of the 5′-region in one or two alleles of HEXB in 15 out of 30 patients with Sandhoff disease. *Hum Genet* **90**:328, 1992.
345. Zhang ZX, Wakamatsu N, Akerman BR, Mules EH, Thomas GH, Gravel RA: A second, large deletion in the HEXB gene in a patient with infantile Sandhoff disease. *Hum Mol Genet* **4**:777, 1995.
346. Wakamatsu N, Kobayashi H, Miyatake T, Tsuji S: A novel exon mutation in the human beta-hexosaminidase beta subunit gene affects 3′ splice site selection. *J Biol Chem* **267**:2406, 1992.
347. McInnes B, Potier M, Wakamatsu N, Melancon SB, Klavins MH, Tsuji S, Mahuran DJ: An unusual splicing mutation in the HEXB gene is associated with dramatically different phenotypes in patients from different racial backgrounds. *J Clin Invest* **90**:306, 1992.
348. Nakano T, Suzuki K: Genetic cause of a juvenile form of Sandhoff disease. Abnormal splicing of beta-hexosaminidase beta chain gene transcript due to a point mutation within intron 12. *J Biol Chem* **264**:5155, 1989.
349. Dlott B, d'Azzo A, Quon DV, Neufeld EF: Two mutations produce intron insertion in mRNA and elongated beta-subunit of human beta-hexosaminidase. *J Biol Chem* **265**:17921, 1990.
350. Dreyfus JC, Poenaru L, Vibert M, Ravise N, Boue J: Characterization of a variant of beta-hexosaminidase: "hexosaminidase Paris." *Am J Hum Genet* **29**:287, 1977.
351. Bolhuis PA, Ponne NJ, Bikker H, Baas F, Vianney de Jong JM: Molecular basis of an adult form of Sandhoff disease: substitution of glutamine for arginine at position 505 of the beta-chain of beta-hexosaminidase results in a labile enzyme. *Biochim Biophys Acta* **1182**:142, 1993.
352. De Gasperi R, Gama Sosa MA, Grebner EE, Mansfield D, Battistini S, Sartorato EL, Raghavan SS, et al: Substitution of alanine543 with a threonine residue at the carboxy terminal end of the beta-chain is associated with thermolabile hexosaminidase B in a Jewish family of Oriental ancestry. *Biochem Molec Med* **56**:31, 1995.
353. Narkis G, Adam A, Jaber L, Pennybacker M, Proia RL, Navon R: Molecular basis of heat labile hexosaminidase B among Jews and Arabs. *Hum Mutat* **10**:424, 1997.
354. Kleiman FE, Oller Ramirez A, Akerman B, Dodelson de Kremer R, Gravel RA, Argarana CE: A frequent TG deletion near the polyadenylation signal of the human HEXB gene: Occurrence of an irregular DNA structure and conserved nucleotide sequence motif in the 3′ untranslated region. *Hum Mutat* **12**:320, 1998.
355. Xie B, Wang W, Mahuran DJ: A Cys_{138} to Arg substitution in the G_{M2} activator protein is associated with the AB variant form of G_{M2} gangliosidosis. *Am J Hum Genet* **50**:1046, 1992.
356. Schroder M, Schnabel D, Suzuki K, Sandhoff K: A mutation in the gene of a glycolipid-binding protein (GM2 activator) that causes GM2-gangliosidosis variant AB. *FEBS Lett* **290**:1, 1991.
357. Xie B, Rigat B, Smiljanic-Georgijev N, Deng H, Mahuran D: Biochemical characterization of the Cys138Arg substitution associated with the AB variant form of GM2 gangliosidosis: Evidence that Cys138 is required for the recognition of the GM2 activator/GM2 ganglioside complex by beta-hexosaminidase A. *Biochemistry* **37**:814, 1998.
358. Schroder M, Schnabel D, Young E, Suzuki K, Sandhoff K: Molecular genetics of GM2-gangliosidosis AB variant: A novel mutation and expression in BHK cells. *Hum Genet* **92**:437, 1993.
359. Schepers U, Glombitza G, Lemm T, Hoffmann A, Chabas A, Ozand P, Sandhoff K: Molecular analysis of a GM2-activator deficiency in two patients with GM2-gangliosidosis AB variant. *Am J Hum Genet* **59**:1048, 1996.
360. Sakuraba H, Itoh K, Shimmoto M, Utsumi K, Kase R, Hashimoto Y, Ozawa T, et al: GM2 gangliosidosis AB variant — Clinical and biochemical studies of a Japanese patient. *Neurology* **52**:372, 1999.
361. Conzelmann E, Nehrkorn H, Kytzia H-J, Macek M, Lehovsky M, Elleder M, Jirasek A, et al: Prenatal diagnosis of GM2 gangliosidosis with high residual hexosaminidase A activity (variant B1; Pheudo AB variant). *Pediatr Res* **19**:1220, 1985.
362. Warner TG, De Kremer RD, Applegarth D, Mock AK: Diagnosis and characterization of GM 2 gangliosidosis type II (Sandhoff disease) by analysis of the accumulating *N*-acetyl- glucosaminyl oligosaccharides with high performance liquid chromatography. *Clin Chim Acta* **154**:151, 1986.
363. Price R, Dance N: The demonstration of multiple heat stable forms of *N*-aceytl-beta-glucosaminidase in normal human serum. *Biochim Biophys Acta* **271**:145, 1972.
364. Dance N, Price RG, Robinson D: Differential assay of human hexosaminidases A and B. *Biochim Biophys Acta* **222**:662, 1970.
365. Young EP, Ellis RB, Lake BD, Patrick AD: Tay-Sachs disease and related disorders: Fractionation of brain *N*-acetyl-β-D-hexosaminidase on DEAE-cellulose. *FEBS Lett* **9**:1, 1970.
366. Kanfer J, Spielvogel C: Hexosaminidase activity of cultured human skin fibroblasts. *Biochim Biophys Acta* **293**:203, 1973.
367. Suzuki Y, Koizumi Y, Togari H, Ogawa Y: Sandhoff disease: Diagnosis of heterozygous carriers of serum hexosaminidase assay. *Clin Chim Acta* **48**:153, 1973.
368. Sandhoff K: Auftrennung der Sauger-*N*-Acetyl-β-D-hexosaminidase in multiple Formen durch Elecktrofokussierung. *Hoppe-Seyler's Z Physiol Chem* **349**:1095, 1968.
369. Harzer K: Analytische isoelektrische Fraktionierung der *N*-Acetyl-β-D- hexosaminidasen. *Z Anal Chem* **252**:170, 1970.
370. Hayase K, Kritchevsky D: Separation and comparison of isoenzymes of *N*-acetyl-β-D-hexosaminidase of pregnant serum by polyacrylamide gel electrofocusing. *Clin Chim Acta* **46**:455, 1973.
371. Christomanou H, Cap C, Sandhoff K: Isoelectric focusing pattern of acid hydrolases in cultured fibroblasts, leukocytes and cell-free amniotic fluid. *Neuropadiatrie* **8**:238, 1977.
372. O'Brien J, Okada S, Fillerup D, Veath M, Adoranto B, Brenner P, Leroy J: Tay-Sachs disease — Prenatal diagnosis. *Science* **172**:61, 1971.
373. Suzuki Y, Suzuki K: Partial deficiency of hexosaminidase component in a juvenile GM2 gangliosidosis. *Neurology* **20**:848, 1970.

374. Klibansky C: Separation of *N*-acetyl-*β*-D-hexosaminidase isoenzymes from human brain and leukocytes by cellulose acetate paper electrophoresis. *J Med Sci* **7**:1086, 1971.
375. Davidson, Rattazzi M: Prenatal diagnosis of genetic disorders. Trials and tribulations. *Clin Chem* **18**:179, 1972.
376. O'Brien J, Okada S, Chem A, Fillerup D: Tay-Sachs disease. Detection of heterozygotes and homozygotes by serum hexosaminidase assay. *N Engl J Med* **283**:15, 1970.
377. Saifer A, Perle G: Automated determination of serum hexosaminidase A by pH inactivation for detection of Tay-Sachs disease heterozygotes. *Clin Chem* **20**:538, 1974.
378. Sandhoff K: Multiple human hexosaminidases. *Birth Defects* **9(2)**:214, 1973.
379. Navon R, Nutman J, Kopel R, Gaber L, Gadoth N, Goldman B, Nitzan M: Hereditary heat-labile hexosaminidase B: Its implications for recognizing Tay-Sachs genotypes. *Am J Hum Genet* **33**:907, 1981.
380. Navon R, Kopel R, Nutman J, Frisch A, Conzelmann E, Sandhoff K, Adam A: Hereditary heat-labile hexosaminidase B: A variant whose homozygotes synthesize a functional HEX A. *Am J Hum Genet* **37**:138, 1985.
381. Inui K, Wenger DA: Usefulness of 4-methylumbelliferyl-6-sulfo-2-acetamido-2-deoxy- beta-D-glucopyranoside for the diagnosis of GM2 gangliosidoses in leukocytes. *Clin Genet* **26**:318, 1984.
382. Fuchs W, Navon R, Kaback MM, Kresse H: Tay-Sachs disease: One-step assay of beta-*N*-acetylhexosaminidase in serum with a sulphated chromogenic substrate. *Clin Chim Acta* **133**:253, 1983.
383. Inui K, Wenger DA, Furukawa M, Suehara N, Yutaka Y, Okada S, Tanizawa O, et al: Prenatal diagnosis of GM2 gangliosidoses using a fluorogenic sulfated substrate. *Clin Chim Acta* **154**:145, 1986.
384. O'Brien JS, Norden AGW, Miller AL, Frost RG, Kelly TE: Ganglioside GM2 *N*-acetyl-*β*-galactosaminidase and asialo GM2 (GA2) *N*-acetyl-*β*-D-galacosaminidase; studies in human skin fibroblasts. *Clin Genet* **11**:171, 1977.
385. Harzer K: Assay of the GM2-ganglioside cleaving hexosaminidase activity of skin fibroblasts for GM2-gangliosidoses. *Clin Chim Acta* **135**:89, 1983.
386. Erzberger A, Conzelmann E, Sandhoff K: Assay of ganglioside GM2-*N*-acetyl-*β*-D-galactosaminidase activity in human fibroblasts employing the natural activator protein — Diagnosis of variant forms of GM2 gangliosidosis. *Clin Chim Acta* **108**:361, 1980.
387. Conzelmann E, Kytzia HJ, Navon R, Sandhoff K: Ganglioside GM2 *N*-acetyl-beta-D-galactosaminidase activity in cultured fibroblasts of late-infantile and adult GM2 gangliosidosis patients and of healthy probands with low hexosaminidase level. *Am J Hum Genet* **35**:900, 1983.
388. Christomanou H, Cap C, Sandhoff K: Prenatal diagnosis of Tay-Sachs disease in cell-free amniotic fluid. *Klin Wochenschr* **56**:1133, 1978.
389. Dreyfus JC, Poenaru L, Svennerholm L: Absence of hexosaminidase A and B in a normal adult. *N Engl J Med* **292**:61, 1975.
390. Banerjee A, Burg J, Conzelmann E, Carroll M, Sandhoff K: Enzyme-linked immunosorbent assay for the ganglioside GM2-activator protein. Screening of normal human tissues and body fluids, of tissues of GM2 gangliosidosis, and for its subcellular localization. *Hoppe Seyler's Z Physiol Chem* **365**:347, 1984.
391. Raghavan S, Krusell A, Lyerla TA, Bremer EG, Kolodny EH: GM2-ganglioside metabolism in cultured human skin fibroblasts: Unambiguous diagnosis of GM2-gangliosidosis. *Biochim Biophys Acta* **834**:238, 1985.
392. Ferlinz K, Hurwitz R, Weiler M, Suzuki K, Sandhoff K, Vanier MT: Molecular analysis of the acid sphingomyelinase deficiency in a family with an intermediate form of Niemann-Pick disease. *Am J Hum Genet* **56**:1343, 1995.
393. Schwarzmann G, Hoffmann-Bleihauer P, Schubert J, Sandhoff K, Marsh D: Incorporation of ganglioside analogues into fibroblasts cell membranes. A spin label study. *Biochemistry* **22**:5041, 1983.
394. Suzuki Y, Berman P, Suzuki K: Detection of Tay-Sachs disease heterozygotes by assay of hexosaminidase A in serum and leukocytes. *J Pediatr* **78**:643, 1971.
395. Okada S, Veath M, Leroy J, O'Brien J: Ganglioside GM2 storage diseases: Hexosaminidase deficiencies in cultured fibroblasts. *Am J Hum Genet* **23**:55, 1971.
396. Carmody P, Rattazzi M, Davidson R: Tay-Sachs disease–The use of tears for the detection of heterozygotes. *N Engl J Med* **289**:1072, 1973.
397. Kaback M, Zeiger R: Heterozygote detection in Tay-Sachs disease: A prototype community screening program for the prevention of recessive genetic disorders, in Volk B, Aronson S (eds): *Sphingolipids, Sphingolipidoses, and Allied Disorders. Advances in Experimental Medicine and Biology.* New York, Plenum, 1972, p 613.
398. Kaback M, Zeiger R, Reynolds L, Sonneborn M: Approaches to the control and prevention of Tay-Sachs disease, in Steinberg AG, Bearn A (eds): *Sphingolipids, Sphingolipidoses, and Allied Disorders.* New York, Grune & Stratton, 1974, p 103.
399. Kaback M, Nathan T, Greenwald S: Tay-Sachs disease: Heterozygote screening and prenatal diagnosis — U.S. experience and world perspective, in Kaback M (ed): *Tay-Sachs Disease: Screening and Prevention.* New York, Alan R. Liss, 1977, p 13.
400. Kaback M: Heterozygote screening and prenatal diagnosis in Tay-Sachs disease: A worldwide update, in Callahan J, Lowden J (eds): *Lysosomes and Lysosomal Storage Diseases.* New York, Raven Press, 1981, p 331.
401. Paw BH, Tieu PT, Kaback MM, Lim J, Neufeld EF: Frequency of three Hex A mutant alleles among Jewish and non-Jewish carriers identified in a Tay-Sachs screening program. *Am J Hum Genet* **47**:698, 1990.
402. Cantor RM, Lim JS, Roy C, Kaback MM: Sandhoff disease heterozygote detection: A component of population screening for Tay-Sachs disease carriers. I. Statistical methods. *Am J Hum Genet* **37**:912, 1985.
403. Schneck L, Friedland J, Valenti C, Adachi M, Amsterdam D, Volk B: Prenatal diagnosis of Tay-Sachs disease. *Lancet* **1**:582, 1970.
404. Navon R, Padeh B: Prenatal diagnosis of Tay-Sachs genotypes. *Br Med J* **4**:17, 1971.
405. Pergament E, Ginsberg N, Verlinsky Y, Cadkin A, Chu L, Truka L, Grebner E, et al: Prenatal Tay-Sachs diagnosis of chronic villi sampling. *Lancet* **2**:286, 1983.
406. Besancon AM, Belon JP, Castelnau L, Dumez Y, Poenaru L: Prenatal diagnosis of atypical Tay-Sachs disease by chorionic villi sampling. *Prenat Diagn* **4**:365, 1984.
407. Triggs Raine BL, Archibald A, Gravel RA, Clarke JT: Prenatal exclusion of Tay-Sachs disease by DNA analysis. *Lancet* **335**:1164, 1990.
408. Myrianthopoulos N: Some epidemiologic and genetic aspects of Tay-Sachs disease, in Aronson S, Volk B (eds): *Cerebral Sphingolipidoses: A Symposium on Tay-Sachs Disease and Allied Disorders.* New York, Academic, 1962, p 375.
409. Aronson S: Epidemiology, in Volk BW (ed): *Tay-Sachs Disease.* New York, Grune & Stratton, 1964, p 118.
410. Petersen GM, Rotter JI, Cantor RM, Field LL, Greenwald S, Lim JS, Roy C, et al: The Tay-Sachs disease gene in North American Jewish populations: Geographic variations and origin. *Am J Hum Genet* **35**:1258, 1983.
411. Triggs Raine BL, Feigenbaum AS, Natowicz M, Skomorowski MA, Schuster SM, Clarke JT, Mahuran DJ, et al: Screening for carriers of Tay-Sachs disease among Ashkenazi Jews. A comparison of DNA-based and enzyme-based tests. *N Engl J Med* **323**:6, 1990.
412. Grebner EE Tomczak J: Distribution of three alpha-chain beta-hexosaminidase A mutations among Tay-Sachs carriers. *Am J Hum Genet* **48**:604, 1991.
413. Landels EC, Ellis IH, Fensom AH, Green PM, Bobrow M: Frequency of the Tay-Sachs disease splice and insertion mutations in the UK Ashkenazi Jewish population. *J Med Genet* **28**:177, 1991.
414. Fernandes MJ, Kaplan F, Clow CL, Hechtman P, Scriver CR: Specificity and sensitivity of hexosaminidase assays and DNA analysis for the detection of Tay-Sachs disease gene carriers among Ashkenazic Jews. *Genet Epidemiol* **9**:169, 1992.
415. Kaback M: Unpublished information, 1993.
416. Kaback M, Lim-Steele J, Dabholkar D, Brown D, Levy N, Zeiger K: Tay-Sachs disease — Carrier screening, prenatal diagnosis, and the molecular era. An international perspective, 1970 to 1993. The International TSD Data Collection Network. *JAMA* **270**:2307, 1993.
417. Aronson S, Valsamis M, Volk B: Infantile amaurotic idiocy. Occurrence, genetic considerations and pathophysiology in the non-Jewish infant. *Pediatrics* **26**:229, 1960.
418. Hanhart E: Uber 27 Sippen mit infantiler amaurotischer Idiotie (Tay-Sachs). *Acta Genet Med Gemellol* **3**:331, 1954.
419. Murakami U: Clinicogenetic study of hereditary diseases of the nervous system. *Folia Psychiatr Neuro Jpn (Suppl)* **1**:1, 1957.
420. Kelly T, Chase G, Kaback M, Kumor K, McKusick V: Tay-Sachs disease: High gene frequency in a non-Jewish population. *Am J Hum Genet* **27**:287, 1975.
421. Anderman E, Scriver C, Wolfe L, Dansky S, Anderman F: Genetic variant of Tay-Sachs disease, in Kaback MM (ed): *Tay-Sachs Disease: Screening and Prevention.* New York, Alan R. Liss, 1977.

422. Brzustowicz LM, Lehner T, Castilla LH, Penchaszadeh GK, Wilhelmsen KC, Daniels R, Davies KE, et al: Genetic mapping of chronic childhood-onset spinal muscular atrophy to chromosome 5q11.2-13.3. *Nature* **344**:540, 1990.
423. Hechtman P, Boulay B, de Braekeleer M, Andermann E, Melancon S, Larochelle J, Prevost C, et al: The intron 7 donor splice site transition: A second Tay-Sachs disease mutation in French-Canada. *Hum Genet* **90**:402, 1992.
424. de Braekeleer M, Hechtman P, Andermann E, Kaplan F: The French Canadian Tay-Sachs disease deletion mutation: Identification of probable founders. *Hum Genet* **89**:83, 1992.
425. Hechtman P, Kaplan F, Bayleran J, Boulay B, Andermann E, de Braekeleer M, Melancon S, et al: More than one mutant allele causes infantile Tay-Sachs disease in French-Canadians. *Am J Hum Genet* **47**:815, 1990.
426. McDowell GA, Mules EH, Fabacher P, Shapira E, Blitzer MG: The presence of two different infantile Tay-Sachs disease mutations in a Cajun population. *Am J Hum Genet* **51**:1071, 1992.
427. Mules EH, Hayflick S, Dowling CE, Kelly TE, Akerman BR, Gravel RA, Thomas GH: Molecular basis of hexosaminidase A deficiency and pseudo-deficiency in the Berks County Pennsylvania Dutch. *Hum Mutat* **1**:298, 1992.
428. Drucker L, Proia RL, Navon R: Identification and rapid detection of three Tay-Sachs mutations in the Moroccan Jewish population. *Am J Hum Genet* **51**:371, 1992.
429. Tanaka A, Sakuraba H, Isshiki G, Suzuki K: The major mutation among Japanese patients with infantile Tay-Sachs disease: A G-to-T transversion at the acceptor site of intron 5 of the β-hexosaminidase α gene. *Biochem Biophys Res Commun* **52**:315, 1993.
430. Mules EH, Dowling CE, Petersen MB, Kazazian HH Jr, Thomas GH: A novel mutation in the invariant AG of the acceptor splice site of intron 4 of the beta-hexosaminidase alpha-subunit gene in two unrelated American black GM2-gangliosidosis (Tay-Sachs disease) patients. *Am J Hum Genet* **48**:1181, 1991.
431. Hechtman P, Boulay B, Bayleran J, Andermann E: The mutation mechanism causing juvenile-onset Tay-Sachs disease among Lebanese. *Clin Genet* **35**:364, 1989.
432. De Kremer R De Levstein I: Enfermedad de Sandhoff o gangliosidosis GM2 tipo 2. alta Frequencia del gen en una problacion Criolla. *Medicina (Buenos Aires)* **40**:55, 1980.
433. De Kremer R, Depetris de Boldini C, Paschini de Capra A, Pons de Veritier P, Goldenhersch H, Corbella L, Sembaj A, et al: Estimacion de la frecuencia de heterocigotes de la enfermedad de Sandhoff en una poblacion argentina de alto riesgo. Asignacion predictiva del genotipo mediante un analisis estadistico. *Medicina (Buenos Aires)* **47**:455, 1987.
434. De Kremer RD, Boldini CD, Capra AP, Levstein IM, Bainttein N, Hidalgo PK, Hliba H: Sandhoff disease: 36 cases from Cordoba, Argentina. *J Inherit Metab Dis* **8**:46, 1985.
435. Lowden J, Ives E, Keene D, Burton A, Skomorowski M, Howard F: Carrier detection in Sandhoff disease. *Am J Hum Genet* **30**:38, 1978.
436. Derkaloustian V, Khoury M, Hallal R, Idriss Z, Deeb M: Sandhoff disease: A prevalent form of infantile GM2 gangliosidosis in Lebanon. *Am J Hum Genet* **33**:85, 1981.
437. Cantor RM, Roy C, Lim JS, Kaback MM: Sandhoff disease heterozygote detection: a component of population screening for Tay-Sachs disease carriers. II. Sandhoff disease gene frequencies in American Jewish and non-Jewish populations. *Am J Hum Genet* **41**:16, 1987.
438. Brown CA, McInnes B, De Kremer RD, Mahuran DJ: Characterization of two HEXB gene mutations in Argentinean patients with Sandhoff disease. *Biochim Biophys Acta* **1180**:91, 1992.
439. Kleiman FE, De Kremer RD, de Ramirez AO, Gravel RA, Argarana CE: Sandhoff disease in Argentina: High frequency of a splice site mutation in the HEXB gene and correlation between enzyme and DNA-based tests for heterozygote detection. *Hum Genet* **94**:279, 1994.
440. Myrianthopoulos N, Aronson S: Population dynamics of Tay-Sachs disease. I. Reproductive fitness and selection. *Am J Hum Genet* **18**:313, 1966.
441. Chase GA, McKusick VA: Founder effect in Tay-Sachs disease. *Am J Hum Genet* **24**:339, 1972.
442. Chase GA: The Tay-Sachs disease gene among Ashkenazic Jews: Founder effect and genetic drift, in Kaback MM (ed): *Tay-Sachs Disease: Screening and Prevention*. New York, Alan R. Liss, 1977, p 107.
443. Myrianthopoulos NC, Melnick M: A genetic-historical view of selective advantage, in Kaback MM (ed): *Tay-Sachs Disease: Screening and Prevention*. New York, Alan R. Liss, 1977, p 95.
444. Rotter JI, Diamond JM: What maintains the frequencies of human genetic diseases? *Nature* **329**:289, 1987.
445. Formisano S, Johnson ML, Lee G, Aloj SM, Edelhoch H: Critical micelle concentrations of gangliosides. *Biochemistry* **18**:1119, 1979.
446. Walkley S, Blakemore W, Purpura D: Alterations in neuron morphology in feline mannosidosis: A Golgi study. *Acta Neuropathol* **53**:75, 1981.
447. Walkley S, Haskins M: Aberrant neurite nad meganeurite development in a feline model of mucopolysaccharidosis (MPS) type 1 as revealed by the Golgi method. *Soc Neurosci Abstr* **8**:1009, 1982.
448. Goodman LA, Livingston PO, Walkley SU: Ectopic dendrites occur only on cortical pyramidal cells containing elevated GM2 ganglioside in alpha-mannosidosis. *Proc Natl Acad Sci U S A* **88**:11330, 1991.
449. Walkley SU: Pathobiology of neuronal storage disease. *Int Rev Neurobiol* **29**:191, 1988.
450. Svennerholm L, Vanier M-T, Mansson JE: Krabbe disease: A galactosylsphingosine (psychosine) lipidosis. *J Lipid Res* **21**:53, 1980.
451. Nilsson O, Mansson J-E, Haskansson G, Svennerholm L: The occurrence of psychosine and other glycolipids in spleen and liver from the three major types of Gaucher's disease. *Biochim Biophys Acta* **712**:453, 1982.
452. Igisu H, Suzuki K: Progressive accumulation of toxic metabolite in a genetic leukodystrophy. *Science* **224**:753, 1984.
453. Neuenhofer S, Conzelmann E, Schwarzmann G, Egge H, Sandhoff K: Occurrence of lysoganglioside lyso-GM2 (II3-Neu-5-Ac-gangliotriaosylsphingosine) in GM2 gangliosidosis brain. *Biol Chem Hoppe-Seyler* **367**:241, 1986.
454. Rosengren B, Mansson JE, Svennerholm L: Composition of gangliosides and neutral glycosphingolipids of brain in classical Tay-Sachs and Sandhoff disease: More lyso-GM2 in Sandhoff disease? *J Neurochem* **49**:834, 1987.
455. Kobayashi T, Goto I, Okada S, Orii T, Ohno K, Nakano T: Accumulation of lysosphingolipids in tissues from patients with GM1 and GM2 gangliosidoses. *J Neurochem* **59**:1452, 1992.
456. Kobayashi T, Goto I: A sensitive assay of lysogangliosides using high-performance liquid chromatography. *Biochim Biophys Acta* **1081**:159, 1991.
457. Hannun Y, Bell R: Lysosphingolipids inhibit protein kinase C: Implications for the sphingolipidoses. *Science* **235**:670, 1987.
458. Norflus F, Tifft CJ, Mcdonald MP, Goldstein G, Crawley JN, Hoffmann A, Sandhoff K, et al: Bone marrow transplantation prolongs life span and ameliorates neurologic manifestations in Sandhoff disease mice. *J Clin Invest* **101**:1881, 1998.
459. Conzelmann E, Sandhoff K: Partial enzyme deficiencies: Residual activities and the development of neurologic disorders. *Dev Neurosci* **6**:58, 1983.
460. Leinekugel P, Michel S, Conzelmann E, Sandhoff K: Quantitative correlation between the residual activity of beta-hexosamindase A and arylsulfatase A and the severity of the resulting lysosomal storage disease. *Hum Genet* **88**:513, 1992.
461. Karbe E, Schiefer B: Familial amaurotic idiocy in male German Shorthair Pointers. *Vet Pathol* **4**:223, 1967.
462. McGrath J, Kelly A, Steinberg S: Cerebral lipidosis in the dog. *J Neuropathol Exp* **27**:41, 1968.
463. Bernheimer H, Karbe E: Morphologishe und Neurochemische Untersuchungen von 2 Formen der amaurotischen Idiotie des Hundesa: nachweis einer GM2-gangliosidose. *Acta Neuropathol* **16**:243, 1970.
464. Cummings JF, Wood PA, Walkley SU, de Lahunta A, DeForest ME: GM2 gangliosidosis in a Japanese spaniel. *Acta Neuropathol (Berl)* **67**:247, 1985.
465. Cork LC, Munnell JF, Lorenz MD, Murphy JV, Baker HJ, Rattazzi MC: GM2 ganglioside lysosomal storage disease in cats with beta-hexosaminidase deficiency. *Science* **196**:1014, 1977.
466. Neuwelt EA, Johnson WG, Blank NK, Pagel MA, Maslen McClure C, McClure MJ, Wu PM: Characterization of a new model of GM2-gangliosidosis (Sandhoff's disease) in Korat cats. *J Clin Invest* **76**:482, 1985.
467. Muldoon LL, Neuwelt EA, Pagel MA, Weiss DL: Characterization of the molecular defect in a feline model for type II GM2-gangliosidosis (Sandhoff disease). *Am J Pathol* **144**:1109, 1994.
468. Read W, Bridges C: Cerebrospinal lipodystrophy in swine: A new disease model in comparative pathology. *Pathol Vet* **5**:67, 1968.

469. Pierce K, Kosanke S, Bay W: Animal model: Porcine cerebrospinal lipodystrophy (GM2 gangliosidosis). *Am J Pathol* **83**:419, 1976.
470. Walkley SU, Wurzelmann S, Rattazzi MC, Baker HJ: Distribution of ectopic neurite growth and other geometrical distortions of CNS neurons in feline GM2 gangliosidosis. *Brain Res* **510**:63, 1990.
471. Siegel DA, Walkley SU: Growth of ectopic dendrites on cortical pyramidal neurons in neuronal storage diseases correlates with abnormal accumulation of GM2 ganglioside. *J Neurochem* **62**:1852, 1994.
472. Walkley SU, Siegel DA, Dobrenis K: GM2 ganglioside and pyramidal neuron dendritogenesis. *Neurochem Res* **20**:1287, 1995.
473. Liu Y, Hoffmann A, Grinberg A, Westphal H, McDonald MP, Miller KM, Crawley JN, et al: Mouse model of GM2 activator deficiency manifests cerebellar pathology and motor impairment. *Proc Natl Acad Sci U S A* **94**:8138, 1997.
474. Cohen-Tannoudji M, Marchand P, Akli S, Sheardown SA, Puech JP, Kress C, Gressens P, et al: Disruption of murine Hexa gene leads to enzymatic deficiency and to neuronal lysosomal storage, similar to that observed in Tay-Sachs disease. *Mamm Genome* **6**:844, 1995.
475. Taniike M, Yamanaka S, Proia RL, Langaman C, Bone-Turrentine T, Suzuki: Neuropathology of mice with targeted disruption of Hexa gene, a model of Tay-Sachs disease. *Acta Neuropathol (Berl)* **89**:296, 1995.
476. Yamanaka S, Johnson MD, Grinberg A, Westphal H, Crawley JN, Taniike, M, et al: Targeted disruption of the Hexa gene results in mice with biochemical and pathologic features of Tay-Sachs disease. *Proc Natl Acad Sci U S A* **91**:9975, 1994.
477. Suzuki K, Sango K, Proia RL, Langaman C: Mice deficient in all forms of lysosomal beta-hexosaminidase show mucopolysaccharidosis-like pathology. *J Neuropath Exp Neurol* **56**:693, 1997.
478. Suzuki K, Proia RL: Mouse models of human lysosomal diseases. *Brain Pathol* **8**:195, 1998.
479. Johnson W, Desnick R, Long D, Sharp M, Krivit W, Brady R: Intravenous injection of purified hexosaminidase A into patients with Tay-Sachs disease, in Desnick R, Bernlohr R, Krivit W (eds): *Enzyme Therapy in Genetic Diseases*. New York, Alan R. Liss, 1973, p 120.
480. von Specht BU, Geiger B, Arnon R, Passwell J, Keren G, Goldman B, Padeh B: Enzyme replacement in Tay-Sachs disease. *Neurology* **29**:848, 1979.
481. Neuwelt EA, Barranger JA, Pagel MA, Quirk JM, Brady RO, Frenkel EP: Delivery of active hexosaminidase across the blood-brain barrier in rats. *Neurology* **34**:1012, 1984.
482. Dobrenis K, Joseph A, Rattazzi MC: Neuronal lysosomal enzyme replacement using fragment C of tetanus toxin. *Proc Natl Acad Sci U S A* **89**:2297, 1992.
483. Wu YY, Lockyer JM, Sugiyama E, Pavlova NV, Li YT, Li SC: Expression and specificity of human GM2 activator protein. *J Bio Chem* **269**:16276, 1994.
484. Krivit W, Lockman LA, Watkins PA, Hirsch J, Shapiro EG: The future for treatment by bone marrow transplantation for adrenoleukodystrophy, metachromatic leukodystrophy, globoid cell leukodystrophy and Hurler syndrome. *J Inherit Metab Dis* **18**:398, 1995.
485. Hoogerbrugge PM, Brouwer OF, Bordigoni P, Ringden O, Kapaun P, Ortega, JJ, et al: Allogeneic bone marrow transplantation for lysosomal storage diseases. The European Group for Bone Marrow Transplantation. *Lancet* **345**:1398, 1995.
486. Walkley SU, Dobrenis K: Bone marrow transplantation for lysosomal diseases. *Lancet* **345**:1382, 1995.
487. Snyder EY, Wolfe JH: Central nervous system cell transplantation: A novel therapy for storage diseases? *Curr Op Pediat* **9**:126, 1996.
488. Snyder EY, Taylor RM, Wolfe JH: Neural progenitor cell engraftment corrects lysosomal storage throughout the MPS VII mouse brain. *Nature* **374**:367, 1995.
489. Lacorazza HD, Flax JD, Snyder EY, Jendoubi M: Expression of human beta-hexosaminidase alpha-subunit gene (the gene defect of Tay-Sachs disease) in mouse brains upon engraftment of transduced progenitor cells. *Nat Med* **2**:424, 1996.
490. Taylor RM, Wolfe JH: Decreased lysosomal storage in the adult MPS VII mouse brain in the vicinity of grafts of retroviral vector-corrected fibroblasts secreting high levels of beta-glucuronidase. *Nat Med* **3**:771, 1997.
491. Guidotti JE, Akli S, Castelnauptakhine L, Kahn A, Poenaru L: Retrovirus-mediated enzymatic correction of Tay-Sachs defect in transduced and non-transduced cells. *Hum Mol Genet* **7**:831, 1998.
492. Akli S, Guidotti JE, Vigne E, Perricaudet M, Sandhoff K, Kahn A, Poenaru L: Restoration of hexosaminidase A activity in human Tay-Sachs fibroblasts via adenoviral vector-mediated gene transfer. *Gene Ther* **3**:769, 1996.
493. Platt FM, Neises GR, Dwek RA, Butters TD: *N*-butyldeoxynojirimycin is a novel inhibitor of glycolipid biosynthesis. *J Biol Chem* **269**:8362, 1994.
494. Platt FM, Neises GR, Reinkensmeier G, Townsend MJ, Perry VH, Proia RL, Winchester B, et al: Prevention of lysosomal storage in Tay-Sachs mice treated with *N*-butyldeoxynojirimycin. *Science* **276**:428, 1997.
495. Jeyakumar M, Butters TD, Cortina-Borja M, Hunnam V, Proia RL, Perry VH, Dwek RA, et al: Delayed symptom onset and increased life expectancy in Sandhoff-disease mice treated with *N*-butyldeoxynojirimycin. *Proc Natl Acad Sci U S A* **96**:6388, 1999.
496. Snyder P, Krivit W, Sweeley C: Generalized accumulation on neutral glycosphingolipids with GM2 ganglioside accumulation in the brain. *J Lipid Res* **13**:128, 1972.
497. Iwamori M, Nagai Y: Ganglioside composition of brain in Tay-Sachs disease: Increased amounts of GD2 and *N*-acetyl-beta-D-galactosaminyl GD1a ganglioside. *J Neurochem* **32**:767, 1979.
498. Sandhoff K, Andreae U, Jatzkewitz H: Deficient hexosaminidase activity in an exceptional case of Tay-Sachs disease with additional storage of kidney globoside in visceral organs. *Pathol Eur* **3**:278, 1968.
499. Itoh T, Li YT, Li SC, Yu RK: Isolation and characterization of a novel monosialosylpentahexosyl ceramide from Tay-Sachs brain. *J Biol Chem* **256**:165, 1981.
500. Iwamori M, Nagai Y: Isolation and characterization of a novel ganglioside, monosialosyl pentahexaosyl ceramide from human brain. *J Biochem* **84**:1601, 1978.
501. Yu RK, Itoh T, Yohe HC, Macala LJ: Characterization of some minor gangliosides in Tay-Sachs brains. *Brain Res* **275**:47, 1983.
502. Conzelmann E, Sandhoff K: Purification and characterization of an activator protein for the degradation of glycolipids GM2 and GA2 by hexosaminidase A. *Hoppe-Seyler's Z Phys Chem* **360**:1837, 1979.
503. O'Brien J: Tay-Sachs disease: From enzyme to prevention. *Fed Proc* **32**:191, 1973.
504. Navon R, Khosravi R, Melki J, Drucker L, Fontaine B, Turpin JC, N'Guyen B: Juvenile-onset spinal muscular atrophy caused by compound heterozygosity for mutations in the HEXA gene. *Ann Neurol* **41**:631, 1997.
505. Harmon DL, Gardner-Medwin D, Stirling JL: Two new mutations in a late infantile Tay-Sachs patient are both in exon 1 of the β-hexosaminidase α subunit gene. *J Med Genet* **30**:123, 1993.
506. Tanaka A, Sakazaki H, Murakami H, Isshiki G, Suzuki K: Molecular genetics of Tay-Sachs disease in Japan. *J Inherit Metab Dis* **17**:593, 1994.
507. Drucker L, Golan A, Boles DJ, el Bedour K, Proia RL, Navon R: Novel HEXA mutation in a Bedouin Tay-Sachs patient associated with exon skipping and reduced transcript level. *Hum Mutat* **9**:260, 1997.
508. Peleg L, Meltzer F, Karpati M, Goldman B: GM2 gangliosidosis B1 variant: Biochemical and molecular characterization of hexosaminidase A. *Biochem Molec Med* **54**:126, 1995.
509. Drucker L, Hemli JA, Navon R: Two mutated HEXA alleles in a Druze patient with late-infantile Tay-Sachs disease. *Hum Mutat* **10**:451, 1997.
510. Nakano T, Nanba E, Tanaka A, Ohno K, Suzuki Y, Suzuki K: A new point mutation within exon 5 of beta-hexosaminidase alpha gene in a Japanese infant with Tay-Sachs disease. *Ann Neurol* **27**:465, 1990.
511. Kaufman M, Grinshpuncohen J, Karpati M, Peleg L, Goldman B, Akstein E, Adam A, et al: Tay-Sachs disease and HEXA mutations among Moroccan Jews. *Hum Mutat* **10**:295, 1997.
512. Ozkara HA, Akerman BR, Ciliv G, Topcu M, Renda Y, Gravel RA: Donor splice site mutation in intron 5 of the HEXA gene in a Turkish infant with Tay-Sachs disease. *Hum Mutat* **5**:186, 1995.
513. Gordon BA, Gordon KE, Hinton GG, Cadera W, Feleki V, Bayleran J, Hechtman P: Tay-Sachs disease: B1 variant. *Pediatr Neurol* **4**:54, 1988.
514. Ainsworth PJ, Coulter-Mackie MB: A double mutation in exon 6 of the Beta-hexosaminidase Alpha subunit in a patient with the B1 variant of Tay-Sachs disease. *Am J Hum Genet* **51**:802, 1992.
515. Hou Y, Vavougios G, Hinek A, Wu KK, Hechtman P, Kaplan F, Mahuran DJ: The Val192Leu mutation in the alpha-subunit of beta-hexosaminidase A is not associated with the B1-variant form of Tay-Sachs disease. *Am J Hum Genet* **59**:52, 1996.
516. Triggs-Raine B, Richard M, Wasel N, Prence EM, Natowicz MR: Mutational analyses of Tay-Sachs disease: Studies on Tay-Sachs carriers of French Canadian background living in New England. *Am J Hum Genet* **56**:870, 1995.

517. Cao Z, Natowicz MR, Kaback MM, Lim-Steele JS, Prence EM, Brown D, Chabot T, et al: A second mutation associated with apparent beta-hexosaminidase A pseudodeficiency: Identification and frequency estimation. *Am J Hum Genet* **53**:1198, 1993.
518. Hechtman P, Boulay B, Bayleran J, Andermann E: The mutation mechanism causing juvenile-onset Tay-Sachs disease among Lebanese. *Clin Genet* **35**:364, 1989.
519. Hechtman P, Boulay B, de Braekeleer M, Andermann E, Melancon S, Larochelle J, Prevost C, et al: The intron 7 donor splice site transition: A second Tay-Sachs disease mutation in French Canada. *Hum Genet* **90**:402, 1992.
520. Ribeiro MG, Pinto R, Miranda MC, Suzuki K: Tay-Sachs disease: Intron 7 splice junction mutation in two Portuguese patients. *Biochim Biophys Acta* **1270**:44, 1995.
521. Akli S, Boue J, Sandhoff K, Kleijer W, Vamos E, Gatti R, Di Natale P, et al: Collaborative study of molecular epidemiology of Tay-Sachs disease in Europe. *Hum Mutat* **1**:229, 1993.
522. Richard MM, Erenberg G, Triggs-Raine BL: An A-to-G mutation at the +3 position of intron 8 of the HEXA gene is associated with exon 8 skipping and Tay-Sachs disease. *Biochem Molec Med* **55**:74, 1995.
523. Brown DH, Triggs-Raine BL, McGinniss MJ, Kaback MM: A novel mutation at the invariant acceptor splice site of intron 9 in the HEXA gene [IVS9-1 G → T] detected by a PCR-based diagnostic test. *Hum Mutat* **5**:173, 1995.
524. Shore S, Tomczak J, Grebner EE, Myerowitz R: An unusual genotype in an Ashkenazi Jewish patient with Tay-Sachs disease. *Hum Mutat* **1**:486, 1992.
525. Tanaka A, Punnett HH, Suzuki K: A new point mutation in the beta-hexosaminidase alpha subunit gene responsible for infantile Tay-Sachs disease in a non-Jewish Caucasian patient (a Kpn mutant). *Am J Hum Genet* **47**:568, 1990.
526. Gil Ribeiro M, Pinto RA, Suzuki K, Sa Miranda MC: Two novel (1334delC and 1363G to A, G455R) mutations in exon 12 of the beta-hexosaminidase alpha-chain gene in two Portuguese patients. *Hum Mutat* **10**:359, 1997.
527. Strasberg P, Warren I, Skomorowski MA, Feigenbaum A: Homozygosity for the common Ashkenazi Jewish Tay-Sachs +1 IVS-12 splice-junction mutation: First report. *Hum Mutat* **10**:82, 1997.
528. Boustany RM, Tanaka A, Nishimoto J, Suzuki K: Genetic cause of a juvenile form of Tay-Sachs disease in a Lebanese child. *Ann Neurol* **29**:104, 1991.
529. Bikker H, van den Berg FM, Wolterman RA, Kleijer WJ, de Vijlder JJ, Bolhuis PA: Distribution and characterization of a Sandhoff disease-associated 50-kb deletion in the gene encoding the human beta-hexosaminidase beta-chain. *Hum Genet* **85**:327, 1990.
530. Hara Y, Ioannou P, Drousiotou A, Stylianidou G, Anastasiadou V, Suzuki K: Mutation analysis of a Sandhoff disease patient in the Maronite community in Cyprus. *Hum Genet* **94**:136, 1994.
531. Fujimaru M, Tanaka A, Choeh K, Wakamatsu N, Sakuraba H, Isshiki G: Two mutations remote from an exon/intron junction in the beta-hexosaminidase beta-subunit gene affect 3′-splice site selection and cause Sandhoff disease. *Hum Genet* **103**:462, 1998.
532. O'Dowd BF, Klavins MH, Willard HF, Gravel R, Lowden JA, Mahuran DJ: Molecular heterogeneity in the infantile and juvenile forms of Sandhoff disease (O-variant GM2 gangliosidosis). *J Biol Chem* **261**:12680, 1986.
533. McInnes B, Brown CA, Mahuran DJ: Two small deletion mutations of the HEXB gene are present in DNA from a patient with infantile Sandhoff disease. *Biochim Biophys Acta* **1138**:315, 1992.
534. Zhang ZX, Wakamatsu N, Mules EH, Thomas GH, Gravel RA: Impact of premature stop codons on mRNA levels in infantile Sandhoff disease. *Hum Mol Genet* **3**:139, 1994.
535. Gomez-Lira M, Sangalli A, Mottes M, Perusi C, Pignatti PF, Rizzuto N, Salviati A: A common beta hexosaminidase gene mutation in adult Sandhoff disease patients. *Hum Genet* **96**:417, 1995.
536. Furihata K, Drousiotou A, Hara Y, Christopoulos G, Stylianidou G, Anastasiadou V, Ueno I, et al: Novel splice site mutation at IVS8 nt 5 of HEXB responsible for a Greek-Cypriot case of Sandhoff disease. *Hum Mutat* **13**:38, 1999.
537. Gomez-Lira M, Perusi C, Mottes M, Pignatti PF, Rizzuto N, Gatti R, Salviati A: Splicing mutation causes infantile Sandhoff disease. *Am J Med Genet* **75**:330, 1998.
538. McInnes B, Potier M, Wakamatsu N, Melancon SB, Klavins MH, Tsuji S, Mahuran DJ: An unusual splicing mutation in the HEXB gene is associated with dramatically different phenotypes in patients from different racial backgrounds. *J Clin Invest* **90**:306, 1992.
539. Kuroki Y, Itoh K, Nadaoka Y, Tanaka T, Sakuraba H: A novel missense mutation (C522Y) is present in the beta-hexosaminidase beta-subunit gene of a Japanese patient with infantile Sandhoff disease. *Biochem Biophys Res Commun* **212**:564, 1995.
540. Gomez-Lira M, Perusi C, Brutti N, Farnetani MA, Margollicci MA, Rizzuto, Pignatti PF, et al: A 48-bp insertion between exon 13 and 14 of the HEXB gene causes infantile-onset Sandhoff disease. *Hum Mutat* **6**:260, 1995.

CHAPTER 154

The Neuronal Ceroid Lipofuscinoses

Sandra L. Hofmann ▪ Leena Peltonen

1. The neuronal ceroid lipofuscinoses (NCL) are a group of progressive hereditary neurodegenerative disorders of children that are distinguished from other neurodegenerative diseases by the accumulation of autofluorescent material ("aging pigment") in the brain and other tissues. The major clinical features include seizures, psychomotor deterioration, blindness, and premature death. Distinct subgroups of NCL have been recognized that differ in the age of onset of symptoms and the appearance of the storage material by electron microscopy. Three major groups—infantile (INCL), classical late infantile (LINCL), and juvenile (JNCL, also referred to as Batten disease)—are caused by autosomal recessive mutations in the CLN1, CLN2, and CLN3 genes, respectively. A small number of adult-onset NCL cases (tentatively designated CLN4), variant late-infantile forms (CLN5, CLN6, and tentatively, CLN7), and a progressive myoclonic epilepsy (CLN8) are also recognized as NCL disorders. The protein products of the CLN1 (palmitoyl-protein thioesterase) and CLN2 (pepinase) genes are soluble lysosomal enzymes, whereas the CLN3 protein (battenin) is a lysosomal membrane protein, as is (tentatively) the CLN5 protein. The identification of mutations in genes encoding lysosomal proteins in several forms of NCL has led to the recognition of the lipofuscinoses as true lysosomal storage disorders.
2. The clinical manifestations of the NCLs are distinctive and vary by age of onset. INCL is characterized by normal development to the age of 6 to 12 months, followed by mental retardation, arrest of cognitive and motor development, microcephaly, myoclonus, and visual deterioration. The EEG is isoelectric by about age 3. Classical LINCL presents between 2 and 4 years of age with severe myoclonic seizures and a slow progression to blindness. Distinctive "giant" visual and somatosensory evoked potentials are seen. Several variant forms of LINCL have clinical presentations intermediate between the classical late infantile and juvenile forms. Juvenile NCL (the most common form of NCL) presents as progressive visual failure between the ages of 4 to 9 years. Cognitive decline and motor deterioration follow inexorably, leading to death in the third or fourth decades. Seizures are a variable feature. Adult NCL (Kufs disease) is distinguished from the other NCL types by the absence of visual failure and an onset at around 30 years of age. A mild progressive myoclonic epilepsy in Finland ("Northern epilepsy") with a nearly normal life span is now also recognized as an NCL disease.
3. All of the NCLs show accumulation of autofluorescent storage material in multiple tissues by light microscopy. In the brain, ballooning of neurons by storage material, macrophage reaction, and cortical astrocytic gliosis may be striking. The cerebral cortex is disproportionately affected. The appearance of the storage material under the electron microscope is highly characteristic for each of the major NCL types: granular osmiophilic deposits (GROD) in INCL, curvilinear profiles in classical LINCL, and fingerprint profiles in JNCL. Variant forms of LINCL usually show a mixture of curvilinear and fingerprint profiles. Adult onset (Kufs) disease shows fingerprint profiles in most cases, but GROD in others. Although the lysosomal storage is present in peripheral tissues, tissue destruction and cell loss are nearly entirely restricted to the central nervous system.
4. In contrast to other lysosomal storage disorders, classical biochemical characterization of NCL storage material has not provided insights sufficient to uncover the underlying biochemical defects. This is probably due to the heterogeneous nature of the storage material. Subunit c of mitochondrial ATP synthase is a major storage protein identified in late infantile, juvenile, and adult forms of NCL, and sphingolipid activator proteins accumulate to a striking degree in INCL. The relationship between the nature of the storage material and the identified molecular defect still remains unclear.
5. Infantile NCL is caused by a deficiency in a lysosomal thioesterase activity (palmitoyl-protein thioesterase, or PPT) that removes fatty acids attached in thioester linkage to cysteine residues in proteins. Accumulation of small fatty acyl-cysteine-containing compounds has been demonstrated in cultured cells from INCL patients by metabolic labeling studies. Classical LINCL is caused by deficiency of a lysosomal protease, pepinase. It is one of the rare lysosomal storage diseases caused by a deficiency of a lysosomal protease. Proteins defective in JNCL, and a Finnish variant late infantile NCL, have also been identified. The protein defective in JNCL (battenin) is a lysosomal membrane protein, as is most probably the protein defective in Finnish variant LINCL. The function of these novel proteins is unknown.
6. With the possible exception of some adult-onset NCL families, the inheritance of the NCLs is autosomal recessive. At least eight genes are involved, and genetic linkage analysis has led to the identification of six confirmed genetic NCL loci. Four of these genes (CLN1, CLN2, CLN3, and CLN5) have been identified and characterized. Over 20 different mutations in the CLN1 and CLN3 genes have been

A list of standard abbreviations is located immediately preceding the index in each volume. Additional abbreviations used in this chapter include: GROD = granular osmiophilic deposits; INCL = infantile neuronal ceroid lipofuscinosis; JNCL = juvenile neuronal ceroid lipofuscinosis; LINCL = late infantile neuronal ceroid lipofuscinosis; NCL = neuronal ceroid lipofuscinosis; PPT = palmitoyl-protein thioesterase; and vLINCL = variant forms of late infantile neuronal ceroid lipofuscinosis.

reported, and phenotype-genotype correlations are beginning to emerge. The molecular genetics have also shown that previous clinical phenotypes do not always correlate with the molecular defect. For example, some JNCL cases ("GROD" variants) are caused by subtle mutations in the CLN1 gene.

7. **The laboratory diagnosis of NCL depends primarily on the recognition of storage material by electron microscopic examination of peripheral blood leukocytes or other accessible tissue. Diagnostic enzymatic assays are available for the infantile and classical late infantile forms. DNA-based diagnostic tests are available for the infantile, late infantile (classical and Finnish variant), and juvenile forms. Prenatal diagnosis is now available for most of the major forms.**
8. **No specific treatment is available for any of the NCL disorders beyond best supportive care. Refractory seizures are a distressing symptom for many patients and require the skilled use of anticonvulsant medications, usually in combination. As infantile and classical late infantile NCL are caused by deficiencies in soluble lysosomal enzymes, strategies designed to replace the defective lysosomal enzymes are appropriately applied to these disorders.**
9. **Naturally occurring NCL disorders have been described in the sheep, dog, and mouse. Syntenic relationships of chromosomal loci suggest that the New Zealand South-hampshire sheep and the *nclf* mouse are models for CLN6. Transgenic mouse models for the major forms of NCL are under development. The use of appropriate animal models will greatly facilitate the development of new therapies for the NCL disorders.**

INTRODUCTION

The neuronal ceroid lipofuscinoses (NCLs) form an interesting group of new lysosomal diseases, showing accumulation of autofluorescent material rich in protein, lipid, and carbohydrate in multiple cells and tissues. The disorders are manifested most dramatically in the brain. In contrast to other known lysosomal storage diseases, classical biochemical characterization of the storage material in NCL has not led to the identification of the underlying biochemical defects, presumably due to the heterogeneous nature of the accumulation. Only recently, molecular and genetic approaches to these disorders, guided by astute clinical and pathologic characterization, have recently provided many new insights into the NCL diseases, which exist both in humans and in animals.

NCL is distributed worldwide, and is probably the most common hereditary progressive neurodegenerative disorder in children, with an estimated carrier frequency of 1 percent of the population. These syndromes were earlier known as late infantile and juvenile types of amaurotic family idiocy, and in the 1970s were expanded to include the adult and infantile types of NCL disorders. Later, further dissection of subtypes took place; currently, four major NCL types, with additional "variant" types are recognized (Table 154-1). The common eponym "Batten disease," strictly applied, refers to the juvenile-onset form of NCL (for Batten-Spielmeyer-Vogt disease), but in some literature, the eponym is used to encompass all the NCLs.

Although molecular characterization is in the initial phase, all currently established NCL genes encode either lysosomal enzymes or lysosomal membrane proteins. Whether these proteins interact, and how the metabolic pathways involving the NCL proteins influence each other, remain open questions. Final characterization of the function of all NCL genes will eventually provide the basis for any treatment strategy for these currently incurable diseases, which dramatically affect the function and life span of neurons in the central nervous system.

CLINICAL MANIFESTATIONS

Infantile Neuronal Ceroid Lipofuscinosis

The clinical manifestations of infantile neuronal ceroid lipofuscinosis (INCL) are well documented in the Finnish population, where the disorder is prevalent. Virtually all Finnish children with the disorder are homozygous for a single point mutation that completely inactivates PPT.[1] Therefore, the Finnish cases reflect the most severe form of disease.[2–4]

Development is normal until the age of 6 to 12 months.[3] Nearly all children are saying single words and about one-third have learned to walk before the onset of symptoms. Typically, a suspicion of mental retardation arises between the ages of 12 and 18 months, after which motor development is arrested and hypotonia and truncal and limb ataxia develop. Microcephaly is universal. Visual deterioration may be noted as early as 1 year and has usually progressed to blindness by 24 months. Myoclonic jerks usually appear between the ages of 16 and 24 months, and characteristic rapid "knitting" movements are observed, but disappear in a few months. The hand movements raise a suspicion of Rett syndrome,[5] especially in girls. Many patients develop hyperexcitability and are difficult to manage during the second year. Generalized convulsions are present in a minority of subjects, and are often difficult to distinguish from frequent myoclonic jerks. A more quiescent stage is entered during the third year, which is characterized by the absence of voluntary movements, hypotonia with episodes of opisthotonos, and myoclonic jerks with any stimulation. After age 5, flexion contractures are common, and generalized hirsutism, acne, and occasional precocious puberty are noted, probably indicating dysfunction of the hypothalamic-pituitary axis. The mean age at death in these most severely affected of children is 6.5 years.

Clinical manifestations outside of the central nervous system have not been reported. Hepatosplenomegaly and bone abnormalities, seen in other lysosomal storage diseases, are noticeably absent. Electromyography and motor nerve conduction velocities are normal.[3] Routine blood, urinary, and cerebrospinal fluid tests are normal, and vacuolated peripheral blood lymphocytes are not seen.

Electroencephalography (EEG), electroretinography (ERG), and visual and somatosensory evoked potentials (VEPs and SEPs) have been used to study the progression of the neuronal dysfunction in this disorder.[6] The EEG is the first of these tests to reveal abnormalities, but may be normal at the preclinical stage. Early EEG abnormalities include attenuated reaction to passive eye opening and closing, disturbances in background activity and diminution in amplitude, and the disappearance of sleep spindles. The EEG is inactive by the age of 3 years. Evoked potentials are normal in the early stages. SEPs show abnormalities at 1.7 years, with ERG and VEP abnormalities by the age of 2.5. All neurophysiological reactions are extinguished by age 4 years.

Computed tomography (CT)[7] and magnetic resonance imaging (MRI) findings[8,9] in INCL have been reported. MRI abnormalities may be detected before clinical symptoms. Signal loss is found in the thalamus in all patients over the age of 12 months. Other important early findings are generalized cerebral atrophy and thin periventricular high-signal rims from 13 months onward on T2-weighted images. Typical late findings are extreme cerebral atrophy and hypointensity of gray matter in relation to white matter on T2-weighted images, which is striking because it gives a pattern that is the reverse of normal. CT and MRI may be of value in distinguishing INCL from Rett syndrome.[4,10] Brain perfusion (SPECT)[11] and localized proton magnetic resonance spectroscopy[12] have been used to document disturbances in brain perfusion and cerebral metabolic disturbances, respectively.

Late Onset and Variant Forms of Neuronal Ceroid Lipofuscinosis with Granular Osmiophilic Deposits

Perhaps 5 to 10 percent of all neuronal ceroid lipofuscinosis cases presenting after the age of 2 years show the granular

Table 154-1 Diagnostic Criteria for the Established Human Forms of Neuronal Ceroid Lipofuscinosis*

Disease Entity† Eponyms:	*Infantile NCL (INCL)* Santavuori-Haltia Disease CLN1 MIM 256730	*Late Infantile NCL (LINCL)* Jansky-Bielschowsky Disease CLN2, "Classical" LINCL MIM 204500	*Late Infantile NCL (LINCL)* Finnish Variant CLN5 MIM 256731	*Late Infantile NCL (LINCL)* Variant/Atypical CLN6 MIM 601780	*Juvenile NCL (JNCL)* Batten-Spielmeyer-Vogt Disease CLN3 MIM 204200	*Adult NCL* Kufs Disease CLN4(?) MIM 204300
Clinical symptoms						
Visual failure—onset and progression	12–22 months	2–3 years Slow progression	5–7 years Blind by 9–10 years	4–5 years	4–9 years Blind by 6–14 years	None
Seizures—onset	6–24 months	2.5–3.5 years (severe)	6–10 years	5–6 years	8–16 years	
Dementia—onset	6–18 months	2.5–3.5 years	4–7 years	5–9 years	6–9 years	30 years
Inability to walk	12–18 months	3.5–6 years	8–10 years	10–20 years	10–20 years	
Motor dysfunction	Stereotypic hand motions	Myoclonus	Myoclonus	Myoclonus	Myoclonus	Facial dyskinesia
Other findings	Choreoathetosis	Ataxia	Ataxia	Ataxia	Slurred speech, echolalia (onset 10–20 years	Myoclonus Psychosis
Age at death	< 14 years	10–15 years	13–30 years	10–30 years	20–40 years	> 20–40 years
Retinal pathology						
Macular degeneration	+	+	+	+	+	—
Pigment aggregation	—	+	—	+	+	—
ERG absent by age	12 months	3–4 years	8 years	4–5 years	5–7 years	—
Neurophysiology						
EEG (helpful findings)	Flattening 18–24 months Isoelectric 3–4 years Photic response absent	Large polyspikes after single flashes (early stage)				
Visual evoked potential	↓, Absent > 12 months	↑↑	↑↑ (early, then ↓)	↑↑	↓	↓
Somatosensory evoked potenial	↓, Absent < 12 months	↑↑	↑↑	↑↑	↓	↓
Neuroimaging						
(CT/MRI)—brain atrophy	++	+	+	?	+	+
Morphology						
LM-vacuolated lymphocytes	—	—	—	—	++	—
EM-predominant inclusions	Granular	Curvillinear	Curvilinear/Fingerprint	Curvilinear/Fingerprint	Fingerprint	Variable

*Adapted from Kohlschütter et al.[29] with additional data from references 14, 27, 38, 40 and 156.
† The classification of NCL types by age of onset, while useful, is imperfect. For example, patients with less severe mutations in the CLN1 gene may overlap with the late infantile and juvenile presentations. In general, this table reflects the most severely affected individuals with a given gene defect.
Abbreviations; LM, light microscopy; EM, electron microscopy

osmiophilic deposits (GROD) that are characteristic of INCL. It is now appreciated that these cases represent milder forms of PPT deficiency caused by certain missense mutations in the PPT (CLN1) gene.[13–15] These patients are indistinguishable on clinical grounds from LINCL or JNCL patients, who have underlying mutations in the CLN2 or CLN3 genes, respectively.

Several independent cases of INCL associated with osteopetrosis have been described.[16,17] Rare congenital cases of neuronal ceroid lipofuscinosis[18–20] have also been reported. The underlying molecular defect in these cases is unknown.

Classical Late Infantile Neuronal Ceroid Lipofuscinosis

Recognition of classical LINCL as a distinct pathologic entity came with the routine examination of storage material by electron microscopy and the description of the pathognomonic type of inclusion, the curvilinear body.[21–23] A number of large series of cases have been described.[24–28]

Classical LINCL typically presents between the ages of 2 and 4 years.[29] Seizures are the earliest and most remarkable feature. Both myoclonic and generalized tonic-clonic convulsions are seen. These are followed by mental retardation, ataxia, and dementia. Only a minority of patients present with clinically evident visual impairment, but blindness eventually develops. Inexorably, the child enters an unresponsive state with continuous myoclonic and occasional grand mal seizures. Death occurs at 10 to 15 years.

As with the other forms of neuronal ceroid lipofuscinosis, the clinical manifestations are limited to the central nervous system. There is no hepatosplenomegaly or bony involvement. Routine blood chemistries are normal.

Neurophysiological studies are well documented and help distinguish classical late infantile from other neuronal ceroid lipofuscinoses.[30–32] The EEG shows large amplitude irregular slow activity and polyphasic spikes that are elicited with low rates of photic stimulation. Visual evoked potentials show grossly enlarged early components ("giant" wave) and, in some cases, a grossly enlarged somatosensory evoked potential is seen. The electroretinogram is said to be normal initially and becomes unrecordable as the disease progresses.

Computed tomography and magnetic resonance imaging have been used to aid in diagnosis and to follow the course of the disease.[33–35] Bilateral, periventricular hyperintensities in the T2-weighted images, without changes in the basal ganglia, are seen. Predominance of cerebral atrophy in the infratentorial area is typical.[33,34] Positron emission tomography was reported in one case.[36] Brain perfusion (SPECT) studies have also shown abnormalities.[37]

Variant Forms of Late Infantile Neural Ceroid Lipofuscinosis

Clinical phenotype in most of the atypical or variant forms of CLN (vLINCL) is intermediate between classic CLN2 and CLN3. A cluster of 16 families in Finland[38] represents one variant vLINCL (CLN5). Another similar clustering of variant cases has been found in Great Britain[39] and a third cluster has been found in Newfoundland.[25] The clinical picture includes motor clumsiness followed by progressive visual failure, mental and motor deterioration, and later by myoclonus and seizures. Visual failure becomes evident after these initial symptoms. Neurophysiological findings of all these forms are virtually identical to those in classic CLN2, except that the onset is at the age of 5 to 7 years. MRI intensity changes appear early, at least in the Finnish variant cases, and they show changes similar to the classical LINCL.[7] The age of death is somewhat later (between 13 and 30 years) than in the classic form.[40] The symptoms are restricted to the central nervous system and there is no hepatosplenomegaly or other tissue involvement. Routine laboratory tests are also normal.

Juvenile Neuronal Ceroid Lipofuscinosis (Batten Disease)

The leading symptom of JNCL is impaired vision, which usually appears between the ages of 4 and 7 years, but occasionally later.[40,41] Mental retardation develops slowly and is often first noticed at school. Some patients have minor psychologic disturbances several years before the impaired vision. Compulsive speaking and mumbling become evident in the first half of the second decade and severe dysarthria develops a few years later. Dementia often becomes profound late in the course of the disease. Motor dysfunction is due to extrapyramidal, slight pyramidal, and cerebellar disturbances, manifesting as Parkinson-like dysfunction and an inability to walk toward the end of the course of the disease. Epileptic seizures of generalized or complex partial type occur at about 10 years, but they may not manifest at all. The ocular fundi show macular degeneration, optic atrophy, and retinal degeneration. At a later stage, the macula may not be clearly visible, and pigment aggregations usually develop after the age of 10.[42]

The EEG shows slow, nonspecific deterioration. Abolished noncorneal electroretinogram (ERG) is an early finding, present in almost all children at the time that the disease is first suspected (5 to 6 years of age). The flash-evoked visual potential is pathologic at the time of the first symptoms and becomes abolished in most patients during the second decade (see reference 43 for a recent review of the electrophysiologic eye findings in the NCLs). The MRI changes in the brain are detectable after the first decade of life, and the patients become nonambulatory between 13 and 30 years of age; the age at death varies within a range of 13 to 40 years. It is thus obvious that, in clinical practice, some patients have a very slow course, while others evolve more rapidly.[40]

PATHOLOGY

To a large extent, each form of NCL has a characteristic ultrastructural appearance to the storage bodies, which characteristic has aided in the dissection of the underlying enzymatic and gene defect. The three major groups, infantile (INCL), classical late infantile (LINCL), and juvenile (JNCL) are characterized by granular osmiophilic deposits (GROD), curvilinear inclusions, or fingerprint profiles, respectively (Fig. 154-1, panels A to C). Variant forms of NCL may show a "mixed" picture with more than one ultrastructural appearance in the same cell (Fig. 154-1, panel D). For example, the finding of GROD in some late infantile and juvenile-onset cases has led to the appreciation that milder defects in the CLN1 gene, normally associated with infantile NCL, may present later in life.

Infantile Neuronal Ceroid Lipofuscinosis

The major findings at autopsy are limited to the central nervous system.[44,45] The brain is very small and atrophic, often weighing less than 500 g (Fig. 154-2). There is diffuse cerebral gyral atrophy and the cerebral cortex is reduced to a thin rim approximately 1 to 2 mm thick. The cerebellum is also atrophic, but the brainstem and spinal cord are less affected. On histologic examination, most of the cerebral cortex is almost entirely depleted of neurons. One exception is the Betz cells of the motor cortex, which are ballooned and filled with granular deposits. Large numbers of macrophages form clusters around large decaying neurons. There is intense cortical fibrillary astrocytic gliosis. In the cerebellar cortex, a total loss of granule cells and Purkinje cells is seen. Most of the remaining areas of the central nervous system show a variable degree of neuronal loss, with ballooning of residual nerve cells bodies with granular material, and macrophage and astrocytic reaction. The thalamic nuclei are largely destroyed, whereas the hypothalamus and subthalamus are relatively spared. In the peripheral and autonomic nervous system, spinal ganglion cells show marked accumulations and some destruction. Cranial nerves (except the optic nerve) and spinal nerve roots are spared. Visceral ganglia, such as the mucosal and myenteric plexuses, are distended with granules.

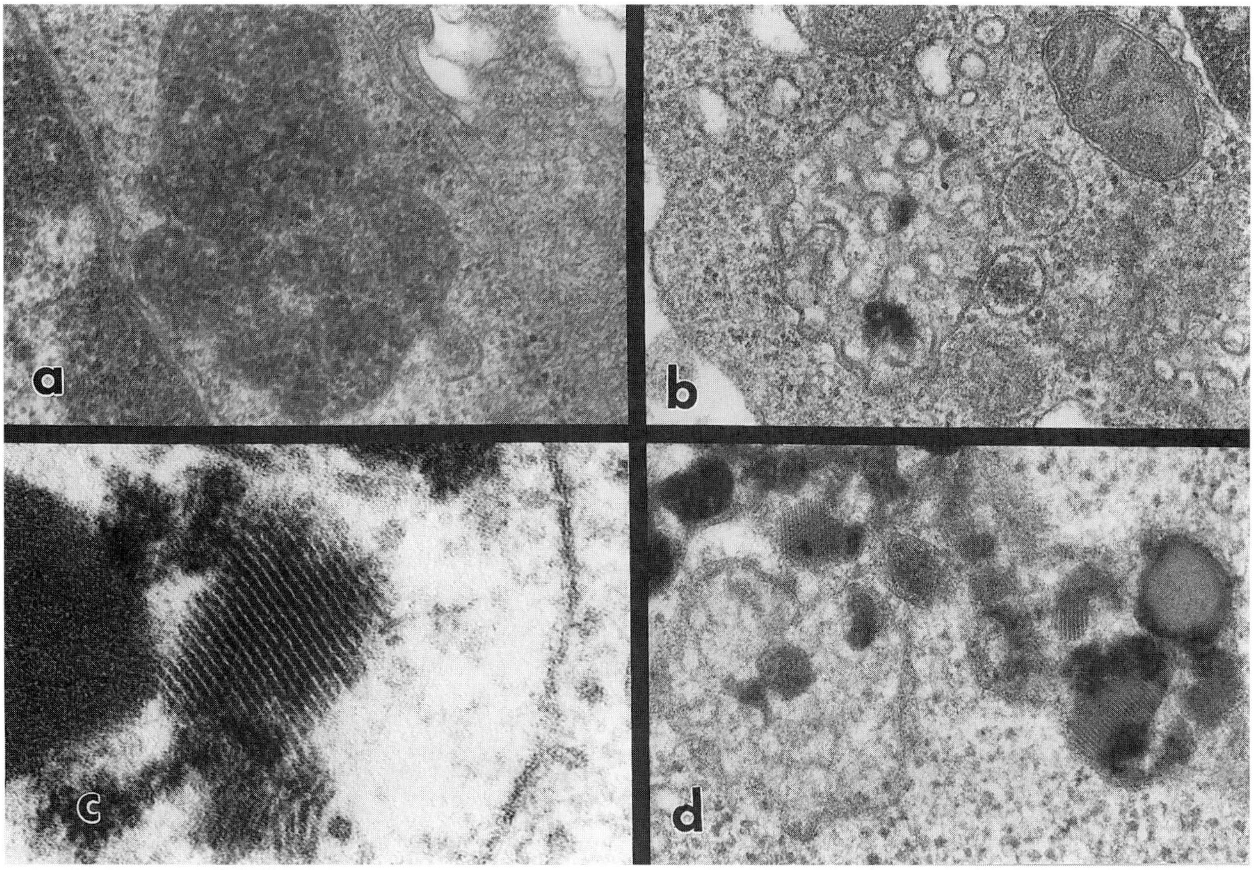

Fig. 154-1 Lysosomal storage material in buffy coat (leukocyte) preparations from subjects with various types of NCL as seen by electron microscopy. *A*, Granular osmiophilic deposits (GRODs) in an INCL (*CLN1−/−*) subject (magnification: ×80,000); *B*, Curvilinear inclusions in a classical LINCL (*CLN2−/−*) subject (magnification: ×63,000); *C*, Fingerprint profiles in a typical JNCL (*CLN3−/−*) subject (magnification: ×185,000); *D*, Mixed granular, curvilinear, and fingerprint inclusions in a juvenile-onset PPT-deficient NCL subject (*CLN1−/−*) (magnification: ×64,500). (*Courtesy of K. Wisniewski, Institute for Basic Research, Staten Island, NY.*)

The neuropathologic changes in INCL assessed by biopsy during the progress of the disease can be roughly divided into three stages. In stage I, there is an accumulation of lipopigment and slight to moderate loss of cortical neurons coupled to severe astrocytosis and invasion of the cortex by macrophages (patients up to 2 years of age). Stage II (2 to 4 years of age) is characterized by a subtotal loss of cortical neurons and extensive astrocytosis. The cortex is infiltrated by macrophages, and the white matter shows loss of the myelin sheath. In stage III (after 4 years of age), the cortex is entirely depleted of neurons, axon, and myelin sheaths. The cortex and convolutional white matter are occupied by astrocytes and macrophages have disappeared. In the retina, the storage material causes atrophy of the optic nerve and loss of its myelin sheath.[46]

Granular material (GROD) is seen in a number of extraneural tissues, but is not associated with tissue destruction,[44] except perhaps in the case of the testis, where extensive accumulation of storage material in the germinal epithelium with cell destruction and macrophage reaction has been described.[44] Striking accumulations also occur in thyroid follicles, exocrine pancreas, and distal convoluted tubules and glomerular podocytes of the kidney. Remarkably, hepatocytes seem to be devoid of storage material. Macrophages in a variety of tissues have marked accumulations. Histochemically, the storage material shows bright yellow-green autofluorescence under ultraviolet light, both in the central nervous system and in extraneural tissues.

Electron microscopic exam shows characteristic membrane-delimited granular osmiophilic deposits.[44,45] The internal structure is electron-dense, homogeneous, and finely granular. In nerve cells and other cell types, globular particles 0.2 μM to 0.5 μM in diameter seem to coalesce into larger aggregates of up to 3 μM in diameter, with an appearance of "snowballs" packed together in some areas. The ultrastructure of the material in renal podocytes is somewhat different, filling more of the cytoplasm with large amounts of material with ill-defined borders.

In the milder forms of "infantile" neuronal ceroid lipofuscinosis caused by PPT deficiency, granular osmiophilic deposits also predominate, but minor amounts of curvilinear or fingerprint inclusions may be seen, causing some diagnostic confusion.[13,14,28]

Late Infantile Neuronal Ceroid Lipofuscinosis

As in all the neuronal ceroid lipofuscinoses, the gross pathology is confined to the central nervous system. Duffy et al.[21] and Gonatas et al.[22] described in detail the gross brain pathology as well as the characteristic ultrastructural findings. Brain weight is severely diminished (<1000 g). There is slight parieto-occipital atrophy and severe atrophy of the cerebellar folia. Light microscopy shows an eosinophilic material within the cytoplasm of almost every nerve cell. A marked decrease in the number of neurons in the cortex is observed with a relative sparing of the molecular and external granular layers. There was a moderate to marked astrocytic proliferation described in one case,[21] but not in two others.[22] Similar changes are present in the basal ganglia, brain stem, cerebellum, and spinal cord. The changes in the thalamus are more marked than in the caudate, putamen, and globus pallidus.

The lysosomal nature of the curvilinear bodies has been demonstrated at the light microscopic level by staining for acid phosphatases.[22] On frozen sections, the periodic acid-Schiff reaction, the Sudan black, and Oil Red O stains are positive. The inclusions are not extractable to chloroform-methanol.[21–23]

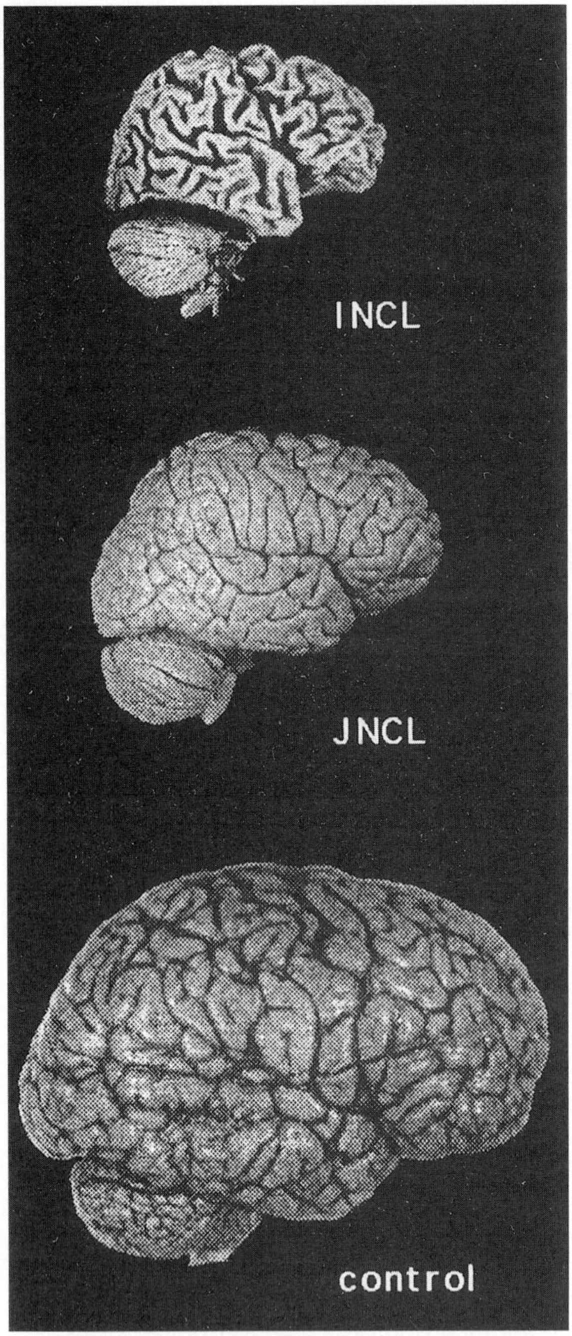

Fig. 154-2 Gross anatomic appearance of brains obtained from infantile and juvenile cases with NCL and an unaffected child. (*Courtesy of J. Tyynelä, University of Helsinki.*)

Curvilinear inclusion bodies are a very distinct ultrastructural hallmark of the disease. The outlines of the bodies are 0.2 to 2.6 μm in diameter and consist of short curvilinear profiles, a few of which form complete circles as seen in cross-section.[21] Inclusions are not only seen in the central nervous system, but can also be seen in cells of the spleen and colon,[21] muscle, peripheral nerve, and skin.[23]

Variant Forms of Late Infantile Neuronal Ceroid Lipofuscinosis

All variant forms of late infantile CLN share similar pathologic findings. Vacuolated lymphocytes are not present and ultrastructural analysis reveals cytosomes with curvilinear profiles, fingerprint profiles, or both. Storage material accumulates in extraneural tissues, often resembling the juvenile form in distribution.[38]

Subunit c of mitochondrial ATP synthase and small quantities of sphingolipid activator proteins (saposins) A and D accumulate in vLINCL tissues. These proteins colocalize in the same storage bodies in all tissues examined, including brain, heart, muscle, and liver. However, in kidney and pancreas, the saposin-containing and ATP-synthase subunit c immunoreactive storage granules are reported to appear in different cell types.[47]

Juvenile Neuronal Ceroid Lipofuscinosis

The classical neuropathology of JNCL was described at the beginning of the century, and the description remains valid today (reviewed in reference 48). The macroscopic appearance of the brain is nearly normal, but with moderately, or even severely, decreased weight. The skull bones are slightly thickened as a reflection of brain atrophy. However, the patients are not microcephalic. The cerebral cortex is narrowed, with yellow-brown discoloration, and the white matter is atrophic. Loss of neurons is observable in all parts of the brains, but the severity of this feature varies, and in some brain areas, it may be difficult to observe. Neuronal loss is associated with reactive astrocytosis.

The most characteristic histologic feature is a change in the cortical neurons known as the Shaffer-Spielmeyer process. The neurons are distended by perikaryonal granular lipopigment, and they become rounded, superficially resembling those in Tay-Sachs and Niemann-Pick diseases; the ballooning, however, never reaches the degree seen in the sphingolipidoses. The accumulation of lipopigment is symmetrical, and the nuclei are pushed to the side of dendritic processes or axon hillocks. In the cortical neurons of the forebrain, the lipopigment aggregations distend the proximal parts of the axons, whereas in the Purkinje cells the dendritic processes are distended. The ballooning and rounding of the neurons are most evident in the cortical neurons of the forebrain and cerebellum. These changes are less obvious, but do exist, in the midbrain, medulla oblongata, and spinal cord. Although the white matter is relatively well preserved with little demyelinization, gliosis is present. Microglia harbor lipopigments, best visualized by staining with PAS. In areas of microgliosis, the capillary endothelial cells contain lipopigments.[46]

The accumulation of lipopigments in extraneural cells in Batten disease was established over 60 years ago.[49] At the light microscopic level, myocardium, liver, spleen, gut wall, and the kidneys are most commonly involved. By electron microscopy, the variety of the cell types showing lipopigment inclusions is much wider. This extraneural manifestation of NCL, first noted in 1948,[50] was very important in the differential diagnosis of the NCL subtypes before the advent of electron microscopy. JNCL is the only NCL subtype in which vacuolated peripheral blood lymphocytes are seen, although they are found in many other lysosome storage disorders.

The progressive visual failure in JNCL has stimulated analyses of the ocular pathology in JNCL.[51] The primary lesion is degeneration of the retinal neuroepithelium, while the remaining neuronal elements of the retina are spared for a long time. In advanced cases, lipopigment-containing cells invade all layers of the retina, and detailed studies show almost complete loss of rods, cones, and both outer nuclear and plexiform layers. The most severe changes are in the central part of the retina, where the peripheral parts are partially preserved. The central part of the pigment epithelium is atrophic and depigmented, but some pigment is preserved in the peripheral parts. Melanin-containing perivascular macrophages are numerous, particularly in the periphery of the fundus. Lipopigment is abundant in the ganglion cells and gliotic astrocytes.[51]

BIOCHEMICAL PATHOLOGY

The NCLs are relative latecomers to the arena of lysosomal storage diseases, because the underlying lysosomal enzyme defects have only recently been identified. In contrast to previously known lysosomal storage diseases (the gangliosidoses and mucopolysaccharidoses, for instance), the nature of the stored material did not provide clues as to the underlying biochemical defect. In retrospect, this may be explained by the heterogeneous nature of the undegraded material. For example, a deficiency of a lysosomal protease is known to cause LINCL, and one might expect that the resulting storage material might contain a complex mixture of undegraded peptides. In addition, it is possible that deficiencies in the NCL lysosomal proteins or enzymes cause a more general dysfunction of lysosomes in which secondary changes, only indirectly related to the primary defect, are more prominent. Previous studies on the biochemical nature of the storage material in the NCLs that were completed before the enzyme or protein defects were known are described in the next section. The relationship between these underlying defects and the observed biochemical storage is still unclear and remains an active area of investigation.

Biochemical Storage

INCL. When examined by histochemistry, the storage material is resistant to lipid solvents and, in unstained sections, is colorless to slightly yellow. The granular deposits are acid-fast, strongly PAS-positive, and stain intensely with Sudan black B, indicating the presence of significant amounts of both carbohydrate and lipid. Strong acid phophatase activity is easily demonstrated, emphasizing the lysosomal nature of the storage bodies.[45] Autofluorescent storage particles with preserved ultrastructure have been purified from INCL brains by homogenization and sucrose[52] or cesium chloride[53] density gradient ultracentrifugation. The storage material consists of 40 percent protein and 35 percent lipid by dry weight.[53] Interestingly, the major identifiable proteins in the storage material are saposins A and D and fragments of glial fibrillary acidic protein.[53] Saposins (sphingolipid activator proteins) accumulate in tissues of patients with several lysosomal storage diseases,[54] and the significance of its striking accumulation in INCL is unknown. Mitochondrial ATPase subunit c accumulation is not a consistent feature, in contrast to late infantile and juvenile-onset NCL.[55] Biochemical studies that have been performed on the brains of patients with INCL largely reflect the severe neuronal loss in the disease. Total lipids are reduced and the yield of myelin is less than 2 percent of normal.[56,57] Long chain polyunsaturated fatty acids are reduced. A marked fall in lipid-bound neuraminic acid is seen.[45] No directed biochemical analysis of INCL brain storage material has been reported in the short time since the discovery of the enzyme defect. Total lack of PPT activity was recorded from autopsy samples of INCL brain.[1]

LINCL. Subunit c of mitochondrial ATP synthase is a major protein component of the storage material in ovine neuronal ceroid lipofuscinosis[59] and in classical LINCL (and to a lesser extent, JNCL).[55] A specific delay in the degradation of subunit c within late infantile cells has been shown.[60,61] Furthermore, the slower degradation is accounted for by a defect in lysosomal proteolysis, as lysosomal extracts from late infantile cells degrade purified subunit c more slowly in vitro.[62] It is not currently known whether subunit c is a substrate for the lysosomal protease defective in classical LINCL, nor whether the defect in this protease directly accounts for the subunit c accumulation. Other biochemical abnormalities in classical LINCL, including the accumulation of dolichol oligosaccharide and oligosaccharyl phosphates, are felt to be secondary to the lysosomal storage.[63]

JNCL. The lipopigments accumulating in JNCL are very similar to the age-related pigments accumulating in normal tissues. The similarity of staining characteristics to those of lipofuscin and ceroid, confirmed by several authors, applies to all types and variants of NCL with insignificant variations. The lipopigments are insoluble in polar and nonpolar solvents, making their study possible in ordinary paraffin sections, where they can be stained for easier detection using PAS, Sudan black B, or acid fuchsin. The material also shows bright yellow autofluorescence under ultraviolet light. The lipopigment granules have an intense activity of acid phosphatase, suggesting an association with lysosomes. This impression has been confirmed by electron microscopic studies and, to some extent later, by the molecular defects identified.

The storage material is already identifiable in the prenatal period, and the typical inclusion profiles have been reported in the first trimester.[64–66] This finding suggests that abnormal levels of accumulated material can be tolerated by cells and tissues to a certain extent. Two fundamental questions that remain unanswered are whether cell death is caused directly by the storage material or for other reasons, and why neuronal cells are most affected while storage material accumulates in multiple cell types.

The major component of the storage material in JNCL inclusions is subunit c of the mitochondrial ATP synthase complex.[55,67] However, cells from JNCL patients show less intense staining for subunit c than cells from patients with LINCL.[67,68] Subunit c is an essential membrane component of the proton channel of the large oligometric complex, ATP synthase, which generates ATP by oxidative phosphorylation. Another protein, subunit c of vacuolar ATPase, is also deposited to some degree in several of the naturally occurring animal models of NCL.[69,70] Vacuolar subunit c (also known as ductin) is a membrane protein that is part of both the vacuolar H^+ translocating ATPase (involved in acidification) and of gap junctions. Mitochondrial ATP synthase subunit c also accumulates in other lysosomal disorders including mucopolysaccharidosis I, II, IIIA, multiple sulfatase deficiency, mucolipidosis I, Niemann-Pick types A and C, and G_{M1} and G_{M2} gangliosidoses.[68,71] However, in these cases, the accumulation is observed only in neurons, whereas in the NCL diseases, cells outside the nervous system also accumulate subunit c, suggesting that the subunit c storage is more specific for NCL diseases than for other lysosomal disorders.

Interestingly, the stored subunit c contains a trimethyllysine residue in the human NCLs[72–74] and in three animal models (mouse, dog, and sheep),[72,75,76] although whether this modified amino acid residue is a direct cause of the accumulation, a result of its accumulation, or even a normal feature remains unknown.

Other minor storage components are two of the sphingolipid activator proteins or saposins.[53] Saposins are small, heat-stable, lysosomal proteins, originating from a single precursor molecule that is cleaved to release four mature saposins.[77] Saposins activate lysosomal hydrolases involved in glycosphingolipid degradation. Saposins A and D are the major accumulating saposins in all NCL diseases, including JNCL,[78] as well as in animal models for NCL.[70] Because both subunit c and saposins are extremely hydrophobic molecules with a tendency to self-aggregate, the underlying problem in the NCLs may be the processing and disposal of these hydrophobic molecules.

In addition to the accumulation of storage material, many other biochemical changes have been reported in tissues from NCL patients or affected animals. Based on the identified defects, various biochemical deficiencies have been proposed. These include a defect in proteases,[79] abnormal lipid/fatty acid peroxidation,[80] abnormal dolichol metabolism,[81–84] and abnormal carnitine biosynthesis.[85] Although the gene defect is now known, the issue of the relationship between the gene defect and these biochemical findings remains unsolved until the cellular function of this membrane protein is clarified.

Enzyme and Protein Deficiencies in the NCLs

Palmitoyl-protein Thioesterase (PPT; CLN1). Virtually all cases of neuronal ceroid lipofuscinosis with predominantly granular osmiophilic deposits, or GROD (which would include all INCL), have an underlying deficiency in PPT activity as a result of mutations in the PPT gene.[1,13,14] Palmitoyl-protein thioesterase [E.C. 3.1.2.22] is a recently described lysosomal enzyme that removes long chain fatty acids (usually palmitate) from cysteine residues in proteins.[87] The covalent linkage involves a thioester bond between the carboxyl end of the fatty acid and the sulfhydryl

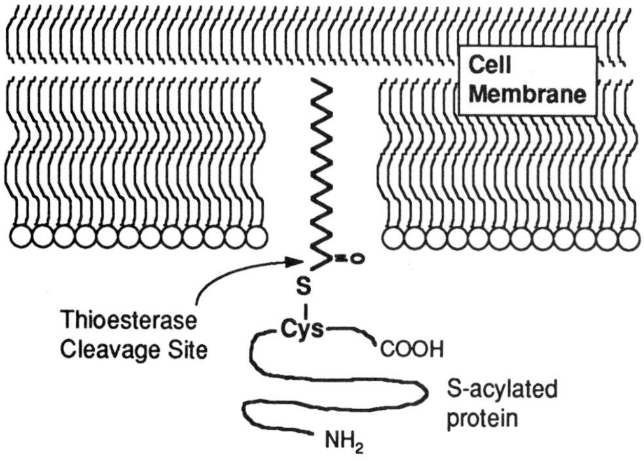

Fig. 154-3 A "typical" palmitoylated protein is normally found in association with the inner surface of the plasma membrane. The thioester bond that is hydrolyzed by palmitoyl-protein thioesterase is shown. The natural substrates of lysosomal palmitoyl-protein thioesterase are palmitoylated proteins and peptides undergoing degradation in the lysosome.

group of the cysteine residue, hence the designation of the enzyme that hydrolyzes this reaction as a thioesterase (Fig. 154-3).

S-acylation at cysteine residues is a common post-translational modification of proteins.[88] The fatty acylated cysteine residue is most often located at the inner surface of the plasma membrane. Cycles of acylation and deacylation of proteins may regulate certain protein-protein or protein-membrane interactions that are important in cellular signal transduction.[89] However, the function of lysosomal PPT appears to be the removal of covalently bound fatty acids from S-acylated proteins that arrive in the lysosome for degradation.[90]

PPT activity was first demonstrated in tissue extracts from bovine brain, a rich source of the enzyme.[87] The substrate for the detection of enzyme activity was H-Ras, a protein that is both palmitoylated and farnesylated near the C-terminus. (Farnesylation is a lipid modification that occurs in a stable thioether linkage to cysteine residues in proteins.) Specific removal of the palmitate (but not the farnesyl group) from the protein could be demonstrated. The enzyme assay was used to guide the purification of PPT to homogeneity.[87] Because the enzyme has a neutral pH optimum for acyl-protein substrates, its lysosomal nature was not suspected until the cloning of the cDNA[91] and subsequent studies of its gene localization[92] and involvement in neuronal ceroid lipofuscinosis, a storage disorder.[1]

cDNAs encoding human,[92] bovine,[91] rat,[91] and mouse[93] PPT have been characterized. A major 2.5-kb mRNA is detected in human, bovine, and rat tissues. (A second 1.4-kb mRNA is detected in the rat, a consequence of use of an alternative polyadenylation site present only in the rat gene.) The human PPT cDNA consists of a short 5′-untranslated region of 14 base pairs, an open reading frame of 918 base pairs, and a 1388-base pair 3′ untranslated region. The amino acid sequence deduced from the cDNA contains 306 amino acids, of which the first 25 amino acids constitute a leader peptide. Sequence motifs characteristic of thioesterases[94] (glycine-X-serine-X-glycine and glycine-aspartic acid-histidine) are present at amino acid residues 113 to 117 and 287 to 289, respectively. Thioesterases contain the classical "catalytic triad" residues of serine, aspartic (or glutamic) acid, and histidine, as do many lipases and proteases.[95,96] Three potential asparagine-linked glycosylation sites are found near the C-terminus of the protein at positions 197, 212, and 232. All of these sites are utilized to some degree in vivo.[91,97]

PPT mRNA is found ubiquitously in a variety of tissues from the human[92] and rat,[91] with fairly high and uniform levels in lung, spleen, brain, and testis, and relatively little mRNA in liver and skeletal muscle. The correlation between mRNA levels and levels of enzyme activity is imperfect, as much higher activity (and protein) levels are found in testis and brain as compared to other tissues.[87] Interestingly, brain and testis are the two most severely affected organs histopathologically in INCL.[44] The analysis of PPT transcript abundance by *in situ* hybridization of mouse brain has revealed that PPT transcripts are expressed widely but not homogeneously in the mouse brain and the expression follows a specific temporal pattern (J. Isosomppi, personal communication). The signal is most intensive in the cerebral cortex (layers II, IV, and V), hippocampal CA1 to CA3 pyramidal cells, dentate gyrus granule cells, and hypothalamus. Localization of PPT transcripts and immunoreactivity is spatially and temporally well correlated. Immunostaining is localized to axons and dendrites, especially in the pyramidal and granular cells of the hippocampus, correlating well, both spatially and temporally, with immunoreactivity of a presynaptic vesicle membrane protein, synaptophysin (J. Isosomppi, personal communication).

The lysosomal targeting and intracellular localization of PPT have been demonstrated through studies of mannose 6-phosphate-mediated cellular uptake[98–100] and immunofluorescence studies.[99] The synthesis and intracellular targeting of PPT are typical for a lysosomal enzyme.[91,98,99] In contrast to a number of other lysosomal enzymes, activation by internal cleavage does not appear to be a feature of the thioesterase. The mature enzyme is a doublet at 37 kDa/35 kDa, due to heterogeneous glycosylation.[91,98,99] Two amino-terminal amino acids (histidine-leucine) that are predicted to be present from analysis of the cDNA, and which are present in the recombinant enzyme, are not present in the mature enzyme purified from brain. This minor processing is probably of little significance, as both unprocessed and amino-terminally processed forms are fully active.[91]

Studies with the purified, recombinant enzyme have shown a preference for long chain fatty acids of 14 to 18 carbons, with virtually no activity using substrates of 6 carbons or less.[91] The enzyme will degrade noncysteine-containing thioesters such as palmitoyl CoA. Sensitivity to diethylpyrocarbonate indicates that an essential histidine residue may be involved in catalysis, and insensitivity to phenylmethanesulfonyl fluoride distinguishes this enzyme from other cellular esterases and was an aid to its identification and purification.[87] The pH optimum is broad and varies with different substrates.

Metabolic labeling studies have provided some insight into the metabolic defect in INCL.[101] When cells from PPT-deficient subjects are incubated with [^{35}S]cysteine and [^{3}H]palmitate, small lipid thioesters containing these labels accumulate in a time-dependent manner (Fig. 154-4). Furthermore, the lipid cysteine thioesters appear to be derived from protein, because cycloheximide blocks their formation. This observation implies that the cysteine must first be incorporated into protein in order to appear in the abnormal products. The fatty acid cysteine thioesters are substrates for the thioesterase in vitro. In addition, their accumulation can be reversed by the addition of PPT to the cell culture medium in cross-correction experiments,[101] especially if the enzyme is modified with mannose 6-phosphate and is therefore competent for uptake through the mannose 6-phosphate receptor pathway.

The mechanism whereby deficiency of PPT leads to severe and selective neurodegeneration is unknown. One possibility is that the lipid-cysteine thioesters consist of small peptides that are resistant to degradation by virtue of their fatty acid modification. This "indigestible" proteolipid material may be particularly harmful to neurons. By analogy, other neurodegenerative disorders, such as Alzheimer disease, the prion diseases, and the polyglutamine disorders, are characterized by the accumulation of unmetabolized peptides. Unfortunately, in none of these diseases is the link between the storage and selective neuronal toxicity well understood.

Pepinase (CLN2; LINCL). Classical LINCL is caused by a deficiency in a novel pepstatin-insensitive lysosomal protease,

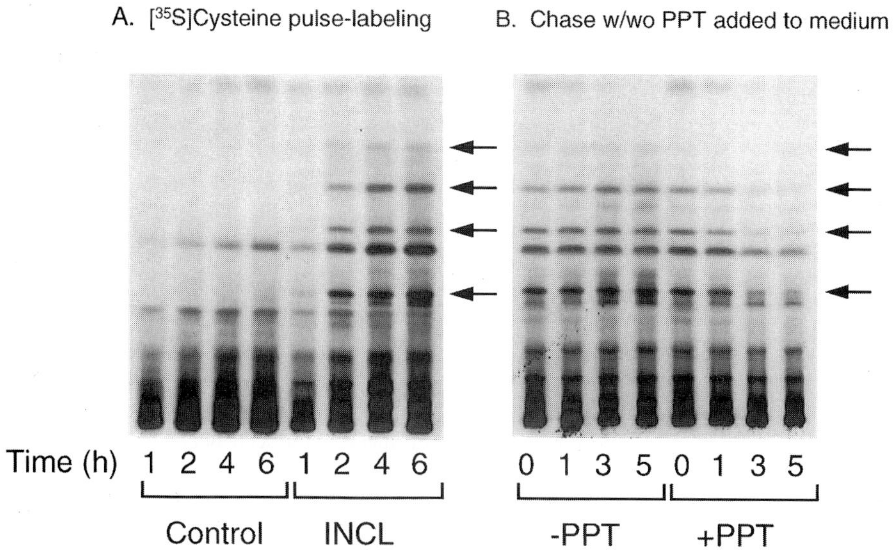

Fig. 154-4 Accumulation of [^{35}S]cysteine-labeled lipids in normal and INCL lymphoblasts and correction of the metabolic defect in INCL lymphoblasts by recombinant PPT. *Panel A*, cells from normal control (lanes 1 to 4) or INCL patients (lanes 5 to 8) labeled with [^{35}S]cysteine for varying times up to 6 h. *Panel B*, cells from INCL patients labeled for 3 h, then incubated with an excess of unlabeled cysteine in the absence (lanes 1 to 4) or presence (lanes 5 to 8) of recombinant human PPT (500 ng/ml) supplied from transfected COS cell-conditioned medium. (*Reprinted with permission from Lu et al.*[101] *Copyright 1996 National Academy of Sciences, U. S. A.*)

pepinase. The deficiency in this enzyme was demonstrated by a technique that may be generally applicable to other lysosomal storage diseases.[102] The mannose 6-phosphate modification of newly synthesized lysosomal enzymes was used as an affinity marker to identify a protein that was absent in brain tissue from a patient with the disorder (Fig. 154-5). (This approach was successful because brain tissue contains relatively high levels of mannose 6-phosphate-modified lysosomal enzymes, whereas in peripheral tissues, the mannose 6-phosphate is normally removed in the lysosome.[102]) Amino acid analysis of this novel 46-kDa protein revealed strong similarity to bacterial proteases, and a deficiency of pepstatin-insensitive protease activity was identified in cells from classical LINCL patients. Furthermore, the gene encoding the enzyme was found to reside on human chromosome 11p15, the site of the CLN2 gene determined by linkage studies in a large number of classical LINCL cases.[27] Mutations in the coding region of the pepinase cDNA were described.[102] Classical LINCL is only the second recognized human lysosomal storage disease to result from the deficiency of a lysosomal protease.

Analysis of cDNA clones encoding pepinase revealed two major transcripts at 3.7 and 2.7 kb, which are the products of alternative use of a polyadenylation signal in the 3′ untranslated region of the message. The mRNA was detected in all tissues examined with highest levels in heart and placenta. The transcripts contain one long, open, reading encoding a 563-residue protein, predicted to contain a 16-residue signal peptide. Amino acid sequencing by Edman degradation of the mature enzyme indicates that a proteolytic cleavage occurs between amino acid residues 194 and 195 during maturation. It was not possible to determine whether the enzyme has a large propiece that is removed, or whether the native enzyme consists of an amino-terminal light chain and a C-terminal heavy chain.

The enzyme has both endoprotease and carboxypeptidase activity[102] (P. Lobel, personal communication). Little is yet known about the substrate specificity of the enzyme, and it will be interesting to see whether its deficiency directly, or indirectly, accounts for the accumulation of subunit c of mitochondrial ATPase or other storage material in this disease.

Battenin (CLN3, JNCL). The CLN3 gene encodes a 438-amino acid protein with a deduced molecular weight of about 48 kDa. The predicted amino acid sequence of the polypeptide shows no homology with any known protein, but computer-based structural analysis indicates the presence of several hydrophobic regions, suggesting that it is an integral transmembrane protein.[103,104] The function of the CLN3 protein remains unknown, but the high degree of evolutionary conservation demonstrated by orthologous genes in *Saccharomyces cerevisiae* (BNT1), *Caenorhabditis elegans,* mouse, and dog, suggests an important role for this protein in eukaryotic cells.[105,106]

Recent in vitro studies in HeLa cells have suggested that the recombinant, expressed CLN3 cDNA encodes a 43-kDa single-chain polypeptide. Analyses of the intracellular synthesis and maturation of the CLN3 polypeptide demonstrate that it is translocated into the ER membrane and is glycosylated on asparagine residues. Based on immunofluorescence studies using confocal microscopy, the polypeptide appears to be localized to lysosomal membranes as it colocalizes with Lamp1, an integral lysosomal membrane protein.[107] However, a mitochondrial location has also been suggested.[72]

Yeast, a simple model organism, has been used to analyze the function of the CLN3 protein. The homologous gene in yeast, BTN1, was deleted in *Saccharomyces cerevisiae*[105] but no obvious disease phenotype was observed. However, mutant strains were resistant to the chemical aminonitrophenyl propanediol (ANP),[108] particularly when grown at low pH, and this resistance could be complemented by the human CLN3 gene, indicating that CLN3 protein functions in yeast. Moreover, the degree of ANP resistance resulting from specific missense mutations was related to the severity of the human disease caused by the same mutations. Interestingly, the gene ANP1, when mutated, makes yeast more sensitive to ANP. The ANP1 gene product is located as part of a complex in the *cis* Golgi where it is implicated in the process of glycosylation.[109–111] Identification of a CLN3 phenotype in yeast will facilitate the identification of genes that will suppress the phenotype, and thereby provide clues to the function of the CLN3 protein.

CLN5 protein (Finnish vLINCL). The causative gene[112] in Finnish variant LINCL is predicted to encode a novel membrane protein of 407 amino acids with a molecular weight of 46 kDa and a calculated pI of 8.41. No homologous proteins exist in protein or DNA databases. It remains to be seen whether the CLN5 protein is a lysosomal membrane protein, as is the CLN3 protein.[107] The tissue expression pattern of the CLN 5 gene is ubiquitous on northern analysis, and a relatively low steady state transcript level is observed. The highest transcript levels have been found in aorta, kidney, lung, and pancreas.[112]

GENETICS

The genetic loci for all of the recognized forms of NCL are given in Table 154-2.

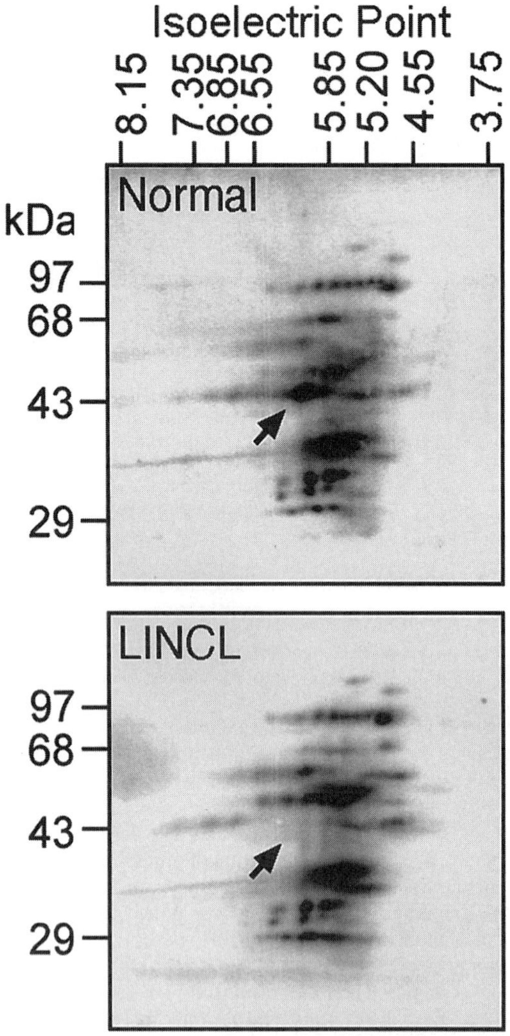

Fig. 154-5 Identification of a protein deficient in LINCL. Detergent-solubilized extracts of gray matter from normal (top) or LINCL (bottom) brain autopsy specimens were fractionated in two dimensions by isoelectric focusing and SDS-polyacrylamide gel electrophoresis, transferred to nitrocellulose, and the mannose 6-phosphorylated glycoproteins were detected with ^{25}I-labeled mannose 6-phosphate receptor. The mannose 6-phosphate glycoprotein (pepinase) that is absent in LINCL extracts is indicated with an arrow. (*Reprinted with permission from Sleat et al.*[102] *Copyright 1997 American Association for the Advancement of Science.*)

Infantile Neuronal Ceroid Lipofuscinosis

The inheritance of INCL is autosomal recessive. The highest incidence is in Finland, where the carrier frequency is 1 in 70 and the incidence in the population is 1 in 20,000.[1] The incidence outside of Finland is unknown, but INCL comprises 11 percent of all neuronal ceroid lipofuscinosis cases in the United States.[28] Because only half of PPT-deficient cases in the United States present as infants,[14] PPT-deficient subjects in the United States probably represent approximately 20 percent of neuronal ceroid lipofuscinosis cases (K. Wisniewski, personal communication).

A random genome scan with the ultimate goal of identifying the INCL mutation began in 1989, with the collection of blood samples from members of 15 INCL families, and CLN1 was linked to the markers D1S57 and D1S7 on 1p32 in 1991.[113] Further linkage analysis of 35 INCL families assigned CLN1 to a 25-cM chromosomal region in the vicinity of the L-*myc* oncogene.[114] Linkage disequilibrium mapping in Finnish alleles assigned the locus to a 300-kb region centromeric to L-*myc*.[115] A physical contig was constructed over this region and positional cloning of the CLN1 gene proceeded with identification of novel transcripts in the genomic clones in the CLN1 region by direct selection, exon trapping, and shotgun sequencing. Simultaneously, FISH mapped the human PPT gene to 1p32 to metaphase chromosomes.[92] Fine mapping of the PPT gene on the constructed physical contig[1] revealed that several of the genomic clones in the CLN1 region contained the PPT gene, and Fiber-FISH was then applied to locate the PPT gene precisely on the map by hybridizing the PPT-containing clones isolated from phage libraries. PPT was found to be located approximately 200 kb centromeric from the L-*myc* gene. Identification of multiple mutations in this gene in INCL patients verified that PPT gene represents the CLN1-gene.[1]

The PPT gene consists of 9 exons spanning 25 kb on human chromosome 1p32.[92] A single mRNA of 2.4 kb is detected on RNA blotting of a variety of human tissues.[92] To date, over 20 different mutations have been described[1,13,14] (Fig. 154-6). The most common mutation, accounting for about 40 percent of alleles in the U.S. population, is a premature stop codon at arginine 151 that results in a severely truncated protein. Another common missense mutation (a threonine to proline substitution at position 75) represents 17 percent of U.S. patients and is associated with juvenile-onset neuronal ceroid lipofuscinosis with granular osmiophilic deposits. A cluster of these patients has been identified in Scotland[13] and all U.S. patients report Scottish or Irish ancestry.[14] All cases of INCL in Finland carry a common missense mutation (R122W) that leads to an unstable protein that is degraded in the endoplasmic reticulum.[99] The remaining mutations are infrequent, and consist of nonsense, missense, and splice-site mutations and small deletions. Large deletions in the PPT gene have not been described.

A second lysosomal thioesterase has been described that shares a 20 percent identity with PPT.[116] The second thioesterase does not complement the metabolic defect in the INCL cells, and its physiological role remains to be determined. The location of the PPT2 gene on human chromosome 6p21.3 does not suggest a major role for the gene in the neuronal ceroid lipofuscinoses.

Late Infantile Neuronal Ceroid Lipofuscinosis

The inheritance of classical late infantile is autosomal recessive. The incidence is not clearly known. A small cluster of cases was reported in British Columbia.[24] Large series have been reported

Table 154-2 Molecular Genetics of the Neuronal Ceroid Lipofuscinoses

NCL Subtype	Locus	Gene Location	Gene Product	Reference(s)
Infantile (INCL)	CLN1	1p32	Palmitoyl-protein thioesterase	1, 114
Classical late infantile (LINCL)	CLN2	11p15	Pepinase	27, 102
Finnish late infantile (vLINCL1)	CLN5	13q22	Membrane protein	112, 122
Variant late infantile (vLINCL2)	CLN6	15q21-q23	Unknown	27
Variant late infantile (vLINCL3)	CLN7	Unknown	Unknown	157
Juvenile (JNCL)	CLN3	16p12	Lysosomal membrane protein	103, 104, 158
Northern epilepsy	CLN8	8p22-ter	Unknown	124, 159
Adult (Kufs disease)	CLN4	Unknown	Unknown	160

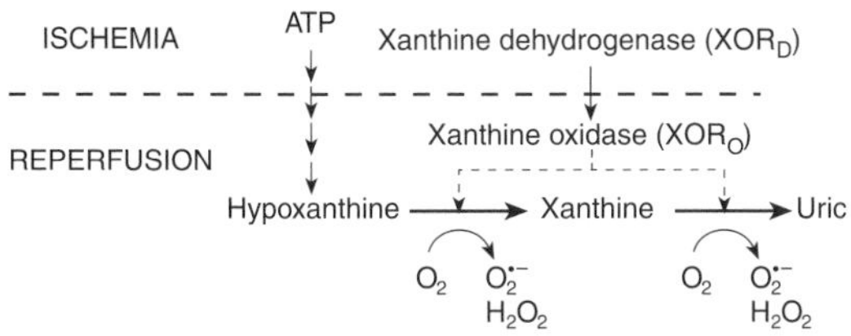

Fig. 154-6 Location of known mutations in the PPT gene in 54 subjects with NCL. The number of times a given allele was observed is shown on the right. A total of 99 mutation-bearing alleles were identified. The analysis in nine patients is incomplete. In some late onset and juvenile-onset subjects, two missense mutations were co-inherited and the relative contribution of either allele to the phenotype is unclear. Genotype-phenotype associations in cases where only one individual was identified should be regarded as provisional until more data are available.

from Newfoundland (32 cases from 24 families),[25] Argentina (24 cases),[26] Italy (8 cases),[117] Northern Europe (38 families from 10 countries),[27] and the United States (116 cases).[28] In the United States, LINCL accounted for 36.3 percent of all neuronal ceroid lipofuscinosis patients in 1992. However, up to 20 percent of these patients were "atypical" and may represent CLN1, 5, 6, or 7 mutations. In addition, milder forms of "classical" LINCL that have less deleterious defects in the pepinase gene may overlap juvenile cases clinically and may go unreported.

Classical LINCL was demonstrated to be distinct from the infantile (Finnish) type, the juvenile type, and a Finnish variant form by genetic linkage studies.[113,118–120] Strong linkage to markers on chromosome 11p15 was found in an initial 5 families and expanded to include 33 families of Northern European origin.[27] A minimum candidate region of 11 cM on 11p15.5 was determined[121] in a group of patients in the United States. Defective genes resulting in variant LINCL have been described (see below).[112]

The structure of the pepinase (CLN2) gene has not been reported as of this writing. Four mutations have been published (a nonsense codon at amino acid residue 208, a splice site mutation, and two different missense mutations, cysteine to arginine and cysteine to tyrosine, at residue 365).[102]

Variant Late Infantile Neuronal Ceroid Lipofuscinosis (Finnish Type)

The Finnish variant of LINCL is recessively inherited and represented a distinct genetic entity when the locus CLN5 was assigned to 13q21-32 by genome-wide scanning for the CLN5 gene in 14 Finnish families.[122] Linkage disequilibrium mapping facilitated the localization of the CLN5 gene to a 200-kb region, which was covered by physical clones.[123] Screening of cDNA libraries, combined with large-scale sequencing and computer-assisted transcript identification, resulted in the identification of the causative gene.[112]

The CLN5 gene spans 13 kb and is transcribed to a 4.1-kb mRNA consisting of four exons with an open reading frame of 1380 bp. Three mutations have been identified in vLINCL patients. One mutation, a 2-bp deletion, is responsible for 98 percent of disease alleles in Finland. This is predicted to change Tyr (392) to a termination codon, and results in a truncated polypeptide of 391 amino acids. The carrier frequency of this mutation is 1 in 200 in this population, and may be as high as 1 in 20 in a subpopulation showing a clustering of cases. Two other mutations have been identified, one resulting in premature termination at amino acid position 75 (W75X) in one Finnish family, and one in a Dutch family resulting in an Asp to Asn change at position 279 (D279N).[112] The cellular consequences of all of these mutations are currently unknown.

Other Variant Forms of Late Infantile Neuronal Ceroid Lipofuscinosis

Another locus for a variant, recessive form of LINCL was recently assigned to chromosome 15q21 by homozygosity mapping in consanguineous families (CLN6).[27] Other loci for variant forms probably await identification, because there are several vLINCL families showing no linkage to either chromosome 13 or 15. These families are currently considered to represent mutations in the CLN7 locus not yet identified.

A new autosomal recessive childhood epilepsy syndrome, designated *Northern* epilepsy, was recently recognized as a new variant form of NCL. It shows striking accumulation of autofluorescent storage material in neurons. The disease is characterized by generalized retardation beginning 2 to 5 years after the first seizures during the first years of life. The life span of Northern epilepsy patients is not severely shortened and vision is not affected. The disease locus has been mapped to chromosome 8p.[124] In autopsies of Northern epilepsy patients, the cerebral cortical and most subcortical neurons showed pronounced intracytoplasmic accumulations of PAS and Sudan black B-positive material. Under electron microscopy these cytosomes consisted of membrane-bound curvilinear profiles and granular material. By immunocytochemistry the storage granules showed a strong positive reaction with antisera raised against subunit c of mitochondrial ATP synthase and sphingolipid activator proteins A and D. Sequence analysis of purified storage cytosomes showed that subunit c is the main storage material (Haltia et al., personal communication). Based on these morphologic and biochemical findings, Northern epilepsy probably represents a new variant of NCL disease (CLN8) with a very protracted course.

Juvenile Neuronal Ceroid Lipofuscinosis

Like other childhood forms of NCL, JNCL is also recessively inherited. Using a genome-wide search strategy, the locus for CLN3 was assigned to 16p12 in 58 European and Canadian families.[125] A classical positional cloning effort by the International Batten Disease Consortium resulted in the identification of the causative gene mutated in patients with JNCL in 1995.[103] The gene covers 15 kb of genomic DNA and contains 15 exons, forming an open reading frame of 1314 bp.

One founder mutation, a 1.02-kb genomic deletion, has been found in 85 percent of the Batten disease alleles worldwide.[126] More than 20 other mutations also have been identified (www.ucl.ac.uk.ncl/). The 1.02-kb mutation shows enrichment in the genetically isolated Finnish population, with an estimated carrier frequency of 1 in 70. In this population, 90 percent of disease alleles carry this mutation.[127]

All CLN3 mutations described to date appear to be of European origin.[103,126,128] The common juvenile mutation is found all over the world in Caucasian populations originating in Europe. With emigration, the mutation has spread to North America, South Africa, and Australia. Because this deletion is also the most common mutation in the Finnish patients, it probably originated over 2000 years ago in the ancestors of one group of immigrants from Europe that was also a part of the founders of the current Finnish population.[129]

GENOTYPE-PHENOTYPE CORRELATIONS

Infantile Neuronal Ceroid Lipofuscinosis

In Finland, virtually all children with INCL are homozygous for a severe missense mutation (tryptophan for an arginine at position 122).[1] This mutation does not seem to be common outside of Finland.[13,14] In the genetically heterogeneous U.S. population, only about half of patients with PPT deficiency are diagnosed as infants.[14] Infantile patients are found to have inherited two severe mutations (usually premature termination or frameshift mutations) and many are homozygous for the common R151X amino acid substitution. Several missense mutations have been associated with late infantile and juvenile-onset phenotypes (Fig. 154-5). The T75P amino acid substitution accounts for most of the juvenile-onset cases. Other mutations unique to JNCL with GROD are D79G, L219Q, and G250V. In families in which more than one sib is affected, the clinical presentation is quite consistent within each family,[14] so that other genes or environmental factors that strongly modify the phenotype are not apparent.

Juvenile Neuronal Ceroid Lipofuscinosis

A total of 25 mutations representing point mutation and deletions at the DNA level have so far been reported in the CLN3 gene[103,126,128,130] (www.ucl.ac.uk/ncl/). The clinical phenotype is relatively homogeneous, although some variation in clinical findings and disease progression occurs even among patients homozygous for the major 1.02-kb deletion mutation. For example, there is one report of a patient homozygous for the common mutation with atypically slow disease progression based on both neuropsychiatric symptoms and MRI findings.[131] The data collected so far would suggest that certain rare point mutations in the CLN3 gene may result in a milder phenotype than the common 1.02-kb deletion.[126,132] In a recent report, 36 patients, either homozygous or heterozygous for the 1.02-kb deletion in the CLN3 gene, were studied to relate their genotype to their clinical phenotype. Suggestive differences emerged. The onset of visual failure and epilepsy was highly concordant in both groups, but there was inter- and intrafamilial heterogeneity in the rate of development of the mental and physical handicap. The homozygous patients uniformly developed mental and physical disabilities, whereas some heterozygous patients with a point mutation in one allele had a more benign disease that did not affect intellectual functioning.[133]

LABORATORY DIAGNOSIS

Infantile Neuronal Ceroid Lipofuscinosis

The diagnosis of INCL is based on a combination of these findings: rapid psychomotor deterioration between 6 and 18 months of age, and retinal degeneration as shown by extinction of the electroretinogram (ERG). In addition, the presence of granular osmiophilic deposits on electron microscopic examination of a suction biopsy of rectal mucosa[2,134] or in peripheral blood leukocytes[28] confirms the diagnosis. However, as many as 15 percent of INCL patients show nondiagnostic findings on initial examination, and serial examination has sometimes been required.[28]

The most direct and precise means of confirming the diagnosis of INCL (or LINCL or JNCL with granular osmiophilic deposits) is the enzymatic assay of PPT from any available cell type (such as leukocytes or skin fibroblasts). Until recently, the release of [^{3}H]palmitate from a palmitate-labeled protein (H-Ras) was measured and a value below 0.2 pmol/min/mg of protein was found to be diagnostic.[13–15] An elegant two-stage thioesterase assay utilizing a 4-methylumbelliferyl derivative of palmitoyl-S-thiogalactose at acidic pH is under development for clinical diagnostic use and will probably replace the more cumbersome protein-based assay (Otto von Diggelen, Erasmus University, personal communication). A DNA-based test is applicable if the causative mutation is known or in isolated populations with one predominant mutation. Population-wide carrier screening is possible for the Finnish population because the $INCL_{FIN}$ major mutation covers 98 percent of disease alleles.[1] The option for DNA-based diagnosis also exists in all Scandinavian countries, which show a predominance of the Finnish mutation (Peltonen, unpublished).

Prenatal testing has been applied successfully in over 30 cases in Finland, first by examination of chorionic villi, which show the characteristic GROD,[66,135] and by linkage studies for families with one affected child. PPT activity can be measured in amniocytes and has been applied successfully in recent cases (Otto van Diggelen, Erasmus University, personal communication). DNA-based mutation detection is available to families seeking prenatal diagnosis for this disorder, but should be considered only when the molecular defect in the specific family at risk is established.

Late Infantile Neuronal Ceroid Lipofuscinosis

Most patients with classical LINCL are diagnosed by histology and electron microscopic exam of leukocytes, skin, or mucosa (such as rectal biopsy). The ultrastructure (curvilinear inclusions) will usually suggest the underlying defect. However, some proportion of patients show nondiagnostic findings on initial examination, and serial biopsies have sometimes been required.[28]

The most direct means of diagnosing classical LINCL is based on the enzymatic assay for pepstatin-insensitive peptidase activity from leukocytes or skin fibroblasts.[102] DNA-based methods are currently under development.

Ultrastructural studies on uncultured amniocytes have been used to diagnose an affected fetus and later to successfully discriminate affected from unaffected fetuses in six pregnancies in one series[136] and in several case reports.[137,138] Considerations concerning morphologic approaches to the prenatal diagnosis of LINCL and JNCL have been reviewed.[138] With the recent discovery of the CLN2 gene and enzyme (pepinase), enzyme and DNA-based prenatal diagnosis should be forthcoming.

Variant Late Infantile Neuronal Ceroid Lipofuscinosis

Until recently, histology and electron microscopy (EM) of tissue biopsies were the only diagnostic methods for diagnosis of the late infantile variants of NCL. For prenatal diagnosis, EM of chorionic villus biopsy in pregnancies at risk is successful. The identification of the CLN5 gene now provides the possibility of DNA-based diagnosis. In the variant LINCL families with established linkage to chromosome 15q, a linkage-based DNA diagnosis can also be offered.

A major problem for the DNA diagnosis of the variant forms of NCL is locus heterogeneity. Until all vLINCL loci are found and corresponding mutations characterized, no reliable estimate of the proportion of vLINCL families linked to different chromosomes (and carrying different mutations) can be made, and this remains a major obstacle for DNA-based diagnosis.

Juvenile Neuronal Ceroid Lipofuscinosis

Unequivocal diagnostic recognition of JNCL is based on electron microscopic examination, which allows identification of the various forms of lipopigments. The best correlation of the structural features of accumulating lipopigments with the clinical subtypes of NCL is seen in circulating lymphocytes, which include both B and T lymphocytes. Numerous lymphocytic vacuoles with fingerprint inclusions are a hallmark feature of classic JNCL. JNCL-related studies show that the number of vacuolated lymphocytes (but not necessarily the abundance of lipopigments or fingerprint patterns) may increase with the duration of the disease. In addition to circulating lymphocytes, which are easily obtainable, skin (and to a less reliable degree, conjunctiva) is the tissue of choice for ultrastructural evidence of NCL, because almost every type of dermal cell may be affected.[139] However, a skin biopsy should not be confined to the epidermis because its cells are relatively poor in NCL-specific lipopigments. Other tissues accessible for biopsy are rectum, bone marrow, tonsils, liver, and urinary sediment.

DNA-based diagnosis is an option, because a 1.02-kb deletion mutation is responsible for 81 percent of affected chromosomes in Batten disease worldwide. A simple, primer extension-based DNA "minisequencing" test was recently reported for rapid detection of this major mutation.[127]

TREATMENT

Infantile Neuronal Ceroid Lipofuscinosis

Treatment of INCL is largely supportive. Early institution of enteral alimentation (per gastrostomy tube) when the child develops difficulty with feedings is recommended. This improves the quality of mealtimes for both child and caregiver. Seizures are often problematic and require combination anticonvulsant therapy, usually with valproate, phenobarbital, and benzodiazepines, as phenytoin and carbamazepine are contraindicated in myoclonic epilepsy.[140] A newer anticonvulsant, lamotrigine, is reported to be a useful adjunct to therapy.[141]

Bone marrow transplantation has been performed in two Finnish infantile cases (P. Santavuori, personal communication), with the rationale that bone marrow-derived migrating microglial cells may provide sufficient normal PPT enzyme to neurons.[142] This approach, utilized with variable success in other lysosomal storage diseases, is supported by the observation that PPT undergoes mannose 6-phosphate-mediated uptake into heterologous cells,[98,99] and that the captured enzyme prevents the accumulation of lipid cysteine thioesters in thioesterase-deficient lymphoblasts.[101] However, whether the production and secretion of the needed enzyme by microglia cells is sufficient to have an impact on the neurodegeneration is unknown. Results in the Finnish cases are not yet available.

Late Infantile Neuronal Ceroid Lipofuscinosis

Treatment of the LINCL forms is supportive, as no specific therapy is available. Seizures are often refractory and require combination anticonvulsant therapy[140] by experts skilled in their use. Bone marrow transplantation has been performed on one patient, once when the patient was asymptomatic (which was rejected) and again at the age of 3 years 9 months, when the EEG became abnormal.[143] The disease progressed, but the course was milder as compared to an older sister. Pepinase is modified by mannose 6-phosphate;[102] therefore, the enzyme should be competent for neuronal uptake through the mannose 6-phosphate receptor pathway. The rationale for bone marrow transplantation in classical LINCL is the same as that for other lysosomal storage diseases.[144,145]

Juvenile Neuronal Ceroid Lipofuscinosis

Just as in other forms of NCL disorders, no effective therapy exists for JNCL, and treatment is largely supportive, including anticonvulsants to control seizures. In JNCL, a combination of two antioxidants (vitamin E and sodium selenite) has been tried in several cases, and some mild benefit has been claimed.[40] Other orally administered treatments have also been tried. Polyunsaturated fatty acids reverse the lysosomal storage and accumulation of subunit c of mitochondrial ATP synthase in cultured lymphoblasts from juvenile NCL patients[146] and provide a rationale for dietary supplements of polyunsaturated fatty acids in patients with JNCL.[146,147] Results from a current uncontrolled trial are too preliminary to permit conclusions at this writing.

Some experimental human bone marrow transplants were performed in JNCL patients in the era before the gene defect was known.[148] Unfortunately, this therapy, which is aimed at replacing the deficient lysosomal enzyme by virtue of its secretion from donor bone marrow-derived cells, would not be expected to be of benefit in JNCL, because CLN3 protein is an intrinsic membrane protein, and is not secreted from cells.[107]

The development of specific therapy applicable to NCLs is at an early stage, partly because not all of the NCL genes have been identified and the biologic role of the known genes is not yet fully elucidated. In addition, treatment of the central nervous system is especially problematic, posing additional challenges in drug delivery. Animal models will be of great importance in testing and refining new and experimental therapies.

ANIMAL MODELS

A summary of the naturally occurring animal models for NCL is given in Table 154-3.

No naturally occurring animal models for PPT deficiency (CLN1) are known. A transgenic mouse model for PPT deficiency (CLN1, INCL) has been established (L. Peltonen, unpublished results). A congenital ovine model of NCL (Swedish Landrace sheep) mimics the clinical presentation and pathology of INCL,[47] but PPT activity in this model is normal.[149]

There are no known animal models for classical LINCL. The New Zealand Southhampshire sheep is the prototype of subunit c-accumulating disease, but pepinase activity is normal (P. Lobel, personal communication). However, linkage studies suggest that this ovine gene defect is located on sheep chromosome 7q13-15, which is syntenic with human chromosome 15q21-23, and therefore corresponds to the human variant late infantile NCL, CLN6 (M. Broom, personal communication). In addition, a spontaneous mouse mutant (nclf) with NCL features linked to mouse chromosome 9 has been described. This chromosomal region is syntenic with human chromosome 15q21 and thus may also represent a homologous gene for human CLN6.[150]

No naturally occurring animal models for JNCL have been shown to have defects in the CLN3 gene. The English setter dog model has been excluded from syntenic loci of both CLN2 and CLN3.[151] Several additional dog models share the JNCL phenotype, but molecular characterization is incomplete (Table 154-3). A knockout mouse model for JNCL was recently developed using a traditional targeting strategy and interruption of the gene by a neomycin expression cassette resulting in a null allele. At the age of 6 months, the mice, homozygotes for the null allele, show no abnormal phenotype (H. Mitchison, personal communication).

Several treatments have been tested in naturally occurring animal models, but because the relationship of any of those models to the human disease is unclear, it is hard to draw conclusions from these studies. Thus far, polyunsaturated fatty acid therapy has been tested in affected English setters, as has been therapy with fish-oil extracts.[152] Both of these failed to show any effect on the disease process. Carnitine supplements in the *mnd* mouse did not prevent the retinal degeneration, but did slow the accumulation of autofluorescent storage material in brain neurons and prolonged the life span of treated mice.[153] Bone marrow transplants have been tested in an English setter dog model, but the results have not

Table 154-3 Animal Models for the Neuronal Ceroid Lipofuscinoses

Model	Age of Onset	Major Storage Protein (Ultrastructure, If Known)	Syntenic Region (Human)	Predicted Human Disease Equivalent	References
Miniature schnauzer	Juvenile	Saposins (GROD)	Unknown	Unknown	47, 161
English setter	Juvenile	Subunit c	Unknown	Unknown	70, 162
Tibetan terrier	Juvenile	Subunit c (mixed)	Unknown	Unknown	70, 163
Border collie	Juvenile	Subunit c	Unknown	Unknown	70
Swedish Landrace sheep	Infantile	Saposins (GROD)	Unknown	Unknown	164
New Zealand Southhampshire sheep	Juvenile	Subunit c	15q	CLN6	165, 166
Mouse (nclf)	Juvenile	Subunit c	15q	CLN6	150, 167
Mouse (mnd)	Juvenile	Subunit c	13q34, 8p11, or 19p13	Unknown	168

been encouraging.[154,155] Small animal models (such as transgenic mice with targeted deletions of the known human CLN genes) will be important in testing future treatment strategies.

ADDENDUM

In the interval since the manuscript for this chapter was submitted, several important new findings have been published and are described below:

1. The EPMR (CLN8) gene has been identified[169] and found to encode a predicted transmembrane protein. The mouse homolog of EPMR was also cloned and found to be located in the same chromosomal region as the mouse mnd locus. A homozygous single base pair insertion was found in the EPMR/CLN8 gene and mnd mice. Therefore, it appears that EPMR and mnd are orthologous genes causing an NCL disorder in mice and humans. Initial data suggest that CLN8 encodes an ER protein (A.-E. Lehesjoki, personal communication).
2. Pepinase (CLN2) has been found to correspond to a recently isolated lysosomal tripeptidyl amino peptidase I (TPPI).[170,171] The amino acid sequences of pepinase and TPPI are the same, and classical late infantile NCL patients are deficient in TPPI activity. TPPI is a lysosomal protease that removes three amino acids processively from the N-terminus of proteins. The enzyme prefers uncharged amino acids in the P1 position.[172]
3. The gene structure of CLN2 (TPPI) has been elucidated.[173] The gene consists of 13 exons and 12 introns and spans 6.65 kb. A large series describing 74 families with two dozen mutations in the CLN2 gene in classical late infantile NCL has been reported.[174] DNA- and enzyme-based prenatal diagnoses for defects in CLN2 have been performed.[175]
4. In vitro expression studies of the CLN3 in a neuronal cell line indicated that the protein co-localizes with synaptophysin, an integral membrane protein of the presynaptic vesicle.[176] Similar co-localization with synaptophysin was also reported for PPT in neuronic cells.[177]
5. Two mouse models for juvenile NCL with targeted deletions in the CLN3 gene have been reported.[178,179] Both models show accumulation of autofluorescent storage material with appropriate ultrastructure in the brain and other tissues.
6. Congenital ovine NCL in Swedish Landrace sheep is due to a homozygous inactivating mutation in the gene encoding cathepsin D (P. Lobel, personal communication). A corresponding human deficiency in cathepsin D has not been described.
7. A clinically useful PPT (CLN1) assay based on the two-stage hydrolysis of a fluorescent substrate is available. The enzymatic diagnosis relies on the ability of an extract of blood leukocytes to cleave a fluorescent thioester substrate (4-methylumbelliferyl-6-thiopalmitoyl-b-D-glucopyranoside).[180] In all affected cases, PPT activity is severely reduced ($>5\%$ of normal).
8. The x-ray crystallographic structure of PPT with and without bound palmitate has been reported.[181] The enzyme adopts an a/b hydrolase fold typical of lipases and utilizes a serine-histidine-aspartic acid catalytic triad. The bound palmitate lies in a deep hydrophobic groove along the surface of the enzyme. Missense mutations associated with a severe phenotype cluster near the active site and palmitate binding site, whereas less severe mutations affect peripheral regions of the structure.
9. Four Finnish infants with INCL have undergone allogeneic bone marrow transplantation. One succumbed to complications of the transplant, and three have done much better than Finnish controls, but the oldest of the children (at 4.5 years) is severely retarded and the disease is progressing (S. L. Vanhanen and P. Santavuori, personal communication).

ACKNOWLEDGMENTS

This work was supported in part by the National Institutes of Health (NS 36867 and NS 35323) and by the Academy of Finland, the Sigrid Juselius Foundation, and the Hjelt Fund of the Pediatric Research Foundation, Finland.

REFERENCES

1. Vesa J, Hellsten E, Verkruyse LA, Camp LA, Rapola J, Santavuori P, Hofmann SL, et al.: Mutations in the palmitoyl protein thioesterase gene causing infantile neuronal ceroid lipofuscinosis. *Nature* **376**:584, 1995.
2. Santavuori P, Haltia M, Rapola J, Raitta C: Infantile type of so-called neuronal ceroid-lipofusinosis. Part I. A clinical study of 15 patients. *J Neurol Sci* **18**:257, 1973.
3. Santavuori P, Haltia M, Rapola J: Infantile type of so-called neuronal ceroid-lipofuscinosis. *Dev Med Child Neurol* **16**:644, 1974.
4. Santavuori P, Vanhanen S-L, Sainio K, Nieminen M, Wallden T, Launes J, Raininko R: Infantile neuronal ceroid-lipofuscinosis (INCL): Diagnostic criteria. *J Inherit Metab Dis* **16**:227, 1993.
5. Hagberg B, Witt-Engerstrom I: Early stages of the Rett syndrome and infantile neuronal ceroid lipofuscinosis—A difficult differential diagnosis. *Brain Dev* **12**:20, 1990.
6. Vanhanen SL, Sainio K, Lappi M, Santavuori P: EEG and evoked potentials in infantile neuronal ceroid-lipofuscinosis. *Dev Med Child Neurol* **39**:456, 1997.
7. Raininko R, Santavuori P, Heiskala H, Sainio K, Palo J: CT findings in neuronal ceroid lipofuscinoses. *Neuropediatrics* **21**:95, 1990.
8. Vanhanen SL, Raininko R, Autti T, Santavuori P: MRI evaluation of the brain in infantile neuronal ceroid-lipofuscinosis. Part 2: MRI findings in 21 patients. *J Child Neurol* **10**:444, 1995.
9. Vanhanen SL, Raininko R, Santavuori P, Autti T, Haltia M: MRI evaluation of the brain in infantile neuronal ceroid-lipofuscinosis. Part 1: Postmortem MRI with histopathologic correlation. *J Child Neurol* **10**:438, 1995.
10. Vanhanen SL, Raininko R, Santavuori P: Early differential diagnosis of infantile neuronal ceroid lipofuscinosis, Rett syndrome, and Krabbe disease by CT and MR. *AJNR Am J Neuroradiol* **15**:1443, 1994.
11. Vanhanen SL, Liewendahl K, Raininko R, Nikkinen P, Autti T, Sainio K, Santavuori P: Brain perfusion SPECT in infantile neuronal ceroid-lipofuscinosis (INCL). Comparison with clinical manifestations and MRI findings. *Neuropediatrics* **27**:76, 1996.
12. Brockmann K, Pouwels PJ, Christen HJ, Frahm J, Hanefeld F: Localized proton magnetic resonance spectroscopy of cerebral metabolic disturbances in children with neuronal ceroid lipofuscinosis. *Neuropediatrics* **27**:242, 1996.
13. Mitchison HM, Hofmann SL, Becerra CH, Munroe PB, Lake BD, Crow YJ, Stephenson JB, et al.: Mutations in the palmitoyl-protein thioesterase gene (PPT; CLN1) causing juvenile neuronal ceroid lipofuscinosis with granular osmiophilic deposits. *Hum Mol Genet* **7**:291, 1998.
14. Das AK, Becerra CHR, Yi W, Lu J-Y, Siakotos AN, Wisniewski KE, Hofmann SL: Molecular genetics of palmitoyl-protein thioesterase deficiency in the U.S. *J Clin Invest* **102**:361, 1998.
15. Wisniewski KE, Connell F, Kaczmarski W, Kaczmarski A, Siakotos A, Becerra CR, Hofmann SL: Palmitoyl-protein thioesterase deficiency in a novel granular variant of late infantile neuronal ceroid lipofuscinosis. *Pediatr Neurol* **18**:119, 1998.
16. Jagadha V, Halliday WC, Becker LE, Hinton D: The association of infantile osteopetrosis and neuronal storage disease in two brothers. *Acta Neuropathol (Berl)* **75**:233, 1988.
17. Takahashi K, Naito M, Yamamura F, Taki T, Sugino S, Taku K, Miike T: Infantile osteopetrosis complicating neuronal ceroid lipofuscinosis. *Pathol Res Pract* **186**:697, 1990.
18. Garborg I, Torvik A, Hals J, Tangsrud SE, Lindemann R: Congential neuronal ceroid lipofuscinosis. A case report. *Acta Pathol Microbiol Immunol Scand [A]* **95**:119, 1987.
19. Barohn RJ, Dowd DC, Kagan-Hallet KS: Congential ceroid-lipofuscinosis [see comments]. *Pediatr Neurol* **8**:54, 1992.
20. Wisniewski KE, Kida E: Congenital ceroid-lipofuscinosis [Letter; Comment]. *Pediatr Neurol* **8**:315, 1992.
21. Duffy PE, Kornfeld M, Suzuki K: Neurovisceral storage disease with curvilinear bodies. *J Neuropath Exp Neurol* **27**:351, 1968.
22. Gonatas NK, Gambetti P, Baird H: A second type of late infantile amaurotic idiocy with multilamellar cytosomes. *J Neuropath Exp Neurol* **27**:371, 1968.
23. Carpenter S, Karpati G, Andermann F: Specific involvement of muscle, nerve, and skin in late infantile and juvenile amaurotic idiocy. *Neurology* **22**:170, 1972.
24. MacLeod PM, Dolman CL, Chang E: The neuronal ceroid-lipofuscinoses in British Columbia. A clinical, epidemiologic and ultrastructural study. *Birth Defects* **12**:289, 1976.

25. Andermann E, Jacob JC, Andermann F, Carpenter S, Wolfe L, Berkovic SF: The Newfoundland aggregate of neuronal ceroid-lipofuscinosis. *Am J Med Genet* **5** **(Suppl)**: 111, 1988.
26. Taratuto AL, Saccoliti M, Sevlever G, Ruggieri V, Arroyo H, Herrero M, Massaro M, et al.: Childhood neuronal ceroid-lipofuscinoses in Argentina. *Am J Med Genet* **57**: 144, 1995.
27. Sharp JD, Wheeler RB, Lake BD, Savukoski M, Järvelä IE, Peltonen L, Gardiner RM, et al.: Loci for classical and a variant late infantile neuronal ceroid lipofuscinosis map to chromosomes 11p15 and 15q21-23. *Hum Mol Genet* **6**: 591, 1997.
28. Wisniewski KE, Kida E, Patxot OF, Connell F: Variability in the clinical and pathological findings in the neuronal ceroid lipofuscinoses: Review of data and observations. *Am J Med Genet* **42**: 525, 1992.
29. Kohlschütter A, Gardiner RM, Goebel HH: Human forms of neuronal ceroid-lipofuscinosis (Batten disease): Consensus on diagnostic criteria, Hamburg 1992. *J Inherit Metab Dis* **16**: 241, 1993.
30. Harden A, Pampiglione G: Neurophysiologic studies (EEG/ERG/VEP/SEP) in 88 children with so-called neuronal ceroid lipofuscinosis, in Armstrong D, Koppang N, Rider JA (eds.) *Ceroid-Lipofuscinosis (Batten's Disease).* Amsterdam, Elsevier Biomedical Press, 1982, p 61.
31. Pampiglione G, Harden A: So-called neuronal ceroid lipofuscinosis. Neurophysiological studies in 60 children. *J Neurol Neurosurg Psychiatry* **40**: 323, 1977.
32. Tackmann W, Kuhlendahl D: Evoked potentials in neuronal ceroid lipofuscinosis. *Eur Neurol* **18**: 234, 1979.
33. Petersen B, Handwerker M, Huppertz HI: Neuroradiological findings in classical late infantile neuronal ceroid-lipofuscinosis. *Pediatr Neurol* **15**: 344, 1996.
34. Autti T, Raininko R, Santavuori P, Vanhanen SL, Poutanen VP, Haltia M: MRI of neuronal ceroid lipofuscinosis. II. Postmortem MRI and histopathological study of the brain in 16 cases of neuronal ceroid lipofuscinosis of juvenile or late infantile type. *Neuroradiology* **39**: 371, 1997.
35. Autti T, Raininko R, Vanhanen SL, Santavuori P: Magnetic resonance techniques in neuronal ceroid lipofuscinoses and some other lysosomal diseases affecting the brain. *Curr Opin Neurol* **10**: 519, 1997.
36. Iannetti P, Messa C, Spalice A, Lucignani G, Fazio F: Positron emission tomography in neuronal ceroid lipofuscinosis (Jansky-Bielschowsky disease): A case report [see comments]. *Brain Dev* **16**: 459, 1994.
37. Liewendahl K, Vanhanen SL, Heiskala H, Raininko R, Nikkinen P, Launes J, Santavuori P: Brain perfusion SPECT abnormalities in neuronal ceroid lipofuscinoses. *Neuropediatrics* **28**: 71, 1997.
38. Santavuori P, Rapola J, Nuutila A, Raininko R, Lappi M, Launes J, Herva R, et al.: The spectrum of Jansky-Bielschowsky disease. *Neuropediatrics* **22**: 92, 1991.
39. Lake B, Cavanagh NPC: Early-juvenile Batten's disease: A recognizable sub-group distinct from other forms of Batten's disease. *J. Neurol Sci* **36**: 265, 1978.
40. Santavuori P: Neuronal ceroid-lipofuscinoses in childhood. *Brain Dev* **10**: 80, 1988.
41. Wisniewski KE, Rapin I, Heaney-Kieras J: Clinicopathological variability in the childhood neuronal ceroid-lipofuscinoses and new observations on glycoprotein abnormalities. *Am J Med Genet* **5**: 27, 1988.
42. Spalton DJ, Taylor DS, Sanders DM: Juvenile Batten's disease: An ophthalmological assessment of 26 patients. *Br J Ophthalmol* **64**: 726, 1980.
43. Weleber RG: The dystrophic retina in multisystem disorders: The electroretinogram in neuronal ceroid lipofuscinoses. *Eye* **12**: 580, 1998.
44. Haltia M, Rapola J, Santavuori P: Infantile type of so-called neuronal ceroid lipofuscinosis. Part II. Histological and electron microscopic studies. *Acta Neuropathol* **26**: 157, 1973.
45. Haltia M, Rapola J, Santavuori P, Keranen A: Infantile type of so-called neuronal ceroid-lipofuscinosis. Part 2. Morphological and biochemical studies. *J Neurol Sci* **18**: 269, 1973.
46. Rapola J: Neuronal ceroid-lipofuscinosis in childhood, in Landing BH, Haust MD, Bernstein J, Rosenberg H, (eds): *Genetic Metabolic Diseases. Perspectives in Pediatric Pathology.* Basel, Karger, 1993, p 7.
47. Tyynelä J, Suopanki J, Baumann M, Haltia M: Sphingolipid activator proteins (SAPs) in neuronal ceroid lipofuscinoses (NCL). *Neuropediatrics* **28**: 49, 1997.
48. Zeman W, Donahue S, Dyken P, Green J: The neuronal ceroid-lipofuscinosis (Batten-Vogt syndrome), in Vinken P, Gruyn G, (eds): *Handbook of Clinical Neurology.* Amsterdam, North-Holland, 1970, p 588.
49. Sjövall E, Ericsson E: The anatomical type in the Swedish cases of juvenile amaurotic idiocy. *Acta Pathol Microbiol Scand* **16** **(Suppl)**: 460, 1933.
50. Van Bagh K, Hortling H: Blodfynd vid juvenil amaurotisk idioti. *Nord Med* **38**: 1072, 1948.
51. Goebel HH, Fix JD, Zeman W: The fine structure of the retina in neuronal ceroid-lipofuscinosis. *Am J Ophthalmol* **77**: 25, 1974.
52. Palo J, Elovaara I, Haltia M, Ng Ying Kin NMK, Wolfe LS: Infantile neuronal ceroid lipofuscinosis: Isolation of storage material. *Neurology* **32**: 1035, 1982.
53. Tyynelä J, Palmer DN, Baumann M, Haltia M: Storage of saposins A and D in infantile neuronal ceroid-lipfuscinosis. *FEBS Lett* **330**: 8, 1993.
54. Tayama M, O'Brien JS, Kishimoto Y: Distribution of saposins (sphingolipid activator proteins) in tissues of lysosomal storage disease patients. *J Mol Neurosci* **3**: 171, 1992.
55. Palmer DN, Fearnley IM, Walker JE, Hall NA, Lake BD, Wolfe LS, Haltia M, et al.: Mitochondrial ATP synthase subunit c storage in the ceroid-lipofuscinoses (Batten disease). *Am J Med Genet* **42**: 561, 1992.
56. Svennerholm L, Hagberg B, Haltia M, Sourander P, Vanier M-T: Polyunsaturated fatty acid lipidosis. II. Lipid biochemical studies. *Acta Pediatr Scand* **64**: 489, 1975.
57. Svennerhol L, Fredman P, Jungbjer B, Mansson JE, Rynmark BM, Bostrom K, Hagberg B, et al.: Large alterations in ganglioside and neutral glycosphingolipid patterns in brains from cases with infantile neuronal ceroid lipofuscinosis/polyunsaturated fatty acid lipidosis [published erratum appears in *J Neurochem* 50(3):996, 1988]. *J Neurochem* **49**: 1772, 1987.
59. Palmer DN, Martinus RD, Cooper SM, Midwinter GG, Reid JC, Jolly RD: Ovine ceroid lipofuscinosis. The major lipopigment protein and the lipid-binding subunit of mitochondrial ATP synthase have the same NH2-terminal sequence. *J Biol Chem* **264**: 5736, 1989.
60. Ezaki J, Wolfe LS, Higuti T, Ishidoh K, Kominami E: Specific delay of degradation of mitochondrial ATP synthase subunit c in late infantile neuronal ceroid lipofuscinosis (Batten disease). *J Neurochem* **64**: 733, 1995.
61. Ezaki J, Wolfe LS, Ishidoh K, Kominami E: Abnormal degradative pathway of mitochondrial ATP synthase subunit c in late infantile neuronal ceroid-lipofuscinosis (Batten disease). *Am J Med Genet* **57**: 254, 1995.
62. Ezaki J, Wolfe LS, Kominami E: Specific delay in the degradation of mitochondrial ATP synthase subunit c in late infantile neuronal ceroid lipofuscinosis is derived from cellular proteolytic dysfunction rather than structural alteration of subunit c. *J Neurochem* **67**: 1677, 1996.
63. Rider JA, Dawson G, Siakotos AN: Perspective of biochemical research in the neuronal ceroid-lipofuscinosis. *Am J Med Genet* **42**: 519, 1992.
64. Conradi NG, Uvebrant P, Hökegård KH, Wahlstrom J, Mellqvist L: First-trimester diagnosis of juvenile neuronal ceroid lipofuscinosis by demonstration of fingerprint inclusions in chorionic villi. *Prenat Diagn* **9**: 283, 1989.
65. Järvelä I, Rapola J, Peltonen L, Puhakka L, Vesa J, Ämmälä P, Salonen R, et al.: DNA-based prenatal diagnosis of the infantile form of neuronal ceroid lipofuscinosis (INCL, CLN1). *Prenat Diagn* **11**: 323, 1991.
66. Rapola J, Salonen R, Ämmälä P, Santavuori P: Prenatal diagnosis of the infantile type of neuronal ceroid lipofuscinosis by electron microscopic investigation of human chorionic villi. *Prenat Diagn* **10**: 553, 1990.
67. Hall NA, Lake BD, Dewji NN, Patrick AD: Lysosomal storage of subunit c of mitochondrial ATP synthase in Batten's disease (ceroid-lipofuscinosis). *Biochem J* **275**: 269, 1991.
68. Lake BD, Hall NA: Immunolocalization studies of subunit c in late-infantile and juvenile Batten disease. *J Inherit Metab Dis* **16**: 263, 1993.
69. Faust JR, Rodman JS, Daniel PF, Dice JF, Bronson RT: Two related proteolipids and dolichol-linked oligosaccharides accumulate in motor neuron degeneration mice (mnd/mnd), a model for neuronal ceroid lipofuscinosis. *J Biol Chem* **269**: 10150, 1994.
70. Palmer DN, Jolly RD, van Mil HC, Tyynelä J, Westlake VJ: Different patterns of hydrophobic protein storage in different forms of neuronal ceroid lipofuscinosis (NCL, Batten disease). *Neuropediatrics* **28**: 45, 1997.
71. Elleder M, Sokolova J, Hrebicek M: Follow-up study of subunit c of mitochondrial ATP synthase (SCMAS) in Batten disease and in unrelated lysosomal disorders. *Acta Neuropathol (Berl)* **93**: 379, 1997.

72. Katz ML, Gao CL, Tompkins JA, Bronson RT, Chin DT: Mitochondrial ATP synthase subunit c stored in hereditary ceroid-lipofuscinosis contains trimethyl-lysine. *Biochem J* **310**:887, 1995.
73. Katz ML, Rodrigues M: Juvenile ceroid lipofuscinosis. Evidence for methylated lysine in neural storage body protein. *Am J Pathol* **138**:323, 1991.
74. Katz ML, Siakotos AN, Gao Q, Freiha B, Chin DT: Late-infantile ceroid-lipofuscinosis:lysine methylation of mitochondrial ATP synthase subunit c from lysosomal storage bodies. *Biochim Biophys Acta* **1361**:66, 1997.
75. Katz ML, Christianson JS, Norbury NE, Gao CL, Siakotos AN, Koppang N: Lysine methylation of mitochondrial ATP synthase subunit c stored in tissues of dogs with hereditary ceroid lipofuscinosis. *J Biol Chem* **269**:9906, 1994.
76. Katz ML, Gerhardt KO: Methylated lysine in storage body protein of sheep with hereditary ceroid-lipofuscinosis. *Biochim Biophys Acta* **1138**:97, 1992.
77. Fürst W, Sandhoff K: Activator proteins and topology of lysosomal sphingolipid catabolism. *Biochim Biophys Acta* **1126**:1, 1992.
78. Tyynelä J, Baumann M, Henseler M, Sandhoff K, Haltia M: Sphingolipid activator proteins in the neuronal ceroid-lipofuscinoses: An immunological study. *Acta Neuropathol (Berl)* **89**:391, 1995.
79. Ivy GO, Shottler F, Wenzel J, Baudry M, Lynch G: Inhibitors of lysosomal enzymes: Accumulation of lipofuscin-like dense bodies in the brain. *Science* **226**:985, 1984.
80. Siakotos AN, Schnippel K, Lin RC, Van Kuijk FJ: Biosynthesis and metabolism of 4-hydroxynonenal in canine ceroid-lipofuscinosis. *Am J Med Genet* **57**:290, 1995.
81. Hall N, Patrick A: Accumulation of dolichol-linked oligosaccharides. *Am J Med Genet* **5**:221, 1988.
82. Keller RK, Armstrong D, Crum FC, Koppang N: Dolichol and dolichyl phosphate levels in brain tissue from English setters with ceroid lipofuscinosis. *J Neurochem* **42**:1040, 1984.
83. Pullarkat RK, Kim KS, Sklower SL, Patel VK: Oligosaccharyl diphosphodolichols in the ceroid-lipofuscinoses. *Am J Med Genet* **5 (Suppl)**:243, 1988.
84. Wolfe LS, Gauthier S, Haltia M, Palo J: Dolichol and dolichyl phosphate in the neuronal ceroid-lipofuscinoses and other diseases. *Am J Med Genet* **5 (Suppl)**:233, 1988.
85. Katz ML, Siakotos AN: Canine hereditary ceroid-lipofuscinosis: evidence for a defect in the carnitine biosynthetic pathway. *Am J Med Genet* **57**:266, 1995.
87. Camp LA, Hofmann SL: Purification and properties of a palmitoyl-protein thioesterase that cleaves palmitate from H-Ras. *J Biol Chem* **268**:22566, 1993.
88. Casey PJ: Protein lipidation in cell signaling. *Science* **268**:221, 1995.
89. Mumby SM: Reversible palmitoylation of signaling proteins. *Curr Opin Cell Biol* **9**:148, 1997.
90. Hofmann SL, Lee LA, Lu JY, Verkruyse LA: Palmitoyl-protein thioesterase and the molecular pathogenesis of infantile neuronal ceroid lipofuscinosis. *Neuropediatrics* **28**:27, 1997.
91. Camp LA, Verkruyse LA, Afendis SJ, Slaughter CA, Hofmann SL: Molecular cloning and expression of palmitoyl-protein thioesterase. *J Biol Chem* **269**:23212, 1994.
92. Schriner JE, Yi W, Hofmann SL: cDNA and genomic cloning of human palmitoyl-protein thioesterase (PPT), the enzyme defective in infantile neuronal ceroid lipofuscinosis [published erratum appears in *Genomics* 38(3):458, 1996]. *Genomics* **34**:317, 1996.
93. Salonen T, Hellsten E, Horelli-Kuitunen N, Peltonen L, Jalanko A: Mouse palmitoyl protein thioesterase: Gene structure and expression of cDNA. *Genome Res* **8**:724, 1998.
94. Naggert J, Witkowski A, Mikkelsen J, Smith S: Molecular cloning and sequencing of a cDNA encoding the thioesterase domain of the rat fatty acid synthetase. *J Biol Chem* **263**:1146, 1988.
95. Witkowski A, Witkowska HE, Smith S: Reengineering the specificity of a serine active-site enzyme: Two active-site mutations convert a hydrolase to a transferase. *J Biol Chem* **269**:379, 1994.
96. Lawson DM, Derewenda U, Serre L, Ferri S, Szittner R, Wei Y, Meighen EA, et al.: Structure of a myristoyl-ACP-specific thioesterase from *Vibrio harveyi*. *Biochemistry* **33**:9382, 1994.
97. Lu J-Y, Hofmann SL: Unpublished observations.
98. Verkruyse LA, Hofmann SL: Lysosomal targeting of palmitoyl-protein thioesterase. *J Biol Chem* **271**:15831, 1996.
99. Hellsten E, Vesa J, Olkkonen VM, Jalanko A, Peltonen L: Human palmitoyl protein thioesterase: Evidence for lysosomal targeting of the enzyme and disturbed cellular routing in infantile neuronal ceroid lipofuscinosis. *EMBO J* **15**:5240, 1996.
100. Sleat DE, Sohar I, Lackland H, Majercak J, Lobel P: Rat brain contains high levels of mannose-6-phosphorylated glycoproteins including lysosomal enzymes and palmitoyl-protein thioesterase, an enzyme implicated in infantile neuronal lipofuscinosis. *J Biol Chem* **271**:19191, 1996.
101. Lu JY, Verkruyse LA, Hofmann SL: Lipid thioesters derived from acylated proteins accumulate in infantile neuronal ceroid lipofuscinosis: Correction of the defect in lymphoblasts by recombinant palmitoyl-protein thioesterase. *Proc Natl Acad Sci U S A* **93**:10046, 1996.
102. Sleat DE, Donnelly RJ, Lackland H, Liu CG, Sohar I, Pullarkat RK, Lobel P: Association of mutations in a lysosomal protein with classical late-infantile neuronal ceroid lipofuscinosis. *Science* **277**:1802, 1997.
103. Anonymous: Isolation of a novel gene underlying Batten disease, CLN3. The International Batten Disease Consortium. *Cell* **82**:949, 1995.
104. Janes RW, Munroe PB, Mitchison HM, Gardiner RM, Mole SE, Wallace BA: A model for Batten disease protein CLN3: Functional implications from homology and mutations. *FEBS Lett* **399**:75, 1996.
105. Pearce DA, Sherman F: BTN1, a yeast gene corresponding to the human gene responsible for Batten's disease, is not essential for viability, mitochondrial function, or degradation of mitochondrial ATP synthase. *Yeast* **13**:691, 1997.
106. Lee RL, Johnson KR, Lerner TJ: Isolation and chromosomal mapping of a mouse homolog of the Batten disease gene CLN3. *Genomics* **35**:617, 1996.
107. Järvelä I, Sainio M, Rantamaki T, Olkkonen VM, Carpén O, Peltonen L, Jalanko A: Biosynthesis and intracellular targeting of the CLN3 protein defective in Batten disease. *Hum Mol Genet* **7**:85, 1998.
108. Pearce DA, Sherman F: A yeast model for the study of Batten disease. *Proc Natl Acad Sci U S A* **95**:6915, 1998.
109. Chapman RE, Munro S: The functioning of the yeast Golgi apparatus requires an ER protein encoded by ANP1, a member of a new family of genes affecting the secretory pathway. *EMBO J* **13**:4896, 1994.
110. Hashimoto H, Yoda K: Novel membrane protein complexes for protein glycosylation in the yeast Golgi apparatus. *Biochem Biophys Res Commun* **241**:682, 1997.
111. Jungmann J, Munro S: Multi-protein complexes in the *cis* Golgi of *Saccharomyces cerevisiae* with alpha-1,6-mannosyltransferase activity. *EMBO J* **17**:423, 1998.
112. Savukoski M, Klockars T, Holmber V, Santavuori P, Lander ES, Peltonen L: CLN5, a novel gene encoding a putative transmembrane protein muated in the Finnish variant late infantile neuronal ceroid lipofuscinosis (vLINCL). *Nat Genet* **19**:286, 1998.
113. Järvelä I, Schleutker J, Haataja L, Santavuori P, Puhakka L, Manninen T, Palotie A, et al.: Infantile neuronal ceroid lipofuscinosis (INCL, CLN1) maps to the short arm of chromosome 1. *Genomics* **9**:170, 1991.
114. Järvelä I: Infantile neuronal ceroid lipofuscinosis (CLN1): Linkage disequilibrium in the Finnish population and evidence that variant late infantile form (variant CLN2) represents a nonallelic locus. *Genomics* **10**:333, 1991.
115. Hellsten E, Vesa J, Heiskanen M, Makela TP, Järvelä I, Cowell JK, Mead S, et al.: Identification of YAC clones for human chromosome 1p32 and physical mapping of the infantile neuronal ceroid lipofuscinosis (INCL) locus. *Genomics* **25**:404, 1995.
116. Soyombo AA, Hofmann SL: Molecular cloning and expression of PPT2, a homolog of lysosomal palmitoyl-protein thioesterase with a distinct substrate specificity. *J Biol Chem* **272**:27456, 1997.
117. Nardocci N, Verga ML, Binelli S, Zorzi G, Angelini L, Bugiani O: Neuronal ceroid-lipofuscinosis: A clinical and morphological study of 19 patients. *Am J Med Genet* **57**:137, 1995.
118. Yan W, Boustany RM, Konradi C, Ozelius L, Lerner T, Trofatter JA, Julier C, et al.: Localization of juvenile, but not late-infantile, neuronal ceroid lipofuscinosis on chromosome 16. *Am J Hum Genet* **52**:89, 1993.
119. Williams R, Vesa J, Järvelä I, McKay T, Mitchison H, Hellsten E, Thompson A, et al.: Genetic heterogeneity in neuronal ceroid lipofuscinosis (NCL): Evidence that the late-infantile subtype (Jansky-Bielschowsky disease; CLN2) is not an allelic form of the juvenile or infantile subtypes. *Am J Hum Genet* **53**:931, 1993.
120. Sharp J, Savukoski M, Wheeler RB, Harris J, Järvelä I, Peltonen L, Gardiner M, et al.: Linkage analysis of late-infantile neuronal ceroid-lipofuscinosis. *Am J Med Genet* **57**:348, 1995.
121. Haines JL, Boustany R-MN, Alroy J, Auger KJ, Shook KS, Terwedow H, Lerner TJ: Chromosomal localization of two genes underlying late-infantile neuronal ceroid lipofuscinosis. *Neurogenetics* **1**:217, 1998.

122. Savukoski M, Kestila M, Williams R, Järvelä I, Sharp J, Harris J, Santavuori P, et al.: Defined chromosomal assignment of CLN5 demonstrates that at least four genetic loci are involved in the pathogenesis of human ceroid lipofuscinoses. *Am J Hum Genet* **55**:695, 1994.
123. Klockars T, Savukoski M, Isosomppi J, Laan M, Järvelä I, Petrukhin K, Palotie A, et al.: Efficient construction of a physical map by fiber-FISH of the CLN5 region: Refined assignment and long-range contig covering the critical region on 13q22. *Genomics* **35**:71, 1996.
124. Tahvanainen E, Ranta S, Hirvasniemi A, Karila E, Leisti J, Sistonen P, Weissenbach J, et al.: The gene for a recessively inherited childhood progressive epilepsy with mental retardation maps to the distal short arm of chromosome 8. *Proc Natl Acad Sci U S A* **91**:7267, 1994.
125. Gardiner M, Sandford A, Deadman M, Poulton J, Cookson W, Reeders S, Jokiaho I, et al.: Batten disease (Spielmeyer-Vogt disease, juvenile onset neuronal ceroid-lipofuscinosis) gene (CLN3) maps to human chromosome 16. *Genomics* **8**:387, 1990.
126. Munroe PB, Mitchison HM, O'Rawe AM, Anderson JW, Boustany RM, Lerner TJ, Taschner PE, et al.: Spectrum of mutations in the Batten disease gene, CLN3. *Am J Hum Genet* **61**:310, 1997.
127. Järvelä I, Mitchison HM, Munroe PB, O'Rawe AM, Mole SE, Syvänen AC: Rapid diagnostic test for the major mutation underlying Batten disease. *J Med Genet* **33**:1041, 1996.
128. Zhong N, Wisniewski KE, Kaczmarski AL, Ju W, Xu WM, Xu WW, McLendon L, et al.: Molecular screening of Batten disease: Identification of a missense mutation (E295K) in the CLN3 gene. *Hum Genet* **102**:57, 1998.
129. Kittles RA, Perola M, Peltonen L, Bergen AW, Aragon RA, Virkkunen M, Linnoila M, et al.: Dual origins of Finns revealed by Y chromosome haplotype variation. *Am J Hum Genet* **62**:1171, 1998.
130. Milá M, Mallolas J, Pineda M, Ferrer I, Vernet A, Badenas C, Sánchez A, et al.: Mutations in CLN3 gene responsible for Batten disease. *Eur J Hum Genet* **6**:145, 1998.
131. Åberg L, Järvelä I, Rapola J, Autti T, Kirveskari E, Lappi M, Sipila L, et al.: Atypical juvenile neuronal ceroid lipofuscinosis with granular osmiophilic deposit-like inclusions in the autonomic nerve cells of the gut wall. *Acta Neuropathol (Berl)* **95**:306, 1998.
132. Wisniewski KE, Zhong N, Kaczmarski W, Kaczmarski A, Kida E, Brown WT, Schwarz KO, et al.: Compound heterozygous genotype is associated with protracted juvenile neuronal ceroid lipofuscinosis. *Ann Neurol* **43**:106, 1998.
133. Järvelä I, Autti T, Lamminranta S, Åberg L, Raininko R, Santavuori P: Clinical and magnetic resonance imaging findings in Batten disease: Analysis of the major mutation (1.02-kb deletion). *Ann Neurol* **42**:799, 1997.
134. Rapola J, Santavuori P, Savilahti E: Suction biopsy of rectal mucosa in the diagnosis of infantile and juvenile types of neuronal ceroid lipofuscinoses. *Hum Pathol* **15**:352, 1984.
135. Rapola J, Santavuori P, Heiskala H: Placental pathology and prenatal diagnosis of infantile type of neuronal ceroid-lipofuscinosis. *Am J Med Genet* **5(Suppl)**:99, 1988.
136. MacLeod PM, L. DC, Nickel RE, Chang E, Nag S, Zonana J, Silvey K: Ultrastructural studies as a method of prenatal diagnosis of neuronal ceroid-lipofuscinosis. *Am J Med Genet* **5(Suppl)**:93, 1988.
137. Chow CW, Borg J, Billson VR, Lake BD: Fetal tissue involvement in the late infantile type of neuronal ceroid lipofuscinosis. *Prenat Diagn* **13**:833, 1993.
138. Lake BD: Morphological approaches to the prenatal diagnosis of late-infantile and juvenile Batten disease. *J Inherit Metab Dis* **16**:345, 1993.
139. Kimura S, Goebel HH: Electron microscopic studies on skin and lymphocytes in early juvenile neuronal ceroid-lipofuscinosis. *Brain Dev* **9**:576, 1987.
140. Aicardi J: Management of the myoclonic epilepsies, in Procopis PG, Rapin I, (eds): *The International Review of Child Neurology Series: Epilepsy in Children*. New York, Raven Press, 1994, p 77.
141. Åberg L, Heiskala H, Vanhanen SL, Himberg JJ, Hosking G, Yuen A, Santavuori P: Lamotrigine therapy in infantile neuronal ceroid lipofuscinosis (INCL): *Neuropediatrics* **28**:77, 1997.
142. Krivit W, Sung JH, Shapiro EG, Lockman LA: Microglia: The effector cell for reconstitution of the central nervous system following bone marrow transplantation for lysosomal and peroxisomal storage diseases. *Cell Transplant* **4**:385, 1995.
143. Lake BD, Steward CG, Oakhill A, Wilson J, Perham TG: Bone marrow transplantation in late infantile Batten disease and juvenile Batten disease. *Neuropediatrics* **28**:80, 1997.
144. O'Marcaigh AS, Cowan MJ: Bone marrow transplantation for inherited diseases. *Curr Opin Oncol* **9**:126, 1997.
145. Kaye EM: Therapeutic approaches to lysosomal storage diseases. *Curr Opin Pediatr* **7**:650, 1995.
146. Bennett MJ, Boriack RL, Boustany RM: Polyunsaturated fatty acids reverse the lysosomal storage and accumulation of subunit 9 of mitochondrial F1F0-ATP synthase in cultured lymphoblasts from patients with Batten disease. *J Inherit Metab Dis* **20**:457, 1997.
147. Bennett MJ, Gayton AR, Rittey CD, Hosking GP: Juvenile neuronal ceroid-lipofuscinosis: Developmental progress after supplementation with polyunsaturated fatty acids. *Dev Med Child Neurol* **36**:630, 1994.
148. Lake BD, Henderson DC, Oakhill A, Vellodi A: Bone marrow transplantation in Batten disease (neuronal ceroid-lipofuscinosis). Will it work? Preliminary studies on coculture experiments and on bone marrow transplant in late infantile Batten disease. *Am J Med Genet* **57**:369, 1995.
149. Tyynelä J, Hofmann SL: Unpublished results.
150. Bronson RT, Donahue LR, Johnson KR, Tanner A, Lane PW, Faust JR: Neuronal ceroid lipofuscinosis (nclf), a new disorder of the mouse linked to chromosome 9. *Am J Med Genet* **77**:289, 1998.
151. Shibuya H, Liu PC, Katz ML, Siakotos AN, Nonneman DJ, Johnson GS: Coding sequence and exon/intron organization of the canine CLN3 (Batten disease) gene and its exclusion as the locus for ceroid-lipofuscinosis in English setter dogs. *J Neurosci Res* **52**:268, 1998.
152. Koppang N: The English setter with ceroid-lipofuscinosis: A suitable model for the juvenile type of ceroid-lipofuscinosis in humans. *Am J Med Genet* **5(Suppl)**:117, 1988.
153. Katz ML, Rice LM, Gao CL: Dietary carnitine supplements slow disease progression in a putative mouse model for hereditary ceroid-lipofuscinosis. *J Neurosci Res* **50**:123, 1997.
154. Deeg HJ, Koppang N, Shulman HM, Albrechtsen D, Graham TC, Storb R: Allogeneic bone marrow transplantation for canine ceroid lipofuscinosis. *Transplant Proc* **21**:3082, 1989.
155. Deeg HJ, Shulman HM, Albrechtsen D, Graham TC, Storb R, Koppang N: Batten's disease: Failure of allogeneic bone marrow transplantation to arrest disease progression in a canine model. *Clin Genet* **37**:264, 1990.
156. Santavuori PJ, Rapola J, Sainio K, Raitta C: A variant of Jansky-Bielschowsky disease. *Neuropediatrics* **13**:135, 1982.
157. Sharp JD, Wheeler RB: Unpublished results.
158. Eiberg H, Gardiner RM, Mohr J: Batten disease (Spielmeyer-Sjögren disease) and haptoglobins (HP): Indication of linkage and assignment to chr. 16. *Clin Genet* **36**:217, 1989.
159. Haltia M et al: CLN8: Northern epilepsy, in Goebel HH, Mole SE and Lake BD (eds): *The Neuronal Ceroid Lipofuscinoses*. Amsterdam, IOS Press, 1999, p 117–121.
160. Berkovic SF, Carpenter S, Andermann F, Andermann E, Wolfe LS: Kufs' disease: A critical reappraisal. *Brain* **111**:27, 1988.
161. Palmer DN, Tyynelä J, van Mil HC, Westlake VJ, Jolly RD: Accumulation of sphingolipid activator proteins (SAPs) A and D in granular osmiophilic deposits in miniature Schnauzer dogs with ceroid-lipofuscinosis. *J Inherit Metab Dis* **20**:74, 1997.
162. Koppang N: English setter model and juvenile ceroid-lipofuscinosis in man. *Am J Med Genet* **42**:599, 1992.
163. Riis RC, Cummings JF, Loew ER, de Lahunta A: Tibetan terrier model of canine ceroid lipofuscinosis. *Am J Med Genet* **42**:615, 1992.
164. Järplid B, Haltia M: An animal model of the infantile type of neuronal ceroid-lipofuscinosis. *J Inherit Metab Dis* **16**:274, 1993.
165. Broom MF, Zhou C, Broom JE, Barwell KJ, Jolly RD, Hill DF: Ovine neuronal ceroid lipofuscinosis: a large animal model syntenic with the human neuronal ceroid lipofuscinosis variant CLN6. *J Med Genet* **35**:717, 1998.
166. Jolly RD, Martinus RD, Palmer DN: Sheep and other animals with ceroid-lipofuscinoses: their relevance to Batten disease. *Am J Med Genet* **42**:609, 1992.
167. Messer A, Plummer J, Maskin P, Coffin JM, Frankel WN: Mapping of the motor neuron degeneration (Mnd) gene, a mouse model of amyotrophic lateral sclerosis. *Genomics* **13**:797, 1992.
168. Bronson RT, Lake BD, Cook S, Taylor S, Davisson MT: Motor neuron degeneration of mice is a model of neuronal ceroid lipofuscinosis (Batten's disease). *Ann Neurol* **33**:381, 1993.
169. Ranta S, Zhang Y, Ross B, Lonka L, Takkunen E, Messer A, Sharp J, et al.: The neuronal ceroid lipofuscinoses in human EPMR and mnd mutant mice are associated with mutations in CLN8. *Nat Genet* **23**:233, 1999.

170. Rawlings ND, Barrett AJ: Tripeptidyl-peptidase I is apparently the CLN2 protein absent in classical late-infantile neuronal ceroid lipofuscinosis. *Biochem Biophys Acta* **1429**:496, 1999.
171. Vines DJ, Warburton MJ: Classical late infantile neuronal ceroid lipofuscinosis fibroblasts are deficient in lysosomal tripeptidyl peptidase I. *FEBS Lett* **443**:131, 1999.
172. Vines D, Warburton MJ: Purification and characterisation of a tripeptidyl aminopeptidase I from rat spleen. *Biochim Biophys Acta* **1384**:233, 1998.
173. Liu CG, Sleat DE, Donnelly RJ, Lobel P: Structural organization and sequence of CLN2, the defective gene in classical late infantile neuronal ceroid lipofuscinosis. *Genomics* **50**:206, 1998.
174. Sleat DE, Gin RM, Sohar I, Wisniewski K, Sklower-Brooks S, Pullarkat RK, Palmer DN, el al.: Mutational analysis of the defective protease in classic late-infantile neuronal ceroid lipofuscinosis, a neurodegenerative lysosomal storage disorder. *Am J Hum Genet* **64**:1511, 1999.
175. Berry-Kravis E, Sleat DE, Sohar I, Meyer P, Donnelly R, Lobel P: Prenatal testing for late infantile neuronal ceroid lipofuscinosis. *Ann Neurol* **47**:254, 2000.
176. Haskell RE, Carr CJ, Pearce DA, Bennett MJ, Davidson BL: Batten disease: Evaluation of CLN3 mutations on protein localization and function. *Hum Mol Genet* **9**:735, 2000.
177. Heinonen O, Kyttälä A, Lehmus E, Paunio T, Peltonen L, Jalanko A: Expression of palmitoyl protein thioesterase in neurons. *Mol Genet Metab* **69**:123, 2000.
178. Katz ML, Shibuya H, Liu PC, Kaur S, Gao CL, Johnson GS: A mouse gene knockout model for juvenile ceroid-lipofuscinosis (Batten disease). *J Neurosci Res* **57**:551, 1999.
179. Mitchison HM, Bernard DJ, Greene ND, Cooper JD, Junaid MA, Pullarkat RK, de Vos N, et al.: Targeted disruption of the Cln3 gene provides a mouse model for Batten disease. *Neurobiol Dis* **6**:321, 1999.
180. Voznyi YV, Keulemans JLM, Mancini GMS, Catsman-Berrevoets CE, Young E, Winchester B, Kleijer WJ, et al.: A new simple enzyme assay for pre- and postnatal diagnosis of infantile neuronal ceroid lipofuscinosis (INCL) and its variants. *J Med Genet* **36**:471, 1999.
181. Bellizzi JJ, Widom J, Kemp C, Lu J-Y, Das AK, Hofmann SL, Clardy J: The crystal structure of palmitoyl-protein thioesterase-1 and the molecular basis of infantile neuronal ceroid lipofuscinosis. *Proc Natl Acad Sci U S A* **97**:4573, 2000.

PART 17

VITAMINS

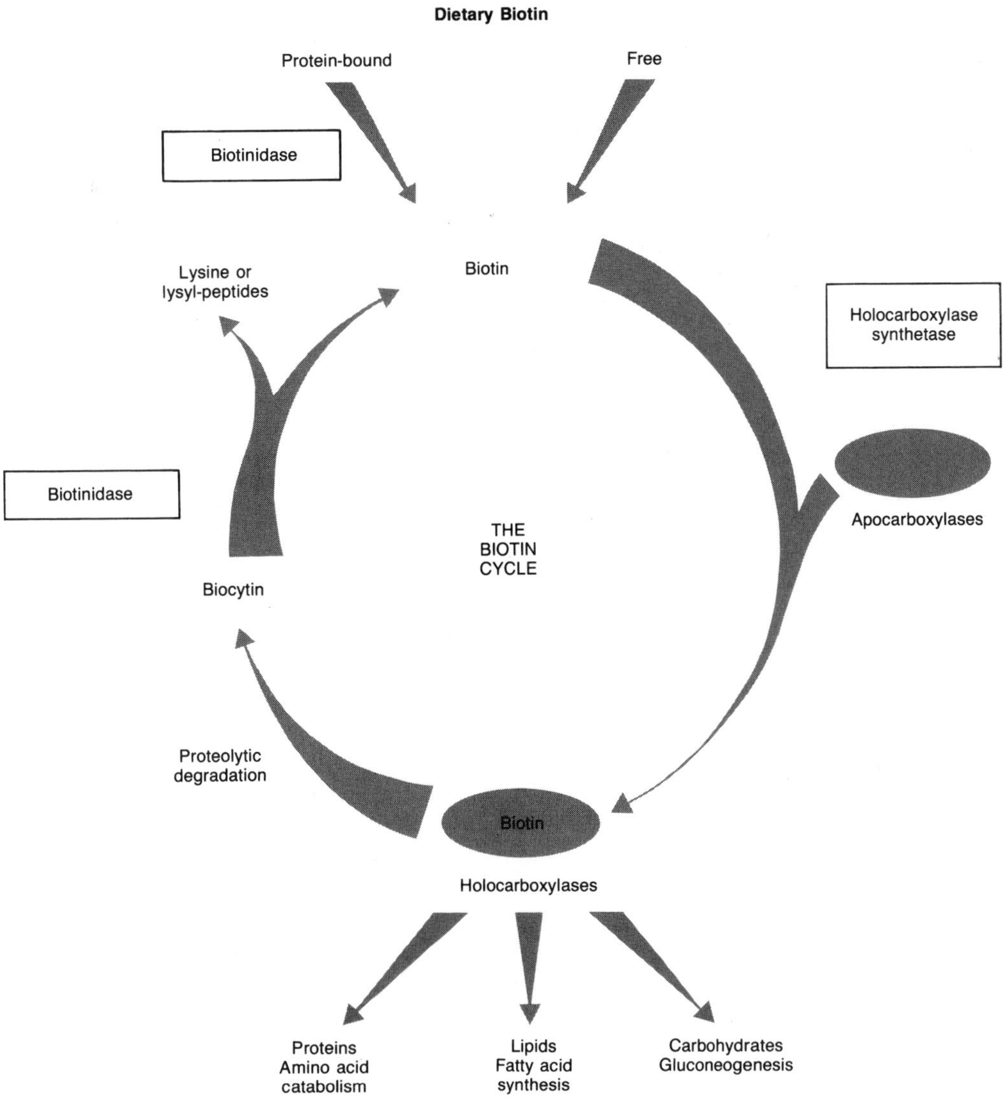

Dietary Biotin
Protein-bound
Free
Biotinidase
Biotin
Lysine or lysyl-peptides
Holocarboxylase synthetase
Apocarboxylases
Biotinidase
THE BIOTIN CYCLE
Biocytin
Proteolytic degradation
Biotin
Holocarboxylases
Proteins Amino acid catabolism
Lipids Fatty acid synthesis
Carbohydrates Gluconeogenesis

CHAPTER 155

Inherited Disorders of Folate and Cobalamin Transport and Metabolism

David S. Rosenblatt ▪ Wayne A. Fenton

1. **Folate coenzymes participate in a number of critical single-carbon transfer reactions, including those involved in the biosynthesis of pyrimidines, purines, serine, and methionine and in the degradation of histidine and purines.**
2. **Five inherited disorders of folate transport and metabolism have been well substantiated: methylene-H_4Folate reductase deficiency (MIM 236250); functional methyltetrahydrofolate (methyl-H_4Folate):homocysteine methyltransferase (methionine synthase) deficiency caused by mutations in the gene for methionine synthase reductase (*cblE*) (MIM 236270) or mutations in the gene for methionine synthase itself (*cblG*) (MIM 250940); glutamate formiminotransferase deficiency (MIM 229100); and hereditary folate malabsorption (MIM 229050).**
3. **Four putative inherited disorders in the literature cannot be considered to be well substantiated: dihydrofolate reductase deficiency; methenyl-H_4Folate cyclohydrolase deficiency; cellular uptake defects; and the original description of primary methyl-H_4Folate: homocysteine methyltransferase deficiency from Japan.**
4. **Methylene-H_4Folate reductase deficiency, the most widely studied of the inherited disorders of folate metabolism, is a condition in which clinical severity correlates with the degree of enzyme deficiency. The clinical symptoms vary, with developmental delay accompanied by motor and gait abnormalities, seizures, and psychiatric manifestations being described. The age of onset has ranged from the neonatal period to adulthood. The major biochemical findings are moderate homocystinuria and hyperhomocysteinemia with low or relatively normal levels of plasma methionine. Most severely affected patients have died. Pathologic findings include vascular changes similar to those seen in classical homocystinuria and demyelination presumably due to low levels of neurotransmitters or methionine in the central nervous system. A variant form of methylene-H_4Folate reductase deficiency resulting in "intermediate homocystinuria" is associated with 50 percent residual activity and enzyme thermolability, and is suggested to be an inherited risk factor for coronary heart disease. In the majority of cases, this variant is due to homozygosity for a common polymorphism, 677C→T, in the methylene-H_4Folate reductase gene. Severe methylene-H_4Folate reductase deficiency is resistant to treatment; folates, methionine, pyridoxine, cobalamin, and carnitine have all been used. Betaine has the theoretical advantage of both lowering homocysteine levels and supplementing methionine levels and has been the most promising therapeutic agent to date, particularly if started immediately after birth. Nevertheless, the prognosis is generally poor.**
5. **Functional methionine synthase deficiency due to the *cblE* and *cblG* mutations is characterized by homocystinuria and defective biosynthesis of methionine. Most patients have presented in the first few months of life with megaloblastic anemia and developmental delay. At least one patient presented in early adulthood with a misdiagnosis of multiple sclerosis. The distribution of cobalamin derivatives was altered in cultured cells, with decreased levels of MeCbl as compared with normal fibroblasts. The *cblE* mutation is associated with low methionine synthase activity when the assay is performed with low levels of thiol, whereas the *cblG* mutation is associated with low activity under all assay conditions. *cblE* and *cblG* represent distinct complementation classes. Both diseases respond to treatment with hydroxocobalamin (OH-Cbl).**
6. **Glutamate formiminotransferase deficiency is a heterogeneous condition associated with elevated excretion of formiminoglutamic acid, 4-amino-5-imidazole-carboxamide, and hydantoin-5-propionate. Clinical findings have varied from mental and physical retardation to massive excretion of formiminoglutamate in the absence of retardation. Therapy with folates and methionine has been described, but given that the correlation between symptoms and formiminoglutamate excretion remains uncertain, the basis for treating these patients is unclear.**
7. **Hereditary folate malabsorption is characterized by the early onset of failure to thrive and severe folate-responsive megaloblastic anemia. All patients have been severely restricted in their ability to absorb oral folic acid or oral reduced folates. Severe mental retardation may be a prominent feature if therapy does not succeed in maintaining adequate levels of folate in the cerebrospinal fluid. Two patients have shown increased susceptibility to**

A list of standard abbreviations is located immediately preceding the index in each volume. Additional abbreviations used in this chapter include: Ado-B_{12} or AdoCbl = 5′ deoxyadenosylcobalamin; AICAR = 5-phosphoribosyl-5-aminoimidazole-4-carboxamide; Cbl = cobalamin; *cbl* = cobalamin metabolism locus (*cblA*, *cblB*, etc.); CN-Cbl = cyanocobalamin; FGAR = α-*N*-formyl-glycinamide ribonucleotide; FIGLU = formiminoglutamate; GAR = 5-phosphoribosylglycinamide; GSCbl = glutathionylcobalamin; H_2PteGlu or H_2Folate = dihydrofolate; H_4PteGlu, H_4Folate, or THF = tetrahydrofolate; IF = intrinsic factor; methyl-B_{12}, CH_3-B_{12}, or MeCbl = methylcobalamin; methyl-H_4Folate = N^5-methyltetrahydrofolate; *mut* = methylmalonyl CoA mutase locus; OH-B_{12} or OH-Cbl = hydroxocobalamin; TC (I, II, or III) = transcobalamin (I, II, or III).

infection. This disorder provides the best evidence for the existence of a specific carrier for folate both at the level of the intestine and at the choroid plexus. Therapy has been attempted with large doses of oral or systemic folates.

8. **All of the clearly delineated disorders of folate metabolism appear to be inherited as autosomal recessive traits. Heterozygotes for methylene-H_4Folate reductase deficiency show decreased enzyme levels in somatic cells. A difference in folate absorption in the heterozygote has been suggested in at least one family with hereditary folate malabsorption.**
9. **Prenatal diagnosis has been successfully performed for methylene-H_4Folate reductase deficiency, methionine synthase reductase deficiency (*cblE*), and methionine synthase (*cblG*) deficiency using cultured amniotic cells.**
10. **Cobalamins (Cbls) are complex organometallic substances consisting of a corrin ring, a central cobalt atom, and various axial ligands. The basic structure, known as vitamin B_{12}, is synthesized exclusively by microorganisms, but most higher animals are capable of converting the vitamin into the two required coenzyme forms, adenosylcobalamin (AdoCbl) and methylcobalamin (MeCbl).**
11. **Dietary Cbl is acquired mostly from animal sources, including meat and milk, and is absorbed in a series of steps that includes proteolytic release from its associated proteins, binding to a gastric secretory protein known as intrinsic factor (IF), recognition of the IF-Cbl complex by cubilin, a receptor on ileal mucosal cells, transport across those cells, and release into the portal circulation bound to transcobalamin II (TC II), the serum protein that carries newly absorbed Cbl throughout the body.**
12. **The cellular metabolism by which the coenzymes are formed involves receptor-mediated binding of the TC II-Cbl complex to the cell surface, adsorptive endocytosis of the complex, intralysosomal degradation of the TC II, release of Cbl into the cytoplasm, enzyme-mediated reduction of the central cobalt atom, and cytosolic methylation to form MeCbl or mitochondrial adenosylation to form AdoCbl.**
13. **Only two enzymes in mammalian cells are known to depend on cobalamin coenzymes: methylmalonyl CoA mutase, which requires AdoCbl; and methionine synthase (also known as N^5-methyltetrahydrofolate:homocysteine methyltransferase), which requires MeCbl.**
14. **Ten different inherited defects are known to impair the pathways of Cbl transport and metabolism in humans (see Fig. 155-12). Three affect absorption and transport; the other seven alter cellular utilization and coenzyme production.**
15. **The defects affecting Cbl absorption and transport generally manifest themselves in infancy or early childhood as developmental delay with megaloblastic anemia. Serum Cbl levels may be reduced (in IF (MIM 261000) or cubilin-protein deficiency (MIM 261100)) or near normal (in TC II deficiency (MIM 275350)). Treatment with periodic injections of Cbl, with or without folate therapy, is generally effective in controlling these problems.**
16. **The clinical manifestations of deficiencies in cellular Cbl utilization and metabolism vary depending on whether one or both coenzymes are affected. Two abnormalities in AdoCbl synthesis only (designated *cblA* (MIM 251100) and *cblB* (MIM 251110) lead to impaired methylmalonyl CoA mutase activity and result in methylmalonic acidemia. In most, but not all, patients with these defects, pharmacologic supplements of Cbl (cyanocobalamin or hydroxocobalamin) produce distinct reductions in methylmalonate accumulation and offer a valuable therapeutic adjunct to dietary protein limitation. Oral antibiotic therapy may be useful to reduce propionate production by gut bacteria. The defect in *cblA* is unknown, while the defect in *cblB* patients is in cob(I)alamin adenosyltransferase, the final step of AdoCbl biosynthesis.**
17. **Three distinct mutations, designated *cblC* (MIM 277400), *cblD* (MIM 277410), and *cblF* (MIM 277380), lead to impaired synthesis of both AdoCbl and MeCbl and, accordingly, to deficient activity of both methylmalonyl CoA mutase and methionine synthase. Children from these groups have methylmalonic aciduria and homocystinuria. Children with the *cblC* mutation appear to be more severely affected clinically than the two known sibs in the *cblD* group or those in the *cblF* group. Major clinical problems in *cblC* patients include failure to thrive, developmental retardation, and such hematologic abnormalities as megaloblastic anemia and macrocytosis. Treatment requires a combination of the therapies for the individual coenzyme deficiencies: protein restriction and pharmacologic doses of hydroxocobalamin, possibly in combination with oral antibiotics and betaine supplements. The precise defects in the *cblC* and *cblD* patients are not yet known, but they must involve early steps in the intracellular metabolism of cobalamins, possibly cytosolic Cbl reduction. The defect in *cblF* appears to be in the transport mechanism by which Cbl is released from lysosomes.**
18. **The discriminating biochemical features of the inherited defects in Cbl transport and metabolism are shown in Table 155-5.**
19. **All the disorders of Cbl metabolism for which there are adequate data are inherited as autosomal recessive traits. Heterozygotes can be detected only for *cblB*. Genetic complementation analyses with somatic-cell heterokaryons have been particularly useful in demonstrating genetic heterogeneity and in confirming the existence of autosomal recessive inheritance among defects in cellular Cbl utilization and metabolism.**
20. **Prenatal detection of fetuses with defects in the complementation groups *cblA*, *cblB*, *cblC*, and *cblF* has been accomplished using cultured amniotic cells and chemical determinations on amniotic fluid or maternal urine. In several cases, *in utero* Cbl therapy was done with apparent success.**

FOLATE

The chemistry, biochemistry, and physiology of folic acid and its derivatives have been extensively reviewed in earlier editions of this book,[1,2] as well as in several excellent monographs.[3,4] A detailed review by Erbe gives a case-by-case analysis in tabular form of each patient who had been reported up to 1986 with verified methylenetetrahydrofolate reductase deficiency or glutamate formiminotransferase deficiency.[5] Other reviews are also available.[6–16]

The pteridine compounds referred to as "folates" participate as coenzymes in a number of critical 1-carbon transfer reactions, including those involved in the biosynthesis of purines, pyrimidines (dTMP), serine, and methionine, and in the degradation of histidine. In the 1930s, at about the same time that pteridine pigments of butterfly wings were being isolated and characterized, Wills and her colleagues determined that the absence of folate from the diet resulted in a macrocytic megaloblastic anemia.[17,18] The structural determination and synthesis of the parent compound were accomplished in the subsequent decade.[19] "Folic acid" and "folate" are the preferred synonyms for pteroylglutamic acid

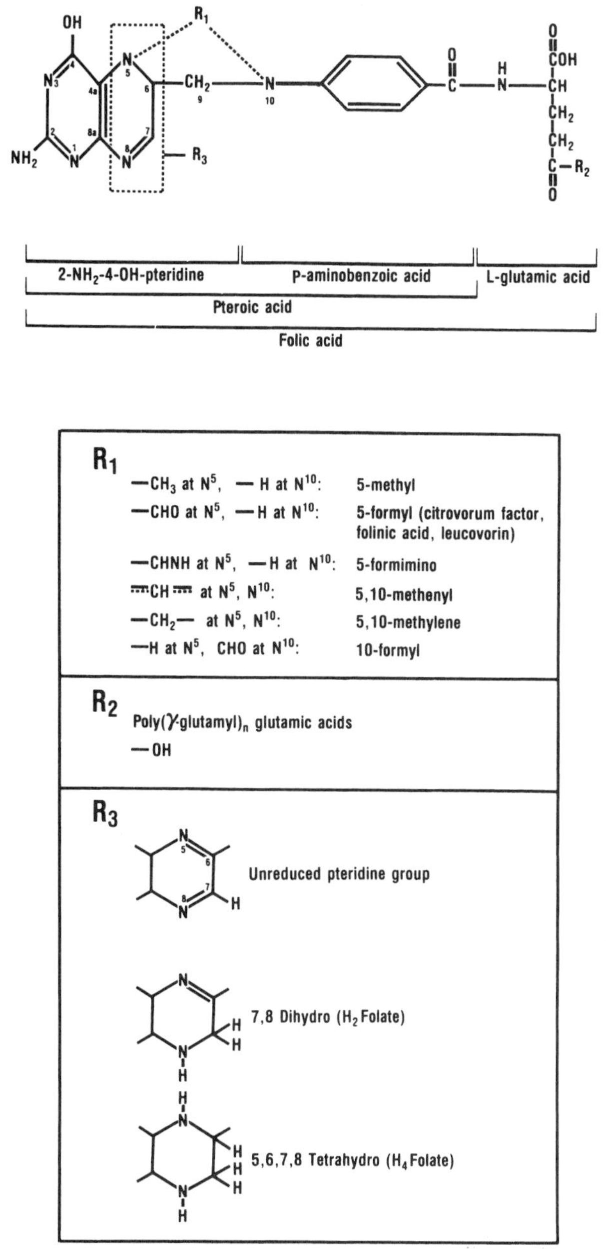

Fig. 155-1 Structure of folic acid and its derivatives. (*Modified from Rowe.[1] Used with permission.*)

(PteGlu) and pteroylglutamate, respectively (Fig. 155-1). The term folate is also used in the generic sense to designate a member of the family of pteroylglutamates, each having a different level of reduction of the pteridine ring, 1-carbon substitution, and number of glutamate residues. In the folate compounds, pteroic acid is conjugated with one or more molecules of L-glutamate, each linked by amide bonds to the preceding molecule of glutamate through the γ-carboxyl group. The terms *pteroylpolyglutamate* and *folate polyglutamate* apply to folate compounds with more than one glutamate residue. The biologically active folates are substituted derivatives of 5,6,7,8-tetrahydrofolic acid (H_4Folate) (Fig. 155-2).

As summarized in Fig. 155-1, there are at least three stages of reduction of the pyrazine ring of the pteridine moiety; at least six different 1-carbon groups substituted at positions N^5, N^{10}, or both; and γ-glutamyl peptide chains of varying length. 5-Methyl-H_4Folate is the predominant form of folate in serum and in many tissues. 5-Formyl-H_4Folate, also known as "folinic acid," "leucovorin," or "citrovorum factor," is a reduced folate that has been used therapeutically because of its chemical stability.

Folate Transport

Two distinct systems have been described for the transport of folates and folate antagonists (antifolates) across mammalian cell membranes.[20,21] One, the reduced folate carrier (RFC), encoded on chromosome 21q22.2-22.3 ([SLC19A1], NM_003056, MIM 600424), has been studied mostly in cancer cells and mediates a low affinity, high-capacity system for the uptake of reduced folates and methotrexate at high (μM) concentrations.[21–25] It shows considerable transcript heterogeneity;[25,26] the putative intestinal folate transporter has an identical cDNA.[27] The second system, a family of membrane-associated folate-binding proteins (FBP) or folate receptors (FR), is coded for by genes on chromosome 11 (q13.3-13.5).[21,28] These glycoproteins mediate a high affinity, low-capacity system and operate at low (nM) concentrations of exogenous folate. The FR-α ([FOLR1], NM_000802, MIM 136430) and FR-β ([FOLR2], NM_000803, MIM 136425) genes have similar structures, but differ in their 5′-untranslated regions and in their transcription regulatory elements. Both FR-α and FR-β are attached to the cell membrane by a glycosylphosphatidylinositol anchor, and there is evidence for receptor-mediated internalization (potocytosis).[29–31] The role of nonclathrin-coated invaginations in the plasma membrane (caveola), the process of "potocytosis," and the linkage of FR and RFC in this process remain debated.[21,32,33] In addition to the above systems, there is evidence that passive diffusion may work together with folate receptors in transplacental folate transport.[34]

Folate Polyglutamates

Human cells need a critical concentration of intracellular folate to allow activity of folate-dependent enzymes. The amount required to maintain an optimal rate of growth in culture varies from about 50 nM in human fibroblasts to about 1 μM in human lymphocytes and certain tumor cells.[35] Although the K_ms for monoglutamate folates of many of the folate-dependent enzymes are greater than 1 μM, those for polyglutamate folates of appropriate chain length are generally much lower, allowing folate metabolism to progress at the concentration of folates present in cells. Both a cytoplasmic and a mitochondrial folylpolyglutamate synthase add glutamate residues to selected folate molecules. A single gene on chromosome 9cen-q34 ([FPGS], NM_004957, MIM 136510) with alternative splice sites codes for the two folylpolyglutamate synthase proteins.[36–38] These enzymes form a peptide bond between the γ-carboxyl of the glutamate already present and the α-amino group of the glutamate to be added. Folylpolyglutamate synthase adds glutamate residues one at a time, requires ATP for its reaction, utilizes H_4Folate and other folates as well as antifolates as substrates with different affinities, and reacts poorly with folic acid and 5-methyl-H_4Folate. There is a unidirectional flow of triglutamate forms from the mitochondria to the cytoplasm, but longer forms cannot exit the mitochondria. Specific instances of channeling of polyglutamate intermediates between active sites of multifunctional proteins have been demonstrated. Thus, they may play a role in maintaining specific protein-protein

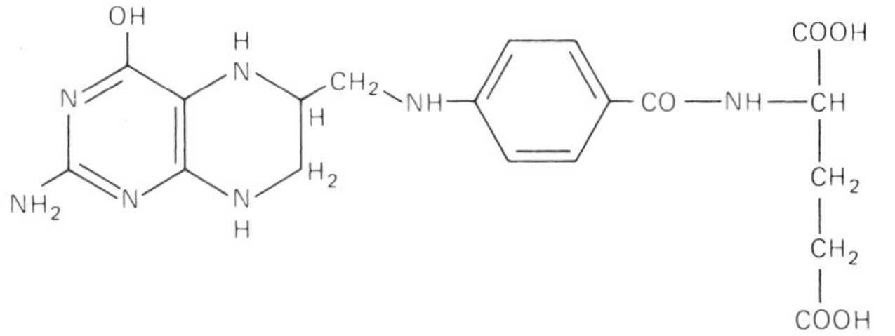

Fig. 155-2 Structure of 5,6,7,8-tetrahydrofolic acid (THF). (*Reproduced from Rowe.[1] Used with permission.*)

interactions.[39] Cell lines defective in folate polyglutamate formation have been reported. A mutant Chinese hamster cell line is auxotrophic for glycine, adenosine, and thymidine, apparently because reactions generating these within the cell require folate polyglutamates.[40,41] A human breast carcinoma cell line is defective in the synthesis of methotrexate polyglutamates and, consequently, is resistant to methotrexate.

Folate polyglutamates must be hydrolyzed in the intestine prior to absorption, and monoglutamates are released into the circulation.[42,43] The γ-glutamyl chain is resistant to digestion by the common proteolytic enzymes and is hydrolyzed by specific pteroylpolyglutamate hydrolase (conjugase) enzymes. Two distinct forms of human conjugase have been described, one in the intestinal brush border, which acts at neutral pH, and another within lysosomes. The lysosomal enzyme may play a role in regulating intracellular polyglutamate levels. Both human ([GGH], NM_003878, MIM 601509) and rat lysosomal conjugases have been cloned.[44,45] Prostate-specific membrane antigen (PSMA) has conjugase activity.[46]

Metabolic Pathways and Enzymes

The major metabolic pathways of the folates are shown in Fig. 155-3. In most cells, because serine and glycine are the major sources of 1-carbon units, entry into the active 1-carbon pool of intermediates is by way of 5,10-methylene-H_4Folate. This compound is used unchanged for the synthesis of thymidylate (Fig. 155-3, reaction 4). 5,10-Methylene-H_4Folate is reduced to 5-methyl-H_4Folate for the biosynthesis of methionine (Fig. 155-3, reaction 1), or is oxidized to 10-formyl-H_4Folate for use in purine synthesis[47] (Fig. 155-3, reactions 6 and 7). All the interconversions of folates involve exchange of side chains between tetrahydrofolates, except for the formation of thymidylate by thymidylate synthase (Fig. 155-3, reaction 4), which results in the oxidation of the folate moiety to dihydrofolate (H_2Folate).

Folic acid, a synthetic vitamin not found in nature, and H_2Folate are reduced by dihydrofolate reductase (Fig. 155-3, reaction 5) to H_4Folate. Dihydrofolate reductase has long been known to be the primary site of action of the chemotherapeutic drug, methotrexate, an antifolate. Unstable gene amplification resulting in resistance to methotrexate is associated with double-minute chromosomes, while in stably amplified cells that are resistant to methotrexate, the amplified genes are associated with elongated chromosomes.[48] The gene for dihydrofolate reductase has been assigned to chromosome 5q11.1-q13.2 ([DHFR], NM_000791, MIM 126060).[49,50]

The major source of single-carbon units in most organisms is carbon 3 of serine, which is derived from glycolytic intermediates. Serine hydroxymethyltransferase catalyzes the cleavage of serine to glycine and 5,10-methylene-H_4Folate (Fig. 155-3, reaction 3). In mitochondria, glycine is also metabolized to 5,10-methylene-H_4Folate, plus carbon dioxide and ammonia, by the glycine cleavage system[16] (also see Chap. 90). There are two separate serine hydroxymethyltransferases, a cytoplasmic form ([SHMT1], cSHMT, NM_004169, MIM 182144) and a mitochondrial form ([SHMT2], mSHMT, NM_005412, MIM 138450). Both have been cloned: cSHMT is on chromosome 17p11.2 (NM_004169), and mSHMT is on chromosome 12q13 (NM_005412).[51–53] The cytosolic form has been crystallized, and its structure solved.[54] A mutant Chinese hamster ovary cell line deficient in the mitochondrial serine hydroxymethyltransferase is auxotrophic for glycine,[55] indicating that the cytoplasmic enzyme cannot take over all the functions of the mitochondrial enzyme. By catalyzing the conversion of glycine in the diet to serine, which then can form pyruvate, cSHMT may also play a role in gluconeogenesis.[16] Both forms of serine hydroxymethyltransferase are capable of catalyzing the hydrolysis of 5,10-methenyl-H_4Folate to 5-formyl-H_4Folate.[56]

Two enzyme systems carry out folate interconversions in mammals.[57] A trifunctional polypeptide bears activities of NADP-dependent methylene-H_4Folate dehydrogenase, methenyl-H_4Folate cyclohydrolase, and 10-formyl-H_4Folate synthase (Fig. 155-3, reactions 6, 7, and 8; [MTHFD], NM_005956).[58] The interconversion of 5,10-methylene-H_4Folate, 5,10-methenyl-H_4Folate, and 10-formyl-H_4Folate links the major source of

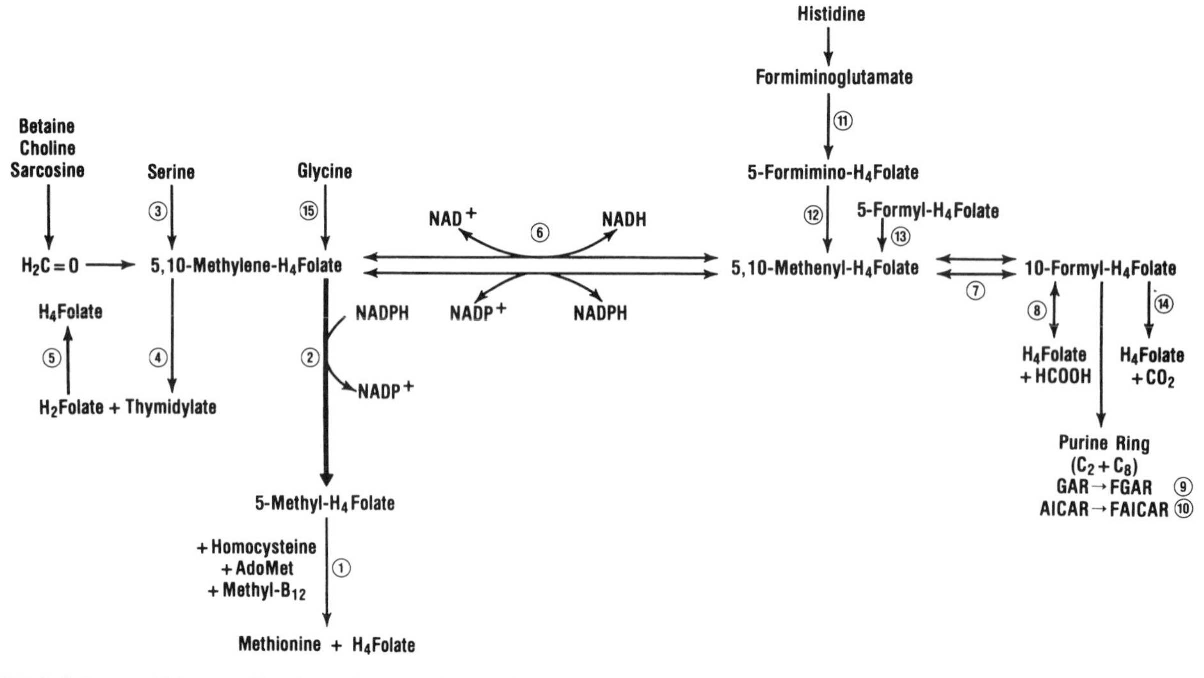

Fig. 155-3 Scheme of folate-mediated 1-carbon transfer reactions: 1. Methionine synthase (methyl-H_4Folate:homocysteine methyltransferase); 2. Methylene-H_4PtGlu reductase; 3. Serine hydroxymethyltransferase; 4. Thymidylate synthase; 5. Dihydrofolate reductase; 6. Methylene-H_4Folate dehydrogenase (NAD and NADP-dependent forms have been described); 7. Methenyl-H_4Folate cyclohydrolase; 8. 10-Formyl-H_4Folate synthase; 9. GAR (5-phosphoribosylglycineamide) transformylase; 10. AICAR (5-phosphoribosyl-5-aminoimidazole-4-carboxamide)transformylase; 11. Glutamate formiminotransferase; 12. Formimino-H_4Folate cycloderaminase; 13. 5,10-Methenyl-H_4Folate synthetase; 14. 10-Formyl-H_4Folate dehydrogenase; 15. Glycine cleavage pathway.

single-carbon units, as methylene-H_4Folate, with synthesis of thymidylate (thymidylate synthase [Fig. 155-3, reaction 4]) or purine (GAR and AICAR transformylase [Fig. 155-3, reactions 9 and 10]). The trifunctional polypeptide also permits either the release of single carbons from folate as formate or, more probably, the scavenging of potentially toxic formate (Fig. 155-3, reaction 8). The trifunctional enzyme is found only in the cytosol,[59] and is encoded by a gene on chromosome 14q24.[60] A separate bifunctional NAD-dependent methylene-H_4Folate dehydrogenase-cyclohydrolase, without synthase activity, also exists ([MTHFD2], NM_006636). This bifunctional enzyme is not detected in normal adult tissue but has been found to be expressed in tissues which contain undifferentiated cells and in transformed mammalian cells.[57,61] It is encoded by a nuclear gene but is found predominantly in the mitochondria of transformed cells.[59] The crystal structure of the dehydrogenase/cyclohydrolase domain of the human trifunctional enzyme has been determined in the presence of NADP,[62] as has that of the bifunctional bacterial enzyme.[63] While the NADP binding site is clear, the folate binding site(s) are only predicted by modeling, and the nature of the cyclohydrolase active site is not apparent.[62]

10-Formyl-H_4Folate dehydrogenase ([Fig. 155-3, reaction 14)]; [10-FTHFDH], AF052732) releases excess active single-carbon fragments from the folate pool and generates carbon dioxide. Its activity is restricted to the liver[64] and serves to maintain sufficient H_4Folate to permit acceptance of single carbons in folate-dependent reactions.

5,10-Methenyl-H_4Folate synthase is an ATP-dependent enzyme ([Fig. 155-3, reaction 13]; [MTHFS], NM_006441)[65–67] which converts 5-formyl-H_4Folate (folinic acid) to 5,10-methenyl-H_4Folate. Thus, this enzyme is important in supporting the clinical use of folinic acid for preventing methotrexate toxicity.

5,10-Methylene-H_4Folate reductase ([Fig. 155-3, reaction 2]; [MTHFR], AJ237672, MIM 236250)[68–70] converts 5,10-methylene-H_4Folate to 5-methyl-H_4Folate and probably uses only polyglutamates as substrates within the cell. The human enzyme binds FAD, uses NADPH as electron donor, and functions as a dimer of 77 kDa subunits.[71,72] It is inhibited by adenosylmethionine, which is bound by the C-terminal regulatory region.[72] The reaction is bidirectional *in vitro*, but *in vivo*, it is essentially unidirectional toward 5-methyl-H_4Folate. It is usually assayed in the reverse direction *in vitro*, using menadione as electron acceptor, but it can be assayed in the physiological direction as well.[68] Under the latter conditions, the concentration of adenosylmethionine required for inhibition is considerably smaller than that required for inhibition of the reverse reaction.[69] The human gene has been cloned and localized to chromosome 1p36.3 (AJ237672) and consists of 11 exons.[73,74] The homologous enzyme from *E. coli* is considerably smaller (33 kDa) by virtue of having no adenosylmethionine-binding regulatory domain. Its crystal structure has been solved.[75]

Methionine synthase, also known as 5-methyl-H_4Folate:L-homocysteine methyltransferase ([MTR], NM_000254, MIM 156570), is a cobalamin-dependent enzyme that catalyzes the transfer of a methyl group from methyl-H_4Folate (or adenosylmethionine) to homocysteine to form methionine (Fig. 155-3, reaction 1). In the complete reaction, the methyl group from methyl-H_4Folate is transferred to enzyme-bound cob(I)alamin to form methylcobalamin. The methyl group is then transferred to homocysteine, producing methionine and regenerating cob(I)alamin. After a number of cycles, the enzyme-bound cob(I)alamin oxidizes spontaneously to inactive, enzyme-bound cob(II)alamin, and a reducing system and adenosylmethionine are required to reform methylcobalamin and reactivate the enzyme.[76–83]

Mammalian methionine synthase is an 85-kDa cytoplasmic enzyme that functions as a monomer. Using the binding of cobalamin to methionine synthase in extracts of human-hamster hybrid cell lines as a marker, methionine synthase was assigned to human chromosome 1.[84] The cloning of the gene for human methionine synthase has confirmed this assignment at 1q43.[85–88] The predicted sequence of the human enzyme is 55 percent identical to the cobalamin-dependent methionine synthase from *E. coli*[86] (bacteria also have a noncobalamin-requiring methionine synthase). The bacterial enzyme has been extensively studied, and the structures of its cobalamin-binding and adenosylmethionine-binding domains have been determined by x-ray crystallography.[89,90] The structure of the cobalamin-binding domain is homologous to that of the C-terminal cobalamin-binding domain of methylmalonyl CoA mutase, the other cobalamin-requiring mammalian enzyme (see Chap. 94).

Because the circulating form of folate in humans is methyl-H_4Folate monoglutamate and because the methylene-H_4Folate reductase reaction is essentially irreversible in the cell, folate entering cells must pass through the methionine synthase reaction in order to generate tetrahydrofolate and the other folate cofactors.[91–95] In cobalamin deficiency (acquired or inherited, see below), or when cobalamin is irreversibly oxidized by nitrous oxide,[96] methionine synthase activity decreases or is absent, methyl-H_4Folate and homocysteine accumulate, and methionine and, especially, adenosylmethionine are reduced. In addition to the folate being "trapped" as methyl-H_4Folate, most of it remains as the monoglutamate because methyl-H_4Folate is a poor substrate for the folylpolyglutamate synthase enzyme. Folic acid or folinic acid can bypass this block until methyl-H_4Folate again accumulates as a result of methylene-H_4Folate reductase activity.

In *E. coli*, the reductive activation system that maintains the active form of the cobalamin cofactor on methionine synthase is a two-component flavoprotein system[97,98] consisting of flavodoxin[99] and flavodoxin reductase.[100] A similar system had been postulated for eukaryotes. Recently, based on the hypothesis that the mammalian enzyme would be a multifunctional protein incorporating both reductase activities, Gravel and colleagues cloned an enzyme called methionine synthase reductase (MSR), which is at least one component of this system.[81,83] MSR is a unique member of the ferredoxin-$NADP^+$ reductase family of electron transferases, combining binding sites for FMN and FAD, along with NADPH. The biochemical details of the reactivation reaction are unknown, and it remains unclear whether another protein may be involved. MSR has a predicted molecular size of 77 kDa and is encoded by a gene on chromosome 5p15.2-15.3 ([MTRR], NM_002454, MIM 602568).[83]

During the catabolism of histidine, a formimino group is transferred to H_4Folate, which transfer is followed by the release of ammonia and generation of 5,10-methenyl-H_4Folate. The two enzyme activities, glutamate formiminotransferase (Fig. 155-3, reaction 11) and formimino-H_4Folate cyclodeaminase (Fig. 155-3, reaction 12), share a single polypeptide which channels folate polyglutamate molecules from one reaction to the next.[101,102] The pathway represents only a minor source of single-carbon folates and may exist only in liver and kidney; the enzymes seem to be absent from fibroblasts and blood cells.

Disorders of Folate Nutrition, Transport, and Metabolism

Nutritional Disorders. Although a number of children born to mothers with a diet deficient in cobalamin have shown evidence of cobalamin deficiency (see "Cobalamin (Vitamin B_{12})" below), folate deficiency in the infant secondary to deficiency in the mother is unusual.[15] In nutritional folate deficiency in adults, as described in Herbert's classic self-study,[103] the peripheral blood and bone marrow changes that occurred after 4 months were preceded by a much-earlier fall in serum folate and a rise in urinary FIGLU levels. Psychologic and mental changes followed, but were rapidly reversed by folic acid supplementation. Red blood cell folate levels fall in folate deficiency significantly later than do serum folate levels. On the other hand, there are some situations in which there are no defects in folate metabolism per se, but in which folate therapy has been suggested. These include supplements of folic acid given to pregnant women to produce an increase in the mean birth weight of infants[104] and, particularly,

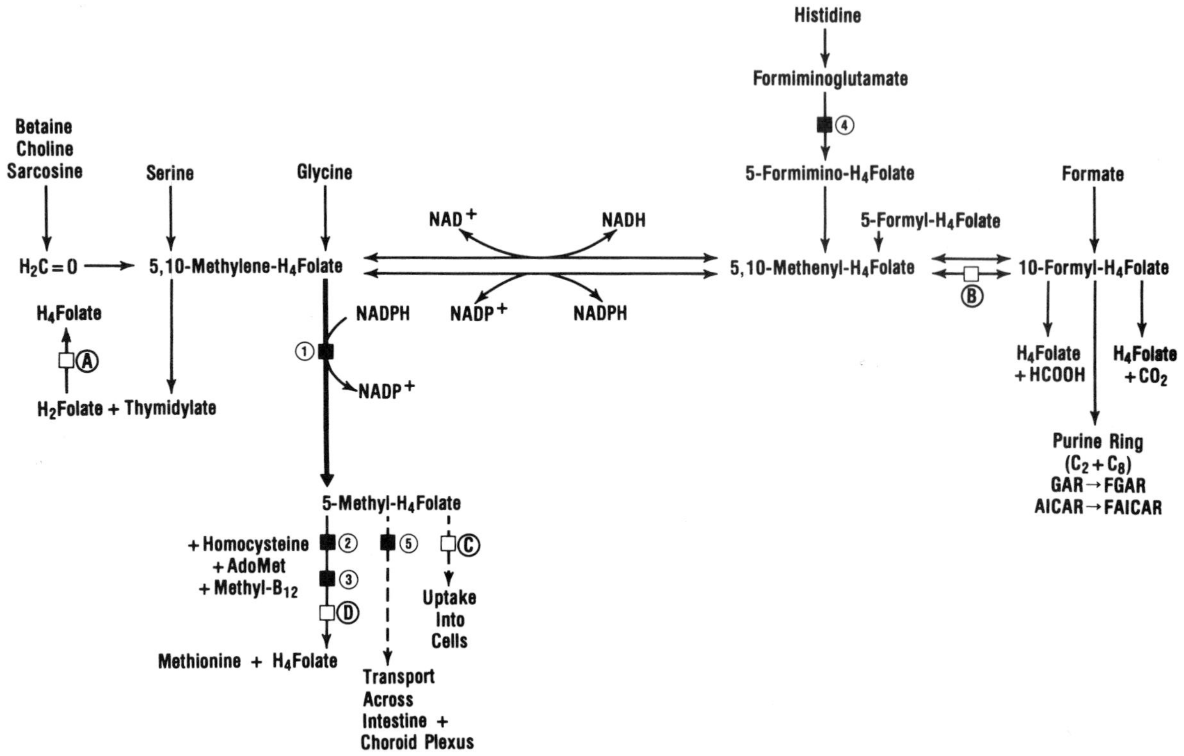

Fig. 155-4 Processes and reactions affected by inherited disorders of folate transport and metabolism; 1. Methylene-H_4Folate reductase deficiency; 2. and 3. Functional methionine synthase deficiency (*cblE*, methionine synthase reductase deficiency; *cblG*, methionine synthase deficiency); see text; 4. Glutamate formiminotransferase deficiency; 5. Hereditary folate malabsorption—*A*, dihydrofolate reductase deficiency; *B*, methenyl-H_4Folate cyclohydrolase deficiency; *C*, cellular uptake defect of folate; and *D*, methyl-H_4Folate:-homocysteine methyltransferase deficiency (original report from Japan[9]). Disorders involving folate transport are indicated by a broken line, whereas those involved in folate metabolism are indicated by a solid line. The numbered steps show the sites of well-characterized inherited disorders of folate transport or metabolism. Steps are the diseases that have been presented in the literature; those that remain in dispute are indicated with letters. AdoMet = adenosylmethionine; H_2folate = dihydrofolate; H_4Folate = tetrahydrofolate; methyl-B_{12} = methylcobalamin; GAR = 5-phosphoribosylglycinamide; FGAR = α-N-Formyl-glycinamide ribonucleotide; AICAR = 5-phosphoribosyl-5-aminoimadazole-4-carboxamide; C_2, C_8 = carbons number 2 and 8 or of purine ring.

supplements given prior to conception to women at risk for bearing a child with neural tube defects to reduce the frequency of these disorders.[105] It has also been suggested that increased folate intake may serve to reduce serum homocysteine concentration, a likely risk factor in peripheral vascular disease (see Chap. 88).[106–108]

The processes and reactions affected by inherited disorders of folate transport and metabolism are shown in Fig. 155-4. Those that are discussed in some detail below include hereditary folate malabsorption (reaction 5); glutamate formiminotransferase deficiency (reaction 4); methylene-H_4Folate reductase deficiency (reaction 1); and functional methionine synthase deficiency (reactions 2 and 3).

Hereditary Folate Malabsorption (MIM 229050)

Clinical and Laboratory Findings. This disorder [Fig. 155-4 (5)], which has also been called congenital malabsorption of folate because of its early clinical presentation, has been described in fewer than 20 patients, mostly females.[109–123] The disease is characterized by severe megaloblastic anemia. Diarrhea, mouth ulcers, and failure to thrive are common, and most patients showed progressive neurologic deterioration. Folinic acid-responsive peripheral neuropathy has been described.[115,123] Among the patients were two pairs of sisters,[111,124] and there may have been additional unrecognized affected patients in these families, because one patient had a sib who died at age 3 months[119] whose sex was not reported. Another patient, who was one of nine children, had sisters who died shortly after birth; in addition, she had a brother who died at the age of 13 years, but no further clinical details were provided.[120] A report from Israel[121] described a boy with this disorder, an infant who presented at age 4 months with severe bilateral pneumonia. He was one of seven siblings, two of whom had died in the first year of life without definitive diagnosis. In contrast to other cases, there was no sign of mental retardation, and correction of the serum folate levels did result in correction of the levels of folate in the cerebrospinal fluid (CSF). There is evidence for parental consanguinity in four families.[112,114,116,121]

The common clinical presentation in hereditary folate malabsorption is megaloblastic anemia in the first few months of life with low serum folates. Laboratory findings may include urinary excretion of formiminoglutamic acid (FIGLU) and orotic acid.[12,120] All patients were severely restricted in their ability to absorb oral folic acid or oral reduced folates. Large doses of oral folates did cause a hematologic response in some patients.[111,112,120] Parenteral therapy with folates has been effective in correcting anemia, but has been of limited effectiveness in correcting the levels of folate in the CSF. Other studies have suggested that folinic acid[118,119] or methyl-H_4Folate is more effective in increasing CSF. There is significant clinical heterogeneity among patients. In some patients, seizures were ameliorated by folate therapy, while in others, they were exacerbated by it. It has been noted[125] that the presence of seizures, with or without cerebral calcifications, is coincident with the ability to respond hematologically to large doses of oral folinic or folic acid; the reason for this is not known.

One of the patients[120] had additional findings, including a relative inability to retain plasma folate after parenteral folate administration, a finding also seen in another patient;[114] high levels of folate in the red blood cells following folate therapy; low normal plasma levels of methionine; the presence of cystathionine in the CSF and a response of the patient to methionine therapy; and increased susceptibility to infections associated with low levels of serum IgM and IgA. One of the affected boys[121] had a partial deficiency in both humoral (surface Ig and response to pokeweed mitogen) and cellular (E-rosette forming and response to hemagglutinin and concanavalin A) immunity.

These patients with hereditary folate malabsorption provide the best evidence for the existence of a specific carrier for folate both at the level of the intestine and the choroid plexus. Oxidized and reduced folates must share this system, because the absorption of both is effectively blocked in these patients. The same gene product must mediate both intestinal transport and transport of folates into the brain because, except in the two affected males,[121,123] levels in the CSF remained low when blood folate levels were raised sufficiently to correct the anemia. As mentioned earlier, a cDNA for the putative intestinal transporter has been cloned, and it is identical to that for the reduced folate carrier.[27] It is likely that uptake of folates into other cells of the body is normal in patients with hereditary folate malabsorption, because a hematologic response occurs in the presence of relatively low blood folate levels. In addition, the content and distribution of folates were normal in cultured fibroblasts from the one patient studied.[120] Thus, it will be interesting whether mutations in the putative gene for intestinal transport will be found in patients with hereditary folate malabsorption.

Treatment. Cooper has stressed[15] that it is essential to maintain folate levels in the serum, red blood cells, and CSF above levels associated with folate deficiency (4, 150, and 15 ng/ml, respectively). As mentioned above, some patients may respond to large oral doses of folic acid, folinic acid, or methyltetrahydrofolic acid. Oral doses may be increased to 100 mg/day or more if necessary.[15] If oral therapy does not work, systemic therapy must be instituted with daily injections (subcutaneous, intramuscular, or intravenous) of folinic acid.[126] If CSF folate levels cannot be normalized, periodic intrathecal injections should be considered.[15]

Genetics. The occurrence of at least one sibship with hereditary folate malabsorption and the documented cases of consanguinity suggest inheritance as an autosomal recessive disorder. All but four of the documented cases[121,123,126] have been female, although in one of the families, there is the suggestion of another possibly affected male.[120] In the father of one patient, the absorption of oral folate was seen to be intermediate,[114] again suggestive of autosomal recessive inheritance.

Cellular Uptake Defects. These disorders (Fig. 155-4 (C)) appear in a group of reported patients with varied clinical findings, some of which were associated with serious hematologic disease. Although the individual abnormalities of folate uptake are well characterized, it remains unclear whether these disorders represent primary inherited abnormalities.

Branda *et al.* reported a patient with severe aplastic anemia that responded to high doses of folate therapy.[127] The patient was part of a large kindred in which there was a high incidence of severe hematologic disease, including anemia, pancytopenia, and leukemia. These diseases were found in 34 individuals in four generations, resulting in the death of 18. The proband showed a marked reduction of the uptake of methyl-H_4Folate in stimulated lymphocytes despite a normal uptake of folic acid. Among eight healthy family members, including three of the proband's children, four were found to have a similar abnormality. In addition, there was a less marked reduction in the uptake of methyl-H_4Folate by bone marrow cells from the proband and his son. Of particular interest, however, was the finding that one son showed initially normal folate uptake, but neutropenia subsequently developed, and then the abnormality was exhibited. This observation has been taken to suggest that this disorder may not be a primary defect in folate uptake.[125] Folate uptake by erythrocytes and the intestinal absorption of folate were found to be normal. Since the original report, the patient died at age 41 due to respiratory failure secondary to pleural effusion and ascites.[128] Three children in the family had an increased incidence of sister chromatid exchange.

An additional family was described with a transport defect which affected red cells and bone marrow, but not lymphocytes.[129] The proband and his daughter had dyserythropoiesis without anemia; three brothers were normal. Erythrocytes from the patient showed abnormalities in the V_{max} and total uptake of methyl-H_4Folate, whereas folic acid uptake was normal; the daughter showed only a possible elevation in the K_m for methyl-H_4Folate, while the three clinically normal brothers resembled the proband kinetically. The status of both of these disorders of cellular uptake remains to be clarified.

An 18-year-old male with progressive neurologic disease, which included sensorineural hearing loss, a cerebellar syndrome, distal spinal muscular atrophy, and pyramidal tract dysfunction, had an isolated folate deficiency in the CSF and normal serum and red blood cell folate levels.[126,130,131] The defect may lie in the isolated transport of folate into the CSF and may turn out to be a variant of hereditary folate malabsorption.

Dihydrofolate Reductase Deficiency — Suspect Disorder. There are two published reports describing three cases of putative dihydrofolate reductase deficiency[132,133] [Fig. 155-4 (A)]. Megaloblastic anemia developed in these patients soon after birth and showed a better clinical response to folinic acid (5-formyl-H_4Folate), a reduced folate, than to folic acid, an oxidized folate. In all three patients, dihydrofolate reductase activity was decreased in liver biopsies.

The original patient[132] had a reduction in dihydrofolate reductase activity in the liver to 35 percent of control values (more than 2 SD lower than autopsy liver samples in seven control subjects). This male had anemia at 6 weeks of age, which subsequently became megaloblastic. Oral doses of 50 to 500 μg/day of folic acid did not produce a clinical response; 5 mg/day of oral folic acid resulted in a sustained 3-year remission. When folate therapy was discontinued, the patient relapsed. Small doses of folinic acid were effective in producing a remission. At age 19 years,[5] he was not grossly mentally retarded but had manifested "sociopathic and frankly criminal behavior that resulted in repeated incarcerations."[5] Although he was still folate-dependent, extracts of cultured fibroblasts showed normal total activity, kinetics, and heat stability of dihydrofolate reductase.

Two unrelated patients were later reported with neonatal megaloblastic anemia that was attributed to dihydrofolate reductase deficiency.[133] Activity in a liver biopsy was not detectable in the routine assay in the first case, but normal levels (1.0 to 1.7 nM of dihydrofolate reduced per min per mg of protein) were found in the presence of 0.6 M potassium chloride. At age 3 years, her bone marrow showed dihydrofolate reductase activity that was 10 percent of control levels and a heat-labile enzyme with a molecular size of 58,000 daltons, considerably higher than that of the normal enzyme.[134] At age 9 years,[1] the child was severely mentally retarded and still showed folate-dependent macrocytic anemia. We have shown that the correct diagnosis in this child is methionine synthase reductase deficiency (*cblE* complementation group, see below).

The second child was first seen at age 26 days because of oral and anal moniliasis and poor feeding. Low neutrophil and platelet counts were seen, and over the next 2 weeks a megaloblastic anemia developed. The serum folate level at 9.5 ng/ml was borderline normal for his age,[1] and the serum cobalamin level was normal. Dihydrofolate reductase activity in a liver biopsy specimen was 20 percent of the normal median value and was activated about twofold by 0.6 M potassium chloride, similar to the control liver samples. Subsequent study revealed that the patient was deficient in functional transcobalamin II[135] (see cobalamin section below). There was absent unsaturated serum cobalamin-binding capacity, although immunoassay did show transcobalamin II protein levels at 39 percent of the normal mean. There was no cobalamin-binding protein corresponding to transcobalamin II on Sephadex-gel chromatography. The patient was reinvestigated because of the development of mental retardation and severe neuropathy after 2 years of treatment.[136] It was concluded that this patient had functionally inactive transcobalamin II of the type described by Seligman.[137]

No additional patients have been described. Although at least two of the reported children had inborn errors of cobalamin metabolism, which were not initially recognized, the low liver values of dihydrofolate reductase remain difficult to explain. Of interest, urinary amino acids were reported to show a normal pattern, and no FIGLU was detected in the urine of the two patients who were reported in the most detail.[133] Thus, although the possibility of dihydrofolate reductase deficiency in an infant with severe megaloblastic anemia must be considered, all other known causes must be ruled out before this diagnosis can be confirmed.

Methenyltetrahydrofolate Cyclohydrolase Deficiency—Suspect Disorder. As previously discussed, methenyl-H_4Folate cyclohydrolase (Fig. 155-3, reaction 7) is part of a trifunctional protein that contains the activities of methylene-H_4Folate dehydrogenase, methenyl-H_4Folate cyclohydrolase, and 10-formyl-H_4Folate synthase.[138,139] Methenyl-H_4Folate cyclohydrolase deficiency [Fig. 155-4 (B)] was proposed in three children who had 44 percent of control enzyme activity on liver biopsy and levels of 58 percent, 36 percent, and 43 percent of control values in erythrocytes.[127] Clinically, the patients had mental retardation, microcephaly, ventricular dilatation, and abnormal electroencephalograms. A later report from the same laboratory[9] essentially retracted the diagnosis, and no additional cases have been reported.

Glutamate Formiminotransferase Deficiency (MIM 229100). As a result of the catabolism of histidine, a formimino group is transferred to tetrahydrofolate, followed by the release of ammonia and the formation of 5,10-methenyl-H_4Folate. The two enzyme activities involved in these steps, glutamate formiminotransferase (EC 2.1.2.5) (Fig. 155-3, reaction 11) and formimino-H_4Folate cyclodeaminase (EC 4.3.1.4) (Fig. 155-3, reaction 12), share a single polypeptide, which forms an octameric enzyme[101,102] that channels polyglutamate folates from one reaction to the next. This pathway represents a minor source of single-carbon units and may be present only in liver and kidney.

Clinical and Laboratory Presentation. Reports on fewer than 20 patients have been published, and it is not clear whether this enzyme deficiency is associated with a disease state or whether the association of clinical findings with FIGLU excretion is a result of bias of ascertainment.[5,126,131,140] Individuals with glutamate formiminotransferase deficiency [Fig. 155-4 (4)] have been described with two distinct phenotypes. In one type, there is mental and physical retardation, cortical atrophy with dilatation of cerebral ventricles, and abnormal electroencephalograms. The second type shows no mental retardation but massive excretion of FIGLU. It has been postulated that the severe form is associated with a major block in the cyclodeaminase activity and the mild form with a block in the formiminotransferase activity,[1] but no direct enzyme measurements have been presented to support this hypothesis.

Diagnosis of these diseases is hampered by the absence of enzyme activity from cultured human cells,[12] and there is dispute as to whether the deficiency can be diagnosed using red blood cells.[5,141] Indeed, in most cases in which the liver has been examined, enzyme activities were higher than would have been expected for a complete block resulting in disease.[9] Erbe[5] has summarized and tabulated most of the known patients with glutamate formiminotransferase deficiency.[124,142–155] The patients have come to medical attention from 3 months to 42 years of age. Three patients presented with delayed speech, two had mental retardation, and two presented with seizures. Two were studied because they were sibs of known cases. Mental retardation was described in most of the original Japanese patients,[9] whereas only three of the eight remaining patients were reported to show evidence of mental retardation.[149,151,152,154] Abnormal electroencephalograms and hypotonia have been described frequently. Several patients showed hematologic findings, including hypersegmentation of neutrophils and macrocytosis. The reported biochemical findings include: increased urinary, as well as serum, FIGLU, especially after a histidine load; normal to high serum folate levels with normal cobalamin levels; hyperhistidinemia; hypomethioninemia; and histidinuria.

In several of the Japanese patients, FIGLU excretion was elevated only after histidine loading. Amino acid levels in plasma, including histidine, were usually normal, but occasionally low methionine levels were seen.[124,154] Urinary excretion of 4-amino-5-imidazolecarboxamide,[149,156] an intermediate metabolite in purine synthesis, has been reported, as has excretion of hydantoin-5-propionate, the stable oxidation product of the FIGLU precursor, 4-imidazolone-5-propionate.[15,154,155]

Three patients of 12 months, 3.3 years, and 5.5 years, with a neuroblastoma, a germ cell tumor, and a fibromatous sarcoma, respectively, were found to have increased excretion of FIGLU and hydantoin propionic acid.[140] High levels persisted after treatment, and it was concluded that the patients had glutamate formiminotransferase deficiency.

Enzyme Activity. Enzyme activity was measured in the livers of five patients and ranged from 14 to 54 percent of the activity in control livers; what these values signify is not yet known. In three families, the level of enzyme activity was said to be low in erythrocytes; on the other hand, several laboratories have been unable to detect enzyme activity in erythrocytes, even in controls.[5]

Treatment. Response to therapy has been judged on the basis of decreased urinary excretion of FIGLU. Two patients in one family responded to treatment with folates;[150] six others did not.[5] One of two patients[152,154] responded to methionine supplementation. Given that the correlation between clinical phenotype and FIGLU excretion remains uncertain, the basis for treating these patients is unclear.

Genetics. Glutamate formiminotransferase deficiency has been found in both male and female offspring of unaffected parents. No consanguinity has been described. The deficiency is presumed to be inherited as an autosomal recessive. In the absence of detectable enzyme activity in cultured cells, definitive resolution of the inheritance of this disorder awaits the cloning of the human gene and the localization of the primary defect, because it is likely that the primary defect could then be detected in DNA from patients. DNA from putative patients should be put aside to await molecular diagnosis.

Differential Diagnosis. The major difficulty in the diagnosis of this disorder lies in the lack of expression of enzyme activity outside of the liver. Aside from FIGLU excretion in the urine and assay of enzyme activity in liver biopsy, which in reported cases has shown unusually high residual activities,[9] definitive diagnosis is difficult. In addition, FIGLU excretion may be caused by other defects in folate or cobalamin metabolism. Indeed, fibroblasts of one patient, who had megaloblastic anemia and folate-responsive homocystinuria,[141] were examined further. This patient has low methionine biosynthesis, low methionine synthase activity, and low MeCbl, and, indeed, has methionine synthase deficiency (*cblG* complementation group, see below). Thus, it is appropriate to study fibroblasts from all patients who show evidence of hypomethioninemia for evidence of a functional deficiency in methionine synthase.

Methylenetetrahydrofolate Reductase Deficiency (MIM 236250). Methylene-H_4Folate reductase (EC 1.5.1.20) is a cytoplasmic enzyme that catalyzes the NADPH-linked reduction of methylene-H_4Folate to methyl-H_4Folate (Fig. 155-3, reaction 2). Methyl-H_4Folate serves as the methyl donor for the methylation of homocysteine in the reaction catalyzed by methionine synthase (5-methyl-H_4Folate:homocysteine methyltransferase [Fig. 155-3, reaction 1]). The combined action of methylene-H_4Folatereductase and methionine synthase supplies single-carbon units for methylation reactions that use adenosylmethionine. The reaction catalyzed by methylene-H_4Folate reductase is essentially irreversible under physiological conditions, and enzyme activity is regulated by levels of adenosylmethionine, which is an inhibitor.[69,157,158]

Clinical and Laboratory Findings. Since the first reports of methylene-H_4Folate reductase deficiency in 1972[159,160] [see Fig. 155-4 (1)], more than 40 cases have been reported.[131,161–197] The major biochemical findings have been moderate homocystinuria and hyperhomocystinemia with low or relatively normal levels of plasma methionine. The clinical severity of this disorder varies greatly from case to case, with most patients being symptomatic in infancy or early childhood, but the age of diagnosis has ranged from before birth to adulthood.[159,182,193,198]. An infant showed extreme progressive brain atrophy and demyelinization on MRI.[197] A 10-year-old male exhibited a developmental history and physical signs compatible with Angelman syndrome.[199] In a family with six sibs, three patients had severe recurrent strokes in their early 20s, resulting in the death of two of them 1 year after clinical onset.[193] Two of these patients were noted to have a marfanoid habitus, although this is not a frequently reported finding. In another family, a younger brother developed limb weakness, incoordination, paresthesias, and memory lapses at age 15 years and was wheelchair-bound by his early 20s, whereas his older brother was asymptomatic at age 37 years.[194]

The most common clinical manifestation in methylene-H_4Folate reductase deficiency is developmental delay. Motor and gait abnormalities, seizures, and psychiatric manifestations have been reported.[195,200,201] In Erbe's 1986 clinical review,[5] about half of the patients were microcephalic; EEG abnormalities were present in most; some abnormalities of gait were described in almost all patients who were old enough to walk. Homocystinuria was present in all patients, with a reported range of 15 to 667 μM/24 h and a mean of 130 μM/24 h. Homocystine, not normally detected in urine or free in plasma, was found in the plasma: mean value 57 μM (range: 12 to 233 μM). Although data on total plasma or serum homocysteine (tHcy) are scarce, levels of 60 to 184 μM (controls: 4 to 14 μM) have been reported.[194,202–204] Plasma methionine levels were low in all patients, ranging from 0 to 18 μM, with a mean of 12 μM; normal is 23 to 35 μM,[5] although values vary among laboratories.

Although homocystinuria was consistently seen in all patients, and indeed is the clinical clue by which the diagnosis of methylene-H_4Folate reductase deficiency is made, the excretion of homocystine in urine is much less than that found in homocystinuria due to cystathionine synthase deficiency (see Chap. 88). Indeed, it may not be detected on spot testing, which, therefore, should not be used in isolation to diagnose the disease.[205] The methionine levels in methylene-H_4Folate reductase deficiency are always low-normal or low. This, again, distinguishes these patients from those with cystathionine synthase deficiency, who generally have hypermethioninemia. In contrast to patients who are functionally deficient in methionine biosynthesis because of abnormalities in methylcobalamin formation (complementation groups *cblC, cblD, cblE, cblF,* and *cblG*; see below), patients with methylene-H_4Folate reductase deficiency do not have megaloblastic anemia. In addition, in contrast to patients with the *cblC, cblD,* and *cblF* disorders, these patients have no methylmalonic aciduria. Although serum folate levels were not always low, many of the patients with methylene-H_4Folate reductase deficiency had serum folate levels that were low on at least one determination. In contrast, serum cobalamin levels were almost always normal. Although the levels of neurotransmitters in the cerebrospinal field have been measured in only a minority of patients, they have usually been low.[5,200]

Studies on Cultured Cells. A deficiency of methylene-H_4Folate reductase has been confirmed on studies of liver, leukocytes, and cultured fibroblasts and lymphoblasts. The enzyme assay routinely used for these studies measures the activity in the nonphysiological direction, using radioactive methyl-H_4Folate. Activity is extremely sensitive to the stage of the culture cycle of fibroblasts, with the specific activity in control cells being highest in confluent cultures.[158] This variability is sufficiently great to allow for the misclassification of controls and heterozygotes if not taken into account. In general, there is rough correlation between residual enzyme activity and the clinical severity. Both the measurement of the proportion of folate present in cultured cells as methyl-H_4Folate[171] and the synthesis of methionine from labeled formate[178,206] provide a better correlation with clinical severity. Studies on cultured fibroblasts[164,171] and liver[177,186] determined the levels and distribution of folate derivatives. In both control and mutant fibroblasts, most of the folates present were polyglutamates, and the proportion of polyglutamates relative to folate monoglutamate was similar; a direct relationship was found in cultured fibroblasts between the proportion of cellular folate which was methyl-H_4Folate and both the clinical severity and the residual enzyme activity, indicating that the distribution of the different folates may be an important control of intracellular folate metabolism.[171]

Control cultured fibroblasts can grow when homocysteine, along with folate and cobalamin, is substituted in the culture medium for methionine, an essential amino acid for these cells. In contrast, fibroblasts from patients with methylene-H_4Folate deficiency do not grow on homocysteine.[160,165] This inability to grow on homocysteine is shared by fibroblasts from patients who are functionally deficient in methionine synthase (*cblC, cblD, cblE, cblF,* and *cblG*; see cobalamin section below).[207]

A differential microbiologic assay that makes use of the fact that *Lactobacillus casei* can utilize methyl-H_4Folate for growth but that *Pediococcus cerevisiae* cannot is a useful screening test for methylene-H_4Folate deficiency, as analysis requires only small numbers of cultured fibroblasts.[164]

Genetic heterogeneity in the severe form of this disorder was suggested by the fact that fibroblast extracts from two of the original families showed differential heat inactivation at 55°C.[165] Although several of the later onset patients had a thermolabile reductase under these conditions, thermolability was also found in patients with early onset disease.[208] In some patients, this was shown to be due to the presence of severe methylene-H_4Folate reductase mutations in combination with the common 677C → T mutation that is responsible for the majority of enzyme thermolability in the general population.[209,210]

Kang and his colleagues originally suggested that thermolability of reductase activity at 46°C for 5 min in lymphocyte extracts of adults may be associated with "intermediate homocystinemia" and an increased risk for vascular disease in adult life.[211–214] Because of the difficulties in performing the assay for methylene-H_4Folate reductase on small cell numbers, there were not many studies designed to test this hypothesis. It is now clear that hyperhomocystinemia is a risk factor for vascular disease.[215–219] The ability to test the role of methylene-H_4Folate reductase thermolability as a contributor to the pathology was greatly aided by the cloning of the gene[220] and the discovery that a common mutation, 677C → T, which converts an evolutionarily conserved alanine at amino acid residue 222 to valine (A222V), is responsible for the thermolability.[209] The T allele was found to have a frequency of 35 to 40 percent in French-Canadians and other North Americans, but the frequency may vary in different ethnic groups.[72,209,221,222] In particular, it was very low in samples from Africa and parts of Asia.[222] The association between homozygosity for the T allele and plasma homocysteine levels in a population was found to be related to the folate status of the population, with elevations of homocysteine being dependent on the presence of lower plasma folate levels.[223–225]. The role of the 677C → T polymorphism as a risk factor for vascular disease and for neural tube defects[226] remains a subject of great interest and debate.[221,225–231] Interestingly, the 677C → T polymorphism was found to be associated with a decreased risk of colon cancer.[232] Another polymorphism, 1298A → C, which converts glutamate to alanine at amino acid residue 429 (E429A), is also associated with decreased enzyme activity.[233–235] A silent genetic variant, 1317T → C in the same exon, is common in Africans and may interfere with detection of the 1298A → C polymorphism;[235] 677C → T and 1298A → C have not been found together in doubly homozygous form.[234,235]

Pathophysiology. The prominent biochemical manifestations of methylene-H_4Folate reductase deficiency include: (a) homocystinuria and homocystinemia; (b) hypomethioninemia; (c) decreased proportion of intracellular folate as methyl-H_4Folate; and (d) decreased neurotransmitter levels. Patients with this disease rarely have megaloblastic anemia, suggesting that there is not a folate-related defect in purine and pyrimidine biosynthesis. The relative importance of homocysteine excess and methionine deficiency in these patients remains a matter of conjecture.

The neurologic findings in monkeys treated with nitrous oxide, an agent that inactivates methionine synthase, are reported to be similar to that caused by cobalamin deficiency;[91–93] this effect is reversed by methionine therapy. Patients with disorders of cobalamin metabolism,[236] who also have a block in methionine biosynthesis, may have neurologic deterioration, but they also have hematologic abnormalities that are absent in methylene-H_4Folate reductase deficiency. The pathologic changes[5,163,166,168,184–186,189,192] in the patients with methylene-H_4Folate reductase deficiency include dilated cerebral ventricles, internal hydrocephalus, microgyria, and low brain weight. Also seen in the brain are perivascular changes, demyelination, macrophage infiltration, gliosis, and astrocytosis. Other major pathologic findings are thromboses of arteries and cerebral veins; these appear to have been major factors in the death of these patients. These thromboses are the only pathologic findings shared with cystathionine synthase deficiency. It has been suggested that the combination of methylene-H_4Folate reductase deficiency and Factor V Leiden may contribute to the vascular pathology in some patients.[237,238] One patient with methylene-H_4Folate reductase deficiency had a fibrosarcoma.[192]

It has been pointed out[192] that the neuropathologic vascular findings in methylene-H_4Folate reductase deficiency are similar to those seen in classical homocystinuria due to cystathionine synthase deficiency. However, in methylene-H_4Folate reductase deficiency, it is necessary to explain the demyelination, astrogliosis, and lipid-filled macrophages, which are associated in many patients with a progressive course of seizures, microcephaly, and severe psychomotor retardation.

Two reports[189,192] have described classical findings of subacute combined degeneration of the cord similar to that observed in patients with untreated cobalamin deficiency in patients dying with methylene-H_4Folate reductase deficiency. It has been proposed that methionine deficiency causes demyelination, presumably by interfering with methylation.

Methylene-H_4Folate reductase is present in mammalian brain.[239,240] Because several authors have suggested that only methyl-H_4Folate among the natural folates can cross the blood-brain barrier,[172,241] methylene-H_4Folate reductase deficiency may result in functionally low folate levels in the brain. Because neurologic symptoms may be observed in patients without very low methionine levels, it has been suggested[77] that the neurologic dysfunction may occur as a result of impaired purine and pyrimidine synthesis in the brain, as opposed to low levels of adenosylmethionine.

The relative importance of low folate levels, low methionine levels, and low levels of neurotransmitters in the pathology of methylene-H_4Folate reductase deficiency is uncertain.[242] Differences seen between functional methionine synthase deficiency[236,243] (*cblC, cblD, cblE, cblF,* and *cblG*) and methylene-H_4Folate reductase deficiency should be useful in sorting out the relative importance of low levels of reduced folates, other than methylene-H_4Folate, and low levels of methionine. These comparisons have the potential of being made more difficult by developmental and tissue differences in the distribution of these enzyme activities.[244,245]

The most important finding in the clinical differential diagnosis is the absence of megaloblastic anemia in patients with methylene-H_4Folate reductase deficiency as compared to patients with functional methionine synthase deficiency (*cblC, cblD, cblE, cblF,* and *cblG* complementation groups), and the absence of methylmalonic aciduria as compared to patients with *cblC, cblD,* and *cblF* disease (see below). It has been shown that levels of methylcobalamin and of methionine synthase may be low in fibroblasts from some patients with methylene-H_4Folate reductase deficiency and that this could lead to the incorrect diagnosis of methionine synthase deficiency (*cblE* or *cblG*).[208]

Treatment. Methylene-H_4Folate reductase deficiency is very resistant to treatment but betaine has improved the overall prognosis.[5,15,126,131,195] The rationale for therapy includes: (a) folates, such as folic acid or folinic acid, in an attempt to maximize any residual enzyme activity; (b) methyl-H_4Folate to replace the missing product; (c) methionine to correct the cellular methionine deficiency; (d) pyridoxine to lower homocysteine levels, because of its role as a cofactor for cystathionine synthase; (e) cobalamin, because of its role as a cofactor for methionine synthase; (f) carnitine, because its synthesis requires *S*-adenosylmethionine; (g) betaine,[176] because it is a substrate for betaine:homocysteine methyltransferase,[245] a liver-specific enzyme that converts homocysteine to methionine; and (h) riboflavin, because of the flavin requirement of methylene-H_4Folate reductase.

Criteria for the success of treatment[5] have included reduction of the plasma homocysteine levels with elevation of plasma methionine levels to normal, along with improvement in the clinical picture. In most cases, several of the agents mentioned above have been used in combination, and it is somewhat difficult to assess the efficiency of a single one.

Cooper[15] suggested a therapeutic regimen consisting of oral betaine, folinic acid, and methionine, with additional vitamin B_6 and cobalamin. Cooper recommended cobalamin because of the observations of subacute combined degeneration of the cord[189] in a child treated with methyl-H_4Folate alone. Interestingly, therapy with methionine alone or with methyl-H_4Folate is not particularly effective in most cases, even though adenosylmethionine deficiency in the central nervous system appears to be playing a major role in the pathogenesis of this disease.[242] Fowler reported that one patient responded to riboflavin.[131] Supplementation with pyridoxine also has been suggested in order to enhance the transsulfuration pathway.[195]

Therapeutic successes include a patient who was treated with a combination of methionine, oral folinic acid and vitamin B_6, and cobalamin,[179,180] and several patients in whom betaine was included in the regimen.[5,181,182,190] One patient who responded to betaine at doses of 20 g/day had not responded to other treatments, including folates and methionine. Cobalamin had not been used in this patient. The two patients who were treated from the first month of life[190] with folic acid and betaine had normal psychomotor testing at around the age of 5 years. Ronge and Kjellman described a 7.5-year-old female, with slight microcephaly, impaired vision, and moderate developmental delay, who was treated from infancy with 3 to 6 g of betaine daily. She developed an unexplained increase in appetite and weight gain from age 4 years. With treatment, her previously undetectable plasma methionine levels normalized, but total plasma homocysteine levels remained elevated.[202]

Thus, betaine[181,190,202,246] appears to be the most promising agent for therapy of methylene-H_4Folate reductase deficiency, although, as mentioned above, some of the other therapies have been partially successful. There is not a great deal of data on the optimum dose of betaine in these patients, but Ronge and Kjellman suggested a dose of 6 g/day (3gb.i.d.) but indicated that they intended to increase the dose to 12 g/day in their patient.[202] Ogier de Baulny and colleagues suggested a dose of 2 to 3 g/day in young infants and 6 to 9 g/day in children and adults.[195] Kakura and colleagues studied the relationship of serum total homocysteine and betaine levels during treatment of a patient with oral betaine in doses of between 20 and 120 mg/kg.[204] They found that serum levels of total homocysteine decreased proportionally until betaine levels reached 400 μM, and suggested that this is the therapeutic threshold for serum betaine.

Many authors[5,12,196,202] have stressed the importance of early diagnosis and therapy because of the poor prognosis in this disorder once there is evidence of neurologic involvement. Even with early diagnosis, it is not clear that any of the therapeutic regimens are universally successful, and it is possible that genetic heterogeneity in the disease itself is responsible for some of the variability in clinical response to therapy.

Genetics. Autosomal recessive inheritance of methylene-H_4Folate reductase deficiency was supported clinically by the occurrence of more than one case in several families, by the presence of both males and females with the disease within the same family, and by the decreased activity of the enzyme in the fibroblasts[165] and lymphocytes[167] of obligate heterozygotes. Consanguinity has been reported.[5,169]

The gene is on chromosome 1p36.3 and has 11 exons.[74] Although nonsense and splice-site mutations have been reported in patients with methylene-H_4Folate reductase deficiency, most mutations have been missense, and each has been reported in only one or two families with severe deficiency.[203,210,220,247] Over 20 different mutations causing severe disease are known, in addition to the polymorphisms described above, which may contribute to disease in the general population; they are shown in Fig. 155-5 in a representation of the methylene-H_4Folate reductase protein. The crystal structure of the *E. coli* enzyme, which is considerably smaller than the mammalian one because it lacks the C-terminal adenosylmethionine-binding regulatory domain, has been reported.[75] Based on this, the possible effect of the common A222V polymorphism on the quaternary structural stability of the enzyme and the role of folates in stabilizing this structure were rationalized.[75] The effects of severe, disease-causing mutations have not yet been accounted for in this model system.

Methylene-H_4Folate reductase deficiency has been diagnosed or excluded prenatally by enzyme assay or by measurement of the incorporation of labeled formate into methionine by cultured amniotic fluid cells.[182,188,190,205,248,249] Enzyme activity is detectable in normal chorionic villi.[182,188] If both mutations segregating in a family are known, molecular analysis allows for early prenatal diagnosis.

Functional Methionine Synthase Deficiency

Three metabolic pathways intersect at methionine synthase: those of folate, cobalamin (Cbl), and sulfur-containing amino acids. Because deficiency of the activity of this enzyme results in diminished or absent methylcobalamin (MeCbl) synthesis, disorders affecting it have been considered and designated genetically as Cbl metabolism defects (symbolized as *cbl*), along with others affecting both MeCbl and adenosylcobalamin (AdoCbl) synthesis or AdoCbl synthesis alone (see cobalamin section below). These designations have been reinforced by the use, in differential diagnosis, of genetic complementation analysis between cell lines from patients with defects in all aspects of Cbl metabolism. Nevertheless, because methyl-H_4Folate participates in the methionine synthase reaction and because methionine synthase deficiency significantly affects folate metabolism, these defects can be considered inborn errors of folate metabolism as well. Here, we discuss the two that directly involve methionine synthase (complementation groups *cblE* (MIM 236270) and *cblG* (MIM 250940). In the subsequent sections on Cbl metabolism, the others indirectly affecting methionine synthase activity (*cblC*, *cblD*, and *cblF*) will be considered in detail. For a full discussion of sulfur amino acid metabolism and transsulfuration pathways, see Chap. 88.

Clinical and Laboratory Findings. Patients from the *cblE* and *cblG* complementation groups are very similar, both clinically and

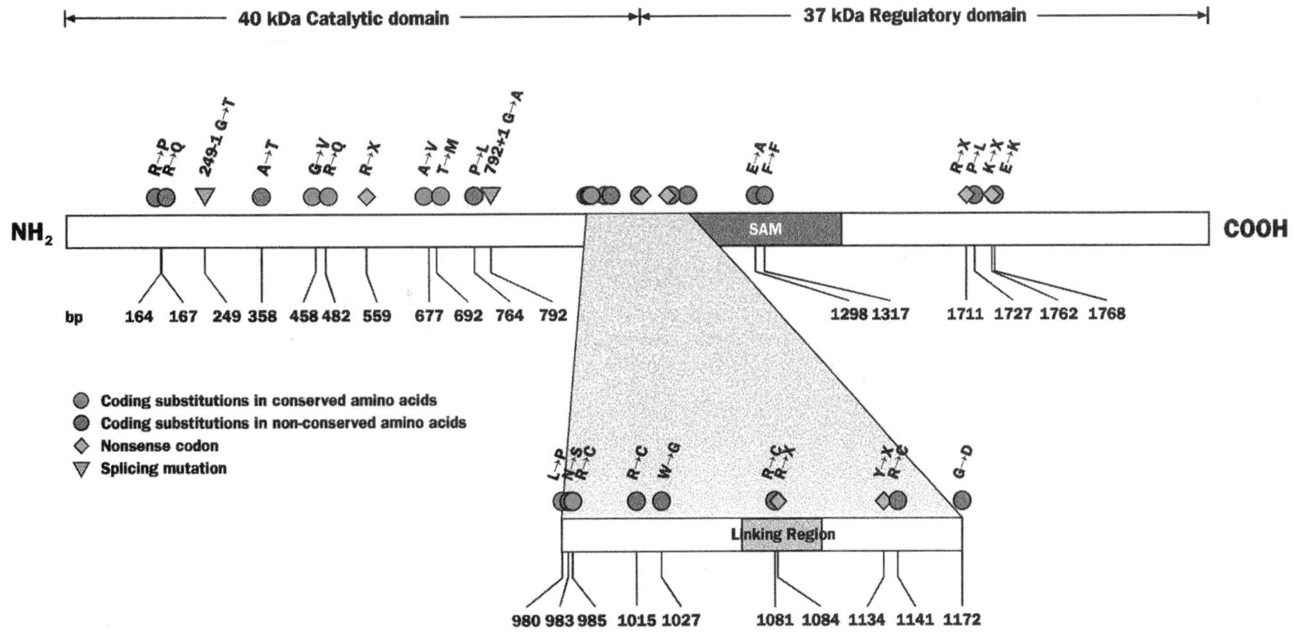

Fig. 155-5 The structures, domains, and mutations of the MTHFR polypeptide. Amino acid changes are indicated above the protein; base pair position is indicated below. An area of the polypeptide is enlarged in order to show all the amino acid changes. (*Courtesy of R. Rozen, McGill University*)

Table 155-1 Clinical and Laboratory Features of Patient with Homocystinemia Due to Defects in MeCbl Synthesis*

Finding	Mutant Class	
	cblE	*cblG*
Megaloblastic anemia	3/4	10/10
Developmental retardation	4/4	10/10
Cerebral atrophy	3/4	7/10
Hypotonia	2/4	8/10
Feeding difficulty	3/4	8/10
Lethargy	2/4	7/10
Seizures	2/4	9/10
Vision abnormalities	2/4	3/10
Skeletal abnormalities	0/4	1/10

*Ratios denote the number of patients showing a particular finding/total nrmber of patients in each mutant class

SOURCE: Compiled from published summaries.[243,259]

biochemically. Most patients so far reported with these disorders presented in the first few months of life with vomiting, poor feeding, and lethargy. Hypotonia, seizures, and developmental delay characterize their severe neurologic dysfunction. There are reports on at least 12 *cblE* and 20 *cblG* patients.[83,243,250–261] Table 155-1 summarizes some of the clinical findings available from the literature. The prevalence of neurologic signs and symptoms is striking. One patient in the *cblG* group presented as an adult with progressively impaired sensory responses and gait disturbances and was initially diagnosed as having multiple sclerosis.[250] Megaloblastic anemia and homocystinuria or homocystinemia are generally present, and hypomethioninemia is often found. Serum Cbl and folate concentrations are normal or elevated, and methylmalonic aciduria is absent, except in one patient, in whom it was a transient finding.[262]

Localization of Defects. The constellation of homocystinuria and hypomethioninemia without methylmalonic aciduria suggested strongly that these patients had isolated deficiencies in the activity of methionine synthase, either primary or secondary to abnormal synthesis or utilization of MeCbl, its cofactor (see Fig. 155-10). Studies of fibroblasts derived from several of these patients have confirmed this hypothesis. Incorporation of [^{14}C]propionate into macromolecules was normal, while incorporation of [^{14}C]methyl-H_4Folate was reduced to 5 to 35 percent of control (average: 15 percent),[243] a value similar to that reported for patients from the *cblC* group (see below). Genetic complementation analysis based on [^{14}C]methyl-H_4Folate incorporation distinguished two complementation groups:[263] *cblE* (index patient reported in reference 264) and *cblG* (index patient reported in reference 252). Accumulation of Cbl by fibroblasts was normal or increased in these groups, as was the fraction recovered as AdoCbl.[243] In contrast, the fraction identified as MeCbl was much reduced.[243]

cblE. When methionine synthase activities were determined under standard conditions in extracts of fibroblasts from *cblE* patients, both holoenzyme and total enzyme were normal or slightly reduced.[243] Under suboptimal assay conditions, namely in the presence of lower concentrations of reducing agents, methionine synthase activities were less than those in controls.[265] These findings have led to the hypothesis that the *cblE* group has defects in an enzyme required either to reduce Cbl so that it can participate in the methionine synthase reaction or to maintain it in its active reduced form [cob(I)alamin] on the methionine synthase.[265] For example, bacterial methionine synthase has accessory reductase proteins[266] that perform these functions. Based on the sequences of these bacterial proteins, Gravel and colleagues cloned a cDNA for a multifunctional human protein called methionine synthase reductase. Sequence analysis of cDNAs for this enzyme from patients in the *cblE* group has revealed a number of likely deleterious mutations in this gene.[83,257] Figure 155-6 is a linear representation of the protein, its cofactor-binding regions, and the localization of the known mutations.

cblG. In the *cblG* complementation group, methionine synthase activities are reduced even under optimal assay conditions,[243] although some heterogeneity has been noted.[255] This finding suggests that patients in this group have primary defects in the catalytic subunit of methionine synthase itself.[263] Moreover, the *cblG* group shows biochemical heterogeneity with respect to binding cellular Cbl to methionine synthase. In extracts of cell lines from most patients, about 75 percent of cellular Cbl migrated at the position of methionine synthase during gel electrophoresis, even though little of it was MeCbl. In a few cell lines (referred to as *cblG* variants), however, no Cbl of any form migrated at this position.[256] This was highly suggestive of mutations in the Cbl-binding domain of methionine synthase or absent methionine synthase protein in these patients, strengthening the possibility that the *cblG* group reflected primary deficiencies in the methionine synthase apoenzyme. Human methionine synthase has now been cloned, and mutations likely to be deleterious have been found by sequence analysis of cDNAs from patients in the *cblG* group.[85,86,267] Based on the crystal structures of the Cbl-binding and adenosylmethionine-binding domains of *E. coli* methionine synthase,[89,90] one of the missense changes uncovered (P1173L) appears to disrupt the adenosylmethionine binding site,[267] while two others, I881Δ[267] and H920D,[85] may affect the pocket in the Cbl-binding domain that accommodates the dimethylbenzimidazole moiety of the cofactor (see cobalamin section). Interestingly,

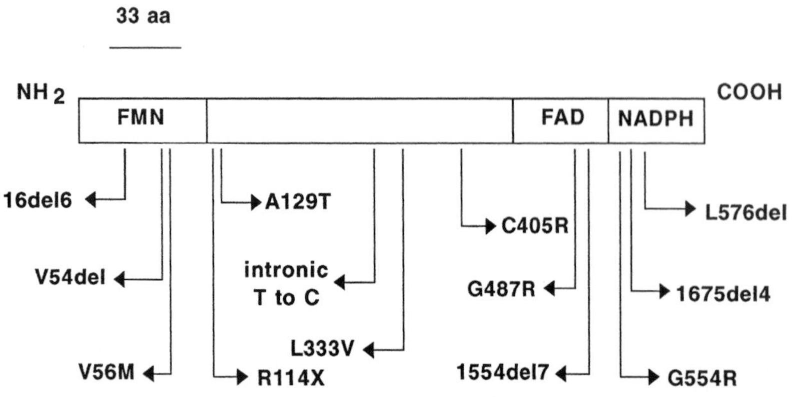

Fig. 155-6 Mutations in the MSR polypeptide. Their relation to the FMN, FAD and NADPH binding sites are shown. (*Modified from Wilson et al.*[257] *Used with permission.*)

the *cblG* variants so far examined all appear to be effectively null for the methionine synthase protein, rather than Cbl-binding mutants.[260]

Pathophysiology and Genetics. The association of isolated functional methionine synthase deficiency with megaloblastic anemia and neurologic defects in these patients provides further strong evidence for the hypothesis outlined in Chap. 94, that these clinical signs are sequelae of defects in the MeCbl-methionine synthase branch of Cbl metabolism, rather than the AdoCbl-methylmalonyl CoA mutase one. Hall[268] and Shevell and Rosenblatt[269] have discussed in detail the relationships between the biochemical defects and their pathophysiologic consequences. As Hall has pointed out, there are three levels at which the impact of these disorders is felt: hematologic, short-term neurologic, and long-term neurodevelopmental. Effects at each of these may result from a different aspect of functional methionine synthase deficiency, and the response of each to treatment may likewise be distinctive. The hematologic problems may reflect disturbed DNA synthesis, while the short-term neurologic symptoms are likely due to either acute toxic effects or aberrant neurotransmitter metabolism.[268] The long-term developmental effects of these disorders appear to be related to defects in myelination in the central nervous system. Abnormal CT scans have been reported for most of the patients on whom the test was performed, with apparent atrophy or hypoplasia of the brain. MRI has been done for only a few patients; in two, myelination was delayed, even after a year of steady clinical improvement with Cbl therapy.[268] Hall has suggested a wide range of possibilities for the disruption of function in the nervous system. They include toxicity of methyl-H_4Folate or homocysteine, the classic folate trap hypothesis or variants of it (discussed above), and reduced methylation of proteins and neurotransmitters due to deficiency in *S*-adenosylmethionine synthesis. DNA methylation, either from *S*-adenosylmethionine or directly from MeCbl,[270] may also play a role. A more complete understanding of the impact of deficiencies in this complex system of interrelated pathways on hematologic and neurologic development requires further study, both of the enzymes involved and of the patients with these and related disorders.

Each of these diseases is inherited as an autosomal recessive trait, with about equal numbers of male and female patients reported.[243,257,268] Both defects act as recessives in complementation analysis in culture.[263] So far, heterozygote detection is possible only by DNA-based techniques.

Diagnosis, Treatment, and Prognosis. The clinical hallmarks of these disorders appear to be developmental delay and megaloblastic anemia, with homocystinuria and without methylmalonic aciduria. Although most patients were diagnosed early in life, one (a *cblG*) did not come to medical attention until age 21.[250] Differentiation from other possible diagnoses such as TC II deficiency (see below), other folate transport or metabolism defects, or cystathionine β-synthase deficiency (Chap. 88) can be accomplished by studies of cultured cells, particularly by incorporation of ^{14}C from [^{14}C]methyl-H_4Folate and complementation analysis. These two assays are especially important because deficiency of methylene-H_4Folate reductase has a similar clinical presentation and may result in decreased cellular MeCbl accumulation and even decreased methionine synthase activity.[208] Prenatal diagnosis using amniotic fluid cells is possible and has been performed for both the *cblE* and *cblG* disorders. With the cloning of both methionine synthase reductase and methionine synthase, molecular diagnosis may be possible in families where the mutations are known.

Because the patients reported to date have responded to hydroxocobalamin (OH-Cbl) therapy with normalization of their biochemical parameters and at least partial resolution of their clinical symptoms[236,243,255,268] and because it seems likely, as in *cblC* patients (below), that delays in treatment may result in incompletely reversible developmental delays or neurologic deficits,[243,250,268] institution of OH-Cbl administration should occur as soon as the diagnosis is made. Dosages of 1 mg OH-Cbl per day (intramuscular injection) have been used initially, then tapered to 1 mg, one to three times a week. Biochemical improvement has been rapid on this regimen, and most clinical symptoms have resolved in a few weeks. In some patients, macrocytic anemia has responded to folinic acid therapy.[259] In general, neurologic symptoms and developmental problems have been slower to improve, sometimes requiring 3 or 4 months of therapy before consistent gains are apparent.[243,268] On the other hand, the *cblE* patient diagnosed prenatally and treated with OH-Cbl both *in utero* and postnatally has developed normally with only minor clinical symptoms,[269,271] suggesting that prenatal therapy may be warranted in these disorders.

As in the case of some *cblC* patients (below), a variety of adjuncts to Cbl therapy have been tried, including supplementation with betaine, methionine, carnitine, and pyridoxine,[269] with variable and poorly documented results. Of these, betaine supplementation to normalize the serum methionine:homocysteine ratio further, beyond what is achieved with OH-Cbl alone, may be justified to avoid the vascular injury and thromboembolism associated with homocystinemia (see Chap. 88). One patient in the *cblE* group (diagnosed postmortem) died at 5 years of age from bilateral renal artery thrombosis and had arteriosclerotic changes elsewhere at autopsy,[243] emphasizing the potentially serious consequences of untreated or poorly controlled homocystinemia.

Because patients with these disorders have been described relatively recently, the long-term prognosis in these conditions remains unknown. The index *cblE* patient is 18 years old and thriving, although he is mildly developmentally delayed,[236] while his prenatally diagnosed and treated brother (14 years old) appears normal, except for a slight speech impediment.[269] In contrast, the index *cblG* patient, although clinically well, remains significantly retarded with major visual defects.[252] It seems likely that patients in the *cblE* and *cblG* groups will show a range of clinical outcomes,[243,268] similar to those of patients in the *cblC* group (below), because the majority of the symptoms of all of these patients arises from the same cause, that is, functional methionine synthase deficiency. Likewise, early diagnosis and treatment may be the only way to avoid permanent neurologic damage and its consequences.[243,268]

Differential Diagnosis of Folate Disorders

A guide to the differential diagnosis of the well-characterized disorders of folate metabolism is shown in Table 155-2. Many of these disorders are associated with normal serum and red blood cell folate levels. Hereditary folate malabsorption is always, and methylene-H_4Folate reductase deficiency is usually, associated with low serum folate levels. Serum folate levels were reported as elevated in most of the original Japanese patients (but none of the subsequent ones) with glutamate formiminotransferase deficiency. Homocystinuria has been described in methylene-H_4Folate reductase deficiency and in the *cblE* and *cblG* disorders. Megaloblastic anemia is seen in hereditary folate malabsorption and in *cblE* and *cblG* patients, but not in glutamate formiminotransferase deficiency, except in the original Japanese patients, and only rarely in methylene-H_4Folate reductase deficiency.

Defects detectable in cultured cells include a decreased incorporation of label from methyl-H_4Folate into protein or from formate into methionine in *cblE* and *cblG* disease, and a decreased content of methyl-H_4Folate in fibroblasts from patients with methylene-H_4Folate reductase deficiency. Cells from patients with *cblE* and *cblG* show decreased levels of MeCbl, as may cells from some patients with methylene-H_4Folate reductase deficiency.[208] In cell extracts from cultured fibroblasts, activity of methylene-H_4Folate reductase is decreased in methylene-H_4Folate reductase deficiency. In extracts of *cblE* and *cblG* cell lines, abnormalities in methionine synthase activity can be detected. Abnormalities of

Table 155-2 Inherited Defects of Folate Metabolism

	Hereditary Folate Malabsorption	Methylene-H_4Floate Reductase Deficiency	Glutamate Formimino-transferase Deficiency	Methionine Synthase Reductase Deficiency *(cblE)*	Methionine Synthase Deficiency *(cblG)*
Clinical findings					
Prevalence	< 20 cases	> 40 cases	< 20 cases	12 cases	20 cases
Megaloblastic anemia	A	N	N*	A	A
Developmental delay	A	A	N*	A	A
Seizures	A	A	N*	A	A
Speech abnormalities	N	N	A*	N	N
Gait abnormalities	N	A	N*	N	A*
Peripheral neuropathy	N*	A	N*	N	A*
Apnea	N	A	N*	N*	N
Biochemical findings					
Homocystinuria/hyperhomocysteinemia	N	A	N	A	A
Hypomethioninemia	N	A	N	A	A
Formiminoglutamic aciduria	A*	N	A	N	N*
Folate absorption	A	N	N	N	N
Serum Cbl	N	N	N*	N	N
Serum folate	A	A	N*	N	N
Red blood cell folate	A	A*	N*	N	N
Defects detectable in cultured whole cells fibroblasts					
Methyl-H_4Folate fixation	N	N	N	A	A
Methyl-H_4Folate content	N	A	N	N	N
MeCbl content	N	N*	N	A	A
Extracts-specific activity					
Methionine synthase holoenzyme	N	N*	N	N**	A
Glutamate formiminotransferase			Activity undetectable in cultured cells ? Abnormal in liver and erythrocytes		
Methylene-H_4Folate reductase	N	A	N	N	N
Treatment	Folic acid, reduced folate	Betaine, folate, methionine	?Folate	OH-Cbl, betaine, reduced folate	

*= exceptions described in some cases.
**= abnormal activity with low concentrations of reducing agent in assay.
N = normal; A = abnormal (i.e., clinical findings or laboratory findings present).

glutamate formiminotransferase have not been detected in any cultured cell system.

COBALAMIN (VITAMIN B_{12})

The structure and function of cobalamins have intrigued students of human biology since Minot and Murphy demonstrated that oral administration of crude liver extract was effective in the treatment of pernicious anemia in 1926.[272] In 1948, this "antipernicious anemia factor" was isolated from liver and kidney[273,274] and was named "vitamin B_{12}." Deficiency of the vitamin leads to an alteration of function or morphology of several organ systems: megaloblastic anemia and defective granulocyte and immune system function; abnormal intestinal function; and neurologic disease, including neurologic degeneration and dementia. Administration of as little as 1 μg of the vitamin daily was shown to prevent relapse of pernicious anemia. Although the vitamin is widely distributed in animal tissues, there is strong evidence that it is synthesized only by microorganisms found in soil and water or in the rumen and intestine of animals. See Dolphin[275] and Banerjee[276] for comprehensive reviews of cobalamin structure, biosynthesis, and chemistry.

Structural Features

The isolation of vitamin B_{12} culminated in the elucidation of its three-dimensional structure by Hodgkin and coworkers using x-ray crystallographic techniques.[277] Cobalamin (Cbl), as it is now officially designated, is composed of a central cobalt atom surrounded by a planar corrin ring, which has a complex side chain extending down from the corrin plane consisting of a phosphoribo-5,6-dimethylbenzimidazolyl group (Fig. 155-7). One of the nitrogens of the benzimidazole group is linked to the cobalt atom by coordination in the "bottom"(α) axial position. The molecule is completed by coordination in the "upper"(β) axial position of several different radicals. Thus, cyanocobalamin (CN-Cbl) (more strictly, α-(5,6-dimethylbenzimidazolyl)-cobamide cyanide) is formed by the complexing of a cyanide ion to the cobalt atom. Although this compound is the most common commercial form of the vitamin, it is an artifact of isolation and does not occur naturally in microorganisms, plants, or animal tissues. Many other Cbls have been formed with other ligands, but only four have been routinely isolated from mammalian tissue: hydroxocobalamin (OH-Cbl), the "natural" form of the vitamin, glutathionylcobalamin (GSCbl), methylcobalamin (MeCbl), and adenosylcobalamin (AdoCbl). Complexes of Cbl with other sulfhydryl compounds have also been reported. MeCbl and AdoCbl are unique for two reasons. They are the only two compounds in nature known to have a direct covalent carbon-cobalt bond, and they are the only two forms of Cbl known to act as specific coenzymes in mammalian systems.

Oxidation and reduction of the cobalt atom further complicate the structure and nomenclature of the Cbls. In OH-Cbl, the cobalt

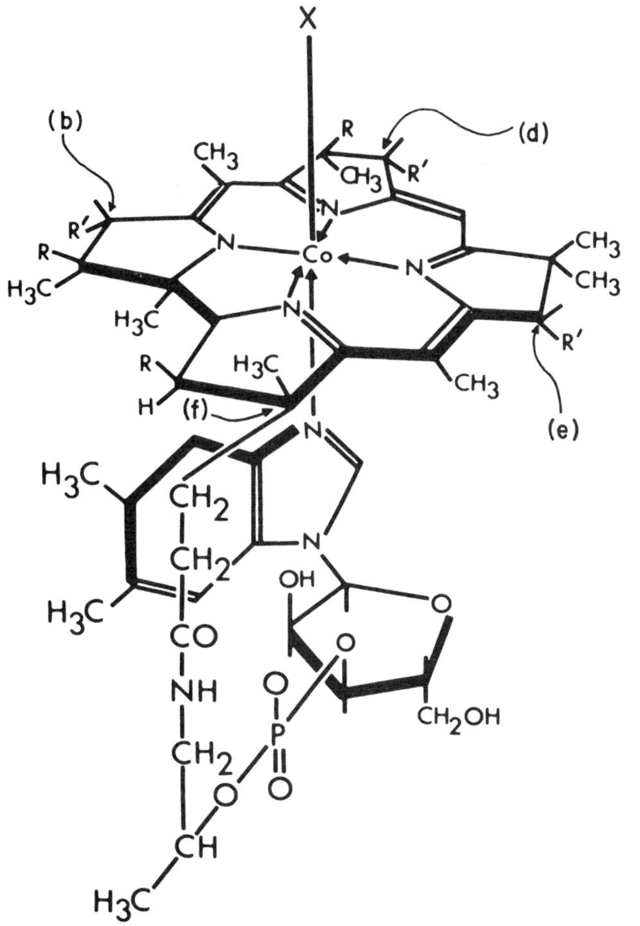

Fig. 155-7 The structure of cobalamin. R = $-CH_2CONH_2$; R′ = $-CH_2CH_2CONH_2$; X = $-OH$ (hydroxocobalamin), $-CN$ (cyanocobalamin), CH_3 (methylcobalamin), or 5′-deoxy-5′-adenosyl (adenosylcobalamin). (*Reproduced from Fenton and Rosenberg.*[343] *Used with permission of the publisher.*)

atom is trivalent (cob(III)alamin), and this compound has been called "vitamin B_{12a}." When the cobalt is reduced to a divalent state (cob(II)alamin), it is called "vitamin B_{12r}," and in the monovalent state (cob(I)alamin), it is called "vitamin B_{12s}." These oxidation-reduction states are important because the cobalt atom must be reduced to its monovalent state prior to formation of MeCbl or AdoCbl, apparently by specific reductase enzymes that sequentially convert cob(III)alamin to cob(I)alamin, with cob(II) alamin as an intermediate.[278]

Cobalamin Coenzymes

In 1958, Barker and his colleagues demonstrated that the glutamate mutase reaction in *Clostridium tetanomorphum* required vitamin B_{12},[279] and, more specifically, that the active coenzyme form of the vitamin was AdoCbl.[280,281] One year later, Smith and Monty reported that the analogous isomerization of methylmalonyl CoA to succinyl CoA was defective in the liver of Cbl-deficient rats.[282] They suggested that Cbl was a cofactor for the latter isomerization system, a thesis borne out by Gurnani *et al.*[283] and Stern and Friedmann,[284] who showed *in vitro* that the activity of methylmalonyl CoA mutase in liver from Cbl-deficient animals could be restored to normal by addition of AdoCbl, but not by CN-Cbl or other vitamin B_{12} analogues. For several years, because AdoCbl was the only known coenzyme form of vitamin B_{12}, it was designated "coenzyme B_{12}." In 1966, Weissbach and colleagues[285] demonstrated that MeCbl is a cofactor in the complex reaction by which homocysteine is methylated to form methionine (Fig. 155-8). This reaction requires *S*-adenosylmethionine and N^5-methyltetrahydrofolate (methyl-H_4Folate), as well as methionine synthase and MeCbl.[286,287] It is relevant to the manifestations of Cbl deficiency and to the interrelationships between folate and Cbl, and is discussed in detail in the folate section above.

The conversion of methylmalonyl CoA to succinyl CoA and the methylation of homocysteine to methionine are the only Cbl-dependent reactions that have been demonstrated conclusively in mammalian systems. Poston reported that AdoCbl acts as a cofactor in the enzymatic reaction by which α-leucine is isomerized to β-leucine,[288] but this has not been confirmed in other laboratories. In microorganisms, several other enzymes require AdoCbl[289,290] such as: glutamate mutase, glycerol dehydratase, ethanolamine ammonia-lyase, and ribonucleotide reductase. In addition, MeCbl participates in the formation of methane and acetic acid and in the fermentation of lysine in bacteria.

Cobalamin Absorption and Distribution

Cbls have a unique and highly specialized mechanism of intestinal absorption that has been reviewed in detail.[236,291,292] The ability to transport physiological quantities of vitamin depends on the combined action of gastric, ileal, and pancreatic components (Fig. 155-9). The gastric substance, called "intrinsic factor" (IF) by Castle,[293] who first demonstrated its existence, is a glycoprotein that binds Cbl in the intestinal lumen. IF, which has been isolated, characterized extensively,[291] and cloned,[294] is synthesized by gastric parietal cells. Evidence obtained *in vitro*[295,296] and *in vivo*[297] suggests that three events precede the formation of IF-Cbl in the gut lumen. First, Cbls are released from dietary protein in the acid environment of the stomach. Second, Cbls bind to "R-binders," or haptocorrins, which are proteins of salivary and gastric origin; these R-binders are members of a family of glycoproteins with a high affinity for Cbl. Third, pancreatic proteases digest the R-binders, thereby liberating Cbls in the upper small intestine, where they form complexes with IF. Subsequently, the IF-Cbl complex interacts through its protein moiety with a specific ileal receptor protein, called cubilin, in the presence of calcium ions. The IF-Cbl-cubilin complex is recognized by megalin, a general transport receptor, and transported into the enterocyte by an endocytic mechanism; the complex is dissociated; and the vitamin is transported across the basal membrane into the portal blood, bound to transcobalamin II (TC II), the transport protein for newly absorbed vitamin.[292] Evidence from cultured adenocarcinoma cells, which behave like polarized intestinal epithelial cells,[298,299] suggests that these latter steps reflect true apical-to-basal transcytosis in which the Cbl is bound to newly synthesized TC II when it is released from the basolateral membrane.[299]

When labeled Cbl is administered intravenously, most of the labeled vitamin is immediately bound to TC II and disappears from the plasma in a few hours.[300,301] Only a small fraction binds to transcobalamin I (TC I) or transcobalamin III (TC III) serum glycoproteins of the R-binder family, even though they carry the majority of the steady state serum Cbl.[302] The Cbl bound to the R-binders turns over very slowly, and its physiological role is still unclear. MeCbl is the major circulating Cbl species, accounting for 60 to 80 percent of total plasma Cbl; OH-Cbl and AdoCbl make up the remainder.[303] Because >90 percent of total plasma Cbl is bound to TC I, it is clear that most of the circulating MeCbl travels with this R-binder. This Cbl distribution pattern is puzzling, particularly in the face of evidence indicating that AdoCbl accounts for ~70 percent of total hepatic Cbl, whereas MeCbl constitutes a mere 1 to 3 percent.[303] This preponderance of AdoCbl is also present in other tissues, such as erythrocytes, kidney, and brain. The physiological significance of these widely different fractional Cbl distributions in extracellular and intracellular compartments remains obscure.

TC II facilitates Cbl uptake by mammalian tissues. Finkler and Hall[304] showed that CN-Cbl bound to TC II was accumulated by HeLa cells much more rapidly than free CN-Cbl or CN-Cbl bound to TC I, IF, or other binding proteins. Such TC II-mediated uptake

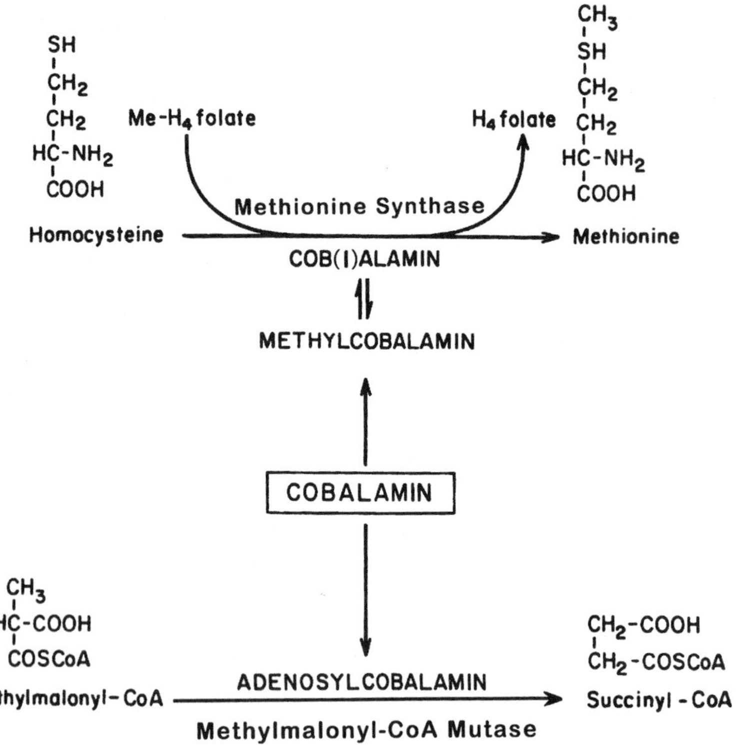

Fig. 155-8 Reactions catalyzed by cobalamin coenzymes in mammalian tissues. Note the specificity of adenosylcobalamin for the isomerization of methylmalonyl CoA and of methylcobalamin for the methylation of homocysteine. Me-H_4Folate = N^5-methyltetrahydrofolate; H_4Folate = tetrahydrofolate.

was subsequently confirmed in a variety of cell types, both *in vivo* and in culture (liver; kidney; heart; spleen; lung; small intestine; cultured fibroblasts; Chinese hamster ovary cells; mouse L cells; lymphoma cells; and phytohemagglutinin-stimulated lymphocytes) (see reference 292 for review). These findings, coupled with the observations *in vivo* that TC II disappeared from plasma as TC II-Cbl was absorbed[305] and appeared in lysosomal fractions of hepatic[306] and kidney cells,[307] led to the proposal that the circulating TC II-Cbl complex is recognized by a specific, widely distributed plasma membrane receptor. This hypothesis has been supported by considerable experimental evidence. Using ^{125}I-labeled TC II-Cbl complexes, Youngdahl-Turner and associates[308] showed that the complex binds to a specific, high-affinity (K_a $\sim 10^{10}$ M^{-1}) cell-surface receptor on cultured skin fibroblasts through a membrane site that recognizes TC II and by a mechanism dependent on Ca^{2+}. They showed further that the TC II-Cbl complex is then internalized intact via adsorptive endocytosis[309] and that the degradation of TC II and release of Cbl from the complex occur as a result of lysosomal protease activity.[308,309] Cbl then exits from the lysosome by a mediated process,[310] and is either converted to MeCbl bound to the methionine synthase in the cytosol or enters the mitochondrion, where, after reduction and adenosylation to AdoCbl, it is bound to methylmalonyl CoA mutase.[311,312]

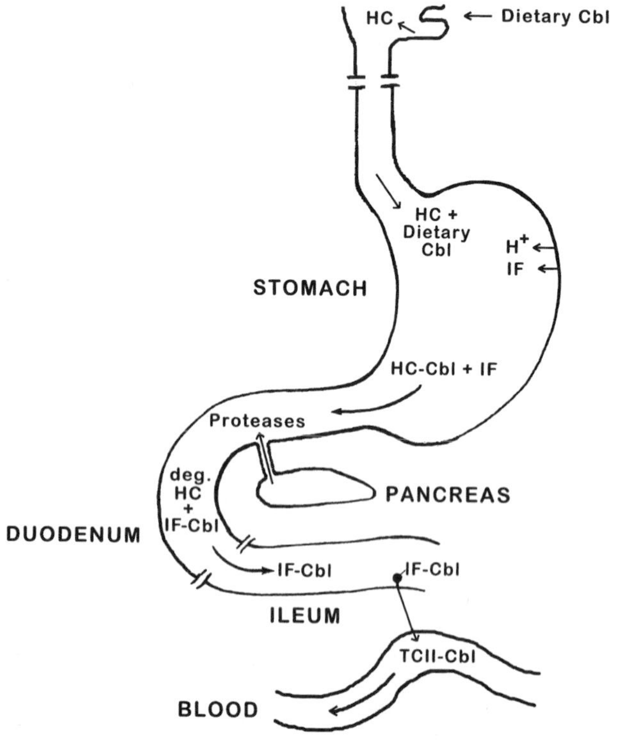

Fig. 155-9 Pathway for the gastrointestinal absorption of dietary cobalamin. Cbl = cobalamin; HC = haptocorrin (transcobalamin I/III); HC-Cbl = haptocorrin-bound cobalamin; degHC = degraded haptocorrin; IF = intrinsic factor; IF-Cbl = intrinsic factor-bound cobalamin; •-IF-Cbl = intrinsic factor-bound cobalamin attached to cubilin, the ileal receptor; TCII-Cbl = cobalamin bound to transcobalamin II. *(Reproduced from Rosenblatt and Fenton.[477] Used with permission.)*

The intricate process just described is the most widely distributed physiological means by which mammalian cells obtain Cbl, but it is not the only one. Hepatocytes, for instance, contain a surface receptor for asialoglycoproteins, and this receptor interacts with TCI-Cbl (and perhaps TC III-Cbl) complexes, thereby providing a second potential means by which this particular tissue obtains Cbl.[313] There is also evidence that at least some tissues are capable of taking up free (unbound) Cbl, if the unbound vitamin is raised to sufficiently high concentrations. In cultured fibroblasts, this uptake process for free Cbl is saturable, Ca^{2+}-independent, and sensitive to inhibitors of protein synthesis and sulfhydryl reagents.[314] Its functional role, under most circumstances, is probably negligible.

Coenzyme Biosynthesis and Compartmentation

Because methylmalonyl CoA mutase, the mammalian enzyme dependent on AdoCbl, is a mitochondrial protein,[315] whereas the MeCbl-dependent methionine synthase is cytoplasmic,[316] it is important to relate the cellular biology of the vitamin to its cellular and molecular chemistry. The chemical pathway of AdoCbl

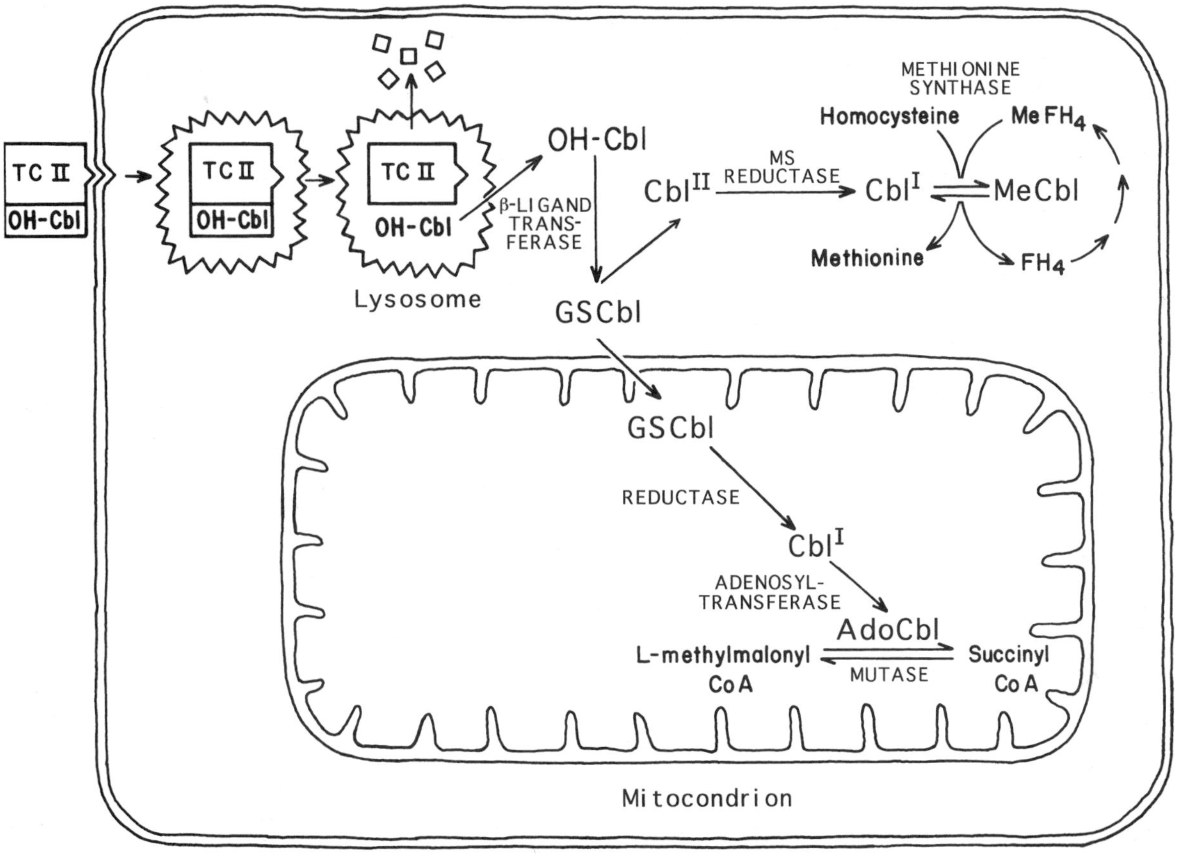

Fig. 155-10 General pathway of the cellular uptake and subcellular compartmentation of cobalamins, and of the intracellular distribution and enzymatic synthesis of cobalamin coenzymes. TC II = transcobalamin II; OH-Cbl = hydroxocobalamin; MeCbl = methylcobalamin; AdoCbl = adenosylcobalamin; Cbl^{III}, Cbl^{II}, Cbl^{I}, = cobalamins with cobalt valences of +3, +2, and +1, respectively.

synthesis was defined initially in bacteria.[278,317] Three enzymes are required for coenzyme synthesis, two reductases and an adenosyltransferase. The reductases are flavoproteins that require NAD as a cofactor. The first (EC 1.6.99.8) is responsible for converting cob(III)alamin, for example, OH-Cbl, to cob(II)alamin, and the second (EC 1.6.99.9) is responsible for catalyzing the further reduction to cob(I)alamin. The latter compound and ATP are substrates for an adenosyltransferase (EC 2.5.1.17) that completes the synthesis of AdoCbl. Neither of the reductases has been purified extensively, but the adenosyltransferase has. It has a pH optimum of 8, requires Mn^{2+}, and has a K_m of 1×10^{-5} M for cob(I)alamin and 1.6×10^{-5} M for ATP.[317] The biosynthetic steps leading to *de novo* MeCbl formation are not as clear. Because maintenance of MeCbl on methionine synthase requires a reductase system to generate cob(I)alamin on methionine synthase itself, this reduction-methylation sequence seems likely for *de novo* MeCbl synthesis as well.[318,319]

Accumulated evidence indicates that mammalian cell metabolism of Cbl proceeds by a very similar set of reactions (Fig. 155-10). In 1964, Pawalkiewicz *et al.*[320] showed that human liver and kidney homogenates could convert CN-Cbl to AdoCbl. Several years later, AdoCbl synthesis from OH-Cbl was observed in HeLa cell extracts incubated with ATP and a reducing system that presumably bypassed the enzymatic reduction of OH-Cbl (cob(III)alamin) to cob(I)alamin.[321] Subsequently, Mahoney and Rosenberg[322] demonstrated the synthesis of both AdoCbl and MeCbl by intact human fibroblasts growing in a tissue culture medium containing OH-[^{57}Co]Cbl. This system was subsequently characterized in cell extracts.[323,324] As with the HeLa cell system, chemical reductants were employed to bypass both cobalamin reductases.[324] Such extracts synthesized AdoCbl, thereby demonstrating that a homologue of the adenosyltransferase found in bacteria also exists in normal human cells. These experiments also revealed that the adenosyltransferase was mitochondrial in location, implying that both the synthesis and cofactor activity of AdoCbl take place in this organelle. The reductive steps in mammalian systems are still poorly understood. Pezacka and colleagues have suggested that GSCbl may be an intermediate in these reactions.[325] Watanabe *et al.* demonstrated both microsomal and mitochondrial reductase activities,[326] but suggested that one or more of these may be nonspecific activities of other enzymes, such as the cytochrome b_5-cytochrome b_5 reductase complex.[327] It seems certain, as shown in Fig. 155-10, that MeCbl synthesis takes place in the cytosol in conjunction with the methionine synthase and methionine synthase reductase (see "Folate" section above).

Metabolic Abnormalities in Cobalamin Deficiency

The biochemical abnormalities in plasma and urine of patients with Cbl deficiency reflect the dysfunction of the enzymes dependent on Cbl coenzymes. The first relevant observation in this context was Cox and White[328] and Barness and his colleagues,[329] demonstration that methylmalonic acid excretion in the urine was distinctly increased in Cbl-deficient patients with classic pernicious anemia. The methylmalonic aciduria in these patients was reversed rapidly by administration of physiologic doses of Cbl, indicating that repletion of Cbl restored the methylmalonyl CoA mutase reaction to normal. Later, Cox *et al.* reported that patients with Cbl deficiency also had distinctly increased amounts of propionic acid in the urine, this abnormality again being reversed by treatment.[330] Interestingly, they also found excessive amounts of acetic acid in the urine of Cbl-deficient subjects. The mechanism leading to this abnormality is not clear because acetate does not participate in the major pathway of propionate catabolism. The finding could, of course, reflect increased utilization of the alternative pathways of propionate metabolism in the face of a block in the major pathway, because each alternative route leads eventually to the formation of acetyl CoA (see Chap. 94). Excessive excretion of homocystine has also been documented in Cbl-deficient patients,[331,332] as has combined methylmalonic aciduria and homocystinuria. Allen and his colleagues examined a large series of patients with suspected or proven Cbl deficiency[333,334] and showed that 95 percent of them have methylmalonic acidemia, homocystinemia, or both, often without hematologic signs. A number of reports now document the occurrence of Cbl deficiency in vegetarian and macrobiotic communities, with accompanying metabolic derangements.[335,336] In some cases, clinical symptoms have been observed as well, particularly in breast-fed offspring of strict vegetarian mothers, who are themselves deficient in the vitamin.[337,338]

Cobalamins and Folic Acid

An interesting, important, and still puzzling aspect of Cbl function concerns its relationship to folic acid.[339] Several lines of evidence bear out this relationship: the appearance of megaloblastic anemia in either Cbl or folate deficiency; the reversal of megaloblastic anemia in Cbl deficiency by large doses of folate; the amelioration of megaloblastic changes in folic acid deficiency by pharmacologic doses of CN-Cbl; the increased plasma concentrations of methyl-H_4Folate in patients with cobalamin deficiency; the excretion of excessive amounts of FIGLU after histidine loading in patients with either Cbl or folate deficiency; and the reduced amounts of total Cbl in the liver of patients with folate deficiency. A plausible explanation for most of these effects was proposed independently by Herbert,[340] Noronha,[341] and Larrabee[342] and their colleagues, and has been referred to as the folate trap hypothesis. This thesis rests on the evidence that the conversion of methyl-H_4Folate to H_4Folate depends on the MeCbl-dependent reaction in which homocysteine is methylated to methionine. If methionine biosynthesis is the only quantitatively significant reaction using methyl-H_4Folate, Cbl deficiency will interfere with the folate cycle and, barring other control mechanisms, will lead to the accumulation of methyl-H_4Folate and the depletion of other folate derivatives. This depletion could become severe enough to interfere with other reactions requiring H_4Folate, such as the synthesis of purines or pyrimidines and the conversion of FIGLU to glutamate. Under these circumstances, H_4Folate deficiency could be relieved by administration of either folates or Cbl, but only the latter would complete the folate cycle. This scheme, if totally correct, would obviate the need for additional Cbl-dependent mechanisms to explain the megaloblastic changes observed in Cbl deficiency and would account for the specific disorders of folate metabolism observed in Cbl-deficient human beings. It does not explain the low Cbl content of livers from folate-deficient subjects or the hematologic response of folate-deficient patients to Cbl (also see "Folate" section above).

INBORN ERRORS OF COBALAMIN TRANSPORT AND METABOLISM

Inherited disorders in the transport and metabolism of Cbl manifest themselves clinically in ways that reflect the underlying defect and, in particular, that depend on which coenzyme is deficient and, hence, which of the two Cbl-dependent enzymes is reduced in activity (see Fig. 155-8). Defects that affect only AdoCbl biosynthesis generally lead to metabolic ketoacidosis in the newborn or infant period, and regularly result in methylmalonic acidemia and methylmalonic aciduria. MeCbl deficiencies present as failure to thrive, megaloblastic changes, and neurologic signs, usually with homocystinuria and hypomethioninemia. Deficiencies of both coenzymes produce a variable combination of these signs and symptoms.

Combined AdoCbl and MeCbl Deficiency

Cbl was first described as "extrinsic factor," an antipernicious anemia factor found in aqueous extracts of raw liver, which combined with "intrinsic factor" (IF), a component of normal gastric secretions, to cure pernicious anemia, an acquired disease resulting from gastric insufficiency. It is recognized, however, that there are several inborn errors of metabolism with presentations similar to pernicious anemia that result from abnormal Cbl transport or from altered cellular Cbl metabolism. Although these diseases share the general clinical phenotype of failure to thrive, developmental delay, neurologic dysfunction, and megaloblastic anemia, the details of their presentations allow them to be differentiated. (For reviews, see references 236, 269, 292, 302, and 343).

Transport Defects: Clinical and Laboratory Findings

Food Cobalamin Malabsorption. Carmel and colleagues described a number of patients, mostly adults, with a condition that includes low serum Cbl concentrations in the face of a normal Schilling test.[344] Neurologic manifestations, with or without megaloblastic changes, appear to be common.[344] These individuals suffer from an inability to release Cbl from the protein-bound state in which it is normally encountered in foodstuffs, usually measured by the absorption of Cbl bound to egg yolk.[345] Because this process requires both an acid gastric pH and peptic activity,[346] any underlying factors that compromise gastric function, including atrophic gastritis or partial gastrectomy, can result in this disorder.[347] However, a significant fraction of patients have shown no evidence of impaired gastric function,[344] suggesting that a more subtle mechanism, whose nature is currently unknown, may be responsible.[348]

Intrinsic Factor (IF) Deficiency. A number of children have been described with a juvenile form of pernicious anemia (see reference 349 for references to case reports). The clinical symptoms, which usually appear after the first year and before the fifth year of age, include developmental delay and the megaloblastic anemia characteristic of pernicious anemia.[236,349] Serum levels of Cbl are markedly deficient, but, in contrast to the adult disease, gastric function and morphology are normal, and serum autoantibodies to IF are absent. Cbl absorption is abnormal in these children, but is restored when the vitamin is mixed with normal human gastric juice as a source of IF. Further investigations of the gastric secretions of these patients have shown that, as expected, they suffer from one of several different classes of functional IF deficiency. One results in failure to produce or secrete any immunologically recognizable IF,[350,351] while another causes production of immunologically reactive protein that is inactive physiologically.[349,352–354] The latter group includes patients whose IF has reduced affinity for the ileal IF receptor,[353] reduced affinity for Cbl,[355] or increased susceptibility to proteolysis.[349] In a few cases with partial deficiency, presentation was delayed into the second decade or later.[352,356] Although a cDNA for human intrinsic factor has been characterized ([GIF], NM_005142, MIM 261000), no mutations have yet been described.[357]

Enterocyte Cbl Malabsorption (Selective Vitamin B_{12} Malabsorption, MGA1, Imerslund-Gräsbeck Syndrome) (MIM 261100). More than 250 cases of a related disorder have been described with the clinical signs of juvenile pernicious anemia, but with normal IF and normal gastrointestinal function, except for specific intestinal Cbl malabsorption.[358–361] In addition to megaloblastic anemia and serum Cbl deficiency, many of these patients have proteinuria. Similarly to IF deficiency, patients usually present between 1 and 5 years of age, although some have been diagnosed much later.[362] In contrast to IF deficiency patients, however, these children's Cbl absorption defect is not corrected by providing normal human IF with the vitamin.[236] There has been a decrease in the number of new cases in recent years, and it has been suggested that there may be dietary or other factors modifying expression.[363]

Most patients are found in Norway, Finland, Saudi Arabia, and among Sephardic Jews. Using microsatellite markers in Finnish and Norwegian families, the disease gene was mapped to a 6-cM region on chromosome 10p12.1.[363] An IF-Cbl-binding protein called cubilin ([CUBN], NM_001081, MIM 602997) was purified from renal proximal tubule, cloned, and localized to the same region.[364,365] This large (~400 kDa) protein comprises a short N-terminal domain, eight EGF repeats, and 27 contiguous, 110-amino acid CUB domains, first identified in certain developmental control proteins. Two mutations in the cubilin gene (*CUBN*) have been found segregating in Finnish families with this disorder.[366] One, P1297L, is found in homozygous form in most Finnish patients (31 of 34 alleles). It changes a highly conserved proline residue, which is predicted by x-ray structural analysis of other CUB domains[367] to be part of a ligand-binding site. Interestingly, this change is in CUB domain 8, suggested by deletion and expression studies to be part of the IF-Cbl binding site (domains 5 to 8).[368] The other change, homozygous in one patient, is a point mutation in an intron in CUB domain 6, resulting in missplicing, insertions containing stop codons in mRNA, and truncated predicted gene products. No cubilin was detected on western blots of proteins from this patient's urine, establishing clearly that *CUBN* is the gene for the IF-Cbl receptor protein.[368] Neither of these mutations has been found in non-Finnish families, and the mutations causing this disorder in other populations are being sought.

Cubilin is a peripheral membrane protein with no clearly defined transmembrane domain. It copurifies with megalin, an even larger receptor protein of the LDL receptor gene family, and colocalizes with it in both intestinal and renal epithelium.[364,369] Megalin appears to be a transporter for many proteins[370] and may be responsible for the endocytosis of the cubilin-IF-Cbl complex. Cubilin itself may have other functions, as suggested by its specific binding of receptor-associated protein[368] and its function in apolipoprotein A-I endocytosis.[371]

Earlier experiments suggested that, in at least some patients, the ileal receptor for IF-Cbl was normal as measured by IF-Cbl binding to homogenates of ileal biopsy specimens.[360] In others, a functional receptor appeared to be absent.[372] Because the mechanism for Cbl transport across the enterocyte is complex, it seems possible that this syndrome encompasses defects at several points in this overall pathway, including cubilin itself (as shown in the Finnish pedigrees), cubilin internalization via megalin, or Cbl transfer to TC II within the enterocyte (also see discussion of *cblF* below). It remains to be seen how many patients with this phenotype will be found to have mutations in the cubilin gene itself.

Transcobalamin II (TC II) Deficiency. At least 36 cases have been described of deficiency of TC II, including both twins and sibs.[236,373] In contrast to the previous two disorders, TC II deficiency has generally presented within the first or second month of life as failure to thrive, with such nonspecific symptoms as vomiting and weakness, accompanied by megaloblastic anemia and, eventually, immunologic deficiency and neurologic disease.[236,373] Because the patients may have immature white blood cell precursors in a marrow that is otherwise hypocellular, they have been misdiagnosed with leukemia. Neurologic disease is not present at the time of diagnosis, but may develop with an extended duration of illness, inadequate cobalamin treatment, or treatment of the anemia with folates and not cobalamin.[373] Interestingly, serum Cbl levels are normal or nearly so in these patients, reflecting the fact that most serum Cbl is carried by TC I and other R-binders.[302] It is essential to measure blood levels of TC II before the patient has been started on cobalamin therapy. Intestinal Cbl absorption has been abnormal in some patients, but not in others.[236]

Most patients have had no immunologically detectable TC II in plasma,[236] although a few had detectable protein,[374,375] and at least one produced a TC II that was able to bind Cbl, although apparently without function.[374] In those patients who do not synthesize TC II, both the diagnosis and prenatal diagnosis can be performed by studying the ability of cultured fibroblasts or amniocytes to synthesize TC II.[376]

Treatment of TC II deficiency requires that serum cobalamin levels be kept very high. It is important to monitor levels carefully and to ensure that the patient is compliant, particularly if oral treatment is used. Serum levels ranging from 1000 to 10,000 pg/ml have been required; these levels have been achieved with oral OH-Cbl or CN-Cbl in doses of 0.5 to 1.0 mg twice weekly or by weekly doses of 1 mg OH-Cbl. Although folic acid or folinic acid can reverse the megaloblastic anemia, folate should never be given as the only therapy because of the danger of hematologic relapse and neurologic deterioration.

The human TC II gene is on chromosome 22, a cDNA has been cloned, and the molecular basis of some variants determined ([TCN2], NM_000355, MIM 275350).[377–380] In a number of patients who have no TC II synthesis, deletions and nonsense mutations have been found.[381,382]

R-Binder Deficiency ([TC I], NM_001062, MIM 193090). Several individuals are known who have deficient or absent R-binder (TC I) in plasma, saliva, and blood cells.[236,383] Although these patients have serum Cbl values in the deficient range, they show no signs of Cbl deficiency, probably because their TC II-Cbl levels are normal. Although several of these patients have had a myelopathy not attributable to other causes,[383,384] the etiology of these symptoms remains unclear, emphasizing our lack of understanding of the role of R-binders in normal Cbl metabolism and homeostasis. It should be noted that R-binders carry Cbl in mother's milk, so the potential exists for Cbl deficiency in breast-fed infants of mothers with this deficiency.

Chemical Abnormalities and Pathophysiology. While megaloblastic anemia is the hallmark of the Cbl transport disorders, the chemical abnormalities expected to accompany functional Cbl deficiency have also been found in many cases. In theory, Cbl deficiency should lead to deficient synthesis of both AdoCbl and MeCbl and, thus, to decreased activities of their respective enzymes, resulting in methylmalonic acidemia(-uria) and homocystinemia(-uria). When examined carefully, most patients with each of the transport deficiencies have these chemical symptoms, although the quantities of both methylmalonate and homocystine excreted have generally been much lower than in patients with abnormalities in cellular Cbl metabolism (see below). On the other hand, some patients do not have one or either of these chemical abnormalities.[236] To a certain extent, these variable findings, which do not appear to correlate well with the nature of the defect or the severity of the general symptoms and hematologic aberrations, may result from the fact that alternative pathways of Cbl transport exist that, although minor in normal individuals, may contribute significantly in patients with these transport defects. For example, receptors for free Cbl have been found on HeLa cells,[385] human fibroblasts,[314] and adenocarcinoma cells,[299] and may permit some Cbl transport even in the absence of one of the transport proteins. In addition, hepatocytes may be able to recover some Cbl from asialo-TC I-Cbl by means of the asialoglycoprotein receptor system.[386] This could be particularly important in TC II deficiency.

One major clinical difference between the two intestinal transport defects and TC II deficiency lies in the different age of onset of these conditions. While neither intestinal Cbl transport deficiency manifests itself before 1 year of age, many TC II-deficient patients are symptomatic within 1 or 2 months of birth, with some exceptions (see above). This appears to be due to two factors. First, the IF-dependent pathway for intestinal Cbl absorption may not become important until later in infancy, when the gastrointestinal tract switches from pinocytotic mechanisms of transport to receptor-mediated ones. IF-Cbl transport falls into the latter category. Interestingly, one report[387] demonstrates that, in rats, expression of IF by the gastric mucosa increases abruptly from the low levels found in the newborn animal to adult levels at about the time of weaning (13 to 20 days), consistent with this hypothesis. Second, the body stores considerable amounts of Cbl beyond daily requirements in blood, liver, and other tissues. Thus, IF-deficient patients and those with Imerslund-Gräsbeck syndrome likely show no signs of deficiency early in infancy both because the IF-dependent mechanism for Cbl transport is not yet operating and because they have acquired sufficient Cbl through other mechanisms or prenatally to sustain themselves for a time after the developmental switch in intestinal absorption has occurred. Conversely, because TC II is presumably necessary for efficient Cbl transport into cells regardless of the mechanism by which it is acquired, TC II-deficient patients have no symptom-free period and become ill as soon as their maternally derived stores of Cbl are exhausted. The observation that most TC II-deficient patients have been normal at birth likely reflects the fact that fetal tissues concentrate Cbl relative to the maternal serum.[388] It is not certain why the neurologic manifestations of TC II deficiency are less severe than those found in the inborn errors of cobalamin metabolism that affect cofactor synthesis.[373]

The megaloblastic anemia characteristic of these disorders likely reflects a deficiency in the activity of methionine synthase brought about by the absence of its cofactor, MeCbl. Because patients with isolated deficiency of AdoCbl (see below) or its partner enzyme, methylmalonyl CoA mutase (see Chap. 94), are usually hematologically normal, this conclusion seems to be solid. Likewise, the severe neurologic manifestations,[373] particularly in patients who are diagnosed long after the onset of their disease, appear more likely to be due to deficient methionine synthase activity. Although isolated mutase deficiency can produce central nervous system dysfunction (see Chap. 94), this is believed to be at least partially a consequence of the severe metabolic ketoacidosis experienced by these patients, a condition not generally present in patients with Cbl transport defects.

The specific etiology of the hematologic and neurologic disturbances in these individuals is not completely understood, but clearly it must derive from the central role of methionine synthase in cellular 1-carbon metabolic pathways, both in terms of folate metabolism (see sections above) and homocysteine-methionine balance (see Chap. 88). Because the folate cycle in mammalian cells requires that methyl-H_4Folate transfer its methyl group to homocysteine, via MeCbl, in order to regenerate tetrahydrofolate, it has been suggested that the accumulation of methyl folate in the absence of the Cbl coenzyme serves as a folate trap, which produces functional folate deficiency intracellularly.[340,342] The effects of this deficiency on the important roles that folate metabolism plays in the synthesis of nucleotides and, hence, of RNA and DNA could easily account for the general disruptions in cellular homeostasis in rapidly dividing tissues, such as the hematopoietic system. Whether this folate trap hypothesis is equally applicable to explaining the neurologic dysfunction in these patients is not clear. An alternative explanation might involve disruption of the interconversion of homocysteine and methionine and of *S*-adenosylhomocysteine and *S*-adenosylmethionine and interference with the role these compounds play in methylation and enzyme regulation in the central nervous system.[270,389] Until more is known about these pathways, however, either hypothesis will be difficult to establish.

Genetics and Molecular Biology. Each of the genetic lesions in Cbl transport appears to be inherited as an autosomal recessive trait on the basis of classic genetic criteria.[236] Because the Imerslund-Gräsbeck syndrome may actually encompass deficiencies in more than one protein (receptor) (see above), it remains possible that other modes of inheritance exist for a subset of families with this disorder. Rat and human IF cDNAs have been cloned,[294,390] and the IF gene has been localized to human chromosome 11.[294] There is suggestive evidence from biochemical analysis of some presumptive heterozygotes for IF deficiency that they express both a normal and an abnormal allele for IF and for the idea that some patients with IF deficiency express two different mutant alleles.[349] The rat IF cDNA has been used to establish that only one cell type — the chief cell of the rat gastric mucosa — expresses IF in the adult animal,[387] in keeping with immunochemical studies that indicate that the parietal cell is the only source of IF in human beings and other mammals.[291] As mentioned above, both cubilin and megalin have been cloned, and deleterious mutations in cubilin have been described in Finnish Imerslund-Gräsbeck patients. TC II has electrophoretic isoforms in normal individuals,[391] and it has been suggested that some cases of TC II deficiency manifest themselves as abnormal isoforms.[392] The structural locus for TC II is on the long arm of chromosome 22,[294,393] linked to the P blood group system locus. Although TC I has been cloned,[394] mutations in it leading to R-binder deficiency have not been described.

Diagnosis and Treatment. The Cbl transport deficiencies, except for food Cbl malabsorption, are usually diagnosed initially by the observation of the combination of macrocytic anemia with developmental delay or failure to thrive.[236] Neurologic symptoms may be present at later times.[373] Serum Cbl levels are low in food Cbl malabsorption, IF deficiency, and Imerslund-Gräsbeck syndrome, but usually normal in TC II deficiency. Schilling tests are normal in the first disorder, abnormal in the second two, and may also be abnormal in some cases of TC II deficiency.[236] The second two disorders can be differentiated by determining whether the Schilling test becomes normal when the test Cbl is incubated with normal human IF before it is administered. Only IF deficiency patients show correction. Confirmation of either of the intestinal malabsorption defects entails demonstration of normal gastric and ileal function other than the specific Cbl absorption deficiency, the absence of antibodies to IF, and, in some cases of IF deficiency, the absence of functional (i.e., Cbl-binding) or immunologically cross-reacting IF in the patient's gastric secretions.[236,349] TC II deficiency can sometimes be differentiated from the other two by an age of onset within the first months (as opposed to years) of life. The diagnosis can often be established by measuring the unsaturated Cbl-binding capacity of the patient's serum; in normal individuals, this largely reflects the amount of TC II present. Gel-filtration chromatography can be used to separate TC II from serum R-binders and thus provides a more accurate assessment of Cbl-binding capacity. Unfortunately, both these tests can be compromised by previous Cbl therapy, possibly even by previous Schilling tests.[395] Because TC II is synthesized by many cell types, including fibroblasts, and because fibroblasts from TC II-deficient patients synthesize a defective protein or none at all,[314] a more satisfactory approach may be to grow patient fibroblasts in medium without TC II and to then determine whether any functional TC II has been synthesized by incubating the cells with radiolabeled Cbl and measuring the extent to which TC II-Cbl accumulates in the medium or in the cells.[314,376]

In the case of sibs or other relatives in families in which one of these defects has been diagnosed, hematologic changes can provide an early sign of the presence of the disease, as can methylmalonic acidemia and homocystinemia. In the two intestinal transport disorders, Schilling tests may prove abnormal before the onset of clinical symptoms. In TC II deficiency, because cord blood contains fetal, not maternal, TC II,[396] it is possible to test immediately for the presence of functional TC II. Biochemical prenatal diagnosis is possible only for TC II deficiency, based on the ability of normal amniocytes to synthesize functional TC II.[376] Because no fetus at risk for TC II deficiency has yet been tested by this method and predicted to be affected, its applicability remains hypothetical. The two intestinal malabsorption syndromes are not expressed in accessible fetal tissues (if, in fact, those proteins are expressed at all during fetal life) and, thus, cannot be diagnosed prenatally by a biochemical test. The cDNA cloning of IF[294] and cubilin[364,365] may make a DNA-based diagnostic procedure, such

Table 155-3 Clinical and Laboratory Features of Patients with Methylmalonic Acidemia and Homocystinuria*

Finding	Mutant Class			
	cblC Early Onset	*cblC* Late Onset	*cblD*	*cblF*
Clinical				
Sex (male/female)			2/0	2/4
Failure to thrive	21/44	1/6	0/2	5/6
Developmental retardation	26/44	2/6	1/2	5/6
Seizures	21/44	2/6	0/2	1/6
Feeding difficulties	32/44	3/6	0/2	3/6
Hypotonia	27/44	3/6		3/6
Microcephaly	19/44	0/6		
Nystagmus	10/44	0/6		
Hydrocephalus	8/44	0/6		
Dementia	1/44	3/6		
Myelopathy	1/44	3/6		
Laboratory				
Normal serum cobalamin	44/44	6/6	2/2	3/6
Hematologic abnormalities	31/44	3/6	0/2	3/6
Acidosis	9/44	0/6	0/6	
Microthrombi	3/44	0/6	1/2	
Pigmentary retinopathy	19/44	1/6		
Decreased visual acuity	15/44	0/6		

*Ratios (except for sex) denote the number of patients showing a particular finding/total number of patients in each mutant class; empty cells indicate data were not available.

SOURCE: Information obtained from published surveys,[420] case reports,[413,417–419,425] and personal communications.

as RFLP analysis, possible in at least some cases involving deficiency of these proteins.

The major treatment regimen for each of these disorders has been pharmacologic doses of Cbl, either CN-Cbl or OH-Cbl, usually administered by injection to avoid dependence on gastric factors and ileal uptake of free Cbl.[236,395] Titration of the dosage used and frequency of therapy should be carried out to ensure resolution of all clinical abnormalities, particularly in TC II-deficient patients with defective immune system function[397,398] or neurologic disorders.[373] The serum Cbl concentration at which patients become asymptomatic has varied widely, especially in TC II deficiency, and should be used as a guide only after the patient has been stabilized. Folate has been administered to some TC II-deficient patients with effective correction of the hematologic signs of the disease.[236] At least one of these patients suffered a relapse, however, and the ability of folate to resolve other symptoms, particularly long-term neurologic dysfunction, has not been determined. Consequently, folate therapy should only accompany effective doses of Cbl.[373]

The prognosis in these diseases appears to be generally very good as long as serum Cbl levels are maintained appropriately.[373,399] Interestingly, while Cbl therapy has been effective in normalizing the hematologic signs in Imerslund-Gräsbeck patients, the proteinuria often observed in this disorder has been unchanged even by many years of therapy.[399] Although one woman with TC II deficiency has borne two normal children,[375] it remains unclear whether Cbl therapy can achieve complete reversal of the neurologic damage and developmental delay that occur if patients remain undiagnosed for an extended period (or if adequate Cbl levels are not maintained) or whether some residual deficit may persist in these cases.[373]

Defects in Cellular AdoCbl and MeCbl Synthesis

Clinical and Laboratory Findings. In comparison to the Cbl transport defects described above, defects in the cellular metabolism of Cbl generally result in clinically more severe metabolic disease. As a consequence, patients with these disorders regularly show the metabolic disturbances that result from deficient synthesis of both AdoCbl and MeCbl, namely methylmalonic acidemia and homocystinuria (Fig. 155-8). Because the amounts of these metabolites detected in these patients generally greatly exceed those found in patients with Cbl transport defects or Cbl deficiency, their measurement has served to distinguish these groups of individuals clinically. We are aware of over 100 patients with inherited combined methylmalonic acidemia and homocystinuria. Many of the early patients were the subjects of individual case reports.[400–413] Cells from these children comprise three biochemically and genetically distinct complementation groups, designated *cblC* (MIM 277400), *cblD* (MIM 277410), and *cblF* (MIM 277380).[323,414–416] The *cblC* group is by far the largest (more than 100 patients), with the *cblD* represented by 2 sibs[400] and the *cblF* group by 6 unrelated individuals.[413,417–419]

cblC. Clinical findings have varied widely among patients in the *cblC* group; Table 155-3 presents a summary of the clinical and laboratory data from a survey of 50 such patients.[420] Most of the early described patients presented in the first few months of life because of failure to thrive, poor feeding, or lethargy. Subsequent reports have emphasized that some patients have a much delayed onset of symptoms: for example, a 4-year-old with fatigue, delirium, and spasticity,[406] and a 14-year-old with the rather sudden onset of dementia and myelopathy.[405] Thus, regardless of age, neurologic manifestations have been prominent. Most, but not all, of these patients have had hematologic abnormalities characterized by megaloblastoid and macrocytic anemia; hypersegmented polymorphonuclear leukocytes and thrombocytopenia have been observed less often. Several patients have had features of hemolytic-uremic syndrome.[421] A few patients have had a characteristic pigmentary retinopathy with perimacular degeneration, as well as other ophthalmologic changes.[404,406,409,412] Hydrocephalus, cor pulmonale, and other congenital malformations also have been seen.[422–424] Moderate to severe developmental delay has been common in the early onset patients, and about a third of early onset patients have died despite treatment.[420]

In addition to the methylmalonic aciduria and homocystinuria that characterize this group of patients, they have hypomethioninemia and cystathioninuria. The methylmalonic aciduria in these children is distinctly less severe than that encountered in children with isolated mutase deficiency (see Chap. 94), although much more severe than that reported for patients with Cbl transport defects. Moreover, neither hyperglycinemia nor hyperammonemia has been reported in any of the *cblC* (or *cblD* or *cblF*) patients. Serum cobalamin and folate concentrations have been normal.

cblD. In sharp contrast with this description, neither of the brothers in the *cblD* group[400] had any clinically significant problems until much later in life. The older brother came to medical attention because of severe behavioral pathology and moderate mental retardation at 14 years of age. He had, as well, a poorly defined neuromuscular problem involving his lower extremities. His then 2-year-old brother was asymptomatic, although biochemically affected. No hematologic abnormalities have been noted in either sib.

cblF. There have been six unrelated patients reported in the *cblF* group.[413,417–419,425] The first two girls presented during the first weeks of life with stomatitis and hypotonia, together with minor facial anomalies. The first patient, who was not diagnosed until 8 months, developed poorly and was clearly delayed.[413] No hematologic abnormalities were found in the first patient, while the second showed macrocytosis and hypersegmented polymorphonuclear neutrophils.[425] The second patient died suddenly at home. Other *cblF* patients have had pancytopenia, neutropenia, or thrombocytopenia.[417,418] Although the first patient had no detectable homocystinuria despite cellular deficits in methionine synthase activity and in MeCbl synthesis, all the others have shown both methylmalonic aciduria and homocystinuria. A male, diagnosed at 11 years of age, had a grossly abnormal Schilling test and low serum Cbl.[417] He had recurrent stomatitis in infancy, arthritis at age 4 years, and confusion and disorientation at age 10 years. He also had a pigmentary skin abnormality.

Localization of Cellular Metabolism Defects

cblC and cblD. It is clear that patients in the *cblC* and *cblD* groups have a defect in cellular metabolism of Cbl based on several criteria: total Cbl content of liver, kidney, and cultured fibroblasts is markedly reduced;[401,426–428] the ability of cultured cells to retain [^{57}Co]-labeled CN-Cbl[429] or to convert [^{57}Co]-labeled CN-Cbl or OH-Cbl to AdoCbl and MeCbl is markedly impaired;[430] activities of methylmalonyl CoA mutase and methionine synthase in cultured cells are deficient, such deficiency being partially reversed by supplementation of the growth medium with OH-Cbl;[415,431,432] and the mutase and the methionine synthase apoenzymes in cells from affected patients appear to be normal.[84,400,415,431]

Because these mutant cells demonstrate normal receptor-mediated adsorptive endocytosis of the TC II-Cbl complex and normal intralysosomal hydrolysis of TC II,[274,309,415,433] perusal of Fig. 155-10 makes it clear that the defects in the *cblC* and *cblD* cells must affect some step or steps subsequent to cellular uptake, common to the synthesis of both coenzymes, and prior to the binding of the Cbl coenzymes to their respective apoproteins. Significantly, *cblC* (and, to a lesser extent, *cblD*) cells use CN-Cbl less well than OH-Cbl[432,434] and are unable to convert CN-Cbl to OH-Cbl, a step shown in normal cells to be a metabolic prerequisite for the synthesis of both AdoCbl and MeCbl.[434] The latter results have been interpreted as evidence for a defect in a cytosolic cob(III)alamin reductase, which is required for reducing the trivalent cobalt prior to alkylation.[434] Partial deficiencies of CN-Cbl β-ligand transferase and of microsomal cob(III)alamin reductase have been described in *cblC* and *cblD* fibroblasts.[435,436] A partial deficiency of mitochondrial NADH-linked aquacobalamin reductase was described by Watanabe and his coworkers in two *cblC* fibroblast extracts.[437] The suggestion by Pezacka and her colleagues that GSCbl may be the product of an intermediate step in this process[325] provides another potential site for the mutation in one of these groups. Finally, it should be mentioned that the distinction between the *cblC* and *cblD* classes is based first and foremost on complementation studies that define the two classes as unique.[415] Their biochemical differences appear to be quantitative rather than qualitative, with the *cblC* group having more severe metabolic derangements than the siblings designated *cblD*. Therefore, it remains possible that the *cblD* mutation is allelic to *cblC* and shows interallelic complementation.

cblF. Studies using cultured fibroblasts from two patients in the *cblF* group[413,416,425] are of particular interest. As with cells from *cblC* and *cblD* patients, both mutase and methionine synthase activities were impaired, and AdoCbl and MeCbl contents were reduced. In contrast to the *cblC* and *cblD* mutants, however, the *cblF* cells accumulated unmetabolized, nonprotein-bound CN-Cbl in lysosomes.[438,439] These findings indicate that *cblF* cells are deficient in the mediated process by which Cbl exits from lysosomes after being taken up by receptor-mediated endocytosis.[310] Two brief reports further indicate that two *cblF* patients had abnormal Schilling tests with both free and IF-bound Cbl,[417,440] suggesting that the putative lysosomal defect affects ileal Cbl transcytosis as well (see Cbl transport section above).

Pathophysiology. The megaloblastic anemia so commonly observed in the *cblC* patients almost surely reflects the disturbance of methionine synthase activity. This can be stated with some assurance because patients with isolated methylmalonyl CoA mutase deficiency (see Chap. 94) more severe than that encountered in the *cblC* patients exhibit no megaloblastic anemia. The early and severe central nervous system abnormalities encountered in the *cblC* group probably reflect the methionine synthase abnormality as well, in that such patients generally do not experience the severe metabolic ketoacidosis that probably accounts for the central nervous system problems in patients with mutase deficiency only. Thus, patients with severe, inherited dysfunction in the synthesis of both Cbl coenzymes resemble closely patients with exogenous Cbl deficiency—both groups having prominent hematologic and neurologic manifestations resulting from the blocked methionine synthase system.

Genetic Considerations. Because equal numbers of affected males and affected females exist in the *cblC* group, because females have been as seriously affected as males, and because cells from affected patients behave as recessives in complementation studies,[414] it seems safe to predict that this disorder is inherited as an autosomal recessive trait. The mode of inheritance of the *cblD* and the *cblF* mutations cannot yet be defined, because of the paucity of known patients (both affected *cblD* patients in the only family yet described are male); both males and females have been identified in the *cblF* group. Identification of heterozygotes for the *cblC*, *cblD*, or *cblF* group has not yet been accomplished.

Diagnosis, Treatment, and Prognosis. The combination of methylmalonic aciduria and homocystinuria with normal serum Cbl concentrations and normal TC II is the set of biochemical parameters needed to distinguish patients in the *cblC*, *cblD*, and, probably, *cblF* groups from those with methylmalonic acidemia caused by isolated methylmalonyl CoA mutase deficiency (see Chap. 94); from those with homocystinuria due to cystathionine synthase deficiency (see Chap. 88), or methylene-H_4Folate reductase deficiency, or isolated methionine synthase deficiency (see "Folate" section above); and from those with Cbl transport defects or exogenous Cbl deficiency (see above). It should be noted that one *cblF* patient had low serum Cbl when diagnosed.[417] Because each of the cellular metabolic defects is expressed in cultured cells from affected individuals, the diagnosis should be confirmed by genetic complementation analysis between patient fibroblasts and fibroblasts from patients whose complementation

Table 155-4 Salient Biochemical Features of Cultured Fibroblasts from Patients with Various Defects in Cellular Cbl Metabolism*

	Mutant Class						
Biochemical Parameter	***cblA***	***cblB***	***cblC***	***cblD***	***cblE***	***cblF***	***cblG***
Studies with intact cells							
[^{14}C]propionate oxidation	−	−	−	−	+	−	+
[^{14}C]Methyl-H_4Folate fixation	+	+	−	−	−	−	−
MeCbl synthesis	+	+	−	−	−	−	−
AdoCbl synthesis	−	−	−	−	+	−	+
Conversion of CN-Cbl to OH-Cbl	+	+	−	±	+	−	+
Lysosomal efflux of free Cbl	+	+	+	+	+	−	+
Enzyme activities in cell extracts†							
Mutase holoenzyme	−	−	−	−	nt	nt	nt
Mutase total enzyme	+	+	+	+	nt	nt	nt
Methionine synthase holoenzyme	+	+	−	−	±**	−	−
Methionine synthase total enzyme	+	+	±	±	+**	±	−
Methionine synthase reductase	+	+	+	+	−	+	+
Cob(I)alamin adenosyltransferase	+	−	+	+	nt	+	nt

*+ = normal; − = markedly deficient or undetectable; ± = partially deficient; nt = not tested.
†*Holoenzyme* is defined as that enzyme activity measured in the absence of added cofactor; *total enzyme* is that activity measured in the presence of saturating concentrations of cofactor.
**Activity dependent on reducing conditions used (see folate section).
Abbreviations: Methyl-H_4Folate = N^5-methyltetrahydrofolate; MeCbl = methylcobalamin; AdoCbl = adenosylcobalamin; CN-Cbl = cyanocobalamin; OH-Cbl = hydroxocobalamin.

groups have been determined previously. This technique also allows the *cblC*, *cblD*, and *cblF* groups to be distinguished from each other. Biochemical studies on cultured cells, such as Cbl uptake, lysosomal Cbl efflux, or AdoCbl and MeCbl synthesis, and direct measurement of mutase and methionine synthase activities in cell extracts can be performed to provide further confirmation (see Table 155-4).

Because normal amniotic fluid cells appear to carry out all the steps of Cbl metabolism observed in cultured fibroblasts, it is be possible to detect each of these defects prenatally by assaying any of these parameters in cultured amniocytes. This has been carried out successfully in both the *cblC* and *cblF*[269] groups.

The distinctions between these cellular metabolic defects and other related conditions are critically important, because appropriate therapy and prognosis depend on them. Whereas exogenous Cbl deficiency responds dramatically to physiologic amounts of Cbl and transport defects to somewhat larger dosages, successful management of *cblC*, *cblD*, and *cblF* demands the administration of large amounts of OH-Cbl (up to 1 mg daily) by intramuscular injection.[195,400,402,404,406,417,440] Such treatment has resulted in dramatic decreases in urinary methylmalonate and in less dramatic, but significant, decreases in urinary homocystine in many patients who have received it. The form of Cbl administered is important, at least in *cblC* patients, because studies on cultured cells from this group have shown that supplementation in culture is much less efficient with CN-Cbl than with OH-Cbl in eliciting an increase in the activity of the affected enzymes.[438] A recently published study of the effects of the chemical form of Cbl administered to two *cblC* patients supports the greater efficacy of OH-Cbl, both biochemically and clinically.[441] A number of adjunctive therapies have been employed for *cblC* patients with variable success, including moderate protein restriction to reduce the load of metabolic end products and, hence, the amount of methylmalonate produced; carnitine supplementation, to improve organic acid excretion and relieve a postulated functional carnitine deficiency (see Chap. 94); folic and folinic acid administration, to bypass the so-called methylfolate trap and restore hematologic function; and betaine administration, to provide substrate for betaine:homocysteine methyltransferase, which is not dependent on a Cbl coenzyme, and thus to return the serum methionine:homocysteine ratio toward normal. Few investigators have evaluated the efficacy of these treatments critically, however. Bartholomew and his colleagues attempted to determine the effects of OH-Cbl dosage schedule and of treatment with carnitine, folinic acid, and betaine on the clinical and biochemical status of two patients with the *cblC* defect.[442] In each case, the OH-Cbl injection schedule could be titrated to control the patient's methylmalonic acidemia and homocystinuria. In addition, betaine administration (250 mg/kg/day) appeared to act synergistically with the OH-Cbl to produce a further reduction in plasma homocystine. No specific clinical improvement accompanied the betaine therapy, however. Neither patient responded clinically or biochemically to folinic acid or carnitine treatment. The overall result in both patients was good metabolic control, as measured by reduced methylmalonic acidemia and normal serum homocysteine and methionine concentrations, and resolution of most of their clinical symptoms, such as lethargy, irritability, vomiting, and failure to thrive, with a treatment regimen of daily betaine administration and biweekly injections of OH-Cbl. Significantly, both patients remained somewhat delayed developmentally, even after a year or more of therapy. In addition, the retinal degeneration present in these patients was not reversed by the therapy, although some improvement in cone response was noted in one of them.

This report serves also to emphasize that early diagnosis and prompt institution of therapy with OH-Cbl (and possibly betaine) may be the only way to change the outcome of these patients, which, at least in the case of the *cblC* group, is dismal thus far (Fig. 155-11). Many have died despite intensive therapy. Severe hemolytic anemia is a major complication in the deceased *cblC* patients, as has congestive heart failure. Thromboemboli, so often encountered in patients with homocystinuria due to cystathionine synthase deficiency, have, thus far, been documented in only a few *cblC* patients[420] and in the older of the two *cblD* brothers, in whom this complication was not noted until he reached 18 years of age. Betaine treatment may reduce this risk by normalizing the serum methionine/homocysteine ratio, even when Cbl-responsiveness is incomplete.[442] Surviving patients, even those under apparently good metabolic control, continue to show signs of neurologic dysfunction, including mild to moderate mental retardation and delayed development of motor skills,[236,420] and, in some cases, the continued presence of abnormal ophthalmologic findings.[442] These problems could be the result of irreversible damage that

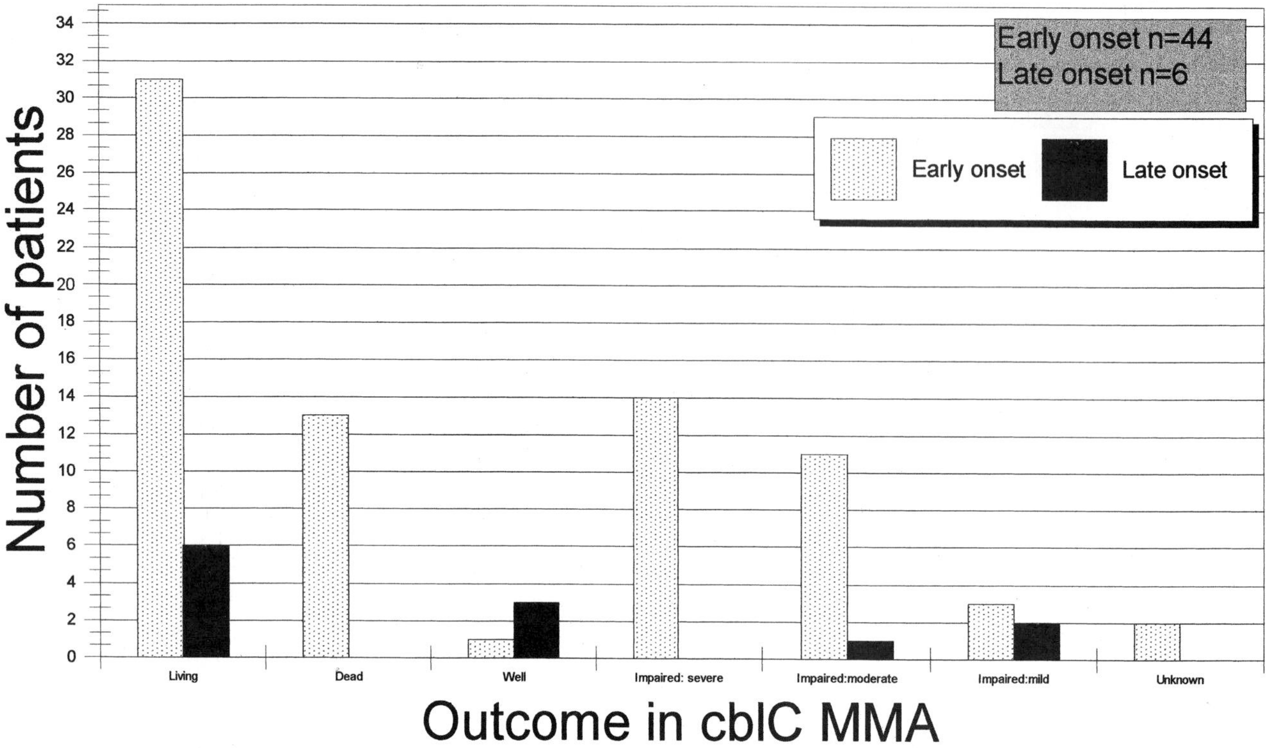

Fig. 155-11 Outcome in *cblC* patients based on age-of-onset less than 1 year (early onset, shaded bars) or greater than 1 year (late onset; solid bars). Late onset patients presented between ages 4 and 14 years. Impairment is classified in functional terms as severe, moderate, or mild according to the expectation for age. (*Reproduced from Rosenblatt et al.*[420] *Used with permission.*)

occurred prior to diagnosis and therapeutic intervention, or could reflect the impossibility of completely correcting the cellular lesion in Cbl metabolism in certain cells whose function is critical in neurologic development. Significantly, patients with apparently later onset or milder disease have done considerably better (Fig. 155-11). Until a number of patients with these defects are diagnosed before birth or soon thereafter, and treated immediately, or even prenatally, with Cbl and betaine supplements, we will not know whether the poor outcome in this group can be modified significantly. Documentation of such experience is particularly important in assessing the clinician's ability to modify the natural history of these disorders.

Defects in AdoCbl Synthesis

In 1968, Rosenberg[443,444] and Lindblad[445,446] and their colleagues described infants with severe metabolic ketoacidosis and developmental delay who accumulated very large amounts of methylmalonate in blood and urine, similar to patients reported earlier by Oberholzer[447] and Stokke[448] and their coworkers. In contrast to the earlier patients, however, these infants responded dramatically to pharmacologic doses of CN-Cbl or AdoCbl with resolution of their clinical symptoms and major reductions in their excretion of methylmalonate. Further studies indicated that the methylmalonyl CoA mutase enzyme was normal in these patients, but that synthesis of AdoCbl was impaired.[430,449] Somewhat later, Kaye *et al.*[450] reported two patients with methylmalonic acidemia who were unresponsive *in vivo* to high doses of CN-Cbl but who also had apparently normal mutase enzyme and defective AdoCbl synthesis. Subsequent biochemical and genetic complementation analysis established that lesions at two genetically distinct loci can be responsible for defective AdoCbl synthesis; they are designated *cblA* (MIM 251100) and *cblB* (MIM 251110)[323,414] Because both groups of patients with deficient AdoCbl synthesis share many clinical features with those with primary defects in the methylmalonyl CoA mutase enzyme, the reader is also referred to Chap. 94 for a discussion of the latter group.

Clinical and Laboratory Presentation. As mentioned above, the clinical findings in patients with methylmalonic acidemia due either to defective mutase enzyme (*mut*) or defective AdoCbl synthesis (*cblA*, *cblB*) are remarkable more for their similarities than for their differences. A survey of the natural history in 45 such patients has been reported:[451] 20 were *mut*; 14 were *cblA*, and 11 were *cblB* (also see Chap. 94). There were approximately equal numbers of males and females in each group. The most common signs and symptoms at the onset of clinical difficulty were lethargy, failure to thrive, recurrent vomiting, dehydration, respiratory distress, and muscular hypotonia. Little interclass difference was observed for these major clinical manifestations or for such less common ones as developmental retardation, hepatomegaly, or coma. The only major clinical distinction between the *mut* group and the groups with defective AdoCbl synthesis was that most of the former group presented very early in life (<1 to 4 weeks), while 60 percent of the *cblA* group and 45 percent of the *cblB* group presented between 1 month and 1 year.[451]

The laboratory findings in *cblA* and *cblB* patients at the time that methylmalonic acidemia was first documented are shown in Table 155-5, with those in *mut* patients for comparison. As expected, serum cobalamin concentrations were routinely normal. Metabolic acidosis, with blood pH values as low as 6.9 and serum bicarbonate concentrations as low as 5 mEq/liter, was observed in the majority of patients. Ketonemia or ketonuria, hyperammonemia, and hyperglycinemia or hyperglycinuria were also observed in many affected patients. Leukopenia, thrombocytopenia, and anemia were the only other manifestations that were noted. Earlier case reports (reviewed in reference 452) found that hypoglycemia occurred in about 40 percent of affected patients. Significantly, the megaloblastic anemia characteristic of functional Cbl deficiency or the inherited disorders of MeCbl synthesis (*cblC*, *cblD*, *cblE*, *cblF*, and *cblG*) was not present in these patients.

Chemical Abnormalities *In Vivo*. Large amounts of methylmalonic acid have appeared in the urine or blood of all reported

Table 155-5 Laboratory Findings in 45 Patients with Methylmalonic Acidemia*

	Mutant Class		
Finding at Clinical Onset	***cblA***	***cblB***	**mut**
Normal serum cobalamin	100	100	100
Metabolic acidosis	100	88	89
Ketonemia and/or ketonuria	78	67	88
Hyperammonemia	50	83	76
Hyperglycinemia and/or -glycinuria	70	83	60
Leukopenia	70	45	69
Anemia	10	45	44
Thrombocytopenia	75	45	40

*Numerical values are the percentages of the patients in each group in whom the particular finding was made.
SOURCE: From Matsui et al.[451]

patients. Whereas normal children and adults excrete less than 0.04 mM (5 mg) methylmalonate daily, children with isolated methylmalonic acidemia have excreted from 2.1 to 49 mM (240 to 5700 mg) in a 24-h period. Their plasma concentrations of methylmalonate, almost undetectable in normal subjects, have ranged from 0.22 to 2.9 mM (2.6 to 34 mg/dl). In the few patients in whom it was measured, the CSF concentration of methylmalonate equaled that of plasma (see reference 392 for references to early case reports). No relationship between the quantities of methylmalonate accumulated in body fluids and the etiology of mutase deficiency (i.e., apoenzyme vs. coenzyme synthesis deficiency) has been reported. Methylmalonate is surely the major, but not the only, abnormal metabolite found in body fluids of these patients. Because propionyl CoA carboxylation is reversible, propionate and some of its precursors (butanone) or metabolites (β-hydroxypropionate and methylcitrate) also accumulate in blood and urine,[443,453,454] their amounts being small compared to that of methylmalonate (see Chap. 94).

Several groups have studied the relationship between protein or amino acid loading and methylmalonate accumulation in these patients. Without exception, administration of protein or amino acids known to be precursors of propionate and methylmalonate, such as methionine, threonine, valine, or isoleucine, has resulted in augmented methylmalonate accumulation and, in some instances, ketosis or acidosis.[443,445,447,448] When Cbl-responsive patients are given supplements of this vitamin, such augmentation by methylmalonate precursors is lessened considerably.[455] All these findings suggest that patients with discrete defects at the mutase step have a major block in the utilization of methylmalonyl CoA, which is expressed as methylmalonate accumulation.

Localization of Enzymatic Defects. Because the conversion of propionate to succinate is blocked in each of the methylmalonic acidemias, whether due to mutase defects or AdoCbl synthesis deficiencies, an early screening test for these disorders measured the ability of intact peripheral blood leukocytes or cultured fibroblasts to oxidize [^{14}C]propionate or [^{14}C]methylmalonate to $^{14}CO_2$ and compared this with the oxidation of [^{14}C]succinate to $^{14}CO_2$.[444] More recently, incorporation of [^{14}C]propionate into trichloroacetic acid-precipitable material by intact cultured cells has replaced the more cumbersome $^{14}CO_2$ evolution technique.[456,457] Further discrimination among the methylmalonic acidemias has depended on studies of cobalamin uptake and AdoCbl formation by intact cultured fibroblasts, on assays of mutase activity in cell extracts, and on genetic complementation studies with cultured cells.

cblA. A series of observations by Rosenberg[449] and Mahoney[430] and their colleagues on the fibroblasts of the index patient with Cbl-responsive methylmalonic acidemia led to the demonstration of a primary defect in AdoCbl synthesis. Such intact cells were unable to convert OH-[^{57}Co]Cbl to Ado[^{57}Co]Cbl, although they took up the labeled vitamin normally and had no abnormality in synthesizing the other cobalamin coenzyme, MeCbl.[430] On the other hand, cell-free extracts from this line synthesized AdoCbl normally when incubated with OH-[^{57}Co]Cbl, ATP, and a reducing system designed to bypass cob(III)alamin reductase and cob(II)-alamin reductase and to measure only cob(I)alamin adenosyltransferase.[323] Fibroblasts from other patients in this clinically defined group had identical findings in similar studies.[323] Genetic complementation analysis established unequivocally that all these patients belonged to a single complementation group, designated *cblA*, and thus presumably had defects in the same enzyme or protein.[414] Because it has been shown that intact mammalian mitochondria can synthesize AdoCbl from OH-Cbl *in vitro* without prior reduction[458] and because Cbl adenosyltransferase activity is normal in this group,[323] it is presumed that the defect must lie in one of the early steps of mitochondrial Cbl metabolism, possibly in a mitochondrial Cbl reductase (see Fig. 155-10). So far, the lack of a specific assay for the reductive step(s) in AdoCbl synthesis[326,327] has prevented a more precise localization of the defect in the *cblA* group.

cblB. Another group of patients with defective AdoCbl synthesis was uncovered when Cbl metabolism was examined in a number of cell lines from patients with methylmalonic acidemia.[323,459] Some of these fibroblasts showed a primary defect in AdoCbl synthesis similar to that described for the *cblA* class (above), except in one aspect. When cell-free extracts from these lines were incubated with OH-[^{57}Co]Cbl, a reducing system, and ATP, no AdoCbl synthesis was detected,[323] in contrast to the result in the *cblA* cell lines. Because this assay is specific for ATP:cob(I)alamin adenosyltransferase, the patients in this group must have defects in this enzyme.[324] Complementation analysis indicates that a single locus, *cblB*, is involved in all these patients and that it is distinct from the *cblA* locus.[414]

Pathophysiology. All studies *in vivo* and *in vitro* in patients with methylmalonic acidemia due to methylmalonyl CoA mutase deficiency, either primary or secondary to AdoCbl synthesis defects, indicate that the block in the conversion of methylmalonyl CoA to succinyl CoA explains fully the accumulation of methylmalonate in blood and urine; the augmentation of methylmalonate excretion and the precipitation of ketosis by protein, amino acids, or propionate; and the excretion of long-chain ketones formed in the catabolism of branched chain amino acids. See Chap. 94 for a complete discussion of methylmalonic acidemia.

By comparing and contrasting the findings in patients with isolated mutase deficiency, whether due to defects in mutase or in AdoCbl synthesis, with those in patients with functional Cbl deficiency (as in classic pernicious anemia or the Cbl transport defects discussed above), it is possible to shed some light on the mechanism responsible for the hematologic and neurologic abnormalities in the latter disorders. Thus, the absence of megaloblastic anemia in any patient with isolated mutase deficiency militates against any involvement of this enzyme in the typical megaloblastoid seen in Cbl deficiency. Similarly, the cerebellar and posterior column abnormalities so often encountered in Cbl-deficient patients have never been observed in patients with methylmalonic acidemia due to specific mutase dysfunction. Therefore, the notion that neurologic dysfunction in pernicious anemia reflects aberrant incorporation of odd-chain or branched chain fatty acids into myelin because of a block in the propionate pathway has little to recommend it. It appears likely, then, that abnormalities in Cbl-dependent methionine synthase account for the hematologic and neurologic abnormalities in Cbl-deficient patients.

Genetic Considerations. Both *cblA* and *cblB* are almost certainly inherited as autosomal recessive traits. This conclusion is based on these observations: (a) approximately equal numbers of affected males and females have been reported in each group; (b) no instance of vertical transmission from affected parent to affected child has been reported; (c) each mutant class behaves as a recessive in culture in complementation experiments;[414,415,431] and (d) cell lines from heterozygotes for the *cblB* mutation show partial adenosyltransferase deficiency.[324]

Diagnosis, Treatment, and Prognosis. Because simple colorimetric assays for urinary methylmalonate and more complex gas chromatography-mass spectrometry assays for serum and urinary methylmalonate are available, it should not be difficult to make a diagnosis of methylmalonic acidemia, once this condition is considered. Other sources of neonatal or infantile ketoacidosis must be ruled out. The quantity of methylmalonate excreted, the absence of megaloblastic changes, and the normal amounts of serum homocysteine, methionine, and Cbl all serve to differentiate these diseases from others that may lead to methylmalonic aciduria. Distinguishing between primary mutase deficiency and primary AdoCbl synthesis defects and between the two causes of the latter ultimately depends on studies with cultured cells B routinely, genetic complementation analysis.[415] Prenatal detection of methylmalonic acidemia has been accomplished in two different ways: by measurement of methylmalonate in amniotic fluid and maternal urine at midtrimester[460,461] and by studies of mutase activity and Cbl metabolism in cultured amniotic fluid cells.[456,461,462] Assays of [^{14}C]propionate utilization[456] in uncultured chorionic villous biopsy specimens have proven unsatisfactory, however. AdoCbl synthesis defects of both complementation groups[461,462] have been identified in these ways.

Two treatment regimens for children with methylmalonic acidemia exist and should be employed in tandem for patients with AdoCbl synthesis deficiencies. A diet restricted in protein (or a special formula restricted in amino acid precursors of methylmalonate) should be instituted as soon as such life-threatening problems as ketoacidosis, hypoglycemia, or hyperammonemia have been addressed; and supplementary Cbl (1 to 2 mg OH-Cbl intramuscularly daily for several days) should be given as soon as the diagnosis of methylmalonic acidemia is made (or even seriously considered). Such measures should decrease the circulating concentrations of methylmalonate and propionate. Even Cbl-unresponsive children with delayed development improve markedly when treated with careful dietary protein restriction.[463,464] In Cbl-responsive patients, titration of Cbl dosage schedules against methylmalonate excretion and clinical status is probably worthwhile. The methylmalonic aciduria is not completely eliminated in even the most responsive patients, even though clinical symptoms such as ketosis and acidosis are completely resolved. As discussed in Chap. 94, Roe and associates[465–467] have pointed out that L-carnitine supplements may be a useful therapeutic adjunct in patients with methylmalonic acidemia, presumably by repleting intracellular and extracellular stores of free carnitine that are depleted in affected patients because of exchange with excess methylmalonyl CoA and propionyl CoA. No trial of this compound has been reported in *cblA* or *cblB* patients. As suggested in Chap. 94, oral antibiotic therapy may prove useful as well. Thompson and his colleagues reported that three Cbl-unresponsive patients showed subjective improvement in alertness and appetite following brief metronidazole therapy;[468] longer treatment periods have resulted in significant improvements in other patients, including decreased number and severity of acidotic episodes, increased appetite, decreased vomiting, growth acceleration, and improved behavior in a *cblB* patient.[469]

The previously mentioned survey[451] suggested that both the response to Cbl supplements and the long-term outcome in affected patients depends considerably on the nature of the biochemical lesion. Whereas more than 90 percent of the *cblA* patients responded to Cbl supplements with a distinct fall in blood or urinary methylmalonate, only ~40 percent of the *cblB* patients showed such a response. Presumably, the ~60 percent of *cblB* patients unresponsive to Cbl supplements have such complete adenosyltransferase deficiency that AdoCbl synthesis cannot be augmented by Cbl supplements, in distinction to the *cblB* patients with apparently "leaky" mutations that permit responsiveness *in vivo*. The uniform responsiveness of patients in the *cblA* group suggests either that the responsible mutations are generally leaky, thereby allowing mass action to result in more AdoCbl synthesis, or that alternative pathways of Cbl reduction, which require high substrate concentrations, exist in cells.[326,327] As in the case of primary mutase deficiency, it should be emphasized that clinical responsiveness *in vivo* does not require complete correction of the functional mutase deficiency or complete normalization of biochemical parameters such as the methylmalonic acidemia (see Chap. 94). Some patients in the *cblB* group, unresponsive to CN-Cbl or OH-Cbl *in vivo,* might be expected to respond to AdoCbl itself, but published reports on two patients suggest that this logical alternative is ineffective.[470,471] Unpublished experiments on cells in culture suggest that AdoCbl is largely converted back to OH-Cbl during transport.

The long-term outlook for affected patients is revealing. The *cblA* patients (i.e., the group biochemically most responsive to Cbl supplements) had the best outcome according to the survey—~70 percent were alive and well at ages up to 14 years and presumably continue to be so. The *cblB* group had about equal fractions in the alive and well, the alive and impaired, and the deceased category. It is interesting, albeit anecdotal, that the index patient in the *cblA* group (now over 30 years old) discontinued Cbl supplements at age 9 years despite advice to the contrary. In the ensuing years, despite accumulation of very large amounts of methylmalonate in the blood and urine, his development and general health have remained excellent, with one exception (see below). Perhaps, as in some other inherited metabolic disorders, treatment of methylmalonic acidemia is most critical early in life. If this experience is borne out, it makes expert clinical management in the early weeks or months of life most important. There have been several reports of "metabolic stroke" in patients following episodes of metabolic decompensation.[472–474] Three of the patients[472,473] belonged to the Cbl-responsive *cblA* group, but were not being treated at the time. Extrapyramidal signs, particularly dystonia, were accompanied by bilateral lucencies of the globus pallidus and persisted after the acute crisis had passed. In one case, the dystonia was gradually progressive over a period of 7 years without visible progression of the neurologic lesions.[474] One complication of long-term survival of some methylmalonic acidemia patients may be chronic renal failure. One report has indicated that 8 of 12 nonresponsive patients (aged 1 to 9 years) had reduced GFR, with 5 severely affected.[475] In one patient "greatly improved metabolic control" over a period of 18 months led to increased, but still impaired, renal function.[475] Significantly, the index *cblA* patient referred to above recently returned to attention following treatment for renal dysfunction due to biopsy-proven interstitial nephritis. The impact of better metabolic control and Cbl supplementation has not been explored in this case.

Finally, the feasibility of prenatal therapy with Cbl supplements has been demonstrated. Ampola *et al.*[461] showed that administration of Cbl supplements to a woman carrying an affected fetus of the *cblA* group resulted in significant reduction in maternal excretion of methylmalonate and the presence of only moderate methylmalonic acidemia(-uria) in the newborn child. She was doing well at the time of the report (20 months) with moderate protein restriction and occasional Cbl therapy, whereas an undiagnosed affected sib had died at 3 months of age.[461] A second, similar case has been reported.[476]

SUMMARY

Tables 155-2 and 155-4 summarize the salient biochemical features of patients with defects in various aspects of folate and

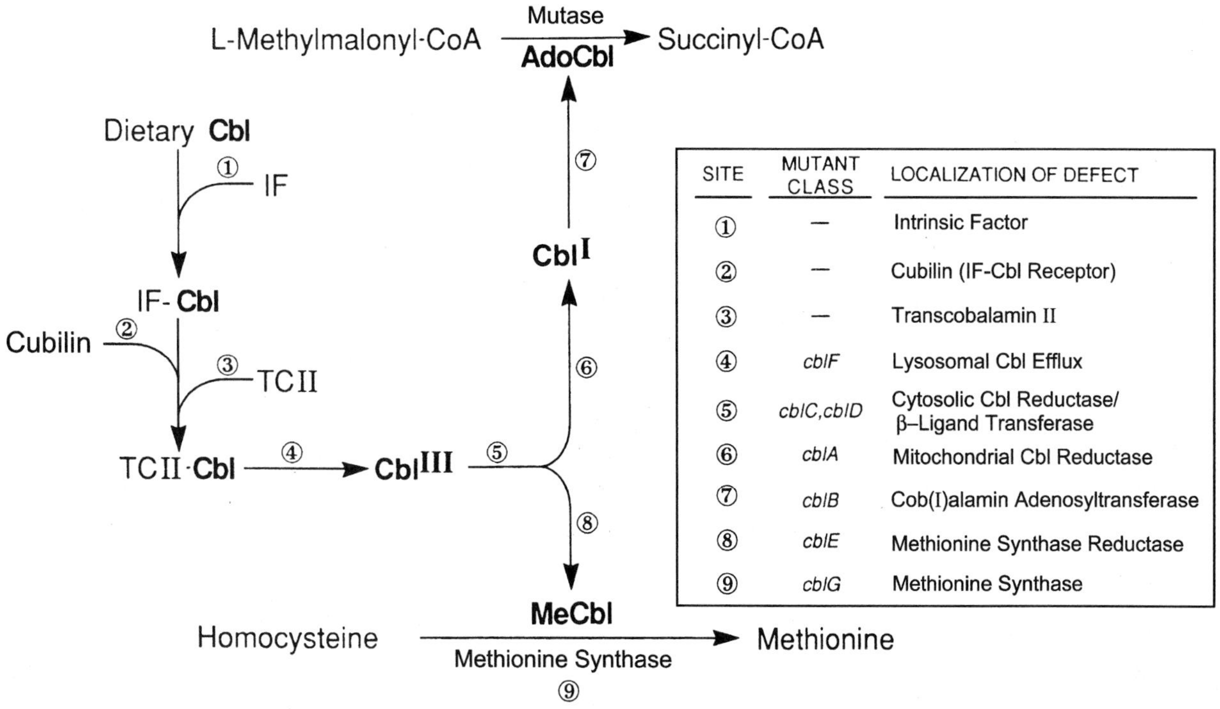

Fig. 155-12 Summary scheme of inherited defects of cobalamin metabolism. The circled numbers and their key signify the general sites at which abnormalities have been identified and the affected protein or process at each site. Cbl^{III} = cob(III)alamin (e.g., OH-Cbl); Cbl^{I} = cob(I)alamin; AdoCbl = adenosylcobalamin; MeCbl = methylcobalamin.

Cbl transport and metabolism and their cultured cells. Figures 155-4 and 155-12 summarize the localization of these defects.

ACKNOWLEDGMENTS

The authors thank L.E. Rosenberg for his contributions to this chapter in previous editions and R. Rozen for the provision of Fig. 155-5. We thank the many clinicians who have provided clinical histories and fibroblasts for analysis.

REFERENCES

1. Rowe PB: Inherited disorders of folate metabolism, in Stanbury JB, Wyngaarden JB, Frederickson DS, Goldstein JL, Brown MS (eds): *The Metabolic Basis of Inherited Disease*. New York, McGraw-Hill, 1983, p 498.
2. Rosenblatt DS: Inherited disorders of folate transport and metabolism, in Scriver CR, Beaudet AL, Sly WS, Valle D (eds): *The Metabolic and Molecular Basis of Inherited Disease*. New York, McGraw-Hill, 1995, p 3111.
3. Blakley RL: *The Biochemistry of Folic Acid and Related Pteridines*. New York, American Elsevier, 1969.
4. Blakley RL, Benkovic SJ: *Folates and Pterins: Chemistry and Biochemistry of Folates*. New York, John Wiley, 1984.
5. Erbe RW: Inborn errors of folate metabolism, in Blakley RL, Whitehead VM (eds): *Nutritional, Pharmacological and Physiological Aspects*, vol 3. New York, John Wiley, 1986, p 413.
6. Shane B: Folylpolyglutamate synthesis and role in the regulation of one-carbon metabolism. *Vitam Horm* **45**:263, 1989.
7. Schirch V, Strong WB: Interaction of folylpolyglutamates with enzymes in one-carbon metabolism. *Arch Biochem Biophys* **269**:371, 1989.
8. Appling DR: Compartmentation of folate-mediated one-carbon metabolism in eukaryotes. *FASEB J* **5**:2645, 1991.
9. Arakawa T: Congenital defects in folate utilization. *Am J Med* **48**:594, 1970.
10. Erbe RE: Inborn errors of folate metabolism (first of two parts). *N Engl J Med* **293**:753, 1975.
11. Cooper BA: Megaloblastic anaemia and disorders affecting utilisation of vitamin B_{12} and folate in childhood. *Clin Haematol* **5**:631, 1976.
12. Erbe RW: Genetic aspects of folate metabolism. *Adv Hum Genet* **9**:293, 1979.
13. Niederweiser A: Inborn errors of pterin metabolism. Folic acid, in Botez MI, Reynolds EH (eds): *Neurology, Psychiatry and Internal Medicine*. New York, Raven, 1979, p 349.
14. Rosenblatt DS: Prenatal diagnosis of inborn errors of folate and cobalamin metabolism and of cystinosis, in Milunsky A, Baltimore MD (eds): *Genetic Disorders and the Fetus: Diagnosis, Prevention, and Treatment*. Baltimore, MD, Johns Hopkins University Press, 1998, p 550.
15. Cooper BA: Anomalies congénitales du métabolisme des folates, in Zittoun J, Cooper BA (eds): *Folates et Cobalamines*. Paris, Doin, 1987.
16. Kisliuk RL: Folate biochemistry in relation to antifolate selectivity, in Jackman A (ed): *Antifolate Drugs in Cancer Therapy*. Totowa, NJ, Humana Press, 1999, p 13.
17. Wills L: Treatment of "pernicious anaemia of pregnancy" and "tropical anaemia" with special reference to yeast extract as curative agent. *Br Med J* **1**:1059, 1931.
18. Wills L, Stewart A: Experimental anemia in monkeys with special reference to macrocytic nutritional anemia. *Br J Exp Pathol* **16**:444; 1935.
19. Angier RB, Booth JH, Mowat JH, Semb J, Stockstad ELR, Subbarow Y, Waller CW, et al: The structure and synthesis of the liver L. casei factor. *Science* **103**:667, 1946.
20. Fan J, Vitols KS, Huennekens FM: Multiple folate transport systems in L1210 cells. *Adv Enzyme Regul* **32**:3, 1992.
21. Antony AC: Folate receptors. *Annu Rev Nutr* **16**:501, 1996.
22. Williams FMR, Flintoff WF: Isolation of a human cDNA that complements a mutant hamster cell defective in methotrexate uptake. *J Biol Chem* **270**:2987, 1995.
23. Moscow JA, Gong M, He R, Sgagias MK, Dixon KH, Anzick SL, Meltzer PS, Cowan KH: Isolation of a gene encoding a human reduced folate carrier (RFC1) and analysis of its expression in transport-deficient, methotrexate-resistant human breast cancer cells. *Cancer Res* **55**:3790, 1995.
24. Wong SC, Proefke SA, Bhushan A, Matherly LH: Isolation of human cDNAs that restore methotrexate sensitivity and reduced folate carrier activity in methotrexate transport-defective chinese hamster ovary cells. *J Biol Chem* **270(29)**:17468, 1995.
25. Tolner B, Roy K, Sirotnak FM: Structural analysis of the human RFC-1 gene encoding a folate transporter reveals multiple promoters and

alternatively spliced transcripts with 5′ end heterogeneity. *Gene* **211**:331, 1998.

26. Zhang L, Wong SC, Matherly LH: Transcript heterogeneity of the human reduced folate carrier results from the use of multiple promoters and variable splicing of alternative upstream exons. *Biochem J* **332**:773, 1998.
27. Nguyen TT, Dyer DL, Dunning DD, Rubin SA, Grant KE, Said HM: Human intestinal folate transport: Cloning, expression, and distribution of complementary RNA. *Gastroenterology* **112**:783, 1997.
28. Wang H, Ross JF, Ratnam M: Structure and regulation of a polymorphic gene encoding folate receptor type (γ/γ). *Nucleic Acids Res* **26**:2132, 1998.
29. Kamen BA, Capdevila A: Receptor-mediated folate accumulation is regulated by the cellular folate content. *Proc Natl Acad Sci U S A* **83**:5983, 1986.
30. Kamen BA, Smith AK, Anderson RGW: The folate receptor works in tandem with a probenecid-sensitive carrier in MA104 cells in vitro. *J Clin Invest* **87**:1442, 1991.
31. Anderson RG, Kamen BA, Rothberg KG, Lacey SW: Potocytosis: Sequestration and transport of small molecules by caveolae [Review]. *Science* **255**:410, 1992.
32. Smart EJ, Mineo C, Anderson RG: Clustered folate receptors deliver 5-methyltetrahydrofolate to cytoplasm of MA104 cells. *J Cell Biol* **134**:1169, 1996.
33. Wu M, Fan J, Gunning W, Ratman M: Clustering of GPI-anchored folate receptor independent of both cross-linking and association with caveolin. *J Membrane Biol* **159**:137, 1997.
34. Henderson GI, Perez T, Schenker S, Mackins J, Antony AC: Maternal-to-fetal transfer of 5-methyltetrahydrofolate by the perfused human placental cotyledon: Evidence for a concentrative role by placental folate receptors in fetal folate delivery. *J Lab Clin Med* **126**:184, 1995.
35. Watkins D, Cooper BA: A critical intracellular concentration of fully reduced non-methylated folate polyglutamates prevents macrocytosis and diminished growth rate of human cell line K562 in culture. *Biochem J* **214**:465, 1983.
36. Garrow TA, Admon A, Shane B: Expression cloning of a human cDNA encoding folylpoly(gamma-glutamate) synthetase and determination of its primary structure. *Proc Natl Acad Sci U S A* **89**:9151, 1992.
37. Taylor SM, Freemantle SJ, Moran RG: Structural organization of the human folylpoly-gamma-glutamate synthetase gene; Evidence for a single genomic locus. *Cancer Res* **55**:6030, 1995.
38. Jones C, Kao F-T, Taylor RT: Chromosomal assignment of the gene for folypolyglutamate synthetase to human chromosome 9. *Cytogenet Cell Genet* **28**:181, 1980.
39. Mackenzie RE: Summary. Pteroylpolyglutamate metabolism, chemistry and biology of pteridines, in Cooper BA, Whitehead VM (eds): *Pteridines and Folic Acid Derivatives*. Berlin, de Gruyter, 1986, p 767.
40. McBurney MW, Whitmore GF: Isolation and biochemical characterization of folate deficient mutants of Chinese hamster cells. *Cell* **2**:173, 1974.
41. Taylor RT, Hanna ML: Folate dependent enzymes in cultured chinese hamster cells. *Arch Biochem Biophys* **181**:331, 1977.
42. Rosenberg IH: Folate absorption and transport in chemistry and biology of pteridines, in Cooper BA, Whitehead VM (eds): *Pteridines and Folic Acid Derivatives*. Berlin, de Gruyter, 1986, p 587.
43. Halsted CH: Intestinal absorption and malabsorption of folates. *Annu Rev Med* **31**:79, 1980.
44. Yao R, Schneider E, Ryan TJ, Galivan J: Human gamma-glutamyl hydrolase; cloning and characterization of the enzyme expressed in vitro. *Proc Natl Acad Sci U S A* **93**:10134, 1996.
45. Yao R, Nimec Z, Ryan TJ, Galivan J: Identification, cloning, and sequencing of a cDNA coding for rat gamma-glutamyl hydrolase. *J Biol Chem* **271**:8525, 1996.
46. Heston WD: Characterization and glutamyl preferring carboxypeptidase function of prostate specific membrane antigen: A novel folate hydrolase. *Urology* **49**:104, 1997.
47. Smith GK, Benkovic PA, Benkovic SJ: L(−)10-formyltetrahydrofolate is the cofactor for glycinamide ribonucleotide transformylase from chicken liver. *Biochemistry* **20**:4036, 1981.
48. Kaufman RJ, Brown PC, Schimke PT: Amplified dihydrofolate reductase genes in unstable methotrexate resistant cells are associated with double minute chromosomes. *Proc Natl Acad Sci U S A* **76**:5669, 1979.
49. Anagnou NP, O'Brien SJ, Shimada T, Nash WG, Chen M, Nienhouse AW: Chromosomal organization of the human dihydrofolate reductase genes: Dispersion, selective amplification, and a novel form of polymorphism. *Proc Natl Acad Sci U S A* **81**:5170, 1984.
50. Funanage VL, Myoda TT, Moses PA, Cowell HR: Assignment of the human dihydrofolate reductase gene to the q11–q22 region of chromosome 5. *Mol Cell Biol* **4**:2010, 1984.
51. Garrow TA, Brenner AA, Whitehead VM, Chen X, Duncan RG, Korenberg JR, Shane B: Cloning of cDNA's encoding mitochondrial and cytosolic serine hydroxymethyltransferases and chromosomal localization. *J Biol Chem* **268**:11910, 1993.
52. Girgis S, Nasrallah IM, Suh JR, Oppenheim E, Zanetti KA, Mastri MG, Stover PJ: Molecular cloning, characterization and alternative splicing of the human cytoplasmic serine hydroxymethyltransferase gene. *Gene* **210**:315, 1998.
53. Stover PJ, Chen LH, Suh JR, Stover DM, Keyomarsi K, Shane B: Molecular cloning, characterization, and regulation of the human mitochondrial serine hydroxymethyltransferase gene. *J Biol Chem* **272**:1842, 1997.
54. Renwick SB, Snell K, Baumann U: The crystal structure of human cytosolic serine hydroxymethyltransferase: a target for cancer chemotherapy. *Structure* **6**:1105, 1998.
55. Chasin LA, Feldman A, Konstam M, Urlaub G: Reversion of a Chinese hamster cell auxotrophic mutant. *Proc Natl Acad Sci U S A* **71**:718,1974.
56. Stover P, Schirch V: Serine hydroxymethyltransferase catalyzes the hydrolysis of 5,10-methenyltetrahydrofolate to 5-formyltetrahydrofolate. *J Biol Chem* **265**:14227, 1990.
57. Mejia N, MacKenzie RE: NAD-dependent methylenetetrahydrofolate dehydrogenase is expressed by immortal cells. *J Biol Chem* **260**:14616, 1985.
58. Tan LUL, Drury EJ, MacKenzie RE: Methylenetetrahydrofolate dehydrogenase-methenyl-tetrahydrofolate cyclohydrolase-formyl-tetrahydrofolate synthetase: A multifunctional protein from porcine liver. *J Biol Chem* **234**:1830, 1977.
59. Mejia NR, MacKenzie RE: NAD-dependent methylenetetrahydrofolate dehydrogenase-methenyltetrahydrofolate cyclohydrolase in transformed cells is a mitochondrial enzyme. *Biochem Biophys Res Commun* **155**:1, 1988.
60. Rozen R, Barton D, Du J, Hum DW, MacKenzie RE, Francke U: Chromosomal localization of the gene for the human trifunctional enzyme, methylenetetrahydrofolate dehydrogenase-methenyltetrahydrofolate cyclohydrolase-formyltetrahydrofolate synthetase. *Am J Hum Genet* **44**:781, 1989.
61. Mejia NR, Rios-Orlandi EM, MacKenzie RE: NAD-dependent methylenetetrahydrofolate dehydrogenase-methenyltetrahydrofolate cyclohydrolase from ascites tumor cells. *J Biol Chem* **261**:9509, 1986.
62. Allaire M, Li Y, MacKenzie RE, Cygler M: The 3-D structure of a folate-dependent dehydrogenase/cyclohydrolase bifunctional enzyme at 1.5 Å resolution. *Structure* **6**:173, 1998.
63. Shen BW, Dyer DH, Huang JY, D'Ari L, Rabinowitz J, Stoddard BL: The crystal structure of a bacterial, bifunctional 5,10 methylene-tetrahydrofolate dehydrogenase/cyclohydrolase. *Protein Sci* **8**:1342, 1999.
64. Krebs HA, Hems R, Tyler B: The regulation of folate and methionine metabolism. *Biochemistry* **158**:341, 1976.
65. Hopkins S, Schirch L: 5,10-methenyltetrahydrofolate synthetase. *J Biol Chem* **259**:5618, 1984.
66. Dayan A, Betrand R, Beauchemin M, Chahla D, Mamo A, Filion M, Skup D, Massie B, Jolivet J: Cloning and characterization of the human 5,10-methenyltetrahydrofolate synthetase-encoding cDNA. *Gene* **165**:307, 1995.
67. Jolivet J: Human 5,10-methenyltetrahydrofolate synthetase. *Methods Enzymol* **281**:162, 1997.
68. Lewis GP, Rowe PB: Methylene tetrahydrofolate reductase: Studies in a human mutant and mammalian liver, in Blair JA (ed): *Chemistry and Biology of Pteridines*. Berlin, de Gruyter, 1983, p 229.
69. Kutzbach C, Stokstad ELR: Feedback inhibition of methylene tetrahydrofolate reductase in rat liver by S-adenosylmethionine. *Biochim Biophys Acta* **139**:217, 1967.
70. Matthews RG, Sheppard C, Goulding C: Methylenetetrahydrofolate reductase and methionine synthase: Biochemistry and molecular biology. *Eur J Pediatr* **157**:S54, 1998.
71. Matthews RG, Vanoni MA, Hainfield JF, Wall J: Methylenetetrahydrofolate reductase. Evidence for spatially distinct subunit domains by scanning transmission electron microscopy and limited proteolysis. *J Biol Chem* **259**:11647, 1984.
72. Rozen R: Molecular genetics of methylenetetrahydrofolate reductase deficiency. *J Inherit Metab Dis* **19**:589, 1996.

73. Goyette P, Milos R, Ducan AM, Rosenblatt DS, Matthews RG, Rozen R: Human methylenetetrahydrofolate reductase: Isolation of cDNA, mapping and mutation identification. *Nat Genet* **7(2)**:195, 1994.
74. Goyette P, Pai A, Milos R, Frosst P, Tran P, Chen ZT, Chan M, Rozen R: Gene structure of human and mouse methylenetetrahydrofolate reductase (MTHFR). *Mamm Genome* **9**:652, 1998.
75. Guenther BD, Sheppard CA, Tran P, Rozen R, Matthews RG, Ludwig ML: The structure and properties of methylenetetrahydrofolate reductase from *Escherichia coli* suggest how folate ameliorates human hyperhomocystinemia. *Nat Struct Biol* **6**:359, 1999.
76. Taylor RT: B_{12}-dependent methionine biosynthesis, in Dolphin D (ed.): *B_{12}*. New York, John Wiley, 1982, p 307.
77. Matthews RG, Jencks DA, Frasca V, Matthews KD: Methionine biosynthesis in chemistry and biology of pteridines, in Cooper BA, Whitehead VM (eds): *Pteridines and Folic Acid Derivatives*. New York, de Gruyter, 1986, p 698.
78. Matthews RG: Methionine Biosynthesis, in Blakley RL, Benkovic SJ (eds): *Folates and Pterins*. New York, John Wiley, 1984, vol 1, p 497.
79. Utley CS, Marcell PD, Allen RH, Asok CA, Kolhouse JF: Isolation and characterization of methionine synthetase from human placenta. *J Biol Chem* **260**:13656, 1985.
80. Ludwig ML, Matthews RG: Structure-based perspectives on B_{12}-dependent enzymes. *Annu Rev Biochem* **66**:269, 1997.
81. Gulati S, Chen Z, Brody LC, Rosenblatt DS, Banerjee R: Defects in auxiliary redox proteins lead to functional methionine synthase deficiency. *J Biol Chem* **272**:19171, 1997.
82. Banerjee R: The yin-yang of cobalamin biochemistry. *Chem Biol* **4**:175, 1997
83. Leclerc D, Wilson A, Dumas R, Gafuik C, Song D, Watkins D, Heng HHQ, Rommens JM, Scherer SW, Rosenblatt DS, Gravel RA: Cloning and mapping of a cDNA for methionine synthase reductase, a flavoprotein defective in patients with homocystinuria. *Proc Natl Acad Sci U S A* **95**:3059, 1998.
84. Mellman IS, Lin P-F, Ruddle FH, Rosenberg LE: Genetic control of cobalamin binding in normal and mutant cells: Assignment of the gene for 5-methyltetrahydrofolate: L-homocysteine S-methyltransferase to human chromosome 1. *Proc Natl Acad Sci U S A* **76**:405, 1979.
85. Leclerc D, Campeau E, Goyette P, Adjalla CE, Christensen B, Ross M, Eydoux P, Rosenblatt DS, Rozen R, Gravel RA: Human methionine synthase: cDNA cloning and identification of mutations in patients of the cblG complementation group of folate/cobalamin disorders. *Hum Mol Genet* **5(12)**:1867, 1996.
86. Li YN, Gulati S, Baker PJ, Brody LC, Banerjee R, Kruger WD: Cloning, mapping and RNA analysis of the human methionine synthase gene. *Hum Mol Genet* **5(12)**:1851, 1996.
87. Kudo H, Ohshio G, Ogawa K, Wakatsuki Y, Inada M: Distribution of vitamin B_{12} R binder in normal tissues: An immunohistochemical study. *J Histochem Cytochem* **35**:855, 1987.
88. Rosenblatt DS, Cooper BA, Pottier A, Lue-Shing H, Matiaszuk N, Grauer K: Altered vitamin B_{12} metabolism in fibroblasts from a patient with megaloblastic anemia and homocystinuria due to a new defect in methionine biosynthesis. *J Clin Invest* **74**:2149, 1984.
89. Drennan CL, Huang S, Drummond JT, Matthews RG, Ludwig ML: How a protein binds B_{12}:A 3.0 Å x-ray structure of B_{12}-binding domains of methionine synthase. *Science* **266**:1669, 1994.
90. Dixon MM, Huang S, Matthews RG, Ludwig M: The structure of the C-terminal domain of methionine synthase: presenting S-adenosylmethionine for reductive methylation of B_{12}. *Structure* **4**:1263, 1996.
91. Scott JM, Wilson P, Dinn JJ, Wier DG: Pathogenesis of subacute combined degeneration as a result of methyl group deficiency. *Lancet* **2**:334, 1981.
92. Scott JM, Weir DG: Hypothesis: The methyl folate trap. *Lancet* **2**:337, 1981.
93. Chanarin I, Deacon R, Lumb M, Muir M, Perry J: Cobalamin-folate interrelations: A critical review. *Blood* **66**:479, 1985.
94. Herbert V, Zalusky R: Interrelationship of vitamin B_{12} and folic acid metabolism: Folic acid clearance studies. *J Clin Invest* **41**:1263, 1962.
95. Norohna JM, Silvermnan MJ: On folic acid, vitamin B_{12}, methionine and formiminoglutamic acid metabolism, in Henrich HC (ed): *Vitamin B_{12} and Intrinsic Factor.* Stuttgart, Verlag, 1962, p 728.
96. Chanarin I: Cobalamin folate interrelationships, in Zittoun J, Cooper BA (eds): *Folates et Cobalamines*. Paris, Doin, 1987, Chapter 3.
97. Fujii K, Huennekens FM: Activation of methionine synthase by a reduced triphosphopyridine nucleotide-dependent flavoprotein system. *J Biol Chem* **249**:6745, 1974.
98. Fujii K, Galivan JH, Huennekens FM: Activation of methionine synthase: Further characterization of the flavoprotein system. *Arch Biochem Biophys* **178**:662, 1977.
99. Osborne C, Chen LM, Matthews RG: Isolation, cloning, mapping, and nucleotide sequencing of the gene encoding flavodoxin in *Escherichia coli. J Bacteriol* **173**:1729, 1991.
100. Bianchi V, Reichard P, Eliasson R, Pontis E, Krook M, Jornvall H, Haggard-Ljungquist E: *Escherichia coli* ferredoxin $NAPD^+$ reductase: Activation of *E. coli* anaerobic ribonucleotide reduction, cloning of the gene (fpr), and overexpression of the protein. *J Bacteriol* **175**:1590, 1993.
101. Beaudet R, MacKenzie RE: Formiminotransferase-cyclohydrolase from porcine liver. An octameric enzyme containing bifunctional polypeptide. *Biochim Biophys Acta* **453**:151, 1976.
102. MacKenzie RE: Formiminotransferase-cyclodeaminase, a bifunctional protein from pig liver, in Kisliuk RL, Brown GM (eds): *Chemistry and Biology of Pteridines*. New York, Elsevier, 1979, p 443.
103. Herbert V: Experimental nutritional folate deficiency in man. *Trans Assoc Am Physicians* **75**:307, 1962.
104. Roschau J, Date J, Kristoffersen K: Folic acid supplements and intrauterine growth. *Acta Obstet Gynecol Scand* **58**:343,1979.
105. Laurence KM, Miller JN, Tennant GB, Campbell H: Double-blind randomized controlled trial of folate treatment before conception to prevent recurrence of neural-tube detects. *Br Med J* **282**:11509, 1981.
106. Malinow MR, Bostom AG, Krauss RM: Homocyst(e)ine, diet, and cardiovascular diseases: A statement for healthcare professionals from the Nutrition Committee, American Heart Association. *Circulation* **99**:178, 1999.
107. Brouwer IA, van Dusseldorp M, West CE, Meyboom S, Thomas CMG, Duran M, van het Hof KH, et al: Dietary folate from vegetables and citrus fruit decreases plasma homocysteine concentrations in humans in a dietary controlled trial. *J Nutr* **129**:1135, 1999.
108. Jacques PF, Selhub J, Bostom AG, Wilson PWF, Rosenberg IH: The effect of folic acid fortification on plasma folate and total homocysteine concentrations. *N Engl J Med* **340**:1449, 1999.
109. Luhby AL, Eagle FJ, Roth E, Cooperman JM: Relapsing megaloblastic anemia in an infant due to a specific defect in gastrointestinal absorption of folic acid. *Am J Dis Child* **102**:482, 1961.
110. Luhby AL, Cooperman JM: Folic acid deficiency in man and its interrelationship with vitamin B_{12} metabolism. *Adv Metab Disord* **1**:263, 1964.
111. Luhby AL, Cooperman JM: Congenital megaloblastic anemia and progressive central nervous system degeneration. Further clinical and physiological characterization and therapy of syndrome due to inborn error of folate transport. *Proceedings of the American Pediatric Society Philadelphia*, Atlantic City, April 26–29, 1967.
112. Lanzkowsky P, Erlandson ME, Bezan AI: Isolated defect of folic acid absorption associated with mental retardation and cerebral calcification. *Blood* **34**:452, 1969.
113. Lanzkowsky P: Congenital malabsorption of folate. *Am J Med* **48**:580, 1970.
114. Santiago-Borrera PJ, Santini R Jr, Perez-Santiago E, Maldonado N, Millan S, Coll-Camalez G: Congenital isolated defect of folic acid absorption. *J Pediatr* **82**:450, 1973.
115. Su PC: Congenital folate deficiency. *N Engl J Med* **294**:1128, 1976.
116. Narisawa K: Personal communication describing siblings reported in the Japanese literature: Kobayashi K and Hoshino M. *Japan J Pediat* **29**:1788, 1976.
117. Konomi H, Kuwajima K, Yanagisawa M, Kamoshita S, Narisawa K: A case of congenital folic acid malabsorption with infantile spasms. *Brain Dev* **3**:234, 1978.
118. Poncz M, Colman N, Herbert V, Schwartz E, Cohen AR: Congenital folate malabsorption. *J Pediatr* **99**:828, 1981.
119. Poncz M, Colman N, Herbert V, Schwartz E, Cohen AR: Therapy of congenital folate malabsorption. *J Pediatr* **98**:76, 1981.
120. Corbeel L, Van Den Berghe G, Jaeken J, Vantornout J, Eeckels R: Congenital folate malabsorption. *Eur J Pediatr* **143**:284, 1985.
121. Urbach J, Abrahamov A, Grossowicz N: Congenital isolated folic acid malabsorption. *Arch Dis Child* **62**:78, 1987.
122. Sakiyama T, Tsuda M, Nakabayashi H, Shimizu H, Owaka M, Kitagawa T: Clinical and biochemical observations in a case with congenital defect of folate absorption. *Annual Meeting of the SSIEM*, Newcastle upon Tyne, September 5–8, 1984.
123. Steinschneider M, Sherbany A, Pavlakis S, Emerson R, Lovelace R, DeVivo DC: Congenital folate malabsorption: Reversible clinical and neurophysiologic abnormalities. *Neurology* **40**:1315, 1990.

124. Russell A, Statter M, Abzug-Horowitz S: Methionine-dependent glutamic acid formiminotransferase deficiency, in Sperling O, de Vries H (eds): *Inborn Errors of Metabolism In Man*, Basel, S Karger, 1978, p 65.
125. Buchanan JA: Fibroblast plasma membrane vesicles to study inborn errors of transport. PhD thesis, McGill University, 1984, p 23.
126. Zittoun J: Congenital errors of folate metabolism, in Wickringamasinghe S (ed): *Megaloblastic Anaemias*, London, Bailière Tindall, 1995, p 603.
127. Branda RF, Moldow CF, MacArthur JR, Wintrobe MM, Anthony BK, Jacob HS: Folate-induced remission in aplastic anemia with familial defect of cellular folate uptake. *N Engl J Med* **298**:469, 1978.
128. Arthur DC, Danzyl TJ, Branda FR: Cytogenetic studies of a family with a hereditary defect of cellular folate uptake and high incidence of hematologic disease: *Nutritional Factors in the Induction and Maintenance of Malignancy*. New York, Academic Press 1983, p 101.
129. Howe RB, Branda RF, Douglas SD, Brunning RD: Hereditary dyserythropoiesis with abnormal membrane folate transport. *Blood* **54**:1080, 1979.
130. Wevers RA, Hansen SI, van Hellenberg Hubar JLM, Holm J, Hoier-Madsen M, Jongen PJH: Folate deficiency in cerebrospinal fluid associated with a defect in folate binding protein in the central nervous system. *J Neurol Neurosurg Psychiatry* **57**:223, 1994.
131. Fowler B: Genetic defects of folate and cobalamin metabolism. *Eur J Pediatr* **157**:S60, 1998.
132. Walters TR: Congenital megaloblastic anemia responsive to N5-formyl tetrahydrofolic acid administration. *J Pediatr* **70**:686, 1987.
133. Tauro GP, Danks DM, Rowe PB, Van der Weyden MB, Schwartz MA, Collins VL, Neal BW: Dihydrofolate reductase deficiency causing megaloblastic anemia in two families. *N Engl J Med* **294**:466, 1976.
134. McGready RK, Tauro GP, Van Der Weyden M: Physical and kinetic characteristics of a mutant dihydrofolate reductase. *Proc Aust Biol Soc* **9**:9, 1976.
135. Hoffbrand AV, Tripp E, Jackson BFA, Luck WE, Frater-Schroder M: Hereditary abnormal transcobalamin II previously diagnosed as congenital dihydrofolate reductase deficiency [Letter]. *N Engl J Med* **310**:789, 1984.
136. Thomas RK, Hoffbrand AV, Smith IS: Neurological involvement in hereditary transcobalamin II deficiency. *J Neurol Neurosurg Psychiatry* **45**:74, 1982.
137. Seligman PA, Steiner LL, Allen RH: Studies of a patient with megaloblastic anemia and an abnormal transcobalamin II. *N Engl J Med* **303**:1209, 1980.
138. Paukert JL, D'Ari-Strauss L, Rabinowitz JC: Formyl-methenyl-methylenetetrahydrofolate synthase (combined). An ovine protein with multiple catalytic activities. *J Biol Chem* **251**:5104, 1976.
139. Tan LU, Drury EJ, MacKenzie RE: Methylenetetrahydrofolate dehydrogenase-methenyltetrahydrofolate cyclohydrolase-formyltetrahydrofolate synthetase. A functional protein from porcine Liver. *J Biol Chem* **252**:1117, 1977.
140. van Gennip AH, Abeling NGGM, Nijenhuis AA, Voute PA, Bakker HD: Formiminoglutamic/hydantoinpropionic aciduria in three patients with different tumours. *J Inherit Metab Dis* **17**:642, 1994.
141. Shin YS, Reiter S, Zelger O, Brunstler I, Vrucker A: Orotic aciduria, homocystinuria, formiminoglutamic aciduria and megaloblastosis associated with the formiminotransferase/cyclodeaminase deficiency, in Nyhan WL, Thompson LF, Watts RWE (eds): *Purine and Pyrimidine Metabolism, Man*. New York, Plenum Press, 1986, p 71.
142. Arakawa T, Ohara K, Kudo Z, Tada K, Hayashi T, Mizuno T: Hyperfolic-acidemia with formiminoglutamic-aciduria following histidine loading: Suggested for a case of congenital deficiency in formiminotransferase. *Tohoku J Exp Med* **80**:370, 1963.
143. Arakawa T, Ohara K, Takahashi Y, Ogasawara J, Hayashi T, Chiba R, Wada Y, Tada K, Mizuno T, Ohamura T, Yoshida T: Formiminotransferase-deficiency syndrome: A new inborn error of folic acid metabolism. *Ann Pediatr* **205**:1, 1965.
144. Arakawa T, Fujii M, Hirono H: Tetrahydrofolate-dependent enzyme activity in formiminotransferase deficiency syndrome. *Tohoku J Exp Med* **88**:305, 1966.
145. Arakawa T, Fujii M, Ohara K: Erythrocyte formiminotransferase activity in formiminotransferase deficiency syndrome. *Tohoku J Exp Med* **88**:195, 1966.
146. Arakawa T, Tamura T, Ohara K, Narisawa K, Tanno K, Honda Y, Higashi O: Familial occurrence of formiminotransferase deficiency syndrome. *Tohoku J Exp Med* **96**:211, 1968.
147. Herman RH, Rosenweig NS, Stifel FB, Herman YF: Adult formiminotransferase deficiency: A new entity. *Clin Res* **17**:304, 1969.
148. Arakawa T, Yoshida T, Konna T, Honda Y: Defect of incorporation of glycine-1-^{14}C into urinary uric acid in formiminotransferase deficiency syndrome. *Tohoku J Exp Med* **106**:213, 1972.
149. Niederwieser A, Giliberti P, Matasovic A, Pluznik S, Steinmann B, Baerlocher K: Folic acid non-dependent formiminoglutamic aciduria in two siblings. *Clin Chim Acta* **54**:293,1974.
150. Perry TL, Applegarth DA, Evans ME, Hansen S: Metabolic studies of a family with massive formiminoglutamic aciduria. *Pediatr Res* **9**:117, 1975.
151. Niederwieser A, Matasovic A, Steinmann B, Baerlocher K, Kempen B: Hydantoin-5-propionic aciduria in folic acid non-dependent formiminoglutamic aciduria observed in two siblings. *Pediatr Res* **10**:215, 1976.
152. Russell A, Statter M, Abzug-Horowitz S: Methionine-dependent formiminoglutamic acid transferase deficiency: Human and experimental studies in its therapy. *Monogr Hum Genet* **9**:65, 1978.
153. Beck B, Christensen E, Brandt NJ, Pederson M: Formiminoglutamic aciduria in a slightly retarded boy with chronic obstructive lung disease. *J Inherit Metab Dis* **14**:225, 1981.
154. Duran M, Ketting D, deBree PK, van Sprang FJ, Wadman SK, Penders TJ, Wilms RHH: A case of formiminoglutamic aciduria. *Eur J Pediatr* **136**:319, 1981.
155. Duran M, Bruinvis L, Wadman SK: Quantitative gas chromatographic determination of urinary hydantoin-5-propionic acid in patients with disorders of folate/vitamin B_{12} metabolism. *J Chromatogr* **381**:401, 1986.
156. Arakawa T, Wada Y: Urinary AICA (4-amino-5-imidazole-carboxamide) following an oral dose of AICA in formiminotransferase deficiency syndrome. *Tohoku J Exp Med* **96**:211, 1968.
157. Jencks DA, Matthews RG: Allosteric inhibition of methylenetetrahydrofolate reductase by adenosylmethionine. *J Biol Chem* **262**:2485,1987.
158. Rosenblatt DS, Erbe RW: Methylenetetrahydrofolate reductase in cultured human cells. I. Growth and metabolic studies. *Pediatr Res* **11**:1137, 1977.
159. Shih VE, Salam MZ, Mudd SH, Uhlendorf BV, Adams RD: A new form of homocystinuria due to *N5,N10*-methylenetetrahydrofolate reductase deficiency. *Pediatr Res* **6**:135, 1972.
160. Mudd SH, Uhlendorf BW, Freeman JM, Finkelstein JD, Shih VE: Homocystinuria associated with decreased methylenetetrahydrofolate reductase activity. *Biochem Biophys Res Commun* **46**:905, 1972.
161. Freeman JM, Finkelstein JD, Mudd SH, Uhlendorf BW: Homocystinuria presenting as reversible "schizophrenia": A new defect in methionine metabolism with reduced 5,10-methylenetetrahydrofolate reductase activity. *Pediatr Res* **6**:423, 1972.
162. Freeman JM, Finkelstein JD, Mudd SH: Folate-responsive homocystinuria and "schizophrenia": A defect in methylation due to deficient 5,10-methylenetetrahydrofolate reductase activity. *N Engl J Med* **292**:491, 1975.
163. Kanwar YS, Manaligod JR, Wong PWK: Morphologic studies in a patient with homocystinuria due to 5,10-methylenetetrahydrofolate reductase deficiency. *Pediatr Res* **10**:598, 1976.
164. Cooper BA, Rosenblatt DS: Folate coenzyme forms in fibroblasts from patients deficient in 5,10-methylenetetrahydrofolate reductase. *Biochem Soc Trans* **4**:921, 1976.
165. Rosenblatt DS, Erbe RW: Methylenetetrahydrofolate reductase in cultured human cells. II. Studies of methylenetetrahydrofolate reductase deficiency. *Pediatr Res* **11**:1141, 1977.
166. Wong PWK, Justice P, Hruby M, Weiss EB, Diamond E: Folic acid non-responsive homocystinuria due to methylenetetrahydrofolate reductase deficiency. *Pediatrics* **59**:749, 1977.
167. Wong PWK, Justice P, Berlow S: Detection of homozygotes and heterozygotes with methylenetetrahydrofolate reductase deficiency. *J Lab Clin Med* **90**:283, 1977.
168. Baumgartner ER, Schweizer K, Wick H: Different congenital forms of defective remethylation in homocystinuria. Clinical, biochemical, and morphological studies. *Pediatr Res* **11**:1015, 1977.
169. Narisawa K, Wada Y, Saito T, Suzuki K, Kudo M, Arakawa TS, Katsushima NA, Tsuboi R: Infantile type of homocystinuria with *N5,10*-methylenetetrahydrofolate reductase defect. *Tohoku J Exp Med* **121**:185, 1977.
170. Rosenblatt DS, Cooper BA: Methylenetetrahydrofolate reductase deficiency: Clinical and biochemical correlations, in Botez MI, Reynolds EH (eds): *Folic Acid in Neurology, Psychiatry, and Internal Medicine*. New York, Raven Press, 1979, p 385.

171. Rosenblatt DS, Cooper BA, Lue-Shing S, Wong PW, Berlow S, Narisawa K, Baumgartner R: Folate distribution in cultured human cells. Studies on 5,10-CH2-H4PteGlu reductase deficiency. *J Clin Invest* **63**:1019, 1979.
172. Narisawa K: Brain damage in the infantile type of 5,10-methylenetetrahydrofolate reductase deficiency, in Botez MI, Reynolds EH (eds): *Folic Acid in Neurology, Psychiatry, and Internal Medicine*. New York, Raven Press, 1979, p 391.
173. Singer HS, Butler I, Rothenberg S, Valle D, Freeman J: Interrelationships among serum folate, CSF folate, neurotransmitters, and neuropsychiatric symptoms. *Neurology* **30**:419, 1980.
174. Baumgartner R, Wick, Ohnacker H, Probst A, Maurer R: Vascular lesions in two patients with congenital homocystinuria due to different defects of remethylation. *J Inherit Metab Dis* **3**:101, 1980.
175. Cederbaum SD, Shaw KNF, Cox DR, Erbe RW, Boss GR, Carrel RE: Homocystinuria due to methylenetetrahydrofolate reductase (MTHFR) deficiency: Response to a high protein diet. *Pediatr Res* **15**:560, 1981.
176. Allen RJ, Wong PWK, Rothenberg SP, Dimauro S, Headington JT: Progressive neonatal leukoencephalomyopathy due to absent methylenetetrahydrofolate reductase, responsive to treatment. *Ann Neurol* **8**:211, 1980.
177. Narisawa K: Folate metabolism infantile type of 5,10-methylenetetrahydrofolate reductase deficiency. *Acta Paediatr Jpn* **23**:82, 1981.
178. Boss G, Erbe RW: Decreased rates of methionine synthesis by methylenetetrahydrofolate reductase-deficient fibroblasts and lymphoblasts. *J Clin Invest* **67**:1659, 1981.
179. Harpey JP, Rosenblatt DS, Cooper BA, Le Moel G, Roy C, Lafourcade J: Homocystinuria caused by 5,10-methylenetetrahydrofolate reductase deficiency: A case in an infant responding to methionine, folinic acid, pyridoxine, and vitamin B_{12} therapy. *J Pediatr* **98**:275, 1981.
180. Harpey JP, Lemoel G, Zittoun J: Follow-up in a child with 5,10-methylenetetrahydrofolate reductase deficiency. *J Pediatr* **103**:1007, 1983.
181. Wendel U, Bremer HJ: Betaine in the treatment of homocystinuria due to 5,10-methylenetetrahydrofolate reductase deficiency. *Eur J Pediatr* **142**:147, 1984.
182. Christensen E, Brandt NJ: Prenatal diagnosis of 5,10-methylenetetrahydrofolate reductase deficiency. *N Engl J Med* **313**:50, 1985.
183. Nishimura M, Yoshino K, Tomita Y, Takashina S, Tanaka J, Narisawa K, Kurobane I: Central and peripheral nervous system pathology of homocystinuria due to 5,10-methylenetetrahydrofolate reductase deficiency. *Pediatr Neurol* **1**:375, 1985.
184. Haan E, Rogers J, Lewis G, Rowe P: 5,10-methylenetetrahydrofolate reductase deficiency: Clinical and biochemical features of a further case. *J Inherit Metab Dis* **8**:53, 1985.
185. Hyland K, Smith I, Howell DW, Clayton PT, Leonard JV: The determination of pterins, biogenic amino metabolites, and aromatic amino acids in cerebrospinal fluid using isocratic reverse phase liquid chromatography within series dual cell coulometric electrochemical and fluorescence determinations — Use in the study of inborn errors of dihydropteridine reductase and 5,10-methylenetetrahydrofolate reductase, in Wachter H, Curtius H, Pfleiderer W (eds): *Biochemical and Clinical Aspects of Pteridines,* vol 4. Berlin, Walter de Gruyter, 1985, p 85.
186. Baumgartner ER, Stokstad ELR, Wick H, Watson JE, Kusano G: Comparison of folic acid coenzyme distribution patterns in patients with methylenetetrahydrofolate reductase and methionine synthetase deficiencies. *Pediatr Res* **19**:1288, 1985.
187. Berlow S: Critical review of cobalamin-folate interrelations [Letter]. *Blood* **67**:1526, 1986.
188. Shin YS, Pilz G, Enders W: Methylenetetrahydrofolate reductase and methylenetetrahydrofolate methyltransferase in human fetal tissues and chorionic villi. *J Inherit Metab Dis* **9**:275, 1986.
189. Clayton PT, Smith I, Harding B, et al: Subacute combined degeneration of the cord, dementia and Parkinsonism due to an inborn error of folate metabolism. *J Neurol Neurosurg Psychiatry* **49**:920, 1986.
190. Brandt NJ, Christensen E, Skovby F, Djernes B: Treatment of methylenetetrahydrofolate reductase deficiency from the neonatal period [Abstract]. *The Society for the Study of Inborn Errors of Metabolism, 24th Annual Symposium*, Amersfoort, The Netherlands, 1986, p 23.
191. Fowler B: Homocystinuria, remethylation defects. Methionine synthesis and cofactor response in cultured fibroblasts [Abstract]. *Society for the Study of Inborn Errors of Metabolism, 24th Annual Symposium, Amersfoort*, The Netherlands, 1986, p 22.
192. Beckman DR, Hoganson G, Berlow S, Gilbert EF: Pathological findings in 5,10-methylenetetrahydrofolate reductase deficiency. *Birth Defects: Original Article Series* **23**:47, 1987.
193. Visy JM, Le Coz P, Chadefaux B, Fressinaud C, Woimant F, Marquet J, Zittoun J, Visy J, Vallat JM, Haguenau M: Homocystinuria due to 5,10-methylenetetrahydrofolate reductase deficiency revealed by stroke in adult siblings. *Neurology* **41**:1313, 1991.
194. Haworth JC, Dilling LA, Surtees RAH, Seargeant LE, Lue-Shing H, Cooper BA, Rosenblatt DS: Symptomatic and asymptomatic methylenetetrahydrofolate reductase deficiency in two adult brothers. *Am J Med Genet* **45**:572, 1993.
195. Ogier de Baulny H, Gerard M, Saudubray JM, Zittoun J: Remethylation defects: Guidelines for clinical diagnosis and treatment. *Eur J Pediatr* **157(12)**:S77, 1998.
196. Abeling NGGM, van Gennip AH, Blom H, Wevers RA, Vreken P, van Tinteren HLG, Bakker HD: Rapid diagnosis: Basis for a favourable outcome in a patient with MTHFR deficiency [Abstract]. *J Inherit Metab Dis* **21**:21, 1998.
197. Sewell AC, Neirich U, Fowler B: Early infantile methylenetetrahydrofolate reductase deficiency: A rare cause of progressive brain atrophy [Abstract]. *J Inherit Metab Dis* 21:22, 1998.
198. Hamano H, Nanba A, Nagayama M, Takizawa S, Shinohara Y: An adult case of homocystinuria probably due to methylenetetrahydrofolate reductase deficiency-treatment with folic acid and the course of coagulation-fibrinolysis parameters [Japanese]. *Rinsho Shinkeigaku* **36**:330, 1996.
199. Arn PH, Williams CA, Zori RT, Driscoll DJ, Rosenblatt DS: Methylenetetrahydrofolate reductase deficiency in a patient with phenotypic findings of Angelman syndrome. *Am J Med Genet* **77**:198, 1998.
200. Kishi T, Kawamura I, Harada Y, Eguchi T, Sakura N, Ueda K, Narisawa K, Rosenblatt DS: Effect of betaine on S-adenosylmethionine levels in the cerebrospinal fluid in a patient with methylenetetrahydrofolate reductase deficiency and peripheral neuropathy. *J Inherit Metab Dis* **17**:560, 1994.
201. Pasquier F, Lebert F, Petit H, Zittoun J, Marquet J: Methylenetetrahydrofolate reductase deficiency revealed by a neuropathy in a psychotic adult [Letter]. *J Neurol Neurosurg Psychiatry* **57**:765, 1994.
202. Ronge E, Kjellman B: Long-term treatment with betaine in methylenetetrahydrofolate reductase deficiency. *Arch Dis Child* **74**:239, 1996.
203. Kluijtmans LAJ, Wendel U, Stevens EMB, van den Heuvel LPWJ, Trijbels FJM, Blom HJ: Indentification of four novel mutations in severe methylenetetrahydrofolate reductase deficiency. *Eur J Hum Genet* **6**:257, 1998.
204. Sakura N, Ono H, Nomura H, Ueda H, Fujita N: Betaine dose and treatment intervals in therapy for homocystinuria due to 5,10-methylenetetrahydrofolate reductase deficiency. *J Inherit Metab Dis* **21**:84, 1998.
205. Fowler B, Jakobs C: Post- and prenatal diagnostic methods for the homocystinurias. *Eur J Pediatr* **157**:S88, 1998.
206. Fowler B, Whitehouse C, Wenzel F, Wraith JE: Methionine and serine formation in control and mutant human cultured fibroblasts: Evidence for methyl trapping and characterization of remethylation defects. *Pediatr Res* **41**:145, 1997.
207. Garovic-Kocic V, Rosenblatt DS: Methionine auxotrophy in inborn errors of cobalamin metabolism. *Clin Invest Med* **15(4)**:395, 1992.
208. Rosenblatt DS, Lue-Shing H, Arzoumanian A, Low-Nang L, Matiaszuk N: Methylenetetrahydrofolate reductase (MR) deficiency: Thermolability of residual MR activity, methionine synthase activity, and methylcobalamin levels in cultured fibroblasts. *Biochem Med Met Biol* **47(3)**:221, 1992.
209. Frosst P, Blom HJ, Milos R, Goyette P, Sheppard CA, Matthews RG, Boers GJH, et al: A candidate genetic risk factor for vascular disease: A common methylenetetrahydrofolate reductase mutation causes thermoinstability. *Nat Genet* **10**:111, 1995.
210. Goyette P, Christensen B, Rosenblatt DS, Rozen R: Severe and mild mutations in *cis* for the methylenetetrahydrofolate (MTHFR) gene, and description of 5 novel mutations in MTHFR. *Am J Hum Genet* **59**:1268, 1996.
211. Kang SS, Zhou J, Wong PWK, Kowalisyn J, Strokosch G: Intermediate homocystinemia: A thermolabile variant of methylenetetrahydrofolate reductase. *Am J Hum Genet* **43**:414, 1988.
212. Kang S-S, Wong PWK, Zhou J, Sora J, Lessick M, Ruggie N, Grcevich G: Thermolabile methylenetetrahydrofolate reductase in patients with coronary artery disease. *Metabolism* **37**:611, 1988.

213. Kang S-S, Wong PWK, Bock H-GO, Horwitz A, Grix A: Intermediate hyperhomocystinemia resulting from compound heterozygosity of methylenetetrahydrofolate reductase mutations. *Am J Hum Genet* **48**:546, 1991.
214. Kang S-S, Wong PWK, Susmano A, Sora J, Norusis M, Ruggie N: Thermolabile methylenetetrahydrofolate reductase: An inherited risk factor for coronary artery disease. *Am J Hum Genet* **48**:536, 1991.
215. McCully KS: Vascular pathology of homocystinemia: Implications for the pathogenesis of arteriosclerosis. *Am J Pathol* **56**:111, 1969.
216. Boushey CJ, Beresford SAA, Omenn GS, Motulsky AG: A quantitative assessment of plasma homocysteine as a risk factor for vascular disease: probable benefits of increasing folic acid intakes. *JAMA* **274**:1049, 1995.
217. Nygard O, Nordrehaug JE, Refsum H, Ueland PM, Farstad M, Vollset SE: Plasma homocysteine levels and mortality in patients with coronary artery disease. *N Engl J Med* **337**:230, 1997.
218. Refsum H, Ueland PM, Nygard O, Vollset SE: Homocysteine and cardiovascular disease. *Annu Rev Med* **49**:31, 1998.
219. Moustapha A, Robinson K: High plasma homocysteine: A risk factor for vascular disease in the elderly. *Coron Artery Dis* **9**:725, 1999.
220. Goyette P, Sumner JS, Milos R, Duncan AM, Rosenblatt DS, Matthews RG, Rozen R: Human methylenetetrahydrofolate reductase: Isolation of cDNA, mapping and mutation identification. *Nat Genet* **7(2)**:195, 1994.
221. Shaw GM, Rozen R, Finnell RH, Wasserman CR, Lammer EJ: Maternal vitamin use, genetic variation of methylenetetrahydrofolate reductase, and risk for spina bifida. *Am J Epidemiol* **148**:30, 1998.
222. Pepe G, Vanegas C, Giusti B, Brunelli T, Marcucci R, Attanasio M, Rickards O, De Stefano GF, et al: Heterogeneity in world distribution of the thermolabile C677T mutation in 5,10-methylenetetrahydrofolate reductase. *Am J Hum Genet* **63**:917, 1998.
223. Jacques PF, Bostom AG, Williams RR, Ellison RC, Eckfeldt JH, Rosenberg IH, Selhub J, Rozen R: Relation between folate status, a common mutation in methylenetetrahydrofolate reductase, and plasma homocysteine concentrations. *Circulation* **93**:7, 1996.
224. Christensen B, Frosst P, Lussier-Cacan S, Selhub J, Goyette P, Rosenblatt DS, Genest JJ, Rozen R: Correlation of a common mutation in the methylenetetrahydrofolate reductase (MTHFR) gene with plasma homocysteine in patients with premature coronary artery disease. *Arterioscler Thromb Vasc Biol* **17**:569, 1997.
225. Blom HJ: Mutated 5,10-methylenetetrahydrofolate reductase and moderate hyperhomocysteinaemia. *Eur J Pediatr* **157**:S131, 1998.
226. van der Put NMJ, Eskes TKAB, Blom HJ: Is the common 677 → T mutation in the methylenetetrahydrofolate reductase gene a risk factor for neural tube defects? A meta-analysis. *Q J Med* **90**:111, 1997.
227. Steegers-Theunissen RPM, Boers GHJ, Trijbels JMF, Finkelstein JD, Blom HJ, Thomas CMG, Borm GR, et al: Maternal hyperhomocystinemia: A risk factor for neural tube defects. *Metabolism* **43**:1475, 1994.
228. van der Put NMJ, Steegers-Theunissen RPM, Frosst P, Trijbels FJM, Eskes TKAB, van den Heuvel LP, Mariman ECM, et al: Mutated methylenetetrahydrofolate reductase as a risk factor for spina bifida. *Lancet* **346**:1070, 1995.
229. Whitehead AS, Gallagher P, Mills JL, Kirke PN, Burke H, Molloy AM, Weir DG, et al: A genetic defect in 5,10 methylenetetrahydrofolate reductase in neural tube defects. *Q J Med* **88**:763, 1995.
230. Eskes TKAB: Neural tube defects, vitamins and homocysteine. *Eur J Pediatr* **157**:S139, 1998.
231. Spence JD, Malinow MR, Barnett PA, Marian AJ, Freeman D, Hegele RA: Plasma homocyst(e)ine concentration, but not MTHFR genotype, is associated with variation in carotid plaque area. *Stroke* **30**:969, 1999.
232. Ma J, Stampfer MJ, Giovannucci E, Artigas C, Hunter DJ, Fuchs C, Willett J, et al: Methylenetetrahydrofolate reductase polymorphism, dietary interactions, and risk of colon cancer. *Cancer Res* **57**:1098, 1997.
233. Viel A, Dall'Agnese L, Simone F, Canzonieri V, Visentin MC, Valle R, Boiocchi M: Loss of heterozygosity at the 5,10-methylenetetrahydrofolate reductase locus in human ovarian carcinomas. *Br J Cancer* **75**:1105, 1997.
234. van der Put NMJ, Gabreels F, Stevens EMB, Smeitink JAM, Trijbels FJM, Eskes TKAB, van der Heuvel LP, Blom HJ: A second common mutation in the methylenetetrahydrofolate reductase gene: An additional risk factor for neural-tube defects? *Am J Hum Genet* **62**:1044, 1998.
235. Weisberg I, Tran P, Christensen B, Sibani S, Rozen R: A second genetic polymorphism in methylenetetrahydrofolate reductase (MTHFR) associated with decreased enzyme activity. *Mol Genet Metab* **64**:169, 1998.
236. Cooper BA, Rosenblatt DS: Inherited defects of vitamin B_{12} metabolism. *Ann Rev Nutr* **7**:291, 1987.
237. Mandel H, Brenner B, Berant M, Rosenberg N, Lanir N, Jakobs C, Fowler B, Seligsohn U: Coexistence of hereditary homocystinuria and factor V Leiden — Effect on thrombosis. *N Engl J Med* **334**:763, 1996.
238. Goyette P, Rosenblatt D, Rozen R: Homocystinuria (methylenetetrahydrofolate reductase deficiency) and mutation of Factor V gene. *J Inherit Metab Dis* **21**:690, 1998.
239. Broderick DS, North JA, Mangum JH: Isolation of N^5,N^{10}-methylene tetrahydrofolate reductase from bovine brain. *Prep Biochem* **2**:207, 1972.
240. Burton EG, Sallach HJ: Methylenetetrahydrofolate reductase in the rat central nervous system: Intracellular and regional distribution. *Arch Biochem Biophys* **166**:483, 1975.
241. Levitt M, Nixon PF, Pincus JH, Bertino JR: Transport of folates in cerebrospinal fluid: A study using doubly labelled 5-methyltetrahydrofolate and 5-formyltetrahydrofolate. *J Clin Invest* **50**:1301, 1971.
242. Hyland K, Smith I, Bottiglieri T, Perry J, Wendel U, Clayton PT, Leonard JV: Demyelination and decreased S-adenosylmethionine in 5,10-methylenetetrahydrofolate reductase deficiency. *Neurology* **38**:459, 1988.
243. Watkins D, Rosenblatt DS: Functional methionine synthase deficiency (cblE and cblG): Clinical and biochemical heterogeneity. *Am J Med Genet* **34**:427, 1989.
244. Kalnitsky A, Rosenblatt DS, Zlotkin S: Differences in liver folate enzyme patterns in premature and full term infants. *Pediatr Res* **16**:628, 1982.
245. Gaull GE, Von Berg W, Raiha NCR, Sturman JA: Development of methyltransferase activities of human fetal tissues. *Pediatr Res* **7**:527, 1973.
246. Holme E, Kjellman B, Ronge E: Betaine for treatment of homocystinuria caused by methylenetetrahydrofolate reductase deficiency. *Arch Dis Child* **64**:1061, 1989.
247. Goyette P, Frosst P, Rosenblatt DS, Rozen R: Seven novel mutations in the methylenetetrahydrofolate reductase gene and genotype/phenotype correlations in severe methylenetetrahydrofolate reductase deficiency. *Am J Hum Genet* **56**:1052, 1995.
248. Wendel U, Claussen U, Dickmann E: Prenatal diagnosis for methylenetetrahydrofolate reductase deficiency. *J Pediatr* **102**:938, 1983.
249. Marquet J, Chadefaux B, Bonnefont JP, Saudubray JM, Zittoun J: Methylenetetrahydrofolate reductase deficiency: Prenatal diagnosis and family studies. *Prenat Diagn* **14(1)**:29, 1994.
250. Carmel R, Watkins D, Goodman SI, Rosenblatt DS: Hereditary defect of cobalamin metabolism (cblG mutation) presenting as a neurologic disorder in adulthood. *N Engl J Med* **318**:1738, 1988.
251. Watkins D, Rosenblatt DS: Heterogeneity in functional methionine synthase deficiency, in Cooper BA, Whitehead VM (eds): *Chemistry and Biology of Pteridines and Folic Acid-Derivatives*. Berlin, Walter de Gruyter, 1986, p 713.
252. Rosenblatt DS, Thomas IT, Watkins D, Cooper BA, Erbe RW: Vitamin B_{12} responsive homocystinuria and megaloblastic anemia: Heterogeneity in methylcobalamin deficiency. *Am J Med Genet* **26**:377, 1987.
253. Hallam L, Clark AL, Van der Weyden MB: Neonatal megaloblastic anemia and homocystinuria with reduced levels of methionine synthetase [Abstract]. *Blood* **66(1)**:44, 1985.
254. McKie VC, Roesal RA, Hommes FA, Watkins D, Rosenblatt DS, Flannery DB: Clinical findings in an infant with methylcobalamin deficiency (cblE variant). *Am J Hum Genet* **39**:A71, 1986.
255. Hall CA, Lindenbaum RH, Arenson E, Begley JA, Chu RC: The nature of the defect in cobalamin G mutation. *Clin Invest Med* **12**:262, 1989.
256. Sillaots SL, Hall CA, Hurteloup V, Rosenblatt DS: Heterogeneity in cblG: Differential retention of cobalamin on methionine synthase. *Biochem Med Meta Biol* **47(3)**:242, 1992.
257. Wilson A, Leclerc D, Rosenblatt DS, Gravel RA: Molecular basis for methionine synthase reductase deficiency in patients belonging to the *cblE* complementation group of disorders in folate/cobalamin metabolism. *Hum Mol Genet* **8**:2009, 1999.
258. Vilaseca MA, Vela E, Cruz O, Fowler B: Functional methionine synthase deficiency without neurologic involvement [Abstract]. *J Inherit Metab Dis* **21**:20, 1998.
259. Harding CO, Arnold G, Barness LA, Wolff JA, Rosenblatt DS: Functional methionine synthase deficiency due to cblG disorder: A report of two patients and a review. *Am J Med Genet* **71**:384, 1997.

260. Wilson A, Leclerc D, Saberi F, Phillips III JA, Rosenblatt DS, Gravel RA: Functionally null mutations in patients with the *cblG* variant form of methionine synthase deficiency. *Am J Hum Genet* **63**:409, 1998.
261. Kvittengen EA, Spangen S, Lindemans J, Fowler B: Methionine synthase deficiency without megaloblastic anemia. *Eur J Pediatr* **156**:925, 1997.
262. Tuchman M, Kelly P, Watkins D, Rosenblatt DS: Vitamin B_{12}-responsive megaloblastic anemia, homocystinuria, and transient methylmalonic aciduria in *cblE* disease. *J Pediatr* **113**:1052, 1988.
263. Watkins D, Rosenblatt DS: Genetic heterogeneity among patients with methylcobalamin deficiency: Definition of two complementation groups, *cblE* and *cblG*. *J Clin Invest* **81**:1690, 1988.
264. Schuh S, Rosenblatt DS, Cooper BA, Schroeder ML, Bishop AJ, Seargeant LE, Haworth JC: Homocystinuria and megaloblastic anemia responsive to vitamin B_{12} therapy. An inborn error of metabolism due to a defect in cobalamin metabolism. *N Engl J Med* **310**:686, 1984.
265. Rosenblatt DS, Cooper BA, Pottier A, Lue-Shing H, Matiaszuk N, Grauer K: Altered vitamin B_{12} metabolism in fibroblasts from a patient with megaloblastic anemia and homocystinuria due to a new defect in methionine biosynthesis. *J Clin Invest* **74**:2149, 1984.
266. Huennekens FM, DiGirolamo PM, Fujii K, Jacobsen DW, Vitols KS: B_{12}-dependent methionine synthetase as a potential target for cancer chemotherapy. *Adv Enzyme Regul* **14**:187, 1976.
267. Gulati S, Baker P, Li YN, Fowler B, Kruger WD, Brody LC, Banerjee R: Defects in human methionine synthase in *cblG* patients. *Hum Mol Genet* **5(12)**:1859, 1996.
268. Hall CA: Function of vitamin B_{12} in the central nervous system as revealed by congenital defects. *Am J Hematol* **34**:121, 1990.
269. Shevell MI, Rosenblatt DS: The neurology of cobalamin. *Can J Neurol Sci* **19**:472, 1992.
270. Pfohl-Leszkowicz A, Keith G, Dirheimer G: Effect of cobalamin derivatives on in vitro enzymatic DNA methylation: Methylcobalamin can act as a methyl donor. *Biochemistry* **30**:8045, 1991.
271. Rosenblatt DS, Cooper BA, Schmutz SM, Zaleski WA, Casey RE: Prenatal vitamin B_{12} therapy of a fetus with methylcobalamin deficiency (cobalamin E disease). *Lancet* **1(8438)**:1127, 1985.
272. Minot GR, Murphy LP: Treatment of pernicious anemia by a special diet. *JAMA* **87**:470, 1926.
273. Smith EL: Purification of anti-pernicious anemia factors from liver. *Nature* **161**:638, 1948.
274. Rickes EL, Brink NG, Koniuszy FR, Wood TR, Folkers K: Crystalline vitamin B_{12}. *Science* **107**:396, 1948.
275. Dolphine D: B_{12}. New York, John Wiley, 1982.
276. Banerjee R (ed): *Chemistry and Biochemistry of* B_{12}. New York, John Wiley, 1999.
277. Hodgkin DC, Kamper J, Mackay M, Pickworth J, Trueblood KN, White JG: Structure of vitamin B_{12}. *Nature* **178**:64, 1956.
278. Walker GA, Murphy S, Heunnekens F: Enzymatic conversion of vitamin B_{12} to adenosyl-B_{12}. Evidence for the existence of two separate reducing systems. *Arch Biochem Biophys* **134**:95, 1969.
279. Barker HA, Smith RD, Wawszkiewicz EJ, Lee MN, Wilson R: Enzymatic preparation and characterization of an α-L-β-methylaspartic acid. *Arch Biochem Biophys* **78**:468, 1958.
280. Barker HA, Weissbach H, Smyth RD: A coenzyme containing pseudovitamin B_{12}. *Proc Natl Acad Sci U S A* **44**:1093, 1958.
281. Weissbach H, Toohey J, Barker HA: Isolation and properties of B_{12} coenzymes containing benzimidazole or dimethylbenzimidazole. *Proc Natl Acad Sci U S A* **45**:521, 1959.
282. Smith RM, Monty KJ: Vitamin B_{12} and propionate metabolism. *Biochem Biophys Res Commun* **1**:105, 1959.
283. Gurnani S, Mistry SP, Johnson BC: Function of vitamin B_{12} in methylmalonate metabolism. 1. Effect of a cofactor form of B_{12} on the activity of methylmalonyl-CoA isomerase. *Biochim Biophys Acta* **38**:187, 1960.
284. Stern JR, Friedmann DC: Vitamin B_{12} and methylmalonyl-CoA isomerase. I. Vitamin B_{12} and propionate metabolism. *Biochem Biophys Res Commun* **2**:82, 1960.
285. Weissbach H, Taylor R: Role of vitamin B_{12} in methionine biosynthesis. *Fed Proc* **25**:1649, 1966.
286. Taylor RT, Weissbach H: Enzymatic synthesis of methionine: Formation of a radioactive cobamide enzyme with N^5-methyl-^{14}C-tetrahydrofolate. *Arch Biochem Biophys* **119**:572, 1967.
287. Taylor RT, Weissbach H: *Escherichia coli* — N^5-methyltetrahydrofolate-homocysteine vitamin-B_{12} transmethylase: Formation and photolability of a methylcobalamin enzyme. *Arch Biochem Biophys* **123**:109, 1968.
288. Poston JM: Leucine 2,3-aminomutase, an enzyme of leucine catabolism. *J Biol Chem* **251**:1859, 1976.
289. Babior BM: Cobamides as cofactors: Adenosylcobamide-dependent reactions, in Babior BM (ed): *Cobalamin: Biochemistry and Pathophysiology*. New York, John Wiley, 1975, p 141.
290. Poston JM, Stadtman TC: Cobamides as cofactors: Methylcobamides and the synthesis of methionine, methane and acetate, in Babior BM (ed): *Cobalamin: Biochemistry and Pathophysiology*. New York, John Wiley, 1975, p 111.
291. Donaldson RMJ: Intrinsic factor and the transport of cobalamin, in Johnson LR (ed): *Physiology of the Gastrointestinal Tract*. New York, Raven, 1981, p 641.
292. Sennett C, Rosenberg LE, Mellman IS: Transmembrane transport of cobalamin in prokaryotic and eukaryotic cells. *Annu Rev Biochem* **50**:1053, 1981.
293. Castle WB, Townsend WC, Heath CW: Observations on the etiologic relationship of achylia gastrica to pernicious anemia. III. The nature of the reaction between normal human gastric juice and beef muscle leading to clinical improvement and increased blood formation similar to the effect liver feeding. *Am J Med Sci* **180**:305, 1930.
294. Hewitt JE, Gordon MM, Taggart RT, Mohandas TK, Alpers DH: Human gastric intrinsic factor: Characterization of cDNA and genomic clones and localization to human chromosome 11. *Genomics* **10**:432,1991.
295. Allen RH, Seetharam B, Podell E, Alpers DH: Effect of proteolytic enzymes on the binding of cobalamin to R protein and intrinsic factor. In vitro evidence that a failure to partially degrade R protein is responsible for cobalamin malabsorption in pancreatic insufficiency. *J Clin Invest* **61**:47, 1978.
296. Allen RH, Seetharam B, Allen NC, Podell ER, Alpers DH: Correction of cobalamin malabsorption in pancreatic insufficiency with a cobalamin analogue that binds with high affinity to R protein but not to intrinsic factor. In vivo evidence that a failure to partially degrade R protein is responsible for cobalamin malabsorption in pancreatic insufficiency. *J Clin Invest* **61**:1628, 1978.
297. Marcoullis G, Parmentier Y, Nicolas J-P, Jimenez M, Gerard P, Dix CJ, Hassan IF, et al: Cobalamin malabsorption due to nondegradation of R proteins in the human intestine: Inhibited cobalamin absorption in exocrine pancreatic dysfunction. The transport of vitamin B_{12} through polarized monolayers of Caco-2 cells. *J Clin Invest* **98**:1272, 1990.
298. Dix CJ, Hassan IF, Obray HY, Shah R, Wilson G: The transport of vitamin B_{12} through polarized monolayers of Caco-2 cells. *Gastroenterology* **98**:1272, 1990.
299. Ramanujam KS, Seetharam S, Ramasamy M, Seetharam B: Expression of cobalamin transport proteins and cobalamin transcytosis by colon adenocarcinoma cells. *Am J Physiol* **260**:G416, 1991.
300. Hall CA, Finkler AE: The dynamics of transcobalamin. II. A vitamin B_{12} binding substance in plasma. *J Lab Clin Med* **65**:459, 1965.
301. Hom BL: Plasma turnover of 57cobalt-vitamin B_{12} bound to transcobalamin I and II. *Scand J Haematol* **4**:321, 1967.
302. Fernandez-Costa F, Metz J: Vitamin B_{12} binders (transcobalamins) in serum. *Crit Rev Clin Lab Sci* **18**:1, 1982.
303. Linnell JC: The fate of cobalamins in vivo, in Babior BM (ed): *Cobalamin: Biochemistry and Pathophysiology*. New York, John Wiley, 1975, p 287.
304. Finkler AE, Hall CA: Nature of the relationship between vitamin B_{12} binding and cell uptake. *Arch Biochem Biophys* **120**:79, 1967.
305. Tan CH, Hansen HJ: Studies on the site of synthesis of transcobalamin II. *Proc Soc Exp Biol Med* **127**:740, 1968.
306. Pletsch QA, Coffey JW: Properties of the proteins that bind vitamin B_{12} in subcellular fractions of rat liver. *Arch Biochem Biophys* **151**:157, 1972.
307. Newmark P, Newman GE, O'Brien JRP: Vitamin B_{12} in the rat kidney: Evidence of an association with lysosomes. *Arch Biochem Biophys* **141**:121, 1970.
308. Youngdahl-Turne P, Rosenberg LE, Allen RH: Binding and uptake of transcobalamin II by human fibroblasts. *J Clin Invest* **61**:133, 1978.
309. Youngdahl-Turner P, Mellman IS, Allen RH, Rosenberg LE: Protein mediated vitamin uptake: Adsorptive endocytosis of the transcobalamin II-cobalamin complex by cultured human fibroblasts. *Exp Cell Res* **118**:127, 1979.
310. Idriss JM, Jonas AJ: Vitamin B_{12} transport by rat liver lysosomal membrane vesicles. *J Biol Chem* **266**:9438, 1991.
311. Mellman IS, Youngdahl-Turner P, Willard HF, Rosenberg LE: Intracellular binding of radioactive hydroxocobalamin to cobalamin-dependent apoenzymes in rat liver. *Proc Natl Acad Sci U S A* **74**:916, 1977.

312. Kolhouse JF, Allen RH: Recognition of two intracellular cobalamin binding proteins and their identification as methylmalonyl-CoA mutase and methionine synthase. *Proc Natl Acad Sci U S A* **74**:921, 1977.
313. Burger RL, Schneider RJ, Mehlman CS, Allen RH: Human plasma R-type vitamin B_{12} binding protein. II. The role of transcobalamin I, transcobalamin III and the normal granulocyte vitamin B_{12}-binding protein in the plasma transport of vitamin B_{12}. *J Biol Chem* **250**:7707, 1975.
314. Berliner N, Rosenberg LE: Uptake and metabolism of free cyanocobalamin by cultured human fibroblasts from controls and a patient with transcobalamin II deficiency. *Metabolism* **30**:230, 1981.
315. Frenkel EP, Kitchens RL: Intracellular localization of hepatic propionyl-CoA carboxylase and methylmalonyl-CoA mutase in humans and normal and vitamin B_{12}-deficient rats. *Br J Haematol* **31**:501, 1975.
316. Wang FK, Koch J, Stokstad EL: Folate coenzyme pattern, folate linked enzymes and methionine biosynthesis in rat liver mitochondria. *Biochemisch Zeitschmift* **246**:458, 1967.
317. Vitols E, Walker GA, Huennekens FM: Enzymatic conversion of vitamin B_{12} to a cobamide coenzyme, αga(5,6-dimethylbenzimidazolyl) deoxyadenosylcobamide (adenosyl-B_{12}). *J Biol Chem* **241**:1455, 1966.
318. Ertel R, Brot N, Taylor R, Weissbach H: Studies on the nature of the bound cobamide in *E. coli* N5-methyltetrahydrofolate-homocysteine transmethylase. *Arch Biochem Biophys* **126**:353, 1968.
319. Taylor RT, Weissbach H: *E. coli*—N5-methyltetrahydrofolate-homocysteine methyltransferase: Sequential formation of bound methylcobalamin with S-adenosyl-l-methionine and N5-methyltetrahydrofolate. *Arch Biochem Bipohys* **129**:728, 1969.
320. Pawalkiewicz J, Gorna M, Fenrych W, Magas S: Conversion of cyanocobalamin in vivo and in vitro into its coenzyme form in humans and animals. *Ann N Y Acad Sci* **112**:641, 1964.
321. Kerwar SS, Spears C, McAuslan B, Weissbach H: Studies on vitamin B_{12} metabolism in HeLa cells. *Arch Biochem Biophys* **142**:231, 1971.
322. Mahoney MJ, Rosenberg LE: Synthesis of cobalamin coenzymes by human cells in tissue culture. *J Lab Clin Med* **78**:302, 1971.
323. Mahoney MJ, Hart AC, Steen VD, Rosenberg LE: Methylmalonicacidemia: Biochemical heterogeneity in defects of 5′-deoxyadenosylcobalamin synthesis. *Proc Natl Acad Sci U S A* **72**:2799, 1975.
324. Fenton WA, Rosenberg LE: The defect in the *cblB* class of human methylmalonic acidemia: Deficiency of cob(I)alamin adenosyltransferase activity in extracts of cultured fibroblasts. *Biochem Biophys Res Commun* **98**:283, 1981.
325. Pezacka E, Green R, Jacobsen DW: Glutathionylcobalamin as an intermediate in the formation of cobalamin coenzymes. *Biochem Biophys Res Commun* **169**:443, 1990.
326. Watanabe F, Nakano Y, Maruno S, Tachikake N, Tamura Y, Kitaoka S: NADH- and NADPH-linked aquocobalamin reductases occur in both mitochondrial and microsomal membranes of rat liver. *Biochem Biophys Res Commun* **165**:675, 1989.
327. Watanabe F, Nakano Y, Saido H, Tamura Y, Yamanaka HT: Cytochrome b_5/cytochrome b_5 reductase complex in rat liver microsomes has NADH-linked aquacobalamin reductase activity. *J Nutr* **122**:940, 1992.
328. Cox EV, White AM: Methylmalonic acid excretion: Index of vitamin-B_{12} deficiency. *Lancet* **2**:853, 1962.
329. Barness LA, Young D, Mellman WJ, Kahn SB, Williams WJ: Methylmalonate excretion in patient with pernicious anemia. *N Engl J Med* **268**:144, 1963.
330. Cox EV, Robertson-Smith D, Small M, White AM: The excretion of propionate and acetate in vitamin B_{12} deficiency. *Clin Sci* **35**:123, 1968.
331. Shipman RT, Townley RRW, Danks DM: Homocystinuria, Addisonian pernicious anaemia, and partial deletion of a G chromosome. *Lancet* **2**:693, 1969.
332. Hollowell JGJ, Hall WK, Coryell ME, McPherson JJ, Hahn DA: Homocystinuria and organic aciduria in a patient with vitamin-B_{12} deficiency. *Lancet* **2**:1428, 1969.
333. Allen RH, Stabler SP, Savage DG, Lindenbaum J: Diagnosis of cobalamin deficiency I: Usefulness of serum methylmalonic acid and total homocysteine concentrations. *Am J Hematol* **34**:90, 1990.
334. Lindenbaum J, Savage DG, Stabler SP, Allen RH: Diagnosis of cobalamin deficiency: II. Relative sensitivities of serum cobalamin, methylmalonic acid, and total homocysteine concentrations. *Am J Hematol* **34**:99, 1990.
335. Miller DR, Specker BL, Ho ML, Norman EJ: Vitamin B-12 status in a macrobiotic community. *Am J Clin Nutr* **53**:524, 1991.
336. Dagnelie PC, Van Staveren WA, Hautvast JG: Stunting and nutrient deficiencies in children on alternative diets. *Acta Paediatr Scand Suppl* **374**:111, 1991.
337. Higginbottom MC, Sweetman L, Nyhan WL: A syndrome of methylmalonic aciduria, homocystinuria, megaloblastic anemia and neurologic abnormalities in a vitamin B_{12}-deficient breast-fed infant of a strict vegetarian. *N Engl J Med* **299**:317, 1978.
338. Specker BL, Miller DR, Norman EJ, Greene H, Hayes KC: Breast-fed infants of vegan mothers. *Am J Clin Nutr* **47**:89, 1988.
339. Beck WS: Metabolic features of cobalamin deficiency in man, in Babior BM (ed): *Cobalamin: Biochemistry and Pathophysiology*. New York, John Wiley, 1975, p 403.
340. Herbert V, Zalusky R: Interrelations of vitamin B_{12} and folic acid metabolism: Folic acid clearance studies. *J Clin Invest* **41**:1263, 1962.
341. Noronha JM, Silverman M: On folic acid, vitamin B_{12}, methionine and formiminoglutamic acid metabolism, in Heinrich HC (ed): *Vitamin B_{12} and Intrinsic Factor*. Stuttgart, Verlag, 1962, p 728.
342. Larrabee AR, Rosenthal S, Cathow RE, Buchanan JM: Enzymatic synthesis of the methyl group of methionine. IV. Isolation, characterization, and role of 5-methyl tetrahydrofolate. *J Biol Chem* **238**:1025, 1963.
343. Fenton WA, Rosenberg LE: Genetic and biochemical analysis of human cobalamin mutants in cell culture. *Annu Rev Genet* **12**:223, 1978.
344. Carmel R, Sinow RM, Siegel ME, Samloff IM: Food cobalamin malabsorption occurs frequently in patients with unexplained low serum cobalamin levels. *Arch Intern Med* **148**:1715, 1988.
345. Doscherholmen A, Silvis S, McMahon J: Dual isotope Schilling test for measuring absorption of food-bound and free vitamin B_{12} simultaneously. *Am J Clin Pathol* **80**:490, 1983.
346. Del Corral A, Carmel R: Transfer of cobalamin from the cobalamin-binding protein of egg yolk to R binder of human saliva and gastric juice. *Gastroenterology* **98**:1460, 1990.
347. Doscherholmen A, Swaim WR: Impaired assimilation of egg Co57 vitamin B_{12} in patients with hypochlorhydria and achlorhydria and after gastric resection. *Gastroenterology* **64**:913, 1973.
348. Carmel R: Subtle and atypical cobalamin deficiency states. *Am J Hematol* **34**:108, 1990.
349. Levine JS, Podell ER, Allen RH: Cobalamin malabsorption in three siblings due to an abnormal intrinsic factor that is markedly susceptible to acid and proteolysis. *J Clin Invest* **76**:2057, 1985.
350. Spurling CL, Sacks MS, Jiji RM: Juvenile pernicious anemia. *N Engl J Med* **271**:995, 1964.
351. McIntyre OR, Sullivan LW, Jeffries GH, Silver RH: Pernicious anemia in childhood. *N Engl J Med* **272**:981, 1965.
352. Katz M, Lee SK, Cooper BA: Vitamin B_{12} malabsorption due to a biologically inert intrinsic factor. *N Engl J Med* **287**:425, 1972.
353. Katz M, Mehlman CS, Allen RH: Isolation and characterization of an abnormal human intrinsic factor. *J Clin Invest* **53**:1274,1974.
354. Levine JS, Allen RH: Intrinsic factor within parietal cells of patients with juvenile pernicious anemia: A retrospective immunohistochemical study. *Gastroenterology* **88**:1132, 1985.
355. Rothenberg SP, Quadros EV, Straus EW, Kapelner S: An abnormal intrinsic factor (IF) molecule: A new cause of "pernicious anemia" (PA). *Blood* **64**:41a, 1984.
356. Carmel R: Gastric juice in congenital pernicious anemia contains no immunoreactive intrinsic factor molecule: Study of three kindreds with variable ages at presentation including a patient first diagnosed in adulthood. *Am J Hum Genet* **35**:67, 1983.
357. Hewitt JE, Gordon MM, Taggart RT, Mohandas TK, Alpers DH: Human gastric intrinsic factor: Characterization of cDNA and genomic clones and localization to human chromosome 11. *Genomics* **10**:432, 1991.
358. Chanarin I: *The megaloblastic anaemias*, 2nd ed. London, Blackwell Scientific, 1979.
359. Gräsbeck R: Familial selective vitamin B_{12} malabsorption. *N Engl J Med* **287**:358, 1972.
360. McKenzie IL, Donaldson RMJ, Trier JS, Mathan VI: Ileal mucosa in familial selective B_{12} malabsorption. *N Engl J Med* **286**:1021, 1972.
361. Gräsbeck R: Selective cobalamin malabsorption and the cobalamin-intrinsic factor receptor. *Acta Biochim Pol* **44**:725, 1997.
362. Chisolm JC: Selective malabsorption of vitamin B_{12} and vitamin B_{12}-intrinsic factor complex with megaloblastic anemia in an adult. *JAMA* **77**:835, 1985.
363. Aminoff M, Tahvanainen E, Gräsbeck R, Weissenbach J, Broch H, de la Chapelle A: Selective intestinal malabsorption of vitamin B_{12}

displays recessive mendelian inheritance: Assignment of a locus to chromosome 10 by linkage. *Am J Hum Genet* **57**:824, 1995.
364. Moestrup SK, Kozyraki R, Kristiansen M, Kaysen JH, Rasmussen HH, Brault D, Pontillon F, et al: The intrinsic factor-vitamin B_{12} receptor and target of teratogenic antibodies is a megalin-binding peripheral membrane protein with homology to developmental proteins. *J Biol Chem* **273**:5235, 1998.
365. Kozyraki R, Kristiansen M, Silahtaroglu A, Hansen C, Jacobsen C, Tommerup N, Verroust PJ, Moestrup SK: The human intrinsic factor-vitamin B_{12} receptor, cubilin: Molecular characterization and chromosomal mapping of the gene to 10p within the autosomal recessive megaloblastic anemia (MGA1) region. *Blood* **91**:3593, 1998.
366. Aminoff M, Carter JE, Chadwick RB, Johnson C, Grasbeck R, Abdelaal MA, Broch H, et al: Mutations in CUBN, encoding the intrinsic factor-vitamin B_{12} receptor, cubilin, cause hereditary megaloblastic anaemia 1. *Nat Genet* **21**:309, 1999.
367. Romero A, Romao MJ, Varela PF, Kolln I, Dias JM, Carvalho AL, Sanz L, et al: The crystal structures of two sperm adhesins reveal the CUB domain fold. *Nat Struct Biol* **4**:783, 1997.
368. Kristiansen M, Kozyraki R, Jacobsen C, Nexo E, Verroust PJ, Moestrup SK: Molecular dissection of the intrinsic factor-vitamin B_{12} receptor, cubilin, discloses regions important for membrane association and ligand binding. *J Biol Chem* **274**:20540, 1999.
369. Birn H, Verroust PJ, Nexo E, Hager H, Jacobsen C, Christensen EI, Moestrup SK: Characterization of an epithelial ~460-kDa protein that facilitates endocytosis of intrinsic factor-vitamin B_{12} and binds receptor-associated protein. *J Biol Chem* **272**:26497, 1997.
370. Christensen EI, Birn H, Verroust P, Moestrup SK: Membrane receptors for endocytosis in the renal proximal tubule. *Int Rev Cytology* **180**:237, 1998.
371. Kozyraki R, Fyfe J, Kristiansen M, Gerdes C, Jacobsen C, Cui S, Christensen EI, et al: The intrinsic factor vitamin B_{12} receptor, cubilin, is a high-affinity apolipoprotein A-I receptor facilitating endocytosis of high-density lipoprotein. *Nat Med* **5**:656, 1999.
372. Burman JF, Waler WF, Smith JA, Phillips AD, Sourial NA, Williams CB, Mollin DL: Absent ileal uptake of IF-bound-vitamin B_{12} in the Imerslund-Gräsbeck syndrome (familial vitamin B_{12} malabsorption with proteinuria). *Gut* **26**:311, 1985.
373. Hall CA: The neurologic aspects of transcobalamin II deficiency. *Br J Haematol* **80**:117, 1992.
374. Haurani FI, Hall CA, Rubin R: Megaloblastic anemia as a result of an abnormal transcobalamin II. *J Clin Invest* **64**:1253, 1979.
375. Seligman PA, Steiner LL, Allen RH: Studies of a patient with megaloblastic anemia and an abnormal transcobalamin II. *N Engl J Med* **303**:1209, 1980.
376. Rosenblatt DS, Hosack A, Matiaszuk N: Expression of transcobalamin II by amniocytes. *Prenat Diagn* **7**:35, 1987.
377. Platica O, Janeczko R, Quadros EV, Regec A, Romain R, Rothenberg SP: The cDNA sequence and the deduced amino acid sequence of human transcobalamin II show homology with rat intrinsic factor and human transcobalamin I. *J Biol Chem* **266**:7860, 1991.
378. Li N, Seetharam S, Lindemans J, Alpers DH, Arwert F, Seetharam B: Isolation and sequence analysis of variant forms of human transcobalamin II. *Biochim Biophys Acta* **1172**:21, 1993.
379. Regec A, Quadros EV, Platica O, Rothenberg SP: The cloning and characterization of the human transcobalamin II gene. *Blood* **85(10)**:2711, 1995.
380. Li N, Seetharam S, Seetharam B: Characterization of the human transcobalamin II promoter: A proximal GC/GT box is a dominant negative element. *J Biol Chem* **273**:16104, 1998.
381. Li N, Rosenblatt DS, Kamen BA, Seetharam S, Seetharam B: Identification of two mutant alleles of transcobalamin II in an affected family. *Hum Mol Genet* **3**:1835, 1994.
382. Li N, Rosenblatt DS, Seetharam B: Nonsense mutations in human transcobalamin II deficiency. *Biochem Biophy Res Com* **204**:1111, 1994.
383. Carmel R: Plasma R binder deficiency. *N Engl J Med* **318**:1401, 1988.
384. Sigal SH, Hall CA, Antel JP: Plasma R binder deficiency and neurologic disease. *N Engl J Med* **317**:1330, 1988.
385. Hall CA, Hitzig WH, Green PD, Begley JA: Transport of therapeutic cyanocobalamin in the congenital deficiency of transcobalamin II (TCII). *Blood* **53**:251, 1979.
386. Lindemans EJM, Dejongh FCM, Brand M, Schoester M, Van Kapel J, Abels J: The uptake of R-type binding protein by isolated rat liver. *Biochim Biophys Acta* **720**:203, 1983.
387. Dieckgraefe BK, Seetharam B, Alpers DH: Developmental regulation of rat intrinsic factor mRNA [Abstract]. *Am J Physiol* **254**:G913, 1988.
388. Giugliani ERJ, Jorge SM, Goncalves AL: Serum vitamin B_{12} levels in parturients, in the intervillous space of the placenta, and in full-term newborns and their interrelationships with folate levels. *Am J Clin Nutr* **41**:330, 1985.
389. Weir DG, Keating S, Molloy A, McPartlin J, Kennedy S, Blanchflower J, Kennedy DG, Rice D, Scott JM: Methylation deficiency causes vitamin B_{12}-associated neuropathy in the pig. *J Neurochem* **51**:1949, 1988.
390. Dieckgraefe BK, Seetharam B, Banaszak L, Leykam JF, Alpers DH: Isolation and structural characterization of a cDNA clone encoding rat gastric intrinsic factor. *Proc Natl Acad Sci U S A* **85**:46, 1988.
391. Daiger SP, Labowe ML, Parsons M, Wang L, Cavalli-Sforza LL: Detection of genetic variation with radioactive ligands. III. Genetic polymorphism of transcobalamin II in human plasma. *Am J Hum Genet* **30**:202, 1978.
392. Frater-Schroder M: Genetic patterns of transcobalamin II and the relationships with congenital defects. *Mol Cell Biochem* **56**:5, 1983.
393. Eiberg H, Moller N, Mohr J, Nielsen LS: Linkage of transcobalamin II (TC2) to the P blood group system and assignment to chromosome 22. *Clin Genet* **29**:354, 1986.
394. Johnston J, Bollekens J, Allen RH, Berliner N: Structure of the cDNA encoding transcobalamin I, a neutrophil granule protein. *J Biol Chem* **264**:15754, 1989.
395. Rosenblatt DS, Cooper BA: Inherited disorders of vitamin B_{12} metabolism. *Blood Rev* **1**:177, 1987.
396. Begley JA, Hall CA, Scott CR: Absence of transcobalamin II from cord blood. *Blood* **63**:490, 1984.
397. Hitzig WH, Dohmann U, Pluss HJ, Vischer D: Hereditary transcobalamin II deficiency: Clinical findings in a new family. *J Pediatr* **85**:622, 1974.
398. Rana SR, Colman N, Goh K-O, Herbert V, Klemperer MR: Transcobalamin II deficiency associated with unusual bone marrow findings and chromosonal abnormalities. *Am J Hematol* **14**:89, 1983.
399. Broch H, Imerslund O, Monn E, Hovig T, Seip M: Imerslund-Gräsbeck anemia: A long-term follow-up study. *Acta Paediatr Scand* **73**:248, 1984.
400. Goodman SI, Moe PG, Schulman JD, Dreyfuss PM, Abeles RH: A derangement in B_{12} metabolism associated with homocystinemia, cystathioninemia, hypomethioninemia and methylmalonic aciduria. *Am J Med* **48**:390, 1970.
401. Dillon MJ, England JM, Gompertz D, Goodey PA, Grant DB, et al. Mental retardation, megaloblastic anemia, methylmalonic aciduria and abnormal homocysteine metabolism due to an error in vitamin B_{12} metabolism. *Clin Sci Mol Med* **47**:43, 1974.
402. Anthony M, McLeay AC: A unique case of derangement of vitamin B_{12} metabolism. *Proc Aust Assoc Neurol* **13**:61, 1976.
403. Baumgartner ER, Wick H, Maurer R, Egli N, Steinmann B: Congenital defect in intracellular cobalamin metabolism resulting in homocystinuria and methylmalonic aciduria. I. Case report and histopathology. *Helv Paediatr Acta* **34**:465, 1979.
404. Carmel R, Bedros AA, Mace JW, Goodman SI: Congenital methylmalonic aciduria—Homocystinuria with megaloblastic anemia: Observations on response to hydroxocobalamin and on the effect of homocysteine and methionine on the deoxyuridine suppression test. *Blood* **55**:570, 1980.
405. Shinnar S, Singer HS: Cobalamin C mutation (methylmalonic aciduria and homocystinuria) in adolescence. A treatable cause of dementia and myelopathy. *N Engl J Med* **311**:451, 1984.
406. Mitchell GA, Watkins D, Melancon SB, Rosenblatt DS, Geoffroy G, Orquin J, Homsy MB, Dallaire L: Clinical heterogeneity in cobalamin C variant of combined homocystinuria and methylmalonic aciduria. *J Pediatr* **108**:410, 1986.
407. Cogan DG, Schulman J, Porter RJ, Mudd SH: Epileptiform ocular movements with methylmalonic aciduria and homocystinuria. *Am J Ophthalmol* **90**:251, 1980.
408. Linnell JC, Miranda B, Bhatt HR, Dowton SB, Levy HL: Abnormal cobalamin metabolism in a megaloblastic child with homocystinuria, cystathioninuria and methylmalonic aciduria. *J Inherit Metab Dis* **6(2)**:137, 1983.
409. Mamlock RJ, Isenberg JN, Rassin DN: A cobalamin metabolic defect with homocystenuria, methylmalonic aciduria and macrocytic anemia. *Neuropediatrics* **17**:94, 1986.
410. Ravindranath Y, Krieger I: Vitamin B_{12} (Cbl) and folate interrelationship in a case of homocysteinuria-methylmalonic (HC-MMA)-uria due to genetic deficiency [Abstract]. *Pediatr Res* **18**:247A, 1984.

411. Ribes A, Vilaseca A, Briones P, Maya A, Sabater J, Pascual P, Alvarez L, Ros J, Gonzalez Pascual E: Methylmalonic aciduria with homocystinuria. *J Inherit Metab Dis* **729**:129, 1984.
412. Robb RM, Dowton SB, Fulton AB, Levy HL: Retinal degeneration in vitamin B_{12} disorder associated with methylmalonic aciduria and sulfur amino acid abnormalities. *Am J Ophthalmol* **97**:691, 1984.
413. Rosenblatt DS, Laframboise R, Pichette J, Langevin P, Cooper BA, Costa T: New disorder of vitamin B_{12} metabolism (cobalamin F) presenting as methylmalonic aciduria. *Pediatrics* **78**:51, 1986.
414. Gravel RA, Mahoney MJ, Ruddle FH, Rosenberg LE: Genetic complementation in heterokaryons of human fibroblasts defective in cobalamin metabolism. *Proc Natl Acad Sci U S A* **72**:3181, 1975.
415. Willard HF, Mellman IS, Rosenberg LE: Genetic complementation among inherited deficiencies of methylmalonyl-CoA mutase activity: Evidence for a new class of human cobalamin mutant. *Am J Hum Genet* **30**:1, 1978.
416. Watkins D, Rosenblatt DS: Failure of lysosomal release of vitamin B_{12}: A new complementation group causing methylmalonic aciduria (*cblF*). *Am J Hum Genet* **39**:404, 1986.
417. MacDonald MR, Wiltse HE, Bever JL, Rosenblatt DS: Clinical heterogeneity in two patients with cblF disease [Abstract]. *Am J Hum Genet* **51**:A353, 1992.
418. Wong LTK, Rosenblatt DS, Applegarth DA, Davidson AGF: Diagnosis and treatment of a child with cblF disease [Abstract]. *Clin Invest Med* **l**:A111, 1992.
419. Waggoner DJ, Ueda K, Mantia C, Dowton SB: Methylmalonic aciduria (*cblF*): Case report and response to therapy. *Am J Med Genet* **79**:373, 1998.
420. Rosenblatt DS, Aspler AL, Shevell MI, Pletcher BA, Fenton WA, Seashore MR: Clinical heterogeneity and prognosis in combined methylmalonic aciduria and homocytinuria (*cblC*). *J Inherit Metab Dis* **20**:528, 1997.
421. Geraghty MT, Perlman EJ, Martin LS, Hayflick SJ, Casella JF, Rosenblatt DS, Valle D: Cobalamin C defect associated with hemolytic-uremic syndrome. *J Pediatr* **120(6)**:934, 1992.
422. Weintraub L, Tardo C, Rosenblatt D, Shapira E: Hydrocephalus as a possible complication of the *cblC* type of methylmalonic aciduria [Abstract]. *Am J Hum Genet* **49**:108, 1991.
423. Caouette G, Rosenblatt D, Laframboise R: Hepatic dysfunction in a neonate with combined methylmalonic aciduria and homocystinuria (cblC) [Abstract]. *Clin Invest Med* **15**:A112, 1992.
424. Andersson HC, Marble M, Shapira E: Long-term outcome in treated combined methylmalonic aciduria and homocystinuria. *Genet Med* **1**:146, 1999.
425. Shih VE, Axel SM, Tewksbury JC, Watkins D, Cooper BA, Rosenblatt DS: Defective lysosomal release of vitamin B_{12} (*cblF*) a hereditary metabolic disorder associated with sudden death. *Am J Med Genet* **33**:555, 1989.
426. Mudd SH, Levy HL, Abeles RH: A derangement in B_{12} metabolism leading to homocystinemia, cystathioninemia and methylmalonicaciduria. *Biochem Biophys Res Commun* **35**:121, 1969.
427. Linnell JC, Matthews DM, Mudd SH, Uhlendorf BW, Wise IJ: Cobalamins in fibroblasts cultured from normal control subjects and patients with methylmalonic aciduria. *Pediatr Res* **10**:179, 1976.
428. Baumgartner ER, Wick H, Linnell JC, Gaull GE, Bachmann C, Steinmann B: Congenital defect in intracellular cobalamin metabolism resulting in homocystinuria and methylmalonic aciduria. II. Biochemical investigations. *Helv Paediatr Acta* **34**:483, 1979.
429. Rosenberg LE, Patel L, Lilljeqvist A: Absence of an intracellular cobalamin binding protein in cultured fibroblasts from patients with defective synthesis of 5′-deoxyadenosylcobalamin and methylcobalamin. *Proc Natl Acad Sci U S A* **72**:4617, 1975.
430. Mahoney MJ, Rosenberg LE, Mudd SH, Uhlendorf BW: Defective metabolism of vitamin B 12 in fibroblasts from children with methylmalonicaciduria. *Biochem Biophys Res Commun* **44**:375, 1971.
431. Willard HF, Rosenberg LE: Inborn errors of cobalamin metabolism: Effect of cobalamin supplementation in culture on methylmalonyl CoA mutase activity in normal and mutant human fibroblasts. *Biochem Genet* **17**:57, 1979.
432. Mudd SH, Uhlendorf BW, Hinds KR, et al: Deranged B_{12} metabolism: Studies of fibroblasts grown in tissue culture. *Biochem Med* **4**:215, 1970.
433. Willard HF, Rosenberg LE: Inherited deficiencies of human methylmalonyl CoA mutase: Biochemical and genetic studies in cultured skin fibroblasts, in Hommes FA (ed): *Methods for the Study of Inborn Errors of Metabolism*. New York, Elsivier, 1979, p 297.
434. Mellman IH, Willard P, Youngdahl-Turner P, Rosenberg LE: Cobalamin coenzyme synthesis in normal and mutant human fibroblasts: Evidence for a processing enzyme activity deficient in cbl C Cells. *J Biol Chem* **254**:11847, 1979.
435. Pezacka EH: Identification and characterization of two enzymes involved in the intracellular metabolism of cobalamin. Cyanocobalamin beta-ligand transferase and microsomal cob(III)alamin reductase. *Biochim Biophys Acta* **1157(2)**:167, 1993.
436. Pezacka EH, Rosenblatt DS: Intracellular metabolism of cobalamin. Altered activities of β-axial-ligand transferase and microsomal cob(III)alamin reductase in *cblC* and *cblD* fibroblasts, in Bhatt HR, James VHT, Besser GM, Bottazzo GF, Keen H (eds): *Advances in Thomas Addison's Diseases*. Bristol, J. of Endocrinology Ltd, 1994, p 315.
437. Watanabe F, Saido H, Yamaji R, Miyatake K, Isegawa Y, Ito A, Yubisui T, et al: Mitochondrial NADH- or NADP-linked aquacobalamin reductase activity is low in human skin fibroblasts with defects in synthesis of cobalamin coenzymes. *J Nutr* **126**:2947, 1996.
438. Rosenblatt DS, Hosack A, Matiaszuk NV, Cooper BA, Laframboise R: Defect in vitamin B_{12} release from lysosomes: Newly described inborn error of vitamin B_{12} metabolism. *Science* **228(4705)**:1319, 1985.
439. Vassiliadis A, Rosenblatt DS, Cooper BA, Bergeron JJ: Lysosomal cobalamin accumulation in fibroblasts from a patient with an inborn error of cobalamin metabolism (cblF complementation group): Visualization by electron microscope radioautography. *Exp Cell Res* **195**:295, 1991.
440. Laframboise R, Cooper BA, Rosenblatt DS: Malabsorption of vitamin B_{12} from the intestine in a child with cblF disease: evidence for lysosomal-mediated absorption [Letter]. *Blood* **80**:291, 1992.
441. Anderson HC, Shapira E: Biochemical and clinical response to hydroxocobalamin versus cyanocobalamin treatment in patients with methylmalonic acidemia and homocystinuria (*cblC*). *J Pediatr* **132**:121, 1998.
442. Bartholomew DW, Batshaw ML, Allen RH, Roe CR, Rosenblatt D, Valle DL, Francomano CA: Therapeutic approaches to cobalamin-C methylmalonic acidemia and homocystinuria. *J Pediatr* **112**:32, 1988.
443. Rosenberg LE, Lilljeqvist A-C, Hsia YE: Methylmalonic aciduria: An inborn error leading to metabolic acidosis, long-chain ketonuria and intermittent hyperglycinemia. *N Engl J Med* **278**:1319, 1968.
444. Rosenberg LE, Lilljeqvist A, Hsia YE: Methylmalonic aciduria: Metabolic block localization and vitamin B-12 dependency. *Science* **162**:805, 1968.
445. Lindblad B, Olin P, Svanberg B, Zetterstrom R: Methylmalonic acidemia. *Acta Paediatr Scand* **57**:417, 1968.
446. Lindblad B, Lindstrand K, Svanberg B, Zetterstrom R: The effect of cobamide coenzyme in methylmalonic acidemia. *Acta Paediatr Scand* **58**:178, 1969.
447. Oberholzer VG, Levin B, Burgess EA, Young WF: Methylmalonic aciduria. An inborn error of metabolism leading to chronic metabolic acidosis. *Arch Dis Child* **42**:492, 1967.
448. Stokke O, Eldjarn L, Norum KR, Steen-Johnsen J, Halvorsen S: Methylmalonic aciduria: A new inborn error of metabolism which may cause fatal acidosis in the neonatal period. *Scand J Clin Lab Invest* **20**:313, 1967.
449. Rosenberg LE, Lilljeqvist AC, Hsia YE, Rosenbloom FM: Vitamin B_{12}-dependent methylmalonicaciduria: Defective B_{12} metabolism in cultured fibroblasts. *Biochem Biophys Res Commun* **37**:607, 1969.
450. Kaye CI, Morrow G 3d, Nadler HL: In vitro "responsive" methylmalonic acidemia: A new variant. *J Pediatr* **85**:55, 1974.
451. Matsui SM, Mahoney MJ, Rosenberg LE: The natural history of the inherited methylmalonic acidemias. *N Engl J Med* **308**:857, 1983.
452. Rosenberg LE: Disorders of propionate, methylmalonate and cobalamin metabolism, in Stanbury JB, Fredrickson DS (eds): *The Metabolic Basis of Inherited Disease*, 4th ed. New York, McGraw-Hill, 1978, p 411.
453. Ando T, Rasmussen K, Wright JM, Nyhan WL: Isolation and identification of methylcitrate, a major metabolic product of propionate in patients with propionic acidemia. *J Biol Chem* **247**:2200, 1972.
454. Stokke OAE, Eldjarn L, Schnitler R: The occurrence of hydroxy-*n*-valeric acid in a patient with propionic and methylmalonic acidemia. *Clin Chim Acta* **45**:391, 1973.
455. Hsia YE, Scully K, Lilljeqvist A-C, Rosenberg LE: Vitamin B_{12} dependent methylmalonicaciduria. *Pediatrics* **46**:497, 1970.
456. Willard HF, Ambani LM, Hart AC, Mahoney MJ, Rosenberg LE: Rapid prenatal and postnatal detection of inborn errors of propionate, methylmalonate, and cobalamin metabolism: A sensitive assay using cultured cells. *Hum Genet* **34**:277, 1976.

457. Morrow G, Revsin B, Mathews C, Giles H: A simple rapid method for prenatal detection of defects in propionate metabolism. *Clin Genet* **10**:218, 1976.
458. Fenton WA, Rosenberg LE: Mitochondrial metabolism of hydroxocobalamin: Synthesis of adenosylcobalamin by intact rat liver mitochondria. *Arch Biochem Biophys* **189**:441, 1978.
459. Morrow G 3d, Mahoney MJ, Mathews C, Lebowitz J: Studies of methylmalonyl coenzyme A carbonylmutase activity in methylmalonic acidemia. I. Correlation of clinical, hepatic, and fibroblast data. *Pediatr Res* **9**:641, 1975.
460. Morrow G, Schwartz RH, Hallock JA, Barness LA: Prenatal detection of methylmalonic acidemia. *J Pediatr* **77**:120, 1970.
461. Ampola M, G., Mahoney MJ, Nakamura E, Tanaka K: Prenatal therapy of a patient with vitamin B_{12} responsive methylmalonic acidemia. *N Engl J Med* **293**:313, 1975.
462. Mahoney MJ, Rosenberg LE, Linblad B, Waldenstrom J, Zetterstrom R: Prenatal diagnosis of methylmalonic aciduria. *Acta Paediatr Scand* **64**:44,1975.
463. Nyhan WL, Fawcett N, Ando T, Rennert OM, Julius RL: Response to dietary therapy in B_{12} unresponsive methylmalonic acidemia. *Pediatrics* **51**:539, 1973.
464. Satoh T, Narisawa K, Igarashi Y, Saitoh T, Hayasaka K, Ichinohazama Y, Onodera H, et al: Dietary therapy in two patients with vitamin B_{12}-unresponsive methylmalonic acidemia. *Eur J Pediatr* **135**:305, 1981.
465. Roe CR, Bohan TP: l-Carnitine therapy in propionic acidemia. *Lancet* **1**:1411, 1982.
466. Roe CR, Millington DS, Maltby DA, Bohan TP: l-Carnitine enhances excretion of propionyl coenzyme A as propionylcarnitine in propionic acidemia. *J Clin Invest* **73**:1785, 1984.
467. Roe CR, Hoppel CL, Stacey TE, Chalmers RA, Tracey BM, Millington DS: Metabolic response to carnitine in methylmalonic aciduria. *Arch Dis Child* **58**:916, 1983.
468. Thompson GN, Chalmers RA, Walter JH, Bresson JL, Lyonnet SL, Reed PJ, Saudubray JM, et al: The use of metronidazole in management of methylmalonic and propionic acidaemias. *Eur J Pediatr* **149**:792, 1990.
469. Bain MD, Jones M, Borriello SP, Reed PJ, Tracey BM, Chalmers RA, Stacey TE: Contribution of gut bacterial metabolism to human metabolic disease. *Lancet* **1**:1078, 1988.
470. Batshaw ML, Thomas GH, Cohen SR, Matalon R, Mahoney MJ: Treatment of the *cblB* form of methylmalonic acidaemia with adenosylcobalamin. *J Inherit Metab Dis* **7**:65, 1984.
471. Chalmers RA, Bain MD, Mistry J, Tracey BM, Weaver C: Enzymologic studies on patients with methylmalonic aciduria: Basis for a clinical trial of deoxyadenosylcobalamin in a hydroxocobalamin-unresponsive patient. *Pediatr Res* **30**:560, 1991.
472. Korf B, Wallman JK, Levy HL: Bilateral lucency of the globus pallidus complicating methylmalonic acidemia. *Ann Neurol* **20**:364, 1986.
473. Morrow G 3d, Burkel GM: Long-term management of a patient with vitamin B_{12}-responsive methylmalonic acidemia. *J Pediatr* **96**:425, 1980.
474. Thompson GN, Christodoulou J, Danks DM: Metabolic stroke in methylmalonic acidemia. *J Pediatr* **115**:499, 1989.
475. Walter JH, Michalski A, Wilson WM, Leonard JV, Barratt TM, Dillon MJ: Chronic renal failure in methylmalonic acidaemia. *Eur J Pediatr* **148**:344, 1989.
476. Van der Meer SB, Spaapen LJM, Fowler B, Jakobs C, Kleijer WJ, Wendel U: Prenatal treatment of a patient with vitamin B_{12}-responsive methylmalonic acidemia. *J Pediatr* **117**:923, 1990.
477. Rosenblatt DS, Fenton WA: Inborn errors of cobalamin metabolism, in Banerjee R (ed): *Chemistry and Biology of B_{12}*. New York, John Wiley, 1999, p 367.

CHAPTER 156

Disorders of Biotin Metabolism

Barry Wolf

1. Biotin, a water-soluble vitamin belonging to the B complex, acts as a coenzyme in each of four carboxylases in humans: pyruvate carboxylase, propionyl CoA carboxylase, β-methylcrotonyl CoA carboxylase, and acetyl CoA carboxylase. These enzymes have important roles in gluconeogenesis, fatty acid synthesis, and amino acid catabolism. Biotin is derived from the diet and possibly also from the synthetic activity of gastrointestinal microflora.
2. Each of the carboxylases is synthesized as an inactive apoenzyme that is subsequently biotinylated through two partial reactions, each of which is catalyzed by the enzyme holocarboxylase synthetase. Acetyl CoA carboxylase functions principally in the cytosol, whereas the other three holocarboxylases function in mitochondria. Ultimately, these enzymes are degraded proteolytically, probably by the lysosomal autophagic system. The biotin-containing products of degradation, biocytin (ε-*N*-biotinyl-L-lysine) and biotinyl peptides, are acted on by biotinidase, which cleaves the amide bond between lysine and biotin. The liberated biotin is recycled and enters the free biotin pool. Biotinidase also has been shown, in presence of biocytin, to transfer biotin to nucleophilic acceptors, such as histones. The physiologic significance of this function remains to be determined.
3. There are two major defects in the cycle of biotin utilization in humans. Both disorders result in multiple carboxylase deficiency. Holocarboxylase synthetase deficiency (OMIM 253270), also known as *early-onset (neonatal) multiple carboxylase deficiency* based on the usual age of onset of symptoms, is a disorder of biotinylation. Biotinidase deficiency (OMIM 253260), also known as *late-onset (juvenile) multiple carboxylase deficiency,* is a disorder of biotin recycling.
4. Holocarboxylase synthetase deficiency has been described in about thirty children. The clinical symptoms include feeding and breathing difficulties, hypotonia, seizures, and lethargy, and there sometimes is progression to developmental delay or coma. Some children exhibit skin rash and alopecia. Affected children exhibit metabolic acidosis, organic aciduria, and mild to moderate hyperammonemia. The organic aciduria includes elevated concentrations of β-hydroxyisovalerate, β-methylcrotonylglycine, β-hydroxypropionate, methylcitrate, lactate, and tiglylglycine.
5. The enzyme defect has been demonstrated in lymphocytes, cultured fibroblasts, and cultured lymphoblasts from affected children. Holocarboxylase synthetase in tissues of most of the children examined have increased K_m values for biotin, although at least one is described with a normal K_m and a decreased V_{max}.
6. Holocarboxylase synthetase deficiency is inherited as an autosomal recessive trait. Heterozygosity cannot be confirmed by measuring enzymatic activity in the tissues of parents but should be determined by mutation analysis.
7. The normal mammalian enzyme has been purified and characterized biochemically. The cDNA for human holocarboxylase synthetase has been isolated and sequenced. Multiple mutations within the synthetase gene have been identified. Some of these mutations occur within the biotin-binding domain and are likely responsible for the increased K_m for biotin, explaining the biotin responsiveness that occurs in this disease. A mutation that results in an enzyme with a normal K_m but decreased V_{max} is speculated to increase in activity sufficiently in the presence of supplemented biotin compared with that at the biotin concentration supplied by the normal diet. A single base deletion/null mutation has always been found in the compound heterozygous state, usually together with a mutation within the biotin-binding domain, but never homozygous, which may be lethal in utero.
8. Children with holocarboxylase synthetase deficiency usually improve clinically following administration of 10 mg of oral biotin per day. One child, whose enzyme had the highest K_m for biotin, continued to have a skin rash and excrete abnormal organic acids even while receiving 60 to 80 mg of biotin per day.
9. Holocarboxylase synthetase deficiency can be diagnosed prenatally by measuring the concentration of abnormal organic acids in the amniotic fluid and/or by measuring and comparing the various mitochondrial carboxylase activities in the amniocytes cultured with and without biotin. Prenatal diagnosis also should be possible by mutation analysis. Prenatal treatment has been performed during two pregnancies. The children were clinically normal at birth and did not have organic aciduria. It is not clear whether treatment of at-risk children with biotin immediately after birth is necessary.
10. Biotinidase deficiency has been described in over 120 symptomatic children. The clinical features commonly include seizures, hypotonia, ataxia, breathing problems, hearing loss, optic atrophy, developmental delay, skin rash, and alopecia. Other symptoms include conjunctivitis and fungal infections, which are probably due to abnormalities in immunoregulation. The clinical expression of the disorder is highly variable. The age at onset of symptoms ranges from several weeks to several years; median and

A list of standard abbreviations is located immediately preceding the index in each volume. Nonstandard abbreviations used in this chapter include: SIDS = sudden infant death syndrome; CRM = cross-reacting material.

mean age of onset are 3 and 5 months, respectively, but onset of symptoms has occurred as late as 10 years of age. Most, but not all, symptomatic children exhibit metabolic ketolactic acidosis and organic aciduria. The organic aciduria commonly manifests as elevated concentrations of β-hydroxyisovalerate, lactate, β-methylcrotonylglycine, β-hydroxypropionate, and methylcitrate.

11. **Biotinidase deficiency is diagnosed by demonstrating deficient enzyme activity in serum. Most symptomatic children have profound biotinidase deficiency (<10 percent of mean normal serum activity). Newborn screening also has identified children with partial biotinidase deficiency (10–30 percent of normal activity). Symptoms of biotinidase deficiency have developed in a small number of children with partial deficiency, usually when they are exposed to a severe infection; the symptoms resolved with biotin treatment. Deficient enzyme activity also was found in other tissues from these children.**
12. **Normal serum contains at least nine isoforms of biotinidase, four major and five minor isoforms, between pH 4.5 and 4.35 on isoelectric focusing immunoblots using antibodies prepared against purified human serum biotinidase. The plasma enzyme has been purified to homogeneity. The enzyme is a glycosylated monomer. Patients with profound biotinidase deficiency can be classified into nine distinct biochemical phenotypes based on the presence or absence of cross-reacting material (CRM) to biotinidase, specific isoforms, and the distribution frequencies of the isoforms. There is no correlation between the age of onset or the severity of symptoms and the CRM status or isoform patterns of the symptomatic children. The isoform patterns of children identified by newborn screening are not different from those of symptomatic children. Children with partial biotinidase deficiency have CRM in their serum and can be classified into six distinct biochemical phenotypes. The isoform patterns observed in these children are not different from those of profoundly deficient patients who have CRM.**
13. **The cDNA for human serum biotinidase has been isolated and sequenced. The genomic structure and organization of the human enzyme also have been determined. The enzyme appears to be a housekeeping gene. Over two dozen mutations have been found in symptomatic children with profound biotinidase deficiency. There are at least two common mutations that occur among children with profound biotinidase deficiency identified by neonatal screening. Partial biotinidase deficiency is usually due to a combination of an allele with a missense mutation, which results in an enzyme having about 50 percent of mean normal activity and is found in about 4 percent of the general population, and an allele for profound biotinidase deficiency.**
14. **Individuals with biotinidase deficiency cannot recycle endogenous biotin and cannot release dietary-protein-bound biotin. The brain may be unable to recycle biotin adequately and may depend on biotin transferred across the blood-brain barrier. This may result in decreased pyruvate carboxylase activity in the brain and in the accumulation of lactate. The localized lactic acidosis may cause the early appearance of neurologic symptoms.**
15. **Biotinidase deficiency is inherited as an autosomal recessive trait. Heterozygotes can be determined in 95 percent of cases by demonstrating that enzyme activity in serum is intermediate between that of normal and deficient individuals. Prenatal diagnosis of biotinidase deficiency by enzymatic and mutation analysis is possible.**
16. **Biotinidase activity can be determined in the same blood-soaked filter paper used in most neonatal screening programs. More than 25 states in the United States and 25 countries are screening for the enzyme deficiency in their newborns. Children with enzyme deficiency identified by screening have been treated with biotin and have remained asymptomatic. The method used in newborn screening also offers a simple, rapid means for the physician to evaluate biotinidase activity in individuals suspected of having the disorder.**
17. **Children with biotinidase deficiency have been treated successfully with between 5 and 20 mg of oral biotin (in the free, unbound form) per day. All patients with the deficiency should respond to biotin therapy. If a child remains undiagnosed for a long time or experiences severe metabolic compromise, some of the neurologic problems, such as hearing loss, optic atrophy, or developmental delay, may not resolve. Doses of biotin only slightly above physiologic requirements eventually may be shown to suffice for treatment.**
18. **The multiple carboxylase deficiencies must be differentiated from other acute-onset metabolic disorders and nutritional deficiencies that result from dietary indiscretion or hyperalimentation with solutions lacking biotin. Because both holocarboxylase synthetase deficiency and biotinidase deficiency are so amenable to biotin therapy, these disorders should be considered in any child with nonspecific neurologic symptoms, especially when cutaneous abnormalities are present. Newborn screening for biotinidase deficiency, followed by prompt initiation of therapy in deficient children, appears to prevent the clinical consequences of this disorder.**

HISTORICAL BACKGROUND

Biotin is a water-soluble B-complex vitamin and, as such, must be provided in the diet of mammals and birds. It was first recognized as an essential factor in living systems in 1936.[1] The biotin molecule consists of a heterocyclic ring attached to an aliphatic side chain terminating in a carboxylic acid group.[2,3] In humans, biotin is directly involved in the vitally important metabolic processes of gluconeogenesis, fatty acid synthesis, and amino acid catabolism via its role as a prosthetic group in each of four carboxylase enzymes (Fig. 156-1).

Three of the enzymes, pyruvate carboxylase (EC 6.4.1.1), propionyl CoA carboxylase (EC 6.4.1.3), and β-methylcrotonoyl CoA carboxylase (EC 6.4.1.4), are mitochondrial, and the fourth, acetyl CoA carboxylase (EC 6.4.1.2), is cytosolic.[4] Pyruvate carboxylase catalyzes the conversion of pyruvate to oxaloacetate, an intermediate in the biosynthesis of phosphoenolpyruvate and, ultimately, glucose. Acetyl CoA carboxylase catalyzes the formation of malonyl CoA from acetyl CoA, the first committed step in the biosynthesis of fatty acids. Propionyl CoA carboxylase is involved in the catabolism of several branched-chain amino acids and fatty acids of odd-carbon chain lengths by converting propionyl CoA to methylmalonyl CoA, which ultimately enters the tricarboxylic acid cycle. β-Methylcrotonoyl CoA carboxylase is involved in leucine catabolism by the conversion of β-methylcrotonoyl CoA to β-methylglutaconyl CoA. Deficiencies of the carboxylases and the consequent accumulation of abnormally high concentrations of metabolic intermediates can have profound effects on other pathways.

The final step in the synthesis and activation of biotin-containing carboxylases is the formation of the active holocarboxylases by means of the covalent attachment of biotin to the various apoenzymes. The biotinyl moiety is attached via an amide linkage through the carboxyl group in its side chain to a lysyl ε-amino group of the apoenzyme. This attachment is catalyzed by

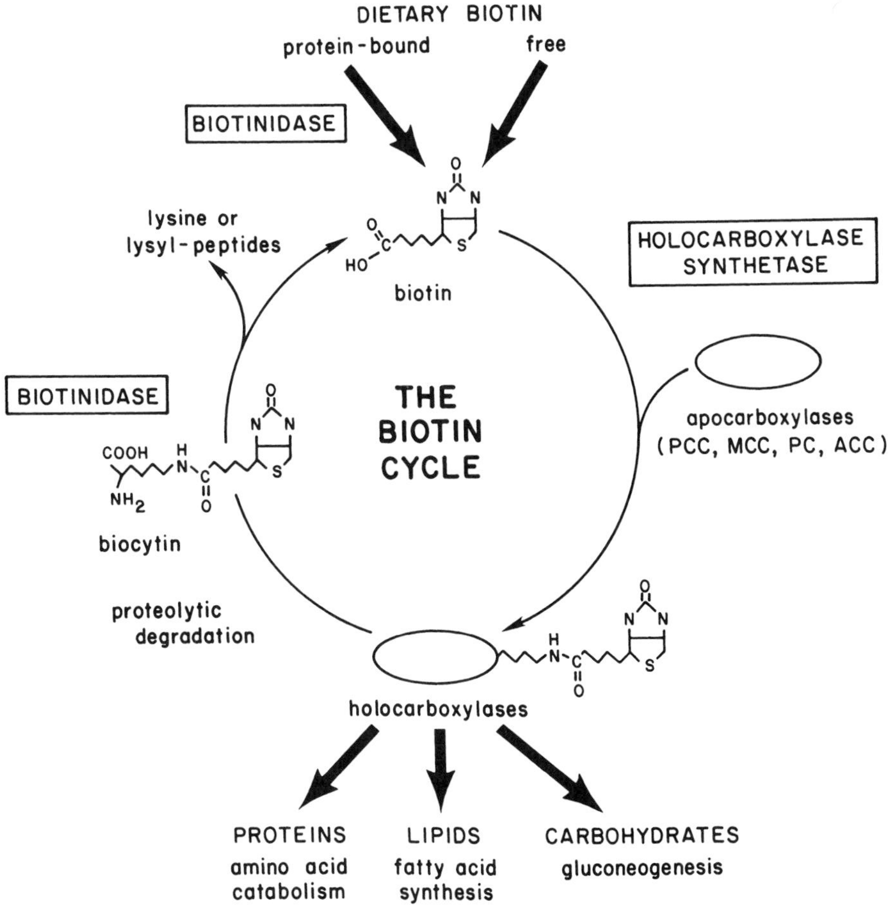

Fig. 156-1 The biotin cycle demonstrates the metabolic recycling of biotin. The two major enzymes involved in this cycle are holocarboxylase synthetase, which covalently attaches biotin to the various apocarboxylases to form holocarboxylases, and biotinidase, the hydrolase that cleaves biotin from biocytin or short biotinyl peptides that are formed from the proteolytic degradation of holocarboxylases and possibly from dietary protein-bond sources. Deficiencies of both these enzymes have been described. (*From Wolf et al.*[86] *Used by permission of Alan R. Liss, Inc.*)

holocarboxylase synthetase.[1,5,6] The terminal step in the degradation of the carboxylases, cleavage of the biotinyl moiety from the ε-amino group of lysine, is catalyzed by biotinidase (EC 3.5.1.12) and results in the release of free biotin,[7] some of which is recycled.

Disorders that result from individual deficiency of each of the three mitochondrial, biotin-dependent carboxylases have been documented[8] (see Chaps. 93, 94, and 100). Each is characterized by an abnormal profile of organic acids in the urine, which is attributable to the accumulation of one or more intermediate compounds in the blood (Fig. 156-2). A single case of acetyl CoA carboxylase deficiency has been reported.[9] Children with the disorders of isolated carboxylases do not respond to treatment with biotin, and the information available indicates that structural alterations of the individual enzymes are responsible for the deficient activity.

Another group of disorders involving deficient activities of the carboxylases was found to be responsive to treatment with biotin. The first patient with such a disorder, reported originally in 1971, was described as having biotin-responsive β-methylcrotonylglycinuria.[10] From birth, the child experienced episodic vomiting; at 6 weeks of age, an erythematous rash developed; and at 5 months, the child exhibited rapid respiration, persistent vomiting, and unresponsiveness. He also had metabolic acidosis and ketosis, and the concentrations of β-methylcrotonic acid and β-methylcrotonylglycine in his urine were greatly elevated. Several days after the commencement of treatment with oral biotin, the symptoms resolved and the urinary metabolites normalized.[11] Later, the excretion of tiglylglycine and β-hydroxyisovaleric acid in the urine was demonstrated.[12] Subsequently, the patient was found to have deficient activity of all three biotin-dependent mitochondrial carboxylases in peripheral blood leukocytes and skin fibroblasts,[13–15] as well as deficient activity of acetyl CoA carboxylase in fibroblasts.[16] These findings prompted the eventual diagnosis of "multiple carboxylase deficiency."

By 1980, several more patients with multiple or combined carboxylase deficiency were reported.[8] Based on the finding of deficient activities of more than one carboxylase in peripheral blood leukocytes and skin fibroblasts, it was suggested that a defect in holocarboxylase synthetase was the probable cause of the disorder.[17] However, the relatively late onset of symptoms in some children prompted the proposal that the absorption and/or transport of biotin was defective.[18]

For several years, patients with multiple carboxylase deficiency were classified as having either the early-onset (also referred to as *neonatal*) form or the late-onset (or *juvenile*) form of multiple carboxylase deficiency, depending on the age at onset of symptoms.[19] Initially, most of the reported patients with the early-onset form of the disorder were shown to have altered holocarboxylase synthetase activity, the K_m of biotin for the enzyme being markedly elevated.[20] Two patients with the late-onset form were reported as having transport defects because of their abnormal responses to oral loading tests with biotin,[21,22] but in 1983 it was shown that the primary biochemical defect in most patients with the late-onset multiple carboxylase deficiency was deficient activity of biotinidase.[23] One of these patients who was described initially as having had a transport defect was shown subsequently to be able to absorb biotin normally if loading tests were performed when tissue biotin concentrations were normal.[24] Biotinidase deficiency was confirmed in both these patients[24] (JM Saudubray, personal communication).

Most patients with holocarboxylase synthetase deficiency (OMIM 253270) have become symptomatic soon after birth,[25] whereas most patients with biotinidase deficiency (OMIM 253260) have not exhibited clinical manifestations prior to 3 months of age.[26] Nevertheless, there is an overlap in the ranges of age of onset. The existence of this overlap raises some intriguing and, as yet unanswered, questions about the role of recycling of biotin.

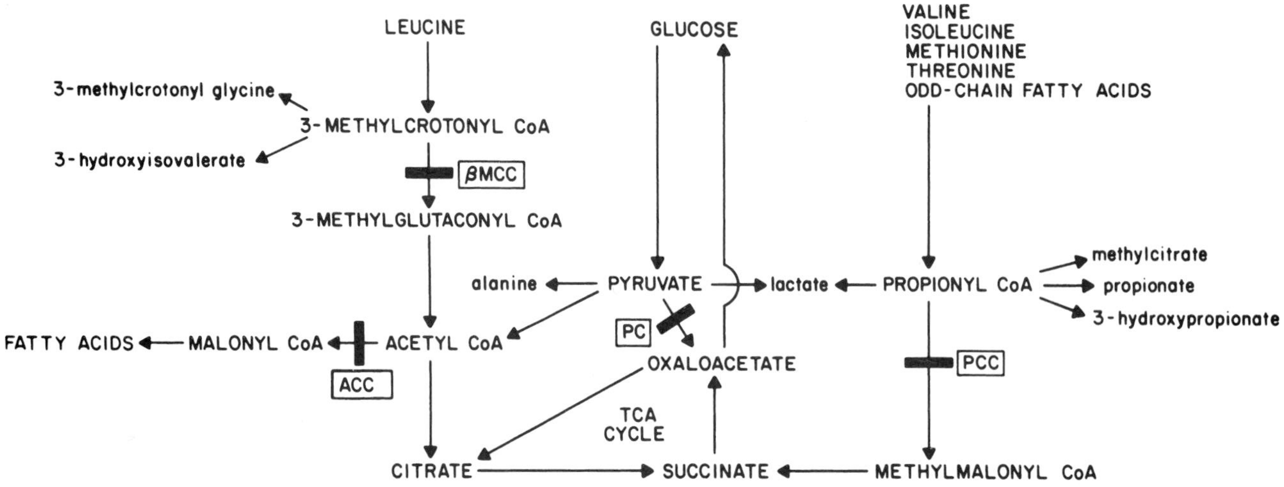

Fig. 156-2 Metabolic pathways in which biotin-dependent enzymes are involved. The solid rectangular blocks indicate the location of the enzymes. PCC, propionyl CoA carboxylase; PC, pyruvate carboxylase; β-MCC, β-methylcrotonyl CoA carboxylase; ACC, acetyl CoA carboxylase. Isolated deficiencies of the first three carboxylases have been established, whereas a deficiency in acetyl CoA carboxylase activity has been reported in only a single case. All four of these enzymes appear to be deficient in holocarboxylase synthetase deficiency and possibly in biotinidase deficiency. Metabolites that are frequently found at elevated concentrations in urine of children with the various isolated and multiple carboxylase deficiencies are indicated by lowercase characters. *(From Wolf et al.*[219] *Used by permission of Pediatrics.)*

This chapter begins with a discussion of biotin metabolism in humans. When appropriate, the results of studies in other species are presented; in some cases they provide the only insight into the use of this essential nutrient. The chapter then describes the cyclic nature of the biochemical pathways involved in the metabolism of biotin and the reaction pathways involving the biotin-dependent carboxylases. The disease states involving the enzymes of biotin metabolism, holocarboxylase synthetase and biotinidase, are described, and their differential diagnosis is discussed. The conclusion considers biotin-responsive disorders of unknown etiology and how these disorders have helped us to better understand normal biotin metabolism.

ACQUISITION AND LOSS OF BIOTIN

In 1916, toxic effects were observed in rats receiving diets that contained a high concentration of dried, raw egg white,[27] and when raw egg white was the sole protein source, a syndrome characterized by neuromuscular disorders, severe dermatitis, and loss of hair developed in rats.[28] The condition was termed *egg white injury* and was shown to be preventable by heating the protein or by administering additional foods such as yeast, liver, or a compound from egg yolk that promoted the growth of yeast.[29] This compound was later shown to be biotin.[1,30] The antagonist for biotin that caused the observed egg white injury is the glycoprotein avidin.[31]

Sources

Foods. Although biotin occurs widely in natural foodstuffs, the absolute concentration even in the richest sources is very low. Liver, kidney, egg yolk, and some vegetables are good sources of biotin, containing 20 to 120 mg/100 g of edible portion, whereas lean meat, fruit, cereals, and bread products contain 1 to 10 mg/100 g.[32]

Intestinal Microflora. For perhaps 40 years it was assumed that the intestinal microflora either synthesized all the biotin required in humans or supplemented the biotin in the diet so that biotin was available in more than adequate quantities.[33] Few attempts have been made to estimate the actual contribution of the microflora. There is now evidence available from several sources to suggest that neither diet nor the microflora alone satisfies the true demand for biotin, even in clinically normal members of the population.[33–36] Debate about the relative importance of the contribution of microflora continues, unfortunately in the almost complete absence of attempts to quantify this contribution. The strongest evidence in favor of a significant contribution by the microflora is the observation that the combined daily output of biotin in urine and stool exceeds the dietary intake.[33,37,38]

Biosynthesis. Mammals cannot synthesize biotin. More than 30 species of bacteria are known to be able to synthesize biotin,[39] and some of these biotin-synthesizing bacteria have been identified in the human gut.[40] Most microorganisms capable of biotin synthesis use a pathway from pimelic acid through 7,8-substituted pelargonic acid and desthiobiotin with subsequent incorporation of sulfur to form biotin.[41] The mechanism of introduction of sulfur into biotin is yet to be determined.

Antibiotics and sulfa drugs alter the intestinal flora and lead to a reduction in the fecal output of biotin.[42–45] The effects of these treatments on the urinary excretion of biotin are unclear. Several of these studies were conducted with very high concentrations of antibiotics or with avidin used in conjunction with the antibiotics, with the result that the urinary output of biotin was reduced.[44,45]

Bioavailability of Biotin

Quantifying Biotin. Knowledge of the concentration of total biotin in a foodstuff is informative but gives little indication of how efficiently biotin may be used for metabolic processes. The concept of bioavailability encompasses this notion of efficiency of utilization of nutrients. Several components affect bioavailability: digestibility, absorption, and availability of the nutrient in an appropriate form in target organs.

The biotin concentrations of foods, tissues, and biologic fluids have been measured using chick and rat growth assays, microbiologic growth assays,[46] and competitive binding assays that involve the use of avidin and radioactively labeled biotin.[47–51] Of these, the methods currently used are the microbiologic and avidin-binding assays. *Lactobacillus plantarum*[52] and the protozoan *Ochromonas danica*[53] are the two microorganisms that are used most frequently to measure biotin in biologic extracts, and several variations of the avidin-binding procedure have been published.[47,48,51–53] It has been shown that biotin accounts for only about half the avidin-binding material in human serum and that some bioassay methods used to quantitate biotin may result in overestimates.[54] Each procedure has its limitations. For example, biotin and biocytin are indistinguishable in most of the avidin-binding methods. It is important to know the method by which a quoted concentration was obtained.

The biotin in foods and biologic materials occurs in different chemical forms,[7,55,56] and selection of the appropriate extraction condition can be as important as selection of an assay technique for obtaining an accurate estimate of true biotin concentration. Vegetables, green plant materials, and fruits contain water-extractable forms of biotin. The biotin in yeast and animal products is abundant but occurs in firmly bound complexes that are insoluble in water. Seeds and nuts also contain large amounts of bound biotin.[56] It is not known if this biotin is covalently bound.

Bound biotin may be freed either by acid hydrolysis or with enzymes such as trypsin, but it is also subject to degradation if the conditions of hydrolysis are severe. For example, treatment with 4 N sulfuric acid destroys some of the biotin in yeast, corn, and soybeans, and hydrolysis with hydrochloric acid also destroys biotin. The optimal conditions for hydrolysis of animal and plant products appear to be autoclaving for 2 hours at 121°C with 6 N and 2 N sulfuric acid, respectively.[56,57]

Selection of the appropriate analytical method depends on the form of biotin in the material to be assayed. The methods based on the avidin-binding reaction are not specific for free biotin. Thus any compounds that have a ureido ring in their structure will react in this assay system,[58] although not necessarily stoichiometrically. Therefore, these methods may overestimate the biotin concentration. *L. plantarum* responds to free biotin and not to biocytin, but oleic acid can replace biotin if it is present at sufficiently high concentrations in the growth medium.[59] *O. danica* responds to free biotin as well as to biocytin.[60] These differences in specificity have led to some confusion about "normal" concentrations, and I stress the importance of establishing how biotin concentrations were obtained.

Release from Foods *in Vivo*. The extent of predigestion required for the uptake of biotin-containing sources in humans remains to be determined, but it has been shown *in vitro* that human plasma biotinidase acts on its natural substrate biocytin much more efficiently than on natural or synthetic biotinylated peptides.[61] The efficiency of release is negatively correlated with the number of amino acid residues in a biotinylated polypeptide. Biotinidase is present in the intestinal mucosa of several species[62] and in pancreatic juice and zymogen granules of rats.[63,64] It may play an important role in the digestion and uptake of dietary biotin in humans.[63,65] Extensive proteolysis is probably required before biotinidase in the gut can be useful in making biotin from biotinylated peptides available for uptake.

Intestinal Absorption. Early studies using everted sacs prepared from the small intestine of rats indicated that free biotin was absorbed by passive diffusion.[66] This finding was confirmed and extended in a study using everted intestinal sacs prepared from rats and several other species.[67] Biotin failed to accumulate against concentration gradients in rats, rabbits, guinea pigs, ferrets, and carps but did accumulate against concentration gradients in hamsters, white mice, chipmunks, gerbils, and squirrels. These studies employed pharmacologic concentrations of biotin (10 μM), whereas the physiologic concentration in rat intestine has been estimated at 0.6 μM.[68] Further studies of intestinal uptake in the hamster indicated that biotin uptake is a saturable sodium-dependent process.[69,70] The uptake of biotin by isolated rat intestinal cells has been shown to be nonsaturable (from 0.01–2 μM), independent of temperature, and not inhibitable by antimycin C.[71] However, studies using ligated loops of rat intestine *in situ,* everted sacs, and membrane vesicles indicated that biotin absorption involved both saturable and nonsaturable components.[72–74] Biotin transport using basolateral membranes of rat intestines[74] and using brush-border membrane vesicles of rabbit intestines is both carrier-mediated and Na^+-gradient-dependent.[75] Transport and plasma concentration of biotin across rat intestine increase with the age of the animal. This increase appears to be due to the increase in activity and/or number of transport carriers but not to the affinity of the biotin transport system.[76] Supplementation of pharmacologic concentrations of biotin in rats caused a significant decrease in biotin transport as compared with unsupplemented rats.[77] These results suggest that biotin transport in rat intestine is regulated by the amount of biotin in the diet. Both biotin and biocytin are actively transported in rat small intestines.[78,79] Biotin uptake by mitochondria isolated from rat liver occurs most rapidly at pH 6.1 and is markedly slower at pH 7.4.[80] Almost certainly some of these inconsistencies can be attributed to methodologic differences, but apparently there are species differences in biotin uptake.

In humans, the vitamin is rapidly absorbed after oral loading, and peak plasma concentrations of biotin are attained 30 to 60 min after administration.[22,24,81] There is one preliminary communication describing experiments in which intracellular concentrations of biotin were measured after jejunal biopsy samples were incubated in medium containing [^{14}C]biotin. The uptake of biotin proceeded against a concentration gradient. The intracellular-to-extracellular concentration ratio was 2.5, and the uptake was sodium-dependent. However, few data were presented, and these results were difficult to interpret.[82] Biotin has been shown to be transported in human intestinal brush-border membranes by a carrier-mediated, sodium-gradient-dependent system.[83] Biotin uptake also has been shown to occur by a carrier-mediated, sodium-gradient-dependent process in human liver basolateral membrane vesicles and HepG2 (human hepatoma) cells.[84,85]

The specificity of site of uptake of biotin has been studied in rats, hamsters, chickens, and, to a limited extent, humans. In rats and hamsters biotin is absorbed more rapidly in the upper half of the intestine than in the lower portion,[67,86] but in chickens there appears to be no site specificity in the small intestine.[87] Biotin introduced at high concentrations in vivo can be absorbed from the large intestine as well as from the small intestine in humans.[88]

Tissue Transport and Cellular Uptake. Biotin binds nonspecifically to serum/plasma proteins,[89] and several specific biotin-binding proteins including biotinidase have been proposed but not well studied.[54,90–94] One study showed that most of the biotin in human plasma is not bound to protein,[94] whereas another showed that at pH 7 biotinidase was the only protein in serum that binds biotin, with two K_d values for biotin, both in the nanomolar range.[93] Recent studies suggest that biotin may be bound covalently to biotinidase at neutral pH,[95] which may be how some or most of the biotin exists in plasma. Confirmation of the existence of specific biotin-binding proteins and elucidation of their role(s) in regulating biotin concentrations in blood and other tissues await further investigation.

In addition to the studies of isolated rat enterocytes already described, the transport of biotin has been studied in cultured HeLa cells, human fibroblasts, mouse fibroblasts, isolated and cultured rat hepatocytes, brush-border and basolateral membrane vesicles prepared from rabbit kidney cortex, perfused rat brain, and isolated rabbit choroid plexus. HeLa cells and human fibroblasts take up protein-bound biotin in the form of an avidin-[^{3}H]biotin complex by a process that is time-dependent, saturable, and energy-dependent. HeLa cells take up free biotin more slowly than bound biotin; the rate of uptake is linear with respect to extracellular concentration of biotin and depends on temperature.[96,97]

Biotin uptake by mouse fibroblasts is sensitive to temperature, shows a nonlinear dependence on external biotin concentration, and demonstrates some substrate specificity. The transport is apparently controlled by two processes: a saturable process, probably carrier-mediated, and a second nonsaturable component that is linear above 75 μM and represents a diffusion-driven process.[98]

Based on the inhibition of transport by ouabain and/or sodium replacement, the uptake of biotin into isolated rat hepatocytes may involve a process that depends on sodium and ATP.[99] The uptake from cultured rat hepatocytes, however, was nonsaturable and was not affected by the extracellular sodium concentration, pH, biotin analogues, or metabolic inhibitors.[100] At least two factors could explain the apparent contradictions in these studies. First, isolated hepatocytes, adipocytes, and fibroblasts are prepared using enzymatic isolation methods that involve potential proteolytic damage to the external receptors. Second, there is evidence from other systems involving biotin and other nutrients to suggest that the gradient of sodium is more important than simply the presence or absence of the cation in the incubation medium.[101]

In brush-border membrane vesicles from the rabbit kidney cortex, biotin uptake is stimulated by an inwardly directed sodium gradient. This gradient-dependent uptake of [^{3}H]biotin is saturable with an apparent K_m of 28 μM and is inhibited by unlabeled biotin and its structural analogues. Biotin is apparently reabsorbed by the sodium/biotin cotransporter in luminal brush-border membranes. The mechanism does not operate in the basolateral membranes of the kidney cortex.[101] These results were confirmed in rat kidney cortex.[102] A sodium-dependent vitamin transporter in human placental choriocarcinoma cells mediates the uptake of biotin in addition to pantothenic and lipoic acids.[103] The transporter has been cloned and sequenced (Genbank AF026554), has a mass of 68.6 kDa, is composed of 634 amino acids, and has 12 putative transmembrane domains.[104] The transport coefficient for biotin and pantothenate is 4.9 μM, whereas the coefficient for lipoate is 15 μM. The transporter is expressed in essentially all tissues.

In the rat brain, biotin is transported through cerebral capillaries by a low-affinity saturable process that depends on the presence of the free carboxylic acid group of the biotin side chain.[105] The choroid plexus appears not to be involved in active transfer of biotin in the brain.[105]

Requirement of Biotin

Recommended Intake. Uncertainty about the contribution of the intestinal microflora has prevented the establishment of a recommended daily allowance of biotin for humans, although safe daily intakes that are assumed to prevent the development of symptoms of biotin deficiency have been suggested in the United States. For infants, the safe daily intake has been set at 35 μg of biotin; that for adults is from 150 to 300 μg.[106] The biotin pool in adults has been estimated to be 675 μg and that of a child to be about 120 μg.[53]

Biotin appears to be relatively nontoxic.[107] Over 200 infants and adults with various disorders have received doses of up to 10 mg daily either orally or intramuscularly for periods exceeding 6 months, and no toxic effects were reported.[33] An adverse effect of biotin on the development of fetuses and placentas in rats has been reported.[107] The dose administered was 50 to 100 times greater than the therapeutic dose for infants, and the results could not be reproduced.[108] In a more recent study, adverse affects were not observed in the offspring of rats given similarly high doses of biotin.[109]

Irreversible Loss. Balance studies with adults on "normal" diets[37,38,110–112] have shown that the total output of biotin in urine and feces is always greater than the dietary intake, suggesting that the excess is due to microbial synthesis. Changes in dietary biotin intake are reflected in urinary excretion.[38,113] The total amount of biotin excreted in urine is usually less than the total intake, but at very low intakes, e.g., less than one-tenth normal, the quantity excreted may exceed that ingested.[38] The quantity of biotin excreted under these conditions is probably an indication of endogenous loss due to normal turnover of the biotin-containing enzymes.[44,45]

Newborn infants excrete biotin in their urine (30 μg/liter), but by the seventh day after birth, it is undetectable.[114] Urinary output of biotin increases subsequently, such that by the age of 2 to 4 weeks it averages 6.5 μg/liter, and by 24 weeks it reaches 31 μg/liter,[115] which is within the range of normal adults. Although serum concentrations of biotin are increased during early pregnancy and then decrease throughout the pregnancy,[116] fetal biotin obtained during amniocentesis (18–24 weeks' gestation) has about sixfold more biotin than does the mother's plasma.[117] This suggests that biotin is actively transported from the mother to the fetus. There is evidence that biotin is taken up by the maternal-side placental membranes by a mediated, carrier-dependent process, but perfusion studies support a passive process.[118] The fetal-side basolateral membrane of human placenta indicates that biotin is taken up by a saturable, carrier-mediated, sodium-dependent process, which is less than the biotin uptake on the maternal-side apical membrane of the placenta.[119]

Catabolism. Degradation of the heterocyclic ureido ring system of biotin does not occur in mammals, but small amounts of biotin sulfoxides are produced through the action of mixed-function oxidase activity in liver.[120] Biotin is also degraded in the mitochondria to bisnorbiotin, which results from β-oxidation of the side chain.[121] Decarboxylation of the intermediate α-keto acid derivatives of biotin leading to the production of methylketones also occurs, and these products are excreted in the urine. Initial studies indicated that human urine contains no D-biotin sulfoxide or biotin sulfone,[122] suggesting that very little modification occurs. More recent studies indicate that biotin sulfone, bisnorbiotin methyl ketone, and tetrabiotin-1-sulfoxide are present in human urine.[123] In fact, bisnorbiotin and biotin sulfoxide increase during acute and chronic supplementation of biotin in serum and urine.[124,125]

Microbial Degradation. Although nothing is known about the catabolism of biotin by the gastrointestinal microflora as an ecologic unit in any mammal, the microbial degradative pathways for biotin have been elucidated.[120] There is a Pseudomonad that can use biotin as its sole source of carbon, nitrogen, sulfur, and energy.[120] Degradation of dietary biotin and biotin synthesized by microorganisms could conceivably be important in conditions in which biotin metabolism is altered.

Biotin Deficiency

The most overt clinical symptoms of biotin deficiency in humans are alopecia and cutaneous abnormalities such as dermatitis, erythematous periorificial rash, dryness, and fungal infection. Neurologic symptoms noted in adults include mild depression progressing to extreme lassitude, somnolence, muscular pain, hyperesthesia, and paresthesia.[126–129] In the absence of dietary biotin and/or the presence in the diet of avidin, the time required for the onset of symptoms depends on the quantity of accessible biotin stored in the body. Even when diets contain large amounts of egg white, symptoms do not appear in adults for 3 or 4 weeks. Although the relatively long interval required to induce deficiencies in humans and other animals[126–130] has been cited as evidence for a contribution by the intestinal microflora, this also may be a reflection of the occurrence of biotin recycling in the body and of the relatively long biologic half-life of biotin.

Spontaneous biotin deficiency in humans is practically unknown, although several reports have appeared in the past decade of biotin-responsive syndromes in intensively reared farm livestock, particularly poultry, swine, and calves.[131–133] The most notable of these describes the fatty liver and kidney syndrome, a biotin-response condition that occurs in young chickens fed diets based on wheat and meat meal without supplementary biotin.[134–136] Many of the birds die when they are subjected to mild stress such as hypothermia or short-term fasting. The syndrome is associated with a marginal deficiency of biotin. Affected chicks have abnormal plasma fatty acid profiles, low concentrations of biotin in the liver, fatty kidneys, and reduced activity of hepatic pyruvate carboxylase, but the classic symptoms of biotin deficiency are not observed. Adults fed an avidin-containing diet for 20 days had increased urinary excretion of β-hydroisovalerate and decreased biotin concentrations.[137] These parameters may be good indicators of early biotin deficiency.

The involvement of marginal biotin deficiency in the etiology of the sudden infant death syndrome (SIDS) in human infants has been proposed,[34] and SIDS victims have had significantly less biotin in their livers than infants who died of known causes.[34,35]

The consumption of raw eggs, which contain avidin, has led to biotin deficiency in several children and adults.[126–128,138] The clinical manifestations of biotin deficiency also have developed in patients receiving long-term total parenteral alimentation without biotin.[129,139,140] These patients also may have decreased serum biotinidase activities, presumably because of nutritional protein deficiency.[141] The prolonged use of anticonvulsants also may lead to biotin deficiency. Phenytoin, primidone, and carbamazepine, but not valproic acid, resulted in decreased serum biotin concentrations relative to control values.[142,143] Biotin transport in human intestine is inhibited by anticonvulsant drugs.[144] Other studies indicate that anticonvulsive therapy accelerates biotin catabolism.[145]

BIOCHEMICAL PATHWAYS

Biotinylation of Apocarboxylases

In active carboxylases, biotin is attached covalently to the ε-amino group of a lysine residue in the active sites.[4] Biotinylation of several apoenzymes has been studied in prokaryotes and eukaryotes[5,20,146–158]; it is catalyzed by holocarboxylase synthetase (see Fig. 156-1). The sequence of amino acids in the region of the biotinylated lysyl residue of the carboxylases (–Ala–Met–biocytin–Met–) is conserved in different species.[159] This region may function as a recognition site for the synthetase.

The mammalian apocarboxylases pyruvate carboxylase and acetyl CoA carboxylase are homopolymeric enzymes, whereas propionyl CoA carboxylase and β-methylcrotonoyl CoA carboxylase are heteropolymeric.[4,160,161] The heteropolymeric enzymes are composed of α and β subunits; biotin is attached to each α subunit. The two nonidentical subunits that comprise the hexamer of propionyl CoA carboxylase are synthesized in the cytosol with leader peptides that facilitate their transport into the mitochondria,[162,163] a feature that they share with other mitochondrial enzymes. Assembly of the subunits occurs after transport and can take place without prior biotinylation.[164] Biotinylation of assembled subunits of the enzyme can occur.[165]

Partial Reactions. Biotinylation of the apocarboxylase requires activation of biotin by ATP (partial reaction 1), which results in the formation of a biotinyl adenylate intermediate (biotinyl AMP synthetase activity).[149,151,152,154] The biotinyl group is then transferred to the apoenzyme to form active carboxylase (partial reaction 2). These two partial reactions are catalyzed by the same enzyme, holocarboxylase synthetase.

Partial reaction 1:

$$\text{Biotin} + \text{ATP} \rightleftharpoons \text{biotinyl 5}'\text{-AMP} + \text{PP}_i$$

Partial reaction 2:

$$\text{Biotinyl 5}'\text{-AMP} + \text{apocarboxylase} \rightleftharpoons \text{holocarboxylase} + \text{AMP}$$

Total reaction:

$$\text{Biotin} + \text{ATP} + \text{apocarboxylase} \rightleftharpoons \text{holocarboxylase} + \text{AMP} + \text{PP}_i$$

Holocarboxylase Synthetase

Bacterial and animal holocarboxylase synthetases are highly specific for biotin, but there is lower specificity for the high-energy phosphate donor and the apoenzyme acceptor.[5,6,147,152,153] Analogues and compounds structurally related to biotin, such as biocytin, homobiotin, norbiotin, and desthiobiotin, fail to substitute for biotin in the biotinylation reaction.[5,147] Holocarboxylase synthetases for propionyl CoA carboxylase from rabbit and rat liver and from various bacteria specifically require ATP and cannot effectively use other nucleoside triphosphates,[5,155] whereas the synthetase for propionyl CoA, pyruvate, and acetyl CoA carboxylases from chicken liver can use nucleoside triphosphates other than ATP.[6,166–168] Holocarboxylase synthetase from one species can effectively biotinylate apocarboxylases from other species.[20,153]

Holocarboxylase synthetase that has been partially purified from the cytosolic fraction of chicken liver biotinylates, mitochondrial apopyruvate carboxylase, and the cytosolic enzyme apoacetyl CoA carboxylase.[6] These findings suggest that, at least in chickens, a single synthetase activates all the apocarboxylases. However, because there are differences in pH optima and nucleotide requirements for the cytosolic and mitochondrial extracts from chicken liver, the existence of two distinct synthetases cannot be excluded.[169] The cytosol and mitochondria contain different apoenzymes, and the differences in the properties of activation simply may reflect differences in the apoenzyme acceptors and not the existence of two separate synthetases.

The synthetase from bovine liver is a monomer with molecular mass of between 60 and 64 kDa[170]; the K_m for biotin is 13 nM. The cDNA of human holocarboxylase synthetase has been cloned and sequenced (Genbank D23672).[171,172] Antiserum prepared against the recombinant protein precipitated human holocarboxylase synthetase, thereby confirming the validity of the gene sequenced. The human enzyme is predicted to be composed of 726 amino acids with a molecular mass of 80,759 Da. The protein sequence has homology to BirA, an enzyme with both biotin ligase and biotin repressor functions in *Escherichia coli,* and with biotin ligase from *Paracoccus denitrifcans.* There are three possible translation initiation sites in the mRNA of holocarboxylase synthetase.[172] Three different cytosolic proteins, 76, 82, and 86 kDa, were identified in placental cytoplasm that reacted with antibody prepared against holocarboxylase synthetase.[173] Synthetase expressed in a cell-free system did not translocate into rat liver mitochondria. These results suggest that the isolated human cDNA encodes cytosolic synthetases. The holocarboxylase synthetase gene was shown to map to chromosome 21q22.1.[171,174]

In 3T3-L1 mouse cells that were fully differentiated into adipocytes and contained high concentrations of pyruvate carboxylase and acetyl CoA carboxylase, 70 percent of holocarboxylase synthetase activity was localized in the cytosolic fraction. The remaining 30 percent of activity was associated with the particulate fraction that contains the mitochondria.[169] Studies of preparations of rat liver yielded similar results.[175]

The best evidence for the existence of a single holocarboxylase synthetase in humans is the demonstration of deficient acetyl CoA carboxylase activity in addition to deficient activities of the three mitochondrial carboxylases in fibroblasts from children with holocarboxylase synthetase deficiency.[176,177] Fibroblasts from children with holocarboxylase synthetase deficiency cultured in biotin-restricted medium have reduced total fatty acid content, especially the percentage of C16:0 and C18:0 fatty acids, whereas the proportion of longer-carbon-chain fatty acids were increased or normal.[178] This reduction in fatty acids is not due to decreased transport of fatty acids into the cells.[179] On Northern blot analysis, several forms of mRNA are seen, consistent with alternative splicing and different possible translation initiation sites.[172] This alternative splicing has been speculated as an explanation for mitochondrial and cytoplasmic expression.

Reactions Involving Biotin-Dependent Carboxylases

The major biochemical pathways and intermediates involving the four biotin-containing carboxylases in humans were depicted in Fig. 156-2. Acetyl CoA carboxylase catalyzes the formation of malonyl CoA from acetyl CoA. Malonyl CoA is the principal substrate in the synthesis and chain elongation of fatty acids. The synthesis of oxaloacetic acid from pyruvate is catalyzed by pyruvate carboxylase. This reaction provides a primary intermediate for the tricarboxylic acid cycle, and it provides a source of carbon skeletons for the synthesis of aspartate and glutamate. Oxaloacetic acid is used in the liver and kidney for gluconeogenesis. Propionyl CoA carboxylase catalyzes the carboxylation of propionyl CoA to form methylmalonyl CoA, which undergoes isomerization to succinyl CoA and subsequently enters the tricarboxylic acid cycle. β-Methylcrotonoyl-CoA carboxylase forms β-methylglutaconyl CoA from β-methylcrotonoyl CoA in the catabolic pathway of leucine. Clearly, altered activity of one or more of the carboxylases would have profound metabolic consequences.

Regulation of Carboxylase Activities. Acetyl CoA carboxylase and pyruvate carboxylase are subject to allosteric regulation; pyruvate carboxylase is activated by catalytic amounts of acetyl CoA.[4,180,181] As carbohydrate is converted to pyruvate during glycolysis, it enters the mitochondria, where it is decarboxylated to form acetyl CoA or carboxylated to form oxaloacetic acid. The increasing concentrations of acetyl CoA and oxaloacetic acid, both derived from pyruvate, lead to increased production of citrate. The fraction of mitochondrial citrate exceeding that which can be catabolized in the tricarboxylic acid cycle can diffuse back into the cytoplasm and activate acetyl CoA carboxylase[4,182] to produce malonyl CoA and, eventually, more fatty acids. Malonyl CoA and derivatives of long-chain fatty acyl CoA are feedback inhibitors because they are negative effectors of acetyl CoA carboxylase.[183]

Removal of Biotin from Partially Degraded Carboxylases

The bulk of cytosolic and membrane-associated proteins is continuously sequestered and digested by lysosomes. Degradation plays an important role in enzyme regulation and cytoplasmic regrowth, facilitates the correction of synthetic errors, and provides a source of free amino acids that can be used for biosynthetic purposes or for essential metabolic reactions when the exogenous supply is limited. The lysosomal system functions as a general pathway for degrading most enzymes and structural proteins to amino acids or dipeptides.[184] Whole mitochondria are degraded in lysosomes, but additional catabolic pathways must be invoked to account for the breakdown of mitochondrial proteins with short half-lives.[185,186]

Degradation of pyruvate carboxylase, and probably also the other mitochondrial carboxylases, is carried out by the autophagic lysosomal system of the cell.[185–187] The biotin-containing products biocytin and/or biotinyl peptides probably then leave the lysosome and perhaps even enter the plasma before being acted on by biotinidase.[185,187]

Biotinidase

Biotinidase catalyzes the cleavage of biotin from biocytin or biotinyl peptides (see Fig. 156-1) but not from intact holocarboxylases.[7,188] Biotinidase probably plays a role in the processing of dietary protein-bound biotin.[63,64] In one study, serum biotinidase was shown to bind biotin, and it was suggested that biotinidase has a role as a biotin carrier protein,[93] but this was not confirmed in another study.[189] Moreover, biotinidase has been shown to exhibit amino-exopeptidase activity with enkephalins and dynorphin (less than a 10-mer) as likely substrates.[190] In 1954, enzymes in hog liver and kidney and in chicken pancreas were described that released free biotin from the proteolytic digests of hog liver. Biotinidase was partially purified from various bacteria, porcine plasma, kidney, and cerebrum,[62,191–193] and it has been purified to homogeneity from human serum[61,194,195] and human milk.[196]

Biotinidase also has been shown to be biotinylated in the presence of biocytin, but not biotin, at neutral and alkaline pH.[95] The biotinylation likely occurred through a thioester bond formed with a cysteine residue in the active site of the enzyme. This raises the possibility that biotinidase acts as a biotin-binding or biotin-carrier protein. Biotinidase has also been shown to have biotinyl-transferase activity resulting in the transfer of biotin from biocytin to nucleophilic acceptors, such as histones.[197] Transferase activity occurs at physiological pH and at physiological concentrations of biocytin and, therefore, may be the main function of the enzyme in serum and other tissues.

Biochemical Characterization of Biotinidase. Mammalian biotinidase is detectable in most tissues, but the highest activities are present in liver, kidney, serum, and adrenal gland.[62] Human biotinidase is a glycoprotein composed of a single polypeptide having a molecular mass of between 67 and 76 kDa.[61,194,195] It contains an essential thiol and possibly a serine residue in or near the active site[61,194,198] and migrates to the α_1-region during the electrophoresis of serum on agarose gel.[195] The K_m values of the artificial substrate, biotinyl *p*-aminobenzoate, and the natural substrate, biocytin, for biotinidase range from 5 to 10 μM.[61,194] Biotin is one of the end products of the reaction and a competitive inhibitor of the enzyme, the K_i being between 225 and 1300 μM.[61,194] The enzyme in human serum has a broad optimal pH (5 to 7) using biotinyl *p*-aminobenzoate as the substrate and a slightly shifted optimal pH (4 to 6) when biocytin is used.[61] Biotinidase is specific for the biotinyl moiety of various substrates; it cleaves at either amide or ester linkages.[191,194] The enzyme hydrolyzes biocytin much more readily than larger biotin-containing peptides comprised of from 5 to 13 amino acid residues. Biocytin is hydrolyzed 83 times faster than such residues derived from bacterial transcarboxylases.[61] Very large biotin-containing peptides (65 to 123 residues) are cleaved at a greatly reduced rate (1200-fold less) as compared with biocytin. It has been suggested that biocytin or very short biotinyl peptides are the primary substrate of biotinidase in vivo.

We have shown that normal serum biotinidase has at least nine isoforms, four major and five minor isoforms, between pH 4.15 by isoelectric focusing[199] (Fig. 156-3). The major isoforms (isoforms 5 to 8) have at least 75 percent of the total enzyme activity. Two additional anodal isoforms (isoforms 10 and 11) have been observed in 20 and 10 percent of healthy control individuals, respectively. All three isoform patterns were found in both whites and blacks and in males and females. Purified enzyme contains all nine isoforms. Serum from a patient with profound biotinidase deficiency lacked all the proteins that reacted with the antibody, indicating that all the proteins detected are isoforms of biotinidase. The isoform pattern in normal plasma is the same as that in serum.

Normal human serum biotinidase is a single band of approximately 76.5 kDa on sodium dodecyl sulfate (SDS)-polyacrylamide gel electrophoresis, suggesting that the relative molecular mass differences between the isoforms are too small to be resolved by this method. Neuraminidase treatment resulted in a shift in the mobility of the enzyme on SDS-polyacrylamide gel electrophoresis to a position corresponding to 71 kDa. Isolectric focusing of neuraminidase-treated biotinidase results in a reduction in the number of isoforms to one major isoform with a pI of 5.27 and three minor isoforms with pI values of 5.01 (doublet) and 5.31. Treatment of biotinidase with *N*-glycanase resulted in a shift in mobility of the enzyme on SDS-polyacrylamide gel electrophoresis corresponding to a relative molecular mass of approximately 60 kDa. Treatment of biotinidase with *N*-glycanase results in a reduction in relative molecular mass, indicating that biotinidase contains 20 to 22 percent carbohydrate by mass. These carbohydrate moieties must be connected by *N*-glycoside linkages because this exoglycosidase specifically cleaves these bonds. The reduction in relative molecular mass of biotinidase after treatment with neuraminidase indicates that biotinidase contains as many as 18 sialic acid residues. Most of the microheterogeneity observed on isoelectric focusing is likely due to differences in the degree of sialylation. Since neuraminidase treatment of biotinidase results in reduction of the isoforms to one major and three minor isoforms, it is possible that some of the

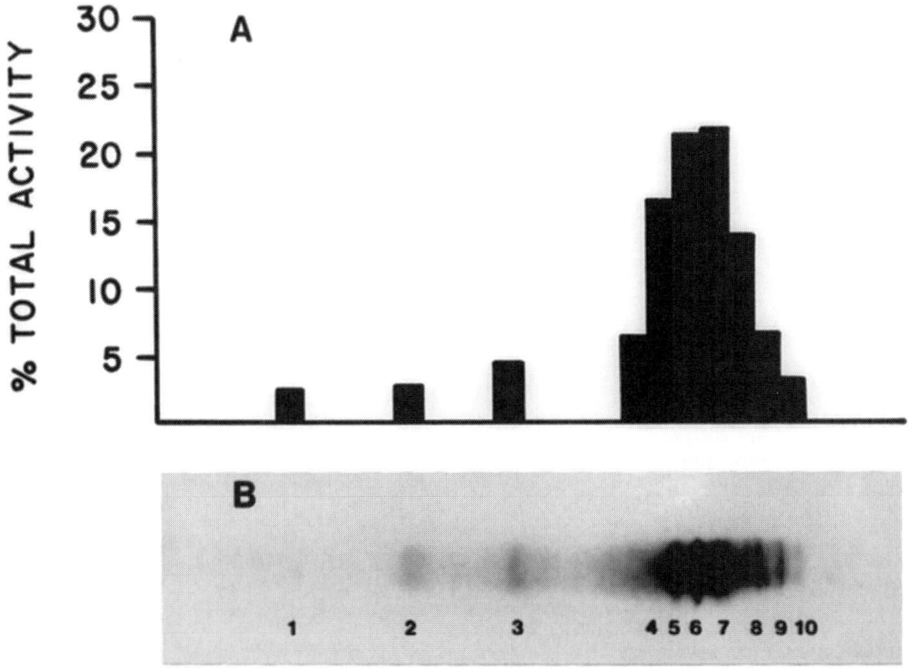

Fig. 156-3 Isoelectric focusing of human serum biotinidase. Serum from a normal individual (80 ml per lane) was focused in two lanes on 7.5 percent hybrid isoelectric focusing gels (pH range of 4.1 to 4.4; 24 cm long). *A.* Biotinidase activity was determined in gel slices of one lane. Position of activity corresponds to the isoforms shown in *B. B.* Immunoblot of the other lane showing isoform pattern with the number of the isoform listed below. (*From Hart et al.*[199] *Used by permission of Elsevier Science Publishers.*)

additional microheterogeneity is due to removal of amino acids from the N-terminus of biotinidase, as seen in other serum glycoproteins.

Increased plasma biotinidase activity, up to two- to threefold that of normal, has been observed in the plasma of individuals with glycogen storage disease type Ia but not in plasma of patients with other forms of glycogen storage disease.[200] The etiology of this increase has not been determined.

Molecular Characterization of the Biotinidase Gene. The cDNA that encodes for normal human serum biotinidase has been cloned from a human liver library using oligonucleotides prepared from the amino acid sequences of purified tryptic peptides of purified biotinidase (Genbank UO3274).[201] Sequence analysis of the cDNA revealed two possible ATG initiator codons and an open reading frame of 1929 bp relative to the first ATG codon and the termination codon. There are 332 bp of 3′ untranslated sequence and a poly(A) addition signal (AATAAA) 24 bp upstream from the 20-bp poly(A) tract. The cDNA encodes for a protein of 543 amino acid residues (molecular mass of 56,661 Da), including 41 amino acids of a potential signal peptide. Comparison of the open reading frame with the tryptic peptides confirmed that this is the cDNA for human serum biotinidase. Expression of the cloned cDNA produced an approximately 53-kDa protein that reacted with monoclonal antibodies prepared against purified human serum biotinidase, thus verifying the validity of this cDNA. Six potential *N*-linked glycosylation sites (Asn–X–Thr/Ser) are present in the deduced amino acid sequence. Glycosylation of the protein could increase its mass by 13 to 19 kDa, assuming that all six of the potential glycosylation sites in the protein were glycosylated and that the glycosylation structures are approximately 2.2 to 3.2 kDa for biantennary and triantennary structures with fucose residues, respectively. The molecular mass of the glycosylated enzyme would be between 70 and 76 kDa, which is consistent with that of the glycosylated serum enzyme. Southern blot analyses suggested that biotinidase is a single-copy gene and that the full-length human cDNA hybridized to single-copy sequences from mammals but not with that from chicken and yeast. Northern blot analyses revealed biotinidase message in human liver, kidney, pancreas, lung, skeletal muscle, heart, brain, and placenta.

The structure of the human biotinidase gene has been determined (Genbank AF018630 and AF018631).[202] The gene is organized into four exons and spans at least 23 kb. The 5′-flanking region of exon 1 contains a CCAAT element, three initiator sequences, an octamer sequence, three methylation consensus sites, two GC boxes, and one HNF-5 site but no TATA element. The region from nucleotides (600 to +400 has features of a CpG island and resembles a housekeeping gene promoter. The biotinidase gene has been mapped to chromosome 3p25.[203]

Forms, Origin, and Sites of Action of Biotinidase. Preliminary studies have shown that serum biotinidase activity correlates positively with the concentration of serum albumin[204]; the concentrations of albumin and the activities of biotinidase in sera of patients with cirrhosis and other hepatic disorders were lowered.[205,206] This suggests that biotinidase in human serum originates principally from the liver. Serum biotinidase activity in rats increases with age and correlates with the increase in serum albumin.[207]

Studies in which hepatotoxic compounds were administered to rats showed that the liver is also the likely source of serum biotinidase in this species.[62] Other tissues with secretory function, such as fibroblasts, leukocytes, and pancreas, as well as the secretory products in pancreatic juice and isolated zymogen granules, have biotinidase activity.[63,208] Biotinidase may be a secretory enzyme that hydrolyzes the products of carboxylase degradation reaching the blood. Because the optimal pH for biotinidase activity is mildly acidic and pyruvate carboxylase is known to be degraded in lysosomes, it is attractive to assume that biotinidase is localized in the lysosome, where it can hydrolyze biotinyl substrates. However, subcellular fractionation studies have revealed that biotinidase activity is enriched in the microsomal fraction and not in the lysosomal fraction.[62,208,209]

The serum enzyme migrates to the α_1-region on agarose gels during electrophoresis. It is sialylated in serum and desialylated in tissues.[194,204] The relatively high specific activity of biotinidase in the serum (about 120 pmol/min/mg of protein as compared with 10 to 50 pmol/min/mg of protein in other tissues) is consistent with the extracellular space being the primary site of action. There is evidence that biotin from degraded carboxylases is not cycled within the cells but rather in the extracellular compartment.[185,187]

Biotinidase in human milk is smaller in size, has a higher pI, has a higher K_i for biotin, and is more markedly activated by β-mercaptoethanol than by the serum enzyme.[196] It is speculated that biotinidase in milk has a role in the intestinal absorption of biotin during infancy.[210] Much remains to be determined about the activities and function of biotinidase.

DISEASE STATES

Isolated deficiencies of each of the mitochondrial carboxylases have been reported. All three isolated mitochondrial carboxylase deficiencies appear to be inherited as autosomal recessive traits.[160] Detailed discussions of these disorders are presented for β-methylcrotonoyl CoA carboxylase deficiency in Chap. 93, for propionyl CoA carboxylase deficiency in Chap. 94, and for pyruvate carboxylase deficiency in Chap. 100. A single case involving an isolated deficiency of the cytosolic enzyme acetyl CoA carboxylase has been reported[9] but has not been substantiated. Our purpose here is to introduce the clinical and biochemical features that may be observed in individuals with isolated carboxylase deficiencies because they may occur in combination in individuals with either of the multiple carboxylase deficiencies caused by holocarboxylase synthetase deficiency or biotinidase deficiency.

Individuals with any one of the isolated mitochondrial carboxylase deficiencies can exhibit vomiting, lethargy, or hypotonia. Some of these children may exhibit seizures and developmental delay. Children with propionyl CoA carboxylase deficiency or pyruvate carboxylase deficiency may become comatose and die. All three disorders are characterized by metabolic ketolactic acidosis. Moderate to severe hyperammonemia may be seen in propionyl CoA carboxylase deficiency, and mild hyperammonemia and hypoglycemia may occur in pyruvate carboxylase deficiency.

All three disorders are characterized by distinctive organic aciduria. Propionyl CoA carboxylase deficiency is characterized by the accumulation of propionic acid in the blood and by the urinary excretion of β-hydroxypropionate, methylcitrate, tiglylglycine, and several other compounds characteristic of ketosis. In pyruvate carboxylase deficiency, the excretion of lactate, alanine, and ketone bodies is elevated. In β-methylcrotonoyl CoA carboxylase deficiency, increased amounts of β-hydroxyisovalerate, β-methylcrotonate, and β-methylcrotonylglycine are excreted.

Children with isolated carboxylase deficiencies do not respond to treatment with biotin.[160,211] Patients with propionyl CoA carboxylase deficiency who were reported to have improved with biotin treatment were shown subsequently to be unresponsive. Most of the children who were reported with biotin-responsive, isolated β-methylcrotonoyl CoA carboxylase deficiency have been shown to have one of the forms of multiple carboxylase deficiency. The biochemical defect in each of the isolated carboxylase deficiencies appears to be an alteration in the structure of the respective carboxylase.[212,213]

The most successful means of treating these children is to restrict their dietary intake of protein and/or the various essential amino acids or odd-chain fatty acids that cannot be catabolized adequately while increasing their caloric intake with carbohydrate and even-chain fatty acids.

There are two biotin-responsive disorders that, because they involve deficient activities of more than one carboxylase, have been known as multiple carboxylase deficiencies. For several years, patients were classified as having either the early-onset (also referred to as *neonatal*) or the late-onset (or *juvenile*) multiple carboxylase deficiency depending on the age at onset of symptoms.[19] Although there is overlap in the age of onset of the two disorders, most individuals with early-onset multiple carboxylase deficiency have altered activity of holocarboxylase synthetase,[20] whereas most individuals with late-onset multiple carboxylase deficiency have deficient activity of biotinidase.[23]

Table 156-1 Frequency of Clinical and Biochemical Features in Children with Biotin Holocarboxylase Synthetase Deficiency*

Percentage of Affected Children	Symptom
100	Ketolactic acidosis
	Organic aciduria
75–100	Hyperammonemia
	Breathing problems; tachypnea and hyperventilation
50–75	Skin rash
25–50	Lethargy
	Irritability
	Feeding problems and vomiting
	Hypotonia/hypertonia
	Seizures
	Odor of urine
	Thrombocytopenia
10–25	Hypothermia
	Hyporeflexia/hyperreflexia
	Developmental delay
	Coma
<10	Ataxia
	Tremor
	Alopecia

*Based on patients reported in the literature.

SOURCE: Data from Wolf,[366] by permission.

Holocarboxylase Synthetase Deficiency

Clinical Manifestations and Biochemical Abnormalities. The clinical and biochemical features of patients with holocarboxylase synthetase deficiency are summarized in Table 156-1.[10,11,13,14,177,214–230] The age of onset of symptoms varied from a few hours after birth to 21 months of age. Most of these children presented with symptoms before reaching 3 months of age.

The most common initial clinical feature was tachypnea or another breathing difficulty. Other common symptoms, which are also observed in children with isolated carboxylase deficiencies, included feeding difficulties, hypotonia, seizures, lethargy, coma, and developmental delay. Many of the children exhibited metabolic acidosis, hyperammonemia, and organic aciduria when they first became symptomatic. Other symptoms that occurred at some time prior to diagnosis included seizures, skin rash, and developmental delay. One child presented with subependymal cysts as a neonate.[229] At 6 months of age following biotin therapy, the child is developmentally normal, and the brain cysts have resolved.

For a time, the absence of a skin rash was thought to distinguish individuals with early-onset multiple carboxylase deficiency from those with the late-onset form, but three of the children with holocarboxylase synthetase deficiency exhibited rashes, and two others had alopecia. Several infants and siblings who probably also were affected became comatose and died before they could be diagnosed and treated. All the children had metabolic ketoacidosis and organic aciduria at some time during the course of their illness.

One affected child had a history of bacteremia. Immunologic studies prior to biotin treatment revealed the absence of lymphocytic response to phytohemagglutinin *in vitro*.[218] The response was restored following the addition of biotin to the culture medium. Abnormalities in immunologic function were attributed to the effects of abnormal accumulations of the metabolites also observed in other organic acidemias.

The gas-liquid chromatographic profiles of organic acids in the urine from these children were characterized by the presence of relatively high concentrations of many of the same metabolites that are elevated in the urine of children with isolated carboxylase deficiencies.[231] These include β-hydroxyisovalerate, β-methylcrotonylglycine, β-hydroxypropionate, methylcitrate, lactate, and tiglylglycine.

Enzyme Defect. In 1971 a child was described with β-methylcrotonylglycinuria.[10] Based on the finding of β-methylcrotonylglycine in the child's urine, it was suspected and later confirmed that the patient had a deficiency of β-methylcrotonoyl CoA carboxylase.[13] Other metabolites, including β-hydroxypropionate and methylcitrate, that were identified subsequently in the urine of this patient were consistent with propionyl CoA carboxylase deficiency. It was found that the activities of both these carboxylases were deficient in the child's fibroblasts.[15] The final concentration of biotin in the medium (Minimal Essential Medium supplemented with 10% fetal calf serum) was 6 nM. Eventually, the third mitochondrial carboxylase, pyruvate carboxylase, was shown to be deficient in this fibroblast line,[232] and the disorder was termed *neonatal* or *early-onset multiple carboxylase deficiency.*[19]

Fibroblasts of patients with this disorder that are incubated in medium containing a low concentration of biotin have deficient activities of the three mitochondrial carboxylases,[15,17,232–235] but when the medium is supplemented with a higher concentration of biotin (> 100 nM), the carboxylase activities increase to within the normal range. The restoration of carboxylase activity is demonstrable even in the presence of cycloheximide (an inhibitor of protein synthesis), which suggests that activation of preexisting apocarboxylases rather than *de novo* protein synthesis is responsible for the increased activity.[17]

Fibroblasts from patients with early-onset multiple carboxylase deficiency complement fibroblasts from children with isolated propionyl CoA carboxylase deficiency.[232,236,237] The propionyl CoA carboxylase activities in the heterokaryons produced in cell fusions of the two enzyme-deficient fibroblast lines increased significantly above those in cultures of mixed, unfused cells. The fibroblasts from the early-onset disorder also complement fibroblasts from patients with isolated pyruvate carboxylase deficiency; pyruvate carboxylase activity in the heterokaryons increases.[232,238] Cultured cells from children with early-onset biotin-responsive multiple carboxylase deficiency do not complement one another, and they have been designated the bio (for *biotin-responsive holocarboxylase synthetase deficiency*) genetic complementation group.[232,236,237] Each of the lines belonging to this bio complementation group appears, therefore, to have a defect in the same enzyme. Several of the fibroblast lines that have been assigned to the bio group also have deficiency of the fourth biotin-dependent enzyme, acetyl CoA carboxylase.[16,176,177] These studies suggest that the enzymatic defect in this disorder is an inability to biotinylate the various apocarboxylases effectively.

The primary defect in early-onset multiple carboxylase deficiency was confirmed in experiments using the apoenzyme substrate apopropionyl CoA carboxylase purified 200-fold from the livers of rats made biotin-deficient by feeding them a diet containing avidin.[20] This apoenzyme preparation was then incubated with fibroblast extracts containing holocarboxylase synthetase in the presence of biotin, ATP, and $Mg.^{2+}$ In normal fibroblast extracts, the holocarboxylase synthetase catalyzed the formation of holopropionyl CoA carboxylase. The activity of the holopropionyl CoA carboxylase was then determined by measuring the fixation of radioactive bicarbonate to propionyl CoA to form labeled methylmalonyl CoA. When extracts of fibroblasts from a patient with early-onset multiple carboxylase deficiency were used, the formation of the methylmalonyl CoA was decreased. The K_m of holocarboxylase synthetase for biotin in the normal fibroblast line was 8.2 nM, whereas the K_m for biotin in cells from the patient was 516 nM (a 63-fold elevation). The V_{max} was only 30 to 40 percent of normal. These findings indicated that the primary defect in early-onset multiple carboxylase deficiency was in holocarboxylase synthetase.

These results were further substantiated by other studies of fibroblasts from patients with early-onset multiple carboxylase deficiency.[239] Cells from a normal and an affected child were made biotin-deficient by maintaining them in medium supplemented with biotin-depleted fetal calf serum. Mitochondria prepared from these cells were incubated with ATP, biotin, and propionyl CoA, and the incorporation of radioactive bicarbonate into methylmalonyl CoA was measured. These studies revealed a K_m of holocarboxylase synthetase for biotin in normal cells of 0.1 mM and a greatly increased K_m of 554 mM in the cells of an affected child. The discrepancy between the K_m values in these two studies may be due to the difference in the species used and/or the sources of apoenzyme.

In a third study, holocarboxylase synthetase activity was determined in extracts of lymphoblasts that had been cultured in biotin-deficient medium.[240] Cell extracts from a normal individual and from a child with early-onset multiple carboxylase deficiency were incubated with ATP and Mg^{2+} in the presence and absence of biotin and then evaluated for propionyl CoA carboxylase activity. Extracts from normal cells, incubated with biotin, showed increased propionyl CoA carboxylase activity above that in extracts from cells that were not incubated with biotin, whereas extracts from the patient showed no change in activity. Moreover, when an extract of normal cells, from which the apocarboxylase had been removed by immunoprecipitation, was incubated with the patient's cell extract, the propionyl CoA carboxylase activity increased about 20-fold.

Holocarboxylase synthetase was characterized in peripheral blood leukocytes and skin fibroblasts from seven children with deficiencies.[25] The activities of the mitochondrial carboxylases varied from 0 to 30 percent of normal in fibroblasts incubated in low-biotin (6 nM) medium. The carboxylase activities increased when the cells were incubated with 220 nM biotin in the medium but failed to increase above 30 percent of normal even when the cells of patient 1 (Table 156-2), who had the highest K_m for biotin, were incubated in medium containing 8000 nM biotin.

The K_m of holocarboxylase synthetase for biotin in these patients ranged from 3 to 70 times the normal concentration. The K_m and the age at onset of symptoms in affected children are strongly negatively correlated, i.e., high K_m with early onset. All but two patients (1 and 7) had a V_{max} of propionyl CoA carboxylase activity in fibroblasts that was below the normal range. Similar results were found in the leukocytes of these two patients. The K_m of ATP for the synthetase in controls ranged from 0.13 to 0.35 mM, whereas the K_m was normal for two patients

Table 156-2 Kinetic Properties of Holocarboxylase Synthetase in Human Fibroblasts

Source of Fibroblasts	K_w Biotin nM	V_{max} of Proprionyl CoA Carboxylase (pmol of Bicarbonate Incorporated/min/mg Protein)
Holocarboxylase synthase deficiency*		
Patient 1	1062	42
Patient 2	718	102
Patient 3	394	124
Patient 4	346	119
Patient 5	322	70
Patient 6	281	95
Patient 7	48	96
Biotinidase deficiency:		
Mean ± 1 SD (n = 6)	15±6	210±196
Normal:		
Mean ± 1 SD (n = 5)	15 ± 3	345±145

*The data for K_w and V_{max} for each patient are single determinations.

SOURCE: Data from Burri et al.,[25] by permission.

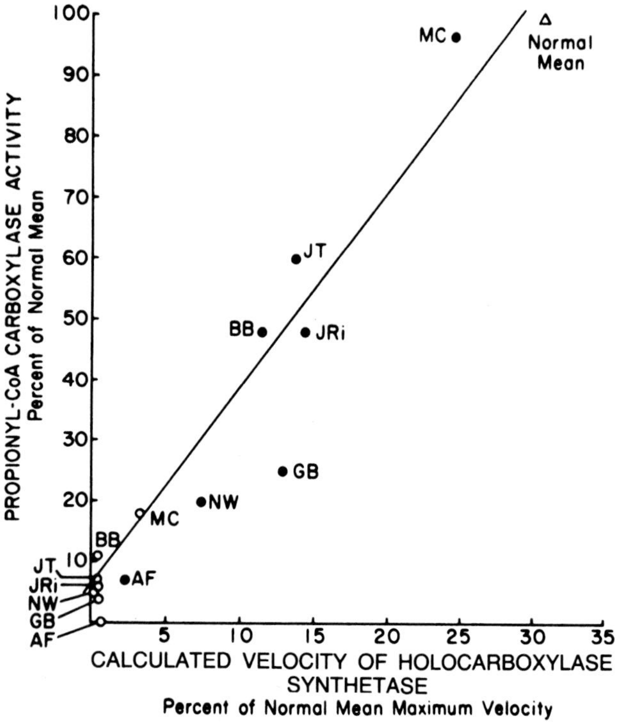

Fig. 156-4 Relationship between propionyl CoA carboxylase activity and holocarboxylase synthetase velocity in fibroblast extracts from patients with holocarboxylase synthetase deficiency. The holocarboxylase synthetase velocities, expressed as the percentage of mean normal maximum activity, were calculated from K_m values determined for biotin, and the concentrations of biotin in the culture medium, using the Michaelis-Menten equation. Open circles represent cells cultured in a low concentration of biotin (6 nM), and the closed circles represent cells cultured in a higher concentration of biotin (220 nM). (*From Burri et al.*[25] *Used by permission of American Journal of Human Genetics.*)

with holocarboxylase synthetase deficiency and was elevated at 1.32 mM for patient 1.

Preliminary studies indicated that the apopropionyl CoA carboxylase concentration that resulted in maximal activity for holocarboxylase synthetase in fibroblast homogenates from two control subjects did not result in maximal activity in cell homogenates from two of the patients. The instability of the apoenzyme in the preparation did not permit quantitation of the K_m for this substrate.

The percentage of mean normal maximum velocity of holocarboxylase synthetase was calculated from the data in Fig. 156-4 using the Michaelis-Menten equation for low (6 nM) and high (220 nM) biotin concentrations. The resulting propionyl CoA carboxylase activity was determined in the patients' fibroblasts that were cultured in one or the other medium. There was a linear relationship between the percentage of mean normal propionyl CoA carboxylase activity and both the calculated velocity of holocarboxylase synthetase activity and the percentage of mean normal maximal velocity (see Fig. 156-4). Thus the kinetic properties of the synthetase *in vitro* appear to be highly positively correlated with the functional activity of its product, holopropionyl CoA carboxylase.

Although the optimal pH of holocarboxylase synthetase in two of the enzyme-deficient fibroblast lines (patients 4 and 5) was the same as in normal lines, the heat stabilities differed. Of the five patients studied, the synthetase was less stable than normal in two (patients 2 and 7) and more stable in three (patients 1, 4, and 5). These findings demonstrate the biochemical heterogeneity of the defect.

The activity of biotinyl AMP synthetase, the first partial reaction in the biotinylation of apocarboxylases, is deficient in all patients with holocarboxylase synthetase deficiency thus far studied.[241] Several new methods have been developed to assay holocarboxylase synthetase activity that use prepared acceptors of biotin. One method measures the incorporation of [^{3}H]biotin into apocarboxyl carrier protein.[242] The K_m for biotin in extracts of normal fibroblasts was 260 nM. Another method measures the biotinylation of bacterial carboxyl carrier protein or the expressed C-terminal fragment of a subunit of human propionyl CoA carboxylase.[172] These assays facilitate the diagnosis of children with holocarboxylase synthetase deficiency.

All patients with holocarboxylase synthetase deficiency have responded to vitamin therapy. Moreover, there is detectable residual synthetase activity in tissues of all affected children. These results suggest that complete deficiency of the enzyme may be lethal in utero.

Mutations Causing Holocarboxylase Synthetase Deficiency. Multiple mutations have been elucidated in the DNA of children with holocarboxylase synthetase deficiency (Fig. 156-5). The first mutations in the holocarboxylase synthetase gene elucidated and the most common in Japanese children (five children of four unrelated families) are a 1-bp deletion (1067delG) that results in premature termination of the enzyme protein and a 1-base substitution (L237P) that, when expressed, results in decreased synthetase activity.[243] Another study demonstrated six different missense mutations in nine children with synthetase

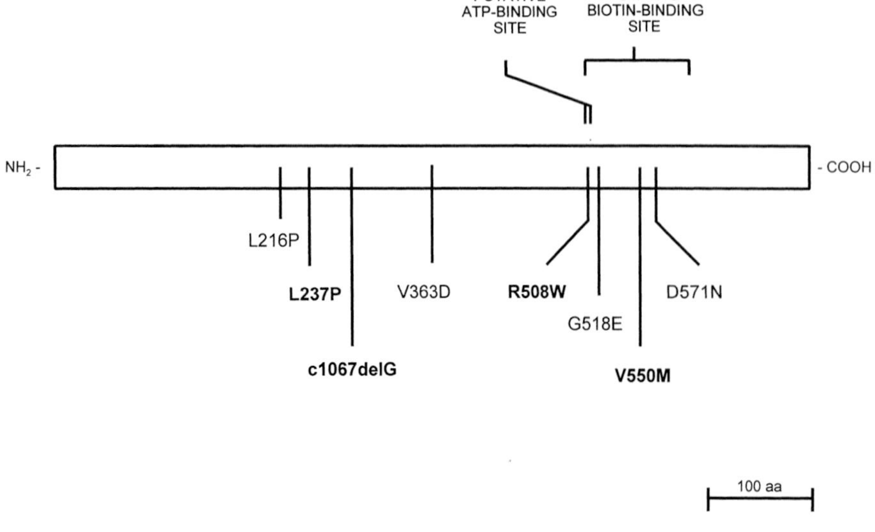

Fig. 156-5 The predicted protein structure of human holocarboxylase synthetase from the cDNA. Mutations and their locations in the enzyme are shown. The more common mutations are shown in boldface. The approximate regions of the putative biotin-binding and ATP-binding sites, based on homology with BirA and avidin, are indicated.

deficiency.[244] Four of the mutations are within the putative biotin-binding domain, including two more common mutations, R508W and V550M. Alterations within this binding domain likely explain the biotin responsiveness in these patients. The missense mutation V550M, which is within the putative biotin-binding domain, and L237P, which is outside the biotin-binding domain, were expressed in holocarboxylase synthetase-deficient fibroblasts.[245] The K_m for biotin was elevated compared with that of the normal enzyme and the enzyme produced with the V550M mutation but was not elevated for the enzyme with the L237P mutation. The V_{max} for the enzyme with the L237P mutation was 4.3 percent of the mean normal value. Biotin responsiveness in patients with the L237P mutation is not due to decreased biotin affinity or restoration of enzyme stability. It is speculated that the enzyme with this alteration has little or no activity at biotin concentrations achieved by normal diet, but the activity increases, but not to normal, when the child is supplemented with pharmacologic doses of biotin. It also has been speculated that a fetus homozygous for the L237P mutation would not be viable. There also has been a child with synthetase deficiency who had a decreased affinity for biotin and a decreased V_{max}.[230] This patient may be a compound heterozygote with one mutation that is identical or similar to the L237P mutation.

Genetics. Holocarboxylase synthetase deficiency has been reported in males and females. Several families have had more than one affected child, but consanguinity has not been demonstrated in any family. These findings are consistent with an autosomal recessive pattern of inheritance. An attempt to demonstrate heterozygosity for the condition in the mother of one patient by studying the activity or kinetic properties of her holocarboxylase synthetase was unsuccessful.[25] Therefore, heterozygotes for holocarboxylase synthetase deficiency may not be identified using the enzyme assays currently available, but this should be possible by mutation analysis.

Treatment. Patients with holocarboxylase synthetase deficiency usually improve with oral administration of 10 mg of biotin per day. Children treated before irreversible neurologic damage occurred generally have shown resolution of the clinical symptoms and biochemical abnormalities. However, the child whose holocarboxylase synthetase in fibroblasts had the highest K_m for biotin continued to excrete abnormal organic acids and to have a mild skin rash even when treated with 60 to 80 mg of biotin per day.[25] Another infant, who had disseminated intravascular coagulopathy and congestive heart failure, died a few days after biotin therapy was begun.[214,215] Biotin that is approved for human use is available from Hoffmann-LaRoche Company in Nutley, New Jersey.

Prenatal Diagnosis. Prenatal diagnosis of holocarboxylase synthetase deficiency has been performed by demonstrating deficient carboxylase activities in cultured amniocytes. The activities increased toward normal values after the cells had been incubated in the presence of biotin.[246] Demonstration of elevated concentrations of β-hydroxyisovalerate and/or methylcitrate in the amniotic fluid by stable isotope dilution techniques appears to be a simpler and more rapid method of prenatal diagnosis.[246,247] The diagnosis can be confirmed by performing both diagnostic procedures on the same sample of amniotic fluid.

Prenatal Therapy. Prenatal treatment of holocarboxylase synthetase deficiency has been performed in two pregnancies in which siblings had been diagnosed previously with the disorder. In the first pregnancy, prenatal diagnosis was not performed.[248] The mother took 10 mg biotin orally beginning at 34 weeks of gestation. The pregnancy resulted in the birth of nonidentical twins. At birth, both twins were clinically normal, both had elevated concentrations of serum biotin, and neither had organic aciduria. Skin fibroblasts from these infants were cultured, and treatment with biotin was withheld pending the outcome of confirmatory enzyme analyses. At 3 months of age one of the twins became clinically and biochemically symptomatic.[216] Fortunately, treatment with 10 mg biotin rapidly reversed the clinical course. This twin was subsequently confirmed to have synthetase deficiency by enzyme analysis, and the other twin was shown to be unaffected.

In the second pregnancy, the fetus was diagnosed prenatally as having holocarboxylase synthetase deficiency.[246] The mother received 10 mg biotin daily beginning at 23.5 weeks of gestation. The infant was clinically normal at birth, and the profile of urinary organic acids was normal. Both synthetase-deficient children have remained asymptomatic and are developing normally while continuing to be treated with biotin. Although the symptoms of holocarboxylase synthetase deficiency can appear soon after birth, it is not clear whether prenatal treatment with biotin is essential. Treatment of at-risk children with biotin immediately after birth until their enzyme status has been determined may be sufficient in this disorder.

Biotinidase Deficiency

Clinical Manifestations and Biochemical Abnormalities. The clinical features of over 120 patients with biotinidase deficiency are summarized in Table 156-3.[6,18,26,34,65,226–228,249–300] About an equal number of females and males are reported. All the children exhibited at least some of the symptoms usually seen in patients with late-onset multiple carboxylase deficiency. The age of onset of symptoms varied from 1 week to years, with median and mean ages of 3 and 5.5 months, respectively. Acute loss of vision, progressive optic neuropathy, and spastic paraparesis have developed in one patient at 10 years of age.[301] The most common initial neurologic symptoms were myoclonic seizures and hypotonia. Several patients exhibited ataxia developmental delay and breathing problems such as hyperventilation, stridor, or apnea. Other common initial symptoms included seborrheic or atopic dermatitis, partial or complete alopecia, and conjunctivitis. Many affected individuals initially showed combinations of these

Table 156-3 Frequency of Clinical and Biochemical Features in Children with Biotinidase Deficiency*

Percentage of Affected Children	Symptom
>50	Alopecia
	Development
	Hypotonia
	Ketolactic acidosis
	Organic aciduria
	Seizures
	Skin rash/skin infection
25–50	Ataxia
	Conjunctivitis
	Hearing loss
	Lethargy
	Mild hyperammonemia
	Tachypnea/apnea/breathing problems
	Visual abnormalities: loss of vision/ optic atrophy
10–25	Coma
	Feeding difficulties/vomiting/diarrhea
	Fungal infections
<10	Hepatomegaly
	Speech problems
	Splenomegaly

*Based on over 80 patients reported in the literature and known to the author.

SOURCE: Data from Wolf,[366] by permission.

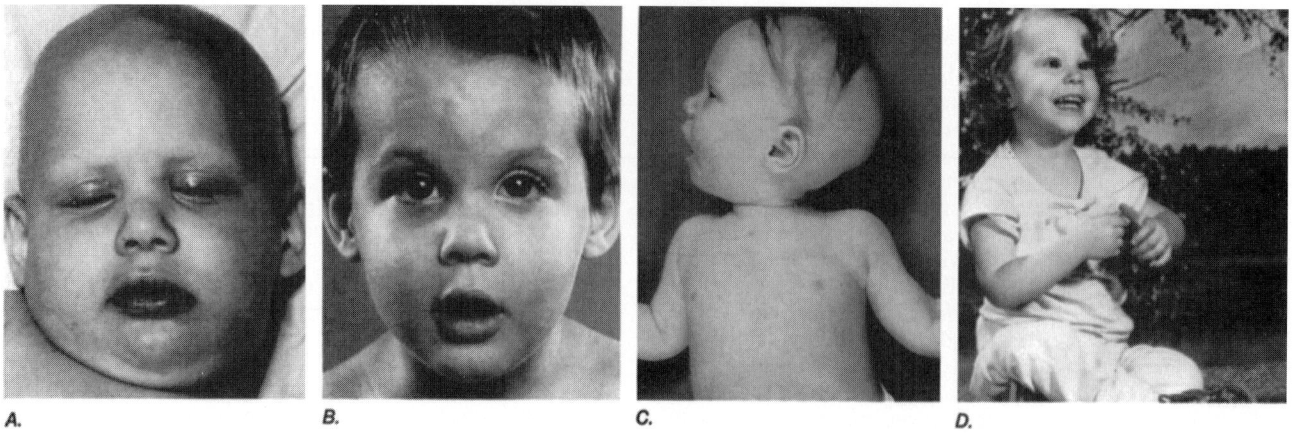

Fig. 156-6 Two children with biotinidase deficiency shown before and after biotin treatment. *A.* Child with biotinidase deficiency at 2 years and 9 months of age with alopecia and periorbital and perioral rash, before biotin therapy. *B.* Same child after 4 months of biotin therapy. *(From Thoene et al.[251] Used by permission of New England Journal of Medicine.)* *C.* Child with biotinidase deficiency at 10 months of age, before biotin therapy. *D.* Same child at 30 months of age, after 20 months of biotin therapy.

neurologic and cutaneous findings. The two children depicted in Fig. 156-6*A* and *C* exhibit several of the symptoms typical of biotinidase deficiency.

More than 70 percent of the patients had seizures[302] or hypotonia or alopecia at some time prior to diagnosis and treatment. About half the children had ataxia, developmental delay, conjunctivitis, and visual problems,[303] including optic atrophy. Hearing loss, which was usually sensorineural in nature, was diagnosed in about 40 percent of the patients. Four of the affected children died while in metabolic coma. In addition, several siblings of biotinidase-deficient children reported in the literature also have died and probably also were affected.

Over 80 percent of the patients had organic aciduria, and 75 percent of the patients had metabolic ketoacidosis at some time. The most frequently observed abnormal urinary metabolite was β-hydroxyisovaleric acid. Other commonly observed metabolites included lactate, β-methylcrotonylglycine, β-hydroxypropionate, and methylcitrate. When looked for, mild hyperammonemia often was found to be present. There is clinical variability among affected individuals from different families, and there is also considerable variability in expression of the disorder among affected individuals within a sibship.[256]

Among 100 Japanese children with intractable seborrheic dermatitis, 2 children were found with serum biotinidase activities of 15 and 30 percent of normal.[304] These children had no neurologic symptoms. The dermatitis resolved after biotin therapy. Because all the biotinidase-deficient patients in whom neurologic symptoms developed in addition to cutaneous symptoms have had less than 5 percent of normal activity, this study may provide further insight into the clinical variability and spectrum of the disorder. Individuals with partial enzyme deficiency may be at risk for developing only cutaneous symptoms.

Abnormalities of the brain, such as cerebral atrophy and ventricular dilation, have been reported in symptomatic children. These alterations resolved in several of these children following biotin therapy[285,296] but persisted in others.

Four children with profound biotinidase deficiency first developed symptoms later in childhood or during adolescence.[305] They had motor limb weakness, spastic paresis, and eye problems, such as loss of visual acuity and scotomata, rather than the more characteristic symptoms observed in young untreated children with the disorder. In addition, a 5-year-old girl developed acute visual loss associated with optic atrophy and disturbance of gait with lower limb pyramidal signs.[300] She was developmentally normal and had no others symptoms.

An adult man and a woman with profound biotinidase deficiency were asymptomatic and were diagnosed only because their biotinidase-deficient children were identified by newborn screening.[306] These adults never exhibited symptoms of the disorder and are homozygous for two different mutations resulting in different abnormal enzymes. There was no evidence of an increased dietary intake of biotin to explain why they have remained asymptomatic. Although these adults may still be at risk for developing symptoms, they may represent a small group of individuals with profound biotinidase deficiency who will never develop clinical problems. Their lack of symptoms suggests that there are epigenetic factors that protect some enzyme-deficient individuals from developing symptoms.

Prior to the elucidation of the primary enzyme defect of late-onset multiple carboxylase deficiency, diagnosis depended in part on the presence of demonstrable organic aciduria. The absence of this finding would have excluded about 17 percent of our cases of biotinidase deficiency. Although the biochemical abnormalities attributed to biotinidase deficiency are often life-threatening, they appear to represent relatively late effects of the disorder. The cutaneous symptoms and some of the neurologic features are similar to those seen in biotin-deficiency states, and they usually occur early in the course of the disease. The skin findings may be associated with fatty acid abnormalities,[307] possibly attributable to deficient activity of acetyl CoA carboxylase.[308]

Immunoregulatory dysfunction has been reported in several children with biotinidase deficiency.[309] Three affected children from one family exhibited *Candida* dermatitis.[249] Two were evaluated and showed absence of delayed hypersensitivity by skin test and by *in vitro* lymphocyte responses to *Candida* challenge.[249,250] The responses to phytohemagglutinin in mixed-lymphocyte cultures were normal. One of these children had IgA deficiency and failed to respond to pneumococcal immunization, whereas the other had subnormal amounts of T-lymphocytes in peripheral blood. A third affected child, who was studied prior to biotin treatment, had normal B- and T-lymphocyte counts and responded normally to a *Candida* skin test.[251] A fourth patient had normal immunoglobulins and B-lymphocyte counts but had only 50 percent of the normal number of T-lymphocytes. Leukocyte killing activity against *Candida* was reduced in this patient, and the neutrophils lacked myeloperoxidase activity. The immunologic functions became normal after the child was treated with biotin. A fifth child was shown to have impaired lymphocyte suppressor activity and prostaglandin E_2 production *in vitro*, in addition to low linoleic acid concentrations in plasma.[310,311] Incubation of the T-lymphocytes with biotin restored the suppressor activity. Since prostaglandin E_2 is synthesized from linoleic acid, it was suggested that a deficiency of acetyl CoA carboxylase resulted in deficient malonyl CoA formation that, in turn, affected prostaglandin E_2 synthesis. Biotin treatment corrected these abnormalities. Another child with biotinidase deficiency was diagnosed initially as having severe combined immunodeficiency and was treated with bone marrow transplantation, but the symptoms were not ameliorated until biotin was given.[269] The clinical features resolved with biotin therapy. The findings in these reports are inconsistent, and further systematic immunologic evaluation of biotinidase-deficient children before and after therapy is needed to characterize better the immunologic dysfunction in this disorder.

Loading tests performed on patients whose tissues are severely biotin depleted apparently result in the rapid entry of the vitamin into these tissues with the result that biotin concentrations in plasma are misleadingly low. In one of two patients described initially as having impaired intestinal transport of biotin,[22] it was shown later that the response to oral biotin was normal when the loading test was conducted when the tissues were not depleted of biotin.[24] We would expect the other patient to respond similarly if the appropriate loading study were performed.[21] Therefore, to date no patient has been confirmed to have abnormal intestinal absorption of biotin.

Pathology. The postmortem findings in the brains of three children with presumptive biotinidase deficiency were similar. In the first patient, aged 3 years at the time of death, there was chronic cerebellar degeneration and atrophy characterized by the absence of the Purkinje cell layer, rarefaction of the granular layer, and proliferation of the Bergmann layer.[250] There was gliosis in the white matter and dentate nucleus. The cerebellar peduncles and brain stem were normal. Focal necrosis with vascular proliferation and infiltration by macrophages characterized the subacute necrotizing myelopathy. There also was acute meningoencephalitis of the entire central nervous system.

The second child died at 3 months of age.[312] Pathologic examination of the brain revealed defective myelination, focal areas of vacuolization, and gliosis in the white matter of the cerebrum and cerebellum. There was mild gliosis in the pyramidal cell layer of the hippocampus, and there were characteristic changes of viral encephalopathy in the putamen and, to a lesser extent, in the caudate nucleus.

The third patient was diagnosed initially as having Leigh syndrome.[313] There was softening and discoloration of the corpus callosum, fornix, periventricular areas of the thalamic nuclei, mammillary bodies, and periaqueductal gray matter. There were spongy lesions in the white matter of the cerebrum, midbrain, pons, medulla, and the cerebellar nuclei. Histologically, the lesions exhibited rarefaction and sponginess of neuropil, increase in the small blood vessels, enlargement of the endothelial cells, astrocytosis, and loss of oligodendrocytic nuclei and myelin sheaths. The axons and nerve cell bodies were less affected, except for a decreased number of axons in the optic nerves and mammillary bodies.

Pathophysiology. Biotin deficiency does not alter biotinidase activity *in vitro*. The activities in the sera of several patients who became biotin deficient while receiving parenteral hyperalimentation were normal.[23,314] Biotin-deficient rats and rats receiving adequate dietary biotin have similar biotinidase activities,[315] and it seems likely that the cutaneous and neurologic symptoms observed early in biotinidase-deficient patients may result from a mild to moderate depletion of biotin. Skin of biotin-deficient rats had 30 percent of the fatty acid content of skin of biotin-replete rats.[316] This loss of protective fatty acids may predispose the skin to alopecia and other abnormalities.

Biotinidase may play a critical role in the processing of dietary protein-bound biotin.[63] We do not know whether biocytin and biotinyl peptides can be absorbed without first being hydrolyzed in the mucosa or in the intestinal lumen by biotinidase originating from bacteria, pancreatic juice, the intestinal mucosa, or all these sources. If the action of biotinidase is a prerequisite, and if the production of biotin and biotinidase by intestinal microorganisms is quantitatively unimportant, then patients with biotinidase deficiency would lack a mechanism for liberating protein-bound biotin from food and would depend entirely on dietary free biotin to meet their requirements for the vitamin.

Biotinidase activity in human brain and cerebrospinal fluid is very low.[193,317] The brain therefore may be unable to recycle biotin and may depend on biotin transferred across the blood-brain barrier. The early stages of biotin deficiency that occur in biotinidase deficiency may cause a moderate decrease in pyruvate carboxylase activity and result in preferential accumulation of lactate in the brain.[263,318,319] This localized lactic acidosis may cause the appearance of neurologic symptoms before many of the other symptoms develop. Ketoacidosis and organic aciduria probably appear only after protracted biotin deficiency occurs.

Usually, the hearing loss in biotinidase-deficient patients has been observed before the initiation of biotin treatment. Rats made biotin-deficient but with normal serum biotinidase activity had abnormal auditory evoked potential studies. This suggests that biotin deficiency alone may cause hearing loss.[320,321] The deficit usually does not appear to improve after biotin therapy.[322–324] Improvement of hearing with biotin treatment has been reported.[271] It is possible that the hearing loss is caused by the accumulation of organic acids or by the accumulation of biocytin or larger biotinyl peptides. Either or both of these events may alter the metabolic pathways involved in the development and/or function of the auditory system. The metabolism of organic acids normalizes after biotin treatment is begun, but biocytin and biotinyl peptides would be expected to accumulate.[325] Although there is no evidence suggesting that hearing loss worsens after treatment is begun, reports of follow-up evaluations are scarce, and it is possible that hearing loss may be progressive. Conversely, it is conceivable that the adverse effects of biocytin and biotinyl peptides on hearing would be prevented in the presence of adequate free biotin.

Although the abnormally high urinary output of biotin by several biotinidase-deficient patients has been attributed to defective reabsorption by the kidney tubules,[81,326,327] this finding also could be caused by the absence of biotinidase functioning as a plasma biotin-binding protein.[63,326] If biotinidase normally acts as a biotin-binding protein in serum, as some have suggested, and if it is absent from the sera of biotinidase-deficient patients or so altered structurally as to be unable to interact with biotin, then the increased excretion of biotin by these patients could be explained by the following mechanism.[63,328] Assuming that in the biotin-replete state normal individuals and biotinidase-deficient patients have similar concentrations of biotin in their sera, the gradient between the serum and the lumen of renal tubules for free biotin would be greater in the patients, and hence they would excrete more biotin.

Enzyme Defect. In 1983, Wolf and colleagues[23] demonstrated that the primary biochemical defect in patients with late-onset multiple carboxylase deficiency was deficient activity of biotinidase. Biotinidase activity has been determined by measuring the release of biotin from biocytin using several microbiologic assays[7,188] and by the release of chromophoric or fluorescent amino compounds from biotinylated substrates. Enzyme activity was determined using a method in which *p*-aminobenzoate released from the artificial substrate *N*-biotinyl *p*-aminobenzoate is diazotized, coupled with a naphthol derivative to form an azo dye, and measured colorimetrically.[191] This assay has been automated.[329] The liberation of *p*-aminobenzoate also can be monitored fluorometrically after the product has been separated from the substrate by high-performance liquid chromatography.[330] Another fluorometric method has been developed that measures the liberation of 6-aminoquinoline from a different artificial substrate, *N*-biotinyl 6-aminoquinoline.[331]

Several assay methods have been developed that use the natural substrate biocytin to measure biotinidase activity. The first, a bioassay, measures the increase in propionyl CoA carboxylase

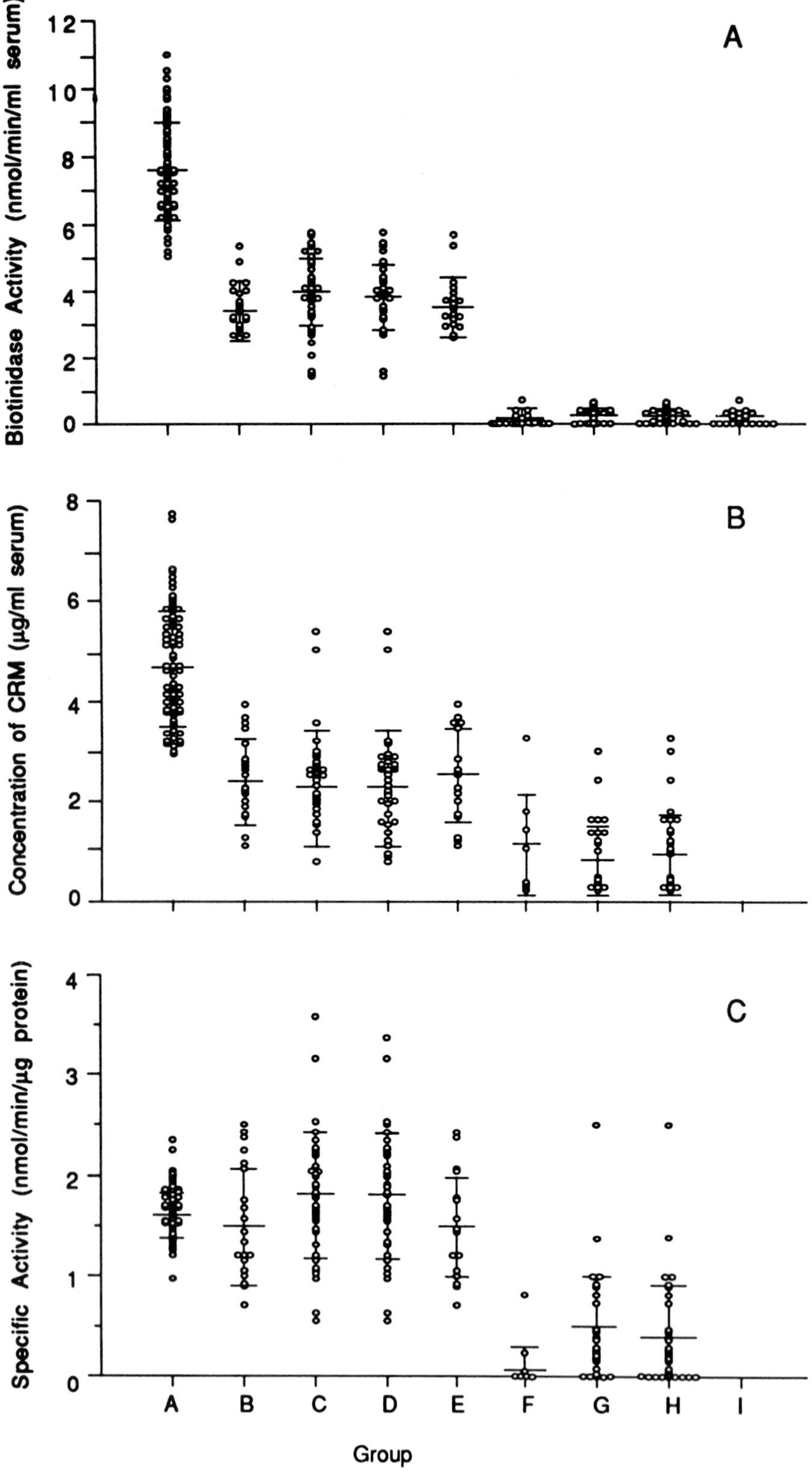

Fig. 156-7 Distribution of biotinidase activity, concentration of CRM, and specific activity in children with profound biotinidase deficiency, their parents, and normal individuals. Bar indicates mean ± SD for each group. *A.* Distribution of biotinidase activity. Group A: Normal individuals (mean = 7.57 ± 1.41 nmol/min/ml serum, *n* = 100). Group B: Parents of children who were ascertained clinically (mean = 3.49 ± 0.72, *n* = 21). Group C: Parents of children who were identified by newborn screening (mean = 3.96 ± 0.99, *n* = 42). Group D: Parents of children who were found to have CRM in their serum (mean = 3.88 ± 0.96, *n* = 45). Group E: Parents of children who lacked CRM in their serum (mean = 3.61 ± 0.85, *n* = 18). Group F: Patients who were symptomatic (mean = 0.12 ± 0.18, *n* = 23). Group G: Patients who were identified by newborn screening (mean = 0.19 ± 0.16, *n* = 41). Group H: Patients who had CRM in their serum (mean = 0.19 ± 0.16, *n* = 42). Group I: Patients who lacked CRM in their serum (mean = 0.13 ± 0.18, *n* = 26). *B.* Distribution of the concentration of CRM in biotinidase. Group A: Mean = 4.7 ± 1.1 mg/ml serum. Group B: Mean = 2.5 ± 0.8. Group C: Mean = 2.4 ± 0.8. Group D: Mean = 2.4 ± 0.8. Group E: Mean = 2.7 ± 0.8. Group F: Mean = 1.1 ± 1.0. Group G: Mean = 0.8 ± 0.7. Group H: Mean = 0.9 ± 0.8. The patients with profound enzyme deficiency who lacked CRM are not shown. *C.* Distribution of the specific activity of biotinidase. Group A: Mean = 1.63 ± 0.22 nmol/min/mg protein. Group B: Mean = 1.53 ± 0.56. Group C: Mean = 1.77 ± 0.60. Group D: Mean = 1.78 ± 0.60. Group E: Mean = 1.47 ± 0.52. Group F: Mean = 0.14 ± 0.28. Group G: Mean = 0.46 ± 0.54. Group H: Mean = 0.37 ± 0.50. (*From Hart et al.*[338] *Used by permission of American Journal of Human Genetics.*)

activity in holocarboxylase synthetase-deficient fibroblasts in response to the liberation of biotin from biocytin by biotinidase from serum.[332] This method was used to confirm that sera from children shown to be biotinidase deficient using the artificial substrate also were deficient using the natural substrate.

Other methods available include a radioassay that measures the liberation of [^{14}C]biotin from [^{14}C]biocytin using separation by ion-exchange chromatography[333] and a fluorometric assay in which the lysine released from biocytin is conjugated with a chromophore after the lysine initially in the sample is removed by dialysis.[334]

The mean biotinidase activity measured by the colorimetric method in the sera of 521 healthy, normal children and adults was 7.1 nmol *p*-aminobenzoate per minute per milliliter, with a range of 3.5 to 12.0 nmol (Fig. 156-7). Biotinidase activity in the sera of children with the clinical features of late-onset multiple carboxylase deficiency was deficient in the range of 0 to 9 percent of mean normal activity. The activities in the sera of obligate

Table 156-4 Biotinidase Activity in Tissues of Individuals with Normal and Deficient Activity in Serum

Tissue	Normal or Serum Enzyme-Deficient Individuals	Biotinidase Activity (pmol of *p*-Aminobenzoate/min/ml or mg Protein)		
		Mean	SD	Range
Serum (ml)	Normal (n=8)	6000	800	4400–7600
	Deficient (n=3)	0		0
Leukocytes* (mg protein)	Normal (n=3)	51	21	29–85
	Deficient (n=2)	0		0
Fibroblasts (mg protein)	Normal (n=6)	29	5	23-36
	Deficient (n=5)	0.1		0–0.3

Prepared from peripheral blood.

SOURCE: Data from Wolf et al.,[314] by permission.

heterozygotes were intermediate between those of affected children and normal controls. We have shown that heterozygosity can be determined with about 95 percent accuracy with this method.[335]

Extracts of fibroblasts from normal individuals have very low detectable activity using the colorimetric assay.[23] Using a more sensitive radioassay based on the liberation of [^{14}C]carboxyl *p*-aminobenzoate from *N*-biotinyl *p*-amino [^{14}C]benzoate, biotinidase activity was demonstrated in extracts of peripheral blood leukocytes and fibroblasts of normal individuals.[336] Extracts of peripheral blood leukocytes and fibroblasts of patients with biotinidase-deficient serum were found to have less than 1 percent of the mean normal activities for these cells (Table 156-4). These studies, and a report of deficient activity in the liver of an affected child,[337] demonstrate that the deficiency of biotinidase activity in patients is not confined to serum. The results also substantiate further that biotinidase deficiency is the primary defect in most patients with late-onset multiple carboxylase deficiency.

Using a specific polyclonal antiserum prepared against human biotinidase, two immunologically cross-reacting material (CRM) were observed.[195] Neither of the proteins was detected by the antiserum in sera from 18 individuals with less than 5 percent of normal enzyme activity in their serum. Only one of these proteins corresponds to the active enzyme in sera from individuals with normal biotinidase activity.

Further biochemical and immunologic characterization of biotinidase was performed in sera from 68 children with profound biotinidase deficiency who were identified symptomatically and by newborn screening and from 63 of their parents[338] (Fig. 156-7). Patients with profound biotinidase deficiency can be classified into at least nine distinct biochemical phenotypes on the basis of the presence or absence of CRM to antibodies against biotinidase, the number of isoforms, and the distribution frequency of the isoforms (Table 156-5). All CRM-positive patients had normal-sized serum biotinidase on SDS-immunoblots. None of the patients with CRM had an abnormal K_m of the substrate for the enzyme. All the parents had normal isoform patterns. The mean activities, CRM concentrations, and specific activities were not significantly different between parents of children who were CRM-positive and CRM-negative. There was no relationship between the age of onset or the severity of symptoms and the isoform patterns or CRM status of the symptomatic children. The isoform patterns of children identified by newborn screening were not different from those of symptomatic children.

Newborn screening for biotinidase deficiency has identified children with profound biotinidase deficiency and about an equal number of children with partial biotinidase deficiency.[275,339,340] Partial biotinidase deficiency was considered initially to be a variant without clinical consequences until in one child, during an episode of gastroenteritis, symptoms of biotinidase deficiency developed that resolved with biotin therapy. We have performed biochemical and immunologic characterization of biotinidase in sera from 23 children with partial biotinidase deficiency from 19 families and from 18 of their parents[341] (Fig. 156-8). As expected, all patients had CRM in their serum. Patients with partial biotinidase deficiency can be classified into six distinct biochemical phenotypes on the basis of the number of isoforms and the distribution frequency of the isoforms (see Table 156-5). Kinetic studies were performed on samples from 17 of the patients and were found to be normal in all cases. The patient with partial deficiency who became symptomatic has an isoform profile that was not different from 10 other symptomatic partially deficient children. The parents had normal isoform patterns. The isoform patterns observed in the patients with partial biotinidase deficiency were not different from those of profoundly deficient patients who have CRM.

To determine if individuals who are deficient in biocytin hydrolase activity are also deficient in biotinyl transferase activity, sera from 103 children (25 identified by exhibiting clinical symptoms and 78 detected by newborn screening) with profound biotinidase deficiency (<10 percent of mean normal biotinyl hydrolase activity) were assessed for biotinyl transferase activity

Table 156-5 Enumeration of the Biochemical Phenotypes of Biotinidase Associated with Enzyme Deficiency

Degree of Enzyme Deficiency	CRM Status	Isoform(s) Missing	Isoform Distribution Frequency
Profound (n=28)	–	All	—
Profound (n=5)	+	None	Normal
Profound (n=8)	+	None	Abnormal
Profound (n=7)	+	9	Similar*
Profound (n=5)	+	9	Dissimilar†
Profound (n=2)	+	8, 9	Dissimilar
Profound (n=4)	+	7–9	Similar
Profound (n=2)	+	7–9	Dissimilar
Partial (n=5)	+	None	Normal
Partial (n=5)	+	None	Abnormal
Partial (n=4)	+	9	Similar
Partial (n=7)	+	9	Dissimilar
Partial (n=1)	+	8, 9	—
Partial (n=1)	+	7–9	—

*Similar to other patients with same isoform pattern.
†Dissimilar to other patients with same isoform pattern.

SOURCE: Data from Hart et al.,[338] with permission.

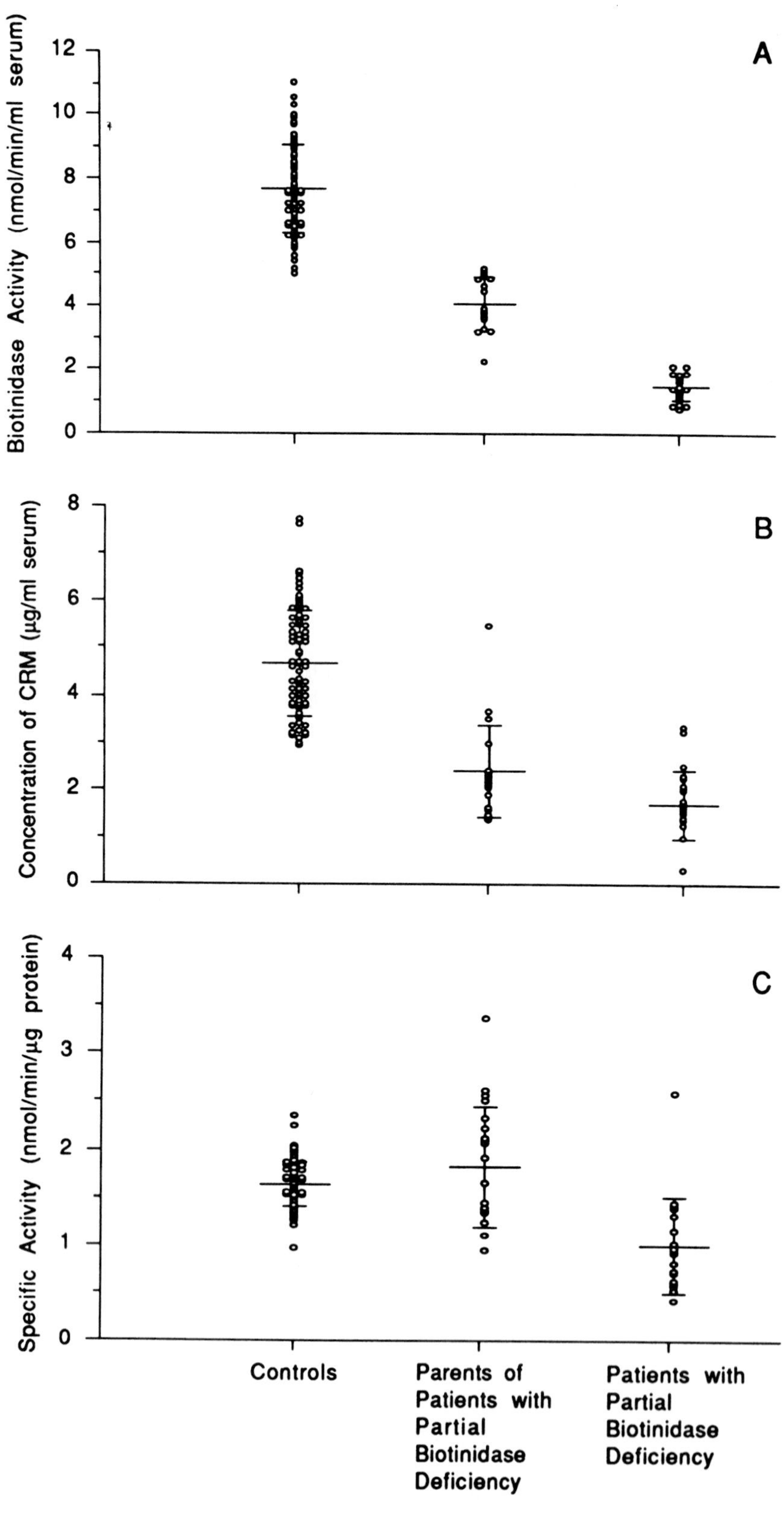

Fig. 156-8 Distribution of biotinidase activity, concentration of CRM, and specific activity in children with partial biotinidase deficiency, their parents, and normal individuals. Bar indicates mean ± SD for each group. *A.* Distribution of biotinidase activity in normal individuals (mean = 7.57 ± 1.41 nmol/min/ml serum, n = 100), parents of children with partial deficiency (mean = 4.07 ± 0.85, n = 18), and patients with partial biotinidase deficiency (mean = 1.47 ± 0.41, n = 23). *B.* Distribution of the concentration of CRM in normal individuals (mean = 4.7 ± 1.1 mg/ml serum), parents of children with partial deficiency of serum biotinidase activity (mean = 1.7 ± 0.7). *C.* Distribution of the specific activity of biotinidase deficiency (mean = 1.6 ± 0.2 nmol/min/mg of enzyme protein), parents of children with partial deficiency (mean = 0.96 ± 0.46), and patients with partial biotinidase deficiency (mean = 0.96 ± 0.46). (*From Hart et al.*[341] *Used by permission of the International Pediatric Research Foundation, Inc.*)

and for the presence of CRM to antibodies prepared against purified serum biotinidase. Sera from all symptomatic patients, both CRM-negative and CRM-positive, had no biotinyl transferase activity. Sera that was CRM-negative from children ascertained by newborn screening also had no biotinyl transferase activity, whereas sera from 67 percent of the CRM-positive children identified by newborn screening had varying degrees of biotinyl transferase activity. These results indicate that there is a large group of enzyme-deficient children detected by newborn screening who are different biochemically from those who are symptomatic.

Two K_m variants of biotinidase were found among 103 children with plasma biotinidase activity that ranged from undetectable to 30 percent of the mean normal activity.[342] The enzymes of three infants had a single elevated K_m for biocytin, 105- to 430-fold. Serum biotinidase activity was 0.2 to 4 percent of mean normal activity, and these children exhibited classic features of the

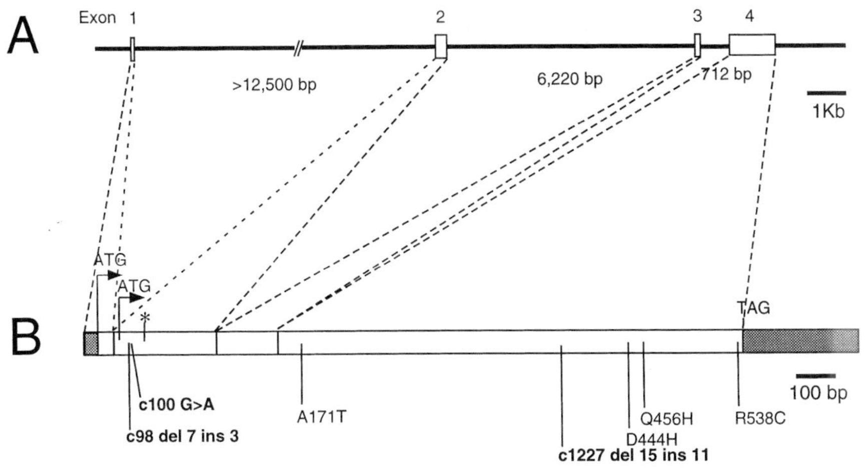

Fig. 156-9 Organization and structure of the biotinidase gene (*A*) and cDNA (*B*). *A*. Genomic organization of BTD. The four exons (1-4) are shown as open boxes separated by three introns. The sizes of the introns are noted. *B*. cDNA of biotinidase. The five common mutations and their locations in the cDNA are indicated. The amino acid changes are below the mutations. The locations of the two putative translation initiation ATG codons, the *N*-terminus of the mature serum enzyme (*), and the TAG stop codon are indicated. The 5′ and 3′ untranslated regions are shaded.

disorder. The enzyme of two children had biphasic kinetics, indicating the presence of one component with a normal K_m and reduced V_{max}, 1.7 and 12 percent, and another with 330- and 59-fold elevated K_m, respectively. The first of these children developed symptoms at 10 to 15 years of age, whereas the second had marginal biotin deficiency but was asymptomatic at 2 years of age. It was recommended that all children with biotinidase deficiency with residual biotinidase activity be evaluated for a K_m mutation by comparing the baseline activity with that after incubating the enzyme in a 10-fold higher substrate concentration.

Mutations. Twenty-one mutations that cause profound biotinidase deficiency were identified in 37 symptomatic children (30 different probands and 7 siblings) in the United States[343] (Fig. 156-9). The two most common mutations (c.98:d7i3 and R538C) were found in 31 of 60 alleles (52 percent), whereas the remainder of the alleles are accounted for by the 19 other unique mutations. The most common mutation, c.98:d7i3, occurs in a region of the gene that encodes the putative signal peptide and results in a frameshift and premature termination of the enzyme.[344] Fifty percent of symptomatic children have this mutation in one of their alleles. The second most common mutation, R538C, is a missense mutation in a CpG dinucleotide in exon 4 of the biotinidase gene.[345] This mutation was found in at least one allele of 30 percent symptomatic children. Aberrant biotinidase protein was not detectable in extracts of fibroblasts from a child who is homozygous for the R538C mutation but was present in less than normal concentration in identical extracts treated with β-mercaptoethanol. Because there is no detectable biotinidase protein in sera of children who are homozygous for the R538C mutation and in combination with the deletion/insertion mutation, the R538C mutation likely results in inappropriate intra- or intermolecular disulfide bond formation, more rapid degradation of the aberrant enzyme, and failure to secrete the residual aberrant enzyme from the cells into blood. Serum samples from these symptomatic children had no detectable CRM to antibody prepared against normal human serum biotinidase, reduced quantities of CRM, or normal quantities of CRM in serum. All these mutations result in complete absence of biotinyl transferase activity in serum.

Among these symptomatic children, a novel point mutation, c.100G > A, was identified 57 bases downstream from the authentic splice acceptor site within the sequence that encodes the signal peptide.[346] This mutation generates a 3′ splice acceptor site. Sequence of the PCR-amplified cDNA from the homozygous child revealed that all the product was shorter than that of normal individuals and was the result of aberrant splicing. The aberrantly spliced transcript lacked 57 bases, including a second in-frame ATG, that encode most of the putative signal peptide and result in an in-frame deletion of 19 amino acids. The mutation results in failure to secrete the aberrant protein into the blood. In addition, a deletion/insertion mutation (c.1227:d15i11) within exon 4 causes a frameshift and premature termination that are predicted to result in a truncated protein.[347] The mutation likely occurred during DNA replication by either of two mechanisms; both involve formation of a quasi-palindromic hairpin loop in the template and dissociation of DNA polymerase α.

The most common cause of profound biotinidase deficiency in children ascertained by newborn screening in the United States is the missense mutation Q456H in exon 4.[348] This mutation was found in at least one allele in 14 unrelated children from 27 different families or 15 of 54 alleles studied (28 percent). This mutation was not identified in 41 normal adults, nor was it found in 296 normal newborns. In addition, biochemical data from a child homozygous for Q456H suggest that the aberrant enzyme has very low biotinyl hydrolase activity, lacks biotinyl transferase activity, and is not recognized by antibody prepared to purified normal human biotinidase. The ethnic backgrounds of the parents contributing the Q456H allele are varied but generally are northern European. The second most common mutation that causes profound biotinidase deficiency in children identified on newborn screening in the United States is a double mutation, A171A (near the 5′ end of exon 4) and D444H (near the 3′ of exon 4), that causes a 52 percent loss of activity in the aberrant enzyme from that allele.[349] Twenty-three individuals with the D444H mutation were found by allele-specific oligonucleotide analysis of DNA from 296 randomly selected anonymous dried-blood spots. We estimate that the frequency of this allele in the general population is 0.039. In contrast, none of the 376 individuals has the A171T mutation. Twelve children (9 probands and 3 siblings) have both the A171T and D444H mutations. Both mutations are inherited from a single parent as a double-mutation allele. The nine families in which this allele was identified are mostly of European ancestry, although the mutation cannot be attributed to a specific nationality or ethnic group. The serum of a child who is homozygous for the double-mutation allele has very little CRM, and the aberrant enzyme has very low biotinyl hydrolase activity and no biotinyl transferase activity.

Eighteen of 19 randomly selected individuals with partial biotinidase deficiency have the D444H mutation.[350] The D444H mutation in biotinidase deficiency appears to be similar to the Duarte variant in galactosemia. The D444H mutation in one allele in combination with a mutation for profound deficiency in the other allele is the common cause of partial biotinidase deficiency.

Genetics. Both males and females have been reported with biotinidase deficiency. Several families had more than one affected child, and consanguinity was found in about 20 percent of the families. These observations, together with the findings that parents of affected children have serum biotinidase activities intermediate between those of normal individuals and those of biotinidase-deficient children, are consistent with biotinidase deficiency being inherited as an autosomal recessive trait.

Prenatal Diagnosis. Biotinidase activity is measurable in both amniotic fluid and cultured amniotic fluid cells obtained by amniocentesis in normal pregnancies.[351] Because the enzymes in amniotic fluid may be of maternal or fetal origin, the definitive diagnosis of biotinidase deficiency in the fetus probably depends on determination of enzyme activity in extracts of amniotic fluid cells. Several prenatal diagnoses were performed experimentally in three pregnancies in which amniocentesis was performed because of advanced maternal age and because the mothers were at risk for a child with biotinidase deficiency.[352] Testing was performed using the colorimetric assay on extracts of amniocytes. The pregnancies resulted in children with biotinidase activities within the heterozygous/normal range. Prenatal diagnosis also was performed in an at-risk pregnancy by measuring biotinidase activity using the colorimetric assay in chorionic villi.[353] The child was shown subsequently to be heterozygous for biotinidase deficiency. Heterozygosity also was diagnosed in another pregnancy using molecular mutation analysis.[352] To date, no children with biotinidase deficiency have been diagnosed prenatally. In our experience, couples who have had a child with biotinidase deficiency identified by newborn screening have not considered prenatal diagnosis in subsequent pregnancies. On the other hand, couples who have had a child with the enzyme deficiency who were diagnosed after the child had developed symptoms are more likely to desire prenatal diagnosis, even after reassurance that immediate diagnosis and institution of biotin therapy will prevent symptoms in an enzyme-deficient child.

Although the sera of heterozygous mothers have half-normal biotinidase activity, neonates with biotinidase deficiency are asymptomatic. This indicates that these mothers can supply the developing infant with adequate free biotin.

Neonatal Screening. A method of neonatal screening for biotinidase deficiency is available. Semiquantitative colorimetric assessment of biotinidase activity is made in the same samples of whole blood spotted on filter paper used in phenylketonuria screening.[354,355] Samples with biotinidase activity show a characteristic purple color on the addition of developing reagents after incubation with biotinyl *p*-aminobenzoate, whereas those with little or no activity remain straw colored. Positive screening tests can be confirmed by a quantitative assay of enzyme activity using additional samples of dried blood or fresh serum.

In 1984, a pilot study was initiated to estimate the incidence of the disorder using samples obtained in the Commonwealth of Virginia for screening for inborn errors of metabolism.[356,357] During the ensuing 2.5-year period, we detected three infants and two siblings of one of these children with biotinidase deficiency.[358] Based on these results, other programs have been initiated in the United States and in several other countries.[359] Of slightly more than 8.5 million newborns screened up to 1990, 142 infants with biotinidase deficiency were identified, 76 infants with profound deficiency and 66 infants with partial deficiency.[360] The estimated incidence of profound deficiency is about 1 in 112,000 (1 in 85,000 to 145,000, 95 percent CI), and the incidence of partial deficiency is about 1 in 129,000 (1 in 113,000 to 177,000). The incidence of combined profound and partial deficiency is about 1 in 60,000 (1 in 50,000 to 73,000). The estimated frequency of alleles for biotinidase deficiency is 0.004, and an estimated 1 in 123 individuals is a heterozygote. Currently, about 25 states in the United States and 25 countries screen their newborns for biotinidase deficiency.

Without biotin treatment, some or most of the symptoms of the disorder are likely to develop in children with the lower range of enzyme activity; the clinical implications of partial enzyme deficiency are still unknown. The preliminary studies from Japan may indicate that these children are at risk for the development of seborrheic dermatitis.[304]

The screening technique also offers a simple, rapid means for the physician to evaluate biotinidase activity in children or adults suspected of having biotinidase deficiency.[26] Because the enzyme activity in the blood spots is stable for at least 18 months at room temperature, the cards may be sent to an appropriate reference laboratory without loss of activity.

Treatment. Children with biotinidase deficiency have been treated successfully with pharmacologic doses of between 5 and 20 mg of biotin per day, an empirically determined dose. There is a report of one patient who required 30 mg/day to resolve his dermatitis.[267] All patients have improved following treatment with pharmacologic doses of biotin.[26,65] The two children depicted in Fig. 156-6*B* and *D* illustrate the dramatic improvements that occur shortly after the commencement of biotin therapy. The cutaneous manifestations usually have resolved quickly, and the seizures and ataxia usually have stopped. However, the hearing loss and optic atrophy appear to be less reversible than the other symptoms. Depending on the severity and frequency of episodes of metabolic and neurologic compromise, many children with developmental delay have rapidly achieved new milestones or regained those which had been lost.

One untreated child with partial biotinidase deficiency became symptomatic after an episode of gastroenteritis.[340] His symptoms resolved shortly after instituting biotin therapy. Since that time, several physicians have communicated to us about children with partial biotinidase deficiency who were not being treated with biotin who developed some mild symptoms, again usually during the course of an infection. All these children improved after biotin treatment. Most children with partial biotinidase deficiency are being treated with biotin, usually 1 to 5 mg/day, and are doing well. Of those who are not being treated, most have remained asymptomatic. These children must be monitored closely to determine the need for biotin supplementation in partial biotinidase deficiency.

It should be stressed that the biotin used in treatment must be in the free form; one patient who was treated with yeast extracts containing large quantities of bound biotin did not improve clinically. However, he improved markedly after treatment with free biotin (B. Wolf, unpublished results).

A biotinidase-deficient child, who apparently had been treated with biotin from birth because a sibling had the disorder became ataxic at 1 year of age.[361] This occurrence has been interpreted to indicate that not all children with biotinidase deficiency respond to biotin therapy. However, there is strong evidence of noncompliance with the prescribed therapeutic regimen in this case (R. Kennedy, personal communication).

Patients with biotinidase deficiency can metabolize carboxylase enzymes to biocytin or biotinyl peptides but no further. Although biocytin or biotinyl peptides are readily excreted in the urine of affected individuals[122,362] and there is no evidence of their accumulation, it is possible that they are toxic. Pharmacologic doses of biotin appear to result in increased concentrations of biocytin or biotinyl peptides in plasma and urine of biotinidase-deficient children.[122,362] It may prove necessary to reduce the therapeutic doses of biotin to limit the production of biocytin. Further evaluation of this possibility is required.

The daily dose of 5 to 20 mg probably supplies more biotin than is actually required to meet the metabolic needs of these patients; one patient remained asymptomatic for 8 years while receiving only 150 μg of biotin daily.[263] An important modifying factor that should be considered in the treatment of this disorder is the amount of free biotin in the diet. It is conceivable that individuals consuming diets containing biotin predominantly in its free form may require less supplemental biotin than those whose diets contain biotin in the bound form. Titration of the doses of

Table 156-6 Comparison of Holocarboxylase Synthetase and Biotinidase Deficiencies

Characteristic	Holocarboxylase Synthetase Deficiency	Biotinidase Deficiency
Clinical features	See Table 156-1	See Table 156-3
Biochemical features	Ketolactic acidosis, hyperammonemia, organic aciduria	Ketolactic acidosis, hyperammonemia, organic aciduria
Biotin concentration in serum	Normal	Low to normal
Carboxylase activities in leukocytes		
Before biotin therapy	Deficient	Deficient
After biotin therapy	Near-normal to normal	Normal
Carboxylase activities in fibroblasts cultured in		
Low-biotin medium (6 nM)	Deficient	Normal
High-biotin medium (>100 nM)	Near-normal to normal	Normal

biotin necessary to treat these children may reveal that doses only slightly above physiologic amounts will be sufficient for treatment.

Differential Diagnosis

Nonspecific clinical symptoms including vomiting, hypotonia, and seizures often characterize treatable disorders such as sepsis, gastrointestinal obstruction, and cardiorespiratory problems. After exclusion of these conditions, or when these findings are accompanied by metabolic ketoacidosis and/or hyperammonemia, the presence of an inborn error of metabolism should be considered. The prompt diagnosis and appropriate treatment of an inherited metabolic disorder may be lifesaving. Both holocarboxylase synthetase deficiency and biotinidase deficiency may present initially with these clinical features (see Tables 156-1 and 156-3) and have been misdiagnosed as other disorders before they were correctly identified.[363]

Other symptoms characteristic of these biotin-responsive multiple carboxylase deficiencies, such as skin rash or alopecia, can occur in children with zinc deficiency or essential fatty acid deficiency. Frequent viral, bacterial, or fungal infections due to abnormal immunologic function may occur in holocarboxylase synthetase deficiency and biotinidase deficiency. Children with either deficiency may have metabolic acidosis and large anion gaps, with elevated concentrations of lactate in the serum and urine. An amino acid analysis may reveal hyperglycinemia, which is also found in other organic acidemias.

The most useful screening technique for determining the type of organic acidemia, and for differentiating isolated carboxylase deficiencies from the biotin-responsive multiple carboxylase deficiencies, is the analysis of urine for abnormal organic acids. Isolated carboxylase deficiency can be confirmed by demonstrating deficient activity of one enzyme and normal activity for the other carboxylases in peripheral blood leukocytes or in cultured fibroblasts. The most common urinary metabolite observed in holocarboxylase synthetase deficiency and biotinidase deficiency is β-hydroxyisovalerate, but it is also seen in isolated β-methylcrotonoyl CoA carboxylase deficiency and biotin deficiency. Elevated urinary concentrations of lactate, methylcitrate, and β-hydroxypropionate, in addition to β-hydroxyisovalerate, are indicative of multiple carboxylase deficiency.

Biotin deficiency usually can be excluded unless there is a history of dietary indiscretion, such as the consumption of a diet containing raw eggs and/or few biotin-containing foods, or a history of protracted parenteral hyperalimentation without biotin supplementation. Low serum biotin concentrations can be useful in differentiating biotin and biotinidase deficiencies from holocarboxylase synthetase deficiency, but it is important to know the method used for the biotin determinations. Only methods that discriminate biotin from biocytin or bound biotin yield reliable estimates of free biotin concentrations.

The symptoms of holocarboxylase synthetase deficiency and biotinidase deficiency are similar, and thus clinical differentiation may be difficult. However, the age of onset of symptoms can be useful in discriminating between these two disorders. Holocarboxylase synthetase deficiency usually manifests before 3 months of age, whereas biotinidase deficiency usually manifests after 3 months of age. Clearly, though, there are exceptions for both disorders, and age of onset alone is not completely reliable. A comparison of the major features of these two disorders is presented in Table 156-6.

Both disorders are characterized by deficient activities of carboxylases in peripheral blood leukocytes prior to biotin administration; the activities of these enzymes increase to near-normal or normal values after biotin treatment.[364] The disorders can be discriminated by determining the activities of the carboxylases in fibroblasts incubated in Minimal Essential Medium containing only the biotin contributed by fetal calf serum (the final concentration is about 6 nM). Fibroblasts from patients with holocarboxylase synthetase deficiency have deficient carboxylase activities when cultured under these conditions, whereas fibroblasts from patients with biotinidase deficiency have activities within the normal range. The activities of the carboxylases are near to or within the normal range of activities when cells from patients having either disorder are cultured in medium supplemented with biotin (final concentration, >200 nM). Definitive diagnosis of holocarboxylase synthetase deficiency is achieved by using one of the several methods detailed previously to measure enzyme activity. Biotinidase deficiency can be determined easily by measuring enzyme activity in the serum of suspected patients. The biotinidase activity in patients with isolated carboxylase deficiency or holocarboxylase synthetase deficiency is normal.

CONCLUSION

Several symptomatic children who have had neither holocarboxylase synthetase deficiency nor biotinidase deficiency have improved clinically after biotin therapy.[365] The nature of the biochemical defect(s) in these patients is unknown. Biotin responsiveness need not be limited to frank biotin deficiency or the two conditions discussed in this chapter, and failure to demonstrate deficiency of one of these two enzymes need not preclude the existence of a condition that is potentially responsive to treatment with biotin.

Since the identification of biotinidase deficiency as the primary defect of late-onset multiple carboxylase deficiency, the number of known and documented symptomatic patients with the disorder has increased greatly. This may be due, in part, to children now known to be biotinidase-deficient who previously had been classified as having idiopathic neurologic disorders. Fortuitously, the first patients to be diagnosed all had near-zero activity, and their parents had half-normal activity. Several children with between 15 and 30 percent of normal activity have been identified through screening programs. The discovery of biotinidase deficiency exemplifies the importance of vitamin recycling in normal nutrition. Biochemical and molecular characterization of both holocarboxylase synthetase and biotinidase and their deficiencies has provided us with a better understanding of the role of biotin in normal metabolism and its role in these two vitamin-responsive disorders.

ACKNOWLEDGMENTS

I thank Dr. Robert Pomponio and Ms. Twyla Booker for the preparation of several figures.

REFERENCES

1. Du Vigneaud V, Hoffmann K, Melville DB: On the structure of biotin. *J Am Chem Soc* **64**:188, 1942.
2. Melville D, Moyer AW, Hofmann K, Du Vigneaud V: The structure of biotin: The formation of thiophenevaleric acid from biotin. *J Biol Chem* **146**:487, 1942.
3. Kogl F, Tonis B: Uber das Bios-Problem: Darstellung und Krystallisiertem biotin aus Eigelb. *Ztschr F Physiol Chem* **242**:43, 1936.
4. Moss J, Lane MD: The biotin-dependent enzymes. *Adv Enzymol* **35**:321, 1971.
5. Lane MD, Young DL, Lynen F: The enzymatic synthesis of holotranscarboxylase from apotranscarboxylase and (+)-biotin: I. Purification of apoenzyme and synthetase: Characteristics of the reaction. *J Biol Chem* **239**:2858, 1964.
6. Achuta Murthy PN, Mistry SP: Synthesis of biotin-dependent carboxylases from their apoproteins and biotin. *Biochem Rev (India)* **43**:1, 1972.
7. Thoma RW, Peterson WH: The enzymatic degradation of soluble bound biotin. *J Biol Chem* **210**:569, 1954.
8. Bonjour JP: Biotin-dependent enzymes in inborn errors of metabolism in humans. *World Rev Nutr Diet* **38**:1, 1981.
9. Blom W, Scholte HR: Acetyl-CoA carboxylase deficiency: An inborn error of *de novo* fatty acid synthesis. *N Engl J Med* **305**:465, 1981.
10. Gompertz D, Draffman GH, Watts JL, Hull D: Biotin-responsive beta-methylcrotonylglycinuria. *Lancet* **2**:22, 1971.
11. Gompertz D, Bartlett K, Blair D, Stern CMM: Child with a defect in leucine metabolism associated with beta hydroxyisovaleric aciduria and beta-methylcrotonylglycinuria. *Arch Dis Child* **48**:975, 1973.
12. Gompertz D, Draffan GH: The identification of tiglylglycine in the urine of a child with beta-methylcrotonylglycinuria. *Clin Chim Acta* **37**:405, 1972.
13. Gompertz D, Goodey PA, Bartlett K: Evidence for the enzymatic defect in beta-methylcrotonylglycinuria. *FEBS Lett* **32**:13, 1973.
14. Sweetman L, Bates SP, Hull D, Nyhan WL: Propionyl-CoA carboxylase deficiency in a patient with biotin-responsive 3-methylcrotonylglycinuria. *Pediatr Res* **11**:1144, 1977.
15. Weyler W, Sweetman L, Maggio DC, Nyhan WL: Deficiency of propionyl-CoA carboxylase and methylcrotonyl-CoA carboxylase in a patient with methylcrotonylglycinuria. *Clin Chim Acta* **76**:321, 1977.
16. Bartlett K, Ghniem HK, Stirk JH, Wastell HJ, Sherrah HSA, Leonard JV: Enzyme studies in combined carboxylase deficiency. *Ann NY Acad Sci* **447**:235, 1985.
17. Bartlett K, Gombertz D: Combined carboxylase defect: Biotin-responsiveness in cultured fibroblasts. *Lancet* **2**:804, 1976.
18. Charles B, Hosking G, Green A, Pollit R, Bartlett K, Taitz LS: Biotin-responsive alopecia and developmental regression. *Lancet* **2**:118, 1979.
19. Sweetman L: Two forms of biotin-responsive multiple carboxylase deficiency. *J Inherited Metab Dis* **4**:53, 1981.
20. Burri BJ, Sweetman L, Nyhan WL: Mutant holocarboxylase synthetase: Evidence for the enzyme defect in early infantile biotin-responsive multiple carboxylase deficiency. *J Clin Invest* **68**:1491, 1981.
21. Munnich A, Saudubray JM, Carre G, Goode FX, Ogier H, Charpentier C, Frezal J: Defective biotin absorption in multiple carboxylase deficiency. *Lancet* **2**:263, 1981.
22. Thoene JG, Lemons RM, Baker H: Impaired intestinal absorption of biotin in juvenile multiple carboxylase deficiency. *N Engl J Med* **308**:639, 1983.
23. Wolf B, Grier RE, Allen RJ, Goodman SI, Kien CL: Biotinidase deficiency: The enzymatic defect in late-onset multiple carboxylase deficiency. *Clin Chim Acta* **131**:273, 1983.
24. Thoene J, Wolf B: Biotinidase deficiency in juvenile multiple carboxylase deficiency. *Lancet* **2**:398, 1983.
25. Burri BJ, Sweetman L, Nyhan WL: Heterogeneity of holocarboxylase synthetase in patients with biotin-responsive multiple carboxylase deficiency. *Am J Hum Genet* **37**:326, 1985.
26. Wolf B, Heard GS, Weissbecker KA, Secor McVoy JR, Grier RE, Leshner RT: Biotinidase deficiency: Initial clinical features and rapid diagnosis. *Ann Neurol* **18**:614, 1985.
27. Bateman WG: The digestibility and utilization of egg protein. *J Biol Chem* **26**:263, 1916.
28. Parsons HT, Lease JG, Kelly E: LIX: The interrelationship between dietary egg white and requirement for a protective factor in the cure of the nutritive disorder due to egg white. *Biochem J* **31**:424, 1937.
29. Gyorgy P: The curative factor (vitamin H) for egg white injury, with particular reference to its presence in different foodstuffs and in yeast. *J Biol Chem* **131**:733, 1939.
30. Gyorgy P: Rachitis und andere avitaminosen. *Z Aerztl Forbild* **28**:377, 1931.
31. Eakin RE, Snell EE, Williams RJ: Concentration and assay of avidin, injury-producting agents in raw egg white. *J Biol Chem* **136**:801, 1940.
32. Harding MG, Crooks H: Lesser known vitamins in foods. *J Am Diet Assoc* **38**:204, 1961.
33. Bonjour J-P: Biotin in man's nutrition and therapy: A review. *Int J Vitam Nutr Res* **47**:107, 1977.
34. Johnson AR, Hood RL, Emery JL: Biotin and the sudden infant death syndrome. *Nature* **285**:159, 1980.
35. Heard GS, Hood RL, Johnson AR: Hepatic biotin and the sudden infant death syndrome. *Med J Aust* **2**:305, 1980.
36. Dostalova L: Vitamin status during puerperium and lactation. *Ann Nutr Metab* **28**:385, 1984.
37. Gardner J, Parsons HT, Peterson WH: Human utilization of biotin from various diets. *Am J Med Sci* **211**:198, 1946.
38. Gardner J, Parsons HT, Peterson WH: Human biotin metabolism on various levels of biotin intake. *Arch Biochem* **8**:339, 1945.
39. Gyorgy P, Langer BW Jr: Biotin VII, in Sebrell WH Jr, Harris RS (eds): *The Vitamins: Chemistry, Physiology, Pathology, Methods*. New York, Academic Press, 1968, p 292.
40. Donaldson RM: *Handbook of Physiology: Alimentary Canal V.* Washington, American Physiological Society, 1968.
41. Eisenberg MA: Biotin: Biogenesis, transport, and their regulation. *Adv Enzymol* **38**:317, 1973.
42. Grundy WE, Freed M, Johnson HC, Henderson CH, Berryman GH, Friedemann TE: The effects of phthalylsulfathiozole (sulfathalidine) on the excretion of B vitamins by normal adults. *Arch Biochem* **15**:187, 1947.
43. Markkanen T: Studies on the urinary excretion of thiamine, riboflavin, nicotinic acid, pantothenic acid and biotin in achlorhydria and after partial gastrectomy. *Acta Med Scand* **169**(suppl):360, 1960.
44. Oppel TW: Studies of biotin metabolism in man: IV. Studies of the mechanism of absorption of biotin and the effect of biotin administration on a few cases of seborrhea and other conditions. *Am J Med Sci* **215**:76, 1948.
45. Sarett HP: Effects of oral administration of streptomycin on urinary excretion of B vitamins in man. *J Nutr* **47**:275, 1952.
46. Gyorgy P, Langer BW Jr: Biotin IV: Estimation in foods and food supplements, in Sebrell WH Jr, Harris RS (eds): *The Vitamins: Chemistry, Physiology, Pathology, and Methods*. New York, Academic Press, 1968, p 261.

47. Dakshinamurti K, Landman AD, Ramamurti L, Constable RJ: Isotope dilution assay for biotin. *Anal Biochem* **61**:225, 1992.
48. Hood RL: A radiochemical assay for biotin in biological materials. *J Sci Food Agric* **26**:1847, 1975.
49. Horsburch T, Gompertz D: A protein-binding assay for measurement of biotin in physiological fluids. *Clin Chim Acta* **82**:215, 1978.
50. Rettenmaier R: Biotin-bestimmung in lebergewebe nach dem prinzip der isopen-verdunnugsanalyse. *Anal Chim Acta* **113**:107, 1980.
51. Sanghvi RS, Lemons RM, Baker H, Thoene JG: A simple method for determination of plasma and urinary biotin. *Clin Chim Acta* **124**:85, 1982.
52. Wright LD, Skeggs HR: Determination of biotin with Lactobacillus arabinosis. *Proc Soc Exp Biol Med* **56**:95, 1944.
53. Baker H, Frank O, Matovitch VB, Pasher I, Aaronson S, Hunter SH, Sobotka H: A new method for biotin in blood, serum, urine and tissues. *Anal Biochem* **3**:31, 1962.
54. Mock DM, lankford GL, Mock NI: Biotin accounts for only half of the total avidin-binding substances in human serum. *J Nutr* **125**:941, 1995.
55. Thompson RC, Eakin RE, Williams RJ: The extraction of biotin from tissues. *Science* **94**:589, 1941.
56. Lampen JO, Bahler GP, Peterson WH: The occurrence of free and bound biotin. *J Nutr* **23**:11, 1942.
57. Scheiner J, Deritter E: Biotin content of feedstuffs. *J Agric Food Chem* **23**:1157, 1975.
58. Green NM: Avidin. *Biochem J* **89**:585, 1963.
59. Williams VR, Fieger EA: Oleic acid as a growth stimulant for Lactobacillus casei. *J Biol Chem* **166**:335, 1946.
60. Baker H: Assessment of biotin status: Clinical implications. *Ann NY Acad Sci* **447**:129, 1985.
61. Craft DV, Goss NH, Chandramouli N, Wood HG: Purification of biotinidase from human plasma and its activity on biotinyl peptides. *Biochemistry* **24**:2471, 1985.
62. Pispa J: Animal biotinidase. *Ann Med Exp Biol Fenn* **43**(suppl 5):1, 1965.
63. Wolf B, Heard GS, McVoy JS, Raetz HM: Biotinidase deficiency: The possible role of biotinidase in the processing of dietary protein-bound biotin. *J Inherit Metab Dis* **7**(suppl 2):121, 1984.
64. Heard GS, Wolf B, Reddy JK: Pancreatic biotinidase activity: The potential for intestinal processing of dietary protein-bound biotin. *Pediatr Res* **18**:198A, 1984.
65. Wolf B, Grier RE, Secor McVoy JR, Heard GS: Biotinidase deficiency: A novel vitamin recycling defect. *J Inherit Metab Dis* **8**(suppl 1):53, 1985.
66. Turner JB, Hughes DE: The absorption of some B-group vitamins by surviving rat intestine preparations. *Q J Exptl Physiol* **47**:107, 1962.
67. Spencer RP, Brody KR: Biotin transport by small intestine of rat, hamster and other species. *Am J Physiol* **206**:653, 1964.
68. Spencer RP, Bow TH: In vitro transport of radiolabeled vitamins by the small intestine. *J Nucl Med* **5**:251, 1964.
69. Berger E, Lang E, Semenza G: The sodium activation of biotin absorption in hamster small intestine in vitro. *Biochim Biophys Acta* **255**:873, 1972.
70. Urban E, Mitchell AM, McKee CR, Hoyumpa A: Biotin transport in rat and hamster small intestine. *Clin Res* **32**:866A, 1984.
71. Gore J, Hoinard C, Maingault P: Biotin uptake by isolated rat intestinal cells. *Biochim Biophys Acta* **856**:357, 1986.
72. Bowman BB, Selhub J, Rosenberg IH: Intestinal absorption of biotin in the rat. *J Nutr* **116**:1266, 1986.
73. Said HM, Redha R: A carrier-mediated system for transport in rat intestine in vitro. *Am J Physiol* **252**:G52, 1987.
74. Said HM: Movement of biotin across the rat intestinal basolateral membrane: Studies with membrane vesicles. *Biochem J* **279**:671, 1991.
75. Said HM, Derweesh I: Carrier-mediated mechanism for biotin transport in rabbit intestine: Studies with brush-border membrane vesicles. *Am J Physiol* **261**:R94, 1991.
76. Said HM, Horne DW, Mock DM: Effect of aging on intestinal biotin transport in the rat. *Exp Gerontol* **25**:67, 1990.
77. Said HM, Mock DM, Collins JC: Regulation of intestinal biotin transport in the rat: Effect of biotin deficiency and supplementation. *Am J Physiol* **256**:G306, 1989.
78. Dakshinamurti K, Chauhan J, Ebrahim H: Intestinal absorption of biotin and biocytin in the rat. *Biosci Rep* **7**:667, 1987.
79. Said H, Thuy LP, Sweetman L, Schatzman B: Transport of the biotin dietary derivative biocytin (*N*-biotinyl-L-lysine) in rat small intestines. *Gastroenterology* **107**:75, 1993.
80. Said HM, McAlister-Henn L, Mahammadkhani R, Horne DW: Uptake of biotin by isolated rat liver mitochondria. *Am J Physiol* **263**:G81, 1992.
81. Baumgartner R, Suormala T, Wick H, Geisert J, Lehnert W: Infantile multiple carboxylase deficiency: Evidence for normal intestinal absorption but renal loss of biotin. *Helv Pediatr Acta* **37**:499, 1982.
82. Munnich A, Grasset E, Gaudry M, Crain AM, Desjeux JF, Saudubray JM: *22nd Annual Symposium of the Society for the Study of Inborn Errors of Metabolism, Newcastle-Upon-Tyne*. Dordrecht, Netherlands, Kluwer Academic Publishers, 1984.
83. Dib C, Faure S, Fizames C, Samson D, Drouot N, Vignal A, Millasseau P, et al: A comprehensive genetic map of the human genome based on 5,264 microsatellites. *Nature* **380**:152, 1996.
84. Said HM, Hoefs J, Mohammadhani R, Horne DW: Biotin transport in human liver basolateral membrane vesicles: A carrier-mediated, sodium gradient-dependent process. *Gastroenterology* **102**:2120, 1992.
85. Said HM, Kamanna VS: Uptake of biotin by human hepatoma cell line, HepG2: A carrier mediated process similar to that of normal liver. *J Cell Physiol* **161**:483, 1994.
86. Wolf B, Heard GS, Jefferson LG, Weissbecker KA, Secor McVoy JR, Nance WE, Mitchell PL, Lambert FW, Linyear AS: Newborn screening for biotinidase deficiency, in Carter TP, Willey AM (eds): *Birth Defect Symposium XVI. Genetic Disease: Screening and Management*. New York, Alan R Liss, 1986, p 175.
87. Heard GS, Bryden WL, Annison EF: Uptake from the gut of pyridoxine, biotin, and their transfer to the egg, in *Proceedings of the 2nd Australian Poultry Stock Feed Convention*. 1978, p 100.
88. Sorrell MF, Frank O, Thomson A, Aquino H, Baker H: Absorption of vitamins from the large intestine in vivo. *Nutr Rep Int* **3**:143, 1971.
89. Frank O, Luisada-Opper AV, Feingold S, Baker H: Vitamin binding by humans and some animal plasma proteins. *Nutr Rep Int* **1**:161, 1970.
90. Vallotton M, Hess-Sander V, Leuthardt F: Fixation spontanee de la biotin a une proteine dans le serum humaine. *Helv Chim Acta* **48**:126, 1965.
91. Gehrig D, Leuthardt F: A biotin-binding glycoprotein from human plasma: Isolation and characterization, in *10th International Congress of Biochemistry, Hamburg*. Frankfurt, Bronners Druckerei Breidenstein, 1976, p 209.
92. Dakshinamurti K, Chalifour LE, Bhullar RP: Requirement for biotin and the function of biotin in cells in culture. *Ann NY Acad Sci* **447**:38, 1985.
93. Chauhan J, Dakshinamurti K: The role of human serum biotinidase as biotin-binding protein. *Biochem J* **256**:265, 1988.
94. Mock D, Malik MI: Distribution of biotin in human plasma: Most of the biotin is not bound to protein. *Am J Clin Nutr* **56**:427, 1992.
95. Hymes J, Fleischhauer K, Wolf B: Biotinylation of biotinidase following incubation with biocytin. *Clin Chim Acta* **233**:39, 1995.
96. Dakshinamurti K, Chalifour LE: The biotin requirement of HeLa cells. *J Cell Physiol* **107**:427, 1981.
97. Chalifour LE, Dakshinamurti K: The biotin requirement of human fibroblasts in culture. *Biochem Biophys Res Commun* **104**:1047, 1982.
98. Cohen ND, Thomas M: Biotin transport into fully differentiated 3T3-L1 cells. *Biochem Biophys Res Commun* **108**:1508, 1982.
99. Weiner D, Wolf B: Biotin uptake in cultured hepatocytes from normal and biotin-deficient rats. *Biochem Med Metab Biol* **44**:271, 1990.
100. Weiner DA, Wolf B: Biotin uptake and efflux in cultured rat hepatocytes: Implications for the treatment of biotinidase deficiency. *Ann NY Acad Sci* **447**:435, 1985.
101. Podevin RA, Barbarat B: Biotin uptake mechanisms in brush-border and basolateral membrane vesicles isolated from rabbit kidney cortex. *Biochim Biophys Acta* **856**:471, 1986.
102. Baur B, Wich H, Baumgartner ER: Sodium-dependent biotin transport into brush-border membrane vesicles from rat kidney. *Am J Physiol* **258**:F840, 1990.
103. Prasad PD, Ramamoorthy S, Leibach FH, Ganapathy V: Characterization of a sodium-dependent vitamin transporter mediating the uptake of pantathenate, biotin and lipoate in human choriocarcinoma cells. *Placenta* **18**:527, 1997.
104. Haagerup A, Andersen JB, Blichfeldt S, Christensen MF: Biotinidase deficiency: Two cases of very early presentation. *Dev Med Child Neurol* **39**:832, 1997.
105. Spector R, Mock D: Biotin transport through the blood-brain barrier. *J Neurochem* **48**:400, 1987.
106. National Resouces Council: *Recommended Dietary Allowances*. Washington, National Academy of Science, 1980.
107. Paul PK: *Effects of Nutrient Toxicities in Animals and Man*. Boca Raton, FL, CRC Press, 1978.

108. Mittelholzer E: Absence of influence of high doses of biotin on reproductive performance in female rats. *Int J Nutr Res* **46**:33, 1976.
109. Watanabe T: Morphological and biochemical effects of excessive amounts of biotin on the embryonic development in mice. *Experientia* **52**:149, 1996.
110. Denko CW, Grundy WE, Porter JW, Berryman GH, Friedemann TE, Youmans JB: The excretion of B-complex vitamins in the urine and feces of several normal adults. *Arch Biochem* **10**:33, 1946.
111. Denko CW, Grundy WE, Wheeler NC, Henderson CR, Berryman GH, Friedemann TE, Youmans JB: The excretion of B-complex vitamins by normal adults on a restricted intake. *Arch Biochem* **11**:109, 1946.
112. Oppel TW: Studies on biotin metabolism in man. *Am J Med Sci* **204**:856, 1942.
113. Hood RL, Johnson AR: Supplementation of infant formulations with biotin. *Nutr Rep Int* **21**:727, 1980.
114. Hamil BM, Coryell MN, Roderuck C: Thiamine, riboflavin, nicotinic acid, pantothenic acid and biotin in urine of newborn infants. *Am J Dis Child* **74**:434, 1947.
115. Berger H: Die Biotinausscheidung im harn bei hautgesunden und hautkranken kingern. *Int Z Vitaminforsch* **22**:190, 1950.
116. Mock DM, Stadler DD, Stratton SL, Mock NI: Biotin status assessed longitudinally in pregnant women. *J Nutr* **127**:710, 1997.
117. Mantagos S, Malamitsi-Puchner A, Antsaklis A, Livaniou E, Evangelatos G, Ithakissios DS: Biotin plasma levels of the human fetus. *Biol Neonate* **74**:72, 1998.
118. Schenker S, Hu ZQ, Johnson RF, Yang Y, Frosto T, Elliott BD, Henderson GI, et al: Human placental biotin transport: Normal characteristics and the effect of ethanol. *Alcohol Clin Exp Res* **17**:566, 1993.
119. Hu ZQ, Henderson GI, Mock DM, Schenker S: Biotin uptake by basolateral membrane vesicles of human placenta: Normal characteristics and role of ethanol. *Proc Soc Exp Biol Med* **206**:404, 1994.
120. McCormick DB: Biotin. *Nutr Rev* **33**:97, 1975.
121. McCormick DB, Wright LD: The metabolism of biotin and analogues, in Florkin M, Stotz EH (eds): *Comprehensive Biochemistry: Metabolism of Vitamins and Trace Elements*. Amsterdam, Elsevier, 1971, p 81.
122. Bonjour JP, Bausch J, Suormala T, Baumgartner ER: Detection of biocytin in urine of children with congenital biotinidase deficiency. *Int J Vitam Nutr Res* **54**:223, 1984.
123. Zempleni J, McCormick DB, Mock DM: Identification of biotin sulfone, bisnorbiotin methyl ketone, and tetranorbiotin-1-sulfoxide in human urine. *Am J Clin Nutr* **65**:508, 1997.
124. Mock DM, Mock NI: Serum concentrations of bisnorbiotin and biotin sulfoxide increase during both acute and chronic biotin supplementation. *J Lab Clin Med* **129**:384, 1997.
125. Mock DM, Heird GM: Urinary biotin analogs increase during chronic supplementation: The analogues are biotin metabolites. *Am J Physiol* **272**:E83, 1997.
126. Sydenstricker VP, Singal SA, Briggs AP, Devaughn NM, Isbell H: Observations on the "egg white injury" in man and its cure with biotin concentrate. *JAMA* **118**:1199, 1942.
127. Williams RH: Clinical biotin deficiency. *N Engl J Med* **228**:247, 1943.
128. Sweetman L, Surh L, Baker H, Peterson RM, Nyhan WL: Clinical and metabolic abnormalities in a boy with dietary deficiency of biotin. *Pediatrics* **68**:553, 1981.
129. Mock DM, Baswell DL, Baker H, Holman RT, Sweetman L: Biotin deficiency complicating parenteral alimentation: Diagnosis, metabolic repercussions and treatment. *Ann NY Acad Sci* **447**:314, 1985.
130. Achuta Murthy PN, Mistry SP: Biotin. *Prog Food Nutr Sci* **2**:405, 1977.
131. Whitehead CC: The assessment of biotin status in man and animals. *Proc Nutr Soc* **40**:165, 1981.
132. Payne CG: Nutritional syndromes of poultry in relation to wheat-based diets, in Haresign W, Swan H, Lewis D (eds): *Nutrition and the Climatic Environment*. London, Butterworth, 1977, p 155.
133. Balnave D: Clinical symptoms of biotin deficiency in animals. *Am J Clin Nutr* **30**:1408, 1977.
134. Payne CG, Gilchrist P, Pearson JA: Involvement of biotin in the fatty liver and kidney syndrome of broilers. *Br Poult Sci* **15**:489, 1974.
135. Hood RL, Johnson AR, Fogarty AC, Pearson JA: Fatty liver and kidney syndrome in chicks: II. Biochemical role of biotin. *Aust J Biol Sci* **29**:429, 1974.
136. Pearson J, Johnson AR, Hood RL, Fogarty AC: Fatty liver and kidney syndrome in chicks: I. Effects of biotin in diet. *Aust J Biol Sci* **29**:419, 1976.
137. Mock NI, Malik MI, Stumbo PJ, Bishop WP, Mock DM: Increased urinary excretion of 3-hydroxyisovaleric acid and decreased urinary excretion of biotin are sensitive early indicators of decreased biotin status in experimental biotin deficiency. *Am J Clin Nutr* **65**:951, 1997.
138. Scott D: Clinical biotin deficiency (egg white injury): Report of a case with some remarks on serum cholesterol. *Acta Med Scand* **162**:69, 1951.
139. Innes SM, Allardya DB: Possible biotin deficiency in adults receiving long-term total parenteral nutrition. *Am J Clin Nutr* **37**:185, 1983.
140. McClain CJ, Baker H, Onstad GR: Biotin deficiency in an adult during home parenteral nutrition. *JAMA* **247**:3116, 1982.
141. Velazquez A, Zamudio S, Baez A, Murguia-Corral R: Indicators of biotin status: A study of patients on prolonged total parenteral nutrition. *Eur J Clin Nutr* **71**:1163, 1989.
142. Krause KH, Berlit P, Bonjour J-P: Impaired biotin status in anticonvulsant therapy. *Ann Neurol* **12**:485, 1982.
143. Krause KH, Bonjour J-P, Berlit P, Kochen W: Biotin status of epileptics. *Ann NY Acad Sci* **447**:297, 1985.
144. Said HM, Redha R, Nylander W: Biotin transport in the human intestine: Inhibition by anticonvulsant drugs. *Am J Clin Nutr* **49**:127, 1989.
145. Mock DM, Mock NI, Nelson RP, Lombard KA: Disturbances in biotin metabolism in children undergoing long-term anticonvulsant therapy. *J Pediatr Gastroenterol Nutr* **26**:245, 1998.
146. Kosow DP, Lane MD: Restoration of biotin-deficiency-induced depression of propionyl CoA carboxylase activity in vivo and in vitro. *Biochem Biophys Res Commun* **4**:92, 1961.
147. Kosow DP, Huang SC, Lane MD: Propionyl holocarboxylase synthesis. *J Biol Chem* **12**:3633, 1962.
148. Foote JL, Christner JE, Coon MJ: Biotin and adenosine triphosphate-dependent activation of propionyl apocarboxylase. *Biochim Biophys Acta* **67**:676, 1963.
149. Siegel L, Foote JL, Christner JE, Coon MJ: Propionyl-CoA holocarboxylase synthesis from biotinyl adenylate and the apocarboxylase in the presence of an activating enzyme. *Biochem Biophys Res Commun* **3**:307, 1963.
150. Lane MD, Rominger KL, Young DL, Lynen F: The enzymatic synthesis of holotranscarboxylase from apotranscarboxylase and (+)-biotin: II. Investigation of the reaction mechanism. *J Biol Chem* **239**:2865, 1964.
151. Christner JE, Schlesinger MJ, Coon MJ: Enzymatic activation of biotin: Biotinyl adenylate formation. *J Biol Chem* **239**:3997, 1964.
152. Siegel L, Foote JL, Coon MJ: The enzymatic synthesis of propionyl coenzyme A holocarboxylase from D-biotinyl 5-adenylate and the apocarboxylase. *J Biol Chem* **240**:1025, 1965.
153. McAllister HC, Coon MJ: Further studies on the properties of liver propionyl coenzyme A holocarboxylase synthetase and the specificity of holocarboxylase formation. *J Biol Chem* **241**:2855, 1966.
154. Cazzulo JJ, Gundaram TK, Dilks SN, Kornberg HL: Synthesis of pyruvate carboxylase from its apoenzyme and (+)-biotin in *Bacillus stearothermophilus:* Purification and properties of the apoenzyme and the holoenzyme synthetase. *Biochem J* **122**:653, 1971.
155. Sundarm TK, Cazzulo JJ, Kornberg HL: Synthesis of pyruvate carboxylase from its apoenzyme and (+)-biotin in *Bacillus stearothermophilus:* Mechanism. *Biochem J* **122**:663, 1971.
156. Chiang GS, Mistry SP: A comparative study of pyruvate holocarboxylase synthesis in rat liver and kidney preparation. *J Biochem* **6**:527, 1975.
157. Wood HG, Harmon FR, Wuhr B, Hubner K, Lynen F: Comparison of the biotination of apotranscarboxylase and its aposubunits. *J Biol Chem* **255**:7397, 1980.
158. Barker DF, Campbell AM: Genetic and biochemical characterization of the bio gene and its product: Evidence for a direct role of biotin holoenzyme synthetase in repression of the biotin operon in *Escherichia coli*. *J Mol Biol* **469**:146, 1981.
159. Rylatt DB, Keech DB, Wallace JC: Pyruvate carboxylase: Isolation of the biotin-containing peptide and the determination of its primary structure. *Arch Biochem Biophys* **183**:113, 1977.
160. Wolf B, Feldman GL: The biotin-dependent carboxylase deficiencies. *Am J Hum Genet* **34**:699, 1982.
161. Hommes FA: Biotin. *World Rev Nutr Diet* **48**:34, 1986.
162. Kraus JP, Kalousek F, Rosenberg LE: Biosynthesis and mitochondrial processing of the beta subunit of propionyl CoA carboxylase from rat liver. *J Biol Chem* **258**:7245, 1983.
163. Kraus JP, Firgaira F, Norotny J, Kalousek F, Williams KR, Williamson C, Ohura T, et al: Coding sequence of the precursor of the beta subunit of rat propionyl-CoA carboxylase. *Proc Natl Acad Sci USA* **83**:8049, 1986.

164. Landman AD: Activation of biotin-enzymes: A possible biochemical rationale. *Life Sci* **19**:1377, 1976.
165. Ahmad PM, Ahmad F: Mammalian pyruvate carboxylase: Effect of biotin on the synthesis and translocation of apoenzyme into 3T3-L adipocyte. *FASEB J* **5**:2482, 1991.
166. Madappally MM, Mistry SP: Synthesis of chicken liver pyruvate holocarboxylase in vivo and in vitro. *Biochim Biophys Acta* **215**:316, 1970.
167. Achuta Murthy PN, Mistry SP: In vitro synthesis of propionyl-CoA holocarboxylase by a partially purified mitochondrial preparation from biotin-deficient chicken liver. *Can J Biochem* **52**:800, 1974.
168. Achuta Murthy PN, Mistry SP: Synthesis of acetyl coenzyme A holocarboxylase in vitro by a cytosolic preparation from chicken liver. *Proc Soc Exp Biol Med* **147**:114, 1974.
169. Chang HI, Cohen ND: Regulation and intracellular regulation of the biotin holocarboxylase synthetase of 3T3-L1 cells. *Arch Biochem Biophys* **225**:237, 1983.
170. Chiba Y, Suzuki Y, Aoki Y, Ishida Y, Nariawa K: Purification and properties of bovine liver holocarboxylase synthetase. *Arch Biochem Biophys* **313**:8, 1995.
171. Suzuki Y, Aoki Y, Ishida Y, Chiba Y, Iwamatsu A, Kishino T, Niikawa N, et al: Isolation and characterization of mutations in the human holocarboxylase synthetase cDNA. *Nature Genet* **8**:122, 1994.
172. Leon-Del Rio A, Leclerc D, Akerman B, Wakamatsu N, Gravel R: Isolation of a cDNA encoding human holocarboxylase synthetase by functional complementation of a biotin auxotroph of *Escherichia coli*. *Proc Natl Acad Sci USA* **92**:4626, 1995.
173. Hiratsuka M, Sakamoto O, Li X, Suzuki Y, Aoki Y, Narisawa K: Identification of holocarboxylase synthetase (HCS) proteins in human placenta. *Biochim Biophys Acta* **1385**:165, 1998.
174. Zhang XX, Leon-Del-Rio A, Gravel RA, Eydoux P: Assignment of holocarboxylase synthetase gene (*HLCS*) to human chromosome band 21q22.1 and to mouse chromosome band 16C4 by *in situ* hybridization. *Cytogenet Cell Genet* **76**:179, 1997.
175. Cohen ND, Thomas M, Stack M: The subcellular distribution of the holocarboxylase synthetase of rat liver. *Ann NY Acad Sci* **447**:393, 1985.
176. Feldman GL, Wolf B: Deficient acetyl-CoA carboxylase activity in multiple carboxylase deficiency. *Clin Chim Acta* **111**:147, 1981.
177. Packman S, Caswell N, Gonzalez-Rios MC, Kaklecek T, Cann H, Rassin D, McKay C: Acetyl CoA carboxylase in cultured fibroblasts: Differential biotin dependence in the two types of biotin-responsive multiple carboxylase deficiency. *Am J Hum Genet* **36**:80, 1984.
178. Packman S, Whitney SC, Fitch M, Fleming SE: Abnormal fatty acid composition of biotin-responsive multiple carboxylase deficiency fibroblasts. *J Inherit Metab Dis* **12**:47, 1989.
179. Packman S, Whitney S: Fatty acid transport in multiple carboxylase deficiency fibroblasts. *J Inherit Metab Dis* **13**:716, 1990.
180. Sols A, Grisolia S (eds): *Metabolic Regulation Enzyme Action*, vol 19. New York, Academic Press, 1970, p 53.
181. Scrutton MC: Pyruvate carboxylase: Studies of activator-independent catalysis and of the specificity of activation by acyl derivatives of coenzyme A for the enzyme from rat liver. *J Biol Chem* **249**:7057, 1974.
182. Wakil SJ (ed): *Lipid Metabolism*. New York, Academic Press, 1970, p 9.
183. Numa S, Bortz WM, Lynen F: Regulation of fatty acid synthesis at the acetyl-CoA carboxylation step. *Adv Enzyme Regul* **3**:407, 1965.
184. Mortimore GE: Regulation of intracellular proteolysis: Introductory remarks. *Fed Proc* **43**:1281, 1984.
185. Chandler CS, Ballard FJ: Inhibition of pyruvate carboxylase degradation and total protein breakdown by lysosomotropic agents in 3T3-L1 cells. *Biochem J* **210**:845, 1983.
186. Chandler CS, Ballard FJ: Distribution and degradation of biotin-containing carboxylases in human cell lines. *Biochem J* **232**:385, 1985.
187. Freytag SO, Utter MF: Regulation of the synthesis and degradation of pyruvate carboxylase in 3T3-L1 cells. *J Biol Chem* **258**:6307, 1983.
188. Wright LD, Driscoll CA, Boger WP: Biocytinase, an enzyme concerned with hydrolytic cleavage of biocytin. *Proc Soc Exp Biol Med* **86**:335, 1954.
189. Mock DM, Lankford G: Studies of the reversible binding of biotin to human plasma. *J Nutr* **120**:375, 1990.
190. Oizumi J, Hayakawa K: Enkephalin hydrolysis by human serum biotinidase. *Biochim Biophys Acta* **1074**:433, 1991.
191. Knappe J, Brommer W, Biederbick K: Reinigung und Eigenschaften der Biotinidase aus Schweinenieren und Lactobacillus casei. *Biochem Z* **228**:599, 1963.
192. Koivusalo M, Pispa J: Biotinidase activity in animal tissue. *Acta Physiol Scand* **58**:13, 1963.
193. Oizumi J, Hayakawa K: Biotinidase in the porcine cerebrum. *Arch Biochem Biophys* **278**:381, 1990.
194. Chauhan J, Dakshinamurti J: Purification and characterization of human serum biotinidase. *J Biol Chem* **261**:4268, 1986.
195. Wolf B, Miller JB, Hymes J, Secor McVoy J, Ishikana Y, Shapira E: Immunological comparison of biotinidase in serum from normal and biotinidase-deficient individuals. *Clin Chim Acta* **164**:27, 1987.
196. Oizumi J, Hayakawa K, Hosoya M: Comparative study of human milk and serum biotinidase. *Biochimie* **71**:1163, 1989.
197. Hymes J, Fleischhauer K, Wolf B: Biotinylation of histones by human serum biotinidase: Assessment of biotinyl-transferase activity in sera from normal individuals and children with biotinidase deficiency. *Biochem Mol Med* **56**:76, 1995.
198. Hayakawa K, Oizumi J: Human serum biotinidase is a thiol-type enzyme. *J Biochem* **103**:773, 1988.
199. Hart PS, Hymes J, Wolf B: Isoforms of human serum biotinidase. *Clin Chim Acta* **197**:257, 1991.
200. Burlina AB, Dermikol M, Mantau A, Piovan S, Grazian L, Zacchello F, Shin Y: Increased plasma biotinidase activity in patients with glycogen storage disease type Ia: Effect of biotin supplementation. *J Inherit Metab Dis* **19**:209, 1996.
201. Cole H, Reynolds TR, Buck GB, Lockyer JM, Denson T, Spence JE, Hymes J, et al: Human serum biotinidase: cDNA cloning, sequence and characterization. *J Biol Chem* **269**:6566, 1994.
202. Knight HC, Reynolds TR, Meyers GA, Pomponio RJ, Buck GA, Wolf B: Structure of the human biotinidase gene. *Mammal Genome* **9**:327, 1998.
203. Cole H, Weremowicz H, Morton CC, Wolf B: Localization of serum biotinidase (BTD) to human chromosome 3 in band p25. *Genomics* **22**:662, 1994.
204. Weiner DL, Grier RE, Watkins P, Heard GS, Wolf B: Tissue origin of serum biotinidase: Implication in biotinidase deficiency. *Am J Hum Genet* **34**:56A, 1983.
205. Grier RE, Heard GS, Watkins P, Wolf B: Low biotinidase activities in the sera of patients with impaired liver function: Evidence that the liver is the source of serum biotinidase. *Clin Chim Acta* **186**:397, 1989.
206. Nagamine T, Saito S, Yamada S, Kaneko M: Clinical evaluation of serum biotin levels and biotinidase activities in patients with various liver diseases. *Nippon Shokakibyo Gakkai Zasshi* **87**:1168, 1990.
207. Heard GS, Tanner RW, Blevins TL, Evans JS: Effects of age and biotin status on postnatal development of plasma biotinidase activity in rats. *Biochem Med Metab Biol* **45**:92, 1991.
208. Heard GS, Grier RE, Weiner DL, Secor McVoy JR, Wolf B: Biotinidase: A possible mechanism for the recycling of biotin. *Ann NY Acad Sci* **447**:259, 1985.
209. Oizumi J, Hayakawa K: Biotinidase and lipoamidase in guinea pig liver. *Biochem Biophys Acta* **991**:410, 1989.
210. Oizumi J, Hirano M, Hayakawa K, Daimatsu T, Zaima K: The significance of breast milk biotinidase. *Acta Paediatr Jpn* **31**:424, 1989.
211. Sweetman L, Nyhan WL: Inheritable biotin-treatable disorders and associated phenomena. *Annu Rev Nutr* **6**:317, 1986.
212. Robinson BH, Oci J, Saunders M, Gravel R: [^{3}H]Biotin-labelled proteins in cultured human skin fibroblasts from patients with pyruvate carboxylase deficiency. *J Biol Chem* **258**:6660, 1983.
213. Lamhonwah AM, Lam KF, Tsui F, Robinson B, Saunders ME, Gravel RA: Assignment of the alpha and beta chains of human propionyl-CoA carboxylase to genetic complementation groups. *Am J Hum Genet* **35**:889, 1983.
214. Roth K, Cohn R, Yandrasitz J, Preti G, Dodd P, Segal S: Beta-methylcrotonic aciduria associated with lactic acidosis. *J Pediatr* **88**:229, 1976.
215. Roth KS, Yang W, Foreman JW, Rothman R, Segal S: Holocarboxylase synthetase deficiency: A biotin-responsive organic acidemia. *J Pediatr* **96**:845, 1980.
216. Roth KS, Allan L, Yang W, Foreman JW, Dakshinamurti K: Serum and urinary biotin levels during treatment of holocarboxylase synthetase during treatment of holocarboxylase synthetase deficiency. *Clin Chim Acta* **109**:337, 1981.
217. Leonard JV, Seakins JWT, Bartlett K, Hyde J, Wilson J, Clayton B: Inherited disorders of 3-methylcrotonyl CoA carboxylation. *Arch Dis Child* **56**:53, 1981.
218. Packman S, Sweetman L, Baker H, Wall S: The neonatal form of biotin responsive multiple carboxylase deficiency. *J Pediatr* **99**:418, 1981.

219. Wolf B, Hsia YE, Sweetman L, Feldman G, Boychuk RB, Bart RD, Crowell DH, et al: Multiple carboxylase deficiency: Cinical and biochemical improvement following neonatal biotin treatment. *Pediatrics* **68**:113, 1981.
220. Narisawa K, Arai N, Igarashi Y, Satoh T, Tada K: Clinical and biochemical findings on a child with multiple biotin-responsive carboxylase deficiencies. *J Inherit Metab Dis* **5**:67, 1982.
221. Sherwood WG, Saunders M, Robinson BH, Brewster T, Gravel RA: Lactic acidosis in biotin-responsive multiple carboxylase deficiency caused by holocarboxylase synthetase deficiency of early and late onset. *J Pediatr* **101**:546, 1982.
222. Briones P, Ribes A, Vilaseca MA, Rodriguez-Valcarcel G, Thuy LP, Sweetman L: A new case of holocarboxylase synthetase deficiency. *J Inherit Metab Dis* **12**:329, 1989.
223. Michalski AJ, Berry GT, Segal S: Holocarboxylase synthetase deficiency: 9-year follow-up of a patient on chronic biotin therapy and a review of the literature. *J Inherit Metab Dis* **12**:312, 1989.
224. Fuchshuber A, Suormala T, Roth B, Duran M, Michalk D, Baumgartner ER: Holocarboxylase synthetase deficiency: Early diagnosis and management of a new case. *Eur J Pediatr* **152**:446, 1993.
225. Livne M, Gibson KM, Amir N, Eshel G, Elpelig ON: Holocarboxylase synthetase deficiency: A treatable metabolic disorder masquerading as cerebral palsy. *J Child Neurol* **9**:170, 1994.
226. Dabbagh O, Brismar J, Gascon GG, Ozand PT: The clinical spectrum of biotin-treatment encephalopathies in Saudi Arabia. *Brain Dev* **16**(suppl):72, 1994.
227. Stigsby B, Yarworth SM, Rahbeeni Z, Dabbagh O, de Gier Munk C, Abdo N, Brismar J, et al: Neurophysiologic correlates of organic acidemias: A survey of 107 patients. *Brain Dev* **16**(suppl):125, 1994.
228. Gascon GG, Ozand PT, Brismar J: Movement disorders in childhood organic acidemias: Clinical, neuroimaging, and biochemical correlations. *Brain Dev* **16**(suppl):94, 1994.
229. Squires L, Betz B, Umfleet J, Kelley R: Resolution of subependymal cysts in neonatal holocarboxylase synthetase deficiency. *Dev Med Child Neurol* **39**:267, 1997.
230. Suormala T, Fowler B, Duran M, Burtscher A, Fuchshuber A, Tratzmuller R, Lenze MJ, et al: Five patients with a biotin-responsive defect in holocarboxylase function: Evaluation of responsiveness to biotin therapy in vivo and comparative biochemical studies in vitro. *Pediatr Res* **41**:666, 1997.
231. Sweetman L, Nyhan WL: Organic aciduria in neonatal multiple carboxylase deficiency. *J Inherit Metab Dis* **5**:49, 1982.
232. Saunders M, Sweetman L, Robinson B, Roth K, Cohn R, Gravel RA: Biotin responsive organicaciduria: Multiple carboxylase defects and complementation studies with propionicacidemia in cultured fibroblasts. *J Clin Invest* **64**:1695, 1979.
233. Bartlett K, Ng H, Dale G, Green A, Leonard JV: Studies on cultured fibroblasts from patients with defects of biotin-dependent carboxylation. *J Inherit Metab Dis* **4**:183, 1981.
234. Feldman GL, Hsia YE, Wolf B: Biochemical characterization of biotin responsive multiple carboxylase deficiency: Heterogeneity within the bio genetic complementation group. *Am J Hum Genet* **33**:692, 1981.
235. Samboni M, Gaudry M, Marquet A, Munnich A, Saudubray JM, Marsac C: Search for the biochemical basis of biotin dependent multiple carboxylase deficiencies: Determination of biotin activation in cultured fibroblasts. *Clin Chim Acta* **122**:241, 1981.
236. Wolf B, Willard HF, Rosenberg LE: Kinetic analysis of complementation in heterokaryons of propionyl CoA carboxylase-deficient human fibroblasts. *Am J Hum Genet* **32**:16, 1980.
237. Wolf B: Molecular basis for genetic complementation in propionyl CoA carboxylase deficiency. *Exp Cell Res* **125**:502, 1980.
238. Feldman GL, Wolf B: Evidence for two genetic complementation groups in pyruvate carboxylase-deficient human fibroblast cell lines. *Biochem Genet* **18**:617, 1980.
239. Ghneim HK, Bartlett K: Mechanism of biotin-responsive combined carboxylase deficiency. *Lancet* **1**:1187, 1982.
240. Saunders ME, Sherwood WG, Dutchie M, Surh L, Gravel RA: Evidence for a defect of holocarboxylase synthetase activity in cultured lymphoblasts from a patient with biotin-responsive multiple carboxylase deficiency. *Am J Hum Genet* **34**:590, 1982.
241. Morita J, Thuy L, Sweetman L: Biotinyl AMP synthetase activities in fibroblasts of patients with abnormal holocarboxylase synthetase activity, in *Proceedings for the Society of Inherited Metabolic Disorder*. Dordrecht, Netherlands,KLuwer Academic Publisher,1989, p 23.
242. Suzuki Y, Aoki Y, Sakamoto O, Li X, Miyabayashi S, Kazuta Y, Kondo H, et al: Enzymatic diagnosis of holocarboxylase synthetase using apocarboxyl carrier protein as a substrate. *Clin Chim Acta* **251**:41, 1996.
243. Aoki Y, Suzuki Y, Li X, Takahashi K, Ohtake A, Sakuta R, Ohura T, et al: Molecular analysis of holocarboxylase synthetase deficiency: A missense mutation and a single base deletion are predominant in Japanese patients. *Biochem Biophys Acta* **1272**:168, 1995.
244. Dupuis L, Leon-Del-Rio A, Leclerc D, Campeau E, Sweetman L, Saudubray JM, Herman G, et al: Clustering of mutations in the biotin-binding region of holocarboxylase synthetase in biotin-responsive multiple carboxylase deficiency. *Hum Mol Genet* **5**:1011, 1996.
245. Aoki Y, Suzuki Y, Li X, Sakamoto O, Chikaoka H, Takita S, Narisawa K: Characterization of mutant holocarboxylase synthetase (HCS): A K_m for biotin was not elevated in a patient with HCS deficiency. *Pediatr Res* **42**:849, 1997.
246. Packman S, Cowan MJ, Golbus MS, Caswell NM, Sweetman L, Burri BJ, Nyhan WL, et al: Prenatal treatment of biotin-responsive multiple carboxylase deficiency. *Lancet* **1**:1435, 1982.
247. Jakobs C, Sweetman L, Nyhan WL: Stable isotope dilution analysis of 3-hydroxyisovaleric acid in amniotic fluid: Contribution to the prenatal diagnosis of inherited disorders of leucine catabolism. *J Inherited Metab Dis* **7**:15, 1984.
248. Roth KS, Yang W, Allen L, Saunders M, Gravel RA, Dakshinamurti K: Prenatal administration of biotin in biotin-responsive multiple carboxylase deficiency. *Pediatr Res* **16**:126, 1982.
249. Cowan MJ, Wana DW, Packman S, Ammann AJ, Yoshino M, Sweetman L, Nyhan WL: Multiple biotin-dependent carboxylase deficiencies associated with defects in T-cell and B-cell immunity. *Lancet* **2**:115, 1979.
250. Sander JE, Malamud N, Cowan MJ, Packman S, Ammann AJ, Wara DW: Intermittent ataxia and immunodeficiency with multiple carboxylase deficiencies: A biotin-responsive disorder. *Ann Neurol* **8**:544, 1980.
251. Thoene J, Baker H, Yoshino M, Sweetman L: Biotin responsive carboxylase deficiency associated with subnormal plasma and urinary biotin. *N Engl J Med* **304**:817, 1981.
252. Munnich A, Saudubray JM, Ogier H, Coude FX, Marsac C, Roccichioli F, Labarthe JC, et al: Deficit multiple des carboxylases. *Arch Fr Pediatr* **38**:83, 1981.
253. Munnich A, Saudubray JM, Cotjsson A, Coude FX, Ogier H, Charpentier C, Marsac C, et al: Biotin dependent multiple carboxylase deficiency presenting as a congenital lactic acidosis. *Eur J Pediatr* **137**:203, 1981.
254. Kien CL, Kohler E, Goodman SI, Berlow S, Hong R, Horowitz SP, Baker H: Biotin-responsive in vivo carboxylase deficiency in two siblings with secretory diarrhea receiving total parenteral nutrition. *J Pediatr* **99**:546, 1981.
255. Packman S, Sweetman L, Yoshino M, Baker H, Cowan M: Biotin-responsive multiple carboxylase deficiency of infantile onset. *J Pediatr* **90**:421, 1981.
256. Wolf B, Grier RE, Allen RJ, Goodman SI, Kien CL, Parker WD, Howell DM, et al: Phenotypic variation in biotinidase deficiency. *J Pediatr* **103**:233, 1983.
257. Swick HM, Kein CL: Biotin deficiency with neurological and cutaneous manifestations but without organic aciduria. *J Pediatr* **103**:265, 1983.
258. Williams ML, Packman S, Cowan MJ: Alopecia and periorficical dermatitis in biotin responsive multiple carboxylase deficiency. *J Am Acad Dermatol* **9**:97, 1983.
259. Schubiger G, Caflisch U, Baumgartner R, Suormala T, Bachmann C: Biotinidase deficiency: Clinical course and biochemical findings. *J Inherit Metab Dis* **7**:129, 1984.
260. Mienie LJ, Reineck CJ: Organic aciduria in neonatal biotin-responsive multiple carboxylase deficiency, in *Proceedings of the 22nd Annual Symposium of the Society for the Study of Inborn Errors of Metabolism*. Dordrecht, Netherlands, Kluwer Academic Publishers, 1984, p 9.
261. Greter J, Holme E, Koivikko M, Lindstedt S: Biotin-responsive 3-methylcrotonylglycinuria with biotinidase deficiency, in *Proceedings of the 22nd Annual Symposium of the Society for the Study of Inborn Errors of Metabolism*. Dordrecht, Netherlands, Kluwer Academic Publishers, 1984, p 8.
262. King M: Biotin-responsive stridor et cetera, in *Proceedings of the 22nd Annual Symposium of the Society for the Study of Inborn Errors of Metabolism*. Dordrecht, Netherlands, Kluwer Academic Publishers, 1984, p 22.
263. Diamantopoulos N, Painter MJ, Wolf B, Heard GS, Roe C: Biotinidase deficiency: Accumulation of lactate in the brain and response to physiologic doses of biotin. *Neurology* **36**:1107, 1986.
264. Baumgartner R, Suormala T, Wick H, Probst A, Vest M, Bachmann C: Biotinidase deficiency with lethal outcome, in *Proceedings from the*

24th Annual Symposium of the Society for the Study of Inborn Errors of Metabolism. Dordrecht, Netherlands, Kluwer Academic Publishers,1986, p 45.
265. Mitchell G, Ogier H, Munnich A, Saudubray JM, Schirrer J, Charpentier C, Rocciccioli F: Neurological deterioration and lactic acidemia in biotinidase deficiency: A treatable condition mimicking Leigh's disease. *Neuropediatrics* **17**:129, 1986.
266. Burton B, Roach ES, Wolf B, Weissbecker KA: Sudden death associated with biotinidase deficiency. *Pediatrics* **79**:482, 1987.
267. Riudor E, Vilaseca MA, Briones P, Ribes A, Sunes J, Martorell R, Macaya A, et al: Requirement of high biotin doses in a case of biotinidase deficiency. *J Inherit Metab Dis* **12**:338, 1989.
268. Colamaria V, Burlina AB, Gaburro D, Pajno-Ferrara F: Biotin-responsive infantile encephalopathy: EEG-polygraphic study of a case. *Epilepsia* **30**:573, 1989.
269. Hurvitz H, Ginat-Israeli T, Elpeleg ON, Klar A, Amir N: Biotinidase deficiency associated with severe combined immunodeficiency. *Lancet* **2**:228, 1989.
270. Nothjunge J, Krageloh-Mann I, Suormala TM, Baumgartner ER: Biotindasemangel: Eine angeborene Stoffwechselerkrankung, die mit Vitamin H erfolgreich behandelt werden kann. *Monatsschr Kinderheilkd* **137**:737, 1989.
271. de Parscau L, Beaufrere B, Vianey-Liaud C, Rolland MO: Biotinidase deficiency: A disease with neurologic and cutaneous expression susceptible to biotin. *Placenta* **44**:383, 1989.
272. Anger H, Lorenz K, Cobet G: Biotinidase deficiency: A progressive metabolic disease in children with seizures and ataxia. *Psychiatr Neurol Med Psychol* **42**:163, 1990.
273. Lara EB, Sansaricq C, Wolf B, Snyderman SE: Biotinidase deficiency in black children. *J Pediatr* **116**:750, 1990.
274. Suormala TM, Baumgartner ER, Wick H, Scheibenreiter S, Schweitzer S: Comparison of patients with complete and partial biotinidase deficiency: Biochemical studies. *J Inherit Metab Dis* **13**:76, 1990.
275. Fois A, Cioni M, Balestri P, Bartalini G, Baumgartner RE, Bachmann C: Biotinidase deficiency: Metabolites in CSF. *J Inherit Metab Dis* **9**:284, 1986.
276. Thuy LP, Zielinska B, Zammarchi E, Pavari E, Vierucci A, Sweetman F, Sweetman L, et al: Multiple carboxylase deficiency due to deficiency of biotinidase. *J Neurogenet* **3**:357, 1986.
277. Campana G, Valentini G, Legnaioli MI, Giovannucci-Uzielli ML, Pavari E: Ocular aspects in biotinidase deficiency: Clinical and genetic original studies. *Ophthalmic Paediatr Genet* **8**:125, 1987.
278. Marandian MH, Soltanabadi A, Lessani M, Kouchanfar A, Fallah A: Deficit en biotinidase: Maladie a manifestations principalement neurocutanees curable par la biotine. *Ann Pediatr* **34**:725, 1987.
279. Schulz PE, Weiner SP, Belmont JW, Fishman MA: Basal ganglia calcifications in a case of biotinidase deficiency. *Neurology* **38**:1326, 1988.
280. Wastell HJ, Bartlett K, Dale G, Shein A: Biotinidase deficiency: A survey of 10 cases. *Arch Dis Child* **63**:1244, 1988.
281. Dionisi-Vici C, Bachmann c, Graziani MC, Sabetta G: Laryngeal stridor as a leading symptom in biotinidase-deficient patient. *J Inherit Metab Dis* **11**:312, 1988.
282. Jaeken J, Casaer P: Cerebral lactic acidosis and biotinidase deficiency (Letter). *Eur J Paediatr* **148**:175, 1988.
283. Erasmus C, Mienie J, Reinecke CJ, Wadman SK: Organic aciduria in late-onset biotin-responsive multiple carboxylase deficiency. *J Inherit Metab Dis* **8**:105, 1985.
284. Schweitzer S, Baumgartner R, Suormala T, Byrd D, Sander J, Moll H, Brodehl J: Biotinidase-Mangel: Fruh- und Spaterkennung. *Monatsschr Kinderheilkd* **136**:562A, 1988.
285. Bousounis DP, Camfield PR, Wolf B: Reversal of brain atrophy with biotin treatment in biotinidase deficiency. *Neuropediatrics* **24**:214, 1993.
286. Lott IT, Lottenberg S, Nyhan WL, Buchsbaum MJ: Cerebral metabolic changes after treatment in biotinidase deficiency. *J Inherit Metab Dis* **16**:399, 1993.
287. Ramaekers VT, Brab M, Rau G, Heimann G: Recovery from neurological deficits following biotin treatment in a biotinidase K_m variant. *Neuropediatrics* **24**:98, 1993.
288. Honavar M, Janota I, Neville BG, Chalmers RA: Neuropathology in biotinidase deficiency. *Acta Neuropathol* **84**:461, 1992.
289. Clauser TA, Bay CA, Hayward JC, Wolf B, Sladsky JT, Kaplan P, Berry GT: Reversible metabolic myopathy and cerebral spinal fluid lactic acidosis in biotinidase deficiency. *Pediatr Res* **28**:344A, 1990.
290. Collins JE, Nichosen NS, Dalton N, Leonard JV: Biotinidase deficiency: Early neurological presentation. *Dev Med Child Neurol* **36**:748, 1994.
291. Kalayci O, Coskun T, Tokatli A, Demir E, Erdem G, Gungor C, Yukselen A, et al: Infantile spasms as the initial symptom of biotinidase deficiency. *J Pediatr* **124**:103, 1994.
292. Heron B, Gautier A, Dulac O, Ponsot G: Biotinidase deficiency: Progressive encephalopathy curable with biotin. *Arch Fr Pediatr* **50**:875, 1993.
293. Ginat-Israeli T, Hurvitz H, Klar A, Blinder G, Branski D, Amir N: Deteriorating neurological and neuroradiological course in treated biotinidase deficiency. *Neuropediatrics* **24**:103, 1993.
294. Ataman M, Sozeri B, Ozalp I: Biotinidase deficiency: A rare cause of laryngeal stridor. *Int J Otorhinolaryngol* **23**:281, 1992.
295. Honaver M, Janota I, Neville BGR, Chalmers RA: Neuropathology of biotinidase deficiency. *Acta Neuropathol* **84**:461, 1992.
296. Bakker HD, Westra M, Overweg-Plandsoen WC, van Waveren G, Sillevis Smitt JH, Abeling NG, Wanders RJ, et al: Normalisation of severe cranial CT scan abnormalities after biotin in a case of biotinidase deficiency. *Eur J Paediatr* **153**:861, 1994.
297. Tokatli A, Coskun T, Ozalp I: Biotinidase deficiency with neurological features resembling multiple sclerosis in a 15-year-old girl. *J Inherit Metab Dis* **20**:707, 1997.
298. Tokatli A, Coskun T, Ozalp I, Gunay M: The major presenting symptom in a biotinidase-deficient patient: laryngeal stridor. *J Inherit Metab Dis* **15**:281, 1992.
299. Wilcken B, Hammond J: Hearing loss in biotinidase deficiency. *Lancet* **2**:1366, 1983.
300. Rahman S, Standing s, Dalton RN, Pike MG: Late presentation of biotinidase deficiency with acute visual loss and gait disturbance. *Dev Med Child Neurol* **39**:830, 1997.
301. Ramaekers VTh, Suormala TM, Brab M, Duran R, Heimann G, Baumgartner ER: A biotinidase K_m variant causing late onset bilateral optic neuropathy. *Arch Dis Child* **67**:115, 1992.
302. Salbert BA, Pellock JM, Wolf B: Characterization of seizures associated with biotinidase deficiency. *Neurology* **43**:1351, 1993.
303. Salbert BA, Astruc J, Wolf B: Ophthalmological findings in biotinidase deficiency. *Ophthalmologica* **206**:177, 1993.
304. Oizumi J, Hayakawa K, Iinuma K, Odajima Y, Iikura Y: Partial deficiency of biotinidase activity. *J Pediatr* **110**:818, 1987.
305. Wolf B, Pomponio RJ, Norrgard KJ, Lott IT, Baumgartner ER, Suormala T, Raemaekers VTh, et al: Delayed-onset profound biotinidase deficiency. *J Pediatr* **132**:362, 1998.
306. Wolf B, Norrgard K, Pomponio RJ, Mock DM, Secor McVoy JR, Fleischhauer K, Shapiro S, et al: Profound biotinidase deficiency in two asymptomatic adults. *Am J Med Genet* **73**:5, 1997.
307. Proud VK, Rizzo WB, Patterson JW, Heard GS, Wolf B: Fatty acid alterations and carboxylase deficiencies in the skin of biotin-deficient rats. *Am J Clin Nutr* **51**:853, 1990.
308. Munnich A, Saudubray JM, Coude FX, Charpentier C, Saurat JH, Frezal J: Fatty acid responsive alopecia in multiple deficiency. *Lancet* **1**:1080, 1980.
309. Williams ML: Biotin-responsive multiple carboxylase deficiency and immunodeficiency. *Curr Probl Dermatol* **18**:89, 1989.
310. Munnich A, Fischer A, Saudubray JM, Griscelli C, Coude FX, Ogier H, Charpentier C, et al: Biotin-responsive immunoregulatory dysfunction in multiple carboxylase deficiency. *J Inherited Metab Dis* **4**:113, 1981.
311. Fischer A, Munnich A, Saudubray JM: Biotin-responsive immunoregulatory dysfunction in multiple carboyxlase deficiency. *J Clin Immunol* **2**:35, 1982.
312. Allen RJ, Wolf B, Grier RE: Infantile seizures in biotinidase deficiency. *Ann Neurol* **2**:386, 1983.
313. Baumgartner ER, Suormala TM, Wick H, Probst A: Biotinidase deficiency: A cause of subacute necrotizing encephalomyelopathy (Leigh syndrome). Report of a case with lethal outcome. *Pediatr Res* **26**:260, 1989.
314. Wolf B, Heard GS, Secor McVoy JR, Grier RE: Biotinidase deficiency. *Ann NY Acad Sci* **447**:252, 1985.
315. Suchy SF, Rizzo WB, Wolf B: Fatty acids in biotin deficiency. *Ann NY Acad Sci* **447**:429, 1985.
316. Proud VK, Rizzo WB, Patterson JW, Heard GS, Wolf B: Fatty acid alterations and carboxylase deficiencies in the skin of biotin-deficient rats. *Am J Clin Nutr* **51**:853, 1990.
317. Suchy SF, Secor McVoy,J.R., Wolf B: Neurologic symptoms of biotinidase deficiency: Possible explanation. *Neurology* **35**:1510, 1985.
318. Sander JE, Packman S, Townsend JJ: Brain pyruvate carboxylase and the pathophysiology of biotin-dependent diseases. *Neurology* **32**:878, 1982.

319. Dirocco M, Superti-Furga A, Durand P, Cerone R, Romano C: Different organic acid patterns in urine and in cerebrospinal fluid in a patient with biotinidase deficiency. *J Inherit Metab Dis* **2**(suppl 7): 119, 1984.
320. Heard GS, Lenhardt ML, Bowie RM, Clarke AM, Harkins SW, Wolf B: Increased central conduction time but no hearing loss in young biotin deficient rats. *FASEB J* **3**: 124, 1989.
321. Rybak LP, Whitworth C, Scott V, Weberg AD, Bhardwaj B: Rat as a potential model for hearing loss in biotinidase deficiency. *Ann Otol Rhinol Laryngol* **100**: 294, 1991.
322. Taitz LS, Green A, Strachan I, Bartlett K, Bennet M: Biotinidase deficiency and the eye and ear. *Lancet* **2**: 918, 1983.
323. Wolf B, Grier RE, Heard GS: Hearing loss in biotinidase deficiency. *Lancet* **2**: 1365, 1983.
324. Taitz LS, Leonard JV, Bartlett K: Long-term auditory and visual complications of biotinidase deficiency. *Early Hum Dev* **11**: 325, 1985.
325. Suormala TM, Baumgartner ER, Bausch J, Holick W, Wick H: Quantitative determination of biocytin in urine of patients with biotinidase deficiency using high-performance liquid chromatography. *Clin Chim Acta* **177**: 253, 1988.
326. Suormala T, Wick H, Bonjour JP, Baumgartner ER: Intestinal absorption and renal excretion of biotin in patients with biotinidase deficiency. *Eur J Paediatr* **144**: 21, 1985.
327. Baumgartner ER, Sourmala T, Wick H, Bonjour JP: Biotin-responsive multiple carboxylase deficiency (MCD): Deficient biotinidase activity associated with renal loss of biotin. *J Inherit Metab Dis* **7**(suppl 2): 123, 1984.
328. Baumgartner ER, Suormala T, Wick H, Bausch J, Bonjour J-P: Biotinidase deficiency associated with renal loss of biocytin and biotin. *Ann NY Acad Sci* **447**: 272, 1985.
329. Weissbecker KA, Gruemer HD, Heard GS, Miller WG: An automated procedure for measuring biotinidase activity in serum. *Clin Chem* **35**: 831, 1989.
330. Hayakawa K, Oizumi J: Determination of biotinidase activity by liquid chromatography with fluorimetric detection. *J Chromatogr* **383**: 148, 1986.
331. Wastell H, Dale G, Bartlett K: A sensitive fluorimetric rate assay for biotinidase using a new derivative of biotin, biotinyl-6-aminoquinoline. *Anal Biochem* **140**: 69, 1984.
332. Weiner DL, Grier RE, Wolf B: A bioassay for determining biotinidase activity and for discriminating biocytin from biotin using holocarboxylase synthetase-deficient cultured fibroblasts. *J Inherit Metab Dis* **8**: 101, 1985.
333. Thuy LE, Zielinska B, Sweetman L, Nyhan WL: Determination of biotinidase activity in human plasma using [^{14}C]biocytin as substrate. *Ann NY Acad Sci* **447**: 434, 1985.
334. Ebrahim H, Dakshinamurti K: A fluorometric assay for biotinidase. *Anal Biochem* **154**: 282, 1986.
335. Weissbecker KA, Nance WE, Eaves LJ, Piussan C, Wolf B: Detection of heterozygotes for biotinidase deficiency. *Am J Hum Genet* **39**: 385, 1991.
336. Wolf B, Secor McVoy JR: A sensitive radioassay for biotinidase activity: Deficient activity in tissues of serum biotinidase-deficient individuals. *Clin Chim Acta* **135**: 275, 1984.
337. Gaudry M, Munnich A, Ogier H, Marsac C, Marquet A, Daudubray JM, Mitchell G, et al: Deficient liver biotinidase activity in multiple carboxylase deficiency. *Lancet* **2**: 397, 1983.
338. Hart PS, Hymes J, Wolf B: Biochemical and immunological characterization of serum biotinidase in profound biotinidase deficiency. *Am J Hum Genet* **50**: 126, 1992.
339. Dunkel G, Scriver CR, Clow CL, Melancon S: Prospective ascertainment of complete and partial serum biotinidase deficiency in the newborn. *J Inherit Metab Dis* **12**: 131, 1989.
340. McVoy JR, Levy HL, Lawler M, Schmidt Ms, Ebers DD, Hart PS, Pettit DD, et al: Partial biotinidase deficiency: Clinical and biochemical features. *J Pediatr* **116**: 78, 1990.
341. Hart PS, Hymes J, Wolf B: Biochemical and immunological characterization of serum biotinidase in partial biotinidase deficiency. *Pediatr Res* **31**: 261, 1992.
342. Suormala T, Ramaekers VT, Schweitzer S, Fowler B, Laub MC, Schwermer C, Bachmann J, et al: Biotinidase K_m-variants: Detection and detailed biochemical investigations. *J Inherit Metab Dis* **18**: 689, 1995.
343. Pomponio RJ, Hymes J, Reynolds TR, Meyers GA, Fleischhauer K, Buck GA, Wolf B: Mutations in the human biotinidase gene that cause profound biotinidase deficiency in symptomatic children: Molecular, biochemical and clinical analysis. *Pediatr Res* **42**: 840, 1997.
344. Pomponio RJ, Reynolds TR, Cole H, Buck GA, Wolf B: Mutational "hotspot" in the human biotinidase gene as a cause of biotinidase deficiency. *Nature Genet* **11**: 96, 1995.
345. Pomponio RJ, Norrgard KJ, Reynolds TR, Hymes J, Buck GA, Wolf B: Arg538 to Cys mutation in a CpG dinucleotide of the human biotinidase gene is the second most common cause of biotinidase deficiency in symptomatic children with biotinidase deficiency. *Hum Genet* **99**: 506, 1997.
346. Pomponio RJ, Reynolds TR, Mandel H, Admoni O, Melone PD, Buck GA, Wolf B: Profound biotinidase deficiency caused by a point mutation that creates a downstream cryptic 3′ splice acceptor site within an exon of the human biotinidase gene. *Hum Mol Genet* **6**: 739, 1997.
347. Pomponio RJ, Narasimhan V, Reynolds TR, Buck GA, Povirk LF, Wolf B: Deletion/insertion mutation that causes biotinidase deficiency may result from the formation of a quasipalindromic structure. *Hum Mol Genet* **5**: 1657, 1996.
348. Norrgard KJ, Pomponio RJ, Swango KL, Hymes J, Reynolds TR, Buck GA, Wolf B: Mutation (Q456H) is the most common cause of profound biotinidase deficiency in children ascertained by newborn screening in the United States. *Biochem Mol Med* **61**: 22, 1997.
349. Norrgard KJ, Pomponio RJ, Swango KL, Hymes J, Reynolds TR, Buck GA, Wolf B: Double mutation (A171T and D444H) is a common cause of profound biotinidase deficiency in children ascertained by newborn screening in United States. *Hum Mutat* **11**: 410, 1998.
350. Swango KL, Demirkol M, Huner G, Pronicka E, Sykut-Cegielska J, Schulze A, Wolf B: Partial biotinidase deficiency is usually due to the D444H mutation in the biotinidase gene. *Hum Genet* **102**: 571, 1998.
351. Secor McVoy JR, Heard GS, Wolf B: The potential for the prenatal diagnosis of biotinidase deficiency. *Prenat Diagn* **4**: 317, 1984.
352. Pomponio RJ, Hymes J, Pandya A, Landa B, Melone P, Javaheri R, Mardach R, et al: Prenatal diagnosis of heterozygosity for biotinidase deficiency by enzymatic and molecular analyses. *Prenat Diagn* **18**: 117, 1998.
353. Chalmers RA, Mistry J, Docherty PW, Stratton D: First trimester prenatal exclusion of biotinidase deficiency. *J Inherit Metab Dis* **17**: 751, 1994.
354. Heard GS, Secor McVoy JR, Wolf B: A screening method for biotinidase deficiency in newborns. *Clin Chem* **30**: 125, 1984.
355. Pettit DA, Amador PS, Wolf B: The quantitation of biotinidase activity in dried blood spots using microtiter transfer plates: Identification of biotinidase-deficient and heterozygous individuals. *Anal Biochem* **179**: 371, 1989.
356. Heard GS, Wolf B, Jefferson LG, Weissbecker KA, Nance WE, Secor McVoy JR, Napolitano A, et al: Neonatal screening for biotinidase deficiency: Results of a 1-year pilot study. *J Pediatr* **108**: 40, 1986.
357. Wolf B, Heard GS, Jefferson LG, Proud VK, Nance WE, Weissbecker KA: Clinical findings in four children with biotinidase deficiency detected through a statewide neonatal screening program. *N Engl J Med* **313**: 16, 1985.
358. Wolf B, Heard GS, Jefferson LG, Weissbecker KA, Secor McVoy JR, Nance WE, Mitchell PL, et al: Neonatal screening for biotinidase deficiency: An Update. *J Inherit Metab Dis* **9**(suppl 2): 303, 1986.
359. Wolf B, Heard GS, Jefferson JG, Bennett G, Mitchell P, Linyear A: Worldwide survey of new born screening for biotinidase deficiency, in Therrell B (ed): *Proceedings of the International Symposium for Neonatal Screening*. Amsterdam, Elsevier, 1992.
360. Wolf B: Worldwide survey of neonatal screening for biotinidase deficiency. *J Inherited Metab Dis* **14**: 923, 1991.
361. Wallace SJ: Biotinidase deficiency: Presymptomatic treatment. *Arch Dis Child* **60**: 574, 1985.
362. Chan PW, Bartlett K: A new solid-phase assay for biotin and biocytin and its application to the study of patients with biotinidase deficiency. *Clin Chim Acta* **159**: 185, 1986.
363. Wolf B, Heard GS: Biotinidase deficiency. *Adv Pediatr* **38**: 1, 1991.
364. Suormala T, Wick H, Bonjour JP, Baumgartner ER: Rapid differential diagnosis of carboxylase deficiencies and evaluation for biotin responsiveness in a single blood sample. *Clin Chim Acta* **145**: 151, 1985.
365. Holme E, Jacobson CE, Kristianson B: Biotin responsive carboxylase deficiency in an 8 year old boy with normal serum biotinidase and fibroblast holocarboxylase synthetase activity. *J Inherit Metab Dis* **11**: 270, 1988.
366. Wolf B: Disorders of biotin metabolism: Treatable neurological syndromes, in Rosenberg R, Prusiner SB, Di Mauro S, Barchi RL, Kunkel LM (eds): *The Molecular and Genetic Basis of Neurological Disease*. Stoneham, MA, Butterworth, 1993.

PART

18

HORMONES

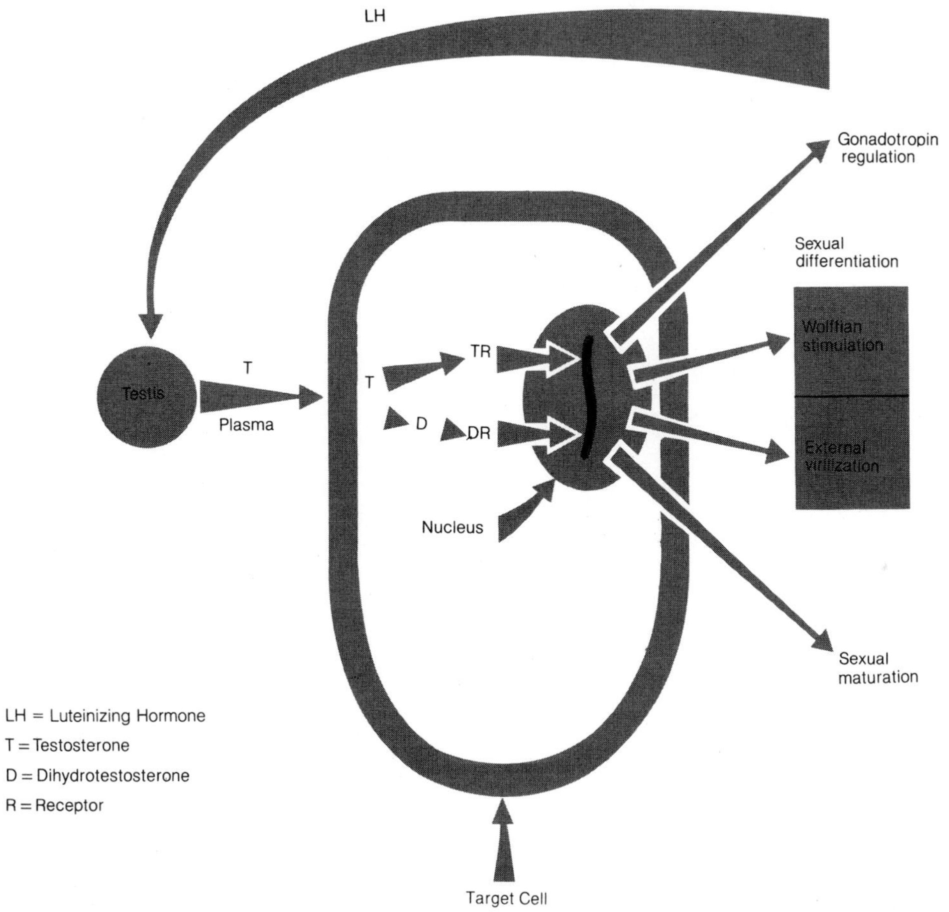

Testosterone

CHAPTER 157

Obesity

Rudolph L. Leibel ▪ Streamson C. Chua ▪ Michael Rosenbaum

1. **Obesity is the presence of excessive amount of adipose tissue. The excessive adipose tissue causes increased blood pressure, hepatic lipid synthesis, insulin resistance, and susceptibility to certain cancers. The anatomic location of the extra body fat has an important effect on the occurrence of these morbidities. Fat located in the intra-abdominal depot appears to convey greater metabolic risk than that in subcutaneous sites. The degree of fatness at which medically significant changes in these quantitative phenotypes occur is variable among individuals and, to some extent, ethnic groups. For example, obesity conveys greater risk of type 2 diabetes in Hispanics, African-Americans and Asians than in Caucasians. Advanced chronologic age may mitigate some of the adverse consequences of an otherwise excessive amount of body fat. For these reasons, no specific absolute amount or fractional content of body fat can be defined as pathologic for all individuals. Finally, adiposity and diminished "metabolic fitness" are not necessarily synonymous. Thus, individuals with high degrees of relative fatness can be physically fit and without apparent metabolic consequence of their adiposity if maintained—with exercise—at sufficient levels of aerobic and strength fitness. For actuarial and public health purposes, recently promulgated World Health Organization Expert Guidelines suggest that overweight and obesity be defined by body mass indices (BMI, a surrogate for adiposity, = Wt(kg)/[Ht(m)]^2) of 25 and 30, respectively.**
2. **Studies of the concordance rates for adiposity among mono- and dizygous twins, and among adoptive children and their family members, and segregation and linkage and association studies, all point to a substantial contribution of genes to the determination of body composition in humans. Relatively rare instances of heritable syndromic obesity (Prader-Willi, Bardet-Biedl, etc.) are well known. More recently, rare mutations of human orthologs of some of the rodent single-gene obesity mutations have been identified (*LEP, LEPR*), as well as mutations in other genes that play a role in the control of body fat (e.g., *POMC, MC4R*, and *PPARG*). However, human obesity is complex and multigenic, with the penetrance of responsible genes showing strong dependence on environmental circumstance. The accelerating prevalence of obesity throughout the world, and especially in developed countries, must be the result of ever more "propitious" environmental circumstances that include high-caloric density foods and labor-saving technologies. The relevant genes determine an individual's adiposity relative to peers in the same environment.**
3. **Experiments in animals and humans point to a dependence of ingestive behavior, reproductive function, somatic growth, and carbohydrate homeostasis on the size of somatic fat stores. Body fat content is "defended" by a complex, coordinated series of metabolic and behavioral responses to reduction of body fat stores below a threshold that is determined by genetic and developmental factors. Clinical evidence of the existence of such regulatory mechanisms is the remarkable long-term constancy of body weight in adults. The average weight gain of 20 pounds between ages 25 and 55 years, considered in the context of energy intake of approximately 900,000 kcal per year, is +0.3 percent. Experimental weight perturbation in closely controlled experimental environment results in compensatory alterations in energy expenditure that can account for much of the relative constancy of body weight over time.**
4. **The neural networks and molecules that mediate control of body composition are now being elucidated. It is clear that the hypothalamus is the center for integration of vegetative endocrine and neural signals arising from adipose tissue, the gastrointestinal tract, various endocrine organs, autonomic nervous system, liver, and other parts of the brain. The hypothalamus also provides efferent signals to higher cortical centers, the brain stem/autonomic nervous system, and the anterior pituitary that affect food intake, energy expenditure, and the partitioning of nutrients between adipose and lean tissues. Within the brain, and especially nuclei of the hypothalamus, a series of orexigenic (NPY, Galanin, MCH, HCRT/Orexin, AGRP) and anorexigenic (MSH, CRF, urocortin, CART) peptides and their cognate receptors mediate the central nervous system processes related to energy homeostasis. Peripheral efferent signals providing information to the central nervous system regarding energy status include signals proportional to fat mass (leptin and possibly insulin) and gut-derived signals (CCK, glucagon, GLP1)**

A list of standard abbreviations is located immediately preceding the index in each volume. Additional abbreviations used in this chapter include: AGRP = agouti-related peptide; ART = agouti-related transcript; AS = Angelman syndrome; ASIP = agouti-signaling peptide; ASP = agouti-signaling protein; BAT = brown adipose tissue; BBS = Bardet Biedl syndrome; BMI = body mass index; CART = cocaine and amphetamine-regulated transcript; CCK = cholecystokinin; CGRP = calcitonin gene-related peptide; CNTF = ciliary muscle neutrotrophic factor; COH1 = Cohen syndrome; CPE = carboxypeptidase E; CRH = corticotrophin-releasing hormone; DA = dopamine; DBH = dopamine beta hydroxylase; DMN = dorsomedial nuclei; DTH = delayed type hypersensitivity; GAL = galanin; GH = growth hormone; GH-R = growth hormone receptor; GLP = glucagon-like peptide; GR = glucocorticoid receptor; GRP = gastrin-releasing peptide; GTG = gold thioglucose; HCRT/ORX = hypocretin/orexin; ICAM-1 = intercellular adhesion molecule 1; ILGH = insulin-like growth factor; LH = lateralhypothalamic area; LPL = lipoprotein lipase; LPS = lipopolysaccharide from bacteria; MAP = mitogen activated protein; MCH = melanin-concentrating hormone; MC1R = melanocortin receptor; MHS = malignant hyperthermia; MR = mineralocorticoid receptor; MSH = melanocyte-stimulating hormone; NPY = neural peptide Y; NTS = nucleus of the solitary tract; OLETF = Otsuka-Long-Evans-Tokushima fatty rat; PBN = parbrachial nucleus; PBSF = pre-B-cell growth-stimulating factor; PC1 = prohormone convertase; PKA = protein kinase A; POMC = proopiomelancoccortin; PPAR = peroxisome proliferator-activated receptor; PVN = paraventricular nucleus; PWS = Prader Willi syndrome; QTL = qualitative trait locus; SDF1 = stromal cell factor 1; SHR = spontaneously hypertensive rat; SRE = sterol regulatory elements; SUR = sulfonylurea receptor; TGF = transforming-growth factor; TH = tyrosine hydroxylase; TNF = tumor-necrosis factor; UCP = uncoupling protein; VMN = ventromedial nuclei; UPD = uniparental disomy; WAT = white adipose tissue; WDF = Wistar diabetic fatty rat; WKY = Wistar Kyoto rat; ZDF = Zucker diabetic fatty rat.

stimulated by single meals. Very short-term neural signals that affect ingestive behavior may be provided by subtle fluctuations in circulating concentrations of glucose (and insulin), and by vagally mediated signals reflecting substrate flux across the gut and hepatic metabolic fuel disposition. The mechanism(s) by which long-term indicators of integrated energy homeostasis (such as leptin) bias short-term feeding decisions (meal size and frequency) is a critical question that remains unsolved.

5. The molecular physiology of weight regulation is profitably viewed through the lens of evolution. Body fat has important permissive effects on reproductive function, somatic growth, and the ability to breast feed progeny. Much of the neural circuitry and many of the molecules alluded to above, function to protect the organism against depletions of energy stores of sufficient severity to impair such critical physiological functions. The higher fractional body fat of females, in a teleological sense, prepares them for the energy costs of pregnancy and lactation. The system for weight regulation evolved in circumstances of restricted, intermittent access to calories, and the need for high levels of physical activity to acquire them. Thus, the system is designed to maximize energy storage, to invoke food seeking, and to reduce energy expenditure in circumstances when energy stores are deemed insufficient. The system is not designed primarily to protect against a phenotype—obesity—not likely to occur in the wild and that would not (unless very severe), either affect reproductive fitness or diminish life span in the reproductive years. The neural pathways and molecules with inhibitory effects on feeding are probably present to prevent the animal from unremitting ingestive behaviors that would interfere with other behaviors necessary for survival and reproduction.
6. Considerations such as those above, and an extensive series of physiological experiments, pointed to the existence of humoral signal(s) from adipose tissue that provide afferent information to the regulatory systems defending body fat content. The *ob* (obese) and *db* (diabetes) mouse mutations display physiologies consistent with this model. A positional cloning strategy was used to clone the *ob* gene whose gene product was named leptin. This molecule was used to identify its cognate receptor in a choroid plexus expression library. The receptor was shown to be the *db* gene. In this way, two important elements (an adipose tissue-derived signal and its hypothalamic receptor) in the regulatory pathway for body fat were identified. The molecular cloning of other rodent single-gene obesities (*Yellow, tubby, fat*) identified other molecules that are components of this system.
7. Leptin is a 146 amino acid peptide which is primarily produced in adipose tissue (but also in placenta and parietal cells of the stomach) and has structural homology to the cytokine family. The molecule is secreted into the blood in proportion to adipose tissue mass, is cleared primarily through the kidneys, and has many of the properties predicted for a feedback signal of somatic fat stores. When administered in the cerebral ventricles of mice and rats, leptin causes reduced food intake, increased energy expenditure (including increased physical activity), and suppresses insulin production while increasing skeletal muscle sensitivity to insulin. Deficiency of leptin action, due either to absence of the peptide (as in the *ob* mutation) or inability to detect the signal (as in the *db* mutation of the receptor) results in extreme obesity and infertility in both rodents and humans. In the hypothalamus, leptin causes coordinate changes in neuropeptide gene expression and release (decreased NPY and HCRT/Orexin; increased CRF, POMC, CART) that reduce food intake. Deficiency of leptin produces the opposite changes. That leptin is not the sole mediator of such responses to the status of energy stores is indicated by the fact that most of these same responses to energy deprivation occur in leptin- (or leptin receptor-) deficient animals.
8. The leptin receptor gene is a member of the cytokine receptor superfamily that includes the interleukin receptors and the growth hormone receptor. LEPR is spliced to at least 5 isoforms, of which the longest (1162 amino acids) is the only one that contains the STAT binding domain required for effects on nuclear transcription. The function of the other isoforms of LEPR is not clear, but the membrane bound isoform may serve as a transporter for leptin across the blood brain barrier, while a soluble isoform without a transmembrane domain, appears to be shed from cells and to act as a binding/transport protein for leptin. The $Lepr^{db}$ mouse has a mutation that interferes only with synthesis of the long form of the receptor. This defect alone is sufficient to produce a phenotype indistinguishable from a leptin deficient (Lep^{ob}) mouse. The long isoform of LEPR functions as a homodimer expressed at highest levels in the hypothalamus. This isoform is expressed at much lower levels in cells outside the central nervous system, including in the pancreatic islets. The role of these peripheral receptors is not clear. Virtually all metabolic effects of leptin can be achieved via central nervous system administration of small amounts of the peptide.
9. The molecular cloning of the extant mouse single-gene obesity mutations, and the identification of many other genes related to energy intake (*NPY, CRF, HCRT/OREXIN*, etc.), energy expenditure (*UCP*'s) and energy partitioning (*GH, LPL, INSULIN, PPARG, MYOSTATIN*) have provided a rich resource for the investigation of the genetic bases for human energy homeostasis. In addition, the availability of reagents and analytic strategies for parametric and nonparametric mapping of phenotypes in human families has enabled the performance of linkage analyses for obesity in humans. In the aggregate, these studies suggest that most human obesity is the result of genetic predisposition mediated by polygenes interacting with the environment. The phenotype that is apparently inherited is adiposity relative to peers within a specific environment. The relevant genes, and allelic variants within them, probably vary among ethnic groups. Approximately 25 mouse quantitative trait loci (QTLs) for aspects of body composition and susceptibility to obesity when provided a high fat diet have been identified. Although no QTL has been cloned, some of them do map to regions of the mouse genome that also contain the major single-gene obesity loci. The same correspondence is noted when human obesity-related phenotypes—treated as qualitative or quantitative traits—are mapped in the human genome.
10. The medical treatment of obesity remains an area of enormous interest and importance, but disappointing efficacy. Based on the molecular physiology of body fat regulation, it is likely that any effective treatment will have to be continued indefinitely because the metabolic/behavioral resistance to maintenance of body composition below "normal" for each individual does not appear, in most instances, to abate with time. It is the maintenance of reduced body weight that is most difficult for patients to

achieve. Behavior modification and drugs that suppress appetite by increasing activity at central noradrenergic and/or serotonergic neurons have limited long-term efficacy. Surgical reduction in gastric capacity has greater long-term efficacy, but carries risks related to surgery. The next generation of drugs—those that impair digestion of dietary fat or increase energy expenditure by activating β_3-adrenoreceptors—are unlikely to have much better efficacy than those that have preceded them because, like their predecessors, they do not interfere with the relevant physiology so centrally as to subvert the compensatory changes that are invoked by alterations in energy intake or expenditure. The pharmacology of obesity at present is in a state similar to that for hypertension 30 years ago. Once the various etiologic mechanisms and contributing genes are better understood, more rational and effective long-term therapy will be possible.

Reproductive efficiency and the suckling of progeny, somatic growth, and ability to withstand extended periods of food deprivation all depend on the availability of somatic stores of chemical energy.[1] The ability to use food energy efficiently, and to store extra calories without impairing mobility or disturbing electrolyte balance, is critical to survival. Adipose tissue was "invented" by evolution to meet these needs.

Triglyceride in adipose tissue is the major physical form in which potential chemical energy is stored in the body (see Table 157-1). The high caloric density and hydrophobicity of triglycerides permit efficient storage of energy without adverse effects on osmotic equilibrium of cytoplasm or plasma. The amount of triglyceride in body adipose tissue stores is the cumulative sum of the difference between energy (food) intake and energy expenditure modified by both endocrine (e.g., growth hormone, insulin, gonadal steroids, the leptin axis) and mechanical factors (e.g., exercise), which affect the partitioning of calories among fat, carbohydrate, or protein.

The prevalence of obesity (excessive adipose tissue stores) in developed and developing countries is increasing rapidly[2] (Table 157-2). Because relevant genetic alterations could not possibly account for such a rapid change in phenotype, the increasing prevalence of obesity may be taken as tacit evidence for potent environmental influences on body fatness. However, as is shown later, there is also strong epidemiologic, physiological, and genetic evidence for the heritability of body fatness.

While there are important examples of single-gene disorders that result in human obesity (discussed later in "Molecular Genetics of Energy Homeostasis"), in most instances body fatness is a continuous quantitative trait reflecting the interaction of developmental processes and environment with genotype. Studies of twins, adoptees, and families[3–6] indicate that as much as 80 percent of the variance in body mass index (BMI = Wt(kg)/[Ht(m)]^2; a surrogate for adiposity) is attributable to genetic factors. That is, the genetic influences on body weight are as potent as those on height, and more potent than those on blood pressure, schizophrenia, and breast cancer[7] (Table 151-3). In twin studies designed to apportion genetic risk variance for obesity (or other phenotypes), phenotypic correspondence is compared in mono- and dizygotic twin pairs.[4,5,7–10] Heritability (H) is defined as $H = 2\ (r_{mz} - r_{dz})$, where r_{mz} refers to the within-pair correlation coefficient of the phenotypic trait in monozygotic twins, and r_{dz} refers to the within-pair correlation coefficient of the trait in dizygous twins.[11] Heritability estimates the fraction of variance in the trait that can be attributed to genotype. Twin studies rely on the assumption that the members of each twin pair share equally the same pre- and postnatal environments, and that, therefore, any greater similarity between mono- versus dizygotic twin pairs reflects mainly the additional 50 percent of genotype shared by the identical twins. This assumption may not be entirely correct because social responses to identical twins may make the environment more concordant between identical than fraternal twins.

By such analytic devices, there is an apparent genetic influence on virtually every aspect of metabolism that relates to somatic energy stores. Heritability of adipose tissue distribution (intra-abdominal versus subcutaneous fat), physical activity, resting metabolic rate, changes in energy expenditure and body composition in response to overfeeding, certain aspects of feeding behavior (including specific food preferences), adipose tissue lipoprotein lipase activity, maximal insulin-stimulated acylglyceride synthesis in adipose tissue, and basal rates of lipolysis are estimated to be as high as 30 to 40 percent.[6,12–14] Segregation analyses in which the familiality of obesity within a population is examined under various inheritance models have found evidence for major genes (allele frequencies 0.14 to 0.26) influencing BMI (20 to 35 percent of variation) in human populations, with an additional approximately 40 percent of the variance being accounted for by polygenic loci.[15] As might be expected, the heritability of early onset obesity appears to be considerably higher than that for adult onset.[3] By virtue of the extremely potent influences of gene x environment interactions in determining the degree of expression of relevant genes, the most strongly inherited trait is probably the rank order of body fatness relative to one's peers within a population sharing the same environment.

Obesity is paradigmatic of phenotypes that are the resolution of complex interactions of genotype with environment and development. Such phenotypes exemplify the important concept that relevant genes mediate *susceptibility* to disease in a specific

Table 157-2 Prevalence of Obesity in the United States from the National Health and Nutrition Education Survey (NHANES)[2]

	NHANES I (1971–74)	NHANES II (1976–80)	NHANES III (1988–91)
Adults —based on BMI >85% from NHANES I	15% (by definition)	24%	33%
Adolescents —based on BMI >85% from NHANES II	No data	15% (by definition)	21%

Table 157-1 Energy Storage Sites in a 70-kg Adult Male and a 30-kg Child*

		70-kg Adult Male		30-kg Child	
Fuel	Tissue	Grams	Kcal	Grams	Kcal
Triglyceride	Adipose	15,000	105,000	4500	31,500
Glycogen	Liver/muscle	70	280	135	540
Glucose	Body fluids	120	480	10	40
Protein	Muscle	6000	25,000	1500	6000

*See references 85 and 938.

Table 157-3 Heritability of Various Medical Conditions Based on Twin Studies[3]

Condition	Heritability
Adiposity in adults based on relative weight at age 45	0.64
Adiposity in adults based on BMI at age 20	0.80
Schizophrenia	0.68
Hypertension	0.57
Epilepsy	0.50
Coronary artery disease	0.49
Breast cancer	0.25

environment, but do not dictate *the inevitable occurrence* of the disease. Individuals with an otherwise potent genetic predisposition to obesity will still be lean (although not as lean as those without such a genetic predisposition to store more calories) in an environment of food deprivation/high demand for physical activity. Individuals not genetically predisposed to obesity may still become so (although not to the extent of those genetically predisposed to store more calories) in an environment that includes readily accessible, highly palatable, calorically dense foods and/or few inducements to physical activity. Thus, in any effort to elucidate the genetic bases for susceptibility to obesity, the "environment" in which the obesity occurs remains a critical determinant of what genes will be identified as contributing to the phenotype. Because the genes that mediate susceptibility to obesity may affect energy intake, energy expenditure, and/or the partitioning of stored calories among lean tissues and fat, the ability to refine phenotypic analysis so as to be able to identify the contribution of each of these subphenotypes is critical to the efficient identification of genes responsible for control of body composition.

Genetic predisposition to obesity is the result of evolution in environments in which food was presumably not easily available, thus favoring selection of metabolically efficient organisms with the ability to store transient caloric excesses as fat.[16] The ability to store excess calories as fat would clearly favor survival in times of restricted nutrient availability, and would also increase the fertility and lactating capacity of females.[17,18] These same evolutionary forces would have little negative effect on the adiposity-related morbidities that are so prevalent in modern Western society—diabetes, hypertension, coronary artery disease, stroke, arthritis—because these morbidities are usually not physiologically important until later in adulthood, that is, after the time of maximal reproductive capacity. It is, therefore, to be expected that the human genome would be enriched for genes that promote the efficient use and storage of the energy in foodstuffs.[16] This chapter reviews the evidence for the existence of such genes, and the neural and molecular mechanisms by which they affect body composition in humans and other animals.

EFFECTS OF EXCESS ADIPOSITY ON HEALTH

Obesity may adversely affect virtually every organ system.[19–21] Between 65 and 75 percent of instances of type 2 diabetes mellitus in the United States are associated with obesity. In addition, obesity remains the most common cause of hypertension in children and adults,[22–24] and is associated with increased frequency of prostate and uterine cancers, mechanical and gouty arthritis and other degenerative joint disease, and a variety of cardiovascular disorders (stroke, coronary artery occlusion).[19] Effects of obesity on various organ systems are summarized in Tables 157-4 and 157-5. The risk of these morbidities and endocrine effects can be substantially reduced by the maintenance of even modest degrees (5 to 10 percent) of weight reduction.[25–30]

Attempts to assess the impact of any measure of body fatness, direct or indirect, on morbidity risk must also take into account related variables such as cigarette smoking, physical activity, diet, and age. In individuals over 55 years of age, body fatness is less predictive of impaired insulin secretion than age per se.[44,45] Therefore, a higher degree of body fatness may be tolerated in an older person without significantly increasing the risk of diabetes mellitus.[46] Similarly, weight gain in men is associated with a significantly greater increase in central (visceral) adipose tissue depot size than similar weight gain in premenopausal women. Because adiposity-related morbidity is closely related to the amount of central body fat, the greater accumulation of central fat in men suggests that more weight gain could be tolerated in premenopausal females than in males.[47] However, weight gain in postmenopausal females assumes more of a male anatomic pattern, and so weight gain in a postmenopausal woman may carry a greater morbidity risk than in a menstruating female (see below).[47]

Table 157-4 Adiposity-Related Morbidities

Skin	Intertrigo; furunculosis; acanthosis nigricans (HAIR-AN syndrome)
Eye	Diabetic eye complications
Respiratory	Increased incidence of upper respiratory infections; abnormalities of central respiratory regulation resulting in sleep apnea; ventilation/perfusion mismatches; respiratory muscle abnormalities; difficulty achieving adequate ventilation during anesthesia
Cardiovascular	Hypertension; atherosclerosis; stroke; syndrome X
Gastrointestinal	Cholecystitis; pancreatitis; colon cancer; hepatic steatosis
Genitourinary	Polycystic ovarian syndrome; infertility; breast cancer; prostate cancer
Musculoskeletal	Coxa vara; slipped capital femoral epiphysis; degenerative arthritis
Neurologic	Stroke; pseudotumor cereberi
Psychologic	Depression; poor self-esteem
Immunologic	Impaired cellular-mediated immunity

Others have suggested that the apparent decline in risk for adiposity-related morbidities with age may reflect the demise of subjects who experienced these morbidities earlier in life.[31,48–50]

From a medical perspective, obesity is perhaps best defined based on the presence of related morbidity and/or the risk of future morbidity, rather than on the basis of an arbitrary BMI (or other) standard. However, the level of energy storage, or "fatness," at which current or future morbidity (e.g., diabetes, dyslipidemia, hypertension) is increased is highly individualized. For example, diabetes, cigarette smoking, hypertension, obesity, and a history of weight gain increase the risk of coronary artery disease in women.[31] Therefore, the risk for this morbidity might be higher in a minimally overweight, hypertensive, diabetic female who

Table 157-5 Adiposity-Related Endocrine Phenotypes[20,939–952]

Somatotroph	Decreased basal and stimulated growth hormone release; normal concentration of somatomedins; accelerated linear growth and bone age
Lactotroph	Decreased prolactin release in response to provocative stimuli; increased basal serum prolactin
Gonadotroph	Early entrance into puberty with normal circulating gonadotropin concentrations
Thyroid	Normal T4 and rT3; normal or increased T3; decreased TSH-stimulated T4 release
Adrenal	Normal (cortisol) but increased cortisol production and excretion; early adrenarche; increased adrenal androgens and DHEA; normal catecholamines
Gonad	Decreased gonadal androgens due to decreased sex-hormone binding globin; dysmenorrhea; dysfunctional uterine bleeding; polycystic ovarian syndrome
Pancreas	Increased insulin and glucagon release; increased resistance to insulin-mediated glucose transport

smokes and has recently gained weight than in a more overweight female without other cardiovascular risk factors. Similarly, in men less than 35 years of age, adiposity is reportedly a better indicator of risk for coronary heart disease than the anatomic distribution of body fat.[32,33] However, in men over 65 years of age, body fat distribution, as measured by waist-to-hip ratio is a much better predictor of coronary risk than body fat mass.[33]

Longitudinal studies of large populations have been used to identify those at increased risk for future morbidity based on measures obtained prospectively in the premorbid state. The relation of body mass index to morbidity related to adiposity illustrates the importance of this approach. In cross-sectional studies, there is a progressive positive correlation of BMI and adiposity-related morbidities.[34] In prospective studies, there is no significant increase in the incidence of future (mean 5 years) adiposity-related morbidities until BMI at entry into the study exceeds 27.5 kg/m^2.[35] Similarly, longitudinal studies have identified obesity in childhood as a risk factor for adult adiposity-related morbidity, independent of whether the obesity persists.[36]

BMI (Wt(kg)/[Ht(m)]^2) is easy to calculate and is commonly used in assessment for obesity.[39] BMI in excess of 28 kg/m^2 is associated with a three- to fourfold increase in overall risk of adiposity-related morbidity (hypertension, dyslipidemia, diabetes mellitus),[40] and a two-fold increase in death rate. Recently, a World Health Organization panel has suggested that individuals with a BMI >25 kg/m^2 should be considered "at-risk" for adiposity-related morbidity while those with a BMI >30 kg/m^2 should be designated as "obese."[34]

BMI is most useful as an epidemiologic tool. However, there are important potential problems that arise from using a specific BMI as a cut off for the "definition" of obesity in an individual, rather than as an indicator of an individual's need to be examined for morbidities that may be related to adiposity. The composition of an individual's body weight is a critical determinant of morbidity risk, and BMI does not provide a direct measure of body composition. Correlation coefficients between BMI and percentage of body fat determined indirectly by skinfold thicknesses[41] vary from 0.23 to 0.89 depending on such factors as age, gender, and ethnicity.[42] BMI is an especially problematic measure in individuals who are at the extremes of adiposity. A muscular athlete may have a high BMI despite low fractional body fat, while an individual with a large intra-abdominal fat depot and resultant high morbidity risk, may have a more normal BMI.[43]

Impact of Body Fat Distribution on Health[36] Relative centrality of distribution of body fat (waist/hip ratio >0.90 in females; >1.0 in males) is associated with a higher risk of stroke, ischemic heart disease, diabetes, and mortality than a more peripheral distribution of body fat (waist/hip ratio <0.75 in females; <0.85 in males), and may be a more sensitive indicator of morbidity risk than absolute fat mass.[51–56] For example, in a 13-year follow-up study of 792 men whose body mass, height, and waist-to-hip ratio had been measured at age 54,[54] the incidence of ischemic heart disease and death were 3.6 and 5.5 times greater, respectively, in subjects who were initially in highest tercile for waist-to-hip ratio but in the lowest tercile for BMI (slender men with an abdominal fat distribution), than subjects who were initially in the lowest tercile for waist-to-hip ratio but in the highest for BMI (overweight men with a peripheral fat distribution).

The physiological mechanisms for the association between body fat distribution and associated morbidities are not known. It has been suggested that the increased flux of free fatty acids through the hepatic portal circulation resulting from large intra-abdominal (visceral) fat depots provides substrates for triglyceride synthesis (some of which are then incorporated in low-density and very-low-density lipoproteins), and also promotes insulin resistance by interfering with first-pass hepatic catabolism of insulin.[56,57] Indirect measures of the size of the visceral adipose tissue depot, such as waist circumference or sagittal diameter, are better correlated with certain cardiovascular morbidities than indices of body fatness (BMI or percentage body fat) or relative fat distribution (waist-to-hip ratio).[58] An interesting alternative mechanistic view of the association between high levels of intra-abdominal fat and increased risk of coronary artery disease, diabetes, and hypertension, suggests that psychologic stress, through effects on the adrenal axis and autonomic nervous system, may cause both the increase in intra-abdominal fat deposition and the associated morbidities.[59]

Just as even modest weight reduction will significantly decrease the risk of these morbidities, weight gain *per se* has been reported to constitute a significant risk factor for hypertension and diabetes mellitus after adjusting for absolute level of body fatness. A woman who is moderately obese but has maintained the same level of body fatness since age 18 years, is at lower risk for hypertension and stroke than a woman who is at the same level of body fatness, but has gained weight in adulthood.[25,50]

Age is also an important factor in assessing morbidity risk related to adiposity. The likelihood that an obese child will become an obese adult increases with chronological age, independent of the number of years that a child has been overweight.[60]

Thus, many factors including age, ethnicity, gender, duration of obesity, as well as individual health history and current morbidities must be included in the evaluation of any individual's risk of subsequent adiposity-related morbiity.[33]

ADIPOSE TISSUE BIOCHEMISTRY AND DEVELOPMENT

Mammals possess both brown and white adipose tissue. Brown adipose tissue (BAT), so named because of the brown color of the cytochrome pigments of its densely packed mitochondria, is probably of neuroectodermal origin.[65] In rodents, BAT is located in the interscapular region, and around the aorta and kidneys. BAT has a very rich vascular and sympathetic nerve supply. BAT's major function appears to be as a thermogenic organ capable of dissipating the energy of its constituent fatty acids as heat rather than capturing their potential chemical energy as ATP. This heat release is achieved by activating a mitochondrial proton shunt (uncoupling protein) which permits protons to descend an energy gradient along the inner mitochondrial membrane, generating heat instead of being transported by F_1F_0 ATP synthase. Facultative invocation of this shunt, by fatty acids either donating protons to the UCP,[61] or themselves being reciprocally translocated through the membrane,[62] enables cold-induced thermogenesis and dietary-induced thermogenesis in rodents.[63,64] There is, however, currently little evidence that BAT plays an important role in thermogenesis in the adult human.[65]

The much more abundant white adipose tissue (WAT) derives from mesenchyme. Fully differentiated adipocytes are first detectable in the human fetus by approximately 15 weeks of gestation. Both adipocyte volume and number continue to increase throughout gestation, with maximal rates of change achieved after about the thirtieth week.[66]

The size of the fetal adipose tissue depot is, to some degree, dependent upon the same factors that determine the size of the adult adipose tissue depot: energy intake (in this case via the placenta); energy expenditure, and the partitioning of stored calories between lean tissues and adipose tissue triglycerides. The infant of the diabetic mother is a model for the influences of fetal overnutrition and partitioning on subsequent adiposity. Exposure of the fetus to high ambient glucose concentrations stimulates endogenous fetal insulin production, and lipogenesis. Because gestationally diabetic women are often obese, it is difficult to separate the metabolic consequences of gestational obesity and/or diabetes *per se* on subsequent adiposity of the infant of a diabetic mother, from the possibility that the mother has transmitted a genetic tendency towards obesity to her offspring. Studies of the obesity-prone Pima Indians of Arizona attempted to distinguish genetic/pregestational and gestational influences on adiposity of progeny. A significantly higher percentage of offspring of gestationally diabetic Pima Indian women are obese (defined as greater than 140 percent "ideal" body weight) at age 15 to 19 years than offspring of nondiabetic women, and these differences in the incidence of obesity are independent of the degree of maternal obesity.[67] This suggests that high rates of fetal fat production and/or other metabolic consequences of the milieu of the diabetic mother may constitute an independent risk factor for subsequent obesity.

Rat pups whose dams are malnourished during the first 2 weeks of a 3-week gestation display hyperphagia and an increase in adult adiposity.[68–70] Epidemiologic studies of the effects of intra- and early extra-uterine malnutrition on the risk of obesity in humans suggest that such effects are subtle in most instances.[71] Males born during or just after the Nazi-imposed Dutch "Winter Hunger" (1944–45) showed slightly higher absolute prevalence of obesity (defined as weight/height greater than 120 percent of the World Health Organization standards) at age 19 (1.32 percent of subjects from famine area vs. 0.82 percent of controls) if malnourished in utero (first two trimesters). These male military inductees showed a slightly reduced incidence of obesity (1.45 percent of subjects from famine area vs. 2.77 percent of controls) if malnourished in the last trimester of pregnancy, or the first 3 to 5 months of extrauterine life.[72] The adipogenic effects of early intrauterine malnutrition might be due to effects on hypothalamic development, while the antiadipogenic effects of early postnatal malnutrition might be due to suppression of adipocyte formation.

In 1968, Knittle and Hirsch reported that underfeeding or overfeeding of preweanling rat pups, by experimental manipulation of litter size, was associated with respective decreases or increases in body size, epididymal fat pad cell number, and cell size that persisted, despite subsequent *ad libitum* feeding of rat chow.[73] In litters of Zucker rat pups in which some of the offspring were homozygous for a *(fa/fa)* mutation in what was subsequently shown to be the leptin receptor,[74] *(fa/fa)* pups subjected to early undernutrition by virtue of large litter size subsequently remained significantly leaner than *(fa/fa)* rats who were not nutritionally deprived, but still fatter than their *(fa/+* or *+/+)* lean littermates, whether they were nutritionally deprived or not, when allowed *ad libitum* access to food.[75] These experiments in Zucker rats demonstrate the profound effects of genotype, environment (in this case, early nutritional plane) and genotype x environment interaction on adiposity.

There is currently no firm evidence that early infant feeding practices significantly affect risk of later obesity in humans. Though formula-fed babies tend to be longer and heavier than their breast-fed peers, these differences do not persist.[77] The age at which specific foods are introduced into the diet[9,78,79] and the relative amount of fat, carbohydrate or protein in the diet of infants[80,81] or adults[82,83] do not appear to exert a significant influence on subsequent adiposity. Consistent with the view that infancy has little long-term effect on adiposity is the observation that obesity in infancy, even in the setting of a strong family history of obesity, is a poor predictor of obesity in adulthood compared to adiposity in adolescence.[84]

During the first year of extrauterine life, most adipose tissue growth occurs via enlargement (hypertrophy) rather than increased adipocyte number (hyperplasia), but after 2 years of age, there is little further increase in adipocyte volume in the nonobese child.[85,86] In nonobese children, there is no significant change in fat cell volume from ages 2 to 14 years and only a slight increase in fat cell number from ages 2 to 10 years. In obese children, there is continual enlargement of adipocytes without hyperplasia during this same period.[87] These observations are consistent with a model of adipose tissue growth (see below) in which adipocyte hyperplasia is triggered by achievement of a critical adipocyte volume.

Most clinically significant obesity in humans effects adipocyte hyperplasia as well as hypertrophy.[76] Adipocyte hyperplasia persists despite weight loss. There is believed to be a virtually unlimited pool of preadipocytes constituted by the pericytes of the pericapillary endothelium. These adipocyte precursors cannot be visually or biochemically distinguished from other fibroblasts, and have no detectable lipogenic or lipolytic enzyme activity. The proximate signal for the start of the differentiation program in these cells is not known. After a cell differentiates into an adipocyte, the differentiation is apparently irreversible except on exposure to unusual hormonal milieus such as the insulin-induced hypersecretion of TNFα, which is present in diabetic lipoatrophy.[88,89] Because adipocytes cannot "de-differentiate," an individual whose obesity was characterized by adipocyte hyperplasia will continue to have an increased number of fat cells, albeit substantially reduced in volume, even after body fat content is reduced to the level of a never-obese individual.[90] The persistence of these small adipocytes and possible changes in adipocyte-related humoral signals due to decreased cell size, may play a role in the metabolic syndrome that characterizes the reduced obese[19] (see "Energy Homeostasis and Regulation of Body Weight" below).

In vitro and *in vivo* studies suggest that there is local control of adipocyte differentiation, perhaps by signals generated from preadipocytes or mature adipocytes in the vicinity. When examined in tissue culture, the fibroblasts from the pericapillary epithelium multiply until a state of confluence is reached. Once confluence has occurred, isolated nests of cells terminally differentiate into groups of adipocytes separated by patches of undifferentiated cells. However, if the remaining undifferentiated cells are stimulated to divide further by creating an "adipocyte-free" space around them, they will also differentiate.[91] In vivo maximal adipocyte lipid content appears to be approximately 1 μg lipid/cell.[76] Once this degree of hypertrophy is reached, recruitment of new adipocytes appears to begin,[92] suggesting that adipocyte hypertrophy may generate signals that promote further differentiation of preadipocytes.[93,94] During therapeutic weight loss in children in early adolescence, the rate at which new fat cells develop is diminished. However, fat cell number apparently continues to increase at a rate significantly greater than that of age-matched controls on an *ad libitum* diet.[95] These data imply that fat cell hyperplasia can be therapeutically restrained, but that the rate of appearance of new fat cells may, to some extent, be genetically or developmentally programmed.

Transcription Factors Affecting Adipogenesis

Several recently described transcription factors have important effects on adipogenesis. PPARγs are members of the Peroxisome Proliferator Activated subfamily of nuclear hormone receptors that form heterodimers with retinoid X receptors (RxRχ) to regulate gene expression.[834] PPARγ exists as two isoforms (γ1, γ2) formed by alternative splicing. The two PPARγ isoforms differ in that PPARγ2 has an NH_2 terminal extension of 28 amino acids.[2] The exact functional significance of these splice variants is not known, but both are important factors in differentiation of fibroblasts to mature adipocytes and differentiation of arterial wall monocytes/macrophages to form cells that scavenge oxidized LDL and promote atherosclerotic lesions.[96,97,835] Thus, these genes may account for some of the associations of body fatness with coronary artery disease (see Effects of Excess Adiposity on Health).

PPARγ gene expression in adipose tissue is diminished during fasting, in hypoleptinemic states (such as that induced by thiazoidinediones), and increased during overfeeding and hyperleptinemic states, glucocorticoid administration, and, as the name implies, in response to the administration of peroxisome-proliferating drugs such as clofibrate.[98] The thiazolidinediones, e.g., troglitzone, which enhance peripheral insulin sensitivity, are also high affinity ligands for the PPARγ receptor[841–843] and induce PPARγ-mediated new adipocyte formation (smaller, more insulin-sensitive adipocytes) and suppерssion of TNF production.[844]

Expression of PPARγ1 converts fibroblasts into fully differentiated adipocytes.[96] PPARγ2, expressed predominantly in fat, is induced very early in adipocyte differentiation and, in turn, controls/induces the expression of adipocyte-specific genes[96,97] by binding to promoters for adipocyte P2 (aP2, encodes fatty acid binding protein) and phosphoenoylyruvate carboxykinase (PEPCK) genes[97,836]), which are themselves important in adipocyte lipid synthesis. Phosphorylation of PPARγ2 at serine 114 reduces the potency of PPARγ2 to promote adipocyte differentiation.[837,838] This serine is a consensus phosphorylation site for mitogen activated protein (MAP) kinase (PXSP motif). Naturally occurring ligands for PPARγ include the members of the prostaglandin D family, 15-deoxyδ 12,14 prostaglandin J2 and, possibly, other saturated fatty acid derivatives.[839,840] If these molecules act as physiological ligands for PPARγ, they presumably do so via mechanisms other than the cell-surface receptors for the prostaglandins.

PPARγ2 interacts in a cooperative manner with other transcription factors in adipogenesis. CCAAT Enhancer Binding Protein Alpha (C/EBPα) is a transcription factor expressed relatively late in adipogenesis. Like PPARγ2, C/EBPα activates adipocyte-specific genes such as aP2.[96,97] Fibroblasts lacking specific activators for PPARγ2 and/or C/EBPα demonstrate reduced adipogenesis and reduced lipid content once differentiated, while cells, such as myoblasts, that do not normally differentiate into adipocytes will undergo adipogenesis if expression of both of these transcription factors is induced by transfection.[99,100] Other CCAAT Enhancer Binding Protein – C/EBPβ and C/EBPδ – are also expressed early in adipogenesis and act to increase expression of PPARγ resulting in further adipocyte generation.[101] Finally, Adipocyte Determination and Differentiation-dependent Factor 1/ Sterol Regulatory Element Binding Protein (ADD/SREBP1, a basic helix-loop-helix protein which is also expressed early in adipogenesis) induces both fatty acid synthetase and lipoprotein lipase expression.[102] Like the C/EBPs, ADD/SREBP1 also induces further expression of PPARγ.[102]

Insulin-mediated changes in C/EBP, ADD/SREBP1 and PPARγ expression and functional activity may provide a connection between nutritional status (energy stores) and rates of adipocyte production.[98] PPARγ induction by C/EBPβ and δ is dependent upon the presence of glucocorticoids.[101] This glucocorticoid-dependence provides a possible explanation for some of the ameliorating effects of adrenalectomy on the obesity phenotype in virtually all models of rodent obesity (genetic, hypothalamic injury).[563] The effects of leptin on these transcription factors have yet to be determined, and may represent another mechanism by which adipocyte metabolism is linked to adipogenesis.

Effects of Metabolite Flux on Leptin Production

Flux through the hexosamine pathway (converts fructose-6-phosphate to UDP-N-acetylglucosamine) has been suggested as a mechanism by which adipose tissue monitors the acute and chronic energy balance status of organisms. Increased flux through this pathway, presumably due to increased availability of fructose-6-phosphate and as reflected in the availability of the end product of the hexosamine pathway (UDP-N-acetylglucosamine), results in increased storage of calories as fat.[998] Transgenic mice overexpressing the rate-limiting enzyme in the hexosamine pathway demonstrate significantly increased leptin production in muscle and adipose tissue.[998,999] Metabolic states, such as hyperglycemia or hyperlipidemia, which increase flux through the hexosamine pathway are also associated with increased leptin production[999] and, like glucose and insulin, glucosamine is capable of inducing expression of C/EBPα, an adipogenic transcription factor, in adipocytes.[1000] Thus, increased flux through the hexosamine pathway (indicative of increased availability of metabolic fuel) may act as a "signal" favoring adipogenesis.

Oral administration of PPARγ_1 ligand, thiazolidinedione BRL49653, to rats, resulted in significant weight gain, increased food intake and a decrease in leptin mRNA expression in epididymal adipose tissue. Incubation of human preadipocytes from subcutaneous depots, but not visceral (omental) depots, with thiazolidinedione, induces adipocyte differentiation.[106] It is likely that some of these proteins play a role in mediating the effects of adipocyte volume on recruitment/differentiation of new adipocytes. Leptin, whose synthesis rate in adipose tissue appears to increase with increased adipocyte volume,[107] is a plausible signal for the recruitment of new adipocytes. In addition, leptin's apparent ability to promote vascularization[108] provides a mechanism for the generation of new blood vessels to perfuse the additional adipose tissue. Leptin, however, cannot be the only signal for such events because *ob* and *db* mice, which lack leptin or its receptor, show abundant adipocyte hyperplasia, and the in vitro conversion rates of preadipocytes to adipocytes do not differ in precursors taken from lean and obese Zucker (leptin-receptor deficient) rats.[109]

ENERGY HOMEOSTASIS AND REGULATION OF BODY WEIGHT

The history of the scientific study of the biology of energy metabolism begins in 1773 with the recognition by Lavoisier and LaPlace that combustion and animal respiratory metabolism are chemically comparable processes: a respiring animal and a burning piece of wood produce the same amount of heat per mass of CO_2 produced.[110] In the ensuing 125 years, a distinguished succession of physicists, chemists, and physiologists established the principles of thermodynamics and their applicability to biologic systems. Much of the struggle to understand the biology of energy metabolism and weight regulation has been conducted in the presence of persisting vitalist misconceptions or misrepresentations regarding bioenergetics, and widely held perceptions of obesity as the "psychologic" product of self-indulgence.[111]

Physiological Evidence of Body Weight Regulation in Humans

Overview of Energy Homeostasis The first law of thermodynamics states that the change in amount of energy stored in a physical system (ΔU) equals the difference between energy input (Q) to the system and work (W) done by the system: $\Delta U = Q - W$. This law is irrevocably applicable to biological systems. In a biological context, U is the chemical energy stored in the organism (mostly as fat, see Table 157-1). Q is food intake and W is metabolic and skeletal muscle work. W can be further compartmentalized into resting energy expenditure, which is the work of maintaining transmembrane ion gradients and cardiovascular/respiratory function at rest; the thermic effect of feeding, which is the work of digestion and transport of ingested molecules and intercurrent oxidation; and nonresting energy expenditure (or physical activity).[112] Resting energy expenditure constitutes about 60 percent of W and is very closely correlated with fat-free mass.[112] The thermic effect of feeding accounts for about 5 to 10 percent of W, and is most affected by the number of calories ingested. Most of the remainder of 24-h energy expenditure is accounted for by nonresting energy expenditure. Another compartment of energy expenditure, sometimes referred to as "thermogenesis" denotes chemical energy used to generate heat rather than metabolic work.[113] Examples of such processes are simultaneous glycolysis and gluconeogenesis, lipolysis and acylglyceride synthesis, and the shunting of mitochondrial protons down an electrochemical gradient into the mitochondrial matrix without generating ATP ("uncoupled oxidation" such as occurs in the mitochondria of brown adipose tissue [see Uncoupling Proteins]). An additional determinant of body fat content is a process referred to as "caloric partitioning." This term denotes the metabolic mechanisms that determine whether an ingested calorie is oxidized, or stored as fat, glycogen, or protein. The ability to convert glucose to fat, nucleotides, or nonessential amino acids is an example of this process. The molecular genetics of partitioning is discussed in detail in "Molecular Genetics of Energy Homeostasis" below.

The amount of fat (triglyceride) in body adipose tissue stores is the cumulative sum of the differences between energy (food) intake and energy expenditure (mainly resting metabolism and physical activity) and effects of partitioning. Although homeostatic mechanisms to be described tend to keep the difference between intake and expenditure very close to zero, very small, long-term imbalances can have large cumulative effects. Given current easy access to highly palatable, calorically dense foods and sedentary lifestyle, it is not surprising that the bias is towards positive energy balance. For example, a nonobese adult ingests about 900,000 kcal of food per annum. A pound of adipose tissue contains about 3500 kcal of potential chemical energy. Thus, a 2 percent cumulative imbalance in intake versus expenditure results in an 18,000-kcal (~5-pound) weight change in 1 year. Because energy expenditure increases as weight increases (energy expenditure is a first-order covariate of body metabolic mass), this imbalance would be, to some extent, compensated for by the additional weight gained. However, based on such calculations, the 20-pound weight gain experienced by the average American adult between 25 and 55 years of age,[114] represents a remarkably small positive imbalance of only about 0.3 percent of ingested calories over such a 30-year period.

Autonomic Nervous System and Thyroid Hormones The autonomic nervous system and the thyroid "axis" provide apparent organism-wide coordination of the various cellular effectors of energy expenditure.[174] Both of these systems are strongly linked to the hypothalamus to provide integration of energy intake and expenditure (see "Neuroanatomy and Neurochemistry of Energy Homeostasis" below). Increased parasympathetic autonomic nervous output slows heart rate, increases pancreatic insulin release, and decreases resting energy expenditure. Increased sympathetic autonomic output has the opposite effects. Noradrenergic and adrenergic transmissions from the sympathetic nervous system modulate vasomotor activity, feeding behavior, and thyroid function. Thyroid hormones alter energy expenditure by effects on mitochondrial respiration and the autonomic nervous system.[175] Obese and never-obese adults studied at usual body weight, during weight loss, and during the maintenance of a reduced body weight, show declines in sympathetic nervous system activity (and increases in parasympathetic activity), and in circulating concentrations of thyroid hormone, when compared to these measures at usual weight both during weight loss and during the maintenance of a reduced body weight.[176,177] Catecholamine release in response to insulin-induced hypoglycemia is diminished in reduced-obese patients,[176,178–180] and serum triiodothyronine is lowered in subjects during the process of weight loss and increased in subjects during dynamic weight gain.[178,181–183] Thus, these systems act in a complementary manner to regulate body weight (Table 157-6).

Mechanisms of Energy Dissipation It is possible that some of the apparent long-term regulation of fat stores occurs via regulated activity of metabolic "futile" cycles that consume ATP without performing net biochemical work. Examples of these include the simultaneous processes of lipolysis and acylglyceride synthesis in adipose tissue, hepatic glycolysis/gluconeogenesis, fatty acid oxidation in BAT uncoupled from ATP generation, and possibly the activity of molecules with structural and functional homology to the uncoupling protein of BAT (UCP1).[113,146–149]

The first uncoupling protein gene cloned (UCP1; located at 4q31) encodes a 307-amino acid mitochondrial-carrier protein expressed primarily in brown adipose tissue.[150] As indicated earlier, UCP1 plays a role in thermogenesis and body weight regulation in rodents and some hibernating species.[63–65] While BAT appears to play a role in nonshivering thermogenesis in the human neonate,[151] there is currently little evidence to support a significant role of UCP1 or other "futile" cycles in energy homeostasis in the adult human.[65,85,152]

The genes encoding uncoupling proteins 2 and 3 (UCP2 and UCP3; located at 11q13) were identified by homology searches to UCP1 among existing mRNA sequences.[153–157] These proteins have 73 percent homology with each other, and 59 percent and 57 percent homology, respectively, with UCP1. UCP2 is expressed in white blood cells, in brown and white adipose tissue, and in skeletal and cardiac muscle.[153] UCP3 is expressed primarily in skeletal muscle.[156] Despite their sequence homology to UCP1, it is not yet clear that UCP2 and UCP3 function primarily (or at all) as true uncoupling proteins. These molecules are members of a family of mitochondrial substrate transport proteins and it is possible that they function primarily as mediators of fuel disposition.[158]

Change in the expression of uncoupling protein(s) is a possible mechanism for the changes in skeletal muscle energy metabolism described above.[153–156,159,160] Administration of a β_3 adrenoreceptor aganist, which induces UCP expression in adipose tissue and skeletal muscle, promotes weight loss in obese yellow KK mice.[160] In rodents, food restriction to 50 percent of usual daily caloric intake causes a significant decline in skeletal muscle UCP3 expression, while UCP2 and UCP3 expression are increased during fasting.[159,161] The decrease in rodent skeletal muscle UCP3 expression during caloric restriction, and paradoxical increase during fasting, may reflect the response of UCP3 to stress hormones, such as glucocorticoids and catecholamines, which are induced by fasting. In humans, fasting is also associated with significant increases in expression of both UCP2 and UPC3 mRNA in skeletal muscle.[162] In humans, skeletal muscle (vastus lateralis) expression of UCP3 mRNA (both long and short isoforms) is decreased by 50 to 75 percent ($P < 0.05$) by maintenance of a reduced body weight (as opposed to fasting); *UCP2* expression is not significantly changed under these circumstances.[163] The observation that maintenance of a reduced body weight is associated with a significant decline in UCP3 mRNA expression, is consistent with the decline in the energy cost of physical activity reported following weight loss, and suggests a possible role for UCP3 as a mediator of the increase in skeletal muscle work efficiency following weight loss in humans.[164] The increase in UCP3 mRNA expression in skeletal muscle noted during fasting in humans may be part of a stress-response to fasting, or a counterregulatory process related to reduced body temperature associated with fasting, rather than a metabolic adaptation to an altered body weight. Further insights into the functional role(s) of UCP3 are afforded by mouse /UCP3/ knockouts and humans with splice mutations of UCP3 (see later).

Diet Composition Some studies in animals and humans suggest that diet composition per se plays an important role in energy homeostasis.[120,171,172] These studies find preferential oxidation of ingested carbohydrates while ingested lipids are stored in adipose tissue. However, in adults, weight-maintenance caloric requirements are not altered by extremely wide variation (10 to 70 percent) of the percentage of the calories derived from fat.[82,173] While diet composition does not appear to affect weight-maintenance caloric requirements, diet composition has potent effects on food intake via palatability and caloric density of food. It is also possible that diet composition affects the partitioning of stored calories in a growing child, but does not have this effect on an organism whose growth has ceased. Likewise, in humans, repeated weight fluctuations ("yo-yoing") does not appear to affect body composition or weight-maintenance caloric requirements at usual body weight.[127]

Genetics of Responses to Weight Perturbation As might be expected, there are genetic influences on the magnitude of responses to weight perturbation. For example, Bouchard et al. and Poehlman et al. demonstrated significantly decreased variance in resting energy expenditure, thermic effect of feeding, and degree of hypermetabolism induced by voluntary overfeeding within monozygotic twin pairs as compared to variance in the

Table 157-6 Changes in Energy Expenditure, Autonomic Nervous System Activity and Thyroid Function During Dynamic Weight Change and Maintenance of an Altered Body Weight[176–183,953]

	Dynamic weight loss	Maintenance of a reduced weight	Dynamic weight gain	Maintenance of an increased weight
24-h energy expenditure	↓↓	↓	↑	↑
Resting energy expenditure	↓	↓	↑	↔
Thermic effect of expenditure	↔	↔	↑	↑
Nonresting energy expenditure	↓	↓	↑	↑
Thyroxine (T4)	↔	↔	↔	↔
Triiodothyronine (T3)	↓	↓	↑	↑
Reverse T3	↑	↑	↔	↔
Thyroid stimulating hormone	↔	↔	↔	↔
Sympathetic nervous system activity	↓	↓	↑	↑
Parasympathetic nervous system	↑	↑	↓	↓

general population or to variance between monozygotic twin pairs.[6,13,140,141]

There is also a strong heritable component to energy intake. Saltzman et al. showed significant heritability of the number of calories consumed, as well as the thermic effect of feeding when subjects are offered diets of varying fat content.[142] Studies comparing mono- and dizygotic twin pairs suggest that 20 to 45 percent of the variance in meal frequency, and 22 to 65 percent of the variance in meal size, as well as food preferences (high-fat vs. low-fat diet) are attributable to genetic factors.[143–145]

Physiological Responses to Weight Change A rapidly growing body of physiological, molecular biologic, and neuroendocrine data indicate that this degree of control of body composition is achieved by coordinate regulation of energy intake and expenditure mediated via endocrine and neural signals emanating from adipose tissue and gut, and integrated by the liver and vegetative central nervous system (hypothalamus and brain stem). The molecular physiology of these systems is discussed in "Neuroanatomy and Neurochemistry of Energy Homeostasis" and "Molecular Genetics of Energy Homeostasis" sections below.

Short-term (daily) food intake is not closely correlated with daily energy expenditure or energy stores in adults[115] or children.[116] Accordingly, some means of biasing these short-term determinants of net energy balance over longer periods of time is needed. Longer term effects on food intake are presumably designed to integrate physiological "knowledge" of the magnitude of somatic energy stores with shorter term ingestive behavior. Some students of this integration see it as mediated by fuel fluxes (circulating free fatty acids, amino acids, glycerol or glucose; or amounts of hepatic glycogen; or rates of hepatic oxidative metabolism) resulting indirectly from changes in adipose tissue mass.[117–121] Others have hypothesized that body fat stores are directly sensed[1,122–126] and that this signal, in turn, biases shorter term ingestive behaviors (and energy expenditure via effects on the autonomic nervous system) so as to hold body energy stores relatively constant over time. These are not, of course, mutually exclusive hypotheses. In fact, it is clear that systems regulating energy intake and expenditure, from the highest cortical centers to the adipocyte, are synergistic and redundant.[1031]

An important clinical observation in support of the concept that body fat content is regulated is the response of human subjects (lean and obese) to experimental perturbations of body weight. At "usual" body weight, 24-h energy expenditure is not significantly different between lean and obese individuals when normalized to body composition. In both obese and lean individuals, relatively small (10 percent) decreases in body weight provoke declines in energy expenditure that are greater than can be accounted for by decreased body size and metabolic mass. This decrease persists, despite return to caloric intake sufficient to maintain the new lower weight and body composition.[127] Thus, a formerly obese individual requires 10 to 15 percent fewer calories to maintain a "lower" body weight than a never-obese individual of the same body weight and body composition.[127–129] This decline in 24-h energy expenditure, corrected for the altered body weight and composition, reflects decreases in resting energy expenditure (~18 percent) and nonresting energy expenditure (~25 percent).[127] There is also metabolic resistance to the maintenance of an elevated body weight. Thus, a lean or obese individual who has overeaten to achieve a body weight 10 percent above usual, requires approximately 15 percent more calories per unit of metabolic mass to maintain the elevated body weight than predicted by energy needs for weight maintenance at usual body weight.[127]

Some investigators have not found such changes in resting energy expenditure following weight loss.[130–133] This discordance may reflect, in part, interstudy differences in how resting energy expenditure was measured (during sleep, awake but before arising from bed, or after arising from bed).[134] Resting energy expenditure is also clearly affected by the process of dynamic weight loss or gain, and lack of precise weight stability in subjects during periods of study may obscure subtle differences in energy expenditure. The subtle nature of the changes in energy metabolism with weight change points to one of the major difficulties in efforts to identify relevant genes in humans: the phenotypes must be ascertained under circumstances in which the environment is fully controlled, and obese individuals show no defect in energy metabolism when obese.

The preeminence of NREE as the component of energy expenditure that is most affected by changes in body weight, suggests that individuals adapt to altered body weight by changing the amount of physical activity (exercise and non-exercise activity such as fidgeting), and/or the efficiency (energy cost) of physical activity.[129,1001,1002] Leibel et al. noted no weight-change associated alteration in the amount of time that subjects spend in physical activity,[127] while the energy cost of physical activity decreases significantly following weight loss, suggesting that the chemomechanical efficiency of skeletal muscle, rather than the time spent in physical activity, is affected by weight change.[129,1001,1002] A number of studies have demonstrated that skeletal muscle mechanical efficiency (ratio of power gnerated to energy expended) is increased in undernourished subjects,[1003–1006] indicating that skeletal muscle is the major effector organ mediating the decline in energy expenditure that occurs with weight loss.

One possible mechanism for the increased chemomechanical efficiency of skeletal muscle following weight loss is that weight change results in alterations in the type of fuel used by muscle to perform low levels of mechanical work. Animal and human studies indicate that a shift towards fatty acid metabolism, as opposed to glucose, is associated with increased skeletal muscle work efficiency *in vivo* and *in vitro*.[1007–1009] Hyperinsulinemia, as might occur following weight gain, has been shown to promote a shift towards greater glycolysis in skeletal muscle[1010] and skeletal muscle glycolytic capacity is negatively correlated with insulin sensitivity.[1011,1012] In contrast, hypocaloric feeding has been reported to favor utilization of fatty acid (over carbohydrate) as fuel by skeletal muscle.[1013,1014]

The differential effects of the process of weight change and of weight maintenance at an altered weight are summarized in Table 157-6.

The mechanisms by which such subtle but significant adjustments in energy expenditure are made are not known. Systems sensitive to somatic energy stores, for example, the leptin axis, may invoke changes in metabolic rate and skeletal muscle chemomechanical efficiency by autonomic or other effector systems. Whatever the mechanism(s), a critical question remains as to why the energy intake in such situations is not decreased to match the lower energy expenditure. It is the persistence of energy intake in excess of energy expenditure that leads to the return of body weight to preperturbation status.[135]

Fig. 157-1 shows the relationships among energy intake, expenditure, and partitioning in determining the amount and proportion of body fat. As indicated earlier, hepatic fuel fluxes and glycogen storage may affect food intake as well as the specific mix of substrates oxidized. In the figure, emphasis is given to the concept that fat mass generates a signal (e.g., leptin) that, acting via the hypothalamus, affects both energy intake and expenditure (and probably partitioning as well).

An important question is whether an individual destined to become obese demonstrates increased metabolic efficiency *before* actually becoming obese. The genetic rodent models of obesity discussed in "Molecular Genetics of Energy Homeostasis" below, demonstrate increased metabolic efficiency within the first few weeks of life.[136,137] Roberts et al.[138] examined resting metabolic rate and 24-h energy expenditure at 3 months of age in infants born to lean and obese mothers. In those infants who became obese by age 1 year, the 24-h energy expenditure was significantly lower at 3 months of age. The finding that 24-h energy expenditure, but not resting metabolic rate, was significantly lower in infants destined to become obese, suggests that the lower 24-h energy expenditure is due to a decrease in the quantity of energy expended in physical activity. Similarly, adults destined to become obese have a lower rate of energy expenditure than nonobese adults.[139] Weight reduction in some obese individuals may "unmask" the metabolic state that predisposes them to become obese. In this sense, the extra body fat of the obese may mediate a metabolic "correction" for low energy expenditure.

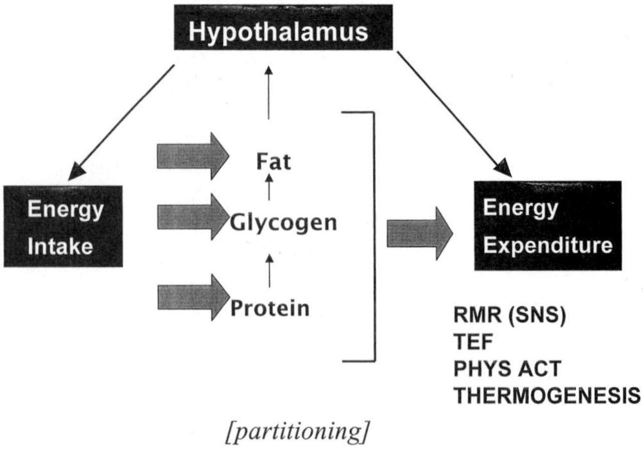

Fig. 157-1 This figure schematizes the mechanisms by which energy stores are held relatively constant over long periods of time, and the concept of fuel partitioning. *Energy intake* is influenced by short-term (e.g. glucose) and longer term (e.g. leptin; insulin) signals that act in the hypothalamus. Psychological (cortical) and environmental factors also have powerful effects. *Energy expenditure* is well matched to intake over extended periods of time in non-growing organisms. Energy expenditure is comprised of *resting metabolic rate* (RMR) which is strongly affected by the tone of the sympathetic nervous system (SNS); *thermic effect feeding* (TEF) which is the energy cost of metabolizing meal related substrates; *physical activity* for which chemical energy is consumed by skeletal muscle; and *thermogenesis*, which is the metabolic cost of maintenance of body temperature and includes the facultative "wastage" of chemical enthalpy by brown fat (UCP1) and possibly other uncoupling proteins. These phenotypes are affected by efferent hypothalamic tracts. Ingested energy can be stored as protein, glycogen or fat. The distribution of chemical energy among these molecules and tissues is influenced by endocrine factors as well as genes expressed in the storage of tissues such as myogenin and PPARγ. The status of the major depot for stored energy (adipose tissue) with regard to mass metabolic flux is signaled to the hypothalamus by effects of fat mass on circulating leptin and insulin concentrations, and probably other as yet unidentified humoral/neural signals related to fat mass.

NEUROANATOMY AND NEUROCHEMISTRY OF ENERGY HOMEOSTASIS

The neural circuitry that subserves energy balance in mammals is complex and redundant. The hypothalamus is the major integrator of disparate signals reporting the status of long-term energy stores and shorter term signals (meal size). The energy cost and the time required to obtain the necessary calories are carefully balanced against the organism's other needs. Although feeding is of paramount importance for the individual organism, reproduction is absolutely necessary for the continued survival of a species. The complexity of the regulation of feeding probably reflects the need for an appropriate balance between feeding and other critical behaviors such as reproduction.

During states of caloric repletion, preferences for specific content, flavors, and textures of foodstuffs may be important factors determining total intake. Termination of meals requires peripheral sensing of amount and quality of food ingested, followed by neural and/or humoral signals to the brain to terminate meal ingestion. While meal termination is a well-studied phenomenon under defined experimental conditions, meal initiation is much more difficult to study. Although it is possible to measure the delay to the initiation of a meal upon presentation of food, it is nearly impossible to quantify foraging and food-seeking behavior related to food identification and acquisition. The effort entailed in these processes is highly dependent on food abundance and quality, as well as on the planning and effort required to obtain food. For example, the effort involved in hunting during periods of low prey abundance is much higher than during periods of high prey abundance. Furthermore, the predominant mode of food acquisition, hunting/gathering versus farming, dictates the costs associated with the initiation of a given meal. Therefore, while meal initiation might seem to be a simple phenomenon to quantify, its relevance to energy balance is highly dependent on prevailing conditions.

The central nervous system integrates neural and humoral signals to imitate consummatory behavior. These signals can be

Table 157-7 Orexigenic and Satiating Molecules

	Abbreviation	Size	Human Chr
Orexigenic			
Neuropeptide Y	NPY	36aa	7p15
Agouti-related transcript	ART/AGRP	132aa	16q22
Melanin-concentrating hormone	MCH	17aa, cyclic	12q23-24
Hypocretin/Orexin	HCRT/ORX	HCRT1-39aa HCRT2-29aa	17q21
Norepinephrine	NE	—	—
Satiating			
Melanin-stimulating hormone	MSH	22aa	2p23.3
Cocaine-amphetamine-regulated transcript	CART	48aa	Unmapped
Corticotrophin-releasing hormone	CRH	41aa	8q12
Cholecystokinin	CCK	8aa/various	3pter-p21
Bombesin	BN	14aa (frog)	Unmapped—not human
Leptin	LEP	167aa	7q32
Insulin	INS	51aa	11p15.5
Dopamine	DA	—	—
Serotonin	5-HT	—	—

classified as orexigenic or satiating (Table 157-7). Neural signals are usually conveyed by neurotransmitters, predominantly monoamines, amino acids, and neuropeptides. Humoral signals are usually peptidergic. However, small molecules, such as glucose, fatty acids, and amino acids may have a role as humoral signals.

The Hypothalamus and the Effects of Specific Lesions

The hypothalamus integrates neuroendocrine systems, such as the thyroid, adrenal, and gonadal axes, as well as the autonomic nervous system. The hypothalamus is comprised of several nuclei that represent aggregations of functionally distinct, cell-rich areas separated by cell-sparse areas (Fig. 157-2). In humans, hypothalamic injury (by head trauma, infection, or surgery) can result in hyperphagia and obesity.[184–186] Such clinical observations led to the initial studies of hypothalamic electrolytic lesions in animals.[187] Bilateral injuries to the hypothalamic ventromedial nuclei (VMN),[187] the arcuate nuclei,[188] the paraventricular nuclei (PVN),[189,190] and the dorsomedial nuclei (DMN)[191] result in hyperphagia, reduced energy expenditure, and obesity. The simultaneous effects of these lesions on both energy intake and expenditure provided further support for the idea that this part of the brain integrates physiological systems subserving multiple aspects of energy homeostasis. Much of what is described in this chapter is, in fact, related to the elucidation, by physiological and genetic techniques, of the components of this control system.

Lesions of the hypothalamus can be made mechanically with electrodes and knife cuts, as well as biochemically with gold thioglucose (GTG) and excitotoxins such as glutamate (MSG).[188,192] In animals, hyperphagia resulting from mechanical lesions is observed almost immediately after recovery from anesthesia. However, the effects of the biochemical lesions take several weeks to be evident, presumably because cell death/disconnection is required to produce the behavioral phenotype. The accessibility of the circumventricular organs, discrete brain areas that are outside the blood-brain barrier, partially explains the anatomic specificity of glutamate lesions.

Bilateral lesions of the lateral hypothalamic area (LH) produce aphagia and adipsia.[193–195] This syndrome is probably due to the injury of both dopaminergic axons carried within the medial forebrain bundle (arising from the ventral tegmental area) as well as intrinsic LH neurons.[196,197] The aphagia and adipsia may be secondary to the physical immobility that is the characteristic result of the loss of dopamine. In addition, the loss of intrinsic LH neurons that secrete orexigenic peptides could also contribute to the aphagia caused by LH lesions. Indeed, LH lesions produced by excitotoxins that only affect neurons with cell bodies within LH injection sites result in hypophagia and hypodipsia similar to that produced by electrolytic lesions.[198–200]

A schematic of the mechanisms by which the hypothalamus integrates the control of energy homeostasis is shown in Fig. 157-3. Many of the neuropeptides alluded to in this section are shown in this figure. Further discussion of these genes is provided below in "Molecular Genetics of Energy Homeostasis" and "Molecular Genetics of Human Obesity."

There is a complex network of connections among the hypothalamic nuclei (Fig. 157-4). Further discussion is provided below regarding connections among various of the chemically defined neuronal populations of the hypothalamus and elsewhere in the body.

Arcuate Nucleus: NPY, POMC, AGRP/ART, CART, and GLP-1

The NPY/AGRP Neuron Colocalization studies of these two orexigenic peptides indicate that most, if not all, AGRP neurons co-express NPY.[1015,1016] Further studies will be needed to determine whether this co-expression results in additive or synergistic effects of behavioral and metabolic processes (Fig. 157-4).

Neuropeptide Y (NPY). Within the arcuate nucleus (ARC), several neuronal subtypes characterized by their secreted neuropeptides have been identified by their respective responses to alterations in the metabolic state of the organism (Fig. 157-4). The neuropeptide Y (NPY) neuron increases synthesis of NPY mRNA and release of NPY in response to net-negative energy balance: fasting,[201] diabetes,[202–204] cold exposure,[205] intense exercise,[206] and lactation.[207,208] Central nervous system infusions of NPY agonists potently stimulate feeding by decreasing latency to feed as well as by increasing calorie intake per meal.[209–211] In addition, NPY infusion into the cerebral ventricles affects autonomic nervous system function, decreasing heart rate, body temperature, and blood pressure in the absence of food.[212] A total deficiency of NPY (via gene knockout) ameliorates the obesity of obese (Lep^{ob})

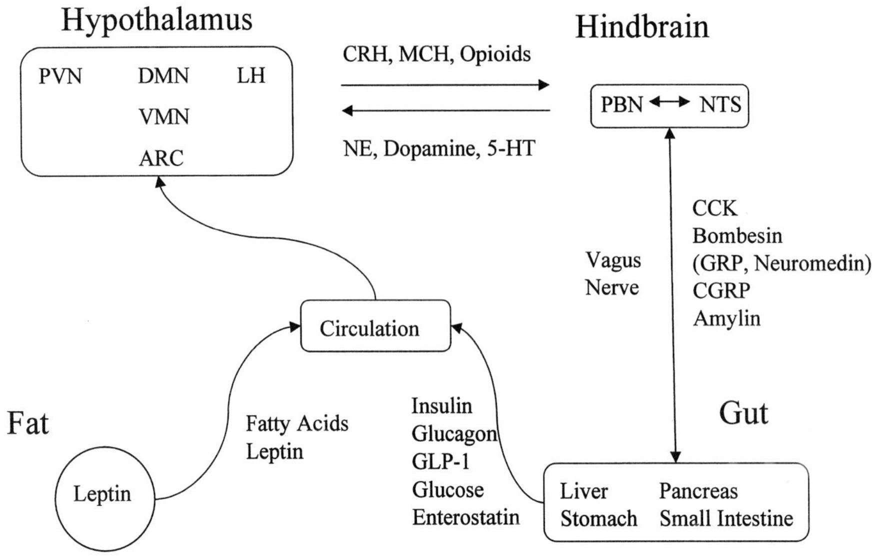

Fig. 157-2 The anatomic components that regulate energy balance. The hypothalamus may be divided functionally into nuclei: paraventricular nucleus (PVN), the dorsomedial nucleus (DMN), the ventromedial nucleus (VMN), the arcuate nucleus (ARC), and the lateral hypothalamic area (LH). The hypothalamus and the hindbrain have reciprocal synaptic connections using neuropeptides and neurotransmitters. Corticotropin-releasing hormone (CRH), melanin-concentrating hormone (MCH), opioids, norepinephrine (NE), dopamine, and serotonin (S-HT). Within the hindbrain, the parabrachial nucleus (PBN) and the nucleus of the solitary tract (NTS) are important modulators of feeding. The hindbrain and the gut have reciprocal connections via the vagus nerve. The gut secretes circulating factors, such as insulin and glucagon, which modulate energy balance. Adipose tissue secretes leptin and fatty acids, among other substances, that circulate to their targets within the brain and the gut.

mice.[213] However, mice that are homozygous for the NPY gene knockout exhibit normal feeding behavior and a robust fasting-induced hyperphagia.[214] This finding is contrary to the report regarding mice with a homozygous knockout of the NPY Y1 receptor[215] in which fasting-induced refeeding is reduced. This discrepancy may be due to redundant systems that compensate for a total loss of NPY during ontogenesis. A partial loss of NPY function, as in the NPY Y1 receptor knockout mouse that has other functional NPY receptor subtypes intact, might not induce such compensatory changes, rendering the functional deficiency more readily apparent.

Agouti-Signaling Protein (ASP)/Agouti Gene-Related Peptide (AGRP)/Agouti-Related Transcript (ART). The observation that overexpression of the agouti protein (ASP), a melanocortin-receptor antagonist not normally expressed in the brain, results in hyperphagia and obesity in yellow mice, led to the search for an endogenous neuronal antagonist of the melanocortin receptor. This search resulted in the discovery of Agouti gene-related peptide/Agouti-related transcript (AGRP/ART).[216,217] Overexpression of AGRP with a transgene causes hyperphagia and obesity. Some neurons express both AGRP and NPY, as *in situ* hybridization studies demonstrate apparent colocalization of both types of neurons within the same subregion of the ARC (Fig. 157-4).

The POMC/CART Neuron Studies regarding these two anorexigenic peptides indicate that most/all arcuate POMC neurons[1017] co-express CART (Fig. 157-4). The symmetry suggested by the two arcuate nucleus populations highlight the balance between processes regulating energy balance.

Proopiomelanocortin (POMC). POMC mRNA expression in POMC neurons is decreased in the food-deprived state.[218] As described in "Molecular Genetics of Energy Homeostasis" below, total deficiency of POMC in humans causes obesity, adrenal insufficiency, and red hair pigmentation.[219] While the POMC gene[220,221] encodes multiple constituent peptides (ACTH, beta- and gamma-lipotropin, alpha-, beta-, and gamma-MSH, beta-endorphin, and CLIP (corticotropin-like intermediate lobe peptide)), it is likely that the melanocyte-stimulating hormone (MSH or melanocortin) peptides are responsible for the effects on feeding and obesity. AGRP/ART, an antagonist of the brain-specific MSH receptor (MC4R), stimulates feeding, while agonists of melanocortin receptors inhibit NPY-stimulated feeding.[222,223] The POMC neurons express NPY receptors, receiving synaptic input from NPY neurons within the ARC, although there are conflicting reports regarding the relevant NPY receptor subtype from mRNA expression and pharmacologic studies.[224,225] It remains to be determined whether NPY and AGRP neurons bear melanocortin receptors.

Cocaine and Amphetamine-Regulated Transcript (CART). Another anorexigenic peptide, CART, is regulated by the metabolic state within the ARC.[226] While also expressed in the DMN and the LH, metabolic regulation of CART expression is less robust than in the ARC. Fasting reduces levels of CART mRNA and leptin injections restore expression to prefasting levels. Infusion of CART peptide inhibits feeding in the dark phase of the circadian cycle as well as during fasting and NPY-induced feeding. It is interesting to note that NPY, by activating the G-protein inhibitory, G_0,[227] and AGRP, acting as an antagonist of melanocortin receptors, exert their orexigenic effects through inhibitory mechanisms, whereas MSH produces anorexia by activating Gs-protein coupled melanocortin receptors.

Both NPY and POMC neurons of the ARCn express the Rb ("long") isoform of the leptin receptor.[228] In obese animals deficient in leptin (e.g., *ob*) or its receptor (e.g., *db, fa*), NPY[229–232] and AGRP[216,217] are overexpressed, whereas POMC mRNA is decreased.[218,233] These derangements in neuropeptide gene expression are normalized by leptin treatment of leptin- (but not leptin receptor-) deficient animals.[229,234] Similarly, the increases of NPY and AGRP expression, and the decrease of POMC expression, caused by caloric deprivation can be prevented by leptin administration in fasting animals. However, these neurons are not solely regulated by ambient leptin concentrations because animals without functional leptin receptors exhibit robust fasting-induced hyperphagia accompanied by increases of NPY mRNA[231] and decreases in POMC mRNA.[218] Both NPY and POMC neurons express the glucocorticoid receptor gene (GR),[235]

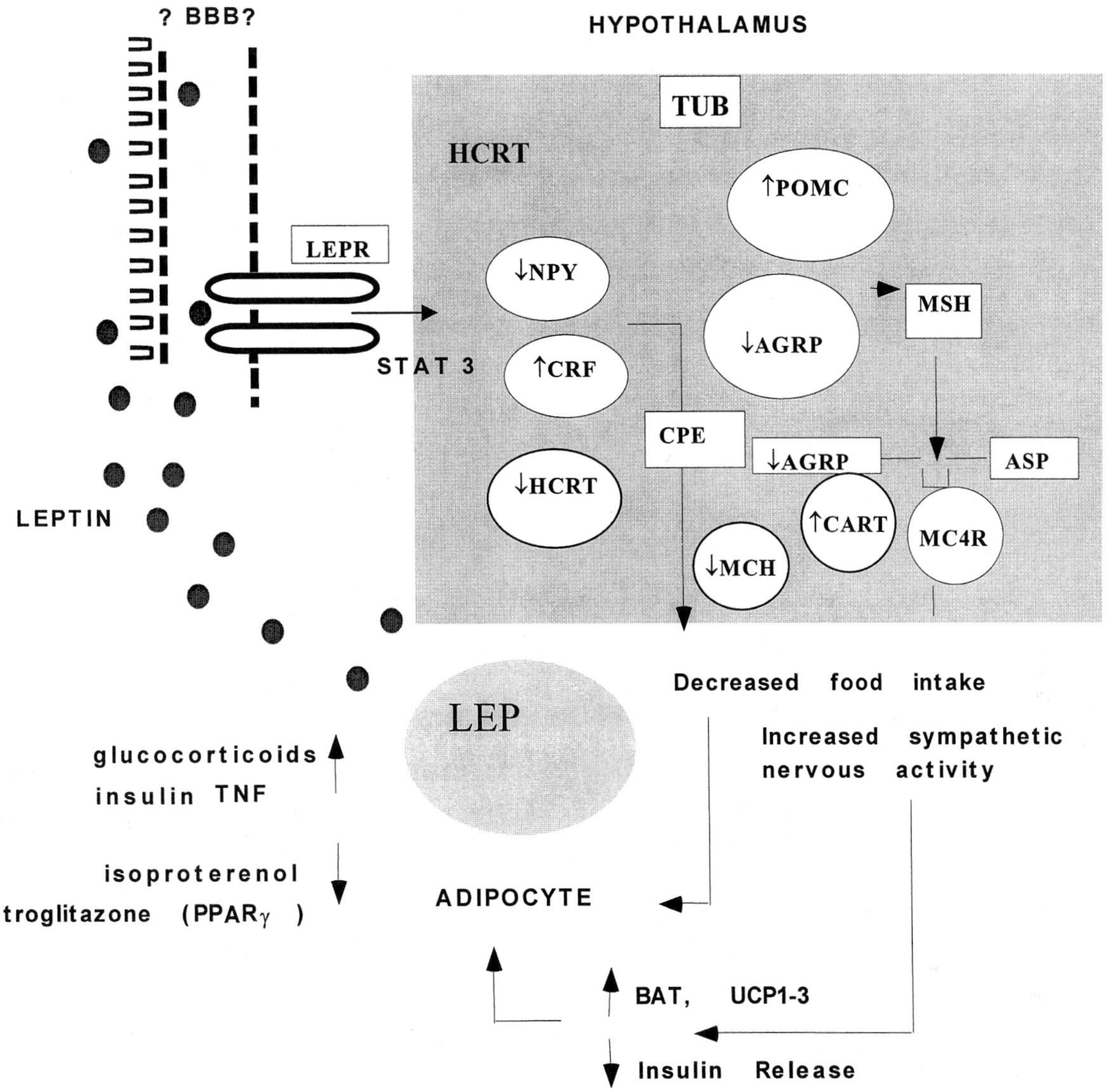

Fig. 157-3 Possible functional relationships among products of the rodent obesity genes. The genes *Lepr, Cpe, tub*, and *agouti* (ASP) in hypothalamus, and *Lep*, which encodes leptin in adipocytes, are depicted in white boxes. Changes in adipocyte volume and fat mass affect leptin production as would be anticipated if leptin were part of a regulatory loop to control body fat by modulating food intake and energy expenditure. Cell size effects may be secondary to changes in substrate fluxes (fatty acids, glucosamine) and/or to associated endocrine changes (e.g. insulin). Leptin production is also experimentally increased by glucocorticoids, TNF, or insulin, and reduced by isoproterenol (β-adrenoreceptor agonist). Leptin may also play a role in peripheral sensitivity to insulin and in insulin synthesis in the islets. Leptin reaches its receptor (LEPR) in the hypothalamus via active transport into CSF (across the blood-brain barrier -(BBB)) and/or by acting upon hypothalamic nuclei that are functionally outside of the BBB. The major signal-transducing form of LEPR in the hypothalamus is probably a dimer of the "long form" (1162aa) of the LEPR protein. Occupation of LEPR causes JAK-mediated activation of STAT3, resulting in decreased production of NPY (a stimulator of food intake) and increased release of CRF, which suppresses food intake. CPE, via its role in processing and intracellular transport proneuropeptides for NPY, CRF, galanin, and CCK, could affect food intake and energy expenditure (autonomic nervous activity). However, there is no direct evidence at present to indicate that the Cpe^{fat} phenotype is conveyed by such effects on central neuropeptides. ASP, which is not normally expressed in the rodent brain, increases food intake in the A^y mouse, apparently through competitive inhibition of the normal ligand for melanocortin receptor 4 (MC4R). The predicted *tub* gene product bears some sequence similarity to a cyclic nucleotide phosphodiesterase. A role in apoptosis of hypothalamic neurons has been suggested because the *tub* mutation results in the death of neurons in the retina and organ of Corti. Sympathetic nervous (SNS) efferent output is affected by the hypothalamic centers in which these peptides act. Intracerebral ventricular leptin administration, for example, increases energy expenditure in BAT and reduces insulin secretion by SNS-mediated mechanisms. UCP3 is a mitochondrial uncoupling protein expressed in skeletal muscle and fat that may play a role in energy expenditure. By analogy to UCP1 in BAT, the sympathetic nervous system would be expected to influence the activity of this pathway. These influences on energy intake and expenditure are shown converging on the amount of fat stored in the adipocyte. For reasons discussed elsewhere, it is most likely that the major role of the "leptin axis" is to prevent excessive depletion of fat stores rather than to prevent obesity.

and glucocorticoids regulate hypothalamic expression of both NPY[236] and POMC[237] genes. Adrenalectomy prevents the induction of NPY mRNA by fasting, and glucocorticoid replacement restores the fasting-induced increase. In the hypothalamus, adrenalectomy increases POMC mRNA and glucocorticoid replacement reduces POMC mRNA to basal levels. Thus, glucocorticoid replacement produces the bias for increased food intake associated with increased NPY and decreased POMC expression. Adrenalectomy ameliorates the obesity of animals deficient in either leptin or the leptin receptor.[186,238,239]

Glucagon-Like Peptide 1 Receptor (GLP-1R). The ARC also contains neurons that express the receptor (GLP-1R) for glucagon-like peptide 1 (GLP-1) and thereby mediate the anorectic effects of

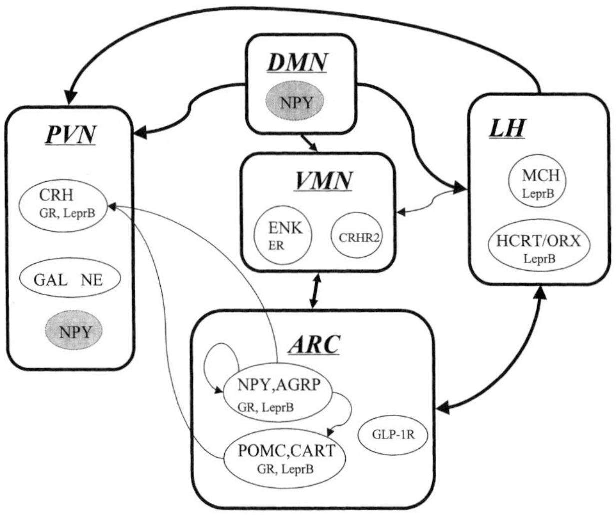

Fig. 157-4 Neuronal populations in the hypothalamic nuclei and their interconnections. There is a reciprocal innervation between the ARC and the VMN.[993,994] The DMN sends projections to the LH, the VMN, and the parvocellular region of the PVN.[995] The LH sends projections to the parvocellular region of the PVN, the DMN, and the VMN.[996,997] Within the arcuate nucleus are neurons that express NPY, POMC, AGRP, CART, and GLP-1R. Some of these neurons have their activity modulated by glucocorticoids and leptin via the glucocorticoid receptor (GR) and the leptin receptor (*LeprB*). The PVN contains CRH neurons that express GR and *LeprB*. A subset of PVN neurons coexpress galanin (GAL) and norepinephrine (NE). The PVN is a site of ectopic NPY expression after endogenous NPY expression in the ARC is ablated by neonatal MSG treatment. The VMN contains enkephalinergic (ENK) neurons that are regulated by estrogen via the estrogen receptor (ER). The DMN of the lethal yellow mouse expresses NPY where it is not found in normal mice. Neurons that secrete hypocretin/orexin (HCRT/OXR) are also found in the LH.

GLP-1.[240–242] The peptide GLP-1 is derived from processing of preproglucagon and is secreted from the endocrine pancreas[243] into the circulation.

Ventromedial Nucleus (VMN): Enkephalin and CRH

Within the VMN, neurons expressing enkephalin also express the estrogen receptor (see Fig. 157-4). Enkephalin gene expression is regulated by estrogen.[244,245] Estrogen withdrawal by ovariectomy reduces enkephalin mRNA, while estrogen replacement restores enkephalin mRNA levels. Because ovariectomy causes a slowly developing obesity,[246–248] and opioidergic peptides can stimulate feeding, it is possible that enkephalin neurons might be involved in the obesity that accompanies ovariectomy. Ovariectomy-induced obesity may not be simply due to hyperphagia, as subtle differences in weight gain are observed in ovariectomized rats that are pair-fed with sham-operated control rats.[249,250] Core temperature is not altered by ovariectomy,[251] although BAT thermogenesis is reduced.[252] We mention the enkephalin neuron due to the paucity of candidate neurons related to energy homeostasis with cell bodies actually within the VMN, the classic anatomic area for electrolytic lesions resulting in obesity. There is a rich reciprocal innervation between the VMN and the ARC although the specific neuropeptides and neurotransmitters subserving these connections have not been identified.

The type 2 corticotrophin-releasing hormone (CRH) receptor (CRHR2) is a G-protein coupled receptor[253–255] that binds members of the CRH family (CRH and urocortin). Expression of CRHR2 mRNA in the VMN is correlated with circulating leptin concentrations and is reduced by fasting.[256] Because some of the anorectic effects of CRH and urocortin[257,258] may be mediated by activation of CRHR2[259] in the VMN, it is possible that the VMN lesions produce obesity, in part, by ablation of CRHR2 signal transduction (see CRH and CRH receptor knockout models). However, the anxiogenic properties of CRH and urocortin[257,260] potentially disqualify them as satiety peptides using the criteria applied to peripheral factors such as CCK.[261] CRH and urocortin are not behaviorally specific, increasing locomotor activity and activating the hypothalamo-pituitary-adrenal axis by promoting the release of ACTH and glucocorticoids.[262] Thus, CRH and urocortin should be regarded as anorexic peptides, rather than satiety peptides.

Paraventricular Nucleus (PVN): Corticotrophin-Releasing Hormone (CRH), and Galanin (GAL)

The parvocellular portion of the PVN (Fig. 157-4) contains CRH neurons that receive innervations from both NPY and POMC neurons of the ARC.[263,264] Intracerebral infusions of CRH can decrease food intake.[265,266] These CRH neurons express the Rb ("long") isoform of the leptin receptor[228] as well as the glucocorticoid receptor,[235] and respond to caloric deprivation by decreasing CRH mRNA.[229] This decrease in CRH mRNA expression can be prevented by leptin infusion.[267,268] There are noradrenergic neurons within the PVN that coexpress galanin. Norepinephrine injected within the PVN consistently increases food intake,[269,270] as does galanin.[271] GAL neurons send projections to the nucleus of the solitary tract.[272] Some PVN neurons express NPY after neonatal ablation of the ARC by glutamate.[273,274]

Dorsomedial Nucleus (DMN)

Ablation of the DMN in adult rats produces mild obesity. DMN lesions of weanling rats produce stunting and mild obesity, similar to ARC nucleus lesions produced by neonatal glutamate administration.[275] However, the neurons responsible for the obesity induced by DMN lesions have not been conclusively identified. The DMN of the obese yellow (A^y) mouse expresses NPY, whereas normal mice do not express NPY within this nucleus.[276] It is possible that the aberrant NPY expression within the DMN and PVN might be used to characterize the neuropeptides/neurotransmitters/receptors expressed by these DMN neurons.

Lateral Hypothalamus Area: Melanin-Concentrating Hormone (MCH) and Hypocretin/Orexin (HCRT/ORX)

Two orexigenic neuropeptides, MCH[277] and HCRT/ORX,[278,279] have been identified in the lateral hypothalamus. These peptides appear to localize to similar areas of the lateral hypothalamus but are not coexpressed in the same neurons. Fasting increases both neuropeptides and their mRNAs, and infusions of the individual peptides into the brain stimulate feeding. However, the maximal feeding response to either peptide is less than the response to NPY on a molar basis. The loss of these orexigenic peptides may partially account for the hypophagia caused by ablative lesions of the LH.

The Hindbrain: Nucleus of the Solitary Tract (NTS) and Parabrachial Nucleus (PBN)

The hindbrain receives innervation from the hypothalamus, as well as from the periphery, via vagal afferents (Fig. 157-2). Several sites within the hindbrain that modulate feeding have been identified. The NTS is innervated by vagal afferents as well as by descending hypothalamic inputs. Lesions of the NTS abolish the satiating effects of cholecystokinin (CCK) and stimulation of CCK receptors within the NTS promotes satiety.[280–282] Bombesin action (see below) is localized to the NTS, as lesions of the NTS abolish the inhibitory effects of bombesin on feeding.[283]

Neurons that bear serotonin receptors within the PBN decrease feeding upon stimulation with specific agonists; serotonin receptor antagonists can block this effect.[284–286] Mice with an induced mutation of the serotonin 5HT-2C receptor subtype exhibit obesity that is due purely to mild hyperphagia.[287] Opioids, specifically μ receptor agonists, can increase feeding by actions within the PBN.[288] Naloxone and naltrexone can block the orexigenic effect of opioids. Interestingly, NPY-induced feeding can be blocked by administration of naltrexone peripherally and within the NTS,[289] and the μ receptor agonist, DAMGO (D-Ala2,N-Me-Phe4,Gly5-ol) enkephalin, increases feeding,[290] suggesting that opioids may be downstream modulators of NPY-induced feeding.

The Gut: Cholecystokinin (CCK) and Bombesin

The gut plays an important role in the control of feeding by modulating meal size and terminating meals (Fig. 157-2).[261] In newborn rodents, filling of the stomach with nonnutritive substances terminates feeding.[291] Stretch receptors presumably are conveying meal-termination signals, because complete denervation of the stomach prevents feeding termination. However, by the second week of life, a rat pup will stop feeding only after infusion into the stomach of nutritive substances, such as milk or glucose.[292] By day 15 in rats, if the passage of ingested food is diverted from the duodenum by an externalized fistula placed in the stomach, feeding time and meal size are both dramatically increased ("sham feeding").[293] Infusions of carbohydrates, proteins, and lipids beyond the point of diversion will terminate sham feeding.[294] One of the meal-terminating signals generated by the gut's intestinal mucosa is CCK.[295,296] Neurons of the enteric nervous system also secrete CCK.[297] CCK is released upon stimulation by the entry of nutrients into the duodenum,[298,299] causing gall bladder contraction (cholecystokinin activity) and the release of pancreatic hormones (pancreozymin activity).[300,301]

Initially produced as a 115-amino acid precursor,[302] CCK is processed and released as multiple molecular weight forms, depending on the species being studied; most species have CCK-33 (33 amino acids) and CCK-8 (8 amino acids).[303–305] The larger form of CCK probably acts at the liver because it is more potent than CCK-8 when administered intravenously and intraportally.[306] CCK-8 probably has a paracrine mode of action[307] because injection into or infusion near the celiac artery is more effective in reducing meal size than administration in any other abdominal artery.[308,309] CCK receptors of vagal afferent fibers and in the circular muscle of the pyloric sphincter may mediate the satiating effects of CCK at the caudal hindbrain.[310]

Systemic administration of CCK agonists decrease meal size while antagonists of CCK increase meal size.[311] These effects of CCK are mediated by the vagus nerve because vagotomy abrogates the effects of CCK on meal size.[312,313] Vagal afferents along the entire gut bearing CCK receptors innervate the nucleus of the solitary tract in the hindbrain, which projects to the PVN of the hypothalamus.[314] Disruption of this neural pathway eliminates the satiety effects of peripherally administered CCK. Compensatory increases of meal frequency appear to counteract the effects of diminished meal size caused by CCK, inicating that robust regulatory mechanisms have been developed at least for CCK-mediated satiety.

Two types of CCK receptors have been characterized[315] and cloned.[316] The CCK-A (A for alimentary) receptor, found in the pancreas, gut, and brain, preferentially binds the sulfated form of CCK. The CCK-B (B for brain) receptor, widely distributed in the rat brain, binds sulfated and nonsulfated CCK-8, gastrin, and CCK fragments. It is unlikely that intestinally secreted CCK has any direct central effects because CCK does not readily cross the blood-brain barrier and has a limited time window for its satiating effect[317].

Otsuka Long-Evans Tokushima fatty (OLETF) rats that lack the CCK-A receptor are obese[318] and their meal patterns are characterized by larger, but less frequent, meals, as would be predicted from the loss of the CCK satiety signal.[319]

A CCK-like peptide, bombesin, has anorectic effects (separate from CCK) when injected systemically or into the brain.[320] Gastrin-releasing peptide (GRP) and neuromedins (NMB, NMC), mammalian homologs of bombesin, are found in the enteric neurons of the gut. Bombesin's site of action is in the upper abdominal organs because bombesin is most potent after infusion at the celiac artery, as opposed to other abdominal arteries.[321–324] Their satiating effect is probably mediated by vagal and spinal visceral afferents. Lesions of both groups of fibers by total abdominal vagotomy and bilateral-dorsal rhizotomies of thoracic ganglia T3 to T5 are required to abolish the satiating effect of bombesin.[325] Simultaneous peripheral administration of GRP and NMB mimics the effects of equimolar doses of bombesin.[326] BRS-3, a bombesin receptor that is structurally related to the CCK receptors, has been identified in a search of orphan receptors. Mice that are homozygous for an induced mutation of BRS-3 ingest more chow than their normal littermates, and develop late onset obesity that appears to be solely due to increased food intake.[327] Mice that are homozygous for an induced mutation of the GRP receptor are resistant to the inhibitory feeding effects of bombesin, but do not appear to develop obesity or hyperphagia.[328] Several other peptides produced by the gut appear to have satiating effects: amylin,[329] calcitonin gene-related peptide (CGRP),[330] and enterostatin.[331] As these peptides have actions when administered peripherally as well as within the central nervous system, the specific sites of action for these peptides remain to be determined.

MOLECULAR GENETICS OF ENERGY HOMEOSTASIS

Obesity can result only from a derangement in one or more of the three components of energy balance: caloric intake, energy expenditure, and caloric partitioning. This section discusses genetic mutations in animals that exemplify the respective roles of these individual components of energy homeostasis. These spontaneous and experimentally-made mutations shed light on the molecular mechanisms by which energy homeostasis is achieved by isolating one or more processes against an otherwise normal genetic and metabolic background. The spontaneous rodent mutations that affect these processes are summarized in Table 157-8 and those that are the result of various experimental genetic manipulations are summarized in Table 157-9.

We first describe mutations that affect one of the three components primarily, then we describe those that affect multiple processes.

Mutations That Mainly Affect Food Intake

Total energy intake is the product of meal energy content and meal frequency. In "Neuroanatomy and Neurochemistry of Energy Homeostasis" above, we identified molecules produced by the brain and the gut that control food intake. Food-seeking behavior can be motivated by the need to replenish caloric stores or by the hedonic reward of ingesting novel or palatable foods. Food deprivation results in a series of metabolic changes that initiate food-seeking behavior: decrease in circulating glucose; changes in circulating hormones (decrease in insulin, increase in glucagon); decline in circulating leptin concentration; decline in the release of satiating gut peptides (CCK, bombesin-related peptides); and alterations in the activity of different populations of hypothalamic neurons (orexigenic: NPY, norepinephrine, AGRP, HCRT/ORX, MCH, opioid peptides; anorexigenic: CRH, MSH, CART, dopamine, serotonin). These chemical changes occur on a time continuum during the course of caloric restriction, and have been examined in isolation by metabolic and genetic manipulations.

The Melanocortin/Agouti System

Melanocyte-Stimulating Hormone (MSH). The POMC gene encodes several peptides (ACTH, α, β, γMSH, βendorphin, CLIP, and others) that are derived from proteolytic processing of the preprohormone. MSH is one of these POMC-derived peptides (αMSH). MSH and its synthetic agonist, SHU9119, inhibit feeding, presumably by activation of the brain melanocortin receptors MC3R and MC4R.[223,332] POMC gene expression in hypothalamic neurons is regulated by nutritional state: repressed in the fasting state, and up-regulated in the fed/refed state. Furthermore, POMC gene expression is repressed in the

Table 157-8 Spontaneous Mutations Related to Energy Balance

Gene name (animal)	Gene symbol	Mutation (name)	Effect of mutation (molecular)	Effect of mutation (physiological)	Chromosome	Age of onset obesity	Human ortholog location
Agouti (mouse)	*A*	A^y (yellow)	Ectopic (brain) overexpression of "agouti-signaling protein (ASP) ? block normal ligand for MC4R	I, ?E, ?P_F	2	Adult	20q11.2
Carboxypeptidase E (mouse)	*Cpe*	Cpe^{fat} (fat)	Processing of prohormones including neuropeptides	?	8	Adult	4q32
Leptin (mouse)	*Lep*	Lep^{ob} (obese)	Deficiency of leptin	I,E, P_F	6	Weanling	7q31.3
Leptin receptor (mouse/rat)	*Lepr*	$Lepr^{db}$ (diabetes)	Deranged leptin-signal transduction	I, E, P_F	4	Weanling	1p31-p22
		$Lepr^{fa}$ (fatty rat)	Deranged leptin-signal transduction	I, E, P_F	5	Weanling	1p31-p22
"Tubby" (mouse)	*tub*	*Tub* (tubby)	? Phosphodiesterase related to apoptosis	?	7	Adult	11p15
OLETF (rat)	*Cckar*	$Cckar^{OLETF}$	Cholecystokinin receptor defect (brain, vagus)	I		Adult	4p16.2-p15.1
Growth hormone releasing hormone receptor	*Ghrhr*	$Ghrhr^{lit}$	Decreased growth hormone	P_F	6	Weanling	7p15-p14
Ryanodine receptor (pig)	*Ryr1*		Skeletal muscle hypersensitivity	P_M	6q12	Adult	19q13.1
Callipyge (sheep)	*Clpg*	*Clpg*	NA	P_M	18	Lambs	NA

Gene and mutation symbols are based on current nomenclature. Gene symbols in animals are italicized in upper- and lowercase. For humans, gene symbols are uppercase, nonitalicized. For animals, mutant alleles are designated as superscripts of the gene symbol. The messenger RNA's and protein products of genes are all capitals, nonitalic. Most investigators will be more familiar with earlier designations; e.g., *ob* for the obese mouse (Lep^{ob}); *db* for the diabetes mouse ($Lepr^{db}$). The *fa* mutation occurred in the 13M rat strain and is frequently referred to as the Zucker mutation. The *f* mutation is allelic to *fa* and arose in the Koletsky rat. The *f* mutation was transferred to other strains (e.g., LA/N) and sometimes referred to as corpulent (*cp*). The preferred gene symbols are *fa* and fa^f because these take account of the sequence of discovery and are the symbols used by the investigators first describing the respective mutations. All mutations shown are recessive except *yellow* (A^y), which is dominant. There is no "official" name for the protein encoded by Agouti. Some investigators refer to this protein as agouti-signaling protein (ASP). The gene symbol for human Agouti is ASIP. In this review, for purpose of brevity, the older gene symbols are generally used. For corresponding human genes, all capital letters are used, although nomenclature for humans for some of these genes is not settled. For physiological effects of these mutations based on the schema presented in the text: I = increased food intake; E = decreased energy expenditure; P_F = partitioning of calories to fat; P_M = partitioning of calories to muscle.

hypothalamus of leptin-deficient and leptin-receptor-deficient rodents.[218,233,234] Two individuals homozygous for "loss of function" mutations of the POMC gene manifest obesity,[219] indicating that POMC, and probably MSH, are important mediators of energy homeostasis (see below, "Leptin and Leptin Receptor Physiology"). Targeted mutation of the POMC gene that disrupts the synthesis of the beta-endorphin peptide (but not MSH produces mice without significant alterations of energy balance.[333] Based on the obese phenotype of the MC4R knockout mouse[334] and humans with POMC mutations, and the suppressive effects of MSH on food intake, it is likely that mice with knockout of the MSH portion of POMC will show hyperphagia and increased body fat.

Mouse POMC Knockout A mouse model of complete POMC deficiency causes obesity in mice, despite some early mortality due to adrenal insufficiency.[1018]

Melanocortin Receptors (*Mc1r*, *Mc2r*, *Mc3r*, and *Mc4r*). The melanocortin receptors are typical G-protein-coupled receptors with seven membrane-spanning domains.[335] The mouse *Mc1r* gene is expressed in skin and encodes the functional MSH receptor in skin. The *Mc2r* gene encodes the ACTH receptor and is expressed in the adrenal gland. The *Mc3r* and *Mc4r* genes are expressed in the brain with high levels of expression in the hypothalamus. Homozygosity for an induced loss of function mutation of the *Mc4r* gene causes obesity and hyperphagia without any alteration in coat color. Heterozygotes for this mutation have an intermediate phenotype.[334] Mice with *Mc3r* deficiency have a metabolically induced obesity accompanied by reduced running wheel activity.[1037] A potent antagonist of MC3R and MC4R, MTII increases food intake when injected into the cerebral ventricles of mice.[223] Humans heterozygous for inactivating mutations of this receptor are obese[336,337] (see below, "Leptin and Leptin Receptor Physiology").

Agouti (A). The agouti protein (agouti signaling protein, ASP) binds to melanocortin receptors and inhibits receptor activation by MSH, possibly as an inverse agonist.[338] Inverse agonists are compounds that decrease a G-protein-coupled receptor's ability to activate G-proteins in the absence of the agonist ligand.[339] In the hair follicle, intermittent expression of ASP causes the alternate black/yellow banding of the agouti hair. ASP blocks the action of MSH on the follicle melanocortin receptor (MC1R), shifting the

Table 157-9 Genetic Manipulations that Alter Body Composition

Gene	Manipulation	Phenotype	Fat content	Intake	Expenditure	Partitioning	Comments	Ref
Energy Intake								
5HT-2c	KO	Obesity	↑	↑	—	—		287
5HT-1B	KO	Normal phenotype	—	—	—	—	Resistant to fenfluramine hypophagia	363
Brs-3	KO	Obesity	↑	↑	↓ activity	↑ WAT	Impaired glucose tolerance	327
Agrp	Overexpression	Obesity	↑	↑	?	?		216
Pomc	KO	Obesity	↑ WAT	↑				1018
Mc3r	KO	Mild Obesity	↑ WAT	—	↓	↑ WAT		1018
Mc4r	KO	Obesity	↑	↑	?	?		334
Npy1r	KO	Mild obesity	↑	↓	↓ activity	?		215
Npy1r + ob/ob	Double KO	Severe obesity	↑	↑	↓	↑ WAT	*ob/ob* phenotype is unchanged	215
Npy5r	KO	Mild obesity	↑	+/−	—	?		378
Npy	KO	Normal phenotype	—	—	—	—		213
Npy + ob/ob	KO	Mild obesity	↑	↑	?	↑ WAT		213
Crh	KO	Normal adult phenotype	—	—	—	—		468
Mch	KO	↓ adiposity	↓	↓	↑	?		379
Tyrosine hydroxylase	KO/substitution	Aphagia	↓	↓	↓ activity	?	Selective dopamine depletion	381
Energy Expenditure								
Ucp1/Diptheria Toxin A chain	Expression in BAT	Obesity	↑	↑	↓	↑ WAT		384
RIIβ of PKA	KO	Small adipocytes	↓	—	↑ temp	↓ WAT	Increased UCP and increased lipolysis	398
Adrb3	KO	Mild obesity	↑	—	?	↑ WAT		388, 389
Ucp1	Overexpression in WAT	↓ subcutaneous fat	↓	—	—	↓ WAT		399
Ucp1	KO	Cold intolerance	—	—	—	?		400
Ucp3	KO	Normal	—	—	—	—		1022-3
Partitioning of stored calories								
Gh	Transgene silencing	Obesity	↑	?	—	↑ WAT		413–415
Ghrhr	KO	Obesity	↑	?	?	↑ WAT		412
Glut4	Overexpression in WAT	Mild obesity	↓	—	—	↑ WAT		429
Gα-q	Antisense transgene	↑ weight	↑	?	?	↑ WAT	Deficiency in WAT and liver	954
Icam-1	KO	Mild obesity	↑	—	?	↑ WAT		431
Mac1	KO	Mild obesity	↑	—	?	↑ WAT		431
aP2/Fabp4	KO	Diet induced obesity	?	?	?	?	Normal weight on regular chow	955
Cebpa	KO	Adipose tissue hypoplasia	↓	?	?	↓ WAT	Neonatal lethal phenotype	100
Cebpb/Cebpd	Double KO	Adipose tissue hypoplasia	↓	?	?	↓ WAT	Neonatal lethal phenotype	432
Glut4 (4)	KO	↓ WAT	↓	?	?	↓ WAT	Cardiomegaly and low free fatty acids	956
aZIP-F1	Dominant Negative Transgene	Reduced WAT	↓	↑	↑	↓ WAT	Severe diabetes	433
Srebp-1c	Dominant Negative Transgene	Reduced WAT	↓	↑	↑	↓ WAT	Severe diabetes	434

(Continued on next page)

Table 157-9 (Continued)

Gene	Manipulation	Phenotype	Fat content	Intake	Expenditure	Partitioning	Comments	Ref
Diptheria Toxin in WAT	Toxic Transgene	Normal	—	—			Resistant to MSG-induced obesity	1024
Myostatin	KO	Hypermuscular	—	?	?	↑ Skeletal muscle		444
Myogenin	KO	Hypomuscular	NA	?	?	↓ Skeletal muscle	Perinatal lethality	461, 462
Myf5 + MyoD	Double KO	Skeletal muscle agenesis	NA	?	?	No skeletal muscle	Perinatal lethality	464
Mrf4 + MyoD	Double KO	Hypomuscular	NA	?	?	↓ skeletal muscle	Perinatal lethality	463
Glucocorticoid receptor	Antisense transgene	Mild obesity	↑	?	?	?		957
Glp1r	KO	Normal phenotype	—	—	—	?	Impaired glucose tolerance	467
Grpr	KO	Normal phenotype	—	—	—	—	Resistant to GRP satiation	328

melanocyte from black (eumelanin) to yellow (pheomelanin) production. While ASP and MSH inhibit each other's binding to melanocortin receptors,[340] their binding sites, to MC1R, appear to be on different domains of the receptor. ASP may interact with one or more extracellular domains of MC1R, whereas MSH may interact with membrane-spanning regions of MC1R.[341,342]

The agouti locus on mouse chromosome 2 is defined by a large allelic series of dominant and recessive mutations that affect coat color and body adiposity.[343] The most dominant allele (A^y) produces yellow pelage by acting as an antagonist of MSH receptors in the hair follicle (MC1R) to block eumelanin (black pigment) synthesis, and in the brain (MC4R), to produce obesity by inducing hyperphagia. The A^y mutation is due to a large interstitial deletion that apposes the promoter of a ubiquitously expressed gene (*Raly*) to the coding sequence of agouti (ASP).[344,345] The loss of *Raly* accounts for the embryonic lethality of the homozygous A^y genotype.[346,347] The agouti gene is normally expressed only in the skin, and ubiquitous expression (including brain) appears to be responsible for producing the obese phenotype in the A^y mouse. Other dominant alleles of agouti also produce yellow pigmentation and obesity. These homozygotes do not die during embryogenesis as the *Raly* gene has not been affected. Most of the other dominant yellow alleles (A^{hvy}, A^i, A^{iapy}, A^{iy}, A^{sy}, A^{vy}, Ay^y) are due to retroviral (intracisternal A particles, IAP) insertions that appose retroviral promoters to the agouti coding sequence, causing ubiquitous, high-level expression of agouti.[348] One unusual feature of the agouti gene that accounts for the high frequency of dominant yellow mutations is the unusually long intron (>100 kbp) prior to the first coding exon. Indeed, one inactivating mutation of agouti (the *a* allele) is the result of a retroviral insertion that inhibits the proper synthesis of several alternatively spliced forms of the agouti gene.[349]

The obesity of the A^y mutant is mainly due to hyperphagia that is accompanied by increased linear (skeletal) growth and a commensurate increase in lean mass. In this regard, the phenotype is similar to that of most obese humans. Pair-feeding experiments suggest that agouti overexpression also affects nutrient partitioning (by preferential deposition of ingested calories in adipose tissue), although not to the same extent as defects in the leptin/leptin-receptor system. Body temperature and BAT function are normal in obese yellow mice. Transgenic studies indicate that overexpression of agouti only in skin and adipocytes does not produce obesity, suggesting that overexpression of agouti within the central nervous system is responsible for the hyperphagia. However, daily insulin injections to transgenic mice expressing agouti protein only in WAT triggered the development of obesity in the transgenic mice but not in control mice.[350] Finally, an inactivating mutation of the MSH receptor gene normally expressed in hair follicles *(Mc1r)* results in a yellow, nonobese mouse.[351] Thus, the yellow coat color can be dissociated from the obese phenotype.

Agouti Gene-Related Peptide/Agouti-Related Transcript (AGRP/ART). This agouti-related gene was found by homology searches to the agouti sequence in brain cDNA libraries and sequence databases.[216,352] The gene is normally expressed predominantly within the hypothalamus. Overexpression of the gene causes obesity, but not yellow coat coloration.[216] Expression of the AGRP/ART gene is repressed in the A^y mouse,[216] possibly due to feedback inhibition of agouti (ASP) on AGRP expression. In addition, AGRP mRNA levels are markedly elevated (approximately tenfold over lean) in the hypothalamus of obese *ob* and *db* mice. The peptide serves as a potent antagonist of both MC3R and MC4R (brain-specific putative MSH-receptors), but is only a poor antagonist for MC1R (the MSH receptor in skin).[216] However, AGRP is not increased in *Lepr*-rats.[101]

Mahogany and Mahoganoid (*mg* and *md*). Spontaneous mutations at two independent loci modulate the expression of the agouti phenotype: mahogany (*mg*) and mahoganoid (*md*). Both of these mutations are recessive and cause extensive darkening of the coat of agouti mice, indicating a shift to eumelanin (black) pigment synthesis. Double-mutant mice, A^y and *mg* or A^y and *md*, are leaner than A^y, indicating that mahogany and mahoganoid suppress both the obesity and the yellow coat color of A^y mice.[353,354]

The gene encoding mahogany has been identified as the murine orthologue of the human attractin protein, a soluble protein produced from activated T cells. The mouse gene encodes a large protein of 1428 amino acids with a single transmembrane domain and a short cytoplasmic tail.[1020,1021]

The *mg* and agouti (*A*) loci are about 0.5 cM apart on mouse chromosome 2. A distinct possibility remains that *mg* may be a regulatory mutation of the agouti gene. Because agouti (ASP) expression is normally suppressed in the skin of nonagouti (*a/a*) black mice without effects on food intake, *mg* and *md* must exert their effects in the brain, perhaps by suppression of AGRP/ART expression or activity. The effects of *mg* and *md* may be independent of the agouti locus because *mg/mg* and *md/md* mice are not obese, despite increased food intake. The increased physical activity that also characterizes these mutants may account, in part, for their resistance to obesity. A loss of function mutation of the *Mc1r* gene suppresses the coat color effects of *mg* and *md*.[353] No effects of *md* or *mg* on plasma levels of MSH or ACTH were observed. Therefore, *mg* and *md* mutations may exert their effects by interfering directly with signaling of agouti (ASP) and AGRP/ART.

Animals homozygous for both an NPY knockout and *ob*, are leaner than *ob/ob* animals.[213] However, *mg/mg ob/ob* mice are just as obese as *ob/ob* mice, indicating that the melanocortin/agouti system is a less important factor than NPY in mediating the phenotypic consequences of leptin deficiency.[213]

Other Components of the Melanocortin/Agouti System. The importance of the *POMC* and *A* and *Art/Agrp* genes in energy homeostasis is clearly demonstrated by the obesity engendered by mutations within these genes. However, it remains to be determined whether the non-MSH peptides derived from the processing of the POMC prohormone play a significant role in energy balance and food intake.

CCK-A Receptor Knockout (OLETF) Rat

Cholecystokinin, which is produced by intestinal mucosa cells, exerts satiety effects by binding to CCK-A receptors expressed in vagal afferent neurons that project to the hindbrain.[355] The OLETF rat develops late onset obesity associated with impaired glucose tolerance in males.[356] A deletion of the promoter and the first two exons for the CCK-A receptor gene in these rats prevents the synthesis of a mature CCK-AR transcript.[357] These rats eat larger meals and the meals are fewer in number, as might be predicted by the loss of a satiating signal from CCK.[358] However, the mutation has not been transferred to a lean inbred strain to prove that the CCK-A receptor mutation is sufficient to cause obesity. As the CCK-A receptor deficiency interacts with more than one gene in OLETF rats to produce an NIDDM syndrome, it is possible that mutations in other genes, in conjunction with the mutant CCK-AR gene, may contribute to the obese phenotype.

The CCK-B/gastrin receptor binds both CCK and gastrin and is expressed mainly in the gut mucosa. Mice with disrupted CCK-B/gastrin receptor genes have alterations in gastric mucosal cell number, diminished acid secretion, and high circulating gastrin levels, but body weight is not altered.[359]

Although the CCK receptors were initially described on a pharmacological basis (A for alimentary and B for brain), the cloning of their respective genes and cDNA's have indicated a much more widespread tissue distribution.

Serotonin Receptor (5HT-2CR and 5HT-1BR) Knockouts

Specific serotonin-receptor subtypes appear to mediate the satiety effects of intracerebroventricular administration of serotonin. Selective 5HT1A/1B/2C receptor agonists induce hypophagia.[360–362] Serotonin reuptake inhibitors (e.g., fenfluramine and sibutramine) also induce hypophagia and weight loss. The loss of 5HT-2C receptor function by gene inactivation causes increased food intake, increased body weight gain, and increased fat pad weights.[287] The increased adiposity is completely reversed by food restriction, suggesting that the weight gain is due purely to hyperphagia. Surprisingly, mice with a knockout of the 5HT-1B receptor gene do not show any alterations in food intake or body weight.[363] However, these mice do not show a hypophagic response to fenfluramine.

Bombesin Receptors (BRS-3 and GRP Receptor) Knockouts

Bombesin, an anorexigenic peptide[364] obtained from amphibian skin, has mammalian homologs with a high degree of amino acid sequence similarity: gastrin-releasing peptide (GRP) and neuromedins B and C. The corresponding receptors, as well other bombesin receptors (BRS3 and BB4), have been identified.[365,366] Mice deficient in BRS3 develop obesity due mainly to hyperphagia.[327] The receptor was identified as an orphan receptor and its endogenous ligand remains unknown. The receptor deficiency induces a small decrease in physical activity that could contribute to the development of obesity.

The GRP receptor knockout mouse shows no alteration in body weight.[359] While spontaneous food intake is unaffected, the GRP-R knockout mice are resistant to the satiety effects of GRP administration.

NPY and NPY receptor (NPY1R and NPY5R) Gene Knockouts

Neuropeptide Y is a potent orexigenic peptide when injected into the third ventricle.[209–211] If food is not available during NPY administration, rats display decreased heart rate, blood pressure, and physical activity.[212] Chronic administration of orexigenic doses of NPY into the brains of rats causes a gain of excess fat, as well as producing hyperinsulinemia.[210,211,367,368] Injection of NPY into the PVN increases lipoprotein lipase activity in WAT, and decreases sympathetic nervous system activity and thermogenesis.[369] These responses indicate that NPY has coordinate effects on energy intake and output which favor weight gain and are similar to the metabolic adaptations to weight loss and maintenance of a reduced body weight seen in humans.[127] NPY mRNA expression in the arcuate is increased during states of negative caloric balance and this increase can be blocked by leptin administration. NPY mediates some of the effects of leptin deficiency because the obesity-diabetes syndrome of obese (*ob/ob*) mice is ameliorated by the loss of a functional *Npy* gene—the mice are less hyperphagic and less obese.[213] However, lean mice that are homozygous for the *Npy* gene knockout exhibit normal growth and development, are fertile, and display a normal fasting-induced hyperphagia. Moreover, *Npy* knockout mice are rendered obese by a high-fat diet, by chemical lesions of the hypothalamus with glutamate or gold thioglucose, and by genetic means (UCP-DTA toxigenic ablation of BAT, and A^y mutation of agouti).[370] These data indicate that NPY is important in the obesity caused by leptin/leptin receptor deficiency, but not in many other models of obesity.

The NPY receptor family is a set of five genes encoding G-protein-coupled receptors: NPY1R, NPY2R, NPY3R/CXCR4, NPY5R, NPY6R. The NPY3R does not respond to NPY[371,372] but may actually be a chemokine receptor for stromal cell derived factor 1 (SDF1), also known as pre-B-cell growth-stimulating factor (PBSF).[373,374] The NPY6R gene is a transcribed pseudogene that encodes a nonfunctional receptor that lacks the seventh transmembrane domain.[375–377] The NPY1R, NPY2R, and NPY5R probably mediate the effects of NPY on food intake, psychomotor activity and vasoactivity. NPY5R was thought to mediate the feeding effects of NPY in the hypothalamus, closely matching the psychoactivity and potency of NPY agonists' and antagonists' effects on feeding. However, gene knockout studies show a role for NPY1R on feeding and body-weight control.

In contrast to the *Npy* knockout mouse, mice with disrupted NPY Y1 receptor genes have multiple subtle defects in energy homeostasis. These Y1 receptor knockout mice are hypophagic under normal conditions and have diminished hyperphagia after a fast. Surprisingly, these mice develop a mild, late onset obesity due to diminished physical activity and oxygen consumption (~20 percent) during the dark (active) phase of the circadian cycle. Their body temperature is normal under normal environmental conditions as well as during a cold challenge. They have no defect in the thermogenic response to adrenergic stimulation.[215]

The NPY Y5 receptor gene has also been disrupted in mice. Similar to the Y1 knockout mice, these mice develop a mild late onset obesity associated with increased fat pad weights. Food intake of these mice does not increase until obesity is apparent at 20 to 25 weeks of age. A normal hyperphagic response to fasting was observed. Body temperature was unaffected. No measures of physical activity have been reported in these animals. The feeding response to central infusions of NPY and PYY (peptide YY, also a member of the pancreatic polypeptide family), was diminished but not completely abolished.[378]

The discrepancies in the phenotypes of the three NPY-related knockout mice, one for the ligand and two for the two receptor subtypes, could be explained by overlapping functions of the various NPY receptor subtypes. For the NPY knockout mice, no NPY is produced, and no compensation among NPY receptors can occur. In the case of single-receptor knockouts, there might be compensation, with NPY overexpression or oversecretion associated with increased stimulation of the remaining NPY receptor subtypes. As NPY affects feeding behavior as well as metabolic rate, it is possible that the late onset obesity in the receptor knockouts may be due to subtle effects on physical activity and/or energy partitioning that are difficult to detect experimentally.

Melanin Concentrating Hormone (MCH) Knockout

Mice with a targeted deletion of the orexigenic lateral hypothalamic peptide *Mch* show reduced body weight (by 24 to 28 percent) and reduced body fat (7 percent vs. 13 percent control) that is due to both reduced food intake and increased energy expenditure.[379] This phenotype is in contradistinction to the normal body weight and fat content of *Npy−/−* mice.[214] Like the *Npy−/−* mouse, *Mch−/−* animals show normal compensatory hyperphagia in response to a fast and are hyperresponsive to the anorexigenic effects of exogenous leptin. Circulating leptin concentrations are reduced proportionately to body fat and yet the animals are hypophagic, suggesting that MCH is required for response to relative leptin deficiency. The −/− animals showed no deficiency in linear growth. The thyroid and gonadal axes of these animals are intact, and hypothalamic expression of *Npy, Hcrt/Orexin*, and *Agrp* are normal. *Pomc* expression is decreased by 63 percent. The effect on *Pomc* could reflect greater sensitivity of POMC neurons to low ambient leptin and/or it could be due to direct effects of MCH neurons on arcuate POMC-expressing neurons. Because the *Mch* gene also encodes the neuropeptides "EI" and "GE," whose physiological roles are unknown, it is possible that the phenotypic effects of the *Mch* knockout are due to deficiency of these peptides. However, neither EI or GE has direct effects on feeding behavior, whereas MCH administration increases food intake.[380]

Heterozygous +/− animals are slightly lower in body weight than +/+ animals. The phenotypes of the *Mch−/−* animals indicate that the redundancies in systems supporting ingestive behaviors are not sufficient to compensate for deficiencies in some neuropeptides under physiological circumstances. However, the compensatory hyperphagia of the animals after fasting shows that MCH is not required for all physiological increases in food intake.

Dopamine Depletion with a Selective Tyrosine Hydroxylase Gene Knockout

Selective loss of dopamine (DA) only within dopaminergic neurons was achieved by gene "knock-in" using homologous recombination.[381] The pathway for dopamine synthesis is:

$$\text{Tyrosine} \xrightarrow{\text{TH}} \text{DOPA} \xrightarrow{\text{DOPA DC}} \text{DA} \xrightarrow{\text{DBH}} \text{NE}$$

TH = Tyrosine hydroxylase

DOPA DC = DOPA decarboxylase

DBH = Dopamine beta hydroxylase

First, the tyrosine hydroxylase (TH) locus was inactivated using standard homologous recombination techniques. Subsequently, tyrosine hydroxylase activity was reconstituted in noradrenergic cells by the insertion of a functional tyrosine hydroxylase construct within the dopamine beta hydroxylase (DBH) locus. Dopamine hydroxylase activity was retained by the remaining functional *Dbh* allele, enabling normal synthesis of noradrenaline. The dopamine- (DA) deficient mice became hypoactive, aphagic, and adipsic several weeks after birth. This phenotype is very similar, if not identical, to the aphagic/adipsic syndrome caused by bilateral lesions of the lateral hypothalamus (see "Neuroanatomy and Neurochemistry of Energy Homeostasis" above). Treatment with L-DOPA (L-dihydroxyphenylalanine), a dopamine precursor that does not require tyrosine hydroxylase, restored food intake. Near-normal growth was achieved with continued L-DOPA treatment.

In contrast to the clear phenotype of the dopamine-deficient mice with regard to energy balance, mice with knockouts for the various dopamine receptor genes (D1, D2, D3, and D4) as well as the dopamine transporter gene, do not have clear deficits in energy homeostasis.[382] Compensatory changes, and mixed genetic backgrounds of the experimental animal models, contribute to the uncertainty regarding the roles of the individual dopamine receptors and the dopamine transporter in food intake and energy homeostasis.

MUTATIONS THAT MAINLY AFFECT ENERGY EXPENDITURE

Toxigenic Targeting of Brown Adipose Tissue (BAT)

BAT accounts for a significant portion of the heat-generated (nonshivering thermogenesis) for maintenance of body temperature in small rodents.[151] Nonshivering thermogenesis is accomplished in BAT by the dissipation of the electrochemical gradient across the mitochondrial membrane by UCP (see sections on UCPs). The 32-kDa protein UCP1 permits protons shuttled out of the mitochondrial matrix by the cytochrome system to return down that gradient without being coupled to the generation of ATP. The potential energy of these protons is released as heat.[383] Mice that are deficient in BAT were generated by a transgenic construct that expressed the diphtheria toxin alpha subunit under the control of the *Ucp1* promoter.[384] The mice show a selective destruction of BAT that is accompanied by decreased body temperature. When these BAT-deficient mice are raised at thermoneutrality (35°C) to circumvent their deficiency in thermogenesis, the increased adiposity, as well as increased food intake, are completely prevented.[385,386] These experiments indicate that BAT is an important component of energy balance in small mammals in specific environments. However, because radiant and convective heat loss are determined by the ratio of surface area to volume, the rate of heat loss dramatically decreases with small increments in body size. Thus, while BAT probably contributes to thermogenesis in human infants, the contribution of BAT to thermogenesis in adult humans is probably minimal[151] (see "Leptin and Leptin Receptor Physiology" below).

β_3-Adrenergic Receptor ($\beta_3$ar) Gene Knockout

The β_3-adrenergic receptor gene is expressed in both brown and white fat cells. Stimulation of the β_3AR with selective agonists can increase thermogenesis in BAT and lipolysis in WAT, decreasing body fat content in rodents.[387] Mice that are deficient in β_3AR activity due to a homozygous knockout of the gene have increased WAT and are of normal weight when fed normal chow, but a high-fat diet induces increased weight gain and increases body fat content (40 percent more fat than nonmutant mice).[388,389] As the receptor functions in both WAT and BAT, it remains to be determined whether the thermogenic defect in BAT, or a lipolytic deficit in WAT, or both contribute to the obese phenotype (see below).

A missense mutation in β_3*AR* (W64R) has been identified in humans. The mutation was initially reported to be associated with obesity and accelerated onset of type 2 diabetes.[390] Subsequent studies have shown weak linkage, or no evidence of linkage, of the mutation to obesity or NIDDM in several populations[391–396]

Protein Kinase A RIIβ Gene Knockout

Protein kinase A (PKA) mediates the effects of cyclic AMP (cAMP) in some tissues.[397] The functional PKA complex is composed of two regulatory and two catalytic subunits. There are four regulatory subunit genes and two catalytic subunit genes in mice that are expressed in a tissue-specific manner. RIIβ is the major R subunit in adipose tissue and brain. Mice homozygous for a knockout of the *RIIβ* gene have diminished fat-pad weights despite normal food intake, and are resistant to the development of obesity when fed a high-fat diet.[398] The loss of RIIβ activity induces a compensatory increase in *RIα* expression, resulting in an isoform switch, as adipose tissue (BAT and WAT) mainly expresses *RIIβ*. Because the RIα subunit has a higher affinity for cAMP, PKA is more readily activated, resulting in increased oxygen consumption and increased body temperature (elevated 0.8°C). In WAT, the increased PKA activity should stimulate lipolysis and inhibit lipogenesis, as was observed in cultured adipocytes from the mutant mice. However, knockout mice do not show the expected elevations in serum glycerol and free fatty acids, suggesting that basal lipolysis is not elevated in vivo in the mutant mice.

GENE Knockouts of Uncoupling Proteins 1 and 3

Given the importance of UCP1 in the thermogenic capacity of BAT, and the development of obesity in BAT-deficient mice, the lack of obesity in *Ucp1* gene knockout mice was surprising.[399] Although *Ucp1*-deficient mice are cold intolerant, their food intakes and body weights are not different from control mice when fed normal chow or a high-fat diet. A compensatory increase in the expression of other uncoupling proteins was proposed to explain the lack of obesity. Indeed, an increase in the expression of *Ucp2*,[153] a ubiquitously expressed gene for a putative uncoupling protein, was observed in *Ucp1* knockout mice. A third putative uncoupling protein gene, *Ucp3*, that is mainly expressed in skeletal muscle (as well as brown fat in rodents) has been described.[155,156] The functions of these new members of the mitochondrial transporter superfamily in energy balance remain to be determined. Mice with UCP3 deficiency exhibit a small uncoupling effect in isolated mitochondria although the mice do not have obesity or cold intolerance.[1022,1023]

Uncoupling Protein (*Ucp1*) Overexpression in WAT

As indicated, UCP1 dissipates the electrochemical gradient created by the mitochondrial cytochromes, generating heat in the process.[383] The *Ucp1* gene is normally expressed in BAT only and is the key component of the thermogenic capacity of BAT. Expression of *Ucp1* in both WAT and BAT with the adipose tissue-specific *aP2* promoter selectively decreases the fat content of mice carrying this transgene.[400] The decreased fat content is probably due to increased thermogenesis from WAT because the BAT is involuted and endogenous *Ucp1* expression is repressed by ~95 percent. Most of the decrease in body fat is due to smaller subcutaneous fat depots. Interestingly, this transgene prevents the development of obesity in dominant yellow (A^y) mice and in mice fed a high-fat diet.[401]

Combined Norepinephrine and Epinephrine Deficiency Due to Dopamine Beta Hydroxylase Gene (*Dbh*) Knockout

Mice that are deficient in both norepinephrine and epinephrine were produced by inactivation of the dopamine beta hydroxylase (*Dbh*) gene.[402] Perinatal lethality can be prevented by provision of a catecholamine precursor in the dam's drinking water. Surprisingly, adult mice with catecholamine deficiency are not obese. They are cold intolerant due to impaired peripheral vasoconstriction and an inability to activate BAT for nonshivering thermogenesis. This failure to activate BAT upon cold challenge was predicted, as BAT is stimulated by the sympathetic nervous system via noradrenergic innervation.[383] Contrary to what was expected based on the well-known hyperphagia induced by intracerebral ventricular norepinephrine infusions, the mutants show increased spontaneous food intake. Excessive body weight gain is prevented by an equally surprising increase in resting metabolic rate. Compensatory changes, such as increased dopaminergic activity (brain dopamine levels are increased) or increased UCP2/UCP3 activity, might be responsible for the paradoxical absence of obesity and hyperphagia in *Dbh* knockout mice. Behavioral abnormalities, such as impaired maternal behavior and deficits in learning, have also been documented in these DBH-deficient mice.[403,404] The phenotypes of these animals are an important reminder of the complexity and redundancy of the systems subserving energy homeostasis.

MUTATIONS THAT MAINLY AFFECT PARTITIONING OF CALORIES BETWEEN ADIPOSE TISSUE AND LEAN TISSUES

Genes that Increase Adipose Tissue Mass

The Growth Hormone System (*Ghrhr, Gh, Ghr, Igf1, Igf2*, and *Igf1r*). Deficiency of growth hormone (GH) results in decreased statural growth and increased adiposity (fractional body fat) in rodents and humans.[405–407] Mutations and genetic manipulations within the genes that affect growth hormone secretion or action also affect body composition. Increased adiposity is seen in several rodent models of growth hormone deficiency: (a) little (*lit/lit*) mice with a spontaneous inactivating mutation of the growth hormone-releasing hormone-receptor gene (*Ghrhr*);[408–410] (b) growth hormone-deficient dwarf (*dw/dw*) rats fed a high-fat diet;[411] (c) growth hormone receptor- (GH-R) deficient mice generated by an induced mutation of the *Ghr* gene;[412] and (d) silencing of endogenous growth hormone secretion due to repression by an overexpressing GH transgene.[413–415] In the GHRHR-deficient mice, increased adipose tissue stores are evident in the postweaning stage, despite normal food intake. In mice with repressed GH secretion by a GH-expressing transgene, increased adiposity is observed with ad libitum feeding as well as with caloric restriction. In these animals, there is no apparent decrease in energy expenditure. Similar results are observed in transgenic rats in which endogenous GH secretion is chronically repressed by low-level expression of a GH transgene.[415] These observations indicate that the loss of GH leads to preferential deposition (partitioning) of calories within WAT, despite normal energy intake and expenditure. This conclusion is supported by the fact that a high-fat diet accelerates the rate of triglyceride deposition in *little* mice and rodents with repressed GH secretion.

As the effects of GH are mediated by insulin-like growth factor 1 (IGF1), it is surprising that mice with *Igf1* and *Igf1r* defects do not recapitulate the phenotype of GH deficiency. Mice deficient in IGF1, IGF2, and IGF1R[416–419] suffer severe intrauterine growth retardation, and are born with body weights ~30 to 60 percent those of normal littermates. Early postnatal lethality is observed (up to 95 percent in one IGF-I-deficient line). Adult mice with IGF1 and IGF2 deficiencies show proportional dwarfing, but no excess adiposity. These knockout mice suggest that the obesity of GH-deficient mice may be mediated by the absence of GH, rather than by the lack of IGF, and imply that GH may have some direct effects independent of IGF. Alternatively, the early growth retardation caused by IGF deficiency may be sufficient to prevent the development of obesity in GH deficiency, perhaps by effects on the production of adipocyte precursor cells (see "Adipose Tissue Biochemistry and Development" above). It is interesting to note that *Stat5b*-deficient mice develop obesity, similar to GH-deficient animals, while *Stat5a/Stat5b* doubly deficient mice mimic the severe growth retardation of mice with deficiencies in *Igfl, Igf1r*, and *Igf2r*.

Stat5a/5b (Signal Transducer and Activator of Transcription 5a/5b) and Jak2 (Janus Kinase 2). JAK2 and STAT 5a/5b mediate the effects of GH. Upon binding of GH, the GH receptor dimerizes and activates JAK2 and STAT5a/5b. Mice homozygous for a deletion of *Stat5b* have a phenotype similar to GH receptor-deficient individuals: proportional dwarfism, obesity, elevated plasma GH, and low circulating IGF1.[420] Surprisingly, mice deficient in STAT5a have only a mild defect in granulocyte macrophage colony stimulating factor (GM-CSF).[421] GM-CSF, like leptin, is a member of the GH/cytokine superfamily and signals via the JAK-STAT pathways. Combined STAT5a/5b deficiency results in severe dwarfism (GH resistance), infertility (deficient progesterone production from the corpora lutea of the ovaries), diminished response to various hematopoietic factors (but not erythropoietin), and diminished fat-pad weights (20 percent of normal). The decreased adiposity of these double mutants is clearly distinct from the increased adiposity associated with GH deficiency, and more closely resembles the somatic stunting seen in mice deficient in IGF1 and IGF1R. Homozygous deletion of the *Jak2* gene results in an embryonic lethal phenotype.[422,423]

Activation of STAT5b by GH is dependent upon a pulsatile pattern of GH exposure. A pulsatile secretory pattern is characteristic of male rats and human males, whereas females (rodents and human) exhibit a relatively constant intermediate level of plasma GH.[424–426] Continuous GH exposure down-regulates activated STAT5b by a rapid dephosphorylation at constituent tyrosines, serines, and threonines.[427] As discussed below in "Leptin and Leptin Receptor Physiology," such down-regulation in the context of exposure to higher/invariant ligand concentrations is a potential model for the apparent leptin insensitivity of some obese humans and rodents.

***GLUT4* Overexpression in WAT.** The expression of the *GLUT4* (glucose transporter 4) gene is normally under the control of ambient insulin levels. Stored within vesicles in the cytoplasm of hepatocytes, adipocytes, and muscle cells, GLUT4 is transported to the plasma membrane upon cell stimulation with insulin. Transcription rates of the *GLUT4* gene are also stimulated by insulin.[428] When GLUT4 is overexpressed in WAT (human GLUT4 cDNA under control of *aP2* promoter), the increased glucose import into adipocytes is associated with increased fractional body fat content without any change in food intake.[429] Presumably, the excess calories provided by the increased transport of glucose into adipocytes increases triglyceride synthesis.

Insulin Receptor Deficiency in Skeletal Muscle. The role of skeletal muscle insulin resistance in the development of obesity has been difficult to address experimentally. A transgenic mouse model of insulin resistance limited to skeletal muscle was developed by the use of a transgene expressing a dominant-negative mutant insulin receptor specifically in striated muscle.[430] While body weights of the transgenic mice were unaltered, carcass analysis revealed increased fat content (22 to 38 percent) accompanied by a decrease in body protein (10 to 15 percent). The transgenic mice had modest elevations in fasting blood glucose (25 percent), triglycerides (29 percent), and free fatty acids (15 percent). The increased fat content and decreased muscle mass of these mice can be attributed to a decrease in the flow of glucose into skeletal muscle, and the resultant partitioning of these calories into adipose tissue and hepatic triglycerides.

ICAM-1 and Mac-1 Leukocyte Adhesion Receptor Gene Knockouts. An unexpected phenotype of mild, late onset obesity[431] was described in mice with knockouts for either of two genes encoding cell adhesion molecules primarily expressed in cells of the immune system (intercellular adhesion molecule 1, ICAM-1) and one of its counterreceptors (Mac-1, CD11b/CD18). Mice deficient in ICAM-1 or Mac-1 exhibit deficits in the inflammatory response (e.g., resistance to septic shock) as well as immune system defects (e.g., reduced contact hypersensitivity). ICAM-1-deficient mice become obese without an increase of food intake on normal or high-fat chow (21 percent fat). Mac-1 deficient mice become obese on a high-fat diet, but the variability of body weights due to genetic heterogenicity (mixed 129/B6 background) does not permit assessment of the development of obesity when fed normal chow. Because energy expenditure was not measured, the increased adiposity could be due to diminished energy expenditure and/or partitioning of calories into fat.

Genes that Decrease White Adipose Tissue Mass

CEBP Isoform Knockouts (*CEBPα*, *CEBPβ*, and *CEBPδ*). Several transcription factors that bind to a common sequence motif, CCAAT, are called CCAAT-enhancer binding proteins. The CEBPα form is expressed mainly in adipocytes and is required for proper differentiation of preadipocytes to adipocytes. Mice with a homozygous knockout of the *Cebpα* gene are born alive but most of the mutant mice die within several hours after birth.[100] The few that do survive for several days have reduced body weights and reduced fat-pad weights. Mice doubly homozygous for knockouts of the *Cebpβ* and *Cebpδ* genes[432] have a phenotype that is similar to *Cebpα* knockout mice: increased neonatal mortality and reduced fat-pad weights (WAT and BAT). The decreased fat content is most likely due to impaired differentiation of preadipocytes.

WAT differentiation is dependent on the coordinate expression of adipocyte differentiation factors (B-ZIP transcription factors) such as CEBPs and SREBP/ADD1.[98] Depletion of WAT was achieved by the expression of a synthetic gene construct, A-ZIP/F-1, in WAT under the control of the aP2 enhancer/promoter.[433] The phenotype of the transgenic mice, characterized by hyperinsulinemia/NIDDM, dyslipidemia, and an anabolic state associated with hyperphagia, mimics that of the human disease congenital lipoatrophic diabetes (Berardinelli-Seip syndrome MIM 269700). The A-ZIP/F-1 transgene encodes a leucine zipper dimerizing domain, allowing heterodimer formation with CEBPs and JUNs, as well as an acidic amphipathic helix replacing the basic DNA binding domain. The acidic and basic domains of the heterodimers (A-ZIP/F-1+CEBPs and A-ZIP/F-1+JUNs) form a stable complex that prevents DNA binding, effectively inhibiting an transcriptional promoting activity of the endogenous transcription factors. The adult transgenic mice were nearly devoid of WAT, with residual fat at sites expected for BAT (interscapular, neck, parasternal, and renal hilum). The lack of WAT was, as expected, associated with leptin deficiency (~5 percent of normal). The transgenic mice had enlarged viscera due to engorgement with triglycerides. Hyperinsulinemia (thirtyfold elevation) was present even at 7 days of age, preceding the onset of hyperglycemia at 3 weeks.

SREBP The differentiation of 3T3-L1 preadipocytes is stimulated by overexpression of a transcription factor that binds to sterol regulatory elements (SREBPs).[102] Overexpression of nSREBP-1c, an engineered form of SREBP-1c that lacks the Golgi membrane attachment domain and that is constitutively targeted to the nucleus, produces transgenic mice that exhibit greatly diminished WAT and BAT, visceromegaly, hyperinsulinemia, and hyperglycemia.[434] This phenotype also mimics Berardinelli-Seip syndrome (MIM 269700). The nSREBP-1c transgenic mice have small fat pads while their enlarged BAT is morphologically and biochemically similar (increased fatty acid synthase and lack of *Ucp1* expression) to normal WAT. The transgenic mice are also hyperinsulinemic and hyperglycemic. Although in vivo insulin tolerance tests indicate that the transgenic mice are insulin resistant, basal and insulin-stimulated skeletal muscle glucose uptake is similar between control and transgenic mice, suggesting that the lack of functional WAT causes insulin resistance due to metabolic changes in WAT per se. This result is consonant with the finding that severe insulin resistance in skeletal muscle is insufficient to precipitate severe hyperinsulinemia or hyperglycemia.[435]

Diptheria Toxin Expression WAT Mice carrying a transgene that drives expression of the diptheria toxin in adipose tissue have been generated.[1024] Transgenic mice expressing high levels of the toxin die prematurely due to the development of chylous ascites. Mice with lower levels of toxin gene expression develop to adults and have normal adiposity. However, these mice are resistant to the development of obesity induced by glutamate.

As more information is collected about the genetic control of adipocyte development, it may be possible to produce depletion of total fat mass or of selected depots such as visceral adipose tissue, an independent risk factor for hypertension and NIDDM. However, the syndrome of NIDDM and dyslipidemia associated with near absence of WAT (Seip syndrome of generalized lipodystrophy) may be an undesirable complication of manipulations that are designed to reduce WAT mass. While reduction of WAT mass by caloric deprivation, as seen in anorexia nervosa or starvation[436] is usually not associated with hyperglycemia or insulin resistance (see Koffler et al.[437] for exceptional cases), manipulations that reduce WAT mass by altering preadipocyte differentiation may cause undesirable metabolic effects. In support of this contention, intrauterine growth retardation due to starvation, which potentially alters preadipocyte differentiation, is associated with decreased glucose tolerance in adult humans and rodents.[438–440] Leptin replacement in A-ZIP/F-1 mice has only a minimal effect on the diabetes phenotype, suggesting that factors other than leptin deficiency are responsible for the metabolic phenotypes associated with virtual absence of body fat.[1025]

HMGIC HMGIC is a DNA binding protein that appears early in development and is not usually expressed in adult tissues. The homozygous knockout mice exhibit a dwarfing phenotype that corresponds to a diminution of cell replication during fetal development. HMGIC also appears to have a role in adipocyte differentiation as HMGIC mice are partially resistant to the obesity-inducing effects of leptin deficiency and a high-fat diet.[1026]

Genes that Increase Skeletal Muscle Mass

Myostatin (*Mstn*) Knockouts in Mice and Cattle. Myostatin is a member of the transforming-growth factor (TGF) family that was discovered during a search with degenerate primers designed to amplify TGF-related genes from mouse genomic DNA.[441] One TGF family member, GDF-8 (growth and differentiation factor 8, subsequently named "myostatin"), is expressed mainly in skeletal muscle with some low-level expression in WAT. Mice homozygous for a myostatin gene knockout display increased weight of all skeletal muscles. Food intake and body compositions have not been reported for these animals (see below for phenotype of cattle with spontaneous mutations of myostatin). The increased muscularity is due to both hypertrophy and hyperplasia of muscles.[441] A spontaneous mutation of the myostatin locus, designated compact, was detected during selective breeding for increased protein content in mice.[442] The compact *(Cmpt)* mutation causes hypermuscularity with an increase in muscle:bone weight (1.61 greater than in nonmutants).[443]

Increased skeletal muscle content is an important trait in the production of cattle for meat production. Several breeds of cattle, such as the Belgian Blue, have been selectively bred for increased muscularity.[444–447] The hypermuscled trait was mapped to bovine chromosome 2 in a region that contains the bovine myostatin gene. Several different mutations of the myostatin gene have been found in various hypermuscled breeds of cattle, indicating independent mutational events.[446] The hypermuscularity of the cattle is accompanied by a decrease in the weights of internal organs. The nominally recessive myostatin mutation has an effect in the heterozygous state, increasing muscle mass and decreasing fat content of muscle.[448] Such heterozygote effects are also seen in mice segregating the Lep^{ob} and $Lepr^{db}$ mutations, and suggest that the interplay of such effects may play a role in human body composition (see"Leptin and Leptin Receptor Physiology" below).

Ryanodine Receptor Gene (RYR1) in Pigs. The ryanodine receptor functions as the calcium release channel in skeletal muscle. The RYR1 gene is mainly expressed in skeletal muscle, whereas the RYR2 gene is expressed in brain. In several breeds of pigs, a dominant mutation in the RYR1 gene is associated with increased dressed carcass weight, a measure of skeletal muscle mass.[449–451] It has been suggested that the increased leanness of the animals may be due to increased muscle tone secondary to the increased isotonic contractions induced by increased skeletal muscle calcium concentrations.[452] If this is true, then expansion of skeletal muscle mass and increased energy expenditure may jointly account for the lean phenotype of the mutant pigs.

While the leaner carcass composition is an advantage for meat production, the mutation is also associated with porcine stress syndrome, in which stress brought about by overcrowding and transport of the pigs, induces a state similar to malignant hyperthermia (MHS) in humans. As a result, the muscles become pale, soft, and unmarketable. The mutation can be detected by in vitro muscle hypercontractility on exposure to caffeine. The in vitro response of skeletal muscles to halothane exposure does not, however, correlate well with the mutation.[453] Halothane exposure during anesthesia precipitates MHS in susceptible humans.[454] Mutations in the RYR1 gene cause susceptibility to MHS in humans. However, MHS is a heterogeneous disorder that is caused by mutations in at least two other loci, CACLN1A3 (α_1 subunit of the dihydropyridine-sensitive L-type voltage-dependent calcium channel receptor), and another gene located on chromosome 3q13.[455] Individuals with mutations in the RYR1 gene show clinical correlation with in vitro muscle contraction tests with caffeine, whereas there is poor association with in vitro halothane exposure.[456]

Callipyge Locus in Sheep. The callipyge mutation is associated with increased muscle mass in the hindquarters of sheep.[457] The mode of transmission is polar overdominance in which the paternally imprinted mutant allele produces an effect only in the heterozygous state.[453] Carcass analysis indicates that there is a clear gradient along the rostral-caudal axis of the body with increasing muscle mass in the hindquarters.[458–460] The forequarters are the least affected, although they are statistically heavier than the equivalent muscles from nonmutant animals. As in the hypermuscled cattle, there is decreased fat content in the individual muscles. The identity of the responsible gene is unknown.

Genes that Decrease Skeletal Muscle Content

Muscle-Specific Regulatory Factors. (*Myogenin, MyoD, Mrf4,* and *Myf5*) are myocyte-specific transcription factors of the basic helix-loop-helix (bHLH) family. Myogenin is responsible for myoblast differentiation, whereas *MyoD* and *Myf5* act earlier to establish myoblast identity. Mice that are myogenin-deficient are born alive but immobile, and die perinatally with a severe lack of skeletal muscle.[461,462] Mice with a combined *Mrf4-MyoD* deficiency[463] exhibit a phenotype very similar to myogenin knockout mice, showing a deficiency of skeletal muscle, but not a complete absence of skeletal muscle differentiation. Mice that are deficient for both *Myf5* and *MyoD* completely lack skeletal muscle.[464] Isolated deficiencies of *Myf5*, *MyoD*, or *Mrf4* do not alter skeletal muscle differentiation. While the extreme phenotypes of mice with deficiencies in these genes suggest that humans with orthologous mutations would be nonviable, it is likely that such muscle-specific factors may act to regulate skeletal muscle mass and muscle capacity to hypertrophy under specific nutritional, exercise or endocrine conditions.

Candidate Genes with Mutations that Do not Alter Body Weight and/or Energy Balance

Glucagon-Like Peptide 1 Receptor (Glp1r). GLP1 (processed from preproglucagon in intestinal L cells) and its longer-acting acting analog, exendin, suppress feeding when introduced into the brain.[465,466] GLP1 receptors have been identified within neurons in the ARC of the hypothalamus. These GLP1 neurons coexpress a glucose transporter (GLUT2) and glucokinase (GK), suggesting that these neurons may be responsive to ambient glucose concentrations. Furthermore, intracerebral GLP1 administration activates CRH neurons within the PVN, indicating that GLP1 probably exerts its anorectic activity via the CRH system. However, knockout mice without the GLP1 receptor exhibit normal feeding behavior and do not become obese.[467]

CRH and CRH Receptors. The CRH neurons within the PVN of the hypothalamus receive important synaptic inputs from NPY and POMC neurons of the ARC. CRH is anorexigenic when infused into the cerebral ventricles. Therefore, it was surprising that mice with knockouts of *Crh*[468] and *Crh1r*[469] did not show significant alterations in body weight, although these mice had diminished responses to stress. Urocortin was discovered as a peptide with significant sequence homology to CRH.[470] Urocortin is more potent than CRH as an anorectic agent and has less anxiogenic activity than CRH.[258,260] It is widely expressed in the brain, including the hypothalamus. A second CRH receptor, CRH2R, with increased affinity for urocortin (over CRH) has been identified.[254] CRH2R is highly expressed in the hypothalamus. Selective down-regulation of CRH2 receptors with CRH2 receptor antisense oligonucleotides blocks the anorectic effect of CRF infusion.[259] It is possible that urocortin and the CRH2 receptor are important modulators of feeding behavior, although specific genetic manipulations of these genes have not been reported.

Crh2r Knockout Mice Recently, mice with a knockout of the *Crh2r* gene have been reported not to have an abese phenotype although more extensive testing regarding energy balance and weight regulation was not reported.[1027–1029]

MUTATIONS AFFECTING MULTIPLE COMPONENTS OF ENERGY BALANCE

The Leptin/Leptin Receptor System

The so-called "lipostatic" model of body-weight regulation[122] was proposed to account for the long-term relative constancy of somatic energy stores in mammals, and to explain the effects of their depletion on ingestive behavior, energy expenditure, linear growth, and fertility.[123,471] The model predicted that a signal from (or related to) adipose tissue would influence behavior and vegetative functions related to energy homeostasis.[1,472,473] Parabiosis studies, in which the circulations of obese and lean mice or rats were surgically joined (see below), gave additional impetus to the validity of this model by developing indirect evidence in favor of a fat-derived humoral signal of adiposity and a central sensing mechanism for that signal.[474–476] As indicated earlier, physiological studies in humans of the metabolic responses to weight perturbation are consistent with the concept of a lipostatic mechanism for defense of somatic energy stores.[127–129,477]

Parabiosis experiments[474,476,478] demonstrated that exchange of small amounts of blood between *ob* mice and wild-type or *db* mice resulted in amelioration of the obesity in the *ob* mouse, while lean mice in parabiosis with *db* mice, or with rats who were obese due to lesions of the ventromedial hypothalamus, died of starvation. Harris et al. reported similar inhibition of growth in lean animals that were parabiosed to obese Zucker rats (*fa*).[475] Based on these experiments, Coleman[474,479,480] suggested that the obesity of the *ob* mouse was due to lack of an afferent humoral signal that could be transmitted by parabiosis, and that this factor was "sensed" by the *db* gene product. The molecular mapping of the rat *fa* gene to a region of synteny-homology with mouse *db* provided strong support for the inference that the *db* and *fa* phenotypes were due to mutations in the same gene.[481] The observation that the parabiosis of rats rendered obese by a lesion of the ventromedial hypothalamus with a nonlesioned animal resulted in a decrease in fat-pad weight and food intake in the nonlesioned member of the parabiosis pair, further supported the belief that the site of action of the *db/fa* gene product might be the hypothalamus.[482,483]

A positional cloning strategy was used to clone the *ob* gene[484–487] whose protein product was named leptin ("leptos" is Greek for thin). Leptin (167 amino acids including 21aa signal sequence) is primarily synthesized in, and secreted from, adipose tissue. Leptin is a member of the cytokine superfamily. It is folded into four helical bundles and has one essential disulfide bond.[488–492] Circulating concentrations of leptin are directly proportional to adipose tissue mass,[493] making it a candidate for the predicted afferent signal regarding fat stores to central and/or peripheral receptors regulating energy homeostasis and endocrine function.

Coleman's initial hypothesis regarding the gene products of *ob* and *db* was proven correct[474] by Zhang et al.'s identification in 1994 of the protein product of the *ob* gene, which was deficient in the Lep^{ob} mouse;[487] by the demonstration that the *db* mutation in the mouse and the *fa* mutation in the rat are mutations in the leptin-receptor gene;[74,481,494,495] and by proof that administration of leptin ameliorates the hyperphagia, obesity, and infertility of Lep^{ob} but not $Lepr^{db}$ mice.[496–499]

The cloning of *ob* enabled the determination of the molecular basis for the two known mouse mutations of this gene:

Leptin (*Lep*) Alleles. The obese mutation (Lep^{ob}) is a recessive mutation due to a premature termination codon in the second (and final) coding exon of the leptin gene.[487] This mutation (R105X) results in a truncated protein that is not secreted. mRNA levels of *Lep* are elevated in adipose tissue. The obese mutation arose in an outbred stock carrying the waltzer (*v*) mutation.[500] To minimize phenotypic variation, the mutation was transferred onto the inbred strain C57BL/6J. Most studies of the obese mutation have been performed with this congenic strain, although *ob* has also been transferred to C57BLKs/J. The Lep^{ob} mouse is characterized by early onset, severe obesity (with increased partitioning of stored calories as fat), stunted growth (skeletal, muscle, brain), extreme insulin resistance, hyperphagia, hypometabolism, infertility, and hypothyroidism.[137,479,501]

Another nonfunctional allele of leptin, *obese2J* (Lep^{ob2J}), is due to a retroviral insertion within the first intron of the leptin gene.[502] The insertion is a transposon of the ETn family and contains multiple splice-acceptor sites that interfere with normal splicing of the first and second exons of the leptin gene. This mutation arose on an inbred background, SM/Ckc, carrying the Dactylaplasia (*Dac*) mutation.

The human OB gene, whose nucleotide sequence and predicted amino acid sequence is 84 percent identical to the murine leptin sequence, is located at 7q31.3[503] and (as in the mouse) consists of 3 exons (2 coding exons) spanning about 18 kb and encoding a 3.5-kb mRNA.[504,505]

Leptin Receptor (*Lepr*). The leptin receptor gene was discovered as a leptin-binding protein expressed at high levels in the choroid plexus.[494] The gene's chromosomal position was in the vicinity of the mouse diabetes and rat fatty mutations.[495] Subsequent analysis found mutations within the leptin receptor gene of all extant diabetes (mouse) and fatty (rat) alleles[137] (see below).

The leptin receptor (Fig. 157-5) is a member of the superfamily of cytokine receptors that includes the growth hormone receptor and the prolactin receptor. There is a large extracellular domain that encodes one intact ligand-binding site, although sequence analysis suggests that the ligand-binding domain was imperfectly duplicated.[506] There is one short membrane spanning domain followed by a variable carboxyl terminus that is dependent on the specific 3′ terminal exon that is spliced into the mature transcript[507]. At least 5 isoforms of the receptor are described for rodents and humans[494,507–511]. The shortest form is encoded by the Re isoform mRNA and lacks the transmembrane and intracytoplasmic domains. The human gene is unable to code for this isoform, as the 3′ terminal exon has lost its polyadenylation signal and no mature Re mRNA is found in human tissues.[507] The soluble receptor in humans is probably made by cleavage of membrane-bound isoforms.

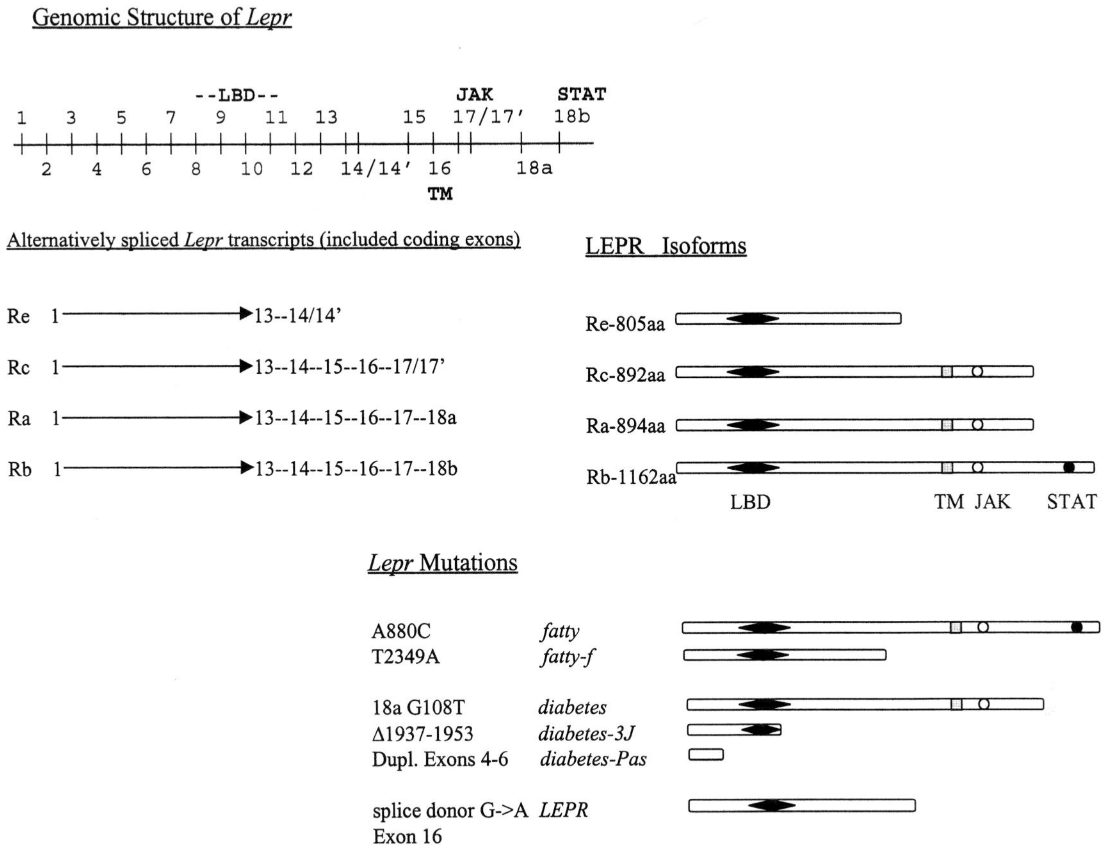

Fig. 157-5 Genomic structure of *LEPR*, alternatively spliced transcripts of *Lepr*, isoforms of LEPR, and inactivating mutations of the leptin-receptor gene in humans, mice, and rats. Sequence motifs of the receptor (in bold) are designated LBD (ligand-binding domain), TM (transmembrane region), JAK (docking site for JAKs) and STAT (activating site for STATs). Exons with a prime designation (14′, 17′) are juxtaposed 3′ terminal exons with termination codons and polyadenylation signals. Exons with a lowercase designation (18a, 18b) are conventional alternatively spliced 3′ terminal exons. Alternatively spliced transcripts are shown with their constituent coding exons. The receptor protein isoforms are shown with the ligand-binding domain (LBD) as a filled elongated diamond, the TM as a shaded square, the JAK docking site as an open circle, and the STAT activation motif as a filled circle. The sizes of the receptor isoforms are shown in amino acids. The known mutations are shown as nucleotide changes beside their allele designations. The effects of the mutations on the receptor are shown schematically; *fatty* (rat), *diabetes* (mouse) *LEPR* (human).

The membrane-bound forms (Ra, Rb, Rc, Rd, and Rf) have a membrane proximal motif that binds JAK proteins. The Rb isoform (1162 amino acids) has a long intracytoplasmic domain that contains another motif near the C-terminus required for STAT activation. Rb is the only isoform that contains a STAT domain. The precise ratios of each isoform in various tissues can vary. The Ra isoform is the most highly expressed type in most tissues, including the choroid plexus; it is also highly expressed in microvessels of the brain, potentially serving a transport function for the entry of leptin to the central nervous system.[512,513] The Rb isoform is most abundant in the hypothalamus and the rat cerebellum. Because loss of only the Rb isoform of the leptin receptor is sufficient to replicate the obesity/diabetes syndrome of leptin deficiency (the *db* mouse), it has been suggested that only Rb isoform-mediated signaling within the hypothalamus is relevant to energy balance. In fact, treatment of *ob/ob* and *db/db* mice with ciliary muscle neurotrophic factor (CNTF), a cytokine superfamily member that activates STAT3 upon binding to its receptor, induces weight loss and increases lipolysis.[514]

Leptin binding to homodimers of Rb on a stoichiometric basis (leptin: leptin receptor monomer) initiates an intracellular phosphorylation cascade of the JAK/STAT pathway.[515–517] The leptin receptor has no intrinsic kinase or phosphatase activity. The Rb isoform activates both JAK2 and STATs, while the Ra isoform, bearing a JAK docking site but lacking a STAT activating domain, can induce the expression of some immediate early genes, such as *c-fos* and *c-jun*.[518] JAK2, a Janus kinase, is important for the phosphorylation of STAT proteins that are activated by leptin binding in vitro. However, within the hypothalamus in vivo, leptin causes phosphorylation and activation of STAT3 only.[519] It is assumed that upon binding leptin and dimerization of the receptors, that JAK2 molecules bound to each of the receptor monomers autophosphorylate each other to initiate the signaling cascade. Activated JAK2 is then capable of phosphorylating and activating STAT3. The targets of STAT3 action specific to leptin receptor activation have not been identified. This specificity may be conferred at a neuronal (cellular) rather than a biochemical (subcellular) level. Termination of the activation signal may be due to leptin-mediated induction of SOCS3 (suppressor of cytokine signaling) as it binds to and inhibits the activity of JAK2.[520] Indicating the importance of this signal transduction pathway, deficiencies of JAK2[422] and STAT3[521] are embryonic lethal mutations.

Because dimerization of the leptin receptor appears to be necessary for signal transduction via JAK/STAT, it is possible that the formation of heterodimers between Ra and Rb would form an inactive receptor-ligand complex. However, cotransfection studies of both Ra and Rb failed to provide evidence of the formation of such heterodimers.[515,522] The nature of the isoform-specific segregation that prevents such heterodimer promotion remains to be determined.

Regulation of leptin-receptor mRNA levels appears to be modulated by ambient leptin levels. Fasting increases overall *Lepr* mRNA levels as well as increasing the fraction of Rb mRNA in the hypothalamus.[523–525] In leptin-resistant *fa/fa* animals that synthesize defective leptin-receptor mRNAs and receptors, there is an overall increase in *Lepr* mRNA, as well as an increase in the fractional content of the Rb isoform in the hypothalamus.[523–525]

As for *ob*, the cloning of *db* enabled the analysis of the molecular bases for the extant mutations of this gene in rodents.

Leptin Receptor (*Lepr*) Alleles. The *diabetes* ($Lepr^{db}$) mutation arose spontaneously in the inbred C57BLKS/J mouse strain.[526] The mutation is a single nucleotide substitution that creates a novel splice donor site such that 106 nucleotides are inserted near the 3′ end of the reading frame for the Rb (long) isoform. No functional Rb (STAT-containing) *Lepr* isoform is made.

The *db3J* ($Lepr^{db3J}$) mutation arose on the inbred 129/J mouse strain.[527] The mutation is due to a 17 bp deletion in coding exon 11, prior to the receptor's transmembrane domain. All isoforms of *Lepr* are affected. The phenotype of the obese 129/J mice is characterized by extreme hyperinsulinemia associated with massive pancreatic islet beta cell proliferation.

The *dbPas* ($Lepr^{dbPas}$) mutation occurred on the DW/Pas inbred mouse strain at the Pasteur Institute.[528] The mutation is due to incomplete duplication of coding exons 4, 5, and 6 that prevents the accumulation of any mature *Lepr* transcript.[529] The obese mice are similar to other leptin-receptor mutants, but the initial report indicated that there was no deficit in nonshivering thermogenesis.

Other *db* alleles have occurred at the Jackson Laboratories and elsewhere. They are/were strains (bearing some lost alleles) characterized by obesity, hyperphagia, and varying degrees of hyperglycemia. The greatest variation occurs in the degree of hyperglycemia (diabetes proneness), which is dependent on the particular strain on which the mutation is carried.[530,531]

Rat Fatty Alleles. The *fatty* mutation ($Lepr^{fa}$) occurred in an outbred rat stock called 13 M that was being used in a selection experiment for the inheritance of body weight.[532] The mutation is a single-nucleotide substitution that causes the substitution of a proline for a glutamine at amino acid 269, near the ligand-binding domain.[74,506,533] This substitution is found in all *Lepr* isoforms. No effects of the substitution are observed on mRNA levels or on ligand binding. Receptor translocation to the cell surface is severely compromised (approximately five- to sevenfold reduction of receptor number at cell surface).[517,534,535] Signal transduction of the mutant receptor is paradoxical because it is capable of ligand-independent activation of transcription.[517] Most of these studies were performed on cell lines transfected with the normal or mutant receptors. Definitive evidence awaits molecular characterization of the mutant receptor *in vivo*. The *fatty* mutation has been maintained on the original outbred 13M stock, widely referred to as the "Zucker fatty" strain. An inbred strain, the Zucker diabetic fatty (ZDF) strain, has been derived from the outbred stock and is characterized by diabetes (due to insulinopenia) in obese males.[536] The fatty mutation was also transferred to the diabetogenic Wistar Kyoto (WKY) inbred rat strain; the resulting congenic is called the "Wistar diabetic fatty" (WDF) strain.[537,538] Although, obese WDF male rats are diabetic, circulating insulin concentrations may be equivalent to normoglycemic obese males of the outbred 13 M stock.

The *fatty-f (corpulent/cp, Koletsky/K)* mutation ($Lepr^{faf}$) was found in an outbred stock created from a cross between a male spontaneously hypertensive rat (SHR) and a female Sprague-Dawley rat.[539] While the original report gave a provisional gene symbol of *f* for the mutation, the mutation was subsequently given other names and gene symbols: corpulent (*cp*)[540] and Koletsky (*k*).[541] The phenotype was obesity with atherosclerosis, diabetes, and a severely shortened life span. The mutation is due to a single nucleotide substitution that causes a premature termination prior to the transmembrane domain.[541,542] All forms of the receptor are truncated. This mutation has been subsequently transferred to two inbred rat strains: SHR, the diabetogenic hypertensive strain, and LA/N, a normotensive, normoglycemic strain.[540]

Phenotypes of Leptin and Leptin receptor Deficiency. Leptin and leptin-receptor deficiencies affect body composition and energy homeostasis, as well as feeding behavior and multiple endocrine systems.[480] The obese rodents resulting from mutation of either gene are characterized by extreme obesity, hyperphagia, decreased core temperature, and diminished physical activity.[543] In addition, these rodents are infertile, have impaired glucose tolerance with strain-specific levels of insulinemia, and oversecrete corticosterone. In the following discussion, we treat leptin deficiency and leptin-receptor deficiency similarly, highlighting those aspects that are significantly different.

The hyperphagia is very marked and is present prior to weaning.[544] Whereas rodents eat most of their meals in the dark phase, feeding patterns in these mutants are chaotic and there does not appear to be a strong influence of the light/dark cycle on them.[545–549] Obese (*ob/ob*) mice and fatty (*fa/fa*) rats exert more effort than lean rodents for a food reward and tolerate a higher concentration of a bitter additive, such as quinine, to their feed.[550–552] This feeding drive distinguishes the mutations of the leptin system from rodents with ventromedial hypothalamic lesions. VMH-lesioned rats are more finicky than normal rats; they work less for a food reward and are more sensitive to adulteration of their feed.[553–557] The molecular mechanisms for this important phenotypic difference are not known.

Obese rodents (*ob*, *db*, and *fa*) have decreased core temperatures due to a defect in the nonshivering component of thermogenesis.[558–561] These rodents have hypotrophic BAT when housed at 20°C ambient temperature. The obese rodents are unable to stimulate thermogenesis from BAT acutely, although prolonged exposure to mild cold (17°C) will increase BAT weight.[562] The deficiency of BAT mass and thermogenic response are due primarily to decreased sympathetic nervous system (tone).[563,564] Mitigating the thermogenic defect of *ob* and *fa* rodents by rearing adults in a thermoneutral environment does not significantly alter the degree of excess of adipose tissue stores.[565] Moreover, when reared in a thermoneutral environment and fed by intragastric infusion of synthetic rat milk, *fa/fa* pups accumulate more adipose tissue than lean littermates.[566,567]

Obese rodents (*ob*, *db*, and *fa*) can easily weigh three or four times as much as a lean control. This excess mass is composed of triglycerides stored in WAT. Although food intake is increased, there is not an accompanying increase in linear growth. Brain weight is reduced, as is skeletal muscle mass, with fast-twitch muscle fibers being proportionately smaller than slow-twitch fibers.[568,569] Forced exercise will decrease adipose tissue stores, although muscle mass does not increase significantly.[570] The increased adipose tissue mass appears to be preferentially spared ("partitioning"),[571] perhaps due to a limited lipolytic response related to functional leptin deficiency. Pair feeding experiments, in which the food intake of obese animals (*ob* and *fa*) is yoked to the intake of normal control animals, show that weight gains are similar between the lean and obese genotypes. However, the genetically obese rodents show a two- to threefold greater increase in fractional body fat content.[572–574] These observations indicate that a deficiency in leptin signaling, due either to deficiencies in leptin or its receptor, causes preferential partitioning of calories into WAT where the calories are stored as triglyceride. These effects on lipid deposition are seen, to a milder degree, in animals heterozygous for these mutations.[575–577]

Obese rodents (*ob*, *db*, and *fa*) are generally infertile due to hypothalamic dysfunction. Obese male *fatty* rats can be selected for fertility such that an outbred colony can be maintained by matings between obese males and heterozygous females. However, obese male mice are less reliable breeders than obese male rats.[497,578,579] The leptin receptor is expressed in both ovarian granulosa cells and in GNRH neurons of the rat.[584] While obese females are also infertile, their ovaries (*ob* and *db*) can be transplanted into histocompatible female hosts. These transplanted ovaries function well and produce normal progeny, indicating that leptin signaling within the ovary is not a necessary component of ovulation. Treatment of obese (*ob*) mice with leptin restores fertility.[580,581] Leptin administration accelerates the onset of puberty (vaginal opening) in normal mice.[582] Incubation of rodent pituitary gonadotrophs with leptin increases the rate of gonadotropin release.[583] In *ob/ob* females, leptin is not required for maintenance of pregnancy, although leptin is required for normal parturition.[581]

The hypercorticosteronemia of obese rodents contributes very importantly to the obese phenotype.[585,586] Adrenalectomy diminishes the excess weight gain of obese rodents (*ob, db*, and *fa*),[587,588] while delivery of corticosterone into the hypothalamus of adrenalectomized obese rodents restores the obese phenotype.[589–591] These effects of adrenal steroids may be mediated in the brain and elsewhere by both the glucacorticoid receptor (GR) and mineralocorticoid receptor (MR). Hypercorticosteronemia, not seen in humans with mutations in *ob* and *db* orthologs (see "Molecular Genetics of Human Obesity" below), may explain the stunting that characterizes the rodent phenotype, but which is absent in humans.

The impaired glucose tolerance of obese rodents is partly due to insulin resistance. Centrally administered leptin has effects on glucose control and insulin sensitivity at low doses that have no effect on feeding,[229] suggesting that leptin may directly affect glucose homeostasis by central nervous system mechanisms rather than conveying its primary effect via causing decreased fat mass. Leptin may also exert some of its effects on insulin secretion by causing hyperpolarization of endocrine pancreas beta cells and inhibiting insulin release.[592–595] This hyperpolarization and inhibition of insulin release can be alleviated by agonists of the sulfonylurea receptor (SUR) such as tolbutamide. A lack of leptin may disinhibit insulin release by both central nervous system and direct beta cell effects, leading to hyperinsulinemia and secondary insulin resistance.[596] The metabolic consequences of insulin resistance are dependent on genes that modulate the response of the pancreatic beta cell to an increased demand for insulin release.[597] In some strains of rodents, such as C57BL/6J and 129/J, this increased demand is met by beta cell hypertrophy/proliferation and a subsequent increase of insulin secretory capacity that meets metabolic demands. These obese rodents have nearly normal glucose control at the expense of hyperinsulinemia. In most rodent strains (e.g., C57BLKS/J, DBA), this increased demand is initially met by beta cell proliferation that is closely followed by beta cell death, resulting in severe hyperglycemia and insulinopenia.[530,598–600] In a third type of response, the beta cell proliferation does not generate a sufficient mass of insulin secreting cells. These rodents (e.g., Wistar-Kyoto rats) display hyperglycemia despite hyperinsulinemia because they are also extremely insulin resistant.[537] The loss of beta cells is probably due to the toxic effects of hyperglycemia because overexpression of the human insulin-regulated glucose transporter (GLUT-4) in the WAT of *db/db* C57BLKS/J mice (obese mice of a diabetogenic strain) significantly improves the diabetes phenotype and increases longevity.[601] These mice are nearly normoglycemic due to the shunting (partitioning) of glucose into WAT by the GLUT4 transgene. The differential response of rodent strains to the diabetogenic stress of obesity has been used to map genetic regions of diabetes susceptibility.[602,1030]

Carboxypeptidase E and the Fat Mutation

The recessive *fat* mutation arose on the HRS/J strain and was subsequently transferred to the C57BLKs/J background.[603] The mutant mice were characterized by late onset obesity and normal glucose control. The lack of diabetes in obese C57BLKs/J mice was surprising, considering the severe insulinopenia that develops in C57BLKs/J mice that are leptin or leptin-receptor deficient.

Mice that are homozygous for the Cpe^{fat} mutation develop obesity between 6 and 8 weeks. The mutants attain body weights at approximately 4–5 months of age that are two to three times greater than normal littermates by mechanisms that are not clear. We have observed hyperphagia in these animals (S. Chua, unpublished observations), while others (J. Naggert, unpublished observations) have not. The animals have no apparent defect in thermoregulation (R.L. Leibel, unpublished data). There are no specific reports regarding caloric partitioning in Cpe^{fat} mutants but their hypercorticosteronemia may favor preferential fat deposition.

Investigations regarding the lack of diabetes in these animals showed that the *fat/fat* mice had circulating hyperproinsulinemia, suggesting a defect in the processing of proinsulin. Genetic mapping of the *fat* locus indicated the close proximity of the mutation to the gene for a prohormone processing enzyme, Carboxypeptidase E. Sequence analysis of the *Cpe* cDNA from *fat/fat* mice indicated the presence of a missense mutation that produces a Ser202Pro substitution.[604] This mutation totally abolishes carboxypeptidase activity[605] as well as the capacity of the protein to sort prohormones into the regulated secretory pathway.[606] Thus, the cause of the obesity in CPE-deficient mice may be due either to the lack of processing of some prohormones/neuropeptides, such as those described earlier in "Neuroanatomy and Neurochemistry of Energy Homeostasis," or the constitutive secretion of these improperly processed peptides.

The Tubby Mutation

Tubby is a recessive mutation that occurred in the C57BL/6J strain.[603] Homozygous affected mice have late onset mild obesity as well as progressive deafness and blindness.[607,608] The *tubby* mutation abolishes a splice-donor site: the mutant transcript bears an intron and lacks the 3′ terminal exon.[609,610] The normal *tubby* transcript has some homology to phosphodiesterase and is neuron-specific, expressed prominently in the hypothalamus, cortex, and hippocampus, as well as in the spiral ganglion of the inner ear and the photoreceptors of the retina.[611] The gene is highly conserved in both plants and animals.

The *tub/tub* mice are not hyperphagic (J. Naggert, personal communication) and there have been no reported studies regarding thermogenesis or caloric partitioning in *tubby* mice. Unlike the *fat* mice, *tub* are not hypercorticosteronemic, but do develop increasing glucose intolerance with age.

Two related genes, TULP1 and TULP2, have been found in the human genome[612] and mutations in TULP1 have been associated with autosomal recessive retinitis pigmentosa in nonobese subjects.[613] The effect of *tub* and *tub*-related mutations on neuronal cell survival in the retina and cochlea suggest that the mutation might affect energy balance by reducing neuronal cell mass in specific regions of the hypothalamus (and elsewhere in the brain). Such a process would recapitulate the effect of mechanical or chemical injury of the VMH.

LEPTIN AND LEPTIN RECEPTOR PHYSIOLOGY

Leptin is expressed primarily in WAT, but it is also found in placenta, stomach, and BAT. Plasma concentrations of leptin are proportional to fat mass, but premenopausal females have circulating concentrations of leptin two- to threefold higher per unit fat mass than males[614] (see below).

Circulating Leptin

Leptin circulates as a higher molecular weight protein complex. In lean individuals, 80 percent of circulating leptin is bound to a carrier protein, whereas in obese individuals, most of the leptin (~80 percent) circulates in the unbound state.[615] The leptin-binding protein is most likely a soluble form of the leptin receptor.[616] Leptin is a cytokine-like molecule and its receptor is structurally in the cytokine receptor superfamily. For the latter, a soluble isoform of the receptor commonly serves as a binding protein for the circulating peptide (cf., growth hormone). The "Re" isoform (soluble receptor) of the leptin receptor is encoded by a leptin-receptor transcript ending in an alternatively spliced 3′ terminal exon. This transcript does not include exons encoding the transmembrane and intracytoplasmic domains. In humans, this 3′ terminal exon is nonfunctional as it has lost its polyadenylation signal, and no Re transcripts are found in human tissues. Therefore, the human soluble receptor in blood is derived from proteolytic cleavage of membrane bound receptors.[507]

In humans, leptin is released from adipose tissue in a pulsatile fashion. The pattern of leptin release in humans shows both diurnal and ultradian frequencies. Plasma leptin concentrations in humans peak at night (range approximately from 10:00 PM to 3:00 AM) and reach their nadir in the morning or afternoon (range approximately from 8:00 AM to 4:00 PM). Ultradian pulse frequencies have been reported in ranges from 3 to 21 pulses per day.[617–620] Pulse frequency is negatively correlated with fat mass and circulating concentrations of insulin.[620] Relative pulse amplitude (expressed as a percentage of baseline) is greater in females than males, and is negatively correlated with age and circulating concentrations of ACTH and cortisol.[617,620] No systematic alterations in pulse frequency or height have been noted in the obese. There is evidence for meal-related entrainment of leptin secretion.[621]

Clearance of leptin from the circulation is primarily (80 percent) by the kidneys; chronic renal failure results in elevated circulating leptin concentrations.[622–624] The remaining clearance is achieved by the liver.

Nutritional and Endocrine Effects on Leptin Synthesis

Leptin synthesis in adipose tissue is modulated by nutritional and hormonal status.[625,626] Fasting causes a rapid decline in circulating concentrations due to diminished gene transcription. Overfeeding increases circulating leptin.[627] Insulin,[614,628–633] and glucocorticoids[634–638] increase leptin gene transcription independently,[639,640] probably via stimulation of regulatory elements in the leptin gene promoter. The decrease in circulating leptin associated with fasting can be prevented by a continuous infusion of glucose, suggesting that either glucose and/or insulin modulates leptin concentrations. While acute manipulations of insulin concentrations do not affect circulating leptin concentrations, manipulations of insulin over several days-to-weeks produce alterations in leptin concentrations independent of changes of fat mass.[628,629] Insulinopenia in individuals with IDDM prior to insulin treatment, and in rats rendered diabetic with streptozotocin, results in circulating leptin concentrations that are lower than predicted for fat mass. Chronic insulin treatment in the insulinopenic state normalizes plasma leptin concentration, and patients with high insulin concentrations due to insulinomas have elevated leptin concentrations that are normalized after surgical resection of the tumor.[629]

Glucocorticoids[634,635] stimulate secretion of leptin, independent of their increase in leptin gene transcription.[641,642] Treatment of human adipocytes with dexamethasone in vitro stimulates leptin secretion from a presynthesized pool, and dexamethasone treatment in vivo stimulates leptin secretion. The high leptin concentrations observed in patients with Cushing's syndrome are consistent with the stimulatory effect of glucocorticoids on leptin release.[643,644] It is interesting to note, in this context, that glucocorticoids produce hyperphagia *despite* this effect on leptin production. Glucocorticoids inhibit the central actions of leptin, and this phenomenon might account for the ability of glucocorticoids to stimulate food intake in the context of higher leptin concentrations.[645]

There is a clear sexual dimorphism in circulating leptin concentrations such that leptin, normalized to fat mass, is two to three times higher in postpubertal females than males.[493,646] This difference is not due primarily to differences in circulating estrogens, as the difference persists in postmenopausal women.[493] In rats, LEP expression is higher in the adipose tissue of females than males.[647] Leptin clearance rates do not differ significantly between males and females.[648] Subcutaneous adipose tissue exhibits higher rates of LEP mRNA expression and leptin protein production than intra-abdominal depots,[649–651] and there is a higher subcutaneous to visceral adipose mass ratio in women.[649–653] Some investigators have suggested that the sexual dimorphism in adipose tissue distribution (visceral vs. subcutaneous depots) is sufficient to account for the sexual dimorphism in circulating concentrations of leptin.[653] However, because visceral adipose tissue typically accounts for <10 percent of total adipose tissue mass,[654] even if females had no visceral adipose tissue (thereby increasing their absolute amount of subcutaneous adipose tissue by as much as 10 percent relative to a fat mass-matched male), such a small increase in the relative amount of subcutaneous fat would not be sufficient to account for the two- to threefold higher circulating leptin concentrations in females. Other studies have reported a significant gender effect on circulating leptin concentration, even when these concentrations are adjusted for the distribution (visceral vs. subcutaneous) of body fat.[654] Leptin concentrations rise during early male puberty, but then fall later in puberty, suggesting that androgens may inhibit leptin production.[655,656,1033] In contrast, leptin concentrations continue to rise throughout puberty in females.[655] Gonadal steroids clearly affect circulating leptin concentrations.[657–662] Hypogonadal men have significantly elevated circulating leptin concentrations compared to eugonadal men, and this elevation is reversed by administration of testosterone.[663] Administration of estrogen increases circulating concentrations of leptin in humans and rodents.[664]

The free fraction of leptin increases to a similar extent during puberty in both sexes[1032] despite a developing sexual dimorphism (females > males) in total circulating concentrations of leptin.[1033] It is not clear whether the relative increase in free leptin as puberty advances is hormonally mediated, is due to an absolute decrease in the production of leptin binding proteins, or simply reflects increased adipose tissue mass resulting in increased leptin production.[1032,1034]

Pregnancy and Neonatal Period

Serum leptin concentrations in umbilical cord blood are approximately two times higher in human female neonates, even though no significant differences are noted in circulating leptin concentrations of mothers of males versus females in the same study.[665] This neonatal dimorphism may be due to the near pubertal levels of circulating androgens that are present in the male fetus and neonate, compared to much lower androgen levels in females.[666,667]

As testosterone establishes a sexual dimorphic pattern of growth hormone secretion from the pituitaries of rats, and perhaps humans, it is possible that the sexual dimorphism in circulating leptin concentrations of humans and rodents might be partially mediated by the ability of testosterone to establish sexually dimorphic patterns of leptin secretion in adipocytes.

Hyperleptinemia occurs during pregnancy in humans and rodents. In humans, placental leptin synthesis is driven by a placenta-specific element of the leptin gene.[668] During gestation in mice, circulating leptin can increase to more than tenfold due to placental production of a soluble leptin receptor.[669] In humans and rats, there is usually a twofold increase in circulating leptin during gestation.[670–672] Leptin does not cross the placenta, as there is no correlation between leptin concentrations of maternal and cord blood.[671,673] Leptin in cord blood does correlate with adiposity indices of neonates.

Cytokine-Mediated Effects

Circulating leptin concentrations are also influenced by the inflammatory cytokines, interleukin 1 (IL-1) and tumor necrosis factor (TNF).[674–677] The inflammatory response induced by injections of lipopolysaccharide from bacteria (LPS) stimulates leptin release and increases circulating leptin concentrations. This response is diminished in IL-1-deficient and TNF-deficient mice. While the anorexia associated with the inflammatory response might be related to hyperleptinemia, LPS induces anorexia in leptin-deficient and leptin receptor-deficient mice.[677] Thus, hyperleptinemia is not absolutely required for inflammation-induced anorexia.

Sympathetic Nervous System

Leptin appears to be produced in adipose tissue in a reciprocal relationship to sympathetic nervous system activity. Agents that increase adipocyte cAMP concentration, such as β_2- or β_3-adrenergic agonists or cAMP itself, depress leptin mRNA expression *in vitro* in rodents, and circulating concentrations of leptin *in vivo* in humans.[678–680] Though the major catecholamine neurotransmitter in sympathetic nervous system nerve endings is norepinephrine, a mixed α- and β- adrenergic agonist, it is clear that the β- adrenergic agonist effect predominates in humans as evidenced by the lipolytic effects of exogenous norepinephrine administration.[1000] Administration of exogenous leptin intravenously or intracerebroventricularly increases sympathetic nervous system output and the expression of UCP1, and hence thermogenesis, in BAT in rodents.[681–684] This reciprocal relationship is consistent with the observation that when adipose tissue mass, and hence circulating concentrations of leptin, is increased, there is a corresponding increase in sympathetic nervous system output and energy expenditure. The reciprocal response occurs in circumstances when leptin concentrations are lowered.[127,614,680]

Central Nervous System Access of Leptin

The access of leptin to brain parenchyma (e.g., the neurons of the hypothalamus) and the CSF probably depends primarily on transport by the so-called "Ra" isoform of the leptin receptor on endothelial cells of the brain[513] and epithelial cells of the choroid plexus.[494] The indirect relationship between brain parenchymal and CSF concentrations of molecules, and the several sources (blood and/or brain) by which molecules may gain access to the CSF, should temper tendencies to consider CSF concentrations a direct window on neuronal levels or activities. It is unlikely that the central nervous system effects of leptin require access to the CSF-per se. Leptin is detectable in the CSF of Zucker ($Lepr^{fa}$) and Koletsky ($Lepr^{fak}$) rats, both of which have mutations in the leptin receptor that either impair or eliminate the Ra isoform of LEPR.[137,542] These findings suggest that leptin can gain access to CSF (and possibly the brain interstitium) via non LEPR-dependent mechanisms. The absence of a blood-brain barrier around the median eminence and the circumvallate/circumventricular organs may provide such a pathway.[685–688] If such CSF diffusion occurs, it must be highly saturable because, in nonobese humans, the ratio of CSF to plasma concentration of leptin is approximately five times that ratio in obese individuals; whereas obese individual have absolute CSF leptin concentrations that are only about 30 percent greater than in nonobese humans.[689] If leptin were freely diffusable into the CSF, then the CSF to plasma leptin ratios should not be curvilinear. It appears that in humans, saturation of the CSF transport system occurs at a plasma leptin concentration of approximately 25 ng/ml, well below the plasma concentration of leptin in most obese individuals.[513,689] The resulting curvilinear relationship between plasma and cerebrospinal fluid leptin concentrations has been proposed as the mechanism for the hypothesized, but so far not directly demonstrated, "leptin resistance" of the obese.

The hyperphagia, hypometabolism, decreased thermogenesis, and hypothyroidism of the leptin-deficient or leptin-resistant rodents mimic the metabolic adaptations of humans to hypocaloric intake.[19,690] Leptin administration reduces food intake and increases energy expenditure per unit of fat-free mass, and time spent in physical activity, resulting in a selective reduction of body fat (i.e., disfavoring partitioning of stored calories to fat) in leptin-deficient (Lep^{ob}) mice when administered systemically or intracerebroventricularly.[496,498,499] Similar effects are seen in nonobese animals when leptin is administered intraperitoneally at high doses (10 to 20 times physiological circulating concentrations).[691,692] Intraperitoneal administration of leptin to mice during starvation rectifies many of the neuroendocrine changes (e.g., suppression of thyroid and gonadal axes, increase in adrenal axis activity) that occur as a result of food deprivation, but does not significantly alter the rate of weight loss.[690,693]

Leptin-Mediated Metabolic Effects

The metabolic and behavioral effects of leptin are most readily observed by replacement of the hormone in leptin-deficient obese mutants. The mutants decrease their food intake (resulting in decreased body weight associated with selective loss of adipose tissue), increase their metabolic rate, and increase their body temperature.[496,498,499,695] Similar changes are observed in lean mice treated with leptin, although the magnitude of the alterations are smaller than in obese mutants. Delivery of leptin into the cerebral ventricles in doses that do not alter circulating concentrations of endogenous leptin produces similar alterations in energy metabolism and behavior,[496] suggesting that nearly all of the metabolic/behavioral disturbances in obese mice are due to lack of leptin action within the central nervous system. However, the leptin receptor has a wide distribution in peripheral tissues,[696] and direct effects on peripheral tissues, such as adipose tissue,[576,697] the endocrine pancreas,[698–701] liver,[702] vascular endothelium,[108] and peripheral leukocytes,[703] may have biologic significance. These findings may be experimentally tested with tissue-specific knockouts of the leptin receptor as well as tissue-specific expression of specific leptin receptor isoforms in LEPR-deficient animals.

Leptin inhibits insulin secretion, probably by a direct effect on beta cells as well as by an indirect neural effect via the autonomic nervous system.[704] Insulin secretion is suppressed by leptin in the perfused pancreas, isolated islets, and insulinoma cell lines.[698,699,705–707] Leptin activates ATP-sensitive potassium channels[595] and hyperpolarizes the beta cell, effectively suppressing insulin release. Tolbutamide, a sulfonylurea inhibitor of ATP-sensitive K^+ channels, relieves the hyperpolarization and leptin-induced suppression of insulin secretion. The absence of this inhibitory action of leptin on insulin secretion may contribute to the progressive hyperinsulinemia of *ob* and *db* mice.

Leptin may modulate the actions of insulin on insulin-sensitive tissues — liver, skeletal muscle, and adipose tissue. The action of insulin on primary hepatocytes and liver-derived cell lines is attenuated by leptin as measured by tyrosine phosphorylation of IRS-1 and down-regulation of gluconeogenesis.[708] However, this finding is in contrast to the observation of enhanced insulin action in rats chronically treated with leptin.[709–713] In white adipose tissue, systemic leptin administration induces lipolysis, and leptin inhibits insulin's lipogenic activity in isolated adipocytes.[697,714] However, there are also reports of a lack of effect of leptin on insulin action in adipose tissue and skeletal muscle.[715,716] Leptin inhibits glycogen synthesis[717] and increases fatty acid oxidation[571] in isolated skeletal muscle. In myotubes formed by C2C12 cells, leptin stimulates glucose transport and glycogen synthesis.[718] These experimental discrepancies may be due to differences in preparation of the animals prior to tissue isolation, as well as to intrinsic differences between cell lines, isolated tissues, and intact organisms.

Leptin may have effects on hematopoietic cells.[511] Leptin treatment of T lymphocytes enhances the response to allogeneic stimulation.[703] Phagocytosis and secretion of inflammatory cytokines by macrophages are stimulated by leptin treatment.[719] Exogenous leptin replacement reversed the immunosuppression induced by a 48-h fast in mice, measured by a delayed type hypersensitivity (DTH) response.[703] These effects of leptin in supporting aspects of the immune response may account, in part, for the immunosuppression that accompanies chronic malnutrition and resulting hypoleptinemia. Bone density of leptin-deficient mice is increased (as it is in *Mc4r* KO mice). ICV leptin causes bone loss in Lep^{ob} and wild-type mice.[1035] It is possible that allelic variation in genes in the leptin MC4R "axis" play a role in predisposition to osteoporosis in humans.

The dramatic effects of leptin administration into the brain at very low doses indicate that the major effects of leptin on energy balance and the endocrine systems are mediated by the central nervous system. Leptin, delivered into the brain or into the periphery, decreases food intake. The major weight-reducing effect of leptin is mediated by reduced food intake, commensurate with the observation that caloric restriction normalizes the body weight of leptin-deficient and leptin receptor-deficient animals. Experiments that address the contributions of central and peripheral effects of leptin on the partitioning defect in leptin- and leptin receptor-deficient animals, independent of leptin's effect on food intake, have not been reported. The extensive sympathetic innervation of WAT[720,721] suggests one mechanism by which central nervous system leptin could have effects on adipose tissue metabolism. It remains to be seen whether the central effects of leptin are the sole mediators of the partitioning defect observed in these animals, or if a lack of direct leptin signaling in adipocytes may be responsible for some part of the metabolic defect causing preferential fat deposition. Similarly, the relative contributions of central and peripheral actions of leptin on the endocrine pancreas and insulin secretion remain to be defined.

Modulation of Leptin Receptor Signaling

STAT-mediated signaling by LEPR is suppressed by SOCS3, a member of the group of Suppressors of Cytokine Signaling (SOCS) molecules. SOCS3 contains an SH2 domain that binds to and inhibits the kinase activity of the JAK activation loop of LEPR. Homozygous deletion of *Socs3* in mice results in fetal demise at ~14 days in association with high levels of erythropoesis.[1036] Peripheral administration of leptin to *ob* mice induces hypothalamic SOCS3 mRNA without affecting peripheral SOCS1 on SOCS2 mRNA.[520] *In vitro* analysis of Chinese Hamster Ovary (CHO) cells expressing the long isoform of LEPR show induction of SOCS-3 mRNA. While leptin pretreatment of CHO-LEPR cells did not affect apparent leptin receptor number (by ^{125}I-binding), the forced expression of SOCS-3 mRNA resulted in inhibition of leptin-induced phosphylation of JAK2 in those cells.[1038] Thus, it is plausible that SOCS3 plays a physiological role in the regulation of leptin signaling. Overactivity of SOCS3 could, in some instances, account for what is detected clinically and experimentally as apparent "leptin resistance".

Role(s) of Leptin in Humans

If obesity in humans were the result of hypoleptinemia, one might anticipate that circulating concentrations of leptin, relative to body fat mass, would be significantly lower in obese humans. However, concentrations of leptin are increased in the plasma of obese humans[493] and rodents[722] (other than *Lep*^{ob}), and this increase is proportional to body fat mass. Within a given fat depot, leptin mRNA expression appears to be proportional to adipocyte volume,[107] and there is no evidence of a primary difference between obese and never-obese individuals in rates of leptin production per unit of fat mass, or of leptin clearance from the circulation.[723] Individuals with hypothalamic obesity secondary to surgical removal of a craniopharyngioma or other central nervous system lesion, do not display an altered relationship between circulating concentrations of leptin and adipose tissue mass when compared to control subjects or to their own preoperative values.[724,725] To the extent that such surgical injury represents a model of the functional consequences of hypothalamic insensitivity to leptin, the compensation for such central "resistance" is by increase in fat mass, not increase in leptin production per unit of fat mass.

Studies relating circulating leptin concentrations to energy expenditure in humans have given equivocal results. Some studies find a significant positive correlation of circulating leptin concentrations with resting energy expenditure or 24-h energy expenditure,[726–728] while others have reported either no correlation[614,662] or a significant negative correlation between circulating leptin and energy expenditure.[729] Some of the discrepancies among these studies are the result of the extreme colinearity of leptin and fat mass ($r^2 > 0.90$ in males and females).[493] In a study in which stepwise multiple regression analysis was used to examine the relationship between leptin and energy expenditure in lean and obese subjects studied at usual body weight, 10 percent above usual body weight and 10 percent below usual body weight, no significant relationship was found between circulating leptin concentrations and 24-h energy expenditure or resting energy expenditure at any weight plateau in lean or obese subjects.[614] In this study, the relationship between fat mass and circulating leptin concentration was generally maintained in weight-stable subjects at, above, and below usual body weight.

The process of weight loss (i.e. sustained negative energy balance) results in a significant decline in leptin concentrations normalized to fat mass in humans[614] and rodents.[730,731] The observation that plasma leptin concentrations are significantly decreased during dynamic weight loss compared to concentrations in the same subjects at the same weight during static weight maintenance, clearly indicates that plasma leptin concentration per unit of fat mass is influenced by intercurrent metabolic and endocrine factors. The process of weight gain due to hypercaloric intake does not produce significant increases in circulating leptin beyond that accounted for by increased fat mass.[614]

Exogenous administration of leptin accelerates sexual maturation in rodents,[580,582] and body fat stores (hence leptin) are related to age at menarche in humans.[732] A rise in serum leptin concentrations may provide a "trigger" for the onset of male puberty.[656] Leptin increases sexual behavior in fed, but not in food-deprived, female hamsters.[733] The observations that leptin administration accelerates pubescence and increases sexual behavior are consistent with a model whereby leptin signals the sufficiency of energy stores to the hypothalamic-pituitary gonadal axis to enhance reproductive activity/capacity during periods of nutritional abundance and to suppress reproduction during periods of nutritional deprivation.[1039,1040]

Stunting of somatic growth is part of the leptin-deficient or leptin-resistant phenotype in mice,[137] and insufficient ambient leptin may be one mechanism by which undernutrition is coupled to reduced statural growth in humans. Leptin concentrations in children are highly correlated with circulating concentrations of growth hormone binding protein, even when corrected for differences in body composition,[734] and administration of leptin to normal rats blunts the fasting-associated diminution in growth hormone release.[735] Leptin receptor gene expression is increased in anterior pituicytes of mice overexpressing a *Ghrhr* transgene.[736] The auxotrophic influence of obesity in children is consistent with a leptin-mediated effect, but the blunted pituitary response to various GH secretogogues suggests that insulin-mediated effects in IGFs may be the more proximate mechanism.[737] Fasting-associated increases in GH, despite low leptin concentrations, indicate that this chronic regulatory relationship can be interrupted by acute metabolic requirements.

Summary Model of Leptin Physiology

Based on available physiology and evolutionary arguments, it appears that leptin's primary role is to conserve a level of body fatness sufficient to insure reproductive function (including lactation) and somatic growth. The central nervous system (hypothalamic) threshold for relevant effects on food intake, energy expenditure, gonadotropin, and growth hormone releasing hormones is probably not the same for each physiological system, and these effects are clearly also influenced by developmental and other factors. For example, higher levels of energy intake per unit metabolic mass are required in growing organisms than in adults; gonadal axis maturation is facilitated by, but not solely dependent upon, body fat content.[1041] The threshold for each leptin-related effect is determined by the response cascade that begins with the leptin receptor and proceeds — by effects on gene expression, peptide phosphorylation, neuromediator release, and receptor activation — to generate the relevant metabolic/behavioral effect. Thus, the "impedance" to response for any physiological effect is determined by the net sensitivity of each response pathway to the signals generated by the LEP-LEPR interaction. In this sense, the obese may be viewed as "leptin resistant" insofar as the metabolic opposition to an altered body weight is invoked at a higher leptin concentration than in the never-obese individual. Those points are summarized in Fig. 157-6. The "threshold" for leptin-mediated effects in the central nervous system is the reflection of aggregate genetic and developmental influences on the cascade of responses triggered by leptin's binding to its central nervous system receptor (see Fig. 157-3). When body fat (hence leptin production) falls below a level required to generate a circulating concentration of leptin sufficient to exceed this threshold, a state of relative leptin-deficiency exists. This state results in the invoking of metabolic adjustments to caloric deprivation. Differences in threshold among individuals—and perhaps over time in the same individual—account for differences in "defended" fat mass.[127,1040]

MOLECULAR GENETICS OF HUMAN OBESITY*

Evidence for Genetic Role in Susceptibility to Obesity in Humans

Human body composition resolves the integrated effects of genetic, developmental, and environmental factors acting over periods of years. Relevant metabolic influences are the result of interactions of allelic variations of a substantial number of genes affecting functions including food intake, nutrient partitioning, and energy expenditure. The striking secular trend towards greater obesity in developed and developing countries[2] proves what is intuitively obvious, that there are also very potent environmental effects on the risk of obesity.

The phenotypic concordance between mono- and dizygous twins, children and their adoptive and biologic parents, and among members of families, indicates that obesity-related phenotypes, such as BMI, skinfold thickness, and body fat mass, are strongly heritable.[9,39,738] Between 30 and 80 percent of risk variance for obesity is heritable.[39] In several segregation analyses, as much as 40 percent of variation in both BMI[15,739] and fat mass[740,741] have been attributable to the apparent effects of single genes. Similar genetic impact on body fat distribution has been reported.[742,743] In addition, estimates of λ (proportional risk among relatives/population risk) show values ranging from 1.7 (parent-offspring) to 5.7 (MZ twins) for BMI above the 90th percentile for the population.[744] However, the importance of the environment in mediating genetic influence can be seen in the substantial phenotypic differences that can exist even between identical twins. For example, in a recent study, Finnish identical twins were found to have substantial differences in body weight (mean difference 14 kg) and glucose metabolism.[745] Another example of the powerful influence of environment is the very different phenotypes of Pima Indians sharing common ancestry but living in very different environments. Among the Pimans living in the Gila River valley near Phoenix, Arizona, and exposed to the full dietary repertoire and mechanical devices of U.S. culture, the prevalence of obesity (BMI $\geq$ 30) in individuals 35 to 44 years of age is 64 percent (males) and 75 percent (females). Approximately 50 percent of all Pimans in this environment who are over age 35 have type II diabetes.[746] The Pimans sharing the same gene pool (separated from the Arizona Pimans 700 to 1000 years ago) but living in the mountains of Northwest Mexico, have much lower rates of obesity and type 2 diabetes.[747] While some of the differences between members of these populations may be due to selection of "thrifty genes" in the Arizona Pimans by a restriction bottleneck imposed by a late nineteenth century drought and famine,[746] the major part of the phenotypic differences between these groups is probably environmental in origin.

The genes involved in the control of body composition are best regarded as having a substantial part of their impact through interaction with the environment. Phenotypes (P) such as body composition and body fat distribution should be thought of as resolvable into genetic (G), environmental (E) and gene × environment (G × E) effects: $P = G + E + (G \times E)$. Such G × E effects probably account for some of the discrepancies among studies of the same candidate gene in different populations. For example, for the W64R sequence variant in the β_3-adrenergic

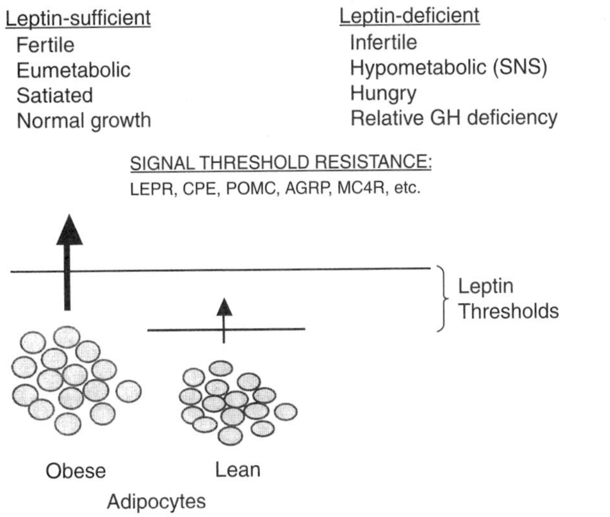

Fig. 157-6 This figure schematizes a hypothetical model of how an apparent "set point" for body fatness might work in response to leptin. Adipocytes from an obese (larger adipocytes) and a lean (same number of smaller adipocytes) individual are shown. The upward arrows are proportional to the concentration of leptin in the blood. Both individuals are producting sufficient leptin (by virtue of different masses of adipose tissue) to exceed their respective signal threshold resistance in the hypothalamus. These thresholds reflect genetic variation, developmental, and possibly environmental influences on the molecular components of the response cascade (LEPR, POMC, etc) that is triggered by leptin.

Leptin "sufficiency" is defined by the threshold (set point), not an absolute concentration of circulating leptin. With regard to energy homeostasis, this "set point" determines the concentration of leptin required to shut off physiological responses to a perceived state of insufficient fat stires. This is the "leptin-sufficient" state. Once this threshold is exceeded, the homeostatic adjustments to perceived insufficiency of fat stores (hunder, food seeking, reduced gonadal axis activity, redued somatic growth, low energy expenditure) cease. Moderate elevations of leptin above these threshold levels has minimal physiological effects, because the system is designed primarily to defend against requced fat stores, not to suppress body fat.

If either the obese or lean individual reduces caloric intake (acute) or fat mass (chronic) sufficiently to result in a lowering of circulating leptin below his/her threshold, the "leptin-deficient" state is achieved.

When an obese individual is therapeutically reduced to a lean body mass, circulating leptin concentration is reduced, and may be below the threshold described above. This reduced-obese individual, despite now having a more "normal" body fat content, will be in a state of relative leptin deficiency. The requced-obese individual would generate leptin proportional to his/her reduced (lean) fat mass, but this would not be sufficient to cross that individual's persisting higher (obese) threshold. Thus, this reduced-obese individual would display a leptin-deficient phenotype (hunger, low energy expenditure, reduced fertility).

Obese and lean individuals differ only in their respective thresholds for leptin effects. Their metabolic/behavioral responses to perceived leptin deficiency are identical. The obese "defend" higher levels of body fat because their thresholds for leptin effects are higher due to genetic and developmental processes affecting the genes and neural pathways that comprise the threshold.

*This is now an area of intense investigation. Any summary of relevant human and rodent studies will be rapidly outdated. Readers are advised to consult the web (http://www.obesity.chair.ulaval.ca/genes.html) and the annual summary of mapping and association studies (all species) published in the Journal of Obesity Research (e.g. reference 755).

receptor (ADRB),[748] in 28 studies of various obesity/diabetes-related phenotypes, there have been 7 positive association/linkages.[749] For the genetic region around the leptin gene, some populations have shown linkage for body composition-related phenotypes,[750,751] while others have not.[752]

Two full genome scans have been published in which the linkage of obesity-related phenotypes with specific genomic intervals were studied in humans. Additional scans are underway. The first was performed on the Pima Indians, described above, living near Phoenix, Arizona. Percent body fat measured by hydrodensitometry was adjusted for age and sex, and mapped as a qualitative trait locus (QTL) versus a 10 cM map in 238 sib pairs (88 nuclear families). Suggestive linkages (two point analysis, LOD = 2.0) were detected for 3p24.2-p22 and 11q21-q22.[753] In the second study, on Mexican Americans living in San Antonio, Texas, 10 families, 459 individuals, 5667 relative pairs were examined for genetic linkages to body composition. QTLs were detected on chromosome 2 (LOD 4.3) and chromosome 8 (LOD 2.2).[754] The chromosome 2 locus includes the *POMC* gene (see below). When these linkages in Pimans and Mexican Americans are subjected to multipoint and/or variance component analysis (for magnitude of gene locus effect on phenotype), LOD scores are generally increased, and these QTLs are found to account for 32 percent and 47 percent of variation in fat mass or serum leptin concentration, respectively.

A larger number of limited scans of human families (usually as sib pairs or other relatives examined for linkage in specific genomic regions) have been performed. The results of these limited analyses are summarized in Table 157-10 where linkages of obesity-related phenotypes to specific genomic intervals are indicated.

Candidate genes and/or genomic regions for human obesity can be derived from analyses of the genes that are known based on physiology (e.g., the potent orexigenic peptide NPY) or genetics (rodent single obesity genes and QTLs) to play a role in energy homeostasis in mammals. Some of these candidate genes and genomic regions (with human homologous regions based on synteny relationships between rodent and human genomes) are indicated in Table 157-11.

As indicated earlier in "Molecular Genetics of Energy Homeostasis," and as discussed below, human orthologs of all extant spontaneous rodent obesity mutations have been identified. Based on mutation analyses to date, however, the great majority of human obesity cannot be attributed to major mutations in these or other known genes.[755] An additional ~55 QTLs for various aspects of body composition have been reported in mice and rats (Table 157-12).[755–760] There is undoubtedly redundancy in this list, so that perhaps 25 unique QTLs are represented. The fact that the same apparent QTLs have been identified in more than one rodent interstrain/species intercross, further supports the likely

Table 157-10 Evidence for the Presence of Linkage with Human Obesity Phenotypes

Gene or marker	Chromosomal location	N-pairs	Phenotype	Inferential statistics	Reference
D1S202	1q31-32	large pedigree	BMI	$P = 4.7 \times 10^{-5}$	958
ACP1	2p25	>300	BMI	P = 0.004	959
GRL	5q31-q32	88	BMI > 27	P = 0.009	960
BF	6p21.3	>168	skinfolds	$0.01 < p < 0.03$	961
TNFA, Tnfir24, D6S273, D6S291	6p21.2	>255	% body fat	$0.002 < p < 0.048$	962
GLO1	6p21.2	>168	skinfolds, relative weight	$0.004 < p < 0.05$	961
SUR (D11S419)	11p15.1	67	BMI > 27	P = 0.0032	963
D1S200 + LEPR region	1p32-p32	137 sibships	BMI	P = 0.009	964
ADA to MC3R	20p12 to 20q13.3	258	% body fat; BMI, fasting insulin	$0.008 > p > 0.0005$	763
POMC (D2S1788)	2p21	Pedigrees	serum leptin	LOD = 4.95; $P \sim 1.8 \times 10^{-6}$	754, 1058
LEP region	7q31.3	>1,000	BMI	$P < 2 \times 10^{-5}$	965, 750
KEL	7q33	402	BMI, skinfolds	P < 0.001	966
ESD	13q14.1-q14.2	194	% body fat, skinfolds	P < 0.04	966
ADA (and ASIP)	20q12-q13.11	428	BMI, skinfolds	$0.02 < p < 0.001$	966
ADA, MC3R, D220S17, 120	20q12-q13	258	BMI, Σ 6 skinfolds, fat mass, % body fat	$0.004 < p < 0.02$	763
P1	22q11.2-qter	>168	Relative weight	P = 0.03	961
D3S2432	3p24.2-p22	874	% body fat	LOD = 2.0	753
ADRB3	8p12-p11.2				967
Glucocorticoid Receptor (GRL)	5q31				960
Na-K ATPase	q21-q23	582 individuals	RQ	P = 0.02	968
D11S2000,2366	11q21-q22	874	% body fat	LOD = 3.1	753
MC5R	18p11.2	242-289	BMI, Σ 6 skinfolds, fat mass, % body fat	$0.001 < p < 0.02$	964
D10S197	10p	158 nuclear families (514 individuals)	BMI	LOD=4.85	1058
CART	5q	158 nuclear families (514 individuals)	Plasma leptin	LOD≈3	1058
ASIP, CEBPB, GNAS1	20q13	Extended pedigrees+Sib pairs, 513 members in 92 nuclear familes	BMI, % body fat	LOD=3.06–3.17	1059

Table 157-11 Selected List of Candidate Genes for Regulation of Human Body Composition

		Chromosomal location (Chr = cM from centromere)		
Gene	Phenotype	Human	Mouse	Ref.
ASIP	obesity	20q11.2-q12	2-88.8	969
CPE	obesity	4q28	8-32	970
LEP	obesity	7q31.3	6-10.5	971
LEPR	obesity	1p31	4-46.7	494
TUB	obesity	11p15.4-p15.5	7-51.45	610
UCP1	energy balance	4q31	8-37	874
UCP2	energy balance	11q13	7-50	153
UCP3	energy balance	11q13	7-50	890
MC3R	feeding behavior	20q13	2-100	972
MC4R	feeding behavior	18q21.3-q22	1 or 18 (predicted)	334
POMC	obesity (serum leptin concentration)	2p23.2	12-4	832, 973
NPYR5	appetite regulation	4q31-q32	8-33	974
MSTN	skeletal muscle growth	2q32.1	1 or 2 (predicted)	444
CCKAR	satiety	4p15.1	5-34.0	975
TNFA	obesity	6p21.3	17-19.1	962
PPAR-γ	adipocyte differentiation	3p25	6-53.0	976
ADRB3	energy expenditure	8p11.1-p12	8-10	977
GAL	obesity, hypogonadism	11q13.3-13.5	19-2	978
GALR1	obesity, hypogonadism	18q23	18E4	979
MCH	obesity	12q23-q24	10-47	980
HCRT (Orexin)	obesity	17q21	11	278
NTS	obesity	12q21	—	981
NTSR1	obesity	20q12	2	982
AGRP	obesity	16q22	8	352
NPY	obesity	7p15.1	6-26	
SNRPN	obesity, hypogonadism (PWS)	15q12	7	983
PC1	Obesity	5q15-q21	2	803

relevance of such QTLs to control of body composition. None of the genes presumably underlying these QTLs has yet been cloned. However, some of these QTLs fall in regions of known single-gene obesities in rodents and/or humans (e.g., *Mob2* in the region of *Lep*^{ob}; *Mob1* in the vicinity of *tub; Pfat3* in the region of *Pc1;* and *Dob3* in Cohen syndrome region). In addition, some of the mouse QTLs are in regions corresponding to other genes that may play important roles in energy homeostasis. For example, *Mob1*[757] is in the vicinity of *Ucp2/Ucp3*,[153,761,762] and *Mob5* (mouse D2Mit50) is syntenic with a region of human chromosome 20q containing genes influencing body fat and insulin homeostasis.[763] These observations, and the finding of linkage of some of obesity-related phenotypes to regions of the genome containing important candidate genes (Table 157-10), raise the possibility that allelic variation in such major genes (either in coding sequence or regulatory elements) may account for some of the variation in the quantitative phenotypes related to body composition, including the tendency to deposit fat in specific anatomic depots. There is precedent for such phenotypic effects of allelic variation at major loci, seen, for example, in the influence on bristle number in *Drosophila melanogaster* of allelic variation at a relatively small number of genes that (by analysis of effects of major mutations) account for most of the interindividual variations in bristle number.[764,765]

Single Genes/Loci

Based on the physiological considerations and the linkage and mutation studies performed to date, it is extremely unlikely that most instances of human obesity will be shown to be due to alterations in a single gene. However, the instances of apparent single-gene/locus obesity in humans, provide both proof of the physiological significance of certain genes (e.g., leptin, leptin receptor, prohormone convertase pathway) and point to a role of yet unknown genes (e.g., Prader-Willi) or pathways (the series of mutations that result in the Bardet-Biedl syndrome) in the regulation of body weight. In this sense, the spontaneous mutations in humans provide insights similar to those that derive from animals with genetically engineered knockouts or overexpression of specific candidate genes (Table 157-13). These human genetic disorders with obesity phenotypes are enumerated in Table 157-13 and are discussed in more detail below.

Prader-Willi Syndrome (PWS; MIM 176270). PWS is an apparent contiguous gene syndrome in which the paternal copies of the imprinted contiguous genes are silenced due either to deletion or uniparental maternal disomy for the interval 15q11.2-q12.[766] Deletion of this interval in maternal chromosomes, or paternal uniparental disomy, results in Angelman syndrome due to effects on UBE3A (E6-AP) which functions in protein ubiquination.[767]

The phenotypes that comprise Angelman syndrome (AS; MIM 105830) (mental retardation, seizures, "happy face," and abnormal gait) are attributable to brain-specific effects. It is likely that the imprinting of UBE3A is tissue-specific. The phenotype of PWS is mainly (hypotonia; hyperphagia; mental retardation; hypogonadotropic hypogonadism; thick saliva; relative pain insensitivity; obsessive compulsive disorder; short stature) but not entirely (narrow frontal skull; almond shaped eyes; small hands and feet; cutaneous depigmentation) attributable to central nervous system effects of the gene or genes affected.[768] No morphologic abnormality of the hypothalamus was noted in a careful analysis of the brain of a single PWS patient.[769] In chimeric mouse embryos containing cells with duplicated paternal and maternal genomes, the paternal cells give rise to hypothalamic but not cortical brain structures, while maternal cells lead to cortical and striatal structures.[770]

Though familial occurrence of PWS has been described repeatedly, the majority of instances of PWS are sporadic. The

Table 157-12 Animal QTLs for Body Composition with Corresponding Human Chromosomes

Animal	Crosses	QTL	LOD score	Phenotype	Chromosome		Ref.
					Animal	Human	
Mouse	C57BJ/6J	Mob 1	4.2	6.5% fat	7	16p12-p11.2	757
	X	Mob 2	4.8	7.1% femoral fat	6	7q21.3-q31.3	
	M. spretus	Mob 3	4.8	7.0% fat	12	14q31-q32	
		Mob 4	3.4	5.9% mesenteric fat	15	5p13	
Mouse	NZB/B1NJ	Mob 5	3.6	36% body fat	2	20p11-q13	763
	X						
	SM/J						
Mouse	AKR/J	Dob 1	4.5	Adiposity	4	1p36.1-p35	758
	X					9p13	
	SWR/J	Dob 2	4.8	7% adiposity	9	3p21	759
		Dob 3	3.9	4% adiposity	15	8q23-q24	
Mouse	A/J X	Bw1	3.4	24% body weight	X	Xp11-q26	984
	M. spretus	Bw2	6.6	(3 QTL together)	X	Xp11-q13	
	X	Bw3	4.3		X	Xp22-q27	
	C57BL/6J						
Mouse	Du6	Qbwl	2.7	6.9% abdominal fat	3	1p22-p21	985
	X					4q23-q25	
	DU6k	Qbw2	7.6	17% body mass	11	17q12-q22	
Mouse	129/Sv	Obq1	8.0	12.3% adiposity	7	19q13.2-13.3	760
	X	Obq2	5.5	6.3% adiposity	1	1q21-q23	
	Le/Suz					2q35-q36.1	
Mouse	AKR/J	Obq3	5.1	7.0% adiposity	2	2q23-q31	986
	X					9q32-q34	
	C57BL/6J					11p12-p11	
						15q13-q14	
						20pter-p11	
						20q11	
		Obq4	4.6	6.1% adiposity	17	6q25-q27	
Mouse	M16I	Pfat1	NA	Adiposity	2	2p13-q21	987
	X					15q11-qter	
	CAST/Ei					20pter-p11	
		Pfat2	NA	Adiposity	2	20qcen-q11	
		Pfat3	NA	Adiposity	13	5q11-q14	
						5q33-qter	
						6p23	
						9q21-q22	
		Pfat4	NA	Adiposity	15	5p14-p12	
						8q22-q24	
		Pfat5	NA	Adiposity	15	8q21-qter	
						22q12-qter	
Mouse	C57BL/6J	Bw6a	3.3	3% 6 weeks' weight	1	1q31-q33	988
	X	Bw6b	3.3	4% 6 weeks' weight	4	9p23-p24	
	DBA/2J	Bw6c	3.2	4% 6 weeks' weight	5	4q12-q13	
		Bw6d	4.3	5% 6 weeks' weight	5	12q24	
		Bw6e	4.0	4% 6 weeks' weight	6	2p12	
		Bw6f	6.9	9% 6 weeks' weight	7	15q11-q13	
						19q13	
		Bw6g	4.4	5% 6 weeks' weight	9	6q12-q16	
		Bw6h	5.7	6% 6 weeks' weight	11	17pter-p13	
		Bw6i	4.1	4% 6 weeks' weight	13	15q23-q25	
		Bw6j	3.0	3% 6 weeks' weight	14	3p21	
						10q22-q24	
						13q14-q22	
						21pter-qter	
		Bw6k	4.9	7% 6 weeks' weight	17	6p21	
Mouse	LG/J	Q1w1	2.3	1.9% late weight gain	1	2q11-q12	989
	X					6p11-p12**	
	SM/J	Q1w2	2.9	2.6% late weight gain	2	20p11	
						20q11	
		Q1w3	2.3	8.4% late weight gain	3	3q25-q26	

Table 157-12 (*Continued*)

Animal	Crosses	QTL	LOD score	Phenotype	Chromosome: Animal	Chromosome: Human	Ref.
		Q1w4	2.4	2.4% late weight gain	4	6q16 8q11-q12	
		Q1w5	2.8	3.4% late weight gain	6	3p26-p24	
		Q1w7	2.0	2.0% late weight gain	7	15q26	
		Q1w9	2.5	2.4% late weight gain	9	11q21 19p13	
		Q1w11	2.6	2.4% late weight gain	11	22q12	
		Q1w12	2.3	2.4% late weight gain	12	2p23-p24**	
		Q1w13	2.4	4.4% late weight gain	13	1pter-q42	
		Q1w14	3.1	2.9% late weight gain	14	8p23 13p12	
		Q1w18	1.6	3.0% late weight gain	18	5q31-q33	
Rat	*Lepr^fa/Lepr^fa* 13M X WKY	Qfa1	2.3 2.5 2.2	5.4% weight (male) 5.8% BMI (male) 6.9% BMI (female)	1	16q13 16q11 11p15 11q13	602
		Qfa12	2.7 3.0	7.8% weight (female) 8.3% BMI (female)	12	7q22	
Rat	GK X BN	Nidd/gk1	NA	13% adiposity	1	3p21	990
		Nidd/gk5	NA	9% bodyweight	8	11q22-q23	
		Nidd/gk6	NA	7% bodyweight	17	1q41-q44	
		Bw/gk1	NA	24% bodyweight	7	8q21-q24 22q12-q13	
Rat	Gk X F	Niddm1	3.2	23.5% bodyweight	1	10q24-q26	991
		Niddm3	3.0	Bodyweight	10	17pter-q23	
		Weight1	6.2	Bodyweight	7	12q22-q23	
Pig	European wild boar X large white	Pig QTL	NA	18% fatness	4	1q21-q25	992

recurrence risk for sibs of affected individuals is about 1:1000 versus a population occurrence rate of about 1:25,000. Seventy to 80 percent of instances of PWS are due to interstitial chromosome deletions that are detectable in prometaphase chromosome preparations. A small number of cases are due to *de novo* balanced translocations, and the remainder to maternal uniparental disomy. Recurrence risk is near zero in siblings of individuals with *de novo* deletions. Based on grandparental haplotypes in the region of the deletions, unequal crossing over in paternal meiosis is the most likely mechanism for the deletion.[771] Formation and excision of an intrachromosomal loop as a somatic event is another possible mechanism. Differences in the methylation (imprinting) pattern of alleles in the PWS interval[772–774] can be used diagnostically in patients suspected of either PWS or AS.

Affection status of disomic PWS patients is approximately equivalent to that of individuals with chromosomal deletions, indicating that there is a limited, contiguous region of imprinting on chromosome 15. However, the frequency of hypopigmentation (presumably due to involvement of the human ortholog of the mouse pink-eyed dilution locus (p)[775] is greater in individuals with deletion (77 percent) than in those with uniparental disomy (UPD) (39 percent), and overall affection status is somewhat milder in females with UPD as compared to those with deletions.[776] Maternal age is increased in disomic patients (as expected for nondisjunction events).[777] The majority (>80 percent) of maternal nondisjunction events leading to uniparental disomy and causing PWS are the result of meiosis I error, whereas most paternal UPD causing AS is due to errors in meiosis II or mitosis.[778]

The molecular classes of PWS subjects breakdown as follows: 70 percent deletion; 25 percent UPD; <5 percent imprinting mutation; 0.1 percent balanced translocation.[766] Unlike AS, in which mutations in a specific gene, UBE3A, encoding ubiquitin-protein ligase E3A, has been shown to cause the phenotype, no single-gene mutation has yet been shown to cause PWS. This situation suggests that PWS requires the loss of expression of two or more paternally expressed genes, and that individuals with single-gene derangements would not have the full PWS phenotype. Such individuals might, however, be obese. Thus, elucidation of the genes involved in PWS will almost certainly generate additional candidate genes for nonsyndromic obesity in humans (see below). Five percent of individuals with PWS (and AS, also) are heterodimeric for chromosome 15, but have abnormal methylation patterns in the imprinted interval on chromosome 15, suggesting the presence of a mutation in the imprinting process per se. About half of the cases with apparent imprinting mutations have a microdeletion that includes exon 1 of *SNRPN*.[766] These microdeletions can be silently transmitted so long as the transmitting sex is female. When passed through a male parent, one half of his progeny will be functionally homozygous for the maternal epigenotype and have the PWS phenotype. The promoter region adjacent to exon 1 of *SNRPN* (deleted in PWS) has been suggested as the imprint switch element that mediates the control of epigenotype in the imprinted region. This inference is supported by the demonstration that a 215-bp portion of the human *SNRPN* promoter human region acts as an imprinting silencer in *Drosophila*.[779]

SNRPN encodes small ribonucleoprotein polypeptide N, a member of a group of peptides associated with small ribonucleoproteins found in spliceosomes. The gene is expressed primarily in the brain. *SNRPN* maps to the minimal deletion interval for PWS and encodes a protein with a possible role as a mediating alternative splicing of central nervous system mRNA transcripts in the central nervous system. Defects in such a protein could

Table 157-13 Human Obesity of Genetic Origin

Disorder	Locus	Gene	Inheritance	Phenotype
Prader-Willi syndrome (PWS)	15q11.2-q12	?SNRPN and other(s)	Uniparental maternal disomy	Intrauterine hypotonia. Floppy infant; early failure to thrive; hyperphagia and increased weight gain by 2–3 years. Hypothalamic hypogonadism. Mental retardation.
Alstrom syndrome	2p14-p13	?	AR	Retinitis pigmentosa, deafness, diabetes mellitus, cirrhosis.
Cohen syndrome (COH1)	8q22-q23	?	AR	Hypotonia, prominent incisors. Benign neutropenia.
Bardet-Biedl syndrome				
BBS1	11q13	?	AR	Mental retardation; pigmental retinopathy, polydactyly, short stature, hypogonadism, renal malformations.
BBS2	16q21	?	AR	Leanest of BBS; Bedouin kindred.
BBS3	3p13-p12	?	AR	Polydactyly of all 4 limbs. Bedouin kindred.
BBS4	15q22.3-q23	?	AR	European kindred; Bedouin kindred Hand-polydactyly, Earliest onset, most obese
BBS6	20p12	MKKS	AR	Mental retardation; pigmentary retinopathy, polydactyly, short stature, hypogonadism, renal malformations
Biemond syndrome II	?	?	—	Iris colomba, hypogonadism, polydactyly, mental retardation
Impaired processing of prohormones	5q15-q21	PC 1	AR	Hyperproinsulinemia, early onset obesity; secondary sexual development with 1° amenorrhea, hypocortisolemia
Choroideremia with deafness	Xq21.2-q21.2	DFN3	XL	Chroroideremia, congenital deafness
Leptin deficiency	7q31.3	LEP	AR	Severe, early onset obesity. Hypothalamic hypogonadism
Leptin Receptor Deficiency	1p31-p22	LEPR	AR	Severe, early onset obesity. Hypothalamic hypogonadism
POMC Deficiency	2p23.2	POMC	AR	Early onset severe obesity. Adrenal insufficiency. Red hair
PPARγ_2Activation	3p25	PPAR-gamma 2	AD	Severe obesity, some with type 2 diabetes
MC4R haploinsufficiency	18q21.3-q22	MC4R	AD	Early onset, moderate-severe obesity

account for many aspects of the complex phenotype of the PWS individuals. Only the paternal allele of *SNRPN* is expressed in the human brain.[780] However, in a PWS patient with a balanced 9:15 translocation of the paternal chromosome, the breakpoint was mapped to the region between *SNRPN* and *PAR1* and in this individual expression of *SNRPN* was unaffected, while the adjacent genes *PAR1* and *IPW* were not expressed.[781] This patient was moderately obese and hypopigmented, had characteristic facies and delayed development of puberty, and met formal criteria for the diagnosis of PWS.[782] However, he was reported not to be hyperphagic. These data suggest that *SNRPN* may play a role in regulating food intake, but not in other somatic and endocrine phenotypes associated with PWS.

Because it is unlikely that PWS occurs as a result of dysfunction of a single gene, animal models may be needed to identify the role of specific genes in the minimal genetic interval. The homologous region on mouse mid chromosome 7 is imprinted, and mice with UPD for this interval have been bred. Maternal UPD for this interval produces an animal with phenotype suggestive of PWS. The animals die before weaning, possibly due to poor suckling and hypotonia that recapitulates the human neonate's phenotype.[783]

Bardet-Biedl Syndrome (BBS; MIM 209900, 209901, 600374, 603650, 600151). BBS is a genetically heterogeneous autosomal recessive disorder characterized by obesity, hypogonadism (apparently at the level of both hypothalamus and the gonads), mental retardation, postaxial polydactyly, renal structural abnormalities (especially cystic dysplasia), and pigmentary retinopathy. These patients may also have an increased incidence of cardiac abnormalities.[784,785] The incidence of hepatic fibrosis and diabetes mellitus is also increased in BBS patients.[786] Mutations in at least four different genes can produce the BBS phenotype. The genes (BBS1 to BBS4) have been mapped to four separate chromosomes (Table 157-13). In no instance is the responsible gene known, but clearly, these genes are likely to be components of a pathway affecting several aspects of organ development and function. Other members of this family of genes may be responsible for the phenotypically closely related Alstrom (and possibly Cohen) syndromes (see below).

Specific chromosomal regions (with preserved interval haplotypes) are implicated in different ethnic groups. BBS1 and BBS4 predominate in European populations, and BBS2 and BBS3 are more common in the Arab-Bedouin kindreds. Some of the phenotypic distinctions among the different mutations are also summarized in Table 157-13. It is important to note that all patients do not have all phenotypic features. For example, while obesity, renal abnormalities, and retinal dystrophy are virtually universal, polydactyly and mental retardation may be present in only one-third to one-half of patients.

In a recent paper, a new BBS locus (BBS6) was mapped and the responsible mutation identified as homozygosity for null alleles of MKKS.[1060,1061]

Alstrom Syndrome (MIM 203800). Alstrom syndrome is an autosomal recessive disorder that resembles BBS (obesity, retinitis pigmentosa, neurosensory hearing loss, and diabetes mellitus), but does not include mental retardation, limb disorders, or hypogonadism.[787] The characteristic phenotype includes severe insulin resistance (sometimes with acanthosis nigricans), and frequent liver disease (chronic active hepatitis).[788] Cardiomyopathy and scoliosis have been reported in some Alstrom patients. Gonadal failure[789] and diabetes insipidus[790] in some patients have suggested that resistance to peptide hormones in addition to insulin may be part of this syndrome. Using homozygosity mapping in a French Canadian kindred, the syndrome was mapped near D2S292 on chromosome 2p14-p13.[791] The close phenotypic similarity of this syndrome to BBS suggests that the responsible gene(s) may also be part of the pathway that is apparently affected in BBS.

Cohen Syndrome (COH1; MIM 216550). Cohen syndrome is an apparently autosomal recessive disorder characterized by obesity; prominent central incisors; hypotonia; moderate mental retardation; slender, elongated fingers and toes; chorioretinal dystrophy; and intermittent, benign neutropenia.[792,793] The disorder is more frequent in Ashkenazi Jews and Finns. In Finns, the syndrome has been mapped to a 10 cM interval on chromosome 8q22.[794] Linkage disequilibrium studies in this population suggest that COH1 gene is near D8S1762.[795]

Prohormone Convertase (PC1) Deficiency (MIM 162150). PC1 is a member of a family of endopeptidases located in acidic secretory vesicles that cleave between pairs of basic amino acids, particularly in prohormones and proneuropeptides.[796] The

C-terminal basic residues remaining after PC1 action are cleaved by carboxypeptidases (e.g., carboxypeptidase E = CPE). CPE is highly expressed in neuroendocrine cells and appears, in addition to its enzymatic role, to act as a membrane-bound sorting receptor for the routing of prohormones in a regulated secretory pathway.[606,797] In the fat (*Cpe^fat^*) mouse, the CPE deficiency results in misprocessing of proinsulin, POMC, GH, CCK, neurotensin, MCH and gastrin.[797–801] Which, if any, of these abnormalities is responsible for the phenotype of the Cpe^{fat} animal is not known. (see section on Mutations Affecting Multiple Components of Energy Balance)

O'Rahilly and his collaborators described a 45-year-old woman with early onset extreme obesity (weight 36 kg at 3 years). She weighed 89.2 kg at 45 years and displayed extremely elevated plasma concentrations of proinsulin but nearly undetectable circulating insulin.[802] She also had hypogonadotropic hypogonadism, hypocortisolism, and elevated circulating POMC. She was subsequently found to be compound heterozygous for mutations in *PC1*: G483R (preventing the processing of proPC1) and A → C^{+4} transversion of the intron 5 donor splice site causing skipping of exon 5 with resultant loss of 26 amino acids, a frameshift and a premature stop in the catalytic domain.[803] PC1 acts just proximal to CPE in the posttranslational processing of prohormones and proneuropeptides described above. The phenotype of this patient confirms the relevance of the pathway deranged in the Cpe^{fat} mouse for human body weight regulation, and anticipates what will certainly be the description of other causal mutations in this pathway in obese humans. However, it is not clear what are the proximate mechanisms by which such mutations lead to obesity, because there is no *a priori* reason to suppose that their effects would be greater on neuropeptides mediating satiety than hunger. The phenotype of the two individuals with POMC mutations described below, however, certainly suggest that disordered processing of POMC and resultant deficiency of αMSH (a suppressor of food intake), probably by effects at the melanocortin 4 receptor (MC4R), might account for some aspects of the phenotype of PC1-deficient individuals. Further characterization of the molecular phenotype of the Cpe^{fat} mouse should help to answer these questions.

Leptin Deficiency (*LEP*; MIM 164160). Montague et al. described the first instances of homozygosity for a mutation that affects leptin bioactivity.[804] Earlier linkage studies had suggested that the region of the leptin gene on human chromosome 7q31.3[805] was linked to measures of body fatness in humans.[750,751] Two children from a highly consanguineous Pakistani family were ascertained on the basis of extreme obesity (female age 8 years; height 137 cm (75th percentile for age); weight 86 kg (40 kg = 98th percentile for age); BMI = 45.8) (male age 2 years; height 89 cm (75th percentile for age); weight 29 kg (15 kg = 98th percentile for age); BMI = 36.6) and found to be homozygous for a frameshift in LEP cDNA due to deletion of a single guanine nucleotide in codon 133 (G_{398}), resulting in the introduction of a new sequence of 14 amino acids after codon 132, followed by a premature stop codon. Transient transfection of CHO cells with the mutant construct led to no detectable secretion of the mutant protein. However, the protein was detected in the lysate of the transfected CHO cells, suggesting that this mutation results in an isoform of leptin that does not traffic normally within the cell. The plasma of both affected children had leptin concentrations at the limits of detection of the assay (1.0 and 0.7 ng per ml, respectively). Given the very high fat mass of both children, these low levels are even more strikingly discordant. No immunoreactive leptin was detectable by western blot analysis of the younger child's plasma, and no immunoreactive material of lower molecular weight was seen in either patient.

The cousins were described as normal in size and adiposity at birth, but both had onset of severe hyperphagia and obesity in the first several months of life. Aside from extreme obesity, both were otherwise nondysmorphic. The endocrine studies obtained are summarized in Table 157-14. Most striking in these studies is the lack of elevated plasma glucocorticoids that are a hallmark of *ob* and *db* mice, and the absence of severe hyperinsulinemia. The lack of statural stunting and the milder hyperinsulinemia may reflect the absence of hypercortisolism in the children. Adrenalectomy in *ob* or *db* mice greatly ameliorates the metabolic and behavioral phenotype of the animals.[563] The reason for this important physiological difference between mouse and human is not known, but probably reflects differences in the regulation of CRH expression by leptin in the two species. The low concentrations of gonadotropins are expected given the hypothalamic hypogonadism of the *ob* and *db* mice. Neither child had any evidence of puberty, but this finding could be attributed to their young age. Hypothalamic hypogonadism was confirmed in subsequent families with mutations of leptin and the leptin receptor (see below).

Table 157-14 Endocrine Biochemistry of Subjects Ob1 and Ob2[804]

	Ob1	Ob2	Reference range
Fasting glucose	4.7	4.4	3.5–5.5 mM^{-1}
insulin	158	46	0–60 pM^{-1}
proinsulin	21	8.1	0–5 pM^{-1}
32–33 split proinsulin	39	11	<13 pM^{-1}
9:00 ACTH	58	28	5–50 ngl^{-1}
9:00 cortisol	420	156	280–650 nM^{-1}
TSH	4.80	4.6	0.4–4 mU^{-1}
Free T4	11.4	12.4	9–20 pM^{-1}
FSH	0.8	0.2	prepubertal 0.6–3.4 ul^{-1}
LH	<0.2	<0.2	prepubertal 0.6–1.7 ul^{-1}
Estradiol	<20	—	prepubertal <60 pM^{-1}
Testosterone	—	<0.2	prepubertal <0.7 nM^{-1}

Levels of testosterone, oestradiol, luteinizing hormone (LH), and follicle-stimulating hormone (FSH) are all consistent with the prepubertal state. Ob1 has marked fasting hyperinsulinemia and a mild elevation in 9:00 levels of adrenocorticotropic hormone (ACTH) and thyrotropic hormone (TSH).

As predicted, striking weight loss has occurred in the child treated with recombinant leptin.[1042]

Strobel et al. described a 22-year-old male (BMI = 55.8) and a 24-year-old female (BMI = 46.9) who are members of a consanguineous Turkish family and homozygous for a missense mutation in the leptin gene.[806] These individuals were ascertained by low serum leptin relative to fat mass, and found to have a C → T transition resulting in R105W and abolishing of an MspI restriction site. Both patients displayed early onset severe hyperphagia. The female had primary amenorrhea, and the nonpubertal adult male displayed clinical and endocrine evidence of hypothalamic hypogonadism. The male also showed a low systolic blood pressure response to the cold pressor test, mild orthostatic hypotension, and reduced sympathetic skin response. These responses were interpreted to indicate a reduction in sympathetic autonomic nervous tone similar to that seen in *ob* mice.[563] Expression of the *LEP* mutant cDNA in COS-1 cells produced no detectable secretion of leptin in the incubation medium, but immunoreactive protein was present in cell lysates. Thus, this mutation appears to affect secretory processing of the peptide, as apparently occurs in the G398 → Del mutation described in the Pakistani family.

It is clear that the majority of obese humans do not have major coding sequence derangements in LEP.[807,808] However, the region of the LEP gene has been linked to skinfold thickness,[750] and an A → G transition at bp26 in a segment of the first exon corresponding to the 5′UT sequence was associated with severe obesity.[809] These linkages/associations suggest that differences in regulation of LEP expression might account for some of the variability in body fat among humans. There is considerable variation in blood leptin concentrations of individuals with the same body fat content.[810,811]

Leptin receptor Defects (*LEPR*; MIM 601007). A Kabilian consanguineous family with high prevalence of severe, early onset obesity was found to be segregating for a recessive mutation (G → A substitution) in the 3′ splice donor site of exon 16 of the leptin receptor.[812] Three affected sisters aged 13, 19, and 19 (deceased) years with BMI's equalling 71.5, 65.5, and 52.5, respectively, were described. None of the three affecteds had any evidence of puberty. Their heights, though in the 25 to 50 percent range for age, were low considering the auxotrophic effects of obesity in nonmutant children.[24] Work-up of the GH axis showed absence of a nighttime GH surge and blunted GH release to secretogogues. Concentrations of IGF-1 and IGF-BP3 were low, and increased after GH administration (as occurs in GH-deficient individuals). Both *ob* and *db* mice have low levels of pituitary GH and hypothalamic GHRH, and the *fa* Zucker rat displays low pituitary GH secretion.[563,813] Circulating leptin concentrations were extremely elevated in the two homozygous affecteds still alive (670 and 600 ng per ml), much higher than accounted for by elevated body fat (as reflected by BMI). Intermediate elevations of serum leptin were seen in proven heterozygotes for the mutation. Whereas in nonmutant individuals 5 to 20 percent of circulating leptin is present as a high MW complex (~450 kDa),[615,814] in the *LEPR* +/− and −/− subjects, about 80 percent of leptin circulated in this high MW complex. The leptin receptor truncated after exon 16 is predicted to be 831 amino acids (830 amino terminal amino acids of the extracellular domain of the normal receptor plus an additional glutamine at the C-terminus). Because it lacks the transmembrane domain, this peptide may be shed from the cell to act — as it does in other cytokine receptor superfamily genes such as GH — as a transport molecule for leptin. A slightly smaller 824-amino acid peptide of *LEPR* dimerizes when expressed in COS cells.[815] The reasons for the apparent discrepancies in phenotypes between *LEP* and *LEPR* mutation subjects are unknown. It is possible the *LEP*-mutant individuals are producing a small amount of functionally impaired ligand, while the receptor mutants are completely null for receptor function. The comparability of the mouse *ob* and *db* mutant animals may be due to the more severe impact of the *Lep* and *Lepr* mutations on ligand/receptor synthesis or function. The *db* mouse is deficient only in the longest known molecular isoform of the receptor (the 1162-amino acid isoform with the STAT binding domain) indicating that absence of this isoform alone is sufficient to produce a phenotype essentially indistinguishable from that of a deficiency of receptor ligand (*ob*). As has been done for *LEP*, careful and extensive searches have been conducted for *LEPR* mutations that might account for variations in human body weight. The individuals described above constitute the only unequivocal examples of *LEPR* mutations leading to human obesity. However, the frequency of allelic variation in exonic sequences of *LEPR* is high in human populations.[816] In the Pima Indians[817] and French Canadians,[818] associations of body composition parameters with several predicted amino acid changes (especially Q223R) have been found. In studies of French obese subjects, no mutation equivalent to the Zucker *fa* mutation[820] (see earlier) or association of obesity with microsatellite polymorphisms flanking the *LEPR* gene were detected.[821] Likewise, association studies in Japanese,[822] British,[823] and Americans (Baltimore)[824] did not show evidence for a role of allelic variation in *LEPR* on adiposity. Also, these variants were also not associated with early onset obesity in a Danish study group.[825] Quantitation and direct sequencing of hypothalamic mRNA for *LEPR* in obese and lean subjects also showed no evidence for a role for quantitative differences or mutation/allelic variation in human obesity.[826]

POMC Defects. Two unrelated Caucasian children with mutations of POMC leading to obesity have been described.[219] Both have central nervous system-mediated (ACTH deficient) adrenal insufficiency, red hair, and onset of hyperphagia and obesity in the first 6 months of life. One of the patients (3-year-old female; 32 kg body weight (~17 kg = 97th percentile for age); normal birth weight; hypoadrenal at 23 days; increased appetite at ~4 months) is a compound heterozygote for mutations in exon 3 ($G_{7013}T$, $C_{7133Del}$). The second (5-year-old male; ~48 kg body weight (~22 kg = 97th percentile for age); normal birth weight; ACTH deficiency diagnosed at age 1 year; onset obesity due to hyperphagia at 5 months) is homozygous for an exon 2 mutation ($C_{3804}A$) that interrupts POMC translation. Both patients have normal pituitary morphology by MRI. In the first patient, the G → T transversion is predicted to result in premature termination at codon 79, causing absence of ACTH, αMSH and β-endorphin. The 1 bp deletion at bp7133 in the other allele produces a frameshift that should disrupt the structure of the receptor-binding core motifs of ACTH and αMSH (HFRW → HFAG), and also introduce a premature termination at codon 131. The 3-year-old female proband had an older brother who died at 7 months of age with severe adrenal hypoplasia. He was shown to have the same genotype at POMC as his affected sister. The mutations predict the complete absence of ACTH, αMSH and β-endorphin, and, accordingly, no POMC peptide, ACTH, or cortisol were detectable in the serum of the 3-year-old female after CRH infusion. Other anterior pituitary hormones were normal. The 5-year-old affected male's C → A transversion in exon 2 is 11 bp 5′ of the normal start site in the 5′UTR. The mutation introduces an additional out-of-frame start codon that probably abolishes translation of the wild type protein. The presence of only trace amounts of POMC-derived peptides in the serum of this patient is consistent with this interpretation of the likely functional consequences of this mutation.

The phenotypes of these patients are consistent with disruption of the synthesis of the cleavage products of pre-POMC: ACTH; α, β, and γMSH; and β-endorphin. Absence of the MSH ligand (probably αMSH) for melanocortin receptor 1 (MC1R) is the probable cause of the red hair, because this receptor mediates black/yellow coat color in mice[351,827] and when mutant results in yellow-coated mice,[827] red-coated cattle,[828,829] and red-haired humans.[830,831] The MC2R has ACTH as its only known ligand, explaining the adrenal insufficiency in these individuals. αMSH acts at the MC4R to suppress food intake.[223,234,832,833] The MC4R knockout animal is obese,[334] and the agouti-signaling peptide (ASIP), over-expressed in the brain of yellow, A^y mice, and Agouti-related peptide (AGRP), apparently produce obesity, at least in part, by competitively blocking MSH activation of MC4R.[332,352] The apparent absence of symptoms referable to β-endorphin deficiency (e.g., increased pain sensitivity)[333] in these patients suggests either that appropriate phenotypic testing was not conducted and/or that other ligands can substitute at the relevant receptors.

Further evidence for a possible role of POMC allelic variation comes from a linkage study listed in Table 157-11 in which a locus on chromosome 2 that includes POMC was estimated to account for 47 percent of variance in serum leptin concentration and 32 percent of variation in fat mass.[754,1043]

MC4R Defects. Obesity, apparently due to haploinsufficiency resulting from heterozygosity for either a 4-bp deletion involving codon 211,[336] or a 4-bp insertion at bp732,[337] was initially described in two unrelated families segregating for early onset, relatively severe obesity as an autosomal dominant phenotype. These mutations result in truncation of this G-protein-coupled 7 transmembrane receptor in the fifth and sixth transmembrane domains respectively. No disorders of hair pigmentation, linear growth, or of the gonadal, adrenal, or thyroid axes are apparent in these individuals. Circulating leptin concentrations are appropriate to the increased fat mass. Other *MC4R* mutations have been described subsequently.[1062,1063] In contrast to the rarity of mutations in *LEP*, *LEPR*, and *POMC*, mutations in *MC4R* are quite common. In some studies, nearly 5% of patients with BMI>40 have been reported to be heterozygous for mutations in *MC4R*. However, not all individuals with such mutations are obese, suggesting that as yet unidentified genetic and developmental factors may influence the expression of the mutation.

Mice homozygous for a knockout of *Mc4r* are severely obese, and those heterozygous for this mutation are less obese, but still fatter than +/+ animals.[334]

The phenotype of humans homozygous for null *MC4R* alleles is not known, but presumably will be more severe than the heterozygotes, consistent with the mouse model. In any event, these mutations of *MC4R* are the first dominantly inherited forms of human obesity.

Peroxisome Proliferator-Activated Nuclear Receptor Gamma (PPARγ; MIM 601487). PPARγ and genes related to it in the adipocyte differentiation process (see Adipose Tissue Biochemistry and Development) are particularly interesting candidate genes for human obesity because they have the potential to influence body fat by mechanisms related primarily to effects on the partitioning of calories to fat. Sequence variants in the PPARγ2 gene, which is located on human chromosome 3[1044] have been linked to body fatness in two caucasian populations.[1045] Lipoprotein lipase (LPL), whose expression, as noted, is induced by ADD1/SREBP1, is also a candidate for this sort of action and has, in fact, been proposed as a "gatekeeper" of adipose tissue stores by virtue of gating effects on the release and uptake by adipocytes of FFAs from circulating triglycerides.[851] However, human mutations that completely inactivate LPL do not affect the size of adipose tissue depot stores.[852]

A silent C$\rightarrow$T substitution in exon 6 of PPARγ was weakly associated ($P<0.03$) with circulating leptin concentration, but not BMI, in 820 French individuals.[103] Leptin is a more accurate surrogate for body fat than BMI, and thus the discrepancy here is not surprising. In light of the results of the mutation analysis described below, it is certainly plausible that allelic variation in PPARγ might influence body fat mass by effects on adipocyte differentiation.

Three hundred fifty-eight unrelated individuals (including 121 obese with BMI >29) were screened for mutations in PPARγ in the region of Ser114 (MAP kinase target).[853] The obese subjects had a mean BMI = 33.9 $\pm$ 4.4 kg/m^2 and a mean age of 57.2 $\pm$ 13.5 years; the nonobese subjects had BMI 25.0 $\pm$ 2.7 kg/m^2 and a mean age of 59.1 $\pm$ 15.5 years. Four of the obese had a missense mutation (P115Q) affecting the amino acid adjacent to Ser114. These four subjects had BMIs ranging from 37.9 to 47.3 kg/m^2, whereas the other 117 obese subjects had a mean BMI of 33.6 kg/m^2. The fasting serum insulin concentration (9.3 $\pm$ 1.5 μu/ml) in the mutant individuals was lower than the nonmutant obese (16.7 $\pm$ 4.6 μu/ml). The mutation was not detected in any nonobese subject. Overexpression of the mutant PPARγ_2 in mouse fibroblasts resulted in defective Ser114 phosphorylation and increased the rates of adipocyte differentiation and triglyceride accumulation compared to the wild-type construct. This activating mutation could increase adipocyte proliferation and enhance insulin sensitivity. Either or both of these partition-related phenotypes could account for increased adiposity of the mutant individuals.[853]

HETEROZYGOSITY FOR RECESSIVE OBESITY MUTATIONS

Although the *ob* and *db* mutations in rodents are correctly described as autosomal recessive, it is clear that the heterozygote of either genotype is not entirely equivalent to the homozygous wild-type animal. Coleman showed that the heterozygote *ob* and *db* animals survived about 20 percent longer in a fast, despite having body weight comparable to that of the +/+ animal.[854] The apparent explanation for this difference is the higher fractional body fat content of the heterozygotes[577] and possibly a difference in ketone metabolism.[855] In addition, gene dosage effects on circulating leptin can be shown for *ob, db*, and *fa*: the *ob*/+ animals having less, and *db*/+ or *fa*/+ more circulating leptin per unit of body fat than +/+ animals.[576,577] C57BLKS/J *db*/+ mice develop gestational diabetes and deliver relatively macrosomic pups.[1046]

Human heterozygotes for the *LEPR* mutation, like the corresponding mice[577] and rats,[576] have plasma leptin concentrations about midway between wild-type and homozygous affecteds. The parents of the individuals with leptin and leptin receptor deficiencies, and the heterozygous sibs of the affecteds, are reported as nonobese in the respective papers. However, detailed longitudinal direct measures of body composition are not available on these proven human heterozygotes. Based on the findings in the rodents, it is likely that heterozygosity for such mutations will have subtle effects to increase body fat in humans. The parents of the *POMC* mutant children are described as normal, as are the children of the patient with the *PC1* mutation, but no data are given. It is relevant to this argument to note that obligate or putative heterozygotes for BBS have increased frequency of obesity, renal disease, hypertension, and type 2 diabetes, consistent with haploinsufficiency for the responsible gene(s).[856,857] As indicated earlier, heterozygosity for inactivating mutations of the melanocortin 4 receptor results in obesity in both mice and humans.

The possibility that heterozygosity for mutations in these and other genes in the regulatory pathways for body composition may have phenotypic effects on these systems is a very important issue. Obviously, heterozygosity for these mutations and other sequence variants will be much more frequent than homozygosity, and it is possible that the conjunction of several such heterozygosities might account for a considerable amount of the body composition variation in a population. Again, in mice, there is evidence for additivity of heterozygosity for mutations of the leptin and leptin-receptor genes.[577] Such possibilities can now be directly examined in humans.

UNCOUPLING PROTEINS

Recent epidemiologic studies in the U.S. indicate that per capita food consumption (and the fraction of calories from fat) has been declining steadily for the past two decades.[858] However, physical activity has been declining as well,[858,859] presumably accounting for the continuing increase in obesity prevalence, despite declining energy intakes. These epidemiologic studies reemphasize what is clear from the studies of metabolic responses to weight perturbation: the energy expenditure compartment plays an important role in determining net energy balance, and energy intake is not perfectly coordinated with expenditure. Interest in genes whose expression might mediate changes in the efficiency with which the enthalpy of ingested molecules is captured as ATP and used in energy-requiring metabolic and mechanical processes derives from this recognition. Mitochondrial proton leak rates are related to body mass and metabolic rate.[860–862]

The uncoupling proteins are members of the mitochondrial carrier superfamily that includes ADP/ATP and Pi carriers, transporters for oxoglutarate, citrate, carnitine, and protons, and (probably) carriers for pyruvate, ornithine, and dicarboxylic acids/malate. Additional members of this group, whose function is unknown, include UCP2 and UCP3, "Graves soluble carrier," and 14 or more genes identified by homology searches in various EST data bases. The uncoupling proteins have predicted structures that include six transmembrane domains encoded by six exons. The terminal exon also encodes a purine nucleotide-binding element that mediates tonic inhibition of UCP activity.[863] UCP2 and UCP3 are 71 percent identical at the amino acid level, 59 percent identical to UCP1, and ~30 percent identical to the oxoglutarate carrier.

Uncoupling Protein 1 (UCP1; MIM 113730)

UCP1 was identified as a 32-kDa mitochondrial protein in BAT,[864] a thermogenic organ in rodents.[865–867] This tissue, whose dark hue is due to the high density of mitochondrial cytochromes, is concentrated in the intrerscapsular region and along the aorta and perirenal areas. The tissue is richly supplied with sympathetic nerves and the constituent adipocytes have a high density of

β_3-adrenergic receptors. Sympathetic activation causes increased lipolysis and the resulting free fatty acids apparently displace GTP from the purine nucleotide binding site at the C-terminus of the molecule,[868] allowing protons pumped out of the mitochondrial matrix by the directional activity of the cytochrome system[869] to descend along that gradient without being coupled to the generation of ATP. The enthalpy of the molecules oxidized is thus released as heat rather than being captured as high-energy phosphate bonds of ATP. The exact mechanism by which these protons are brought back across the mitochondrial membrane into the matrix is not completely understood.[383]

Clones for rat and mouse *Ucp1* CDNAs were isolated by several labs[150,871,872] and the human cDNA by Bouillaud et al.[873] The human gene is ~13 kb on chromosome 4q31 and has 6 exons and encodes a 305-amino acid protein (32.8 kDa).[874]

When the quantity of BAT is limited by transgenic insertion of an expressing toxigene (diptheria toxin behind a UCP-specific promoter) the resulting transgenic animals are obese primarily due to reduced energy expenditure.[384] However, complete knockout of *Ucp1* in mice results in animals that are not obese when fed standard chow or a high-fat diet. These animals do, however, show reduced thermogenic response to a β_3-adrenergic agonist or to reduced ambient temperature.[399]

The catecholamines, norepinephrine and epinephrine, are the primary neurotransmitters for sympathetic nervous system impulses in BAT and elsewhere. Both of these catecholamines require the activity of dopamine beta hydroxylase (DBH) for synthesis. Mice segregating for a knockout of DBH show the expected cold intolerance and hypoactivity of BAT, but are not obese despite being hyperphagic. An unexpected elevation of basal metabolic rate accompanying this knockout may be responsible for failure to gain weight.[402]

The phenotypes of these rodent models altering various components in the energy expenditure pathway demonstrates both the importance of the sympathetic nervous system and its effector organs in energy homeostasis, but also emphasize the redundancy of the systems subserving energy balance.

UCP1 mRNA has been detected at low levels in human WAT, and such levels are, in fact, lower in intraperitoneal adipose tissue of obese as compared to lean individuals.[875] Some of this difference in expression levels is attributable to allelic variation of an intronic sequence variant at or near the *UCP1* locus.[876] Several efforts have been made to associate the *UCP1* locus with differences in energy-related phenotypes in humans. In a French Canadian population, a Bcl1 RFLP (A382G) was associated with gains in body fat over 12 years.[877] This polymorphism was also associated in French Caucasians with weight gain, in morbidly obese patients,[878] and in velocity of weight loss in therapeutic regimens.[879] However, no association was found in a case-control study of obesity in Swedish subjects.[880]

Although UCP1 protein and mRNA are detectable in human WAT,[873,881,882] amounts are small and it seems unlikely that BAT and/or UCP1 plays a significant role in the control of human body weight.[883] If UCP's do play such a role, *UCP2* and *UCP3* seem more likely candidates by virtue of the location and quantities of their expression.

Uncoupling Protein 2 (UCP2; MIM 601693)

This gene was identified by differential display[154] and by homology searches based upon the sequence of *UCP1*.[153,155] *UCP2* is widely expressed in human tissue (lung, liver, spleen, placenta, kidney, pancreas macrophages, WAT, and skeletal muscle). Expression of *UCP2* in yeast results in growth inhibition under aerobic, but not anaerobic, conditions, and reduces mitochondrial membrane potential as determined by $DiOC_6$ fluorescent dye staining.[154] Expression of *UCP2* is highest in WAT, and its expression is increased in *Ucp1* knockout mice,[399] *ob* and *db* mice,[154] and in mice overexpressing leptin,[412] suggesting that *UCP2* may be compensating for defects in thermogenesis (*UCP1* deficiency) and responding to ambient leptin concentrations in a direction consistent with leptin's effects on energy expenditure. *UCP2* message abundance is greater in intraperitoneal (omental) than abdominal subcutaneous fat, and intraperitoneal (but not subcutaneous) levels are lower in obese subjects than in lean subjects. These lower levels persist in omental depots of weight-reduced obese subjects.[884] Levels of *Ucp2* expression in WAT correlate inversely with weight gain efficiency in A/J (resistant to weight gain) and C57BL/6J (susceptible to weight gain) mouse strains.[153]

Surprisingly, both *UCP2* and *UCP3* expression are increased in skeletal muscle and WAT of obese and lean subjects who are fasted,[162] suggesting that these molecules may be induced to compensate for the reduced body temperature that accompanies fasting. Neither β_3-adrenergic agonists nor insulin induce *UCP2* expression.[153]

The genetic region of *UCP2* (chromosome 11q13, which also contains *UCP3*) has been linked to resting metabolic rate and obesity in a French Canadian population,[762] but not to obesity and type 2 diabetes phenotypes in a Danish[885] or French population.[886] In an association study of the *UCP2/UCP3* gene cluster in Pima Indians, three polymorphisms in strong linkage disequilibrium were detected (Ala → Val in exon 4 *UCP2*; 45 bp Ins/Del in the 3′ UTR of *UCP2*; and C → T silent polymorphisms in exon 3 UCP3). The *UCP2* variants were associated with sleeping metabolic rate and 24-h metabolic rate. An overdominant pattern of effects was shown, with heterozygotes for the *UCP2* variants having higher metabolic rates than homozygotes.[887] The region of mouse chromosome 7 that contains *Ucp2* and *Ucp3*, also contains a QTL for type 2 diabetes and obesity.[760,888,889]

Uncoupling Protein 3 (UCP3; MIM 602044)

UCP3 is located about 50 kb from *UCP2* in the same reading orientation,[890,891] suggesting that the pair arose from a gene duplication. *UCP3* is expressed primarily in skeletal muscle and heart, although transcripts are also found in WAT and BAT (in rats).[155,156] The gene has 7 exons and encodes two RNA isoforms UCP3L (312aa) and UCP3S (275aa), which differ only by the absence of the terminal 37 amino acids in the latter. UCP3L is predicted to encode six transmembrane domains and the C-terminus consensus purine nucleotide-binding domain. The short isoform (UCP3S) uses a polyadenylation signal in the sixth intron to terminate the 275aa peptide that lacks sequence encoded by the sixth exon and, hence, the putative terminal transmembrane domain and purine nucleotide-binding domain.[890] Thus, UCP3S, if functional, might be constitutively active due to the absence of a regulatory domain. However, instability due to the absence of a transmembrane domain could also disrupt (impair) function.

UCP3S is approximately five times as abundant as UCP3L in human skeletal muscle,[163] and this proportionality does not appear to be different between lean and obese subjects. *UCP3* expression is increased by T3, β_3-adrenergic agonists, and leptin.[157] As indicated, fasting induces *UCP3* expression. However, maintenance of a reduced body weight by formerly obese subjects is associated with decreased expression of *UCP3* (both isoforms).[163,892] The reduction of *UCP3* in the reduced obese is fully consistent with the decreased resting metabolic rate and TEE reported in these subjects, and may account for the apparent enhancement of skeletal muscle chemomechanical coupling noted during exercise in these individuals.[127]

A splice site mutation in intron 5 of UPC3 has been described in African-Americans.[158,1047] This mutation eliminates the UCP3L isoform. The functional consequences with regard to obesity of a deficiency of UCP3L appear to be small. An increase in RQ (reduced fat oxidation) was found in heterozygous humans by one group.[1047] Cheng et al found no effect on RQ or cytochrome coupling in skeletal muscle mitochondria in a homozygous female and association of this splice mutation with RQ or BMI in a large African-American population.[158] The apparently small phenotypic effect of congenital absence of UCPL is consistent with the non obese phenotype of mice with UCP3 knockouts.[1022,1023] These findings suggest that UCP3L does not function primarily as a mitochondrial uncoupling protein, or that its congenital absence can be compensated for by other genes. The recent description of hypermetabolism, hyperphagia, low body fat, and resistance to weight gain in mice over-expressing human UCP3 in skeletal muscle suggests that UCP3 can uncouple oxidation metabolism *in vivo*.[1050]

TREATMENT

Few would disagree that the best treatment for obesity is to prevent it. However, while we know that genetic and environmental factors interact to convert potential to actuality, we still have only rudimentary understanding of the former and great difficulty in manipulating the latter in directions (e.g., increasing physical activity/reducing caloric-intake) that would be helpful.

Until we solve these problems, hopefully by devising tests of susceptibility and more effective methods of prophylaxis, we will continue to encounter large numbers of patients requiring medical intervention for obesity.

Treatment of the obese individual should be directed toward reducing current morbidity and the risks of future morbidities. The majority of adiposity-related morbidity and mortality from coronary artery disease is attributable to intermediate phenotypes such as diabetes, hyperlipidemia, and hypertension.[31] In large prospective studies, there is little, if any, direct effect of adiposity on mortality risk once outcomes are adjusted for the effects of such secondary morbidities.[48,893] The maintenance of even modest degrees (5 to 10 percent) of weight reduction is associated with significant improvement in glucose tolerance, hyperlipidemia, and hypertension in many morbidly obese individuals.[29,30,894–897] These secondary adiposity-related morbidities are potentially worsened or improved by modification of other lifestyle factors such as diet, exercise, and limiting cigarette or alcohol intake.[19,898–901] Thus, the adoption of a healthier lifestyle may substantially reduce the risk of cardiovascular disease, even if body composition per se does not change.[19] Furthermore, because maintenance of a lower body weight usually requires prolonged restriction of caloric intake,[127,128] the treatment period does not end once a patient has achieved a prescribed degree of body fatness.

Benefits of Exercise

Large population studies and longitudinal studies of individuals have demonstrated that cardiovascular morbidity and morbidity risks are actually higher in sedentary "unfit" never-obese individuals than in physically active "fit" (defined as engaging in at least 30 min of regular exercise twice per week) overweight individuals.[899,902] Inclusion of exercise in weight-reduction and weight-maintenance programs enhances the amount of weight loss and likelihood of maintaining a reduced body weight,[902] and decreases overall morbidity and age-related weight gain, even if the reduced body weight is not maintained.[898,902–904] Both dietary modification to a *Heart Healthy* diet (less than 30 percent of total calories as fat, less than 10 percent as saturated fat)[897,905] and regular exercise should be an integral part of any attempt to lose weight or to maintain a reduced body weight.[906–909]

Drug Treatments

Theoretically, obesity pharmacotherapy could act functionally to decrease food intake, decrease nutrient absorption, or alter the partitioning of stored calories between fat, protein, and carbohydrate. Because so many more calories are stored as adipose tissue than as muscle or glycogen (especially in obese individuals, see Table 157-1) and because of the relatively greater caloric density of triglyceride, it is unlikely that an agent affecting partitioning of stored calories would provide significant efficacy if functioning without affects on energy intake and/or expenditure. Due to the hydrophobic and calorically dense nature of triglyceride, the caloric density (kcal/gm) of adipose tissue is at least 4–5 times that of muscle protein/glycogen or liver glycogen. Thus, an individual would have to gain at least 40 kg of muscle to store the same number of calories contained in 10kg of fat.

Current drug treatments of obesity tend either to decrease nutrient availability (either by appetite suppression or blockade of nutrient absorption) or to increase energy expenditure (thermogenesis). Anorexiant drugs have been used in the treatment of obesity for over 30 years. Currently available anorexiants incclude serotonin reuptake inhibitors, such as fluoexitine, central adrenergic agonists, such as amphetamines, phentermine, or nisoxetine (a noradrenergic reuptake inhibitor), and the drug sibutramine which acts both as a serotonin- and norepinephrine- uptake inhibitor and may also increase thermogenesis.[910,911,1002,1051–1053] Fluoxetine and sibutramine both have been shown to promote some weight loss (average less than 10% of pre-treatment weight) for 6–18 months.[910,911,917–919,1053] Obese subjects treated with sibutramine for more than 1 year maintained only a small degree (~5%) of weight loss.[918,919] These medications may increase heart rate and exacerbate hypertension and, if used, subjects need to be monitored closely for exacerbation of underlying cardiovascular disease. Until recently, fenfluramine and dexfenfluramine, whose metabolite D-norfenfluramine binds to and activates the 5HT2c serontonin receptor on the post sympatic neuron, were used alone or in combination with the sympathomimetic agent, phentermine, as pharmacotherapy for obesity. However, reported side-effects of dexfenfluramine, including pulmonary hypertension and valvular heart disease,[912–916] have resulted in the removal of fenfluramine and dexfenfluramine from pharmacies in the United States by order of the Food and Drug Administration.

Sympathomimetic agents, designed to increase energy expenditure, also have potential cardiovascular side effects (tachycardia, hypertension) that make them unsuitable for the treatment of many morbidly obese patients. Studies of the administration of ephedrine (also available in herbal weight-loss preparations containing ma-huang) and caffeine have demonstrated that the majority of the weight loss induced by these drugs may be due to appetite suppression rather than to increased thermogenesis.[1053,1054]

The pancreatic lipase inhibitor, tetrahydrolipostatin (orlistat), blocks digestion of fat and has been shown to augment both weight loss and the likelihood of sustaining at least some degree of weight reduction for 1–2 years after weight loss. Inhibition of lipase may result in steatorrhea if excessive quantities of fat are ingested. Increased fat excretion necessitates dietary supplementation with fat soluble vitamins (A, D, E, and K). Even with combined therapy of counseling to decrease caloric intake and to increase exercise, and orlistat, only approximately 1/3 of patients are able to lose more than 5% of their usual weight (versus 1/5 of subjects receiving placebo) and of those who successfully lose weight, less than 1/2 have maintained more than 25% of their weight loss 1 year later (versus approximately 1/3 of subjects receiving placebo)[1055,1056] even though they continue to use the lipase inhibitor.

Some have argued that pharmacological weight reduction (or weight reduction by other means) so reduces the hazard of type 2 diabetes – especially in morbidly obese individuals – that the improvement in health is worth taking drugs with relatively small hazards of side-effects.[917] Whether or not this is so must be evaluated on a highly individualized basis and take account of factors such as likelihood of adiposity-related morbidity (based on current morbidity and family history) in a given patient. It is also important that such drug regimens be administered in association with dietary recommendations to reduce caloric intake and, usually, exercise regiments to increase energy expenditure. In general, currently available drugs may make it easier for some individuals to adhere to a hypocaloric diet, at least in the short term.

The "ideal" obesity pharmacotherapy would address the central nervous system feedback loop linking energy stores to energy expenditure and adipogenesis such that weight reduction would occur without invoking the hypometabolic and hyperphagic responses discussed above which characterize the reduced-obese individual. Unfortunately, this ideal has not yet been realized, and the anti-obesity drugs currently available tend to target the "symptoms" of hypometabolism or hyperphagia that characterize both dynamic weight loss and the maintenance of a reduced body weight rather than the underlying molecular genetic physiology that lead to and perpetuate the obesity. Candidate systems for future pharmacotherapy include leptin, melanocortin, neuropeptide Y, MCH, orexin, urocortin, CART, as well as adrenergic, serotinergic, and opioidergic afferent and efferent pathways. Given the importance of systemic energy homeostasis to survival, it is not surprising that attempts to disrupt any single system are, in the long run, largely ineffective due to the synergy and redundancy of systems regulating body weight. Suppression of caloric intake or increases in energy expenditure will not promote weight loss unless the net balance between energy intake and expenditure remains negative. Maintenance of a reduced body weight will not occur unless this balance remains at zero. It is likely that effective pharmacotherapy will need to target multiple systems of energy homeostasis simultaneously and/or act at the most central control points in the regulation of body weight to promote successful and sustained weight reduction.

Surgery

Most surgical treatment of obesity has consisted of efforts to decrease gastric volume (e.g., gastroplasty) in order to induce earlier satiety, and/or intestinal bypass to decrease absorption of calories. The jejunoileal shunt, which bypasses a large portion of the ileum involved in food absorption, was commonly performed until the mid-1980s. The jejunoileal bypass, however, frequently leads to symptoms related to the presence of a blind gut loop. These include liver disease (cholecystitis, liver failure) in approximately 10 percent of patients, diarrhea resulting in electrolyte disturbances in approximately 29 percent of patients, and renal disease, including nephrolithiasis and renal failure, in as many as 37 percent of patients over a 15-year period.[923,924]

The more commonly performed procedures at this time are gastric reduction operations (gastroplasty), with or without a smaller partial small bowel bypass, rather than the jejunoileostomy described above. The procedure results in substantial (10 to 40 percent) weight reduction, and approximately 80 percent of these patients remain at least 10 percent below their preoperative body weight 10 years following surgery.[920] Weight loss is due to earlier satiety secondary to gastroplasty, and perhaps neurohumoral signals emanating from the distal gut,[921] and increased gastrointestinal tract caloric wastage, especially of fat, secondary to the "dumping" that occurs with direct passage of gastric contents into the ileum.[920,922] The reduction in gastric volume and the "dumping" that occurs with passage of gastric contents into the small intestine act as deterrents to food intake. There may also be direct anorexiant effects of the passage of partially digested foodstuff into the distal small bowel.[921] Patients who have such procedures must have careful medical supervision because it is possible to overeat liquid or semisolid diets or to develop intestinal obstruction and electrolyte disturbances.

Behavior Modification

While psychologic disturbances are not often the primary etiology of obesity, behavior modification based on analysis of the circumstances under which subjects tend to eat, and the particular meaning of food intake, can be helpful in weight reduction. Experts in these manipulations recommend that subjects receive such advice or counseling in member-stable group settings over long periods of time. Frequent contacts with the group and therapist after weight is lost are also considered important.[925] Involvement of the entire family in long-term psychologic and behavioral therapy appears to increase the likelihood of maintaining weight-reduction in obese adults and children.[926,927] However, a 10-year study of a family-based treatment program showed only a modest degree of weight loss. The average subject was 140 percent above ideal body weight at the start of the study and maintained a weight 130 percent above ideal.[926] However, as indicated above, even a small degree of weight loss may result in significant decline in morbidity and psychologic support clearly has a role to play in the therapy of obesity. It should be clear that behavior alone, disarticulated from nutritional and endocrine factors, is generally not the sole determinant of obesity. The obese, while in the obese state, do not overeat relative to the nonobese if food intake is appropriately calculated on the basis of active metabolic mass.[127] But after weight reduction, the almost inevitable recidivist behavior is characterized by intermittent marked hyperphagia leading to a rapid regain of weight.[928] While some subtle behavioral theories might attempt to explain these events, it seems more plausible that the behavior of eating is secondary to overwhelming forces that act to maintain "usual" body weight, even when this body weight is obese.

Long-Term Results

The long-term results of medical weight reduction therapies are poor. Ninety to 95 percent of adults and children who lose weight return to their previous state of fatness.[24,928] Long-term treatment successes by any technique are few. Yet, it is hard to know how many individuals have lost weight and successfully managed their obesity without resorting to surgery, drugs, or medically administered diets. In general, it is believed that this is more likely to occur with those of lesser degrees of obesity than the morbidly obese (BMI > 35). The redundancy and synergism in systems regulating body composition probably account for the overall poor long-term success.

Future Therapies

As knowledge of the biology of the development and control of adipose tissue mass increases, new therapeutic targets will be suggested. The proliferation of neuropeptides that affect ingestive behavior provides a growing, attractive set of potential targets. The recent identification of an inhibitor (butabinidide) of the CCK-inactivating peptidase is a very recent example of a "prosatiater" developed from an understanding of the neurohormonal mediation of ingestive behavior.[929]

A preliminary report of the effects of subcutaneous leptin administration (0.01 to 0.3 mg/kg) combined with dietary restriction, suggests that leptin administration may aid in weight reduction in some obese subjects.[930] Whether such weight loss can be sustained is yet to be determined. The "threshold" model of leptin-mediated control of body weight (see "Leptin and Leptin Receptor Physiology" above) suggests that administration of leptin to weight-reduced persons would relieve the metabolic opposition to maintenance of a reduced weight by "tricking" the central nervous system and other organs into sensing that the lost fat is still present.[931] Leptin administration has been shown to result in earlier sexual maturation in rodents.[580,932] A rise in circulating leptin just prior to the onset of puberty in girls and boys has been proposed as a "signal" for the onset of puberty.[656,661,933,934] Thus, the administration of leptin to prepubertal children for stimulation or maintenance of weight loss would probably be inappropriate.

Other drugs being tested or under development include β_3-agonists,[935] which increase metabolic rate, and a pancreatic lipase inhibitor,[936,937] which prevents the digestion and absorption of ingested fat. It is too soon to know whether such drugs will be useful in the treatment of obesity. The growing understanding of the molecular genetic basis for regulation of body fat stores is likely to lead to better delineation of the pathogenesis of human obesity. New information and insight carries the possibility that totally different pharmacologic approaches than those currently available may come to the market.

ACKNOWLEDGMENTS

The work of this laboratory is supported in part by NIH grants DK30583, DK52431, DK26687 and RR00645. Assistance in preparation of the manuscript was provided by Mary Prudden and Alyssa Schabloski.

REFERENCES

1. Leibel RL: A biologic radar system for the assessment of body mass: The model of a geometry sensitive endocrine system is presented. *J Theor Biol* **66**:297, 1977.
2. Kuczmarski RJ, Flegal KM, Campbell SM, Johnson CL: Increasing prevalence of overweight among US adults: The National Health and Nutrition Examination Surveys, 1960 to 1991. *JAMA* **272**:205, 1994.
3. Stunkard AJ, Sorensen TI, Hanis C, Teasdale TW, Chakraborty R, Schull WJ, Schulsinger F. An adoption study of human obesity: *N Engl J Med* **314**:193, 1986.
4. Stunkard AJ, Harris JR, Pedersen NL, McClean GE: The body-mass index of twins who have been reared apart. *N Engl J Med* **322**:1483, 1990.
5. Hewlitt JK, Stunkard AJ, Carroll D, Sims J, Turner JR: A twin study approach towards understanding genetic contributions to body size and metabolic rate. *Acta Genet Med Gemellol (Roma)* **40**:133, 1991.
6. Bouchard C, Tremblay A, Despres JP, Nadeau A, Lupien PJ, Theriault G, Dussault J, Moorjani S, Pinault S, Fournier G: The response to long-term overfeeding in identical twins. *N Engl J Med* **322**:1477, 1990.
7. Stunkard AJ, Foch TT, Hrubec Z: A twin study of human obesity. *JAMA* **256**:51, 1986.
8. Selby JV, Newman B, Jr CPQ, Fabsitz RR, King MM, Meaney FJ: Evidence of genetic influence on central body fat in middle-aged twins. *Hum Biol* **61**:179, 1989.
9. Borjeson M: The aetiology of obesity in children. *Acta Pediatr Scand* **65**:279, 1976.
10. Price RA, Gottesman II: Body fat in identical twins reared apart: roles for genes and environment. *Behav Genet* **21**:1, 1991.
11. Falconer DS. *Introduction to Quantitative Genetics*. New York, John Wiley, 1989.
12. Komi PV, Viitasalo JHT, Havu M, Thorstensson A, Sjodin B, Karlsson J: Skeletal muscle fibres and muscle enzyme activities in monozygous and dizygous twins of both sexes. *Acta Physiol Scand* **100**:385, 1977.
13. Poehlman ET, Tremblay A, Despres JP, Fontaine E, Perusse L, Theriault G, Bouchard C: Genotype-controlled changes in body composition and fat morphology following overfeeding in twins. *Am J Clin Nutr* **43**:723, 1986.
14. Barnett AH, Eff C, Leslie DG, Pyke DA: Diabetes in identical twins. *Diabetologia* **20**:87, 1981.
15. Moll PP, Burns TL, Lauer RM: The genetic and environmental sources of body mass index variability: The Muscatine ponderosity family study. *Am J Hum Genet* **49**:1243, 1991.
16. Neel JV: Diabetes mellitus: A "thrifty" genotype rendered detrimental by "progress"? *Am J Hum Genet* **14**:353, 1962.
17. Frisch RE: Fatness, menarche and female fertility. *Perspect Biol Med* **28**:611, 1985.
18. Frisch RE: Body fat, menarche, fitness and fertility. *Hum Reprod* **2**:521, 1987.
19. Rosenbaum M, Leibel RL, Hirsch J: Medical Progress: Obesity. *N Engl J Med* **1337**:396, 1997.
20. Glass AR, Burman KD, Dahms WT, Boehm TM: Endocrine function in human obesity. *Metabolism* **30**:89, 1981.
21. Pi-Sunyer FX: Medical hazards of obesity. *Ann Intern Med* **119**:655, 1993.
22. Michaelis OE, Carswell N, Velasquez MT, Hansen CT: The role of obesity, hypertension and diet in diabetes and its complications in the spontaneous hypertensive/NIH-corpulent rat. *Nutrition* **5(1)**:56, 1989.
23. Kaplan N: The deadly quartet: upper-body obesity, glucose intolerance hypertriglyceridemia, and hypertension. *Arch Intern Med* **149**:1514, 1989.
24. Rosenbaum M, Leibel RL: Pathophysiology of childhood obesity. *Adv Pediatr* **35**:73, 1988.
25. Huang Z, Willett WC, Manson JE, Rosner B, Stampfer MJ, Speizer FE, Colditz GA: Body weight, weight change, and risk for hypertension in women. *Ann Intern Med* **128**:81, 1998.
26. Henry RR, Wallace P, Olfesky JM: Effects of weight loss on mechanisms of hyperglycemia in obese non-insulin-dependent diabetes mellitus. *Diabetes* **35(9)**:990, 1986.
27. Long SD, O'Brien K Jr, MacDonald KG Jr, Leggett-Frazier N, Swanson MS, Pories WJ, Caro JF: Weight loss in severely obese subjects prevents the progression of impaired glucose tolerance to type II diabetes. A longitudinal interventional study. *Diabetes Care* **17(5)**:372, 1994.
28. Rossner S: Defining success in obesity management. *Int J Obes Relat Metab Disord* **21(Suppl)**:S2, 1997.
29. Goldstein DJ: Beneficial health effects of modest weight loss. *Int J Obes Relat Metab Disord* **16**:397, 1992.
30. Blackburn GL: Effect of degree of weight loss on health benefits. *Obes Res* **3**:211S, 1995.
31. Manson J, Colditz G, Stampfer M, Willett W, Rosner B, Monson R, Speizer F: A prospective study of obesity and risk of coronary heart disease in women. *N Engl J Med* **322**:882, 1990.
32. Seidell JC, Andres R, Sorkin JD, Muller DC: The sagittal waist diameter and mortality in men: The Baltimore Longitudinal Study on Aging. *Int J Obes Relat Metab Disord* **18**:61, 1994.
33. Rimm EB, Stampfer MJ, Giovannucci E, Acherio A, Spiegelman D, Colditz GA, Willett WC: Body size and fat distribution as predictors of coronary heart disease among middle-aged and older US men. *Am J Epidemiol* **141**:1117, 1995.
34. WHO: Obesity: Preventing and Managing the Global Epidemic. Geneva: World Health Organization, 1998.
35. Sorkin JD, Muller D, Andres R: Body mass index and mortality in Seventh-Day Adventist men. A critique and re-analysis. *Int J Obes Relat Metab Disord* **18**:752, 1994.
36. Must A, Jacques P, Dallai G, Bajema D, Deitz W: Long-term morbidity and mortality of overweight adolescents. *N Engl J Med* **327**:1350, 1992.
37. Deleted in proof.
39. Bouchard C (ed): *The Genetics of Obesity.* Boca Raton, CRC Press, 1994.
40. VanItallie TB: Health implications of overweight and obesity in the United States. *Ann Intern Med* **103**:983, 1985.
41. Durnin JV, Womersley J: Body fat assessed from total body density and its estimation from skinfold thickness: Measurements on 481 men and women aged from 16 to 72 years. *Br J Nutr* **32**:77, 1974.
42. Norgan N: Population differences in body composition in relation to body mass index. *Eur J Clin Nutr* **48(Suppl)**:S10, 1994.
43. Himes JH, Bouchard C, Pheley AM: Lack of correspondence among measures identifying the obese. *Am J Prevent Med* **7(2)**:107, 1991.
44. Shimokata H, Muller DC, Fleg JL, Sorkin J, Ziemba AW, Andres R: Age as independent determinant of glucose tolerance. *Diabetes* **40**:44, 1991.
45. Muller DC, Elahi D, Tobin JD, Andres R: The effect of age on insulin resistance and secretion: A review. *Semin Nephrol* **16**:289, 1996.
46. Andres R, Elahi D, Tobin JD, Muller DC, Brant L: Impact of age on weight goals. *Ann Intern Med* **103**:1030, 1985.
47. Shimokata H, Tobin J, Muller D, Elahi D, Coon P, Andres R: Studies in the distribution of body fat: I. Effects of age, sex, and obesity. *J Geron* **44**:M66, 1989.
48. Manson JE, Meir J, Stampfer MJ, Hennekens CH, Willett WC: Body weight and longevity: A reassessment. *JAMA* **257**:353, 1987.
49. Manson JE, Willett WC, Stampfer MJ, Colditz GA, Hunter DJ, Hankinson SE, Hennekens CH, Speizer FE: Body weight and mortality among women. *N Engl J Med* **333(11)**:677, 1995.
50. Rexrode KM, Hennekens CH, Willett WC, Colditz GA, Stampfer MH, Rich-Edwards JW, Speizer FE, Manson JE: A prospective study of body mass index, weight change, and risk of stroke in women. *JAMA* **277**:1539, 1997.
51. Kissebah AH, Vydelingum N, Murray R, Evans DJ, Hartz AJ, Kalkhoff RK, Adams PW: Relation of body fat distribution to metabolic complications of obesity. *J Clin Endocrinol Metab* **54**:254, 1982.
52. Krotkiewski M, Bjorntorp P, Sjostrom L, Smith U: Impact of obesity on metabolism in men and women: Importance of regional adipose tissue distribution. *J Clin Invest* **72**:1150, 1983.
53. Lapidus L, Bengtsson C, Larsson B, Pennert K, Rybo E, Sjostrom L. Distribution of adipose tissue and risk of cardiovascular disease and death: A 12-year follow up of participants in the population study of women in Gothenburg, Sweden. *Br Med J* **289**:1257, 1984.
54. Larsson B, Svarsudd K, Welin L, Wilhelmsen L, Bjorntorp P, Tibblin G: Abdominal adipose tissue distribution, obesity, and risk of cardiovascular disease and death: 13-year follow up of participants in the study of men born in 1913. *Br Med J* **288**:1401, 1984.
55. Bjorntorp P: "Portal" adipose tissue as a generator of risk for cardiovascular disease and diabetes. *Arteriosclerosois* **10**:493, 1990.
56. Kissebah AH, Krakower GR: Regional adiposity and morbidity. *Physiol Rev* **74**:761, 1994.
57. Stromblad G, Bjorntorp P: Reduced hepatic insulin clearance in rats with dietary induced obesity. *Metabolism* **35**:323, 1986.
58. Pouliot MC, Despres JP, Lemieux S, Moorjani S, Bouchard C, Tremblay A, Nadeau A, Lupien PJ: Waist circumference and abdominal sagittal diameter: Best simple anthropometric indexes

of abdominal visceral adipose tissue accumulation and related cardiovascular risk in men and women. *Am J Cardiol* **73**:460, 1994.
59. Rosmond R, Dallman MF, Bjorntorp P. Stress-related cortisol secretion in men: Relationships with abdominal obesity and endocrine, metabolic and hemodynamic abnormalities. *J Clin Endocrinol Metab* **83**:1853, 1998.
60. Braddon FEM, Rodgers B, Wadsworth MEJ, Davies JMC. Onset obesity in a 36-year birth cohort study. *Br Med J* **293**:299, 1986.
61. Winkler E, Klingenberg M: Effect of fatty acids on H^+ transport activity of the reconstituted uncoupling protein. *J Biol Chem* **269**:2508, 1994.
62. Garlid KD, Orsz DE, Modriansky M, Vassanelli S, Jezek P: On the mechanism of fatty acid-induced proton transport by mitochondrial uncoupling protein. *J Biol Chem* **271**:2615, 1996.
63. Rothwell NJ, Stock MJ: A role for brown adipose tissue in diet-induced thermogenesis. *Nature* **281**:31, 1979.
64. Himms-Hagen J: Brown adipose tissue metabolism and thermogenesis. *Ann Rev Nutr* **5**:69, 1985.
65. Lean ME: Brown adipose tissue in humans. *Proc Nutr Soc* **48**:243, 1989.
66. Knittle JL: *Adipose Tissue Development in Man*. New York, Plenum Press, 1978, p 295.
67. Pettit DJ, Baird HR, Allech KA, Knowler WC: Excessive obesity in offspring of Pima Indian women with diabetes during pregnancy. *N Engl J Med* **308**:242, 1983.
68. Aubert R, Suquet JP, Lemmonier O: Long-term morphological and metabolic effects of early under- and over-nutrition in mice. *J Nutr* **110**:649, 1980.
69. Jones AP, Assimon SA, Friedman MI: The effect of diet on food intake and adiposity in rats made obese by gestational undernutrition. *Physiol Behav* **37**:381, 1986.
70. Anguita RM, Sigulen DM, Sawaga AL: Intrauterine food restriction is associated with obesity in young rats. *J Nutr* **123**:1421, 1993.
71. Whitaker RC, Dietz WH: Role of the prenatal environment in the development of obesity. *J Pediatr* **132**:78, 1998.
72. Ravelli GP, Stein Z, Susser MW: Obesity in young men after famine exposure in utero and early infancy. *N Engl J Med* **295**:349, 1976.
73. Knittle J, Hirsch J: Effect of early nutrition on the development of rat epididymal fat pads: Cellularity and metabolism. *J Clin Invest* **47**:2091, 1968.
74. Chua SC, White DW, Wu-Peng XS, Liu S-M, Okada N, Kershaw EE, Chung WK, Power-Kehoe L, Chua M, Tartaglia LA, et al: Phenotype of *fatty* due to Gln269Pro mutation in the Leptin Receptor (*Lepr*). *Diabetes* **45(8)**:1141, 1996.
75. Johnson PR, Stern JS, Greenwood MRC, Zucker LM, Hirsch J: Effect of early nutrition on adipose cellularity and pancreatic insulin release in the Zucker rat. *J Nutr* **103**:738, 1973.
76. Hirsch J, Batchelor BR: Adipose tissue cellularity in human obesity, in: Albrink M (ed): *Clinics in Endocrinology and Metabolism*, vol. 5, no. 2. London, WB Saunders, 1976, p 299.
77. Fomon S, Rogers R, Ziegler E, Nelson S, Thomas L: Indices of fatness and serum cholesterol at age eight years in relation to feeding and growth during early infancy. *Pediatr Res* **18**:1233, 1984.
78. DeSwiet M, Fayers P, Cooper L: Effect of feeding habit on weight in infancy. *Lancet* **II**:892, 1977.
79. DuBois S, Hill D, Beaton G: An examination of factors believed to be associated with infantile obesity. *Am J Clin Nutr* **32**:1997, 1979.
80. Butte C, Garza C, Smith E, Nichols B: Human milk intake and growth in exclusively breast fed infants. *J Pediatr* **104(2)**:187, 1984.
81. Enzi G, Inelman E, Rubaltelli F, Zinardo V, Favaretto L: Postnatal development of adipose tissue in normal children on strictly controlled caloric intake. *Metabolism* **31**:1029, 1982.
82. Leibel RL, Hirsch J, Appel BE, Checani GC: Energy intake required to maintain body weight is not affected by wide variation in diet composition. *Am J Clin Nutr* **55**:350, 1992.
83. Willett WC: Is dietary fat a major determinant of body bat? *Am J Clin Nutr* **67(Suppl)**:556, 1998.
84. Whitaker RC, Wright J, Pepe MS, Seidel KD, Deitz WH: Predicting obesity in young adulthood from childhood and parental obesity. *N Engl J Med* **337**:869, 1997.
85. Leibel RL, Berry EM, Hirsch J: Biochemistry and development of adipose tissue in man, in Conn HL, DeFelice EA, Kuo EA: (eds): *Pediatric Health and Obesity*. New York, Raven Press, 1983, p 21.
86. Johnston FE: Sex differences in fat patterning in children and youth, in Bouchard C, Johnston FE: (eds): *Fat Distribution During Growth and Later Health Outcomes*. New York, Alan R. Liss, 1988, p 85.
87. Knittle JL, Timmers K, Ginsberg-Fellner F, Brown RE, Katz DP: The growth of adipose tissue in children and adolescents. *J Clin Invest* **63**:239, 1979.
88. Atlan-Gepner C, Bongrand P, Farnarier C, Xerri L, Choux R, Gauthier JF, Brue T, Vague P, Grob JJ, Vialettes B: Insulin-induced lipoatrophy in type diabetes. A possible tumor necrosis factor-alpha-medicated dedifferentiation of adipocytes. *Diabetes Care* **19**:1283, 1996.
89. Prins JB, O'Rahilly S: Regulation of adipose cell number in man. *Clin Sci* **92**:3, 1997.
90. Hirsch J, Batchelor B: Adipose tissue cellularity in human obesity. *Clin Endocrinol Metab* **5**:299, 1976.
91. Ailhaud G: Adipose cell differentiation in culture. *Mol Cell Biochem* **49**:17, 1982.
92. Doglio A, Amri E, Dani C, Grimaldi P, Deslex S, Negrel R, Ailhaud G: Effects of growth in the differentiation process of preadipose cells, in Isaksson O (ed): *Nordisk Insulin Symposium "Growth Hormone Basic and Clinical Aspects" Stockholm, Sweden 29 June 1 July 1987*, New York, Elsevier Science, 1987, p 299.
93. Faust IM, Miller WH: *Hyperplastic Growth of Adipose Tissue in Obesity*. New York, Raven Press, 1983, p 41.
94. Ailhaud G, Grimaldi P, Negrel R: Cellular and molecular aspects of adipose tissue development. *Annu Rev Nutr* **12**:207, 1992.
95. Hager A, Sjostrom L, Arvidsson B, Bjorntorp P, Smith U: Adipose tissue cellularity in obese school girls before and after dietary treatment. *Am J Clin Nutr* **31**:68, 1978.
96. Tontonoz P, Hu E, Spiegelman BM: Stimulation of adipogenesis in fibroblasts by PPAR gamma 2, a lipid-activated transcription factor. *Cell* **79**:1147, 1994.
97. Tontonoz P, Hu E, Graves RA, Budavari A, Spiegelman BM: mPPAR gamma 2: Tissue-specific regulator of an adipocyte enhancer. *Genes Dev* **8**:1224, 1994.
98. Spiegelman BM, Flier JS: Adipogenesis and obesity: Rounding out the big picture. *Cell* **87**:377, 1996.
99. Hu E, Tontonoz P, Spiegelman BM: Transdifferentiation of myoblasts by the adipogenic transcription factors PPAR gamma and C/EBP alpha. *Proc Natl Acad Sci U S A* **92**:9856, 1995.
100. Wang ND, Finegold MJ, Bradley A, Ou CN, Abdelsayed SV, Wilde MD, Taylor LR, Wilson DR, Darlington GJ: Impaired energy homeostasis in C/EBP alpha knockout mice. *Science* **269**:1108, 1995.
101. Wu Z, Bucher NL, Farmer SR: Induction of peroxisome proliferator-activated receptor gamma during the conversion of 3T3 fibroblasts into adipocytes is mediated by C/EBPbeta, C/EBPdelta and glucocorticoids. *Mol Cell Biol* **16**:4128, 1996.
102. Kim JB, Spiegelman BM: ADD1/SREBP1 promotes adipocyte differentiation and gene expression linked to fatty acid metabolism. *Genes Dev* **10**:1096, 1996.
103. Meirhaeghe A, Fajas L, Helbecque N, Cottel D, Lebel P, Dallongeville J, Deeb S, Auwerx J, Amouyel P: A genetic polymorphism of the peroxisome proliferator-activated receptor gamma gene influences plasma leptin levels in obese humans. *Hum Mol Genet* **7**:435, 1998.
106. Adams M, Montague CT, Prins JB, Holder JC, Smith SA, Sanders L, Digby JE, Sewter CP, Lazar MA, Chatterjee VK, et al: Activators of peroxisome proliferator-activated receptor gamma have depot-specific effects on human preadipocyte differentiation. *J Clin Invest* **100**:3149, 1997.
107. Hamilton BS, Paglia D, Kwan AYM, Deitel M: Increased obese mRNA expression in omental fat cells from massively obese humans. *Nat Med* **9**:953, 1995.
108. Sierra-Honigmann MR, Nath AK, Murakami C, Garcia-Cardena G, Papapetropoulos A, Sessa WC, Madge LA, Schechner JS, Schwabb MB, Polverini PJ, et al: Biological action of leptin as an angiogenic factor. *Science* **281**:1683, 1998.
109. Gregoire FM, Johnson PR, Greenwood MR. Comparison of the adipoconversion of preadipocytes derived from lean and obese Zucker rats in serum-free cultures. *Int J Obes Relat Metab Disord* **19**:664, 1995.
110. Kleiber M: *The Fire of Life*. Malabar, FL, Robert E. Krieger, 1975.
111. Staffieri JR: A study of social stereotype of body image in children. *J Pers Soc Psychol* **10**:337, 1969.
112. Ravussin E, Lillioja S, Anderson TE, Christin L, Bogardus C: Determinants of 24-hour energy expenditure in man. Methods andresults using a respiratory chamber. *J Clin Invest* **78**:1568, 1986.
113. Newsholme EA. Substrate cycles: Their metabolic, energetic and thermic consequences in man. *Biochem Soc Symp* **43**:183, 1978.

114. Belanger BA, Cupples LA, D'Agostino RB. The Framingham Study: An epidemiologic study investigation of cardiovascular disease. Section 36: Measures at each examination and interexamination consistency of specified characteristics. Framingham publicationNo. 88-2970, 1988.
115. Edholm O: Energy balance in man. *J Hum Nutr* **31**:413, 1977.
116. Birch LL, Johnson SL, Andersen G, Peters JC, Schulte MC. The variability of young children's energy intake. *N Engl J Med* **324**:233, 1991.
117. Russek M: Demonstration of the influence of an hepatic glucosensitive mechanism on food intake. *Physiol Behav* **5**:1207, 1970.
118. Campfield LA, Smith FJ: Systemic factors in control of food intake, in *Handbook of Behavioral Neurobiology*. New York: Plenum Press, 1990, p 183.
119. VanItallie TB: The glucostatic theory 1953–1988: Roots and branches. *Int J Obes* **14**:1, 1990.
120. Flatt J: Dietary fat, carbohydrate balance, and weight maintenance. *Ann N Y Acad Sci* **683**:122, 1993.
121. Friedman MI, Tordoff MG, Ramirez I: Integrated metabolic control of food intake. *Brain Res Bull* **17**:855, 1991.
122. Kennedy GC: The role of depot fat in the hypothalamic control of food intake in the rat. *Proc Royal Soc Biol Sci* **140**:578, 1953.
123. Hervey GR: Regulation of energy balance. *Nature* **222**:629, 1969.
124. Hervey GR: A hypothetical mechanism for the regulation of food intake in relation to energy balance. *Proc Nutr Soc* **28**:54A, 1969.
125. Hervey GR: Physiological mechanisms for the regulation of energy balance. *Proc Nutr Soc* **30**:109, 1971.
126. Parameswaran SV, Steffens AB, Hervey GR, deRuiter L: Involvement of a humoral factor in regulation of body weight in parabiotic rats. *Am J Physiol* **232**:R150, 1977.
127. Leibel RL, Rosenbaum M, Hirsch J: Changes in energy expenditure resulting from altered body weight in man. *N Engl J Med* **332**:621, 1995.
128. Leibel RL, Hirsch J: Diminished energy requirements in reduced-obese patients. *Metabolism* **33**:164, 1984.
129. Weigle DS, Sande KJ, Iverius PH, Monsen ER, Brunzell JD: Weight loss leads to a marked decrease in nonresting energy expenditure in ambulatory human subjects. *Metabolism* **37**:930, 1988.
130. Amatruda J, Statt M, Welle S: Total and resting energy expenditure in obese women reduced to ideal body weight. *J Clin Invest* **92**:1236, 1993.
131. McCargar LJ, Sale J, Crawford SM: Chronic dieting does not result in a sustained reduction in resting metabolic rate in overweight women. *J Am Diet Assoc* **96**:1175, 1996.
132. Ballor DL, Poehlman ET: A meta-analysis of the effects of exercise and/or dietary restriction on resting metabolic rate. *Eur J Appl Physiol* **71**:535, 1995.
133. dePeuter R, Withers RT, Brinkman M, Tomas FM, Clark DG: No differences in rates of energy expenditure between post-obese women and their matched, lean controls. *Int J Obes Relat Metab Disord* **16**:801, 1992.
134. Rosenbaum M, Ravussin E, Matthews DE, Gilker C, Ferraro R, Heysmfield SB, Hirsch J, Leibel RL: A comparative study of different means of assessing long-term energy expenditure in humans. *Am J Physiol* **270**:R496, 1996.
135. Hirsch J, Leibel RL: A biologic basis for human obesity. *J Clin Endocrinol Metab* **73**:1153, 1991.
136. Bray GA, York DA: Genetically transmitted obesity in rodents. *Physiol Rev* **51**:598, 1971.
137. Leibel RL, Chung WK, Chua SC: The molecular genetics of rodent single gene obesities. *J Biol Chem* **272**:31937, 1997.
138. Roberts SB, Savage J, Coward WA: Energy expenditure and intake in infants born to lean and over-weight mothers. *N Engl J Med* **318**:461, 1988.
139. Ravussin E, Lillioja S, Knowler WC, Christin L, Freymond D, Abbott WG, VBoyce, Howard BV, Bogardus C: Reduced rate of energy expenditure as a risk factor for body-weight gain. *N Engl J Med* **318**:467, 1988.
140. Poehlman ET, Tremblay A, Fontaine E: Genotype dependency of the thermic effect of a meal and associated hormonal changes following short-term overfeeding. *Metabolism* **35**:30, 1986.
141. Poehlman ET, Despres JP, Marcotte M, Tremblay A, Theriault G, Bouchard C: Genotype dependency of adaptation in adipose tissue metabolism after short-term overfeeding. *Am J Physiol* **250**:E480, 1986.
142. Saltzman E, Dallal GE, Roberts SB. Effect of high-fat and low-fat diets on voluntary energy intake and substrate oxidation: Studies in identical twins consuming diets matched for energy density, fiber and palatability. *Am J Clin Nutr* **66**:1332, 1997.
143. deCastro JM: Independence of genetic influences of body size, daily intake, and meal patterns of humans. *Physiol Behav* **54**:633, 1993.
144. deCastro JM: Genetic influences on daily intake and meal patterns of humans. *Physiol Behav* **53**:777, 1993.
145. Falciglia GA, Norton PA: Evidence for a genetic influence on preference for some foods. *J Am Diet Assoc* **94**:154, 1994.
146. Katz J, Rognstad R: Futile cycles in the metabolism of glucose. *Curr Top Cell Regul* **10**:237, 1976.
147. Himms-Hagen J: Thermogenesis in brown adipose tissue as an energy buffer. *N Engl J Med* **311**:1549, 1984.
148. Nicholls DG, Locke RM: Thermogenic mechanisms in brown fat. *Physiol Rev* **64**:1, 1984.
149. Boss O, Muzzin P, Giacobino J-P: The uncoupling proteins, a review. *Eur J Endocrinol* **139**:1, 1998.
150. Jacobsson A, Stadler U, Glotzer MA, Kozak LP: Mitochondrial uncoupling protein from mouse brown fat. Molecular cloning, genetic mapping and mRNA expression. *J Biol Chem* **260**:16250, 1985.
151. Himms-Hagen J: Brown adipose tissue thermogenesis: interdisciplinary studies. *FASEB J* **4**:2890, 1990.
152. Wolfe RR, Klein S, Herndon DN, Jahoor F: Substrate cycling in thermogenesis and amplification of net substrate flux in human volunteers and burned patients. *J Trauma* **30**:S6, 1990.
153. Fleury C, Neverova M, Collins S, Raimbault S, Champigny O, Levi-Meyrueis C, Bouillaud F, Seldin ME, Surwit RS, Ricquier D, et al.: Uncoupling protein-2: A novel gene linked to obesity and hyperinsulinemia. *Nat Genet* **15**:269, 1997.
154. Gimeno RE, Dembski M, Weng X, Deng N, Shyjan AW, Gimeno CJ, Iris F, Ellis SJ, Woolf EA, Tartaglia LA: Cloning and characterization of an uncoupling protein homolog: A potential molecular mediator of human thermogenesis. *Diabetes* **46**:900, 1997.
155. Boss O, Samec S, Paolini-Giacobino A, Rossier C, Dulloo A, Seydoux J, Muzzin P, Giacobino JP: Uncoupling protein-3: A new member of the mitochondrial carrier family with tissue-specific expression. *FEBS Lett* **408**:39, 1997.
156. Vidal-Puig A, Solanes G, Grujic D, Flier JS, Lowell BB: UCP3: An uncoupling protein homologue expressed preferentially and abundantly in skeletal muscle and brown adipose tissue. *Biochem Biophys Res Commun* **235**:79, 1997.
157. Gong DW, He Y, Karas M, Reitman M: Uncoupling protein-3 is a mediator of thermogenesis regulated by thyroid hormone, beta3-adrenergic agonists, and leptin. *J Biol Chem* **272**:24129, 1997.
158. Chung WK, Luke A, Cooper RS, Rotini C, Vidal-Puig A, Rosenbaum M, Chua M, Solanes G, Zheng M, Zhao L, et al: Genetic and physiological analysis of the role of ucp3 in human obesity and energy homeostasis. Submitted for Publication, *Diabetes* **48**: 1890, 1999.
159. Boss O, Samec S, Dulloo A, Seydouz J, Muzzin P, Giacobino JP: Tissue-dependent upregulation of rat uncoupling protein-2 expression in response to fasting or cold. *FEBS Lett* **412**:111, 1997.
160. Nagase I, Yoshida T, Kumamoto K, Umekawa T, Sakane N, Nikami H, Kawada T, Saito M: Expression of uncoupling protein in skeletal muscle and white fat of obese mice treated with thermogenic beta 3-adrenergic agonist. *J Clin Invest* **97**:2898, 1996.
161. Boss O, Samec S, Kuhne F, Bijlenga P, Jeannet-Assimacopoulos F, Seydoux J, Giacobino JP, Muzzin P: Uncoupling protein-3 expression in rodent skeletal muscle is modulated by food intake but not by changes in environmental temperature. *J Biol Chem* **273**:5, 1998.
162. Millet L, Vidal H, Andreelli F, Larrouy D, Riou JP, Ricquier D, Laville M, Langin D: Increased uncoupling protein-2 and -3 mRNA expression during fasting in obese and lean humans. *J Clin Invest* **100**:2665, 1997.
163. Vidal-Puig A, Rosenbaum M, Considine R, Leibel RL, Lowell BB: Effects of obesity and stable weight reduction on UCP2 and UCP3 gene expression in humans. *Obes Res* **7**:133, 1999.
164. Segal KR, Simoneau J-A, Rosenbaum M, Hirsch J, Leibel RL: Impact of body weight perturbation in energy efficiency during exercise. Submitted for publication, 1998.
170. Zurlo F, Nemeth PM, Choksi RM, Sesodia S, Ravussin E: Whole-body energy *Metabolism* and skeletal muscle biochemical characteristics. *Metabolism* **43**:481, 1994.
171. Schutz Y, Flatt JP, Jequier E: Failure of dietary fat intake to promote fat oxidation: A factor favoring the development of obesity. *Am J Clin Nutr* **50**:307, 1989.
172. Flatt JP: The difference in the storage capacities for carbohydrate and for fat, and its implications in the regulation of body weight. *Ann N Y Acad Sci* **499**:104, 1987.

173. Hill JO, Drougas H, Peters JC: Obesity treatment: Can diet composition play a role. *Ann Intern Med* **120**:520, 1994.
174. Bray GA: Integration of energy intake and expenditure in animals and man: The autonomic and adrenal hypothesis. *J Clin Endocrinol Metab* **13**:521, 1984.
175. Harper ME, Ballantyne JS, Leach M, Brand MD: Effects of thyroid hormones on oxidative phosphorylation. *Biochem Soc Trans* **21**:785, 1993.
176. Jung RT, Campbell RG, James WP, Callingham BA: Altered hypothalamic and sympathetic response to hypoglycaemia in familial obesity. *Lancet* **1(8280)**:1043, 1982.
177. Aronne LJ, Mackintosh R, Rosenbaum M, Leibel RL, Hirsch J: Autonomic nervous system activity in weight gain and weight loss. *Am J Physiol* **269**:R222, 1995.
178. Jung RT, Shetty PS, James WPT: Nutritional effects on thyroid and catecholamine metabolism. *Clin Sci* **58**:97, 1980.
179. Landsberg L, Young JB: The role of the sympathoadrenal system in modulating energy expenditure. *J Clin Endocrinol Metab* **13**:475, 1984.
180. Leibel RL, Berry EM, Hirsch J: Metabolic and hemodynamic responses to endogenous and exogenous catecholamines in formerly obese subjects. *Am J Physiol* **260**:R785, 1991.
181. Vagenakis AG, Burger A, Portnoy GI, Rudolph M, OBrien JR, Azizi F, Arky RA, Nicod P, Ingbar SH, Braverman LE: Diversion of peripheral thyroxine metabolism from activating to inactivating pathways during complete fasting. *J Clin Endocrinol Metab* **41**:191, 1975.
182. Danforth E, Burger A: The role of thyroid hormones in the control of energy expenditure. *Clin Endocrinol Metab* **13**:581, 1984.
183. Wimpfheimer C, Saville E, Voirol MJ, Danforth E, Burger AG: Starvation-induced decreased sensitivity of resting metabolic rate to triiodothyronine. *Science* **205**:1272, 1979.
184. Ono N, Kohga H, Zama A, Inoue HK, Tamura M. A comparison of children with suprasellar germ cell tumors and craniopharyngiomas: Final height, weight, endocrine and visual sequelae after treatment. *Surg Neurol* **46**:370, 1996.
185. Curtis J, Daneman D, Hoffman HJ, Ehrlich RM: The endocrine outcome after surgical removal of craniopharyngiomas. *Pediatr Neurosurg* **21(Suppl)**:24, 1994.
186. Bray GA, Gallagher TF: Manifestations of hypothalamic obesity in man: A comprehensive investigation of eight patients and a review of the literature. *Medicine* **54**:301, 1975.
187. Hetherington AW, Ranson SW: Hypothalamic lesions and adiposity in the rat. *Anat Rec* **78**:149, 1940.
188. Olney JW: Brain lesions, obesity, and other disturbances in mice treated with monosodium glutamate. *Science* **164**:719, 1969.
189. Kirchgessner AL, Sclafani A: Histochemical identification of a PVN-hindbrain feeding pathway. *Physiol Behav* **42**:529, 1988.
190. Kirchgessner AL, Sclafani A: PVA-hindbrain pathway involved in the hypothalamic hyperphagia-obesity syndrome. *Physiol Behav* **42**:517, 1988.
191. Bernardis LL, Bellinger LL: Production of weanling rat ventromedial and dorsomedial hypothalamic syndromes by electrolytic lesions with platinum-iridium electrodes. *Neuroendocrinology* **22**:97, 1976.
192. Debons AF, Krimmsky I, Maayan ML, Fani K, Jimenez FA: Gold thioglucose obesity syndome. *Federation Proc* **36**:143, 1977.
193. Kennedy GC: Food intake, energy balance and growth. *Br Med Bull* **22**:216, 1966.
194. Keesey RE, Hirvonen MD: Body weight set-points: Determination and adjustment. *J Nutr* **127**:1875S, 1997.
195. Anand BK, Brobeck JR: Nutrition classics: The Yale Journal of Biology and Medicine, vol. XXIV, 1951-1952, hypothalamic control of food intake in rats and cats. *Nutr Rev* **42**:354, 1984.
196. Nadaud D, Simon H, Herman JP, LeMoal M: Contributions of the mesencephalic dopaminergic system and the trigeminal sensory pathway to the ventral tegmental aphagia syndrome in rats. *Physiol Behav* **33**:879, 1984.
197. Lenard L, Jando G, Karadi Z, Hajnal A, Sandor P. Lateral hypothalamic feeding mechanisms: Iontophoretic effects of kainic acid, ibotenic acid and 6-hydroxydopamine. *Brain Res Bull* **20**:847, 1988.
198. Markowska A, Bakke HK, Walther B, Ursin H: Comparison of electrolytic and ibotenic acid lesions in the lateral hypothalamus. *Brain Res* **328**:313, 1985.
199. Oltmans GA, Harvey JA: Lateral hypothalamic syndrome in rats: A comparison of the behavioral and neurochemical effects of lesions placed in the lateral hypothalamus and nigrostriatal bundle. *J Comp Physiol Psychol* **90**:1051, 1976.
200. Grossman SP, Dacey D, Halaris AE, Collier T, Routtenberg A: Aphagia and adipsia after preferential destruction of nerve cell bodies in hypothalamus. *Science* **202**:537, 1978.
201. Chua SC, Leibel RL, Hirsch J: Food deprivation and age modulate neuropeptide gene expression in the murine hypothalamus and adrenal gland. *Mol Brain Res* **9**:95, 1991.
202. Williams G, Gill JS, Lee YC, Cardoso HM, Okpere BE, Bloom SR: Increased neuropeptide Y concentrations in specific hypothalamic regions of streptozocin-induced diabetic rats. *Diabetes* **38**:321, 1989.
203. White JD, Olchovsky D, Kershaw M, Berelowitz M: Increased hypothalamic content of preproneuropeptide-Y messenger ribonucleic acid streptozotocin diabetic rats. *J Endocrinol* **126**:765, 1990.
204. Sahu A, Sninski CA, Kalra PS, Kalra SP: Neuropeptide-Y concentration in microdissected hypothalamic regions and in vitro release from the medial basal hypothalamus-preoptic area of streptozotocin-diabetic rats with and without insulin substitution therapy. *Endocrinology* **126**:192, 1990.
205. Mercer JG, Moar KM, Rayner DV, Trayhurn P, Hoggard N: Regulation of leptin receptor and NPY gene expression in hypothalamus of leptin-treated obese (*ob/ob*) and cold-exposed lean mice. *FEBS Lett* **402**:185, 1997.
206. Lewis DE, Shellard L, Koeslag DG, Boer DE, McCarthy HD, McKibbin PE, Russell JC, Williams G: Intense exercise and food restriction cause similar hypothalamic neuropeptide Y increases in rats. *Am J Physiol* **264**:E279, 1993.
207. Wilding JP, Ajala MO, Lambert PD, Bloom SR: Additive effects of lactation and food restriction to increase hypothalamic neuropeptide Y mRNA in rats. *J Endocrinol* **152**:365, 1997.
208. Pickavance L, Dryden S, Hopkins D, Bing C, Frankish H, Wang Q, Vernon RG, Williams G: Relationships between hypothalamic neuropeptide Y and food intake in the lactating rat. *Peptides* **17**:577, 1996.
209. Clark JT, Kalra PS, Kalra SP: Neuropeptide Y stimulates feeding but inhibits sexual behavior in rats. *Endocrinology* **117**:2435, 1985.
210. Levine AS, Morley JE: Neuropeptide Y: A potent inducer of consummatory behavior in rats. *Peptides* **5**:1025, 1984.
211. Stanley BG, Leibowitz SF: Neuropeptide Y: Stimulation of feeding and drinking by injection into the paraventricular nucleus. *Life Sci* **35**:2635, 1984.
212. Jolicoeur FB, Michaud JN, Rivest R, Menard D, Gaudin D, Fournier A, St-Pierre S: Neurobehavioral profile of neuropeptide Y. *Brain Res Bull* **26**:265, 1991.
213. Erickson JC, Hollopeter G, Palmiter RD: Attenuation of the obesity syndrome of *ob/ob* mice by the loss of neuropeptide Y. *Science* **274**:1704, 1996.
214. Erickson JC, Clegg KE, Palmiter RD: Sensitivity to leptin and susceptibility to seizures of mice lacking neuropeptide Y. *Nature* **381**:415, 1996.
215. Pedrazzini T, Seydouz J, Kunstner P, Aubert JF, Grouzmann E, Beermann F, Brunner HR: Cardiovascular response, feeding behavior and locomotor activity in mice lacking the NPY Y1 receptor. *Nat Medi* **4**:722, 1998.
216. Ollmann MM, Wilson BD, Yang YK, JKerns JA, Chen Y, Gantz I, Barsh GS: Antagonism of central melanocortin receptors in vitro and in vivo by agouti-related protein. *Science* **278**:135, 1997.
217. Fong TM, Mao C, MacNeil T, Kalyani R, Smith T, Weinberg D, Tota MR, VanderPloeg LH: ART (protein product of agouti-related transcript) as an antagonist of MC-3 and MC-4 receptors. *Biochem Biophys Res Commun* **237**:629, 1997.
218. Mizuno TM, Kleppoulos SP, Bergen HT, Roberts JL, PRiest CA, Mobbs CV: Hypothalamic pro-opiomelanocortin mRNA is reduced by fasting and (corrected) in *ob/ob* and *db/db* mice, but is stimulated by leptin. *Diabetes* **47**:294, 1998.
219. Krude H, Biebermann H, Luck W, Horn R, Brabant G, Gruters A: Severe early-onset obesity, adrenal insufficiency and red hair pigmentation caused by POMC mutations in humans. *Nat Genet* **19**:155, 1998.
220. Nakanishi S, Teranishi Y, Noda M, Notake M, Watanabe Y, Kakidami H, Jingami H, Numa S: The protein-coding sequence of the bovine ACTH-beta-LPH precursor gene is split near the signal peptide region. *Nature* **287**:752, 1980.
221. Chang AC, Cochet M, Cohen SN: Structural organization of human genomic DNA encoding the pro-opiomelanocortin peptide. *Proc Natl Acad Sci U S A* **77**:489, 1980.
222. Thiele TE, VanDijk G, Campfield LA, SMith FJ, Burn P, Woods SC, Bernstein IL, Seeley RJ: Central infusion of GLP-1, but not leptin,

produces conditioned taste aversions in rats. *Am J Physiol* **272**:R726, 1997.
223. Fan W, Boston BA, Kesterson RA, Hruby VJ, Cone RD: Role of melanocortinergic neurons in feeding and the agouti obesity syndrome. *Nature* **385**:165, 1997.
224. Broberger C, Landry M, Wond H, Walsh JN, Hokfelt T: Subtypes Y1 and Y2 of the neuropeptide Y receptor are respectively expressed in pro-opiomelanocortin- and neuropeptide-Y-containing neurons of the rat hypothalamic arcuate nucleus. *Neuroendocrinology* **66**:393, 1997.
225. Garcia-de-Yebenes E, Li S, Fournier A, St-Pierre S, Pelletier G: Regulation of proopiomelanocortin gene expression by neuropeptide Y in the rat arcuate nucleus. *Brain Res* **674**:112, 1995.
226. Kristensen P, Judge ME, Thim L, Ribel U, Christjjansen KN, Wulff BS, Clausen JT, Jensen PB, Madsen OD, Vrang N, et al: Hypothalamic CART is a new anorectic peptide regulated by leptin. *Nature* **393**:72, 1998.
227. Perney TM, Miller RJ: Two different G-proteins mediate neuropeptide Y and bradykinin-stimulated phospholipid breakdown in cultured rat sensory neurons. *J Biol Chem* **264**:7317, 1989.
228. Hakansson ML, Brown H, Ghilardi N, Skoda RC, Meister B: Leptin receptor immunoreactivity in chemically defined target neurons of the hypothalamus. *J Neurosci* **18**:559, 1998.
229. Schwartz MW, Baskin DG, Bukowski TR, Kuijper JL, Foster D, Lasser G, Prunkard DE, Porte D, Woods SC, Seeley RJ, et al: Specificity of leptin action on elevated blood glucose levels and hypothalamic neuropeptide Y gene expression in *ob/ob* mice. *Diabetes* **45**:531, 1996.
230. Sanacora G, Kershaw M, Finkelstein JA, White JD: Increased hypothalamic content of preproneuropeptide Y messenger ribonucleic acid in genetically obese Zucker rats and its regulation by food deprivation. *Endocrinology* **127**:730, 1990.
231. Jhanwar-Uniyal M, Chua SC: Critical effects of aging and nutritional state on hypothalamic neuropeptide Y and galanin gene expression in lean and genetically obese Zucker rats. *Mol Brain Res* **19**:195, 1993.
232. Chua SC, Brown AW, Kim J, Hennessey KL, Leibel RL, Hirsch J: Food deprivation and hypothalamic neuropeptide gene expression: Effects of strain background and the diabetes mutation. *Mol Brain Res* **11**:291, 1991.
233. Thornton JE, Cheung CC, Clifton DK, Steiner RA: Regulation of hypothalamic proopiomelanocortin mRNA by leptin in *ob/ob* mice. *Endocrinology* **138**:5063, 1997.
234. Schwartz MW, Seeley RJ, Woods SC, Weigle DS, Campfield LA, Burn P, Baskin DG: Leptin increases hypothalamic pro-opiomelanocortin mRNA expression in the rostral arcuate nucleus. *Diabetes* **46**:2119, 1997.
235. Fuxe K, Cintra A, Agnati LF, Harfstrand A, Wikstrom A-C, Okret S, Zoli M, Miller LS, Greene JL, Gustafsson J-A: Studies on the cellular localization and distribution of glucocorticoid receptor and estrogen receptor immunoreactivity in the central nervous system of the rat and their relationship to the monoaminergic and peptidergic neurons of the brain. *J Steroid Biochem* **27**:159, 1987.
236. Watanabe Y, Akabayaski A, McEwen BS. Adrenal steroid regulation of neuropeptide Y (NPY) mRNA: Differences between dentate hilus and locus ceruleus and arcuate nucleus. *Brain Res Mol Brain Res* **28**:135, 1995.
237. Wardlaw SL, McCarthy KC, Conwell IM: Glucocorticoid regulation of hypothalamic proopiomelanocortin. *Neuroendocrinology* **67**:51, 1998.
238. Dubuc PU, Carlisle HJ: Food restriction normalizes somatic growth and diabetes in adrenalectomized *ob/ob* mice. *Am J Physiol* **255**:R787, 1988.
239. Marchington D, Rothwell NJ, Stock MJ, York DA: Energy balance, diet-induced thermogenesis and brown adipose tissue in lean and obese (*fa/fa*) Zucker rats after adrenalectomy. *J Nutr* **113**:1395, 1983.
240. Turton MD, O'Shea D, Gunn I, Beak SA, Edwards CM, Meeran K, Choi SJ, Taylor GM, Heath MM, Lambert PD, et al: A role for glucagon-like peptide-1 in the central regulation of feeding. *Nature* **379**:69, 1996.
241. Tang-Christensen M, Vrang N, Larsen PJ: Glucagon-like peptide 1(7-36) amide's central inhibition of feeding and peripheral inhibition of drinking are abolished by neonatal monosodium glutamate treatment. *Diabetes* **47**:530, 1998.
242. Navarro M, Rodriquez-de-Fonseca F, Alvarez E, Chowen JA, Zueco JA, Gomez R, Eng J, Blazquez E: Colocalization of glucagon-like peptide-1 (GLP-1) receptors, glucose transporter GLUT-2 and glucokinase mRNAs in rat hypothalamic cells: Evidence for a role of GLP-1 receptor agonists as an inhibitory signal for food and water intake. *J Neurochem* **67**:1982, 1996.
243. Bell GI, Sanchez-Pescador R, Laybourn PJ, Najarian RC: Exon duplication and divergence in the human preproglucagon gene. *Nature* **304**:368, 1983.
244. Priest CA, Borsook D, Pfaff DW: Estrogen and stress interact to regulate the hypothalamic expression of a human proenkephalin promoter-beta-galactosidase fusion gene in a site-specific and sex-specific manner. *J Neuroendocrinol* **9**:317, 1997.
245. Zhang C, Pfaff DW, Kow LM: Functional analysis of opioid receptor subtypes in the ventromedial hypothalamic nucleus of the rat. *Eur J Pharmacol* **308**:153, 1996.
246. Gale SK, Sclafani A: Comparison of ovarian and hypothalamic obesity syndromes in the female rat: Effects of diet palatability on food intake and body weight. *J Comp Physiol Psychol* **91**:381, 1977.
247. Beatty WW, O'Briant DA, Vilberg TR: Effects of ovariectomy and estradiol injections on food intake and body weight in rats with ventromedial hypothalamic lesions. *Pharmacol Biochem Behav* **3**:539, 1975.
248. Wade GN: Some effects of ovarian hormones on food intake and body weight in female rats. *J Comp Physiol Psychol* **88**:183, 1975.
249. Mueller K, Hsaio S: Estrus- and ovariectomy-induced body weight changes: Evidence for two estrogenic mechanisms. *J Comp Physiol Psychol* **94**:1126, 1980.
250. Shimomura Y, Shimizu H, Kobayashi I, Kobayashi S: Importance of feeding time in pair-fed, ovariectomized rats. *Physiol Behav* **45**:1197, 1989.
251. Shimizu H, Shimomura Y, Sato N, Uehara Y, Kobayashi I: Colonic temperature was not changed in the development of obesity after ovariectomy. *Exp Clin Endocrinol* **99**:99, 1992.
252. Yoshioka K, Yoshida T, Wakabayashi Y, Nishioka H, Kondo M: Reduced brown adipose tissue thermogenesis of obese rats after ovariectomy. *Endocrinol Jpn* **35**:537, 1988.
253. Liaw CW, Lovenberg TW, Barry G, Oltersdorf T, Grigoriadis DE, deSouza EB: Cloning and characterization of the human corticotropin-releasing factor-2 receptor complementary deoxyribonucleic acid. *Endocrinology* **137**:72, 1996.
254. Lovenberg TW, Liaw CW, Grigoriadis DE, Clevenger W, Chalmers DT, deSouza EB, Oltersdorf T: Cloning and characterization of a functionally distinct corticotropin-releasing factor receptor subtype from rat brain. *Proc Natl Acad Sci U S A* **92**:836, 1995.
255. Perrin M, Donaldson C, Chen R, Blount A, Berggren T, Bilezikjian L, Sawchenko P, Vale W: Identification of a second corticotropin-releasing factor receptor gene and characterization of a cDNA expressed in heart. *Proc Natl Acad Sci U S A* **92**:2969, 1995.
256. Makino S, Nishiyama M, Asaba K, Gold PW, Hashimoto K: Altered expression of type 2 CRH receptor mRNA in the VMH by glucocorticoids and starvation. *Am J Physiol* **275**:R1138, 1998.
257. Jones DN, Kortekaas R, Slade PD, Middlemiss DN, Hagan JJ: The behavioural effects of corticotropin-releasing factor-related peptides in rats. *Psychopharmacology (Berl)* **138**:124, 1998.
258. Spina M, Merlo-Pich E, Chan RK, Basso AM, Rivier J, Vale W, Koob GF: Appetite-suppressing effects of urocortin, a CRF-related neuropeptide. *Science* **273**:1561, 1996.
259. Smagin GN, Howell LA, Rayn DH, DeSouza EB, Harris RB: The role of CRF2 receptors in corticotropin-releasing factor- and urocortin-induced anorexia. *Neuroreport* **9**:1601, 1998.
260. Moreau JL, Kilpatrick G, Jenck F: Urocortin, a novel neuropeptide with anorexigenic-like properties. *Neuroreport* **8**:1697, 1997.
261. Koopmans HS, Deutsch JA, Branson PJ: The effect of cholecystokinin-pancreozymin on hunger and thirst in mice. *Behav Biol* **7**:441, 1972.
262. Asaba K, Makino S, Hashimoto K: Effect of urocortin on ACTH secretion from rat anterior pituitary in vitro and in vivo: Comparison with corticotropin-releasing hormone. *Brain Res* **806**:95, 1998.
263. Liposits Z, Sievers L, Paull WK: Neuropeptide-Y and ACTH-immunoreactive innervation of corticotropin releasing factor (CRF)-synthesizing neurons int he hypothalamus of the rat. An immunocytochemical analysis at the light and electron microscopic levels. *Histochemistry* **88**:227, 1988.
264. Baker RA, Herkenham M, Brady LS: Effects of long-term treatment with antidepressant drugs on proopiomelanocortin and neuropeptide Y mRNA expression in the hypothalamic arcuate nucleus of rats. *J Neuroendocrinol* **8**:337, 1996.
265. Drescher VS, Chen HL, Romsos DR: Corticotropin-releasing hormone decreases feeding, oxygen consumption and activity of genetically obese (*ob/ob*) and lean mice. *J Nutr* **124**:524, 1994.

266. Gosnell BA, Morley JE, Levine AS: A comparison of the effects of corticotropin-releasing factor and sauvagine on food intake. *Pharmacol Biochem Behav* **19**:771, 1983.
267. Uehara Y, Shimizu H, Ohtani K, Sato N, Mori M: Hypothalamic corticotropin-releasing hormone is a mediator of the anorexigenic effect of leptin. *Diabetes* **47**:890, 1998.
268. Huang Q, Rivest R, Richard D: Effects of leptin on corticotropin-releasing factor (CSF) synthesis and CRF neuron activation in the paraventricular hypothalamic nucleus of obese (*ob/ob*) mice. *Endocrinology* **139**:1524, 1998.
269. Hajnal A, Mark GP, Rada PV, Lenard L, Hoebel BG: Norepinephrine microinjections in the hypothalamic paraventricular nucleus increase extracellular dopamine and decrease acetylcholine in the nucleus accumbens: Relevance to feeding reinforcement. *J Neurochem* **68**:667, 1997.
270. Leibowitz SF, Hammer NJ, Chang K: Feeding behavior induced by central norepinephrine injection is attenuated by discrete lesions in the hypothalamic paraventricular nucleus. *Pharmacol Biochem Behav* **19**:945, 1983.
271. Rada P, Mark GP, Hoebel BG: Galanin in the hypothalamus raises dopamine and lowers acetylcholine release in the nucleus accumbens: A possible mechanism for hypothalamic initiation of feeding behavior. *Brain Res* **798**:1, 1998.
272. Koegler FH, Ritter S: Galanin injection into the nucleus of the solitary tract stimulates feeding in rats with lesions of the paraventricular nucleus of the hypothalamus. *Physiol Behav* **63**:521, 1998.
273. Bai FL, Yamano M, Shiotani Y, Emson PC, Smith AD, Powell JF, Tohyama M: An arcuato-paraventricular and -dorsomedial hypothalamic neuropeptide Y-containing system which lacks noradrenaline in the rat. *Brain Res* **331**:172, 1985.
274. Kerkerian L, Pelletier G: Effects of monosodium L-glutamate administration on neuropeptide Y-containing neurons in the rat hypothalamus. *Brain Res* **369**:388, 1986.
275. Bernardis LL, Bellinger LL: The dorsomedial hypothalamic nucleus revisited: 1998 update. *Proc Soc Exp Biol Med* **218**:284, 1998.
276. Kesterson RA, Huszar D, Lynch CA, Simerly RB, Cone RD: Induction of neuropeptide Y gene expression in the dorsal medial hypothalamic nucleus of two models of the agouti obesity syndrome. *Mol Endocrinol* **11**:630, 1997.
277. Nahon JL: The melanin-concentrating hormone: From the peptide to the gene. *Crit Rev Neurobiol* **8**:221, 1994.
278. Sakurai T, Amemiya A, Ishii M, Matsuzaki I, Chemelli RM, Tanaka H, Williams SC, Richardson JA, Kozlowski GP, Wilson S, et al: Orexins and orexin receptors: A family of hypothalamic neuropeptides and G protein-coupled receptors that regulate feeding behavior. *Cell* **92**:573, 1998.
279. deLecea L, Kilduff TS, Peyron C, Gao X, Foye PE, Danielson PE, Fukuhara C, Battenberg EL, Gautvik VT, Bartlett FS, et al: The hypocretins: Hypothalamus-specific peptides with neuroexcitatory activity. *Proc Natl Acad Sci U S A* **95**:322, 1998.
280. Schick RR, Harty GJ, Yaksh TL, Go VL: Sites in the brain at which cholecystokinin octapeptide (CCK-8) acts to suppress feeding in rats: A mapping study. *Neuropharmacology* **29**:109, 1990.
281. Crawley JN, Kiss JZ: Paraventricular nucleus lesions abolish the inhibition of feeding induced by systemic cholecystokinin. *Peptides* **6**:927, 1985.
282. Palkovits M, Kiss JZ, Beinfeld MC, Williams TH: Cholecystokinin in the nucleus of the solitary tract of the rat: Evidence for its vagal origin. *Brain Res* **252**:386, 1982.
283. Ladenheim EE, Ritter RC: Caudal hindbrain participation in the suppression of feeding by central and peripheral bombesin. *Am J Physiol* **264**:R1229, 1993.
284. Lee MD, Aloyo VJ, Fluharty SJ, Simansky KJ: Infusion of the serotonin 1B (5-HT1B) agonist CP-93, 129 into the parabrachial nucleus potently and selectively reduces food intake in rats. *Psychopharmacology* **136**:304, 1998.
285. Halford JC, Blundell JE: The 5-HT1B receptor agonist CP-94,253 reduces food intake and preserves the behavioural satiety sequence. *Physiol Behav* **60**:933, 1996.
286. Kitchener SJ, Dourish C: An examination of the behavioural specificity of hypophagia induced by 5-HT1B, 5-HT1C and 5-HT2 receptor agonists using the post-prandial satiety sequence in rats. *Psychopharmacology* **113**:369, 1994.
287. Tecott LH, Sun LM, Akana SF, Strack AM, Lowenstein DH, Dallman MF, Julius D: Eating disorder and epilepsy in mice lacking 5-HT2c serotonin receptors. *Nature* **374**:542, 1995.
288. Carr KD, Aleman DO, Bak TH, Simon EJ: Effects of parabrachial opioid antagonism on stimulation-induced feeding. *Brain Res* **545**:283, 1991.
289. Kotz CM, Grace MK, Briggs J, Levine AS, Billington CJ: Effects of opioid antagonists naloxone and naltrexone on neuropeptide Y-induced feeding and brown fat thermogenesis in the rat. Neural site of action. *J Clin Invest* **96**:163, 1995.
290. Kotz CM, Billington CJ, Levine AS: Opioids in the nucleus of the solitary tract are involved in feeding in the rat. *Am J Physiol* **272**:R1028, 1997.
291. Epstein AN: The ontogeny of neurochemical systems for control of feeding and drinking. *Proc Soc Exp Biol Med* **175**:127, 1984.
292. Swithers SE, Hall WG: A nutritive control of independent ingestion in rat pups emerges by nine days of age. *Physiol Behav* **46**:873, 1989.
293. Phifer CB, Hall WG: Ingestive behavior in preweanling rats: Emergence of postgastric controls. *Am J Physiol* **255**:R191, 1988.
294. Gibbs J, Smith GP: Gut peptides and food in the gut produce similar satiety effects. *Peptides* **3**:553, 1982.
295. Eysselein VE, Eberlein GA, Schaeffer M, Grandt D, Goebell H, Niebel W, Rosenquist GL, Meyer HE, Reeve JR: Characterization of the major form of cholecystokinin in human intestine: CCK-58. *Am J Physiol* **258**:G253, 1990.
296. Turkelson CM, Solomon TE: Molecular forms of cholecystokinin in rat intestine. *Am J Physiol* **259**:G364, 1990.
297. Ritter RC, Brenner LA, Tamura CS: Endogenous CCK and the peripheral neural substrates of intestinal satiety. *Ann N Y Acad Sci* **713**:255, 1994.
298. Ivy AC, Oldberg E: Contraction and evacuation of gall bladder caused by highly purified "secretin" preparation. *Proc Soc Exp Biol Med* **25**:113, 1927.
299. Harper AA, Raper HS: Pancreozymin, a stimulant of secretion of pancreatic enzymes in extracts of the small intestine. *J Physiol (Lond)* **102**:115, 1943.
300. Jorpes JE, Mutt V: Cholecystokinin and pancreozymin, one single hormone? *Acta Physiol Scand* **66**:196, 1966.
301. Mutt V, Jorpes E: Hormonal polypeptides of the upper intestine. *Biochem J* **125**:57, 1971.
302. Deschenes RJ, Lorens LJ, Haum RS, Roos BA, Collier KJ, Dixon JE: Cloning and sequence analysis of a cDNA encoding rat preprocholecystokinin. *Proc Natl Acad Sci U S A* **81**:726, 1984.
303. Calam J, Ellis A, Dockray CJ: Identification and measurement of molecular variants of cholecystokinin in duodenal mucosa and palma. *J Clin Invest* **69**:218, 1982.
304. Walsh JH, Lamer CB, Valenzuela JE: Cholecystokinin octapeptide-like immunoreactivity in human plasma. *Gastroenterology* **82**:438, 1982.
305. Eberlien GA, Eysselein VE, Boebell H: Cholecystokinin-58 is the major molecular form in man, dog and cat but not in pig, beef and rat intestine. *Peptides* **9**:993, 1988.
306. Smith GP, Dorre P, Melville L: CCK-33 inhibits food intake after intraportal and intravenous administration. *Soc Neurosci Abstr* **22**:17, 1996.
307. Greenberg D, Smith GP, Gibbs J: Infusion of CCK-8 into the hepatic-portal vein fails to reduce food intake in rats. *Am J Physiol* **252**:1015, 1987.
308. Cox JE, Perdue GS, Tyler WJ: Suppression of sucrose intake by continuous near-celiac and intravenous cholecystokinin infusions in rats. *Am J Physiol* **268**:R150, 1995.
309. Calingasan N, Ritter S, Ritter R, Brenner L: Low-dose near-celiac arterial cholecystokinin suppresses food intake in rats. *Am J Physiol* **263**:R572, 1992.
310. Moran TH, Ladenheim EE: Identification of receptor populations mediating the satiating actions of brain and gut peptides, in Smith GP (ed): *Satiation: From Gut to Brain*. New York, Oxford University Press, 1998, pp 126–163.
311. Weller A, Smith GP, Gibbs J: Endogenous cholecystokinin reduces feeding in young rats. *Science* **247**:1589, 1990.
312. Joyner K, Smith GP, Gibbs J: Abdominal vagotomy decreases the satiating potency of CCK-8 in sham and real feeding. *Am J Physiol* **264**:R912, 1993.
313. LeSauter J, Goldberg B, Geary N: CCK inhibits real and sham feeding in gastric vagotomized rats. *Physiol Behav* **44**:527, 1988.
314. Monnikes H, Lauer G, Arnold R: Peripheral administration of cholecystokinin activates c-fos expression in the locus coeruleus/subcoeruleus nucleus, dorsal vagal complex and paraventricular nucleus via capsaicin-sensitive vagal afferents and CCK-A receptors in the rat. *Brain Res* **770**:277, 1997.

315. Moran TH, Robinson PH, Goldrich MS, McHugh P: Two brain cholecystokinin receptors: Implications for behavioral actions. *Brain Res* **362**:175, 1986.
316. Wank SA, Pisgena JR, DeWeerth A: Brain and gastrointestinal cholecystokinin receptor family: Structure and functional expression. *Proc Natl Acad Sci U S A* **89**:8691, 1992.
317. Passaro E, Debas H, Oldendorf W, Yamada T: Rapid appearance of intraventricularly administered neuropeptides in the peripheral circulation. *Brain Res* **241**:335, 1982.
318. Takiguchi S, Takata Y, Funakoshi A, Miyasaka K, Kataoka K, Fujimura Y, Goto T, Kono A: Disrupted cholecystokinin type-A receptor (CCKAR) gene in OLETF rats. *Gene* **197**:169, 1997.
319. Moran TH, Katz LF, Plata-Salaman CR, Schwartz GJ: Disordered food intake and obesity in rats lacking cholecystokinin A receptors. *Am J Physiol* **274**:R618, 1998.
320. Gibbs J, Fauser DJ, Rowe EA, Rolls BJ, Rolls ET, Maddison SP: Bombesin suppresses feeding in rats. *Nature* **282**:208, 1979.
321. Yen EI, Miesner J, Gibbs J, Weller A, Smith GP: Intravenous bombesin reduces food intake in the rat. *Soc Neurosci Abstr* **15**:1280, 1989.
322. Miesner JA, Yen EI, Gibbs J, Weller A, Smith GP: Intravenous administration of cholecystokinin antagonist increases food intake in the rat. *Soc Neurosci Abstr* **15**:1280, 1989.
323. Greenberg D, Torres NI, Smith GP, Gibbs J: The satiating effects of fats is attenuated by the cholecystokinin antagonist proglumide. *Ann N Y Acad Sci* **575**:517, 1989.
324. Kirkham TC, Gibbs J, Smith GP: The satiating effect of bombesin is mediated by receptors perfused by the coeliac artery. *Am J Physiol* **261**:R614, 1991.
325. Stuckey JA, Gibbs J, Smith GP: Neural disconnection of gut from brain blocks bombesin-induced satiety. *Peptides* **6**:1249, 1985.
326. Stratford TR, Gibbs J, Smith GP: Simultaneous administration of neuromedin B-10 and gastrin-releasing peptide (1-27) reproduces the satiating and microstructural effects of bombesin. *Peptides* **17**:107, 1996.
327. Ohki-Hamazaki H, Watase K, Yamamoto K, Ogura H, Yamano M, Yamada K, Maeno H, Imaki J, Kikuyama S, Wada E, et al.: Mice lacking bombesin receptor subtype-3 develop metabolic defects and obesity. *Nature* **390**:165, 1997.
328. Hampton LL, Ladeheim EE, Way MAJM, Weber HC, Sutliff VE, Jensen RT, Wine LJ, Arnheiter H, Battey JF: Loss of bombesin-induced feeding suppression in gastrin-releasing peptide receptor-deficient mice. *Proc Natl Acad Sci U S A* **95**:3188, 1998.
329. Morley JE, Flood JF, Farr SA, Perry HJ, Kaiser FE, Morley PM: Effects of amylin on appetite regulation and memory. *Can J Physiol Pharmacol* **73**:1042, 1995.
330. Lutz TA, Rossi R, Althaus J, DelPrete E, Scharrer E: Evidence for a physiological role of central calcitonin gene-related peptide (CGRP) receptors int he control of food intake in rats. *Neurosci Lett* **230**:159, 1997.
331. Erlanson-Albertsson C, York D: Enterostatin — A peptide-regulating fat intake. *Obes Res* **5**:360, 1997.
332. Lu D, Willard D, Patel IR, Kadwell S, Overton L, Kost T, Luther M, Chen W, Woychik RP, Wilkison WO, et al.: Agouti protein is an antagonist of the melanocyte-stimulating-hormone receptor. *Nature* **371**:799, 1994.
333. Rubinstein M, Mogil JS, Japon M, Chan EC, Allen RG, Low MJ: Absence of opioid stress-induced analgesia in mice lacking beta-endorphin by site-directed mutagenesis. *Proc Natl Acad Sci U S A* **93**:3995, 1996.
334. Huszar D, Lynch CA, Fairchild-Huntress V, Dunmore JH, Fang Q, Berkemeier LR, Gu W, Kesterson RA, Boston BA, Cone RD, et al.: Targeted disruption of the melanocortin-4 receptor resulting in obesity in mice. *Cell* **88**:131, 1997.
335. Cone RD, Lu D, Koppula S, Vage DI, Klungland H, Boston B, Chen W, Orth DN, Pouton C, Kesterson RA: The melanocortin receptors: Agonists, antagonists, and the hormonal control of pigmentation. *Recent Prog Horm Res* **51**:287, 1996.
336. Yeo GS, Farooqi IS, Aminian S, Halsall DJ, Stanhope RG, O'Rahilly S: A frameshift mutation in MC4R associated with dominantly inherited human obesity. *Nat Genet* **20**:111, 1998.
337. Vaisse C, Clement K, Guy-Grand B, Forguel P: A frameshift mutation in human MC4R is associated with a dominant form of obesity. *Nat Genet* **20**:113, 1998.
338. Siegrist W, Drozdz R, Cotti R, Willard DH, Wilkison WO, Eberle AN: Interactions of alpha-melanotropin and agouti on B16 melanoma cells: Evidence for inverse agonism of agouti. *J Recep Signal Transduct Res* **17**:75, 1997.
339. Leff P, Scaramellini C, Law C, McKechnie K: A three-state receptor model of agonist action. *Trends Pharmacol* **18**:355, 1997.
340. Ollmann MM, Kamoreaux ML, Wilson BD, Barsh GS: Interaction of Agouti protein with the melanocortin receptor in vitro and in vivo. *Genes Dev* **12**:316, 1998.
341. Miwa H, Gantz I, Konda Y, Shimoto Y, Yamada T. Structural determinants of the melanocortin peptides required for activation of melanocortin-3 and melanocortin-4 receptors. *J Pharmacol Exp Ther* **273**:1248, 1995.
342. Prusis P, Frandberg PA, Muceniece R, Kalvinsh I, Wikberg JE: A three-dimensional model for the interaction of MSH with the melanocortin-1 receptor. *Biochem Biophys Res Commun* **210**:205, 1995.
343. Silvers WK: The agouti and extension series of alleles, umbrous and sable, in Silvers, Willys, eds: *The Coat Colors of Mice*. New York, Springer-Verlag, 1979, p 6.
344. Bultman SJ, Michaud EJ, Woychik RP: Molecular characterization of the mouse agouti locus. *Cell* **71**:1195, 1992.
345. Miller MW, Duhl DM, Vrieling H, Cordes SP, Ollmann MM, Winkes BM, Barsh GS: Cloning of the mouse agouti gene predicts a secreted protein ubiquitously expressed in mice carrying the lethal yellow mutation. *Genes Dev* **7**:454, 1993.
346. Duhl DM, Stevens ME, Vrieling H, Miller MW, Epstein CJ, Barsh GS: Pleiotropic effects of the mouse lethal yellow (A^y) mutation explained by deletion of a maternally expressed gene and the simultaneous production of agouti fusion RNAs. *Development* **120**:1695, 1994.
347. Michaud EJ, Bultman SJ, Stubbs LJ, Woychik RP: The embryonic lethality of homozygous lethal yellow mice (A^y/A^y) is associated with the disruption of a novel RNA-binding protein. *Genes Dev* **7**:1203, 1993.
348. Miltenberger RJ, Mynatt RL, Wilkinson JE, Woychik RP: The role of the agouti gene in the yellow obese syndrome. *J Nutr* **127**:1902S, 1997.
349. Bultman SJ, Klebig ML, Michaud EJ, Sweet HO, Davisson MT, Woychik RP: Molecular analysis of reverse mutations from nonagouti (a) to black-and-tan (a(t)) and white-bellied agouti (Aw) reveals alternative forms of agouti transcripts. *Genes Dev* **8**:481, 1994.
350. Mynatt RL, Miltenberger RJ, Klebig ML, Zemel MB, Wilkinson JE, Wilkinson WO, Woychik RP: Combined effects of insulin treatment and adipose tissue-specific agouti expression on the development of obesity. *Proc Natl Acad Sci U S A* **94**:919, 1997.
351. Robbins L, Nadeau J, Johnson K, Kelly M, Roselli-Rehfuss L, Baack E, Mountjoy K, Cone R: Pigmentation phenotypes of variant extension locus alleles result from point mutations that alter MSH receptor function. *Cell* **72**:827, 1993.
352. Shutter JR, Graham M, Kinsey AC, Scully S, Luthy R, Stark KL: Hypothalamic expression of ART, a novel gene related to agouti, is up-regulated in obese and diabetic mutant mice. *Genes Dev* **11**:593, 1997.
353. Miller KA, Gunn TM, Carrasquillo MM, Lamoreaux ML, Galbraith DB, Barsh GS, et al: Genetic studies of the mouse mutations mahogany and mahoganoid. *Genetics* **146**:1407, 1997.
354. Dinulescu DM, Fan W, Boston BA, McCall K, Lamoreuz ML, Moore KJ, Montagno J, Cone RD: *Mahogany (mg)* stimulates feeding and increases basal metabolic rate independent of its suppression of *agouti*. *Proc Natl Acad Sci U S A* **95**:12707, 1998.
355. Wank SA: Cholecystokinin receptors. *Am J Physiol* **269**:G628, 1995.
356. Miyasaka K, Kanai S, Ohta M, Kawanami T, Kono A, Funakoshi A: Lack of satiety effect of cholecystokinin (CCK) in a new rat model not expressing the CCK-A receptor gene. *Neurosci Lett* **180**:143, 1994.
357. Funakoshi A, Miyasaka K, Shinozaki H, Masuda M, Kawanami T, Takata Y, Kono A: An animal model of congenital defect of gene expression of cholecystokinin (CCK)-A receptor. *Biochem Biophys Res Commun* **210**:787, 1995.
358. Moran TH, Katz LF, Plata-Salaman CR, Schwartz GJ: Disordered food intake and obesity in rats lacking cholecystokinin A receptors. *Am J Physiol* **274**:R618, 1998.
359. Langhans N, Rindi G, Chiu M, Rehfeld JF, Ardman B, Beinborn M, Kopin AS: Abnormal gastric histology and decreased acid production in cholecystokinin-B/gastrin receptor deficient mice. *Gastroenterology* **112**:280, 1997.
360. Ebenezer IS: Effects of buspirone on operant and nonoperant food intake in food-deprived rats. *Methods Find Exp Clin Pharmacol* **18**:475, 1996.
361. Lee MD, Aloyo VJ, Fluharty SJ, Simansky KJ: Infusion of serotonin1B (50HT1B) agonists CP-93,129 into the parabrachial

nucleus potentially and selectively reduces food intake in rats. *Psychopharmacology (Berl)* **136**:304, 1998.

362. Kennett GA, Wood MD, Bright F, Trail B, Riley G, Holland V, Avenell KY, Stean T, Upton N, Bromidge S, et al: SB 242084, a selective and brain penetrant 5-HT2C receptor antagonist. *Neuropharmacology* **36**:609, 1997.
363. Lucas JJ, Yamamoto A, Scearce-Levie K, Saudou F, Hen R: Absence of fenfluramine-induced anorexia and reduced c-Fos induction in the hypothalamus and central amygdaloid complex of serotonin 1B receptor knock-out mice. *J Neurosci* **18**:5537, 1998.
364. McCoy JG, Avery DD: Bombesin: Potential integrative peptide for feeding and satiety. *Peptides* **11**:595, 1990.
365. Battey J, Wada E: Two distinct receptor subtypes for mammalian bombesin-like peptides. *Trends Neurosci* **14**:524, 1991.
366. Nagalla SR, Barry BJ, Creswick KC, Eden P, Taylor JT, Spindel ER: Cloning of a receptor for amphibian (Phe13) bombesin distinct from the receptor for gastrin-releasing peptide: Identification of a fourth bombesin receptor subtype (BB4). *Proc Natl Acad Sci U S A* **92**:6205, 1995.
367. Beck B, Stricker-Krongrad A, Nicholas JP, Burlet C: Chronic and continuous intracerebroventricular infusion of neuropeptide Y in Long-Evans rats mimics the feeding behaviour of obese Zucker rats. *Int J Obes Relat Metab Disord* **16**:295, 1992.
368. Zarjevski N, Cusin I, Vettor F, Rohner-Jeanrenaud F: Chronic intracereberoventricular neuropeptide-Y administration to normal rats mimics hormonal and metabolic changes of obesity. *J Endocrinol* **133**:1753, 1993.
369. Billington C, Briggs J, Harker S, Grace M, Levine A: Neuropeptide Y in hypothalamic paraventricular nucleus: A center coordinating energy metabolism. *Am J Physiol* **266**:R1765, 1994.
370. Hollopeter G, Erickson JC, Palmiter RD: Role of neuropeptide Y in diet-, chemical- and genetic-induced obesity of mice. *Int J Obes Relat Metab Disord* **22**:506, 1998.
371. Herzog H, Hort YJ, Shine J, Selbie LA: Molecular cloning, characterization and localization of the human homolog to the reported bovine NPY Y3 receptor: Lack of NPY binding and activation. *DNA Cell Biol* **12**:465, 1993.
372. Jazin EE, Yoo H, Blomqvist AG, Yee A, Weng G, Walker MW, Salon J, Larhammar D, Wahlestedt C: A proposed bovine neuropeptide Y (NPY) receptor cDNA clone, or its human homologue, confers neither NPY binding sites nor NPY responsiveness on transfected cells. *Regul Pept* **47**:247, 1993.
373. Bleul CC, Farzan M, Choe H, Parolin C, Clark-Lewis I, Sodroski J, Springer TA: The lymphocyte chemoattractant SDF-1 is a ligant for LESTR/fusin and blocks HIV-1 entry. *Nature* **382**:829, 1996.
374. Oberlin E, Amara A, Bachelerie F, Bessia C, Virelizier J-L, Arenzana-Seisdedos F, Schwartz O, Heard J-M, Clark-Lewis I, Legler DF, et al: The CXC chemokine SDF-1 is the ligant for LESTR/fusin and prevents infection by T cell-line-adapted HIV-1. *Nature* **382**:833, 1996.
375. Rose PM, Lynch JS, Frazier ST, Fisher SM, Chung WK, Battaglino P, Fathi Z, Leibel RL, Fernandes P: Molecular genetic analysis of a human neuropeptide Y receptor. *J Biol Chem* **272**:3622, 1997.
376. Matsumoto M, Nomura T, Momose K, Ikeda Y, Kondou Y, Akiho H, Togami J, Kimura Y, Okada M: Inactivation of a novel neuropeptide Y/peptide YY receptor gene in primate species. *J Biol Chem* **271**:27217, 1996.
377. Gregor P, Feng Y, DeCarr LB, Cornfield LJ, McCaleb ML: Molecular characterization of a second mouse pancreatic polypeptide receptor and its inactivated human homologue. *J Biol Chem* **271**:27776, 1996.
378. Marsh DJ, Hollopeter G, Kafer KE, Palmiter RD: Role of the Y5 neuropeptide Y receptor in feeding and obesity. *Nat Med* **4**:718, 1998.
379. Shimada M, Tritos NA, Lowell BB, Flier JS, Maratos-Flier E: Mice lacking melanin-concentrating hormone are hypophagic and lean. *Nature* **396**:670, 1998.
380. Qu D, Ludwig DS, Gammeltoft S, Piper M, Pelleymounter MA, Cullen MJ, Mathes WF, Przypek J, Kanarek R, Maratos-Filer E: A role for melanin-concentrating hormone in the central regulation of feeding behaviour. *Nature* **380**:243, 1996.
381. Zhou QY, Palmiter RD: Dopamine-deficient mice are severely hypoactive, adipsic, and aphagic. *Cell* **83**:1197, 1995.
382. Drago J, Padungchaichot P, Accili D, Fuchs S: Dopamine receptors and dopamine transporter in brain function and additive behaviors: Insights from targeted mouse mutants. *Dev Neurosci* **20**:188, 1998.
383. Ricquier D, Casteilla L, Bouillaud F: Molecular studies of the uncoupling protein. *FASEB J* **5**:2237, 1991.
384. Lowell BB, S-Susulic V, Hamann A, Lawitts JA, Himms-Hagen J, Boyer BB, Kozak LP, Flier JS: Development of obesity in transgenic mice after genetic ablation of brown adipose tissue. *Nature* **366**:740, 1993.
385. Klaus S, Munzberg H, Truloff C, Heldmaier G: Physiology of transgenic mice with brown fat ablation: Obesity is due to lowered body temperature. *Am J Physiol* **274**:R287, 1998.
386. Melnyk A, Harper ME, Himms-Hagen J: Raising at thermoneutrality prevents obesity and hyperphagia in BAT-ablated transgenic mice. *Am J Physiol* **272**:R1088, 1997.
387. Lowell BB, Flier JS: Brown adipose tissue, beta 3-adrenergic receptors, and obesity. *Annu Rev Med* **48**:307, 1997.
388. Revelli JP, Preitner F, Samec S, Muniesa P, Kuehne F, Boss O, Vasalli JD, Dulloo A, Seydoux J, Giacobino JP, et al: Targeted gene disruption reveals a leptin-independent role for the mouse beta3-adrenoceptor in the regulation of body composition. *J Clin Invest* **100**:1098, 1997.
389. Susulic VS, Frederich RC, Lawitts J, Tozzo E, Kahn BB, Harper ME, Himms-Hagen J, Flier JS, Lowell BB: Targeted disruption of the beta 3-adrenergic receptor gene. *J Biol Chem* **270**:29483, 1995.
390. Walston J, Silver K, Bogardus C, Knowler WC, Celi FS, Austin S, Manning B, Strosberg AD, Stern MP, Raben N, et al: Time of onset of non-insulin-dependent diabetes mellitus and genetic variation in the beta 3-adrenergic-receptor gene. *N Engl J Med* **333**:343, 1995.
391. Sun L, Ishibashi S, Osuga J, Harada K, Ohashi K, Gotoda T, Fukuo Y, Yazaki Y, Yamada N: Clinical features associated with the homozygous Trp64Arg mutation of the beta3-adrenergic receptor: No evidence for its association with obesity in Japanese. *Arterioscler Thromb Vasc Biol* **18**:941, 1998.
392. Kadowaki H, Yasuda K, Iwamoto K, Otabe S, Shimokawa K, Silver K, Walston J, Yoshinaga H, Kosaka K, Yamada N: A mutation in the beta 3-adrenergic receptor gene is associated with obesity and hyperinsulinemia in Japanese subjects. *Biochem Biophys Res Commun* **215**:555, 1995.
393. Nagase T, Aoki A, Yamamoto M, Yasuda H, Kado S, Nishikawa M, Kugai N, Akatsu T, Nagata N: Lack of association between the Trp64 Arg mutation in the beta 3-adrenergic receptor gene and obesity in Japanese men: A longitudinal analysis. *J Clin Endocrinol Metab* **82**:1284, 1997.
394. Silver K, Walston J, Wang Y, Dowse G, Zimmet P, Shuldiner AR: Molecular scanning for mutations int he beta 3-adrenergic receptor gene in Nauruans with obesity and non-insulin dependent diabetes mellitus. *J Clin Endocrinol Metab* **81**:4155, 1996.
395. Widen E, Lehto M, Kanninen T, Walston J, Shuldiner AR, Groop LC: Association of a polymorphism in the beta 3-adrenergic receptor gene with features of the insulin resistance syndrome in Finns. *N Engl J Med* **333**:348, 1995.
396. Zhang Y, Wat N, Stratton IM, Warren-Perry MG, Orho M, Groop L, Turner RC: UKPDS 19: Heterogeneity in NIDDM: Separate contributions of IRS-1 and beta 3-adrenergic receptor mutations to insulin resistance and obesity respectively with no evidence for glycogen synthase gene mutations. UK Prospective Diabetes Study. *Diabetologia* **39**:1505, 1996.
397. Lowell BB: Slimming with a leaner enzyme. *Nature* **382**:585, 1996.
398. Cummings DE, Brandon EP, Planas JV, Motamed K, Idzerda RL, McKnight GS: Genetically lean mice result from targeted disruption of the RII-beta subunit of protein kinase A. *Nature* **382**:622, 1996.
399. Enerback S, Jacobsson A, Simpson EM, Guerra C, Yamashita H, Harper ME, Kozak LP: Mice lacking mitochondrial uncoupling protein are cold-sensitive but not obese. *Nature* **387**:90, 1997.
400. Kopecky J, Clarke G, Enerback S, Spiegelman B, Kozak LP: Expression of the mitochondrial uncoupling protein gene from the aP2 gene promoter prevents genetic obesity. *J Clin Invest* **96**:2914, 1995.
401. Kopecky J, Hodny Z, Rossmeisl M, Syrovy I, Kozak LP: Reduction of dietary obesity in a P2-Ucp transgenic mice: Physiology and adipose tissue distribution. *Am J Physiol* **270**:E768, 1996.
402. Thomas SA, Palmiter RD: Thermoregulatory and metabolic phenotypes of mice lacking noradrenaline and adrenaline. *Nature* **387**:94, 1997.
403. Thomas SA, Palmiter RD: Impaired maternal behavior in mice lacking norepinephrine and epinephrine. *Cell* **91**:583, 1997.
404. Thomas SA, Palmiter RD: Disruption of the dopamine beta-hydroxylase gene in mice suggests roles for norepinephrine in motor function, learning, and memory. *Behav Neurosci* **111**:579, 1997.
405. Binnerts A, Deurenberg P, Swart GR, Wilson JH, Lamberts SW: Body composition in growth hormone-deficient adults. *Am J Clin Nutr* **55**:918, 1992.

406. Hoffman DM, O'Sullivan AJ, Freund J, Ho KK: Adults with growth hormone deficiency have abnormal body composition but normal energy metabolism. *J Clin Endocrinol Metab* **80**:72, 1995.
407. Toogood AA, Adams JE, O'Neill PA, Shalet SM: Body composition in growth hormone deficient adults over the age of 60 years. *Clin Endocrinol (Oxf)* **45**:399, 1996.
408. Donahue LR, Beamer WG: Growth hormone deficiency in "little" mice results in aberrant body composition, reduced insulin-like growth factor-I and insulin-like growth factor-binding protein-3 (IGFBP-3), but does not affect IGFBP-2, -1, or -4. *J Endocrinol* **136**:91, 1993.
409. Chua SC, Hennessey KL, Zeitler P, Leibel RL: The little mutation (lit) cosegregates with the growth hormone releasing factor receptor on mouse chromosome 6. *Mamm Genome* **4**:555, 1993.
410. Wajnrajch M, Gertner JM, Harbison MD, Chua SC, Leibel RL: Nonsense mutation in the human growth hormone releasing hormone receptor (GHRHR) causes growth failure analogous to that of the little (lit) mouse. *Nat Genetics* **12**(1–90), 1996.
411. Clark RG, Mortensen DL, Carlsson LM, Carlsson B, Carmignac D, Robinson IC: The obese growth hormone (GH)-deficient dwarf rat: Body fat responses to patterned delivery of GH and insulin-like growth factor-I. *Endocrinology* **137**:1904, 1996.
412. Zhou YT, Shimabukuro M, Koyama K, Lee Y, Wang MY, Trieu F, Newgard CB, Unger RH: Induction by leptin of uncoupling protein-2 and enzymes of fatty acid oxidation. *Proc Natl Acad Sci U S A* **94**:6386, 1997.
413. Oberbauer AM, Stern JS, Johnson PR, Horwitz BA, German JB, Phinney SD, Beermann DH, Pomp D, Murray JD: Body composition of inactivated growth hormone (oMt1a-oGH) transgenic mice: Generation of an obese phenotype. *Growth Dev Aging* **61**:169, 1997.
414. Pomp D, Oberbauer AM, Murray JD: Development of obesity following inactivation of a growth hormone transgene in mice. *Transgenic Res* **5**:13, 1996.
415. Ikeda A, Chang KT, Matsumoto Y, Furuhata Y, Nishihara M, Sasaki F, Takahashi M: Obesity and insulin resistance in human growth hormone transgenic rats. *Endocrinology* **139**:3057, 1998.
416. Liu JP, Baker J, Perkins AS, Robertson EJ, Efstratiadis A: Mice carrying null mutations of the genes encoding insulin-like growth factor I (Igf-1) and type IGF receptor (Igf1r). *Cell* **75**:59, 1993.
417. Baker J, Liu JP, Robertson EJ, Efstratiadis A: Role of insulin-like growth factors in embryonic and postnatal growth. *Cell* **75**:73, 1993.
418. DeChiara TM, Efstratiadis A, Robertson EJ: A growth-deficiency phenotype in heterozygous mice carrying an insulin-like growth factor II gene disrupted by targeting. *Nature* **345**:78, 1990.
419. Powell-Braxton L, Hollingshead P, Warburton C, Dowd M, Pitts-Meek S, Dalton D, Gillett N, Stewart TA: IGF-1 is required for normal embryonic growth in mice. *Genes Dev* **7**:2609, 1993.
420. Udy GB, Towers RP, Snell RG, Wilkins RJ, Park SH, Ram PA, Waxman DJ, Davey HW: Requirement of STAT5b for sexual dimorphism of body growth rates and liver gene expression. *Proc Natl Acad Sci U S A* **94**:7239, 1997.
421. Feldman GM, Rosenthal LA, Liu X, Hayes MP, Wynshaw-Boris A, Leonard WJ, Hennighausen L, Finbloom DS: STAT5A-deficient mice demonstrate a defect in granulocyte-macrophage colony-stimulating factor-induced proliferation and gene expression. *Blood* **90**:1768, 1997.
422. Neubauer H, Cumano A, Muller M, Wu H, Huffstadt U, Pfeffer K: Jak2 deficiency defines an essential development checkpoint in definitive hematopoiesis. *Cell* **93**:397, 1998.
423. Parganas E, Wang D, Stravopodis D, Topham DJ, Marine JC, Teglund S, Vanin EF, Bodner S, Colaminici OR, van Deursen JM, et al: Jak2 is essential for signaling through a variety of cytokine receptors. *Cell* **93**:385, 1998.
424. Jaffe CA, Ocampo-Lim B, Guo W, Krueger K, Sugahara I, DeMott-Friberg R, Bermann M, Barkan AL: Regulatory mechanisms of growth hormone secretion are sexually dimorphic. *J Clin Invest* **102**:153, 1998.
425. Hartman ML, Veldhuis JD, Thorner MO: Normal control of growth hormone secretion. *Horm Res* **40**:37, 1993.
426. Jansson JO, Eden S, Isaksson O: Sexual dimorphism in the control of growth hormone secretion. *Endocr Rev* **6**:128, 1985.
427. Gebert CA, Park SH, Waxman DJ: Regulation of signal transducer and activator of transcription (STAT) 5b activation by the temporal pattern of growth hormone stimulation. *Mol Endocrinol* **11**:400, 1997.
428. Kahn BB: Lilly Lecture 1995. Glucose transport: Pivotal step in insulin action. *Diabetes* **45**:1644, 1996.
429. Shepherd PR, Gnudi L, Tozzo E, Yang H, Leach F, Kahn BB: Adipose cell hyperplasia and enhanced glucose disposal in transgenic mice overexpressing GLUT4 selective in adipose tissue. *J Biol Chem* **268**:22243, 1993.
430. Moller DE, Chang PY, Yaspelkis BB, Flier JS, Wallberg-Henriksson H, Ivy JL: Transgenic mice with muscle-specific insulin resistance develop increased adiposity, impaired glucose tolerance, and dyslipidemia. *J Endocrinology* **137(6)**:2397, 1996.
431. Dong ZM, Gutierrez-Ramos J-C, Coxon A, Mayuadas TN, Wagner DD: A new class of obesity genes encodes leukocyte adhesion receptors. *Proc Natl Acad Sci U S A* **94**:7526, 1997.
432. Tanaka T, Yoshida N, Kishimoto T, Akira S: Defective adipocyte differentiation in mice lacking the C/EBPbeta and/or C/EBPdelta gene. *EMBO J* **16**:7432, 1997.
433. Moitra J, Mason MM, Olive M, Krylov D, Gavrilova O, Marcus-Samuels B, Feigenbaum L, Lee E, Aoyama T, Eckhaus M, et al: Life without white fat: A transgenic mouse. *Genes Dev* **12**:3168, 1998.
434. Shimomura I, Hammer RE, Richardson JA, Ikemoto S, Bashmakov Y, Goldstein JL, Brown MS: Insulin resistance and diabetes mellitus in transgenic mice expressing nuclear SREBP-1c in adipose tissue: Model for congenital generalized lipodystrophy. *Genes Dev* **12**:3182, 1998.
435. Lauro D, Kido Y, Castle AL, Zarnowski MJ, Hayashi H, Ebina Y, Accili D: Impaired glucose tolerance in mice with targeted impairment of insulin action in muscle and adipose tissue. *Nat Genet* **20**:294, 1998.
436. Casper RC: Carbohydrate metabolism and its regulatory hormones in anorexia nervosa. *Psychiatry Res* **62**:85, 1996.
437. Koffler M, Kisch ES: Starvation diet and very-low-calorie diets may induce insulin resistance and overt diabetes mellitus. *J Diabetes Complications* **10**:109, 1996.
438. Holemans K, Verhaeghe J, Dequeker J, VanAssche FA: Insulin sensitivity in adult female rats subjected to malnutrition during the perinatal period. *J Soc Gynecol Investig* **3**:71, 1996.
439. Phipps K, Berker DJ, Hales CN, Fall CH, Osmond C, Clark PM: Fetal growth and impaired glucose tolerance in men and women. *Diabetologia* **36**:225, 1993.
440. Ravelli AC, vanderMeulen JH, Michaels RP, Osmond C, Barker DJ, Hales CN, Bleker OP: Glucose tolerance in adults after prenatal exposure to famine. *Lancet* **351**:173, 1998.
441. McPherron AC, Lawler AM, Lee SJ: Regulation of skeletal mass in mice by a new TGF-beta superfamily member. *Nature* **387**:83, 1997.
442. Szabo G, Dallmann G, Muller G, Patthy L, Soller M, Varga L: A deletion in the myostatin gene causes the compact (Cmpt) hypermuscular mutation in mice. *Mamm Genome* **9**:671, 1998.
443. Varga L, Szabo G, Darvasi A, Muller G, Sass M, Soller M: Inheritance and mapping of Compact (*Cmpt*), a new mutation causing hypermuscularity in mice. *Genetics* **147**:755, 1997.
444. McPherron AC, Lee SJ: Double muscling in cattle due to mutations in myostatin gene. *Proc Natl Acad Sci U S A* **94**:12457, 1997.
445. Kambadur R, Sharma M, Smith TP, Bass JJ: Mutations in myostatin (GDF8) in double-muscled Belgian Blue and Piedmontese cattle. *Genome Res* **7**:910, 1997.
446. Grobet L, Poncelet D, Royo LJ, Brouwers B, Pirottin D, Michaux C, Menissier F, Zanotti M, Dunner S, Georges M: Molecular definition of an allelic series of mutations disrupting the myostatin function and causing double-muscling in cattle. *Mamm Genome* **9**:210, 1998.
447. Grobet L, Martin LJ, Poncelet D, Pirottin D, Brouwers B, Riquet J, Schoeberlein A, Dunner S, Menissier F, Massabanda J, et al: A deletion in the bovine myostatin gene causes double-muscled phenotype in cattle. *Nat Genet* **17**:71, 1997.
448. Casas E, Keele JW, Shackelford SD, Koohmaraie M, Sonstegard TS, Smith TP, Kappes SM, Stone RT: Association of the muscle hypertrophy locus with carcass traits in beef cattle. *J Anim Sci* **76**:468, 1998.
449. Fujii J, Otsu K, Zorzato F, deLeon S, Khanna VK, Weiler JE, O'Brien PJ, MacLennan DH: Identification of a mutation in porcine ryanodine receptor associated with malignant hyperthermia. *Science* **253**:448, 1991.
450. Otsu K, Khanna VK, Archibald AL, MacLennan DH: Cosegregation of porcine malignant hyperthermia and a probable causal mutation in the skeletal muscle ryanodine receptor gene in backcross families. *Genomics* **11**:744, 1991.
451. Vogeli P, Bolt R, Fries R, Stranzinger G: Co-segregation of the malignant hyperthermia and the Arg615-Cys516 mutation in the skeletal muscle calcium release channel protein in five European Landrace and Pietrain pig breeds. *Anim Genet* **25(Suppl)**:59, 1994.

452. MacLennan DH: Malignant hyperthermia. *Science* **256**:789, 1992.
453. Fletcher JE, Calvo PA, Rosenberg H: Phenotypes associated with malignant hyperthermia susceptibility in swine genotyped as homozygous or heterozygous for the ryanodine receptor mutation. *Br J Anaesth* **71**:410, 1993.
454. Allen GC, Larach MG, Kunselman AR: The sensitivity and specificity of the caffeine-halothane contracture test: A report from the North American Malignant Hyperthermia Registry. *Anesthesiology* **88**:579, 1998.
455. Richter M, Schleitihoff L, Deufel T, Lehmann-Horn F, Hermann-Frank A: Functional characterization of a distinct ryanodine receptor mutation in human malignant hyperthermia-susceptible muscle. *J Biol Chem* **272**:5256, 1997.
456. Manning BM, Quane KA, Ording H, Urwyler A, Tegazzin V, Lehane M, O'Halloran J, Hartung E, Giblin LM, Lynch PJ, et al: Identification of novel mutations in the ryanodine-receptor (RYR1) in malignant hyperthermia: genotype-phenotype correlation. *Am J Hum Genet* **62**:599, 1998.
457. Cockett NE, Jackson SP, Shay TL, Nielsen D, Moore SS, Steele MR, Barendse W, Green RD, Georges M: Chromosomal localization of the callipyge gene in sheep (Ovis aries) using bovine DNA markers. *Proc Natl Acad Sci U S A* **91**:3019, 1994.
458. Jackson SP, Green RD, Miller MF: Phenotypic characterization of rambouillet sheep expressing the callipyge gene: I. Inheritance of the condition and production characteristics. *J Anim Sci* **75**:14, 1997.
459. Jackson SP, Miller MF, Green RD. Phenotypic characterization of rambouillet sheep expression the callipyge gene: II. Carcass characteristics and retail yield. *J Anim Sci* **75**:125, 1997.
460. Jackson SP, Miller MF, Green RD: Phenotypic characterization of rambouillet sheep expression the callipyge gene: III. Muscle weights and muscle weight distribution. *J Anim Sci* **75**:133, 1997.
461. Hasty P, Bradley A, Morris JH, Edmondson DG, Venuti JM, Olson EN, Klein WH: Muscle deficiency and neonatal death in mice with a targeted mutation in the myogenin gene. *Nature* **364**:501, 1993.
462. Nabeshima Y, Hanaoka K, Mayasaka M, Esumi E, Li S, Nonaka I, Nabeshima Y: Myogenin gene disruption results in perinatal lethality because of severe muscle defect. *Nature* **364**:532, 1993.
463. Rawls A, Valdez MR, Zhang W, Richardson J, Klein WH, Olson EN. Overlapping functions of the myogenic bHLH genes MRF4 and MyoD revealed in double mutant mice. *Development* **125**:2349, 1998.
464. Rudnicki MA, Schnegelsberg PN, Stead RH, Braun T, Arnold HH, Jaenisch R: MyoD or Myf-5 is required for the formation of skeletal muscle. *Cell* **75**:1351, 1993.
465. McMahon LR, Wellman PJ: Decreased intake of a liquid diet in nonfood-deprived rats following intra-PVN injections of GLP-1(7-36) amide. *Pharmacol Biochem Behav* **58**:673, 1997.
466. Turton MD, O'Shea D, Gunn I, Beak SA, Edwards CM, Meeran K, Choi SJ, Taylor GM, Heath MM, Lambert PD, et al: A role for glucagon-like peptide-1 in the central regulation of feeding. *Nature* **379**:69, 1996.
467. Scrocchi LA, Borwn TJ, MaClusky N, Brubaker PL, Auerbach AB, Joyner AL, Drucker DJ: Glucose intolerance buy normal satiety in mice with a null mutation in the glucagon-like peptide receptor gene. *Nat Med* **2**:1254, 1996.
468. Muglia L, Jacobson L, Kikkes P, Majzoub JA: Corticotropin-releasing hormone deficiency reveals major fetal but not adult glucocorticoid need. *Nature* **373**:427, 1995.
469. Timpl P, Spanagel R, Sillaber I, Kresse A, Reul JM, Stalla GK, Blanquet V, Steckler T, Holsboer F, Wurst W: Impaired stress response and reduced anxiety in mice lacking a functional corticotropin-releasing hormone receptor 1110ee. *Nat Genet* **19**:162, 1998.
470. Vaughan J, Donaldson C, Bittencourt J, Perrin MH, Lewis K, Sutton S, Chan R, Turnbull AV, Lovejoy D, Rivier C: Urocortin, a mammalian neuropeptide related to fish urotensin I and to corticotropin-releasing factor. *Nature* **378**:287, 1995.
471. Frisch R, Revelle R: Height and weight at menarche and a hypothesis of critical body weights and adolescent events. *Science* **169**:397, 1970.
472. Faust IM, Johnson PR, Hirsch J: Surgical removal of adipose tissue alters feeding behavior and the development of obesity in rats. *Science* **197**:393, 1977.
473. Faust IM, Johnson PR, Hirsch J: Adipose tissue regeneration following lipectomy. *Science* **197**:391, 1977.
474. Coleman DL: Effects of parabiosis of obese with diabetes and normal mice. *Diabetologia* **9**:294, 1973.
475. Harris RB, Hervey E, Hervey GR, Tobin G: Body composition of lean and obese Zucker rats in parabiosis. *Int J Obes* **11**:275, 1987.
476. Hausberger F: Parabiosis and transplantation experiments in hereditarily obese mice. *Anat Rec* **130**:313, 1959.
477. Astrup A, Buemann B, Toubro S, Ranneries C, Raben A: Low resting metabolic rate in subjects predisposed to obesity: A role for thyroid status. *Am J Clin Nutr* **63**:879, 1996.
478. Hervey GR: The effects of lesions in the hypothalamus in parabiotic rats. *J Physiol (Lond)* **145**:336, 1959.
479. Coleman DL: Obese and diabetes: Two mutant genes causing diabetes-obesity syndromes in mice. *Diabetologia* **14**:141, 1978.
480. Coleman DL. Diabetes-obesity syndromes in mice. *Diabetes* **31**:1, 1982.
481. Truett GE, Bahary N, Friedman JM, Leibel RL: Rat obesity gene fatty (*fa*) maps to chromosome 5: Evidence for homology with the mouse gene diabetes (*db*). *Proc Natl Acad Sci U S A* **88(17)**:7806, 1991.
482. Nishizawa Y, Bray GA: Evidence for a circulating ergostatic factor: Studies on parabiotic rats. *Am J Physiol* **239**:R344, 1980.
483. Harris RB: Factors influencing body weight regulation. *Dig Dis* **11**:133, 1993.
484. Friedman JM, Leibel RL, Siegel DA, Walsh J, Bahary N: Molecular mapping of the mouse *ob* mutation. *Genomics* **11**:1054, 1991.
485. Bahary N, Zorich G, Pachter JE, Leibel RL, Friedman JM: Molecular genetic linkage maps of mouse chromosomes 4 and 6. *Genomics* **11**:33, 1991.
486. Friedman JM, Leibel RL: Tackling a weighty problem. *Cell* **69**:217, 1992.
487. Zhang Y, Proenca R, Maffei M, Barone M, Leopold L, Friedman JM: Positional cloning of the mouse obese gene and its human homologue. *Nature* **372(6505)**:425, 1994.
488. Giese K, Fantl WJ, Vitt C, Stephans JC, Cousens L, Wachowicz M, Williams LT: Reduction of food intake and weight gain by the ob protein requires a specific secondary structure and is reversible. *Mol Med* **2**:50, 1996.
489. Kline AD, Becker GW, Churgay LM, Landen BE, Martin DK, Muth WL, Rathnachalam R, Richardson JM, Schoner B, Ulmer M, et al.: Leptin is a four-helix bundle: Secondary structure by NMR. *FEBS Lett* **407**:239, 1997.
490. Madej T, Boguski MS, Bryant SH: Threading analysis suggests that the obese gene product may be a helical cytokine. *FEBS Lett* **373**:13, 1995.
491. Zhang F, Basinski MB, Beals JM, Briggs SL, Churgay LM, Clawson DK, Marchi RDD, Furman TC, Hale JE, Hsiung HM, et al.: Crystal structure of the obese protein leptin-E100. *Nature* **387**:206, 1997.
492. Rock FL, Altmann SW, vanHeek M, Kastelein RA, Bazan JF: The leptin haemopoietic cytokine fold is stabilized by an intrachain disulfide bond. *Horm Metab Res* **28**:649, 1996.
493. Rosenbaum M, Nicolson M, Hirsch J, Heymsfield SB, Gallagher D, Chu F, Leibel RL: Effects of gender, body composition, and menopause on plasma concentrations of leptin. *J Clin Endocrinol Metab* **81**:3424, 1996.
494. Tartaglia LA, Dembski M, Weng X, Deng N, Culpepper J, Devos R, Richards GJ, Campfield LA, Clark FT, Deeds J, et al.: Identification and expression cloning of a leptin receptor, OB-R. *Cell* **83**:1263, 1995.
495. Chua SC, Chung WK, Wu-Peng XS, Zhang Y, Liu S-M, Tartaglia L, Leibel RL: Phenotypes of mouse *diabetes* and rat *fatty* due to mutations in the OB (leptin) receptor. *Science* **27**:994, 1996.
496. Campfield LA, Smith FJ, Guisez Y, Devos R, Burn P: Recombinant mouse OB protein: Evidence for a peripheral signal linking adiposity and central neural networks. *Science* **269**:546, 1995.
497. Mounzih K, Lu R, Chehap FF: Leptin treatment rescues the sterility of genetically obese *ob/ob* males. *Endocrinology* **138**:1190, 1997.
498. Halaas JL, Gajiwala KS, Maffei M, Cohen SL, Chait BT, Rabinowitz D, Lallone RL, Burley SK, Friedman JM: Weight-reducing effects of the plasma protein encoded by the *obese* gene. *Science* **269**:543, 1995.
499. Pelleymounter MA, Cullen MJ, Baker MB, Hecht R, Winters D, Boone T, Collins F: Effects of the *obese* gene product on body weight regulation in *ob/ob* mice. *Science* **269**:540, 1995.
500. Ingalls A, Dickie M, Coleman D: Obese, a new mutation in the house mouse. *J Hered* **41**:317, 1950.
501. Ohtake M, Bray GA, Azukizawa M: Studies on hypothermia and thyroid function in the obese (*ob/ob*) mouse. *Am J Physiol* **233**:R110, 1977.
502. Moon BC, Friedman JM: The molecular basis of the obese mutation in ob^{2J} mice. *Genomics* **42**:152, 1997.
503. Green ED, Maffei M, Braden VV, Procenca R, DeSilva U, Zhang Y, S C Chua J, Leibel RL, Weissenbach J, Friedman JM: The human obese (OB) gene: RNA expression pattern and mapping on the physical, cytogenetic, and genetic maps of chromosome 7. *Genet Res* **5**:5, 1995.

504. Isse N, Ogawa Y, Tamura N, Masuzaki H, Mori K, Okazaki T, Satoh M, Shigemoto M, Yoshimasa Y, Nishi S: Structural organization and chromosomal assignment of the human obese gene. *J Biol Chem* **270**:27728, 1995.
505. Gong D-W, Bi S, Pratley RE, Weintraub BD: Genomic structure and promoter analysis of the human *obese* gene. *J Biol Chem* **271**:3971, 1996.
506. Phillips MS, Liu Q, Hammond HA, Dugan V, Hey PJ, Caskey CT, Hess JF: Leptin receptor missense mutation in the *fatty* Zucker rat. *Nat Genet* **13**:18, 1996.
507. Chua SC, Koutras IK, Han L, Liu S-M, Kay J, Young SJ, Leibel RL: Fine structure of the murine leptin receptor gene: Splice site suppression is required to form two alternatively spliced transcripts. *Genomics* **45**:264, 1997.
508. Chen H, Charlat O, Tartaglia LA, Woolf EA, Weng X, Ellis SJ, Lakey ND, Culpepper J, Moore KJ, Breitbart RE, et al.: Evidence that the *diabetes* gene encodes the leptin receptor: Identification of a mutation in the leptin receptor gene in *db/db* mice. *Cell* **84**:491, 1996.
509. Lee G-H, Proenca R, Montez JM, Carroll KM, Darvishzadeth JG, Lee JI, Friedman JM: Abnormal splicing of the leptin receptor in diabetic mice. *Nature* **379**:632, 1996.
510. Wang MY, Zhou YT, Newgard CB, Unger RH: A novel leptin receptor isoform in rat. *FEBS Lett* **392**:87, 1996.
511. Cioffi JA, Shaper AW, Zupancic TJ, Smith-Gbur J, Mikhail A, Platika D, Snodgrass HR: Novel B219/OB receptor isoforms: Possible role of leptin in hematopoiesis and reproduction. *Nat Med* **2(5)**:585, 1996.
512. Bjorbaek C, Elmquist JK, Michl P, Ahima RS, vanBueren A, McCall AL, Flier JS: Expression of leptin receptor isoforms in rat brain microvessels. *Endocrinology* **139**:3485, 1998.
513. Golden PL, Maccagnan TJ, Pardridge WM: Human blood-brain barrier leptin receptor. Binding and endocytosis in isolated human brain microvessels. *J Clin Invest* **99**:14, 1997.
514. Gloaguen I, Costa P, Demartis A, Lazzaro D, DiMarco A, Graziani R, Paonessa G, Chen F, Rosenblum CI, Ploeg LHTVd, et al.: Ciliary neurotropic factor corrects obesity and diabetes associated with leptin deficiency and resistance. *Proc Natl Acad Sci U S A* **94**:6456, 1997.
515. Devos R, Guisez Y, VanderHeyden J, White DW, Kalai M, Fountoulakis M, Plaetinck G: Ligand-independent dimerization of the extracellular domain of the leptin receptor and determination of the stoichiometry of leptin binding. *J Biol Chem* **272**:18304, 1997.
516. Ghilardi N, Skoda RC: The leptin receptor activates Janus kinase 2 and signals for proliferation in a factor-dependent cell line. *Mol Endocrinol* **11**:393, 1997.
517. White DW, Wang Y, Chua SC, Morgenstern JP, Leibel RL, Baumann H, Tartaglia LA: Constitutive and impaired signaling of leptin receptors containing the Gln → pro extracellular domain fatty mutation. *Proc Natl Acad Sci U S A* **94**:10657, 1997.
518. Murakami T, Yamashita T, Iida M, Kuwajima M, Shima K: A short form of leptin receptor performs signal transduction. *BBRC* **231**:26, 1997.
519. Vaisse C, Halaas JL, Horvath CM, Darnell JEJ, Stoffel M, Friedman JM: Leptin activation of Stat3 in the hypothalamus of wild-type and *ob/ob* mice but not *db/db* mice. *Nat Genet* **14**:95, 1996.
520. Bjorbaek C, Elmquist JK, Frantz JD, Shoelson SE, Flier JS: Identification of SOCS-3 as a Potential Mediator of Central Leptin Resistance. *Mol Cells* **1**:619–625, 1998.
521. Takeda K, Noguchi K, Shi W, Tanaka T, Matsumoto M, Yoshida N, Kishimoto T, Akira S. Targeted disruption of the mouse Stat3 gene leads to early embryonic lethality. *Proc Natl Acad Sci U S A* **94**:3801–3804, 1997.
522. White DW, Kuropatwinski KK, Devos R, Baumann H, Tartaglia LA: Leptin receptor (OR-R) signaling. Cytoplasmic domain mutational analysis and evidence for receptor homo-oligomerization. *J Biol Chem* **272**:4065, 1997.
523. Lin S, Huang XF: Fasting increases leptin receptor mRNA expression in lean but not obese (*ob/ob*) mouse brain. *Neuroreport* **8**:3625, 1997.
524. Bennett PA, Lindell K, Karlsson C, Robinson IC, Carlsson LM, Carlsson B: Differential expression and regulation of leptin receptor isoforms in the rat brain: Effects of fasting and oestrogen. *Neuroendocrinology* **67**:29, 1998.
525. Baskin DG, Seeley RJ, Kuijper JL, Lok S, Weigle DS, Erickson JC, Palmiter RD, Schwartz MW: Increased expression of mRNA for the long form of the leptin receptor in the hypothalamus is associated with leptin hypersensitivity and fasting. *Diabetes* **47**:538, 1998.
526. Hummel KP, Dickie MM, Coleman DL: Diabetes, a new mutation in the mouse. *Science* **153**:1127, 1966.
527. Leiter EH, Coleman DL, Eisenstein AB, Strack I: A new mutation (db3J) at the diabetes locus in strain 129/J mice I. Physiological and histological characterization. *Diabetologia* **19**:58, 1980.
528. Aubert R, Herzog J, Camus M-C, Guenet J-L, Lemonnier D: Description of a new model of genetic obesity: The db^{pas} mouse. *J Nutr* **115**:327, 1985.
529. Liu SM, Leibel RL, Chua SC: Partial duplication in the $Lepr^{db\text{-}Pas}$ mutation is a result of unequal crossing over. *Mamm Genome* **9**:780, 1998.
530. Leiter EH, Coleman DL, Hummel KP: The influence of genetic background on the expression of mutations at the diabetes locus in the mouse III. Effect of H-2 haplotype and sex. *Diabetes* **30**:1029, 1981.
531. Leiter EH, Chapman HD: The obesity mutation diabetes (*db*) in mice: Diabetogenic virilization of hepatic metabolism entails transcriptional induction of an estrogen sulfotransferase gene. *Diabetes* **42(Suppl 1)**:52, 1993.
532. Zucker LM, Zucker TF: Fatty, a new mutation in the rat. *J Hered* **52**:275, 1961.
533. Takaya K, Ogawa Y, Isse N, Okazaki T, Satoh N, Masuzaki H, Mori K, Tamura N, Hosoda K, Nakao K: Molecular cloning of rat leptin receptor isoform complementary DNAs—Identification of a missense mutation in Zucker fatty (*fa/fa*) rats. *Biochem Biophys Res Commun* **225**:75, 1996.
534. Crouse JA, Elliott GE, Burgess TL, Chiu L, Bennett L, Moore J, Nicolson M, Pacifici RE: Altered cell surface expression and signaling of leptin receptors containing the *fatty* mutation. *J Biol Chem* **273**:18365, 1998.
535. Rosenblum CI, Tota M, Cully D, Smith T, Collum R, Qureshi S, Hess JF, Phillips MS, Hey PJ, Vongs A, et al.: Functional STAT and 3 signaling by the leptin receptor (OB-R): Reduced expression of the rat fatty leptin receptor in transfected cells. *Endocrinology* **137**:5178, 1996.
536. Friedman JE, deVente JE, Peterson RG, Dohm GL: Altered expression of muscle glucose transporter GLUT-4 in diabetic fatty Zucker rats (ZDF/Drt-fa). *Am J Physiol* **261**:E782, 1991.
537. Ikeda H, Shino A, Matsuo T, Iwatsuka H, Suzuoki Z: A new genetically obese-hyperglycemic rat (Wistar fatty). *Diabetes* **30**:1045, 1981.
538. Kava RA, West DB, Lukasik VA, Greenwood MRC: Sexual dimorphism of hyperglycemia and glucose tolerance in Wistar fatty rats. *Diabetes* **38**:159, 1989.
539. Koletsky S: Obese spontaneous hypertensive rats: A model for the study of atherosclerosis. *Exp Mol Pathol* **19**:53, 1973.
540. Recant L, Voyles NR, Timmers KI, Bhathena SJ, Solomon D, Wilkins S, Michaelis OE: Comparison of insulin secretory patterns in obese nondiabetic LA/N-cp and obese diabetic SHR/N-cp rats. Role of hyperglycemia. *Diabetes* **38**:691, 1989.
541. Takaya K, Ogawa Y, Hiraoka J, Hosoda K, Yamori Y, Nakao K, Koletsky RJ: Nonsense mutation of leptin receptor in the obese spontaneously hypertensive Koletsky rat [letter]. *Nat Genet* **14**:130, 1996.
542. Wu-Peng XS, Chua SC, Okada N, Liu S-M, Nicolson M, Leibel RL: Phenotype of the obese Koletsky (f) rat due to Tyr763Stop mutation in the extracellular domain of the leptin receptor (Lepr): Evidence for deficient plasma-to-CSF transport of leptin in both the Zucker and Koletsky obese rat. *Diabetes* **46**:513, 1997.
543. Dauncey MJ, Brown D: Role of activity-induced thermogenesis in 24-hour energy expenditure of lean and genetically obese (*ob/ob*) mice. *Q J Exp Physiol* **72**:549, 1987.
544. Kowalski TJ, Houpt TA, Jahng J, Okada N, Chua SC, Smith GP: Ontogeny of neuropeptide Y expression in response to deprivation in lean Zucker rat pups. *Am J Physiol* **275**:R466, 1998.
545. Strohmayer AJ, Smith GP: The meal pattern of genetically obese (*ob/ob*) mice. *Appetite* **8**:111, 1987.
546. Ho A, Chin A: Circadian feeding and drinking patters of genetically obese mice fed solid chow diet. *Physiol Behav* **43**:651, 1988.
547. Castonguay TW, Upton DE, Leung PM, Stern JS: Meal patterns in the genetically obese Zucker rat: A reexamination. *Physiol Behav* **28**:911, 1982.
548. Enns MP, Grinker JA: Dietary self-selection and meal patterns of obese and lean Zucker rats. *Appetite* **4**:281, 1983.
549. Alingh-Prins A, deJong-Nagelsmit A, Keijser J, Strubbe JH: Daily rhythms of feeding in the genetically obese and lean Zucker rats. *Physiol Behav* **38**:423, 1986.
550. Cruce JA, Greenwood MR, Johnson PR, Quatermain D: Genetic versus hypothamatic obesity: Studies of intake and dietary manipulation in rats. *J Comp Physiol Psych* **87**:265, 1974.

551. Slafani A, Springer D, Kluge L: Effects of quinine adulterated diets on the food intake and body weight of obese and non-obese hypothalamic hyperphagic rats. *Physiol Behav* **16**:631, 1976.
552. Greenwood MR, Quartermain D, Johnson PR, Cruce JAF, Hirsch J: Food-motivated behavior in genetically obese and hypothalamic-hyperphagic rats and mice. *Physiol Behav* **13**:687, 1974.
553. Nisbett RE: Hunger, obesity, and the ventromedial hypothalamus. *Psychol Rev* **79**:433, 1972.
554. Kent MA, Peters RH: Effects of ventromedial hypothalamic lesions on hunger-motivated behavior in rats. *J Comp Physiol Psychol* **83**:92, 1973.
555. Sclafani A, Kluge L: Food motivation and body weight levels in hypothalamic hyperphage rats: A duel lipostat model of hunger and appetite. *J Comp Physiol Psychol* **86**:28, 1974.
556. Franklin KBJ, Herberg LJ: Ventromedial syndrome: The rats "finickiness" results from the obesity, not from the lesions. *J Comp Physiol Psychol* **87**:410, 1974.
557. Peters RH, Luttmers LL, Gunion MW, Wellman PJ: Ventromedial hypothalamic syndrome: Finickiness? *Physiol Behav* **20**:279, 1978.
558. Kaul R, Schmidt I, Carlisle H: Maturation of thermoregulation in Zucker rats. *Int J Obes* **9**:401, 1985.
559. Himms-Hagen J: Defective brown adipose tissue thermogenesis in obese mice. *Int J Obes* **9**:17, 1985.
560. Atgie C, Marette A, Desautels M, Tulp O, Bukowiecki LJ: Specific decrease of mitochondrial thermogenic capacity in brown adipose tissue of obese SHR/N-cp rats. *Am J Physiol* **265**:C1674, 1993.
561. Trayhurn P, James WP: Thermoregulation and non-shivering thermogenesis in the genetically obese (*ob/ob*) mouse. *Pflugers Arch* **373**:189, 1978.
562. Milner RE, Tayhurn P: Cold-induced changes in uncoupling protein and GDP-binding sites in brown fat of *ob/ob* mice. *Am J Physiol* **257**:R292, 1989.
563. Bray GA, York DA: Hypothalamic and genetic obesity in experimental animals: An autonomic and endocrine hypothesis. *Physiol Rev* **59**:719, 1979.
564. Trayhurn P, James WP, Gurr MI: Studies on the body composition, fat distribution and fat cell size and number of "Ad", a new obese mutant mouse. *Br J Nutr* **41(1)**:211, 1979.
565. Romsos DR, Ferguson D, VanderTuig JG: Effects of a warm environment on energy balance in obese (*ob/ob*) mice. *Metabolism* **34**:931, 1985.
566. Markewicz B, Kuhmichel G, Schmidt I: Onset of excess fat deposition in Zucker rats with and without decreased thermogenesis. *Am J Physiol* **265**:E478, 1993.
567. Kaul R, Heldmaier G, Schmidt I: Defective thermoregulatory thermogenesis does not cause onset of obesity in Zucker rats. *Am J Physiol* **259**:E11, 1990.
568. Purchas RW, Romsos DR, Allen RE, Merkel RA: Muscle growth and satellite cell proliferative activity in obese (*ob/ob*) mice. *J Anim Sci* **60**:644, 1985.
569. Campion DR, Purchas RW, Merkel RA, Romsos DR: Genetic obesity and the muscle satellite cell. *Proc Soc Exp Biol Med* **176**:143, 1984.
570. Strickland NC, Batt RA, Crook AR, Sutton CM: Inability of muscles in the obese mouse (*ob/ob*) to respond to changes in body weight and activity. *J Anat* **184**:527, 1994.
571. Muoio DM, Dohm GL, Fiedorek FT, Tapscott EB, Coleman RA: Leptin directly alters lipid partitioning in skeletal muscle. *Diabetes* **48**:1360, 1997.
572. Coleman DL, Hummel KP: The effects of hypothalamics lesions in genetically diabetic mice. *Diabetologia* **6**:263, 1976.
573. Dubuc PU, Cahn PJ, Willis P: The effects of exercise and food restriction on obesity and diabetes on young *ob/ob* mice. *Int J Obes Relat Metab Disord* **8**:271, 1984.
574. Deb S, Martin RJ: Effects of exercise and of food restriction on the development of spontaneous obesity in rats. *J Nutr* **105**:543, 1975.
575. Truett GE, Tempelman RJ, Walker JA: Codominant effects of the fatty (*fa*) gene during early development of obesity. *Am J Physiol* **268**:E15, 1995.
576. Zhang Y, Olbort M, Schwarzer K, Nuesslein-Hildescheim B, Nicholson M, Murphy E, Kowalski TJ, Schmidt I, Leibel RL: The leptin receptor mediates apparent autocrine regulation of leptin gene expression. *Biochem Biophys Res Commun* **240**:492, 1997.
577. Chung WK, Belfi K, Chua M, Wiley J, Mackintosh R, Nicolson M, Boozer CN, Leibel RL: Heterozygosity for $Lepr^{ob}$ and $Lepr^{db}$ affects body composition and leptin homeostasis in adult mice. *Am J Physiol* **274**:R985, 1998.
578. Swerdloff RS, Batt RA, Bray GA: Reproductive hormonal function in the genetically obese (*ob/ob*) mouse. *Endocrinology* **98**:1359, 1976.
579. Barash IA, Cheung CC, Weigle DS, Ren H, Kabigting EB, Kuiper JL, Clifton DK, Steiner RA: Leptin is a metabolic signal to the reproductive system. *Endocrinology* **137**:3144, 1996.
580. Ahima RS, Dushay J, Flier SN, Prabakaran D, Flier JS: Leptin accelerates the onset of puberty in normal female mice. *J Clin Invest* **99**:391, 1997.
581. Chehab FE, Lim ME, Lu RH: Correction of the sterility defect in homozygous obese female mice by treatment with the human recombinant leptin. *Nat Genet* **12**:318, 1996.
582. Chehab FF, Mounzih K, Lu R, Lim ME: Early onset of reproductive function in normal female mice treated with leptin. *Science* **275(5296)**:88, 1997.
583. Yu WH, Kimura M, Walczewska A, Karanth S, McCann SM: Role of leptin in hypothalamic-pituitary function. *Proc Natl Acad Sci U S A* **94**:1023, 1997.
584. Zamorano PL, Mahesh VB, DeSevilla LM, Chorich LP, Bhat GK, Brann DW: Expression and localization of the leptin receptor in endocrine and neuroendocrine tissues of the rat. *Neuroendocrinology* **65**:223, 1997.
585. Coleman DL, Burkart DL: Plasma corticosterone concentrations in diabetic (*db*) mice. *Diabetologia* **13**:25, 1977.
586. Saito M, Bray GA. Diurnal rhythm for corticosterone in obese (ob/ob) diabetes (db/db) and gold theoglucose-induced obesity in mice. *Endocrinology* **113**:21818, 1983.
587. Shimomura Y, Bray GA, Lee M: Adrenalectomy and steroid treatment in obese (*ob/ob*) and diabetic (*db/db*) mice. *Horm Metab Res* **19**:295, 1987.
588. Solomon J, Bradwin G, Chocchia MA, Coffey D, Condon T, Garrity W, Grieco W: Effects of adrenalectomy on body weight and hyperglycemia in five-month-old *ob/ob* mice. *Horm Metab Res* **9**:152, 1977.
589. Chen HL, Romsos DR: A single intracerebroventricular injection of dexamethasone elevates food intake and plasma insulin and depresses metabolic rates in adrenalectomized obese (*ob/ob*) mice. *J Nutr* **125**:540, 1995.
590. Tokuyama K, Himms-Hagen J: Enhanced acute response to corticosterone in genetically obese (*ob/ob*) mice. *Am J Physiol* **257**:E133, 1989.
591. Yukimura Y, Bray GA, Wolfsen AR: Some effects of adrenalectomy in the fatty rat. *Endocrinology* **103**:1924, 1978.
592. Poitout V, Rouault C, Guerre-Millo M, Briaud O, Reach G: Inhibition of insulin secretion by leptin in normal rodent islets of Langerhans. *Endocrinology* **139**:822, 1998.
593. Harvey J, McKenna F, Herson PS, Spanswick D, Ashford ML: Leptin activates ATP-sensitive potassium channels in the rat insulin-secreting cell line, CRi-G1. *J Physiol (Lond)* **504**:527, 1997.
594. Spanswick D, Smith MA, Groppi VE, Logan SD, Ashford ML: Leptin inhibits hypothalamic neurons by activation of ATP-sensitive potassium channels. *Nature* **390**:521, 1997.
595. Kieffer TJ, Heller RS, Leech CA, Holz GG, Habener JF: Leptin suppression of insulin secretion by the activation of ATP-sensitive K^+ channels in pancreatic beta-cells. *Diabetes* **46**:1087, 1997.
596. Wang MY, Koyama K, Shimabukuro M, Newgard CB, Unger RH: OB-Rb gene transfer to leptin-resistant islets reverses diabetogenic phenotype. *Proc Natl Acad Sci U S A* **95**:714, 1998.
597. Leiter EH: Obesity genes and diabetes induction in the mouse. *Crit Rev Food Sci Nutr* **33**:333, 1993.
598. Leiter EH, Le PH, Coleman DL: Susceptibility to *db* gene and streptozotocin-induced diabetes in C57BL mice: Control by gender-associated, MHC-unlinked traits. *Immunogenetics* **26**:6, 1987.
599. Leiter EH: Genetic control of pathogenesis of diabetes in C3H mice. Influence of the major histocompatibility complex. *Diabetes* **33**:1068, 1984.
600. Clark JB, Palmer CJ, Shaw WN: The diabetic Zucker fatty rat. *Proc Soc Exp Biol Med* **173**:68, 1983.
601. Gibbs EM, Stock JL, McCoid SC, Stukenbrok HA, Pessin JE, Stevenson RW, Milici AJ, McNeish JD: Glycemic improvement in diabetic *db/db* mice by overexpression of the human insulin-regulatable glucose transporter (GLUT4). *J Clin Invest* **95**:1512, 1995.
602. Chung WK, Zheng M, Chua M, Power-Kehoe L, Tsuij I, Wu-Peng XS, Williams J, Chua SC, Leibel RL: Genetic modifiers of $Lepr^{fa}$ which alter susceptibility to NIDDM. *Genomics* **41**:332, 1997.
603. Coleman DL, Eicher EM: Fat (fat) and tubby (tub): Two autosomal recessive mutations causing obesity syndromes in the mouse. *J Hered* **81(6)**:424, 1990.
604. Naggert JK, Fricker LD, Varlamov O, Nishin RM, Rouille T, Steiner DF, Carroll RJ, Raigen BJ, Leiter EH: Hyperproinsulinaemia in obese

fat/fat mice associated with a carboxypeptidase E mutation which reduces enzyme activity. *Nat Genet* **10(2)**:135, 1995.

605. Fricker L, Berman Y, Leiter E, Devi L: Carboxypeptidase E activity is deficient in mice with the *fat* mutation. *J Biol Chem* **271**:30619, 1996.
606. Cool DR, Normant E, Shen F, Chen H-C, Pannell L, Zhang Y, Loh YP: Carboxypeptidase E is regulated secretory pathway sorting receptor: Genetic obliteration leads to endocrine disorders in Cpe^{fat} mice. *Cell* **88**:73, 1997.
607. Ohlemiller KK, Hughes RM, Mosinger-Ogilvie J, Speck JD, Grosof DH, Silverman MS: Cochlear and retinal degeneration in the tubby mouse. *Neuroreport* **6(6)**:845, 1995.
608. Heckenlively JR, Chang B, Erway LC, Peng C, Hawes NL, Hageman GS, Roderick TH: Mouse model for usher syndrome: Linkage mapping suggests homology to Usher type I reported at human chromosome 11p15. *Proc Natl Acad Sci U S A* **42**:11100, 1995.
609. Noben-Trauth K, Naggert JK, North MA, Nishina PM: A candidate gene for the mouse mutation *tubby*. *Nature* **380(6574)**:534, 1996.
610. Kleyn PW, Fan W, Kovats SG, Lee JJ, Pulido JC, Wu Y, Berkemeier LR, Misumi DJ, Holmgren L, Charlet O, et al.: Identification and characterization of the mouse obesity gene *tubby*: A member of a novel gene family. *Cell* **85**:281, 1996.
611. Sahly I, Gogat K, Kobetz A, Marchant D, Menasche M, Castel M, Revah F, Dufier J, Guerre-Millo M, Abitbol MM: Prominent neuronal-specific tub gene expression in cellular targets of tubby mice mutation. *Hum Mol Genet* **7**:1437, 1998.
612. North MA, Naggert JK, Yan Y, Noben-Trauth K, Nishina PM: Molecular characterization of TUB, TULP1, and TULP2, members of the novel tubby gene family and their possible relation to ocular diseases. *Proc Natl Acad Sci U S A* **94**:3128, 1997.
613. Hagstrom SA, North MA, Nishina PL, Berson EL, Dryja TP: Recessive mutations in the gene encoding the tubby-like protein TULP1 in patients with retinitis pigmentosa. *Nat Genet* **18**:174, 1998.
614. Rosenbaum M, Nicolson M, Hirsch J, Murphy E, Leibel RL: Effects of weight change on plasma leptin concentrations and energy expenditure. *J Clin Endoc Metab* **82**:3647, 1997.
615. Houseknecht KL, Manzoros CS, Kuliawit R, Hadro E, Flier JS, Kahn BB: Evidence for leptin binding to proteins in serum of rodents and humans: Modulation with obesity. *Diabetes* **45**:1638, 1996.
616. Sinha MK, Opentanova I, Ohannesian JP, Kolacynski JW, Heiman ML, Hale J, Becker GW, Bowsher RR, Stephens TW, Caro JF: Evidence of free and bound leptin in human circulation. Studies in lean and obese subjects and during short-term fasting. *J Clin Invest* **98(6)**:1277, 1996.
617. Licinio J, Mantzoros C, Negrao AB, Cizza G, Wong ML, Bongiorno PB, Chrousos GP, Karp B, Allen C, Flier JS, et al.: Human leptin levels are pulsatile and inversely related to pituitary-adrenal function. *Nat Med* **3**:575, 1997.
618. Licinio J, Mantzoros C, Kaklamani V, Wong ML, Bongiorno PB, Mulla A, Cearnal L, Veldhuis JD, Flier JS, McCann SM, et al.: Synchronicity of frequently sampled, 24-h concentrations of circulating leptin, luteinizing hormone, and estradiol in healthy women. *Proc Natl Acad Sci U S A* **95**:2541, 1998.
619. Sinha MK, Sturis J, Ohannesian J, Magosin S, Stephens T, Heiman ML, Polonsky KS, Caro JF: Ultradian oscillations of leptin secretion in humans. *Biochem Biophysl Res Commun* **228(3)**:733, 1996.
620. Saad MF, Riad-Gabriel MG, Khan A, Sharma A, Michael R, Jinagouda SD, Boyadijian R, Steil GM: Diurnal and ultradian rhythmicity of plasma leptin: Effects of gender and adiposity. *J Clin Endocrinol Metab* **83**:453, 1998.
621. Schoeller DA, Cella LK, Sinha MK, Caro JF: Entrainment of the diurnal rhythm of plasma leptin to meal timing. *J Clin Invest* **100**:1882, 1997.
622. Heimburger O, Lonnqvist F, Danielsson A, Nordenstrom J, Stenvinkel P: Serum immunoreactive leptin concentration and its relation to the body fat content in chronic renal failure. *J Am Soc Nephrol* **8**:1423, 1997.
623. Iida M, Murakami T, Tamada M, Sei M, Kuwajima M, Mizuno A, Noma Y, Aono T, Shima K: Hyperleptinemia in chronic renal failure. *Horm Metab Res* **28**:724, 1996.
624. Daschner M, Tonshoff B, Blum WF, Englaro P, Wingen AM, Schaefer F, Wuhl E, Rascher W, Mehls O: Inappropriate elevation of serum leptin levels in children with chronic renal failure. European Study Group for Nutritional Treatment of Chronic Renal Failure in Childhood. *J Am Soc Nephrol* **9**:1074, 1998.
625. Ahren B, Pacini G: Impaired adaption of first-phase insulin secretion in postmenopausal women with glucose intolerance. *Am J Physiol* **273**:E701, 1997.
626. Boden G, Chen X, Mozzoli M, Ryan I: Effect of fasting on serum leptin in normal human subjects. *J Clin Endocrinol Metab* **81**:3419, 1996.
627. Kolaczynski JW, Ohannesian J, Considine RV, Marco C, Caro JF: Response to leptin to short-term and prolonged overfeeding in humans. *J Clin Endocrinol Metab* **81**:4162, 1996.
628. Havel PJ, Uriu-Hare JY, Liu T, Stanhope KL, Stern JS, Keen CL, Ahren B: Marked and rapid decreases of circulating leptin in streptozotocin diabetic rats: Reversal by insulin. *Am J Physiol* **274**:R1482, 1998.
629. Popovic V, Micic D, Danjanovic S, Zoric S, DJurovic M, Obradovic S, Petakov M, Dieguez C, Casaneuva FF: Serum leptin and insulin concentrations in patients with insulinoma before and after surgery. *Eur J Endocrinol* **138**:86, 1998.
630. Kolaczynski JW, Nyce MR, Considine RV, Boden G, Nolan JJ, Henry R, Mudaliar SR, Olefsky J, Caro JF: Acute and chronic effect of insulin on leptin production in humans: Studies in vivo and in vitro. *Diabetes* **45**:699, 1996.
631. Wabitsch M, Jensen PB, Blum WF, Christoffersen CT, Englaro P, Heinze E, Rascher W, Teller W, Tornqvist H, Hauner H: Insulin and cortisol promote leptin production in cultured human fat cells. *Diabetes* **45**:1435, 1996.
632. Malmstrom R, Taskinen MR, Karonen SL, Yki-Jarvinen H: Insulin increases plasma leptin concentrations in normal subjects and patients with NIDDM. *Diabetologia* **39**:993, 1996.
633. Pratley RE, Nicolson M, Bogardus C, Ravussin E: Effects of acute hyperinsulinemia on plasma leptin concentrations in insulin-sensitive and insulin-resistant Pima Indians. *J Clin Endocrinol Metab* **81**:4418, 1996.
634. DeVos P, Lefebvre AM, Shrivo I, Fruchart JC, Auwerx J: Glucocorticoids induce the expression of the leptin gene through a non-classical mechanism of transcriptional activation. *Eur J Biochem* **253**:619, 1998.
635. Halleux CM, Servais I, Reul BA, Dentry R, Brichard SM: Multihormonal control of ob gene expression and leptin secretion from cultured human visceral adipose tissue: Increased responsiveness to glucocorticoids in obesity. *J Clin Endocrinol Metab* **83**:902, 1998.
636. Papaspyrou-Rao S, Schneider SH, Peterson RN, Fried SK: Dexamethasone increases leptin expression in humans in vivo. *J Clin Endocrinol Metab* **82**:1635, 1997.
637. Larsson H, Ahren B: Short-term dexamethasone treatment increases plasma leptin independently of changes in insulin activity in health women. *J Clin Endocrinol Metab* **81**:4428, 1996.
638. Slieker LJ, Sloop KW, Surface PL, Kriaciunas A, Laquier F, Manetta J, Buevalleskey J, Stephens TW: Regulation of expression of OBmRNA proteins by glucocorticoids and cAMP. *J Biol Chem* **271**:5301, 1996.
639. Mason MM, He Y, Chen H, Quon MJ, Reitman M: Regulation of leptin promoter function by Spl, C/EBP, and a novel factor. *Endocrinology* **139**:1013, 1998.
640. Kim JB, Sarraf P, Wright M, Yao KM, Mueller E, Solanes G, Lowell BB, Spiegelman BM: Nutritional and insulin regulation of fatty acid synthetase and leptin gene expression through ADD1/SREBP1. *J Clin Invest* **101**:1, 1998.
641. Hardie LJ, Guilhot N, Trayhurn P: Regulation of leptin production in cultured mature white adipocytes. *Horm Metab Res* **28**:685, 1996.
642. Miell JP, Englaro P, Blum WF: Dexamethasone induces an acute and sustained rise in circulating leptin levels in normal human subjects. *Horm Metab Res* **28**:704, 1996.
643. Leal-Cerro A, Considine RV, Peino R, Venegas E, Astorga R, Casaneuva FF, Dieguez C: Serum immunoreactive-leptin levels are increased in patients with Cushing's syndrome. *Horm Metab Res* **28**:711, 1996.
644. Masuzaki H, Ogawa Y, Hosoda K, Miyawaki T, Hanaoka I, Hiraoka J, Yasuno A, Nishimura H, Yoshimasa Y, Nishi S, et al.: Glucocorticoid regulation of leptin synthesis and secretion in humans: Elevated plasma leptin levels in Cushing's syndrome. *J Clin Endocrinol Metab* **82**:2542, 1997.
645. Zakrzewska KE, Cusin I, Sainsbury A, Rohner-Jeanenaud F, Jeanenaud B: Glucocorticoids as counterregulatory hormones of leptin: Toward an understanding of leptin resistance. *Diabetes* **46**:717, 1997.
646. Saad MF, Damini S, Gingerich RL, Riad-Gabriel MG, Khjan A, Boyadjian R, Jinagouda SD, el-Tawil K, Rude RK, Kamdar V: Sexual dimorphism in plasma leptin concentration. *J Clin Endocrinol Metab* **82**:579, 1997.

647. Wu-Peng S, Rosenbaum M, Nicolson M, Chua SC, Leibel RL: Effects of exogenous gonadal steroids on leptin homeostasis in rats. *Obes Res* **7**:586, 1999.
648. Meyer C, Robson D, Rackovsky N, Nadkarni V, Gerich J: Role of the kidney in human leptin metabolism. *Am J Physiol* **273**:E903, 1997.
649. Hube F, Lietz U, Igel M, Jensen PB, Tornqvist H, Joost HG, Hauner H: Difference in leptin mRNA levels between omental and subcutaneous abdominal adipose tissue from obese humans. *Horm Metab Res* **28**:690, 1996.
650. Takahashi M, Funahashi T, Shimomura I, Miyaoka K, Matsuzawa Y: Plasma leptin levels and body fat distribution. *Horm Metab Res* **28**:751, 1996.
651. Montague CT, Prins JB, Sanders L, Digby JE, O'Rahilly S: Depot- and sex-specific differences in human leptin mRNA expression: Implications for the control of regional fat distribution. *Diabetes* **46**:342, 1997.
652. Kotani K, Tokunaga K, Fujioka S, Kobatake T, Keno Y, Yoshida S, Shimomura I, Tarui S, Matsuzawa Y. Sexual dimorphism of age-related changes in whole-body fat distribution in the obese. *Int J Obes Relat Metab Disord* **18**:207, 1994.
653. Nagy TR, Gower BA, Trowbridge CA, Dezenberg C, Shewchuk RM, Goran MI: Effects of gender, ethnicity, body composition, and fat distribution on serum leptin concentrations in children. *J Clin Endocrinol Metab* **82**:2148, 1997.
654. Rosenbaum M, Pietrobelli A, Vasselli JR, Heymsfield SB, Leibel RL: Sexual dimorphism in circulating leptin concentrations is not accounted for by dimorphism in adipose tissue distribution. Submitted for publication, *Intl J Obes*, 2000.
655. Clayton PE, Gill MS, Hall CM, Tillman V, Wahtmore AJ, Price DA: Serum leptin through childhood and adolescence. *Clin Endocrinol (Oxf)* **46**:727, 1997.
656. Mantzoros CS, Flier JS, Rogol AD: A longitudinal assessment of hormonal and physical alterations during normal puberty in boys. V. Rising leptin levels may signal the onset of puberty. *J Clin Endocrinol Metab* **82**:1066, 1997.
657. Wabitsch M, Blum WF, Muche R, Braun M, Hube F, Rascher W, Heinze E, Teller W, Hauner H: Contribution of androgens to the gender difference in leptin production in obese children and adolescents. *J Clin Invest* **100**:808, 1997.
658. Hassink SG, Sheslow DV, deLancey E, Opentanova I, Considine RV, Caro JF: Serum leptin in children with obesity: Relationship to gender and development. *Pediatrics* **98**:201, 1996.
659. Blum WF, Englaro P, Hanitsch S, Juul A, Hertel NT, Muller J, Skakkebaek NE, Heiman ML, Birkett M, Attanasio AM, et al.: Plasma leptin levels in health children and adolescents: Dependence on body mass index, body fat mass, gender, pubertal stage and testosterone. *J Clin Endocrinol Metab* **82**:2904, 1997.
660. Falorni A, Bini V, Molinari D, Papi F, Celi F, DiStefano G, Berioli MG, Bacosi ML, Contessa G: Leptin serum levels in normal weight and obese children and adolescents: Relationship with age, sex, pubertal development, body mass index and insulin. *Int J Obes Relat Metab Disord* **21**:881, 1997.
661. Arslanian S, Suprasongsin C, Kalhan SC, Drash AL, Brna R, Janosky JE: Plasma leptin in children: Relationship to puberty, gender, body composition, insulin sensitivity, and energy expenditure. *Metabolism* **47**:309, 1998.
662. Kennedy A, Gettys TW, Watson P, Wallace P, Ganaway E, Pan Q, Garvey WT: The metabolic significance of leptin in humans: Gender - based differences in relationship to adiposity, insulin sensitivity and energy expenditure. *J Clin Endocrinol Metab* **82**:1293, 1997.
663. Jockenhovel F, Blum WF, Vogel E, Englaro P, Muller-Wieland D, Reinwein D, Rascher W, Krone W: Testosterone substitution normalizes elevated serum leptin levels in hypogonadal men. *J Clin Endocrinol Metab* **82**:2510, 1997.
664. Shimizu H, Shimonmura Y, Nakanishi Y, Futawatari T, Ohtani K, Sato N, Mori M: Estrogen increases in vivo leptin production in rats and human subjects. *J Endocrinol* **154**:285, 1997.
665. Tome MA, Lage M, Camina JP, Garcia-Mayor RV, Dieguez C, Casanueva FF: Sex-based differences in serum leptin concentrations from umbilical cord blood at delivery. *Eur J Endocrinol* **137**:655, 1997.
666. Speroff L: The ovary, in Felig P, Baxter J, Broadus A, Frohman L (eds):*Endocrinology and Metabolism*. New York, McGraw Hill, 1981, pp. 669–724.
667. Troen P, Oshima H: The testis, in Felig P, Baster J, Broadus A, Frohman L (eds): *Endocrinology and Metabolism*. New York, McGraw Hill, 1981, pp. 627–668.
668. Bi S, Gavrilova O, Gong DW, Mason MM, Reitman M: Identification of a placental enhancer for the human leptin gene. *J Biol Chem* **272**:30583, 1997.
669. Gavrilova O, Barr V, Marcus-Samuels B, Reitman M: Hyperleptinemia of pregnancy associated with the appearance of a circulating form of the leptin receptor. *J Biol Chem* **272**:30546, 1997.
670. Highman TJ, Friedman JE, Huston LP, Wong WW, Catalano PM: Longitudinal changes in maternal serum leptin concentrations, body composition, and resting metabolic rate in pregnancy. *Am J Obstet Gynecol* **178**:1010, 1998.
671. Schubring C, Kiess W, Englaro P, Rascher W, Dotsch J, Hanitsch S, Attanasio A, Blum WF: Levels of leptin in maternal serum, amniotic fluid, and arterial and venous cord blood: Relation to neonatal and placental weight. *J Clin Endocrinol Metab* **82**:1480, 1997.
672. Tamura T, Goldenberg RL, Johnston KE, Cliver SP: Serum leptin concentrations during pregnancy and their relationship to fetal growth. *Obstet Gynecol* **91**:389, 1998.
673. Gross GA, Solenberger T, Philpott T, Holcomb WL, Landt M: Plasma leptin concentrations in newborns of diabetic and nondiabetic mothers. *Am J Perinatol* **15**:243, 1998.
674. Sarraf P, Frederich RC, Turner EM, Ma G, Jaskowiak NT, Rivet DJ, Flier JS, Lowell BB, Fraker DL, Alexander HR: Multiple cytokines and acute inflammatory anorexia. *J Exper Med* **185(1)**:171, 1997.
675. Faggioni R, Fantuzzi G, Fuller J, Dinarello CA, Feingold KR, Grunfeld C: IL-1 beta mediates leptin induction during inflammation. *Am J Physiol* **274**:R204, 1998.
676. Janik JE, Curti BD, Considine RV, Rager HC, Powers GC, Alvord WG, Smith JW, Gause BL, Kopp WC: Interleukin alpha increases serum leptin concentrations in humans. *J Clin Endocrinol Metab* **82**:3084, 1997.
677. Faggioni R, Fuller J, Moser A, Feingold KR, Grunfeld C: LPS-induced anorexia in leptin-deficient (*ob/ob*) and leptin receptor-deficient (*db/db*) mice. *Am J Physiol* **273**:R181, 1997.
678. Donahoo WT, Jensen DR, Yost TJ, Eckel RH: Isoproterenol and somatostatin decrease plasma leptin in humans: A novel mechanism regulating leptin secretion. *J Clin Endocrinol Metab* **82**:4139, 1997.
679. Li H, Matheny M, Scarpace PJ: β3-Adrenergic-mediated suppression of leptin gene expression in rats. *Am J Physiol* **272**:E1031, 1997.
680. Trayhurn P, Duncan JS, Rayner DV, Hardie LJ: Rapid inhibition of *ob* gene expression and circulating leptin levels in lean mice by the beta 3-adrenoceptor agonists BRL 35135A and ZD2079. *Biochem Biophys Res Commun* **228**:605, 1996.
681. Scarpace PJ, Matheny M, Pollock BH, Tumer N: Leptin increases uncoupling protein expression and energy expenditure. *Am J Physiol* **273**:E226, 1997.
682. Dunbar JC, Hu Y, Lu H: Intracerebroventricular leptin increases lumbar and renal sympathetic nerve activity and blood pressure in normal rats. *Diabetes* **46**:2040, 1997.
683. Elmquist JK, Ahima RS, Maratos-Flier E, Flier JS, Saper CB: Leptin activates neurons in ventrobasal hypothalamus and brainstem. *J Endocrinol* **138(2)**:839, 1997.
684. Haynes WG, Sivitz WI, Morgan DA, Walsh SA, Mark AL: Sympathetic and cardiorenal actions of leptin. *Hypertension* **30**:619, 1997.
685. Mezey E, Palkovits M: Meningeal relations of the rat hypothalamo-hypophyseal system. Extravascular fluid spaces in and around the median eminence. *Brain Res* **250**:21, 1982.
686. Broadwall RD, Balin BJ, Salcman M, Kaplan RS: Brain-blood barrier? Yes and no. *Proc Natl Acad Sci U S A* **80**:7352, 1983.
687. Rethelyi M: Diffusional barrier around the hypothalamic arcuate nucleus in the rat. *Brain Res* **307**:355, 1984.
688. McKinley MJ, Oldfield BJ: The brain as an endocrine target for peptide hormones. *Trends Endocrinol Metab* **9**:349, 1998.
689. Caro JF, Kolaczynski JW, Nyce MR, Ohannesian JP, Opentanova I, Goldman WH, Lynn RB, Zhang PL, Sinha MK, Considine RV: Decreased cerebrospinal-fluid/serum leptin ratio in obesity: A possible mechanism for leptin resistance. *Lancet* **348**:159, 1996.
690. Ahima RS, Prabakaran D, Mantzoros C, Qu DQ, Lowell B, Matos-Flier E, Flier JS: Role of leptin in the neuroendocrine response to fasting. *Nature* **382**:250, 1996.
691. Collins S, Kuhn CM, Petro AE, Swick AG, Chrunyk BA, Surwit RS: Role of leptin in fat regulation. *Nature* **380**:677, 1996.
692. Halaas JL, Boozer C, Blair-West J, Fidahusein N, Denton DA, Friedman JM: Physiological response to long-term peripheral and central leptin infusion in lean and obese mice. *Proc Natl Acad Sci U S A* **94**:8878, 1997.
693. Legradi G, Emerson CH, Ahima RS, Flier JS, Lechan RM: Leptin prevents fasting-induced suppression of prothyrotropin-releasing

hormone messenger ribonucleic acid in neurons of the hypothalamic paraventricular nucleus. *Endocrinology* **138**:2569, 1997.
694. Campfield LA, Smith FJ, Burn P: Strategies and potential molecular targets for obesity treatment. *Science* **280**:1383, 1998.
695. Weigle DS, Bukowski TR, Foster DC, Holderman S, JKramer JM, Lasser G, Lofton-Day CD, Prunkard DE, Raymond C, Kuijper JL: Recombinant ob protein reduces feeding and body weight in the *ob/ob* mouse. *J Clin Invest* **96**:2065, 1995.
696. Ghilardi N, Ziegler S, Wiestner A, Stoffel R, Heim MH: Defective STAT signaling by the leptin receptor in *diabetic* mice. *Proc Natl Acad Sci U S A* **93**:6231, 1996.
697. Siegrist-Kaiser CA, Pauli V, Juge-Aubry CE, Boss O, Pernin A, Chin WW, Cusin I, Pohner-Jeanrenaud F, Burger AG, Zapf J, et al.: Direct effects of leptin on brown and white adipose tissue. *J Clin Invest* **100**:2858, 1997.
698. Fehmann HC, Peiser C, Bode HP, Stamm M, Staats P, Hedetoft C, Lang RE, Goke B: Leptin: A potent inhibitor of insulin secretion. *Peptides* **18**:1267, 1997.
699. Emilsson V, Liu YL, Cawthorne MA, Morton NM, Davenport M: Expression of the functional leptin receptor mRNA in pancreatic islets and direct inhibitory action of leptin on insulin secretion. *Diabetes* **46**:313, 1997.
700. Kulkarni RN, Wang ZL, Wang RM, Hurley JD, Smith DM, Ghatei MA, Withers DJ, Gardiner JV, Bailey CJ, Bloom SR: Leptin rapidly suppresses insulin release from insulinoma cells, rat and human islets and, in vivo, in mice. *J Clin Invest* **100**:2729, 1997.
701. Shimabukuro M, Koyama K, Chen G, Wang M-Y, Trieu F, Lee Y, Newgard CB, Unger R: Direct antidiabetic effect of leptin through triglyceride depletion of tissues. *Proc Natl Acad Sci U S A* **94**:4637, 1997.
702. Cohen B, Novick D, Rubinstein M: Modulation of insulin activities by leptin. *Science* **274**:1185, 1996.
703. Lord GM, Matarese G, Howard JK, Baker RJ, Bloom SR, Lechler RI: Leptin modulates the T-cell immune response and reverses starvation-induced immunosuppression. *Nature* **394**:897, 1998.
704. Mizuno A, Murakami T, Otani S, Kuwajima M, Shima K: Leptin affects pancreatic endocrine functions through the sympathetic nervous system. *Endocrinology* **139**:2863, 1998.
705. Ishida K, Murakami T, Mizuno A, Iida M, Kuwajima M, Shima K: Leptin suppresses basal insulin secretion from rat pancreatic islets. *Regul Pept* **70**:179, 1997.
706. Tanizawa Y, Okuya S, Ishihara H, Asano T, Yada T, Oka Y: Direct stimulation of basal insulin secretion by physiological concentrations of leptin in pancreatic beta cells. *Endocrinology* **138**:4513, 1997.
707. Pallett AL, Morton NM, Cawthorne MA, Emilsson V: Leptin inhibits insulin secretion and reduces insulin mRNA levels in rat isolated pancreatic islets. *Biochem Biophys Res Commun* **238**:267, 1997.
708. Cohen B, Novick D, Rubinstein M: Modulation of insulin activities by leptin. *Science* **274(5290)**:1185, 1996.
709. Barzilai N, Wang J, Massilon D, Vuguin P, Hawkins M, Rossetti L: Leptin selectively decreases visceral adiposity and enhances insulin action. *J Clin Invest* **100**:3105, 1997.
710. Shi ZQ, Nelson A, Whitcomb L, Wang J, Cohen AM: Intracerebroventricular administration of leptin markedly enhances insulin sensitivity and systemic glucose utilization in conscious rats. *Metabolism* **47**:1274, 1998.
711. Sivitz WI, Walsh SA, Morgan DA, Thomas MJ, Haynes WG: Effects of leptin on insulin sensitivity in normal rats. *Endocrinology* **138**:3395, 1997.
712. Cusin I, Zakrzewska KE, Boss O, Muzzin P, Giocobino JP, Ricquier D, Jeanrenaud B, Rohner-Jeanrenaud F: Chronic central leptin infusion enhances insulin-stimulated glucose *Metabolism* and favors the expression of uncoupling proteins. *Diabetes* **47**:1014, 1998.
713. Kamohara S, Burcelin R, Halaas JL, Friedman JM, Charron MJ: Acute stimulation of glucose metabolism in mice by leptin treatment. *Nature* **389**:374, 1997.
714. Muller G, Ertl J, Gerl M, Preibisch G: Leptin impairs metabolic actions of insulin in isolated rat adipocytes. *J Biol Chem* **272**:10585, 1997.
715. Ranganathan S, Ciaraldi TP, Henry RR, Mudaliar S, Kern PA: Lack of effect of leptin on glucose transport, lipoprotein lipase, and insulin action in adipose and muscle cells. *Endocrinology* **139**:2509, 1998.
716. Zierath JR, Frevert EU, Ryder JW, Berggren PO, Kahn BB: Evidence against a direct effect of leptin on glucose transport in skeletal muscle and adipocytes. *Diabetes* **47**:1, 1998.
717. Liu YL, Emilsson V, Cawthorne MA: Leptin inhibits glycogen synthesis in the isolated soleus muscle of obese (*ob/ob*) mice. *FEBS Lett* **411**:351, 1997.
718. Berti L, Kellerer M, Capp E, Haring HU: Leptin stimulates glucose transport and glycogen synthesis in C2C12 myotubes: Evidence for a P13-kinase mediated effect. *Diabetologia* **40**:606, 1997.
719. Loffreda S, Yang SQ, Lin HZ, Karp CL, Brengman ML, Wang DJ, Klein AS, Bulkley GB, Bao C, Noble PW, et al.: Leptin regulates proinflammatory immune responses. *FASEB J* **12**:57, 1998.
720. Bamshad M, Aoki VT, Adkison MG, Warren WS, Bartness TJ: Central nervous system origins of the sympathetic nervous system outflow to white adipose tissue. *Am J Physiol* **275**:R291, 1998.
721. Bartness TJ, Bamshad M: Innervation of mammalian white adipose tissue: Implications for the regulation of total body fat. *Am J Physiol* **275**:R1399, 1998.
722. Frederich RC, Hamann A, Anderson S, Lollmann BB, Lowell BB, Flier JS: Leptin levels reflect body lipid content in mice: Evidence for diet-induced resistance to leptin action. *Nat Med* **1**:1311, 1995.
723. Klein S, Coppack SW, Mohamed-Ali V, Landt M: Adipose tissue leptin production and plasma leptin kinetics in humans. *Diabetes* **45**:984, 1996.
724. Brabant G, Horn R, Mayr B, VonZurMuhlen A, Honegger J, Buchfelder M: Serum leptin levels following hypothalamic surgery. *Horm Metab Res* **28**:728, 1996.
725. Carlsson B, Lindell K, Gabrielsson B, Karlsson C, Bjarnason R, Westphal O, Karlsson U, Sjorstrom L, Carlsson LM: Obese (ob) gene defects are rare in human obesity. *Obes Res* **5**:30, 1997.
726. Salbe AD, Nicolson M, Ravussin E: Total energy expenditure and the level of physical activity correlate with plasma leptin concentrations in five-year old children. *J Clin Invest* **99**:592, 1997.
727. Toth MJ, Gottlieb SS, Fisher ML, Ryan AS, Nicklas BJ, Poehlman ET: Plasma leptin concentrations and energy expenditure in heart failure patients. *Metabolism* **46**:450, 1997.
728. Tuominen JA, Ebeling P, Heiman ML, Stephens T, Koivisto VA: Leptin and thermogenesis in humans. *Acta Physiol Scand* **160**:83, 1997.
729. Niskanen L, Haffner S, Karhunen LJ, Turpeinen AK, Miettinen H, Uusitupa MI: Serum leptin in relation to resting energy expenditure and fuel metabolism in obese subjects. *Int J Obes Relat Metab Disord* **21**:309, 1997.
730. Weigle DS, Bukowski TR, Foster DC, Holderman S, Kramer JM, Lasser G, Lofton-Day CE, Prunkard DE, Raymond C, Kuijper JL: Recombinant *ob* protein reduces feeding and body weight in *ob/ob* mouse. *J Clin Invest* **96**:2065, 1995.
731. Maffei M, Halaas J, Ravussin E, Pratley RE, Lee GH, Zhang Y, Fei H, Kim S, Lallone R, Ranganathan S, et al.: Leptin levels in human and rodents: Measurement of plasma leptin and *ob* RNA in obese and weight-reduced subjects. *Nat Med* **1**:1155, 1995.
732. Frisch RE, McArthur JW: Menstrual cycles: Fatness as a determinant of minimum weight for height necessary for their maintenance or onset. *Science* **185**:949, 1974.
733. Wade GN, Lempicki RL, Panicker AK, Frisbee RM, Blaustein JD: Leptin facilitates and inhibits sexual behavior in female hamsters. *Am J Physiol* **272**:R1354, 1997.
734. Bjarnason R, Boguszewski M, Dahlgren J, Gelander L, Kristrom B, Rosberg S, Carlsson B, Albertsson-Wikland K, Carlsson LM: Leptin levels are strongly correlated with those of GH-binding protein in prepubertal children. *Eur J Endocrinol* **137**:68, 1997.
735. Carro E, Senaris R, Considine RV, Casanueva FF, Dieguez C: Regulation of in vivo growth hormone secretion by leptin. *Endocrinology* **138**:2203, 1997.
736. Cai A, Hyde J: Upregulation of leptin receptor gene expression in the anterior pituitary of human growth hormone-releasing hormone transgenic mice. *J Endocrinol* **139**:420, 1998.
737. Rosenbaum M, Fried JK, Leibel RL: Effects of systemic growth hormone (GH) on regional adipose tissue distribution and metabolism in GH-deficient children. *J Clin Endocrinol Metab* **69**:1274, 1989.
738. Stunkard AL, Sorensen TI: Obesity and socioeconomic status — A complex relation. *N Engl J Med* **329(14)**:1036, 1993.
739. Price R: Within birth cohort segregation analyses support recessive inheritance of body mass index in white and African-American families. *Int J Obes Relat Metab Disord* **20**:1044, 1996.
740. Comuzzie AG, Blangero J, Mahaney MC, Mitchell BD, Hixson JE, Samollow PB, Stern MP: Major gene with sex-specific effects influences fat mass in Mexican Americans. *Genet Epidemiol* **12**:475, 1995.
741. Rice T, Borecki I, Bouchard C, Rao D: Segregation analysis of fat mass and other body composition measures derived from underwater weighing. *Am J Hum Genet* **52**:967, 1993.
742. Borecki IB, Rice T, Perusse L, Bouchard C, Rao DC: Major gene influence on the propensity to store fat in trunk versus extremity

depots: Evidence from the Quebec Family Study. *Obes Res* **3**:1, 1995.
743. Hasstedt SJ, Ramirez ME, Kuida H, Williams RR: Recessive inheritance of a relative fat pattern. *Am J Hum Genet* **45(6)**:917, 1989.
744. Allison DB, Faith MS, Nathan JS: Risch's lambda values for human obesity. *Int J Obes Relat Metab Disord* **20**:990, 1996.
745. Ronnemaa T, Koskenvuo M, Marniemi J, Koivunen T, Sajantila A, Rissanen A, Kaitsaari M, Bouchard C, Kaprio J: Glucose metabolism in identical twins discordant for obesity: The critical role of visceral fat. *J Clin Endocrinol Metab* **82**:383, 1997.
746. Knowler WC, Pettitt DJ, Saad MF, Charles MA, Nelson RG, Howard BV, Bogardus C, Bennett PH: Obesity in the Pima Indians: Its magnitude and relationship with diabetes. *Am J Clin Nutr* **53**:1543S, 1991.
747. Ravussin E, Valencia ME, Esparza J, Bennett PH, Schulz LO: Effects of a traditional lifestyle on obesity in Pima Indians. *Diabetes Care* **17**:1067, 1994.
748. Shuldiner AR: Transgenic animals. *N Engl J Med* **334**:653, 1996.
749. Chagnon YC, Perusse L, Bouchard C: Familial aggregation of obesity, candidate genes and quantitative trait loci. *Curr Opin Lipidol* **8**:205, 1997.
750. Duggirala R, Stern MP, Mitchell BD, Reinhart LJ, Shipman PA, Uresandi OC, Chung WK, Leibel RL, Hales CN, O'Connell P, et al.: Quantitative variation in obesity-related traits and insulin precursors linked to *OB* gene region on human chromosome 7. *Am J Hum Genet* **59**:694, 1996.
751. Reed DR, Ding Y, Xu W, Cather C, Green ED, Price RA: Extreme obesity may be linked to markers flanking the human *OB* gene. *Diabetes* **45(5)**:691, 1996.
752. Norman R, Chung W, Power-Kehoe L, Chua S, Leibel R, Devoto M, Fann C, Ott J, Bogardus C, Ravussin E: Genetic linkage studies of homologues to rodent obesity genes in Pima Indians. *Diabetes* **45**:1229, 1996.
753. Norman RA, Thompson DB, Foroud T, Garvey WT, Bennett PH, Bogardus C, Ravussin E: Genomewide search for genes influencing percent body fat in Pima Indians: suggestive linkage at chromosome 11q21-q22. *Am J Hum Genet* **60**:166, 1997.
754. Comuzzie AG, Hixson JE, Almasy L, Mitchell BD, Mahaney MC, Dyer TD, Stern MP, MacCluer JW, Blangero J: A major quantitative trait locus determining serum leptin levels and fat mass is located on human chromosome 2. *Nat Genet* **15**:273, 1997.
755. Chagnon YC, Perusse L, Bouchard C: The human obesity gene map: The 1997 update. *Obes Res* **6**:76, 1998.
756. Mehrabian M, Wen P, Fisler J, Davis R, Lusis A: Genetic loci controlling body fat, lipoprotein metabolism, and insulin levels in a multifactorial mouse model. *J Clin Invest* **101**:2485, 1998.
757. Warden CH, Fisler JS, Shoemaker SM, Wen PZ, Svenson KL, Pace MJ, Lusis AJ: Identification of four chromosomal loci determining obesity in a multifactorial mouse model. *J Clin Invest* **95**:1545, 1995.
758. West DB, Goudey-Lefevre J, York B, Truett GE: Dietary obesity linked to genetic loci on chromosomes 9 and 15 in a polygenic mouse model. *J Clin Invest* **94**:1410, 1994.
759. West DB, Waguespack J, York B, Goudey-Lefevre J, Price RA: Genetics of dietary obesity in AKR/J x SWR/J mice: Segregation of the trait and identification of a linked locus on chromosome 4. *Mamm Genome* **5**:546, 1994.
760. Taylor BA, Phillips SJ: Detection of obesity QTLs on mouse chromosome and 7 by selective DNA pooling. *Genomics* **34**:389, 1996.
761. Hashimoto L, Habita C, Beressi JP, Delepine M, Besse C, Cambon-Thomsen A, Deschamps I, Rotter JI, Djoulah S, James MR: Genetic mapping of a susceptibility locus for insulin-dependent diabetes mellitus on chromosome 11q. *Nature* **1371**:161, 994.
762. Bouchard C, Perusse L, Chagnon YC, Warden C, Ricquier D: Linkage between markers in the vicinity of the uncoupling protein 2 gene and resting metabolic rate in humans. *Hum Mol Genet* **6**:1887, 1997.
763. Lembertas AV, Perusse L, Chagnon YC, Fisler JS, Warden CH, Purcell-Huynh DA, Dionne FT, Gagnon J, Nadeau A, Lusis AJ, et al.: Identification of an obesity quantitative trait locus on mouse chromosome 2 and evidence of linkage to body fat and insulin on the human homologous region 20q. *J Clin Invest* **100**:1240, 1997.
764. Lai C, Lyman R, Long A, Langley C, Mackay T: Naturally occurring variation in bristle number and DNA polymorphisms at the *scabrous* locus of *Drosophila melanogaster. Science* **266**:1697, 1994.
765. Long A, Mullaney S, Reid L, Fry J, Langley C, Mackay T: High resolution mapping of genetic factors affecting abdominal bristle number in *Drosophila melanogaster. Genetics* **139**:1273, 1995.
766. Nicholls R, Saitoh S, Horsthemke B: Imprinting in Prader-Willi and Angelman syndromes. *Trends Genet* **14**:194, 1998.
767. Kishino T, Lalande M, Wagstaff J: UBE3A/E6-AP mutations cause Angelman syndrome. *Nat Genet* **15**:70, 1997.
768. Cassidy SB, Schwartz S: Prader-Willi and Angelman syndromes: Disorders of genomic imprinting. *Medicine (Baltimore)* **77**:140, 1998.
769. Warkany J: Cited in MIM 176270, 1970.
770. Keverne E, Fundele R, Narasimha M, Barton S, Surani M: Genomic imprinting and the differential roles of parental genomes in brain development. *Brain Res Dev Brain Res* **92**:91, 1996.
771. Carrozzo R, Rossi E, Christian S, Kittikamron K, Livieri C, Corrias A, Pucci L, Fois A, Simi P, Bosio L, et al.: Inter- and intrachromosomal rearrangements are both involved in the origin of 15q11-q13 deletions in Prader-Willi syndrome. *Am J Hum Genet* **61**:228, 1997.
772. Driscoll D, Waters M, Williams C, Zori R, Glenn C, Avidano K, Nicholls R: A DNA methylation imprint, determined by the sex of the parent, distinguishes the Angelman and Prader-Willi syndromes. *Genomics* **13**:917, 1992.
773. Dittrich B, Robinson W, Knoblauch H, Buiting K, Schmidt K, Gillessen-Kaesbach G, Horsthemke B: Molecular diagnosis of the Prader-Willi and Angelman syndromes by detection of parent-of-origin specific DNA methylation in 15q11-13. *Hum Genet* **90**:313, 1992.
774. Kubota T, Sutcliffe J, Aradhya S, Gillessen-Kaesbach G, Christian S, Horsthemke B, Beaudet A, Ledbetter D: Validation studies of SNRPN methylation as a diagnostic test for Prader-Willi syndrome. *Am J Med Genet* **66**:77, 1996.
775. Rinchik E, Bultman S, Horsthemke B, Lee S, Strunk K, Spritz R, Avidano K, Jong M, Nicholls R: A gene for the mouse pink-eyed dilution locus and for human type II oculocutaneous albinism. *Nature* **361**:72, 1993.
776. Mitchell J, Schinzel A, Langlois S, Gillessen-Kaesbach G, Schuffenhauer S, Michaelis R, Abeliovich D, Lerer I, Christian S, Guitart M, et al.: Comparison of phenotype in uniparental disomy and deletion Prader-Willi syndrome: Sex specific differences. *Am J Med Genet* **65**:133, 1996.
777. Robinson W, Bottani A, Yagang X, Balakrishman J, Binkert F, Machler M, Prader A, Schinzel A: Molecular, cytogenetic, and clinical investigations of Prader-Willi syndrome patients. *Am J Hum Genet* **49**:1219, 1991.
778. Robinson W, Bernasconi F, Mutirangura A, Ledbetter D, Langlois S, Malcolm S, Morris M, Schinzel A: Nondisjunction of chromosome 15: Origin and recombination. *Am J Hum Genet* **53**:740, 1993.
779. Lyko F, Buiting K, Horsthemke B, Paro R: Identification of a silencing element in the human 15q11-q13 imprinting center by using transgenic *Drosophila. Proc Natl Acad Sci U S A* **95**:1698, 1998.
780. Reed ML, Leff SE: Maternal imprinting of human SNRPN, a gene deleted in Prader-Willi syndrome. *Nat Genet* **6**:163, 1994.
781. Schulze A, Hansen C, Skakkebaek NE, Brondum-Nielsen K, Ledbeter DH, Tommerup N: Exclusion of SNRPN as a major determinant of Prader-Willi syndrome by a translocation breakpoint. *Nat Genet* **12**:452, 1996.
782. Holm VA, Cassidy SB, Butler MG, Hanchett JM, Greenswag LR, Whitman BY, Greenberg F: Prader-Willi syndrome: consensus diagnostic criteria. *Pediatrics* **91**:398, 1993.
783. Cattanach B, Barr J, Evans E, Burtenshaw M, Beechey C, Leff S, Brannan C, Copeland N, Jenkins N, Jones J: A candidate mouse model for Prader-Willi syndrome which shows an absence of Snrpn expression. *Nat Genet* **2**:270, 1992.
784. Kwitek-Black AE, Carmi R, Duyk GM, Buetow KH, Elbedour K, Parvari R, Yandava CN, Stone EM, Sheffield VC: Linkage of Bardet-Biedl syndrome to chromosome 16q and evidence for non-allelic genetic heterogeneity. *Nat Genet* **5**:392, 1993.
785. Elbedour K, Zucker N, Zalzstein E, Barki Y, Carmi R: Cardiac abnormalities in the Bardet-Biedl syndrome: Echocardiographic studies of 22 patients. *Am J Med Genet* **52**:164, 1994.
786. Green J, Parfrey P, Harnett J, Farid N, Cramer B, Johnson G, Heath O, McManamon P, O'Leary E, Pryse-Phillips W: The cardinal manifestations of Bardet-Biedl syndrome, a form of Laurence-Moon-Biedl syndrome. *N Engl J Med* **321**:1002, 1989.
787. Alstrom CH, Hallgren B, Nilsson LB, Asander H: Retinal degeneration combined with obesity, diabetes mellitus and neurogenous deafness: A specific syndrome (not hitherto described) distinct form the Laurence-Moon-Biedl syndrome. A clinical endocrinological and genetic examination based on a large pedigree. *Acta Psychiatr Neurol Scand* **34**:1, 1959.
788. Connolly M, JHan J, Couch R, Wong L, Dimmick J, Rigg J: Hepatic dysfunction in Alstrom disease. *Am J Med Genet* **40**:421, 1991.

789. Alter C, Moshang T: Growth hormone deficiency in two siblings with Alstrom syndrome. *Am J Dis Child* **147**:97, 1993.
790. Aynaci F, Okten A, Mocan H, Gedik Y, Sarpkaya A: A case of Alstrom syndrome associated with diabetes insipidus. *Clin Genet* **48**:164, 1995.
791. Collin G, Marshall J, Cardon L, Nishina P: Homozygosity mapping at Alstrom syndrome to chromosome 2p. *Hum Mol Genet* **6**:213, 1997.
792. Cohen MM, Hall BD, Smith DW, Graham CB, Lampert KJ: A new syndrome with hypotonia, obesity, mental deficiency, and facial, oral, ocular and limb anomalies. *J Pediatr* **83**:280, 1973.
793. Friedman E, Sack J. The Cohen syndrome: Report of five new cases and a review of the literature. *J Craniofac Genet Dev Biol* **2**:193, 1982.
794. Tahvanainen E, Norio R, Karila E, Ranta S, Weissenbach J, Sistonen P, Chapelle ADL: Cohen syndrome gene assigned to the long arm of chromosome 8 by linkage analysis. *Nat Genet* **7**:201, 1994.
795. Kolehmainen J, Norio R, Kivitie-Kallio S, Tahvanainen E, Chapelle ADL, Lehesjoki A: Refined mapping of the Cohen syndrome gene by linkage disequilibrium. *Eur J Hum Genet* **5**:206, 1997.
796. Davidson H, Pashavaria M, Hutton J: Proteolytic conversion of proinsulin into insulin. Identification of a Ca^{2+}-dependent acidic endopeptidase in isolated insulin-secretory granules. *Biochem J* **246**:279, 1987.
797. Normant E, Loh Y: Depletion of carboxypeptidase E, a regulated secretory pathway sorting receptor, causes misrouting and constitutive secretion of proinsulin and proenkephalin, but not chromogranin A. *Endocrinology* **139**:2137, 1998.
798. Rovere C, Viale A, Nahon JL, Kitabgi P: Impaired processing of brain proneurotensin and promelanin-concentrating hormone in obese *fat/fat* mice. *J Endocrinol* **137(7)**:2954, 1996.
799. Udupi V, Gomez P, song L, Varlamov O, Reed J, Leiter E, Fricker L, Greeley G: Effect of carboxypeptidase E deficiency on progastrin processing and gastrin messenger ribonucleic acid expression in mice with the fat mutation. *Endocrinology* **138**:1959, 1997.
800. Shen F-S, Loh Y: Intracellular misrouting and abnormal secretion of adrenocorticotropin and growth hormone in Cpe^{fat} mice associated with a carboxypeptidase E mutation. *Proc Natl Acad Sci U S A* **94**:5314, 1997.
801. Cain B, Wang W, Beinfeld M: Cholecystokinin (CCK) levels are greatly reduced in the brains but not the duodenums of Cpe (fat)/Cpe(fat) mice: A regional difference in the involvement of carboxypeptidase E (Cpe) in pro-CCK processing. *Endocrinology* **138**:4034, 1997.
802. O'Rahilly S, Gray H, Humphreys P, Krook A, Polonsky K, White A, Gibson S, Taylor K, Carr C: Brief report: Impaired processing of prohormones associated with abnormalities of glucose homeostasis and adrenal function. *N Engl J Med* **333**:1386, 1995.
803. Jackson RS, Creemers JWM, Ohagi S, Raffin-Sanson M-L, Sanders L, Montague CT, Hutton JC, O'Rahilly S: Obesity and impaired prohormone processing associated with mutations in the human prohormone convertase gene. *Nat Genet* **16**:303, 1997.
804. Montague CT, Farooqi IS, Whitehead JP, Soos MA, Rau H, Wareham NJ, Swewter CP, Digby JE, Mohammed SN, Hurst JA, et al.: Congenital leptin deficiency is associated with severe early-onset obesity in humans. *Nature* **387**:903, 1997.
805. Green ED, Maffei M, Braden VV, Procena R, DeSilva U, Zhang Y, Chua S, Leibel RL, Weissenbach J, Friedman JM: The human obese (OB) gene: RNA expression pattern and mapping on the physical, cytogenic and genetic maps of chromosome 7. *Genome Res* **5**:5, 1995.
806. Strobel A, Issad T, Camoin L, Ozata M, Strosberg A: A leptin missense mutation associated with hypogonadism and morbid obesity. *Nat Genet* **18**:213, 1998.
807. Considine RV, Considine EL, Williams CJ, Nyce MR, Magosin SA, Bauer TL, Rosato EL, Colberg J, Caro JF: Evidence against either a premature stop codon or the absence of obese gene mRNA in human obesity. *J Clin Invest* **95**:2986, 1995.
808. Maffei M, Stoffel M, Barone M, Moon B, Dammerman M, Ravussin E, Bogardus C, Ludwig DS, Flier JS, Talley M, et al.: Absence of mutations in the human OB gene in obese/diabetic subjects. *Diabetes* **45**:679, 1996.
809. Clement K, Garner C, Hager J, Philippi A, Leduc C, Carey A, Harris TJR, Jury C, Cardon LR, Basdevant A, et al.: Indication for linkage of the human *OB* gene region with extreme obesity. *Diabetes* **45(5)**:687, 1996.
810. Lonnqvist F, Arner P, Nordfors L, Schalling M: Overexpression of the obese (ob) gene in human obese subjects. *Nat Med* **1**:950, 1995.
811. Lonnqvist F, Wennlund A, Arner P: Relationship between circulating leptin and peripheral fat distribution in obese subjects. *Int J Obes Relat Metab Disord* **21**:255, 1997.
812. Clement K, Vaisse C, Lahlou N, Cabrol S, Pelloux V, Cassuto D, Gourmelen M, Dina C, Chambaz J, Lacorte JM, et al.: A mutation in the human leptin receptor gene causes obesity and pituitary dysfunction. *Nature* **392**:398, 1998.
813. Tannenbaum G, Lapointe M, Gud W, Finkelstein J: Mechanisms of impaired growth hormone secretion in genetically obese Zucker rats: Roles of growth hormone-releasing factor and somatostatin. *Endocrinology* **127**:3087, 1990.
814. Diamond F, Eichler D, Duckett G, Jorgensen EV, Shulman D, Root A: Demonstration of a leptin binding factor in human serum. *Biochem Biophysl Res Commun* **233**:818, 1997.
815. Liu C, Liu X, Barry G, Ling N, Maki R, DeSouza E: Expression and characterization of a putative high affinity human soluble leptin receptor. *Endocrinology* **138**:3548, 1997.
816. Chung WK, Power-Kehoe L, Chua M, Chu F, Aronne L, Huma Z, Sothern M, Udall JN, Kahle EB, Leibel RL: Exonic and intronic allelic variation in the leptin receptor (OBR) of obese humans. *Diabetes* **46**:1509, 1997.
817. Thompson DB, Ravussin E, Bennett PH, Bogardus C: Structure and sequence variation at the human leptin receptor gene in lean and obese Pima Indians. *Hum Mol Genet* **6**:675, 1997.
818. Chagnon YC, Chung WK, Perusse L, Chagnon M, Leibel RL, Bouchard C: Linkages and associations between the leptin receptor (LEPR) gene and human body composition in the Quebec Family Study. *Int J Obes Relat Metab Disord* **23**:278, 1999.
820. Rolland V, Clement K, Dugail I, Guy-Grand B, Basdevant A, Froguel P, Lavau M: Leptin receptor gene in a large cohort of massively obese subjects: No indication of the *fa/fa* rat mutation. Detection of an intronic variant with no association with obesity. *Obes Res* **6**:122, 1998.
821. Francke S, Clement K, Dina C, Inoue H, Behn P, Vatin V, Basdevant A, Guy-Grand B, Permutt MA, Froguel P, et al.: Genetic studies of the leptin receptor gene in morbidly obese French Caucasian families. *Hum Genet* **100**:491, 1997.
822. Matsuoka N, Ogawa Y, Hosoda K, Matsuda J, Masuzaki H, Miyawaki T, Azuma N, Natsui K, Nishimura H, Yoshimasa Y, et al.: Human leptin receptor gene in obese Japanese subjects: Evidence against either obesity-causing mutations or association of sequence variants with obesity. *Diabetologia* **40**:1204, 1997.
823. Gotoda T, Manning BS, Goldstone AP, Imrie H, Evans AL, Stroberg AD, KcKeigue PM, Scott J, Aitman TJ: Leptin receptor gene variation and obesity: Lack of association in a white British male population. *Hum Mol Genet* **6**:869, 1997.
824. Silver K, Walston J, Chung WK, Yao F, Parikh VV, Anderson R, Cheskin LJ, Eliahi D, Muller D, Leibel RL, et al.: The Gln223Arg and Lys656Asn polymorphisms in the human leptin receptor do not associate with traits related to NIDDM or obesity. *Diabetes* **46**:1898, 1997.
825. Echwald SM, Sorensen TD, Sorensen TI, Tybjaerg-Hansen A, Chung WK, Leibel RL, Pedersen O: Amino acid variants in the human leptin receptor: Lack of association to juvenile onset obesity. *Biochem Biophysl Res Commun* **233**:248, 1997.
826. Considine RV, Considine EL, Williams CJ, Hyde TM, Caro JF. The hypothalamic leptin receptor in humans: Identification of incidental sequence polymorphisms and absence of the *db/db* mouse and *fa/fa* rat mutations. *Diabetes* **45**:992, 1996.
827. Poole T, Silvers W: An experimental analysis of the recessive yellow coat color mutant in the mouse. *Dev Biol* **48**:377, 1976.
828. Klungland H, Vage D, Gomez-Raya L, Adalsteinsson S, Lien S: The role of melanocyte-stimulating hormone (MSH) receptor in bovine coat color determination. *Mamm Genome* **6**:636, 1995.
829. Joerg H, Fries H, Meijerink E, Stranzinger G: Red coat color in Holstein cattle is associated with a deletion in the *MSHR* gene. *Mamm Genome* **7**:317, 1996.
830. Valverde P, Healy E, Jackson I, Rees JL, Thody AJ: Variants of the melanocyte-stimulating hormone receptor gene are associated with red hair and fair skin humans. *Nat Genet* **11(3)**:328, 1995.
831. Box N, Wyeth J, O'Gorman L, Martin N, Sturm R: Characterization of melanocyte stimulating hormone receptor variant alleles in twins with red hair. *Hum Mol Genet* **6**:1891, 1997.
832. Boston BA, Blaydon KM, Varnerin J, Cone RD: Independent and additive effects of central pomc and leptin pathways on murine obesity. *Science* **278**:1641, 1997.
833. Seeley R, Yagaloff K, Fisher S, Burn P, Thiele T, vanDijk G, Baskin D, Schwartz M: Melanocortin receptors in leptin effects. *Nature* 390:349, 1997.

834. Latruffe N, Vamecq J: Peroxisome proliferators and peroxisome proliferator activated receptors (PPARs) as regulators of lipid metabolism. *Biochimie* **79**:81, 1997.
835. Tontonoz P, Nagy L, Alvarez J, Thomazy V, Evans R: PPARy promotes monocyte/macrophage differentiation and uptake of oxidized LDL. *Cell* **93**:241, 1998.
836. Tontonoz P, Hu E, Devine J, Beale E, Spiegelman B: PPAR gamma 2 regulates adipose expression of the phosphoenolpyruvate carboxykinase gene. *Mol Cell Biol* **15**:351, 1995.
837. Hu E, Kim JB, Sarraf P, Spiegelman BM: Inhibition of adipogenesis through MAP kinase-mediated phosphorylation of PPARgamma. *Science* **274**:2100, 1996.
838. Adams M, Reginato MJ, Shao D, Lazar MA, Chatterjee VK: Transcriptional activation by peroxisome proliferator-activated receptor gamma is inhibited by phosphorylation at a consensus mitogen-activated protein kinase site. *J Biol Chem* **272**:5128, 1997.
839. Forman BM, Tontonoz P, Chen J, Brun RP, Spiegelman BM, Evans RM: 15-Deoxy-delta 12, 14-prostaglandin J2 is a ligand for the adipocyte differentiation factor PPAR gamma. *Cell* **83**:803, 1995.
840. Green S, Wahli W: Peroxisome proliferator-activated receptors: Finding the orphan a home. *Mol Cell Endocrinol* **100**:149, 1994.
841. Lehmann JM, Moore LB, Smith-Oliver TA, Wilkison WO, Willson TM, Kliewer SA: An antidiabetic thiazolidinedione is a high affinity ligand for peroxisome proliferator-activated receptor gamma (PPAR gamma). *J Biol Chem* **270**:12953, 1995.
842. Nolan J, Ludvik B, Beerdsen P, Joyce M, Olefsky J: Improvement in glucose tolerance and insulin resistance in obese subjects treated with troglitazone. *N Engl J Med* **331**:1188, 1994.
843. Saltiel AR, Olefsky JM: Thiazolidinediones in the treatment of insulin resistance and type II diabetes. *Diabetes* **45**:1661, 1996.
844. Hofmann C, Lorenz K, Braithwaite S, Colca J, Palazuk B, Hotamisligil G, Spiegelman B: Altered gene expression for tumor necrosis factor-alpha and its receptors during drug and dietary modulation of insulin resistance. *J Endocrinol* **134**:264, 1994.
845. Vidal-Puig A, Jimenez-Linan M, Lowell BB, Hamann A, Hu E, Spiegelman B, Flier JS, Moller DE: Regulation of PPAR gamma gene expression by nutrition and obesity in rodents. *J Clin Invest* **97**:2553, 1996.
846. Qian H, Hausman GJ, Compton MM, Azain MJ, Hartzell DL, Baile CA: Leptin regulation of peroxisome proliferator-activated receptor-gamma, tumor necrosis factor, and uncoupling protein-2 expression in adipose tissue. *Biochem Biophys Res Commun* **246**:660, 1998.
847. MacDougald OA, Lane MD: Transcriptional regulation of gene expression during adipocyte differentiation. *Annu Rev Biochem* **64**:345, 1995.
848. Yeh W, Cao Z, Classon M, McKnight S: Cascade regulation of terminal adipocyte differentiation by three members of the C/EBP family of leucine zipper proteins. *Genes Dev* **9**:168, 1995.
849. Tontonoz P, Kim J, Graves R, Spiegelman B: ADD1: A novel helix-loop-helix transcription factor associated with adipocyte determination and differentiation. *Mol Cell Biol* **13**:4753, 1993.
850. Yokoyama C, Wang X, Briggs M, Admon A, Wu J, Hua X, Goldstein J, Brown M: SREBP-1, a basic-helix-loop-helix-leucine zipper protein that controls transcription of the low density lipoprotein receptor gene. *Cell* **75**:187, 1993.
851. Greenwood M: The relationship of enzyme activity to feeding behavior in rats: Lipoprotein lipase as the metabolic gatekeeper. *Int J Obes* **9(Suppl)**:67, 1985.
852. Brunzell JD: Familial lipoprotein lipase deficiency and other causes of the chylomicronemia syndrome, in Scriver CR, Beaudet AL, Sly WS, Valle D: (eds):*The Metabolic Basis of Inherited Disease*, vol. 1. New York, McGraw-Hill, 1989, p 1165.
853. Ristow M, Muller-Wieland D, Pfeiffer A, Krone W, Kahn CR: Human obesity associated with a mutation in PPARγ2, a regulator of adipocyte differentiation. *N Engl J Med* **339**:953, 1998.
854. Coleman DL: Obesity genes: Beneficial effects in heterozygous mice. *Science* **203**:663, 1979.
855. Coleman DL: Acetone *Metabolism* in mice: Increased activity in mice heterozygous for obesity genes. *Proc Natl Acad Sci U S A* **77**:290, 1980.
856. Croft J, Morrell D, Chase C, Swift M: Obesity in heterozygous carriers of the gene for Bardet-Biedl syndrome. *Am J Med Genet* **55**:12, 1995.
857. Croft J, Swift M: Obesity, hypertension and renal disease in relatives of Bardet-Biedl syndrome sibs. *Am J Med Genet* **36**:37, 1990.
858. Ching PL, Willett WC, Rimm EB, Colditz GA, Gortmaker SL, Stampfer MJ: Activity level and risk of overweight in male health professionals. *Am J Public Health* **86**:25, 1996.
859. Prentice AM, Jebb SA: Obesity in Britain: Gluttony or sloth? *BMJ* **311**:437, 1995.
860. Porter RK, Brand MD: Body mass dependence of H^+ leak in mitochondria and its relevance to metabolic rate. *Nature* **362**:628, 1993.
861. Porter RK, Brand MD: Causes of differences in respiration rate of hepatocytes from mammals of different body mass. *Am J Physiol* **269**:R1213, 1995.
862. Rolfe DE, Brand MD: Contribution of mitochondrial proton leak to skeletal muscle respiration and to standard metabolic rate. *Am J Physiol* **271**:C1380, 1996.
863. Jezek P, Orosz DE, Modriansky M, Garlid KD: Transport of anions and protons by the mitochondrial uncoupling protein and its regulation by nucleotides and fatty acids. A new look at old hypotheses. *J Biol Chem* **269**:26184, 1994.
864. Klaus S, Casteilla L, Bouillaud F, Ricquier D: The uncoupling protein UCP: A membraneous mitochondrial ion carrier exclusively expressed in brown adipose tissue. *Int J Biochem* **23**:791, 1991.
865. Himms-Hagen J: Brown adipose tissue thermogenesis and obesity. *Prog Lipid Res* **28**:67, 1989.
866. Nicholls DG, Locke RM: Thermogenic mechanisms in brown fat. *Physiol Rev* **64**:1, 1984.
868. Gonzalez-Barroso MM, Fleury C, Arechaga I, Zaragoza P, Levi-Meyrueis C, Raimbault S, Ricquier D, Bouillaud F, Rial E: Activation of the uncoupling protein by fatty acids is modulated by mutations in the C-terminal region of the protein. *Eur J Biochem* **239**:445, 1996.
869. Mitchell P, Moyle J: Chemiosmotic hypothesis of oxidative phosphorylation. *Nature* **213**:137, 1967.
870. Cunningham S, Leslie P, Hopwood D, Illingsworth P, Jung RT, Nicholls DG, Peden N, Rafael J, Rial E: The characterization and energetic potential of brown adipose tissue in man. *Clin Sci* **69**:343, 1985.
871. Ridley RG, Patel HV, Gerber GE, Morton RC, Freeman KB: Complete nucleotide and derived amino acid sequence of cDNA encoding the mitochondrial uncoupling protein of rat brown adipose tissue: Lack of a mitochondrial targeting presequence. *Nucleic Acids Res* **14**:4025, 1986.
872. Bouillaud F, Weissenbach J, Ricquier D: Complete cDNA-derived amino acid sequence of rat brown fat uncoupling protein. *J Biol Chem* **261**:1487, 1986.
873. Bouillaud F, Villarroya F, Hentz E, Raimbault S, Cassard A, Ricquier D: Detection of brown adipose tissue uncoupling protein mRNA in adult patients by a human genomic probe. *Clin Sci* **75**:21, 1988.
874. Cassard AM, Bouillaud F, Mattei MG, Hentz E, Raimbault S, Thomas M, Ricquier D: Human uncoupling protein gene: structure, comparison with rat gene, and assignment to the long arm of chromosome 4. *J Cell Biochem* **43**:255, 1990.
875. Oberkofler H, Dallinger G, Liu YM, Hell E, Krempler F, Patsch W: Uncoupling protein gene: Quantification of expression levels in adipose tissues of obese and non-obese humans. *J Lipid Res* **38**:2125, 1997.
876. Esterbauer H, Oberkofler H, Liu YM, Breban D, Hell E, Krempler F, Patsch W: Uncoupling protein-1 mRNA expression in obese human subjects: the role of sequence variations at the uncoupling protein-1 gene locus. *J Lipid Res* **39**:834, 1998.
877. Oppert JM, Vohl MC, Chagnon M, Dionne FT, Cassard-Doulcier AM, Ricquier C, Perusse L, Bouchard C: DNA polymorphism in the uncoupling protein (UCP) gene and human body fat. *Int J Obes Relat Metab Disord* **18**:526, 1994.
878. Clement K, Ruiz J, Cassard-Doulcier AM, Bouillaud F, Ricquier D, Basdevant A, Guy-Grand B, Froguel P: Additive effect of A$\rightarrow$G ($-$3826) variant of the uncoupling protein gene and the Trp64Arg mutation of the beta 3-adrenergic receptor gene on weight gain in morbid obesity. *Int J Obes Relat Metab Disord* **20**:1062, 1996.
879. Fumeron F, Durack-Brown I, Betoulle D, Cassard-Doulcier AM, Tuzet S, Bouillaud F, Melchior JC, Ricquier D, Apfelbaum M: Polymorphisms of uncoupling protein (UCP) and beta 3 adrenoreceptor genes in obese people submitted to a low calorie diet. *Int J Obes Relat Metab Disord* **20**:1051, 1996.
880. Gagnon J, Lago F, Chagnon YC, Perusse L, Naslund I, Lissner L, Sjostrom L, Bouchard C: DNA polymorphism in the uncoupling protein (UCP1) gene has no effect on obesity related phenotypes in

the Swedish obese subjects cohorts. *Int J Obes Relat Metab Disord* **22**:500, 1998.
881. Lean ME, James WP, Jennings G, Trayhurn P: Brown adipose tissue uncoupling protein content in human infants, children and adults. *Clin Sci* **71**:291, 1986.
882. Garruti G, Ricquier D: Analysis of uncoupling protein and its mRNA in adipose tissue deposits of adult humans. *Int J Obes Relat Metab Disord* **16**:383, 1992.
883. Astrup A, Bulow J, Madsen J, Christensen NJ: Contribution of BAT and skeletal muscle to thermogenesis induced by ephedrine in man. *Am J Physiol* **248**:E507, 1985.
884. Oberkofler H, Liu YM, Esterbauer H, Hell E, Krempler F, Patsch W: Uncoupling protein-2 gene: Reduced mRNA expression in intraperitoneal adipose tissue of obese humans. *Diabetologia* **41**:940, 1998.
885. Urhammer SA, dalgaard LT, Sorensen TI, Moller AM, Anderson T, Tybjaerg-Hansen A, Hansen T, Clausen JO, Vestergaard H, Pederson O: Mutational analysis of the coding region of the uncoupling protein 2 gene in obese NIDDM patients: Impact of a common amino acid polymorphism on juvenile and maturity onset forms of obesity and insulin resistance. *Diabetologia* **40**:1227, 1997.
886. Otabe S, Clement K, Dubois S, Lepretre F, Pelloux V, Leibel RL, Chung WK, Boutin P, Guy-Grand B, Froguel P, et al.: Mutation screening and association studies of the human UCP3 gene in normoglycemic and diabetic morbidly obese patients. *Diabetes* **48**:206, 1999.
887. Walder K, Norman RA, Hanson RL, Schrauwen P, Neverova M, Jenkinson CP, Easlick J, Warden CH, Pecqueur C, Raimbault S, et al.: Association between uncoupling protein polymorphisms (UCP2-UCP3) and energy metabolism/obesity in Pima Indians. *Hum Mol Genet* **7**:1431, 1998.
888. Warden CH, Fisler JS, Pace MJ, Svenson KL, Lusis AJ: Coincidence of genetic loci for plasma cholesterol levels and obesity in a multifactorial mouse model. *J Clin Invest* **92**:773, 1993.
889. Seldin MF, Mott D, Bhat D, Petro A, Kuhn CM, Kingsmore SF, Bogardus C, Opara E, Feinglos MN, Surwit S: Glycogen synthase: A putative locus for diet-induced hyperglycemia. *J Clin Invest* **94**:269, 1994.
890. Solanes G, Vidal-Ouig A, Grujic D, Flier JS, Lowell BB: The human uncoupling protein-3 gene. Genomic structure, chromosomal localization, and genetic basis for short and long form transcripts. *J Biol Chem* **272**:25433, 1997.
891. Boss O, Giacobino JP, Muzzin P: Genomic structure of uncoupling protein-3 (UCP3) and its assignment to chromosome 11q13. *Genomics* **47**:425, 1998.
892. Esterbauer H, Oberkofler H, Dallinger G, Breban D, Hell E, Krempler F, Patsch W: Uncoupling protein-3 gene expression: Reduced skeletal muscle mRNA levels in obese humans after pronounced weight loss. *Diabetologia* **42**:302, 1999.
893. Walker SP, Rimm EB, Ascherio A, Kawachi I, Stampfer MJ, Willett WC: Body size and fat distribution as predictors of stroke among US men. *Am J Epidemiol* **144**:1143, 1996.
894. Suskind R, Sothern M, Faris R, Almen TV, Schumacher H, Carlisle L, Vargas A, Escobar O, Loftin M, Fuchs G: Recent advances in the treatment of childhood obesity. *Ann N Y Acad Sci* **699**:181, 1993.
895. Knip M, Nuutinen O: Long-term effects of weight reduction on serum lipids and plasma insulin in obese children. *Am J Clin Nutr* **57**:490, 1993.
896. Endo H, Takagi Y, Nozue T, Kuwahata K, Uemasu F, Kobayashi A: Beneficial effects of dietary intervention on serum lipid and apoprotein levels in obese children. *Am J Dis Child* **146**:303, 1992.
897. Frank G, Berenson G, Webber L: Dietary studies and the relationship of diet to cardiovascular disease risk factor variables in 10-year old children: The Bogalusa Heart Study. *Am J Clin Nutr* **31**:328, 1978.
898. Wei M, Macera CA, Hornung CA, Blair SN: Changes in lipids associated with change in regular exercise in free-living men. *J Clin Endocrinol Metab* **50**:1137, 1997.
899. Blair S, Kohn H, Gordon W, Pafenberger R: How much physical activity is good for health? *Ann Rev Pub Health* **13**:99, 1992.
900. Gordon NF, Scott CB, Wilkinson WJ, Duncan JJ, Blair SN: Exercise and mild essential hypertension. Recommendations for adults. *Sports Med* **10**:390, 1990.
901. Dunn AL, Marcus BH, Kampert JB, Garcia ME, Kohn HW, Blair SN: Reduction in cardiovascular disease risk factors: Six month results from Project Active. *Prev Med* **26**:883, 1997.
902. Blair SN: Evidence for success of exercise in weight loss and control. *Ann Intern Med* **119(7pt 2)**:706, 1993.
903. Kriska AM, Blair SN, Pereira MA: The potential role of physical activity in the prevention of non-insulin-dependent diabetes mellitus: The epidemiological evidence. *Exerc Sport Sci Rev* **22**:121, 1994.
904. DiPietro L, Kohn HW, Barlow CE, Blair SN: Improvements in cardiorespiratory fitness attenuate age-related weight gain in healthy men and women: The Aerobics Center Longitudinal Study. *Int J Obes Relat Metab Disord* **22**:55, 1998.
905. Dobrin-Seckler BE, Deckelbaum RJ: Safety of the American Heart Association Step Diet in childhood. *Ann N Y Acad Sci* **623**:263, 1991.
906. Eckel RH, Krauss RM: American Heart Association call to action: Obesity as a major risk factor for coronary heart disease. *Circulation* **97**:2099, 1998.
907. Eckel RH: Obesity and heart disease: A statement for healthcare professionals from the Nutrition Committee, American Heart Association. *Circulation* **96**:3248, 1997.
908. American Heart Association: American Heart Association guidelines for weight management programs for healthy adults. *Heart Dis Stroke* **3**:221, 1994.
909. Strong WB, Deckelbaum RJ, Gidding SS, Kavey RE, Washington R, Wilmore JH, Perry CL: Integrated cardiovascular health promotion in childhood. A statement for health professionals. *Circulation* **85**:1638, 1992.
910. Weiser M, Frishman W, Michaelson M, Abdeen M: The pharmacologic approach to the treatment of obesity. *J Clin Pharmacol* **37**:453, 1997.
911. Pi-Sunyer FX, Laferrere B, Aronne LJ, Bray GA: Obesity: A modern day epidemic. *J Clin Endocrinol Metab* (In press), 1999.
912. Abenhaim L, Moride Y, Brenot F, Rich S, Benichou J, Kurz X, Higenbottam T, Oakley C, Wouters E, Aubier M, et al.: Appetite-suppressant drugs and the risk of primary pulmonary hypertension. *N Engl J Med* **335**:609, 1996.
913. Connolly HM, Crary JL, McGoon MD, Hensrud DD, Edwards BS, Edwards WD, Schaff HV: Valvular heart disease associated with fenfluramine-phentermine. *N Engl J Med* **337**:581, 1997.
914. Khan MA, Herzog CA, StPeter JV, Hartley GG, Madlon-Kay R, Dick CD, Asinger RW, Vessey JT: The prevalence of cardiac valvular insufficiency assessed by transthoracic echocardiography in obese patients treated with appetite-suppressant drugs. *N Engl J Med* **339**:713, 1998.
915. Jicks H, Vasilakis C, Weinrauch LA, Meier CR, Jick SS, Derby LE: A population-based study of appetite-suppressant drugs and the risk of cardiac-valve regurgitation. *N Engl J Med* **339**:719, 1998.
916. Weissman NJ, Tighe JF, Gottdeiner JS, Gwynne JT: An assessment of heart-valve abnormalities in obese patients taking Dexfenfluramine, sustained-release Dexfenfluramine or placebo. *N Engl J Med* **339(339)**:725, 1998.
917. Manson JE, Faich GA: Pharmacotherapy for obesity—Do the benefits outweigh the risks? *N Engl J Med* **335**:659, 1996.
918. Stock MJ: Sibutramine: A review of the pharmacology of a novel anti-obesity agent. *Int J Obes Relat Metab Disord* **21(Suppl)**:S25, 1997.
919. Lean ME: Sibutramine: A review of clinical efficacy. *Int J Obes Relat Metab Disord* **21(Suppl)**:S30, 1997.
920. Kral JG: Surgical interventions for obesity, in Brownell KD, Fairburn CG: (eds): *Eating Disorders and Obesity*. New York, Guilford Press, p 510, 1995.
921. Koopmans HS: The effect of infused nutrients and absorbed foods on daily food intake in rats. *Obes Res* **3(Suppl)**:675S, 1995.
922. Glenny AM, O'Meara S, Melville A, Sheldon TA, Wilson C: The treatment and prevention of obesity: A systemic review of the literature. *Int J Obes Relat Metab Disord* **21**:715, 1997.
923. Alpers DH: Surgical therapy for obesity. *N Engl J Med* **308**:1026, 1983.
924. Sax H: Long-term morbidity following jejunoileal bypass: The continuing potential need for surgical reversal. *Arch Surg* **130**:318, 1995.
925. Perri MG, Nezu AM, Patti ET, McCann KL: Effect of length of treatment on weight loss. *J Consult Clin Psych* **57**:450, 1989.
926. Epstein LH, Valoski A, Wing RR, McCurley J: Ten-year follow-up of behavioral, family-based treatment of obese children. *JAMA* **264**:2519, 1990.
927. Epstein LH: Family-based behavioural intervention for obese children. *Int J Obese Relat Metab Disord* **20**:S14, 1996.
928. Wadden TA: Treatment of obesity by moderate and severe caloric restriction. Result of clinical research trials. *Ann Intern Med* **119**:688, 1993.

929. Rose C, Vargas F, Facchinetti P, Bourgeat P, Bambal RB, Bishop PB, Chan SMT, Moore ANJ, Ganellin CR, Schwartz J-C: Characterization and inhibition of a cholecystokinin-inactivating serine peptidase. *Nature* **380**:403, 1996.
931. Rosenbaum M, Leibel RL: Leptin: A molecule integrating somatic energy stores, energy expenditure and fertility. *Trends Endocrinol Metabol* **9**:117, 1998.
932. Cheung CC, Thornton JE, KJuijper JL, Weigle DS, Clifton DK, Steiner RA: Leptin is a metabolic gate for the onset of puberty in the female rat. *Endocrinology* **138**:855, 1997.
933. Matkovic V, Ilich JZ, Skugor M, Badenhop NE, Goel P, Clairmont A, Klisovic D, Nahhas RW, Landoll JD: Leptin is inversely related to age at menarche in human females. *J Clin Endocrinol Metab* **82**:3239, 1997.
934. Garcia-Mayor RV, Andrade MA, Rios M, Lage M, Dieguez C, Casaneuva FF: Serum leptin levels in normal children: Relationship to age, gender, body mass index, pituitary-gonadal hormones, and pubertal age. *J Clin Endocrinol Metab* **82**:2849, 1997.
935. Arch JR, Wilson S: Prospects for beta 3-adrenoceptor agonists in the treatment of obesity and diabetes. *Int J Obes Relat Metab Disord* **20**:191, 1996.
936. Drent ML, VanDerVeen EA: First clinical studies with orlistat: A short review. *Obes Res* **3**:553S, 1995.
937. James WP, Avenell A, Broom J, Whitehead J: A one-year trial to assess the value of orlistat in the management of obesity. *Int J Obes Relat Metab Disord* **21(Suppl)**:S24, 1997.
938. Cahill G: Starvation in man. *N Engl J Med* **282**:668, 1970.
939. Carnelutti M, Guercio MD, Chiumello G: Influence of growth hormone on the pathogenesis of obesity in children. *J Pediatr* **77**:285, 1970.
942. Forbes BG: Nutrition and growth. *J Pediatr* **91**:40, 1977.
943. Cacciari E, Cicognani A, Pirazzoli P, Zappulla F, Tassoni P, Bernardi F, Salardi S, Mazzanti L: Effect of obesity on the hypothalamo-pituitary-gonadal function in childhood. *Acta Paediatr Scand* **66**:345, 1977.
944. Cacciari E, Frejaville E, Balsamo A, Cicognani A, Pirazzoli P, Bernardi F, Zappulla F: Disordered prolactin secretion in the obese child and adolescent. *Arch Dis Child* **56**:386, 1981.
945. Schmitt T, Luceman W, McCool C, Lenz F, Ahmad U, Nolan S, Stephan T, Sundar J, Danowski T: Unresponsiveness to exogenous TSH in obesity. *Int J Obes* **1**:185, 1977.
946. Genazzani AR, Pintor C, Corda R: Plasma level of gonadotropins, prolactin, thyroxine, and adrenal and gonadal steroids in obese prepubertal girls. *J Clin Endocrinol Metab* **45**:974, 1978.
947. Slavnov VN, Epshtein EV: Somatotrophic, thyrotrophic, and adrenocorticotrophic functions of the anterior pituitary in obesity. *Endocrinology* **15**:213, 1977.
948. Dunkel L, Sorva R, Voutilainen R: Low levels of sex hormone-binding globulin in obese children. *J Pediatr* **107**:95, 1985.
949. Glass AR, Swedloft RS, Bray GA, Dahms WT, Atkinson RL: Low serum testosterone and sex hormone-binding globulin in massively obese men. *J Clin Endocrinol Metab* **45**:1211, 1977.
950. Hartz AJ, Kalkhoff RK, Rimm AA, McCall RJ: A study of factors associated with the ability to maintain weight loss. *Prev Med* **8(4)**:471, 1979.
951. Atkinson RL, Kaiser DL: Effects of calorie restriction and weight loss on glucose and insulin levels in obese humans. *J Am Coll Nutr* **4**:411, 1985.
952. Chiumello G, DelGuercio MJ, Carnelutti M, Bidone G: Relationship between obesity, chemical diabetes, and beta pancreatic function in children. *Diabetes* **18**:238, 1969.
953. Aronne LJ, Mackintosh RM, Rosenbaum M, Leibel RL, Hirsch J: Cardiac autonomic nervous system activity in obese and never-obese young men. *Obes Res* **5**:354, 1997.
954. Galvin-Parton PA, Chun X, Moxhan CM, Malban CC: Induction of Galphaq-specific antisense RNA in vivo causes increased body mass and hyperadiposity. *J Biol Chem* **272**:4335, 1997.
955. Hotamisligil GS, Peraldi P, Budvari A, Ellis H, White MF, Spiegelman BM: IRS-1 mediated inhibition of insulin receptor tyrosine kinase activity in TNF-alpha- and obesity-induced insulin resistance. *Science* **271**:665, 1996.
956. Katz EB, Stenbit AE, Hatton K, DePinho R, Charron MJ: Cardiac and adipose tissue abnormalities but not diabetes in mice deficient in GLUT4. *Nature* **377**:151, 1995.
957. Pepin M-C, Pothier F, Barden N: Impaired type II glucocorticoid-receptor function in mice bearing antisense RNA transgene. *Nature* **355**:725, 1992.
958. Murray J, Buetow K, Weber J, Ludwigsen S, Scherpbier-Heddema T, Manion F, Quillen J, Sheffield V, Sunden S, Duyk G: A comprehensive human linkage map with centimorgan density. Cooperative human linkage center (CHLC). *Science* **265**:2049, 1994.
959. Bailey-Wilson J, Wilson A, Bamba V: Linkage analysis in a large pedigree ascertained due to essential familial hypercholesterolemia. *Genet Epidemiol* **10**:665, 1993.
960. Clement K, Philippi A, Jury C, Pividal R, Hager J, Demenais F, Basdevant A, Guy-Grand B: Candidate gene approach of familial morbid obesity: Linkage analysis of the glucocorticoid receptor gene. *Int J Obes Relat Metab Disord* **20**:507, 1996.
961. Wilson AF, Elston RC, Tran LD, Siervogel RM: Use of the robust sib-pair method to screen for single-locus, multiple-locus and pleiotropic effects: Application to traits related to hypertension. *Am J Hum Genet* **48**:862, 1991.
962. Norman RA, Bogardus C, Ravussin E: Linkage between obesity and a marker near the tumor necrosis factor-α locus in Pima Indians. *J Clin Invest* **96**:158, 1995.
963. Hani EH, Clement K, Velho G, Vionnet N, Hager J, Philippi A, Dina C, Inoue H, Permut MA, Basdevant A, et al.: Genetic studies of the sulfonylurea receptor gene locus in NIDDM and in morbid obesity among French Caucasians. *Diabetes* **46**:688, 1997.
964. Chagnon YC, Lamothe M, Perusse L, Chagnon M, Gagnon J, Nadeau A, Chung WK, Power-Kehoe L, Chua SC, Leibel RL, et al.: Suggestive linkages between markers on human 1p32-p22 and body fat and insulin levels in the Quebec Family Study. *Obes Res* **5**:115, 1997.
965. Allison DB, Heo M: Meta-analysis of linkage data under worst-case conditions: A demonstration using the human OB region. *Genetics* **148**:859, 1998.
966. Borecki IB, Rice T, Perusse L, Bouchard C, Rao DC: An exploratory investigation of genetic linkage with body composition and fatness phenotypes: the Quebec family study. *Obes Res* **2**:213–9, 1994.
967. Widen E, Lehto M, Kanninen T, Walston J, Shulcnier AR, Groop LC: Association of a polymorphism in the β3-adrenergic-receptor gene with features of the insulin resistance syndrome in Finns. *N Engl J Med* **333(6)**:348, 1995.
968. Deriaz O, Dionne F, Perusse L, Tremblay A, Vohl MC, Cote G, Bouchard C: DNA variation in the genes of the Na, K-adenosine triphosphatase and its relation with resting metabolic rate, respiratory quotient, and body fat. *J Clin Invest* **93**:838, 1994.
969. Michaud EJ, Mynatt RL, Miltenberger RJ, Klebig ML, Wilkinson JE, Zemel MB, Wilkison WO, Woychik RP: Role of the agouti gene in obesity. *J Endocrinol* **155**:207, 1997.
970. Hall C, Manser E, Spurr NK, Lim L: Assignment of the human carboxypeptidase E (CPE) gene to chromosome 4. *Genomics* **15**:461, 1993.
971. Geffroy S, Vos PD, Staels B, Duban B, Auwerx J, Martinville BD: Localization of the human OB gene (OBS) to chromosome 7q32 by fluorescence in situ hybridization. *Genomics* **28(3)**:603, 1995.
972. Magenis RE, Smith L, Nadeau JH, Johnson KR, Mountjoy KG, Cone RD: Mapping of the ACTH, MSH and neural (MC3 and MC4) melanocortin receptors in the mouse and human. *Mamm Genome* **5**:503, 1994.
973. Mountjoy KG, Wong J: Obesity, diabetes and functions for proopiomelanocortin-deprived peptides. *Mol Cell Endocrinol* **128**:171, 1997.
974. Nakamura M, Yokoyama M, Watanabe H, Matsumoto T: Molecular cloning, organization and localization of the gene for the mouse neuropeptide Y-Y5 receptor. *Biochim Biophys Acta* **1328**:83, 1997.
975. Huppi K, Siwarski D, Pisegna JR, Wank S: Chromosomal localization of the gastric and brain receptors for cholecystokinin (CCKAR and CCKBR) in human and mouse. *Genomics* **25**:727, 1995.
976. Chawla A, Schwarz EJ, Dimaculangan DD, Lazar MA: Peroxisome proliferator-activated receptor (PPAR) gamma: Adipose-predominant expression and induction early in adipocyte differentiation. *Endocrinology* **135**:798, 1994.
977. Mitchell BD, Blangero J, Comuzzie AG, Almasy LA, Shuldiner AR, Silver K, Stern MP, MacCluer JW, Hixson JE: A paired sibling analysis of the beta-3 adrenergic receptor and obesity in Mexican Americans. *J Clin Invest* **101**:584, 1998.
978. Evans H, Baumgartner M, Shine J, Herzog H: Genomic organization and localization of the gene encoding human preprogalanin. *Genomics* **18**:473, 1993.

979. Nicholl J, Kofler B, Sutherland GR, Shine J, Iismaa TP: Assignment of the gene encoding human galanin receptor (GALNR) to 18q23 by in situ hybridization. *Genomics* **30**:629, 1995.
980. Pedeutour F, Szpirer C, Nahon JL. Assignment of the human pro-melanin-concentrating hormone gene (PMCH) to Chr. 12q23-24 and two variant genes (PMCH1 and PMCHL2) to Chr. 5p14 and 5q12-13. *Genomics* **19**:31, 1994.
981. Marondel I, Renault B, Lieman J, Ward D, Kucherlapati R: Physical mapping of the human neurotensin gene (NTS) between markers D12S1444 and D12S81 on Chr. 12q21. *Genomics* **38**:243, 1996.
982. Laurent P, Clerc P, Mattei MG, Forgez P, Dumont X, Ferrara P, Caput D, Rostene W: Chromosomal localization of mouse and human neurotensin receptor genes. *Mamm Genome* **5**:303, 1994.
983. Ozcelik T, Leff S, Robinson W, Donlon T, Lalande M, Sanjines E, Sanjines A, Schinzel A, Francke U: Small nuclear ribonucleoprotein polypeptide N (SNRPN), an expressed gene in the Prader-Willi syndrome critical region. *Nat Genet* **2**:265, 1992.
984. Dragani TA, Zeng ZB, Canzian F, Gariboldi M, Ghilarducci MT, Manenti G, Pierotti MA: Mapping of body weight loci on mouse chromosome X. *Mamm Genome* **6**:778, 1995.
985. Brockmann G, Timtchenko D, Das P, et al.: Detection of QTL for body weight and body fat content in mice using genetic markers. *J Anim Breed Genet* **113**:373, 1996.
986. Taylor BA, Phillips SJ: Obesity QTLs on mouse chromosomes 2 and 17. *Genomics* **43**:249, 1997.
987. Pomp D: Genetic dissection of obesity in polygenic animals models. *Behav Genet* **27**:285, 1997.
988. Keightley PD, Hardge T, May L, Bulfield G: A genetic map of quantitative trait loci for body weight in the mouse. *Genetics* **142**:227, 1996.
989. Cheverud JM, Routman EJ, Duarte FA, Swinderen BV, Cothran K, Perel C: Quantitative trait loci for murine growth. *Genetics* **142**:1305, 1996.
990. Gauguier D, Froguel P, Parent V, Bernard C, Bihoreau M-T, Porta B, James MR, Penicaud L, Lathrop M, Ktorza A: Chromosomal mapping of genetic loci associated with non-insulin dependent diabetes in the GK rat. *Nat Genet* **12**:38, 1996.
991. Galli J, Li L-S, Glaser A, Ostenson C-G, Jiao H, Fakhrai-Rad H, Jacob HJ, Lander ES, Luthman H: Genetic analysis of non-insulin dependent diabetes mellitus in the GK rat. *Nat Genet* **12**:31, 1996.
992. Anderson L, Haley CS, Ellegren H, et al.: Genetic mapping of quantitative trait loci for growth and fatness in pigs. *Science* **263**:1771, 1994.
993. Bodoky M, Rethelyi M: Dendritic arborization and axon trajectory of neurons in the hypothalamic arcuate nucleus of the rate. *Exp Brain Res* **28**:543, 1977.
994. Zaborszky L, Makara GB: Intrahypothalamic connections: An electron microscopic study in the rat. *Exp Brain Res* **34**:201, 1979.
995. terHorst GJ, Luiten PG: The projection of the dorsomedial hypothalamic nucleus in the rat. *Brain Res Bull* **16**:231, 1986.
996. Saper CB, Swanson LW, Cowan WM: An autoradiographic study of the efferent connections of the lateral hypothalamic area in the rat. *J Comp Neurol* **183**:689, 1979.
997. Berk ML, Finkelstein JA: Efferent connections of the lateral hypothalamic area of the rat: An autoradiographic investigation. *Brain Res Bull* **8**:511, 1982.
998. McClain D, Alexander T, Cooksey R, Considine R: Hexosamines stimulate leptin production in transgenic mice. *Endocrinol* **141**:1999, 2000.
999. Wang J, Liu R, Hawkins M, Barzilai N, Rossetti L: A nutrient-sensing pathway regulates leptin gene expression in muscle and fat. *Nature* **393**:684, 1998.
1000. Wang Y, Lee-Kwon W, Martindale J, Adams L, Heller P, Egan J, Bernier M: Modulation of CCAAT/enhancer-binding protein-alpha gene expression by metabolic signals in rodent adipocytes. *Endocrinol* **140**:2938, 1999.
1001. Levine J, Eberhardy N, Jensen M: Role of nonexercise activity thermogenesis in resistance to fat gain in humans. *Science* **283**:212, 1999.
1002. Shetty P: Adaptation to low energy intakes: the responses and limits to intakes in infants, children, and adults. *Eur J Clin Nutr* **53**:S14, 1999.
1003. Kulkarni R, Shetty P: Net mechanical efficiency during stepping in chronically energy deficient human subjects. *Ann Hum Biol* **19**:421, 1992.
1004. Ashworth A: An investigation of very lower calorie intake in Jamaica. *Br Med J* **22**:341, 1968.
1005. Satyanarayana K, Venkataramana Y, Rao S: Nutrition and work performance studies carried out in India. Proceedings of XIVth International Congress of Nutrition. Seoul, Korea: Korean Nutrition Society, 1989:98.
1006. Rosenbaum M, Vandenborne K, Goldsmith R, Simoneau J, Hirsch J, Segal K, Joanisse D, Leibel R: Effects of weight change on skeletal muscle fuel utilization and chemomechanical coupling. Submitted for publication, 2000.
1007. Rall JA: Energetic aspects of skeletal muscle contraction: implications of fiber types. *Exercise & Sport Sci Rev* **13**:33, 1985.
1008. Phillips S, Wiseman R, Woledge R, Kushmerick M: The effect of metabolic fuel on force production and resting inorganic phosphate levels in mouse skeletal muscle. *J Physiol* **463**:135, 1993.
1009. Barclay C, Constable J, Gibbs C: Energetics of fast- and slow-twitch muscle fibers of the mouse. *J Physiol* **472**:61, 1993.
1010. Holmang A, Brzezinska Z, Bjorntorp P: Effects of hyperinsulinemia on muscle fiber composition and capillarization in rats. *Diabetes* **42**:1073, 1993.
1011. Simoneau JA, Colberg SR, Thaete FL, Kelley DE: Skeletal muscle utilization of free fatty acids in women with visceral obesity. *J Clin Invest* **95**:1846, 1995.
1012. Simoneau JA, Colberg SR, Thaete FL, Kelley DE: Skeletal muscle glycolytic and oxidative enzyme capacities are determinants of insulin sensitivity and muscle composition in obese women. *FASEB J* **9**:273, 1995.
1013. Russell DM, Walker PM, Leiter LA, Sima AA, Tanner WK, Mickle DA, Whitwell J, Marliss EB, Jeejeebhoy KN: Metabolic and structural changes in skeletal muscle during hypocaloric dieting. *Am J Clin Nutr* **39**:503, 1984.
1014. de la Torre AM, Madapallimattam A, Cross A, Armstrong RL, Jeejeebhoy KN: Effect of fasting, hypocaloric feeding, and refeeding on the energetics of stimulated rat muscle as assessed by nuclear magnetic resonance spectroscopy. *J Clin Invest* **92**:114, 1993.
1015. Broberger C, Johansen J, Johansson C, Schalling M, Hokfelt T: The neuropeptide Y/agouti gene-related protein (AGRP) brain circuitry in normal, anorectic, and monosodium glutamate-treated mice. *Proc Natl Acad Sci USA* **95**:15043–8, 1998.
1016. Hahn TM, Breininger JF, Baskin DG, Schwartz MW: Coexpression of Agrp and NPY in fasting-activated hypothalamic neurons. *Nat Neurosci* **1**:271–2, 1998.
1017. Elias CF, Lee C, Kelly J, Aschkenasi C, Ahima RS, Couceyro PR, Kuhar MJ, Saper CB, Elmquist JK: Leptin activates hypothalamic CART neurons projecting to the spinal cord. *Neuron* **21**:1375–85, 1998.
1018. Yaswen L, Diehl N, Brennan MB, Hochgeschwender U: Obesity in the mouse model of pro-opiomelanocortin deficiency responds to peripheral melanocortin. *Nat Med* **5**:1066–70, 1999.
1019. Korner J, Wardlaw SL, Liu SM, Conwell IM, Leibel RL, Chua SC Jr.: Effects of leptin receptor mutation on Agrp gene expression in fed and fasted lean and obese (LA/N-faf) rats. *Endocrinology* **141**:2465–71, 2000.
1020. Gunn TM, Miller KA, He L, Hyman RW, Davis RW, Azarani A, Schlossman SF, Duke-Cohan JS, Barsh GS. *Nature* **398**:152–6, 1999.
1021. Nagle DL, McGrail SH, Vitale J, Woolf EA, Dussault BJ Jr, DiRocco L, Holmgren L, Montagno J, Bork P, Huszar D, Fairchild-Huntress V, Ge P, Keilty J, Ebeling C, Baldini L, Gilcrist J, Burn P, Carlson GA, Moore KJ: The mahogany protein is a receptor involved in suppression of obesity. *Nature* **398**:148–52, 1999.
1022. Gong DW, Monemdjou S, Gavrilova O, Leon LR, Marcus-Samuels B, Chou CJ, Everett C, Kozak LP, Li C, Deng C, Harper ME, Reitman ML: Lack of obesity and normal response to fasting and thyroid hormone in mice lacking uncoupling protein-3. *J Biol Chem* **275**:16251–7, 2000.
1023. Vidal-Puig AJ, Grujic D, Zhang CY, Hagen T, Boss O, Ido Y, Szczepanik A, Wade J, Mootha V, Cortright R, Muoio DM, Lowell BB: Energy metabolism in uncoupling protein 3 gene knockout mice. *J Biol Chem* **275**:16258–66, 2000.
1024. Ross SR, Graves RA, Spiegelman BM: Targeted expression of a toxin gene to adipose tissue: transgenic mice resistant to obesity. *Genes Dev* **7**:1318–24, 1993.
1025. Gavrilova O, Marcus-Samuels B, Leon LR, Vinson C, Reitman ML: Leptin and diabetes in lipoatrophic mice. *Nature* **403**:850, 2000.
1026. Andand A, Chada K: In vivo modulation of Hmgic reduces obesity. *Nat Genet* **24**:377–80, 2000.
1027. Kishimoto T, Radulovic J, Radulovic M, Lin CR, Schrick C, Hooshmand F, Hermanson O, Rosenfeld MG, Speiss J: Deletion of

crhr2 reveals an anxiolytic role for corticotorpin-releasing hormone receptor-2. *Nat Genet* **4**:415–9, 2000.

1028. Bale TL, Contarino A, Smith GW, Chan R, Gold LH, Sawchenko PE, Koob GF, Vale WW, Lee KF. Mice deficient for corticotropin-releasing hormone receptor-2 display anxiety-like behavior and are hypersensitive to stress. *Nat Genet* **4**:410–4, 2000.
1029. Coste SC, Kesterson RA, Heldwein KA, Stevens SL, Heard AD, Hollis JH, Murray SE, Hill JK, Pantely GA, Hohimer AR, Hatton DC, Phillips TJ, Finn DA, Low MJ: Abnormal adaptations to stress and impaired cardiovascular function in mice lacking corticotropin-releasing hormone receptor-2. *Nat Genet* **4**:403–9, 2000.
1030. Coleman DL. The influence of genetic background on the expression of mutations at the diabetes (db) locus in the mouse. VI: Hepatic malic enzyme activity is associated with diabetes severity. *Metabolism* **41**:1134–6, 1992.
1031. Rosenbaum M, Leibel RL, Hirsch J: Medical Progress: Obesity. *N Engl J Med* **334**:396, 1997.
1032. Sinha MK, Opentanova I, Ohannesian JP, Kolaczynski JW, Heiman ML, Hale J, Becker G, Bowsher RR, Stephens TW, Caro JF: Evidence of free and bound leptin in human circulation. Studies in lean and obese subjects and during shortterm fasting. *J Clin Invest* **98**:1277–82, 1996.
1033. Horlick MB, Rosenbaum M, Nicolson M, Levine LS, Fedun B, Wang J, Pierson RN Jr, Leibel RL. Effect of puberty on the relationship between circulating leptin and body composition. *J Clin Endo Metab* **85**:2509–18, 2000.
1034. Houseknecht KL, Mantzoros CS, Kuliawat R, Hadro E, Flier JS, Kahn GG. Evidence for leptin binding to proteins in serum of rodents and humans: modulation with obesity. *Diabetes* **45**:1638–43, 1996.
1035. Ducy P, Amling M, Takeda S, Priemel M, Schilling AF, Beil FT, Shen J, Vinson C, Rueger JM, Karsenty G. Leptin inhibits bone formation through a hypothalamic relay: a central control of bone mass. *Cell* **100**:197–207, 2000.
1036. Marine JC, Topham DJ, McKay C, Wang D, Parganas E, Stravopodis D, Yoshimura A, Ihle JN: SOCS1 deficiency causes a lymphocyte-dependent perinatal lethality. *Cell* **98**:609–616, 1999.
1037. Butler. In press. *Endocrinol*, 2000.
1038. Bjorbaek C, El-Haschimi K, Frantz JD, Flier JS: The role of SOCS-3 in leptin signaling and leptin resistance. *J Biol Chem* **274**:30059–65, 1999.
1039. Flier JS. Clinical review 94: What's in a name? In search of leptin's physiological role. *J Clin Endocrinol Metab* **83**:1407–13, 1998.
1040. Rosenbaum M, Leibel RL: The role of leptin in human physiology. *N Engl J Med* **341**:913–5, 1999.
1041. Frisch RE: Pubertal adipose tissue: is it necessary for normal sexual maturation? Evidence from the rat and human female. *Fed Proc* **39**:2395–400, 1980.
1042. Farooqi IS, Jebb SA, Langmack G, Lawrence E, Cheetham CH, Prentice AM, Hughes IA, McCamish MA, O'Rahilly S: Effects of recombinant leptin therapy in a child with congential leptin deficiency. *N Engl J Med* **341**:879–84, 1999.
1043. Hixson JE, Almasy K, Cole S, Birnbaum S, Mitchell BD, Mahaney MC, Stern MP, MacCluer JW, Blangero J, Comuzzie AG: Normal variation in leptin levels in associated with polymorphisms in the proopiomelanocortin gene, POMC. *J Clin Endocrinol Metab* **84**:3187–91, 1999.
1044. Beamer B, Negri C, Yen C, Gavrilova O, Rumberger J, Durcan M, Yarnall D, Hawkins A, Griffin C, Burns D: Chromosomal localization and partial genomic structure of the human peroxisome proliferator activated receptor-gamma (hPPAR gamma) gene. *Biochem Biophys Res Comm* **233**:756–59, 1997.
1045. Beamer B, Yen C, Andersen R, Muller D, Elahi D, Cheskin L, Andres R, Roth J, Shuldiner A: Association of the Pro12Ala variant in the peroxisome proliferator-activated receptor-g2 gene with obesity in two Caucasian populations. *Diabetes* **47**:1806–08, 1998.
1046. Ishizuka T, Klepcyk P, Liu S, Panko L, Liu S, Gibbs EM, Friedman JE: Effects of overexpression of human GLUT4 gene on maternal diabetes and fetal growth in spontaneous gestational diabetic C57BLKS/J Lepr (db/+) mice. *Diabetes* **48**:1061–9, 1999.
1047. Argyropoulos G, Brown AM, Willi SM, Zhu J, He Y, Reitman M, Gevao SM, Spruill I, Garvey WT: Effects of mutations in the human uncoupling protein 3 gene on the respiratory quotient and fat oxidation in severe obesity and type 2 diabetes. *J Clin Invest* **102**:1345–51, 1998.
1050. Clapham JC, Arch JRS, Chapman H, Haynes A, Lister C, Moore GBT, Piercy V, Carter SA, Lehner I, Smith SA, Beeley LJ, Godden RJ, Herrity N, Skehel M, Kumar Changani K, Hockings PD, Reid DG, Squires SM, Hatcher J, Trail B, Latcham J, Rastan S, Harper AJ, Cadenas S, Buckingham JA, Brand MD, Abuin A: Mice over-expressing human uncoupling protein-3 in skeletal muscle are hyperphagic and lean. *Nature* **406**:415–8, 2000.
1051. Weiser M, Frishman WH, Michaelson MD, Abdeen MA: The pharmacological approach to the treatment of obesity. *J Clin Pharmacol* **37**:453–73, 1997.
1052. Pi-Sunyner FX, Laferre B, Aronne LJ, Bray GA: Therapeutic controversy: Obesity – a modern-day epidemic. *J Clin Endocrinol Metab* **84**:3–12, 1999.
1053. Bray GA, Tartaglia LA: Medicinal strategies in the treatment of obesity. *Nature* **404**:672–77, 2000.
1054. Astrup A, Buemann B, Christensen NJ, Toubro S, Thorbek G, Victor OJ, Quaade F: The effect of ephedrine/caffeine mixture on energy expenditure and body composition in obese women. *Metabolism* **41**:686–8, 1992.
1055. Finer N, James WP, Kopelman PG, Lean ME, Williams G: One-year treatment of obesity: a randomized, double-blind, placebo-controlled, multicentre study of orlistat, a gastrointestinal lipase inhibitor. *Int J Obes* **24**:306–13, 2000.
1056. Hill JO, Hauptman J, Anderson JW, Fujioka K, O'Neil PM, Smith DK, Zavoral JH, Aronne LJ: Orlistat, a lipase inhibitor, for weight maintenance after conventional dieting: a 1-y study. *Am J Clin Nutr* **69**:1108–16, 1999.
1057. Katzmarzyk PT, Rankinen T, Perusse L, Deriaz O, Tremblay A, Borecki I, Rao DC, Bouchard C: Linkage and association of the sodium potassium-adenosine triphosphatase alpha2 and betal genes with respiratory quotient and resting metabolic rate in the Quebec Family Study. *J Clin Endocrinol Metab* **84**:2093–7, 1999.
1058. Hager J, Dina C, Francke S, Dubois S, Houari M, Vatin V, Vaillant E, Lorentz N, Basdevant A, Clement K, Guy-Grand B, Froguel P: A genome-wide scan for human obesity genes reveals a major susceptibility locus on chromosome 10. *Nat Genet* **20**:304–8, 1998.
1059. Lee JH, Reed DR, Li WD, Xu W, Joo EJ, Kilker RL, Nanthakumar E, North N, Sakul H, Bell C, Price RA: Genome scan for human obesity and linkage to markers in 20q13.. *Am J Hum Genet* **64**:196–209, 1999.
1060. Katsanis N, Beales PL, Woods MO, Lewis RA, Green JS, Parfrey PS, Ansley SJ, Davidson WS, Lupski JR: Mutations in MKKS cause obesity, retinal dystrophy and renal malformations associated with Bardet-Biedl syndrome. *Net Genet*, **26**:67–70, 2000.
1061. Slavotinek AM, Stone EM, Mykytyn K, Heckenlively JR, Green JS, Heon A, Musarella MA, Parfrey PS, Sheffield VS, Biesecker LG: Mutations in MKKS cause Bardet-Biedl syndrome. *Nat Genet* **26**:15–6, 2000.
1062. Hinney A, Schmidt A, Nottebom K, Heibult O, Becker I, Ziegler A, Gerber G, Sina M, Gorg T, Mayer H, Siegfried W, Fichter M, Remschmidt H, Hebebrand J: Several mutations in the melanocortin-4 receptor gene including a nonsense and a frameshift mutation associated with dominantly inherited obesity in humans. *J Clin Endocrinol Metab* **84**:1483–6, 1999.
1063. Sina M, Hinney A, Ziegler A, Neupert T, Mayer H, Siegfried W, Blum WF, Remschmidt H, Hebebrand J: Phenotypes in three pedigrees with autosomal dominant obesity casued by haploinsufficiency mutations in the melanocortin-4 receptor gene. *Am J Hum Gene*. **65**:1501–1507, 1999.

CHAPTER 158

Thyroid Disorders

Samuel Refetoff ▪ Jacques Dumont ▪ Gilbert Vassart

1. **Synthesis, storage, secretion, delivery, action, and metabolism of the thyroid hormones involve a complex sequence of molecular events, for which a number of the genes involved are known. Thyroid diseases may result from impairments at many steps in this process. Defects may be classified as resulting from anomalies within the thyroid gland (dyshormonogenesis), in the development of the thyroid anlage (thyroid dysgenesis), in the transport of thyroid hormones, in target tissues of thyroid hormones (thyroid hormone resistance), or in the regulatory hypothalamo-pituitary circuit.**
2. **Defects involving genes expressed in the thyroid gland may be responsible for a series of different phenotypes. Gain of function mutations of the thyrotropin receptor cause autosomal dominant toxic thyroid hyperplasia, or sporadic (neonatal) toxic thyroid hyperplasia, depending on whether the mutation is transmitted from one parent or is a new mutation. Loss-of-function mutations in any of the genes encoding proteins implicated directly or indirectly in thyroid hormone synthesis, cause hypothyroidism, usually associated with goiter secondary to hyperstimulation by thyrotropin (congenital goiter). Mutations of this type have been found in the sodium-iodide symporter (trapping defects), thyroglobulin (coupling defects), and thyroperoxidase and pendrin (organification defects). In all these instances, transmission is autosomal recessive and, except for the last one, the disease is nonsyndromic. Mutations of pendrin cause hypothyroidism associated with sensorineural deafness. Additional mutations are expected to be found in the genes responsible for H_2O_2 generation (an additional cause of organification defect), and in iodotyrosine deiodinase.**
3. **Inadequate regulation of thyroid function by thyrotropin causes a decrease in thyroid function (synthesis and secretion of thyroid hormone) and growth (thyroid hypoplasia). This may result from defects at the hypothalmo-pituitary level (central hypothyroidism), secondary to mutations in a series of developmental genes (*PIT1*, *PROP1*) required for normal growth and function of thyrotrophs. Mutations directly affecting the TRH receptor or thyrotropin beta genes also cause congenital hypothyroidism with thyroid hypoplasia. Similarly, but at the thyroid level, loss-of-function mutations of the TSH receptor gene cause variable levels of resistance to thyrotropin, the more severe cases presenting with congenital hypothyroidism and thyroid hypoplasia.**
4. **Thyroid dysgenesis is responsible for the majority of cases with congenital hypothyroidism (85%). It encompasses a series of developmental defects affecting the thyroid gland, whose common characteristic is an inadequate amount of functional thyroid tissue. The situation is anatomically (and probably genetically) heterogeneous, presenting as thyroid aplasia (agenesis), hypoplasia, ectopy, or hemiagenesis. Most cases are sporadic (~1/3500 newborn) which poses the unresolved problem of the genetic or environmental cause of the disease. In a handful of cases, a mutation has been identified in genes implicated in the development of the gland: *PAX8* and *TTF2*. In the latter, hypothyroidism is part of a complex syndrome with choanal atresia, cleft palate, and kinky hairs (Bamforth syndrome), reflecting the multiple sites of normal *TTF2* expression.**
5. **Since only free thyroid hormones are responsible for the effects on target tissues (including the hypothalamus and the thyrotrophs), mutations in the proteins implicated in the transport of thyroid hormones in the blood (thyroid binding globulin, TBG; transthyretin; albumin) are responsible only for anomalies of the concentration of circulating thyroxine or triodothyronine, without any other biological or clinical sign of thyroid dysfunction. Mutations have been described leading to quantitative (complete/partial TBG deficiency, TBG excess) or qualitative anomalies in thyroxin binding globulin, the most frequent situation being defective production of the protein secondary to loss-of-function mutations in this X-linked gene. Increase in serum total thyroxine is observed in patients with mutations resulting in the production of transthyretin with increased affinity for the hormone. Similarly, variant albumin molecules have been described and the mutations identified, with increased affinity for iodothyronines, the result being euthyroid hyperthyroxinemia or hyper-triodothyroninemia. Values of thyroid hormones may reach extremely high values in some cases.**
6. **Resistance to thyroid hormone of variable severity and tissue distribution has been identified. In the majority of**

A list of standard abbreviations is located immediately preceding the index in each volume. Additional abbreviations used in this chapter include: ADHD = attention deficit hyperactivity disorder; ALB = albumin; BAT = brown adipose tissue; BMR = basal metabolic rate; CG = chorionic gonadotropin; CGr = CG receptor; CPK = creatine kinase; CoA = Coactivator; CoR = Corepressor; CPHD = combined pituitary hormone deficiency; DIT = diiodotyrosine; dnTBG = denatured TBG; DBD = DNA-binding domain; DIO = deiodinase; DRA = down-regulated in adenoma (a gene); FSH = follicle-stimulating hormone; FSHr = FSH receptor; FT_3 = free T_3; FT_4 = free T_4; GH = growth hormone; G-protein = guanine nucleotide-binding protein; GPCR = G protein-coupled receptor; HAT = histone acetylation; hCG = human CG; HDAC = histone deacetylase; HTTH = hereditary toxic thyroid hyperplasia; I^- = iodide; IEF = isoelectric focusing; LBD = ligand-binding domain; LH = luteinizing hormone; LHr = LH receptor; LST-1 = liver-specific organic anion transporter; MIT = monoiodotyrosine; NCoR = nuclear corepressor; NIS = sodium/iodide symporter; oatp = organic anion transporter; PDS = Pendred syndrome; p/CAF = CREB binding protein-associated factor; PRL = prolactin; RAIU = radioactive iodide uptake; RTH = resistance to thyroid hormone; RXR = retinoid X receptor; rT_3 = reverse triiodothyronine or 3,3′,5′-triiodothyronine; sin3 = single minded (a corepressor); S/P = saliva to plasma ratio; SHBG = sex hormone-binding globulin; SRC-1 = steroid receptor coactivator (see CoA); STTH = sporadic toxic thyroid hyperplasia; T_1 = monoiodothyronine; T_2 = diiodothyronine; T_3 = 3,3′,5-triiodothyronine; T_4 = thyroxine of 3,3′,5,5′-tetraiodothyronine; TBG = thyroxine binding globulin; TBPA = thyroxine-binding prealbumin; Tg = thyroglobulin; TETRAC = tetraiodothyroacetic acid; TPO = thyroid peroxidase; TR = thyroid hormone receptor; TRAP = TR associated protein; TRE = thyroid hormone response element; TRH = thyrotropin releasing hormone; TRIAC = triiodothyroacetic acid; TSAb = thyroid stimulating antibodies; TSH = thyroid stimulating hormone or thyrotropin; TSHr = TSH receptor; TT_4 = total T_4; TTF 1 = thyroid transcription factor 1; TTF 2 = thyroid transcription factor 2; TTR = transthyretin; WT = wild-type.

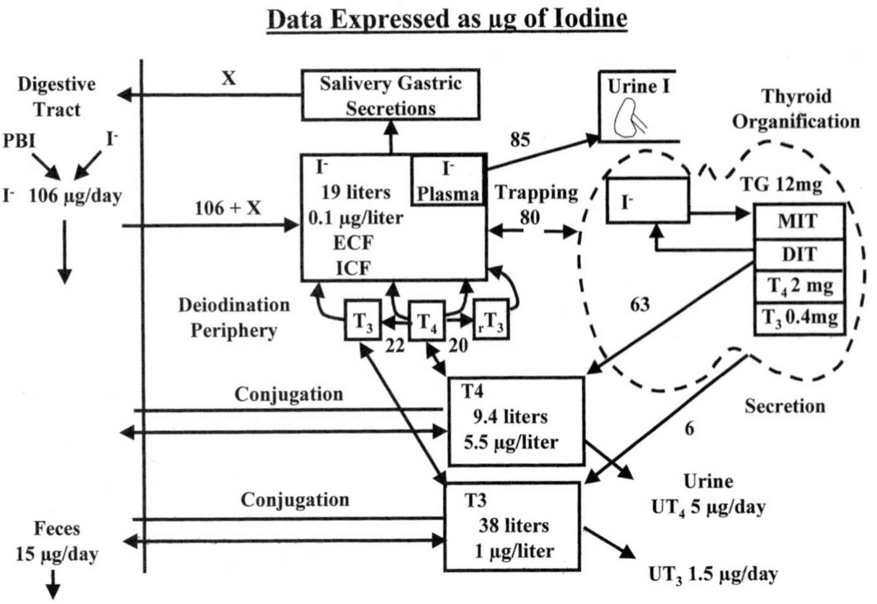

Fig. 158-1 Compartments in iodine metabolism in man. The data within boxes indicate volume of compartment and iodine concentration except for the thyroid where total iodine is given. The data on the arrows joining the compartments indicate fluxes as µg per day. All the fluxes have been corrected to insure equality of total inward and outward fluxes. ECF = extracellular fluid; ICF = intracellular fluid.

cases it is caused by mutations in the thyroid hormone receptor beta gene. The more common form is inherited dominantly because the mutant receptors, with decreased ligand binding or abnormal interaction with transcription cofactors, interfere with the function of the normal receptor. Resistance caused by receptor deletion is inherited recessively while a third form, without thyroid hormone receptor abnormalities, may be caused by defects in any of the cofactors involved in the mediation of thyroid hormone action.

Laboratory investigations of subjects with familial thyroid disease have resulted in classification of most patients according to their biochemical defect in specialized thyroid metabolism. In each of the categories reviewed here, the lesion affects one of the proteins involved. However, the net effect of most defects is the same: reduced thyroid hormone action through defective synthesis, delivery, or action of hormone. In the case of congenital hyperthyroidism activating mutation of the TSH receptor leads to thyroid hyperfunction, goiter, and thyrotoxicosis. Before considering each defect, it is appropriate to review relevant aspects of thyroid and iodine metabolism. A scheme of the metabolic pathway of iodine appears in Fig. 158-1. For a relevant older bibliography, earlier editions of this chapter may be consulted.[1,2]

THYROID PHYSIOLOGY AND METABOLISM: AN OVERVIEW

Iodide* ion is absorbed through the gastrointestinal tract and is rapidly distributed throughout the extracellular fluid of the body. The volume of distribution is approximately 30 percent of body weight. Except in the postprandial state, the iodide concentration in the plasma is less than 0.2 µg/dl. The kidney and the thyroid gland remove the iodide from plasma almost entirely. Renal clearance of iodide is normally about 35 ml/min and is independent of the iodine supply. Thyroid clearance varies widely. It depends on the functional state of the gland and on the iodine supply in the diet, but is normally between 10 and 35 ml/min. The iodide taken by the salivary and gastric glands is returned to plasma after absorption in the small intestine. Small amounts of iodide are removed by the mammary glands during lactation, and some organic iodine is lost in the feces and urine.

The function of the thyroid follicle cell is to trap iodide from the blood and to use it for the synthesis of the thyroid hormones T_4 and T_3. Iodide is trapped at the basal membrane of the cell and concentrated in the lumen; it is oxidized and bound to the tyrosyl residues of thyroglobulin by thyroperoxidase at the apical membrane of the cell (Fig. 158-2). The H_2O_2 required by the peroxidase is supplied by a still poorly defined H_2O_2-generating system. Thyroperoxidase also catalyzes the oxidative coupling of iodotyrosines into iodothyronines T_4 and T_3 within the matrix of thyroglobulin. Thyroglobulin slowly diffuses within the follicular lumen to ensure the relative homogeneity of the luminal content, the colloid. Thyroid colloid thus constitutes a store of sequestered iodine, the iodotyrosyls, and thyroid hormones contained in thyroglobulin. In the secretory process, follicular cells internalize thyroglobulin by micropinocytosis or macropinocytosis and digest it in constituent amino acids in secondary lysosomes. While the iodothyronines are released, presumably by diffusion, the iodotyrosines are deiodinated in the cell by a still unknown iodotyrosine deiodinase, thus allowing the reutilization of their iodine. Part of the thyroxine is deiodinated to triiodothyronine by iodothyronine deiodinase type II.

TSH (thyroid-stimulating hormone, or thyrotropin) controls all the metabolic steps of the follicular cell, as well as its growth. The level of TSH in the plasma is mainly the result of positive hypothalamic control exerted through TRH (thyrotropin-releasing hormone) and negative control on TSH and TRH synthesis and secretion exerted by circulating iodothyronines.

Iodinated thyronines and tyrosines may be absorbed intact by the gut but are partially (T_3 and T_4 less than 5 percent) or almost totally (iodotyrosines = 95 percent) deiodinated prior to absorption. On absorption or secretion, T_4, and to some extent T_3, are first confined to the vascular compartment because of binding to carrier proteins in the plasma.

They are transported mostly bound to serum proteins: thyroxine-binding globulin (TBG), transthyretin (TTR; previously known as "thyroxine-binding prealbumin"), and albumin. T4, which must be considered a prohormone, is deiodinated to the active hormone, 3,5,3′-triiodothyronine (T3), or to an inactive species, 3,3′,5′-triiodothyronine, or reverse T3 (rT3), in peripheral tissues. The action of thyroid hormone on peripheral cells, which is mediated through thyroid hormone receptors exerting their effects mostly at the level of gene expression, is to enhance certain

*Note: In this chapter, iodine is used in a generic sense to encompass all forms and oxidation states unless otherwise indicated; iodide designates the

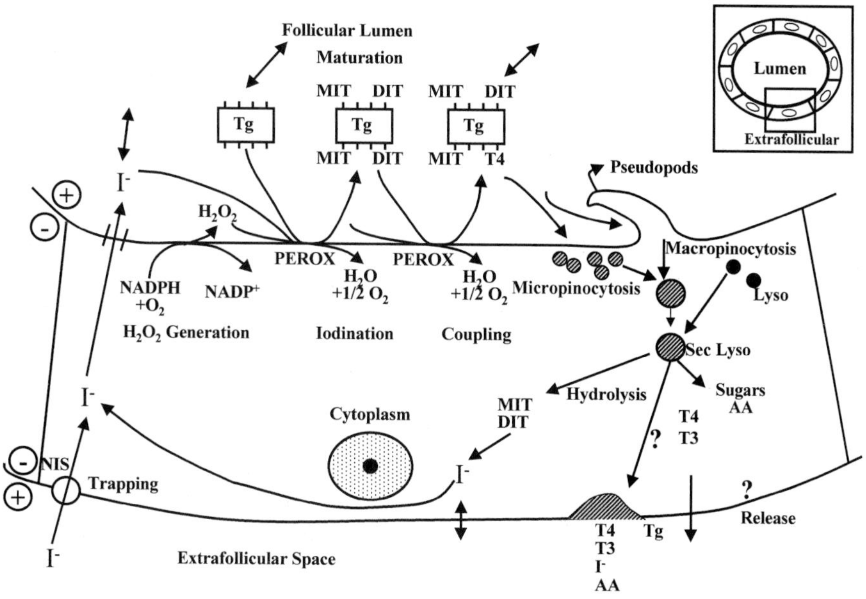

Fig. 158-2 Cellular physiology of iodine metabolism in the thyroid cell. + and − indicate the electrical polarity of the membranes. −⊕→ Active transport of iodide by the Na^+/I^- symporter. =→ Diffusion of iodide through the apical channel (probably pendrin, see text). Peroxi = peroxidase.

components of cellular intermediary metabolism and thus the general whole body basal metabolic rate and to sustain body and brain growth and development.

Most of the metabolic steps and controls outlined here involve several different proteins. Structural or regulatory defects may be expected for any of the proteins involved in each step, but the phenotypic expression of such defects will be virtually identical: clinical and biologic hypothyroidism in all cases except those of resistance to thyroid hormones, and goiter in all thyroid-specific iodine metabolism defects downstream from the TSH receptor cAMP cascade. In this chapter, defects are classified based on the function involved, that is, according to the phenotypic expression. It is understood that each of these classes may encompass several different genetic defects.

THE THYROID SYSTEM

The thyroid system is controlled at five levels: the brain, hypothalamus, hypophysis, thyroid, and periphery by the conversion of prohormone T4 to T3 (Fig. 158-3).

Control at the Hypothalamic Pituitary Level

Effects at the level of the hypothalamus are of the neural type, that is, immediate and of short duration. At the lower levels, effects are more delayed and of longer duration. For example, the first effects of T_3 take place hours after hormone administration and persist for days. Desensitization to TRH and TSH actions contributes to termination of their action. Impulses from the brain influence the hypophysiotropic TRH secretory neurons through an ill-defined neural network. Adrenergic neurons, through α receptors, probably constitute the final common activating pathway for diverse positive (e.g., cold), negative (e.g., stress, morphine), or periodic (e.g., nychthemeral rhythms) stimuli. Thyroid hormones exert a negative feedback on these neurons and on TRH secretion.[3]

TRH is a tripeptide (pyroglutamylhistidylprolinamide). It results from the hydrolysis and posttranslational processing (cyclization) of a large protein prohormone (27 kDa) containing 5 Gln-His-Pro-Gly sequences. TRH neurons are located in the thyrotropic area of the hypothalamus where electrical excitation causes TSH release. They extend from the paraventricular and supraoptic nuclei to the anterior border of the median eminence. TRH granules are transported down the axon by axoplasmic flow and are secreted at the level of the median eminence, where TRH

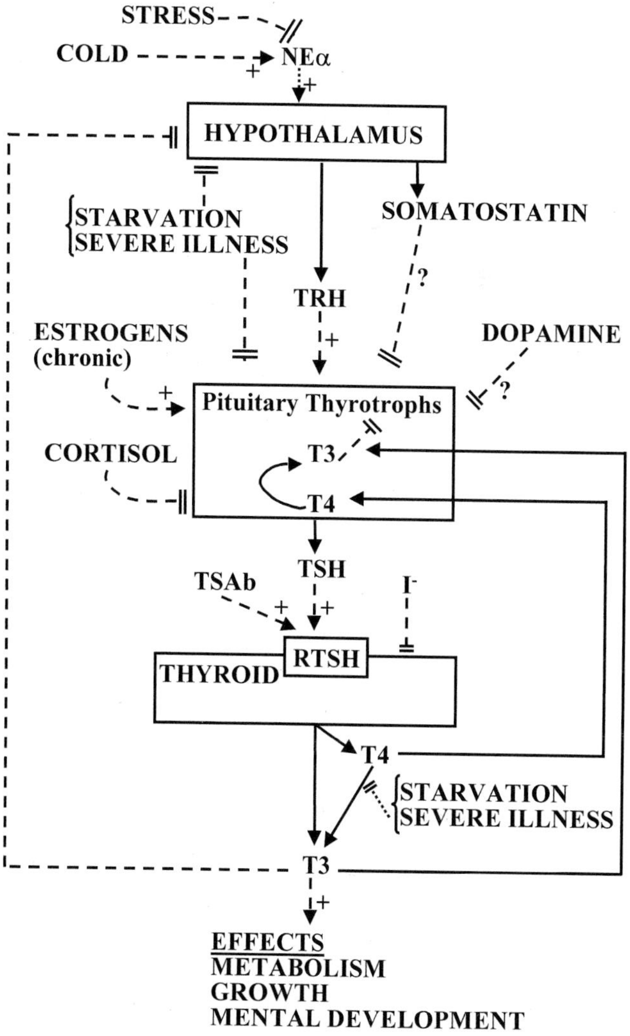

Fig. 158-3 Physiological control of the thyroid gland. → indicates metabolism or transport; - - - - -→+ indicates stimulation; and - - - - | | indicates inhibition. NEα = norepinephrine acting through α-adrenergic receptors.

penetrates fenestrated capillaries into the hypophyseal portal venous system, to be carried to the anterior lobe of the hypophysis. TRH is also a general neurotransmitter found in various areas of the brain and in the periphery (e.g., in the pancreas). It is inactivated in the serum within minutes.

The action of TRH on the thyrotrophs is very rapid. Binding to its receptor[4] triggers a depolarization and an influx of calcium into the cytosol and an activation of the Ca^2-phosphatidylinositol cascade. Calcium and diacylglycerol by the classic stimulus-secretion coupling mechanism cause TSH secretion. TRH also activates the synthesis and glycosylation of α and β subunits of TSH. It activates prolactin secretion, but whether this effect has a physiological meaning remains controversial.[5]

TSH is a glycoprotein of molecular weight 28,000. It is composed of two noncovalently linked subunits, α (M_r = 14,700, two oligosaccharide moieties) and β (M_r = 15,600, one oligosaccharide moiety). The α subunit is common to TSH, follicle-stimulating hormone (FSH), hCG, and LH, while the β subunit is specific for each of these hormones. This subunit confers on the hormone its biologic specificity and is the major determinant of immunologic specificity. Separate α and β subunits have no thyroid effect. The α and β subunits are coded on different genes, and there is no common precursor protein. Their biosynthesis is comparable to that of other glycoproteins, with synthesis of a preprotein with a signal sequence in the ER, cleavage of the signal sequence in the lumen of the ER, core glycosylation of dolichol phosphate intermediates, transfer to asparagine residues in the proteins, removal of some glucose residues, and further glycosylation in the ER and Golgi apparatus. The α subunits are synthesized in great excess as compared with the β subunits, but the β subunits have to be glycosylated in order to combine. In normal humans, TSH and its α and β subunits are secreted, but when the thyrotrophs are stimulated, as in hypothyroidism, both α- and β-subunit levels may increase. The final processed structure of secreted TSH carbohydrates varies depending on the physiological conditions, and it is important in determining the intrinsic biologic activity, that is, the biologic versus immunologic activity ratio, as well as the clearance rate of the hormone.[6,7] Because of its carbohydrate composition, TSH of hypothyroid patients has a prolonged half-life and a greater specific activity.[8]

The thyrotrophs are mainly controlled by the antagonistic control of TRH and thyroid hormones. Hypothalamic control accounts for the TSH nychthemeral rhythm, with its nocturnal maximum, and for the cold-induced TSH, T_4, and T_3 secretion which in man operates only for a short time after birth. TRH has only a small effect on transcription of the TSH gene, but stimulates the processing and glycosylation of the subunits and selectively increases the bioactivity of the secreted TSH. It also represses the expression of T_3 receptors and thus decreases the sensitivity of the thyrotrophs to the thyroid hormone negative feedback.[9]

The level of free thyroid hormone tightly controls TSH secretion. Small relative changes result in altered TSH secretion over the entire physiological range. The inhibiting effect of thyroid hormone is exerted both acutely and chronically on the number of TRH receptors, transcription of the TSH subunit genes, TSH synthesis, TSH secretion, the relative bioactivity of circulating TSH, and even the growth and multiplication of thyrotrophs. The inhibition of secretion is faster and will induce TSH accumulation in a first phase.

T_3 inhibits the thyrotrophs directly, but at the physiological level, the main external agent of control is T_4, which, through deiodination in the thyrotrophs themselves, provides the inhibiting cellular T_3. Chronic primary hypothyroidism leads not only to increased TSH levels but also to hypertrophy and multiplication of the thyrotrophs (which normally represent about 2 percent of the cell population of the anterior lobe) and to enlargement of the sella turcica.

Estrogens enhance the responsiveness of the thyrotrophs to TRH in animals and possibly in humans. Dopamine exerts negative control on TSH secretion in humans, probably at the level of the thyrotrophs. The metabolism of TSH is rapid (half-life about 1 h). It is accelerated by hyperthyroidism and decreased in hypothyroidism. TSH is principally metabolized in the kidney. Control of the hypothalamohypophyseal thyroid system fully matures only at the end of fetal life and the beginning of neonatal life.

Control at the Thyroid Level (Fig. 158-4)

Thyroid function and growth are stimulated by TSH and inhibited by iodine. Several accessory circuits involving neurotransmitters (ATP, norepinephrine, and TRH) and prostaglandins are superimposed on these main regulations but their physiological or pathologic significance remains to be demonstrated.[10] TSH acutely stimulates the binding of iodide to proteins, iodotyrosine oxidative coupling, thyroid hormone release, and many pathways of intermediary metabolism. With a delay of several hours, TSH enhances the trapping of iodide, gene expression and cell growth, and division. Over the long-term, it induces cell hypertrophy and thyroid hyperplasia.

TSH interacts with the thyroid follicular cell at the level of the plasma membrane by binding to a specific seven-transmembrane receptor coupled to G proteins, the TSH receptor. A recent extensive review is available.[11]

The TSH receptor is characterized by a long (398 amino acids) extracellular N-terminal, seven-transmembrane α helices, short intracellular and extracellular loops joining the α helices, and a rather short intracellular C-terminal. TSH binds to the extracellular part of the receptor and presumably to the transmembrane part. The C-terminal part, which in other receptors contains the phosphorylation sites involved in receptor desensitization, is short. It does not contain putative phosphorylation sites for G-protein receptor-coupled kinases or cyclic AMP-dependent protein kinase, which fits in well with the weak desensitization of this receptor. The TSH receptor is located at the basal and on the lateral membranes of the thyroid cell. It is able to couple to several G proteins in membranes G_s, $G_{i/o}$, G_{q11}, G_{12}. In human intact cells, there is only evidence for coupling to G_s, G_q, and $G_{i/o}$. That the dog TSH receptor is able to couple to G_q in isolated membranes but not in the intact cell, shows that all the possible interactions do not necessarily take place in the intact cell. The human TSH receptor, therefore, activates G_s and adenylate cyclase, and G_q and PIP_2 phospholipase C, and thus the cAMP and the PIP_2 PLC cascades. The former effect is obtained at 10 times lower concentrations of TSH than the latter. The role of G_i activation is unknown. The interaction of the TSH receptor and Gs involves the N- and C-terminals of the third intracellular loop.[11] Most of the effects of TSH on the human thyroid cell, the induction of $Na^+/I-$ symporter, the secretion of thyroid hormone, and the growth and proliferation of the cell are mediated by cAMP. However the generation of H_2O_2, the oxidation of iodide, and the synthesis of thyroid hormones are inhibited by cAMP and only activated by Ca^{++} and protein kinase C.[12]

In the cytosol, cAMP binds to cAMP-dependent protein kinases by the following reaction: $R_2C_2 + 4cAMP = R_2(cAMP)_4 + 2\ C$. R, the regulatory subunit of the kinases, blocks enzyme activity, while the binding of cAMP to R releases the active catalytic (C) subunits that phosphorylate specific protein substrates in the cell. Several such proteins are phosphorylated in response to TSH, but only a few of these, the histone H1, high-mobility-group protein HMG14, p70 S6 protein kinase, and the CREB and CREM transcription factors, have been identified, and the relation of the first phosphorylations to the physiologic effects of the hormone are still unknown. CREB and CREM phosphorylations may lead to several gene inductions (e.g., cfos, ICER) and appear to be necessary for cell cycle triggering. Early immediate gene induction by TSH and cyclic AMP involves cmyc, cfos, fosB, junB, ICER ornithine decarboxylase, and NGFIB.[10] The direct causal upstream and downstream consequent events of these inductions are unknown. Certainly, thyroglobulin and thyroperoxidase induction must involve mechanisms other than CRE

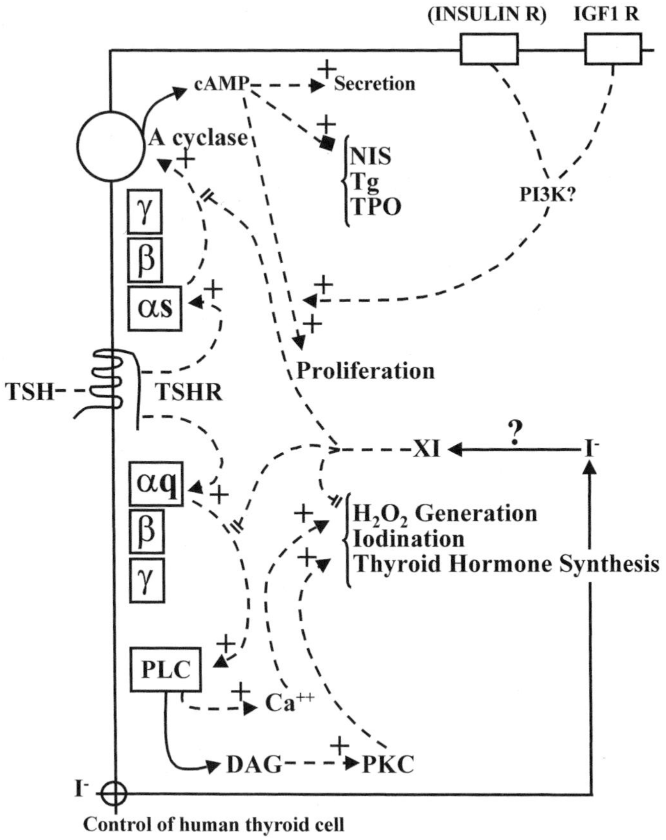

Fig. 158-4 Regulatory pathways of the human thyroid follicular cell. → indicates metabolism or transport; - - - - - →+ indicates stimulation; - - - - - || indicates inhibition; and - - - -◆+ indicates induction of protein. Controls may bear directly on a target or on the control of a target. α, β, and γ are the subunits of the G proteins G_s and G_q. DAG = diacylglycerol; PI3K = phosphatidylinositol-3 kinase.

activation and in the case of thyroglobulin the induction of an intermediary protein. The action of protein kinase A is necessary for most of the effects of TSH and cAMP but it is not sufficient for proliferation and induction of thyroglobulin synthesis. Other targets of cAMP must therefore be postulated. The recently discovered EPAC or GEF1, a GTP exchanger protein for Rap1, which binds to and is directly activated by cAMP, is one such target.[13]

The expression of the TSH-receptor gene is extremely "robust"; it is reduced but persists in the presence of agents (or after several steps in tumor progression) that promote extinction of the other markers of thyroid-cell differentiation. This leads to the conclusion that a basic marker of the thyroid phenotype is probably the TSH receptor itself. In a teleologic perspective, this makes sense: the gene encoding the sensor of TSH—the major regulator of thyroid function, growth, and expression of the fully differentiated phenotype—is virtually constitutive in thyrocytes.[14]

Long-term stimulation of the thyroid gland by TSH leads to a relative decrease in the secretory response (desensitization). Several mechanisms account for this: acute decrease in the stimulation of adenylate cyclase, exhaustion of the apical membranes available for macropinocytosis, and a later mild down-regulation of the TSH receptors.

Several other physiologic agents activate thyroid adenylate cyclase; among them are norepinephrine acting on β-adrenergic receptors and E prostaglandins. Compared to those of TSH, their effects are in general of lower amplitude, shorter duration, and unknown functional significance. The thyroid-stimulating immunoglobulins found in the serum of patients with Graves disease bind to the TSH receptor, activate adenylate cyclase, and reproduce the effects of TSH. TSH receptor-blocking antibodies, on the other hand, cause hypothyroidism.[15]

The thyroid cAMP system is negatively controlled by iodide at the level of adenylate cyclase and downstream. The effect is relieved by inhibitors of iodide trapping and iodide oxidation and presumably mediated by a still unknown signal molecule termed XI, which may contain iodine. Iodohexadecanal is a candidate XI. The same or a similar mechanism may also account for the inhibition by iodide of its own oxidation (Wolff-Chaikoff effect), the Ca^{2+}-PIP_2 cascade, of several transports including that of iodide itself, and perhaps of growth and secretion. Iodide inhibits thyroperoxidase and NIS expression, as well as thyroid cell proliferation in vivo.[16]

Specific gene expression in the thyroid and embryonic differentiation of the tissue requires several thyroid relatively specific transcription factors: TTF1, TTF2, and PAX8. During embryogenesis, these genes are expressed before thyroglobulin and thyroperoxidase (see "Thyroid Hypoplasia" below). However, no convincing role of these factors in the induction of differentiation or specific gene induction by TSH cAMP has been demonstrated.

Iodide Transport

The first step of iodine metabolism in the thyroid is the trapping of iodide by the follicles. The uptake, which takes place even in the absence of any further metabolism of iodide, requires an active transport mechanism. At normal plasma iodide concentrations, trapping is generally the limiting step of iodine metabolism in the thyroid. Iodide uptake, as measured by its clearance, depends on blood flow through the thyroid gland and on the iodide extraction ratio, $(A - V)/A$, where A and V are the arterial and venous concentrations, respectively, of iodide. Because the blood transit time in the thyroid gland is shorter than the half-life of iodide in red cells, this extraction ratio cannot be greater than 0.55 to 0.60, even if 99 percent of the plasma iodide is eventually taken up. Such ratios are obtained in iodine-deficient dogs, in which iodide trapping is limited by the thyroid blood flow. In normal humans, the extraction ratio is estimated at around 0.20, which suggests that blood flow is not limiting.

Under normal circumstances, the iodide extraction ratio in the thyroid reflects the activity of an iodide transport mechanism commonly called the iodide pump. Pump efficiency is generally evaluated, in tissues in which iodide oxidation has been blocked, as the ratios T/M, T/S, or C/M, where T, C, M, and S are the radioactivities per unit volume of labeled iodide in the thyroid, in isolated cells, in the incubation medium, and in the serum, respectively. At equilibrium, and if the thyroid is considered as one compartment, these ratios are equal to C/M/KTB, where C/M is the unidirectional iodide clearance per unit of tissue weight and KTB is the rate constant for unidirectional iodide efflux.[17]

Autoradiography, as well as compartmental analysis of uptake kinetics, shows that the thyroid follicle concentrates radioiodide in its lumen. This requires follicle integrity and implies a flux through both the basal and apical membranes of the cell. The potential difference across the membrane is about −20 mV, with the interior negative. Iodide has to overcome an electrical gradient to enter the cell, but it may flow downhill with the gradient, to accumulate in the lumen. This, and the fact that isolated cells also concentrate iodide, indicated the existence of an active transport mechanism in the basal membrane. Kinetic and autoradiographic experiments showing that under certain conditions perchlorate and radioiodide first accumulate in the cell and, more recently, direct measurements in polarized thyroid cells in culture suggest a permeability barrier and a transport at the apical membrane. This efflux is accelerated by TSH through Ca^{2+} in humans. The sodium iodide symporter cDNA has been cloned. It is a Na^+/I^- symporter (NIS) with 12 or 13 transmembrane helices (see "Dyshormonogenesis-Congenital Hypothyroidism with Goiter" below).[18]

Iodide transport is inhibited by thiocyanate perchlorate and inhibitors of the Na^+, K^+-activated ATPase such as ouabain. Iodide trapping with similar characteristics has been demonstrated in the salivary gland, gastric mucosa, mammary gland, and choroid plexus. The fact that these epithelia are unable to concentrate iodide in subjects with congenital cretinism due to a thyroidal defect of iodide trapping supports the hypothesis that the same mechanism is involved in other tissues. NIS has indeed been demonstrated in these tissues. Iodide is, however, not oxidized or bound to proteins in tissues other than thyroid.

Iodide trapping is first decreased and then increased by TSH. The former effect reflects an accelerated efflux presumably caused by increased cell permeability; the latter effect reflects an increased influx by enhancement of the V_{max} of the pump. This TSH action results from an induction by the cAMP cascade of the NIS mRNA and protein at the level of transcription. Long-term treatment with TSH considerably increases iodide trapping, while excess iodine depresses it, even in hypophysectomized animals.

Iodide trapping can be evaluated in vivo by measurement of iodide clearance under treatment with methimazole or, more conveniently, by the uptake of $^{99m}TcO_4-$, a nonmetabolized analogue. The transport mechanism can also be studied in other glands with iodide-concentrating ability, such as the salivary gland, as the salivary to plasma (S/P) radioiodide or thiocyanate (SCN−) ratios (see below).

Iodine Metabolism

Most of the iodine stored in the thyroid is covalently bound to amino acids within 19 S thyroglobulin in the form of thyroid hormones (T_3, T_4) and their iodotyrosine precursors, monoiodotyrosine (MIT) and diiodotyrosine (DIT). Thyroglobulin also contains small amounts of 3,3′,5′-iodothyronine (rT_3), 3,3′-diiodothyronine (T′2), and monoiodohistidine. Other organic forms are found, including particulate insoluble iodoproteins (a small percent of the iodine) and traces of iodinated lipids. The role of these forms is unknown. The concentrations of iodide (less than 0.25 percent) and of free hormones or iodotyrosines are very low. The synthesis of thyroid hormones requires several elements: iodide and thyroglobulin as substrates, an H_2O_2-generating system, and thyroperoxidase. At least three steps are involved: generation of H_2O_2, oxidation of iodide and binding to the tyrosyl residues of thyroglobulin, and the oxidative coupling of these iodotyrosyls into iodothyronines. The last two steps take place in a sequential manner within the matrix of thyroglobulin; they are catalyzed by the same enzymes and will be considered together in this section. Iodination and oxidative coupling are posttranslational processes. They are independent of protein synthesis.[19]

When iodination is allowed to proceed, the normal thyroid gland accumulates little iodide. Iodide transport is therefore the limiting step in iodide uptake; the machinery of protein iodination is geared to lock iodide trapped by the gland efficiently into covalent linkage.

Iodination occurs at the interface between the follicular cells and the colloid lumen, that is, at the level of the apical membrane and its microvilli. Light and electron microscopy can demonstrate rings of radioiodine-labeled proteins at the periphery of the colloid and on the apical cell membrane early after administration of radioiodide. This apical localization fits the location of the substrates for protein iodination (iodide and thyroglobulin), which are concentrated in the lumen, and of the cytosol coenzyme NADPH of the H_2O_2-generating system. It explains the correlation between iodinating capacity and follicular structure during ontogenesis and in cell cultures. This arrangement allows the thyroid cells to sequester H_2O_2 and possibly oxygen radicals and the iodinating system extracellularly, thus preventing iodination or oxidation of cell lipids and proteins in the absence of the proper substrate, thyroglobulin. Under some circumstances, iodination can take place inside the follicular cells, for example, in isolated cells and in some tumors. In these cases, the major iodination sites are microfollicular spaces inside the cell or in a few cells. Although such a mechanism may be operative in some pathological conditions, its physiological significance is questionable.

All the peroxidases need H_2O_2 in order to oxidize I^- and to bind it to proteins. The nature of the H_2O_2-generating system is poorly understood. As in leukocytes, NADH and predominantly NADPH stimulate iodination in broken cell systems. Two such NAPH oxidases have now been cloned.

In intact cells, as in broken cell systems, H_2O_2 greatly enhances iodination. Catalase inhibits iodination, and stimulation by TSH of iodination in dog and human thyroid slices is accompanied by a stimulation of H_2O_2 formation. These facts suggest that H_2O_2 generation may be the limiting step regulating iodination at least at high iodide levels. Iodination and H_2O_2 generation are stimulated by any agent that increases intracellular free Ca^{2+} and is inhibited by blockers of Ca^{2+} influx and by the cAMP cascade. This suggests that intracellular Ca^{2+} controls the rate-limiting step in iodination.[15]

Inorganic iodide must lose an electron before it can displace hydrogen from tyrosyl residues. This is accomplished in the presence of H_2O_2 by thyroid peroxidase. Most antithyroid drugs and goitrogens, which inhibit protein iodination in vivo or in intact cells, inhibit the peroxide-peroxidase system. Thyroid peroxidase exhibits a rather broad specificity. It is active only in the presence of H_2O_2, but excess H_2O_2 inhibits it. The enzyme catalyzes the iodination of free or bound tyrosines, and it also catalyzes the oxidation of I^- to I_2 and that of tyrosine to bityrosine. These reactions involve two closely related binding sites, which bind either tyrosine or iodide and oxidize iodide to iodonium (I^+) or hypoiodous ion (OI^-).[19] This explains why each time I_2 is formed in the reaction, iodination is inhibited, and thus why high levels of iodide inhibit iodination. Inhibition of iodination by thiourea and similar drugs is attributed to competition with iodide.

Thyroid peroxidase, like other peroxidases, is also able to catalyze the intramolecular coupling of iodotyrosyl groups in thyroglobulin. The same antithyroid agents that inhibit iodination in intact cells and in broken cell systems also inhibit oxidative coupling. Results obtained with thyroperoxidase and lactoperoxidase support the idea that the iodination and the coupling reactions are catalyzed by two different peroxidase-H_2O_2 species of the same enzyme. The formation of these different species would depend on the respective levels of H_2O_2 and iodide. The coupling results in the replacement of one iodotyrosine by an iodothyronine and the other by a dehydroalanine in the peptide chains of thyroglobulin. Thyroid peroxidase is the only enzyme that catalyzes iodination and coupling at physiological pH. Other peroxidases catalyze the two reactions at different pHs. Coupling requires iodotyrosines and H_2O_2, as well as iodide and free DIT. Thyroperoxidase may also oxidatively cleave peptides at the level of tyrosyl and tryptophan peptide bonds.

The kinetics of formation of iodotyrosines and iodothyronines in thyroglobulin suggest that iodination and coupling proceed in a rigid sequential manner. Only four to eight tyrosyl groups per thyroglobulin chain are among the first to be iodinated and coupled into iodothyronines. T_3 is preferentially formed at low levels of iodination, but never exceeds 0.4 mol of T_3 per mole of thyroglobulin. About 100 of the 144 tyrosyl groups in thyroglobulin are not iodinated, while only part of the MIT can be transformed into DIT. There is a maximal number of iodothyronines synthesized in thyroglobulin (potentially up to eight). All these facts indicate that there are rigid structural and spatial requirements for tyrosyl iodination and coupling imposed by the thyroglobulin structure itself (with a normal iodine diet, the average is 2.3 mol of T_4 and 0.3 mol of T_3 per molecule of thyroglobulin).[6]

Iodination of thyroglobulin is accompanied by important structural changes in the protein. There is an increase in the sedimentation coefficient (17 to 19 S), lower dissociability into its protomers, and so on. These changes reflect the effects of the addition of iodine, the effects of cystine formation and conformational changes in the protein.

The inhibitory effect of iodide, after its oxidation to an unknown intermediate, on adenylate cyclase, phospholipase C, and H_2O_2 generation, certainly inhibits iodination.[20] Thyroid peroxidase itself is also inhibited by excess iodide, which competes with tyrosine for the second substrate site of the enzyme. These effects could explain the well-known Wolff-Chaikoff effect, in which excess iodide inhibits protein iodination in intact cells. No evidence has been found for an action of TSH or cAMP on thyroid peroxidase activity and no consensus site for phosphorylation by protein kinase A exists in the enzyme structure.

In normal humans, radioiodide is organified immediately after trapping. The thyroidal radioactivity rises, while that in plasma decreases, and no radioiodide can be chased from the thyroid gland by thiocyanate or perchlorate. In the case of a complete block of protein iodination, thyroidal radioactivity declines in parallel with plasma radioiodide; this radioactivity is completely released within minutes after administration of anions such as SCN^- and ClO_4^-. It is thus easy to detect in vivo a complete block of protein iodination (see "Dyshormonogenesis–Congenital Hypothyroidsm with Goiter" below). With partial defects, the perchlorate discharge test is not very sensitive, and quantitative measurements in vivo of protein iodination capacity are needed. This requires a protocol in which this variable could be measured (as radioiodide uptake or clearance) under conditions in which this step becomes rate limiting, such as at relatively high ($\pm 10^{-5}$ M) iodide concentrations.

Thyroglobulin is secreted by the thyrocyte into the lumen of the thyroid follicle. It provides three functions: a thyroid hormone precursor, storage of iodine, and storage of inactive thyroid hormones (covalently bonded within the protein structure). Strictly speaking, thyroglobulin is the homodimeric glycosylated iodoprotein of sedimentation coefficient 19 S that accumulates in the follicular lumen. Its abundance and degree of iodination vary greatly depending on the activity of the gland. It may constitute 75 percent of total protein and contribute up to 50 percent of protein synthesis in the gland. Dimers (27 S) or trimers (37 S) of 19 S thyroglobulin are formed in variable amounts during the oxidative iodination of the molecule by thyroperoxidase. Recent data, complementing extensive discussion of thyroglobulin function and regulation provided in previous editions,[1,2] are presented in "Dyshormonogenesis–Congenital Hypothyroidism with Goiter" below.

Secreted iodothyronines and iodide appear in the venous outflow, and thyroglobulin appears mostly in the thyroid lymphatics. The turnover of the colloid in humans is normally about 1 percent per day, but this may be increased or decreased, depending on the level of activity of the gland. In the chronically stimulated gland, the colloid lumen virtually disappears, and the thyroglobulin pool is almost nonexistent. This suggests that the whole storage process is short-circuited and that thyroglobulin is iodinated and hydrolyzed within a very short time.

The endocytosis of the colloid in the follicular cells takes place by macropinocytosis and micropinocytosis. Macropinocytosis accounts for thyroid secretion after an acute stimulation by TSH. Within minutes pseudopods develop, mostly at the margin of follicular cells. Their size and number depend on the level of TSH. The lateral and apical borders of the pseudopods progressively fuse, engulfing the colloid indiscriminately in a process similar to phagocytosis. Tubulin and actomyosin are involved in the process. The resulting colloid droplets are interiorized and later fuse with primary lysosomes to form secondary lysosomes in which hydrolysis can take place. In fully stimulated dog follicular cells, the lifetime of the colloid droplet may extend to 40 min. Although endocytosis is obviously the limiting step in secretion, lysis of thyroglobulin may become limiting during acute stimulation of cells filled with colloid droplets. Thyroid secretion is not fully accounted for by macropinocytosis. For example, the very active secretion of chronically hyperstimulated follicular cells is not inhibited by inhibitors of macropinocytosis; moreover, it is not accompanied by morphologic evidence of this process (pseudopods, colloid droplets, and so on, as shown by transmission or scanning EM). On the other hand, micropinocytosis of proteins (ferritin, for example) has been demonstrated in follicular cells by EM. Micropinocytosis plays an important (probably the major) role in basal thyroid secretion. Experiments in vitro suggest some selectivity in this process, with the mature and more iodinated molecules being taken up more rapidly.

During endocytosis of colloid, a large surface of the apical membrane is interiorized. This is possible only because exocytosis of newly formed thyroglobulin by fusion of secretory microvesicles with the membrane supplies the necessary membranes. In fact, the two processes of exocytosis and endocytosis are coupled, with exocytosis preceding endocytosis after TSH stimulation. Under several circumstances, such as after long-term thyroid hormone treatment, the supply of secretory vesicles becomes limiting for endocytosis. Thus, the secretory cycle is similar in the follicular cell to that in other protein-secreting cells if one considers that protein secretion is directed toward the follicular lumen. Endocytosis and iodination take place at the periphery of the colloid lumen. It is clear that more recently iodinated thyroglobulin molecules have more chance to be taken up and hydrolyzed than the others. Slow diffusion of the colloid enhances this phenomenon, which is referred to as the "last come, first served" hypothesis. That excretory vesicles as well as apical membranes at the bases of microvilli, but not pseudopod or colloid droplet membranes, contain peroxidase, shows that extensive membrane reshuffling takes place in both exocytosis and endocytosis.

The hydrolysis of thyroglobulin droplets resulting from micropinocytosis as well as macropinocytosis takes place in the lysosomes. These organelles contain all the enzymes necessary to hydrolyze glycoproteins at acid pH, that is, proteases, glycoside hydrolases, peptidyl amino acid hydrolases, dipeptide hydrolases, and so on. Lysis of thyroglobulin in intact lysosomes is activated by glutathione, suggesting that reduction of disulfide bonds in the protein could be a limiting step. The released amino acids are probably mixed with the cellular pools, causing a dilution of exogenous amino acids taken up by the cells. After intense stimulation, a spillover of amino acids into venous blood is observed. The carbohydrate moieties of thyroglobulin are digested, as evidenced by the loss of PAS staining. The released carbohydrates are presumably recycled in the cells, although some sialic acid is released into the blood.

Free iodotyrosines are rapidly deiodinated by a deiodinase constituted of a ferredoxin — NADPH ferredoxin reductase — and a flavin mononucleotide-containing deiodinase. The same system operates in thyroid and in peripheral tissues (e.g., kidney, liver). It is inhibited competitively by dinitrotyrosine and blocked by any agent that oxidizes NADPH, such as menadione. The exact localization of this "microsomal" system has not been elucidated. The iodide released from iodotyrosines is largely reutilized in the thyroid, mixing with the trapped exogenous iodide. Part of this iodide leaks out of the gland. The importance of this leakage is related to the intrathyroidal iodine content. In cases of intense or acute TSH stimulation, some iodotyrosines escape the deiodinase and spill into the venous effluent of the gland. The iodothyronines (T_4, T_3, and small amounts of rT_3) are excreted by an unknown mechanism. Because there is no evidence of lysosomal exocytosis at the basal membrane, it is believed that the iodothyronines are secreted by passive diffusion or, since they are charged amino acids, by passive mediated transport. The T_4:T_3 ratio in the thyroid secretion is lower than in thyroglobulin, especially early after TSH stimulation. This reflects two mechanisms, an earlier release of T_3 during lysis of thyroglobulin and a partial deiodination of T_4 by the peripheral type of 5′deiodinase I (5′DIO1) inhibited by propylthiouracil.

Thyroid secretion is controlled by TSH. In the dog, basal secretion, mostly involving micropinocytosis of thyroglobulin, may not require cAMP, while secretion after short-term TSH administration, involving macropinocytosis, is mediated by cAMP. Secretion is inhibited by iodide even in patients treated with antiperoxidase drugs.

DEFECTS INVOLVING GENES EXPRESSED IN THE THYROID GLAND

Gain of Function Mutations of the cAMP Regulatory Cascade

For a hormone receptor, gain-of-function may have three different meanings: activation in the absence of ligand (constitutivity), or increased sensitivity to its normal agonist, or broadening of its specificity. When the receptor is part of a chemostat, as is the case for the TSHr, the first situation is expected to lead to tissue "autonomy," whereas the second is expected to cause adjustment of the agonist concentration to a lower value. In the third case, inappropriate stimulation of the gland is expected to occur because the promiscuous agonist is not expected to be subjected to the normal negative feedback. If a gain-of-function mutation of the first category occurs in a single cell expressing normally the receptor (somatic mutation), it will only become symptomatic if the regulatory cascade controlled by the receptor is mitogenic in this particular cell type. Autonomous activity of the receptor will cause clonal expansion of the mutated cell. If the regulatory cascade also activates function, the resulting tumor will progressively take over the function of the normal tissue, leading ultimately to autonomous hyperfunction. If the mutation is present in all cells of an organism (germ line mutation), autonomy will be displayed by the whole tissue expressing the receptor. In cases where the regulatory cascade is both mitogenic and activates function, the expected result is hyperplasia associated with hyperfunction.

From what we know of thyroid cell physiology (see "Thyroid Physiology and Metabolism" above) it is easy to predict the phenotypes that would result from gain-of-function of the cAMP-dependent regulatory cascade. Two observations provide pertinent models of this situation. Transgenic mice made to express the adenosine A2a receptor in their thyroid glands display severe hyperthyroidism associated with thyroid hyperplasia.[21] As the A2a adenosine receptor is coupled to the G protein $G_{\alpha s}$ and displays constitutive activity due to its continuous stimulation by ambient adenosine,[22] this model mimics closely the situation expected for a gain-of-function germ line mutation of the TSHr. Patients with the McCune-Albright syndrome are mosaic for mutations in G_s (G_{sp} mutations), leading to the constitutive stimulation of adenylylcyclase.[23] Hyperfunctioning thyroid adenomas develop in these patients from cells harboring the mutation, making them a model for gain-of-function somatic mutations of the TSHr. A transgenic model in which Gsp mutations are targeted for expression in the mouse thyroid gland has been constructed[24] and exhibits a similar, but milder, phenotype.

TSH Receptor (TSHr). TSHr belongs to the large family of G protein-coupled receptors (GPCRs).[12,25–27] More precisely, it is one of the three glycoprotein hormone receptors (LH/CGr, FSHr, and TSHr) that are structurally and evolutionary related by their serpentine portion to the large subfamily of opsin-related GPCRs. The primary structure of the TSHr has been deduced from the sequence of the cDNA: it is composed of a serpentine C-terminal moiety typical of GPCRs that is encoded in a single exon (exon 10).[28] In contrast to other GPCRs, but in common with the LH/CGr and FSHr, the TSHr has a long (398 residues) N-terminal extracellular domain encoded in multiple exons (1 to 9, for the TSHr).[28] This domain has sequence similarity with proteins containing leucine repeats, the prototype of which is the ribonuclease inhibitor.[29,30] The TSHr gene is located on chromosome 14q24.[28] Amongst GPCRs, the TSHr has the unique characteristic to undergo posttranslational cleavage within a segment close to the border between the leucine-repeat-containing domain and the beginning of the serpentine domain.[11,31,32] This segment has no counterpart in the LH/CG and FSH receptors. A still unidentified metalloprotease is involved in the cleavage, which does not necessarily involve all molecules at the cell surface. Cleavage probably takes place around Ser 314 and results in further removal of amino acid residues from the N-terminal end of the serpentine segment.[32] The two domains remain connected by disulfide bonds. The functional significance of this proteolytic step is still unknown.

The modular structure of the glycoprotein hormone receptors reflects a dichotomy in their structure-function relationships. The extracellular N-terminal domains are responsible for high affinity binding of the hormones, the serpentine portion being the "effector" transducing the binding signal to the G protein.[26,33–36] For GPCRs of the opsin family, the serpentine molecule itself carries out ligand binding and activation of G proteins. For the glycoprotein hormone receptors, the observation that the N-terminal domain made of leucine repeats is enough to bind the hormone with high affinity,[36] opens the question of how the binding signal is translated into a conformational change in the serpentine portion. Spontaneous mutants of the TSHr may help answering this question (see "Structure-Function Relationships," below).

The modular structure of the glycoprotein hormone receptors appeared very early in evolution. Receptors with a similar structure and highly significant sequence similarity have been cloned from cnidarians (*Anthopleura elegantissima*)[37] and *Drosophila*.[38] Very recently, sequences with the potential to encode orphan GPCRs displaying extensive similarity with glycoprotein hormone receptors have been identified.[39] Their functions remain totally unknown.

The detailed tridimensional structure of the GPCRs is still unknown. Models of the serpentine portion have been proposed for the glycoprotein hormone receptors.[40] The recent availability of the tridimensional structure of the porcine ribonuclease inhibitor[30] has provided a starting point to model the leucine repeat portion of the extracellular domain of the TSHr.[41] This consists in a sector of a doughnut, with the concave and convex surfaces made of β sheets and α helices, respectively. Although they provide a potentially helpful basis for the interpretation of experimental observations, only the future will tell whether present models are close to reality.

Familial Nonautoimmune Hyperthyroidism or Hereditary Toxic Thyroid Hyperplasia (HTTH) (MIM 603372). The major cause of hyperthyroidism in adults is Graves disease in which an autoimmune reaction is mounted against the thyroid gland and thyroid stimulating antibodies are produced (TSAb) that recognize and stimulate the TSHr. The mechanisms leading to autoimmune thyroid diseases are still unknown, but genetic factors are certainly involved as familial clustering is frequently observed (see "Multigenic-Multifactorial Thyroid Diseases," below). This may explain why the initial description by the group of Leclère of a family showing segregation of thyrotoxicosis as an autosomal dominant trait in the absence of signs of autoimmunity was met with skepticism.[42] Reinvestigation of this family, together with another family from Reims (France), identified two mutations of the TSHr gene, which segregated in perfect linkage with the disease.[43] A series of additional families have been studied since and, surprisingly, each showed a different mutation of the TSHr gene.[44,45] Functional characterization of these mutant receptors confirms that they are constitutively stimulated (see "Structure-Function Relationships," below). This new nosological entity, sometimes called Leclère disease, has these clinical characteristics: autosomal dominant transmission; hyperthyroidism with a variable age of onset (from infancy to adulthood, even within a given family); hyperplastic goiter of variable size, but with a steady growth; and absence of clinical or biologic stigmata of autoimmunity. An observation common to the cases described to date is the need for drastic ablative therapy (surgery or radioiodine) in order to control the disease, once the patient has become hyperthyroid. Incomplete thyroidectomies are indeed followed by recurrences. The autonomous nature of the thyroid tissue from these patients has been elegantly demonstrated by grafting it in nude mice.[46] Contrary to tissue from Graves disease patients, HTTH cells continue to grow in the absence of stimulation by TSH or TSAb.

The prevalence of HTTH is difficult to estimate. It is likely that many cases have been (and still are) mistaken for Graves disease. This may be explained by the relative insensitivity and lack of specificity of TSAb assays, together with the high frequency of the other thyroid autoantibodies (antithyroglobulin, antithyroperoxidase) in the general population. It is expected that wider knowledge of the existence of the disease will lead to better diagnosis. Presymptomatic diagnosis in children of affected families may prevent the developmental or psychologic complications associated with infantile or juvenile hyperthyroidism.

Sporadic Toxic Thyroid Hyperplasia (STTH). Cases with toxic thyroid hyperplasia have been described in children born from unaffected parents.[47–52] Conspicuously, congenital hyperthyroidism was present in most cases and required aggressive treatment. Mutations of one TSHr allele were identified in the children, but were absent in the parents. Because mini- or microsatellite testing confirmed paternity, these cases qualify as true neomutations. When comparing the amino acid substitutions implicated in hereditary and sporadic cases, the majority of the substitutions do not overlap (Fig. 158-5). Whereas most of the sporadic cases harbor mutations that are also found in toxic adenomas, most of the hereditary cases have "private" mutations. The analysis of the functional characteristics of the individual mutant receptors in COS cells, and the clinical course of individual patients, suggest an explanation for this observation: "sporadic" mutations seem to have a much stronger activating effect than "hereditary" mutations. From their severe phenotypes, it is likely that newborns with neomutations would not have survived if not treated efficiently. On the contrary, from inspection of the available pedigrees, it seems that the milder phenotype of patients with "hereditary" mutations has only limited effect on reproductive fitness. The fact that hereditary mutations are rarely observed in toxic adenomas is compatible with the suggestion that they would cause extremely slow tissue growth and, accordingly, would rarely cause thyrotoxicosis. If this explanation holds true, one may predict that mutations of the hereditary type may be found in the older patients with toxic adenomas.

Somatic Mutations: Autonomous Toxic Adenomas. Somatic gain-of-function mutations of the cAMP regulatory pathway have played an important role in the identification of their germinal counterparts. As such, and for their importance in delineating structure-function relationships of the TSHr, they deserve a brief mention.

$G_{s\alpha}$ Mutations. Soon after mutations of $G_{s\alpha}$ had been found in adenomas of the pituitary somatotrophs, similar mutations (also called Gsp mutations) were found in some toxic thyroid adenomas and follicular carcinomas.[53] The mutated residues (Arg201, Glu227) are homologous to mutations found in the ras protooncogenes; that is, the mutations decrease the endogenous GTPase activity of the G protein, resulting in a constitutively active molecule.

Mutations in the TSHr. The demonstration by site-directed mutagenesis that GPCRs can be constitutively activated by amino acid substitutions in the third cytoplasmic loop[54–56] led to a search for similar mutations in the TSHr.[57,58] Toxic adenomas were found to be a fruitful source of somatic mutations activating the TSHr, probably because the phenotype is very conspicuous and easy to diagnose. Most of the mutations are located in the third cytoplasmic loop or in the adjacent sixth transmembrane segment of the receptor (see Fig. 158-5). The clustering reflects the pivotal role of this portion of the molecule in the activation mechanisms.[59] However amino acid substitutions were found over most of the serpentine portion of the receptor,[57,58,60–63] and even in the extracellular N-terminal domain.[64]

Despite disagreement about the prevalence of TSHr mutations in toxic adenomas, which may be due to the different origin of patients[65,66] or to different sensitivity of the methodology, we conclude that in countries with a moderate shortage of iodine, activating mutations of the TSHr are the major cause of solitary toxic adenomas.[63,67] In some patients with a multinodular goiter and two anatomically distinct areas of autonomy, a different mutation of the TSHr was identified in each nodule.[64] Finally, the involvement of TSHr mutations in thyroid cancers has been implicated in a limited proportion of follicular thyroid carcinoma selected for their high basal activity of adenylylcyclase.[68,69]

Structure-Function Relationships of the TSHr as Deduced from Activating Mutations. The majority of the activating mutations of the TSHr have been studied by transient expression in COS cells. By the built-in amplification of the transfected construct, it is possible to detect even slight increases in the constitutive activity of the TSHr. An important observation has been that the wild-type receptor itself displays significant constitutive activity.[43,70] This characteristic is not unique to the TSHr[71–73] but, interestingly, it is not shared by its close relative the LH/CG receptor.[74] The effect of activating mutations must, accordingly, be interpreted in terms of increase in constitutive activity.

Most amino acid substitutions found in toxic adenomas and/or toxic thyroid hyperplasia share common characteristics: (a) they increase the constitutive activity of the receptor towards stimulation of adenylylcyclase; (b) with a few notable exceptions,[61] they do not display constitutive activity towards the inositolphosphate/diacylglycerol pathway; (c) their expression at the cell surface is decreased to a variable degree; (d) most, but not all of them, keep responding to TSH for stimulation of cAMP and inositolphosphate generation, with a tendency to do so with decreased EC_{50}; and (e) they bind TSH with an apparent affinity higher than the wild-type receptor.

There is no simple relationship between the position of the mutations or the nature of the amino acid substitution and their functional characteristics. All mutations so far identified in transmembrane segments II, III, VI, and VII and the third

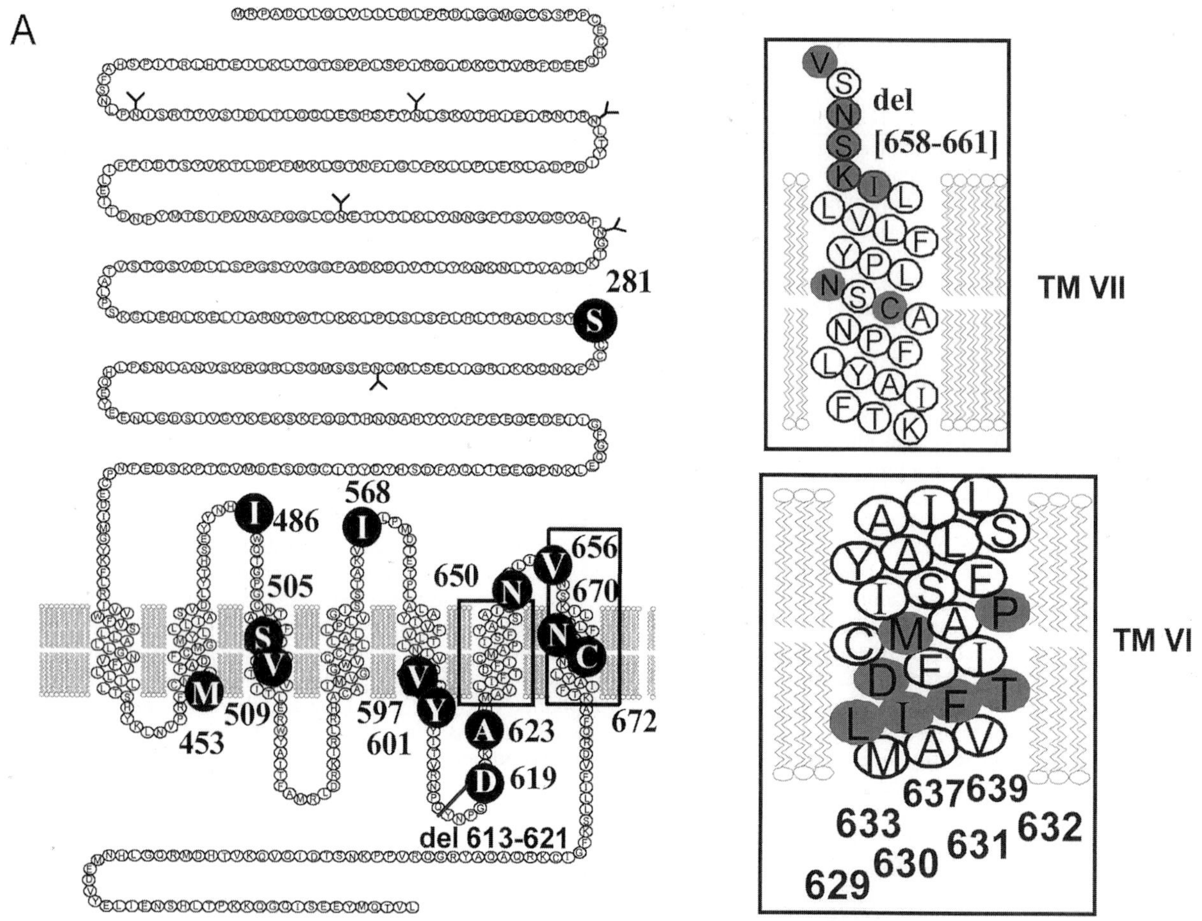

B CODON	Substitution	Somatic mutation	Germline Neomutation (STTH)	Germline Familial (HTTH)	Stimulation of [cAMP]	Stimulation of [IP]	References
Ser 281	Asn	+			+	-	67
	Thr	+	+		+	-	49, 75
	Ile	+			+	-	52
Met453	Thr	+	+		+	-	48, 67
Ile 486	Phe	+			+	+	61
	Met	+			+	+/-	61
Ser505	Arg			+	+	-	44
	Asn		+		+	-	
Val509	Ala			+	+	-	43
Ile568	Thr	+			+	+/-	61
Del613-631		+			+	-	62
Asp619	Gly	+			+	-	57
Ala623	Ile	+			+	+/-	57
	Val	+			+	-	63
	Ser	+			+	-	476
Leu629	Phe	+		+	+	-	67, 476, 45
Ile630	Leu	+			+	-	476
Phe631	Leu	+	+		+	-	47
	Cys	+					58
Thr632	Ile	+	+		+	-	58, 60
	Ala	+					69
Asp633	Tyr	+			+	-	67, 58
	Glu	+			+	-	67, 63, 476, 58
	His	+			+	-	68
	Ala	+			+	-	67
Pro639	Ser	+		+	+	+	476
Asn650	Tyr			+	+	-	44
Val656	Phe	+			+	-	63
Del658-661		+			+	-	67
Asn670	Ser			+	+	-	44
Cys672	Tyr			+	+	-	43

Fig. 158-5 Representation of the TSH receptor. *Panel A*: The locations of known activating mutations are indicated. *Panel B*: The nature of the mutations is indicated with their origins (somatic, germ line sporadic, germline familial), effects on intracellular regulatory cascades, and references.

cytoplasmic loop have similar phenotypes; they affect amino acids belonging to all classes (charged, polar, and hydrophobic), with substitutions not necessarily involving a shift to another class. Mutations of Ile486 and Ile568 in the first and second extracellular loops, respectively, and Pro639 in transmembrane segment VI are exceptional in that, in addition to stimulating adenylylcyclase, they cause constitutive activation of the inositolphosphate pathway.[61] Three additional mutations deserve special mention because of their unexpected nature or location: the four-amino-acid deletion (residues 658 to 661) in the third extracellular loop;[67] the nine-amino-acid deletion in the third intracellular loop;[62] and the substitutions at Ser281 in the N-terminal extracellular domain.[75]

There is no direct relation between the level of cAMP achieved by different mutant TSHrs in transfected COS cells and their level of expression at the cell membrane.[76] This means that individual mutants have widely different specific constitutive activity (cAMP accumulation/receptor number at the cell surface ratio). While this specific activity may tell us something about the mechanisms of receptor activation, it is not a measure of the actual phenotypic effect of the mutation in vivo, which depends on both the specific activity of individual receptors and their number. Indeed, C672Y, a relatively mild mutation, observed up to now only in an HTTH family, is among the strongest according to this measurement. It would be logical to expect the best correlation to be found between the phenotype and the actual level of cAMP achieved, irrespective of the level of receptor expression. However, differences between the effects of the mutants in COS cells and thyrocytes in vivo may render these correlations a futile exercise. According to a current model for GPCR activation, the TSHr would exist under at least two interconverting conformations: R (silent conformation) and R* (the active forms).[55] The unliganded receptor would shuttle between both forms, the equilibrium being in favor of R. Binding of the ligand, to the slit between the transmembrane segments (for biogenic amines) and/or residues of the N-terminal segment or extracellular loops (for neuropeptides), is believed to stabilize the R* conformation. The resulting R to R* transition is supposed to involve a conformational change modifying the relative position of transmembrane helices. In turn, this would translate into conformational changes of the cytoplasmic domains interacting with trimeric G proteins. Seminal studies with the α_{1b}-adrenergic receptor have shown that a variety of amino acid substitutions in the C-terminal portion of the third intracellular loop led to their constitutive activation.[54] The observation that all amino acid substitutions at Ala293 were effective in activating the receptor led to the concept that the silent form of GPCRs would be submitted to a structural constraint, requiring the wild-type primary structure of the third intracellular loop. This constraint could be released by a wide spectrum of amino acid substitutions in this segment.[54,55,77,78]

The observation that amino acid substitutions in a large number of residues scattered over the serpentine portion of the TSHr causes an increase in its constitutive activity is fully compatible with the above model, and provides arguments for its extension. That mutations in residues distributed over most of the serpentine portion of the receptor are equally effective in activating it (which does not seem to be a general characteristic in all GPCRs) suggests that the unliganded TSHr might be less constrained than others. The readily measurable constitutive activity of the wild-type receptor is compatible with this contention. Being already "noisy," the TSHr would be more prone to further destabilization by a variety of mutations.

The precise effects of individual mutations in structural terms are difficult to predict: the sixth transmembrane segment and its continuation in the C-terminal portion of the third cytoplasmic loop is clearly a hot region (Fig. 158-5), with at least 20 residues potentially implicated in keeping the receptor inactive. That consecutive residues in transmembrane helix VI are implicated (residues 631, 632, and 633) is against a simple model in which activation would result from the rupture of an interaction with specific residues in another transmembrane helix (e.g., TM III). Nevertheless, it is likely that the common consequence of activating mutations is the stabilization of a conformation of the serpentine with individual helices in a different relative position. The identification of activating amino acid substitutions in TM II, III, and VII also fits well with this notion. The deletion of 9 residues in the third cytoplasmic loop is believed to activate the receptor by facilitating binding of G_{sa} to portions of the transmembrane domains.[62]

The activating mutations identified in the extracellular loops and the N-terminal extracellular domain are more difficult to interpret in the lights of a simple model based on constraint involving only the serpentine portion of the receptor. They are compatible with an extension of this model, in which the unliganded N-terminal domain would contribute to the constraint keeping silent the serpentine portion. According to this model activation would result from the release of a silencing interaction between the extracellular loops and the N-terminal domain.

Familial Gestational Hyperthyroidism (MIM 603373). Some degree of stimulation of the thyroid gland by human chorionic gonadotrophin (hCG) is commonly observed during early pregnancy. It is usually responsible for the decrease in serum TSH with relative increases in the free T_4 concentration that, nevertheless, remains within the normal range.[79,80] When the concentrations of hCG are abnormally high, as in molar pregnancy, true hyperthyroidism may ensue. The pathophysiological mechanism is believed to be the promiscuous stimulation of the TSHr by excess hCG, as suggested by the rough correlation between serum hCG and free T_4 concentrations.[81,82] A convincing rationale is provided by the close structural relationships of the glycoprotein hormones and their receptors, respectively.[8]

A new syndrome was described in 1998, in a family with dominant transmission of hyperthyroidism limited to pregnancy.[83] The propositus and her mother had severe thyrotoxicosis together with hyperemesis gravidarum during the course of each of their pregnancies. When not pregnant they were euthyroid clinically and by laboratory tests. Both patients were heterozygous for a K183R mutation in the extracellular N-terminal domain of the TSHr. When tested by transient transfection in COS cells, the mutant receptor responded normally to TSH. However, it showed higher sensitivity to stimulation by hCG, when compared with wild-type TSHr, providing a convincing explanation to the phenotype.

The amino acid substitution responsible for the promiscuous stimulation of the TSHr by hCG is surprisingly conservative. Also surprising is the observation that residue 183 is a lysine in both the TSH and LH/CG receptors. When placed on the available three-dimensional model of the hormone-binding domain of the TSHr,[41] residue 183 belongs to one of the beta sheets that constitute the putative surface of interaction with the hormones.[84] It is likely that an arginine in position 183 would confer a slight increase in stability to the illegitimate hCG-TSHr complex.[85] This would be enough to cause signal transduction by the hCG concentrations achieved in pregnancy, but not by the LH concentrations observed after menopause. Indeed, the mother of the propositus remained euthyroid after menopause. This is compatible with a relatively modest gain-of-function of the K183R mutant for stimulation by hCG.

Contrary to other mammals, human and primates rely on chorionic gonadotropin for maintenance of corpus luteum in early pregnancy.[86] The frequent partial suppression of TSH observed at peak hCG levels during normal pregnancy indicates that evolution has selected physiological mechanisms operating very close to the border of thyrotoxicosis. This may provide a rationale to the observation that, in comparison to other species, the glycoprotein hormones of primates display a lower biological activity due to positive selection by evolution of specific amino acid substitutions in their alpha subunits.[8] If this reasoning is correct, it is likely that further cases of hereditary gestational thyrotoxicosis will be

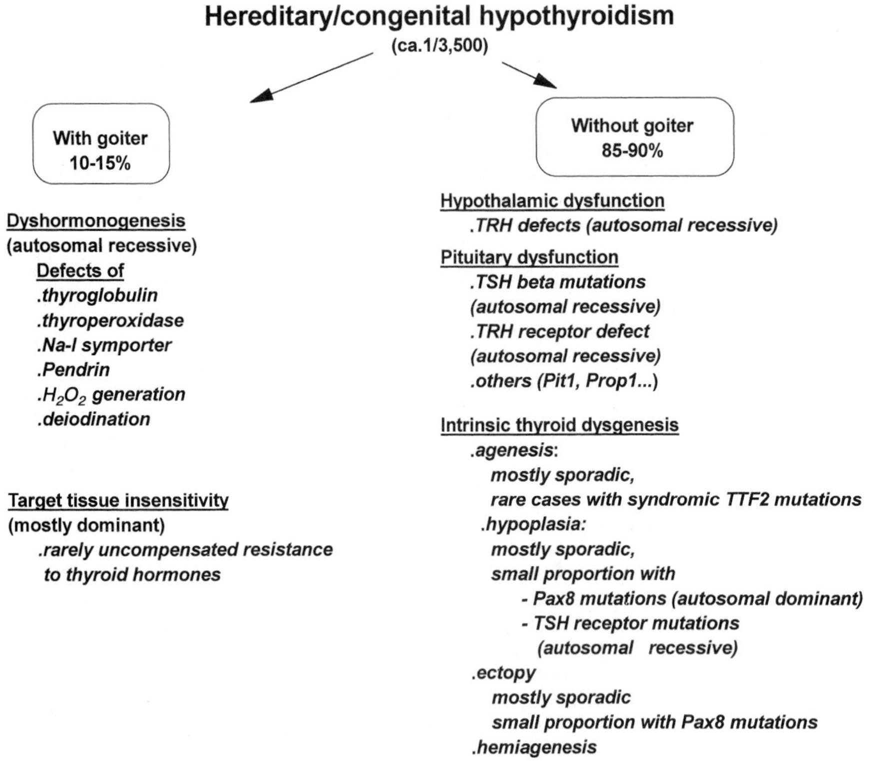

Fig. 158-6 Classification of the various causes of congenital hypothyroidism.

identified with mutations in the alpha or beta subunits of hCG of the fetus.

Loss-of-Function: From Hypothyroidism with Congenital Goiter to Thyroid Agenesis

Heritable or congenital situations with loss-of-function of the thyroid gland due to intrinsic molecular alterations expand over a broad spectrum of diseases. In an attempt to classify them on a pathophysiological basis, they are usually subdivided into diseases with or without goiter (Fig. 158-6). In the former, the loss-of-function affects one of the many steps leading to thyroid hormone synthesis (hormonogenesis defects). The hypothalamic-pituitary-thyroid chemostat responds to a reduction in thyroid hormone level by increasing TSH release, which overstimulates the growth of a partially or completely nonfunctional gland. The resulting goiter may be present at birth, or develop progressively, depending on the severity of the metabolic block, the efficiency of the maternal supply of hormones during fetal life and the iodine supply from the diet. Since the introduction of routine neonatal screening for congenital hypothyroidism in the mid-1970s, most neonates with a high TSH are detected and treated early, so that a goiter may never develop. This makes sometimes difficult the distinction between hormonogenesis defects and the other category of loss-of-function thyroid diseases in which, even if not treated, a goiter would never develop. The latter are grouped under the term dysembryogenesis or dysgenesis, reflecting the belief that the underlying cause is an alteration of the program required for the normal development and function of the gland. Data collected during the last 5 years suggest that nongoitrous loss-of-function of the thyroid is a heterogenous group of diseases in which the common characteristic is diminished or absent growth of the thyroid gland or its anlage due to a faulty stimulus or abnormal responses to normal stimuli. If this happens during embryonic life, when the normal stimuli for growth and differentiation are poorly characterized, it may lead to thyroid agenesis, ectopy, or hypoplasia. If it occurs later, it results in a normally located (eutopic) gland, hyporesponsive to TSH, the physiological thyroid stimulator for growth and maintenance of differentiation during fetal and postnatal life. Absence or structural alterations of TSH itself, is dealt with under a separate heading.

Dyshormonogenesis–Congenital Hypothyroidism with Goiter. In agreement with the autosomal location of the pertinent genes and the functional reserve observed in the majority of metabolic pathways, all inheritable dyshormonogenic disorders of the thyroid gland segregate as autosomal recessive traits. This also means that no dominant negative mechanisms are at work, suggesting that the protein/enzymes involved are abundant and behave functionally as monomers even if, as for the thyroglobulin molecule, they may actually be homodimers. In the past, many cases presented with a goiter and variable degrees of mental retardation (cretinism). Nowadays, in developed countries, most cases are detected neonatally and, when treated adequately, do not show goiter and have normal intellectual quotients (IQ).[87]

The quasi-uniform presentation of neonates with congenital hypothyroidism (screened as positive on the basis of an elevated TSH) makes it sometimes difficult to achieve a correct molecular diagnosis. Although this does not affect the choice of the treatment (immediate hormone administration), or its efficacy, it does make it impossible to subsequently identify fetuses at risk in the pertinent families. In spite of the success of the neonatal screening programs, it is certainly advisable to know in advance whether a newborn is affected or not, in order to initiate treatment without any delay. Figure 158-7 proposes an algorithm which may help identifying the defect when confronted with an isolated case of congenital hypothyroidism.

Key elements of the clinical investigation of a newborn with congenital hypothyroidism are scintigraphy, echography, and the perchlorate discharge test. Scintigraphy will indicate whether (partially) functional thyroid tissue is present or not and, if positive, will anatomically localize the tissue. If scintigraphy is negative, echography may allow identification of putative thyroid tissue, whether in place or not. It must be stressed, however, that echography of the newborn neck may be difficult to interpret and requires proper equipment and an experienced echographist. A helpful addition to these image analyses is measurement of

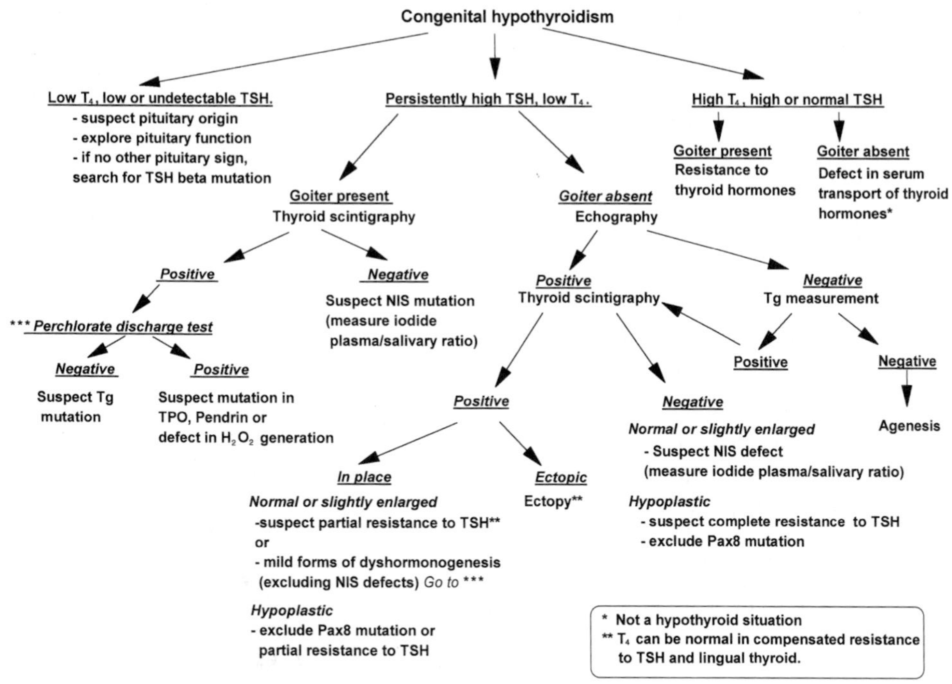

Fig. 158-7 Conceptual algorithm for the exploration of cases with congenital hypothyroidism. The figure should be considered a help in approaching diagnosis, rather than a rigid decision tree.

circulating thyroglobulin (Tg). If positive, even in the absence of demonstrable thyroid tissue by scintigraphy or echography, it excludes the diagnosis of athyreosis. Negative scintigraphy with a normally located thyroid is compatible with defective iodide trapping or resistance to TSH. In case of a positive scintigraphy, the perchlorate discharge test enables differentiation between organification defects and a putative Tg or deiodinase defect. The test is based on the observation that administered radioiodide is almost quantitatively and immediately organified by being covalently linked to thyroglobulin or to other intrathyroidal proteins. If organification is defective, retention of radioiodide in the gland depends on the continuous activity of the Na-I symporter (NIS). In these cases, inhibition of NIS by administration of perchlorate 2 h after that of radioiodide results in discharge of a large proportion of the radioactivity from the gland. The test is considered positive if more than 10 percent of the radioactivity is released within a 60 min period and the defect is complete when >90 percent is discharged. While a negative perchlorate test indicates that the organification machinery is working, it does not rule out qualitative or quantitative defects in Tg production because the misfolded Tg molecule, or other proteins including serum albumin, become iodinated. A positive perchlorate discharge test is diagnostic of an organification defect; this may be due to defects in thyroperoxidase (TPO) activity, H_2O_2 generation, or apical transport of iodide.

If not treated adequately, patients with dyshormonogenesis disorders will develop goiters that may become extremely large. Initially a homogenous hyperplasia, the goiter evolves towards nodularity and malignant transformation of some of the nodules could occur.[88,89]

Thyroglobulin (Tg). The structure of the protein and its gene were described in much detail in the previous edition of this work.[1,2] A summary, including new data, is presented here (see also Fig. 158-8). Tg is synthesized as a homodimeric glycoprotein of 2 × 330,000 daltons.[1,2] The primary structure of human Tg monomers was recently revised and a compilation of polymorphisms detectable at the cDNA level provided.[90] The molecule comprises 2750 amino acids. Of 20 sites for *N*-glycosylation, 16 are actually used,[91] resulting in a protein with about 10 percent of its weight accounted for by carbohydrates. Tg is also subjected to additional posttranslational modifications whose significance is not clear; it is sulfated and phosphorylated.[92,93] In addition to its obvious role as the template for thyroid hormone synthesis, Tg has the important function of storing hormones in an inactive form (as an integral part of its polypeptide backbone) as well as iodine (as iodotyrosine residues of the protein). This is achieved within the colloid of the follicular lumen, where Tg concentration reaches extremely high values (100 to 400 mg/ml). The necessity to remain soluble at such concentrations imposes additional constrains on the molecule that may be related to some of the posttranslational modifications, including sulfation. In addition to soluble 19S Tg dimers, the follicular lumen contains molecules with a higher iodine content constituting the 27S tetramers[1,2] and insoluble Tg.[94] The metabolism of these insoluble, highly iodinated molecules is poorly understood, but the possibility that they can be degraded, and their iodine released by the TPO/H_2O_2-generating system has been proposed.[95]

Under condition of normal iodine availability, the yield of T_4 per dimeric Tg molecule is close to 2.[1,2] The tyrosine residues implicated in the hormonogenesis reactions are the first to be iodinated at low iodide concentrations. The specificity for this choice is encoded within Tg primary structure, rather that in TPO.[96] They are of two different types: the donor monoiodo- or diiodo-tyrosines, as their names indicate, give their iodinated phenolic ring to acceptor diiodotyrosine to yield the triiodo- or tetraiodo-thyronines, respectively. The location of the two kinds of tyrosine residues within Tg primary structure is still debated. In human Tg, tyrosines 130, 847, and 1488 have been proposed as donor sites and positions 5, 1291, 2554, and 2747 as acceptor sites.[97] The consensus that a major acceptor site is tyrosine 5 is not disputed. The corresponding major donor tyrosine is probably tyrosine 130. The study of patients or animals with mutations identified in the Tg primary structure has helped locate the functionally important sites (see "Tg Gene Defects," below). The other residues with putative acceptor or donor functions are distributed over the molecule, with some clustering close to the C-terminus. Additional sites have been suggested by studies with animal Tgs. The precise identification of all hormonogenic residues in human Tg will require analysis by mass spectrometry, as was recently initiated for the bovine molecule.[98] When iodinated Tg is isolated from normal glands, a fraction of its

A

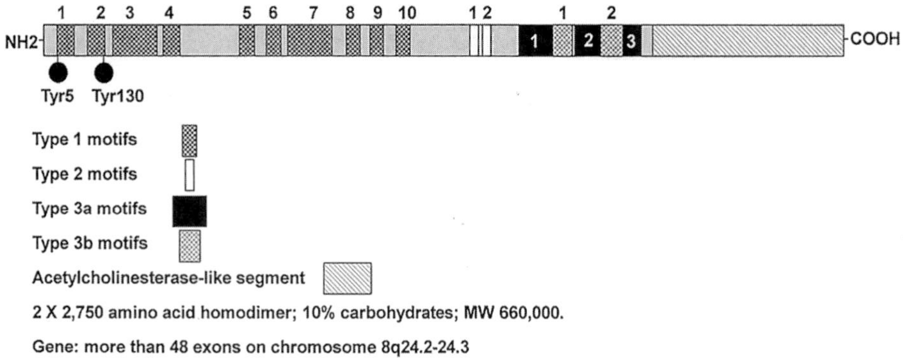

B

Loss-of-function mutations identified in human thyroglobulin

Mutations	References
C to G transversion IVS3 -3 acceptor site	106
R 277 Stop	90
C1,263Rg	477
R 1,510 Stop	116
Splicing defect removing segment 1,831-1,876	478

Fig. 158-8 Representation of thyroglobulin monomer, with indication (*panel A*) of structural repetition motifs and major hormonogenic tyrosines. *Panel B*: List of known mutations with references.

subunits is found cleaved, generating N-terminal fragments that remain attached to the molecule by disulfide bonds. Arguments have been proposed that link this posttranslational modification to the hormonogenic reaction.[99]

The Tg gene is located in 8q24.2-24.3. It spans more than 300 kb and is subdivided in at least 48 exons.[100] It is an example of a large gene made of a limited number of building blocks encoding repeated motifs or entire copies of ancestral genes. Three different motifs, encoded each in multiple exons, are repeated respectively 10 (type I), 2 (type II), and 5 times (type III) to constitute about 80 percent of the polypeptide. The type I motif is found in a large family of proteins.[101] The remaining 20 percent is made of an entire copy of an acetylcholinesterase homolog, with the intron-exon junctions perfectly conserved. A putative role for the type I repeated motif has recently been proposed. It is based on the observation that a similar motif is endowed with potent cysteine-protease inhibitor (ECI) activity in a protein from salmon egg.[102] Accordingly, the 10 type I motifs would protect Tg molecules with a low iodine content from being degraded, and allow their recycling.

Tg Gene Defects (MIM 188450). Mutations in the Tg gene have been suspected in a large number of cases during the precloning era. Their detailed clinical descriptions can be found in the previous editions of this book[1,2] and in a review.[103] Here is a brief outline of common clinical and laboratory findings in such patients.

The patient should be hypothyroid or show a compensated hypothyroidism with elevated TSH, trap iodide excessively, have no MIT or DIT in the urine, and usually a negative perchlorate discharge test. When thyroid tissue has been analyzed, some Tg-related antigens are almost invariably found in the glands, and ultrastructural evidence for defective secretion or folding of Tg is frequently present in the form of overdistension of rough endoplasmic reticulum (RER). Findings of abnormal iodoproteins in the plasma and of abnormal low-molecular-weight iodinated compounds in the urine complete the picture.[104] Urinary iodohistidine[105] is diagnostic of iodination of protein material unrelated to Tg within the thyroid gland. Albumin is most likely the substrate for iodohistidine production, as well as for the abnormal iodinated protein found in the blood. However, iodination of albumin is very nonspecific, being observed in a series of situations leading to goiter formation.

In the more recent years, a limited number of cases have been described with their mutations identified (see Fig. 158-8). The phenotype varies in severity, depending on the location of the mutation in Tg primary structure, and on the iodine supply in the diet. A characteristic, common to most, but not all cases, where it has been studied, is the decrease in circulating Tg as measured by conventional immunoassays. This decrease may be absolute or relative, taking into consideration the overstimulation of the gland by TSH. In a few cases, stimulation by exogenous TSH was performed and proposed as a diagnostic procedure.[103] It must be understood that the results from such kind of measurements are highly variable and depend on the nature of the mutation (missense, truncation by nonsense or frameshift, amputation by missplicing, and so forth) and the characteristics of the antibodies used in the immunoassay.

Considering that no prevalent mutation has been identified to date and that there is no indication that frequent mutations do exist, except for the preferential implication of CpG dinucleotides, there is no point describing in details the individual studies. In a few patients, however, the location of the mutations may tell us something about structure-function relationships of this large molecule. This was the case with the first mutation identified in man.[106] A transversion of C to G at position −3 of the acceptor splice site of intron 3 of the Tg gene caused skipping of exon 4. Because amputation of exon 4 does not affect the reading frame, this gave a strong argument in favor of Tyr130 (encoded in exon 4) being a important hormonogenic residue.[107,108] Although there is still room for debate regarding the respective roles of Tyr5 and Tyr130,[109] independent biochemical[110] and genetic studies have since consolidated this conclusion.

Detailed investigation of a large Brazilian kindred,[111] together with studies of the *cog/cog* mouse[112], lead to the conclusion that mutations affecting the Tg gene may frequently be the cause of endoplasmic reticulum storage disease (ERSD), where the misfolded protein remains trapped in the RER in association with molecular chaperones (GRP94, BiP).[113]

Animal models of Tg gene defects were available before the era of homologous recombination and knockout mice. They have been identified in a variety of species including the merino sheep, the Africander cattle, the Dutch goat, the Bongo antelope, and the *cog/cog* mouse. The phenotypes are quite variable. In the Africander cattle, animals are euthyroid but display a huge goiter. The mutation creates a nonsense codon at position 697 in exon 9. Detailed analysis of this model has revealed the first case of a "salvage" phenomenon by which alternative splicing removes the mutated exon from a proportion of the mature transcripts.[114,115] A similar phenomenon has been demonstrated in some of the human cases.[116] The Dutch goat is spontaneously hypothyroid except if supplemented with excess iodine in the diet. The mutation creates also a nonsense codon at position 296 in exon 8, the result being production of a 35-kDa N-terminal peptide. These two models provide strong support to the notion that the extreme N-terminal portion of Tg contains the major hormonogenic domain. When iodine in the diet is normal or high, the animals achieve euthyroidism despite the lower amounts of handicapped Tg present in their glands. Indeed, in both cases, the amounts of Tg mRNA, and of Tg antigens in the glands were much reduced, reflecting the destabilization associated with the presence of the nonsense mutation. The mutation of the *cog/cog* mouse has recently been identified.[112] It involves Leucine 2263 of the acetylcholinesterase-like domain, a residue highly conserved in the family of molecules containing the "α/β hydrolase fold."[117] The resulting phenotype in homozygous mice is trapping of Tg molecules in the RER. This identifies the acetylcholinesterase-like segment of Tg as an important structural motif, which has been implicated in the normal trafficking and dimerization of this family of molecules.[118]

Mutation of the Tg gene has been proposed as a cause of familial euthyroid goiter transmitted in an autosomal dominant manner.[119] The hypothesis is tempting and agrees with predictions from the studies of Kim and Arvan.[113] Misfolded Tg molecules translated from the mutated allele would interfere with routing through the ER of both the mutated and part of the normal molecules. Considering the large functional reserve of the hormonogenic machinery, the defect would become symptomatic only in areas of limited iodine supply. This notion will require independent confirmation before gaining recognition as a cause of familial goiter.

Sodium/Iodide Symporter (NIS). Active iodide (I^-) transport is the first step in the biosynthesis of thyroid hormone. This process is mediated through NIS, a protein located in the basolateral membrane of the thyroid follicle cell. Furthermore, the process requires energy because I^- is transported into the cell against concentration and electrical gradients. NIS couples the energy that is released by the transport of sodium (Na^+) downhill to its electrochemical gradient with I^- transport, thereby maintaining the I^- concentration inside the thyroid cell up to twenty- to fortyfold higher than in serum.[17,18] Active I^- transport is stimulated by TSH and inhibited, in a dose-dependent manner, by thiocyanate (SCN^-), perchlorate (ClO_4^-), or ouabain.[120] mRNA analyses suggest that the human NIS is not only expressed in the known iodide concentrating tissues, namely, the thyroid, salivary glands, gastric mucosa, choroid plexus and mammary glands, but is also present in the colon, ovary, omentum, and gall bladder.[121,122]

The mechanism of I^- delivery to the colloid, which is the site of thyroid peroxidase (TPO)-catalyzed I^- organification, is different. The anion is transported via an I^- channel at the apical membrane,[123] the molecular nature of which likely corresponds to the protein encoded by the pendrin gene.[124]

The human NIS gene was mapped to chromosome 19p13.2-p12. It has 15 exons that encode a protein of 643 amino acids with a molecular mass of ~65 kDa.[121] Of serpentine structure, NIS has a transmembrane domain believed to consist of 13 segments.[125] However, it is possible that there are as few as 12 segments[126] or as many as 14. The former structure is similar to the glucose transporter family[127] and the latter is akin to the sodium/glucose transporter-1 protein[128] with which NIS shares 30 percent

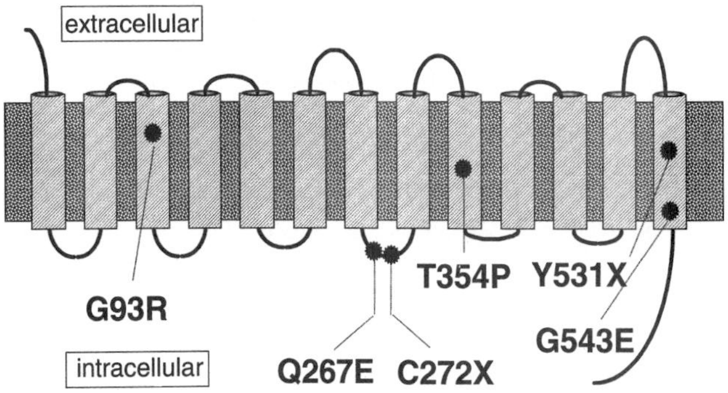

Fig. 158-9 Structure of the human NIS based on a model predicting a transmembrane domain of 13 segments. The location and nature of known mutations are indicated. (*From Pohlenz and Refetoff.*[479] *Used with permission.*)

homology. Thus, it is uncertain whether the N-terminus of the molecule is located inside or outside the cell. In contrast, the C-terminus, having a potential cAMP-dependent phosphorylation site,[126] is located intracellularly. The protein has three potential sites for *N*-linked glycosylation. Based on the molecular model of a 13-segment transmembrane domain, one glycosylation site is located in the fourth and two are in the last extracellular loop[125] (Fig. 158-9).

NIS Gene Defects (MIM 601843 and 27440). The failure of the thyroid gland to actively accumulate I^- ("iodide-trapping defect") under conditions of normal I^- supply, produces congenital hypothyroidism. About 40 patients with a phenotype compatible with iodide-trapping defect have been described since 1958, the year this defect was first suspected.[129]

As with other primary thyroid defects, newborns are brought to medical attention because of a high blood TSH level detected during neonatal screening. In children, attention is drawn by growth retardation and by the appearance of neck enlargement. In adults, frank hypothyroidism, enlargement of the thyroid gland or a thyroid nodule may be the reason for further investigation. The clinical phenotype is, however, quite variable, a phenomenon not simply due to the degree of loss-of-function of the mutant NIS.

The prevalence of iodide-trapping defect is unknown. Because heterozygous individuals do not express the phenotype, NIS gene defects can be detected only when both alleles are affected. Furthermore, under conditions of high I^- intake, mutations causing partial loss of NIS function may not be detected even in the homozygous individual. For these reasons, and because congenital hypothyroidism in the absence of positive radionuclide scan is often misdiagnosed as thyroid agenesis, the actual prevalence of NIS gene mutations may be higher than heretofore suspected. The defect appears to be as frequent in males as in females.

Goiters can be large or small, diffuse or nodular. The degree of hypothyroidism is also variable. Severe hypothyroidism with growth and mental retardation has been observed in several instances. More rarely, subjects have been found to be clinically and biochemically euthyroid.[129] The reduction of thyroid hormone levels and increase in TSH concentration in serum are usually consistent with the degree of clinical hypothyroidism. When measured, serum thyroglobulin Tg concentrations have been high.[130]

Histologic examination of thyroid tissue is not helpful in the diagnosis. Specimens obtained from nodules by fine needle aspiration or biopsy are often erroneously interpreted as representing malignancies because of extreme nuclear pleomorphism associated with marked follicular hyperplasia. Such findings can lead to thyroid surgery.

The laboratory hallmarks of iodide-trapping defect are markedly reduced or absent radioactive thyroidal uptake of radioiodide or pertechnetate, reduced I^- saliva to plasma ratio

(S/P), and restoration of euthyroid state by treatment with pharmacologic doses of iodide (1 to 5 mg/day). Absence of thyroidal radioactive iodide uptake (RAIU) is also typical for thyroid agenesis, a diagnosis erroneously assigned to some patients with iodide-trapping defect, especially when goiter was not present. Furthermore, depending on the timing of measurements following the administration of radioiodide, RAIU values can be low in other forms of congenital thyroid defects. In contrast, a low I^- S/P is pathognomonic of the iodide-trapping defect and can be carried out without interruption of thyroid hormone treatment.

The test is based on the observation that all tissues that normally concentrate iodide are affected by the iodide-trapping defect.[131] Saliva is collected, preferably without stimulation, over a period of 5 to 10 min, 1 h after the oral administration of 5 μCi of $Na^{125}I$. At the same time, a venous blood sample is obtained. After defrothing of the saliva and removal of the cell debris by centrifugation, the S/P ratio of radioiodide is determined by counting equal volumes of these fluids in a gamma-scintillation counter. A normal I^- S/P is 25 or greater, whereas the salivary glands of affected individuals are not able to concentrate iodide and therefore cannot secrete it in the saliva, resulting in a very low S/P. An I^- S/P in the vicinity of 1 is considered to be the consequence of a complete iodide-trapping defect, while an I^- S/P of up to 20 is considered to represent a partial defect.

Definitive diagnosis is based on the identification of a mutation in the NIS gene and on the in vitro demonstration of the resulting functional impairment. Six mutations of the NIS gene have been so far identified (Fig. 158-9). The first mutation was reported by Fujiwara et al.,[132] 9 months after cloning of the human NIS was published. It occurred in an individual born to consanguineous parents that presented as a homozygous missense mutation (T354P). A Brazilian patient with congenital hypothyroidism due to iodide-trapping defect was homozygous for a nonsense mutation in the NIS gene (C272X).[133] Another patient with iodide-trapping defect was compound heterozygote for two mutations in the NIS gene (Q267E and Y531X).[134] The latter mutation creates a new 3′-splice acceptor site that is used preferentially with the consequence that the mutant NIS has a stop at codon 515, resulting in a protein that lacks 129 amino acids from its C-terminus. Three additional families and two new missense mutations (G93R and G543E) were reported from Japan.[135,136] The G93R mutation was identified in a compound heterozygous association with T354P. The latter mutation appears to occur more frequently in the Japanese population because it has been identified in both alleles of affected individuals in five apparently unrelated families.[132,135,136] The small amounts of NIS mRNA present in circulating mononuclear cell is sufficient for the study of splice variants of NIS through the synthesis of cDNA.[134]

When expressed in HEK-293 cells, the mutant NIS354P had no detectable I^- transport activity above background, measured 60 min after the addition of I^-.[132] However, measurement of the initial velocity of iodide uptake, 5 min after the addition of radioiodide to COS-7 cells expressing NIS354P, demonstrated a small difference in specific I^- uptake above to the negative, untransfected, control.[135] Functional analysis of the NIS mutants 93R, 354P, and 543G transfected into COS-7 showed minimal transport activity, the statistical significance of which has not been determined.[136] No iodide transport activity was found in the mutants 267E, 272X, and 531X. None interfered with the function of the cotransfected WT-NIS.

Thyroid tissue from a patient expressing NIS354P showed a marked increase in the mRNA.[135] Cells transfected with NIS 267E, 515X, and 272X, express these mutant NIS molecules as effectively as the WT-NIS. While the mutant NIS354P appears to be targeted to the plasma membrane, even though it is virtually devoid of iodide transport activity,[137] 267E and 515X remain trapped intracellularly.[137a]

There are treatment options for NIS defects. The reversible consequences of iodide-trapping defect should, by definition, be corrected with by the administration of an excess if I^-. Indeed, I^- supplementation has been effective in restoring euthyroidism. The recommended dosage is 14 mg of I^-/day.[138] Treatment with replacement doses of thyroid hormone is also effective and more practical.

Thyroperoxidase (TPO). TPO is a glycosylated hemoprotein bound to the apical plasma membrane of thyroid follicular cells, with its catalytic domain facing the colloid space.[19,139] It corresponds to the major antigenic component of the thyroid "microsomal antigen" implicated in thyroid autoimmunity.[140–142] The primary structure of human thyroid peroxidase has been deduced from cloned cDNA.[142–144] Two cDNAs differing by 171 nucleotides have been obtained; they encode TPO1, the complete polypeptide corresponding to the protein as extracted from the gland, and TPO2, which is translated from an mRNA missing exon 10.[143] When expressed by transfection in CHO cells, TPO2 remains trapped in the ER and is devoid of enzymatic activity.[145] TPO extracted from thyroid glands displays 105- and 110-kDa protein species upon analysis by western blotting. Once believed to correspond to TPO1 and TPO2, both species are clearly encoded by TPO1 cDNA[146] and the functional significance of TPO2 is unknown. In addition to the major 3.2-kb TPO mRNA, shorter species have been demonstrated corresponding to misspliced primary transcripts.[147] Their significance, if any, is also unknown. Analysis of hydropathy profiles of the polypeptides encoded by the major messages indicates that the protein is anchored in the membrane by a segment close to its C-terminus. The extracellular domain has similarity with myeloperoxidase and other peroxidases (42 percent identity over 745 residues with myeloperoxidase),[142] indicating a common evolutionary origin. Candidate histidine residues (His 239 and 494)[148] implicated in the binding of the heme moiety have tentatively been identified and placed on a molecular model elaborated on the basis of the tridimensional structure of myeloperoxidase.[149]

TPO gene is located on the short arm of chromosome 2 (2p25).[150] It contains 17 exons and spans more than 150 kb. Exon 10 is the one subjected to alternative splicing. As is the case for Tg, the promoter of the TPO gene is the target for the three transcription factors TTF1, TTF2, and Pax8.[151,151] Pax8 plays a particularly important role because it can transactivate the proximal promoter in the nonthyroid environment of the Hela cells.[152] A tissue-specific enhancer, which binds TTF1, has also been identified 5.5 kb upstream.[153]

TSH increases both TPO enzymatic activity and steady state mRNA level in the thyrocytes of all species studied.[154] This effect is mimicked by cAMP analogs and by forskolin, and is likely to be mainly transcriptional.[155] In contrast to the regulation of the Tg gene, activation of TPO gene transcription by cAMP is rapid and does not require ongoing protein synthesis.[155] The TPO gene thus behaves as a series of other genes under rapid control by cAMP. However, the intermediate steps and all actors of this regulation have not been elucidated.

TPO Gene Defects (MIM 274500). A comprehensive list of organification defects described since 1950 has been published.[156] The first mutation responsible for the phenotype of a patient presenting with typical congenital goiter, organification defect, and hypothyroidism was identified in 1992.[104] It is worth describing because it is the only recurrent mutation described to date.[104,157,158] It consists in the duplication of a GGCC tetranucleotide in exon 8 of the TPO gene, resulting in the truncation of the normal reading frame. The patient was homozygous for the mutation. Translation of the mutated mRNA would yield a polypeptide less than half the length of normal TPO and devoid of the putative proximal and distal histidine residues implicated in heme binding (see "Thyroperoxidase," above). Analysis by RT-PCR of the RNA extracted from the goitrous tissue demonstrated accumulation of a misspliced mRNA resulting from the use of a cryptic acceptor splice site in exon 9. The normal

A

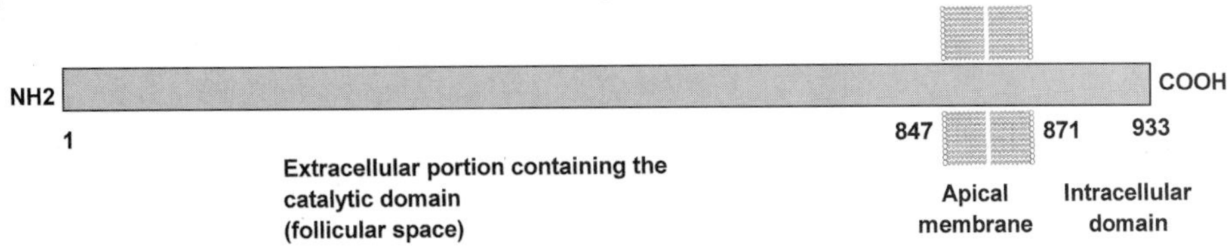

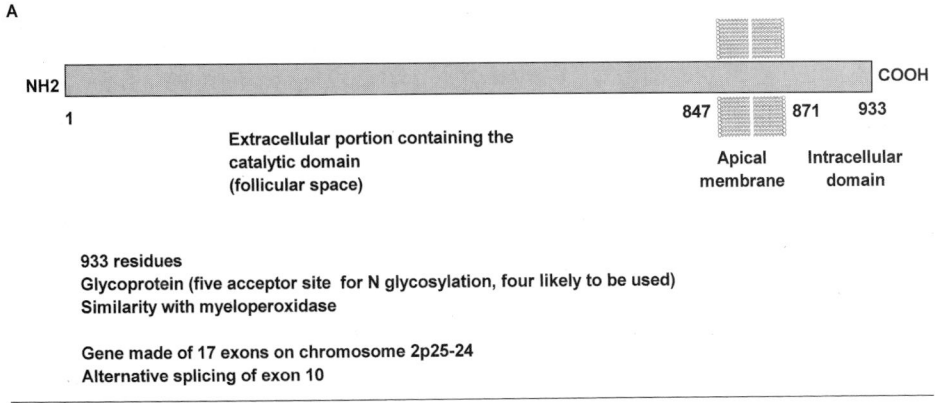

933 residues
Glycoprotein (five acceptor site for N glycosylation, four likely to be used)
Similarity with myeloperoxidase

Gene made of 17 exons on chromosome 2p25-24
Alternative splicing of exon 10

B

Mutations	References
Frameshift (20 bp duplication, pos.141)	157
Frameshift (GGCC duplication pos.1277)	104, 157
Y 453 D	157
R 540 Stop	157
G 590 S	157
R 648 Q	164
Frameshift (7C=>8C, pos2505-2511)	157
E 799 K	157, 164

Fig. 158-10 Representation of thyroperoxidase (*panel A*). *Panel B*: List of known mutations with references.

reading frame was restored in exon 9 downstream of the alternative splicing, which means that mRNA in the goiter has the potential to encode a near full-length TPO with 51 unrelated residues in its middle. The unmasking of alternative splicing as the result of nonsense or frameshift mutations is not unusual (e.g., see "Tg Gene Defects" above).

A series of additional mutations were subsequently identified (see Fig. 158-10).[157–163] They are distributed along most of the TPO molecule and, as expected for loss-of-function mutations, they comprise missense, nonsense, and frameshift mutations. Of particular interest, two different TPO mutations have been found to segregate within a large inbred pedigree of Amish, which had been screened with the hope of identifying defects in the H_2O_2-generating system.[164] This unusual observation illustrates the strength, as well as possible pitfalls, associated with homozygosity mapping of autosomal recessive mutations in inbred populations. A compilation of polymorphic sites in TPO cDNA has been published.[157]

Pendred Syndrome (PDS; MIM 274600). Pendred syndrome is a "syndromic" hereditary goiter associated with sensorineural hearing loss and transmitted in an autosomal recessive manner. Patients are usually euthyroid or present with compensated hypothyroidism (i.e., low-normal serum thyroid hormone levels with elevated TSH). Expression is variable, both in terms of thyroid and hearing defects. Deafness is often associated with the Mondini cochlear defect (lack of the normal coiled structure)[165] and may be present at birth or develop in childhood.[166] As with other hormonogenesis defects, the goiter is quite variable in size ranging from virtual absence (in this case patients present with deafness only) to voluminous masses requiring surgery for tracheal decompression. Diagnosis requires demonstration of sensorineural hearing defect together with a positive perchlorate discharge test. The disease thus qualifies as an organification defect with normal iodide trapping. It is only recently that mutations in a single gene were found to account for the syndrome. The gene was named pendrin after the syndrome.[167]

Pendrin gene was first localized to chromosome 7q31 by homozygosity mapping in inbred pedigrees.[168–170] A thorough investigation of candidate genes and exons in the interval identified the gene on the basis that it was found mutated in the families under study.[167] The pendrin gene is made of 20 exons encoding an mRNA of approximately 5 kb containing a 2343-bp open-reading frame. The conceptual protein of 780 amino acids has strong similarities with a family of sulfate transporters, amongst which is DRA (down-regulated in adenoma),[171] whose gene is contiguous to pendrin. Mutations in DRA are responsible for a congenital chloride diarrhea syndrome. A proposed model for sulfate transporters and pendrin includes 11 putative transmembrane segments, with the N- and C-termini in the cytoplasmic and extracellular spaces, respectively (Fig. 158-11A). The homology with sulfate transporters together with a putative role for sulfation of Tg in hormonogenesis (see above) made it tenable that pendrin would function as a sulfate transporter. However, the "sulfate transporter signature" of pendrin (a series of residues shared by the primary structure of sulfate transporters) is not canonical, and a possible role in the transport of iodide at the apical membrane of the thyrocyte is an appealing alternative hypothesis. The first functional studies of pendrin performed in *Xenopus oocyte* and *Sf9* cells did not show evidence for a role in sulfate transport; rather they demonstrate convincingly its ability to transport iodide and chloride.[124] Further studies are required to determine whether pendrin is the apical iodide transporter that has been characterized functionally.[172,173] The role of pendrin in iodide transport at the apical membrane would provide a satisfactory explanation for its role in thyroid hormone synthesis and a rationale to the positive perchlorate discharge test demonstrated by patients with pendrin gene mutations. Its role in the development of the cochlea is presently less clear. It has been repeatedly proposed that the hearing loss of Pendred patients might be secondary to intrauterine hypothyroidism.[1] However, recent evidence points to a direct role of the protein in the development of the inner ear.[174]

Putative loss-of-function mutations have been identified in a series of patients and kindreds.[167,175–177] As expected for loss-of-functions mutations, the mutations are quite diverse in nature (missense, nonsense, frameshift, splicing defects) and scattered along the primary structure of the protein (see Fig. 158-11B). As indicated above, the phenotypes display a broad spectrum of expressivity. Most interesting is the evidence that a significant proportion of deaf people with no clinically obvious thyroid

A

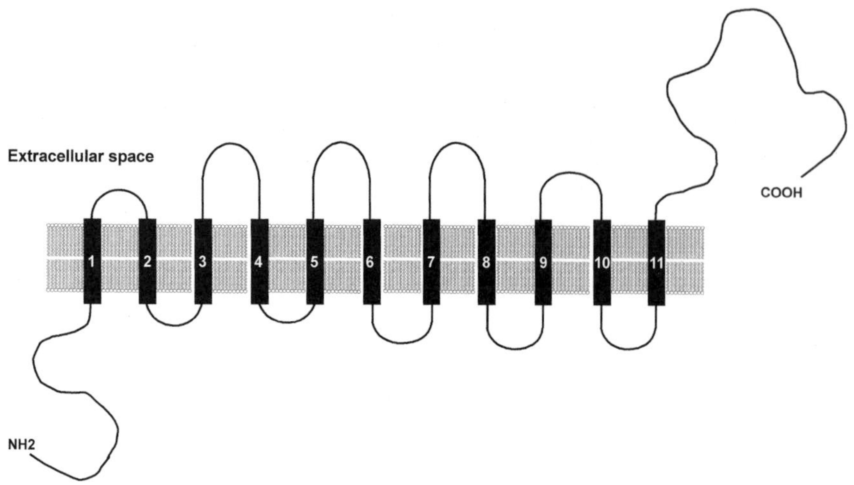

B

Mutations	References
Frameshift 279 del T, Stop 96	177
V 138 F	175, 176
G 139 A	176
Frameshit 560-561 ins T, Stop 180	175
G 209 V	176
L 236 P	175, 176
Frameshift 977-981 del CTCT , Stop 286	175
D 271 H	176
1225+1 G>A donor splice site	175
Frameshift 1370 del C, Stop 383	176
E 384 G	175
Frameshift 1421 del T, Stop 430	167, 176
R 4O9 H	175, 176
T 410 M	175
T 416 P	175, 176
1508-10 del TGC, minus A 429	175
L 445 W	176
Frameshift 1558-59, ins AGTC, Stop 467	175
Frameshift 1565 del T, Stop 453	167
Frameshift 1760-62 del AG, Stop 524	175
Y 513 H	175
Y 556 C	175
C 565 Y	176
Frameshift 2122 del A, Stop 634	176
F 667 C	167
G 672 E	175
Frameshift 2351 del T, Stop 719	175
H 723 R	176

Fig. 158-11 Representation of pendrin according to Everett et al.[167] *(panel A)*. *Panel B*: List of known mutations with 194 references.

disorder (i.e., without goiter) may have mutations in the pendrin gene. However, the number of cases analyzed in molecular terms is presently too low to draw definitive conclusion.

H_2O_2-Generating System. Defects in iodide oxidation that cannot be explained by abnormalities in thyroperoxidase expression or function could be attributed to the H_2O_2-generating system. On that basis, they could account for a small but definite proportion of such defects.

That defects in the similar O_2^--generating system of the leucocyte and macrophages in X-linked chronic granulomatous disease are not accompanied by thyroid insufficiency indicates the existence of a distinct system in the thyroid. One element of a system has been cloned, but no mutant has yet been characterized. In the absence of genetic tools, deficiency in H_2O_2 production has been suggested in cases where restoration of normal organification of iodide is observed after addition of H_2O_2 to the thyroid homogenate or medium of incubation of thyroid slices.[178] This has been demonstrated in one congenital iodide organification defect and in one cold nodule.[179]

Failure of Iodotyrosine Deiodinase (MIM 274800). Failure of iodotyrosine deiodinase activity does not interfere directly with thyroid hormone synthesis or secretion. However, it leads to leakage of iodotyrosines into the circulation, with a failure of iodine recirculation in the thyroid and loss of the iodotyrosines in the urine. The iodine in the serum iodotyrosines, of course, cannot be recovered by the thyroid iodide-trapping mechanism. The main consequence of this defect is, therefore, a great loss of iodine, which steps up a vicious circle of thyroid stimulation, hyperplasia, goiter, and increased synthesis and leakage of hormone precursors. The severity of the defect is, therefore, inversely proportional to the iodine content of the diet.

The clinical picture of patients affected by the iodotyrosine deiodinase defect is that of congenital hypothyroidism with goiter. The severity of hypothyroidism and goiter and of their possible consequences depends on the severity of the defect and on the supply of iodine. The decrease in serum T_4 and T_3 levels and increase in serum TSH will vary accordingly. Radiodiodide or $^{99}TCO_4^-$ uptakes are high and fast, and radioiodine release is rapid.

Trichloroacetic acid treatment of serum precipitates partially the iodotyrosines and thus part of the released radiodione. Chromatography of extracts of the serum and the urine demonstrates radioiodine in the iodotyrosines. Demonstration of the defect is achieved by the in vivo diiodotyrosine test. Radioiodine-labeled DIT is injected intramusculary or intravenously, and urine is collected at 1-h intervals for a few hours. Chromatography of the urine demonstrates less than 5 percent of the radioactivity in the iodotyrosines in normal controls, but up to 80 percent in patients.[180–186] Alternatively, urinary DIT may be measured by radioimmunoassay after its immunoprecipitation from urine. Its secretion is considerably increased in deficient patients (1.2 to 17.7 nM/mM creatine versus 0.108 ± 0.048 in normal individuals).[187] Thyroid slices from these patients will not deiodinate labeled DIT; to validate such a finding, positive deiodination by human and/or animal thyroid slices should be demonstrated at the same time. The latter activity should be inhibited by dinitrotyrosine (mM), an inhibitor of the enzyme. Finally, demonstration of the defect and of the proposed pathogenic mechanism requires that iodine medication alone should be sufficient to reestablish euthyroidism.[184,188] An isolated defect in the deiodinating capacity of peripheral tissues, but not of the thyroid, should not cause the syndrome, as iodotyrosines as such are released only as traces by the thyroid.

The genetics of this kind of goitrous cretinism was studied by Hutchison and McGirr.[189,190] It behaves as a simple autosomal recessive trait. There is no sex prediclection. Carriers of the trait[185] are less efficient in deiodinating the DIT. When given 20 to 25 mg of stable DIT along with labeled DIT, the best discrimination was achieved during the first 2 h of excretion of undeiodinated labeled DIT. The relatives of patients excreted an average of 20.4 percent as diiodotyrosine during this time, whereas normal subjects excreted 11.4 percent and the patients with dehalogenase deficiency excreted 52 to 79 percent.

Developmental Defects: Thyroid Dysgenesis. The mammalian thyroid anlage develops from a group of cells forming a thickening of the floor of the pharynx (embryonic day E8.5 in mouse).[191] These cells migrate caudally while multiplying and forming a two-lobe structure to reach their destination on both sides of the trachea (by E13 to E14 in the mouse).[191] A complement of cells coming laterally from the neural crest join the thyroid primordium. These cells are believed to contribute the ultimobranchial body in lower species and the C-cells of the adult thyroid. In humans, the median thyroid primordium is visible around day 16 to 17 of gestation and has reached its definitive location in the anterior neck by 6 to 7 weeks.[192] Induction and migration of the thyroid rudiment do not seem to be under control of the pituitary gland. Embryos with congenital absence of the anterior pituitary develop a thyroid rudiment,[192] as do mutants lacking TSH or the TSHr. Nevertheless, in the absence of stimulation by TSH, the thyroid, while in eutopic position, remains hypoplastic and virtually nonfunctional (see "Resistance to Thyrotropin," below). Three transcription factors play a key role in the differentiation and growth of the thyroid anlage: thyroid transcription factor 1 (TTF1 or T/ebp or Nkx2.1),[151,193] thyroid transcription factor 2 (TTF2 or FKHL15),[194,195] and Pax8.[196] Their structures and implications in hereditary/congenital hypothyroidism are presented in detail below. Figure 158-12 summarizes their expression pattern in relation with embryonic thyroid development. In the present state of knowledge, TTF1, TTF2, and Pax8 are the earliest markers of thyroid differentiation. They can already be detected at the site of the invagination of the pharynx that will form the thyroid bud (E8.5 in the mouse), and their expression continues uninterrupted thereafter.[194] The other markers of thyrocyte differentiation — Tg, TPO and TSHr — are not detectable before the thyroid has reached its final position (E14 to E15 in the mouse). TTF1, together with TTF2 and Pax8 genes, is expressed in the adult thyroid, where its role as a *positive* regulator of thyroid gland-specific gene expression by TSH and insulin is debated.[197,198]

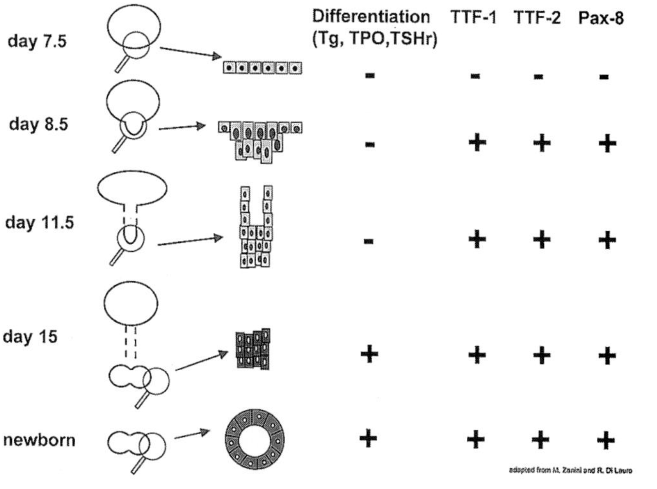

Fig. 158-12 Representation of the pattern of expression of genes involved in the control the development of the thyroid during mouse embryogenesis. For each mouse embryonal developmental stage (E7.5 to E15) and newborn, the status of expression of differentiation markers (Tg, TPO, TSHr) and developmental genes (TTF1, TTF2, Pax8) is indicated (+ or −). (*Adapted with permission from M. Zanini and R. Di Lauro*[194] *(Naples, Italy).*)

Thyroid dysgenesis can be classified into agenesis or athyreosis, hemiagenesis, ectopy, and hypoplasia. When a newborn screens positive based on a high TSH but is found to have no detectable thyroid tissue by both scintigraphy and echography, then the diagnosis of thyroid agenesis or athyreosis should be straightforward. Athyreosis accounts for about 15 percent of newborns with permanent congenital hypothyroidism.[199] The differential diagnosis of agenesis versus hypoplasia or even a normal-sized thyroid gland that is unable to concentrate iodide or pertechnetate, depends very much on technical skill and interpretation of scintiscans and echograms. An important additional parameter is the serum level of Tg. When detectable it signs the presence of thyroid tissue. Cases initially misclassified as athyreosis have been correctly diagnosed as hypoplasia on the basis of a normal or even elevated value for serum Tg.[200] An undetectable Tg, while TSH values are still high, is compatible with true thyroid agenesis or defective Tg synthesis (see "Tg Gene Defects," above).

Thyroid ectopy is defined as the presence of thyroid tissue outside its normal location on both sides of the trachea. It accounts for about 60 percent of permanent congenital hypothyroidism.[199,201] The tissue is detected by its ability to trap iodide or 99m pertechnetate, which is frequently enhanced secondary to the overstimulation by the high circulating TSH concentrations. It may be found anywhere from the foramen caecum at the base of the tongue (sublingual thyroid), under the chin (submental) to the mediastinum, on the midline, or laterally. In most cases, the tissue is both ectopic and hypoplastic, which accounts for the hypofunction. In some cases, however, ectopy is compatible with euthyroidism or compensated hypothyroidism (elevated TSH, normal thyroid hormone levels). An indication that different pathogenetic mechanisms may be implicated in agenesis, and ectopy is given by the different sex ratio observed in the two situations. A clear excess of females is found in ectopy (3:1),[199] while agenesis and hypoplasia seem to affect both sexes equally.[199]

Thyroid hemiagenesis is a rare situation that also affects females preferentially.[202] The mechanism responsible for agenesis more frequently affecting the left lobe (80 percent of cases) is presently unknown.

Thyroid hypoplasia is the diagnosis when echography detects thyroid tissue in its normal location but in insufficient amounts to achieve euthyroidism despite hyperstimulation by TSH.

Hypoplasia may be associated with absent or detectable trapping of iodide. In the first instance, identification of the tissue relies solely on echography and may be problematic.

Several studies have addressed the association of congenital hypothyroidism with other developmental defects.[199,203,204] Most report an overall increase of a variety of malformations. Except for the well-defined Bamforth syndrome (see "Thyroid Transcription Factor 2," below) and for an association with Down syndrome, the most common abnormality is cardiac septal defects,[205], fivefold higher than in the general population in one study.[199] Patients with Down syndrome have a thirty-fivefold increased risk for congenital hypothyroidism.[203]

The cause of thyroid dysgenesis in the majority of cases is unknown. Most are sporadic, although familial occurrence has been occasionally described. Therefore, except for a minority of patients in who it is clearly transmitted as a mendelian trait (see next three sections), even the genetic nature of the disease may be questioned. It is conceivable, but not demonstrated, that many cases are due to new mutations and that, before the implementation of routine neonatal screening, the affected individuals would display a severe decrease in reproductive fitness. This would lead to misclassification of the disease as sporadic. The situation may soon clarify as the generation of "rescued cretins" enters the reproduction age. Another possibility is that the disease would be multigenic. The discovery that mutated alleles of the Pax8 genes are the cause of thyroid hypoplasia transmitted in an autosomal dominant manner, but with incomplete penetrance would fit with this hypothesis (see *Pax8*, below).

During the past few years, mutations have been identified in a small proportion of cases with thyroid dysgenesis. They were logically screened for abnormalities in the genes suspected to be implicated in the development or regulation of thyroid function: TTF1, TTF2, PAX8, and the TSHr.

Thyroid Transcription Factor 1 (TTF1, or TITF1, or NKX2.1; MIM 600635). TTF1 is the prototype of a subfamily of transcription factors containing a homeobox domain.[193,206] It comprises the *Drosophila* tinman gene and the Nkx family of factors in vertebrates. TTF1, also called Nkx2.1, is expressed in the fetal brain, the pituitary, the developing and adult thyroid gland, and in lung.[207,208] The gene is encoded by two exons, on chromosome 14q13.[209] In the adult lung and thyroid, it acts as a tissue-specific transcription factor, controlling positively expression of the surfactant proteins in the former and Tg and TPO genes in the latter.[206] Multiple target sites for TTF1 binding have been identified in the proximal promoters of the Tg and TPO genes, and in more distant upstream enhancers. Interestingly, a similar arrangement of TTF1 and Pax8 sites has been described in the promoters of both genes. TTF1 gene is probably controlled in turn by another homeobox protein that remains unidentified.[206] The role of TTF1 in embryonic development can be appreciated from the analysis of knockout mice.[208] While heterozygous animals are completely normal, TTF1 −/− mice die in the neonatal period. They lack thyroid tissue completely, both thyrocytes and C cells being absent. In addition, they suffer from profound hypoplasia of the lungs and display brain malformations. This phenotype is in good agreement with expression of TTF1 in the developing thyroid gland (see above), the lung buds and the fetal forebrain. From this picture, it is expected that severe loss-of-function mutations of TTF1 in humans would be lethal, and that the gross pulmonary and brain malformations would mask the thyroid phenotype. No report fitting the description of the TTF1 −/− mouse has been reported yet in humans, and no mutation of TTF1 has been reported in a series of congenital hypothyroid patients.[210,211] One case of compensated hypothyroidism (elevated TSH, normal T_4) with eutopic thyroid gland was described in a child with respiratory failure harboring a heterozygotous deletion spanning less than 13 cM on chromosome 14q13 and including the TTF1 locus.[212] However, the large size of the monosomic segment, which certainly encompasses other genes (Pax9 gene is included in the deletion) does not allow one to conclude that hemizygosity of TTF1 alone was responsible for the phenotype.

Thyroid Transcription Factor 2 (TTF2, TITF2, or FKHL15); Bamforth Syndrome (MIM 241850). TTF2 was identified and cloned initially in the mouse on the assumption that a factor resembling HNF3 should be present in thyroid tissue. This hypothesis was based on the identification of *cis*-acting elements characteristic of the forkhead gene family in the promoters of thyroid-specific genes.[194,206] TTF2 gene is encoded by a single exon on chromosome 9q22.[195] It is expressed in the developing thyroid, the foregut endoderm, the craniopharyngeal ectoderm and Rathke's pouch.[213] The human cDNA was cloned independently from a skin cDNA library and was named FKHL15.[195] In addition to its putative role as a repressor of thyroid-specific genes during thyroid embryogenesis and in the development of the thyroid anlage, TTF2 plays a role in the positive control of thyroid-specific gene expression by insulin and possibly by TSH in the adult thyroid gland.[214] TTF2 knockout mice provided the phenotype to look for in humans.[213] The −/− mice are profoundly hypothyroid with undetectable T_4 in their blood. They die shortly after birth, most probably because of an inability to suckle due to severe cleft palate. Two different thyroid phenotypes—complete absence of thyroid tissue and sublingual ectopy—are observed with about equal frequency.[213] When studied in the embryo, development of the thyroid gland is completely normal in the heterozygous mice. In −/− embryos, budding of the thyroid primordium takes place normally at day E8 to 8.5. The bud expresses TTF1 and Pax8 normally. Thereafter, no migration of the bud is observed, and at day E11.5, in 50 percent of the mice, there is no more thyroid tissue to be seen. In the other half of the animals, the tissue remains in its original position. Absence of TTF2 is thus mainly characterized by absence of migration of the thyroid primordium, which is associated with hypoplasia or complete involution of the misplaced tissue. As expected, elevated TSH levels accompany hypothyroidism. This indicates that TTF2, while expressed in Rathke's pouch, is not required for normal development of the pituitary gland. In humans, Bamforth et al. described siblings with congenital hypothyroidism, cleft palate, choanal atresia, and kinky hairs.[215] Ten years after the original description, a homozygous loss-of-function mutation of TTF2 (A65V) was identified in the same two patients.[216] No trace of thyroid tissue could be detected by ultrasonography. The parents were healthy and euthyroid, which classifies Bamforth syndrome as an autosomal recessive cause of congenital hypothyroidism. In agreement with one of the phenotypes of TTF2 −/− mice, it remains to be seen whether cases of Bamforth syndrome will be identified with sublingual ectopic thyroid.

Pax8 (MIM 167415). The Pax8 cDNA was cloned originally as a member of the paired domain transcription factors expressed in both the kidney and the thyroid gland.[196] Its gene is encoded by at least 10 exons on chromosome 2q12-q14.[217,218] Together with TTF1, Pax8 was shown to be implicated in the tissue-specific expression of the thyroid genes Tg and TPO.[151,206] More recently, it was shown to play a key role in the embryonic development of the gland. Transgenic mice homozygous for a null Pax8 allele display profound hypoplasia of their thyroid glands, the heterozygotes being morphologically normal.[219] The thyroid anlage appears at the normal time and is positive for TTF1 transcripts. Thereafter, while starting to migrate caudally, it fails to grow and endures almost complete involution. Interestingly, and contrary to what happens in TTF1 knockouts, the calcitonin-secreting cells develop normally and reach a position similar to that of the normal thyroid lobes. The thyroids of the Pax8 −/− mice are composed almost completely of C cells. They display expression of TTF1, but show no Tg or TPO.[219]

In a series of 145 human cases with congenital hypothyroidism and thyroid dysgenesis, 2 sporadic cases and 3 members of 1 family were found to harbor loss-of-function mutations in their

Pax8 gene.[220] The mutations were shown to affect Pax8 function, as evidenced from transfection experiments: the mutants had lost the ability to transactivate a luciferase reporter gene expressed in Hela cells under the control of the TPO gene promoter.[220] Contrary to the situation in the mouse model, the patients were heterozygous for the mutation and in the familial cases, transmission was autosomal dominant. The two sporadic cases were neomutations. The patients displayed variable degrees of thyroid gland dysgenesis with hypoplasia as the common denominator. In the family with three affected individuals, expressivity was extremely variable, ranging from frank hypothyroidism associated with a cystic thyroid rudiment, to compensated hypothyroidism with a thyroid gland of close to normal size. Plasma Tg was detectable or even elevated in some of the cases, which may be due to leakage from an abnormally differentiated gland. A similar observation has been made in thyroid hypoplasia caused by TSHr mutations (see next section). The reason for the difference between transmission in the mouse model and man is not clear. The variability of the phenotypes observed in man, even within the same family, suggests that the genetic background plays an important role in the expression of Pax8 defects. It is likely that recessive transmission in the knockout mice is a peculiarity associated with the genetic background of the animal strain used.

TSH Receptor: Resistance to Thyrotropin (MIM 275200). Loss-of-function mutations in the TSHr gene are expected to cause a syndrome of resistance to TSH. The expected phenotype is likely to resemble that of patients with mutations in TSH itself (see "Isolated Central Hypothyroidism" below). A mouse model of resistance to TSH is available in the *hyt/hyt* line. Homozygous *hyt/hyt* mice are hypothyroid due to a developmental anomaly of their thyroid glands, which remain hypoplastic.[221] The cause has been traced to a mutation of the TSHr gene (P556L).[221,222] From this information one would expect patients with two mutated alleles to exhibit a degree of hypothyroidism in relation with the extent of the loss-of-function. Heterozygous carriers are expected to be normal or to display minimal increase in plasma TSH.

Clinical cases with documented mutations in the TSH receptor have been identified (Fig. 158-13). A few patients with convincing resistance to TSH had been described before molecular genetics allowed for identification of the mutations.[223,224] Another family was described more recently, but no mutation was found in the receptor gene.[225] The first cases described in molecular terms were euthyroid sibs with elevated serum TSH levels.[226] They were compound heterozygotes for mutations in the extracellular N-terminal portion of the receptor (maternal allele: P162A; paternal allele: I167N). The functional characteristics of the mutant receptors were studied by transient expression in COS cells; the paternal allele was almost completely nonfunctional, whereas the maternal allele displayed an increase in EC_{50} for stimulation of cAMP production by TSH. The I167N paternal allele is expressed in normal amounts in COS cells, but it remains trapped intracellularly and does not reach the cell surface. When both mutations are displayed on a tentative model of the extracellular domain, their location is compatible with the observed phenotype: the P162A mutation affects a residue predicted to be at the surface of the molecule, which may explain its interference with effects of TSH. The I167N mutation affects a residue protruding within the hydrophobic tunnel between the alpha helices and the beta sheets in the doughnut-shaped model.[41] It is expected that a polar residue would be incompatible with such position and result in severe misfolding of the whole extracellular domain. Coexpression in COS cells of the wild-type and mutated receptors did not show evidence for dominant negative effects of the mutants.

Familial cases with loss-of-function mutations of the TSHr have been identified in the frame of screening programs for congenital hypothyroidism (Fig. 158-13).[200,226–229] All infants have high serum TSH levels; depending upon the severity of the TSHr defect, however, some are euthyroid,[226,229] while others display hypothyroidism of variable magnitude.[200,227,228] Also

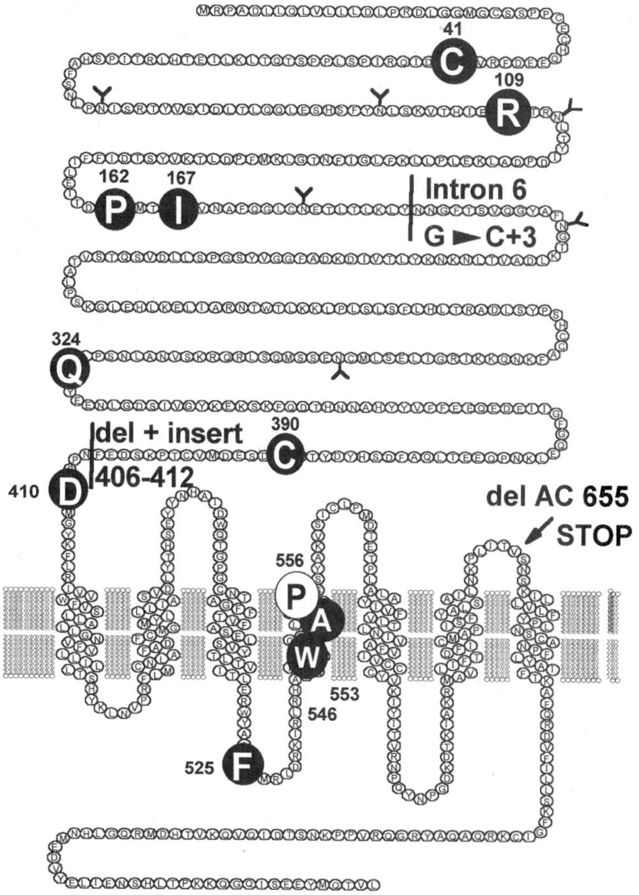

Position	Substitution	Loss-of-function	References
Cys 41	Ser	partial (?)	229
Arg 109	Gln	partial	480
Pro 162	Ala	partial	226
Ile 167	Asn	complete	226
Gln 324	Stop	complete	229
Cys 390	Trp	partial (?)	228, 229
406 - 412	del + insert	complete	228
Asp 410	Asn	partial	229
Phe 525	Leu	partial (?)	229
Trp 546	Stop	complete	229, 480
Ala 553	Thr	complete	200
655 del AC		complete	227
+3 IVS 6	G > C	complete	227
Pro 556 (hyt/hyt mouse)	Leu	complete	222

Fig. 158-13 Representation of the TSH receptor. ***Panel A*: The locations of known loss-of-function mutations are indicated. *Panel B*: The natures of the mutations are indicated with the extent of their effects and references.**

depending upon the severity of the defect, thyroidal uptake of $^{99}TcO_4^-$ can be normal or absent. All thyroids were small and normally located at echography. Surprisingly, in some of the cases, serum Tg levels were high. It is likely that, similar to what is observed in hypoplasia due Pax8 mutations (see above), the hypoplastic glands would suffer a differentiation defect that may have as a consequence the leakage of Tg from abnormal follicles or its misrouting to the basolateral membrane.

As may be expected for loss-of-functions, mutations were diverse and patients were mainly compound heterozygotes, except when consanguinity was present. In one instance, the patients were sibs born from consanguineous parents and were homozygous for a mutation in transmembrane segment IV of the serpentine portion of the receptor (A553T), close to the *hyt* mutation of the mouse. When transiently expressed in COS cells, the mutants were barely expressed at the cell surface. However, the residual expression was compatible with some TSH binding and stimulation of cAMP production by TSH.[200] When the phenotypes of these cases is known in more detail, they will provide a means to understand the role of the receptor on thyroid organogenesis. Indeed, the difference in phenotype between people with mutations abolishing the hormone or the receptor will tell us whether the mere expression of a functional receptor and of its constitutive activity on adenylyl-cyclase stimulation (see "Structure-Function Relationships of the TSHr," above) plays a role in the development of a structurally normal thyroid gland.

Others. Families with autosomal dominant transmission of apparent partial resistance to TSH where the phenotype does not cosegregate with the TSHr gene have been described.[230] In some of these families, linkage was also excluded with candidate genes known to be implicated in the normal development of the thyroid gland (TTF1, TTF2, Pax8) (unpublished results from the authors' laboratories). The underlying pathophysiological mechanism is still unknown.

DEFECTS INVOLVING EXTRATHYROIDAL GENE EXPRESSION

Central Hypothyroidism

Combined Pituitary Hormone Deficiency (CPHD). As the name indicates, CPHD is characterized by concomitant deficiency of more than one type of pituitary hormones. Causal mechanisms have been traced to developmental anomalies secondary to mutations in transcription factors required for the normal differentiation and growth of specific pituitary cell lineages. Two such transcription factors are implicated in the development of thyrotrophs: POU1F1 (or Pit1, or GHF1) and PROP1.

POU1F1 (MIM 173110) is the human homolog of the murine Pit1 gene. It is a pituitary-specific transcription factor with a positive effect, both on the expression of genes encoding GH, PRL, and TSH-β, and on the development of somatotrophs, lactotrophs, and thyrotrophs.[231–233] The protein has 291 amino acids; it belongs to the POU family, which is characterized by a highly conserved bipartite DNA-binding domain — a POU-homeodomain implicated in low-affinity binding to DNA and the POU-specific domain responsible for binding specificity and possible interaction with other factors.[233] The transactivating domain of POU1F1 is located in the N-terminal segment. POU1F1 gene is comprised of six exons and is located on human chromosome 3p11.[234] Spontaneous mice models with loss-of-function mutations of Pit1 have been described — Snell and Jackson dwarf (*dw*) mice. Since the first description in humans,[231] a series of mutations has been described in familial and sporadic cases with combined deficiency of TSH, PRL, and GH (see Table 158-1). In the absence of treatment, the patient phenotype is characterized by severe growth retardation secondary to combined GH deficiency and hypothyroidism. When loss-of-function is complete GH, PRL, and TSH are undetectable and the pituitary is profoundly hypoplastic. As expected for loss-of-function mutations with no apparent benefit for heterozygote carriers, the spectrum of mutations is quite heterogenous (Table 158-1). However, a mutation hot spot has been identified that affects the CpG dinucleotide: CGG to TGG (R271W). This mutation has been observed in several unrelated families and in one documented neomutation.[235] While most mutations are transmitted on the autosomal recessive mode, some, including Arg271Trp (R271W), have a dominant negative effect and are transmitted on the autosomal dominant mode.[236] It is important to note that in patients with POU1F1 mutations, gonadotropin production is not affected. When treated for their hypothyroidism and GH problems, they undergo normal puberty.

Table 158-1 Mutations Causing Central Hypothyroidism

Gene	Mutation	References
PROP1	R120Y	239
	301del AG frameshift stop 109	239
	F117I	239
	149del GA	502
	296del GA	502
PIT1/POU1F1	R172X	503
	F135Y	504
	R271W	505
		506
		507
		508
	A158P	231
	P24L	505
	R143Q	505
	E250X	509
	P239S	510
TRH receptor	343del 9: del [S115, I116, T117] + A118T	240
	R49X	240
TSH beta	G29R	245
	E32X	246
	313delT	242, 246

PROP1 (MIM 601538) encodes a 226-amino-acid paired-like homeodomain protein expressed specifically in the embryonic pituitary. It was initially cloned as the gene responsible for the dwarfism (*df*) in Ames mice (Prop1 for "prophet of Pit1"), the phenotype of which is similar to that of Snell and Jackson dwarfs.[237,238] Prop1 is epistatic to Pit1 as its pituitary expression is required for Pit1 expression. The coding region of PROP1 gene contains three exons and is located on human chromosome 5q. Loss-of-function mutations of PROP1 have been identified in patients with CPHD who, in addition to GH, PRL, and TSH deficiency, display defective basal and GnRH-stimulated production of gonadotropins.[239] The disease is transmitted on the autosomal recessive mode and displays variability in its expressivity, depending on the nature of the mutations (Table 158-1). The phenotype of patients with CPHD and PROP1 mutations provide a strong argument in favor of the hypothesis that during pituitary development gonadotrophs originate from a precursor of the lineage that gives also birth to somatotrophs, lactotrophs, and thyrotrophs.[239]

Isolated Central Hypothyroidism. Loss-of-function mutations in any gene implicated in the hypothalamopituitary TRH-TSH pathway is theoretically expected to cause isolated central hypothyroidism. To date, only mutations in the TRH receptor and TSHβ have been identified.

The TRH receptor (MIM 188545) belongs to the large family of serpentine G protein-coupled receptors.[5] It is a 398-amino-acid protein encoded by a gene on chromosome 8q23. TRH receptor expressed in thyrotrophs and lactotrophs is coupled to the generation of diacylglycerol and inositolphosphates via G_q. A patient has been identified with two different loss-of-function mutations in the TRH receptor.[240] His phenotype was that of relatively mild hypothyroidism (presenting symptoms at 9 years of age were short stature and delayed bone age) with normal basal TSH and prolactin concentrations that fail to rise after TRH administration. The absence of extrathyroidal symptoms in this natural human TRH receptor knockout indicates that extrapituitary expression of TRH[241] is of little functional significance or does not exerts its effects through the known TRH receptor.

The TSHβ gene is comprised of three exons on chromosome 1p13 (MIM 188540). Loss-of-function mutations have been identified in several patients with severe congenital hypothyroidism and mental retardation with low or undetectable TSH[242–246] (Table 158-1). The disease is transmitted on the autosomal recessive mode. In most cases, serum TSH is undetectable and does not rise after TRH. The normal response of PRL to TRH allows differentiation of this situation from defective TRH receptor. The absence of immunoassayable TSH may be secondary to structural alterations caused by the mutations and interfering with recognition of the epitope(s), or to the inability of the mutant β subunit to associate with the α subunit and be secreted. In cases described recently, a single base deletion leading to substitution of Cys105 by Val and causing truncation at codon 114 was compatible with detection by some immunoassays, but not by others.[243] This indicates that diagnosis of isolated TSH β deficiency must be considered not only in cases of low thyroid hormones associated with undetectable TSH, but also in cases with measurable TSH devoid of biologic activity.

Transport of Thyroid Hormones in Blood

Thyroxine (T_4) and its metabolites are transported in blood bound to three serum proteins: thyroxine-binding globulin (TBG); transthyretin (TTR), formerly known as thyroxine-binding prealbumin (TBPA); and albumin (ALB). All circulating iodothyronines are associated in various proportions to these three carrier proteins, which are synthesized in the liver. Their concentrations in serum can be measured by colorimetric electrophoretic, radioimmunometric and ligand-binding techniques. The normal distribution of T_4 among these proteins is 75 to 80 percent bound to TBG, 15 to 20 percent bound to TTR, and 5 to 10 percent bound to ALB. Several other serum proteins, such as α- and β-lipoproteins have a minor contribution to thyroid hormone transport.[247,248] In pathologic conditions, variable amounts of a specific iodothyronine may circulate bound to γ-globulins.[249]

Iodothyronine interactions with each of the binding proteins are noncovalent, reversible, and obey the law of mass action. The concentration of free (unbound) iodothyronine (FT_i) can be calculated from the total concentration of the iodothyronine (TT_i), that of the binding protein (BP_j), and their association constant ($K_{i,j}$). The concentration of FT_i is very small relative to the TT_i, under normal circumstances being 0.03 percent for T_4 and 0.3 percent for T_3.

Because only a minute fraction of free thyroid hormone is diffusible, and thus immediately available to tissues, it has been speculated that the large extrathyroidal pool of dissociable protein-bound hormone serves as a reservoir readily available to tissues as well as to safeguard the body from the effects of abrupt changes in hormonal secretion or metabolism. It can be estimated that in the absence of binding proteins, a small extrathyroidal pool of free hormone would be completely depleted in a matter of hours after a sudden cessation of hormone secretion. However, in the presence of a normally functioning hypothalamic-pituitary-thyroid axis, free hormone concentration, and thus the metabolic status, can be maintained even with profound alterations in circulating thyroid hormone-binding proteins.[250] The maintenance of stable supply of thyroid hormone is then dependent on the rapidity with which the hypothalamus and pituitary respond to changes of thyroid hormone concentrations as evidenced by the higher Tg concentrations in individuals with congenital TBG deficiency, a measure that indirectly reflects the degree of thyroid stimulation by TSH.[251] Another role of the serum thyroid hormone-binding proteins may be to facilitate even distribution of T_4 and T_3 throughout all body tissues.[252]

TBG is a 54-kDa acidic glycoprotein composed of a single polypeptide chain of 395 amino acids (44 kDa) and 4 heterosaccharide units with 5 to 9 terminal sialic acids.[253,254] The polypeptide core, encoded by a single gene copy located in the long arm of the human X-chromosome (Xq22.2),[255,256] has a striking homology to cortisol binding globulin (CBG) and to glycoproteins belonging to the family of serum protease inhibitors (α_1-antitrypsin, antichymotrypsin, antithrombin).[254,257] As with other members of this gene family, TBG has four coding exons and a promoter that contains a hepatocyte transcription factor-1 binding motif that imparts to the gene a strong liver-specific transcriptional activity.[258] The carbohydrate moieties appear to be important for the correct posttranslational folding and secretion of the molecule,[259] are responsible for the multiple TBG isoforms (microheterogeneity) detected by isoelectric focusing (IEF),[260] and affect the stability of TBG and its clearance by the liver.[261] Improper folding of the molecule due to faulty glycosylation or to changes in the polypeptide core alters not only the secretion of TBG but also its ability to bind the iodothyronine ligands and its immunoreactivity.[262,263] In contrast, cleavage of the carbohydrate moieties from a properly folded and secreted TBG does not affect its ligand-binding and immunogenic properties.[264,265]

The TBG molecule has a single iodothyronine binding site with affinity of approximately 10^{10} M^{-1} for T_4 and 10^9 M^{-1} for T_3.[266] It is stable at room temperature and in dilute alkali, but rapidly undergoes irreversible denaturation at temperatures above 55°C and pH below 4. Denatured TBG does not bind the ligands but retains its molecular weight and can be detected with antibodies that recognize the primary structure of the molecule.[264]

In the serum of normal euthyroid adults, about one-third of the TBG molecules carry iodothyronines, mainly T_4; the remaining two-thirds circulates unbound (without ligand). At full saturation, the 1.6 mg of TBG/dl of serum (about 260 nM) can carry 20 µg of T_4. The biologic half-life of TBG is about 5 days.[267] A number of compounds may alter its concentration in serum. The most common, estrogen, during pregnancy or given for birth control, increases TBG concentration mainly through reduction of its rate of degradation caused by an increase in complexity of the oligosaccharide residues.[261] Many more compounds compete with T_4 at its binding site on TBG owing to their structural similarities to the iodothyronines.[268]

TTR is a stable tetramer composed of 4 identical subunits, each containing 127 amino acids encoded by a single gene copy located on chromosome 18 (18q11.2-12.1)[269,270] and synthesized in the liver. The gene is 7 kb long with 4 exons of approximately 200 bp. The complete molecule has the molecular mass of 55,000 and is highly acidic, but contains no carbohydrate. The four subunits form a symmetric, double trumpet-shaped channel that traverses the molecule, forming two iodothyronine-binding sites. However, only a single T_4 is usually bound with a Ka of approximately 10^8 M^{-1} because the binding affinity for the second, identical site is greatly reduced through negative cooperativity of the first ligand interaction.[271] TTR complexes with retinol-binding protein and thus also plays a role in the transport of vitamin A. This interaction does not influence T_4-binding.[272]

Although on a molar basis the normal TTR concentration is twentyfold that of TBG, due to its relatively lower association constant for all iodothyronines, it plays a minor role in thyroid hormone transport. Thus, despite its relatively short half-life of 2 days, and high propensity for wide fluctuation in response to a variety of physiological and pathologic factors, its effect on the concentration of circulating thyroid hormones is minor and of no practical consequence.

Albumin is a monomer composed of 585 amino acids encoded by a single gene copy located on chromosome 4 (4q11-q13) and synthesized in the liver.[273,274] It associates with a variety of natural and exogenous substances having a hydrophobic domain. In this sense, the association of iodothyronines with ALB can be viewed as nonspecific. Despite its high abundance (two thousandfold that of TBG) and multiple iodothyronine binding sites, their relative low affinities (less than 10^6 M^{-1}) are responsible for the negligible contribution of normal ALB to thyroid hormone transport.[275]

Disorders of thyroid hormone transport are caused by inherited abnormalities of each of the three hormone carrier proteins. They produce variable degrees of alterations in the concentration of circulating iodothyronines with no effect on the free hormone

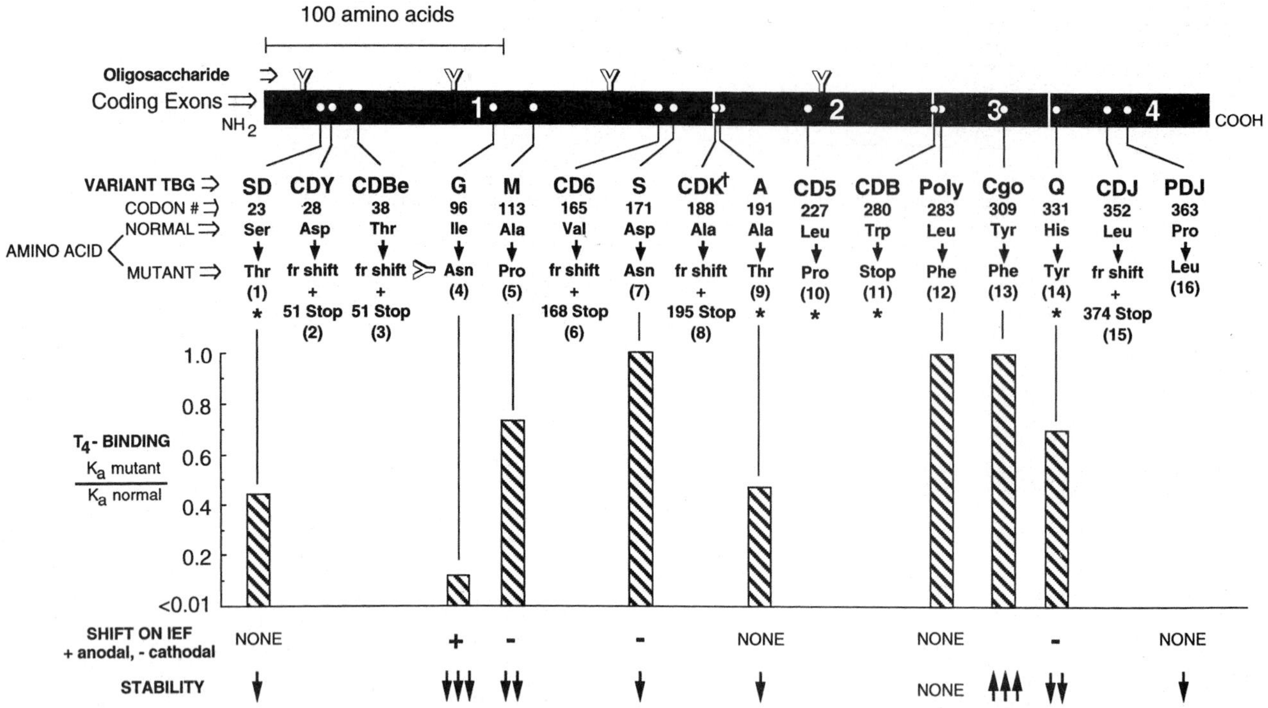

Fig. 158-14 Known mutations in the TBG gene, their location, and their effect on the properties of the molecule. The TBG variants are: -SD = San Diego; -CDY = complete deficiency Yonago; -CDBe = complete deficiency Bedouin; -G = Gary; -M = Montreal, -CD6 = complete deficiency 6; -S = slow; -CDK = complete deficiency Kankakee; -A = Aborigine; -CD5 = complete deficiency 5; -CDB = complete deficiency Buffalo; -Poly = polymorphic; -Cgo = Chicago; -Q = Quebec; -CDJ = complete deficiency Japan; and -PDJ = partial deficiency Japan. For detailed description, see (1) Sarne etal.[298] and Bertenshaw et al.;[481] (2) Ueta et al.;[290] (3) Miura et al.;[291] (4) Murata et al.;[282] Mori et al.[300] and Kambe et al.;[262] (5) Takamatsu et al.;[299] and Janssen et al.;[263] (6) Li et al.;[287] (7) Takamatsu et al.[305] and Waltz et al.;[295] (8) Carvalho et al.;[292] (9) Murata et al.[297] and Takeda et al.;[294] (10) Mori et al.[284] and Janssen et al.;[263] (11) Carvalho et al.;[286] (12) Mori et al.[284] and Takeda et al.;[293] (13) Takamatsu et al.[308] and.;[309] (14) Takamatsu et al.[299] and Bertenshaw et al.;[482] (15) Yamamori et al.[288,289] and Miura et al.;[483] (16) Miura et al.[301,484] * = Coexistence of TBG-Poly; † = Mutation in the acceptor splice site of intron II.

concentrations, the activity of the thyroid gland, or the metabolic status of the patient.[276] Despite changes in the fractional turnover rates of extrathyroidal iodothyronines, their daily production and metabolism remain unaltered.[267,277] Nevertheless, because these thyroid hormone transport defects manifest as alterations in total T_3 and/or T_4 concentration, failure of their recognition often leads to inappropriate treatments aimed at normalizing the serum hormone level to the detriment of the affected subject. Because TTR and ALB serve to fulfill additional functions to thyroid-hormone transport, some inherited defects of these proteins can cause specific illnesses, such as familial amyloidotic polyneuropathy associated with TTR gene mutations[278] (see Chap. 209). In contrast, even extreme abnormalities of TBG, such as complete deficiency, do not affect the health or survival of affected individuals. This probably accounts for their high overall frequency in the populations of varied racial and ethnic background.[276] The associations of inherited TBG defects with thyrotoxicosis,[279], goiter,[280], and Turner's syndrome[281,282] are most likely fortuitous.

Inherited TBG Abnormalities (MIM 314200). Inheritance of most TBG defects in humans follows an X-linked pattern[276,283] in agreement with the chromosomal localization of the TBG gene. Thus, there is no male-to-male transmission, and all female offspring of affected males are heterozygous. Clinically, TBG defects are divided into three groups according to level of TBG in serum in hemizygotes (XY males or 45X females) who express only the mutant allele: complete TBG deficiency (TBG-CD), partial TBG deficiency (TBG-PD), and TBG excess (TBG-E). Inherited TBG defects can be further characterized according to the level of denatured TBG in serum and the properties of the variant molecule. The properties of variant TBG that are easily determined without the need of purification from serum are: (a) immunologic identity; (b) isoelectric focusing (IEF) pattern; (c) rate of inactivation at various temperatures or pHs; and (d) affinity for the ligands T_4 and T_3. More precise identification of TBG defects requires sequencing of the variant TBG gene. This has been accomplished in 17 different TBG variants (Fig. 158-14).

Complete TBG Deficiency (TBG-CD). TBG-CD is defined as undetectable TBG in serum of affected hemizygous subjects. The current limit of detection is 0.5 μg/dl, which corresponds to 0.03 percent of the average TBG concentration in serum of normal adults.[284] Heterozygous females have approximately half the normal concentration of TBG and thyroid hormone levels intermediate to those of affected hemizygous subjects and normal individuals. This suggests an equal contribution of cells expressing the normal and mutant TBG genes. On rare occasions, selective inactivation of the X-chromosome has been the cause for the complete defect (hemizygous phenotype) to manifest in heterozygous females.[285] The prevalence of TBG-CD is approximately 1:15,000 newborn males.[276]

Seven distinct mutant TBGs have been identified in subjects with TBG-CD (Fig. 158-14). Six have truncated molecules due to early termination of translation caused by a single nucleotide substitution ($\text{TBG-CDB}_{\text{BUFFALO}}$[286]), by a frameshift due to a nucleotide deletion (TBG-CD6,[287], $\text{TBG-CDJ}_{\text{JAPAN}}$,[288,289] $\text{TBG-CDY}_{\text{YONAGO}}$,[290] $\text{TBG-CDBe}_{\text{BEDOUIN}}$[291]), or an addition caused by a mutation in an acceptor splice junction ($\text{TBG-CDK}_{\text{KANKAKEE}}$[292]). TBG-CDK is the only known TBG defect caused by a mutation outside the coding region of the gene. The replacement of the normal Leu227 with Pro in TBG-CD5[284] results in the failure of its secretion due to aberrant posttranslational processing.[263] All subjects with TBG-CDJ so far identified have been

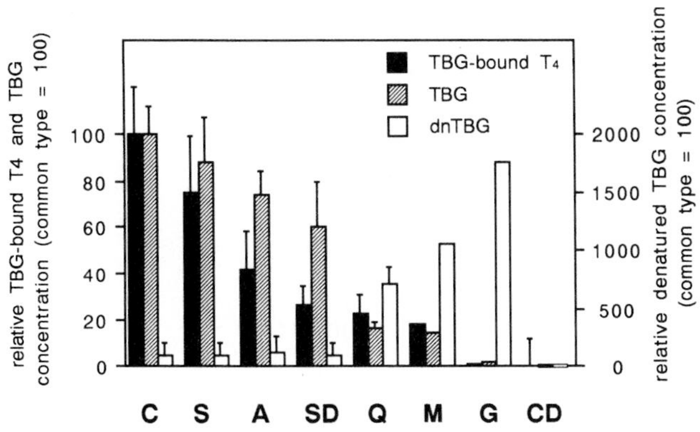

Fig. 158-15 Serum TBG-bound T_4 and the concentrations of TBG and denatured (dn) TBG in hemizygous subjects expressing the different TBG variants. The results, expressed as mean ±SD, are normalized relative to the mean normal values for the common type TBG (TBG-C; 16 mg/liter). Abbreviations for the TBG variants are given in the legend to Fig. 158-14 (*From Janssen et al.*[485] *Used with permssion.*)

Japanese. However, the allele frequency of this TBG variant in the Japanese population is not known.[289,293]

Partial TBG Deficiency (TBG-PD). Variant TBGs comprised in this category are detected in serum of hemizygotes, albeit at a reduced level. When TBG levels in affected males are above 15 percent of the mean normal value, those in heterozygous females often overlap the normal range, invalidating the assignment of phenotype based solely on serum TBG concentration. This is the most common form of TBG-deficiency, having a prevalence of 1:4,000 newborns.[276] Six variants manifesting as TBG-PD have been identified (Fig. 158-14). Two have high frequency in some population. TBG-Aborigine (TBG-A), presenting with moderate TBG deficiency has an allele frequency of 50 percent in Australian Aborigines,[294] and TBG-Slow (TBG-S), associated with a very mild TBG deficiency, has an allele frequency of 2 to 16 percent in Black African and Pacific Islands populations.[295]

While the reduction in total T_4 and T_3 concentrations is generally proportional to that of TBG, this is not the case in TBG variants, which, in addition, have reduced affinity for these hormone ligands. Most notable for such discrepancies are TBG-A and $TBG_{SAN\ DIEGO}$ (TBG-SD) (Fig. 158-15).[296–298]

The decreased stability at 37°C and increased concentration of denatured TBG in serum of subjects expressing three TBG variants [TBG_{GARY} (TBG-G), $TBG_{MONTREAL}$ (TBG-M) and TBG_{QUEBEC} (TBG-Q)] suggested that an accelerated rate of degradation is responsible for their markedly low concentration in serum.[282,299] In vitro expression of TBG-M confirmed this hypothesis.[263] However, in the case of TBG-G, transfection experiments indicate that impaired secretion leading to excessive intracellular degradation is responsible for the low concentrations of TBG in subjects expressing this variant molecule.[262] This is caused by improper folding and faulty intracellular processing of the molecule due to the presence of an additional carbohydrate at a new site of *N*-linked glycosylation created by the replacement of the normal Ile96 with an Asn.[300] The additional carbohydrate chain in TBG-G increases its overall content in sialic acid and produces a characteristic anodal shift on IEF. Data suggest that association of the GRP78 molecular chaperon with TGB-PDJ is responsible for the impaired secretion of this variant TBG.[301]

Autosomal dominant inheritance with transmission of the TBG-PD phenotype from father to son was recently reported in a Japanese family.[302] The concentration of TBG in affected males and females was approximately half the normal mean value and the molecule had normal IEF, heat lability, and affinity for T_4. All coding areas of the gene or in the promoter region had normal sequences. Although the mechanism of TBG-CD in this family is unknown, an abnormality in one of the factors regulating TBG gene transcription is a distinct possibility.

TBG Excess (TBG-E). Inherited TBG-E has a lower prevalence than TBG deficiency. It is detected in 1:25,000 newborns.[276] For many years, the molecular basis of TBG-E had been elusive and complete sequencing of the coding and promoter regions failed to show any defects.[258] However, in 1995, Mori et al.[303] found that gene amplification was the cause of TBG-E in two families. Gene triplication and duplication were demonstrated by gene dosage studies using HPLC measurements of the PCR-amplified product. As expected, affected males with triplication or duplication had approximately three- and twofold the average normal serum TBG concentration, respectively. *In situ* hybridization of prometaphase and interphase chromosomes from an affected male confirmed the presence of multiple TBG gene copies in tandem.

TBG Variants with Unaltered Biologic Properties and Concentrations. Six TBG variants have been identified with clinically insignificant alteration in concentration and biologic properties (Fig. 158-14), four of which occur with high frequency in some population groups. TBG-Poly, with no alterations of its physical or biologic properties, has been found in 16 percent and 20 percent of the French Canadian and Japanese populations, respectively.[284,293] TBG-S is detected by a cathodally shifted IEF pattern[304,305] caused by the loss of a negative change owing to the substitution of the negatively charged Asp171 by a neutral Asn.[295] The molecule also has a reduced stability when exposed at 60°C, but a normal affinity for T_4. TBG-S has an allele frequency of 5 to 16 percent in Black populations of African origin and 2 to 10 percent in Pacific Islanders. The molecular structure of two other polymorphic TBG variants has not been identified. TBG-F has an allele frequency of 3.2 percent in Eskimos residing on the Kodac and St. Lawrence islands. It has a slight anodal (fast) mobility on IEF.[306] TBG-C1 has been identified in subjects inhabiting two Mali villages.[307] It has a small cathodal shift on IEF, and an allele frequency of 5.1 percent. TBG-Poly, harboring a Phe283 instead of Leu, is found with high frequency in some populations, but has normal binding and physical properties. TBG-Cgo is probably a rare variant, found fortuitously during the screening of TBG for reduced heat stability. This variant TBG is relatively resistant to high temperature ($t_{\frac{1}{2}}$ at 60°C of 90 min compared to 6.8 ± 1.1 min for TBG-C) and low pH.[308] Its concentration in serum is normal, as are its association constant for T_4 and IEF pattern. The replacement of the normal Tyr309 with a Phe ties the internal α-helixes to the molecule, thus stabilizing its tertiary structure.[309]

Inherited TTR Abnormalities (MIM 176300). Sequencing of the TTR gene has identified a large number of variant molecules.[310] Only those few with altered binding affinity for iodothyronines are herein presented (Table 158-2).

Moses et al.[311] described a family in which affected members had elevated serum total T_4 that was predominantly bound to TTR. They were clinically euthyroid and had normal free T_4 levels measured by equilibrium dialysis. In accordance with the thyroid hormone-binding properties of the wild-type molecule, serum T_3 concentration was normal and tetraiodothyroacetic acid bound to TTR with higher affinity than T_4. The defect is caused by a single nucleotide substitution producing a replacement of the normal Ala109 for Thr in the TTR and the inheritance is autosomal dominant.[312] Crystallographic analysis of this variant TTR revealed an alteration in the size of the T_4-binding pocket.[313] The same mutation, with the characteristic serum T_4 elevation, was found in 1 of 5000 Portuguese subjects screened for TTR variants.[314] Another TTR gene mutation involving the same codon was more recently described.[315] This mutant TTR with Val109 has an increased affinity for T_4 that is similar to that of TTR Thr109, about one order of magnitude higher than the affinity of wild-type TTR.

Table 158-2 TTR Variants with Altered Affinity for T_4 and Potentially an Effect on Tests of Thyroid Function in Serum

Affinity for T_4 Mutant/Normal					
Homozygous	Heterozygous	TTR Concentration	Codon Number	Amino Acid (Normal → Variant)	References
Decreased					
<0.1	0.17–0.41	N	30	Val→Met	318, 511
	0.54		58	Leu → His	511
	0.45		77	Ser → Tyr	511
	0.19–0.46	N	84	Ile → Ser	318, 511
~ 1.0	0.44		122	Val → Ile	511
Increased					
	3.5*	N	6	Gly → Ser	317, 512, 513
8.3–9.8†	3.2–4.1	N	109	Ala → Thr	312, 315, 511, 514
	7.3†	N	109	Ala → Val	315
	1–2.1+	↑ or N	119	Thr → Met	316, 515–517

* Probably overestimated since the subjects harboring this TTR variant have normal serum TT_4 concentrations.
Affinity of recombinant TTR *Thr109* is nine fold that of the normal TTR;[514] Affinity for *Val109* component of serum TTR.[318]
Variant TTR tested and shown not to have altered affinity to T_4 are: *Ala60* (hetero).[318,511]
N, normal; ↑, increased
Endonucleases useful in the identification of TTR variants: *Msp*I$^-$ for Ser6 in exon 2 associated PHA; *Bso*FI$^-$ and *Fnu* 4H$^+$ for Thr109; *Bso*FI$^-$ for *Val109* and *Nco*I$^+$ for *Met119*, all in exon 4.

A more common mutation found in subjects with prealbumin-associated hyperthyroxinemia (PAH), is a point mutation in exon 4 of the TTR gene replacing the normal Thr119 with a Met.[316] Although the majority of heterozygous individuals harboring Met119 have an increase in fraction of T_4 and reverse T_3 (rT_3) associated with TTR, only few had T_4 levels above the upper limit of normal.[316] Furthermore, the hyperthyroxinemia in subjects with Met119 appears to be transient and associated with nonthyroidal illness. It remains unknown whether under such circumstances the variant TTR contributes to the hyperthyroxinemia, possibly through the formation of an increased proportion of mutant-normal heterotetramers of TTR. Akbari et al.[317] observed the absence of a normal *Msp*I site in exon 2 of the TTR gene of an individual with PAH. This abnormality has not been further characterized. The variant TTRs associated with PAH are not amyloidogenic.

A growing list of variant TTRs have been shown to produce dominantly inherited familial amyloidotic polyneuropathy (FAP)[278] (see Chap. 209). Several of these variant TTRs also have reduced affinity for T_4 (Table 158-2). The increased incidence of hypothyroidism in patients with FAP is probably due to the destruction of the thyroid gland by amyloid deposits.[318] Studies carried out in the TTR-null mouse indicate that, as in the case of TBG, TTR is not essential for the supply of T_4 to body tissues, and that mice maintain an euthyroid status despite significant reduction in serum total T_4 concentration.[277,319]

Another genetic defect, giving rise to a striking TTR polymorphism, has been found in monkeys but not in humans.[320] Its biologic significance has not been fully explored.[321]

Inherited Albumin (ALB) Abnormalities that Alter Serum Iodothyronine Concentrations (MIM 103600). Another form of dominantly inherited euthyroid hyperthyroxinemia, later to be linked to the albumin gene on chromosome 4 (4q11-q13), was familial dysalbuminemic hyperthyroxinemia (FDH).[322] It is the most common cause of inherited increase in total T_4 in serum in the Caucasian population, producing on the average a twofold increase in the serum total T_4 concentration. First described in 1979,[323,324] it was found in 12 percent of subjects with euthyroid hyperthyroxinemia.[325] The overall prevalence varies from 0.01 to 1.8 percent, depending on the ethnic origin, the highest being in Hispanics.[326,327] This form of FDH has not been reported in subjects of African or Asian origin. Subjects have normal basal serum TSH levels that respond normally to TRH, and normal free T_4 concentration measured by equilibrium dialysis using appropriate buffer systems.[322,323,328] However, the falsely elevated free T_4 values, when estimated by standard clinical laboratory techniques, have often resulted in inappropriate thyroid gland ablative or drug therapy.[325,329,330] The concentration of albumin is invariably normal.

FDH is suspected when serum total T_4 concentration is increased without proportional elevation in total T_3 level and nonsuppressed serum TSH (Table 158-3). Because the same combination of test results are found in subjects with the Thr109 TTR variant, the diagnosis of FDH should be confirmed by the demonstration that an increased proportion of the total serum T_4 migrates with ALB on nondenaturing electrophoresis or precipitates with anti-ALB serum.

A tight linkage between FDH and the ALB gene (lod score 5.25) was found in a large Swiss-Amish family using two polymorphic markers.[331] This was followed by the identification of a missense mutation replacing the normal Arg218 with His.[332,333] Its association with a Sac I$^+$ polymorphism in 11 families, though unrelated, suggested a founder effect based on the ethnic predilection of FDH.[333]

Two additional mutations of the ALB gene that increased the affinity of the molecule for iodothyronines were recently identified. One is located also in codon 218, but the mutant amino acid is Pro.[334,520] This variant ALB results in serum total T_4 concentrations that are 14 to 20 times the mean normal, the highest observed under any circumstances (Table 158-3). The other mutation, a replacement of the normal Leu66 with a Pro, produces a fortyfold increase in the affinity for T_3, but only 50 percent increase in the affinity for T_4[335] (Table 158-3). Consequently, patients have hypertriiodothyroninemia but not hyperthyroxinemia. In this FDH-T_3, serum T_3 concentrations are falsely low, or even undetectable, when T_3 is measured using as a tracer an analog of T_3 rather than T_3-labeled with a radioisotope. It has resulted in inappropriate treatment with thyroid hormone.[335]

Variable binding of T_4 to the two ALB components in bisalbuminemia have been reported.[336,337] However, this does not seem to be associated with gross alterations in thyroid hormone concentration in serum. The effect of analbuminemia on thyroid hormone transport has been studied only in two

Table 158-3 Serum Iodothyronine Levels and Their Affinities for Variant Albumins

Variant	Serum Concentration			Albumin-binding (K_a)	
	T_4 µg/dl	T_3 ng/dl (% of the normal mean)	rT_3 ng/dl	T_4 fold of normal mean	T_3
A218H	16.0 (200)	147 (120)	29 (138)	10–15	4
A218P	146 (1820)	253 (230)	135 (612)	11–13*	1*
L66P	8.7 (113)	320 (330)	22 (101)	1.5	40

*Determined at saturation. Affinities are higher at the concentrations of T_4 and T_3 found in serum.[519,520]

subjects.[338] The virtual absence of ALB had no clear effect on the concentration of serum iodothyronines as judged by protein-bound iodine determination.

Transport of Thyroid Hormone into Cells

It is generally accepted that thyroid hormones enter cells in an unbound or "free" form. Such concept is in agreement with the observation that the concentration of free rather than total (protein-bound) hormone in serum best correlates with the thyroid hormone-dependent metabolic status of the organism. Because the amounts of T_4 and T_3 metabolized each day represent 150 to 300 times that available in the circulation in free form, continuous dissociation of protein-bound hormone must occur in the capillary bed. While this mechanism of hormone supply to cells is realistic, both on analytical and theoretical grounds,[339,340] Pardridge has postulated that a major source of thyroid hormone for cellular uptake is protein-bound.[341] Whatever the mechanism, at equilibrium, it is the rate of irreversible thyroid hormone metabolism that influences the net efflux of thyroid hormone from the circulation.

A more critical issue concerning thyroid hormone transfer into cells which has not been fully resolved, is the requirement of a specific transport system at the level of the cell membrane. A saturable and energy-dependent system involving a plasma membrane protein and ATP has been described in rat hepatocytes.[342] The transport process is also temperature dependent and is inhibited by hormone analogs and compounds that disturb the Na^+ gradient across the plasma membrane.[343] A mechanism of hormone internalization through coated pits has also been suggested.[344] Finally, even less is known of the processes that determine the intracellular distribution of thyroid hormones. A stereospecific pump acting at the nuclear membrane has been suggested.[345]

A human liver-specific organic anion transporter (LST-1) cDNA has been recently isolated.[346] This 691-amino-acid-protein, with a putative 12-transmembrane-segments structure, has 42 percent homology with other members of the organic anion transporter (oatp) family. LST-1, as rat oatp2 and oatp3,[347,348] transports T_4 and T_3 in a Na^+-independent manner and with a K_m of ~3 µM. LTS-1 also transports taurocholate, conjugated steroids, and eicosanoids. Na^+-dependent cotransporters have been also identified.[349]

A defect in the plasma membrane transport of T_4 has been suggested in a 74-year-old woman, based on an apparent reduction in the ratio of cytosol to total T_4 uptake in the subject's red blood cells.[350] Other members of the family were euthyroid despite high serum T_4 and T_3 concentrations without a defect of the thyroid hormone-binding serum proteins. However, the postulated plasma membrane defect of T_4 but not T_3 transport cannot explain the high serum T_3 and rT_3 levels. A mutation in the thyroid hormone receptor (TR)-β gene in affected members of this family[351] was subsequently identified, explaining the discrepancy between the clinical presentation and serum hormone values (see "Resistance to Thyroid Hormone (RTH)" below).

Recently, 6 families were identified in which with the syndrome of RTH was not associated with mutations in the TR genes.[352,353] Such individuals are candidates for defects at other gene loci including the putative LST-1 or other genes encoding proteins with a more specific thyroid hormone membrane transport function.

Iodothyronine Metabolism

While the principal secretory product of the thyroid gland is T_4, this "prohormone" needs to undergo "activation" by conversion to T_3 through specific intracellular 5′-monodeiodination. In fact, 80 percent of T_4 is metabolized through a process of stepwise deiodination that eventually strips the four iodine atoms from the molecule (Fig. 158-16).

Minor pathways of iodothyronine metabolism include conjugation with glucuronic or sulfuric acid at the phenolic hydroxyl, deamination and decarboxylation of the alanine side chain, and cleavage of the ether bond.[354,355]

The only source of T_4 is the thyroid gland, which, in an average size adult, secretes from 80 to 90 µg/day (approximately 110 nM). The rate of T_4 production in the healthy adult is remarkably constant with a 25 to 50 percent increase during pregnancy. The deiodination pathway of T_4 metabolism yields about equal amounts (45 nM) of T_3 (3,5,3′-T_3) and rT_3 (3,3′,5′-T_3) by 5′- and 5-monodeiodination, respectively. About 80 percent of the T_3 is derived from T_4, while the remaining 20 percent is secreted by the thyroid gland. T_4 has a large extrathyroidal pool that is predominantly extracellular. The smaller pool of T_3 is mainly localized in the intracellular compartment and is metabolized 20 times more rapidly than the pool of T_4 (Table 158-4).

Iodothyronine Deiodinases (DIO) (MIM 147892 and 601413). The ability of peripheral tissues to generate through T_4 monodeiodination either a metabolically active (T_3) or inactive (rT_3) hormone, provides target cells with a mechanism of thyroid hormone autoregulation. Two enzymes are involved in outer ring 5′-monodeiodination: type I 5′-deiodinase (DIO1) and type II 5′-deiodinase (DIO2). DIO1 has a high K_m for T_4 (500 nM), is inhibited by propylthiouracil (PTU) and is present in liver, kidney, muscle, and skin, thus providing T_3 for the whole body. In contrast, DIO2 has a low K_m for T_4 (<5 nM), is not inhibited by PTU, and is present mainly in the anterior pituitary, cerebral cortex, and brown adipose tissue (BAT) controlling locally the intracellular T_3 concentration.[355] Both enzymes are inhibited by iopanoic acid. While DIO1 also mediates inner ring deiodination of T_4 and T_3 in liver and kidney, a third deiodinase (DIO3) specifically catalyzes 5-deiodination and is present in large quantities in placenta, brain and fetal liver. The subcellular localization of the enzymes varies somewhat from tissue to tissue

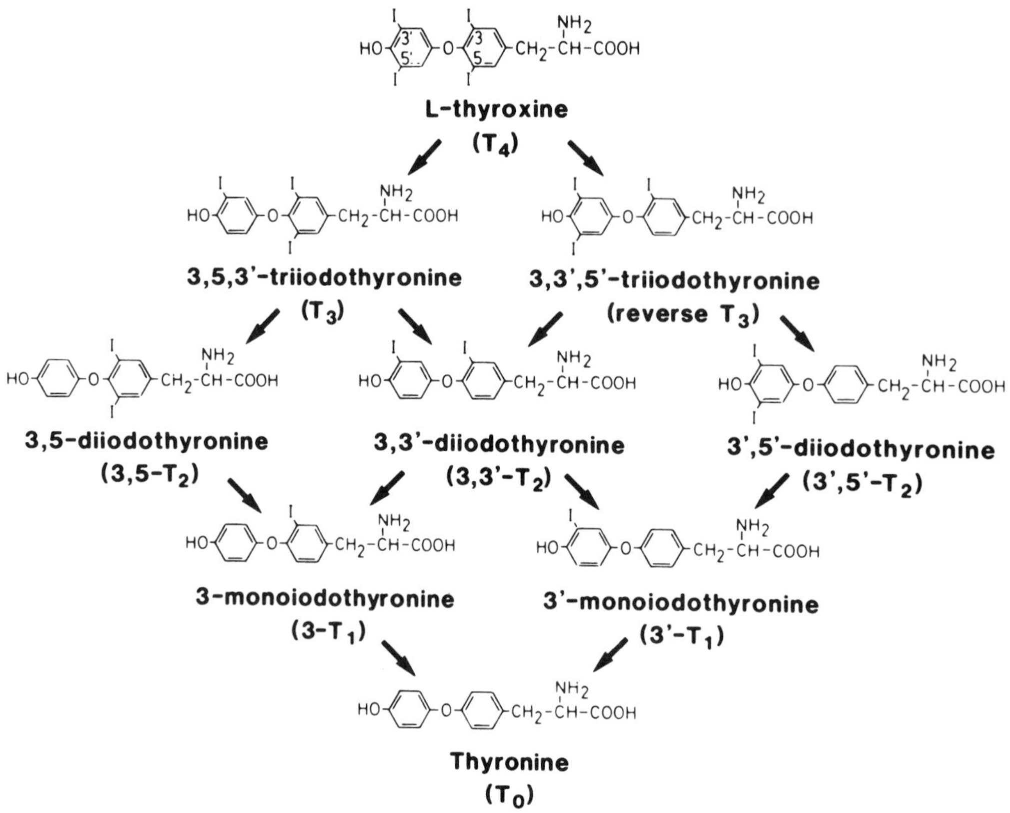

Fig. 158-16 The pathway of monodeiodination of iodothyronines. The process involves stepwise monodeiodination eventually stripping the molecule of all iodines. (*From Engler and Burger.*[354] *Used with permission.*)

and includes microsomes, endoplasmic reticulum, and plasma membrane. The deiodination reaction is reductive in nature, and probably involves selenyl iodide intermediate.[355]

The amino acid sequence and molecular structure of all three DIOs was deduced from their respective cDNA sequences.[356–358] Of 29- to 32-kDa with only 30 percent amino acid identity, the three isoforms share important structural homology. All contain selenocysteine as a reactive residue at the catalytic cleft, conserved histidine residues, and a hydrophobic transmembrane region near the N-terminus. The substitution of the selenocysteine with a cysteine decreases the enzymatic activity to 1 percent.[359] Incorporation of selenocysteine at the time of translation is directed by a specific insertion sequence (SECIS) located at the 3′-untranslated region of the mRNAs. The DIO genes, 1, 2, and 3 contain 4, 2, and 1 exons, respectively, and are located on chromosomes 1p33-p32 (DIO1),[360] 14q24.3 (DIO2),[361] and 14q32 (DIO3).[362]

Autoregulation of hormonal activity is largely mediated through the selective effect on the iodothyronine deiodinases

Table 158-4 Metabolic Parameters of T_4, T_3, and rT_3

		T_4	T_3	rT_3
Concentration in serum	μg/dl	8	0.125	0.025
	(nM)	(103)	(0.19)	(0.038)
Distribution volume	Liters	10	42	90
Metabolic clearance rate	Liters/day	1.1	24	110
Disposal (production)	μg/d	88	30	28
	(nmol/d)	(113)	(46)	(43)
Fraction derived from T_4	%		80	98
Fraction of T_4	%		40	38

Mean values for a 70-kg man.

expression. Hyperthyroidism is associated with reduced DIO2 and increased DIO1 activity. In contrast, reciprocal changes are observed in hypothyroidism. The net effect, mediated through actual changes in tissue enzyme content, is an apparent protection of the central nervous system by increasing T_3 supply when thyroid hormone supply is restricted and disposal of T_3 by increased metabolism in peripheral tissues when thyroid hormone is available in excess. During carbohydrate deprivation and in systemic illnesses, DIO1 activity is greatly reduced through a decrease in tissue cofactors, which accounts for the diminished T_3 production and for a decrease in T_3 and an increase in rT_3 levels in serum. This situation, referred to as the low T_3 syndrome,[363] is believed to safeguard the body from the catabolic effect of thyroid hormone, and thus serves the purpose of energy conservation in the face of decreased caloric supply or increased metabolic demands. 5′-Deiodinase activity is also very low in the fetus, producing low T_3 and high rT_3 levels at birth.

DIO Defects. While reduced conversion of T_4 to T_3 is common in nonthyroidal illness and in response to a variety of drugs, inherited defects in iodothyronine deiodination have not been clearly demonstrated in humans. They should be distinguished from decreases in enzyme activity due to selenium deficiency. Maxon et al.[364] reported the occurrence of familial elevation of serum T_4 and rT_3 but not T_3 concentration in subjects who were clinically euthyroid. Although this finding is compatible with a primary abnormality in the deiodination of T_4 in peripheral tissues, direct proof could not be obtained owing to the refusal of the subjects to undergo turnover studies or ingestion of thyroid hormone. Kleinhaus et al.[365] reported a sporadic case with similar findings. Elevated serum TT_4 and FT_4 levels were accompanied by high concentrations of rT_3 and 3′,5′-T_2 but low 3,3′-T_2, indicating a reduced 5′- monodeiodination but not a reduced 5-monodeiodination. This impression is supported by the ability to suppress serum TSH with 50 μg L-T_3 as compared to 200 μg of L-T_4.

The most compelling evidence for an inherited 5′-deiodinase deficiency was presented by Rösler et al. in 1982.[366] Six affected women, belonging to three generations, presented with classic symptoms and signs of hyperthyroidism, high serum levels of T_4 and T_3, but nonsuppressed TSH. This apparent pituitary resistance to thyroid hormone responded to the administration of physiologic doses of L-T_3 but not to doses of L-T_4. Until recently, this family represented the only example of deficiency in DIO2, the enzyme present in the pituitary, but not in most peripheral tissues. However, a mutation in the TRβ gene (R320L) was identified in affected members of the family, explaining the apparent partial resistance to thyroid hormone (DJ Goss, PR Larsen, and WW Chin, personal communication).

DIO1 deficiency has been demonstrated in an inbred mouse strain, C3H/HeJ.[367,368] In these mice, hepatic enzyme activity is less than 20 percent the WT level as is the enzyme concentration and its mRNA. As a consequence, serum total and free T_4 and rT_3 levels are elevated while the concentrations of T_3 and TSH remain in the normal range.

Thyroid Hormone Action

Thyroid hormone plays an important role in growth and development and acts on peripheral tissues of the adult to regulate their level of metabolism. The effects of thyroid hormone are not confined to mammals and even extend to nonvertebrate species, such as the regulation of the life cycle of coelenterates.[369] Some of the most dramatic effects of thyroid hormone involve the metamorphosis of amphibians. In an extraordinary sequence of events involving simultaneous inhibition and stimulation of synthesis of specific proteins, the tail of the larval tadpole is resorbed, which, together with budding of the limbs, results in the acquisition of the adult form, freed of dependence on the aquatic environment. The biochemical changes of this metamorphosis are even more dramatic and include conversion from ammonotelism to ureotelism.[370]

Although the impact of thyroid hormone is, in comparison, less dramatic in man, the hormone is necessary for the sustenances of normal body growth and maturation, including brain development. Although it is still debated whether the hormone is absolutely required for intrauterine fetal development,[371–373] thyroid hormone deficiency during early neonatal life leads to reversible growth retardation and to delayed bone development, but, more importantly, results in an irreversible failure of brain maturation. Supply of thyroid hormone during the perinatal period appears to be most important for mental development[374] with severe and more prolonged deficiency resulting in cretinism, the full blown syndrome of congenital hypothyroidism.

The TR Gene. The intranuclear localization of thyroid hormone[375] and the demonstration of a nuclear protein that fulfills the criteria of a hormone-receptor[376] was followed by the cloning of two thyroid hormone receptors (TRα and TRβ),[377,378] mapped to the human chromosomes 17 and 3, respectively. They share structural and functional similarities with a family of nuclear receptors, which include the glucocorticoid, mineralocorticoid, estrogen, progesterone, androgen, vitamin D, and retinoic acid receptors.[379] Nuclear receptors possess a well-conserved DNA-binding domain (DBD) separated from the C-terminal ligand (hormone)-binding domain (LBD) by a short segment that constitutes the "hinge" region. The DBD of TRs contains two stretches of 13 and 12 amino acids separated by pairs of cysteines that interact with zinc to create two peptide loops.[379] These "zinc fingers," projecting from the surface of the protein, interact with specific DNA sequences (hormone response elements) that are usually located near the transcription start point of genes regulated by thyroid hormone. Transactivation of these genes requires activation of the receptor by hormone bound to the LBD and the presence of additional cofactors. A highly conserved region within the distal C-terminus of the LBD, termed activation function-2 (AF-2), has little effect on ligand binding or dimerization, but is necessary for transcriptional activation.[380] TRα and TRβ genes have substantial structural and sequence similarities (Fig. 158-17).

Each generates two TR proteins (α1 and α2; β1 and β2) by alternative splicing. TRα2 binds to thyroid hormone response

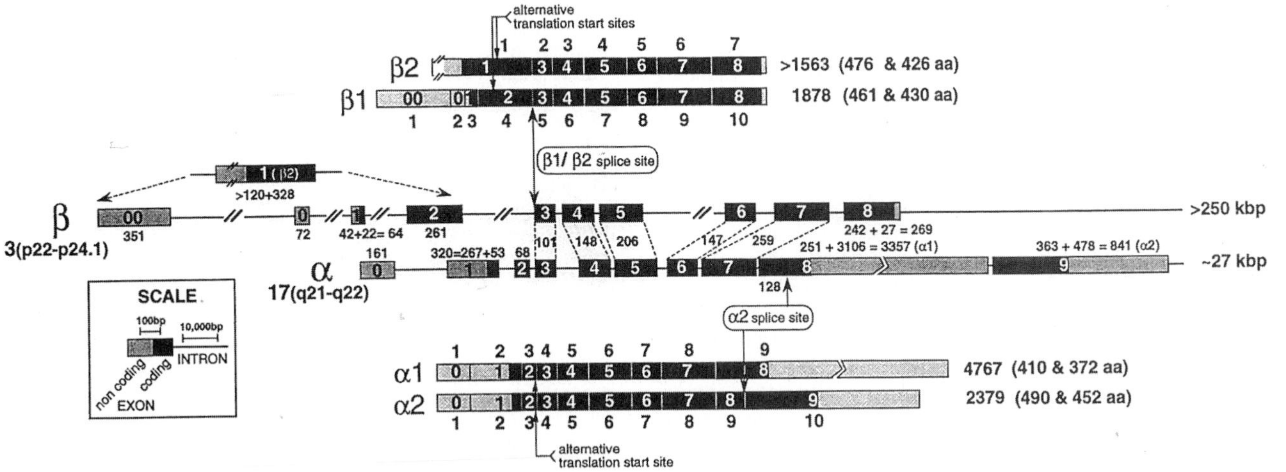

Fig. 158-17 Structures of the α and β thyroid receptor (TR) genes and their transcription and translation products. The genomic organization is shown in the center of the figure and the mRNA products of each TR gene, β2 and β1, and α1 and α2, above and below, respectively. Alternative splicing at the indicated sites generates them. The TRα1 mRNA is much larger due to its long 3′-untranslated sequence. The coding sequences corresponding to the amino acids (aa) of the products of translation are represented by the black nonstippled areas. Alternative translation start points result in further diversification of the TRs. The sizes of the exons are indicated. The boxes represent exons. The numbers within these boxes, beginning with number 1 for the first coding exon, provide common numbering for identical exons in splice variants of the same gene and for homologous exons of the α and β genes. Consecutive exon numbering, including noncoding exons, which is commonly used in publications, is given next to each exon box represented in the product of gene translation. The number of coding and noncoding nucleotides in each exon are indicated under the TRβ and above the TRα gene. Exons 3 through 7 of the α and β TRs, enclosed within the two alternative splice sites of the two genes, are identical in size. The much larger size of the TRβ gene is due to larger introns. Information for the construction of this figure is contained in references 378, 381 486, 487, 415, 488, 489, 490, and 408, as well as in unpublished information provided by Dr. V.K.K. Chatterjee and from the authors' laboratory. The numbering of TRβ codons takes into account the corrections of the sequence,[488] and thus include five additional amino acids at the N-terminus of the molecule (a total of 461 residues for the TRβ1 protein). This correction is reflected in the nomenclature of mutant TRβ genes shown in Fig. 158-20.

elements (TREs), but due to a sequence difference at the LBD site, it does not bind thyroid hormone and thus does not function as a TR proper.[381] It is of interest that nuclear receptors, which arose from two waves of gene duplication during the evolution of metazoans, were initially orphan receptors that subsequently acquired ligand-binding ability.[382] The relative expression of the two TR genes and the distribution of their products vary among tissues and during different stages of development.[383–385]

TREs, located in thyroid hormone regulated genes, consist of half-sites having the consensus sequence of AGGTCA, and vary in number, spacing, and orientation.[386,387] Each half-site usually binds a single TR molecule (monomer) and two half-sites bind two TRs (dimer) or one TR and a heterologous partner (heterodimer), the most prominent being the retinoid X receptor (RXR). The latter belong to the nuclear receptor superfamily; its ligand is 9 *cis*-retinoic acid.[388,389] Dimer formation is facilitated by the presence of an intact "leucine zipper" motif located in the middle of the LBD of TRs. Occupation of TREs by unliganded (without hormone) TRs inhibits the constitutive expression of genes that are positively regulated by thyroid hormone[390] through association with corepressors, such as the nuclear corepressor (NCoR) or the silencing mediator of retinoic acid and thyroid hormone receptors (SMRT).[391] Transcriptional repression is mediated through the recruitment of the mammalian homologue of the *Saccaromyces* transcriptional corepressor (mSin3A) and histone deacetylases (HDAC).[392] This latter activity compacts nucleosomes into a tight and inaccessible structure, effectively shutting down gene expression. This effect is relieved by the addition of thyroid hormone, which releases the corepressor, reduces the binding of TR dimers to TRE, enhances the occupation of TREs by TR/RXR heterodimers,[393] and recruits coactivators (CoA) such as p/CAF (CREB-binding protein-associated factor) and NCoA [steroid receptor coactivator-1 (SRC-1)] with HAT (histone acetylation) activity.[391,394] This results in the loosening of the nucleosome structure making the DNA more accessible to transcription factors. More than 20 additional proteins, collectively known as TR-associated proteins are involved. These proteins, in conjunction with the general coactivators PC2 and PC4, act to mediate transcription by RNA polymerase II and general initiation factors[395] (Fig. 158-18). TR dimerization is not required for hormone binding nor is the hormone needed for dimerization. Furthermore, it is believed that T_3 exerts its effect by inducing conformational changes of the TR molecule and that RXR stabilizes the association of TR with TRE.

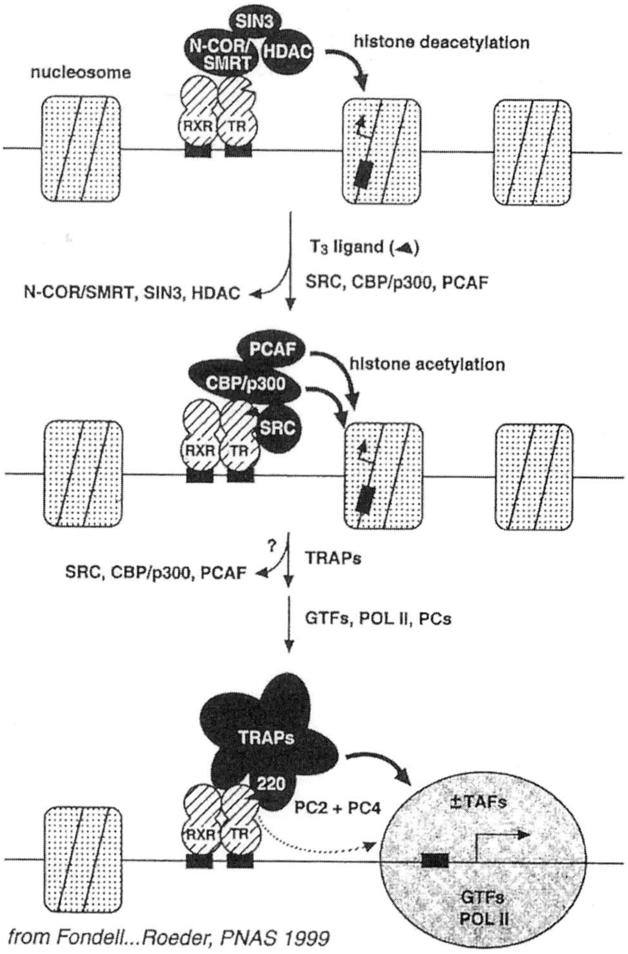

Fig. 158-18 Representation of the steps and substances involved in the control of genes positively regulated by thyroid hormone. (1) Gene Silencing (Repression): unliganded TR RXR heterodimers or TR homodimers (not shown) bind to TRE sequences, usually located in the promoter region, and through interaction with corepressors (SMRT/NCoR, SIN3) and the associated HDAC repress gene expression (top diagram). (2) Derepression: binding of ligand (T_3) to TR dissociates the corepressors and recruits coactivators (CBP/p300, SRC-1, PCAF) with intrinsic HAT activity (middle diagram). (3) Gene Activation: the cooperative functions of TR auxillary proteins (TRAPs), in conjunction with the general coactivators PC2 and PC4s mediate DNA template transcription by RNA polymerase II and general initiation factors. (*From Fundell et al.*[395] *Used with permission.*)

Resistance to Thyroid Hormone (RTH); Refetoff Syndrome (MIM 188570). RTH encompasses a clinically heterogeneous group of conditions characterized by reduced responses of target tissues to a supply of thyroid hormone that, under normal circumstances, would be excessive. Detailed reviews are available.[396,397] In all subjects so far identified, the defect has been partial. Usually RTH is first suspected when serum thyroid hormone levels are found to be elevated in association with nonsuppressed TSH, and in the absence of intercurrent illness, drugs, or alterations of thyroid hormone transport serum proteins. More importantly, full replacement doses of thyroid hormone fail to produce the expected suppressive effect on the secretion of TSH and/or induce the appropriate responses in peripheral tissues.

Classification. Until recently, RTH was subdivided into three forms based on clinical observations: generalized tissue resistance to thyroid hormone (GRTH); isolated pituitary resistance to thyroid hormone (PRTH); and peripheral tissue (but not pituitary) resistance to thyroid hormone (PTRTH).[397] The majority of subjects appeared to be eumetabolic and have been classified as having GRTH. The presence of symptoms and signs suggestive of hypermetabolism, and sinus tachycardia in particular, has lead to the diagnosis of PRTH. Recent studies show that the distinction between GRTH and PRTH has no genetic or physiological basis. In fact, the same TRβ gene mutations are found in association with GRTH and PRTH not only in individuals belonging to different kindreds, but also in affected subjects from the same family.[398,399] Clinical studies have failed to demonstrate that the peripheral tissues of patients with presumed PRTH have different sensitivity to thyroid hormone than those of patients with GRTH. Even more compelling is the observation that the clinical features may fluctuate so that at different times the same individual can be classified as having GRTH or PRTH.[400] The possible reasons for the phenotypic differences in this single genetic entity are discussed below.

PTRTH has been reported in only one individual.[401] The diagnosis was based on the requirement of supraphysiological doses of L-T_3 to maintain an eumetabolic state without adverse effect on cardiac and hepatic function. Because the pituitary thyrotrophs are spared, such patients have normal serum TSH and thyroid hormone levels and it has been argued that this is the reason for the failure to recognize other individuals with PTRTH. Yet, sequencing the TRβ gene from peripheral tissue DNA of the original case showed no abnormalities.[402] Caution should be exerted in making the diagnosis of PTRTH in individuals ingesting excessive amounts of thyroid hormone. This commonly encountered subjective requirement for supraphysiologic doses of thyroid hormone may involve a desensitization process whose mechanism is not well understood.

Prevalence and Inheritance. The exact incidence of RTH is unknown. A limited neonatal survey suggested the occurrence of one case per 50,000 life births.[403] Since the first report in 1967,[404] more than 600 cases belonging to approximately 200 families have been recognized. Contrary to most thyroid diseases, which predominantly affect females, RTH is found with equal frequency in both genders.[397]

The condition appears to have a broad geographical distribution and has been reported in Caucasians, Orientals, and Blacks. However, the prevalence may vary among different ethnic groups. Inheritance in the majority of families appears to be autosomal dominant. Nevertheless, transmission was clearly recessive in one family.[404] Consanguinity in a family with dominance of RTH has produced a homozygous child with very severe resistance to thyroid hormone who died at the age of 7 years.[405]

Pathophysiology and Clinical Features. The reduced sensitivity to thyroid hormone in subjects with RTH is shared to a variable extent by all tissues. The hyposensitivity of the pituitary thyrotrophs results in nonsuppressed serum TSH, which, in turn, increases the synthesis and secretion of thyroid hormone. This apparent paradoxic dissociation between thyroid hormone and TSH is responsible for the wide use of the phrase "inappropriate secretion of TSH" to designate the syndrome. However, TSH hypersecretion is not at all inappropriate given that the response to thyroid hormone is reduced. It is compensatory and appropriate for the level of thyroid hormone action mediated through a defective TR. Consequently, most patients are eumetabolic, although the compensation is variable among affected individuals and among tissues in the same individual. However, the level of tissue responses does not correlate with the level of thyroid hormone, probably owing to a discordance between the hormonal effect on the pituitary and other body tissues. Thyroid gland enlargement occurs with chronic, though minimal, TSH hypersecretion due to increased biologic potency of this glycoprotein through increased sialylation.[406] Administration of supraphysiologic doses of thyroid hormone is required to suppress TSH secretion without induction of thyrotoxic changes in peripheral tissues.

While the paucity of clinical manifestations is characteristic of RTH, when clinical manifestations are present, they are variable, and symptoms and signs of thyroid hormone deficiency and excess often coexist. Compatible with thyroid hormone deficiency are growth retardation, delayed bone maturation, learning disabilities, mental retardation, sensorineural deafness, and nystagmus. Those suggestive of thyroid hormone excess are tachycardia, hyperactivity, and increased BMR. Frank symptoms of hypothyroidism are more common in individuals who, because of erroneous diagnosis, have received treatment to normalize their thyroid hormone levels. A list of clinical features and their frequency is provided in Table 158-5.

Goiter is by far the most common finding, which has prompted further investigation in most of the key cases. It is of variable size and has a high propensity to recur after ablation. Delayed bone maturation resulting in significant growth retardation occurred in 15 to 25 percent of cases. Severe growth retardation is usually the consequence of inappropriate treatment, attempting to maintain all thyroid hormone levels within the normal range.

A common finding is learning disability, often associated with the attention deficit/hyperactivity disorder (ADHD; 30 to 60 percent of cases). Some children have been found to have RTH through testing because of the suspicion of thyrotoxicosis based on hyperactive behavior. Although children with RTH and ADHD have a lower intellectual quotient (IQ) than those with ADHD only,[407] mental retardation (IQ = 60) was found in < 10 percent of subjects with RTH.

Table 158-5 Clinical Features of Resistance to Thyroid Hormone

Symptoms/Clinical Findings/Test Results	Frequency (%)
Pathognomonic	
Elevated serum free T_4 and T_3 concentrations	98
Normal or slightly elevated serum TSH level	100
Common	
Enlarged thyroid gland (goiter)	66–95
Attention deficit hyperactivity disorder (ADHD)	26–60
Emotional disturbances	60
Recurrent ear and throat infections	55
Variable	
Tachycardia	16–75
Hyperkinesis	33–68
Delayed bone age (> 2 sd)	29–47
Less frequent	
Learning disability	30
Mental retardation (IQ < 70)	4–16
Short stature (< 5% percentile)	18–25
Hearing loss	10–22
Low body mass index (children)	33

Data derived from references 397,400, and 518.

Sinus tachycardia is also very common with a frequency range of 16 to 75 percent in three studies. While tachycardia is second to goiter as the reason for thyroid investigation, it is the most common reason for reaching the erroneous diagnosis of autoimmune thyrotoxicosis and that of PRTH.

While almost total hearing loss that results in deaf-mutism is typical of complete TRβ deficiency,[408] significant, but less severe, hearing loss has been found in 21 percent of subjects with RTH.[409] Detection of conductive defects in half of these individuals suggests that frequent ear infections is as common a cause as cochlear dysfunction.

Diagnosis. Diagnostic procedures need to be initiated only after persistence of elevated serum T_4 and T_3 concentrations in association with nonsuppressed TSH levels is confirmed on samples obtained several weeks apart. The differential diagnosis encompasses all causes of elevated serum thyroid hormone levels in association with a normal TSH concentration. Normal T_3 levels are typical of FDH (see preceding section). This condition, as well as TBG excess or the presence of antibodies to T_3 and T_4, can be excluded by specific tests and by measurement of the free T_4 and T_3 levels.

Because the occurrence of subclinical thyrotoxicosis can be overlooked and because failure to demonstrate a pituitary gland abnormality by imaging does not exclude the presence of a small TSH-secreting microadenoma, current diagnostic evaluation relies on a number of dynamic tests. Diagnosis is based on the responses to substances known to either stimulate or suppress TSH. Any of the following results are strongly suggestive of a TSH-producing adenoma: (a) failure of serum TSH to appropriately increase in response to thyrotropin-releasing hormone (TRH); (b) failure of serum TSH to decrease in response to supraphysiologic doses of thyroid hormone; and (c) an increase of the α subunit to whole TSH ratio.[410]

Several tests that are altered by thyroid hormone through its effects on peripheral tissues have potential diagnostic value, including: serum sex hormone-binding globulin (SHBG), ferritin, cholesterol, creatine kinase (CPK), angiotensin-converting enzyme, triglycerides, carotene, osteocalcin, pyridinium crosslinks and alkaline phosphatase; urine hydroxyproline, carnitine, and magnesium; measurement of sleeping pulse, basal metabolic rate

(BMR), cardiac contractility by echography, and deep tendon reflex relaxation time. Unfortunately, none are specific; more importantly, none are sensitive enough to clearly discriminate patients with RTH from subjects with a mild degree of thyrotoxicosis, in whom the tests are not altered. Nor are the tests sensitive enough to determine the presence of other factors that may affect the results of these tests. In fact, considerable overlap of results has been observed between hyperthyroid, euthyroid, and hypothyroid subjects. The value of these tests and their interpretation is much enhanced if measured during the administration of thyroid hormone as compared to the individual's baseline results.

At the University of Chicago, diagnostic tests are carried out before and at three-day intervals, each interval following the administration of a replacement and two incremental supraphysiologic doses of L-T_3. These doses for an adult of average size are 50, 100, and 200 µg/day. L-T_3, rather than L-T_4, is given because the more rapid onset and shorter duration of its action reduce the period of evaluation and shorten the duration of symptoms that may arise in individuals with normal responses to the hormone. Valuable information can be obtained on the anabolic versus catabolic effect of thyroid hormone, reflecting physiologic versus toxic effects, respectively, by following body weight and urea nitrogen excretion under a diet constant in calorie and protein nitrogen. Using this protocol, significant responses are observed in 95 percent of nonresistant subjects irrespective of their baseline thyroid state, while subjects with RTH show a blunted response and/or paradoxic changes[411–413] (Fig. 158-19).

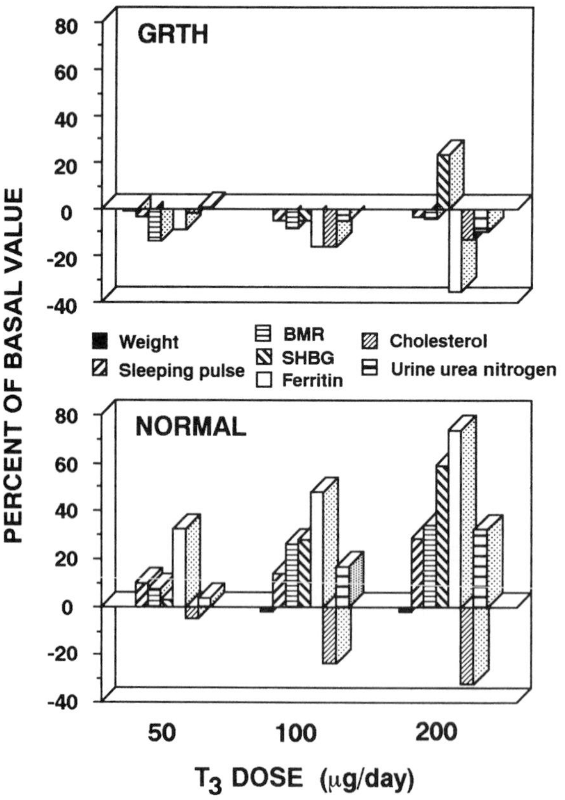

Fig. 158-19 Responses of peripheral tissues to the administration of L-T_3. Each L-T_3 dose level was given for 3 consecutive days and was administered in 6 doses, every 12 h. Average responses for each parameter and treatment period are expressed as percent increment (+) or decrement (−) from the corresponding mean basal value. Results of a patient with RTH are compared to those of a normal relative. Serum levels of T_3 achieved on each dose of L-T_3 were comparable or higher to those of the normal subject. Yet, the responses in the patient with RTH are clearly attenuated. (*Modified from Sakurai et al.*[415] *Used with permission.*)

Etiology and Genetics. Using the technique of restriction fragment length polymorphism (RFLP), Usala et al.[414] demonstrated linkage between a TRβ locus on chromosome 3 and the RTH phenotype, 21 years after description of the syndrome.[404] Subsequent studies at the University of Chicago and at the National Institutes of Health identified distinct point mutations in the TRβ gene of two unrelated families with RTH.[415,416] In both families, only one of the two TRβ alleles was involved, compatible with the apparent dominant mode of inheritance. These mutations resulted in the substitutions of single amino acids in the T_3-binding domain of the TRβ.

Mutations in the TRβ gene have now been identified in subjects with RTH who belong to 158 families (Fig. 158-20). They comprise 99 different mutations. With the exception of the index family, which has a complete deletion of the TRβ gene[408] and which is not shown on Fig. 158-20, all others harbor minor alterations at the DNA level. Five have trinucleotide deletions producing the loss of single amino acids; 1 has a single nucleotide deletion resulting in a premature stop; 3 have single nucleotide insertions and 1 has a duplication of 7 nucleotides producing frameshifts and proteins containing two extra amino acids; 88 have single nucleotide substitutions resulting in single amino acid replacements in 84 instances and stop codons in 4 others, producing truncated molecules of 433 to 450 amino acids. Given that there are 59 more families than the number of different mutations, 25 of the mutations are shared by more than 1 family. Haplotyping of intragenic polymorphic markers showed that in most instances, identical mutations have developed independently in different families. Ten of these occur in more than five apparently unrelated families and, with the exception of two, all others occur in mutagenic CpG dinucleotide hot spots. The mutation R338W (CGG → TGG) was identified in 18 different families. In agreement with this finding is the relatively high prevalence (16 percent) of neomutations. In addition, different mutations producing more than one amino acid substitution at the same codon have been found at 20 different sites; mutations at codon 345 have produced five different amino acid replacements, G345R, S, A, V, and D.

All TRβ gene mutations are localized in the functionally relevant domain of T_3-binding and its adjacent hinge region (Fig. 158-20). Three mutational clusters with intervening cold regions were identified (Fig. 158-20). With the exception of the family with TRβ gene deletion, inheritance is autosomal dominant. No mutations have been so far detected in the TRα gene, probably because its products play a minor role in the regulation of TSH and other genes of physiological relevance (see "Animal Models of RTH" below). The significance of somatic TRα gene mutations identified in nonfunctioning pituitary adenomas[417] is unclear.

In a few patients, the RTH occurs without defects in the TRα or TRβ genes.[352,418] The phenotype is indistinguishable from that in subjects harboring TRβ gene mutations, although the tissue resistance to the hormone tends to be more severe than the average. Such individuals may have a defect in one of the cofactors involved in the mediation of TH action[352] (see "Animal Models of RTH" below) and represent 10 percent of individuals with RTH.

Properties of Mutant TRβ Receptors and Dominant Negative Effect. TRβ gene mutations produce two forms of RTH. The less common form, described in only one family,[404] is caused by deletion of all coding sequences of the TRβ gene and is inherited as an autosomal recessive trait.[408] In addition to the hormonal and metabolic abnormalities typical to the syndrome of RTH, these individuals have severe deafness resulting in mutism, probably because of the complete lack of TRβ in specific areas of the brain during embryonic development.[419] Heterozygous individuals that express a single TRβ gene have no clinical or laboratory abnormalities. This is not due to compensatory overexpression of the single normal allele of the TRβ gene nor to that of the TRα gene.[420] However, because some responses to thyroid hormone

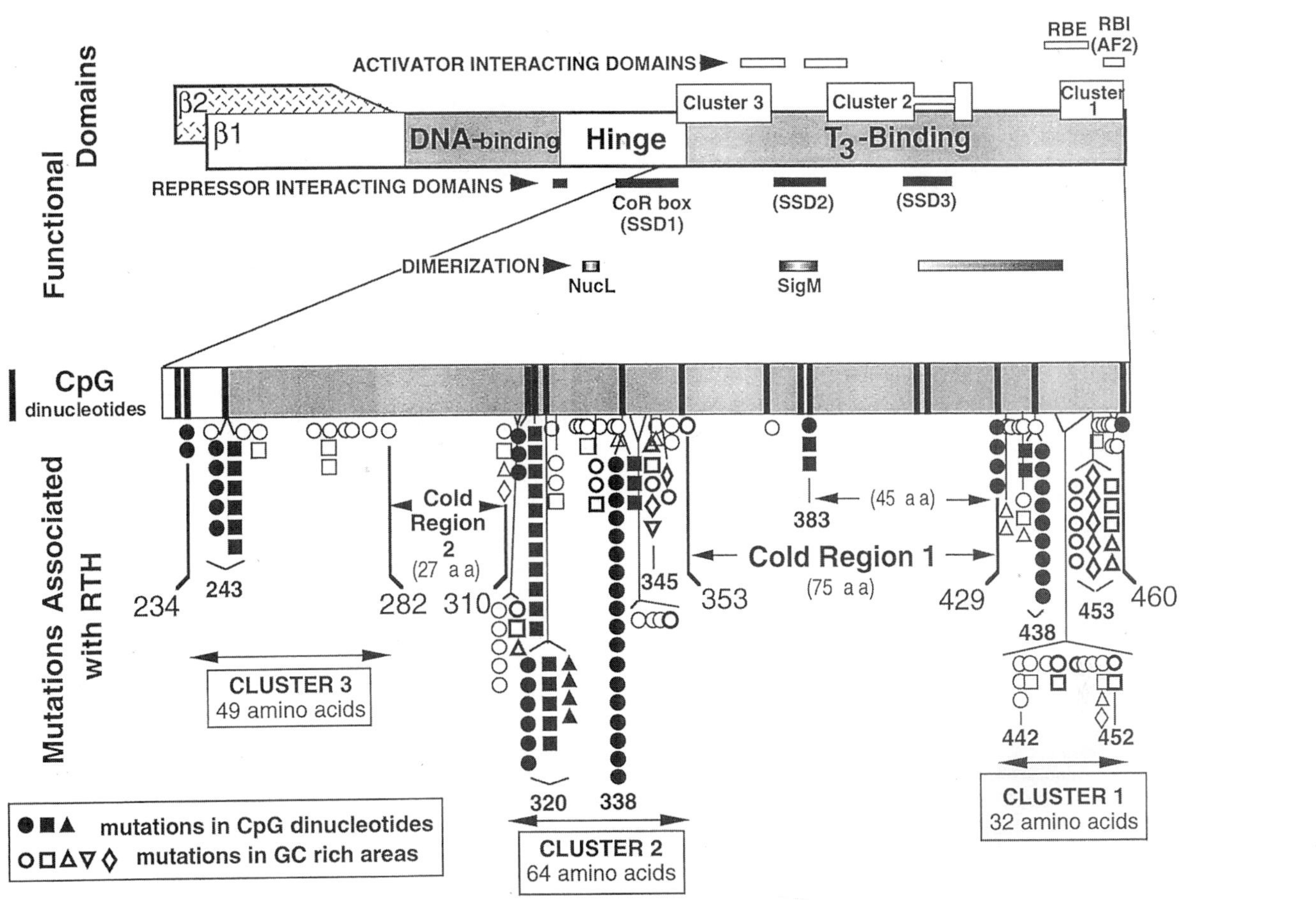

Fig. 158-20 Location of natural mutations in the TRβ molecule associated with RTH. ***Top portion*****: Representation of the TRβ and its functional domains for interaction with TREs (DNA-binding), with hormone (T_3-binding), with activating[491] and repressing[492–494] cofactors, and with nuclear receptor partners (dimerization).[427,495–497] Their relationship to the three clusters of natural mutations is also indicated.** ***Bottom portion*****: The T_3-binding domain and distal end of the hinge region which contain the three mutation clusters are expanded and show the positions of CpG dinucleotide mutational "hot spots" in the corresponding TRβ gene. The location of the 99 different mutations detected in 158 unrelated families (published and our unpublished data) are each indicated by a symbol. Identical mutations in members of unrelated families are represented by the same shading pattern of vertically placed symbols. "Cold regions" are areas devoid of mutations associated with RTH. Amino acids are numbered consecutively starting at the amino terminus of the TRβ1 molecule according to the consensus statement of the First International Workshop on RTH.*[498]* *TRβ2* has 15 additional residues at the N-terminus. AF2 = Hormone-dependent activation function (12th amphipathic helix);[380,499] RBE = corepressor-binding enhancer; RBI = corepressor-binding inhibitor;[499] SSD = silencing subdomain;*[494]* and NucL = nuclear localization;[500] SigM = signature motif.[501]**

could be demonstrated in subjects homozygous for TRβ gene deletion, it is logical to conclude that TRα_1 is capable of partially substituting for the function of TRβ (see "Animal Models of RTH" below).

The second, most common form of RTH is inherited in a dominant fashion and is characterized by minor defects in one allele of the TRβ gene, principally missense mutations. This is in contrast to individuals who lack one allele of the TRβ and who do not exhibit the TRH phenotype. These findings indicate that RTH is not simply the consequence of reduced amount of functional TR (haploinsufficiency), but that it is caused by the interference of the mutant TR (mTR) with the function of the WT-TR (dominant negative effect). This was clearly demonstrated in experiments in which mTRs are coexpressed with WT-TRs.[421,422] The most severe resistance to thyroid hormone observed in one child homozygous for a TRβ mutation[423] underscores the role of the dominant negative effect exerted by the expression of two mTR alleles in the pathogenesis of RTH.

Studies carried out during the last decade have established two basic requirements for mTRs to exert a dominant negative effect: (a) preservation of binding to TREs on DNA and (b) the ability to dimerize with a homologous[424–426] or heterologous[427,428] partner. These criteria apply to mTRs with predominantly impaired T_3-binding activity (Fig. 158-21). In addition, a dominant negative effect can be exerted through impaired association with a cofactor even in the absence of important impairment of T_3-binding. Increased affinity of a mTR to a corepressor (CoR)[429,430] or reduced association with a coactivator (CoA)[431–433] were found to play a role in the dominant expression of RTH. These conclusions are based on direct experimental evidence, as well as on observations that correlate the location of mutations on the receptor molecule and the clinical consequences. In the first instance, the introduction in a mTR of an additional artificial mutation that abolishes either DNA binding, dimerization, or the association with a CoR, results in the abrogation of its dominant negative effect.[428,434,435] Examination of the distribution of TRβ mutations associated with RTH reveals conspicuous absence of mutations in regions of the molecule that are important for dimerization, for the binding to DNA and for the interaction with CoR (Fig. 158-20). These "cold regions" are not devoid of CpG hot spots, which suggests that these regions of the molecule may not be devoid of natural mutations. However, they would escape detection owing to their failure to produce clinically significant RTH in heterozygotes. This has been indirectly deduced from in vitro studies with mTRβs harboring artificial mutations placed in the CpGs of the cold region 1.[436] Structural studies of the DBD

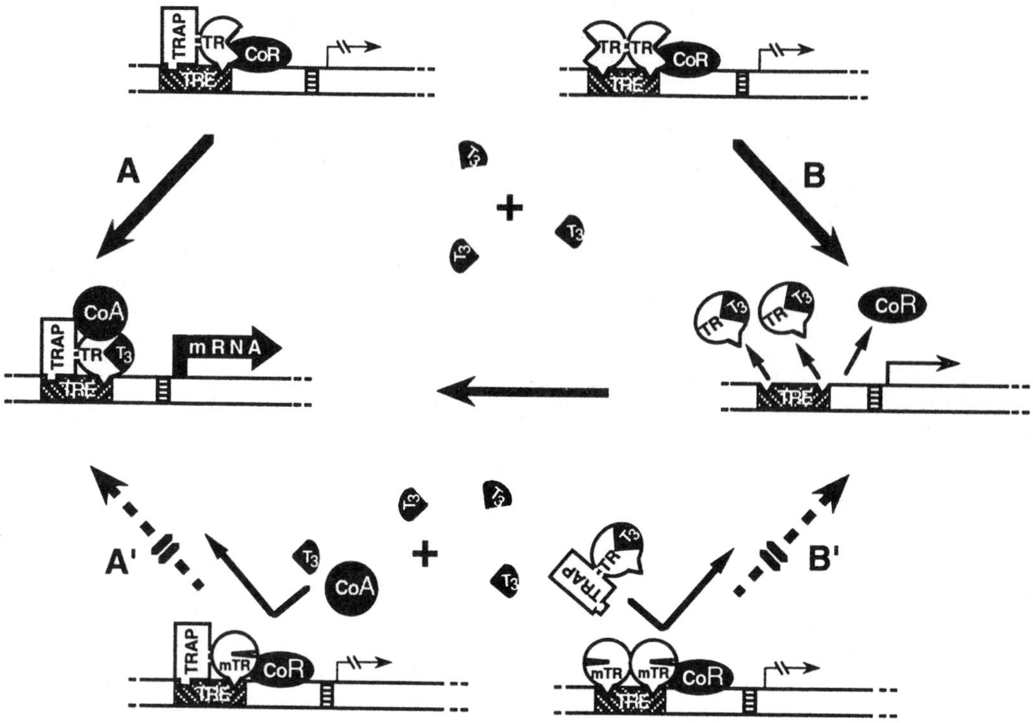

Fig. 158-21 Mechanism of the dominant expression of RTH: In the absence of T_3, occupancy of TRE by TR heterodimers (TR-TRAP) or dimers (TR-TR) suppresses transactivation through association with a corepressor (CoR). *A*, T_3-activated transcription mediated by TR-TRAP heterodimers involves the release of the CoR and association with coactivators (CoA). *B*, The removal of TR dimers from TRE releases their silencing effect and liberates TREs for the binding of active TR-TRAP heterodimers. The dominant negative effect of a mutant TR (mTR) that does not bind T_3 can be explained by the inhibitory effect of mTR-containing-dimers and heterodimers that occupy TRE. Thus, T_3 is unable to activate the mTR-TRAP heterodimer (A′) or relieve TREs from the inactive mTR homodimers (B′). TRAP refers here to TR-auxiliary protein or RXR. (*Modified from Refetoff et al.*[397] *Used with permission.*)

and LBD have provided further understanding about the clustered distribution of mTRβs associated RTH.[437,438]

Based on the early finding that RTH is associated with mutations confined to the LBD of the TRβ it was anticipated that the clinical severity of RTH would correlate with the degree of T_3-binding impairment. Some studies appeared to be in agreement with this hypothesis.[439] Other investigators found a better correlation with the potency of the dominant negative effect of the mTR assessed in vitro.[426,440] Examination of 18 different mTRβs suggested that both opinions are correct.[413] The serum-free T_4 concentration, used as indicator of thyrotroph hyposensitivity to thyroid hormone, correlated with the degree of T_3-binding impairment of the corresponding mutant receptor in 12 of these mTRβs, designated as group I. This correlation was not found in six of the mTRβs studied, a discrepancy explained in some of the studied mTRβs by the demonstration of reduced dominant negative potency due to diminished ability to form homodimers (for example R316H and E338W).[413,426] Weakened association with DNA of CoR can produce the same effect.

While reduced dominant negative effect can explain a mild impairment of function in the heterozygote despite severe impairment of T_3-binding, the reason for the occurrence of the reverse situation was less readily apparent. Indeed, more severe RTH and interference with the function of the WT-TRβ despite very mild impairment of T_3-binding or no binding defect at all has been also observed.[441] Two such mTRβs, R243Q and R243W, which are located in the hinge region of the receptor, have no significant impairment of T_3-binding when tested in solution, yet both clinically and in vitro they manifested relatively severe RTH and impairment of transactivation function, respectively. The demonstration of normal nuclear translocation but reduced ability of T_3 to dissociate homodimers formed on TRE suggested that these mutant TRβs have reduced affinity for T_3 only after they bound to DNA.[441] This was confirmed by measurement of T_3-binding after complexing to TRE.[442] Another mTRβ, L454V, which is located in the AF2 domain (Fig. 158-20), that has near normal T_3-binding, exhibited altered transcriptional function and RTH because of attenuated interaction with the CoA.[431] Finally, some mTRβs, such as R383H, exhibit a delay in CoR release despite minimal reduction of T_3-binding.[443]

In general, the relative degree of impaired function among various mTRβs is similar whether tested using TRE-controlled reporter genes that are negatively or positively regulated by T_3. Exceptions to this rule are the mTRβs R383H and R429Q that show greater impairment of transactivation on negatively regulated promoters than on positively regulated promoters.[413,443,444] The reason for this discrepancy is a matter of conjecture. Given that R429Q binds normally T_3, it is possible that T3-binding to these mTRβs is allosterically modulated by the different TREs and cofactors.[445,446]

Molecular Basis of the Variable Phenotype of RTH. The very extremes of the RTH phenotypes have a clear molecular basis. Subjects heterozygous for a TRβ gene deletion are normal because the expression of a single TRβ allele is sufficient for normal function. RTH manifests in homozygotes completely lacking the TRβ gene and in heterozygotes that express an mTRβ with dominant negative effect. The most severe form of RTH, with extremely high thyroid hormone levels and signs of both hypothyroidism and thyrotoxicosis, occurred in a homozygous individual expressing only a mutant TRs.[405,423] The severe hypothyroidism manifested in bone and brain of this subject can be explained by the silencing effect of a double-dose mTR and its strong interference with the function of TRα, a situation that does not occur in homozygous subjects with TRβ deletion. In contrast, manifestations of thyrotoxicosis in other tissues, such as the heart, may be explained by the effect high thyroid hormone levels have on tissues that normally express predominantly TRα1. It is for the same reason that tachycardia is a relatively common finding in RTH.

Table 158-6 Possible Mechanisms for the Variation in Clinical Phenotype of Resistance to Thyroid Hormone

Differences in the Sensitivity to Thyroid Hormone Among Tissues
1. Differences in tissue distribution of TR isoforms (level of TRβ expression)
2. Relative expression of mTRβ and WT-TRβ
3. Variability in the potency of a particular mTRβ to exert dominant negative effect on different target genes due to
   (a) TRE configuration
   (b) Formation of heterodimers vs. homodimers
4. Differences in the expression or interaction with cofactors (CoR and CoA)

Differences among individuals
1. Relative level of mTRβ expression
2. Genetic variability of TRE
3. Genetic variability of cofactors

Various mechanisms can be postulated to explain the tissue differences in thyroid hormone resistance within the same subject and among individuals (Table 158-6). The distribution of receptor isoforms varies from tissue to tissue.[383,447,448] This likely accounts for greater hormonal resistance of the liver as compared to the heart. Differences in the degree of resistance among individuals harboring the same mTRβ could be explained by the relative level of mutant and WT-RT expression. Such differences have been found in one study,[449] but not in another.[420]

Although in a subset of mTRβs a correlation was found between their functional impairment and the degree of thyrotroph hyposensitivity to thyroid hormone, it is surprising that this correlation was not maintained with regard to the hormonal resistance of peripheral tissues.[413] Subjects with the same mutations, even those belonging to the same family, showed a different degree of RTH. A most striking example is that of family GH in which the mTRβR316H did not cosegregate with the RTH phenotype in all family members.[450] This variability of clinical and laboratory findings was not observed in affected members of two other families with the same mutation.[399,451] A study in a large family with the mTRβR320H, suggests that genetic variability of factors other than TR may modulate the phenotype of RTH.[452]

Animal Models of RTH. The features of RTH found in patients homozygous for TRβ deletion also manifest in the TRβ-deficient mouse.[453–455] In particular, the presence of sensorineural deafness[456] indicates that the lack of TRβ per se, rather than deletion of other genetic material, is responsible for the deaf mutism in affected members of the family.[408] Mice deficient in TRβ have increased heart rate that can be decreased to the level of the WT mouse by reduction on the thyroid hormone level.[455] This finding, together with the lower heart rate in mice selectively deficient in TRα1,[457] indicates that thyroid hormone dependent changes in heart rate are mediated through TRα, and explain the tachycardia observed in some patients with RTH.

In mice, the combined deletion of TRα1 and α2, produces no important alterations in thyroid hormone or TSH concentrations in serum.[373] However, expression of the C-terminal fragment of the TRα, due to the presence of a natural promoter and a transcription start site in intron 5, produces in the context of deficient intact TRα, severe neonatal hypothyroidism that is lethal but that can be rescued by short-term treatment with thyroid hormone.[458] The combined TRβ- and TRα-deficient mice have serum TSH levels that are five hundredfold higher those in WT mice, and T_4 concentrations twelvefold above the average normal mean.[373] Thus, the total absence of TR is compatible with life, but it is not yet known whether thyroid hormone can exert any effect on these animals.

A true animal model of the common form of RTH has not yet been produced. A partial model of the dominantly inherited RTH was developed by somatic gene transfer of the mTRβ1, G345R, by means of a recombinant adenovirus.[459] The liver of these mice was resistant to thyroid hormone as demonstrated by the reduced responsiveness of thyroid hormone controlled genes to the administration of T_3. Overexpression of the WT-TRβ increased the severity of hypothyroidism in the thyroid hormone deprived mouse, confirming that the unliganded TR has a constitutive effect in vivo as in vitro. Similarly, the response to thyroid hormone is enhanced in animals that overexpress the WT-TR. Transgenic mice have been also developed that express a mTRβ1.[460] Although these mice have minimal changes in thyroid hormone values, they display reduced body weight and hyperactivity. Mutant TRβs have also been targeted to the pituitary thyrotrophs, resulting in mild phenotype of PRTH.[461,462]

Finally, recent work has shown that NcoA (SRC-1)-deficient mice have RTH manifesting with elevated T_4, T_3, and TSH concentrations.[463] These data indicate that abnormalities in cofactors can produce RTH.

Treatment. No specific treatment is available to fully correct the defect. The ability to identify mutations in the TRβ gene provides a mean for prenatal diagnosis and family counseling. In subjects adequately compensated by an increase of the endogenous supply of thyroid hormone, no further treatment is required. In those subjects in whom compensation appears to be incomplete, judicious administration of supraphysiologic doses of the hormone is indicated. Requirements should be determined on individual basis by assessing tissue responses to incremental doses of the hormone. In children, particular attention must be paid to growth, bone maturation, and mental development. The emergence of a catabolic state is an indication of overtreatment. Adults who have received ablative therapy due to erroneous diagnosis, and who thus have limited thyroidal reserve, also need treatment with thyroid hormone. Suppression of the elevated serum TSH values is an appropriate guide to therapy.

Subjects with RTH that complain of symptoms suggestive of thyrotoxicosis, and in particular have tachycardia, should be treated symptomatically with the β-blocking agent, atenolol. Somatostatin and TRIAC have been used to reduce the thyroid hormone levels by the suppression of TSH. The former loses effect when given chronically, and long-term experience with the latter is limited.[464]

MULTIGENIC-MULTIFACTORIAL THYROID DISEASES

The respective roles of genetic versus environmental factors in the most prevalent thyroid diseases are still under intensive investigation. Endemic goiter is a paradigmatic environmental disease related to the supply of iodine in the diet. The large size of the populations exposed for centuries to the shortage of iodine together with the expected reduction of reproductive fitness of the affected individuals (severe for hypothyroid cretinism, moderate for goitrous hypothyroidism) makes this situation a good candidate for the positive selection of alleles with advantageous effects. Alternatively, it may unmask defective alleles that would be neutral in an iodine-sufficient environment. Despite this kind of reasoning, no convincing evidence has yet been presented in favor of the existence of such type of alleles. The genes that should be looked for are now in hand (Tg, TPO, NIS, pendrin) or will be soon available (the H_2O_2-generating system). A variant Tg was found to segregate with simple goiter in a dominant pedigree.[119] The future will tell whether this observation can be related to a peculiar functional characteristic of this variant. Recently, whole-genome mapping endeavors have been initiated to identify genes responsible for plain or multinodular goiter.

After iodine deficiency, autoimmunity is the second major cause of thyroid diseases. As with most of the other autoimmune disorders, familial clustering is observed, but transmission is clearly nonmendelian. For both Graves disease and Hashimoto thyroiditis, *associations* with distinct HLA and CTLA-4 alleles have been described.[465] The associations are quite loose and involve different alleles in populations with different genetic backgrounds. However, no significant *linkage* with these loci could be demonstrated, suggesting that their effects in the development of the diseases are only marginal.[466] The results of studies with twins indicate that environmental factors play an important role in thyroid autoimmunity. Concordance rates of monozygotic twins have recently been scaled down from more than 50 percent to about 20 percent, and those of dizygotic twins from up to 20 percent to 0 percent.[465] Not unexpectedly in this context, linkage studies for Graves disease, whether by whole-genome mapping, or the candidate-gene approach, have met with difficulties. No linkage to the TSHr gene could be found in a large sample of families with Graves disease.[467] A limited number of genomic segments have been identified (on chromosome 14q31 and 20q11.2) displaying cosegregation with the phenotypes, but no genes have been found yet.[468,469] These studies are only beginning and will certainly receive a strong boost from the future use of SNP markers.

NEONATAL SCREENING

In many programs, neonatal screening involves T_4 and TSH measurements, some TSH measurements only, and a few T_4 measurements only. Except for absence or abnormality of TSH and resistance to thyroid hormone, all the defects described should lead to hypothyroidism and, therefore, high TSH levels. If already hypothyroid at birth, such patients should be detected by the TSH screening. False positive tests might result from heavy iodine contamination and consequent thyroid inhibition around birth.[470] TSH measurements miss the cases for which lack of TSH or defective TSH is the cause of hypothyroidism.

Similarly, T_4 screening should detect all cases with hypothyroidism at birth except those with resistance to thyroid hormones. It is, however, less sensitive than TSH measurements. It may miss hypothyroidism compensated by high TSH stimulation especially in dysgenesis cases (the most frequent cause of congenital hypothyroidism).[470] In some cases, the detection by echography of a goiter in the fetus in utero may signal a defect.

TSH screening or the use of both tests should be preferred (day 2 to day 6).[470,471] Any result above 20 mU/liter should be followed by T_4 determinations, further investigation (serum T_3 and thyroglobulin, urinary concentration of iodine in mother and infant, and, eventually, ^{99}Tc pertechnetate scan and determination of the degree of bone maturation),[470] to be followed by immediate treatment.

TREATMENT

Treatment should begin as early as possible as any delay will decrease the final mental status achieved. With treatment started no later than 2 weeks after birth, no decrease[472] of IQ has been observed, but slight disturbances in motor development may remain. Small differences in IQ are observed only when treatment is begun after 3 weeks and clear differences when it is started after 3 months.[473,474]

As most brain T_3 is derived in the brain from thyroxine mainly, thyroxine (10 μg/kg/day, i.e., 25 to 37.5 μg/day) should be administered orally,[474] but preparations with some T_3 might better correct deficits in all organs.[475] Detailed search for the cause of hypothyroidism can be postponed until 3 years of age.

ACKNOWLEDGMENTS

S. Refetoff and his work are supported in part by grants RR-55 and DK-15070 from the National Institutes of Health, USA.

REFERENCES

1. Dumont JE, Vassart G, Refetoff S: Thyroid disorders, in Scriver CR, Beaudet AL (ed): *The Metabolic Basis of Inherited Diseases*, 6th ed. New York, McGraw-Hill, 1989, p 1843.
2. Vassart G, Refetoff S, Dumont JE: Thyroid disorders, in Scriver CR, Beaudet AL, Sly WS, Vale D (eds): *The Metabolic and Molecular Basis of Inherited Diseases*, 7th ed. New York, McGraw-Hill, 1995, p 2883.
3. Polk DH, Reviczky A, Lam RW, et al: Thyrotropin-releasing hormone in ovine fetus: Ontogeny and effect of thyroid hormone. *Am J Physiol* **260**:E53, 1991.
4. Straub RE, Frech GC, Joho RH, et al: Expression cloning of a cDNA encoding the mouse pituitary thyrotropin-releasing hormone receptor. *Proc Natl Acad Sci U S A* **87**:9514, 1990.
5. Gershengorn MC, Osman R: Molecular and cellular biology of thyrotropin-releasing hormone receptors. *Physiol Rev* **76**:175, 1996.
6. Magner JA: Thyroid-stimulating hormone: Biosynthesis, cell biology, and bioactivity. *Endocr Rev* **11**:354, 1990.
7. Weintraub BD, Stannard BS, Magner JA, et al: Glycosylation and posttranslational processing of thyroid-stimulating hormone: Clinical implications. *Recent Prog Horm Res* **41**:577, 1985.
8. Grossmann M, Weintraub BD, Szkudlinski MW: Novel insights into the molecular mechanisms of human thyrotropin action: Structural, physiological, and therapeutic implications for the glycoprotein hormone family. *Endocr Rev* **18**:476, 1997.
9. Jones KE, Chin WW: Differential regulation of thyroid hormone receptor messenger ribonucleic acid levels by thyrotropin-releasing hormone. *Endocrinology* **128**:1763, 1991.
10. Dumont JE, Lamy F, Roger P, et al: Physiological and pathological regulation of thyroid cell proliferation and differentiation by thyrotropin and other factors. *Physiol Rev* **72**:667, 1992.
11. Rapoport B, Chazenbalk GD, Jaume JC, et al: The thyrotropin (TSH) receptor: Interaction with TSH and autoantibodies [Citation]. *Endocr Rev* **19**:673, 1998.
12. Vassart G, Dumont JE: The thyrotropin receptor and the regulation of thyrocyte function and growth. *Endocr Rev* **13**:596, 1992.
13. de Rooij J, Zwartkruis FJT, Verheijen MHG, et al: Epac is a Rap1 guanine-nucleotide-exchange factor directly activated by cyclic AMP. *Nature* **396**:474, 1998.
14. Maenhaut C, Brabant G, Vassart G, et al: In vitro and in vivo regulation of thyrotropin receptor mRNA levels in dog and human thyroid cells. *J Biol Chem* **15**:3000, 1992.
15. Uyttersprot N, Allgeier A, Baptist M, et al: The cAMP in Thyroid From the TSH receptor to mitogenesis and tumorigenesis, in Corbin J, Francis S (eds): *Signal Transduction in Health and Disease, Advances in Second Messenger and Phosphorylation Research.* Philadelphia, Lippincott-Raven Publishers, 1997, p 125.
16. Uyttersprot N, Pelgrims N, Carrasco N, et al: Moderate doses of iodide in vivo inhibit cell proliferation and the expression of thyroperoxidase and Na+/I− symporter mRNAs in dog thyroid. *Mol Cell Endocrinol* **131**:195, 1997.
17. Wolff J: Transport of iodide and other anions in the thyroid gland. *Physiol Rev* **44**:45, 1964.
18. Dai G, Levy O, Amzel LM, et al: The mediator of thyroidal iodide accumulation: The sodium/iodide symporter, in Konings WN, Kaback HR, Lolkema JS (eds): *Handbook of Biological Physics.* Amsterdam, Elsevier Science, 1996, p 343.
19. Nunez J, Pommier J: Formation of thyroid hormones. *Vitam Horm* **39**:175, 1982.
20. Corvilain B, Laurent E, Lecomte M, et al: Role of the cyclic adenosine 3′,5′-monophosphate and the phosphatidylinositol-Ca2+ cascades in mediating the effects of thyrotropin and iodide on hormone synthesis and secretion in human thyroid slices. *J Clin Endocrinol Metab* **79**:152, 1994.
21. Ledent C, Dumont JE, Vassart G, et al: Thyroid expression of an A2 adenosine receptor transgene induces thyroid hyperplasia and hyperthyroidism. *EMBO J* **11**:537, 1992.
22. Maenhaut C, Van Sande J, Libert F, et al: RDC8 codes for an adenosine A2 receptor with physiological constitutive activity. *Biochem Biophys Res Commun* **173**:1169, 1990.
23. Weinstein LS, Shenker A, Gejman PV, et al: Activating mutations of the stimulatory G protein in the McCune-Albright syndrome. *N Engl J Med* **325**:1688, 1991.
24. Michiels FM, Caillou B, Talbot M, et al: Oncogenic potential of guanine nucleotide stimulatory factor alpha subunit in thyroid glands of transgenic mice. *Proc Natl Acad Sci U S A* **91**:10488, 1994.

25. Strader CD, Fong TM, Tota MR, et al: Structure and function of G protein-coupled receptors. *Annu Rev Biochem* **63**:101, 1994.
26. Nagayama Y, Rapoport B: The thyrotropin receptor 25 years after its discovery: New insight after its molecular cloning. *Mol Endocrinol* **6**:145, 1992.
27. Vassart G, Parma J, Van Sande J, et al: The thyrotropin receptor and the regulation of thyrocyte function and Growth: update 1994. *Endocr Rev* **3**:77, 1994.
28. Gross B, Misrahi M, Sar S, et al: Composite structure of the human thyrotropin receptor gene. *Biochem Biophys Res Commun* **177**:679, 1991.
29. Kobe B, Deisenhofer J: A structural basis of the interactions between leucine-rich repeats and protein ligands. *Nature* **374**:183, 1995.
30. Kobe B, Deisenhofer J: The leucine-rich repeat: A versatile binding motif. *TIBS* **19**:415, 1994.
31. Misrahi M, Ghinea N, Sar S, et al: Processing of the precursors of the human thyroid-stimulating hormone receptor in various eukaryotic cells (human thyrocytes, transfected L cells and baculovirus-infected insect cells). *Eur J Biochem* **222**:711, 1994.
32. de Bernard S, Misrahi M, Huet JC, et al: Sequential cleavage and excision of a segment of the thyrotropin receptor ectodomain. *J Biol Chem* **274**:101, 1999.
33. Nagayama Y, Russo D, Wadsworth HL, et al: Eleven amino acids (Lys-201 to Lys-211) and 9 amino acids (Gly-222 to Leu-230) in the human thyrotropin receptor are involved in ligand binding. *J Biol Chem* **266**:14926, 1991.
34. Nagayama Y, Wadsworth HL, Chazenbalk GD, et al: Thyrotropin-luteinizing hormone/chorionic gonadotropin receptor extracellular domain chimeras as probes for thyrotropin receptor function. *Proc Natl Acad Sci U S A* **88**:902, 1991.
35. Braun T, Schofield PR, Sprengel R: Amino-terminal leucine-rich repeats in gonadotropin receptors determine hormone selectivity. *EMBO J* **10**:1885, 1991.
36. Segaloff DL, Ascoli M: The lutropin/choriogonadotropin receptor—4 years later. *Endocr Rev* **14**:324, 1993.
37. Nothacker HP, Grimmelikhuijzen CJ: Molecular cloning of a novel, putative G protein-coupled receptor from sea anemones structurally related to members of the FSH, TSH, LH/CG receptor family from mammals. *Biochem Biophys Res Commun* **197**:1062, 1993.
38. Hauser F, Nothacker HP, Grimmelikhuizen C: Molecular cloning, genomic organization and developemental regulation of a novel receptor from *Drosophila melanogaster* structurally related to members of the TSH, FSH, LH/CG receptor family from mammals. *J Biol Chem* **10**:1002, 1997.
39. Hsu SY, Liang SG, Hsueh AJ: Characterization of two LGR genes homologous to gonadotropin and thyrotropin receptors with extracellular leucine-rich repeats and a G protein-coupled, seven-transmembrane region [Citation]. *Mol Endocrinol* **12**:1830, 1998.
40. Hoflack J, Hibert MF, Trumpp Kallmeyer S, et al: Three-dimensional models of gonado-thyrotropin hormone receptor transmembrane domain. *Drug Des Discov* **10**:157, 1993.
41. Kajava AV, Vassart G, Wodak SJ: Modeling of the three-dimensional structure of proteins with the typical leucine-rich repeats. *Structure* **3**:867, 1995.
42. Thomas JS, Leclere J, Hartemann P, et al: Familial hyperthyroidism without evidence of autoimmunity. *Acta Endocrinol Copenh* **100**:512, 1982.
43. Duprez L, Parma J, Van Sande J, et al: Germline mutations in the thyrotropin receptor gene cause nonautoimmune autosomal dominant hyperthyroidism. *Nat Genet* **7**:396, 1994.
44. Tonacchera M, Van Sande J, Cetani F, et al: Functional characteristics of three new germline mutations of the thyrotropin receptor gene causing autosomal dominant toxic thyroid hyperplasia. *J Clin Endocrinol Metab* **81**:547, 1996.
45. Fuhrer D, Wonerow P, Willgerodt H, et al: Identification of a new thyrotropin receptor germline mutation (Leu629Phe) in a family with neonatal onset of autosomal dominant nonautoimmune hyperthyroidism. *J Clin Endocrinol Metab* **82**:4234, 1997.
46. Leclere J, Béné MC, Duprez A, et al: Behavior of thyroid tissue from patients with Graves' disease in nude mice. *J Clin Endocrinol Metab* **59**:175, 1984.
47. Kopp P, Van Sande J, Parma J, et al: Congenital non-autoimmune hyperthyroidism caused by a neomutation in the thyrotropin receptor gene. *N Engl J Med* **332**:150, 1995.
48. de Roux N, Polak M, Couet J, et al: A neomutation of the thyroid-stimulating hormone receptor in a severe neonatal hyperthyroidism [Comment]. *J Clin Endocrinol Metab* **81**:2023, 1996.
49. Gruters A, Schoneberg T, Biebermann H, et al: Severe congenital hyperthyroidism caused by a germ-line neo mutation in the extracellular portion of the thyrotropin receptor. *J Clin Endocrinol Metab* **83**:1431, 1998.
50. Kopp P, Jameson JL, Roe TF: Congenital nonautoimmune hyperthyroidism in a nonidentical twin caused by a sporadic germline mutation in the thyrotropin receptor gene. *Thyroid* **7**:765, 1997.
51. Holzapfel HP, Wonerow P, von Petrykowski W, et al: Sporadic congenital hyperthyroidism due to a spontaneous germline mutation in the thyrotropin receptor gene. *J Clin Endocrinol Metab* **82**:3879, 1997.
52. Kopp P, Muirhead S, Jourdain N, et al: Congenital hyperthyroidism caused by a solitary toxic adenoma harboring a novel somatic mutation (serine281→isoleucine) in the extracellular domain of the thyrotropin receptor. *J Clin Invest* **100**:1634, 1997.
53. Farfel Z, Bourne HR, Iiri T: Review articles: Mechanisms of disease: The expanding spectrum of g protein diseases. *N Engl J Med* **340**:1012, 1999.
54. Kjelsberg MA, Cotecchia S, Ostrowski J, et al: Constitutive activation of the alpha 1B-adrenergic receptor by all amino acid substitutions at a single site. Evidence for a region which constrains receptor activation. *J Biol Chem* **267**:1430, 1992.
55. Samama P, Cotecchia S, Costa T, et al: A mutation-induced activated state of the beta 2-adrenergic receptor. Extending the ternary complex model. *J Biol Chem* **268**:4625, 1993.
56. Cotecchia S, Exum S, Caron MG, et al: Regions of the alpha 1-adrenergic receptor involved in coupling to phosphatidylinositol hydrolysis and enhanced sensitivity of biological function. *Proc Natl Acad Sci U S A* **87**:2896, 1990.
57. Parma J, Duprez L, Van Sande J, et al: Somatic mutations in the thyrotropin receptor gene cause hyperfunctioning thyroid adenomas. *Nature* **365**:649, 1993.
58. Porcellini A, Ciullo I, Laviola L, et al: Novel mutations of thyrotropin receptor gene in thyroid hyperfunctioning adenomas. *J Clin Endocrinol Metab* **79**:657, 1994.
59. Gether U, Lin S, Ghanouni P, et al: Agonists induce conformational changes in transmembrane domains III and VI of the beta2 adrenoceptor. *EMBO J* **16**:6737, 1997.
60. Paschke R, Tonacchera M, Van Sande J, et al: Identification and functional characterization of two new somatic mutations causing constitutive activation of the TSH receptor in hyperfunctioning autonomous adenomas of the thyroid. *J Clin Endocrinol Metab* **79**:1785, 1994.
61. Parma J, Van Sande J, Swillens S, et al: Somatic mutations causing constitutive activity of the TSH receptor are the major cause of hyperfunctional thyroid adenomas: Identification of additional mutations activating both the cAMP and inisitolphosphate-Ca++ cascades. *Mol Endocrinol* **9**:725, 1995.
62. Wonerow P, Schoneberg T, Schultz G, et al: Deletions in the third intracellular loop of the thyrotropin receptor. A new mechanism for constitutive activation. *J Biol Chem* **273**:7900, 1998.
63. Fuhrer D, Holzapfel HP, Wonerow P, et al: Somatic mutations in the thyrotropin receptor gene and not in the Gs alpha protein gene in 31 toxic thyroid nodules. *J Clin Endocrinol Metab* **82**:3885, 1997.
64. Duprez L, Parma J, Dumont JE, et al: Diversity and prevalence of somatic mutations in the TSH receptor gene as a cause of toxic adenoma. *J Endocrinol Invest* **19**:69, 1996.
65. Takeshita A, Nagayama Y, Yokoyama N, et al: Rarity of oncogenic mutations in the thyrotropin receptor of autonomously functioning thyroid nodules in Japan. *J Clin Endocrinol Metab* **80**:2607, 1995.
66. Russo D, Arturi F, Wicker R, et al: Genetic alterations in thyroid hyperfunctioning adenomas. *J Clin Endocrinol Metab* **80**:1347, 1995.
67. Parma J, Duprez L, Van Sande J, et al: Diversity and prevalence of somatic mutations in the TSH receptor and Gs alpha genes as a cause of toxic thyroid adenomas. *J Clin Endocrinol Metab* **82**:2695, 1997.
68. Russo D, Arturi F, Schlumberger M, et al: Activating mutations of the TSH receptor in differentiated thyroid carcinomas. *Oncogene* **11**:1907, 1995.
69. Spambalg D, Sharifi N, Elisei R, et al: Structural studies of the TSH receptor and G_{sa} in human thyroid cancers: Low prevalence of mutations predicts infrequent involvement in malignant transformation. *J Clin Endocrinol Metab* **81**:3898, 1996.
70. Kosugi S, Okajima F, Ban T, et al: Mutation of Alanine 623 in the third cytoplasmic loop of the rat TSH receptor results in a loss in the phosphoinositide but not cAMP signal induced by TSH and receptor autoantibodies. *J Biol Chem* **267**:24153, 1992.

71. Eggerickx D, Denef JF, Labbe O, et al: Molecular cloning of an orphan G-protein-coupled receptor that constitutively activates adenylate cyclase. *Biochem J* **309**:837, 1995.
72. Westphal RS, Backstrom JR, Sanders Bush E: Increased basal phosphorylation of the constitutively active serotonin 2C receptor accompanies agonist-mediated desensitization. *Mol Pharmacol* **48**:200, 1995.
73. Tiberi M, Caron MG: High agonist-independent activity is a distinguishing feature of the dopamine D1B receptor subtype. *J Biol Chem* **269**:27925, 1994.
74. Shenker A: G protein-coupled receptor structure and function: The impact of disease-causing mutations. *Baillieres Clin Endocrinol Metab* **9**:427, 1995.
75. Duprez L, Parma J, Costagliola S, et al: Constitutive activation of the TSH receptor by spontaneous mutations affecting the N-terminal extracellular domain. *FEBS Lett* **409**:469, 1997.
76. Chazenbalk GD, Rapoport B: Expression of the extracellular domain of the thyrotropin receptor in the baculovirus system using a promoter active earlier than the polyhedrin promoter. Implications for the expression of functional highly glycosylated proteins. *J Biol Chem* **270**:1543, 1995.
77. Ren Q, Kurose H, Lefkowitz RJ, et al: Constitutively active mutants of the a2-adrenergic receptor. *J Biol Chem* **268**:16483, 1993.
78. Lefkowitz RJ, Cotecchia S, Samama P, et al: Constitutive activity of receptors coupled to guanine nucleotide regulatory proteins. *TIPS* **14**:303, 1994.
79. Glinoer D: The regulation of thyroid function in pregnancy: Pathways of endocrine adaptation from physiology to pathology. *Endocr Rev* **18**:404, 1997.
80. Burrow GN: Thyroid function and hyperfunction during gestation. *Endocr Rev* **14**:194, 1993.
81. Goodwin TM, Montoro M, Mestman JH, et al: The role of chorionic gonadotropin in transient hyperthyroidism of hyperemesis gravidarum. *J Clin Endocrinol Metab* **75**:1333, 1992.
82. Swaminathan R, Chin RK, Lao TT, et al: Thyroid function in hyperemesis gravidarum. *Acta Endocrinol Copenh* **120**:155, 1989.
83. Rodien P, Bremont C, Sanson ML, et al: Familial gestational hyperthyroidism caused by a mutant thyrotropin receptor hypersensitive to human chorionic gonadotropin. *N Engl J Med* **339**:1823, 1 998.
84. Nagayama Y, Russo D, Chazenbalk GD, et al: Extracellular domain chimeras of the TSH and LH/CG receptors reveal the mid-region (amino acids 171–260) to play a vital role in high affinity TSH binding. *Biochem Biophys Res Commun* **173**:1150, 1990.
85. Mrabet NT, Van den Broeck A, Van den brande I, et al: Arginine residues as stabilizing elements in proteins. *Biochemistry* **31**:2239, 1992.
86. Stewart HJ, Jones DSC, Pascall JC, et al: The contribution of recombinant DNA technology to reproductive biology. *J Reprod Fertil* **83**:1, 1988.
87. Illig R, Largo RH, Qin Q, et al: Mental development in congenital hypothyroidism after neonatal screening. *Arch Dis Child* **62**:1050, 1987.
88. Medeiros-Neto G, Gil-Da-Costa MJ, Santos CL, et al: Metastatic thyroid carcinoma arising from congenital goiter due to mutation in the thyroperoxidase gene. *J Clin Endocrinol Metab* **83**:4162, 1998.
89. Cooper DS, Axelrod L, DeGroot LJ, et al: Congenital goiter and the development of metastatic follicular carcinoma with evidence for a leak of nonhormonal iodide: Clinical, pathological, kinetic, and biochemical studies and a review of the literature. *J Clin Endocrinol Metab* **52**:294, 1981.
90. van de Graaf SA, Pauws E, de Vijlder JJ, et al: The revised 8307 base pair coding sequence of human thyroglobulin transiently expressed in eukaryotic cells. *Eur J Endocrinol* **136**:508, 1997.
91. Yang SX, Pollock HG, Rawitch AB: Glycosylation in human thyroglobulin: Location of the N-linked oligosaccharide units and comparison with bovine thyroglobulin. *Arch Biochem Biophys* **327**:61, 1996.
92. Sakurai S, Fogelfeld L, Schneider AB: Anionic carbohydrate groups of human thyroglobulin containing both phosphate and sulfate. *Endocrinology* **129**:915, 1991.
93. Blode H, Heinrich T, Diringer H: A quantitative assay for tyrosine sulfation and tyrosine phosphorylation in peptides. *Biol Chem Hoppe Seyler* **371**:145, 1990.
94. Berndorfer U, Wilms H, Herzog V: Multimerization of thyroglobulin (TG) during extracellular storage: isolation of highly cross-linked TG from human thyroids. *J Clin Endocrinol Metab* **81**:1918, 1996.
95. Baudry N, Lejeune PJ, Delom F, et al: Role of multimerized porcine thyroglobulin in iodine storage. *Biochem Biophys Res Commun* **242**:292, 1998.
96. Xiao S, Dorris ML, Rawitch AB, et al: Selectivity in tyrosyl iodination sites in human thyroglobulin. *Arch Biochem Biophys* **334**:284, 1996.
97. Dunn JT: Thyroglobulin: chemistry and biosynthesis, in Braverman LE, Utiger D (eds): *Werner's & Ingbar's The Thyroid*. Philadelphia, JB Lippincott, 1996, p 85.
98. Gentile F, Ferranti P, Mamone G, et al: Identification of hormonogenic tyrosines in fragment 1218-1591 of bovine thyroglobulin by mass spectrometry. Hormonogenic acceptor TYR-12 donor TYR-1375. *J Biol Chem* **272**:639, 1997.
99. Marriq C, Lejeune PJ, Venot N, et al: Hormone synthesis in human thyroglobulin: Possible cleavage of the polypeptide chain at the tyrosine donor site. *FEBS Lett* **242**:414, 1989.
100. Mendive F, Rivolta CM, Vassart G, et al: Genomic organization of the 3′ region of the human thyroglobulin gene. *Thyroid* **9**:903, 1999.
101. Molina F, Bouanani M, Pau B, et al: Characterization of the type-1 repeat from thyroglobulin, a cysteine-rich module found in proteins from different families. *Eur J Biochem* **240**:125, 1996.
102. Molina F, Pau B, Granier C: The type-1 repeats of thyroglobulin regulate thyroglobulin degradation and T3, T4 release in thyrocytes. *FEBS Lett* **391**:229, 1996.
103. Medeiros-Neto G, Targovnik HM, Vassart G: Defective thyroglobulin synthesis and secretion causing goiter and hypothyroidism [erratum published in *Endocr Rev* 15(4):438, 1994]. *Endocr Rev* **14**:165, 1993.
104. Abramowicz MJ, Targovnik HM, Varela V, et al: Identification of a mutation in the coding sequence of the human thyroid peroxidase gene causing congenital goiter. *J Clin Invest* **90**:1200, 1992.
105. Savoie JC, Massin JP, Savoie F: Studies on mono- and diiodohistidine. II. Congenital goitrous hypothyroidism with thyroglobulin defect and iodohistidine-rich iodoalbumin production. *J Clin Invest* **52**:116, 1973.
106. Ieiri T, Cochaux P, Targovnik H, et al: A 3′ splice-site mutation in the thyroglobulin gene responsible for congenital goitre with hypothyroidism. *J Clin Invest* **88**:1901, 1991.
107. Dunn AD, Corsi CM, Myers HE, et al: Tyrosine 130 is an important outer ring donor for thyroxine formation in thyroglobulin. *J Biol Chem* **273**:25223, 1998.
108. Marriq C, Lejeune PJ, Venot N, et al: Hormone formation in the isolated fragment 1–171 of human thyroglobulin involves the couple tyrosine 5 and tyrosine 130. *Mol Cell Endocrinol* **81**:155, 1991.
109. Xiao S, Pollock HG, Taurog A, et al: Characterization of hormonogenic sites in an N-terminal, cyanogen bromide fragment of human thyroglobulin. *Arch Biochem Biophys* **320**:96, 1995.
110. den Hartog MT, Sijmons CC, Bakker O, et al: Importance of the content and localization of tyrosine residues for thyroxine formation within the N-terminal part of human thyroglobulin. *Eur J Endocrinol* **132**:611, 1995.
111. Medeiros-Neto G, Kim PS, Yoo SE, et al: Congenital hypothyroid goiter with deficient thyroglobulin. Identification of an endoplasmic reticulum storage disease with induction of molecular chaperones. *J Clin Invest* **98**:2838, 1996.
112. Kim PS, Hossain SA, Park YN, et al: A single amino acid change in the acetylcholinesterase-like domain of thyroglobulin causes congenital goiter with hypothyroidism in the cog/cog mouse: A model of human endoplasmic reticulum storage diseases. *Proc Natl Acad Sci U S A* **95**:9909, 1998.
113. Kim PS, Arvan P: Endocrinopathies in the family of endoplasmic reticulum (ER) storage diseases: Disorders of protein trafficking and the role of ER molecular chaperones. *Endocr Rev* **19**:173, 1998.
114. Ricketts MH, Simons MJ, Parma J, et al: A nonsense mutation causes hereditary goiter in the Afrikander cattle and unmasks alternative splicing of thyroglobulin transcripts. *Proc Natl Acad Sci U S A* **84**:3181, 1987.
115. Chelly J, Gilgenkrantz H, Lambert M, et al: Effect of dystrophin gene deletions on mRNA levels and processing in Duchenne and Becker muscular dystrophies. *Cell* **63**:1239, 1990.
116. Targovnik HM, Medeiros-Neto G, Varela V, et al: A nonsense mutation causes human hereditary congenital goiter with preferential production of a 171 nucleotide deleted thyroglobulin RNA messenger. *J Clin Endocrinol Metab* **77**:219, 1993.
117. Cousin X, Hotelier T, Giles K, et al: aCHEdb: The database system for ESTHER, the alpha/beta fold family of proteins and the cholinesterase gene server. *Nucleic Acids Res* **26**:226, 1998.

118. Bourne Y, Taylor P, Bougis PE, et al: Crystal structure of mouse acetylcholinesterase. A peripheral site-occluding loop in a tetrameric assembly. *J Biol Chem* **274**:2963, 1999.
119. Corral J, Martin C, Perez R, et al: Thyroglobulin gene point mutation associated with non-endemic simple goitre. *Lancet* **341**:462, 1993.
120. Ajjan RA, Findlay C, Metcalfe RA, et al: The modulation of the human sodium iodide symporter activity by Graves' disease sera. *J Clin Endocrinol Metab* **83**:1217, 1998.
121. Smanik PA, Ryu K-Y, Theil KS, et al: Expression, exon-intron organization, and chromosome mapping of the human sodium iodide symporter. *Endocrinology* **138**:3555, 1997.
122. Venkataraman GM, Yatin M, Ain KB: Cloning of the human sodium/iodide symporter promoter and characterization in a differentiated human thyroid cell line, KAT-50. *Thyroid* **8**:63, 1998.
123. Golstein PE, Sener A, Beauwens R: The iodide channel of the thyroid: II. Selective iodide conductance inserted into liposomes. *Am J Physol* **268**:C111, 1995.
124. Scott DA, Wang R, Kreman TM, et al: The Pendred syndrome (PDS) gene encodes a chloride, iodide transport protein. *Nat Genet* **21**:440, 1999.
125. Levy O, De la Vieja A, Ginter CS, et al: N-linked glycosylation of the thyroid Na+/I− symporter (NIS): Implications for its secondary structure model. *J Biol Chem* **273**:22657, 1998.
126. Smanik PA, Liu Q, Furminger TL, et al: Cloning of the human sodium iodide symporter. *Biochem Biophys Res Commun* **226**:339, 1996.
127. Mueckler M, Caruso C, Baldwin SA, et al: Sequence and structure of a human glucose transporter. *Science* **229**:941, 1985.
128. Turk E, Kerner CJ, Lostao MP, et al: Membrane topology of the Na^+/glucose cotransporter SGLT1. *J Biol Chem* **271**:1925, 1996.
129. Medeiros-Neto G, Stanbury JB: *Inherited Disorders of the Thyroid System.* Boca Raton, FL, CRC Press, 1994, p 1.
130. Vulsma T, Rammeloo JA, Gons MH, et al: The role of serum thyroglobulin concentration and thyroid ultrasound imaging in the detection of iodide transport defects in infants. *Acta Endocrinol Copenh* **124**:405, 1991.
131. Stanbury JB, Chapman EM: Congenital hypothyroidism with goitre: Absence of an iodide-concentrating mechanism. *Lancet* **1**:1162, 1960.
132. Fujiwara H, Tatsumi K, Miki K, et al: Congenital hypothyroidism caused by a mutation in the Na^+/I^- symporter. *Nat Genet* **16**:124, 1997.
133. Pohlenz J, Medeiros-Neto G, Gross JL, et al: Hypothyroidism in a Brazilian kindred due to iodide trapping defect caused by a homozygous mutation in the sodium/iodide symporter gene. *Biochem Biophys Res Commun* **240**:488, 1997.
134. Pohlenz J, Rosenthal IM, Weiss RE, et al: Congenital hypothyroidism due to mutations in the sodium/iodide symporter: Identification of a nonsense mutation producing a downstream cryptic 3′ splice site. *J Clin Invest* **101**:1028, 1998.
135. Matsuda A, Kosgi S: A homozygous missense mutation in the sodium/iodide symporter gene causing iodide transport defect. *J Clin Endocrinol Metab* **82**:3966, 1997.
136. Kosugi S, Inoue S, Matsuda A, et al: Novel, missense and loss-of-function mutations in the sodium/iodide symporter gene causing iodide transport defect in three Japanese patients. *J Clin Endocrinol Metab* **83**:3373, 1998.
137. Levy O, Ginter CS, De la Vieja A, et al: Identification of a structural requirement for thyroid Na^+/I^- symporter (NIS) function from analysis of a mutation that causes human congenital hypothyroidism. *FEBS Lett* **429**:36, 1998.
137a. Pohlenz J, Duprez L, Weiss RE, et al: Failure of membrane targeting causes the functional defect of two mutant sodium iodide symporters. *J Clin Endocrinol Metab* **85**:2366, 2000.
138. Wolff J: Congenital goiter wit defective iodide transport. *Endocr Rev* **4**:240, 1983.
139. Rawitch AB, Pollock G, Yang SX, et al: Thyroid peroxidase glycosylation: The location and *Nature* of the N-linked oligosaccharide units in porcine thyroid peroxidase. *Arch Biochem Biophys* **297**:321, 1992.
140. Czarnocka B, Ruf J, Ferrand M, et al: Purification of the human thyroid peroxidase and its identification as the microsomal antigen involved in autoimmune thyroid diseases. *FEBS Lett* **190**:147, 1985.
141. Portmann L, Hamada N, Heinrich G, et al: Anti-thyroid peroxidase antibody in patients with autoimmune thyroid disease: Possible identity with anti-microsomal antibody. *J Clin Endocrinol Metab* **61**:1001, 1985.
142. Libert F, Ruel J, Ludgate M, et al: Thyroperoxidase, an auto-antigen with a mosaic structure made of nuclear and mitochondrial gene modules. *EMBO J* **6**:4193, 1987.
143. Kimura S, Kotani T, McBride OW, et al: Human thyroid peroxidase: Complete cDNA and protein sequence, chromosome mapping, and identification of two alternately spliced mRNAs. *Proc Natl Acad Sci U S A* **84**:5555, 1987.
144. Seto P, Hirayu H, Magnusson RP, et al: Isolation of a complementary DNA clone for thyroid microsomal antigen. Homology with the gene for thyroid peroxidase. *J Clin Invest* **80**:1205, 1987.
145. Niccoli P, Fayadat L, Panneels V, et al: Human thyroperoxidase in its alternatively spliced form (TPO2) is enzymatically inactive and exhibits changes in intracellular processing and trafficking. *J Biol Chem* **272**:29487, 1997.
146. Cetani F, Costagliola S, Tonacchera M, et al: The thyroperoxidase doublet is not produced by alternative splicing. *Mol Cell Endocrinol* **115**:125, 1995.
147. Nagayama Y, Seto P, Rapoport B: Characterization, by molecular cloning, of smaller forms of thyroid peroxidase messenger ribonucleic acid in human thyroid cells as alternatively spliced transcripts. *J Clin Endocrinol Metab* **71**:384, 1990.
148. Taurog A, Wall M: Proximal and distal histidines in thyroid peroxidase: Relation to the alternatively spliced form, TPO-2. *Thyroid* **8**:185, 1998.
149. Zeng J, Fenna RE: X-ray crystal structure of canine myeloperoxidase at 3 A resolution. *J Mol Biol* **226**:185, 1992.
150. de Vijlder JJ, Dinsart C, Libert F, et al: Regional localization of the gene for thyroid peroxidase to human chromosome 2pter-p12. *Cytogenet Cell Genet* **47**:170, 1988.
151. Damante G, Di Lauro R: Thyroid-specific gene expression. *Biochim Biophys Acta* **1218**:255, 1994.
152. Zannini M, Francis Lang H, Plachov D, et al: Pax-8, a paired domain-containing protein, binds to a sequence overlapping the recognition site of a homeodomain and activates transcription from two thyroid-specific promoters. *Mol Cell Biol* **12**:4230, 1992.
153. Kikkawa F, Gonzalez FJ, Kimura S: Characterization of a thyroid-specific enhancer located 5.5 kilobase pairs upstream of the human thyroid peroxidase gene. *Mol Cell Biol* **10**:6216, 1990.
154. Damante G, Chazenbalk G, Russo D, et al: Thyrotropin regulation of thyroid peroxidase messenger ribonucleic acid levels in cultured rat thyroid cells: Evidence for the involvement of a nontranscriptional mechanism. *Endocrinology* **124**:2889, 1989.
155. Gerard CM, Lefort A, Christophe D, et al: Control of thyroperoxidase and thyroglobulin transcription by cAMP: Evidence for distinct regulatory mechanisms. *Mol Endocrinol* **3**:2110, 1989.
156. Medeiros-Neto GA, Billerbeck AE, Wajchenberg BL, et al: Defective organification of iodide causing hereditary goitrous hypothyroidism. *Thyroid* **3**:143, 1993.
157. Bikker H, Vulsma T, Baas F, et al: Identification of five novel inactivating mutations in the human thyroid peroxidase gene by denaturing gradient gel electrophoresis. *Hum Mutat* **6**:9, 1995.
158. Gruters A, Kohler B, Wolf A, et al: Screening for mutations of the human thyroid peroxidase gene in patients with congenital hypothyroidism. *Exp Clin Endocrinol Diabetes* **104(Suppl 4)**:121, 121, 1996.
159. Bikker H, den Hartog MT, Baas F, et al: A 20-basepair duplication in the human thyroid peroxidase gene results in a total iodide organification defect and congenital hypothyroidism. *J Clin Endocrinol Metab* **79**:248, 1994.
160. Bikker H, Waelkens JJ, Bravenboer B, et al: Congenital hypothyroidism caused by a premature termination signal in exon 10 of the human thyroid peroxidase gene. *J Clin Endocrinol Metab* **81**:2076, 1996.
161. Bikker H, Baas F, de Vijlder JJ: Molecular analysis of mutated thyroid peroxidase detected in patients with total iodide organification defects. *J Clin Endocrinol Metab* **82**:649, 1997.
162. de Vijlder JJ, Ris-Stalpers C, Vulsma T: Inborn errors of thyroid hormone biosynthesis. *Exp Clin Endocrinol Diabetes* **105(Suppl 4)**:32, 1997.
163. Kotani T, Umeki K, Yamamoto I, et al: A novel mutation in the human thyroid peroxidase gene resulting in a total iodide organification defect. *J Endocrinol* **160**:267, 1999.
164. Pannain S, Weiss RE, Jackson CE, et al: Two different mutations in the thyroid peroxidase gene of a large inbred Amish kindred: Power and limits of homozygosity mapping. *J Clin Endocrinol Metab* **84**:1061, 1999.

165. Johnsen T, Jorgensen MB, Johnsen S: Mondini cochlea in Pendred's syndrome. A histological study. *Acta Otolaryngol (Stockh)* **102**:239, 1986.
166. Johnsen T, Sorensen MS, Feldt-Rasmussen U, et al: The variable intrafamiliar expressivity in Pendred's syndrome. *Clin Otolaryngol* **14**:395, 1989.
167. Everett LA, Glaser B, Beck JC, et al: Pendred syndrome is caused by mutations in a putative sulphate transporter gene (PDS). *Nat Genet* **17**:411, 1997.
168. Coyle B, Coffey R, Armour JA, et al: Pendred syndrome (goitre and sensorineural hearing loss) maps to chromosome 7 in the region containing the nonsyndromic deafness gene DFNB4. *Nat Genet* **12**:421, 1996.
169. Sheffield VC, Kraiem Z, Beck JC, et al: Pendred syndrome maps to chromosome 7q21-34 and is caused by an intrinsic defect in thyroid iodine organification. *Nat Genet* **12**:424, 1996.
170. Coucke P, Van Camp G, Demirhan O, et al: The gene for Pendred syndrome is located between D7S501 and D7S692 in a 1.7-cM region on chromosome 7q. *Genomics* **40**:48, 1997.
171. Haila S, Hoglund P, Scherer SW, et al: Genomic structure of the human congenital chloride diarrhea (CLD) gene. *Gene* **214**:87, 1998.
172. Nilsson M, Bjorkman U, Ekholm R, et al: Iodide transport in primary cultured thyroid follicle cells: Evidence of a TSH-regulated channel mediating iodide efflux selectively across the apical domain of the plasma membrane. *Eur J Cell Biol* **52**:270, 1990.
173. Golstein PE, Sener A, Colin F, Beauwens R: Iodide channel of the thyroid: Reconstitution of iodide conductance in proteoliposomes. *Methods Enzymol* **294**:304, 1999.
174. Li XC, Everett LA, Lalwani AK, et al: A mutation in PDS causes non-syndromic recessive deafness [Letter]. *Nat Genet* **18**:215, 1998.
175. Coyle B, Reardon W, Herbrick JA, et al: Molecular analysis of the PDS gene in Pendred syndrome (sensorineural hearing loss and goiter). *Hum Mol Genet* **7**:1105, 1998.
176. Van Hauwe P, Everett LA, Coucke P, et al: Two frequent missense mutations in Pendred syndrome. *Hum Mol Genet* **7**:1099, 1998.
177. Kopp P, Arseven OK, Sabacan L, et al: Phenocopies for deafness and goiter development in a large inbred Brazilian kindred with Pendred's syndrome associated with a novel mutation in the PDS gene. *J Clin Endocrinol Metab* **84**:336, 1999.
178. Niepomniszcze H, Targovnik HM, Gluzman B, et al: Abnormal H2O2 supply in the thyroid of a patient with goiter and iodine organification defect. *J Clin Endocrinol Metab* **65**:344, 1987.
179. Demeester-Mirkine N, Van Sande J, Corvilain B, et al: Benign thyroid nodule with normal iodide trap and iodine organification defect. *J Clin Endocrinol* **41**:1169, 1975.
180. Stanbury JB, Dumont JE: Familial goiter and related disorders, in Stanbury JB, Wyngaarden J, Fredrickson D, Goldstein J, Brown MB (eds): *in The Metabolic Basis of Inherited Disease*. New York, McGraw-Hill, 1983, p 231.
181. Stanbury JB, Kassenaar AAH, Meijer JWA, et al: The occurrence of mono- and diiodotyrosine in the blood of a patient with congenital goiter. *J Clin Endocrinol Metab* **15**:1216, 1955.
182. Stanbury JB, Kassenaar AAH, Meijer JWA: The metabolism of iodotyrosines. I. The fate of mono- and diiodotyrosine in normal subjects and in patients with various diseases. *J Clin Endocrinol Metab* **16**:735, 1956.
183. Stanbury JB, Meijer JWA, Kassenaar AAH: The metabolism of iodotyrosines. II. The metabolism of mono- and diiodotyrosine in certain patients with familial goitre. *J Clin Endocrinol Metab* **16**:848, 1956.
184. Choufoer JC, Kassenaar AAH, Querido A: The syndrome of congenital hypothyroidism with defective dehalogenation of iodotyrosines: Further observations and discussion of the pathophysiology. *J Clin Endocrinol Metab* **20**:983, 1960.
185. Rochiccioli P, Dufau G: Trouble de l'hormonosynthèse thyroïdienne par déficit en iodotyrosine-deshalogenase. *Arch Fr Pediatr* **31**:25, 1974.
186. Kusakabe Y, Miyake T: Thyroidal deiodination defect in three sisters with simple goiter. *J Clin Endocrinol Metab* **24**:456, 1964.
187. Meinhold H, Olbricht T, Schwartz PD: Turnover and urinary excretion of circulating diiodotyrosine. *J Clin Endocrinol Metab* **64**:794, 1987.
188. Vague J, Codaccioni JL: Results of 7 years of iodine treatment in a first case of infantile hypothyroidism due to defective deiodination of iodotyrosines. *Ann Endocrinol (Paris)* **31**:1156, 1970.
189. McGirr EM, Hutchison JH, Clement WE: Sporadic goitrous cretinism: Dehalogenase deficiency in the thyroid gland of a goitrous cretin and in the heterozygous carriers. *Lancet* **2**:823, 1959.
190. Murray P, Thomson JA, McGirr EM, et al: Absent and defective iodotyrosine deiodination in a family some of whose members are goitrous cretins. *Lancet* **1**:183, 1965.
191. Theiler K: *The House Mouse, Atlas of Embryonic Development*. New York, Springer-Verlag, 1989.
192. Toran-Allerand CD: Normal development of the hypothalamic-pituitary-thyroid axis: Ontogeny of the neuroendocrine unit, in Ingbar SH, Braverman LE (eds): *Werner's The Thyroid*, 5th ed. New York, Lipincott, 1986, p 7.
193. Guazzi S, Price M, de Felice M, et al: Thyroid nuclear factor 1 (TTF-1) contains a homeodomain and displays a novel DNA binding specificity. *EMBO J* **9**:3631, 1990.
194. Zannini M, Avantaggiato V, Biffali E, et al: TTF-2, a new forkhead protein, shows a temporal expression in the developing thyroid which is consistent with a role in controlling the onset of differentiation. *EMBO J* **16**:3185, 1997.
195. Chadwick BP, Obermayr F, Frischauf AM: FKHL15, a new human member of the forkhead gene family located on chromosome 9q22. *Genomics* **41**:390, 1997.
196. Poleev A, Fickenscher H, Mundlos S, et al: PAX8, a human paired box gene: Isolation and expression in developing thyroid, kidney and Wilms' tumors. *Development* **116**:611, 1992.
197. Pouillon V, Pichon B, Donda A, et al: TTF-2 does not appear to be a key mediator of the effect of cyclic AMP on thyroglobulin gene transcription in primary cultured dog thyrocytes. *Biochem Biophys Res Commun* **242**:327, 1998.
198. Ortiz L, Zannini M, Di Lauro R, et al: Transcriptional control of the forkhead thyroid transcription factor TTF-2 by thyrotropin, insulin, and insulin-like growth factor I. *J Biol Chem* **272**:23334, 1997.
199. Devos H, Rodd C, Gagne N, et al: A search for the possible molecular mechanisms of thyroid dysgenesis: Sex ratio and associated malformations. *J Clin Endocrinol Metab* **84**:2502, 1999.
200. Abramowicz MJ, Duprez L, Parma J, et al: Familial congenital hypothyroidism due to inactivating mutation of the thyrotropin receptor causing profound hypoplasia of the thyroid gland. *J Clin Invest* **99**:3018, 1997.
201. Van Vliet G: Neonatal hypothyroidism: Treatment and outcome. *Thyroid* **9**:79, 1999.
202. Melnick JC, Stemkowski PE: Thyroid hemiagenesis (hockey stick sign): A review of the world literature and a report of four cases. *J Clin Endocrinol Metab* **52**:247, 1981.
203. Roberts HE, Moore CA, Fernhoff PM, et al: Population study of congenital hypothyroidism and associated birth defects, Atlanta, 1979–1992. *Am J Med Genet* **71**:29, 1997.
204. Law WY, Bradley DM, Lazarus JH, et al: Congenital hypothyroidism in Wales (1982–1993): Demographic features, clinical presentation and effects on early neurodevelopment. *Clin Endocrinol (Oxf)* **48**:201, 1998.
205. Siebner R, Merlob P, Kaiserman I, et al: Congenital anomalies concomitant with persistent primary congenital hypothyroidism. *Am J Med Genet* **44**:57, 1992.
206. Missero C, Cobellis G, de Felice M, et al: Molecular events involved in differentiation of thyroid follicular cells. *Mol Cell Endocrinol* **140**:37, 1998.
207. Lazzaro D, Price M, de Felice M, et al: The transcription factor TTF-1 is expressed at the onset of thyroid and lung morphogenesis and in restricted regions of the foetal brain. *Development* **113**:1093, 1991.
208. Kimura S, Hara Y, Pineau T, et al: The T/ebp null mouse: Thyroid-specific enhancer-binding protein is essential for the organogenesis of the thyroid, lung, ventral forebrain, and pituitary. *Genes Dev* **10**:60, 1996.
209. Ikeda K, Clark JC, Shaw-White JR, et al: Gene structure and expression of human thyroid transcription factor-1 in respiratory epithelial cells. *J Biol Chem* **270**:8108, 1995.
210. Lapi P, Macchia PE, Chiovato L, et al: Mutations in the gene encoding thyroid transcription factor-1 (TTF-1) are not a frequent cause of congenital hypothyroidism (CH) with thyroid dysgenesis. *Thyroid* **7**:383, 1997.
211. Perna MG, Civitareale D, De Filippis V, et al: Absence of mutations in the gene encoding thyroid transcription factor-1 (TTF-1) in patients with thyroid dysgenesis. *Thyroid* **7**:377, 1997.
212. Devriendt K, Vanhole C, Matthijs G, et al: Deletion of thyroid transcription factor-1 gene in an infant with neonatal thyroid dysfunction and respiratory failure [Letter]. *N Engl J Med* **338**:1317, 1998.
213. de Felice M, Ovitt C, Biffali E, et al: A mouse model for hereditary thyroid dysgenesis and cleft palate. *Nat Genet* **19**:395, 1998.

214. Aza Blanc P, Di Lauro R, Santisteban P: Identification of a *cis*-regulatory element and a thyroid-specific nuclear factor mediating the hormonal regulation of rat thyroid peroxidase promoter activity. *Mol Endocrinol* **7**:1297, 1993.
215. Bamforth JS, Hughes IA, Lazarus JH, et al: Congenital hypothyroidism, spiky hair, and cleft palate. *J Med Genet* **26**:49, 1989.
216. Clifton-Bligh RJ, Wentworth JM, Heinz P, et al: Mutation of the gene encoding human TTF-2 associated with thyroid agenesis, cleft palate and choanal atresia. *Nat Genet* **19**:399, 1998.
217. Poleev A, Wendler F, Fickenscher H, et al: Distinct functional properties of three human paired-box-protein, PAX8, isoforms generated by alternative splicing in thyroid, kidney and Wilms' tumors. *Eur J Biochem* **228**:899, 1995.
218. Nothwang HG, Strahm B, Denich D, et al: Molecular cloning of the interleukin-1 gene cluster: Construction of an integrated YAC/PAC contig and a partial transcriptional map in the region of chromosome 2q13. *Genomics* **41**:370, 1997.
219. Mansouri A, Chowdhury K, Gruss P: Follicular cells of the thyroid gland require Pax8 gene function. *Nat Genet* **19**:87, 1998.
220. Macchia PE, Lapi P, Krude H, et al: PAX8 mutations associated with congenital hypothyroidism caused by thyroid dysgenesis. *Nat Genet* **19**:83, 1998.
221. Stein SA, Shanklin DR, Krulich L, et al: Evaluation and characterization of the hyt/hyt hypothyroid mouse. II. Abnormalities of TSH and the thyroid gland. *Neuroendocrinology* **49**:509, 1989.
222. Stein SA, Oates EL, Hall CR, et al: Identification of a point mutation in the thyrotropin receptor of the *hyt/hyt* hypothyroid mouse. *Mol Endocrinol* **8**:129, 1994.
223. Stanbury JB, Rocmans P, Buhler UK, et al: Congenital hypothyroidism with impaired thyroid response to thyrotropin. *N Engl J Med* **279**:1132, 1968.
224. Codaccioni JL, Carayon P, Michel Bechet M, et al: Congenital hypothyroidism associated with thyrotropin unresponsiveness and thyroid cell membrane alterations. *J Clin Endocrinol Metab* **50**:932, 1980.
225. Takeshita A, Nagayama Y, Yamashita S, et al: Sequence analysis of the TSH receptor gene in congenital primary hypothyroidism associated with TSH unresponsiveness. *Thyroid* **4**:255, 1994.
226. Sunthornthepvarakul T, Gottschalk ME, Hayashi Y, et al: Resistance to thyrotropin caused by mutations in the thyrotropin-receptor gene. *N Engl J Med* **332**:155, 1995.
227. Gagne N, Parma J, Deal C, et al: Apparent congenital athyreosis contrasting with normal plasma thyroglobulin levels and associated with inactivating mutations in the thyrotropin receptor gene: Are athyreosis and ectopic thyroid distinct entities? *J Clin Endocrinol Metab* **83**:1771, 1998.
228. Biebermann H, Schoneberg T, Krude H, et al: Mutations of the human thyrotropin receptor gene causing thyroid hypoplasia and persistent congenital hypothyroidism. *J Clin Endocrinol Metab* **82**:3471, 1997.
229. de Roux N, Misrahi M, Brauner R, et al: Four families with loss of function mutations of the thyrotropin receptor. *J Clin Endocrinol Metab* **81**:4229, 1996.
230. Xie J, Pannain S, Pohlenz J, et al: Resistance to thyrotropin (TSH) in three families is not associated with mutations in the TSH receptor or TSH. *J Clin Endocrinol Metab* **82**:3933, 1997.
231. Pfaffle RW, DiMattia GE, Parks JS, et al: Mutation of the POU-specific domain of Pit-1 and hypopituitarism without pituitary hypoplasia. *Science* **257**:1118, 1992.
232. Schonemann MD, Ryan AK, Erkman L, et al: POU domain factors in neural development. *Adv Exp Med Biol* **449**:39, 1998.
233. Treier M, Rosenfeld MG: The hypothalamic-pituitary axis: Co-development of two organs. *Curr Opin Cell Biol* **8**:833, 1996.
234. Ohta K, Nobukuni Y, Mitsubuchi H, et al: Characterization of the gene encoding human pituitary-specific transcription factor, Pit-1. *Gene* **122**:387, 1992.
235. Arnhold IJ, Nery M, Brown MR, et al: Clinical and molecular characterization of a Brazilian patient with Pit-1 deficiency. *J Pediatr Endocrinol Metab* **11**:623, 1998.
236. Radovick S, Cohen LE, Wondisford FE: The molecular basis of hypopituitarism. *Horm Res* **49**(Suppl 1):30, 1998.
237. Andersen B, Pearse RV2, Jenne K, et al: The Ames dwarf gene is required for Pit-1 gene activation. *Dev Biol* **172**:495, 1995.
238. Sornson MW, Wu W, Dasen JS, et al: Pituitary lineage determination by the Prophet of Pit-1 homeodomain factor defective in Ames dwarfism. *Nature* **384**:327, 1996.
239. Wu W, Cogan JD, Pfaffle RW, et al: Mutations in PROP1 cause familial combined pituitary hormone deficiency. *Nat Genet* **18**:147, 1998.
240. Collu R, Tang J, Castagne J, et al: A novel mechanism for isolated central hypothyroidism: Inactivating mutations in the thyrotropin-releasing hormone receptor gene. *J Clin Endocrinol Metab* **82**:1561, 1997.
241. Wilber JF, Xu AH: The thyrotropin-releasing hormone gene 1998: Cloning, characterization, and transcriptional regulation in the central nervous system, heart, and testis. *Thyroid* **8**:897, 1998.
242. Doeker BM, Pfaffle RW, Pohlenz J, et al: Congenital central hypothyroidism due to a homozygous mutation in the thyrotropin beta-subunit gene follows an autosomal recessive inheritance. *J Clin Endocrinol Metab* **83**:1762, 1998.
243. Medeiros-Neto G, Herodotou DT, Rajan S, et al: A circulating, biologically inactive thyrotropin caused by a mutation in the beta subunit gene. *J Clin Invest* **97**:1250, 1996.
244. Hayashizaki Y, Hiraoka Y, Tatsumi K, et al: Deoxyribonucleic acid analyses of five families with familial inherited thyroid stimulating hormone deficiency [Comment]. *J Clin Endocrinol Metab* **71**:792, 1990.
245. Hayashizaki Y, Hiraoka Y, Endo Y, et al: Thyroid-stimulating hormone (TSH) deficiency caused by a single base substitution in the CAGYC region of the beta-subunit [erratum published in *EMBO J* 8(11):3542, 1989]. *EMBO J* **8**:2291, 1989.
246. Dacou-Voutetakis C, Feltquate DM, Drakopoulou M, et al: Familial hypothyroidism caused by a nonsense mutation in the thyroid-stimulating hormone beta-subunit gene. *Am J Hum Genet* **46**:988, 1990.
247. Hoch H, Lewallen CG: Low affinity binding of thyroxine to proteins of human serum. *J Clin Endocrinol Metab* **38**:663, 1974.
248. Benvenga S, Cahnmann HJ, Rader D, et al: Thyroid hormone binding to isolated human apolipoproteins A-II, C-I, C-II, and C-III: homology in thyroxine binding sites. *Thyroid* **4**:261, 1994.
249. Ikekubo K, Konishi J, Endo K, et al: Anti-thyroxine and anti-triiodothyronine antibodies in three cases of Hashimoto's thyroiditis. *Acta Endocrinol* **89**:557, 1978.
250. Robbins J, Cheng SY, Gerschengorn MC, et al: Thyroxine transport proteins of plasma. Molecular properties and biosynthesis. *Recent Prog Horm Res* **34**:477, 1978.
251. Sarne D, Barokas K, Scherberg NH, et al: Elevated serum thyroglobulin level in congenital thyroxine-binding globulin (TBG) deficiency. *J Clin Endocrinol Metab* **57**:665, 1983.
252. Mendel CM, Weisiger RA: Thyroxine uptake by perfused rat liver: No evidence for facilitation by five different thyroxine-binding proteins. *J Clin Invest* **86**:1840, 1990.
253. Zinn AB, Marshall JS, Carlson DM: Carbohydrate structures of thyroxine-binding globulin and their effects on hepatocyte membrane binding. *J Biol Chem* **253**:6768, 1978.
254. Flink IL, Bailey TJ, Gustefson TA, et al: Complete amino acid sequence of human thyroxine-binding globulin deduced from cloned DNA: Close homology to the serine antiproteases. *Proc Natl Acad Sci U S A* **83**:7708, 1986.
255. Trent JM, Flink IL, Morkin E, et al: Localization of the human thyroxine-binding globulin gene to the long arm of the X chromosome (Xq21-22). *Am J Hum Genet* **41**:428, 1987.
256. Mori Y, Miura Y, Oiso Y, et al: Precise localization of the human thyroxine-binding globulin gene to chromosome Xq22.2 by fluorescence in situ hybridization. *Hum Genet* **96**:481, 1995.
257. Hammond GL, Smith CL, Goping IS, et al: Primary structure of human corticosteroid binding globulin, deduced from hepatic and pulmonary cDNAs, exhibits homology with serine protease inhibitors. *Proc Natl Acad Sci U S A* **84**:5153, 1987.
258. Hayashi Y, Mori Y, Janssen OE, et al: Human thyroxine-binding globulin gene: Complete sequence and transcriptional regulation. *Mol Endocrinol* **7**:1049, 1993.
259. Murata Y, Magner J, Refetoff S: The role of glycosylation in the molecular conformation and secretion of thyroxine-binding globulin. *Endocrinology* **118**:1614, 1986.
260. Gärtner R, Henze R, Horn K, et al: Thyroxine-binding globulin: Investigation of microheterogeneity. *J Clin Endocrinol Metab* **52**:657, 1981.
261. Ain KB, Mori Y, Refetoff S: Reduced clearance rate of thyroxine-binding globulin (TBG) with increased sialylation: A mechanism for estrogen induced elevation of serum TBG concentration. *J Clin Endocrinol Metab* **65**:689, 1987.

262. Kambe F, Seo H, Mori Y, et al: An additional carbohydrate chain in the variant thyroxine-binding globulin-Gary (TBG^{Asn-96}) impairs its secretion. *Mol Endocrinol* **6**:443, 1992.
263. Janssen OE, Refetoff S: In vitro expression of thyroxine-binding globulin (TBG) variants: Impaired secretion of $TBG^{PRO-227}$ but not $TBG^{PRO-113}$. *J Biol Chem* **267**:13998, 1992.
264. Refetoff S, Murata Y, Vassart G, et al: Radioimmunoassays specific for the tertiary and primary structures of thyroxine-binding globulin (TBG): Measurement of denatured TBG in serum. *J Clin Endocrinol Metab* **59**:269, 1984.
265. Cheng SY, Morrone S, Robbins J: Effect of deglycosylation on the binding and immunoreactivity of human thyroxine-binding globulin. *J Biol Chem* **254**:8830, 1979.
266. Korcek L, Tabachnick M: Thyroxine-protein interactions: Interaction of thyroxine and triiodothyronine with human thyroxine-binding globulin. *J Biol Chem* **251**:3558, 1976.
267. Refetoff S, Fang VS, Marshall JS, et al: Metabolism of thyroxine-binding globulin (TBG) in man: Abnormal rate of synthesis in inherited TBG deficiency and excess. *J Clin Invest* **57**:485, 1976.
268. Sarne DH, Refetoff S: Thyroid function tests, in DeGroot LJ (ed): *Endocrinology*, 3rd ed. Philadelphia, WB Saunders, 1995, p 617.
269. Tsuzuki T, Mita S, Maeda S, et al: Structure of human prealbumin gene. *J Biol Chem* **260**:12224, 1985.
270. LeBeau MM, Geurts van Kessel G: Report of the committee on the genetic constitution of chromosome 18. *Cytogenet Cell Genet* **58**:739, 1991.
271. Irace G, Edelhoch H: Thyroxine induced conformational changes in prealbumin. *Biochemistry* **17**:5729, 1978.
272. Van Jaarsveld PP, Edelhoch H, Goodman DS, et al: The interaction of human plasma retinol binding protein with prealbumin. *J Biol Chem* **248**:4698, 1973.
273. Peters T Jr: Serum albumin. *Adv Protein Chem* **37**:161, 1985.
274. Murray JC, Van Ommen GJB: Report of the committee on the genetic constitution of chromosome 4. *Cytogenet Cell Genet* **58**:231, 1991.
275. Tabachnick M, Giorgio NA Jr: Thyroxine-protein interactions. II. The binding of thyroxine and its analogues to human serum albumin. *Arch Biochem Biophys* **105**:563, 1964.
276. Refetoff S: Inherited thyroxine-binding globulin (TBG) abnormalities in man. *Endocr Rev* **10**:275, 1989.
277. Palha JA, Hays MT, Morreale de Escobar G, et al: Transthyretin is not essential for thyroxine to reach the brain and other tissues in transthyretin-null mice. *Am J Physiol* **272**:E485, 1997.
278. Gertz MA, Kyle RA, Thibodeau SN: Familial amyloidosis: A study of 52 North American-born patients examined during a 30-year period. *Mayo Clin Proc* **67**:428, 1992.
279. Horwitz DL, Refetoff S: Graves' disease associated with familial deficiency of thyroxine-binding globulin. *J Clin Endocrinol Metab* **44**:242, 1977.
280. Shane SR, Seal US, Jones JE: X-chromosome-linked inheritance of elevated thyroxine-binding globulin in association with goiter. *J Clin Endocrinol Metab* **32**:587, 1971.
281. Refetoff S, Selenkow HA: Familial thyroxine-binding globulin deficiency in a patient with Turner's syndrome (X0): Genetic study of a kindred. *N Engl J Med* **278**:1081, 1968.
282. Murata Y, Takamatsu J, Refetoff S: Inherited abnormality of thyroxine-binding globulin with no demonstrable thyroxine-binding activity and high serum levels of denatured thyroxine-binding globulin. *N Engl J Med* **314**:694, 1986.
283. Burr WA, Ramsden DB, Hoffenberg R: Hereditary abnormalities of thyroxine-binding globulin concentration. *QJM* **49**:295, 1980.
284. Mori Y, Takeda K, Charbonneau M, et al: Replacement of Leu^{227} by Pro in thyroxine-binding globulin (TBG) is associated with complete TBG deficiency in three of eight families with this inherited defect. *J Clin Endocrinol Metab* **70**:804, 1990.
285. Okamoto H, Mori Y, Tani Y, et al: Molecular analysis of females manifesting thyroxine-binding globulin (TBG) deficiency: Selective X-chromosome inactivation responsible for the difference between phenotype and genotype in TBG-deficient females. *J Clin Endocrinol Metab* **81**:2204, 1996.
286. Carvalho GA, Weiss RE, Vladutiu AO, et al: Complete deficiency of thyroxine-binding globulin (TBG-CD Buffalo) caused by a new nonsense mutation in the thyroxine-binding globulin gene. *Thyroid* **8**:161, 1998.
287. Li P, Janssen OE, Takeda K, et al: Complete thyroxine-binding globulin (TBG) deficiency caused by a single nucleotide deletion in the TBG gene. *Metabolism* **40**:1231, 1991.
288. Yamamori I, Mori Y, Seo H, et al: Nucleotide deletion resulting in frameshift as a possible cause of complete thyroxine-binding globulin deficiency in six Japanese families. *J Clin Endocrinol Metab* **73**:262, 1991.
289. Yamamori I, Mori Y, Miura Y, et al: Gene screening of 23 Japanese families with complete thyroxine-binding globulin deficiency: Identification of a nucleotide deletion at codon 352 as a common cause. *Endocr J* **40**:563, 1993.
290. Ueta Y, Mitani Y, Yoshida A, et al: A novel mutation causing complete deficiency of thyroxine binding globulin. *Clin Endocrinol* **47**:1, 1997.
291. Miura Y, Inagaki A, Hershkovitz E, et al: Gene analysis of complete thyroxine-binding globulin deficiency in Bedouin in southern Israel. *Thyroid* **7**(Suppl 1):S-98, 1997.
292. Carvalho GA, Weiss RE, Refetoff S: Complete thyroxine-binding globulin (TBG) deficiency produced by a mutation in the acceptor splice site causing frameshift and early termination of translation (TBG-Kankakee). *J Clin Endocrinol Metab* **83**:3604, 1998.
293. Takeda K, Iyota K, Mori Y, et al: Gene screening in Japanese families with complete deficiency of thyroxine-binding globulin demonstrates that a nucleotide deletion at codon 352 may be a race specific mutation. *Clin Endocrinol* **40**:221, 1994.
294. Takeda K, Mori Y, Sobieszczyk S, et al: Sequence of the variant thyroxine-binding globulin of Australian Aborigines: Only one of two amino acid replacements is responsible for its altered properties. *J Clin Invest* **83**:1344, 1989.
295. Waltz MR, Pullman TN, Takeda K, et al: Molecular basis for the properties of the thyroxine-binding globulin-slow variant in American Blacks. *J Endocrinol Invest* **13**:343, 1990.
296. Sarne DH, Refetoff S, Murata Y, et al: Variant thyroxine-binding globulin in serum of Australian Aborigines. A comparison with familial TBG deficiency in Caucasians and American Blacks. *J Endocrinol Invest* **8**:217, 1985.
297. Murata Y, Refetoff S, Sarne DH, et al: Variant thyroxine-binding globulin in serum of Australian Aborigines: Its physical, chemical and biological properties. *J Endocrinol Invest* **8**:225, 1985.
298. Sarne DH, Refetoff S, Nelson JC, et al: A new inherited abnormality of thyroxine-binding globulin (TBG-San Diego) with decreased affinity for thyroxine and triiodothyronine. *J Clin Endocrinol Metab* **68**:114, 1989.
299. Takamatsu J, Refetoff S, Charbonneau M, et al: Two new inherited defects of the thyroxine-binding globulin (TBG) molecule presenting as partial TBG deficiency. *J Clin Invest* **79**:833, 1987.
300. Mori Y, Seino S, Takeda K, et al: A mutation causing reduced biological activity and stability of thyroxine-binding globulin probably as a result of abnormal glycosylation of the molecule. *Mol Endocrinol* **3**:575, 1989.
301. Miura Y, Mori Y, Kambe F, et al: Impaired intracellular transport contributes to partial thyroxine-binding globulin (TBG) deficiency in a Japanese family. *J Clin Endocrinol Metab* **79**:740, 1994.
302. Kobayashi H, Sakurai A, Katai M, et al: Autosomally transmitted low concentration of thyroxine-binding globulin. *Thyroid* **9**:159, 1999.
303. Mori Y, Miura Y, Takeuchi H, et al: Gene amplification as a cause for inherited thyroxine-binding globulin excess in two Japanese families. *J Clin Endocrinol Metab* **80**:3758, 1995.
304. Daiger SP, Rummel DP, Wang L, et al: Detection of genetic variation with radioactive ligands. IV. X-linked, polymorphic genetic variation of thyroxin-binding globulin (TBG). *Am J Hum Genet* **33**:640, 1981.
305. Takamatsu J, Ando M, Weinberg M, et al: Isoelectric focusing variant thyroxine-binding globulin (TBG-S) in American Blacks: Increased heat lability and reduced concentration in serum. *J Clin Endocrinol Metab* **63**:80, 1986.
306. Kamboh MI, Ferrell RE: A sensitive immunoblotting technique to identify thyroxine-binding globulin protein heterogeneity after isoelectric focusing. *Biochem Genet* **24**:273, 1986.
307. Constans J, Ribouchon MT, Gouaillard C, et al: A new polymorphism of thyroxin-binding globulin in three African groups (Mali) with endemic nodular goitre. *Hum Genet* **89**:199, 1992.
308. Takamatsu J, Refetoff S: Inherited heat stable variant thyroxine-binding globulin (TBG-Chicago). *J Clin Endocrinol Metab* **63**:1140, 1986.
309. Janssen EO, Chen B, Büttner C, et al: Molecular and structural characterization of the heat-resistant thyroxine-binding globulin-Chicago. *J Biol Chem* **270**:28234, 1995.
310. Saraiva MJM: Transthyretin mutations in health and disease. *Hum Mutat* **5**:191, 1995.

311. Moses AC, Lawlor J, Haddow J, et al: Familial euthyroid hyperthyroxinemia resulting from increased thyroxine binding to thyroxine-binding prealbumin. *N Engl J Med* **306**:966, 1982.
312. Moses C, Rosen HN, Moller DE, et al: A point mutation in transthyretin increases affinity for thyroxine and produces euthyroid hyperthyroxinemia. *J Clin Invest* **86**:2025, 1990.
313. Steinrauf LK, Hamilton JA, Braden BC, et al: X-ray crystal structure of the Ala-109→Thr variant of human transthyretin which produces euthyroid hyperthyroxinemia. *J Biol Chem* **268**:2425, 1993.
314. Alves IL, Altland K, Almeida MR, et al: Screening for biochemical characterization of transthyretin variants in Portuguese population. *Hum Mutat* **9**:226, 1997.
315. Refetoff S, Marinov VSZ, Tunca H, et al: A new family with hyperthyroxinemia due to transthyretin Val109 misdiagnosed as thyrotoxicosis and resistance to thyroid hormone. *J Clin Endocrinol Metab* **81**:3335, 1996.
316. Scrimshaw BJ, Fellowes AP, Palmer BN, et al: A novel variant of transthyretin (prealbumin), Thr119 to Met, associated with increased thyroxine binding. *Thyroid* **2**:21, 1992.
317. Akbari MT, Fitch NJ, Farmer M, et al: Thyroxine-binding prealbumin gene: A population study. *Clin Endocrinol* **33**:155, 1990.
318. Refetoff S, Dwulet FE, Benson MD: Reduced affinity for thyroxine in two of three structural thyroxine-binding prealbumin variants associated with familial amyloidotic polyneuropathy. *J Clin Endocrinol Metab* **63**:1432, 1986.
319. Palha JA, Episckopou V, Maeda S, et al: Thyroid hormone metabolism in a transthyretin-null mouse strain. *J Biol Chem* **269**:33135, 1994.
320. Alper CA, Robin NI, Refetoff S: Genetic polymorphism of Rhesus thyroxine-binding prealbumin: Evidence for tetrameric structure in primates. *Proc Natl Acad Sci U S A* **63**:775, 1969.
321. Van Jaarsveld PP, Branch WT, Edelhoch H, et al: Polymorphism of Rhesus monkey serum prealbumin. Molecular properties and binding of thyroxine and retinol-binding protein. *J Biol Chem* **248**:4706, 1973.
322. Ruiz M, Rajatanavin R, Young RA, et al: Familial dysalbuminemic hyperthyroxinemia: A syndrome that can be confused with thyrotoxicosis. *N Engl J Med* **306**:635, 1982.
323. Henneman G, Krenning EP, Otten M, et al: Raised total thyroxine and free thyroxine index but normal free thyroxine. A serum abnormality due to inherited increased affinity of iodothyronines for serum binding protein. *Lancet* **1**:639, 1979.
324. Lee WNP, Golden MP, Van Herle AJ, et al: Inherited abnormal thyroid hormone-binding protein causing selective increase of total serum thyroxine. *J Clin Endocrinol Metab* **49**:292, 1979.
325. Croxson MS, Palmer BN, Holdaway IM, et al: Detection of familial dysalbuminaemic hyperthyroxinaemia. *BMJ* **290**:1099, 1985.
326. DeCosimo DR, Fang SL, Braverman LE: Prevalence of familial dysalbuminemic hyperthyroxinemia in Hispanics. *Ann Intern Med* **107**:780, 1987.
327. Arevalo G: Prevalence of familial dysalbuminemic hyperthyroxinemia in serum samples received for thyroid testing. *Clin Chem* **37**:1430, 1991.
328. Barlow JW, Csicsmann JM, White EL, et al: Familial euthyroid thyroxine excess: Characterization of abnormal intermediate affinity thyroxine binding to albumin. *J Clin Endocrinol Metab* **55**:244, 1982.
329. Fleming SJ, Applegate GF, Beardwell CG: Familial dysalbuminemic hyperthyroxinemia. *Postgrad Med J* **63**:273, 1987.
330. Wood DF, Zalin AM, Ratcliffe WA, et al: Elevation of free thyroxine measurement in patients with thyrotoxicosis. *QJM* **65**:863, 1987.
331. Weiss RE, Angkeow P, Sunthornthepvarakul T, et al: Linkage of familial dysalbuminemic hyperthyroxinemia to the albumin gene in a large Amish family. *J Clin Endocrinol Metab* **80**:116, 1995.
332. Petersen CE, Ha C-E, Jameson DM, et al: Mutations in a specific human serum albumin thyroxine binding site define the structural basis of familial dysalbuminemic hyperthyroxinemia. *J Biol Chem* **271**:19110, 1996.
333. Sunthornthepvarakul T, Angkeow P, Weiss RE, et al: A missense mutation in the albumin gene produces familial disalbuminemic hyperthyroxinemia in 8 unrelated families. *Biochem Biophys Res Commun* **202**:781, 1994.
334. Wada NHC, Shimizu C, et al: A novel missense mutation in codon 218 of the albumin gene in a distinct phenotype of familial dysalbuminemic hyperthyroxinemia in a Japanese kindred. *J Clin Endocriol Metab* **82**:3246, 1997.
335. Sunthornthepvarakul T, Likitmaskul S, Ngowngarmratana S, et al: Familial dysalbuminemic hypertriiodothyroninemia: A new dominantly inherited albumin defect. *J Clin Endocrinol Metab* **83**:1448, 1998.
336. Sarcione EJ, Aungst CW: Bisalbuminemia associated with albumin thyroxine-binding defect. *Clin Chim Acta* **7**:297, 1962.
337. Andreoli M, Robbins J: Serum proteins and thyroxine-protein interaction in early human fetuses. *J Clin Invest* **41**:1070, 1962.
338. Hollander CS, Bernstein G, Oppenheimer JH: Abnormalities of thyroxine binding in analbuminemia. *J Clin Endocrinol Metab* **28**:1064, 1968.
339. Robbins J, Rall JE: The iodine containing hormones, in Grey CH, James VHT (eds): *Hormones in Blood*. London, Academic Press, 1983, p 219.
340. Ekins R, Edwards P, Newman B: The role of binding-proteins in hormone delivery, in Albertini A, Ekins RP (eds): *Free Hormones in Blood*. Amsterdam, Elsevier Biomedical, 1982, p 45.
341. Pardridge WM: Transport of protein-bound hormones into tissues in vivo. *Endocr Rev* **2**:103, 1981.
342. Krenning E, Docter R, Bernard B, et al: Characteristics of active transport of thyroid hormone into rat hepatocytes. *Biochem Biophys Acta* **676**:314, 1981.
343. Kragie L: Membrane iodothyronine transporters. I. Review of physiology. *Endocr Res* **20**:319, 1994.
344. Maxfield ER, Willingham MC, Pastan I, et al: Binding and mobility of the cell surface receptors for 3,3′,5-triiodo-l-thyronine. *Science* **211**:63, 1981.
345. Oppenheimer JH, Schwartz HL: Stereospecific transport of triiodothyronine from plasma to cytosol and from cytosol to nucleus in rat liver, kidney, brain and heart. *J Clin Invest* **75**:147, 1985.
346. Abe T, Kakyo M, Tokui T, et al: Identification of a novel gene family encoding human liver-specific organic anion transporter LST-1. *J Biol Chem* **274**:17159, 1999.
347. Noé B, Hagenbuch B, Stieger B, et al: Isolation of a multispecific organic anion and cardiac glycoside transporter from rat brain. *Proc Natl Acad Sci U S A* **94**:10346, 1997.
348. Abe T, Kakyo M, Sakagami H, et al: Molecular characterization and tissue distribution of a new organic anion transporter subtype (oatp3) that transports thyroid hormones and taurocholate and comparison with oatp2. *J Biol Chem* **273**:22395, 1998.
349. Friesema ECH, Docter R, Moerings EPCM, et al: Identification of thyroid hormone transporters. *Biochem Biophys Res Commun* **254**:497, 1999.
350. Wortsman J, Premachandra BN, Williams K, et al: Familial resistance to thyroid hormone associated with decreased transport across the plasma membrane. *Ann Intern Med* **98**:904, 1983.
351. Takeda K, Weiss RE, Refetoff S: Rapid localization of mutations in the thyroid hormone receptor-β gene by denaturing gradient gel electrophoresis in 18 families with thyroid hormone resistance. *J Clin Endocrinol Metab* **74**:712, 1992.
352. Weiss RE, Hayashi Y, Nagaya T, et al: Dominant inheritance of resistance to thyroid hormone not linked to defects in the thyroid hormone receptors α or β genes may be due to a defective co-factor. *J Clin Endocrinol Metab* **81**:4196, 1996.
353. Pohlenz J, Weiss RE, Macchia PE, et al: Five new families with resistance to thyroid hormone not caused by mutations in the thyroid hormone receptor genes. *J Clin Endocrinol Metab* **84**:3919, 1999.
354. Engler D, Burger AG: The deiodination of iodothyronines and of their derivatives in man. *Endocr Rev* **5**:151, 1984.
355. St.Germain DL, Galton VA: The deiodinase family of selenoproteins. *Thyroid* **7**:655, 1997.
356. Mandel SJ, Berry MJ, Kieffer JD, et al: Cloning and in vitro expression of the human selenoprotein, Type I iodothyronine deiodinase. *J Clin Enocrinol Metab* **75**:1133, 1992.
357. Croteau W, Davey JC, Galton VA, et al: Cloning of the mammalian type II iodothyronine deiodinase: A selenoprotein differentially expressed and regulated in the human brain and other tissues. *J Clin Invest* **98**:405, 1996.
358. Salvatore D, Low SC, Berry M, et al: Type 3 iodothyronine deiodinase: cloning, in vitro expression, and functional analysis of the placental selenoenzyme protein. *J Clin Invest* **96**:2421, 1995.
359. Berry ML, Maia AL, Kieffer JD, et al: Substitution of cysteine for selenocysteine in type I iodothyronine deiodinase reduces the catalytic efficiency of the protein but enhances translation. *Endocrinology* **131**:1848, 1992.
360. Jakobs TC, Koehler MR, Schmutzler C, et al: Structure of human type I iodothyronine 5′-deiodinase gene and location to chromosome 1p32-p33. *Genomics* **42**:361, 1997.

361. Celi FS, Canettieri G, Yarnall DP, et al: Genomic characterization of the coding region of the human type II 5′-deiodinase. *Mol Cell Endocrinol* **141**:49, 1998.
362. Hernndez A, Park J, Lyon GJ: Localization of type 3 iodothyronine deiodinase (DIO3) gene to human chromosome 14q32 and mouse chromosome 12F1. *Genomics* **53**:119, 1998.
363. Wartofsky L, Burman KD: Alterations in thyroid function in patients with systemic illness: The "euthyroid sick syndrome." *Endocr Rev* **3**:164, 1982.
364. Maxon HR, Burman KD, Premachandra BN, et al: Familial elevation of total and free thyroxine in healthy, euthyroid subjects without detectable binding protein abnormalities. *Acta Endocrinol* **100**:224, 1982.
365. Kleinhaus N, Faber J, Kahana L, et al: Euthyroid hyperthyroxinemia due to a generalized 5′-deiodinase defect. *J Clin Endocrinol Metab* **66**:684, 1988.
366. Rösler A, Litvin Y, Hage C, et al: Familial hyperthyroidism due to inappropriate thyrotropin secretion successfully treated with triiodothyronine. *J Clin Endocrinol Metab* **54**:76, 1982.
367. Berry MJ, Grieco D, Taylor BA, et al: Physiological and genetic analyses of inbred mouse strains with type I iodothyronine 5′ deiodinase deficiency. *J Clin Invest* **92**:1517, 1993.
368. Schoenmakers CH, Pigmans IG, Poland A, et al: Impairment of the selenoenzyme type I iodothyronine deiodinase in C3H/He mice. *Endocrinology* **132**:357, 1993.
369. Spangenberg DB: Thyroxine in early strobilation in *Aurelia aurita*. *Ann Zool* **14**:825, 1974.
370. Frieden E: Thyroid hormones and the biochemistry of amphibian metamorphosis. *Recent Progr Horm Res* **23**:139, 1967.
371. Morreale de Escobar G, Obergon MJ, Escobar del Rey F: Transfer of thyroid hormone from the mother to the fetus, in Delange F, Fisher DA, Glinoer D (eds): *Research in Congenital Hypothyroidism. Nato-ASI Series A*, New York, Plenum Press, 1989, p 15.
372. Seo H, Wunderlich C, Vassart G, et al: Growth hormone responses to thyroid hormone in the neonatal rat: Resistance and anamnestic response. *J Clin Invest* **67**:569, 1981.
373. Gauthier K, Chassande O, Platerotti M, et al: Different functions for the thyroid hormone receptors TRα and TRβ in the control of thyroid hormone production and post-natal development. *EMBO J* **18**:623, 1999.
374. Glorieux J, Dussault JH, Letarte J, et al: Preliminary results on the mental development of hypothyroid infants detected by the Quebec screening program. *J Pediatr* **102**:19, 1982.
375. Oppenheimer JH, Koerner D, Schwartz HL, et al: Specific-nuclear triiodothyronine binding sites in rat liver and kidney. *J Clin Endocrinol Metab* **35**:330, 1972.
376. Oppenheimer JH: The nuclear receptor-triiodothyronine complex: Relationship to thyroid hormone distribution, metabolism and biological action, in Oppenheimer JH, Samuels HH (eds): *Molecular Basis of Thyroid Hormone Action*. New York, Academic Press, 1983, p 1.
377. Sap J, Muñoz A, Damm K, et al: The *c-erb*-A protein is a high-affinity receptor for thyroid hormone. *Nature* **324**:635, 1986.
378. Weinberger C, Thompson CC, Ong ES, et al: The *c-erb*-A gene encodes a thyroid hormone receptor. *Nature* **324**:641, 1986.
379. Evans RM: The steroid and thyroid hormone receptor superfamily. *Science* **240**:889, 1988.
380. Tone Y, Collingwood TN, Adams M, et al: Functional analysis of a transactivation domain in the thyroid hormone β receptor. *J Biol Chem* **269**:31157, 1994.
381. Mitsuhashi T, Tennyson GE, Nikodem VM: Alternative splicing generates messages encoding rat c-erbA proteins that do not bind thyroid hormones. *Proc Natl Acad Sci U S A* **85**:5804, 1988.
382. Escriva H, Safi R, Hänni C, et al: Ligand binding was acquired during evolution of nuclear receptors. *Proc Natl Acad Sci U S A* **94**:6803, 1997.
383. Hodin RA, Lazar MA, Chin WW: Differential and tissue-specific regulation of the multiple rat c-erbA messenger RNA species by thyroid hormone. *J Clin Invest* **85**:101, 1990.
384. Macchia E, Nakai A, Janiga A, et al: Characterization of site-specific polyclonal antibodies to c-erbA peptides recognizing human thyroid hormone receptors α_1, α_2, and β and native 3,5,3′-triiodothyronine receptor, and study of tissue distribution of the antigen. *Endocrinology* **126**:3232, 1990.
385. Strait KA, Schwartz HL, Perez-Castillo A, et al: Relationship of c-erbA mRNA content to tissue triiodothyronine nuclear binding capacity and function in developing and adult rats. *J Biol Chem* **265**:10514, 1990.
386. Forman BM, Casanova J, Raaka BM, et al: Half-site spacing and orientation determines whether thyroid hormone and retinoic acid receptors and related factors bind to DNA response elements as monomers, homodimers, or heterodimers. *Mol Endocrinol* **6**:429, 1992.
387. Glass CK: Differential recognition of target genes by nuclear receptor monomers, dimers and heterodimers. *Endocr Rev* **15**:391, 1994.
388. Darling DS, Beebe JS, Burnside J, et al: 3,5,3′-triiodothyronine (T3) receptor-auxiliary protein (TRAP) binds DNA and forms heterodimers with the T3 receptor. *Mol Endocrinol* **5**:73, 1991.
389. Zhang X-K, Hoffmann B, Tran PBV, et al: Retinoid X receptor is an auxiliary protein for thyroid hormone and retinoic acid receptors. *Nature* **355**:441, 1992.
390. Brent GA, Dunn MK, Harney JW, et al: Thyroid hormone apo receptor represses T_3-inducible promoters and blocks activity of the retinoic acid receptor. *New Biologist* **1**:329, 1989.
391. Koenig RJ: Thyroid hormone receptor coactivators and corepressors. *Thyroid* **8**:703, 1998.
392. Pazin MJ, Kadonaga JT: What's up and down with histone deacetylation and transcription? *Cell* **89**:325, 1997.
393. Yen PM, Darling DS, Carter RL, et al: Triiodothyronine (T3) decreases binding to DNA by T3-receptor homodimers but not receptor-auxiliary protein heterodimers. *J Biol Chem* **267**:3565, 1992.
394. Glass CK, Rose DW, Rosenfeld MG: Nuclear receptor coactivators. *Curr Opin Cell Biol* **9**:222, 1997.
395. Fondell JD, Guermah M, Malik S, et al: Thyroid hormone receptor-associated proteins and general positive cofactors mediate thyroid hormone receptor function in the absence of the TATA box-binding protein-associated factors of TFIID. *Proc Natl Acad Sci U S A* **96**:1959, 1999.
396. Refetoff S, Weiss RE: Resistance to thyroid hormone, in Thakker TV (ed): *Molecular Genetics of Endocrine Disorders*. London, Chapman & Hill, 1997, p 85.
397. Refetoff S, Weiss RE, Usala SJ: The syndromes of resistance to thyroid hormone. *Endocr Rev* **14**:348, 1993.
398. Weiss RE, Weinberg M, Refetoff S: Identical mutations in unrelated families with generalized resistance to thyroid hormone occur in cytosine-guanine-rich areas of the thyroid hormone receptor beta gene: Analysis of 15 families. *J Clin Invest* **91**:2408, 1993.
399. Adams M, Matthews C, Collingwood TN, et al: Genetic analysis of 29 kindreds with generalized and pituitary resistance to thyroid hormone: Identification of thirteen novel mutations in the thyroid hormone receptor β gene. *J Clin Invest* **94**:506, 1994.
400. Beck-Peccoz P, Chatterjee VKK: The variable clinical phenotype in thyroid hormone resistance syndrome. *Thyroid* **4**:225, 1994.
401. Kaplan J-C, Kahn A, Chelly J: Illegitimate transcription: Its use in the study of inherited diseases. *Hum Mutat* **1**:357, 1992.
402. Usala SJ: Molecular diagnosis and characterization of thyroid hormone resistance syndromes. *Thyroid* **1**:361, 1991.
403. Snyder D, Sesser D, Skeels M, et al: Thyroid disorders in newborn infants with elevated screening T4. *Thyroid* **7**:S29, 1997.
404. Refetoff S, DeWind LT, DeGroot LJ: Familial syndrome combining deaf-mutism, stippled epiphyses, goiter, and abnormally high PBI: Possible target organ refractoriness to thyroid hormone. *J Clin Endocrinol Metab* **27**:279, 1967.
405. Ono S, Schwartz ID, Mueller OT, et al: Homozygosity for a "dominant negative" thyroid hormone receptor gene responsible for generalized resistance to thyroid hormone. *J Clin Endocrinol Metab* **73**:990, 1991.
406. Persani L, Borgato S, Romoli R, et al: Changes in the degree of sialylation of carbohydrate chain modify the biological properties of circulating thyrotropin isoforms in various physiological and pathological states. *J Clin Endocrinol Metab* **83**:2486, 1998.
407. Stein MA, Weiss RE, Refetoff S: Neurocognitive characteristics of individuals with resistance to thyroid hormone: Comparisons to individuals with attention deficit hyperactivity disorder only. *J Dev Behav Pediatr* **16**:406, 1995.
408. Takeda K, Sakurai A, DeGroot LJ, et al: Recessive inheritance of thyroid hormone resistance caused by complete deletion of the protein-coding region of the thyroid hormone receptor-β gene. *J Clin Endocrinol Metab* **74**:49, 1992.
409. Brucker-Davis F, Skarulis MC, Pikus A, et al: Prevalence and mechanisms of hearing loss in patients with resistance to thyroid hormone. *J Clin Endocrinol Metab* **81**:2768, 1996.

410. Beck-Peccoz P, Persani L, Faglia G: Glycoprotein hormone α-subunit in pituitary adenomas. *Trends Endocrinol Metab* **3**:41, 1992.
411. Sarne DH, Refetoff S, Rosenfield RL, et al: Sex-hormone binding globulin in the diagnosis of peripheral tissue resistance to thyroid hormone: The value of changes following short-term triiodothyronine administration. *J Clin Endocrinol Metab* **66**:740, 1988.
412. Sarne DH, Sobieszczyk S, Ain KB, et al: Serum thyrotropin and prolactin in the syndrome of generalized resistance to thyroid hormone: Responses to thyrotropin-releasing hormone stimulation and triiodothyronine suppression. *J Clin Endocrinol Metab* **70**:1305, 1990.
413. Hayashi Y, Weiss RE, Sarne DH, et al: Do clinical manifestations of resistance to thyroid hormone correlate with the functional alteration of the corresponding mutant thyroid hormone-β receptors? *J Clin Endocrinol Metab* **80**:3246, 1995.
414. Usala SJ, Bale AE, Gesundheit N, et al: Tight linkage between the syndrome of generalized thyroid hormone resistance and the human c-erbAb gene. *Mol Endocrinol* **2**:1217, 1988.
415. Sakurai A, Takeda K, Ain K, et al: Generalized resistance to thyroid hormone associated with a mutation in the ligand-binding domain of the human thyroid hormone receptor β. *Proc Natl Acad Sci U S A* **86**:8977, 1989.
416. Usala SJ, Tennyson GE, Bale AE, et al: A base mutation of the c-erbAb thyroid hormone receptor in a kindred with generalized thyroid hormone resistance. Molecular heterogeneity in two other kindreds. *J Clin Invest* **85**:93, 1990.
417. McCabe CJ, Gittoes NJ, Sheppard MC, et al: Thyroid receptor α1 and α2 mutations in nonfunctioning pituitary tumors. *J Clin Endocrinol Metab* **84**:649, 1999.
418. Pohlenz J, Weiss RE, Macchia PE, et al: Five new families with resistance to thyroid hormone not caused by mutations in the thyroid hormone receptor β gene. *J Clin Endocrinol Metab* **84**:3919, 1999.
419. Bradley DJ, Towle HC, Young III WS: A and β thyroid hormone receptor (TR) gene expression during auditory neurogenesis: Evidence for TR isoform-specific transcriptional regulation *in vivo*. *Proc Natl Acad Sci U S A* **91**:439, 1994.
420. Hayashi Y, Janssen OE, Weiss RE, et al: The relative expression of mutant and normal thyroid hormone receptor genes in patients with generalized resistance to thyroid hormone determined by estimation of their specific messenger ribonucleic acid products. *J Clin Endocrinol Metab* **76**:64, 1993.
421. Sakurai A, Miyamoto T, Refetoff S, et al: Dominant negative transcriptional regulation by a mutant thyroid hormone receptor β in a family with generalized resistance to thyroid hormone. *Mol Endocrinol* **4**:1988, 1990.
422. Chatterjee VKK, Nagaya T, Madison LD, et al: Thyroid hormone resistance syndrome. Inhibition of normal receptor function by mutant thyroid hormone receptors. *J Clin Invest* **87**:1977, 1991.
423. Usala SJ, Menke JB, Watson TL, et al: A homozygous deletion in the c-erbAβ thyroid hormone receptor gene in a patient with generalized thyroid hormone resistance: isolation and characterization of the mutant receptor. *Mol Endocrinol* **5**:327, 1991.
424. Yen PM, Sugawara A, Refetoff S, et al: New insights on the mechanism(s) of the dominant negative effect of mutant thyroid hormone receptor in generalized resistance to thyroid hormone. *J Clin Invest* **90**:1825, 1992.
425. Piedrafita FJ, Ortiz MA, Pfahl M: Thyroid hormone receptor-β mutants, associated with generalized resistance to thyroid hormone show defects in their ligand-sensitive repression function. *Mol Endocrinol* **9**:1533, 1995.
426. Hao E, Menke JB, Smith AM, et al: Divergent dimerization properties of mutant β1 thyroid hormone receptors are associated with different dominant negative activities. *Mol Endocrinol* **8**:841, 1994.
427. Au-Fliegner M, Helmer E, Casanova J, et al: The conserved ninth C-terminal heptad in thyroid hormone and retinoic acid receptors mediates diverse responses by affecting heterodimer but not homodimer formation. *Mol Cell Endocrinol* **13**:5725, 1993.
428. Nagaya T, Jameson JL: Thyroid hormone receptor dimerization is required for the dominant negative inhibition by mutations that cause thyroid hormone resistance. *J Biol Chem* **268**:15766, 1993.
429. Yoh SM, Chatterjee VKK, Privalsky ML: Thyroid hormone resistance syndrome manifests as an aberrant interaction between mutant T_3 receptor and transcriptional corepressor. *Mol Endocrinol* **11**:470, 1997.
430. Tagami T, Gu W-X, Peairs PT, et al: A novel natural mutation in the thyroid hormone receptor defines a dual functional domain that exchanges nuclear receptor corepressors and coactivators. *Mol Endocrinol* **12**:1888, 1998.
431. Collingwood TN, Rajanayagam O, Adams M, et al: A natural transactivation mutation in the thyroid hormone β receptor: Impaired interaction with putative transcriptional mediators. *Proc Natl Acad Sci U S A* **94**:248, 1997.
432. Liu Y, Takeshita A, Misiti S, et al: Lack of coactivator interaction can be a mechanism for dominant negative activity by mutant thyroid hormone receptors. *Endocrinology* **139**:4197, 1998.
433. Collingwood TN, Wagner R, Matthews CH, et al: A role for helix 3 of the TRβ ligand-binding domain in coactivator recruitment identified by characterization of a third cluster of mutations in resistance to thyroid hormone. *EMBO J* 16:4760, 1998.
434. Nagaya T, Madison LD, Jameson JL: Thyroid hormone receptor mutants that cause resistance to thyroid hormone. Evidence for receptor competition for DNA sequences in target genes. *J Biol Chem* **267**:13014, 1992.
435. Nagaya T, Fujieda N, Seo H: Requirement of corepressor binding of thyroid hormone receptor mutants for dominant negative inhibition. *Biochem Biophys Res Commun* **247**:620, 1998.
436. Hayashi Y, Sunthornthepvarakul T, Refetoff S: Mutations of CpG dinucleotides located in the triiodothyronine (T_3)-binding domain of the thyroid hormone receptor (TR) β gene that appears to be devoid of natural mutations may not be detected because they are unlikely to produce the clinical phenotype of resistance to thyroid hormone. *J Clin Invest* **94**:607, 1994.
437. Rastinejad F, Perlmann T, Evans F, et al: Structural determinants of nuclear receptor assembly on DNA direct repeats. *Nature* **375**:203, 1995.
438. Wagner RL, Apriletti JW, McGrath ME, et al: A structural role for hormone in the thyroid hormone receptor. *Nature* **138**:690, 1995.
439. Meier CA, Dickstein BM, Ashizawa K, et al: Variable transcriptional activity and ligand binding of mutant β1 3,5,3′-triiodothyronine receptors from four families with generalized resistance to thyroid hormone. *Mol Endocrinol* **6**:248, 1992.
440. Nagaya T, Eberhardt NL, Jameson JL: Thyroid hormone resistance syndrome: correlation of dominant negative activity and location of mutations. *J Clin Endocrinol Metab* **77**:982, 1993.
441. Yagi H, Pohlenz J, Hayashi Y, et al: Resistance to thyroid hormone caused by two mutant thyroid hormone receptor β, R243Q and R243W, with marked impairment of function that cannot be explained by altered in-vitro 3,5,3′-triiodothyronine binding affinity. *J Clin Endocrinol Metab* **82**:1608, 1997.
442. Safer JD, Cohen RN, Hollenberg AN, et al: Defective release of corepressor by hinge mutants of the thyroid hormone receptor found in patients with resistance to thyroid hormone. *J Biol Chem* **273**:30175, 1998.
443. Clifton-Bligh RJ, de Zegher F, Wagner RL, et al: A novel mutation (R383H) in resistance to thyroid hormone syndrome predominantly impairs corepressor release and negative transcriptional regulation. *Mol Endocrinol* **12**:609, 1998.
444. Flynn TR, Hollenberg AN, Cohen O, et al: A novel C-terminal domain in the thyroid hormone receptor selectively mediates thyroid hormone inhibition. *J Biol Chem* **629**:32713, 1994.
445. Kurokawa R, DiRenzo J, Boehm M, et al: Regulation of retinoid signaling by receptor polarity and allosteric control of ligand binding. *Nature* **371**:528, 1994.
446. Zamir I, Zhang J, Lazar MA: Stoichiometric and steric principles governing repression by nuclear hormone receptors. *Genes Dev* **11**:835, 1997.
447. Lazar MA: Thyroid hormone receptors: Multiple forms, multiple possibilities. *Endocr Rev* **14**:184, 1993.
448. Falcone M, Miyamoto T, Fierro-Renoy F, et al: Antipeptide polyclonal antibodies specifically recognize each human thyroid hormone receptor isoform. *Endocrinology* **131**:2419, 1992.
449. Mixson AJ, Hauser P, Tennyson G, et al: Differential expression of mutant and normal beta T_3 receptor alleles in kindreds with generalized resistance to thyroid hormone. *J Clin Invest* **91**:2296, 1993.
450. Geffner ME, Su F, Ross NS, et al: An arginine to histidine mutation in codon 311 of the C-erbAβ gene results in a mutant thyroid hormone receptor that does not mediate a dominant negative phenotype. *J Clin Invest* **91**:538, 1993.
451. Weiss RE, Stein MA, Duck SC, et al: Low intelligence but not attention deficit hyperactivity disorder is associated with resistance to thyroid hormone caused by mutation R316H in the thyroid hormone receptor β gene. *J Clin Endocrinol Metab* **78**:1525, 1994.

452. Weiss RE, Marcocci C, Bruno-Bossio G, et al: Multiple genetic factors in the heterogeneity of thyroid hormone resistance. *J Clin Endocrinol Metab* **76**:257, 1993.
453. Forrest D, Hanebuth E, Smeyne RJ, et al: Recessive resistance to thyroid hormone in mice lacking thyroid hormone receptor β: Evidence for tissue-specific modulation of receptor function. *EMBO J* **15**:3006, 1996.
454. Weiss RE, Forrest D, Pohlenz J, et al: Thyrotropin regulation by thyroid hormone in thyroid hormone receptor β-deficient mice. *Endocrinology* **138**:3624, 1997.
455. Weiss RE, Murata Y, Cua K, et al: Thyroid hormone action on liver, heart and energy expenditure in thyroid hormone receptor β deficient mice. *Endocrinology* **139**:4945, 1998.
456. Forrest D, Erway LC, Ng L, et al: Thyroid hormone receptor β is essential for development of auditory function. *Nat Genet* **13**:354, 1996.
457. Wikstsöm L, Johansson C, Salto C, et al: Abnormal heart rate and body temperature in mice lacking thyroid hormone receptor $\alpha 1$. *EMBO J* **17**:455, 1998.
458. Fraichard A, Chassande O, Plateroti M, et al: The $T_3R\alpha$ gene encoding a thyroid hormone receptor is essential for post-natal development and thyroid hormone production. *EMBO J* **16**:4412, 1997.
459. Hayashi Y, Mangoura D, Refetoff S: A mouse model of resistance to thyroid hormone produced by somatic gene transfer of a mutant thyroid hormone receptor. *Mol Endocrinol* **10**:100, 1996.
460. Wong R, Vasilyev VV, Ting Y-T, et al: Transgenic mice bearing a human mutant thyroid hormone $\beta 1$ receptor manifest thyroid function anomalies, weight reduction, and hyperactivity. *Mol Med* **3**:303, 1997.
461. Hayashi Y, Xie J, Weiss RE, et al: Selective pituitary resistance to thyroid hormone produced by expression of a mutant thyroid hormone receptor β gene in the pituitary gland of transgenic mice. *Biochem Biophys Res Commun* **245**:204, 1998.
462. Abel ED, Kaulbach HC, Campos-Barros A, et al: Novel insight from transgenic mice into thyroid hormone resistance and the regulation of thyrotropin. *J Clin Invest* **103**:271, 1998.
463. Weiss RE, Xu J, Ning G, et al: Mice deficient in the steroid receptor co-activator 1 (SRC-1) are resistant to thyroid hormone. *EMBO J* **18**:1900, 1999.
464. Weiss RE: Management of patients with resistance to thyroid hormone. *Thyroid Today* **12**:1, 1999.
465. Brix TH, Kyvik KO, Hegedus L: What is the evidence of genetic factors in the etiology of Graves' disease? A brief review. *Thyroid* **8**:727, 1998.
466. Barbesino G, Tomer Y, Concepcion E, et al: Linkage analysis of candidate genes in autoimmune thyroid disease: 1. Selected immunoregulatory genes. International Consortium for the Genetics of Autoimmune Thyroid Disease. *J Clin Endocrinol Metab* **83**:1580, 1998.
467. DE Roux N, Shields DC, Misrahi M, et al: Analysis of the thyrotropin receptor as a candidate gene in familial Graves' disease. *J Clin Endocrinol Metab* **81**:3483, 1996.
468. Tomer Y, Barbesino G, Keddache M, et al: Mapping of a major susceptibility locus for Graves' disease (GD-1) to chromosome 14q31. *J Clin Endocrinol Metab* **82**:1645, 1997.
469. Tomer Y, Barbesino G, Greenberg DA, et al: A new Graves disease-susceptibility locus maps to chromosome 20q11.2. International Consortium for the Genetics of Autoimmune Thyroid Disease. *Am J Hum Genet* **63**:1749, 1998.
470. Delange F: Neonatal screening for congenital hypothyroidism: Result and perspectives. *Horm Res* **48**:51, 1997.
471. Dussault JH: Screening for congenital hypothyroidism. *Clin Obstet Gynecol* **40**:117, 1997.
472. Simons WF, Fuggle PW, Grant DB, et al: Educational progress, behaviour, and motor skills at 10 years in early treated congenital hypothyroidism. *Arch Dis Child* **77**:219, 1997.
473. Rovet JF, Ehrlich RM: Long-term effects of l-thyroxine therapy for congenital hypothyroidism. *J Pediatr* **126**:380, 1995.
474. Dubuis JM, Glorieux J, Richer F, et al: Outcome of severe congenital hypothyroidism: Closing the development gap with early high-dose levothyroxine treatment. *J Clin Endocrinol Metab* **81**:222, 1996.
475. Van Wassenaer AG, Kok JH, Dekker FW, et al: Thyroxine administration to infants of less than 30 weeks gestational age decreases plasma tri-iodothyronine concentrations. *Eur J Endocrinol* **139**:508, 1998.
476. Tonacchera M, Chiovato L, Pinchera A, et al: Hyperfunctioning thyroid nodules in toxic multinodular goiter share activating thyrotropin receptor mutations with solitary toxic adenoma. *J Clin Endocrinol Metab* **83**:492, 1998.
477. Hishinuma A, Kasai K, Masawa N, et al: Missense mutation (C1263R) in the thyroglobulin gene causes congenital goiter with mild hypothyroidism by impaired intracellular transport. *Endocr J* **45**:315, 1998.
478. Targovnik HM, Vono J, Billerbeck AE, et al: A 138-nucleotide deletion in the thyroglobulin ribonucleic acid messenger in a congenital goiter with defective thyroglobulin synthesis. *J Clin Endocrinol Metab* **80**:3356, 1995.
479. Pohlenz J, Refetoff S: Mutations in the sodium/iodide symporter (NIS) gene as a cause for iodide transport defects and congenital hypothyroidism. *Biochimie* **81**:469, 1999.
480. Clifton-Bligh RJ, Gregory JW, Ludgate M, et al: Two novel mutations in the thyrotropin (TSH) receptor gene in a child with resistance to TSH. *J Clin Endocrinol Metab* **82**:1094, 1997.
481. Bertenshaw R, Sarne D, Tornari J, et al: Sequencing of the variant thyroxine-binding globulin (TBG)-San Diego reveals two nucleotide substitutions. *Biochim Biophys Acta* **1139**:307, 1992.
482. Bertenshaw R, Takeda K, Refetoff S: Sequencing of the variant thyroxine-binding globulin (TBG)-Quebec reveals two nucleotide substitutions. *Am J Hum Genet* **48**:741, 1991.
483. Miura Y, Kambe F, Yamamori I, et al: A truncated thyroxine-binding globulin due to a frameshift mutation is retained within the rough endoplasmic reticulum: A possible mechanism of complete thyroxine-binding globulin deficiency in Japanese. *J Clin Endocrinol Metab* **78**:283, 1994.
484. Miura Y, Mori Y, Yamamori I, et al: Sequence of a variant thyroxine-binding globulin (TBG) in a family with partial TBG deficiency in Japanese (TBG-PDJ). *Endocr J* **40**:127, 1993.
485. Janssen OE, Bertenshaw R, Takeda K, et al: Molecular basis of inherited thyroxine-binding globulin defects. *Trends Endocrinol Metab* **3**:49, 1992.
486. Nakai A, Seino S, Sakurai A, et al: Characterization of a thyroid hormone receptor expressed in human kidney and other tissues. *Proc Natl Acad Sci U S A* **85**:2781, 1988.
487. Miyajima N, Horiuchi R, Shibuya Y, et al: Two *erbA* homologs encoding proteins with different T3 binding capacities are transcribed from opposite DNA strands of the same genetic locus. *Cell* **57**:31, 1989.
488. Sakurai A, Nakai A, DeGroot LJ: Structural analysis of human thyroid hormone receptor β gene. *Mol Cell Endocrinol* **71**:83, 1990.
489. Sakurai A, Miyamoto T, DeGroot LJ: Cloning and characterization of the human thyroid hormone receptor $\beta 1$ gene promoter. *Biochem Biophys Res Commun* **185**:78, 1992.
490. Laudet V, Begue A, Henry-Duthoit C, et al: Genomic organization of the human thyroid hormone receptor α (c-erbA-1) gene. *Nucleic Acids Res* **19**:1105, 1991.
491. Feng W, Ribeiro RCJ, Wagner RL, et al: Hormone-dependent coactivator binding to a hydrophobic cleft on nuclear receptors. *Science* **280**:1747, 1998.
492. Chen JD, Evans RM: A transcriptional co-repressor that interacts with nuclear hormone receptors. *Nature* **377**:454, 1995.
493. Hörlein AJ, Näär AM, Heinzel T, et al: Ligand-independent repression by the thyroid hormone receptor mediated by a nuclear receptor co-repressor. *Nature* **377**:397, 1995.
494. Busch K, Martin B, Baniahmad A, et al: At least three subdomains of v-erbA are involved in its silencing function. *Mol Endocrinol* **11**:379, 1997.
495. Forman BM, Samuels HH: Interactions among a subfamily of nuclear hormone receptors: The regulatory zipper model. *Mol Endocrinol* **4**:1293, 1990.
496. O'Donnell AL, Koenig RJ: Mutational analysis identifies a new functional domain of the thyroid hormone receptor. *Mol Endocrinol* **4**:715, 1990.
497. Kurokawa R, Yu VC, Naar A, et al: Differential orientations of the DNA-binding domain and carboxy-terminal dimerization interface regulate binding site selection by nuclear receptor heterodimers. *Genes Dev* **7**:1423, 1993.
498. Beck-Peccoz P, Chatterjee VKK, Chin WW, et al: Nomenclature of thyroid hormone receptor β-gene mutations in resistance to thyroid hormone: Consensus statement from the first workshop on thyroid hormone resistance, July 10–11, 1993, Cambridge, United Kingdom. *J Clin Endocrinol Metab* **78**:990, 1993.

499. Baniahmad A, Leng X, Burris TP, et al: The T_4 activation domain of the thyroid hormone receptor is required for release of a putative corepressor(s) necessary for transcriptional silencing. *Mol Cell Biol* **15**:76, 1995.
500. Hamy F, Helbeque NJ, Henichart P: Comparison between synthetic nuclear localisation signal peptides from the steroid thyroid hormone receptor superfamily. *Biochem Byophys Res Commun* **183**:289, 1992.
501. Wurtz J-M, Bourguet W, Renaud J-P, et al: A canonical structure for the ligand-binding domain of the nuclear receptors. *Nature Struct Biol* **3**:97, 1966.
502. Fofanova O, Takamura N, Kinoshita E, et al: Compound heterozygous deletion of the PROP-1 gene in children with combined pituitary hormone deficiency. *J Clin Endocrinol Metab* **83**:2601, 1998.
503. Tatsumi K, Miyai K, Notomi T, et al: Cretinism with combined hormone deficiency caused by a mutation in the PIT1 gene. *Nat Genet* **1**:56, 1992.
504. Pellegrini-Bouiller I, Belicar P, Barlier A, et al: A new mutation of the gene encoding the transcription factor Pit-1 is responsible for combined pituitary hormone deficiency. *J Clin Endocrinol Metab* **81**:2790, 1996.
505. Ohta K, Nobukuni Y, Mitsubuchi H, et al: Mutations in the Pit-1 gene in children with combined pituitary hormone deficiency. *Biochem Biophys Res Commun* **189**:851, 1992.
506. Radovick S, Nations M, Du Y, et al: A mutation in the POU-homeodomain of Pit-1 responsible for combined pituitary hormone deficiency. *Science* **257**:1115, 1992.
507. Okamoto N, Wada Y, Ida S, et al: Monoallelic expression of normal mRNA in the PIT1 mutation heterozygotes with normal phenotype and biallelic expression in the abnormal phenotype. *Hum Mol Genet* **3**:1565, 1994.
508. Aarskog D, Eiken HG, Bjerknes R, et al: Pituitary dwarfism in the R271W Pit-1 gene mutation. *Eur J Pediatr* **156**:829, 1997.
509. Irie Y, Tatsumi K, Ogawa M, et al: A novel E250X mutation of the PIT1 gene in a patient with combined pituitary hormone deficiency. *Endocr J* **42**:351, 1995.
510. Pernasetti F, Milner RD, al Ashwal AA, et al: Pro239Ser: A novel recessive mutation of the Pit-1 gene in seven Middle Eastern children with growth hormone, prolactin, and thyrotropin deficiency. *J Clin Endocrinol Metab* **83**:2079, 1998.
511. Rosen HN, Moses AC, Murrell JR, et al: Thyroxine interactions with transthyretin: A comparison of 10 naturally occurring human transthyretin variants. *J Clin Endocrinol Metab* **77**:370, 1993.
512. Lalloz MR, Byfield PG, Goel KM, et al: Hyperthyroxinemia due to the coexistence of two raised affinity thyroxine-binding proteins (albumin and prealbumin) in one family. *J Clin Endocrinol Metab* **64**:346, 1987.
513. Fitch NJS, Akbary MT, Ramsden DB: An inherited non-amyloidogenic transthyretin variant, [Ser^6]-TTR, with increased thyroxine-binding affinity, characterized by DNA sequencing. *J Endocrinol* **129**:309, 1991.
514. Rosen HN, Murrell JR, Liepnieks JL, et al: Threonine for alanine substitution at position 109 of transthyretin differentially alters human transthyretin's affinity for iodothyronines. *J Clin Endocrinol Metab* **134**:27, 1994.
515. Harrison HH, Gordon ED, Nichols WC, et al: Biochemical and clinical characterization of prealbumin^{CHICAGO}: An apparently benign variant of serum prealbumin (transthyretin) discovered with high-resolution two-dimensional electrophoresis. *Am J Med Gen* **39**:442, 1991.
516. Alves IL, Divino CM, Schussler GC, et al: Thyroxine binding in a TTR met 119 kindred. *J Clin Endocrinol Metab* **76**:484, 1993.
517. Curtis AL, Scrimshaw BL, Topliss DJ, et al: Thyroxine binding by human transthyretin variants: Mutations at position 119, but not 54, increase thyroxine binding affinity. *J Clin Endocrinol Metab* **78**:459, 1994.
518. Brucker-Davis F, Skarulis MC, Grace MB, et al: Genetic and clinical features of 42 kindreds with resistance to thyroid hormone. The National Institutes of Health prospective study. *Ann Intern Med* **123**:573, 1995.
519. Petersen CE, HA CE, Harohalli K, et al: Structural investigations of a new familial dysalbuminemic hyperthyroxinemia genotype. *Clin Chem* **45**:1248, 1999.
520. Pannain S, Feldman M, Eiholzer U, et al: Familial dysalbuminemic hyperthyroxinemia in a Swiss family caused by a mutant albumin (R218P) shows an apparent discrepancy between serum concentration and affinity for thyroxine. *J Clin Endocrinol Metab* **85**:2786, 2000.

CHAPTER 159

Congenital Adrenal Hyperplasia

Patricia A. Donohoue ▪ Keith L. Parker ▪ Claude J. Migeon

1. **Congenital adrenal hyperplasia (CAH, MIM 300200) is a group of diseases whose common feature is an enzymatic defect in the steroidogenic pathway leading to the biosynthesis of cortisol. This relative decrease in cortisol production causes an increase in adrenocorticotropic hormone (ACTH) secretion and consequent hyperplasia of the adrenal cortex. All forms of CAH are inherited in an autosomal recessive manner. The variable phenotypes are determined by the effects produced by deficient hormones and by excess production of steroids unaffected by the enzymatic block.**
2. **The biochemical pathways of adrenal steroid production are interrelated. The three zones of the adrenal cortex produce three classes of steroid hormones: glucocorticoids and androgens (zona fasciculata/reticularis) and mineralocorticoids (zona glomerulosa). All but one of the enzymatic steps are mediated by members of the cytochrome P_{450} (CYP) family of mixed-function oxidases. The first step in the production of all steroid hormones, mediated by CYP11A, is the conversion of cholesterol to pregnenolone. Pregnenolone may then be acted on by CYP17 to form 17-hydroxypregnenolone and then dehydroepiandrosterone (DHEA), or it may be converted to progesterone by the non-P_{450} enzyme 3β-hydroxysteroid dehydrogenase (3β-HSD). 3β-HSD also converts 17-hydroxypregnenolone to 17-hydroxyprogesterone and DHEA to androstenedione, an androgen precursor. Progesterone and 17-hydroxyprogesterone are then converted by CYP21 to 11-deoxycorticosterone (a mineralocorticoid) and 11-deoxycortisol, respectively. These two products are then converted by CYP11B1 to corticosterone and cortisol (the major glucocorticoid), respectively. Aldosterone, the major mineralocorticoid, is produced from corticosterone by the enzyme CYP11B2 (aldosterone synthase).**
3. **Control of adrenal steroid production is multifaceted. Glucocorticoid production is stimulated primarily by the anterior pituitary hormone ACTH, which itself is controlled by the hypothalamic corticotropin-releasing hormone (CRH). Aldosterone secretion is modulated by the renin-angiotensin system. Adrenal androgen secretion is stimulated by excessive ACTH, but physiologic control is through an unidentified factor.**
4. **In keeping with their different physiologic regulations, the secretion rates of the various adrenocortical hormones vary independently. The cortisol secretion rate is approximates 12 mg/m^2 of body surface area per day. This rate is somewhat higher—but quite variable—in newborn infants and significantly higher during periods of physiologic stress, such as fever and surgery. The aldosterone secretion rate (approximately 100 µg/day) remains fairly constant throughout life. Adrenal androgen secretion is quite low during infancy and childhood and increases gradually to maximal levels during puberty and early adulthood, with age-related declines thereafter.**
5. **21-Hydroxylase (CYP21) deficiency is the most common form of CAH, accounting for over 90 percent of cases. The incidence varies from 1 in 10,000 to 18,000 live births. There is a continuum of degrees of CYP21 deficiency that results in a continuum of severity of clinical presentations. The most marked deficiency results in the salt-losing form of CAH, characterized by both mineralocorticoid and glucocorticoid deficiencies. The steroid precursors prior to the enzymatic block (progesterone and 17-hydroxyprogesterone) accumulate due to excessive ACTH stimulation of the gland and are shunted into the androgen biosynthetic pathway, which is unaffected by the block. The resulting androgen excess produces prenatal masculinization (ambiguous genitalia) in females and postnatal virilization in both sexes. In the simple virilizing form, milder CYP21 deficiency results in androgen excess (prenatal masculinization in females and postnatal virilization in both sexes), but salt loss does not occur. In the attenuated or late onset form, minimal CYP21 deficiency results in androgen excess that becomes clinically significant only in pubertal or adult females. Genetic studies in CYP21 deficiency have identified two 21-hydroxylase genes within the class III region of the major histocompatibility complex on chromosome 6p. The disease is therefore HLA-linked. The active gene (*CYP21*) and the pseudogene (*CYP21P*) lie in tandem duplication with the genes encoding the C4A and C4B complement proteins. Most of the mutations in CYP21 deficiency are caused by events to which duplicated loci are predisposed, such as unequal crossovers and gene conversions.**
6. **11β-Hydroxylase (CYP11B1) deficiency is the second most common form of CAH, representing approximately 5 percent of cases. Deficiency of CYP11B1 causes accumulation of the mineralocorticoid 11-deoxycorticosterone, resulting in hypertension. In the glucocorticoid pathway, 11-deoxycortisol accumulates. The androgen pathway is unaffected by the enzymatic deficiency; thus prenatal masculinization occurs in females, and postnatal**

A list of standard abbreviations is located immediately preceding the index in each volume. Nonstandard abbreviations used in this chapter include: CAH = congenital adrenal hyperplasia; ACTH = adrenocorticotropic hormone; SF-1 = steroidogenic factor 1; StAR = steroidogenic acute regulatory protein; 3β-HSD = 3β-hydroxysteroid dehydrogenase; DHEA = dehydroepiandrosterone; DOC = 11-deoxycorticosterone; POMC = proopiomelanocortin; CRH = corticotropin-releasing hormone; 11β-HSD = 11β-hydroxysteroid dehydrogenase; PCO = polycystic ovary; MHC = major histocompatibility complex.

virilization occurs in both sexes. A late onset form exists that is similar in its clinical presentation to attenuated CYP21 deficiency. Genetic studies in CYP11B1 deficiency have mapped two homologous genes, *CYP11B1* and *CYP11B2*, to chromosome 8q. The product of *CYP11B1* catalyzes 11β-hydroxylation in the glucocorticoid pathway in the zona fasciculata/reticularis, and the product of *CYP11B2* (aldosterone synthase) converts corticosterone to aldosterone in the zona glomerulosa. Mutations of *CYP11B1* cause CAH due to 11β-hydroxylase deficiency; mutations of *CYP11B2*, which do not impair glucocorticoid production, cause autosomal recessive aldosterone deficiencies without CAH; and intergenic recombinations producing fusion of the 5′ end of *CYP11B1* and the 3′ end of *CYP11B2* produce autosomal dominant glucocorticoid-remediable aldosteronism.

7. **CAH due to CYP17 deficiency occurs less frequently than that due to CYP11B1 deficiency, and the clinical features vary depending on the enzymatic activity affected. In severe CYP17 deficiency, both 17β-hydroxylase and 17,20-lyase activities are reduced or absent. This results in mineralocorticoid excess and hypertension and in absent sex steroid production in both the adrenal and gonad, producing female external genitalia in all patients. Partial CYP17 deficiencies may cause ambiguous sexual development in genetic males. Mutations within specific regions of *CYP17*, a single-copy gene on chromosome 10q, produce deleterious effects on 17β-hydroxylase and/or 17,20-lyase activities.**
8. **Deficiency of 3β-HSD is a rare cause of CAH, and the varying degrees of defective enzymatic activity produce a continuum of clinical effects. In severe 3β-HSD deficiency, there is absent production of all three classes of steroid hormones, with accumulation of 17-hydroxypregnenolone and DHEA. Patients suffer from renal salt loss, insufficient cortisol, and deficient sex steroid production. Excess DHEA can act as the substrate for peripheral conversion to androgen, which may cause some virilization in females; however, there is insufficient androgen production for normal virilization in male patients. Although it has been reported that mild 3β-HSD deficiency can cause a late onset form of CAH in postpubertal females with symptoms of excessive androgen derived from DHEA, mutations in the different 3β-HSD genes have not been demonstrated; thus the pathogenesis of late onset 3β-HSD deficiency remains unknown.**
9. **There are no reported cases of CAH due to CYP11A deficiency. This may reflect the obligatory requirement for steroidogenesis by the fetal component of the placenta in maintaining pregnancy. A phenotype closely resembling that predicted for deficiency of CYP11A, however, is seen in patients with congenital lipoid adrenal hyperplasia (lipoid CAH), which results from mutations in the gene encoding the steroidogenic acute regulatory protein (StAR). These patients have established definitively that StAR is essential for the delivery of substrate cholesterol into the steroidogenic pathway. There is no production of steroid hormones, and cholesterol accumulates in the adrenocortical cells, producing lipoid adrenal hyperplasia. Patients have renal salt loss, cortisol deficiency, and sex steroid deficiency; thus all patients have a female phenotype.**
10. **The mainstay of treatment in all forms of CAH is glucocorticoid replacement therapy, which corrects the cortisol deficiency and reverses the abnormal hormonal patterns resulting from excessive ACTH secretion. Patients with deficiencies of mineralocorticoids and sex steroids require the appropriate replacement therapies. Glucocorticoid replacement must be increased during periods of stress. The majority of female patients with prenatal masculinization require surgical correction. Heterozygous carrier detection, prenatal diagnosis, and prenatal therapy are routinely available in families with CYP21 deficiency and are often used in CYP11B1 deficiency. They are being explored in other forms of CAH.**
11. **Long-term follow-up studies of large numbers of patients are limited to results in CYP21 deficiency. These studies show normal adult health and subnormal adult stature in both sexes, normal fertility in males, and some degree of decreased fertility in females. A prenatal effect of androgens on the developing female brain is suspected. There may be an increased prevalence of homosexuality among females with CYP21 deficiency.**

HISTORICAL BACKGROUND

Thomas Addison is generally credited with demonstrating the importance of the "suprarenal capsules" in human homeostasis. While working at Guy's hospital in London in 1855, Addison reported the case of a patient who presented with chronic adrenal insufficiency due to progressive lesions of tuberculosis of the glands.[1] One year later, Brown-Sequard in Paris reported that bilateral adrenalectomy in rabbits and dogs resulted in rapid death.[2] Following these observations, more than 70 years elapsed before adrenocortical extracts were shown to prolong the survival of adrenalectomized dogs[3] and of patients with Addison disease.[4] In 1939, 11-deoxycorticosterone acetate (DOCA) was isolated, synthesized, and used successfully to treat patients with hypoadrenocorticism.[5] Although cortisone was isolated in 1936,[6] its biologic activity was recognized only in 1949, when it was used in the treatment of rheumatoid arthritis.[7]

Following recognition of syndromes due to total absence of adrenocortical function, syndromes of hypersecretion of adrenocortical hormones were described. In 1932, Harvey Cushing reported several cases of basophilic adenoma of the anterior pituitary, which resulted in hyperplasia of the adrenal cortex and a clinical syndrome that bears his name.[8] Despite this discovery, there remained a great deal of confusion in relation to the syndromes of adrenocortical hyperfunction that resulted in virilism. In 1942, Fuller Albright clearly delineated the differences between children with Cushing syndrome and those with congenital adrenal hyperplasia (adrenogenital syndrome).[9] In particular, he contrasted the increased catabolism resulting from excess secretion of "sugar hormone" (cortisol) in Cushing syndrome and the increased protein anabolism due to excessive androgen secretion in congenital adrenal hyperplasia (CAH). In the first condition he described delay in growth and bone age with characteristic truncal obesity, whereas in the second condition he emphasized accelerated statural growth and bone maturation along with the masculinization of the external genitalia.[9] DeCrecchia[10] is usually credited with the first pathologic description of a female subject with marked masculinization, ambiguous external genitalia, presence of Müllerian ducts, and bilateral adrenal hyperplasia, reported in 1865. The clinical aspects of the salt-losing form of CAH were reported in 1939 and 1940,[11,12] but it is probable that a similar condition was reported previously both in 1905[13] and in 1925.[14] As to the therapy for CAH, it was devised simultaneously from 1950 to 1952 at the Johns Hopkins hospital[15,16] and the Massachusetts General hospital.[17]

Tremendous advances have been made in our understanding of the pathophysiology and the genetic aspects of CAH. Its therapy also has been well established. Nonetheless, any disorder that requires a lifetime of treatment is associated with problems. In this case, these include therapeutic compliance, reproductive function, and gender identity of some female patients.

PHYSIOLOGY OF THE ADRENAL CORTEX

Anatomy, Histology, and Embryology of the Adrenal Gland

Anatomy. The human adrenal gland is composed of two organs—the cortex and the medulla—each embryologically and functionally distinct. The adrenal glands are located at the upper pole of each kidney and are surrounded by perirenal fat. Perhaps because of the proximity and common origin of the embryonic precursors of the adrenal cortex, gonads, and kidneys, ectopic nodules (rests) of hormonally active adrenocortical tissue may occur in the broad ligaments of the female or in the testes or spermatic cords of the male.[18]

The adrenal glands vary in size, depending on the age or the gestational stage of the individual. This variation results mostly from growth and regression of zones within the adrenal cortex (Fig. 159-1). At birth, the adrenal glands—which account for 0.5 percent of total body weight—are much larger relative to body weight than during adulthood, and the absolute weight of the glands is nearly that seen in adults. During the first postnatal year, the fetal component of the cortex involutes, causing a greater than 50 percent reduction in size. The adrenal glands then grow to a weight of 8 to 12 g throughout childhood and adolescence.[18,19]

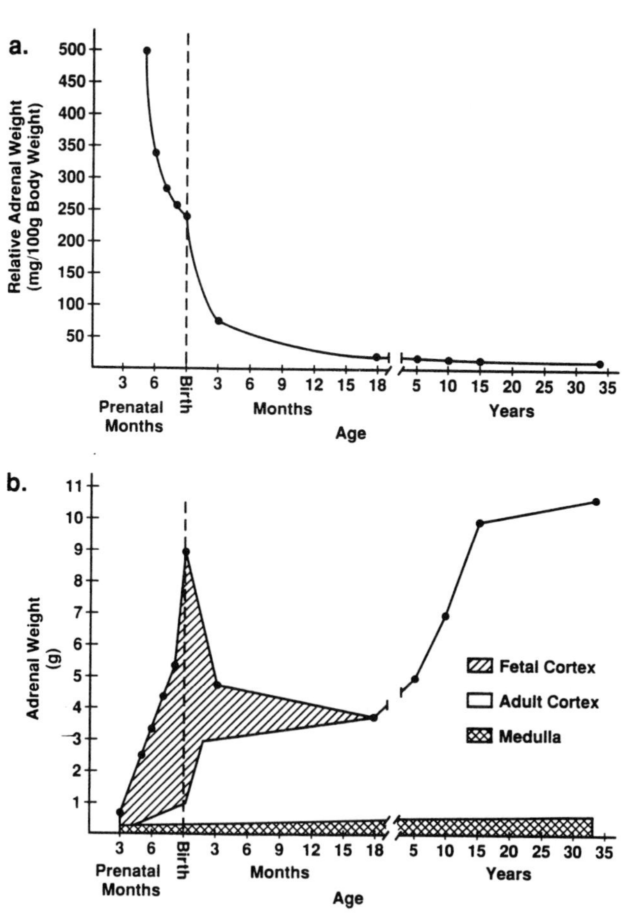

Fig. 159-1 Size of the human adrenal gland at various ages. *A.* **Weight of the adrenal relative to the weight of the body.** *B.* **Contribution of the so-called fetal cortex and the adult cortex to the absolute weight of the adrenal gland. (*From Migeon and Donohoue.*[322] *Used by permission from Charles C Thomas Publishers.*)**

Histology. In the adult, the adrenal cortex contains three zones—the outer zona glomerulosa, the middle zona fasciculata, and the inner zona reticularis; each has characteristic histologic features. The zona glomerulosa is the site of mineralocorticoid synthesis and contains clusters of relatively small cells with minimal cytoplasm. There is a gradual transition to the largest zone, the zona fasciculata, which contains columns of larger cells occupied by cytoplasmic lipid vacuoles that store cholesterol. There is an area of transition to the zona reticularis that contains compact, anastomosing cells with relatively lipid-free cytoplasm. It is believed that these clear cells of the zona fasciculata and the cells of the zona reticularis work together in the synthesis of glucocorticoids and androgens.[18,19]

Embryology. The adrenal cortex is derived from mesodermal tissue, whereas the adrenal medulla arises from neuroectoderm. At approximately the fifth week of gestation, mesothelial cells migrate into the underlying mesenchyme near the developing bipotential gonad to form the adrenal primordium. A second group of mesothelial cells then arrives to form the smaller definitive or adult zone. The inner fetal zone remains distinct from the adult zone throughout fetal life and then regresses postnatally. Cells that are destined to form the adrenal medulla, the chromaffin cell precursors, also migrate into the adrenal primordium at about the eighth week of gestation. During the first trimester, the adrenal cortex responds to adrenocorticotropic hormone (ACTH) with increased synthesis of steroids, as evidenced by the resulting ambiguity of the external genitalia in female infants with virilizing forms of CAH. Studies are beginning to identify some of the mechanisms that underlie differentiation of the adrenal cortex. One gene that plays a critical role in adrenal development is that encoding steroidogenic factor 1 (SF-1). This protein and its effects are described in detail below under "Control of Adrenal Steroid Secretion." In brief, SF-1, a member of the nuclear hormone receptor family of zinc finger transcription factors, was first described as a regulator of the tissue-specific expression of P_{450} steroid hydroxylases and subsequently of 3β-hydroxysteroid dehydrogenase, the ACTH receptor, the steroidogenic acute regulatory protein (StAR), and Müllerian-inhibiting substance. SF-1 transcripts are present in the gonads and adrenals from the very earliest stages of development, suggesting that SF-1 plays a critical role in their differentiation. Besides the steroidogenic organs, SF-1 transcripts were detected in the anterior pituitary and hypothalamus. Collectively, these findings indicate that SF-1 regulates the expression of both hormones critical for male sexual differentiation (androgens and Müllerian-inhibiting substance) and also raise the possibility that SF-1 plays additional roles at other levels of the endocrine axis.[20]

A second transcription factor implicated in adrenal differentiation is *DAX-1*. *DAX-1* encodes an atypical member of the nuclear receptor family that retains the conserved ligand-binding domain but lacks the typical zinc finger DNA-binding motif,[21] suggesting that *DAX-1* regulates gene expression through protein-protein interactions. *DAX-1* was isolated initially by positional cloning of the gene responsible for X-linked adrenal hypoplasia congenita (AHC), a disorder in which patients present with ACTH-insensitive adrenal insufficiency due to impaired development of the definitive zone of the adrenal cortex. If kept alive with corticosteroids, most AHC patients later exhibit features of hypogonadotrophic hypogonadism, reflecting a mixed phenotype of hypothalamic and pituitary gonadotropin deficiencies. The association of impaired adrenal development and hypogonadotrophic hypogonadism somewhat resembles the phenotype in *SF-1* knockout mice, suggesting that *DAX-1* and *SF-1* also may act in the same developmental pathway. In support of this model, recent studies have shown that both genes are expressed in many of the same sites during embryogenesis, including the gonads, adrenal cortex, pituitary gonadotropes, and ventromedial hypothalamus,[22] and that *DAX-1* is stimulated by *SF-1*.[23]

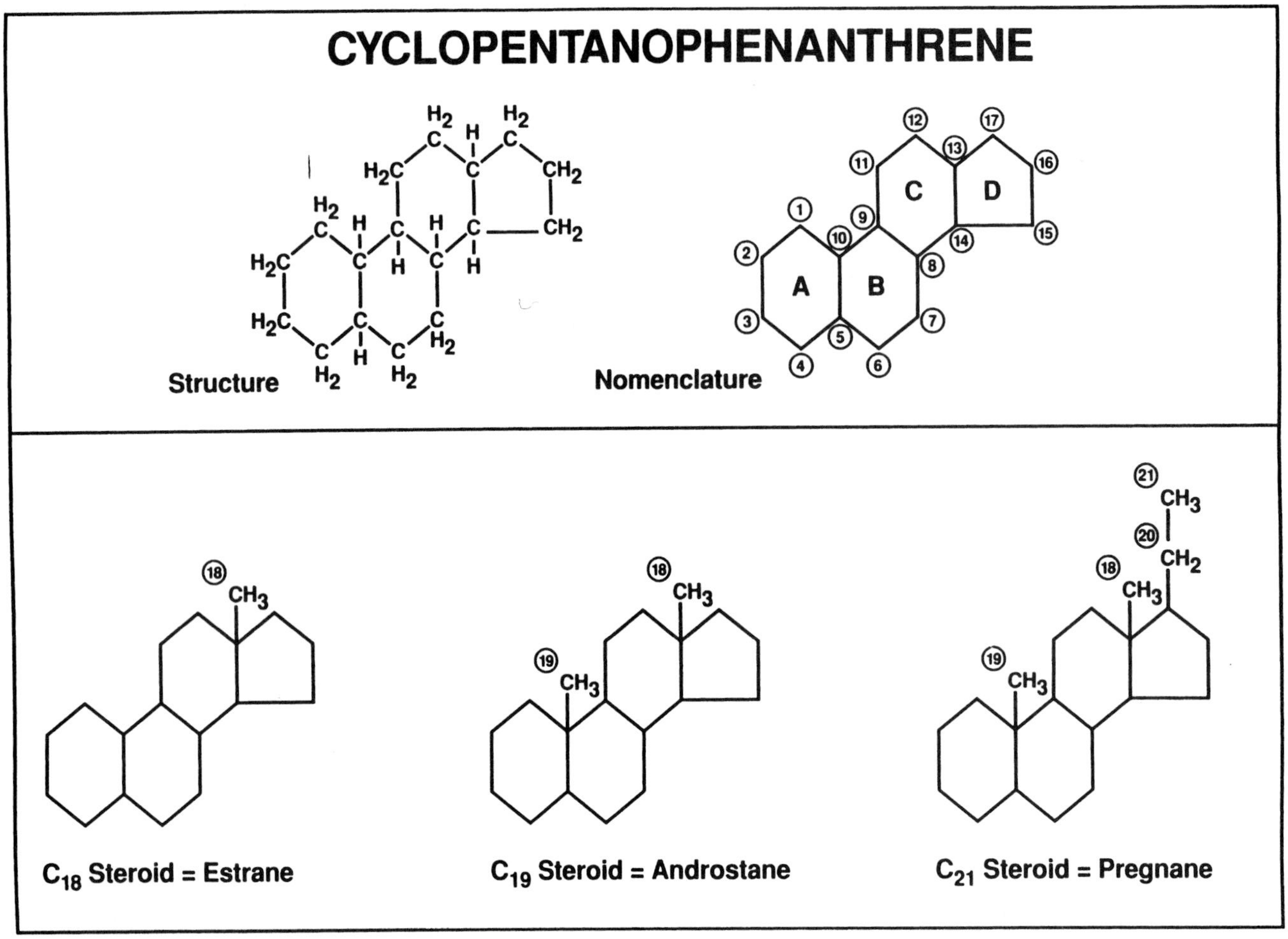

Fig. 159-2 Structure of cyclopentanophenanthrene and the numeration of its various carbons as used in the nomenclature of steroids. The lower panel shows the structure of the various types of steroids, specifically estrogen (C-18 steroid, estrane), androgens (C-19 steroid, androstane), and glucocorticoids and mineralocorticoids (C-21 steroid, pregnane). (*From Migeon and Donohoue.*[322] *Used by permission from Charles C Thomas Publishers.*)

Biochemical and Molecular Basis of Synthesis of Adrenal Steroids

All endogenous steroids are derived from cholesterol; they therefore have the same basic structural backbone, the cyclopentanophenanthrene structure (see Fig. 159-2 for a diagram of the basic steroid nucleus and numbering system). The bioactivity of each steroid hormone is determined by modifications of this basic nucleus that alter its affinity for specific receptors within target tissues. For example, C-21 (pregnane) derivatives can have progestational, glucocorticoid, or mineralocorticoid activities. Cleavage of the C-17 to C-20 bond in the C-21 steroids results in C-19 androstanes, which have androgenic activity. Finally, C-19 steroids can be converted to C-18 estrogens by aromatization of the A ring and removal of the C-19 methyl group, reactions that occur outside the adrenal cortex.

The stepwise conversion of cholesterol to corticosteroids requires the sequential action of a series of enzymes (Fig. 159-3); all but one are members of the cytochrome P_{450} superfamily of mixed-function oxidases. This diverse group of heme-containing proteins metabolizes a wide variety of exogenous and endogenous substrates.[24] Some P_{450} enzymes in the liver and lung can metabolize substances such as carcinogens and drugs. Endogenous compounds metabolized by P_{450} enzymes include steroid hormones, bile acids, prostaglandins, nitric oxide, and the various physiologic forms of vitamin D. Within adrenocortical cells, the steroidogenic cytochromes P_{450} are localized into either the mitochondria (class I enzymes) or the microsomes (endoplasmic reticulum) (class II enzymes) (Fig. 159-4). Besides differing in their locations within the cell, the steroidogenic cytochromes P_{450} use two distinct electron-transfer systems. The mitochondrial enzymes require both an iron-sulfur protein, adrenodoxin, and a flavoprotein, adrenodoxin reductase; in contrast, the microsomal enzymes use cytochrome P_{450} reductase (Fig. 159-5). Despite these differences, both mitochondrial and microsomal P_{450} enzymes acquire electrons from NADPH.

Certain structural features are common to all cytochromes P_{450} and thus are shared by all the steroidogenic cytochromes P_{450}. A highly conserved heme-binding region, which includes a cysteine that forms the fifth ligand with the heme iron, is located near the C-terminus.[25] Also conserved is a positively charged region centered over the heme-binding cysteine, which apparently is critical for interaction with the electron donor(s). In addition, all microsomal cytochromes P_{450} have a highly hydrophobic region of approximately 20 residues at their N-termini followed by a short cationic stretch; these hydrophobic regions play important roles in proper insertion and orientation of the protein in the membrane, whereas the cationic residues serve as a halt-transfer signal. As for the mitochondrial cytochromes P_{450}, they are targeted to the mitochondria by an N-terminal signal sequence of approximately 24 to 39 amino acids that is cleaved proteolytically on insertion into the mitochondrial membrane.[26] Outside these shared domains, the structures of the various steroidogenic cytochromes P_{450} diverge significantly. In particular, the substrate-recognition

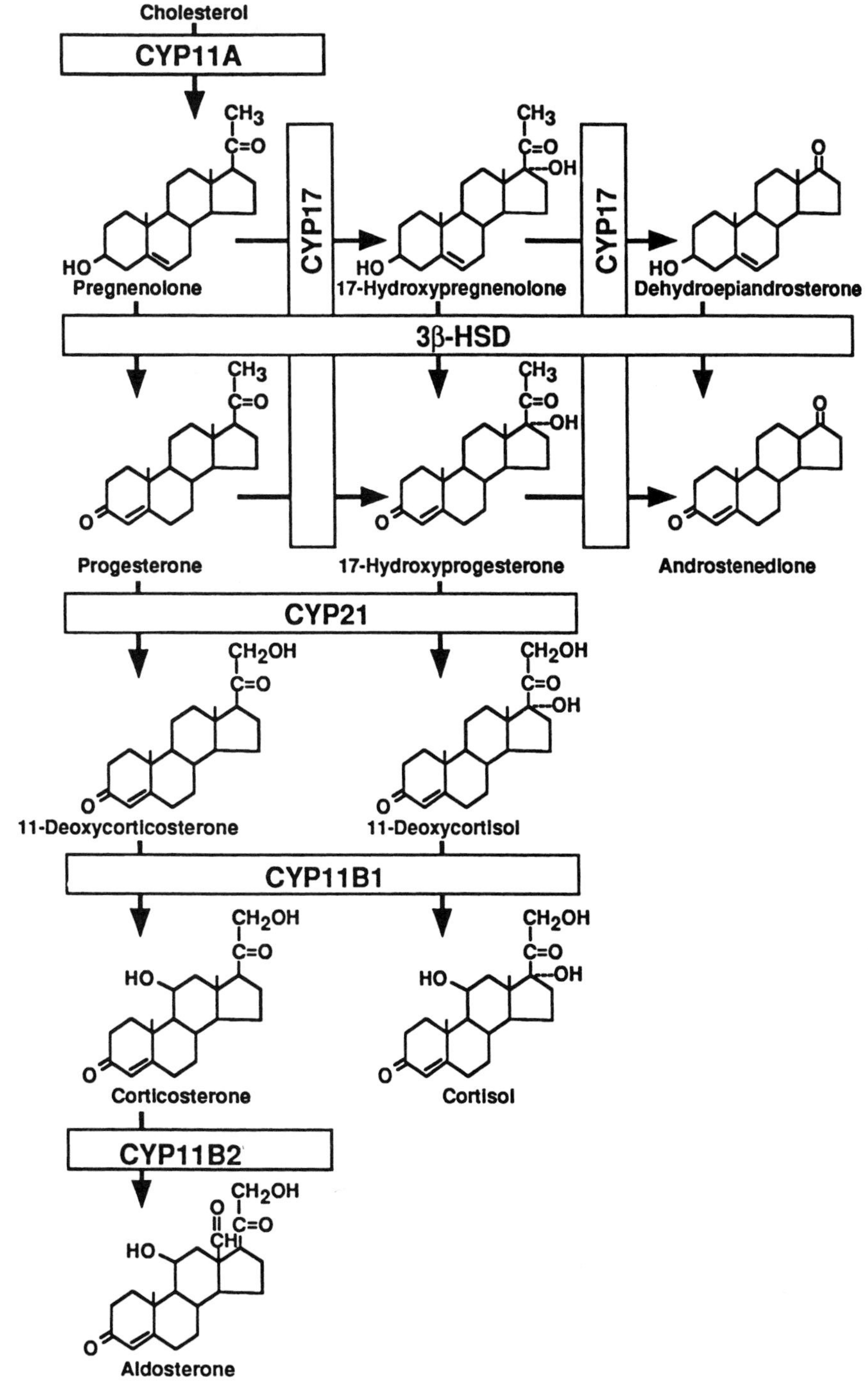

Fig. 159-3 Biosynthesis of adrenocortical steroids from cholesterol (the nomenclature for the various enzyme activities and their respective genes was outlined at the beginning of this chapter). The usual name of the various steroids and their biochemical names are as follows: pregnenolone = 3β-hydroxy-pregn-5-ene-20-one; 17-hydroxypregnenolone = 3β,17α-dihydroxy-pregn-5-ene-20-one; progesterone = pregn-4-ene-3,20-dione; 17-hydroxyprogesterone = 17α-hydroxy-pregn-4-ene-3,20-dione; 11-deoxycorticosterone = 21-hydroxy-pregn-4-ene-3,20-dione; 11-deoxycortisol = 17α,21-dihydroxy-pregn-4-ene-3,20-dione; corticosterone = 11β,21-dihydroxy-pregn-4-ene-3,20-dione; cortisol = 11β,17α,21-trihydroxy-pregn-4-ene-3,20-dione; aldosterone = 11β,21-dihydroxy-pregn-4-ene-3,18,20-trione; dehydroepiandrosterone = 3β-hydroxy-androst-5-ene-17-one; androstenedione = androst-4-ene-3,17-dione.

regions are extremely heterogeneous, suggesting that sequence alignments of various cytochromes P_{450} will not reliably predict substrate contact residues.[27]

A summary of the pathways of steroid hormone biosynthesis in the adrenal cortex is shown in Fig. 159-3. As discussed previously under "Anatomy, Histology, and Embryology of the Adrenal Gland," the adrenal cortex is divided anatomically and functionally into two discrete compartments — the outer zona glomerulosa, which makes mineralocorticoids, and the inner zonae fasciculata/reticularis, where glucocorticoid and androgen synthesis occur. Despite differences in steroid products and regulators, the enzymes that produce these steroid classes are quite similar, and the pathways will be described together where possible.

Conversion of Cholesterol to Pregnenolone. This initial step in adrenal steroidogenesis is mediated by the cholesterol side-chain cleavage enzyme CYP11A, which catalyzes the three distinct reactions that convert cholesterol to pregnenolone. These three reactions, 20α-hydroxylation, 22-hydroxylation, and cleavage of the cholesterol side chain at C-20 to C-22, are all performed at a single active site in the CYP11A molecule.[28] As a mitochondrial cytochrome P_{450}, CYP11A obtains electrons from adrenodoxin and adrenodoxin reductase. As expected for the initial step in the biosynthesis of all physiologic steroids, CYP11A is expressed in all primary steroidogenic tissues, including the adrenal cortex, ovary, testicular Leydig cells, and placenta.

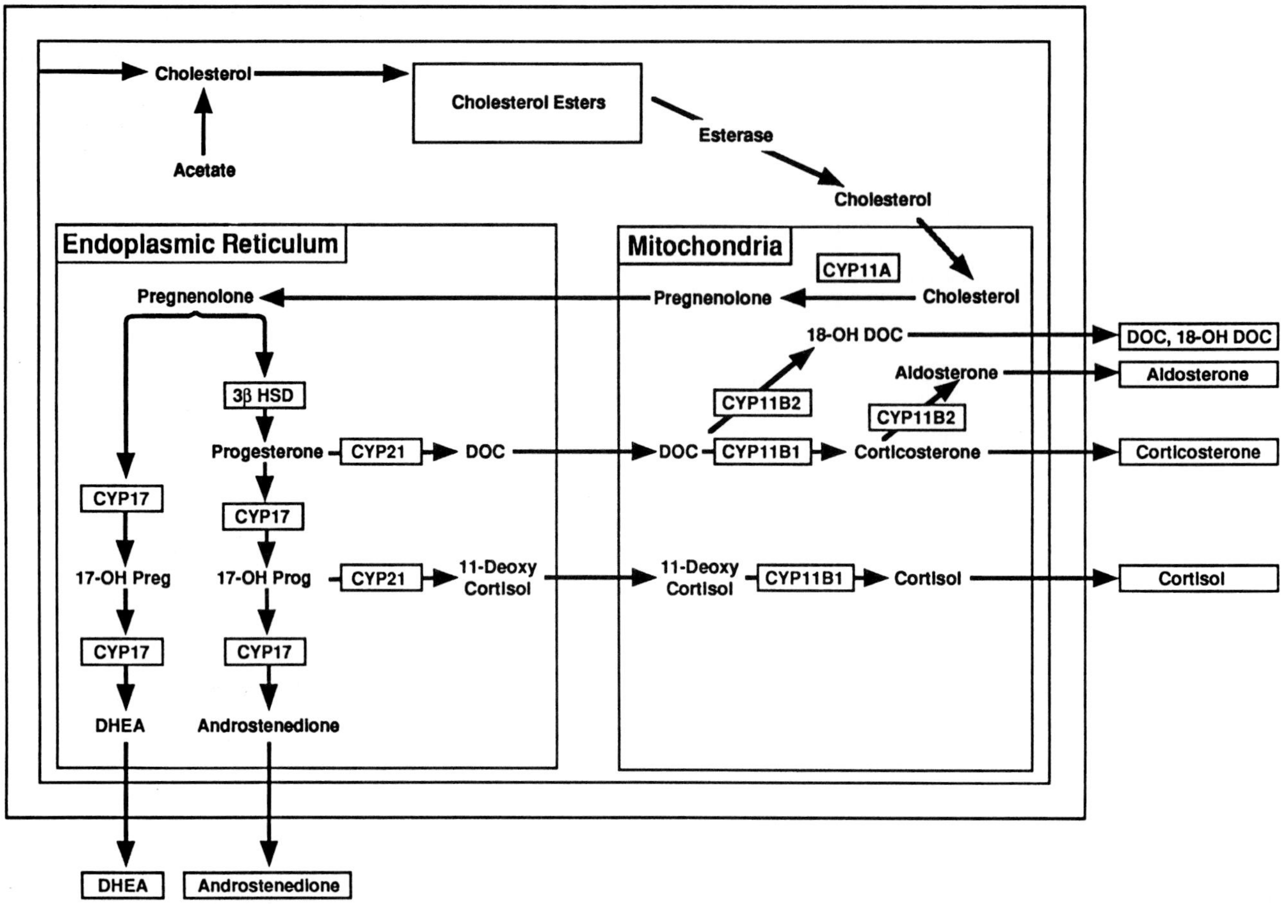

Fig. 159-4 Subcellular localization of the various enzymatic activities involved in the biosynthesis of adrenal steroids. As shown in the figure, mitochondria include the enzymatic activities related to the products of *CYP11A, CYP11B1,* and *CYP11B2.* The ER includes the rest of the other enzymatic activities. (*From Migeon and Donohoue.*[322] *Used by permission from Charles C Thomas Publishers.*)

3β-Hydroxysteroid Dehydrogenase. The enzyme 3β-hydroxysteroid dehydrogenase (3β-HSD) mediates the conversion of pregnenolone to progesterone, of 17-hydroxypregnenolone to 17-hydroxyprogesterone, and of dehydroepiandrosterone (DHEA) to androstenedione (see Fig. 159-3). This microsomal enzyme is the only steroidogenic enzyme that is not a cytochrome P_{450}. It uses a diphosphopyridine nucleotide cofactor and successively reduces the 3β-hydroxyl group to a 3-ketone and isomerizes the C-5,6 double bond to the C-3,4 position. These conversions are required for the production of glucocorticoids and mineralocorticoids, the two essential classes of corticosteroids, as well as for the production of adrenal androgens. The 3β-HSD activity is found not only in steroidogenic tissues (adrenal cortex, gonads, placenta) but also in breast, prostate, liver, and skin. As discussed below, distinct isozymes of 3β-HSD are expressed differentially in the various tissues, and one form (type II) is specifically required for adrenal and gonadal steroidogenesis.

17β-Hydroxylase and 17,20-Lyase Reactions. The enzymatic conversions of pregnenolone to 17-hydroxypregnenolone and of progesterone to 17-hydroxyprogesterone require hydroxylation at the 17β position. Thereafter, these intermediates can be converted by 17,20-lyase to DHEA and androstenedione, respectively. It has been shown conclusively that a single microsomal cytochrome P_{450}, steroid 17β-hydroxylase (CYP17), performs both these conversions. CYP17 is expressed in the inner zones of the adrenal cortex, where it participates in the formation of both glucocorticoids and adrenal androgens, but it is not expressed in the outer zona glomerulosa. In gonadal tissues, the same protein participates in the biosynthesis of androgens and estrogens.

21-Hydroxylase Reaction. Within the inner, glucocorticoid-producing zones, the conversion of 17-hydroxyprogesterone to 11-deoxycortisol is mediated by steroid 21-hydroxylase (CYP21). Steroid 21-hydroxylation was the first biologic function attributed to a cytochrome P_{450}.[29] CYP21 is located in adrenal microsomes and thus obtains electrons from cytochrome P_{450} reductase. Biochemical analyses have shown that 17-hydroxyprogesterone is the preferred substrate for this reaction. CYP21 also is required for the production of mineralocorticoids in the zona glomerulosa, converting progesterone to 11-deoxycorticosterone (DOC). Hydroxylation at C-21 is unique to corticosteroids, and CYP21 is expressed to a significant degree only in the adrenal cortex. As discussed in considerable detail below, a deficiency of CYP21 is the most common inherited disorder of steroid hormone biosynthesis.

Terminal Reactions in Corticosteroid Biosynthesis. The terminal reactions in the biosynthesis of both mineralocorticoids and glucocorticoids are catalyzed by two closely related mitochondrial enzymes—steroid 11β-hydroxylase, encoded by the *CYP11B1* gene, and aldosterone synthase, encoded by the *CYP11B2* gene. In the zona glomerulosa, aldosterone synthase performs successive 11β-hydroxylation, 18-hydroxylation (corticosterone methyloxidase type I, or CMO I), and 18-oxidation (CMO II) reactions to convert DOC to aldosterone (Fig. 159-6). In the inner zones, steroid 11β-hydroxylase performs only a single reaction, converting 11-deoxycortisol to cortisol.[30] The expression of these functionally distinct CYP11B isozymes in the appropriate cortical zones plays an essential role in the gland's ability to regulate separately the biosynthesis of mineralocorticoids and glucocorticoids.

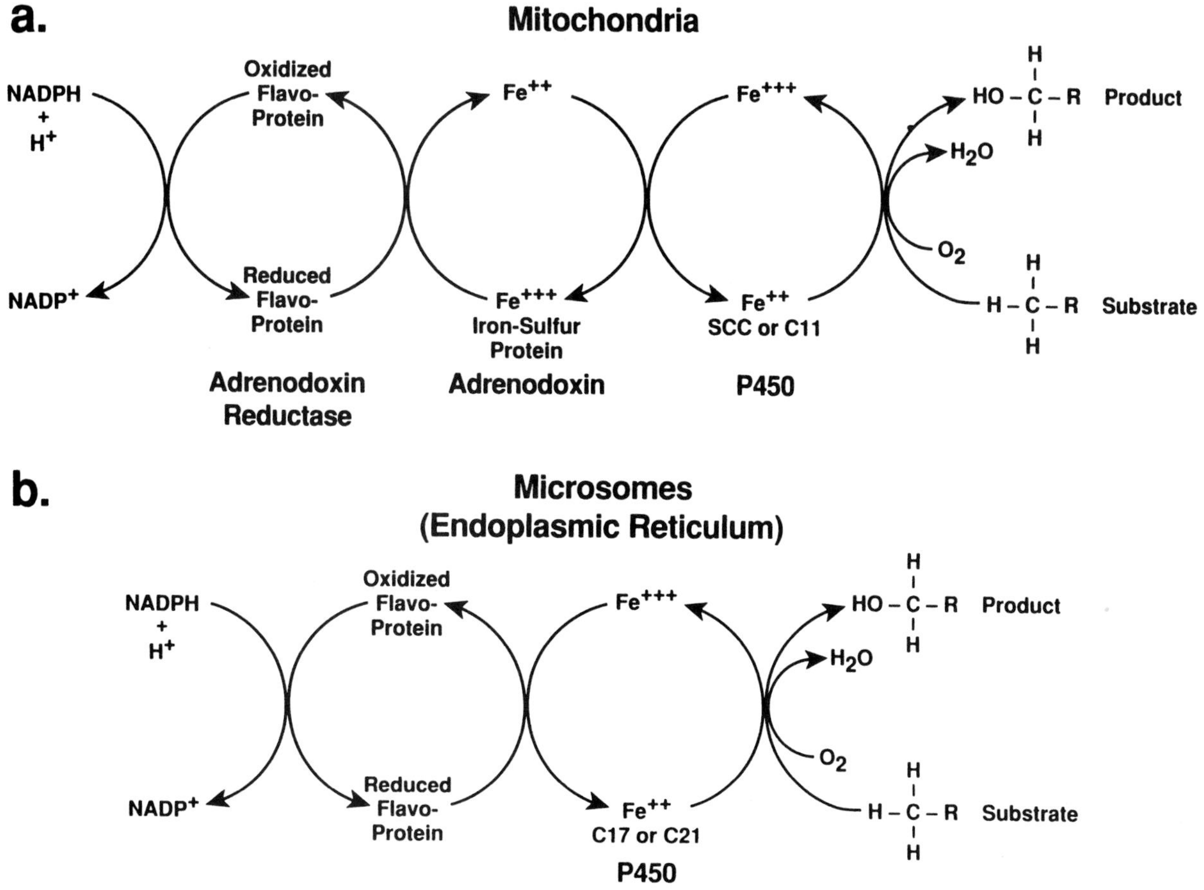

Fig. 159-5 Outline of the electron transport in mitochondria from NADPH to cytochrome P_{450} (*A*) and in the microsomes (*B*). (*From Migeon and Donohoue.*[322] *Used with permission from Charles C Thomas Publishers.*)

Control of Adrenal Steroid Secretion

In contrast to cells that secrete peptide or catecholamine hormones, steroidogenic cells do not contain intracellular reservoirs of preformed hormone. Moreover, steroids, once formed, are freely permeable to the cell membrane, and specific secretory processes have not been identified. Thus *de novo* production of steroids from cholesterol is of paramount importance in controlling steroid hormone concentrations. The regulation of steroidogenesis can be viewed at two separate levels. First, steroid hormone production is considered at the level of the organism, with emphasis on regulation by complex feedback loops involving other organs such as the hypothalamus, pituitary, and kidney. We then consider the specific biochemical events within adrenocortical cells that regulate steroidogenesis.

Steroid Production in the Intact Organism

Regulation of Cortisol Secretion by Adrenocorticotropic Hormone and Corticotropin-Releasing Hormone. It has been known for over 60 years that secretion of glucocorticoid by the adrenal cortex is controlled by pituitary ACTH,[31] a 39-amino-acid peptide.[32] The 1-24 N-terminal amino acid sequence of ACTH has the same steroidogenic stimulatory activity despite its slightly shorter half-life than the 7 to 12 min of the native peptide. ACTH is one of the proteolytic products of the preprohormone proopiomelanocortin (POMC). Several other fragments derive from the same POMC protein and are secreted in equimolar amounts,[33] but the physiologic importance of some of these peptides is unclear. It has been suggested that γ-melanocyte-stimulating hormone (γ-MSH), one of these POMC fragments, stimulates aldosterone production.[34] Other POMC cleavage products include α-MSH and β-endorphin.

ACTH and cortisone became available for therapeutic purposes in 1949–1950. Since ACTH was more abundant in supply than cortisone, many of the therapeutic effects of cortisone were first revealed by the use of ACTH. In 1948, it was demonstrated that the secretion of pituitary hormones is controlled by the central nervous system[35]; soon thereafter the critical role of the hypothalamus in this system was established. In 1955, it was shown conclusively that a hypothalamic factor, the corticotropin-releasing hormone (CRH), increases ACTH secretion.[36,37] More than 25 years later, CRH was characterized as a 41-amino-acid peptide.[38] Subsequent studies showed that most mammals secrete CRH; rat CRH is similar to that of both humans and sheep, whereas goat CRH differs from human CRH by 7 amino acids.[39] Circulating CRH is bound to some degree by a specific CRH-binding protein, which is unusual for neuropeptides.[40]

CRH production is located mainly in the paraventricular nuclei of the hypothalamic median eminence.[41] Lesser amounts of CRH have been detected in the cerebral cortex, brain stem, and spinal cord. It is also present in nonneural tissues such as liver, pancreas, and placenta. The concentration of CRH in cerebrospinal fluid is several times higher than that observed in peripheral blood.

CRH secretion is modulated by glucocorticoids, sex steroids, stress, adrenergic agents, and aging, as well as by peptides of the immune system.[42,43] CRH exerts its effects by interaction with type I or type II CRH receptors.[44] The type I receptors on anterior pituitary corticotrophs mediate ACTH release through increases in intracellular cAMP and calcium levels. These in turn activate a series of protein kinases that eventually result in increased transcription of the POMC gene and the processing of its mRNA. The stimulation of POMC gene transcription is mediated by a number of transcription factors, including c-fos and NGFI-B.[45,46] CRH is the major factor controlling ACTH secretion, but

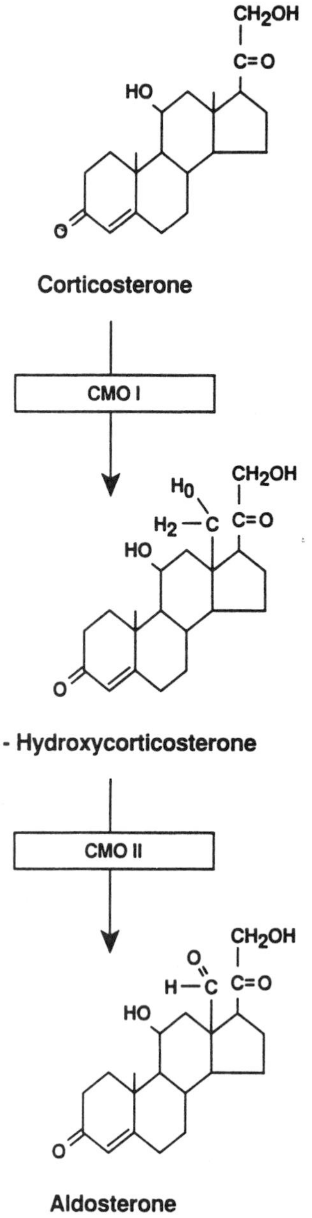

Fig. 159-6 Biosynthesis of aldosterone from corticosterone. Aldosterone synthase is encoded by *CYP11B2* and has three distinct enzymatic activities. In addition to the 11β-hydroxylation of 11-deoxycorticosterone to corticosterone in the zona glomerulosa, it performs activities termed *corticosterone methyloxidase type I* (CMO I) and *cortiscosterone methyloxidase type II* (CMO II). CMO I activity results in the formation of 18-hydroxycorticosterone, and CMO II activity results in aldosterone. (*From Migeon and Donohoue.*[322] *Used by permission from Charles C Thomas Publishers.*)

other substances also modulate ACTH secretion. Arginine vasopressin (AVP) is a weak secretagogue by itself, but it markedly potentiates the effect of CRH on ACTH secretion by corticotrophs. Stressful conditions such as insulin-induced hypoglycemia and pyrogen-induced fever appear to act directly on ACTH secretion.[47] The factors that control basal and stress-induced CRH release are complex, and CRH effects are widespread.[48] Evidence has suggested that noradrenergic input to CRH/AVP cells mediates the increased CRH and AVP release in response to acute stress, and chronic stress alters this noradrenergic input in ways that may facilitate long-term maintenance of the stress response. Serotonin appears to play a stimulatory role in CRH secretion. Cyproheptadine, a serotonin antagonist, partially blocks ACTH secretion and is used therapeutically for this purpose in patients with Cushing disease.

In normal individuals, ACTH is secreted episodically, with an average of 8 to 10 bursts per day; these bursts are most frequent just prior to awakening and correlate with peak serum cortisol levels, which occur in the early morning. Because of this episodic release, single serum levels of ACTH or cortisol, even if obtained in the morning when bursts are most frequent, may not accurately reflect activity of the hypothalamic-pituitary-adrenal axis.

ACTH increases steroidogenesis by stimulating the activity of CYP11A (P_{450scc}), which mediates the first and rate-limiting step of cortisol synthesis. The enzymatic activities of the other steroidogenic enzymes are increased by ACTH in cell culture.[49] Chronic stimulation by endogenous or exogenous ACTH eventually results in hyperplasia of adrenocortical tissue, including adrenal rests. These rests are generally anatomically inconsequential, but in CAH, chronic stimulation by ACTH causes enlargement of adrenal rests that may raise concerns about possible testicular tumors. In one such case, studies of nodular adrenocortical tissue within the testes of a patient with 21-hydroxylase deficiency showed that they were responsive to ACTH stimulation. *In vitro* studies of these cells demonstrated the presence of angiotensin II receptors and undetectable 21-hydroxylase activity.[50] The CRH-ACTH axis is involved in other activities in addition to its major role in stimulation of adrenal steroidogenesis. These are varied and include control of feeding behavior through interaction with the leptin system.[51–54]

In summary, three major factors influence the rate of production of glucocorticoids—stress, diurnal rhythm, and negative feedback inhibition by glucocorticoids. Negative feedback by excess glucocorticoids inhibits ACTH secretion and abolishes diurnal rhythm. In contrast, stress increases ACTH levels and thus glucocorticoid production, even in the presence of high levels of glucocorticoids. High-affinity glucocorticoid receptors in both pituitary corticotrophs and specific neurons of the hypothalamus are believed to play major roles in this negative feedback inhibition.

Control of Aldosterone Secretion by the Renin-Angiotensin System. An appreciation of the relationship between renin-angiotensin and aldosterone secretion emerged from research in a variety of disciplines, including cardiology, nephrology, and endocrinology.[2,6,55–59] As a result of these studies, it now is clear that the major regulator of mineralocorticoid biosynthesis is the renin-angiotensin system (Fig. 159-7). In response to changes in volume and electrolyte concentrations, the juxtaglomerular cells of the kidney release renin, a proteolytic enzyme that cleaves angiotensinogen produced by the liver to form angiotensin I. Thereafter, angiotensin-converting enzyme, which is most abundant in vascular endothelial cells of the pulmonary system, cleaves the C-terminal dipeptide from angiotensin I to produce angiotensin II. This cleavage converts angiotensin I, a mild vasopressor, into angiotensin II, a potent vasoconstrictor that also increases the secretion of aldosterone by the adrenal cortex. Three factors regulate the rate of renin release by the juxtaglomerular cells—renal baroreceptors, adrenergic innervation, and circulating ion concentrations. The renal baroreceptors monitor renal perfusion pressure; any decrease in pressure—whether related to decreased cardiac output, hypovolemia, or decreased peripheral resistance—induces the secretion of renin. Factors that increase sympathetic tone, such as hypotension or pain, also increase renin release through stimulation of β-adrenergic receptors on juxtaglomerular cells. Finally, changes in the filtered load of sodium within the renal tubule are sensed by the macula densa, which then alters juxtaglomerular renin release. Renin secretion is reduced indirectly by the effects of aldosterone on fluid and electrolyte balance. Thus an increase in aldosterone stimulates sodium and water retention by the kidney, thereby increasing blood volume. The stretching of the renal arterioles then results in decreased secretion of renin.

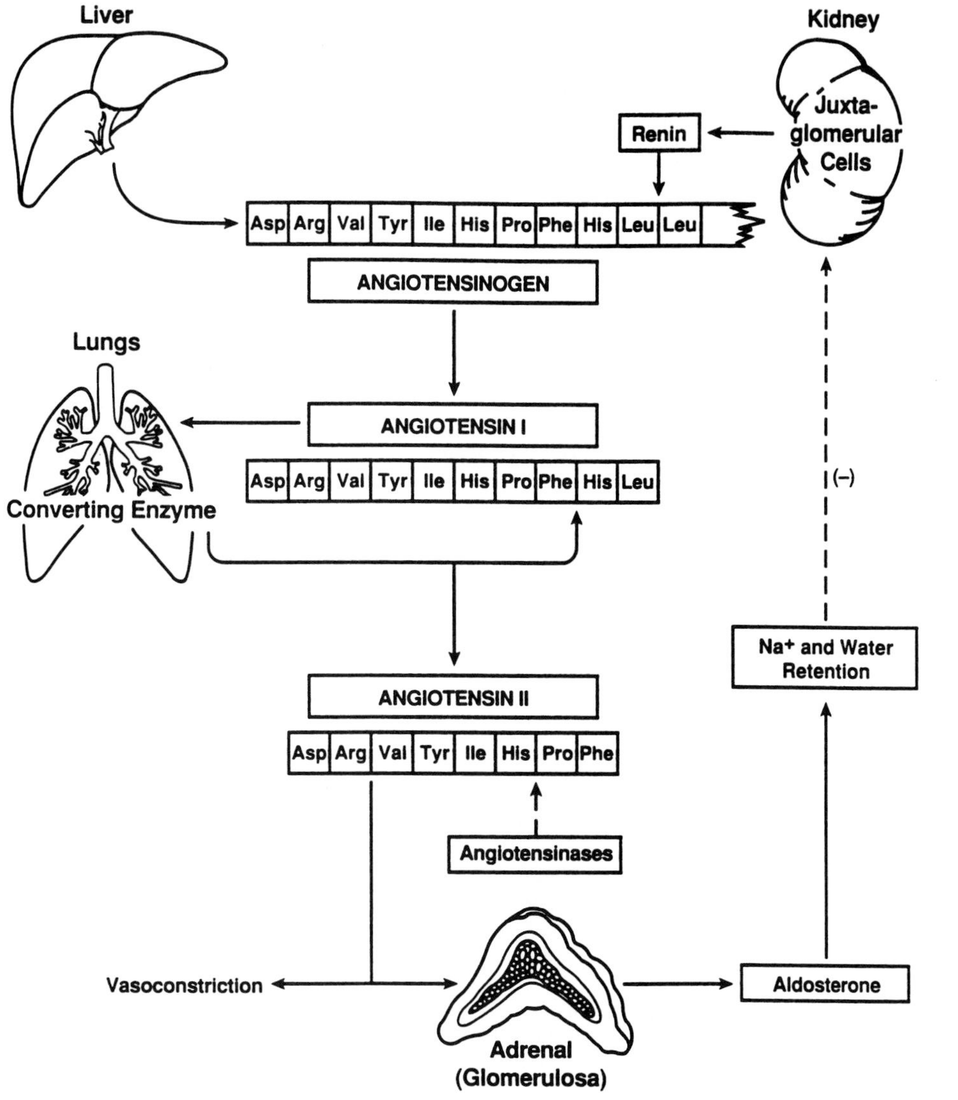

Fig. 159-7 The renin-angiotensin-aldosterone system. Renin produced by the kidney hydrolyzes angiotensinogen secreted by the liver into a decapeptide, angiotensin I. Under the effects of a converting enzyme in the lungs, angiotensin I is transformed into an octapeptide, angiotensin II. In itself, angiotensin II has vasoconstrictive properties, but it also binds to a membrane receptor of the cells of the zona glomerulosa of the adrenal cortex in order to activate the secretion of aldosterone. (*From Migeon and Donohoue.*[322] *Used by permission from Charles C Thomas.*)

Hyperkalemia directly stimulates aldosterone production, whereas hypokalemia markedly impairs the response of glomerulosa cells to angiotensin II. Studies with anephric patients and with isolated adrenocortical cells have confirmed that potassium affects mineralocorticoid production directly rather than through the renin-angiotensin system.[60,61] The precise mechanisms for potassium effects are unknown, but changes in K^+ levels affect the membrane potential of glomerulosa cells and presumably alter the activity of voltage-dependent Ca^{2+} channels.

In contrast, atrial natriuretic factor (ANF) potently inhibits both basal and angiotensin II-induced aldosterone production.[62] After binding to specific membrane receptors, ANF increases intracellular cGMP levels; this increase in cGMP is probably involved in the mechanism by which ANF inhibits aldosterone production.

Acutely, ACTH also directly stimulates aldosterone secretion. Bolus IV injection of 1-24 ACTH (Cortrosyn) rapidly increases plasma aldosterone levels.[63] On the other hand, although prolonged treatment with ACTH leads to a sustained increase in cortisol levels, there is a progressive fall in aldosterone concentrations. Furthermore, aldosterone secretion is maintained in hypopituitary patients receiving glucocorticoid replacement, indicating that ACTH is not necessary for this regulation (Fig. 159-8).

Control of Secretion of Adrenal Androgens. Although the essential adrenocorticosteroids are the mineralocorticoids and glucocorticoids, the human adrenal cortex also produces androgens. The predominant adrenal androgens are DHEA and androstenedione, as well as the sulfated conjugate of DHEA, DHEA-S. Of interest, the first two androgens isolated in human peripheral blood were DHEA and androsterone.[64,65] Both were present as sulfated conjugates, and both arose predominantly from the adrenal cortex. Although DHEA-S has the highest concentration of any steroid in human peripheral blood, largely because of its markedly prolonged half-life, its biologic effects remain unclear. These adrenal androgens require the action of CYP17, which is expressed only in the inner zones of the adrenal cortex; hence adrenal androgens are exclusively produced in the zonae fasciculata/reticularis.

Clinical observations have demonstrated that the secretion of glucocorticoids and androgens is not tightly coupled. Plasma levels of androgens are virtually undetectable during childhood, increasing markedly at puberty without any change in ACTH or cortisol secretion rates. With early aging (after 30 to 40 years of age), the levels of adrenal androgens decline significantly, whereas cortisol secretion relative to body size remains fairly constant throughout the human life cycle. In premature adrenarche, during which time adrenal androgens reach adult concentrations abnormally early and produce androgenic effects, the cortisol secretion remains normal for size.

This dissociated secretion of glucocorticoids and adrenal androgens has led to the proposal that extra-adrenal factors

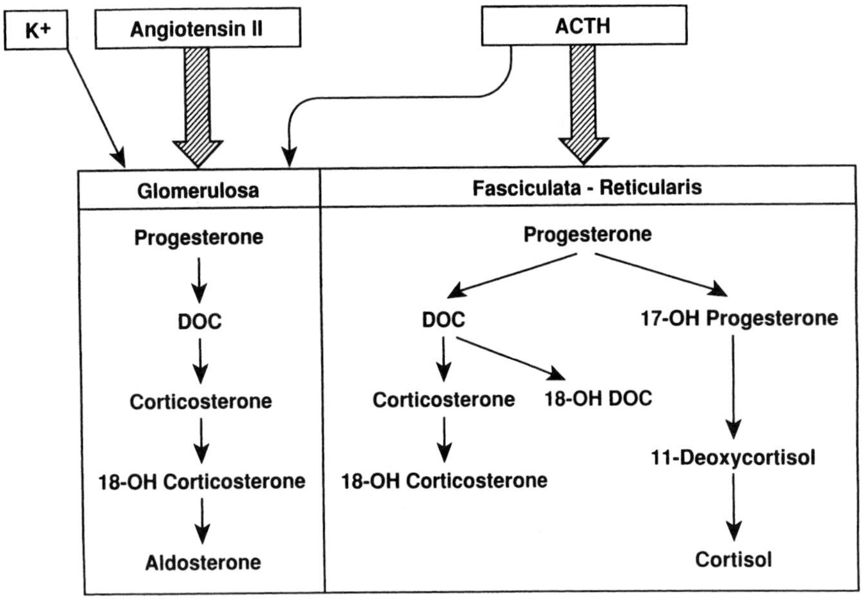

Fig. 159-8 Regulation of the secretion of glucocorticoids and mineralocorticoids. ACTH acts mainly on the zonae fasciculata/reticularis by increasing the production of cortisol and corticosterone. It also transiently increases the secretion of aldosterone by the glomerulosa. The major inducers of mineralocorticoid secretion are angiotensin II and the serum concentration of potassium. *(From Migeon and Donohoue.[322] Used by permission from Charles C Thomas Publishers.)*

modulate the production of adrenal androgens.[66] Cultured human adrenocortical tumor cells (NCI-H295) independently produce either cortisol or androgens depending upon the type of hormonal stimulation.[67] In these cells, ACTH preferentially stimulates cortisol production, whereas Forskolin stimulates androstenedione production. Although a provocative report attributed androgen stimulation to a joining peptide comprising amino acids 79 to 96 of POMC, [68] other studies have refuted this observation.[69,70] The existence of a pituitary regulator of adrenal androgen production thus remains unresolved. Other studies have focused on the effect of cytochrome P_{450} reductase to modulate the ratio of 17β-hydroxylase and 17,20-lyase activities with purified protein[71] or in transfection studies[72]; it is therefore possible that variations in the relative activities reflect accessibility of cofactors.[73]

Control at the Cellular Level. Temporally, trophic hormones stimulate steroidogenesis biphasically. The acute response occurs within seconds to minutes and largely reflects increased delivery of cholesterol substrate to the mitochondria, where CYP11A carries out the initial rate-limiting reaction.[74] The chronic phase, in contrast, requires hours to days and largely reflects increased transcription of the cytochrome P_{450} steroid hydroxylases and other components of the steroidogenic apparatus.

Acute Response. The primary event in the acute response to trophic hormones is the translocation of cholesterol to the inner mitochondrial membrane, where CYP11A carries out the initial step in steroidogenesis. As shown in Fig. 159-4, this cholesterol comes from a number of sources, including endocytotic uptake and degradation of circulating lipoproteins by the low-density lipoprotein (LDL) receptor, *de novo* synthesis of cholesterol from acetate, and cleavage of cholesterol esters by cholesterol ester hydrolase. Regardless of the source of cholesterol, trophic hormones apparently act by increasing its delivery to CYP11A. This translocation system is induced by cAMP, the second messenger for most actions of ACTH, and requires ongoing protein synthesis, suggesting that a labile protein mediates the stimulation. Studies have implicated specialized contact sites in the mitochondrial membrane in these events.[75]

A number of candidates have been proposed as the labile factor that activates steroidogenesis. Recent studies have shown that the mitochondrial phosphoprotein StAR plays essential roles in this acute steroidogenic response.[76] StAR was identified initially as a structurally related group of mitochondrial phosphoproteins, designated pp37 and pp30, found only in steroidogenic cells. These proteins have the short half-life predicted for the labile mediator and are phosphorylated in response to trophic hormones.[77,78] A considerable breakthrough came with the cloning of a cDNA encoding StAR.[79] StAR is expressed specifically in steroidogenic cells of the adrenal glands and gonads, and the onset of its expression during development correlates with steroidogenic capacity. Perhaps most significantly, as described below, mutations in StAR have been identified in patients with congenital lipoid adrenal hyperplasia (lipoid CAH), proving definitively that StAR is required for steroidogenesis. Although these studies have established that StAR is essential, the mechanisms by which it acts remain unknown. Expression studies and analyses of patients with lipoid CAH have shown that the C-terminal region is required for steroidogenesis, but it is unclear if StAR binds cholesterol directly or instead interacts with other proteins to facilitate cholesterol delivery to CYP11A. Moreover, StAR is not expressed in the placenta and probably not to a significant degree in the ovary, suggesting that it is not essential for cholesterol delivery in this site[80–83] and thus is not the sole peptide with this function.

The peripheral benzodiazepine receptor (PBR), a widely expressed mitochondrial protein, and its endogenous ligand diazepam-binding inhibitor (DBI) also have been implicated in the acute steroidogenic response.[84] Several lines of evidence support a role of DBI and the PBR in steroidogenesis. Initially isolated as an activator of steroidogenesis, DBI subsequently was found to be closely related to the brain protein endozepine when its primary structure was determined. When added to isolated mitochondria, DBI stimulates the conversion of cholesterol to pregnenolone in a dose-dependent manner and augments cholesterol transfer to inner membrane sites. In addition, various benzodiazepine agonists activate steroidogenesis with a rank order that correlates with their affinity for the PBR.[85] Finally, inactivation of DBI by treating steroidogenic cells with antisense oligonucleotides[86] or of PBR by targeted gene disruption[87] markedly impairs steroidogenesis. Thus these data suggest that PBR contributes to the acute induction of steroidogenesis in response to trophic hormones. It is probable that the acute steroidogenic response involves a number of regulators that act cooperatively to bring about the full response.

Chronic Response. The chronic response of steroidogenic cells to trophic hormones largely reflects increased transcription of the steroid hydroxylases. With the availability of cloned genes encoding the steroidogenic enzymes, a number of laboratories have studied the molecular mechanisms that regulate their transcription. These studies have addressed two major levels of gene regulation: cell-selective and hormonally induced expression. Although not yet complete, intriguing insights into these mechanisms are emerging.

One important aspect of the gene regulation of the steroidogenic cytochromes P_{450} is their cell specificity, exhibiting distinct but overlapping patterns of expression. CYP11A is expressed in all classic steroidogenic tissues (adrenal cortex, testicular Leydig cells, ovarian theca cells, and placenta). CYP17 likewise is expressed in multiple steroidogenic tissues. In contrast, CYP21, CYP11B1, and CYP11B2 are expressed only in the adrenal cortex, with the latter two enzymes displaying zone-specific expression. These overlapping profiles of expression suggested that certain promoter elements coordinately regulate adrenocortical expression of the steroid hydroxylases, whereas other elements direct expression of CYP11A and CYP17 in nonadrenal tissues.

One essential regulator of the steroidogenic enzymes is SF-1. As described earlier under "Embryology," SF-1 first was described as an important regulator of the tissue-specific expression of the cytochrome P_{450} steroid hydroxylases.[88] Thereafter, the isolation of an SF-1 cDNA showed that this critical regulator of the steroidogenic enzymes belonged to the nuclear hormone receptor family of zinc finger transcription factors that mediate transcriptional activation by steroid hormones, thyroid hormone, vitamin D, and retinoids.[89,90] Following its initial isolation and characterization, a number of groups have shown that SF-1 regulates adrenal and gonadal expression of multiple genes that are required for steroidogenesis, including the steroid hydroxylases, 3β-HSD, the ACTH receptor, and StAR.[20,91] Analyses in transfected Sertoli cells and transgenic mice further have implicated SF-1 as an important regulator of the gene encoding the Müllerian-inhibiting substance.[92,93] Besides the steroidogenic organs, SF-1 transcripts were detected in the anterior pituitary and hypothalamus.[94] Thus SF-1 regulates hormones that are critical for male sexual differentiation and possibly plays additional roles at other levels of the endocrine axis.[95]

Production of mice with targeted disruption of the *SF-1* gene confirmed that this transcription factor plays key roles at all three levels of the hypothalamic-pituitary-steroidogenic organ axis. Strikingly, these *SF-1* knockout mice lacked adrenal glands and gonads, undergoing loss of the primordial organs via programmed cell death precisely when gonadal events in sexual differentiation normally occur (Fig. 159-9). These findings demonstrate unequivocally that SF-1 has essential roles in the early development of both adrenal and gonadal precursors. In keeping with the loss of the testes at relatively early developmental stages-before androgens and Müllerian Inhibiting Substance (MIS) are produced-*SF-1* knockout mice have male-to-female sex reversal of both their internal and external genitalia.[96] They also have impaired expression of a number of markers of the differentiated phenotype of pituitary gonadotropes, the pituitary cell type that secretes gonadotropins and regulates gonadal steroidogenesis.[97] Finally, they lack the ventromedial hypothalamic nucleus, a medial hypothalamic nucleus implicated in ingestive and reproductive behaviors.[98]

These findings in mice, which reveal multiple essential roles of SF-1 in endocrine development and function, raised the possibility that *SF-1* mutations are associated with human genetic disorders. The human gene encoding SF-1 maps to chromosome 9q33,[99] and shares extensive homology with its mouse counterpart and is expressed in many of the same sites, suggesting that SF-1 functions in humans as it does in mice. A patient with a female phenotype, 46 XY karyotype, and neonatal adrenal insufficiency has been identified as having a heterozygous *SF-1* mutation.[99a] The phenotype is less severe than that of the SF-1 null mouse.

The second major level of regulation of the steroid hydroxylases is their response to trophic hormones. As noted earlier, the induction of steroid hydroxylase gene transcription is an essential

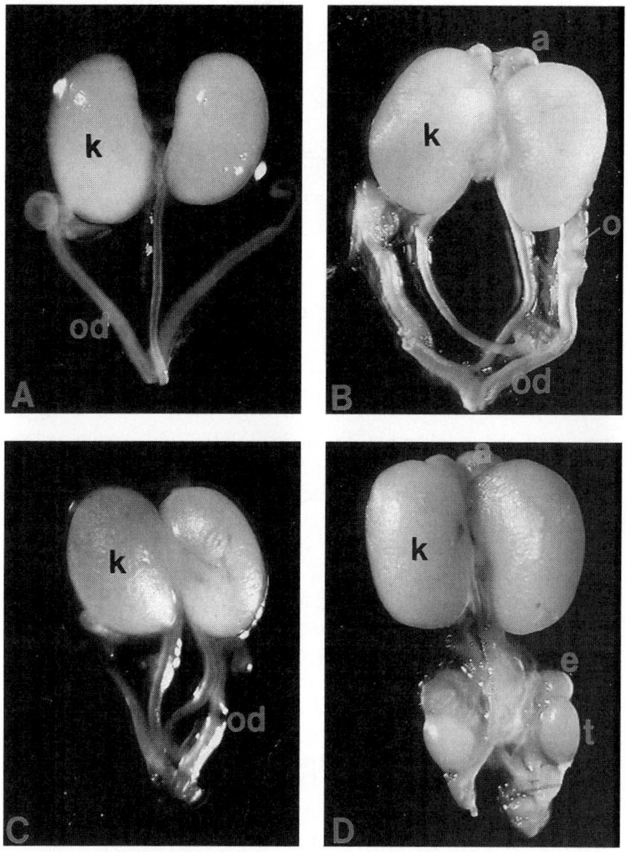

Fig. 159-9 Newborn *SF-1* knockout mice lack adrenal glands and gonads and have female internal genitalia. *SF-1* knockout pups and wild-type littermates were sacrificed, and the genitourinary tracts were isolated by dissection. *A. SF-1* knockout female. *B.* Wild-type female. *C. SF-1* knockout male. *D.* Wild-type male. The scale bar equals 1 mm. Abbreviations: *k,* kidney; *a,* adrenal; *o,* ovary; *t,* testis; *e,* epididymis; *od,* oviduct. (*Reprinted with permission from Luo et al.*[323])

component of the chronic response to trophic hormones, and identifying the underlying mechanisms remains an important goal. Several different promoter elements and transcriptional regulators have been proposed to confer responsiveness to trophic hormones, and it appears probable that several systems contribute to this induction. Among candidates are the cAMP-responsive element binding protein (CREB), the general transcription factor Sp1,[100] the orphan nuclear receptors NGFI-B[101] and SF-1, and c-fos.[102] Further studies are needed to ascertain the precise roles that these regulators play in mediating the induction by trophic hormone.

Metabolism and Action of Adrenocortical Hormones

Glucocorticoids

Metabolism. Cortisol, the major circulating glucocorticoid, is more than 90 percent protein bound in blood. Seventy percent is bound avidly to a specific glycosylated α-globulin known as *transcortin* or *corticosteroid-binding globulin (CBG),* and a smaller portion is bound less avidly to albumin. Transcortin also has a high affinity for progesterone and is capable of binding prednisolone and aldosterone but not dexamethasone.[103] Approximately 8 percent of the total circulating cortisol is free and biologically active.

The metabolism of glucocorticoids and of all steroid hormones occurs mostly in the liver. A number of different enzymes are involved in the conversion of glucocorticoids into inactive metabolites that then are excreted in urine or bile. Therefore, these metabolizing enzymes have not received much attention, probably because they generate inactive products. The predominant inactive products include tetrahydrocortisol and tetrahydrocortisone, which

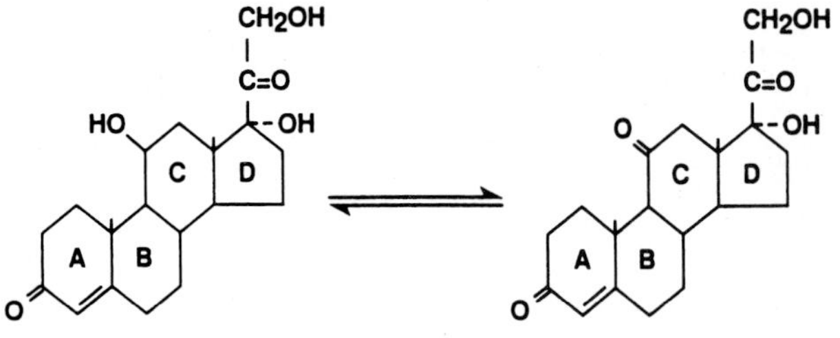

Fig. 159-10 Interconversion of cortisol and cortisone by 11β-hydroxysteroid dehydrogenase.

then undergo conversion to more soluble glucuronidated or sulfated compounds. These steroids then enter the circulation or are excreted into the bile. Glucocorticoids and their metabolites and conjugates are excreted mainly by the kidney (approximately 90 percent), and the remainder are excreted in the intestine. The kidney also converts cortisol to cortisone, as described in more detail later. The excreted steroids are mainly conjugated. The tetrahydro metabolites are measured as urinary 17-hydroxycorticosteroids by the Porter-Silber reaction. The urinary 17-hydroxycorticosteroids measured by this method represent one-third of the urinary metabolites of cortisol.[104]

One steroid-metabolizing enzyme that has been studied extensively is 11β-hydroxysteroid dehydrogenase (11β-HSD). This enzyme interconverts cortisol, a potent glucocorticoid, and its 11-keto derivative cortisone, which lacks biologic activity (Fig. 159-10). Several different roles for this enzyme in maintaining steroid hormone homeostasis have been proposed. *In utero*, placental 11β-HSD is proposed to protect the fetus from potentially deleterious effects of large amounts of maternal cortisol. A second role derives from the demonstration that the mineralocorticoid receptor binds glucocorticoids and mineralocorticoids with comparable affinities.[105] To explain the specific action of small quantities of mineralocorticoids in the face of vast excesses of glucocorticoids, it was proposed that 11β-HSD protects the mineralocorticoid receptor by converting glucocorticoids to inactive derivatives.[106] As discussed later in this chapter, a clinical abnormality of fluid and electrolyte handling in human patients strikingly supports such a role: the syndrome of apparent mineralocorticoid excess (AME).

Action. Glucocorticoid actions are mediated by the interaction of steroid hormones with the glucocorticoid receptor. The term *glucocorticoid* is derived from its effects on carbohydrate metabolism — mainly production and storage of glucose. Cortisol inhibits cellular glucose uptake and utilization. Amino acids from muscle and free fatty acids from adipocytes are mobilized, providing increased substrates for gluconeogenesis. In addition to this increased substrate supply, gluconeogenesis is increased through induction of the gluconeogenic enzymes. The breakdown of proteins causes increased urinary nitrogen excretion and induction of urea cycle enzymes. Glycogen synthesis is also stimulated.

At supraphysiologic concentrations, such as when used pharmacologically or in patients with Cushing disease, glucocorticoid effects are widespread and include anti-inflammatory and immunosuppressive actions, retardation of wound healing, interference with linear growth, inhibition of vitamin D-mediated intestinal calcium absorption, psychiatric disturbances (depression, psychosis), and fluid and electrolyte abnormalities that may be mediated by the mineralocorticoid receptor.

Mineralocorticoids

Metabolism. The major circulating mineralocorticoid is aldosterone, with DOC having some mineralocorticoid activity. Aldosterone binds to transcortin with 10 percent of the affinity of cortisol. By contrast, DOC and corticosterone bind transcortin with affinities of 50 and 100 percent, respectively, relative to cortisol.[104] Essentially all the aldosterone entering the hepatic circulation is catabolized by the liver. The primary metabolites, tetrahydroaldosterone and aldosterone-18-glucuronide, are excreted in the urine.

Action. Mineralocorticoid actions are mediated by the interaction of steroid hormones with the mineralocorticoid receptor. Mineralocorticoids, as the name implies, control the excretion of electrolytes, mainly in the kidney, but also in the colon and sweat glands. Aldosterone enhances the reabsorption of sodium in the cortical collecting duct. This effect is accompanied by chloride and water retention, resulting in expansion of extracellular volume. Aldosterone also enhances the excretion of hydrogen and potassium ions from the medullary collecting duct. The increased potassium excretion depends on adequate sodium intake.

Excess mineralocorticoid causes hypokalemia, metabolic alkalosis, and hypertension. These effects are seen most frequently in primary hyperaldosteronism, mineralocorticoid-secreting tumors, and glucocorticoid-remediable aldosteronism (see "Glucocorticoid-Remediable Aldosteronism" below).

Androgens

Metabolism. Circulating androstenedione and DHEA are bound to sex hormone-binding globulin (SHBG) to a much greater degree than to transcortin. Binding of androstenedione and DHEA, on the other hand, is of lower affinity than the binding of testosterone and dihydrotestosterone, the biologically active androgens. A portion of circulating adrenal androgens is metabolized in the liver, but a significant degree of production and interconversion of the sex steroids also occurs in the gonads, skin, and adipose tissue. The major metabolite of DHEA is DHEA-S, which is produced rapidly in the liver and in the adrenal cortex. DHEA-S has a relatively long half-life of 8 to 11 h and undergoes minimal hepatic extraction or renal clearance. DHEA is also conjugated in the liver to form DHEA-glucuronide. Androstenedione undergoes reversible conversion to testosterone by the enzyme 17-ketosteroid reductase. Androstenedione also may be irreversibly converted to estrone by the aromatase enzyme (Fig. 159-11).

The determination of urinary excretion of 17-ketosteroids has long been used to assess adrenal androgen production. Because the assay for 17-ketosteroids by the Zimmermann reaction detects conjugated and unconjugated C-19 compounds with a 17-ketone, DHEA, DHEA-S, and androstenedione are the major precursors of the urinary 17-ketosteroids, whereas testosterone metabolites contribute very little.

Action. Adrenal androgen effects are mediated by the potent metabolites produced in extraadrenal tissues. These products, testosterone and dihydrotestosterone, then interact with the androgen receptor within androgen target tissues.

Life Cycle of Adrenocortical Function

Since the treatment of CAH is basically a replacement of the missing hormones, it is important to understand the life cycle of adrenocortical function in order to establish appropriate therapy.

Adulthood

Cortisol Secretion. As described earlier, cortisol secretion is controlled by the rate of output of pituitary ACTH, which itself is controlled by the rate of secretion of CRH. The output of these three hormones is in homeostatic equilibrium. Specifically, CRH increases the secretion of ACTH, and ACTH increases cortisol production; conversely, cortisol has a negative-feedback effect on the secretion of both CRH and ACTH. These positive and negative effects are transmitted to the adrenal cortex. Careful studies of cortisol concentration in blood have demonstrated rapid fluctuations due to a pulsatile secretion of the steroid.[107] In addition, there

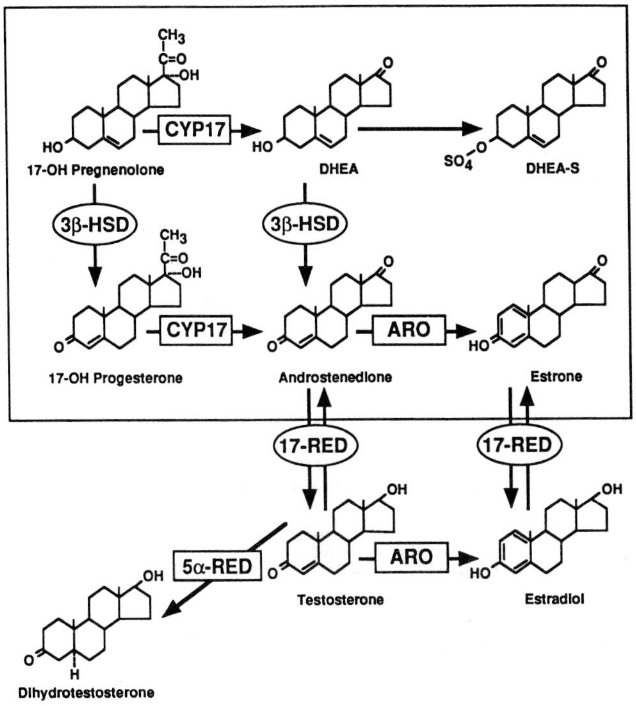

Fig. 159-11 Biosynthetic pathway for the formation of androgens and estrogens by the adrenal cortex. The box represents the adrenal cortex. Sex steroids secreted include DHEA and its sulfate, androstenedione, and estrone. It should be noted that androstenedione is metabolized peripherally to testosterone and dihydrotestosterone, whereas estrone can be metabolized to estradiol. Enzyme activities: 3β-HSD = 3β-hydroxysteroid dehydrogenase; CYP17 = 17α-hydroxylase/17,20-lyase; ARO = aromatase; 17RED = 17-ketoreductase; 5α-RED = 5α-reductase. *(From Migeon and Donohoue.[322] Used by permission from Charles C. Thomas Publishers.)*

is a diurnal or circadian variation of cortisol concentration in plasma due to an episodic secretion of the steroid. This variation is characterized by a major surge of secretion between 2 to 6 AM, followed by a slow decrease during the rest of the day; the lowest cortisol concentrations are observed in late evening and early night. This circadian rhythm predominantly is related to sleep-wake cycles, as long as the cycles are fairly constant.[100,108] This diurnal pattern parallels that of ACTH. In fungi, *Drosophila,* and mammals, circadian rhythms are believed to be controlled by products of so-called CLOCK genes.[109]

Although studies of the cortisol secretion rate have some definite limitations, they permit us to approximate the total output in a 24-h period and thus the daily requirement of replacement therapy. Normally, cortisol secretion increases with body size.[110] When the various values are corrected for body surface area, cortisol secretion is similar in both sexes and at all ages with an average ±SD of 12.1 ± 1.5 mg/m^2/24 h. The only exception is in the first week of life, when the cortisol secretion is about 11/2 times that of children and adults.[111] Subsequent studies, which employed a slightly different method of analysis, suggest a lower but more variable cortisol production rate.[112,113] Regardless of which methods produced the most reliable data, the ideal doses for cortisol replacement therapy must be individualized for each patient.

Aldosterone Secretion. Like cortisol, the plasma concentration of aldosterone varies diurnally, although the fluctuations are not quite as marked.[63] Numerous factors can influence the plasma concentrations of aldosterone. Changes in body position, such as standing versus lying down, bring about rapid but unsustained variations. In contrast, variation in sodium or potassium intake results in changes that occur 12 to 24 h later. Overall, there are fairly large variations in plasma aldosterone concentrations, both throughout the day and among individuals. However, the range tends to be similar throughout childhood and adulthood.[114] In infancy, plasma concentrations of aldosterone and plasma renin activity are somewhat more elevated than later on in life.

In contrast with the changes in cortisol secretion rate due to body size, aldosterone daily secretion rates are similar in infants, children, and adults at approximately 100 μg. As a consequence, the dosage of salt-retaining hormone replacement therapy is relatively constant throughout life, whereas that of cortisol must be adjusted with growth.

Androgen Secretion. Traditionally, it has been believed that the major adrenal androgens, androstenedione, DHEA, and DHEA-S, have very little biologic significance in adult males. Considerable attention has recently been directed at DHEA as a component of aging and other physiologic processes; however, its role in these areas is poorly understood. It is known, however, that adrenal androgens contribute more than 75 percent of blood testosterone in adult women. Indeed, adrenal androgens are responsible for development of axillary and pubic hair in females at puberty. DHEA-S is by far the steroid with the greatest concentration in the blood of adult subjects. This is related to the fact that steroid sulfates have a prolonged half-life of about 12 h, as discussed previously. Neither androstenedione nor DHEA binds to the androgen receptor, and therefore, both are void of direct biologic activity mediated by this nuclear receptor. Approximately 10 percent of androstenedione is metabolized peripherally into testosterone, a highly potent androgen. It is of interest that DHEA-S concentrations in blood are at the maximum in early adulthood and tend to decrease by 30 years of age in both sexes.

Pregnancy. The markedly elevated production of estrogen during pregnancy results in an increased synthesis of transcortin. Because of this increased binding capacity for cortisol in blood, plasma concentrations of cortisol rise above normal. In addition, there is some degree of increase in the concentration of unbound cortisol, the fraction of the steroid considered to be active at the level of the target cells. Therefore, there is a mild degree of hyperadrenocorticism during pregnancy. The increase in cortisol concentration in plasma is related more to its prolonged half-life rather than to an increased secretion. Indeed, there is a slight but significant decrease in cortisol secretion during pregnancy.[115] A consequence of these observations is that the treatment of CAH in pregnancy consists of the usual or slightly decreased dose of cortisol replacement.

Labor and delivery are important stresses that result in markedly increased cortisol secretion. Hence, at the time of labor, patients with CAH must receive an increased dose of glucocorticoid.

Pregnancy increases plasma renin activity, plasma aldosterone concentration, and aldosterone secretion rate. A low-sodium diet increases further the concentrations of aldosterone.[116] The markedly elevated secretion of progesterone during pregnancy is thought to cause a mild salt-losing tendency, which in turn is corrected by an increase in renin, angiotensin, and aldosterone. The concentrations of DHEA-S in pregnancy are significantly decreased.

Fetal Life. The fetal adrenal cortex starts producing cortisol by about 10 weeks of gestation. The evidence is based on the fact that the female fetus with CAH undergoes masculinization of its external genitalia by that time, suggesting that the homeostatic regulation of the hypothalamic-pituitary-adrenal axis is already active. The deficiency in 21-hydroxylase results in decreased cortisol secretion, increased output of ACTH, and increased androgen secretion. At the same time, it is well established that the fetal adrenal is deficient in 3β-HSD, the enzyme required for the

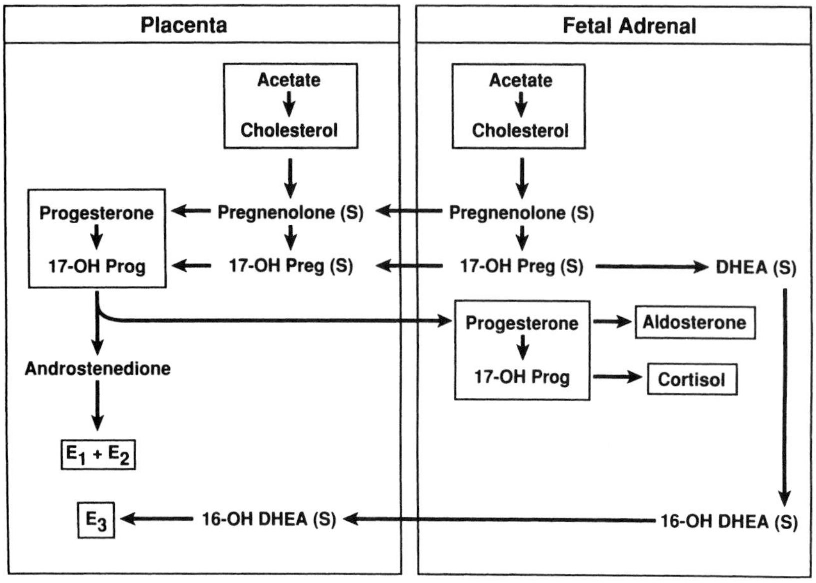

Fig. 159-12 Steroid biosynthesis in the placental-fetal unit. The fetal adrenal has low 3β-HSD activity. For this reason, it produces large amounts of pregnenolone, 17-hydroxypregnenolone, and DHEA, all of which are conjugated as sulfates. These products cross into the placenta, which is rich in sulfatase and 3β-HSD, resulting in the formation of progesterone and 17α-hydroxyprogesterone. These two products are returned to the fetus, which then can complete the biosynthesis of aldosterone and cortisol. Note that DHEA is metabolized to 16α-hydroxy-DHEA, which, after it is returned to the placenta, is the substrate for the formation of estriol. (*From Migeon and Donohoue.*[322] *Used by permission from Charles C Thomas Publishers.*)

transformation of Δ5-3β-hydroxysteroid into Δ4-3-ketosteroid. This paradox is explained by the existence of a "placental-fetal unit" (Fig. 159-12). The Δ5-3β-hydroxysteroids and their sulfates are produced in large amounts by the fetus and are transferred to the placenta, which is rich in both sulfatase and 3β-HSD. In the next step, progesterone and 17-hydroxyprogesterone are returned to the fetus, where they are metabolized to cortisol.

Maternal cortisol can be transferred to the fetus, but in very small amounts because only unbound cortisol can cross the placenta. Furthermore, both fetus and placenta are rich in 11β-HSD, which metabolizes cortisol to cortisone (see Fig. 159-10). Studies of steroid transfer in pregnancy have shown that the mother contributes 20 percent of the fetal concentration of cortisol and about 75 percent of the fetal concentration of cortisone.[117] For this reason, when glucocorticoid therapy of the fetus is considered, one must administer a steroid such as dexamethasone that is not sequestered by binding to maternal plasma protein and that is not metabolized into inactive products. This issue will be discussed further in the section describing prenatal treatment of CAH.

Like cortisol, aldosterone also is secreted by the fetal adrenal cortex. The maternal contribution to the fetal concentration is about 10 to 20 percent.[118]

Neonatal Period. When corrected for body surface area, the secretion rate of cortisol in the first 10 to 15 days of life is about 11/2 times that observed later in infancy and childhood. It also has been noted that aldosterone concentration and secretion rate, in contrast to those of cortisol, are similar in infancy and childhood, without correction for body size. Consequently, the treatment of patients with salt-losing 21-hydroxylase deficiency includes a dose of cortisol based on body size, whereas the dose of salt-retaining hormone is more or less constant throughout life. The only exception is the frequent need for higher doses of salt-retaining hormone during early infancy.

At birth and during the first 4 to 8 weeks of life, the secretion of adrenal androgens continues to be quite high. Thereafter, the concentration of adrenal androgens decreases concomitantly with the involution of the fetal zone of the adrenal cortex.

Childhood and Puberty. Diurnal variation of cortisol appears in infants as they start to establish a sleep-wake cycle similar to that of older children and adults. At that time, plasma cortisol concentrations are also similar to those of adults, whereas their secretion rate continues to be related to body size.

After the neonatal period, the secretion of adrenal androgens drops to extremely low levels and does not rise again until early puberty.

Adrenocortical Function in Stress

It was Hans Selye who first introduced the concepts of *stress, alarm reaction,* and the *adaptation syndrome.*[119] Initially these concepts were somewhat confusing and certainly unproven; progress clarified this field. When it became possible to measure cortisol concentration in plasma by biochemical methods, a large body of information demonstrated that various types of stress result in increased cortisol concentration. Conditions of stress were found to be numerous, including surgical stress (anesthesia, tissue destruction, blood loss, etc.)[120] and medical stress (particularly acute disorders with fever).[121] It also was noted that diabetic ketoacidosis and hypoglycemia profoundly increased cortisol concentrations. These stressful conditions have in common a cellular reaction to a variety of noxious agents. Emotional stress in certain individuals also results in an increase in cortisol secretion.

Hormones of the hypothalamic-pituitary-adrenal axis interact with components of the immune system in a complex manner. The cytokine interleukin 1 (IL-1) is secreted by macrophages in response to microbial invasion, inflammation, immunologic reaction, and tissue injury.[122] IL-1 initiates a proinflammatory cascade, activating resting T cells, accelerating hematopoesis, clonally expanding activated T cells, and accelerating the transformation of B cells into plasma cells, which then produce antibodies. Simultaneously, IL-1 activates the CRH-ACTH-cortisol system[123]; the increased cortisol concentration in plasma results in a negative feedback on the macrophages. Other cytokines, including tumor necrosis factor α and IL-6, as well as IL-1, stimulate CRH release but are inhibited by cortisol.[124] The endocrine immune system interactions are influenced reciprocally by the autonomic nervous system.[125] In summary, it is well demonstrated that the body's response to immune stress is intimately related to cortisol secretion.

In view of the important role of cortisol in the body's response to stress, including a negative-feedback function, it is clear that a lack of cortisol secretion can create major problems in patients with hypoadrenocorticism. This was recognized empirically quite early, but the progress in understanding of the stress reaction has given a biologic basis to our knowledge of adrenocortical function in stress.

Table 159-1 Classification of Hypoadrenocorticism

Primary adrenocortical insufficiency
- Congenital adrenal aplasia/hypoplasia (may include SF-1* defect)
- X-linked adrenal hypoplasia (AHC)
- Autosomal recessive adrenal hypoplasia
- Congenital adrenal hyperplasia (CAH)
  - Deficiency of CYP21 (21-hydroxylase)
  - Deficiency of CYP11B1 (11β-hydroxylase)
  - Deficiency of CYP17 (17α-hydroxylase)
  - Deficiency of 3β-HSD (3β-hydroxysteroid dehydrogenase)
  - Deficiency of CYP11A (cholesterol side-chain cleavage) due to StAR† defect
- Adrenoleukodystrophy/adrenomyeloneuropathy
- Wolman disease (acid lipase deficiency)
- Bilateral adrenal hemorrhage of the newborn
- Bilateral adrenal hemorrhage of acute infection
- Chronic hypoadrenocorticism (Addison disease)
- Isolated mineralocorticoid deficiency due to CMO I or CMO II (CYP11B2) deficiency

Secondary to deficient ACTH secretion
- Hypopituitarism, ACTH or CRH deficiency
- Cessation of glucocorticoid therapy
- Resection of unilateral cortisol-producing tumor
- Infants born to glucocorticoid-treated mothers
- Starvation, anorexia nervosa

Related to end-organ unresponsiveness
- Pseudohypoaldosteronism (mineralocorticoid resistance)
- Cortisol resistance
- ACTH resistance

* SF-1 = steroidogenic factor-1.
† StAR = steroidogenic acute regulatory protein.

CLINICAL IMPORTANCE AND CLASSIFICATION OF HYPOADRENOCORTICISM

Maintenance of normal adrenocortical function is vital to physiologic homeostasis. Glucocorticoids preserve normal blood levels of glucose for metabolic fuel, permit normal free water clearance, and mediate the body's response to stress. Mineralocorticoids are required for preservation of sodium, potassium, and hydrogen ion balance, ultimately maintaining sufficient intravascular volume. The clinical manifestations of adrenocortical insufficiency vary depending on the missing hormone(s). In addition, the steroid precursors that accumulate in the various inborn errors of steroid biosynthesis may produce clinical effects.

The causes of hypoadrenocorticism are classified on the basis of whether the etiology is an intrinsic defect within the adrenal cortex (primary hypoadrenocorticism), secondary to CRH or ACTH deficiency (secondary hypoadrenocorticism), or unresponsiveness to an adrenocortical hormone (Table 159-1).

Because this chapter focuses on CAH, the other forms of hypoadrenocorticism will not be described further. The different forms of CAH are described, with the most common disorders presented first. Specific features for each are presented, including pathogenesis, clinical manifestations, diagnosis, treatment, and genetics. Finally, diseases resulting from inborn errors of mineralocorticoid synthesis will be described. Table 159-2 summarizes the adrenal steroidogenic enzymes and the clinical entities resulting from their deficient or abnormal activities.

CONGENITAL ADRENAL HYPERPLASIA DUE TO 21-HYDROXYLASE DEFICIENCY

Of the various disorders of adrenal steroidogenesis, the greatest progress has been made in our understanding of 21-hydroxylase deficiency. This reflects the preeminent role of 21-hydroxylase

Table 159-2 Human Adrenal Steroidogenic Enzymes and Cofactors

Name	Location/Action	Chromosomal Location	Result of Markedly Altered Activity
CYP11A ($P_{450\ scc}$)	(Mitochondrial) 20-hydroxylase, 22-hydroxylase, 20, 22-desmolase (cholesterol side-chain cleavage)	15q23-q24	Congenital lipoid adrenal hyperplasia (female phenotype in all) resulting from StAR* defect
3β-HSD	(Microsomal) 3β-hydroxysteroid dehydrogenase, Δ4-Δ5 isomerase	1p13.1	Salt-losing congenital adrenal hyperplasia (male or female pseudohermaphroditism)
CYP17 (P_{450c17})	(Microsomal) 17α-hydroxylase, 17,20-lyase	10q24-q25	Hypertensive congenital adrenal hyperplasia (male pseudohermaphroditism)
CYP21 CYP21P (P_{450c21})	(Microsomal) 21-hydroxylase	6p21—active gene and pseudogene	Congenital virilizing adrenal hyperplasia (female pseudohermaphroditism)
CYP11B1 (p_{450c11})	(Zona fasciculata/reticularis, mitochondrial) 11β-hydroxylase	8q22—two homologous *CYP11B* genes	Hypertensive virilizing adrenal hyperplasia (female pseudohermaphroditism)
CYP11B2 (aldosterone synthase)	(Zona glomerulosa, mitochondrial) 11β-hydroxylase, 18-hydroxylase (CMO† I) 18-dehydrogenase (CMO† II)	8q22	Aldosterone deficiency (renal salt loss) Dexamethasone-remediable aldosteronism (*CYP11B1/B2* fusion gene)
Adrenodoxin	Iron-sulfur protein intermediate	11q22: active gene 20: pseudogenes	Unknown
Adrenodoxin reductase	(Mitochondrial) flavoprotein intermediate for $P_{450\ scc}$ and P_{450c11}	17q24-q25	Unknown

* StAR = Steroidogenic acute regulatory protein.
† CMO = Corticosterone methyl oxidase.

deficiency as a cause of clinical disorders of steroidogenesis and the location of its gene (*CYP21*) within the HLA complex on human chromosome 6. The molecular basis for the majority of cases of 21-hydroxylase deficiency is now established. Moreover, studies have provided a correlation between severity of the clinical disorder and the effect of specific mutations on enzymatic activity.[126] These studies have been summarized in several reviews.[127–135]

Clinically, it is useful to differentiate 21-hydroxylase deficiency into three forms, depending on the initial presentation. Two of these forms, which reflect severe deficiencies in P_{450c21} activity, present early in life. The most severe impairment in enzyme activity results in the salt-losing form of CAH. Male patients with this form present with acute adrenal crisis in the neonatal period or early infancy and are designated as having the *salt-losing form.* Females with the salt-losing form are usually detected at birth due to ambiguity of the external genitalia. Female patients who present with milder masculinization of the external genitalia but no evidence of acute adrenal crisis or males who show virilism during early life are considered to have the *simple virilizing form.* Finally, the *attenuated form* (also called *late onset* or *nonclassic*) is manifested only in female patients. At puberty or shortly thereafter, signs and symptoms consistent with mild androgen excess develop, including hirsutism, amenorrhea, and infertility.[18,136] In males, the mild androgen excess is clinically silent, since the effects of testicular testosterone override the masculinizing effects of adrenal androgens. It is important to remember that individual patients with the various forms of 21-hydroxylase deficiency represent a continuum of clinical manifestations secondary to impaired adrenal production of cortisol.

Simple Virilizing Form of 21-Hydroxylase Deficiency

Pathogenesis

Decreased Efficiency in Cortisol Secretion. As noted previously, 21-hydroxylase deficiency results in decreased secretion and plasma concentration of cortisol. This decreases negative feedback at the hypothalamic-pituitary level, which is translated into increased secretion of CRH and ACTH. The high concentrations of plasma ACTH are responsible for the adrenocortical hyperplasia characteristic of the syndrome. Since 21-hydroxylase deficiency is not complete in the simple virilizing form, the increased ACTH activity is capable of restoring cortisol secretion to an approximately normal rate.[137]

Increased Secretion of Cortisol Precursors. The increased ACTH concentration required to normalize cortisol secretion markedly elevates production of cortisol precursors. As shown in Fig. 159-3, the immediate precursor is 17α-hydroxyprogesterone.[138] To a lesser degree, there is also increased secretion of progesterone and 17-hydroxypregnenolone, as well as the product of an alternate pathway from 17-hydroxyprogesterone to cortisol—21-deoxycortisol.

Increased Activity of the Renin-Angiotensin-Aldosterone System. The major precursor of cortisol, 17α-hydroxyprogesterone, has limited biologic activity in normal subjects, although in excess it has the ability to produce a mild salt-losing tendency. Its massive hypersecretion in CAH results in definite sodium loss and potassium retention and is accompanied by water loss. To compensate for this situation, a greater amount of angiotensin II is formed. In salt-losing CAH, the marked deficiency in 21-OH does not permit the secretion of any aldosterone (see below). In the simple virilizing form of CAH, the fact that the 21-hydroxylase deficiency is only partial permits an increased secretion of aldosterone, which reestablishes a normal sodium balance.[139]

Increased Secretion of Androgens. In normal infants and prepubertal children, the concentration of ACTH in blood is insufficient to activate the secretion of adrenal androgens. In CAH, however, the high ACTH secretion, in conjunction with the enzymatic block, results in an abnormally elevated secretion of adrenocortical androgens,[140,141] specifically, androstenedione, DHEA, and DHEA-S. There also is increased secretion of 11β-hydroxy- and 11-keto-androstenedione. These androgens may reflect 11β-hydroxylation of androstenedione or the action of 17,20-lyase on 21-deoxycortisol.

Adrenal androgens are felt to lack intrinsic biologic activity, since they do not bind to the androgen receptor. Androstenedione is metabolized peripherally into testosterone, as described earlier, and this is responsible for the androgenic symptoms characteristic of CAH.

Clinical Manifestations. Patients with simple virilizing CAH have a partial 21-hydroxylase deficiency. The increased ACTH secretion results in normal cortisol plasma concentrations, and there are no symptoms of glucocorticoid deficiency. The salt-losing tendency caused by the marked hypersecretion of 17α-hydroxyprogesterone is compensated by increased aldosterone levels; therefore, these patients do not normally have electrolyte abnormalities.

Secretion of excess androgens produces somewhat different symptoms in males and females. Increased androgen activity starts early in fetal life, between 6 and 10 weeks of gestation. In the female fetus, this results in a variable degree of posterior fusion of the labia majora, as well as variable degrees of hypertrophy of the clitoris. In most cases, the enlarged phallus is held down by chordee and somewhat hidden by a hood of redundant skin. The labial fusion usually results in formation of a urogenital sinus located at the base of the phallus. The degree of masculinization of the external genitalia of female fetuses is usually classified as described by Prader[142] (Fig. 159-13). In the male fetus, testicular androgens carry out the normal masculinization of the external genitalia, and the addition of adrenal androgens has no effect.

Later in life, hypersecretion of androgen in either sex results in the early appearance of pubic hair (usually between 6 months and 2 years of age). This is followed by early appearance of axillary

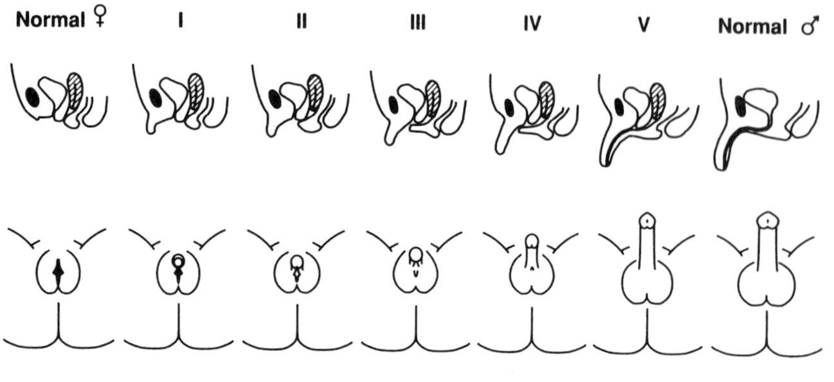

Fig. 159-13 Classification of the stages of masculinization of the female external genitalia as described by Prader.[142] The sagittal view of the genitalia shows, from left to right, a dark area as the pubic symphysis, the bladder as a clear space, the uterus as a shaded area, and the rectum.

hair (between 2 and 4 years of age) and facial hair (between 8 and 14 years of age). Acne appears at a variable time, in most cases before the appearance of facial hair. Deepening of the voice also will occur usually between 8 and 12 years of age. In many cases, parents report frequent erection of the phallus in infancy and early childhood.

The secretion of adrenal androgens in infancy and early childhood creates an anabolic condition that results in rapid osseous development. Bone age and height age are markedly advanced. Premature closure of the epiphyseal plates will result in short adult stature in untreated or inadequately treated patients. As a result, the adult height of female subjects is between 140 and 150 cm,[143,144] whereas that of male subjects is between 145 and 155 cm.[145]

In males, the anabolic effects of adrenal androgens generally result in advanced somatic growth and skeletal age, enlargement of the penis, and development of pubic hair; however, the testes remain small. If a patient's skeletal age is advanced to that of a child of pubertal age, subsequent suppression of adrenal androgen secretion with glucocorticoid therapy may be followed by the onset of true gonadotropin-mediated precocious puberty. This would result in the need to treat both the CAH and the true precocious puberty.

In females, the hypersecretion of adrenal androgens interferes with the maturation of the hypothalamic-pituitary axis. Only after complete suppression of adrenal androgen secretion can the female patient expect normal menstruation. Females also may be at risk for the development of true precocious puberty if inadequate therapy results in significant advancement of skeletal age.

In males, one frequently can observe hypertrophic adrenal rests located either in the body of the testes, near the epididymis, or in the spermatic cord. Such findings reflect the fact that adrenal rests are frequent in the normal population but are detected only when they are hypertrophic. Females also may have adrenal rests, usually in the broad ligament and, on occasion, in the ovary.

Laboratory Diagnosis. Increased plasma concentrations of cortisol precursors and of adrenal androgens are characteristic of CAH due to 21-hydroxylase deficiency. As already noted, the main cortisol precursor is 17α-hydroxyprogesterone and, to a lesser extent, progesterone, 17α-hydroxypregnenolone, and 21-deoxycortisol. In addition, androstenedione, DHEA, DHEA-S, and, to a lesser degree, testosterone concentrations will be elevated. 17α-Hydroxyprogesterone is metabolized to pregnanetriol, which is detected in large amounts in the urine of patients. Urinary excretion of 17-ketosteroids, the metabolites of adrenal androgens, also will be markedly elevated. The elevation of the plasma concentrations of ACTH is often difficult to demonstrate. Finally, as discussed earlier under "Pathogenesis," cortisol secretion is normal and that of aldosterone is increased in untreated patients. In contrast, both cortisol and aldosterone secretion is low or nil in salt-losing congenital adrenal hyperplasia.

Positive and Differential Diagnosis. In female patients, the diagnosis of simple virilizing CAH is made by the presence of ambiguous external genitalia with 46,XX karyotype and markedly increased concentrations of 17-hydroxyprogesterone and androstenedione that are reduced by glucocorticoid-suppressive therapy. Ambiguous external genitalia and a 46,XX karyotype also can be seen in infants without CAH who have been masculinized either by maternal androgens (virilizing adrenal or ovarian tumor of the mother) or by maternal ingestion of androgenic preparations.

In very mild cases of the simple virilizing CAH, the masculinization of the external genitalia of the newborn female can be minimal (slight clitoral hypertrophy and mild posterior labial fusion) and unnoticed at birth. In such patients, the first symptom is the appearance of pubic hair between 6 months and 2 years of age; the differential diagnosis includes virilizing adrenal tumor, ovarian tumor, and premature adrenarche. In virilizing adrenal tumors, the main androgens secreted are DHEA and DHEA-S and, to a lesser degree, androstenedione; in contrast, 17α-hydroxyprogesterone concentrations are normal or only slightly elevated. In addition, a dexamethasone-suppression test will fail to suppress the adrenal hypersecretion of androgens by the virilizing tumor. The diagnosis is confirmed by computed tomography (CT) or magnetic resonance imaging (MRI) of the abdomen showing a mass in one of the adrenal glands. In premature adrenarche, one observes an increase of DHEA and DHEA-S as well as androstenedione above the low level expected in prepubertal children but never above the concentration observed in normal adults. In addition, the concentration of 17α-hydroxyprogesterone is normal in premature adrenarche.

In male infants, the diagnosis of simple virilizing 21-hydroxylase deficiency is usually missed at birth and is considered only after premature appearance of pubic hair later in life, along with advanced bone and height ages. The testes remain prepubertal in size. The diagnosis of CAH is confirmed by the extremely high plasma concentrations of 17α-hydroxyprogesterone and androstenedione or the elevated urinary excretion of pregnanetriol and 17-ketosteroids. The differential diagnosis of early appearance of pubic hair in a boy includes complete sexual precocity of idiopathic origin or related to a benign or malignant tumor. In sexual precocity, the androgen responsible for the masculinization is testosterone; the concentrations of androstenedione, DHEA, and DHEA-S, on the other hand, are only slightly elevated above the prepubertal concentration but never exceeding the values found in normal adult subjects. The presence of a hamartoma or a central nervous system tumor will be diagnosed by MRI of the head. In true precocious puberty (gonadotropin-mediated), the testes enlarge as opposed to the small testes typical of CAH. Sexual precocity also can be related to a human chorionic gonadotropin-producing tumor such as a dysgerminoma or hepatoma, to a unilateral Leydig cell tumor, or to a virilizing adrenal tumor. Leydig cell tumors usually can be palpated in one of the testes; a sonogram of the scrotum confirms the diagnosis. Leydig cell tumors produce mainly testosterone, in contrast to virilizing adrenal tumors, which produce huge amounts of DHEA-S and DHEA.

Medical Treatment. Prior to 1949, the year in which cortisol became available for therapy, there was no treatment for CAH.[146] Patients with the simple virilizing form would show rapid and progressive virilization, whereas those with the salt-losing form would die during the neonatal period.[147] The principle of the treatment is to administer a dose of cortisol equal to that normally secreted. This exogenous steroid produces a negative feedback on the hypothalamic-pituitary axis reducing CRH and ACTH secretion, which, in turn, suppresses the secretion of cortisol precursors and adrenal androgens. In summary, treatment provides exogenous cortisol in amounts equal to the endogenous production, eliminates the salt-losing tendency, returns aldosterone secretion to normal, and suppresses androgen production and its virilizing effects.

Maintenance Therapy. Based on the normal cortisol secretion rate,[111] a child with a body surface area of 1 m^2 requires a dose of 8 to 16 mg/day of intramuscular cortisol or constant intravenous infusion (mean of 12 mg). Unfortunately, intramuscular cortisone acetate is a preparation that is in short supply. We formerly recommended intramuscular therapy during the first 1 or 2 years of life because it avoided problems resulting from regurgitation of an oral dose.

Because of the short half-life of cortisol given orally and its partial destruction by gastric acidity, the daily oral replacement dose is approximately twice that of the normal daily cortisol secretion rate (i.e., 24 $mg/m^2/24$ h). Furthermore, the total daily oral dose must be divided in three equal fractions, given approximately every 8 h. Instead of oral cortisol (e.g., hydrocortisone), one can use oral prednisolone or prednisone. These steroids are about five times more potent than cortisol (daily dose 4–5 mg/m^2/24 h). In addition, they have a longer half-life than cortisol, which makes it possible to give the daily dose in two fractions, every 12 h. Other synthetic glucocorticoid preparations even more potent than prednisolone are not useful as replacement therapy. Their great potency makes it difficult to titrate the appropriate dosage of each patient.

Experience has shown that the dose of glucocorticoid must be adjusted to the requirement of individual subjects. The criteria for determining the appropriate dose include the measurement of the concentration of 17-hydroxyprogesterone and androstenedione in plasma or the excretion of pregnanetriol and 17-ketosteroids in urine, as well as a close follow-up of somatic growth (bone age and height age). In children, levels of plasma androstenedione and urinary 17-ketosteroids should be undetectable or in the prepubertal range. However, fully suppressed urinary pregnanetriol and prepubertal concentrations of 17-hydroxyprogesterone are indicative of overtreatment (normal prepubertal 17-hydroxyprogesterone is 0–80 ng/dl; acceptable values for treated CAH patients are up to 500 ng/dl; concentrations of more than 1000 ng/dl indicate insufficient therapy). Patients with simple virilizing CAH have normal serum electrolytes and do not have an absolute requirement for mineralocorticoid replacement therapy. However, in the clinical setting of difficulty in suppressing adequately the adrenal androgen excess combined with an elevated plasma renin activity, mineralocorticoid treatment may be beneficial[148] and avoid the deleterious effects of high cortisone doses. The use of antagonists of androgens and aromatase is investigational.[149]

Therapy under Stress Conditions. After approximately 4 weeks of exogenous cortisol therapy, the CRH-ACTH system is suppressed and unable to respond normally to stress. Under such conditions, it is necessary to provide the patient with increased cortisol therapy. Minor infection and/or low-grade fever (temperature up to 38°C) may not require a change in dosage. During conditions of moderate stress (upper respiratory infections, with lung congestion and temperature above 38°C), the dosage should be doubled, whereas in major stress, the cortisol requirement may be three to four times the normal replacement.

Under stress conditions, infants and children are frequently unable to retain oral therapy. In such cases, the parents are advised to administer an intramuscular injection of approximately 50 mg/m^2 of cortisol sodium succinate (SoluCortef). This measure will give the parents up to 6 h to get in touch with a physician.

Therapy during Surgical Procedures. Since surgery does not permit oral therapy, we advise the following schedule of treatment: A dose of 25 mg/m^2 of SoluCortef is given intravenously stat just prior to anesthesia and is followed by a dose of approximately 50 mg/m^2 as a constant infusion for the period of the surgical procedure; finally, a third dose of approximately 50 mg/m^2 of SoluCortef is given at a constant intravenous rate for the rest of the first 24 h of the surgical day. This is a total of 125 mg/m^2 of SoluCortef over a 24-h period or approximately 10 times replacement therapy. This is followed the next day by approximately four times replacement therapy (50 mg/m^2/24 h) by constant intravenous infusion of SoluCortef. Eventually, oral therapy is resumed as appropriate.

Surgical Treatment of CAH. We believe that it is important to correct the ambiguous genitalia of female patients early in life. Usually, surgeons prefer to wait at least until 6 to 12 weeks of age. Appropriate administration of intravenous SoluCortef must be given as described earlier. The size of the phallus is reduced by removing its posterior part (corpora) but keeping the glans, which is recessed. In cases of mild posterior fusion of the labia majora, it is usually quite easy to exteriorize the vaginal opening at the same time. When the fusion is extensive and the vaginal canal opens in the posterior part of the urethra, the exteriorization of the vagina is much more difficult. Some surgeons feel that correction of the vaginal opening can be done successfully early in life. Others prefer to postpone surgery at least until the patient is going through puberty. The latter is our personal recommendation.

Early vaginal correction often results in formation of a ring of scar tissue at the level of the introitus that interferes with sexual intercourse. The use of dilators postoperatively may prevent this problem. However, their use in infants and children is often painful and psychologically traumatic for both patient and parents.

Salt-Losing Form of 21-Hydroxylase Deficiency

Pathogenesis. The pathogenesis of the salt-losing form of CAH due to 21-hydroxylase deficiency is similar to that of the simple virilizing form. The only difference is that the 21-hydroxylase deficiency is more severe or even complete. Hence secretion of cortisol is almost nil. In addition, the adrenal cortex cannot secrete sufficient aldosterone to respond to the salt-losing tendency created by the large production of 17α-hydroxyprogesterone. This results in an acute adrenal crisis, which will be described below.

Simultaneously, the complete or almost complete absence of secretion of cortisol results in a maximal activity of the CRH-ACTH axis, inducing maximal secretion of adrenal androgens and maximal masculinization of the external genitalia in females.

Clinical Manifestations. In female infants, attention is attracted first to the markedly ambiguous genitalia. The extremely elevated secretion of adrenal androgen is responsible for this finding. On occasion, the masculinization is so extreme that there is complete fusion of the labia and formation of a penile urethra (Fig. 159-14). In such cases, the external genitalia are similar to those of a normal male except that no gonads can be palpated in the rugated scrotal folds.[150] The extreme secretion of pituitary ACTH is accompanied by a large secretion of melanocyte-stimulating hormone (MSH); in both male and female infants, there is often a marked pigmentation of the external genitalia.

The total or almost complete absence of secretion of cortisol and aldosterone results in an acute adrenal crisis usually between the fourth and fifteenth days of life but occasionally as late as 6 to 12 weeks of age. As a prelude to the crisis, the infants feed poorly, vomit excessively, contract diarrhea, and lose a significant amount of weight. The serum electrolytes generally first show an increase in serum potassium concentration followed shortly thereafter by a fall in sodium. The loss of body weight is related to the negative sodium balance and concomitant dehydration. In the absence of treatment, the acute adrenal crisis readily develops into cardiovascular collapse, cardiac arrest, and death.

On occasion, salt loss is first noted in early childhood, usually at the time of a major infection. Such patients probably carry a degree of deficiency of 21-hydroxylase that is intermediate between that of the simple virilizing form and that of the salt-losing form. It is also interesting that the salt-losing tendency

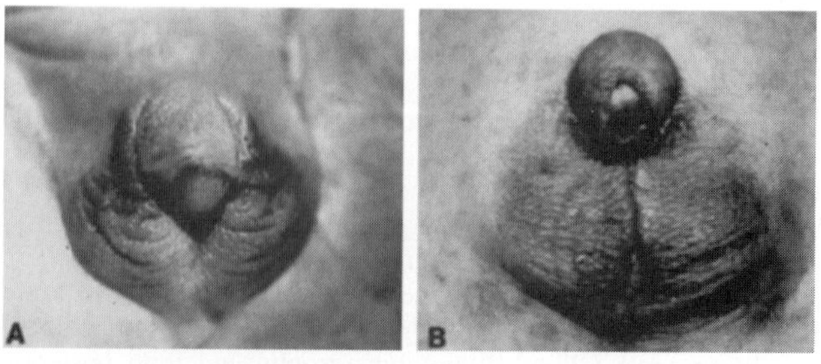

Fig. 159-14 Appearance of the external genitalia of two 46,XX infants with 21-hydroxylase deficiency and salt loss. *A.* Large clitoris with chordee surrounded by rugated labial folds. *B.* Large phallus with penile urethra and complete fusion of labia into a scrotum-like structure.

seems to be somewhat less marked after 4 or 5 years of age and even less in late childhood and adulthood. Despite this, it has been shown that such patients cannot sustain a prolonged low-sodium diet without experiencing a major sodium and water loss.[151] There are many patients with salt-losing CAH who tolerate discontinuation of their mineralocorticoid treatment in later life.[152,153]

Diagnosis. In female infants with ambiguous external genitalia or with completely masculinized genitalia without palpable gonads, the diagnosis of the salt-losing form of 21-hydroxylase deficiency is made on the basis of a normal female karyotype of 46,XX, the characteristic pattern of serum electrolytes (hyponatremic, hypochloremic, hyperkalemic acidosis), and markedly elevated plasma concentrations of plasma 17-hydroxyprogesterone and androstenedione. Because of the dehydration, there is usually a decrease in plasma volume resulting in hemoconcentration. Low plasma concentration of aldosterone along with elevated plasma renin activity confirms the primary adrenal insufficiency.

In male infants, the absence of ambiguous genitalia makes the diagnosis somewhat more difficult. The clinical symptoms can be confused with those of pyloric stenosis. The typical pattern of serum electrolytes of CAH will contrast with that of pyloric stenosis (hyponatremic, hypochloremic, hypokalemic alkalosis). Furthermore, the diagnosis will be confirmed by demonstrating elevated concentrations of plasma 17-hydroxyprogesterone and androstenedione. A family history of an older sibling with CAH or one who died in the neonatal period from a syndrome of dehydration without a specific diagnosis is of further help in recognizing the salt-losing form of CAH.

Treatment of Adrenal Crisis. The rapid recognition and prompt therapy of the salt-losing crisis are critical to survival of these infants. Electrolyte and fluid therapy must be instituted as soon as possible. In this first stage of therapy, appropriate blood samples must be obtained for the measurement of steroids and determination of karyotype.

During the first hour, we administer 20 ml/kg of body weight of a solution of 5% dextrose and 0.9% sodium chloride. Although this will correct the plasma sodium and chloride concentrations, as well as hypoglycemia if present, the potassium concentration usually remains elevated, and the acidosis may persist. After the first hour of treatment, the condition usually improves, and the same intravenous solution is continued for the next 24 h at a rate of approximately 100 ml/kg of body weight. During this time, it is helpful to obtain an additional blood sample for confirmation of the concentration of plasma steroids. A 12- to 18-h urine sample, for measurement of pregnanetriol and 17-ketosteroids, can aid in the diagnosis.

If the electrolytes do not improve after the first hour of treatment and the vital signs remain critical, it is necessary to dispense with additional blood and urine collections for confirmatory diagnosis and start therapy with replacement of glucocorticoid and mineralocorticoids. In newborn infants we advise adding to the intravenous fluid a dose of 20 mg of cortisol sodium succinate (SoluCortef) administered at a constant rate over a 24-h period. This 20-mg dose of cortisol is the equivalent of about six times replacement therapy for an infant with a normal body surface area (approximately 0.25 m^2) and has a salt-retaining activity of approximately 0.1 mg of Florinef (9α-fluorocortisol).

During treatment of the salt-losing crisis, the use of sedatives or the addition of potassium to the intravenous fluid is contraindicated. Throughout the treatment, electrolytes and water balance must be monitored very carefully to avoid hypernatremia, water retention, and possible pulmonary edema.

Maintenance Therapy. After the acute adrenal crisis has been controlled, it is then appropriate to start maintenance therapy.

Glucocorticoid Replacement Therapy. Previously, the treatment of choice was intramuscular cortisone acetate. Unfortunately, this

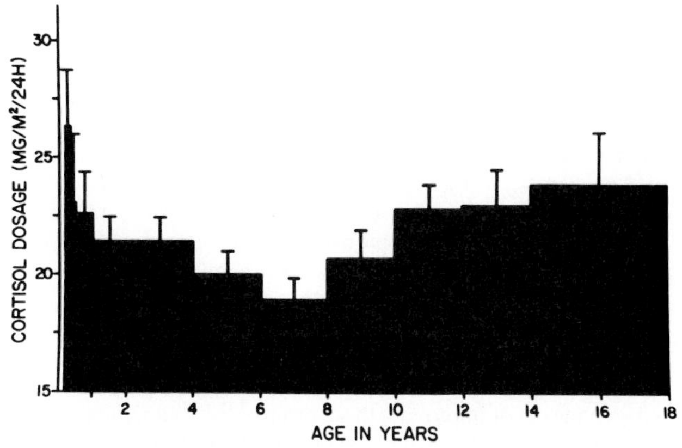

Fig. 159-15 Cortisol dosage (mg/m²/24 h) in patients with the salt-losing form of CAH due to 21-hydroxylase deficiency. The dark area represents the mean dose, and the bar is the SEM. The dosage, which was maximum very early in life, dropped rapidly by 1 year of age and was minimum between 6 and 8 years, before it returned to a higher adult level. (*From Sandrini et al.*[154] *Used by permission from Acta Paediatrica.*)

preparation is in limited supply. Cortisol liquid for oral use is occasionally difficult to obtain in pharmacies, and one might have to resort to a prednisolone syrup (Pediapred 1 mg/ml). Although this is a perfectly good preparation, it can be difficult to adjust the dose required precisely because of the five times greater potency of prednisolone over cortisol.

Mineralocorticoid Replacement Therapy. The only medication currently available for this specific purpose is Florinef given orally at a dose of 0.05 to 0.15 mg/24 h.

In infancy, breast milk or prepared formula provides a very low salt intake (8–10 meq of sodium per 24 h). For this reason, one-fifth of a teaspoon of table salt (about 18 meq sodium or 1 g of sodium chloride) is added to the formula once or twice daily. When the diet of the child becomes more varied and includes solid food, which is usually rich in sodium, the salt supplement is no longer required.

During the growth period of the child, it is important to adjust the glucocorticoid dose in relation to body size, as described for the simple virilizing form. It is also important to adjust the dose to individual requirements. It is of interest that even when dose is adjusted to body size, there appears to be a temporal variation of requirement (Fig. 159-15); in infancy, the dose is much higher than it is in childhood; then there is another increase at the time of puberty.[154]

During stress, whether medical or surgical, the rules outlined for the simple virilizing form also apply to patients with the salt-losing form. Since the only mineralocorticoid preparation available is Florinef, which must be given orally, the salt-retaining replacement can be obtained by giving extra intravenous cortisol, with 20 mg SoluCortef having the same sodium-retaining effect as 0.1 mg Florinef.

Surgical Treatment

Correction of the External Genitalia of Female Patients. It is important to correct the appearance of the external genitalia of female infants with the salt-losing form, just as it is for female infants with the simple virilizing form. Although it is appropriate to wait for the infant to recover fully from the original acute adrenal crisis and to begin normal weight gain, it remains of great importance to feminize the appearance of the external genitalia. This is often done between 2 and 6 months of age. In reducing the size of the phallus, the glans of the clitoris must be saved. As noted earlier, salt-losing females may present extremely marked degrees of virilization, with a vagina that opens by a narrow passage to the posterior part of the urethra sometimes at the neck of the bladder.

In such cases, we advise a two-step correction. In a first step, the size of the phallus is reduced and the labioscrotal folds are corrected. The second step, at the time the patient reaches puberty, consists of exteriorizing the vagina. Some families may desire to delay surgery until the patient is old enough to participate in the decision-making process.

Alternative Therapies. In some females with salt-losing CAH, results of therapy are suboptimal, and androgen excess is quite problematic and refractory to suppression with physiologic cortisol replacement dosages. For this reason, adrenalectomy has been proposed for specific patients. Because of this, and because in general the long-range results of replacement therapy have not been perfect, bilateral adrenalectomy has been proposed as a possible means of improving these results.[155,156] Other approaches to treatment have included peripheral blockade of androgen action and estrogen production with testalactone and flutamide.[149] It is important to emphasize that such alternatives are presently experimental and many years of follow-up will be required to judge their validity. In the realm of even more esoteric possibilities, one could mention agents to block adrenal androgen secretion and 21-hydroxylase gene therapy.

Psychological Treatment. In all patients with CAH, it is important to explain — first to the parents and later to the patient — the pathogenesis of the disorder. Emphasis is put on the nature of the therapy, which is the replacement of a deficient secretion of glucocorticoids and mineralocorticoids. In females, it is important to point out that the abnormalities of the external genitalia are related to excessive androgens of adrenal origin. Appropriate glucocorticoid treatment will remediate this situation. There is some evidence that prenatal androgen exposure influences postnatal behavior in some females with CAH, but this is highly variable.[157–159]

Attenuated Form of 21-Hydroxylase Deficiency

This form of CAH presents the mildest degree of 21-hydroxylase deficiency. Because the symptomatology in the female appears at puberty, it was formerly wrongly called *acquired adrenal hyperplasia.* The terminology *late onset* also has been used. In the recent past, the term *nonclassic form* has been proposed[160] to contrast with the *classic forms* (simple virilizing and the salt-losing forms). Because the terms *classic* and *nonclassic* do not carry a specific meaning in relation to the disorder, we use and prefer the term *attenuated form* for minimal 21-hydroxylase deficiency. There also exists an *asymptomatic* or *cryptic form* of 21-hydroxylase deficiency manifested by the steroid pattern diagnostic of CAH in the complete absence of symptoms of the disorder.

Pathogenesis. The pathogenesis is similar to that of the other two forms except that the mildness of the 21-hydroxylase deficiency results in small changes in steroidogenesis and therefore an attenuation of the symptoms of the disorder.

The absence of masculinization of the female genitalia during fetal life reflects the low degree of fetal adrenal androgen secretion. Similarly, there are little or no signs of androgen effects during childhood. The effect of hypersecretion of adrenal androgens is noted only in females, at the time of puberty.

Clinical Manifestations. There is no expression of the attenuated form of CAH in males, since at puberty the testicular secretion of testosterone overrides the effects of increased adrenal androgen output. In females, there is no abnormality of the external genitalia at birth. It is generally thought that the virilization that occurs at puberty is triggered by the same mechanism that normally produces adrenarche, the difference in CAH being an excessive response of adrenal androgens.

Most girls have some breast development but with exaggerated development of body hair, including facial hair. The androgen excess causes either primary or secondary amenorrhea. Another androgenic effect is the frequent presence of multiple, small ovarian cysts.

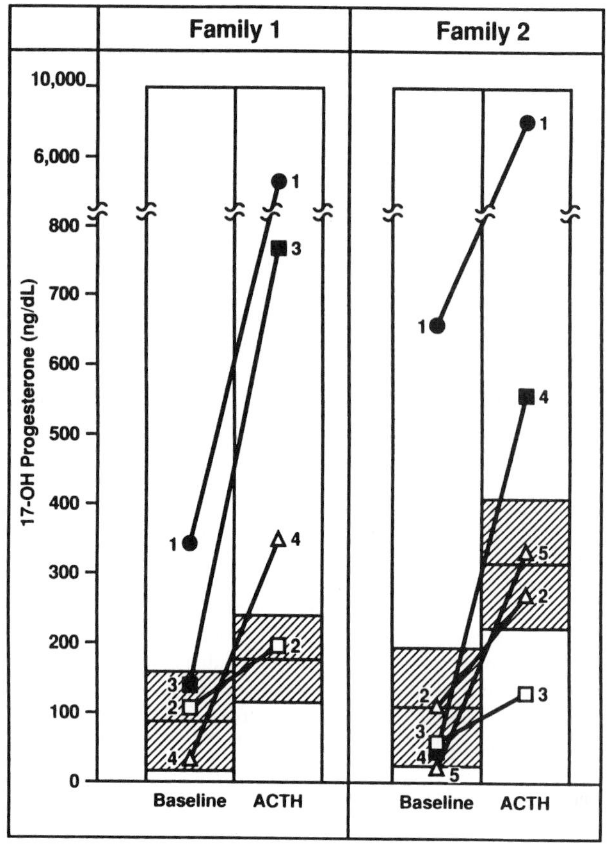

Fig. 159-16 Plasma concentration of 17α-hydroxyprogesterone (ng/dl) at baseline and 30 min after intravenous ACTH administration (1 mg Cortrosyn). In the left panel, the shaded area represents the means ± 2 SD of a normal subject at baseline and 30 minutes after ACTH injection. In the right panel, the shaded area represents the mean ± 2 SD of an obligate heterozygote for the CAH trait at baseline and 30 min after intravenous ACTH administration. In family 1, subject 1 is the proband, subjects 3 and 4 are her parents, and subject 2 is her homozygous normal brother. In family 2, subject 1 is the proband, subjects 4 and 5 are her parents, subject 3 is a homozygous normal brother, and subject 2 is her heterozygous sister. (*Data adapted from Migeon et al.*[161] *Used with permission from the* Journal of Clinical Endocrinology and Metabolism.)

Laboratory Diagnosis. In female patients of pubertal age, the baseline concentrations of plasma 17-hydroxyprogesterone and androstenedione are quite elevated.[161,162] The urinary excretions of pregnanetriol and 17-ketosteroids are increased concordantly with the secretion of 17-hydroxyprogesterone and androstenedione.

Administration of 1 mg of 1,24-ACTH (Cortrosyn) intravenously over a 1- to 2-min period results in an exaggerated increase of 17α-hydroxyprogesterone and also of progesterone (Fig. 159-16).

Differential Diagnosis of the Attenuated Form of 21-Hydroxylase Deficiency. The polycystic ovary (PCO) syndrome, also called *Stein-Leventhal syndrome,* presents clinical symptoms that are very similar to those found in the attenuated form of CAH. In both conditions, there are signs of excessive androgens, including hirsutism and acne, and menstrual abnormalities. In some cases the androgenic effects are more marked, resulting in a slight enlargement of the clitoris, some increase in muscle mass, and mild deepening of the voice.

Although the pathophysiology of PCO syndrome is not completely understood, the starting abnormality may be an increased secretion of ovarian estrone, which in turn produces a positive feedback on the secretion of luteinixing hormone (LH) but not of follicle-stimulating hormone (FSH) so that the LH/FSH ratio is greater than 2 (normal, ≤ 1). In turn, LH activates the ovarian hilar cells, which secrete large amounts of androstenedione. This steroid is metabolized peripherally to testosterone. The precursor of androstenedione is 17α-hydroxyprogesterone, which itself is secreted in increased amounts. Therefore, both PCO syndrome and attenuated CAH present a similar pattern of basal steroids. In both conditions, cortisol secretion is normal, but androstenedione, testosterone, and 17α-hydroxyprogesterone concentrations are elevated. Plasma concentrations of DHEA and DHEA-S are usually normal in PCO syndrome but tend to be above normal in attenuated CAH.

The intravenous ACTH test is the best means to distinguish the two conditions. In PCO syndrome, the rate of increase of 17-hydroxyprogesterone and progesterone is either normal or similar to that of obligate heterozygotes for CAH.[163] In contrast, in attenuated CAH, the rates of increase of 17-hydroxyprogesterone and progesterone are markedly above normal (see Fig. 159-16).

To complicate the differential diagnosis further, ovarian cysts are found in both conditions, and both respond to glucocorticoid-suppressive treatment. Some confusion about the two disorders is present in the literature. Strict definitions should include the elements discussed below.

In the attenuated form of CAH, there is a major increase of 17-hydroxyprogesterone and progesterone concentrations in response to ACTH administration with somewhat elevated baseline concentrations of these two steroids, an ACTH response in both parents typical for CAH heterozygotes, and ideally, a family study showing linkage of the *CYP21* mutation and HLA haplotypes.

In PCO syndrome, the ACTH response of 17-hydroxyprogesterone and progesterone concentrations should be either normal or similar to that of CAH heterozygotes, and the clinical phenotype does not segregate with HLA haplotype.

Treatment. Treatment of the attenuated form of CAH is similar to that of the simple virilizing form of CAH. Prednisone is usually preferred, since it can be administered in only two daily doses. Dexamethasone, in one daily dose, also may be used. Appropriate treatment should result in resumption of menstrual periods. Unfortunately, because of problems with compliance or perhaps other factors, results are usually not perfect.

Results of therapy for PCO syndrome are also imperfect. Some patients respond to glucocorticoid therapy. Suppression of ovulation by treatment with contraceptive pills generally produces good results in establishing menstrual cycles and reducing ovarian androgen production.

Long-Term Results of Therapy

Because the Pediatric Endocrine Clinic of the Johns Hopkins Children's Center started glucocorticoid therapy of CAH due to 21-hydroxylase deficiency in 1949 and has maintained interest in this field, this center was the first to publish analysis of the results of long-range treatment.

Adult Male Patients. A group of 30 male subjects with CAH who had reached adulthood was studied.[145] Several patients whose therapy had been well controlled by their parents in childhood admitted to poor compliance in later adulthood. In fact, four of them had stopped therapy for 7 to 15 years at the time of the evaluation. The reason for cessation of treatment was usually that the patients noted no difference on or off treatment. Two patients with the simple virilizing form of CAH were never treated, for unclear reasons. At the other end of the spectrum, a few patients had maintained a strict compliance, reporting development of general malaise and headache when therapy was interrupted for a short time. In the remainder of patients, compliance was variable.

There were no major health complaints among the 30 patients whether they were on or off therapy. Their adult height was significantly below the normal for American males, ranging from 150 to 178.6 cm. Steroid studies were performed in 18 of the 30 subjects (2 who were never treated, 4 who had interrupted therapy, and 12 who were still treated). Only 5 had normal concentrations of plasma 17-hydroxyprogesterone, and only 8 had normal levels of androstenedione. Concentration of plasma testosterone was within the normal range in all, including the 6 patients who were off therapy at the time of the study. Interestingly, concentrations of serum luteinizing hormone were significantly lower than normal but ranged between the mean and −2 SD of the mean. Using sperm count and reproductive history as criteria for fertility, all patients appeared to be fertile; a large number of them were married with several children. A later study showed that among Finnish males treated for 21-hydroxylase deficiency, diagnosis at a later age correlated with reduction in adult height.[164]

Adult Female Patients. In a survey of 98 adult female patients,[143] the height of those who were treated late in life was 150.9 ± 4.3 cm (mean ± 1 SD), whereas the height of those who were treated prior to 1 year of age was significantly greater (157.4 ± 7.3 cm). The age at pubarche was about 3 years earlier than normal, thelarche occurred at a normal age, and menarche usually was delayed by 2 or more years.[143] Other studies have confirmed the risk for reduced adult height.[164–166] More recently, we carried out a survey of 80 adult women with CAH; of the 40 patients with the simple virilizing form, 17.5 percent had an introitus inadequate for sexual intercourse (a finding seen in only 2 percent of normal women), 30 percent reported no sexual activity (only 5 percent in the female population), and 50 percent never married (10 percent in American females). Among the 40 patients with the salt-losing form, 52 percent had an inadequate introitus, 45 percent reported no sexual activity, and 87.5 percent never married.

The fertility rate was low among the 40 women who had an adequate introitus and had reported heterosexual activity. This rate was about 60 percent in the simple virilizing form and 7 percent in the salt-losing form.[144] Reduced fertility has been reported in other female CAH patient populations as well.[165,166]

In our study, among 28 patients with an inadequate introitus, 18 reported no sexual activity, 3 were homosexual, and 7 had some degree of heterosexual activity.[144] The lack of sexual activity reported by a large number of patients, even when the vaginal opening was adequate, is not readily explained. It has been suggested that androgen hyperactivity in fetal life may have an influence on adult sexuality.[167]

Genetic Aspects of 21-Hydroxylase Deficiency

Inheritance. CAH due to 21-hydroxylase deficiency is inherited as an autosomal recessive trait[168] and is expressed clinically only in homozygous subjects. Following recognition of the trait as autosomal recessive, a major breakthrough occurred when Dupont and colleagues discovered and subsequently reported a tight linkage between 21-hydroxylase deficiency and the HLA major histocompatibility complex (MHC) on chromosome 6.[169]

Genetic Linkage Disequilibrium. Studies of genetic linkage positioned the locus of the 21-hydroxylase genes in the HLA complex[169] among the genes of the class III products of the MHC.[170,171] Simultaneously, isolation of the cytochrome P_{450} involved in the 21-hydroxylase activity permitted later the isolation and sequencing of the *CYP21* gene and *CYP21P* pseudogene.[172,173]

The study of linkage of CAH alleles with HLA and fourth component of complement (C4) alleles has been particularly useful in demonstrating that one of the two 21-hydroxylase genes (*CYP21P*) is actually a pseudogene. The extended haplotype HLA-A3,Bw47,C6,DR7,GLO1/BfF,C2C,C4A1,C4BQO (so-called HLA-Bw47) was found to be linked to a large deletion including one of the 21-hydroxylase genes and one of the C4 genes; the remaining 21-hydroxylase gene was inactive,[174] as demonstrated by the clinical phenotype of the patient. It is of interest that the deletion of the 21-hydroxylase gene linked to the Bw47 haplotype was observed with great frequency in various countries of northern Europe as well as in the United States among subjects originating from northern Europe.

A similar haplotype containing Bw47 was found in subjects of the Old-Order Amish who immigrated from Switzerland and southern Germany to Lancaster County in Pennsylvania. Their HLA haplotype is linked to normal 21-hydroxylase activity,[175] suggesting that the Amish HLA-Bw47 haplotype, including a normal *CYP21,* was the precursor of the CAH-linked HLA-Bw47 haplotype.[176]

In the attenuated form of 21-hydroxylase deficiency, a genetic linkage disequilibrium has been noted with the HLA-B14,DR1 haplotype. This haplotype includes three C4 genes (*C4A2, C4B1, C4B2*) in tandem with three 21-hydroxylase genes, two of them being pseudogenes and one being a *CYP21* gene with a missense mutation in exon 7 (*P281L*).[177] The frequency of the HLA-B14 haplotype is 8 to 9 percent of the population of the United States, but probably only half of these HLA B14 haplotypes are linked to the *CYP21* mutation mentioned above.[178] Studies in Israel have shown that the frequency of the B14 haplotype may be slightly above 12 percent.[179] Based on the frequency of the HLA-B14 haplotype with a mutant *CYP21* gene and the frequency of all other *CYP21* mutations, one could calculate that the number of women with the attenuated form of CAH could be very large. However, the expression of this particular mutant *CYP21* has a variable penetrance.[180]

Molecular Studies of the Normal Gene. As was reported in 1985,[174,181] two homologues of 21-hydroxylase genes (*CYP21* and *CYP21P*) reside within the class III region of the MHC, immediately adjacent to two genes encoding the fourth component of complement, *C4A* and *C4B* (Fig. 159-17). Although sequencing has revealed that *CYP21* and *CYP21P* are 98 percent homologous in their coding regions, several deleterious mutations preclude activity of one of them (pseudogene *CYP21P,* previously called *21-hydroxylase A gene*), and all enzymatic activity derives from the product of the other gene (*CYP21,* previously called *21-hydroxylase B gene*).[172,173] The mutations of the *CYP21P* gene include several missense mutations as well as an 8-bp deletion in exon 3 and a single-base insertion in exon 7, both of which alter the reading frame and generate premature termination codons. Although the *CYP21P* gene was thought previously to be nontranscribed, *CYP21P* transcripts of unknown function have been identified.[182] The *CYP21P* gene promoter contains sequence variants that render it much less efficient than that of the active *CYP21* gene.[183–185]

A gene termed *TN-X* (formerly *XB*) overlaps human *CYP21* and is transcribed on the strand opposite that which transcribes *CYP21. TN-X* encodes a predicted peptide that resembles the extracellular matrix protein tenascin and is thus called *tenascin-X.* Its mRNA is found in multiple human fetal tissues.[127] Tenascin-X deficiency has been associated with Ehlers-Danlos syndrome (MIM 130000).[186]

The duplicated *CYP21/C4* configuration is found in a number of other animal species, including mice, cattle, great apes, and sheep. The 8-bp deletion of the human *CYP21P* pseudogene is also present in the *CYP21P* genes of some great apes.[187] On the other hand, there appears to be only one porcine *CYP21* gene copy.[188] In sheep, both 21-hydroxylase genes are transcribed.[189] In the murine MHC (the so-called H_2 region), the gene-pseudogene alignment is the reverse of that in humans; the more upstream gene is functional, and the more downstream gene is the pseudogene. *CYP21* expression is stimulated by ACTH and cAMP. In mice[190] and humans,[191] the region upstream of *CYP21* contains three copies of the hexanucleotide motif AGGTCA, which may mediate cAMP stimulation. In studies with transgenic mice, the 3′ region of murine *C4* gene SLP (sex-limited protein) contains sequences necessary for optimal *CYP21* expression.[192]

Frequency of *CYP21* Mutations in the General Population. The establishment of the frequency of mutation of the *CYP21* gene is quite difficult. Clearly, it is not practical to sequence and express *CYP21* alleles on a large scale for an extended population. For this reason, the approach has been to estimate the incidence of cases of CAH. Frequency of the disorder can be obtained indirectly by establishing the number of patients diagnosed in a specific geographic area in relation to the total number of births during a specific period. The technique has the drawback of tending to underestimate the frequency because even though the number of births is quite precise, the number of CAH cases diagnosed may be below the occurrence of CAH, particularly in males who have normal-appearing external genitalia. Indeed, many clinics have reported a ratio of 2:1 or 3:1 in favor of female patients when the ratio should be close to 1. Another approach has been the screening of a large number of newborns for their 17-hydroxyprogesterone blood concentration using a microfilter paper method for blood collection.[193] This technique may have a tendency to overestimate cases of CAH. In addition, it is clear that the frequency will be much greater in some inbred populations than in outbred populations.

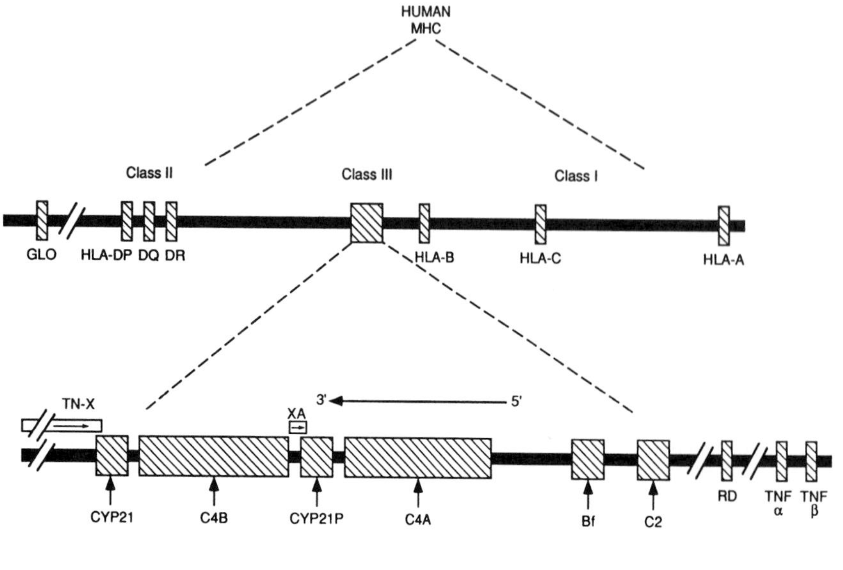

Fig. 159-17 Mapping of the short arm of chromosome 6 in the region of the major histocompatibility (MHC) genes. Between HLA-B and HLA-D are the loci of class III genes [*C2,* factor B (*Bf*), *C4A,* and *C4B*]. The 21-hydroxylase genes (*CYP21* and *CYP21P*) and the *C4* genes are in tandem duplication. In addition, two genes, *TN-X* and *XA,* which are transcribed 3′ to 5′, overlap *CYP21* and *CYP21P.*[127]) A total of at least 11 overs lapping transcriptional units have now been mapped to this locus.[324]

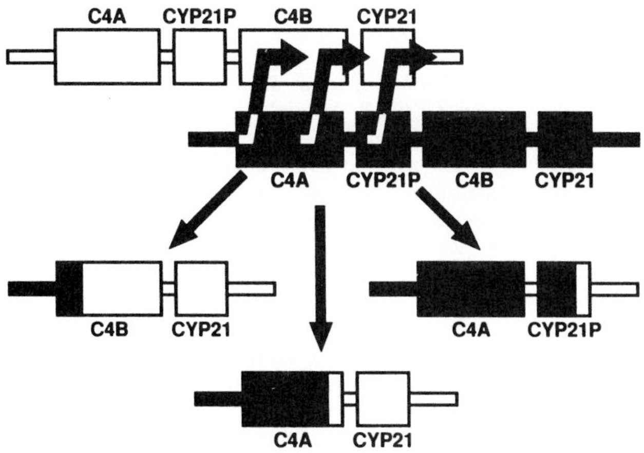

Fig. 159-18 Theoretical representation of crossing-over events involving the loci of the genes for the C4 complement and 21-hydroxylase. Depending on the level of unequal crossing over, one can obtain one complement gene made mainly of *C4B* sequences in its 3′ area with one *CYP21,* or one complement gene made mainly of *C4A* in its 5′ area with one *CYP21,* or one *C4A* and a 21-hydroxylase gene that includes mainly the 5′ part of *CYP21P.* In the third type of crossing over, the 21-hydroxylase gene, although it contains some sequences of the 3′ part of *CYP21,* is made mainly of the 5′ part of *CYP21P,* including deleterious mutations characteristic of *CYP21P.* (*From Migeon and Donohoue.*[129] *Used by permission from Endocrinology and Metabolism Clinics of North America.*)

The report of a case survey in the state of Maryland[168] definitely underestimated the incidence of the disorder. Various other surveys in Europe and North America reported an incidence of the disorder ranging from 1 in 10,000 to 1 in 25,000 births, giving a frequency of carriers for the mutant gene of 1 in 50 to 1 in 80. The incidence of CAH found in various screenings was slightly higher than that obtained by case surveys, with values between 1 in 10,000 and 1 in 18,000 births.[194] In the state of Texas, the incidence based on newborn screen is 1 in 16,000, with a ratio of salt-losing to non-salt-losing forms of 2.7:1.[195]

Much higher incidences were found in markedly inbred populations such as the Yupik Eskimo of Alaska, in whom the incidence by case survey was 1 in 490 births[196] and by screening[194] was 1 in 684 births. Another example of the effect of inbreeding was found in the island of La Reunion in the Indian Ocean, where the incidence by screening was 1 in 2000 births.[197]

The frequency of the attenuated form of 21-hydroxylase deficiency is even more difficult to determine in view of the frequent complaint of hirsutism and virilism in female subjects. Nomograms charting the values of 17-hydroxyprogesterone in basal conditions versus those 60 min after administration of intravenous ACTH have been used.[198] With this technique, the frequency of the attenuated form of CAH is high.[199] It is probable, though, that the frequency of the attenuated form is much lower than that expected from steroid studies. One also must consider that some cases of adrenal virilism may not represent mutation of the *CYP21* gene as reported in some familial cases not linked to HLA type.

Types of Mutations

Deletions of the 21-Hydroxylase B gene (CYP21). The presence of highly homologous, tandemly arranged genes provides an opportunity for meiotic mispairing and unequal crossing over between sister chromatids, thus leading to gene duplication in one chromatid and deletion in the other (Fig. 159-18). Obviously, loss of the *CYP21* gene on both chromosomes would lead to a complete loss of 21-hydroxylase activity. Although the precise frequency with which deletion causes clinical 21-hydroxylase deficiency has been the subject of some controversy, it is clear that abnormal numbers of 21-hydroxylase genes are found frequently both in the normal population and in patients with 21-hydroxylase deficiency. A reasonable consensus from a number of studies suggests that deletion events may account for approximately 20 to 25 percent of all 21-hydroxylase-deficient chromosomes (Table 159-3). Of these, the most frequent is deletion of a 30-kb region that includes the 3′ portion of *CYP21P,* all of *C4B,* and the 5′ end of *CYP21.* This deletion always appears to involve homologous bases within the *CYP21* gene and the *CYP21P* pseudogene such that no bases were added or deleted from the fusion gene. Because *CYP21P* includes a TaqI restriction site in its 5′ flanking region that is not shared by *CYP21* the hybrid or fusion gene almost always has a characteristic 3.2-kb TaqI fragment that is indistinguishable from that normally derived from *CYP21P.* The deletion boundary varies on different chromosomes but is generally between exons 3 and 8 of *CYP21.*[200] The 5′ end of the fusion gene thus contains sequences derived from *CYP21P* that include deleterious mutations that preclude enzymatic activity of the product, including those within the promoter region.[201] The deletion linked to HLA-Bw47 appears to be a more complicated genetic rearrangement rather than a single unequal crossover.[176]

Gene Conversion Events. Gene conversion is another mechanism that frequently produces *CYP21* mutations. Gene conversion

Table 159-3 Frequency of Various Mutations Among Haplotypes Carrying 21-Hydroxylase Deficiency in Certain Nationalities

	Nationality (Reference)									
Types of Mutation	American (312)	American (313)	American (314)	British (315)	Swedish (316)	French (317)	Dutch (318)	Italian (319)	Irish (320)	Spanish (321)
Deletion of *CYP21*	17[a]	38[a]	26	25	35	8[a]	23	11	33[c]	20
Large conversion of *CYP21* to *CYP21P*	11	8	15	NR	3	13	12	3	3	13
Duplication of *CYP21P*	3	NR	NR	NR	3	9	2	14	0	NR
Point mutation of *CYP21*[b]	57	35	59	42	53	68	65	86[d]	67	67
Number of pedigrees	14	13	17	11	17	53	29	33	15	38
Form of CAH[e]	SL	SL,SV	SL	SL,SV	SL,SV	SL,SV	SL,SV	SL,SV, AT	SL,SV	SL,SV, AT
Most prevalent HLA-B	Bw47	Bw47	NR	NR	B40	B12	NR	B5	B40	NR

[a] Percentage hyplotypes containing *CYP21* deletions, if all HLA-Bw47-linked deletions are counted as one haplotype, in order to correct for the preponderance of this haplotype in these populations.
[b] *CYP21* genes that had normal restriction patterns on Southern analysis were presumed to contain point mutations.
[c] Ten of 30 haplotypes contained *CYP21* deletions. Of these, 8 had the same HLA haplotype (A3, Bw60, Cw3, DRI).
[d] The high percentage of point mutations in this study is likely due to the inclusion of patients with attenuated CAH.
[e] SL, Salt-losing; SV, simple virilizing.

Table 159-4 Deleterious Point Mutations of *CYP21* Genes in 21-Hydroxylase Deficiency

Site of Mutation	Type of CAH
Base −4, C → T	AT
Exon 1, codon 30, C → T* (Pro → Leu)	AT
Second intron, C → T* (Aberrant splicing, frameshift)	SL, SV (Yupik Eskimos)
Exon 3, 8-bp deletion* (frameshift, premature termination) (Ile → Asn)	SL, SV
Exon 4, codon 172, G → C*	SL, SV
Exon 6, cluster of 3 T → A substitutions (Ile → Asn, Val → Glu, Met → Lys)	SL
Intron 7, splice donor site G → C†	SL
Exon 7, codon 292, G → A† (Gly → Ser)	SL
Exon 7, codon 281, G → T* (Val → Leu)	AT (HLA-B14)
Exon 7, codon 306, T insertion	SL or SV
Exon 8, codon 318, G → T (nonsense, Gln → stop)	SL
Exon 8, codon 339, G → A (Arg → His)	AT
Exon 8, codon 356, C → T (Arg → Trp)	SL, SV
Exon 9, codon 380, C → G† (Glu → Asp)	SL
Exon 9, codon 406, G → A† (Trp → stop)	SL
Exon 10, codon 453, C → T*,† (Pro → Ser)	AT
Exon 10, codon 483, G → C† (Arg → Pro)	SV
Exon 10, codon 484, GG → C† (frameshift)	SL
Exon 10, codon 494, A → G (Asn → Ser)†	SL

* Mutations that were confirmed as deleterious with in vitro expression studies.
† Mutations that were *not* characteristically found in the *CYP21P* pseudogene.
NOTE: AT, attenuated (late onset); SL, salt-losing; SV, simple virilizing.

involves a nonreciprocal exchange of homologous genetic information; the sequence of one gene (the target) is "converted" to that of a related gene (the source). These gene conversion events probably involve incorrect meiotic alignment of the two 21-hydroxylase genes followed by mismatch repair converting a segment of the sequence of the *CYP21* to that of the *CYP21P* pseudogene. The net result of such gene conversion events is the transfer of deleterious mutations from *CYP21P* to *CYP21*, thus leading to alterations in enzymatic activity of the encoded product. The various positions at which these small gene conversions are known to affect activity of the *CYP21* gene are summarized in Table 159-4. It is readily apparent that these gene conversion events generate the full spectrum of clinical phenotypes of 21-hydroxylase deficiency. In fact, gene conversions can account for a large number of mutations that alter the enzymatic activity of the *CYP21* product.[126,202–206] The most common point mutation of *CYP21* is the intron 2 mutation that occurs normally in the *CYP21P* gene and alters splicing. This is the presumed cause of CAH in the Yupik Eskimos; however, it has been associated with a broad range of phenotypes.[207,208] Expression studies have also confirmed the synergistic effects of a number of point mutations on 21-hydroxylase enzyme activity.[209]

In some patients, the *C4B/CYP21* tandem appears to be replaced by a *C4A/CYP21P* tandem, a so-called large gene conversion.[180] This accounts for up to 15 percent of mutations in the salt-losing form (see Table 159-3) and may have arisen as a result of two unequal crossing over events.

***De Novo* Point Mutations and Mutations That Were Not Transferred from *CYP21P*.** As discussed earlier, some of the apparent point mutations in *CYP21* reflect gene conversion events that introduce mutations from *CYP21P* into *CYP21*. In nearly all the reported cases, these mutations also were demonstrated in the heterozygous parents. One study revealed a patient with attenuated 21-hydroxylase deficiency who had two missense mutations (*R339H* and *P453S*) that are not found in *CYP21P* and that presumably represent *de novo* point mutations. When these mutations were analyzed in an expression system, they both resulted in mild impairment of 21-hydroxylase activity, consistent with the patient's phenotype.[210] Additional *de novo* mutations have been described but remain rare.[211] A *de novo* gene conversion involving the transfer of 390 nucleotides from *CYP21P* to *CYP21* in a maternal chromosome produced 21-hydroxylase deficiency in her offspring.[128] Point mutations within *CYP21* that were not derived from *CYP21P* have been identified in Swedish and American families.[212,213] These mutations showed Mendelian segregation patterns within the families.

Frequency of the Various Types of Mutations. As shown in Table 159-3, the frequency of various types of *CYP21* mutations and their corresponding HLA haplotypes is variable in the literature. As expected, point mutations of *CYP21* are the most frequent in all series reported. The frequency of deletion of *CYP21* and of its conversion to *CYP21P* is rather high; this is probably related to the tandem duplication of the complement and 21-hydroxylase genes.

Detection of heterozygotes for the CAH Trait. Attempts to determine carrier status by biochemical techniques were first made on obligate CAH heterozygotes. Carriers showed normal basal concentrations of steroids but abnormally elevated production of cortisol precursors (17-hydroxyprogesterone, progesterone) in response to ACTH stimulation. New *et al.*[198] have used plasma concentrations of 17-hydroxyprogesterone prior to and 60 min after intravenous ACTH administration. We advocate[214,215] measurement of the rate of increase of 17-hydroxyprogesterone and progesterone, the immediate precursors of cortisol, following intravenous ACTH administration and using the following formula:

$$(17\text{-OHP}_{30} - 17\text{-OHP}_0) + (P_{30} - P_0)/30 = \text{ng/dl/min}$$

where 17-OHP_{30} and 17-OHP_0 are the concentrations of 17-hydroxyprogesterone 30 min after and just before the administration of intravenous ACTH, and P_{30} and P_0 are the plasma concentrations of progesterone 30 min after and just before the injection of ACTH. Because the ovaries produce large amounts of 17-hydroxyprogesterone and progesterone late in the menstrual cycle, it is necessary to carry out the tests of adult females during the first 5 days after the beginning of the menstrual flow. A rate of increase of cortisol precursors of less than 7 ng/dl/min is found in subjects who are homozygous for two normal *CYP21* genes. Values of 9 to 30 ng/dl/min are found in heterozygotes for CAH. However, there is a 5 to 10 percent overlap between normal individuals and carriers. When biochemical tests were compared with genotyping to determine carrier status in one study, the latter method was felt to be more reliable.[216]

The biochemical techniques are the least expensive way to provide genetic counseling information to members of CAH families. Knowledge of the HLA typing of the index case also can be used in determining the carrier status, so long as no recombination occurs in the HLA locus. Molecular techniques can supplement these methods in families in whom the specific molecular defect in the proband can be determined.

Prenatal Diagnosis of 21-Hydroxylase Deficiency. The prenatal diagnosis of CAH is particularly useful if the index case presents the salt-losing form. This information may be used rarely for the purpose of terminating pregnancy in view of the often troublesome clinical course of these patients. It also can be useful in preparing for appropriate therapy if the fetus is affected.

A biopsy of chorionic villi can be obtained during the first trimester. This material can be used for HLA typing, karyotyping, and characterization of *CYP21* mutations.[217,218] All these methods imply that an index case has already been studied and that information is known about the HLA type and *CYP21* mutation.[218] Sources of error can arise from recombination in the HLA locus,[219] possibility of contamination of the fetal material by maternal tissue, and generation of unauthentic sequences by the polymerase chain reaction (PCR) amplification.

Amniocentesis can be performed at 15 to 18 weeks of gestation. Cells can be used for a karyotype, as well as for HLA type and *CYP21* genotype in some cases, whereas the fluid permits measurement of steroid concentrations. In affected fetuses, the levels of 17-hydroxyprogesterone and androstenedione are markedly elevated, and the concentrations of cortisol, progesterone, DHEA, and DHEA-S show no significant abnormalities.[220–223]

Prenatal Therapy of 21-Hydroxylase Deficiency. Although prenatal treatment of affected males is unnecessary, the most compelling reason for treating affected female fetuses is to reduce the masculinization of the genitalia.[224] Of major importance is the fact that corrective surgery of the external genitalia is not always satisfactory. In addition, many patients have difficulty in maintaining regular menses; this may be related to exposure of the fetal hypothalamus to abnormal androgen concentrations that disrupt the female cyclic secretion of luteinizing hormone and follicle-stimulating hormone. It also has been suggested that problems of gender identity encountered by a number of adult female patients may be due to fetal brain exposure to abnormal concentrations of androgens.

Requirements for effective therapy are well established. Since cortisol does not cross the placenta readily, it is necessary to use dexamethasone. Because the masculinization of the external genitalia takes place between 5 and 12 weeks of gestation, for therapy to be maximally effective, it must be started at 5 to 6 weeks. Treatment has been shown to normalize the external genitalia of affected females.[217,218,225] The dose of dexamethasone usually used is 20 μg/kg of body weight per 24 h, with a daily dose varying between 1 and 1.5 mg/day. Treatment is monitored by study of the suppression of cortisol secretion (concentration of maternal plasma cortisol, measurement of urinary excretion of free cortisol). As reviewed in the section entitled, "Physiology of the Adrenal Cortex," the fetal adrenal gland secretes large amounts of DHEA-S and its 16α-hydroxy derivative; the latter is metabolized by the placenta into 16α-hydroxyandrostenedione and estriol. Full suppression of fetal adrenal secretion results in suppression of estriol in maternal plasma and maternal urine. Hence estriol measurement is also used for monitoring therapy.

Since the chance of heterozygous parents having an affected child is 1 in 4, and since about half the fetuses will be male, the risk of an affected female fetus is only 12.5 percent, and dexamethasone therapy is given unnecessarily in 87.5 percent of pregnancies. Attempts to decrease the length of unnecessary therapy are made by prenatal diagnosis of CAH. Because of the slightly greater risk of abortion when biopsying the chorionic villi as compared with performing amniocentesis, we have adopted the following protocol of therapy (Danish RK, Migeon CJ, unpublished data):

1. Treatment is started at 5 to 7 weeks of gestation (at 8–11 weeks, results are less favorable; after 12 weeks, it is too late to start treatment).
2. The dose of dexamethasone is 0.5 mg orally every 12 h.
3. Dexamethasone therapy is stopped 10 days prior to amniocentesis. Immediately after amniotic fluid has been obtained, dexamethasone treatment is resumed.
4. Amniotic cells are used for determination of the karyotype, and the amniotic fluid is used for determination of 17α-hydroxyprogesterone, androstenedione, and testosterone concentrations. Results are obtained 3 to 7 days after the amniocentesis. Therapy is stopped if steroid concentrations are normal or if the karyotype is 46,XY. If the studies show the presence of an affected female, therapy is continued to the end of the pregnancy. At the time of labor and delivery, intravenous SoluCortef is administered to the mother. In three cases of affected female infants, only one infant showed a mild clitoral hypertrophy, and no side effects were observed.

Protocols for treatment and outcomes of therapy are similar in other centers,[217,226] and many centers also employ CYP21 genotyping.

In general, few side effects of therapy have been observed,[227] but abnormal weight gain, fluid retention, and hypertension may occur.[228] At this time, our opinion is that the potential advantages of treatment outweigh the possible risk of side effects.

Neonatal Screening. The concentration of 17α-hydroxyprogesterone can be determined on neonatal screening blood spots.[194] Using this method, studies of various groups of infants have determined the frequency of the disorder and of the mutant *CYP21* in the general population.

Neonatal screening also has been proposed to avoid complications occurring when CAH is unrecognized and untreated. Specifically, the purpose of screening would be to treat appropriately an acute adrenal crisis and to avoid potential death. At birth, females with the salt-losing form attract attention because of their ambiguous genitalia. Hence the major problem is related to male newborns who may be misdiagnosed or may be mistakenly thought to have pyloric stenosis. Based on an incidence of 1 salt-losing CAH infant per 20,000 births, and therefore, 1 affected male per 40,000 births, one can question the relative cost-benefit analysis. Although CAH screening does not appear worthwhile for many populations, it is certainly helpful in inbred populations who are at high risk. Many American states and other countries have included screening for CAH in their newborn screening panels. The major benefit has been the identification of affected males while they are still healthy. The pitfalls have been false-positive results in premature infants[229] and false-negative results as well as difficulty in differentiating the salt-losing and non-salt-losing forms in affected patients.[195,230]

CAH DUE TO DEFICIENCY OF 11β-HYDROXYLASE (CY11B1 DEFICIENCY)

Steroid 11β-hydroxylase deficiency was described initially as a hypertensive form of CAH in 1951,[146,231] and the biochemical defect was identified in 1956.[232] This form of CAH is relatively rare, accounting for approximately 5 percent of all cases of CAH. Given a frequency of 21-hydroxylase deficiency of 1 in 10,000 births, and assuming that one-half of 11β-hydroxylase–deficient patients are undetected, the calculated frequency of 11β-hydroxylase deficiency would be about 1 in 100,000 births.

Pathogenesis. In the zona fasciculata, the 11β-hydroxylase deficiency impairs decreased cortisol and corticosterone secretion. As in 21-hydroxylase deficiency, the consequent loss of negative feedback increases ACTH release, which in turn increases the production of the steroid precursors 11-deoxycortisol, DOC, and 18-hydroxy DOC. The hypertension seen in this form of CAH is attributed to the increased secretion of DOC. Secretion of 17-hydroxyprogesterone and progesterone also is increased, but to a lesser extent than in 21-hydroxylase deficiency. The mineralocorticoid effect of high DOC concentrations suppresses renin and angiotensin, resulting in very low aldosterone secretion. Thus this disorder is a genetically defined cause of "low renin hypertension."

Table 159-5 Urinary Steroid Profiles and Blood Pressure in Two Sibs with 11β-Hydroxylase Deficiency

Urinary Steroids (mg/24 h)	Patient JJ (Female, 29 yrs)	Patient AA (Female, 47 yrs)
Tetrahydro-11-deoxycortisol	22.0	3.5
Tetrahydro-11-deoxycorticosterone	0.3	0.5
Tetrahydro-cortisol and cortisone	4.5	0.8
Total 17-ketosteroids	3.8	4.6
Androsterone	0.4	0.1
Etiocholanolone	2.5	3.8
Dehydroisoandrosterone	0	0
11-Oxy-17-ketosteroids	0.2	0.7
Blood pressure (mmHg)		
Systolic	212–190	175
Diastolic	150–134	110

SOURCE: Data adapted by permission from David *et al.*[236]

Clinical Manifestations. The CYP11B1 deficiency, by impairing 11β-hydroxylase, leads to hypersecretion of ACTH. The hypersecretion of ACTH, in conjunction with the block in the normal corticosteroid biosynthetic pathway, causes an overproduction of adrenal androgens. Therefore, 11β-hydroxylase deficiency, like 21-hydroxylase deficiency, is characterized by masculinization of the female fetus and by early virilization postnatally. Females present at birth with variable degrees of ambiguity of the external genitalia, which can lead to male-appearing genitalia, with a phallic urethra and complete fusion of the labial-scrotal folds but no palpable gonads. On occasion, the virilism is not evident until puberty or adulthood,[233] thus resulting in a late onset form of the disease generally diagnosed only in females. Although mutations in *CYP11B1* were detected in two such patients, *CYP11B1* coding sequences were normal in several other patients with clinical manifestations suggestive of attenuated 11β-hydroxylase deficiency. These findings suggest that some caution should be used in making this diagnosis.[234]

Male newborns have normal external genitalia with descended testes. As with 21-hydroxylase deficiency, it is not unusual to find nodules of hyperplastic ectopic adrenal tissue in the spermatic cord, epididymis, or testes. Gynecomastia also has developed in several patients prior to puberty.[235] Deficient cortisol production and the consequent ACTH hypersecretion lead to significant increases in 11-deoxycortisol and DOC (see Fig. 159-3). Although 11-deoxycortisol has little biologic activity, DOC is a potent salt-retaining steroid that causes a high-mineralocorticoid, low-renin form of hypertension. This hypertension is usually moderate but occasionally can be sufficiently severe to cause cardiomegaly and eventual cardiac failure. For reasons that are not apparent, a few patients exhibit only minimal or no hypertension.

Diagnosis. In the appropriate clinical setting, the diagnosis of 11β-hydroxylase deficiency is made by detecting increased levels of DOC and 11-deoxycortisol in blood and/or their tetrahydro derivatives in urine. It must be remembered that these levels vary considerably in different patients, with significant variation even among sibs who are expected to have the same genotype[236] (Table 159-5). Prenatal diagnosis of 11β-hydroxylase deficiency is now available,[237] based on measurement of maternal urinary tetrahydro-11-deoxycortisol. This is of greatest benefit in populations at risk, such as Jews of Moroccan origin.[238]

Genetics. Initial descriptions of 11β-hydroxylase deficiency were consistent with autosomal recessive inheritance. A gene encoding 11β-hydroxylase was cloned in 1987.[239] Subsequent gene mapping studies suggested that the disorder was tightly linked to a locus encoding *CYP11B1* on chromosome 8q21-q22,[240] a finding consistent with the functional and anatomic segregation of the 11β-hydroxylase isozymes discussed below.

Subsequent advances have improved our understanding of the genetics and function of steroid 11β-hydroxylase. It is now apparent that two homologous adjacent 11β-hydroxylase genes, designated *CYP11B1* and *CYP11B2,* encode two distinct proteins.[240] Although the two genes encode proteins with 93 percent identity in their amino acid sequences, they differ in their sites of expression and in the enzymatic activities of their protein products. The product of the *CYP11B1* gene, termed *11β-hydroxylase,* is expressed at high levels in the inner zones of the adrenal cortex and can convert DOC to corticosterone but not to aldosterone. Thus this protein mediates 11β-hydroxylation but does not perform the terminal reactions required for aldosterone biosynthesis. The other gene, *CYP11B2,* encodes a protein that has been designated aldosterone synthase. This protein is uniquely expressed in the zona glomerulosa, where mineralocorticoids are produced, and catalyzes all reactions needed for the conversion of deoxycorticosterone to aldosterone (11β-hydroxylation, 18-hydroxylation, and 18-dehydrogenation; see Fig. 159-6).[240,241] A similar *CYP11B1/CYP11B2* gene arrangement has been described in mice.[242] The first genetic studies were of six families of Moroccan Jewish ancestry. When analyzed at the molecular level, 11 of 12 mutant *CYP11B1* genes contained a missense mutation (*R448H*) in exon 8.[243] As shown in Fig. 159-19, several other mutations that cause classic 11β-hydroxylase deficiency have been identified. Nonsense mutations, missense mutations, and small insertions and deletions, as well as a 5-bp duplication, have been identified.[241,244–246] All the nonsense and frameshift mutations result in truncated proteins lacking regions known to be essential for cytochrome P_{450} function, such as the heme-binding domain. With respect to the patients with attenuated 11β-hydroxylase

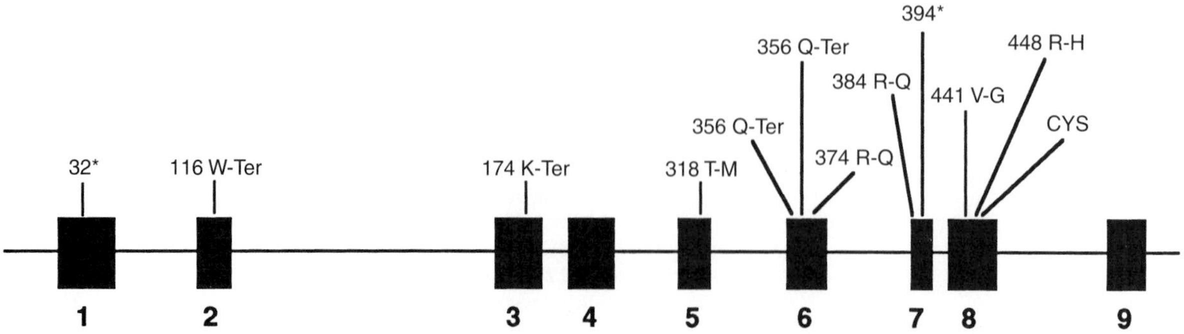

Fig. 159-19 Several mutations that cause 11β-hydroxylase deficiency. The positions of mutations in *CYP11B1* that are associated with 11β-hydroxylase deficiency are shown relative to the gene structure. CYS indicates the conserved cysteine that coordinates the heme group. The asterisks indicate the position of frameshift mutations.

deficiency described earlier, one was a compound heterozygote for missense mutations *N133H* and *T319M,* and the other was a compound heterozygote for a nonsense mutation (*Y423X*) on one allele and a missense mutation (*P42S*) on the other.[234] The precise mechanisms by which the missense mutations inactivate 11β-hydroxylase remain to be elucidated. When analyzed in an expression system, all the missense mutations abolished enzymatic activity, indicating their importance in the disease state. The *V441G* and *R448H* mutations cluster in close proximity to C-450, a residue that is conserved in all cytochromes P_{450} and serves as the fifth ligand to the heme iron. This proximity suggests that they may interfere with this essential domain. The *T318* residue also is highly conserved and is postulated to facilitate the proton transfer that cleaves molecular oxygen. Important insights into the structure-function relationships of *CYP11B1* mutations have been elucidated by *in vitro* studies of mutant enzyme activities.[246] Despite the duplicated *CYP11B1/CYP11B2* gene arrangement and its presumed predilection for unequal crossing over and gene deletion, such mutations have not yet been noted in 11β-hydroxylase deficiency.

Treatment. Cortisol replacement therapy corrects the secretion of excessive 11-deoxycortisol, DOC, and androgens so that the hypertension and hyperandrogenemia resolve. As expected, these patients do not require mineralocorticoid replacement therapy despite the block in aldosterone secretion because they are able to synthesize DOC and because their *CYP11B2* gene is intact.[247] As in 21-hydroxylase deficiency, affected females may require corrective surgery of their genitalia.

CONGENITAL ADRENAL HYPERPLASIA DUE TO DEFICIENCY OF 17α-HYDROXYLASE (CYP17 DEFICIENCY)

Like the aldosterone synthase enzyme discussed earlier, steroid 17α-hydroxylase catalyzes more than one enzymatic conversion on steroid intermediates, performing both the 17α-hydroxylase and 17,20-lyase reactions.[248] Dissociation of these two enzymatic functions was reported by using site-directed mutations in the rat *CYP17* gene.[249] The studies demonstrated amino acids in the *CYP17* protein product that are essential specifically for 17α-hydroxylation or for side-chain removal (17,20-lyase activity) and are illustrated in Fig. 159-20.

Current evidence suggests that a single human gene encodes steroid 17α-hydroxylase, since the cDNAs cloned from human testis and adrenal cortex were identical.[250] Moreover, in expression studies, a single cDNA isolated from the bovine adrenal gland exhibited both 17α-hydroxylase and 17,20-lyase activities.[251] Computer-based structural modeling of human CYP17 protein supports the presence of both enzyme activities.[251a]

Pathophysiology and Clinical Manifestations. The description of the first case of 17-hydroxylase deficiency in 1966[252] suggested a deficiency of both 17-hydroxylation and 17,20-desmolase. A severe deficiency of 17α-hydroxylase is relatively rare, although the reported number of patients now exceeds 120,[248] at least 14 of whom exhibited only 17,20-lyase deficiency. As with all forms of CAH, the underlying clinical manifestations result from the inability to produce normal levels of glucocorticoids and the consequent increase in ACTH secretion. Although cortisol is not produced, patients with 17α-hydroxylase deficiency produce large amounts of corticosterone, which binds the glucocorticoid receptor with an affinity approximately one-hundredth that of cortisol. The manifestations of glucocorticoid deficiency are thus less severe than in other forms of CAH. DOC, the precursor of corticosterone, is also secreted in abnormally large amounts (see Fig. 159-3). By virtue of the significant intrinsic mineralocorticoid activity of DOC, patients with 17α-hydroxylase deficiency present with hypertension. Although the biochemical pathways for aldosterone production in the zona glomerulosa are intact, the presence of high circulating concentrations of DOC suppresses the renin-angiotensin system, thus leading to decreased aldosterone levels.

In addition to 17α-hydroxylase deficiency preventing glucocorticoid biosynthesis, the deficiency of 17,20-lyase causes an

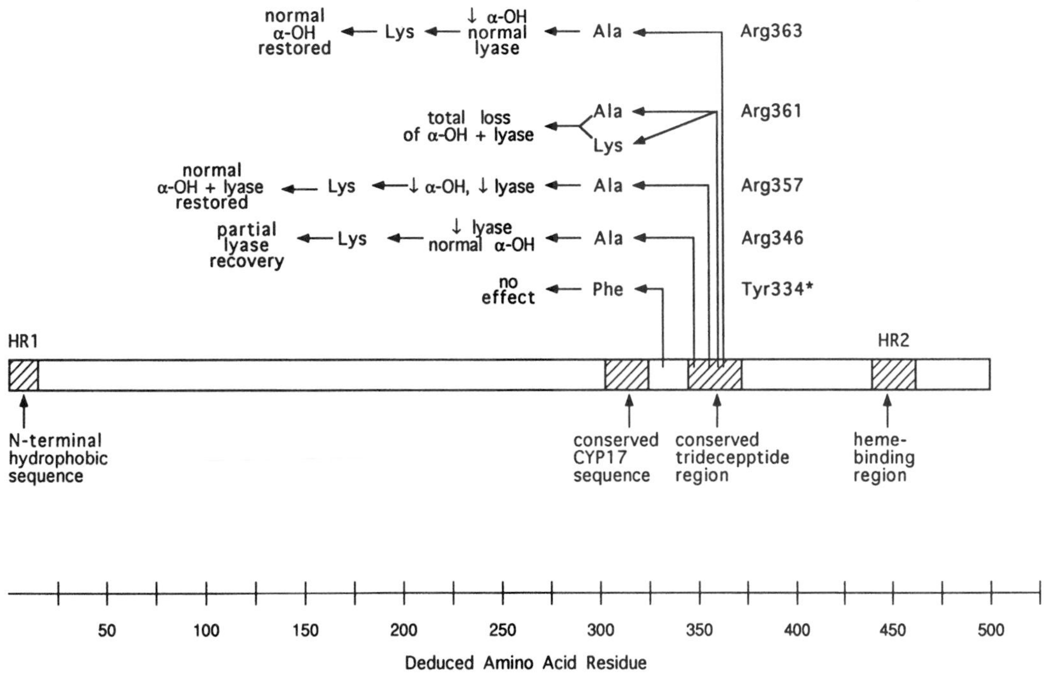

Fig. 159-20 Map of site-directed mutations of the rat *CYP17* cDNA. Schematic scale diagram shows the locations of conserved regions and of mutations tested in the P_{450c17} protein. The *CYP17* cDNA underwent site-directed mutagenesis to produce the codon changes shown. The mutants were expressed in COS-1 cells, and 17α-hydroxylase (α-OH) and 17,20-lyase (lyase) activities were measured. The mutations at arginine 346, 357, and 363 were corrected by a second mutation replacing the mutant alanine with lysine. * The only residue tested that is not conserved between the rat and human; HR1 and HR2-, homologous regions 1 and 2; both contain highly conserved critical cysteine residues.

inability to form C-19 and C-18 steroids from C-21 precursors, thus impairing the production of androgens and estrogens. Since normal development of external genitalia in males requires testosterone biosynthesis *in utero*, affected males have incomplete genital development and present with ambiguous external genitalia (pseudohermaphroditism) and in some cases with completely female-appearing genitalia. Müllerian regression occurs normally because production of Müllerian-inhibiting substance is not affected by the CYP17 deficiency. Because *in utero* development of female fetuses does not require endogenous sex steroid production, the external genitalia of affected females are normal at birth. In both females and in males with pseudohermaphroditism, the inability to produce sex steroids is manifested later in life, at the time of puberty. Female patients usually present with primary amenorrhea and clinical signs of hypogonadism, including scant or absent axillary and pubic hair due to adrenal androgen deficiency, as well as infantile breast and genital development. Male pseudohermaphrodites present with ambiguous genitalia and failure of masculinization at puberty.

Diagnosis. As in all forms of CAH, 17α-hydroxylase deficiency results in decreased cortisol secretion and increased ACTH output. However, changes in cortisol secretion are difficult to demonstrate.

From 3 to 4 months of age until puberty, plasma concentrations of 17-hydroxyprogesterone and 17-hydroxypregnenolone are normally low; thus demonstration of decreased concentrations in patients with 17α-hydroxylase deficiency is not always possible. The same is true for concentrations of androgens (DHEA, DHEA-S, androstenedione, testosterone) and estrogens (estradiol).

By contrast, increased levels of pregnenolone, progesterone, DOC, 18-hydroxy DOC, and corticosterone will be characteristic. These steroid concentrations can be determined in plasma or in urine (as their respective glucuronidated tetrahydro derivatives). Because of the increased DOC, 18-hydroxy DOC, and corticosterone secretion, the renin and aldosterone levels are below normal.

The steroid patterns so far described apply to patients with combined 17α-hydroxylase and 17,20-lyase deficiencies. In isolated 17,20-lyase deficiency, there is an increase in 17-hydroxyprogesterone and 17-hydroxypregnenolone concentrations. Thus an adequate flow of precursors results in normal cortisol and aldosterone secretion, and the levels of corticosterone and DOC are approximately normal.

In newborn patients with 46,XY karyotype and ambiguous genitalia, the measurement of cortisol and androgen precursors elucidates the enzymatic defect. It must be noted that the diagnosis may be missed in infants with completely female-appearing genitalia whether the karyotype is 46,XX or 46,XY. At the age when puberty is expected, 17α-hydroxylase deficiency will be detected because of elevated gonadotropin levels, low gonadal steroid concentrations, elevated levels of precursors, and low-renin hypertension.

Genetics. The gene encoding 17α-hydroxylase, *CYP17*, has been mapped to chromosome 10q24.3.[248,253] Its nucleotide sequence and gene structure most closely resemble those of *CYP21*, the other microsomal steroid hydroxylase. Analyses of *CYP17* alleles from patients with 17α-hydroxylase deficiency have defined the causal mutations in a number of patients.[248,254–261] A summary of the various mutations producing CYP17 deficiency is provided in Table 159-6. In contrast to 21-hydroxylase deficiency, large-scale deletions are not an important cause of 17α-hydroxylase deficiency. Rather, the deleterious mutations include missense and nonsense mutations as well as small insertions or deletions that alter the reading frame or splice sites. A quite interesting mutation was identified in an Italian patient with combined 17α-hydroxylase/17,20-lyase deficiency. The patient was homozygous for an insertion of 469 bp of foreign DNA into the site of a 518-bp deletion spanning exon II, intron 2, and part of exon III of the *CYP17* gene. Because of the similarity in sizes of the insertion and deletion, Southern blotting showed no detectable abnormality. The foreign DNA shared 95.5 percent sequence similarity with the nuclear antigen-binding site on Marek disease virus DNA and with sequences of rearranged mitochondrial DNA of rat hepatoma cells, and it shared 99 percent sequence similarity with part of the *Escherichia coli* lac operon. The inserted DNA contained an in-frame stop codon, resulting in a severely truncated P_{450C17} molecule.[262] A small deletion of three codons, D487-S488-F489, has been identified in a Thai patient with combined 17α-hydroxylase/17,20-lyase deficiency and was proven to be deleterious with *in vitro* studies.[263] In a Japanese patient previously thought to have glucocorticoid-remediable aldosteronism (GRA) hypertension (see below), detection of a *CYP17* gene mutation resulted in a change in diagnosis.[264] A patient with isolated 17,20-lyase deficiency was a compound heterozygote for a missense mutation causing loss of 17,20-lyase activity but normal 17α-hydroxylase activity *in vitro*.[265] The patient's other mutation truncated the product, thus rendering it nonfunctional. The molecular basis in another patient with isolated 17,20-lyase deficiency also has been described.[266]

Treatment. Cortisol replacement therapy, as in the other forms of CAH, will suppress ACTH output and the excessive mineralo-

Table 159-6 Mutations of the *GYP17* Gene in Patients with 17α-Hydroxylase/17, 20-Lyase Deficiency

Karyotype	External Genitalia	Sex of Rearing	Mutations	Codon (Exon)
46,XY	F	F	4-bp (CATC) duplication (frameshift with early stop)	480 (8)
46,XX	F	F	TGG → TGA (Trp → stop)	17 (1)
46,XX	F	F	TTC deletion (loss of phenylalanine)	53 (1)
46,XY	F	F	7-bp (GCGCACA) duplication	120 (2)
46,XY	Ambiguous	F	ACA → CCA (Pro → Thr)	342 (6)
			CGA → TGA (Arg → stop)	239 (4)
46,XY	F	F	CAG → TAG (Gln → stop)	461 (8)
			CGC → TGC (Arg → Cys)	496 (8)
46,XY	F	F	518-bp deletion containing 469-bp insertion of foreign DNA	Involves the 3′ end of exon 2, intron 2, and 5′ end of exon 3
46,XY*	F	F	TCC → CCC (Ser → Pro)	106 (2)
46,XX†	F	F	In-frame 9-bp deletion	487/488/489 (8)
46,XX	F	F	1-base deletion → frameshift	483 (8)

* Described in two unrelated patients, both homozygous for the same mutation.
† In-frame deletion demonstrated to be deleterious in an in vitro system.

SOURCE: Data are compiled from published reports.[248,254,256,261–263] Many additional point mutations have been described,[257–260] including one altering only 17,20-lyase activity.[266]

corticoid secretion. This treatment generally causes the blood pressure to normalize.

Adult females and genetic male patients reared as females require estrogen replacement therapy. Removal of abdominal testes is recommended because of the risk of malignant transformation. Adult genetic males reared as males need surgical correction of their external genitalia and androgen replacement therapy.

CONGENITAL ADRENAL HYPERPLASIA DUE TO DEFICIENCY OF 3β-HYDROXYSTEROID DEHYDROGENASE

Pathogenesis and Clinical Manifestations. CAH due to 3β-HSD deficiency represents less than 1 percent of all CAH cases. In severe 3β-HSD deficiency there is a nearly total absence of secretion of biologically active adrenal steroids. This is due to an inability to synthesize steroids with the Δ4-3 ketone group characteristic of the biologically active glucocorticoids, mineralocorticoids, and androgens. The only accumulated precursors prior to the enzymatic blocks are pregnenolone and its 16α-, 17α-, and 20α-hydroxylated derivatives, as well as DHEA and several of its hydroxylated derivatives (see Fig. 159-3). Thus there are deficiencies of glucocorticoids, mineralocorticoids, and active androgens. The first report of cases of this type of deficiency was in 1962.[267] Five of the six patients in this report were salt-losers, and four of them died despite seemingly adequate replacement therapy. By 1970, there were approximately 20 patients reported.[268,269] The mapping of a gene encoding 3β-HSD to chromosome 1p13 was consistent with the clinical observation that the disorder is inherited as an autosomal recessive manner.[270]

The main androgens secreted in this form of CAH are DHEA and its 16-hydroxylated derivative. Neither binds to the androgen receptor, and thus neither has biologic androgenic activity. Regardless of this, patients with severe 3β-HSD deficiency exhibit some androgenic effects (females present with slight labial fusion and clitoral enlargement; males present with ambiguous genitalia). This suggests that the enzyme deficiency is not complete and that biologically active androgens are produced and cause mild masculinization of the external genitalia in females.[140] On the other hand, there is inadequate androgen production to result in complete masculinization of the genitalia in males. As with 21-hydroxylase deficiency, the impaired corticosteroid production is manifested by signs and symptoms of adrenal insufficiency that may be fatal if left untreated in the neonatal period. Less severe defects may lead to a variant that is akin to the non-salt-wasting 21-hydroxylase-deficiency patients, who produce sufficient mineralocorticoid to avoid salt-wasting crises. In contrast to 21-hydroxylase deficiency, in which gonadal steroid production is unimpaired, 3β-HSD deficiency also prevents gonadal steroidogenesis, and patients exhibit abnormal genital development, as discussed earlier.

Studies have suggested that a milder 3β-HSD deficiency may be the cause of minimal androgen excess in some females.[271–273] Indeed, analysis of steroid profiles, particularly following ACTH infusion, have suggested a mild defect in 3β-HSD activity in some patients presenting with hirsutism, oligomenorrhea, or infertility.[274] Population studies suggest that this milder form of 3β-HSD deficiency may be a relatively common disorder of steroid hormone biosynthesis. These milder manifestations are seen only in females, presumably because the effects of mild androgen excess in males are not readily detected. Of note, analyses of the various isoforms of 3β-HSD in these patients with late onset 3β-HSD deficiency have not revealed any mutations (see below). Thus the role of the 3β-HSD genes in these patients remains to be determined.

Diagnosis. Deficiency of 3β-HSD may be diagnosed by demonstrating elevated levels of Δ5 steroids—pregnenolone, 17α-hydroxypregnenolone, DHEA, and 16α-hydroxy-DHEA—in serum and urine. The typical finding is an elevated ratio of Δ5 to Δ4 steroids. However, the interpretation of baseline steroid profiles can be complicated by the peripheral conversion of Δ5 steroids by the type I enzyme (see "Genetics" below), which is expressed normally in various tissues such as liver, skin, and mammary gland. Therefore, patients with the attenuated form are best diagnosed by provocative testing with ACTH, with particular attention to absolute 17α-hydroxypregnenolone concentrations and to the ratio of 17α-hydroxypregnenolone to 17α-hydroxyprogesterone.

Newborn infants normally secrete relatively high amounts of DHEA, DHEA-S, and pregnenolone and its metabolites. Newborns with 21-hydroxylase deficiency also may secrete increased amounts of Δ5 steroids. Thus the steroid concentrations must be interpreted with caution, and sometimes it may be difficult to establish the diagnosis in mild deficiencies.

Genetics. Major advances have been made in our understanding of the molecular genetics of 3β-HSD. These studies have identified two distinct human genes that encode isozymes of 3β-HSD, designated *type I* and *type II,* both of which localize to chromosome 1p13.[275,276] Although the products of these two genes differ slightly in the kinetics with which they metabolize steroids, both forms convert C-21 and C-19 steroids with Δ5-3β-hydroxyl groups into corresponding Δ4-3 ketones, arguing against distinct roles of the two isozymes in the production of glucocorticoids and androgens. Of particular interest, the type II gene is expressed only in the typical steroidogenic tissues (adrenal and gonads), whereas the type I gene is expressed predominantly in nonsteroidogenic tissues such as placenta, skin, and mammary gland. This finding explains the previous demonstration that patients with CAH secondary to 3β-HSD deficiency had intact peripheral 3β-HSD activity despite severe impairment in adrenal and gonadal steroidogenesis. In mice, at least three isoforms of 3β-HSD exist, two of which are male-specific.[277,278]

The molecular defects responsible for salt-losing CAH in association with 3β-HSD deficiency have been defined using approaches similar to those employed with 21-hydroxylase. The first molecular characterization defined two different mutations in the type II gene—a nonsense mutation at codon 171 and a frameshift mutation in which insertion of a C at codon 186 altered the reading frame.[279] To date, analyses of these patients have identified many point mutations that include nonsense and frameshift mutations.[280–282] In a non-salt-wasting patient, an interesting missense mutation (*A245P*) was described[280]; the cDNA encoded by this mutated allele retained approximately 10 percent of normal activity in transfected cells, suggesting that sufficient enzymatic activity was retained *in vivo* to permit mineralocorticoid biosynthesis. Other studies of non-salt-wasting patients revealed additional missense mutations and splice-site alterations.[283,284] As more patients with deficiency of 3β-HSD have been studied, structure-function relationships of mutations in the salt-losing and non-salt-losing forms have been determined.[285] To date, no 3β-HSD gene mutations have been identified in the milder, late onset form.[286,287]

Treatment. As with other forms of CAH, cortisol replacement therapy will correct the abnormal steroid secretion and the cortisol deficiency. When electrolytes and water balance are disturbed, mineralocorticoid replacement therapy also must be administered.

In the fairly complete form, it is expected that sex-steroid replacement will be needed after puberty, but in many cases androgen and estrogen secretion is normal.

CONGENITAL LIPOID ADRENAL HYPERPLASIA (StAR DEFICIENCY)

Pathogenesis, Clinical Manifestations, and Diagnosis. This is an extremely rare but interesting form of CAH. Initially described in 1957,[287a] the underlying defect in lipoid CAH is an inability to convert cholesterol to pregnenolone, precluding the biosynthesis of all major steroid classes. Because of a failure to produce androgens in utero, genetic males present with normal-appearing female external genitalia; because of unimpaired production of Müllerian-inhibiting substance, the internal ducts develop along male patterns. In contrast, females appear completely normal at birth. Because of their inability to produce glucocorticoids and mineralocorticoids, patients present postnatally with symptoms and signs of adrenocortical insufficiency, including poor feeding, vomiting, lethargy, volume depletion, respiratory distress, and hyponatremic, hyperkalemic acidosis. In contrast to patients with salt-wasting 21-hydroxyase deficiency, the age of presentation varies, and patients may not be diagnosed until several months of age. Moreover, there are reports of genetic females (46,XX) with lipoid CAH who, at the time of puberty, underwent menarche, strongly suggesting some capacity for gonadal steroidogenesis.[80,82]

The adrenal glands in patients with lipoid CAH show marked hyperplasia, with cortical cells engorged with lipoid material containing cholesterol and cholesterol esters. This histologic picture and the failure to produce significant amounts of any steroids led to the hypothesis that congenital lipoid adrenal hyperplasia results from a mutation in *CYP11A*. Recent studies have shown definitively that lipoid CAH results from mutations in StAR that impair cholesterol delivery to the inner mitochondrial membrane where *CYP11A* carries out the initial step in steroidogenesis. Based on the finding that males exhibit evidence for androgen action in their internal genital structures and the onset of menses in some XX patients at puberty, a two-stage model for the pathogenesis of lipoid CAH has been proposed.[83] According to this model, some steroidogenesis can occur in the absence of StAR, allowing virilization of male internal genitalia and initiation of menses in females.[81] Persistent exposure to trophic hormones, however, leads to severe deposits of cholesterol and cholesterol esters within steroidogenic cells, ultimately leading to their death. It is at this point that the capacity for steroid production is lost completely. The recent development of a knockout mouse model of StAR deficiency should provide a model system in which to verify this two-stage model.[288]

Genetics. The human StAR gene maps to chromosome 8p11.2. StAR mutations causing lipoid CAH include frameshift, nonsense, missense, and splicing mutations that interfere with StAR activity.[83,289,290] Strikingly, many of the missense mutations cluster at the C-terminal region of the protein, suggesting that these residues are essential for cholesterol delivery.

The genes encoding the three peptides required for the conversion of cholesterol to pregnenolone (CYP11A and its cofactors, adrenodoxin, and adrenodoxin reductase) have been cloned and mapped (see Table 159-2). CYP11A is encoded by a single gene[211] that maps to chromosome 15q23-q24.[253] A rabbit model of CYP11A deficiency is clinically similar to this form of CAH in humans. CAH in the rabbit model is due to a *CYP11A* deletion.[291] Adrenodoxin is encoded by a gene on chromosome 11q22, and adrenodoxin pseudogenes map to chromosome 20.[253] Two alternatively spliced human adrenodoxin reductase mRNA molecules are encoded by a single gene on chromosome 17q24-q25.[248] Both species of mRNA are present in human testis and adrenal cortex.[292]

Treatment. The presentation with overt adrenal crisis necessitates aggressive initial therapy, as described for the salt-losing crisis of 21-hydroxylase deficiency. Lifelong replacement therapy with glucocorticoid and mineralocorticoid is required, and estrogen replacement is needed at puberty. Long-term follow-up is available in only a limited number of patients.[80,81,293]

CYP11A Deficiency. There are no documented cases of CYP11A deficiency. As discussed earlier, lipoid CAH initially was believed to result from *CYP11A* mutations, but it is now clear that these patients have mutations in StAR that abrogate steroidogenesis. Based on the known importance of placental steroids in the maintenance of human pregnancy, it has been proposed that mutations in *CYP11A* are incompatible with fetal survival *in utero*. The proposal that placentally derived progesterone—and thus CYP11A—is essential to maintain human pregnancy suggests that some cases of recurrent miscarriage may result from mutations of *CYP11A* that preclude placental steroidogenesis.

DEFECTS IN ALDOSTERONE PRODUCTION

Strictly speaking, isolated defects in the production of mineralocorticoids do not cause the hyperplasia of the adrenal glands seen with deficient glucocorticoid biosynthesis and consequent elevated ACTH secretion. Nonetheless, important advances have been made in our understanding of the molecular basis of certain of these disorders, and it is appropriate to consider them in this chapter. There are three major genetic disorders of mineralocorticoid biosynthesis. Deficiencies in CYP11B2 are associated with two of these disorders. A third genetic disorder of this locus is a rare form of autosomal dominant hypertension caused by a hybrid *CYP11B1/CYP11B2* gene.

Defects in Aldosterone Synthase

A genetic defect in the *CYP11B2* gene impairs the production of mineralocorticoids without compromising glucocorticoid production. Because the unimpaired glucocorticoid production provides normal negative-feedback inhibition, the adrenal cortex is not chronically exposed to high ACTH concentrations, and this disorder is not associated with adrenal hyperplasia. It was hypothesized previously that two distinct enzymes carried out 18-hydroxylation and 18-oxidation, now known to be performed by CYP11B2, and two deficiencies were characterized clinically—corticosterone methyloxidase I (CMO I) deficiency and corticosterone methyloxidase II (CMO II) deficiency. More recent analyses have shown definitively that a single protein, encoded by the *CYP11B2* gene, catalyzes both these reactions, as well as the initial 11β-hydroxylation required for aldosterone production.[294]

Pathophysiology, Clinical Features, and Diagnosis. Deficient CMO I or CMO II causes aldosterone deficiency and elevated renin, accompanied by accumulation of steroid precursors prior to the biosynthetic block: DOC and corticosterone in CMO I deficiency; DOC, corticosterone, and 18-hydroxycorticosterone in CMO II deficiency (see Fig. 159-6). These precursors possess some mineralocorticoid activity, which compensates partially for the aldosterone deficiency. Thus patients with CMO I or CMO II deficiency generally present with partial salt loss, rather than with the typical salt-losing crisis of complete mineralocorticoid deficiency. Infants may present only with failure to thrive.

18-Hydroxylase (CMO I) Deficiency. This was first described as the etiology of isolated aldosterone deficiency in a Dutch family with three affected children.[295,296] Renal salt-wasting and decreased growth velocity developed in these children. Laboratory evaluation revealed undetectable urinary aldosterone with elevated excretion of DOC and corticosterone. Postmortem histopathologic specimens from one patient showed poor development of the adrenal zona glomerulosa and hyperplasia of the renal juxtaglomerular apparatus. Treatment of the surviving sibs with mineralocorticoid supplementation resulted in resumption of normal growth along with decreased excretion of DOC and corticosterone.

Genetics. Molecular analyses of patients with CMO I deficiency showed that mutations within *CYP11B2* totally preclude aldosterone synthase activity rather than selectively impairing 18-hydroxylation.[244,295]

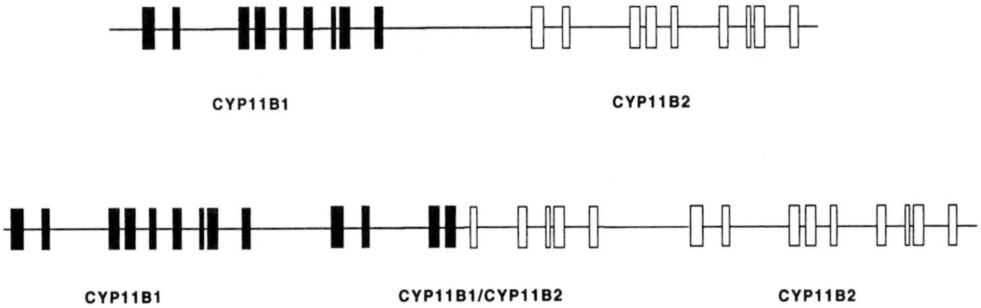

Fig. 159-21 Molecular basis of glucocorticoid-remediable aldosteronism. The normal gene organization of the *CYP11B1* and *CYP11B2* genes is shown above. Below is the hybrid *CYP11B1/CYP11B2* gene that results from meiotic mismatch and unequal crossing over. In all instances, the crossover is located 5′ to intron 4 of the *CYP11B* genes.

18-Oxidase (CMO II) Deficiency. This is more common than CMO I deficiency, based on a greater number of reported cases. The earliest descriptions were in 1964,[297] with additional cases reviewed in 1980.[298] Because of their selective inability to produce mineralocorticoids, patients with CMO II deficiency present with typical abnormalities of electrolyte and water metabolism. Severe electrolyte abnormalities can occur in the neonatal period, with potentially life-threatening hyponatremia and hyperkalemia. However, adrenal crisis as seen in 21-hydroxylase deficiency is rare, probably because the normal secretion of cortisol can compensate partially for the lack of mineralocorticoids. Although electrolyte abnormalities and poor growth persist throughout early childhood, symptoms later in life are attenuated and eventually disappear. At the time of diagnosis, there are increased concentrations of corticosterone and 18-hydroxycorticosterone in plasma, accompanied by an increased ratio of urinary 18-hydroxycorticosterone to aldosterone.

Genetics. Like CMO I deficiency, CMO II deficiency is caused by mutations residing within the *CYPIIB2* structural gene. In the first case described, the mutated gene contained two missense mutations—*R181W* and *V386A*.[299] When analyzed by expression studies, these two mutations together resulted in the loss of both 18-hydroxylase and 18-oxidase activities. The presence of either mutation alone does not lead to clinical manifestations, since apparently asymptomatic patients have been found with either mutation in isolation. Other complex mutations in *CYPIIB2* also have been associated with CMO II deficiency.[294,300,301]

Glucocorticoid-Remediable Aldosteronism (GRA)

An important determinant of normal corticosteroid regulation is the zone-specific expression of CYP11B2, which carries out the terminal steps in mineralocorticoid production. The clinical syndrome of GRA (also termed *dexamethasone-suppressible hypertension*) provides a striking example of the consequences of alterations in zonally segregated expression.

Pathogenesis and Clinical Manifestations. Clinical studies identified a form of hypertension with symptoms and laboratory findings that resembled those seen with an aldosterone-secreting adrenal adenoma.[302,303] These findings included hypokalemia in the setting of high aldosterone and low renin levels. However, elevated urinary excretions of 18-hydroxy- and 18-oxocortisol (steroids not normally found in appreciable amounts) also were observed. In contrast to primary aldosteronism, the hypertension in these patients was suppressed by short-term treatment with dexamethasone, and this disease was therefore termed GRA. Careful analyses of families by screening for elevated 18-hydroxy- and 18-oxocortisol showed a surprisingly large variation in serum potassium levels of individual patients, some of them maintaining normal levels. The lack of consistent hypokalemia, which is commonly used as a screening test to identify hypertensive patients with abnormal mineralocorticoid production, suggests that a number of patients with GRA may be missed.[304]

The pathogenesis of GRA is a persistent and unregulated overproduction of mineralocorticoids, eventually leading to hypertension and hypokalemia. In the setting of prolonged hyperaldosteronism, the hypertension can produce secondary changes in the renal vasculature, thus causing a fixed form of hypertension.

Genetics. GRA is an autosomal dominant disorder whose degree of penetrance varies depending on whether the diagnosis is based on hypokalemia and hypertension, which are relatively insensitive indexes, or analyses of abnormal steroid metabolites in urine that are hallmarks of GRA. These abnormal cortisol derivatives and the favorable effects of glucocorticoid treatment suggested that inner cortical zones, which express CYP17 and are ACTH-responsive, produced the excess mineralocorticoids. The recognition that two distinct gene products perform the terminal steps in biosynthesis of mineralocorticoid (CYP11B2) and glucocorticoid (CYP11B1) prompted the proposal that a hybrid *CYP11B1/CYP11B2* gene caused the disorder. As shown in Fig. 159-21, the promoter-regulatory sequences derived from *CYP11B1* would direct ACTH-responsive expression of the chimeric gene in the inner (fasciculata and reticularis) cortical zones. The chimeric protein, by virtue of critical amino acids encoded by *CYP11B2,* should perform all reactions required for aldosterone production, thus causing ACTH-dependent hyperaldosteronism. Ectopic expression of the chimeric protein in the inner cortical zones, which also express CYP17, would permit the formation of 18-hydroxy- and 18-oxocortisol, the biochemical hallmarks of GRA. Finally, treatment with glucocorticoids, by suppressing the steroidogenesis of the zona fasciculata and reticularis, should alleviate the hypertension.

Studies have elegantly verified this model. At least 13 independently derived chimeric genes have been identified at the molecular level,[305–308] all of which contain 5′ sequences derived from the *CYP11B1* gene and 3′ sequences derived from the *CYP11B2* gene. All crossovers occurred downstream of exon 2 and upstream of exon 5, a region identified in transfection studies as essential for aldosterone synthase activity.[305]

Treatment. In contrast to patients with essential hypertension, a pathophysiologically sound and effective treatment for GRA exists. Replacement doses of glucocorticoids, by suppressing steroidogenesis by the zonae fasciculata and reticularis, alleviate the mineralocorticoid excess. Although initial studies used dexamethasone, this potent glucocorticoid has caused hypercortisolism in some patients. Determining the optimal dose of glucocorticoid can be difficult, especially in children, in whom glucocorticoid requirements vary markedly at different stages of development. Alternative therapies include mineralocorticoid antagonists such as spironolactone, which competitively inhibits the mineralocorticoid receptor, and amiloride, which indirectly inhibits mineralocorticoid actions in the kidney. As noted earlier, prolonged hypertension can produce a fixed hypertension that is less amenable to treatment with glucocorticoids.

SYNDROME OF APPARENT MINERALOCORTICOID EXCESS

With the cloning of the mineralocorticoid receptor, it became apparent that its affinity for cortisol equals that for aldosterone. This raises a paradox, because specificity of mineralocorticoid action is maintained *in vivo* despite circulating levels of cortisol that exceed those of aldosterone by at least 100-fold. Insights into the mechanisms that maintain this specificity came from analyses of patients with the syndrome of apparent mineralocorticoid excess (AME). AME is a rare inherited disorder of steroid metabolism in which patients exhibit manifestations of a high mineralocorticoid state, including hypertension, hypokalemia, and suppressed plasma renin. Serum aldosterone levels are paradoxically very low, with the major abnormality in steroid hormone levels being a markedly elevated ratio of cortisol to cortisone.[309,310] It was proposed that AME patients have a deficiency of 11β-HSD that inactivates cortisol by converting it to cortisone and thus were subject to persistent activation of the mineralocorticoid receptor by circulating glucocorticoids. A very similar clinical picture results from ingestion of large amounts of licorice or from treatment with carbenoxalone, and subsequent studies demonstrated that the active ingredient in licorice (glycyrrhetinic acid) and carbenoxalone both inhibit 11β-HSD.[311]

The molecular explanation for AME came with the cloning of 11β-HSD. Two distinct 11β-HSD cDNAs were isolated: type I (*HSD11B1*), which is expressed predominantly in the liver and catalyzes NADP-dependent dehydrogenation and reduction, and type II (*HSD11B2*), which is expressed in the kidney and placenta and catalyzes NAD-dependent dehydrogenation. Strikingly, analyses of multiple kindreds with AME demonstrated mutations in the *HSD11B2* gene that preclude the production of functional 11β-HSD activity. These studies provide compelling evidence for the essential role of the type II isozyme of 11β-HSD in protecting the mineralocorticoid receptor from cortisol.[311a]

Note added in proof: Educational materials for families of patients with disorders of sexual differentiation or congenital adrenal hyperplasia are available at www.med.jhu.edu/pedendo/ml.patient.htw

REFERENCES

1. Addison T: *On the Constitutional and Local Effects of the Suprarenal Capsules*. London, Samuel Higley, 1855.
2. Brown-Sequard GE: Recherche experimentale sur la physiologie et pathologie des capsules surrenales. *CR Seances Soc Biol* **43**:422, 1856.
3. Rogoff JM, Stewart GN: Supra cortical extracts in suprarenal insufficiency. *JAMA* **92**:1569, 1929.
4. Hartman FA, Aaron AH, Culp JE: The use of cortin in Addison syndrome. *Endocrinology* **14**:438, 1930.
5. Thorn GW, Howard RP, Emerson KJ: Treatment of Addison syndrome with dexoxycorticosterone acetate. *J Clin Invest* **18**:449, 1939.
6. Mason HL, Myers CS, Kendall EC: The chemistry of crystalline substances isolated from suprarenal gland. *J Biol Chem* **114**:613, 1936.
7. Hench PS, Kendall EC, Slocumb CH, Polley HF: Effect of hormone of adrenal cortex (17-hydroxy-11-dehydrocortisone; compound E) and of pituitary adrenocorticotropic hormone on rheumatoid arthritis: Preliminary report. *Proc Staff Meetings Mayo Clin* **24**:181, 1949.
8. Cushing H: Basophil adenoma of the pituitary body. *Bull Johns Hopkins Hosp* **50**:1371932.
9. Albright F: Cushing syndrome: Its pathological physiology, its relationship to the adrenogenital syndrome and its connection with the problem of the reaction of the body to injurious agents ("alarm reaction" of Selye). *Harvey Lect* **38**:123,1942.
10. DeCrecchia L: Sopra un caso di apparence virili in una donna. *Il Morgani* **7**:151, 1865.
11. Butler AM, Ross RA, Talbot NB: Probable adrenal insufficiency in an infant. *J Pediatr* **15**:831, 1939.
12. Wilkins L, Fleischmann W, Howard JE: Macrogenitosomia precox associated with hyperplasia of the androgenic tissue of the adrenal and death from adrenocorticoadrenal insufficiency. *Endocrinology* **26**:385, 1940.
13. Fibiger J: Beitrage zur kenntniss des weiblichen schweinzwittertums. *Virchows Arch Pathol Anat* **181**:1,1905.
14. Debre R, Semelaigne G: Hypertrophie considerable des capsules surrenales chez un nourrison mort a 10 mois sans avoir agumente de poids depuis sa naissance. *Bull Soc Paediatr Paris* **23**:270, 1925.
15. Wilkins L, Lewis RA, Klein R, Rosemberg E: The suppression of androgen secretion by cortisone in a case of congenital adrenal hyperplasia. *Bull Johns Hopkins Hosp* **86**:249, 1950.
16. Wilkins L, Gardner LI, Crigler JF, Silverman SH, Migeon CJ: Further studies on the treatment of congenital adrenal hyperplasia with cortisone. *J Clin Endocrinol* **12**:257, 1952.
17. Bartter FC, Albright F, Forbes AP: The effects of adrenocorticotropic hormone and cortisone in adrenogenital syndrome associated with congenital adrenal hyperplasia: An attempt to explain and correct its disordered hormonal pattern. *J Clin Invest* **30**:237, 1951.
18. Donohoue PA, Parker KL, Migeon CJ: Congenital adrenal hyperplasia, in Scriver CR, Beaudet AL, Sly WS, Valle D (eds): *The Metabolic and Molecular Basis of Inherited Disease*. New York, McGraw-Hill, 1995, pp 2929–2966.
19. Mesiano S, Jaffe RB: Developmental and functional biology of the primate fetal adrenal cortex. *Endocr Rev* **18**:378, 1997.
20. Parker KL, Schimmer BP: Steroidogenic factor 1: A key determinant of endocrine development and function. *Endocr Rev* **18**:361, 1997.
21. Guo W, Burris TP, Zhang Y-H, Huang B-L, Mason J, Copeland KC, Kupfer SR, Pagon RA, McCabe ERB: Genomic sequence of the *DAX1* gene: An orphan nuclear receptor responsible for X-linked adrenal hypoplasia congenita and hypogonadotropic hypogonadism. *J Clin Endocrinol Metab* **81**:2481, 1996.
22. Ikeda Y, Swain A, Weber T, Hentges KE, Zanaria E, Lalli E, Tamai KT, Sassone-Corsi P, Lovell-Badge R, Camerino G, Parker KL: Steroidogenic factor 1 and Dax-1 colocalize in multiple cell lineages: Potential links in endocrine development. *Mol Endocrinol* **10**:1261, 1996.
23. Yu RN, Ito M, Jameson JL: The murine Dax-1 promoter is stimulated by SF-1 (steroidogenic factor-1) and inhibited by COUP-TF (chicken ovalbumin upstream promoter-transcription factor) via a composite nuclear receptor-regulatory element. *Mol Endocrinol* **12**:1010, 1998.
24. Nebert DW, Gonzalez FJ: P450 genes and evolutionary genetics. *Hosp Pract* March 15:63, 1987.
25. Gotoh O, Tagashira Y, Iizuka T, Fujii-Kuriyama Y: Structural characteristics of cytochrome P-450: Possible location of the heme-binding cysteine in determined amino-acid sequences. *J Biochem* **93**: 807, 1983.
26. Black SD: Membrane topology of the mammalian P450 cytochromes. *FASEB J* **6**:680, 1992.
27. Hasemann CA, Kurumbail RG, Boddupalli SS, Peterson JA, Deisenhofer J: Structure and function of cytochromes P450: A comparative analysis of three crystal structures. *Structure* **2**:41, 1995.
28. Miller WL: Structure of genes encoding steroidogenic enzymes. *J Steroid Biochem* **27**:759, 1987.
29. Cooper DY, Levin S, Narashimhulu S, Rosenthal O, Estabrook RW: Photochemical action spectrum of the terminal oxidase of mixed function oxidase systems. *Science* **145**:400, 1965.
30. Curnow KM, Tusie-Luna MT, Pascoe L, Natarajan R, Gu JL, Nadler JL, White PC: The product of the *CYP11B2* gene is required for aldosterone biosynthesis in the human adrenal cortex. *Mol Endocrinol* **5**:1513, 1991.
31. Smith PE: Hypophysectomy and a replacement therapy in the rat. *Am J Anat* **45**:205, 1930.
32. Li CH, Geschwind II, Cole RD, Raacke ID, Harris JI, Dixon JS: Amino acid sequence of alpha corticotropin. *Nature* **176**:687, 1955.
33. Whitfield PL, Seeburg PH, Shine J: The human pro-opiomelanocortin gene: Organisation, sequence and interspersion with repetitive DNA. *DNA* **1**:133, 1982.
34. Griffing GT, Berelowitz B, Hudson M, Salzman R, Manson JA, Aurrechia S, Melby JC: Plasma immunoreactive gamma melanotropin in patients with idiopathic hyperaldosteronism, aldosterone-producing adenomas, and essential hypertension. *J Clin Invest* **76**:163, 1985.
35. Harris GW: Neural control of the pituitary gland. *Physiol Rev* **28**:139, 1948.

36. Saffran M, Schally AV, Benfey BG: Stimulation of the release of corticotropin from the adenohypophysis by neurohypophysical factor. *Endocrinology* **57**:439,1955.
37. Guillemin R, Rosenberg B: Humoral hypothalamic control of anterior pituitary: A study with combined tissue cultures. *Endocrinology* **57**: 599, 1955.
38. Vale W, Spiess J, Rivier C, Rivier J: Characterization of a 41-residue ovine hypothalamic peptide that stimulates secretion of corticotropin and β-endorphin. *Science* **213**:1394, 1981.
39. Gillies G, Linton E, Lowry P: The physiology of corticotropin releasing factor, in DeGroot LJ et al (eds): *Endocrinology*. Philadelphia, Saunders, 1989, p 167.
40. Petraglia F, Florio P, Gallo R, Salvestroni C, Lombardo M, Genazzani AD, Di Carlo C, Stomati M, D'Ambrogio G, Artini PG: Corticotropin-releasing factor-binding protein: Origins and possible functions. *Hormone Res* **45**:187, 1996.
41. Nieuwenhuyzen-Kruseman AC, Linton EA, Ackland J, Besser GM, Lowry PJ: Heterogeneous immunocytochemical reactivities of oCRF-41-like material in the human hypothalamus, pituitary, and gastrointestinal tract. *Neuroendocrinology* **38**:212, 1984.
42. Xia L, Matera C, Ferin M, Wardlaw SL: Interleukin-1 stimulates the central release of corticotropin-releasing hormone in the primate. *Neuroendocrinology* **63**:79, 1996.
43. Vamvakopoulos NC, Chrousos GP: Hormonal regulation of human corticotropin-releasing hormone gene expression: Implications for the stress response and immune/inflammatory reaction. *Endocr Rev* **15**:409, 1994.
44. Liaw CW, Lovenberg TW, Barry G, Oltersdorf T, Grigoriadis DE, DeSouza EB: Cloning and characterization of the human corticotropin releasing-factor-2 receptor complementary deoxyribonucleic acid. *Endocrinology* **137**:72, 1996.
45. Parkes D, Rivest S, Lee S, Rivier C, Vale W: Corticotropin-releasing factor activates *c-fos, NGFI-B,* and corticotropin-releasing factor gene expression within the paraventricular nucleus of the rat hypothlalmus. *Mol Endocrinol* **7**:1357, 1993.
46. Boutillier AL, Monnier D, Lorang D, Lundblad JR, Roberts JL, Loeffler JP: Corticotropin-releasing hormone stimulates proopiomelanocortin transcription by cFos-dependent and -independent pathways: Characterization of an AP1 site in exon 1. *Mol Endocrinol* **9**:745, 1995.
47. Taylor AL, Fishman LM: Corticotropin-releasing hormone. *N Engl J Med* **319**:213, 1988.
48. Johnson EO, Kamilaris TC, Chrousos GP, Gold PW: Mechanisms of stress: A dynamic overview of hormonal and behavioral homeostasis. *Neurosci Biobehav Rev* **16**:115, 1992.
49. John M, John MC, Boggaram V, Simpson ER, Waterman MR: Transcriptional regulation of steroid hydroxylase genes by corticotropin. *Proc Natl Acad Sci USA* **83**:4715, 1986.
50. Clark RV, Albertson BD, Munabi A, Cassorla F, Aguilera G, Warren DW, Sherins RJ, Loriaux DL: Steroidogenic enzyme activities, morphology, and receptor studies of a testicular adrenal rest in a patient with congenital adrenal hyperplasia. *J Clin Endocrinol Metab* **70**:1408, 1990.
51. Boston B, Blaydon KM, Varnerin J, Cone RD: Independent and additive effects of central POMC and leptin pathways on murine obesity. *Science* **278**:1641, 1997.
52. Uehara Y, Shimizu H, Ohtani K, Sato N, Mori M: Hypothalamic corticotropin-releasing hormone is a mediator of the anorexigenic effect of leptin. *Diabetes* **47**:890, 1998.
53. Woods SC, Seeley RJ, Porte D Jr, Schwartz MW: Signals that regulate food intake and energy homeostasis. *Science* **280**:1378, 1998.
54. Mizuno TM, Kleopoulos SP, Bergen HT, Roberts JL, Priest CA, Mobbs CM: Hypothalamic pro-opiomelanocortin mRNA is reduced by fasting in ob/ob and db/db mice, but is stimulated by leptin. *Diabetes* **47**:294, 1997.
55. Berman LB, Vertes V: The pathophysiology of renin, in Shapter RK (ed): *Clinical Symposia*. Sommit, NJ, CIBA Pharmaceutical Corporation, 1973, p 3
56. Tigerstadt R, Bergman PG: Niere and kreislaug. *Scand Arch Physiol* **8**:223, 1898.
57. Goldblatt H: Studies on experimental hypertension: I. The production of persistent elevation of systolic blood pressure by means of renal ischemia. *J Exp Med* **59**:347,1934.
58. Laragh JH, Angers M, Kelly WG, Lieberman S: Hypotensive agents and pressor substances: The effects of epinephrine, norepinephrine, angiotensin II and others on the secretion rate of aldosterone in man. *JAMA* **17**:234,1960.
59. Simpson SAS, Tait JF, Wettstein A, Neher R, Von Euw J, Schindler O, Reichstein T: Konstitution des aldosterons, das neuen mineralocorticoid. *Experientia* **10**:132, 1952.
60. Bayard F, Cooke CR, Tiller DJ, Beitins IA, Kowarski A, Walker WG, Migeon CJ: The regulation of aldosterone secretion in anephric man. *J Clin Invest* **50**:1585, 1971.
61. Kaplan NM: The biosynthesis of adrenal steroids: Effects of angiotensin II, adrenocorticotropin and potassium. *J Clin Invest* **44**:2029, 1965.
62. Needleman P, Greenwald JE: Atriopeptin: A cardiac hormone intimately involved in fluid, electrolyte, and blood-pressure homeostasis. *N Engl J Med* **314**:828, 1986.
63. Kowarski A, Lacerda L, Migeon CJ: Integrated concentration of plasma aldosterone in normal subjects: Correlation with cortisol. *J Clin Endocrinol Metab* **40**:205, 1975.
64. Migeon CJ, Player JE: Identification and isolation of dehydroisoandrosterone from peripheral human plasma. *J Biol Chem* **209**:767, 1954.
65. Migeon CJ: Identification and isolation of androsterone from peripheral human plasma. *J Biol Chem* **218**:941, 1956.
66. McKenna TJ, Fearon U, Clarke D, Cunningham SK: A critical review of the origin and contol of adrenal andogens. *Ballieres Clin Obstet Gynaecol* **11**:229, 1997.
67. Rainey WE, Bird IM, Sawetawan C, Hanley NA, McCarthy JL, McGee EA, Wester R, Mason JI: Regulation of human adrenal carcinoma cell (NCI-H295) production C_{19} steroids. *J Clin Endocrinol Metab* **77**:731, 1993.
68. Parker L, Lifrak E, Shively J, Lee T, Kaplan B, Walker P, Calacay J, Florsheim W, Soon-Shiong P: Human adrenal gland cortical androgen-stimulating hormone (CASH) is identical with a portion of the joining peptide of pituitary pro-opiomelanocortin (POMC) (abstract 299), in *Proceedings of the 71st Annual Meeting of the Endocrine Society*, The Endocrine Society, Bethesda, Md, 1989 (abstract).
69. Mellon SH, Shively JE, Miller WL: Human proopiomelanocortin (79–96), a proposed androgen stimulatory hormone, does not affect steriodogenesis in cultured human fetal adrenal cells. *J Clin Endocrinol* **72**:19, 1991.
70. Penhoat A, Sanchez P, Jaillard C, Langlois D, Begeot M, Saez JM: Human proopiomelanocortin-(79–96), a proposed cortical androgen-stimulating hormone, does not affect steroidogenesis in cultured human adult adrenal cells. *J Clin Endocrinol Metab* **72**:23, 1991.
71. Yanagibashi K, Hall PF: Role of electron transport in the regulation of the lyase activity of C-21 side-chain cleavage P450 from porcine adrenal and testicular microsomes. *J Biol Chem* **261**:8429, 1986.
72. Lin D, Black SM, Nagahama Y, Miller WL: Steroid 17α-hydroxylase and 17,20-lyase activities of P450c17: Contributions of serine106 and P450 reductase. *Endocrinology* **132**:2498, 1993.
73. Sakai Y, Yanase T, Takayanagi R, Nakao R, Nishi Y, Haji M, Nawata H: High expression of cytochrome b5 in adrenocortical adenomas from patients with Cushing's syndrome associated with high levels of adrenal androgens. *J Clin Endocrinol Metab* **76**:1286, 1993.
74. Privalle CT, Crivello JF, Jefcoate CR: Regulation of intramitochondrial cholesterol transfer to side-chain cleavage P-450 in rat adrenal gland. *Proc Natl Acad Sci USA* **80**:702, 1983.
75. Jefcoate CR, McNamara BC, Artemenko I, Yamazaki T: Regulation of cholesterol movement to cytochrome P450scc in steroid hormone synthesis. *J Steroid Biochem Mol Biol* **43**:751, 1992.
76. Lin D, Sugawara T, Strauss III JF, Clark BJ, Stocco DM, Saenger P, Rogol A, Miller WL: Role of steroidogenic acute regulatory protein in adrenal and gonadal steroidogenesis. *Science* **267**:1828, 1995.
77. Alberta JA, Epstein LF, Pon LA, Orme-Johnson NR: Mitochondrial localization of a phosphoprotein that rapidly accumulates in adrenal cortex cells exposed to adrenocorticotrophic hormone or to cAMP. *J Biol Chem* **264**:2368, 1989.
78. Epstein LF, Orme-Johnson NR: Regulation of steroid hormone biosynthesis: Identification of precursors of a phosphoprotein targeted to the mitochondrion in stimulated rat adrenal cells. *J Biol Chem* **266**:19739, 1991.
79. Clark BJ, Wells J, King SR, Stocco DM: Purification, cloning, and expression of a novel LH-induced mitochondrial protein from the MA-10 mouse leydig tumor cells: Characterization of the steroidogenic acute regulatory (StAR) protein. *J Biol Chem* **269**:28314, 1994.
80. Fujeida K, Tajima T, Nakae J, Sageshima S, Tachibana K, Suwa S, Sugawara T, Strauss III JF: Spontaneous puberty in 46,XX subjects with congenital lipoid adrenal hyperplasia: Ovarian steroidogenesis is

spared to some extent despite inactivating mutations in the steroidogenic acute regulatory protein (StAR) gene. *J Clin Invest* **99**:1265, 1977.
81. Arakane F, Sugawara T, Nishino H, Liu Z, Holt JA, Pain D, Stocco DM, Miller WL, Strauss JF III: Steroidogenic acute regulatory protein (StAR) retains activity in the absence of mitochondrial import: Implications for the mechanism of StAR action. *Proc Natl Acad Sci USA* **93**:13731, 1996.
82. Bose HS, Pescovitz OH, Miller WL: Spontaneous feminization in a 46,XX female patient with congenital lipoid adrenal hyperplasia due to a homozygous frameshift mutation in the steroidogenic acute regulatory protein. *J Clin Endocrinol Metab* **82**:1511, 1997.
83. Bose HS, Sugawara T, Strauss JF III, Miller WL: The pathophysiology and genetics of congenital lipoid adrenal hyperplasia. *N Engl J Med* **335**:1870, 1998.
84. Besman MJ, Yanagibashi K, Lee TD, Kawamura M, Hall PF, Shively JE: Identification of des-(Gly-Ile)-endozepine as an effector of corticotropin-dependent adrenal steroidogenesis: Stimulation of cholesterol delivery is mediated by the peripheral benzodiazepine receptor. *Proc Natl Acad Sci USA* **86**:4897, 1989.
85. Papadopoulos V: Structure and function of the peripheral-type benzodiazepine receptor in steroidogenic cells. *Proc Soc Exp Biol Med* **217**:130, 1998.
86. Boujrad N, Hudson JR, Jr., Papadopoulos V: Inhibition of hormone stimulates steroidogenesis in cultured Leydig tumor cells by a cholesterol-linked phosphothioate oligodeoxynycleotide antisense to diazepam-binding inhibitor. *Proc Aatl Acad Sci USA* **90**:5728, 1993.
87. Papadopoulos V, Amri H, Li H, Boujrad N, Vidic B, Garnier M: Targeted disruption of the peripheral-type benzodiazepine receptor gene inhibits steroidogenesis in the R2C Leydig tumor cell line. *J Biol Chem* **272**:32129, 1997.
88. Lala DS, Rice DA, Parker KL: Steroidogenic factor I, a key regulator of steroidogenic enzyme expression, is the mouse homolog of fushi tarazu-factor I. *Mol Endocrinol* **6**:1249, 1992.
89. Honda S, Morohashi K, Nomura M, Takeya H, Kitajima M, Omura T: Ad4BP regulating steroidogenic P-450 gene is a member of steroid hormone receptor superfamily. *J Biol Chem* **268**:7494, 1993.
90. Evans RM: The steroid and thyroid hormone superfamily. *Science* **240**:889, 1988.
91. Hatano O, Takayama K, Imai T, Waterman MR, Takayanagi R, Omura T, Morohashi K: Sex-dependent expression of a transcription factor, AdBP, regulating steroidogenic P-450 genes in the gonads during prenatal and postnatal rat development. *Development* **120**:2787, 1994.
92. Giuili G, Shen WH, Ingraham HA: The nuclear receptor SF-1 mediates sexually dimorphic expression of Mullerian inhibiting substance, in vivo. *Development* **124**:1799, 1997.
93. Shen WH, Moore CC, Ikeda Y, Parker KL, Ingraham HA: Nuclear receptor steroidogenic factor 1 regulates the mullerian inhibiting substance gene: A link to the sex determination cascade. *Cell* **77**(5):651, 1994.
94. Ramayya MS, Zhou J, Kino T, Segars JH, Bondy CA: Steroidogenic factor 1 messenger ribonucleic acid expression in steroidogenic and nonsteroidogenic human tissues: Northern blot and in situ hybridization studies. *J Clin Endocrinol Metab* **82**:1799, 1997.
95. Ingraham HA, Lala DS, Ikeda Y, Luo X, Shen WH, Nachtigal MW, Abbud R, Nilson JH, Parker KL: The nuclear receptor steroidogenic factor 1 acts at multiple levels of the reproductive axis. *Genes Dev* **8**:2302, 1994.
96. Sadovsky Y, Crawford PA, Woodson KG, Polish JA, Clements MA, Tourtellotte LM, Simburger K, Milbrandt J: Mice deficient in the orphan nuclear receptor steroidogenic factor 1 lack adrenal glands and gonads but express P450 side-chain cleavage enzyme in the placenta and have normal embryonic serum levels of corticosteroids. *Proc Natl Acad Sci USA* **92**:10939, 1995.
97. Shinoda K, Lei H, Yoshii H, Nomura M, Nagano M, Shiba H, Sasaki H, Osawa Y, Niwa O, et al: Developmental defects of the ventromedial hypothalamic nucleus and pituitary gonadotroph in the Ftz-F1-disrupted mice. *Dev Dynamics* **204**:22, 1995.
98. Ikeda Y, Luo X, Abbud R, Nilson JH, Parker KL: The nuclear receptor steroidogenic factor 1 is essential for the formation of the ventromedial hypothalamic nucleus. *Mol Endocrinol* **9**:478, 1995.
99. Taketo M, Parker KL, Howard TA, Tsukiyama T, Wong M, Niwa O, Morton CC, Miron PM, Seldin MF: Homologs of *Drosophila* fushi tarazu factor 1 map to mouse chromosome 2 and human chromosome 9q33. *Genomics* **25**:565, 1995.
99a. Achermann J, Ito M, Ito M, Hindmarsh PC, Jameson JL: A mutation in the gene encoding steroidogenic factor-1 causes xy sex reversal and adrenal failure in humans. *Nat Genet* **22**:125, 1999.
100. Orth DN, Island DP, Liddle GW: Experimental alteration of the circadian rhythm in plasma cortisol (17-OHCS) concentration in man. *J Clin Endocrinol Metab* **29**:4791967.
101. Wilson TE, Mouw AR, Weaver CA, Milbrandt J, Parker KL: The orphan nuclear receptor NGFI-B regulates expression of the gene encoding steroid 21-hydroxylase. *Mol Cell Biol* **13**(2):861, 1993.
102. Kimura E, Armelin HA: Phorbol ester mimics ACTH action in corticoadrenal cells stimulating steroidogenesis, blocking cell shape, and inducing *c-fos* protooncogene expression. *J Biol Chem* **265**:3518, 1990.
103. Orth DN, Kovacs WJ, DeBold CR: The adrenal cortex, in Wilson JD, Foster DW (eds): *Williams Textbook of Endocrinology*, 8th ed. Philadelphia, Saunders, 1992, p 489.
104. Meikle AW: Secretion and metabolism of the corticosteroids and adrenal function testing, in DeGroot LJ et al (eds): *Endocrinology*. Philadelphia, Saunders, 1989, p 1610.
105. Arriza JL, Weinberger C, Cerelli G, Glaser TM, Handelin BL, Housman DE, Evans RM: Cloning of human mineralocorticoid receptor complementary DNA: Structural and functional kinship with the glucocorticoid receptor. *Science* **237**:268,1987.
106. Funder JW, Pearce PT, Smith R, Smith AI: Mineralocorticoid action: Target tissue specificity is enzyme, not receptor, mediated. *Science* **242**:583, 1988.
107. Weitzman ED, Fukushima D, Nogeire C, Roffwarg H, Gallagher TF, Hellman L: Twenty-four hour pattern of the episodic secretion of cortisol in normal subjects. *J Clin Endocrinol Metab* **33**:14, 1971.
108. Migeon CJ, Tyler FH, Mahoney JP, Florentin AA, Castle H, Bliss EL, Samuels LT: The diurnal variation of plasma levels and urinary excretion of 17-hydroxycorticosteroids in normal subjects, night workers, and blind subjects. *J Clin Endocrinol Metab* **16**:6221956.
109. Dunlap J: Circadian rhythms: An end in the beginning. *Science* **280**:1548, 1998.
110. Migeon CJ, Green OC, Eckert JP: Study of adrenocortical function in obesity. *Metabolism* **12**:718, 1963.
111. Kenny FM, Preeyasombat C, Migeon CJ: Cortisol production rate: II. Normal infants, children and adults. *Pediatrics* **37**:34, 1966.
112. Lindr BL, Esteban NV, Yergey AL, Winterer JC, Loriaux DL, Cassorla F: Cortisol production rate in childhood and adolescence. *J Pediatr* **117**:892, 1990.
113. Esteban NV, Loughlin T, Yergey AL, Zawadki JK, Booth JD, Winterer JC, Loriaux DL: Daily cortisol production rate in man determined by stable isotope dilution/mass spectrometry. *J Clin Endocrinol Metab* **71**:39, 1991.
114. Kowarski A, Katz H, Migeon CJ: Plasma aldosterone concentration in normal subjects from infancy to adulthood. *J Clin Endocrinol Metab* **38**:489, 1974.
115. Migeon CJ, Kenny FM, Taylor FH: Cortisol production rate: VIII. Pregnancy. *J Clin Endocrinol Metab* **28**:661, 1968.
116. Beitins IZ, Bayard F, Levitsky L, Ances IG, Kowarski A, Migeon CJ: Plasma aldosterone concentration at delivery and during the neonatal period. *J Clin Invest* **51**:386, 1972.
117. Beitins IZ, Bayard F, Ances IG, Kowarski A, Migeon CJ: The metabolic clearance rate, blood production, interconversion and transplacental passage of cortisol and cortisone in pregnancy near term. *Pediatr Res* **7**:509, 1973.
118. Bayard F, Ances IG, Tapper AJ, Weldon VV, Kowarski A, Migeon CJ: Transplacental passage and fetal secretion of aldosterone. *J Clin Invest* **49**:1389, 1970.
119. Selye H: Stress, in Heusor G (ed): *Fifth Annual Report*. New York, MD Publications, 1956.
120. Oyama T: Influence of general anesthesia and surgical stress on endocrine function, in Brown BR (ed): *Anesthesia and the Patient with Endocrine Disease*. Philadelphia, FA Davis, 1980, pp 173–184.
121. Levine A, Cohen D, Zadik Z: Urinary free cortisol values in children under stress. *J Pediatr* **125**:853, 1994.
122. Dinarello CA, Mier JW: Current concepts: Lymphokines. *N Engl J Med* **317**:940, 1987.
123. Sapolsky R, Rivier C, Yamamoto G, Plotsky P, Vale W: Interleukin-1 stimulates the secretion of hypothalamic corticotropin-releasing factor. *Science* **238**:522, 1987.
124. Chrousos GP: The hypothalamic-pituitary-adrenal axis and immune-mediated inflammation. *N Engl J Med* **332**:1351, 1995.

125. Besedovsky HO, Del Ray A: Immune-neuroendocrine interactions: Facts and hypotheses. *Endocr Rev* **17**:64, 1996.
126. Speiser PW, Dupont J, Zhu D, Serrat J, Buegelesein M, Tusie-Luna MT, Lesser M, New MI, White PC: Disease expression and molecular genotype in congenital adrenal hyperplasia due to 21-hydroxylase deficiency. *J Clin Invest* **90**:584, 1992.
127. Bristow J, Tee MK, Gitelman SE, Mellon SH, Miller WL: Tenascin-X: A novel extracellular matrix protein encoded by the human *XB* gene overlapping P450c21B. *J Cell Biol* **122**:265, 1993.
128. Collier S, Tassabehju M, Strachan T: A *de novo* pathological point mutation at the 21-hydroxylase locus: Implications for gene conversion in the human genome. *Nature Genet* **3**:260, 1993.
129. Migeon CJ, Donohoue PA: Congenital adrenal hyperplasia caused by 21-hydroxylase deficiency: Its molecular basis and its remaining therapeutic problems. *Endocrinol Metab Clin North Am* **20**:277, 1991.
130. Strachan T, White PC: Molecular pathology of steroid 21-hydroxylase deficiency. *J Steroid Biochem Mol* **40**:537, 1991.
131. Morel Y, Miller WL: Clinical and molecular genetics of congenital adrenal hyperplasia due to 21-hydroxylase deficiency, in Harris H, Hirschhorn K (eds): *Advances in Human Genetics*. New York, Plenum Press, 1991, p 1.
132. Gitelman SE, Bristow J, Miller WL: Mechanism and consequences of the duplication of the human C4/P450c21/gene X locus. *Mol Cell Biol* **12**(5):2124, 1992.
133. Jääskeläinen J, Levo A, Voutilainen R, Partanen J: Population-wide evaluation of disease manifestation in relation to molecular genotype in steroid 21-hydroxylase (CYP21) deficiency: Good correlation in a well defined population. *J Clin Endocrinol Metab* **82**:3293, 1998.
134. Wedell A, Stengler B, Luthman H: Characterization of mutations on the rare duplicated C4/CYP21 haplotype in steroid 21-hydroxylase deficiency. *Hum Genet* **94**:50, 1994.
135. Shen L, Wu LC, Sanlioglu S, Chen R, Mendoza AR, Dangel AW, Carroll MC, Zipf WB, Yu CY: Structure and genetics of the partially duplicated gene *RP* located immediately upstream of the complement *C4A* and the *C4B* genes in the HLA class III region: Molecular cloning, exon-intron structure, composite retroposon, and breakpoint of gene deletion. *J Biol Chem* **269**:8466, 1994.
136. Rosenwaks Z, Lee PA, Jones GS, Migeon CJ, Wentz AC: An attenuated form of congenital virilizing adrenal hyperplasia. *J Clin Endocrinol Metab* **49**:335, 1979.
137. Migeon CJ, Kenny FM: Cortisol production rate: V. Congenital virilizing adrenal hyperplasia. *J Pediatr* **69**:779, 1966.
138. Jailer JW, Gold JJ, Vande Wiele R, Lieberman S: 17α-hydroxyprogesterone and 21-desoxyhydrocortisone: Their metabolism and possible role in congenital adrenal virilism. *J Clin Invest* **34**:1639, 1955.
139. Kowarski A, Finkelstein JW, Spaulding JS, Holman GS, Migeon CJ: Aldosterone secretion rate in congenital adrenal hyperplasia: A discussion of the theories on pathogenesis of the salt-losing form of the syndrome. *J Clin Invest* **44**:1505, 1965.
140. Rivarola MA, Saez JM, Migeon CJ: Studies of androgens in patients with congenital adrenal hyperplasia. *J Clin Endocrinol Metab* **7**:624, 1967.
141. Pang S, Levine LS, Chow DM, Faiman C, New MI: Serum androgen concentrations in neonates and young infants with congenital hyperplasia due to 21-hydroxylase deficiency. *Clin Endocrinol* **11**:575, 1979.
142. Prader A: Vollkommen mannliche auBere Genitalentwicklung und Salzverlustsyndrom bei Madchen mit kongenitalem adrenogenitalem Syndrom. *Helv Paediat Acta* **13**:5, 1958.
143. Klingensmith GJ, Garcia SC, Jones HW Jr, Migeon CJ, Blizzard RM: Glucocorticoid treatment of girls with congenital adrenal hyperplasia: Effects on height, sexual maturation and fertility. *J Pediatr* **90**:996, 1977.
144. Mulaikal RM, Migeon CJ, Rock JA: Fertility rates in female patients with congenital adrenal hyperplasia due to 21-hydroxylase deficiency. *New Engl J Med* **316**:178, 1987.
145. Urban MD, Lee PA, Migeon CJ: Adult height and fertility in man with congenital virilizing adrenal hyperplasia. *N Engl J Med* **299**:1392, 1978.
146. Wilkins L, Lewis RA, Klein R, Gardner LI, Crigler JF, Rosemberg E, Migeon CJ: Treatment of congenital adrenal hyperplasia with cortisone. *J Clin Endocrinol Metab* **11**:1, 1951.
147. Iversen T: Congenital adrenocortical hyperplasia with disturbed electrolyte regulation. *Pediatrics* **16**:875, 1955.
148. Miller WL: Clinical review 54: Genetics, diagnosis and management of 21-hydroxylase deficiency. *J Clin Endocrinol Metab* **78**:241, 1994.
149. Laue L, Merke DP, Jones JV, Barnes KM, Hill S, Cutler GB Jr: A preliminary study of flutamide, testalactone, and reduced hydrocortisone dose in the treatment of congenital adrenal hyperplasia. *J Clin Endocrinol Metab* **81**:3535, 1996.
150. Weldon VV, Blizzard RM, Migeon CJ: Newborn girls misdiagnosed as bilaterally cryptorchid males. *New Engl J Med* **274**:829, 1966.
151. Edwin C, Lanes R, Migeon CJ, Lee PA, Plotnick LP, Kowarski AA: Persistence of the enzymatic block in adolescent patients with salt-losing congenital adrenal hyperplasia. *J Pediatr* **95**:534, 1979.
152. Hoffman WH, Shin MY, Donohoue PA, Helman SW, Brown SL, Rosculet G, Mahesh VB: Phenotypic evolution of classic 21-hydroxylase deficiency. *Clin Endocrinol* **45**:103, 1996.
153. Speiser PW, Agsere L, Ueshiba H, White PC, New MI: Aldosterone sysnthesis in salt-wasting congenital adrenal hyperplasia with complete absence of adrenal 21-hydroxylase. *N Engl J Med* **324**:145, 1991.
154. Sandrini R, Jospe N, Migeon CJ: Temporal and individual variations in the dose of glucocorticoid used for the treatment of salt-losing congenital virilizing adrenal hyperplasia due to 21-hydroxylase deficiency. *Acta Paediatr Suppl* **388**:56, 1993.
155. Van Wyk JJ, Gunther DFJ, Ritzén M, Wedell A, Cutler GB Jr, Migeon CJ, New MI: Therapeutic controversies: The use of adrenalectomy as a treatment for congenital adrenal hyperplasia. *J Clin Endocrinol Metab* **81**:3180, 1996.
156. Gunther DFJ, Bukowski TP, Ritzén M, Wedell A, Van Wyk JJ: Prophylactic adrenalectomy of a three-year-old girl with congenital adrenal hyperplasia: Pre- and postoperative studies. *J Clin Endocrinol Metab* **82**:3324, 1997.
157. Resnick SM, Berenbaum SA, Gottesman II, Bouchard TJ: Early hormonal influences on cognitive functioning in congenital adrenal hyperplasia. *Dev Psychol* **22**:191, 1986.
158. Tirosh E, Rod R, Cohen A, Hochberg Z: Congenital adrenal hyperplasia and cerebral lateralizations. *Pediatr Neurol* **9**:198, 1993.
159. Berenbaum SA, Hines M: Early androgens are related to childhood sex-typed toy preferences. *Psychol Sci* **3**:203, 1992.
160. Speiser PW, New MI: Genotype and hormonal phenotype in nonclassical 21-hydroxylase deficiency. *J Clin Endocrinol Metab* **64**:86, 1987.
161. Migeon CJ, Rosenwaks Z, Lee PA, Urban MD, Bias WB: The attenuated form of congenital adrenal hyperplasia is an allelic form of 21-hydroxylase deficiency. *J Clin Endocrinol Metab* **51**:647, 1980.
162. Chrousos GP, Loriaux DL, Mann D, Cutler GB Jr: Late-onset 21-hydroxylase deficiency is an allelic variant of congenital adrenal hyperplasia characterized by attenuated clinical expression and different HLA haplotype associations. *Horm Res* **16**:193, 1982.
163. Azziz R, Rafi A, Smith GG, Bradley EL Jr, Zacur HA: On the origin of the elevated 17-hydroxyprogesterone levels after adrenal stimulation in hyperandrogenism. *J Clin Endocrinol Metab* **70**:431, 1990.
164. Jääskeläinen J, Voutilainen R: Growth of patients with 21-hydroxylase deficiency: An analysis of the factors influencing adult height. *Pediatr Res* **41**:30, 1997.
165. Kuhnle U, Bullinger M: Outcome of congenital adrenal hyperplasia. *Pediatr Surg Int* **12**:511, 1997.
166. Premawardhana LDKE, Hughes IA, Read GF, Scanlon MF: Longer outcome in females with congenital adrenal hyperplasia (CAH): The Cardiff experience. *Clin Endocrinol* **46**:327, 1997.
167. Federman DD: Psychosexual adjustment in congenital adrenal hyperplasia. *N Engl J Med* **316**:209, 1987.
168. Childs B, Grunbach MM, Van Wyk JJ: Virilizing adrenal hyperplasia: A genetic and hormonal study. *J Clin Invest* **35**:213, 1956.
169. Dupont B, Oberfield SE, Smithwick ER, Lee TD, Levine LS: Close genetic linkage between HLA and congenital adrenal hyperplasia (21-hydroxylase deficiency). *Lancet* **2**:1309, 1977.
170. O'Neill GJ, Dupont B, Pollack MS, Levine LS, New MI: Complement C4 allotypes in congenital adrenal hyperplasia due to 21-hydroxylase deficiency: Further evidence for different allelic variants at the 21-hydroxylase locus. *Clin Immunol Immunopathol* **23**:312, 1982.
171. Fleischnick E, Awdeh ZL, Raum D, Granados J, Alosco SM, Crigler JF Jr, Gerald PS, Giles CM, Yunis EJ, Alper CM: Extended MHC haplotypes in 21-hydroxylase deficiency congenital adrenal hyperplasia: Shared genotypes in unrelated patients. *Lancet* **1**:152, 1983.
172. Higashi Y, Yoshioka H, Yamane M, Gotoh O, Fujii-Kuriyama Y: Complete nucleotide sequence of two steroid 21-hydroxylase genes tandemly arranged in human chromosome: A pseudogene and a genuine gene. *Proc Natl Acad Sci USA* **83**:2841, 1986.

173. White PC, New MI, Dupont B: Structure of human steroid 21-hydroxylase genes. *Proc Natl Acad Sci USA* **83**:5111, 1986.
174. White PC, Grossberger D, Onufer BJ, Chaplin DD, New MI, Dupont B, Strominger JL: Two genes encoding steroid 21-hydroxylase are located near the genes encoding the fourth component of complement in man. *Proc Natl Acad Sci USA* **82**:1089, 1985.
175. Donohoue PA, Van Dop C, Migeon CJ, McLean RH, Bias WB: Coupling of HLA-A3, Cw6, Bw47, DR7 and a normal CA21HB steroid 21-hydroxylase gene in the Old Order Amish. *J Clin Endocrinol Metab* **65**:980, 1987.
176. Donohoue PA, Guethlein L, Collins MM, Van Dop C, Migeon CJ, Bias WB, Schmeckpeper BJ: The HLA-A3, Cw6, Bw47, DR7 extended haplotypes in salt-losing 21-hydroxylase deficiency and in the Old Order Amish: Identical MHC class I antigens and class II alleles with at least two crossover sites in the class III region. *Tissue Antigens* **46**:163, 1995.
177. Tusie-Luna MT, Speiser PW, Dumic M, New MI, White PC: A mutation (Pro-30 to Leu) in CYP21 represents a potential nonclassic steroid 21-hydroxylase deficiency allele. *Mol Endocrinol* **5**:685, 1991.
178. Libber SM, Migeon CJ, Bias WB: Ascertainment of 21-hydroxylase deficiency in individuals with HLA-B14 haplotype. *J Clin Endocrinol Metab* **60**:727, 1985.
179. Laron Z, Pollack MS, Zamir R, Roitman A, Dickerman Z, Levine LS, Lorenzen F, O'Neil GK, Pang S, New MI, Dupont B: Late onset 21-hydroxylase deficiency and HLA in the Ashkenazi population: A new allele at 21-hydroxylase locus. *Hum Immunol* **1**:55, 1980.
180. Donohoue PA, Van Dop C, McLean RH, White PC, Jospe N, Migeon CJ: Gene conversion in salt-losing congenital adrenal hyperplasia with absent complement C4B protein. *J Clin Endocrinol Metab* **62**:995, 1986.
181. Carroll MC, Campbell RD, Porter RR: Mapping of steroid 21-hydroxylase genes adjacent to complement component *C4* genes in HLA, the major histocompatibility complex in man. *Proc Natl Acad Sci USA* **82**:521, 1985.
182. Bristow J, Gitelman SE, Tee MK, Staels B, Miller WL: Abundant adrenal-specific transcription of the human P450c21A "pseudogene." *J Biol Chem* **268**:12919, 1993.
183. Kyllo JH, Collins MM, Donohoue PA: Constitutive steroid 21-hydroxylase promoter gene and pseudogene activity in steroidogenic and nonsteroidogenic cells with the luciferase gene as a reporter. *Endocr Res* **21**:777, 1995.
184. Kyllo JH, Collins MM, Donohoue PA: Human steroid 21-hydroxylase promoter activity is greater than 21-hydroxylase pseudogene reporter activity in steroidogenic cells, in *Proceedings of the 77th Annual Meeting of the Endocrine Society* (abstract). Betheseda, MD, The Endocrine Society, 1995, p 2–550.
185. Chang S-F, Chung B: Difference in transcriptional activity of two homologous *CYP21A* genes. *Mol Endocrinol* **9**:1330, 1995.
186. Burch GH, Gong Y, Liu W, Dettman RW, Curry CJ, Smith L, Miller WL, Bristow J: Tenascin-X deficiency is associated with Ehlers-Danlos syndrome. *Nature Genet* **17**:5, 1997.
187. Kawaguchi H, O'hUigin C, Klein J: Evolutionary origin of mutations in the primate cytochrome *P450c21* gene. *Am J Hum Genet* **50**:766, 1992.
188. Burghelle-Mayeur C, Geffrotin C, Vaiman M: Sequences of the swine 21-hydroxylase gene (*CYP21*) and a portion of the opposite-strand overlapping gene of unknown function previously described in human. *Biochim Biophys Acta* **1171**:153, 1992.
189. Crawford RJ, Hammond VE, Connell JMC, Coghlan JP: The structure and activity of two cytochrome P450c21 proteins encoded in the ovine adrenal cortex. *J Biol Chem* **267**(23):16212, 1992.
190. Schimmer BP, Parker KL: Promoter elements of the mouse 21-hydroxylase (*Cyp-21*) gene involved in cell-selective and cAMP-dependent gene expression. *J Steroid Biochem Mol Biol* **43**(8):937, 1992.
191. Donohoue PA, Collins MM: The human complement C4B/steroid 21-hydroxylase (*CYP21*) and complement C4A/21-hydroxylase pseudogene (*CYP21P*) intergenic sequences: Comparison and identification of possible regulatory elements. *Biochem Biophys Res Commun* **186**: 256–262, 1992.
192. Millstone DS, Shaw SK, Parker KL, Szyf M, Siedman JG: An element regulating adrenal-specific steroid 21-hydroxylase expression is located within the *slp* gene. *J Biol Chem* **267**:21924, 1992.
193. Pang S, Hotchkiss J, Drash AL, Levine LS, New MI: Microfilter paper method for 17α-progesterone radioimmunoassay: Its application for rapid screening for congenital adrenal hyperplasia. *J Clin Endocrinol Metab* **45**:1003, 1977.
194. Pang S, Wallace MA, Hofman L, Thuline MA, Dorche C, Lyon ICT, Dobbins RH, Kling S, Fujieda K, Suwa S: Worldwide experience in newborn screening for classical congenital adrenal hyperplasia due to 21-hydroxylase deficiency. *Pediatrics* **81**:866, 1988.
195. Therell BL, Berenbaum SA, Manter-Kapanke V, Simmank J, Korman K, Prentice L, Gonzalez J, Gunn S: Results of screening 1.9 million Texas newborns for 21-hydroxylase-deficient congenital adrenal hyperplasia. *Pediatrics* **101**:583, 1998.
196. Hirschfeld AJ, Fleishman JK: An unusually high incidence of salt-losing congenital adrenal hyperplasia in the Alaskian Eskimo. *J Pediatr* **75**:492, 1969.
197. Dorche C, Dhoudt SL, Bozon D: Systematic neonatal screening for congenital adrenal hyperplasia: Report of a pilot study in two centers in France, in Therrell BL (ed): *Advances in Neonatal Screening* (Excerpta Medica International Congress Series). Amsterdam, Elsevier, 1987, p 289
198. New MI, Lorenzen F, Lerner AJ, Kohn B, Oberfield SE, Pollack MS, Dupont B, Stoner E, Levy DJ, Pang S, Levine LS: Genotyping steroid 21-hydroxylase deficiency: Hormonal reference data. *J Clin Endocrinol Metab* **57**:320, 1983.
199. Speiser PW, Dupont B, Rubinstein P, Piazza A, Kastelan a, New MI: High frequency of nonclassical steroid 21-hydroxylase deficiency. *Am J Hum Genet* **37**:650, 1985.
200. Donohoue PA, Jospe N, Migeon CJ, Van Dop C: Two distinct areas of unequal crossingover within the steroid 21-hydroxylase genes produce absence of CYP21B. *Genomics* **5**:397, 1989.
201. Donohoue PA, Wedell A: Normal and mutant 21-hydroxylase promoter activities differ in an in vitro luciferase reporter assay (abstract). *Hormone Res* **48** (suppl 2):97, 1997.
202. Tusie-Luna MT, Traktman P, White PC: Determination of functional effects of mutations in the steroid 21-hydroxylase gene (CYP21) using recombinant vaccinia virus. *J Biol Chem* **265**:20916, 1990.
203. Higashi Y, Hiromasa T, Tanae A, Miki T, Nakura J, Kondo T, Ohura T, Ogawa E, Nakayama K, Fujii-Kuriyama Y: Effects of individual mutations in the P-450(C21) pseudogene on the P-450(C21) activity and their distribution in the patient genomes of congenital steroid 21-hydroxylase deficiency. *J Biochem* **109**:638, 1991.
204. Wu D-A, Chung B: Mutations of P450c21 (steroid 21-hydroxylase) at Cys428, Val281, and Ser268 result in complete, partial, or no loss of enzymatic activity, respectively. *J Clin Invest* **88**:519, 1991.
205. Hsu L-C, Hsu N-C, Guzova JA, Guzov VM, Chang S-F, Chung B: The common *I172N* mutation causes conformational change of cytochrome P450c21 revealed by systematic mutation, kinetic, and structural studies. *J Biol Chem* **271**:3310, 1996.
206. Chung B, Hu M-C, Govoz VM, Wu D-A: Structure and expression of the *CYP21* (P450c21, steroid 21-hydroxylase) gene with respect to its deficiency. *Endocr Res* **21**:343, 1995.
207. Witchel SF, Bhamidipati DK, Hoffman EP, Cohen JB: Phenotypic heterogeneity associated with the splicing mutation in congenital adrenal hyperplasia due to 21-hydroxylase deficiency. *J Clin Endocrinol Metab* **81**:4081, 1996.
208. Shulze E, Scharer G, Rogatzki A, Priebe S, Lewicka S, Bettendorf M, Hoepffner W, Heinrick UE, Schwabe U: Divergence between genotype and phenotype in relatives of patients with the intron 2 mutation of steroid 21-hydroxylase. *Endocr Res* **21**:359, 1995.
209. Nikoshkov A, Lajic S, Holst S, Holst M, Wedell A, Luthman H: Synergistic effect of partially inactivating mutations in steroid 21-hydroxylase deficiency. *J Clin Endocrinol Metab* **82**:194, 1997.
210. Helmberg A, Tusie-Luna MT, Tabarelli M, Kofler R, White PC: R339H and P453S: *CYP21* mutations associated with nonclassic steroid 21-hydroxylase deficiency that are not apparent gene conversions. *Mol Endocrinol* **6**:1318, 1992.
211. Tajima T, Fujieda K, Fujii-Kuriyama Y: *De novo* mutation causes steroid 21-hydroxylase deficiency in one family of HLA-identical affected and unaffected siblings. *J Clin Endocrinol Metab* **77**:86, 1993.
212. Wedell A, Luthman H: Steroid 21-hydroxylase deficiency: two additional mutations in salt-wasting disease and rapid screening of disease-causing mutations. *Hum Mol Genet* **2**:499, 1993.
213. Kirby-Keyser L, Porter CC, Donohoue PA: E380D: A novel point mutation of *CYP21* in an HLA-homozygous patient with salt-losing congenital adrenal hyperplasia due to 21-hydroxylase deficiency. *Hum Mutat* **9**:181, 1997.
214. Gutai JP, Kowarski AA, Migeon CJ: The detection of the heterozygote carrier for congenital virilizing adrenal hyperplasia. *J Pediatr* **90**:924, 1977.

215. Gutai JP, Lee PA, Johnsonbaugh RE, Gareis F, Urban MD, Migeon CJ: Detection of the heterozygous state in siblings of patients with CAH due to 21-hydroxylase deficiency. *J Pediatr* **94**:770, 1979.
216. Wichel SF, Lee PA: Identification of heterozygote carriers of 21-hydroxylase defiency: Sensitivity of stimulation tests. *Am J Med Genet* **76**:337, 1998.
217. Mercado AB, Wilson RC, Cheng KC, New MI: Extensive personal experience: prenatal treatment and diagnosis of congenital adrenal hyperplasia owing to steroid 21-hydroxylase deficiency. *J Clin Endocrinol Metab* **80**:2014, 1995.
218. Speiser PW, Laforgia N, Kato K, Pareira J, Khan R, Yang SY, Whorwood C, White PC, Elias S, Schriock E, Simpson JL, Taslimi M, Najjar J, May S, Mills G, Crawford C, New MI: First trimester prenatal treatment and molecular genetic diagnosis of congenital adrenal hyperplasia (21-hydroxylase deficiency). *J Clin Endocrinol Metab* **70**:838, 1990.
219. Pang S, Pollack MS, Loo M, Green O, Nussbaum R, Clayton G, Dupont B, New MI: Pitfalls of prenatal diagnosis of 21-hydroxylase deficiency congenital adrenal hyperplasia. *J Clin Endocrinol Metab* **61**:89, 1985.
220. Frasier SD, Thorneycroft IH, Weiss BA, Horton R: Elevated amniotic fluid concentrations of 17α-hydroxyprogesterone in congenital adrenal hyperplasia. *J Pediatr* **86**:310, 1975.
221. Pang S, Levine LS, Cederqvist LL, Fuentes M, Riccardi VM, Holcombe JH, Nitowsky HM, Sachs G, Anderson CE, Duchon MA, Owens R, Merkatz I, New MI: Amniotic fluid concentrations of delta 5 and delta 4 steroids in fetuses with congenital adrenal hyperplasia due to 21-hydroxylase deficiency and anencephalic fetuses. *J Clin Endocrinol Metab* **51**:223, 1980.
222. Carson DJ, Okuno A, Lee PA, Stetten G, Didolkar SM, Migeon CJ: Amniotic fluid steroid levels: Fetuses with adrenal hyperplasia, 46,XXY fetuses, and normal fetuses. *Am J Dis Child* **136**:218, 1982.
223. Forest M, Bétuel H, Couillin P, Boué A: Prenatal diagnosis of congenital adrenal hyperplasia (CAH) due to 21-hydroxylase deficiency by steroid analysis in the amniotic fluid of mid pregnancy: Comparison with HLA typing in 17 pregnancies at risk for CAH. *Prenat Diagn* **1**:197, 1981.
224. Migeon CJ: Editorial: Comments about the need for prenatal treatment of congenital adrenal hyperplasia due to 21-hydroxylase defiency. *J Clin Endocrinol Metab* **70**:836, 1990.
225. David M, Forest M: Prenatal treatment of congenital adrenal hyperplasia resulting from 21-hydroxylase deficiency. *J Pediatr* **90**:799, 1984.
226. Pang S, Pollack MS, Marshall RN, Immken L: Prenatal treatment of congenital adrenal hyperplasia due to 21-hydroxylase deficiency. *N Engl J Med* **322**:111, 1990.
227. Forest MG, Dorr H, Gobo E: Prenatal treatment of congenital adrenal hyperplasia (CAH) due to 21-hydroxylase deficiency: European experience in 223 pregnancies at risk. *Pediatr Res* **33**(5):S3, 1993.
228. Pang S, Clark A, Dolan L, Schulman D: Hormonal monitoring and side effects of prenatal dexamethasone (DEX) treatment for 21-hydroxylase deficiency congenital adrenal hyperplasia (CAH). *Pediatr Res* **33**(5):S3, 1993.
229. Saedi SA, Dean H, Dent W, Stockl E, Cronin C: Screening for congenital adrenal hyperplasia: The Delphia screening test overestimates serum 17-hydroxyprogesterone in preterm infants. *Pediatrics* **97**:100, 1996.
230. Cutfield WS, Webster D: Newborn screening for congenital adrenal hyperplasia in New Zealand. *J Pediatr* **126**:118, 1998.
231. Shepard TH, Clausen SW: Case of adrenogenital syndrome with hypertension treated with cortisone. *Pediatrics* **8**:805, 1951.
232. Eberlein WR, Bongiovanni AM: Plasma and urinary corticosteroids in the hypertensive form of congenital adrenal hyperplasia. *J Biol Chem* **223**:85, 1956.
233. Gabrilove JL, Sharma DC, Dorfman RI: Adrenocortical 11β-hydroxylase deficiency and virilism first manifest in the adult woman. *N Engl J Med* **72**:1189, 1965.
234. Joehrer K, Geley S, Strasser-Wozak EM, Azziz R, White PC: CYP11B mutations causing nonclassic adrenal hyperplasia due to 11β-hydroxylase deficiency. *Hum Mol Genet* **6**:1829, 1997.
235. Maclaren NK, Migeon CJ, Raiti S: Gynecomastia with congenital virilizing adrenal hyperplasia (11β-hydroxylase deficiency). *J Pediatr* **86**:579, 1975.
236. David RR, Bergada C, Migeon CJ: Effect of age on urinary steroid excretion in congenital adrenal hyperplasia. *Bull Johns Hopkins Hosp* **117**:16, 1965.
237. Rösler A, Weshler N, Leiberman E, Hochberg Z, Weidenfeld J, Sack J, Chemke J: 11β-Hydroxylase deficiency congenital adrenal hyperplasia: Update of prenatal diagnosis. *J Clin Endocrinol Metab* **66**:830, 1988.
238. Rösler A, Leiberman E, Cohen T: High frequency of congenital adrenal hyperplasia (classic 11β-hydroxylase deficiency) among Jews from Morocco. *Am J Med Genet* **42**:827, 1992.
239. Chua SC, Szabo P, Vitek A, Grzeschik KH, John M, White PC: Cloning of cDNA encoding steroid 11β-hydroxylase (P450c11). *Proc Natl Acad Sci USA* **84**:7193, 1987.
240. Mornet E, Dupont J, Vitek A, White PC: Characterization of two genes encoding human steroid 11β-hydroxylase (P-45011β). *J Biol Chem* **264**:20961, 1989.
241. Curnow KC, Slutsker L, Vitek J, Cole T, Speiser PW, New MI, White PC, Pascoe L: Mutations in the *CYP11B1* gene causing congenital adrenal hyperplasia and hypertension cluster in exons 6, 7, and 8. *Proc Natl Acad Sci USA* **90**:4552, 1993.
242. Domalik LJ, Chaplin DD, Kirkman MS, Wu RC, Liu W, Howard TA, Sedlin MF, Parker KL: Different isozymes of mouse 11β-hydroxylase produce mineralocorticoids and glucocorticoids. *Mol Endocrinol* **5**:1853, 1991.
243. White PC, Dupont J, New MI, Leiberman E, Hochberg Z, Rosler A: A mutation in *CYP11B1* (Arg448His) associated with steroid 11β-hydroxylase deficiency in Jews of Moroccan origin. *J Clin Invest* **87**:1664, 1991.
244. White PC, Curnow KC, Pascoe L: Disorders of steroid 11β-hydroxylase isozymes. *Endocr Rev* **15**:421, 1995.
245. Merke DP, Tajima T, Chhabra A, Barnes K, Mancilla E, Baron J, Cutler GB Jr: Novel *CYP11B1* mutations in congenital adrenal hyperplasia due to steroid 11β-hydroxylase deficiency. *J Clin Endocrinol Metab* **83**:270, 1998.
246. Geley S, Kapelari K, Jöhrer K, Peter M, Glatzl J, Vierhapper H, Schwarz S, Helmberg A, Sippell WG, White PC, Kofler R: *CYP11B1* mutations causing congenital adrenal hyperplasia due to 11β-hydroxylase deficiency. *J Clin Endocrinol Metab* **81**:2896, 1996.
247. Boon WC, Coghlan JP, Curnow KC, McDougall JG: Aldosterone secretion. *Trends Endocrinol Metab* **8**:346, 1997.
248. Yanase T, Simpson ER, Waterman MR: 17-Hydroxylase/17,20-desmolase deficiency: From clinical investigation to molecular definition. *Endocr Rev* **12**:91, 1991.
249. Kitamura M, Buczko E, Dufau ML: Dissociation of hydroxylase and lyase activities by site-directed mutagenesis of the rat P45017α. *Mol Endocrinol* **5**:1373, 1991.
250. Chung BC, Picado-Leonard J, Haniu M, Bienkowski M, Hall PF, Shively JF, Miller WL: Cytochrome P450c17 (steroid 17α-hydroxylase/17,20-lyase): Cloning of human adrenal and testis cDNAs indicates the same gene is expressed in both tissues. *Proc Natl Acad Sci USA* **84**:407, 1987.
251. Zuber MX, Simpson ER, Waterman MR: Expression of bovine 17α-hydroxylase cytochrome P-450 cDNA in nonsteroidogenic (COS 1) cells. *Science* **234**:1258, 1986.
251a. Auchus RJ, Miller WL: Molecular modeling of human P450c17 (17α-hydroxylase 17,20-lyase): Insights into reaction mechanisms and effects of mutations. *Mol Endocrinol* **13**:1169, 1999.
252. Biglieri EG, Herron MA, Brust N: 17α-Hydroxylase deficiency in men. *J Clin Invest* **45**:1946, 1966.
253. Sparkes RS, Klisak I, Miller WL: Regional mapping of genes encoding human steroidogenic enzymes: P450scc to 15q23-q24; adrenodoxin to 11q22; adrenodixin reductase to 17q24-q25; and P450c17 to 10q24-q25. *DNA Cell Biol* **10**:359,1991.
254. Lin D, Harikrishna JA, Moore CCD, Jones KL, Miller WL: Missense mutation serine106 proline causes 17α-hydroxylase deficiency. *J Biol Chem* **266**:15992, 1991.
255. Suzuki Y, Nagashima T, Nomura Y, Onigata K, Nagashima K, Morikawa A: A new compound heterozygous mutation (W17X, 436 + 5G $\rightarrow$ T) in the cytochrome *P450c17* gene causes 17α-hydroxylase/17,20-lyase deficiency. *J Clin Endocrinol Metab* **83**:199, 1998.
256. Yamaguchi H, Nakazato M, Kangawa K, Matsukura S: A 5′ splice mutation in the cytochrome P450 steroid 17α-hydroxylase gene in 17α-hydroxylase deficiency. *J Clin Endocrinol Metab* **82**:1934, 1997.
257. Laflamme N, Leblanc G, Maillouz J, Faure N, Labrie C, Simard J: Mutation R96W in cytochrome *P450c17* gene causes combined 17α-hydroxylase/17,20-lyase defiency in two French Canadian patients. *J Clin Endocrinol Metab* **81**:264, 1996.
258. Monno S, Ogawa H, Date T, Fujioka M, Miller WL, Kobayashi M: Mutation of histidine 373 to leucine in cytochrome P450c17 causes 17α-hydroxylase deficiency. *J Biol Chem* **268**:25811, 1993.

259. Rumsby G, Skinner C, Lee HA, Honour JW: Combined 17α-hydroxylase/17,20-lyase deficiency caused by heterozygous stop codons in the cytochrome P450 17α-hydroxylase gene. *Clin Endocrinol* **39**:483, 1993.
260. Fardella CE, Hum DW, Homoki J, Miller WL: Point mutation of Arg440 to His in cytochrome P450c17 causes severe 17α-hydroxylase deficiency. *J Clin Endocrinol Metab* **79**:160, 1994.
261. Oshiro C, Takasu N, Wakugami T, Komiya I, Yamada T, Eguchi Y, Takei H: 17α-hydroxylase deficiency with one base pair deletion of the cytochrome P450c17 (*CYP17*) gene. *J Clin Endocrinol Metab* **80**:2526, 1995.
262. Biason A, Mantero F, Scaroni C, Simpson ER, Waterman MR: Deletion within the *CYP17* gene together with insertion of foreign DNA is the cause of combined complete 17α-hydroxylase/17,20-lyase deficiency in an Italian patient. *Mol Endocrinol* **5**:2037, 1991.
263. Fardella CE, Zhang LH, Mahachoklertwattana P, Lin D, Miller WL: Deletion of amino acids Asp487-Ser488-Phe489 in human cytochrome P450c17 causes severe 17α-hydroxylase deficiency. *J Clin Endocrinol Metab* **77**:489, 1993.
264. Miura K, Yasuda K, Yanase T, Yamakita N, Sasano H, Nawata H, Inoue M, Fukaya T, Shizuta Y: Mutation of cytochrome P-45017α gene (*CYP17*) in a Japanese patient previously reported as having glucocorticoid-responsive hyperaldosteronism: With a review of Japanese patients with mutations of *CYP17*. *J Clin Endocrinol Metab* **81**:3797, 1996.
265. Biason-Lauber A, Leiberman E, Zachmann M: A single amino acid substitution in the putative redox partner-binding site of P450c17 as cause of isolated 17,20-lyase deficiency. *J Clin Endocrinol Metab* **82**:3807, 1997.
266. Geller DH, Auchus RJ, Mendoca BB, Miller WL: The genetic and functional basis of isolated 17,20-lyase deficiency. *Nature Genet* **17**:201, 1997.
267. Bongiovanni AM: The adrenogenital syndrome with deficiency of the 3β-hydroxysteroid dehydrogenase. *J Clin Invest* **41**:2086, 1962.
268. Zachmann M, Vollmin JA, Murset G, Curtius H-CH, Prader A: Unusual type of congenital adrenal hyperplasia probably due to a deficiency of 3β-hydroxysteroid dehydrogenase: Case report of a surviving girl and steroid studies. *J Clin Endocrinol Metab* **30**:719, 1970.
269. Janne O, Perheentupa J, Vihko R: Plasma and urinary steroids in an eight-year-old boy with 3β-hydroxysteroid dehydrogenase deficiency. *J Clin Endocrinol Metab* **31**:162, 1970.
270. Bérubé D, The VL, Lachance Y, Agné R: Assignment of the human 3β-hydroxysteroid dehydrogenasene (HSDB3) to the 1p13 band of chromosome 1. *Cytogenet Genet* **52**:199, 1989.
271. Pang S, Lerner AJ, Stoner E, Levine LS, Oberfield SE, Engel I, New MI: Late-onset adrenal steroid 3β-hydroxysteroid dehydrogenase deficiency: A cause of hirsutism in pubertal and postpubertal women. *J Clin Endocrinol Metab* **60**:428, 1985.
272. Rosenfield RL, Rich BH, Wolfsdorf JL, Cassorla F, Parka JS, Bongiovanni AM, Wu CH, Shackelton CHL: Pubertal presentation of congenital 3-beta-hydroxysteroid dehydrogenase deficiency. *J Clin Endocrinol Metab* **51**:345, 1980.
273. Bongiovanni AM: Acquired adrenal hyperplasia: With special reference to 3β-hydroxysteroid dehydrogenase. *Fertil Steril* **35**:599, 1981.
274. Zerah M, Schram P, New MI: The diagnosis and treatment of nonclassical 3β-HSD deficiency. *Endocrinologist* **1**:75, 1991.
275. Luu-The V, Lachance Y, Labrie C, Leblanc G, Thomas JL, Strickler RC, Labrie F: Full-length cDNA structure and deduced amino sequence of human 3β-hydroxy-5-ene steroid dehydrogenase. *Mol Endocrinol* **3**:1310, 1989.
276. Rhéaume E, Lachance Y, Zhao H-F, Breton N, Dumont M, de Launoit Y, Trudel C, Luu-The V, Simard J, Labrie F: Structure and expression of a new complementary DNA encoding the almost exclusive 3β-hydroxysteroid dehydrogenase/D5-D4-isomerase in human adrenals and gonads. *Mol Endocrinol* **5**:1147, 1991.
277. Fardella CE, Zhang LH, Mahachoklertwattana P, Lin D, Miller WL: Multiple isoforms of 3β-hydroxysteroid dehydrogenase/delta-5-4-isomerase in mouse tissues: Male-specific isoforms are expressed in the gonads and liver. *Endocrinology* **133**:39, 1993.
278. Abbaszade IG, Clarke TR, Park C-HJ, Payne A: The mouse 3β-hydroxysteroid dehydrogenase multigene family includes two functionally distinct groups of proteins. *Mol Endocrinol* **9**:1214, 1998.
279. Rhéaume E, Simard J, Morel Y, Mebarki F, Zachmann M, Forest MG, New MI, Labrie F: Congenital adrenal hyperplasia due to point mutations in the type II 3β-hydroxysteroid dehydrogenase gene. *Nature Genet* **1**:239, 1992.
280. Simard J, Rhéaume E, Sanchez R, Laflamme N, de Launoit Y, Luu-The V, Van Seters AP, Gordon RD, Bettendorf M, Heinrich U, Moshang T, New MI, Labrie F: Molecular basis of congenital adrenal hyperplasia due to 3β-hydroxysteroid dehydrogenase deficiency. *Mol Endocrinol* **7**:716, 1993.
281. Zhang L, Sakkal-Alkaddour H, Chang YT, Yang X, Pang S: A new compond heterozygous frameshift mutation in the type II 3β-hyroxysteroid dehydrogenase (3β-HSD) gene causes salt-wasting 3β-HSD deficiency congenital adreanl hyperplasia. *J Clin Endocrinol Metab* **81**:291, 1996.
282. Chang YT, Kappy MS, Iwamoto K, Wang J, Yang X, Pang S: Mutations in the type II 3β-hydroxysteroid dehydrogenase gene in a patient with classic salt-wasting 3β-hydroxysteroid dehydrogenase deficiency congenital adrenal hyperplasia. *Pediatr Res* **34**:698, 1993.
283. Rhéaume E, Snachez R, Simard J, Chang YT, Wang J, Pang S, Labrie C: Molecular basis of congenital adrenal hyperplasia in two siblings with classical nonsalt-losing 3β-hydroxysteroid dehydrogenase deficiency. *J Clin Endocrinol Metab* **79**:1012, 1994.
284. Mébarki F, Sanchez R, Rhéaume E, Laflamme N, Simard J, Forest M, Bey-Omar R, David M, Labrie C, Morel Y: Nonsalt-losing male pseudohermaphroditism due to the novel homozygous *N100S* mutation in the type II 3β-hydroxysteroid dehydrogenase gene. *J Clin Endocrinol Metab* **80**:2127, 1995.
285. Simard J, Sanchez R, Durocher F, Rhéaume E, Turgeon C, Labrie C, Luu-The V, Mebarki F, Morel Y, de Launoit Y, Labrie F: Structure-function relationships and molecular genetics of the 3β-hydroxysteroid dehydrogenase gene family. *J Steroid Biochem Mol Biol* **55**:489, 1995.
286. Chang YT, Zhang L, Alkaddour HS, Mason JI, Lin.K., Yang X, Garibaldi LR, Bourdony CJ, Dolan LM, Donaldson DL, Pang S: Absence of molecular defect in the type II 3β-hydroxysteroid dehydrogenase (*3β-HSD*) gene in premature pubarche children and hirsute female patients with moderately decreased adrenal 3β-HSD activity. *Pediatr Res* **37**:820, 1995.
287. Zerah M, Rhéaume E, Mani P, Schram P, Simard J, Labrie C, New MI: No evidence of mutations in the genes for type I and type II 3β-hydroxysteroid dehydrogenase (3βHSD) in nonclassical 3βHSD deficiency. *J Clin Endocrinol Metab* **79**:1811, 1994.
287a. Prader A, Siebenmann RE: Nebennireninsuffiziene be kongenitaler lipoid hyperplasia der nebennierin. *Helv Paediatr Acta* **12**:569, 1957.
288. Caron KM, Soo S-C, Clark BJ, Stocco DM, Wetzel W, Parker KL: Targeted disruption of the mouse gene encoding the steroidogenic acute regulatory protein provides insights into congenital lipoid adrenal hyperplasia. *Proc Natl Acad Sci USA* **94**:11540, 1997.
289. Okuyama E, Nishi N, Onishi S, Itoh S, Ishii Y, Miyanaka H, Fujita K, Ichikawa Y: A novel splicing junction mutation in the gene for the steroidogenic acute regulatory protein causes congeital lipod adrenal hyperplasia. *J Clin Endocrinol Metab* **82**:2337, 1997.
290. Tee M-K, Lin D, Sugawara T, Holt JA, Guiguen Y, Buckingham B, Strauss III JF, Miller WL: T→A transversion 11 bp from a splice donor site in the human gene for steroidogenic acute regulatory protein causes congenital lipoid adrenal hyperplasia. *Hum Mol Genet* **12**:2299, 1995.
291. Yang X, Iwamoto K, Wang M, Artwohl J, Mason JI, Pang S: Inherited congenital adrenal hyperplasia in the rabbit is caused by a deletion in the gene encoding cytochrome P-450 cholesterol side-chain cleavage enzyme. *Endocrinology* **132**:1977, 1993.
292. Solish SB, Picado-Leonard J, Morel Y, Kuhn RW, Mohandas TK, Hanukoglu I, Miller WL: Human adrenodoxin reductase: Two mRNAs encoded by a single gene on chromosome 17cenq25 are expressed in steroidogenic tissues. *Proc Natl Acad Sci USA* **85**:7104, 1988.
293. Hauffa BP, Miller WL, Grumbach MM, Conte FA, Kaplan SL: Congenital adrenal hyperplasia due to deficient cholesterol side-chain cleavage activity (20,22-desmolase) in a patient treated for 18 years. *Clin Endocrinol* **23**:481, 1985.
294. Shizuta Y, Kawamoto T, Mitsuuchi Y, Toda K, Miyahara K, Ichikawa Y, Imura H, Ulick S: Molecular genetic studies on the biosynthesis of aldosterone in humans. *J Steroid Biochem* **8**:981, 1992.
295. Degenhart HJ, Frankena L, Visser HKA, Cost WS, Van Setters AP: Further investigation of a new hereditary defect in the biosynthesis of aldosterone: Evidence for a defect in the 18-hydroxylation of corticosterone. *Acta Physiol Pharmacol Neerl* **14**:88, 1966.
296. Visser HKA, Cost WS: A new hereditary defect in the biosynthesis of aldosterone: Urinary C21-corticosteroid pattern in three related

patients with a salt-losing syndrome, suggesting an 18-oxidation defect. *Acta Endocrinol (Oxf)* **47**:589, 1964.

297. Ulick S, Gautier E, Vetter KK, Markello JR, Yaffe S, Lowe CV: An aldosterone biosynthesis defect in a salt-losing disorder. *J Clin Endocrinol Metab* **24**:669, 1964.
298. Veldhuis JD, Kulin HE, Santen RJ, Wilson TE, Melby JC: Inborn error in the terminal step of aldosterone biosynthesis: corticosterone methyl oxidase type II deficiency in a North American pedigree. *N Engl J Med* **303**:117, 1980.
299. Mitsuuchi Y, Kawamoto T, Rösler A, Naiki Y, Miyahara K, Toda K, Kuribayashi I, Orii T, Yasuda K, Miura K, Nakao K, Imura H, Ulick S, Shizuta Y: Congenitally defective aldosterone biosynthesis in humans: The involvement of point mutations of the P-450c18 gene (*CYP11B2*) in CMOII deficient patients. *Biochem Biophys Res Commun* **182**:974, 1992.
300. Fardella CE, Hum DW, Rodriguez H, Zhang G, Barry FL, Ilicki A, Bloch CA, Miller WL: Gene conversion in the *CYP11B2* gene encoding P450c11AS is associated with, but does not cause, the syndrome of corticosterone methyloxidase II deficiency. *J Clin Endocrinol Metab* **81**:321, 1996.
301. Pascoe L, Curnow KM, Slutsker L, Rösler A, White PC: Mutations in the human *CYP11B2* (aldosterone synthase) gene causing corticosterone methyloxidase II deficiency. *Proc Natl Acad Sci USA* **89**:4996, 1992.
302. Sutherland DJ, Ruse JL, Laidlaw JC: Hypertension, increased aldosterone secretion, and low plams renin activity relieved by dexamethasone. *Can Med Assoc J* **95**:1109, 1966.
303. New MI, Peterson RE: A new form of congenital adrenal hyperplasia. *J Clin Endocrinol Metab* **27**:300, 1967.
304. Rich GM, Ulick S, Cook S, Wang JZ, Lifton RP, Dluhy RG: Glucocorticoid-remediable hypertension in a large kindred: Clinical spectrum and diagnosis using a characteristic biochemical phenotype. *Ann Intern Med* **116**:813, 1992.
305. Pascoe L, Curnow KM, Slutsker L, Connell JMC, Speiser PW, New MI, White PC: Glucocorticoid-suppressible hyperaldosteronism results from hybrid genes created by unequal crossovers between *CYP11B1* and *CYP11B2*. *Proc Natl Acad Sci USA* **89**:8327, 1992.
306. Lifton RP, Dluhy RG, Powers M, Rich GM, Cook S, Ulick S, Lalouel J-M: A chimaeric 11β-hydroxylase/aldosterone synthase gene causes glucocorticoid-remediable aldosteronism and human hypertension. *Nature* **355**:262, 1992.
307. Lifton RP, Dluhy RG, Powers M, Rich GM, Gutkin M, Fallo F, Gill JR Jr, Feld L, Ganguly A, Laidlaw JC, Murnaghan DJ, Kaufman C, Stockigt JR, Ulick S, Lalouel J-M: Hereditary hypertension caused by chimaeric gene duplications and ectopic expression of aldosterone synthase. *Nature Genet* **2**:66, 1992.
308. Miyahara K, Kawamoto T, Mitsuuchi Y, Toda K, Imura H, Gordon RD, Shizuta Y: The chimeric gene linked to glucocorticoid-suppressible hyperaldosteronism encodes a fused P-450 protein possessing aldosterone synthase activity. *Biochem Biophy Res Commun* **189**: 885, 1992.
309. Monder C: Corticosteroids, receptors, and the organ-specific function of 11β-hydroxysteroid dehydrogenase. *FASEB J* **5**:3047, 1991.
310. Stewart PM, Corrie JET, Shackleton CHL: Syndrome of apparent mineralocorticoid excess: A defect in the cortisol-cortisone shuttle. *J Clin Invest* **82**:340, 1988.
311. Farese RV Jr, Biglieri EG, Shackleton CHL, Irony I, Gomez-Fontes R: Licorice-induced hypermineralocorticoidism. *N Engl J Med* **325**: 1223, 1991.
311a. White PC, Mune T, Agarwal AK: 11β-Hydroxysteroid dehydrogenase and the syndrome of apparent mineralocorticoid excess. *Endocr Rev* **18**: 135, 1997.
312. Jospe N, Donohoue PA, Van Dop C, McLean RH, Bias WB, Migeon CJ: Prevelance of polymorphic 21-hydroxylase gene (*CA21HB*) mutations in salt-losing congenital adrenal hyperplasia. *Biochem Biophys Res Commun* **142**:798, 1987.
313. White PC, Vitek A, Dupont B, New MI: Characterization of frequent deletions causing steroid 21-hydroxylase deficiency. *Proc Natl Acad Sci USA* **85**:4436, 1988.
314. Owerbach D, Crawford YM, Draznin MB: Direct analysis of *CYP21B* genes in 21-hydroxylase deficiency using polymerase chain reaction amplification. *Mol Endocrinol* **4**:125, 1990.
315. Rumsby G, Fielder AH, Hague WM, Honour JW: Heterogeneity in the gene locus for steroid 21-hydroxylase deficiency. *J Med Genet* **25**:596, 1988.
316. Partanen J, Koskimies S, Sipilä I, Lipsanen V: Major-histocompatibility-complex gene markers and restriction-fragment analysis of steroid 21-hydroxylase (*CYP21*) and complement C4 genes in classical congenital adrenal hyperplasia patients in a single population. *Am J Hum Genet* **44**:660, 1989.
317. Morel Y, André J, Uring-Lambert B, Hauptmann G, Bétuel H, Tossi M, Forest MG, David M, Bertrand J, Miller WL: Rearrangements and point mutations of P450c21 genes are distinguished by five restriction endonuclease haplotypes identified by a new probing strategy in 57 families with congenital adrenal hyperplasia. *J Clin Invest* **83**:527, 1989.
318. Koppens PFJ, Hoogenboezem T, Halley DJJ, Barendse CAM, Oostenbrink AJ, Degenhart HJ: Family studies of the steroid 21-hydroxylase and complement C4 genes define 11 haplotypes in classical congenital adrenal hyperplasia in The Netherlands. *Eur J Pediatr* **151**:885, 1992.
319. Sinnott PJ, Livieri C, Sampietro M, Marconi M, Harris R, Severi F, Strachan T: *CYP21/C4* gene organisation in Italian 21-hydroxylase deficiency families. *Hum Genet* **88**:545, 1992.
320. Sinnot PJ, Costigan C, Dryer PA, Harris R, Strachan T: Extended MHC haplotypes and *CYP21/C4* gene organisation in Irish 21-hydroxylase deficiency families. *Hum Genet* **87**:361, 1991.
321. Ezquieta B, Oliver A, Gracia R, Gancedo P: Analysis of steroid 21-hydroxylase gene mutations in the Spanish population. *Hum Genet* **96**:198, 1995.
322. Migeon CJ, Donohoue PA: Adrenal disorders. In Kappy MS, Blizzard RM, Migeon CJ (eds): *Wilkins' The Diagnosis and Management of Endocrine Disorders in Childhood and Adolescence*. Springfield, IL, Charles C Thomas, 1994, pp 717–856.
323. Luo X, Ikeda Y, Parker KL: A cell-specific nuclear receptor is essential for adrenal and gonadal development and sexual differentiation. *Cell* **77**(4):481, 1994.
324. Wijesuriya SD, Zhang G, Dardis A, Miller WL: Transcriptional regulatory elements of the human gene for cytochrome P450c21 (steroid 21-hydroxylase) lie within intron 35 of the linked C4B gene. *J Biol Chem* **274**: 38097, 1999.

CHAPTER 160

The Androgen Resistance Syndromes: Steroid 5α-Reductase 2 Deficiency, Testicular Feminization, and Related Disorders

James E. Griffin ▪ Michael J. McPhaul
David W. Russell ▪ Jean D. Wilson

1. Androgens act within target cells by mechanisms similar to those of other hormones of the steroid-thyroid-retinoid class. The hormone combines with a receptor protein, and the androgen-receptor complex interacts with other proteins to form transcription regulatory complexes that control the formation of messenger RNA. However, androgen action differs from that of other steroid hormones in two important ways. First, testosterone, the major circulating androgen, must be converted to dihydrotestosterone before exerting many of its actions. Second, during embryogenesis, androgens act to convert the undifferentiated urogenital tract into the male phenotype. In this manner, androgens promote differentiation of the organs that serve as major target tissues for the hormone in later life.

2. Inherited defects that impede androgen action cause resistance to the action of the hormone and produce manifestations that range from undervirilized or infertile men to individuals with ambiguous genitalia to phenotypic women. In molecular terms, these disorders can be classified on the basis of the step in androgen action that is impeded by the individual mutations.

3. Steroid 5α-reductase 2 deficiency (MIM 264600) is an autosomal recessive disorder that impairs the conversion of testosterone to dihydrotestosterone. In affected males, the internal urogenital tract virilizes normally, but formation of the male external genitalia is variably impaired and is usually female in character. In affected 46,XY males raised as women, this disorder is commonly associated with a change to male gender role behavior after the time of expected puberty.

4. Mutations of the receptor that mediates the action of both testosterone and dihydrotestosterone cause at least four syndromes in 46,XY individuals: women with complete and incomplete testicular feminization, the Reifenstein syndrome, and the undervirilized or infertile male (MIM 300068, 312300, 308370). Most of the defects are due to point mutations that result in premature termination codons or amino acid substitutions in the hormone- or DNA-binding domains of the receptor; partial or complete deletions of the coding sequence and splicing abnormalities are less common.

5. The fact that mutations of the androgen receptor are more common than mutations in all other receptors of this class is due to three factors. First, the gene that encodes the androgen receptor is located on the X chromosome, and hence mutations are always expressed in males. Second, normal androgen action is essential for reproduction but not for the life of individuals, so the total absence of receptor function is compatible with life. Third, even slight abnormalities in androgen action can cause anatomic or functional abnormalities (and hence usually come to the attention of physicians). As a consequence, the androgen resistance syndromes have provided a remarkable opportunity to use mutations for the analysis of normal hormone action and of abnormal sexual development.

The fact that endocrine disease can result from resistance to hormone action at the cellular level was first recognized by Albright and colleagues, who deduced that pseudohypoparathyroidism is caused by peripheral resistance to the action of parathyroid hormone.[1] The next disorder shown to result from resistance to hormone action was the testicular feminization syndrome, a form of male pseudohermaphroditism in which genetic males with testes differentiate as phenotypic women as a result of a single-gene defect.[2] In 1957, Wilkins showed that the administration of androgen to a woman with testicular feminization did not induce virilization, and he deduced that this disorder is caused by resistance to androgen action during embryogenesis and postnatal life.[3] Additional syndromes of androgen resistance have been delineated subsequently in which the manifestations vary from phenotypic women with so-called incomplete testicular feminization to men with infertility or undervirilization.[4]

A list of standard abbreviations is located immediately preceding the index in each volume. Nonstandard abbreviations used in this chapter include: hCG = human chorionic gonadotropin; LH = luteinizing hormone; FSH = follicle-stimulating hormone; LHRH = luteinizing hormone-releasing hormone.

Investigations of several types have provided insight into the pathophysiology of these disorders:

1. The role of androgens in the formation of the male phenotype during embryogenesis has been defined.[5]
2. Quantitative assessment of androgen and estrogen metabolism in intact subjects has provided insight into the feminization that occurs with the more severe disorders.[6,7]
3. Analysis of the patterns of inheritance made it possible to recognize distinct subgroups of the disorders.[8]
4. The molecular processes by which androgens act within cells have been identified,[9,10] and techniques have been developed to assess these processes in biopsy material from affected subjects and in fibroblasts cultured from skin biopsies.[4]
5. The cDNAs for two key proteins in the pathway of androgen action, steroid 5α-reductase 2[11,12] and the androgen receptor, have been cloned,[13–16] and many of the mutations that cause androgen resistance have been defined.

The principal focus of this chapter is to describe the mechanisms by which androgens virilize the normal male during fetal development and in postnatal life and to summarize the current concepts of the pathogenesis of the syndromes of androgen resistance.

DYNAMICS OF ANDROGEN AND ESTROGEN METABOLISM IN NORMAL MEN

The principal androgen secreted by the testis and present in male plasma is the 19-carbon steroid testosterone. Testosterone also serves as the precursor (or prohormone) for two other active hormones — dihydrotestosterone and estradiol[6,7,9] (Fig. 160-1). Dihydrotestosterone is the intracellular mediator of many androgen actions and circulates in blood at about one-tenth the level of testosterone.[9] Dihydrotestosterone is derived primarily by formation from testosterone in extraglandular tissues and to a lesser extent by direct secretion by the testes.

In normal men, estrogen formation appears to play a role in closure of the epiphyses,[17,18] control of growth hormone secretion at puberty,[19] regulation of gonadotropin secretion by testosterone,[20,21] and possibly control of high-density lipoprotein levels.[22] Excess estrogen in men — either relative or absolute — causes feminization, particularly enlargement of the breasts (gynecomastia),[23] and increased estradiol formation is responsible for feminization in several disorders of androgen action.[7] The dynamics of estrogen and androgen production and metabolism are summarized in Fig. 160-2*A*.[7] As determined by isotope dilution techniques, the production rates of estrone and estradiol, respectively, average about 65 and 45 μg/day in normal men, and production rates of testosterone and the 19-carbon adrenal steroid androstenedione, respectively, average about 5000 and 3000 μg/day,[7] so the ratio of the production rate of testosterone to estradiol is normally about 100:1. All of estrone and about 85 percent of estradiol are formed by extraglandular conversion of androstenedione and testosterone. Thus, in normal men, at best only 6 to 10 μg estradiol are secreted directly into the circulation by the testes.[6,7] Kelch et al.[24] and Weinstein et al.[25] also concluded that estrogen in men is synthesized predominantly in extraglandular tissues as the result of direct measurements of estrogen levels in testicular venous blood of normal men. However, when large amounts of human chorionic gonadotropin (hCG) are administered [or when plasma luteinizing hormone (LH) levels are elevated in pathologic states], direct secretion of estrogen by the testes increases in proportion to the enhancement of testosterone secretion.[25] In summary, whereas most estrogen in normal men is formed by extraglandular aromatization of circulating 19-carbon steroids, the testes may secrete large amounts of estrogen into the circulation when gonadotropin concentrations are elevated. Feminization of men results when the normal hundredfold excess of androgens to estrogens is disturbed either by an increase in estrogen production or by a decrease in testosterone formation (or action) under circumstances in which estrogen production remains appreciable.[23]

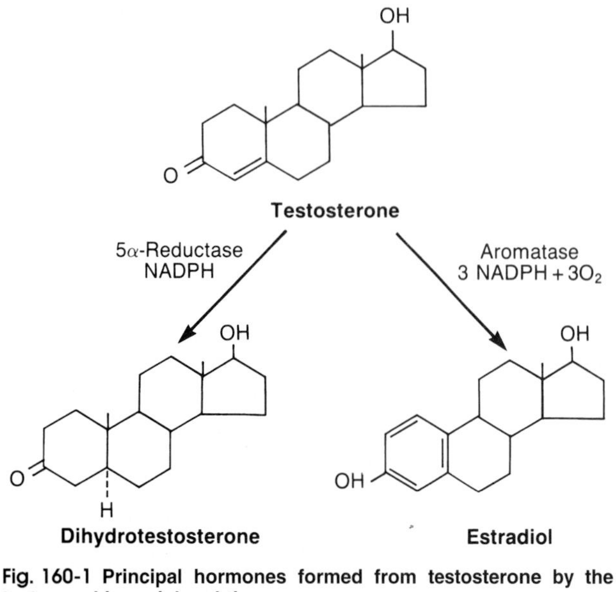

Fig. 160-1 Principal hormones formed from testosterone by the testes and in peripheral tissues.

MECHANISMS OF ANDROGEN ACTION

The current concepts of the mechanisms by which androgens act are schematized in Fig. 160-3. Testosterone, the principal androgen secreted by the testis and the major androgen in the plasma of men, circulates for the most part bound to two proteins, sex hormone-binding globulin (also termed *testosterone-binding globulin*) and albumin.[26] Protein-bound steroid is in dynamic equilibrium with unbound or free hormone, the latter comprising 1 to 3 percent of the total.[26] The entry of unbound testosterone into cells is not energy-dependent and probably occurs by passive diffusion,[27] so the concentration of testosterone in most androgen target tissues is lower than that in plasma.[28]

Inside the cell, testosterone can be reduced to dihydrotestosterone by 5α-reductase enzymes or aromatized to estradiol. Dihydrotestosterone and testosterone bind to the same receptor. Androgen receptors are located predominantly in the nucleus in the unbound state, and binding of androgen results in their transformation to a state with greater affinity for specific DNA sequences (hormone response elements) in the promoter regions of target genes.[29] Like other members of the superfamily of steroid, thyroid, and retinoid receptors, the androgen receptor has DNA- and hormone-binding domains in the C-terminal region; the amino acid sequence in these regions is closely related to comparable domains of the glucocorticoid, progesterone, and mineralocorticoid receptors. The N-terminal region is only weakly homologous to comparable regions of other steroid hormone receptors and contains glutamine, proline, and glycine homopolymeric sequences[13–16] (Fig. 160-4; see also Chap 161). The length of the glutamine repeat is polymorphic, and more than 90 percent of normal women are heterozygous at this locus.[30] The pathologic consequences of very long glutamine repeat sequences at this locus are discussed in Chap. 161. As with other receptors of this class, the active form of the androgen receptor is a homodimer that forms as a result of interacting sites in the N-terminal and C-terminal steroid-binding domains of the protein.[31] The homodimer in turn is believed to interact with other proteins to form the active transcripition regulatory complex.[10]

Although dihydrotestosterone and testosterone bind to the same receptor,[32] the two receptor-hormone complexes have distinct physiologic roles. The testosterone-receptor complex is respon-

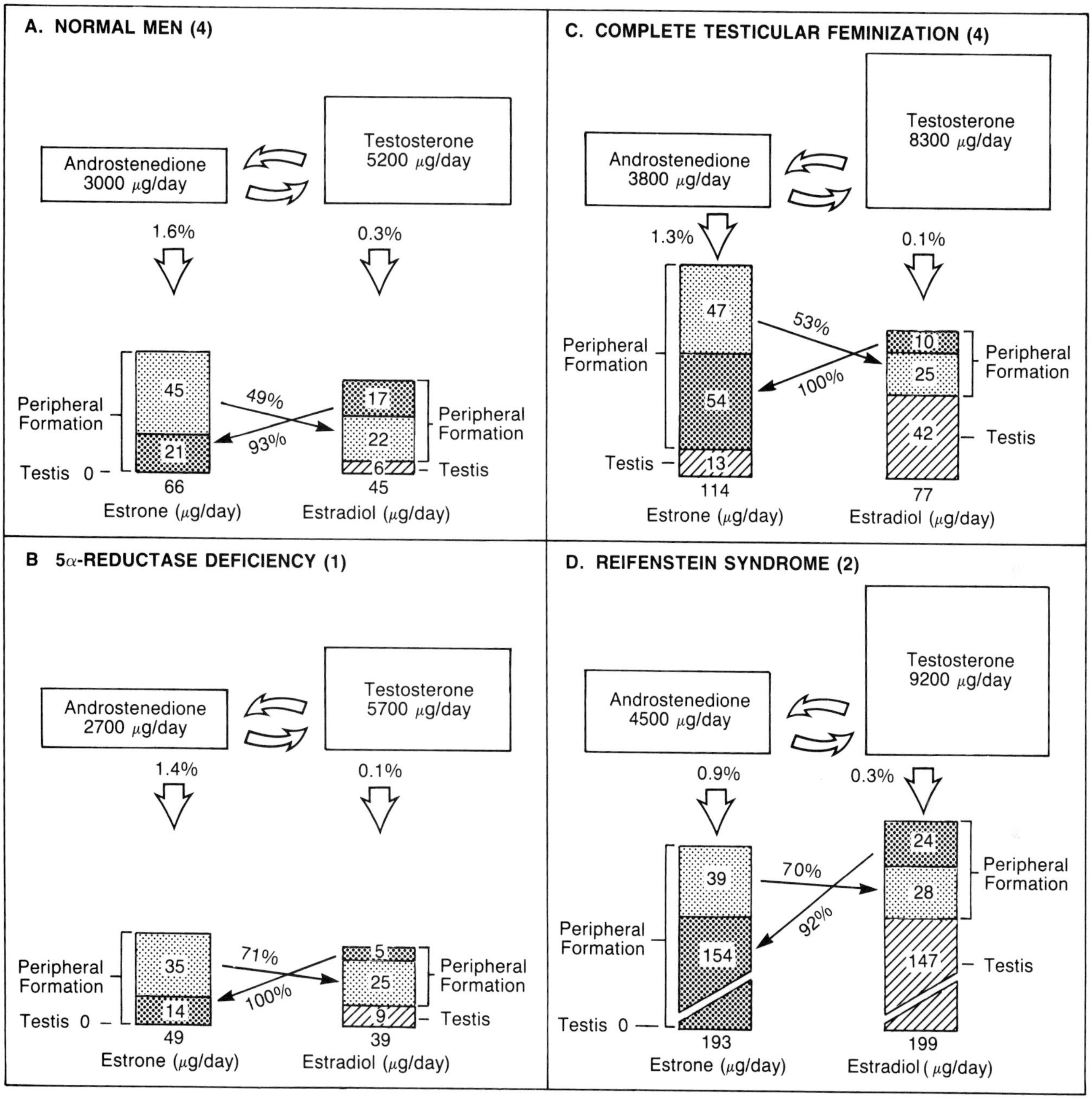

Fig. 160-2 Dynamics of androgen and estrogen production in normal men and in 46,XY subjects with androgen resistance. *A.* Four normal men. *B.* One subject with 5α-reductase 2 deficiency. *C.* Four subjects with complete testicular feminization. *D.* Two men with Reifenstein syndrome. Average production rates of androgen are indicated in the upper boxes, and the production rates of estrogen are shown below the vertical bar. Extent of conversion of plasma testosterone and androstenedione to estradiol and estrone is indicated by the vertical arrows, and interconversion of estrone and estradiol and of testosterone and androstenedione are indicated by the horizontal arrows. The sources of estradiol and estrone are indicated in the vertical bars. Thus estradiol arises from plasma testosterone, from estrone, and from direct secretion by the testis, and estrone arises from plasma androstenedione, from estradiol, and in some instances from direct secretion by the testis. (*From MacDonald et al.,*[7] *Walsh et al.,*[71] *and Wilson et al.*[204] *Used by permission.*)

sible for regulation of the secretion of LH by the hypothalamic-pituitary system, for virilization of the Wolffian ducts during male phenotypic sex differentiation, and probably for the regulation of spermatogenesis.[9,33] The dihydrotestosterone-receptor complex, in turn, promotes development of the male external genitalia and prostate during embryogenesis and most of the androgen-mediated events of sexual maturation at the time of male puberty (growth of facial and body hair, temporal hair recession, maturation of external genitalia).[9,33] The reason that different species of one hormone perform different functions is twofold: Dihydrotestosterone binds more avidly to the receptor than testosterone,[32] and the dihydrotestosterone-receptor complex is much more readily transformed to the DNA-binding state[34] and activates a reporter gene system more efficiently.[35] The net consequence is that dihydrotestosterone formation amplifies the androgenic signal. In addition, the dihydrotestosterone-receptor complex may be required for the activation of some gene networks.[36]

In summary, the process by which all steroid hormones act is believed to involve passive entry of the hormone into target tissue, binding of the hormone to a receptor, attachment of the

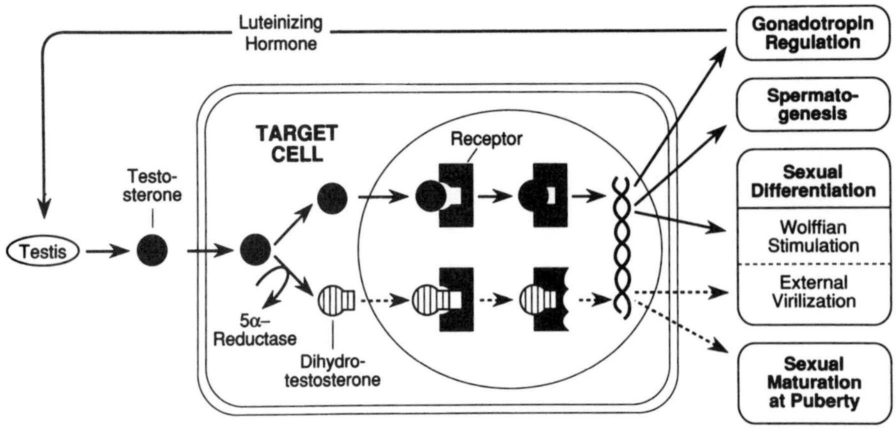

Fig. 160-3 Normal androgen physiology. Testosterone, secreted by the testis, binds to the androgen receptor in a target cell, either directly or after conversion to dihydrotestosterone. Dihydrotestosterone binds more tightly than testosterone, and the complex of dihydrotestosterone and the androgen receptor can bind more efficiently to the chromatin. The major actions of androgens, shown on the right, are mediated by testosterone (*solid lines*) or by dihydrotestosterone (*broken lines*). (*From Griffin.[4] Used by permission.*)

receptor-hormone complex to the nuclear chromatin, and regulation of the transcription of mRNA. Androgen action differs from that of other steroid hormones in at least two ways: (1) Many effects of testosterone, the major circulating androgen, are mediated by intracellular metabolites of testosterone — dihydrotestosterone and (possibly) estradiol. Thus the physiologic effects of testosterone comprise the actions of testosterone itself and of its 5α-reduced and estrogenic metabolites. Since dihydrotestosterone cannot be converted to estrogen, its actions are purely androgenic. (2) During embryogenesis, androgen promotes differentiation of the tissues that will be major sites of action for the hormone in postnatal life. In performing this critical role in normal male sexual development, androgens exert their most fundamental action.

NORMAL MALE SEXUAL DEVELOPMENT

Sexual development during embryogenesis consists of three sequential, ordered, and interrelated processes.[5] The first involves the establishment of chromosomal sex at fertilization. In the mammal, the heterogametic sex (XY) is male and the homogametic sex (XX) is female. In the second phase, chromosomal sex is translated into gonadal sex. The mechanisms by which the genetic information determines that an indifferent gonad differentiates into a testis in the male or an ovary in the female and secretes the hormones characteristic of the testis or ovary are incompletely understood,[33] but the SRY (sex-determining region on the Y) locus near the pseudoautosomal region of the short arm of the Y chromosome encodes a DNA-binding protein[37] that is sufficient to cause the indifferent gonad to develop into a testis when the protein is expressed as a transgene in female mice.[38] The third phase, the translation of gonadal sex into phenotypic sex, is the direct consequence of the type of gonad formed and the resulting hormonal secretions of the fetal testis. In the formation of phenotypic sex, indifferent internal and external genital anlagen are converted to male or female forms, and the behavioral and functional characteristics of the two sexes ultimately are determined.

The anatomic processes involved in the development of phenotypic sex are summarized in Fig. 160-5. The internal urogenital tracts in the two sexes arise from different anlagen, namely, the Wolffian and Müllerian ducts.[33] The Wolffian ducts are the excretory ducts of the mesonephric kidney system and are connected anatomically with the indifferent gonad. The Müllerian ducts form adjacent to the Wolffian ducts and are not contiguous with the gonad.[39] In males, the Wolffian ducts give rise to the epididymides, vasa deferentia, and seminal vesicles, and the Müllerian ducts disappear. In females, the Müllerian ducts give rise to the fallopian tubes, uterus, and upper vagina, and the Wolffian ducts either disappear or persist in vestigial form as Gartner's ducts.

In contrast, the external genitalia in the two sexes develop from common anlagen, the genital tubercle, genital folds, and genital swellings. In females, the system enlarges but does not fundamentally change; the genital tubercle becomes the clitoris, the genital folds become the labia minora, and the genital swellings become the labia majora. In males, fusion and elongation of the genital folds cause formation of the urethra and shaft of the penis and bring the urethral orifice to the genital tubercle (glans penis). The fused genital swellings become the scrotum, and a prostate forms in the wall of the urogenital sinus.[33]

Under ordinary conditions, development of the sexual phenotype conforms to chromosomal sex — that is, chromosomal sex determines gonadal sex, and gonadal sex in turn determines phenotypic sex. In the absence of the testes, as in the normal female or in rabbit embryos of either sex castrated prior to the onset of phenotypic differentiation, the development of phenotypic sex proceeds along female lines.[5] Thus masculinization of the fetus is the positive result of action by testicular hormones, whereas female phenotypic development does not require hormone from the fetal ovary.

Three hormones regulate the development of the male phenotype[30] (Table 160-1). Two of the hormones — Müllerian-inhibiting hormone (also called *anti-Müllerian hormone*) and testosterone — are secretory products of the fetal testes. Müllerian-inhibiting hormone is a large (140-kDa) dimeric glycoprotein that is formed by the Sertoli cells of the fetal and newborn testis[40,41] and that acts locally to suppress Müllerian duct development and prevent formation of the uterus and fallopian tubes in the male.

Testosterone is the principal androgen secreted by both fetal and adult testes.[42] Testosterone secretion begins just prior to the onset of virilization of the male embryo (at about the eighth week

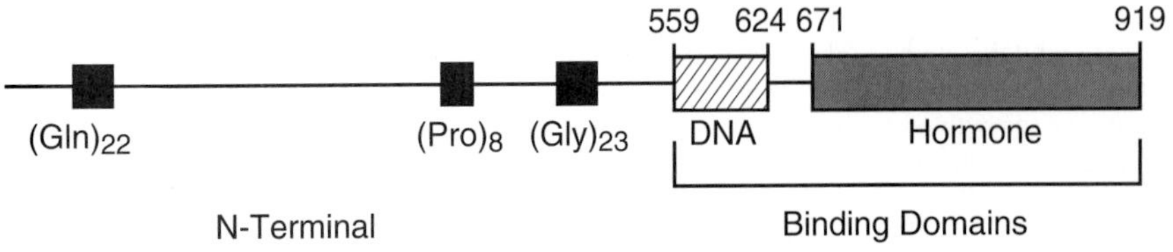

Fig. 160-4 Schematic diagram of the normal androgen receptor.

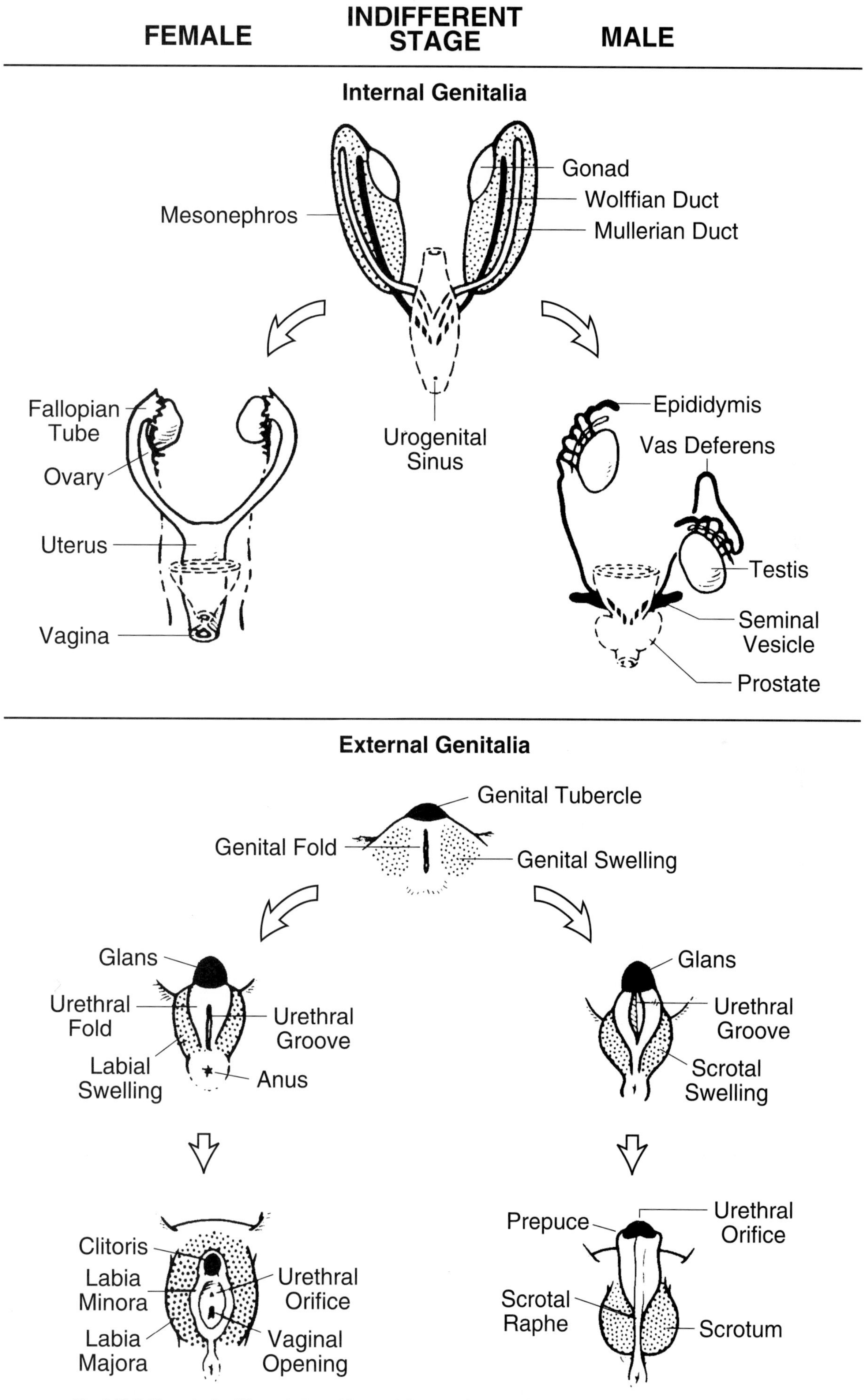

Fig. 160-5 Phenotypic differentiation of internal ducts and external genitalia in male and female embryos.

Table 160-1 Hormonal Control of Male Phenotypic Sex Differentiation

Gonadal Hormone	Active Hormone	Phase of Phenotypic Differentiation: Müllerian Duct Regression	Wolffian Duct Differentiation	Virilization of Urogenital Sinus and External Genitalia
Müllerian-inhibiting hormone	Müllerian-inhibting hormone	+		
Testosterone	Testosterone		+	
	Dihydrotestosterone			+

of human embryogenesis). The factors that regulate the initial secretion of testosterone have not been defined, but Leydig cell function may be autonomous at first and come under the control of pituitary gonadotropins later in embryogenesis.[43] The fact that loss-of-function mutations of the LH receptor cause male pseudohermaphroditism,[44] whereas loss-of-function mutations of the β subunit of LH cause undervirilization but not male pseudohermaphroditism[45] suggests that hCG, which acts via the LH receptor, may be critical for the initiation of testosterone synthesis.

In several species, including humans, virilization of the urogenital tract during embryogenesis occurs by two distinct processes. Testosterone acts directly to stimulate the Wolffian ducts and induce development of the epididymides, vasa deferentia, and seminal vesicles.[33] Differentiation of the Wolffian ducts into seminal vesicle and epididymis is complete in the human male embryo at about 13 weeks of development, before the capacity to form dihydrotestosterone is acquired by these tissues.[42] In contrast, in the urogenital sinus and external genitalia, testosterone acts as a prohormone for dihydrotestosterone—the third hormone of fetal virilization.[33] Dihydrotestosterone is synthesized in small amounts by the human fetal testis at the time of male phenotypic development,[46] but most is formed by enzymatic reduction of testosterone within the urogenital sinus and anlage of the external genitalia.[42,46] Dihydrotestosterone acts in the urogenital sinus to induce development of the male urethra and prostate and in the urogenital tubercle, swelling, and folds to promote the midline fusion, elongation, and enlargement that result in the male external genitalia. The deduction that testosterone and dihydrotestosterone perform separate roles in male embryogenesis has been substantiated by studies of human mutations that impair the steroid 5α-reductase 2 enzyme (see below) and by studies of the effects of specific inhibitors of 5α-reductase during embryogenesis in the rat [47,48] and rhesus monkey.[49]

Despite attempts in several laboratories, 5α-reductase enzymes have not been solubilized or purified successfully,[50] but two types of enzyme activities were characterized on the basis of different pH optima.[51] The technique of expression cloning was used to characterize the cDNA for rat steroid 5α-reductase 1, and the analogous human 5α-reductase 1 was cloned by taking advantage of the homology between the two enzymes.[11] Expression cloning was again used to identify the cDNA for steroid 5α-reductase 2, an enzyme with a pH optimum similar to that of the principal enzyme expressed in the urogenital tract.[12]

The characteristics of the two human 5α-reductases are summarized in Table 160-2. Enzyme 1 is encoded on chromosome 5, and enzyme 2 is encoded on chromosome 2. 5α-Reductase 2 is expressed primarily in androgen target tissues, and 5α-reductase 1 is expressed principally in liver and skin. Enzyme 2 has a lower K_m for testosterone and is more sensitive to inhibition by the 5α-reductase inhibitor finasteride. The two enzymes have about a 50 percent sequence homology, are expressed at low levels, and are hydrophobic (explaining the failure to solubilize). The gene structures are similar, with five coding exons and four introns each. The androgen-binding domain is encoded in the N-terminal end of the molecule.[52] Two 5α-reductase enzymes analogous to human enzymes 1 and 2 appear to be expressed in all animal species studied to date.[53,54] It is of particular interest in this regard that 5α-reductase deficiency in a plant species (arabidopsis) causes dwarfism due to the impairment of 5α-reduction of a brassinosteroid to form an active plant growth hormone.[55]

Two common polymorphisms of the steroid 5α-reductase 2 gene have been described. A TA dinucleotide repeat polymorphism in the 3′ untranslated region of the gene may or may not be associated with an increased risk for development of prostate cancer,[56,57] and a homozygous polymorphism of the coding sequence (V89L) is present in 5 percent of a Mexican population.[58]

Because of the small amounts of embryonic tissues available for study, the fetal androgen receptor was characterized after that for adult tissues. As a result of direct studies[59] and of studies of single-gene defects that impede androgen action,[4] the schema shown in Fig. 160-3 is valid for both embryonic and postnatal androgen action—namely, a single receptor is responsible for mediating the actions of both testosterone and dihydrotestosterone, and the androgen receptor is the same in male and female embryos. Thus, when female embryos are exposed to androgens at the appropriate time in embryonic development, both the Wolffian ducts and the external genitalia virilize in characteristic male fashion[60] (see also Chap. 159). The differences in male and female phenotypic development, therefore, are due solely to the hormones produced by the fetal testes at the critical period of embryonic development and not to differences in receptor expression.

Table 160-2 Comparison of Human Steroid 5α-Reductases 1 and 2

	5α-Reductase 1	5α-Reductase 2
pH optimum	7.5	5.0
Location of gene	Chromosome 5	Chromosome 2
Tissue distribution	Liver and skin	Male urogential tract
K_m for testosterone	4 μM	<1 μM
K_i for finasteride	~300 nM	<3–5 nM
Activity in 5α-reductase deficiency	Normal	Impaired
Sequence homology	50%	

DISORDERS OF SEXUAL DEVELOPMENT

A disturbance of sexual differentiation at any step during embryogenesis can impair sexual development. Disorders of sexual development can be classified in terms of the initial developmental stage influenced, namely, as errors in chromosomal sex, errors in gonadal sex, or errors in phenotypic sex.[8,61] Such abnormalities may arise by several mechanisms, including environmental insults (e.g., maternal ingestion of a virilizing drug during pregnancy), sporadic aberrations in the sex chromosomes (e.g., 45,X gonadal dysgenesis), developmental birth defects of multifactorial etiology (as in most cases of hypospadias), or a single-gene mutations (as in the testicular feminization syndrome). A number of simply inherited disorders of sexual development are recognized.

Male pseudohermaphroditism is a disorder of phenotypic sex in which 46,XY males with testes do not develop as normal men. Three general categories of such disorders have been delineated: the persistent Müllerian duct syndrome, deficiency of testosterone formation, and the androgen resistance syndromes.

The persistent Müllerian duct syndrome is a rare disorder characterized by normal male virilization but failure of Müllerian regression so that affected men have a uterus and fallopian tube(s) in addition to normal Wolffian structures. Some instances are due to mutations that impair the production of Müllerian-inhibiting hormone,[62] and others are due to mutations in the receptor for the hormone.[63]

Disorders of testosterone formation result either from developmental abnormalities in the testis or from impairment of any of the enzymatic steps necessary for testosterone synthesis from cholesterol; such mutations can cause defects in one of four enzymatic reactions involved in testosterone biosynthesis [3β-hydroxysteroid dehydrogenase II (3β-HSD II), 17α-hydroxylase/17,20-lyase (CYP17), or 17β-hydroxysteroid dehydrogenase 3 (17β-HSD 3)] or in the steroidogenic acute regulatory protein (StAR) that delivers substrate to the cholesterol side-chain cleavage enzyme (CYP11A1). These disorders result in variable defects in virilization in affected males and are discussed in Chap. 159.

The third type of disorder, and the focus of this chapter, androgen resistance, appears to be the most common cause of male pseudohermaphroditism because testosterone formation and Müllerian duct regression are normal in the majority of such men.[64–66] Instead, these men are resistant to androgen during embryogenesis and in the postnatal state because of a defect in some aspect of androgen action. This category of disorders was delineated originally by studying patients in whom profound defects in virilization were associated with normal male (or high) production rates of testosterone. Subsequently, it was recognized that partial defects in androgen action do not necessarily result in anatomic abnormalities or enhanced testosterone secretion but can be manifested only as impairment of virilization or of spermatogenesis in otherwise phenotypically normal men. Indeed, some affected men are fertile. Thus the spectrum of androgen resistance syndromes is broader than envisioned originally. Molecular defects responsible for androgen resistance have been identified in the cDNAs for steroid 5α-reductase 2 and for the androgen receptor.

THE ANDROGEN RESISTANCE SYNDROMES

Steroid 5α-Reductase 2 Deficiency

Clinical Features. A specific form of hereditary male pseudohermaphroditism termed *pseudovaginal perineoscrotal hypospadias* was defined on clinical and genetic grounds in 1961 by Nowakowski and Lenz[67,68] and subsequently by Simpson et al.[69] and by Opitz et al.[70] This entity also has been called *familial incomplete male pseudohermaphroditism type 2*.[71] Affected 46,XY males have an autosomal recessive disorder characterized by an external female phenotype at birth, bilateral testes, and normally virilized Wolffian structures that terminate in or empty into the vagina. While this eponym encompassed more than one disorder, the fact that the phenotype is usually the result of deficient production of dihydrotestosterone was established in 1974 by studies of two families with the disorder, one in Dallas[71] and the other in the Dominican Republic.[72,73] The entity is now termed *steroid 5α-reductase 2 deficiency.*

The initial studies in Dallas were performed in a 13-year-old 46,XY phenotypic girl with primary amenorrhea. She was partially virilized (Fig. 160-6*A*), and plasma testosterone values were in the adult male range. Because of the virilization, the decision was made to remove the testes and to repair the external genitalia. The finding at surgery of normal male Wolffian duct structures—epididymides, vasa deferentia, seminal vesicles, and ejaculatory ducts that terminated in a blind-ending vagina—was characteristic of the phenotype of pseudovaginal perineoscrotal hypospadias (see Fig. 160-6*B*). Dihydrotestosterone formation in tissue slices of foreskin, epididymis, and labia majora obtained at the time of surgery was virtually undetectable, establishing that deficiency in dihydrotestosterone formation was the cause.[71] This interpretation was confirmed by studies of the 5α-reductase enzyme in fibroblasts cultured from the skin of affected individuals.[51,74]

A similar conclusion as to the pathogenesis was reached by Imperato-McGinley and colleagues as the result of analyses of

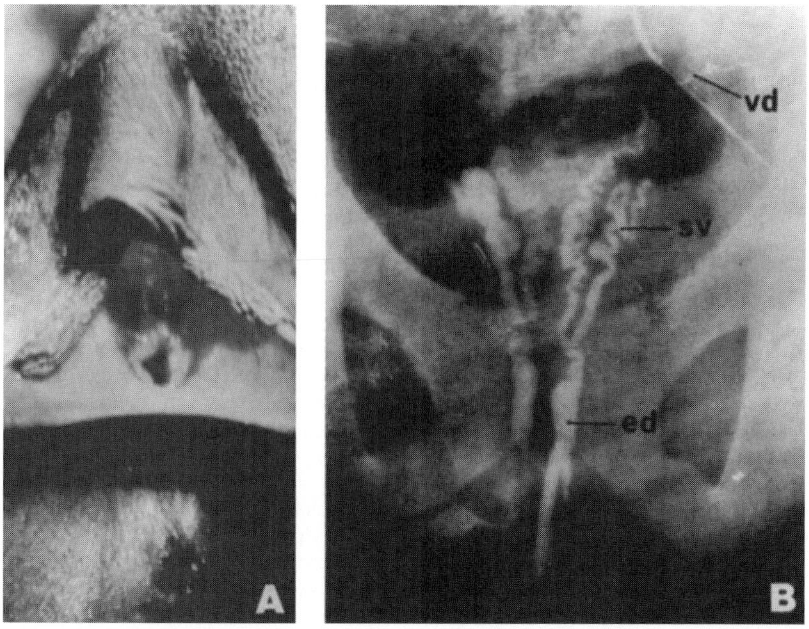

Fig. 160-6 External genitalia and internal ducts of a patient with 5α-reductase 2 deficiency; the patient is the propositus from Walsh et al.[71] *A*. Photograph of external genitalia showing clitoromegaly and the opening of a blind-ending vagina. *B*. X-ray of the abdomen after the injection of diatrizoate sodium into the vasa deferentia at the time of abdominal exploration (vd = vas deferens; sv = seminal vesicles; ed = ejaculatory duct). The dye emptied into the vagina.

Table 160-3 Features of Steroid 5α-Reductase 2 Deficiency

External phenotype: Female genitalia with some clitoromegaly at birth and variable virilization at expected time of puberty; normal male breast development
Urogenital tract: Testes; epididymides, vasa deferentia, and seminal vesicles empty into vagina; no Müllerian duct derivatives
Karyotype: 46,XY
Inheritance: Autosomal recessive
Endocrinology
Testosterone: Normal male plasma levels and production rates
Dihydrotestosterone: Low or low normal male plasma levels and production rates
Estrogen: Normal male plasma levels and production rates
Gonadotropin: Normal to slightly elevated plasma LH levels
Pathogenesis: Inability to form dihydrotestosterone

Table 160-4 Clinical Features in Steroid 5α-Reductase 2 Deficiency

Feature	Number Affected	Percent
Documented consanguinity	16/47	39
Positive family history	20/49	41
Anatomic features		
Pseudovagina	18/33	55
Urogenital Sinus	12/33	36
Hypospadias	6/33	16
Testes in inguinal canals, labia, or scrotum	43/43	100
Spermatogenesis, absent or profoundly impaired	9/9	100
Gynecomastia	1/50	2
How diagnosis established		
Ratios of 5β/5α metabolites in urine	13/46	28
Ratios of testosterone: dihydrotestosterone in plasma (before or after hCG)	46/47	98
5α-Reductase measurements in biopsy tissue or fibroblasts	31/47	66
Gonadotropin values		
Elevated luteinizing hormone	10/23	43
Elevated follicle-stimulating hormone	12/23	52
Gender role behaviour		
Raised as male	6/40	15
Changed from female to male	19/40	48
Female	9/40	22
Too young to ascertain	6/40	16
Homozygotes	23/37	61
Compound heterozygotes or presumed compound heterozygotes	13/37	32

SOURCE: Reprinted from Wilson et al.[118] Used by permission

plasma and urinary steroids in a large family in the Dominican Republic with autosomal recessive male pseudohermaphroditism.[72,73] Namely, the urinary excretion of 5α-androstanediol and androsterone (the end products of dihydrotestosterone metabolism) was low, as would be predicted if dihydrotestosterone formation were deficient.

The usual clinical features are summarized in Table 160-3 and include autosomal recessive inheritance; severe perineoscrotal hypospadias with a dorsal, hooded prepuce and a ventral urethral groove that opens at the base of the phallus; a blind-ending vaginal pouch of variable length; well-developed and histologically differentiated testes with normal epididymides, vasa deferentia, and seminal vesicles; absent Müllerian duct derivatives; and variable masculinization and no breast enlargement at the time of expected puberty.

Most affected individuals are raised as females, despite the clitoromegaly that may be present at birth. It was recognized in the first two families evaluated by us that the phenotype can be variable; one affected sister in each family had a pseudovagina, whereas the other was more virilized and had only a single perineal orifice — a urethra that provided the outlet for a urogenital sinus.[71,75,76] A sufficient number of families subsequently have been reported in the literature to make possible certain generalizations about the variability of manifestations[71–73,75–99] (Table 160-4). Consanguinity is present in about a third, and the family history is positive in about 40 percent of families. Approximately 55 percent of patients have a blind-ending vagina (pseudovagina), as originally described by Lenz[67,68]; in 12 families, a urogenital sinus was present; and in 6 families, the phallus was sufficiently large at birth that the children were identified as males with hypospadias and raised as males. Occasional affected individuals have only a microphallus with a normal male urethra,[100] but 5α-reductase deficiency is an unusual cause of microphallus.[101]

The testes in all patients are extraabdominal — present in the inguinal canals, labia majora, or scrotum. Although sperm production is profoundly impaired or absent in most subjects in whom it has been examined, one affected man from the Dominican Republic family fathered a child after intrauterine insemination,[102] and fertility has been reported in a family in which the disorder is associated with a male phenotype.[103]

In summary, the anatomic features range from minor to profound impairment of virilization of the external genitalia. The most consistent features are a small phallus and absence of the prostate. The nature of the variability in expression (even within families) is not clear, but one implication of this analysis is that this disorder must now be considered in the differential diagnosis of hypospadias (at least familial hypospadias).

Imperato-McGinley and colleagues reported that 18 of 19 individuals from the Dominican Republic who were raised as females changed gender role behavior to male at the time of expected puberty.[77,104] A similar phenomenon has been described in 19 of the 40 families summarized in Table 160-4. Change in gender role behavior from female to male has been described in people with 17β-hydroxysteroid dehydrogenase 3 deficiency, in subjects with 45,X/46,XY gonadal dysgenesis, and in one individual with 3β-hydroxysteroid dehydrogenase II deficiency.[105–107] It is of interest that change in gender role behavior is not characteristic of mutations of the androgen receptor in which gender behavior usually conforms to the sex of rearing.

The gender role reversal in 5α-reductase deficiency has been described in different ethnic groups and in different social settings. This finding suggests that androgen action in utero, during the neonatal period, and/or at puberty has an impact on the determination of male gender identity that is so pervasive that it can override female sex assignment and female rearing.[77,104] Whether these individuals actually undergo a true change of gender identity rather than a change in gender role behavior is not clear. Individuals with ambiguous genitalia may be aware of their abnormalities from an early age and consequently uncertain about their exact gender role prior to puberty.[83] Furthermore, many individuals in whom gender role has changed from female to male at puberty have been raised in cultures in which the sexes have fairly rigid stereotypes as to sexual role and in which being male might be viewed as desirable.[105] It seems safe to assume that psychosocial forces interact with hormonal factors in determining the sexual behavior of humans, but definitive studies into this problem are difficult because of limitations in the methods available for studying human behavior.

Two ancillary aspects of this phenomenon deserve comment. First, the New Guinean cluster of subjects with 5α-reductase deficiency[108–111] includes some people raised initially as females and some raised from the first as males. In this group, the disorder is sufficiently common that affected individuals are frequently recognized at birth and assigned initially to a third sex, but they eventually have the same type of difficulties fitting into adult life as do subjects with intersex in other parts of the world. Second, the first case of gender role reversal and indeed of steroid 5α-reductase 2 deficiency may have been Herculine Barbin, a nineteenth-century woman who changed her legal sex from female to male and whose phenotype, including evidence from autopsy, is compatible with the diagnosis.[112]

Endocrinology. Simpson et al.[69] showed that testosterone secretion in 5α-reductase deficiency is normal and is under normal feedback control. Subsequent studies have supported this interpretation. The characteristic endocrine features are as follows:

1. Normal male levels of plasma testosterone and low levels of plasma dihydrotestosterone[71–73]
2. Elevation in the ratio of the concentration of plasma testosterone to dihydrotestosterone in adulthood and after stimulation with hCG in childhood[73,89,93,113,114]
3. Elevated ratios of urinary 5β- to 5α-metabolites of androgen[73,87,88,93,113,114]
4. Diminished conversion of testosterone to dihydrotestosterone in biopsied tissues[71]
5. Elevated ratios of urinary 5β- to 5α-metabolites of C-21 steroids[87,95,114]
6. Increased ratio of plasma testosterone to dihydrotestosterone after the administration of testosterone[83,113]

Levels of plasma LH are either normal[71,83,88,97] or slightly elevated (although never as high as in men with primary testicular failure or in subjects with male pseudohermaphroditism due to abnormalities of the androgen receptor).[72,73,79,95,96] In one study, elevation of plasma LH level was due to increased amplitude of LH pulses in the face of normal frequency of pulses.[115] It is of interest in this regard that elevated LH was present in 10 of the 23 and elevated follicle-stimulating hormone (FSH) was described in 12 of the 23 subjects summarized in Table 160-4. This finding implies that dihydrotestosterone plays a role, probably minor, in the regulation of gonadotropin secretion.

Androgen and estrogen dynamics were studied in detail in the index case in the Dallas family[71] (see Fig. 160-2*B*); plasma levels of androstenedione (1.1 ng/ml) and testosterone (6.9 ng/ml) and the plasma production rates of androstenedione (2.7 mg/day) and testosterone (5.2 mg/day) were in the normal range for men. Estradiol production also was in the range for normal men (45 μg/day). The finding that androgen and estrogen production is in the normal male range explains the failure of patients to undergo female breast development at the time of puberty; in contrast, in subjects with mutations of the androgen receptor, variable feminization at the expected time of puberty correlates with increased estrogen secretion by the testes.

Pathogenesis. The enzymatic features of 5α-reductase deficiency were characterized in fibroblasts cultured from the genital skin, and two categories were recognized, namely, one group of patients with profound deficiency/absence of enzyme activity and another group in whom a normal amount of kinetically abnormal enzyme was synthesized.[51,74–76] The meaning of these functional studies became apparent only when the cDNAs for the 5α-reductases were cloned. Steroid 5α-reductase 1, the first of the cDNAs to be cloned, was established in formal genetic studies to be normal in patients with 5α-reductase deficiency.[116] Subsequently, the cDNA for 5α-reductase 2 was cloned, and a number of mutations of the cDNAs for this protein have been documented in these families.[12,117,118]

Although plasma dihydrotestosterone levels are low,[69–71] they are always measurable and may fall within the low-normal range. The circulating dihydrotestosterone in this disorder could be synthesized by the residual activity of the mutant enzyme or derived from 5α-reductase 1. Studies of two groups of affected individuals clearly indicate that the latter source predominates. Indeed, New Guinean subjects who have a deletion of the entire coding sequence for 5α-reductase 2 enzyme[12] and who, as a consequence, make no functional enzyme nevertheless have measurable plasma dihydrotestosterone.[111] Likewise, one subject from a family with a splice junction abnormality that precludes synthesis of a functional steroid 5α-reductase 2 enzyme[117] had basal plasma dihydrotestosterone levels in the low-normal range and supraphysiologic levels after he was given large amounts of testosterone propionate by injection for 3 days.[83] These findings indicate that steroid 5α-reductase 1 contributes to plasma dihydrotestosterone, recognizing that in some patients dihydrotestosterone also may be formed in small amounts from the residual activity of mutated steroid 5α-reductase 2.[117] The fact that 5α-reductase activity is normal in hair follicles from the scalps of patients with 5α-reductase deficiency[119] suggests that androgen action in some tissues may be mediated by steroid 5α-reductase 1. Elucidation of the role of steroid 5α-reductase 1 in androgen physiology is a major imperative.

The degree of virilization at expected puberty can be striking, and in some subjects the habitus becomes masculine, although affected subjects virilize less completely than their unaffected brothers. This virilization could be mediated by the circulating dihydrotestosterone that is measurable in all subjects or could be due to the actions of testosterone itself over a long period; attempts to resolve this question have yielded inconclusive results.[83] Namely, in four affected men, the parenteral administration of sufficient amounts of testosterone esters to elevate testosterone levels above normal for several months did promote virilization but simultaneously raised plasma dihydrotestosterone levels to normal. Consequently, it was not possible to deduce whether the virilization at puberty is mediated by testosterone or dihydrotestosterone. Testosterone can enhance transcription of some androgen-responsive reporter genes,[35] but the fact that dihydrotestosterone is formed in men with 5α-reductase 2 deficiency and the fact that it binds more tightly to the androgen receptor[32] suggest that dihydrotestosterone itself is the principal mediator of virilization at puberty, even in subjects with steroid 5α-reductase 2 deficiency.

Women in the Dominican Republic family who have homozygous mutations of the 5α-reductase 2 gene are endocrinologically normal,[120] and two affected women who are endocrinologically normal (one homozygote and one compound heterozygote) were identified in another study.[121] In those affected women in whom it was measured, plasma levels of 5α-reduced progesterone (5α-dihydroprogesterone) were normal during the luteal phase despite the 5α-reductase 2 deficiency.[121] Since 5α-dihydroprogesterone is a major metabolite in the blood of women during the luteal phase[122] and during pregnancy,[123] the fact that the levels are normal in these women implies that this metabolite is formed by 5α-reductase 1. The physiologic role of 5α-reductase in women is still to be defined. It is of interest in this regard that steroid 5α-reductase 1 activity is necessary for normal gestation and delivery in the female mouse.[124,125]

Molecular Genetics. Cloning of the 5α-reductase 2 cDNA made it possible to analyze the mutations in the disorder. Forty-five different mutations have been described to date, including 35 different missense mutations, 3 premature stop codons, 3 small deletions, 1 insertion of a nucleotide, and 1 change from a stop codon to a missense codon[12,117,118,120,121,126–141] (Fig. 160-7). In the New Guinea cluster, the entire coding sequence is deleted.[12] Approximately two-thirds of patients have homozygous mutations (see Table 160-4), and one-fourth are compound heterozygotes. Mutations of only one allele have been found in some individuals, and no mutations were detected in one family with convincing endocrinologic evidence of 5α-reductase deficiency.[119] We believe that the latter two groups are compound heterozygotes and homozygotes, respectively, for mutations that map outside the coding exons and the immediate flanking intron sequences.

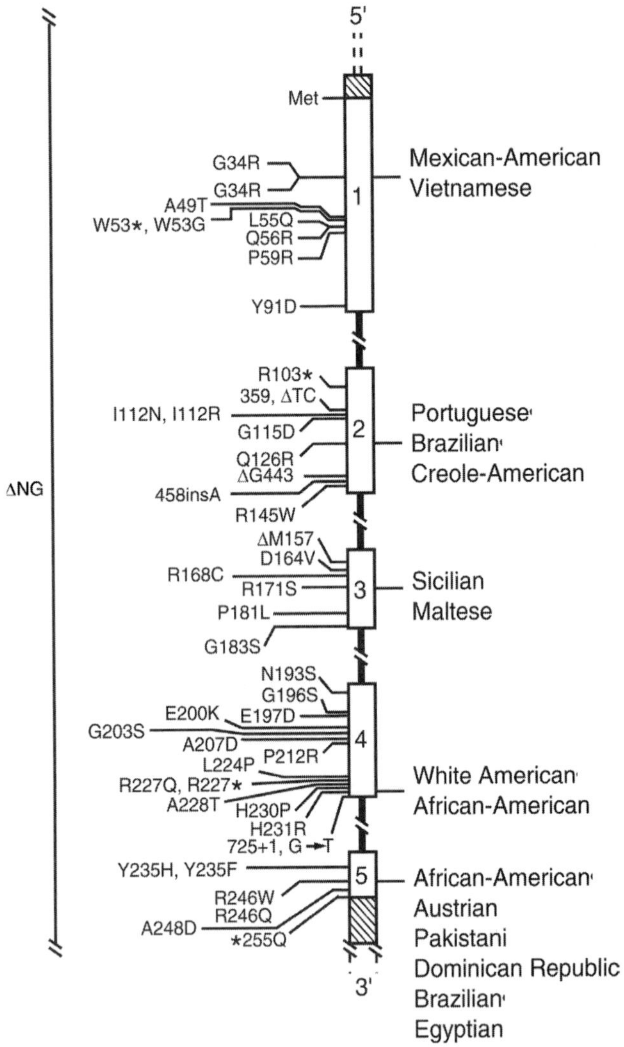

Fig. 160-7 Mutations in the steroid 5α-reductase 2 gene and protein. A schematic diagram of the 5α-reductase 2 gene is shown in the middle. On the left are the locations of 45 different mutations, and the sites of several recurring mutations are shown on the right. (NG represents the deletion of the gene in the New Guinea cohort. The initiating methionine is designated *Met* in exon 1, and the normal termination codon is designated with an asterisk in exon 5.) The various mutations have been reported as follows: G34R,G → A,[117,126,127] G34R,G → C,[117,126] L55Q[117,126,128,129] Q56R,[117,126] P59R,[126] Y91D,[126] R103*,[126], 359ΔTC,[117] I112N,[128,130] G115D,[117,126,127,131] Q126R,[117,126,128,130,132,133] R145W,[126] M157Δ,[128,130134,136] D164V,[117,126,132] R168C,[132] R171S,[117,126] P181L,[126] G183S,[117,120,126,131,132] N193S,[117,126,133] G196S,[117,126,128,130,135] E197D,[117,126] E200K,[137] G203S,[127] A207D,[117,126,127] L224P,[117,126] R227Q,[128,130,135] R227*,[117,132,138] A228T,[128,130,135] H230P,[126] H231R,[117,126,128,130,133,139] 725 + 1,G → T,[117,120] Y235F,[126,] R246W,[117,120,121,126,131,132,140] R246Q,[117,121,126] *255Q,[132,141] ΔNG.[12] Several of these mutations are being reported for the first time: A49T, W53*, W53G, I112R, ΔG443, 458insA, Y235H, A248D (*D Davis, DW Russell, unpublished observations.*)

The mutations are distributed throughout the coding sequence. No affected individual had more than two of the mutations shown in Fig. 160-7, and none of these mutations has been detected in the normal individuals screened to date. Most missense mutations cause abnormalities of NADPH binding or impair binding of testosterone to the enzyme. Other mutations cause a premature termination codon, gene deletions (both complete and partial), or splice-junction abnormalities. The cDNAs for several of the missense mutations have been expressed in cultured cells, and the residual enzyme activities have been characterized in detail.[126]

Identical mutations have been discovered in different ethnic groups (see Fig. 160-7). In some instances, this recurrence is probably due to a founder effect. For example, the same missense mutation (*R171S*) has been described in both Sicily and Malta, and it is likely that a heterozygous carrier from one of these islands was responsible for the spread of the *R171S* mutation. In other instances, for example, the appearance of the *R246W* mutation in Egypt, Brazil, and the Dominican Republic may be due to recurring mutations. Formal genetic testing to establish which mutations are recurrent and which are ancient has not been performed.

Three large clusters of patients with 5α-reductase deficiency have been described in different parts of the world — the Dominican Republic family involving some 38 members,[68,69] the Turkish cluster of 12 subjects,[95,141] and 13 affected members of the Sambia tribe in the New Guinea highlands.[108–111] The high incidence of the disorder in these groups is probably due to a founder effect in geographic isolates of people with a high coefficient of inbreeding. It is of interest in this regard that the Turkish kindred also has a high incidence of another rare autosomal recessive trait, 17β-hydroxysteroid dehydrogenase 3 deficiency.[141]

Diagnosis. The diagnosis of 5α-reductase deficiency is usually made either at the time of expected puberty or in infancy. In the adolescent or young adult, diagnosis is usually straightforward — a 46,XY male pseudohermaphrodite with the characteristic phenotype, male plasma testosterone levels, and abnormal ratios of plasma testosterone to dihydrotestosterone or abnormal ratios of urinary 5β- to 5α-steroid metabolites (see Table 160-4). Because the phenotypes can overlap, it is necessary to distinguish 5α-reductase deficiency from defects in testosterone biosynthesis on the one hand and partial defects of the androgen receptor on the other. In all three types of disorders, virilization of the Wolffian ducts can be more complete than that of the external genitalia. Defects in testosterone biosynthesis usually cause low plasma testosterone levels, but in men with partial enzyme defects, testosterone can be normal at the expense of high LH values and increased levels of precursor steroids. The most common hereditary defect in testosterone biosynthesis, 17β-hydroxysteroid dehydrogenase 3 deficiency, can be recognized on the basis of elevated androstenedione levels,[142] and it is our practice to measure androstenedione routinely in suspected cases of 5α-reductase deficiency. Separation of the disorder from the Reifenstein syndrome also can be perplexing, since defects of the androgen receptor can impair the development of tissues that are major sites of dihydrotestosterone biosynthesis and hence cause *secondary* 5α-reductase deficiency and high ratios of plasma testosterone to dihydrotestosterone.[143,144] In this situation, detailed family histories indicating the pattern of inheritance, careful phenotypic characterization to determine whether gynecomastia is present, and measurements of the ratios of urinary 5β- to 5α-glucocorticoid metabolites (which mainly reflect hepatic metabolism) usually establish the true diagnosis.

Recognition of 5α-reductase deficiency in infants and prepubertal children presents special problems, particularly when the family history is uninformative. In this situation, determination of the ratios of plasma testosterone to dihydrotestosterone before and after administration of hCG generally serves to establish the diagnosis.[132,135,145] When the testes have been removed, the diagnosis can be established either by determining the ratio of urinary 5β- to 5α-glucocorticoid metabolites[114,145] or by determining the ratio of plasma testosterone to dihydrotestosterone after the administration of testosterone esters by injection.[85]

Management. For individuals raised as males or who elect to function as males, several procedures are appropriate. First, urologic consultation should be obtained regarding appropriate corrective surgery to repair chordee, correct hypospadias, and bring cryptorchid testes as low as possible into the labioscrotal

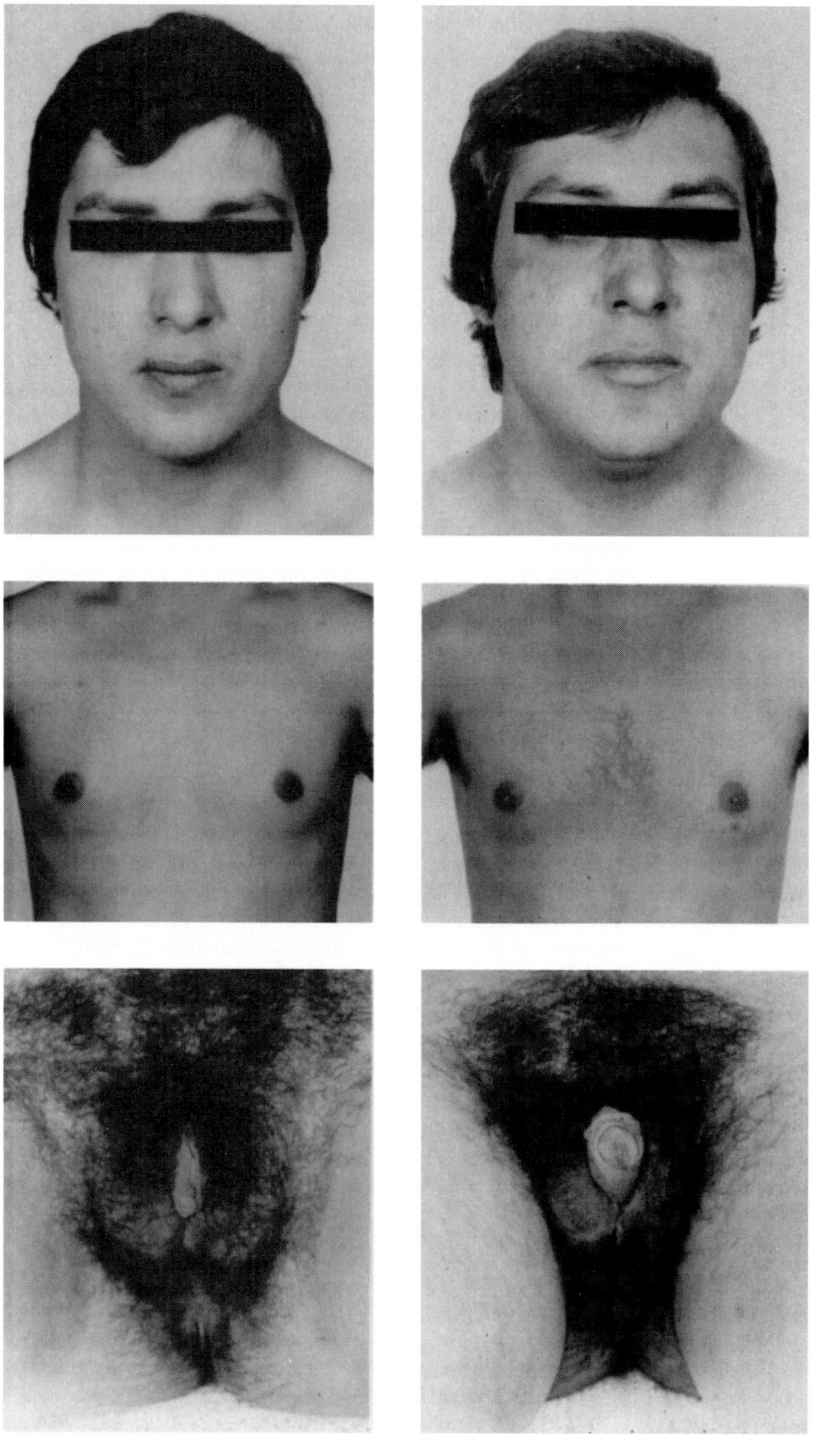

Fig. 160-8 Patient with 5α-reductase 2 deficiency before and after high-dose androgen therapy. *Left.* Before treatment (June 1976). *Right.* After treatment with a mixture of testosterone esters 500 mg intramuscularly weekly (March 1980). Correction of chordee was performed between these dates. (*From Price et al.*[83] *Used by permission.*)

folds. Second, since the degree of virilization is generally unsatisfactory, supplemental androgen therapy may be indicated. The ideal agent would be one that replaces the missing dihydrotestosterone; in experimental studies, the administration of dihydrotestosterone enanthate by injection at 4- to 6-week intervals results in a sustained elevation of plasma dihydrotestosterone levels,[146] but at present the agent is not available for general use. A second approach is to administer testosterone esters in quantities sufficient to elevate the plasma testosterone to supraphysiologic levels; in patients with 5α-reductase deficiency, such regimens bring dihydrotestosterone levels to the normal male range and promote virilization[83] (Fig. 160-8); it is not known whether such high doses of testosterone are safe over the long term. A third approach is to administer an androgen that does not require 5α-reduction to be active. For example, 19-nortestosterone can be given by injection in an esterified form such as nandrolone decanoate.[147] A fourth approach is the administration of a dihydrotestosterone cream by inunction; this regimen raises plasma dihydrotestosterone levels and can cause considerable phallic growth in infants.[80] Although administration of dihydrotestosterone cream appears to be safe over the short term, the long-term efficacy and safety have not been established.[148] While these regimens do promote virilization, most men in whom androgen therapy is instituted in adulthood do not have growth of the phallus into the normal range; whether earlier diagnosis and treatment will result in more successful virilization is not clear at present.[132]

Table 160-5 Clinical Features of Complete Testicular Feminization

External phenotype: Female external genitalia with underdevelopment of the labia and a blind-ending vagina, female habitus and breast development, paucity of axillary and pubic hair
Urogenital tract: Testes that may be intraabdominal, along the course of the inguinal canal, or in the labia; absent Wolffian and Müllerian derivatives
Karyotype: 46,XY
Inhertance: X-linked recessive
Endocrinology:
- Testosterone: Normal or high male plasma levels and production rates
- Estrogen: Plasma levels and production rates higher than in normal men
- Gonadotropin: Elevated plasma LH levels

Pathogenesis: Complete resistance to all actions of testosterone and dihydrotestosterone

In subjects who elect to live as women, the management is similar to that in women with testicular feminization and allied syndromes (see below) but should be undertaken only after rigorous psychiatric and psychological evaluation to establish beyond reasonable doubt the presence of a female gender identity. In such women, the testes should be removed to preclude (or stop) virilization, estrogen-progestogen therapy should be instituted at an appropriate age to feminize, and when appropriate, vaginoplasty should be undertaken either by surgical or medical means.[61]

Disorders of the Androgen Receptor

Disorders of the androgen receptor can cause several distinct phenotypes. Despite differences in the clinical manifestations, these disorders are similar with regard to endocrinology, genetics, and basic pathophysiology.

Clinical Features of Complete Testicular Feminization (Complete Androgen Insensitivity Syndrome). The clinical features of complete testicular feminization are summarized in Table 160-5. The syndrome has been recognized for many years (the early literature has been reviewed by Hauser[149]). The initial insight into the pathogenesis was provided by two pioneering studies. First, in 1937, Pettersson and Bonnier deduced from family studies that affected individuals are genetic males, that the pattern of inheritance is consistent with X-linked transmission, and that the syndrome could best be explained by a failure of male development in an embryo in which the fundamental trend is toward the female phenotype.[150] Second, soon after Morris introduced the term *testicular feminization* to describe the disorder,[2] Wilkins deduced that the pathogenesis is due to resistance to the action of androgen.[3]

The clinical manifestations have been reviewed.[149,151] The typical subject is seen by a physician either because of primary amenorrhea (postpubertally) or an inguinal hernia (prepubertally). In a 2-year survey in the United Kingdom, 76 percent of cases in infants were ascertained on the basis of unilateral or bilateral inguinal hernias, and one or two gonads could be palpated in most of these babies.[152] On occasion, the diagnosis is not established until late in life.[153] Breast development is that of a normal woman, and the general body habitus and distribution of body fat are female in character (Fig. 160-9*A*). Axillary and pubic hair is absent or scanty, but some vulvar hair (albeit diminished in amount) is usually present. Facial and scalp hair is that of normal women. The external genitalia are unambiguously female (Fig. 160-10*A*). The labia and clitoris are normal or somewhat underdeveloped. Although usually adequate for successful coitus, the vagina may be absent or shallow. The vagina, if present, is blind-ending, and the internal genitalia are absent except for gonads that have the histologic features of undescended testes (i.e., normal or increased Leydig cells and seminiferous tubules without spermatogenesis). The testes may be located in the abdomen, along the course of the inguinal canal, or in the labia majora. Remnants of Müllerian or Wolffian duct origin can be identified in the paratesticular fascia or

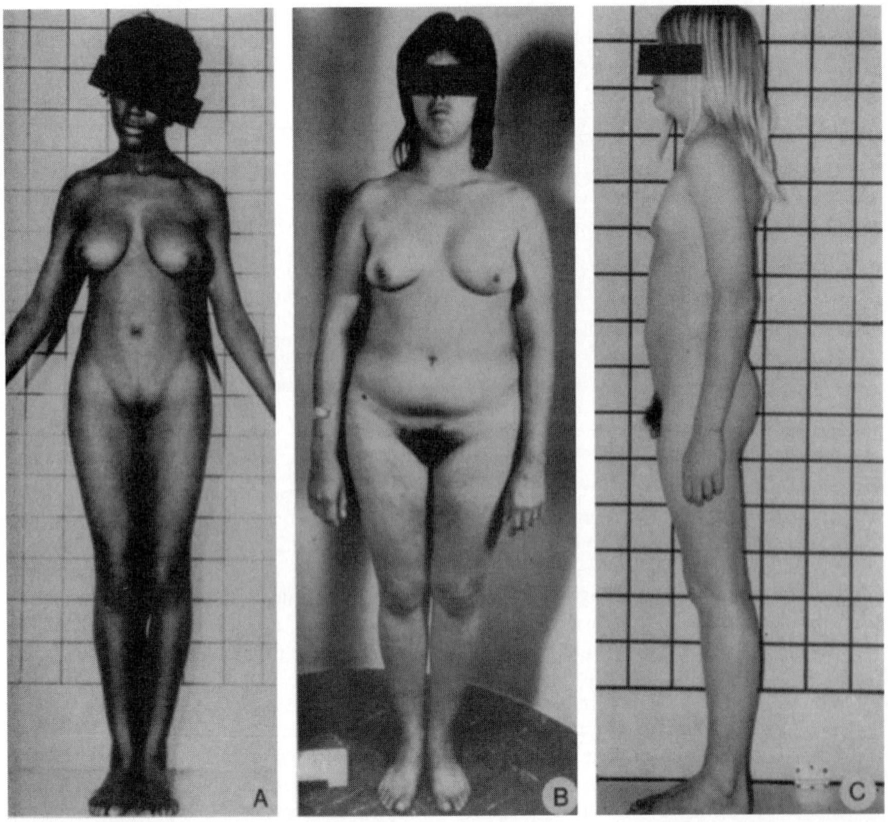

Fig. 160-9 ***A.*** **Complete testicular feminization.** ***B.*** **Incomplete testicular feminization.** ***C.*** **Reifenstein syndrome. *(From Griffin and Wilson.[61] Used by permission.)***

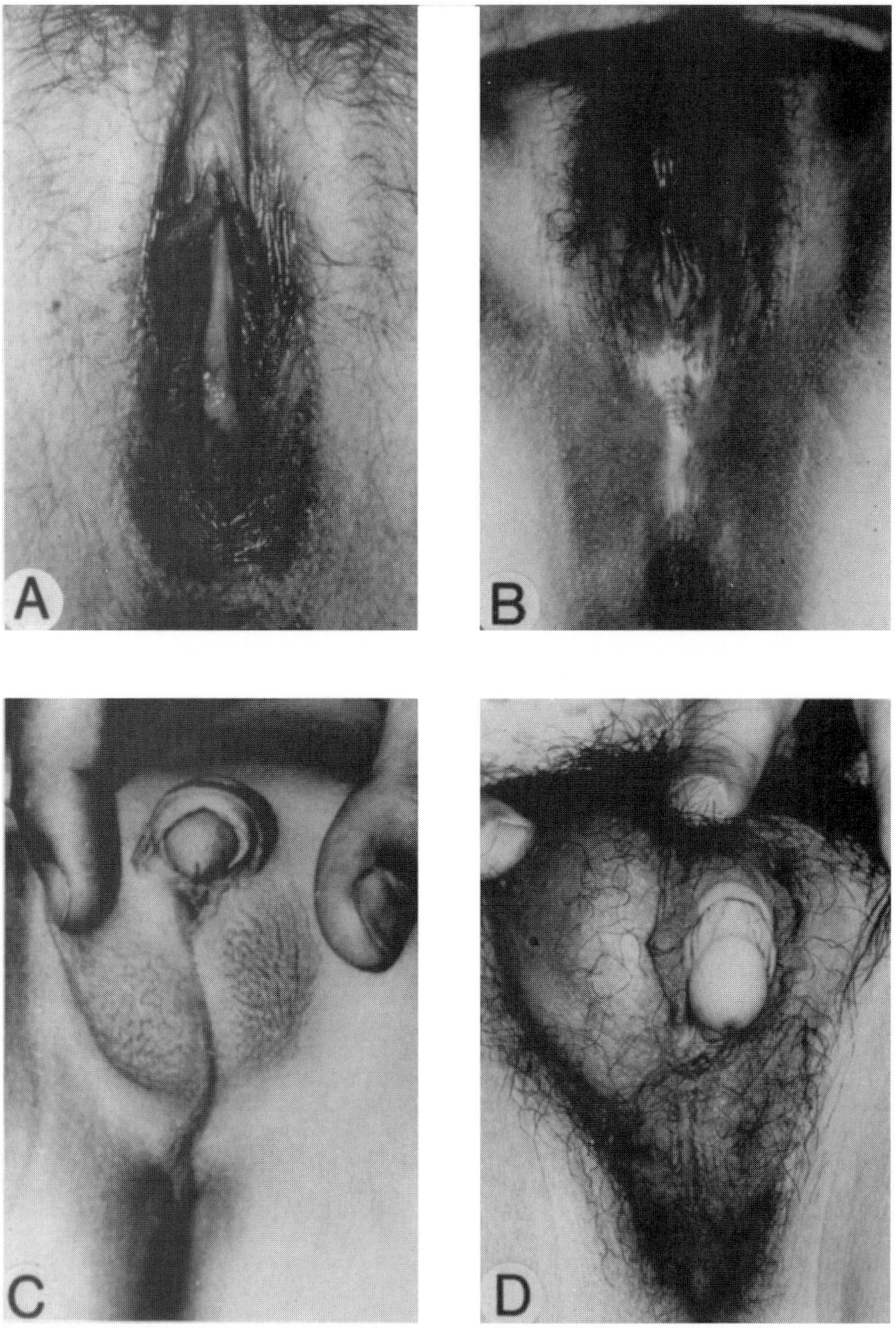

Fig. 160-10 External genitalia of four subjects with disorders of androgen receptor function. *A.* Complete testicular feminization. *B.* Incomplete testicular feminization. *C.* Reifenstein syndrome (prepubertal). *D.* Reifenstein syndrome (adult). (*From Griffin and Wilson.*[61] *Used by permission.*)

in fibrous bands extending from the testes,[149,154,155] and rarely, uterine remnants are present.[156–159] It is of interest in this regard that levels of anti-Müllerian hormone are elevated in affected children.[160]

Documentation that nuclear chromatin is male in character[161,162] and that the chromosomal complement is 46,XY[163–165] confirmed the deductions from pedigree analysis and gonadal histology that affected individuals are genetic males. Affected subjects tend to be rather tall for women, averaging 171.5 cm in height in one series[166]; bone age corresponds to chronologic age[149]; body size is larger than average[166]; tooth size is as large as in normal men (and larger than in normal women)[167]; and the cranial dimensions and dental arch dimensions and occlusion are larger than in normal women.[168,169] The fact that these parameters are larger than in normal women indicates that the Y chromosome may have direct effects on the teeth and skeleton that are not mediated by androgens. A possible role of estrogens has been postulated to explain the acceleration of linear growth.[170] Adrenal and thyroid function are normal, and there are no commonly associated somatic anomalies.[149] Intelligence is normal,[171] and psychological development is feminine in regard to behavior, outlook, and maternal instincts.[172]

Estimates of incidence vary from 1 in 20,000 to 1 in 64,000 male births.[149,173] On the basis of studies of buccal smears, as many as 1 to 2 percent of girls with inguinal hernias may have the disorder.[173,174] In a survey in Japan, testicular feminization was the most common form of primary resistance to hormone action, with some 390 patients having been ascertained in a 10-year period.[175] In one series this disorder was the third most frequent cause of primary amenorrhea in women after gonadal dysgenesis and congenital absence of the vagina.[176]

Except for psychological problems related to the infertility and the complications of cryptorchid testes, these women are usually healthy and have normal life spans. However, in one study a decrease in trabecular bone density was observed in eight women with testicular feminization,[177] and in another study five adult women had decreased density of the lumbar spine.[178] Most of the women in these studies had been castrated so that the extent to which these changes are due to estrogen deprivation and/or inadequate estrogen replacement is not clear, but one 17-year-old subject with intact testes had decreased bone density.[179]

These women have a profound resistance to the action of both exogenous and endogenous androgens. Wilkins[3] gave methyltestosterone in large doses to women with testicular feminization after castration and showed that there was no growth of pubic or axillary hair (despite documentation of pubic hair follicles by biopsy), no enlargement of the clitoris, no change in the voice, and no other detectable virilizing effect. Subsequent work confirmed the lack of response of pubic hair to androgen treatment[180,181] and also demonstrated resistance to androgen in regard to sebum production,[181] failure of the expected decrease in thyroxine-binding globulin levels in plasma,[182,183] diminished feedback on LH secretion by the pituitary,[184] and lack of effect on phosphorus and nitrogen balance.[185–187] Thus resistance to the action of androgen appears to be virtually absolute in complete testicular feminization.

The histologic features of the testes are similar to those of testes in other forms of cryptorchidism but differ in that spermatogenesis is consistently absent (whereas spermatogenesis is present in half of age-matched cryptorchid testes due to other causes), germinal elements are detected rarely, and Sertoli cell adenomas are frequent.[188–190] Although the number of Leydig cells per high-power field is increased,[189] the total volume and number of Leydig cells are probably normal.[191] Malignant tumors are usually germ cell tumors, particularly seminomas,[192] but malignant sex cord stromal tumors also occur.[193] It is probable that the incidence of tumors is no greater than in other cryptorchid testes.[189]

Clinical Features of Incomplete Testicular Feminization. The term *incomplete testicular feminization* was introduced to characterize a phenotype similar to that of complete testicular feminization but associated with partial virilization of the external genitalia and mixed virilization and feminization at expected puberty.[194] The term was used subsequently to characterize several types of incomplete male pseudohermaphroditism, including defects of testosterone synthesis, the Reifenstein syndrome, and some subjects for whom data are insufficient to determine the diagnosis. Nevertheless, certain of these subjects with abnormalities of the androgen receptor constitute a distinct phenotype[195–198] (Table 160-6).

Affected individuals have the habitus and general appearance of women and, as in the complete form of the disorder, usually present because of primary amenorrhea (see Fig. 160-9*B*). The karyotype is 46,XY; the testes are in the abdomen or in the inguinal canals and are histologically indistinguishable from those in complete testicular feminization. The external genitalia are distinctive in that the labioscrotal folds are partially fused, and clitoromegaly may be present (see Fig. 160-10*B*). The vagina is short and ends blindly.

Table 160-6 Clinical Features of Incomplete Testicular Feminization

External phenotype: Clitoromegaly and/or partial fusion of the labioscrotal folds, female habitus and breast development, normal axillary and pubic hair

Urogenital tract: Testes that may or may not be cryptorchid, Wolffian duct derivatives emptying into the vagina, no Müllerian duct derivatives

Karyotype: 46,XY

Inheritance: X-linked recessive

Endocrinology:

- Testosterone: Normal or high male plasma levels and production rates
- Estrogen: Plasma levels and production rates higher than in normal men
- Gonadotropin: Elevated plasma LH level

Pathogenesis: Partial resistance to the action of testosterone and dihydrotestosterone

At the expected time of puberty, variable degrees of feminization and virilization may occur. Müllerian duct derivatives are usually absent, but Wolffian duct structures are present; this latter feature, together with the partial virilization of the external genitalia, separates the phenotype from that of testicular feminization. Not only are upper Wolffian duct structures present (epididymides and vasa deferentia), but in addition, terminal Wolffian duct derivatives, including the ampullae of the vasa deferentia, the seminal vesicles, and the ejaculatory ducts, are male in character (although underdeveloped in comparison with normal men). The ejaculatory ducts empty into the vagina. Thus certain features resemble testicular feminization (female breast development), some resemble 5α-reductase deficiency (presence of male Wolffian duct derivatives and ambiguous external genitalia), and some resemble the Reifenstein syndrome (mixed virilization and feminization at expected puberty). The frequency of this disorder is uncertain, but in most series (including our experience) it is about one-tenth as common as complete testicular feminization.

Clinical Features of the Reifenstein Syndrome (Partial Androgen Insensitivity Syndrome). In some families, male pseudohermaphroditism that is typically less severe than in incomplete testicular feminization is inherited as an X-linked recessive trait. Although the usual phenotype is male, affected men within a given family may have a spectrum of abnormalities ranging from almost complete failure of virilization to nearly complete masculinization. The disorder has been described under a variety of terms, including *Reifenstein syndrome*,[199–200] *Lubs syndrome*,[201] *Gilbert-Dreyfus syndrome*,[202] *Rosewater syndrome*,[203] and *familial incomplete male pseudohermaphroditism type 1*,[204] but the common appellation is *Reifenstein syndrome*. The fact that these disorders are variable manifestations of similar mutations was deduced from pedigree analyses. The most extensive family reported is the one studied by Ford[205] and by Walker et al.[206] In this family, the manifestations in 12 affected men ranged from moderate abnormalities (microphallus and gynecomastia) to intermediate defects of virilization (hypospadias) to such severe defects of virilization (complete failure of scrotal fusion) that three affected family members were identified initially as females.[206] In another family reported originally by Bowen et al.[200] and subsequently by Wilson et al.,[204] the phenotype also ranged from a moderate defect in virilization in two (microphallus and bifid scrotum) to a more severe abnormality in eight (perineoscrotal hypospadias) to almost complete male pseudohermaphroditism in one (perineoscrotal hypospadias, no vas deferens, and a vaginal orifice). The phenotypic variability in this family is illustrated in Fig. 160-11. In a third family, described by Gardo and Papp,[207] three of four affected individuals were phenotypic females, whereas the fourth had perineoscrotal hypospadias, bifid scrotum, and gynecomastia typical of the Reifenstein syndrome. Variability in phenotypic expression also has been noted in other families with the disorder.[208,209]

The features are summarized in Table 160-7. The most common presentation is a 46,XY male with perineoscrotal hypospadias, azoospermia with infertility, incomplete virilization, and gynecomastia that develops at expected puberty (see Fig. 160-9*C*). The external genitalia of an affected child and an affected adult are shown in Fig. 160-10*C* and *D*, respectively. Axillary and pubic hair is normal, but chest and facial hair is absent or sparse. Temporal recession of the hairline is minimal, and the voice tends to be somewhat high-pitched. Less severely affected men may exhibit only a bifid scrotum, infertility, and incomplete virilization at puberty. More severely affected individuals can have incomplete

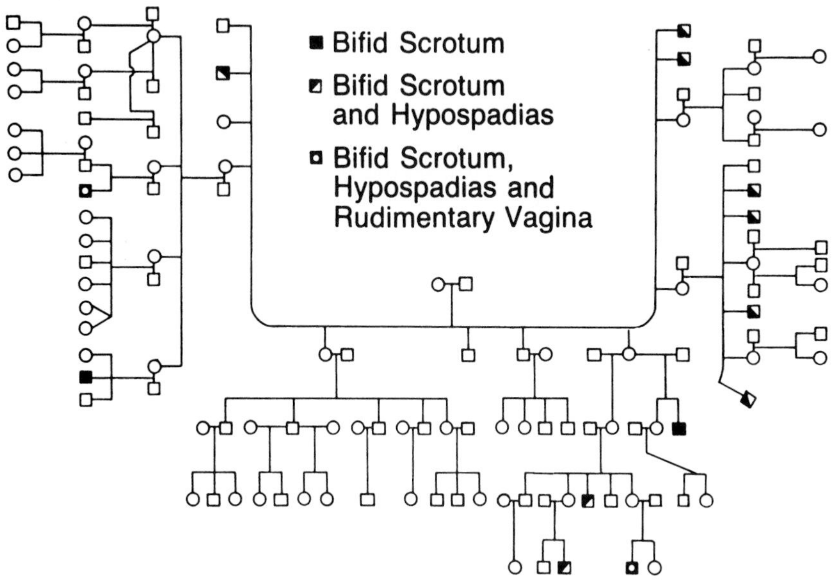

Fig. 160-11 Pedigree of a family with Reifenstein syndrome. (*From Grino et al.*[263] *Used by permission.*)

Wolffian duct structures and formation of a vagina; only by identification of less severely affected members within the same family can severely affected subjects be distinguished from those with incomplete testicular feminization. Partial virilization of the urogenital sinus results in a prostatic utricle but no true prostate. The lower ejaculatory duct system has not been characterized in detail.

Cryptorchidism is common, and the testes on average are small (although usually larger than in Klinefelter syndrome). Leydig cells are usually normal by histologic examination, but Leydig cell neoplasia has been described.[210] Spermatogenic tubules contain both Sertoli cells and germinal epithelium, but the germ cells do not mature beyond the primary spermatocyte stage. Hyaline degeneration of the tubules is often present.[200]

Most affected individuals are raised as men. Although the number of reported subjects is small and no in-depth psychological studies have been performed, gender identity/behavior in affected subjects raised as men seems to be unambiguously male, and some have had successful marriages. Presumably because of incomplete development of the prostate and ejaculatory system, however, ejaculate volume is characteristically small. Infertility is a consistent feature and appears to be the result of defective spermatogenesis and possibly of the anatomic abnormalities of the ejaculatory system.

Clinical Features of Men with Infertility or Undervirilization due to Androgen Resistance. In a study of a family with the Reifenstein syndrome, some affected men were identified who were infertile but otherwise phenotypically normal. They had the same apparent degree of androgen resistance, as assessed by endocrinologic criteria,[204] and the same abnormality of the androgen receptor in cultured skin fibroblasts as the more severely affected relatives.[211] Gynecomastia was variable and late in appearance. Thus the Reifenstein syndrome can encompass both mild and severe phenotypic evidence of androgen receptor deficiency. Subsequently, it was recognized that some men with infertility or undervirilization but without a family history of the Reifenstein syndrome have endocrine evidence of androgen resistance and androgen receptor abnormalities similar to those in individuals with familial Reifenstein syndrome.[212–221] The clinical features are summarized in Table 160-8. Such men have normal male external genitalia, apparently normal Wolffian duct structures, and variable sperm production. Some have a small phallus, minimal beard and body hair, and gynecomastia. The prevalence of this form of androgen resistance as a cause of male infertility in normally virilized men is not established, but in some series it accounts for a significant fraction of male infertility associated with idiopathic azoospermia or severe oligospermia.[222,223] Some affected men are fertile.[218]

Table 160-7 Clinical Features of the Reifenstein Syndrome

External phenotype: Usually a male with perineoscrotal hypospadias, normal axillary and pubic hair, but scant beard and body hair; breast enlargement at time of expected puberty
Urogenital tract: Testes often cryptorchid, Wolffian duct structures vary in the degree of the male development, no Müllerian duct derivatives
Karyotype: 46,XY
Inheritance: X-linked recessive
Endocrinology:
- Testosterone: Normal or high male plasma levels and production rates
- Estrogen: Plasma levels and production rates higher than those in normal men
- Gonadotropin: Elevated plasma LH levels

Pathogenesis: Variable resistance to the action of testosterone and dihydrotestosterone

Table 160-8 Clinical Features of Men with Infertility or Undervirilization Due to Androgen Resistance

External phenotype: Normal man, variable small phallus, beard and body hair, and gynecomastia
Urogenital tract: Testes, fertility with variable sperm density or infertility associated with azoospermia or extreme oligospermia, Wolffian duct structures of normal men, no Müllerian duct derivatives
Karyotype: 46,XY
Inheritance: X-linked recessive
Endrocrinology:
- Testosterone: Plasma levels and production rates of normal men or slightly higher
- Estrogen: Production rates usually higher than in normal men
- Gonadotropin: Plasma LH levels normal or elevated

Pathogenesis: Resistance to the action of androgen varies in different tissues

Endocrinology. The endocrine features are similar in all forms of androgen receptor disorders but have been characterized best in subjects with complete testicular feminization. The early deductions by Morris[2] and Wilkins[3] that androgen production is normal in patients with testicular feminization have been confirmed and extended. Plasma levels of testosterone are either in the normal male range or somewhat higher than those of normal men,[7,224–228] a phenomenon that is probably due to two factors: (1) the subjects have elevated estrogen production rates (see below) that result in an increase in the level of testosterone-binding globulin in plasma, and (2) production rates of testosterone tend to be somewhat higher than in normal men.[7] As in normal men, testosterone is produced in the testes.[24,225,229] In one study, testosterone production in women with testicular feminization averaged about 50 percent higher than in normal men (8.3 versus 5.7 mg/day) but was only higher in women with inguinal testes and not in those with intraabdominal testes[7] (see Fig. 160-2*C*).

The elevated testosterone production rate is presumably secondary to high levels of LH in plasma, which in turn are the consequence of defective feedback regulation because of resistance at the hypothalamic-pituitary level to the feedback effects of androgen on LH production.[184,227,228,230] In addition, elevated estradiol levels in the disorder may cause positive feedback on LH production.[231] The elevated plasma LH levels are due both to more frequent and greater amplitude of LH secretory pulses than in normal men.[228] Further increase in plasma LH levels after the administration of luteinizing hormone-releasing hormone (LHRH) is within the normal range.[228] Plasma levels of FSH are usually normal.[228] Although the negative-feedback regulation of LH secretion by androgens is defective in testicular feminization, LH secretion in these patients is influenced by estradiol—the administration of the antiestrogen clomiphene citrate causes a further increase in plasma LH, and plasma LH also rises further after castration.

The origin of estrogen in four women with testicular feminization is illustrated in Fig. 160-2*C*[7]; the mean production rates of estrone and estradiol, respectively, were 114 and 77 μg/day (versus 66 and 45 μg/day, respectively, in normal men). Testicular estradiol secretion in these women averaged 42 μg/day (versus 6 μg/day in normal men). Thus most of the increased estradiol production is due to secretion by the testes. This finding is in keeping with the reports by Kelch et al.[24] and by Laatikainen et al.[229] that levels of estradiol in spermatic vein blood are high in women with testicular feminization.

To summarize, resistance to the feedback regulation of LH production by circulating androgen results in elevated plasma LH levels, and this in turn results in the enhanced secretion of both testosterone and estradiol by the testes. The fact that hCG levels rise even higher (and that symptoms of menopausal flushing develop) when the testes are removed is consistent with the view that gonadotropin secretion is under some type of regulatory control; presumably, in the steady state and in the absence of an effect of androgen, estrogen regulates LH secretion in subjects with testicular feminization. This feedback control is accomplished at the expense of a higher plasma estrogen level than in normal men.[184,232]

Endocrine findings in individuals with less severe forms of androgen resistance are similar to those in women with complete testicular feminization. In women with incomplete testicular feminization, plasma levels of testosterone are similar to those of normal men,[233,234] and in one such subject the daily production rate of testosterone was greater (12.0 mg/day)[198] than the average in normal men.[7] Plasma LH levels[198,233,234] and estrogen production rates and estrogen secretion by the testes[198] are also elevated. Interestingly, administration of a large amount of estradiol benzoate to a subject with incomplete testicular feminization (to simulate the preovulatory surge of estradiol in normally cycling women) resulted in an LH surge similar to that of normal women.[235] Urinary gonadotropin excretion is elevated in men with the Reifenstein syndrome,[206] and plasma LH and testosterone levels are high on average,[204] indicating defective feedback control of LH secretion at the hypothalamic-pituitary level. When LHRH is administered to subjects with Reifenstein syndrome, the surge in plasma LH is either normal or high.[228,236,237] Furthermore, plasma LH does not decrease after the administration of medroxyprogesterone acetate,[204] testosterone,[238] or dihydrotestosterone.[228] As in complete testicular feminization, steady-state control of LH secretion is regulated by estradiol.[237] The production rates for plasma testosterone (9.2 mg/day) and for estradiol (199 μg/day) are high; three-fourths of the estradiol (147 (g/day, 10 times the normal amount) is secreted directly into the circulation, presumably from the testes[204] (see Fig. 160-2*D*).

The endocrine changes in infertile or undervirilized men with androgen resistance are similar to but less marked than those in men with other types of androgen receptor defects. Specifically, plasma production rates of testosterone and plasma levels of LH are normal to high, and estradiol production rates are normal or slightly elevated.[212,218,220]

The mechanism by which feminization occurs in individuals with receptor defects is clear. In each disorder, androgen resistance can cause a high mean level of plasma LH, elevated estradiol secretion by the testes, and feminizing signs at puberty. However, there is no direct relation between the absolute amount of estrogen secretion and the degree of feminization. Indeed, two phenotypic men with Reifenstein syndrome had higher estrogen secretion rates[166] than any found to date in either complete or incomplete testicular feminization. We conclude that feminization in subjects with androgen resistance requires increased estradiol production but that the degree of feminization is influenced by the severity of the androgen resistance. It follows that the failure to feminize in some infertile men with androgen resistance is due both to less severe resistance to the action of androgen and to an inconsistent increase in estradiol formation.

Dihydrotestosterone formation is low on average in skin slices from patients with complete testicular feminization,[71,195,239] and in some testicular feminization patients the excretion of dihydrotestosterone metabolites in urine is also decreased.[240,241] This decrease in dihydrotestosterone formation is believed to be secondary to a decrease in the mass of the androgen target tissues that normally form dihydrotestosterone.[143] Dihydrotestosterone formation is normal in fibroblasts cultured from most biopsies of genital skin from such individuals.[51] Furthermore, in genital skin biopsies from subjects with incomplete testicular feminization[198] and the Reifenstein syndrome[204] and in fibroblasts cultured from the skin of such individuals, dihydrotestosterone formation is normal.[51,242] Thus, on endocrine, genetic, and phenotypic grounds, these individuals are distinct from subjects with 5α-reductase 2 deficiency.

Pathogenesis. The basic study that allowed the pathogenesis of these disorders to be unraveled was the observation by Keenan and coworkers that the androgen receptor is present in fibroblasts cultured from the skin of normal subjects.[243,244] Receptor content is greater in fibroblasts cultured from genital skin (foreskin, scrotum, labia majora) than from nongenital sites.[211] The receptor in normal fibroblasts has a dissociation constant of approximately 0.2 nM for dihydrotestosterone and is the same intracellular androgen receptor as in androgen target tissues. Keenan et al. showed that fibroblasts grown from some women with complete testicular feminization showed no detectable dihydrotestosterone binding,[244] a finding that was confirmed in other laboratories.[211,245] The finding of absent receptor binding in fibroblasts from some women with testicular feminization provided an explanation for the profound androgen resistance in this disorder.

Other subjects with complete testicular feminization have receptor binding that is demonstrable but qualitatively abnormal. Identification of such a phenomenon came first from studies of thermolability of binding in two sisters with complete testicular feminization,[246] and similar thermolability was reported in other

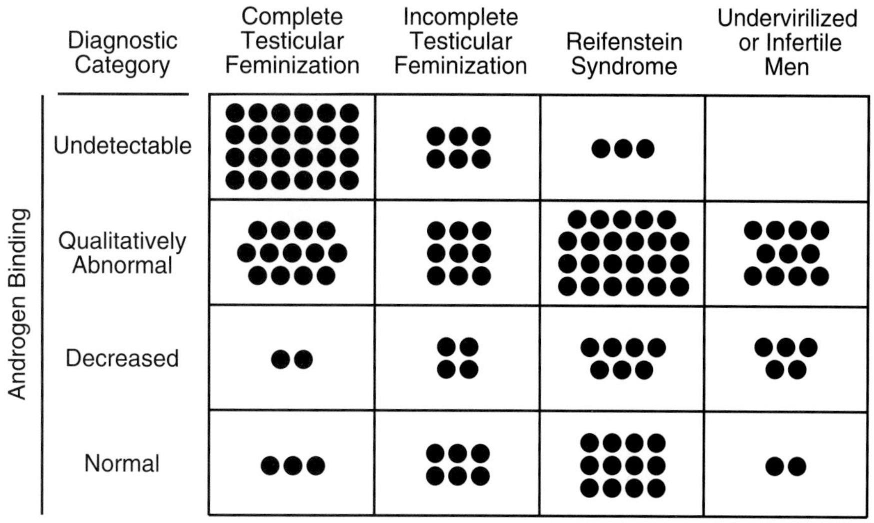

Fig. 160-12 Androgen binding in cultured genital skin fibroblasts from 130 families with androgen resistance of the receptor type. The type of androgen binding in clinical syndromes of androgen resistance is shown. Each dot represents a family in which one or more persons were found to have a particular type of androgen binding, as measured by saturation analysis of dihydrotestosterone binding in cultured genital skin fibroblasts. Androgen binding was considered undetectable if it measured less than 4 fmol/mg protein. Binding was considered qualitatively abnormal if the androgen receptor in cultured fibroblasts was thermolabile or unstable or if the dihydrotestosterone-androgen receptor complex in intact cells dissociated at an increased rate. Binding was considered to be decreased if the amount was less than normal but no qualitative abnormality could be detected. (*Adapted with permission from Griffin.*[4])

patients.[216,247,248] Qualitative abnormalities of the receptor were identified subsequently by a variety of tests of receptor function in individuals with androgen resistance, including failure of molybdate to stabilize the 8S androgen receptor complex,[216,249,250] decreased affinity of ligand binding to the receptor,[144,214,247,251–253] impairment of nuclear retention of the binding ligand,[254] failure of androgens to up-regulate the level of androgen receptor,[216,251,252,255–258] increased rate of dissociation of ligand from receptor,[216,220,247–252,259–262] and lability of the androgen receptor under transforming conditions.[34]

The characteristics of the androgen receptor binding in fibroblasts grown from biopsies of individuals from 130 families studied in our laboratory who fulfill the phenotypic and endocrine requirements to be designated androgen resistant are summarized in Fig. 160-12.[4] Receptor binding is designated qualitatively abnormal when it is measurable in intact cells and exhibits thermolability, instability in cytosol on sucrose gradients, or increased dissociation. In 33 families, binding was absent or nearly absent, most commonly in association with complete testicular feminization. Qualitatively abnormal receptor binding was the most common binding abnormality identified (56 families) and was present in each of the four clinical syndromes. A decreased amount of apparently normal receptor was present in subjects in 18 families, usually in individuals with a predominant male phenotype.[263] In 23 families with endocrine and phenotypic evidence of androgen resistance, androgen receptor binding was normal both in quality and quantity. Androgen resistance with normal androgen binding was originally called *receptor-positive resistance* or *postreceptor resistance*.[264–273] Some families reported in this category[264] were shown subsequently to have qualitatively abnormal receptor binding.[247] The most important deduction drawn from the functional studies of the receptors was the recognition that the mutated androgen receptors have different characteristics in almost every family.

In 1937, Pettersson and Bonnier concluded on the basis of pedigree analysis that testicular feminization could be due either to an X-linked recessive trait or to an autosomal trait that is manifested only in genetic males,[150] and it was deduced subsequently that the disorder is X-linked. Similar mutations have been described in dogs,[274] cows,[275] rats,[276] mice,[277,278] horses,[279] chimpanzees,[280] raccoon dogs,[281] and cats.[282] In mice, X-linkage of the mutant gene was established by mapping techniques.[277] Because all known instances in which genes are X-linked in one species are also X-linked in other species,[283] documentation of X-linkage for the gene in mice suggested that the mutation is on the X chromosome in other species as well. Meyer et al.[284] reported that skin fibroblasts cloned from an obligate heterozygote for complete testicular feminization consisted of two populations, some with deficient androgen binding and others with normal binding. This finding was consistent with random inactivation of one X-linked allele in each cell, as would be predicted by the Lyon hypothesis,[285] and indicated X-linkage for the gene that encodes the androgen receptor. X-linkage for this gene was confirmed by Migeon and coworkers with the use of mouse-human hybrid cells[286] and by similar studies in a family with a qualitatively abnormal androgen receptor.[287] Evidence for X-linkage of the syndrome of incomplete testicular feminization[246] and the Reifenstein syndrome[199,200,204–209] provided support for the concept that these disorders have a common pathogenesis. More important, using an informative restriction-fragment polymorphism, the mutant gene in one large family with Reifenstein syndrome was shown to be either tightly linked to or to involve the same gene responsible for testicular feminization.[288] Demonstration of qualitatively abnormal receptor binding in some Reifenstein families[254,289] and in some infertile and/or undervirilized men[216,220,222] also indicated that these disorders involve the same gene product as testicular feminization.

Molecular Genetics. The cloning of the cDNA for the human androgen receptor and confirmation of the X-linkage of the gene[13–16] made it possible to develop techniques to characterize mutations,[290–292] including Southern blot analyses to detect large deletions, exon amplification by the polymerase chain reaction followed by sequencing to detect point mutations, measurements of androgen receptor mRNA,[291,293] immunoblots of receptor protein,[294] assessment of functional capacity using reporter genes fused to androgen response elements,[295,296] estimation of receptor function in intact cells infected with an adenovirus containing an androgen-responsive reporter gene,[297] and single-strand DNA conformational polymorphism analysis.[298]

The mutations in this gene have been the subject of reviews,[299,300] and as of February 1999, more than 321 different

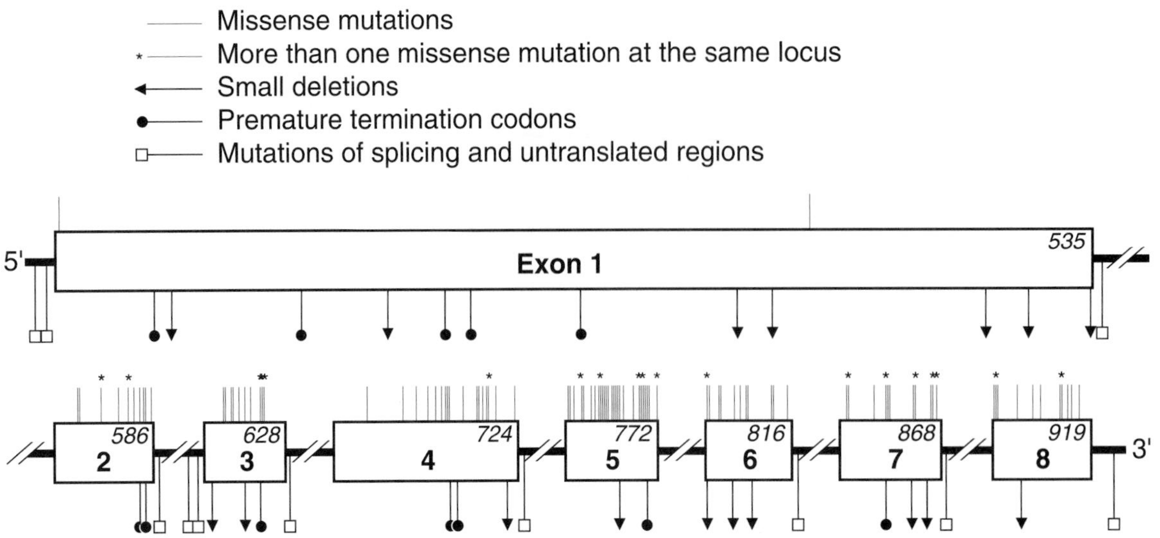

Fig. 160-13 Schematic representation of the mutations of the human androgen receptor that cause androgen resistance states as registered in the McGill University database. (*As of 1998. An update is available in Gottlieb et al.*[301] *and on the Internet at http://www.mcgill.ca/androgendb.*) The eight coding exons are numbered and are separated by seven introns. Missense mutations are indicated above the exons, and premature termination codons, small deletions, and splicing defects are shown below the exons. Large deletions and mutations that have only been reported in prostate cancer are not shown.

mutations of the androgen receptor had been reported to be associated with androgen resistance and recorded in the McGill University database, as reported by Gottlieb et al.[301] (available on the Internet at *http://www.mcgill.ca/androgendb/*) (Fig. 160-13 and Table 160-9). Mutations that have been described only in prostate cancer (and hence may not cause androgen resistance)[301] and the various expansions of the polyglutamine tract associated with the Kennedy syndrome (see Chap. 161) are not shown. It is noteworthy that most cDNAs sequenced to date are from patients with complete testicular feminization rather than from patients with less severe forms of androgen resistance, and consequently, the tentative mutation map shown in Fig. 160-13 may not be representative of all disease categories. Nevertheless, the mutations described to date are diverse and include partial or complete gene deletions, mutations that result in aberrant splicing of androgen receptor mRNA, mutations in the untranslated region of the gene, and nucleotide replacements that cause either the introduction of premature termination codons or amino acid substitutions.

Table 160-9 Mutations of the Androgen Receptor that Cause Androgen Resistance as Recorded in the Database.

28	Structural Defects	Different Mutants
	Complete gene deletions	3
	Partial gene deletions	9
	1–4-bp deletions	9
	Intron deletions	1
	Splice-junction deletion	1
	Insertions	4
	Bp duplications	1
245	**Single-Base Mutations**	**Different Mutants**
	Amino acid subsitutions	218
	Multiple amino acid subtitution	3
	Splice-junction abnormalities	6
	Premature termination codons	18
	TOTAL	271

SOURCE: Reformulated from McGill database in 1998. Later version in ref.[301]

The large deletions of the androgen receptor gene[301] are not shown in Fig. 160-13. Complete deletion of the gene has been described in three families[302–304]; in the two families in which the deletion extends the farthest, complete testicular feminization is associated with mental retardation.[303,304] This finding suggests that a gene that causes mental retardation is located near the androgen receptor gene. In several patients, other large deletions have been characterized.[301] In most instances, fibroblasts from these patients do not express androgen receptor that is detectable by assays of hormone binding, but a deletion of exon 3 described by Quigley et al.[305] led to the synthesis of a receptor protein that bound hormone but was unable to activate an androgen-responsive gene. Other small-scale deletions that remove single or multiple nucleotides can either cause a shift in the translational reading frame and premature termination of the receptor protein (as occurs in the *tfm* mouse.[306–308]) or, if multiples of three nucleotide residues are deleted, maintain the open reading frame. The size (single or multiple nucleotides) and position of these deletions (within the hormone or DNA-binding domains) determine the type of receptor defect (absent ligand binding or detectable ligand binding) in such individuals. Insertions are less common.

Single nucleotide substitutions in either the DNA- or hormone-binding domains can disrupt the primary structure of the androgen receptor in a variety of ways. First, premature termination codons cause the formation of truncated receptors that are defective in hormone or DNA binding or in assays of transcriptional activation. In one instance, a premature termination codon in the N-terminal region was associated with the formation of a small amount of a shorter receptor that was initiated at a downstream methionine[309]; this shorter isoform is formed in all tissues and functions similarly to the longer, more abundant receptor.[310,311] Second, single-nucleotide substitutions (or deletions) can cause aberrant splicing of androgen receptor mRNA.[301] Third, missense mutations that cause single-amino-acid substitutions in the DNA-binding domain comprise a category of androgen resistance previously termed *receptor-positive resistance* or *normal androgen binding* (see Fig. 160-12) in which hormone binding is normal but binding to DNA is impaired.[295,296] Fourth, amino acid substitutions in the hormone-binding domain of the receptor can result in the synthesis of androgen receptor that is unable to bind ligand (absent androgen binding) or that exhibits one or more evidences of impaired hormone binding, such as thermal instability or accelerated ligand dissociation; these substitutions cause a spectrum of phenotypic effects and of alterations in assays using reporter genes.[312–315] Fifth, amino acid substitutions can impair dimerization of the receptor.[31]

The functional categorization of the androgen resistance syndromes on the basis of the binding characteristics in cultured fibroblasts in some instances has predictive value as to the underlying mutations involved (see Fig. 160-12). Namely, the "normal ligand binding" category consists primarily of individuals with mutations of the DNA-binding domain and one individual with a deletion of exon 3.[305] Likewise, the "qualitatively abnormal' category largely consists of missense mutations in the androgen-binding domain. There are multiple causes for "undetectable" binding, including gene deletions (large and small), single-amino-acid substitutions in the androgen-binding domain, premature termination codons, and splicing defects. Likewise, the category of "decreased" amount of receptor that is qualitatively normal has several causes, including single-amino-acid substitutions in the hormone-binding domain,[299] intronic mutations that result in the formation of small amounts of normal receptor,[316,317] and mosaicism in which the mutation of the androgen receptor is assumed to have occurred shortly after fertilization and in which some cells have a normal gene.[318] In all cases, however, mutations in the androgen receptor gene cause different phenotypes by interfering with receptor function to different degrees. Mutations that markedly decrease receptor abundance, receptor function, or both result in complete testicular feminization. Mutations that have lesser effects on receptor quantity and function cause the spectrum of disorders from incomplete testicular feminization to the infertile or undervirilized male. It should be noted that in some families with clear-cut androgen resistance, no mutation has been identified in the gene itself or in its flanking sequences.[319]

In most instances, the phenotypes of patients with identical mutations of the androgen receptor are similar, whereas individuals with generalized resistance to thyroid hormone, in which individuals carry a specific mutation — even from within a single pedigree — commonly exhibit different manifestations.[320] This feature suggests that the level of androgen receptor abundance and function is the principal determinant of phenotype in most patients with androgen resistance. This relation is not uniform, however, because in some families patients with androgen resistance have distinctive phenotypes. In the case of mutations that cause quantitative defects in the formation of normal receptor,[263] it is logical that small variations in receptor level could influence phenotype (see Fig. 160-11), but in the case of missense mutations, it is not clear how phenotypic variation arises from the same mutation.[321] Factors that may affect phenotype could influence the androgen receptor gene itself (e.g., genes that control the level and timing of androgen receptor expression) or could affect the level of testosterone synthesis or metabolism (e.g., level or timing of 5α-reductase expression). Additional studies will have to be performed to distinguish among these possibilities.

An unexpected feature of androgen receptor disorders is the distribution of mutations in the androgen receptor gene. Although premature termination codons and deletions can occur in all segments of the androgen receptor gene, amino acid substitutions are present predominately in the DNA- and hormone-binding domains. Furthermore, the amino acid substitutions in the hormone-binding domain appear to be particularly common in exon 5.[321] Namely, almost one-fifth of the amino acid substitutions shown in Fig. 160-13 are present in an area that includes less than 6 percent of the coding sequence of the receptor. Whether this localization occurs because these segments are particularly vital to the formation of a functional receptor or because the DNA encoding these segments is more prone to mutation remains to be determined. The fact that few amino acid substitutions have been identified in the N-terminal portion of the receptor may be due to ascertainment bias in the types of patients who have been studied or to the complex nature of the domains contained in this region. In vitro mutagenesis of the N-terminus has demonstrated that large segments of the region must be removed before function is altered significantly.[322–324]

Approximately 40 percent of individuals with androgen resistance have an uninformative family history, and their disorder is presumed to be due to new mutations. Hiort and colleagues[325] studied 30 families in which a mutation in the androgen receptor gene was present in only one family member and found that in 22 the mothers and grandmothers were heterozygous carriers, indicating that the mutation in these families had occurred remotely and was passed through several generations before becoming manifest. In the other 8 instances, a *de novo* mutation was identified, including 3 individuals with somatic mosaicism, indicating that the mutation occurred after the zygote stage. In another study, evidence was obtained for germ-line mosaicism for a mutation of the androgen receptor in the mother of two individuals with the Reifenstein syndrome.[326] These findings are in keeping with the concept that new mutations must be frequent in X-linked disorders that impair reproduction.[327]

Patients with spinobulbar muscular atrophy (Kennedy syndrome), an X-linked disorder characterized by progressive degeneration of anterior motor neurons and the late onset of mild androgen resistance, have large expansions of the polyglutamine repeat sequences in exon 1 (see Chap. 161). Lesser expansions (28 or more glutamines) are associated with a higher incidence of infertility,[221] and very short glutamine repeat sequences also may impair receptor function.[314]

Diagnosis. Suspicion of the presence of an androgen receptor disorder can either occur at birth (genital ambiguity or girls with inguinal hernias or palpable testes in the labia) or after the time of expected puberty (primary amenorrhea in women or unexplained undervirilization or infertility in men). It is necessary to separate these disorders from steroid 5α-reductase 2 deficiency (see above) and from defects in testosterone biosynthesis (see Chap. 159). In the adolescent or adult, the diagnosis of complete testicular feminization is straightforward. A phenotypic woman with primary amenorrhea, a 46,XY karyotype, male levels of testosterone, and bilateral testes (abdominal or inguinal) is found to have absence of Müllerian derivatives by ultrasound[328] or by computed tomography (CT) of the abdomen.[329] However, separation of incomplete testicular feminization in the adolescent or adult from steroid 5α-reductase 2 deficiency (see above), defects in testosterone biosynthesis (see Chap. 159), and mixed gonadal dysgenesis[61] can be a diagnostic problem. In each of these disorders, defects in virilization of the external genitalia may be more severe than that of the Wolffian ducts. Mixed gonadal dysgenesis is often diagnosed by chromosomal analysis. Defects in testosterone biosynthesis usually can be excluded by the presence of normal male testosterone levels, but patients with partial deficiencies may have plasma testosterone levels in the normal or near-normal range; such partial defects, however, are accompanied by elevations in the plasma levels of androgen precursors.[142] Steroid 5α-reductase 2 deficiency in this age group is usually diagnosed on the basis of measurement of plasma or urinary 5α-reduced steroids (see above). In resolving these issues, careful analysis of the family history, the phenotype, the endocrine profile, and androgen metabolism in cultured fibroblasts may be required (see Table 160-10). Rarely, women with testicular feminization are not diagnosed until late in life.[153]

The diagnosis is a special problem in the neonate and young infant, particularly when the family history is uninformative. A presumptive diagnosis of androgen resistance can be made in neonates in whom plasma LH and/or testosterone levels are elevated.[330,331] In most circumstances, a more extensive evaluation is necessary, including evaluation of karyotype, measurement of plasma steroids after stimulation with hCG, evaluation of the genitourinary tract by radiographic or endoscopic procedures, and on occasion, assessment of androgen metabolism in cultured skin fibroblasts.[61,332] It is of particular importance to establish the correct diagnosis of incomplete testicular feminization as early as

Table 160-10 **Summary of Androgen Resistance Syndromes**

			Phenotype					
Category	**Inheritance**	**Horomonal Profile**	**Spermatogenesis**	**Müllerian Derivatives**	**Wolffian Derivatives**	**Urogenital Sinus**	**External Genitalia**	**Breasts**
Steroid 5α-reductase 2 deficiency	Autosomal recessive	Normal male testosterone and estrogen production	Decreased	Absent	Male	Female	Female (may virilize at puberty)	Male
Receptor disorders								
Complete testicular feminization	X-linked recessive	Increased testosterone and estrogen production (usually)	Absent	Absent	Absent	Female	Female	Female
Incomplete testicular feminization	X-linked recessive	Increased testosterone and estrogen production (usually)	Absent	Absent	Male	Female	Posterior fusion and/or clitoromegaly	Female
Reifenstein syndrome	X-linked recessive	Increased testosterone and estrogen production (usually)	Absent	Absent	Male	Underdeveloped male	Perineoscrotal hypospadias	Gynecomastia
Undervirlized or infertile men	X-linked recessive	Increased testosterone and estrogen production (usually)	Absent or decreased	Absent	Male	Male	Male	Gynecomastia in some

possible so that castration can be performed early enough in life to prevent partial virilization at puberty.

It is disappointing that diagnosis of androgen receptor mutations has not been made easier by the techniques of molecular biology; indeed, the profound heterogeneity of the mutations of the androgen receptor, the size of the protein, and technical problems involving the use of the polymerase chain reaction to amplify DNA segments containing polyglutamine repeat sequences have impeded the development of techniques for the diagnosis of new mutations in clinical laboratories. Even in research laboratories the sequencing is so slow that it is rarely useful for intrauterine diagnosis. However, once the diagnosis of an androgen receptor defect is established in a specific family, three techniques have been used for carrier detection and/or prenatal diagnosis in individuals at risk. First, the diagnosis can be made in subsequent fetuses at risk early in gestation by sequencing the appropriate exon in DNA prepared from chorionic villus sampling or amniotic fluid cells.[309,333] Second, in some families it is possible to use an informative HindIII restriction fragment polymorphism for making the prenatal diagnosis even in the absence of knowing the specific mutation.[334] Third, the glutamine repeat polymorphism in exon 1 of the gene also can be used for linkage diagnosis.[314,335,336]

A functional diagnostic test to aid in the diagnosis of androgen resistance would be particularly useful in children of prepubertal age, but the available tests, including measuring the response of sex hormone-binding globulin levels in plasma to the administration of hCG[337] or a nonaromatizable androgen[338] and the measurement of sebum production and/or nitrogen balance after the administration of high-dose androgen therapy,[339] are both cumbersome and imprecise.

Management. Since no specific therapy is available to circumvent or reverse the abnormal development that takes place during embryogenesis, treatment is directed toward correction of the external genitalia, prevention of complications and adverse secondary effects of the mutations (including psychological support), and appropriate hormone replacement or supplementation when necessary

The External Genitalia. Surgical correction of hypospadias and creation of neovaginas by medical or surgical means should be undertaken when appropriate but only at the appropriate age. Usually hypospadias is repaired before boys start school so that they can stand upright when urinating. Vaginal repair should be undertaken only when women are ready to lead an active sex life because of the tendency for the vagina to restenose unless it is dilated regularly and can involve surgical or medical procedures.[340] Long-term follow-up studies indicate that neovaginas created by medical means (the Frank procedure) are more likely to function normally than those created surgically.[341] Women with incomplete testicular feminization may require correction of the deep posterior forchette, and in some, recession of the clitoris is appropriate.

The Psychological Problems. Undervirilized or infertile men and women with complete testicular feminization, respectively, have unambiguous male and female phenotypes at birth and are raised accordingly. Individuals with incomplete testicular feminization and the Reifenstein syndrome have varying degrees of abnormal external genitalia, and the correct diagnosis usually can be made in the newborn or child. Because gender identity is critical to psychological development and normal mental health, it is mandatory that gender assignment be made as early as possible, preferably at the time of birth in newborns with ambiguous external genitalia. A detailed discussion of the diagnostic procedures and of the various problems encountered in reaching a decision about gender assignment in infants with ambiguous genitalia is given elsewhere.[61,332,342] Once gender assignment is made, the central obligation is to perform any indicated surgery as early as feasible to provide the appropriate hormonal environment at expected puberty and to assist affected individuals in adjusting to their inevitable infertility. With appropriate counseling, women with testicular feminization accept their infertility and make successful adoptive mothers. Indeed, such women have a high record of success in many arenas.

The question of exactly how much and when such women should be told about their diagnosis is an unresolved issue. The argument has been advanced that with appropriate education, sufficient information should be provided so that subjects understand the complete pathophysiology of the condition.[343,344] One strong argument for complete disclosure is to prevent the worse alternative of learning the diagnosis inadvertently. However, gender and gender identity are considered by society at large and by many individuals to be rigidly polarized, and subjects with intersex conditions are subjected to discrimination and prejudice. Consequently, it is not surprising that some women with testicular feminization have had severe psychiatric problems, including suicidal behavior after being informed of the true diagnosis. Consequently, no matter how desirable complete disclosure may be in the abstract, the decision to disclose should be made on an individual basis, usually only after consultation with family and after the development of an appropriate support network to aid in helping subjects to make appropriate decisions.[345] A support group for individuals with androgen resistance and their parents publishes three newsletters a year and provides valuable psychological support; the address is AIS Support Group, 4203 Genesee Ave., #103-436, San Diego CA 92117.

The Cryptorchid Testis. The most serious complication of the undescended testis in testicular feminization is the development of tumors.[2,149,346,347] It likely that tumor incidence in patients with this disorder is similar to that in cryptorchidism of other causes. Approximately 1 in 64 undescended testes becomes malignant, and the frequency of tumor is about four times greater in abdominal than in inguinal testes.[348] The natural history of the tumors in women with testicular feminization is not entirely clear, but some behave as true malignancies.[347] Therefore, it is generally accepted that the testes should be removed in these women. Since these patients undergo a normal pubertal growth spurt and feminize successfully at the time of expected puberty,[2,149] and since tumors usually do not develop in cryptorchid testes until after this time,[349] it is customary to delay castration until secondary sexual maturation is complete. Carcinoma *in situ* of the testes has been described in prepubertal children with testicular feminization, but the functional significance of lesions in unclear.[350–352] If, however, hernia repair is indicated in the prepubertal years, or if testes that are located in the inguinal region or the labia majora cause discomfort, some physicians prefer to perform castration at the time of herniorrhaphy. When testes are removed prepubertally, estrogen therapy is required at the appropriate age to ensure normal growth and breast development. If castration is performed after pubescence, menopausal symptoms and other evidence of estrogen withdrawal supervene,[2,149] and suitable estrogen replacement is indicated.

Tumors also can develop in intraabdominal testes in women with incomplete testicular feminization.[352] The testes in these subjects should be removed prior to the time of expected puberty to prevent disfiguring virilization that can occur when the plasma testosterone level rises. As above, feminization should be induced in such women with estrogens at the appropriate time.

Cryptorchidism is frequent in the Reifenstein syndrome[204] and should be corrected surgically. The Reifenstein case material is small, but in other forms of cryptorchidism, development of tumors is rare following successful repair.[348]

Gynecomastia in Men with Defects of the Androgen Receptor. Gynecomastia in these disorders is histologically indistinguishable from other forms of estrogen-induced gynecomastia.[200] In men with the Reifenstein syndrome[204] and in some infertile men[212] or undervirilized men,[220] gynecomastia develops as a result both of increased estrogen production and of androgen resistance, as in testicular feminization.[7,198] The gynecomastia may be disfiguring as well as disturbing. The appropriate therapy is surgical removal. As in normal men who are castrated,[23] gynecomastia occasionally can develop following castration of individuals with androgen resistance.[353] This is presumably due to the fact that estrogen formation from adrenal precursors continues unabated following removal of the testes.[23]

Carcinoma of the breast has been described in men with the Reifenstein syndrome,[354,355] whereas mutations in the androgen receptor were not detected in 11 breast cancers of men not associated with an androgen resistance syndrome,[356] and it is likely that gynecomastia itself rather than the mutation in the androgen receptor is the predisposing factor.[357] Nevertheless, the overall risk in men with gynecomastia is believed to be small.[358]

Hormone Treatment. Appropriate estrogen treatment is indicated in all phenotypic women after removal of the testes[2,149,151]; such therapy supports or promotes breast development and lubrication of the vagina and promotes feminization in general, but it is not clear whether such regimens prevent the development of osteopenia.[179] Testosterone (which can be converted to estrogen in peripheral tissues) also has been used for replacement therapy in women with testicular feminization following castration but has no advantage.[359]

Supplemental androgen has been administered with success in some[83] but not all[228,262] men with Reifenstein syndrome. In two instances the fact that the function of the mutant androgen receptor in vitro was enhanced by increased levels of androgen was used to predict successful virilization after the administration of supraphysiologic doses of androgen in two patients with amino acid substitutions in the hormone-binding domain.[314,360] Positive responses to androgen also have been described in men with missense mutations of the DNA-binding domain.[361,362] However, the value of long-term androgen supplementation in this disorder is not clear. In one man with oligospermia associated with a missense mutation of the hormone-binding domain, treatment with a nonaromatizable androgen caused an increase in sperm count from 2.3 to 3.7 to 28 million/ml.[363]

THE NATURE OF ANDROGEN RESISTANCE

The concept of resistance to hormone action was formulated originally by Albright and colleagues to describe the defect in pseudohypoparathyroidism in which there was a lack of response to endogenous and exogenous parathyroid hormone,[1] and the term *resistance* is now used widely throughout the endocrinology literature to describe subnormal responses to many hormones, including insulin, cortisol, LH, etc. Consequently, in this chapter we have referred to *androgen resistance* rather than to *androgen insensitivity*, a term introduced many years later to characterize the disorder in mice.[277] In the case of androgen resistance, it was assumed originally that the degree of resistance to the hormone is equal in all tissues at all times of life and that the inevitable phenotypic expression of such a disorder was male pseudohermaphroditism. As the complexity of androgen action has been elucidated further, the spectrum of the manifestations of androgen resistance has expanded beyond the original formulation. Not only do different androgen metabolites have different physiologic effects, but any one androgen may have different actions during different phases of life — from embryogenesis to old age. Furthermore, at the clinical level, androgen resistance can be documented in some but not all tissues of the same affected subject, and the clinical manifestations of androgen resistance can vary from mild defects in virilization to individuals with a female phenotype. Finally, the identical mutation in the androgen receptor can have different manifestations in different families. Therefore, we use a complex classification of androgen resistance that depends on a combination of molecular, genetic, phenotypic, and endocrine characteristics.

As in other forms of genetic disease, elucidation of the pathophysiology of the androgen resistance syndromes has provided insight into the normal pathway of androgen action. Each new type of androgen resistance that is recognized provides an opportunity for defining the nature of a specific reaction essential for the action of the hormone.

Subjects with steroid 5α-reductase 2 deficiency have a special type of androgen resistance in which certain target tissues that are resistant to the action of testosterone would have responded normally to the missing end product (dihydrotestosterone) if it had been administered at the appropriate time during embryogenesis. This condition is analogous to hereditary resistance to the action of vitamin D; in one form of this disorder—so-called vitamin D-dependent rickets type I—the subject is unable to synthesize the 1,25-dihydroxyvitamin D. In contrast, persons with androgen receptor abnormalities appear to be equally unresponsive to all androgens, with the degree of resistance varying with the severity of the mutation.

Androgen resistance associated with male pseudohermaphroditism is relatively common, and if androgen resistance is the cause of a significant fraction of male infertility, it may prove to be more frequent than all other forms of steroid hormone resistance combined. There are several possible reasons for this frequency. First, expression of androgen activity is required for reproduction but not for the life of the individual. As a consequence, those with complete androgen resistance have a normal life span. In contrast, severe mutations affecting the action of hormones essential for life (such as cortisol) are lethal. Second, defects in androgen action result either in abnormal sexual development, in reproductive failure, or in undervirilization. As a consequence, there is a high probability that even subtle defects in androgen action eventually come to the attention of physicians. Third, since the gene that specifies the androgen receptor is X-linked, defects in the androgen receptor become clinically manifest in the hemizygous (XY) state. As a consequence, there is a high probability that a new mutation in the androgen receptor will be clinically evident.

Characterization of the molecular defects that cause steroid 5α-reductase 2 deficiency and androgen receptor abnormalities has provided additional insight into the pathogenesis of androgen resistance. In particular, specific domains in each protein have been identified—for example, the NADPH- and ligand-binding domains of steroid 5α-reductase 2 and the ligand- and DNA-binding domains of the androgen receptor. More important, techniques have been developed for prenatal diagnosis of infants at risk and for identification of heterozygous carriers.

In the case of mutations that prevent the formation of the enzyme or receptor (major gene deletions, premature termination codons, splice-junction abnormalities), impairment of protein function is absolute, and the phenotype within families is constant. In most instances, however, the mutations cause single-amino-acid substitutions, some of which cause profound impairment of protein function and some of which impair function to a lesser extent. The latter types of mutations frequently are associated with blunted phenotypes and variable manifestations within the same families; this variability implies that other genes (proteins) influence the expression of the normal and mutant proteins. The identification of these secondary genes in androgen action is a major challenge.

In certain regards, the results from molecular analysis are disappointing. In particular, the mutations in both proteins, like those in many other human disorders, are heterogeneous—approximately 45 different mutations of steroid 5α-reductase 2 and more than 321 mutations of the androgen receptor have been identified to date. The consequence of this heterogeneity is that molecular diagnosis requires full-scale sequencing of the coding sequence of the genes, not currently a practical diagnostic alternative. Therefore, for the near future, diagnosis, as before, will depend on a combination of phenotypic, genetic, and endocrine studies supplemented with functional studies of the enzyme and receptor in cultured skin fibroblasts when available. More specific and more cost-effective means of diagnosing defects of 5α-reductase and the androgen receptor are needed. However, even when the 5α-reductase and androgen receptor cDNAs are sequenced, many individuals with clinical and endocrine features of androgen resistance do not have identifiable abnormalities in either of these molecules, implying that defects in additional, possibly unidentified steps in androgen action during embryogenesis also may cause androgen resistance syndromes.

REFERENCES

1. Albright F, Burnett CH, Smith PH, Parson W: Pseudohypoparathyroidism—An example of "Seabright-Bantam" syndrome. *Endocrinology* **30**:922, 1942.
2. Morris JM: The syndrome of testicular feminization in male pseudohermaphrodites. *Am J Obstet Gynecol* **65**:1192, 1953.
3. Wilkins L: Abnormal sex differentiation: Hermaphroditism and gonadal dysgenesis, in *The Diagnosis and Treatment of Endocrine Disorders in Childhood and Adolescence*. Springfield, IL, Charles C Thomas, 1957, p 258.
4. Griffin JE: Androgen resistance—The clinical and molecular spectrum. *New Engl J Med* **326**:611, 1992.
5. Jost A: Hormonal factors in the sex differentiation of the mammalian foetus. *Philos Trans R Soc Lond [Biol]* **259**:119, 1970.
6. Siiteri PK, MacDonald PC: Role of extraglandular estrogen in human endocrinology, in Greep RO, Astwood EB (eds): *Handbook of Physiology*, vol 2: *Endocrinology*. Washington, American Physiological Society, 1973, p 615.
7. MacDonald PC, Madden JD, Brenner PF, Wilson JD, Siiteri PK: Origin of estrogen in normal men and in women with testicular feminization. *J Clin Endocrinol Metab* **49**:905, 1979.
8. Wilson JD, Goldstein JL: Classification of hereditary disorders of sexual development. *Birth Defects* **11**:1, 1975.
9. Wilson JD: Metabolism of testicular androgens, in Greep RO, Astwood EB (eds): *Handbook of Physiology*, vol 5: *Endocrinology*, sec 7: *Male Reproductive System*. Washington, American Physiological Society, 1975, p 491.
10. Tsai M-J,Clark JH, Schrader WT, O'Malley BW: Mechanisms of action of hormones that act as transcription regulatory factors, in Wilson JD, Foster DW, Kronenberg HM, Larsen PR (eds): *Williams' Textbook of Endocrinology*, 9th ed. Philadelphia, Saunders, 1998, p 55.
11. Andersson S, Russell DW: Structural and biochemical properties of cloned and expressed human and rat steroid 5α-reductases. *Proc Natl Acad Sci USA* **87**:3640, 1987.
12. Andersson S, Berman DM, Jenkins EP, Russell DW: Deletion of steroid 5α-reductase 2 gene in male pseudohermaphroditism. *Nature* **354**:159, 1991.
13. Chang C, Kokontis J, Liao S: Molecular cloning of human and rat complementary DNA encoding androgen receptors. *Science* **240**:324, 1988.
14. Lubahn DB, Joseph DR, Sullivan PM, Willard HF, French FS, Wilson EM: Cloning of human androgen receptor complementary DNA and localization to the X chromosome. *Science* **240**:327, 1988.
15. Trapman J, Klaassen P, Kuiper GGJM, Van der Korput JAGM, Faber PW, van Rooij HCJ, van Kessel AG, Voorhorst MM, Mulder E, Brinkmann AO: Cloning, structure, and expression of a cDNA encoding the human androgen receptor. *Biochem Biophys Res Commun* **153**:241, 1988.
16. Tilley WD, Marcelli M, Wilson JD, McPhaul MJ: Characterization and expression of a cDNA encoding the human androgen receptor. *Proc Natl Acad Sci USA* **86**:327, 1989.
17. Smith EP, Boyd J, Frank GR, et al: Estrogen resistance caused by a mutation in the estrogen receptor gene in man. *New Engl J Med* **331**:1056, 1994
18. Morishima A, Grumbach MM, Simpson ER, et al: Aromatase deficiency in male and female siblings caused by a novel mutation and the physiological role of estrogens. *J Clin Endocrinol Metab* **80**:3689, 1995.
19. Keenan BS, Richards GE, Ponder SW, et al: Androgen-stimulated pubertal growth: The effects of testosterone and dihydrotestosterone on growth hormone and insulin-like growth factor I in the treatment of short stature and delayed puberty. *J Clin Endocrinol Metab* **76**:996, 1993.

20. Bagatell CJ, Dahl KD, Bremner WJ: The direct pituitary effect of testosterone to inhibit gonadotropin secretion in men is partially mediated by aromatization to estradiol. *J Androl* **15**:15, 1994.
21. Bhatnagar AS, Muller P, Shenkel L, et al: Inhibition of estrogen biosynthesis and its consequences on gonadotropin secretion in the male. *J Steroid Biochem Mol Biol* **41**:457, 1992.
22. Bagatell CJ, Knopp RH, Rivier JE, et al: Physiological levels of estradiol stimulate plasma high density lipoprotein cholesterols in normal men. *J Clin Endocrinol Metab* **78**:855, 1994.
23. Wilson JD, Aiman J, MacDonald PC: The pathogenesis of gynecomastia. *Adv Intern Med* **25**:1, 1980.
24. Kelch RP, Jenner MR, Weinstein R, Kaplan SL, Grumbach MM: Estradiol and testosterone secretion by human, simian, and canine testes, in males with hypogonadism and in male pseudohermaphrodites with the feminizing testes syndrome. *J Clin Invest* **51**:824, 1972.
25. Weinstein RL, Kelch RP, Jenner MR, Kaplan SL, Grumbach MM: Secretion of unconjugated androgens and estrogens by the normal and abnormal human testis before and after human chorionic gonadotropin. *J Clin Invest* **53**:1, 1974.
26. Pardridge WM: Serum bioavailability of sex hormones. *J Clin Endocrinol Metab* **15**:259, 1986.
27. Lasznitzki I, Franklin HR, Wilson JD: The mechanism of androgen uptake and concentration by rat ventral prostate in organ culture. *J Endocrinol* **60**:81, 1974.
28. McConnell JD, Wilson JD, George FW, Geller J, Pappas F, Stoner E: Finasteride, an inhibitor of 5α-reductase, suppresses prostatic dihydrotestosterone in men with benign prostatic hyperplasia. *J Clin Endocrinol Metab* **74**:505, 1992.
29. Wilbert DM, Griffin JE, Wilson JD: Characterization of the cytosol androgen receptor of the human prostate. *J Clin Endocrinol Metab* **56**:113, 1983.
30. Edwards A, Hammond HA, Jin L, Caskey CT, Chakraborty R: Genetic variation of five trimeric and tetrameric tandem repeat loci in four human population groups. *Genomics* **12**:241, 1992.
31. Langley E, Kemppainen JA, Wilson EM: Intermolecular NH_2-carboxyl-terminal interactions in androgen receptor dimerization revealed by mutations that cause androgen insensitivity. *J Biol Chem* **273**:92, 1998.
32. Grino PB, Griffin JE, Wilson JD: Testosterone at high concentrations interacts with the human androgen receptor similarly to dihydrotestosterone. *Endocrinology* **126**:1165, 1990.
33. George FW, Wilson JD: Sex determination and differentiation, in Knobil E, Neill JD, (eds): *The Physiology of Reproduction,* 2d ed. New York, Raven Press, 1994, pp 3–28.
34. Kovacs WJ, Griffin JE, Weaver DD, Carlson BR, Wilson JD: A mutation that causes lability of the androgen receptor under conditions that normally promote transformation to the DNA-binding state. *J Clin Invest* **73**:1095, 1984.
35. Deslypere J-P, Young M, Wilson JD, McPhaul MJ: Testosterone and 5β-dihydrotestosterone interact differently with the androgen receptor to enhance transcription of the MMTV-CAT reporter gene. *Mol Cell Endocrinol* **88**:15, 1992.
36. George FW, Russell DW, Wilson JD: Feed-forward control of prostate growth: Dihydrotestosterone induces expression of its own biosynthetic enzyme, steroid 5α-reductase. *Proc Natl Acad Sci USA* **88**:8044, 1991.
37. Sinclair AH, Berta P, Palmer MS, Hawkins JR, Griffiths BL, Smith MJ, Foster JW, Frischauf AM, Lovell-Badge R, Goodfellow PN: A gene from the human sex-determining region encodes a protein with homology to a conserved DNA-binding motif. *Nature* **346**:240, 1990.
38. Koopman P, Gubbay J, Vivian N, Goodfellow P, Lovell-Badge R: Male development of chromosomally female mice transgenic for *Sry. Nature* **351**:117, 1991.
39. Lawrence WD, Whitaker D, Sugimura H, Cunha GR, Dickersin GR, Robboy SJ: An ultrastructural study of the developing urogenital tract in early human fetuses. *Am J Obstet Gynecol* **167**:185, 1992.
40. Josso N, Boussin L, Knebelmann B, Nihoul-Fekete C, Picard J-Y: Anti-Müllerian hormone and intersex states. *Trends Endocrinol Metab* **2**:227, 1991.
41. Donahoe PK, Cate RL, MacLaughlin DT, Epstein J, Fuller AF, Takahashi M, Coughlin JP, Ninfa EG, Taylor LA: Müllerian inhibiting substance: Gene structure and mechanism of action of a fetal regressor. *Recent Prog Horm Res* **43**:431, 1987.
42. Siiteri PK, Wilson JD: Testosterone formation and metabolism during male sexual differentiation in the human embryo. *J Clin Endocrinol Metab* **38**:113, 1974.
43. George FW, Simpson ER, Milewich L, Wilson JD: Studies on the regulation of the onset of steroid hormone biosynthesis in fetal rabbit gonads. *Endocrinology* **105**:1100, 1979.
44. Themmen APN, Martens JWM, Brunner HG: Gonadotropin receptor mutations. *J Endocrinol* **153**:179, 1997.
45. Weiss J, Axelrod L, Whitcomb RW, Harris PE, Crowley WF, Jameson JL: Hypogonadism caused by a single amino acid substitution in the β subunit of the luteinizing hormone. *New Engl J Med* **326**:179, 1992.
46. George FW, Carr BR, Noble JF, Wilson JD: 5α-Reduced androgens in the human fetal testis. *J Clin Endocrinol Metab* **64**:628, 1987.
47. Imperato-McGinley J, Binienda Z, Arthur A, Mininberg DT, Vaughan ED Jr, Quimby FW: The development of a male pseudohermaphroditic rat using an inhibitor of the enzyme 5α-reductase. *Endocrinology* **116**:807, 1985.
48. George FW, Peterson K: 5α-Dihydrotestosterone formation is necessary for embryogenesis of the rat prostate. *Endocrinology* **122**:1159, 1988.
49. Prahalada S, Tarantal AF, Harris GS, Ellsworth KP, Clarke AP, Skiles GL, MacKenzie KI, Kruk LF, Ablin DS, Cukierski MA, Peter CP, van Zwieten MJ, Hendricks AG: Effects of finasteride, a type 2 5α-reductase inhibitor, on fetal development in the rhesus monkey (*Cacaca mulatta*). *Teratology* **55**:119, 1997.
50. Moore RJ, Wilson JD: Extraction of the reduced nicotinamide adenine dinucleotide phosphate: Δ^4-3keto-5α-oxidoreductase rat prostate with digitonin and potassium chloride. *Biochemistry* **13**:450, 1974.
51. Moore RJ, Wilson JD: Steroid 5α-reductase in cultured human fibroblasts: Biochemical and genetic evidence for two distinct enzyme activities. *J Biol Chem* **251**:5895, 1976.
52. Thigpen AE, Russell DW: Four amino acid segments in steroid 5α-reductase 1 confers sensitivity to finasteride, a competitive inhibitor. *J Biol Chem* **267**:8577, 1992.
53. Span PN, Shalken JA, Sweep FG, Smals AG: Identification and partial characterization of two steroid 5α-reductase isozymes in the canine prostate. *Prostate* **34**:222, 1998.
54. Levy MA, Brandt M, Sheedy KM, Holt DA, Heaslip JI, Trill JJ, Ryan PJ, Morris RA, Garrison LM, Bergsma DJ: Cloning, expression and functional characterization of type 1 and type 2 steroid 5α-reductases from *Cynomolgus* monkey: Comparison with human and rat isoenzymes. *J Steroid Biochem Mol Biol* **52**:307, 1995.
55. Li J, Biswas MG, Chao A, Russell DW, Chory J: Conservation of function between mammalian and plant steroid 5α-reductases. *Proc Natl Acad Sci USA* **94**:3554, 1997.
56. Makridakis N, Ross RK, Pike MC, Chang L, Stanczyk FZ, Kolonel LN, Shi CY, Yu MC, Henderson BE, Reichardt JK: A prevalent missense substitution that modulates activity of prostatic steroid 5α-reductase. *Cancer Res* **57**:1020, 1997.
57. Kantoff PW, Febbo PG, Giovannucci E, Krithivas K, Dahl DM, Chang G, Hennekens CH, Brown M, Stampfer MJ: A polymorphism of the 5α-reductase gene and its association with prostate cancer: A case-control analysis. *Cancer Epidemiol Biomark Prevent* **6**:189, 1997.
58. Vilchis G, Hernandez D, Canto P, Mendez JP, Chavez B: Codon 89 polymorphism of the human 5α-steroid reductase type 2 gene. *Clin Genet* **51**:399, 1997.
59. George FW, Noble JF: Androgen receptors are similar in fetal and adult rabbits. *Endocrinology* **115**:1451, 1984.
60. Schultz FM, Wilson JD: Virilization of the wolffian duct in the rat fetus by various androgens. *Endocrinology* **94**:979, 1974.
61. Griffin JE, Wilson JD: Disorders of sexual differentiation, in Walsh PC, Retik AB, Stamey TA, Vaughan ED Jr (eds): *Campbell's Urology.* Philadelphia, Saunders, 1992, p 1509.
62. Imbeaud S, Carre-Eusebe D, Rey R, Belville C, Josso N, Picard J-Y: Molecular genetics of the persistent mullerian duct syndrome: A study of 19 families. *Hum Mol Genet* **3**:125, 1994.
63. Imbeaud S, Bellville C, Messika-Zeitoun L, Re R, di Clemente N, Josso N, Picard J-Y: A 27 base-pair deletion of the anti-mullerian type II receptor gene is the most common cause of the persistent Müllerian duct syndrome. *Hum Mol Genet* **5**:1259, 1996.
64. Savage MO, Chaussain JL, Evain D, Roger M, Canlorbe P, Job JC: Endocrine studies in male pseudohermaphroditism in childhood and adolescence. *Clin Endocrinol (Oxf)* **8**:219, 1978.
65. Campo S, Stivel M, Nicolau G, Monteagudo C, Rivarola M: Testicular function in postpubertal male pseudohermaphroditism. *Clin Endocrinol (Oxf)* **11**:481, 1979.
66. Campo S, Monteagudo C, Nicolau G, Pellizzari E, Belgorosky A, Stivel M, Rivarola M: Testicular function in prepubertal male pseudohermaphroditism. *Clin Endocrinol (Oxf)* **14**:11, 1981.

67. Nowakowski H, Lenz W: Genetic aspects in male hypogonadism. *Recent Prog Horm Res* **17**:53, 1961.
68. Lenz W: Genetisch bedingte Storungen der weiblichen Fortpflanzungsfunktionen. *Med Welt* **1**:16, 1962.
69. Simpson JL, New M, Peterson RE, German J: Pseudovaginal perineoscrotal hypospadias (PPSH) in sibs. *Birth Defects* **7**(6):140, 1971.
70. Opitz JM, Simpson JL, Sarto GE, Summitt RL, New M, German J: Pseudovaginal perineoscrotal hypospadias. *Clin Genet* **3**:1, 1972.
71. Walsh PC, Madden JD, Harrod MJ, Goldstein JL, MacDonald PC, Wilson JD: Familial incomplete male pseudohermaphroditism type 2: Decreased dihydrotestosterone formation in pseudovaginal perineoscrotal hypospadias. *New Engl J Med* **291**:944, 1974.
72. Imperato-McGinley J, Guerrero L, Gautier T, Peterson RE: Steroid 5α-reductase deficiency in man: An inherited form of male pseudohermaphroditism. *Science* **186**:1213, 1974.
73. Peterson RE, Imperato-McGinley J, Gautier T, Sturla E: Male pseudohermaphroditism due to steroid 5α-reductase deficiency. *Am J Med* **62**:170, 1977.
74. Wilson JD: Dihydrotestosterone formation in cultured human fibroblasts: Comparison of cells from normal subjects and patients with familial incomplete male pseudohermaphroditism, type 2. *J Biol Chem* **250**:3498, 1975.
75. Fisher LK, Kogut MD, Moore RJ, Goebelsmann U, Weitzman JJ, Isaacs H Jr, Griffin JE, Wilson JD: Clinical, endocrinological, and enzymatic characterization of two patients with 5α-reductase deficiency: Evidence that a single enzyme is responsible for the 5α-reduction of cortisol and testosterone. *J Clin Endocrinol Metab* **47**:653, 1978.
76. Leshin M, Griffin JE, Wilson JD: Hereditary male pseudohermaphroditism associated with an unstable form of 5α-reductase. *J Clin Invest* **62**:685, 1978.
77. Imperato-McGinley J, Peterson RE, Gautier T, Sturla E: Male pseudohermaphroditism secondary to 5α-reductase deficiency: A model for the role of androgens in both the development of the male phenotype and the evolution of a male gender identity. *J Steroid Biochem* **11**:637, 1979.
78. Maes M, Sultan C, Zerhouni N, Rothwell SW, Migeon CJ: Role of testosterone binding to the androgen receptor in male sexual differentiation of patients with 5α-reductase deficiency. *J Steroid Biochem* **11**:1385, 1979.
79. Imperato-McGinley J, Peterson RE, Leshin M, Griffin JE, Cooper G, Draghi S, Berenyi M, Wilson JD: Steroid 5α-reductase deficiency in a 65 year old male pseudohermaphrodite: The natural history, ultrastructure of the testes and evidence for inherited enzyme heterogeneity. *J Clin Endocrinol Metab* **50**:15, 1980.
80. Carpenter TO, Imperato-McGinley J, Boulware SD, Weiss RM, Shackleton C, Griffin JE, Wilson JD: Variable expression of 5α-reductase deficiency: Presentation with male phenotype in a child of Greek origin. *J Clin Endocrinol Metab* **71**:318, 1990.
81. Johnson L, George FW, Neaves WB, Rosenthal IM, Christensen RA, Decristoforo A, Schweikert H-U, Sauer MV, Leshin M, Griffin JE, Wilson JD: Characterization of the testicular abnormality in 5α-reductase deficiency. *J Clin Endocrinol Metab* **63**:1091, 1986.
82. Saenger P, Goldman AS, Levine LS, Korthschutz S, Muecke EC, Katsumata M, Doberne Y, New MI: Prepubertal diagnosis of steroid 5α-reductase deficiency. *J Clin Endocrinol Metab* **46**:627, 1978.
83. Price P, Wass JAH, Griffin JE, Leshin M, Savage MO, Large DM, Bu'Lock DE, Anderson DC, Wilson JD, Besser GM: High dose androgen therapy in male pseudohermaphroditism due to 5α-reductase deficiency and disorders of the androgen receptor. *J Clin Invest* **74**:1496, 1984.
84. Deslypere J-P, Coucke W, Robbe N, Vermeulen A: 5α-Reductase deficiency: An infrequent cause of male pseudohermaphroditism. *Acta Clin Belg* **40**:240, 1985.
85. Corrall RJM, Wakelin K, O'Hare JP, O'Brien IAD, Ishmail AAA, Honour J: 5α-Reductase deficiency: Diagnosis via abnormal plasma levels of reduced testosterone derivatives. *Acta Endocrinol (Copenh)* **107**:538, 1984.
86. Bartsch G, Decristoforo A, Schweikert H-U: Pseudovaginal perineoscrotal hypospadias: Clinical, endocrinological and biochemical characterization of a patient. *Eur Urol* **13**:386, 1987.
87. Peterson RE, Imperato-McGinley J, Gautier T, Shackleton C: Urinary steroid metabolites in subjects with male pseudohermaphroditism due to 5α-reductase deficiency. *Clin Endocrinol (Oxf)* **23**:43, 1985.
88. Savage MO, Preece MA, Jeffcoate SL, Ransley PG, Rumsby G, Mansfield MD, Williams DI: Familial male pseudohermaphroditism due to deficiency of 5α-reductase. *Clin Endocrinol (Oxf)* **12**:397, 1980.
89. Cantu JM, Hernandez-Montes H, del Castillo V, Cortes-Gallegos V, Sandoval R, Armendares S, Parra A: Potential fertility in incomplete male pseudohermaphroditism type 2. *Rev Invest Clin* **28**:177, 1976.
90. Cantu JM, Corona-Rivera E, Diaz M, Medina C, Esquinca E, Cortes-Gallegos V, Vaca G, Hernandez A: Post-pubertal female psychosexual orientation in incomplete male pseudohermaphroditism type 2 (5α-reductase deficiency). *Acta Endocrinol (Copenh)* **94**:273, 1980.
91. Jaffiol C, Robin M, Corratge P, Mirouze J: Un cas de pseudohermaphrodisme masculin par defaut de conversion de testosterone en dihydrotestosterone. *Ann Endocrinol (Paris)* **39**:47, 1978.
92. Greene SA, Symes E, Brook CGD: 5α-Reductase deficiency causing male pseudohermaphroditism. *Arch Dis Child* **53**:751, 1978.
93. Kuttenn F, Mowszowicz I, Wright F, Baudot N, Jaffiol C, Robin M, Mauvais-Jarvis P: Male pseudohermaphroditism: A comparative study of one patient with 5α-reductase deficiency and three patients with the complete form of testicular feminization. *J Clin Endocrinol Metab* **49**:861, 1979.
94. Mauvais-Jarvis P, Kuttenn F, Mowszowicz I, Wright F: Different aspects of 5α-reductase deficiency in male pseudohermaphroditism and hypothyroidism. *Clin Endocrinol (Oxf)* **14**:459, 1981.
95. Akgun S, Ertel NH, Imperato-McGinley J, Sayli BS, Shackleton C: Familial male pseudohermaphroditism due to 5α-reductase deficiency in a Turkish village. *Am J Med* **81**:267, 1986.
96. Okon E, Livni N, Rosler A, Yorkoni S, Segal S, Kohn G, Schenker JG: Male pseudohermaphroditism due to 5α-reductase deficiency: Ultrastructure of the gonads. *Arch Pathol Lab Med* **104**:363, 1980.
97. Mendonca BB, Batista MC, Arnhold IJP, Nicolau W, Madureira G, Lando VS, Kohek MBF, Carvalho DG, Bloise W: Male pseudohermaphroditism due to 5α-reductase deficiency associated with gynecomastia. *Rev Hosp Clin Fac Med Sao Paulo* **42**:66, 1987.
98. El Awady MK, Salam MA, Temtamy SA: Deficient 5α-reductase due to mutant enzyme with reduced affinity to steroid substrate. *Enzyme* **32**:116, 1984.
99. Iudice GL, Esposito V, Federico P, D'Alessandro B: Male pseudohermaphroditism due to 5-α-reductase deficiency: Clinical and endocrinological data in a 17-year-old patient. *Minerva Endocrinol* **11**:7, 1986.
100. Ng WK, Taylor NF, Hughes IA, Taylor J, Ransley PG, Grant DB: 5α-Reductase deficiency without hypospadias. *Arch Dis Child* **65**:1166, 1990.
101. Gad YZ, Nasr H, Mazen I, Salah, El-Ridi R: 5α-Reductase deficiency in patients with micropenis. *J Inherit Metab Dis* **20**:95, 1997.
102. Katz MD, Kligman I, Cai LQ, Zhu YS, Fratianni CM, Zervoudakis I, Rosenwaks Z, Imperato-McGinley J: Paternity by intrauterine insemination with sperm from a man with 5α-reductase 2 deficiency. *New Engl J Med* **336**:994, 1997.
103. Ivarsson SA: 5α-Reductase deficient men are fertile. *Eur J Pediatr* **155**:425, 1996.
104. Imperato-McGinley J, Peterson RE, Gautier T, Sturla E: Androgens and the evolution of male-gender identity among male pseudohermaphrodites with 5α-reductase deficiency. *New Engl J Med* **300**:1233, 1979.
105. Wilson JD: Gonadal hormones and sexual behavior, in Besser GM, Martini L (eds): *Clinical Neuroendocrinology,* vol 2. New York, Academic Press, 1982, p 1.
106. Rosler A, Kohn G: Male pseudohermaphroditism due to 17β-hydroxysteroid dehydrogenase deficiency: studies on the natural history of the defect and effect of androgens on gender role. *J Steroid Biochem* **19**:663, 1983.
107. Mendonca BB, Bloise W, Arnhold IJP, Batista MC, de Almeida Toledo SP, Drummond MCF, Nicolau W, Mattrar E: Male pseudohermaphroditism due to non-salt-losing 3β-hydroxysteroid dehydrogenase deficiency: Gender role change and absence of gynecomastia at puberty. *J Steroid Biochem* **28**:669, 1987.
108. Gadjusek DC: Urgent opportunistic observations: The study of changing transient and disappearing phenomena of medical interest in disrupted health communities. *Ciba Found Symp* **49**:69, 1976.
109. Herdt GH, Davidson J: The Sambia "turnin-man": Sociocultural and clinical aspects of gender formation in male pseudohermaphrodites with 5-alpha-reductase deficiency in Papua New Guinea. *Arch Sex Behav* **17**:33, 1988.
110. Herdt G: Mistaken gender: 5α-Reductase, hermaphroditism and biological reductionism in sexual identity reconsidered. *J Am Anthropol Assoc* **92**:433, 1990.
111. Imperato-McGinley J, Miller M, Wilson JD, Peterson RE, Shackleton C, Gadjusek DC: A cluster of male pseudohermaphroditism with

5α-reductase deficiency in Papua New Guinea. *Clin Endocrinol (Oxf)* **34**:293, 1991.
112. Foaucault MHB: *Being the Recently Discovered Memories of a Nineteenth Century French Hermaphrodite*. New York, Panther, 1980.
113. Greene S, Zachmann M, Manella B, Hesse V, Hoepffner W, Willgerodt H, Prader A: Comparison of two tests to recognize or exclude 5α-reductase deficiency in prepubertal children. *Acta Endocrinol (Copenh)* **114**:113, 1987.
114. Imperato-McGinley J, Peterson RE, Gautier T, Arthur A, Shackleton C: Decreased urinary C19 and C21 steroid 5α-metabolites in parents of male pseudohermaphrodites with 5α-reductase deficiency: Detection of carriers. *J Clin Endocrinol Metab* **60**:553, 1985.
115. Cantovatchel WJ, Wolquez D, Huang S, Wood E, Lesser ML, Gautier T, Imperato-McGinley J: Luteinizing hormone pulsatility in subjects with 5α-reductase deficiency and decreased dihydrotestosterone production. *J Clin Endocrinol Metab* **78**:916, 1994.
116. Jenkins EP, Andersson S, Imperato-McGinley J, Wilson JD, Russell DW: Genetic and pharmacological evidence for more than one human steroid 5α-reductase. *J Clin Invest* **89**:293, 1992.
117. Thigpen AE, Davis DL, Milatovich A, Mendonca BB, Imperato-McGinley J, Griffin JE, Francke U, Wilson JD, Russell DW: Molecular genetics of steroid 5α-reductase 2 deficiency. *J Clin Invest* **90**:799, 1992.
118. Wilson JD, Griffin JE, Russell DW: Steroid 5α-reductase 2 deficiency. *Endocr Rev* **14**:577, 1993.
119. Schmidt JA, Schweikert H-U: Testosterone and epitestosterone metabolism of single hairs in 5 patients with 5α-reductase deficiency. *Acta Endocrinol (Copenh)* **113**:588, 1986.
120. Katz MD, Cai L-Qm, Zhu Y-S, Herrera C, DeFillo-Ricart M, Shackleton CHL, Imperato-McGinley J: The biochemical and phenotypic characterization of females homozygous for 5α-reductase 2 deficiency. *J Clin Endocrinol Metab* **80**:3160, 1995.
121. Milewich L, Mendonca BB, Arnhold I, Wallace AM, Donaldson MDC, Wilson JD, Russell D: Women with steroid 5α-reductase 2 deficiency have normal concentrations of plasma 5α-dihydrotestosterone during the luteal phase. *J Clin Endocrinol Metab* **80**:3136, 1996.
122. Milewich L, Gomez-Sanchez C, Crowley G, Porter JC, Madden JD, MacDonald PC: Progesterone and 5α-pregnane-3,20-dione in peripheral blood of normal young women: Daily measurements throughout the menstrual cycle. *J Clin Endocrinol Metab* **45**:617, 1977.
123. Milewich L, Gomez-Sanchez C, Madden JD, MacDonald PC: Isolation and characterization of 5α-pregnane-3,20-dione and progesterone in peripheral blood of pregnant women: Measurements throughout pregnancy. *Gynecol Invest* **6**:291, 1975.
124. Mahendroo MS, Cala KM, Landrum DP, Russell DW: Fetal death in mice lacking 5α-reductase type 1 is caused by estrogen excess. *Mol Endocrinol* **11**:917, 1997.
125. Mahendroo MS, Cala KM, Russell DW: 5α-Reduced androgens play a key role in murine parturition. *Mol Endocrinol* **19**:380, 1996.
126. Wigley WC, Prihoda JS, Mowszowicz I, Mendonca BB, New MI, Wilson JD, Russell DW: Natural mutagenesis study of the human steroid 5α-reductase 2 isoenzyme. *Biochemistry* **33**:1265, 1994.
127. Canto P, Vilchis F, Chavez B, Mutchinick O, Imperato-McGinley J, Perez-Palacios G, Ulloa-Aguire A, Mendez JP: Mutations of the 5α-reductase type 1 gene in eight Mexican patients from six different pedigrees with 5α-reductase-2 deficiency. *Clin Endocrinol* **46**:155, 1997.
128. Hiort O, Sinnecker HG, Willenbring H, Lehners A, Zollner A, Struve D: Nonisotopic single strand conformation analysis of the 5α-reductase type 2 gene for the diagnosis of 5α-reductase deficiency. *J Clin Endocrinol Metab* **81**:3415, 1996.
129. Hochberg, Z, Chayen R, Reiss N, Falik Z, Makler A, Munichor M, Farkas A, Goldfarb H, Ohana N, Hiort O: Clinical, biochemical, and genetic findings in a large pedigree of male and female patients with 5α-reductase 2 deficiency. *J Clin Endocrinol Metab* **81**:2821, 1996
130. Sinnecker GHG, Hiort O, Dibbelt L, Albers N, Dorr HG, Hauss H, Heinrich U, Hemminghaus M, Hoepffner W, Holder M, Schnabel, Kruse K: Phenotypic classification of male pseudohermaphroditism due to steroid 5α-reductase 2 deficiency. *Am J Med Genet* **63**:223, 1996.
131. Cai LQ, Zhu YS, Katz MD, Herrera C, Baez J, Defillo-Ricart M, Shackleton, Imperato-McGinley J: 5α-Reductase 2 gene mutations in the Dominican Republic. *J Clin Endocrinol Metab* **81**:1730, 1996.
132. Mendonca BB, Inacio M, Costa EMF, Arnhold IVP, Silva FAQ, Nicolau W, Bloise W, Russell DW, Wilson JD: Male pseudohermaphroditism due to steroid 5α-reductase 2 deficiency: Diagnosis, psychological evaluation, and management. *Medicine* **75**:64, 1996.
133. Boudon C, Lumbroso S, Lobaccaro JM, Szarras-Czapnik M, Romer TE, Garrandeau P, Montoya P, Sultan C: Molecular study of the 5α-reductase type 2 gene in three European families with 5α-reductase deficiency. *J Clin Endocrinol Metab* **80**:2149, 1995.
134. Boudon C, Lobaccaro JM, Lumbroso S, Ogur G, Ocal G, Belon C, Sultan C: A new deletion of the 5α-reductase type 2 gene in a Turkish family with 5α-reductase deficiency. *Clin Endocrinol* **43**:183, 1995.
135. Hiort O, Willenbring H, Albers N, Hecker W, Engert J, Dibbelt L, Sinnecker GHG: Molecular genetic analysis and human chorionic gonadotropin stimulation tests in the diagnosis of prepubertal patients with partial 5α-reductase deficiency. *Eur J Pediatr* **155**:445, 1996.
136. Walden U, Rauch R, Hiort O, Sinnecker GH, Dorr HG: Diagnosis of 5α-reductase deficiency in a teenage Turkish girl. *J Pediatr Adolesc Gynecol* **11**:39, 1998.
137. Anwar R, Gilbey SG, New JP, Markham AF: Male pseudohermaphroditism resulting from a novel mutation in the human steroid 5α-reductase type 2 gene (*SRD5A2*). *J Clin Pathol Mol Pathol* **50**:51, 1997.
138. Vilchis F, Canto P, Chavez B, Ulloa-Aguirre A, Mendez JP: Molecular analysis of the 5α-steroid reductase type 2 gene in a family with deficiency of the enzyme. *Am J Med Genet* **69**:69, 1997.
139. Forti G, Falchetti A, Sanforo S, Davis DL, Wilson JD, Russell DW: Steroid 5α-reductase 2 deficiency: Virilization in early infancy may be due to partial function of mutant enzyme. *Clin Endocrinol* **44**:477, 1996.
140. Thigpen AE, Davis DL, Gautier T, Imperato-McGinley J, Russell DW: Brief report: The molecular basis of steroid 5α-reductase deficiency in a large Dominican kindred. *New Engl J Med* **327**:1216, 1992.
141. Can S, Zhu YS, Cai LQ, Ling Q, Katz MD, Akgun S, Shackleton CH, Imperato-McGinley J: The identification of 5α-reductase-2 and 17β-hydroxysteroid dehydrogenase-3 gene defects in male pseudohermaphrotites from a Turkish kindred. *J Clin Endocrinol Metab* **83**:560, 1998
142. Givens JR, Wiser WL, Summitt RL, Kerber IJ, Andersen RN, Pittaway DE, Fich SA: Familial male pseudohermaphroditism without gynecomastia due to deficient testicular 17-ketosteroid reductase activity. *New Engl J Med* **291**:938, 1974.
143. Imperato-McGinley J, Peterson RE, Gautier T, Cooper G, Danner R, Arthur A, Morris PL, Sweeney WJ, Shackleton C: Hormonal evaluation of a large kindred with complete androgen insensitivity: Evidence for secondary 5α-reductase deficiency. *J Clin Endocrinol Metab* **54**:931, 1982.
144. Jukier L, Kaufman M, Pinsky L, Peterson RE: Partial androgen resistance associated with secondary 5α-reductase deficiency: Identification of a novel qualitative androgen receptor defect and clinical implications. *J Clin Endocrinol Metab* **59**:679, 1984.
145. Imperato-McGinley J, Gautier T, Pichardo M, Shackleton C: The diagnosis of 5α-reductase deficiency in infancy. *J Clin Endocrinol Metab* **63**:1313, 1986.
146. Keenan BS, Eberle AJ, Sparrow JT, Greger NG, Panko WB: Dihydrotestosterone heptanoate: Synthesis, pharmacokinetics, and effects on hypothalamic-pituitary-testicular function. *J Clin Endocrinol Metab* **64**:557, 1987.
147. Liao S, Liang T, Fang S, Castaneda E, Shao T-C: Steroid structure and androgenic activity: Specificities involved in the receptor binding and nuclear retention of various androgens. *J Biol Chem* **248**:6154, 1973.
148. Kuhn JM, Rieu M, Laudat MH, Forest MG, Pugeat M, Bricaire H, Luton JP: Effects of 10 days administration of percutaneous dihydrotestosterone on the pituitary-testicular axis of normal men. *J Clin Endocrinol Metab* **58**:231, 1992.
149. Hauser GA: Testicular feminization, in Overzier C (ed): *Intersexuality*. London, Academic Press, 1963, p 255.
150. Pettersson G, Bonnier G: Inherited sex-mosaic in man. *Hereditas* **23**:49, 1937.
151. Simmer HH, Pion RJ, Dignam WJ: *Testicular Feminization: Endocrine Function of Feminizing Testes, Comparison with Normal Testes*. Springfield, IL, Charles C Thomas, 1965, p 1.
152. Viner RM, Teoh Y, Williams DM, Patterson, Hughes IA: Androgen insensitivity syndrome: A survey of diagnostic procedures and management in the U.K. *Arch Dis Child* **77**:305, 1997.
153. Khodr GS: An elderly patient with testicular feminization. *Fertil Steril* **32**:708, 1979.
154. Ulloa-Aguirre A, Mendez JP, Angeles A, del Castillo CE, Chavez B, Perez-Palacios G: The presence of mullerian remnants in the complete androgen insensitivity syndrome: A steroid hormone-mediated defect? *Fertil Steril* **45**:302, 1986.

155. Rutgers JL, Scully RE: The androgen insensitivity syndrome (testicular feminization): A clinicopathologic study of 43 cases. *Int J Gynecol Pathol* **10**:126, 1991.
156. Oka M, Katabuchi H, Munemura M, Mizumoto J, Maeyama M: An unusual case of male pseudohermaphroditism: Complete testicular feminization associated with incomplete differentiation of the mullerian duct. *Fertil Steril* **41**:154, 1984.
157. Dodge ST, Finkelston MS, Miyazawa K: Testicular feminization with incomplete mullerian regression. *Fertil Steril* **43**:937, 1985.
158. Swanson ML, Coronel EH: Complete androgen insensitivity with persistent Müllerian structures. *J Reprod Med* **38**:565, 1993
159. Chen F-P: Testicular feminization with incomplete Müllerian regression in twin patients: Laparoscopic diagnosis and treatment. *Acta Obstet Gynaecol Scand* **75**:304, 1996.
160. Rey R, Mebarki F, Forest MG, Mowszowicz I, Cate RL, Morel Y, Chaussain J-L, Josso N: Anti-Müllerian hormone in children with androgen insensitivity. *J Clin Endocrinol Metab* **79**:960, 1994.
161. Stern ON, Vandervort WJ: Testicular feminization in the male pseudohermaphrodite: Report of a case. *New Engl J Med* **254**:787, 1956.
162. Grumbach MM, Barr ML: Cytologic tests of chromosomal sex in relation to sexual anomalies in man. *Recent Prog Horm Res* **14**:255, 1958.
163. Jacobs PA, Baikie AG, Court Brown WM, Forrest H, Roy JR, Steard JSS, Lennox B: Chromosomal sex in the syndrome of testicular feminisation. *Lancet* **2**:519, 1959.
164. Puck TT, Robinson A, Tjio JH: Familial primary amenorrhea due to testicular feminization: A human gene affecting sex differentiation. *Proc Soc Exp Biol Med* **103**:192, 1960.
165. Ehy C, Grumbach MM, Morishima A: Karyotypic analysis of a male pseudohermaphrodite with the syndrome of feminizing testes. *J Clin Endocrinol Metab* **20**:1608, 1960.
166. Varrela J, Alvesalo L, Vinkka H: Body size and shape in 46,XY females with complete testicular feminization. *Ann Hum Biol* **2**:291, 1984.
167. Alvesalo L, Varrela J: Permanent tooth sizes in 46,XY females. *Am J Hum Genet* **32**:736, 1980.
168. Gron M, Alvesalo L: Dental occlusion and arch size and shape in karyotype 46,XY females. *Eur J Orthod* **19**:329, 1997.
169. Pietila K, Gron M, Alvesalo L: The craniofacial complex in karyotype 46,XY females. *Eur J Orthod* **19**:383, 1997.
170. Zachmann M, Prader A, Sobel EH, Crigler JF Jr, Ritzen EM, Atares M, Ferrandez A: Pubertal growth in patients with androgen insensitivity: Indirect evidence for the importance of estrogens in pubertal growth of girls. *J Pediatr* **108**:694, 1986.
171. Masica DN, Money J, Ehrhardt AA, Lewis VG: IQ, fetal sex hormones and cognitive patterns: Studies in the testicular feminizing syndrome of androgen insensitivity. *Johns Hopkins Med J* **124**:34, 1969.
172. Money J, Ehrhardt AA, Masica DN: Fetal feminization induced by androgen insensitivity in the testicular feminizing syndrome: Effect on marriage and maternalism. *Johns Hopkins Med J* **123**:105, 1968.
173. German J, Simpson JL, Morillo-Cucci G, Passarge E, Demayo AP: Testicular feminisation and inguinal hernia. *Lancet* **1**:891, 1973.
174. Pergament E, Heimler A, Shah P: Testicular feminisation and inguinal hernia. *Lancet* **2**:740, 1973.
175. Imura H, Matsumoto K, Ogata E, Yoshida S, Igarashi Y, Kono T, Matsukura S: "Hormone receptor diseases" in Japan: A nation-wide survey for testicular feminization syndrome, pseudohypoparathyroidism, nephrogenic diabetes insipidus, Bartter's syndrome and congenital adrenocortical unresponsiveness to ACTH. *Folia Endocrinol Jpn* **56**:1031, 1980.
176. Ross GT: Disorders of the ovary and female reproductive tract, in Wilson JD, Foster DW (eds): *Williams' Textbook of Endocrinology.* Philadelphia, Saunders, 1985, p 206.
177. Finkelstein JS, Klibanski A, Neer R: Cortical and trabecular bone density in patients with the complete form of androgen insensitivity syndrome, in *Abstracts of the 9th International Congress of Endocrinology, Nice*, France, August 30–September 5, 1992, p 256.
178. Soule SG, Conway G, Prelevic GM, Prentice M, Ginsburg J, Jacobs HS: Osteopenia as a feature of the androgen insensitivity syndrome. *Clin Endocrinol* **43**:671, 1995.
179. Munoz-Torres M, Jodar E, Quesada M, Escobar-Jiminez F: Bone mass in androgen-insensitivity syndrome: Response to hormonal replacement therapy. *Calcif Tissue Int* **57**:94, 1995.
180. Schreiner WE: On a hereditary form of male pseudohermaphroditism ("testicular feminization"). *Geburtshilfe Frauenheikld* **19**:1110, 1959.
181. Gwinup G, Wieland RG, Besch PK, Hamwi GJ: Studies on the mechanism of the production of the testicular feminization syndrome. *Am J Med* **41**:448, 1966.
182. Vagenakis AG, Hamilton C, Maloof F, Braverman LE, Ingbar SH: The concentration and binding of thyroxine in the serum of patients with the testicular feminization syndrome: Observations on the effects of ethinyl estradiol and norethandrolone. *J Clin Endocrinol Metab* **34**:327, 1972.
183. Tremblay RR, Schlaeder G, Dussault JH: Effects de l'ethynil estradiol et des androgenes sur les parametres de la fonction throidienne dans le syndrome de pseudohermaphrodisme male avec feminisation testiculaire. *Union Med Can* **103**:421, 1974.
184. Faiman C, Winter JSD: The control of gonadotropin secretion in complete testicular feminization. *J Clin Endocrinol* **39**:631, 1974.
185. French FS, Van Wyk JJ, Baggett V, Esterling WE, Talbert LM, Johnston FR, Forchielli E, Dey AC: Further evidence of a target organ defect in the syndrome of testicular feminization. *J Clin Endocrinol Metab* **26**:493, 1966.
186. Volpe R, Knowlton TG, Foster AD, Conen PE: Testicular feminization: A study of two cases, one with a seminoma. *Can Med Assoc J* **98**:438, 1968.
187. Castaneda E, Perez AE, Guillen MA, Ramirez-Robles S, Gual C, Perez-Palacios G: Metabolic studies in a patient with testicular feminization syndrome. *Am J Obstet Gynecol* **110**:1002, 1971.
188. Siegler RW, Beecham JB, Schned AR: Corpus albicans-like structures in the gonads in androgen insensitivity syndrome. *Int J Gynaecol Pathol* **15**:177, 1996.
189. O'Leary JA: Comparative studies of the gonad in testicular feminization and cryptorchidism. *Fertil Steril* **16**:813, 1965.
190. Justrabo E, Cabanne F, Michiels R, Bastien H, Dusserre P, Pansiot F, Cayot F: A complete form of testicular feminisation syndrome: A light and electron microscopy study. *J Pathol* **126**:165, 1978.
191. Faulds JS, Lennoz B: Leydig-cell hyperplasia in testicular feminisation. *Lancet* **1**:344, 1971.
192. Collins GM, Kim DU, Logrono R, Rickert RB, Zablow A, Breen JL: Pure seminoma arising in androgen insensitivity syndrome (testicular feminization syndrome): A case report and review of the literature. *Mod Pathol* **6**:89, 1993
193. McNeill SA, O'Donnell M, Donat R, Lessels A, Hargreave TB: Estrogen secretion from a malignant sex cord stromal tumor in a patient with complete androgen insensitivity. *Am J Obstet Gynecol* **177**:1542, 1997,
194. Morris JM, Mahesh VB: Further observations on the syndrome, "testicular feminization." *Am J Obstet Gynecol* **87**:731, 1963.
195. Rosenfeld RL, Lawrence AM, Liao S, Landau RL: Androgens and androgen responsiveness in the feminizing testis syndrome: Comparison of complete and "incomplete" forms. *J Clin Endocrinol Metab* **32**:625, 1971.
196. Crawford JD, Adams RD, Kliman B, Federman DD, Ulfelder HS, Holmes LH: Syndromes of testicular feminization. *Clin Pediatr (Phila)* **9**:165, 1970.
197. Winterborn MH, France NE, Raiti S: Incomplete testicular feminization. *Arch Dis Child* **45**:811, 1970.
198. Madden JD, Walsh PC, MacDonald PC, Wilson JD: Clinical and endocrinological characterization of a patient with the syndrome of incomplete testicular feminization. *J Clin Endocrinol Metab* **40**:751, 1975.
199. Reifenstein EC Jr: Hereditary familial hypogonadism. *Clin Res* **3**:86, 1947.
200. Bowen P, Lee CSN, Migeon CJ, Kaplan NM, Whalley PJ, McKusick VA, Reifenstein EC Jr: Hereditary male pseudohermaphroditism with hypogonadism, hypospadias, and gynecomastia (Reifenstein's syndrome). *Ann Intern Med* **62**:252, 1965.
201. Lubs HA Jr, Vilar O, Bergenstal DM: Familial male pseudohermaphroditism, hypospadias, and gynecomastia (Reifenstein's syndrome). *Ann Intern Med* **62**:252, 1965.
202. Gilbert-Dreyfus S, Sebaoun CA, Belaisch J: Etude d'un cas familial d'androgynoidisme avec hypospadias grave, gynecomastie et hyperoestrogenie. *Ann Endocrinol (Paris)* **18**:93, 1957.
203. Rosewater S, Gwinup G, Hamwi GJ: Familial gynecomastia. *Ann Intern Med* **63**:377, 1965.
204. Wilson JD, Harrod MJ, Goldstein JL, Hemsell DL, MacDonald PC: Familial incomplete male pseudohermaphroditism, type I: Evidence for androgen resistance and variable clinical manifestations in a family with the Reifenstein syndrome. *New Engl J Med* **290**:1097, 1974.
205. Ford E: Congenital abnormalities of the genitalia in related Bathurst Island natives. *Med J Aust* **1**:450, 1941.

206. Walker AC, Stack EM, Horsfall WA: Familial male pseudohermaphroditism. *Med J Aust* **1**:156, 1970.
207. Gardo S, Papp Z: Clinical variations of testicular intersexuality in a family. *J Med Genet* **11**:267, 1974.
208. Perez-Palacios G, Ortiz S, Lopez-Amor E, Morato T, Febres F, Lisker R, Scaglia H: Familial incomplete virilization due to partial end organ insensitivity to androgens. *J Clin Endocrinol Metab* **41**:946, 1975.
209. Pittaway DE, Stage AH: Familial male pseudohermaphroditism with incomplete virilization. *Obstet Gynecol* **51**:82S, 1978.
210. Jockenhovel JKL, Rutgers JS, Griffin JE, Swerdloff RS: Leydig cell neoplasia in a patient with Reifenstein syndrome. *Exp Clin Endocrinol* **101**:365, 1993.
211. Griffin JE, Punyashthiti K, Wilson JD: Dihydrotestosterone binding by cultured human fibroblasts: Comparison of cells from control subjects and from patients with hereditary male pseudohermaphroditism due to androgen resistance. *J Clin Invest* **57**:1342, 1976.
212. Aiman J, Griffin JE, Gazak JM, Wilson JD, MacDonald PC: Androgen insensitivity as a cause of infertility in otherwise normal men. *New Engl J Med* **300**:223, 1979.
213. Warne GL, Khalid BAK, Gyorki S, Funder JW, Risbridger GP: Correlations between fibroblast androgen receptor levels and clinical features in abnormal male sexual differentiation and infertility. *Aust NZ J Med* **13**:335, 1983.
214. Pinsky L, Kaufman M, Killinger DW, Burko B, Shatz D, Volpe RP: Human minimal androgen insensitivity with normal dihydrotestosterone-binding capacity in cultured genital skin fibroblasts: Evidence for an androgen-selective qualitative abnormality of the receptor. *Am J Hum Genet* **36**:965, 1984.
215. Migeon CJ, Brown TR, Lanes R, Palcios A, Amrhein JA, Schjoen EJ: A clinical syndrome of mild androgen insensitivity. *J Clin Endocrinol Metab* **59**:672, 1984.
216. Smallridge RC, Vigersky R, Glass AR, Griffin JE, White BJ, Eil C: Androgen receptor abnormalities in identical twins with oligospermia. *Am J Med* **77**:1049, 1984.
217. Cundy TF, Rees M, Evans BAJ, Hughes IA, Butler J, Wheeler MJ: Mild androgen insensitivity presenting with sexual dysfunction. *Fertil Steril* **46**:721, 1986.
218. Grino PB, Griffin JE, Cushard WG Jr, Wilson JD: A mutation of the androgen receptor associated with partial androgen resistance, familial gynecomastia, and fertility. *J Clin Endocrinol Metab* **66**:754, 1982.
219. Pinsky L, Kaufman M, Killinger DW: Impaired spermatogenesis is not an obligate expression of receptor-defective androgen resistance. *Am J Med Genet* **32**:100, 1989.
220. Tsukada T, Inoue M, Tachibana S, Nakai Y, Takebe H: An androgen receptor mutation causing androgen resistance in undervirilized male syndrome. *J Clin Endocrinol Metab* **79**:1202, 1994.
221. Tut TG, Ghadessy FJ, Trifiro MA, Pinsky L, Yong EL: Long polyglutamine tracts in the androgen receptor are associated with reduced trans-activation, impaired sperm production, and male infertility. *J Clin Endocrinol Metab* **82**:3777, 1997.
222. Aiman J, Griffin JE: The frequency of androgen receptor deficiency in infertile men. *J Clin Endocrinol Metab* **54**:725, 1982.
223. Morrow AF, Gyorki S, Warne GL, Burger HG, Bangah ML, Outch KH, Mirovics A, Baker HWG: Variable androgen receptor levels in infertile men. *J Clin Endocrinol Metab* **64**:1115, 1987.
224. Southren AL, Ross H, Sharma DC, Gordon G, Weingold AB, Dorfman RI: Plasma concentration and biosynthesis of testosterone in the syndrome of feminizing testes. *J Clin Endocrinol Metab* **23**:1044, 1963.
225. Jeffcoate SL, Brooks RV, Prunty FTG: Secretion of androgens and oestrogens in testicular feminization: Studies in vivo and in vitro in two cases. *Br Med J* **1**:208, 1968.
226. Tremblay RR, Foley TP Jr, Corvol P, Park IJ, Kowarski A, Blizzard RM, Jones HW Jr, Migeon CJ: Plasma concentration of testosterone, dihydrotestosterone, testosterone-oestradiol binding globulin, and pituitary gonadotropins in the syndrome of male pseudohermaphroditism with testicular feminization. *Acta Endocrinol (Copenh)* **70**:331, 1972.
227. Tremblay RR, Kowarski A, Park IJ, Migeon CJ: Blood production rate of dihydrotestosterone in the syndrome of male pseudohermaphroditism with testicular feminization. *J Clin Endocrinol Metab* **35**:101, 1972.
228. Boyar RM, Moore RJ, Rosner W, Aiman J, Chipman J, Madden JD, Marks JF, Griffin JE: Studies of gonadotropin-gonadal dynamics in patients with androgen insensitivity. *J Clin Endocrinol Metab* **47**:1116, 1978.
229. Laatikainen T, Apter D, Wahlstrom T: Steroids in spermatic and peripheral vein blood in testicular feminization. *Fertil Steril* **34**:461, 1980.
230. Zarate A, Canales ES, Soria J, Carballo O: Studies on the luteinizing hormone- and follicle-stimulating hormone-releasing mechanism in the testicular feminization syndrome. *Am J Obstet Gynecol* **119**:971, 1974.
231. Schmitt S, Knorr D, Schwarz HP, Kuhnle U: Gonadotropin regulation during puberty in complete androgen insensitivity syndrome with testicles in situ. *Horm Res* **42**:253, 1994.
232. Medina M, Ulloa-Aguirre A, Fernandez MA, Perez-Palacios G: The role of oestrogens on gonadotropin secretion in the testicular feminization syndrome. *Acta Endocrinol (Copenh)* **95**:314, 1980.
233. Gunasegaram R, Loganath A, Peh KL, Sinniah R, Kottegoda SR, Ratnam SS: Altered hypothalamic-pituitary-testicular function in incomplete testicular feminization syndrome. *Aust NZ J Obstet Gynaecol* **24**:288, 1984.
234. Fredricsson B, Carlstrom K, Kjessler B, Lindstedt J, Ploen L, Ritzen M, de la Torre B: Incomplete androgen insensitivity: Asymmetry in morphology and steroid profile and metabolism of the gonads. An analysis of a case. *Acta Endocrinol (Oxf)* **110**:564, 1985.
235. Hochman J, Ganguly M, Weiss G: Induction of an LH surge with estradiol benzoate in a patient with incomplete testicular feminization syndrome. *Obstet Gynecol* **49**:17S, 1977.
236. Flatau E, Josefsberg Z, Prager-Lewin R, Markman-Halabe E, Kaufman H, Laron Z: Response to LH-RH and HCG in two brothers with the Reifenstein syndrome. *Helv Paediatr Acta* **30**:377, 1975.
237. Medina M, Castorena G, Herrera J, Bermudez JA, Zarate A: Modulation of luteinizing hormone secretion by estrogens in patients with Reifenstein's syndrome. *Fertil Steril* **52**:239, 1989.
238. Leonard JM, Bremner WJ, Capell PT, Paulsen CA: Male hypogonadism: Klinefelter and Reifenstein syndromes. *Birth Defects* **11(4)**:17, 1975.
239. Northcutt RC, Island DP, Liddle GW: An explanation for the target organ unresponsiveness to testosterone in the testicular feminization syndrome. *J Clin Endocrinol Metab* **24**:422, 1969.
240. Mauvais-Jarvis P, Floch HH, Bercovici J-P: Studies on testosterone metabolism in human subjects with normal and pathological sexual differentiation. *J Clin Endocrinol Metab* **29**:422, 1969.
241. Mauvais-Jarvis P, Vercovici JP, Crepy O, Gauthier F: Studies on testosterone metabolism in subjects with testicular feminization syndrome. *J Clin Invest* **49**:31, 1970.
242. Pinsky L, Kaufman M, Staisfeld C, Zilahi B, Hall CSt-G: 5α-Reductase activity of genital and nongenital skin fibroblasts from patients with 5α-reductase deficiency, androgen insensitivity, or unknown forms of male pseudohermaphroditism. *Am J Med Genet* **1**:407, 1978.
243. Keenan BS, Meyer WJ III, Hadjian AJ, Jones HW, Migeon CJ: Syndrome of androgen insensitivity in man: Absence of 5α-dihydrotestosterone binding protein in skin fibroblasts. *J Clin Endocrinol Metab* **38**:1143, 1974.
244. Keenan BS, Meyer WJ III, Hadjian AJ, Migeon CJ: Androgen receptor in human skin fibroblasts: Characterization of a specific 17β-hydroxy-5α-androstan-3-one-protein complex in cell sonicates and nuclei. *Steroids* **25**:535, 1975.
245. Kaufman M, Straisfeld C, Pinsky L: Male pseudohermaphroditism presumably due to target organ unresponsiveness to androgens: Deficient 5α-dihydrotestosterone binding in cultured skin fibroblasts. *J Clin Invest* **58**:345, 1976.
246. Griffin JE: Testicular feminization associated with a thermolabile androgen receptor in cultured human fibroblasts. *J Clin Invest* **64**:1624, 1979.
247. Brown TR, Maes M, Rothwell SW, Migeon CJ: Human complete androgen insensitivity with normal dihydrotestosterone receptor binding capacity in cultured genital skin fibroblasts: Evidence for a qualitative abnormality of the receptor. *J Clin Endocrinol Metab* **55**:61, 1982.
248. Evans BAJ, Jones TR, Hughes IA: Studies of the androgen receptor in dispersed fibroblasts: Investigation of patients with androgen insensitivity. *Clin Endocrinol (Oxf)* **20**:93, 1984.
249. Griffin JE, Durrant JL: Qualitative receptor defects in families with androgen resistance: Failure of stabilization of the fibroblast cytosol androgen receptor. *J Clin Endocrinol Metab* **55**:465, 1982.
250. Schweikert H-U, Weissbach L, Stangenberg C, Leyendecker G, Kley H-K, Griffin JE, Wilson JD: Clinical and endocrinological characterization of two subjects with Reifenstein syndrome associated with qualitative abnormalities of the androgen receptor. *Horm Res* **25**:72, 1987.

251. Kaufman M, Pinsky L, Bowin A, Au MWS: Familial external genital ambiguity due to a transformation defect of androgen-receptor complexes that is expressed with 5α-dihydrotestosterone and the synthetic androgen methyltrienolone. *Am J Med Genet* **18**:493, 1984.
252. Pinsky L, Kaufman M, Chudley AE: Reduced affinity of the androgen receptor for 5α-dihydrotestosterone but not methyltrienolone in a form of partial androgen resistance. *J Clin Invest* **75**:1291, 1985.
253. Bals-Pratsch M, Schweikert H-U, Nieschlag E: Androgen receptor disorder in three brothers with bifid prepenile scrotum and hypospadias. *Acta Endocrinol (Copenh)* **123**:271, 1990.
254. Eil C: Familial incomplete male pseudohermaphroditism associated with impaired nuclear androgen retention. *J Clin Invest* **71**:850, 1983.
255. Kaufman M, Pinsky L, Feder-Hollander R: Defective up-regulation of the androgen receptor in human androgen insensitivity. *Nature* **293**:735, 1981.
256. Kaufman M, Pinsky L, Hollander R, Bailey JD: Regulation of the androgen receptor by androgen in normal and androgen-resistant genital skin fibroblasts. *J Steroid Biochem* **18**:383, 1983.
257. Kaufman M, Pinsky L, Killinger DW: Ligand-specific thermal misbehavior of synthetic androgen-receptor complexes in genital skin fibroblasts of subjects with familial ligand-sensitive androgen resistance. *J Steroid Biochem* **25**:323, 1986.
258. Evans BAJ, Hughes IA: Augmentation of androgen-receptor binding in vitro: Studies in normals and patients with androgen insensitivity. *Clin Endocrinol (Oxf)* **23**:567, 1985.
259. Jukier L, Kaufman M, Pinsky L, Peterson RE: Partial androgen resistance associated with secondary 5α-reductase deficiency: Identification of a novel qualitative androgen receptor defect and clinical implications. *J Clin Endocrinol Metab* **59**:679, 1984.
260. Kaufman M, Pinsky L, Simard L, Wong SC: Defective activation of androgen-receptor complexes: A marker of androgen insensitivity. *Mol Cell Endocrinol* **25**:151, 1982.
261. Pinsky L, Kaufman M, Summitt RL: Congenital androgen insensitivity due to a qualitatively abnormal androgen receptor. *Am J Med Genet* **10**:91, 1981.
262. Grino PB, Isidro-Gutierrez RF, Griffin JE, Wilson JD: Androgen resistance associated with a qualitative abnormality of the androgen receptor and responsive to high dose androgen therapy. *J Clin Endocrinol Metab* **68**:578, 1989.
263. Grino PB, Griffin JE, Wilson JD: Androgen resistance due to decreased amounts of androgen receptor: A reinvestigation. *J Steroid Biochem* **35**:647, 1990.
264. Amrhein JA, Meyer WJ III, Jones HW Jr, Midgeon JC: Androgen insensitivity in man: Evidence for genetic heterogeneity. *Proc Natl Acad Sci USA* **73**:891, 1976.
265. Collier ME, Griffin JE, Wilson JD: Intranuclear binding of [^{3}H]dihydrotestosterone by cultured human fibroblasts. *Endocrinology* **103**:1499, 1978.
266. Keenan BS, Kirkland JL, Kirkland RT, Clayton GW: Male pseudohermaphroditism with partial androgen insensitivity. *Pediatrics* **59**:224, 1977.
267. Maes M, Lee PA, Jeffs RD, Sultan C, Migeon CJ: Phenotypic variation in a family with partial androgen insensitivity syndrome. *Am J Dis Child* **134**:470, 1980.
268. Kaufman M, Pinsky L, Baird PA, McGillivray BC: Complete androgen insensitivity with a normal amount of 5α-dihydrotestosterone-binding activity in labium majus skin fibroblasts. *Am J Med Genet* **4**:401, 1979.
269. Brown TR, Rothwell SW, Migeon CJ: Human androgen insensitivity mutation does not alter oligonucleotide recognition by the androgen receptor-DHT complex. *Mol Cell Endocrinol* **32**:215, 1983.
270. Grunstein HS, Warne GL, Gyorki S, Clifton-Gligh P, Posen S: "Receptor positive" androgen insensitivity: Report of a case with brief review of the literature. *Aust NZ J Med* **12**:289, 1982.
271. Brown TR, Migeon CJ: Androgen binding in nuclear matrix of human genital skin fibroblasts from patients with androgen insensitivity syndrome. *J Clin Endocrinol Metab* **62**:542, 1986.
272. Gyorki S, Warne GL, Khalid BAK, Funder JW: Defective nuclear accumulation of androgen receptors in disorders of sexual differentiation. *J Clin Invest* **72**:819, 1983.
273. Hughes IA, Evans BAJ, Ismail R, Matthews J: Complete androgen insensitivity syndrome characterized by increased concentration of a normal androgen receptor in genital skin fibroblasts. *J Clin Endocrinol Metab* **63**:309, 1986.
274. Schultz MG: Male pseudohermaphroditism diagnosed with aid of sex chromatin technique. *J Am Vet Med Assoc* **140**:241, 1962.
275. New N: Testikulaer feminisering hos storfe. *Nord Vet Med* **18**:19, 1966.
276. Bardin CW, Bullock L, Schneider G, Allison JE, Stanley AJ: Pseudohermaphrodite rat: End-organ insensitivity to testosterone. *Science* **167**:1136, 1970.
277. Lyon MF, Hawkes SG: X-linked gene for testicular feminization in the mouse. *Nature* **227**:1217, 1970.
278. Politch JA, Fox TO, Houben P, Bullock L, Lovell D: *TfmLac*: A second isolation of testicular feminization in mice. *Biochem Genet* **26**:213, 1988.
279. Kieffer NM, Burns SJ, Judge NG: Male pseudohermaphroditism of the testicular feminizing type in a horse. *Equine Vet J* **8**:38, 1976.
280. Eil C, Merriam GR, Bowen J, Ebert J, Tabor E, White B, Douglass EC, Loriaux DL: Testicular feminization in the chimpanzee. *Clin Res* **28**:624A, 1980.
281. van Vlissingen JMF, Blankenstein MA, Thijssen JHH, Colenbrander B, Verbruggen AJEP, Wensing CJG: Familial male pseudohermaphroditism and testicular descent in the racoon dog (*Nyctereutes*). *Anat Rec* **222**:350, 1988.
282. Meyers-Wallen VN, Wilson JD, Griffin JE, Fisher S, Moorhead PH, Goldschmidt MH, Haskins ME, Patterson DF: Testicular feminization in a cat. *J Am Vet Med Assoc* **195**:631, 1989.
283. Ohno S: *Major Sex-Determining Genes*. New York, Springer-Verlag, 1979.
284. Meyer WJ III, Migeon BR, Migeon CJ: Locus on human X chromosome for dihydrotestosterone receptor and androgen insensitivity. *Proc Natl Acad Sci USA* **72**:1469, 1975.
285. Lyon MF: X-chromosome inactivation and developmental patterns in mammals. *Biol Rev* **14**:1, 1972.
286. Migeon BR, Brown TR, Axelman J, Migeon CJ: Studies of the locus for androgen receptor: Localization on the human X chromosome and evidence for homology with the *Tfm* locus in the mouse. *Proc Natl Acad Sci USA* **78**:6339, 1981.
287. El Awady MK, Allman DR, Griffin JE, Wilson JD: Expression of a mutant androgen receptor in cloned fibroblasts derived from a heterozygous carrier for the syndrome of testicular feminization. *Am J Hum Genet* **35**:376, 1983.
288. Wieacker P, Griffin JE, Wienker T, Lopez JM, Wilson JD, Breckwoldt M: Linkage analysis with RFLPs in families with androgen resistance syndromes: Evidence for close linkage between the androgen receptor locus and the DXS1 segment. *Hum Genet* **76**:248, 1987.
289. Wilson JD, Carlson BR, Weaver DD, Kovacs WJ, Griffin JE: Endocrine and genetic characterization of cousins with male pseudohermaphroditism: Evidence that the Lubs phenotype can result from a mutation that alters the structure of the androgen receptor. *Clin Genet* **26**:363, 1984.
290. Lubahn DB, Brown TR, Simental JA, Higgs JA, Migeon CJ, Wilson EM: Sequence of the intron/exon junctions of the coding region of the human androgen receptor gene and identification of a point mutation in a family with complete androgen insensitivity. *Proc Natl Acad Sci USA* **86**:9534, 1989.
291. Marcelli M, Tilley WD, Wilson CM, Griffin JE, Wilson JD, McPhaul MJ: Definition of the human androgen receptor gene structure permits the identification of mutations that cause androgen resistance: Premature termination of the receptor protein at amino acid residue 588 causes complete androgen resistance. *Mol Endocrinol* **4**:1105, 1990.
292. Kuiper GGJM, Faber PW, van Rooij HCJ, van der Korput JA, Ris-Stalpers C, Klaassen P, Trapman J, Brinkmann AO: Structural organization of the androgen receptor gene. *J Mol Endocrinol* **2**:R1, 1989.
293. Marcelli M, Tilley WD, Zoppi S, Griffin JE, Wilson JD, McPhaul MJ: Androgen resistance associated with a mutation of the androgen receptor at amino acid 772 (Arg-Cys) results from a combination of decreased messenger ribonucleic acid levels and impairment of receptor function. *J Clin Endocrinol Metab* **73**:318, 1991.
294. Wilson CM, Griffin JE, Wilson JD, Marcelli M, Zoppi S, McPhaul MJ: Immunoreactive androgen receptor expression in patients with androgen resistance. *J Clin Endocrinol Metab* **75**:1474, 1992.
295. Marcelli M, Zoppi S, Grino PB, Griffin JE, Wilson JD, McPhaul MJ: A mutation in the DNA-binding domain of the androgen receptor gene causes complete testicular feminization in a patient with receptor-positive androgen resistance. *J Clin Invest* **87**:1123, 1991.
296. Zoppi S, Marcelli M, Deslypere J-P, Griffin JE, Wilson JD, McPhaul MJ: Amino acid substitutions in the DNA-binding domain of the human androgen receptor are a frequent cause of receptor-binding positive androgen resistance. *Mol Endocrinol* **6**:409, 1992.
297. McPhaul MJ, Sehweikert H-U, Allman DR: Assessment of androgen receptor function in genital skin fibroblasts using a recombinant

adenovirus to deliver an androgen-responsive-reporter gene. *J Clin Endocrinol Metab* **82**:1944, 1997.
298. Ris-Stalpers C, Hoogenboezem T, Sleddens, HFBM, Verleun-Mooijman MCT, Degenhart HJ, Drop SLS, Halley DJJ, Oosterwijk JC, Hodgins MB, Trapman J, Brinkmann AO: A practical approach to the detection of androgen receptor gene mutations and pedigree analysis in families with X-linked androgen insensitivity. *Pediatr Res* **36**:227, 1994.
299. McPhaul MJ, Marcelli M, Zoppi S, Griffin JE, Wilson JD: The spectrum of mutations in the androgen receptor gene that causes androgen resistance. *J Clin Endocrinol Metab* **76**:17, 1993.
300. Quigley CA, DeBellis A, Marschke KB, El-Awady MK, Wilson EM, French FS: Androgen receptor defects: Historical, clinical, and molecular perspectives. *Endocrine Rev* **16**:271, 1995.
301. Gottlieb B, Beitel LK, Lumbroso R, Pinsky, Trifiro M: Update of the androgen receptor gene mutations database. *Hum Mut* **14**:103, 1999.
302. Quigley CA, Friedman KJ, Johnson A, Lafreniere RG, Silverman LM, Lubahn DB, Brown TR, Wilson EM, Willard HF, French FS: Complete deletion of the androgen receptor gene: Definition of the null phenotype of the androgen insensitivity syndrome and determination of carrier status. *J Clin Endocrinol Metab* **74**:927, 1992.
303. Trifiro M, Gottlieb B, Pinsky L, et al: The 56/58 kDa androgen-binding protein in male genital skin fibroblasts with a deleted androgen receptor gene. *Mol Cell Endocrinol* **75**:37, 1991.
304. Davies HR, Hughes IA, Savage MO, Quigley CA, Trifiro M, Pinsky L, Brown TR, Patterson MN: Androgen insensitivity with mental retardation: A contiguous gene syndrome? *J Med Genet* **34**:158, 1997.
305. Quigley CA, Evans BAJ, Simental JA, Marschke KB, Sar M, Lubahn DB, Davies P, Hughes IA, Wilson EM, French FS: Complete androgen insensitivity due to deletion of exon C of the androgen receptor gene highlights the functional importance of the second zinc finger of the androgen receptor in vivo. *Mol Endocrinol* **6**:1103, 1992.
306. He WW, Kumar MV, Tindall DJ: A frame-shift mutation in the androgen receptor gene causes complete androgen insensitivity in the testicular-feminized mouse. *Nucl Acids Res* **19**:2373, 1991.
307. Gaspar M-L, Meo T, Bourgarel P, Guenet J-L, Tosi M: A single base deletion in the *Tfm* androgen receptor gene creates a short-lived messenger RNA that directs internal translation initiation. *Proc Natl Acad Sci USA* **88**:8606, 1991.
308. Charest NJ, Zhou Z-X, Lubahn DB, Olsen KL, Wilson EM, French FS: A frameshift mutation destabilizes androgen receptor messenger RNA in the *Tfm* mouse. *Mol Endocrinol* **5**:573, 1991.
309. Zoppi S, Wilson CM, Harbison MD, Griffin JE, Wilson JD, McPhaul MJ, Marcelli M: Complete testicular feminization caused by an amino terminal truncation of the androgen receptor with downstream initiation. *J Clin Invest* **91**:1105, 1993.
310. Gao T, McPhaul MJ: Functional activities of the A and B forms of the human androgen receptor in response to androgen receptor agonists and antagonists. *Mol Endocrinol* **12**:654, 1998.
311. Wilson CM, McPhaul MJ: A and B forms of the androgen receptor are expressed in a variety of human tissues. *Mol Cell Endocrinol* **12**:51, 1996.
312. Nakao R, Haji M, Yanase T, et al: A single amino acid substitution (Met786-Val) in the steroid-binding domain of the human androgen receptor leads to complete androgen insensitivity syndrome. *J Clin Endocrinol Metab* **74**:1152, 1992.
313. Ris-Stalpers C, Trifiro MA, Kuiper GGJM, Jenster G, Romalo G, Sai T, van Rooij HCJ, Kaufman M, Rosenfield RL, Liao S, Schweikert H-U, Trapman J, Pinsky L, Brinkmann AO: Substitution of aspartic acid-686 by histidine or asparagine in the human androgen receptor leads to a functionally inactive protein with altered hormone-binding domain characteristics. *Mol Endocrinol* **5**:1562, 1991.
314. McPhaul MJ, Marcelli M, Tilley WD, Griffin JE, Isidro-Guiterrez RF, Wilson JD: Molecular basis of androgen resistance in a family with a qualitative abnormality of the androgen receptor and responsive to high-dose androgen therapy. *J Clin Invest* **87**:1413, 1991.
315. Prior L, Bordet S, Trifiro MA, Mhatre A, Kaufman M, Pinsky L, Wrogeman K, Belsham DD, Pereira F, Greenberg C, Trapman J, Brinkmann AO, Chang C, Liao S: Replacement of arginine 773 by cysteine or histidine in the human androgen receptor causes complete androgen insensitivity with different receptor phenotypes. *Am J Hum Genet* **51**:143, 1992.
316. Ris-Stalpers C, Verleun-Mooijman MCT, De Blaeij TJP, Degenhart HG, Trapman J, Brinkmann AO: Differential splicing of human androgen receptor pre-mRNA in X-linked Reifenstein syndrome, because of a deletion involving a putative branch site. *Am J Hum Genet* **54**:609, 1994.
317. Bruggenwirth HT, Boehmer AKM, Ramnarain S, Verleun-Mooijman, Satijn DPE, Trapman J, Grootegoed JA, Brinkmann AO: Molecular analysis of the androgen-receptor gene in a family with receptor-positive partial androgen insensitivity: An unusual type of intronic mutation. *Am J Hum Genet* **61**:1067, 1997.
318. Holterhus P-M, Bruggenwirth HT, Hiort O, Kleinkauf-Houcken A, Kruse K, Sinnecker GHG, Brinkmann AO: Mosaicism due to a somatic mutation of the androgen receptor gene determines phenotype in androgen insensitivity syndrome. *J Clin Endocrinol* **82**:3584, 1997.
319. Choong CS, Sturm MJ, Strophair JA, Mc Cullough RK, Hurley DM: Reduced expression and normal nucleotide sequence of androgen receptor gene coding and promoter regions in a family with partial androgen insensitivity syndrome. *Clin Endocrinol* **46**:281, 1997.
320. Meier CA, Dickstein BM, Ashizawa K, Mc Claskey JH, Muchmore P, Ransom SC, Menke JB, Hao E-H, Usala SJ, Bercu BB, Cheng S-Y, Weintraub BD: Variable transcriptional activity and ligand binding of mutant β13,5,3′-triiodothyronine receptors from four families with generalized resistance to thyroid hormone. *Mol Endocrinol* **6**:248, 1992.
321. McPhaul MJ, Marcelli M, Zoppi S, Wilson CM, Griffin JE, Wilson JD: Mutations in the ligand-binding domain of the androgen receptor gene cluster in two regions of the gene. *J Clin Invest* **90**:2097, 1992.
322. Jenster g, Van der Korput HA, van Vroonhoven C, van der Swast TH, Trapman J, Brinkman AO: Domains of the human androgen receptor involved in steroid binding, transcription activation, and subcellular localization. *Mol Endocrinol* **5**:1396, 1991.
323. Simental JA, Sar M, Lane MV, French FS, Wilson EM: Transcriptional activation and nuclear targeting sigfnals of the human androgen receptor. *J Biol Chem* **266**:510, 1991.
324. Gao TS, Marcelli M, McPhaul MJ: Transcriptional activation and transient expression of the human androgen receptor. *J Steroid Biochem Mol Biol* **59**:9, 1996.
325. Hiort O, Sinnecker HG, Holterbus P-M, Nitsche EM, Kruse K: Inherited and *de novo* androgen receptor gene mutations: Investigation of single-case families. *J Pediatr* **131**:939, 1998.
326. Boehmer ALM, Brinkmann AO, Niermeijer MF, Bakker L, Halley DJJ, Drop SLS: Germ-line and somatic mosaicism in the androgen insensitivity syndrome: Implications for genetic counseling. *Am J Hum Genet* **60**:1003, 1997.
327. Leslie ND: Haldane was right: *De novo* mutations in androgen insensitivity syndrome. *J Pediatr* **131**:917, 1998.
328. Griffin JE, Edwards C, Madden JD, Harrold MJ, Wilson JD: Congenital absence of the vagina: The Mayer-Rokitansky-Kuster-Howard syndrome. *Ann Intern Med* **85**:224, 1976.
329. Hales ED, Rosser SB: Computed tomography of testicular feminization. *J Comput Assist Tomogr* **8**:772, 1984.
330. Nagel BA, Lippe BM, Griffin JE: Androgen resistance in the neonate: Use of hormones of hypothalamic-pituitary-gonadal axis for diagnosis. *J Pediatr* **109**:486, 1986.
331. Lee PA, Brown TR, Latorre HA: Diagnosis of the partial androgen insensitivity syndrome during infancy. *JAMA* **255**:2207, 1986.
332. Berkovitz GD, Lee PA, Brown TR, Migeon CJ: Etiologic evaluation of male pseudohermaphroditism in infancy and childhood. *Am J Dis Child* **138**:755, 1984.
333. Lumbroso S, Lobaccaro J-M, Belon C, et al: Molecular prenatal exclusion of familial partial androgen insensitivity (Reifenstein syndrome). *Eur J Endocrinol* **130**:327, 1994.
334. Lobaccaro J-M, Belon C, Lumbroso S, Olewniczack G, Carre-Pigeon F, Job J-C, Chaussain J-L, Toublanc J-E, Sultan C: Molecular prenatal diagnosis of partial androgen insensitivity syndrome. *Clin Endocrinol* **40**:297, 1994.
335. Batch JA, Davies HR, Evans BAJ, Hughes IA, Patterson MN: Phenotypic variation and detection of carrier status in the partial androgen insensitivity syndrome. *Arch Dis Child* **68**:453, 1993.
336. Lobaccaro JM, Lumbroso S, Pigeon FC, et al: Prenatal prediction of androgen insensitivity syndrome using exon 1 polymorphism of the androgen receptor gene. *J Steroid Biochem* **43**:659, 1992.
337. Bertelloni S, Federico G, Baroncelli GI, Cavallo L, Corsello G, Liotta A, Rigon F, Saggese G: Biochemical selection of prepubertal patients with androgen insensitivity syndrome by sex hormone-binding response to human chorionic gonadotropin test. *Pediatr Res* **41**:266, 1997.
338. Sinnecker GHG, Hiort O, Nitsche EM, Holterhus P-M, Kruse K: Functional assessment and clinical classification of androgen sensitivity in patients with mutations of the androgen receptor gene. *Eur J Pediatr* **156**:7, 1997.

339. Tincello DG, Saunders PTK, Hodgins MB, Simpson NB, Edwards CRW, Hargreaves TB, Wu FCW: Correlation of clinical, endocrine and molecular abnormalities with in vivo responses to high-dose testosterone in patients with partial androgen insensitivity syndrome. *Clin Endocrinol* **46**:497, 1997.
340. Wabrek AJ, Millard PR, Wilson WB Jr, Pion RJ: Creation of a neovagina by the Frank nonoperative method. *Obstet Gynecol* **37**:408, 1971.
341. Costa EMF, Arnhold IJP, Mendonca BB, Silva FAQ, Inacio M, Lodovici O: Management of ambiguous genitalia in pseudohermaphrodites: New perspectives on vaginal dilatation. *Fertil Steril* **67**:229, 1997.
342. Donahoe PK, Powell DM, Lee MM: Clinical management of intersex abnormalities. *Curr Probl Surg* **28**:513, 1991.
343. Goodall J: Helping a child to understand her own testicular feminisation. *Lancet* **1**:33, 1991.
344. Minogue BP, Taraszewski R, Elias S, Annas GJ: The whole truth and nothing but the truth? *Hastings Cent Rep* **18**:34, 1988.
345. Warne GL, Zajac JD, MacLean HE: Androgen insensitivity syndrome in the era of molecular genetics and the internet: a point of view. *J Pediatr Endocrinol Metab* **11**:3, 1998.
346. Dewhurst CJ, Ferreira HP, Gillett PG: Gonadal malignancy in XY females. *J Obstet Gynaecol Br Commonw* **78**:1077, 1971.
347. O'Connell MJ, Ramsey HE, Whang-Peng J, Wiernik PH: Testicular feminization syndrome in three sibs: Emphasis on gonadal neoplasia. *Am J Med Sci* **265**:321, 1973.
348. MacNab GH: Maldescent of the testicle. *J R Coll Surg Edinb* **1**:126, 1955.
349. Hurt WG, Bodurtha JN, McCall JB, Ali MM: Seminoma in pubertal patient with androgen insensitivity syndrome. *Am J Obstet Gynecol* **161**:530, 1989.
350. Muller J: Morphometry and histology of gonads from twelve children and adolescents with the androgen insensitivity (testicular feminization) syndrome. *J Clin Endocrinol Metab* **59**:785, 1984.
351. Muller J, Skakkebaek NE: Testicular carcinoma in situ in children with the androgen insensitivity (testicular feminisation) syndrome. *Br Med J* **288**:1419, 1984.
352. Cassio A, Cacciari E, D'Errico A, Balsamo A, Grigioni FW, Pascucci MG, Bacci F, Tacconi M, Mancini AM: Incidence of intratubular germ cell neoplasia in androgen insensitivity syndrome. *Acta Endocrinol (Copenh)* **123**:416, 1990.
353. Andler W, Zachmann M: Spontaneous breast development in an adolescent girl with testicular feminization after castration in early childhood. *J Pediatr* **94**:304, 1979.
354. Wooster R, Mangion J, Eeles R, Smith S, Dowsett M, Averill D, Barrett-Lee P, Easton DF, Ponder BAJ, Stratton MR: A germline mutation in the androgen receptor gene in two brothers with breast cancer and Reifenstein syndrome. *Nature Genet* **2**:132, 1992.
355. Lobaccaro J-M, Lumbroso S, Belon C, Galtier-Dereure F, Bringer J, Lesimple T, Namer M, Curuli BF, Pujol H, Sultan C: Androgen receptor gene mutation in male breast cancer. *Hum Mol Genet* **2**:1799, 1993.
356. Hiort O, Naber SP, Lehners A, Muletta-Feurer S, Sinnecker GHG, Zollner A, Komminoth P: The role of androgen receptor gene mutations in male breast carcinoma. *J Clin Endocrinol Metab* **81**:2404, 1996.
357. Mabuchi K, Bross DS, Kessler II: Risk factors for male breast cancer. *J Natl Cancer Inst* **74**:371, 1985.
358. Dexter CJ: Benign enlargement of the male breast. *New Engl J Med* **254**:996, 1956.
359. Slob AK, van der Werff ten Bosch JJ, van Hall EV, de Jong FH, Weijmar Schultz WCM, Eikelboom FA: Psychosexual functioning in women with complete testicular feminization: Is androgen replacement therapy preferable to estrogen? *J Sex Marital Ther* **19**:201, 1993.
360. Radmayr C, Culig Z, Hobisch A, Corvin S, Bartsch G, Klocker H: Analysis of a mutant androgen receptor offers a treatment modality in a patient with partial androgen insensitivity syndrome. *Eur Urol* **33**:222, 1998.
361. Weidemann W, Peters B, Romalo G, Spindler K-D, Schweikert H-U: Response to androgen treatment in a patient with partial androgen insensitivity and a mutation in the deoxyribonucleic acid-binding domain of the androgen receptor. *J Clin Endocrinol Metab* **83**:1173, 1998.
362. Tincello DG, Saunders PTK, Hodgins MB, Simpson NB, Edwards CRW, Hargreaves TB, Wu FCW: Correlation of clinical, endocrine, and molecular abnormalities in patients with partial androgen insensitivity syndrome. *Clin Endocrinol* **46**:497, 1997.
363. Yong EL, Ng SC, Roy AC, Yun G, Ratnam SS: Pregnancy after hormonal correction of severe spermatogenic defect due to mutation in androgen receptor gene. *Lancet* **344**:826, 1994.

CHAPTER 161

Spinobulbar Muscular Atrophy

Leonard Pinsky ▪ Lenore K. Beitel ▪ Mark A. Trifiro

1. **X-linked spinobulbar muscular atrophy (SBMA, Kennedy disease, McKusick no. 313200) is an adult-onset motor neuronopathy that typically causes slowly progressive, symmetric wasting and weakness, initially of the proximal muscles of the hip and shoulder. Muscle cramps, hand tremors, and fasciculations are often associated. Eventually, motor nuclei of the brain stem become involved, leading to speech and swallowing difficulties. Male hypogonadism, usually represented by gynecomastia and testicular atrophy and attributable to mild androgen insensitivity, is not infrequent. Variable expressivity is prominent.**
2. **SBMA is the archetype and prototype of the class of Mendelian, adult-onset neuronodegenerative diseases caused by proteins with expanded polyglutamine (polyGln) tracts. It is archetypical for two reasons: (a) it was the first member of the class to be identified when it was discovered that exon 1 of the androgen receptor gene (*AR*) in SBMA patients had an expanded $(CAG)_n$ tract, and (b) it was the first member of the class in which the normal functions of the culpable protein were well known. Since subjects with complete androgen insensitivity, including those with complete *AR* deletions, do not develop SBMA, this knowledge mandated the logic that the polyCAG-expanded *AR* or the polyGln-expanded AR protein is somehow motor neuronotoxic by a gain, not a loss, of function.**
3. **SBMA is prototypical of the class for several reasons: (a) it is now clear that the polyGln-expanded AR protein, and probably the expanded polyGln tracts themselves, with certain flanking segments of the various parental proteins, are the essential pathogenetic agents in this class of neuronodegenerative disease, (b) the preferential death of certain motor neurons in SBMA exemplifies the fact that selective death of certain neuronal populations is responsible for the clinical diversity among the eight known diseases in the class, (c) there is extremely variable clinical expressivity (age of onset, rate and pattern of progression) of SBMA, and compared with other members of the class, relatively little of this variability is attributable to different degrees of polyGln expansion generated by meiotic or mitotic instability of $(CAG)_n$-repeat size, and (d) SBMA illustrates that 38 or more repeats endow a polyGln tract with a threshold property (or more than one) that is selectively lethal to certain neurons. The biochemical, histopathologic, and neurophysiologic features of SBMA are, unremarkably, those secondary to motor denervation. Endocrine laboratory evidence of mild androgen insensitivity (normal or elevated serum testosterone and luteinizing hormone levels) is not generally found.**
4. **The mild androgen insensitivity component of SBMA is clearly due to a loss of function by the polyGln-expanded AR protein. The loss may be attributable to one or more of the following: decreased steady-state levels of AR, decreased androgen-binding affinity of the mutant AR, or decreased transcriptional regulatory competence of the mutant AR. These factors may contribute to different extents in various androgen target cells. Since androgens are both motor neuro*notropic* and motor neuro*notrophic*, it is possible that the polyGln-expanded AR protein loses a function that is necessary, but not sufficient, for the motor neuronopathy of SBMA generally or for death of certain motor neurons specifically.**
5. **As of mid-1999, data bearing on the pathogenesis of SBMA, and of the polyGln-expanded neuronopathies as a group, are accumulating rapidly. These data are being generated by research with the following underlying themes: (a) polyGln expansion alters the folding of a parental protein and therefore its sensitivity to proteosomes, proteases, or chaperones and, therefore, the nature or extent of the polyGln-expanded fragments derived from it, (b) these polyGln-expanded fragments oligomerize, directly or through intermediates, either noncovalently (by hydrogen-bonded *polar zippering*) or covalently (by transglutaminase-catalyzed isodipeptide formation), to yield cellular inclusions that accumulate in or around the nucleus of certain neurons, (c) the entire process is slow, so it takes years to see the clinical consequences. Why neurons are selectively vulnerable to the toxicity of polyGln-expanded proteins when these proteins (e.g., the AR) are widely distributed in many nonneuronal cells and why, as in SBMA, only certain motor neurons are affected remain entirely speculative.**
6. **It is reasonable to postulate that cells that are spared are "protected" in one or more ways. Such protection may be due to the paucity of a particular protease (perhaps one of the caspases that become active during apoptosis), to the abundance of certain chaperones (either proteins or small molecules) that ensure the proper proteolysis of certain polyGln-expanded fragments and thus avert their pathogenicity, or to other defense mechansims that flow logically from the aforementioned current research themes.**
7. **Such pathogenetic concepts favor the development of certain approaches to the prophylaxis of SBMA. These include inhibitors of transglutaminases or caspases and**

A list of standard abbreviations is located immediately preceding the index in each volume. Nonstandard abbreviations used in this chapter include: AR = androgen receptor; SBMA = spinobulbar muscular atrophy; MAI = mild androgen insensitivity; AIS = androgen insensitivity syndrome; SAPs = sensory nerve action potentials; ALS = amyotrophic lateral sclerosis; PSMA = progressive spinal muscular atrophy; LH = luteinizing hormone; CK = creatinine kinase; DHT = 5α-dihydrotestosterone; GSFs = genital skin fibroblasts; LBD = ligand-binding domain; DRPLA = dentatorubral-pallidoluysian atrophy; SCA1 = spinocerebellar ataxia type 1.

potentiators of proteosomes or chaperones. Indeed, there does not seem to have been a proper clinical trial of prophylaxis using prolonged androgen or antiandrogen supplementation. Since androgen promotes nuclear localization of the AR protein, the strategy of such a trial would be to sequester the parental polyGln-expanded AR in the nucleus of motor neurons, away from the processes of abnormal protein turnover that would otherwise take place in the cytoplasm.

INTRODUCTION AND HISTORICAL BACKGROUND

An entirely new frontier of biomedical research was created when La Spada *et al.*[1] discovered that expansion of the CAG trinucleotide repeat encoding the polymorphic polyglutamine (polyGln) tract in the human androgen receptor (AR) was absolutely associated with the neurodegenerative disease spinobulbar muscular atrophy (SBMA). In the next 5 years, CAG-repeat expansion within coding regions of other genes was identified as the cause of seven more neurodegenerative diseases[2] (see Chaps. 223 and 226). Except for the α_{1A} calcium-channel protein in SCA6,[3] the extremely diverse proteins encoded by the other six genes, and their respective functions, are largely unknown (as of mid-1999). In contrast, the AR is well known to be an intracellular androgen-binding protein that regulates the rates of transcription of genes subject to androgenic control. As such, it is responsible for primary male sexual morphogenesis (masculinization), for secondary male sexual development at puberty (virilization), and for a variety of other sexually dimorphic features. Like other steroid receptors, it has separate C-terminal and central domains for androgen and DNA binding, respectively (Fig. 161-1). Its N-terminal modulatory domain is distinguished by several polyamino acid tracts. The one composed of glutamines is encoded by a series of CAG triplets followed by a single CAA (henceforth, the *CAG repeat*). The normal *AR* CAG repeat ranges from 9 to 36 CAGs; in SBMA subjects, the mutant repeat contains 38 to 62 CAGs.[4] Thus there is no overlap. The properties of the normal AR and the behavior of a wide variety of other mutant ARs are fully discussed in Chap. 160.

SBMA is characterized by progressive weakness and wasting (atrophy) of muscles that lose their motor nerve supply as a result of death of motor neurons in various brain and spinal cord nuclei (see "Clinical Features of the Spinobulbar Component" below) and by expressions of mild androgen insensitivity (MAI) that include breast enlargement (gynecomastia) and infertility (see "Clinical Features of the Mild Androgen Insensitivity Component" below). No individual with any other form of *AR* mutation, including complete *AR* deletion leading to complete androgen insensitivity, has developed SBMA. This fact mandated the postulate that expansion of the CAG repeat, and consequently, of the polyglutamine (polyGln) tract, is selectively neuronotoxic by a gain of function. Furthermore, it strongly suggested that the other translated CAG-repeat-expansion diseases also reflect gain-of-function mutations. The exact mechanism by which the parental polyGln-expanded AR or one of its polyGln-expanded derivative(s) causes degeneration of certain motor neurons is not known at this writing. In fact, the polyGln-expanded AR does suffer a loss of function that is responsible for the MAI component of SBMA. Indeed, there are substantive reasons to believe that this loss, or another form of lost function, may contribute to the motor neuronotoxic process in SBMA. These pathogenetic concepts are considered fully below (see "Pathogenetic Concepts").

SBMA is also known as *Kennedy disease* in deference to Kennedy, Alter, and Sung,[5] who are usually credited with the first full description of the disease. In the same year, three similar patients were described by Stefanis *et al.*[6] In retrospect, case reports of SBMA were published as early as 1932 in the Western literature[7] and, evidently, in 1897 by Dr. H. Kawahara of Aichi Medical University, Japan.[8]

Arbizu *et al.*[9] first suggested that hereditary AR failure involving mainly the spinal and bulbar motor neurons and germinal cells could cause SBMA. In fact, some of the clinical and laboratory features of male hypogonadism in these patients were eminently compatible with androgen insensitivity rather than androgen deficiency. However, causality between the *AR* gene and SBMA seemed dubious in view of the fact that no subject with complete androgen insensitivity (due to loss of function of the AR) had ever been reported to develop SBMA. In 1986, Fischbeck *et al.*[10] found that SBMA was linked to the *DXYS1* locus on a proximal portion of the long arm of the X chromosome. Soon after, Wieacker *et al.*[11] demonstrated close linkage between *DXYS1* and AR-defective androgen insensitivity syndrome (AIS). This strengthened the candidacy of *AR* as the SBMA locus. In 1989, *AR* was mapped to the proximal long arm of the X chromosome, at Xq11-12.[12] La Spada *et al.*[1] then wisely pursued the candidacy of *AR* by sequencing its entire coding region in SBMA patients. This revealed an absolute association between SBMA and an *AR* allele with a CAG-repeat length of 40 or more. Not surprisingly for an intragenic marker, the likelihood of such a strong association by chance alone was 10^{-13}; thus the Lod score was 13. This dramatic finding had several immediate consequences: It stimulated a sucessful search for CAG-repeat expansion in other adult-onset, selective neuronodegenerative diseases, it suggested the gain-of-function postulate, and it provided clues to the mechanism of the gain of function (see "Pathogenetic Concepts" below).

EPIDEMIOLOGY AND PREVALENCE

SBMA is a rare, X-linked recessive, panethnic disease affecting fewer than 1 in 40,000 men.[4] Initial linkage studies[1] included families of English, Irish, Polish, French, Italian, German, Norwegian, Japanese, Chinese, Turkish, and Mexican ancestry; Greek[13] and Australian[14] subjects also have been described.

Based on linkage disequilibrium between $(GGN)_n$-repeat size (see Fig. 161-1) and the mutant $(CAG)_n$ repeat in exon 1 of *AR*, a founder effect was proposed for Japanese SBMA patients.[15] This effect may explain the apparently high frequency of SBMA

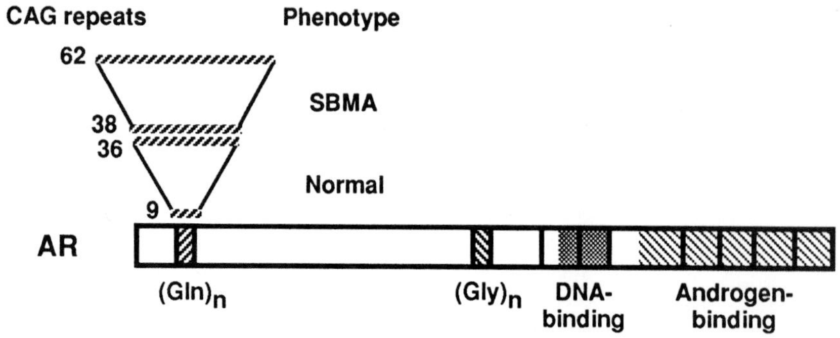

Fig. 161-1 Schematic diagram of the androgen receptor (AR) protein showing the location of the CAG (glutamine, Gln)$_n$ and GGN (glycine, Gly)$_n$ tracts, and the DNA- and androgen-binding domains. The range of *AR* CAG-repeat lengths (hatched lines) and corresponding phenotype are indicated.

in Japan. It could not be found in Caucasian SBMA subjects.[16]

CLINICAL FEATURES AND NATURAL HISTORY OF SBMA

Clinical Features of the Spinobulbar Component

The typical course of SBMA (McKusick Catalogue MIM 313200) is slowly progressive atrophy (wasting) and weakness of the proximal musculature (the muscles of the pelvic and shoulder girdles) starting in the third to fifth decades (middle adulthood) (Fig. 161-2). Unusually, the weakness may appear in the second[17] or sixth decade. Muscle cramps occur in about 70 percent of patients; they may precede the onset of weakness by 10 or more years. With time, there is involvement of the peripheral limb muscles (so that muscle stretch and deep tendon reflexes are reduced or lost) and those served by certain cranial motor nerves in the brain stem (the bulb) of the central nervous system. The latter results in speech (dysphonia, dysarthria) and swallowing (dysphagia) impairment and myopathic facies with lower lip sagging. Fasciculation (muscle twitching) is common, especially of the tongue and the perioral muscles; it may be generalized and sufficiently severe to interfere with sleep. Tremor of the hands is not infrequent, it is postural and fine-rapid in character, and it seems to be family-specific.[18] Tremor and fasciculation also may precede atrophy and weakness.[19]

Atypically, onset may occur in the seventh decade. Remarkably, in two such patients recently described by Igarashi *et al.*,[20] late onset was followed by relatively rapid ("subacute") progression. Speech difficulty was the first abnormality noted by one of these patients. Dyspnea appeared soon after; it exacerbated his stair-climbing impairment. Acute respiratory failure caused his death within 1 year. The other patient presented with rapidly worsening difficulty in standing up and climbing stairs. Both patients had tongue fasciculation and atrophy, and reduced deep tendon reflexes, but neither experienced muscle cramps or sensory abnormalities.

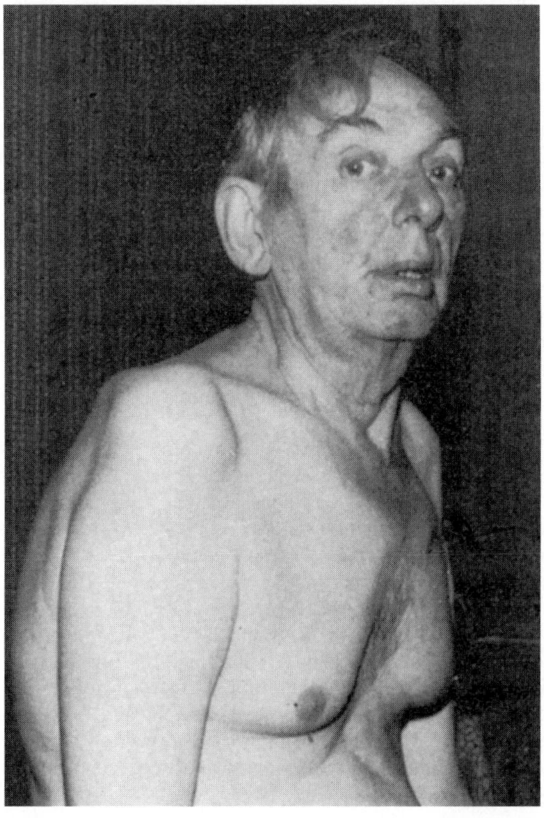

Fig. 161-2 Case 2 from Harding *et al.*[24] showing marked wasting of the proximal upper arm and shoulder girdle muscles and less prominent facial atrophy. There is obvious gynecomastia. (*Reproduced with permission from Harding et al.*[24] *and the BMJ Publishing Group.*)

Sensory Neuron Involvement. It is not widely appreciated that sensory neurons in the dorsal root ganglia are affected in SBMA.[21] It may thus be thought of as a motor-sensory neuronopathy.[22] In some patients, vibratory and tactile sensation and joint position sense are mildly or moderately impaired[23]; others have complained of numbness or tingling in the hands and feet or a burning sensation in the soles of the feet.[22] Small or absent sensory action potentials (SAPs) of the sural nerve can be found, even in the absence of clinical sensory loss.[5,6,19,24–26] These sensory deficits, albeit mild, may be differentially diagnostic because they are atypical of amyotrophic lateral sclerosis (ALS).[19,22]

Expression in Carriers. Heterozygous female carriers seldom display any overt signs of SBMA; very mild symptoms and subclinical signs have been noted. A maternal aunt of one SBMA patient had a history of mild muscle aching with exertion, and her electromyogram (EMG) demonstrated mild chronic denervation in upper and lower limb muscles.[27] Several carriers in the family reported by Ferlini *et al.*[28] had mild weakness and fatigue cramps in the legs, and the EMG indicated lower motor neuron involvement. Sobue *et al.*[29] also noted EMG abnormalities in four of eight neurologically intact carriers. It is probable that motor neuron death at a given level of the spinal cord must exceed a critical threshold before it can have a clinical effect on related muscles. Presumably, random inactivation of the X chromosome bearing the *AR* CAG-repeat expansion permits this level to be reached seldomly in carrier females. It also has been proposed that the relatively low levels of circulating androgens in females may provide a protective effect.[30]

Clinical Features of the Mild Androgen Insensitivity Component

Gynecomastia is the single most common sign of MAI, and it is frequently the first such sign. Decreased libido and impotence usually appear next. Testicular atrophy and infertility typically appear last. Testicular atrophy represents impaired spermatogenesis and corresponds to oligospermia (reduced sperm production) or azoospermia (no sperm production) on semen analysis. Interestingly, otherwise normal males with 28 or more CAG repeats in their *AR* have been reported to have more than a fourfold increased risk of impaired spermatogenesis, and the longer the CAG repeat, the more severe the spermatogenic defect.[31]

Because impotence, reduced libido, and impaired spermatogenesis appear relatively late, often between 40 and 50 years of age,[32] males affected with SBMA are usually fertile. In fact, of the patients described by Warner *et al.*,[33] 72 percent had children.

Differential Diagnosis

Knowing the underlying genetic defect in SBMA permits a definitive diagnosis to be made by DNA analysis. This eliminates ALS, progressive spinal muscular atrophy (PSMA), and occasionally, polymyositis[20] from the differential diagnosis. The polymerase chain reaction (PCR) is used to amplify the CAG-containing region,[1] and the product(s) is analyzed by electrophoresis on agarose or sequencing-type polyacrylamide gels. A larger than normal DNA fragment indicates an expanded CAG-repeat allele in males with SBMA or carrier females (Fig. 161-3). This analysis also may be used for presymptomatic testing, for identifying carrier woman, and debatably, for prenatal diagnosis.[34,34a]

SBMA has been underrecognized in males without a family history suggestive of X-linked inheritance,[27] and it can be misdiagnosed. In a series of 25 unrelated patients with motor neuron disease,[28] DNA analysis exposed an increased number of

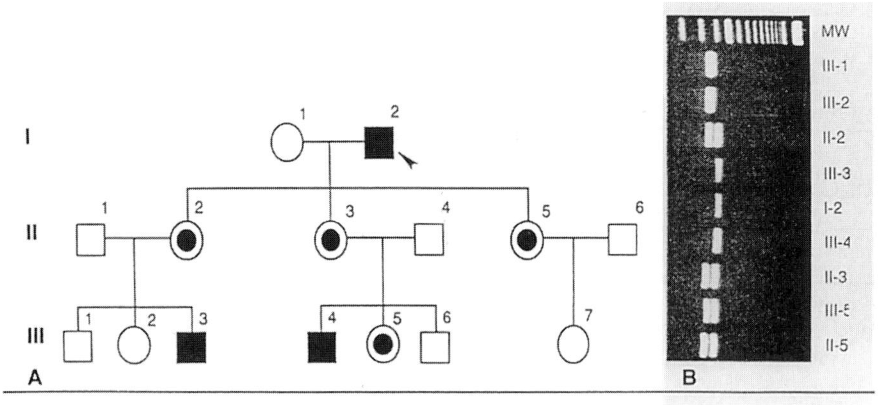

Fig. 161-3 (*A*) Pedigree of family A. (*B*) Ethidium bromide-stained 2.5 percent agarose gel showing the amplification of the *AR* CAG repeat from members of family A. Unaffected individuals show approximately 450 basepair (bp) products. Affected family members have an increased fragment size of approximately 500 bp. Female carriers have both an expanded and a normal fragment. The molecular weight markers (MW) range from low (left) to high (right). (*Reproduced with permission of Lippincott-Raven Publishers from Amato et al.*[38])

CAG repeats in the *AR* of two patients previously diagnosed with PSMA, found a normal repeat size in an individual thought to have SBMA, and confirmed the diagnosis of SBMA in another. Parboosingh *et al.*[22] identified *AR* CAG-repeat expansions in 2 percent of "ALS" families and male patients classified as having ALS, implying that 2 percent of ALS patients are clinically misdiagnosed and actually suffer from SBMA. This is prognostically important: ALS disease progression is typically rapid, death occurring within 2 to 5 years of onset, whereas the life expectancy of patients with SBMA is generally not reduced.[22] Conversely, only 7 of 20 suspected SBMA patients could be confirmed to have a CAG-repeat expansion.

LABORATORY FEATURES

Endocrine and Biochemical Findings

Random plasma testosterone levels are frequently normal but may be low and seldom are high. Random luteinizing hormone (LH) levels may or may not be high. Thus concurrently elevated levels of testosterone and LH, the classic expectation for diminished androgen feedback due to androgen insensitivity of the hypothalamic-pituitary-testis axis, are seldom seen in random sampling. It is likely that frequent periodic sampling (to accommodate pulsatility) would reveal an increased number and amplitude of secretory spikes and increased mean circulating levels of testosterone and LH in some SBMA patients with normal random levels of testosterone and/or LH. Importantly, patients with SBMA may have elevated follicle-stimulating hormone (FSH) levels in response to impaired spermatogenesis, elevated LH responses to gonadotrophin-releasing hormone (GnRH), reflecting diminished androgenic feedback (due to androgen insensitivity) on the hypothalamic-pituitary gonadotrope axis and an increased estradiol level. The latter probably represents increased aromatization of androgen to estrogen due to enhanced androgen secretory dynamics (despite apparently normal random levels of testosterone and/or LH).

Creatine kinase (CK) levels in the blood are usually mildly elevated as a secondary sign of slowly progressive muscle atrophy. Rarely, as in the two late onset patients described recently,[20] markedly elevated CK levels reflected rapid progression of muscle atrophy. Hypobetalipoproteinemia has been reported,[33] almost certainly as a chance concurrence; however, Sobue[8] mentions "fatty liver" in most of his 95 Japanese patients. Some patients have glucose intolerance and/or elevated serum glutamate-pyruvate transaminase activity. The "metabolic" aspects of SBMA need formal evaluation.

Histopathology

Brain Stem and Spinal Cord. The oculomotor, trochlear, and abducens nuclei have a normal density of neurons; this accounts for the sparing of the extraocular muscles. In contrast, neurons in the trigeminal, facial, glossopharyngeal, and hypoglossal nuclei are atrophic or lost; these deficits contribute to the dysarthria, dysphonia, dysphagia, and myopathic facies of SBMA.

There is severe depletion of ventral horn cells and large myelinated fibers at all levels of the spinal cord.[8] The lateral nuclear groups are affected most. In a study on the fourth lumbar ventral horn of seven patients, the medial group, and the intermediate group of small interneurons, also were affected.[35] In the same study, the density and size distribution of myelinated fibers in the lateral corticospinal tract were unremarkable. Accordingly, upper motor neuron signs are rare. There are no special features of the motor neuron atrophy under light microscopy; however, electron microscopy has revealed polyribosome disaggregation in the motor neurons of one patient.[36]

The dorsal root ganglia have a lower density of large neurons but a higher density of small neurons; thus neuron number is maintained at the expense of neuron size.[23] There is a reduced number of large myelinated fibers; demyelination and distal axonal degeneration are prominent. Together with those of the sural nerve described below, these abnormalities explain the sensory deficits observed relatively frequently in SBMA patients.

Nerve, Muscle, and Testis. Sural nerve biopsy reveals reduced density of large myelinated fibers; small myelinated and unmyelinated fibers are relatively protected.[23,33,37] Axonal atrophy is prominent; segmental remyelination is not infrequent.

In muscle, typically one sees type 1 or type 2 fiber-type groupings, the occasional hypertrophic fiber, groups of fibers with internal nuclei or pycnotic nuclear clumping, and adipose tissue replacing muscle fibers.[5,33,38]

Testicular atrophy usually reflects impaired spermatogenesis in otherwise normal seminiferous tubules. Occasionally, the tubules become hyalinized. The Leydig cells may be hyperplastic in a diffuse or nodular pattern[39,40] as a consequence of overstimulation by LH.

Electrophysiology

Motor nerve conduction is not severely impaired, but terminal motor latencies are prolonged.[8] In contrast, the sural nerve often exhibits small or absent SAPs and normal or mildly reduced conduction velocities.[19] Electromyographically, denervation potentials of various kinds ("positive sharp waves," fibrillations, fasciculations) and a decreased number of high-amplitude motor unit potentials are seen frequently.[8]

Androgen Binding in Genital Skin Fibroblasts

The AR is expressed widely but not ubiquitously; scrotal skin and foreskin fibroblasts have relatively high concentrations of AR, allowing for characterization of AR function in the mild AIS of

SBMA. Curiously, diverse abnormal androgen-binding properties of the AR have been demonstrated in certain SBMA patients. For example, decreased 5α-dihydrotestosterone (DHT) binding was found in scrotal skin fibroblasts from three patients of one SBMA family but not in those of five patients from three other families.[40] Low maximum specific receptor binding (B_{max}) (decreased androgen-binding capacity) was found in the genital skin fibroblasts (GSFs) of one patient with a normal equilibrium dissociation constant (apparent binding affinity; K_d)[41] but not in four others.[42] In contrast, MacLean *et al.*[43] demonstrated abnormal K_d values, with normal B_{max}, in suprapubic skin fibroblasts from five of six SBMA patients. Furthermore, they found a significant correlation between the AR K_d and the severity of gynecomastia and testicular atrophy. Immunohistochemistry using an antibody against the ligand-binding domain (LBD) of the AR revealed no immunoreactive AR in scrotal skin of three SBMA patients.[44] Since androgen binding has been found in the GSF of other SBMA patients, this observation implied that polyGln expansion alters the LBD such that it fails to bind antibody.

GENOTYPE AND ITS RELATION TO PHENOTYPE

Genotype-Phenotype Correlation

Initially, equal attention was paid to two widely different pathogenetic hypotheses. One was that CAG-repeat expansion of *AR* into the pathogenic range would cause some form of misbehavior at the DNA or RNA level (perhaps aberrant nucleic acid–protein binding) that generated a mild loss of AR function to account for MAI but also a gain of function whose neuronotoxicity resulted in SBMA. Another hypothesis was that the loss and gain of function occurred at the level of the polyGln-expanded AR protein. For either hypothesis, it was reasonable to question whether the extent of expansion might correlate with age of onset or rate of progression of the disease. Several groups of investigators[28,38,45,46] have found no correlation between the number of CAG repeats and the severity of clinical symptoms. La Spada *et al.*[47] reported that the age of onset of weakness and the age at which stair-climbing difficulty began did correlate inversely with CAG-repeat length. However, they also noted intrafamilial variation in disease severity with the same number of repeats and intrafamilial variation in repeat length without variation in disease severity. Igarashi *et al.*[17] and Doyu *et al.*[48] found that CAG-repeat length was strongly correlated with age of onset of muscular weakness ($r = 0.801$ and 0.596, respectively) but not with such other clinical parameters as muscle cramps, hand tremor, serum CK value, or endocrine abnormalities. Recently, it was shown that, in general, patients with a higher number of CAG repeats had earlier ages of onset ($r = 0.68$) but no greater disease severity; in fact, CAG-repeat size could only account for 46 percent (r^2) of the age-of-onset variance.[22] Weak correlation between genotype (CAG-repeat length) and clinical phenotype emphasizes that genetic background and environmental factors[8] affect the overall severity of expanded CAG-repeat disorders; reduced penetrance, as a function of adult age of onset, also may complicate genotype-phenotype correlation.[4]

Anticipation

Anticipation is defined as a worsening of clinical symptoms and earlier age of onset in successive generations due to expansion of the CAG repeat on transmission from parent to offspring.[49] This phenomenon may be difficult to observe in SBMA for several reasons: (1) the CAG repeat in *AR* appears to be more stable than comparably sized CAG repeats in other genes, with small expansions during meiosis (see "*AR* CAG-Repeat Stability" below), (2) SBMA is an X-linked recessive disease, and therefore carrier females who are daughters of an affected individual may have no overt expression of SBMA (grandsons, rather than sons, of an affected individual could exhibit an SBMA phenotype), and (3) it has become apparent that additional factors besides CAG length must influence the age of onset and disease progression in SBMA.[8]

AR CAG-Repeat Stability

The CAG repeat in *AR* appears to be more stable, both meiotically and mitotically, than CAG-triplet repeats in other genes. Meiotic instability has been assessed both by following transmission of expanded alleles through successive generations and by typing individual sperm. La Spada *et al.*[47] demonstrated that 27 percent of the 45 meioses of an expanded CAG repeat yielded a change in CAG-repeat length, with greater instability in male (4/7) relative to female (4/31) meiotic events. Biancalana *et al.*[45] also showed increased instability of male compared with female transmission, with average expansions of 2 and 0.3 repeats, respectively. Meiotic instability (66 percent expansions, 15 percent contractions) was found to be increased in sperm from an SBMA patient with 47 CAG repeats.[50] This was in contrast to sperm from individuals with 20 to 22 repeats (1.3 percent change) or 28 to 31 repeats (3.2 percent change).[51]

Somatic instability of the *AR* CAG repeat was reported initially by Biancalana *et al.*[45]; others consider these results to be PCR artifacts.[52] CAG-repeat length was identical in DNA from leukocytes and skeletal muscle of eight men,[53] and no tissue-specific variation in the major bands of CAG repeats was found in a number of neural (including the cerebellum) and nonneural tissues from an SBMA patient at either the DNA[15] or mRNA level[54] or a male fetus carrying an expanded CAG repeat.[34a] In contrast, individuals with dentatorubral-pallidoluysian atrophy (DRPLA) and Machado-Joseph disease (MJD), two other CAG-repeat diseases, clearly have somatic instability.[15,54] The *AR* CAG-repeat length in tissues from two cousins whose CAG repeats differed by one (due to meiotic instability) did not differ in each individual, nor were their respective cultured fibroblast *AR* CAG repeats mitotically unstable.[52] Furthermore, as determined by automated sequence analysis of PCR products, the level of mosaicism in a SBMA sperm sample was found to be higher than that in leukocytes but lower than seen for spinocerebellar ataxia type 1 (SCA1) and DRPLA patients. Further analysis indicates that a tissue-specific pattern of somatic mosaicism may be present in SBMA patients, with greater mosaicism in cardiac and skeletal muscles, skin, prostate, and testis than in CNS, liver, and spleen.[54a,54b] Nevertheless, the evidence indicates that the CAG repeat in SBMA is relatively stable mitotically and meiotically compared with other CAG-repeat diseases.[53]

Mouse Models

Transgenic mouse models that mimic SBMA are in development. Bingham *et al.*[55] developed several lines of transgenic mice containing the AR cDNA with an expanded repeat. However, expression of the polyGln-expanded AR was low, the CAG-repeat length did not change with transmission, and the mice had no SBMA-like signs. Nevertheless, when a yeast artificial chromosome (YAC) containing a human CAG-expanded *AR* with 45 CAG repeats was used to generate transgenic mice, intergenerational repeat instability (preferentially maternal) was observed, but somatic mosaicism was not. This suggests that flanking DNA may play a role in repeat instability and that mouse models may be useful in elucidating how CAG-repeat expansions and/or contractions are generated during meiosis.[56] Transgenic mice with the prion protein promoter driving expression of a truncated AR containing 112 Gln develop a neurologic phenotype with progressive gait difficulty, circling behavior, tremors, and seizures.[56a] This model may serve to answer questions on the basic mechanisms of expanded-polyGln diseases; it remains to be seen if mice expressing the full-length polyGln-expanded AR will develop SBMA-like neurodegeneration.

PATHOGENETIC CONCEPTS

Protein-Protein Interaction

The recognition that an expanded *AR* CAG repeat, or its product, had to gain a function in order to be neuronotoxic meant that a rapidly growing number of other polyGln-expanded diseases very probably share the same pathogenetic basis. The fundamental problem, therefore, became to explain what was the shared gain of function and how different sets of neurons are targeted in the different diseases.

The first approach to the problem was to postulate that polyGln-expanded proteins or their respective polyGln-expanded derivatives are prone to conjugate with another protein, including themselves, either covalently or noncovalently. Such conjugates might then be neuronotoxic (Fig. 161-4*A*). One view of this postulate is that transglutaminase catalyzes covalent isodipeptide crosslinks between the Glns of a polyGln-expanded protein and the lysines (or other attacking nucleophiles) of their target protein (or peptide).[57–59] Such isodipeptide bonds are difficult to cleave, and it was reasoned that their rate of formation and accumulation might be slow enough to account for the adult onset of SBMA. It also was considered that neuronotoxic selectivity among the different polyGln diseases might stem from differences in the combinatorial properties of the isodipeptides composed of different lysine-containing targets. Perutz[60] pointed out that polyGln proteins tended to organize themselves into β strands that could be linked (oligomerized) into β-pleated sheets by hydrogen bonds according to the model of a *polar zipper.* In fact, under certain conditions, hetero-oligomer formation might predominate.

The postulate of protein-protein interaction as the basis for neuronotoxicity prompted searches for such interaction involving the polyGln-expanded AR using the yeast two-hybrid system and affinity chromatography. By both approaches,[61] glyceraldehyde-3-phosphate dehydrogenase (GAPDH) has been found to associate with the AR, albeit in a polyGln-length-independent fashion. The interaction of ARA24, a nuclear RAS-related G-protein, with AR and the ability of ARA24 to function as an AR coactivator, however, decrease with increasing polyGln length.[61] This could contribute to AR loss of function and MAI in SBMA; gain-of-function interactions remain to be identified.

Protein Aggregates and Nuclear Inclusions

More recently, greater emphasis has been placed on the way polyGln-expanded fragments may be derived from parental polyGln-expanded proteins and the role such fragments may

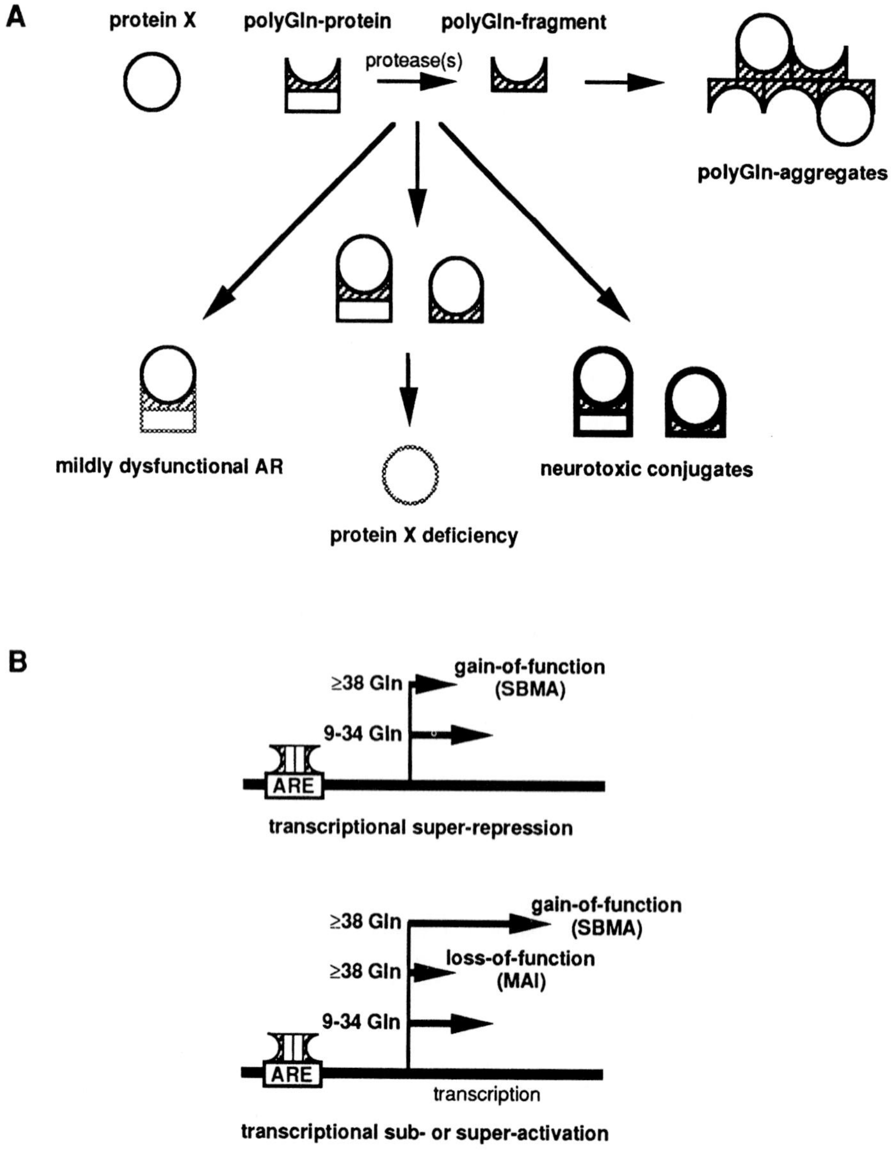

Fig. 161-4 Postulated mechanisms of neurotoxicity in SBMA. (*A*) A polyGln-expanded AR or a polyGln-expanded derivative of it may conjugate (cross-link, hydrogen-bond) with protein X. Abnormal conjugation with protein X or altered interaction with a usual factor may impair the ability of the AR to perform its "neurosupportive" function(s); the conjugates (complexes) may be combinatorially neuronotoxic, or conjugation may consume sufficient protein X so that the residual amount of free protein X is insufficient to perform its normal neuronotrophic function(s). The polyGln-expanded fragment may form neuronotoxic aggregates alone or in association with other proteins. (*B*) Aberrant androgen-dependent transcription regulation may result in decreased transcription to give a loss of function; a gain of function could represent increased transactivation or transrepression ("super-repression"). ARE, androgen response element; a sequence of nucleotides with which an AR dimer interacts in order to regulate transcription of a gene that is under androgenic control.

play in the formation of various peptide-protein aggregates that may be selectively neuronotoxic (see Fig. 161-4*A*). In particular, the action of proapoptotic proteases (caspases, cysteine active site aspartate cleavage enzymes) in generating the fragments is the subject of much study.[62,62a,63] Another focus is the idea that aggregates containing polyGln-expanded peptides become neuronotoxic because they accumulate in or around the nucleus or affect normal cell function.[63a]

We have recently found that when COS-1 cells are transfected with a polyGln-expanded AR, they produce an unconventional polyGln-expanded 75-kDa fragment that is nuclear-associated and are twice as likely to undergo apoptotic death as cells transfected with the normal AR. The normal AR does not yield a homologous fragment with a normal-sized Gln tract. Furthermore, when *in vitro*–synthesized polyGln-expanded AR is exposed to partial-progressive denaturant proteolysis, it generates polyGln-expanded fragments that are proteolytically resistant.[64]

The 75-kDa fragment is "unconventional" because its expanded polyGln tract (beginning at residue 58) allows it to react against monoclonal antibody (mAb) 1C2,[65] yet it does not react against mAb F39.4.1, whose epitope is composed of amino acids 301 to 320 (as numbered by ref. 66). In a standard western blot assay, a conventional linear peptide of approximately 75 kDa should react against both antibodies. This unusual immunologic behavior led us to postulate either atypical proteolytic processing of the parental polyGln-expanded AR or adoption of an atypical conformation by the polyGln-expanded 75-kDa fragment that conceals its epitope from mAb F39.4.1.

A similar sized ($\approx$74 kDa) polyGln-expanded AR fragment also was found in COS-7 and mouse neuroblastoma NB2a/d1 cells expressing the polyGln-expanded AR. Western blotting demonstrated that this fragment lacked the AR LBD, leading Butler *et al.*[67] to propose that hormone-independent constitutive transactivation of specific genes by the C-terminal truncated AR could be a pathogenetic component of SBMA. They also found the polyGln-expanded AR mainly in cytoplasmic aggregates even after androgen treatment of the cells. Merry *et al.*[68] showed that truncated polyGln-expanded AR proteins could form high-molecular-weight aggregates both *in vitro* and *in vivo*. The polyGln-expanded AR fragments were toxic to cells and formed aggregates (cytoplasmic in COS-7 cells and nuclear in MN-1 motor neuronal cells) in a repeat-length-dependent manner (65 CAG repeats or longer). Our own experiments with green fluorescent protein-tagged normal and polyGln-expanded AR confirm the production of protein aggregates in cultured cells containing the mutant AR (Fig. 161-5). Indeed, nuclear inclusions containing the AR recently have been seen in motor neurons of SBMA patients.[69] These ubiquitinated inclusions were immunoreactive with antibodies specific for the first 20 or 21 N-terminal amino acids of the AR but not with antibodies directed to the N-terminal 321 amino acids, the DNA-binding domain, or C-terminal sequences. Thus certain AR epitopes may be unavailable in SBMA nuclear inclusions due to altered AR conformation, masking of certain AR epitopes by other proteins, or proteolytic cleavage of the AR.[69] Nuclear inclusions have not been considered pathognomonic of polyGln protein diseases because they were not revealed by routine (nonimmunologic) neurohistochemistry.[70]

The association of expanded CAG repeats with aggregation of polyGln-expanded proteins or their fragments, has been observed repeatedly (reviewed in refs. 2 and 70a). For example, mice transgenic for the *HD* mutation developed neuronal intranuclear inclusions containing the huntingtin protein and ubiquitin,[71] and insoluble high-molecular-weight aggregates have been generated *in vitro* from truncated polyGln-expanded huntingtin[72] and SCA3 proteins.[73] A model for formation of intranuclear inclusions in polyGln-expanded diseases, by association of fragments through β-sheet formation, is depicted by Ross.[2] Insertion of a long polyGln tract (146 Gln) into a non-CAG-repeat-disease protein (hypoxanthine phosphoribotransferase) and its expression in mice resulted in a neurologic phenotype and formation of nuclear inclusions.[74] Strikingly, expression of a segment of the polyGln-expanded SCA3/MJD protein in *Drosophila* led to the formation of nuclear inclusions and late onset cell degeneration. However, nuclear inclusions were found in cells other than neurons, indicating that polyGln protein aggregation is not sufficient to cause degeneration in every cell type.[75] Similarly, nuclear inclusions have been observed in nonneuronal tissues, as well as in the neurons that degenerate in SBMA.[75a] Although nuclear inclusions have been postulated to be directly noxious to neurons, and thus to play a key role in the pathogenesis of CAG-repeat diseases,[71] alternative views hold that they are merely markers for other processes actually responsible for neuronal cell death or that they represent a cellular defense mechanism to sequester toxic polyGln-expanded protein fragments.[74,75b]

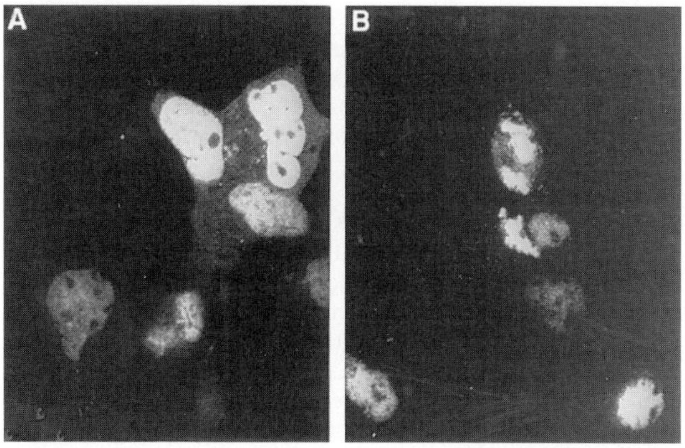

Fig. 161-5 Subcellular localization of the normal and SBMA AR tagged with green fluorescent protein (GFP). AR cDNAs containing 20 or 50 CAG repeats (20 or 50 Gln) were cloned in frame with GFP in pS65T-C1. COS-1 cells were transiently transfected with (*A*) pS65T-C1:hAR20Gln or with (*B*) pS65T-C1:hAR50Gln and incubated with 100 nM mibolerone, a synthetic androgen, 1 h prior to fixation. Bright nuclear staining is seen in the cells transfected with normal human AR. Cells transfected with SBMA human AR show large inclusion bodies in the cytoplasm. (*Courtesy of Valerie Panet-Raymond.*)

The potential involvement of caspases in the generation of truncated proteins was explored by Wellington *et al.*,[62] who demonstrated that AR, as are huntingtin, atrophin-1, and ataxin-3, can be cleaved by apoptotic cell extracts. Purified caspases 1, 3, and 8 efficiently cleaved normal and polyGln-expanded AR, while caspase 7 did not. Two specific caspase 3 sites were found in the AR: mutation of one of them (Asp146) blocked the ability of the polyGln-expanded AR to form perinuclear aggregates and reduced apoptosis.[63] As Wellington *et al.*[62] pointed out, abnormal levels of caspase or other protease activity need not be invoked for production of truncated proteins. Basal levels of caspase activity may be sufficient to cleave proteins into smaller polyGln-expanded peptides toxic to neurons. Accumulation of toxic fragments could further stress the cell in a feed-forward fashion, resulting in additional caspase activation, protein cleavage and aggregation, and neuronal death.[62] It is likewise easy to imagine that a series of otherwise innocent apoptotic-inducing insults may activate certain proteases or caspases[62,76] sufficiently to cleave the polyGln-expanded AR into a fragment(s) that is directly or indirectly, but cumulatively, motor neuronotoxic, thereby representing the mysterious gain of function (see Fig. 161-4*A*).

Protein misfolding is seen as a central feature in certain neurodegenerative diseases, and misfolding of expanded-polyGln domains is viewed as a novel toxic property.[70a] Experimentally, HeLa cells transfected with an polyGln-expanded AR develop both cytoplasmic and nuclear aggregates in a hormone-dependent manner.[63a] Aggregates also were shown to contain the Hsp70, Hsp90, and HDJ-2/HSDJ chaperone proteins; the ubiquitin-like

NEDD8 protein; steroid receptor coactivator (SRC-1); PA700 proteosome caps; and mitochondria. It is proposed that failure to proteolyse misfolded polyGln-expanded AR protein results in aggregate formation and that subsequent sequestration of chaperones, proteosomes, and coactivators adversely affects neuronal cell function.[63a]

Altered Transregulation by the AR

Although men with an expanded *AR* CAG allele have sufficient AR function to ensure normal development of the primary and, usually, the secondary sexual characteristics, one component of the SBMA phenotype is MAI, indicative of some AR loss of function. The expanded polyglutamine tract, by itself, could render the AR transcriptionally dysfunctional (see Fig. 161-4*B*). In COS or CV-1 cells transiently transfected with normal or polyGln-expanded AR and an androgen-inducible reporter gene, the polyGln-expanded AR expressed reduced transactivation compared with the normal AR.[77–80] The androgen-binding properties of the expanded AR, such as the equilibrium dissociation constant (K_d) and the dissociation rate constant, were normal. In transiently transfected neuronal cells, transactivation was slightly reduced with SBMA-sized *AR* alleles and more so with still longer repeats.[81] McPhaul *et al.*[42] used an adenovirus-based reporter gene assay to demonstrate that AR transactivation was markedly reduced in cultured GSF from SBMA patients, despite their normal levels of AR binding and immunoreactivity. Others[82,83] have attributed loss of AR transactivation to lower expression of the polyGln-expanded AR or segregation of the polyGln-expanded AR into cytoplasmic aggregates.[67] Contrarily, Neuschmid-Kaspar *et al.*[84] found no loss of transactivation or transrepression function with the polyGln-expanded AR.

PolyGln expansion may alter interactions with coregulators (coactivators or corepressors) and thereby expression of AR-regulated genes.[61a,63a] It has not escaped our attention that polyGln expansion may increase the extent to which the AR *represses* a target gene to the point where the product of that gene may not reach a concentration critical for the survival of certain motor neurons (see Fig. 161-4*B*). Another gain of function to consider is transcriptional superactivation by a polyGln-expanded AR, resulting in the neuronotoxic accumulation of a gene product that is under androgenic control.

Neurons and Androgens

Androgens concentrate selectively in those bulbar and spinal motor neurons that are affected in SBMA.[85] Androgens can reduce degeneration or promote regeneration of mammalian motor neurons.[86–89] Lustig *et al.*[90] found that AR-transfected PC12 cells respond to androgen and nerve growth factor additively by increasing neurite outgrowth, whereas androgen alone increases neurite branching. NG108-15 mouse glioma-neuroblastoma hybrid cells stably transfected with normal AR but not polyGln-expanded AR demonstrated an androgen-dependent increase in cell number.[91] Perez and Kelley[92] recently reported that DHT exerts its trophic effect on axotomized laryngeal motor neurons of juvenile *Xenopus laevis* by maintaining calbindin expression. Presumably, this serves to counteract the elevation of cytoplasmic calcium that is associated with neuronal death caused by the lesion.

AR is expressed in many parts of the brain, including the brain stem, hypothalamus, cerebellum, and amygdala,[93] as well as the spinal cord.[94] AR appears in the rat lumbar spinal cord just before androgen exerts its initiating action on the process of testicular descent.[94] Appropriately, antiandrogen-induced cryptorchidism in rats is associated with a reduced number of motor neurons in the genitofemoral nucleus, a portion of the lumbar spinal cord that is sexually dimorphic.[94] *AR* mRNA has been detected in motor neurons of the fifth, seventh, tenth, and twelfth cranial nerves,[95] in the sciatic nerve, sympathetic, and dorsal root ganglia,[96] and in a wide variety of nonneuronal tissues, including the testis, scrotal skin, liver, and skeletal and cardiac muscle. The level of *AR* mRNA and protein was decreased in spinal cord from an SBMA patient.[97] Perhaps this contributes to AR loss of function.

As for all polyGln-expansion neuronodegenerative diseases, the vexing question is how to explain selective neuronal death when the abnormal AR is expressed in many different cell types. Furthermore, since androgens are motor neuronotrophic, there is a strong basis for believing that a polyGln-expanded AR may lose a function that is *not* sufficient by itself to cause SBMA but that predisposes certain motor neurons to the harmful gain of function that is necessary for the pathogenesis of SBMA.[98] Additional contributory factors in motor neuron selectivity of SBMA could include the availability of caspases, the vulnerability of the polyGln-expanded AR to those caspases, the presence of transglutaminases, the levels of chaperone proteins (see below), and susceptibility of certain motor neurons to the toxic effects of polyGln-expanded fragments directly or of the aggregates/inclusions derived from these fragments.

Prophylactic/Therapeutic Strategies

Given the association between the formation of polyGln aggregates and neurodegenerative diseases, several different strategies have been suggested to prevent or reduce nuclear inclusions and presumably disease progression. For instance, certain transglutaminase inhibitors partially suppressed aggregate formation and apoptotic cell death of COS-7 cells expressing a truncated polyGln-expanded DRPLA protein.[99] Likewise, overexpression of a dnaJ-like chaperone protein (HDJ-2/HSDJ) decreased nuclear aggregation in HeLa cells transfected with either polyGln-expanded ataxin-1 (SCA1)[100] or polyGln-expanded AR,[63a] possibly by increasing refolding or ubiquitin-dependent degradation of the mutant protein. The involvement of caspases in producing polyGln-expanded protein fragments[62,63,76] suggests that specific caspase inhibitors, or inhibitors of other still unidentified proteases, could be ameliorative. For SBMA specifically, androgen treatment may be helpful (but see "Management" below), since DHT and testosterone counter motor neuron insults,[86–89,92] whereas testosterone suppresses aggregate formation[63] and apoptosis in motor neuron-like cells expressing polyGln-expanded AR.[63,101] Obviously, a multitargeted approach may be necessary to accomplish prophylaxis or treatment of SBMA.

MANAGEMENT

No treatment for SBMA has been proven beneficial. Propranolol improved tremor in one patient,[24] and fluoxymesterone treatment temporarily improved the muscle weakness of the four extremities in another.[102] Two affected brothers, 55 and 66 years old, were treated daily with 37.5 mg of oral testosterone for 18 months or with 25 mg for 6 months, respectively, both with concurrent exercise therapy.[103] The younger brother improved his muscle work output appreciably; the older brother exercised less and did not improve, suggesting that androgen and exercise may be complementary. However, Danek *et al.*[41] and Neuschmid-Kaspar *et al.*[84] found no benefit of androgens to several SBMA patients. Thus androgen therapy is, at least, not harmful, even if its benefits are, at best, uncertain. Currently, there is no clear rationale for treatment of the neuronopathy component of SBMA with antiandrogen, and antiandrogen could worsen the MAI component of SBMA. For instance, there is no evidence that antiandrogen can retard the production of polyGln-expanded AR fragments from full-length mutant AR. On the other hand, androgen therapy potentially could ameliorate the symptoms of MAI, and it might counteract any loss-of-function component contributing to the neuronopathy. However, androgen stabilizes the AR; thus it also could exacerbate the spinobulbar component of SBMA by increasing the concentration of a neuronotoxic fragment derived from the polyGln-expanded AR. In patients with advanced disease, various assistive devices may be necessary for locomotion and respiration, and precautions against aspiration pneumonia must be installed. Unraveling the pathogenetic pathway(s) in SBMA should lead to development of rational approaches to the prevention, if not the treatment, of SBMA.

REFERENCES

1. La Spada AR, Wilson EM, Lubahn DB, Harding AE, Fischbeck KH: Androgen receptor gene mutations in X-linked spinal and bulbar muscular atrophy. *Nature* **352**:77, 1991.
2. Ross CA: Intranuclear neuronal inclusions: A common pathogenic mechanism. *Neuron* **19**:1147, 1997.
3. Zhuchenko O, Bailey J, Bonnen P, Ashizawa T, Stockton DW, Amos C, Dobyns WB, et al: Autosomal dominant cerebellar ataxia (SCA6) associated with small polyglutamine expansions in the α_{1A}-voltage-dependent calcium channel. *Nature Genet* **15**:62, 1997.
4. Andrew SE, Goldberg YP, Hayden MR: Rethinking genotype and phenotype correlations in polyglutamine expansion disorders. *Hum Mol Genet* **6**:2005, 1997.
5. Kennedy WR, Alter M, Sung JH: Progressive proximal spinal and bulbar muscular atrophy of late onset: A sex-linked recessive trait. *Neurology* **18**:671, 1968.
6. Stefanis C, Papapetropoulos T, Scarpalezos S: A peculiar form of X-linked hereditary degenerative motor neuron disease. Presented at the Annual Meeting of the Hellenic Association of Neurology and Psychiatry, November 26, 1968.
7. Mollen GA: Familial progressive muscular atrophy. *Arch Neurol Psychiatr* **27**:645, 1932.
8. Sobue G: X-linked recessive bulbospinal neuronopathy (SBMA). *Nagoya J Med Sci* **58**:95, 1995.
9. Arbizu T, Santamaria J, Gomez JM, Quilez A, Serra JP: A family with adult spinal and bulbar muscular atrophy, X-linked inheritance and associated testicular failure. *J Neurol Sci* **59**:371, 1983.
10. Fischbeck KH, Ionasescu V, Ritter AW, Ionasescu R, Davies K, Ball S, Bosch P, et al: Localization of the gene for X-linked spinal muscular atrophy. *Neurology* **36**:1595, 1986.
11. Wieacker P, Griffin JE, Wienker T, Lopez JM, Wilson JD, Breckwoldt M: Linkage analysis with RFLPs in families with androgen resistance syndromes: Evidence for close linkage between the androgen receptor locus and the *DXS1* segment. *Hum Genet* **76**:248, 1987.
12. Brown CJ, Goss SJ, Lubahn DB, Joseph DR, Wilson EM, French FS, Willard HF: Androgen receptor locus on the human X chromosome: Regional localization to Xq11-12 and description of a DNA polymorphism. *Am J Hum Genet* **44**:264, 1989.
13. Stefanis C, Papapetropoulos T, Scarpalezos S, Lygidakis G, Panayiotopoulos CP: X-linked spinal and bulbar muscular atrophy of late onset: A separate type of motor neuron disease? *J Neurol Sci* **24**:493, 1975.
14. Choi WT, MacLean HE, Chu S, Warne GL, Zajac JD: Kennedy's disease: Genetic diagnosis of an inherited form of motor neuron disease. *Aust N Z J Med* **23**:187, 1993.
15. Tanaka F, Doyu M, Ito Y, Matsumoto M, Mitsuma T, Abe K, Aoki M, et al.: Founder effect in spinal and bulbar muscular atrophy (SBMA). *Hum Mol Genet* **5**:1253, 1996.
16. Parboosingh JS, Goto J, Meininger V, Leonard D, Mandel JL, Rouleau GA: Haplotype analysis of Caucasian spinobulbar muscular atrophy chromosomes. *Am J Hum Genet* **61**(suppl):A317, 1997.
17. Igarashi S, Tanno Y, Onodera O, Yamazaki M, Sato S, Ishikawa A, Miyatani N, et al: Strong correlation between the number of CAG repeats in androgen receptor genes and the clinical onset of features of spinal and bulbar muscular atrophy. *Neurology* **42**:2300, 1992.
18. Ringel SP, Lava NS, Treihaft MM, Lubs ML, Lubs HA: Late-onset X-linked recessive spinal and bulbar muscular atrophy. *Muscle Nerve* **1**:297, 1978.
19. Olney RK, Aminoff MJ, So YT: Clinical and electrodiagnostic features of X-linked recessive bulbospinal neuronopathy. *Neurology* **41**:823, 1991.
20. Igarashi S, Yonemochi Y, Tanaka K, Inuzuka T, Oyanagi S, Ikuta F, Horikawa Y, et al: Atypical clinical presentations of X-linked spinal and bulbar muscular atrophy in patients with mild CAG expansions in androgen receptor gene. *Eur Neurol* **38**:310, 1997.
21. Sobue G, Hashizume Y, Mukai E, Hirayama M, Mitsuma T, Takahashi A: X-linked recessive bulbospinal neuronopathy: A clinicopathological study. *Brain* **112**:209, 1989.
22. Parboosingh JS, Figlewicz DA, Krizus A, Meininger V, Azad NA, Newman DS, Rouleau GA: Spinobulbar muscular atrophy can mimic ALS: The importance of genetic testing in male patients with atypical ALS. *Neurology* **49**:568, 1997.
23. Li M, Sobue G, Doyu M, Mukai E, Hashizume Y, Mitsuma T: Primary sensory neurons in X-linked recessive bulbospinal neuropathy: Histopathology and androgen receptor gene expression. *Muscle Nerve* **18**:301, 1995.
24. Harding AE, Thomas PK, Baraitser M, Bradbury PG, Morgan HJ, Ponsford JR: X-linked recessive bulbospinal neuronopathy: A report of ten cases. *J Neurol Neurosurg Psychiatry* **45**:1012, 1982.
25. Penisson-Besnier I, Dubas F, Delestre F, Emile J: Sensory nerve involvement in X-linked bulbospinal amyotrophy (Kennedy syndrome): Contributions of electrophysiologic and histologic data. *Neurophysiol Clin* **19**:163, 1989.
26. Polo A, Teatini F, D'Anna S, Manganotti P, Salviati A, Dallapiccola B, Zanette G, et al: Sensory involvement in X-linked spino-bulbar muscular atrophy (Kennedy's syndrome): An electrophysiological study. *J Neurol* **243**:388, 1996.
27. Belsham DD, Yee WC, Greenberg CR, Wrogemann K: Analysis of the CAG repeat region of the androgen receptor gene in a kindred with X-linked spinal and bulbar muscular atrophy. *J Neurol Sci* **112**:133, 1992.
28. Ferlini A, Patrosso MC, Guidetti D, Merlini L, Uncini A, Ragno M, Plasmati R, et al: Androgen receptor gene $(CAG)_n$ repeat analysis in the differential diagnosis between Kennedy disease and other motoneuron disorders. *Am J Med Genet* **55**:105, 1995.
29. Sobue G, Doyu M, Kachi T, Yasuda T, Mukai E, Kumagai T, Mitsuma T: Subclinical phenotypic expressions in heterozygous females of X-linked recessive bulbospinal neuronopathy. *J Neurol Sci* **117**:74, 1993.
30. MacLean HE, Warne GL, Zajac JD: Spinal and bulbar muscular atrophy: Androgen receptor dysfunction caused by a trinucleotide repeat expansion. *J Neurol Sci* **135**:149, 1996.
31. Tut TG, Ghadessy FJ, Trifiro MA, Pinsky L, Yong EL: Long polyglutamine tracts in the androgen receptor are associated with reduced *trans*-activation, impaired sperm production, and male infertility. *J Clin Endocrinol Metab* **82**:3777, 1997.
32. Guidetti D, Motti L, Marcello N, Vescovini E, Marbini A, Dotti C, Lucci B, et al: Kennedy disease in an Italian kindred. *Eur Neurol* **25**:188, 1986.
33. Warner CL, Servidei S, Lange DJ, Miller E, Lovelace RE, Rowland LP: X-linked spinal muscular atrophy (Kennedy's syndrome): A kindred with hypobetalipoproteinemia. *Arch Neurol* **47**:1117, 1990.
34. Wang Z, Thibodeau SN: A polymerase chain reaction-based test for spinal and bulbar muscular atrophy. *Mayo Clin Proc* **71**:397, 1996.

34a. Jedele K, Wahl D, Chahrokh-Zadeh S, Wirtz A, Murken J, Holinski-Feder E: Spinal and bulbar muscular atrophy (SBMA): Somatic stability of an expanded CAG repeat in fetal tissues. *Clin Genet* **54**:148, 1998.

35. Terao S, Sobue G, Li M, Hashizume Y, Tanaka F, Mitsuma T: The lateral corticospinal tract and spinal ventral horn in X-linked recessive spinal and bulbar muscular atrophy: A quantitative study. *Acta Neuropathol* **93**:1, 1997.
36. Oyanagi K, Aoki K, Morita T, Igarashi S, Inuzuka T, Horikawa Y: Disaggregation of polyribosomes in the spinal anterior horn cells in a patient with X-linked spinal and bulbar muscular atrophy. *Acta Neuropathol* **91**:444, 1996.
37. Nagashima T, Seko K, Hirose K, Mannen T, Yoshimura S, Arima R, Nagashima K, et al: Familial bulbo-spinal muscular atrophy associated with testicular atrophy and sensory neuropathy (Kennedy-Alter-Sung syndrome): Autopsy case report of two brothers. *J Neurol Sci* **87**:141, 1988.
38. Amato AA, Prior TW, Barohn RJ, Snyder P, Papp A, Mendell JR: Kennedy's disease: A clinicopathologic correlation with mutations in the androgen receptor gene. *Neurology* **43**:791, 1993.
39. Hausmanowa-Petrusewicz I, Borkowska J, Janczewski Z: X-linked adult form of spinal muscular atrophy. *J Neurol* **229**:175, 1983.
40. Warner CL, Griffin JE, Wilson JD, Jacobs LD, Murray KR, Fischbeck KH, Dickoff D, et al: X-linked spinomuscular atrophy: A kindred with associated abnormal androgen receptor binding. *Neurology* **42**:2181, 1992.
41. Danek A, Witt TN, Mann K, Schweikert HU, Romalo G, La Spada AR, Fischbeck KH: Decrease in androgen binding and effect of androgen treatment in a case of X-linked bulbospinal neuronopathy. *Clin Investig* **72**:892, 1994.
42. McPhaul MJ, Schweikert H-U, Allman DR: Assessment of androgen receptor function in genital skin fibroblasts using a recombinant adenovirus to deliver an androgen-responsive reporter gene. *J Clin Endocrinol Metab* **82**:1944, 1997.
43. MacLean HE, Choi WT, Rekaris G, Warne GL, Zajac JD: Abnormal androgen receptor binding affinity in subjects with Kennedy's disease

(spinal and bulbar muscular atrophy). *J Clin Endocrinol Metab* **80**:508, 1995.

44. Matsuura T, Demura T, Aimoto Y, Mizuno T, Moriwaka F, Tashiro K: Androgen receptor abnormality in X-linked spinal and bulbar muscular atrophy. *Neurology* **42**:1724, 1992.
45. Biancalana V, Serville F, Pommier J, Julien J, Hanauer A, Mandel JL: Moderate instability of the trinucleotide repeat in spino bulbar muscular atrophy. *Hum Mol Genet* **1**:255, 1992.
46. Yamamoto Y, Kawai H, Nakahara K, Osame M, Nakatsuji Y, Kishimoto T, Sakoda S: A novel primer extension method to detect the number of CAG repeats in the androgen receptor gene in families with X-linked spinal and bulbar muscular atrophy. *Biochem Biophys Res Commun* **182**:507, 1992.
47. La Spada AR, Roling DB, Harding AE, Warner CL, Spiegel R, Hausmanowa-Petrusewicz I, Yee WC, et al: Meiotic stability and genotype-phenotype correlation of the trinucleotide repeat in X-linked spinal and bulbar muscular atrophy. *Nature Genet* **2**:301, 1992.
48. Doyu M, Sobue G, Mukai E, Kachi T, Yasuda T, Mitsuma T, Takahashi B: Severity of X-linked recessive bulbospinal neuronopathy correlates with size of tandem CAG repeat in androgen receptor gene. *Ann Neurol* **32**:707, 1992.
49. Kaytor MD, Burright EN, Duvick LA, Zoghbi HY, Orr HT: Increased trinucleotide repeat instability with advanced maternal age. *Hum Mol Genet* **6**:2135, 1997.
50. Zhang L, Fischbeck KH, Arnheim N: CAG repeat length variation in sperm from a patient with Kennedy's disease. *Hum Mol Genet* **4**:303, 1995.
51. Zhang L, Leeflang EP, Yu J, Arnheim N: Studying human mutations by sperm typing: Instability of CAG trinucleotide repeats in the human androgen receptor gene. *Nature Genet* **7**:531, 1994.
52. Spiegel R, La SA, Kress W, Fischbeck KH, Schmid W: Somatic stability of the expanded CAG trinucleotide repeat in X-linked spinal and bulbar muscular atrophy. *Hum Mutat* **8**:32, 1996.
53. Watanabe M, Abe K, Aoki M, Yasuo K, Itoyama Y, Shoji M, Ikeda Y, et al: Mitotic and meiotic stability of the CAG repeat in the X-linked spinal and bulbar muscular atrophy gene. *Clin Genet* **50**:133, 1996.
54. Ito Y, Tanaka F, Yamamoto M, Doyu M, Nagamatsu M, Riku S, Mitsuma T, et al: Somatic mosaicism of the expanded CAG trinucleotide repeat in mRNAs for the responsible gene of Machado-Joseph disease (MJD), dentatorubral-pallidoluysian atrophy (DRPLA), and spinal and bulbar muscular atrophy (SBMA). *Neurochem Res* **23**:25, 1998.

54a. Ansved T, Lundin A, Anvret M: Larger CAG expansions in skeletal muscle compared with lymphocytes in Kennedy disease but not in Huntington disease. *Neurology* **51**:1442, 1998.

54b. Tanaka F, Ito Y, Sobue G: Somatic mosaicism of expanded CAG trinucleotide repeat in spinal and bulbar muscular atrophy (SBMA). *Jpn J Clin Med* **57**:862, 1999.

55. Bingham PM, Scott MO, Wang S, McPhaul MJ, Wilson EM, Garbern JY, Merry DE, Fischbeck KH: Stability of an expanded trinucleotide repeat in the androgen receptor gene in transgenic mice. *Nature Genet* **9**:191, 1995.
56. La Spada AR, Peterson KR, Meadows SA, McClain ME, Jeng G, Chmelar RS, Haugen HA, et al: Androgen receptor YAC transgenic mice carrying CAG 45 alleles show trinucleotide repeat instability. *Hum Mol Genet* **7**:959, 1998.

56a. Fischbeck KH, Lieberman A, Bailey CK, Abel A, Merry DE: Androgen receptor mutation in Kennedy's disease. *Philos Trans R Soc Lond [Biol]* **354**:1075, 1999.

57. Green H: Human genetic diseases due to codon reiteration: Relationship to an evolutionary mechanism. *Cell* **74**:955, 1993.
58. Kahlem P, Terre C, Green H, Djian P: Peptides containing glutamine repeats as substrates for transglutaminase-catalyzed cross-linking: Relevance to diseases of the nervous system. *Proc Natl Acad Sci USA* **93**:14580, 1996.
59. Cooper AJ, Sheu KF, Burke JR, Onodera O, Strittmatter WJ, Roses AD, Blass JP: Polyglutamine domains are substrates of tissue transglutaminase: Does transglutaminase play a role in expanded CAG/poly-Q neurodegenerative diseases? *J Neurochem* **69**:431, 1997.
60. Perutz MF: Glutamine repeats and inherited neurodegenerative diseases: Molecular aspects. *Curr Opin Struct Biol* **6**:848, 1996.
61. Koshy B, Matilla T, Burright EN, Merry DE, Fischbeck KH, Orr HT, Zoghbi HY: Spinocerebellar ataxia type-1 and spinobulbar muscular atrophy gene products interact with glyceraldehyde-3-phosphate dehydrogenase. *Hum Mol Genet* **5**:1311, 1996.

61a. Hsiao PW, Lin DL, Nakao R, Chang C: The linkage of Kennedy's neuron disease to ARA24, the first identified androgen receptor polyglutamine region-associated coactivator. *J Biol Chem* **274**:20229, 1999.

62. Wellington CL, Ellerby LM, Hackam AS, Margolis RL, Trifiro MA, Singaraja R, McCutcheon K, et al: Caspase cleavage of gene products associated with triplet expansion disorders generates truncated fragments containing the polyglutamine tract. *J Biol Chem* **273**:9158, 1998.

62a. Kobayashi Y, Miwa S, Merry DE, Kume A, Mei L, Doyu M, Sobue G: Caspase-3 cleaves the expanded androgen receptor protein of spinal and bulbar muscular atrophy in a polyglutamine repeat length-dependent manner. *Biochem Biophys Res Commun* **252**:145, 1998.

63. Ellerby L, Hackman A, Propp S, Ellerby H, Rabizadeh S, Trifiro M, Pinsky L, et al: Kennedy's disease: Caspase cleavage of the androgen receptor is a crucial event in cytotoxicity. *J Neurochem* **72**:185, 1999.

63a. Stenoien DL, Cummings CJ, Adams HP, Mancini MG, Patel K, DeMartino GN, Marcelli M, et al: Polyglutamine-expanded androgen receptors form aggregates that sequester heat shock proteins, proteasome components and SRC-1, and are suppressed by the HDJ-2 chaperone. *Hum Mol Genet* **8**:731, 1999.

64. Abdullah AAR, Trifiro MA, Panet-Raymond V, Alvarado C, de Tourreil S, Frankel D, Schipper HM, et al: Spinobulbar muscular atrophy: Polyglutamine-expanded androgen receptor is proteolytically resistant in vitro and processed abnormally in transfected cells. *Hum Mol Genet* **7**:379, 1998.
65. Trottier Y, Lutz Y, Stevanin G, Imbert G, Devys D, Cancel G, Saudou F et al: Polyglutamine expansion as a pathological epitope in Huntington's disease and four dominant cerebellar ataxias. *Nature* **378**:403, 1995.
66. Zegers ND, Claassen E, Neelen C, Mulder E, van Laar JH, Voorhorst MM, Berrevoets CA, et al: Epitope prediction and confirmation for the human androgen receptor: Generation of monoclonal antibodies for multiassay performance following the synthetic peptide strategy. *Biochim Biophys Acta* **1073**:23, 1991.
67. Butler R, Leigh PN, McPhaul MJ, Gallo JM: Truncated forms of the androgen receptor are associated with polyglutamine expansion in X-linked spinal and bulbar muscular atrophy. *Hum Mol Genet* **7**:121, 1998.
68. Merry DE, Kobayashi Y, Bailey CK, Taye AA, Fischbeck KH: Cleavage, aggregation and toxicity of the expanded androgen receptor in spinal and bulbar muscular atrophy. *Hum Mol Genet* **7**:693, 1998.
69. Li M, Miwa S, Kobayashi Y, Merry DE, Yamamoto M, Tanaka F, Doyu M, et al: Nuclear inclusions of the androgen receptor protein in spinal and bulbar muscular atrophy. *Ann Neurol* **44**:249, 1998.
70. Becher MW, Kotzuk JA, Sharp AH, Davies SW, Bates GP, Price DL, Ross CA: Intranuclear neuronal inclusions in Huntington's disease and dentatorubral and pallidoluysian atrophy: Correlation between the density of inclusions and *IT15* CAG triplet repeat length. *Neurobiol Dis* **4**:387, 1998.

70a. Paulson HL: Protein fate in neurodegenerative proteinopathies: Polyglutamine diseases join the (mis)fold. *Am J Hum Genet* **64**:339, 1999.

71. Davies SW, Turmaine M, Cozens BA, DiFiglia M, Sharp AH, Ross CA, Scherzinger E, et al: Formation of neuronal intranuclear inclusions underlies the neurological dysfunction in mice transgenic for the HD mutation. *Cell* **90**:537, 1997.
72. Scherzinger E, Lurz R, Turmaine M, Mangiarini L, Hollenbach B, Hasenbank R, Bates GP, et al: Huntingtin-encoded polyglutamine expansions form amyloid-like protein aggregates in vitro and in vivo. *Cell* **90**:549, 1997.
73. Paulson HL, Perez MK, Trottier Y, Trojanowski JQ, Subramony SH, Das SS, Vig P, et al: Intranuclear inclusions of expanded polyglutamine protein in spinocerebellar ataxia type 3. *Neuron* **19**:333, 1997.
74. Ordway JM, Tallaksen GS, Gutekunst CA, Bernstein EM, Cearley JA, Wiener HW, Dure LS, et al: Ectopically expressed CAG repeats cause intranuclear inclusions and a progressive late onset neurological phenotype in the mouse. *Cell* **91**:753, 1997.
75. Warrick JM, Paulson HL, Grayboard GL, Bui QT, Fischbeck KH, Pittman RN, Bonini NM: Expanded polyglutamine protein forms nuclear inclusions and causes neural degeneration in *Drosophila*. *Cell* **93**:939, 1998.

75a. Li M, Nakagomi Y, Kobayashi Y, Merry DE, Tanaka F, Doyu M, Mitsuma T, Hashizume Y, Fischbeck KH, Sobue G: Nonneural nuclear inclusions of androgen receptor protein in spinal and bulbar muscular atrophy. *Am J Pathol* **153**:695, 1998.

75b. Saudou F, Finkbeiner S, Devys D, Greenberg ME: Huntingtin acts in the nucleus to induce apoptosis but death does not correlate with the formation of intranuclear inclusions. *Cell* **95**:55, 1998.

76. Goldberg YP, Nicholson DW, Rasper DM, Kalchman MA, Koide HB, Graham RK, Bromm M, et al: Cleavage of huntingtin by apopain, a proapoptotic cysteine protease, is modulated by the polyglutamine tract. *Nature Genet* **13**:442, 1996.
77. Brinkmann AO, Jenster G, Ris-Stalpers C, van der Korput JAGM, Bruggenwirth HT, Boehmer ALM, Trapman J: Androgen receptor mutations. *J Steroid Biochem Mol Biol* **53**:443, 1995.
78. Chamberlain NL, Driver ED, Miesfeld RL: The length and location of CAG trinucleotide repeats in the androgen receptor N-terminal domain affect transactivation function. *Nucl Acids Res* **22**:3181, 1994.
79. Kazemi-Esfarjani P, Trifiro MA, Pinsky L: Evidence for a repressive function of the long polyglutamine tract in the human androgen receptor: Possible pathogenetic relevance for the $(CAG)_n$-expanded neuronopathies. *Hum Mol Genet* **4**:523, 1995.
80. Mhatre AN, Trifiro MA, Kaufman M, Kazemi EP, Figlewicz D, Rouleau G, Pinsky L: Reduced transcriptional regulatory competence of the androgen receptor in X-linked spinal and bulbar muscular atrophy. *Nature Genet* **5**:184, 1993.
81. Nakajima H, Kimura F, Nakagawa T, Furutama D, Shinoda K, Shimizu A, Ohsawa N: Transcriptional activation by the androgen receptor in X-linked spinal and bulbar muscular atrophy. *J Neurol Sci* **142**:12, 1996.
82. Brooks BP, Paulson HL, Merry DE, Salazar GE, Brinkmann AO, Wilson EM, Fischbeck KH: Characterization of an expanded glutamine repeat androgen receptor in a neuronal cell culture system. *Neurobiol Dis* **3**:313, 1997.
83. Choong CS, Kemppainen JA, Zhou ZX, Wilson EM: Reduced androgen receptor gene expression with first exon CAG repeat expansion. *Mol Endocrinol* **10**:1527, 1996.
84. Neuschmid-Kaspar F, Gast A, Peterziel H, Schneikert J, Muigg A, Ransmayr G, Klocker H, et al: CAG-repeat expansion in androgen receptor in Kennedy's disease is not a loss of function mutation. *Mol Cell Endocrinol* **117**:149, 1996.
85. Sar M, Stumpf WE: Androgen concentration in motor neurons of cranial nerves and spinal cord. *Science* **197**:77, 1977.
86. Nordeen EJ, Nordeen KW, Sengelaub DR, Arnold AP: Androgens prevent normally occurring cell death in a sexually dimorphic spinal nucleus. *Science* **229**:671, 1985.
87. Perez J, Kelley DB: Trophic effects of androgen: Receptor expression and the survival of laryngeal motor neurons after axotomy. *J Neurosci* **16**:6625, 1996.
88. Tanzer L, Jones KJ: Gonadal steroid regulation of hamster facial nerve regeneration: Effects of dihydrotestosterone and estradiol. *Exp Neurol* **146**:258, 1997.
89. Yu WH: Administration of testosterone attenuates neuronal loss following axotomy in the brain-stem motor nuclei of female rats. *J Neurosci* **9**:3908, 1989.
90. Lustig RH, Hua P, Smith LS, Wang C, Chang C: An in vitro model for the effects of androgen on neurons employing androgen receptor-transfected PC12 cells. *Mol Cell Neurosci* **5**:587, 1994.
91. Nakajima H, Kimura F, Nakagawa T, Ikemoto T, Furutama D, Shinoda K, Kato S, et al: Effects of androgen receptor polyglutamine tract expansion on proliferation of NG108-15 cells. *Neurosci Lett* **222**:83, 1997.
92. Perez J, Kelley DB: Androgen mitigates axotomy-induced decreases in calbindin expression in motor neurons. *J Neurosci* **17**:7396, 1997.
93. Clancy AN, Bonsall RW, Michael RP: Immunohistochemical labeling of androgen receptors in the brain of rat and monkey. *Life Sci* **50**:409, 1992.
94. Cain MP, Kramer SA, Tindall DJ, Husmann DA: Expression of androgen receptor protein within the lumbar spinal cord during ontologic development and following antiandrogen induced cryptorchidism. *J Urol* **152**:766, 1994.
95. Simerly RB, Chang C, Mutamatsu M, Swanson LW: Distribution of androgen and estrogen receptor mRNA-containing cells in the rat brain: An *in situ* hybridization study. *J Comp Neurol* **294**:76, 1990.
96. Doyu M, Sobue G, Kimata K, Yamamoto K, Mitsuma T: Androgen receptor mRNA with increased size of tandem CAG repeat is widely expressed in the neural and nonneural tissues of X-linked recessive bulbospinal neuronopathy. *J Neurol Sci* **127**:43, 1994.
97. Nakamura M, Mita S, Matuura T, Nagashima K, Tanaka H, Ando M, Uchino M: The reduction of androgen receptor mRNA in motoneurons of X-linked spinal and bulbar muscular atrophy. *J Neurol Sci* **150**:161, 1997.
98. Trifiro M, Kazemi-Esfarjani P, Pinsky L: X-linked muscular atrophy and the androgen receptor. *Trends Endocrinol Metab* **5**:416, 1994.
99. Igarashi S, Koide R, Shimohata T, Yamada M, Hayashi Y, Takano H, Date H, et al: Suppression of aggregate formation and apoptosis by transglutaminase inhibitors in cells expressing truncated DRPLA protein with an expanded polyglutamine stretch. *Nature Genet* **18**:111, 1998.
100. Cummings CJ, Mancini MA, Antalffy B, Defranco DB, Orr HT, Zoghbi HY: Chaperone suppression of aggregation and altered subcellular proteasome localization imply protein misfolding in SCA1. *Nature Genet* **19**:148, 1998.
101. Simeoni S, Mancini MA, Stenoien DL, Marcelli M, Weigel NL, Zanisi M, Mancini L, Poletti A: Motoneuronal cell death is not correlated with aggregate formation of androgen receptors containing an elongated polyglutamine tract. *Hum Mol Genet* **9**:133, 2000.
102. Harad T, Ishizaki F, Yamamura Y, Tokunaga J, Kito S: A case of Kennedy-Alter-Sung syndrome associated with external ophthalmoplegia: Therapeutic efficacy of fluoxymesterone (in Japanese). *No to Shinkei* **41**:143, 1989.
103. Goldenberg JN, Bradley WG: Testosterone therapy and the pathogenesis of Kennedy's disease (X-linked bulbospinal muscular atrophy). *J Neurol Sci* **135**:158, 1996.

CHAPTER 162

Inherited Defects in Growth Hormone Synthesis and Action

Joy D. Cogan ▪ John A. Phillips III

1. Human growth hormone (hGH, or somatotropin) is essential for normal postnatal growth. It is a 191-amino acid protein that is released from the anterior pituitary gland on stimulation by growth hormone-releasing hormone (GHRH, or somatocrinin), a factor produced by the hypothalamic region of the brain. Like other pituitary hormones, hGH acts on target tissues, in this case primarily the liver, to cause synthesis and release of a second hormone mediator, insulin-like growth factor (IGF) I, also called somatomedin C, into the systemic circulation. IGF-I is a growth-accelerating peptide that acts directly on cartilage to promote bone growth.

2. Deficiency of hGH production causes metabolic alterations and growth failure. While most cases of hGH deficiency are idiopathic, 17 known single gene disorders as well as a variety of other genetic disorders and syndromes are associated with deficiency of hGH or defective action. These genetic disorders are caused by alterations in the hGH gene, alterations of distant loci (such as Pit-1, Prop-1, or GHRHR) that cause hGH deficiency through epistatic effects, or alterations of genes (such as the growth hormone receptor gene (GHR)) that affect the response to hGH.

3. Deficiency of hGH was treated in the past by replacement with exogenous hGH isolated from cadaver pituitaries. Because of the accompanying danger of transmission of infectious neurodegenerative disease (Creutzfeldt-Jakob disease; MIM 123400), alternative methods of treatment are now used. These include replacement with biosynthetic hGH or, in some cases, treatment with GHRH. The potential for hGH gene therapy has been demonstrated in animals.

4. Human chorionic somatomammotropin (hCS, or human placental lactogen) has similar biologic activities, but it is much less potent than hGH. During pregnancy, maternal hCS levels are very high and approximately 300 times greater than fetal levels. While hCS is thought to be important in maternal carbohydrate and fat metabolism, normal fetal growth occurs in pregnancies in which it is absent.

5. Two genetic disorders of the hCS loci have been described. While these alterations lead to deficiency or absent hCS production, affected individuals are thought to be asymptomatic.

HUMAN GROWTH AND CHORIONIC SOMATOMAMMOTROPIN HORMONES

Structure of Human Growth Hormone

Human growth hormone (hGH, or somatotropin) is a globular protein with a molecular mass of 22 kDa. It consists of a single polypeptide chain of 191 amino acid residues, with two disulfide bridges and no carbohydrate moieties (Fig. 162-1).[1–3] Growth hormones (GH) from cattle, sheep, and pigs are very similar, although not identical in structure, to hGH, but all are sufficiently different to render them inactive in humans.[4] The hGH molecule is predominantly α-helical in its secondary structure. While most of the hGH contained in the pituitary gland is the 22-kDa form shown in Fig. 162-1, four other variants (one 45 kDa, two 24 kDa, and one 20 kDa) have been identified.[4] The 45-kDa variant is an aggregate or dimer that probably arises during synthesis of the 22-kDa form in the anterior pituitary.[4–8] It can be converted to the 22-kDa form by treatment with mercaptoethanol and constitutes about 1 percent of the hGH isolated from pituitary glands.[9,10] One 24-kDa variant results from proteolytic cleavage of the 22-kDa molecule between residues 139 and 140. Removal of this peptide bond converts the hGH molecule to a two-chain form, thereby altering its secondary and tertiary structure and increasing its apparent molecular mass.[4,11] A second 24-kDa variant of GH represents pre-hGH, which retains the amino-terminal signal peptide sequence of 26 amino acids (molecular mass, ~2 kDa). This signal or leader sequence is important in directing the transport of the nascent protein molecule across the membrane of the rough endoplasmic reticulum (RER) into its cisternae for packaging.[12] The final hGH variants found in the anterior pituitary are 20 and 17.5 kDa (see Fig. 162-2). These variants, unlike the others, arise from alternative splicing that deletes amino acid residues 32 through 46 or all residues (32 through 71) of exon 3, respectively, during processing of hGH pre-mRNA. The 20-kDa variant constitutes 5 to 10 percent of total pituitary hGH and the 17.5-kDa variant is much less.[13,14]

hGH is synthesized by the somatotropic cells of the anterior pituitary (see Fig. 162-2). It is the most abundant hormone in the pituitary, and the content of a single pituitary gland ranges from 5 to 15 mg, which corresponds to 1 to 3 percent of the weight of the gland.[15]

Structure of Human Chorionic Somatomammotropin and Prolactin

Two other known hormones are similar in structure to hGH. The first, chorionic somatomammotropin (hCS, or human placental lactogen), also contains 191 amino acids, of which 85 percent are

A list of standard abbreviations is located immediately preceding the index in each volume. Additional abbreviations used in this chapter include: CPHD = combined pituitary hormone deficiency; EEC = ectrodactyly-ectodermal dysplasia-clefting syndrome; FSH = follicle-stimulating hormone; GHBP = growth hormone binding protein; GHIF = growth hormone inhibiting factor (somatostatin); GHR = growth hormone receptor; GHRH = human growth hormone-releasing hormone, or somatocrinin; GHRHR = human growth hormone-releasing hormone receptor; hCS = human chorionic somatomammotropin, or human placental lactogen; hGH = human growth hormone, or somatotropin; hPrL = human prolactin; IGF = insulin-like growth factor; IGHD = isolated growth hormone deficiency; LH = luteinizing hormone; Pit-1 = pituitary transcription factor 1; PrL = prolactin; Prop-1 = prophet of Pit-1; RER = rough endoplasmic reticulum RIA = radioimmunoassay; TRH = thyroid-releasing hormone; TSH = thyroid-stimulating hormone.

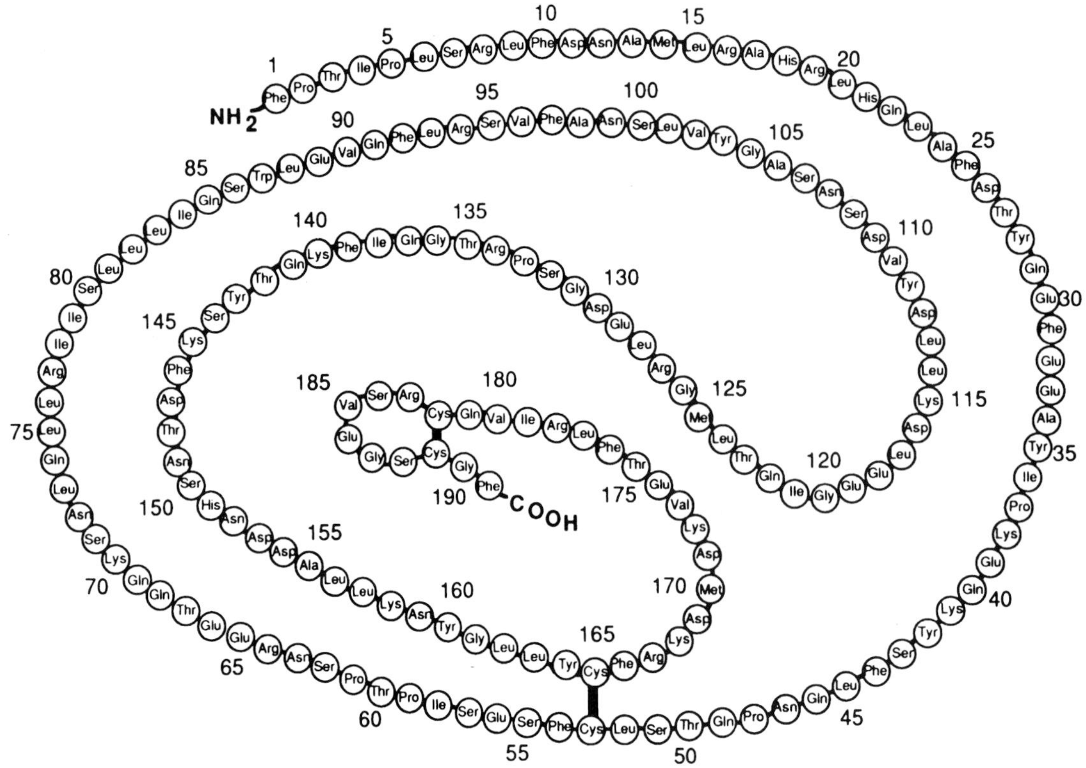

Fig. 162-1 Amino acid sequence of 22-kDa hGH.

identical to hGH, and it also has two disulfide bonds that occur at the same positions as in hGH.[16,17] hCS is synthesized by the syncytiotrophoblastic cells of the fetal placenta, and it is secreted into the maternal circulation. The second hormone that is structurally similar to hGH is prolactin (hPrL), which contains 199 amino acids, of which 35 percent are identical to hGH and 13 percent are identical to hCS.[18,19] hPrL, like hGH, is produced and secreted by the anterior pituitary gland but differs in that hPrL acts to initiate and maintain lactation. hGH, hCS, and hPrL are thought to share sequence homologies because of their evolution from a common ancestral protein through gene duplication events followed by sequence divergence.[18–20]

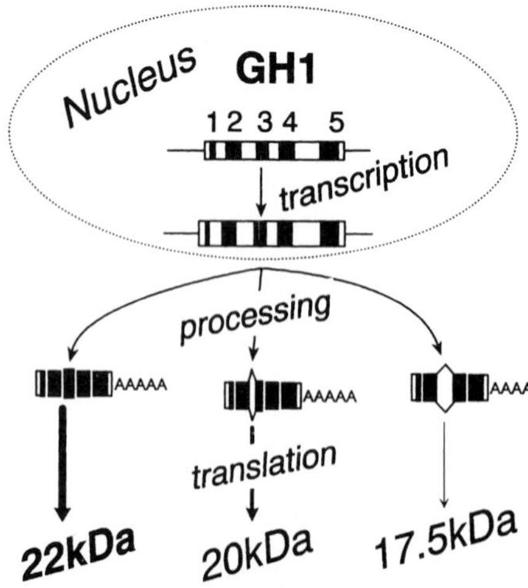

Fig. 162-2 Schematic representation of hGH biosynthesis. The GH1 gene is transcribed to produce pre-mRNA-containing intron sequences. Processing of the pre-mRNA includes removal of introns I to V and the addition of a polyA tail. In 90 percent of the GH1 pre-mRNA molecules, intron II is removed. Alternative splicing of 10 percent of the pre-mRNA molecules also removes the first 15 codons of exon III. In a trace amount of pre-MRNA, all 40 codons of exon III are removed by alternative splicing. The translation products of the major and minor species of pre-mRNA yield 22-, 20-, and 17.5-kDa hGH, respectively. Solid and open rectangles represent exons and introns.

Functional Properties of hGH and hCS

hGH promotes postnatal growth of skeletal and soft tissues through a variety of effects. Controversy remains about the contribution of direct and indirect actions of hGH in this process. On the one hand, direct effects of hGH have been demonstrated in a variety of tissues and organs and the presence of hGH receptors has been documented on a variety of cell types.[4,21–23] On the other hand, a large amount of data indicate that at least a major portion of the effects of hGH are mediated by hGH-dependent insulin-like growth factors (IGF) called "somatomedins."[21,24,25] IGF-I, also called somatomedin C, is highly dependent on the circulating level of hGH.[26] It is a 7649-dalton peptide containing 70 amino acid residues and three disulfide bonds.[27] Traditionally, the liver was thought to be the primary site of IGF-I synthesis, but evidence now suggests that IGF-I is synthesized in many organs and tissues.[28] IGF-II is less dependent on the level of hGH.[27] The protein sequences of both IGF-I and IGF-II have a homology with proinsulin.[29] Preparations of IGF devoid of hGH, insulin, testosterone, or thyroxin have been shown to have somatic and cartilage growth-stimulating potential equivalent to that of hGH.[24,30] Regulation of IGF-I levels is a complex process that is influenced by hGH, hCS, hPrL, steroid hormones (including glucocorticoids, estrogens, and androgens), thyroid hormones, and insulin, as well as the nutritional status and certain disease states.[24,25]

While the biologic functions of hCS and hGH are similar, hCS is a much less potent hormone. Interestingly, hCS is present in very high concentrations in maternal serum and is thought to be partially responsible for the rise in maternal IGF-I levels that occur during pregnancy.[31] hCS shares an anti-insulin effect with hGH, and it is probably important in maternal carbohydrate and fat metabolism during pregnancy.[32,33] Interestingly, studies of two pregnancies associated with an absence of hCS indicate that the

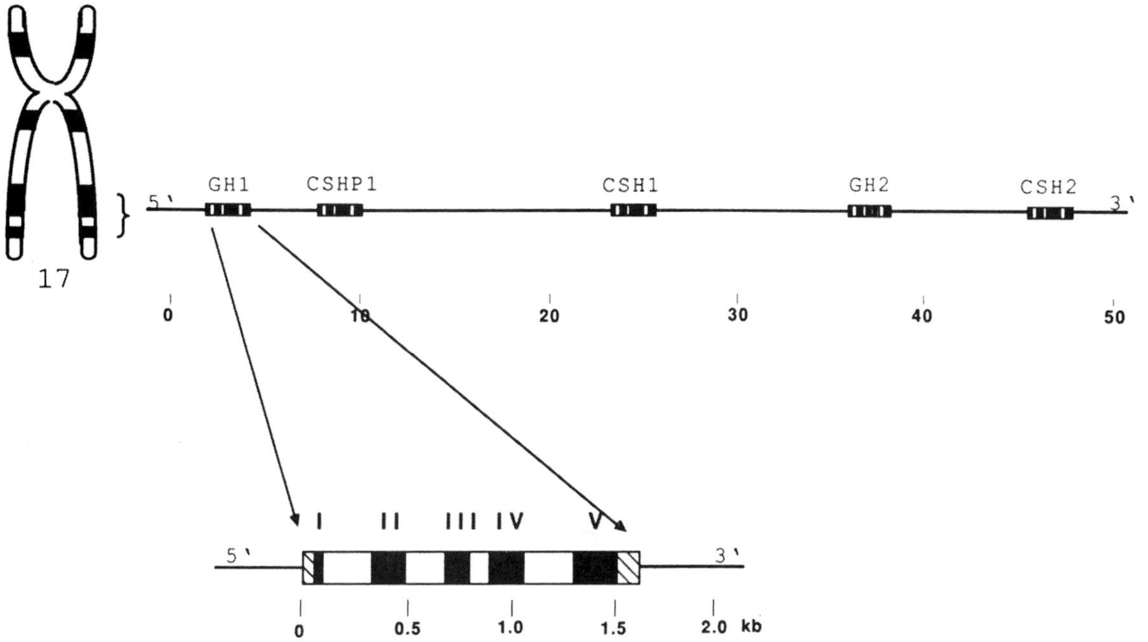

Fig. 162-3 Schematic representation of the GH gene cluster and its localization on human chromosome 17. Exons, introns, and nontranslated sequences are depicted by solid, open, and shaded rectangles, respectively. GH1 encodes hGH; GH2 encodes a variant protein that differs from hGH by 13 amino acids; CSH1 and CSH2 both encode hCS. While CSHP1 has homology, no functional status has been shown.

hormone is not essential for fetal growth, maintenance of pregnancy, or postpartum lactation.[34,35]

hGH AND hCS BIOSYNTHESIS

Genetics

Chromosomal Localizations of hGH and hCS Genes. The genes for hGH and hCS lie within a 50-kb portion of human chromosome 17 (Fig. 162-3). The hGH gene cluster has been assigned to the 17q22-q24 region, whereas the hPrL gene has been mapped to 6p23-q12.[36–39]

hGH Gene Cluster. Previous estimates of the number of hGH-related loci within the 50-kb limits of the hGH gene cluster have ranged from 5 to 7.7.[40–47] Studies of the nucleotide sequences of isolated genomic DNA fragments containing hGH or hCS alleles, as well as studies of large genomic fragments cloned into cosmid vectors, currently indicate that only five loci (two hGH, two hCS, and one hCS-like) reside within the hGH gene cluster (see Fig. 162-3).[45–47] In the case of the hGH genes, one locus (GH1)

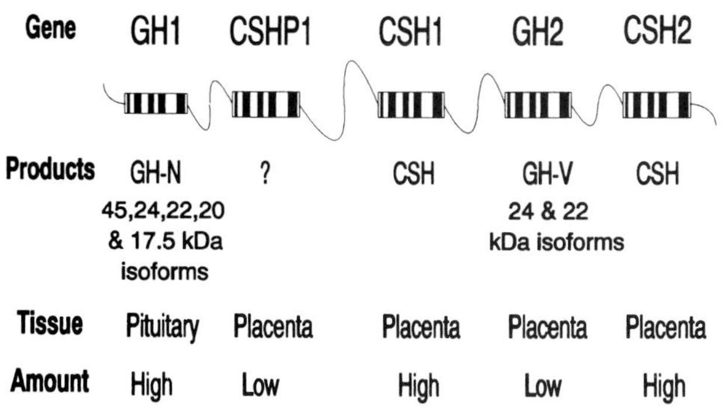

Fig. 162-4 The hGH gene cluster is shown above and the corresponding protein products and the sites of expression are shown below.

encodes the known protein sequence, while the other locus (GH2) encodes a protein that differs from the primary sequence of hGH (Fig. 162-4) at 13 amino acid residues.[41–48] In the case of the hCS genes, there are three loci. The CHS1 and CSH2 loci encode proteins of identical sequence, while the CSHP1 locus encodes a protein that differs by 13 amino acids.[47] Unusual features of the hGH gene cluster include the very high degree of sequence homology retained between its component loci and their flanking regions and the large number (≥27) of *Alu*-type middle repetitive sequences that occur throughout the cluster.[47]

Gene Structure. The nucleotide sequences of the GH1, CSHP1, CSH1, GH2, and CSH2 genes, as well as allelic variants of CSH1 and CSH2, have been reported.[41,47,48] Cloned *Eco*RI-derived genomic DNA fragments of 2.6 kb contain the 2 nonallelic GH1 and GH2 genes. The 2.9-kb *Eco*RI-derived fragments contain the nonallelic CSH1 and CSH2 genes, while the 9.5-kb fragment contains the CSHP1 gene. All five genes are very similar in organization (see Figs. 162-3 and 162-4), each with five exons interrupted at identical positions by small introns. These genes retain 92 to 98 percent homology in their immediate flanking, intervening, and coding sequences.[18] An important exception to the conserved intron-exon organizational homology is CSHP1, which contains 25 nucleotide substitutions in its exons, of which 13 give rise to amino acid substitutions.[47] Another important feature of CSHP1 is the presence of a G-to-A transition in the 5′ or donor splice site of its second intron.[47] This substitution would prevent pre-mRNA processing at the same 5′ splice site utilized by the GH1, CSH1, GH2, and CSH2 loci.[49] While CSHP1 has a cryptic splice site located 45 nucleotides downstream that would yield a protein having 15 additional amino acids, this alternative splice site does not appear to be utilized, because CSHP1-specific oligonucleotides do not detect cDNA clones in libraries derived from human pituitary or placental mRNAs.[47] These data suggest that either CSHP1 is a pseudogene (an inactive gene), hence the designation CSHP1, or that it is only expressed in human tissues other than pituitary or placenta.

The GH1, GH2, CSH1, CSH2, and CSHP1 genes all have CATAAA and TATAAA promoter sequences located 85 and 30 bp,

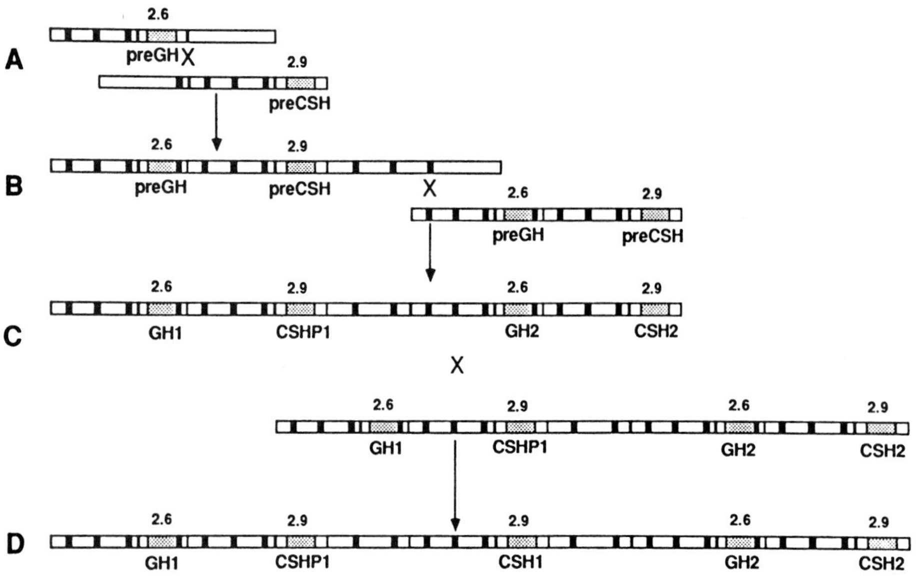

Fig. 162-5 Schematic of the evolution of the hGH gene cluster. The GH/CS precursor gene contained in a 2.6-kb *Eco*RI fragment is shown in A. The product of the first duplication event and the resulting GH and CS genes are shown in B. The GH1-CSHP1-GH2-CSH2 products of the second duplication event are shown in C. Mechanism of the final duplication event which yielded the complete GH gene cluster is shown in D with the partial *Eco*RI restriction map noted above the cluster.

respectively, upstream from their 5′-transcription initiation sites (see Fig. 162-2). In addition, all have the AATAAA sequence in their 3′-flanking regions 20 bp upstream from their polyadenylate (polyA) addition sites.[41,47] The first four genes encode protein products of 217 amino acids (see Fig. 162-4). The length of any possible protein encoded by CSHP1 remains in question because of the gene's possible alternative splice sites and the lack of identified transcripts.[47] The 26 additional amino acids at the N-terminal of each 217-amino acid product constitute signal peptides, or leader sequences, that are important in directing transport through the membrane of the RER.[12] Following transport to this compartment, the signal peptides are cleaved from the 24-kDa prehormones to yield the 191-amino acid (20-kDa) mature hormones.

Introns I, II, III, and IV of GH1 are 256, 209, 93, and 253 bp in length (see Figs. 162-2 and 162-3).[4] Each intron has a 5′-GT and 3′-AG dinucleotide as seen in other eukaryotic intervening sequences. Exon I contains 60 bp of 5′-untranslated sequences, codons −26 through −24 and the first nucleotide of codon −23 (codons −26 through −1 encode the 26 amino acids of the leader sequence with codon −26 encoding the initial methionine residue). Exon II encodes the remainder of the signal peptide sequence and amino acids 1 through 31 of mature hGH (see Fig. 162-1). Exons III, IV, and V encode amino acids 32 through 71, 72 through 126, and 127 through 191, respectively.[4,47] The last exon includes 112 bp of 3′-flanking sequence that extends to the polyA addition site. An AATAAA sequence lies 20 bp upstream from the polyA addition site. The hGH and hCS genes diverge in their 3′-nontranscribed regions, where the genes for GH1 and GH2 contain complete members of an *Alu* family repeat, while the hCS genes all contain a truncated *Alu* sequence of 25-bp length.[41,47]

Evolution of the hGH Gene Cluster. The extensive homology between the various loci within the hGH gene cluster suggests that this multigene family arose through a series of gene duplication events. The finding of a middle-dispersed *Alu* repeat 100 bp downstream from the polyA site of GH1 and GH2, but only a truncated *Alu* repeat in the corresponding region of CS1 and CS2 and CSHP1, suggests that the truncated *Alu* repeat represents the 3′ end point of homology.[46,47] The presence of an *Alu* repeat at the breakpoint also suggests that the mechanism of duplication involved unequal recombination between two nonallelic *Alu* repeats as has been reported for nonreciprocal recombination events in the globin and LDL receptor genes.[50,51] Interestingly, sequences extending at least 500 bp upstream from the hGH and hCS genes show very high homology. This homology includes a 5′-*Eco*RI-derived fragment of 4.7 to 5.3 kb flanking each of the hGH and hCS loci. These *Eco*RI-derived fragments contain three *Alu* repeats located in analogous positions.[46,47] The hGH gene cluster is hypothesized to have arisen by serial unequal crossover events involving copies of these repeated segments.[18,20,46,47] *Alu*-*Alu* recombination probably constituted the first duplication event that yielded a GH-CS unit (Fig. 162-5). The second hypothesized duplication event created a 5′-GH1-CSHP1-GH2-CSH2-3′ cluster. Subsequently, the CSH1 locus probably arose by another unequal crossover between *Alu* repeats to give the final 5′-GH1-CSHP1-CSH1-GH2-CSH2-3′ cluster (see Fig. 162-5).[18,20,46,47]

DNA Polymorphisms. Six RFLPs have been reported in the hGH gene cluster (Fig. 162-6).[20] Of these 6 RFLPs, five (two *Bgl*II, two *Msp*I, and one *Hinc*II) occur in blacks, Mediterraneans, and Northern Europeans.[20,45] The sixth, a *Bam*HI-derived RFLP, occurs predominantly in blacks. Haplotypes constructed for these RFLPs display strong nonrandom associations. Interestingly, the strongest associations are found between the RFLPs closely related by evolution rather than between those that are in closest physical proximity.[20] The observations of strong linkage disequilibrium between GH1 and GH2 and between CSHP1 and CSH1 and CSH2 support the idea of an evolution of the hGH gene

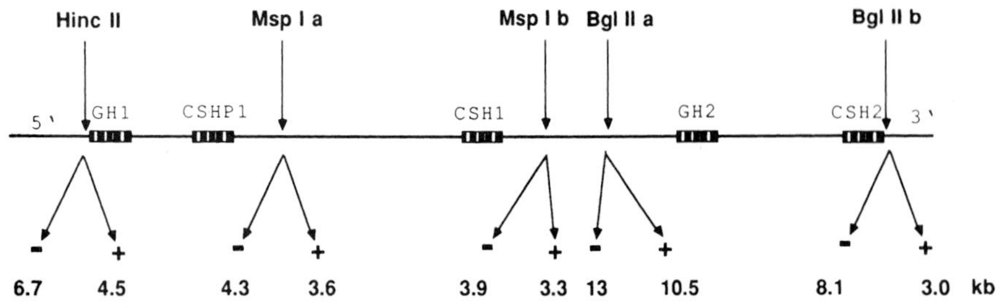

Fig. 162-6 Locations of five polymorphic restriction endonuclease cleavage sites in the hGH gene cluster detected with GH1 cDNA as a probe. The size (kb) of the alternative alleles is shown below.

cluster through the serial duplications described above (see Fig. 162-5).

Ontogeny and Disease Manifestation

The hGH and hCS genes are expressed in different tissues in different relative amounts and at different times during human development (see Fig. 162-4). Fetal production of hCS is roughly proportional to the syncytiotrophoblastic cell mass.[52] The amount synthesized at 34 to 37 weeks of gestation is four- to fivefold higher than at the end of the first trimester. At term, 15 to 20 percent of polyA+ placental RNA is hCS mRNA, and 1 g/day hCS is produced.[53,54] Maternal serum hCS levels reach 3 to 8 μg/ml, about 300 times fetal levels. The CSH1 and CSH2 genes are expressed in an approximately 1:1 ratio at term.[55] Because production of hCS is normally limited to placental tissue, none is produced after birth. Complete deficiency of hCS production has been detected during pregnancy by monitoring maternal serum levels.[34,35] The presence of a normal growth pattern during fetal life and infancy in these cases suggests that hCS is not required for fetal or extrauterine growth.[56]

Synthesis of hGH in the fetal pituitary occurs by 7 to 9 weeks of gestation.[57,58] hGH appears in fetal serum at the end of the first trimester, and its level increases rapidly to reach a peak of 100 to 150 ng/ml at about 20 weeks gestation.[58] Mean fetal plasma levels then decline to about 30 ng/ml at term. Levels of hGH continue to decline for the first several months after birth, and in childhood the basal levels of hGH are similar to those of adults. Secretion of hGH occurs in pulses, and the frequency and amplitude of these increase during puberty. Secretion continues throughout life, declining in old age.

While hGH production occurs in the fetus, its presence seems to be less important to fetal growth than maternal and nutritional factors.[57–59] For example, anencephalic fetuses and those with aplasia of the pituitary gland, as well as those with absent hGH production due to genetic defects, are of relatively normal size at birth. Hormonal and familial factors, as well as nutrition, affect growth between birth and puberty. Growth retardation may occur due to deficiencies in hGH or other hormonal deficiencies, as well as chronic illness. The combined actions of hGH, sex steroids, and IGF-I are required for the pubertal growth spurt.[60] HGH production continues throughout life and is limited to the anterior pituitary.[61]

The onset of growth retardation due to hGH deficiency usually occurs after birth. Fetuses who are homozygous for GH1 gene deletions have relatively normal fetal growth, suggesting that other gene products are primarily responsible for stimulation of embryonic and fetal growth.[62] Infants with severe congenital hGH deficiency manifest growth retardation by 4 to 6 months of age. Children with acquired or progressive hGH deficiency may appear to have had relatively normal growth until several months or years of age, but their growth data often reveal a decreased growth velocity in infancy. Finally, certain growth disorders may not present until puberty. The short stature of African pygmies, for example, is due to absence of the normal pubertal increase in IGF-I levels with resultant lack of a pubertal growth spurt.[63]

hGH and hCS Biosynthesis

Normal and Alternative Transcription Initiation. The primary transcripts of GH1, CSHP1, CSH1, GH2, and CSH2 genes are about 1650 nucleotides in length (see Figs. 162-2 and 162-3). In the case of the CSH1 and CSH2 genes, two different initiation sites for transcription have been demonstrated.[64] While the majority of transcripts initiate 30 bp downstream from the TATAAA sequence, about 5 percent of the transcripts initiate 30 bp downstream from a CATAAA sequence that is located 55 bp upstream of the TATAAA sequence. A second initiation site, 196 bp upstream from the cap site, is also known for the GH1 gene. The gene product, called GH gene-derived transcriptional activator (GHDTA), does not resemble GH but instead shares sequence homology with hepatic nuclear factor-1α.[65]

Normal and Alternative Splicing. Processing of the transcripts, including excision of intervening sequences and splicing of the five exons, yields mRNA that encodes the prehormones of 217 amino acids. The mRNA sizes expected to correspond to unprocessed and processed hCS RNA have been documented in northern blot analysis of term placental RNA.[54] Placental total RNA contained a predominance of hCS mRNA that was about 860 nucleotides in length, while nuclear RNA also contained species that were 990, 1200, 1460, and 1760 nucleotides in length. These higher-molecular-weight nuclear RNA species represent intermediate and unspliced transcripts of hCS mRNA.

Alternative splicing of the primary GH1 transcripts is the basis of the 20-kDa and 17.5-kDa hGH-variant peptides (see Figs. 162-2 and 162-4)[11,13] in contrast to the 22-kDa standard hGH. The 20-kDa variant constitutes between 5 and 10 percent of the total hGH in pituitary extracts, and it differs from the major 22-kDa hGH polypeptide by having an internal deletion of 15 amino acids (residues 32 through 46).[13,14] The triplets that encode these 15 amino acids begin precisely at the 5′ end of exon III (see Fig. 162-2). In addition, 45 bp downstream from this point the sequence preceding the codon for amino acid 47 corresponds to consensus sequences for splice acceptor sites.[44,66–68] Thus, the 45 nucleotides contained in the 5′ end of exon III are deleted by alternative splicing at the cryptic splice acceptor site that precedes codon 47, which results in the deletion of codons 32 through 46. The 17.5-kDa variant is the result of splicing out or "skipping" of exon 3 which encodes amino acids 32 to 71. Production of the 22-kDa hGH relative to the 17.5-kDa variant is determined by an IVS3 splice enhancer which modulates selection of the IVS3 5′ splice site. Mutations within the IVS3 splice enhancer cause increased "skipping" of exon 3, overproduction of the 17.5-kDa isoform, and IGHD II in humans (see "IGHD II" below).[69]

Variant Peptides. Multiple size and charge variants of hGH have been described in addition to the 20-kDa alternative splice product (see Fig. 162-4). These include the 45-kDa dimers and two 24-kDa variants that result from posttranslational modifications of hGH. One 24-kDa variant results from retention of the 26-amino acid signal-peptide sequence of pre-hGH. The other 24-kDa variant results from cleavage between amino acids residues 139 and 140 of the normal 22-kDa form of hGH.[4] While each may represent a unique hormone with specific receptors and physiological functions, only in the case of the 24-kDa variant is a specialized function reported. This variant may be responsible for the lactogenic activity of hGH.[70] While none of these variants are thought to represent products of the CSHP1 or GH2 genes, specific radioimmunoassays to detect these products in serum are not available. An alternative method of detection of expression of these gene products is to screen cDNA libraries derived from various tissues. Using this approach, GH2-specific mRNA has been detected in placental tissue.[44,47]

Physiological Regulation

Gene Structure. hGH production and secretion by the anterior pituitary gland is under complex regulatory control (see Figs. 162-2 and 162-7). At the level of transcription hGH production is increased by thyroid hormone, glucocorticoids, and growth hormone-releasing hormone (GHRH).[71,72] The DNA sequences required for the effects of thyroid and glucocorticoid hormone induction appear to be different. The thyroid hormone receptor complex binds to GH1 flanking sequences −290 to −129 bp upstream from the transcription initiation site.[73] Additional studies of the local effects of thyroid hormone on GH1 chromatin indicate that four sites may function in transcription: one is located over 1000 bp upstream from the GH1 promoter; a second is located in the first 200 bp upstream from the origin of transcription; a third at the position of the TATA sequence; and the fourth is located in the first intron.[74] Sequences of hGH that preferentially bind to glucocorticoid receptor complexes also include immediate 5′-flanking sequences as well as a portion of the first intron.[75] The

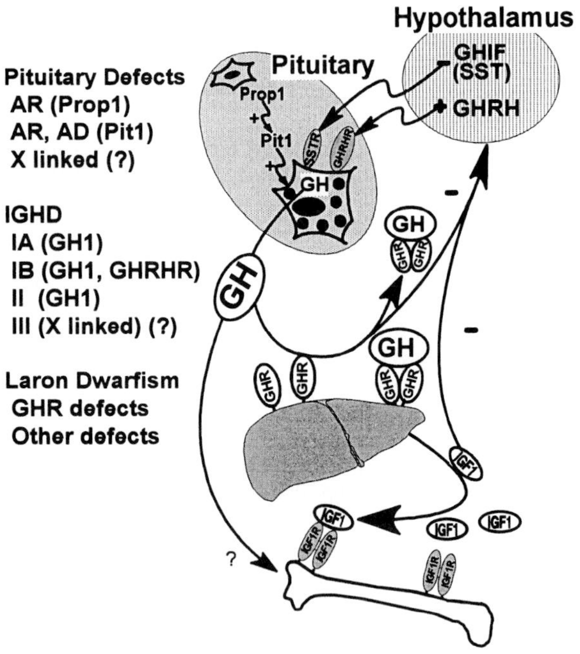

Fig. 162-7 The hGH secretory pathway showing regulatory factors. The sites of derangements responsible for various familial disorders of the hGH axis are indicated on the left. AR = autosomal recessive; AD = autosomal dominant.

effects of thyroid and glucocorticoid hormones appear to be independent and additive.[71] In addition to inducing GH1 transcription, glucocorticoids may also enhance hGH expression through stabilization of the mRNA.[76]

In contrast to hGH, relatively little is known about the regulation of hCS secretion. Synthesis of hCS is normally limited to the syncytiotrophoblastic cells of the placenta. Thyroid hormone may also enhance hCS transcription, because the thyroid hormone-receptor complex binds to analogous promoter regions of the CSH genes.[73]

Hormonal Modulators and Interactions. Secretion of hGH into the peripheral circulation is controlled by at least two hypothalamic factors—growth hormone-releasing hormone (GHRH or somatocrinin) and somatostatin (GHIF) (Fig. 162-7).[77,78] Secretion of hGH into the general circulation is promoted by the 44-amino acid GHRH, and pulsatile release of hypothalamic GHRH is the principal cause of the pulsatile pattern of hGH secretion.[79] Somatostatin is a 14-amino acid neuropeptide that inhibits release of hGH.[78,80,81] In turn, GHRH and GHIF are modulated by the effects of various environmental and biologic factors including stress, sleep, hypoglycemia, chemicals (L-dopa, chlorpromazine), and hormones (androgens, estrogens, hGH, and vasopressin) on the central nervous system and hypothalamus.[77] Apart from sleep, most physiological stimuli of hGH release are inhibited by α-adrenergic blocking agents such as phentolamine, and release is stimulated by α-adrenergic agonists such as clonidine. β-Adrenergic blockade increases hGH secretion and propranolol is used to stimulate hGH secretion in provocative tests. Stimulation of hGH release by L-dopa is mainly through its conversion to norepinephrine. Estrogens enhance hGH secretion, and hGH responses in males increase with the onset of puberty due to androgens.[77] High hGH levels are thought to inhibit hGH release by negative feedback. In conditions in which the level of IGF-I is low, such as severe malnutrition, these low levels may function to increase hGH release.[25,27]

The complex interactions of various factors that modulate hGH synthesis and secretion result in its pulsatile secretion pattern. After the neonatal period, basal plasma levels of hGH are low throughout most of the 24-h daily cycle. Intermittent pulses of secretion occur in response to physiological stimuli, and a consistent surge lasting about 2 h occurs 1 to 2 h after sleep begins. Additional pulses of secretion occur with exercise, stress, or high-protein meals, while hyperglycemia suppresses hGH release. The mean concentration of hGH in plasma calculated from continuous 24-h monitoring is 2 to 4 ng/ml in young adults and 5 to 8 ng/ml in children and adolescents. Based on mean hGH plasma levels and calculated clearance of hGH, the 24-h secretion rate in young men is about 1 to 2 mg/day.[82]

GENETIC DISORDERS OF hGH OR hCS SYNTHESIS AND ACTION

Background

Because neither hGH nor hCS is essential for fetal growth, newborns with complete deficiency of either are usually of normal length and weight. The presence of micropenis or fasting hypoglycemia in some affected infants may be early diagnostic clues to hGH deficiency.[83] Linear growth of affected individuals continues at a low rate, falling into the subnormal range by 6 to 12 months of age, and the height becomes progressively retarded with advancing age. In isolated hGH deficiency (IGHD), the skeletal maturation or bone development age usually exhibits a delay that is proportional to the retardation in height. The presence of a fine, wrinkled skin similar to that of premature aging often occurs in adult patients.[84] Puberty may be delayed until the late teens, but IGHD is quite compatible with fertility in both sexes. Concomitant deficiency of luteinizing hormone (LH), follicle-stimulating hormone (FSH), thyrotropin (TSH), and/or ACTH along with hGH deficiency is called combined pituitary hormone deficiency (CPHD) or panhypopituitarism. Due to these additional hormone deficiencies, the retardation of growth and skeletal maturation in CPHD tends to be more severe, and spontaneous puberty may not occur.

Diagnosis of hGH Deficiency

Basal levels of hGH are high in normal newborns. Very low or undetectable levels during the neonatal period are significant, and hypoglycemia in the neonatal period without abnormalities in insulin or cortisol levels should be evaluated by determining an hGH level. Serum hGH levels of < 10 ng/ml in the presence of hypoglycemia and low insulin concentrations should be considered highly suggestive of hGH deficiency. In such cases, thyroxine and TSH should be measured, because primary hypothyroidism can impair the response to hGH. The small genitalia of males with hGH deficiency may or may not be associated with gonadotropin deficiency. If an infant does not have hypoglycemia or other signs that make IGHD likely, provocative tests may be delayed to permit observations of the growth velocity over several months.

During early childhood the presence of short stature and decreased growth velocity are important clinical clues to hGH deficiency. Most children with hGH deficiency have truncal obesity in addition to significant short stature, and their facial appearance often suggests that they are younger than their chronologic age. Secondary dentition is often delayed, and the voice is usually high-pitched. Small genitalia in males and features associated with deficiencies of other pituitary hormones may also be present in those with CPHD.

In the school-aged child with IGHD the height is usually 2.5 to 3 SD below the mean.[85,86] This may not be true for those with deficiency of recent onset, such as that caused by craniopharyngioma or other central nervous system tumors, head trauma, histiocytosis X, meningitis, or head irradiation.[77,82] The parental heights should be used to calculate a target range for the child's height appropriate for the genetic background. Also, the weight-for-height percentile should be determined, because IGHD children, in contrast to those with short stature due to non-endocrine causes, tend to be obese. Finally, determinations of upper to lower segment body ratios and skeletal radiographs are helpful in detecting the various skeletal dysplasias. While most school-aged children with IGHD will have bone ages that are 2 or more SD below the mean for their age, untreated patients with CPHD may have even greater retardation of the bone age with epiphyseal closure delayed beyond the third decade.

Confirmatory Tests of hGH Deficiency

There is no single laboratory test or procedure that establishes with 100 percent accuracy the presence or absence of hGH deficiency. Most tests require the measurement of stimulated serum levels of hGH by radioimmunoassay. Because levels of hGH are low throughout most of the 24-h period, results of single, random blood samples usually are not helpful. For this reason, provocative tests of hGH secretory reserve are utilized. Those most frequently used include stimulation of hGH release by exercise, L-dopa, insulin, arginine, clonidine, glucagon, or combinations of exercise plus L-dopa or insulin plus arginine.[82,87,88] An inadequate hGH response (peak plasma levels < 7 ng/ml) following two or more of the provocative tests suggests hGH deficiency. Peak levels between 7 and 15 ng/ml are compatible with partial deficiency, and levels over 15 ng/ml exclude deficiency.[88]

Patients should be carefully evaluated for other systemic diseases prior to testing for hGH deficiency. The usual screening tests for evaluation of a child with significant short stature include determination of levels of serum electrolytes, creatinine, thyroid and thyroid-stimulating hormone, chromosome analysis in females, lateral skull films, and bone age determinations. Disorders that should be considered include Bartter syndrome, craniopharyngioma, hypothyroidism, renal tubular acidosis or chronic renal failure, Turner syndrome, and systemic diseases such as congenital heart disease and cystic fibrosis.[88] Selected testing procedures for hGH status include those discussed below.

Postexercise Test. A blood sample for hGH is taken 25 min after strenuous exercise—for example, after 15 min on a bicycle ergometer or after climbing stairs. About 80 percent of healthy children will have normal hGH levels.[89]

L-Dopa Tests. Following administration of an oral dose of L-dopa (125 mg for patients under 10 kg, 250 mg for those weighing 10 to 30 kg, and 500 mg for those over 30 kg, or 50 mg/1.75 m^2 to a maximum of 500 mg), about 80 percent of normal children will respond.[87,90]

Insulin-Tolerance Test. Blood samples for hGH levels are taken at 0, 20, 30, 45, 60, 90, 120, and 150 min after IV administration of insulin (0.1 U/kg).[87,88] About 90 percent of normal children respond.[91] For a valid test, the blood glucose level must fall to less than half the fasting level. Precautions must be taken to prevent severe hypoglycemia. The insulin dose should be decreased to 0.05 U/kg in those with suspected CPHD.

Intravenous Arginine Test. Blood samples for hGH are taken at 0, 30, 60, 90, 120, and 150 min after IV administration of arginine (0.5 g/kg; maximum dose 40 g) over 30 min.[92] Between 80 and 90 percent of normal children respond.[87,88,92] This test is contra-indicated in children with diabetes insipidus or severe renal disease.

Oral Clonidine Test. Blood samples for hGH are taken at 0, 30, 60, 90, 120, and 150 min after oral administration of clonidine (0.15 mg/m^2).[88,93–96] This test has a comparable reliability (about 90 percent) to the insulin-tolerance test but may be safer.[96] Side effects include hypotension and drowsiness.

Intramuscular Glucagon Test. Blood samples for hGH are taken 0, 30, 60, 90, 120, and 150 min after the administration of glucagon (30 to 100 μg/kg; maximum dose 1 mg) intramuscularly.[88,95] About 55 percent of normal adults respond. Reliability is improved with oral administration of propranolol prior to glucagon administration; however, this increases the danger of hypoglycemia.[96]

Exercise and L-Dopa Test. Following 20 min of climbing stairs, blood samples are drawn 0, 30, 60, 90, and 120 min after administration of 10 mg/kg L-dopa orally.[97] This test is reported to increase the sensitivity of either component test.

Insulin Plus Arginine Test. Blood samples for hGH are taken at 0, 20, 30, 45, 60, and 90 min after the IV administration of insulin (0.1 or 0.05 U/kg; see above). Immediately after obtaining the 90-min sample, IV arginine (0.5 g/kg) is given over 30 min, and samples are taken at 30, 45, 60, 90, and 120 min.[88] The combination of these two tests provokes response in about 95 percent of normal children.[98]

Etiology of hGH Deficiency

Estimates of the frequency of hGH deficiency range from 1 in 4000 to 1 in 10,000 births in the British Isles.[99–101] Most cases are sporadic and are presumed to be secondary to a wide variety of etiologies, including central nervous system insults or defects, such as septo-optic dysplasia, head trauma, meningitis, cerebral edema, congenital infections, histiocytosis X, chromosome anomalies, cranial tumors, or cranial radiation.[77,82,102–109] In families in which there is consanguinity or a second case occurs, a genetic etiology should be suspected. Estimates of the number of cases having an affected first-degree relative (parent or sib) range from 3 to 30 percent in different series.[100,110,111] There are 17 recognized Mendelian disorders that can cause decreased hGH or hCS production or action (Table 162-1). These disorders differ in their phenotypes (degree of hGH or other hormonal deficiencies) as well as their modes of inheritance.

Isolated hGH Deficiency (IGHD; MIM 262400). There are four known Mendelian types of IGHD (see Table 162-1). These disorders differ in their degree of hGH deficiency, mode of inheritance, or responsiveness to hGH replacement.

IGHD Type IA. Of the Mendelian types of IGHD, type IA (originally referred to as type A) is the most severe. Patients with IGHD type IA occasionally have short body length at birth and hypoglycemia, but severe dwarfism by 6 months of age is a consistent finding. In response to exogenous hGH, they have a strong initial anabolic response that is frequently followed by the development of anti-hGH antibodies in sufficient titer to cause an arrest of response to hGH replacement.[112–114] These features led Illig *et al.* to hypothesize that individuals affected with IGHD-IA had prenatal deficiency of endogenous hGH secretion causing a lack of immune tolerance to exogenous hGH.[114]

The pedigrees of 11 unrelated families, each with one or more individuals with several of these clinical features, are shown in Fig. 162-8. To determine whether the GH1 genes were altered in these patients, genomic DNA was isolated from the leukocytes and each subject's GH1 gene complement was determined by Southern blotting and hybridization with ^{32}P-labeled GH1 cDNA.[115–118] The affected individuals were found to be homozygous for GH1 gene deletions (Fig. 162-9).[46,119] Additional studies of DNA from affected individuals in pedigrees from other countries (see Fig. 162-8) also revealed homozygous deletions of their GH1 genes.[120–123] Additional patients from Israel and France have been described, so that more than 25 cases are reported.[124,125]

To determine whether the deletions were heterogeneous in affected individuals whose pedigrees are shown in Fig. 162-8, aliquots of DNA were digested with *Hind*III and analyzed by Southern blot. These studies showed differences in the sizes of the DNA deletions (6.7, 7.0, or 7.6 kb) with the majority (14 of 19, or ~75 percent) being 6.7 kb (see Fig. 162-10 and Table

Table 162-1 Genetic Disorders of hGH or hCS Biosynthesis or Action

Disorder	Gene	Inheritance	Endogenous hGH	Response to hGH
Isolated hGH deficiency				
IA	GH	AR	Absent	Often temporary
IB	GH	AR	Decreased	Present
	GHRHR	AR	Decreased	Present
II	GH	AD	Decreased	Present
III	?	X-linked	Decreased	Present
"Bioinactive" hGH	GH	?	?Inactive	?Present
Laron dwarfism I	GHR	AR	Normal or increased	Absent
Laron dwarfism II	IGF-1	AR	Normal or increased	Absent
Combined pituitary hormone deficiency				
I	Pit-1	AR or AD	Decreased*	Present
	Prop-1	AR	Decreased*	Present
II	Xq25-q26	X-linked	Decreased*	Present
EEC syndrome	?	AD	Decreased*	Present
Fanconi pancytopenia	?	AR	Decreased	Present
Holoprosencephaly	?	AR or AD	Absent or decreased*	NA
Pituitary aplasia	?	?AR	Absent*	Present
Rieger syndrome	?	AD	Decreased*	?Present
Isolated hCS deficiency	?			
1A	CSH	AR	Absent	NA
1B	CSH	AR	Decreased	NA

AR = autosomal recessive; AD = autosomal dominant; NA = nonapplicable.
*Conditions in which deficiencies of hGH and other anterior pituitary hormones occur.

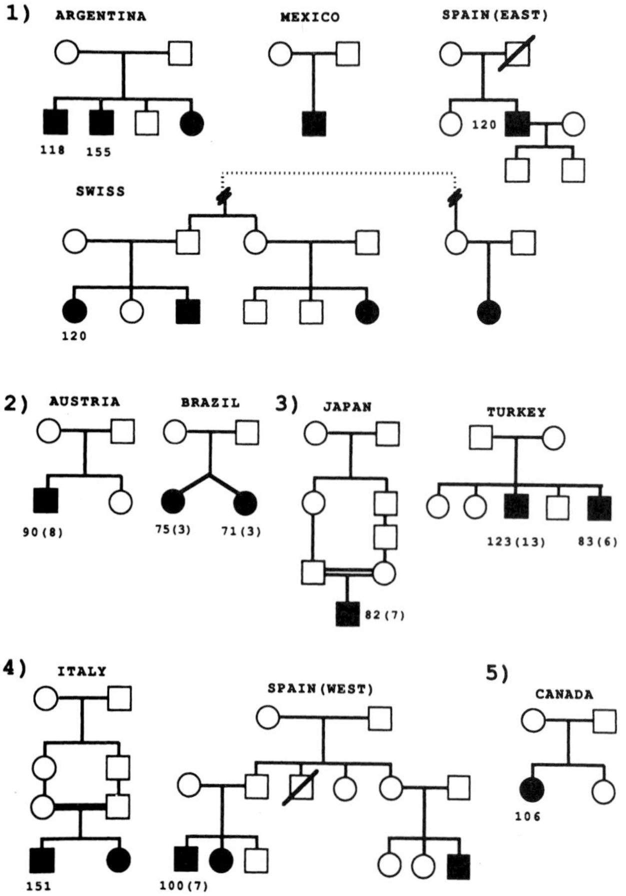

Fig. 162-8 Pedigrees of families each having one or more individuals affected (solid symbols) with IGHD-IA. The country of origin and adult heights are given above and below the pedigree symbols.

162-2).[121,123,126] Several cases of patients with 45 kb deletions (deletion of the GH1, CSHP1, CSH1, and GH2 genes) have also been reported in unrelated families from Turkey, Italy, and Asia (see Table 162-2).[127–131]

DNA sequence analysis of the fusion fragments associated with GH1 gene deletions has shown that homologous recombination between sequences flanking GH1 causes these deletions.[132,133] Using oligonucleotide primers that match both flanking sequences, the 5′ and 3′ homologous sequences that normally flank the GH1 gene and the fusion fragments associated with GH1 gene deletions can be PCR-amplified (Fig. 162-11).[133] Because the 5′, 3′, and fused sequences differ in their restriction enzyme sites, such as *Sma*I, the fusion fragments associated with deletions can be easily detected by enzyme digestion of PCR products (Fig. 162-12).[133,134] Using this method Mullis *et al.* surveyed 78 patients with severe IGHD (≥4.5 SD in height) and found that 13 percent had GH1 gene deletions.[135]

The levels of hGH for patients with hGH deletions are extremely low and the majority have high titers of anti-hGH antibodies during replacement, which block the growth response to exogenous hGH (see Table 162-2).[119,122,136,137] Interestingly, one patient in whom blocking antibodies to pituitary-derived hGH developed has subsequently shown a good initial response when treated with recombinant DNA-derived methionyl-hGH.[138] In addition, some patients have shown fair to good long-term growth responses despite high titers of anti-hGH antibodies. Interestingly, Laron *et al.* reported cases of IGHD-IA in which no anti-hGH antibodies were detected following hGH replacement.[124] In 10 GH gene-deletion patients who were identified by PCR analysis of 78 patients with severe IGHD (height ≤4.5 SD) (see Figs. 162-11 and 162-12), 30 percent developed anti-GH antibodies following treatment with exogenous GH.[135]

Finally, the clinical response to treatment with hGH as determined by height increments ranged widely from poor to good. The growth responses are shown on composite growth charts (Figs. 162-13 and 162-14) in which the solid lines represent growth without and the dotted lines represent growth during hGH

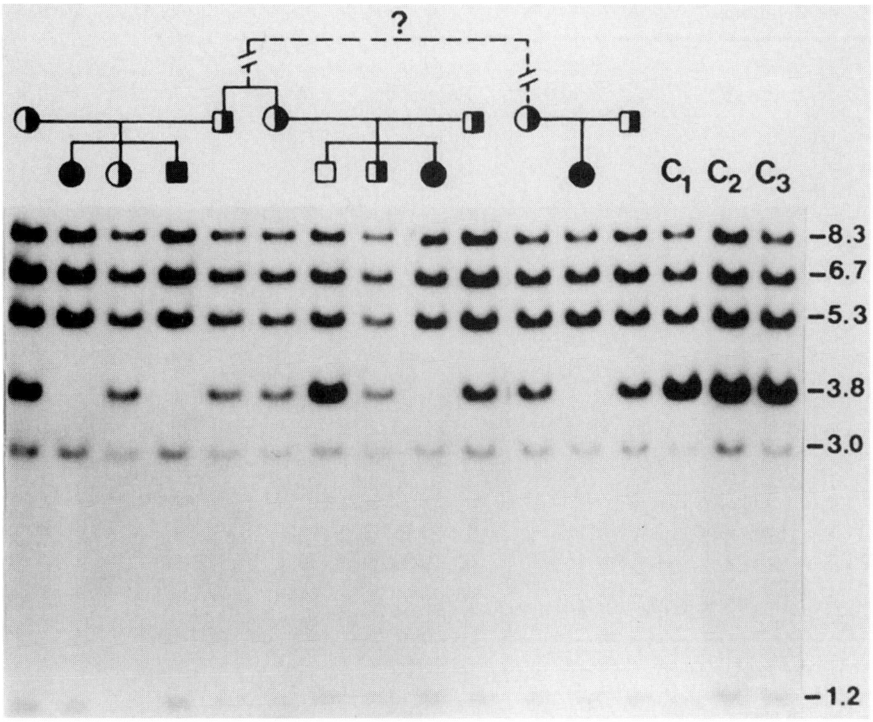

Fig. 162-9 Autoradiogram patterns of DNA from three Swiss families and three controls (C_1-C_3) following digestion with *Bam*HI and hybridization to the GH1 cDNA probe. The multiple bands seen correspond to DNA fragments containing the various genes that comprise the GH gene cluster (see Figs. 162-3 to 162-6). In decreasing order of size the fragments and genes included are 8.3-kb CSHP1, 6.7-kb CSC2, 5.3-kb CSH1, 3.8-kb GH1, and 3.0- plus 1.2-kb GH2.[46,117] The affected individuals lack and their parents have decreased amounts of the 3.8-kb fragment as compared with the controls (C_1-C_3).[117]

replacement therapy.[120,124,126] It is interesting that better growth responses occurred in the patients with the larger 7.6-kb deletion.[121,122] Normal adult height was achieved in one subject with this deletion who was begun on hGH replacement within the first 3 months after birth (Fig. 162-14).[123]

Studies utilizing DNA sequence analysis of PCR amplification products have detected point mutations causing IGHD-IA.[139–141] In a consanguineous Turkish family, a G → A transition in the twentieth codon of GH1 signal peptide was found that converts a TGG (Trp) → TAG (stop) codon and generates a new *Alu*I recognition site. *Alu*I digestion of PCR amplification products of the GH1 alleles of family members segregates with the IGHD phenotype (see Fig. 162-15 and Table 162-3).[139,140] Interestingly, the responses to exogenous GH replacement differed between two affected cousins due to the development of anti-GH antibodies in one.[140] In another patient, Duquesnoy *et al.* found a deletion that was inherited from one parent and a frameshift in the signal peptide of the GH1 gene that was inherited from the other (see Table 162-3).[141]

IGHD Type IB. A second autosomal recessive type of IGHD (IGHD-IB) is characterized by the production of deficient but detectable amounts of hGH after provocative stimuli. This contrasts with the absence of hGH secretion that occurs in IGHD-IA. In contrast to IGHD-IA patients, those with IGHD-IB have no detectable GH1 gene deletions.[45]

GH1 Gene Defects. Using DNA sequence analysis of PCR amplification products Cogan et al. detected a point mutation causing IGHD-IB.[140] In a Saudi Arabian family a G → C transversion was found that alters the first base of the 5′ splice site of intron 4 (IVS4) (see Figs. 162-3 and Table 162-3).[140,142] This substitution perturbs GH1 mRNA splicing and destroys an *Hph*I site that was used to demonstrate cosegregation of the G → C transversion with the IGHD-IB phenotype. Interestingly, Miller-Davis *et al.* identified another mutation (G → T) at the same base of the IVS4 5′ splice site that also causes IGHD-IB (see Table 162-3).[143]

Abdul-Latif *et al.* identified a G → C transversion of the fifth base of the 5′ splice site of IVS4 in a consanguineous family with IGHD-IB (see Table 162-3).[144] This substitution created an additional *Mae*II site, which was used to screen all family members. RT-PCR analysis of mRNA transcripts from lymphoblasts of an affected patient demonstrated that the IVS4 +5G → C had the same effect on splicing as the IVS4 +1G → C.

Igarashi *et al.* found that a fourth IGHD-IB patient with severe growth retardation had two different GH gene defects One allele had a 6.7-kb GH gene deletion and the other had a 2-bp deletion in exon 3 (see Table 162-3).[145] The 2-bp deletion causes a frameshift in exon 3, generating a premature stop codon in exon 4. The patient responded well to GH replacement therapy and did not produce anti-GH antibodies.

The clinical criteria used to classify the IGHD-IB phenotype includes an accelerated growth response to exogenous hGH replacement.[45,137] This observation and lack of anti-hGH antibodies in those studied suggests that sufficient endogenous hGH secretion occurs to prevent the anti-hGH antibody production that characterizes IGHD-IA. Interestingly, some patients with IGHD-IB have been shown to have intact secretory granules in their somatotropes and to exhibit normal hGH responses to GHRH infusions.[146,147] This observation indicates that the GH1 allele(s)

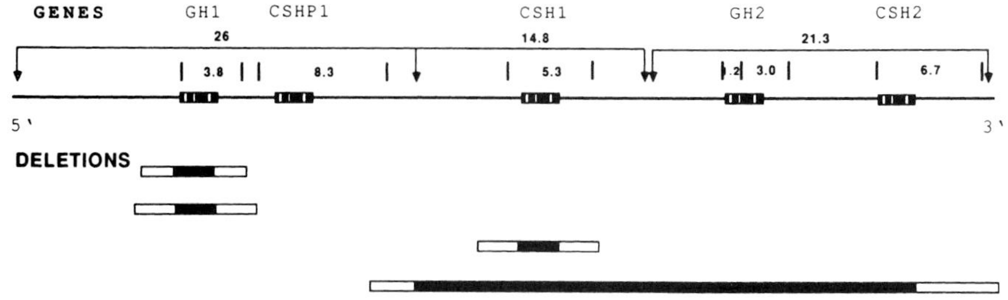

Fig. 162-10 Schematic representation of the hGH gene cluster showing the location of *Hind*III (arrows) and selected *Bam*HI (vertical lines) restriction sites. The locations of four known deletions of various loci in the hGH gene cluster are shown at the bottom, with dark and open rectangles indicating obligatory deletions and ranges of end points, respectively.

Table 162-2 GH1 Gene Deletions

Origin	Size, Kb	Loci involved	hGH Ab	Reference
Switzerland	6.7	GH1	+	Phillips et al. (1981)
Japan	6.7	GH1	+	Nishi et al. (1984)
Argentina	6.7	GH1	+	Rivarola et al. (1984) Kamijo and Phillips (1992)
Austria	6.7	GH1	+	Frisch and Phillips (1986) Schwartz et al. (1987)
Brazil	6.7	GH1	+	Kamijo and Phillips (1992)
Canada	7.0	GH1	+	Kamijo and Phillips (1992)
Mexico	7.0	GH1	+	Kamijo and Phillips (1992)
China	7.0	GH1	NT	He et al. (1990)
Iraq, Iran	7.6	GH1	−	Laron et al. (1985)
Italy	7.6	GH1	+	Braga et al. (1986)
Italy, Turkey	7.6	GH1	+	Kamijo and Phillips (1992)
Spain	7.6	GH1	−	Kamijo and Phillips (1992)
Turkey	45	GH1, CSHP1, CSH1, GH2	+	Akinci et al. (1992)
Italy	45	GH1, CSHP1, CSH1, GH2	+	Baroncini et al. (1993) Cacciari et al. (1994)
Italy	45	GH1, CSHP1, CSH1, GH2	+	Ghizzoni et al. (1994)
Asia	45	GH1, CSHP1, CSH1, GH2	−	Wagner et al. (1998)

(+) Presence of anti-GH antibodies after treatment with exogenous GH.
(−) Absence of anti-GH antibodies after treatment with exogenous GH.
(NT) Not treated with exogenous GH.

are capable of expression and suggests that defects in GHRH synthesis or secretion may underlie this disorder.

GHRHR Gene Defects. The defect in the "little" (lit) mouse is a point mutation in the GHRHR gene that results in an Asp → Gly substitution at residue 60.[148] A nonsense mutation has been reported in the human GHRHR gene in two first cousins of a consanguineous Indian Moslem family with profound IGHD.[149] Both cousins were homozygous for a G → T transversion in exon 3, which converted a Glu → Stop in their GHRHR genes. Subsequently, the same mutation was identified in an isolate from the Indus valley of Pakistan.[150] A second mutation was identified in a large isolate from Brazil that was diagnosed with an autosomal recessive form of IGHD. Affected patients were found to be homozygous for a G → A transition of the first base of IVS1, which is predicted to alter splicing and results in an inactive protein product.[151]

IGHD-II (MIM 173100). A third type of IGHD (IGHD-II) has an autosomal dominant mode of inheritance. Patients diagnosed with IGHD-II have a single affected parent, respond well to exogenous GH, but differ in the severity of hGH deficiency and in their propensity for developing hypoglycemia.[152–155] Nearly all of the IGHD-II GH gene defects reported to date are mutations in IVS3 that alter splicing of GH mRNA and cause skipping of exon 3. The mechanism by which the mutant GH protein interferes with the normal GH protein is not proven but may involve the formation of GH heterodimers or aggregates.

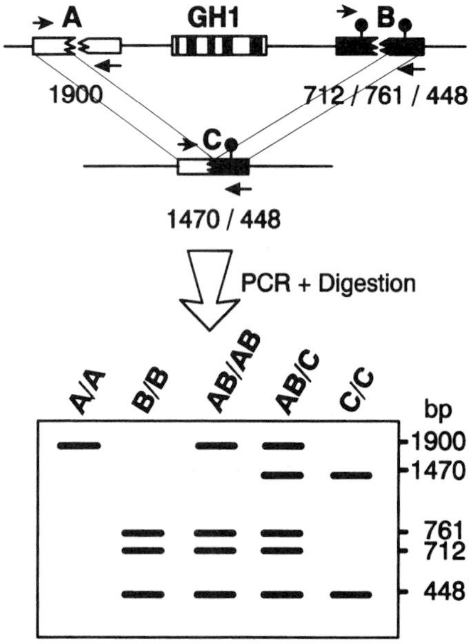

Fig. 162-11 PCR amplification of homologous sequences that flank the GH1 gene using a single set of oligonucleotide primers. Note that the 5′ and 3′ homologous sequences (labeled A and B) differ in the location of restriction sites (indicated by •). The sites also differ from those on junction or fusion fragments (labeled C) shown below that arise during recombination events that produce GH1 gene deletions.[125,126]

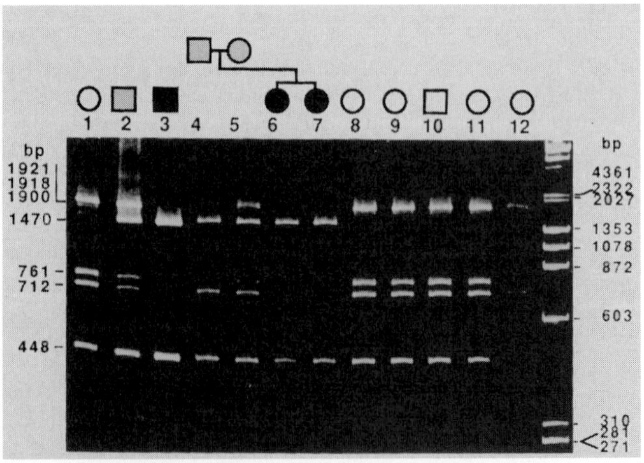

Fig. 162-12 Patterns of DNA fragments seen after PCR amplification using primers shown in Fig. 162-11 followed by digestion with *Sma*I, gel electrophoresis, and ethidium bromide staining. Lanes 3, 6, and 7 show results obtained from DNA of individuals homozygous for the deletion that is illustrated in Fig. 162-11 while 2, 4, and 5 are heterozygous and 1 and 8 to 12 are homozygous for the absence of this deletion.[126]

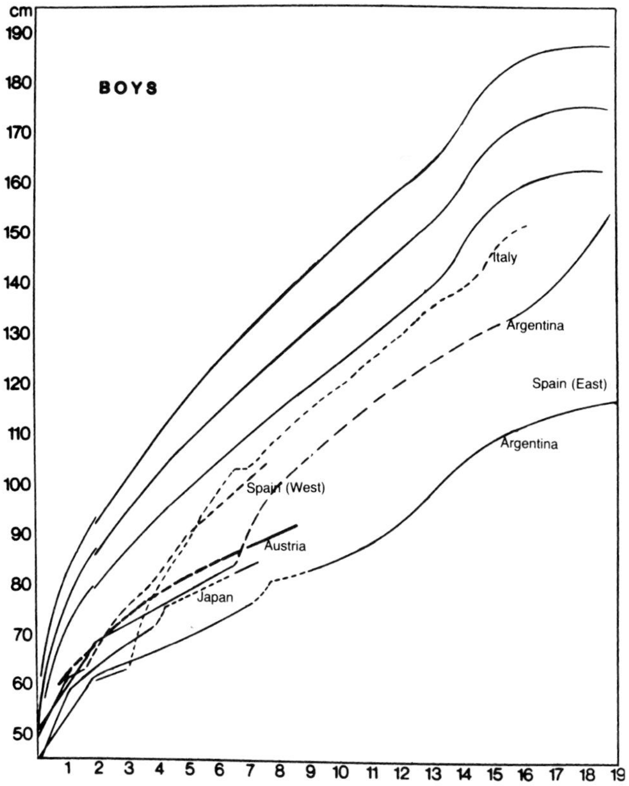

Fig. 162-13 Composite growth charts of males homozygous for GH1 gene deletions whose pedigrees are shown in Fig. 162-8. Solid lines indicate growth without and dotted lines growth during treatment with exogenous hGH.

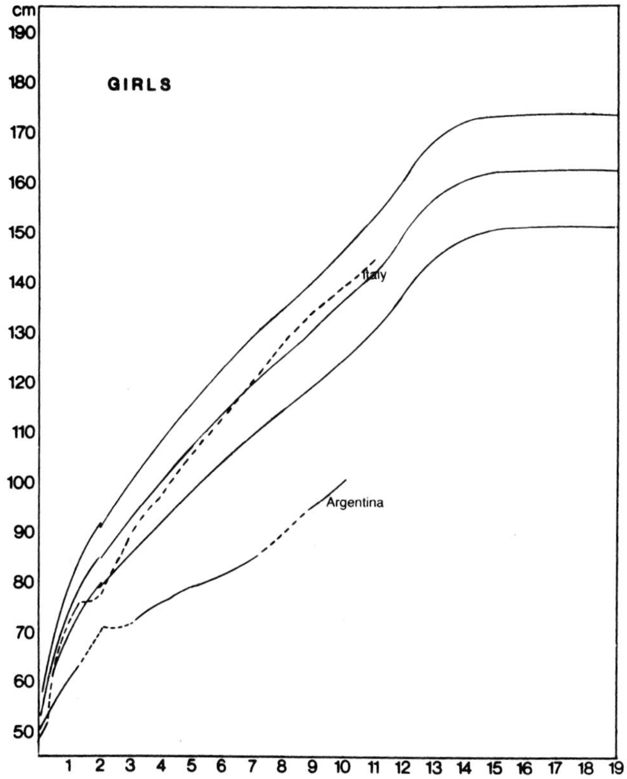

Fig. 162-14 Composite growth charts of females homozygous for GH1 gene deletions whose pedigrees are shown in Fig. 162-8. Solid lines indicate growth without and dotted lines growth during treatment with exogenous hGH.

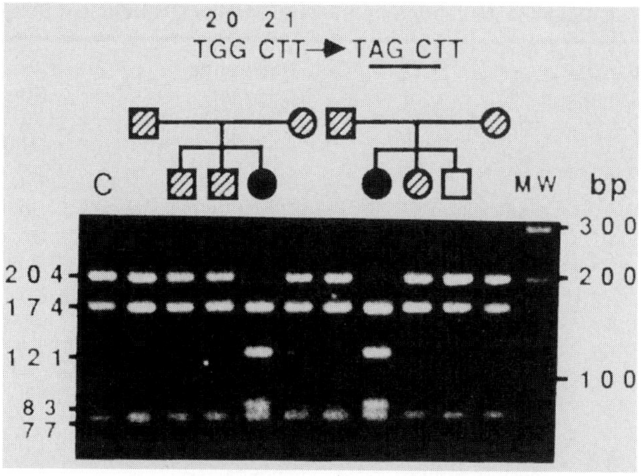

Fig. 162-15 Electrophoretic analysis of PCR-amplified segments of GH1 genes from a normal control and a family with a codon 20 (TGG→TAG) mutation following digestion with *Alu*I. The presence of the mutation generates an additional *Alu*I site (see above). The presence of this *Alu*I site converts a 204-bp product to 181- and 83-bp restriction fragments. Solid symbols = homozygous affected; open = homozygous normal; hatched = heterozygotes.

The first GH1 gene defect was identified in an IGHD-II kindred that showed segregation with a marker tightly linked to the GH1 gene (see Fig. 162-16).[142,156] DNA sequence analysis of PCR amplification products of four affected relatives showed a change in the sixth base of the IVS3 5′ splice site (see Fig. 162-17 and Table 162-3). This mutation causes skipping or deletion of exon 3, which codes for amino acids 32 to 71, including one of the four cysteines (amino acid 53, see Figs. 162-1 and 162-18) necessary for intramolecular disulfide bonding. The resulting truncated GH protein product retains the signal peptide and exons 4-5 sequences thought to be important for transport to the secretory granules. The presence of the mutant and normal GH protein products within the secretory granules may possibly result in formation of intermolecular disulfide bridges that inhibit expression of the normal GH molecule.[142]

Two additional IGHD-II mutations alter the first base of the IVS3 5′ splice site. One is a G → C transversion (IVS3 +1G → C), and the other is a recurring G → A transition (IVS3 +1G → A) (see Table 162-3).[157,158] The latter was found in three nonrelated families and is thought to be caused by the high mutation frequency at CpG dinucleotides that result in C → T and G → A transitions (discussed further under GHR point mutations). Both IGHD-II mutations were proven to cause exon 3 skipping in lymphoblastoid cells and transfections studies, respectively.

Subsequently, other IGHD-II mutations in IVS3 that also cause skipping of exon 3 but do not occur within the branch consensus 5′ or 3′ splice sites have been identified.[69] The first deletes 18 bp (IVS3 del+28–45) and the second is a G → A transition (IVS3 + 28G → A) (see Table 162-3). RT-PCR amplification of GH1 gene transcripts from transient expression studies, using IGHD-II mutant constructs in mammalian cells, yielded DNAs showing dramatic increases in exon 3 skipping relative to normal controls. The shift towards exon 3 skipping is caused by the disruption of an intronic XGGG repeat, which regulates mRNA splicing by some unknown mechanism.

One IGHD-II mutation has been reported that does not occur within IVS3 or affect splicing. This mutation is a G → A transition that results in an Arg → His substitution at residue 183 (Arg183His) of the mature GH protein (see Table 162-3).[159] This substitution is believed to alter the intracellular processing of the normal GH molecules by binding zinc and thereby deranging the zinc associated presecretory packaging of GH.

IGHD-III (MIM 307200). A fourth reported type of IGHD (IGHD-III) has an X-linked recessive mode of inheritance (see

Table 162-3 Mutations in the GH Genes of GH Deficient Subjects

IGHD Type	Location	Nucleotide Change*	Effect of Mutation	References
IA	Exon II	5536 del C	Frameshift after 17th aa of signal peptide	Duquesnoy et al. (1990)
	Exon II	5543 G → A	Stop codon after 19th aa of signal peptide	Cogan et al. (1993)
IB	Intron IV	6242 G → C	Donor splice site mutation; frameshift	Cogan et al. (1994)
	Intron IV	6242 G → T	Donor splice site mutation; frameshift	Miller-Davis et al. (1993)
	Intron IV	6246 G → C	Donor splice site mutation; frameshift	Abdul-Latif (1995)
	Exon III	5938-39 del AG	Frameshift after 55th aa of mature GH	Igarashi et al. (1993)
II	Intron III	5955 G → A	Donor splice site mutation; exon 3 skip	Cogan et al. (1995)
	Intron III	5955 G → C	Donor splice site mutation; exon 3 skip	Binder et al. (1995)
	Intron III	5960 T → C	Donor splice site mutation; exon 3 skip	Cogan et al. (1994)
	Intron III	5982-99 del	Splicing mutation; exon 3 skip	Cogan et al. (1997)
	Intron III	5982 G → A	Splicing mutation; exon 3 skip	Cogan et al. (1997)
	Exon IV	6664 G → A	Arginine 183 to Histidine	Wajnrach et al. (1996)

*Nucleotide numbering according to Chen et al., 1989.

Table 162-1). In the reported kindred, all four affected males had hypogammaglobulinemia (deficient IgG, IgA, IgM, and IgE) and peak hGH responses of ≤5 ng/ml hGH to various provocative tests.[160] Interestingly, one of these patients was treated with exogenous hGH and developed detectable circulating B lymphocytes as well as higher levels of IgA, IgM, and IgE than his affected relatives. Because hGH replacement in other hGH-deficient children who do not have IGHD-III is associated with a decrease in B lymphocytes, it seems plausible that IGHD-III is caused by a mutation (perhaps a deletion) of a portion of the X chromosome that contains two loci, one necessary for normal immunoglobulin production and the other for hGH expression.[160,161]

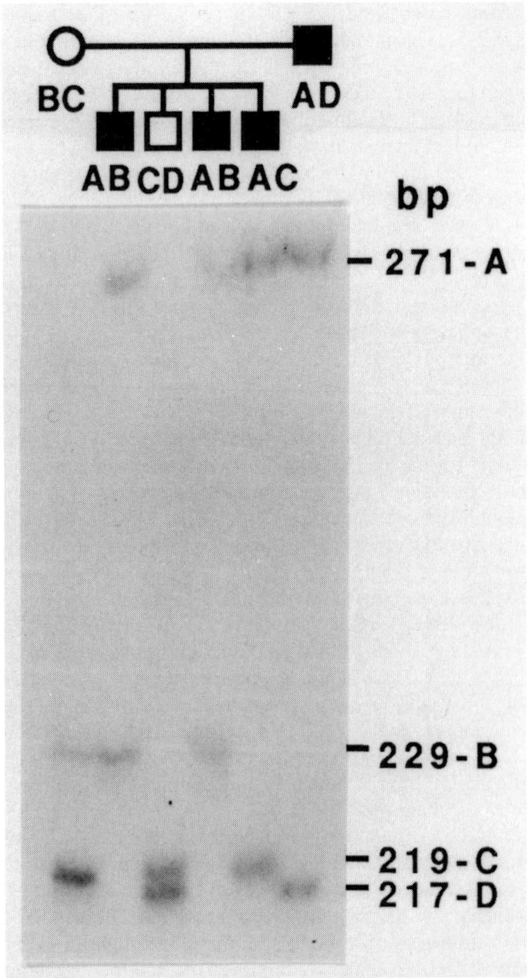

Fig. 162-16 Pedigree of an IGHD II family showing segregation of a dinucleotide repeat tightly linked with the GH1 gene. Open circles (female) or squares (male) represent unaffected individuals. Solid squares (male) represent IGHD II patients.

Bioinactive hGH

Some children with short stature comparable to that seen in hGH deficiency have low levels of IGF-I but normal levels of hGH assayed by radioimmunoassay (RIA).[162–166] In such cases, the administration of exogenous hGH is reported to produce an increase in IGF-I levels and a growth response. In some, the concentration of hGH, as measured by radioimmunoassay, greatly exceeds the concentration measured by radioreceptor assay. These results suggest that the primary defect could be production of an abnormal hGH polypeptide whose alteration causes a reduced somatogenic activity but enables it to react with anti-hGH antibodies.[4]

Takahashi *et al.* identified a C → T transition in codon 77 which results in an Arg → Cys substitution in the GH1 gene of a subject diagnosed with bioinactive GH. The patient was heterozygous for the mutation and isoelectric focusing of his serum showed an abnormal GH peak in addition to a normal peak.

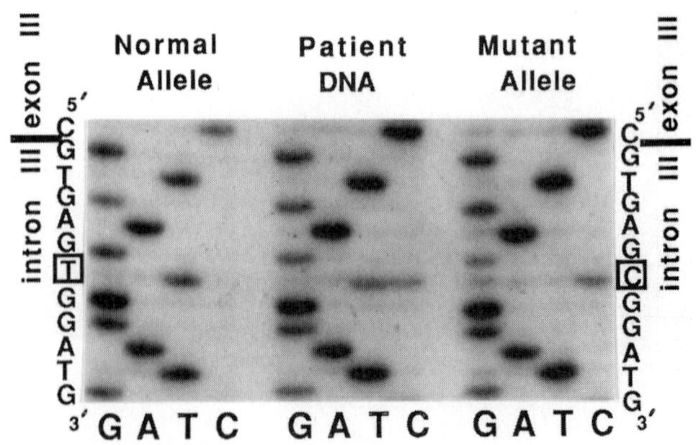

Fig. 162-17 Comparison of DNA sequencing ladders of IGHD-II patient 3 derived from direct sequencing of PCR-amplified GH genes (middle) and sequencing of cloned PCR-amplified normal and mutant GH genes (left and right panels, respectively). The T→C substitution that affects the sixth nucleotide of intron III is bracketed. (Published with permission from Cogan JD, Phillips JA III, Shenkman SS, Milner, RDG, Sakati N: Familial growth hormone deficiency: A model of dominant and recessive mutations affecting a monomeric protein. *J Clin Endocrinol Metab* 79:1261, 1994. The Endocrine Society.)

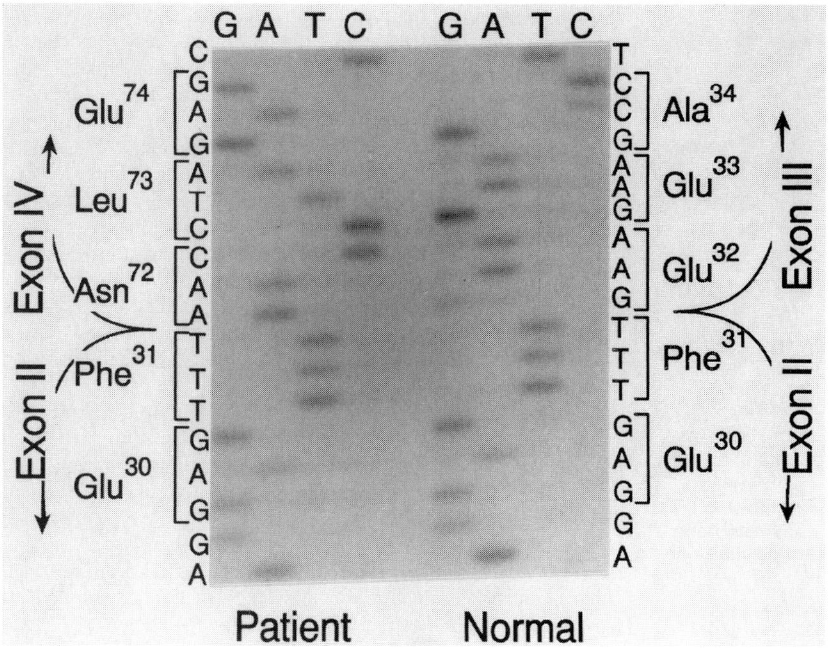

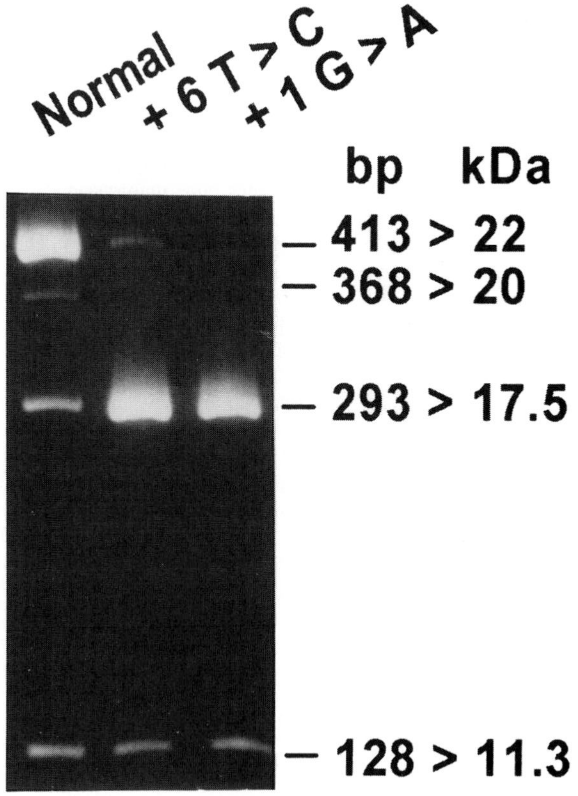

Fig. 162-18 *A*, DNA sequence results of reverse-transcribed cDNA using mRNA extracted from HeLa cells transfected with normal and IGHD-II patient GH expression plasmids. (Published with permission from Cogan JD, Phillips JA III, Shenkman SS, Milner, RDG, Sakati N: Familial growth hormone deficiency: a model of dominant and recessive mutations affecting a monomeric protein. *J Clin Endocrinol Metab* 79:1261, 1994. The Endocrine Society.) *B*, Electrophoretic analysis of RT-PCR products derived from GH1 mRNA extracted from HeLa cells transfected with normal (lane 1), +6T→C IGHD-II (lane 2), and +1G→A IGHD-II (lane 3) GH expression plasmids. (Published with permission from Cogan JD, Ramel B, Lehto M, Phillips JA III, Prince M, Blizzard RM, deRavel TJL, Brammert M, Groop L: A recurring dominant-negative mutation causes autosomal dominant growth hormone deficiency—A clinical research center study. *J Clin Endocrinol Metab* 80:3591, 1995.)

Surprisingly, his father was also heterozygous for the C→T transition but was of normal height and had normal isoelectric focusing results.[167] The disparate findings in the father and his affected child were not explained.

Laron Dwarfism. Laron dwarfism is an autosomal recessive disorder characterized by low IGF-I levels but normal to high levels of hGH by RIA.[168] While the majority of reported patients are Jewish, the disorder has been described in other ethnic groups.[152,169] Laron dwarfs have the clinical appearance of severe IGHD with very delayed growth, abnormal facial appearance, high-pitched voice, and small male genitalia.[168–171] Length at birth may be short in relation to the birth weight, and tooth eruption and fontanelle closure are delayed. Laron dwarfs have the truncal obesity and the increased upper-lower segment body ratios typical of pituitary dwarfs. While spontaneous hypoglycemia can occur, the production of other anterior pituitary hormones (ACTH, TSH, and gonadotropins) remains intact. Fasting hGH levels are usually increased and range from normal to greater than 100 ng/ml. Plasma IGF-I levels are low and, in contrast to those of hGH-deficient patients, do not respond to exogenous hGH.[170,171]

Laron Dwarfism I (MIM 262500). Studies indicate that hGH produced by Laron dwarfs reacts normally in radioreceptor assays with the hGH receptors of normal hepatic cells.[170] This, along with their lack of response to exogenous hGH, suggests the primary

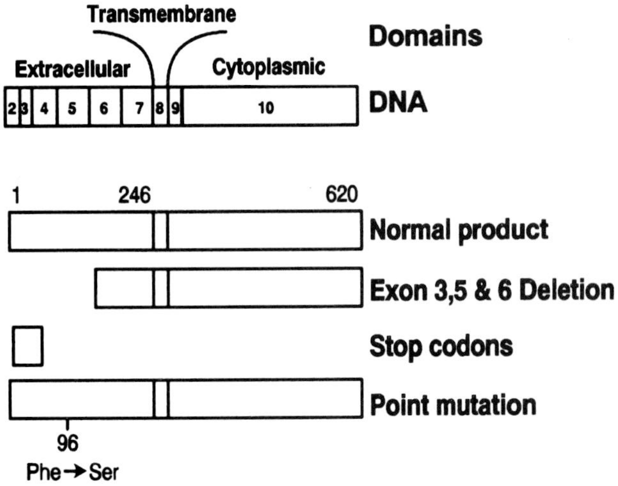

Fig. 162-19 Schematic representation of the GHR gene showing the relationship of various exons to the extracellular, transmembrane, and cytoplasmic GHR domains. Locations of selected deletions or point mutations are shown below.[154]

defect may be an abnormality of membrane receptors for hGH. Molecular analysis of GH receptor (GHR) genes has shown deletions, point mutations, and splicing defects.

GHR Deletions. The first examples of GHR mutations reported were deletions of portions of the gene encoding the extracellular domain (see Fig. 162-19).[172,173] Southern blotting showed altered restriction patterns of the GHR genes from patients with Laron syndrome who had no detectable GH binding protein (GHBP) and very low levels of IGF-I. While these and other studies were interpreted as showing deletions of exons 3, 5, 6, and part of 4 from the GHR gene, the mechanism by which these two noncontiguous deletions arose remains unclear. In two of nine patients studied by Godowski *et al.* GHR deletions were found, and Parks detected GHR deletions in five of nine of the Laron syndrome probands studied.[172,173]

GHR Point Mutations. Multiple point mutations have been detected within the GHR gene (see Human Gene Mutation Database at www.uwcm.ac.uk/uwcm/mg/search/119984.html).[174–176] Amselem *et al.* detected a T → C transition that converts the 96th residue of the extracellular domain from phenylalanine to serine.[175] Duquesnoy *et al.* demonstrated that cells transfected with this mutant cDNA lacked GH binding activity.[176]

Two different stop codon mutations of GHR genes in Laron dwarf patients have been reported.[174] In a patient of Northern European origin, a TGC (Cys) → TGA (stop) mutation was detected at codon 38 in exon 4, and a CGA (Arg) → TGA (stop) mutation was found at codon 43 in exon 4 of two Mediterranean patients who were products of consanguineous marriages. Both stop codons truncate the GHR protein and delete most of its GHBP domain and all of its transmembrane and intracellular domains. These findings are consistent with the lack of GHBP in each patient with Laron syndrome. The mechanism of the CGA to TGA mutation is consistent with deamination of 5-methylcytosine that preferentially occurs in CpG dinucleotides. Such dinucleotides often represent "hotspots" for CG to TG or CG to CA mutations, and 17 occur in the GHR gene. Two of these, at nucleotides 181 and 703, occur in CGA codons that could yield stop codons.[172,174,175]

A GAT (Asp) → CAT(His) mutation was identified in exon 6 of two unrelated kindreds with growth deficiency but normal GHBP levels. Conversion of the highly conserved aspartic acid residue to histidine was shown to prevent dimerization of the GH receptor which is necessary for GH action.[177,178]

GHR Splicing Defects. Rosenbloom *et al.* identified 20 patients with Laron syndrome in an inbred population of Spanish extraction in Southern Ecuador.[179] These patients were −6.7 to −10 SD below the mean height and had limited elbow extension, blue sclera, short limbs, hip degeneration, acrohypoplasia, and normal or superior intelligence. To determine the associated defect in the GHR gene, Berg *et al.* used denaturing gradient gel electrophoresis to analyze each exon of the GHR gene.[180] Unusual fragments derived from exon 6 showed abnormal mobility and DNA sequencing showed an A → G transition in the third position of codon 180, which is 24 nucleotides from the 3′ end of exon 6. While this mutation does not cause an amino acid substitution, it produces a consensus 5′ splice site sequence within exon 6. The resulting near consensus 5′ splice site within exon 6 causes aberrant splicing and deletion of eight amino acids of the 3′ end of exon 6. Deletion of these residues is thought to reduce the function of the GHBP molecule.[180]

Two cousins of Pakistani descent were found to have a G → C transversion at the 5′ splice site of exon 8 resulting in exon skipping. The mutant protein lacks the transmembrane and intracellular domains and results in elevated circulating levels of GH binding protein in the affected patients.[181]

Laron Dwarfism II (MIM 245590). Patients with Laron dwarfism II have elevated serum GH, normal GHBP levels, and respond well to treatment with IGF-1 indicating their growth deficiency is due to a post-GHR defect.

IGF1 Gene Deletions. Woods *et al.* described a patient with severe growth failure, sensorineural deafness, and mental retardation.[182] The patient was found to be homozygous for a partial deletion of the IGF-1 gene. RT-PCR analysis confirmed the deletion of exons 4-5, which would result in a severely truncated mature IGF-1 peptide. Interestingly, this patient had only a slightly delayed bone age indicating that GH directly stimulates bone maturation.

Combined Pituitary Hormone Deficiency (CPHD). CPHD, or panhypopituitary dwarfism, is characterized by the presence of a deficiency of one or more of the other pituitary trophic hormones (ACTH, FSH, LH, or TSH) in addition to hGH deficiency. While the great majority of cases are sporadic, at least two Mendelian forms are known (see Table 162-1). These two types differ in their modes of inheritance, with type I having an autosomal recessive and type II an X-linked recessive mode of inheritance.[126,154,160]

The clinical features of familial CPHD are identical to those of cases of nongenetic etiology. The phenotype varies with the specific trophic hormone deficiencies, which occur in decreasing order: gonadotropins (FSH, LH) > ACTH > TSH.[160] Associated gonadotropin deficiency causes sexual immaturity and primary amenorrhea in females, and small external genitalia and lack of beard growth in males. TSH deficiency may become severe after GH replacement and ACTH deficiency may contribute to recurrent hypoglycemia. The severity of deficiencies of various trophic hormones exhibits interfamilial and intrafamilial variability in CPHD types I and II. Furthermore, the hGH secretory responses to GHRH infusions vary from deficient to normal in different related individuals from the same families.[146]

CPHD-I (MIM 262600). Mutations of either the PIT1 or PROP1 genes can cause CPHD-I. Both of these genes are members of the POU (Pit-1, Oct-1, Unc-86) homeodomain family of transcription factors and they each play an important role in pituitary development. Pit-1 gene defects were first identified in Snell and Jackson dwarf mice, which lack somatotropes, lactotropes, and thyrotropes, and have severe deficiencies of GH, prolactin (PrL), and TSH.[183] The Pit-1 (or GHF-1) gene whose product binds to and activates GH, PrL, and TSH promoters was found to have a T → G substitution at codon 261 giving a TGG (tryptophan) to TGT (cysteine) in the Snell and a gross rearrangement in the Jackson dwarf mouse. The deficiencies seen in these mice differ from most humans with CPHD, who have GH, TSH, gonadotropin, and ACTH deficiencies but increased PrL. In examining a subset of patients with GH, PrL, and TSH deficiency, eight different PIT1 mutations were found in humans.

Autosomal Recessive Pit-1 Mutations. The first Pit-1 mutation reported to cause CPHD was a T → C transition in codon 172, which changes a CGA (Arg) → TGA (stop).[184] The second Pit-1 mutation reported was an A → G transition in codon 143 changing a CGA (Arg) → CAA (Gln).[185] Both mutations occur in the POU-specific domain of Pit-1 and are thought to affect binding of the Pit-1 protein to DNA. The third and fourth Pit-1 mutations were found in two Dutch families who had postnatal growth failure with complete deficiencies of GH and PrL, and T_4 levels that fell after treatment with GH in one case and were low prior to treatment in the other.[186,187] One Dutch family had affected sibs whose T_4 levels were initially normal. These sibs were homozygous for a C → G transversion in codon 158 which encoded a GCA (Ala) → CCA (Pro) substitution. This Ala158Pro mutation interferes with formation of Pit-1 homodimers and greatly reduces transcription activation. The second Dutch family had affected sibs whose initial T_4 levels were low. These sibs were genetic compounds with one deleted and one Ala158Pro Pit-1 allele. Interestingly, this combination of defects was associated with more severe hypothyroidism and small anterior pituitary glands.[187] These cases emphasize the importance of determining T_4 and PrL levels and TSH responses to TRH administration in those with CPHD. Because GH and TSH deficiency often occur together, failure of patients to have PrL and TSH responses to TRH should raise the question of their having Pit-1 gene defects. A fifth Pit-1 mutation was identified in a Thai patient who was homozygous for a G → T transversion in codon 25 converting a GAA (Glu) → TAA (stop) codon. This mutation resulted in complete loss of the POU-homeodomain, which is necessary for DNA binding.[188] The sixth Pit-1 mutation was found in a consanguineous family of Tunisian decent. All of the affected sibs were found to be homozygous for a T → G transversion in codon 135 converting a TTT (Phe) → TGT (Cys) in the POU-specific domain of Pit-1.[189]

Autosomal Dominant Pit-1 Mutations. Two dominant negative Pit-1 mutations have been reported. While the mechanism of action is not completely understood, neither of these mutations appears to inhibit binding of the mutant Pit-1 protein to its target DNA. The first mutation, located in the POU-homeodomain, is a C → T transition in codon 271 converting a CGG (Arg) → TGG (Trp).[190] Three unrelated patients (two adults and one infant) were reported to be heterozygous for this Arg271Trp mutation. Both adults had pituitary hypoplasia and the 2-month-old had a normal pituitary by imaging. These findings suggest that Pit-1 may be necessary for anterior pituitary survival and that the 2-month-old will develop pituitary hypoplasia with age. The second dominant negative mutation was a C → T transition of the 24th codon converting a CCT (Pro) → CTT (Leu). This mutation resides within the major transactivating domain of PIT1, which is highly conserved in different species.[185]

PROP1 Mutations. Ames dwarf (df/df) mice have CPHD and hypocellular anterior pituitaries that lack somatotropes, lactotropes, thyrotropes, and GH transcripts. The genetic defect associated with the Ames dwarf phenotype was recently found in the gene called Prophet of Pit-1 (Prop-1) that encodes a pituitary specific homeodomain factor.[191] Sequence analysis of the Prop-1 cDNA in the df/df mouse revealed a T → C transition in codon 83 that causes a Ser → Pro amino acid change in the first α-helix of its homeodomain. While Prop-1 is required for expression of Pit-1, how Prop-1 regulates Pit-1 expression remains uncertain.

Four Prop-1 gene mutations that cause autosomal recessive CPHD in humans (MIM 601538) have been identified.[192] In addition to deficiencies of GH, PrL, and TSH that are seen in those with Pit-1 defects, patients with Prop-1 defects also have deficiencies of LH and FSH which prevent the onset of spontaneous puberty. The first mutation was a C → T transition

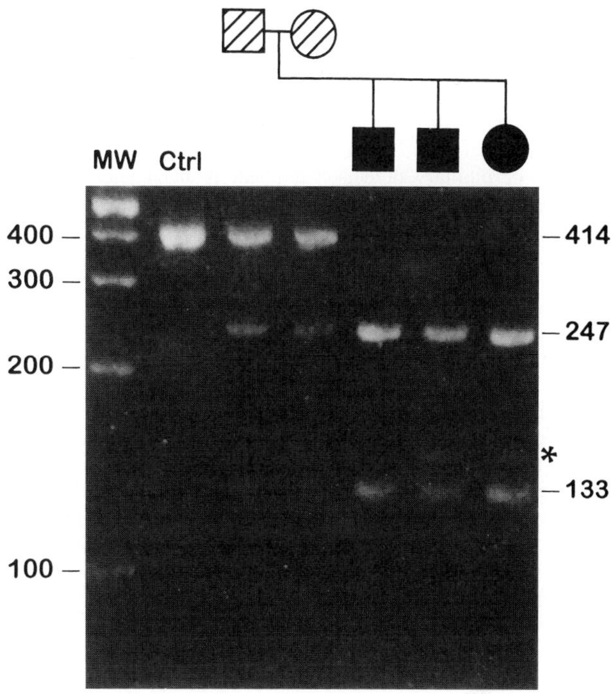

Fig. 162-20 Electrophoretic analysis of PCR amplification products, derived from exon 2 of the Prop-1 genes, of subjects with Prop-1 2-bp deletions following digestion with *BcgI*. The normal 414-bp fragments are cleaved to 247 bp when the 2-bp deletion is present. The asterisk shows size of an artifactual PCR product that was seen in most products before and after digestion with *BcgI*. MW = molecular weight standard; Ctrl = unaffected control. (Published with permission from Cogan JD, Wu W, Phillips JA III, Arnhold IJP, Fofanova OV, Osorio MGF, Bircan I, Moreno A, Mendonca BB: The Prop-1 2-bp deletion is a common cause of combined pituitary hormone deficiency. *J Clin Endocrinol Metab* 83(9):3346–3349, 1998. The Endocrine Society.)

in codon 120 of the Prop-1 gene which encoded a TGC (Arg) → CGC (Cys) substitution in the third helix of the homeodomain. The second mutation was a T → A transversion that encodes a TTC (Phe) → ATC (Ile) substitution at codon 117. The third mutation was a 2-bp AG deletion in codon 101 (101delAG) that causes a frameshift and results in a premature stop at codon 109 (Fig. 162-20). The resulting protein products from all three Prop-1 mutations have been shown to have greatly reduced DNA binding and transactivating abilities. The 2-bp AG deletion is a recurring mutation and is estimated to occur in about 55 percent of familial and 12 percent of sporadic CPHD cases.[193] The fourth mutation reported is a 2-bp GA deletion in codon 51 (51delGA).[194] Like the 101delAG mutation, 51delGA causes a frameshift and results in a premature stop at codon 109. This mutation was found in familial (12 percent) and sporadic (21 percent) CPHD cases.

CPHD-II (MIM 312000). A family with four cases of X-linked recessive CPHD was found to show linkage with markers in the Xq25-q26 region (peak lod score of 4.12). Further examination revealed an extra copy of the marker DXS102, suggesting a duplication in this region.[195]

African Pygmies. Peripheral unresponsiveness to exogenous hGH and normal levels of hGH have been documented in African pygmies. These individuals resemble pituitary dwarfs in size and proportions, but they lack the truncal obesity, typical facies, and skin findings of pituitary dwarfs.[152]

Serum concentrations of IGF-I are decreased in African pygmies.[196] Because levels of hGH and IGF-II were normal, an isolated deficiency of IGF-I was hypothesized. Examinations of children, as well as adult, pygmies indicate that the short stature of the adults is due mainly to a failure of pubated growth acceleration due to the absence of an increase in IGF-I during puberty.[63]

Developmental Anomalies and Genetic Syndromes

A variety of complex genetic syndromes associated with hypothalamic or pituitary defects that result in hGH and/or trophic hormone deficiencies have been described.[152] Some that are better characterized or that are reported to have genetic etiologies are briefly discussed.

Congenital Absence of the Pituitary. Complete absence of the pituitary causes adrenal insufficiency, hGH deficiency, hypothyroidism, and hypoglycemia. The thyroid and adrenal glands are usually hypoplastic, and the penis is small.[152] Occurrence of the disorder in multiple sib pairs suggests that it can be inherited as an autosomal recessive trait.

Anencephaly (MIM 206500). Anencephaly is associated with absence of the hypothalamus and hypoplasia of the pituitary. Often, the adrenals are hypoplastic and plasma hGH levels may be absent to low-normal.[152] Anencephaly is due to multifactorial inheritance, and the recurrence risk for a subsequent sib of an affected proband is 2 to 4 percent.[197]

Holoprosencephaly (MIM 236100). Holoprosencephaly is characterized by the presence of median cleft lip and palate. Cases are usually sporadic but can be familial with either autosomal dominant or recessive modes of inheritance in different families.[197] Those due to chromosome anomalies (trisomy 13, 13q-, 18p-, and triploidy) usually have a variety of additional congenital anomalies.[152,197] Associated abnormalities of the hypothalamus can cause IGHD or CPHD.

Septo-Optic Dysplasia (MIM 182230). This disorder, also referred to as de Morsier syndrome, is characterized by hypoplastic optic disks, absent septum pellucidum, and hGH deficiency.[197] A missense mutation in the HESX1 gene was found in two sibs with septo-optic dysplasia. Both sibs were found to be homozygous for a C → T transition in codon 53 converting a highly conserved Arg → Cys.[198]

Cleft Lip and Palate. While over 200 syndromes, including many that are either chromosomal or Mendelian in etiology, have cleft lip and/or palate as components, the great majority of cases with isolated cleft lip and/or cleft palate are due to multifactorial inheritance.[152,197] Associated developmental defects of the pituitary causing IGHD or CPHD occur in about 4 percent of cases.[199]

Rieger Syndrome (MIM 180500). Rieger syndrome is characterized by iris dysplasia, hypodontia, and occasional optic atrophy and pituitary insufficiency.[152,197] It has an autosomal dominant mode of inheritance and variable expression.

CPHD with Abnormal Sella Turica. Familial cases of pituitary insufficiency with hGH, TSH, and ACTH deficiency associated with an abnormally small or large sella turcica have been reported.[152,197] Both disorders have an apparently autosomal recessive mode of inheritance. Recently Prop-1 gene mutations have been reported in some individuals with large sella turcica.[200]

Fanconi Pancytopenia Syndrome (MIM 227650). This syndrome is inherited as an autosomal recessive trait, and it is characterized by short stature, anomalies of the thumbs, hyperpigmentation, pancytopenia, and occasional hGH deficiency.[152,197] Studies suggest that there may be eight or more complementation groups. Thus, autosomal recessive inheritance due to defects at multiple loci, and probably multiple alleles, should be considered.

Ectrodactyly-Ectodermal Dysplasia-Clefting (EEC) Syndrome (MIM 122900). EEC syndrome features include defects in the hands and feet varying from syndactyly to ectrodactyly, ectodermal dysplasia causing fair, thin skin and partial anodontia, and cleft lip and/or palate. The disorder has an autosomal dominant mode of inheritance and locus heterogeneity. Patients with EEC and hGH deficiency associated with absent septum pellucidum have been reported.[201]

Achondroplasia with Obstructive Sleep Apnea (MIM 100800). Obstructive sleep apnea due to upper airway obstruction is a common complication of achondroplasia. When the obstructive sleep apnea is severe, it can cause secondary hGH deficiency due to deficient hGH release during sleep.[202] This mechanism should be considered for other skeletal dysplasias that have associated airway obstruction and disturbed sleep patterns.

Isolated hCS Deficiency (ICSD; MIM 150200)

ICSD Type IA. Complete antenatal deficiency of hCS is called ICSD-IA. Its molecular basis was first determined in a Danish child who produced no detectable hCS prior to birth and had normal height at 4.5 years of age.[34,56] Restriction analysis revealed that the CSH1-GH2-CSH2 gene cluster was deleted from both homologs of 17 chromosomes, while the GH1 and CSHP1 genes were retained.[56] Analysis of DNA following digestion with *Hinc*II and *Msp*I detected identical RFLP haplotypes, suggesting that the gene deletions were identical.

ICSD Type IB. Partial deficiency of hCS is termed ICSD-IB and was described in a normal Danish infant who was the product of a pregnancy in which peak maternal hCS levels were 1.1 μg/ml (normal is 3 to 9.2 μg/ml).[203] Analysis of DNA from the child revealed heterozygosity for the CSH1-GH2-CSH2 deletion described above and a deletion of only the CSH1 gene on the second chromosome 17 homolog. Thus, the child retained only one of the four normal CSH genes in agreement with the roughly one-quarter normal levels of hCS that were observed. Interestingly, Orlando *et al.*[204] found that 3 of 66 CSH1 alleles were deleted in a cohort of Spanish patients with IGHD.

Mouse Models of hGH Deficiency

In the mouse, three nonallelic recessive mutant genes have been identified that cause dwarfism as a result of decreased GH production. These mutant genes, referred to as Little (lit), Snell dwarf (dw), and Ames dwarf (df), are assigned to three different chromosomes.[205] The GH deficiency is isolated in the case of Little mice, while Snell and Ames dwarfs have deficiencies of additional anterior pituitary hormones and are models of CPHD. Restriction analysis studies suggest that the GH genes are grossly intact in all three types of dwarfs. Ultrastructural studies of the anterior pituitary gland of Little mice showed a deficiency of secretory granules within somatotropes, while Snell and Ames dwarf pituitaries lacked identifiable somatotropes. Furthermore, GH precursor RNA and mRNA were decreased in the total RNA from Little pituitaries, while GH transcripts appeared to be absent in the total RNA from Snell or Ames dwarf pituitaries.[206] Little (lit/lit) mice have IGHD due to a G → T transversion causing a Glu → stop at codon 72 of the GHRHR gene.[148] The CPHD phenotype of the Snell and Ames dwarf mice are due to point mutations in the Pit-1 and Prop-1 genes, respectively. The Snell dwarf mutation is a G → T transversion in codon 261 of the Pit-1 gene converting a Trp → Cys.[183] The Prop-1 mutation identified in the Ames dwarf mouse is a T → C transition in codon 83 converting a Ser → Pro in the first α-helix of the homeodomain.[191]

TREATMENT OF hGH DEFICIENCY

hGH Replacement

Dose and Route of Administration. hGH extracted from pituitary glands was first administered to humans in 1958.[207] By 1964, it was clear that replacement with exogenous hGH could stimulate linear growth in patients with hGH deficiency. The effectiveness of replacement therapy depended on the chronologic age, height, weight, and bone age, as well as possibly the pretreatment growth rate, peak hGH response to stimuli, and degree of obesity.[208] The linear growth response to hGH treatment during the first year of therapy depended on both the dose of hGH used and the schedule of its administration. Frazier *et al.*[209] demonstrated a significant dose-response increment as the dose of hGH was increased from 0.03 IU/kg three times a week to 0.05 IU/kg three times a week to 0.10 IU/kg three times a week. A trial of 0.3 IU/kg three times a week suggested that a dose-response relationship continues with higher amounts.[210] The conventional route of administration is intramuscular, although subcutaneous injection is reported to achieve the same growth rate without detected differences in antibody production or lipodystrophy.[211] If glucocorticoid replacement is indicated because of CPHD, the dose should be limited to 10 to 15 mg/m^2/day to avoid blunting the growth response to exogenous hGH.[208]

Results of Long-Term Treatment. The effectiveness of long-term treatment with hGH for children with short stature due to hGH deficiency has been well documented.[107,203,207,208,212,213] While the average final height improved from 6 SD below the mean in untreated patients to 2.3 SD below the mean in treated patients, only half the males and 15 percent of the females had final heights above the third percentile.[213] The patients studied had relatively severe growth retardation and were 9 to 14 years old before treatment was begun. While better outcomes occur when treatment is begun earlier, before the growth retardation becomes severe, it remains unclear whether optimal replacement therapy can consistently ameliorate the growth deficit.

Cassorla *et al.* studied the effect of delaying epiphyseal fusion on the growth of GH-deficient children. Patients treated with GH and an LHRH analogue had suppression of their pituitary-gonadal axis and a marked delay in bone age progression. After 3 years of treatment a greater gain in height prediction was observed in these patients than in patients treated with GH and placebo. The authors concluded that delaying epiphyseal fusion with an LHRH analogue in pubertal GH-deficient children treated with GH increased the final height prediction and may increase final height compared to treatment with GH alone.[214]

Cuneo *et al.* reported the results of a multicenter, randomized, trial of the effects of exogenous hGH treatment in adults with GH deficiency. GH treatment produced these results: prominent increases in serum IGF1 at the doses employed, in some cases to supraphysiologic levels; modest decreases in total and low-density lipoprotein cholesterol, together with substantial reductions in total-body and truncal fat mass consistent with an improved cardiovascular risk profile; substantial increases in lean tissue mass; and modest improvements in perceived quality of life.[215]

Side Effects of hGH Therapy. The development of hypothyroidism during hGH therapy occurs in a small percentage of euthyroid children treated with hGH.[178] The decreased thyroxine concentrations observed reflect the inhibition by hGH of TSH responsiveness to TRH as well as the natural history of CPHD.[208,216]

Antibodies to hGH. The development of anti-hGH antibodies following hGH replacement occurs in 30 to 60 percent of treated patients.[208,217] However, antibodies of sufficient titer to inhibit responsiveness to hGH treatment occur in no more than 5 percent of treated cases and in less than 15 percent of those in whom antibodies develop.[208] While some patients who become refractory to hGH therapy due to antibody production may respond to higher doses of hGH,[218] most with IGHD-IA have antibody titers that preclude response to even very-high-dose hGH treatment.[112–114,119–126,136–138]

Creutzfeldt-Jakob Disease. hGH purified from cadaver pituitaries had been used in treatment for 27 years before the first recipient to contract with degenerative neurologic disease was detected.[219] The first patient was a 22-year-old who died of Creutzfeldt-Jakob disease, a brain infection caused by a "slow virus." The patient's death occurred 6 years after completion of a 13-year course of treatment with hGH supplied by the National Hormone and Pituitary Program.[219] The discovery of additional cases suggested that the infections arose by contamination of one or more hGH preparation lots with the Creutzfeldt-Jacob disease agent.[219–221] Because of this discovery the National Institutes of Health halted distribution of hGH derived from cadaver pituitaries in 1985. Due to the potential for a long latency period and contamination of multiple batches of hGH, it is doubtful that distribution of this material will be resumed.

Biosynthetic hGH

Following withdrawal of hGH derived from cadaver pituitaries in 1985, hGH-deficient children, adolescents, and adults were left without treatment.[220–222] This problem was solved by approval of the Food and Drug Administration to market genetically engineered versions of hGH.[222]

The original report of successful expression of hGH in bacteria was in 1979.[223] *Escherichia coli* containing the recombinant vector produced an altered hGH (methionyl-hGH, or met-hGH) that contained an additional N-terminal methionine encoded by the AUG or start codon of the cloned hGH segment.[224] Treatment with this product resulted in production of antibodies that were later found to be induced by small amounts of contaminating *E. coli* proteins rather than the recombinant hGH itself. These antibodies were demonstrated in 21 of 22 treated subjects.[225] Subsequent refinements were successful in lowering this contamination so that met-hGH was equivalent to pituitary hGH in potency and had a much lower incidence of antibody formation. These improvements and subsequent production of recombinant hGH, which lacks the extra methionine residue, now provide a plentiful supply of hGH that has the full biologic activity of pituitary hGH. The availability of recombinant hGH in large amounts has raised concern that it will be misused to make normal children taller and for other "cosmetic endocrinology" applications.[222,225]

Somatocrinin (GHRH)

Treatment of hGH deficiency with GHRH is an alternative to hGH replacement for some hGH-deficient children. In two different studies, about 40 percent of hGH-deficient subjects had increases of over 5 ng/ml in plasma hGH after IV injection of GHRH preparations.[226,227] Subsequent trials of intermittent or constant infusions of GHRH have demonstrated restoration of endogenous hGH secretion and growth in hGH-deficient children.[228,229] The utility of this approach is limited by the need for frequent doses and the lack of response by a majority of hGH-deficient subjects.

Synthetic GH Secretagogues

A number of orally or nasally administered synthetic GH secretagogues have been tried as alternatives to parental GH replacement. These include the GH-releasing peptide-mimetic MK-0677, which can be given orally. Chapman *et al.* found that GH-deficient men had increases in IGF1 and 24-h mean GH levels of ~80 percent following treatment with 50 mg MK-0677/day.[230] Subsequently other synthetic secretagogues, including GHRP-2, have been shown to be well tolerated and to cause a modest but significant increase in growth velocity in children.[231]

Gene Therapy

The successes in attaining integration and expression of GH and GHRH genes in animals have provided dramatic models for studies of the biologic effects of these gene products and the potential for correcting genetic diseases.[232–234] The method utilized is microinjection of DNA fragments encoding GH or GHRH into pronuclei of fertilized mouse, rabbit, pig, or sheep eggs, and reimplantation of these eggs into appropriate females. Many of the resulting offspring produce high levels of GH or GHRH and manifest enhanced growth. While this approach has potential for producing transgenic livestock, applications to humans have four major limitations: First, the levels of plasma or GHRH that result vary from animal to animal. Second, because synthesis may not occur in the appropriate tissue (anterior pituitary or hypothalamus), levels may not be under normal regulatory control (see Fig. 162-7). Third, the mutagenic potential of integration of recombinant DNA into the host genome can result in disruption of mature genes and cause lethal mutations in the homozygous state.[235] Fourth, infertility is frequently found in transgenic animals, especially among females.[234] While potential applications of gene therapy to somatic cells of humans are feasible, the potential for achieving appropriate hormonal regulation less dangerously than with exogenous hormone replacement given under standard conditions seems remote.

ACKNOWLEDGMENTS

This work was supported in part by National Institutes of Health grants DK-52312 (JDC) and DK-35592 (JAP), and grants from the Genentech Foundation for Growth and Development (JDC and JAP).

REFERENCES

1. Li CH, Dixon JS: Human pituitary growth hormone XXXII. The primary structure of the hormone. *Rev Arch Biochem Biophys* **146**:233, 1971.
2. Niall HD: Revised primary structure for human growth hormone. *Nature* **23**:90, 1971.
3. Li CH: Human growth hormone: 1974–1981. *Mol Cell Biochem* **46**:31, 1982.
4. Chawla RK, Parks JS, Rudman D: Structural variants of human growth hormone: Biochemical, genetic, and clinical aspects. *Annu Rev Med* **34**:519, 1983.
5. Ferguson KA, Wallace ALC: Prolactin activity of human growth hormone. *Nature* **190**:632, 1961.
6. Cheever EV, Lewis UJ: Estimation of the molecular weights of the multiple components of growth hormone and prolactin. *Endocrinology* **85**:465, 1969.
7. Chrambach A, Yardley RA, Ben-David M, Rodbard D: Isohormones of human growth hormone. *Endocrinology* **93**:848, 1973.
8. Hummel BCW, Brown GM, Hwang P, Friesen HG: Human and monkey prolactin and growth hormone: Separation of polymorphic forms by isoelectric focusing. *Endocrinology* **97**:855, 1975.
9. Frohman LA, Burek L, Stachura ME: Characterization of growth hormone different molecular weights in rat, dog, and human pituitaries. *Endocrinology* **91**:262, 1972.
10. Lewis UJ, Peterson SM, Bonewald LF, Seavey BK, Vanderlaan WP: An interchain disulfide dimer of human growth hormone. *J Biol Chem* **252**:3697, 1977.
11. Lewis UJ, Singh RNP, Tutwiler GF, Sigel MB, Vanderlaan EF, Vanderlaan WP: Human growth hormone: A complex of proteins. *Recent Prog Horm Res* **36**:477, 1980.
12. Lingappa VR, Blobel G: Early events in the biosynthesis of secretory and membrane proteins: The signal hypothesis. *Recent Prog Horm Res* **36**:451, 1980.
13. Lewis UJ, Bonewald LF, Lewis LJ: The 20,000-dalton variant of human growth hormone: Location of the amino acid deletions. *Biochem Biophys Res Commun* **92**:511, 1980.
14. Denoto F, Moore DD, Goodman HM: Human growth hormone DNA sequence and mRNA structures: Possible alternative splicing. *Nucleic Acids Res* **9**:3719, 1981.
15. Wilhelmi AE: Fractionation of human pituitary glands. *Can J Biochem Physiol* **39**:1659, 1961.
16. Li CH, Dixon JS, Chung D: Primary structure of the human chorionic somatomammotropin (HCS) molecule. *Science* **173**:56, 1971.
17. Sherwood LM, Handweger S, McLaurin WD: Amino-acid sequence of human placental lactogen. *Nature* **233**:59, 1971.
18. Miller WL, Eberhardt NL: Structure and evolution of the growth hormone gene family. *Endocr Rev* **4**:97, 1983.
19. Cooke NE, Coit D, Shine J, Baxter JD, Martial JA: Human prolactin cDNA structural analysis and evolutionary comparisons. *J Biol Chem* **255**:4007, 1981.
20. Chakravarti A, Phillips JA III, Mellits KB, Buetow KH, Seeburg PH: Patterns of polymorphism and linkage disequilibrium suggest independent origins of the human growth hormone gene cluster. *Proc Natl Acad Sci U S A* **81**:6085, 1984.
21. Van Buul-Offers S, Dumoleijn L, Hacking W, et al: The Snell dwarf mouse: Interrelationship of growth in length and weight, serum somatomedin activity and sulfate incorporation in costal cartilage during growth hormone, thyroxine and somatomedin treatment, in Giordano G, Van Wyk JJ, Minuto F (eds): *Somatomedins and Growth: Proceedings of the Serono Symposia*. New York, Academic, 1979, vol 23, pp 281–283.
22. Isaksson OGP, Jansson J-O, Gause IAM: Growth hormone stimulates longitudinal bone growth directly. *Science* **216**:1237, 1982.
23. Grichting G, Levy LK, Goodman HM: Relationship between binding and biological effects of human growth hormone in rat adipocytes. *Endocrinology* **113**:1111, 1983.
24. Phillips LS, Vassilopoulou-Sellin R: Somatomedins (first of two parts). *N Engl J Med* **302**:371, 1980.
25. Phillips LS, Vassilopoulou-Sellin R: Somatomedins (second of two parts). *N Engl J Med* **302**:438, 1980.
26. D'Ercole AJ, Underwood LE, Van Wyk JJ: Serum somatomedin-C in hypopituitarism and in other disorders of growth. *J Pediatr* **90**:375, 1977.
27. D'Ercole AJ: Somatomedins/insulin-like growth factors: Relationship to insulin and diabetes, in Oh W, Gabbe SG (eds): *Infants of the Diabetic Mother, Report of the 93rd Ross Conference on Pediatric Research*. Columbus, OH, Ross Laboratories, pp 50–65.
28. Han VKM, D'Ercole AJ, Lund PK: Cellular localization of somatomedin (insulin-like growth factor) messenger RNA in the human fetus. *Science* **236**:193, 1987.
29. Rindernecht E, Humbel RE: The amino acid sequence of human insulin-like growth factor 1 and its structural homology with proinsulin. *J Biol Chem* **253**:2769, 1978.
30. Underwood LE, D'Ercole AJ: Insulin and insulin-like growth factors/somatomedins in fetal and neonatal development. *Clin Endocrinol Metab* **13**:69, 1984.
31. Merimee TJ, Zapf J, Froesch ER: Insulin-like growth factor in pregnancy: Studies in a growth hormone-deficient dwarf. *J Clin Endocrinol Metab* **54**:1101, 1982.
32. Grumbach MM, Kaplan SL, Vinik A: *Peptide Hormones*. New York, North Holland, 1974.
33. Rosenfeld RG, Wilson DM, Dollar LA, Bennett A, Hintz RL: Both human pituitary growth hormone and recombinant DNA-derived human growth hormone cause insulin resistance at a postreceptor site. *J Clin Endocrinol Metab* **54**:1033, 1982.
34. Nielsen PV, Pedersen H, Kampmann EM: Absence of human placental lactogen in an otherwise uneventful pregnancy. *Am J Obstet Gynecol* **135**:322, 1979.
35. Borody IB, Carlton MA: Isolated defect in human placental lactogen synthesis in a normal pregnancy. *Br J Obstet Gynecol* **88**:44, 1981.
36. Owerbach D, Rutter WJ, Martial JA, Baxter JD, Shows TB: Genes for growth hormone, chorionic somatomammotropin, and growth hormone-like gene on chromosome 17 in humans. *Science* **209**:289, 1980.
37. George DL, Phillips JA III, Francke U, Seeburg PH: The genes for growth hormone and chorionic somatomammotropin are on the long arm of human chromosome 17 in region q21 to qter. *Hum Genet* **57**:138, 1981.
38. Harper ME, Barrera-Saldana HA, Saunders GF: Chromosomal localization of the human placental lactogen-growth hormone gene cluster to 17q22-24. *Am J Hum Genet* **34**:227, 1982.
39. Owerbach D, Rutter WJ, Cooke NE, Martial JA, Shows TB: The prolactin gene is located on chromosome 6 in humans. *Science* **212**:815, 1981.
40. Fiddes JC, Seeburg PH, Denoto FM, Hallewell RA, Baxter JD, Goodman HM: Structure of genes for human growth hormone and chorionic somatomammotropin. *Proc Natl Acad Sci U S A* **76**:4294, 1979.
41. Seeburg PH: The human growth hormone gene family: Nucleotide sequences show recent divergence and predict a new polypeptide hormone. *DNA* **1**:239, 1982.
42. Moore DD, Conkling MA, Goodman HM: Human growth hormone: A multigene family. *Cell* **29**:285, 1982.
43. Kidd VJ, Saunders GJ: Linkage arrangement of human placental lactogen and growth hormone genes. *J Biol Chem* **157**:10673, 1982.
44. Moore DD, Walker MD, Diamond DJ, Conkling MA, Goodman HM: Structure, expression, and evolution of growth hormone genes. *Recent Prog Horm Res* **38**:197, 1982.
45. Phillips JA III, Parks JS, Hjelle BL, Herd JE, Plotnick LD, Migeon CJ, Seeburg PH: Genetic basis of familial isolated growth hormone deficiency type I. *J Clin Invest* **70**:489, 1982.
46. Barsh GS, Seeburg PH, Gelinas RE: The human growth hormone gene family: Structure and evolution of the chromosomal locus. *Nucleic Acids Res* **11**:3939, 1983.

47. Hirt K, Kimelman J, Birnbaum MJ, Chen EY, Seeburg PH, Eberhardt NL, Barta A: The human growth hormone gene locus: Structure, evolution, and allelic variations. *DNA* **6**:59, 1987.
48. Pavlakis GN, Hizuka N, Gorden P, Seeburg P, Hamer DH: Expression of two human growth hormone genes in monkey cells infected by simian virus 40 recombinants. *Proc Natl Acad Sci U S A* **78**:7398, 1981.
49. Wieringa B, Meyer F, Reiser J, Weissman C: Unusual splice sites revealed by mutagenic inactivation of an authentic splice site of the rabbit. β-globin gene. *Nature* **301**:38, 1983.
50. Vanin EF, Henthon PS, Kioussi D, Grosveld I, Smithies O: Unexpected relationships between four large deletions in the human β-globin cluster. *Cell* **35**:701, 1983.
51. Lehrman MA, Schneider WJ, Sudhof TC, Brown MS, Goldstein JL, Russell DW: Mutation in LDL receptor: *Alu-Alu* recombination deletes exons encoding transmembrane and cytoplasmic domains. *Science* **227**:140, 1985.
52. McWilliams D, Boime I: Cytological localization of placental lactogen messenger ribonucleic acid in syncytiotrophoblast layers of human placenta. *Endocrinology* **107**:761, 1980.
53. McWilliams D, Callahan RC, Boime I: Human placental lactogen mRNA and its structural gene during pregnancy: Quantitation with a complementary DNA. *Proc Natl Acad Sci U S A* **71**:1024, 1977.
54. Barrera-Saldana HA, Robberson DL, Sauncers GF: Transcriptional products of the human placental lactogen gene. *J Biol Chem* **257**:12399, 1982.
55. Barrera-Saldana HA, Seeburg PH, Saunders GF: Two structurally different genes produce the same placental lactogen hormone. *J Biol Chem* **258**:3787, 1983.
56. Wurzel JM, Parks JS, Herd JE, Nielsen PV: A gene deletion is responsible for absence of human chorionic somatomammotropin. *DNA* **1**:251, 1982.
57. Siler-Khodr TM, Morgenstern LL, Greenwood FC: Hormone synthesis and release from human fetal adenohypophyses in vitro. *J Clin Endocrinol Metab* **39**:891, 1974.
58. Gluckman PD, Grumbach MM, Kaplan SL: The neuroendocrine regulation and function for growth hormone and prolactin in the mammalian fetus. *Endocr Rev* **2**:363, 1981.
59. Rechler MM, Nissley SP, Roth J: Hormonal regulation of human growth. *N Engl J Med* **316**:941, 1987.
60. Hall K, Sara VR: Somatomedin levels in childhood, adolescence and adult life. *Clin Endocrinol Metab* **13**:91, 1984.
61. Meites J: Changes in neuroendocrine control of anterior pituitary function during aging. *Neuroendocrinology* **34**:151, 1982.
62. Sara VR, Hall K, Rodeck CH, Wetterberg L: Human embryonic somatomedin. *Proc Natl Acad Sci U S A* **78**:3175, 1981.
63. Merimee TJ, Zapf J, Hewlett B, Cavalli-Sforza LL: Insulin-like growth factors in pygmies: The role of puberty in determining final stature. *N Engl J Med* **316**:906, 1987.
64. Selby MJ, Barta A, Baxter JD, Bell GI, Eberhardt NL: Analysis of a major human chorionic somatomammotropin gene. Evidence for two-functional promoter elements. *J Biol Chem* **259**:13131, 1984.
65. Labarriere N, Selvais PL, Lemaigre FP, Michel A, Maiter DM, Rousseau GG: A novel transcriptional activator originating from an upstream promoter in the human growth hormone gene. *J Biol Chem* **270**:19205, 1995.
66. Seif I, Khoury G, Dhar R: BKV splice sequences based on analysis of preferred donor and acceptor sites. *Nucleic Acids Res* **6**:3387, 1979.
67. Lerner M, Boyle J, Mount S, Wolin S, Steitz J: Are snRNPs involved in splicing? *Nature* **283**:220, 1980.
68. Rodgers J, Wall R: A mechanism for RNA splicing. *Proc Natl Acad Sci U S A* **77**:1877, 1980.
69. Cogan JD, Prince MA, Lekhakula S, Bundey S, Futrakul, A, McCarthy EMS, Phillips JA III: A novel mechanism of aberrant pre-mRNA splicing in humans. *Hum Molec Genet* **6**:909, 1997.
70. Lewis UJ, Singh RNP, Tutwiler GF, Sigel MB, Vanderlaan EF, Vanderlaan WP: Human growth hormone: A complex of proteins. *Recent Prog Horm Res* **36**:477, 1980.
71. Evans RM, Birnberg NC, Rosenfeld MG: Glucocorticoid and thyroid hormones transcriptionally regulate growth hormone gene expression. *Proc Natl Acad Sci U S A* **79**:7659, 1982.
72. Barinaga M, Yamonoto G, Rivier C, Vale W, Evans E, Rosenfeld MG: Transcriptional regulation of growth hormone gene expression by growth hormone-releasing factor. *Nature* **306**:84, 1983.
73. Barlow JW, Voz MLJ, Eliard PH, Mathy-Hartert M, Denayer P, Economidis JV, Belayew A, Martial JA, Rousseau GG: Thyroid hormone receptors bind to defined regions of the growth hormone and placental lactogen genes. *Proc Natl Acad Sci U S A* **83**:9021, 1986.
74. Nyborg JK, Spindler SR: Alterations in local chromatin structure accompany thyroid hormone induction of growth hormone gene transcription. *J Biol Chem* **261**:5685, 1986.
75. Slater EP, Rabenau O, Karin M, Baxter JD, Beato M: Glucocorticoid receptor binding and activation of a heterologous promoter by dexamethasone by the first intron of the human growth hormone gene. *Mol Cell Biol* **5**:2984, 1985.
76. Paek I, Axel R: Glucocorticoids enhance stability of human growth hormone mRNA. *Mol Cell Biol* **7**:1496, 1987.
77. Martin JB: Neural regulation of growth hormone secretion. *N Engl J Med* **288**:1384, 1973.
78. Wehrenberg WB, Ling N, Bohlen P, Esch F, Brazeau P, Guillemin R: Physiological roles of somatocrinin and somatostatin in the regulation of growth hormone secretion. *Biochem Biophys Res Commun* **109**:562, 1982.
79. Grossman A, Savage MO, Besser GM: Growth hormone releasing hormone. *Clin Endocrinol Metab* **15**:607, 1986.
80. Brazeau P, Epelbaum J, Tannenbaum GS, Rorstad O, Martin JB: Somatostatin: Isolation, characterization, distribution, and blood determination. *Metabolism* **27**:1133, 1978.
81. Kasting NW, Martin JB, Arnold MA: Pulsatile somatostatin release from the median eminence of the unanesthetized rat and its relationship to plasma growth hormone levels. *Endocrinology* **109**:1739, 1981.
82. Daughaday WH: The anterior pituitary, in Wilson JD, Foster DW (eds): *Textbook of Endocrinology*, 7th ed. Philadelphia, Saunders, 1985, pp 568–613.
83. Wolfsdorf JI, Sadeghi-Nejad A, Senior B: Hypoketonemia and age-related fasting hypoglycemia in growth hormone deficiency. *Metabolism* **32**:457, 1983.
84. Abramovici A, Josefsberg Z, Mimouni M, Liban E, Laron Z: Histopathological features of the skin in hypopituitarism and Laron-type dwarfism. *Isr J Med Sci* **19**:515, 1983.
85. National Centre for Health Statistics: NCHS growth curves for children, birth to 18 years. *United States Vital and Health Statistics*, Series 11, No 165, November 1977.
86. Tanner JM, Whitehouse RH: Clinical longitudinal standards for height, weight, height velocity, weight velocity and stages of puberty. *Arch Dis Child* **51**:170, 1976.
87. Eddy RL, Gilliland PF, Ibarra JD Jr, McMurry JF Jr, Thompson JQ: Human growth hormone release: Comparison of provocative tests procedures. *Am J Med* **56**:179, 1974.
88. Milner RDG, Burns EC: Investigation of suspected growth hormone deficiency. *Arch Dis Child* **57**:944, 1982.
89. Lacey KA, Hewison A, Parkin JM: Exercise as a screening test for growth hormone deficiency in children. *Arch Dis Child* **48**:508, 1973.
90. Collu R, Brun G, Milsant F, Leboeuf G, Letarte J: Reevaluation of levodopapropranolol as a test of growth hormone reserve in children. *Pediatrics* **61**:242, 1978.
91. Roth J, Glick SM, Yalow RS, Berson SA: Hypoglycemia: A potent stimulus to secretion of growth hormone. *Science* **140**:987, 1963.
92. Parker ML, Hammond JM, Daughaday WH: The arginine provocative tests: An aid to the diagnosis of hyposomatotropism. *J Clin Endocrinol* **27**:1129, 1967.
93. Gil-Ad I, Topper E, Laron Z: Oral clonidine as a growth hormone stimulation test. *Lancet* **2**:278, 1979.
94. The Health Services Human Growth Hormone Committee: Comparison of the intravenous insulin and oral clonidine tolerance tests for growth hormone secretion. *Arch Dis Child* **56**:852, 1981.
95. Vandershuerin-Lodeweyckx MWR, Malvaux P, Eggermont E, Eeckels R: The glucagon stimulation test: Effect on plasma growth hormone and on immunoreactive insulin, cortisol and glucose in children. *J Pediatr* **85**:182, 1974.
96. Parks JS: Growth hormone response to propanol-glucagon stimulation: A comparison with other tests of growth hormone reserve. *J Clin Endocrinol* **37**:85, 1973.
97. Liberman B, Cesar FP, Wajchenberg BL: Human growth hormone (hGH) stimulation tests: The sequential exercise and L-dopa procedure. *Clin Endocrinol* **10**:649, 1979.
98. Penny R, Blizzard RM, Davis WT: Sequential study of arginine and insulin tolerance tests on the same day. *J Clin Endocrinol Metab* **29**:1499, 1969.
99. Vimpani GV, Vimpani AF, Lidgard GP, Cameron EHD, Farquhar JW: Prevalence of severe growth hormone deficiency. *Br Med J* **2**:427, 1977.
100. Rona RJ, Tanner JM: Aetiology of idiopathic growth hormone deficiency in England and Wales. *Arch Dis Child* **52**:197, 1977.
101. Lacey KA, Parkin JM: Causes of short stature—A community study of children in New Castle upon Tyne. *Lancet* **1**:42, 1974.

102. Ishihara M: Optic hypoplasia with pituitary dwarfism (Kaplan-Grumbach-Hoyt syndrome, or DeMorsier syndrome). *Endocrinology* **30**:7, 1983.
103. Keller RJ, Wolfsdorf JI: Isolated growth hormone deficiency alters cerebral edema complicating diabetic ketoacidosis. *N Engl J Med* **316**:857, 1987.
104. Preece MA, Kearney PJ, Marshall WC: Growth-hormone deficiency in congenital rubella. *Lancet* **2**:842, 1977.
105. Butenandt O: Growth hormone deficiency and growth hormone therapy in Ullrich-Turner-Syndrome. *Klin Wochenschr* **58**:99, 1980.
106. Shalet SM, Beardwell CG, Morris Jones PH, Pearson D: Growth hormone deficiency after treatment of acute leukemia in children. *Arch Dis Child* **51**:489, 1976.
107. Burns EC, Tanner JM, Preece MA, Cameron N: Growth hormone treatment in children with craniopharyngioma: Final growth status. *Clin Endocrinol* **14**:587, 1981.
108. Richards GE, Wara WM, Grumbach MM, Kaplan SL, Sheline GE, Conte FA: Delayed onset of hypopituitarism: Sequelae of therapeutic irradiation of central nervous system, eye, and middle ear tumors. *J Pediatr* **89**:553, 1976.
109. Romshe CA, Zipf WB, Miser A, Miser J, Sotos JF, Newton WA: Evaluation of growth hormone release and human growth hormone treatment in children with cranial irradiation-associated short stature. *J Pediatr* **104**:177, 1984.
110. Tanner JM: Human growth hormone. *Nature* **237**:433, 1972.
111. Seip M, Trygstad O, Aarskog D: Comment on pituitary dwarfism in Norway, 1961–1970. *Birth Defects* **7**:33, 1971.
112. Illig R: Growth hormone antibodies in patients treated with different preparations of human growth hormone (hGH). *J Clin Endocrinol Metab* **31**:679, 1970.
113. Illig R, Prader A, Ferrandez A, Zachmann M: Hereditary prenatal growth hormone deficiency with increased tendency to growth hormone antibody formation, in Kracht J (ed): *Endokrinologie der Entwicklung und Reifung*. Berlin, Springer-Verlag, 1970, p 246.
114. Illig R, Prader A, Ferrandez A, Zachmann M: Hereditary prenatal growth hormone deficiency with increased tendency to growth hormone antibody formation ("A-type" isolated growth hormone deficiency). *Acta Pediatr Scand Suppl* **60**:607, 1971.
115. Kunkel LM, Smith KD, Boyer SH, Borgaonkor DS, Wachtel SS, Miller OJ, Breg WR, Jones HW, Rary JM: Analysis of human Y-chromosome specific reiterated DNA in chromosome variants. *Proc Natl Acad Sci U S A* **74**:1245, 1977.
116. Martial JA, Hallewell RA, Baxter JD, Goodman HM: Human growth hormone: Complementary DNA cloning and expression in bacteria. *Science* **205**:602, 1979.
117. Southern EM: Detection of specific sequences among DNA fragments separated by gel electrophoresis. *J Mol Biol* **98**:503, 1975.
118. Jeffreys AJ, Flavell RA: A physical map of the DNA regions flanking the rabbit β-globin gene. *Cell* **12**:429, 1977.
119. Phillips JA III, Hjelle BL, Seeburg PH, Zachmann M: Molecular basis for familial isolated growth hormone deficiency. *Proc Natl Acad Sci U S A* **78**:6372, 1981.
120. Rivarola MA, Phillips JA III, Migeon CJ, Heinrich JJ, Hjelle BJ: Phenotypic heterogeneity in familial isolated growth hormone deficiency (IGHD) type A. *J Clin Endocrinol Metab* **59**:34, 1984.
121. Nishi Y, Aihara K, Usui T, Phillips JA III, Mallonee RL, Migeon CJ: Isolated growth hormone deficiency type 1A in a Japanese family. *J Pediatr* **104**:885, 1984.
122. Frisch H, Phillips JA III: Growth hormone deficiency due to GH-N gene deletion in an Austrian family. *Acta Endocrinol* **113**:107, 1986.
123. Braga S, Phillips JA III, Joss E, Schwarz H, Zuppinger K: Familial growth hormone deficiency resulting from a 7.6 kb deletion within the growth hormone gene cluster. *Am J Med Genet* **25**:443, 1986.
124. Laron Z, Kelijman M, Pertzelan A, Keret R, Shoffner JM, Parks JS: Human growth hormone gene deletion without antibody formation or growth arrest during treatment — A new disease entity? *Isr J Med Sci* **21**:999, 1985.
125. Goossens M, Brauner R, Czernichow P, Duquesnoy P, Rappaport R: Isolated growth hormone (GH) deficiency type 1A associated with a double deletion in the human GH gene cluster. *J Clin Endocrinol Metab* **62**:712, 1986.
126. Phillips JA III, Ferrandez A, Frisch H, Illig R, Zuppinger K: Defects of GH genes: Clinical syndromes, in Raiti S (ed): *Human Growth Hormone*. New York, Plenum, 1986, pp 211–226.
127. Akinci A, Kanaka C, Eble A, Akar N, Vidinlisan S, Mullis PE: Isolated growth hormone (GH) deficiency type 1A associated with a 45-kilobase gene deletion within the human GH gene cluster. *J Clin Endocrinol Metab* **75**:437, 1992.
128. Baroncini C, Baldazzi L, Pirazzoli P, Marchetti G, Capelli M, Cacciari E, Bernardi F: Deletion breakpoints in a 32bp perfect repeat located 45.1 kb apart in the human growth hormone gene cluster. *Hum Molec Genet* **2**:2151, 1993.
129. Cacciari E, Pirazzoli P, Gualandi S, Baroncini C, Baldazzi L, Treviaani B, Capelli M, et al: Molecular study of human growth hormone gene cluster in three families with isolated growth hormone deficiency and similar phenotype. *Eur J Pediatr* **153**:635, 1994.
130. Ghizzoni L, Duquesnoy P, Torresani T, Vottero A, Goossens M, Bernasconi S: Isolated growth hormone deficiency type 1A associated with a 45-kilobase gene deletion within the human growth hormone gene cluster in an Italian family. *Paediatr Res* **36**:654, 1994.
131. Wagner JK, Eble A, Hindmarsh PC, Mullis PE: Prevalence of human GH-1 gene alterations in patients with isolated growth hormone deficiency. *Pediatr Res* **43**:105, 1998.
132. Vnencak-Jones CL, Phillips JA III: Hot spots for growth hormone gene deletions in homologous regions outside of *Alu* repeats. *Science* **250**:1745, 1990.
133. Vnencak-Jones CL, Phillips JA III, De-fen W: Use of polymerase chain reaction in detection of growth hormone gene deletions. *J Clin Endocrinol Metab* **70**:1550, 1990.
134. Kamijo T, Phillips JA III: Detection of molecular heterogeneity in GH-1 gene deletions by analysis of polymerase chain reaction amplification products. *J Clin Endocrinol Metab* **74**:786, 1992.
135. Mullis PE, Akinci A, Kanaka CH, Eble A, Brook CGD: Prevalence of human growth hormone-1 gene deletions among patients with isolated growth hormone deficiency from different populations. *Pediatr Res* **31**:532, 1992.
136. Phillips JA III: Genetic diagnosis: Differentiating growth disorders. *Hosp Pract (Off Ed)* **20**:85, 1985.
137. Schwarz S, Berger P, Frisch H, Moncayo R, Phillips JA III, Wick G: Growth hormone blocking antibodies in a patient with deletion of the GH-N gene. *Clin Endocrinol* **27**:213, 1987.
138. Hauffa BP, Illig R, Torresani T, Stolecke H, Phillips JA III: Discordant immune and growth response to pituitary and biosynthetic growth hormone in siblings with isolated growth hormone deficiency type IA. *Acta Endocrinol (Copenh)* **121**:609, 1989.
139. Cogan JD, Phillips JA III, Sakati NA, Frisch H, Milner D, Burr IM: Molecular analysis of familial growth hormone deficiency. *The Endocrine Society, Program and Abstracts*, 321, 1992.
140. Cogan JD, Phillips JA III, Sakati N, Frisch H, Schober E, Milner RDG: Heterogeneous growth hormone (GH) gene mutations in familial GH deficiency. *J Clin Endocrinol Metab* **76**:1224, 1993.
141. Duquesnoy P, Amselem S, Gourmelen M, Le Bouc Y, Goossens M: A frameshift mutation causing isolated growth hormone deficiency type 1A. *Am J Hum Genet* **47**:A110, 1990.
142. Cogan JD, Phillips JA III, Sakati NA, Schenkman SS, Milner D: Molecular basis of autosomal recessive and autosomal dominant inheritance in familial GH deficiency. *Endocrine Society, Program and Abstracts*, 376, 1993.
143. Miller-Davis S, Phillips JA III, Milner RDG, Al-Ashwal A, Sakati NA, Summar ML: Detection of mutations in GH genes and transcripts by analysis of DNA from dried blood spots and mRNA from lymphoblastoid cells of GH deficient subjects. *Endocrine Society, Program and Abstracts*, 1131, 1993.
144. Abdul-Latif HD, Brown MR, Parks JS, Carmi R, Leiberman E: Mutation of intron 4 of the GH-1 gene causes GH deficiency. *Endocrine Society, Program and Abstracts*, 470, 1995.
145. Igarashi Y, Ogawa M, Kamijo T, Iwatani N, Nishi Y, Kohno H, Masumura T, et al: A new mutation causing inherited growth hormone deficiency: A compound heterozygote of a 6.7-kb deletion and two base deletion in the third exon of the GH-1 gene. *Hum Mol Genet* **2**:1073, 1993.
146. Rogol AD, Blizzard MR, Foley TP Jr, Furlanetto R, Selden R, Mayo K, Thorner MO: Growth hormone releasing hormone and growth hormone: Genetic studies in familial growth hormone deficiency. *Pediatr Res* **19**:489, 1985.
147. Rimoin DL, Schechter JE: Histological and ultrastructural studies of isolated growth hormone deficiency. *J Clin Endocrinol Metab* **37**:725, 1973.
148. Lin SC, Lin CR, Gukovsky I, Lusis AJ, Sawchenko PE, Rosenfeld MG: Molecular basis of the little mouse phenotype and implications for cell type-specific growth. *Nature* **364**:208, 1993.
149. Wajnrajch MP, Gertner JM, Harbison MD, Chua SC Jr, Leibel RL: Nonsense mutation in the human growth hormone-releasing hormone

receptor causes growth failure analogous to the little (lit) mouse. *Nat Genet* **12**:88-90, 1996.
150. Bauman G, Maheshwari H: The dwarfs of Sindh: Severe growth hormone deficiency caused by a mutation in the GH-releasing hormone receptor gene. *Acta Paediatr Suppl* **423**:33, 1997.
151. Salvatori R, Gondo RG, Oliveira MHA, Phillips JA III, Souza AH, Hayashida CY, Toledo SP, et al: Familial isolated growth hormone deficiency due to a novel mutation in the growth hormone-releasing hormone receptor. *Endocrine Society, Program and Abstracts,* OR4-5, 1998.
152. Rimoin DL: Genetic disorders of the pituitary gland, in Emery AEH, Rimoin DL (eds): *Principles and Practice of Medical Genetics.* Edinburgh, Churchill Livingstone, 1983, pp 1134–1151.
153. Sheikholislam BM, Stempfell RS Jr: Hereditary isolated somatotropin deficiency: Effects of human growth hormone administration. *Pediatrics* **49**:362, 1972.
154. Poskitt EME, Rayner PHW: Isolated growth hormone deficiency: Two families with autosomal dominant inheritance. *Arch Dis Child* **49**:55, 1974.
155. Van Gelderen HH, Van Der Hoog CE: Familial isolated growth hormone deficiency. *Clin Genet* **20**:173, 1981.
156. Polymeropoulos, MH, Rath DS, Xiao H, Merril CR: A simple sequence repeat polymorphism at the human growth hormone locus. *Nucleic Acids Res* **19**:689, 1991.
157. Binder G, Ranke MB: Screening for growth hormone (GH) gene splice-site mutations in sporadic cases with severe isolated GH deficiency using ectopic transcript analysis. *J Clin Endocrinol Metab* **80**:1247, 1995.
158. Cogan JD, Ramel B, Lehto M, Phillips JA III, Prince M, Blizzard RM, deRavel TJL, et al: A recurring dominant-negative mutation causes autosomal dominant growth hormone deficiency. *J Clin Endocrinol Metab* **80**:3591, 1995.
159. Wajnrajch MP, Gertner JM, Moshang T, Saenger P, Leibel RL. Isolated growth hormone (GH) deficiency, type II (IGHD II) caused by substitution of arginine by histidine in C-terminal portion of the GH molecule. *Endocrine Society, Programs and Abstracts*, P2-313, 1996.
160. Fleisher TA, White RM, Broder S, Nissley SP, Blaese RM, Mulvihill JJ, Olive G, Waldmann TA: X-linked hypogammaglobulinemia and isolated growth hormone deficiency. *N Engl J Med* **302**:1429, 1980.
161. Rapaport R, Oleske J, Ahdieh H, Solomon S, Delfaus C, Denny T: Suppression of immune function in growth hormone-deficient children during treatment with human growth hormone. *J Pediatr* **109**:434, 1986.
162. Kowarski AA, Schneider J, Ben-Galim E, Weldon VV, Daughaday WH: Growth failure with normal serum RIA-GH and low somatomedin activity: Somatomedin restoration and growth acceleration after exogenous GH. *J Clin Endocrinol Metab* **47**:461, 1978.
163. Rudman D, Kutner MH, Goldsmith MA, Kenny J, Jennings H, Bain RP: Further observations on four subgroups of normal variant short stature. *J Clin Endocrinol Metab* **51**:1378, 1980.
164. Rudman K, Kutner MH, Blackston RD, Cushman RA, Bain RP, Patterson JH: Children with normal-variant short stature: Treatment with human growth hormone for six months. *N Engl J Med* **305**:123, 1981.
165. Hayek A, Peake GT: Growth and somatomedin-C responses to growth hormone in dwarfed children. *J Pediatr* **99**:868, 1981.
166. Frazer T, Gavin JR, Daughaday WH, Hillman RE, Weldon V: Growth hormone-dependent growth failure. *J Pediatr* **101**:12, 1982.
167. Takahashi Y, Kaji H, Okimura Y, Goji K, Abe H, Chihara K. Brief report: Short stature caused by a mutant growth hormone. *N Engl J Med* **334**:432, 1996.
168. Pertzelan A, Adam A, Laron Z: Genetic aspects of pituitary dwarfism due to absence or biological inactivity of growth hormone. *Isr J Med Sci* **4**:895, 1968.
169. Adam A, Josefsberg Z, Pertzelan A, Zadik Z, Chemke JM, Laron Z: Occurrence of four types of growth hormone-related dwarfism in Israeli communities. *J Pediatr* **137**:35, 1981.
170. Jacobs LS, Sneid SD, Garland JT, Laron Z, Daughaday WH: Receptor-active growth hormone in Laron dwarfism. *J Clin Endocrinol Metab* **42**:403, 1976.
171. Laron Z, Pertzelan A, Karp M, Kowadlo-Silbergeld A, Daughaday WH: Administration of growth hormone to patients with familial dwarfism with high plasma immunoreactive growth hormone: Measurement of sulfation factor, metabolic and linear growth response. *J Clin Endocrinol Metab* **33**:332, 1971.
172. Phillips JA III: Molecular biology of growth hormone receptor dysfunction. *Acta Paediatr Scand Suppl* **383**:127, 1992.
173. Godowski PJ, Leung DW, Meacham LR, Galgani JP, Hellmiss R, Keret R, Rotwein PS, Parks JS, Laron Z, Wood WI: Characterization of the human growth hormone receptor gene and demonstration of a partial gene deletion in two patients with Laron-type dwarfism. *Proc Natl Acad Sci U S A* **86**:8083, 1989.
174. Amselem S, Sobrier ML, Duquesnoy P, Rappaport R, Postel-Vinay M-C, Gourmelen M, Dallapiccola B, Goossens M: Recurrent nonsense mutations in the growth hormone receptor from patients with Laron dwarfism. *J Clin Invest* **87**:1098, 1991.
175. Amselem S, Duquesnoy P, Attree O, Novelli G, Bousnina S, Postel-Vinay M-C, Goossens M: Laron dwarfism and mutation of the growth hormone-receptor gene. *N Engl J Med* **321**:989, 1989.
176. Duquesnoy P, Sobrier ML, Amselem S, Goossens M: Defective membrane expression of human growth hormone (GH) receptor causes Laron-type GH insensitivity syndrome. *Proc Natl Acad Sci U S A* **88**:10272, 1991.
177. Buchanan CR, Maheshwari HG, Norman MR, Morrell DJ, Preece MA: Laron-type dwarfism with apparently normal high affinity serum growth hormone-binding protein. *Clin Endocrinol* **35**:179, 1991.
178. Duquesnoy P, Sobrier ML, Duriez B, Dastot F, Buchanan CR, Savage MO, Preece MA, et al: A single amino acid substitution in the exoplasmic domain of the human growth hormone (GH) receptor confers familial GH resistance (Laron syndrome) with positive GH-binding activity by abolishing receptor homodimerization. *EMBO J* **13**:1386, 1994.
179. Rosenbloom AL, Guevara-Aguirre J, Rosenfeld RG, Fielder PJ: The little women of Loja — Growth hormone-receptor deficiency in an inbred population of southern Ecuador. *N Engl J Med* **323**:1367, 1990.
180. Berg MA, Guevara-Aguirre J, Rosenbloom AL, Rosenfeld RG, Francke U: Mutation creating a new splice site in the growth hormone receptor genes of 37 Ecuadorian patients with Laron syndrome. *Hum Mutat* **1**:24, 1992.
181. Woods KA, Fraser NC, Postel-Vinay MC, Savage MO, Clark AJ: A homozygous splice site mutation affecting the intracellular domain of the growth hormone (GH) receptor resulting in Laron syndrome with elevated GH-binding protein. *J Clin Endocrinol Metab* **81**:1686, 1996.
182. Woods KA, Camacho-Hubner C, Savage MO, Clark AJL: Intrauterine growth retardation and postnatal growth failure associated with deletion of the insulin-like growth factor 1 gene. *N Engl J Med* **335**:1363, 1996.
183. Li S, Crenshaw EB III, Rawson EJ, Simmons DM, Swanson LW, Rosenfeld MG: Dwarf locus mutants lacking three pituitary cell types result form mutations in the POU-domain gene Pit-1. *Nature* **347**:527, 1990.
184. Tatsumi K-i, Miyai K, Notomi T, Kaibe K, Amino N, Mizuno Y, Kohno H: Cretinism with combined hormone deficiency caused by a mutation in the Pit-1 gene. *Nat Genet* **1**:56, 1992.
185. Ohta K, Nobukuni Y, Mitsubuchi, Mitsubichi H, Fujimoto S, Matsuo N, Inagaki H, Endo F, et al: Mutations in the Pit-1 gene in children with combined pituitary hormone deficiency. *Biochem Biophys Res Comm* **189**:851, 1992.
186. Wit JM, Drayer NM, Jansen M, Walenkamp MJ, Hackeng WHL, Thijssen JHH, Van den Bunde JL: Total deficiency of growth hormone and prolactin, and partial deficiency of thyroid stimulating hormone in two Dutch families: A new variant of hereditary pituitary deficiency. *Horm Res* **32**:170, 1989.
187. Pfaffl RW, DiMattia GE, Parks JS, Brown MR, Wit JM, Jansen M, Van der Nat H, Van den Brande JL, Rosenfeld MG, Ingraham HA: Mutation of the POU-specific domain of Pit-1 and hypopituitarism without pituitary hypoplasia. *Science* **257**:1118, 1992.
188. Irie Y, Tatsumi K, Ogawa M, Kamijo T, Preeyasombat C, Suprasongsin C, Amino N: A novel E250X mutation of the Pit-1 gene in a patient with combined pituitary hormone deficiency. *Endocr J* **42**:351, 1995.
189. Pelligrini-Bouiller I, Belicar P, Barlier A, Gunz G, Charvet JP, Jauet P, Brue T, et al: A new mutation of the gene encoding the transcription factor Pit-1 is responsible for combined pituitary hormone deficiency. *J Clin Endocrinol Metab* **81**:2790, 1996.
190. Radovick S, Nations M, Du Y, Berg LA, Weintraub BD, Wondisford FE: A mutation in the POU-homeodomain of Pit-1 responsible for combined pituitary hormone deficiency. *Science* **257**:1115, 1992.
191. Sornson MW, Wu W, Dasen JS, Flynn SE, Norman DJ, O'Connell SM, Gukovsky I, et al: Pituitary lineage determination by the Prophet of Pit-1 homeodomain factor defective in Ames dwarfism. *Nature* **384**:327, 1996.

192. Wei W, Cogan JD, Pfaffle RW, Dasen JS, Frisch H, O'Connell SM, Flynn SE, et al: Mutations in Prop-1 cause familial combined pituitary hormone deficiency. *Nat Genet* **18**:147, 1998.
193. Cogan JD, Wu W, Phillips JA III, Arnhold IJP, Fofanova OV, Osorio MGF, Bircan I, et al: The Prop-1 2-bp deletion is a common cause of combined pituitary hormone deficiency. *J Clin Endocrinol Metab* **83**:3346, 1998.
194. Fofanova O, Takamura N, Kinoshita E, Parks JS, Brown MR, Peterkova VA, Evgrafov OV, et al: Compound heterozygous deletion of the PROP-1 gene in children with combined pituitary hormone deficiency. *J Clin Endocrinol Metab* **83**:2601, 1998.
195. Lagerstrom-Fermer M, Sundvall M, Johnsen E, Warne GL, Forrest SM, Zajac JD, Rickards A, et al: X-linked recessive panhypopituitarism associated with a regional duplication in Xq25-q26. *Am J Hum Genet* **60**:910, 1997.
196. Merimee TJ, Zapf J, Froesch ER: Dwarfism in the pygmy: An isolated deficiency of insulin-like growth factor I. *N Engl J Med* **305**:965, 1981.
197. McKusick VA: *Mendelian Inheritance in Man*, 7th ed. Baltimore, Johns Hopkins University Press, 1986.
198. Dattani MT, Marinez-Barbera JP, Thomas PQ, Brickman JM, Gupta R, Martensson IL, Toresson H, et al: Mutations in the homeobox gene HESX1/Hesx1 associated with septo-optic dysplasia in human and mouse. *Nat Genet* **19**:125, 1998.
199. Rudman D, Davis GT, Priest JH, Patterson JH, Kutner MH, Heymsfield SB, Bethel RA: Prevalence of growth hormone deficiency with cleft lip or palate. *J Pediatr* **93**:378, 1978.
200. Parks JS, Brown MR, Baumbach L, Sanchez JC, Stanley CA, Gianella-Neto D, Wu W, et al: Natural history and molecular mechanisms of hypopituitarism with large sella turcica. *Endocrine Society, Program and Abstracts*, P3-409, 1998.
201. Knudtzon J, Aarskog D: Growth hormone deficiency associated with the ectrodactyly-ectodermal dysplasia-clefting syndrome and isolated absent septum pellucidum. *Pediatrics* **79**:410, 1987.
202. Goldstein SJ, Sphrintzen RJ, Wu RHK, Thorpy MJ, Hahm SY, Marion R, Sher AE, Saenger P: Achondroplasia and obstructive sleep apnea: Correction of apnea and abnormal sleep-entrained growth hormone release by tracheostomy. *Birth Defects* **21(2)**:83, 1985.
203. Parks JS, Nielsen PV, Sexton LA, Jorgensen EH: An effect of gene dosage on production of human chorionic somatomammotropin. *J Clin Endocrinol Metab* **60**:994, 1985.
204. Orlando PJ, Phillips JA III, Ferrandez AN, Arnal JM, Woodard MJ, Bueno M: Frequency and types of deletions in the growth hormone (GH) gene clusters of Spanish subjects with GH deficiency. *Am J Hum Genet* **41**:A105, 1987.
205. Phillips JA III, Beamer WG, Bartke A: Analysis of growth hormone genes in mice with genetic defects of growth hormone expression. *J Endocrinol* **92**:405, 1982.
206. Cheng TC, Beamer WG, Phillips JA III, Bartke A, Mallonee RL, Dowling C: Etiology of growth hormone deficiency in Little, Ames, and Snell dwarf mice. *Endocrinology* **113**:1669, 1983.
207. Raben MS: Treatment of pituitary dwarf with human growth hormone. *J Clin Endocrinol Metab* **18**:901, 1958.
208. Frazier SD: Human pituitary growth hormone (hGH) therapy in growth hormone deficiency. *Endocr Rev* **4**:155, 1983.
209. Frasier SD, Costin G, Lippe BM, Aceto T, Bunger PF: A dose-response curve for human growth hormone. *J Clin Endocrinol Metab* **53**:1213, 1981.
210. Gertner JM, Tamborlane WV, Gianfredi SP, Genel M: Renewed catch-up growth with increased replacement doses of human growth hormone. *Clin Lab Obs* **110**:425, 1987.
211. Russo L, Moore WV: A comparison of subcutaneous and intramuscular administration of human growth hormone in the therapy of growth hormone deficiency. *J Clin Endocrinol Metab* **55**:1003, 1982.
212. Soyka LF, Bode HH, Crawford JD, Flynn FJ: Effectiveness of long-term human growth hormone therapy for short stature in children with growth hormone deficiency. *Growth Horm Ther Short Stature* **30**:1, 1970.
213. Burns EC, Tanner JM, Preece MA, Cameron N: Final height and pubertal development in 55 children with idiopathic growth hormone deficiency, treated for between 2 and 15 years with human growth hormone. *Eur J Pediatr* **137**:155, 1981.
214. Cassorla F, Mericq V, Eggers M, Avila A, Garcia C, Fuentes A, Rose SR, et al: Effects of luteinizing hormone-releasing hormone analog-induced pubertal delay in growth hormone (GH)-deficient children treated with GH: Preliminary results. *Metabolism* **82**:3989, 1997.
215. Cuneo RC, Judd S, Wallace JD, Perry-Keene D, Burger H, Lim-Tio S, Strauss B, et al: The Australian multicenter trial of growth hormone (GH) treatment in GH-deficient adults. *J Clin Endocrinol Metab* **83**:107, 1998.
216. Lippe BM, Van Herle AJ, LaFranchi SH, Uller RP, Lavin N, Kaplan SA: Reversible hypothyroidism in growth hormone-deficient children treated with human growth hormone. *J Clin Endocrinol Metab* **40**:612, 1975.
217. Frasier SD, Aceto T, Hayles AB, Parker ML, Meyer-Bahlburg HFL: Collaborative study of the effects of human growth hormone in growth hormone deficiency. II. Development and significance of antibodies to human growth hormone during the first year of therapy. *J Clin Endocrinol Metab* **38**:14, 1974.
218. Winterer J, Chousos G, Cassorla F, Loriaux DL: Acquired refractoriness to growth hormone in a patient with isolated growth hormone deficiency: Growth and plasma somatomedin-C response to high-dose growth hormone therapy. *J Pediatr* **104**:908, 1984.
219. Report of the Committee on Growth Hormone Use of the Lawson Wilkins Pediatric Endocrine Society, May 1985: Degenerative neurologic disease in patients formerly treated with human growth hormone. Special article. *J Pediatr* **107**:10, 1985.
220. Virus scare halts hormone research. Three deaths attributed to a brain virus have halted distribution of human growth hormone and other products of the pituitary gland. *Science* **228**:1176, 1985.
221. Preece MA: Creutzfeldt-Jakob disease: Implications for growth hormone deficient children. *Neuropathol Appl Neurobiol* **12**:509, 1986.
222. Kolata G: New growth industry in human growth hormone. *Science* **234**:22, 1986.
223. Goeddel DV, Heynecker HL, Hozumi T, Arentzen R, Itakura K, Yansura DG, Ross MJ, Miozzari G, Crea R, Seeburg PH: Direct expression in *Escherichia coli* of a DNA sequence coding for human growth hormone. *Nature* **281**:544, 1979.
224. Olson KC, Fenno J, Lin N, Harkins RN, Snider C, Kohr WH, Ross MJ, Fodge D, Prender G, Stebbing N: Purified human growth hormone from *E. coli* is biologically active. *Nature* **293**:408, 1981.
225. Kaplan SL, August GP, Blethen SL, Brown DR, Hintz RL, Johansen A, Plotnick LP, Underwood LE, Bell JJ, Blizzard RM, Foley TP, Hopwood NJ, Kirkland RT, Rosenfeld RG, Van Wyk JJ: Clinical studies with recombinant-DNA derived methionyl human growth hormone in growth hormone deficient children. *Lancet* **1**:697, 1986.
226. Rogol AD, Blizzard RM, Johanson AJ, Furlanetto RW, Evans WS, Rivier J, Vale WW, Thorner MO: Growth hormone release in response to human pancreatic tumor growth hormone-releasing hormone-40 in children with short stature. *J Clin Endocrinol Metab* **59**:580, 1984.
227. Takano K, Hizuka N, Shizume K, Asakawa K, Miyokawa M, Herose N, Shibasaki T, Ling NC: Plasma growth hormone (GH) response to GH-releasing factor in normal children with short stature and patients with pituitary dwarfism. *J Clin Endocrinol Metab* **58**:236, 1984.
228. Thorner MO, Reschke J, Chitwood J, Rogol AD, Furlanetto R, Rivier J, Vale W, Blizzard RM: Acceleration of growth in two children treated with human growth hormone-releasing factor. *N Engl J Med* **312**:4, 1985.
229. Rochiccioli PE, Tauber M-T, Uboldi F, Coude F-X, Morre M: Effect of over night constant infusion of human growth hormone (GH)-releasing hormone-(1-44) on 24-hour GH secretion in children with partial GH deficiency. *J Clin Endocrinol Metab* **63**:1100, 1986.
230. Chapman IM, Pescovitz OH, Murphy G, Treep T, Cerchio KA, Krupa D, Gertz B, et al: Oral administration of growth hormone (GH)-releasing peptide-mimetic MK-677 stimulates the GH/insulin-like growth factor-I axis in selected GH-deficient adults. *J Clin Edocrinol Metab* **82**:3455, 1997.
231. Pihoker C, Badger TM, Reynolds GA, Bowers CY: Treatment effects of intranasal growth hormone releasing peptide-2 in children with short stature. *J Endocrinol* **155**:79, 1997.
232. Palmiter RD, Brinster RL, Hammer RE, Trumbauer ME, Rosenfeld MG, Birnberg NC, Evans RM: Dramatic growth of mice that develop from eggs microinjected with metallothionein-growth hormone fusion genes. *Nature* **300**:611, 1982.
233. Hammer RE, Pursel VG, Rexroad CE Jr, Wall RJ, Bolt DJ, Ebert KM, Palmiter RD, Brinster RL: Production of transgenic rabbits, sheep and pigs by microinjection. *Nature* **315**:680, 1985.
234. Hammer RE, Brinster RL, Rosenfeld MG, Evans RM, Mayo KE: Expression of human growth hormone-releasing factor in transgenic mice results in increased somatic growth. *Nature* **315**:413, 1985.
235. Wagner EF, Covarrubias L, Stewart TA, Mintz B: Prenatal lethalities in mice homozygous for human growth hormone gene sequences integrated in the germ line. *Cell* **35**:647, 1983.

CHAPTER 163

Nephrogenic Diabetes Insipidus

Daniel G. Bichet ■ T. Mary Fujiwara

1. **Nephrogenic diabetes insipidus (NDI), which can be inherited or acquired, is characterized by an inability to concentrate urine despite normal or elevated plasma concentrations of the antidiuretic hormone, arginine vasopressin (AVP). Polyuria, with hyposthenuria and polydipsia are the cardinal clinical manifestations of the disease.**
2. **About 90 percent of patients with congenital NDI are males with X-linked recessive NDI (MIM 304800) who have mutations in the arginine-vasopressin receptor 2 (*AVPR2*) gene that codes for the vasopressin V_2 receptor. The gene is located in chromosome region Xq28.**
3. **In less than 10 percent of the families studied, congenital NDI has an autosomal recessive or autosomal dominant mode of inheritance (MIM 222000 and 125800). Mutations have been identified in the aquaporin-2 gene (*AQP2*), which is located in chromosome region 12q13 and codes for the vasopressin-sensitive water channel.**
4. **When studied in vitro, most *AVPR2* mutations lead to receptors that are trapped intracellularly and are unable to reach the plasma membrane. A few mutant receptors reach the cell surface but are unable to bind AVP or to properly trigger an intracellular cAMP signal. Similarly, AQP2 mutant proteins are misrouted and cannot be expressed at the luminal membrane.**
5. **Prior knowledge of *AVPR2* or *AQP2* mutations in NDI families and perinatal mutation testing is of direct clinical value because early diagnosis and treatment can avert the physical and mental retardation associated with repeated episodes of dehydration.**
6. **NDI is clinically distinguishable from neurogenic diabetes insipidus (MIM 125700) by a lack of response to exogenous AVP and by plasma levels of AVP that rise normally with increase in plasma osmolality. Neurogenic diabetes insipidus is secondary to mutations in the prepro-arginine-vasopressin-neurophysin II (*prepro-AVP-NPII*) gene. Neurogenic diabetes insipidus is also a component of Wolfram syndrome (MIM 222300), an autosomal recessive disorder.**
7. **Other inherited disorders with mild to moderate inability to concentrate urine include Bartter syndrome (MIM 601678) and cystinosis (MIM 219800), while long-term lithium administration is the main cause of acquired NDI.**

Nephrogenic failure to concentrate urine maximally may be due to a defect in vasopressin-induced water permeability of the distal tubules and collecting ducts, to insufficient build-up of the corticopapillary interstitial osmotic gradient, or to a combination of these two factors.[1] Thus, the broadest definition of the term NDI embraces any antidiuretic hormone-resistant urinary-concentrating defect, including medullary disease with low interstitial osmolality, renal failure, and osmotic diuresis. The antidiuretic hormone in humans and most mammals is 8-arginine vasopressin (AVP). In its narrower sense, NDI describes only those conditions in which AVP release fails to induce the expected increase in water permeability of the cortical and medullary collecting ducts (Table 163-1).[2]

URINE CONCENTRATION AND THE COUNTERCURRENT SYSTEM

Urine is not concentrated by active transport of water from tubule fluid to blood because such a system would require a tremendous expenditure of metabolic energy. It has been estimated that more than 300 times the energy needed by an active salt transport and passive water equilibration system would be required, as salt concentrations are about 0.15 mM, whereas water concentrations are about 55 mM. Instead, urine is concentrated with relatively little expenditure of metabolic energy by a complex interaction among the loops of Henle, the medullary interstitium, the medullary blood vessels or vasa recta, and the collecting tubules. This mechanism of urine concentration is called the countercurrent mechanism because of the anatomic arrangement of the tubules and vascular elements (Fig. 163-1). Tubular fluids move from the cortex toward the papillary tip of the medulla via the proximal straight tubule and the thin descending limbs. The tubules then loop back toward the cortex so that the direction of the fluid movement is reversed in the ascending limbs. Similarly, the vasa recta descend to the tip of the papilla and then loop back toward the cortex. This arrangement of tubule segments and vasa recta allows the two fundamental processes of the countercurrent mechanism to take place—countercurrent multiplication and countercurrent exchange.[1,3]

For the following descriptions, osmolality within the medulla is considered to range from 300 mOsm/kg at the corticomedullary tip junction to 1400 mOsm/kg at the papillary tip (Fig. 163-1). In keeping with tissue analysis,[4] approximately half the medullary hypertonicity is assigned to NaCl and half to urea. It is also assumed that the secretion of the antidiuretic hormone, AVP, is intact and that it will interact with specific receptors on the collecting tubule (*vide infra*).

The permeability and structural characteristics of the tubular and vascular segments responsible for the countercurrent mechanism are now described at a molecular level. The presence and abundance of the water channels of the aquaporin family seem to determine whether tubular or vascular structure is highly permeable or impermeable to water. Aquaporin 1 (AQP1), the first aquaporin to be characterized,[5,6] is present in both apical and basolateral plasma membranes of proximal tubules, in thin

---

A list of standard abbreviations is located immediately preceding the index in each volume. Additional abbreviations used in this chapter include: AVP = arginine vasopressin; dDAVP = 1-desamino[8-D-arginine]vasopressin; PKA = protein kinase A; PKC = protein kinase C.

GenBank accession numbers: *AQP2* (D31846, S73196, Z29491); *AVPR2* (L22206, U04357, U52112, Z11687); *prepro-AVP-NPII* (M11166, M25647).

Table 163-1 Causes of Nephrogenic Diabetes Insipidus

Narrow definition of NDI: water permeability of the collecting duct not increased by AVP
Congenital (idiopathic)
Hypercalcemia
Hypokalemia
Drugs:
Lithium
Demeclocycline
Amphotericin B
Methoxyflurane
Diphenylhydantoin
Nicotine
Alcohol
Broad definition of NDI: defective medullary countercurrent function
Renal failure, acute or chronic (especially interstitial nephritis or obstruction)
Medullary damage:
Sickle-cell anemia and trait
Amyloidosis
Sjögren syndrome
Sarcoidosis
Hypercalcemia
Hypokalemia
Protein malnutrition
Cystinosis

Modified from Magner and Halperin[2] with permission.

descending limbs of Henle epithelia, and in descending vasa recta endothelia.[7]

The facilitated urea transporter (UT2) is located in the late part of descending thin limbs of short loops of Henle[8] (Fig. 163-2). Isotonic fluid containing 280 mOsm/kg NaCl entering the highly water permeable (but urea and Na^+ impermeable) descending thin limb is concentrated almost entirely by water abstraction, so that fluid entering the ascending limb has a higher NaCl concentration and a lower urea concentration than the medullary interstitium. These passive driving forces between lumen and interstitium poise the system for fluid dilution.[9]

Thin and thick ascending loops of Henle are impermeable to water because they bear no water channels. The urea transporter present in the thin ascending segment is not precisely characterized but, as fluid moves up the water-impermeable thin limb, NaCl efflux from lumen to interstitium exceeds passive urea influx from interstitium to tubular fluid resulting in tubular fluid dilution. The recently characterized chloride channel CLC-K1[10,11] is critically involved in active chloride transport in the thin ascending part of Henle's loop (see references 12 and 13, and *vide infra*). This kidney-specific member of the CLC chloride channel family is found exclusively in the thin ascending limb of Henle's loop in both apical and basolateral membranes.[11]

In the thick ascending limb, tubular fluid is diluted further by the active transport of NaCl from tubule to interstitium (Fig. 163-3). The NaCl reabsorption mechanisms for the thick ascending loop of Henle and the distal convoluted tubule depend on low intracellular Na^+ activity maintained by active extrusion of Na^+ from the cell by the basolateral Na^+-K^+-ATPase (Na^+ pump). K^+ that enters the thick ascending loop of Henle by the Na-K-2Cl cotransporter recycles back to the tubular urine through potassium channels[14] (Fig. 163-3). This has two major consequences: it replenishes the urinary K^+ that would otherwise be lost through absorption by the Na-K-2Cl cotransporter; and it also results in a lumen-positive transepithelial voltage that provides the driving force for paracellular transport of one half of Na^+ reabsorption.[14] It is now recognized that loss-of-function mutations in the genes coding for the Na-K-2Cl cotransporter, the apical K^+ channel, or the basolateral chloride channel are responsible for Bartter syndrome[15–18] (Fig. 163-3). Bartter syndrome (MIM 601678) is a hereditary disease characterized by salt wasting, hypokalemic alkalosis, and deficits in diluting and concentrating capacity.

In the collecting duct, the first step in the antidiuretic action of AVP is its binding to the vasopressin V2 receptor (Fig. 163-4) located on the basolateral membrane of collecting duct cells. This step initiates a cascade of events—receptor-linked activation of the cholera toxin-sensitive G-protein (G_s), activation of adenylyl cyclase, production of cAMP, and stimulation of protein kinase A (PKA)—that leads to the final step in the antidiuretic action of AVP. That is, the exocytic insertion of specific water channels, AQP2, into the luminal membrane thereby increases the permeability of the luminal membrane. AQP2 is the vasopressin-regulated water channel in renal collecting ducts. It is exclusively

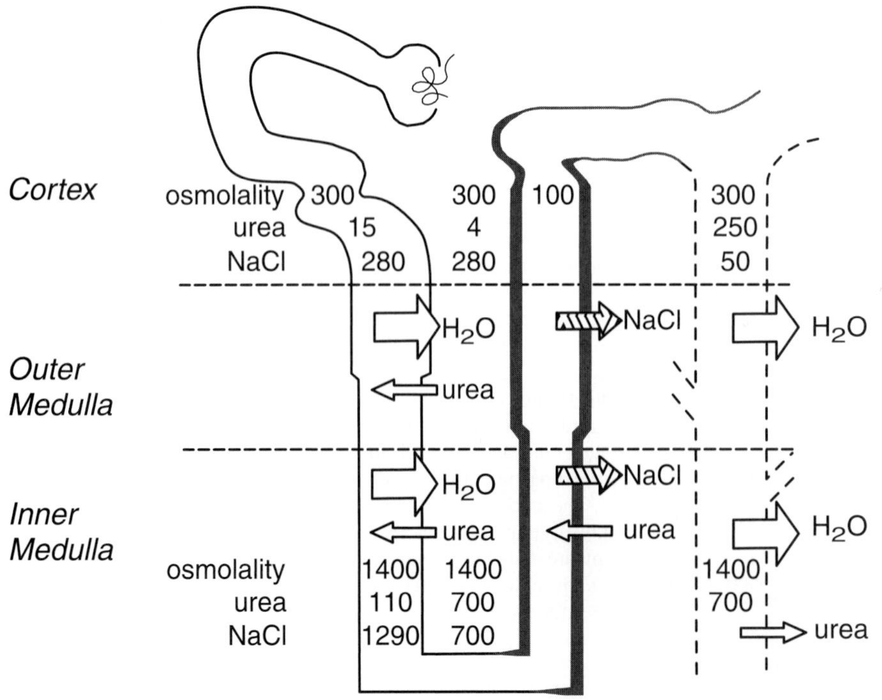

Fig. 163-1 Illustration of the model of Kokko and Rector for the renal concentrating mechanism. Heavy boundaries indicate very low permeability to water. Arrows indicate relative magnitudes of solute and water fluxes in the various segments. Note that active chloride transport in the thin ascending part of Henle's loop is now demonstrated.[13] (*Modified from Reeves and Andreoli.[83] Used with permission.*)

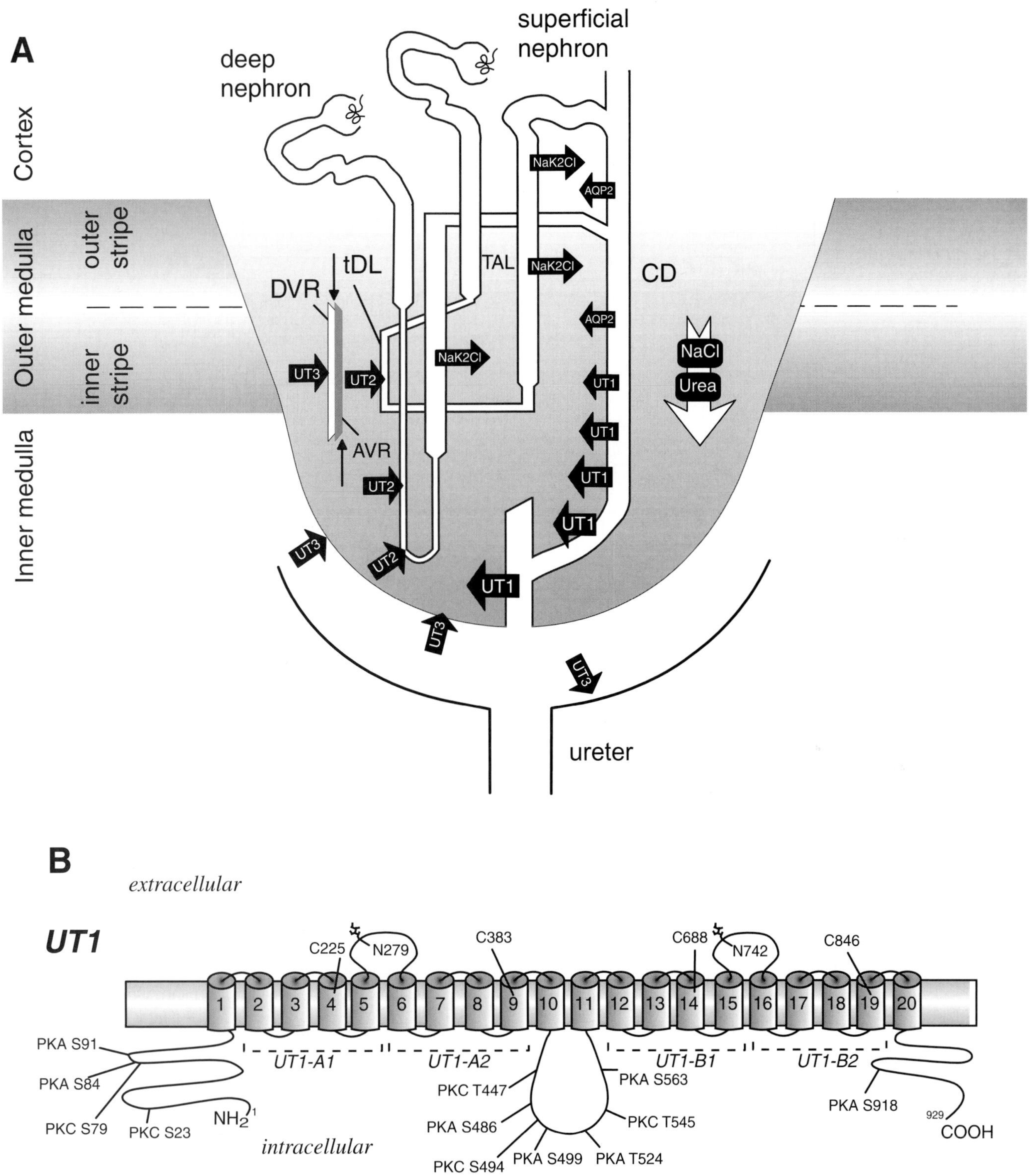

Fig. 163-2 *A*, Representation of urea transporters in the rat kidney. A superficial nephron with a short loop and a deep nephron with a long loop of Henle are represented. UT1 is present in the apical membrane of the terminal inner medullary collecting duct and is involved in vasopressin-regulated urea reabsorption. UT2 is located in the late part of descending thin limbs of short loops and participates in urea recycling. In the inner stripe of the outer medulla, vascular structures of ascending vasa recta (AVR), descending vasa recta (DVR), and tubule components of thin descending limb (tDL) are arranged together to form vascular bundles. UT3 is present in DVR and allows efficient countercurrent exchange between AVR and DVR, as well as between DVR and dTL. The vertical arrow on the right indicates the corticopupillary osmolality gradient which is primarily formed by NaCl and urea. TAL = thick ascending limb; CD = collecting duct. (*Modified from Tsukaguchi et al.*[8] *Used with permission.*) *B*, Hypothetical structural model and hydropathy analysis of UT1, the vasopressin-regulated urea channel. *UT1* cDNA encodes a 929-amino acid residue protein that consists of 2 similar halves, each composed of 2 extended hydrophobic membrane spanning stretches (UT1A and UT1B). In addition, each half of UT1 can be further subdivided into two homologous hydrophobic domains (UT1-A1/UT1-A2 and UT1-B1/UT1-B2). UT1 has 12 potential phosphorylation sites, 7 for PKA and 5 for PKC. Although there is no significant homology between water channels and urea transporters, the urea transporter repeats UT1-A1, UT1-A2, UT1-B1, and UT1-B2 contain a similar motif: Asn-Pro-Leu/Trp. This motif could conceivably form part of the urea translocation pathway. (*Modified from Shayakul et al.*[33] *Used with permission.*)

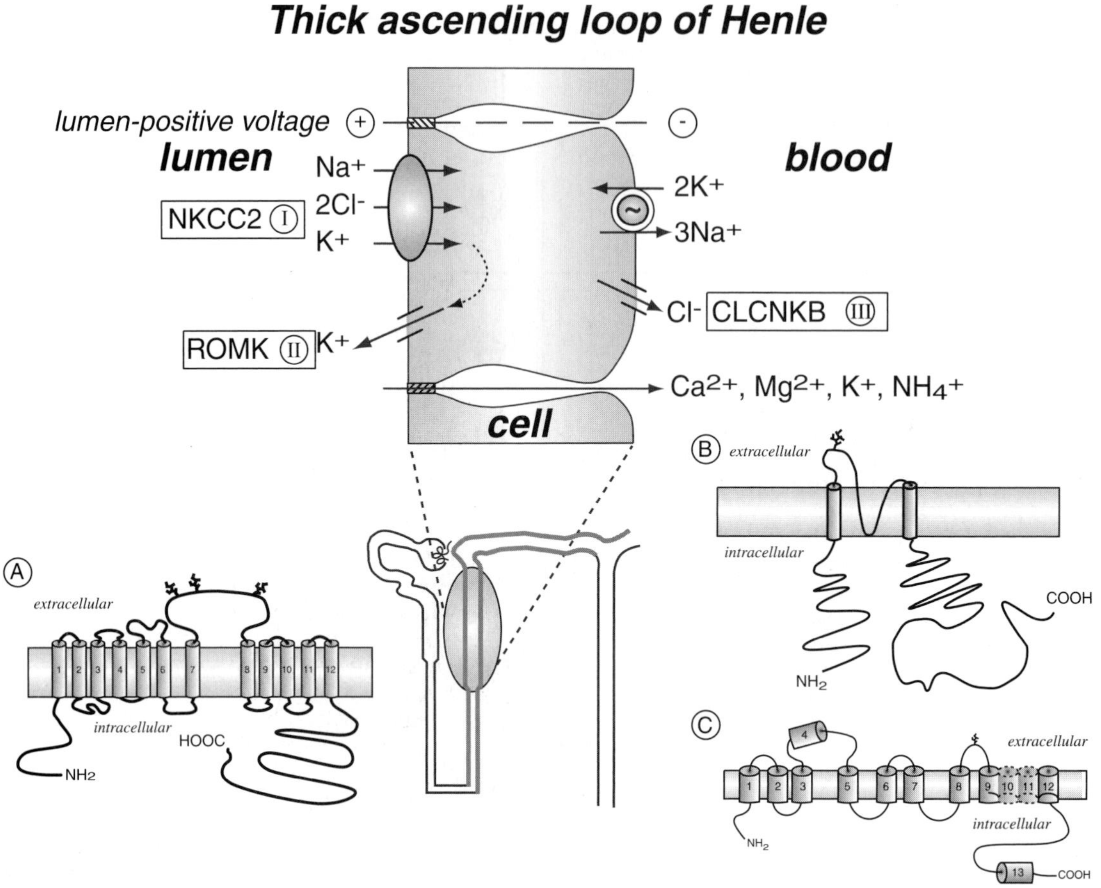

Fig. 163-3 Polyuria-polydipsic symptoms are frequently observed in patients with Bartter syndrome. Bartter syndrome is secondary to loss-of-function mutations in three different genes. Mutations in the bumetanide-sensitive Na-K-2Cl cotransporter gene (*NKCC2*) cause Bartter syndrome type I.[15] *NKCC2* is expressed exclusively in apical membranes of thick ascending limb cells. NKCC2 (*A*) is a large protein with a core molecular weight of about 120 kDa and its topology includes a large hydrophobic central region that includes at least 12 membrane-spanning helices. Sugar residues are linked to an extracellular loop between the seventh and eighth membrane-spanning segments, making this cotransporter a glycoprotein and increasing its apparent molecular weight on western blotting to 150 to 165 kDa. Mutations in the gene that encodes the inwardly rectifying renal potassium channel ROMK (*B*) cause Bartter syndrome type II.[16,17] Mutations in the gene that encodes the renal chloride channel CLCNKB (*C*) cause Bartter syndrome type III.[18]

present in principal cells of inner medullary collecting duct cells and is diffusely distributed in the cytoplasm in the euhydrated condition, whereas apical staining of AQP2 is intensified in the dehydrated condition or after administration of 1-desamino[8-D-arginine]vasopressin (dDAVP), a synthetic structural analog of AVP. The short-term AQP2 regulation by AVP involves the movement of AQP2 from intracellular vesicles to the plasma membrane, a confirmation of the shuttle hypothesis of AVP action that was proposed two decades ago.[19] In the long-term regulation, which requires a sustained elevation of circulating AVP levels for 24 h or more, AVP increases the abundance of water channels. This is thought to be a consequence of increased transcription of the *AQP2* gene.[20] The activation of PKA leads to phosphorylation of AQP2 on serine residue 256 in the cytoplasmic carboxyl terminus. This phosphorylation step is essential for the regulated movement of AQP2-containing vesicles to the plasma membrane upon elevation of intracellular cAMP.[21,22] A second G-protein (the first being the cholera-toxin sensitive G-protein G_s) has also been shown to be essential for the AVP-induced shuttle of AQP2. This G-protein is sensitive to pertussis toxin and is involved in the pathway downstream of the cAMP/cAMP-dependent protein kinase signal.[23] The molecular basis for the translocation process of the AQP2 containing vesicles remains incompletely known but it is thought to be analogous to neuronal exocytosis.[24] This is supported by the identification in the vesicles of various proteins known to be involved in regulated exocytosis, for example, Rab3a and synaptobrevin II (VAMP2) or synaptobrevin II-like protein.[25–27] In contrast to neuronal exocytosis, which is triggered by Ca^2, cAMP and PKA appear to be crucial for the translocation process.[28,29] Vesicle trafficking probably involves the interaction of AQP2-containing vesicles with the cytoskeleton (Fig. 163-4).[30] Drugs that disrupt microtubules or actin filaments have long been known to inhibit the hormonally induced permeability response in target epithelia.[31] More recently, Sabolic and coworkers have shown that microtubules are required for the apical polarization of AQP2 in principal cells.[32] AQP3 and AQP4 are the constitutive water channels in the basolateral membranes of renal medullary collecting ducts.

AVP also increases the water reabsorptive capacity of the kidney by regulating the urea transporter UT1 (Fig. 163-2) which is present in the inner medullary collecting duct, predominantly in its terminal part (Fig. 163-5).[33]

Knockout Mice with Urinary Concentration Defects

A useful strategy to establish the physiological function of a protein is to determine the phenotype produced by pharmacologic inhibition of protein function or by gene disruption. Transgenic knockout mice deficient in AQP1, AQP4, or CLCNK1 have been engineered.[13,34–36] To date, descriptions of knockout mice with inactivation of *Avpr2* or *Aqp2* have not been published.

Aqp1 knockout mice were normal in terms of survival, physical appearance, and organ morphology. However, they became severely dehydrated and lethargic after water deprivation for 36 h. Body weight decreased by 35 ± 2 percent (Fig. 163-6),

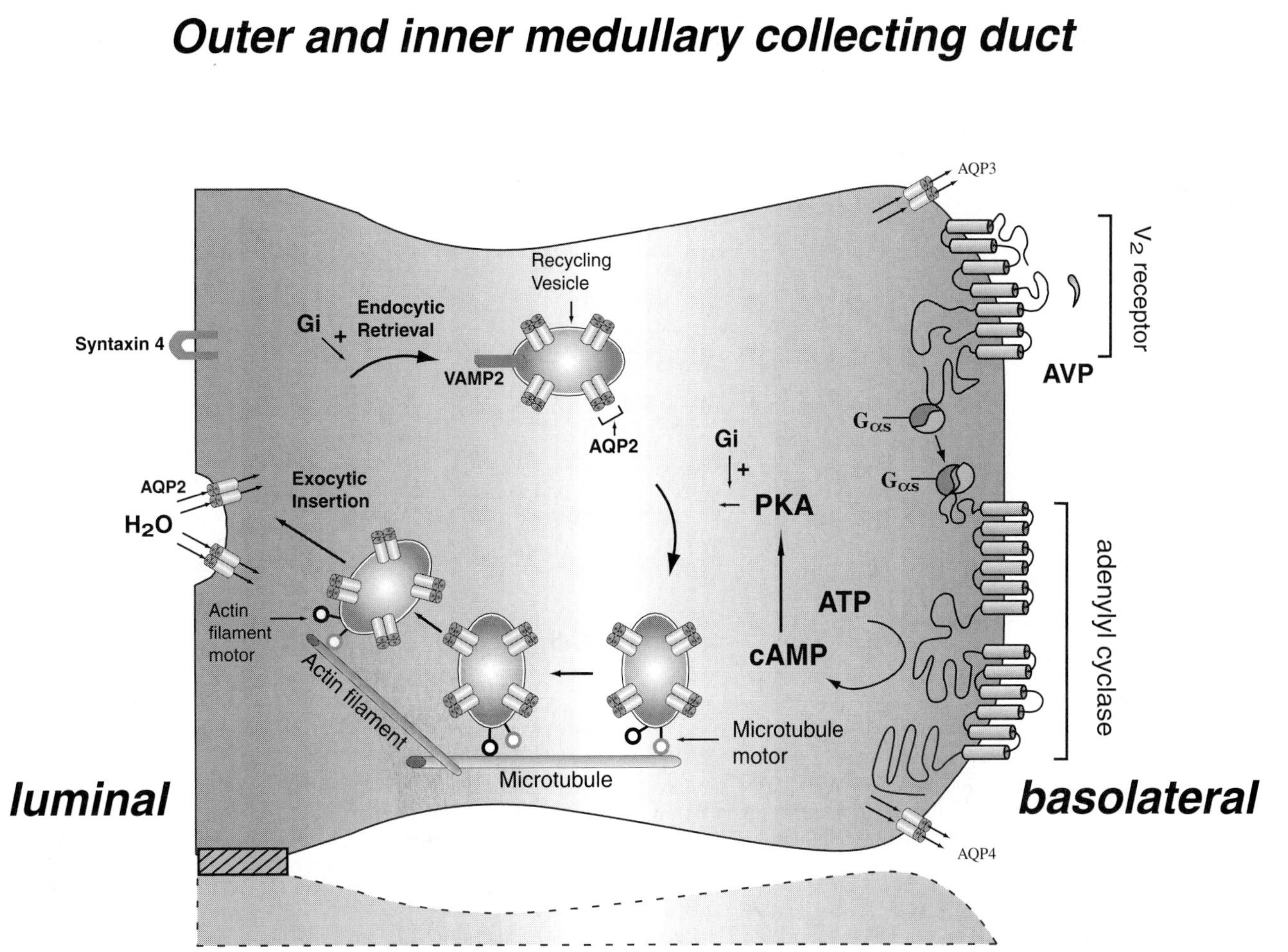

Fig. 163-4 Representation of the effect of AVP to increase water permeability in the principal cells of the collecting duct. AVP is bound to the V_2 receptor (a G-protein-linked receptor) on the basolateral membrane. The basic process of G-protein-coupled receptor signaling consists of three steps: a hepta-helical receptor that detects a ligand (in this case, AVP) in the extracellular milieu, a G-protein that dissociates into α subunits bound to GTP and $\beta\gamma$ subunits after interaction with the ligand-bound receptor, and an effector (in this case, adenylyl cyclase) that interacts with dissociated G-protein subunits to generate small-molecule second messengers. AVP activates adenylyl cyclase increasing the intracellular concentration of cAMP. The topology of adenylyl cyclase is characterized by two tandem repeats of six hydrophobic transmembrane domains separated by a large cytoplasmic loop and terminates in a large intracellular tail. Generation of cAMP follows receptor-linked activation of the heteromeric G-protein (G_s) and interaction of the free $G_{\alpha s}$-chain with the adenylyl cyclase catalyst. PKA is the target of the generated cAMP. Cytoplasmic vesicles carrying the water channel proteins (represented as homotetrameric complexes) are fused to the luminal membrane in response to AVP, thereby increasing the water permeability of this membrane. Microtubules and actin filaments are necessary for vesicle movement toward the membrane. The mechanisms underlying docking and fusion of AQP2 bearing vesicles are not known. The detection of the small GTP binding protein Rab3a, synaptobrevin 2, and syntaxin 4 in principal cells suggests that these proteins are involved in AQP2 trafficking.[23] When AVP is not available, water channels are retrieved by an endocytic process, and water permeability returns to its original low rate. AQP3 and AQP4 water channels are expressed on the basolateral membrane.

serum osmolality increased to about 500 mOsm/kg (a value not compatible with life in humans) and urinary osmolality (657 ± 59 mOsm/kg) did not change from that before water deprivation (Fig. 163-6).[35] In the *Aqp1* knockout mice, a decrease in superficial glomerular filtration rate was responsible for normal distal flow despite decreased proximal reabsorption.[37] This decrease in single nephron glomerular filtration rate was most probably caused by activation of a tubuloglomerular feedback mechanism. The increased urinary flow rate despite normal distal delivery suggests that the diuresis seen in *Aqp1* knockout mice results primarily from reduced fluid absorption in the collecting duct. This defect is secondary to a low interstitium medullary tonicity as suggested more recently by Chou et al.[36] Freeze fracture electron microscopy of rat thin descending limbs of Henle demonstrated an exceptionally high density of intramembranous particles which may represent tetramers of AQP1.[38] A striking decrease in the density of these intramembranous particles was observed in the thin descending limbs of Henle of *Aqp1*-deficient mice.[36] Transepithelial osmotic water permeability (Pf) in isolated perfused segments in thin descending limbs of Henle of wild-type mice was very high and was reduced 8.5-fold by the *Aqp1* knockout mice. These results demonstrate that osmotic equilibration along the thin descending limb of Henle by water transport plays a key role in the renal concentrating mechanism. By contrast, inactivation of *Aqp4*[34] has little or no effect on development, survival, and growth, and only causes a small defect in urinary concentrating ability[39] consistent with *AQP4* expression in the medullary collecting duct. The relative mild defect in urinary concentrating ability in the *Aqp4* knockout mice suggests that other water channels (e.g., AQP3) may have a significant functional role in more proximal segments of the collecting duct.

The *Aqp1* knockout mouse, has no human counterpart because *AQP1* null individuals have no obvious symptoms.[40] Three women bearing loss-of-function mutations of *AQP1* were identified because of the presence of high titers of circulating antibodies to the Colton blood group that apparently developed during pregnancy. Linkage between the Colton blood group and *AQP1*

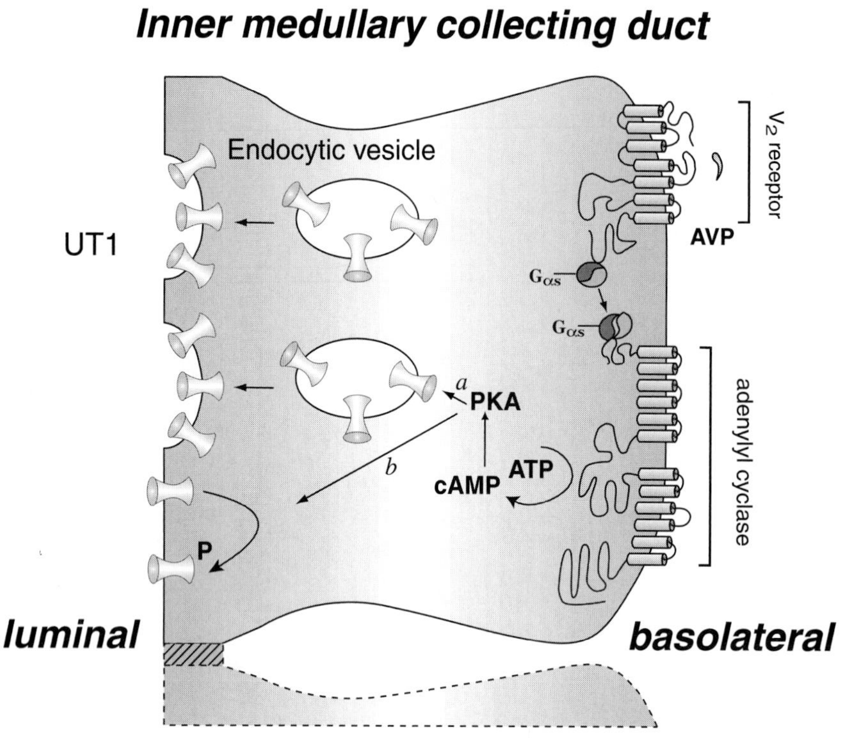

Fig. 163-5 Potential mechanisms of urea transporter (UT1) activation by AVP in the inner medullary collecting duct. AVP binds to the V_2 receptor in the basolateral membrane. This results in the activation of the $G_{\alpha s}$ subunit, activation of adenylyl cyclase, production of cAMP, and stimulation of PKA. Two potential mechanisms for UT1 activation by PKA are indicated (*a*) by increasing the insertion of vesicles containing the urea transporter and (*b*) by direct phosphorylation of urea transporter molecules. Current experimental evidence suggests that mechanism *b* is mainly involved in UT1 activation. (*Modified from Tsukaguchi et al.*[8] *Used with permission.*)

was demonstrated[41] and subsequent sequencing of DNA samples from individuals with defined Colton phenotypes demonstrated that the Colton antigen results from a missense mutation at residue 45 of the first extracellular loop of *AQP1* (Fig. 163-7).[42] Members of five kindreds were identified with a total lack of the Colton antigen. Blood and urine specimens were obtained from three probands from three different kindreds, and DNA analysis confirmed that each was homozygous for a different *AQP1*

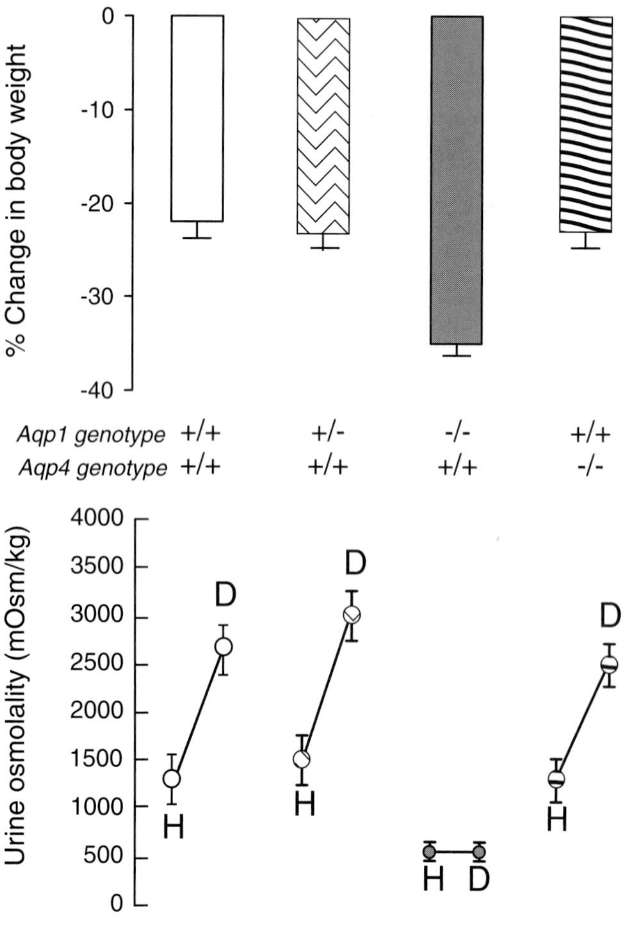

Fig. 163-6 Urinary concentrating ability in transgenic mice lacking AQP1 (*Aqp1* genotype = −/−) or AQP4 (*Aqp4* genotype = −/−) water channels. Change in body weight and urine osmolality in mice before (H) versus after (D) water deprivation for 36 h. (*Modified from Ma et al.*[35] *Used with permission.*)

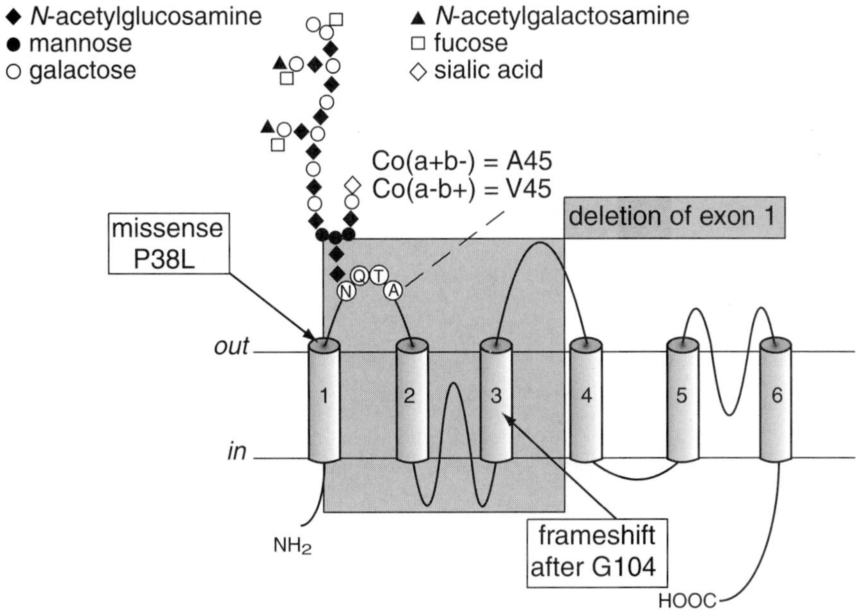

Fig. 163-7 Model representing the membrane topology of an AQP1 monomer. The site of glycosylation and the Colton (Co) blood group are represented as well as three mutations observed in Colton-null individuals (see text).[40,42] A45, V45 = arginine or valine at residue 45; G104 = glycine at residue 104; P38L = proline to leucine substitution at residue 38.

mutation.[40] Two Colton-null individuals had no detectable AQP1 in red cells or renal sediment: the first was homozygous for deletion of the entire exon 1; the second was homozygous for a frameshift mutation after glycine residue 104. A third Colton-null individual was homozygous for the missense mutation P38L at the top of the first bilayer-spanning domain (Fig. 163-7). This mutation resulted in unstable AQP1 protein when expressed in oocytes and corresponded to a 99 percent reduction in AQP1 in red cells.[40] The reasons for the difference between *Aqp1* knockout mice and AQP1-null humans are unknown.

Clcnk-1 knockout mice ($Clcnk^{-/-}$) when dehydrated were also lethargic with a decrease of 27 percent in body weight as compared to 13 percent in wild-type mice.[13] Serum osmolality increased to 360 to 381 mOsm/kg in $Clcnk^{-/-}$ mice as compared to 311 to 323 mOsm/kg in heterozygous ($Clcnk^{+/-}$) and wild-type ($Clcnk^{+/+}$) mice, and urinary osmolality was minimally increased after dDAVP administration (636 ± 31 mOsm/kg pre; 828 ± 25 mOsm/kg post).

VASOPRESSIN BIOSYNTHESIS, RECEPTORS AND CONTROL OF WATER TRANSPORT

Vasopressin Biosynthesis

Nonapeptides of the vasopressin family are the key regulators of water homeostasis in amphibia, reptiles, birds, and mammals. Because these peptides reduce urinary output, they are also referred to as antidiuretic hormones. Oxytocin (OT) and AVP (Fig. 163-8) are synthesized in separate populations of magnocellular neurons of the supraoptic and paraventricular nuclei.[43] OT is most recognized for its key role in parturition and milk letdown in mammals.[44] The axonal projections of AVP and OT-producing neurons from supraoptic and paraventricular nuclei reflect the dual function of AVP and OT as hormones and as neuropeptides because they project their axons to several brain areas and to the neurohypophysis. Another pathway from parvocellular neurons to the hypophysial portal system transports high concentration of

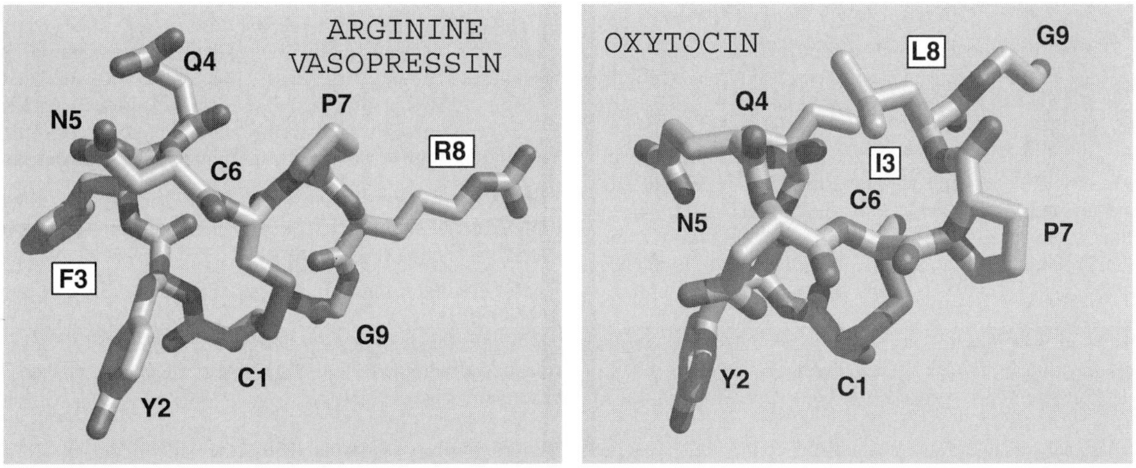

Fig. 163-8 Contrasting structures of AVP and OT. The peptides differ only by two amino acids (F3 → I3 and R8 → L8 in AVP and OT, respectively). At the receptor level (see Fig. 163-13), Y115 in the first extracellular loop of the V_{1a} receptor (equivalent to D103 in the human V_2 receptor and to F103 in the human OT receptor) is not only crucial for agonist high affinity but also for receptor selectivity.[62] The conformation of AVP was obtained from Mouillac et al.[61] and the conformation of OT was obtained from the Protein Data Bank (PDB Id 1XY1).

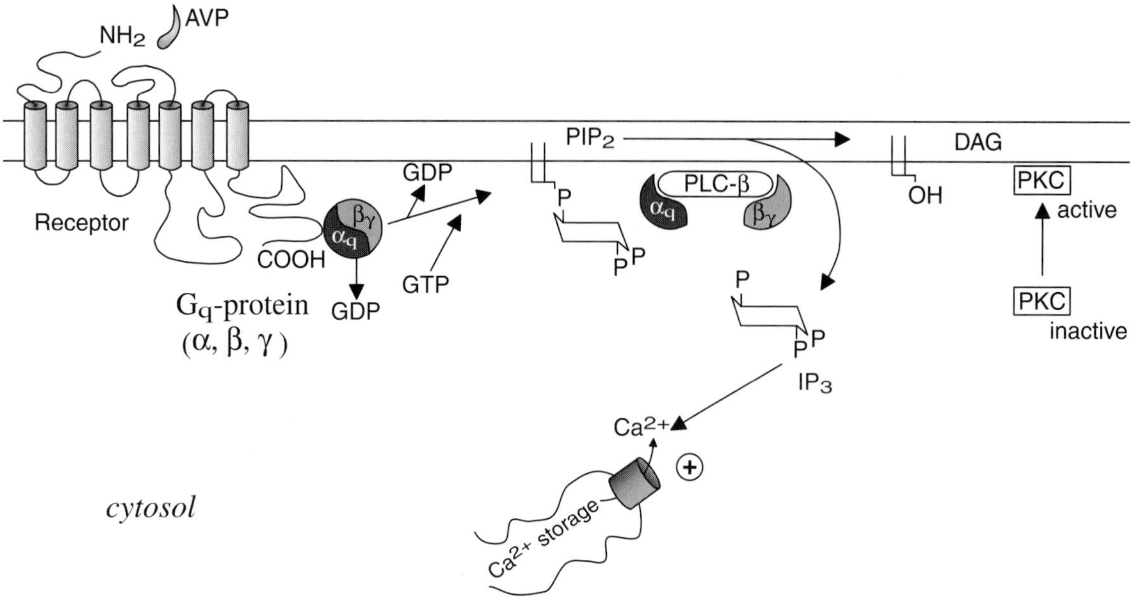

Fig. 163-9 Interaction of AVP with V_{1a}, V_{1b}, or OT receptors and representation of receptor-linked phosphoinositide hydrolysis by phospholipase C-β (PLC-β) isoform. AVP binding stimulates G-protein dissociation and α-chains of the G_q class (pertussis-toxin insensitive) mediate activation of PLC-β1 to hydrolyze membrane phosphatidylinositol 4,5-biphosphate (PIP_2). This degradation generates the second messenger inositol 1,4,5-triphosphate (IP_3) and diacylglycerol (DAG) which elevate cytosolic Ca^{2+} and activate PKC. (*Modified from Watson and Arkinstall.*[56] *Used with permission.*)

AVP to the anterior pituitary gland. AVP produced by this pathway together with the corticotropin-releasing hormone are two major hypothalamic secretagogues regulating the secretion of adrenocorticotropic hormone by the anterior pituitary[45] (see also Fig. 20.6 at page 851 in reference 46).

AVP and its corresponding carrier protein, neurophysin II, are synthesized as a composite precursor by the magnocellular and parvocellular neurons described previously. Proteolytic processing takes place in the producing neurons and during axonal transport to the posterior pituitary, where AVP is stored in vesicles. Exocytotic release is stimulated by minute increases in serum osmolality (hypernatremia, osmotic regulation) and by more pronounced decreases of extracellular fluid (hypovolemia, nonosmotic regulation) (see also Fig. 163-12). OT and neurophysin I are released from the posterior pituitary by the suckling response in lactating females.

Vasopressin Receptors

AVP binds to at least four distinct subtypes of receptors: the vasopressin receptors subtypes V_{1a}, V_{1b}, and V_2, and to the OT receptor. These receptors are now cloned and sequenced.[47–55] They belong to the G-protein coupled-receptor superfamily characterized by seven putative transmembrane helices. An extraordinarily large number of neurotransmitters, peptide hormones, neuromodulators, and autocrine and paracrine factors exert their physiological actions via binding to specific plasma membrane receptors that are coupled to distinct classes of heterotrimeric G-proteins.[56] The V_{1a}, V_{1b}, V_2, and OT receptors are strikingly similar in both size and amino acid sequence. However, the V_{1a}, V_{1b}, and OT receptors are selectively coupled to G-proteins of the $G_{q/11}$ family that mediates the activation of distinct isoforms of phospholipase C_β resulting in the breakdown of phosphoinositide lipids (Fig. 163-9). The V_2 receptor, on the other hand, preferentially activates the G-protein G_s, resulting in the activation of adenylyl cyclase (Fig. 163-4).

The classical vascular smooth muscle contraction, platelet aggregation, and hepatic glycogenolysis actions of AVP are mediated by the V_{1a} receptor that increases cytosolic calcium. *In situ* hybridization histochemistry using ^{35}S-labeled cRNA probes specific for the V_{1a} receptor mRNA showed high levels of V_{1a} receptor transcripts in the liver among hepatocytes surrounding central veins and in the renal medulla among the vascular bundles, the arcuate and interlobular arteries.[57] V_{1a} receptor mRNA was extensively distributed throughout the brain where AVP may act as a neurotransmitter or a neuromodulator in addition to its classical role on vascular tone.[58] Brain AVP receptors have been proposed to mediate the effect of AVP on memory and learning, antipyresis, brain development, selective aggression, and partner preference in rodents; cardiovascular responsivity, blood flow to the choroid plexus and cerebrospinal fluid production; regulation of smooth muscle tone in superficial brain vasculature; and analgesia. It is, however, not known whether V_{1a} brain receptors respond to AVP released within the brain proper or whether the receptors also respond to AVP from the peripheral circulation.[58]

V_{1b} receptors are not only expressed in the anterior pituitary[52] and kidney[51] as originally reported, but also in brain, uterus, thymus, heart, breast, and lung.[54] The physiological role of these extrapituitary V_{1b} receptors remains unknown, but some functions of AVP attributed in the past to V_{1a} receptors or OT receptors may be due to the activation of V_{1b} receptors.[54] In the rat adrenal medulla, AVP may regulate the adrenal functions by paracrine/autocrine mechanisms involving distinct AVP receptor subtypes: V_{1a} in the adrenal cortex and V_{1b} in the adrenal medulla.[59]

V_2 transcripts are heavily expressed in cells of the renal collecting ducts (in humans and rodents) and in cells of the thick ascending limbs of the loops of Henle (in rodents only).[57]

Receptor Functional Domains Underlying Binding of Vasopressin and Oxytocin to Their Receptors and G-Protein Coupling

A three-dimensional model of the human V_2 receptor was constructed by Ala et al.[60] using the model of the rat V_{1a} receptor as a template.[61] AVP was completely embedded in a 15 to 20 Å deep cleft defined by the transmembrane helices 2 to 7 of the receptor (Fig. 163-10).

Extracellular Domains. Only the side chain of the arginine residue at position 8 of AVP projects outside the transmembrane core of the V_2 receptor and possibly interacts with an aspartic acid residue at position 103 (D103) in the second extracellular domain connecting helices 2 and 3 (Fig. 163-11). D103 likely determines V_2 versus V_{1a} selectivity because the replacement by a tyrosine or

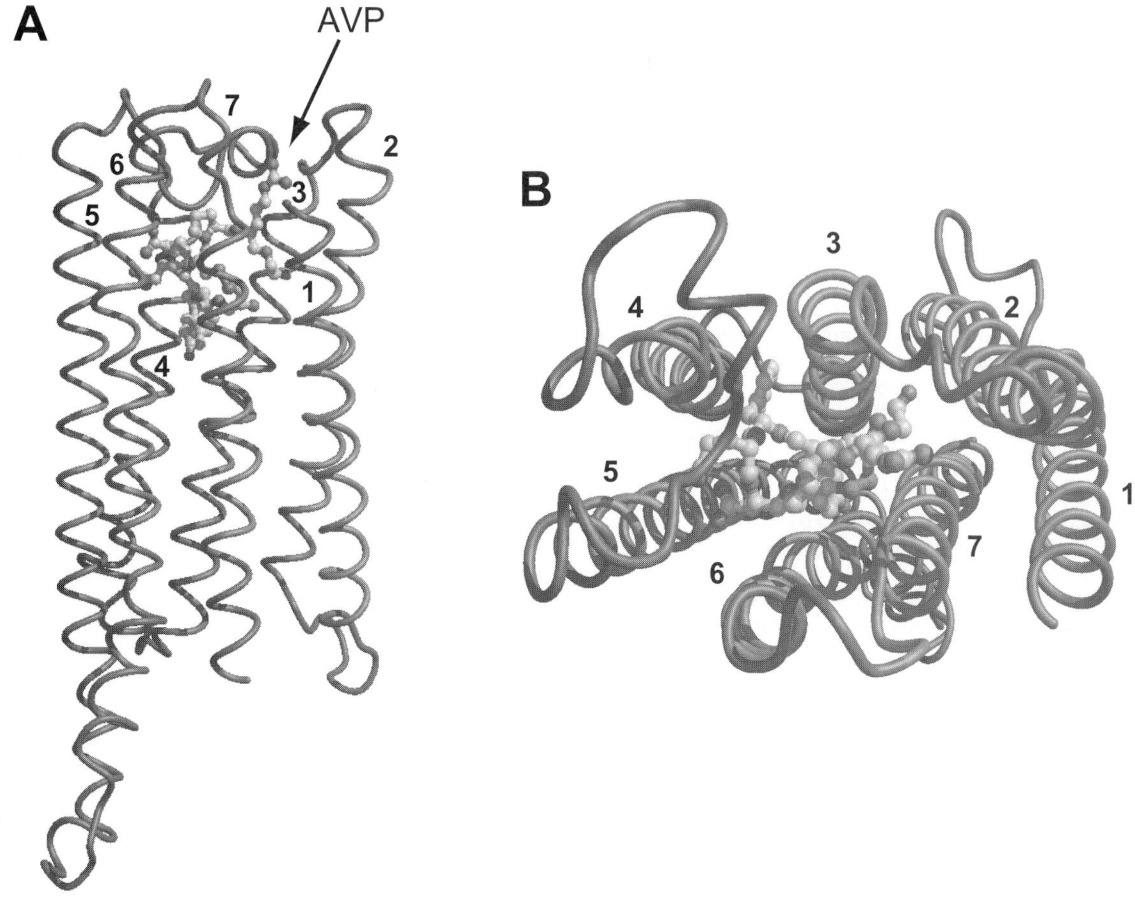

Fig. 163-10 Ribbon representation of the V_2 receptor.[60] *A*, Side view from a direction parallel to the cell membrane surface. The positioning of the transmembrane domains 1 to 7 is counterclockwise when viewed from the extracellular surface of the receptor. The model is oriented such that the extracellular side is at the top of the image. *B*, An upper view from a direction perpendicular to the outside of the cell membrane surface. This hypothetical model of interaction between AVP and the V_2 receptor is constructed according to the model published by Mouillac et al.[61] pertaining to the V_{1a} receptor. These images were produced using the MidasPlus program from the Computer Graphics Laboratory, University of California, San Francisco (supported by NIH RR-01081).

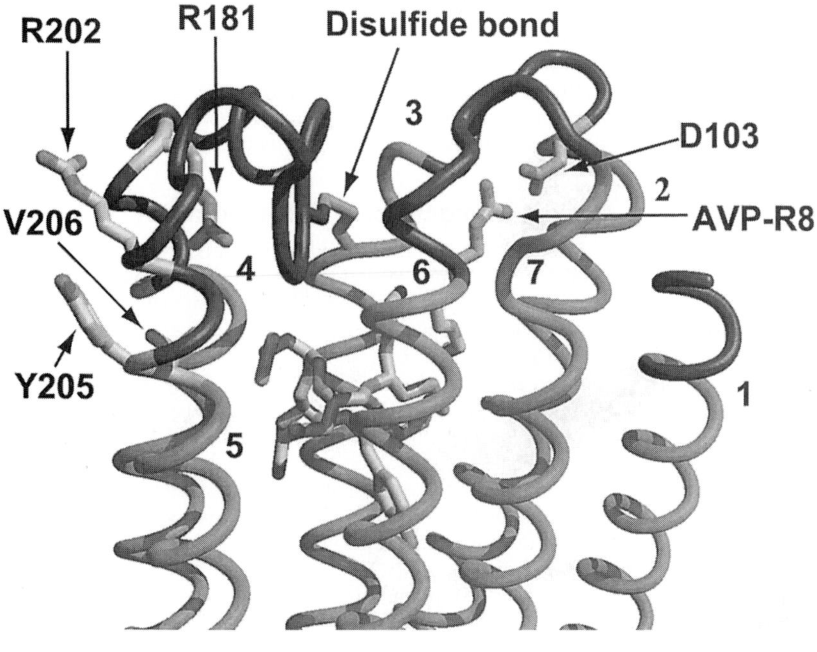

Fig. 163-11 Ribbon representation of the V_2 receptor similar to Fig. 163-10*A* showing important exofacial residues. Amino acid residue D103 in the V_2 receptor is important for high-affinity binding and receptor selectivity; it is shown to be in close contact with residue 8 of AVP (AVP-R8). Missense mutations have occurred at V_2 residues 181, 202, and 205 in families with X-linked NDI: arginine-to-cysteine substitutions (R181C and R202C) and tyrosine-to-cysteine substitution (Y205C). If these mutants are expressed on the cell surface, these new residues could possibly form additional cysteine bridges and alter the conformation of the V_2 receptor.

a phenylalanine (the amino acids naturally occurring in the V_{1a} and the OT receptor subtypes) changed the agonist selectivity accordingly.[62] The slight change in conformation induced by these different residues might change the arrangement of helices thereby influencing the activation process.

Transmembrane Domains. Mouillac et al.[61] also proposed that residues highly conserved in V_{1a} and OT transmembrane domains (glutamine at residues 14 and 18 within the second transmembrane domain) formed the same agonist-binding site shared by all members of this receptor family. These conserved residues were mutated to alanine, which decreased the affinity of the receptor for agonists but not for antagonists. These results indicate a different binding mode for agonists and antagonists in the vasopressin receptor, a theme pertinent to the development of nonpeptide V_1 and V_2 receptor agonists and antagonists.[63]

The vasopressin receptor family is unique among all classes of peptide receptors because its individual members couple to different subsets of G-proteins.[64] Hybrid receptors with different intracellular domains exchanged between V_{1a} and V_2 receptors were expressed in COS-7 cells by Liu and Wess.[64] All mutant receptors containing V_{1a} receptor sequence in the second intracellular loop were able to stimulate the phosphatidyl inositol pathway. On the other hand, only those hybrid receptors containing V_2 receptor sequence in the third intracellular loop were capable of stimulating cAMP production. These studies could lead to three-dimensional models of the vasopressin receptor G-protein binding/activation interactions.

Vasopressin Control of Water Transport

In the presence of AVP, the entire collecting tubule system becomes permeable to water and the kidney is able to take advantage of the osmotic pressure gradient between the concentrated medullary interstitium and the dilute collecting tubule fluid. In the human kidney, the maximum achievable osmolality is around 1200 mOsm/kg (Fig. 163-1) and because the obligatory excretion of waste products, such as urea, sulfate, and phosphate, amounts to about 600 mOsm/day, at least 0.5 liters of water per day must be excreted by the kidney.

The regulation of AVP release from the posterior pituitary is dependent primarily on two mechanisms involving the osmotic and nonosmotic pathways.[65] The osmotic regulation of AVP is dependent on osmoreceptor cells. In magnocellular neurons, stretch-inactivating cationic channels transduce osmotically evoked changes in cell volume and results in functionally relevant changes in membrane potential; hypertonicity will trigger a membrane depolarization of these cells and AVP secretion.[66,67] Cell volume is decreased most readily by substances that are restricted to the extracellular fluid, such as hypertonic saline or hypertonic mannitol, which not only enhance osmotic water movement from the cells, but also very effectively stimulate AVP release. In contrast, hypertonic urea, which moves rapidly into the cells, neither readily alters cell volume nor effectively stimulates AVP release.[68] The osmoreceptor cells are very sensitive to changes in extracellular fluid osmolality. With fluid deprivation a 1 percent increase in extracellular fluid osmolality stimulates AVP release, whereas with water ingestion a 1 percent decrease in extracellular fluid osmolality suppresses AVP release.

AVP release can also be caused through a nonosmotic mechanism. Large decrements in blood volume or blood pressure (>10 percent) sensed by stretch and baroreceptors in the central venous and arterial system stimulate AVP release. A variety of hypothalamic neurotransmitters, including monoamines and neuropeptides, are involved in the control of AVP release.[69] Noradrenaline in the supraoptic nuclei, as well as in the paraventricular nuclei, has a primary excitatory effect on AVP release, most probably mediated through α_1-adrenergic receptors.[70] Angiotensin II is also a potent stimulant of AVP release.[71] Knockout mice with loss-of-function of angiotensinogen (a precursor peptide of angiotensin II) or of the angiotensin-receptor type 1A do not demonstrate obvious alterations in thirst or in water balance.[72–74] Mice that lack the gene encoding the angiotensin receptor type 2 have a mild impairment in drinking response to water deprivation.[75] β-Adrenergic receptors[69] and opioid receptors[76] may be involved in the inhibition of AVP release.

The osmotic stimulation of AVP release by dehydration or hypertonic saline infusion, or both, is regularly used to test the AVP secretory capacity of the posterior pituitary. This secretory capacity can be assessed directly by comparing the plasma AVP concentration measured sequentially during a dehydration procedure with the normal values and then correlating the plasma AVP with the urinary osmolality measurements obtained simultaneously (Fig. 163-12).[77]

The AVP release can also be assessed indirectly by measuring plasma and urine osmolalities at regular intervals during the dehydration test.[78] The maximum urinary osmolality obtained during dehydration is compared with the maximum urinary osmolality obtained after the administration of dDAVP.

CONGENITAL X-LINKED NDI

History

Forssman[79] provides an anecdotal account of the independent discovery by himself[80] and Waring et al.[81] of the recognition of NDI as a disease entity. Forssman[80] also established that NDI segregated as an X-linked recessive disease. In two large pedigrees, there were affected males in four to six consecutive generations. It is tempting to assume that the family described in 1892 by McIlraith,[82] and discussed by Reeves and Andreoli,[83] was a family with X-linked NDI. By 1967, only a few families were reported in the literature; no cases were identified among 875,000 living males in the Oxford Regional Hospital Board area, and the birth frequency was estimated to be less than 1 in 1 million male births.[84]

In 1988, the locus for X-linked NDI (MIM 304800) was mapped to the distal region of the long arm of the X chromosome (Xq28) by linkage analysis[85,86] and confirmed by additional studies.[87–89] In 1989, it was observed that the administration of dDAVP had no effect on plasma cAMP concentration in 14 males with X-linked NDI, whereas it increased in normal males.[90] Intermediate responses were observed in obligate female carriers of the disease, corresponding to about half of the normal receptor response. Based on these results, it was suggested that the defective gene in patients with X-linked NDI was likely to code for a defective V_2 receptor. Jans et al.[91] also identified the V_2 receptor as a candidate gene on the basis of examining V_2 receptor binding activity and induction of cAMP production in response to AVP in somatic cell hybrids.[91] In 1992, 100 years after the description by McIlraith,[82] the human V_2 receptor was cloned[47] and the first two mutations were identified.[92] To date, 155 putative disease-causing *AVPR2* mutations have been identified in the 239 families (Fig. 163-13).[93]

Clinical Characteristics of X-Linked NDI

The natural history of untreated X-linked NDI includes hypernatremia, hyperthermia, mental retardation, and repeated episodes of dehydration in early infancy.[80,81,94,95] Mental retardation, a consequence of repeated episodes of dehydration, was prevalent in the Crawford and Bode study,[95] in which only 9 of 82 patients (11 percent) had normal intelligence. Early recognition and treatment of X-linked NDI, with an abundant intake of water allows a normal lifespan with normal physical and mental development.[96] Familial occurrence among males and mental retardation in untreated patients are two characteristics suggestive of X-linked NDI. Skewed X-inactivation is the most likely explanation for clinical symptoms of NDI in female carriers[97,98] (see Chap. 61).

The early symptoms of NDI and its severity in infancy are clearly described by Crawford and Bode.[95] The first manifesta-

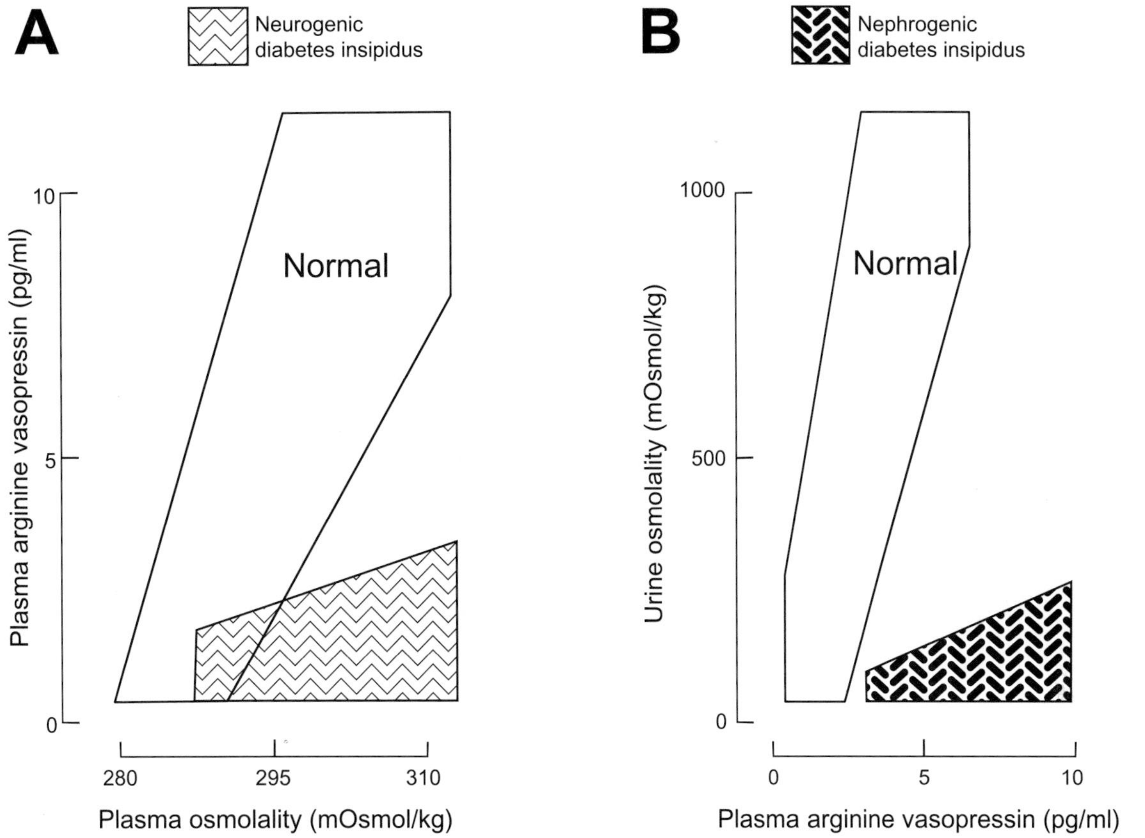

Fig. 163-12 *A*, **Diagram of the relationship between plasma AVP and plasma osmolality during hypertonic saline infusion. In patients with neurogenic diabetes insipidus, plasma AVP is almost always subnormal relative to plasma osmolality. In contrast, patients with primary polydipsia or NDI have values within the normal range (data not shown).** *B*, **Relationship between urine osmolality and plasma AVP during a dehydration test. Patients with NDI have hypotonic urine despite high plasma AVP. In contrast, patients with neurogenic diabetes insipidus or primary polydipsia have values within the normal range (data not shown). (*Modified from Zerbe and Robertson.*[187] *Used with permission.*)**

tions of the disease can be seen during the first week of life. The infants are irritable, cry almost constantly, and, although eager to suck, will vomit milk soon after ingestion unless prefed with water. The history given by the mothers often includes persistent constipation, erratic unexplained fever, and failure to gain weight. Even though the patients characteristically show no visible evidence of perspiration, increased water loss during fever, or warm weather, exacerbates the symptoms.

Unless the condition is recognized early, children will experience frequent bouts of hypertonic dehydration, sometimes complicated by convulsions or death. Mental retardation is a frequent consequence of these episodes. The intake of large quantities of water, combined with the patient's voluntary restriction of dietary salt and protein intake, leads to hypocaloric dwarfism, beginning in infancy. Children frequently develop lower urinary tract dilatation and obstruction, which are secondary to the large volume of urine produced.[99] Chronic renal insufficiency due to thrombosis of the glomerular tufts may occur by the end of the first decade of life, and could be the result of episodes of dehydration.[95]

Abnormal Renal and Extrarenal V_2 Receptor Responses in Males with X-linked NDI. In male patients with X-linked NDI, urinary osmolality does not change after administration of dDAVP, and maximum urinary osmolality remains less than 290 mOsm/kg. The plasma endogenous AVP concentrations also remain within the normal range and increase normally during dehydration or hypertonic saline infusion. These results indicate that the renal V_2 receptor responses are abnormal.[90,100]

Two extrarenal actions of dDAVP have been described: the release of two coagulation factors—factor VIIIc and von Willebrand factor—by stimulation with dDAVP;[101,102] and a decrease in blood pressure and peripheral resistance, and an increase in plasma renin activity, induced by dDAVP or [4-valine,8-D-arginine]vasopressin (VDAVP), another V_2 selective agonist.[103,104] These hemodynamic responses to VDAVP have been observed in anephric dogs,[105] and an increase in coagulation factors has been observed in anephric patients.[101] Thus, these hemodynamic and coagulation responses to dDAVP or VDAVP are probably mediated by extrarenal V_2 receptors.

Bichet et al.[90,100] found that blood pressure did not decrease, plasma renin activity did not increase, and coagulation factors (factor VIIIc, von Willebrand factor, and tissue plasminogen activator) were not released in response to the administration of dDAVP in 14 male patients with congenital NDI. Similar results were obtained by other investigators.[106,107] The lack of hemodynamic and coagulation factor responses to the administration of dDAVP in patients with congenital NDI indicate that extrarenal V_2 receptor responses are also abnormal.

In addition, dDAVP administration increased plasma cAMP concentrations in normal individuals but had no effect in congenital NDI patients.[90] Intermediate responses were observed in obligate female carriers, corresponding to half-normal receptor responses. These results suggested an altered pre-cAMP stimulation mechanism in patients with congenital NDI, a result now confirmed because X-linked NDI is secondary to mutations in the *AVPR2* gene that codes for the V_2 receptor.

Normal V_1 Receptor Responses in Males with X-linked NDI. The abnormal V_2 receptor responses are in contrast to the apparently normal V_1 receptor vascular or pressor responses to AVP in patients with X-linked NDI. In these patients, AVP,

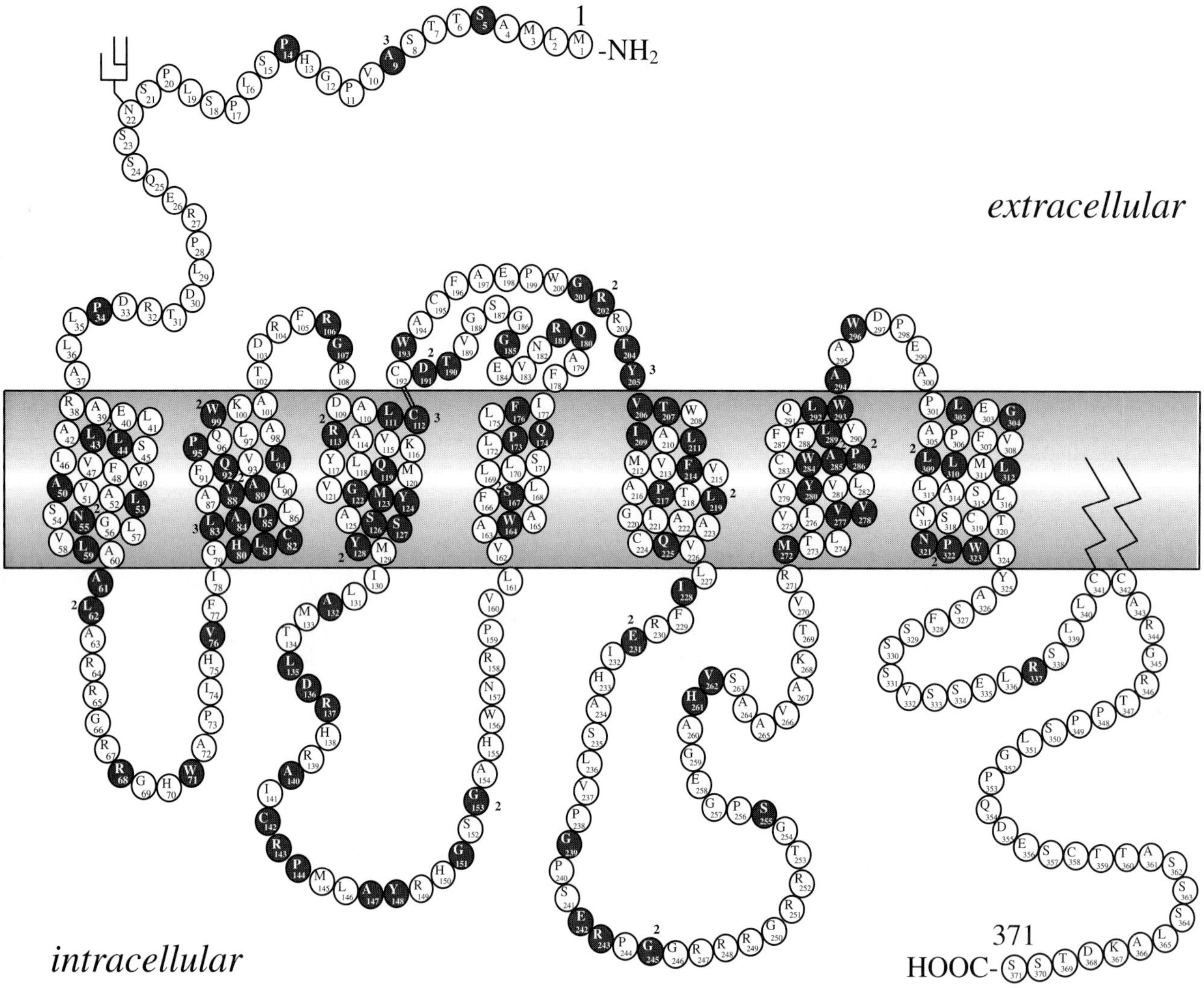

Fig. 163-13 Representation of the V_2 receptor and identification of 155 putative disease-causing *AVPR2* mutations. Predicted amino acids are given as the one-letter code. A solid symbol indicates the location (or the closest codon) of a mutation; a number indicates more than one mutation in the same codon. The names of the mutations were assigned according to recommended nomenclature.[188] The extracellular, transmembrane, and cytoplasmic domains are defined according to Mouillac et al.[61] The common names of the mutations are listed by type. *78 missense*: L43P, L44F, L44P, L53R, N55D, N55H, L59P, L62P, H80R, L81F, L83P, L83Q, A84D, D85N, V88L, V88M, Q92R, L94Q, P95L, W99R, R106C, G107E, C112R, R113W, G122R, M123K, S126F, S127F, Y128S, A132D, L135P, R137H, [C142W; R143G], R143P, A147V, W164S, S167L, S167T, Q174L, R181C, G185C, D191G, G201D, R202C, T204N, Y205C, V206D, T207N, I209F, F214S, P217T, L219P, L219R, M272K, V277A, Y280C, A285P, P286L, P286R, P286S, L289P, L292P, A294P, L309P, S315R(AGC > AGA), S315R(AGC > AGG), N317K, C319R, N321D, N321K, N321Y, P322H, P322S, W323R, W323S; *17 nonsense*: W71X, Q119X, Y124X, W164X, S167X, Q180X, W193X(TGG > TAG), W193X(TGG > TGA), Q225X, E231X, E242X, W284X, W293X, W296X, L312X, W323X, R337X; *42 frameshift*: in E_{I}—15delC, 27-54del, 46-47delCT, 54-55ins28, 102delG; in TMI—137-138delTA; in C_{I}—185-219del, 206-207insG, [225delC; 223C > A]; in TM_{II}—247-248ins7, 268-269delCT, 295delT; in TM_{III}—331-332delCT, 335-336delGT, 340delG, 407-446del; in C_{II}—418delG, 430-442del, 442-443insG, 452delG, 457-463del, 460delG; in E_{III}—567-568insC, 572-575del, 612-613insC, 614-615delAT; in TM_{V}—631delC; C_{III}—682-683insC, 692delA, 717delG, 727-728delAG, 738delG, 738-739insG, 763delA, 784delG, 785-786insT; in TM_{VI}—838-839insT, 847-851del, 851-852ins5; in TM_{VII}—907delG, 930delC, 969delG; *6 inframe deletions or insertions*: in C_{I}—185-193del; in TM_{II}—252-253ins9; in TM_{III}—Y128del; in TM_{IV}—F176del; in E_{III}—R202del; in TM_{VI}—V279del; *3 splice-site*: IVS2+1delG, IVS2+1G > A, IVS2-2A > G[60,92,97,98,111–114,116,120,121,130,172–177,189–204] (B. Chini, personal communication). 8 large deletions and 1 complex mutation are not shown.[97,114,173,198,201] See also http://www.medcon.mcgill.ca/nephros/.

through a V_1-mediated effect, induced skin blanching and abdominal cramps, and increased arterial blood pressure and prostaglandin E_2 excretion.[90] These patients also have normal platelet V_1 receptors because their platelet binding (to tritiated AVP) and functional (aggregation by AVP) characteristics are normal.[108,109]

AVPR2 Gene and Mutations

X-linked NDI (MIM 304800) is secondary to *AVPR2* mutations that result in loss-of-function or dysregulation of the V_2 receptor. The *AVPR2* gene has three exons and two small introns.[47,110] The cDNA sequence predicts a polypeptide with seven transmembrane, four extracellular, and four cytoplasmic domains that belong to the family of G-protein coupled receptors (Fig. 163-13).

To date, 155 putative disease-causing *AVPR2* mutations have been identified in 239 NDI families (Fig. 163-13).[93] Half of the mutations are missense mutations. Frameshift mutations due to nucleotide deletions or insertions (27 percent), nonsense mutations (11 percent), large deletions (5 percent), inframe deletions or insertions (4 percent), splice-site mutations (2 percent), and one complex mutation account for the remainder of the mutations. Mutations have been identified in every domain, but on a per nucleotide basis, about twice as many mutations occur in transmembrane domains compared to the extracellular or intra-

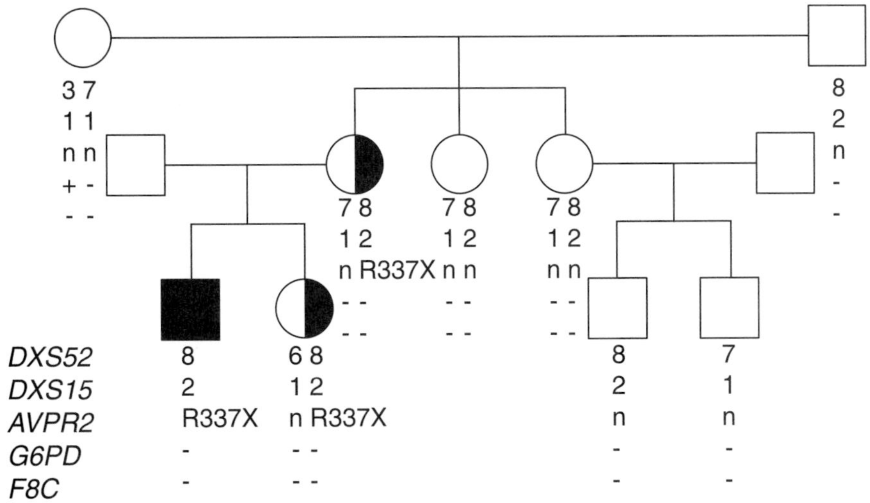

Fig. 163-14 Example of a *de novo* mutation inferred to have arisen during spermatogenesis in the maternal grandfather. Haplotypes consist of markers (*DXS52*, *DXS15*, *G6PD*, and *F8C*) that flank the *AVPR2* gene.[87,173]

cellular domains. Mechanisms of mutagenesis have been discussed[111–113] (see also Chap. 13). Additional information is available in the NDI Mutation Database at www.medcon.mcgill.ca/nephros/.

A family history of affected maternal uncles or great-uncles often provides the evidence for a presumptive diagnosis of X-linked NDI in an affected infant. A number of *de novo* mutations have been described (Fig. 163-14). In a worldwide collection of 117 NDI families with 82 different putative disease-causing mutations, the origin of a *de novo* mutation was deduced or inferred on the basis of mutation and haplotype analysis in 26 percent of the families.[114] About half of the *de novo* mutations were considered to have arisen during spermatogenesis in the maternal grandfather and 35 percent during oogenesis in the mother of an affected child. As a guide for investigating sporadic families, that is, a family that presents with one affected boy and no other family history of NDI, 76 percent of the mothers may be carriers whereas a *de novo* mutation may have arisen during oogenesis in the mother in 20 percent of these families. Thus, the absence of a family history of X-linked NDI does not rule out the disease, and DNA of a sporadic case (especially a newborn or young male infant) and the mother should be analyzed for *AVPR2* mutations. In general, low urinary osmolality unresponsive to dDAVP should be documented before performing DNA analysis (see Table 163-2).

Table 163-2 Differential Diagnosis of Diabetes Insipidus

1. Measure plasma osmolality and/or sodium concentration under conditions of *ad libitum* fluid intake. If plasma osmolality is >295 mOsm/kg and sodium is >143 mOsm/liter, the diagnosis of primary polydipsia is excluded and the workup should proceed to step (5) and/or (6) to distinguish between NDI and neurogenic diabetes insipidus. *Otherwise:*
2. Perform a dehydration test. If urinary concentration does not occur before plasma osmolality reaches 295 mOsm/kg and/or sodium reaches 143 mOsm/liter, the diagnosis of primary polydipsia is again excluded and the workup should proceed to step (5) and/or (6). *Otherwise:*
3. Determine the ratio of urine to plasma osmolality at the end of the dehydration test. If it is <1.5, the diagnosis of primary polydipsia is again excluded and the workup should proceed to step (5) and/or (6). *Otherwise:*
4. Perform a hypertonic saline infusion with measurement of plasma AVP and osmolality at intervals during the procedure. If the relationship between these two variables falls below the normal range, the diagnosis of neurogenic diabetes insipidus is established (Fig. 163-12***A***). *Otherwise:*
5. Perform a dDAVP infusion test. If urine osmolality increases by <150 mOsm/kg above the value obtained at the end of the dehydration test, the diagnosis of NDI is established. *Alternatively:*
6. Measure urine osmolality and plasma AVP at the end of the dehydration test. If the relationship falls below the normal range, the diagnosis of NDI is established (Fig. 163-12***B***).

Data from Robertson.[168]

Incidence and Population Genetics

A recent estimate of the incidence of X-linked NDI in the general population is about 1 in 152,000 male births.[114] This estimate was based on the ascertainment of 3 affected boys who were born in the province of Quebec, Canada during the 10-year period 1988 to 1997 among 455,000 male births. Thus, in general, X-linked NDI is a rare disorder. One exception is in Nova Scotia, where NDI was known to be a common disorder.[115] An estimate of the incidence of X-linked NDI in Nova Scotia and New Brunswick is 1 in 17,000 males.[114] Moreover, the prevalence in two small villages in Nova Scotia was estimated to be 24/1000 males.[87] These affected males are descendants of the pedigree studied by Bode and Crawford[115] and carry the nonsense mutation, W71X (Fig. 163-15).[111,116] This is the largest known pedigree with X-linked NDI and has been referred to as the Hopewell kindred, named after the Irish ship *Hopewell*, which arrived in Halifax, Nova Scotia, in 1761.[115] Affected males in four additional extended families from Nova Scotia and New Brunswick also carry the W71X mutation on the same haplotype as that of the affected males in the Hopewell kindred.[111] The W71X mutations in these different families are assumed to be identical by descent from a common ancestor. The four additional families have Scottish ancestry but are not known to be related to each other or to the Hopewell kindred within six to seven generations. Descendants of Scottish Presbyterians who migrated to the Ulster Province of Ireland in the 17th century, emigrated from Ireland in 1718 and settled in northern Massachusetts. A later group of immigrants were passengers on the ship *Hopewell* and settled in Colchester County, Nova Scotia. Members of the two groups were subsequently united in Colchester County.[115] Thus, it is likely that Ulster Scot immigrants, perhaps on more than one occasion, brought the W71X mutation to North America.

The diversity of *AVPR2* mutations found in many different ethnic groups, and the rareness of the disease, is consistent with an X-linked recessive disease that in the past was lethal for affected males. In general, each NDI family is likely to have an

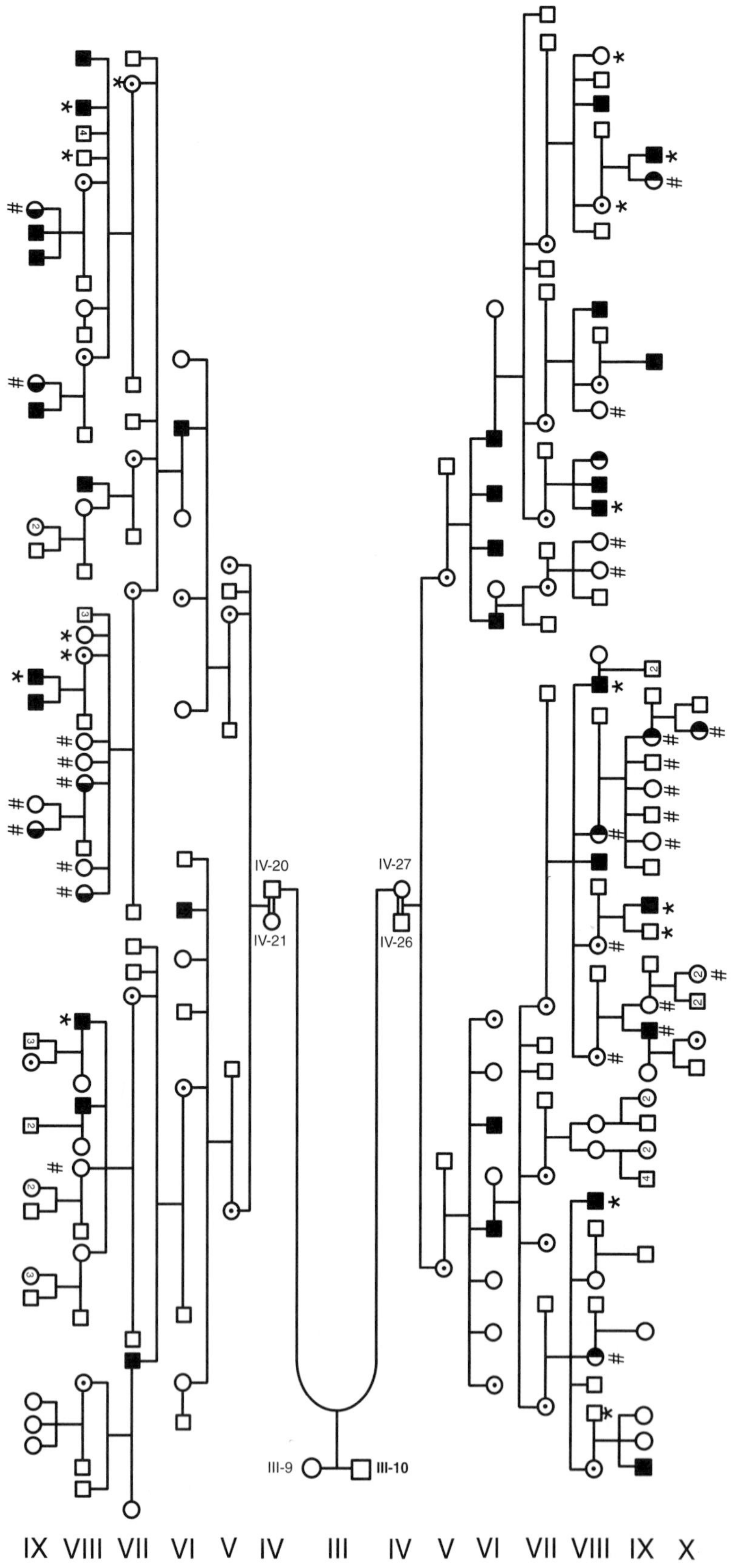

Fig. 163-15 Partial pedigree of the Hopewell kindred with the W71X mutation. Mutation analysis was done by DNA sequencing (★) or by restriction enzyme or allele specific oligonucleotide analysis (#). ■ = affected male; □ = unaffected male; ● = obligate carrier female; ◐ = carrier by DNA analysis; ○ = noncarrier or unknown; a number within a symbol indicates the number of male or female siblings. (*Modified from Bichet et al.*[111] *Used with permission.*)

independent mutation that occurred at random on existing genetic backgrounds of normal X chromosomes. Haplotype analysis confirms this expectation in that the same mutation in unrelated families was found on different haplotypes and the most frequent recurrent mutations occurred at potential mutational hotspots.[114] An exception, as mentioned above, is the W71X mutation, which is the oldest known *AVPR2* mutation and has segregated for at least seven generations (Fig. 163-15).[111]

Molecular Basis of X-Linked NDI

The basis of loss-of-function or dysregulation of 46 different mutant V_2 receptors (including nonsense, frameshift, deletion, or

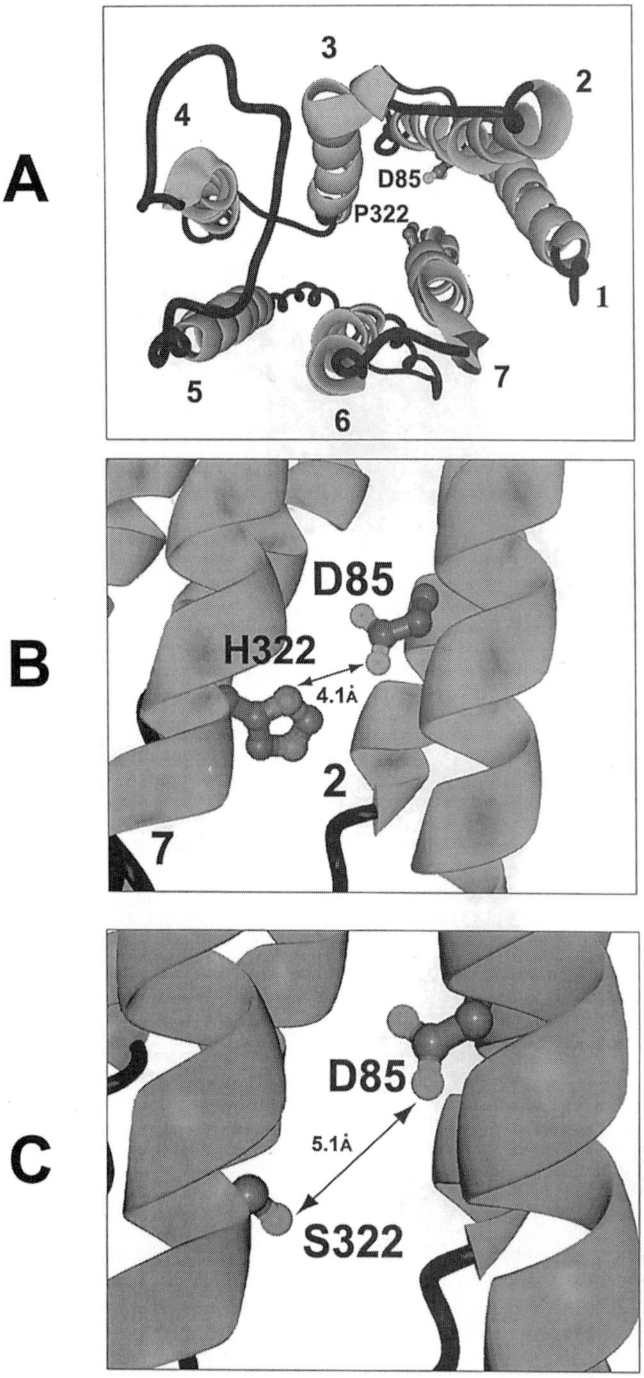

Fig. 163-16 *A*, View of the V_2 receptor from a direction perpendicular to the cell membrane surface.[60] The positioning of the transmembrane domains 1 to 7 is counterclockwise when viewed from the extracellular surface of the receptor. Amino acid residues D85 and P322 are labeled. *B* and *C* are close-up side views of the complex from a direction parallel to the cell-surface membrane. *B*, The mutant receptor with histidine at residue 322 (H322) is expressed at the cell membrane surface but is unable, in vitro, to stimulate cAMP after AVP stimulation. A hydrogen bond between H322 and D85 could result in a conformational constraint resulting in an inability of the mutant receptor to activate the G_s/adenylyl cyclase system. *C*, The mutant receptor with serine at residue 322 (S322) is also expressed normally at the cell-surface membrane but the serine side chain may be too far away to interact with D85 and would not form the same interaction, thus allowing the receptor to be partially activated.[60]

missense mutations) has been studied using in vitro expression systems. The classification of defects for the V_2 receptor is based on that of the LDL receptor.[117] Most of the mutant V_2 receptors tested were not transported to the cell membrane, and were thus retained within the intracellular compartment.[60] Schöneberg et al.[118,119] pharmacologically rescued truncated or missense V_2 receptors by coexpression of a polypeptide consisting of the last 130 amino acids of the V_2 receptor in COS-7 cells. Four of the six truncated receptors (E242X, 804delG, 834delA, and W284X), and the missense mutant Y280C, regained considerable functional activity, as demonstrated by an increase in the number of binding sites and stimulation of adenylyl cyclase activity. However, the absolute number of receptors expressed at the cell surface is low.

Only three *AVPR2* mutations (D85N, G201D, and P322S) have been associated with a mild or partial phenotype.[60,120,121] Males bearing these missense mutations were identified later in life, and the classical episodes of dehydration were less severe. This mild phenotype is consistent with expression studies (Fig. 163-16). The mutant proteins are expressed on the plasma membrane of cells transfected with these mutants, and demonstrate more stimulation of cAMP at higher concentrations of agonists compared with other *AVPR2* mutations.[60,120]

CONGENITAL AUTOSOMAL NDI

History

On the basis of phenotypic characteristics of both males and females affected with NDI and dDAVP infusion studies, a non-X-linked form of NDI with a postreceptor defect was suggested.[122–124] In contrast to males affected with X-linked NDI[90,100], two males and two females with NDI experienced a normal rise, for example, two- to threefold, in plasma concentrations of factor VIII and von Willebrand factor after dDAVP infusion, but urinary osmolality remained low.[125] X-linked NDI was excluded for two sisters with vasopressin-resistant hypotonicity because they inherited different alleles of an Xq28 marker from their mother; autosomal recessive inheritance was suggested on the basis of gender, parental consanguinity, and normal urine concentration in the parents.[123]

In 1993, the cloning of the cDNA that encodes a water channel in the rat and its exclusive expression in the collecting duct provided a strong candidate gene for non-X-linked NDI.[126] The cDNA and gene of the human homolog, designated aquaporin-2 (*AQP2*), was cloned and two missense mutations were found in a male NDI patient.[10,127,128] To date, patients in 13 of 19 families with autosomal recessive NDI were homozygous for an *AQP2* mutation[121,127,129–135] (D.G. Bichet, unpublished data). Consanguinity was known in 12 of these 13 families. This is consistent with a rare deleterious autosomal recessive disease. Thus, being homozygous for an *AQP2* mutation or being a compound heterozygote for two different *AQP2* mutations is the cause of autosomal recessive NDI (MIM 222000 and 107777).

In 1998, an affected mother and daughter were identified who were heterozygous for a missense mutation, E258K, in the intracellular C-terminus (Fig. 163-17).[136] This was the first example of autosomal dominant NDI (MIM 125800 and 107777) due to heterozygosity for an *AQP2* mutation. Five additional families have been identified that are consistent with autosomal dominant NDI due to an *AQP2* mutation[137] (D.G. Bichet, unpublished data).

AQP2 Gene and Mutations

The human *AQP2* gene is located in chromosome region 12q13, and has four exons and three introns.[127,128,138] It is predicted to code for a polypeptide of 271 amino acids that is organized into two repeats oriented at 180° to each other, and to have six transmembrane, three extracellular, and four cytoplasmic domains. AQP2 is a member of the major intrinsic protein (MIP) family of transmembrane channel proteins, and has the characteristic NPA

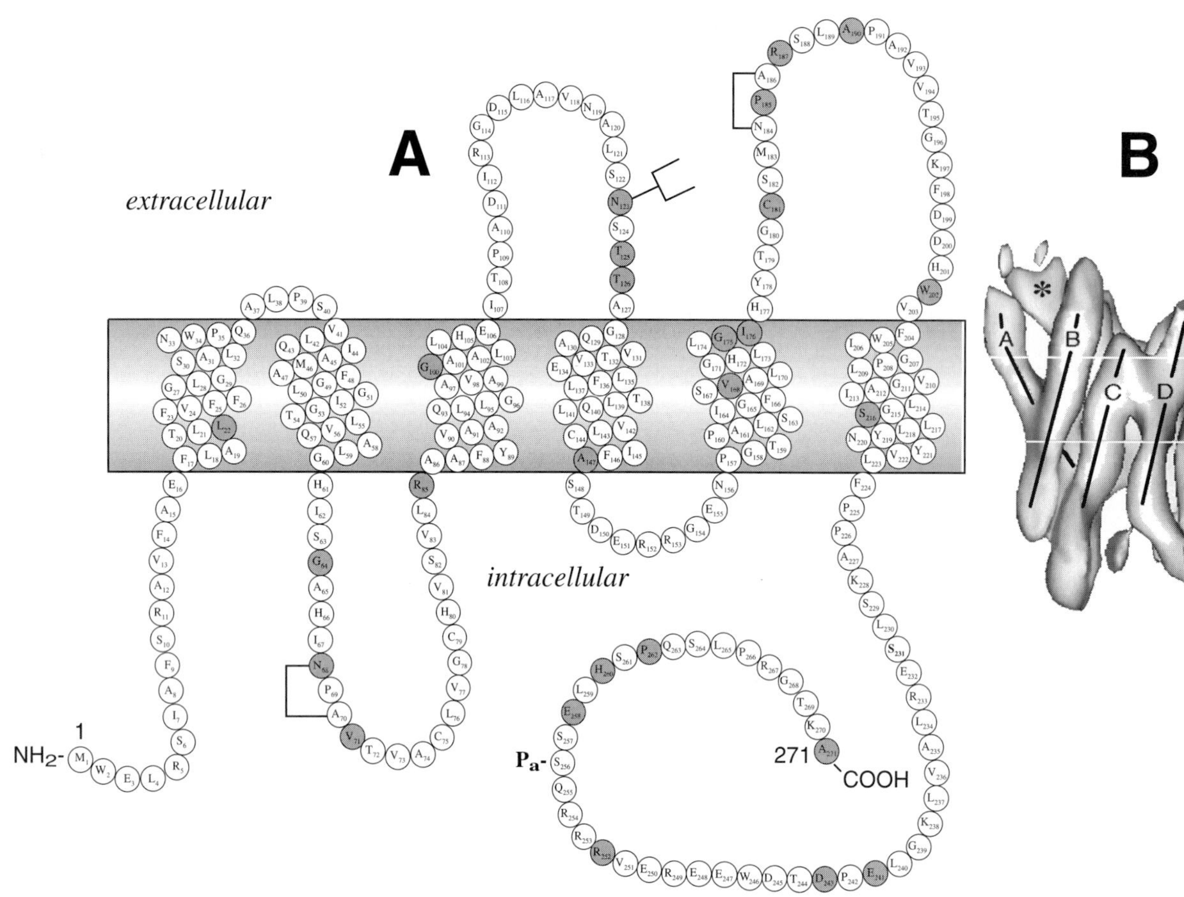

Fig. 163-17 *A*, **Representation of the aquaporin-2 (AQP2) protein and identification of 26 putative disease-causing *AQP2* mutations. A monomer is represented with six transmembrane helices. The location of the PKA phosphorylation site (P_a) is indicated. This site is possibly involved in the AVP induced trafficking of AQP2 from intracellular vesicles to the plasma membrane and in the subsequent stimulation of endocytosis.[21,22] The extracellular (E), transmembrane (TM), and cytoplasmic (C) domains are defined according to Deen et al.[127] As in Fig. 163-13, solid symbols indicate the location of the mutations. The common names of the mutations are listed by domain. TM_{I}: L22V; C_{II}: G64R, N68S, V71M, R85X; TM_{III}: G100X; E_{II}: 369delC, T125M, T126M; TM_{IV}: A147T; TM_{V}: V168M, G175R, IVS2-1G > A; E_{III}: C181W, P185A, R187C, A190T, W202C; TM_{VI}: S216P; C_{IV}: 721delG, 727delG, 756-765del, E258K, 779-780insA, P262L, 812-816del[121,127,129–136] (D.G. Bichet, unpublished data). See also http://www.medcon.mcgill.ca/nephros/.** ***B*, A surface-shaded representation of the six-helix barrel of the AQP1 protein viewed parallel to the bilayer; black lines indicate the approximate helix axes. (*Modified from Cheng et al.*[205] *Used with permission.*)**

motifs at residues 68 to 70 and 134 to 136 (Fig. 163-17).[128] Aquaporin-1 (AQP1), and by analogy, AQP2, are homotetramers containing four independent water channels. To date, 26 putative disease-causing *AQP2* mutations have been identified in 25 NDI families (Fig. 163-17). By type of mutation, there are 65 percent missense, 23 percent frameshift due to small nucleotide deletions or insertions, 8 percent nonsense, and 4 percent splice-site mutations. Additional information is available in the NDI Mutation Database at www.medcon.mcgill.ca/nephros/.

Molecular Basis of Autosomal Recessive and Dominant NDI

The oocytes of the African clawed frog *Xenopus* have provided a useful system for looking at the function of many channel proteins.[139] Oocytes are large cells, which are just about to become mature eggs ready for fertilization. They have all the normal translation machinery of living cells, and respond to the injection of mRNA by making the protein for which it codes. Functional expression studies showed that *Xenopus* oocytes injected with mutant cRNA had a reduced coefficient of water permeability, whereas *Xenopus* oocytes injected with both normal and mutant cRNA had a coefficient of water permeability similar to that of normal constructs alone. These findings provide conclusive evidence that NDI can be caused by homozygosity for mutations in the *AQP2* gene.

A patient with a partial phenotype was a compound heterozygote for the L22V and C181W mutations.[131] Immunolocalization of AQP2-transfected CHO cells showed that the C181W mutant had an endoplasmic reticulum-like intracellular distribution, whereas L22V and wild-type AQP2 showed endosome and plasma membrane staining. It was suggested that the L22V mutation was key to the patient's unique response to dDAVP. The leucine at position 22 might be necessary for proper conformation, or for binding of another protein that is important for normal targeting and trafficking of the molecule. Reminiscent of expression studies done with AVPR2 proteins, misrouting of AQP2 mutant proteins is the major cause underlying autosomal recessive NDI.[133,139,140] To determine whether the severe AQP2 trafficking defect observed with the naturally occurring mutations T126M, R187C, and A147T is correctable, CHO and Madin-Darby canine kidney cells, were incubated with the chemical chaperone glycerol for 48 h. Using immunofluorescence, redistribution of AQP2 from the endoplasmic reticulum to the plasma membrane-endosome fractions was observed. This redistribution was correlated with improved water permeability measurements.[139] It is important to correct this defective AQP2 trafficking in vivo.

In contrast to the *AQP2* mutations in autosomal recessive NDI, which are located throughout the gene, the dominant mutations are predicted to affect the C-terminus of AQP2[141] (D.G. Bichet, unpublished data). One dominant mutation, E258K, has been analyzed in detail in vitro; AQP2-E258K had reduced water permeability compared to wild-type AQP2.[136] In addition, AQP2-E258K was retained in the Golgi apparatus, which differs from mutant AQP2 in recessive NDI that is retained in the endoplasmic reticulum. The dominant action of *AQP2* mutations can be explained by the formation of heterotetramers of mutant and wild-type AQP2 that are impaired in their routing after oligomerization.[136]

OTHER FORMS OF INHERITED DIABETES INSIPIDUS

Neurogenic Diabetes Insipidus

Lacombe[142] and Weil[143] described a familial non-X-linked form of diabetes insipidus without any associated mental retardation. The descendants of the family described by Weil were later found to have autosomal dominant neurogenic diabetes insipidus.[144–146] Neurogenic diabetes insipidus (MIM 125700) is a well-characterized entity, secondary to mutations in the *prepro-AVP-NPII* (MIM 192340). This disorder is also referred to as central, cranial, pituitary or neurohypophyseal diabetes insipidus. Patients with autosomal dominant neurogenic diabetes insipidus retain some limited capacity to secrete AVP during severe dehydration, and the polyuria-polydipsic symptoms usually appear after the first year of life,[147] when the infant's demand for water is more likely to be understood by adults. Two families with autosomal recessive neurogenic diabetes insipidus have been identified in which the patients were homozygous or compound heterozygotes for *prepro-AVP-NPII* mutations.[148] These families are characterized phenotypically by severe and early onset in the first 3 months of life, polyuria, polydipsia, and dehydration. Consequently, early hereditary diabetes insipidus can be neurogenic or nephrogenic.

Wolfram Syndrome

Diabetes insipidus is also a component of Wolfram syndrome (MIM 222300), an autosomal recessive disorder characterized by juvenile diabetes mellitus, diabetes insipidus, optic atrophy, and a number of neurologic symptoms including deafness, ataxia, and peripheral neuropathy. Wolfram syndrome is also referred to as DIDMOAD (diabetes insipidus, diabetes mellitus, optic atrophy, and deafness). This disease is secondary to mutation in the *WFS1* gene (chromosome region 4p16), which codes for a transmembrane protein expressed in various tissues including brain and pancreas.[149,150]

ACQUIRED NDI

Acquired NDI is much more common than congenital NDI but it is rarely as severe. The ability to produce hypertonic urine is usually preserved in spite of inadequate concentrating ability of the nephron. Polyuria and polydipsia are therefore moderate (3 to 4 liters/day).

The more common causes of acquired NDI are listed in Table 163-1. Lithium administration is the most frequent cause; 54 percent of 1105 unselected patients on chronic lithium therapy developed NDI.[151] Nineteen percent of these patients had polyuria, as defined by a 24-h urine output exceeding 3 liters. The mechanism whereby lithium causes polyuria has been extensively studied. Lithium inhibits adenylyl cyclase in a number of cell types including renal epithelia.[152,153] The concentration of lithium in urine of patients on well-controlled lithium therapy (i.e., 10 to 40 mOsm/liter) is sufficient to exert this effect. Measurement of adenylyl cyclase activity in membranes isolated from a cultured pig kidney cell line ($LLC\text{-}PK_1$) revealed that lithium in the concentration range of 10 mOsm/liter interfered with the hormone-stimulated guanyl nucleotide regulatory unit (G_s).[154] The effect of chronic lithium therapy has been studied in rat kidney membranes prepared from the inner medulla. It caused a marked down-regulation of AQP2, only partially reversed by cessation of therapy, dehydration or dDAVP treatment, consistent with clinical observations of slow recovery from lithium-induced urinary concentrating defects.[155] Down-regulation of AQP2 has also been shown to be associated with the development of severe polyuria due to other causes of acquired NDI (hypokalemia,[156] release of bilateral ureteral obstruction,[157] and hypercalciuria[158]). Thus, AQP2 expression is severely down-regulated in both congenital[159] and acquired NDI. More studies are needed to determine whether nonpeptide vasopressin agonists, permeable cAMP-like compounds, or other signaling molecules will be able to restore AQP2 expression and function. For patients on long-term lithium therapy, amiloride has been proposed to prevent the uptake of lithium in the collecting ducts, thus preventing the inhibitory effect of intracellular lithium on water transport.[160]

INVESTIGATION OF A PATIENT WITH POLYURIA

Plasma sodium and osmolality are maintained within normal limits (136 to 143 mOsm/liter for plasma sodium; 275 to 290 mOsm/kg for plasma osmolality) by a thirst-AVP-renal axis. Thirst and AVP release, both stimulated by increased osmolality, is a double-negative feedback system.[161] Even when the AVP component of this double-negative regulatory feedback system is lost, the thirst mechanism still preserves the plasma sodium and osmolality within the normal range, but at the expense of pronounced polydipsia and polyuria. Thus, the plasma sodium concentration or osmolality of an untreated patient with diabetes insipidus may be slightly greater than the mean normal value, but these small increases have no diagnostic significance.

Theoretically, it should be relatively easy to differentiate between neurogenic diabetes insipidus, NDI and primary polydipsia by comparing the osmolality of urine obtained during dehydration with that of urine obtained after the administration of dAVP. Patients with neurogenic diabetes insipidus should reveal a rapid increase in urinary osmolality whereas it should increase normally in response to moderate dehydration in patients with primary polydipsia.

These distinctions, however, may not be as clear as one might expect, owing to several factors.[162] First, chronic polyuria due to any cause interferes with the maintenance of the medullary concentration gradient and this "washout" effect diminishes the maximum concentrating ability of the nephron. The extent of the blunting varies in direct proportion to the severity of the polyuria. Hence, for any given basal urine output, the maximum urine osmolality achieved in the presence of saturating concentrations of AVP is depressed to the same extent in patients with primary polydipsia, neurogenic diabetes insipidus or NDI (Fig. 163-18). Second, most patients with neurogenic diabetes insipidus maintain a small, but detectable, capacity to secrete AVP during severe dehydration and urinary osmolality may then increase to greater than the plasma osmolality. Third, patients referred to as partial diabetes insipidus (either neurogenic or nephrogenic) and patients with acquired NDI have an incomplete response to AVP and are able to concentrate their urine to varying degrees in a dehydration test. Finally, all polyuric states (whether neurogenic, nephrogenic or psychogenic) can induce large dilatations of the urinary tract and bladder.[163,164] As a consequence, the urinary bladder of these patients has an increased residual capacity and changes in urinary osmolality induced by diagnostic maneuvers might be difficult to demonstrate.

Indirect Tests for Diabetes Insipidus

The measurement of urinary osmolality after dehydration and dDAVP administration is usually referred to as indirect testing because AVP secretion is indirectly assessed through changes in urinary osmolalities.[78] The patient is maintained on a complete fluid-restriction regimen until urinary osmolality reaches a plateau, as indicated by an hourly increase of less than 30 mOsm/kg for at least three successive hours. After measuring the plasma

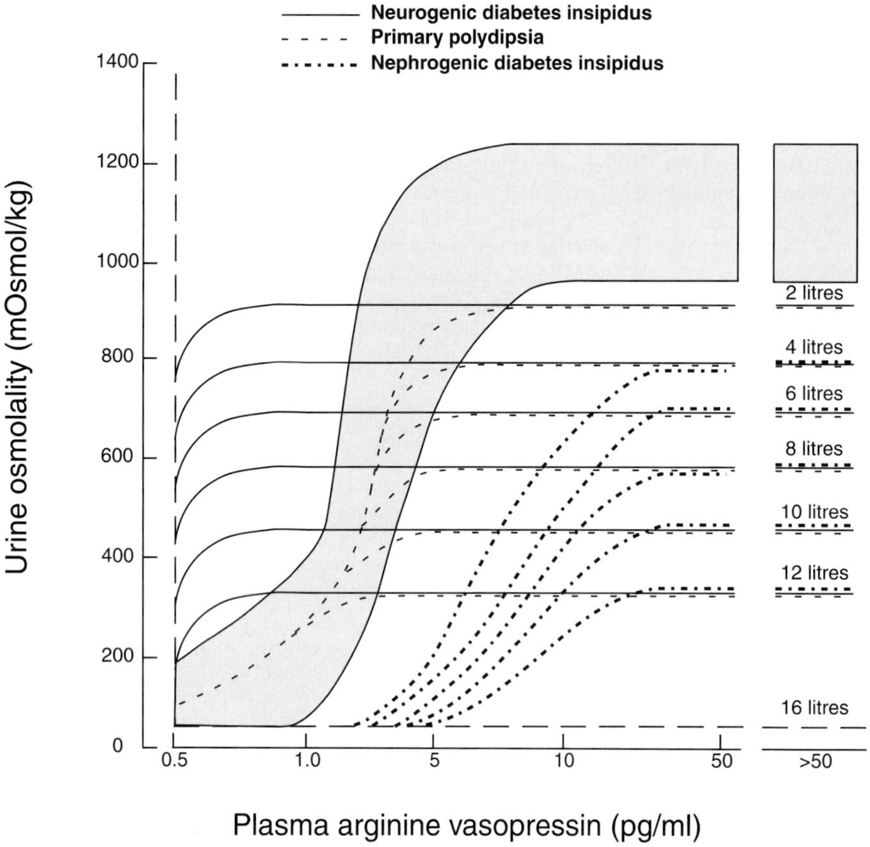

Fig. 163-18 Diagram of the relationship between urine osmolality and plasma AVP in patients with polyuria of diverse cause and severity. The shaded area represents the normal range. For each of the three categories of polyuria, a family of sigmoid curves that differ in height describes the relationship. These differences in height reflect differences in maximum concentrating capacity due to "washout" of the medullary concentration gradient. They are proportional to the severity of the underlying polyuria (indicated in liter/day at the right-hand side of each plateau) and are largely independent of the cause. The three categories of diabetes insipidus differ principally in the submaximal or ascending portion of the dose-response curve. In patients with neurogenic diabetes insipidus, this part of the curve lies to the left of normal, reflecting increased sensitivity to the antidiuretic effects of very-low concentrations of plasma AVP. In contrast, in patients with NDI, this part of the curve lies to the right of normal, reflecting decreased sensitivity to the antidiuretic effects of normal concentrations of plasma AVP. In primary polydipsia, this relationship is relatively normal. (*Modified from Robertson.*[162] *Used with permission.*)

osmolality, 2 μg dDAVP are administered subcutaneously. Urinary osmolality is measured 30 and 60 min later. The last urinary osmolality value obtained before the dDAVP injection and the highest value obtained after the injection are compared. In patients with severe neurogenic diabetes insipidus, urinary osmolality after dehydration is usually low (<200 mOsm/kg) and increases more than 50 percent after dDAVP administration. In patients with severe NDI, urinary osmolality after dehydration is also low (<200 mOsm/kg) but does not increase after dDAVP administration (<20 percent). Urinary osmolality increases to variable degrees (10 to 50 percent) after dDAVP administration to patients with partial neurogenic or partial nephrogenic diabetes insipidus. In patients with primary polydipsia, maximum urinary osmolality is obtained after dehydration (>295 mOsm/kg), and does not increase after dDAVP administration (<10 percent).

Alternatively, plasma sodium and plasma and urinary osmolalities can be measured at the beginning of the dehydration procedure and at regular intervals (usually hourly) thereafter depending on the severity of the polyuria.[165] For example, an 8-year-old patient (body weight 31 kg) with a clinical diagnosis of congenital NDI (later found to bear an *AVPR2* mutation) continued to excrete large volumes of urine (300 ml/h) during a short 4-h dehydration test. During this time, the patient suffered from severe thirst, his plasma sodium was 155 mOsm/l, plasma osmolality was 310 mOsm/kg, and urinary osmolality was 85 mOsm/kg. The patient received 1 μg of dDAVP intravenously and was allowed to drink water. Repeated urinary osmolality measurements demonstrated a complete urinary resistance to dDAVP. It would have been dangerous and unnecessary to prolong the dehydration further in this young patient. Thus, the usual prescription of overnight dehydration should not be used in patients, and especially children, with severe polyuria and polydipsia (more than 30 ml/kg body weight per day). Great care should be taken to avoid any severe hypertonic state, arbitrarily defined as plasma sodium greater than 155 mOsm/l.

Direct Tests of Diabetes Insipidus

The two approaches of Zerbe and Robertson are used[77] although they are expensive, time-consuming, and difficult to do on young patients. First approach: During the dehydration test, plasma is collected hourly and assayed for AVP. The results are plotted on a nomogram depicting the normal relationship between plasma sodium or osmolality and plasma AVP in normal individuals (Fig. 163-12*A*). If the relationship falls below the normal range, the disorder is diagnosed as neurogenic diabetes insipidus.

Second approach: NDI can be differentiated from primary polydipsia by analyzing the relationship between plasma AVP and urinary osmolality at the end of the dehydration period (Fig. 163-12*B*). However, definitive differentiation might be impossible because a normal or even supranormal AVP response to increased plasma osmolality occurs in polydipsic patients. None of the patients with psychogenic or other forms of severe polydipsia studied by Robertson showed any evidence of pituitary suppression.[162]

In a comparison of diagnoses based on indirect versus direct tests of AVP function in 54 patients with polyuria of diverse cause, Robertson[162] found that the indirect test was reliable only for patients with severe defects. Three severe NDI patients and 16 of 17 patients with severe neurogenic diabetes insipidus were accurately diagnosed. However, the error rate of the indirect test was about 50 percent in diagnosing patients, who were able to concentrate their urine to varying degrees when water deprived, as partial neurogenic diabetes insipidus, partial NDI or primary polydipsia. Stern and Valtin discussed the benefits of combined direct and indirect testing of AVP function.[166] The diagnosis of primary polydipsia remains one of exclusion and the cause could be psychogenic[167] or inappropriate thirst.[168,169] Psychiatric patients with polydipsia and hyponatremia have unexplained defects in urinary dilution, the osmoregulation of water intake, or the secretion of vasopressin.[170]

Therapeutic Trial of dDAVP

In selected patients with an uncertain diagnosis, a closely monitored therapeutic trial of dDAVP (10 μg intranasally twice a day for 2 to 3 days) may be used to distinguish partial NDI from partial neurogenic diabetes insipidus or primary polydipsia. If dDAVP at this dosage causes a significant antidiuretic effect, NDI is effectively excluded. If polydipsia as well as polyuria is abolished and plasma sodium does not fall below the normal range, the patient probably has neurogenic diabetes insipidus. Conversely, if dDAVP causes a reduction in urine output without reduction in water intake and hyponatremia appears, the patient probably has primary polydipsia. Because fatal water intoxication is a remote possibility, the dDAVP trial should be closely monitored.

The methods of differential diagnosis of diabetes insipidus are described in Table 163-2.

MOLECULAR DIAGNOSIS OF CONGENITAL NDI

Over the past few years it has become clear that congenital NDI is caused by an inactivating mutation(s) in the genes that code for the V_2 receptor or the AQP2 water channel. The time of onset of the disease (shortly after birth) and the clinical symptoms are similar regardless of the molecular defect. The defective gene can be deduced by clinical testing: dDAVP elicits extrarenal (coagulation and vasodilatory) responses in patients with NDI due to *AQP2* mutations, whereas patients with *AVPR2* mutations lack extrarenal responses.[100,122,127] Because this test is difficult to do in young infants, it has been replaced by *AVPR2* and *AQP2* mutation analysis.

Identification of the molecular defect underlying congenital NDI is of immediate clinical significance because early diagnosis and treatment of affected infants can avert the physical and mental retardation associated with repeated episodes of dehydration. Diagnosis of X-linked NDI was accomplished by mutation testing of chorionic villus samples, cultured amniotic cells, or cord blood.[171] These infants were immediately treated with abundant water intake, a low-sodium diet, and hydrochlorothiazide. They have not experienced episodes of dehydration and their physical and mental development remains normal.

DNA analysis should be performed on newborns with a family history of NDI and on patients of any age with a firm diagnosis of congenital NDI, with or without a family history. It may also be considered in babies presenting with continuing fever of unknown origin, vomiting, constantly low urine osmolality, and failure to thrive. DNA analysis is also important for the identification of female carriers in families with X-linked NDI. Most females who are heterozygous for a mutation in the V_2 receptor do not present with clinical symptoms; few are severely affected.[97,98,114] Benign variants in *AVPR2* or *AQP2*[114,121,172–176] (D.G. Bichet, unpublished data) and/or flanking markers[87,177] might be useful to determine the segregation of mutant alleles in a family prior to mutation analysis.

TREATMENT OF CONGENITAL NDI

Knoers and Monnens reviewed the treatment of congenital NDI.[178] An abundant, unrestricted water intake should always be provided and affected patients should be carefully followed during their first few years of life.[96,179] Water should be offered every 2 h day and night, and temperature, appetite, and growth should be monitored.[180] The parents of these children accept the setting of their alarm clock every 2 h during the night! Admission to hospital may be necessary for continuous gastric feeding. A low osmolar and sodium diet, hydrochlorothiazide (1 to 2 mg/kg/day) and indomethacin (1.5 to 3 mg/kg) substantially reduce water excretion[107,181–184] and are helpful in the treatment of children. The advantageous effect of these drugs has to be weighed against the side effects (thiazides: electrolyte disturbances; indomethacin: reduction of the glomerular filtration rate and gastrointestinal symptoms). Many adult patients receive no treatment. In our experience, prior knowledge of the *AVPR2* mutation in NDI families and perinatal mutation testing has been of direct clinical value for early treatment and prevention of dehydration episodes.[173]

Future Therapeutic Developments

With the identification of the genes responsible for congenital NDI, treatment based on somatic cell gene transfer is possible. Two prerequisites crucial for somatic gene therapy seem to be fulfilled. First, the defect in the kidney appears to be restricted to water reabsorption with no other functional or histologic defects. Unlike neurogenic diabetes insipidus,[147] retinitis pigmentosa and many other diseases, deterioration of kidney function due to progressive structural changes is not observed. Thus, the integrity of the organ seems to be preserved. Second, recent experiments with rats show that adenoviral-mediated gene transfer to the tubular system of the kidney can be achieved either by selective perfusion of the renal artery or by retrograde infusion through a catheter placed into the pelvic cavity.[185] Depending on the route, expression of the reporter gene (β-galactosidase) is observed in proximal tubule cells (kidney perfusion via renal artery) or tubular cells of the papilla and medulla (retrograde infusion).

The mutations in the *AVPR2* gene associated with X-linked NDI were the first naturally occurring mutations found in the very large group of G-protein coupled receptors. Within the last few years however, a number of diseases were shown to be due to mutations in genes encoding other G-protein coupled receptors. In addition to retinitis pigmentosa and X-linked NDI, examples of such diseases or traits are stationary night blindness; color blindness/altered color perception; primary adrenocortical deficiency; hypocalciuric hypercalcemia/hyperparathyroidism; hypercalcemia/metaphyseal chondrodysplasia; hypocalcemia; male precocious puberty; male pseudohermaphroditism; hyperfunctioning thyroid adenoma; and Hirschsprung disease (reviewed in reference 186). The main defect of many inactivating mutations is the reduced expression of mutant receptors on the cell surface. Here the loss of receptor function occurs regardless of the remaining biological activity of the individual protein. At present, very little is known about the cellular routing of G-protein coupled receptors. Progress in this field is crucial for the understanding of the clinical phenotypes of receptor diseases on a molecular level and for the development of therapeutic strategies based on gene transfer to somatic cells.

ACKNOWLEDGMENTS

The authors' work cited in this chapter was supported by the Medical Research Council of Canada, the Canadian Kidney Foundation, and the Fonds de la Recherche en Santé du Québec, and by funds to Kenneth Morgan from the Canadian Genetic Diseases Network (Federal Networks of Centres of Excellence Program). We thank our coworkers, Marie-Françoise Arthus, Danielle Binette, Joyce Crumley, Michèle Lonergan, and Kenneth Morgan, and many colleagues who contributed families and ideas to our work.

REFERENCES

1. Valtin H, Schafer JA: Concentration and dilution of urine: H_2O balance, in Valtin H, Schafer JA, (eds): *Renal Function*, 3rd ed. Boston, MA, Little, Brown, 1995, p 151.
2. Magner PO, Halperin ML: Polyuria-a pathophysiological approach. *Med North Am* **15**:2987, 1987.
3. Jamison RL, Oliver RE: Disorders of urinary concentration and dilution. *Am J Med* **72**:308, 1982.

4. Valtin H: Sequestration of urea and nonurea solutes in renal tissues of rats with hereditary hypothalamic diabetes insipidus: Effect of vasopressin and dehydration on the countercurrent mechanism. *J Clin Invest* **45**:337, 1966.
5. Agre P, Preston GM, Smith BL, Jung JS, Raina S, Moon C, Guggino WB, et al: Aquaporin CHIP: The archetypal molecular water channel. *Am J Physiol* **34**:F463, 1993.
6. Lee MD, King LS, Agre P: The aquaporin family of water channel proteins in clinical medicine. *Medicine* **76**:141, 1997.
7. Nielsen S, Smith BL, Christensen EI, Knepper MA, Agre P: CHIP28 water channels are localized in constitutively water-permeable segments of the nephron. *J Cell Biol* **120**:371, 1993.
8. Tsukaguchi H, Shayakul C, Berger UV, Hediger MA: Urea transporters in kidney: Molecular analysis and contribution to the urinary concentrating process. *Am J Physiol* **275**:F319, 1998.
9. Reeves WB, Bichet DG, Andreoli TE: Posterior pituitary and water meatbolism, in Wilson JD, Foster DW, Kronenberg H, Larsen PR (eds): *Williams Textbook of Endocrinology*, 9th ed. Philadelphia, WB Saunders, 1998, p 341.
10. Uchida S, Sasaki S, Furukawa T, Hiraoka M, Imai T, Hirata Y, Marumo F: Molecular cloning of a chloride channel that is regulated by dehydration and expressed predominantly in kidney medulla [published erratum appears in *J Biol Chem* 1994 **269(29)**:19192]. *J Biol Chem* **268**:3821, 1993.
11. Uchida S, Sasaki S, Nitta K, Uchida K, Horita S, Nihei H, Marumo F: Localization and functional characterization of rat kidney-specific chloride channel, ClC-K1. *J Clin Invest* **95**:104, 1995.
12. Kere J: Kidney kinetics and chloride ion pumps [News]. *Nat Genet* **21**:67, 1999.
13. Matsumura Y, Uchida S, Kondo Y, Miyazaki H, Ko SB, Hayama A, Morimoto T, et al: Overt nephrogenic diabetes insipidus in mice lacking the CLC-K1 chloride channel. *Nat Genet* **21**:95, 1999.
14. Hebert SC: Roles of Na-K-2Cl and Na-Cl cotransporters and ROMK potassium channels in urinary concentrating mechanism. *Am J Physiol* **275**:F325, 1998.
15. Simon DB, Karet FE, Hamdan JM, DiPietro A, Sanjad SA, Lifton RP: Bartter's syndrome, hypokalaemic alkalosis with hypercalciuria, is caused by mutations in the Na-K-2Cl cotransporter NKCC2. *Nat Genet* **13**:183, 1996.
16. Simon DB, Karet FE, Rodriguez-Soriano J, Hamdan JH, DiPietro A, Trachtman H, Sanjad SA, et al: Genetic heterogeneity of Bartter's syndrome revealed by mutations in the K^+ channel, ROMK. *Nat Genet* **14**:152, 1996.
17. Karolyil L, Konrad M, Kockerling A, Ziegler A, Zimmerman DK, Roth B, Wieg C, et al: Mutations in the gene encoding the inwardly-rectifying renal potassium channel, ROMK, cause the antenatal variant of Bartter syndrome: Evidence for genetic heterogeneity. International Collaborative Study Group for Bartter-like Syndromes [published erratum in *Hum Mol Genet* **6(4)**:650, 1997]. *Hum Mol Genet* **6**:17, 1997.
18. Simon DB, Bindra RS, Mansfield TA, Nelson-Williams C, Mendonca E, Stone R, Schurman S, et al: Mutations in the chloride channel gene, CLCNKB, cause Bartter's syndrome type III. *Nat Genet* **17**:171, 1997.
19. Wade JB, Stetson DL, Lewis SA: ADH action: Evidence for a membrane shuttle mechanism. *Ann N Y Acad Sci* **372**:106, 1981.
20. Knepper MA: Molecular physiology of urinary concentrating mechanism: Regulation of aquaporin water channels by vasopressin. *Am J Physiol* **272**:F3, 1997.
21. Fushimi K, Sasaki S, Marumo F: Phosphorylation of serine 256 is required for cAMP-dependent regulatory exocytosis of the aquaporin-2 water channel. *J Biol Chem* **272**:14800, 1997.
22. Katsura T, Gustafson C, Ausiello D, Brown D: Protein kinase A phosphorylation is involved in regulated exocytosis of aquaporin-2 in transfected LLC-PK1 cells. *Am J Physiol* **272**:F817, 1997.
23. Valenti G, Procino G, Liebenhoff U, Frigeri A, Benedetti PA, Ahnert-Hilger G, Nurnberg B, et al: A heterotrimeric G protein of the Gi family is required for cAMP-triggered trafficking of aquaporin 2 in kidney epithelial cells. *J Biol Chem* **273**:22627, 1998.
24. Mandon B, Nielsen S, Kishore BK, Knepper MA: Expression of syntaxins in rat kidney. *Am J Physiol* **273**:F718, 1997.
25. Jo I, Harris HW, Amendt-Raduege AM, Majewski RR, Hammond TG: Rat kidney papilla contains abundant synaptobrevin protein that participates in the fusion of antidiuretic hormone-regulated water channel-containing endosomes in vitro. *Proc Natl Acad Sci U S A* **92**:1876, 1995.
26. Liebenhoff U, Rosenthal W: Identification of Rab3-, Rab5a- and synaptobrevin II-like proteins in a preparation of rat kidney vesicles containing the vasopressin-regulated water channel. *FEBS Lett* **365**:209, 1995.
27. Nielsen S, Marples D, Birn H, Mohtashami M, Dalby NO, Trimble M, Knepper M: Expression of VAMP-2-like protein in kidney collecting duct intracellular vesicles. Colocalization with Aquaporin-2 water channels. *J Clin Invest* **96**:1834, 1995.
28. Star RA, Nonoguchi H, Balaban R, Knepper MA: Calcium and cyclic adenosine monophosphate as second messengers for vasopressin in the rat inner medullary collecting duct. *J Clin Invest* **81**:1879, 1988.
29. Snyder HM, Noland TD, Breyer MD: cAMP-dependent protein kinase mediates hydroosmotic effect of vasopressin in collecting duct. *Am J Physiol* **263**:C147, 1992.
30. Brown D, Katsura T, Gustafson CE: Cellular mechanisms of aquaporin trafficking. *Am J Physiol* **275**:F328, 1998.
31. Taylor A, Mamelak M, Reaven E, Maffly R: Vasopressin: Possible role of microtubules and microfilaments in its action. *Science* **181**:347, 1973.
32. Sabolic I, Katsura T, Verbabatz JM, Brown D: The AQP2 water channel: Effect of vasopressin treatment, microtubule disruption, and distribution in neonatal rats. *J Membr Biol* **143**:165, 1995.
33. Shayakul C, Steel A, Hediger MA: Molecular cloning and characterization of the vasopressin-regulated urea transporter of rat kidney collecting ducts. *J Clin Invest* **98**:2580, 1996.
34. Ma T, Yang B, Gillespie A, Carlson EJ, Epstein CJ, Verkman AS: Generation and phenotype of a transgenic knockout mouse lacking the mercurial-insensitive water channel aquaporin-4. *J Clin Invest* **100**:957, 1997.
35. Ma T, Yang B, Gillespie A, Carlson EJ, Epstein CJ, Verkman AS: Severely impaired urinary concentrating ability in transgenic mice lacking aquaporin-1 water channels. *J Biol Chem* **273**:4296, 1998.
36. Chou C-L, Knepper MA, van Hoek AN, Brown D, Yang B, Ma T, Verkman AS: Reduced water permeability and altered ultrastructure in thin descending limb of Henle in aquaporin-1 null mice. *J Clin Invest* **103**:491, 1999.
37. Schnermann J, Chou CL, Ma T, Traynor T, Knepper MA, Verkman AS: Defective proximal tubular fluid reabsorption in transgenic aquaporin-1 null mice. *Proc Natl Acad Sci U S A* **95**:9660, 1998.
38. Verbavatz JM, Brown D, Sabolic I, Valenti G, Ausiello DA, Van Hoek AN, Ma T, et al: Tetrameric assembly of CHIP28 water channels in liposomes and cell membranes: A freeze-fracture study. *J Cell Biol* **123**:605, 1993.
39. Chou CL, Ma T, Yang B, Knepper MA, Verkman AS: Fourfold reduction of water permeability in inner medullary collecting duct of aquaporin-4 knockout mice. *Am J Physiol* **274**:C549, 1998.
40. Preston GM, Smith BL, Zeidel ML, Moulds JJ, Agre P: Mutations in aquaporin-1 in phenotypically normal humans without functional CHIP water channels. *Science* **265**:1585, 1994.
41. Zelinski T, Kaita H, Gilson T, Coghlan G, Philipps S, Lewis M: Linkage between the Colton blood group locus and ASSP11 on chromosome 7. *Genomics* **6**:623, 1990.
42. Smith BL, Preston GM, Spring FA, Anstee DJ, Agre P: Human red cell aquaporin CHIP. I. Molecular characterization of ABH and Colton blood group antigens. *J Clin Invest* **94**:1043, 1994.
43. Richter D: Molecular events in the expression of vasopressin and oxytocin and their cognate receptors. *Am J Physiol* **255**:F207, 1988.
44. Williams PD, Pettibone DJ: Recent advances in the development of oxytocin receptor antagonists. *Curr Pharm Design* **2**:41, 1996.
45. Kalogeras KT, Nieman LN, Friedman TC, Doppman JL, Cutler GBJ, Chrousos GP, Wilder RL, et al: Inferior petrosal sinus sampling in healthy human subjects reveals a unilateral corticotropin-releasing hormone-induced arginine vasopressin release associated with ipsilateral adrenocorticotropin secretion. *J Clin Invest* **97**:2045, 1996.
46. Litwack G, Schmidt TJ: Biochemistry of hormones I: Polypeptide hormones, in Devlin TM, (ed) *Textbook of Biochemistry with Clinical Correlations*, 4th ed. New York, Wiley-Liss, 1997, p 839.
47. Birnbaumer M, Seibold A, Gilbert S, Ishido M, Barberis C, Antaramian A, Brabet P: Molecular cloning of the receptor for human antidiuretic hormone. *Nature* **357**:333, 1992.
48. Kimura T, Tanizawa O, Mori K, Brownstein MJ, Okayama H: Structure and expression of a human oxytocin receptor. *Nature* **356**:526, 1992.
49. Lolait SJ, O'Carroll A-M, McBride OW, Konig M, Morel A, Brownstein MJ: Cloning and characterization of a vasopressin V2 receptor and possible link to nephrogenic diabetes insipidus. *Nature* **357**:336, 1992.
50. Morel A, O'Carroll A-M, Brownstein MJ, Lolait SJ: Molecular cloning and expression of a rat V1a arginine vasopressin receptor. *Nature* **356**:523, 1992.

51. de Keyzer Y, Auzan C, Lenne F, Beldjord C, Thibonnier M, Bertagna X, Clauser E: Cloning and characterization of the human V3 pituitary vasopressin receptor. *FEBS Lett* **356**:215, 1994.
52. Sugimoto T, Saito M, Mochizuki S, Watanabe Y, Hashimoto S, Kawashima H: Molecular cloning and functional expression of a cDNA encoding the human V1b vasopressin receptor. *J Biol Chem* **269**:27088, 1994.
53. Thibonnier M, Auzan C, Madhun Z, Wilkins P, Berti-Mattera L, Clauser E: Molecular cloning, sequencing, and functional expression of a cDNA encoding the human V1a vasopressin receptor. *J Biol Chem* **269**:3304, 1994.
54. Lolait SJ, O'Carroll A-M, Mahan LC, Felder CC, Button DC, Young III WS, Mezey E: Extrapituitary expression of the rat V1b vasopressin receptor gene. *Proc Natl Acad Sci U S A* **92**:6783, 1995.
55. Rozen F, Russo C, Banville D, Zingg H: Structure, characterization, and expression of the rat oxytocin receptor gene. *Proc Natl Acad Sci U S A* **92**:200, 1995.
56. Watson S, Arkinstall S: *The G-Protein Linked Receptor Factsbook.* London, Academic Press, 1994.
57. Ostrowski NL, Young II WS, Knepper MA, Lolait ST: Expression of vasopressin V1a and V2 receptor messenger ribonucleic acid in the liver and kidney of embryonic, developing, and adult rats. *Endocrinol* **133**:1849, 1993.
58. Ostrowski NL, Lolait SJ, Young III WS: Cellular localization of vasopressin V1a receptor messenger ribonucleic acid in adult male rat brain, pineal, and brain vasculature. *Endocrinol* **135**:1511, 1994.
59. Grazzini E, Lodboerer AM, Perez-Martin A, Joubert D, Guillon G: Molecular and functional characterization of V1b vasopressin receptor in rat adrenal medulla. *Endocrinol* **137**:3906, 1996.
60. Ala Y, Morin D, Mouillac B, Sabatier N, Vargas R, Cotte N, Déchaux M, et al: Functional studies of twelve mutant V2 vasopressin receptors related to nephrogenic diabetes insipidus: Molecular basis of a mild clinical phenotype. *J Am Soc Nephrol* **9**:1861, 1998.
61. Mouillac B, Chini B, Balestre M-N, Elands J, Trumpp-Kallmeyer S, Hoflack J, Hibert M: The binding site of neuropeptide vasopressin V1a receptor. *J Biol Chem* **270**:25771, 1995.
62. Chini B, Mouillac B, Ala Y, Balestre M-N, Trumpp-Kallmeyer S, Hoflack J, Elands J, et al: Tyr 115 is the key residue for determining agonist selectivity in the V1a vasopressin receptor. *EMBO J* **14**:2176, 1995.
63. Serradeil-Le Gal C, Lacour C, Valette G, Garcia G, Foulon L, Galindo G, Bankir L, et al: Characterization of SR 121463A, a highly potent and selective, orally active vasopressin V2 receptor antagonist. *J Clin Invest* **98**:2729, 1996.
64. Liu J, Wess J: Different single receptor domains determine the distinct G protein coupling profiles of members of the vasopressin receptor family. *J Biol Chem* **271**:8772, 1996.
65. Robertson GL, Berl T: Pathophysiology of water metabolism, in Brenner BM, Rector FC (eds): *The Kidney*, 5th ed. Philadelphia, WB Saunders, 1996, p 873.
66. Bourque CW, Oliet SHR, Richard D: Osmoreceptors, osmoreception, and osmoregulation. *Front Neuroendocrinol* **15**:231, 1994.
67. Bourque CW, Oliet SHR: Osmoreceptors in the central nervous system. *Annu Rev Physiol* **59**:601, 1997.
68. Zerbe RL, Robertson GL: Osmoregulation of thirst and vasopressin secretion in human subjects: Effect of various solutes. *Am J Physiol* **244**:E607, 1983.
69. Leibowitz SF: Impact of brain monoamines and neuropeptides on vasopressin release, in Cowley AWJ, Liard JF, Ausiello DA (eds): *Vasopressin. Cellular and Integrative Functions*. New York, Raven, 1988, p 379.
70. Randle JC, Mazurek M, Kneifel D, Dufresne J, Renaud LP: Alpha 1-adrenergic receptor activation releases vasopressin and oxytocin from perfused rat hypothalamic explants. *Neurosci Lett* **65**:219, 1986.
71. Fitzsimons JT: Angiotensin, thirst, and sodium appetite. *Physiol Rev* **78**:583, 1998.
72. Ito M, Oliverio MI, Mannon PJ, Best CF, Maeda N, Smithies O, Coffman TM: Regulation of blood pressure by the type 1A angiotensin II receptor gene. *Proc Natl Acad Sci U S A* **92**:3521, 1995.
73. Nimura F, Labosky P, Kakuchi J, Okubo S, Yoshida H, Oikawa T, Ichiki T, et al: Gene targeting in mice reveals a requirement for angiotensin in the development and maintenance of kidney morphology and growth factor regulation. *J Clin Invest* **96**:2947, 1995.
74. Sugaya T, Nishimatsu S, Tanimoto K, Takimoto E, Yamagishi T, Imamura K, Goto S, et al: Angiotensin II type 1a receptor-deficient mice with hypotension and hyperreninemia. *J Biol Chem* **270**:18719, 1995.
75. Hein L, Barsh GS, Pratt RE, Dzau VJ, Kobilka BK: Behavioural and cardiovascular effects of disrupting the angiotensin II type-2 receptor gene in mice. *Nature* **377**:744, 1995.
76. Robertson GL, Oiso Y, Vokes TP, Gaskill MB: Diprenorphine inhibits selectively the vasopressin response to hypovolemic stimuli. *Trans Assoc Am Physicians* **98**:322, 1985.
77. Zerbe RL, Robertson GL: A comparison of plasma vasopressin measurements with a standard indirect test in the differential diagnosis of polyuria. *N Engl J Med* **305**:1539, 1981.
78. Miller M, Dalakos T, Moses AM, Fellerman H, Streeten DH: Recognition of partial defects in antidiuretic hormone secretion. *Ann Intern Med* **73**:721, 1970.
79. Forssman H: The recognition of nephrogenic diabetes insipidus. A very small page from the history of medicine. *Acta Med Scand* **197**:1, 1975.
80. Forssman H: On the mode of hereditary transmission in diabetes insipidus. *Nordisk Med* **16**:3211, 1942.
81. Waring AG, Kajdi L, Tappan V: Congenital defect of water metabolism. *Am J Dis Child* **69**:323, 1945.
82. McIlraith CH: Notes on some cases of diabetes insipidus with marked family and hereditary tendencies. *Lancet* **2**:767, 1892.
83. Reeves WB, Andreoli TE: Nephrogenic diabetes insipidus, in Scriver CR, Beaudet AL, Sly WS, Valle D (eds): *The Metabolic and Molecular Bases of Inherited Disease*, 7th ed. New York, McGraw-Hill, 1995, p 3045.
84. Stevenson AC, Kerr CB: On the distributions of frequencies of mutation to genes determining harmful traits in man. *Mutat Res* **4**:339, 1967.
85. Kambouris M, Dlouhy SR, Trofatter JA, Conneally PM, Hodes ME: Localization of the gene for X-linked nephrogenic diabetes insipidus to Xq28. *Am J Med Genet* **29**:239, 1988.
86. Knoers N, van der Heyden H, van Oost BA, Ropers HH, Monnens L, Willems J: Nephrogenic diabetes insipidus: Close linkage with markers from the distal long arm of the human X chromosome. *Hum Genet* **80**:31, 1988.
87. Bichet DG, Hendy GN, Lonergan M, Arthus M-F, Ligier S, Pausova Z, Kluge R, et al: X-linked nephrogenic diabetes insipidus: From the ship *Hopewell* to restriction fragment length polymorphism studies. *Am J Hum Genet* **51**:1089, 1992.
88. Knoers N, van der Heyden H, van Oost BA, Monnens L, Willems J, Ropers HH: Three-point linkage analysis using multiple DNA polymorphic markers in families with X-linked nephrogenic diabetes insipidus. *Genomics* **4**:434, 1989.
89. van den Ouweland AM, Knoop MT, Knoers VV, Markslag PW, Rocchi M, Warren ST, Ropers HH, et al: Colocalization of the gene for nephrogenic diabetes insipidus (DIR) and the vasopressin type 2 receptor gene (AVPR2) in the Xq28 region. *Genomics* **13**:1350, 1992.
90. Bichet DG, Razi M, Arthus M-F, Lonergan M, Tittley P, Smiley RK, Rock G, et al: Epinephrine and dDAVP administration in patients with congenital nephrogenic diabetes insipidus. Evidence for a pre-cyclic AMP V2 receptor defective mechanism. *Kidney Int* **36**:859, 1989.
91. Jans DA, van Oost BA, Ropers HH, Fahrenholz F: Derivatives of somatic cell hybrids which carry the human gene locus for nephrogenic diabetes insipidus (NDI) express functional vasopressin renal V2-type receptors. *J Biol Chem* **265**:15379, 1990.
92. Rosenthal W, Seibold A, Antaramian A, Lonergan M, Arthus M-F, Hendy GN, Birnbaumer M, et al: Molecular identification of the gene responsible for congenital nephrogenic diabetes insipidus. *Nature* **359**:233, 1992.
93. Fujiwara TM, Crumley J, Morin D, Lonergan M, Arthus M-F, Morgan K, Bichet DG: Nephrogenic diabetes insipidus mutation database. http://www.medcon.mcgill.ca/nephros.
94. Williams RM, Henry C: Nephrogenic diabetes insipidus transmitted by females and appearing during infancy in males. *Ann Int Med* **27**:84, 1947.
95. Crawford JD, Bode HH: Disorders of the posterior pituitary in children, in Gardner LI (ed): *Endocrine and Genetic Diseases of Childhood and Adolescence*, 2nd ed. Philadelphia, WB Saunders, 1975, p 126.
96. Niaudet P, Dechaux M, Trivin C, Loirat C, Broyer M: Nephrogenic diabetes insipidus: Clinical and pathophysiological aspects. *Adv Nephrol Necker Hosp* **13**:247, 1984.
97. van Lieburg AF, Verdijk MAJ, Schoute F, Ligtenberg MJL, van Oost BA, Waldhauser F, Dobner M, et al: Clinical phenotype of nephrogenic diabetes insipidus in females heterozygous for a vasopressin type 2 receptor mutation. *Hum Genet* **96**:70, 1995.
98. Nomura Y, Onigata K, Nagashima T, Yutani S, Mochizuki H, Nagashima K, Morikawa A: Detection of skewed X-inactivation in

two female carriers of vasopressin type 2 receptor gene mutation. *J Clin Endocrinol Metab* **82**:3434, 1997.

99. Streitz JMJ, Streitz JM: Polyuric urinary tract dilatation with renal damage. *J Urol* **139**:784, 1988.
100. Bichet DG, Razi M, Lonergan M, Arthus M-F, Papukna V, Kortas C, Barjon JN: Hemodynamic and coagulation responses to 1-desamino[8-d-arginine]vasopressin (dDAVP) infusion in patients with congenital nephrogenic diabetes insipidus. *N Engl J Med* **318**:881, 1988.
101. Mannucci PM, Aberg M, Nilsson IM, Robertson B: Mechanism of plasminogen activator and factor VIII increase after vasoactive drugs. *Br J Haematol* **30**:81, 1975.
102. Richardson DW, Robinson AG: Desmopressin. *Ann Intern Med* **103**:228, 1985.
103. Schwartz J, Liard JF, Ott C, Cowley AW Jr: Hemodynamic effects of neurohypophyseal peptides with antidiuretic activity in dogs. *Am J Physiol* **249**:H1001, 1985.
104. Williams TD, Lightman SL, Leadbeater MJ: Hormonal and cardiovascular responses to DDAVP in man. *Clin Endocrinol (Oxf)* **24**:89, 1986.
105. Liard JF: Effects of a specific antidiuretic agonist on cardiac output and its distribution in intact and anephric dogs. *Clin Sci* **74**:293, 1988.
106. Derkx FHM, Brink HS, Merkus P, Smiths J, Brommeer EJR, Schalekamp MADH: Vasopressin V2-receptor-mediated hypotensive response in man. *J Hypert* **5**:S107, 1987.
107. Knoers N, Brommer EJ, Willems H, van Oost BA, Monnens LA: Fibrinolytic responses to 1-desamino-8-d-arginine-vasopressin in patients with congenital nephrogenic diabetes insipidus [Comment]. *Nephron* **54**:322, 1990.
108. Bichet DG, Arthus MF, Lonergan M: Platelet vasopressin receptors in patients with congenital nephrogenic diabetes insipidus. *Kidney Int* **39**:693, 1991.
109. Knoers N, Janssens PM, Goertz J, Monnens LA: Evidence for intact V1-vasopressin receptors in congenital nephrogenic diabetes insipidus. *Eur J Pediatr* **151**:381, 1992.
110. Seibold A, Brabet P, Rosenthal W, Birnbaumer M: Structure and chromosomal localization of the human antidiuretic hormone receptor gene. *Am J Hum Genet* **51**:1078, 1992.
111. Bichet DG, Arthus M-F, Lonergan M, Hendy GN, Paradis AJ, Fujiwara TM, Morgan K, et al: X-linked nephrogenic diabetes insipidus mutations in North America and the Hopewell hypothesis. *J Clin Invest* **92**:1262, 1993.
112. Holtzman EJ, Kolakowski LFJ, Geifman-Holtzman O, O'Brien DG, Rasoulpour M, Guillot AP, Ausiello DA: Mutations in the vasopressin V2 receptor gene in two families with nephrogenic diabetes insipidus. *J Am Soc Nephrol* **5**:169, 1994.
113. Wildin RS, Antush MJ, Bennett RL, Schoof JM, Scott CR: Heterogeneous AVPR2 gene mutations in congenital nephrogenic diabetes insipidus. *Am J Hum Genet* **55**:266, 1994.
114. Arthus M-F, Lonergan M, Crumley MJ, Naumova AK, Morin D, De Marco LA, Kaplan BS, et al: Report of 33 novel *AVPR2* mutations and analysis of 117 families with X-linked nephrogenic diabetes insipidus. *J Am Soc Nephrol* **11**:1044, 2000.
115. Bode HH, Crawford JD: Nephrogenic diabetes insipidus in North America: The Hopewell hypothesis. *N Engl J Med* **280**:750, 1969.
116. Holtzman EJ, Kolakowski LF, O'Brien D, Crawford JD, Ausiello DA: A null mutation in the vasopressin V2 receptor gene (AVPR2) associated with nephrogenic diabetes insipidus in the Hopewell kindred. *Hum Mol Genet* **2**:1201, 1993.
117. Hobbs HH, Brown MS, Goldstein JL: Molecular genetics of the LDL receptor gene in familial hypercholesterolemia. *Hum Mutat* **1**:445, 1992.
118. Schöneberg T, Yun J, Wenkert D, Wess J: Functional rescue of mutant V2 vasopressin receptors causing nephrogenic diabetes insipidus by a coexpressed receptor polypeptide. *EMBO J* **15**:1283, 1996.
119. Schöneberg T, Sandig V, Wess J, Gudermann T, Schultz G: Reconstitution of mutant V2 vasopressin receptors by adenovirus-mediated gene transfer. *J Clin Invest* **100**:1547, 1997.
120. Sadeghi H, Robertson GL, Bichet DG, Innamorati G, Birnbaumer M: Biochemical basis of partial NDI phenotypes. *Mol Endocrinol* **11**:1806, 1997.
121. Vargas-Poussou R, Forestier L, Dautzenberg MD, Niaudet P, Déchaud M, Antignac C: Mutations in the vasopressin V2 receptor and aquaporin-2 genes in 12 families with congenital nephrogenic diabetes insipidus. *J Am Soc Nephrol* **8**:1855, 1997.
122. Knoers N, Monnens LA: A variant of nephrogenic diabetes insipidus: V2 receptor abnormality restricted to the kidney. *Eur J Pediatr* **150**:370, 1991.
123. Langley JM, Balfe JW, Selander T, Ray PN, Clarke JT: Autosomal recessive inheritance of vasopressin-resistant diabetes insipidus. *Am J Med Genet* **38**:90, 1991.
124. Lonergan M, Birnbaumer M, Arthus M-F, Bichet DG: Non-X-linked nephrogenic diabetes insipidus: Phenotype and genotype features. *J Am Soc Nephrol* **4**:264A, 1993.
125. Brenner B, Seligsohn U, Hochberg Z: Normal response of factor VIII and von Willebrand factor to 1-deamino-8-D-arginine vasopressin in nephrogenic diabetes insipidus. *J Clin Endocrinol Metab* **67**:191, 1988.
126. Fushimi K, Uchida S, Hara Y, Hirata Y, Marumo F, Sasaki S: Cloning and expression of apical membrane water channel of rat kidney collecting tubule. *Nature* **361**:549, 1993.
127. Deen PMT, Verdijk MAJ, Knoers NVAM, Wieringa B, Monnens LAH, van Os CH, van Oost BA: Requirement of human renal water channel aquaporin-2 for vasopressin-dependent concentration of urine. *Science* **264**:92, 1994.
128. Sasaki S, Fushimi K, Saito H, Saito F, Uchida S, Ishibashi K, Kuwahara M, et al: Cloning, characterization, and chromosomal mapping of human aquaporin of collecting duct. *J Clin Invest* **93**:1250, 1994.
129. van Lieburg AF, Verdijk MAJ, Knoers NVAM, van Essen AJ, Proesmans W, Mallmann R, Monnens LAH, et al: Patients with autosomal nephrogenic diabetes insipidus homozygous for mutations in the aquaporin 2 water-channel gene. *Am J Hum Genet* **55**:648, 1994.
130. Oksche A, Moller A, Dickson J, Rosendahl W, Rascher W, Bichet DG, Rosenthal W: Two novel mutations in the aquaporin-2 and the vasopressin V2 receptor genes in patients with congenital nephrogenic diabetes insipidus. *Hum Genet* **98**:587, 1996.
131. Canfield MC, Tamarappoo BK, Moses AM, Verkman AS, Holtzman EJ: Identification and characterization of aquaporin-2 water channel mutations causing nephrogenic diabetes insipidus with partial vasopressin response. *Hum Mol Genet* **6**:1865, 1997.
132. Hochberg Z, van Lieburg A, Even L, Brenner B, Lanir N, van Oost BA, Knoers NVAM: Autosomal recessive nephrogenic diabetes insipidus caused by an aquaporin-2 mutation. *J Clin Endocrinol Metab* **82**:686, 1997.
133. Mulders SB, Knoers NVAM, van Lieburg AF, Monnens LAH, Leumann E, Wühl E, Schober E, et al: New mutations in the AQP2 gene in nephrogenic diabetes insipidus resulting in functional but misrouted water channels. *J Am Soc Nephrol* **8**:242, 1997.
134. Goji K, Kuwahara M, Gu Y, Matsuo M, Marumo F, Sasaki S: Novel mutations in aquaporin-2 gene in female siblings with nephrogenic diabetes insipidus: Evidence of disrupted water channel function. *J Clin Endocrinol Metab* **83**:3205, 1998.
135. Kuwahara M: Aquaporin-2, a vasopressin-sensitive water channel, and nephrogenic diabetes insipidus. *Intern Med* **37**:215, 1998.
136. Mulders SM, Bichet DG, Rijss JPL, Kamsteeg E-J, Arthus M-F, Lonergan M, Fujiwara M, et al: An aquaporin-2 water channel mutant which causes autosomal dominant nephrogenic diabetes insipidus is retained in the Golgi complex. *J Clin Invest* **102**:57, 1998.
137. Kuwahara M, Iwai K, Uchida S, Gu Y, Terada Y, Sato K, Asai T, et al: A novel mutation in the aquaporin-2 (AQP2) gene causing autosomal dominant nephrogenic diabetes insipidus (NDI). *J Am Soc Nephrol* **9**:390A, 1998.
138. Deen PMT, Weghuis DO, Sinke RJ, Geurts van Kessel A, Wieringa B, van Os CH: Assignment of the human gene for the water channel of renal collecting duct aquaporin 2 (AQP2) to chromosome 12 region q12 → q13. *Cytogenet Cell Genet* **66**:260, 1994.
139. Tamarappoo BK, Verkman AS: Defective aquaporin-2 trafficking in nephrogenic diabetes insipidus and correction by chemical chaperones. *J Clin Invest* **101**:2257, 1998.
140. Deen PMT, Croes H, van Aubel RAMH, Ginsel LA, van Os CH: Water channels encoded by mutant aquaporin-2 genes in nephrogenic diabetes insipidus are impaired in their cellular routing. *J Clin Invest* **95**:2291, 1995.
141. van Os CH, Deen PM: Aquaporin-2 water channel mutations causing nephrogenic diabetes insipidus. *Proc Assoc Am Physicians* **110**:395, 1998.
142. Lacombe UL: De la polydipsie [Thesis of Medicine, no. 99]. Imprimerie et Fonderie de Rignoux, 1841.
143. Weil A: Ueber die hereditare form des diabetes insipidus. *Virchows Arch* **95**:70, 1884.
144. Weil A: Ueber die hereditare form des diabetes insipidus. *Deutches Archiv fur Klinische Medizin* **93**:180, 1908.
145. Camerer JW: Eine ergänzung des Weilschen diabetes-insipidus-stammbaumes. *Archiv für Rassen und Gesellschaftshygiene Biologie* **28**:382, 1935.

146. Dölle W: Eine weitere ergänzung des Weilschen diabetes-insipidus-stammbaumes. *Zeitschrift für Menschliche Vererbungs und Konstitutionslehre* **30**:372, 1951.
147. Rittig R, Robertson GL, Siggaard C, Kovacs L, Gregersen N, Nyborg J, Pedersen EB: Identification of 13 new mutations in the vasopressin-neurophysin II gene in 17 kindreds with familial autosomal dominant neurohypophyseal diabetes insipidus. *Am J Hum Genet* **58**:107, 1996.
148. Bichet DG, Arthus M-F, Lonergan M, Morgan K, Fujiwara TM: Hereditary central diabetes insipidus: autosomal dominant and autosomal recessive phenotypes due to mutations in the *prepro-AVP-NPII* gene. *J Am Soc Nephrol* **9**:386A, 1998.
149. Inoue H, Tanizawa Y, Wasson J, Behn P, Kalidas K, Bernal-Mizrachi E, Mueckler M, et al: A gene encoding a transmembrane protein is mutated in patients with diabetes mellitus and optic atrophy (Wolfram syndrome). *Nat Genet* **20**:143, 1998.
150. Strom TM, Hortnagel K, Hofmann S, Gekeler F, Scharfe C, Rabl W, Gerbitz KD, et al: Diabetes insipidus, diabetes mellitus, optic atrophy and deafness (DIDMOAD) caused by mutations in a novel gene (wolframin) coding for a predicted transmembrane protein. *Hum Mol Genet* **7**:2021, 1998.
151. Boton R, Gaviria M, Batlle DC: Prevalence, pathogenesis, and treatment of renal dysfunction associated with chronic lithium therapy. *Am J Kidney Dis* **10**:329, 1987.
152. Christensen S, Kusano E, Yusufi AN, Murayama N, Dousa TP: Pathogenesis of nephrogenic diabetes insipidus due to chronic administration of lithium in rats. *J Clin Invest* **75**:1869, 1985.
153. Cogan E, Svoboda M, Abramow M: Mechanisms of lithium-vasopressin interaction in rabbit cortical collecting tubule. *Am J Physiol* **252**:F1080, 1987.
154. Goldberg H, Clayman P, Skorecki K: Mechanism of Li inhibition of vasopressin-sensitive adenylate cyclase in cultured renal epithelial cells. *Am J Physiol* **255**:F995, 1988.
155. Marples D, Christensen S, Christensen EI, Ottosen PD, Nielsen S: Lithium-induced downregulation of aquaporin-2 water channel expression in rat kidney medulla. *J Clin Invest* **95**:1838, 1995.
156. Marples D, Frokiaer J, Dorup J, Knepper MA, Nielsen S: Hypokalemia-induced downregulation of aquaporin-2 water channel expression in rat kidney medulla and cortex. *J Clin Invest* **97**:1960, 1996.
157. Frokiaer J, Marples D, Knepper MA, Nielsen S: Bilateral ureteral obstruction downregulates expression of vasopressin-sensitive AQP-2 water channel in rat kidney. *Am J Physiol* **270**:F657, 1996.
158. Sands JM, Flores FX, Kato A, Baum MA, Brown EM, Ward DT, Hebert SC, et al: Vasopressin-elicited water and urea permeabilities are altered in IMCD in hypercalcemic rats. *Am J Physiol* **274**:F978, 1998.
159. Kanno K, Sasaki S, Hirata Y, Ishikawa S, Fushimi K, Nakanishi S, Bichet DG, et al: Urinary excretion of aquaporin-2 in patients with diabetes insipidus [Comment]. *N Engl J Med* **332**:1540, 1995.
160. Batlle DC, von Riotte AB, Gaviria M, Grupp M: Amelioration of polyuria by amiloride in patients receiving long-term lithium therapy. *N Engl J Med* **312**:408, 1985.
161. Leaf A: Neurogenic diabetes insipidus. *Kidney Int* **15**:572, 1979.
162. Robertson GL: Diagnosis of diabetes insipidus, in Czernichow P, Robinson AG (eds): *Frontiers of Hormone Research*, vol 13. Basel, Karger, 1985, p 176.
163. Boyd SD, Raz S, Ehrlich RM: Diabetes insipidus and nonobstructive dilatation of urinary tract. *Urology* **16**:266, 1980.
164. Gautier B, Thieblot P, Steg A: Mégauretère, mégavessie et diabète insipide familial. *Semin Hop* **57**:60, 1981.
165. Bichet D: Nephrogenic diabetes insipidus, in Davison A, Cameron J, Grünfeld J, Kerr D, Ritz E, Winearls C (eds): *Oxford Textbook of Clinical Nephrology*, vol 2. New York, Oxford University Press, 1998, p 1095.
166. Stern P, Valtin H: Verney was right, but... [Editorial]. *N Engl J Med* **305**:1581, 1981.
167. Barlow ED, de Wardener HE: Compulsive water drinking. *QJM (New Series)* **28**:235, 1959.
168. Robertson GL: Dipsogenic diabetes insipidus: a newly recognized syndrome caused by a selective defect in the osmoregulation of thirst. *Trans Assoc Am Physicians* **100**:241, 1987.
169. Robertson GL: Differential diagnosis of polyuria. *Annu Rev Med* **39**:425, 1988.
170. Goldman MB, Luchins DJ, Robertson GL: Mechanisms of altered water metabolism in psychotic patients with polydipsia and hyponatremia. *N Engl J Med* **318**:397, 1988.
171. Bichet DG, Fujiwara TM: Diversity of nephrogenic diabetes insipidus mutations and importance of early recognition and treatment. Proceedings of the Second International Forum "The Frontiers of Nephrology," Japan, 9–12 May 1998. *Clin Exper Nephrol* **2**:253, 1998.
172. Pan Y, Metzenberg A, Das S, Jing B, Gitschier J: Mutations in the V2 vasopressin receptor gene are associated with X-linked nephrogenic diabetes insipidus. *Nat Genet* **2**:103, 1992.
173. Bichet DG, Birnbaumer M, Lonergan M, Arthus M-F, Rosenthal W, Goodyer P, Nivet H, et al: Nature and recurrence of AVPR2 mutations in X-linked nephrogenic diabetes insipidus. *Am J Hum Genet* **55**:278, 1994.
174. Pan Y, Wilson P, Gitschier J: The effect of eight V2 vasopressin receptor mutations on stimulation of adenylyl cyclase and binding to vasopressin. *J Biol Chem* **269**:31933, 1994.
175. Wenkert D, Merendino JJJ, Shenker A, Thambi N, Robertson GL, Moses AM, Spiegel AM: Novel mutations in the V2 vasopressin receptor gene of patients with X-linked nephrogenic diabetes insipidus. *Hum Mol Genet* **3**:1429, 1994.
176. Wildin RS, Cogdell DE, Valadez V: AVPR2 variants and V2 vasopressin receptor function in nephrogenic diabetes insipidus. *Kidney Int* **54**:1909, 1998.
177. Knoers NV, van den Ouweland AM, Verdijk M, Monnens LA, van Oost BA: Inheritance of mutations in the V2 receptor gene in thirteen families with nephrogenic diabetes insipidus. *Kidney Int* **46**:170, 1994.
178. Knoers N, Monnens LA: Nephrogenic diabetes insipidus: Clinical symptoms, pathogenesis, genetics and treatment. *Pediatr Nephrol* **6**:476, 1992.
179. Niaudet P, Dechaux M, Leroy D, Broyer M: Nephrogenic diabetes insipidus in children, in Czernichow P, Robinson AG, (eds): *Frontiers of Hormone Research, Diabetes Insipidus in Man*, vol 13. Basel, Karger, 1985, p 224.
180. Behrman RE, Vaughan VC, Nelson WE: Nephrogenic diabetes insipidus, in Behrman RE, Vaughan VC, Nelson WE (eds): *Nelson Textbook of Pediatrics*. Philadelphia, WB Saunders, 1987, p 1136.
181. Blalock T, Gerron G, Quiter E, Rudman D: Role of diet in the management of vasopressin-responsive and -resistant diabetes insipidus. *Am J Clin Nutr* **30**:1070, 1977.
182. Alon U, Chan JC: Hydrochlorothiazide-amiloride in the treatment of congenital nephrogenic diabetes insipidus. *Am J Nephrol* **5**:9, 1985.
183. Libber S, Harrison H, Spector D: Treatment of nephrogenic diabetes insipidus with prostaglandin synthesis inhibitors. *J Pediatr* **108**:305, 1986.
184. Jakobsson B, Berg U: Effect of hydrochlorothiazide and indomethacin treatment on renal function in nephrogenic diabetes insipidus. *Acta Paediatr* **83**:522, 1994.
185. Moullier P, Friedlander G, Calise D, Ronco P, Perricaudet M, Ferry N: Adenoviral-mediated gene transfer to renal tubular cells in vivo. *Kidney Int* **45**:1220, 1994.
186. Coughlin SR: Expanding horizons for receptors coupled to G-proteins: Diversity and disease. *Curr Biol* **6**:191, 1994.
187. Zerbe RL, Robertson GL: Disorders of ADH. *Med North Am* **13**:1570, 1984.
188. Antonarakis S, and the Nomenclature Working Group: Recommendations for a nomenclature system for human gene mutations. Nomenclature Working Group. *Hum Mutat* **11**:1, 1998.
189. van den Ouweland AM, Dreesen JC, Verdijk M, Knoers NV, Monnens LA, Rocchi M, van Oost BA: Mutations in the vasopressin type 2 receptor gene (AVPR2) associated with nephrogenic diabetes insipidus. *Nat Genet* **2**:99, 1992.
190. Holtzman EJ, Harris HWJ, Kolakowski LFJ, Guay-Woodford LM, Botelho B, Ausiello DA: Brief report: A molecular defect in the vasopressin V2-receptor gene causing nephrogenic diabetes insipidus. *N Engl J Med* **328**:1534, 1993.
191. Merendino JJJ, Speigel AM, Crawford JD, O'Carroll AM, Brownstein MJ, Lolait SJ: Brief report: A mutation in the vasopressin V2-receptor gene in a kindred with X-linked nephrogenic diabetes insipidus. *N Engl J Med* **328**: 1538, 1993.
192. Tsukaguchi H, Matsubara H, Aritaki S, Kimura T, Abe S, Inada M: Two novel mutations in the vasopressin V2 receptor gene in unrelated Japanese kindreds with nephrogenic diabetes insipidus. *Biochem Biophys Res Commun* **197**:1000, 1993.
193. Faa V, Ventruto ML, Loche S, Bozzola M, Podda R, Cao A, Rosatelli MC: Mutations in the vasopressin V2-receptor gene in three families of Italian descent with nephrogenic diabetes insipidus. *Hum Mol Genet* **3**:1685, 1994.
194. Friedman E, Bale AE, Carson E, Boson WL, Nordenskjold M, Ritzen M, Ferreira PC, et al: Nephrogenic diabetes insipidus: An X chromosome-linked dominant inheritance pattern with a vasopressin

type 2 receptor gene that is structurally normal. *Proc Natl Acad Sci U S A* **91**:8457, 1994.

195. Oksche A, Dickson J, Schülein R, Seyberth HW, Müller M, Rascher W, Birnbaumer M, et al: Two novel mutations in the vasopressin V2 receptor gene in patients with congenital nephrogenic diabetes insipidus. *Biophys Biochem Res Com* **205**:552, 1994.
196. Yuasa H, Ito M, Oiso Y, Kurokawa M, Watanabe T, Oda Y, Ishizuka T, et al: Novel mutations in the V2 vasopressin receptor gene in two pedigrees with congenital nephrogenic diabetes insipidus. *J Clin Endocrinol Metab* **79**:361, 1994.
197. Tsukaguchi H, Matsubara H, Inada M: Expression studies of two vasopressin V2 receptor gene mutations, R202C and 804insG, in nephrogenic diabetes insipidus. *Kidney Int* **48**:554, 1995.
198. Jinnouchi H, Araki E, Miyamura N, Kishikawa H, Yoshimura R, Isami S, Yamaguchi K, et al: Analysis of vasopressin receptor type II (V2R) gene in three Japanese pedigrees with congenital nephrogenic diabetes insipidus: identification of a family with complete deletion of the V2R gene. *Eur J Endocrinol* **134**:689, 1996.
199. Tajima T, Nakae J, Takekoshi Y, Takahashi Y, Yuri K, Nagashima T, Fujieda K: Three novel AVPR2 mutations in three Japanese families with X-linked nephrogenic diabetes insipidus. *Pediatr Res* **39**:522, 1996.
200. Yokoyama K, Yamauchi A, Izumi M, Itoh T, Ando A, Imai E, Kamada T, et al: A low-affinity vasopressin V2-receptor gene in a kindred with X-linked nephrogenic diabetes insipidus. *J Am Soc Nephrol* **7**:410, 1996.
201. Cheong HI, Park HW, Ha IS, Moon HN, Choi Y, Ko KW, Jun JK: Six novel mutations in the vasopressin V2 receptor gene causing nephrogenic diabetes insipidus. *Nephron* **75**:431, 1997.
202. Szalai C, Molnár E, Sallay P, es Czinner A: Nephrogen diabetes insipidusos betegek molekuláris biológia vizsgálata. *Orvosi Hetilap* **139**:883, 1998.
203. Schöneberg T, Schulz A, Biebermann H, Grüters A, Grimm T, Hübschmann K, Filler G, et al: V2 vasopressin receptor dysfunction in nephrogenic diabetes insipidus caused by different molecular mechanisms. *Hum Mutat* **12**:196, 1998.
204. Shoji Y, Takahashi T, Suzuki Y, Suzuki T, Komatsu K, Hirono H, Shoji Y, et al: Mutational analyses of AVPR2 gene in three Japanese families with X-linked nephrogenic diabetes insipidus: Two recurrent mutations, R137H and delta V278, caused by the hypermutability at CpG dinucleotides. *Hum Mutat* **1(Suppl)**:S278, 1998.
205. Cheng A, van Hoek AN, Yeager M, Verkman AS, Mitra AK: Three-dimensional organization of a human water channel. *Nature* **387**:627, 1997.

CHAPTER 164

Pseudohypoparathyroidism

Allen M. Spiegel ▪ Lee S. Weinstein

1. **_Pseudohypoparathyroidism_ is a term applied to a heterogeneous group of disorders whose common feature is resistance to parathyroid hormone.**
2. **Most patients with pseudohypoparathyroidism are hypocalcemic and hyperphosphatemic despite elevated concentrations of parathyroid hormone in plasma. Hypocalcemia and hyperphosphatemia are due to loss of the phosphaturic action of parathyroid hormone and reduced formation of 1,25-dihydroxyvitamin D with resultant defective mobilization of calcium from bone and reduced gastrointestinal absorption of calcium.**
3. **Clinical features and location of the putative defect causing hormone resistance permit separation of pseudohypoparathyroidism into distinct subtypes.**
4. **_Pseudohypoparathyroidism type Ia_ is associated with resistance to multiple hormones in addition to parathyroid hormone, and with a constellation of physical abnormalities collectively termed "Albright hereditary osteodystrophy." Patients with pseudohypoparathyroidism Ia may show clinical signs of, or even present with, endocrinopathies other than hypoparathyroidism, presumably due to generalized hormone resistance. Relatives of patients with pseudohypoparathyroidism may show features of Albright hereditary osteodystrophy without overt hormone resistance, a condition termed _pseudopseudohypoparathyroidism_. The molecular defect causing hormone resistance in most, but not all, patients with pseudohypoparathyroidism Ia is a deficiency in a guanine nucleotide-binding protein (Gs) that couples hormone receptors to stimulation of adenylyl cyclase. Distinct mutations in the gene encoding the Gs-α subunit have been identified in affected individuals from many families with pseudohypoparathyroidism Ia. The disease is inherited in autosomal dominant fashion in most families, but there is also evidence for paternal imprinting of the Gs-α gene. Thus, offspring who inherit the mutant gene from their mother are affected with pseudohypoparathyroidism, whereas those who inherit the mutant gene from their father show the pseudopseudohypoparathyroidism phenotype. A defect in some other general component of the receptor-Gs-adenylyl cyclase complex is postulated in patients with the identical phenotype of pseudohypoparathyroidism Ia but normal Gs activity.**
5. **In _pseudohypoparathyroidism type Ib_, physical appearance is normal, and resistance is limited to the renal response to parathyroid hormone. As in pseudohypoparathyroidism Ia, the defect is located proximal to cAMP formation, but unlike pseudohypoparathyroidism Ia, the defect is likely to involve a signal transduction component specific to the kidney. Although the parathyroid hormone receptor is an obvious candidate gene, several studies have excluded mutations in this receptor as a cause of this disease, and the molecular pathogenesis remains to be defined. The disease may be both sporadic and familial, and in the latter case, the mode of inheritance has not been defined.**
6. **_Pseudohypoparathyroidism type II_ is rarely if ever familial. Resistance is limited to parathyroid hormone and is due to a defect distal to cAMP formation.**

A list of standard abbreviations is located immediately preceding the index in each volume. Nonstandard abbreviations used in this chapter include: Gs = guanine nucleotide binding protein coupled to stimulation of adenylyl cyclase; PHP = pseudohypoparathyroidism; PPHP = pseudopseudohypoparathyroidism; PTH = parathyroid hormone; TRF = thyrotropin-releasing factor; TSH = thyrotropin.

HISTORICAL BACKGROUND

In 1942, Albright and colleagues described three patients with hypocalcemia, hyperphosphatemia, and normal renal function, characteristic findings in hypoparathyroidism.[1] All three subjects showed reduced calcemic and phosphaturic responses (by comparison with other hypoparathyroid subjects) to injected bovine parathyroid extract. This led Albright to postulate that hypoparathyroidism in the three reported subjects was due to resistance to parathyroid hormone (PTH) action rather than to PTH deficiency and to term the disorder "pseudohypoparathyroidism" (PHP).* Albright's formulation of the pathogenesis of the disorder in these subjects is notable as perhaps the first description of the concept of hormone resistance as a basis for reduced hormone action.

In the original report,[1] Albright noted certain abnormal physical features in the patients with pseudohypoparathyroidism. These included short stature, obesity, rounded face and short neck, and shortened metacarpals. No obvious connection between these features and the abnormality in calcium metabolism was apparent, nor was familial occurrence noted. In a subsequent report,[2] Albright and colleagues described a 29-year-old woman with physical features similar to those of the subjects with PHP but with no evident abnormality in calcium metabolism. Albright considered this a distinct syndrome, which he termed "pseudopseudohypoparathyroidism" (PPHP).

Albright's postulate of end-organ resistance to PTH action as the basis for PHP was confirmed by subsequent studies. Parathyroid hyperplasia was found on biopsy of untreated subjects with PHP,[3] and biologically active PTH was found in gland extracts.[4] Elevation in immunoreactive PTH in plasma of untreated subjects with PHP has been found in numerous studies. Chase, Melson, and Aurbach defined the locus of the defect in most patients with PHP.[5] These authors showed that in the normal subject, PTH stimulates formation of the second messenger, cAMP, in bone and kidney. The latter action is reflected in urinary

*The OMIM numbers corresponding to the eponyms are: #103580, pseudohypoparathyroidism; #300800, Albright hereditary osteodystrophy; #174800, McCune-Albright syndrome. (The # symbol indicates mutant alleles identified in the *GNAS1* gene on chromosome 20q13.2.) There are additional MIM entries for: (a) guanine nucleotide-binding protein, α-stimulating activity polypeptide 1 (*GNAS1*) locus and gene (MIM #139320); and (b) parathyroid hormone receptor 1 (*PTHR1*) locus and gene (MIM #168468). [Comment: The MIM entries indicate the confusion that has long existed when trying to link phenotype to genotype; the text of this chapter is clarifying. The Editors] excretion of cAMP. Subjects with PHP showed a markedly reduced rise in urinary cAMP excretion in response to infused bovine PTH compared with normal subjects and subjects with other forms of hypoparathyroidism. Subsequently, a 22-month-old child was described in whom resistance to PTH was associated with a normal urinary cAMP response to PTH.[6] This, and other observations, emphasized the heterogeneity of PHP. Recent efforts are aimed at elucidating the biochemical and genetic basis for this heterogeneity. In one subtype of PHP, deficient activity was found of Gs, a guanine nucleotide-binding protein that couples hormone receptors to stimulation of cAMP formation.[7,8] This defect could help explain resistance to PTH and to other agents that act by stimulating production of cAMP in subjects with this form of PHP. In subjects with deficient Gs activity, mutations that are predicted to disrupt formation of normal protein have been identified in the gene encoding the Gs-α subunit.[9,10]

CONTROL OF CALCIUM AND PHOSPHORUS METABOLISM BY PARATHYROID HORMONE AND VITAMIN D

A brief review of the actions of PTH and vitamin D in regulating calcium and phosphorus metabolism is necessary before a discussion of the pathophysiology of PHP. Together, PTH and vitamin D control the flux of calcium and phosphate into and out of the kidney, the gastrointestinal tract, and bone. The concerted actions of these two hormones maintain the serum ionized calcium concentration within narrow limits and permit normal skeletal growth and remodeling.

Parathyroid Hormone Synthesis and Secretion

PTH is synthesized in the parathyroid glands as preproPTH, a 115-amino acid polypeptide. The hydrophobic 25-amino acid *pre*, "leader," sequence, and the basic hexapeptide *pro* sequence are cleaved before secretion of the native hormone (amino acids 1–84).[11] The intact hormone is rapidly cleaved in the peripheral circulation into biologically inactive fragments. There is an inverse relationship between PTH secretion and the extracellular fluid concentration of ionized calcium.[12] A decrease in the latter provokes secretion of PTH, which, through direct actions on kidney and bone and indirect actions on the gastrointestinal tract, raises extracellular fluid calcium concentration (Fig. 164-1).

Parathyroid Hormone Actions on Kidney

Effect on Phosphate Clearance. PTH acts on sites in the proximal, and probably also the distal, nephron to increase phosphate clearance.[12] The phosphaturic action of PTH counteracts the hormone-induced release of phosphate from bone into extracellular fluid. The net effect of the hormone in subjects with normal renal function is to lower serum phosphate concentration. Elevations in serum phosphate concentration depress serum calcium by reducing bone resorption and by decreasing synthesis of 1,25-dihydroxyvitamin D, the active metabolite of vitamin D. The phosphaturic action of PTH thus serves indirectly to maintain normal serum calcium concentration.

Effect on Calcium Clearance. PTH enhances calcium reabsorption by the kidney through an action on sites beyond the proximal tubule.[12] Increased PTH secretion releases calcium from bone into extracellular fluid, thereby increasing the filtered load of calcium; but for any filtered load, PTH reduces net calcium excretion.

Increased Formation of 1,25-Dihydroxyvitamin D. (See also Chap. 165 for additional information on vitamin D metabolism, its effect on target organs, and Mendelian disorders impairing its action.) Vitamin D (cholecalciferol) is formed by the action of ultraviolet light on skin or is ingested as the plant sterol ergocalciferol. These precursor forms of the active hormone are hydroxylated in the 25 position in the liver to form 25-hydroxyvitamin D, the major circulating form. The active metabolite, 1,25-dihydroxyvitamin D, is formed by hydroxylation in the 1α position by a microsomal enzyme in the kidney. The 1-hydroxylation reaction is under the direct (or indirect, through lowering of the serum phosphate level) control of PTH. By increasing formation of 1,25-dihydroxyvitamin D, PTH acts indirectly on the gastrointestinal tract to increase calcium absorption. 1,25-dihydroxyvitamin D is also required for PTH to release calcium from bone. Loss of PTH action on the kidney impairs normal calcium homeostasis both through loss of the direct effects (phosphaturic) of PTH and through the indirect effects mediated by 1,25-dihydroxyvitamin D.

PTH Actions on Bone. PTH has dual actions on bone. The hormone acutely mobilizes calcium from bone to the extracellular fluid. Osteocytes are the presumed target cells for the acute effect of PTH, which serves to maintain normal serum calcium concentration.[12] PTH also stimulates bone resorption. Available evidence suggests that PTH acts directly on osteoblasts to alter their shape and function.[13] There is no cogent evidence for a direct action of PTH on osteoclasts.[14] Instead, PTH may stimulate osteoclastic resorption indirectly by causing osteoblasts to release factors that activate osteoclasts.[13,14] Coupling of bone formation to bone resorption (possibly through release of paracrine factors) is reflected in increased bone formation that follows PTH-stimulated resorption.[15] The long-term effects of excess PTH action on bone are increased resorption (osteitis fibrosa cystica in the most extreme form) and a secondary increase in bone formation by osteoblasts reflected by increased serum alkaline phosphatase activity. The dual effects of PTH on bone, the calcemic effect and the skeletal remodeling effect, can be dissociated. 1,25-Dihydroxyvitamin D is required for the normal calcemic response to PTH, but is not essential for the skeletal remodeling effect.[16] In states of PTH excess and 1,25-dihydroxyvitamin D deficiency (e.g., chronic renal failure), osteitis fibrosa cystica and hypocalcemia may coexist.

MECHANISM OF PARATHYROID HORMONE ACTION

Understanding resistance to PTH action requires an understanding of the mechanism of action of the hormone. Several steps in

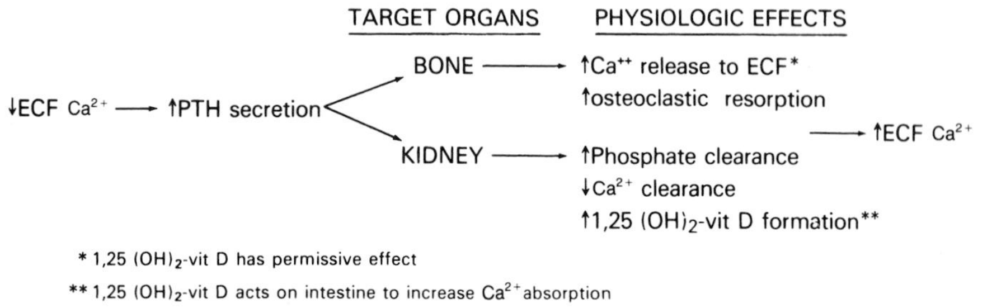

Fig. 164-1 Control of calcium and phosphorus metabolism by PTH. A fall in the concentration of extracellular fluid ionized calcium (ECF Ca^{2+}) provokes PTH secretion from the parathyroid glands. The actions of PTH (discussed in the text) on its principal targets, bone and kidney, lead to an increase in ECF Ca^{2+}.

the pathway of PTH action are now defined in considerable detail, but major gaps remain. PTH acts by binding to specific receptors on the surface of its target cells in bone and kidney.[12] Receptor activation triggers formation of intracellular second messengers.

Second Messengers of Parathyroid Hormone Action in Kidney and Bone

PTH stimulates formation of the second messenger, cAMP, in kidney and bone.[12] Whether cAMP is the exclusive, or even the most important, mediator of all PTH actions in kidney and bone is unclear. Urinary cAMP excretion reflects PTH action on the kidney.[5,12] Administration of PTH increases urinary excretion of cAMP and increases the concentration of cAMP in plasma.[17] Both effects result from PTH action on the kidney and are useful clinically as tests of renal responsiveness to PTH.[5,17]

cAMP appears to mediate the phosphaturic action of PTH,[18] and is probably the second messenger for PTH action on the renal 25-hydroxycholecalciferol-1α-hydroxylase as well.[19] There is no definitive evidence that cAMP mediates PTH's anticalciuric effect.[20] In bone, because of the heterogeneity of cell types and the likelihood of important cell-cell interactions via local mediators,[13] identification of second messengers for PTH action is particularly difficult. PTH binds to and stimulates cAMP formation in osteoblasts.[13] It is not clear, however, that cAMP mediates PTH-stimulated bone resorption.[21] cAMP itself has complex effects on bone resorption in organ culture studies.[21] PTH may also utilize a signal transduction pathway involving changes in cytosolic calcium concentration in bone cells.[22] Many polypeptide hormones (including PTH[23]), in addition to stimulating cAMP formation, stimulate breakdown of phosphoinositides. The latter leads to release of two second messengers, diacylglycerol which activates protein kinase C, and inositol triphosphate, which increases cytosolic calcium by releasing calcium from intracellular stores. Increased cytosolic calcium secondary to PTH modulation of plasma membrane calcium channels is also a theoretical possibility. The precise relationship between the cAMP and intracellular calcium signal transduction pathways and the actions of PTH in both bone and kidney remains to be elucidated.

Components of Signal Transduction Pathway for Parathyroid Hormone

The first step in the action of PTH, as for many other polypeptide hormones and amine neurotransmitters, is binding to specific cell surface receptors. Activated receptors interact with one or more members of a family of guanine nucleotide-binding proteins (G proteins) to facilitate release of GDP and binding of GTP.[24] GTP-bound G proteins, in turn, interact with specific effectors, often enzymes that catalyze formation of second messengers. The latter mediate the effects of first messengers on cell function, generally by causing specific protein kinases to phosphorylate key proteins within the cell.

As discussed above, PTH action is mediated by cAMP and possibly also by other second messengers, such as products of phosphoinositide breakdown. Because the cAMP cascade is the best-characterized signal transduction pathway for PTH action, the components of this pathway are presented in greater detail. In addition to receptors, this pathway includes adenylyl cyclase, the enzyme that catalyzes formation of cAMP from ATP and Mg^{2+} and is under dual regulation by distinct G proteins: Gs and Gi.[24] Gs couples receptors for many agonists, including PTH, that stimulate cAMP formation, whereas Gi couples receptors for agonists that inhibit cAMP formation to adenylyl cyclase (Fig. 164-2). cAMP is degraded by cyclic nucleotide phosphodiesterase. The concentration of cAMP in the cell controls the activity of a specific cAMP-dependent protein kinase, which, in turn, regulates the function of key substrates through phosphorylation.

The components of the cAMP cascade may be divided into those unique to a given hormone and cell and those common to all hormones and cells. Receptors and substrates for cAMP-dependent protein kinase are in the first category. Gs, adenylyl cyclase, cAMP phosphodiesterase, and cAMP-dependent protein kinase are in the latter category. Specificity in hormone action resides in the first (receptor binding) and last (cAMP-dependent phosphorylation of specific cellular substrates) steps of the cAMP cascade.[25] The existence of multiple subtypes of adenylyl cyclase and

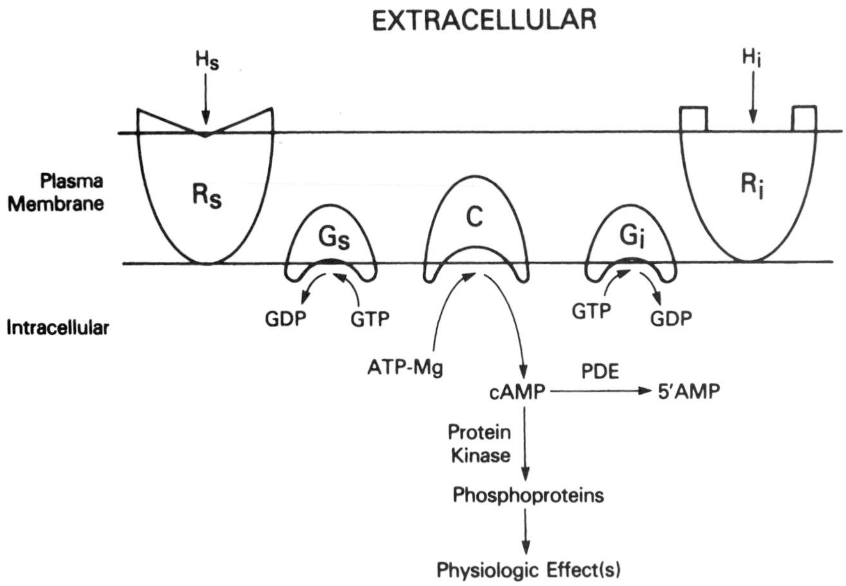

Fig. 164-2 Outline of the signal transduction system using cAMP as second messenger. H_s and H_i denote stimulatory and inhibitory agonists, respectively; Rs and Ri, stimulatory and inhibitory receptors; G_s and G_i, the stimulatory and inhibitory guanine nucleotide-binding proteins. C denotes adenylyl cyclase, and PDE refers to phosphodiesterase. Details of the interactions between these components are discussed in the text. (*From Spiegel et al.*[25] Used by permission.)

phosphodiesterase, which differ in their regulation and tissue-specific expression, may also contribute to differences in hormone responsiveness between different tissues.[26–28]

Structure of Components of the cAMP Transduction Pathway

Receptors. A PTH receptor cDNA has been cloned from an opossum kidney cell line.[29] † The cDNA encodes a predicted 585-amino acid protein with seven potential membrane-spanning domains similar in overall topography to other members of the G protein-coupled receptor family.[30] An approximately 200-amino acid N-terminal portion contains a putative signal peptide and four potential glycosylation sites. The seven putative membrane-spanning domains would produce three extracellular and three intracellular loops, as well as a C-terminal tail on the cytoplasmic side of the plasma membrane. The expressed receptor binds PTH and the PTH-related peptide with equal affinity, and binding of either ligand to the expressed receptor stimulates adenylyl cyclase activity.[29] This makes it likely that the cloned receptor couples to Gs, but does not exclude the possibility that the same receptor could couple to other G proteins such as members of the Gq subfamily that stimulate phosphoinositide breakdown.[24]

A second receptor that binds only PTH has been cloned, but its expression is limited to the central nervous system; therefore, it is unlikely to be relevant to the pathogenesis of renal resistance to PTH in PHP.[31] It is theoretically possible that distinct forms of PTH receptor could exist in bone and kidney. Differences in the binding and activity of certain analogues of PTH in kidney and bone suggest that renal and skeletal PTH receptors may differ.[32,33] The 3-34 analogue of PTH is an antagonist of PTH-stimulated cAMP formation in the kidney, but shows agonist activity in bone *in vitro*[32] and when administered *in vivo*.[34] Photoaffinity labeling of PTH in bone- and kidney-derived cells, however, identifies a single protein with identical molecular size (70 kDa) in bone and kidney.[35] A second PTH receptor expressed in either bone or kidney remains to be identified.

Guanine Nucleotide Binding Protein. Gs couples receptors for the many agents that stimulate cAMP formation, including PTH, to adenylyl cyclase.[24] Gs has also been shown to stimulate the opening of specific calcium channels. Like other G proteins, Gs consists of three subunits, α, β, and γ, each the product of a separate gene. The α subunit binds guanine nucleotides with high affinity, and shows intrinsic GTPase activity that serves to terminate Gs activation. Activation of Gs by GTP binding is dependent on interaction with an agonist-bound receptor. Interaction of Gs with receptor confers on the receptor a higher affinity for agonist binding. The β and γ subunits, which behave as a tightly bound complex under native conditions, facilitate Gs interaction with receptors and dissociate from the α subunit on Gs activation. The activated Gs-α subunit alone can bind to and activate adenylyl cyclase. It is the α subunit that clearly differs among G protein heterotrimers, and is believed to confer specificity in receptor and effector coupling.

Gs is ubiquitously distributed. The stoichiometry between Gs and the other components of the receptor-adenylyl cyclase complex has not been rigorously defined, nor is it clear which is the rate-limiting component. This could vary from tissue to tissue. The α subunit of Gs is a substrate for ADP-ribosylation by cholera toxin. This covalent modification has profound effects on Gs function. By lowering the activity of the "turn-off" GTPase reaction, cholera toxin activates Gs constitutively and provokes increased cAMP formation. Mutations of the arginine residue that is the target of cholera toxin modification, and mutation of certain other key amino acids, cause similar reduction in GTPase activity and constitutive Gs activation. Such mutations were identified in certain benign endocrine tumors and in tissues from subjects with the McCune-Albright syndrome, a sporadic disorder characterized by hyperfunction of multiple endocrine glands.[36]

With radioactive NAD as cofactor, the cholera toxin-catalyzed reaction can be used to identify and quantitate Gs-α in cell membranes. Specific antibodies can also be used.[37,38] At least two forms of Gs-α (approximate sizes 45 and 52 kDa) have been identified in most cells by this method. Human red blood cells contain only the 45-kDa form. cDNAs for Gs-α from several species, including human,[39] have been cloned. The amino acid and nucleotide sequences show extremely high (>94 percent) conservation. Multiple forms of Gs-α mRNA, corresponding to the multiple forms of Gs-α protein, have been identified.[39] mRNA heterogeneity arises via alternative splicing of a single, approximately 20-kb gene (*GNAS1*)[40] located on the distal long arm of chromosome 20.[41] The functional significance of Gs-α heterogeneity has yet to be defined.

Adenylyl Cyclase. There are multiple subtypes of adenylyl cylase, including calmodulin-sensitive (predominantly in brain) and insensitive forms. cDNAs encoding several of the subtypes have been cloned.[12,26,42] These predict a large (110 to 150 kDa) protein with multiple putative membrane-spanning domains, and an overall topography placing it within the ATP-binding transporter family to which the cystic fibrosis gene product also belongs (see Chap. 201). No transport function has yet been identified for adenylyl cyclase. Biochemical studies are beginning to define differences in regulation of adenylyl cyclase subtypes,[26,43] but the physiological significance of this heterogeneity is still unclear.

cAMP-Phosphodiesterase. Multiple forms of cyclic nucleotide phosphodiesterase, differing in both substrate (cAMP vs cGMP) specificity and affinity and hormonal regulation, are found within the same cell.[27,28,44] Phosphodiesterases have been classified into

---

†There is no complete genomic sequence for the human *GNAS1* gene. The following are GenBank accession numbers for the nucleotide sequences of portions of this gene; accession numbers for the human parathyroid hormone receptor gene; and accession numbers for tissue-specific expressed forms of both genes.

L04308
  Human parathyroid hormone receptor mRNA, complete cds,
  gi|190721|gb|L04308|HUMPTHR [190721]
X68596
  H. sapiens mRNA for parathyroid hormone receptor
  gi|396812|emb|X68596|HSPHR [396812]
GNASI:
AJ224868
  H. sapiens GNASI gene
  gi|3297876|emb|AJ224868|HSA224868 [3297876]
AJ224867
  H. sapiens mRNA for GNAS1 protein (IMAGE cDNA clone 359933 (827-k06))
  gi|3297870|emb|AJ224867|HSA224867 [3297870]
U12466
  Human guanine nucleotide regulatory protein (GNAS1) gene, exon 13, partial cds
  gi|527670|gb|U12466|HSU12466 [527670]
SEG_HUMGNAS
  Human guanine nucleotide-binding protein alpha-subunit gene (G-s-alpha)
  gi|183403|gb||SEG_HUMGNAS [183403]
M21142
  Human guanine nucleotide-binding protein alpha-subunit gene (G-s-alpha), exons 7 through 13
  gi|183402|gb|M21142|HUMGNAS6 [183402]
M21141
  Human guanine nucleotide-binding protein alpha-subunit gene (G-s-alpha), exon 6
  gi|183401|gb|M21141|HUMGNAS5 [183401]
M21741
  Human guanine nucleotide-binding protein alpha-subunit gene (G-s-alpha), exons 4 and 5
  gi|183400|gb|M21741|HUMGNAS4 [183400]
M21140
  Human guanine nucleotide-binding protein alpha-subunit gene (G-s-alpha), exon 3
  gi|183399|gb|M21140|HUMGNAS3 [183399]
M21740
  Human guanine nucleotide-binding protein alpha-subunit gene (G-s-alpha), exon 2
  gi|183398|gb|M21740|HUMGNAS2 [183398]
M21139
  Human guanine nucleotide-binding protein alpha-subunit gene (G-s-alpha), exon 1

five families based on their kinetic and regulatory characteristics, with multiple isozymes within each family. Amino acid and cDNA sequencing identify conserved domains among the different forms of phosphodiesterase, but differences between several of the forms make it likely that these are products of separate genes. The numerous isozymes also vary in their tissue-specific distribution.[27] The number and identity of forms responsible for physiological regulation of intracellular cAMP concentration have not been unequivocally established.

cAMP-Dependent Protein Kinase and Kinase Substrates. cAMP-dependent protein kinase is a tetramer, consisting of two regulatory (cAMP-binding) and two catalytic subunits. Binding of cAMP promotes regulatory subunit dissociation and activation of catalytic subunits. At least two forms of regulatory subunits, differing in tissue distribution, have been identified, and there are likely at least two closely related forms of catalytic subunit.[45] In only a few cases have specific substrates for cAMP-dependent protein kinase been identified and functionally characterized. PTH can be shown to modulate cAMP-dependent protein kinase activity in its target organs[46] and to stimulate phosphorylation of renal brush border membrane proteins, but the structure and function of substrates for phosphorylation in kidney and bone cells have not been well characterized.

PATHOPHYSIOLOGY OF PSEUDOHYPOPARATHYROIDISM

As originally proposed by Albright,[1] defective target organ response to PTH should lead to the same consequences, hypocalcemia and hyperphosphatemia, as deficiency of the hormone (Fig. 164-1). In theory, resistance could involve either of the target organs of the hormone (kidney and bone), or both. Renal resistance to PTH would cause loss of the phosphaturic response and lead to hyperphosphatemia. The latter and/or primary resistance to PTH would lead to diminished formation of 1,25-dihydroxyvitamin D. By reducing gastrointestinal absorption of calcium, 1,25-dihydroxyvitamin D deficiency also contributes to hypocalcemia. Because the skeletal calcium-mobilizing effect of PTH is dependent on 1,25-dihydroxyvitamin D,[16] a blunted calcemic response to PTH could be caused by renal resistance to PTH with resultant reduction in 1,25-dihydroxyvitamin D formation, without invoking primary skeletal resistance to PTH. Primary skeletal resistance to PTH should cause loss of both the calcemic and bone-remodeling responses to the hormone.

Resistance to PTH action could, in theory, be due to defects at any one of the multiple steps in the pathway of hormone action. If PTH actions are mediated through second messengers other than, or in addition to, stimulation of cAMP formation (Fig. 164-2), selective lesions causing incomplete forms of PTH resistance are possible. Heterogeneity of PTH receptors, either in a given target organ or between kidney and bone, could provide another theoretical basis for selectivity in hormone resistance.

Within the cAMP pathway (Fig. 164-2), certain lesions (e.g., specific PTH receptor antagonists, abnormal receptors, abnormal substrate(s) for cAMP-dependent protein kinase) would be expected to cause isolated resistance to PTH. In contrast, defects in Gs, adenylyl cyclase, cAMP phosphodiesterase, or cAMP-dependent protein kinase could cause generalized resistance to agonists acting through the cAMP pathway.[25,47] Even for these "general" components of the cAMP transduction pathway, cDNA cloning has revealed substantial heterogeneity at the gene and/or mRNA level. Differences in range of expression and function for subtypes of each of these components have not yet been fully defined, so that it is possible that defects in one or more of these components could cause more selective forms of hormone resistance.

Genetic defects in several components of the cAMP transduction pathway have been identified in eukaryotic cells. Discrete mutations in the α subunit of Gs in mouse S49 lymphoma cells can lead to partial or total deficiency of Gs activity, to receptor uncoupling, or to failure to undergo activation by GTP.[48] Mutations in cAMP phosphodiesterase causing excessive activity in S49 cells have also been described.[49] Mutations causing deficient cAMP phosphodiesterase activity[50] and calmodulin-sensitive adenylyl cyclase activity[51] have been identified in *Drosophila*, and interestingly, both are associated with learning defects. A naturally occurring mouse mutant, barrelless, disrupts patterning of the somatosensory cortex, and was identified as an adenylyl cyclase type I mutation.[52] Mutants deficient in adenylyl cyclase activity or showing constitutive activation of cAMP-dependent protein kinase due to a regulatory subunit defect have been described in yeast,[53] whereas a catalytic subunit mutation abolishes kinase activity in S49 cells.[48] Each of these mutations causes generalized abnormalities in cellular response to extracellular signals.

Available evidence suggests that defects at different sites in the PTH response pathway are responsible for distinct forms of PHP. The majority of patients with PHP tested show a markedly lower increase in urinary cAMP excretion in response to PTH infusion than do normal controls or patients with PTH-deficient forms of hypoparathyroidism (Fig. 164-3). These data indicate that a defect (or defects) in the pathway that is proximal to cAMP generation is responsible for the majority of cases of PHP. Rarely, patients with PHP[6] show a normal rise in urinary cAMP excretion in response to PTH. Their defect is presumptively located distal to cAMP generation.

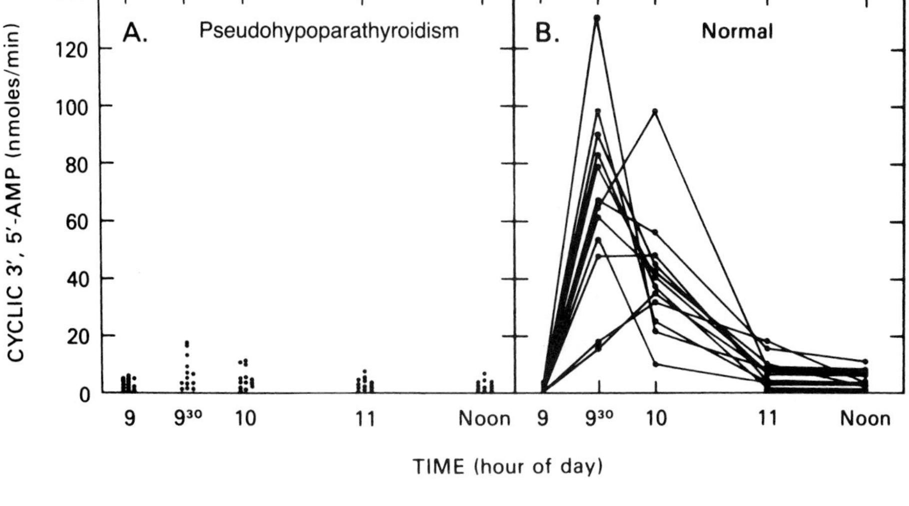

Fig. 164-3 Deficient urinary cAMP excretion in response to PTH infusion in PHP. Two hundred USP units of purified bovine PTH were infused intravenously between 9:00 and 9:15 AM. Urine was collected hourly (one-half-hourly immediately after infusion) before and after infusion for measurement of cAMP. The individual responses in a group of 13 subjects with PHP and a group of normal controls are shown. (*From Chase et al.*[5] Used by permission.)

In the sections that follow, PHP is classified according to the presumed locus of the defect that causes PTH resistance. PHP is divided into type I (defect proximal to cAMP production) and type II (defect distal to cAMP generation). PHP type I may be further subdivided into Ia (generalized hormone resistance due to a defect in a common component of the receptor-cyclase complex, such as Gs) and Ib (resistance limited to PTH). Pseudopseudohypoparathyroidism (PPHP) is the term applied to individuals who are first-degree relatives of subjects with PHP Ia and who show Gs deficiency and features of Albright osteodystrophy, but who are not overtly resistant to hormones.

Pseudohypoparathyroidism Type Ia

This is a familial form of PHP characterized by generalized resistance to agents that stimulate adenylyl cyclase and by the phenotypic features of Albright osteodystrophy. Patients with PHP Ia show a blunted rise in urinary cAMP excretion in response to PTH.[5,54] This implicates a defect in the receptor-G protein-adenylyl cyclase complex. Clinical observations compatible with resistance to hormones other than PTH suggested the possibility of a defect in a general (e.g., Gs) rather than a specific (e.g., PTH receptor) component of the complex.[25] Thus, primary hypothyroidism, particularly a subtle form detectable by thyrotropin-releasing factor stimulation of thyrotropin, is extremely common in this form of PHP.[55] Primary hypothyroidism is not associated with thyroid enlargement in these patients, nor are thyroid antibodies detectable.[55] Primary thyroid resistance to thyrotropin could explain these results. Similarly, a patient with PHP and phenotypic features of Albright osteodystrophy was reported to show resistance to gonadotropins and glucagon.[56]

Renal tissue obtained at autopsy from a woman with a familial form of PHP associated with Albright osteodystrophy showed qualitatively normal stimulation of adenylyl cyclase activity by PTH.[57] Studies of renal biopsy material from a similar patient confirmed that the PTH receptor and adenylyl cyclase were qualitatively normal, but revealed a subtle abnormality compatible with a defect in Gs.[58] Because Gs is ubiquitously distributed, the hypothesis that Gs deficiency causes generalized hormone resistance in certain patients with PHP could be tested by assays of accessible tissues rather than of relatively inaccessible PTH target organs, bone and kidney.

Two groups,[7,8] using a functional assay based on stimulation of adenylyl cyclase activity by Gs in membrane extracts and an assay based on cholera toxin-catalyzed incorporation of radioactive ADP-ribose into Gs-α, measured Gs in membranes from patients with PHP and normal controls. An approximately 50 percent reduction in Gs activity was found in red cell membranes from almost all patients with PHP and Albright osteodystrophy (Fig. 164-4), and normal activity was seen in membranes from patients with PHP lacking the physical features of Albright osteodystrophy.[7,8] Platelet,[59] fibroblast,[60,61] and lymphoblast[62] membranes from subjects with PHP and Albright osteodystrophy are also deficient in Gs activity. Renal membranes from the patient with PHP that showed a subtle defect in adenylyl cyclase stimulation[58] were also found to contain about half the Gs activity of renal membranes taken from three normal controls.[63]

Reduced Gs activity in membranes from patients with PHP, in particular those showing features of Albright osteodystrophy, has been confirmed in studies of patients in Japan[64] and Europe.[65] Gi, the G protein associated with inhibition of adenylyl cyclase (Fig. 164-2), is a gene product distinct from Gs[24] and a substrate for ADP-ribosylation by pertussis toxin. Two studies, using cholera and pertussis toxin-catalyzed ADP-ribosylation, indicate that Gs is deficient in red cell membranes from patients with PHP and Albright osteodystrophy, but that Gi concentration is normal.[66,67] Deficient Gs activity is also reflected in reduced formation of the high affinity ternary complex between agonist, receptor, and Gs in membranes from patients with PHP Ia.[68]

Deficient Gs activity in membranes from patients with PHP Ia could be due to reduced synthesis of Gs protein or to synthesis of a defective form of one of the subunits of Gs. Immunoblot analysis of cell membranes from patients with PHP Ia shows reduced Gs-α protein in most patients.[38] In most cases, reduction in amount of Gs-α protein appears to be due to reduction at the mRNA level. Blot hybridization analysis of RNA from cultured skin fibroblasts shows a significant reduction (to less than 50 percent of normal) in steady state content of Gs-α mRNA in most patients with PHP Ia.[69,70] No abnormality in mRNA size was observed; also, S-1 nuclease analysis showed that all forms of Gs-α mRNA (see above) are proportionately reduced in patients with PHP Ia.[69] Genomic blots show no gross deletions or rearrangements of the Gs-α gene in most subjects studied.[69,70] The data are compatible with subtle lesions in the gene that either reduce transcription or prevent formation of stable mRNA.

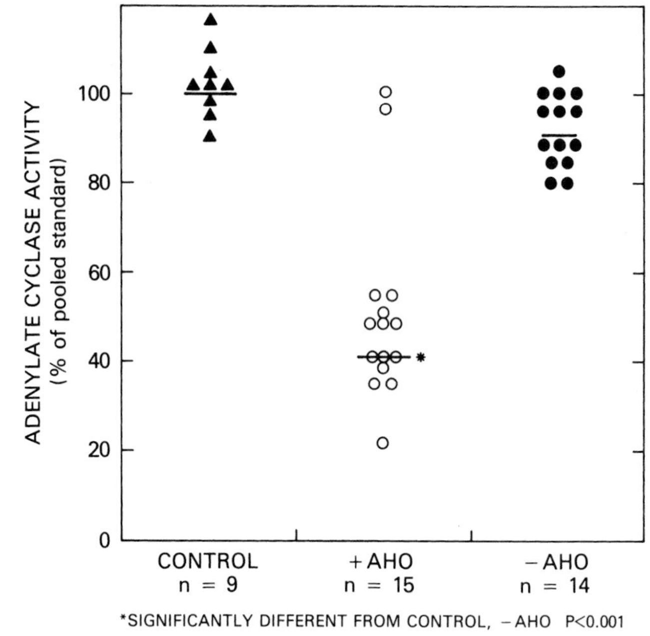

Fig. 164-4 Gs activity in erythrocyte membranes of control subjects and subjects with PHP with (+AHO) or without (−AHO) the phenotypic features of Albright hereditary osteodystrophy. Membrane extracts to be assayed for Gs activity were added to a preparation of avian erythrocyte membranes containing adenylyl cyclase. Resultant activity (referred to as "adenylate cyclase" in the figure) is a function of Gs activity in the added extract of human erythrocyte membranes. Activity is expressed as percent of the activity (defined as 100 percent) of a pooled membrane standard from normal subjects. (*From Levine et al.*[90] Used by permission.)

The genetic defect in patients with PHP Ia (and PPHP) has been confirmed by the identification of multiple heterozygous loss-of-function mutations within the *GNAS1* gene (see Table 164-1). With two exceptions (see below), each *GNAS1* mutation associated with PHP Ia and/or PPHP has been identified in a single kindred. In many cases, the mutations result in abnormal RNA processing and lack of expression of the mutant allele (i.e., base substitution at a splice junction site; coding frameshift mutations, premature stop codons, and large deletions) (see references 10, 71–82 and L.S.W., unpublished data; for an example, see Fig. 164-5). One specific 4 bp deletion within exon 7 of *GNAS1* was identified in affected members from multiple unrelated PHP Ia kindreds.[71,77–80] This deletion hotspot coincides with a consensus sequence for arrest of DNA polymerase α, and likely results from arrest of polymerization and slipped-strand mispairing during DNA replication.[78]

Missense mutations in *GNAS1* have also been identified. In some cases, the encoded amino acid substitution (L99P and R165C;[72] S250R[83]) appears to globally alter tertiary structure, or intracellular trafficking of the Gs-α protein, because in each case, the level of Gs-α mRNA is normal, but the level of membrane Gs-α

Table 164-1 *GNAS1* **Mutations in PHP Ia and PPHP**

	Systematic name*	Trivial Name†	mRNA	Protein	Comments	Reference
Exon 1	c.1A > G	M1V	NI‡	Abnormal 70K form; NI form↓	Cyc-assay↓¶	9
Exon 1	c.92C > T	N31X	ND§	↓		82
Exon 1	c.111C > G	Y37X	ND	↓		82
Exon 1/Intron 1	g.119-156del	Deletion	ND	ND	Cyc-assay ↓	81
Intron 3	IVS3-2A > G	Acceptor splice junction	ND	ND		73
Exon 4/Intron 4	c.278del43nt (including some of IVS4)	Deletion	ND	ND		75
Exon 4	c.292-294del	N98del	ND	ND		Unpublished (LSW)
Exon 4	c.296T > C	L99P	ND	↓		72
Exon 4	c.301-302del	Frameshift	↓	ND		191
Exon 5	c.343C > T	P115S	ND	ND		77
Exon 5	c.348delC	Frameshift	ND	ND	Cyc- assay ↓	74
Intron 5	IVS5+1G > A	Donor splice junction	ND	ND		76
Exon 6	c.493C > T	R165C	NI	↓		72
Exon 7	c.565-568del	Frameshift	↓	ND	Present in several kindreds; Cyc-assay ↓	71, 77–80
Exon 7	c.568T > G	Y190D	ND	ND		73
Exon 8	c.617-618del	Frameshift	ND	ND		191
Exon 8	c.640-643del	Frameshift	NI	↓		72
Exon 9	c.692G > A	R231H	ND	ND	Defective receptor-dependent signaling	86
Exon 10	c.750C > G	S250R	NI	↓	Cyc- assay ↓ ↑ GDP release ↑ GTP hydrolysis	83
Exon 10	c.772C > T	R258W	NI	↓	Cyc-assay ↓	88, 192
Exon 10	c.776A > G	E259V	ND	ND	Decreased stability and signaling	77, 193
Exon 10	c.798-799insC	Frameshift	ND	ND	Cyc- assay ↓	74
Exon 10	c.814delC	Frameshift	ND	ND		10
Intron 10	IVS10+1G > C	Donor splice junction	↓	ND		10
Exon 13	c.1096G > C	A366S	ND	ND	PHP Ia and testotoxicosis; Cyc-assay ↓ at 37°C; rapid GDP release and activation at low temp	85
Exon 13	c.1147-1149del	I383del	ND	ND		73
Exon 13	c.1154G > A	R385H	ND	Moderate ↓	Cyc-assay ↓; uncoupled from receptor	84

*Reference sequence for mutations in coding regions (denoted c.) is the Gsα-1 cDNA (GenBank accession no. SEG_HUMGNAS; reference 40), while the reference sequence for g.119-156del is the *GNAS1* genomic sequence (same accession number and reference).

†Reference sequence for assigning amino acid residues is Gsα-1 cDNA.

‡NI = normal.

§ND = not determined or not available.

¶Denotes decreased Gs bioactivity in membranes based on reconstitution assays with cyc- membranes.

protein is decreased. In one kindred, a mutation at the translational start site codon results in the expression of an abnormally large form of Gs-α protein which is presumed to be nonfunctional.[9] For several missense mutations (ΔN98, P115S, Y190D, ΔI383) the biochemical defect remains to be determined.[73,77]

Some *GNAS1* missense mutations associated with PHP Ia or PPHP produce specific biochemical defects in the Gs-α protein. One missense mutation (R385H) identified in the C-terminus region results in a specific defect in receptor coupling.[84] Another missense mutation (A366S) in a region encoding a portion of the highly conserved guanine nucleotide binding site was identified in two unrelated males who presented with Albright osteodystrophy and PTH resistance in association with gonadotropin-independent precocious puberty.[85] This mutation was shown to decrease the protein's affinity for GDP. At internal body temperature (37°C), Gs-α unbound to guanine nucleotide is unstable, leading to decreased expression of Gs-α protein and to the clinical expression of AHO and hormone resistance. At slightly lower temperatures (the ambient temperature of the testes), this mutation leads to Gs activation, increased intracellular cAMP, and gonadotropin-

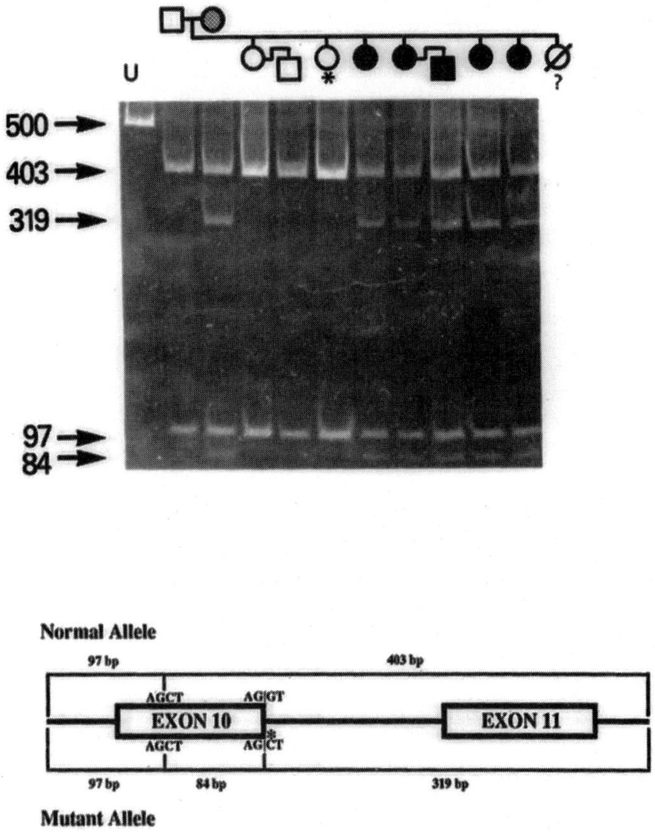

Fig. 164-5 *Upper panel:* **Pedigree of kindred with PHP Ia with *Alu I* restriction analysis of genomic DNA. The genomic fragment including exons 10 and 11 of Gs-α was amplified using the polymerase chain reaction and digested with *Alu I* restriction endonuclease. The digests were electrophoresed in a nondenaturing 5% acrylamide gel. Symbols of pedigree members with PHP are blackened and that for the member with PPHP is stippled. The asterisk denotes an unaffected member with four unaffected sons who were not analyzed. One subject who died in infancy and whose disease status is unknown is listed with a question mark. The size of the restriction fragments is depicted on the left with the 500-base pair undigested fragment shown in lane U. Unaffected members show 403- and 97-base pair fragments, whereas affected subjects show 2 additional fragments of 319 and 84 base pairs, as predicted if these individuals are heterozygous for the mutation discussed below.**

Lower panel: **Genomic fragment including exons 10 and 11 and showing *Alu I* restriction sites. The 500-base pair genomic fragment contains an *Alu I* restriction site 97 base pairs from the 5′ end within the normal sequence of exon 10, predicting 97- and 403-base pair fragments in the normal allele as shown above the diagram. As shown below the diagram a G-to-C base substitution at the donor splice junction site of intron 10 creates a new *Alu I* restriction site, which leads to 319-, 97-, and 84-base pair fragments. (*From Weinstein et al.*[10] Used by permission.)**

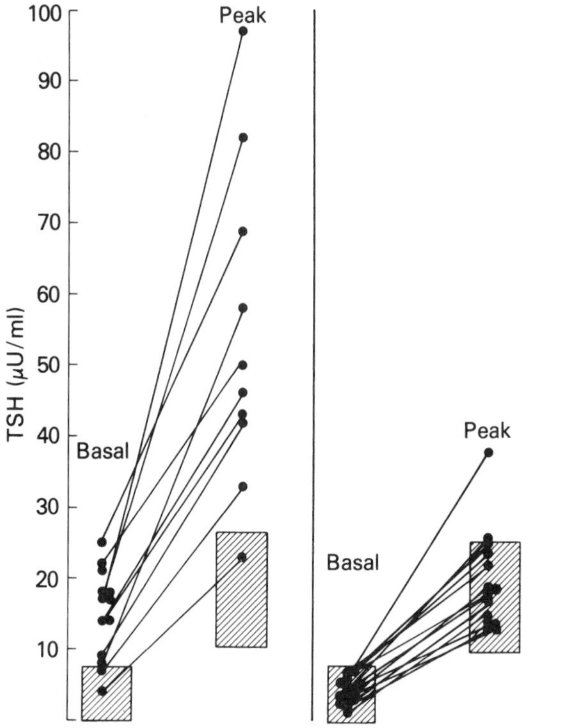

Fig. 164-6 Basal and peak serum thyrotropin (TSH) concentrations following intravenous administration of 500 μg thyrotropin-releasing factor (TRF) to subjects with PHP. The normal range for basal and peak TSH is shown in the hatched boxes. Most subjects with deficient Gs activity (left) show hyperresponsiveness to TRF, indicative of primary hypothyroidism. With one exception, subjects with PHP and normal Gs activity (right) show normal responses. (*From Levine et al.*[90] Used by permission.)

independent precocious puberty, because GDP release is normally the rate-limiting step in G protein activation. A mutation (R231H) in a region of Gs-α that undergoes a major conformational shift upon receptor-activation (switch 2 region) was shown to have a specific defect in activation by receptor or the transition state analog aluminum fluoride.[86,87] A mutation (R258W) in the switch 3 region was demonstrated to have an increased rate of GDP release.[88]

Deficient Gs activity might be expected to reduce adenylyl cyclase responsiveness to stimulation by a wide variety of agonists. Indeed, the S49 mouse lymphoma mutant CYC-, which is totally deficient in Gs activity[48] and in Gs-α mRNA,[39] fails to respond to prostaglandins and β-adrenergic agonists, potent stimulators of adenylyl cyclase activity in wild-type cells. An S49 cell mutant with partial deficiency of Gs shows reduced adenylyl cyclase stimulation by agonists.[48] Fibroblasts and platelets from patients with PHP Ia have shown reduction in agonist-stimulated cAMP formation in some,[60,89] but not all, studies.[59,61]

Impaired adenylyl cyclase stimulation due to Gs deficiency should lead to generalized resistance to agents acting via cAMP. Clinical studies of patients with PHP Ia provide evidence for resistance to hormones other than PTH. Primary thyroid resistance to thyrotropin appears to be extremely common, if not universal, in patients with PHP Ia (Fig. 164-6).[55,90] Defective adenylyl cyclase stimulation by GTP and thyrotropin in thyroid membranes obtained from a patient with PHP Ia, provides direct evidence for thyroid resistance to thyrotropin, presumably secondary to Gs deficiency, in this disease.[91] Gonadotropin,[56,90,92–94] glucagon,[56,90,95] and isoproterenol[96,97] resistance were also documented in patients with PHP Ia, particularly when proximal responses such as plasma cAMP concentration were measured. Distal responses to hormones, for example, glycemic response to glucagon,[90,95] free fatty acid response to isoproterenol,[98] and antidiuretic response to arginine vasopressin,[99] however, are often normal in patients with PHP Ia.

Olfactory dysfunction was documented by objective testing in patients with PHP Ia, but not in patients with PPHP or PHP Ib (normal Gs).[100,101] This was attributed to a possible role for Gs in transduction of odorant stimuli, but it is now likely that a unique G protein (termed G*olf,* as it is expressed primarily in olfactory neuroepithelium) is responsible for primary odorant signal transduction. Apparent olfactory dysfunction, as well as sensorineural hearing dysfunction reported in PHP Ia,[102] may actually reflect effects of neuronal Gs deficiency on higher-order signal processing rather than primary sensory impairment. The mild

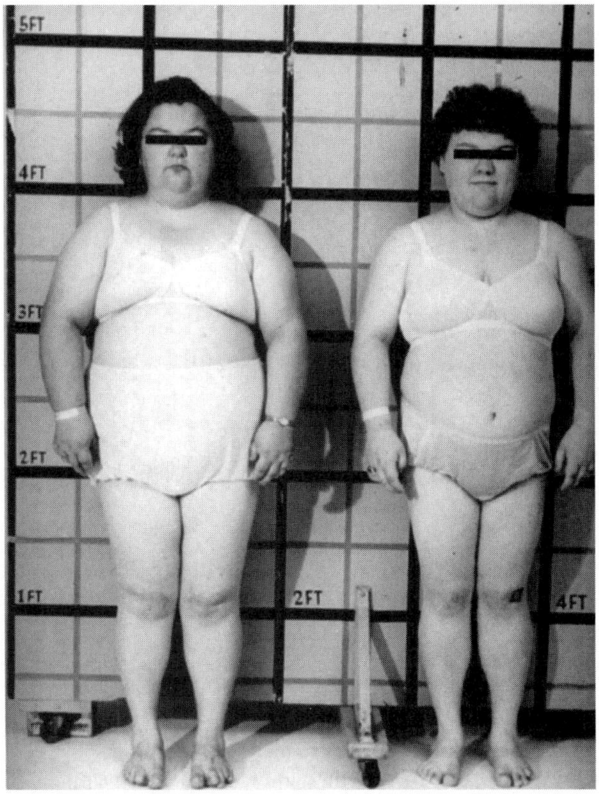

Fig. 164-7 Mother (left) and daughter with PHP Ia. Several features of Albright osteodystrophy are evident, including obesity, short stature, round face, and short neck. Short fourth and fifth fingers (particularly on the right hand of both subjects) and short fourth toes on the left feet of both subjects are due to short metacarpal and metatarsal bones, respectively.

mental retardation often seen in patients with PHP Ia[103] could also complicate interpretation of sensory testing.

While resistance to PTH, TSH, and gonadotropins is common in PHP Ia, resistance to other hormones, such as vasopressin or adrenocorticotropin, which also stimulate Gs-coupled pathways, is almost never observed in this disorder.[90,99,104] The basis for variability in clinical expression of hormone resistance in PHP Ia is unclear. Differences in the absolute concentrations of cAMP needed to achieve physiologic responses to agonists could influence the impact of Gs deficiency. One may also speculate that the degree of clinically evident hormone resistance is a function of tissue- and hormone-specific variations in the components of the cAMP signal transduction pathway. Recent data in mice suggest that the tissue-specific nature of hormone resistance in PHP Ia might be caused by tissue-specific imprinting of the gene encoding Gs-α (see section on Genetics and reference 105).

The phenotypic features of Albright osteodystrophy (Fig. 164-7) are an important component of PHP Ia, but their underlying basis is not understood. One possibility is that Gs deficiency, through limitation in cAMP formation or perhaps through some other mechanism, is the proximate cause of some or all of the features of Albright osteodystrophy. This is a plausible, but unproven, mechanism for the obesity and mental retardation often seen in patients with PHP Ia, because lipolytic factors act by stimulating cAMP formation,[97] and abnormalities in cAMP metabolism are associated with learning defects in invertebrate[51,63] and vertebrate[106] model systems. Subjects with PPHP (see below) by definition manifest some features of Albright osteodystrophy. Because such individuals are deficient in Gs, but do not show impaired cAMP formation (at least in terms of renal response to PTH), reduced cAMP formation may not be the principal cause of all features of Albright osteodystrophy. Short stature and metacarpal and metatarsal shortening are typical features of Albright osteodystrophy and may be due to premature skeletal maturation and closure of epiphyses.[107] Defects in the PTH/PTHrP receptor are also associated with premature skeletal maturation.[108] Data on growth hormone secretion in PHP Ia are limited to anecdotal reports; some suggesting normal growth hormone secretion,[104,109] others consistent with growth hormone deficiency.[93,110] The relationship of either Gs or growth hormone deficiency to the skeletal abnormalities of Albright osteodystrophy, including the soft tissue ossification and calcification (Fig. 164-8), remains unclear. Prolactin deficiency has also been reported in PHP Ia,[111–113] but the cause of this abnormality has not been elucidated.

Pseudopseudohypoparathyroidism. Since its initial description by Albright,[2] the entity PPHP has generated much confusion. In part, this stems from the relative lack of objective specificity of certain features of the Albright phenotype, including short stature, obesity, "round face," and even shortening of fourth metacarpals. Diagnosis of normocalcemic individuals with some or all of these features as having PPHP is almost certain to lead to inaccuracy; for example, patients with Turner syndrome may be included. Genetic linkage between PHP and PPHP was recognized early,[3] and reemphasized more recently.[114] The term PPHP is best restricted to relatives of patients with PHP Ia who show phenotypic features of Albright osteodystrophy and a normal rise in urinary cAMP excretion in response to PTH infusion.[5,115]

Diagnosis of PHP or PPHP based on serum calcium concentration (Albright's original criterion) may be misleading. Patients with clear-cut resistance to PTH (elevated serum PTH, blunted urinary cAMP response to PTH) may be normocalcemic.[116] Hypocalcemia is not present from birth in patients with PHP Ia; instead, it may develop during the first decade and be preceded by other signs of PTH resistance, including hyperphosphatemia and elevated serum PTH.[54,117] Serum calcium, moreover, may fluctuate between low and normal concentrations in patients with PHP.[118] Because Gs deficiency is likely present from birth, and unlikely to fluctuate during life, variations in serum calcium must reflect other factors such as 1,25-dihydroxyvitamin D synthesis. Estrogens and placental synthesis of 1,25-dihydroxyvitamin D in pregnancy are among the factors that can alter serum calcium in PHP.[119]

Within a family with PHP Ia, multiple members may show features of Albright osteodystrophy and yet show wide variation in degree of hormone resistance. Unaffected family members (no hormone resistance, no features of Albright osteodystrophy) show normal Gs activity,[115,120] and lack mutations in the Gs-α gene (Fig. 164-5).[10] Subjects with Albright osteodystrophy show similar reductions in Gs activity and identical mutations in the Gs-α gene whether (with PHP Ia) or not (with PPHP) they are overtly resistant to hormones.[9,10,63,115,121] Recent clinical genetic studies,[76,80,122] as well as studies in mice with a targeted mutation of the Gs-α gene,[105] suggest that imprinting of *GNAS1* is the likely basis for the variable presentation of patients with Albright osteodystrophy (PHP Ia vs. PPHP), although this has not been formally proven[94,123] (see "Genetics" below).

Pseudohypoparathyroidism with Albright Osteodystrophy, Generalized Hormone Resistance, and Normal Guanine Nucleotide-Binding Protein Activity

This form of PHP could be termed "Ia or Ib" depending on whether the Albright osteodystrophy phenotype or Gs activity is used for classification; PHP type "Ic" is an alternative term that has been proposed.[12] Although most patients with generalized hormone resistance and Albright osteodystrophy are deficient in Gs, several groups have reported normal Gs activity in a small number of patients with this phenotype.[65,90,120] It is possible that subtle defects in Gs in such individuals are not detected by

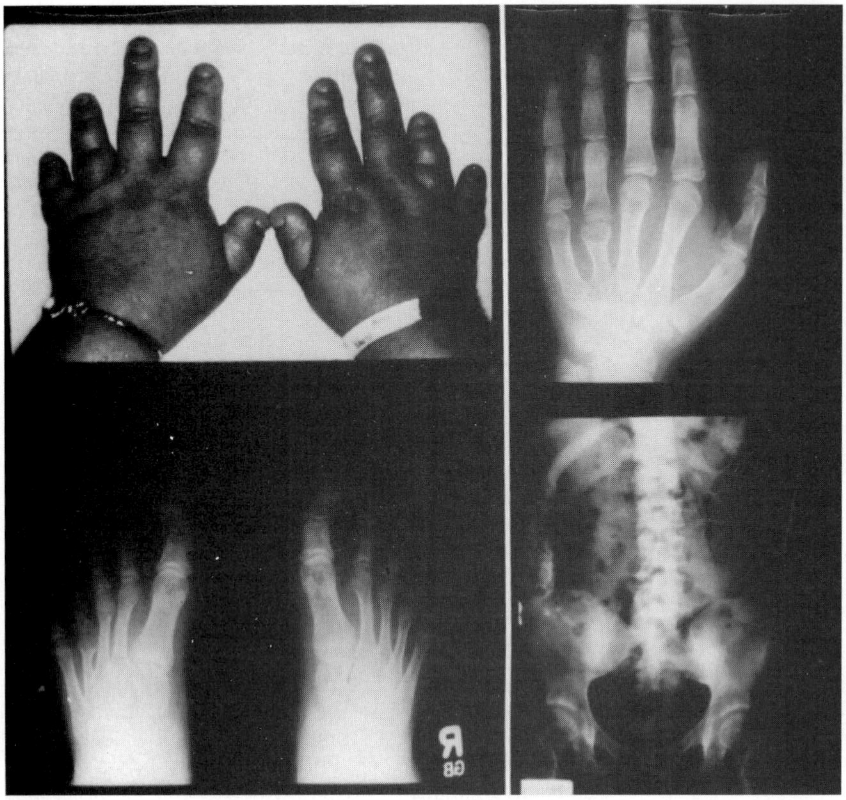

Fig. 164-8 Features of Albright osteodystrophy (clockwise from upper left) include: (a) short stubby fingers, particularly the fourth and fifth and the distal phalanx of the thumb; (b) shortening of the fourth metacarpal; (c) subcutaneous calcification, shown here in the abdominal wall (lower-right quadrant); and (d) shortening of the left fourth metatarsal on the right.

available assays, but in at least two families, such a Gs defect (receptor uncoupling) was specifically excluded.[120] Elevation in Gi, another theoretical explanation for this phenomenon, has not been observed using pertussis toxin-catalyzed ADP-ribosylation.[66] A single patient was reported with this phenotype and biochemical data compatible with an adenylyl cyclase defect.[124] With the cloning of cDNAs encoding adenylyl cyclase,[42] molecular genetic studies of such patients should be feasible. Defects in other general components of the cAMP pathway, for example, cAMP phosphodiesterase, also should be sought, as these could lead to a similar phenotype. The occurrence of Albright osteodystrophy in this form of PHP suggests the possibility that different defects in the cAMP transduction pathway could cause this phenotype, with deranged synthesis, degradation, or action of cAMP as the underlying mechanism.

Pseudohypoparathyroidism Type Ib

In this form of PHP, physical appearance is normal, resistance is limited to PTH, and Gs activity in peripheral (e.g., red blood cell) cell membranes is normal.[90,125] The presumed site of the defect in the pathway is proximal to cAMP generation, as in PHP Ia, because urinary cAMP excretion in response to PTH infusion is abnormally low.[90] The specificity of hormone resistance suggests a defect involving a unique component of the transduction mechanism. This form of PHP may itself be heterogenous, with reports of both familial[111,126] and apparently sporadic[127] cases. In one study,[127] cultured skin fibroblasts from 7 of 10 patients with PHP Ib showed selective resistance to PTH in terms of cAMP formation. The persistence of abnormal PTH response in cells cultured *in vitro* is consistent with an intrinsic abnormality in the PTH receptor, a candidate gene for PHP Ib. In a subsequent study of fibroblasts from subjects with PHP Ib, however, the reduction in cAMP response to PTH could be corrected by treatment of cells with dexamethasone and correlated with an increase in receptor mRNA after dexamethasone treatment.[128] Subsequent molecular genetic studies failed to identify mutations in the PTH receptor gene in subjects with PHP Ib.[129,130] Given the lethal phenotype of homozygous disruption of the PTH receptor gene in mice and in the human disease Blomstrand chondrodysplasia,[108] it appears unlikely that PHP Ib could be caused by homozygous loss of function mutation of the PTH receptor. However, subtler abnormalities have yet to be completely excluded.[129] An analysis of the promoter region of the PTH receptor gene revealed a general as well as a renal-specific promoter, but no specific defect in the promoter regions could be identified in seven PHP Ib subjects.[131] A defect in a renal-specific signal transduction component proximal to cAMP generation in response to PTH remains the most likely cause of PHP Ib but the identity of this component is unknown.

In common with PHP type Ia, prolactin deficiency has been reported in PHP type Ib.[111–113] Defective prolactin response to various stimuli occurs in some, but not all, patients with both PHP Ia and Ib.[90,112] Primary hypothyroidism in a family with PHP Ib[111] was associated with antithyroid antibodies, in distinction to the form of hypothyroidism associated with PHP Ia, in which antithyroid antibodies are generally not found.

Pseudohypoparathyroidism Type II

This form of PHP involves a defect distal to PTH-stimulated cAMP production. It was originally described in a child of normal appearance who was hypocalcemic and hyperphosphatemic, who showed elevated serum PTH concentration, and who had normal renal function, all consistent with PTH-resistant hypoparathyroidism.[6] Urinary cAMP response to PTH infusion, however, was completely normal, and the phosphaturic response was equivocal. Such a phenotype could be caused by a defect in a PTH and cAMP-sensitive renal phosphate transport mechanism, but this hypothesis has not been directly tested. Because the phosphaturic response to PTH is often equivocal even in normal subjects,[6] the diagnosis rests on finding clear elevations in serum PTH in association with hypocalcemia, normal renal function, and a normal urinary cAMP response to PTH infusion.

PHP type II may be an acquired disease;[132] only a single instance of familial PHP II (in two brothers) has been reported.[132] Calcium infusion may normalize the phosphaturic response to PTH in patients with PHP type II.[133] This effect is not due to suppression of endogenous PTH secretion, and may reflect calcium dependence of PTH-stimulated phosphaturia.[133] Findings compatible with PHP type II also occur in some patients with vitamin D deficiency.[132,134] Urinary cAMP excretion in response to PTH is normal in such patients, but the phosphaturic response is defective. Treatment with vitamin D restores a normal phosphaturic response.[132,134] The mechanism of vitamin D action involves more than restoration of normocalcemia, because hypocalcemic patients with PTH-deficient hypoparathyroidism show a normal phosphaturic response to PTH.

PHP type II in association with Sjögren syndrome was reported in a patient with antirenal tubular plasma membrane autoantibodies.[135] Whether such antibodies were relevant to the pathogenesis of the phosphate transport defect is not clear, but this case emphasizes that PHP type II may be an acquired defect caused by diverse mechanisms.

Parathyroid Hormone Inhibitors as a Cause of Pseudohypoparathyroidism

Potent antagonists to PTH action on its target organs could, in theory, cause PHP. Inhibitors could be abnormal forms of PTH itself or unrelated molecules, such as antibodies to PTH receptors. An abnormal form of PTH, lacking biologic activity, could not by itself account for the resistance to exogenous PTH characteristic of PHP. Thus, in cases with secretion of a putatively ineffective form of PTH, renal responsiveness to exogenous PTH was normal.[136–138] To date, there is no evidence that an altered form of PTH could function as a potent inhibitor of normal PTH action in vivo.[34] Molecular genetic analysis of the PTH gene, moreover, failed to reveal abnormalities in most families with hypoparathyroidism that were studied.[139] In one family with isolated hypoparathyroidism, a mutation in the PTH gene was found, but this involved the signal peptide-encoding region and presumptively impaired processing of preproPTH to proPTH.[140]

Using an ultrasensitive renal cytochemical assay for PTH, one group reported a dissociation between PTH biologic activity and immunoreactivity in patients with PHP type I.[141] Whereas immunoreactivity was supranormal, biologic activity was in the normal range. These results were interpreted to indicate the existence of an inhibitor of PTH action in the serum of patients with PHP type I. Another group, using the same assay, reported similar findings in vitamin D-treated patients with PHP, but observed that patients treated for nutritional vitamin D deficiency showed a similar discrepancy between immunoreactive PTH and biologic activity.[142] Reports of improved PTH responsiveness after correction of hypocalcemia with vitamin D treatment[143] or after parathyroidectomy (in one of Albright's original patients[144]) have prompted speculation that secretion of an abnormal form of PTH could lead to PTH resistance in PHP. Given the difficulty in synthesizing PTH analogues that function as potent antagonists *in vivo*,[34] it seems unlikely that secretion of an altered form of PTH could explain resistance to pharmacologic doses of exogenous PTH in patients with PHP. There is no evidence, moreover, that vitamin D treatment restores a normal urinary cAMP response to PTH in PHP. Also, the parathyroidectomized patient with PHP showed a deficient urinary cAMP response to PTH infusion even after parathyroidectomy.[5] The hypothesis remains unproven that an inhibitor of PTH action, related to PTH itself or not, could explain some cases of PHP. In any event, PTH inhibitors cannot explain the resistance to other hormones commonly seen in PHP Ia.

Skeletal Resistance to Parathyroid Hormone in Pseudohypoparathyroidism

Studies of vitamin D metabolites in patients with PHP suggest that the deficient calcemic response to PTH reflects 1,25-dihydroxyvitamin D deficiency rather than primary skeletal resistance to PTH. Bone cells isolated from two PHP patients demonstrated normal responsiveness to PTH *in vitro*.[145,146] Serum 1,25-dihydroxyvitamin D is often low in untreated patients with PHP type I, and treatment with vitamin D restores calcemic responsiveness to PTH without changing the deficient urinary cAMP response.[16,147–149] Selective deficiency of 1,25-dihydroxyvitamin D was invoked as the cause of isolated skeletal resistance to PTH in an unusual variant of PHP.[150] Deficient 1,25-dihydroxyvitamin D formation in response to PTH was directly demonstrated in patients with PHP,[151,152] and reflects renal resistance to PTH. Dibutyryl cAMP, a metabolically stable analogue, can bypass the site of resistance in PHP type I, increase 1,25-dihydroxyvitamin D formation, and correct other abnormalities secondary to renal resistance to PTH.[153–155]

The bone-remodeling response to PTH is relatively intact in many patients with PHP. Decreased bone density, increased urinary hydroxyproline excretion, and increased resorption on bone biopsy have been reported.[16,156] These findings reflect the difference in requirement for normal 1,25-dihydroxyvitamin D concentration of the remodeling, as opposed to the calcemic response to PTH. Patients with PHP may actually show rickets[157,158] or osteomalacia[148] that improves on treatment with vitamin D.

Overt osteitis fibrosa cystica is rare in PHP, but some patients with hypocalcemia, hyperphosphatemia, normal renal function, renal resistance to PTH, and skeletal manifestations of excessive PTH secretion have been reported.[159,160] These have virtually all been patients with PHP type Ib. Although subtle findings compatible with bony demineralization can be seen in patients with PHP Ia,[156] radiographically visible parathyroid bone disease is rare.[160] One group has postulated that there is a spectrum of skeletal responsiveness to PTH in PHP.[160] It is possible, though, that patients with PHP and signs of osteitis fibrosa cystica (so-called pseudohypo-hyper-parathyroidism) represent a unique variant of the disease with a distinctive pathogenesis. Potential differences in the transduction mechanisms of the skeletal calcemic and remodeling responses to PTH and in the PTH receptors of kidney and bone provide a theoretical basis for lesions that spare the bone-remodeling response to PTH. PTH hypersecretion secondary to renal resistance could then lead to the characteristic findings of osteitis fibrosa cystica.

GENETICS

Most reports on the mode of inheritance of PHP have not considered the heterogeneity of the disease. PHP type II is rarely, if ever, familial, and many cases of PHP type Ib appear to be sporadic. Small kindred size and lack of a definitive genetic marker preclude clear-cut identification of the mode of inheritance in the few reported kindreds with PHP Ib.[111,126]

The pattern of inheritance of PHP type Ia was initially considered to be X-linked dominant[3] based on a 2:1 ratio of female/male cases and a presumed lack of well-documented cases of male-to-male transmission. Kindreds with PHP Ia tend to be relatively small, perhaps in part because of impaired fertility in patients expressing the full defect, including generalized hormone resistance. Recent evidence argues in favor of autosomal dominant transmission as the most common pattern.[114,120,161] Male-to-male transmission does occur in PHP Ia;[162] in one family, father-to-son transmission of Gs deficiency was observed.[163] Gs deficiency and heterozygous mutations in the Gs-α gene (mapped to the distal long arm of chromosome 20[41]) cosegregate with phenotypic features of Albright osteodystrophy in families with PHP Ia.[9,10,12,120] Gs-deficient patients expressing the full phenotypic defect and patients with Gs deficiency, features of Albright osteodystrophy, but no overt hormone resistance (PPHP), often occur in the same family,[115,121] and show identical mutations in the Gs-α gene.[9,10,12] For example, in one family,[164] four affected sisters show Gs deficiency, Albright osteodystrophy, and generalized hormone resistance.[90] Two sisters are normal. The father was said to show PPHP based on a single, short fifth metacarpal bone.[164] Reevaluation of this kindred indicates that the mother and four affected daughters, but not the father and two unaffected daughters, show the identical mutation in the Gs-α gene[10]

(Fig. 164-5). Only one affected daughter has had a child, a son who is clinically severely affected and who shows the identical mutation. The father's fifth metacarpal abnormality is due to an old traumatic fracture, whereas the mother shows very subtle but definite (short stature, broadening of the first distal phalanx, subcutaneous calcifications) features of Albright osteodystrophy. Heterozygous mutation in the Gs-α gene alone leads to Albright osteodystrophy, but not the full phenotypic expression of PHP Ia. These observations, as well as the localization of the Gs-α gene to chromosome 20, are most consistent with an autosomal dominant mode of inheritance of Albright osteodystrophy with variable expressivity (PHP vs. PPHP).

It is proposed that genomic imprinting of the *GNAS1* gene might explain the variable phenotypes (PHP Ia vs. PPHP) associated with *GNAS1* mutations, based on the observation that maternal transmission of Albright osteodystrophy leads to offspring with PHP Ia while paternal transmission leads to PPHP.[122] This pattern of inheritance is also observed in kindreds in which *GNAS1* mutations are documented.[76,80] If the paternal *GNAS1* allele is imprinted (poorly expressed) in specific tissues, such as the proximal renal tubule, inheritance of a loss-of-function mutation from the mother should result in minimal Gs-α expression and, therefore, hormone resistance (due to imprinting of the paternal allele and mutation within the maternal allele). In contrast, inheritance of a mutation from the father should have little effect on Gs-α expression and hormone action, because the mutation is on the paternal allele, which is normally not expressed due to imprinting. This is consistent with the observed response of urinary cAMP to exogenous PTH, which is almost fully blunted in PHP Ia, but totally normal in PPHP.[115]

Direct evidence for imprinting of a Gs-α gene comes from studies in mice. The mouse homolog *Gnas* maps within a defined "imprinted" region in the distal portion of chromosome 2.[165–167] Mice with a targeted disruption of *Gnas* on the maternal allele showed evidence of renal resistance to PTH, including decreased PTH-stimulated cAMP generation and decreased Gs-α expression in isolated proximal tubules.[105] In contrast, disruption of the *Gnas* paternal allele had no effect on PTH action or Gs-α expression in proximal tubules. This is consistent with the inheritance pattern observed in humans and is consistent with imprinting of the *Gnas* paternal allele in proximal tubules. Mice with maternal and paternal inheritance of the mutation also had many other phenotypic differences, consistent with imprinting of *Gnas*.

Similar to PHP Ia patients (who have maternal inheritance of *GNAS1* mutations), mice with disruption of the *Gnas* maternal allele showed no evidence of resistance to vasopressin.[105] In mice with disruption of the maternal or paternal *Gnas* allele, Gs-α expression was equally reduced by about 50 percent in the renal inner medulla (the major site of vasopressin action), demonstrating lack of imprinting of the gene in this tissue. It is likely that lack of imprinting of *Gnas* in the inner medulla leads to the absence of vasopressin resistance in *Gnas* mutant mice, because a 50 percent defect in cAMP generation may still lead to a full physiological response.[95,98] If *GNAS1* is imprinted in humans, it is presumed to be in a tissue-specific manner, because there are no differences in Gs-α expression between PHP Ia and PPHP patients in accessible tissues.[115] As in *Gnas* knockout mice, tissue-specific imprinting of *GNAS1* could be an explanation for why PHP Ia patients demonstrate resistance to some (e.g., PTH, thyrotropin, gonadotropins) hormones, but not to others (e.g., vasopressin, adrenocorticotropin), even though all activate Gs-coupled pathways. In PHP Ia patients, PTH actions on the proximal tubule (increased 1,25 dihydroxyvitamin D synthesis, decreased phosphate reabsorption) are diminished, while PTH actions on distal portions of the nephron (increased calcium reabsorption) are maintained.[168] Imprinting of *GNAS1* in the proximal tubule, but not in more distal portions of the nephron, could explain this clinical observation.

Despite strong evidence for imprinting of the Gs-α in humans, however, molecular studies have not yet proven this.[94,123] One study which examined multiple human fetal tissues showed no evidence for monoallelic expression of Gs-α, although specific targets of hormone action were not tested.[123] A single case report describes the apparent expression of PHP type Ia in an infant in which Gs deficiency was inherited from his father.[169] The diagnosis was based on a blunted cAMP response to exogenous PTH. Baseline calcium, phosphorus, and PTH, as well as thyroid function tests, however, were all normal, making the diagnosis of PHP type Ia somewhat equivocal.

There may be additional genetic heterogeneity within the PHP Ia subtype. A family originally reported to show autosomal recessive inheritance of Albright osteodystrophy and hormone resistance[170] was restudied in terms of Gs assay, and was shown to inherit Gs deficiency in an autosomal recessive manner.[120] Further work is needed to identify other potential lesions in signal transduction components in kindreds with PHP Ia.

CLINICAL FEATURES

The clinical features of PHP may be divided into those that are common to all patients with hypoparathyroidism and those that are unique to different subtypes of PHP. The former include the characteristic chemical findings of hypoparathyroidism, hypocalcemia, and hyperphosphatemia with normal renal function; symptoms of neuromuscular irritability secondary to hypocalcemia, such as paresthesias, tetany, seizures, and prolonged QT interval on electrocardiogram; dental defects, such as enamel hypoplasia and failure of teeth to erupt, particularly in patients with onset of disease in childhood; cataracts; and basal ganglion calcification.[171,172] As noted earlier, hypocalcemia may not be evident immediately after birth in PHP Ia but may develop later in the first decade.[117] Patients with PHP type Ib may show unique clinical features, such as overt skeletal demineralization, even osteitis fibrosa cystica, which are not found in patients with hormone-deficient hypoparathyroidism.[160]

In addition to the findings common to all forms of hypoparathyroidism, patients with PHP type Ia show clinical features of Albright osteodystrophy (Fig. 164-8) and generalized hormone resistance. The features of Albright osteodystrophy include short stature (usually first evident in late childhood[107]), obesity, mental retardation,[103] subcutaneous ossification,[173] and a number of bony abnormalities, most commonly metacarpal and metatarsal shortening.[174,175] The expression of the bony abnormalities is often asymmetric and variable, even within the same family. The fourth and fifth metacarpals are most commonly short; the second metacarpal is least commonly short. Shortening of distal phalanges, particularly relative to increased width, is another common finding.[175] Patients without hypocalcemia and hyperphosphatemia may show all these features, including subcutaneous ossification. This suggests that the features are not directly caused by abnormal calcium homeostasis.

Clinical features of generalized hormone resistance are also unique to PHP Ia. These include primary hypogonadism and chemical or overt hypothyroidism. Screening for congenital hypothyroidism has led to the diagnosis of PHP Ia in several cases.[176–178] These cases emphasize that resistance to thyrotropin may be clinically evident before resistance to PTH in patients with PHP Ia. In several of these cases, hypocalcemia developed only after clinically apparent hypothyroidism. These cases also raise the question of whether mental retardation in PHP Ia is due to congenital hypothyroidism. This appears unlikely, because patients may show mental retardation unassociated with overt hypothyroidism, but further studies of the contribution of hypothyroidism, as well as seizures secondary to untreated hypocalcemia, to the mental retardation seen in PHP Ia are needed.

DIAGNOSIS

Hypocalcemia, hyperphosphatemia, and normal renal function establish the diagnosis of hypoparathyroidism. Other causes of hypocalcemia are generally associated with low or normal serum phosphorus with the exception of renal failure, where renal function is obviously abnormal.[12] Distinction between hormone-deficient and hormone-resistant forms of hypoparathyroidism in patients with hypocalcemia depends primarily on immunoassay of PTH in plasma. In theory, patients could show elevated plasma immunoreactive PTH without being resistant to PTH, for example, biologically inactive PTH,[136–138] but this is rare. Increased plasma-immunoreactive PTH in a patient with hypocalcemia, hyperphosphatemia, and normal renal function is generally diagnostic for PHP. Testing responsiveness to exogenous PTH can confirm this diagnosis and distinguish between PHP types I and II. In the former, the urinary cAMP response to PTH is deficient; in the latter, it is normal. The phosphaturic response to PTH is deficient in both PHP type I and type II, but this response may be equivocal even in normal subjects. A deficient rise in plasma 1,25-dihydroxyvitamin D in response to PTH in PHP type I also permits distinction from hormone-deficient hypoparathyroidism; this test has not been evaluated in subjects with PHP type II.[179]

The features of Albright osteodystrophy and evidence of resistance to hormones other than PTH help distinguish PHP Ia from PHP Ib. Gs measurement also distinguishes between these two subtypes of PHP I, but this test is performed in only a few laboratories. No simple genetic test is available for diagnosis of PHP Ia, because different mutations in *GNAS1* were found in most families studied to date. Patients with PHP Ia, as discussed earlier, may present with signs of other endocrinopathies, for example, hypothyroidism,[176–178] rather than hypocalcemia. Phenotypic features of Albright osteodystrophy and blunted urinary cAMP response to PTH infusion (even when patients are normocalcemic) may still permit diagnosis of PHP Ia in patients presenting with other endocrinopathies.

Relatives of patients with PHP Ia may also show features of Albright osteodystrophy without overt signs of hormone resistance and with relatively normal urinary cAMP response to PTH infusion (PPHP). The diagnosis of PPHP should not be made indiscriminately. Isolated shortening of the fourth metacarpal is a relatively nonspecific finding, insufficient by itself for a diagnosis of Albright osteodystrophy.[180] A variety of familial disorders share certain features in common with PHP Ia, but, in general, are readily distinguished from it. Soft tissue ossification is present in myositis ossificans but differs in location (muscle) from that in PHP Ia (subcutaneous). The pattern of metacarpal shortening differs in PHP Ia and in Turner syndrome,[175] and the latter is not associated with resistance to PTH. Acrodysostosis is an apparently sporadic syndrome with metacarpal abnormalities similar to those of Albright osteodystrophy.[175] Nasal hypoplasia may be a distinctive feature of acrodysostosis, but this finding was present in at least one patient with other features characteristic of PHP Ia.[181] Thus, the distinction between acrodysostosis and PHP Ia may not be clear-cut. In a study of two unrelated patients with acrodysostosis, neither deficient red cell membrane Gs bioactivity nor mutation in the Gs-α gene was found.[182]

The Kenney-Caffey syndrome is associated with short stature, hypocalcemia, and bony anomalies, but unlike PHP Ia, hypocalcemia in the Kenney-Caffey syndrome is of the PTH-deficient type, skeletal involvement consists of medullary stenosis of the long bones, and there are distinctive ophthalmologic abnormalities.[183] Several types of familial brachydactyly show metacarpal abnormalities said to be similar, and in some instances identical, to those in Albright osteodystrophy.[175,184] The suggestion that familial brachydactyly and PHP Ia represent variable expressions of the same genetic defect is interesting but unproven. A report of the coexistence of brachydactyly D and PHP in the same family[184] lacked conclusive evidence to support a diagnosis of PHP. Definition of the relationship between PHP Ia and familial brachydactyly requires analysis of the molecular genetic defect in the latter. A deletion localized to 2q37 was identified in patients with brachydactyly and mental retardation, suggesting that genes important for skeletal and neurodevelopment are located in this region.[185,186]

TREATMENT

Treatment of hypocalcemia associated with PHP is generally similar to treatment of other forms of hypoparathyroidism.[12] Chronic therapy with vitamin D, ergocalciferol, or one of its more active metabolites, such as 1,25-dihydroxyvitamin D, should be given in an effort to maintain the patient free of symptoms of tetany and to prevent cataract formation. The serum calcium should be maintained at least in the low-normal range. There is some evidence that high levels of PTH coupled with relatively greater renal than skeletal resistance to PTH can lead to bony demineralization in PHP.[187] This may justify efforts to give sufficient vitamin D to maintain serum calcium in the high-normal range, thereby suppressing high PTH levels. In contrast to PTH-deficient forms of hypoparathyroidism, correction of hypocalcemia in patients with PHP type Ia does not typically lead to hypercalciuria.[187–189] Oral calcium supplements in addition to vitamin D may be useful, but depending on dietary calcium intake, may not be essential. Vitamin D therapy and correction of hypocalcemia generally cause lowering of serum phosphorus. Acetazolamide causes phosphaturia and lowering of serum phosphorus in patients with PHP.[190] Treatment with acetazolamide could lessen requirements for vitamin D, but this probably does not justify adding this agent to the treatment regimen. Patients receiving vitamin D treatment must be closely monitored (including measurement of urinary calcium excretion) to avoid under- or overtreatment. The latter can lead to hypercalcemia and renal damage. Compliance, particularly in patients with subnormal intelligence, must be ensured. Treatment with vitamin D is less expensive than with 1,25-dihydroxyvitamin D, and for this reason may be preferred for chronic use. 1,25-Dihydroxyvitamin D has the theoretical advantage of more rapid onset of action (and more rapid offset in the event of intoxication), but treatment with vitamin D can achieve control of serum calcium at least as adequate as that with 1,25-dihydroxyvitamin D. With vitamin D treatment, serum 25-hydroxyvitamin D can be used to monitor compliance, whereas with 1,25-dihydroxyvitamin D, serum 1,25-dihydroxyvitamin D must be measured.

In patients with PHP Ia, treatment of associated endocrinopathies, in particular hypothyroidism, may be needed. Some patients with hypogonadism may require sex steroid treatment.

ADDENDUM

Recently the *GNASI* gene was shown to have two alternative promoters generating transcripts encoding the proteins NESP55 and XLα that are imprinted in an opposite manner.[194–196]

PHP Ib was mapped in four families to 20q13, in the vicinity of *GNASI*, and in these families PTH resistance was only evident when the trait was inherited from the mother, suggesting that PHP Ib might be asociated with a defect involving *GNASI*.[197]

REFERENCES

1. Albright F, Burnett CH, Smith PH, et al: Pseudohypoparathyroidism: An example of "Seabright-Bantam syndrome." *Endocrinology* **30**:922, 1942.
2. Albright F, Forbes AP, Henneman PH: Pseudopseudohypoparathyroidism. *Trans Assoc Am Physicians* **65**:337, 1952.
3. Mann JB, Alterman S, Hills AG: Albright's hereditary osteodystrophy comprising pseudohypoparathyroidism and pseudopseudohypoparathyroidism. *Ann Intern Med* **56**:315, 1962.
4. Tashjian AH Jr, Frantz AG, Lee JB: Pseudohypoparathyroidism: assays of parathyroid hormone and thyrocalcitonin. *Proc Natl Acad Sci U S A* **56**:1138, 1966.
5. Chase LR, Melson GL, Aurbach GD: Pseudohypoparathyroidism: defective excretion of 3′,5′-AMP in response to parathyroid hormone. *J Clin Invest* **48**:1832, 1969.

6. Drezner M, Neelon FA, Lebovitz HE: Pseudohypoparathyroidism type II: A possible defect in the reception of the cyclic AMP signal. *N Engl J Med* **289**:1056, 1973.
7. Levine MA, Downs RW Jr, Singer M, et al: Deficient activity of guanine nucleotide regulatory protein in erythrocytes from patients with pseudohypoparathyroidism. *Biochem Biophys Res Commun* **94**:1319, 1980.
8. Farfel Z, Brickman AS, Kaslow HR, et al: Defect of receptor-cyclase coupling protein in pseudohypoparathyroidism. *N Engl J Med* **303**:237, 1980.
9. Patten JL, Johns DR, Valle D, et al: Mutation in the gene encoding the stimulatory G protein of adenylate cyclase in Albright's hereditary osteodystrophy. *N Engl J Med* **322**:1412, 1990.
10. Weinstein LS, Gejman PV, Friedman E, et al: Mutations of the Gs α-subunit gene in Albright hereditary osteodystrophy detected by denaturing gradient gel electrophoresis. *Proc Natl Acad Sci U S A* **87**:8287, 1990.
11. Vasicek TJ, McDevitt BE, Freeman MW, et al: Nucleotide sequence of the human parathyroid hormone gene. *Proc Natl Acad Sci U S A* **80**:2127, 1983.
12. Weinstein LS. Albright hereditary osteodystrophy, pseudohypoparathyroidism, and Gs deficiency, in Spiegel, AM (ed): *G Proteins, Receptors, and Disease*. Totowa, NJ: Humana Press, 1998, pp 23–56.
13. Rodan GA, Rodan SB: Hormone-adenylate cyclase coupling in osteosarcoma clonal cell lines. *Adv Cyclic Nucleotide Protein Phosphorylation Res* **17**:127, 1984.
14. Jilka RL: Are osteoblastic cells required for the control of osteoclast activity by parathyroid hormone. *Bone Miner* **1**:261, 1986.
15. Howard GA, Bottemiller BL, Turner RT, et al: Parathyroid hormone stimulates bone formation and resorption in organ culture: Evidence for a coupling mechanism. *Proc Natl Acad Sci U S A* **78**:3204, 1981.
16. Drezner MK, Neelon FA, Haussler M, et al: 1,25-dihydroxycholecalciferol deficiency: The probable cause of hypocalcemia and metabolic bone disease in pseudohypoparathyroidism. *J Clin Endocrinol Metab* **42**:621, 1976.
17. Lewin IG, Papapoulos SE, Tomlinson S, et al: Studies of hypoparathyroidism and pseudohypoparathyroidism. *Q J Med* **47**:533, 1978.
18. Caverzasio J, Rizzoli R, Bonjour JP: Sodium-dependent phosphate transport inhibited by parathyroid hormone and cyclic AMP stimulation in an opossum kidney cell line. *J Biol Chem* **261**:3233, 1986.
19. Shigematsu T, Horiuchi N, Ogura Y, et al: Human parathyroid hormone inhibits renal 24-hydroxylase activity of 25-hydroxyvitamin D3 by a mechanism involving adenosine 3′,5′-monophosphate in rats. *Endocrinology* **118**:1583, 1986.
20. Puschett JB: Are all of the renal tubular actions of parathyroid hormone mediated by the adenylate cyclase system. *Miner Electrolyte Metab* **7**:281, 1982.
21. Peck WA: Cyclic AMP as a second messenger in the skeletal actions of parathyroid hormone: A decade-old hypothesis. *Calcif Tissue Int* **29**:1, 1979.
22. Löwik CWGM, van Leeuwen JPTM, van der Meer JM, et al: A two-receptor model for the action of parathyroid hormone on osteoblasts: A role for intracellular free calcium and cAMP. *Cell Calcium* **6**:311, 1985.
23. Cosman F, Morrow B, Kopal M, et al: Stimulation of inositol phosphate formation in ROS 17/2.8 cell membranes by guanine nucleotide, calcium, and parathyroid hormone. *J Bone Miner Res* **4**:413, 1989.
24. Spiegel AM, Jones TLZ, Simonds WF, Weinstein LS. G Proteins. Austin, TX: RG Landes, 1994.
25. Spiegel AM, Gierschik P, Levine MA, et al: Clinical implications of guanine nucleotide-binding proteins as receptor-effector couplers. *N Engl J Med* **312**:26, 1985.
26. Tang W-J, Gilman AG: Type-specific regulation of adenylyl cyclase by G protein $\beta\gamma$ subunits. *Science* **254**:1500, 1991.
27. Nicholson CD, Chaliss RAJ, Shahid M: Differential modulation of tissue function and therapeutic potential of selective inhibitors of cyclic nucleotide phosphodiesterase isoenzymes. *Trends Pharmacol Sci* **12**:19, 1991.
28. Conti M, Jin S-LC, Monaco L, et al: Hormonal regulation of cyclic nucleotide phosphodiesterases. *Endocrine Rev* **12**:218, 1991.
29. Jüppner H, Abou-Samra A-B, Freeman M, et al: A G protein-linked receptor for parathyroid hormone and parathyroid hormone-related peptide. *Science* **254**:1024, 1991.
30. Dohlman HG, Thorner J, Caron MG, et al: Model systems for the study of seven-transmembrane-segment receptors. *Annu Rev Biochem* **60**:653, 1991.
31. Usdin TB, Gruber C, Bonner TI: Identification and functional expression of a receptor selectively recognizing parathyroid hormone, the PTH2 receptor. *J Biol Chem* **270**:15455, 1995.
32. Demay M, Mitchell J, Goltzman D: Comparison of renal and osseous binding of parathyroid hormone and hormonal fragments. *Am J Physiol* **249**:E437, 1985.
33. Martin KJ, Bellorin-Font E, Morrissey JJ, et al: Relative sensitivity of kidney and bone to the amino-terminal fragment b-PTH (1-30) of native bovine parathyroid hormone: Implications for assessment of bioactivity of parathyroid hormone fragments in vivo and in vitro. *Calcif Tissue Int* **35**:520, 1983.
34. Horiuchi N, Rosenblatt M, Keutmann HT, et al: A multiresponse parathyroid hormone assay: An inhibitor has agonist properties in vivo. *Am J Physiol* **244**:E589, 1983.
35. Goldring SR, Tyler GA, Krane SM, et al: Photoaffinity labeling of parathyroid hormone receptors: Comparison of receptors across species and target tissues and after desensitization to hormone. *Biochemistry* **23**:498, 1984.
36. Weinstein LS, Shenker A, Gejman PV, et al: Activating mutations of the stimulatory G protein in the McCune-Albright syndrome. *N Engl J Med* **325**:1688, 1991.
37. Spiegel AM, Simonds WF, Jones TL, et al: Antibodies against synthetic peptides as probes of G protein structure and function. *Soc Gen Physiol Ser* **45**:185, 1990.
38. Patten JL, Levine MA: Immunochemical analysis of the α-subunit of the stimulatory G-protein of adenylyl cyclase in patients with Albright's hereditary osteodystrophy. *J Clin Endocrinol Metab* **71**:1208, 1990.
39. Bray P, Carter A, Simons C, et al: Human cDNA clones for four species of Gαs signal transduction protein. *Proc Natl Acad Sci U S A* **83**:8893, 1986.
40. Kozasa T, Itoh H, Tsukamoto T, et al: Isolation and characterization of the human Gs α gene. *Proc Natl Acad Sci U S A* **85**:2081, 1988.
41. Gejman PV, Weinstein LS, Martinez M, et al: Genetic mapping of the Gs-α subunit gene (*GNAS1*) to the distal long arm of chromosome 20 using a polymorphism detected by denaturing gradient gel electrophoresis. *Genomics* **9**:782, 1991.
42. Krupinski J, Coussen F, Bakalyar HA, et al: Adenylyl cyclase amino acid sequence: Possible channel- or transporter-like structure. *Science* **244**:1558, 1989.
43. Taussig R, Gilman AG: Mammalian membrane-bound adenylyl cyclases. *J Biol Chem* **270**:1, 1995.
44. Charbonneau H, Beier N, Walsh KA, et al: Identification of a conserved domain among cyclic nucleotide phosphodiesterases from diverse species. *Proc Natl Acad Sci U S A* **83**:9308, 1986.
45. Adavani SR, Schwarz M, Showers MO, et al: Multiple mRNA species code for the catalytic subunit of the cAMP-dependent protein kinase from LLC-PK1 cells. Evidence for two forms of the catalytic subunit. *Eur J Biochem* **167**:221, 1987.
46. Ausiello DA, Rosenblatt M, Dayer JM: Parathyroid hormone modulates protein kinase in giant cell tumors of human bone. *Am J Physiol* **239**:E144, 1980.
47. Spiegel AM: Albright's hereditary osteodystrophy and defective G proteins. *N Engl J Med* **322**:1461, 1990.
48. Farfel Z, Salomon MR, Bourne HR: Genetic investigation of adenylate cyclase: Mutations in mouse and man. *Annu Rev Pharmacol Toxicol* **21**:251, 1981.
49. Brothers VM, Walker N, Bourne HR: Increased cyclic nucleotide phosphodiesterase activity in a mutant S49 lymphoma cell. Characterization and comparison with wild-type enzyme activity. *J Biol Chem* **257**:9349, 1982.
50. Chen CN, Denome S, Davis RL: Molecular analysis of cDNA clones and the corresponding genomic coding sequences of the Drosophila dunce+ gene, the structural gene for cAMP phosphodiesterase. *Proc Natl Acad Sci U S A* **83**:9313, 1986.
51. Levin LR, Han P-L, Hwang PM, et al: The *Drosophila* learning and memory gene *rutabaga* encodes a Ca^{2+}/calmodulin-responsive adenylyl cyclase. *Cell* **68**:479, 1992.
52. Abdel-Majid RM, Leong WL, Schallkwyk LC, et al: Loss of adenylyl cyclase I activity disrupts patterning of mouse somatosensory cortex. *Nat Genet* **19**:289, 1998.
53. Matsumoto K, Uno I, Oshima Y, et al: Isolation and characterization of yeast mutants deficient in adenylate cyclase and cAMP-dependent protein kinase. *Proc Natl Acad Sci U S A* **79**:2355, 1982.
54. Werder EA, Fischer JA, Illig R, et al: Pseudohypoparathyroidism and idiopathic hypoparathyroidism: Relationship between serum calcium and parathyroid hormone levels and urinary cyclic adenosine-3′,5′-

monophosphate response to parathyroid extract. *J Clin Endocrinol Metab* **46**:872, 1978.

55. Werder EA, Illig R, Bernasconi S, et al: Excessive thyrotropin response to thyrotropin-releasing hormone in pseudohypoparathyroidism. *Pediatr Res* **9**:12, 1975.
56. Wolfsdorf JI, Rosenfield RL, Fang VS, et al: Partial gonadotrophin-resistance in pseudohypoparathyroidism. *Acta Endocrinol (Copenh)* **88**:321, 1978.
57. Marcus R, Wilber JF, Aurbach GD: Parathyroid hormone-sensitive adenyl cyclase from the renal cortex of a patient with pseudohypoparathyroidism. *J Clin Endocrinol Metab* **33**:537, 1971.
58. Drezner MK, Burch WM Jr: Altered activity of the nucleotide regulatory site in the parathyroid hormone-sensitive adenylate cyclase from the renal cortex of a patient with pseudohypoparathyroidism. *J Clin Invest* **62**:1222, 1978.
59. Farfel Z, Bourne HR: Deficient activity of receptor-cyclase coupling protein in platelets of patients with pseudohypoparathyroidism. *J Clin Endocrinol Metab* **51**:1202, 1980.
60. Levine MA, Eil C, Downs RW Jr, et al: Deficient guanine nucleotide regulatory unit activity in cultured fibroblast membranes from patients with pseudohypoparathyroidism type I. A cause of impaired synthesis of 3′,5′-cyclic AMP by intact and broken cells. *J Clin Invest* **72**:316, 1983.
61. Bourne HR, Kaslow HR, Brickman AS, et al: Fibroblast defect in pseudohypoparathyroidism, type I: Reduced activity of receptor-cyclase coupling protein. *J Clin Endocrinol Metab* **53**:636, 1981.
62. Farfel Z, Abood ME, Brickman AS, et al: Deficient activity of receptor-cyclase coupling protein in transformed lymphoblasts of patients with pseudohypoparathyroidism type I. *J Clin Endocrinol Metab* **55**:113, 1982.
63. Downs RW Jr, Levine MA, Drezner MK, et al: Deficient adenylate cyclase regulatory protein in renal membranes from a patient with pseudohypoparathyroidism. *J Clin Invest* **71**:231, 1983.
64. Saito T, Akita Y, Fujita H, et al: Stimulatory guanine nucleotide binding protein activity in the erythrocyte membrane of patients with pseudohypoparathyroidism type I and related disorders. *Acta Endocrinol (Copenh)* **111**:507, 1986.
65. Radeke HH, Auf'mkolk B, Jüppner H, et al: Multiple pre- and postreceptor defects in pseudohypoparathyroidism (a multicenter study with twenty-four patients). *J Clin Endocrinol Metab* **62**:393, 1986.
66. Downs RW, Sekura RD, Levine MA, et al: The inhibitory adenylate cyclase coupling protein in pseudohypoparathyroidism. *J Clin Endocrinol Metab* **61**:351, 1985.
67. Akita Y, Saito T, Yajima Y, et al: The stimulatory and inhibitory guanine nucleotide-binding proteins of adenylate cyclase in erythrocytes from patients with pseudohypoparathyroidism type I. *J Clin Endocrinol Metab* **61**:1012, 1985.
68. Heinsimer JA, Davies AO, Downs RW, et al: Impaired formation of beta-adrenergic receptor-nucleotide regulatory protein complexes in pseudohypoparathyroidism. *J Clin Invest* **73**:1335, 1984.
69. Carter A, Bardin C, Collins R, et al: Reduced expression of multiple forms of the α subunit of the stimulatory GTP-binding protein in pseudohypoparathyroidism type Ia. *Proc Natl Acad Sci U S A* **84**:7266, 1987.
70. Levine MA, Ahn TG, Klupt SF, et al: Genetic deficiency of the α subunit of the guanine nucleotide-binding protein Gs as the molecular basis for Albright hereditary osteodystrophy. *Proc Natl Acad Sci U S A* **85**:617, 1988.
71. Weinstein LS, Gejman PV, De Mazancourt P, et al: A heterozygous 4-bp deletion mutation in the $G_s\alpha$ gene (*GNAS1*) in a patient with Albright hereditary osteodystrophy. *Genomics* **13**:1319, 1992.
72. Miric A, Vechio JD, Levine MA: Heterogeneous mutations in the gene encoding the α subunit of the stimulatory G protein of adenylyl cyclase in Albright hereditary osteodystrophy. *J Clin Endocrinol Metab* **76**:1560, 1993.
73. Ringel MD, Schwindinger WF, Levine MA: Clinical implications of genetic defects in G proteins. The molecular basis of McCune-Albright syndrome and Albright hereditary osteodystrophy. *Medicine (Baltimore)* **75**:171, 1996.
74. Shapira H, Mouallem M, Shapiro MS, et al: Pseudohypoparathyroidism type Ia: Two new heterozygous frameshift mutations in exons 5 and 10 of the Gs α gene. *Hum Genet* **97**:73, 1996.
75. Oude Luttikhuis MEM, Wilson LC, Leonard JV, et al: Characterization of a *de novo* 43-bp deletion of the Gsα gene (*GNAS1*) in Albright hereditary osteodystrophy. *Genomics* **21**:455, 1994.
76. Wilson LC, Oude Luttikhuis ME, Clayton PT, et al: Parental origin of Gs α gene mutations in Albright's hereditary osteodystrophy. *J Med Genet* **31**:835, 1994.
77. Ahmed SF, Dixon PH, Bonthron DT, et al: *GNAS1* Mutational analysis in pseudohypoparathyroidism. *Clin Endocrinol* (oxf) **49**:525, 1998.
78. Yu S, Yu D, Hainline BE, et al: A deletion hot-spot in exon 7 of the $G_s\alpha$ gene (*GNAS1*) in patients with Albright hereditary osteodystrophy. *Hum Mol Genet* **4**:2001, 1995.
79. Yokoyama M, Takeda K, Iyota K, et al: A 4-base pair deletion mutation of Gs α gene in a Japanese patient with pseudohypoparathyroidism. *J Endocrinol Invest* **19**:236, 1996.
80. Nakamoto JM, Sandstrom AT, Brickman AS, et al: Pseudohypoparathyroidism type Ia from maternal but not paternal transmission of a Gsα gene mutation. *Am J Med Genet* **77**:261, 1998.
81. Fischer JA, Egert F, Werder E, et al: An inherited mutation associated with functional deficiency of the α-subunit of the guanine nucleotide-binding protein Gs in pseudo- and pseudopseudohypoparathyroidism. *J Clin Endocrinol Metab* **83**:935, 1998.
82. Jan de Beur SM, Deng Z, Ding C, et al: Amplification of the GC-rich exon 1 of GNAS1 and identification of three novel nonsense mutations in Albright's hereditary osteodystrophy [Abstr.]. *Program and Abstracts of the 80th Annual Meeting of the Endocrine Society* 62, 1998.
83. Warner DR, Gejman PV, Collins RM, et al: A novel mutation adjacent to the switch III domain of *Gsα* in a patient with pseudohypoparathyroidism. *Mol Endocrinol* **11**:1718, 1997.
84. Schwindinger WF, Miric A, Zimmerman D, et al: A novel Gsα mutant in a patient with Albright hereditary osteodystrophy uncouples cell surface receptors from adenylyl cyclase. *J Biol Chem* **269**:25387, 1994.
85. Iiri T, Herzmark P, Nakamoto JM, et al: Rapid GDP release from Gs-α in patients with gain and loss of endocrine function. *Nature* **371**:164, 1994.
86. Farfel Z, Iiri T, Shapira H, et al: Pseudohypoparathyroidism, a novel mutation in the βγ-contact region of Gsα impairs receptor stimulation. *J Biol Chem* **271**:19653, 1996.
87. Iiri T, Farfel Z, Bourne HR: Conditional activation defect of a human Gsα mutant. *Proc Natl Acad Sci U S A* **94**:5656, 1997.
88. Warner DR, Weng G, Yu S, et al: A novel mutation in the switch 3 region of Gsα in a patient with Albright hereditary osteodystrophy impairs GDP binding and receptor activation. *J Biol Chem* **273**:23976 1998.
89. Motulsky HJ, Hughes RJ, Brickman AS, et al: Platelets of pseudohypoparathyroid patients: Evidence that distinct receptor-cyclase coupling proteins mediate stimulation and inhibition of adenylate cyclase. *Proc Natl Acad Sci U S A* **79**:4193, 1982.
90. Levine MA, Downs RW Jr, Moses AM, et al: Resistance to multiple hormones in patients with pseudohypoparathyroidism. Association with deficient activity of guanine nucleotide regulatory protein. *Am J Med* **74**:545, 1983.
91. Mallet E, Carayon P, Amr S, et al: Coupling defect of thyrotropin receptor and adenylate cyclase in a pseudohypoparathyroid patient. *J Clin Endocrinol Metab* **54**:1028, 1982.
92. Shapiro MS, Bernheim J, Gutman A, et al: Multiple abnormalities of anterior pituitary hormone secretion in association with pseudohypoparathyroidism. *J Clin Endocrinol Metab* **51**:483, 1980.
93. Shima M, Nose O, Shimizu K, et al: Multiple associated endocrine abnormalities in a patient with pseudohypoparathyroidism type 1a. *Eur J Pediatr* **147**:536, 1988.
94. Namnoum AB, Merriam GR, Moses AM, et al: Reproductive dysfunction in women with Albright's hereditary osteodystrophy. *J Clin Endocrinol Metab* **83**:824, 1998.
95. Brickman AS, Carlson HE, Levin SR: Responses to glucagon infusion in pseudohypoparathyroidism. *J Clin Endocrinol Metab* **63**:1354, 1986.
96. Carlson HE, Brickman AS: Blunted plasma cyclic adenosine monophosphate response to isoproterenol in pseudohypoparathyroidism. *J Clin Endocrinol Metab* **56**:1323, 1983.
97. Kaartinen JM, Käär M-L, Ohisalo JJ: Defective stimulation of adipocyte adenylate cyclase, blunted lipolysis, and obesity in pseudohypoparathyroidism 1a. *Pediatr Res* **35**:594, 1994.
98. Carlson HE, Brickman AS, Burns TW, et al: Normal free fatty acid response to isoproterenol in pseudohypoparathyroidism. *J Clin Endocrinol Metab* **61**:382, 1985.
99. Moses AM, Weinstock RS, Levine MA, et al: Evidence for normal antidiuretic responses to endogenous and exogenous arginine vasopressin in patients with guanine nucleotide-binding stimulatory protein-deficient pseudohypoparathyroidism. *J Clin Endocrinol Metab* **62**:221, 1986.
100. Weinstock RS, Wright HN, Spiegel AM, et al: Olfactory dysfunction in humans with deficient guanine nucleotide-binding protein. *Nature* **322**:635, 1986.

101. Doty RL, Fernandez AD, Levine MA, et al: Olfactory dysfunction in type I pseudohypoparathyroidism: Dissociation from Gs alpha protein deficiency. *J Clin Endocrinol Metab* **82**:247, 1997.
102. Koch T, Lehnhardt E, Böttinger H, et al: Sensorineural hearing loss owing to deficient G proteins in patients with pseudohypoparathyroidism: Results of a multicentre study. *Eur J Clin Invest* **20**:416, 1990.
103. Farfel Z, Friedman E: Mental deficiency in pseudohypoparathyroidism type I is associated with Ns-protein deficiency. *Ann Intern Med* **105**:197, 1986.
104. Faull CM, Welbury RR, Paul B, et al: Pseudohypoparathyroidism: Its phenotypic variability and associated disorders in a large family. *Q J Med* **78**:251, 1991.
105. Yu S, Yu D, Lee E, et al: Variable and tissue-specific hormone resistance in heterotrimeric G protein α-subunit ($G_s\alpha$) knockout mice is due to tissue-specific imprinting of the $G_s\alpha$ gene. *Proc Natl Acad Sci U S A* **95**:8715, 1998.
106. Wu ZL, Thomas SA, Villacres EC, et al: Altered behavior and long-term potentiation in type I adenylyl cyclase mutant mice. *Proc Natl Acad Sci U S A* **92**:220, 1995.
107. de Wijn EM, Steendijk R: Growth and maturation in pseudohypoparathyroidism: A longitudinal study in five patients. *Acta Endocrinol (Copenh)* **101**:223, 1982.
108. Jobert AS, Zhang P, Couvineau A, et al: Absence of functional receptors for parathyroid hormone and parathyroid hormone-related peptide in Blomstrand chondrodysplasia. *J Clin Invest* **102**:34, 1998.
109. Urdanivia E, Mataverde A, Cohen MP: Growth hormone secretion and sulfation factor activity in pseudohypoparathyroidism. *J Lab Clin Med* **86**:772, 1975.
110. Scott DC, Hung W: Pseudohypoparathyroidism type Ia and growth hormone deficiency in two siblings. *J Pediatr Endocrinol Metab* **8**:205, 1995.
111. Carlson HE, Brickman AS, Bottazzo GF: Prolactin deficiency in pseudohypoparathyroidism. *N Engl J Med* **296**:140, 1977.
112. Brickman AS, Carlson HE, Deftos LJ: Prolactin and calcitonin responses to parathyroid hormone infusion in hypoparathyroid, pseudohypoparathyroid, and normal subjects. *J Clin Endocrinol Metab* **53**:661, 1981.
113. Kruse K, Gutekunst B, Kracht U, et al: Deficient prolactin response to parathyroid hormone in hypocalcemic and normocalcemic pseudohypoparathyroidism. *J Clin Endocrinol Metab* **52**:1099, 1981.
114. Fitch N: Albright's hereditary osteodystrophy: A review. *Am J Med Genet* **11**:11, 1982.
115. Levine MA, Jap TS, Mauseth RS, et al: Activity of the stimulatory guanine nucleotide-binding protein is reduced in erythrocytes from patients with pseudohypoparathyroidism and pseudopseudohypoparathyroidism: Biochemical, endocrine, and genetic analysis of Albright's hereditary osteodystrophy in six kindreds. *J Clin Endocrinol Metab* **62**:497, 1986.
116. Balachandar V, Pahuja J, Maddaiah VT, et al: Pseudohypoparathyroidism with normal serum calcium level. *Am J Dis Child* **129**:1092, 1975.
117. Tsang RC, Venkataraman P, Ho M, et al: The development of pseudohypoparathyroidism. Involvement of progressively increasing serum parathyroid hormone concentrations, increased 1,25-dihydroxyvitamin D concentrations, and "migratory" subcutaneous calcifications. *Am J Dis Child* **138**:654, 1984.
118. Breslau NA, Notman DD, Canterbury JM, et al: Studies on the attainment of normocalcemia in patients with pseudohypoparathyroidism. *Am J Med* **68**:856, 1980.
119. Breslau NA, Zerwekh JE: Relationship of estrogen and pregnancy to calcium homeostasis in pseudohypoparathyroidism. *J Clin Endocrinol Metab* **62**:45, 1986.
120. Farfel Z, Brothers VM, Brickman AS, et al: Pseudohypoparathyroidism: Inheritance of deficient receptor-cyclase coupling activity. *Proc Natl Acad Sci U S A* **78**:3098, 1981.
121. Fischer JA, Bourne HR, Dambacher MA, et al: Pseudohypoparathyroidism: Inheritance and expression of deficient receptor-cyclase coupling protein activity. *Clin Endocrinol (Oxf)* **19**:747, 1983.
122. Davies SJ, Hughes HE: Imprinting in Albright's hereditary osteodystrophy. *J Med Genet* **30**:101, 1993.
123. Campbell R, Gosden CM, Bonthron DT: Parental origin of transcription from the human *GNAS1* gene. *J Med Genet* **31**:607, 1994.
124. Barrett D, Breslau NA, Wax MB, et al: New form of pseudohypoparathyroidism with abnormal catalytic adenylate cyclase. *Am J Physiol* **257**:E277, 1989.
125. Farfel Z, Bourne HR: Pseudohypoparathyroidism: Mutation affecting adenylate cyclase. *Miner Electrolyte Metab* **8**:227, 1982.
126. Winter JS, Hughes IA: Familial pseudohypoparathyroidism without somatic anomalies. *Can Med Assoc J* **123**:26, 1980.
127. Silve C, Santora A, Breslau N, et al: Selective resistance to parathyroid hormone in cultured skin fibroblasts from patients with pseudohypoparathyroidism type Ib. *J Clin Endocrinol Metab* **62**:640, 1986.
128. Suarez F, Lebrun JJ, Lecossier D, et al: Expression and modulation of the parathyroid hormone (PTH)/PTH-related peptide receptor messenger ribonucleic acid in skin fibroblasts from patients with type Ib pseudohypoparathyroidism. *J Clin Endocrinol Metab* **80**:965, 1995.
129. Schipani E, Weinstein LS, Bergwitz C, et al: Pseudohypoparathyroidism type Ib is not caused by mutations in the coding exons of the human parathyroid hormone (PTH)/PTH-related peptide receptor gene. *J Clin Endocrinol Metab* **80**:1611, 1995.
130. Fukumoto S, Suzawa M, Takeuchi Y, et al: Absence of mutations in parathyroid hormone (PTH)/PTH-related protein receptor complementary deoxyribonucleic acid in patients with pseudohypoparathyroidism type Ib. *J Clin Endocrinol Metab* **81**:2554, 1996.
131. Bettoun JD, Minagawa M, Kwan MY, et al: Cloning and characterization of the promoter regions of the human parathyroid hormone (PTH)/PTH-related peptide receptor gene: Analysis of deoxyribonucleic acid from normal subjects and patients with pseudohypoparathyroidism type 1b. *J Clin Endocrinol Metab* **82**:1031, 1997.
132. Rao DS, Parfitt AM, Kleerekoper M, et al: Dissociation between the effects of endogenous parathyroid hormone on adenosine 3′,5′-monophosphate generation and phosphate reabsorption in hypocalcemia due to vitamin D depletion: An acquired disorder resembling pseudohypoparathyroidism type II. *J Clin Endocrinol Metab* **61**:285, 1985.
133. Rodriguez HJ, Villarreal H Jr, Klahr S, et al: Pseudohypoparathyroidism type II: Restoration of normal renal responsiveness to parathyroid hormone by calcium administration. *J Clin Endocrinol Metab* **39**:693, 1974.
134. Matsuda I, Takekoshi Y, Tanaka M, et al: Pseudohypoparathyroidism type II and anticonvulsant rickets. *Eur J Pediatr* **132**:303, 1979.
135. Yamada K, Tamura Y, Tomioka H, et al: Possible existence of antirenal tubular plasma membrane autoantibody which blocked parathyroid hormone-induced phosphaturia in a patient with pseudohypoparathyroidism type II and Sjögren's syndrome. *J Clin Endocrinol Metab* **58**:339, 1984.
136. Nusynowitz ML, Klein MH: Pseudoidiopathic hypoparathyroidism. Hypoparathyroidism with ineffective parathyroid hormone. *Am J Med* **55**:677, 1973.
137. Connors MH, Irias JJ, Golabi M: Hypo-hyperparathyroidism: Evidence for a defective parathyroid hormone. *Pediatrics* **60**:343, 1977.
138. McElduff A, Wilkinson M, Lackmann M, et al: Familial hypoparathyroidism due to an abnormal parathyroid hormone molecule. *Aust N Z J Med* **19**:22, 1989.
139. Ahn TG, Antonarakis SE, Kronenberg HM, et al: Familial isolated hypoparathyroidism: A molecular genetic analysis of 8 families with 23 affected persons. *Medicine (Baltimore)* **65**:73, 1986.
140. Arnold A, Horst SA, Gardella TJ, et al: Mutation of the signal peptide-encoding region of the preproparathyroid hormone gene in familial isolated hypoparathyroidism. *J Clin Invest* **86**:1084, 1990.
141. de Deuxchaisnes CN, Fischer JA, Dambacher MA, et al: Dissociation of parathyroid hormone bioactivity and immunoreactivity in pseudohypoparathyroidism type I. *J Clin Endocrinol Metab* **53**:1105, 1981.
142. Allgrove J, Chayen J, Jayaweera P, et al: An investigation of the biological activity of parathyroid hormone in pseudohypoparathyroidism: comparison with vitamin D deficiency. *Clin Endocrinol (Oxf)* **20**:503, 1984.
143. Stögmann W, Fischer JA: Pseudohypoparathyroidism. Disappearance of the resistance to parathyroid extract during treatment with vitamin D. *Am J Med* **59**:140, 1975.
144. Loveridge N, Fischer JA, Nagant De Deuxchaisnes C, et al: Inhibition of cytochemical bioactivity of parathyroid hormone by plasma in pseudohypoparathyroidism type I. *J Clin Endocrinol Metab* **54**:1274, 1982.
145. Murray TM, Rao LG, Wong M-M, et al: Pseudohypoparathyroidism with osteitis fibrosa cystica: Direct demonstration of skeletal responsiveness to parathyroid hormone in cells cultured from bone. *J Bone Miner Res* **8**:83, 1993.
146. Ish-Shalom S, Rao LG, Levine MA, et al: Normal parathyroid hormone responsiveness of bone-derived cells from a patient with pseudohypoparathyroidism. *J Bone Miner Res* **11**:8, 1996.
147. Drezner MK, Haussler MR: Normocalcemic pseudohypoparathyroidism. Association with normal vitamin D3 metabolism. *Am J Med* **66**:503, 1979.
148. Epstein S, Meunier PJ, Lambert PW, et al: 1α,25-dihydroxyvitamin D3 corrects osteomalacia in hypoparathyroidism and pseudohypoparathyroidism. *Acta Endocrinol (Copenh)* **103**:241, 1983.

149. Sinha TK, DeLuca HF, Bell NH: Evidence for a defect in the formation of 1α,25-dihydroxyvitamin D in pseudohypoparathyroidism. *Metabolism* **26**:731, 1977.
150. Metz SA, Baylink DJ, Hughes MR, et al: Selective deficiency of 1,25-dihydroxycholecalciferol. A cause of isolated skeletal resistance to parathyroid hormone. *N Engl J Med* **297**:1084, 1977.
151. Lambert PW, Hollis BW, Bell NH, et al: Demonstration of a lack of change in serum 1α,25-dihydroxyvitamin D in response to parathyroid extract in pseudohypoparathyroidism. *J Clin Invest* **66**:782, 1980.
152. Braun JJ, Birkenhäger JC, Visser TJ, et al: Lack of response of 1,25-dihydroxycholecalciferol to exogenous parathyroid hormone in a patient with treated pseudohypoparathyroidism. *Clin Endocrinol (Oxf)* **14**:403, 1981.
153. Bell NH, Avery S, Sinha T, et al: Effects of dibutyryl cyclic adenosine 3′,5′-monophosphate and parathyroid extract on calcium and phosphorus metabolism in hypoparathyroidism and pseudohypoparathyroidism. *J Clin Invest* **51**:816, 1972.
154. Yamaoka K, Seino Y, Ishida M, et al: Effect of dibutyryl adenosine 3′,5′-monophosphate administration on plasma concentrations of 1,25-dihydroxyvitamin D in pseudohypoparathyroidism type I. *J Clin Endocrinol Metab* **53**:1096, 1981.
155. Breslau NA, Weinstock RS: Regulation of 1,25(OH)2D synthesis in hypoparathyroidism and pseudohypoparathyroidism. *Am J Physiol* **255**:E730, 1988.
156. Breslau NA, Moses AM, Pak CY: Evidence for bone remodeling but lack of calcium mobilization response to parathyroid hormone in pseudohypoparathyroidism. *J Clin Endocrinol Metab* **57**:638, 1983.
157. Wilson JD, Hadden DR: Pseudohypoparathyroidism presenting with rickets. *J Clin Endocrinol Metab* **51**:1184, 1980.
158. Dabbagh S, Chesney RW, Langer LO, et al: Renal-nonresponsive, bone-responsive pseudohypoparathyroidism. A case with normal vitamin D metabolite levels and clinical features of rickets. *Am J Dis Child* **138**:1030, 1984.
159. Frame B, Hanson CA, Frost HM, et al: Renal resistance to parathyroid hormone with osteitis fibrosa: "Pseudohypohyperparathyroidism." *Am J Med* **52**:311, 1972.
160. Kidd GS, Schaaf M, Adler RA, et al: Skeletal responsiveness in pseudohypoparathyroidism. A spectrum of clinical disease. *Am J Med* **68**:772, 1980.
161. Van Dop C, Bourne HR: Pseudohypoparathyroidism. *Annu Rev Med* **34**:259, 1983.
162. Weinberg AG, Stone RT: Autosomal dominant inheritance in Albright's hereditary osteodystrophy. *J Pediatr* **79**:996, 1971.
163. Van Dop C, Bourne HR, Neer RM: Father to son transmission of decreased Ns activity in pseudohypoparathyroidism type Ia. *J Clin Endocrinol Metab* **59**:825, 1984.
164. Kinard RE, Walton JE, Buckwalter JA: Pseudohypoparathyroidism: Report on a family with four affected sisters. *Arch Intern Med* **139**:204, 1979.
165. Wilkie TM, Gilbert DJ, Olsen AS, et al: Evolution of the mammalian G protein α subunit multigene family. *Nat Genet* **1**:85, 1992.
166. Peters J, Beechey CV, Ball ST, et al: Mapping studies of the distal imprinting region of mouse chromosome 2. *Genet Res* **63**:169, 1994.
167. Cattanach BM, Kirk M: Differential activity of maternally and paternally derived chromosome regions in mice. *Nature* **315**:496, 1985.
168. Stone MD, Hosking DJ, Garcia-Himmelstine C, et al: The renal response to exogenous parathyroid hormone in treated pseudohypoparathyroidism. *Bone* **14**:727, 1993.
169. Schuster V, Kress W, Kruse K: Paternal and maternal transmission of pseudohypoparathyroidism type Ia in a family with Albright hereditary osteodystrophy: No evidence of genomic imprinting. *J Med Genet* **31**:84, 1994.
170. Cederbaum SD, Lippe BM: Probable autosomal recessive inheritance in a family with Albright's hereditary osteodystrophy and an evaluation of the genetics of the disorder. *Am J Hum Genet* **25**:638, 1973.
171. Aurbach GD, Marx SJ, Spiegel AM. Parathyroid hormone, calcitonin, and the calciferols, in Wilson JD, Foster DW (eds): *Williams Textbook of Endocrinology*. Philadelphia, WB Saunders, 1992, pp 1397–1476.
172. Illum F, Dupont E: Prevalences of CT-detected calcification in the basal ganglia in idiopathic hypoparathyroidism and pseudohypoparathyroidism. *Neuroradiology* **27**:32, 1985.
173. Eyre WG, Reed WB: Albright's hereditary osteodystrophy with cutaneous bone formation. *Arch Dermatol* **104**:634, 1971.
174. Poznanski AK, Werder EA, Giedion A, et al: The pattern of shortening of the bones of the hand in pseudohypoparathyroidism and pseudopseudohypoparathyroidism — A comparison with brachydactyly E, Turner syndrome, and acrodysostosis. *Radiology* **123**:707, 1977.
175. Steinbach HL, Young DA: The roentgen appearance of pseudohypoparathyroidism (PH) and pseudo-pseudohypoparathyroidism (PPH). Differentiation from other syndromes associated with short metacarpals, metatarsals, and phalanges. *Am J Roentgenol Radium Ther Nucl Med* **97**:49, 1966.
176. Levine MA, Jap TS, Hung W: Infantile hypothyroidism in two sibs: An unusual presentation of pseudohypoparathyroidism type Ia. *J Pediatr* **107**:919, 1985.
177. Weisman Y, Golander A, Spirer Z, et al: Pseudohypoparathyroidism type Ia presenting as congenital hypothyroidism. *J Pediatr* **107**:413, 1985.
178. Yokoro S, Matsuo M, Ohtsuka T, et al: Hyperthyrotropinemia in a neonate with normal thyroid hormone levels: The earliest diagnostic clue for pseudohypoparathyroidism. *Biol Neonate* **58**:69, 1990.
179. Miura R, Yumita S, Yoshinaga K, et al: Response of plasma 1,25-dihydroxyvitamin D in the human PTH(1-34) infusion test: An improved index for the diagnosis of idiopathic hypoparathyroidism and pseudohypoparathyroidism. *Calcif Tissue Int* **46**:309, 1990.
180. Slater S: An evaluation of the metacarpal sign (short fourth metacarpal). *Pediatrics* **46**:468, 1970.
181. Ablow RC, Hsia YE, Brandt IK: Acrodysostosis coinciding with pseudohypoparathyroidism and pseudo-pseudohypoparathyroidism. *AJR Am J Roentgenol* **128**:95, 1977.
182. Wilson LC, Oude Luttikhuis ME, Baraitser M, et al: Normal erythrocyte membrane Gs α bioactivity in two unrelated patients with acrodysostosis. *J Med Genet* **34**:133, 1997.
183. Larsen JL, Kivlin J, Odell WD: Unusual cause of short stature. *Am J Med* **78**:1025, 1985.
184. Graudal N, Milman N, Nielsen LS, et al: Coexistent pseudohypoparathyroidism and D brachydactyly in a family. *Clin Genet* **30**:449, 1986.
185. Wilson LC, Leverton K, Oude Luttikhuis MEM, et al: Brachydactyly and mental retardation: An Albright hereditary osteodystrophy-like syndrome localized to 2q37. *Am J Hum Genet* **56**:400, 1995.
186. Phelan MC, Rogers RC, Clarkson KB, et al: Albright hereditary osteodystrophy and del(2)(q37.3) in four unrelated individuals. *Am J Med Genet* **58**:1, 1995.
187. Kruse K, Kracht U, Wohlfart K, et al: Biochemical markers of bone turnover, intact serum parathyroid hormone and renal calcium excretion in patients with pseudohypoparathyroidism and hypoparathyroidism before and during vitamin D treatment. *Eur J Pediatr* **148**:535, 1989.
188. Yamamoto M, Takuwa Y, Ogata E: Effects of endogenous and exogenous parathyroid hormone on tubular reabsorption of calcium in pseudohypoparathyroidism. *J Clin Endocrinol Metab* **66**:618, 1988.
189. Mizunashi K, Furukawa Y, Sohn HE, et al: Heterogeneity of pseudohypoparathyroidism type I from the aspect of urinary excretion of calcium and serum levels of parathyroid hormone. *Calcif Tissue Int* **46**:227, 1990.
190. Baran DT, Klahr S, Slatopolsky E, et al: Effect of acetazolamide on calcium and phosphate metabolism in type I pseudohypoparathyroidism: interaction with parathyroid hormone. *J Clin Endocrinol Metab* **48**:766, 1979.
191. Yu D, Schuster V, et al: Identification of two novel deletion mutations within the Gsα gene (*GNAS1*) in Albright hereditary osteodystrophy. *J Clin Endocrinol Metab* **84**:3254, 1999.
192. Warner DR, Weinstein LS: A mutation in the heterotrimeric stimulatory guanine nucleotide binding protein α-subunit with impaired receptor-mediate activation because of elevated GTPase activity. *Proc Natl Acad Sci U S A* **96**:4268, 1999.
193. Warner DR, Romanowski R, Yu S, et al: Mutagenesis of the conserved residue Glu^{259} of Gsα demonstrates the importance of interactions between switches 2 and 3 for activation. *J Biol Chem* **274**:4977, 1999.
194. Hayward BE, Kamiya M, Strain L, et al: The human *GNAS1* gene is imprinted and encodes distinct paternally and biallelically expressed G proteins. *Proc Natl Acad Sci U S A* **95**:10038, 1998.
195. Hayward BE, Moran V, Strain L, et al: Bidirectional imprinting of a single gene: *GNAS1* endodes maternally, paternally, and biallelically derived proteins. *Proc Natl Acad Sci U S A* **95**:15475, 1998.
196. Peters J, Wroe SF, Wells CA, et al: A cluster of oppositely imprinted transcripts at the *Gnas* locus in the distal imprinting region of mouse chromosome 2 *Proc Natl Acad Sci U S A* **96**:3830, 1999.
197. Jüppner H, Schipani E, Bastepe M, et al: The gene responsible for pseudohypoparathyroidism type Ib is paternally imprinted amd maps in four unrelated kindreds to chromosome 20q13.3. *Proc Natl Acad Sci U S A* **95**:11798, 1998.

CHAPTER 165

Vitamin D and Other Calciferols

Uri A. Liberman ▪ Stephen J. Marx

1. **Normal calciferol physiology includes activation through 25-hydroxylation in the liver and 1α-hydroxylation in the renal proximal tubule; the most active metabolite is 1α,25-dihydroxyvitamin D [1α,25$(OH)_2$D], which acts on target tissues by a mechanism analogous to that of the true steroid hormones. Two distinct hereditary defects have been recognized: (1) selective deficiency (which implies normal concentrations of the immediate precursor) and simple deficiency (which implies that other metabolic pathways are not abnormal) of 1α,25$(OH)_2$D, and (2) generalized resistance (which means that all target tissues are affected) to 1α,25$(OH)_2$D. Hereditary defects in calciferol metabolism or action show all the features of the calciferol deficiency states beginning early in life. These features are intestinal malabsorption of calcium, hypocalcemia, secondary hyperparathyroidism, increased renal clearance of phosphorus, and hypophosphatemia. The combination of hypocalcemia and hypophosphatemia results in impaired mineralization of bone (rickets and osteomalacia).**
2. **Hereditary selective and simple deficiency of 1α,25$(OH)_2$D is an autosomal recessive trait (MIM 264700). Patients respond to any doses of calciferol analogues that maintain normal circulating bioactivity of equivalents of 1α,25$(OH)_2$D. The cellular basis is a deficiency of the renal 25-hydroxyvitamin D [25(OH)D] 1α-hydroxylase.**
3. **Hereditary selective deficiency of 1α,25$(OH)_2$D also can occur as part of complex disorders that affect additional metabolic pathways not related to calciferols. Examples include X-linked hypophosphatemia, pseudohypoparathyroidism, and some forms of Fanconi syndrome.**
4. **Hereditary generalized resistance to 1α,25$(OH)_2$D is an autosomal recessive trait (MIM 277440). The cellular basis is an abnormality in the vitamin D receptor. Point mutations in the vitamin D receptor gene have been implicated in almost every kindred studied and, depending on its location, will affect DNA binding, hormone binding, heterdimerization with the retinoid X receptors, or all of the above. The type of defect is not correlated with the clinical features, and it seems likely that each defect could produce varying severity of clinical dysfunction. Approximately half of patients show alopecia; these are usually the more severely affected patients. Depending on the severity of the defect, patients may respond to treatment with (1) calciferol analogues that allow for endogenous regulation of 1α,25$(OH)_2$D production, (2) calcium plus high doses of calciferol analogues that bypass 25(OH)D 1α-hydroxylase, or (3) extremely high doses of calcium orally or intravenously (for patients unresponsive to maximal doses of all calciferols).**

A list of standard abbreviations is located immediately preceding the index in each volume. Nonstandard abbreviations used in this chapter include: 1α,25$(OH)_2D_3$, = 1α,25-dihydroxyvitamin D_3; PTH = parathyroid hormone; RXR, retinoid X receptor; VDRE, vitamin D–responsive element.

HISTORY

Rickets and osteomalacia were widespread problems until the discovery of the calciferols in 1919.[1] This discovery resulted in the use of calciferols for the prevention and treatment of rickets and osteomalacia. Some patients did not respond to the usual doses of calciferols, and multiple causes of rickets or osteomalacia resistant to vitamin D subsequently were recognized. In 1937, Albright et al.[2] reported detailed studies of a child with this problem and suggested a hereditary resistance to the actions of calciferols. Rickets resistant to calciferols subsequently was recognized as a common cause of hereditary dwarfism. Most cases showed biochemical features different from those of nutritional deficiency of calciferols and are now classified as phosphate diabetes or X-linked hypophosphatemia (see Chap. 197).

In 1961, Prader et al.[3] characterized a distinctive form of hereditary rickets that they called "pseudodeficiency rickets." Features that distinguished pseudodeficiency rickets from X-linked hypophosphatemia were hypocalcemia, the potential for complete remission with high doses of calciferols, and a different transmission pattern. In 1970 it was shown that untreated patients with pseudodeficiency rickets had intestinal malabsorption of calcium[4] and secondary hyperparathyroidism[5] and that both these abnormalities could be corrected by high doses of calciferols.

In 1971, three groups identified 1α,25-dihydroxyvitamin D_3 [1α,25$(OH)_2D_3$]* as the active metabolite of vitamin D_3 that accumulated in the nuclei of vitamin D_3 target tissues.[6,7] This discovery accelerated further exploration of calciferol metabolism, including the development of methods to measure active metabolites in blood, characterization of defects in 1α,25$(OH)_2$D synthesis and action, and understanding the roles of 1α-hydroxylated and other analogues for therapy. In 1973, Fraser et al.[8] showed that a patient with pseudodeficiency rickets could be treated with a physiologic dose of 1α,25$(OH)_2D_3$; they suggested that this disorder represented a defect in the 25(OH)D 1-hydroxylase enzyme. In 1978, Brooks et al.[9] described a patient with similar clinical features but high serum levels of 1α,25$(OH)_2$D before and during treatment and suggested that pseudodeficiency rickets be subclassified as type I [deficient production of 1,25$(OH)_2$D] or type II [impaired end-organ response to 1,25$(OH)_2$D].

*D_3 refers to a metabolite of cholecalciferol (vitamin D_3); D_2 refers to a metabolite of ergocalciferol (vitamin D_2); and D refers to a metabolite of vitamin D_3 and/or vitamin D_2. For tests in vitro, a pure D_2 or D_3 isoform is usually used. For clinical tests, the two isoforms are often not separated.

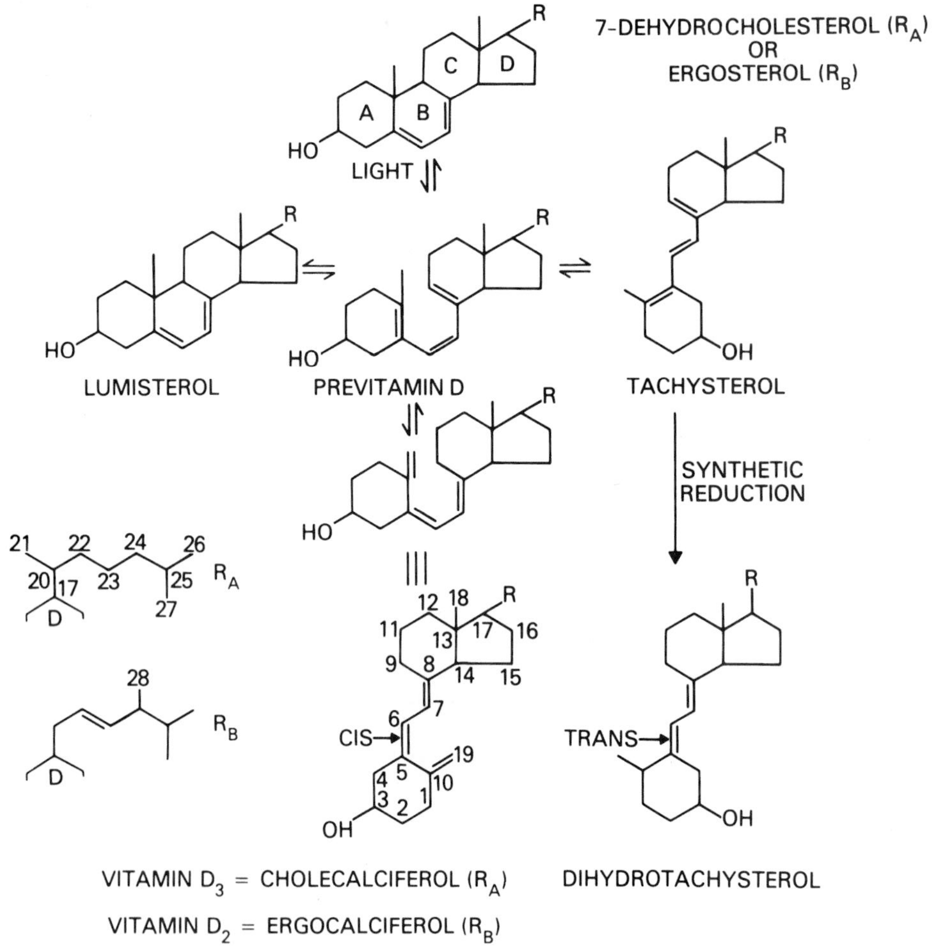

Fig. 165-1 Synthesis of cholecalciferol, ergocalciferol, and dihydrotachysterol.

NORMAL PHYSIOLOGY OF CALCIFEROLS

Normal Metabolism

Vitamin D Sources. Cholecalciferol (vitamin D_3)[10] is a secosteroid that is formed by opening the B ring of 7-dehydrocholesterol (Fig. 165-1). In human beings, this reaction occurs in the basal layers of the epidermis[11] and is driven by ultraviolet radiation (from sunlight). Skin pigment in blacks can decrease the amount of cholecalciferol synthesized in response to a submaximal dose of ultraviolet radiation.[12] Ergocalciferol (vitamin D_2) is a secosteroid formed by opening the B ring of ergosterol, a sterol found in plants and fungi. Plants do not contain pharmacologically important amounts of ergocalciferol, but this chemical is synthesized in bulk for use as a nutritional supplement. Human beings obtain calciferols either as an endogenous metabolite in skin, as a natural dietary component, or as a dietary supplement. The metabolism and actions of vitamin D_3 and vitamin D_2 are similar in human beings.

Vitamin D 25 Hydroxylation. Cholecalciferol and ergocalciferol are inert when exposed directly to calciferol target tissues. They must be hydroxylated at positions 25 and 1α to become maximally active (Fig. 165-2). The initial hydroxylation at carbon 25 is carried out only in the liver by a mitochondrial cytochrome P_{450} monooxygenase.[13] This same cytochrome P_{450} mediates 27-hydroxylation of cholestanetriol, a cholesterol metabolite.[14,15] A different 25-hydroxylase system has been purified from rat liver microsomes, but absence of this system in microsomes from females makes its physiologic significance doubtful.[16] 25-Hydroxylation of vitamin D is not highly regulated; the principal determinant of its rate is the circulating level of vitamin D.

1α-Hydroxylation. 25(OH)D is 1α-hydroxylated to 1α,25$(OH)_2$D[17] by a mitochondrial cytochrome P_{450} enzyme system in the kidney. 25(OH)D 1α-hydroxylase activity is also found in placenta, in certain cultured cells of diverse origin, and in certain pathologic tissues (such as granulomas, certain solid tumors, and activated T cells). Virtually all 1α,25$(OH)_2$D in blood normally derives from renal

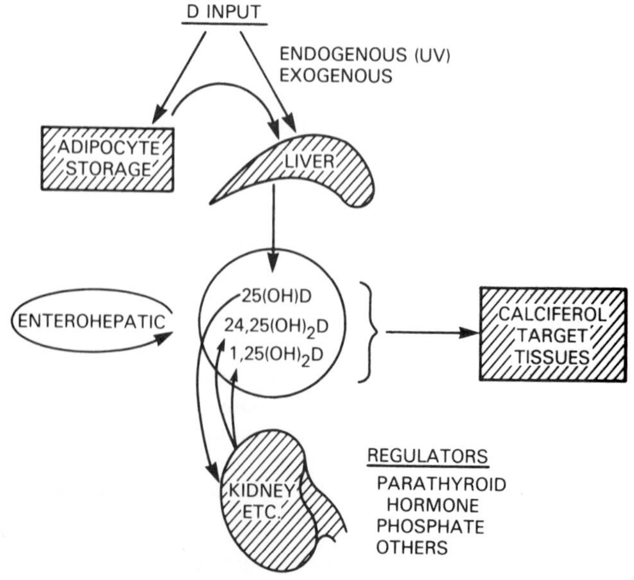

Fig. 165-2 Metabolic pathways for activation of cholecalciferol or ergocalciferol.

secretion.[18] The renal 1α-hydroxylase enzyme is stringently regulated. Parathyroid hormone activates it in the renal proximal tubule through a cAMP-medicated pathway[19]; calcitonin activates it in a more distal region of the proximal tubule, apparently without a rise in cAMP.[20] 25(OH)D 1α-hydroxylase activity is inhibited by 1α,25$(OH)_2$D (through its receptor) and by calcium and phosphate by unknown mechanisms. Recently, cloning of cDNA for mouse, rat, and human 25(OH)D 1α-hydroxylase has been reported.[21a–21c] The human cDNA consists of 2469 base pairs and encodes a protein of 508 amino acids that shows more than 80 percent sequence identity with the rat enzyme. Sequence analysis of the 25(OH)D 1α-hydroxylase has revealed homology to the liver vitamin D 25-hydroxylase and the ubiquitously expressed vitamin D 24-hydroxylase (44 and 34 percent identity, respectively). The gene for the human 25(OH)D 1α-hydroxylase consists of 9 exons spanning approximately 6 kb and is present as a single copy.[21c,21d] The 25(OH)D 1α-hydroxylase gene is being regulated at the transcriptional level by parathyroid hormone (PTH) and calcitonin (positive regulation) and by 1α,25$(OH)_2$D via its receptor (negative regulation).[22]

24-Hydroxylation. 25(OH)D, 1α,25$(OH)_2$D, and other metabolites are substrates for 24-hydroxylation. The 24-hydroxylase enzyme shares many properties with the 25(OH)D 1α-hydroxylase enzymes. Both are mitochondrial enzymes containing cytochrome P_{450}.[23] Both are modulated (though in opposing directions) by cAMP and the receptor for 1α,25(OH)D.[24] Their anatomic distributions, however, are different; the 1α-hydroxylase is confined to the proximal renal tubule; the 24-hydroxylase occurs in a wide range of normal tissues. Their many similarities have raised the possibilities that they may share certain components. The 24-hydroxylase from rat, mouse, human, and chicken has been analyzed by molecular cloning.[25,25a–25c] The full-length complementary DNA of the mouse vitamin D 24-hydroxylase consists of 3309 base pairs encoding a protein of 514 amino acids that shows 82 and 95 percent sequence identity with the human and rat enzymes.[25b] The gene for rat and human vitamin D 24-hydroxylase is transcriptionally regulated by 1α,25$(OH)_2$D via its receptor binding to two specific vitamin D response elements.[25d,25e] The importance of 24-hydroxylation has not been fully determined; it may be the only route to a group of calciferols with unique actions not obtainable with 1α,25$(OH)_2$D [see "Specific Role of 24,25$(OH)_2$D," below], and it may be the most important step in 1α,25$(OH)_2$D removal. Induction of 24-hydroxylase by 1α,25$(OH)_2$D in target tissues[23] and preference of this enzyme for 1α,25$(OH)_2$D rather than 25(OH)D as substrate suggest an important role in ending the action of 1α,25$(OH)_2$D.

5,6-*Cis-Trans* Isomerization. 25(OH)D also may be converted to 5,6-*trans*-25(OH)D. This pathway has so far been documented only with rat plasma after the animals were treated with pharmacologic amounts of vitamin D_3.[26] However, the pathway is of interest because it produces a metabolite analogous to 25(OH)dihydrotachysterol (Fig. 165-3) (dihydrotachysterol is a synthetic calciferol analogue used in therapy). These metabolites have the A ring rotated 180°, brining the 3β-hydroxyl group into a pseudo-1α-hydroxyl position. This rotation increases the agonist potency of the parent metabolite on the vitamin D receptor, and 5,6-*trans*-25(OH)D may have important roles in states in which the renal 1α-hydroxylase enzyme is severely deficient.

Other Calciferol Metabolites. A series of hydroxylations and other oxidations of the C-17 side chain has been characterized by studies in vivo and in vitro. The 24-hydroxyl group can be oxidized to a ketone. 23-Hydroxylation[27] is the initial step in conversion of 25$(OH)D_3$ to 25$(OH)D_3$-23,26-lactone, the principal circulating metabolite. Multiple oxidations can be followed by cleavage of the C-17 side chain.

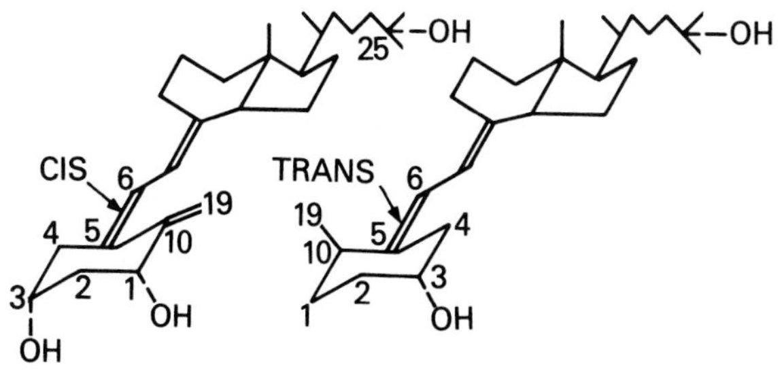

1α, 25-$(OH)_2$-D_3 25-(OH)-DHT_3

Fig. 165-3 Steric conformation of two activated calciferol analogues. 1α,25$(OH)_2D_3$ has the 5–6 double bond in *cis* configuration. 25(OH)dihydrotachysterol$_3$ has the 5–6 double bond in *trans* configuration; the 180° rotation of the A ring (lowest ring in the figure) brings the 3β-hydroxyl group into a pseudo-1α configuration.

Transcalciferin as a Calciferol Binder. All calciferols are fat-soluble and circulate principally bound to transcalciferin, an α-globulin of 58 kDa.[28] Transcalciferin, also known as *group-specific component*, or Gc, is structurally homologous to albumin and α-fetoprotein.[29] It has one high-affinity sterol-binding site with preferential affinity for 25(OH)D. Detailed affinity testing shows the following series: 25$(OH)D_3$-26,23-lactone > 25(OH)D = 24,25$(OH)_2$D > 1,25$(OH)_2$D ≫ vitamin D. It is a major component of plasma protein (normal concentration 10^{-5} M) that has multiple isoforms[30] that had been studied extensively for their genetic diversity long before a function in calciferol transport was recognized.

Calciferol Turnover and Requirements. Most of the body pool of vitamin D is in body fat, whereas only a small fraction of the pools of 25(OH)D or 1α,25$(OH)_2$D are in fat.[31] In the circulation, more than 99 percent of each metabolite is bound to transcalciferin. Normal daily turnover of vitamin D is approximately 30 μg/day; most of this is cleared through catabolic pathways, with only 1 μg/day contributing to daily production of 1α,25$(OH)_2$D (Table 165-1). In the vitamin D–deficient state, the fractional conversion of vitamin D to 1α,25$(OH)_2$D is maximized to near 100 percent. The recommended daily allowance for vitamin D in the United States is 200 to 400 IU (5–10 μg).

Normal Actions

Vitamin D Receptors. 1α,25$(OH)_2D_3$ is the most potent natural calciferol metabolite, with a median effective dose (ED_{50}) of approximately one-thousandth that of 25(OH)D in most test systems. 1α,25$(OH)_2$D acts by binding to its nuclear receptor (VDR), a member of the superfamily of nuclear receptors that includes the receptors for steroid and thyroid hormones, retinoid,

Table 165-1 Serum Levels and Body Pools of Calciferol Metabolites in Adults

Metabolite	Concentration in Serum, ng/ml	Half-time in Serum, days	Pool Size in Body, μg	Turnover in Body, μg/day
D_3	10*	30	1000	30
25(OH)D	25	14	500	15
1α,25$(OH)_2$D	0.03	0.2	0.5	1
24,25$(OH)_2$D	1	2	10	10

*Typical summer mean in temperate climate; normal winter mean is below 0.5 mg/ml. D_2 concentration (not tabulated) depends largely on diet supplements.

NOTE: With the exception of serum concentration, these numbers are based on limited data.

as well as orphan receptors whose natural ligands are unknown.[32] These receptors posses a well-defined and conserved DNA binding domain and a less well defined hormone-binding domain.[32,33] The VDR is a 50-kDa nuclear phosphoprotein that binds the hormone with high affinity and regulates the expression of genes via a zinc finger–mediated DNA-binding domain and protein-protein interaction.[32]

Structure-function studies with a series of calciferol analogues[34] indicate that in vivo the receptor may be occupied by a mixture of metabolites including $1\alpha,25(OH)_2D$, 25(OH)D, and 5,6-*trans*-25(OH)D. The vitamin D receptor is found in many tissues[35] and can be induced by increased cell proliferation, by exposure to $1\alpha,25(OH)_2D$, and by the ontogenetic state. The vitamin D receptor is encoded by a single gene on chromosome 12, and the protein may undergo important posttranslational modifications, such as phosphorylation.[36]

Transcriptional Effects of $1\alpha,25(OH)_2D$. The VDR is presumed to stimulate or inhibit transcription of many genes in target tissues.[32,37] The basic model of $1\alpha,25(OH)_2D_3$ transcriptional activity consists of a hormone-liganded Vitamin D receptor (VDR) that binds to DNA as a heterodimer with another nuclear receptor, the retinoid X receptors (RXRs).[32] This is analogous to the action of the receptors of the thyroid hormone *trans*-retinoic acid and peroxisome proliferator-activator and in contrast to the classic steroid hormone receptor that forms homodimers. The heterodimer binds to vitamin D–responsive elements (VDREs) consisting of 2 direct hexanucleotides repeats separated by three nucleotides that have been identified in the promoter regions of vitamin D–responsive genes such as osteoclacin, osteopontin, β_3-integrin, and vitamin D 24(OH)-hydroxylase. The consensus sequence for VDREs as obtained by random selection is GGGTCA NNG
A
GGTTCA. (Different DNA motives that interact with liganded
A
VDR were found on VDREs).

From analogous studies with other heterodimeric receptors, it appears that the RXR binds the 5′ half site and the VDR binds the 3′ half site of the VDRE. While $1\alpha,25(OH)_2D_3$ promotes VDR-RXR heterodimerization and specific high-affinity VDRE binding, the natural RXR ligand, 9-*cis*-retinoic acid is not required for these interactions and was even shown to suppress $1,25(OH)_2D_3$-stimulated transcription by diverting RXR to form homodimers.

Studies of protein-protein interactions recently revealed that the VDR also binds to the basal transcription factor IIB (TFIIB). Transfection experiments indeed demonstrated a strong synergistic interaction between VDR and TFIIB in the induction of expression of a luciferase reporter gene containing a VDRE. For transcriptional activation by $1\alpha,25(OH)_2D_3$, both VDR and RXR require an intact short amphipathic α-helix known as AF-2 positioned at their extreme C-termini. Because the AF-2 domain participates neither in VDR-RXR heterodimerization nor in TFIIB association, it is postulated that it participates in ligand-dependent interactions with transcriptional coactivators, as shown for other members of the nuclear receptor family.[32]

Nongenomic Effects of $1\alpha,25(OH)_2D$. $1\alpha,25(OH)_2D$ may have some cellular effects not mediated by the genomic pathway. These include rapid effects on calcium translocation, intracellular calcium, and intracellular cyclic GMP.[38,39]

Calbindin and Intestinal Transport of Calcium. The most important physiologic action of $1\alpha,25(OH)_2D$ is stimulation of active calcium transport across the duodenum from lumen to bloodstream. Surprisingly few details are known about the molecular details of this process.[40] In particular, the roles of calbindin (also called *cholecalcin* or *vitamin D–dependent calcium-binding protein*) are not known; this is despite the facts that it binds calcium with high affinity (the calcium-binding regions are homologous to those of the calmodulin family), that it constitutes approximately 2 percent of duodenal mucosal cell protein in the vitamin D–replete state, and that it is undetectable in duodenum in the vitamin D–deficient state. Proposed roles of calbindin in duodenum include a buffer of intracellular calcium[41] and a regulator of calcium ATPase.[42] There are at least two calbindin genes in the rat; one codes for a 9-kDa protein concentrated in the duodenum, whereas the other codes for a homologous 28-kDa protein concentrated in kidney, brain, and many other tissues.

A wide tissue distribution of vitamin D receptors and of a family of calbindin proteins indicates that $1\alpha,25(OH)_2D$ may have direct actions in many tissues. Several potential targets outside the intestine will be discussed here.

$1\alpha,25(OH)_2D$ Actions on Bone. Most of the antirachitic actions of calciferols are secondary to maintenance of adequate calcium and phosphate concentrations in extracellular fluid to allow mineralization.[43,44] Many of the direct actions of $1\alpha,25(OH)_2D$ in bone seem to be catabolic. For example, $1\alpha,25(OH)_2D_3$ inhibits proliferation and collagen synthesis in fetal bone and in fetal osteoblasts.[45] In osteoblast-like cells from adult humans, $1\alpha,25(OH)_2D_3$ stimulates collagen synthesis.[46] Differing effects on alkaline phosphatase have been reported in several systems; however, there is general agreement that in rapidly growing osteoblast-like cells, alkaline phosphatase levels are low and will rise in response to $1\alpha,25(OH)_2D_3$.[47] $1\alpha,25(OH)_2D_3$ stimulates synthesis and secretion of osteocalcin by osteoblast-like cells.[45] Based on data from osteocalcin knockout mice, it seems to be that the normal function of oteocalcin is to curtail bone matrix formation.[47]

$1\alpha,25(OH)_2D_3$ is a potent activator of osteoclasts in vivo and in organ culture. However, isolated osteoclasts have shown no response to $1\alpha,25(OH)_2D_3$[48]; this results from the absence of vitamin D receptors in these cells.[49] At least three mechanisms have been suggested for $1\alpha,25(OH)_2D_3$ activation of osteoclasts: (1) $1\alpha,25(OH)_2D_3$ may stimulate differentiation of osteoclast precursors, related to monocytes and macrophages,[50,51] (2) $1\alpha,25(OH)_2D_3$ may stimulate fusion and metabolism of the immediate precursor of the multinucleated osteoclast,[52] and (3) $1\alpha,25(OH)_2D_3$ may stimulate adjacent cells such as osteoblasts to activate osteoclasts (adjacent cells could help make bone surfaces more accessible to osteoclasts or could release mediators such as osteopontin that may activate osteoclasts).[53]

$1\alpha,25(OH)_2D$ Actions on Skin and Hair. Vitamin D receptors have been documented directly by in vivo autoradiography in basal layers of the epidermis and in the outer root sheath cells of the rat hair follicle.[54] Furthermore, $1\alpha,25(OH)_2D_3$ stimulates differentiation of epidermal keratinocytes in tissue culture.

$1\alpha,25(OH)_2D$ Actions on the Parathyroid Gland. $1\alpha,25(OH)_2D$ decreases transcription of mRNA for preproparathyroid hormone.[55] It may also inhibit parathyroid gland function at other steps.

$1\alpha,25(OH)_2D$ Actions on Calciferol Metabolism. $1\alpha,25(OH)_2D_3$ can increase the levels of 7,8-didehydrocholesterol in skin.[56] $1\alpha,25(OH)_2D_3$ is a potent inhibitor of the renal 25(OH)D 1α-hydroxylase enzyme[17,22] (see above). $1\alpha,25(OH)_2D$ activates the 24-hydroxylase enzyme in kidney and in many other tissues.[24,25d,25e] $1\alpha,25(OH)_2D_3$ stimulates the clearance of 25(OH)D and $1\alpha,25(OH)_2D$; this regulated clearance is a combination of 24-hydroxylation, 23-hydroxylation, and less well defined processes.[57]

Specific Role of $24,25(OH)_2D$. It has been reported that $24,25(OH)_2D_3$ shows unique actions on cartilage from fetal or newborn animals not reproduced by any dosage of $1\alpha,25(OH)_2D_3$.[58,59] These actions include stimulation of proliferation and stimulation of creatine kinase BB isoenzyme. However, extensive efforts have failed to show an important role for 24,25$(OH_2)D_3$ in vivo.[60] For example, rats can be raised through two generations without this metabolite. This has been accomplished by raising them on a vitamin D–free diet supplemented with 24,24(F)-25$(OH)D_3$, a metabolite that precludes the formation of the 24-hydroxylated metabolite [though it may not preclude formation of other metabolites that may activate a putative receptor for 24,25$(OH)_2D$].

NOMENCLATURE IN CALCIFEROL DEFICIENCY STATES

Hormones or Vitamins

The calciferols traverse a metabolic pathway that could justify their being described as normal metabolites, vitamins (a metabolic component required in trace amounts in states of limited skin exposure to ultraviolet light), or hormones [1α,25$(OH)_2D$ is a secosteroid secreted by a "gland" at a regulated rate and acting on distant targets]. The term *calciferol* refers to the entire family of secosteroid metabolites in this pathway. The letter *D*, as in 25(OH)D, refers to the sum of D_2 and D_3 forms.

Deficiency States

Prior terminology applied to calciferol deficiency states has led to much confusion; this is principally because the terms were first used prior to our detailed understanding of calciferol pathophysiology. Since widely used terms to characterize calciferol pathophysiology are ambiguous and likely to remain in use, it is helpful to understand the limitations of these terms.

It is important to specify the location of a defect as precisely as possible. Thus the description of a deficiency state should indicate the most proximal metabolite in the biosynthetic pathway that is deficient. Deficiency of 1α,25$(OH)_2D$ could result from deficiency of vitamin D or 25(OH)D. We use the term *selective deficiency* to emphasize that a deficiency is associated with normal levels of the immediate precursor of the metabolite specified.

Several terms related to the term *deficiency* have been used, including *pseudodeficiency, dependency*, and *resistance*. The term *vitamin D deficiency* should be reserved for states in which blood and tissue levels of vitamin D are abnormally low. Because of difficulty in measuring vitamin D in blood, the diagnosis is usually established by measuring 25(OH)D. Vitamin D deficiency can be associated with normal or even high circulating levels of 1α,25$(OH)_2D$ (see below).

The term *pseudo-vitamin D deficiency* refers to a state with biochemical and tissue features of vitamin D deficiency (i.e., calcium deficiency, secondary hyperparathyroidism, impaired skeletal mineralization) but no deficiency in vitamin D levels or diet calcium. Pseudo-vitamin D deficiency has been subdivided into type I [deficiency of 1α,25$(OH)_2D$] and type II [resistance to 1α,25$(OH)_2D$].

The term *vitamin D dependency* has been used interchangeably with pseudo-vitamin D deficiency. However, it should be reserved for patients capable of responding to (i.e., dependent on) supraphysiologic doses of vitamin D. It has been applied to but does not accurately describe patients responding to high doses of 1α,25$(OH)_2D$ but not to vitamin D or patients completely unresponsive to vitamin D or 1α,25$(OH)_2D$ but responsive to high doses of calcium.

The term *resistance* specifies a metabolite proximal to a defect, whereas *deficiency* characterizes a metabolite distal to the defect (assuming the latter defect is in production, not clearance). *Resistance* should only be used with the most distal metabolite to which there is resistance.

Some descriptions (of deficiency or resistance) include a bioeffect, such as rickets or osteomalacia.[61] This can be particularly confusing because not all causes of rickets or osteomalacia involve primary problems in calciferol metabolism

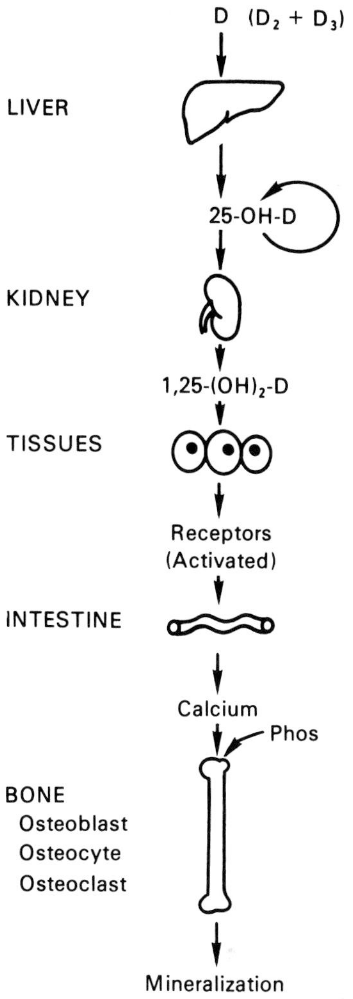

Fig. 165-4 Calciferol activation as a component of the bone mineralization pathway.

or action. For example, rickets resistant to 1α,25$(OH)_2D$ could include primary bone defects such as hypophosphatasia.[62] The most helpful bioeffect to include in a description is the most proximal one(s) known to be abnormal; thus calcium malabsorption is more useful than osteomalacia to characterize defects in calciferol metabolism or action. The term *vitamin D–resistant rickets* combines all the problems addressed earlier. It could be applied to a defect (associated with normal vitamin D intake) anywhere in the bone mineralization pathway (Fig. 165-4).

Since defects in calciferol metabolism or action can be associated with or even secondary to defects in other pathways, disease categories also should indicate if dysfunction extends to other pathways. We use the term *simple* to specify that a calciferol defect is not associated with defects in other pathways and *complex* to specify the converse. Other important qualifying terms can indicate if a defect is hereditary or acquired or if a defect is anatomically localized (tissue selective) or generalized (tissue nonselective).[63] In this chapter we will use precise terms (Table 165-2), consistent with our current understanding of calciferol metabolism. As our understanding increases, these terms will need to be replaced.

Two hereditary defects limited to the calciferol pathway (i.e., simple defects) have been recognized. The first is selective* and

*By *selective* deficiency of a metabolite, we mean deficiency of this metabolite without deficiency of its immediate precursor.

Table 165-2 Classification of Calciferol Deficiency States by Theoretically Possible Etiology

Vitamin D deficiency
Deficient input
Deficient diet
Deficient synthesis
Increased clearance
Selective* 25(OH)D deficiency
Deficient vitamin D 25-hydroxylase
Increased clearance
Selective $1\alpha,25(OH)_2D$ deficiency
Deficient 25(OH)D 1α-hydroxylase
Increased clearance
Resistance to $1\alpha,25(OH)_2D$
Local
Generalized
Deficient vitamin D receptor function
Defects proximal or distal to vitamin D receptor

**Selective* means that the immediate precursor of the metabolite is not deficient.

NOTE: In theory, each category except deficient diet could have a hereditary or acquired etiology, and each subcategory could be further partitioned into simple (implying that the defect is localized only to the step in calciferol metabolism) or complex (implying that the fundamental defect also involves other metabolic pathways). At present, the only recognized hereditary and simple defects are selective deficiency of $1\alpha,25(OH)_2D$ and generalized resistance to $1\alpha,25(OH)_2D$.

simple† deficiency of $1\alpha,25(OH)_2D$. The second is generalized simple resistance to $1\alpha,25(OH)_2D$. It seems likely that all cases in the first category result from defects of 25(OH)D 1α-hydroxylase and that all in the second category reflect simple deficiency of vitamin D receptor function.

GENERAL FEATURES OF CALCIFEROL DEFICIENCY

Clinical Presentation

The general features of vitamin D deficiency will be reviewed[64] because almost all are shown in patients with hereditary defects in calciferol metabolism [selective deficiency of $1\alpha,25(OH)_2D$ or generalized resistance to $1\alpha,25(OH)_2D$]. The clinical features of calciferol deficiency are weakness, bone pain, bone deformity, and fracture. The most rapidly growing bones show the most striking abnormalities. In the first year of life, the most rapidly growing bones are in the cranium, ribs, and wrists. Calciferol deficiency at this time leads to widened cranial sutures, frontal bossing, posterior flattening of the skull, bulging of costochondral junctions, and enlargement of the wrists. The rib cage may be so deformed that it contributes to respiratory failure. Dental eruption is delayed, and teeth show enamel hypoplasia. Muscular weakness and hypotonia are severe and result in a protuberant abdomen. Muscular weakness can contribute to respiratory failure. Linear growth may be adequate, but the child may be unable to walk without support. Tetany is unusual because the degree of hypocalcemia is mild and its onset is slow. After age 1, deformities are most prominent in the legs because of their weight-bearing function.

The clinical features of calciferol deficiency states depend principally on age of onset. Calcium and phosphate levels in fetal plasma are sustained by placental transport from maternal plasma, and this transport is not regulated by calciferols.[65] A fetus with a hereditary abnormality in calciferol metabolism that develops in a mother with normal calciferol metabolism is presumed to have normal calcium and phosphate levels in plasma and bone until birth. In children, mineralization defects result in abnormalities of diaphyses, metaphyses, and epiphyses. In particular, deficient mineralization of the epiphyseal growth plate results in distorted (bulging) epiphyses and bone deformity.

Calciferol deficiency that begins after epiphyseal fusion causes less deformity. Calciferol deficiency in adults causes less severe features. In the mature, remodeling skeleton, less than 5 percent of the calcium is newly deposited per year. Thus a mineralization defect must be present for several years to be manifested. The earliest symptom is bone pain, particularly low in the back. Proximal muscle weakness may be so prominent as to suggest a primary neurologic disturbance.

Radiographs

The radiographic features of calciferol deficiency states in children are quite uniform. Delayed opacification of epiphyses causes widening and distortion of growth plates; the usually straight ends of the mineralizing metaphyses are irregular (frayed). The bone cortex is abnormally thin, and bone trabeculae are sparse. Pseudofractures are uncommon in children. Secondary hyperparathyroidism may cause subperiosteal erosions, but bone cysts are unusual in children.

Response to Therapy

During the first 1 to 4 months of treatment, endogenous production of $1\alpha,25(OH)_2D$ is regulated to rates above normal.[66,67] The minimal vitamin D requirement for treatment of vitamin D deficiency is 2 to 5 μg/day, but much larger amounts are usually given (100–200 μg/day) both to accelerate repletion of body vitamin D pools and because the extra vitamin D is not converted to excessive $1\alpha,25(OH)_2D$. Successful initiation of therapy is evidenced by diminution of secondary hyperparathyroidism; that is, PTH and urinary cAMP levels fall, serum phosphate level rises, and serum alkaline phosphatase level falls.

Pathophysiology

Virtually all the features of calciferol deficiency can be understood as direct or remote consequences of deficient calciferol effect on duodenal transport of calcium. Malabsorption of calcium results in hypocalcemia. Hypocalcemia and perhaps also the deficient calciferol effect on the parathyroid gland[68] result in increased secretion of PTH (i.e., secondary hyperparathyroidism). If this process continues for many months, the parathyroid glands develop hypertrophy and hyperplasia. PTH acts on the proximal renal tubule to decrease reabsorption of phosphate and bicarbonate, resulting in hypophosphatemia and hyperchloremic acidosis. However, the phosphaturic effect of PTH is not inevitable; hypocalcemia that is severe and long-standing paradoxically can inhibit the phosphaturic effect of PTH. This can result in a confusing picture of secondary hyperparathyroidism with high urinary cAMP but not hypophosphatemia[69] (so-called pseudohypoparathyroidism type II). In children, secondary hyperparathyroidism also causes generalized aminoaciduria. The combination of hypocalcemia and hypophosphatemia results in a slowed rate of mineralization of bone matrix. PTH also has direct actions on bone. It increases osteoclastic resorption (but the release of calcium and phosphate from bone does not fully compensate for the hypocalcemia or hypophosphatemia), and osteoblastic activity rises because it is "coupled" with osteoclast activity.

The response to therapy in calciferol deficiency states can be clearly understood by considering the changes in calcium homeostasis. The principal goal of therapy is provision of enough calcium and calciferol in plasma to allow normalization of bone mineralization and suppression of secondary hyperparathyroidism. A chronic deficiency of calciferol is associated with skeletal

†By *simple* deficiency, we mean a defect that involves only the calciferol metabolic pathway. The alternative is *complex* deficiency, involving other pathways as well. Most acquired disturbances in calciferol metabolism are complex (e.g., malabsorption or chronic renal disease). Some hereditary deficiencies are also complex. For example, 25(OH)D 1α-hydroxylase deficiency can occur as a part of a Fanconi syndrome, pseudohypoparathyroidism, or X-linked hypophosphatemia.

calcium deficiency that can withdraw calcium from plasma for many months after treatment begins. In children, normal bone mass may be produced after recovery from calciferol deficiency, but in adults, bone mass may remain low after "recovery."[70] In simple nutritional deficiency of vitamin D, therapy with vitamin D allows the PTH–1α-hydroxylase axis to generate high and appropriate amounts of 1α,25(OH)$_2$D during this remineralization phase.

Remineralization entails large fluxes of calcium and phosphate from blood into undermineralized bone; during this phase, serum contains low calcium, high PTH, low phosphate, and normal or high 25(OH)D levels, all of which promote synthesis of 1α,25(OH)$_2$D. In patients with deficiency of the 1α-hydroxylase or with target resistance to, 1α,25(OH)$_2$D therapy should be designed to compensate for the defect and manage the phase of "hungry bones."

Table 165-3 Daily Calciferol Doses for Maintenance Treatment of Patients with Hereditary Defects in Calciferol Metabolism

Calciferol Analogue	In Deficient 25(OH)D 1α-Hydroxylase, μg/day	In Generalized Resistance to 1α,25(OH)$_2$D, μg/day
D$_3$ or D$_2$	500–3000	500–?*
25(OH)D$_3$	30–200	30–?*
1α,25(OH)$_2$D$_3$	0.3–2	5–60†
1α(OH)D$_3$	0.5–3	5–60†
Dihydrotachysterol	150–1000	2000–20,000†

*Patients with milder grades of resistance to 1α,25(OH)$_2$D (usually with normal hair) can respond to analogues requiring 1α-hydroxylation. Maximal useful doses have not been defined. Serum 1α,25(OH)$_2$D must be maintained in the range of 200 to 10,000 pg/ml.

†Maximal doses are limited only by cost and patient acceptance; some patients have shown no response to maximal doses tested.

NOTE: Dose requirements as μg/day (i.e., uncorrected for body size) are similar in children and adults.

HEREDITARY DEFECTS IN CALCIFEROL METABOLISM

Hereditary Selective Deficiency of 1α,25(OH)$_2$D (MIM 264700)

Clinical Features. Deficiency of 1α,25(OH)$_2$D occurs as a component of several hereditary disorders (e.g., X-linked hypophosphatemia, some variants of Fanconi syndrome, and pseudohypoparathyroidism), but selective and simple (as defined earlier) deficiency of 1α,25(OH)$_2$D is a distinctive state to be described later. This disorder (formerly called *hereditary vitamin D dependency type I* or *hereditary pseudo-vitamin D deficiency type I*) is an unusual cause of hereditary rickets.[71,72] Patients appear normal at birth but have recognizable dysfunction between the ages of 2 and 24 months, suggesting lack of calciferol effect (see above) that began at the time of birth. Muscle weakness is prominent, radiographic features are striking, and responsivity to calciferols is complete (see below).

Serum shows low calcium, high PTH, but low or even undetectable 1α,25(OH)$_2$D.[73,74] The latter can be associated with normal or even modestly increased 25(OH)D [reflecting vitamin D supplementation and/or diminished clearance of 25(OH)D]. During therapy with vitamin D or 25(OH)D, serum 1α,25(OH)$_2$D continues to be low or undetectable. During successful maintenance therapy with 1α-hydroxylated vitamin D metabolites, serum 1α,25(OH)$_2$D is normal; random serum determinations may be hard to interpret during therapy with 1α,25(OH)$_2$D$_3$ because of the rapid turnover of this drug. Serum calcium and phosphate determinations in the partially treated patient also can be difficult to interpret. With partial treatment or early after discontinuation of treatment, secondary hyperparathyroidism can be associated with hypophosphatemia and a normal serum calcium level[75]; this can cause confusion with X-linked hypophosphatemia, particularly because some patients with that disorder also show secondary hyperparathyroidism.

Inheritance. Several sibships show features highly suggestive of autosomal recessive inheritance. No biochemical abnormalities have been recognized in obligate heterozygotes. The homozygous state is relatively common in the Saguenay region of Quebec (estimated gene frequency 0.02), and this has been attributed to a founder effect rather than to a high rate of consanguinity.[76] Genetic linkage analysis in this population established a locus on the long arm of chromosome 12.[77] It is of interest to note that the gene for 25(OH)D 1α-hydroxylase was mapped to chromosome 12q13.3.[83a–83c]

Therapy. Patients with this disorder have been treated successfully with all widely available calciferol analogues.[75,78–80] During the early phases of therapy (initial 3–6 months), they respond best to therapy with two to five times the expected long-term maintenance dose (Table 165-3) because of the high calcium requirements of the undermineralized skeleton. Long-term maintenance therapy is accomplished with any regimen that establishes normal circulating activity of metabolites that will activate vitamin D receptors. Based on the primary defect, it is obvious that physiologic replacement doses of 1α-hydroxylated metabolites are sufficient, whereas high doses of vitamin D or 25(OH)D are required to achieve remission (see Table 165-3). During successful treatment with vitamin D or 25(OH)D$_3$, serum 25(OH)D levels are in the range of 250 ng/ml, but serum 1α,25(OH)$_2$D may remain low or undetectable.[73,74] This has several important implications. First, the degree of 1α-hydroxylase deficiency in these patients is severe; second, the indicated concentration of 25(OH)D is insufficient to be associated with normal activation of the vitamin D receptor. The second implication does not establish whether 25(OH)D is acting directly or through other metabolites [such as 5,6,-*trans*-25(OH)D]. During long-term maintenance therapy, the serum total 1α,25(OH)$_2$D bioactivity is prevented by the deficiency of 1α-hydroxylase. Thus the patient must adapt to fluctuations in calcium availability through direct actions of PTH alone. Since intestinal fractional absorption of calcium cannot be regulated by endogenous mechanisms, all the external calcium balance must be regulated at the renal level. Thus these patients may show a more rapid fall of urine calcium or a rise of urine calcium at times of calcium deficiency or excess, respectively. The best way to minimize such fluctuations is to include a fixed calcium supplement (1000 mg/day as elemental calcium). Treatment must be continued indefinitely. Although relapses may be slow to develop after withdrawing treatment in an adult, relapses are inevitable and should be prevented.

Cellular Defect. The presumption is that hereditary selective deficiency of 1α,25(OH)$_2$D results, in all cases, from defects in 25(OH)D 1α-hydroxylase. It seems inconceivable that accelerated clearance of 1α,25(OH)$_2$D could produce this state. Deficient activity of the decidual enzyme 25(OH)D 1α-hydroxylase in cells isolated from the placenta of two women with this disease was reported.[81] It is noteworthy that it was well documented that human decidual cells do produce 1α,25(OH)$_2$D that was regulated by feedback mechanisms.[82,83] The recent availability of sequence information for the 25(OH)D 1α-hydroxylase gene enabled screening for mutations in patients with hereditary selective deficiency of 1α,25(OH)$_2$D and their obligate carriers. Close to 20 different mutations were documented in 26 kindreds with this disease.[83a–83e] All patients were homozygous for the genetic defect, whereas the obligate carriers had one copy of the mutant allele. The cellular defect does not seem to impair 25(OH)D 24-hydroxylase. Serum levels of 24,25-(OH$_2$)D are appropriate for the level of 25(OH)D, and cultured skin fibroblasts show a normal 25(OH)D 24-hydroxylase response to $1\alpha,25(OH)_2D_3$.[84] These data suggested nonidentity of the 25(OH)D 1α- and 24-hydroxylase enzyme systems.

Animal Models for Hereditary Selective Deficiency of $1\alpha,25(OH)_2D$. Ploniat[85] reported an autosomal recessive rachitic disorder in pigs. More recent studies[86] have shown that the animals had hypocalcemic rickets responsive to "physiologic" doses of $1\alpha,25(OH)_2D$ or $1\alpha(OH)D_3$. A similar trait was transferred to miniature pigs for detailed study. Direct assay of renal homogenates of homozygotes from both strains of pig established undetectable $25(OH)D_3$ 1α-hydroxylase activity.[87,88] Both strains also exhibited low circulating 24,25(OH)D and undetectable renal $25(OH)D_3$ 24-hydroxylase activity. Furthermore, renal homogenate from a rachitic pig rendered normocalcemic by $1,25(OH)_2D_3$ treatment showed no detectable 25(OH)D 24-hydroxylase activity. This seemed different from the findings of normal 25(OH)D 24-hydroxylase in affected humans.[84] There are several possible explanations for this apparent inconsistency.[84]

States Resembling Hereditary Selective Deficiency of $1\alpha,25(OH)_2D$. In several hereditary or acquired disorders, 25(OH)D 1α-hydroxylase deficiency is one component of a more complex disturbance. These disorders affecting the proximal renal tubule include X-linked hypophosphatemia[89,90] (see Chap. 197), renal tubular acidosis[91,92] (see Chap. 195), some forms of Fanconi syndrome[93,94] (see Chap. 196), and tumor-associated osteomalacia[95] (in which a humoral factor seems to cause impairment of 1α-hydroxylase and renal wasting of phosphate; see Chap. 197). Replacement of $1\alpha,25(OH)_2D$ is often an important component in therapy of these disorders.

Hereditary Generalized Resistance to $1\alpha,25(OH)_2D$ (MIM 277440)

Clinical Features. Hereditary generalized resistance to $1\alpha,25(OH)_2D$ (also called *vitamin D dependency type II* or *pseudo-vitamin D deficiency type II*) was first recognized in 1977 and is a rare disorder. There are fewer than 50 known kindreds (a partial list in refs. 9 and 96–132 and personal communications). The clinical features are almost identical to those in hereditary selective deficiency of $1\alpha,25(OH)_2D$ with the exception that hereditary generalized resistance to $1,25(OH)_2D$ has been associated with alopecia in about half the kindreds. Patients with hereditary generalized resistance to $1\alpha,25(OH)_2D$ appear normal at birth but develop the clinical and biochemical features of calciferol deficiency (see above) with hypocalcemia and rickets over the first 2 to 8 months of life. In many cases, hair loss occurs between the ages of 2 and 12 months. The hair loss may be complete (Fig. 165-5) or incomplete; sometimes there is selective sparing of the eyelashes. Light microscopic examination of a scalp biopsy showed normal numbers and morphology of hair follicles in a patient with total alopecia.[98] Alopecia occurs in patients with the most severe resistance to $1\alpha,25(OH)_2D$ (see below).[133] Without therapy, this disorder leads to inanition, severe skeletal deformity, recurrent respiratory infections, and death. Although therapy with calciferols can sustain complete biochemical remission in some patients, the alopecia does not improve. Other ectodermal defects have been reported in small numbers of patients and have an uncertain relation to the syndrome; these include oligodentia[98] and papular skin rash.[98,134] All patients suffer from the consequences of intestinal malabsorption of calcium. Attempts to show vitamin D receptor–mediated dysfunctions outside the intenstine in vivo have so far been inconclusive. Basal and stimulated concentrations of insulin, thyrotropin, prolactin, growth hormone, and testosterone have been normal (aside from deficiencies in insulin stimulation attributable to hypocalcemia).[135] Bone biopsies have shown normal or increased numbers of osteoclasts (suggesting that the vitamin D receptor is not essential for osteoclast formation), but their resportive activity was suggested to be impaired.[136]

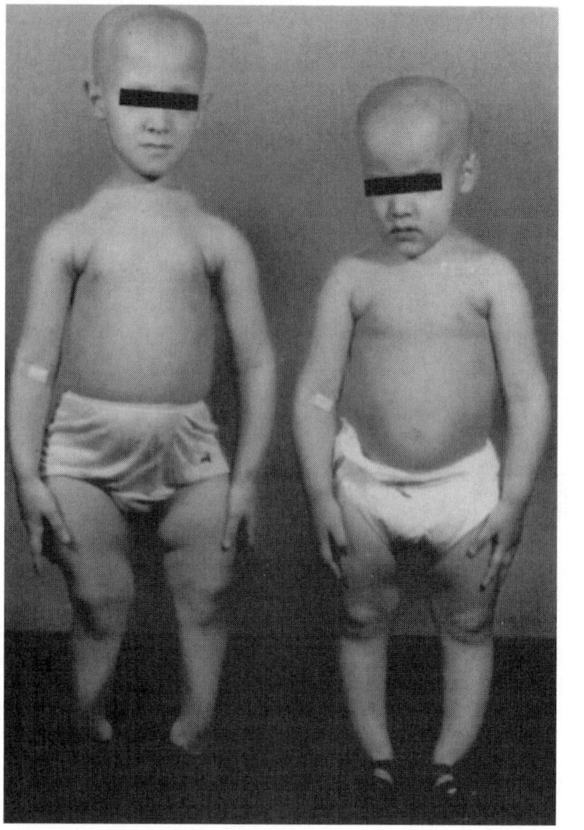

Fig. 165-5 Sisters (aged 7 and 3) with alopecia and rickets from hereditary generalized resistance to $1\alpha,25(OH)_2D$. (*Used with permission from Rosen et al.*[97])

In several cases, early postnatal development was apparently normal, and dysfunction was not evident until late in childhood[101] or even in adulthood[99] [in the latter case, serum $1\alpha,25(OH)_2D$ was not measured, so alternate etiologies such as noncompliance were not excluded]. These patients did not show alopecia and responded to high doses of calciferols, indicating a mild variant of the syndrome. None showed clear features of a genetic etiology (that is to say, there was no parental consanguinity and no affected siblings; unfortunately, cultured cells were not evaluated in any).

Several patients have shown unexplained fluctuations in disease severity. Two patients without any clear calcemic response to calciferols experienced lessening of secondary hyperparathyroidism and improved bone mineralization around the ages of 7 to 9. One patient showed a prolonged remission of biochemical and radiographic abnormalities that subsequently seemed completely unresponsive to much higher doses of calciferols.[104] Another patient showed amelioration of resistance to $1\alpha,25(OH)_2D$ following a brief trial of $24,25(OH)_2D$.[98]

Measurement of calciferol metabolites in plasma usually provides useful information for diagnosis. Serum concentrations of $1\alpha,25(OH)_2D$ are 50 to 1000 pg/ml (normal in children is 30–100 pg/ml) before treatment. During treatment with calciferols, typical concentrations are 200 to 10,000 pg/ml[133] (Fig. 165-6).

Inheritance. There usually have been strong suggestions of autosomal recessive transmission (parental consanguinity, etc.). Most patients have been recognized in a broad region centered on the Mediterranean shores, and this may relate to a high consanguinity rate in the receptor-disease source population.[137] No clinical abnormalities have been reported in obligate heterozygotes.

Treatment. Some patients show complete remission while receiving high doses of calciferols[109] (see Table 165-3). The

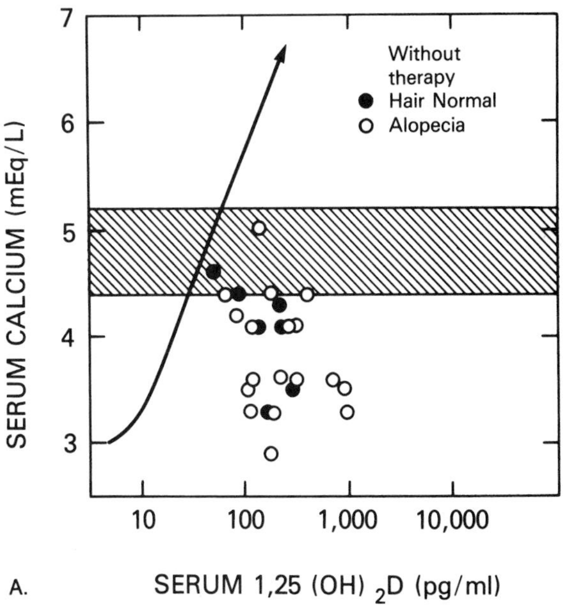

A.

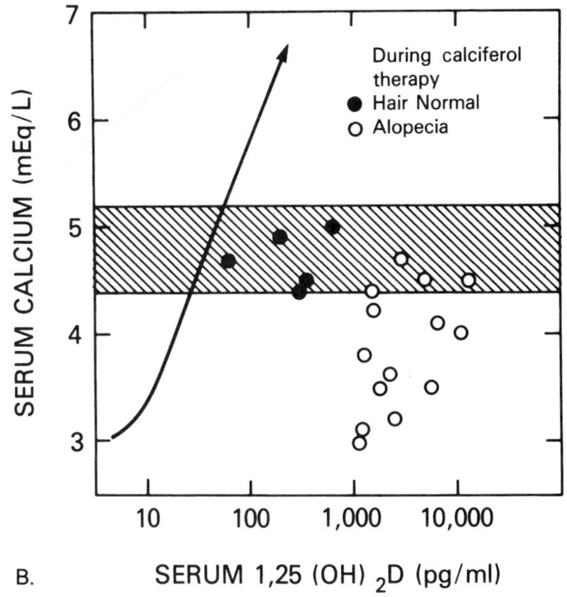

B.

Fig. 165-6 Relations between serum concentrations of calcium and 1α,25(OH)$_2$D in patients with generalized resistance to 1α,25(OH)$_2$D. Stippled area is normal range for calcium. Solid curve is theoretical normal relation between calcium and 1α,25(OH)$_2$D. Each symbol depicts data from one patient with generalized resistance to 1α,25(OH)$_2$D: (*A*) Without calciferol therapy. (*B*) During calciferol therapy. Solid circle, hair normal; open circle, alopecia. (*Used with permission from Marx et al.*[133])

presence or absence of alopecia is one simple predictor of potential for response to therapy.[133] Virtually all patients with normal hair can sustain remission when given high doses of analogues not requiring 1α-hydroxylation. Among patients with alopecia, approximately half have not responded to the highest doses of calciferols available; half have shown satisfactory calcemic response, but the dose requirement [deduced from serum 1,25(OH)$_2$D during therapy] is typically tenfold higher than in patients with normal hair (see Fig. 165-6). Maintenance treatment is based on four considerations: (1) the most mildly affected patients can be treated with calciferols [vitamin D$_3$, vitamin D$_2$, 25(OH)D$_3$] that provide substrate for a high renal secretion of 1α,25(OH)$_2$D, (2) more severely affected patients may respond only to extremely high doses of analogues [1α,25(OH)$_2$D, 1α-(OH)D$_3$, dihydrotachysterol] that do not require 1α-hydroxylation, (3) some patients may not respond to maximal doses of any calciferols, and (4) the role of calcium supplements is different in each of the prior three therapy categories (see below).

Several patients have shown remissions while receiving high doses of vitamin D$_2$ or 25(OH)D$_3$[9,96]; they respond to this because their tissue resistance is only moderate, and they can produce sufficient 1α,25(OH)$_2$D endogenously if presented with a high level of substrate for 1α-hydroxylation. It is uncertain if this mechanism of therapy requires pathologic elevations of PTH; it seems possible that near-normal parathyroid function may be sufficient because of deficient feedback suppression of 1α-hydroxylation (Fig. 165-7) (resulting from the defect of vitamin D receptors in the proximal renal tubule). In this group, calcium supplements may have little or no role, since serum concentrations of both PTH and 1α,25(OH)$_2$D can compensate for fluctuations in calcium availability. High levels of 1α,25(OH)$_2$D in an affected female can permit a normal pregnancy[138]; this is important because of concern that a high level of 1α,25(OH)$_2$D may disturb fetal tissues (see "Calciferol Excess States," below).

Patients unable to produce sufficient 1α,25(OH)$_2$D endogenously [because of a requirement for particularly high 1α,25(OH)$_2$D concentrations] may still respond to extraordinarily high doses of analogues not requiring 1α-hydroxylation [i.e., 1α,25(OH)$_2$D$_3$, 1α-(OH)D$_3$, dihydrotachysterol]. Patients in this group requiring therapy that bypasses 1α-hydroxylation should receive fixed calcium supplements (1000 mg/day elemental calcium) for the same reasons as patients with hereditary selective deficiency of 1α,25(OH)$_2$D [see "Hereditary Selective Deficiency of 1α,25(OH)$_2$D," above].

Some patients may have little or no response to maximal calciferol doses. But it is difficult to identify these patients. There are no widely available indexes of intestinal responsivity to calciferols; fractional calcium absorption is the most relevant index, but this test may be unavailable because of the inconvenience of balance studies or because of radiation exposure from calcium-47. It is possible to measure this parameter with stable calcium isotopes.[139] Most studies have relied on the calcemic response to a therapeutic trial (Fig. 165-8). These trials may be unsatisfactory, first, because of the time required for repletion of underminerealized bones (i.e., as long as the bones retain the increased calcium input, this will not result in normalization of serum calcium). Second, therapeutic trials with high calciferol doses are limited by available drug formulations and drug cost. Patients with an undetectable response to calciferols can receive substantial benefit if large amounts of calcium can be delivered to the bloodstream. The most rapid way to accomplish this is by intravenous infusions[136,139–141]; high calcium doses (1000 mg elemental calcium per day infused over 12 h) can be tolerated even by young children with this disorder. Since normal positive calcium balance during childhood growth is approximately 300 mg/day, and since the total deficit may be several hundred grams of elemental calcium, such infusions must be given repeatedly over many months to accomplish significant results. This form of therapy requires methods similar to those used in hyperalimentation programs. Another way to increase calcium input to the bloodstream is to increase net absorption independent of calciferols. This can be accomplished by increasing calcium intake to the point of intolerance.[134] Unfortunately, the upper limit of oral intake is around 6000 mg/day and requires great cooperation; in the absence of calciferol bioeffect, the fractional calcium absorption (virtually all of which is retained) is approximately 10 percent, implying that up to 600 mg/day can be delivered to the bloodstream by oral supplements. With high doses of calcium intravenously or orally, the serum phosphate level may decrease further; oral phosphate supplements should then be added. The utility of therapy with intravenous or oral calcium confirms the centrality of the intestine as a target tissue for 1α,25(OH)$_2$D.

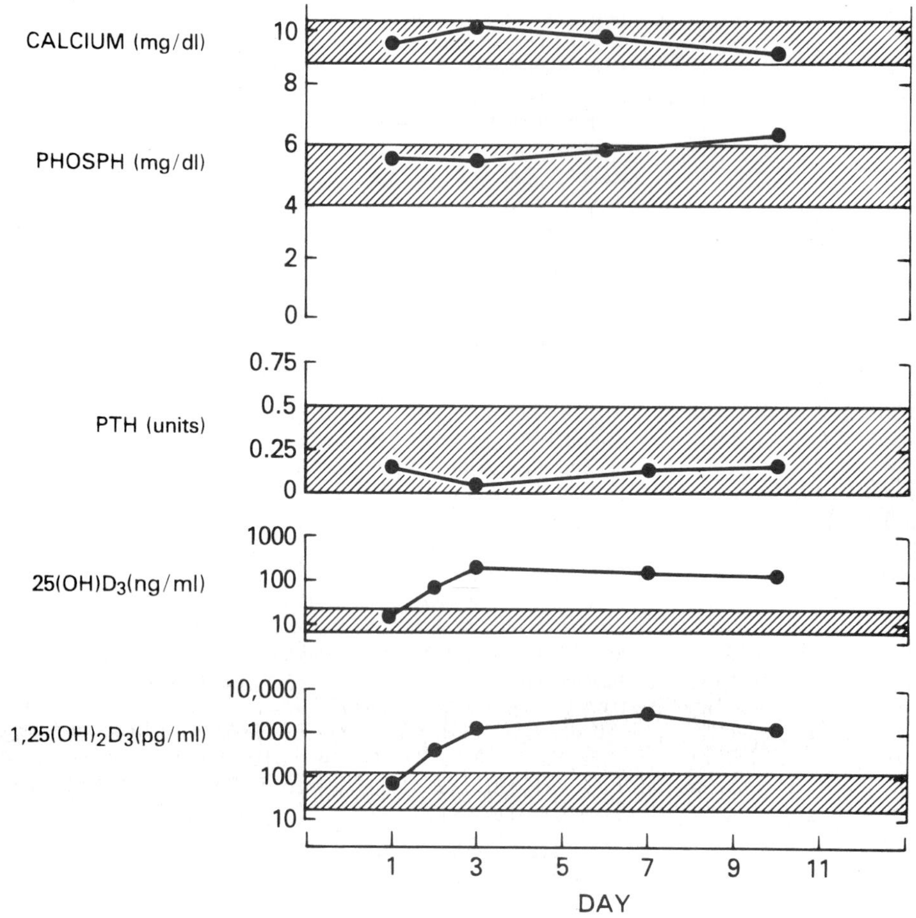

Fig. 165-7 Abnormal regulation of $1\alpha,25(OH)_2D$ in serum of a patient with hereditary generalized resistance to $1\alpha,25(OH)_2D$. Serum calcium, phosphate, and PTH had been normalized by treatment with $1\alpha(OH)D_3$. $1\alpha(OH)D_3$ was stopped for 2 days, and the patient received $25(OH)D_3$ as sole therapy. Stippled zones indicate normal ranges. Note logarithmic scales for calciferols. Serum $1\alpha,25(OH)_2D$ reaches extremely high concentrations without the usual stimuli (low calcium, high PTH, low phosphate) for its production. PHOSPH, phosphorus. (*Used with permission from Marx et al.*[109])

Detailed studies of the interactions of calciferol dose with calcium dose have not been done. However, it seems possible that some patients (e.g., those with 90 percent deficiency in hormone-binding capacity[104,109]) would have a diminished maximal response to calciferols; such patients with partial responses may obtain unique benefits from combinations of calciferols and calcium, both at high doses.

As in the calciferol deficiency states, total-body calcium requirements are highest at the onset of treatment. Thus the doses of calcium, the doses of calciferols, and even the type of approach judged necessary to initiate therapy (e.g., intravenous calcium) may not prove the same as those used for maintenance therapy.

Cellular Defects. Cells from patients with hereditary generalized resistance to $1\alpha,25(OH)_2D$ have been used to characterize the defect presumed to be present in all target tissues. Because of the widespread expression of the $1\alpha,25(OH)_2D$ effector system in many tissues, these studies have been possible with skin fibroblasts in most studies, keratinocytes,[105] bone cells,[142] peripheral lymphocytes,[144,145] and virally transformed lymphocytes.[146] These cells were used to assess most of the steps in $1,25(OH)_2D$ action from cellular uptake to bioresponse and to elucidate the molecular aberrations in the hormone-receptor protein and the nuclear DNA that encodes for it.[116–121,123–132] The latter became feasible with cloning and sequencing of the human VDR chromosomal gene.

Several methods have been used to characterize the hormone-receptor interaction, including binding capacity and affinity of $[^3H]1,25(OH)_2D_3$ to intact cells, nuclei, or high-salt-soluble extract cytosol,[102,103,106] measurements of receptor content by monoclonal antibodies,[117,119,124] and characterization of the hormone-receptor complex on continuous sucrose gradient and heterologous DNA-cellulose columns.[111,112,117]

Based on the hormone-receptor-nuclear interaction, three different classes of intracellular defects have been identified in these cells, as presented below:

1. *Hormone binding defects*
   a. *No (negative) hormone binding.* Unmeasurable specific binding of $[^3H]1,25(OH)_2D_3$ to either high-salt-soluble cell extract and/or intact cells or nuclei[106,107] is the most common abnormality observed. In the majority of these patients, high concentrations of $1,25(OH)_2D$ in serum or culture medium did not evoke a biologic or biochemical response in vivo or in vitro (see below).
   b. *Decreased maximal capacity of hormone binding.* This abnormality has been reported in only one kindred.[104] Cell extracts showed a hormone-binding capacity only 10 percent of normal but a hormone-binding affinity that was normal. The patient did not respond to prolonged treatment with high doses of active vitamin D metabolites.
   c. *Decreased affinity of hormone binding.* A selective abnormality in hormone-binding affinity with normal hormone-binding capacity has been suggested but not proven conclusively in one kindred.[106] An additional patient, recently described, had a modest decrease of the affinity of the receptor for $1,25(OH)_2D_3$ when measured at 0°C.[130] A complete remission of the disease in all these patients could be achieved with high doses of active calciferol metabolites.[106,130]
2. *Defective receptor translocation to nucleus.* Extracts of cells from two kindreds have shown normal capacity and affinity of hormone binding; however, high-affinity uptake of hormone into the nucleus of intact cells was undetectable.[102,106] The receptors from both kindreds showed a normal affinity for nonspecific DNA.[112] Analysis by immunocytology showed that

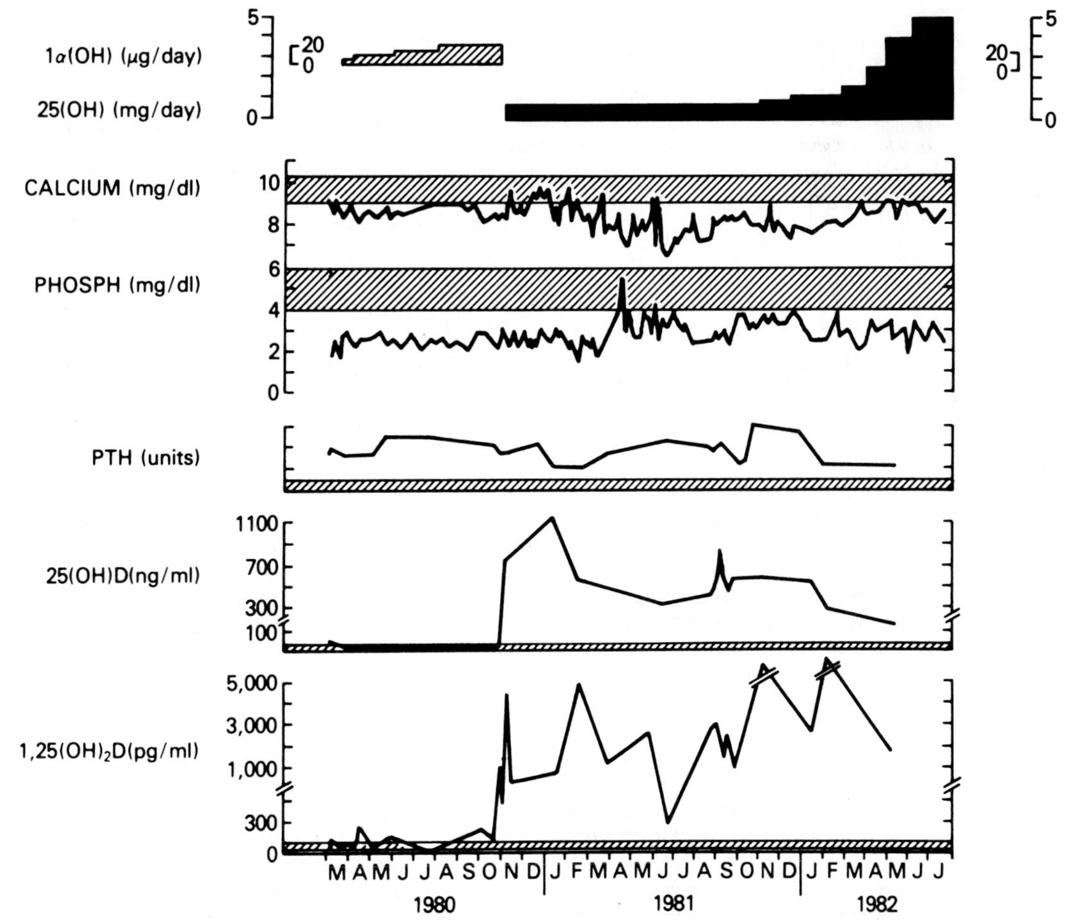

Fig. 165-8 Absent calcemic response during a long therapeutic trial with calciferols. Calciferol therapy is in upper panel: 1α(OH) refers to 1α(OH)D_3. Stippled zones indicate normal ranges. Not only is hypocalcemia persistent, but also secondary hyperparathyroidism persists (high PTH and low phosphate), and very high serum levels of 1α,25$(OH)_2D$ are documented. PHOSPH, phosphorus. (*Used with permission from Marx et al.*[109])

vitamin D receptors from these patients accumulated along the nuclear membrane after addition of 1α,25$(OH)_2D_3$, unlike normal receptors, which rapidly translocated from cytoplasm into nucleus.[147] Recently, two additional unrelated patients were described with a lowered 1,25$(OH)_2D_3$ retention in intact cells incubated at 37°C.[129] All these patients were treated successfully with high doses of vitamin D and its active metabolites.[96,102,129]

3. *Defective receptor binding to DNA*. With cells from several kindreds the 1α,25$(OH)_2D$ receptor showed abnormal elution from nonspecific DNA[111,112,117]; in each the receptor eluted from the DNA at lower salt concentration than normal (Fig. 165-9). No biologic response to high doses of vitamin D or its active metabolites either in vivo or in vitro (see below) was documented in almost all patients with this type of defect.[98,111,112,117]

To summarize, no patient has met the strict criteria for a possible prereceptor or postreceptor defect. Wherever detailed testing of vitamin D receptor properties has been done, abnormalities have been found. The class of cellular defect has shown no correlation with clinical features. Rather, these patients seem to fit along one continuous spectrum of severity of disease.

1α,25$(OH)_2D_3$ Bioeffect in Patients' Cells. Several assays have tested posttranscriptional actions of 1α,25$(OH)_2D_3$ in cells from these patients. In all assays, each patient's cells have shown severely deficient responses. The most extensively tested response

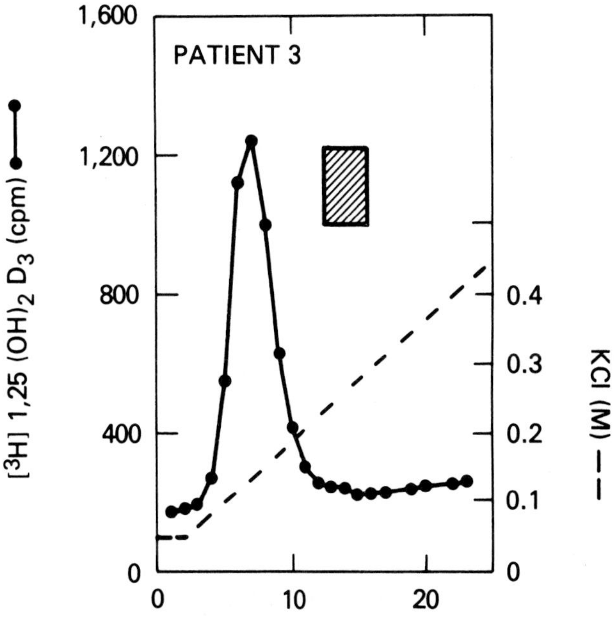

Fig. 165-9 Elution of vitamin D receptor from a column of DNA-cellulose. Shaded area shows location of elution peak for normal receptors. Solid circle, elution profile for receptors from patient with hereditary resistance to 1α,25$(OH)_2D$ and receptors with a DNA-binding defect. (*Used with permission from Liberman et al.*[112])

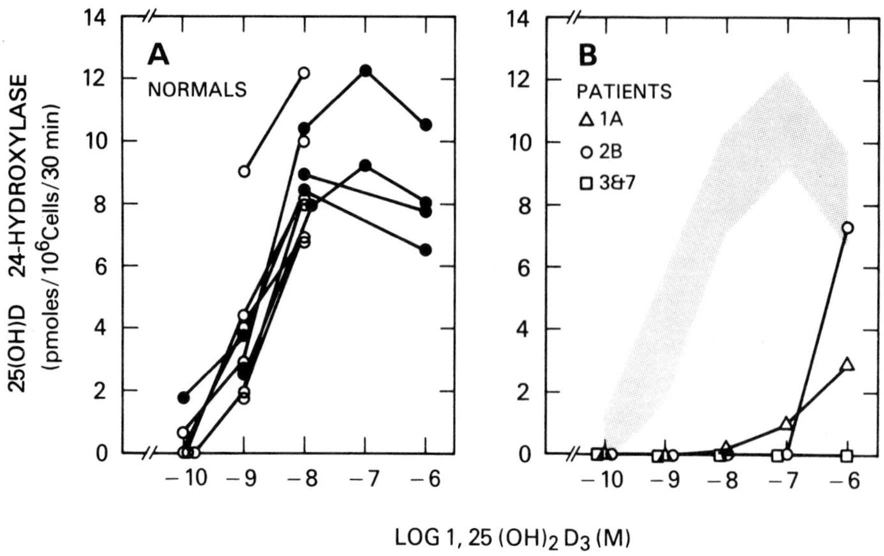

Fig. 165-10 25(OH)D_3 24-hydroxylase in skin fibroblasts preincubated with indicated concentrations of 1α,25$(OH)_2D_3$. (*A*) Normal subjects. (*B*) Patients with hereditary generalized resistance to 1α,25$(OH)_2$D. Patients 1A and 2B each showed a satisfactory calcemic response to high doses of 1α,25$(OH)_2D_3$, but patients 3 and 7 showed no calcemic response. Shaded area in *B* indicates normal response. (*Modified with permission from Gamblin et al.*[149])

is 1,25$(OH)_2D_3$ induction of 25(OH)D_3 24-hydroxylase activity in cultured skin fibroblasts.[148,149] In general, patients with milder disease (normal hair, calcemic response to high doses of calciferols) show inducible 24-hydroxylase with supraphysiologic concentrations of 1α,25$(OH)_2D_3$ (Fig. 165-10), but patients with the severest disease (alopecia, no calcemic response to maximal doses of calciferols) show no 24-hydroxylase response to maximal concentrations of 1α,25$(OH)_2D_3$. Five of six obligate heterozygotes showed no abnormality[107]; the sixth showed a 50 percent decrease in hormone-binding capacity and a similar decrease in maximal induction of 24-hydroxylase. Similar severe defects have been identified with other bioassays or different cells, including inhibition of cell proliferation by 1α,25$(OH)_2$D (cultured skin fibroblasts, keratinocytes,[105] peripheral mononuclear cells[144,145]), 1,25$(OH)_2D_3$-mediated stimulation of 24-hydroxylase and of osteocalcin secretion in osteoblast-like bone cells,[142] and rapid stimulation of cGMP accumulation by 1,25$(OH)_2D_3$ in fibroblasts.[39]

If the predictive therapeutic value of the in vitro bioresponse to 1,25$(OH)_2D_3$ could be substantiated, it may eliminate the need for expensive and time-consuming therapeutic trials with high doses of vitamin D and its metabolites (as discussed before).

Gene Defects. Studies on the molecular defects have used isolation, amplification, and sequencing of genomic VDR DNA, as well as cloning and sequencing of VDR cDNA, recreation of the mutant VDR in vitro, and testing transcriptional activity of patients and artificially created mutant VDR. Mutations in the VDR gene have been identified in almost every patient with this disease who was investigated (Fig. 165-11). Four of these genetic alterations resulted in a nonsense change that introduced a stop condon predicting a truncated VDR that lacks hormone-binding or both hormone- and DNA-binding domains.[124,131,132]

Recently, two unrelated patients were described in whom two different point mutations led to a frameshift in translation resulting in a premature stop codon that would produce a VDR lacking both DNA- and hormone-binding sites in one patient and the ligand-binding site in the second.[128,131]

Missense VDR mutations were documented in cells derived from almost all other patients or kindreds examined. The functional characterization of the patient's VDR reflected the localization of the point mutation: (1) mutations localized to the DNA-binding, N-terminal, and zinc-finger region[111,118,120,123,125–127] (these mutations typically are found in residues conserved across the entire receptor family, and most lie within α-helices on the C-terminal side of the zinc fingers, which are involved in DNA base recognition and phosphate backbone interaction, respectively), (2) mutations localized to the C-terminal hormone-binding domain confirming defects in ligand binding,[119–121] and (3) mutations in a subregion of the C-terminal domain that affect heterodimerization of the VDR and RXR.[129–131] In two of these patients, some impairment of hormone binding to whole cells was observed at 37°C with no abnormality in 1α,25$(OH)_2D_3$ high-affinity binding to cytosol at

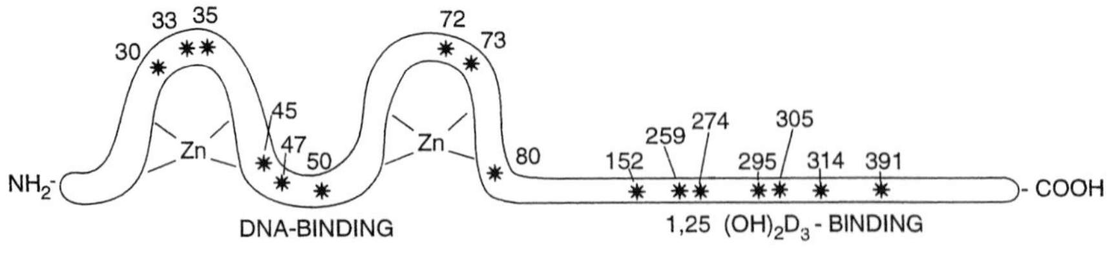

NORMAL	MUTANT	NORMAL	MUTANT
30 Arg (CGA)	Stop (TGA)	**152** Gln (CAG)	Stop (TAG)
33 Gly (GGC)	Asp (GAC)	**259** Gln (CAG)	Pro (CCG)
35 His (CAC)	Gln (CAG)	**274** Arg (CGC)	Leu (CTC)
45 Lys (AAA)	Glu (GAA)	**295** Tyr (TAC)	Stop (TAA)
47 Phe (TTC)	Lle (ATC)	**305** His (CAC)	Gln (CAG)
50 Arg (CGA)	Gln (CAA)	**314** Lle (ATC)	Ser (AGC)
72 Arg (CGC)	Stop (TGA)	**391** Arg (CGC)	Cys (TGC)
73 Arg (CGG)	Gln (CAA)		
80 Arg (CGG)	Gln (CAG)		

Fig. 165-11 Schematic presentation of the homozygous mutation in the vitamin D receptor in patients with hereditary generalized resistance to 1α,25$(OH)_3$D. The asterisks depict sites of amino acid substitutions due to point mutations and codon changes using the numbering system of Baker et al.[143]

4°C (the so-called functional defect in receptor translocation to nucleus, described before). These receptors do not bind RXRs with normal affinity, and in cotransfection assays with normal exogenous RXR, the mutant VDR could be rescued, although it required higher concentrations of 1α,25$(OH)_2D_3$. This showed that, as expected, the hormone-binding and heterodimerization functions of VDR are not entirely separable.

In every kindred in which more than one patient was examined, the same genetic defects were identified. Obligatory heterozygotes were found to have one normal and one mutant allele. The same mutation was observed in some unrelated patients.

Animal Models for Hereditary Generalized Resistance to 1α,25$(OH)_2D$. A state resembling hereditary generalized resistance to 1α,25$(OH)_2D$ is present in New World primates (marmosets and tamarins). Osteomalacia sometimes develops in these animals in captivity, and they are known to have high nutritional requirements for calciferols.[150] New World primates have high circulating concentrations of 1α,25$(OH)_2D$.[151] Intestinal and other cells form these animals have shown deficient calcitriol-binding capacity (in comparison with cells from Old World primates)[152,153] and deficient calcitriol-binding affinity.[154] These New World primates also exhibit hereditary generalized resistance to the true steroid hormones, including glucocorticoids, estrogens, and progestogens.[155] Thus their special metabolic features appear to involve elements shared by many of the nuclear-active steroids and secosteroids. Extracts from New World primate cells are capable of inhibiting 1α,25$(OH)_2D$ binding to Old World primate vitamin D receptors.[156] Nuclear extracts from β-lymphoblastoid cell lines of New World primates contain a VDRE-binding protein(s) that is capable of inhibiting normal VDR-RXR heterodimer binding to the VDRE.[157]

Recently, VDR knockout mice have been created by targeted ablation of the first zinc finger[158] or the second zinc finger.[159] Only the homozygote mice were affected. Although phenotypically normal at birth, they become hypocalcemic and develop secondary hyperparathyroidism, rickets, osteomalacia and progressive alopecia. The mice with ablation of the first zinc finger are infertile and die within 15 weeks after birth, whereas the mice with ablation of the second zinc finger survive at least until 6 months.

States Resembling Hereditary Generalized Resistance to 1α,25$(OH)_2D$. There are multiple causes of rickets or osteomalacia in which calciferol metabolism is normal or is abnormal only as an appropriate response to a primary disturbance in mineral flux (see Fig. 165-4). These include hereditary and acquired causes. Rickets or osteomalacia with high circulating 1α,25$(OH)_2D$ is found in generalized resistance to 1α,25$(OH)_2D$ and in two additional states (calcium deficiency and phosphate deficiency).

Calcium Deficiency. Severe deficiency of calcium has been recognized as a common dysfunction in Bantu adolescents, who consume a diet severely deficient in calcium.[160] Of course, calcium repletion cures all abnormalities. Osteopetrosis (marble-bones disease) results from a spectrum of defects in osteoclast function. Both in humans and in animal models of this disease, serum 1α,25$(OH)_2D$ is increased, and subtle histologic changes of osteomalacia have been noted.[161] At least one patient has been treated with a low-calcium diet plus high doses of 1α,25$(OH)_2D$ with apparent improvement in osteoclast function.[162] Other patients with osteopetrosis have not responded to similar treatment, and at least one cellular defect (carbonic anhydrase II deficiency) unlikely to be overcome by 1α,25$(OH)_2D$ has been discovered.[162]

Phosphate Deficiency. Severe deficiency of phosphate also can cause rickets with high serum levels of 1α,25$(OH)_2D$. In hereditary hypophosphatemic rickets with hypercalciuria, the primary renal loss of phosphate causes osteomalacia and activation of the renal 1α-hydroxylase.[163] High 1α,25$(OH)_2D$ results in absorptive hypercalciuria; therefore, parathyroid function is suppressed in this condition, unlike in hereditary generalized resistance to 1α,25$(OH)_2D$.

Survivors of extreme prematurity can pass through a phase when their growing bones (deprived of the placental pump) are severely deficient in both calcium and phosphate, resulting in neonatal rickets with high serum 1α,25$(OH)_2D$.[164,165] In this group, immaturity of the intestinal response to 1α,25$(OH)_2D$ may contribute to the disturbance.[166]

Deficient Bone Mineralization with Normal Calcium and Phosphate in Serum. There are several causes of deficient bone mineralization with otherwise normal calcium and phosphate fluxes. These include hypophosphatasia,[62] the chondrodystrophies (which can disturb epiphyseal function), and skeletal accumulation of aluminum, bisphosphonates, or fluoride.[64]

OTHER HEREDITARY DEFECTS IN CALCIFEROL METABOLISM

Calciferol Deficiency States

The only hereditary defects in calciferol metabolism proven to date are selective deficiency of and generalized resistance to 1α,25$(OH)_2D$. Although antigenic variation in transcalciferin is common, no differences in its function for calciferol transport have been identified in human beings.[167] However, in the chicken this protein shows tenfold higher affinity for vitamin D_3 metabolites than for vitamin D_2 metabolites, and this seems to account for a higher requirement for vitamin D_2 than for vitamin D_3 in this species.[168]

Deficient 25-hydroxylation of vitamin D was suggested as an additional defect in one patient with hereditary generalized resistance to 1α,25$(OH)_2D$.[169] Increased clearance of 25(OH)D is an alternative explanation for these observations.

Deficient 24-hydroxylation of 25(OH)D was suggested in another patient with hereditary generalized resistance to 1α,25$(OH)_2D$.[98] This patient has low concentrations of 24,25$(OH)_2D$ and showed partial remission of resistance to 1α,25$(OH)_2D$ when given a therapeutic trial of 24,25$(OH)_2D$. These observations remain unexplained, but a point mutation in the vitamin D receptor gene has been documented in this patient, suggesting that any deficiency of 24,25$(OH)_2D$ was a secondary feature.[112] Decreased production of 24,25$(OH)_2D$ could be secondary to the abnormality in 1α,25$(OH)_2D$ action, since one of its actions is induction of 25(OH)D 24-hydroxylase.

CALCIFEROL EXCESS STATES

Lightwood,[170] Williams et al.,[171] and Beuren et al.[172] described a syndrome of infantile hypercalcemia, elfin facies, mental retardation, and supravalvular aortic stenosis (also termed *idiopathic hypercalcemia of infancy*). The characteristic dysmorphology includes the following: wide, slack mouth, malocclusion, prominent upper lip, underdeveloped mandible, depressed nasal bridge, hypertelorism, epicanthic folds, low-set ears, increased bone density, craniostenosis, and osteosclerosis, especially of the base of the skull. Patients showing portions of the phenotype have sometimes been grouped within this syndrome without implying identical pathophysiology for all.[173] Most cases have been sporadic, but several patients have had similarly affected siblings.[174] Autosomal dominant transmission was suggested in one kindred.[175] The hypercalcemia has many features suggesting excess vitamin D effect; there is increased calcium absorption, hypercalciuria, and nephrocalcinosis. In some cases glucocorticoids have lessened the hypercalcemia. Early strides suggested that calciferol bioactivity was increased in plasma,[176] but assays of specific calciferol metabolites have not provided a consistent explanation of these findings. Taylor et al.[177] found that these patients and their phenotypically normal relatives show an abnormal accumulation of 25(OH)D when given a test dose of vitamin D_2. However, serum $25(OH)D_2$ and $25(OH)D_3$ have been normal in most other patients during the normocalcemic or hypercalcemic phase.[178] Serum $24,25(OH)_2D$ and $25,26(OH)_2D$ also have been normal.[178] Garabedian et al.[179] evaluated serum $1\alpha,25(OH)_2D$ in four patients and found inappropriate increases. However, other patients have shown clear suppression of $1\alpha,25(OH)_2D$,[178,180,181] suggesting more than one mechanism for the hypercalcemia.[182]

The implication of factors related to calciferols is strengthened by an animal model for this disorder. The offspring of rabbits with vitamin D intoxication show similar skeletal features (mandibular hypoplasia and characteristic dental abnormalities)[183] and typical supravalvular aortic lesions.[184]

To summarize, it is unclear that the syndrome of idiopathic hypercalcemia with its associated abnormalities can result from a defect in calciferol metabolism or action.

REFERENCES

1. Mellanby E: An experimental investigation on rickets. *Lancet* **1**:407, 1919.
2. Albright F, Butler AM, Bloomberg E: Rickets resistant to vitamin D therapy. *Am J Dis Child* **54**:531, 1937.
3. Prader VA, Illig R, Heide E: Eine besondere form der primaren vitamin-D-resintenten rachitis mit hypocalcamie und autosomal-dominantem erbgang: Der hereditare pseudomangelrachitis. *Helv Paediatr Acta* **5/6**:452, 1961.
4. Hamilton R, Harrison J, Fraser D, Radde I, Morecki R, Paunier L: The small intestine in vitamin D–dependent rickets. *Pediatrics* **45**:364, 1970.
5. Arnaud C, Maijer R, Reade T, Scriver CR, Whelan DT: Vitamin D dependency: An inherited postnatal syndrome with secondary hyperparathyroidism. *Pediatrics* **46**:871, 1970.
6. Holick MF, Schnoes HK, Deluca HF: Identification of 1,25-dihydroxycholecalciferol, a form of vitamin D_3 metabolically active in the intestine. *Proc Natl Acad Sci USA* **68**:803, 1971.
7. Norman AW, Midgett RJ, Myrtle JF, Nowicki HG, Williams W, Popjack G: 1,25-Dihydroxycholecalciferol: Identification of the proposed active form of vitamin D_3 in the intestine. *Science* **173**:51, 1971.
8. Fraser D, Kooh SW, Kind HP, Holick MF, Tanaka Y, Deluca HF: Pathogenesis of hereditary vitamin D–dependent rickets: An inborn error of vitamin D metabolism involving defective coversion of 25-hydroxyvitamin D to 1α,25-dihydroxyvitamin D. *New Engl J Med* **289**:817, 1973.
9. Brooks MH, Bell NH, Love L, Stern PH, Orfei E, Queener SF, Hamstra AJ, et al: Vitamin D–dependent rickets type II: Resistance of target organs to 1,25-dihydroxyvitamin D. *New Engl J Med* **298**:996, 1978.
10. Aurbach GD, Marx SJ, Spiegel AM: Parathyroid hormone, calcitonin, and the calciferols, in Wilson JD, Foster DW (eds): *Williams Textbook of Endocrinology*, 8th ed. Philadelphia, Saunders, 1992; p 1397.
11. Holick MF, MacLaughlin JA, Clark MB, Holick SA, Potts JT Jr, Anderson RR, Blank IH, et al: Photosynthesis of previtamin D_3 in human skin and the physiological consequences. *Science* **210**:203, 1980.
12. Clemens TL, Adams JS, Henderson LS, Holick MF: Increased skin pigment reduces the capacity of skin to synthesize vitamin D_3. *Lancet* **1**:74, 1982.
13. Saarem K, Bergseth S, Oftebro H, Pedersen JR: Subcellular localization of vitamin D_3 25-hydroxylase in human liver. *J Biol Chem* **259**:10936, 1984.
14. Usui E, Noshiro M, Ohyama Y, Okuda K: Unique property of liver mitochondrial P-450 to catalyze the two physiologically important reactions involved in both cholesterol catabolism and vitamin D activation. *FEBS Lett* **274**:175, 1990.
15. Ohyama Y, Masumoto O, Usui E, Okuda K: Multifunctional property of rat liver mitochondrial cytochrome P-450. *J Biochem* **109**:389, 1991.
16. Dahlback H, Wikvall K: 25-Hydroxylation of vitamin D_3 in rat liver: Roles of mitochondrial and microsomal cytochrome P-450. *Biochem Biophys Res Commun* **142**:999, 1987.
17. Turner RT: Mammalian 25-hydroxyvitamin D-1α-hydroxylase: Measurement and regulation, in Kumar R (ed): *Vitamin D: Basic and Clinical Aspects*. Boston, Martinus Nijhoff, 1984; p 175.
18. Reeve L, Tanaka Y, Deluca HF: Studies on the site of 1,25-dihydroxyvitamin D_3 synthesis in vivo. *J Biol Chem* **258**:3615, 1983.
19. Trechsel U, Bonjour JP, Fleisch H: Regulation of the metabolism of 25-hydroxyvitamin D_3 in primary cultures of chick kidney cells. *J Clin Invest* **64**:206, 1979.
20. Kawashima H, Torikai S, Kurokawa K: Calcitonin selectively stimulates 25-hydroxyvitamin D_3-1α-hydroxylase in proximal straight tubule of rat kidney. *Nature* **291**:327, 1981.
21a. Takeyama K, Kitanaka S, Sato T, Kobori M, Yanagisawa J, Kato S: 25-Hydroxyvitamin D_3 1α-hydroxylase and vitamin D synthesis. *Science* **277**:1827, 1997.
21b. Shinki T, Shimada H, Wakino S, Anazawa H, Hayashi M, Saruta T, DeLuca HF, Suda T: Cloning and expression of rat 25-hydroxyvitamin D_3 1α-hydroxylase cDNA. *Proc Natl Acad Sci USA* **94**:12920, 1997.
21c. Monkawa T, Yoshida T, Wakino S, Shinki T, Anazawa H, DeLuca HF, Suda T, Hayashi M, Saruta T: Molecular cloning of cNDA and genomic DNA for human 25-hydroxyvitamin D_3 1α-hydroxylase. *Biochem Biophys Res Commun* **239**:527, 1997.
21d. Fu GK, Portale AA, Miller WL: Complete structure of the human gene for the vitamin D 1α-hydroxylase. *Cell Biol* **16**:1499, 1997.
21e. Jones G, Ramshaw H, Zhang A, Cook R, Byford V, White J, Petkovich M: Expression and activity of vitamin D–metabolizing cytochrome P450s (CYP1α and CYP 24) in human nonsmall cell lung carcinomas. *Endocrinology* **140**:3303, 1999.
22. Murayama A, Takeyama K, Kitanaka S, Kodera Y, Kawaguchi Y, Hosoya T, Kato S: Positive and negative regulations of the renal 25-hydroxyvitamin D_3 1α-hydroxylase gene by parathyroid hormone, calcitonin and 1α, 25 $(OH)_2D_3$ in intact animals. *Endocrinology* **140**:2224, 1999.
23. Burgos-Trinidad M, Brown AJ, DeLuca HF: Solubilization and reconsititution of chick renal mitochondrial 25-hydroxyvitamin D_3 receptors and functions in cultured pig kidney cells (LLCPK1): Regulation of 24,25-dihydroxyvitamin D_3 production. *Biochemistry* **25**:2692, 1985.
24. Colston K, Feldman D: 1,25-Dihydroxyvitamin D_3 receptors and functions in cultured pig kidney cells (LLCPK1): Regulation of 24,25-dihydroxyvitamin D_3 production. *J Biol Chem* **257**:2504, 1982.
25. Ohyama Y, Noshiro M, Okuda K: Cloning and expression of cDNA encoding 25-hydroxyvitamin D_3 24-hydroxylase. *FEBS Lett* **278**:195, 1991.
25a. Ohyama Y, Noshiro M, Eggersten G, Gotoh O, Kato Y, Bjorkhem I, Okuda K: Structural characterization of the gene encoding rate 25-hydroxyvitamin D_3 24-hydroxylase. *Biochemistry* **32**:76, 1993.
25b. Akeno N, Saikatsu S, Kawane T, Horiuchi N: Mouse vitamin D 24-hydroxylase: Molecular cloning, tissue distribution, a transcriptional regulation by 1α,25-dihydroxyvitamin D_3. *Endocrinology* **138**:2233, 1997.
25c. Jehan F, Ismail R, Hanson K, DeLuca HF: Cloning and expression of the chicken 25-hydroxyvitamin D_3 24-hydroxylase cDNA. *Biochem Biophys Acta* **1395**:259, 1998.
25d. Ozono K, Yamagata M, Ohyama Y, Nakajima S: Direct repeat 3-type element lacking the ability to bind to the vitamin D receptor enhances the function of a vitamin D-response element. *J Steroid Biochem Mol Biol* **66**:263, 1998.
25e. Chen KS, DeLuca HF: Cloning of the human 1α,25-dihydroxyvitamin D_3 24-hydroxylase gene promoter and identification of two vitamin D-responsive elements. *Biochem Biophys Acta* **25**:1263, 1995.
26. Kumar R, Nagubandi S, Jardine I, Londowski JM, Bollman S: The isolation and identification of 5,6-*trans*-25-hydroxyvitamin D_3 from the plasma of rats dosed with vitamin D_3. *J Biol Chem* **256**:9389, 1981.
27. Engstrom GW, Reinhart TA, Horst RL: 25-Hydroxyvitamin D_3 23-hydroxylase, a renal enzyme in several species. *Arch Biochem Biophys* **250**:86, 1986.
28. Haddad JF: Nature and functions of the plasma binding protein for vitamin D and its metabolites, in Kumar R (ed): *Vitamin D: Basic and Clinical Aspects*. Boston, Martinus Nijhoff, 1984; p 383.
29. Cooke NE: Rat vitamin D binding protein: Determination of the full-length primary structure from cloned cDNA. *J Biol Chem* **261**:3441, 1985.
30. Coppenhaver DH, Sollenne NP, Bowman BH: Posttranslational heterogeneity of the human vitamin D–binding (group-specific component). *Arch Biochem Biophys* **226**:218, 1983.
31. Lawson DEM, Douglas J, Lean M, Sedrani S: Estimation of vitamin D_3 and 25-hydroxyvitamin D_3 in muscle and adipose tissue of rats and man. *Clin Chim Acta* **157**:175, 1986.
32. Haussler MR, Haussler CA, Jurutka PW, Thompson PD, Hsieh J-C, Remus LS, Selznick SH, et al: The vitamin D hormone and its nuclear

receptor: Molecular actions and disease states. *J Endocrinol* **154**:557, 1997.
33. Evans RM: The steroid and thyroid hormone receptor super family. *Science* **240**:889, 1986.
34. Procsal DA, Okamura WH, Norman AW: Structural requirements for interaction of 1α,25-(OH)2-vitamin D_3 with its chick intestinal receptor system. *J Biol Chem* **250**:8382, 1975.
35. Stumpf WE, Sar M, Reid FA, Tanaka Y, Deluca HF: Target cells for 1,25-dihydroxyvitamin D_3 in intestinal tract, stomach, kidney, skin, pituitary, and parathyroid. *Science* **206**:1188, 1979.
36. Hsieh J-C, Juruta PW, Galligan MA, Terpening CM, Haussler CA, Samuels DS, Shimizu Y, et al: Human vitamin D receptor is selectively phosphorylated by protein kinase C on serine 51, a residue crucial to its trans-activation function. *Proc Natl Acad Sci USA* **88**:9315, 1991.
37. Ozono K, Sone T, Pike JW: The genomic mechanism of action of 1,25-dihydroxyvitamin D_3. *J Bone Miner Res* **6**:1021, 1991.
38. Nemere I, Yoshimoto Y, Norman AW: Calcium transport in perfused duodena from normal chicks: Enhancement within fourteen minutes of exposure to 1,25-dihydroxyvitamin D_3. *Endocrinology* **115**:1476, 1984.
39. Barsony J, Marx SJ: Receptor-mediated rapid action of 1α,25-dihydroxycholecalciferol: Increase of intracellular cGMP in human skin fibroblasts. *Proc Natl Acad Sci USA* **85**:1223, 1988.
40. Wasserman RH, Fullmer CS, Shimura F: Calcium absorption and the molecular effects of vitamin D_3, in Kumar R (ed): *Vitamin D: Basic and Clinical Aspects*. Boston, Martinus Nijhoff, 1984; p 223.
41. Feher JJ: Facilitated calcium diffusion by intestinal calcium-binding protein. *Am J Physiol* **224**:C303, 1983.
42. Morgan DW, Welton AF, Heick AE, Christakos S: Specific in vitro activation of Ca,Mg-ATPase by vitamin D–dependent rat renal calcium binding protein (calbindin D28K). *Biochem Biophys Res Commun* **138**:547, 1986.
43. Underwood JL, DeLuca HF: Vitamin D is not directly necessary for bone growth and mineralization. *Am J Physiol* **246**:E493, 1984.
44. Holtrop ME, Cox KA, Carnes DL, Holick MF: Effects of serum calcium and phosphate on skeletal mineralization in vitamin D–deficient rats. *Am J Physiol* **251**:E234, 1986.
45. Lian JB, Coutts M, Canalis E: Studies of hormonal regulation of osteocalcin synthesis in cultured fetal rat calvariae. *J Biol Chem* **260**:8706, 1985.
46. Beresford JN, Gallagher JA, Russel RGG: 1,25-Dihydroxyvitamin D_3 and human bone-derived cells in vitro: Effects on alkaline phosphatase, type I collagen, and proliferation. *Endocrinology* **119**:1776, 1986.
47. Majeska RJ, Rodan GA: The effect of $1,25(OH)_2D_3$ on alkaline phosphatase in osteoblastic osteosarcoma cells. *J Biol Chem* **257**:3362, 1982.
47a. Ducy P, Desbois C, Boyce B, Pinero G, Story B, Dunstan C, Smith E, et al: Increased bone formation in osteocalcin-deficient mice. *Nature* **382**:448, 1996.
48. Chambers TJ, McSheehy PMJ, Thomson BM, Fuller K: The effect of calcium-regulating hormones and prostaglandins on bone resorption by osteoclasts disaggregated from neonatal rabbit bones. *Endocrinology* **60**:234, 1985.
49. Merke J, Hughel U, Waldherr R, Ritz E: No 1,25-dihydroxyvitamin D_3 receptors on osteoclasts of calcium-deficient chickens despite demonstrable receptors on circulating monocytes. *J Clin Invest* **77**:312, 1986.
50. Bar-Shavit Z, Kahn AJ, Stone KR, Trial J, Hilliard T, Reitsma PH, Teitelbaum SL: Reversibility of vitamin D–induced human leukemia cell-line maturation. *Endocrinology* **118**:679, 1986.
51. Roodman GD, Ibbotson KJ, MacDonald BR, Kuehl TJ, Mundy GR: 1,25-Dihydroxyvitamin D_3 causes formation of multinucleated cells with several osteoclast characteristics in cultures of primate marrow. *Proc Natl Acad Sci USA* **82**:8213, 1985.
52. Abe E, Shina Y, Miyaura C, Tanaka H, Hayashi T, Kanegasaki S, Saito M, et al: Activation and fusion induced by 1α,25-dihydroxyvitamin D_3 and their relation in alveolar macrophages. *Proc Natl Acad Sci USA* **81**:7112, 1984.
53. Chambers TJ: The pathobiology of the osteoclast. *J Clin Pathol* **38**:241, 1985.
54. Stumpf WE, Clark SA, Sar M, DeLuca HJ: Topographical and developmental studies on target sites of $1,25(OH)_2$ vitamin D_3 in skin. *Cell Tissue Res* **238**:489, 1984.
55. Cantley LK, Russell J, Lettieri D, Sherwood LM: 1,25-Dihydroxyvitamin D_3 suppresses parathyroid hormone secretion from bovine parathyroid cells in tissue culture. *Endocrinology* **117**:2114, 1985.
56. Esvelt RP, DeLuca HF, Wichman JK, Yoshizawa S, Zurcher J, Sar M, Stumpf WE: 1,25-Dihydroxyvitamin D_3 stimulated increase of 7,8-didehydrocholesterol levels in rat skin. *Biochemistry* **19**:6158, 1980.
57. Clements MR, Johnson L, Fraser DR: A new mechanism for induced vitamin D deficiency in calcium deprivation. *Nature* **325**:62, 1987.
58. Binderman I, Somjen D: 24,25-Dihydroxycholecalciferol induced the growth of chick cartilage in vitro. *Endocrinology* **115**:430, 1984.
59. Somjen D, Kaye AM, Binderman I: 24R,25-Dihydroxyvitamin D stimulates creatine kinase BB activity in chick cartilage cells in culture. *FEBS Lett* **167**:281, 1984.
60. Brommage R, DeLuca HF: Evidence that 1,25-dihydroxyvitamin D_3 is the physiologically active metabolite of vitamin D_3. *Endocr Rev* **6**:491, 1985.
61. Marel GM, McKenna MJ, Frame B: Osteomalacia. *J Bone Miner Res* **4**:335, 1986.
62. Opshaug O, Maurseth K, Howlid H, Aksnes L, Aarskog D: Vitamin D metabolism in hypophosphatasia. *Acta Pediatr Scand* **71**:517, 1982.
63. Marx SJ, Barsony J: Tissue-selective 1,25-dihydroxyvitamin D_3 resistance: Novel applications of calciferols. *J Bone Miner Res* **3**:481, 1988.
64. Aurbach GD, Marx SJ, Spiegel AM: Metabolic bone disease, in Wilson JD, Foster DW (eds): *Williams Textbook of Endocrinology*, 8th ed. Philadelphia, Saunders, 1992; p 1477.
65. Brommage R, DeLuca HF: Placental transport of calcium and phosphate is not regulated by vitamin D_3. *Am J Physiol* **246**:F526, 1984.
66. Papapoulos SE, Clemens TL, Fraher LJ, Gleed J, O'Riordan JLH: Metabolites of vitamin D in human vitamin D deficiency: Effect of vitamin D_3 or 1,25-dihydroxycholecalciferol. *Lancet* **2**:612, 1980.
67. Garabedian M, Vainsel M, Mallet E, Guillozo H, Toppet M, Grimberg R, Nguyen TM, et al: Circulating vitamin D metabolite concentrations in children with nutritional rickets. *J Pediatr* **103**:381, 1983.
68. Lopez-Hilker S, Galceren T, Chan YL, Rapp N, Martin KJ, Slatopolsky E: Hypocalcemia may not be essential for the development of hyperparathyroidism in chronic renal failure. *J Clin Invest* **78**:1097, 1986.
69. Rao DS, Parfitt AM, Kleerekoper M, Pumo BS, Frame B: Dissociation between the effects of endogenous parathyroid hormone on adenosine 3′,5′-monophosphate generation and phosphate reabsorption in hypocalcemia due to vitamin D depletion: An acquired disorder resembling pseudohypoparathyroidism type II. *J Clin Endocrinol Metab* **61**:285, 1985.
70. Parfitt AM, Rao DS, Stanciu J, Villanueva AR, Kleerekoper M, Frame B: Irreversible bone loss in osteomalacia: Comparison of radial photon absorptiometry with iliac bone histomorphometry during treatment. *J Clin Invest* **76**:2403, 1985.
71. Dommergues J-P, Garabedian M, Gueris J, Ledeunff M-J, Creignou L, Courtecuisse V, Balsan S: Effects des principaux derives de la vitamine D: Chez trois enfants d'une fratrie atteints de rachitisme "pseudo-carentiel." *Arch Fr Pediatr* **35**:1050, 1978.
72. Bravo H, Almedia S, Tato IG, Bustillo JM, Tojo R: Early pseudo-deficiency or Prader's hypocalcemia familial type I rickets. *An Esp Pediatr* **25**:121, 1986.
73. Scriver CR, Reade TM, Deluca HF, Hamstra AJ: Serum 1,25-dihydroxyvitamin D levels in normal subjects and in patients with hereditary rickets or bone disease. *New Engl J Med* **299**:976, 1978.
74. Garabedian M, N'guyen TM, Guillozo H, Grimberg R, Balsan S: Mesure des taux circulants des metabolites actifs de la vitamine D chez l'enfant; interet et limites. *Arch Fr Pediatr* **38**:857, 1981.
75. Delvin EE, Glorieux FH, Marie PJ, Pettifor JM: Vitamin D dependency: Replacement therapy with calcitriol. *J Pediatr* **99**:26, 1981.
76. Bouchard G, Laberge C, Scriver CR: La tyrosinemie hereditarie et le rachitisme vitamino-dependent au Saguenay. *Union Med Can* **114**:633, 1985.
77. Labuda M, Morgan K, Glorieux FH: Mapping autosomal recessive vitamin D dependency type I to chromosome 12q14 by linkage analysis. *Am J Hum Genet* **47**:28, 1990.
78. Balsan S, Garabedian M: 25-Hydroxycholecalciferol: A comparative study in deficiency rickets and different types of resistant rickets. *J Clin Invest* **51**:749, 1972.
79. Reade TM, Scriver CR, Glorieux FH, Nogrady B, Delvin E, Poirier R, Holick MF, DeLuca HF: Response to crystalline 1α-hydroxyvitamin D_3 in vitamin D dependency. *Pediatr Res* **9**:593, 1975.
80. Marx SJ: Rickets and osteomalacia, in Conn HF (ed): *Current Therapy*. Philadelphia, Saunders, 1983, pp 451–456.
81. Glorieux FH, Arabian A, Delvin EE: Pseudo-vitamin D deficiency: Absence of 25-hydroxyvitamin D 1α-hydroxylase activity in human placenta decidual cells. *J Clin Endocrinol Metab* **80**:2255, 1995.

82. Weisman Y, Harell A, Edlestein S, David M, Spirer Z, Golander A: 1α,25-Dihydroxyvitamin D_3 and 24,25-dihydroxyvitamin D_3 in vitro synthesis by human decidua and placenta. *Nature* **281**:317, 1979.
83. Delvin EE, Arabian A: Kinetics and regulation of 25-hydroxycholecalciferol 1α-hydroxylase from cells isolated form human term decidua. *Eur J Biochem* **163**:659, 1987.
83a. St. Arnaud R, Messerlian S, Moir JM, Omdahl JL, Glorieux FH: The 25-hydroxyvitamin D 1α-hydroxylase gene maps to the pseudovitamin D deficiency rickets (PDDR) disease locus. *J Bone Miner Res* **12**:1552, 1997.
83b. Fu GK, Lin D, Zhang MY, Bikle DD, Shackleton CH, Miller WL, Portale AA: Cloning of human 25-hydroxyvitamin D 1α-hydroxylase and mutations causing vitamin D–dependent rickets type 1. *Endocrinology* **11**:1961, 1997.
83c. Kitanaka S, Takeyama K, Murayama A, Sato T, Okumura K, Nogami M, Hasegawa Y, Niimi H, Yanagisawa J, Tanaka T, Kato S: Inactivating mutations in the 25-hydroxyvitamin D_3 1α-hydroxylase gene in patients with pseudo-vitamin D–deficiency rickets (see comments). *New Engl J Med* **338**:653, 1998.
83d. Yoshida T, Monkawa T, Tenenhouse HS, Goodyear P, Shinki T, Suda T, Wakino S, Hayashi M, Saruta T: Two novel 1α-hydroxylase in French-Canadians with vitamin D dependency rickets type II (see comments). *Kidney Int* **54**:1437, 1998.
83e. Wang JT, Lin CJ, Burridge Sm, Fu GK, Labuda M, Portale AA, Miller WL: Genetics of vitamin D 1α-hydroxylase deficiency in 17 families. *Am J Hum Genet* **63**:1694, 1998.
84. Mandla S, Jones G, Tenehouse HS: Normal 24-hydroxylation of vitamin D metabolites in patients with vitamin D–dependency rickets type I: Structural implications for the vitamin D hydroxylases. *J Clin Endocrinol Metab* **74**:814, 1992.
85. Ploniat H: Klinsche fragen der calciumstoff wechselstorungen beim scnwein. *Dtsch Tierarztl Wochenschr* **69**:198, 1962.
86. Harmeyer J, Grabe V, Winkler I: Pseudo-vitamin D deficiency rickets in pigs: An animal model for the study of familial vitamin D dependency. *Exp Biol Med* **7**:117, 1981.
87. Fox J, Maunder FMW, Randall VR, Care AD: Vitamin D–dependent rickets type I in pigs. *Clin Sci* **69**:541, 1985.
88. Winkler, I, Schreiner F, Harmeyer J: Absence of 25-hydroxycholecalciferol 1 hydroxylase activity in pig strain with vitamin D–dependent rickets. *Calcif Tissue Int* **38**:87, 1986.
89. Lyles KW, Clark AG, Drezner MK: Serum 1,25-dihydroxyvitamin D levels in subjects with X-linked hypophosphatemic rickets and osteomalacia. *Calcif Tissue Int* **34**:125, 1982.
90. Nesbitt T, Lobaugh B, Drezner M: Calcitonin stimulation of renal 25-hydroxyvitamin D 1α-hydroxylase activity in hypophosphatemic mice: Evidence that regulation of calcitriol production is not universally abnormal in X-linked hypophosphatemia. *J Clin Invest* **79**:15, 1987.
91. Brenner RJ, Spring DB, Sebastian A, McSherry EM, Genant HK, Palubinskas AJ, Morris RC Jr: Incidence of radiographically evident bone disease, nephrocalcinosis, and nephrolithiasis in various types of renal tubular acidosis. *New Engl J Med* **307**:217, 1982.
92. Chesney RW, Kaplan BS, Phelps M, DeLuca HF: Renal tubular acidosis does not alter circulating values of calcitriol. *J Pediatr* **104**:51, 1984.
93. Steinherz R, Chesney RW, Schulman JD, Deluca HF, Phelps M: Circulating vitamin D metabolites in nephropathic cystinosis. *J Pediatr* **102**:592, 1983.
94. Kitagawa T, Akatsuka A, Owada M, Mano T: Biologic and therapeutic effects of 1α-hydroxycholcalciferol in different types of Fanconi syndrome. *Contrib Nephrol* **22**:107, 1980.
95. Ryan EQ, Reiss E: Oncogenous osteomalacia: A review of the world literature of 42 cases and report of two new cases. *Am J Med* **77**:501, 1984.
96. Marx SJ, Spiegel AM, Brown EM, Gardner DG, Downs RW Jr, Attie M, Hamstra AJ, DeLuca HF: A familial syndrome of decrease in sensitivity to 1,25-dihydroxyvitamin D. *J Clin Endocrinol Metab* **47**:1303, 1978.
97. Rosen JF, Fleischman AR, Finberg L, Hamstra A, DeLuca HF: Rickets with alopecia: An inborn error of vitamin D metabolism. *J Pediatr* **94**:729, 1979.
98. Liberman UA, Samuel R, Halabe A, Kauli R, Edelstein S, Weisman Y, Papapoulos SE, Clemens TL, Fraher LJ, O'Riordan JLH: End-organ resistance to 1,25-dihydroxy-cholecalciferol. *Lancet* **1**:504, 1980.
99. Fujita T, Normura M, Okajima S, Furuya H: Adult-onset vitamin D–resistant osteomalacia with the unresponsiveness to parathyroid hormone. *J Clin Endocrinol Metab* **50**:927, 1980.
100. Tsuchiya Y, Matsuo N, Cho H, Kumagai M, Yasaka A, Suda T, Orimo H, et al: An unusual form of vitamin D–dependent rickets in a child: Alopecia and marked end-organ hyposensitivity to biological active vitamin D. *J Clin Endocrinol Metab* **51**:685, 1980.
101. Kudoh T, Kumagai T, Uetsuji N, Tsugawa S, Oyanagi K, Chiba Y, Minami R, et al: Vitamin D–dependent rickets: Decreased sensitivity to 1,25-dihydroxyvitamin D. *Eur J Pediatr* **137**:307, 1981.
102. Eil C, Liberman UA, Rosen JF, Marx SJ: A cellular defect in hereditary vitamin D–dependent rickets type II: Defective nuclear uptake of 1,25-dihydroxyvitamin D in cultured skin fibroblasts. *New Engl J Med* **304**:1588, 1981.
103. Feldman D, Chen T, Cone C, Hirst M, Shari S, Benderli A, Hochberg Z: Vitamin D resistant rickets with alopecia: Cultured skin fibroblasts exhibit defective cytoplasmic receptors and unresponsiveness to 1,25-$(OH)_2D_3$. *J Clin Endocrinol Metab* **55**:1020, 1982.
104. Balsan S, Garabedian M, Liberman UA, Eil C, Bourdeau A, Guillozo H, Grimberg R, et al: Rickets and alopecia with resistance to 1,25-dihydroxyvitamin D: Two different clinical courses with two different cellular defects. *J Clin Endocrinol Metab* **57**:803, 1983.
105. Clemens TL, Adams JS, Horiuchi N, Gilchrest BA, Cho H, Tsuchiya Y, Matsuo N, et al: Interaction of 1,25-dihydroxyvitamin-D_3 with keratinocytes and fibroblasts from skin of normal subjects and a subject with vitamin D–dependent rickets, type II: A model for study of the mode of action of 1,25-dihydroxyvitamin D_3. *J Clin Endocrinol Metab* **56**:824, 1983.
106. Liberman UA, Eil C, Marx SJ: Resistance to 1,25-dihydroxyvitamin D: Association with heterogeneous defects in cultured skin fibroblasts. *J Clin Invest* **71**:192, 1983.
107. Chen TL, Hirst MA, Cone CM, Hochberg Z, Tietze H-U, Feldman D: 1,25-Dihydroxyvitamin D resistance rickets, and alopecia: Analysis of receptors and bioresponse in cultured fibroblasts from patients and parents. *J Clin Endocrinol Metab* **59**:383, 1984.
108. Hochberg Z, Benderli A, Levy J, Vardi P, Weisman Y, Chen T, Feldman D: 1,25-Dihydroxyvitamin D resistance, rickets, and alopecia. *Am J Med* **77**:805, 1984.
109. Marx SJ, Liberman UA, Eil C, Gamblin GT, DeGrange DA, Balsan S: Hereditary resistance to 1,25-dihydroxyvitamin D. *Recent Prog Horm Res* **40**:589, 1984.
110. Hochberg Z, Gilhar A, Haim S, Friedman-Birnbaum R, Levy J, Benderly A: Calcitriol-resistant rickets with alopecia. *Arch Dermatol* **121**:646, 1985.
111. Hirst M, Hockman H, Feldman D: Vitamin D resistance and alopecia: A kindred with normal 1,25-dihydroxyvitamin D binding, but decreased receptor affinity for deoxyribonucleic acid. *J Clin Endocrinol Metab* **60**:490, 1985.
112. Liberman UA, Eil C, Marx SJ: Receptor-positive hereditary resistance to 1,25-dihydroxyvitamin D: Chromatography of hormone-receptor complexes on deoxyribonucleic acid-cellulose shows two classes of mutation. *J Clin Endocrinol Metab* **62**:122, 1986.
113. Fraher LJ, Karmali R, Hinde FRJ, Hendy GN, Jani H, Nicholson L, Grant D, et al: Vitamin D–dependent rickets type II: Extreme end organ resistance to 1,25-dihydroxyvitamin D_3 in a patient without alopecia. *Eur J Pediatr* **145**:389, 1986.
114. Castells S, Greig F, Fusi MA, Finberg L, Yasumura S, Liberman UA, Eil C, et al: Severely deficient binding of 1,25-dihydroxyvitamin D to its receptors in a patient responsive to high doses of this hormone. *J Clin Endocrinol Metab* **63**:252, 1986.
115. Tajikda E, Kuroda Y, Saijo T, Naito E, Kobashi H, Yokota I, Miyao M: 1α-hydroxyvitamin D_3 treatment of three patients with 1,25-dihydroxyvitamin D–receptor-defect rickets and alopecia. *Pediatrics* **80**:97, 1987.
116. Hughes MR, Malloy PJ, Kieback DG, Kesterson RA, Pike JW, Feldman D, O'Malley BW: Point mutations in the human vitamin D receptor gene associated with hypocalcemic rickets. *Science* **242**:1702, 1988.
117. Malloy PJ, Hochberg Z, Pike JW, Feldman D: Abnormal binding of vitamin D receptors to deoxyribonucleic acid in a kindred with vitamin D–dependent rickets, type II. *J Clin Endocrinol Metab* **68**:263, 1989.
118. Stone T, Marx SJ, Liberman UA, Pike JW: A unique point mutation in the human vitamin D receptor chromosomal gene confers hereditary resistance to 1,25-dihydroxyvitamin D_3. *Mol Cell Endocrinol* **4**:623, 1990.
119. Malloy PJ, Hochberg Z, Tiosano D, Pike JW, Hughes MR, Feldman D: The molecular basis of hereditary 1,25 dihydroxyvitamin D_3 resistant rickets in seven related families. *J Clin Invest* **86**:2071, 1990.
120. Saiijo T, Ito M, Takeda E, Mahbubul Huq AHM, Naito E, Yokota I, Sine T, et al: A unique mutation in the vitamin D receptor gene in three

Japanese patients with vitamin D–dependent rickets type II: Utility of single-strand conformation polymorphism analysis for heterozygous carrier detection. *Am J Hum Genet* **49**:668, 1991.

121. Kristjansson K, Rut AR, Hewison M, O'Riordan, Hughes MR: Two mutations in the hormone binding domain of the vitamin D receptor cause tissue resistance to 1,25-dihydroxyvitamin D_3. *J Clin Invest* **92**:12, 1993.
122. Hewison M, Rut AR, Kristjansson K, Walker RE, Dillon MJ, Hughes MR, O'Riordan JLH: Tissue resistance to 1,25-dihydroxyvitamin D without a mutation in the vitamin D receptor gene. *Clin Endocrinol* **39**:663, 1993.
123. Yagi H, Ozono K, Miyake H, Nagashima K, Kuraum T, Pike JW: A new point mutation in the deoxyribonucleic acid-binding domain of the vitamin D receptor in a kindred with hereditary 1,25-dihydroxyvitamin D resistant rickets. *J Clin Endocrinol Metab* **76**:509, 1993.
124. Weise RJ, Goto H, Prahl JM, Marx SJ, Thomas M, Al-Aqeel A, DeLuca HF: Vitamin D–dependency rickets type II: Truncated vitamin D receptor in three kindred. *Mol Cell Endocrinol* **90**:197, 1993.
125. Rut AR, Hewison K, Kristjansson K, Luisi B, Hughes MR, O'Riordan JLH: Two mutations causing vitamin D–resistant rickets modeling on the basis of steroid hormone receptor DNA-binding domain crystal structures. *Clin Endocrinol* **41**:581, 1994.
126. Malloy PJ, Weisman Y, Feldman D: Hereditary 1,25-dihydroxyvitamin D–resistant rickets resulting from a mutation in the vitamin D receptor deoxyribonucleic acid binding domain. *J Clin Endocrinol Metab* **78**:313, 1994.
127. Lin Nu-T, Malloy PJ, Sakati N, Al-Ashwal A, Feldman D: A novel mutation in the deoxyribonucleic acid-binding domain of the vitamin D receptor causes hereditary 1,25-dihydroxyvitamin D–resistant rickets. *J Clin Endocrinol Metab* **81**:2564, 1996.
128. Hawa NS, Cockerill FJ, Vodher S, Hewison M, Rut AR, Pike JW, O'Riordan JLH, et al: Identification of a novel mutation in hereditary vitamin D resistant rickets causing exon skipping. *Clin Endocrinol* **45**:85, 1996.
129. Whitfield GK, Selznick SH, Haussler CA, Hsieh JC, Galligan MA, Jurutka PW, Thompson PD, et al: Vitamin D receptors from patients with resistance to 1,25-dihydroxyvitamin D_3: Point mutations confer reduced transactivation in response to ligand and impaired interaction with the retinoid X receptor heterodimeric partner. *Mol Endocrinol* **10**:1617, 1996.
130. Malloy PJ, Eccleshall TR, Gross C, van Maldergem L, Bouillion R, Feldman D: Hereditary vitamin D–resistant rickets caused by a novel mutation in the vitamin D receptor that results in decreased affinity for hormone and cellular hyporesponsiveness. *J Clin Invest* **99**:297, 1997.
131. Cockerill FJ, Hawa NS, Yousaf N, Hewison M, O'Riordan JFL, Farrow SM: Mutations in the vitamin D receptor gene in three kindreds associated with hereditary vitamin D–resistant rickets. *J Clin Endocrinol Metab* **82**:3156, 1997.
132. Mechica JB, Leite MOR, Mendonca BB, Frazzatto EST, Borelli A, Latronico AC: A novel nonsense mutation in the first zinc finger of the vitamin D receptor causing hereditary 1,25-dihydroxyvitamin D–resistant rickets. *J Clin Endocrinol Metab* **82**:3892, 1997.
133. Marx SJ, Bliziotes MM, Nanes M: Analysis of the relation between alopecia and resistance to 1,25-dihydroxyvitamin D. *Clin Endocrinol* **25**:373, 1986.
134. Sakati N, Woodhouse NJY, Niles N, Harfi H, DeGrange DA, Marx S: Hereditary resistance to 1,25-dihydroxyvitamin D: Clinical and radiological improvement during high-dose oral calcium therapy. *Horm Res* **24**:280, 1986.
135. Hochberg Z, Borochowitz Z, Benderli A, Vardi P, Oren S, Spirer Z, Heyman I, et al: Does 1,25-dihydroxyvitamin D participate in the regulation of hormone release from endocrine glands. *J Clin Endocrinol Metab* **60**:57, 1985.
136. Balsan S, Garabedian M, Larchet M, Gorski AM, Cournot G, Tau C, Bourdeau A, et al: Long-term nocturnal calcium infusions can cure rickets and promote normal mineralization in hereditary resistance to 1,25-dihydroxyvitamin D. *J Clin Invest* **77**:1661, 1986.
137. Al-Awadi SA, Moussa MA, Naguib KK, Farag TI, Teebi AS, El-Khalifa M, El-Dossary L: Consanguinity among the Kuwaiti population. *Clin Genet* **27**:483, 1985.
138. Marx SJ, Swart EG Jr, Hamstra AJ, Deluca HF: Normal intrauterine development of the fetus of a woman receiving extraordinarily high doses of 1,25-dihydroxyvitamin D_3. *J Clin Endocrinol Metab* **51**:1138, 1980.
139. Bliziotes M, Yergey AL, Nanes MS, Muenzer J, Begley MG, Vieira NE, Kher KK, et al: Absent intestinal response to calciferols in hereditary resistance to 1,25-dihydroxyvitamin D: Documentation and effective therapy with high dose intravenous calcium infusions. *J Clin Endocrinol Metab* **66**:294, 1988.
140. Weisman Y, Bab I, Gazit D, Spirer Z, Jaffe M, Hochberg Z: Long term intracaval calcium infusion therapy in end-organ resistance to 1,25-dihydroxyvitamin D. *Am J Med* **83**:984, 1987.
141. Lin JP, Uttley WS: Intraarterial calcium infusions, growth, growth and development in end-organ resistance to vitamin D. *Arch Dis Child* **69**:689, 1993.
142. Liberman UA, Eil C, Holst P, Rosen JF, Marx SJ: Hereditary resistance to 1,25-dihydroxyvitamin D: Defective function of receptors for 1,25-dihydroxyvitamin D in cells cultured from bone. *J Clin Endocrinol Metab* **57**:958, 1983.
143. Baker AR, McDonnell DP, Hughes M, Crisp TM, Mangelsdorf DJ, Haussler MR, Pike JW, et al: Cloning and expression of full-length cDNA encoding human vitamin D receptor. *Proc Natl Acad Sci USA* **85**:3294, 1988.
144. Koren R, Ravid A, Liberman UA, Hochberg Z, Weisman Y, Novogrodsky A: Defective binding and function of 1,25-dihydroxyvitamin D_3 receptors in peripheral mononuclear cells of patients with end-organ resistance to 1,25-dihydroxyvitamin D. *J Clin Invest* **76**:2012, 1985.
145. Takeda E, Kuzoda Y, Saiijo T, Toshima K, Naito E, Kobashi H, Iwakuni Y, et al: Rapid diagnosis of vitamin D-dependent rickets type II by use of phytohemagglutinin-stimulated lymphoctyes. *Clin Chim Acta* **155**:245, 1986.
146. Koeffler HP, Bishop JE, Reichel H, Singer F, Nagler A, Tobler A, Walka M, et al: Lymphocyte cell lines from vitamin D-dependent rickets type II show functional defects in the 1α,25-dihydroxyvitamin D_3 receptor. *Mol Cell Endocrinol* **70**:1, 1990.
147. Barsony J, Pike JW, Deluca HF, Marx SJ: Immunocytology with microwave-fixed fibroblasts shows 1 alpha,25-dihydroxyvitamin D_3–dependent rapid and estrogen-dependent slow reorganization of vitamin D receptors. *J Cell Biol* **111**:2385, 1990.
148. Griffin JE, Chandler JS, Haussler MR, Zerwekh JE: Receptor-positive resistance to 1,25-dihydroxyvitamin D: A new cause of osteomalacia associated with impaired induction of 24-hydroxylase in fibroblasts. *J Clin Invest* **72**:1190, 1983.
149. Gamblin GT, Liberman UA, Eil C, Downs RW Jr, DeGrange DA, Marx SJ: Vitamin D–dependent rickets type II. Defective induction of 25-hydroxyvitamin D_3-24-hydroxylase by 1,25-dihydroxyvitamin D_3 in cultured skin fibroblasts. *J Clin Invest* **75**:954, 1985.
150. Yamaguchi A, Kohno Y, Yamazaki T, Takahashi N, Shinki T, Horiuchi N, Suda T, et al: Bone in the marmoset: A resemblance to vitamin D–dependent rickets, type II. *Calcif Tissue Int* **39**:22, 1986.
151. Adams JS, Gacad MA, Baker AJ, Gonzales B, Rude RK: Serum concentrations of 1,25 dihydroxyvitamin D_3 in platyrrhini and catarrhini: A phylogenetic appraisal. *Am J Primatol* **9**:219, 1985.
152. Takahashi N, Suda S, Shinki T, Horiuchi N, Shina Y, Tanioka Y, Koizumi H, et al: The mechanism of end-organ resistance to 1α,25-dihydroxycholecalciferol in the common marmoset. *Biochem J* **227**:555, 1985.
153. Adams JS, Gacad MA: D_3-receptor interaction among different genera of new world primates. *J Clin Endocrinol Metab* **66**:224, 1988.
154. Liberman UA, DeGrange D, Marx SJ: Low affinity of the receptor for 1α,25-dihydroxyvitamin D_3 in the marmoset, a New World monkey. *FEBS Lett* **182**:385, 1985.
155. Lipsett MB, Chrousos GP, Tomita M, Brandon DD, Loriaux DL: The defective glucocorticoid receptor in man and nonhuman primates. *Recent Prog Horm Res* **41**:199, 1985.
156. Gacad MA, Adams JS: Endogenous blockade of 1,25-dihydroxyvitamin D-receptor binding in New World primate cells. *J Clin Invest* **87**:996, 1991.
157. Arbelle JE, Chen H, Gacad MA, Allegretto EA, Pike JW, Adams JS: Inhibition of vitamin D receptor-retinoid X receptor-vitamin D response element complex formation by nuclear extracts of vitamin D–resistant New World primate cells. *Endocrinology* **137**:786, 1996.
158. Yoshizawa T, Handa Y, Uematsu Y, Takeda S, Sekine K, Yoshihara Y, Kawakami T, et al: Mice lacking the vitamin D receptor exhibit impaired bone formation, uterine hypoplasia and growth retardation after weaning. *Nature Genet* **16**:391, 1997.
159. Li YC, Pirro AE, Amling M, Delling G, Baron R, Bronson R, Demay MB: Targeted ablation of the vitamin D receptor: An animal model of vitamin D–dependent rickets type II with alopecia. *Proc Natl Acad Sci USA* **94**:9831, 1997.

160. Pettifor JM, Ross FP, Travers R, Glorieux FH, Deluca HF: Dietary calcium deficiency: A syndrome associated with bone deformities and elevated serum 1,25-dihydroxyvitamin D concentrations. *Metab Bone Dis Relat Res* **2**:301, 1981.
161. Marks SC Jr: Osteopetrosis—Multiple pathways for the interruption of osteoclast functions. *Appl Pathol* **5**:172, 1987.
162. Key L, Carnes D, Cole S, Holtrop M, Barshavit Z, Shapiro F, Arceci R, et al: Treatment of congenital osteopetrosis with high-dose calcitriol. *New Engl J Med* **310**:409, 1984.
163. Tieder M, Modai D, Samuel R, Arie R, Halabe A, Bab I, Gabizon D, et al: Hereditary hypophosphatemic rickets with hypercalciuria. *New Engl J Med* **312**:611, 1985.
164. Chesney RW, Hamstra AJ, Deluca HF: Rickets of prematurity: Supranormal levels of serum 1,25-dihydroxyvitamin D. *Am J Dis Child* **135**:34, 1981.
165. Steichen JJ, Tsang RC, Greer FR, Ho M, Hug G: Elevated serum 1,25-dihydroxyvitamin D concentrations in rickets of very low-birth-weight infants. *J Pediatr* **99**:293, 1981.
166. Halloran BP, Deluca HF: Appearance of the intestinal cytosolic receptor for 1,25-dihydroxyvitamin D_3 during neonatal development in the rat. *J Biol Chem* **256**:7338, 1981.
167. Kawakami M, Imawari M, Goodman DS: Quantitative studies of the interaction of cholecalciferol (vitamin D_3) and its metabolites with different genetic variants of the serum binding protein for these sterols. *Biochem* **179**:413, 1979.
168. Belsey R, Deluca HF, Potts JT Jr: Selective binding properties of the vitamin D transport protein in chick plasma in vitro. *Nature* **247**:208, 1974.
169. Zerwekh JE, Glass K, Jowsey J, Pak CYC: An unique form of osteomalacia associated with end organ refractoriness to 1,25-dihydroxyvitamin D and apparent defective synthesis of 25-hydroxyvitamin. *J Clin Endocrinol Metab* **49**:171, 1979.
170. Lightwood R: Idiopathic hypercalcemia with failure to thrive. *Proc R Soc Med* **45**:401, 1952.
171. Williams JCP, Barratt-Boyes BG, Lowe JB: Supravalvular aortic stenosis. *Circulation* **24**:1311, 1961.
172. Beuren AJ, Apitz J, Harmjanz D: Supravalvular aortic stenosis in association with mental retardation and a certain facial appearance. *Circulation* **26**:1235, 1962.
173. Jones KL, Smith DW: The Williams elfin facies syndrome: A new perspective. *J Pediatr* **86**:718, 1975.
174. Wiltse HE, Goldbloom RB, Antia AU, Ottesen OE, Towe RD, Cooke RE: Infantile hypercalcemia syndrome in twins. *New Engl J Med* **275**:1157, 1966.
175. Mehes K, Szelid A, Toth P: Possible dominant inheritance of the idiopathic hypercalcemic syndrome. *Hum Hered* **25**:30, 1975.
176. Fellers FX, Schwartz R: Etiology of the severe form of idiopathic hypercalcemia of infancy. *New Engl J Med* **259**:1050, 1958.
177. Taylor AB, Stern PH, Bell NH: Abnormal regulation of circulating 25-hydroxyvitamin D in the Williams syndrome. *New Engl J Med* **306**:972, 1982.
178. Martin NDT, Snodgrass GJAI, Cohen RD, Porteous CE, Coldwell RD, Trafford DJH, Makin HLJ: Vitamin D metabolites in idiopathic infantile hypercalcemia. *Arch Dis Child* **60**:1140, 1985.
179. Garabedian M, Jacqz E, Guillozo H, Grimberg R, Guillot M, Gagnadoux MF, Broyer M, et al: Elevated plasma 1,25-dihydroxyvitamin D concentrations in infants with hypercalcemia and an elfin facies. *New Engl J Med* **312**:948, 1985.
180. Aarskog D, Aksnes L, Markestad T: Vitamin D metabolism in idiopathic infantile hypercalcemia. *Am J Dis Child* **135**:1021, 1981.
181. Chesney RW, Deluca HF, Gertner JM, Genel M: Increased plasma 1,25-dihydroxyvitamin D in infants with hypercalcemia and elfin facies. *New Engl J Med* **313**:889, 1985.
182. Culler FL, Jones KL, Deftos LJ: Impaired calcitonin secretion in patients with Williams syndrome. *J Pediatr* **107**:720, 1985.
183. Friedman WF, Mills LF: The relationship between vitamin D and the craniofacial and dental anomalies of the supravalvular aortic stenosis syndrome. *Pediatrics* **43**:12, 1969.
184. Friedman WF, Roberts WC: Vitamin D and the supravalvular aortic stenosis syndrome: The transplacental effects of vitamin D on the aorta of the rabbit. *Circulation* **34**:77, 1966.

CHAPTER 166

Steroid Sulfatase Deficiency and X-Linked Ichthyosis

Andrea Ballabio ▪ Larry J. Shapiro

1. Steroid sulfatase (STS) deficiency (MIM 308100) is an inborn error of metabolism causing X-linked ichthyosis, a skin disorder inherited as an X-linked trait. The condition affects between 1 in 2000 and 1 in 6000 males in many different populations from a range of geographic locations and racial and ethnic backgrounds.

2. The phenotype of STS deficiency is characterized by the presence of dark scaly skin starting between birth and 4 months of age. Mild corneal opacities, which do not affect vision, are present in approximately one quarter of patients. In fetal life, placental deficiency of STS causes a diminished estrogen biosynthesis by the maternal-fetal-placental pregnancy unit. This often results in prolonged labor due to difficulty in cervical effacement, which leads to cesarean section in many cases. Patients with STS deficiency have increased levels of cholesterol sulfate in both plasma and stratum corneum. The increase of cholesterol sulfate levels in the stratum corneum appears to be responsible for the ichthyotic changes observed in patients with STS deficiency.

3. STS is localized primarily in the rough endoplasmic reticulum. The human STS polypeptide is composed of 583 amino acids encoded by a gene located on the distal short arm of the X chromosome (Xp22.3). It is composed of 10 exons spanning approximately 140 kb of DNA. The gene shares significant homology with all the other members of the sulfatase gene family. The sequence and organization of the *STS* gene appear to be particularly similar to that of a cluster of three sulfatase genes also located in the Xp22.3 region, suggesting the occurrence of duplication events in this region during recent mammalian evolution.

4. A highly homologous unprocessed STS pseudogene is located on the proximal long arm of the human Y chromosome. In human females, the *STS* gene escapes X chromosome inactivation (at least partially), being expressed by both the active and the inactive X chromosomes. This lack of dosage compensation and the presence of a Y-linked homologue suggests an ancestral pseudoautosomal location for the *STS* gene. This hypothesis is supported by the pseudoautosomal location of the murine *STS* gene. Human and murine *STS* genes share a low degree of sequence similarity (only 63 percent in the coding region), consistent with a high evolutionary divergence of pseudoautosomal regions in mammals.

5. Most patients with STS deficiency (85 to 90 percent) have submicroscopic deletions spanning the entire *STS* gene and flanking markers. Most of these deletions appear to be due to abnormal recombination caused by the presence of low-copy-number repeats. Approximately 10 percent of patients with STS deficiency have point mutations in the *STS* gene. Rare patients with STS deficiency (~5 percent) have a complex phenotype resulting from the presence of a contiguous gene syndrome involving a deletion of additional disease genes located in the Xp22.3 region, such as the Kallmann syndrome gene, the gene for X-linked recessive chondrodysplasia punctata, and that for ocular albinism. Some of these patients with Xp22.3 contiguous gene syndromes have cytogenetically visible abnormalities such as large terminal Xp deletions or X/Y translocations. STS deficiency also occurs as a manifestation of multiple sulfatase deficiency, an extremely rare autosomal recessive disorder affecting the activity of many sulfatases and resulting in a very severe and complex phenotype.

6. STS deficiency may be readily diagnosed either prenatally or postnatally by a combination of enzymatic, endocrinologic, and molecular methods. Treatment of STS deficiency focuses on the ichthyosis. The topical application of 12 percent ammonium lactate provides considerable benefit.

In 1969, France and Liggins described a novel inborn error of metabolism characterized by absence of neutral steroid sulfatase (STS) activity from the placenta in a pregnancy associated with very low estrogen production.[1] Following the recognition of additional cases in ensuing years, further attention focused on this condition, on the STS enzyme protein, and on the gene that encodes it. These studies have been carried out by geneticists, endocrinologists, and dermatologists, and have provided a rich collection of data with implications extending far beyond what was originally anticipated. The findings have yielded insight into the mechanism of steroid hormone metabolism and estrogen biosynthesis and into the interconversion and role of sterols in the skin. The identification of the *STS* gene has advanced our understanding of the evolution and regulation of gene expression on the mammalian X chromosome, of the homology between different sulfatase genes, and of the mechanisms of chromosomal rearrangements.

A list of standard abbreviations is located immediately preceding the index in each volume. Additional abbreviations used in this chapter include: *ARSD*/ARSD = arylsulfatase D gene/protein; *ARSE*/ARSE = arylsulfatase E gene/protein; *ARSF*/ARSF = arylsulfatase F gene/protein; CDPX = X-linked recessive chondrodysplasia punctata; *Clcn4* = mouse gene for chloride channel voltage-gated 4; DHEA = dehydroepiandrosterone; DHEAS = dehydroepiandrosterone sulfate; GS1 = gene designated by CpG island near steroid sulfatase equivalent to *DXF681E*; *KAL*/KAL = Kallman syndrome gene/protein; *MIC2* = gene for surface antigen recognized by Monoclonal Imperial Cancer Institute 2; *MIC2R* = *MIC2*-related gene; *Mid1* = mouse gene for midline 1 ring finger protein; MRX = X-linked mental retardation mapping to Xp22.3; MSD = multiple sulfatase deficiency; MyrBP = million years before present; PAR = pseudoautosomal region; *PHOG* = pseudoautosomal homeobox-containing osteogenic gene, same as *SHOX*; SS = steroid sulfatase; *SHOX* = short stature homeobox X-containing gene, same as *PHOG*; *STS*/STS = steroid sulfatase gene/protein; TDF = testis-determining factor; XLI = X-linked ichthyosis.

BIOCHEMISTRY

Sulfated Steroids

Sulfated steroids are ubiquitously distributed compounds found in abundance in mammalian tissues and body fluids.[2] They have unique biologic and chemical properties, which are conferred by their relative water solubility (as compared to the parent steroids) and by their capacity for lipophilic interactions owing to their cyclopentanophenanthrene ring structure. These molecules have in common a 3β-hydroxysteroid sulfate ester linkage. The first sulfated steroid to be isolated and structurally characterized was estrone sulfate, which was found in urine of pregnant mares.[3] Shortly afterwards, androsterone sulfate and dehydroepiandrosterone sulfate (DHEAS) were identified in human urine.[4,5] Relatively little further work was done with these compounds until the 1950s and 1960s, when adequate chemical methods for separating and quantitating these steroids were developed. In addition to methodologic constraints, a general feeling prevailed that steroid sulfates were merely water-soluble storage or excretory forms of active hormones and thus were uninteresting. With the development of chromatographic separation methods and the availability of isotopically labeled steroid sulfates, this view gradually changed. A comprehensive summary of the chemistry, distribution, and physiology of the steroid sulfates is beyond the scope of this chapter, but several excellent reviews are available.[2,6]

The 3β-hydroxysteroid sulfates are formed from free steroids by the action of the sulfotransferase activity present in the adrenal glands, liver, skin, testis, ovary, and placenta (Fig. 166-1). The high-energy sulfate donor is 3′-phosphoadenosine-5′-phosphosulfate (PAPS), which is formed by the sequential action of ATP sulfurylase and adenosine phosphosulfate phosphokinase. Whether a single enzyme or gene product mediates all sulfotransferase reactions is not known. The 3β-hydroxysteroid sulfates can be interconverted along pathways analogous to those used for the unconjugated steroids. This was elegantly verified by infusion into experimental subjects of sulfated steroids labeled with tritium in the sterol nucleus and ^{35}S in the sulfate moiety. When doubly labeled substrates were given, a variety of metabolites could be isolated with the same $^{35}S/^{3}H$ ratio as the starting material.[7] That indicates that these compounds are metabolized without prior desulfation. In spite of the conclusive demonstration of the existence of these pathways of biotransformation, their relative importance in normal steroid hormone economy is still largely unknown (Fig. 166-1).

For a number of years, several investigators endeavored to explain the apparent paradox of large quantities of circulating sulfated steroids in the face of their relative biologic inactivity. Pregnenolone sulfate is not active per se. DHEAS fails to cause changes in the activities of several enzymes that are modulated by free dehydroepiandrosterone (DHEA), and large doses of DHEAS given to human subjects are generally without effect. Estrogen sulfates apparently cannot interact with the estrogen receptor without prior hydrolysis.[8,9] It was suggested that sulfated steroids are a reservoir or a source of precursors for the production of active hormones, and this point of view may have some merit. It has been shown that the circulating half-life of most plasma steroid sulfates is longer than that of the corresponding free steroids, so that the sulfates must be more slowly metabolized or excreted. In addition, sulfated steroids may be hydrolyzed in situ by the ubiquitously distributed STS enzyme to yield free active hormones in target tissues (Fig. 166-1).

Cholesterol sulfate (CS) has been identified in considerable abundance in plasma, urine, seminal fluid, feces, gallstones, aortic plaques, and cell membranes, and is an important component of the stratum corneum of the epidermis.[10–14] CS is among the least soluble of the 3β-hydroxysteroid sulfates, and, by virtue of its amphiphilic nature, it can act as a detergent and form micelles or mixed micelles in aqueous solution. Normal plasma contains 150 to 350 µg/dl of CS, most of which is associated with low-density lipoprotein (LDL). Very large amounts of CS in plasma can alter the electrophoretic charge of plasma LDL, but there is no evidence that this affects the interaction of LDL with its receptor. However, Williams et al. showed that cholesterol sulfate is a very potent inhibitor of 3-hydroxy-3-methylglutaryl coenzyme A (HMG-CoA) reductase activity, the rate-limiting step in the de novo sterol biosynthetic pathway.[15,16] This inhibition of HMG-CoA reductase activity might account for the somewhat reduced level of total plasma cholesterol seen in these individuals (see "Ichthyosis and Lipid Metabolism" below).

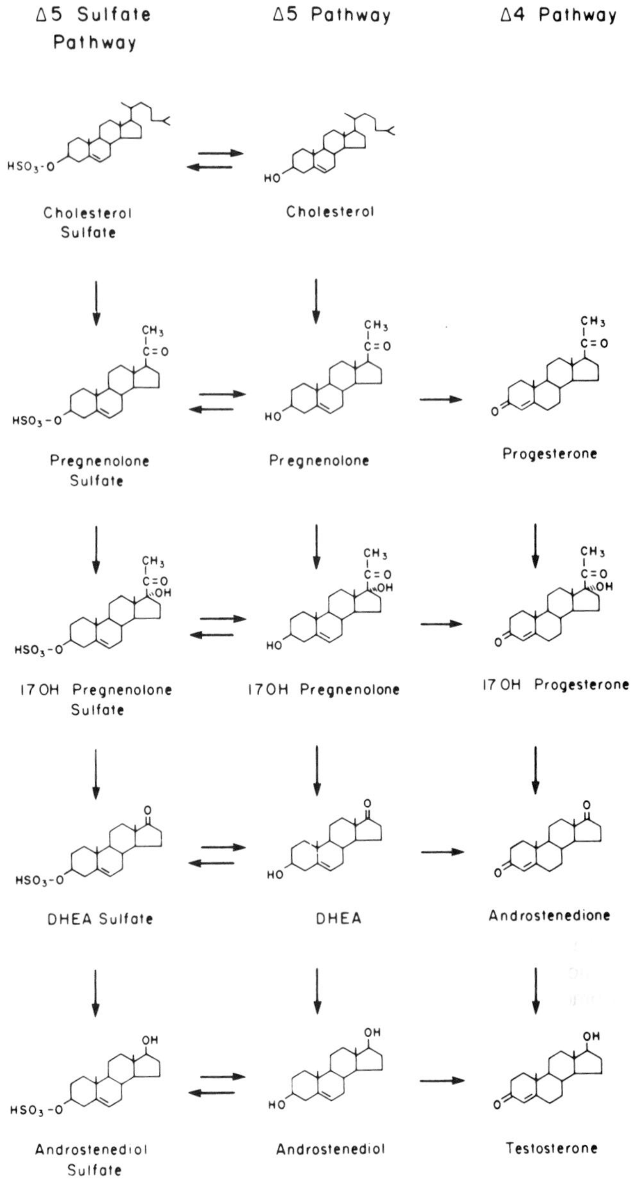

Fig. 166-1 Interrelationships of sulfated steroids with other metabolic pathways. Δ^5 Steroid sulfates are interconverted exactly as their parent Δ^5 free steroids are metabolized. For each compound, the sulfate can be converted to free steroid by STS, and the sulfate esters can be regenerated by the sulfotransferase reaction. Δ^5 Steroids can be transformed to Δ^4 steroids in some tissues by the action of 3β-hydroxysteroid dehydrogenase. Testosterone can potentially be derived via either the Δ^5 or the Δ^4 pathway.

DHEAS is another quantitatively important sulfated steroid. It has a clear role as a precursor for estrogen production during human pregnancies, and it may be important in the overall metabolism of androgen by the testis as well. It is the most abundant secretory product of the human adrenal gland. DHEAS is present at relatively high levels in cord blood, but rapidly diminishes in concentration during the first few months of life.

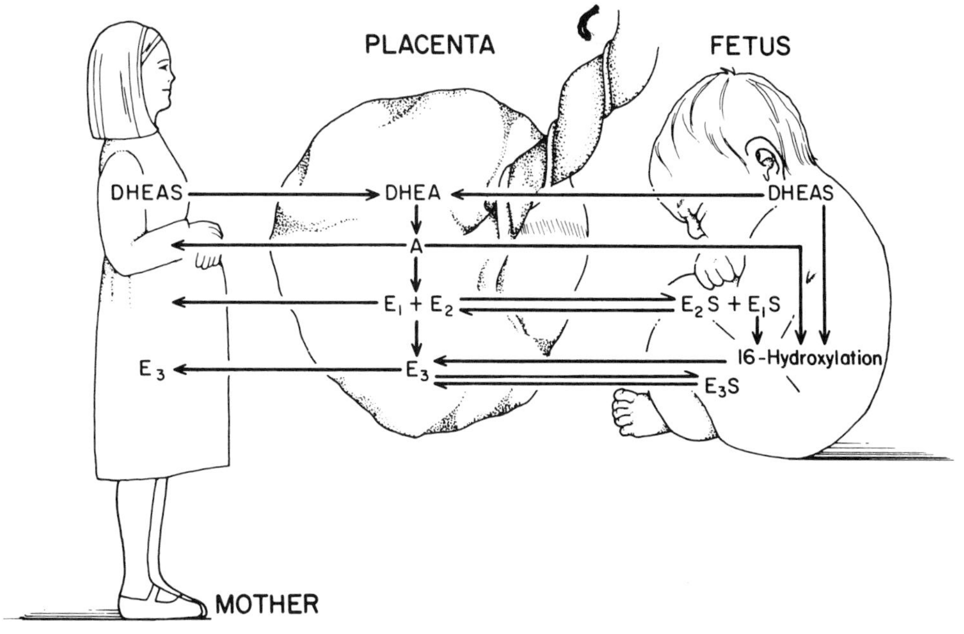

Fig. 166-2 Outline of fetal-maternal-placental estrogen biosynthesis. Total estrogen production increases several hundredfold during the normal course of pregnancy. The primary substrates for this biosynthetic activity are C_{19} steroids, particularly DHEA, 16-hydroxy-DHEA, and their sulfates. Early in pregnancy, DHEAS supplied by the maternal adrenals is important; in later gestation, fetally derived DHEAS and 16-hydroxy-DHEAS are most significant. These precursors are supplied to the placenta, where they are hydrolyzed by STS and metabolized by 3β-hydroxysteroid dehydrogenase, Δ^5-isomerase, and aromatase enzyme systems to give rise to estrogens. The estrogen present in largest quantities in normal pregnancy is estriol. E_1 = estrone; E_2 = estriol.

Plasma levels begin to rise again 1 to 2 years prior to the onset of puberty.[17–19] Adult production rates of DHEAS are on the order of 6 to 10 mg/day. Although an arteriovenous difference (increase) in DHEAS concentration across the testis can be demonstrated, studies of surgically adrenalectomized patients and subjects with exogenously induced adrenal suppression confirm that most of the circulating plasma DHEAS is derived from adrenal secretion.

DHEAS secreted by the maternal adrenal glands early in pregnancy and by the fetal adrenal glands later in gestation appears to be the substrate for the very large amounts of estrogen produced in normal human pregnancies (Fig. 166-2).[20,21] When pregnant women are given adrenocorticotropic hormone (ACTH), augmentation of estrogen production is observed, and when maternal adrenal glands are suppressed by dexamethasone, estrogen production diminishes.[22] Isolated fetal adrenal hypoplasia or fetal adrenal hypoplasia associated with anencephaly impairs DHEAS availability and leads to diminished estrogen production. Administration of exogenous DHEAS loads to pregnant women stimulates estrogen biosynthesis.[23] DHEAS that traverses the fetal compartment is subject to 16-hydroxylation by the fetal liver and can ultimately be converted to estriol.

The principal site of conversion of DHEAS to estrogen is probably the placenta, specifically the syncytiotrophoblast.[24–26] This metabolic transformation requires desulfation of DHEAS prior to aromatization to estrogen. The placenta contains very high levels of both STS and aromatase activities, and both are localized to the endoplasmic reticulum of the outer syncytiotrophoblast layer.[27] Perfused placentas can efficiently carry out desulfation and aromatization whether the DHEAS is supplied to the maternal surface (intervillous space) or via the umbilical circulation. The mechanism and kinetics of steroid transport across the placenta still require further investigation. However, the near complete inability of genetically STS-deficient placentas to support estrogen production is one of the strongest pieces of evidence regarding the importance of STS in estrogen production.

DHEAS may also play a significant role in androgen metabolism. Because the half-life in plasma of DHEAS is considerably greater than the half-life of DHEA, and as DHEAS is present at about 1000 times the concentration of DHEA, continual desulfation of DHEAS may ensure a basal level of DHEA in plasma between the episodic bursts that characterize DHEA secretion.[28] Circulating DHEAS could also be a potential precursor of testosterone via the sequence DHEAS → DHEA → androstenedione → testosterone (Fig. 166-1). Several investigators have attempted to assess the hormone flux through this pathway. The results of these studies, plus determinations of testosterone levels in adrenalectomized patients, makes it unlikely that adrenally secreted, circulating DHEAS is a quantitatively important precursor for testosterone biosynthesis.[29–31]

The possible role of DHEAS and other sulfated steroids as entirely intratesticular intermediates in the testosterone biosynthetic pathway have also been considered (Fig. 166-1).[32–41] The Δ5-3β-hydroxysteroid sulfates have been thought to be important intermediates in testosterone synthesis. On the other hand, to the extent to which the synthesis of testosterone from progesterone predominates (Δ4 pathway), sulfated steroids may not be of significant quantitative importance. Supporting this latter model is the finding that patients with inherited STS deficiency have normal values of testosterone, follicle-stimulating hormone (FSH), and luteinizing hormone (LH), are normally virilized; and have normal fertility (see "STS Deficiency and Androgen Metabolism" below).[41,42]

Steroid Sulfatase and Arylsulfatase C

Most mammalian tissues have a 3β-hydroxysteroid sulfate sulfatase activity that has a neutral pH optimum and is capable of hydrolyzing the sulfate ester bonds of a variety of sulfated sterols.[6,43] In addition, sulfate ester hydrolase activity against a variety of artificial chromogenic and fluorogenic compounds can be observed. The latter activities are conventionally referred to as "arylsulfatases." STS is one of the arylsulfatases. Several arylsulfatases are clearly distinct from one another: they can be independently purified; they have unique pH optima; they have different susceptibilities to inhibitors; and they are genetically separable, as they map to different chromosomes and have their function disrupted by distinct genetic entities. Arylsulfatases A and B are lysosomal in subcellular localization, have acidic pH optima, are inhibited by sulfate, phosphate, and barium, and are deficient in metachromatic leukodystrophy (see Chap. 148) and mucopolysaccharidosis VI (Maroteaux-Lamy syndrome), (see Chap. 136) respectively.[44,45] Both hydrolyze nitrocatechol sulfate and 4-methylumbelliferyl sulfate. The natural substrate for arylsulfatase A is galactosyl sulfatide and that of arylsulfatase B is the *N*-acetylgalactosamine-4-sulfate linkage in dermatan sulfate. In contrast, arylsulfatase C is microsomal in location, has a neutral-to-alkaline pH optimum, is inhibited preferentially by CN −, and is deficient in X-linked ichthyosis (STS deficiency). Arylsulfatase C hydrolyzes *p*-nitrophenylsulfate

Table 166-1 Enzymatic Properties or Purified STS from Human Placenta Toward a Variety of Steroid Sulfate and Aryl Sulfate Substrates

Steryl Sulfate/Aryl Sulfate	K_m (μM)	Specific Activity (mU/mg Protein)
Estrone sulfate	0.8	2900
Pregnenolone sulfate	0.6	1600
Cholesterol sulfate	2.0	1400
Dehydroepiandrosterone sulfate	1.7	1000
16α-Hydroxydehydroepiandrosterone sulfate	12	900
11-Deoxycorticosterone sulfate	40	150
Testosterone sulfate	40	1
Vitamin D_3 sulfate	—	<1*
4-Acetylphenyl sulfate	400	7000
4-Methylumbelliferyl sulfate	800	7000
4-Nitrocatechol sulfate	500	5000
4-Nitrophenyl sulfate	400	4000
Phenolphthalein bisulfate	—	<10*
4-Nitrophenyl phosphate	—	<20*

* Below the given limit of detection.

SOURCE: Dibbelt and Kuss.[48] Used by permission of *Biol Chem Hoppe-Seyter.*

and 4-methylumbelliferyl sulfate at the appropriate pH and ionic conditions. Positional cloning efforts have led to the identification of a cluster of three novel genes encoding arylsulfatases, namely arylsulfatase D, E, and F (*ARSD*, *ARSE*, and *ARSF*), whose natural substrates are still unknown. Similar to arylsulfatase C, these novel arylsulfatases are microsomal and have neutral pH optima; therefore, their activities toward artificial substrates, such as *p*-nitrophenylsulfate and 4-methylumbelliferyl sulfate, are difficult to separate from that of ARSC.[46,47] Arylsulfatase E is involved in the pathogenesis of X-linked recessive chondrodysplasia punctata and warfarin embryopathy.[46]

Table 166-1 shows a number of compounds that have been tested as substrates of highly purified STS.[48] Several investigators have questioned the number of discrete forms of STS that may exist and that could be necessary to hydrolyze the full range of structurally disparate steroid sulfates.[43,49–54] Using kinetic data, it has been observed that many sulfated steroids inhibit the hydrolysis of one another but do so noncompetitively, as assessed from Lineweaver-Burk plots. In addition, the relative activities toward different substrates are not always equally enriched during enzyme purification, and the pH optima and thermal stabilities of enzyme activity differ for various substrates.[49] These data should be viewed with some caution. First, most of these studies were conducted using relatively crude microsomal preparations or partially purified enzyme. Such impure systems may contain a variety of other factors that affect apparent activities. Second, a number of the substrates used have limited solubility and may in fact exist as micelles in aqueous media.

There are a number of compelling reasons to believe that all of the STS activities are associated with a single gene product in humans. First, all of the activities copurify to homogeneity and are competitively inhibited by all steroid sulfates.[55] Second, antibodies (including several monoclonal antibodies) raised against STS precipitate all of the enzyme's activities.[56,57] Third, all of the STS activities map to the same region of the X chromosome short arm in somatic cell genetic experiments. Fourth, a patient with an entirely intragenic deletion of the *STS* gene (see "The Molecular Basis of STS Deficiency" below)[58] shows a loss of all of the various enzyme activities. Finally, transfection of a mammalian expression plasmid containing a full-length *STS* cDNA construct confers all the 3β-hydroxysteroid sulfatase activities on recipient cells.[56] Thus, it is highly probable that this single protein is somewhat promiscuous with regard to the steroid sulfates it will hydrolyze. On the other hand, there is some degree of specificity, in that 3α-hydroxy steroid sulfates, vitamin D sulfate, phenolphthalein bisulfate, and tyrosine sulfate cannot serve as substrates.[48,59]

It has long been debated whether STS and arylsulfatase C activities reside in the same enzyme molecule. Vaccaro et al. showed that the activity of purified estrone sulfatase and dehydroepiandrosterone sulfatase to hydrolyze 4-nitrophenyl sulfate was competitively inhibited by both estrone sulfate and DHEAS.[60]

Chang et al. reported on the identification of two variants of arylsulfatase C by both electrophoresis and immunoprecipitation. These two variants were designated F (fast migrating) and S (slow migrating). Only the latter of these two variants appeared to correspond to STS, the other being a separate entity.[61,62] The two variants showed a different tissue-specific pattern of expression. The S form appears to be more abundant in placenta, while the F form is found mostly in liver.[57,63,64] Both the biochemical features and tissue distribution of the F form strongly suggest that it corresponds to arylsulfatase E.[46]

There is evidence for the presence of extensive variation in the number and types of molecules contributing to STS and arylsulfatase C enzymatic activities in different species.[55,65–67] Ruoff and Daniel performed a systematic comparative study on the biochemical features of hepatic STS and arylsulfatase C in 11 mammals.[68] Their data indicate that in some species these two activities are contributed by the same enzyme, while in other species the two activities are contributed by multiple loci and mechanisms.[57,64]

Immunocytochemical studies provide insights into the tissue distribution and ultrastructural localization of STS. Electron microscopy performed in human fibroblasts using anti-STS polyclonal antibodies localized STS to the rough endoplasmic reticulum, Golgi cisternae, trans-Golgi reticulum, plasma membrane, and endocytic pathway.[69] Within these sites, the distribution of STS was similar to that of lysosomal enzymes and the mannose-6-phosphate receptor. A similar subcellular distribution was observed after transfection of a full-length *STS* cDNA into baby hamster kidney cells (BHK-21).[70] Studies performed in human placenta using STS monoclonal antibodies revealed a more specific distribution of STS protein, the immunoreactivity being limited to the rough endoplasmic reticulum of the syncytiotrophoblast, where *STS* mRNA was also found to be most abundant.[27] These data suggest that STS is an integral endoplasmic reticulum protein with both membrane-spanning and lumen-oriented domains.

STS can be solubilized and released from the microsomal fraction by a variety of detergents. Detergents have proven necessary to maintain solubility during all purification procedures. Several groups report partial purification[49,71,72] or the preparation of apparently homogeneous STS from human placentas.[48,55,56,73–75] The active enzyme is a multimer of identical subunits, each with a molecular mass of approximately 63 kDa. The smallest aggregate that has activity appears to be a 126-kDa dimer (by gel-filtration analysis). A variety of the other molecular masses for the native enzyme have been suggested, including an estimate of 533 kDa achieved by neutron inactivation analysis[71] and 1000 kDa by chromatography.[76] The enzyme appears to be a glycoprotein, as it binds to concanavalin A-sepharose and can be specifically eluted.[56] The amino acid sequence of the protein predicted from the cDNA sequence includes four potential *N*-glycosylation sites as well as a number of possible *O*-glycosylation sites.[56,70] Digestion of in-vivo-synthesized STS by endoglycosidase H provided evidence that only two of the *N*-glycosylation sites are used.[70] The enzyme is remarkably stable to heat, to alterations of pH, and to exposure to urea. SDS-PAGE experiments indicate that there are no intermolecular disulfide bonds. Studies of STS biosynthesis and processing showed that newly synthesized STS is converted within 2 days into a mature 61-kDa form by processing of the oligosaccharide chains, which are cleavable by endoglycosidase H.[70,75,77] The half-life of STS polypeptides appears to be approximately 4 days.[75] The enzyme has no apparent cofactor requirements and is unaffected by divalent cation concentration.

Using antibodies prepared against the purified enzyme and partial amino acid sequence data, *STS* cDNA clones have been obtained from expression libraries.[56,70,78–80] Sequencing studies predict a mature protein of 583 amino acids.[70] There is a 22-amino-acid hydrophobic signal sequence that is probably cleaved after translocation across the endoplasmic reticulum membrane. There is a relatively long core hydrophobic region, as well as two potential membrane-spanning domains. Based on computer analysis, resistance toward proteinase K, and localization of *N*-glycosylation sites, Stein et al. proposed a three-domain model for the topology of STS, with the N- and C-terminal domains located at the luminal side of the membrane.[70]

GENETICS

Mapping the *STS* Gene

Much excitement has been generated by the elucidation of some unique aspects of the genetics of the STS system. In addition to the clear X-linked inheritance of STS deficiency, strong evidence for linkage with the polymorphic blood group antigen Xg located near the distal end of Xp was obtained.[81–86] A variety of approaches have been used to further map the *STS* gene to the distal tip of the X chromosome short arm (Fig. 166-3). Somatic cell genetic studies provided extensive verification of this assignment. Standard somatic cell fusion studies with hybrids segregating intact human X chromosomes, or portions of the human X derived from X/autosome and X/Y translocation chromosomes, permitted the assignment of the *STS* structural gene to Xp22.3,[87–89] and then the localization was refined by deletion-mapping studies of patients who are nullisomic for portions of distal Xp.[90,91] Analysis of genomic DNA from the relevant cell lines and hybrids with *STS* molecular probes and by chromosomal in situ hybridization using an *STS* cDNA probe confirms these observations.[56,78]

The *STS* Gene and Its Y-Encoded Pseudogene

The availability of human *STS* cDNA clones (GenBank J04964, M16505) made it possible to determine the size of *STS* mRNA

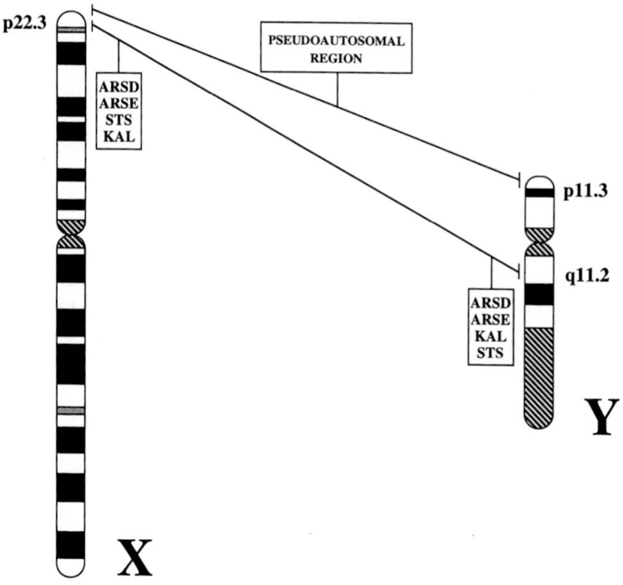

Fig. 166-3 Localization of the *STS* gene on the human sex chromosomes. The *STS* gene maps proximal to the pseudoautosomal region on the short arm of the X chromosome near the Kallmann syndrome (*KAL*), arylsulfatase D (*ARSD*), and arylsulfatase E (*ARSE*) genes. Similar to *STS*, all of these genes have a nonfunctional copy on the Y chromosome long arm.

transcripts and to characterize the genomic organization of the *STS* gene. *STS* mRNA transcripts of 2.7, 5.2, and 7.2 kb have been identified in different tissues and are the result of alternate poly(A) addition site usage with consequent variation in the length of the 3′ untranslated portion of the mRNA.[56,78] Whether or not these various transcripts have functionally different properties remains to be established. A representation of the X-encoded gene was obtained from overlapping phage genomic clones that span approximately 146 kb (Fig. 166-4).[92] Sequences corresponding to the cDNA have been localized to 10 individual exons, with the longest intron being about 37 kb in length.

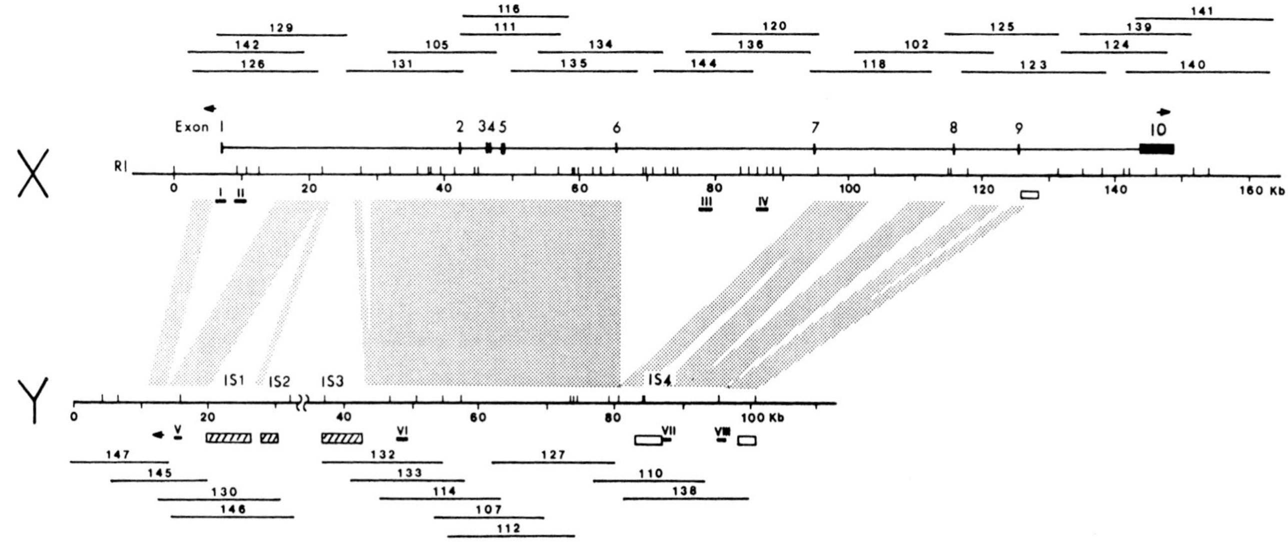

Fig. 166-4 Structural organization of human *STS* gene sequences on the X (top) and Y (bottom) chromosomes. The restriction maps show only *Eco*RI sites as vertical lines. Recombinant phages with overlapping human inserts from *STS-X* and *STS-Y* loci are shown above and below the respective maps. The positions of exons 1 through 10 are indicated above the *STS-X* map. The arrows above exons 1 and 10 in *STS-X* and below *STS-Y* at 13 kb represent the 1.6-kb inverted repeats and their orientations.[92] Single-copy probes used in the studies (probes I through VIII) are indicated below the maps. IS1 and IS4 are insertions in *STS-Y* that are absent in *STS-X*. The shaded areas between the *STS-X* and *STS-Y* maps indicate regions of high homology. (*From Yen et al.[96] Used by permission of Cell.*)

The 5′ region of the *STS* gene was studied to characterize the STS promoter. Four transcription start sites scattered over a 50-bp region were found. A putative promoter was identified and found to be TATA-less and GC poor. Several regulatory elements acting as enhancers and repressors were also found.[93]

Sequences that cross-hybridize to the *STS* cDNA were also found on the human Y chromosome.[56,94] The Y locus was cloned and has been mapped to the Yq11.2 region by both somatic cell genetic and deletion mapping methods.[56,95] The Y locus is a pseudogene, because a number of single-nucleotide changes and small deletions interrupt the open-reading frame. However, the positions of intron-exon boundaries appear to be similar to those of the X copy, and there is approximately 90 percent sequence similarity between the X and Y copies in both intron-like and exon-like areas (Fig. 166-4).[96]

Physical mapping studies in the region surrounding the *STS* locus have been performed by several groups. Long-range restriction mapping by pulsed field-gel electrophoresis determined the distance between *STS* and adjacent loci.[97,98] Overlap cloning using yeast artificial chromosome (YAC) clones defined the location of linked genes and anonymous loci in the region of the *STS* locus.[99,100] This provided essential reagents for gene identification and for the characterization of breakpoints from patients carrying chromosomal rearrangements in the region (see "The Molecular Basis of STS Deficiency" below).

The Escape of *STS* from X Chromosome Inactivation

X chromosome inactivation is an example of a developmentally programmed pattern of regulation of early embryonic gene expression.[101–103] This phenomenon has been extensively documented and studied, and occurs in all somatic cells of female mammals. The inactivation of one of the two X chromosomes in normal females results in dosage compensation (as compared to XY males) for the expression of X-linked gene products, and females who are detectably heterozygous for any X-linked locus are rendered mosaic at a cellular level. X chromosome inactivation is extensively described in Chap. 61.

It has long been suspected that there might be portions of the X chromosome that are not inactivated. If some X-encoded genes normally escape inactivation, that might explain some of the abnormalities observed clinically in X-chromosome aneuploid states.[104] If, on the other hand, the inactivation of the inactivated X chromosome is complete, one would expect to find no genetic difference between XY males (one copy of the X chromosome material), XO Turner syndrome individuals (one copy of the X chromosome material), and normal XX females (two copies of the X chromosome material with one copy inactivated). Similarly, if the second X in Klinefelter (47,XXY) individuals is completely inactivated, one would not anticipate the clinical abnormalities characteristic of this condition. Finally, based on genetic and evolutionary considerations, it seems likely that some genes have functional counterparts on both the X and Y chromosomes. Molecular evidence indicating partial or complete lack of inactivation has now been obtained for several genes from both within and outside the pseudoautosomal region (see "The Pseudoautosomal Region and Sex Chromosome Evolution" below). Such genes may well have evolved in such a way as not to require X inactivation for dosage compensation. Genes that are equally expressed from the X and Y would result in equivalent dosage between males and females only if the X-encoded locus escaped X inactivation in XX female somatic cells.

There are now strong data indicating the lack of inactivation of a number of human X-encoded genes (see reviews in references 102 and 103). The evidence supporting this conclusion is heterogeneous, including lack of mosaic expression of gene product, dosage of gene product, gene expression pattern in somatic cell hybrids, lack of mosaic clinical expression of X-linked traits, clonal selection in vivo, and variable phenotype in heterozygotes. The ability to detect STS expression in interspecific hybrids made it appropriate to study the inactivation of the STS locus. At least three lines of evidence support the conclusion that *STS* does not undergo full X inactivation. These include fibroblast cloning studies, somatic cell genetic experiments, and gene dosage determinations. When fibroblast cultures from females who were obligate heterozygotes for STS null alleles were diluted and single-cell-derived clones were isolated, all expressed significant amounts of STS activity.[105,106] This is in contrast to the recovery of fully STS-deficient clones that would be expected if the *STS* locus did undergo inactivation. A number of the women studied were also heterozygous for glucose-6-phosphate dehydrogenase (G-6-PD) electrophoretic or activity variants. This marker made it possible to distinguish clones in which the paternal X was active from those in which the maternal X was active. Furthermore, it was possible through pedigree analysis to assign the phase relationship between the two X chromosomes in each subject and the STS^+ and STS^- alleles. Carefully controlled measurements indicated that there was slight repression of expression of the intact STS allele on the inactive X relative to the one on the active X.[106] These studies provided the first indication that *STS* genes could be expressed from an otherwise inactive X chromosome.

Further support for this model comes from studies in which inactive human X chromosomes were segregated from any active X-genetic material in murine-human hybrid cell lines through appropriate selective culture conditions. It is interesting to note that the inactive X chromosome in such hybrids continues to demonstrate the properties of late DNA replication and extinction of gene expression even in this unusual heterologous background and even when the inactive X is separated from most of the human genetic complement.[107] The persistent expression of human *STS* in these cell lines which contain only an "inactive" X chromosome provides the second major piece of evidence that STS escapes inactivation. A final line of evidence supporting the lack of inactivation of the human *STS* locus derives from gene-dosage studies. Although data from X aneuploid individuals have not provided consistent results, a clear difference in STS activity between normal males and females has been documented in a variety of tissues and by a number of laboratories. The ratio of female to male activities ranges from 1.6 to 1.8 in fibroblasts, leukocytes, and placenta, and more careful quantitation of STS levels in fibroblasts from obligate heterozygotes is consistent with the view that some partial repression of STS expression may occur on the inactive X chromosome.[54,108–113]

Genes on the X chromosome that escape inactivation might conceivably do so through one of two general mechanisms. Either the position of these genes in some way protects them from being inactivated, or intrinsic aspects of the individual gene structure (e.g., a promoter) render them resistant to X inactivation. Current data seem to favor the latter, gene-specific model. This conclusion derives from studies of patients with X chromosome translocations and inversions. Autosomal segments positioned at the distal end of Xp may be inactivated if the X chromosome to which they are attached undergoes such regulation.[114] Thus, other genes translocated to a position comparable to *STS* may be inactivated. Conversely, when the *STS* and *MIC2* loci are relocated to a site within the long arm of the X and are flanked by other DNA sequences that are inactivated, they continue to be expressed.[115] These two genes appear to escape inactivation by a mechanism independent of their chromosomal location. However, characterization of the regulatory regions (i.e., promoter, enhancers) of the *STS* gene has failed to identify any specific feature differentiating it from genes undergoing X inactivation.[93]

The Pseudoautosomal Region and Sex Chromosome Evolution

It is generally believed that the X and Y chromosomes evolved from an ancestral homologous chromosome pair.[104,116] Some differential functions related to sex determination then became localized to the X, the Y, or both. During evolution, there has been very efficient selection for alterations that would suppress recombination between the X and Y so that the sex-determining and associated genes would not "inadvertently" be transposed to the wrong sex chromosome by crossing over or other genetic exchanges. The mechanism of this recombination suppression has probably involved a number of inversions, deletions, and other gross chromosomal alterations which had the end effect of isolating the X and Y. When these two chromosomes ceased exchanging DNA during meiosis, they became free to diverge rapidly from one another. There appear to be few functional genes on the mammalian Y chromosome. As X inactivation equalizes gene expression of X-encoded genes in XX and XY individuals, and because any mutations of the Y-encoded copy of genes shared by the X would be "covered" functionally, the Y has been freed of selective constraints and has developed extensive deletions and other mutations.

For more than 50 years, however, it has been predicted that the X and Y chromosomes would retain a segment of persistent homology.[117] The two sex chromosomes must somehow recognize one another in order to pair during meiotic division in spermatogenesis. It is believed that actual chiasma formation is required to assure proper segregation of chromosome pairs and to avoid nondisjunction. Such a region of the X and Y has been identified in both human[118–121] and mouse[122–127] sex chromosomes and is called the *pseudoautosomal region*. The major pseudoautosomal region of the human X and Y is located at the distal ends of their respective short arms, while, in the mouse, this area corresponds to the telomeres of the single chromosome arms (Fig. 166-3). More recently, a second small pseudoautosomal region was identified in humans, located at the distal ends of the X and Y long arms.[128]

Cytogenetic demonstration of chiasmata and synaptonemal complexes in the major (Xp/Yp) pseudoautosomal region complements genetic and molecular evidence. The importance of this region for proper sex chromosome pairing and recombination is evident from the study of an individual carrying a terminal Xp deletion. Primary spermatocytes from this individual showed failure of sex-chromosome pairing and absence of X-Y synaptonemal complexes.[129]

By definition, pseudoautosomal DNA sequences should be identical at the corresponding loci of the X and Y because of the relatively frequent recombination that would transfer sequences between these two chromosomes in succeeding generations. Because a given allele at a pseudoautosomal locus might be on the X in one generation and on the Y in another, such markers would either demonstrate partial or no sex linkage on pedigree analysis, depending on how telomeric the marker is and, therefore, how frequently recombination is observed relative to the X- and Y-unique portions of the chromosomes. Such frequently recombining genes could be readily confused with autosomally inherited loci, hence the term *pseudoautosomal*.[116]

A number of noncoding DNA segments have been used to identify pseudoautosomal loci in humans. These sequences are identical in males and females, map to the distal tip of Xp and Yp, and can be used to detect restriction fragment length polymorphisms (RFLP). Study of the segregation of RFLPs in families documents a gradient of recombination increasing from proximal to distal sites, such that the most telomeric loci show absolutely no sex linkage.[130] Comparison of recombination frequency using these RFLPs in XX and XY individuals indicates that the latter have a tenfold higher recombination rate than the former, as well as a very high rate of recombination relative to physical distance between markers. It seems that there must be an obligatory recombination event in any functional male meiotic division which is constrained to occur within a relatively small region of homology between the X and the Y, while recombination events between the two X chromosomes in female meiosis can occur anywhere along the length of the X chromosomes. This high frequency of recombination observed in both human and mouse pseudoautosomal regions[126,131] (see review in reference 132) gives rise to a far greater frequency of crossing-over per unit physical length than is the case for most of the rest of the genome. While these exchange events are supposed to be confined to the homologous segments of the X and Y, there is growing evidence that occasional recombination can be initiated in nearby regions. The most dramatic clinical consequence of aberrant X-Y exchange is seen in XX males (see Chap. 62).

Several genes have been isolated from the major (Xp/Yp) pseudoautosomal region on the human sex chromosomes (see review in reference 132). As previously discussed, one might speculate that some of these genes may be responsible for certain features of the Turner syndrome phenotype. In particular, patients carrying deletions involving the pseudoautosomal region have short stature. This conclusion is supported by the finding of short stature in patients monosomic for the pseudoautosomal region as the result of terminal X deletions or unbalanced X/Y translocations (see review in reference 90). A homeobox-containing gene, isolated by two different groups and named *SHOX* and *PHOG*, was isolated from this region and proposed as a candidate gene for the growth retardation observed in Turner syndrome.[133,134]

Homology between the human X and Y chromosomes is not limited to the pseudoautosomal region. The human *STS* gene is not pseudoautosomal and is located, together with the Kallmann syndrome gene (*KAL*),[135,136] the *GS1* gene,[137] and the recently identified cluster of arylsulfatase genes (*ARSD*, *ARSE*, and *ARSF*)[46,47] in the Xp22.3 region just proximal to the pseudoautosomal boundary. These genes lie in a region sharing high sequence identity with a region of the Y chromosome long arm (Yq11.2). It has been proposed that this region of homology was originally part of an ancestral pseudoautosomal region that was disrupted initially by a pericentric inversion followed by a series of other chromosomal rearrangements which occurred on the Y chromosome recently in evolution.[56,94]

Conservation of the genomic organization among the four Xp22.3 arylsulfatases strongly suggest that the *ARSD*, *ARSE*, *ARSF*, and *STS* genes originated from a common ancestral gene through a series of duplication events which occurred recently during evolution.[138,139]

An ancestral pseudoautosomal location of this cluster of genes is consistent with their origin through duplication events. These may have been caused by the high frequency of recombination present in this region, with one obligatory crossing over occurring at each male meiosis. The same mechanisms may have generated another cluster of genes, *MIC2*, *MIC2R*, and *Xg*, which are located only 150 kb apart from the *ARSD* gene, but within the present-day pseudoautosomal region (PAR).[140,141]

According to this hypothesis, at an earlier point in evolution the *STS*, *ARSD*, *ARSE*, *ARSF*, and *KAL* genes were present as functional genes on both X and Y, and these loci exchanged so as to maintain sequence similarity. Owing to the presence of two functional copies of these genes in both males and females, dosage compensation was not required and, therefore, these genes escaped X inactivation. Later in evolution, a complex series of rearrangements on the Y chromosome led to the repositioning of the pseudoautosomal boundary and to the relocation of the sulfatase gene cluster, together with *KAL-Y* and, presumably, other Xp22.3 genes, on the long arm of the Y chromosome, abruptly halting pseudoautosomal exchange. These Y loci started to diverge and degenerate in the absence of selective pressure, and the functional X genes, which were no longer pseudoautosomal, still maintained their ability to escape X inactivation.

To test this hypothesis, the sequences of Xp22.3 loci, including *STS*, *ARSD*, *ARSE*, and *KAL*, were compared to those of their Y-derived homologs.[138,142] Figure 166-5 shows arylsulfatase D and E sequence analysis indicating that each gene is more similar to its Y-homolog than to other members of the cluster.[138] These data strongly support the hypothesis that duplication events occurred before the X and Y copies of these genes started to diverge, that is, while they were still pseudoautosomal (Fig. 166-6). Altogether, X/Y comparison analysis suggests the occurrence of complex evolutionary changes, rather than a single pericentric inversion event on the Y chromosome. These rearrangements

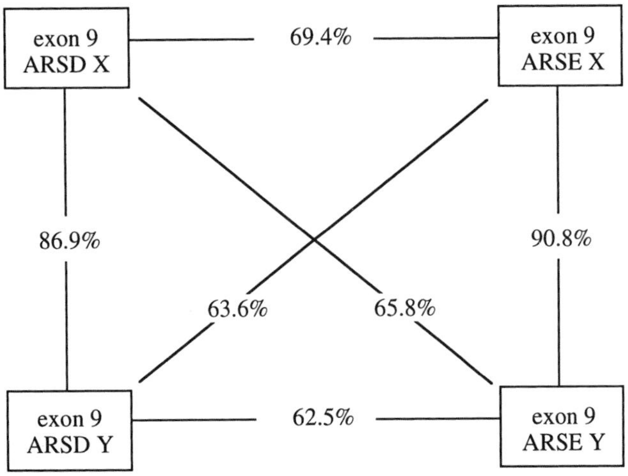

Fig. 166-5 Identity values among *ARSD* and *ARSE* exon 9 sequences and their Y-linked counterparts. (*From Meroni et al.*[138] *Used by permission of Human Molecular Genetics.*)

presumably led to the loss of *ARSF*, for which no Y homolog has been identified, and to lack of conservation of the order of these genes on Yq. It is tempting to speculate that, in addition to chromosomal rearrangements such as inversions, deletions, and transpositions, other mechanisms, including gene conversion, have contributed to the organization of the contemporary human sex chromosomes.

STS Genetics in Mice and Other Mammals

The study of STS in the mouse has generated several interesting and unexpected results. An insightful observation was made by Balazs et al., who noted that the murine A9 cell line, which had been so useful for somatic cell genetic studies because it was deficient in STS activity, was derived from the C3H/An inbred mouse strain. When tissues of these animals were examined, they were also found to be essentially devoid of STS activity.[143] Subsequently, other investigators documented interstrain variation in STS activity in several other inbred mouse lines, although none of them were nearly as deficient in STS as the C3H/An.[66,67,144–146] In contrast to human patients with genetic STS defects, the C3H/An mice are healthy, have normal skin and reproduction, and have only a twofold increase in plasma cholesterol sulfate levels compared to other mice (Bergner and Shapiro, unpublished). In initial test crosses and backcrosses, these STS variations behaved like single-gene Mendelian traits, but showed no sex linkage and were therefore assumed to represent autosomal genes affecting STS activity. However, further experiments suggested that the mouse *STS* gene in fact represents a true pseudoautosomal gene with frequent recombination between functional X and Y loci.

Cloning the mouse *Sts* gene has been a very difficult task. Initial attempts using human reagents such as *STS* cDNA and anti-STS antibodies were unsuccessful. An important tool was the purification of a rat enzyme with estrone sulfatase activity, which showed a high degree of similarity with human STS in the 24 amino-acid residues that could be sequenced.[55] Degenerate oligonucleotides based on this sequence permitted isolation of a small fragment of the rat *Sts* cDNA, which was then successfully used as a probe to identify rat and mouse *Sts* cDNAs.[147]

The overall amino acid sequence of the mouse Sts was found to be only 73 percent and 59 percent identical to the rat and human STSs, respectively. Despite this low level of conservation, the gene corresponds to a functional *Sts* gene, as demonstrated by restoring enzyme activity on transfection of the STS-deficient A9 cells. Mapping of the mouse *Sts* gene demonstrated that it is indeed pseudoautosomal, and placed it distal to the obligatory cross-over in male meiosis.[147] As expected for its location, the mouse *Sts* gene escapes X inactivation. In contrast, mapping of the rat *Sts* gene indicated that it is a nonpseudoautosomal, X-linked gene that undergoes X inactivation.[148]

The remarkable low sequence similarity between human and mouse STS is not a unique feature, but involves other genes located in Xp22.3. For many of the human pseudoautosomal genes, a mouse homologue could not be identified at all, owing to the complete lack of cross-hybridization to mouse DNA. This lack of homology between the human and mouse extends beyond the pseudoautosomal boundary into the more proximal X-specific portion of the human X chromosome, containing the *STS*, *KAL*, *ARSD*, *ARSE*, and *ARSF* genes. Both hybridization- and PCR-based approaches have failed to identify the mouse homologues for the *KAL*, *ARSD*, *ARSE*, and *ARSF* genes. A high degree of sequence divergence in this region of the human and mouse X

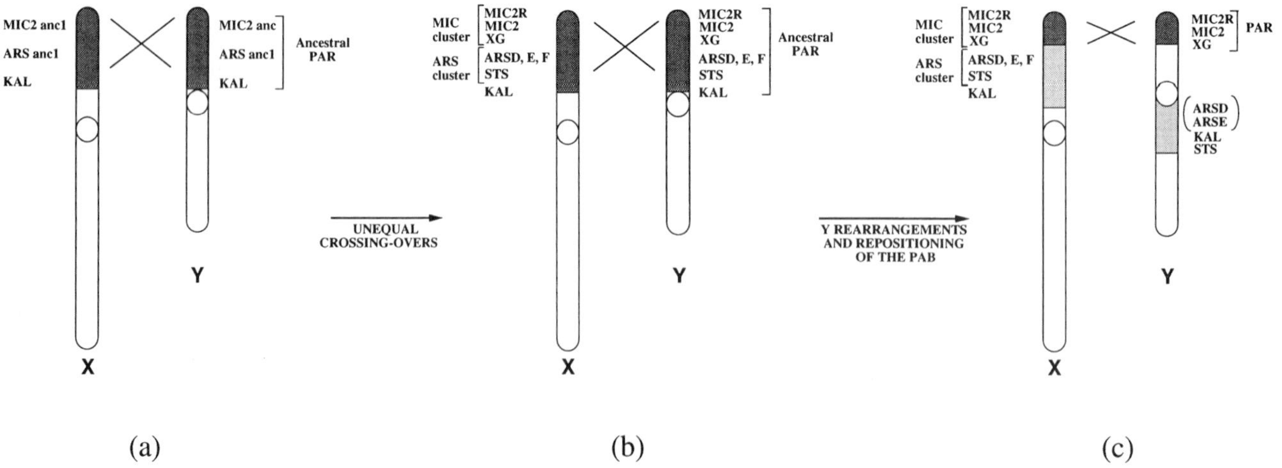

Fig. 166-6 Tentative model of the origin of sulfatase and *MIC2* gene clusters in an ancestral pseudoautosomal region. A hypothetical ancestral pseudoautosomal region (a), whose boundary was situated somewhere proximal to the *KAL* gene, is shown in dark gray. Two ancestral genes, *MIC2anc1* and *ARSanc1*, one for each of the two families, were present within this ancestral PAR. Due to a series of unequal crossing-over events, each of these genes gave rise to a cluster of genes (b) on both the X and Y chromosomes. A complex series of events led to the repositioning of the PAB to a more distal location on Yp and to the transfer of the cluster of sulfatase gene homologs to Yq (gray region), together with the KAL-Y. In parentheses are loci whose relative order is unknown. (*Modified figure from Meroni et al.*[138] *Used by permission of Human Molecular Genetics.*)

chromosomes may be due to the pseudoautosomal region being subject to obligatory crossing over in male meiosis, which may lead to a higher frequency of double-strand breakage and repair, and, consequently, to a high mutation rate.

Kipling et al. showed that the murine PAR is subject to a very high frequency of de novo rearrangements. New *Pac*I restriction fragments were found to occur at a sex-averaged rate of 30 percent per allele[149] in C57BL/6 × C57BL/6 crosses. Further molecular evidence for major rearrangements occurred close to the pseudoautosomal boundary during mammalian evolution was obtained by mapping the *Clcn4* gene in the mouse. This gene was in fact found to map to the X chromosome close to the PAR boundary in the wild Mediterranean mouse, *Mus spretus*, as well as in humans, but it mapped to chromosome 7 in the inbred strain C57BL/6 mouse.[150] Finally, the murine *Mid1* gene, which spans the pseudoautosomal boundary was found to be subject to spontaneous deletion/duplication events, due to the high frequency of unequal cross-over in the murine PAR.[151] Together these data indicate that this region of mammalian sex chromosomes has been changing very rapidly during evolution.

Further insights into the evolution of the *STS* gene come from the study of higher mammals. Phylogenetic studies on the organization of the *STS* gene on the X and Y chromosomes have been performed in great apes and in Old World and New World monkeys.[92] These studies suggest that great apes and Old World monkeys have an *STS-X* gene and *STS-Y* pseudogene configuration similar to humans, whereas New World monkeys appear to lack the Y-linked copy of the gene (or have a highly divergent Y copy). Interestingly, *STS* is autosomal in prosimian lemurs.[152]

Additional comparative research on *STS* expression and mapping has been carried out in the wood lemming,[153] the root vole,[154] carnivores and ungulates,[155] and several marsupials.[156] In the wood lemming, STS activity parallels the number of X chromosomes present, providing indirect evidence for X-linkage and escape from inactivation in this species. In the root vole, STS activity is higher in the male than in the female for reasons that are not clear. In both dog and sheep, *STS* was found to be located in the X-Y pairing region. In contrast, the *STS* locus is autosomal in marsupials.

Overall, these data suggest that the human *STS* gene is located in a region of the X chromosome that was originally autosomal, as demonstrated by its autosomal location in marsupials. This region of the X chromosome (Xp22.3) was then added to the eutherian X after the divergence of eutherians and marsupials (130 MyrBP) and before the radiation of eutherians (80MyrBP), consistent with its pseudoautosomal location in mouse, carnivores, and ungulates. In humans and Old World Monkeys, this ancestral pseudoautosomal region was disrupted by a complex rearrangement that occurred on the Y chromosome, which placed STS-X in the more proximal X-specific region of Xp22.3 and STS-Y to Yq11.2 (see previous section). The finding that *STS* is autosomal in prosimians probably reflects a loss of this gene from the sex chromosomes of a prosimian ancestor.

STS DEFICIENCY

Placental STS Deficiency

In 1969, France and Liggins reported studies of a single pregnancy in which estriol production was strikingly impaired despite the normal growth and viability of the fetus.[1] Labor was prolonged, and after delivery the placental extracts were assayed for activities for several enzymes thought to be important in estrogen biosynthesis. A specific and virtually complete absence of STS was found. These investigators were subsequently able to study another pregnancy in vivo by loading techniques.[157] Intravenously administered DHEAS could not be converted to estrogen in a normal fashion, while exogenous free DHEA could serve as an effective substrate. This suggested a metabolic block in the conversion of DHEAS to DHEA, which was again confirmed by biochemical studies of the placenta.

During the ensuing years, a number of similar cases were described in the obstetrical literature (see reviews in references 158 and 159). This was in part due to the growing popularity of the use of radioimmunoassay determination of maternal urinary and serum estriol levels as an index of fetal-placental-maternal integrity and well-being during pregnancy. In many of these earlier cases, there was an ascertainment bias, because estriol measurements were done routinely only in complicated obstetrical situations. However, with the advent of large-scale estriol screening programs, many more cases of apparent "placental" STS deficiency were identified, and, by the mid-1970s, this was a well-established clinical entity. The total 24-h urinary estrogen excretion of women carrying affected pregnancies is generally less than 3 mg, and serum estriol levels are dramatically reduced to less than 10 percent of normal values controlled for gestational age.

In the initial reports of the clinical features of STS deficiency, a relative refractoriness to the onset of labor was noted, particularly in primigravidas. Further evaluation suggests that this may be due to some difficulty in cervical effacement with prolongation of labor. Despite that many of the women carrying affected fetuses require cesarian section, many do deliver vaginally.[160] Some women have had a history of prior pregnancy losses with death of full-term or postmature infants. There was one report of placental sulfatase deficiency associated with intrauterine fetal death.[161] A single pregnancy in which STS deficiency was present in a fetus as the result of autosomal recessive multiple sulfatase deficiency disease also had marked impairment of estriol production.[162] Diminished maternal-fetal-placental estrogen production is also seen in substrate deficiency conditions such as fetal adrenal hypoplasia (with or without anencephaly). Infants born of pregnancies complicated by STS deficiency are usually clinically normal at birth, and their placentas lack any anatomic defects. Maternal urinary excretion of a number of sulfated steroids is detectably abnormal during the latter half of pregnancy, with the 16-hydroxy-DHEAS level averaging 20 times normal.[163] DHEAS levels in amniotic fluid from affected pregnancies are also strikingly increased.[164,165] In contrast, cord blood levels of DHEAS and 16-hydroxy-DHEAS are usually normal in affected infants.[1,158,163,166] It is hypothesized that the local estrogen/progesterone ratio in chorion and decidua influence myometrium contractility, and that this ratio is abnormal in STS deficiency.[167]

Most of the earlier studies of STS deficiency focused on obstetrical aspects. Because cord blood and neonatal urinary steroid levels were normal in infants born of affected pregnancies and because these children looked well clinically, it was speculated that STS deficiency was an enzymopathy that was confined to the placenta. This view changed with the development of sensitive enzyme assays, which could be applied to cultured skin fibroblasts, leukocytes, and hair follicles.[168] It then became clear that STS deficiency is a generalized metabolic disturbance that affects essentially all tissues in the fetus and newborn. Furthermore, a visible phenotypic manifestation of ichthyosis made it clear that there was a specific postnatal phenotype associated with this inborn error of metabolism. The availability of the fibroblast assay has facilitated widespread case finding and the performance of family studies that would not have been possible were it necessary to have placental tissue in order to recognize affected individuals. The first reports of STS deficiency noted recurrence in families and the fact that all affected fetuses were males. Application of the cell culture assay to postnatally derived samples permitted the rigorous confirmation of X-linked inheritance in several families.[169,170]

STS Deficiency as the Cause of X-Linked Ichthyosis

Ichthyosis describes a number of genetic and acquired skin disorders.[171] The clinical hallmark is hyperkeratosis or increased thickness of the stratum corneum (Fig. 166-7). A number of complex syndromes have been described with ichthyosis as one component. In addition, distinct hereditary disorders have been

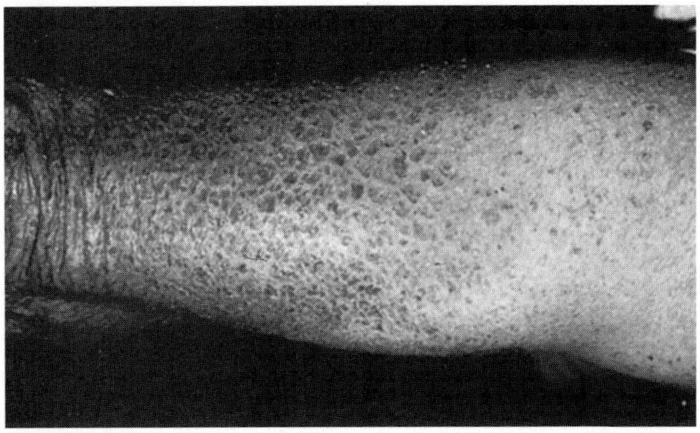

Fig. 166-7 Photograph of the arm of a 45-year-old adult with X-linked ichthyosis due to STS deficiency. The scales are thick and dark and are present on the neck, trunk, and lower soles. This individual had two affected grandsons and an affected brother and uncle.

delineated in which ichthyosis is the principal feature, including the relatively severe autosomal recessively inherited conditions known as lamellar ichthyosis and congenital ichthyosiform erythroderma, the somewhat milder disorder autosomal dominant ichthyosis vulgaris, various types of autosomal dominant bullous ichthyosis, and X-linked ichthyosis. Table 166-2 lists the features that should be considered in the differential diagnosis of the major types of ichthyosis. Reviews on the clinical, histopathologic, and biochemical features of the ichthyoses are available.[172–175]

It has been known for more than 100 years that ichthyosis can segregate in some families as an X-linked trait.[164] The work of Wells, Kerr, and Jennings in the early and middle 1960s provided clear genetic and clinical delineation of these various forms of ichthyosis.[165,176–179] These workers were able to demonstrate that autosomal dominant and X-linked ichthyosis were relatively common disorders, with the latter condition being present in approximately 1 in 6000 males studied in their population. They had reason to believe that they had complete ascertainment within the geographic area under consideration. They were able to show that X-linked ichthyosis differed from autosomal dominant

Table 166-2 Differential Diagnosis of the Major Types of Ichthyosis

Disorder	Inheritance*	Incidence	Onset/Natural Course	Scale	Distribution	Associated Features	Histology	Biochemical Findings
Ichthyosis vulgaris	AD	1:250	3–12 months, improves with age	Fine, like bran flakes, mostly adherent	Extensor extremities, palms and soles: face spared	Keratosis pilaris, atopy	Thickened stratum corneum: diminished or absent granular layer	Unknown
X-linked ichthyosis	XL	1:2000–6000 (males)	0–3 months, improves with age	Large, dark, adherent	Both extensor and flexor extremities, trunk, lateral face, neck; palms and soles spared (in most cases)	Corneal opacities, cryptorchidism, testicular cancer	Thickened stratum corneum; normal to thickened granular layer	Steroid sulfate deficiency; abnormal, mobility of serum β lipoprotein, increased cholesterol sulfate in serum and stratum corneum
Lamellar ichthyosis	AR, AD (rare)	1:300.000	birth, persistent	Large, thick, plate-like, raised borders	Generalized, palms and soles	Ectropion, eversion of lip; collodion baby; hyperpyrexia	Hyperkeratosis; granular layer present	Increased free sterols and ceramides stratum corneum
Congenital ichthyosiform erythroderma	AR	1:300.000	birth, presistent	Fine white scale	Generalized	Erythroderma, collodion baby; scarring alopecia; nail dystrophy	Hyperkeratosis; granular layer present	Unknown
Bullous ichthyoses	AD	1:300.000	birth, may improve with age	Verrucous, thick, dark	Generalized with blisters, accentuated in flexures, face spared	Generalized bacterial overgrowth; foul body odor; nail dystrophy	Vacuolization of the granular and upper epidermal cell layers with variable keratosis	Unknown

*AD = autosomal dominant: XL = X-linked: AR = autosomal recessive.

SOURCE: Modified from Shwayder and Ott.[175] *(Used by permission of WB Saunders.)*

Table 166-3 Clinical Abnormalities Associated with STS Deficiency

Prenatal	Postnatal
Consistent Features	
Low maternal urinary and serum estriol	Ichthyosis with onset from birth to 3–4 months
Elevated DHEAS and 16-hydroxy-DHEAS in maternal urinary and amniotic fluid	Corneal opacities
Absent placental STS activity	Increased cholesterol sulfate in plasma, red blood cells, and skin with rapidly migrating LDL
	Absent STS activity
Variable Features	
Delayed onset of labor	Undescended testis
Relative refractoriness of cervical dilatation	Testicular tumors (?)

ichthyosis vulgaris in age of onset, relative distribution of disease, severity, and a variety of histopathologic features.

The clinical features of X-linked ichthyosis are listed in Table 166-3. Aside from the obvious differences in inheritance patterns, X-linked ichthyosis is characterized by onset between birth and 4 months of age and involvement of the upper and lower limbs and trunk. There is frequent involvement of the scalp and neck but, in most cases, the palms and soles are spared. The nails and hair are normal. The scales are large, dark, and prominent. Histologically, there is hyperkeratosis, with a normal or increased granular layer. Finally, characteristic corneal opacities may be observed on slit-lamp examination. These opacities are found in Descemet's membrane or in the deep stroma anterior to it (Fig. 166-8), and they have no effect on visual acuity.[174,180–182] A survey of 38 patients with X-linked ichthyosis and of female heterozygotes found an incidence of corneal opacities of approximately 25 percent in both groups.[181] Aside from the eye findings, most female heterozygotes are asymptomatic and do not show any cutaneous abnormalities.

Two groups independently observed that patients with STS deficiency, as ascertained by low estrogen production, had clinically apparent ichthyosis.[169,170] Furthermore, in a number of the extended families of probands, a clear history of X-linked ichthyosis could be obtained. When family studies of STS activity in cultured fibroblasts were conducted, complete concordance between enzyme deficiency and ichthyosis was demonstrated. Finally, many studies of families ascertained solely on the basis of the X-linked inheritance of ichthyosis showed them all to be associated with STS deficiency, while enzyme assays done on patients with other types of ichthyosis revealed normal activity levels.[183,184]

It was suggested that STS deficiency might not be causally related to ichthyosis but that the *STS* gene and the "ichthyosis" gene might be contiguous and included in deletion events. Although STS deficiency is often the result of a gene deletion (see "The Molecular Basis of STS Deficiency" below), it is clear that STS deficiency per se does cause the ichthyosis. There are several reasons for coming to this conclusion. First, there is an invariant association between ichthyosis and STS deficiency. All patients lacking STS activity have this phenotypic finding. Second, there is good pathophysiological reason to suspect that disordered sulfated sterol metabolism might interfere with epidermal function (see "Ichthyosis and Lipid Metabolism" below). The third line of evidence supporting the causal relationship of X-linked ichthyosis and STS deficiency is genetic. At least seven patients with point mutations in the *STS* gene,[185–188] and an additional subject with an entirely intragenic deletion at the STS locus,[58] have ichthyosis. In addition, patients with the rare autosomal recessive disorder multiple sulfatase deficiency have reduced STS activity as the result of a non-X–linked mutation, and still have clinically apparent ichthyosis. Finally, somatic transfer of the *STS* gene to keratinocytes from patients with STS deficiency leads to a partial correction of the phenotypic abnormalities observed in tissue culture and in xenotransplants.[189,190]An exceptional pedigree with XLI was published by Robledo et al.[191] Affected individuals from this pedigree show the classical clinical features of XLI but appear to have normal levels of STS enzymatic activity. Consistently, molecular analysis of patients' DNA failed to detect any abnormality of the *STS* gene. Partial linkage data appear to exclude linkage of the disease locus to markers from the Xp22.3 region, suggesting that XLI may also be caused by mutation of another gene located in a different region of the X chromosome.[191]

To date, the only sulfated 3β-hydroxy steroid observed to accumulate in STS-deficient patients in amounts comparable to the increases of substrates seen in other inborn errors of metabolism is CS. CS is strikingly elevated in plasma, red blood cell membranes, and the stratum corneum of STS-deficient individuals.[192,193] The amounts may be as much as 20 times the normal levels. Determination of plasma CS content by either radioimmunoassay,[192,193] gas chromatography,[194] or HPLC/mass spectrometry[195] may be of use for diagnostic purposes. As in normal individuals, most of the CS is physically associated with the LDL plasma fraction and gives the LDL an abnormal electronegativity. In patients with STS deficiency, an increase of the CS content leads to an abnormal electrophoretic mobility of LDL.[193] A systematic study of LDL mobility in 14 patients with STS deficiency and in normal individuals, demonstrated that LDL migrated consistently faster in patients with STS deficiency than in normal individuals.[196] The relative contents of apoB, cholesterol, and triglyceride were also altered in LDL from patients with STS deficiency. Female heterozygotes and individuals with autosomal dominant ichthyosis vulgaris showed no abnormalities. This and other studies[194]

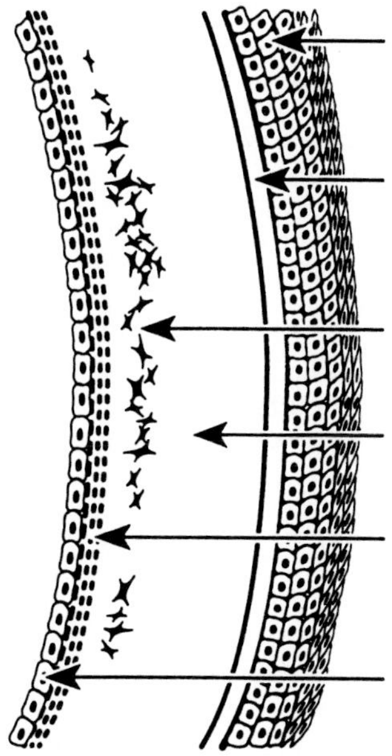

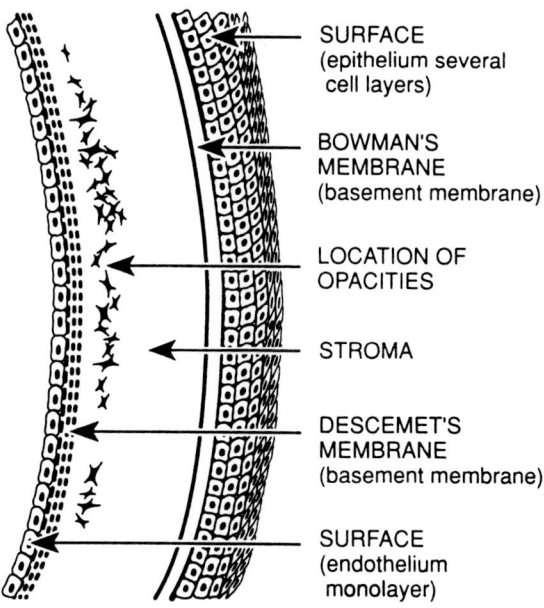

Fig. 166-8 Eye lesions in X-linked ichthyosis. Corneal opacities associated with X-linked ichthyosis are found in Descemet's membrane or in the deep stroma anterior to Descemet's membrane. (*From Ghadially and Chong.*[174] *Used by permission of Dermatologic Clinics.*)

suggest that lipoprotein electrophoresis could also represent a simple, readily available screening test for X-linked ichthyosis.

Ichthyosis and Lipid Metabolism

The end product of epidermal differentiation is the stratum corneum, which functions primarily as a barrier against transepidermal water loss.[197] This barrier function is provided by a unique two-compartment system composed of protein-enriched corneocytes that are "glued" together by a hydrophobic, lipid-enriched intercellular matrix. Corneocytes, desmosomes, hydrolytic enzymes, and both locally synthesized and essential lipids are critical components of the stratum corneum.[197] Disorders affecting any of these components may cause inflammation, hyperkeratosis, and scaling.[198,199]

Under normal conditions, epidermal desquamation is a continuous process resulting from detachment of individual corneocytes from the skin surface. It is known that alterations of the stratum corneum lipid content cause abnormal desquamation and scaling. In this pathologic condition, corneocytes are shed in clusters that appear as scales (the term ichthyosis derives from the Greek ichthys, "fish").[197–199]

Several studies demonstrated that drug-induced imbalances of lipid metabolism may cause scaling. Topical application of cholesterol sulfate to hairless mice can induce ichthyosis.[200] Drugs inhibiting de novo cholesterol synthesis, such as lovastatin, triparanol, and nicotinic acid, have been shown to produce scaling and abnormalities of barrier function in experimental animals.[197,199,201] However, the precise pathogenetic sequence of this phenomenon has not been determined. For the most part, the cholesterol, sphingolipids, and most of the fatty acids in the stratum corneum are synthesized locally by the epidermis. However, essential fatty acids, such as linoleic acids derive from dietary sources and reach the skin through systemic delivery. Elimination of these essential lipid components from the diet can cause scaling. Experimental fatty acid deficiency caused by elimination of linoleic acid from the diet causes abnormal barrier function, scaling, and alopecia. These are the consequences of alterations in the fatty composition of stratum corneum lipids, such as the substitution of oleic acid for linoleic acid in epidermal acylsphingolipids (see reviews in references 197 and 199).

X-linked ichthyosis caused by STS deficiency is an example of a human-inherited lipid abnormality resulting in a scaling disorder. Studies of the lipid content of skin scales from individuals with STS deficiency revealed a fivefold increase in cholesterol sulfate and a 50 percent decrease in free sterol content.[13] It has been shown that cholesterol sulfate inhibits cholesterol synthesis.[16] STS may, therefore, act as a regulator for epidermal sterologenesis. It is not clear whether scaling in STS deficiency is caused by an alteration of the ratio of cholesterol sulfate to cholesterol or by an overall reduction of free sterol content. Studies of the [^{3}H]thymidine labeling index in the epidermis of patients with STS deficiency gave normal results, suggesting that scaling is not due to hyperproliferation but to delayed desquamation.[202] However, in vitro studies using fluorescence-activated cell sorting combined with [^{3}H]thymidine labeling revealed a significant increase in the labeling of S-phase undifferentiated cells in cultures from patients with either X-linked or autosomal dominant ichthyosis, indicating the presence of hyperproliferation.[203] This was particularly evident in cultures in which regeneration was induced by stripping of the suprabasal cells from the multilayered culture. These in vitro data are in conflict with the in vivo data and might result from the lack of hyperkeratosis under in vitro conditions. Nevertheless, the in vitro system is an excellent model for studying keratinocyte differentiation.[203] Recent studies indicate that restoration of STS activity in cells from patients with STS deficiency after transfection with a recombinant *STS* gene causes an increase in the number of differentiated cells and, therefore, a shift toward a normal epidermal maturation pattern.[189] Freiberg et al. developed a model of corrective *STS* gene delivery in vivo. Primary keratinocytes from STS-deficient patients were transduced using a new retroviral expression vector containing the *STS* cDNA. Transduced XLI keratinocytes were then grafted onto immunodeficient mice and regeneration of a full thickness epidermis, histologically indistinguishable from that formed by normal keratinocytes, was achieved. Transduced XLI epidermis also showed a return of barrier function parameters to normal.[190] These experiments represent the first attempt to genetically correct an inherited defect of keratinocytes.

Ichthyosis is also found in other genetic disorders of lipid metabolism (Table 166-4).[204] Refsum syndrome, in which ichthyosis is a prominent feature, is the result of a defect in

Table 166-4 Genetic Disorders of Lipid Metabolism Producing Ichthyosis

Disorder (Chap.)	Enzyme Defect	Pathogenesis	Inheritance	Other Features
X-linked ichthyosis (166)	Steroid sulfatase deficiency	Elevated cholesterol sulfate in stratum corneum	X-linked recessive	See text
Refsum syndrome (132)	Phytanic acid oxidase deficiency	Accumulation of phytanic acid and phytanic acid–cholesteryl esters	Autosomal recessive	Retinitis pigmentosa, polyneuritis, ataxia, deafness
Sjögren-Larsson syndrome (98)	Fatty alcohol oxidoreductase deficiency	Accumulation of long-chain fatty alcohols	Autosomal recessive	Spasticity, mental retardation, short stature, brittle hair, hypoplasia of teeth, metaphyseal dysplasia
Neutral lipid storage disease*	Unknown	Triglyceride storage of unknown cause	Autosomal recessive	Cataracts, deafness, ataxia, droplets in many cells
Multiple sulfatase deficiency (149)†	Conversion of Cys to 2-amino-3-oxopropionic acid	STS deficiency (along with other sulfatase deficiencies)	Autosomal recessive	Neurodegeneration, hepatosplenomegaly, and skeletal disorders
Harlequin ichthyosis	Unknown	Increased cholesterol and triglycerides in stratum corneum	Uncertain	Ectropion, malformations, absent eyebrows and lashes, ? developmental delay

*MIM 275630. †MIM 242500.

phytanic acid oxidation with the accumulation of phytanic acid cholesterol esters.[204] Abnormal fatty alcohol metabolism has been reported in Sjögren-Larsson syndrome, in which ichthyosis also occurs,[205] and harlequin ichthyosis fetuses have been found to have various abnormalities of epidermal lipids.[206]

STS Deficiency in Patients with Contiguous Gene Syndromes

Following the demonstration that STS deficiency is a systemic disorder affecting all tissues and organs, several centers undertook a systematic search for phenotypic and biochemical abnormalities. In addition to the ichthyosis and corneal opacities already mentioned, several patients with STS deficiency have a complex phenotype characterized by the association of multiple monogenic X-linked disorders. These complex phenotypes are the hallmark of a contiguous gene syndrome[207] resulting from deletions or translocations involving the Xp22.3 region and spanning the *STS* gene (see Chap. 65).[90,208] Some of these chromosomal rearrangements are detectable by cytogenetic analysis, although an appreciable percentage of them are submicroscopic and can only be detected by molecular analysis.[90] Table 166-5 shows the full spectrum of clinical features of Xp22.3 contiguous gene syndromes. The single-gene phenotypes include short stature (SS), X-linked recessive chondrodysplasia punctata (CDPX), mental retardation (MRX), X-linked ichthyosis (XLI), Kallmann syndrome (KAL), and X-linked ocular albinism (OA1) (see review in reference 90 and Chap. 65).

Figure 166-9 shows the phenotype of a patient with X-linked ichthyosis and Kallmann syndrome, carrying a deletion of both genes. The recognition of a contiguous gene syndrome has important clinical implications. A patient with STS deficiency showing a complex phenotype should be carefully examined to rule out the presence of clinical manifestations of all the other diseases listed in Table 166-5. In addition, cytogenetic and molecular analysis will determine which of the Xp22.3 disease genes is involved in the deletion event. In some cases, this has helped predict the final outcome of the phenotype in young patients.[208]

In addition to the clinical implications, the study of individuals with Xp22.3 contiguous gene syndromes has been extremely valuable for the mapping of several disease loci and for the positional cloning of the Kallmann syndrome (Chap. 225), chondrodysplasia punctata and ocular albinism genes.[46,135,136,209] The consensus order of disease loci in this region is this: telomere-SS-CDPX-MRX-STS-KAL-OA1-centromere.

Table 166-5 Spectrum of Clinical Manifestations in Patients with Xp22.3 Contiguous Gene Syndromes Associated with STS Deficiency

Disease Entities	Main Features
Short stature (MIM312865)	Short stature
X-linked recessive chondrodysplasia punctata (MIM302950)	Nasal hypoplasia, focal calcification of cartilage, distal phalangeal hypoplasia
X-linked mental retardation (MIM309530)	Mental retardation, usually mild to moderate
X-linked ichthyosis (MIM308100)	Scaly skin
X-linked Kallmann syndrome (MIM308700)	Hypogonadotropic hypogonadism and anosmia
X-linked ocular albinism (MIM300500)	Impaired visual acuity, nystagmus, strabismus, photophobia

NOTE: Individuals with Xp22.3 deletions or translocations can have one or more of the above disease. Deletions may be invisible on cytogenetic analysis. Diseases are listed following a telomere-to-centromere order of the corresponding genetic loci.

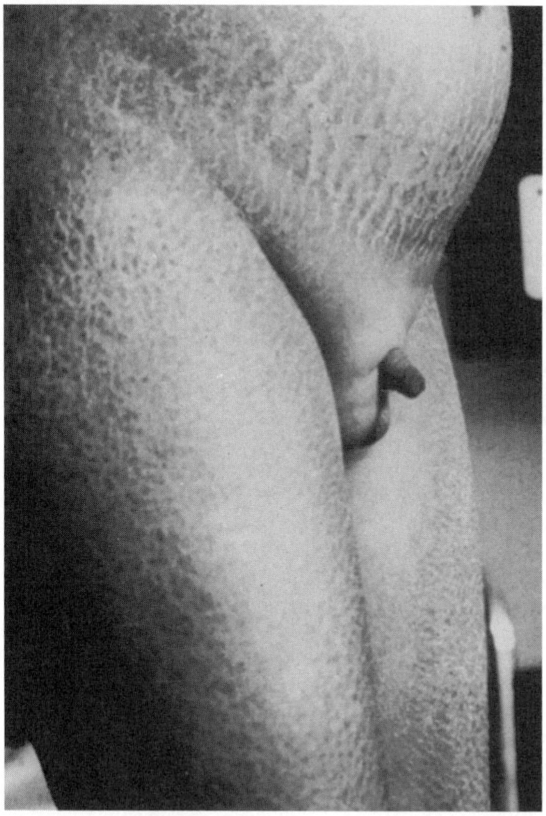

Fig. 166-9 A boy affected by X-linked ichthyosis associated with Kallmann syndrome. The presence of dark brown scales on the skin is a feature of X-linked ichthyosis due to STS deficiency. Micropenis and microtestes are features of Kallmann syndrome and are the result of hypogonadotropic hypogonadism due to gonadotropin releasing hormone deficiency. This patient was completely unable to smell.[237]

STS Deficiency and Androgen Metabolism

In addition to the above-mentioned association of STS deficiency with Kallmann syndrome, which is characterized by hypogonadotropic hypogonadism and inability to smell (anosmia), several gonadal abnormalities have been identified in some patients who appeared to have the common type of STS deficiency and X-linked ichthyosis. At least four such patients with testicular neoplasms have been seen, including one unfortunate man with an embryonal cell carcinoma and seminoma discovered five years apart.[210,211] What the precise relationship between these tumors and STS deficiency might be is unknown. In addition, Lykkesfeldt et al. observed testicular cancer in three patients with ichthyosis and normal STS activity.[211]

Traupe and Happle have called attention to the possible association of cryptorchidism and STS deficiency.[212] They observed unilateral or bilateral testicular maldescent in 7 of 25 patients examined and found a total of 30 cases of cryptorchidism with STS deficiency described in the literature. One other series of patients has also shown this association.[210] It may be hypothesized that abnormal STS function per se is responsible in some cases for hypogonadism and cryptorchidism. The relative importance of STS in testicular testosterone biosynthesis has not been definitively established; it could conceivably be implicated. It is possible that there is some degree of polymorphism in the flux through various potential steroidogenic pathways, and while testosterone biosynthesis appears to be normal in most STS-deficient patients studied, there may be a subset of patients in whom it is not, with consequent testicular abnormality. Alternatively, at different stages of ontogeny, the relative importance of various steroidogenic pathways may change.

There is probably no gross alteration of testosterone biosynthesis or secretion in STS deficiency.[41,42] Several groups have measured serum levels of testosterone, follicle stimulating hormone, and luteinizing hormone in adults with STS deficiency and have found these parameters to be normal. Furthermore, several subjects who received human chorionic gonadotropin (hCG) stimulation responded with abnormal augmentation of testosterone levels. DHEAS, 17-hydroxy-pregnenolone sulfate, and androstenediol sulfate are moderately increased in the circulation of STS-deficient individuals, and their corresponding free steroids are, on average, slightly reduced.[43] This suggests that STS has some physiological role in the desulfation of these steroids, but, quantitatively, the production of the free steroids must not be terribly dependent on sulfated intermediates. Conversely, there must be active systemic pathways capable of disposing of or metabolizing the sulfated compounds without the necessity for hydrolysis.

Although the quantitative importance of desulfation in the metabolism of DHEAS cannot be great, the question can be raised as to whether any desulfation of this major adrenal secretory product can be demonstrated in vivo. To clarify this issue, [^{3}H]DHEAS and [^{14}C]DHEA have been administered to a series of STS-deficient subjects and controls.[43] The conversion of [^{14}C]DHEA to either DHEAS or DHEA glucuronide occurred normally in STS-deficient patients, indicating no impairment of conjugation. Furthermore, the plasma half-life of [^{3}H]DHEAS infused into STS-deficient patients was essentially normal. However, when the conversion of DHEAS to DHEA glucuronide was examined, an unexpected result was obtained. A significant amount of labeled DHEAS was converted to the glucuronide in two of three STS-deficient individuals. Presumably, the exchange of sulfate for glucuronide at the 3β-hydroxy position requires desulfation to the free intermediate and reconjugation, although it is possible that a "transconjugase" activity might exist, which could carry out this exchange without hydrolysis.

Milone et al. used gas chromatography to measure the serum levels of CS and DHEAS in normal individuals and in 15 patients with STS deficiency.[194] A significant increase of both CS and DHEAS was observed in all the individuals with STS deficiency ($p < 0.001$). They pointed out that inconsistencies of DHEAS levels described in previous studies could be due to the much greater spread of the values obtained by radioimmunoassay compared to gas chromatography, the latter being a much more reliable method for measuring DHEAS.[194] The observation that some STS-deficient subjects can apparently hydrolyze some DHEAS in vivo can be explained by the presence of some cryptic STS activity situated in an anatomic site not previously anticipated. Because most patients with STS deficiency have gene deletions, it is unlikely that there are tissue differences in the expression of the authentic STS gene product. However, it is possible that there are separately encoded enzymes capable of hydrolyzing DHEAS that are expressed in a tissue-specific fashion. There is no evidence to support a second *STS* gene or enzyme, but a detailed autopsy survey of STS activity in organs and tissues of STS-deficient subjects has not been undertaken.

The Molecular Basis of STS Deficiency

The large majority of patients with STS deficiency do not have microscopically detectable cytogenetic abnormalities. Typically, these patients are affected by the "classical" type of STS deficiency, which is characterized exclusively by the X-linked ichthyosis phenotype. The cloning of human *STS* cDNAs and the characterization of the *STS* gene provide the basis for elucidating the molecular defects in these individuals.

Hundreds of independently ascertained patients with classical STS deficiency have been tested by Southern blotting analysis using both partial and full-length *STS* cDNA probes and various DNA markers flanking the gene.[56,58,78–80,213–215] The large majority (85 to 90 percent) of these subjects, regardless of their ethnic origin, have submicroscopic deletions detectable by either

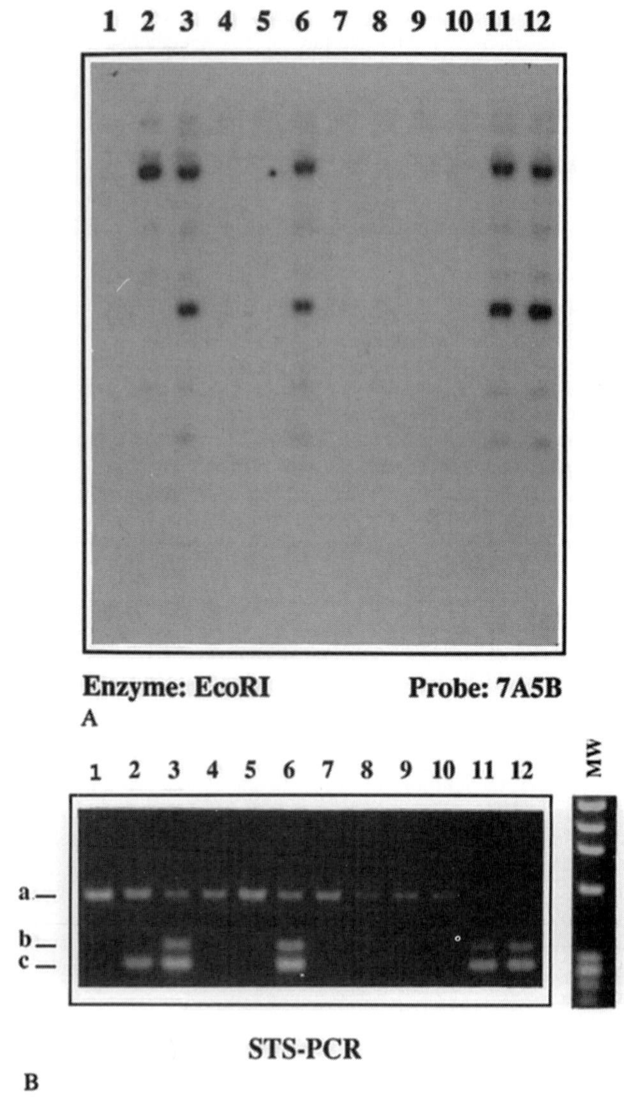

Primer set	Sequence	Amplified
(1) 5′STS gene	F-5′GGCCTAGAAGAAGGTTGAAGGTCCC R-5′AAGAGGTTGGATGAGATGGGCATAC	292 bp
(2) 3′STS gene	F-5′GAAATCCTCAAAGTCATGCAGGAAG R-5′CCTCCAGTTGAGTAGCTGTTGAGCT	363 bp

C

Fig. 166-10 DNA analysis on patients with STS deficiency. Panel A: Southern analysis of *Eco*RI-digested DNA samples from 11 patients (lanes 1 to 11) and one male control (lane 12) using an *STS* full-length cDNA clone. Panel B: Multiplex DNA amplification of the *STS* gene (STS-PCR) in 11 patients with STS deficiency (lanes 1 to 11, loaded in the same order as in A) and one male control (lane 12). Band a corresponds to an exon of the *DMD* gene and was used as an internal control for the amplification. Bands b and c correspond to the 3′ and the 5′ ends of the *STS* gene, respectively. MW = molecular weight marker. Panel C: Sequence of oligonucleotide primers for PCR amplifications of STS. F = forward primer; R = reverse primer. (*From Ballabio et al.*[216] *Used by permission of Human Genetics.*)

Southern blotting or polymerase chain reaction (PCR) analysis.[58,214] Figure 166-10 shows the results of Southern blot analysis and of a multiplex PCR test for the detection of *STS* gene deletions.[216] Most of these deletions span the entire 146-kb *STS* gene and flanking sequences on Xp22.3 and are also detectable by flow cytometry.[217] Two patients have been identified with partial deletions of the gene.[58,214] In the first case, the deletion starts within intron 7 of the gene and extends over 150 kb downstream toward the centromere, spanning the last three exons of the gene (Fig. 166-10).[214] The other patient has an intragenic deletion of about 40 kb including exons II-V. This subject's cells made reduced amounts of shortened RNA transcripts.[58]

A minority of patients with STS deficiency (10 to 15 percent) do not show any abnormality with Southern blotting analysis using the full-length *STS* cDNA probe. In seven of these patients, point mutations in the coding region of the *STS* gene were identified. These were a nonsense mutation at nucleotide 1236; a change of a serine to a leucine at codon 1243 (S1243L); a change of a tryptophan to an arginine at codon 1335 (W1335R), which changes a hydrophobic to a basic hydrophilic amino acid; a change of a tryptophan to a proline at codon 1336 (W1336P); a splice site mutation at nucleotide 1477; a change of a histidine to an arginine at codon 1552 (H1552R); and a change of a cysteine to a tyrosine at codon 1558 (C1558Y), which potentially prevents a disulfide bond.[185,187,188] These mutations may allow insights into functionally important domains of the protein. All of these mutations resulted in lack of a functionally active STS polypeptide when expressed in COS7 cells. The mutations also appeared to affect mRNA stability.

All patients with STS deficiency tested so far, including both deletion and "nondeletion" cases, display absence of cross-reacting material by Western blot analysis using anti-STS polyclonal antibodies on patients' fibroblast extracts.[72,214,218] Finally, one patient with alleged partial deficiency of STS activity has been reported.[53]

With the possible exception of the α-thalassemias (Chap. 181) and del(22)(q11.2q11.2) causing DiGeorge/velocardiofacial syndrome (Chap. 65), gene deletions in STS deficiency represent the highest frequency of deletion among mutations reported at a single Mendelian disease locus. In the case of the α-thalassemias, it is likely that the original mutations occurred relatively rarely but were expanded in frequency in certain populations by selection. STS deficiency is a common and equally frequent disorder in many racial and ethnic groups and geographic areas. Furthermore, no obvious selective advantage for homozygosity or heterozygosity has been suggested. Thus, it is tempting to speculate that the lesions involving the *STS* locus are fairly frequent de novo events. Most patients with STS deficiency carry deletions of approximately 2 Mb of DNA. It is remarkable that nullisomy of such large regions of the human genome in male individuals is viable and results in such a relatively mild clinical condition as X-linked ichthyosis. In addition to the *STS* gene, these deletions involve at least one other gene, *GS1*, whose function is still unknown.[137]

Two families of low-copy-number repeats, the G1.3 and the CRI-S232 families, have been found to be interspersed in the Xp22.3 region and clustered on either side of the *STS* gene.[219–221] This suggested that the frequent occurrence of interstitial deletions in this region was due, at least in some patients, to abnormal pairing and homologous recombination between different repeat units.[220,222] This hypothesis was strongly supported by the finding of CRI-S232 repeat units at the deletion breakpoints of most patients with STS deficiency.[222] It is difficult to establish whether these unequal recombination events occur during meiotic or mitotic cell divisions of primordial germ cells, or whether they involve recombination between two discrete chromosomes, between sister chromatids, or between CRI-S232-like sequences on the same chromatid. Sequence analysis of several of these repeat units revealed the presence of two elements containing a variable number of tandem repeats (VNTR) in each of the units.[223] CRI-S232 repeats are also present on the long arm of the human Y chromosome (Yq11.2). The main difference between the X-linked and the Y-linked CRI-S232 repeats is the great variation in the number of elements of the X-linked units versus the constant nature of the Y-linked ones. Furthermore, the Y-linked units appeared to have a much higher intrarepeat sequence variation.

Although most *STS* gene deletions appear to be due to unequal recombination between CRI-S232 repeats, there is evidence that this mechanism does not apply to all STS deletions. Physical mapping studies indicate that at least in some cases the deletion breakpoints are not located near CRI-S232 repeat units. In two of these cases the deletion breakpoint was cloned and sequenced. A 3-bp homology was found at the site of the deletion junction in one case,[224] while no repeat sequences were identified in the second case (P. Yen and A. Ballabio, unpublished data).

Some patients with STS deficiency have detectable cytogenetic abnormalities, which include large terminal deletions and X/Y translocations resulting in loss of the terminal Xp region. As mentioned previously, Xp22.3 rearrangements may result in contiguous gene syndromes in male individuals. Female individuals carrying these rearrangements have terminal Xp monosomy and typically do not have any of the recessive diseases described in affected males because they have a normal X chromosome. However, almost invariably they have short stature. This observation is consistent with the putative presence of a gene affecting height in the pseudoautosomal region, two active copies of which are needed for normal growth.[208,225,226] It has been proposed that this gene is the homeobox-containing gene, which maps to this region.[133,134]

Many patients with X/Y translocations involving breaks in Xp22.3 have been described (see reviews in references 90 and 227). These translocations can be divided into two major groups: Xp/Yq and Xp/Yp translocations. Xp/Yq translocations are the most common type of X/Y translocation, and some multigenerational families segregating this chromosomal abnormality have been reported. These translocations can be recognized cytogenetically because of the presence of the highly fluorescent Y heterochromatic region (Yq11.2-qter) located at the distal Xp region. Male subjects carrying these rearrangements have no normal X chromosome, but do have an additional intact Y chromosome.

In some Xp/Yq translocations, abnormal pairing and exchange within a 1 to 1.5 Mb region of close sequence identity shared by Xp22.3 and Yq11.2 takes place. The result is a translocation of Yq11.2-qter to distal Xp with the concomitant production of a terminal Xp22.3-pter deletion. Sequence analysis of the X/Y junction fragment from two of these translocations suggests the occurrence of abnormal pairing and homologous recombination between Xp and Yq homologous regions.[228,229] This distinctive mechanism may play an important role in most Xp/Yq translocations, although other mechanisms, such as nonhomologous recombination, may also be involved.

Xp/Yp translocations usually involve the testis-determining factor (*TDF*) on Yp and are found in sex-reversed individuals (XX males). These are probably the result of unequal exchanges within and outside the pairing region of the human sex chromosomes.[230] Usually these translocations are not visible by cytogenetic analysis and can therefore only be detected using molecular probes. The breakpoint on the X chromosome in most individuals carrying this type of X/Y translocation is distal to the *STS* gene, leaving two intact copies of the *STS* gene, one on the normal and one on the derivative X chromosome. However, in rare cases, the X breakpoint may lie proximal to *STS* with a consequent loss of the *STS* gene from the derivative X chromosome.[231–233]

Terminal deletions involving the *STS* gene can be detected by both cytogenetic and molecular analysis (see review in reference 90). The name terminal deletion may not be used in a strict sense in these cases, because the deleted Xp arm presumably retains a functional telomere, which may or may not correspond to the normal Xp telomere. However, chromosomes in which Xp subtelomeric markers are deleted are usually referred to as "terminal deletions." The position of the breakpoints in the various patients with terminal deletions, and consequently the sizes of the deleted regions, are highly variable. The molecular mechanisms underlying these types of Xp rearrangements are unknown.

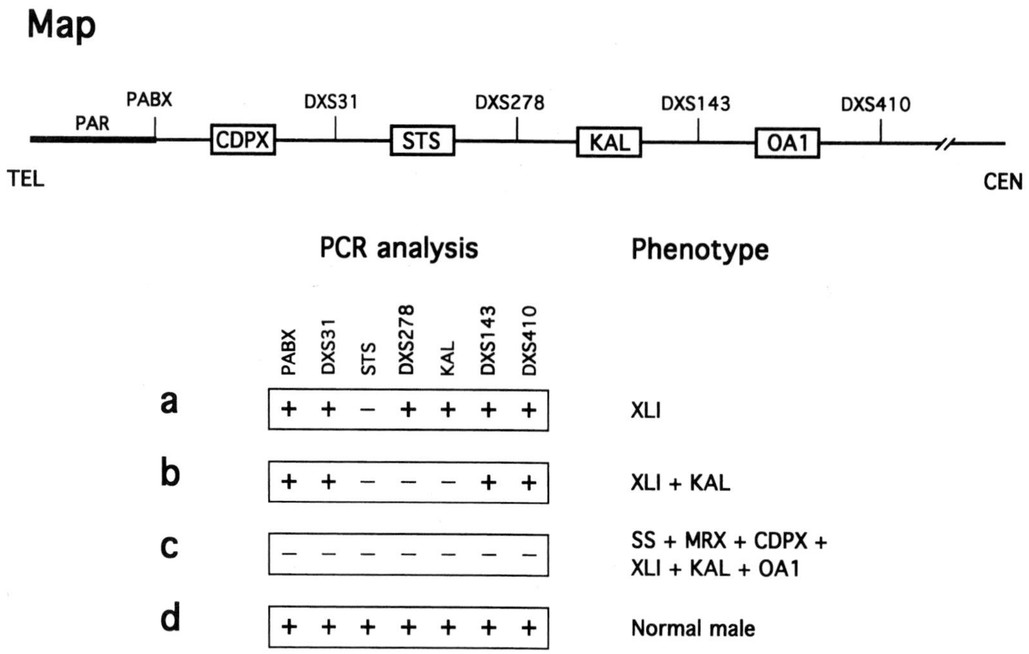

Fig. 166-11 PCR test for Xp22.3 CGS. The order of some of the disease genes and DNA markers in the Xp22.3 region is shown at the top. PAR = pseudoautosomal region; PABX = pseudoautosomal boundary on the X chromosome. A seven loci-PCR test has been designed for the detection and partial characterization of Xp22.3 CGS. *a*, Pattern observed in most males with isolated X-linked ichthyosis; *b*, pattern observed in most males with X-linked ichthyosis associated with Kallmann syndrome; *c*, pattern observed in males with very complex phenotypes, including features of all Xp22.3 diseases; and *d*, normal male pattern.

The study of patients with chromosomal rearrangements in the Xp22.3 region has been essential for the construction of deletion maps of the region.[91] This has made possible the ordering of several DNA markers and of the six disease loci mentioned previously. It could be anticipated that other genes in the region will be isolated as the map becomes more refined. The large number of patients with complex phenotypes due to various types of chromosomal rearrangements makes the distal short arm of the human X chromosome a very attractive region for positional cloning of disease genes. A close interaction between the clinician, the cytogeneticist, and the molecular biologist is essential in these efforts. The successful cloning of disease genes will then be of great help for the understanding of the molecular mechanisms involved in the disease pathogenesis and would possibly provide new diagnostic and therapeutic tools. Figure 166-11 shows a PCR-based diagnostic test for Xp22.3 contiguous gene syndromes.

Incidence, Clinical Diagnosis, Carrier Identification, and Prenatal Diagnosis

STS deficiency a common inborn error of metabolism. It has been described in all racial backgrounds and in a diversity of ethnic populations. Frequency estimates reported by Wells and Kerr, who identified patients on the basis of X-linked ichthyosis, were about 1 in 6000 males.[176] There may have been some biases in these families and others because of the use of ichthyosis as the discriminant, which could lead to underreporting. First, in cases where no extensive pedigree information is available to support a diagnosis of an X-linked disorder, dermatologists who are consulted might be less inclined to consider this diagnostic possibility. Second, because of the non-life–threatening nature of the condition, its variation in severity, seasonal fluctuations, and the lack of responsiveness (until recently) to therapy, many affected individuals have probably not sought medical care. Lykkesfeldt et al. have suggested that when patients are identified through maternal estriol screening, the incidence may be as high as 1 in 2000 males in Western Europe.[234] This seems to apply also to the U.S. population, because an increased ascertainment has been observed as a result of the antenatal triple marker (including estriol) screening test. The true population incidence needs to be determined through suitable large-scale prospective studies. Similarly, the relative homogeneity or heterogeneity of mutations at this locus requires prospective assessment by molecular studies to determine whether mutations have arisen on a common haplotype background and whether deletion end points are unique or recurrent. No studies have been performed on the origin of new mutations in families with STS deficiency because sporadic cases of STS deficiency are extremely rare.

Confirmation of a suspected diagnosis is now relatively straightforward. Affected males can have STS activity assayed using one of a variety of substrates in fibroblasts, leukocytes, hair follicles, etc. Because 85 to 90 percent of patients have sub-microscopic gene deletions, DNA testing is a rapid and effective way to establish a diagnosis in many instances, although STS deficiency obviously cannot be excluded on the basis of a normal result. Simple PCR tests are available for isolated STS deficiency (Fig. 166-10) and for patients with contiguous gene syndromes involving STS (Fig. 166-11).[216] Molecular detection of *STS* gene deletions can also be performed by fluorescence in situ hybridization (FISH) on metaphase spreads using genomic clones (usually cosmids) from within the *STS* gene as probes.[235] This method is particularly useful for the detection of female heterozygotes. A frequent *Xmn*I RFLP has also been identified in the *STS* gene and can be used for family studies.[236]

Assessment of substrate levels may also be of use because elevated plasma CS levels do appear to be diagnostic for STS deficiency.[192–195] The finding of abnormal lipoprotein electrophoresis caused by incorporation of CS into LDL is also of great value because of the wide availability of this test in clinical laboratories.[193,196] Heterozygote identification is somewhat more problematic. While it is clear that there is normally a gene dosage effect on STS enzyme activity between subjects bearing one X-encoded copy of STS (XY, XO, or XX heterozygotes for *STS* mutations) and those with two copies (XX), there is considerable overlap between these two groups. This is largely the result of poorly understood variations in enzyme activity measurements. Thus, it may be difficult to be absolutely certain about heterozygote status in any single individual. FISH is clearly the best method for carrier identification if a deletion has been identified in the proband.[235]

As with postnatal diagnosis, many methods are potentially applicable to the prenatal diagnosis of STS deficiency. Syncytiotrophoblast tissue is normally very rich in STS activity, and this is particularly true in the first trimester, when STS specific activity is highest. Thus, chorionic villus biopsy can be performed for early prenatal assessment. Again, when a deletion has been identified in the proband, PCR testing and/or FISH can be performed. Midtrimester diagnosis is also readily made by careful assessment of serum estriol levels (using gestational-age–appropriate standards) and by measurement of amniotic fluid DHEAS concentrations. Cultured amniocytes normally express STS and can be used for either DNA or enzymatic analysis. Finally, in the third trimester, maternal urinary estriol and sulfated steroid excretion can be monitored in addition to the other studies already described. The purpose of establishing a third-trimester diagnosis of STS deficiency might be to exclude a more serious cause of incidentally detected low estriol levels. In addition, it might be argued that such diagnostic information would be of use in obstetrical management, so that prolonged labor might be anticipated and suitable intervention planned if needed.

Once a diagnosis of STS deficiency is made, a critical issue, particularly in prenatal and early postnatal diagnosis, is to rule out the presence of a contiguous gene syndrome, because this has very important clinical implications. A contiguous gene syndrome can be detected by both cytogenetic and molecular analysis using *STS* and flanking markers as probes (see Chap. 65). In the absence of a contiguous gene syndrome, the rationale for prenatal diagnosis in simple, uncomplicated STS deficiency (X-linked ichthyosis) should be carefully considered with at-risk families from a medical and ethical standpoint. The overall severity and impact on quality of life is usually minimal and can now be quite effectively managed. It is therefore important to be sure that parents have an adequate understanding of the nature of this dermatologic disorder before proceeding with prenatal studies. In addition, experimental models for corrective *STS* gene transfer into patients' keratinocytes have been developed (see above).[189,190]

Treatment

Treatment of X-linked ichthyosis is now quite satisfactory. Lac-Hydrin (12 percent ammonium lactate) is a well-tolerated and effective keratolytic agent that gives good cosmetic results if applied once or twice daily. Older preparations seemed to be associated with unacceptable stinging and itching. Use of *cis*-retinoic acid is probably contraindicated, although it is useful in the treatment of some other forms of ichthyosis. The risks of teratogenesis are not of direct concern in the male patients under treatment, although reports of hypertriglyceridemia are of note. Furthermore, patients with X-linked ichthyosis seem not to respond to this treatment and may even become worse. In any event, the simple application of a topical keratolytic agent is quite effective and without apparent side effects. The only other point worthy of mention is the possible increased risk of testicular neoplasms in STS-deficient patients. Although the data supporting this association are not compelling at present, it may be appropriate to instruct patients in testicular self-examination and to employ other efforts at prospective diagnosis without unduly alarming these subjects. Because the general health of STS-deficient patients is otherwise good, no other specific management is indicated.

ACKNOWLEDGMENTS

We thank Germana Meroni for helpful discussion and Melissa Smith for help with the manuscript preparation.

REFERENCES

1. France JT, Liggins GC: Placental sulfatase deficiency. *J Clin Endocrinol Metab* **29**:138, 1969.
2. Roberts DR, Lieberman S: The biochemistry of the 3β-hydroxy- Æ5-steroid sulfates, in Bernstein S, Solomon S (eds): *Chemical and Biological Aspects of Steroid Conjugation.* New York, Springer-Verlag, 1970, p 219.
3. Schachter B, Marrian GF: The isolation of estrone sulfate from the urine of pregnant mares. *J Biol Chem* **126**:663, 1938.
4. Venning EH, Hoffman MM, Browne JSL: Isolation of androsterone sulfate. *J Biol Chem* **146**:369, 1942.
5. Munson PL, Gallagher TF, Kock FC: Isolation of dehydroisoandrosterone sulfate from normal male urine. *J Biol Chem* **152**:67, 1944.
6. Roy AB: Enzymological aspects of steroid conjugation, in Bernstein S, Solomon S (eds): *Chemical and Biological Aspects of Steroid Conjugation.* New York, Springer-Verlag, 1970, p 74.
7. Roberts KD, Bandi L, Calvin HI, Drucker WD, Lieberman S: Evidence that steroid sulfates serve as biosynthetic intermediates. IV. Conversion of cholesterol sulfate in vivo to urinary C19 and C21 steroidal sulfates. *Biochemistry* **3**:1983, 1964.
8. Payne AH, Lawrence CC, Foster DL, Jaffee RB: Intranuclear binding of 17-estradiol and estrone in female ovine pituitaries following incubation with estrone sulfate. *J Biol Chem* **248**:1598, 1973.
9. Vignon F, Terqui M, Westley B, Derocq D, Rochefort H: Effects of plasma estrogen sulfates in mammary cancer cells. *Endocrinology* **106**:1079, 1980.
10. Drayer NM, Lieberman S: Isolation of cholesterol sulfate from human blood and gallstones. *Biochem Biophys Res Commun* **18**:126, 1965.
11. Drayer NM, Lieberman S: Isolation of cholesterol sulfate from human aortas and adrenal tumors. *J Clin Endocrinol Metab* **27**:136, 1967.
12. Moser HW, Moser AB, Orr JC: Preliminary observations on the occurrence of cholesterol sulfate in man. *Biochim Biophys Acta* **116**:146, 1966.
13. Williams ML, Elias PM: Stratum corneum lipids in disorders of cornification. I. Increased cholesterol sulfate content of stratum corneum in recessive X-linked ichthyosis. *J Clin Invest* **68**:1404, 1981.
14. Elias PM, Williams ML, Maloney MB, Bonifas JA, Brown BE, Grayson S, Epstein EH: Stratum corneum lipids in disorders of cornification. II. Steroid sulfatase and cholesterol sulfate in normal desquamation and the pathogenesis of recessive of X-linked ichthyosis epidermis. *J Clin Invest* **74**:1414, 1984.
15. Williams ML, Wiley M, Elias PM: Inhibition of 3-hydroxymethylglutaryl coenzyme A reductase activity and sterol synthesis by cholesterol sulfate in cultured fibroblasts. *Biochim Biophys Acta* **845**:349, 1985.
16. Williams ML, Rutherford SA, Feingold KR: Effects of cholesterol sulfate on lipid metabolism in cultured human keratinocytes and fibroblasts. *J Lipid Res* **28**:955, 1987.
17. Korth-Schultz S, Levine LS, New I, Chow DM: Dehydroepiandrosterone sulfate (DS) levels, a rapid test for abnormal adrenal androgen secretion. *J Clin Endocrinol Metab* **42**:1005, 1976.
18. Riiter EO, Fuldauer VG, Root AW: Secretion of the adrenal androgen, dehydroepiandrosterone sulfate during normal infancy, childhood, and adolescence, in sick infants, and in children with endocrinologic abnormalities. *J Pediatr* **90**:766, 1977.
19. Peretti E, Forest MG: Patterns of plasma dehydroepiandrosterone sulfate levels in humans from birth to adulthood: Evidence for testicular production. *J Clin Endocrinol Metab* **47**:572, 1978.
20. Frandsen VA, Stakeman G: The site of production of oestrogenic hormones in human pregnancy. Hormone excretion in pregnancy with anencephalic fetus. *Acta Endocrinol* **38**:383, 1961.
21. Frandsen VA, Stakeman G: The site of production of oestrogenic hormones in human pregnancy. II. Experimental investigations on the role of the fetal adrenal. *Acta Endocrinol* **43**:184, 1963.
22. Siiteri PK, MacDonald PC: Placental estrogen biosynthesis during human pregnancy. *J Clin Endocrinol Metab* **26**:751, 1966.
23. Siiteri PK, MacDonald PC: The utilization of circulating dehydroisoandrosterone sulfate for estrogen synthesis during human pregnancy. *Steroids* **2**:713, 1963.
24. Warren JC, Timberlake CE: Steroid sulfatase in the human placenta. *J Clin Endocrinol Metab* **22**:1148, 1962.
25. Warren JC, Timberlake CE: Biosynthesis of estrogens in pregnancy: Precursor role of plasma dehydroisoandrosterone. *Obstet Gynecol* **23**:689, 1964.
26. Ryan KJ: Biological aromatization of steroids. *J Biol Chem* **234**:268, 1959.

27. Salido EC, Yen PH, Barajas L, Shapiro LJ: Steroid sulfatase expression in human placenta: Immunocytochemistry and in situ hybridization study. *J Clin Endocrinol Metab* **70**:1564, 1990.
28. Rosenfeld RS, Hellman L, Gallagher TF: Metabolism and interconversion of dehydroisoandrosterone and dehydroisoandrosterone sulfate. *J Clin Endocrinol Metab* **35**:187, 1972.
29. MacDonald PC, Chapdelaine A, Gonzalez O, Gurpide E, Van DeWiele RL, Lieberman S: Studies on the secretion and interconversion of the androgens. III. Results obtained after the injection of several radioactive C19 steroids, singly or as mixtures. *J Clin Endocrinol* **25**:1557, 1965.
30. Chapdelaine A, MacDonald PC, Gonzalez O, Gurpide E, Van De Wiele RL, Lieberman S: Studies on the secretion and interconversion of the androgens. IV. Quantitative results in a normal man whose gonadal and adrenal function were altered experimentally. *J Clin Endocrinol* **25**:1569, 1965.
31. Horton R, Tait JF: In vivo conversion of dehydroisoandrosterone to plasma androstenedione and testosterone in man. *J Clin Endocrinol* **27**:79, 1967.
32. Domínguez OV, Valencia SA, Loza AC: On the role of steroid sulfates in hormone biosynthesis. *J Steroid Biochem* **6**:301, 1975.
33. Huhtaniemi I: Studies on steroidogenesis and its regulation in human fetal adrenal and testis. *J Steroid Biochem* **8**:491, 1977.
34. Notation AD: Regulatory interactions for the control of steroid sulfate metabolism. *J Steroid Biochem* **6**:311, 1975.
35. Payne AH: Testicular steroid sulfotransferases: Comparison to liver and adrenal steroid sulfotransferases of the mature rat. *Endocrinology* **106**:1365, 1980.
36. Siiteri PK, Wilson JD: Testosterone formation and metabolism during male sexual differentiation in the human embryo. *J Clin Endocrinol Metab* **38**:113, 1974.
37. Vihko R, Ruokonen A: Regulation of steroidogenesis in testis. *J Steroid Biochem* **5**:843, 1974.
38. Vihko R, Ruokonen A: Steroid sulphates in human adult testicular steroid synthesis. *J Steroid Biochem* **6**:353, 1975.
39. Ruokonen A, Lukkarinen O, Vihko R: Secretion of steroid sulfates from human testis and their response to a single intramuscular injection of 5000 IU hCG. *J Steroid Biochem* **14**:1357, 1981.
40. Ruokonen A, Vihko R: Quantitative changes of endogenous unconjugated and sulfated steroids in human testis in relation to synthesis of testosterone in vitro. *J Androl* **4**:104, 1983.
41. Ruokonen A, Oikarinen A, Vihko R: Regulation of serum testosterone in men with steroid sulfatase deficiency: Response to human chorionic gonadotropin. *J Steroid Biochem* **25**:113, 1986.
42. Lykkesfeldt G, Bennet P, Lykkesfeldt AE, Nicic S, Muller S, Svenstrup B: Abnormal androgen and oestrogen metabolism in men with steroid sulfatase deficiency and recessive X-linked ichthyosis. *Clin Endocrinol* **23**:385, 1985.
43. Bergner EA, Shapiro LJ: Metabolism of ^{3}H-Dehydroepiandrosterone sulphate by subjects with steroid sulphatase deficiency. *J Inherit Metab Dis* **11**:403, 1988.
44. Rose FA: The mammalian sulphatases and placental sulfatase deficiency in man. *J Inherit Metab Dis* **5**:145, 1982.
45. Iwamori M, Moser HW, Kishimoto Y: Solubilization and partial purification of steroid sulfatase from rat liver: Characterization of estrone sulfatase. *Arch Biochem Biophys* **174**:199, 1976.
46. Franco B, Meroni G, Parenti G, Levilliers J, Bernard L, Gebbia M, Cox L, Maroteaux P, Sheffield L, Rappold GA, Andria G, Petit C, Ballabio A: A cluster of sulfatase genes on Xp22.3: Mutations in chondrodysplasia punctata (CDPX) and implications for Warfarin embryopathy. *Cell* **81**:15, 1995.
47. Puca A, Zollo M, Repetto M, Andolfi G, Guffanti A, Simon G, Ballabio A, Franco B: Identification by shotgun sequencing, genomic organization, and functional analysis of a fourth arylsulphatase gene (ARSF) from the Xp22.3 region. *Genomics* **42**:192, 1997.
48. Dibbelt L, Kuss E: Human placental sterylsulfatase: Interaction of the isolated enzyme with substrates, products, transition-state analogues, amino-acid modifiers and anion transport inhibitors. *Biol Chem Hoppe-Seyler* **372**:173, 1991.
49. Gauthier R, Vigneault N, Bleau G, Chapdelaine A, Roberts KD: Solubilization and partial purification of steroid sulfatase of human placenta. *Steroids* **31**:783, 1978.
50. Zuckerman NA, Hagerman DD: The hydrolysis of estrone sulfate by rat kidney microsomal sulfatase. *Arch Biochem Biophys* **135**:410, 1969.
51. French AP, Warren JC: Properties of steroid sulphatase and arylsulphatase activities of human placenta. *Biochem J* **105**:233, 1967.
52. Bleau G, Chapdelaine A, Roberts KD: Studies on mammalian and molluscan steroid sulfatase. Solubilization and properties. *Can J Biochem* **49**:234, 1971.
53. Hameister H, Wolff G, Lauritzen CH, Lehmann WO, Hauser A, Ropers HH: Clinical and biochemical investigations on patients with partial deficiency of placental steroid sulfatase. *Hum Genet* **46**:199, 1979.
54. Craig IW, Tolley E: Steroid sulphatase and the conservation of mammalian X chromosomes. *Trends Genet* **2**:201, 1986.
55. Kawano J-I, Kotani T, Ohtaki S, Minamino N, Matsuo H, Oinuma T, Aikawa E: Characterization of rat and human steroid sulfatases. *Biochim Biophys Acta* **997**:199, 1989.
56. Yen PH, Allen E, Marsh B, Mohandas T, Wang N, Taggart RT, Shapiro LJ: Cloning and expression of steroid sulfatase cDNA and the frequent occurrence of deletions in STS deficiency: Implication for X-Y interchange. *Cell* **49**:443, 1987.
57. Shankaran R, Ameen M, Daniel WL, Davidson RG, Chang PL: Characterization of arylsulfatase C isozymes from human liver and placenta. *Biochim Biophys Acta* **1078**:251, 1991.
58. Shapiro LJ, Yen P, Pomerantz D, Martin E, Rolewic L, Mohandas T: Molecular studies of deletions at the human steroid sulfatase locus. *Proc Natl Acad Sci U S A* **86**:8477, 1989.
59. Epstein EH, Allen A, Shackleton HL: Failure of steroid sulfatase to desulfate vitamin D3 sulfate. *J Invest Dermatol* **80**:514, 1983.
60. Vaccaro AM, Salvioli R, Muscillo M, Renola L: Purification and properties of arylsulfatase C from human placenta. *Enzyme* **37**:115, 1987.
61. Chang PL, Varey PA, Rosa NE, Ameen M, Davidson RG: Association of steroid sulfatase with one of the arylsulfatase C isozymes in human fibroblasts. *J Biol Chem* **261**:14443, 1986.
62. Chang PL, Mueller OT, Lafrenie RM, Varey PA, Rosa NE, Davidson RG, Henry WM, Shows TB: The human arylsulfatase-C isoenzymes: Two distinct genes that escape from X inactivation. *Am J Hum Genet* **46**:729, 1990.
63. Munroe DG, Chang PL: Tissue-specific expression of human arylsulfatase-C isozymes and steroid sulfatase. *Am J Hum Genet* **40**:102, 1987.
64. Daniel WL, Chang PL: Comparison of arylsulfatase C and steroid sulfatase from human placenta and liver. *Enzyme* **43**:212, 1990.
65. Mathew J, Balasubramanian AS: Arylsulphatase C and estrone sulphatase of sheep hypothalamus, preoptic area, and midbrain: Separation by hydrophobic interaction chromatography and evidence for differences in their lipid environment. *J Neurochem* **39**:1205, 1982.
66. Nelson K, Keinanen BM, Daniel WL: Murine arylsulfatase C: Evidence for two isozymes. *Experientia* **39**:740, 1983.
67. Keinanen BM, Nelson K, Daniel WL, Roque JM: Genetic analysis of murine arylsulfatase C and steroid sulfatase. *Genetics* **105**:191, 1983.
68. Ruoff BM, Daniel WL: Comparative biochemistry of mammalian arylsulfatase C and steroid sulfatase. *Comp Biochem Physiol* **98B**:313, 1991.
69. Willemsen R, Kroos M, Hoogeveen AT, van Dongen JM, Parenti G, van der Loos CM, Reuser AJJ: Ultrastructural localization of steroid sulphatase in cultured human fibroblasts by immunocytochemistry: A comparative study with lysosomal enzymes and the mannose 6-phosphate receptor. *Histochem J* **20**:41, 1988.
70. Stein C, Hille A, Seidel J, Rijnbout S, Waheed A, Schmidt B, Geuze H, von Figura K: Cloning and expression of human steroid-sulfatase. *Bio Chem* **264**:13865, 1989.
71. Noel H, Beauregard G, Potier M, Bleau G, Chapedelaine A, Roberts KD: The target sizes of the in situ and solubilized forms of human placental steroid sulfatase as measured by radiation inactivation. *Biochim Biophys Acta* **758**:88, 1983.
72. Epstein EH, Bonifas JM: Recessive X-linked ichthyosis: Lack of immunologically detectable steroid sulfatase enzyme protein. *Hum Genet* **71**:201, 1985.
73. van der Loos CM, van Breda AJ, van den Berg FM, Walboomers JMM, Jöbsis AC: Human placental steroid sulphatase—Purification and monospecific antibody production in rabbits. *J Inherit Metab Dis* **7**:97, 1984.
74. Burns GRJ: Purification and partial characterization of arylsulphatase C from human placental microsomes. *Biochim Biophys Acta* **759**:199, 1983.
75. Conary J, Nauerth A, Burns G, Hasilik A, von Figura K: Steroid sulfatase. Biosynthesis and processing in normal and mutant fibroblasts. *Eur J Biochem* **158**:71, 1986.
76. McNaught RW, France JT: Studies of the biochemical basis of steroid sulphatase deficiency: Preliminary evidence suggesting a defect in membrane-enzyme structure. *J Steroid Biochem* **13**:363, 1980.

77. Horwitz AL, Warshawsky L, King J, Burns G: Rapid degradation of steroid sulfatase in multiple sulfatase deficiency. *Biochem Biophys Res Commun* **135**:389, 1986.
78. Ballabio A, Parenti G, Carrozzo R, Sebastio G, Andria G, Buckle V, Fraser N, Craig I, Rocchi M, Romeo G, Jobsis AC, Persico MG: Isolation and characterization of a steroid sulphatase cDNA clone: Genomic deletions in patients with X-chromosome-linked ichthyosis. *ProcNat Acad Sci U S A* **84**:4519, 1987.
79. Conary J, Lorkowski G, Schmidt B, Pohlmann R, Nagel G, Meyer HE, Krentler C, Cully J, Hasilik A, von Figura K: Genetic heterogeneity of steroid sulfatase deficiency revealed with cDNA for human steroid sulfatase. *Biochem Biophys Res Commun* **144**:1010, 1987.
80. Bonifas JM, Morley BJ, Oakey RE, Kan YW, Epstein EHJ: Cloning of a cDNA for steroid sulfatase: Frequent occurrence of gene deletions in patients with recessive X chromosome-linked ichthyosis. *Proc Natl Acad Sci U S A* **84**:9248, 1987.
81. Kerr CB, Wells RS, Sanger R: X-linked ichthyosis and the Xg groups. *Lancet* **2**:1369, 1964.
82. Adam A, Ziprkowski L, Feinstein A, Sanger R, Race RR: Ichthyosis, Xg blood groups, and protan. *Lancet* **1**:877, 1966.
83. Wells RS, Jennings MC, Sanger R, Race RR: Xg blood groups and ichthyosis. *Lancet* **2**:493, 1966.
84. Filippi G, Meera Khan P: Linkage studies on X-linked ichthyosis in Sardinia. *Am J Hum Genet* **20**:564, 1968.
85. Adam A, Ziprokowki L, Feinstein A, Sanger R, Tippet P, Gavin J, Race RR: Linkage relations of X-borne ichthyosis to Xg blood groups and to other markers of the X in Israelis. *Ann Hum Genet* **32**:323, 1969.
86. Went LN, De Groot WP, Sanger R, Tippet P, Gavin J: X-linked ichthyosis: Linkage relationship with the Xg blood groups and other studies in a large Dutch kindred. *Ann Hum Genet* **32**:333, 1969.
87. Mohandas T, Shapiro LJ, Sparkes RS, Sparkes MC: Regional assignment of the steroid sulfatase-X-linked ichthyosis locus: Implications for a non-inactivated region on the short arm of human X chromosome. *Proc Natl Acad Sci U S A* **76**:5779, 1979.
88. Müller CR, Westerveld A, Migl B, Franke W, Ropers HH: Regional assignment of the gene locus for steroid sulfatase. *Hum Genet* **54**:197, 1980.
89. Tiepolo L, Zuffardi O, Fraccaro M, di Natale D, Gargantini L, Müller CR, Ropers H-H: Assignment by deletion mapping of the steroid sulfatase X-linked ichthyosis locus to Xp22.3. *Hum Genet* **54**:205, 1980.
90. Ballabio A, Andria G: Deletions and translocations involving the distal short arm of the human X chromosome: review and hypotheses. *HumMolGene* **1**:221, 1992.
91. Schaefer L, Ferrero GB, Grillo A, Bassi MT, Roth EJ, Wapenaar MC, van Ommen GJB, Mohandas TK, Rocchi M, Zoghbi HY, Ballabio A: A high resolution deletion map of human chromosome Xp22. *Nat Genet* **4**:272, 1993.
92. Yen PH, Marsh B, Allen E, Mohandas T, Shapiro LJ: Organization of the human steroid sulfatase gene and sequence homology between the X and the Y chromosomes. *Am J Hum Genet* **41**:A248, 1987.
93. Li X-M, Alperin ES, Salido E, Gong Y, Yen P, Shapiro LJ: Characterization of the promoter region of human steroid sulfatase: a gene which escapes X inactivation. *Somat Cell Mol Genet* **22**:105, 1996.
94. Fraser N, Ballabio A, Zollo M, Persico G, Craig I: Identification of incomplete coding sequences for steroid sulphatase on the human Y chromosome: evidence for an ancestral pseudoautosomal gene? *Development* **101**(Suppl):127, 1987.
95. Bardoni B, Zuffardi O, Guioli S, Ballabio A, Simi P, Cavalli P, Grimoldi MG, Fraccaro M, Camerino G: A deletion map of the human Yq11 region: Implications for the evolution of the Y chromosome and tentative mapping of a locus involved in spermatogenesis. *Genomics* **11**:443, 1991.
96. Yen PH, Marsh B, Allen E, Tsai SP, Ellison J, Connolly L, Neiswanger K, Shapiro LJ: The human X-linked steroid sulfatase gene and a Y-encoded pseudogene: Evidence for an inversion of the Y chromosome during primate evolution. *Cell* **55**:1123, 1988.
97. Ross MT, Ballabio A, Craig IW: Long-range physical mapping around the human steroid sulfatase locus. *Genomics* **6**:528, 1990.
98. Li X-M, Yen P, Mohandas T, Shapiro LJ: A long range restriction map of the distal human X chromosome short arm around the steroid sulfatase locus. *Nucleic Acids Res* **18**:2783, 1990.
99. Carrozzo R, Ellison J, Yen P, Taillon-Miller P, Brownstein BH, Persico G, Ballabio A, Shapiro L: Isolation and characterization of a yeast artificial chromosome (YAC) contig around the human steroid sulfatase gene. *Genomics* **12**:7, 1992.
100. Lee W-C, Ferrero GB, Chinault AC, Yen PH, Ballabio A: A yeast artificial chromosome contig linking the steroid sulfatase and Kallmann syndrome loci on the human X chromosome short arm. *Genomics* **18**:1, 1993.
101. Gartler SM, Riggs AD: Mammalian X-chromosome inactivation. *Annu Rev Genet* **17**:155, 1983.
102. Ballabio A, Willard HF: Mammalian X-chromosome inactivation and the *XIST* gene. *Curr Opin Genet Dev* **2**:439, 1992.
103. Borsani G, Ballabio A: X chromosome gene dosage compensation in female mammals. *Dev Biol* **4**:129, 1993.
104. Polani PE: Pairing of X and Y chromosomes, non-inactivation of X-linked genes, and the maleness factor. *Hum Genet* **60**:207, 1982.
105. Shapiro LJ, Mohandas T, Weiss R, Romeo A: Noninactivation of an X chromosome locus in man. *Science* **204**:1224, 1979.
106. Migeon BR, Shapiro LJ, Norum RA, Mohandas T, Axelman J, Dabora RC: Differential expression of the steroid sulfatase locus on the active and inactive human X chromosome. *Nature* **299**:838, 1982.
107. Shapiro LJ, Mohandas T: DNA methylation and the control of gene expression on the human X chromosome. *Cold Spring Harbor Symp Quant* **47**:631, 1983.
108. Müller CR, Migl B, Ropers HH, Happle R: Heterozygote detection in steroid sulfatase deficiency. *Lancet* **1**:546, 1980.
109. Müller CR, Migl B, Traupe H, Ropers HH: X-linked steroid sulfatase: Evidence for different gene dosage in males and females. *Hum Genet* **54**:197, 1980.
110. Bedin M, Weil D, Fournier T, Cedar L, Frezal J: Biochemical evidence for the non-inactivation of the steroid sulfatase locus in human placenta and fibroblasts. *Hum Genet* **59**:256, 1981.
111. Lykkesfeldt G, Bock E, Lykkesfeldt AE: Sex specific difference in placental steroid sulphatase activity. *Lancet* **2**:255, 1981.
112. Chance PF, Gartler SM: Evidence for a dosage effect at the X-linked steroid sulfatase locus in human tissues. *Am J Hum Genet* **35**:234, 1983.
113. Dancis J, Jansen V, Hutzler J: Hair root analysis in X-linked ichthyosis. *J Inherit Metab Dis* **6**:173, 1983.
114. Mohandas T, Sparkes RS, Shapiro LJ: Genetic evidence for the inactivation of a human autosomal locus attached to an inactive X chromosome. *Am J Hum Genet* **34**:811, 1982.
115. Mohandas T, Geller RL, Yen PH, Rosendorff J, Bernstein R, Yoshida A, Shapiro LJ: Cytogenetic and molecular studies on a recombinant human X chromosome: Implications for the spreading of X chromosome inactivation. *Proc Natl Acad Sci U S A* **84**:4954, 1987.
116. Burgoyne PS: Genetic homology and crossing over in the X and Y chromosomes of mammals. *Hum Genet* **61**:85, 1982.
117. Koller PD, Darlington CD: Genetical and mechanical properties of sex-chromosomes; *Rattus norvegicus*. *J Genet* **29**:159, 1934.
118. Cooke HJ, Brown WRA, Rappold GA: Hypervariable telomeric sequences from the human sex chromosomes are pseudoautosomal. *Nature* **317**:687, 1985.
119. Simmler M-C, Rouyer F, Vergnaud G, Nyström-Lahti M, Ngo KY, de la Chapelle A, Weissenbach J: Pseudoautosomal DNA sequences in the pairing region of the human sex chromosomes. *Nature* **317**:692, 1985.
120. Buckle V, Mondello C, Darling S, Craig IW, Goodfellow PN: Homologous expressed genes in the human sex chromosome pairing region. *Nature* **317**:739, 1985.
121. Rouyer F, Simmler MC, Page DC, Weissenbach J: A sex chromosome rearrangement in a human XX male caused by Alu-Alu recombination. *Cell* **51**:417, 1987.
122. Singh L, Jones KW: Sex reversal in the mouse (*Mus musculus*) is caused by a recurrent non-reciprocal crossover involving the X and an aberrant Y chromosome. *Cell* **28**:205, 1982.
123. Evans EP, Burtenshaw MD, Cattanach BM: Meiotic crossover between the X and Y chromosomes of male mice carrying the sex-reversing (Sxr) factor. *Nature* **300**:443, 1982.
124. Keitges E, Rivest M, Siniscalco M, Gartler SM: X-linkage of steroid sulphatase in the mouse is evidence for a functional Y-linked allele. *Nature* **315**:226, 1985.
125. Keitges EA, Schorderet DF, Gartler SM: Linkage of the steroid sulfatase gene to the sex-reversed mutation in the mouse. *Genetics* **116**:465, 1987.
126. Soriano P, Keitges EA, Schorderet DF, Harbers K, Gartler SM, Jaenisch R: High rate of recombination and double crossovers in the mouse pseudoautosomal region during male meiosis. *Proc Natl Acad Sci U S A* **84**:7218, 1987.
127. Harbers K, Soriano P, Müller U, Jaenisch R: High frequency of unequal recombination in pseudoautosomal region shown by proviral insertion in transgenic mouse. *Nature* **324**:682, 1986.

128. Freije D, Helms C, Watson MS, Donis-Keller H: Identification of a second pseudoautosomal region near the Xq and Yq telomeres. *Science* **258**:1784, 1992.
129. Mohandas TK, Speed RM, Passage MB, Yen PH, Chandley AC, Shapiro LJ: Role of the pseudoautosomal region in sex-chromosome pairing during male meiosis: Meiotic studies in a man with a deletion of distal Xp. *Am JHum Genet* **51**:526, 1992.
130. Rouyer F, Simmler MC, Johnsson C, Vergnaud G, Cooke HJ, Weissenbach J: A gradient of sex linkage in the pseudoautosomal region of the human sex chromosomes. *Nature* **319**:291, 1986.
131. Henke A, Fischer C, Rappold GA: Genetic map of the human pseudoautosomal region reveals a high rate of recombination in female meiosis at the Xp telomere. *Genomics* **18**:478, 1993.
132. Rappold GA: The pseudoautosomal regions of the human sex chromosomes. *Hum Genet* **92**:315, 1993.
133. Rao E, Weiss B, Fukami M, Rump A, Niesler B, Mertz A, Muroya K, Binder G, Kirsch S, Winkelmann M, Nordsiek G, Heinrich U, Breuning MH, Ranke MB, Rosenthal A, Ogata T, Rappold GA: Pseudoautosomal deletions encompassing a novel homeobox gene cause growth failure in idiopathic short stature and Turner syndrome. *Nat Genet* **16**:54, 1997.
134. Ellison JW, Wardak Z, Young MF, Gehron Robey P, Laig Webster M, Chiong W: PHOG, a candidate gene for involvement in the short stature of Turner syndrome. *Hum Mol Genet* **6**:1341, 1997.
135. Franco B, Guioli S, Pragliola A, Incerti B, Bardoni B, Tonlorenzi R, Carrozzo R, Maestrini E, Pieretti M, Taillon-Miller P, Brown CJ, Willard HF, Lawrence C, Persico MG, Camerino G, Ballabio A: A gene deleted in Kallmann's syndrome shares homology with neural cell adhesion and axonal path-finding molecules. *Nature* **353**:529, 1991.
136. Legouis R, Hardelin J-P, Levilliers J, Claverie J-M, Compain S, Wunderle V, Millasseau P, Le Paslier D, Cohen D, Caterina D, Bougueleret L, Delemarre-Van de Waal H, Lutfalla G, Weissenbach J, Petit C: The candidate gene for the X-linked Kallmann syndrome encodes a protein related to adhesion molecules. *Cell* **67**:423, 1991.
137. Yen PH, Ellison J, Salido EC, Mohandas T, Shapiro L: Isolation of a new gene from the distal short arm of the human X chromosome that escapes X-inactivation. *Hum Mol Genet* **1**:47, 1992.
138. Meroni G, Franco B, Archidiacono N, Messali S, Andolfi G, Rocchi M, Ballabio A: Characterization of a cluster of sulfatase genes on Xp22.3 suggests gene duplications in an ancestral pseudoautosomal region. *Hum Mol Genet* **5**:423, 1996.
139. Parenti G, Meroni G, Ballabio A: The sulfatase gene family. *Curr Opin Genet Dev* **7**:386, 1997.
140. Ellis NA, Ye T-Z, Patton S, German J, Goodfellow PN, Weller P: Cloning of *PBDX*, an *MIC2*-related gene that spans the pseudoautosomal boundary on chromosome Xp. *Nat Genet* **6**:394, 1994.
141. Ellis NA, Tippett P, Petty A, Reid M, Weller PA, Ye TZ, German J, Goodfellow PN, Thomas S, Banting G: *PBDX* is the *XG* blood group gene. *Nat Genet* **8**:285, 1994.
142. Incerti B, Guioli S, Pragliola A, Zanaria E, Borsani G, Tonlorenzi R, Bardoni B, Franco B, Wheeler D, Ballabio A, Camerino G: Kallmann syndrome gene on the X and Y chromosomes: implications for evolutionary divergence of human sex chromosomes. *Nat Genet* **2**:311, 1992.
143. Balazs I, Purrello M, Rocchi M, Siniscalco M: Is the gene for steroid sulfatase X-linked? An appraisal of data from humans, mice, and their hybrids. *Cytogenet Cell Genet* **32**:251, 1982.
144. Nelson K, Daniel WL: Interstrain variation of murine arylsulfatase C1. *Experientia* **35**:309, 1979.
145. Erickson RP, Harper K, Kramer JM: Identification of an autosomal locus affecting steroid sulfatase activity among inbred strains of mice. *Genetics* **105**:181, 1983.
146. Crocker M, Craig I: Variation in regulation of steroid sulphatase locus in mammals. *Nature* **303**:721, 1983.
147. Salido EC, Li XM, Yen PH, Martin N, Mohandas TK, Shapiro LJ: Cloning and expression of the mouse pseudoautosomal steroid sulphatase gene *(Sts)*. *Nat Genet* **13**:83, 1996.
148. Li XM, Salido EC, Gong Y, Kitada K, Serikawa T, Yen PH, Shapiro LJ: Cloning of the rat steroid sulfatase gene (Sts), a non-pseudoautosomal X-linked gene that undergoes X inactivation. *Mamm Genome* **7**:420, 1996.
149. Kipling D, Salido EC, Shapiro LJ, Cooke HJ: High frequency de novo alterations in the long-range genomic structure of the mouse pseudoautosomal region. *Nat Genet* **13**:78, 1996.
150. Rugarli E, Adler DA, Borsani G, Tsuchiya K, Franco B, Hauge X, Disteche C, Chapman V, Ballabio A: Different chromosomal localization of the *Clcn4* gene in *Mus spretus* and C57BL/6J mice. *Nat Genet* **10**:466, 1995.
151. Dal Zotto L, Quaderi NA, Elliott R, Lingerfelter PA, Carrel L, Valsecchi V, Montini E, Yen C-H, Chapman V, Kalcheva I, Arrigo G, Zuffardi O, Thomas S, Willard H, Ballabio A, Disteche CM, Rugarli EI: The mouse *Mid1* gene: Implications for the pathogenesis of Opitz syndrome and the evolution of the mammalian pseudoautosomal region. *Hum Mol Genet* **7**:489, 1998.
152. Toder R, Rappold GA, Schiebel K, Schempp W: ANT3 and STS are autosomal in prosimian lemurs: Implications for the evolution of the pseudoautosomal region. *Hum Genet* **95**:22, 1995.
153. Ropers HH, Wiberg U: Evidence for X-linkage and non-inactivation of steroid sulphatase locus in wood lemmings. *Nature* **296**:766, 1982.
154. Wiberg UH, Fredge K: Steroid sulphatase levels are higher in males than in females of the root vale (*Microtus oeconomus*). *Hum Genet* **77**:6, 1987.
155. Toder R, Glaser B, Schiebel K, Wilcox SA, Rappold G, Graves JA, Schempp W: Genes located in and near the human pseudoautosomal region are located in the X-Y pairing region in dog and sheep. *Chromosome Res* **5**:301, 1997.
156. Toder R, Marshall Graves JA: CSF2RA, ANT3, and STS are autosomal in marsupials: implications for the origin of the pseudoautosomal region of mammalian sex chromosomes. *Mamm Genome* **9**:373, 1998.
157. France JT, Seddon RJ, Liggins GC: A study of a pregnancy with low estrogen production due to placental sulfatase deficiency. *J Clin Endocrinol Metab* **36**:1, 1973.
158. Taylor NF: Review: Placental sulphatase deficiency. *J Inherit Metab Dis* **5**:164, 1982.
159. Crawfurd MD: Review: Genetics of steroid sulfatase deficiency and X-linked ichthyosis. *J Inherit Metab Dis* **5**:153, 1982.
160. Harkness RA: Current clinical problems in placental steroid or arylsulphatase-C deficiency and the related "cervical dystocia" and X-linked ichthyosis. *J Inherit Metab Dis* **5**:142, 1982.
161. Rizk DEE, Johansen KA: Placental sulfatase deficiency and congenital ichthyosis with intrauterine fetal death: Case report. *Am J Obstet Gynecol* **168**:570, 1993.
162. Steinmann B, Mieth D, Gitzelmann R: A newly recognized cause of low urinary estriol in pregnancy: Multiple sulfatase deficiency of the fetus. *Gynecol Obstet Invest* **12**:107, 1981.
163. Taylor NF, Shackleton CHL: Gas chromatographic steroid analysis for diagnosis of placental sulfatase deficiency: A study of nine patients. *J Clin Endocrinol Metab* **49**:78, 1979.
164. Sedgwick W: On the influence of sex in hereditary disease. *Br Foreign Med-Churg Rev* **31**:445, 1863.
165. Kerr CB, Wells RS: Sex-linked ichthyosis. *Ann Hum Genet* **29**:33, 1965.
166. Tabei T, Heinrichs WL: Diagnosis of placental sulfatase deficiency. *Am J Obstet Gynecol* **124**:409, 1976.
167. Chibbar R, Mitchell BF: Steroid sulfohydrolase in human chorion and decidua: Studies using pregnenolone sulfate and dehydroepiandrosterone sulfate as substrate. *J Clin Endocrinol Metab* **70**:1693, 1990.
168. Shapiro LJ, Cousins L, Fluharty AL, Stevens RL, Kihara H: Steroid sulfatase deficiency. *Pediatr Res* **11**:894, 1977.
169. Shapiro LJ, Weiss R, Webster D, France JT: X-linked ichthyosis due to steroid sulfatase deficiency. *Lancet* **1**:70, 1978.
170. Koppe JG, Marinkovic-Ilsen A, Rijken Y, De Groot WP, Jobsis AC: X-linked ichthyosis. A sulphatase deficiency. *Arch Dis Child* **53**:803, 1978.
171. Marks R, Dykes PJ: *The Ichthyoses*. New York: Spectrum Publications, 1978.
172. Bousema M, van Diggelen O, van Joost T, Stolz E, Naafs B: Reliability of clinical signs in the differentiation between autosomal dominant and sex-linked forms. *Int J Dermatol* **28**:240, 1989.
173. Mevorah B, Krayenbuhl A, Bovey EH, van Melle GD: Autosomal dominant ichthyosis and X-linked ichthyosis. *Acta Derm Venereol (Stockh)* **71**:431, 1991.
174. Ghadially R, Chong LP: Ichthyoses and hyperkeratotic disorders. *Dermatol Clin* **10**:597, 1992.
175. Shwayder T, Ott F: All about ichthyosis. *Pediatr Clin North Am* **38**:835, 1991.
176. Wells RS, Kerr CB: Clinical features of autosomal dominant and sex-linked ichthyosis in an English population. *Br Med J* **1**:947, 1966.
177. Wells RS, Kerr CB: The histology of ichthyosis. *J Invest Dermatol* **46**:530, 1966.
178. Merrett JD, Wells RS, Kerr C, Barr A: Discriminant function analysis of phenotype variates in ichthyosis. *Am J Hum Genet* **19**:575, 1967.

179. Wells RS, Jennings MC: X-linked ichthyosis and ichthyosis vulgaris. *JAMA* **202**:485, 1967.
180. Sever RJ, Frost P, Weinstein G: Eye changes in ichthyosis. *JAMA* **206**:2283, 1968.
181. Costagliola C, Fabbrocini G, Illiano GMP, Scibelli G, Delfino M: Ocular findings in X-linked ichthyosis: A survey on 38 cases. *Ophthalmologica* **202**:152, 1991.
182. Marano RPC, Ortiz MA, Stradtmann O, Uxo M, Iglesias E: Ocular findings associated with congenital X-linked ichthyosis. *Ann Ophthalmol* **23**:167, 1991.
183. Shapiro LJ, Buxman MM, Weiss R, Vidgoff J, Dimond RL, Roller JA, Wells RS: Enzymatic basis of typical X-linked ichthyosis. *Lancet* **2**:756, 1978.
184. Shapiro LJ: X-linked ichthyosis. *Int J Dermatol* **20**:26, 1981.
185. Basler E, Grompe M, Parenti G, Yates J, Ballabio A: Identification of point mutations in the steroid sulfatase gene of three patients with X-linked ichthyosis. *Am J Hum Genet* **50**:483, 1992.
186. Martin ES, Yen P, Shapiro LJ: A splice junction mutation in a patient with X-linked ichthyosis and steroid sulfatase deficiency. *Am J Hum Genet* **47**:A228, 1990.
187. Alperin ES, Shapiro LJ: Characterization of point mutations in patients with X-linked ichthyosis. *J BioChem* **272**:20756, 1997.
188. Morita E, Katoh O, Shinoda S, Hiragun T, Tanaka T, Kameyoshi Y, Yamamoto S: A novel point mutation in the steroid sulfatase gene in X-linked ichthyosis. *J Invest Dermatol* **109**:244, 1997.
189. Jensen TG, Jensen UB, Jensen PKA, Ibsen HH, Brandrup F, Ballabio A, Bolund L: Correction of steroid sulfatase deficiency by gene transfer into basal cells of tissue cultured epidermis from patients with recessive X-linked ichthyosis. *Exp Cell Res* **209**:392, 1993.
190. Freiberg RA, Choate KA, Deng H, Alperin ES, Shapiro LJ, Khavari PA: A model of corrective gene transfer in X-linked ichthyosis. *Hum Mol Genet* **6**:927, 1997.
191. Robledo R, Melis P, Schillinger E, Casciano I, Balazs I, Rinaldi A, Siniscalco M, Filippi G: X-linked ichthyosis without STS deficiency: Clinical, genetical, and molecular studies. *AmJ Med Genet* **59**:143, 1995.
192. Bergner E, Shapiro LJ: Increased cholesterol sulfate in plasma and red blood cell membranes of steroid sulfatase-deficient patients. *J Clin Endocrinol Metab* **53**:221, 1981.
193. Epstein EH, Krauss RM, Shackleton CHL: X-linked ichthyosis: Increased blood cholesterol sulfate and electrophoretic mobility of low-density lipoprotein. *Science* **214**:659, 1981.
194. Milone A, Delfino M, Piccirillo A, Illiano GMP, Aloj SM, Bifulco M: Increased levels of DHEAS in serum of patients with X-linked ichthyosis. *J Inherit Metab Dis* **14**:96, 1991.
195. Shackleton CHL, Reid S: Diagnosis of recessive X-linked ichthyosis: Quantitative HPLC/Mass spectrometric analysis of plasma for cholesterol sulfate. *Clin Chem* **35**:1906, 1989.
196. Nakamura T, Matsuzawa Y, Okano M, Kitano Y, Funahashi T, Yamashita S, Tarui S: Characterization of low-density lipoproteins from patients with recessive X-linked ichthyosis. *Atherosclerosis* **70**:43, 1988.
197. Jackson SM, Williams ML, Feingold KR, Elias PM: Pathobiology of the stratum corneum. *West J Med* **158**:279, 1993.
198. Williams ML: Ichthyosis: Mechanisms of disease. *Pediatr Dermatol* **9**:365, 1992.
199. Williams ML: Epidermal lipids and scaling diseases of the skin. *Semin Dermatol* **11**:169, 1992.
200. Maloney ME, Williams ML, Epstein EH Jr, Law MY, Fritsch PO, Elias PM: Lipids in the pathogenesis of ichthyosis: Topical cholesterol sulfate-induced scaling in hairless mice. *J Invest Dermatol* **83**:252, 1984.
201. Williams ML, Feingold KR, Grubauer G, Elias PM: Ichthyosis induced by cholesterol-lowering drugs: Implications for epidermal cholesterol homeostasis. *Arch Dermatol* **123**:1535, 1987.
202. Frost P: Ichthyosiform dermatoses. *J Invest Dermatol* **60**:541, 1973.
203. Jensen PKA, Herrmann FH, Hadlich J, Bolund L: Proliferation and differentiation of cultured epidermal cells from patients with X-linked ichthyosis and ichthyosis vulgaris. *Acta Derm Venerol (Stockh)* **70**:99, 1990.
204. Williams ML, Kock TK, O'Donnell JJ, Frost PN, Epstein LB, Grizzard WS, Epstein CJ: Ichthyosis and neural lipid storage disease. *Am J Med Genet* **20**:711, 1985.
205. Rizzo WB, Dammann AL, Craft DA: Sjögren-Larsson. Impaired fatty alcohol oxidation in cultured fibroblasts due to deficient fatty alcohol: Nicotinamide adenine dinucleotide oxidoreductase activity. *J Clin Invest* **81**:738, 1988.
206. Buxman MM, Goodkin PE, Fahrenbach WH, Dimond RL: Harlequin ichthyosis with epidermal lipid abnormality. *Arch Dermatol* **115**:189, 1979.
207. Schmickel RD: Contiguous gene syndromes: a component of recognizable syndromes. *J Pediatr* **109**:231, 1986.
208. Ballabio A, Bardoni B, Carrozzo R, Andria G, Bick D, Campbell L, Hamel B, Ferguson-Smith MA, Gimelli G, Fraccaro M, Maraschio P, Zuffardi O, Guioli S, Camerino G: Contiguous gene syndromes due to deletions in the distal short arm of the human X chromosome. *Proc Natl Acad Sci U S A* **86**:10001, 1989.
209. Bassi MT, Schiaffino MV, Renieri A, De Nigris F, Galli L, Bruttini M, Gebbia M, Bergen AAB, Lewis RA, Ballabio A: Cloning of the gene for ocular albinism type 1 from the distal short arm of the X chromosome. *Nat Genet* **10**:13, 1995.
210. Lykkesfeldt G, Hoyer H, Ibsen HH, Brandrup: Steroid sulphatase deficiency disease. *Clin Genet* **28**:231, 1985.
211. Lykkesfeldt G, Bennett P, Lykkesfeldt AE, Micic S, Rorth M, Skakkebaek NE: Testis Cancer. Ichthyosis constitutes a significant risk factor. *Cancer* **67**:730, 1991.
212. Traupe H, Happle R: Clinical spectrum of steroid sulftatase deficiency: X-linked recessive ichthyosis, birth complications and cryptorchidism. *Eur J Pediatr* **140**:19, 1983.
213. Gillard EF, Affara NA, Yates JRW, Goudie DR, Lambert J, Aitken DA, Ferguson-Smith MA: Deletion of a DNA sequence in eight of nine families with X-linked ichthyosis (steroid sulfatase deficiency). *Nucleic Acids Res* **15**:3977, 1987.
214. Ballabio A, Carrozzo R, Parenti G, Gil A, Zollo M, Persico MG, Gillard E, Affara N, Yates J, Ferguson-Smith MA, Frants RR, Eriksson AW, Andria G: Molecular heterogeneity of steroid sulfatase deficiency: A multicenter study on 57 unrelated patients, at DNA and protein levels. *Genomics* **4**:36, 1989.
215. Cuevas-Covarrubias SA, Kofman-Alfaro SH, Maya-Núnez G, Días-Zagoya JC, Orozco Orozco E: X-linked Ichthyosis in Mexico: High frequency of deletions in the steroid sulfatase encoding gene. *Am J MedGenet* **72**:415, 1997.
216. Ballabio A, Ranier JE, Chamberlain JS, Zollo M, Caskey CT: Screening for steroid sulfatase (STS) gene deletions by multiplex DNA amplification. *Hum Genet* **84**:571, 1990.
217. Cooke A, Gillard EF, Yates JRW, Mitchell MJ, Aitken DA, Weir DM, Affara NA, Ferguson-Smith MA: X chromosome deletions detectable by flow cytometry in some patients with steroid sulphatase deficiency (X-linked ichthyosis). *Hum Genet* **79**:49, 1988.
218. Parenti G, Ballabio A, Hoogeveen AT, van der Loos CM, Jobsis AC, Andria G: Studies on cross-reacting material to steroid sulphatase in fibroblasts from patients affected by different types of steroid sulphatase deficiency. *J Inherit Metab Dis* **10**:224, 1987.
219. Bardoni B, Guioli S, Raimondi E, Heilig R, Mandel JL, Ottolenghi S, Camerino G: Isolation and characterization of a family of sequences dispersed on the human X chromosome. *Genomics* **3**:32, 1988.
220. Ballabio A, Bardoni B, Guioli S, Basler E, Camerino G: Two families of low-copy-number repeats are interspersed on Xp22.3: Implications for the high frequency of deletions in this region. *Genomics* **8**:263, 1990.
221. Knowlton RG, Nelson CA, Brown VA, Page DC, Donis-Keller H: An extremely polymorphic locus on the short arm of the human X chromosome with homology to the long arm of the Y chromosome. *Nucleic Acids Res* **17**:423, 1989.
222. Yen PH, Li X-M, Tsai S-P, Johnson C, Mohandas T, Shapiro LJ: Frequent deletions of the human X chromosome distal short arm result from recombination between low copy repetitive elements. *Cell* **61**:603, 1990.
223. Li X-M, Yen PH, Shapiro LJ: Characterization of a low copy repetitive element S232 involved in the generation of frequent deletions of the distal short arm of the human X chromosome. *Nucleic Acids Res* **20**:1117, 1992.
224. Bernatowicz LF, Li X-M, Carrozzo R, Ballabio A, Mohandas T, Yen PH, Shapiro LJ: Sequence analysis of a partial deletion of the human steroid sulfatase gene reveals 3 bp of homology at deletion breakpoints. *Genomics* **13**:892, 1992.
225. Henke A, Wapenaar M, van Ommen GJ, Maraschio P, Camerino G, Rappold G: Deletions within the pseudoautosomal region help map three new markers and indicate a possible role of this region in linear growth. *Am J Hum Genet* **49**:811, 1991.
226. Ogata T, Goodfellow P, Petit C, Aya M, Matsuo N: Short stature in a girl with a terminal Xp deletion to *DXYS15*: Localisation of a growth gene(s) in the pseudoautosomal region. *J Med Genet* **29**:455, 1992.

227. Bernstein R: X, Y chromosome translocations and their manifestations, in Sandberg AA (eds): *Progress and Topics in Cytogenetics: The Y Chromosome,* Vol. 6B New York, Alan R Liss, 1985, p 171.
228. Yen PH, Tsai SP, Wenger SL, Steele MW, Mohandas TK, Shapiro LJ: X/Y translocations resulting from recombination between homologous sequences on Xp and Yq. *Proc Natl Acad Sci U S A* **88**:8944, 1991.
229. Guioli S, Incerti B, Zanaria E, Bardoni B, Franco B, Taylor K, Ballabio A, Camerino G: Kallmann syndrome due to a translocation resulting in an X/Y fusion gene. *Nat Genet* **1**:337, 1992.
230. Petit C, de la Chapelle A, Levilliers J, Castillo S, Noel B, Weissenbach J: An abnormal Terminal X-Y interchange accounts for most but not all cases of human XX maleness. *Cell* **49**:595, 1987.
231. Ropers HH, Migl B, Zimmer J, Muller CR: Steroid sulfatase activity in cultured fibroblasts of XX males. *Cytogenet Cell Genet* **30**:168, 1981.
232. Mohandas TK, Stern HJ, Meeker CA, Passage MB, Müller U, Page DC, Yen PH, Shapiro LJ: Steroid sulfatase gene in XX males. *Am J Hum Genet* **46**:369, 1990.
233. Lindsay EA, Grillo A, Ferrero GB, Roth EJ, Magenis E, Grompe M, Hultén M, Gould C, Baldini A, Zoghbi HY, Ballabio A: Microphthalmia with linear skin defects (MLS) syndrome: clinical, cytogenetic and molecular characterization. *Am J Med Genet* **49**:229, 1994.
234. Lykkesfeldt G, Nielsen MD, Lykkesfeldt AE: Placental steroid sulfatase deficiency: biochemical diagnosis and clinical review. *Obstet Gynecol* **64**:49, 1984.
235. Lebo RV, Lynch ED, Golbus MS, Flandermeyer RR, Yen PH, Shapiro LJ: Prenatal in situ hybridization test for deleted steroid sulfatase gene. *Am J Med Genet* **46**:652, 1993.
236. Wirth B, Gal A: XmnI polymorphism of the human STS gene. *Nucleic Acids Res* **17**:3326, 1989.
237. Andria G, Ballabio A, Parenti G, Di Maio S, Piccirillo A: Steroid sulphatase deficiency is present in patients with the syndrome "Ichthyosis and male hypogonadism" and with "Rud syndrome." *J Inherit Metab Dis* **7**:159, 1984.

CHAPTER 167

Adrenal Hypoplasias and Aplasias

Edward R.B. McCabe

1. **Adrenal hypoplasia congenita (AHC) has an estimated incidence of 1:12,500 live births and two distinct histological patterns to the adrenal cortices, the miniature adult and cytomegalic forms.**
2. **In the miniature adult form of AHC, the small amount of residual adrenal cortex is composed primarily of permanent adult cortex with normal structural organization. The miniature adult form is either sporadic or inherited in an autosomal recessive manner, and is frequently associated with abnormal central nervous system development, including anencephaly or pituitary gland abnormalities.**
3. **In the cytomegalic form of AHC, the residual adrenal cortex is structurally disorganized with scattered irregular nodular formations of eosinophilic cells, with the adult permanent zone absent or nearly absent. Enlarged cells are present, some with abundant vacuolated cytoplasm. The cytomegalic form is generally considered to be X-linked, but there may be one or more autosomal genes associated with this phenotype.**
4. **X-linked AHC (MIM 300200) is caused by intragenic mutations or complete deletion of the Xp21 DAX1 gene (*DSS-AHC* critical region on the X chromosome, gene 1). Associated with deletion of DAX1, the Duchenne muscular dystrophy (DMD) and glycerol kinase (GK) genes may also be deleted as part of a contiguous gene syndrome. Patients with DAX1 mutations have adrenal insufficiency with glucocorticoid and mineralocorticoid deficiency, and hypogonadotropic hypogonadism (HH) of mixed hypothalamic and pituitary origin. Gonadal mosaicism for a DAX1 mutation has been reported in one family with X-linked AHC.**
5. **DAX1 is an unusual member of the nuclear hormone receptor superfamily with a characteristic C-terminal putative ligand-binding domain (LBD), but an atypical N-terminal portion that is a DNA-binding domain (DBD) in the typical receptor. Because DAX1 has the structure of a transcription factor and maps to the 160 kb critical region for dosage sensitive sex reversal (DSS) within the tandem duplications among XY individuals with female or ambiguous genitalia, it is a candidate gene for the DSS locus. XY transgenic mice with overexpression of the murine homologue, Dax1, and reduced expression of *SRY* (sex determining region, Y chromosome) are phenotypically female. These observations suggest that DAX1 may be the hypothetical X-linked negative regulator of male gene expression that is antagonized by SRY in normal XY males.**
6. **There are at least six single-gene disorders associated with adrenal hypoplasia/aplasia that have definite or apparent autosomal recessive inheritance: ACTH deficiency (MIM 201400); AHC with absent pituitary LH (MIM 202150); cytomegalic form of AHC with autosomal recessive inheritance (MIM 202155); Pena-Shokeir syndrome, type 1 (MIM 208150); holoprosencephaly 1, alobar (MIM 236100); hypoadrenocorticism, familial (MIM 240200); and Meckel syndrome (MIM 249000).**
7. **A number of chromosomal abnormalities have been associated with adrenal hypoplasia. These include tetraploidy, triploidy, trisomy 18, trisomy 21, 5p duplication, monosomy 7 and the $11q^-$ syndrome. Because these patients frequently have central nervous system abnormalities, the adrenal hypoplasia is often the miniature adult form.**

INTRODUCTION AND HISTORICAL PERSPECTIVE

The terms hypoplasia and aplasia derive from the Greek verb, *plassein*, meaning to mold or to form, and, therefore, the adrenal hypoplasias and aplasias are disorders associated with underdevelopment or absent formation, respectively, of the adrenal glands. The diagnosis of adrenal aplasia should be viewed with caution in the absence of an exhaustive pathologic examination, because there may be small amounts of residual tissue present in the perirenal fat that may be missed by imaging or routine autopsy. However, adrenal aplasia does occur in humans, and there are animal models — for example, the murine knockout for the mouse homologue of steroidogenic factor 1, *SF1* — that may result in complete absence or aplasia of the adrenals (see below). For the purpose of this chapter, the term adrenal hypoplasia will be used inclusively for all forms of adrenal gland underdevelopment, including adrenal aplasia.

We follow the convention of referring to adrenal cortical underdevelopment as adrenal hypoplasia congenita (AHC), in order to distinguish this diagnosis from the similar-sounding but very different diagnosis, congenital adrenal hyperplasia (CAH) (see Chap. 159).

The incidence of AHC has been estimated to be 1:12,500 live births.[1] There are two distinct histological patterns of the adrenal cortices seen among patients with AHC, the miniature adult and the cytomegalic forms.[2] In the miniature adult form, the small amount of cortical tissue is made up primarily of permanent adult cortex that is normal in structural organization, with absent or

A list of standard abbreviations is located immediately preceding the text in each volume. Additional abbreviations used in this chapter include: AHC = adrenal hypoplasia congenita; Ahch = adrenal hypoplasia congenita, mouse homologue of DAX1; BMD = Becker muscular dystrophy; CAH = congenital adrenal hyperplasia; DAXI = DSS-AHC critical region on the X chromosome, gene 1; DBD = DNA-binding domain; DHEA = dehydroepiandrosterone; DHEAS = dehydroepiandrosterone sulfate; DMD = Duchenne muscular dystrophy; DSS = dosage sensitive sex reversal; FSH = follicle stimulating hormone; FtzF1 = murine homologue of steroidogenic factor 1; GK = glycerol kinase; GKD = glycerol kinase deficiency; HH = hypogonadotropic hypogonadism; LBD = ligand-binding domain; MIS = Müllerian inhibiting substance; MR = mental retardation; N-CoR = nuclear receptor corepressor; RE = response element; SF1 = steroidogenic factor 1; SHP = small heterodimer partner; StAR = steroidogenic acute regulatory protein; WAGR = Wilms tumor, aniridia, genitourinary abnormalities, and mental retardation; WT1 = Wilms tumor 1 gene.

Table 167-1 Disorders Catalogued in MIM[2] Associated with Adrenal Hypoplasia Congenita

*201400	ACTH deficiency
202150	Adrenal hypoplasia, congenital, with absent pituitary luteinizing hormone (miniature adult type)
202155	Adrenal hypoplasia, cytomegalic type
*208150	Pena-Shokeir syndrome, type I; arthrogryposis multiplex congenita with pulmonary hypoplasia (miniature adult type)
*236100	Holoprosencephaly 1, alobar
*240200	Hypoadrenocorticism, familial (miniature adult form)
*249000	Meckel syndrome; Meckel-Gruber syndrome; dysencephalia splanchnocystica
*300200	Adrenal hypoplasia, congenital (cytomegalic form)

minimal fetal cortex.[3–6] In the cytomegalic form of AHC, the following features are observed: the cells are enlarged, some with abundant vacuolated cytoplasm; the permanent adult zone is absent or nearly absent; and the cortical tissue evidences structural disorganization with scattered irregular nodular formations of eosinophilic cells.[7–13] The miniature adult pathologic form is frequently associated with abnormal development of the central nervous system, including anencephaly or pituitary gland abnormalities, and therefore is presumed to have multiple etiologies.[2] This miniature adult form of AHC is either sporadic or inherited in an autosomal recessive manner.[2,14] The cytomegalic form is generally considered to be inherited in an X-linked fashion.[2] As discussed below, however, a significant proportion of patients with the clinical diagnosis of AHC and no abnormalities of the central nervous system have no identified mutations in the gene responsible for X-linked AHC, *DAX1*. This suggests that there may be one or more additional genes, possibly autosomal, that cause this phenotype. MIM[2] recognizes the possibility of a cytomegalic form of AHC with autosomal recessive inheritance (MIM 202155).

There are at least eight single-gene disorders associated with adrenal hypoplasia, seven with definite or apparent autosomal recessive inheritance, and one with definite X-linked inheritance[2] (Table 167-1). For five of these disorders, the mode of inheritance is considered as conclusively shown, but, for two, the mode of inheritance remains inconclusive. One of the latter is the putative autosomal recessive cytomegalic form of AHC (MIM 202155). These disorders are considered in more detail below.

AHC may also be seen in patients with chromosomal abnormalities, including tetraploidy, triploidy, trisomy 18, trisomy 21, 5p duplication, monosomy 7, and the $11q^-$ syndrome.[6,15,16] The AHC in these patients is frequently associated with pituitary or other central nervous system abnormalities, and therefore is often the miniature adult form.

NORMAL DEVELOPMENT OF THE ADRENAL GLAND

The adrenal gland is made up of two distinct tissues, the cortex and the medulla, with different embryologic origins. The cells that give rise to the fetal and adult adrenal cortex derive from the posterior abdominal wall mesenchyme, and the adrenal medulla develops from neural crest cells.[13,17]

The adrenal cortical primordia are mesodermal in origin and develop near the cephalic portion of the mesonephros.[13,17] The primordial cells are first recognized at approximately 32 days postfertilization (Carnegie stage 14, 5 to 7 mm) in the adrenal ridge of the coelomic epithelium. By approximately 33 days (Carnegie stage 15, 7 to 9 mm) cellular proliferation in the mesenchyme ventral to the mesonephros gives rise to a population of cells that migrate to the adrenal area. At a similar stage of development, cells that will become the capsule and the underlying structural framework for the endocrine cells in the gland begin to migrate from the mesonephric glomerular medial wall epithelium, a migration that continues for approximately two weeks (until Carnegie stage 19). A second migratory wave of coelomic epithelium cells enters the adrenal area at approximately 37 days (Carnegie stage 16, 8 to 10 mm). The adrenal cortex grows in a centrifugal fashion, with new cells added to the periphery in the subcapsular region. The fetal (provisional) cortex lies deep to the subcapsular adult (permanent or definitive) cortex.

Each adrenal medulla primordium migrates to, and then through, the adrenal cortex primordium, eventually taking a position centrally within this compound organ.[13,17] The adrenal medullary primordial cells develop in the sixth week, at approximately 41 days (Carnegie stages 16 to 17, 11 to 14 mm), and migrate as paired large neural complexes, containing better-developed sympathetic nerve fibers as well as more primitive sympathicoblasts, from paraaortic sympathetic ganglia to the dorsomedial aspects of the adrenal cortical primordia. As each medullary primordium migrates through its respective adrenal cortical primordium, beginning at approximately weeks 7 to 8 and completing the process by approximately weeks 10 to 14, some disorganization of the cortex results. Cellular arrests, represented by clusters of small primitive sympathicoblasts, known as neuroblastic nodules, are commonly seen in the fetal adrenal and are considered normal. While it remains controversial whether or not these neuroblastic nodules represent the origin of neuroblastoma *in situ*,[13,18] it is important to distinguish the normal neuroblastic nodules from early malignancies.[18]

Adrenal cortical tissues may also be seen in ectopic sites that may be predicted in part by the normal embryological development of this tissue from mesenchymal cells in the lining of the posterior coelomic cavity immediately adjacent to the urogenital ridge.[19] These ectopic sites include the celiac plexus in the retroperitoneum, the hilum of the spleen, positions around the ovaries, near the epididymis and spermatic cord in the scrotum, and, rarely, within the liver, the gallbladder wall, the ovary, or surrounding the brain.

From the time that the adrenal is first recognizable grossly, at approximately 2 months gestation, when the medullary neuroectodermal cells begin to invade the cortex, its size grows rapidly. At midgestation the normal adrenal is larger than the kidney. The inner fetal zone is larger than the outer definitive zone by the second trimester, representing most of the adrenal tissue at that stage of development. The fetal zone accounts for 75 to 80 percent of the adrenal cortex at birth, followed by a rapid decrease. This loss of the fetal cortex is reflected by a 50 percent reduction in adrenal weight by 2 weeks of age.[13] Because of the dramatic decrease in the fetal zone, it represents only 25 percent of the adrenal cortex at 2 months of age, and has disappeared by the end of the first year of life.[19] While it used to be thought that the decrease in the fetal zone was due to complete involution, it now appears that cells from the fetal cortex give rise to the inner fasciculata and reticularis.[13,20] The mechanism for decreased fetal-zone cell mass remains to be determined, but we would speculate that this may be due to apoptosis.

Observations in the adrenal of the anencephalic fetus provide insight into the role of ACTH in early adrenal development.[21] Because the adrenal glands of these fetuses develop normally for the first 15 weeks, and because the fetal pituitary does not produce ACTH during that period, then the early development of the fetal adrenal is considered to be independent of fetal pituitary ACTH. ACTH is necessary, but may not be sufficient, for later growth and development of the fetal adrenal.[19] Other growth factors that are involved in maintenance of the adult adrenal include the proopiomelanocortin amino-terminal fragment, epidermal growth factor, fibroblast growth factor, and insulin-like growth factor-1.[19]

The adrenal cortex appears to be maintained by division and centripetal migration of putative stem cells that originate in the capsule or subcapsular region of the zona glomerulosa. Cell division is more frequently seen in the glomerulosa, whereas cell division is rare and cell death is more frequently observed in the reticularis.[22] Apoptosis should be considered as a possible mechanism for the cell death at the corticomedullary junction. Centripetal cell "streaming" was demonstrated by radiolabeling cells in living animals.[23] Additional evidence consistent with a subcapsular stem cell is the observation of regeneration of cortical tissue from subcapsular remnants.[24,25]

There is general correlation between the anatomic zones of the adrenal cortex and steroid production.[19] In the fetal adrenal gland, the fetal zone produces pregnenolone sulfate and DHEAS, beginning at approximately week 25 of gestation. Because the fetal zone is deficient in 3β-hydroxysteroid dehydrogenase, large amounts of DHEAS and only small amounts of cortisol are produced. The DHEAS is converted by peripheral fetal tissues to a substrate for placental estrogen production. The definitive zone of the fetal gland synthesizes primarily cortisol. In the adult adrenal gland, the glomerulosa and outer portion of the fasciculata produce the mineralocorticoid aldosterone, the fasciculata and, to a much lesser extent, the reticularis produce the glucocorticoid cortisol, DHEA, and other adrenal androgens and estrogens are produced by the fasciculata and reticularis, with only the reticularis carrying out sulfation.

X-LINKED ADRENAL HYPOPLASIA CONGENITA (MIM 300200)

Clinical Aspects

The familial occurrence of adrenal cortical insufficiency due to adrenal hypoplasia, with a pattern of inheritance consistent with X-linkage, is well recognized.[7,26–39] Most patients present within the first days, weeks, or months of life, but occasionally affected individuals with family histories compatible with X-linked AHC may develop acute adrenal insufficiency as late as 10 years,[27,34] and, in one family of two brothers and their maternal uncles, between 17 and 32 years of age.[26] The two brothers who we originally described with AHC, GKD, and a dystrophic myopathy,[40,41] who we now know to be completely deleted for *DAX1*,[42,43] did not present with acute adrenal insufficiency until 33 months and 6 years of age. The younger boy died at 33 months, 12 hours into an episode of gastroenteritis following 2 days after surgery for esotropia, and his older brother presented 11 months later, at 6 years of age, 29 hours into an episode of gastroenteritis, with dehydration, acidemia, hyponatremia, and hyperkalemia. In a series of 18 patients from 16 families, among the 17 who presented clinically, the range in age for first acute symptoms was 1 week to 3 years, with a median age of 3 weeks.[44] In this series, the younger of two brothers with a deletion of *DAX1* and *GK* presented with salt wasting at 1 month, and the older boy was diagnosed at 3 years of age with a similar episode. Peter et al. reviewed other reports of delayed-onset and intrafamilial variability,[44] but the explanation for why some patients have a significantly longer period of residual function from their hypoplastic adrenal cortices remains unknown.

The hypoplastic adrenals with X-linked AHC evidence cytomegalic pathologic changes with absence or near-absence of the permanent zone, and cortical disorganization with nodular formations of eosinophilic cells in the residual cortex.[7–13,29–31,45,46] Occasionally, in families with pedigrees consistent with X-linked inheritance, no adrenal tissue could be identified, despite thorough autopsy, including a careful search for adrenal vascular supply.[28,33,36,47] This suggests adrenal aplasia.

HH is known to be associated with the X-linked form of AHC.[11,32,34,35,37,38,44,48–66] While some investigators suggested that there was a distinct locus telomeric to the AHC gene,[67,68] with the cloning of the gene responsible for X-linked AHC, *DAX1* (see below), intragenic mutations in this gene were found to be responsible for HH.[59,60] The data were contradictory regarding whether the HH in patients with *DAX1* mutations was hypothalamic or pituitary in origin,[56,57] until the controversy was resolved by showing that the HH in these patients had mixed hypothalamic and pituitary origins.[62,63] This explanation of the HH in these patients fit well with the observation that *DAX1* is expressed in the hypothalamus and the pituitary.[69] The "mini-puberty" of infancy appears to be normal in affected boys, suggesting loss of functional integrity over time or differences in the mechanisms responsible for hypothalamic-pituitary-gonadal axis regulation in infancy and adolescence.[44,70,71] Despite the usual association of X-linked AHC and HH, four male cousins, whose maternal grandmothers were sisters, had androgenic precocity of varying degrees, one with nonprogressive virilization at birth, and the other three with advanced growth and/or skeletal maturation and elevated testosterone levels.[36]

The majority of patients with AHC are not recognized clinically until they develop an adrenal crisis. Some may be misdiagnosed with congenital adrenal hyperplasia (CAH)[44] (E.R.B. McCabe, unpublished finding). In a series of 18 patients from one center, 16 presented with salt-wasting, one had an initial hypoglycemic seizure, and one was treated presymptomatically, based on the results of prenatal diagnostic testing.[44] Acute deterioration may be preceded by nonspecific features, such as feeding difficulties, vomiting, poor weight gain, and dehydration. Hyperpigmentation resulting from excessive proopiomelanocortin production is usually present and may be quite profound, with the increased keratinocyte melanin giving a coal-black coloration to the skin, except on the palms and soles.[72] Wheezing, which may be attributed initially to asthma, may represent a mild form of Addisonian crisis in patients with AHC.[73]

Neurologic abnormalities and developmental delay may be observed in patients with AHC. Progressive high-frequency hearing loss beginning at about 14 years of age has been observed in three brothers.[58] Among those who present later, personality changes may be seen.[32,53] Seizures are often seen at presentation or as a consequence of Addisonian crises, and acute adrenal insufficiency may also result in other neurologic sequelae and developmental abnormalities. Bilateral infantile striatal necrosis has been observed in AHC.[74]

AHC may be due to deletion of *DAX1*, as part of an Xp21 contiguous gene syndrome (Chap. 97), or it may be an isolated disorder, due to intragenic mutations within the *DAX1* gene. Patients with large deletions will have complex phenotypes depending on the other loci involved, most often the *GK* and Duchenne muscular dystrophy (*DMD*) loci along with the *DAX1* gene. There appears to be one or more MR loci telomeric to *DAX1* that may be deleted in some patients (reviewed in Chap. 97). The observation of developmental delay in patients with isolated AHC from acute episodes of adrenal insufficiency may make it difficult to determine the etiology of the MR in individual patients. However, the observations of MR in female carriers for deletions in this region[75] and of a patient with MR and an interstitial deletion telomeric to and not involving *DAX1*,[76] support the presence of one or more MR loci independent of AHC. In addition, a patient with a contiguous gene syndrome involving *DAX1*, *GK*, and *DMD*, who also has agenesis of the corpus callosum, suggests the localization of a gene for this midline defect to Xp22.11 to p21.1.[77]

Treatment

Acute presentation with suspected adrenal crisis frequently will require parenteral glucose, saline, and glucocorticoid. The mineralocorticoid activity of a glucocorticoid, such as cortisol sodium succinate (Solu-Cortef), often will be adequate for acute management. Clinical status, blood glucose, electrolytes, and hydration must be monitored closely. If the electrolytes do not respond, the only mineralocorticoid available at this time is fludrocortisone (Florinef), which is an oral preparation. Therefore, if the patient will not tolerate oral medication, the dose of parenteral glucocorticoid should be increased to take advantage of its mineralocorticoid activity. For example, 20 mg of Solu-Cortef has the same effect on sodium retention as approximately 0.1 mg of Florinef or 1 mg of deoxycorticosterone (DOC) acetate (see Chap. 159). The patient's electrolyte and water balance must be closely monitored to prevent hypernatremia, overhydration, and pulmonary edema.

Maintenance therapy involves physiological replacement doses of a glucocorticoid, such as hydrocortisone, and titration of the mineralocorticoid fludrocortisone (Florinef). Increased sodium chloride intake may also be required. During times of stress, such as significant intercurrent illnesses, the dose of glucocorticoid should be increased three to four times. The dosage should be 5 to 10 times maintenance for surgeries and significant traumas, and these should be managed in centers where a pediatric endocrinologist is available. Education of the parents, patients, and primary care physicians is extremely important, because deaths in diagnosed patients occur when steroid doses are subtherapeutic, particularly during times of stress. Parenteral Solu-Cortef may be provided for home use with appropriate education. Dosages must be increased appropriately to accommodate the growth of the child, without overdosing. A medical information bracelet or necklace should be used by the patient.

HH should be anticipated in patients with AHC, and treated with testosterone for initiation of secondary sexual characteristics.

Future directions in therapy for AHC, as well as other disorders of the adrenal cortex, may include gene therapy and stem-cell therapy. A promoter that would provide tissue specific expression, alone or in combination with other promoter elements to enhance expression efficiency in the adrenal cortex could be used to drive *DAX1* expression in an in vivo gene therapy vector. If the *DAX1* promoter is shown to be sufficiently specific and efficient, then it may be a candidate for a gene therapy vector designed to target adrenal cortical expression of *DAX1* or other adrenal disease genes.[78] If DAX1 dimerization is required for normal function, then the possibility of a dominant negative effect by endogenously expressed mutant protein must be considered.[79] Alternative targeting strategies, such as introducing proteins or smaller molecule ligands that would interact with a specific receptor or docking molecule on the surface of the targeting vector, would also be possible.[80–85] Identification of one or more adrenal cortical stem cells[24,25] would open the possibility of stem-cell therapy for AHC and other adrenal disorders.

Diagnosis

My initial screen for a patient suspected of having AHC includes plasma ACTH, which is consistently elevated in AHC, whereas cortisol may be within the normal range; serum triglyceride level and/or urinary organic acids prepared by the solvent extraction method, for evaluation of GKD by pseudohypertriglyceridemia and glyceroluria, respectively; and a serum creatine phosphokinase (CPK) level to rule out DMD or Becker muscular dystrophy (BMD). With this assessment, one will determine whether additional work-up for AHC is indicated and whether the AHC is part of the most common form of the Xp21 contiguous gene syndrome, complex GKD (cGKD), involving the AHC, GKD, and DMD loci (see Chap. 97).

If the ACTH level is elevated and there is evidence of GKD and/or DMD/BMD, then it is most likely that this patient has AHC. For isolated AHC, other work-up may be indicated. In contrast to CAH due to 21-hydroxylase deficiency, in which urinary 17-ketosteroids and pregnanetriol, and plasma cortisol precursors and adrenal androgens typically are elevated (see Chap. 159), these compounds usually will be low or normal in patients with AHC. The patient with AHC will not have a normal cortisol response to an ACTH stimulation test.

Molecular genetic diagnosis of *DAX1* is also possible. The *DAX1* gene consists of only two exons and is easily sequenced (see section on Genetics, below). It should be noted, however, that not all individuals with a clinical diagnosis of AHC will have mutations in *DAX1*.[44,60] In our own experience, the number of samples referred with an AHC diagnosis but no *DAX1* mutation detectable by sequencing has been significant.

Imaging studies may be helpful to attempt to evaluate adrenal size. The normal position of the adrenal gland within the perirenal fat, and the potential for aberrant locations for adrenals, may make it difficult to interpret a study that does not detect normal adrenals. The imaging results must be interpreted in the context of the other clinical and molecular investigations.

If the patient comes to autopsy, the weights of the adrenal glands will be low compared with the normal range for age.[86–89] The histologic appearance of the adrenals from an individual with the X-linked cytomegalic form is characteristic, with disorganization of the cortex and large eosinophilic cells (see "Introduction and Historical Perspective" above).

Prenatal diagnostic testing may use a variety of approaches. Maternal plasma estriol levels are low in pregnancies of a fetus with AHC.[8,44,47,90–93] If there is a family history of a *DAX1* deletion, then fluorescence *in situ* hybridization (FISH) may be used to determine whether the fetus is at risk for AHC.[43] Mutation analysis is well established for identification of affected individuals (see "Genetics" below); however, to our knowledge, this approach has not been used for prenatal diagnosis at this time.

Genetics

AHC was originally mapped to Xp21 by clinical characterization of patients who had deletions that also involved GKD and DMD/BMD (reviewed in Chap. 97). Not all of the deletions result in loss of the *DAX1* coding region. Patient TM, who has AHC, GKD, and DMD,[42] is not deleted for *DAX1*,[59] and has a telomeric breakpoint that is estimated to be approximately 100 kb centromeric of the *DAX1* coding sequence (Guo and McCabe, unpublished observations). The observations in this patient indicate that deletions in this region may lead to position effects on *DAX1* expression.

A series of 18 patients with AHC in 16 families ascertained clinically by a German group gives insight into the approximate proportion of individuals with *DAX1* deletions, intragenic mutations, or no detectable gene alteration.[44] Seven families had large deletions, four involving AHC, GKD, and DMD (only two of which were analyzed), one with AHC and GKD, and two with deletion of *DAX1*. Seven families exhibited intragenic mutations, five with frameshift and two with nonsense mutations. One family with isolated AHC had no *DAX1* mutation detected, and another did not have mutation analysis performed.

In a review of intragenic *DAX1* mutations, we tabulated 42 mutations from 48 families, to determine the types of mutations responsible for AHC and to identify the positions of single amino acid changes in a DAX1 structural model.[94] Fourteen new mutations were identified in that report, with the other 28 described previously.[43,59,60,62,64,65,70,95,96] One nonsense mutation (W235X) was found in three families, and one frameshift mutation (1292delG), two nonsense mutations (W171X and Y91X), and one in-frame deletion (V269del) were observed in two families each. To our knowledge, the families with identical mutations were unrelated, and we confirmed this by showing substantial differences between the mitochondrial D-loop sequences[97] in the two families with the frameshift mutation. The 23 frameshift and 12 nonsense mutations were distributed throughout the DAX1 protein, but all seven of the mutations resulting in single amino acid changes (six missense mutations and one single codon in-frame deletion) mapped to the C-terminal half of DAX1 in the region of similarity with the LBDs of other members of the nuclear hormone receptor superfamily[78] (Fig. 167-1). When the seven single amino acid changes were mapped to a three-dimensional model of the DAX1, putative LBD developed by homology with the known structures of rat $\alpha 1$ thyroid hormone receptor[98] and human retinoid-X receptor RXRα,[99] they all clustered in the hydrophobic core of the LBD (Fig. 167-2). These seven mutations all involved amino acids that were identical in human DAX1 and the homologous murine protein, Ahch, and were predicted to provide a major disruption of receptor folding, dimerization, and overall DAX1 function.[94] Subsequent to this tabulation of *DAX1* mutations, additional reports that include intragenic mutations

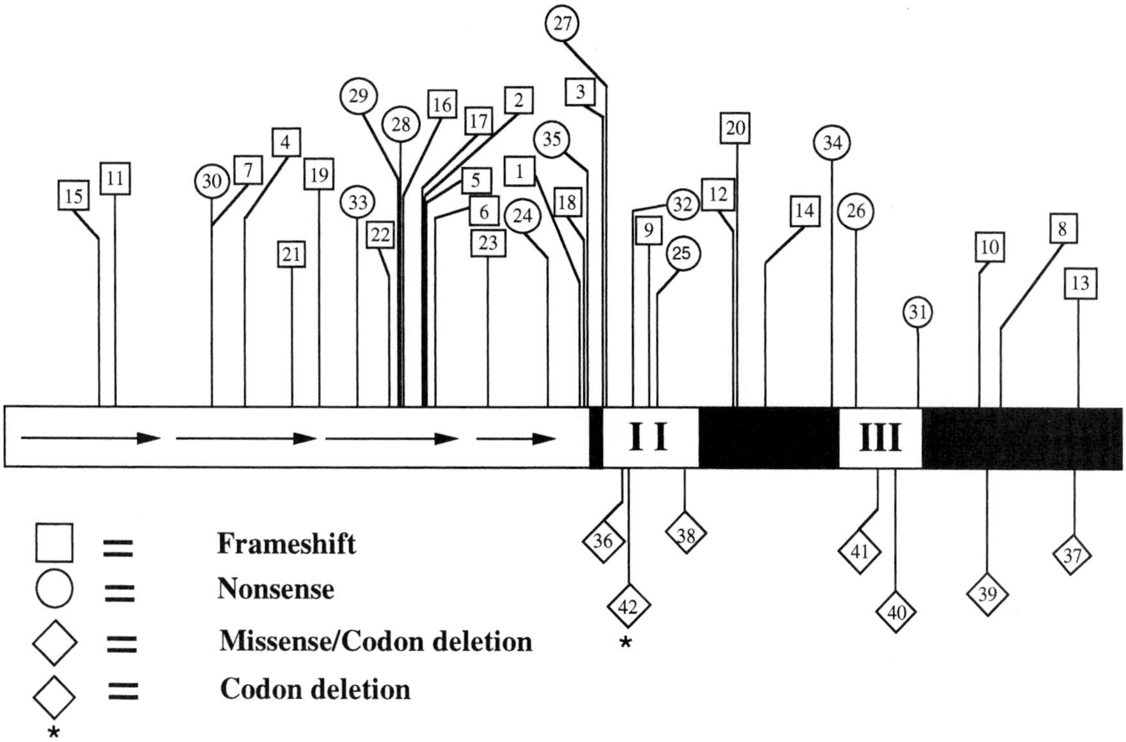

Fig. 167-1 Diagram tabulating 42 intragenic mutations within the DAX1 protein as more specifically identified elsewhere.[94] Although the frameshift and nonsense mutations were distributed throughout the protein molecule, the mutations resulting in single amino acid changes were localized to the C-terminal half of the protein in the putative ligand-binding domain (LBD). (*From Zhang et al.[94] Used by permission.*)

have been published,[44,100–103] and two new missense mutations have been reported, W291C and K382N.[103] Both of these missense mutations map to the same hydrophobic core of the putative LBD as those in our report proposing the model.[94]

Gonadal mosaicism for a *DAX1* mutation has been described (Fig. 167-3), which has important implications for genetic counseling.[94] The matriarch of a three-generation family had a carrier daughter and an affected son with a 23 bp frameshift deletion in *DAX1*, but she did not carry this mutation in her blood. The results were confirmed on independent blood samples redrawn from each of the family members, and two additional buccal brushings from the matriarch did not identify a mutation in her by PCR. The matrilineal relationships within the family were affirmed by mitochondrial D-loop sequencing.[97] Based on the observation of gonadal mosaicism in this family, if a boy with AHC and a *DAX1* mutation is the son of a noncarrier female, she must be counseled that there is the possibility that she may have other offspring with this mutation, either affected males or carrier females, despite the absence of a detectable mutation in the genomic DNA from her somatic cells.

While AHC associated with *DAX1* mutations is clearly an X-linked disease, early experience showed that girls may occasionally be affected.[104] In a family with AHC and GKD, a 7.5-month-old girl was hypoglycemic and unarousable after a nap. She had a large amount of glycerol in her urine and hypoplastic adrenals at autopsy. Based on this, as well as experience with Lyonization in

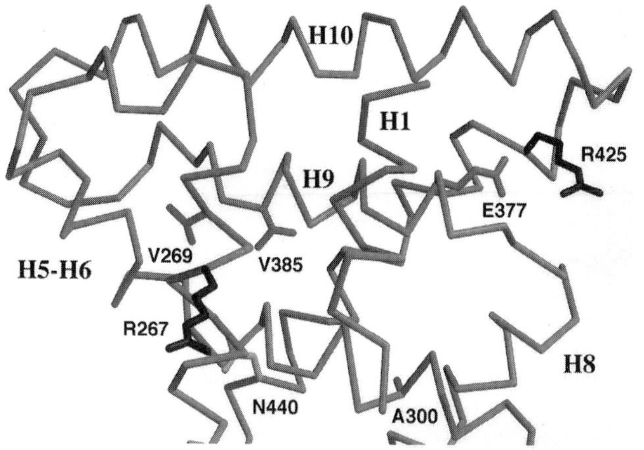

Fig. 167-2 Model of the DAX1 putative LBD hydrophobic core showing the residues altered by mutations involving single amino acids that cause AHC.[94] The model was generated by homology with the solved structures of rTRα_1[98] and hRXRα.[99] (*From Zhang et al.[94] Used by permission.*)

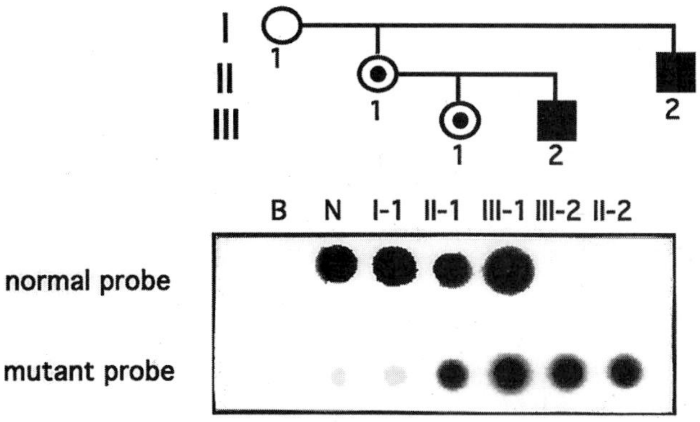

Fig. 167-3 Gonadal mosaicism in a family with a 23 bp frameshift deletion.[94] DNA sequencing data were confirmed by allele-specific oligonucleotide (ASO) hybridization of PCR amplification products. The mother (I-1) of a carrier daughter (II-1) and an affected son (II-2) did not carry the deletion. B = blank control and N = normal individual. (*From Zhang et al.[94] Used by permission.*)

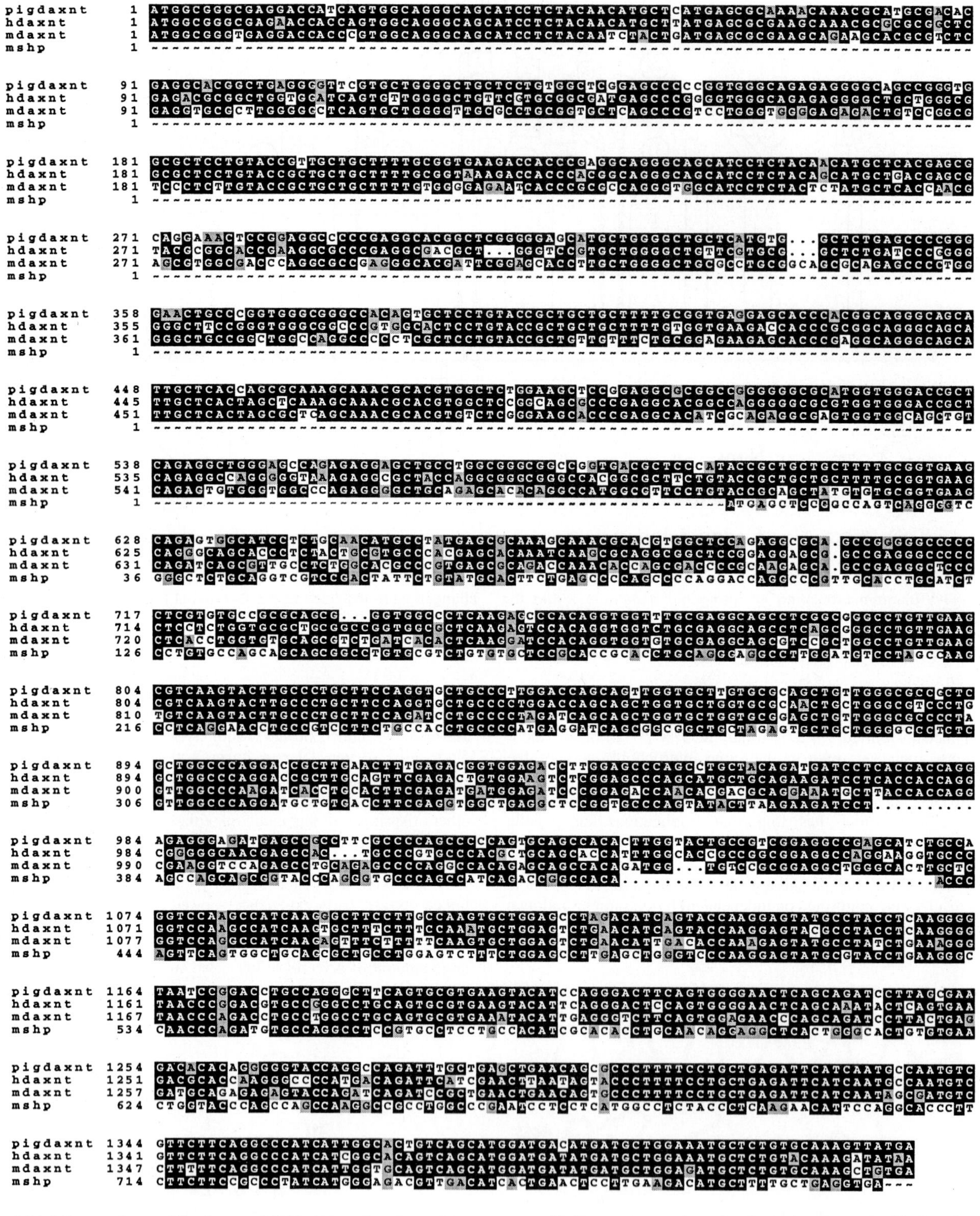

Fig. 167-4 Comparison of the human DAX1 deduced amino acid sequence with its porcine and murine homologues and with the closely related nuclear hormone receptor, SHP. (*Adapted from Vilain et al.*[66] *Drawn by M. Patel.*)

other X-linked disorders, one should counsel a family that a pregnancy with a female carrier fetus has a low but not impossible risk for developing AHC, and one may wish to consider a plasma ACTH level test for such girls in the neonatal period.

Pathogenesis of AHC

DAX1 is an unusual member of the nuclear hormone receptor superfamily with closest resemblance to other superfamily members in the C-terminal portion coding for the putative LBD.[43,59,78,105] The deduced amino acid sequences of the porcine homologue, pDAX1, and the murine homologue, Ahch, show 79 percent and 66 percent identity, and 80 percent and 69 percent similarity, respectively, with the human sequence[66,106–109] (Fig. 167-4). The N-terminal half of DAX1, which differs strikingly from most other nuclear hormone receptors,[78] does not include a canonical zinc finger structure, but does contain cysteine residues

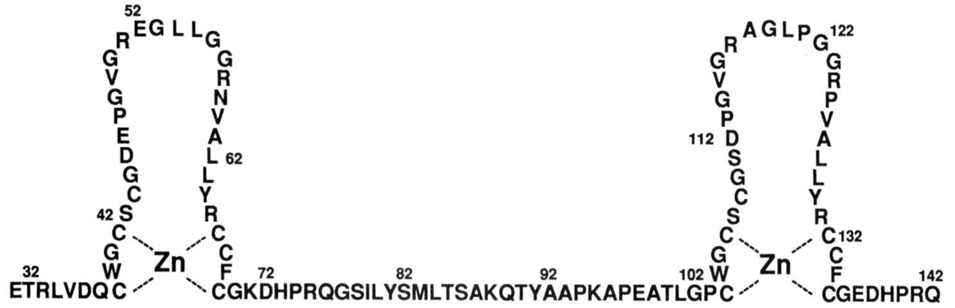

Fig. 167-5 Putative zinc finger domain in the N-terminal half of DAX1. The interaction of the zinc ions was drawn arbitrarily with residues 41 and 107, but the interaction could be with cysteines 41 or 43 and 107 or 109. (*From Guo et al.*[43] *Used by permission.*)

that are located appropriately for interaction with zinc ions (Fig. 167-5). All ten of these cysteine residues are conserved in the human, porcine, and murine deduced sequences.[66]

The closest relative to DAX1 is the SHP,[110] which also lacks a conventional DBD, but has one of the 3.5 N-terminal repeats found in DAX1. SHP interacts with several other nuclear hormone receptors to serve as a negative regulator in receptor-dependent signaling pathways.

DAX1 is expressed in the human hypothalamus, pituitary, fetal and adult adrenals, ovaries and testes,[59,69] and in these same tissues in the developing mouse.[108] *In situ* hybridization in fetal mouse shows that the mouse *DAX1* homologue, *Ahch*, is expressed in the adrenals on day 12.5 days post coitum (dpc), one day following the development of the adrenal primordium from the urogenital ridge, and expression persists.[108] In the gonads of male and female mouse fetuses, *Ahch* is expressed initially at 11.5 dpc, which corresponds to the first expression of *Sry* and the initial appearance of differentiation in the testes. Subsequently, ovarian expression of *Ahch* persists at similar levels, but testicular expression is reduced considerably.

The tissue profile of expression for *Ftz-F1* is similar to *Ahch*, but the temporal profiles differ.[111,112] *Ftz-F1* is the murine homologue of steroidogenic factor 1 (*SF1*), a nuclear receptor that regulates expression of a number of steroidogenic genes. *Ftz-F1* is expressed in the ventromedial nucleus of the hypothalamus, the anterior pituitary, the adrenal cortex, and the gonads of both sexes. However, *Ftz-F1* appears 3.5 days earlier than *Ahch*, at 9 dpc in the urogenital ridge. Development of the ventromedial nucleus and expression of LH and FSH are disrupted in *Ftz-F1* knockout mice, and these animals completely lack adrenal tissue.[113,114] These observations led to the hypothesis that SF1 and DAX1 may act in a concerted fashion during the normal development of the hypothalamic-pituitary-gonadal axis.[115]

There are conflicting data regarding a hypothetical interaction between SF1 and DAX1. The identification of potential SF1 response elements (REs) in similar positions in the human *DAX1*[95,105] and murine *Ahch* promoters[108] is consistent with the temporal pattern of expression suggesting that SF1 would act upstream of DAX1. SF1 binds specifically to this RE.[105] Transfection experiments have been contradictory. Transfection with a reporter construct containing various portions of the *DAX1* promoter in an adrenal cortical cell line that normally expresses DAX1 and SF1 showed the importance of the SF1 RE, and cotransfection with an SF1-expressing vector stimulated *DAX1* promoter expression in the presence of the SF1 RE.[116] Transfections in adrenal cortical cells that do not normally express DAX1 or in Leydig-derived cells, however, suggested that the SF1 RE was not required for DAX1 expression.[111] *DAX1* expression was not impaired in *SF1* knockout mice,[111] leading to the conclusion that DAX1 and SF1 interact in a common developmental pathway, but that SF1 is not required for the expression of *DAX1*. These contradictory observations may reflect tissue-dependent differences in the regulation of *DAX1* expression, perhaps with the involvement of additional factors in various tissues.[66]

DAX1 has the structure of a transcription factor,[43,59,78] and its nearest relative identified to date is a negative regulator in other nuclear receptor signaling pathways.[110] DAX1 also acts as an inhibitory regulator. Coexpression of DAX1 and SF1 inhibits transactivation mediated by SF1.[117] This does not appear to involve DAX1-SF1 heterodimerization. Although residues in the N-terminal portion of DAX1 interact directly with SF1, the heterodimerization does not alter SF1 binding to DNA containing the SF1 RE. A C-terminal portion of DAX1, however, contains a transcriptional-silencing domain.[117,118] Naturally occurring C-terminal mutations and single amino acid changes (R267P and V269del) reduce transcriptional silencing.[117,119] Silencing by the C-terminal DAX1 residues varies with promoter and cell type, suggesting involvement of additional factors, the abundance of which may vary with the cell type.[119] One such factor that is involved is the N-CoR, which is recruited by DAX1 to SF1.[118] DAX1 transcriptional repression is mediated by DAX1 binding to DNA hairpin structures that are found in the human steroidogenic acute regulatory protein (*StAR*) and murine *Dax1* promoters, and DAX1 decreases *StAR* RNA expression and steroidogenesis in murine Y-1 adrenocortical tumor cells.[120] The close proximity of the SF1 and DAX1 REs in the *Dax1* and *StAR* promoters suggests that DAX1 alters SF1 binding through an allosteric inhibition mechanism.[120]

ASSOCIATION OF DAX1 TANDEM DUPLICATIONS WITH DOSAGE-SENSITIVE SEX REVERSAL (DSS)

Tandem duplication of a 160 kb region in Xp21 that includes *DAX1* results in DSS, specifically, ambiguous genitalia or phenotypically female external genitalia in XY individuals.[121–123] *DAX1* was a candidate for DSS, because it was within the critical region and coded for a putative transcription factor expressed in the hypothalamic-pituitary-adrenal/gonadal axis.[59,69,109,122] *DAX1* is evolving extremely rapidly,[106,109,124] although not quite as rapidly as *SRY*.[125,126] The evolutionary rate for *DAX1* may be coincidental or it may reflect the importance of DAX1 as a possible SRY antagonist in the principal pathway for sex determination.[127] The use of structural motifs as REs by both DAX1 and SRY is intriguing.[120]

One model for mammalian sex determination hypothesizes that a gene product, unknown at the time the model was proposed and designated Z, is a negative regulator of male-specific gene expression, and SRY antagonizes the activity of Z.[128,129] According to this model, if Z is on the X chromosome, then a normal 46,XX individual would be genotype Z/Z, the expression of male-specific genes would be inhibited, and the phenotype would be female. A normal 46, XY individual would be genotype Z/SRY, the inhibition of male-specific genes would be antagonized, and the phenotype would be male. A tandem duplication of Z would have no effect on an XX individual who would be ZZ/Z, but in an XY individual with the ZZ/SRY genotype, the extra dose of Z would exceed the antagonistic function of SRY and the phenotype would be ambiguous or female.

It appears that DAX1 may be Z. When *Ahch* is overexpressed transgenically in *Mus musculus musculus* carrying a Y chromosome from the *Poschiavinus* strain of *Mus musculus domesticus*, which has a low level of SRY expressed, XY mice are phenotypically female.[130] In *Mus musculus musculus* animals, which do not carry the "weak" Y, sex reversal is not observed. The results suggest DAX1 antagonizes SRY. The requirement of a mouse strain with diminished SRY expression for observation of the sex reversal may be due to the nature of the model, but also could relate to rapid evolution of sex-determining mechanisms between mouse and human, or by the presence of one or more additional genes within the DSS locus acting in concert with *DAX1*.

DAX1 is involved in testis development. It is expressed in Leydig[110] and Sertoli cells.[130] In the rat testis, Sertoli *DAX1* gene expression varies during the spermatogenic cycle, peaking in the androgen-sensitive phase.[131] In cultured Sertoli cells, FSH down-regulates *DAX1* expression in a transcription- and translation-dependent fashion. Disruption of murine *Ahch* expression by Cre-mediated targeted deletion of exon 2 results in progressive testicular germinal epithelial regression, indicating a critical role for this gene product in maintaining spermatogenesis.[132] The targeted disruption of *Ahch* by this construct had no effect on ovarian development or female fertility, effects that would be anticipated if DAX1 is Z[127] and if the intact exon 1 did not influence the phenotype. Whether the absence of ovarian changes represents evidence that DAX1 is not Z, or is due to partial disruption of Ahch expression generated by the murine construct or recognized differences in sex determination between mouse and human, remains to be determined.

SF1 and WT1 act synergistically to promote expression of the Müllerian inhibiting substance gene, *MIS*, in male sexual development, and DAX1 antagonizes this synergy, possibly by direct SF1-DAX1 interaction.[133] Interestingly, human *WT1* mutations result in the WAGR contiguous gene syndrome, and the Denys-Drash and Frasier syndromes. In all three syndromes, 46, XX individuals generally develop as normal phenotypic females, but most 46, XY individuals have features of hypogonadism, sexual ambiguity, or male pseudohermaphroditism.[2] These human mutations of the autosomal *WT1* would decrease the ratio of WT1/DAX1, inhibiting the SF1-WT1 synergy, favoring SF1-DAX1 interaction and antagonizing male-specific gene expression.[133] Targeted disruption of the murine homologue of *SF1* results in apoptosis of cells in the embryonic gonads of both sexes beginning about E12.0 and eventually the absence of gonads, after initial normal migration of the primordial germ cells.[112]

In summary, *DAX1* is contained within the DSS critical region, is involved in gonadal development, is evolving extremely rapidly like *SRY*, and, when its murine homologue is expressed transgenically in mice with diminished SRY expression, is associated with DSS. Therefore, *DAX1* is a candidate gene for human DSS.[126,134–137]

OTHER CAUSES OF AHC

In addition to the X-linked form of AHC that is due to deletion of, or mutations in, *DAX1*, there are at least six other disorders catalogued in MIM[2] that are associated with AHC, all of which are presumed to be, or definitely are, inherited in an autosomal recessive manner (Table 167-1).

ACTH Deficiency (MIM 201400)

Children of both sexes have been reported with isolated ACTH deficiency.[138–144] Linkage to the corticotropin-releasing hormone gene has been demonstrated.[145]

In one patient, who presented with hypoglycemia as a neonate, a defect in the enzymatic cleavage of ACTH from proopiomelanocortin was considered.[144,146] The ACTH was not measurable at baseline or after corticotropin-releasing hormone stimulation. However, ACTH precursors were present and were responsive to corticotropin-releasing hormone stimulation and glucocorticoid suppression. No mutation was detected in the proopiomelanocortin coding region.

Prenatal diagnosis for ACTH deficiency has been carried out by measuring maternal plasma estriol levels.[143]

AHC with Absent Pituitary LH (MIM 202150)

AHC with selective absence of pituitary LH was reported in three of four sibs in one family, two girls and a boy, and therefore was considered to be an autosomal recessive disorder.[6] The AHC was the miniature adult form. The male had a micropenis and cryptorchidism. GK activity was reduced in two of the infants, but it was not consistent using two different assays in one patient and was not in the GKD range. Haplotype analysis excluded linkage to Xp21.

Cytomegalic Form of AHC with Autosomal Recessive Inheritance (MIM 202155)

Two sisters were reported with AHC.[147] The first girl was small-for-dates and died at 7 weeks of age. Her severely hypoplastic adrenals were made up of a fetal zone with large eosinophilic cells, irregularly organized and extending to the capsule, without a clear definitive zone. The second girl also showed intrauterine growth retardation and had AHC clinically and biochemically, with no adrenals identified by CT scan at 1 year of age. She was treated with hydrocortisone and fludrocortisone.

Pena-Shokeir Syndrome, Type 1 (MIM 208150)

Pena-Shokeir syndrome, type 1, also known as arthrogryposis multiplex congenita with pulmonary hypoplasia, the fetal akinesia sequence, or the fetal akinesia deformation sequence,[2] is a heterogeneous disorder.[148] In addition to the multiple contractures, ankyloses, pulmonary hypoplasia, and cryptorchidism, these patients have dysmorphic facial features including hypertelorism, depressed nasal tip, micrognathia, and poorly folded, posteriorly rotated ears.[149–151] The reduction in anterior horn cells and diffuse muscle atrophy suggest a primary motor neuropathy.[152] Adrenal hypoplasia of the miniature adult type has been reported.[152] The association of AHC with cryptorchidism, suggesting hypogonadism, is intriguing.

Holoprosencephaly, Alobar (MIM 236100)

Holoprosencephaly 1, alobar type, or HPE1 maps to 21q 22.3, and may be associated with endocrine dysgenesis (see Chap. 250).[2] Two brothers were reported with this association and with micropenis.[153] The boy who died and was autopsied had adrenal hypoplasia and no pituitary gland. The association with central nervous system abnormalities and the reported absence of the fetal cortex in a boy who died at 1 day of age[153] are consistent with the miniature adult form of AHC.

Hypoadrenocorticism, Familial (MIM 240200)

This is probably a heterogeneous group of patients who share common adrenal pathological features, specifically those of the miniature adult form of adrenal hypoplasia.[2] Another characteristic feature is the lack of hypoaldosteronism,[28,154] and the endocrine defect may be limited to the glucocorticoid pathway.[2] Hyperplasia of basophilic pituitary cells has been reported.[7]

Meckel Syndrome (MIM 249000)

First reported by Meckel in 1822,[155] this disorder was called dysencephalia splanchnocystica by Gruber,[156] and is referred to as Meckel syndrome or Meckel-Gruber syndrome.[2] The features are numerous and quite variable, but a characteristic constellation is a posterior encephalocele, polydactyly, and cystic dysplasia of the kidneys.[2,151] Cryptorchidism, and incompletely developed and ambiguous genitalia are frequently observed, and adrenal hypoplasia and aplasia are occasional abnormalities.[2,151] The Meckel syndrome locus maps to a 1 cM interval in 17q22 in Finnish families, in which affected patients share a common haplotype,[157,158] and examination of linkage in families from other ethnic groups suggests locus heterogeneity, which may explain, at least in part, the clinical heterogeneity.[159]

REFERENCES

1. Kelch RP, Virdis R, Rapaport R, Greig F, Levine LS, New MI: Congenital adrenal hypoplasia. *Pediatr Adolesc Endocrinol* **13**:156, 1984.
2. Online Mendelian Inheritance in Man, MIM. Center for Medical Genetics, Johns Hopkins University (Baltimore, MD) and National Center for Biotechnology Information, National Library of Medicine (Bethesda, MD). www.ncbi.nim.nih.gov/OMIM. 1996.
3. Benirischke K: Adrenals in anencephaly and hydrocephaly. *Obstet Gynecol* **8**:412, 1956.
4. O'Donohoe NV, Holland PD: Familial congenital adrenal hypoplasia. *Arch Dis Child* **43**:717, 1968.
5. Laverty CRA, Fortune DW, Beischer NA: Congenital idiopathic adrenal hypoplasia. *Obstet Gynecol* **41**:655, 1973.
6. Burke BA, Wick M, King R, Thompson T, Hansen J, Darras BT, Francke U, et al.: Congenital adrenal hypoplasia and selective absence of pituitary luteinizing hormone — A new autosomal recessive disorder. *Am J Med Genet* **31**:75, 1988.
7. Boyd JF, MacDonald AM: Adrenal cortical hypoplasia in siblings. *Arch Dis Child* **35**:561, 1960.
8. Hensleigh PA, Moore WV, Wilson K, Tulchinsky D: Congenital X-linked adrenal hypoplasia. *Obstet Gynecol* **52**:228, 1978.
9. Marsden HB, Zakhour HD: Cytomegalic adrenal hypoplasia with pituitary cytomegaly. *Virchows Arch Abt A Path Anat Histol* **378**:105, 1978.
10. Bartley JA, Hayford JT, Perkins J, Firminger HI, McCabe ERB: Glycerol kinase deficiency: An X-linked disorder associated with congenital adrenal hypoplasia, myopathy and developmental delay. *Proc Greenwood Gen Ctr* **2**:110, 1983.
11. Renier WO, Nabbe FAE, Hustinx TWJ, Veerkamp JH, Otten BJ, Ter Laak HJ, Ter Haar BGA, et al.: Congenital adrenal hypoplasia, progressive muscular dystrophy, and severe mental retardation, in association with glycerol kinase deficiency, in male sibs. *Clin Genet* **24**:243, 1983.
12. Seltzer WK, Firminger H, Klein J, Pike A, Fennessey P, McCabe ERB: Adrenal dysfunction in glycerol kinase deficiency. *Biochem Med* **33**:189, 1985.
13. Lack EE, Kozakewich HPW: Embryology, developmental anatomy, and selected aspects of non-neoplastic pathology, in Lack EE (ed): *Pathology of the Adrenal Glands*. New York, Churchill Livingstone, 1990, p 1.
14. Favara BE, Franciosi RA, Miles V: Idiopathic adrenal hypoplasia in children. *Am J Clin Pathol* **57**:287, 1972.
15. Le SQ, Kutteh WH: Monosomy 7 syndrome associated with congenital adrenal hypoplasia and male pseudohermaphroditism. *Obstet Gynecol* **87**:854, 1996.
16. Chen H, Hoffman WH, Kusyk CJ, Tuck-Miller M, Hoffman MG, Davis LS: De novo dup (5p) in a patient with congenital hypoplasia of the adrenal gland. *Am J Med Genet* **55**:489, 1995.
17. Matsumura G, England MA: *Embryology Colouring Book*. London, Wolfe, 1992.
18. Lack EE, Kozakewich HPW: Adrenal neuroblastoma, ganglioneuroblastoma, and related tumors, in Lack EE (ed): *Pathology of the Adrenal Glands*. New York, Churchill Livingstone, 1990, p 277.
19. Orth DN, Kovacs WJ, DeBold CR: The adrenal cortex, in Wilson JD, Foster DW (eds): *Williams Textbook of Endocrinology, 8th ed.* Philadelphia, WB Saunders, 1992, p 489.
20. Sucheston ME, Cannon MS: Development of zonular patterns in the human adrenal gland. *J Morphol* **126**:477, 1968.
21. Carr BR, Parker CR Jr, Porter JC, MacDonald PC, Simpson ER: Regulation of steroid secretion by adrenal tissue of a human anencephalic fetus. *J Clin Endocrinol Metab* **50**:870, 1980.
22. Vinson GP, Whitehouse B, Hinson J: *The Adrenal Cortex*. Englewood Cliffs, NJ, Prentice Hall, 1992.
23. Zajicek G, Ariel I, Arber N: The streaming adrenal cortex: Direct evidence of centripetal migration of adenocytes by estimation of cell turnover rate. *J Endocrinol* **111**:477, 1986.
24. Skelton FR: Adrenal regeneration and adrenal regeneration hypertension. *Physiol Rev* **39**:162, 1959.
25. Belloni AS, Neri G, Musajo FG, Andreis PA, Boscaro M, D'Agostino D, Rebuffat P, et al.: Investigations on the morphology and function of adrenocortical tissue regenerated from gland capsular fragments autotransplanted in the musculus gracilis of the rat. *Endocrinology* **126**:3251, 1990.
26. Brochner-Mortensen K: Familial occurrence of Addison's disease. *Acta Med Scand* **156**:205, 1956.
27. Meakin JW, Nelson DH, Thorn GW: Addison's disease in two brothers. *J Clin Endocrinol Metab* **19**:726, 1959.
28. Stempfel RS Jr, Engel FL: A congenital, familial syndrome of adrenocortical insufficiency without hypoaldosteronism. *J Pediatr* **57**:443, 1960.
29. Uttley WS: Familial congenital adrenal hypoplasia. *Arch Dis Child* **43**:724, 1968.
30. Migeon CJ, Kenny FM, Kowarski A, Snipes CA, Spaulding JS, Finkelstein JW, Blizzard RM: The syndrome of congenital adrenocortical unresponsiveness to ACTH. Report of six cases. *Pediatr Res* **2**:501, 1968.
31. Weiss L, Mellinger RC: Congenital adrenal hypoplasia — An X-linked disease. *J Med Genet* **7**:27, 1970.
32. Martin MM: Familial Addison's disease. *Birth Defects Orig Art Ser* **VII**:98, 1971.
33. Sperling MA, Wolfsen AR, Fisher DA: Congenital adrenal hypoplasia: An isolated defect of organogenesis. *J Pediatr* **82**:444, 1973.
34. Golden MP, Lippe BM, Kaplan SA: Congenital adrenal hypoplasia and hypogonadotropic hypogonadism. *Am J Dis Child* **131**:1117, 1977.
35. Zachmann M, Illig R, Prader A: Gonadotropin deficiency and cryptorchidism in three prepubertal brothers with congenital adrenal hypoplasia. *J Pediatr* **97**:255, 1980.
36. Wittenberg DF: Familial X-linked adrenocortical hypoplasia association with androgenic precocity. *Arch Dis Child* **56**:633, 1981.
37. Hay ID, Smail PJ, Forsyth CC: Familial cytomegalic adrenocortical hypoplasia: An X-linked syndrome of pubertal failure. *Arch Dis Child* **56**:715, 1981.
38. Petersen KE, Bille T, Jacobsen BB, Iversen T: X-linked congenital adrenal hypoplasia: A study of five generations of a Greenlandic family. *Acta Paediatr Scand* **71**:947, 1982.
39. Preeyasombat C, Sriphrapradang A, Chaubtam L: X-linked congenital adrenal hypoplasia: Proposal pathogenesis. *J Med Assoc Thai* **72**:164, 1989.
40. McCabe ERB, Fennessey PV, Guggenheim MA, Miles BS, Bullen WW, Sceats DJ, Goodman SI: Human glycerol kinase deficiency with hyperglycerolemia and glyceroluria. *Biochem Biophys Res Commun* **78**:1327, 1977.
41. Guggenheim MA, McCabe ERB, Roig M, Goodman SI, Lum GM, Bullen WW, Ringel SP: Glycerol kinase deficiency with neuromuscular, skeletal and adrenal abnormalities. *Ann Neurol* **7**:441, 1980.
42. Worley KC, Ellison KA, Zhang Y-H, Wang D-F, Mason J, Roth EJ, Adams V, et al.: Yeast artificial chromosome cloning in the glycerol kinase and adrenal hypoplasia congenita region of Xp21. *Genomics* **16**:407, 1993.
43. Guo W, Mason JS, Stone CG, Morgan SA, Madu SI, Baldini A, Lindsay EA, et al.: Diagnosis of X-linked adrenal hypoplasia congenita by mutation analysis of the DAX-1 gene. *JAMA* **274**:324, 1995.
44. Peter M, Viemann M, Partsch C-J, Sippell WG: Congenital adrenal hypoplasia: Clinical spectrum, experience with hormonal diagnosis, and report on new point mutations of the DAX-1 gene. *J Clin Endocrinol Metab* **83**:2666, 1998.
45. Baker WDC, Wise G, Mezger ML: Cytomegalic adrenal hypoplasia in a 4 $\frac{1}{2}$-year-old boy. *Am J Dis Child* **114**:180, 1967.
46. Zondek LH, Zondek T: Congenital adrenal hypoplasia in two infants. *Acta Paediatr Scand* **57**:250, 1968.
47. Pakravan P, Kenny FM, Depp R, Allen AC: Familial congenital absence of the adrenal glands: Evaluation of the glucocorticoid, mineralocorticoid and estrogen metabolism in the perinatal period. *J Pediatr* **84**:74, 1974.
48. Prader A, Zachman M, Illig R: Luteinizing hormone deficiency in hereditary congenital adrenal hypoplasia. *J Pediatr* **86**:421, 1975.
49. Hay ID: Pubertal failure in congenital adrenocortical hypoplasia. *Lancet* **II**:1035, 1977.
50. Chaussain JL, Roger M, Job JC: Insuffisance gonadotrope associee a l'hypoplasie surrenale congenitale a forme cytomegalique. *Arch Fr Pediatr* **39**:109, 1982.
51. Cohen HN, Hay ID, Beastall GH, Thomson JA: Failure of adrenal androgen to induce puberty in familial cytomegalic adrenocortical hypoplasia. *Lancet* **II**:1471, 1982.
52. Virdis R, Levine LS, Levy D, Pang S, Rapaport R, New MI: Congenital adrenal hypoplasia: Two new cases. *Endocrinol Invest* **6**:51, 1983.
53. Martin MM, Martin ALA: The syndrome of congenital hereditary adrenal hypoplasia and hypogonadotropic hypogonadism. *Int J Adol Med Health* **1**:119, 1985.

54. Kikuchi K, Kaji M, Momoi T, Mikawa H, Shigematsu Y, Sudo M: Failure to induce puberty in a man with X-linked congenital adrenal hypoplasia and hypogonadotropic hypogonadism by pulsatile administration of low-dose gonadotropin-releasing hormone. *Acta Endocrinol* **114**:153, 1987.
55. Wise JE, Matalon R, Morgan AM, McCabe ERB: Phenotypic features of patients with congenital adrenal hypoplasia and glycerol kinase deficiency. *Am J Dis Child* **141**:744, 1987.
56. Partsch C-J, Sippell WG: Hypothalamic hypogonadism in congenital adrenal hypoplasia. *Horm Metab Res* **21**:623, 1989.
57. Kletter GB, Gorski JL, Kelch RP: Congenital adrenal hypoplasia and isolated gonadotropin deficiency. *Trends Endocrinol Metab* **2**:123, 1991.
58. Zachmann M, Fuchs E, Prader A: Progressive high frequency hearing loss: An additional feature in the syndrome of congenital adrenal hypoplasia and gonadotropin deficiency. *Eur J Pediatr* **151**:167, 1992.
59. Zanaria E, Muscatelli F, Bardoni B, Strom TM, Guioli S, Guo W, Lalli E, et al.: A novel and unusual member of the nuclear hormone receptor superfamily is responsible for X-linked adrenal hypoplasia congenita. *Nature* **372**:635, 1994.
60. Muscatelli F, Strom TM, Walker AP, Zanaria E, Recan D, Meindl A, Bardoni B, et al.: Mutations in the DAX-1 gene give rise to both X-linked adrenal hypoplasia congenita and hypogonadotropic hypogonadism. *Nature* **372**:672, 1994.
61. Matfin G, Sheaves R, Muscatelli F, Walker A, Monaco A, Grant D, Nwose O, et al.: Gene deletion causing adrenal hypoplasia congenita and hypogonadotropic hypogonadism. *Clin Endocrinol* **40**:807, 1994.
62. Habiby RL, Boepple P, Nachtigall L, Sluss PM, Crowley WF Jr, Jameson JL: Adrenal hypoplasia congenita with hypogonadotropic hypogonadism: Evidence that DAX1 mutations lead to combined hypothalamic and pituitary defects in gonadotropin production. *J Clin Invest* **98**:1055, 1996.
63. McCabe ERB: Sex and the single DAX1: Too little is bad, but can we have too much? *J Clin Invest* **98**:881, 1996.
64. Yanase T, Takayanagi R, Oba K, Nisiji Y, Ohe K, Nawata H: New mutations of DAX1 genes in two Japanese patients with X-linked congenital adrenal hypoplasia and hypogonadotropic hypogonadism. *J Clin Endocrinol Metab* **81**:530, 1996.
65. Schwartz M, Blichfeldt S, Muller J: X-linked adrenal hypoplasia in a Greenlandic family. Detection of a missense mutation (N440I) in the DAX-1 genes: Implication for genetic counseling and carrier diagnosis. *Hum Genet* **99**:83, 1997.
66. Vilain E, Guo W, Patel M, McCabe ERB: X-linked adrenal hypoplasia congenita (AHC): A DAX1 deficiency disorder, in Chrousos G, Olefsky J, Samols E (eds): *Hormone Resistance*. Philadelphia, Lippincott-Raven, (In press), .
67. Matsumoto T, Kondoh T, Yoshimoto M, Fujieda K, Matsuura N, Matsuda I, Miike T, et al.: Complex glycerol kinase deficiency: Molecular genetic, cytogenetic, and clinical studies of five Japanese patients. *Am J Med Genet* **31**:603, 1988.
68. Goonewardena P, Dahl N, Ritzen M, van Ommen GJ, Pettersson U: Molecular Xp deletion in a male: Suggestion of a locus for hypogonadotropic hypogonadism distal to the glycerol kinase and adrenal hypoplasia loci. *Clin Genet* **35**:5, 1989.
69. Guo W, Burris TP, McCabe ERB: Expression of DAX-1, the gene responsible for X-linked adrenal hypoplasia congenita and hypogonadotropic hypogonadism, in the hypothalamic-pituitary-adrenal/gonadal axis. *Biochem Molec Med* **56**:8, 1995.
70. Takahashi T, Shoji Y, Haraguchi N, Takahashi I, Takada G: Active hypothalamic-pituitary-gonadal axis in an infant with X-linked adrenal hypoplasia congenita. *J Pediatr* **130**:485, 1997.
71. Kaiserman KB, Nakamoto JM, Geffner ME, McCabe ERB: Minipuberty of infancy and adolescent pubertal function in adrenal hypoplasia congenita. *J Pediatr* **133**:300, 1998.
72. Jones D, Kay M, Craigen W, McCabe ERB, Hawkins H, Dominey A: Coal-black hyperpigmentation at birth in a child with congenital adrenal hypoplasia. *J Am Acad Dermatol* **33**:323, 1995.
73. Sakura N, Nishimura S, Kawahara N, Komazawa Y, Yamaguchi S: Asthma as the first presenting symptom of complex glycerol kinase deficiency. *Acta Paediatr Scand* **80**:723, 1991.
74. van der Ent CK, de Vroede MA, Augustijn PB, Wit JM: A special case of congenital adrenal hypoplasia and acute bilateral infantile striatal necrosis. *Acta Paediatr* **84**:957, 1995.
75. Fries MH, Lebo RV, Schonberg SA, Golabi M, Seltzer WK, Gitelman SE, Golbus MS: Mental retardation locus in Xp21 chromosome microdeletion. *Am J Med Genet* **46**:363, 1993.
76. Billuart P, Vinet MC, des Portes V, Llense S, Richard L, Moutard ML, Recan D, et al.: Identification by STS PCR screening of a microdeletion in Xp21.3-22.1 associated with non-specific mental retardation. *Hum Mol Genet* **5**:977, 1996.
77. Baranzini SE, del Rey G, Nigro N, Szijan I, Chamoles N, Cresto JC: Patient with an Xp21 contiguous gene deletion syndrome in association with agenesis of the corpus callosum. *Am J Med Genet* **70**:216, 1997.
78. Burris TP, Guo W, McCabe ERB: The gene responsible for adrenal hypoplasia congenita, DAX1, encodes a nuclear hormone receptor that defines a new class within the superfamily, in Conn PM (ed): *Recent Progress in Hormone Research*. Bethesda, MD, The Endocrine Society, 1996, p 241.
79. Herskowitz I: Functional inactivation of genes by dominant negative mutations. *Nature* **329**:219, 1987.
80. Kasahara N, Dozy AM, Kan YW: Tissue-specific targeting of retroviral vectors through ligand-receptor interactions. *Science* **266**:1373, 1994.
81. Han X, Kasahara N, Kan YW: Ligand-directed retroviral targeting of human breast cancer cells. *Proc Natl Acad Sci U S A* **92**:9747, 1995.
82. Douglas JT, Rogers BE, Rosenfeld ME, Michael SI, Feng M, Curiel DT: Targeted gene delivery by tropism-modified adenoviral vectors. *Nat Biotechnol* **14**:1574, 1996.
83. Feero WG, Li S, Rosenblatt JD, Sirianni N, Morgan JE, Partridge TA, Huang L, et al.: Selection and use of ligands for receptor-mediated gene delivery to myogenic cells. *Gene Ther* **4**:664, 1997.
84. Yajima T, Kanda T, Yoshiike K, Kitamura Y: Retroviral vector targeting human cells via c-Kit-stem cell factor interaction. *Hum Gene Ther* **9**:779, 1998.
85. Sawai K, Meruelo D: Cell-specific transfection of choriocarcinoma cells by using Sindbis virus hCG expressing chimeric vector. *Biochem Biophys Res Commun* **248**:315, 1998.
86. Tahka H: On the weight and structure of the adrenal glands and the factors affecting them, in children of 0–2 years. *Acta Paediatr Scand* **40**:1, 1951.
87. Spector WS (ed.): *Handbook of Biological Data*. Philadelphia, WB Saunders, 1956.
88. Schulz DM, Giordano DA, Schulz DH: Weights of organs of fetuses and infants. *Arch Pathol* **74**:244, 1962.
89. Eberlein WR: The fetal adrenal cortex, in Christy HP (ed.): *The Human Adrenal Cortex*. New York, Harper & Row, 1971, p 317.
90. Williamson R, Patil S, Bartley J, Greenberg F: Prenatal evaluation for glycerol kinase deficiency (GKD) associated with congenital adrenal hypoplasia. *Am J Hum Genet* **36**:200S, 1984.
91. Batch JA, Montalto J, Yong ABW, Gold H, Goss P, Warne GL: Three cases of congenital adrenal hypoplasia: A cause of salt-wasting and mortality in the neonatal period. *J Paediatr Child Health* **27**:108, 1991.
92. Akkurt I, Haagen M, Blunck W: Konnatale Nebennierenrindenhypoplasie. *Monatsschr Kinderheilkd* **141**:103, 1993.
93. Peter M, Partsch C-J, Dorr HG, Sippell WG: Prenatal diagnosis of congenital adrenal hypoplasia. *Horm Res* **46**:41, 1996.
94. Zhang Y-H, Guo W, Wagner RL, Huang B-L, McCabe L, Vilain E, Burris TP, et al.: DAX1 mutations map to putative structural domains in a deduced three-dimensional model. *Am J Hum Genet* **62**:855, 1998.
95. Guo W, Burris TP, Zhang Y-H, Huang B-L, Mason J, Copeland KC, Kupfer SR, et al.: Genomic sequence of the DAX1 gene: An orphan nuclear receptor responsible for X-linked adrenal hypoplasia congenita and hypogonadotropic hypogonadism. *J Clin Endocrinol Metab* **81**:2481, 1996.
96. Nakae J, Tajima T, Kusuda S, Kohda N, Okabe T, Shinohara N, Kato M, et al.: Truncation at the C-terminus of the DAX-1 protein impairs its biological actions in patients with X-linked adrenal hypoplasia congenita. *J Clin Endocrinol Metab* **81**:3680, 1996.
97. Mumm S, White MP, Thakker RV, Buetow KH, Schlessinger D: Mitochondrial DNA analysis shows common ancestry in two kindreds with X-linked recessive hypoparathyroidism and reveals a heteroplasmic silent mutation. *Am J Hum Genet* **60**:153, 1997.
98. Wagner RL, Apriletti JW, McGrath ME, West BL, Baxter JD, Fletterick RJ: A structural role for hormone in the thyroid hormone receptor. *Nature* **378**:690, 1995.
99. Bourguet W, Ruff M, Chambon P, Gronemeyer H, Moras D: Crystal structure of the ligand-binding domain of the human nuclear receptor RXR-alpha. *Nature* **375**:377, 1995.
100. Kinoshita E, Yoshimoto M, Motomura K, Kawaguchi T, Mori R, Baba T, Nishijo K, et al.: DAX-1 gene mutations and deletions in Japanese patients with adrenal hypoplasia congenita and hypogonadotropic hypogonadism. *Horm Res* **48**:29, 1997.

101. Hamaguchi K, Arikawa M, Yasu S, Kakuma T, Fukagawa K, Yanase T, Nawata H, et al.: Novel mutation of the DAX1 gene in a patient with X-linked adrenal hypoplasia congenita and hypogonadotropic hypogonadism. *Am J Med Genet* **76**:62, 1998.
102. Meloni A, Cao A, Rosatelli MC: New frameshift mutation in the DAX-1 gene in a patient with X-linked adrenal hypoplasia and hypogonadotropic hypogonadism. *Hum Mut* **8**:183, 1996.
103. Nakae J, Abe S, Tajima T, Shinohara N, Murashita M, Igarashi Y, Kusuda S, Suzuki J, Fujieda K: Three novel mutations and a de novo deletion mutation of the DAX-1 gene in patients with X-linked adrenal hypoplasia congenita. *J Clin Endo Metab* **82**:3835, 1997.
104. Bartley JA, Miller DK, Hayford JT, McCabe ERB: The concordance of X-linked glycerol kinase deficiency with X-linked adrenal hypoplasia in two families. *Lancet* **2**:733, 1982.
105. Burris TP, Guo W, Le T, McCabe ERB: Identification of a putative steroidogenic factor-1 response element in the DAX-1 promoter. *Biochem Biophys Res Commun* **214**:576, 1995.
106. Lahbib-Mansais Y, Barbosa A, Yerle M, Parma P, Milan D, Pailhoux E, Gellin J, et al.: Mapping in pigs of genes involved in sexual differentiation: AMH, WT1, FTZF1, SOX2, SOX9, AHC, and placental and embryonic CYP19. Accession Number U82466. *Cytogenet Cell Genet* **76**:109, 1997.
107. Guo W, Lovell RS, Zhang Y-H, Huang B-L, Burris TP, Craigen WJ, McCabe ERB: Ahch, the mouse homologue of DAX1: Cloning, characterization and synteny with GyK, the glycerol kinase locus. *Gene* **178**:31, 1996.
108. Bae DS, Schaefer ML, Partan BW, Muglia L: Characterization of the mouse DAX1 gene reveals evolutionary conservation of a unique amino-terminal motif and widespread expression in mouse tissue. *Endocrinology* **137**:3921, 1996.
109. Swain A, Zanaria E, Hacker A, Lovell-Badge R, Camerino G: Mouse Dax1 expression is consistent with a role in sex determination as well as in adrenal and hypothalamus function. *Nat Genet* **12**:404, 1996.
110. Seol W, Choi H-S, Moore DD: An orphan nuclear hormone receptor that lacks a DNA binding domain and heterodimerizes with other receptors. *Science* **272**:1336, 1996.
111. Ikeda Y, Swain A, Weber TJ, Hentges KE, Zanaria E, Lalli E, Tamai KT, et al.: Steroidogenic factor 1 and Dax-1 colocalize in multiple cell lineages: Potential links in endocrine development. *Mol Endocrinol* **10**:1261, 1996.
112. Ikeda Y, Shen W-H, Ingraham HA, Parker KL: Developmental expression of mouse steroidogenic factor-1, an essential regulator of the steroid hydroxylases. *Mol Endocrinol* **8**:654, 1994.
113. Luo X, Ikeda Y, Parker KL: A cell-specific nuclear receptor is essential for adrenal and gonadal development and sexual differentiation. *Cell* **77**:481, 1994.
114. Ikeda Y, Luo X, Abbud R, Nilson JH, Parker KL: The nuclear receptor steroidogenic factor 1 is essential for the formation of the ventromedial hypothalamic nucleus. *Mol Endocrinol* **9**:478, 1995.
115. Parker KL, Schimmer BP: The roles of the nuclear hormone receptor steroidogenic factor 1 in endocrine differentiation and development. *Trends Endocrinol Metab* **7**:203, 1996.
116. Vilain E, Guo W, Zhang Y-H, McCabe ERB: DAX1 gene expression upregulated by steroidogenic factor 1 in an adrenocortical carcinoma cell line. *Biochem Molec Med* **61**:1, 1997.
117. Ito M, Yu R, Jameson JL: DAX-1 inhibits SF-1-mediated transactivation via a carboxy-terminal domain that is deleted in adrenal hypoplasia congenita. *Mol Cell Biol* **17**:1476, 1997.
118. Crawford PA, Dorn C, Sadovsky Y, Milbrandt J: Nuclear receptor DAX-1 recruits nuclear receptor corepressor N-CoR to steroidogenic factor 1. *Mol Cell Biol* **18**:2949, 1998.
119. Lalli E, Bardoni B, Zazopoulos E, Wurtz JM, Strom TM, Moras D, Sassone-Corsi P: A transcriptional silencing domain in DAX-1 whose mutation causes adrenal hypoplasia congenita. *Mol Endocrinol* **11**:1950, 1997.
120. Zazopoulos E, Lalli E, Stocco DM, Sassone-Corsi P: DNA binding and transcriptional repression by DAX-1 blocks steroidogenesis. *Nature* **390**:311, 1997.
121. Arn P, Chen H, Tuck Muller CM, Mankinen C, Wachtel G, Li S, Shen CC, et al.: A sex-reversing locus in Xp21.2 to p22.11. *Hum Genet* **93**:389, 1994.
122. Bardoni B, Zanaria E, Guioli S, Floridia G, Worley KC, Tonini G, Ferrante E, et al.: A dosage sensitive locus at chromosome Xp21 is involved in male to female sex reversal. *Nat Genet* **7**:497, 1994.
123. Baumstark A, Barbi G, Djalali M, Geerkens C, Mitulla B, Mattfeldt T, Cabra del Almeida JC, et al.: Xp-duplications with and without sex reversal. *Hum Genet* **97**:79, 1996.
124. Patel M, Vilain E, Dorman K, Zhang Y-H, Huang B-L, Arnold A, Sinsheimer J, et al.: DAX1: Rapid evolution in primates suggests a role early in the sex determination pathway. *Am J Hum Genet* **63**:A188, 1998.
125. Whitfield S, Lovell-Badge R, Goodfellow PN: Rapid evolution of the sex-determining gene SRY. *Nature* **364**:713, 1993.
126. Tucker PK, Lundrigan BL: Rapid evolution of the sex determining locus in Old World mice and rats. *Nature* **364**:715, 1993.
127. Vilain E, McCabe ERB: Mammalian sex determination: From gonads to brain. *Mol Genet Metab* **65**:74, 1998.
128. Vilain E, McElreavey K, Herskowitz I, Fellous M: La determination du sexe: Faits et nouveaux concepts. *Medecine/Sciences* **8**:I, 1992.
129. McElreavey K, Vilain E, Abbas N, Herskowitz I, Fellous M: A regulatory cascade hypothesis for mammalian sex determination: SRY represses a negative regulator of male development. *Proc Natl Acad Sci U S A* **90**:3368, 1993.
130. Swain A, Narvaez V, Burgoyne P, Camerino G, Lovell-Badge R: Dax1 antagonizes Sry action in mammalian sex determination. *Nature* **364**:713, 1998.
131. Tamai KT, Monaco L, Alastalo TP, Lalli E, Parvinen M, Sassone-Corsi P: Hormonal and developmental regulation of DAX-1 expression in Sertoli cells. *Mol Endocrinol* **10**:1561, 1996.
132. Yu RN, Ito M, Saunders TL, Camper SA, Jameson JL: Role of Ahch in gonadal development and gametogenesis. *Nat Genet* **20**:353, 1998.
133. Nachtigal MW, Hirokawa Y, Enyeart-VanHouten DL, Flanagan JN, Hammer GD, Ingraham HA: Wilms' Tumor 1 and Dax-1 modulate the orphan nuclear receptor SF-1 in sex-specific gene expression. *Cell* **93**:445, 1998.
134. Zanaria E, Bardoni B, Dabovic B, Calvari V, Fraccaro M, Zuffardi O, Camerino G: Xp duplication and sex reversal. *Philos Trans R Soc Lond B Biol Sci* **350**:291, 1995.
135. Ramkissoon Y, Goodfellow P: Early steps in mammalian sex determination. *Curr Opin Genet Dev* **6**:316, 1996.
136. Ogata T, Matsuo N: Sex determining gene on the X chromosome short arm: Dosage sensitive sex reversal. *Acta Paediatr Jpn* **38**:390, 1996.
137. Capel B: Sex in the 90s: SRY and the switch to the male pathway. *Annu Rev Physiol* **60**:497, 1998.
138. O'Dell WD, Green GM, Williams RH: Hypoadrenotropism: The isolated deficiency of adrenotropic hormone. *J Clin Endocrinol* **20**:1017, 1960.
139. Hung W, Migeon CJ: Hypoglycemia in a two-year-old boy with adrenocorticotropic hormone (ACTH) deficiency (probably isolated) and adrenal medullary unresponsiveness to insulin-induced hypoglycemia. *J Clin Endocrinol* **28**:146, 1968.
140. Lucking T, Willig RP: Selektiver ACTH-Mangel bei zwei Gecshwistern. *Dtsch Med Wochenschr* **100**:2646, 1975.
141. Aynsley-Green A, Moncrieff MW, Ratter S, Benedict CR, Stotts CN, Wilkinson RH: Isolated ACTH deficiency: Metabolic and endocrine studies in a 7-year-old boy. *Arch Dis Child* **53**:499, 1978.
142. Ichiba Y, Goto T: Isolated corticotropin deficiency. *Am J Dis Child* **137**:1202, 1983.
143. Malpuech G, Vanlieferinghen P, Dechelotte P, Gaulme J, Labbe A, Guiot F: Isolated familial adrenocorticotropin deficiency: Prenatal diagnosis by maternal plasma estriol assay. *Am J Med Genet* **29**:125, 1988.
144. Nussey SS, Soo S-C, Gibson S, Gout I, White A, Bain M, Johnstone AP: Isolated congenital ACTH deficiency: A cleavage enzyme defect? *Clin Endocrinol* **39**:381, 1993.
145. Kyllo JH, Collins MM, Vetter KL, Cuttler L, Rosenfield RL, Donohoue PA: Linkage of congenital isolated adrenocorticotropic hormone deficiency to the corticotropin releasing hormone locus using simple sequence repeat polymorphisms. *Am J Med Genet* **62**:262, 1996.
146. Funder JW, Smith AI: Isolated ACTH deficiency: Enzyme defect or chimaeric enzyme? *Clin Endocrinol* **39**:385, 1993.
147. Kruger G, Mix M, Pelz L, Dunker H: Cytomegalic type of congenital adrenal hypoplasia due to autosomal recessive inheritance. *Am J Med Genet* **46**:475, 1993.
148. Hall JG: Analysis of Pena-Shokeir phenotype. *Am J Med Genet* **25**:99, 1986.
149. Pena SDJ, Shokeir MHK: Syndrome of camptodactyly, multiple ankyloses, facial anomalies and pulmonary hypoplasia: A lethal condition. *J Pediatr* **85**:373, 1974.

150. Pena SDJ, Shokeir MHK: Syndrome of camptodactyly, multiple ankyloses, facial anomalies and pulmonary hypoplasia—Further delineation and evidence for autosomal recessive inheritance. *Birth Defects Orig Art Ser* **XII**:201, 1976.
151. Jones KL: *Smith's Recognizable Patterns of Human Malformation, 5th ed.* Philadelphia, WB Saunders, 1997.
152. Moerman P, Fryns JP, Goddeeris P, Lauweryns JM: Multiple ankyloses, facial anomalies, and pulmonary hypoplasia associated with severe antenatal spinal muscular atrophy. *J Pediatr* **103**:238, 1983.
153. Begleiter ML, Harris DJ: Holoprosencephaly and endocrine dysgenesis in brothers. *Am J Med Genet* **7**:315, 1980.
154. Shepard TH, Landing BH, Mason DG: Familial Addison's disease: Case reports of two sisters with corticoid deficiency unassociated with hypoaldosteronism. *Am J Dis Child* **97**:154, 1959.
155. Mecke S, Passarge E: Encephalocele, polycystic kidneys, and polydactyly as an autosomal recessive trait simulating certain other disorders: The Meckel syndrome. *Ann Genet* **14**:97, 1971.
156. Gruber GB: Beitrage zur Frage "gekoppelter" Missbildungen. (Akrocephalo-Syndactylie und Dysencephalia splanchnocystica.) *Beitr Path Anat* **93**:459, 1934.
157. Paavola P, Salonen R, Weissenbach J, Peltonen L: The locus for Meckel syndrome with multiple congenital anomalies maps to chromosome 17q21-q24. *Nat Genet* **11**:213, 1995.
158. Salonen R, Paavola P: Meckel syndrome. *J Med Genet* **35**:497, 1998.
159. Paavola P, Salonen R, Baumer A, Schinzel A, Boyd PA, Gould S, Meusburger H, et al.: Clinical and genetic heterogeneity in Meckel syndrome. *Hum Genet* **101**:88, 1997.

CHAPTER 168

Nitric Oxide Synthases

David S. Bredt

1. **Modern molecular biology has revealed vast numbers of large and complex proteins and nucleic acids that regulate body function. By contrast, discoveries over the past 10 years indicate that crucial features of neuronal communication, blood vessel modulation, and immune response are mediated by a remarkably simple chemical, nitric oxide (NO).**
2. **Endogenous NO is generated from arginine by a family comprised of three distinct calmodulin-dependent NO synthase (NOS) enzymes. NOS from endothelial cells (eNOS) and neurons (nNOS) are both constitutively expressed enzymes, whose activities are stimulated by increases in intracellular calcium. Immune functions for NO are mediated by a calcium-independent inducible NOS (iNOS). Expression of iNOS protein requires transcriptional activation, which is mediated by specific combinations of cytokines. All three NOSs use NADPH as an electron donor and employ five enzyme cofactors to catalyze a five-electron oxidation of arginine to NO with stoichiometric formation of citrulline.**
3. **Highest levels of NO throughout the body are found in neurons, where NO functions as a unique messenger molecule. In the autonomic nervous system NO functions as a major nonadrenergic noncholinergic (NANC) neurotransmitter. This NANC pathway plays a particularly important role in producing relaxation of smooth muscle in the cerebral circulation and the gastrointestinal, urogenital, and respiratory tracts. Disregulation of NOS activity in autonomic nerves plays a major role in diverse pathophysiological conditions, including migraine headache, hypertrophic pyloric stenosis, and male impotence. In the brain, NO functions as a neuromodulator and appears to mediate aspects of learning and memory.**
4. **Although endogenous NO was originally appreciated as a mediator of smooth muscle relaxation, NO also plays a major role in skeletal muscle. Physiologically, muscle-derived NO regulates skeletal muscle contractility and exercise-induced glucose uptake. nNOS occurs at the plasma membrane of skeletal muscle, which facilitates diffusion of NO to the vasculature to regulate muscle perfusion. nNOS protein occurs in the dystrophin complex in skeletal muscle and NO may therefore participate in the pathophysiology of muscular dystrophy.**
5. **NO signaling in excitable tissues requires rapid and controlled delivery of NO to specific cellular targets. This tight control of NO signaling is largely regulated at the level of NO biosynthesis. Acute control of nNOS activity is mediated by allosteric enzyme regulation, by posttranslational modification, and by subcellular targeting of the enzyme. nNOS protein levels are also dynamically regulated by changes in gene transcription, which affords long-lasting changes in tissue NO levels.**
6. **While NO normally functions as a physiological neuronal mediator, excess production of NO mediates brain injury. Overactivation of glutamate receptors associated with cerebral ischemia and other excitotoxic processes results in massive release of NO. As a free radical, NO is inherently reactive and mediates cellular toxicity by damaging critical metabolic enzymes and by reacting with superoxide to form peroxynitrite, an even more potent oxidant. Through these mechanisms, NO appears to play a major role in the pathophysiology of stroke, Parkinson disease, Huntington disease, and amyotrophic lateral sclerosis.**

INTRODUCTION AND HISTORICAL PERSPECTIVE

Nitric oxide, whose chemical formula is NO, is a gas under ambient conditions. It is distinct from nitrous oxide, the "laughing gas" used as anesthetic, whose formula is N_2O. NO is notoriously noxious because of its free-radical structure: it possesses an extra electron, making it highly chemically reactive. Although NO has long been known to occur in bacteria, no one anticipated that such a reactive agent would have vital functions in mammals. Yet, discoveries over the past 10 years reveal that NO is one of the major messenger molecules of biology, enabling white blood cells to kill certain pathogens, enabling neurotransmitters to dilate blood vessels, and serving as a neuronal messenger molecule.

Discovery of Endogenous NO as an Immune Mediator

NO is extraordinarily labile, with a half-life of only about 3 to 5 sec, after which it is converted by oxygen and water into nitrates and nitrites. While humans excrete nitrates, these were generally thought to derive from dietary sources. In 1981, Steven Tannenbaum and associates noted that humans and rats fed diets with low levels of nitrates still excreted substantial amounts of nitrates in the urine.[1-3] A clue to one source of nitrate formation came from studies showing increased levels of urinary nitrates in patients with diarrhea and fever.[4] Inflammatory processes associated with the diarrhea seemed to be responsible for the nitrate formation. Indeed, it was noted that injections of bacterial endotoxin or lipopolysaccharide stimulated nitrate excretion.[5]

The determination of the source of the nitrate formation and its biologic role in inflammatory responses is derived primarily from the work of Michael Marletta and Dennis Stuehr and John Hibbs and associates. Marletta and Stuehr noted that mice with genetically determined deficiency of macrophages had very low

A list of standard abbreviations is located immediately preceding the index in each volume. Additional abbreviations used in this chapter include: ACh = acetylcholine; AChR = acetylcholine receptor; CaM = calmodulin binding; CPR = cytochrome P450 reductase; EDRF = endothelial-derived relaxing factor; eNOS = endothelial nitric oxide synthase; Glu = glutamate; H_4B = tetrahydrobiopterin; iNOS = inducible nitric oxide synthase; LHRH = luteinizing hormone-releasing hormone; L-NAA = L-N^{ω}-aminoarginine; LNMA = L-N^{ω}-methylarginine; L-NNA = L-N^{ω}-nitroarginine; LTD = long-term depression; LTP = long-term potentiation; MCA = middle cerebral artery; Myr = myristoyation; NANC = nonadrenergic noncholinergic; NHA = L-N^{ω}-hydroxyarginine; NMDA = *N*-methyl-D-aspartate; nNOS = neuronal nitric oxide synthase; NO = nitric oxide; NOS = nitric oxide synthase; O_2^- = superoxide; $ONOO^-$ = peroxynitrite; Palm = palmitoylation; PIN = protein inhibitor of nNOS; SOD = superoxide dismutase; SR = sarcoplasmic reticulum; and VIP = vasoactive intestinal polypeptide.

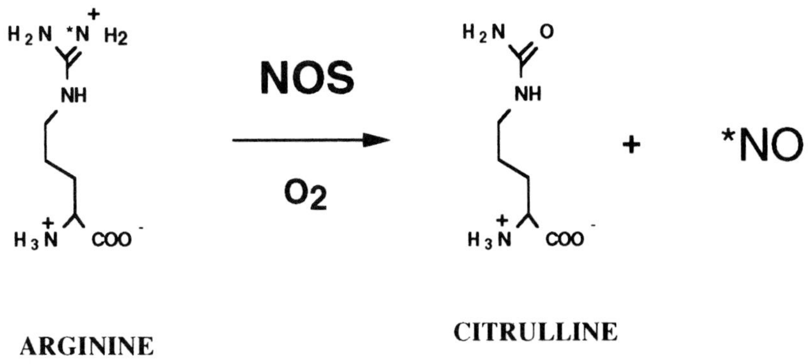

Fig. 168-1 NO biosynthesis. NOS forms NO from L-arginine with a stoichiometric generation of L-citrulline. The nitrogen in NO (*) derives from one of the two equivalent chemically equivalent guanidino-nitrogens (*) in L-arginine. The oxygen in NO derives from molecular oxygen (O_2).

levels of nitrate excretion.[6] Utilizing isolated cultures of macrophages they found that the combination of lipopolysaccharide and interferon-γ stimulated nitrate formation by the macrophages.[7,8] They also noted that nitrate formation by macrophages was abolished when arginine was removed from the incubation medium. This indicated that a specific enzyme in macrophages converts arginine into an intermediate chemical that turned out to be NO,[9] which, in turn, is transformed into nitrites and nitrates.

Independently, Hibbs was evaluating the capability of macrophages to kill tumor cells and bacteria. He cultured tumor cells together with macrophages and noted that the tumor-killing effects of the macrophages were abolished when arginine was removed from the medium.[10] He demonstrated that arginine is converted to both nitrates and to the amino acid citrulline.[11] This work provided independent evidence that a specific enzyme of activated macrophages generates NO from arginine (Fig. 168-1). Hibbs also identified the first inhibitor of the NO synthesizing enzyme, when he showed that certain methyl derivatives of arginine blocked the formation of nitrates, as well as the tumoricidal activity of macrophages.[10]

Discovery of NO as an Endogenous Messenger Molecule

A completely unrelated line of investigation independently led to the identification of NO as a messenger molecule. There are two arms to this story, one relating to mechanisms whereby neurotransmitters dilate blood vessels and the other dealing with drugs that relieve the symptoms of angina.

NO as the Endothelial Derived Relaxing Factor. For much of this century it was assumed that acetylcholine acted directly on vascular smooth muscle cells to cause vasodilation. However, in 1980, Robert Furchgott demonstrated that acetylcholine acts on receptors located on endothelial cells to provoke the release of a small molecule that diffuses to and relaxes the adjacent muscle.[12] Numerous investigators, including Furchgott, tried to isolate this "endothelial-derived relaxing factor," also called EDRF, but were unsuccessful, because EDRF seemed to be extremely labile.[13,14] Even without knowing the chemical identity of the factor, researchers were able to show that it acted by stimulating the formation of cyclic GMP,[15] a second messenger related to the better known cyclic AMP.

Quite independently, other investigators were trying to understand how nitroglycerin exerts its extraordinarily potent and dramatic alleviation of cardiac angina. Nitroglycerin is the active chemical in dynamite, which was invented by Alfred Nobel. Nitroglycerin's therapeutic effects in angina were sufficiently well known in the late nineteenth century that in 1885, Nobel, who had cardiac symptoms, wrote a friend, "It sounds like the irony of fate that I should be ordered by my doctor to take nitroglycerin internally." The great success of nitroglycerin resulted in numerous derivatives, the organic nitrates, which are still mainstays in anginal therapy. Insight into the molecular mechanism of action of organic nitrates came in the late 1970s, based on research of Ferid Murad and Louis Ignarro, who showed that nitroglycerin and the organic nitrates are themselves inactive, but elicit blood vessel relaxation after they are converted to an active metabolic product, NO.[16,17] Moreover, Murad showed that NO relaxes the muscle by stimulating the formation of cyclic GMP.[15] NO augments cGMP levels by binding to iron in the heme that is part of soluble guanylyl cyclase, stimulating the formation of cGMP.[18,19]

By 1986, it was predicted that NO or some closely related derivative may account for EDRF activity.[20–22] Definitive proof that EDRF is identical to NO was provided by Salvador Moncada and his associates. Using cultured endothelial cells as a source, they monitored the release of EDRF activity and, at the same time, chemically quantitated NO release. They found that the endothelium releases sufficient NO to fully account for relaxation of adjacent muscle cells.[23] Moncada's group also found that endothelium synthesizes NO from arginine[24] with the stoichiometric formation of citrulline.[25] Besides relaxing blood vessels, endothelium-derived NO was also shown to inhibit blood clotting by preventing the aggregation of platelets.[26–29]

How important is NO as a normal regulator of blood pressure? Other substances, such as angiotensin and norepinephrine, were previously assumed to be the major determinants of blood pressure. However, physiological studies using inhibitors of NO synthase (NOS) demonstrate a primary role for NO in regulating vascular tone. Intravenous administration of NOS inhibitors, such as monomethyl arginine, to animals[30–32] or humans[33,34] provokes a rapid and marked increase in vascular resistance. NOS inhibitors also cause a more notable increase in blood pressure than do drugs that influence norepinephrine or angiotensin. Thus, NO may be the principal regulator of basal blood pressure.

NO as a Neuronal Messenger Molecule. The third major site of NO messenger activities is in neurons. The first hint for a neuronal role for NO dates to 1977 when Takeo Deguchi noticed that activation of cyclic GMP formation in the brain requires a low molecular weight substance, which he subsequently identified as the amino acid arginine.[35,36] Once EDRF was shown to be NO, Moncada reasoned that arginine's role in cyclic GMP formation in the brain likely relates to NO formation.[37] Moncada directly demonstrated a NO forming enzyme in brain preparations.[37] Independently, John Garthwaite observed the formation of a short-lived substance that had the properties of NO when he stimulated cultured neurons by administering the glutamate.[38] The regulation of NOS by neurotransmitters was first examined in the cerebellum. The cerebellum contains the highest levels of cGMP in the brain with its formation stimulated by glutamate acting on *N*-methyl-D-aspartate (NMDA) receptors.[39,40] By monitoring the conversion of arginine to NO or to citrulline, David Bredt and Solomon Snyder demonstrated in cerebellar slices that NOS activity is enhanced 300 percent in response to NMDA receptor stimulation.[41] The concentration-response relationship for NOS activation was the same as for the stimulation of cGMP levels (Fig. 168-2). The enhanced NOS activity is responsible for the increased levels

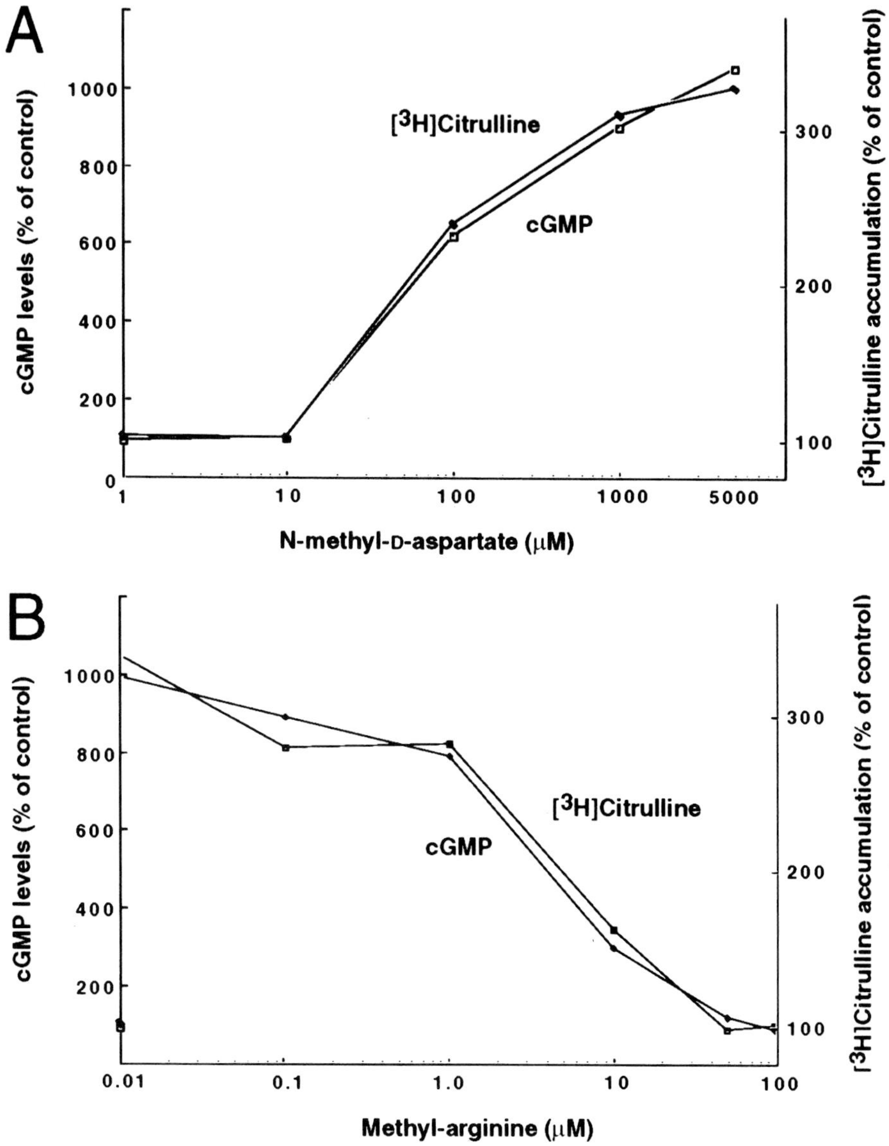

Fig. 168-2 Nitric oxide mediates glutamate-linked enhancement of cGMP levels in cerebellum. *A*, NMDA treatment of cerebellar slices simultaneously augments both cGMP levels and NOS activity, which is reflected by [^{3}H]citrulline accumulation. *B*, Methyl-arginine, a NOS inhibitor, blocks NMDA-stimulated cGMP formation and NOS activation cerebellar slices. All slices in *B* were stimulated with 500 μM NMDA. (Adapted from Bredt and Snyder.[41])

of cGMP, because methyl-arginine, an inhibitor of NOS, completely prevents the stimulation of cGMP formation in brain.[41,42]

CHARACTERIZATION OF NO SYNTHASE

Because NO cannot be stored, released, or inactivated by conventional regulatory mechanisms, biosynthetic regulation is more important for NO than for other mediators. Indeed, NO synthase (NOS), the NO biosynthetic enzyme, is one of the most regulated enzymes in biology. Initial efforts to purify the enzyme were unsuccessful because of a rapid loss of enzyme activity on purification. Observations that calmodulin is required for NOS activity in the brain led to a simple purification of neuronal NOS (nNOS) to homogeneity.[43] Using this approach, other groups purified nNOS,[44,45] inducible NOS[46–49] (iNOS), and endothelial NOS (eNOS).[50] Molecular cloning of the cDNA for neuronal,[51,52] endothelial,[53–55] and inducible[56–59] forms of NOS has helped elucidate NOS function. The structure of NOS reveals numerous regulatory mechanisms.

NOS oxidizes the guanidine group of L-arginine in a process that consumes five electrons and results in the formation of NO with stoichiometric formation of L-citrulline. L-N^{ω}-substituted arginine analogues such as L-N^{ω}-nitroarginine (L-NNA) and L-N^{ω}-methylarginine (L-NMA), function as NOS inhibitors.[60] The inhibition of NOS by these substrate analogues can initially be reversed by simultaneous application of excess arginine consistent with their competitive blockade of the active site. However, following prolonged exposure NOS is irreversibly inhibited by some of these agents. The irreversible inactivation of the macrophage enzyme and brain enzymes by L-NMA requires simultaneous incubation with NOS cofactors suggesting "mechanism-based" inhibition.[61,62] The time-dependent inactivation of the brain enzyme by L-NNA[63] is independent of NOS enzymatic turnover.[64]

NOS isoforms display modest differences in their sensitivity to various arginine analogs. L-NNA is a more potent inhibitor of the brain and endothelial enzymes (K_i = 200–500 nM), and L-N^{ω}-aminoarginine (L-NAA) is a more potent blocker of the inducible enzyme (K_i = 1–5 μM). Clinically useful inhibitors of NOS will likely need to be isoform specific. Intensive work by numerous pharmaceutical companies has focused on discovery of such selective antagonists. High throughput drug screening yielded a highly selective nNOS antagonist[65] that appears useful for mitigating neuronal injury in an animal model of cerebral ischemia (see below).

NOS Cofactors

Flavins. Oxidative enzymes generally employ redox active cofactors. NOS is unprecedented in employing five. The cloning of NOS's oxidative enzymes (discussed below) indicates a close homology of the C-terminal half of NOS with cytochrome P450 reductase (CPR) including consensus sequences for NADPH, FAD, and FMN binding.[51] While NADPH is a stoichiometric substrate, the two flavins copurify with NOS in a ratio of 1 eq each of FAD and FMN per NOS monomer.[46,66] FAD slowly dissociates from NOS and must be exogenously supplied for maximal activity. The close homology of NOS with CPR suggests that electrons follow the same path through NOS as they do through CPR; that is, NADPH initially reduces FAD, which, in turn, reduces FMN. In fact, NOS and CPR share a domain thought to be involved in this electron transfer.[51]

Heme. CPR supplies the reducing equivalents from NADPH to the heme-containing cytochrome P450 enzymes. This mechanism is apparently shared by NOS isoforms, which contain 1 eq of iron-protoporphyrin IX per NOS monomer.[67–69] Furthermore, NOS displays reduced CO difference spectra typical of cytochrome P450 with wavelength absorbance maximum at 445 nM, which provided that first indication of a heme-binding cysteinyl ligand. CO inhibits purified NOS, which is also consistent with the participation of a cytochrome P450-type heme in the reaction. NO itself appears to exert feedback inhibition of NOS,[70–72] perhaps by interacting with the enzyme's heme prosthetic group. Optical-difference spectroscopy indicates that heme binds to the substrate arginine prior to participating in the oxygenation reactions.[73] Heme-substrate binding is also the initial event in catalysis with the various cytochrome P450s. Unlike other mammalian cytochrome P450 enzymes, NOSs are unique because they are soluble and their flavin (reductase) and heme (oxygenase)-containing domains are fused in a single polypeptide. A bacterial fatty acid monooxygenase, P450BM3, also has been identified as a soluble, self-contained P450 system.[74]

H_4B. NOS is also regulated by tetrahydrobiopterin (H_4B). While isolated iNOS and eNOS are absolutely dependent on H_4B,[50,75,76] purified nNOS retained substantial activity in the absence of added H_4B.[43,77] This discrepancy is explained by the tight binding of H_4B to nNOS such that H_4B copurifies with the enzyme.[78] It was initially assumed that H_4B functions directly in the hydroxylation of arginine by analogy to its role in aromatic amino acid hydroxylase enzymes. Kaufman and coworkers[79] challenged this notion in experiments, proposing that H_4B stabilizes NOS. Their conclusion was based on experiments with nNOS that showed that H_4B functions catalytically, is not recycled, and does not affect the initial rate of NOS. Marletta and colleagues,[80] based on experiments with pterin analogues used to probe the iNOS reaction, also suggested that H_4B stabilizes NOS.

In many cell types, the availability of H_4B is rate limiting for NO biosynthesis. Resting macrophages, smooth muscle cells, and hepatocytes contain only minute amounts of H_4B. However, following stimulation with cytokines, cellular H_4B levels dramatically increase to support NO synthesis.[81,82] The mechanism for this increase is that immunostimulants selectively induce expression of GTP cyclohydrolase I, the first and rate-limiting enzyme for the synthesis of H_4B. This increase in GTP cyclohydrolase I occurs at the transcriptional level and follows a time course that closely parallels the induction of iNOS transcription.[81,82] These findings suggest that pterin synthesis inhibitors may offer a strategy for antagonizing iNOS activity.

The recent 3D structural characterization of the N-terminal half of iNOS by x-ray crystallography determines, at atomic resolution, the location of cofactors in the oxygenase domain.[83,84] This work reveals an unusual fold and heme environment in NOS that resembles a baseball catcher's mitt, and which helps stabilize activated oxygen intermediates that are key for catalysis. Confirming mutagenesis work, the heme is axially coordinated to proximal cysteine-194. In the dimeric crystal, arginine is bound to glutamate-371 and stacks with heme in a hydrophobic pocket near the dimer interface. The iNOS dimer structure supports previous proposals that H_4B plays a primary role in regulating NOS dimerization and active site formation, but that H_4B does not appear to play a direct redox role in catalysis. [83]

NO Formation

The conversion of arginine to NO is catalyzed in two independent steps (Fig. 168-3). The first step is a two-electron oxidation of arginine to N^{ω}-hydroxyarginine (NHA).[85] Although this hydroxylated intermediate is tightly bound to NOS, under certain conditions NHA can be isolated as a product.[64] This hydroxylation step resembles a classical P450 type monooxygenation reaction utilizing 1 eq of NADPH and 1 eq of O_2.[85] The hydroxylation reaction is accelerated by H_4B, requires calcium and calmodulin as activators, and is blocked by CO.[64,68,85]

The steps in the pathway from NHA to NO and citrulline are less clear. Any proposed mechanism should account for experiments which find that this oxidation (a) utilizes 0.5 eq NADPH, (b) requires O_2 and calcium/calmodulin, (c) is accelerated by H_4B, and (d) is inhibited by CO and arginine analogues with a pharmacology similar to that seen in the initial hydroxylation reaction.[64,68,85] In one model consistent with these data, NOS would use both its reductase and heme domains for successive independent oxidations of arginine at a common active site with heme directly functioning in the activation of molecular oxygen. For the first hydroxylation, both reducing equivalents for oxygen

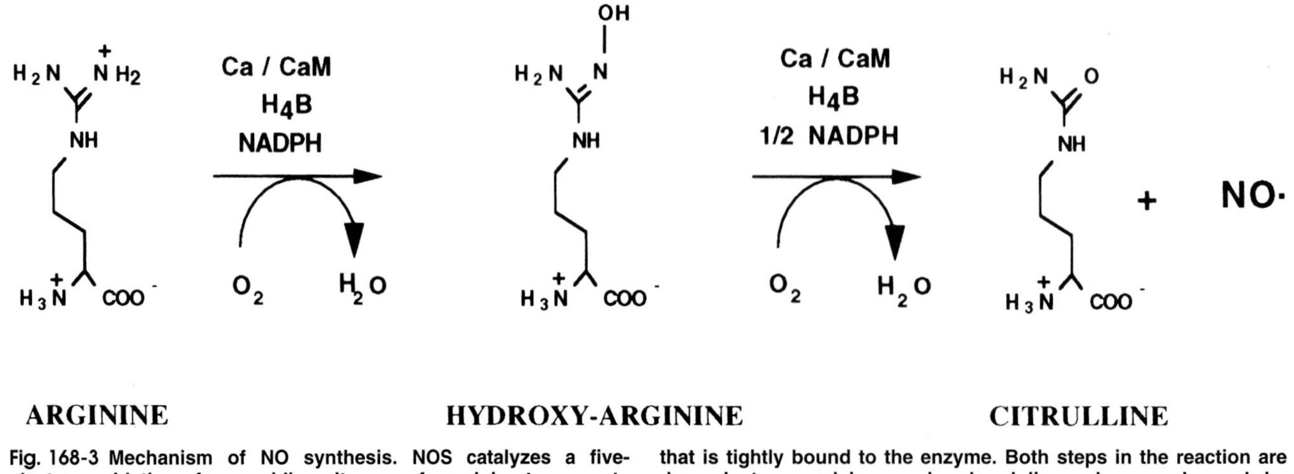

Fig. 168-3 Mechanism of NO synthesis. NOS catalyzes a five-electron oxidation of a guanidine nitrogen of L-arginine to generate NO and L-citrulline. L-Hydroxyarginine is formed as an intermediate that is tightly bound to the enzyme. Both steps in the reaction are dependent on calcium and calmodulin and are enhanced by tetrahydrobiopterin.

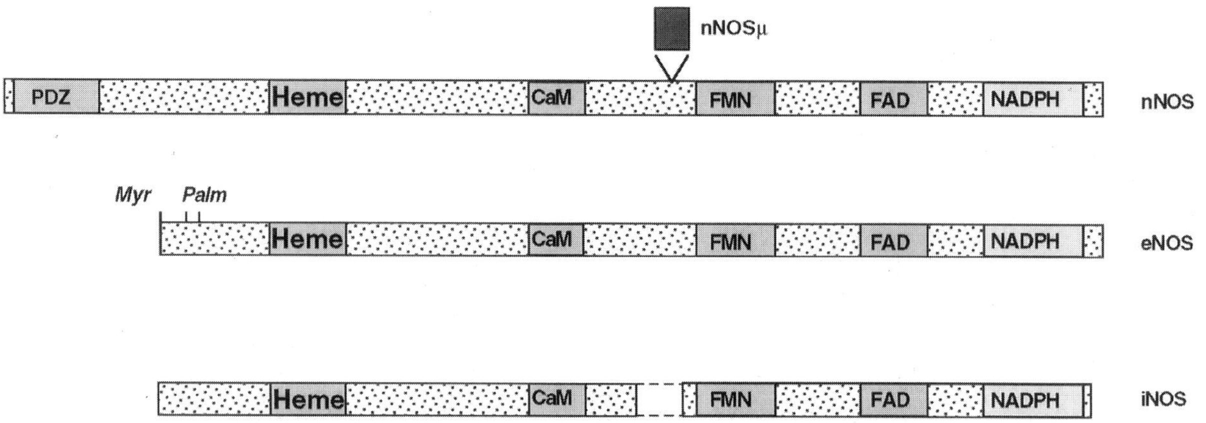

Fig. 168-4 Alignment of the co-factor recognition sites within NOS enzymes. Predicted sites for binding heme, calmodulin (CaM), FMN, FAD, and NADPH are noted. The N-terminal PDZ domain in nNOS, and the myristoylation (Myr) and palmitoylation (Palm) sites in eNOS are marked. The unique alternatively spliced region in nNOS*μ* from skeletal muscle corresponds to the domain not present in iNOS.

activation derive from NADPH. It has been speculated that NHA and NADPH each provide one electron for the second oxidation step.[86] This explains both the 0.5 stoichiometry of NADPH utilization and accounts for the unusual five-electron chemistry of NO biosynthesis. The crystallographic structure of dimeric iNOS oxygenase domain is consistent with this proposed mechanism. Indeed, these ligand-bound NOS crystal structures suggest that the different protonation state of arginine vs. *N*-hydroxyarginine differentiates the two chemical steps of NO synthesis.[83]

Molecular Cloning of NOS Isoforms

Neuronal NOS. Isolation of the brain isoform[43] permitted its molecular cloning.[51] The cDNA predicts a polypeptide of 160 kD and was striking in having 36 percent identity to CPR in its C-terminal half, the NOS reductase domain, which contains the binding sites of NADPH, FAD, and FMN (Fig. 168-4). This homology to CPR is shared by all NOSs cloned to date, and reflects the oxidative mechanism of NO biosynthesis. The sequence of the N-terminal half of NOSs, the heme domains, is not similar to any cloned gene. Although the classic P450 heme-binding cysteinyl peptide sequence is absent, the amino acids surrounding cysteine-414 showed some of the expected homology. Indeed, mutagenesis and x-ray crystallographic studies have definitively demonstrated cysteine-414 of nNOS as the site for heme coordination.

The reductase domain of NOS shares many functional properties with CPR. nNOS catalyzes a rapid NADPH-dependent reduction of cytochrome c. In the absence of arginine, NOS can transfer electrons from NADPH to $O_2{}^-$ and form $O_2{}^-$ and H_2O_2.[87] The formation of these reactive oxygen intermediates may contribute to glutamate neurotoxicity and neurodegeneration as discussed below. Near the middle of the nNOS cDNA there is an amphipathic alpha helix domain, which conforms to the consensus sequence for calmodulin binding.[51] This assignment was confirmed by experiments showing that peptides corresponding to this region bind calmodulin with low nanomolar affinity in a calcium-dependent manner.[88] Cloning of nNOS from human cerebellum predicts 94 percent acid identity with the rat protein.[89]

nNOS Gene. Genomic cloning has shown that nNOS is a huge and complex gene that occupies at least 160 kb[90] and maps to chromosome position 12q24.2.[91,92] The most common mRNA isolated from brain derives from 29 exons, but several alternatively spliced forms of nNOS mRNA in brain have been described. Esumi and coworkers[93] reported the first example of alternative splicing of nNOS. These investigators found that, in mouse cerebellum and in human neuroblastoma cell lines, a small percentage of nNOS mRNA has a 315-nucleotide deletion corresponding to nucleotides 1510–1824. Structural analysis of the corresponding part of the nNOS gene indicated that the deletion corresponds to exons 9 and 10. The greatest diversity of nNOS transcripts occurs in the 5′ untranslated region. Molecular cloning of nNOS from human brain cDNA identified two distinct 5′-terminal exons that are spliced to a common exon 2. Genomic cloning demonstrated that the unique exons occur within 300 bp of each other. Transcriptional analyses revealed that expression of the 5′-terminal exons is regulated by separate upstream promoter regions.[94] Independent analysis by Marsden *et al.* indicates that at least eight different examples of exon 1 of nNOS are expressed in human tissues.[95] Again, the diverse 5′ ends are spliced into a common exon 2. Despite this immense diversity of 5′ mRNA variants of nNOS, most transcripts encode the same 155-kD protein. What might be the biologic advantage of such a system? Clearly, this complexity could allow for tissue- and stage-specific gene expression. It is also possible that the multiple nNOS mRNAs have different functional properties. The distinct 5′ termini may either influence mRNA translational efficiency or alter mRNA localization or stability.

Endothelial NOS. eNOS was cloned independently by three labs using low stringency screening strategies based on the DNA sequence of nNOS.[53–55] Overall, the predicted sequence shares 60 percent identity with nNOS. Consensus binding sites for FAD, FMN, NADPH, and calmodulin are conserved between the brain and endothelial isoforms. A unique feature of the eNOS gene is a consensus sequence for N-terminal myristoylation. [^{3}H]Myristate is directly incorporated into eNOS, and mutation of the myristoylation sequence renders eNOS soluble.[96,97] Insertion of the myristoyl[RHA4] group into the plasma membrane presumably accounts for the enzyme's particulate location.

Near its N-terminus, the eNOS protein also contains an unusual glycine/leucine penta-repeat that is flanked on both sides by cysteine residues. These cysteines are sites of palmitoylation, which is another posttranslational fatty acid modification of the enzyme.[98,99] Palmitoylation of eNOS refines the subcellular target of the enzyme and helps recruit the protein both to the Golgi complex and to caveolae, small cave-like invaginations of the plasma membrane.[100,101] Palmitoylation of eNOS appears to be a dynamic process that contributes to enzyme activation and recycling following agonist stimulation.[102]

eNOS Gene. Human eNOS is a large gene that contains 25 exons spanning 21 kb on the 7q35-36 region of chromosome number 7, the same chromosome that contains CPR.[91,103] Characterization of 5′-flanking genomic regions indicates that the endothelial NO synthase promoter is "TATA-less" and contains proximal promoter elements that are commonly found in constitutively expressed endothelial transcripts, including Sp1 and GATA elements.[91] Functional analysis shows that the canonical Sp1 site is required for basal promoter activity.[104] The 5′ promoter region of the human gene contains AP-1, AP-2, NF-1, heavy metal, acute-phase response shear stress, and sterol-regulatory elements.[91] This complex array of 5′ sequence motifs fit with work showing eNOS expression is regulated by diverse physiological stimuli including shear stress,[105] physical exercise,[106] hypoxia,[107,108] estrogen treatment,[109] and low levels of oxidized low-density lipoproteins.[110,111]

Inducible NOS. Cloning of iNOS from rodent macrophages was independently achieved by three labs. Two groups used nNOS cDNA as a homologous probe,[56,58] while the third used an iNOS antibody for expression cloning.[57] Overall, the amino acid sequence is 50 percent identical to nNOS and 51 percent identical to eNOS. The iNOS cDNA predicts a protein of 133 kD with consensus binding sequences for NADPH, FAD, FMN, and calmodulin.

An inducible calcium-independent NOS activity is well characterized in human hepatocytes following treatment with LPS, γ-interferon, tumor necrosis factor-α, and interleukin-1β.[112] Cloning of this cDNA indicated 82 percent identity with mouse iNOS, suggesting that it represents the human-inducible isoform.[59] Independently, a nearly identical human-inducible NOS gene was cloned from articular chondrocytes activated with interleukin-1β.[113] The human iNOS gene maps to chromosome 17qcen-q12.[114–116]

iNOS Promoter. For inducible NOS, one would expect the regulatory region of the gene to determine the rate of synthesis of enzyme protein. Initial characterization of the promoter region of the gene for iNOS revealed a pattern for complex regulation.[117] There appear to be two distinct regulatory regions upstream of the TATA box, which is 30 base pairs upstream of the transcription start site. One of these, region 1, lies 50 to 200 base pairs upstream of the start site. Region 1 contains LPS-related response elements, such as the binding site for NF-IL6 and the κB binding site for NF-κB,[118] indicating that this region regulates the LPS induced expression of iNOS. Region 2, which is 900 to 1000 base pairs upstream of the start site, does not itself directly regulate NOS expression, but provides a tenfold increase above the 75-fold increase in NOS expression provided by region 1. Region 2 contains motifs for interferon regulatory factor-1 and is responsible for interferon-γ-mediated regulation.[119,120] In sum, LPS and interferon-γ responsive elements occur in two distinct regulatory genes with LPS directly stimulating iNOS expression while interferon-γ acts only in the presence of LPS.

This unique organization of gene enhancers may explain important aspects of inflammation. In sepsis, LPS is released from Gram-negative bacterial cell walls and circulates throughout the body to stimulate inflammatory responses. By contrast, interferon-γ is released locally and serves to augment inflammatory responses in specific cell populations close to its release. LPS alone stimulates macrophages to a limited extent. Interferon-γ elaborated by infiltrating lymphocytes can prime the macrophages for a maximal response to LPS. Thus, maximal production of NO is restricted to those cells needed to kill the invader, thereby minimizing damage to adjacent tissue.

Similar to iNOS in rodents, human iNOS is regulated in a complex manner by specific cytokine combinations. Characterization of the proximal human iNOS promoter region demonstrates major differences in sequence and potential *cis*-acting elements as compared to the rodent iNOS promoter.[114] At a functional level, the human iNOS promoter also contrasts markedly from mouse iNOS. Whereas the proximal 1 kb of the murine iNOS promoter mediates responses to cytokines, reporter constructs containing the first 4 kb upstream of human iNOS show no cytokine-inducible activity.[121,122] Instead, cytokine-responsive regions, containing functional NF-κB sites,[123] occur 5 to 10 kb upstream of the transcriptional start site.[124] This absence of inducible promoter elements near the transcription start site is very unusual for a cytokine-regulated gene and helps explain the unique regulation of iNOS by diverse inflammatory stimuli.

PHYSIOLOGICAL FUNCTIONS FOR NEURON-DERIVED NO

Regulation of Intestinal Function

Physiological functions for neuron-derived NO were first demonstrated in the gastrointestinal tract. These studies resolved pharmacologic observations that had puzzled physiologists for over 20 years. Following the development of adrenergic-blocking agents in the early 1960s it became clear that certain actions of the autonomic nervous system are mediated by nonadrenergic, noncholinergic (NANC) nerves. This NANC pathway plays a particularly important role in producing relaxation of smooth muscle in the cerebral circulation and the gastrointestinal, urogenital, and respiratory tracts.[125] Parallel studies by several investigators in the late 1980s demonstrated that the NANC transmitter in several of these pathways is identical to the endothelial-derived relaxing factor (EDRF) described by Furchgott.[126,127] Molecular biological studies helped detail the mechanisms for NO-mediated neurotransmission. In the intestine, neuronal NOS (nNOS) is selectively concentrated in axon varicosities of myenteric neurons.[128] Adjacent intestinal smooth muscle cells contain an "NO receptor," the soluble guanylyl cyclase. During intestinal peristalsis, myenteric neurons fire action potentials. The resulting calcium influx activates calmodulin, which stimulates nNOS. The NO then diffuses into adjacent smooth muscle cells and augments accumulation of cGMP, which mediates intestinal relaxation. Definitive evidence that neuron-derived NO regulates intestinal motility derives from studies of genetically engineered mutant mice. nNOS knockout mice, which selectively lack the neuronal NOS isoform from conception, display a grossly enlarged stomach that histologically resembles the human disease hypertrophic pyloric stenosis.[129] Alterations in NOS may play a causal role in some newborns with this disorder, as recent genetic studies indicate that nNOS is a susceptibility locus for infantile pyloric stenosis.[130]

Regulation of Blood Flow

Neuron-derived NO also plays a major role in regulation of blood flow. In brain, neuronal activity is associated with an increase in local blood flow and this response is prevented by NOS inhibitors.[131] Particularly high levels of nNOS occur in vasodilator nerves that innervate the large cerebral blood vessels.[132] Abnormal reactivity of these vessels appears to mediate migraine headache as sumatriptan constricts these large vessels and controls headache.[133] Sumatriptan is also effective in treatment of nitroglycerin-induced headache, suggesting a role for endogenous NO in migraine.[134] Pharmacologic manipulations of nNOS may, therefore, offer an avenue for migraine therapy.

Therapeutic modulation of NO levels for treatment of migraine or other recurring disorders may be complicated by adaptive responses to the therapy. Control of cerebral blood flow involves complex and overlapping physiological pathways regulated by NO and a variety of other vasoactive compounds. Alterations in NO biosynthesis are often compensated by changes in the levels of other mediators. An illustrative example involves the increase in cerebral blood flow that normally occurs in response to hypercapnia. This local vascular reflex to hypercapnia is NO dependent, as it is acutely blocked by NOS inhibitors.[131] Surprisingly, hypercapnic cerebral blood flow responses are intact in nNOS knockout mice, and NOS inhibitors do not block the response in the nNOS knockouts.[135] Therefore, the maintenance of hypercapnic blood flow response in the nNOS knockout mice is not due to up-regulation of other NOS isoforms, but is instead mediated by an NO-independent mechanism. Compensation by such alternative pathways appears to be a common physiological

Table 168-1 Effect of NOS Inhibition on Penile Erection in Intact Rats

Agent	Dose (mg/kg)	% Intracavernous pressure (±SEM)	*n*
L-Nitroarginine methyl ester	1.0	75±7	3
	2.5	47±5	10
	5.0	16±1	4
	10.0	10±10.3	3
	40.0	0	5
N-Methyl-L-arginine	10.0	63±3	11
	20.0	17±2	2
	40.0	15±5	4
N-Methyl-D-arginine	40.0	128±5	2

Penile erection was induced electrically with a Grass S48 square wave stimulator in anesthetized male rats with optimal stimulation parameters. Intracavernous pressures were measured with a 25-gauge needle inserted unilaterally at the base of the penis and connected to a pressure transducer. (From Burnett et al.[137] Used with permission.)

reaction to deficiencies in NO biosynthesis and has been observed in several systems.

Regulation of Penile Erection

Through regulation of blood flow, neuron-derived NO also mediates penile erection. nNOS is enriched in neurons of the pelvic plexus and is concentrated in their axonal varicosities that ramify in the trabecular smooth muscle of the penis and about the adventitia of the penile arteries.[136] Activation of these nerves causes increased blood flow and engorgement of the erectile tissue. NOS inhibitors block penile erection in animal models *in vivo* (Table 168-1)[137] and in strips of human cavernosal tissue *in vitro*.[138] nNOS mutant mice, however, display normal erectile function.[139] Apparently NO derived from other NOS isoforms compensates for the loss of nNOS as NOS inhibitors block penile erection in nNOS mutant mice.

Recent studies demonstrate that abnormalities in NO biosynthesis may also underlie erectile dysfunction. Diabetes mellitus is associated with impaired NOS-dependent erectile function.[140] NOS levels in the penis are also decreased in aging rats, and this age-related decrease correlates with impaired erectile responses.[141] Androgens are essential for penile reflexes in the rat and are essential for normal libido. Similarly, nNOS expression in penis is dependent on active androgens as nNOS levels decrease by 60 percent 1 week after castration and are restored to normal levels with testosterone replacement.[142] Pharmacologic manipulation of NO or NOS expression may, therefore, offer a viable strategy for treatment for some causes of erectile dysfunction. Indeed, sildenafil (Viagra), an inhibitor of cGMP-specific phosphodiesterase type 5[143,144] enhances male sexual function by promoting the actions of NO to relax corpora cavernosum smooth muscle.[145,146]

Functions for NO in the Central Nervous System

Functions for NO in brain remain less certain. Because NO is a uniquely diffusible mediator, it was proposed on theoretical grounds that NO may mediate neuronal plasticity, which underlies aspects of both development and information storage in brain. Evidence for NO involvement in synaptic plasticity has accumulated steadily. At the cellular level, NO signaling appears to be essential for two forms of neuronal plasticity: long-term potentiation (LTP) in the hippocampus[147] and long-term depression (LTD) in the cerebellum.[148] In these cellular models, repeated neuronal stimulation yields long-lasting changes in synaptic strength, and NOS inhibitors prevent these changes. Studies with NOS inhibitors have been controversial because these arginine analogues often have nonspecific effects. This controversy may now be resolved by studies of NOS knockout mice. Both endothelial NOS (eNOS) and nNOS activities are found in hippocampus. Mice that lack either eNOS or nNOS have essentially normal LTP, whereas mutant mice deficient in both eNOS and nNOS have substantially decreased LTP.[149]

Regulation of Neurotransmitter Release

NO appears to mediate synaptic plasticity by potentiating neurotransmitter release. In several model systems, NOS inhibitors, such as nitroarginine, block the release of neurotransmitters.[150–152] In brain synaptosomes, the release of neurotransmitter evoked by stimulation of NMDA receptors is blocked by nitroarginine.[150,153,154] Presumably, glutamate acts at NMDA receptors on NOS terminals to stimulate the formation of NO, which diffuses to adjacent terminals to enhance neurotransmitter release so that blockade of NO formation inhibits release. In addition to regulating glutamate release, NO can also regulate secretion of hormones and neuropeptides. Regulation of hormone secretion by NO was most convincingly demonstrated in the hypothalamus.[155] An elegant series of experiments by McCann and colleagues showed that NO directly stimulates release of luteinizing hormone-releasing hormone (LHRH) from hypothalamic explants.[156] These findings explain physiological studies showing the NOS inhibitors block mating behavior *in vivo*, as this behavior requires LHRH release.[157] NO formation in hypothalamic explants can be stimulated by oxytocin, which also induces mating behavior in an NO-dependent manner *in vivo*.[157,158]

Behavioral Roles for NO

Through regulation of synaptic plasticity and transmitter release, NO mediates complex influences on brain development, memory formation, and behavior. Inhibition of NOS prevents the precise targeting of retinal axons to their proper location in the optic tectum.[159] In adult animals, NOS inhibitors hinder motor learning[160] and the formation of olfactory memories.[161] NOS inhibitors also prevent the long-lasting hyperalgesia that follows tissue injury.[162] In rodent experimental models using formalin injection to the paw to induce hyperalgesia, inhibitors of NOS prevent the subsequent augmented response triggered by noxious inputs. nNOS knockout mice, however, display normal sensitization to peripheral tissue damage in this model, and NOS inhibitors do not block sensitization in the nNOS knockouts.[163] Again, the deficiency of nNOS is compensated by an NO-independent pathway. Any potential development of nNOS inhibitors for chronic pain or other neurologic disorders must be prepared to tackle this recurring phenomenon of compensation following chronic removal of NOS activity.

ROLES FOR NO IN SKELETAL MUSCLE

Although endogenous NO was originally appreciated as a mediator of smooth muscle relaxation, recent studies indicate a role for NO in skeletal muscle. nNOS mRNA is expressed at high levels in human skeletal muscle,[52] where nNOS mRNA is alternatively spliced yielding a muscle specific isoform, nNOSμ.[164] nNOSμ contains an additional 102-bp exon, which is inserted between exons 16 and 17 and encodes a 34-amino acid insert between the calmodulin- and FMN-binding domains.[164] Regulation of nNOSμ activity by calcium/calmodulin and other biochemical cofactors is indistinguishable from that of nNOS purified from brain, suggesting that the alternative splicing may instead regulate nNOS interactions with specific skeletal muscle proteins.

Physiological Functions for NO in Skeletal Muscle

Understanding functions for nNOS in skeletal muscle is facilitated by the discrete localization of nNOS in myofibers. In rodent muscle, nNOS is specifically enriched beneath the sarcolemma of fast-twitch muscle fibers.[165] NOS activity stimulated during muscle membrane depolarization inhibits contractile force in fast-twitch fibers. Depression of contractile force also occurs

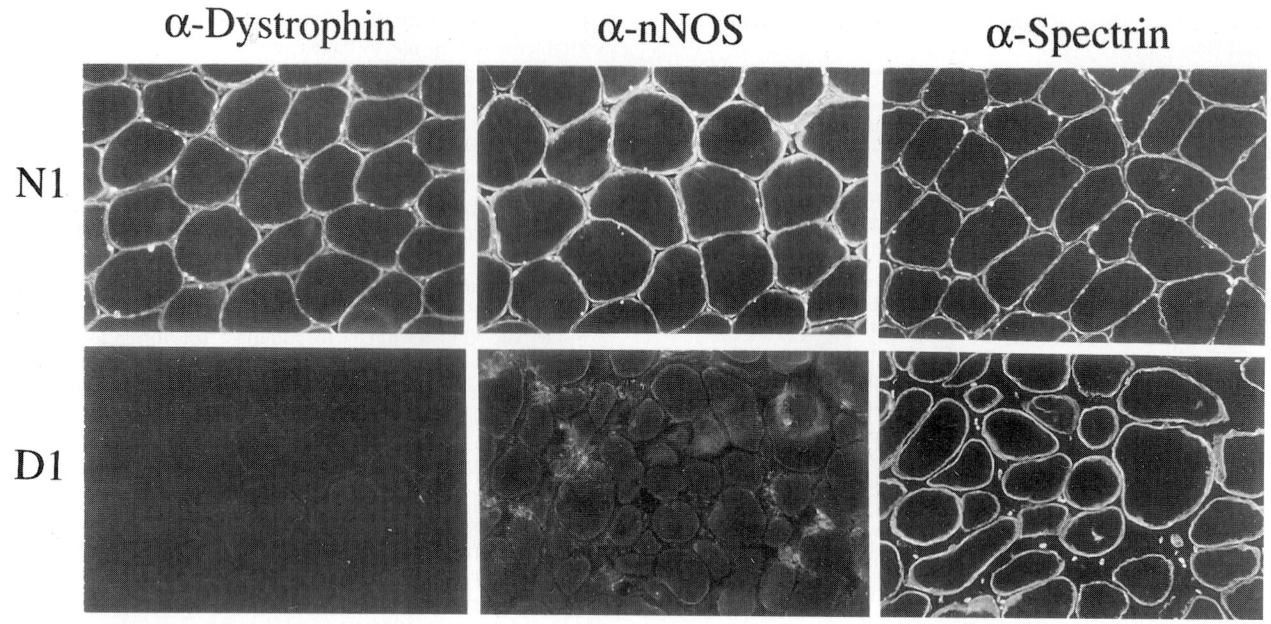

Fig. 168-5 nNOS is absent from sarcolemma in Duchenne dystrophy muscle biopsies. Skeletal muscle cryosections of biopsies from normal (N1) or Duchenne muscular dystrophy (D1) skeletal muscle were immunostained with antibodies to dystrophin, nNOS, and spectrin. In healthy muscle, all three proteins occur at the sarcolemma or plasma membrane of skeletal muscle. The absence of dystrophin in Duchenne muscular dystrophy disrupts nNOS localization to the sarcolemma but has no influence on spectrin, which is not part of the dystrophin complex. (*From Brenman et al.*[172] *Used with permission.*)

following induction of iNOS in skeletal muscle. iNOS protein is expressed in diaphragm 12 hours following LPS inoculation of rat.[166] The decrease in diaphragmatic tone that accompanies sepsis is rapidly reversed by a NOS inhibitor. NO derived from skeletal muscle iNOS therefore appears to mediate a critical component of the respiratory depression associated with sepsis.

In addition to modulating contractile force, NO derived from sarcolemmal nNOS regulates physiological functions at the muscle membrane. During muscle development, myocytes fuse to form muscle myotubes and this membrane fusion is blunted by NOS inhibitors.[167] In myocyte/motor neuron cocultures, NOS produced at the postsynaptic muscle membrane functions as a retrograde messenger to regulate myotube innervation.[168] In mature muscle fibers, NOS regulates glucose uptake across the sarcolemma.[169] Glucose uptake in skeletal muscle is regulated by both acute exercise and by insulin. NOS inhibitors selectively blunt exercise-induced uptake, but have no effect on insulin-stimulated glucose transport.[170] Interestingly, chronic exercise increases nNOS protein expression in muscle,[171] which might be expected to have long-lasting enhancing effects on glucose transport in heavily used muscle.

NO in Muscular Dystrophy

A striking aspect of skeletal muscle nNOS is that the synthase is quantitatively associated with the sarcolemma. nNOS occurs at skeletal muscle sarcolemma owing to its association with the dystrophin complex.[172] Detailed biochemical studies determined the specific protein in the dystrophin complex that binds to nNOS. This work shows that the PDZ protein motif at the N-terminus of nNOS binds to a similar PDZ motif near the N-terminus of syntrophin,[173] a dystrophin-associated protein. Syntrophin directly binds to dystrophin and links nNOS to the dystrophin complex.

Both patients with Duchenne muscular dystrophy and *mdx* mice that lack dystrophin evince a loss of nNOS from the sarcolemma (Fig. 168-5). Certain mutations in the rod-like domain of dystrophin that cause Becker's dystrophy result in loss of sarcolemmal nNOS but not other components of the dystrophin complex.[173] The specific cause of muscle pathology that results from dystrophin deficiency is unknown. One model proposes that the loss of dystrophin in Duchenne dystrophy disrupts the normal link between the extracellular matrix and the myofiber cytoskeleton.[174] This results in sarcolemmal damage and myofiber necrosis. Other evidence suggests that disruptions of intracellular calcium homeostasis and subsequent free radical-induced oxidative damage contribute to muscle pathology in Duchenne dystrophy.[175] nNOS represents a possible source for free radical injury in Duchenne dystrophy. On the other hand, because NO also plays a role in myofiber differentiation, the loss of sarcolemmal nNOS signaling may contribute to failed muscle regeneration in Duchenne dystrophy.

Future work will determine whether manipulation of skeletal muscle NO levels represents a valuable therapeutic approach to Duchenne dystrophy or other muscle diseases. Whether NO plays a primary role in a muscular dystrophy remains unknown. Linkage analysis has mapped an autosomal dominant scapuloperoneal spinal muscular atrophy locus to 12q24.1-q24.31, a region that includes the nNOS gene.[176] It is important to determine whether this or other muscular dystrophies are due to mutations in nNOS.

CELLULAR MECHANISMS REGULATING nNOS

NO signaling in excitable tissues requires rapid and controlled delivery of NO to specific cellular targets. Other neurotransmitters are packed in secretory vesicles that are released at synaptic sites. Enzymes and pumps that eliminate the active transmitter from the synapse mediate signal termination. Regulation of NO signaling is complicated by the physical properties of NO that prevent storage of NO in lipid-lined vesicles or metabolism of NO by hydrolytic degradative enzymes. In addition, excessive production of NO is toxic to neurons and other cells. NO signaling must therefore allow for rapid and localized NO production and immediate termination of biosynthesis. This tight control of NO signaling is largely regulated at the level of NO biosynthesis. Indeed, the NOS proteins are among the most highly regulated of all neuronal enzymes. Acute control of nNOS activity is mediated by allosteric regulation, by posttranslational modification, and by subcellular targeting of the enzyme. nNOS protein levels are also dynamically

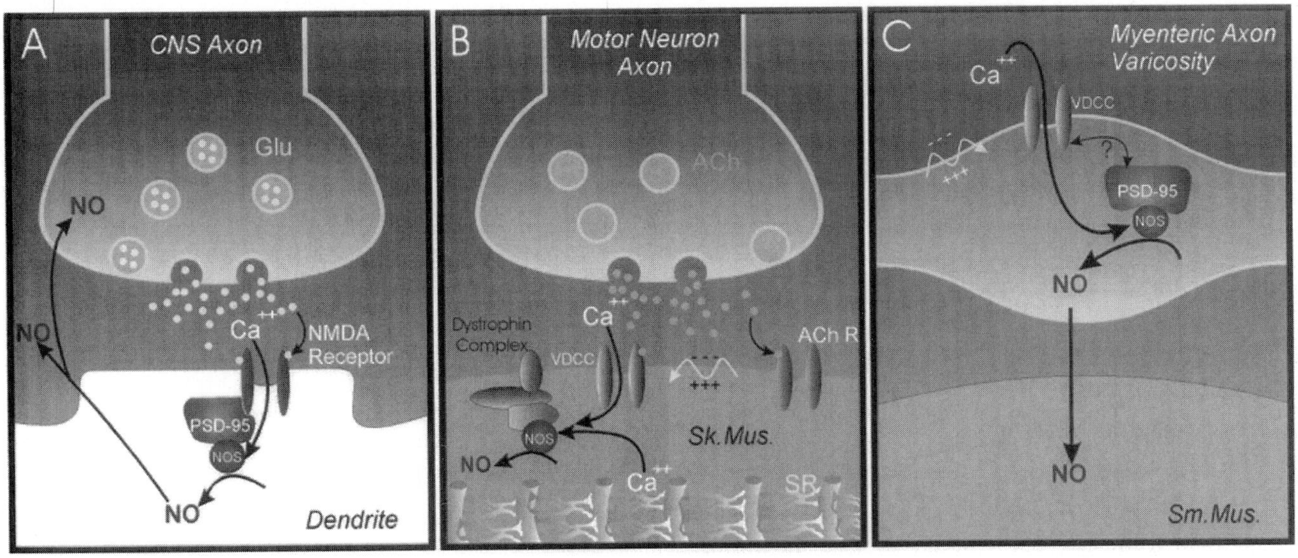

Fig. 168-6 Synaptic regulation of neuronal nitric oxide synthase. Protein interactions with nNOS target the synthase to discrete sites in neurons and skeletal muscle. These interactions likely account for differential regulation of nNOS by specific calcium influx pathways. *A*, Association with PSD-95 mediates coupling of nNOS to NMDA receptor activity in the CNS. *B*, In skeletal muscle (Sk. Mus.) nNOS occurs at the sarcolemma owing to interaction of nNOS with the dystrophin complex. Accordingly, nNOS activity is regulated by calcium influx associated with sarcolemmal depolarization. *C*, Myenteric axon varicosities contain both nNOS and PSD-95. Calcium influx through voltage-dependent calcium channels (VDCC) regulates nNOS activity in myenteric neurons and the NO relaxes the adjacent smooth muscle (Sm. Mus.) cells. Abbreviations: ACh, acetylcholine; AChR, acetylcholine receptor; Glu, glutamate; SR, sarcoplasmic reticulum. (Adapted from Christopherson and Bredt.[214])

regulated by changes in gene transcription, and this affords long-lasting changes in tissue NO levels.

Regulation of nNOS by Specific Calcium Channels

nNOS activity is primarily regulated by local increases in intracellular calcium, which stimulates nNOS through interaction with calmodulin.[43] Distinct cellular calcium influx pathways specifically regulate nNOS in various tissues. In the myenteric nervous system, where NO functions as a neurotransmitter, NOS activity is primarily regulated by calcium influx through voltage-dependent calcium channels (Fig. 168-6). Intestinal relaxation mediated by NO is suppressed by the N-type calcium channel antagonist, ω-conotoxin.[177] Vasoactive intestinal polypeptide (VIP) also appears to play an important role in regulating NO synthesis in intestinal neurons.[178] In the brain, calcium influx through the *N*-methyl-D-aspartate (NMDA)-type glutamate receptor potently activates nNOS in brain.[38] NMDA receptors are also known to play a critical role in learning and memory; the intimate relationship of NMDA receptors with nNOS helps to explain the role of NO in memory consolidation.

Selective regulation of NOS activity by distinct calcium stores is mediated by targeting nNOS protein to specific intracellular regions. nNOS protein contains an N-terminal PDZ protein motif that mediates subcellular targeting of the enzyme.[172] In the brain, the PDZ domain of nNOS targets the enzyme to postsynaptic sites by binding to PDZ domains in PSD-95 and PSD-93 proteins.[179] Importantly, NMDA receptors also occur at postsynaptic densities through binding to PSD-95.[180,181] PSD-95 and related proteins thereby function as molecular scaffolds and physically link nNOS to NMDA receptors (Fig. 168-6). Internalization of peptides that antagonize the interaction of nNOS with PSD-95 block NMDA-coupled increases in NOS activity. Some nNOS protein in brain occurs outside the postsynaptic density and can be regulated by calcium influx through voltage-dependent calcium channels. The molecular mechanisms that link nNOS to these voltage-dependent channels are unknown.

In skeletal muscle, nNOS activity is linked to muscle acetylcholine receptors and also to membrane depolarization. nNOS protein in skeletal muscle occurs at the endplate and at the plasma membrane owing to association with the dystrophin glycoprotein complex.[172] Again, the nNOS protein is targeted to the cellular domain that regulates the enzyme's activity (Fig. 168-6). Additional protein interactions appear to regulate NOS activity directly. A small molecular weight protein inhibitor of nNOS (PIN) that is enriched in both brain and testes and is highly conserved between species has been described.[182] PIN binds specifically to the neuronal isoform of NOS and acts by destabilizing the nNOS dimer, which is the active form of the enzyme.

Transcriptional Regulation of NOS in the Nervous System

The calcium-dependent NOS in normal brain was originally termed "constitutive" to distinguish the activity from "inducible" NOS that is present only in cells stimulated with cytokines or similar factors. However, it is now clear that transcription of all three forms of NOS is dynamically regulated in the nervous system. Induction of nNOS appears to be an adaptive response to permit sustained increases in NO biosynthesis. For example, in sensory pathways NO participates in processing of nociceptive inputs.[162] nNOS protein is induced in sensory neurons following tissue damage or peripheral nerve lesion, and this nNOS induction appears to participate in the prolonged nociceptive responses that follow these injuries.[183] Dramatic regulation of nNOS also occurs in the central nervous system following certain traumatic neuronal insults. Because nNOS is transiently expressed at high levels during brain development,[184] it is interesting to speculate that neurons recover from physical damage by reactivating cellular developmental paradigms. The induction of nNOS in the injured central nervous system can also be a maladaptive response, which mediates neuronal cell death. Avulsion of nerve roots from the ventral spinal cord causes induction of nNOS in motor neurons. The ensuing death of the nNOS positive motor neurons can be prevented with NOS inhibitors demonstrating the toxic role for NO in this response.[185] The specific transcriptional pathways that regulate nNOS induction are uncertain. However, neurotrophic growth factors, whose levels can change following nerve injury, may play a central role as NGF, BDNF, NT-3, and NT-4 have all been shown to induce nNOS expression in specific pathways.[186,187]

Expression of iNOS in Brain

While traumatic injury is associated with up-regulation of nNOS in neurons, inflammatory processes in brain often cause induction of iNOS in brain astrocytes and microglia. In *Toxoplasma gondii* induction, iNOS induction prevents parasite invasion into the brain, as iNOS knockout mice are uniquely susceptible to colonization of the central nervous system following peripheral inoculation with *T. gondii.*[188] Although iNOS induction can protect brain from certain infectious diseases, the excessive levels of NO that result can be toxic to neurons. In patients with multiple sclerosis, high levels of iNOS are found in reactive astrocytes in active demyelinating lesions and at the edge of chronic active demyelinating lesions.[189] Excess NO biosynthesis may mediate the inflammatory demyelination as NOS inhibitors decrease pathology in an experimental autoimmune encephalomyelitis model of multiple sclerosis.[190] iNOS protein levels are also increased in patients with severe AIDS dementia compared to seropositive individuals displaying no or mild impairment.[191] Purified viral gp41 from HIV increases iNOS expression and induces cell death in neuronal cultures and this cell death is prevented by an NOS inhibitor. Defining the potential role of iNOS inhibitors as therapy in AIDS dementia and other inflammatory brain disorders is an area of active research.

ROLE OF NO IN EXCITOTOXIC PROCESSES IN BRAIN

Inappropriate induction of NOS protein in brain and other tissues clearly mediates injury in diverse disease states. In a similar way, excess stimulation of nNOS at the synapse has the potential to mediate neurotoxicity in brain. Many causes of neuronal injury, including those associated with stroke and certain neurotoxins, are due to excess release of glutamate, which acts at synaptic NMDA receptors to cause neurotoxicity.[192] Accordingly, NMDA receptor antagonists are protective in animal models of cerebral ischemia.[193] The first experimental evidence that endogenous NO mediates brain injury associated with NMDA receptor activity derived from studies in cultured neurons.[194] This work showed that inhibition of NOS attenuates glutamate toxicity in primary neuronal cultures from rat cerebral cortex. Initially, this work was controversial, as subsequent studies concerning the role of NO in glutamate toxicity yielded contradictory results. These discrepancies were difficult to resolve due to the use of different neuronal cell types and culture conditions, which can have large effects on nNOS protein levels. nNOS knockout mice have helped clarify the role of nNOS in glutamate neurotoxicity. Cultured neurons derived from these knockout mice are resistant to glutamate toxicity, establishing that NO derived from nNOS can be toxic.[195]

NO Toxicity in Stroke

By mediating toxicity associated with excess glutamate release, NO plays a central role in stroke and other neurodegenerative diseases *in vivo*.[196] Decisive evidence that *neuron-derived* NO mediates injury in stroke comes from studies of nNOS knockout mice. Compared to littermate controls, nNOS knockouts show similar changes in regional blood flow following focal ischemia, but have 38 percent smaller infarcts (Fig. 168-7).[197] In contrast, eNOS-deficient mice show decreased blood flow at the periphery of the ischemic region, where NO-mediated excitotoxicity is most prevalent, and suffer an increased infarct size.[198] iNOS protein is not present in normal brain, so this isoform does not participate in the acute phase following ischemia. iNOS expression is induced, however, in reactive astrocytes and in infiltrating neutrophils following cerebral ischemia.[199] iNOS levels peak within 48 hours suggesting that postischemic inflammation and iNOS induction may contribute to a late phase of neuronal death. Indeed, mice deficient in iNOS display decreased infarct size in models of cerebral ischemia.[199]

Because eNOS activity protects the ischemic brain by maintaining blood flow, initial pharmacologic studies showed that nonspecific NOS inhibitors, which block both nNOS and eNOS, do not effectively protect from injury following stroke. The recent development of specific nNOS antagonists, such as ARL17477, 7-nitroindazole, and *S*-methyl-isothioureido-L-norvaline demonstrate that selective blockade of nNOS offers a useful pharmacologic strategy for controlling brain injury following stroke in rodent models.[199] Protective actions by NOS inhibitors are clearly mediated by antagonism of nNOS, as nonspecific NOS blockers paradoxically increase infarct volume in nNOS knockouts due to inhibition of eNOS.

Mechanisms for NO Toxicity

The molecular targets mediating NO toxicity are uncertain. Unlike the NO pathways that regulate intestinal motility and hippocampal LTP, cGMP is almost certainly not involved in toxicity. Instead, NO neurotoxicity is likely mediated by its free radical character, which makes NO reactive with certain proteins containing heme-

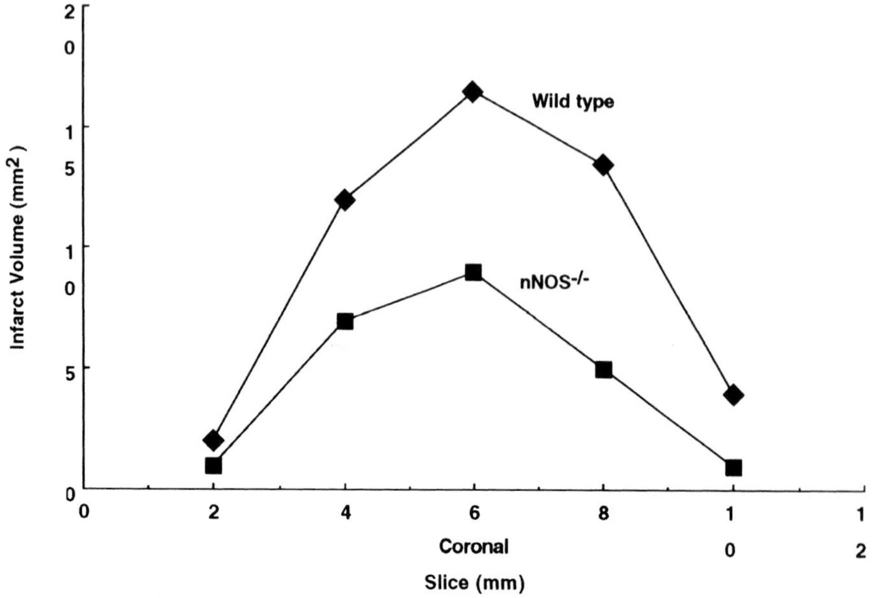

Fig. 168-7 Reduced infarct volume in nNOS$^{-/-}$ (knockout) mice. Wild-type or NOS$^{-/-}$ mice were subjected to middle cerebral artery occlusion for 24 h. Infarction area for each of five coronal sections from rostral to caudal (2 to 10 mm) is shown for wild-type and mutants. (Adapted from Huang et al.[197])

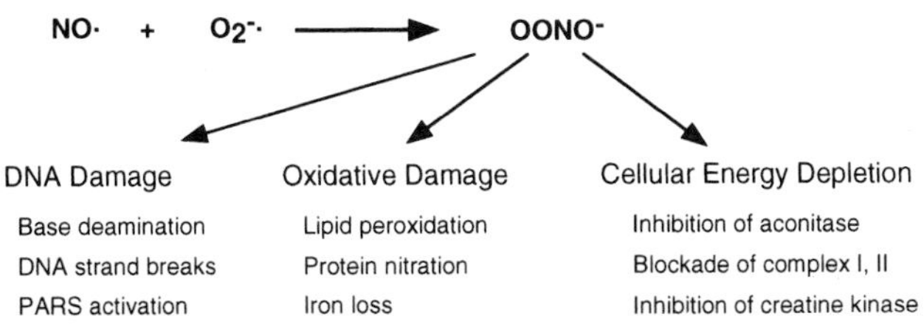

Fig. 168-8 Mechanisms for NO neurotoxicity. NO reacts rapidly with superoxide (O_2^-) to form a peroxynitrite ($OONO^-$), which is a potent oxidant. NO and peroxynitrite mediate cytotoxicity by causing oxidative damage, DNA damage and by depleting cellular energy stores.

iron prosthetic groups, iron sulfur clusters, or reactive thiols.[200] Cellular energy depletion is a hallmark of neuronal cell death associated with ischemic injury and NO can attenuate oxidative phosphorylation by inhibiting mitochondrial iron-sulfur cluster enzymes including NADH-ubiquinone oxidoreductase and NADH succinate:oxidoreductase. NO can also inhibit glycolysis by reactions with *cis*-aconitase[201] and by competing with oxygen at cytochrome oxidase.[202]

In addition to directly reacting with protein prosthetic groups, NO also reacts readily with superoxide (O_2^-) to produce peroxynitrite ($ONOO^-$) (Fig. 168-8), which may mediate much of the NO neurotoxicity.[203] Peroxynitrite is a powerful oxidant, but is sufficiently stable to diffuse through a cell to react with a target. Peroxynitrite is particularly efficient at oxidizing iron-sulfur clusters, zinc-fingers, and protein thiols, and these reactions would contribute to cellular energy depletion. Peroxynitrite will also react with superoxide dismutase (SOD) and this combination catalyzes the 3-nitration of protein tyrosine residues, particularly those in cytoskeletal proteins. The accumulation of 3-nitrotyrosine-containing proteins, detected with antisera to 3-nitrotyrosine, is a convenient marker of peroxynitrite formation.[203]

Direct evidence that NO and O_2^- conspire in neuronal toxicity derives from studies of transgenic animals. Cu/Zn SOD is a cytosolic scavenging enzyme that removes reactive O_2^- and prevents formation of peroxynitrite. Overexpression of Cu/Zn SOD in transgenic mice reduces the infarct volume in the middle cerebral artery (MCA) occlusion model of focal ischemia compared to wild-type mice.[204] Cu/Zn SOD overexpressing mice have now been bred with nNOS knockout mice and the resulting double transgenics acquire even less ischemic damage than either single-transgenic parental strain.[205]

NO in Neurodegenerative Diseases

While NO clearly participates in neuronal injury following vascular stroke, the role of NO in human neurodegenerative disease is not as easily understood. The slow progression of these diseases, perhaps occurring over 50 years or more, complicates experimental approaches to modeling their pathophysiological mechanism. Histopathologic evidence, however, suggests that certain neurodegenerative diseases, including Huntington disease, may also be mediated by NO and glutamate toxicities (Table 168-2). NADPH-diaphorase-positive neurons in the corpus striatum, which are the NOS neurons, are selectively spared in Huntington disease.[206] This selective pathology can be replicated in striatal culture models and *in vivo* following lesions with NMDA, but not with other classes of glutamate agonists.[207] The spared NADPH diaphorase neurons are uniquely endowed with high levels of SOD, which may protect the cells from peroxynitrite-mediated NO neurotoxicity.[208] Indeed, 3-nitrotyrosine, the footprint of peroxynitrite, is detected in striatal neurons in animals models of Huntington disease.[209]

While stigmata of NO toxicity correlate with Huntington disease pathology, a more causal role for NO and peroxynitrite toxicity has been established in some forms of Parkinson disease. MPTP, which contaminated batches of illicit drugs in the 1970s, produces parkinsonian-like symptoms in humans. MPTP causes pathology by targeting the destruction of nigrostriatal dopaminergic neurons, the same cells that are selectively lost in idiopathic Parkinson disease. Treatment of experimental animals, including mice and primates, with MPTP replicates this selective toxicity and results in accumulation of 3-nitrotyrosine in the nigrostriatal pathway. Inhibition of NOS prevents both the neurotoxicity of MPTP and the associated formation of 3-nitrotyrosine.[210] Definitive evidence that NO and peroxynitrite mediate toxicity in the MPTP model of Parkinson disease again derives from studies of transgenic mice.[211] Both nNOS knockouts and mice that overexpress Cu/Zn SOD are resistant to MPTP toxicity.

While nNOS inhibitors can prevent acute toxicity associated with MPTP, it remains less clear whether long-term treatment would be therapeutic for slowly developing neurodegenerative disorders. Chronic animal models for these diseases will first need to be established, and then the role of NO can then be rigorously evaluated. The recent identification of a Parkinson disease gene,[212] and the development of transgenic animal model for Huntington

Table 168-2 Diseases Associated with nNOS

Disease	Expression/Regulation of NOS in Diseased Tissue	Role of NO in Disease Pathogenesis
Stroke	nNOS activity acutely increases during cerebral ischemia. iNOS expression and activity are upregulated 12–48 h following ischemia.	Excessive NO causes free radical injury. Mice treated with NOS inhibitors and nNOS mutant mice have decreased infarct volume.
Parkinson disease	Axons from the degenerating substantia nigra project to the corpus striatum, which contains a rich density of nNOS neurons.	NO mediates nigral injury in the MPTP model of Parkinson disease. NOS inhibitors and nNOS mutant mice have decreased neuronal loss after MPTP.
Huntington disease	nNOS neurons are selectively spared in the otherwise degenerating corpus striatum.	NO may mediate neurodegeneration as NOS inhibitors prevent glutamate toxicity in cultures of striatal neurons.
Hypertrophic pyloric stenosis	nNOS neurons are absent from the pylorus in diseased infants.	Absence of NO results in increased tone of pyloric sphincter. nNOS is a susceptibility locus for infantile pyloric stenosis.
Muscular dystrophy	nNOS is absent from myofiber membranes in Duchenne and Becker dystrophies.	Role of NO in pathophysiology unclear.

disease,[213] suggests it will not be long until these issues are decisively addressed.

ACKNOWLEDGMENTS

Original studies were supported by grants from the Muscular Dystrophy Association, the National Association for Research on Schizophrenia and Depression, the National Institutes of Health, and the National Science Foundation.

REFERENCES

1. Green LC, Tannenbaum SR, Goldman P: Nitrate synthesis in the germfree and conventional rat. *Science* **212**:56, 1981.
2. Green LC, Ruiz de Luzuriaga K, Wagner DA, Rand W, Istfan N, Young VR, Tannenbaum SR: Nitrate biosynthesis in man. *Proc Natl Acad Sci U S A* **78**:7764, 1981.
3. Wagner DA, Young VR, Tannenbaum SR, Schultz DS, Deen WM: Mammalian nitrate biochemistry: Metabolism and endogenous synthesis. *IARC Sci Publ* **34**:247, 1984.
4. Hegesh E, Shiloah J: Blood nitrates and infantile methemoglobinemia. *Clin Chim Acta* **125**:107, 1982.
5. Wagner DA, Young VR, Tannenbaum SR: Mammalian nitrate biosynthesis: Incorporation of $^{15}NH_3$ into nitrate is enhanced by endotoxin treatment. *Proc Natl Acad Sci U S A* **80**:4518, 1983.
6. Stuehr DJ, Marletta MA: Mammalian nitrate biosynthesis: Mouse macrophages produce nitrite and nitrate in response to *Escherichia coli* lipopolysaccharide. *Proc Natl Acad Sci U S A* **82**:7738, 1985.
7. Stuehr DJ, Marletta MA: Synthesis of nitrite and nitrate in murine macrophage cell lines. *Cancer Res* **47**:5590, 1987.
8. Stuehr DJ, Marletta MA: Induction of nitrite/nitrate synthesis in murine macrophages by BCG infection, lymphokines, or interferon-gamma. *J Immunol* **139**:518, 1987.
9. Marletta MA, Yoon PS, Iyengar R, Leaf CD, Wishnok JS: Macrophage oxidation of L-arginine to nitrite and nitrate: Nitric oxide is an intermediate. *Biochemistry* **27**:8706, 1988.
10. Hibbs JB, Jr, Vavrin Z, Taintor RR: L-Arginine is required for expression of the activated macrophage effector mechanism causing selective metabolic inhibition in target cells. *J Immunol* **138**:550, 1987.
11. Hibbs JB Jr, Taintor RR, Vavrin Z: Macrophage cytotoxicity: Role for L-arginine deiminase and imino nitrogen oxidation to nitrite. *Science* **235**:473, 1987.
12. Furchgott RF, Zawadzki JV: The obligatory role of endothelial cells in the relaxation of arterial smooth muscle by acetylcholine. *Nature* **288**:373, 1980.
13. Griffith TM, Edwards DH, Lewis MJ, Newby AC, Henderson AH: The nature of endothelium-derived vascular relaxant factor. *Nature* **308**:645, 1984.
14. Cocks TM, Angus JA, Campbell JH, Campbell GR: Release and properties of endothelium-derived relaxing factor (EDRF) from endothelial cells in culture. *J Cell Physiol* **123**:310, 1985.
15. Rapoport RM, Murad F: Agonist-induced endothelium-dependent relaxation in rat thoracic aorta may be mediated through cGMP. *Circ Res* **52**:352, 1983.
16. Arnold WP, Mittal CK, Katsuki S, Murad F: Nitric oxide activates guanylate cyclase and increases guanosine 3′:5′-cyclic monophosphate levels in various tissue preparations. *Proc Natl Acad Sci U S A* **74**:3203, 1977.
17. Ignarro LJ, Lippton H, Edwards JC, Baricos WH, Hyman AL, Kadowitz PJ, Gruetter CA: Mechanism of vascular smooth muscle relaxation by organic nitrates, nitrites, nitroprusside and nitric oxide: Evidence for the involvement of S-nitrosothiols as active intermediates. *J Pharmacol Exp Ther* **218**:739, 1981.
18. Craven PA, DeRubertis FR: Restoration of the responsiveness of purified guanylate cyclase to nitrosoguanidine, nitric oxide, and related activators by heme and hemeproteins. Evidence for involvement of the paramagnetic nitrosyl-heme complex in enzyme activation. *J Biol Chem* **253**:8433, 1978.
19. Ignarro LJ, Degnan JN, Baricos WH, Kadowitz PJ, Wolin MS: Activation of purified guanylate cyclase by nitric oxide requires heme. Comparison of heme-deficient, heme-reconstituted and heme-containing forms of soluble enzyme from bovine lung. *Biochim Biophys Acta* **718**:49, 1982.
20. Furchgott RF: Studies on relaxation of rabbit aorta by sodium nitrite: the basis for the proposal that the acid-activatable inhibitory factor from retractor penis is inorganic nitrite and the endothelium derived relaxing factor is nitric oxide, in Vanhoutte PM (ed): *Vasodilation: Vascular Smooth Muscle, peptides, Autonomic Nerves and Endothelium.* New York, Raven Press, 1988, p 401.
21. Ignarro LJ, Buga GM, Wood KS, Byrns RE, Chaudhuri G: Endothelium-derived relaxing factor produced and released from artery and vein is nitric oxide. *Proc Natl Acad Sci U S A* **84**:9265, 1987.
22. Ignarro LJ, Byrns RE, Wood KS: Biochemical and pharmacological proteins of EDRF and its similarity to NO radical, in Vanhoutte PM (ed): *Vasodilation: Vascular Smooth muscle, peptides, Autonomic Nerves and Endothelium.* New York, Raven Press, 1988, p 427.
23. Palmer RM, Ferrige AG, Moncada S: Nitric oxide release accounts for the biological activity of endothelium-derived relaxing factor. *Nature* **327**:524, 1987.
24. Palmer RM, Ashton DS, Moncada S: Vascular endothelial cells synthesize nitric oxide from L-arginine. *Nature* **333**:664, 1988.
25. Palmer RM, Moncada S: A novel citrulline-forming enzyme implicated in the formation of nitric oxide by vascular endothelial cells. *Biochem Biophys Res Commun* **158**:348, 1989.
26. Azuma H, Ishikawa M, Sekizaki S: Endothelium-dependent inhibition of platelet aggregation. *Br J Pharmacol* **88**:411, 1986.
27. Furlong B, Henderson AH, Lewis MJ, Smith JA: Endothelium-derived relaxing factor inhibits in vitro platelet aggregation. *Br J Pharmacol* **90**:687, 1987.
28. Radomski MW, Palmer RM, Moncada S: Endogenous nitric oxide inhibits human platelet adhesion to vascular endothelium. *Lancet* **2**:1057, 1987.
29. Radomski MW, Palmer RM, Moncada S: The anti-aggregating properties of vascular endothelium: Interactions between prostacyclin and nitric oxide. *Br J Pharmacol* **92**:639, 1987.
30. Aisaka K, Gross SS, Griffith OW, Levi R: NG-methylarginine, an inhibitor of endothelium-derived nitric oxide synthesis, is a potent pressor agent in the guinea pig: Does nitric oxide regulate blood pressure in vivo? *Biochem Biophys Res Commun* **160**:881, 1989.
31. Whittle BJ, Lopez-Belmonte J, Rees DD: Modulation of the vasodepressor actions of acetylcholine, bradykinin, substance P and endothelin in the rat by a specific inhibitor of nitric oxide formation. *Br J Pharmacol* **98**:646, 1989.
32. Rees DD, Palmer RM, Moncada S: Role of endothelium-derived nitric oxide in the regulation of blood pressure. *Proc Natl Acad Sci U S A* **86**:3375, 1989.
33. Vallance P, Collier J, Moncada S: Effects of endothelium-derived nitric oxide on peripheral arteriolar tone in man [see comments]. *Lancet* **2**:997, 1989.
34. Vallance P, Collier J, Moncada S: Nitric oxide synthesised from L-arginine mediates endothelium dependent dilatation in human veins in vivo. *Cardiovasc Res* **23**:1053, 1989.
35. Deguchi T: Endogenous activating factor for guanylate cyclase in synaptosomal-soluble fraction of rat brain. *J Biol Chem* **252**:7617, 1977.
36. Deguchi T, Yoshioka M: l-Arginine identified as an endogenous activator for soluble guanylate cyclase from neuroblastoma cells. *J Biol Chem* **257**:10147, 1982.
37. Knowles RG, Palacios M, Palmer RM, Moncada S: Formation of nitric oxide from L-arginine in the central nervous system: A transduction mechanism for stimulation of the soluble guanylate cyclase. *Proc Natl Acad Sci U S A* **86**:5159, 1989.
38. Garthwaite J, Charles SL, Chess-Williams R: Endothelium-derived relaxing factor release on activation of NMDA receptors suggests role as intercellular messenger in the brain. *Nature* **336**:385, 1988.
39. Ferrendelli JA, Chang MM, Kinscherf DA: Elevation of cyclic GMP levels in central nervous system by excitatory and inhibitory amino acids. *J Neurochem* **22**:535, 1974.
40. Garthwaite J, Balazs R: Excitatory amino acid-induced changes in cyclic GMP levels in slices and cell suspensions from the cerebellum. *Adv Biochem Psychopharmacol* **27**:317, 1981.
41. Bredt DS, Snyder SH: Nitric oxide mediates glutamate-linked enhancement of cGMP levels in the cerebellum. *Proc Natl Acad Sci U S A* **86**:9030, 1989.
42. Garthwaite J, Garthwaite G, Palmer RM, Moncada S: NMDA receptor activation induces nitric oxide synthesis from arginine in rat brain slices. *Eur J Pharmacol* **172**:413, 1989.
43. Bredt DS, Snyder SH: Isolation of nitric oxide synthetase, a calmodulin-requiring enzyme. *Proc Natl Acad Sci U S A* **87**:682, 1990.
44. Mayer B, John M, Böhme E: Purification of a Ca^{2+}/calmodulin-dependent nitric oxide synthase from porcine cerebellum. Cofactor role of tetrahydrobiopterin. *FEBS Lett* **277**:215, 1990.

45. Schmidt HH, Pollock JS, Nakane M, Gorsky LD, Förstermann U, Murad F: Purification of a soluble isoform of guanylyl cyclase-activating-factor synthase. *Proc Natl Acad Sci U S A* **88**:365, 1991.
46. Hevel JM, White KA, Marletta MA: Purification of the inducible murine macrophage nitric oxide synthase. Identification as a flavoprotein. *J Biol Chem* **266**:22789, 1991.
47. Yui Y, Hattori R, Kosuga K, Eizawa H, Hiki K, Kawai C: Purification of nitric oxide synthase from rat macrophages. *J Biol Chem* **266**:12544, 1991.
48. Stuehr DJ, Cho HJ, Kwon NS, Weise MF, Nathan CF: Purification and characterization of the cytokine-induced macrophage nitric oxide synthase: An FAD- and FMN-containing flavoprotein. *Proc Natl Acad Sci U S A* **88**:7773, 1991.
49. Evans T, Carpenter A, Cohen J: Purification of a distinctive form of endotoxin-induced nitric oxide synthase from rat liver. *Proc Natl Acad Sci U S A* **89**:5361, 1992.
50. Pollock JS, Förstermann U, Mitchell JA, Warner TD, Schmidt HH, Nakane M, Murad F: Purification and characterization of particulate endothelium-derived relaxing factor synthase from cultured and native bovine aortic endothelial cells. *Proc Natl Acad Sci U S A* **88**:10480, 1991.
51. Bredt DS, Hwang PM, Glatt CE, Lowenstein C, Reed RR, Snyder SH: Cloned and expressed nitric oxide synthase structurally resembles cytochrome P-450 reductase. *Nature* **351**:714, 1991.
52. Nakane M, Schmidt HH, Pollock JS, Förstermann U, Murad F: Cloned human brain nitric oxide synthase is highly expressed in skeletal muscle. *FEBS Lett* **316**:175, 1993.
53. Sessa WC, Harrison JK, Barber CM, Zeng D, Durieux ME, D'Angelo DD, Lynch KR, Peach MJ: Molecular cloning and expression of a cDNA encoding endothelial cell nitric oxide synthase. *J Biol Chem* **267**:15274, 1992.
54. Lamas S, Marsden PA, Li GK, Tempst P, Michel T: Endothelial nitric oxide synthase: Molecular cloning and characterization of a distinct constitutive enzyme isoform. *Proc Natl Acad Sci U S A* **89**:6348, 1992.
55. Janssens SP, Shimouchi A, Quertermous T, Bloch DB, Bloch KD: Cloning and expression of a cDNA encoding human endothelium-derived relaxing factor/nitric oxide synthase [published erratum appears in *J Biol Chem* **267(31)**:22694, 1992]. *J Biol Chem* **267**:14519, 1992.
56. Lyons CR, Orloff GJ, Cunningham JM: Molecular cloning and functional expression of an inducible nitric oxide synthase from a murine macrophage cell line. *J Biol Chem* **267**:6370, 1992.
57. Xie QW, Cho HJ, Calaycay J, Mumford RA, Swiderek KM, Lee TD, Ding A, Troso T, Nathan C: Cloning and characterization of inducible nitric oxide synthase from mouse macrophages. *Science* **256**:225, 1992.
58. Lowenstein CJ, Glatt CS, Bredt DS, Snyder SH: Cloned and expressed macrophage nitric oxide synthase contrasts with the brain enzyme. *Proc Natl Acad Sci U S A* **89**:6711, 1992.
59. Geller DA, Lowenstein CJ, Shapiro RA Nussler AK, Di Silvio M, Wang SC, Nakayama DK, Simmons RL, Snyder SH, Billiar TR: Molecular cloning and expression of inducible nitric oxide synthase from human hepatocytes. *Proc Natl Acad Sci U S A* **90**:3491, 1993.
60. Moncada S, Palmer RM, Higgs EA: Nitric oxide: physiology, pathophysiology, and pharmacology. *Pharmacol Rev* **43**:109, 1991.
61. Pufahl RA, Nanjappan PG, Woodard RW, Marletta MA: Mechanistic probes of N-hydroxylation of L-arginine by the inducible nitric oxide synthase from murine macrophages. *Biochemistry* **31**:6822, 1992.
62. Feldman PL, Griffith OW, Hong H, Stuehr DJ: Irreversible Inactivation of macrophage and brain nitric oxide synthase by L-NG-methylarginine requires NADPH-dependent hydroxylation. *J Med Chem* **36**:491, 1993.
63. Dwyer MA, Bredt DS, Snyder SH: Nitric oxide synthase: Irreversible inhibition by L-NG-nitroarginine in brain in vitro and in vivo. *Biochem Biophys Res Commun* **176**:1136, 1991.
64. Klatt P, Schmidt K, Uray G, Mayer B: Multiple catalytic functions of brain nitric oxide synthase. Biochemical characterization, cofactor-requirement, and the role of N omega-hydroxy-L-arginine as an intermediate. *J Biol Chem* **268**:14781, 1993.
65. Zhang ZG, Reif D, Macdonald J, Tang WX, Kamp DK, Gentile RJ, Shakespeare WC, Murray RJ, Chopp M: ARL 17477, a potent and selective neuronal NOS inhibitor decreases infarct volume after transient middle cerebral artery occlusion in rats. *J Cereb Blood Flow Metab* **16**:599, 1996.
66. Mayer B, John M, Heinzel B, Werner ER, Wachter H, Schultz G, Böhme E: Brain nitric oxide synthase is a biopterin- and flavin-containing multi-functional oxido-reductase. *FEBS Lett* **288**:187, 1991.
67. McMillan K, Bredt DS, Hirsch DJ, Snyder SH, Clark JE, Masters BS: Cloned, expressed rat cerebellar nitric oxide synthase contains stoichiometric amounts of heme, which binds carbon monoxide. *Proc Natl Acad Sci U S A* **89**:11141, 1992.
68. White KA, Marletta MA: Nitric oxide synthase is a cytochrome P-450 type hemoprotein. *Biochemistry* **31**:6627, 1992.
69. Stuehr DJ, Ikeda-Saito M: Spectral characterization of brain and macrophage nitric oxide synthases. Cytochrome P-450-like hemeproteins that contain a flavin semiquinone radical. *J Biol Chem* **267**:20547, 1992.
70. Rogers NE, Ignarro LJ: Constitutive nitric oxide synthase from cerebellum is reversibly inhibited by nitric oxide formed from L-arginine. *Biochem Biophys Res Commun* **189**:242, 1992.
71. Rengasamy A, Johns RA: Regulation of nitric oxide synthase by nitric oxide. *Mol Pharmacol* **44**:124, 1993.
72. Assreuy J, Cunha FQ, Liew FY, Moncada S: Feedback inhibition of nitric oxide synthase activity by nitric oxide. *Br J Pharmacol* **108**:833, 1993.
73. McMillan K, Masters BS: Optical difference spectrophotometry as a probe of rat brain nitric oxide synthase heme-substrate interaction. *Biochemistry* **32**:9875, 1993.
74. Narhi LO, Fulco AJ: Characterization of a catalytically self-sufficient 119,000-dalton cytochrome P-450 monooxygenase induced by barbiturates in *Bacillus megaterium*. *J Biol Chem* **261**:7160, 1986.
75. Kwon NS, Nathan CF, Stuehr DJ: Reduced biopterin as a cofactor in the generation of nitrogen oxides by murine macrophages. *J Biol Chem* **264**:20496, 1989.
76. Tayeh MA, Marletta MA: Macrophage oxidation of L-arginine to nitric oxide, nitrite, and nitrate. Tetrahydrobiopterin is required as a cofactor. *J Biol Chem* **264**:19654, 1989.
77. Schmidt HHHW, Pollock JS, Nakane M, Gorsky LD, Forstermann U, Murad F: Purification of a soluble isoform of guanylyl cyclase-activating-factor synthase. *Proc Natl Acad Sci U S A* **88**:365, 1991.
78. Schmidt HH, Smith RM, Nakane M, Murad F: Ca^{2+}/calmodulin-dependent NO synthase type I: A biopteroflavoprotein with Ca^{2+}/calmodulin-independent diaphorase and reductase activities. *Biochemistry* **31**:3243, 1992.
79. Giovanelli J, Campos KL, Kaufman S: Tetrahydrobiopterin, a cofactor for rat cerebellar nitric oxide synthase, does not function as a reactant in the oxygenation of arginine. *Proc Natl Acad Sci U S A* **88**:7091, 1991.
80. Hevel JM, Marletta MA: Macrophage nitric oxide synthase: Relationship between enzyme-bound tetrahydrobiopterin and synthase activity. *Biochemistry* **31**:7160, 1992.
81. Hattori Y, Gross SS: GTP cyclohydrolase I mRNA is induced by LPS in vascular smooth muscle: Characterization, sequence and relationship to nitric oxide synthase. *Biochem Biophys Res Commun* **195**:435, 1993.
82. Di Silvio M, Geller DA, Gross SS, Nussler A, Freeswick P, Simmons RL, Billiar TR: Inducible nitric oxide synthase activity in hepatocytes is dependent on the coinduction of tetrahydrobiopterin synthesis. *Adv Exp Med Biol* **338**:305, 1993.
83. Crane BR, Arvai AS, Ghosh DK, Wu C, Getzoff ED, Stuehr DJ, Tainer JA: Structure of nitric oxide synthase oxygenase dimer with pterin and substrate. *Science* **279**:2121, 1998.
84. Crane BR, Arvai AS, Gachhui R, Wu C, Ghosh DK, Getzoff ED, Stuehr DJ, Tainer JA: The structure of nitric oxide synthase oxygenase domain and inhibitor complexes [see comments]. *Science* **278**:425, 1997.
85. Stuehr DJ, Kwon NS, Nathan CF, Griffith OW, Feldman PL, Wiseman J: N omega-hydroxy-L-arginine is an intermediate in the biosynthesis of nitric oxide from L-arginine. *J Biol Chem* **266**:6259, 1991.
86. Griffith OW, Stuehr DJ: Nitric oxide synthases: Properties and catalytic mechanism. *Annu Rev Physiol* **57**:707, 1995.
87. Pou S, Pou WS, Bredt DS, Snyder SH, Rosen GM: Generation of superoxide by purified brain nitric oxide synthase. *J Biol Chem* **267**:24173, 1992.
88. Vorherr T, Knöpfel L, Hofmann F, Mollner S, Pfeuffer T, Carafoli E: The calmodulin binding domain of nitric oxide synthase and adenylyl cyclase. *Biochemistry* **32**:6081, 1993.
89. Nakane M, Schmidt HH, Pollock JS, Förstermann U, Murad F: Cloned human brain nitric oxide synthase is highly expressed in skeletal muscle. *FEBS Lett* **316**:175, 1993.
90. Hall AV, Antoniou H, Wang Y, Cheung AH, Arbus AM, Olson SL, Lu WC, Kau CL, Marsden PA: Structural organization of the human

neuronal nitric oxide synthase gene (NOS1). *J Biol Chem* **269**:33082, 1994.
91. Marsden PA, Heng HH, Scherer SW, Stewart RJ, Hall AV, Shi XM, Tsui LC,, Schappert KT: Structure and chromosomal localization of the human constitutive endothelial nitric oxide synthase gene. *J Biol Chem* **268**:17478, 1993.
92. Xu W, Gorman P, Sheer D, Bates G, Kishimoto J, Lizhi L,, Emson P: Regional localization of the gene coding for human brain nitric oxide synthase (NOS1) to 12q24.2 → 24.31 by fluorescent in situ hybridization. *Cytogenet Cell Genet* **64**:62, 1993.
93. Ogura T, Yokoyama T, Fujisawa H, Kurashima Y, Esumi H: Structural diversity of neuronal nitric oxide synthase mRNA in the nervous system. *Biochem Biophys Res Commun* **193**:1014, 1993.
94. Xie J, Roddy P, Rife TK, Murad F, Young AP: Two closely linked but separable promoters for human neuronal nitric oxide synthase gene transcription. *Proc Natl Acad Sci U S A* **92**:1242, 1995.
95. Wang Y, Marsden PA: Nitric oxide synthases: Gene structure and regulation. *Adv Pharmacol* **34**:71, 1995.
96. Busconi L, Michel T: Endothelial nitric oxide synthase. N-terminal myristoylation determines subcellular localization. *J Biol Chem* **268**:8410, 1993.
97. Sessa WC, Barber CM, Lynch KR: Mutation of N-myristoylation site converts endothelial cell nitric oxide synthase from a membrane to a cytosolic protein. *Circ Res* **72**:921, 1993.
98. Robinson LJ, Michel T: Mutagenesis of palmitoylation sites in endothelial nitric oxide synthase identifies a novel motif for dual acylation and subcellular targeting. *Proc Natl Acad Sci U S A* **92**:11776, 1995.
99. Liu J, Garcia-Cardena G, Sessa WC: Biosynthesis and palmitoylation of endothelial nitric oxide synthase: Mutagenesis of palmitoylation sites, cysteines-15 and/or -26, argues against depalmitoylation-induced translocation of the enzyme. *Biochemistry* **34**:12333, 1995.
100. Shaul PW, Smart EJ, Robinson LJ, German Z, Yuhanna IS, Ying Y, erson RG, Michel T: Acylation targets endothelial nitric-oxide synthase to plasmalemmal caveolae. *J Biol Chem* **271**:6518, 1996.
101. Garcia-Cardena G, Oh P, Liu J, Schnitzer JE, Sessa WC: Targeting of nitric oxide synthase to endothelial cell caveolae via palmitoylation: Implications for nitric oxide signaling. *Proc Natl Acad Sci U S A* **93**:6448, 1996.
102. Robinson LJ, Busconi L, Michel T: Agonist-modulated palmitoylation of endothelial nitric oxide synthase. *J Biol Chem* **270**:995, 1995.
103. Robinson LJ, Weremowicz S, Morton CC, Michel T: Isolation and chromosomal localization of the human endothelial nitric oxide synthase (NOS3) gene. *Genomics* **19**:350, 1994.
104. Tang JL, Zembowicz A, Xu XM, Wu KK: Role of Sp1 in transcriptional activation of human nitric oxide synthase type III gene. *Biochem Biophys Res Commun* **213**:673, 1995.
105. Nadaud S, Philippe M, Arnal JF, Michel JB, Soubrier F: Sustained increase in aortic endothelial nitric oxide synthase expression in vivo in a model of chronic high blood flow. *Circ Res* **79**:857, 1996.
106. Sessa WC, Pritchard K, Seyedi N, Wang J, Hintze TH: Chronic exercise in dogs increases coronary vascular nitric oxide production and endothelial cell nitric oxide synthase gene expression. *Circ Res* **74**:349, 1994.
107. Zhang ZG, Chopp M, Zaloga C, Pollock JS, Förstermann U: Cerebral endothelial nitric oxide synthase expression after focal cerebral ischemia in rats. *Stroke* **24**:2016, 1993.
108. Arnet UA, McMillan A, Dinerman JL, Ballermann B, Lowenstein CJ: Regulation of endothelial nitric-oxide synthase during hypoxia. *J Biol Chem* **271**:15069, 1996.
109. Weiner CP, Lizasoain I, Baylis SA, Knowles RG, Charles IG, Moncada S: Induction of calcium-dependent nitric oxide synthases by sex hormones. *Proc Natl Acad Sci U S A* **91**:5212, 1994.
110. Hirata K, Miki N, Kuroda Y, Sakoda T, Kawashima S, Yokoyama M: Low concentration of oxidized low-density lipoprotein and lysophosphatidylcholine upregulate constitutive nitric oxide synthase mRNA expression in bovine aortic endothelial cells. *Circ Res* **76**:958, 1995.
111. Zembowicz A, Tang JL, Wu KK: Transcriptional induction of endothelial nitric oxide synthase type III by lysophosphatidylcholine. *J Biol Chem* **270**:17006, 1995.
112. Stadler J, Curran RD, Ochoa JB, Harbrecht BG, Hoffman RA, Simmons RL, Billiar TR: Effect of endogenous nitric oxide on mitochondrial respiration of rat hepatocytes in vitro and in vivo. *Arch Surg* **126**:186, 1991.
113. Charles IG, Palmer RM, Hickery MS, Bayliss MT, Chubb AP, Hall VS, Moss DW, Moncada S: Cloning, characterization, and expression of a cDNA encoding an inducible nitric oxide synthase from the human chondrocyte. *Proc Natl Acad Sci U S A* **90**:11419, 1993.
114. Chartrain NA, Geller DA, Koty PP, Sitrin NF, Nussler AK, Hoffman EP, Billiar TR, Hutchinson NI, Mudgett JS: Molecular cloning, structure, and chromosomal localization of the human inducible nitric oxide synthase gene. *J Biol Chem* **269**:6765, 1994.
115. Marsden PA, Heng HH, Duff CL, Shi XM, Tsui LC, Hall AV: Localization of the human gene for inducible nitric oxide synthase (NOS2) to chromosome 17q11.2-q12. *Genomics* **19**:183, 1994.
116. Xu W, Charles IG, Moncada S, Gorman P, Sheer D, Liu L, Emson P: Mapping of the genes encoding human inducible and endothelial nitric oxide synthase (NOS2 and NOS3) to the pericentric region of chromosome 17 and to chromosome 7, respectively. *Genomics* **21**:419, 1994.
117. Xie QW, Whisnant R, Nathan C: Promoter of the mouse gene encoding calcium-independent nitric oxide synthase confers inducibility by interferon gamma and bacterial lipopolysaccharide. *J Exp Med* **177**:1779, 1993.
118. Xie QW, Kashiwabara Y, Nathan C: Role of transcription factor NF-kappa B/Rel in induction of nitric oxide synthase. *J Biol Chem* **269**:4705, 1994.
119. Martin E, Nathan C, Xie QW: Role of interferon regulatory factor 1 in induction of nitric oxide synthase. *J Exp Med* **180**:977, 1994.
120. Kamijo R, Harada H, Matsuyama T, Bosland M, Gerecitano J, Shapiro D, Le J, Koh SI, Kimura T, Green SJ, et al: Requirement for transcription factor IRF-1 in NO synthase induction in macrophages. *Science* **263**:1612, 1994.
121. de Vera ME, Shapiro RA, Nussler AK, Mudgett JS, Simmons RL, Morris SM Jr, Billiar TR, Geller DA: Transcriptional regulation of human inducible nitric oxide synthase (NOS2) gene by cytokines: Initial analysis of the human NOS2 promoter. *Proc Natl Acad Sci U S A* **93**:1054, 1996.
122. Zhang X, Laubach VE, Alley EW, Edwards KA, Sherman PA, Russell SW, Murphy WJ: Transcriptional basis for hyporesponsiveness of the human inducible nitric oxide synthase gene to lipopolysaccharide/interferon-gamma. *J Leukoc Biol* **59**:575, 1996.
123. Taylor BS, de Vera ME, Ganster RW, Wang Q, Shapiro RA, Morris SM Jr, Billiar TR, Geller DA: Multiple NF-kappaB enhancer elements regulate cytokine induction of the human inducible nitric oxide synthase gene. *J Biol Chem* **273**:15148, 1998.
124. Linn SC, Morelli PJ, Edry I, Cottongim SE, Szabó C, Salzman AL: Transcriptional regulation of human inducible nitric oxide synthase gene in an intestinal epithelial cell line. *Am J Physiol* **272**:G1499, 1997.
125. Burnstock G: Review lecture. Neurotransmitters and trophic factors in the autonomic nervous system. *J Physiol (Lond)* **313**:1, 1981.
126. Gillespie JS, Liu XR, Martin W: The effects of L-arginine and NG-monomethyl L-arginine on the response of the rat anococcygeus muscle to NANC nerve stimulation. *Br J Pharmacol* **98**:1080, 1989.
127. Li CG, Rand MJ: Evidence for a role of nitric oxide in the neurotransmitter system mediating relaxation of the rat anococcygeus muscle. *Clin Exp Pharmacol Physiol* **16**:933, 1989.
128. Bredt DS, Hwang PM, Snyder SH: Localization of nitric oxide synthase indicating a neural role for nitric oxide. *Nature* **347**:768, 1990.
129. Huang PL, Dawson TM, Bredt DS, Snyder SH, Fishman MC: Targeted disruption of the neuronal nitric oxide synthase gene. *Cell* **75**:1273, 1993.
130. Chung E, Curtis D, Chen G, Marsden PA, Twells R, Xu W, Gardiner M: Genetic evidence for the neuronal nitric oxide synthase gene (NOS1) as a susceptibility locus for infantile pyloric stenosis. *Am J Hum Genet* **58**:363, 1996.
131. Iadecola C, Zhang F, Xu X: Role of nitric oxide synthase-containing vascular nerves in cerebrovasodilation elicited from cerebellum. *Am J Physiol* **264**:R738, 1993.
132. Nozaki K, Moskowitz MA, Maynard KI, Koketsu N, Dawson TM, Bredt DS, Snyder SH: Possible origins and distribution of immunoreactive nitric oxide synthase-containing nerve fibers in cerebral arteries. *J Cereb Blood Flow Metab* **13**:70, 1993.
133. Welch KM: Drug therapy of migraine [see comments]. *N Engl J Med* **329**:1476, 1993.
134. Iversen HK, Olesen J: Headache induced by a nitric oxide donor (nitroglycerin) responds to sumatriptan. A human model for development of migraine drugs [see comments]. *Cephalalgia* **16**:412, 1 996.
135. Irikura K, Huang PL, Ma J, Lee WS, Dalkara T, Fishman MC, Dawson TM, Snyder SH, Moskowitz MA: Cerebrovascular alterations in mice

lacking neuronal nitric oxide synthase gene expression. *Proc Natl Acad Sci U S A* **92**:6823, 1995.
136. Burnett AL, Tillman SL, Chang TS, Epstein JI, Lowenstein CJ, Bredt DS, Snyder SH, Walsh PC: Immunohistochemical localization of nitric oxide synthase in the autonomic innervation of the human penis. *J Urol* **150**:73, 1993.
137. Burnett AL, Lowenstein CJ, Bredt DS, Chang TS, Snyder SH: Nitric oxide: A physiologic mediator of penile erection. *Science* **257**:401, 1992.
138. Rajfer J, Aronson WJ, Bush PA, Dorey FJ, Ignarro LJ: Nitric oxide as a mediator of relaxation of the corpus cavernosum in response to nonadrenergic, noncholinergic neurotransmission. *N Engl J Med* **326**:90, 1992.
139. Burnett AL, Nelson RJ, Calvin DC, Liu JX, Demas GE, Klein SL, Kriegsfeld LJ, Dawson VL, Dawson TM, Snyder SH: Nitric oxide-dependent penile erection in mice lacking neuronal nitric oxide synthase. *Mol Med* **2**:288, 1996.
140. Vernet D, Cai L, Garban H, Babbitt ML, Murray FT, Rajfer J, Gonzalez-Cadavid NF: Reduction of penile nitric oxide synthase in diabetic BB/WORdp (type I) and BBZ/WORdp (type II) rats with erectile dysfunction. *Endocrinology* **136**:5709, 1995.
141. Carrier S, Nagaraju P, Morgan DM, Baba K, Nunes L, Lue TF: Age decreases nitric oxide synthase-containing nerve fibers in the rat penis. *J Urol* **157**:1088, 1997.
142. Penson DF, Ng C, Cai L, Rajfer J, Gonzalez-Cadavid NF: Androgen and pituitary control of penile nitric oxide synthase and erectile function in the rat. *Biol Reprod* **55**:567, 1996.
143. Boolell M, Allen MJ, Ballard SA, Gepi-Attee S, Muirhead GJ, Naylor AM, Osterloh IH, Gingell C: Sildenafil: An orally active type 5 cyclic GMP-specific phosphodiesterase inhibitor for the treatment of penile erectile dysfunction. *Int J Impot Res* **8**:47, 1996.
144. Ballard SA, Gingell CJ, Tang K, Turner LA, Price ME, Naylor AM: Effects of sildenafil on the relaxation of human corpus cavernosum tissue in vitro and on the activities of cyclic nucleotide phosphodiesterase isozymes. *J Urol* **159**:2164, 1998.
145. Goldstein I, Lue TF, Padma-Nathan H, Rosen RC, Steers WD, Wicker PA: Oral sildenafil in the treatment of erectile dysfunction. Sildenafil Study Group [see comments]. *N Engl J Med* **338**:1397, 1998.
146. Chuang AT, Strauss JD, Murphy RA, Steers WD: Sildenafil, a type-5 CGMP phosphodiesterase inhibitor, specifically amplifies endogenous cGMP-dependent relaxation in rabbit corpus cavernosum smooth muscle in vitro. *J Urol* **160**:257, 1998.
147. Schuman EM, Madison DV: Nitric oxide and synaptic function. *Annu Rev Neurosci* **17**:153, 1994.
148. Shibuki K, Okada D: Endogenous nitric oxide release required for long-term synaptic depression in the cerebellum. *Nature* **349**:326, 1991.
149. Son H, Hawkins RD, Martin K, Kiebler M, Huang PL, Fishman MC, Kandel ER: Long-term potentiation is reduced in mice that are doubly mutant in endothelial and neuronal nitric oxide synthase. *Cell* **87**:1015, 1996.
150. Hirsch DB, Steiner JP, Dawson TM, Mammen A, Hayek E, Snyder SH: Neurotransmitter release regulated by nitric oxide in PC-12 cells and brain synaptosomes. *Curr Biol* **3**:749, 1993.
151. Lonart G, Wang J, Johnson KM: Nitric oxide induces neurotransmitter release from hippocampal slices. *Eur J Pharmacol* **220**:271, 1992.
152. Dickie BG, Lewis MJ, Davies JA: NMDA-induced release of nitric oxide potentiates aspartate overflow from cerebellar slices. *Neurosci Lett* **138**:145, 1992.
153. Montague PR, Gancayco CD, Winn MJ, Marchase RB, Friedlander MJ: Role of NO production in NMDA receptor-mediated neurotransmitter release in cerebral cortex. *Science* **263**:973, 1994.
154. Hanbauer I, Wink D, Osawa Y, Edelman GM, Gally JA: Role of nitric oxide in NMDA-evoked release of [3H]-dopamine from striatal slices. *Neuroreport* **3**:409, 1992.
155. McCann SM, Rettori V: The role of nitric oxide in reproduction. *Proc Soc Exp Biol Med* **211**:7, 1996.
156. Rettori V, Belova N, Dees WL, Nyberg CL, Gimeno M, McCann SM: Role of nitric oxide in the control of luteinizing hormone-releasing hormone release in vivo and in vitro. *Proc Natl Acad Sci U S A* **90**:10130, 1993.
157. Mani SK, Allen JM, Rettori V, McCann SM, O'Malley BW, Clark JH: Nitric oxide mediates sexual behavior in female rats. *Proc Natl Acad Sci U S A* **91**:6468, 1994.
158. Rettori V, Canteros G, Renoso R, Gimeno M, McCann SM: Oxytocin stimulates the release of luteinizing hormone-releasing hormone from medial basal hypothalamic explants by releasing nitric oxide. *Proc Natl Acad Sci U S A* **94**:2741, 1997.
159. Wu HH, Williams CV, McLoon SC: Involvement of nitric oxide in the elimination of a transient retinotectal projection in development. *Science* **265**:1593, 1994.
160. Hawkins RD: NO honey, I don't remember. *Neuron* **16**:465, 1996.
161. Kendrick KM, Guevara-Guzman R, Zorrilla J, Hinton MR, Broad KD, Mimmack M, Ohkura S: Formation of olfactory memories mediated by nitric oxide. *Nature* **388**:670, 1997.
162. Meller ST, Gebhart GF: Nitric oxide (NO) and nociceptive processing in the spinal cord [see comments]. *Pain* **52**:127, 1993.
163. Crosby G, Marota JJ, Huang PL: Intact nociception-induced neuroplasticity in transgenic mice deficient in neuronal nitric oxide synthase. *Neuroscience* **69**:1013, 1995.
164. Silvagno F, Xia H, Bredt DS: Neuronal nitric oxide synthase-m, an alternatively spliced isoform expressed in differentiated skeletal muscle. *J Biol Chem* **271**:11204, 1996.
165. Kobzik L, Reid MB, Bredt DS, Stamler JS: Nitric oxide in skeletal muscle. *Nature* **372**:546, 1994.
166. Boczkowski J, Lanone S, Ungureanu-Longrois D, Danialou G, Fournier T, Aubier M: Induction of diaphragmatic nitric oxide synthase after endotoxin administration in rats: Role on diaphragmatic contractile dysfunction. *J Clin Invest* **98**:1550, 1996.
167. Lee KH, Baek MY, Moon KY, Song WK, Chung CH, Ha DB, Kang MS: Nitric oxide as a messenger molecule for myoblast fusion. *J Biol Chem* **269**:14371, 1994.
168. Wang T, Xie Z, Lu B: Nitric oxide mediates activity-dependent synaptic suppression at developing neuromuscular synapses. *Nature* **374**:262, 1995.
169. Balon TW, Nadler JL: Nitric oxide release is present from incubated skeletal muscle preparations [see comments]. *J Appl Physiol* **77**:2519, 1994.
170. Roberts CK, Barnard RJ, Scheck SH, Balon TW: Exercise-stimulated glucose transport in skeletal muscle is nitric oxide dependent. *Am J Physiol* **273**:E220, 1997.
171. Balon TW, Nadler JL: Evidence that nitric oxide increases glucose transport in skeletal muscle. *J Appl Physiol* **82**:359, 1997.
172. Brenman JE, Chao D S, Xia H, Aldape K, Bredt DS: Nitric oxide synthase complexed with dystrophin and absent from skeletal muscle sarcolemma in Duchenne muscular dystrophy. *Cell* **82**:743, 1995.
173. Chao DS, Gorospe RM, Brenman JE, Rafael JA, Peters MF, Froehner SC, Hoffman EP, Chamberlain JS, Bredt DS: Selective loss of sarcolemmal nitric oxide synthase in Becker Muscular Dystrophy. *J Exp Med* **184**:609, 1996.
174. Campbell KP: Three muscular dystrophies: Loss of cytoskeleton-extracellular matrix linkage. *Cell* **80**:675, 1995.
175. Brown RH: Free radicals, programmed cell death and muscular dystrophy [Editorial]. *Curr Opin Neurol* **8**:373, 1995.
176. Isozumi K, DeLong R, Kaplan J, Deng HX, Iqbal Z, Hung WY, Wilhelmsen KC, Hentati A, Pericak-Vance MA, Siddique T: Linkage of scapuloperoneal spinal muscular atrophy to chromosome 12q24.1-q24.31. *Hum Mol Genet* **5**:1377, 1996.
177. Daniel EE, Haugh C, Woskowska Z, Cipris S, Jury J, Fox-Threlkeld JE: Role of nitric oxide-related inhibition in intestinal function: Relation to vasoactive intestinal polypeptide. *Am J Physiol* **266**:G31, 1994.
178. Mashimo H, He XD, Huang PL, Fishman MC, Goyal RK: Neuronal constitutive nitric oxide synthase is involved in murine enteric inhibitory neurotransmission. *J Clin Invest* **98**:8, 1996.
179. Brenman JE, Chao DS, Gee SH, McGee AW, Craven SE, Santillano DR, Huang F, Xia H, Peters MF, Froehner SC, Bredt DS: Interaction of nitric oxide synthase with the postsynaptic density protein PSD-95 and α-1 syntrophin mediated by PDZ motifs. *Cell* **84**:757, 1996.
180. Kornau H-C, Seeburg PH, Kennedy MB: Interaction of ion channels and receptors with PDZ domains. *Curr Opin Neurobiol* **7**:368, 1997.
181. Sheng M: PDZs and receptor/channel clustering: Rounding up the latest suspects [Comment]. *Neuron* **17**:575, 1996.
182. Jaffrey SR, Snyder SH: PIN: An associated protein inhibitor of neuronal nitric oxide synthase. *Science* **274**:774, 1996.
183. Wiesenfeld-Hallin Z, Hao JX, Xu XJ, Hokfelt T: Nitric oxide mediates ongoing discharges in dorsal root ganglion cells after peripheral nerve injury. *J Neurophysiol* **70**:2350, 1993.
184. Bredt DS, Snyder SH: Transient nitric oxide synthase neurons in embryonic cerebral cortical plate, sensory ganglia, and olfactory epithelium. *Neuron* **13**:301, 1994.
185. Wu W, Li L: Inhibition of nitric oxide synthase reduces motoneuron death due to spinal root avulsion. *Neurosci Lett* **153**:121, 1993.

186. Holtzman DM, Kilbridge J, Bredt DS, Black SM, Yiwen L, Clary DO, Reichardt LF, Mobley WC: NOS induction by NGF in basal forebrain cholinergic neurons suggests novel mechanism for NGF effects on learning and memory. *Neurobiol Dis* **1**:51, 1994.
187. Huber KA, Krieglstein K, Unsicker K: The neurotrophins BDNF, NT-3 and -4, but not NGF, TGF-beta 1 and GDNF, increase the number of NADPH-diaphorase-reactive neurons in rat spinal cord cultures. *Neuroscience* **69**:771, 1995.
188. Scharton-Kersten TM, Yap G, Magram J, Sher, A: Inducible nitric oxide is essential for host control of persistent but not acute infection with the intracellular pathogen *Toxoplasma gondii. J Exp Med* **185**:1261, 1997.
189. Bo L, Dawson TM, Wesselingh S, Mork S, Choi S, Kong PA, Hanley D, Trapp BD: Induction of nitric oxide synthase in demyelinating regions of multiple sclerosis brains. *Ann Neurol* **36**:778, 1994.
190. Cross AH, Misko TP, Lin RF, Hickey WF, Trotter JL, Tilton RG: Aminoguanidine, an inhibitor of inducible nitric oxide synthase, ameliorates experimental autoimmune encephalomyelitis in SJL mice. *J Clin Invest* **93**:2684, 1994.
191. Adamson DC, Wildemann B, Sasaki M, Glass JD, McArthur JC, Christov VI, Dawson TM, Dawson VL: Immunologic NO synthase: Elevation in severe AIDS dementia and induction by HIV-1 gp41. *Science* **274**:1917, 1996.
192. Choi DW: Glutamate receptors and the induction of excitotoxic neuronal death. *Prog Brain Res* **100**:47, 1994.
193. Simon RP, Swan JH, Griffiths T, Meldrum BS: Blockade of *N*-methyl-D-aspartate receptors may protect against ischemic damage in the brain. *Science* **226**:850, 1984.
194. Dawson VL, Dawson TM, London ED, Bredt DS, Snyder SH: Nitric oxide mediates glutamate neurotoxicity in primary cortical cultures. *Proc Natl Acad Sci U S A* **88**:6368, 1991.
195. Dawson VL, Kizushi V, M, Huang PL, Snyder SH, Dawson TM: Resistance to neurotoxicity in cortical cultures from neuronal nitric oxide synthase-deficient mice. *J Neurosci* **16**:2479, 1996.
196. Dawson VL, Dawson TM: Nitric oxide in neuronal degeneration. *Proc Soc Exp Biol Med* **211**:33, 1996.
197. Huang Z, Huang PL, Panahian N, Dalkara T, Fishman MC, Moskowitz MA: Effects of cerebral ischemia in mice deficient in neuronal nitric oxide synthase. *Science* **265**:1883, 1994.
198. Huang Z, Huang PL, Ma J, Meng W, Ayata C, Fishman MC, Moskowitz MA: Enlarged infarcts in endothelial nitric oxide synthase knockout mice are attenuated by nitro-L-arginine. *J Cereb Blood Flow Metab* **16**:981, 1996.
199. Iadecola C: Bright and dark sides of nitric oxide in ischemic brain injury. *Trends Neurosci* **20**:132, 1997.
200. Stamler JS: Redox signaling: nitrosylation and related target interactions of nitric oxide. *Cell* **78**:931, 1994.
201. Drapier JC, Hibbs JB Jr: Aconitases: A class of metalloproteins highly sensitive to nitric oxide synthesis. *Methods Enzymol* **269**:26, 1996.
202. Brown GC: Nitric oxide regulates mitochondrial respiration and cell functions by inhibiting cytochrome oxidase. *FEBS Lett* **369**:136, 1995.
203. Beckman JS, Koppenol WH: Nitric oxide, superoxide, and peroxynitrite: The good, the bad, and ugly. *Am J Physiol* **271**:C1424, 1996.
204. Kinouchi H, Epstein CJ, Mizui T, Carlson E, Chen SF, Chan PH: Attenuation of focal cerebral ischemic injury in transgenic mice overexpressing CuZn superoxide dismutase. *Proc Natl Acad Sci U S A* **88**:11158, 1991.
205. Samdani AF, Dawson TM, Dawson VL: Nitric oxide synthase in models of focal ischemia. *Stroke* **28**:1283, 1997.
206. Ferrante RJ, Kowall NW, Beal MF, Richardson EP Jr, Bird ED, Martin JB: Selective sparing of a class of striatal neurons in Huntington's disease. *Science* **230**:561, 1985.
207. Koh JY, Peters S, Choi DW: Neurons containing NADPH-diaphorase are selectively resistant to quinolinate toxicity. *Science* **234**:73, 1986.
208. Inagaki S, Suzuki K, Taniguchi N, Takagi H: Localization of Mn-superoxide dismutase (Mn-SOD) in cholinergic and somatostatin-containing neurons in the rat neostriatum. *Brain Res* **549**:174, 1991.
209. Galpern WR, Matthews RT, Beal MF, Isacson O: NGF attenuates 3-nitrotyrosine formation in a 3-NP model of Huntington's disease. *Neuroreport* **7**:2639, 1996.
210. Hantraye P, Brouillet E, Ferrante R, Palfi S, Dolan R, Matthews RT, Beal MF: Inhibition of neuronal nitric oxide synthase prevents MPTP-induced parkinsonism in baboons. *Nat Med* **2**:1017, 1996.
211. Przedborski S, Jackson-Lewis V, Yokoyama R, Shibata T, Dawson VL, Dawson TM: Role of neuronal nitric oxide in 1-methyl-4-phenyl-1,2,3,6-tetrahydropyridine (MPTP)-induced tetrahydropyridine (MPTP)-induced dopaminergic neurotoxicity. *Proc Natl Acad Sci U S A* **93**:4565, 1996.
212. Polymeropoulos MH, Lavedan C, Leroy E, Ide SE, Dehejia A, Dutra A, Pike B, Root H, Rubenstein J, Boyer R, Stenroos ES, Chandrasekharappa S, Athanassiadou A, Papapetropoulos T, Johnson WG, Lazzarini AM, Duvoisin RC, Di Iorio G, Golbe LI, Nussbaum RL: Mutation in the alpha-synuclein gene identified in families with Parkinson's disease [see comments]. *Science* **276**:2045, 1997.
213. Davies SW, Turmaine M, Cozens BA, DiFiglia M, Sharp AH, Ross CA, Scherzinger E, Wanker EE, Mangiarini L, Bates GP: Formation of neuronal intranuclear inclusions underlies the neurological dysfunction in mice transgenic for the HD mutation. *Cell* **90**:537, 1997.
214. Christopherson KS, Bredt DS: Nitric oxide in excitable tissues: Physiological roles and disease. *J Clin Invest* **100**:2424, 1997.

PART 19

BLOOD

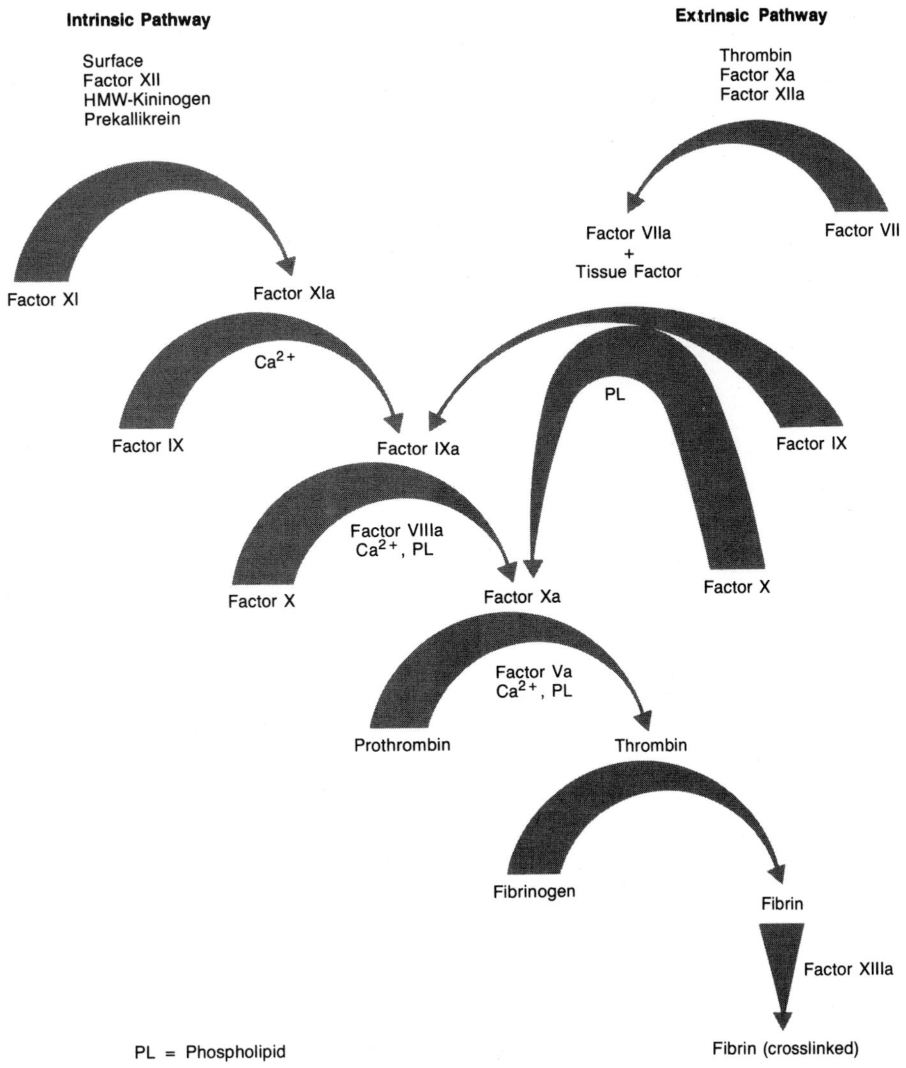

Intrinsic Pathway
Surface
Factor XII
HMW-Kininogen
Prekallikrein
Extrinsic Pathway
Thrombin
Factor Xa
Factor XIIa
Factor VIIa
+
Tissue Factor
Factor VII
Factor XI
Factor XIa
Ca2+
Factor IX
Factor IXa
PL
Factor IX
Factor VIIIa
Ca2+, PL
Factor X
Factor Xa
Factor X
Factor Va
Ca2+, PL
Prothrombin
Thrombin
Fibrinogen
Fibrin
Factor XIIIa
Fibrin (crosslinked)
PL = Phospholipid

CHAPTER 169

Introduction to Hemostasis and the Vitamin K-Dependent Coagulation Factors

Daniel L. Greenberg ▪ Earl W. Davie

1. Six plasma proteins— prothrombin, factor VII, factor IX, factor X, protein C, and protein S—require vitamin K for their biosynthesis in the liver. Each contains 9 to 12 γ-carboxyglutamic acid residues in the N-terminal portion of their molecule, and these residues are formed by vitamin K-dependent carboxylation of specific glutamic acid residues. The γ-carboxyglutamic acid residues are required for the calcium-dependent binding of the vitamin K-dependent proteins to phospholipid surfaces.

2. Prothrombin, factor VII, factor IX, factor X, and protein C circulate in blood as precursor molecules to serine proteases. When the blood coagulation cascade is initiated by exposure to tissue factor, prothrombin, factor VII, factor IX, and factor X are converted to serine proteases by minor proteolysis. Each protease in turn then cleaves a specific protein substrate(s). These reactions eventually lead to the generation of thrombin and fibrin at the site of vascular injury. Protein C is also converted to a serine protease by minor proteolysis during the coagulation cascade. This enzyme, however, plays a regulatory role in blood coagulation in that it inactivates factor Va and factor VIIIa in the presence of protein S, which helps bring the coagulation cascade to a halt.

3. Reduced levels of prothrombin (MIM 176930), factor VII (MIM 227500), factor IX (MIM 306900), and factor X (MIM 227600) result in bleeding complications in patients with these deficiencies. Reduced levels of protein C or protein S, however, may be associated with thrombotic risk because the regulation of the coagulation pathway is impaired.

4. The genes for prothrombin, factor VII, factor IX, protein C, and protein S have been well characterized and their chromosomal locations established. Abnormalities in the genes for the vitamin K-dependent proteins have been identified and range from partial gene deletions to single nucleotide changes or deletions. These abnormalities were observed in the exons coding for the mature protein and the leader sequence, as well as in the intron-exon boundaries and regulatory regions of the genes for these proteins.

A list of standard abbreviations is located immediately preceding the index in each volume. Additional abbreviations used in this chapter include: APTT = activated partial thromboplastin time; ARE = androgen response element; C/EBP = CCAAT/enhancer binding protein; DBP = D site (of albumin) binding protein; DGGE = denaturing gradient gel electrophoresis; DIC = disseminated intravascular coagulation; FFP = fresh frozen plasma; FXP1, FXP2, etc. = factor X promoter element 1, 2, etc.; Gla = γ-carboxyglutamic acid; HCV = hepatitis C virus; PT = prothrombin time; HNF-1, 2, etc. = hepatic nuclear factor 1, 2, etc.; NF-1 = nuclear factor 1; PACE = pulmonary angiotensin I converting enzyme; RVV-X = Russell's viper venom.

GENERAL INTRODUCTION TO HEMOSTASIS

Hemostasis in humans involves a number of plasma proteins and platelets, and their interaction with the vascular endothelium. Initially, a platelet plug is formed followed by a fibrin clot at the site of vascular injury. Platelet plug formation requires von Willebrand factor, a plasma protein that forms a bridge between the activated platelet and the subendothelium. This reaction, which is called *platelet adhesion*, involves a specific platelet membrane receptor (glycoprotein Ib) that binds to von Willebrand factor. Platelet adhesion is immediately followed by platelet aggregation. In this reaction, fibrinogen forms a bridge between platelets by binding one activated platelet to another. Another platelet membrane receptor, called *glycoprotein IIb/IIIa*, is involved in this reaction. During platelet plug formation, phospholipid is made available and the blood coagulation cascade is initiated. The precise events that trigger the coagulation cascade are not known, but it appears that tissue factor, a subendothelial-cell surface glycoprotein, plays an important role in the process.

The plasma proteins that participate in the coagulation cascade circulate in blood in precursor or inactive forms. When blood coagulation is initiated, these proteins are converted to active enzymes, or cofactors, which eventually leads to the generation of thrombin and fibrin. The plasma and cellular proteins and their cofactors have been assigned Roman numerals and are listed in Table 169-1 along with their common names. The terms *fibrinogen*, *prothrombin*, *tissue factor*, and *calcium* are employed by most investigators working in the field, while the remaining proteins (factors V through XIII) are usually referred to by their Roman numerals alone. No protein has been assigned as factor VI.

The amino acid sequences for all of the proteins shown in Table 169-1 were established by a combination of protein sequence analysis and cDNA cloning. Furthermore, the chromosomal location, gene organization, and DNA sequence also have been determined for these proteins. These data show that the plasma proteins involved in fibrin formation and its regulation often share considerable amino acid sequence homology, physiological function, and mechanism of action. For example, the vitamin K-dependent proteins (prothrombin, factors VII, IX, and X, protein C, and protein S) all share common domains, and all but protein S are converted to serine proteases by minor proteolysis. Likewise, factors V and VIII are large single-chain glycoproteins with considerable sequence homology. These two proteins also participate in the coagulation cascade as cofactors in the presence of calcium and phospholipid following their activation by minor

Table 169-1 Nomenclature and Chapter Assignment for the Blood Coagulation Factors, Associated Proteins, and Platelets

Roman Numeral Designation	Common Name	Chapter
Factor I	Fibrinogen	171
Factor II	Prothrombin	169
Factor III	Tissue factor	169
Factor IV	Calcium ions	—
Factor V	Proaccelerin	170
Factor VII	Proconvertin	169
Factor VIII	Antihemophilic factor	172
Factor IX	Christmas factor	169,173
Factor X	Stuart factor	169
Factor XI	Plasma thromboplastin antecedent	175
Factor XII	Hageman factor	178
Factor XIII	Fibrin-stabilizing factor	170
—	Prekallikrein (Fletcher factor)	178
—	HMW kininogen (high-molecular weight-kininogen)	178
—	Protein C	169,170
—	Protein S	169,170
—	Antithrombin III	176
—	Heparin cofactor II	176
—	von Willebrand factor	174
—	Platelets	177

proteolysis. Similarly, factor XI and plasma prekallikrein are highly homologous molecules that share common domains and are converted to serine proteases by minor proteolysis.

In this chapter and the chapters that follow (170 to 178), the plasma proteins and the platelet surface glycoproteins that are involved in hemostasis are discussed and their gene structures described.

INTRODUCTION TO VITAMIN K-DEPENDENT COAGULATION PROTEINS

The vitamin K-dependent proteins that participate in blood coagulation and its regulation include prothrombin, factor VII, factor IX, factor X, protein C, and protein S. These glycoproteins are synthesized in the liver and are secreted into the blood. They circulate in the blood as trace proteins with plasma concentrations that range from 0.47 μg/ml for factor VII to 80 to 90 μg/ml for prothrombin (Table 169-2). Their half-lives in blood also vary considerably, with those for factor VII and protein C being the shortest. Prothrombin, factor VII, factor IX, factor X, and protein C circulate in blood as precursor or zymogen molecules and are converted to active serine proteases during the coagulation cascade (Fig. 169-1). Protein S, however, participates as a cofactor to activated protein C, and these two proteins are involved in the regulation of the coagulation pathway by the inactivation of factor Va and factor VIIIa in the presence of phospholipid (Fig. 169-2).

Each of the six human vitamin K-dependent coagulation factors consists of a series of homologous structural domains. The N-terminal region of each of the vitamin K-dependent coagulation proteins contains from 9 to 12 γ-carboxyglutamic acid (Gla) residues. These residues are formed by carboxylation of glutamic acid residues located within the first 40 to 45 amino acids in the amino-terminal region of each protein.[1–3] The γ-carboxyglutamic acid residues constitute the Gla domains in each of the vitamin K-dependent proteins and are required for the calcium-dependent binding of these proteins to phospholipid surfaces.[4] Based on three-dimensional x-ray crystallographic analysis of the N-terminal region of prothrombin, in the presence of calcium ions, the Gla domain maintains a highly ordered structure, with nine Gla residues interacting with seven calcium ions.[5] This creates an environment in which some of the positively charged calcium ions presumably form an electrostatic bridge between the negatively charged Gla residues and the negatively charged phospholipid of a membrane surface. This binding localizes the vitamin K-dependent coagulation factors at the site of vascular injury where platelet plug formation has occurred and an active phospholipid surface has been made available.

Two kringle domains follow the Gla domain in prothrombin.[6] These kringle domains are composed of approximately 80 amino acids with disulfide bonds linking the six Cys residues in a pattern of $1 \rightarrow 6$, $2 \rightarrow 4$, and $3 \rightarrow 5$. Kringle structures are also present in factor XII,[7] plasminogen,[8] tissue plasminogen activator,[9] and urokinase.[10] In factor VII,[11] factor IX,[12–14] factor X,[15–17] and protein C,[18,19] the kringle domains are replaced by two growth factor domains. These domains are composed of 40 to 50 amino acids with disulfide bonds linking the 6 Cys residues in a characteristic pattern of $1 \rightarrow 3$, $2 \rightarrow 4$, and $5 \rightarrow 6$ (Fig. 169-3). These domains show considerable structural similarity to epidermal growth factor (EGF) and EGF precursor.[20–22] Protein S contains four growth factor domains present as tandem repeats following the amino-terminal Gla domain.[23,24] Homologous growth factor structures are also present in several other hemostatic proteins (factor XII, urokinase, tissue plasminogen activator), as well as a number of functionally unrelated extracellular and membrane-bound proteins.[25,26] A comparison of two-dimensional NMR spectroscopic studies of the growth factor domains of human,[27,28] mouse,[29] and rat[30] EGF, human transforming growth factor (TGF)-α-[28,31–33] human factor IX,[34,35] and bovine factor X[36,37] indicates considerable similarity in overall secondary structure. The structure of these growth factor domains is highly constrained by the three conserved disulfide loops and consists of one major and one minor β-sheet and five β-turns (Fig. 169-3). In contrast to EGF and TGF-α-, however, the N-terminal portion of the growth factor domains of the vitamin K-dependent proteins does not form a third strand of the major β-sheet. Instead, these N-terminal residues apparently constitute Gla-independent high-affinity calcium-binding sites[38–41] that have been demonstrated in factor IX,[42] factor X,[43] protein C,[44] and protein S.[45] In factors IX and X in particular, residues 47 to 50 and 64 and 65 (factor IX numbering) have been implicated in

Table 169-2 Properties of the Vitamin K-Dependent Proteins

Protein	Molecular Weight	Number of Chains	Number of Gla Residues	Plasma Conc., μg/ml	Plasma Half-Life
Prothrombin	71,600	One	10	80–90	2–5 days
Factor VII	50,000	One	10	0.47	2–5 h
Factor IX	56,800	One	12	4	20–24 h
Factor X	58,800	Two	11	6.4	32–48 h
Protein C	62,000	Two	9	3.9–5.9	6–8 h
Protein S	70,700	One	11	25–35	–

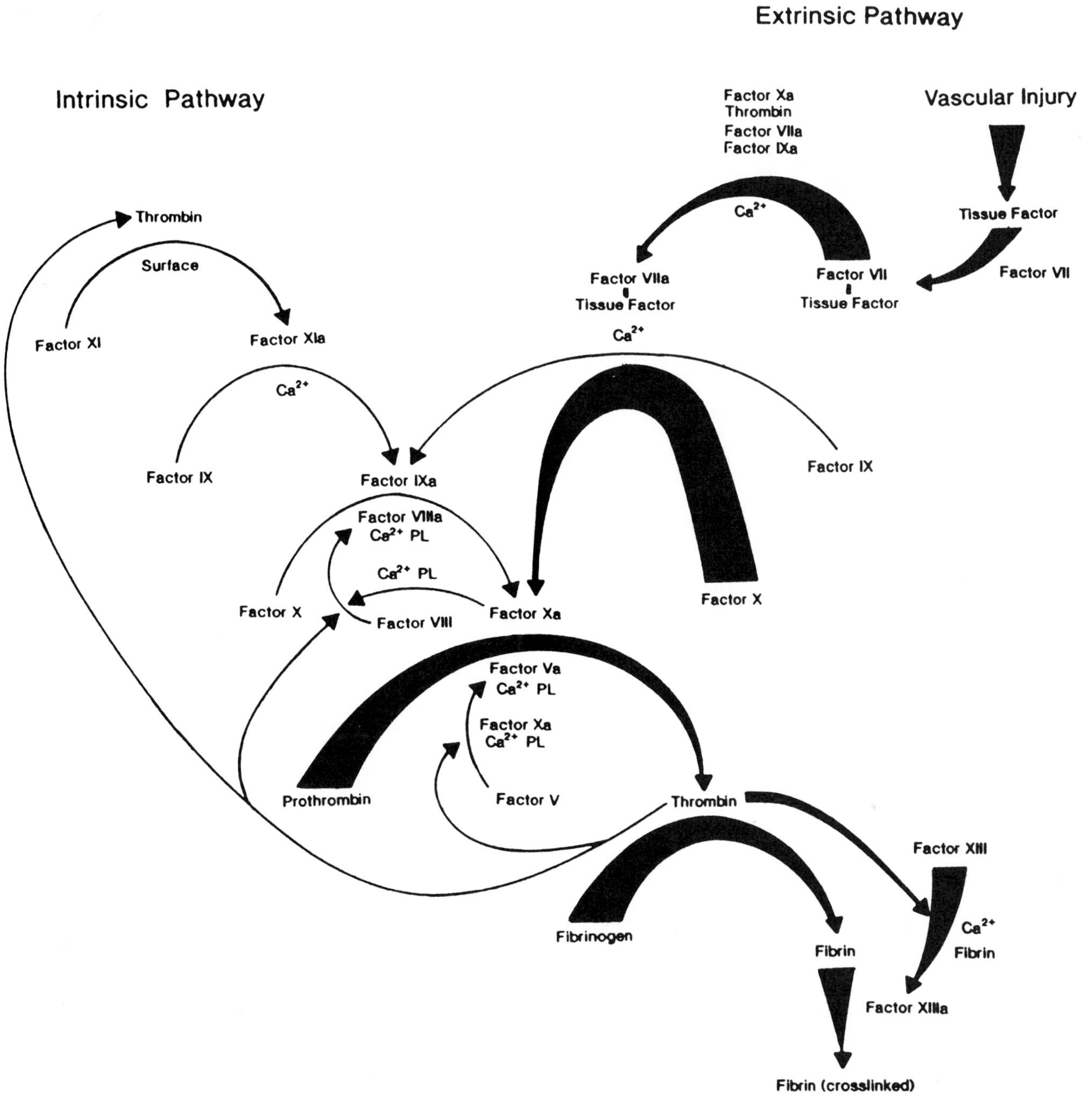

Fig. 169-1 Coagulation cascade and fibrin formation by the intrinsic and extrinsic pathways. The initiation of the coagulation cascade occurs following vascular injury and the exposure of tissue factor to the blood. This triggers the extrinsic pathway (right side), shown in heavy arrows. The intrinsic pathway (left side) can be triggered when thrombin is generated, leading to the activation of factor XI. The two pathways converge by the formation of factor Xa. The activated clotting factors (except thrombin) are designated by lowercase a; that is, IXa, Xa, XIa, and so on. PL refers to phospholipid. The phospholipid bound to tissue factor is not shown. (*From Davie et al.*[122] *Reproduced with permission.*)

calcium-binding.[34,46,47] Both the Gla and the growth factor domains have been implicated in the specific interactions and assembly of the vitamin K-dependent factors and their cofactors on membrane surfaces.[48–65]

The C-terminal region of prothrombin, factor VII, factor IX, factor X, and protein C contains the catalytic or serine protease domain that includes the active site residues, Asp, His, and Ser. The amino acid sequence in this domain shows considerable sequence and structural similarity to pancreatic trypsin and chymotrypsin, and is responsible for hydrolysis of specific Arg-containing peptide bonds. The serine proteases that are generated during blood coagulation have a high degree of substrate specificity and cleave only one or two peptide bonds in their protein substrates. Thus, they are far more substrate-specific than the pancreatic serine proteases that are involved in protein digestion. Based on computer modeling[66] and x-ray crystallographic comparisons[67] with the pancreatic enzymes, several unique insertion loop structures surrounding the active site center are responsible for the substrate specificity of the coagulation serine proteases.

BIOSYNTHESIS OF THE VITAMIN K-DEPENDENT COAGULATION PROTEINS

A number of steps are required for the biosynthesis of the vitamin K-dependent proteins in liver. Initially, large mRNAs are

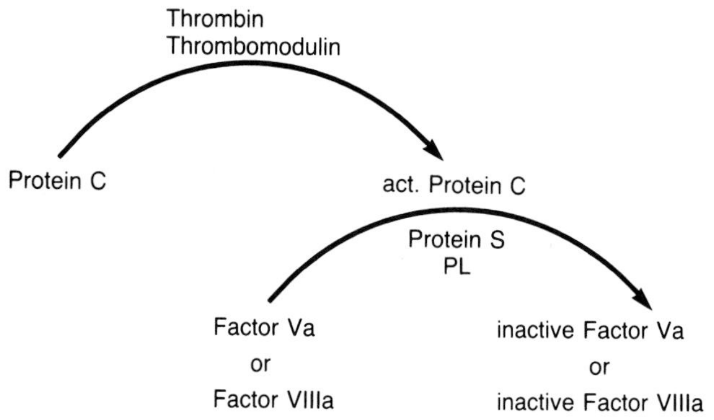

Fig. 169-2 Activation of protein C and the inactivation of factors Va and VIIIa. PL = phospholipid.

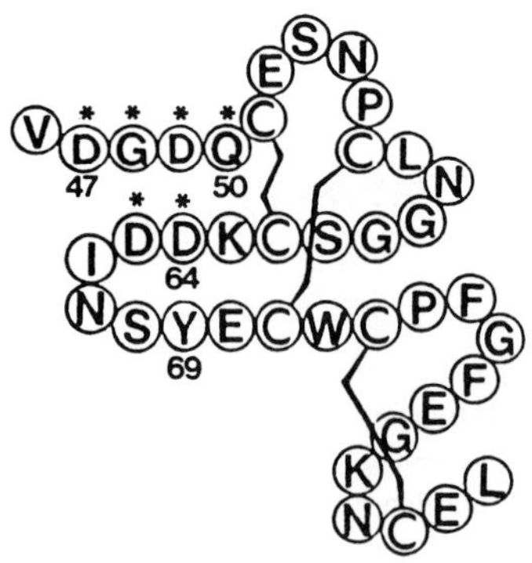

Fig. 169-3 The first growth factor domain of human factor IX (residues 46 to 84) based on the NMR structure of human EGF.[27] Single-letter amino acid code is used. Asp64 is β-hydroxylated. The structure consists of three disulfide loops and two β-sheets (see text). The amino acids denoted by an asterisk indicate residues that have been implicated in a Gla-independent calcium-binding site.[34,46,47] *(Modified from Handford et al.[46] Used by permission.)*

synthesized in the nucleus of the hepatocyte for each of these proteins and processed by a capping reaction at the 5′ end, removal of the RNA corresponding to the introns, and polyadenylation at the 3′ end of the mRNA. This results in a mature mRNA that is transported from the nucleus into the cytoplasm of the cell. Translation of the mature mRNA on the ribosomal machinery results in an immature polypeptide chain that contains a prepro leader sequence of approximately 40 amino acids (Fig. 169-4). Removal of the prepro leader sequence by proteolytic processing gives rise to the mature protein that circulates in plasma.

The prepro leader sequences of the human vitamin K-dependent proteins show considerable amino acid sequence similarity[11,12,16–19,23,24,68,69] (Fig. 169-4). Each contains an initiator methionine followed by a very hydrophobic region of 13 to 17 residues, which is required to transport these proteins to the lumen of the rough endoplasmic reticulum during polypeptide elongation. The pre or signal peptides are 28, 23, and 18 amino acids in factor IX,[69] factor X,[70] and protein C,[71] respectively. The length of the signal peptides for prothrombin, factor VII, and protein S have not been established.

A propeptide ranging from 17 to 24 residues in length follows the signal peptide sequence in the vitamin K-dependent proteins. This region is important for the carboxylation of the vitamin K-dependent proteins and serves as a recognition site for the carboxylase complex.[69,71–75] The carboxylation reaction is carried out posttranslationally[76–78] by a membrane-bound enzyme[79,80] in a reaction requiring CO_2, O_2, polypeptide substrate, NADH, and vitamin K.[81,82] Vitamin K antagonists, such as dicumarol or warfarin, inhibit the carboxylation of the vitamin K-dependent proteins.[83,84]

The carboxyl end of the propeptide contains highly conserved basic residues and serves as a recognition site for a processing protease(s) that preferentially cleaves peptide bonds, which generally follow an -Arg-X-Lys/Arg-Arg- motif (Fig. 169-4), which defines the substrate specificity for the endoprotease furin/PACE of the Golgi apparatus.[89] Cleavage of the propeptide gives rise to an N-terminal Ala in the mature polypeptide chain of prothrombin, factor VII, factor X, protein C, and protein S, and to a Tyr in factor IX. Failure of factor IX propeptide cleavage due to naturally-occurring point mutations of the conserved basic residues at either the −1, −2, or −4 positions results in a circulating factor IX molecule that is devoid of clotting activity.[85–87,90,91] The enzyme(s) responsible for propeptide processing of the vitamin K-dependent proteins are unknown, but several candidate proteases also have been identified.[88,89,92,93]

In addition to γ-carboxylation, several of the vitamin K-dependent coagulation proteins undergo a second type of enzymatic modification of certain amino acid residues during synthesis. A specific aspartic acid residue within the first growth factor domains of factor IX, factor X, protein C, and protein S, and a specific Asn residue in the last three growth factor domains of protein S undergo β-hydroxylation to form β-erythro-hydroxy-asparatic acid or β-erythro-hydroxyasparagine, respectively.[94–98] Interestingly, hydroxylated aspartic acid or asparagine residues have also been identified in other proteins containing growth factor domains, such as thrombomodulin, uromodulin, the LDL receptor, transforming growth factor-β1, and the complement proteins C1r and C1s.[26] The β-hydroxylation reaction occurs independently of γ-carboxylation and does not require vitamin K.[72,84] The enzyme responsible for β-hydroxylation has been characterized as an α-ketoglutarate-dependent dioxygenase that requires Fe^{2+} for activity.[99,100] The β-hydroxylase is functionally similar to, but structurally distinct from the collagen prolyl- and lysyl-hydroxylases.[101] The β-hydroxylase modifies specific Asp or Asn

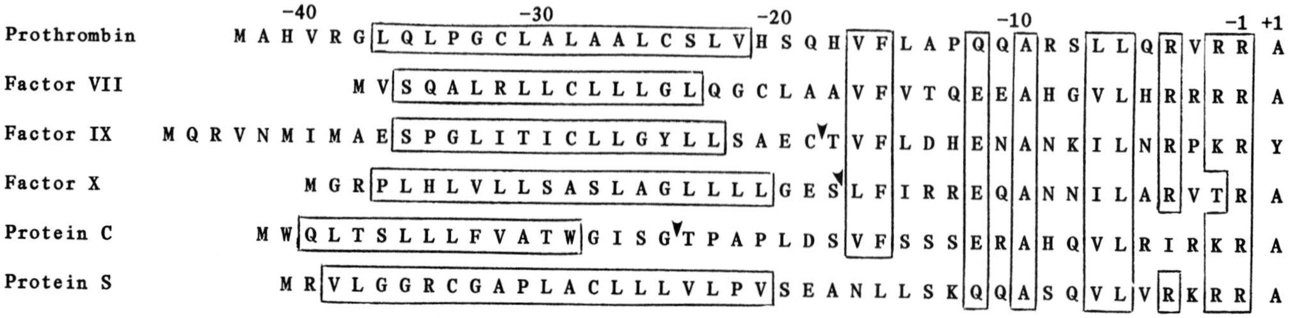

Fig. 169-4 Prepro leader sequences of the vitamin K-dependent proteins present in human plasma. The apparent hydrophobic core of each signal or presequence is boxed. Arrowheads indicate the known signal peptidase cleavage sites. Identical or homologous amino acid residues within the propeptide regions of each protein are also boxed. Numbering of the residues is relative to the N-terminus of the mature proteins circulating in plasma. *(Modified from Foster et al.[71] Used with permission.)*

residues within an eight-residue epidermal growth factor consensus sequence.[98,100] Other sequence or structural requirements for β-hydroxylation must exist, however, because the first growth factor domain of factor VII conforms to this sequence but does not undergo hydroxylation.[102] Furthermore, in contrast to factor X and protein C, human factor IX and protein S are only partially hydroxylated.[98,103,104] The functional significance of the β-hydroxyaspartic acid and β-hydroxyasparagine residues within the vitamin K-dependent proteins is not yet determined.

Like many other newly synthesized proteins, the vitamin K-dependent protein precursors are modified by the addition of carbohydrate chains to certain Asn (N-linked) and Ser or Thr (O-linked) residues. Cotranslational glycosylation of specific Asn residues within the consensus sequence -Asn-X-Ser/Thr- occurs in the endoplasmic reticulum and is catalyzed by the enzyme oligosaccharyltransferase. Subsequently, the N-linked oligosaccharides undergo further processing by various glycosidases and glycosyltransferases within the endoplasmic reticulum and Golgi to generate complex carbohydrate structures that often terminate in sialic acid residues. Each vitamin K-dependent coagulation protein contains two to four potentially glycosylated Asn residues per molecule. These N-linked carbohydrate structures may be important for efficient secretion, proteolytic processing, and proper functioning of the newly synthesized proteins.[77,105,106]

In addition to the N-linked carbohydrate, two unique O-linked carbohydrate moieties were identified within the first growth factor domain of several of the vitamin K-dependent proteins. Specifically, Xyl-Glc or Xyl-Xyl-Glc structures are attached to a conserved serine residue in factor VII (Ser52) and factor IX (Ser53), as well as to the homologous serine residue within the first growth factor domains of vitamin K-dependent protein Z.[107,108] Secondly, O-linked fucose is attached to Ser60 or Ser61 in factor VII[109] and factor IX,[110] respectively, as well as to homologous serine or threonine residues in the growth factor domains of prourokinase,[111] tissue plasminogen activator,[112] and factor XII.[113] The function of these unusual O-linked sugar chains is not yet conclusively determined, but thus far they are identified only in proteins containing growth factor domains. Interestingly, desialated factor IX and factor X have full anticoagulant activity.[114] However, the glycosyl moieties attached to Ser52 and Ser60 of factor VII are important in the rapid association of factor VII/VIIa with tissue factor.[115]

Prothrombin, factor VII, factor IX, and protein S circulate in plasma as single polypeptide chains, wheras factor X and protein C undergo proteolysis of an internal arginyl bond and circulate in plasma as mature two-chain proteins. Analogous to propeptide processing, this internal cleavage occurs following basic residues, that is, the dibasic sequence -Lys-Arg- in protein C and the tetrabasic sequence -Arg-Arg-Lys-Arg- in factor X. Proteolytic processing at these internal basic sequences is a calcium-dependent event that occurs late in the secretion pathway.[77,116,117] While secreted factor X is fully processed to the two-chain form, approximately 10 to 15 percent of plasma protein C exists in the unprocessed single-chain form.[118] Interestingly, the efficiency of proteolytic processing of recombinant protein C to the two-chain form can be increased either by introducing a basic residue at the −4 position[119] or by coexpression of a yeast-processing protease (Kex2) that is capable of cleaving the peptide bond following dibasic sequences.[120] Thus, an enzyme(s) recognizing basic sequences identical or similar to that responsible for propeptide processing of the vitamin K-dependent proteins may also cleave factor X and protein C to their mature forms.

The two-chain forms of factor X and protein C, as well as the activated forms of factor VII, factor IX, and prothrombin, are linked by interchain disulfide bonds between cysteine residues of the N-terminal light chain and the C-terminal heavy chain containing the catalytic domain. In addition, each vitamin K-dependent protein contains several intrachain disulfide bonds in highly conserved positions throughout the molecule. Disulfide bond formation is catalyzed within the endoplasmic reticulum lumen during protein synthesis by the enzyme protein disulfide isomerase.[121]

PROTHROMBIN

Prothrombin participates in the final stages of the blood coagulation cascade[122] where it is converted to thrombin in the presence of factor Xa, factor Va, calcium ions, and phospholipid (Fig. 169-1). Thrombin then cleaves fibrinopeptides A and B from the N-terminal end of the two α and two β chains of fibrinogen leading to the formation of the fibrin clot. Thrombin also activates factor V,[123,124] factor VIII,[125–128] factor XIII,[129,130] and protein C[131–133] by limited proteolysis (Fig. 169-2). In addition, thrombin is capable of factor XI activation in the presence of a negatively charged surface, such as sulfatide, heparin, or dextran sulfate.[134,135] Finally, thrombin is capable of a number of cellular interactions.[136] Of particular importance among these interactions, thrombin binds to and cleaves specific membrane receptors on platelets, endothelium, and other cells,[137–140] resulting in a wide range of cellular functions, including platelet activation, aggregation, and release of intracellular granule contents.

Prothrombin is a single-chain glycoprotein with a molecular weight of 71,600 and an N-terminal sequence of Ala-Asn-Thr-Phe-Leu[141] (Fig. 169-5). The mature protein circulating in plasma contains 579 amino acids, including 10 residues of γ-carboxyglutamic acid that constitute the Gla domain.[142] The two kringle structures in prothrombin are located between the Gla domain and the serine protease portion of the molecule. Prothrombin also contains 8.2 percent carbohydrate, which is apparently attached to asparagine residues 78 and 100 located in kringle 1 and Asn373 in the catalytic domain of the molecule. The catalytic domain also contains the three active site residues that include His363, Asp419, and Ser525.

The activation of human prothrombin involves the cleavage of internal Arg271-Thr and Arg320-Ile peptide bonds by factor Xa[143] (Figs. 169-5 and 169-6). The reaction requires calcium ions and is accelerated about 20,000-fold by the addition of phospholipid and factor Va.[144,155] The principal effect of the phospholipid is to decrease the K_m for the substrate about 150-fold, while factor Va, in a complex with factor Xa at a molar ratio of 1:1, increases the V_{max} of the reaction approximately 1000-fold. In the presence of factor Va, the activation of human prothrombin proceeds by the initial cleavage of the Arg320-Ile bond, generating a meizothrombin intermediate.[146] Meizothrombin has peptidase activity toward small synthetic substrates and incorporates diisopropylfluoridate in its active site serine. It is unable, however, to convert fibrinogen to fibrin. A second cleavage occurs in meizothrombin at the Arg271-Thr bond. This cleavage generates thrombin by the liberation of fragment 1.2, which contains amino acids 1 to 271 and includes the Gla and kringle domains. The thrombin generated is composed of a light chain of 49 amino acids and a heavy chain of 259 amino acids. These two chains are held together by a disulfide bond. This molecule undergoes further cleavage at Arg284-Thr in the light chain to form a thrombin molecule with a light chain of 36 amino acids. These reactions reduce the molecular weight of the precursor from 71,600 to about 34,500.

In the absence of factor Va, the activation of prothrombin proceeds by a prethrombin-2 intermediate generated by the initial cleavage at the Arg271-Thr bond[146] (Fig. 169-6). In whole plasma, the cleavage in prothrombin occurs primarily at Arg284-Thr in the light chain as well as the Arg320-Ile bond.[147] This latter pathway generates a thrombin molecule with an initial light chain of 36 amino acids rather than 49 amino acids, and a Gla-kringle fragment of 284 amino acids (fragment 1.2.3). This latter pathway may well represent a major avenue for thrombin generation under physiological conditions.

Activation of prothrombin occurs on phospholipid surfaces where the protein substrate is concentrated.[148] It appears that factor Va enhances the binding of factor Xa to membrane

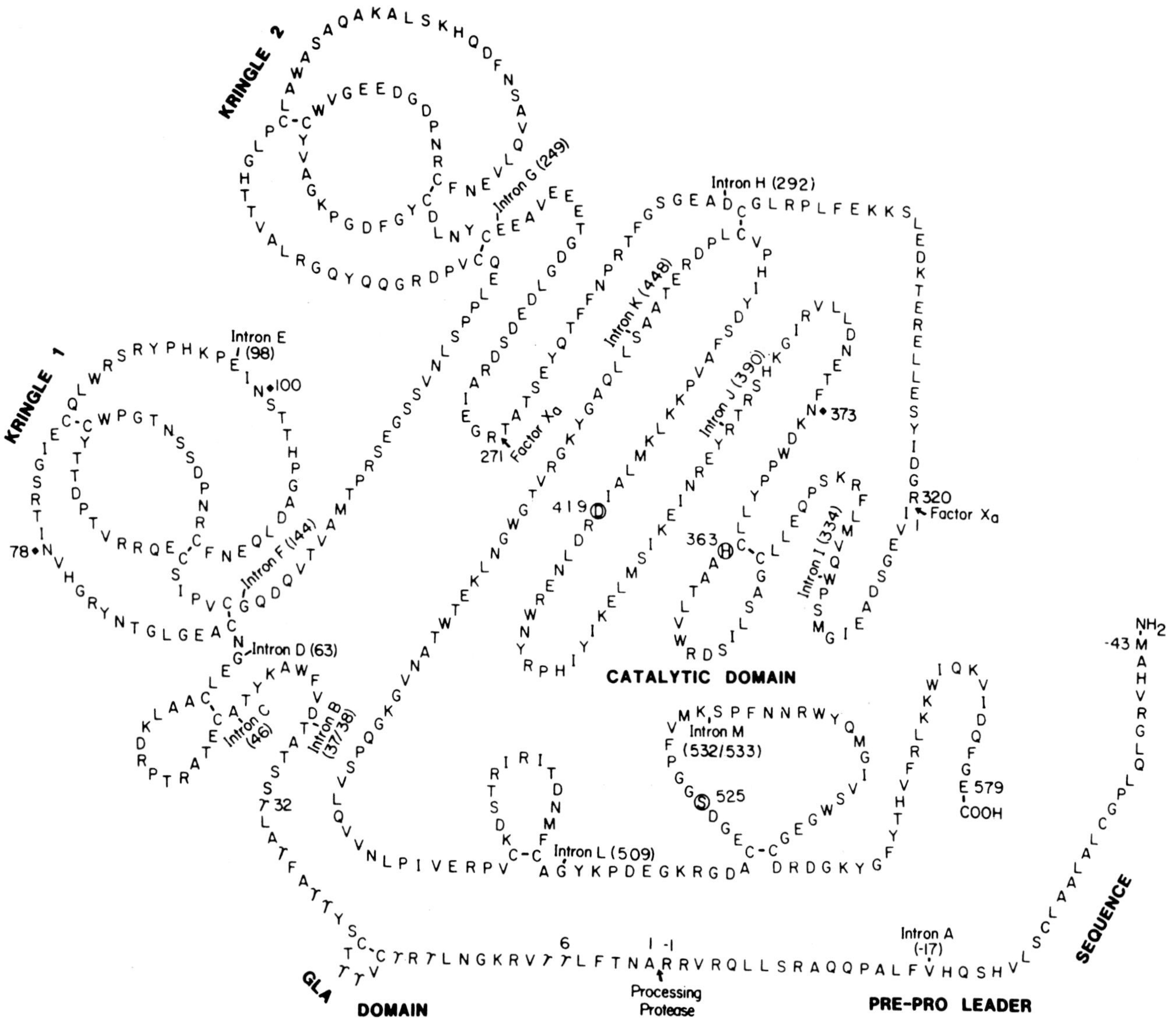

Fig. 169-5 Amino acid sequence and tentative structure of human prepro prothrombin. The locations of the 13 introns (A to M) are shown in the various regions of the protein. The prepro leader sequence is cleaved during protein biosynthesis to give rise to mature protein with an amino-terminal sequence of A-N-T-F-. The two peptide bonds cleaved by factor Xa during the activation reaction are shown with small arrows. The three amino acids in the catalytic domain (H363, D419, S525) that participate in catalysis are circled, while the three carbohydrate attachment sites are shown with solid diamonds. The amino acids are numbered as follows starting with the N-terminal end of the protein: −43 to −1, prepro leader sequence; (+)1 to 271, prothrombin fragment 1.2; 272 to 320, light chain of thrombin; 321 to 579, catalytic chain of thrombin. The single-letter code for amino acids is as follows: A = Ala; R = Arg; N = Asn; D = Asp; C = Cys; Q = Gln; E = Glu; G = Gly; H = His; I = Ile; L = Leu; K = Lys; M = Met; F = Phe; P = Pro; S = Ser; T = Thr; W = Trp; Y = Tyr; V = Val; γ = γ-carboxyglutamic acid. (*From Degen et al.*[68,142] *Reproduced with permission.*)

surfaces[149] and that this association modulates the orientation and conformation of the bound factor Xa and prothrombin.[150,151] The calcium-dependent binding of prothrombin to the phospholipid surfaces involves the Gla region[4,152] and possibly the first kringle structure.[153] In vivo, the phospholipid component of the reaction may be provided by platelets,[154,155] endothelial cells,[156] or leukocytes.[155] When the newly generated thrombin is formed, it is released from the phospholipid surface and is then free to interact with its various substrates, such as fibrinogen and factor XIII.

X-ray crystallographic studies of thrombin[67,157] and its complexes with hirudin,[158] fibrinopeptide A,[159,160] prothrombin fragment F2 (kringle 2),[161] and thrombin receptor peptides[162] have been reported. Prothrombin fragment F1 (Gla domain and kringle 1) has also been studied by x-ray crystallography.[163,164] These data have been instrumental in understanding the structural aspects and allosteric regulation of this multifunctional protein. Thrombin exhibits the characteristic fold of the trypsin-like serine proteases.[157] The active site residues (see Fig. 169-7) are sandwiched between two β-barrel domains of the thrombin heavy chain. The disulfide-linked light chain forms an integral structural part of the enzyme, but is not directly involved in catalysis.[67,157] The heavy chain is 27 residues longer than chymotrypsin, and most of these residues occur as loops that border and shape the active site cleft, making the cleft deep and narrow, with the catalytic residues at the base.[159,160,165] These insertion loops limit the accessibility of many substrates or inhibitors to the catalytic residues. Unique to thrombin is the presence of two exosites, or allosteric binding sites, which can modulate the specificity of the active site.[67,157,165] The two exosites are surface patches composed of mostly positively charged residues. Exosite II, which is located "northwest" of the active site, binds heparin, thereby accelerating complex formation with the serpins antithrombin III and heparin cofactor II.[165,166] Exosite I, the fibrinogen recognition site, is

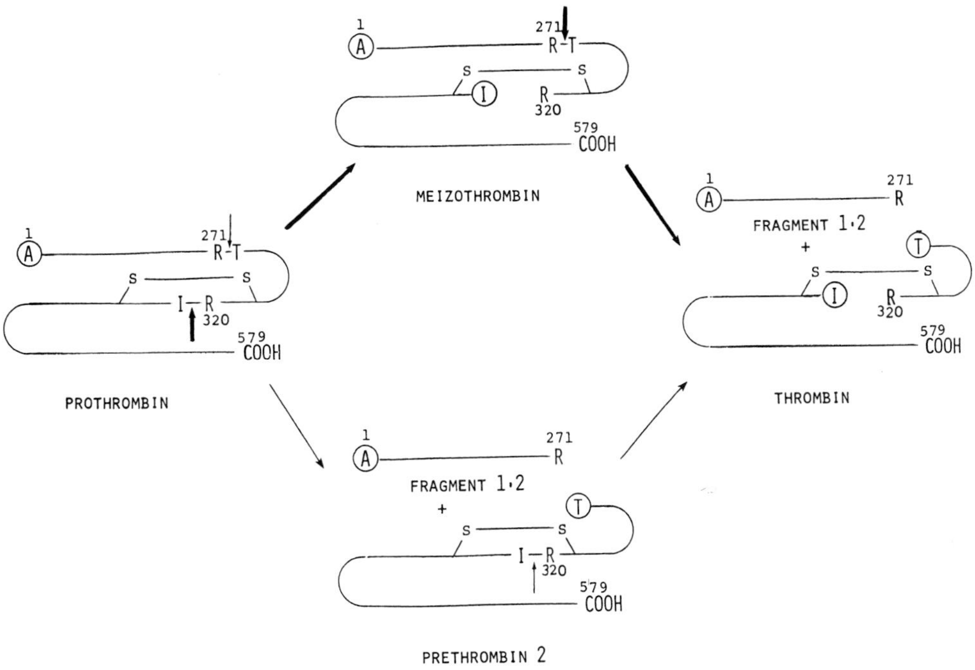

Fig. 169-6 Activation scheme for human prothrombin. In the presence of factor Va, the initial cleavage by factor Xa occurs at R320 to I321 (heavy vertical arrow) generating thrombin and fragment 1.2. In the absence of factor Va, the initial cleavage by factor Xa occurs at R271 to T272 (thin vertical arrow), generating prethrombin 2 and fragment 1.2. The second cleavage then occurs at R320 to I321 (thin vertical arrow) generating thrombin. Amino-terminal amino acids are circled.

located to the "east" of the active site and interacts with fibrinogen, fibrin, hirudin, thrombomodulin, and thrombin receptor peptides.[158–160,162] Accordingly, the crystallographic structure of thrombin reveals a division of the protein into several functional regions. These observations have pointed the way to the design of novel antithrombotic drugs and inhibitors, which bind the active site and the fibrinogen recognition exosite.[167,166]

Prothrombin Gene

The gene for human prothrombin is located on chromosome 11 at p11-q12.[167] It contains about 21 kilobases of DNA and its complete sequence has been established (GenBank V00595 and NM 000506).[68] The gene is composed of 14 exons separated by 13 introns. The introns range in size from 84 to 9447 nucleotides, while the exons range in size from 25 to 315 nucleotides (Table 169-3). The intron-exon splice junction sequences follow the GT-AG rule[170] and the typical splice junction consensus,[171] except for the splice site at the 5′ end of intron L (Table 169-4). The exons in the gene for prothrombin code for 579 amino acids comprising the mature protein that circulates in plasma, in addition to a prepro leader sequence of 43 amino acids. The first intron (intron A) is located in the prepro leader sequence (Val −17), while the second intron is located just after the Gla domain (between Thr37 and Asp38). The third intron occurs nine residues later (Ala46), while the fourth intron occurs just prior to the first kringle (Gly63). The fifth intron is located within the first kringle (Glu98), and the sixth intron is located between kringles 1 and 2 (Gly144). The second kringle in prothrombin, in contrast to the first kringle, is coded by a single exon. Accordingly, the seventh intron is present immediately following kringle 2 (Glu249). The remaining introns in the gene for prothrombin occur throughout the molecule, including five in the catalytic domain (Fig. 169-5).

The gene for human prothrombin contains 30 copies of Alu repetitive DNA and two copies of partial *Kpn*I repeats. These repeats comprise approximately 40 percent of the human gene for prothrombin. The Alu sequences occur in clusters with 20 being present in the twelfth intron (intron L). The human haploid genome contains about 300,000 copies of Alu repetitive sequences

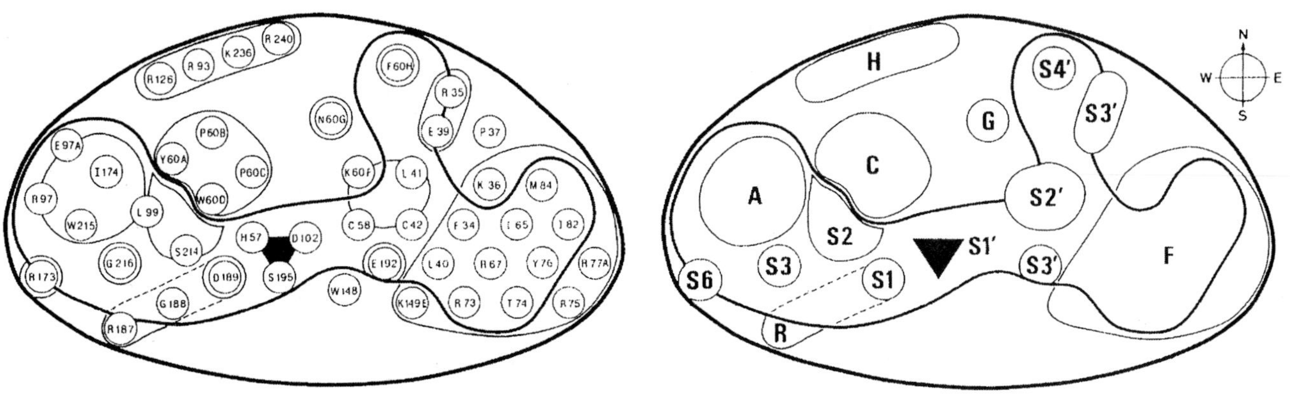

Fig. 169-7 Diagram derived from x-ray crystal structure of α-thrombin showing residues involved in the various subsites. Surface residues appear in their approximate locations in the standard orientation (left). The right-hand side shows the division of the surface into functional regions. Key: active site triad; S1-S6 = specificity sites N-terminal to cleavage; A = aryl-binding site (the aryl binding site and the S2 site together form the "apolar binding site"); F = fibrinogen recognition exosite; H = heparin-binding site; G = glycosylation site; S1′-S3′ = putative specificity sites carboxy-terminal to cleavage; C = chemotactic region; R = RGD sequence; compass defines orientation relative to the active site.

Table 169-3 Location and Size of Exons and Introns in the Gene for Human Prothrombin

Exon	Nucleotide Positions	Length, bp	Amino Acids	Intervening Sequence	Nucleotide Positions	Length, bp	Number of *Alu* Repeats
I	+1–79	79+*	−43 to −17	A	80–465	386	
II	466–626	161	−17 to 37	B	627–1285	659	
III	1286–1310	25	38–46	C	1311–1552	242	
IV	1553–1603	51	46–63	D	1604–3929	2326	4
V	3930–4035	106	63–98	E	4036–4131	96	
VI	4132–4268	137	98–144	F	4269–6606	2338	3
VII	6607–6921	315	144–249	G	6922–7245	324	
VIII	7246–7374	129	249–292	H	7375–7458	84	
IX	7459–7585	127	292–334	I	7586–8742	1157	2
X	8743–8910	168	334–390	J	8911–9407	497	
XI	9408–9581	174	390–448	K	9582–10123	542	1
XII	10124–10305	182	448–509	L	10306–19752	9447	20†
XIII	19753–19823	71	509–532	M	19824–19969	146	
XIV	19970–20210	241	533–polyA site				

*The length of the 5′ noncoding region of the mRNA for human prothrombin is unknown; therefore, the length of exon I is measured from the initiator methionine.

†This intervening sequence also has two copies of partial "*Kpn*" repeats.

SOURCE: Degen and Davie.[68]

that are about 300 nucleotides in length and show about 80 percent sequence homology.[172,173] This is equivalent to about one Alu repetitive sequence in every 6 kilobases of human DNA. Thus, the prothrombin gene has an unusually high concentration of these repetitive sequences whose function is presently unknown.

The 5′ region of the prothrombin gene lacks a typical TATA or CCAAT sequence, but appears to have a weak promoter immediately upstream from a heterogeneous transcription initiation site.[174,175] In addition, a bidirectional liver-specific enhancer element is located between nucleotides −940 and −860.[175] The prothrombin enhancer region contains a putative HNF-1 binding site flanked by an inverted CCTCCC sequence that is present in other HNF-1 liver-specific promoters such as the fibrinogen β-chain and α_1-antitrypsin promoters.

Several common polymorphisms have been identified within the prothrombin gene. An 800-bp insertion resulting in a *Pst*I RFLP occurs in intron D with a frequency of about 30 percent in Caucasians.[176,177] In Japanese individuals, two common polymorphisms occur within 71 bp: an *Nco*I RFLP due to a T to C substitution in exon VI resulting in a Thr/Met polymorphism at residue 122,[178] and a *Mbo*II RFLP in intron E due to a C/G polymorphism at nucleotide 4125.[179] A common G to A substitution at nucleotide 20210 in the 3′ untranslated end of the prothrombin gene was recently described.[180] Individuals who are heterozygous for this mutation have a slightly elevated level of circulating prothrombin and are at a 2.8-fold increased risk for venous thrombosis relative to persons homozygous for the G allele.[180] The estimated frequency of the heterozygous G to A substitution is reported to be about 2 percent in the general population, with an increased frequency in southern Europeans and a decreased frequency among those of Asian and African descent.[181,182] The mechanism by which this mutation causes the observed increase in prothrombin expression and the associated increased risk of thrombosis is not clear at this time.

Prothrombin Deficiency

Prothrombin deficiency (MIM 176930) is a very rare abnormality with about 50 reported cases. Patients with this deficiency have been placed in two broad categories: (a) those with normal plasma levels of an abnormal protein that has decreased biologic activity

Table 169-4 Intron–Exon Splice Junction Sequences in the Gene for Human Prothrombin

		Splice Junction Sequences			
Intron	Exon	5′	Intron	3′	Exon
A	ATG	GTAAGG	----	CCACCGCCTTTACAG	T
B	ACG	GTGAGC	----	GCCCTTGTTTTTCAG	G
C	CAG	GTGAGC	----	CTGGGTCTTTTCCAG	C
D	AAG	GTGAGC	----	GTGGGGTCTCCGCAG	G
E	TGA	GTGAGT	----	AATTTCCTCTTCCAG	A
F	GTG	GTAGGC	----	CCCCTCACCCACCAG	G
G	GTG	GTGAGC	----	CCTGGGTCCCAACAG	A
H	CAG	GTGAGG	----	TGGCTTGCTCTGCAG	A
I	TTG	GTGTGT	----	TGCTGCCCCTCCCAG	G
J	AAG	GTACAG	----	TTGGGGTCTCTGCAG	G
K	CAG	GTGGGC	----	CTTCCTTCCCCAAAG	C
L	CTG	GCAAGT	----	CTGTTCTCTTTCAAG	G
M	AAG	GTAAGC	----	ATCTTTCTTCTTCAG	A
Consensus sequence*	$^{C}_{A}$AG	GT$^{A}_{G}$AGT	----	$^{T}_{C}$$^{T}_{C}$$^{T}_{C}$$^{T}_{C}$$^{T}_{C}$$^{T}_{C}$$^{T}_{C}$$^{T}_{C}$$^{T}_{C}$$^{T}_{C}$$^{T}_{C}N^{T}_{C}$AG	G

*From Mount.[171]

SOURCE: Degen and Davie.[68]

(dysprothrombinemia), and (b) those with decreased biosynthesis and reduced plasma levels (hypoprothrominemia). Hypoprothrombinemia has been described as an autosomal recessive disorder and most reported cases have been of individuals of Mediterranean descent.[183,184] Patients who are homozygous have bleeding complications and their prothrombin coagulant activity ranges from 2 to 25 percent of normal. Bleeding complications include bruising easily, epistaxis, gingival hemorrhage, menorrhagia, and postoperative hemorrhage; spontaneous hemarthrosis is rare. Individuals who are heterozygous have prothrombin activity levels of 50 percent or greater and are asymptomatic.

Congenital dysprothrombinemia is also inherited in an autosomal recessive manner and bleeding manifestations are similar to those of congenital hypoprothombinemia.[185] The severity of bleeding, however, does not necessarily correlate with residual prothrombin clotting activity. Thus far, more than 20 abnormal prothrombins have been reported. Ten have been isolated and characterized, but specific molecular abnormalities have been identified in only six of these. Of the six different molecular abnormalities in prothrombin identified to date, four are the result of C to T transitions within codons containing CGX. This type of nucleotide transition occurs fairly commonly, because CG is a major site of methylation in genomic DNA and the deamination of methyl cytosine to thymidine would give rise to this mutation.

Prothrombin$_{\text{BARCELONA}}$,[186] prothrombin$_{\text{MADRID}}$,[187] and prothrombin$_{\text{DHAHRAN}}$[188] have been shown to be due to the replacement of an Arg by a Cys residue at position 271.*

The Arg271-Thr bond is one of two peptide bonds that must be cleaved by factor Xa during the conversion of prothrombin to thrombin, and the replacement of an Arg by a Cys residue prevents this cleavage. The Cys residue in prothrombin Barcelona and prothrombin Madrid apparently results from a base change of C to T in the triplet of CGT originally coding for arginine in the gene for human prothrombin. Mutations at the analogous arginine activation sites in factor IX and factor X have also been described in patients with these respective deficiencies (see below).

Prothrombin$_{\text{TOKUSHIMA}}$ is an abnormal protein that is readily converted to thrombin by factor Xa in the presence of factor Va, phospholipid, and calcium ions.[192] The newly generated thrombin, however, shows only 21 percent clotting activity relative to normal thrombin. The abnormal thrombin also exhibits reduced platelet aggregating activity. Amino acid sequence analysis indicates that the reduced clotting activity in this protein is due to the replacement of Agr418 by Trp in the catalytic region of the abnormal molecule. This mutation can be explained by a single base change of C to T in the triplet of CGG coding for arginine in the normal molecule.[193] The reduced fibrinogen clotting activity for thrombin$_{\text{TOKUSHIMA}}$ also suggests that Arg418, located adjacent to the essential Asp419 (Fig. 169-5), is important for the binding of fibrinogen to the enzyme, and is consistent with the increased K_m and decreased catalytic rate constant for the abnormal enzyme.

Prothrombin$_{\text{QUICK}}$ was recently separated into two components designated thrombin$_{\text{QUICK I}}$ and thrombin$_{\text{QUICK II}}$.[194] In thrombin$_{\text{QUICK I}}$, a substitution of Arg382 to Cys (presumably due to a mutation of CGC to TGC) in the putative fibrinogen binding site results in decreased thrombin clotting activity, normal amidolytic activity toward chromogenic substrates, decreased platelet aggregating activity, and markedly reduced platelet binding affinity.[195,196] Thrombin$_{\text{QUICK II}}$, on the other hand, is characterized by a substitution of Gly558 to Val (corresponding to a mutation of GGC to GTC) in the primary substrate binding pocket that completely abolishes both clotting and amidolytic activity as well as platelet aggregation, but has less effect on high-affinity platelet binding.[196,197]

Prothrombin$_{\text{SALAKTA}}$[198] and prothrombin$_{\text{FRANKFURT}}$[190] results in asymptomatic individuals with about 15 percent clotting activity and reduced substrate binding affinity. The molecular abnormality has been identified as a substitution of Glu (GAG) to Ala (GCG) at residue 466 of the thrombin heavy chain. Presumably, this substitution affects the conformation of a surface loop surrounding Trp468 that is thought to be necessary for specific substrate binding.[199]

Although the precise molecular abnormalities involved have not been confirmed, prothrombin$_{\text{CARDEZA}}$[184] and prothrombin$_{\text{CLAMART}}$[200] appear to be due to defects similar to prothrombin$_{\text{BARCELONA}}$ and prothrombin$_{\text{MADRID}}$ in that the zymogen is not converted to thrombin by factor Xa. In contrast, prothrombin$_{\text{HI-MI}}$,[201] prothrombin$_{\text{METZ}}$,[202] and prothrombin$_{\text{MOLISE}}$[203] apparently have abnormalities in the thrombin portion of the molecule, whereas prothrombin$_{\text{SAN JUAN I}}$[184] shows an abnormality in the calcium binding domain. Prothrombin$_{\text{GREENVILLE}}$[189] may result in the disruption of a novel Na+ binding site.

Treatment of bleeding episodes in patients with congenital prothrombin deficiency consists of plasma transfusions to maintain plasma prothrombin levels above 30 percent of normal (30 U/dl). Fresh frozen plasma (FFP) contains 1 unit per ml of prothrombin, which has a circulating half-life of approximately 3 days. For major bleeding episodes or surgical procedures, prothrombin complex concentrates can be used, but these products carry an increased risk of viral transmission and thromboembolic complications.

COMBINED DEFICIENCY OF THE VITAMIN K-DEPENDENT COAGULATION FACTORS

Combined deficiency of the vitamin K-dependent coagulation factors usually occurs because of vitamin K deficiency. Common clinical settings include newborns, liver disease, and malabsorption. A few patients, however, have been described with congenital deficiency of prothrombin as well as factor VII, factor IX, and factor X.[204–210] In some instances, levels of protein C and protein S were also reduced, but generally not as greatly as the procoagulant proteins. Clinical severity has varied in that some patients presented with severe bleeding episodes from early childhood,[204,205,208,210] while others were diagnosed later in life, following postsurgical or mucocutaneous bleeding.[206,207,209] The lack of γ-carboxylation of the vitamin K-dependent proteins[205,207,209,210] and the response to parenteral vitamin K[205,207,208,210] suggest an abnormality in vitamin K-dependent γ-carboxylation in these patients. One patient had associated skeletal abnormalities and was found to have a congenital deficiency of vitamin K epoxide reductase.[209] An abnormality of the liver carboxylase enzyme has been proposed in other patients.[210]

FACTOR VII

Factor VII participates in the extrinsic pathway of blood coagulation[122] where it is converted to factor VIIa by a trace amount of a circulating protease (e.g., thrombin, factor IXa, factor Xa, factor XIIa, or factor VIIa) or by some as yet unidentified plasma or cellular enzyme (Fig. 169-1).[211–217] Factor VIIa, in turn, converts factor IX to factor IXa[218] and/or factor X to factor Xa. These reactions require a cofactor called *tissue factor*.[219] Tissue factor is an integral membrane protein that is present in the vascular subendothelium as well as other extravascular sites.[220–222] It binds circulating factor VII at sites of vascular injury.[223–225] The binding of exposed tissue factor to factor VII or to factor VIIa greatly increases the catalytic efficiency of these reactions,[226–228] apparently by causing a conformational change in the catalytic site of factor VIIa.[229,230] Tissue factor is not accessible to factor VII without prior tissue damage. Thus, generation of the factor VII/tissue factor complex is critical for

*This residue was originally assigned to position 273 according to the early protein sequence analysis of prothrombin.[191] In these studies a Glu-Glu peptide was reported at positions 266 and 267. Subsequent amino acid sequence analysis and sequence analysis of the cDNA and the gene coding for human prothrombin indicated the absence of this peptide in the normal molecule.

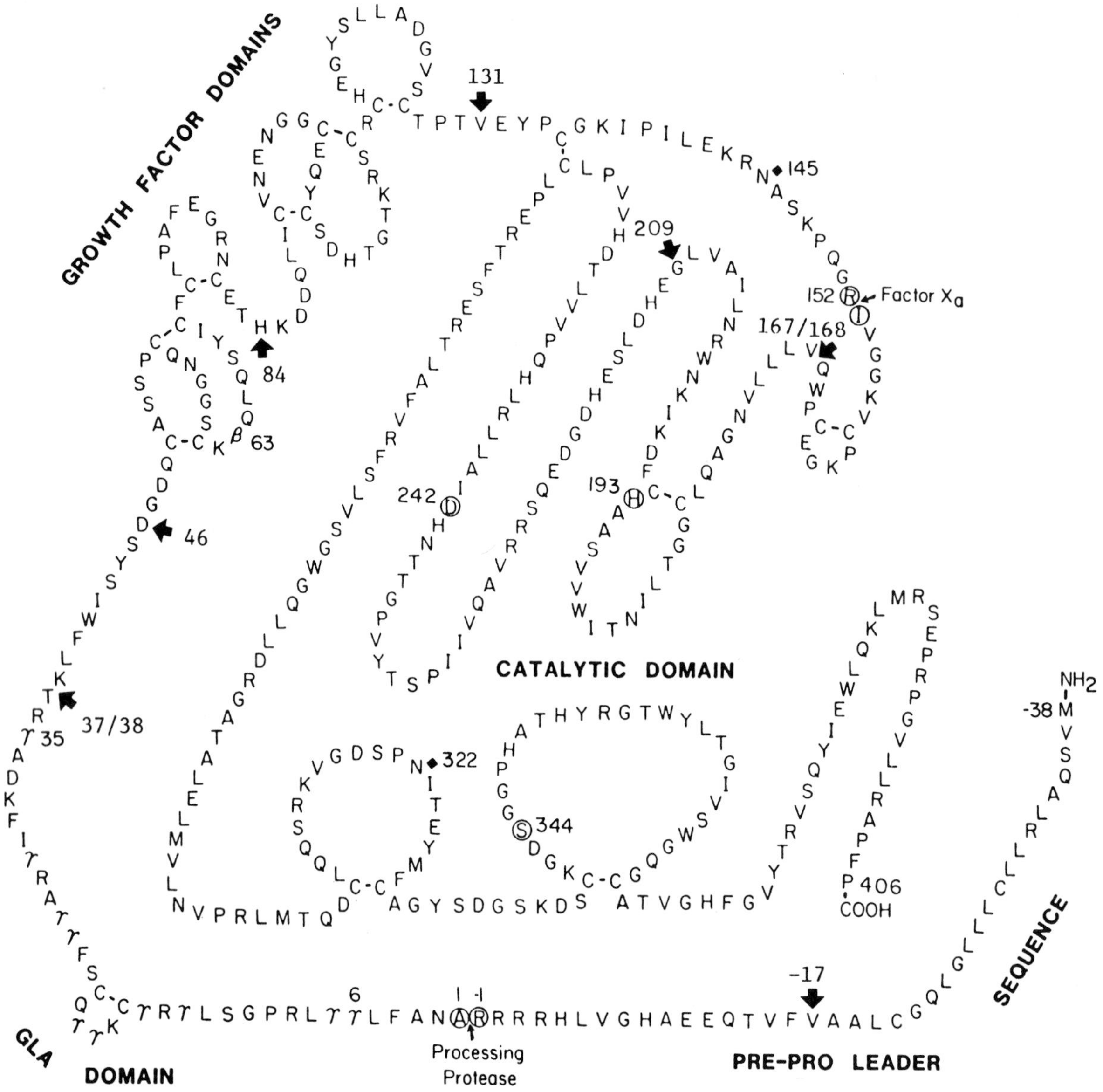

Fig. 169-8 Amino acid sequence and tentative structure of human prepro factor VII. Heavy arrows show the locations of the seven introns. The prepro leader sequence is cleaved during protein biosynthesis to give rise to the mature protein with an N-terminal sequence of A-N-A-F-. The single peptide bond cleaved by factor Xa during the activation reaction is shown with a small arrow. The three amino acids in the catalytic domain (H193, D242, S344) that participate in catalysis are circled, while the tentative carbohydrate attachment sites are shown with solid diamonds. The amino acids are numbered as follows, starting with the amino-terminal end of the protein: −38 to −1 = prepro leader sequence; +1 to 152 = light chain of factor VIIa; 153 to 406 = catalytic chain of factor VIIa. The single-letter code for amino acids is shown in the legend to Fig. 169-5. β = β-hydroxyaspartic acid. *(Modified from Hagen et al.[11] and O'Hara et al.[264] Used with permission.)*

initiating the blood coagulation cascade leading to fibrin formation. After the factor VIIa/tissue factor complex is formed and factor Xa is generated, a lipoprotein-associated inhibitor that forms a quaternary complex with factor VIIa/tissue factor/factor Xa rapidly inactivates the extrinsic pathway.[231,232]

Human factor VII is a single-chain glycoprotein with a molecular weight of 50,000 and an N-terminal sequence of Ala-Asn-Ala-Phe-Leu[11,233] (Fig. 169-8). The protein is initially synthesized with a prepro leader sequence of 38 amino acids. Signal peptidase and a processing protease remove this prepropeptide, resulting in a mature protein of 406 amino acids. The Gla-containing region contains ten γ-carboxyglutamic acid residues and is followed by two growth factor domains. Factor VII also contains carbohydrate, a portion of which is attached to Asn145 in the light chain and Asn322 in the heavy chain of the activated molecule.[102] In addition, factor VII contains two unique O-linked carbohydrate chains, glucose-(xylose)$_2$ at Ser52 and fucose at Ser60.[108,109] These carbohydrate moieties may be important in the association of factor VII/VIIa with tissue factor.[114,115]

The activation of human factor VII involves the cleavage of an internal Arg152-Ile peptide bond (Fig. 169-8). This generates factor VIIa, which is composed of a light chain of 152 amino acids and a heavy chain of 254 amino acids. These two chains are held together by a single disulfide bond. The heavy chain of the molecule contains the catalytic domain, including the active site residues of His193, Asp242, and Ser344. No activation peptide is liberated during the activation reaction; thus, factor VII and factor VIIa have essentially the same molecular weight.

Human tissue factor (M_r 44,000) is a single-chain glycoprotein composed of 263 amino acids.[252–255] It is initially synthesized with a signal peptide of 32 amino acids that is cleaved from the growing polypeptide chain by signal peptidase. This generates the mature membrane-bound glycoprotein with an N-terminal sequence of Ser-Gly-Thr-Thr. The extracellular domain at the

N-terminal end of the protein is 219 residues in length and contains the factor VII or factor VIIa binding sites,[228,256] as well as a possible recognition site for factor X.[257] This region is followed by a membrane-spanning region of 23 hydrophobic residues and a cytoplasmic region of 21 residues at the carboxyl end of the molecule. The membrane-spanning region, in addition to the extracellular domain, appears to be required for full cofactor activity.[258–260] The extracellular domain of tissue factor consists of two fibronectin type III repeats.[237] The crystal structure of the extracellular domain of tissue factor shows the fibronectin repeats are arranged end to end, creating a rigid structure with a bend of 120° between each repeat.[238,239] This structure is similar to that of the interferon-γ receptor.[240] This rigid conformation is largely preserved when tissue factor is bound to factor VIIa.[243,244] These data suggest a true receptor function of the factor VIIa/tissue factor complex in addition to its role in coagulation. Recently, the factor VIIa/tissue factor complex was shown to play a role in transmembrane signaling,[241,242] presumably through an additional protease activated cofactor or receptor, but the cellular function corresponding to these observations is not yet understood.

The binding of factor VII/VIIa to tissue factor is calcium-dependent. The crystal structure of factor VIIa bound to the extracellular domain of tissue factor has been determined.[243,244] These studies show that the binding of tissue factor occurs via an extensive interface, which may be divided into three major contact sites.[244,245] The first contact site is between the second fibronectin type III repeat domain and the factor VIIa Gla-domain. The second contact site involves the boundary residues of the fibronectin type III domains and the EGF-1 domain of factor VIIa, and makes the largest contribution to the tissue factor/factor VIIa binding affinity. The third contact site is between the top of the first fibronectin type III domain and the EGF-2 and catalytic domains of factor VIIa. These interactions suggest that tissue factor imposes a constraint on the otherwise flexible factor VIIa molecule, thereby stabilizing an active conformation. Additionally, these structural data agree with previous functional observations that several discrete regions within both the light chain (Gla and growth factor domains) and heavy chain (catalytic domain) are required for this specific interaction.[48–52,234–236,246–250]

Factor VII and Tissue Factor Genes

The gene for factor VII is located on chromosome 13 in the region q34-qter, which is very close to the gene for factor X.[261–263] The complete sequence for the gene for factor VII has been determined and spans about 12.8 kb of DNA (GenBank J02933 and U14580).[264] The mRNA for factor VII can undergo alternative splicing, forming a major transcript from eight exons and a very minor transcript utilizing nine exons. The additional exon located in the 5′ end of the gene results in a prepro leader sequence of 60 amino acids rather than the usual 38 amino acids. The smallest exon in the gene for factor VII codes for 9 amino acids (residues 38 to 46 in the light chain), while the largest exon codes for 198 amino acids (residues 57 to 254 in the heavy chain). The introns range in size from 68 nucleotides (intron C) to 2574 nucleotides (intron A). All the intron/exon splice junctions follow the GT-AG rule.[170] The gene for factor VII is free of *Alu* repetitive sequences. It does contain, however, five regions of tandem repeats that are also similar to hypervariable minisatellite DNA.[264,265] A prevalent polymorphism due to the presence or absence of a 37-bp monomer element is present in intron G and is readily detected by PCR.[266,267] In addition, an *Msp*I RFLP in exon VIII is present in about 10 percent of Caucasian factor VII alleles;[268] this G/A dimorphism results in substitution of Gln for Arg353.

The essential transcription regulatory elements in the 5′-flanking region of the factor VII gene have been characterized.[269,270] The absence of a CCAAT box in the factor VII promoter contrasts with the promoter structures of factor IX, which has a functional CCAAT box, and factor X, which contains a putative CCAAT box that binds the ubiquitous transcription factor NF-Y.[271,272,521] The major transcription start site is located approximately 50 bp upstream from the initiation Met and is close to the binding sites for an Sp1-like transcription factor and HNF-4. The factor VII HNF-4 recognition sequence, ACTTG, is also present in the promoters for factor X and factor IX. A naturally occurring mutation in the factor IX HNF-4 site causes the hemophilia B Leyden phenotype (see below), while a similar mutation in the factor VII promoter causes lifelong bleeding and absence of factor VII in the circulation.[23–32,273]

Five of the seven introns in the gene for factor VII are located in the regions coding for the N-terminal half of the protein (Fig. 169-8 and Table 169-5). The first intron occurs in the prepro leader sequence (Val −17), while the second follows the Gla domain (between Thr37 and Lys38). The third intron is located just prior to the first growth factor domain (Asp46). The fourth intron is located between the two growth factor domains (His84), while the fifth intron is found just after the second growth factor domain (Val131). The last two introns are present within the catalytic domain (between Gln167 and Val168 and Gly209). The remaining portion of the protein (from Gly209 to Pro406) is coded by a single exon. These seven introns in the gene for factor VII are located in the same position as the seven introns in factor IX, factor X, and protein C, and in the same position as the first three introns in prothrombin relative to the amino acid sequence of each of these proteins[13,17,68,264,274,275] (Table 169-5). The introns in the genes of

Table 169-5 Comparison of the Location, Splice Junction Type, and Size of the Introns in the Genes for Human Factors VII, IX, and X, Protein C, and Prothrombin

Intron	Protein	Location* (Amino Acid)	Splice Junction Type	Size, bp
A	Factor VII	−17	I	2574
	Factor IX	−17	I	6206
	Factor X	−17	I	≈5000
	Protein C	−19	I	1263
	Prothrombin	−17	I	386
B	Factor VII	37/38	0	1919
	Factor IX	38/39	0	188
	Factor X	37/38	0	≈7400
	Protein C	37/38	0	1462
	Prothrombin	37/38	0	659
C	Factor VII	46	I	68
	Factor IX	47	I	3689
	Factor X	46	I	≈950
	Protein C	46	I	92
	Prothrombin	46	I	242
D	Factor VII	84	I	1908
	Factor IX	85	I	7163
	Factor X	84	I	≈1800
	Protein C	92	I	102
E	Factor VII	131	I	971
	Factor IX	128	I	2565
	Factor X	128	I	≈2900
	Protein C	137	I	2668
F	Factor VII	15/16	0	595
	Factor IX	15/16	0	9473
	Factor X	15/16	0	≈3400
	Protein C	15/16	0	873
G	Factor VII	57	I	816
	Factor IX	54	I	668
	Factor X	55	I	≈1700
	Protein C	55	I	1129

*Numbering for introns A through E refers to light chain and for introns F and G refers to heavy chain.

NOTE: Type 0 splice junctions have introns between the triplets coding for two amino acids; type I splice junctions have introns between the first and second nucleotides of the triplet coding for one amino acid.

this family of vitamin K-dependent proteins differ greatly, however, in their size and DNA sequence, with the exception of intron C in factor VII and protein C. The similarity of the amino acid sequence and the organization of the genes in this family of proteins has led to the proposal that the vitamin K-dependent proteins have evolved from a common ancestor through gene duplication and exon shuffling.[276]

The gene for tissue factor is located on region p21-22 of chromosome 1[277,278] and includes 12.4 kb.[279] It contains six exons separated by five introns with typical consensus intron-exon boundaries (GenBank J02846). The first exon encodes the 32-residue signal peptide, while the second through fifth exons encode the N-terminal extracellular domain. The sixth exon contains 1278 bp and includes the transmembrane and cytoplasmic domains as well as a long 3′ untranslated region. The gene for tissue factor also contains three full-length and one partial *Alu* repeat and a single major transcription initiation site 26 bp downstream of a TATA box. Transcription of the tissue factor gene in activated monocytes results in a 2.2-kb mRNA encoding the tissue factor protein and a 3.1-kb mRNA due to an alternative splice site in intron 1 that terminates in a premature stop codon.[280]

Tissue factor is expressed constitutively in a differentiation-dependent manner in extravascular cells and tumor cells, and is inducible in fibroblasts, monocytes, and endothelial cells in response to a variety of cytokines and inflammatory mediators.[220,281] Regulation of cell-surface tissue factor expression is complex and probably occurs at both the transcriptional and posttranscriptional levels.[281] The tissue factor promoter region is divisible into two functional regions: (a) a downstream minimal promoter region responsible for maintaining low baseline levels of expression that contains the TATA box and an Sp1 binding site, and (b) an upstream modulator/enhancer region that amplifies transcription to high levels in response to lipopolysaccharide, and which contains AP-1 and NF-KB binding sites.

Clinical Aspects of Factor VII

Elevated levels of factor VII are associated with a number of clinical conditions. Levels of factor VII rise during pregnancy, delivery, and puerperium, most likely occurring in a complex of factor VII and phospholipid.[282] Elevated levels of factor VII have also been associated with increasing age,[283] hyperglycemia,[284] dietary fat intake,[285] and hyperlipidermia,[284,286,287] particularly large triglyceride-rich lipoproteins such as VLDL and chylomicrons. The effect of lipids on factor VII:C levels may be due to the contact surface activation of factor XII by negatively charged plasma lipid particles, with the subsequent activation of factor VII.[288,289] Finally, raised plasma factor VII:C activity was associated retrospectively and prospectively with an increased risk of ischemic heart disease.[290–292] Interestingly, the Gln353 allele of the *Msp*I RFLP in exon VIII correlates strongly with lower plasma factor VII:C levels.[268]

Congenital factor VII deficiency (MIM 227500) is a very rare condition. It is inherited as an autosomal recessive disorder with variable expression and high penetrance.[293–295] There is no absolute correlation between a decreased plasma level of factor VII and bleeding symptoms. Cerebral hemorrhage has been reported to occur in 16 percent of factor VII-deficient patients.[296] Other common bleeding manifestations include easy bruising, epistaxis, gingival hemorrhage, and menorrhagia. Hemarthroses generally occur only in severely affected individuals. Paradoxically, some patients with factor VII deficiency have been reported to suffer from thromboembolism.[297–299]

Factor VII deficiency is usually characterized by an isolated prolonged prothrombin time (PT) and normal partial thromboplastin time (APTT). Several molecular variants of factor VII have been described that show variable patterns with regard to the level of factor VII coagulant activity (factor VII:C) and factor VII antigen (factor VII:Ag).[300,301] Furthermore, the factor VII activity may vary depending upon the thromboplastin used in the coagulation assay.[302]

Several factor VII variants have been characterized at the molecular level.[303] A symptomatic patient with severe factor VII deficiency (factor VII:C < 1 percent; factor VII:Ag normal) was found to be homozygous for a G $\rightarrow$ A mutation resulting in the substitution of Gln for Arg79 within the first growth factor domain. This patient was also heterozygous for a second mutation of G $\rightarrow$ A, resulting in the substitution of Gln for Arg152 at the factor VII activation site.[306] Secondly, an asymptomatic individual was found to have an Arg (CCG) to Gln (CAG) mutation at codon 304 within the catalytic domain.[307] This individual had a factor VII:C level that was undetectable using rabbit tissue factor, but was 30 percent of normal using human tissue factor. The factor VII:Ag level in this patient was normal. A homozygous Cys310 to Phe mutation (TGC to TTC) was found in an Italian patient with 4 percent factor VII:C activity and a mild bleeding disorder.[267] A severely affected patient (factor VII:C and factor VII:Ag = 1 percent) was a compound heterozygote for two different single base deletions at codons 260/261 and 289/290, respectively.[308] A substitution of Phe38 to Ser, known as factor $VII_{CENTRAL}$,[304] results in reduced tissue factor binding and impairs the activation of factors IX and X. The factor VII variant Gln100 to Arg[305] is likewise characterized by reduced tissue factor binding and procoagulant function. Finally, substitution of G for T at nucleotide -61[273] disrupts the HNF-4 binding site in the factor VII promoter and results in severe factor VII deficiency.

When bleeding episodes occur, factor VII deficient patients may be treated with plasma or a prothrombin complex concentrate that contains significant amounts of all the vitamin K-dependent plasma proteins, including factor VII. Concentrates of purified factor VII have also been prepared for this purpose, but are less readily available.

Recombinant human factor VIIa has been successfully used to treat patients with hemophilia A who have antibodies against factor VIII (see Chap. 172).[309,310] The administered recombinant factor VIIa presumably forms a complex with exposed tissue factor at the site of injury that directly activates factor X (Fig. 169-1) independently of the presence of factors VIII and IX.

Recombinant factor VIIa has also been used to treat a variety of hemostatic disorders including factor VII deficiency,[311] coagulopathy secondary to cirrhosis of the liver,[312] antibody-mediated acquired hemophilia,[313] and thrombocytopenia.[314] Recently, localized infusions of active site-inhibited recombinant factor VIIa to freshly injured vessels in a rabbit model was shown to have a significant antithrombotic effect without causing bleeding.[315] Accordingly, the uses of recombinant factor VIIa and its derivatives continue to be investigated in a wide spectrum of clinical settings.

FACTOR IX

As is true of most coagulation factors, factor IX was first recognized as a special entity by the revelation that hemophilia could be caused by a deficiency of two different plasma proteins. In 1947, Pavlovsky found that the prolonged coagulation time of plasma from one hemophilia patient normalized the clotting time of another hemophilic plasma. Further studies[316,317] clearly showed two types of hemophilia, both of which were inherited as sex-linked recessive disorders that were clinically indistinguishable from each other. One was called *hemophilia A* and was caused by a deficiency of factor VIII. The other was designated *hemophilia B* and was defined as a deficiency of factor IX (Christmas factor, plasma thromboplastin component, β-prothromboplastin).

Factor IX participates in the middle stages of the blood coagulation cascade[122] and is converted to factor IXa in the presence either of factor XIa and calcium ions[318] or of factor VIIa, tissue factor, and calcium ions[218] (Fig. 169-1). Factor IXa then activates factor X in the presence of factor VIIIa, calcium ions, and phospholipid.

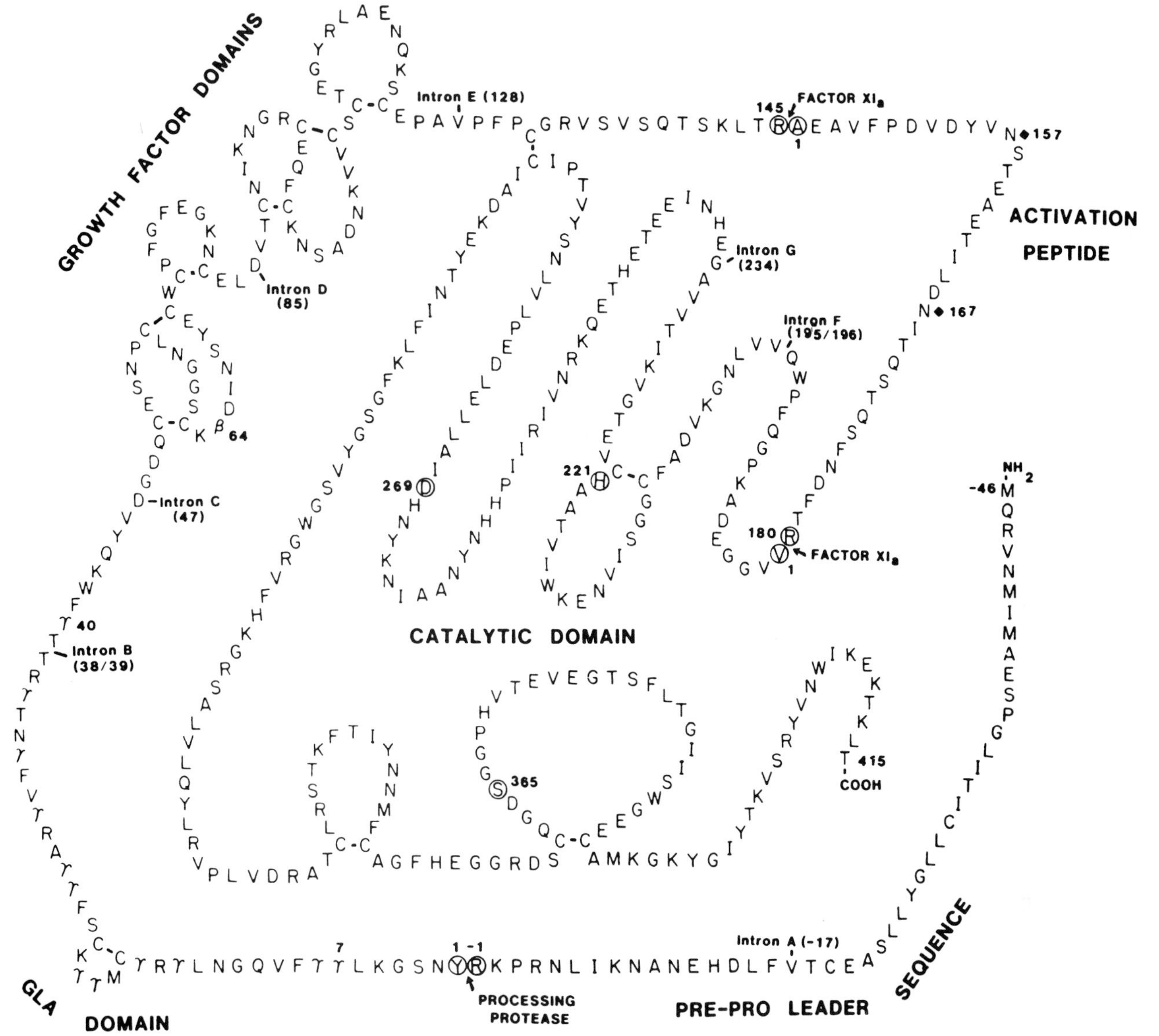

Fig. 169-9 Amino acid sequence and tentative structure for human prepro factor IX. The locations of the seven introns (A to G) are shown in the various regions of the protein. The prepro leader sequence is cleaved during protein biosynthesis to give rise to the mature protein with an amino-terminal sequence of Y-N-S-G-. The two peptide bonds cleaved by factor XIa (or factor VIIa) during the activation reaction are shown with small arrows. The three amino acids in the catalytic domain (H221, D349, and S365) that participate in catalysis are circled, while the two potential N-linked carbohydrate attachment sites in the activation peptide are shown with solid diamonds. The amino acids are numbered as follows, starting with the amino-terminal end of the protein: −46 to −1 = prepro leader sequence; +1 to 145 = light chain of factor IXa; 146 to 180 = activation peptide; 181 to 415 = catalytic chain of factor IXa. The single-letter code for amino acids is shown in the legend to Fig. 169-5. β = β-hydroxyaspartic acid. (*Modified from Yoshitake et al.*[13] *Used with permission.*)

Human factor IX is a single-chain glycoprotein with a molecular weight of 56,800 and an N-terminal sequence of Tyr-Asn-Ser-Gly-Lys[319] (Fig. 169-9). The mature protein circulating in plasma contains 415 amino acids, including 12 residues of γ-carboxyglutamic acid.[12] The human protein also contains 0.3 equivalents of β-hydroxyaspartic acid at position 64 in the first of the two growth factor domains [96,97]. The function of β-hydroxyaspartic acid in factor IX has not been established. Equilibrium dialysis experiments show that it does not participate in the high-affinity calcium-binding sites present in factor IX.[320,104] In addition, nonhydroxylated recombinant factor IX retains full procoagulant activity.[321] Factor IX also contains 17 percent carbohydrate, a portion of which is attached to asparagine residues 157 and 167 in the activation peptide. Like factor VII, human factor IX also contains two unique O-linked carbohydrate structures including Xyl-Glc at Ser53 in the first growth factor domain[107,108] and a tetrasaccharide at Ser61 which is O-linked through a fucose residue.[110]

Human factor IX is converted to a serine protease during the coagulation process by the cleavage of two internal peptide bonds[318] (Figs. 169-9 and 169-10). Cleavage occurs initially at the Arg145-Ala bond with the formation of factor IXa followed by cleavage of the Arg180-Val bond leading to the generation of factor IXab. The second cleavage releases an activation glycopeptide of 35 amino acids. The light chain of factor IXab contains the Gla domain and the two growth factor domains, while the heavy chain contains the catalytic domain that includes the active site residues of His221, Asp269, and Ser365. The light chain and the heavy chain of factor IXab are linked together by a single disulfide bond involving Cys132 in the light chain and Cys289 in the heavy chain (Fig. 169-9). The cleavage of the two internal arginine peptide bonds is catalyzed either by factor XIa in the presence of

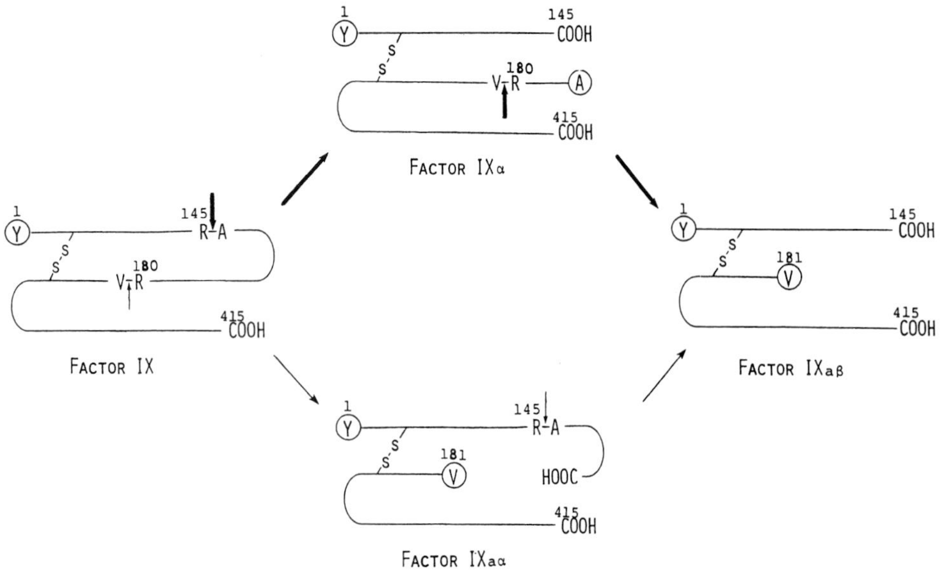

Fig. 169-10 Activation scheme for human factor IX. In the presence of factor XIa or factor VIIa, the principal cleavage occurs initially at R145 to A146 (heavy vertical arrow) generating the factor IXa intermediate. The second cleavage then occurs at R180 to V181 (heavy vertical arrow) generating factor IXab and an activation peptide. Factor IX can also be cleaved initially at R180 to V181 (thin vertical arrow) by factor XIa, generating factor IXaa. The second cleavage then occurs at R145 to A146 (thin vertical arrow), generating factor IXab and an activation peptide. Amino-terminal amino acids are circled.

calcium ions, or by factor VIIa in the presence of tissue factor, phospholipid, and calcium ions. Cleavage of only the Arg180-Val bond gives rise to factor IXaa, an enzyme with markedly reduced biologic activity. This activation reaction occurs in the presence of a protease from Russell's viper venom (RVV-X).[322]

The binding of calcium ions to the Gla domain is required for the interaction of factor IX with phospholipid membrane surfaces.[323,324] Factor IX contains two additional calcium-binding sites located within the first growth factor domain[39,42,46,320] and within the N-terminal portion of the catalytic domain.[325] In addition to binding calcium and phospholipid, the Gla and growth factor domains of the factor IX/IXa light chain are implicated in the binding of the protein to specific receptors on platelets[60] and endothelial cells.[53,54,58,59,326,327] In contrast, interaction of factor IXa with its cofactor (factor VIIIa) and substrate (factor X) appears to require determinants within both the light and heavy chains of factor IXa.[55–57,328]

Factor IX Gene

The genes for human factor IX and factor VIII are located close to each other at the tip of the long arm of the X chromosome at Xq26-Xq27.[329,330] The gene for factor IX is about 34 kb in size, and its complete nucleotide sequence is established (GenBank M11309).[13] The gene contains seven introns and eight exons in the coding and 3′ noncoding regions of the gene (Table 169-6). The 8 exons code for 415 amino acids comprising the mature protein that circulates in plasma. The first 2 exons also code for a prepro leader sequence of 46 amino acids (Figs. 169-4 and 169-9), and the intron/exon splice junction sequences follow the GT-AG rule.[170] The introns contain four Alu repetitive sequences and range in size from 188 nucleotides (intron B) to 9473 nucleotides (intron F).

Initiation sites for the transcription of the gene for human factor IX appears to be heterogeneous, reflecting the absence of a well-defined or typical TATA-like promoter element in the 5′ end of the gene.[334] The 5′ region also contains three Met codons at −46, −41, and −39 bp for polypeptide initiation. The Met at −39 bp is the only one conserved in the human, monkey, dog, and murine factor IX genes,[335] suggesting that the Met at −39 bp is the most probable initiation site for human factor IX biosynthesis. Several *cis*-acting regulatory elements have been identified in the 5′-untranslated region of the factor IX gene. A consensus androgen response element (ARE) is located between nucleotides −36 and −17.[331] This sequence overlaps a functional HNF-4 binding site.[332,336] Three C/EBP elements are located between nucleotides −220 and +18.[337] The distal and proximal C/EBP sites partially overlap with a D-site binding protein (DBP) element, while the middle C/EBP site is close to a nuclear factor 1 (NF-1) site.[271,337,338] The upstream region of the 5′-flanking sequence of the factor IX gene contains a putative negative regulatory or

Table 169-6 Location and Size of Exons and Introns in the Gene for Human Factor IX

Exon	Nucleotide Positions*	Nucleotide Length*	Amino Acids†	Intron	Nucleotide Position	Nucleotide Length
I	1–117	117	−46 to −17	A	118–6325	6206‡
II	6326–6489	164	−17 to 37	B	6490–6677	188
III	6678–6702	25	38–47	C	6703–10391	3689
IV	10392–10505	114	47–85	D	10506–17668	7163
V	17669–17797	129	85–128	E	17798–20362	2565
VI	20363–20565	203	128–195	F	20566–30038	9473
VII	30039–30153	115	196–234	G	30154–30821	668
VIII	30822–32757	1935	234–415			

*Includes 30 nucleotides at the 5′ end and 1390 nucleotides at the 3′ end that are not translated.
†Amino acids coded for by each exon; negative numbers refer to amino acids in the prepro leader sequence.
‡Includes 50 extra nucleotides present in some polymorphic forms of the gene.
Source: Yoshitake et al.[13]

silencer element ATCCTCTCC in the region spanning −1700 to −1400 bp.[271] This sequence is associated with silencer activity in several genes expressed primarily in the liver.[339]

The x-ray crystal structure of porcine factor IXa complexed with D-phenylalanyl-prolyl-arginine chloromethyl ketone (PPACK) has been described.[340] The overall structure of factor IXa resembles a tulip: the catalytic domain represents the flower, the two interlaced EGF domains represent a bent stalk-like structure, and the N-terminal Gla domain represents the bulb. Like the crystal structures of thrombin,[157] factor X,[341] and factor VII,[244] the specificity pocket of factor IXa containing the catalytic site has similar features to the trypsin-like serine proteases. The data from the crystal structure of factor IXa helped give a structural context to the properties of naturally occurring and experimentally introduced mutations, which have already been functionally characterized.

Normal Variants of Factor IX

Several RFLPs have been identified within the gene for human factor IX,[342,343] including a *Bam*HI site in the 5′ untranslated region; a *Dde*I/*Hin*fI site in intron A; an *Xmn*I site in intron C; a *Taq*I site in intron D; an *Msp*I site in intron D; an *Mnl*I site in exon VI; and an *Hha*I site in the 3′ untranslated region. The allelic frequencies of these seven RFLPs vary considerably among different ethnic groups. The *Bam*HI and *Msp*I sites are more polymorphic in African-Americans, whereas the *Dde*I/*Hin*fI, *Xmn*I, *Taq*I, and *Mnl*I sites are more polymorphic in Caucasians. The two polymorphic sites in Asians are the *Hha*I site in the 3′ flanking region, and the *Mse*I site in the 5′ flanking region.[344] Most of the known factor IX polymorphisms are in some degree of linkage dysequilibrium with one another. The exon VI *Mnl*I polymorphism results in an amino acid polymorphism of Thr/Ala at residue 148 in the factor IX activation peptide that has no effect on biologic activity,[345] but which can be detected by an immunoassay using a monoclonal antibody that only recognizes the more common threonine allele.[346,347]

Abnormal Variants of Factor IX

All patients with hemophilia B have a prolonged coagulation time and decreased factor IX clotting activity (factor IX:C) in their plasma. In 1956, however, two distinct phenotypes of hemophilia B were described. In one case, barium sulfate-absorbed plasma from one patient's blood blocked a specific inhibitor against factor IX in the assay plasma, whereas, in a second case, a similar fraction from another patient had no effect.[348] Later it was shown that approximately 10 percent of all factor IX-deficient patients have factor IX antigenic material (factor IX:Ag) or cross-reacting material (CRM^+) in their plasma.[349] The remaining 90 percent of patients deficient in factor IX either lack cross-reacting material (CRM^-) or have reduced amounts (CRM^R). Patients with severe factor IX deficiency (factor IX:C < 1 percent) have lower factor IX:Ag levels, while those patients with milder defects fall in the low, intermediate, or normal range.[350]

The phenotypic heterogeneity of factor IX deficiency is reflected by the identification of a large number of molecular abnormalities in hemophilia B patients. As of 1998, 652 unique factor IX mutations had been identified in 1713 hemophilia B pedigrees worldwide.[342,351] Of the mutations identified, 12 percent are gross gene alterations (complete or partial gene deletions, insertions, or rearrangements), 3 percent are short nucleotide deletions or insertions, and 85 percent are single base substitutions (point mutations). Of the point mutations, over 75 percent are missense mutations and the 25 percent are nonsense mutations. Molecular abnormalities responsible for factor IX deficiency have been identified in the 5′ noncoding region, at intron/exon splice junctions, and in the eight exons of the coding sequence. Over half of the identified point mutations, however, are located in exons VII or VIII (i.e., the catalytic domain).

Gross transcriptional abnormalities, such as complete or partial factor IX gene deletions, insertions, frameshift mutations, and nonsense mutations, are almost invariably associated with severe hemophilia B (factor IX:C < 1 percent) and levels of circulating factor IX antigen that are markedly reduced or undetectable. In addition, severely affected patients who develop factor IX inhibitors usually have one of these gross gene abnormalities. Also associated with CRM^- factor IX deficiency are single base substitutions (missense mutations) that cause mRNA or protein instability or degradation.

Hemophilia B_{LEYDEN} is a particularly interesting CRM^- variant characterized by moderate to severe factor IX deficiency during childhood followed by clinical improvement and near-normalization of factor IX clotting and antigen levels with the onset of puberty.[352] This phenotype is associated with point mutations in a region of approximately 54 bp (−40 to +13) surrounding the putative transcription initiation site of the factor IX gene.[332,333,336,353–355,359] The developmental timing of the expression of the factor IX gene characterized by these mutations suggests that the transcription of the factor IX gene is, in part, hormonally mediated. A consensus ARE was identified between nucleotides −36 and −17 of the factor IX promoter.[331] This sequence is partially overlapped by a functional HNF-4 binding site. Interestingly, a substitution of C for G at −26 bp (hemophilia $B_{BRANDENBURG}$) causes lifelong severe hemophilia B, presumably by disruption of the ARE, while substitutions at −21 and −20 bp (A, G, or C for T in the sequence ACTTTG) result in disruption of HNF-4 binding alone and the Leyden phenotype.[331,332,336] These data suggest that androgen binding can partially overcome the negative effect of impaired HNF-4 binding to the promoter. Other Leyden mutations include nucleotide substitutions at positions −6, −5, and +13 relative to the transcription start site.[351] These mutations correspond to a disruption in the proximal C/EBP binding site and a disruption in the binding site (−15 to −1) of an uncharacterized *trans*-acting regulatory factor.[333,337] Experiments investigating the molecular mechanisms explaining Leyden-specific mutations outside the putative ARE have identified interactions between C/EBP and the hormonally regulated transcription factors DBP and hepatic leukemia factor (HLF).[338,358] Accordingly, the hormonal sensitivity of the expression of these factor IX mutants may be mediated by both direct androgen receptor binding to the factor IX ARE and the indirect regulatory effects of androgen receptor on the expression of developmentally regulated transcription factors.[356–358]

Of the many CRM^+ and CRM^R variants of factor IX described, several provide means for understanding the relationship between the factor IX amino acid sequence, protein structure, and coagulant function. Several patients have severe CRM^+ to CRM^R hemophilia B (factor IX:C usually < 1 percent) caused by a mutation of one of several highly conserved basic amino acids within the carboxyl end of the 18-residue propeptide.[351] These include mutations of Arg −4 to Gln (factor IX Oxford 3,[85] factor $IX_{SAN\ DIMAS}$,[87] and factor $IX_{KAWACHINAGANO}$[90]), Arg −1 to Ser (factor $IX_{CAMBRIDGE}$),[86] and Lys −2 to Asn.[91] These mutations prevent removal of the propeptide prior to secretion from the hepatocyte and result in a circulating dysfunctional factor IX molecule with an 18-amino acid N-terminal extension. Recently, an Ala10 to Val or Thr was described,[360] which results in a reduced affinity of the carboxylase enzyme to the propeptide that results in excessive bleeding during anticoagulant therapy with warfarin.

Several CRM^+ variants are caused by mutations within the Gla or first growth factor domains and are characterized by reduced factor IX procoagulant activity; this is presumably due to abnormal calcium binding. Mutations of glutamic acid residues that are normally γ-carboxylated include Gla7 to Ala (factor $IX_{OXFORD\ B2}$),[361] Gla21 to Lys (factor $IX_{NAGOYA\ 4}$),[365] and Gla27 to Lys (factor $IX_{SEATTLE\ 3}$)[366] or Val (factor $IX_{CHONGQUING}$).[367] The two Gla27 variants are characterized by severe factor IX deficiency (factor IX:C < 1 percent) and reduced factor IX:Ag levels, especially when measured using a calcium-dependent antibody. In addition, site-directed mutagenesis of the equivalent Gla21 and Gla27 residues in protein C completely abolishes protein C calcium-dependent anticoagulant activity.[368] A Gly12 to Arg variant[362] has been characterized and shows normal activation by factor XIa, but diminished activation by factor VIIa/tissue factor. Substitution of Cys18 to Arg (factor $IX_{ZUTPHEN}$)[363] disrupts the disulfide bond normally present in the Gla domain between residues Cys18 and Cys23. The remaining free Cys results in the formation of a 95-kDa complex between factor IX and α_1-microglobulin through an intermolecular disulfide bond. These conserved Gla residues and the structural integrity of the Gla domain are thus important for the calcium-dependent interaction of the vitamin K-dependent proteins with their associated activators, cofactors and phospholipid membrane surfaces. Several residues within the N-terminal region of the first growth factor domain of factor IX also are involved in calcium binding and factor IX function.[34,46] Factor $IX_{ALABAMA}$ was isolated from a patient with moderately severe CRM$^+$ hemophilia B (factor IX:C = 10 percent).[369] The mutation was later identified as Asp47 to Gly, which results in reduced factor IX clotting activity, most notably in the presence of calcium and factor VIIIa.[370] Factor $IX_{NEW\ LONDON}$, described in a severely affected patient (factor IX:C < 1 percent; normal factor IX:Ag), is due to a substitution of Gln50 by Pro, which results in markedly reduced activation of factor IX by factor XIa.[371] Mutation of the normally β-hydroxylated Asp64 to Gly (factor IX London 6)[372] or Asn (factor $IX_{OXFORD\ DL}$)[361] results in moderately severe CRM$^+$ hemophilia B; the latter variant demonstrated impaired calcium-binding affinity. Substitution of Asn92 by His in the second growth factor domain[364] results in severe hemophilia B due to defective interaction with factors VIIa and X.

Factor IX variants caused by mutations at either of the two activation sites have been described. Factor $IX_{CHAPEL\ HILL}$ was first reported in a patient with a mild bleeding disorder (factor IX:Ag = 100 percent; factor IX:C = 20 percent).[373] The molecular defect was later shown to be a substitution of a His for Arg145, the first, or a, cleavage site necessary for factor IX conversion to factor IXa[373] (Fig. 169-9). Factor $IX_{CHAPEL\ HILL}$ is cleaved by factor XIa, however, only at the second, or b, cleavage site (Arg180-Val), giving rise to factor IXaa.[375] In this molecule, the activation peptide remains attached to the light chain. Factor $IXaa_{CHAPEL\ HILL}$ has only about 20 percent of the clotting activity of normal factor IXab, but is essentially the same as normal factor IXaa. This indicates that both activation cleavages are required for normal factor IXa activity. In factor $IX_{ALBUQUERQUE}$ (factor IX:C = 1 percent; factor IX:Ag = 30 percent), the Arg145 is replaced by Cys, which similarly results in reduced factor IX activation.[376] A number of mutations involving the b activation site (Arg180-Val) have also been reported. As opposed to the Arg145 mutations, the Arg180-Val mutations are manifested by severe CRM$^+$ hemophilia B (factor IX:C < 1 percent) indicating that the b cleavage is essential for factor IX procoagulant activity. Examples include Arg180 to Trp (factor $IX_{DEVENTER/NAGOYA}$),[377,378] Gln (factor $IX_{HILO/NOVARA}$),[377,379] or Gly (factor IX_{MADRID})[380] and Val181 to Phe (factor IX_{MILANO}).[377]

Over half of the identified point mutations associated with factor IX deficiency are located within the catalytic domain or factor IXa heavy chain. Mutations in the catalytic domain characterized by a circulating dysfunctional factor IX protein can interfere with factor IX catalytic activity by several different mechanisms. Once factor IX is activated, the new N-terminus formed at Val181 of the factor IXa heavy chain forms an ion pair with Asp364 adjacent to the active center Ser365 (Fig. 169-9). By analogy with chymotrypsin, formation of the ion pair results in a conformational change in the active site required for catalysis. Thus, a substitution of Asp364 with Val[31] or His (factor $IX_{MECHTAL}$)[382] results in severe factor IX deficiency (factor IX:C < 1 percent) with normal levels of a circulating dysfunctional protein caused by the lack of ion pair formation. Likewise, mutations at two highly conserved glycine residues, Gly309 to Val and Gly311 to Glu (factor $IX_{AMAGASAKI}$), both result in undetectable factor IX clotting activity and normal factor IX:Ag levels. Computer modeling of the catalytic domain predicts that both mutations disrupt the active site conformational change accompanying ion pair formation.[383,384]

Several mutations directly affect the catalytic site. Mutations of the active site serine itself (Ser365 to Gly,[382] Ile,[382] or Arg[386]) result in a severely dysfunctional factor IX molecule (factor IX:C < 1 percent) incapable of catalytic activity. Replacement of Gly363 with Val (factor $IX_{EAGLE\ ROCK}$) is associated with a moderately severe bleeding disorder (factor IX:C = 1 to 5 percent; factor IX:Ag = 100 percent), because the highly conserved glycine residue is required for stabilization of the factor IXa active site and substrate binding during catalysis.[387]

Another set of CRM$^+$ variants interfere with the extended or secondary substrate binding site(s) within the factor IXa heavy chain. In factor IX_{ANGERS}, substitution of Arg for the highly conserved Gly396 results in severe hemophilia (factor IX:C < 1 percent; factor IX:Ag = 100 percent). It is assumed that this is caused by the positively charged arginine amino group binding to the negatively charged side chain of Asp359 at the base of the substrate binding pocket, thus forming a "self-inhibited" enzyme.[388,389] Similarly, mutation of Ile397 to Thr (factor $IX_{VANCOUVER}$,[389] factor $IX_{LONG\ BEACH}$,[390] and factor $IX_{LOS\ ANGELES}$[391]) causes moderately severe to severe hemophilia (factor IX:C = 1 to 5 percent; factor IX:Ag = 50 to 100 percent). Computer modeling predicts that the new side chain hydroxyl group of Thr397 forms a hydrogen bond with the carbonyl oxygen of Trp385, thus disrupting the factor X binding site.[392,393] Another moderately severe CRM$^+$ variant, factor $IX_{LAKE\ ELSINORE/NIIGATA}$,[394,395] results from an Ala390 to Val substitution, which also may inhibit macromolecular substrate binding.

Hemophilia B_M, a phenotypic variant of CRM$^+$ factor IX deficiency, was initially described by Hougie and Twomey,[396] who found that the one-stage ox brain prothrombin time was prolonged in some patients. Patients with hemophilia B_M synthesize a factor IX that is devoid of clotting activity (factor IX:C usually < 1 percent), but is capable of inhibiting the activation of factor X catalyzed by factor VIIa and bovine tissue factor.[377,397] At the molecular level, two groups of abnormalities have been found in patients with the B_M phenotype. The first group involves the b activation site (Arg180-Val), and includes Arg180 to Trp (factor IX $B_{M\ DEVENTER/NAGOYA}$),[377,378] Gly (factor IX_{MADRID}),[380] or Gln (factor $IX_{HILO/NOVARA}$),[377,379] Val181 to Phe (factor IX_{MILANO}),[377] and Val182 to Phe (factor $IX_{KASHIHARA}$)[398] or Leu (factor $IX_{CARDIFF\ 2}$).[399] The second group of B_M mutations are located near the catalytic center or substrate binding site. These include Gly311 to Glu (factor $IX_{AMAGASAKI}$),[384] Val313 to Asp (factor IX_{KIRYU}),[385] Pro368 to Thr (factor $IX_{BERGAMO}$),[378] Ala390 to Val (factor $IX_{LAKE\ ELSINORE/NIIGATA}$),[394,395] Gly396 to Arg (factor IX_{ANGERS}),[388,389] and Ile397 to Thr (factor $IX_{VANCOUVER}$).[389]

Overall, about 40 percent of the point mutations identified in patients with hemophilia B are located within CG dinucleotides,[342,351,381] where deamination of methylcytosine results in a transition of CG to TG or CG to CA depending on whether the mutation occurs in the DNA coding strand or complementary strand, respectively. Thus, CG-type transitions account for most of the mutations that recur in more than one pedigree.[400] The remaining "recurrent" mutations identified in multiple hemophilic families appear to represent a "founder effect;" that is, they result from a distant common ancestor. These include factor $IX_{VANCOUVER}$ (Ile397 to Thr),[401,402] as well as mutations of Thr296 to Met[91,403] and Gly60 to Ser[91,404] that are associated with moderately severe (factor IX:C about 5 percent) and mild (factor IX:C = 10 to 15 percent) hemophilia, respectively.

Genetic Counseling for Hemophilia B

Recent developments in the molecular biology of factor IX, as well as advances in the field of molecular genetics, have greatly facilitated genetic counseling of families with hemophilia B.

Detection of female carriers and prenatal diagnosis of affected males can now be accomplished in the vast majority of families either indirectly by linkage analysis using RFLPs or by direct identification of the causative mutation in the particular hemophilia B pedigree.[405] Linkage analysis is based on the cosegregation of an intragenic factor IX RFLP (see above) with the hemophilic mutation; this approach requires female heterozygosity for the particular RFLP, as well as the availability and cooperation of key family members for testing. Most of the known factor IX RFLPs were initially detected by Southern blotting.[329,406–409] This technique employs a radiolabeled DNA fragment or probe prepared from factor IX cDNA or genomic DNA. More recently, the polymerase chain reaction (PCR) simplified detection of previously known factor IX RFLPs and also enabled the identification of new RFLPs.[410,411] RFLP linkage analysis by PCR requires only minute amounts of DNA, is nonradioactive, and can be performed much more rapidly than Southern blotting. Taking into account the ethnic frequencies (see above) and degree of linkage equilibrium of the various factor IX RFLPs, carrier detection by linkage analysis should be successful in about 90 percent, 80 percent, and 50 percent of African-American, Caucasian, and Asian families, respectively.

Because linkage analysis by RFLP testing is not successful in every family, identification of the actual hemophilic mutation is the ultimate goal for genetic counseling. Furthermore, for the relatively high proportion of families with "sporadic"hemophilia due to a recent or de novo mutation (30 to 50 percent), direct detection of the hemophilic mutation is required for accurate assignment of carrier status. The identification of causative factor IX mutations, however, is complicated by the genetic heterogeneity of hemophilia B (see above). Nevertheless, relatively rapid and efficient screening procedures using PCR-based techniques have recently been applied to detection of hemophilic mutations.[412] These include denaturing gradient gel electrophoresis (DGGE),[388] chemical cleavage of mismatches,[413] single-strand conformation polymorphism (SSCP),[414] and direct sequencing of PCR-amplified genomic DNA fragments[372,381] or transcripts.[386] Once the particular mutation in an affected individual is identified by DNA sequencing, family members can be rapidly tested by restriction enzyme digestion of the appropriate PCR-amplified DNA fragment.[91,415,416]

Clinical Aspects

Like hemophilia A, hemophilia B (Christmas disease) occurs in a severe, moderate, or mild form according to the level of factor IX activity in plasma. Clinical symptoms reflect the factor IX:C level in plasma regardless of the level of factor IX:Ag. Severe factor IX deficiency (factor IX:C < 0.01 U/ml) is characterized by spontaneous bleeding, especially in the joints. A unit (U) of factor IX is defined as the amount of coagulant activity in 1 ml of normal pooled plasma. The disease is usually diagnosed when the affected male infant starts crawling or walking. A typical symptom at this stage is the development of large hematomas on the forehead. The hematomas may become the size of a golf ball and cause a dangerous strain on the skin. These hematomas must be watched carefully to avoid skin necrosis or any trauma to the skin. A typical feature for the superficial, subcutaneous hematomas that are often seen in hemophilia patients is the easily palpable subcutaneous infiltrate. These characteristics are otherwise found only in very severely thrombocytopenic patients and never occur in normal individuals.

When the afflicted youngster begins to stand and walk, recurrent joint bleeding is the most obvious clinical manifestation, appearing as swollen, very painful joint regions. The joints most often affected are the large joints, such as knees as ankles. Muscle bleeding may occur both spontaneously and after trauma in severely affected patients.[417,418] Large flexor muscle groups (i.e., ileopsoas, calf, and forearm) are most commonly affected. Large volumes of blood may be extravasated in the muscle tissue, resulting in compression of blood vessels and nerves. Muscle necrosis occurs rapidly due to ischemia. Bleeding into the ileopsoas muscle is rather common and presents with pain in the groin associated with local swelling. The patient is unable to stretch the hip joint. Retroperitoneal bleeding is also rather common and may be difficult to diagnose. Ultrasound, computed tomography, and MRI are of great help in these situations. Muscle and tissue hematomas should never be aspirated or treated surgically. A serious sequela to deep tissue bleeding is the development of pseudotumors (hemophilic blood cysts).[419] The incidence of such cysts has been reported as about 1 percent. Further bleeding will occur with gradual increase in size, resulting in pressure on surrounding structures. These formations may assume enormous dimensions and erode bone and even destroy adjacent joints and muscles. Finally, they may perforate into the abdomen or intestines. Infections may then supervene. Treatment should be aimed at prevention and all deep hematomas should be treated vigorously with plasma factor IX concentrates. Established pseudotumors may require surgical removal under the protection of adequate substitution therapy.[420] Gastrointestinal bleeding and bleeding from the urinary tract are also common. With the development of better plasma concentrates, surgical intervention in the case of peptic ulcers is often recommended. Central nervous system hemorrhage can occur in severe hemophiliacs following relatively minor trauma, and until recently, was the major cause of death in hemophiliacs.[421] Thus, any severe hemophiliac with neurologic symptoms should receive replacement therapy and observed closely until a head CT scan is obtained.

It should be remembered that bleeding might imitate any disease in hemophiliacs. Thus, a hematoma in the wall of the bowel mimicked acute appendicitis in a patient, and similar bleeding caused acute hepatic stasis in another patient.[422] A rule of thumb is to regard any symptom in a hemophiliac as caused by bleeding, and substitution therapy should be started immediately as the diagnostic work proceeds.

Patients with moderate hemophilia B (factor IX:C = 0.01 to 0.05 U/ml) most often have less-severe bleeding, and massive joint bleeding occurs less frequently. Patients with a factor IX:C level of 0.01 to 0.03 U/ml, however, require substitution treatment to almost the same extent as severe hemophiliacs.

Mild hemophiliacs (factor IX:C = 0.05 to 0.30 U/ml) usually do not develop spontaneous joint bleeding. However, they present some special problems. Mild hemophilia often is not diagnosed until adulthood and is then detected at times of surgery or trauma. Such patients may be difficult to manage because they might have unexpected heavy bleeding, and mild hemophilia should be kept in mind as a diagnostic possibility. It should be stressed that gastrointestinal bleeding and hematuria are almost as common in mild hemophilia as in the severe form. After trauma, mild hemophiliacs may develop life-threatening bleeding such as intracranial bleeding and muscle bleeding. Both the patients and their physicians may tend to underestimate the risk, resulting in an unnecessary delay in starting treatment.

Joint Disease. Typical joint disease is seen mainly in severely affected hemophiliacs. Its clinical pattern is the same in hemophilia A and B. In adults, acute hemarthrosis is most frequent in the knee joints, followed by the elbow, ankle, and wrist.[417,418] The hip is most often spared, probably because it is protected by the large muscle cuff.[423] Repeated joint bleeding leads to chronic changes of hyperplasia and hyperemia of the synovium, which makes the joint more susceptible to recurrent bleeding. This stresses the need for adequate substitution treatment for each joint bleed to minimize the development of chronic synovitis.

Chronic Arthritis. The chronic degenerative lesions of the joints in hemophilia are characterized by the presence of gross deformity with fixed flexion contractures. The muscle cuffs around the joint are often severely atrophied. Often there are also chronic effusions and pain. Microscopically, the synovium is greatly hypertrophied and heavily infiltrated with inflammatory cells and deposits of iron. Extensive fibrosis and bone cysts are seen. The radiologic findings have been described in detail.[424] Osteoporosis is invariable. Loss of cartilage results in loss of joint space, and underlying bone is resorbed with formation of subchondral cysts. Later, osteophytic outgrowth may be marked. Resorption of bone occurs especially in the knee joint with production of an enlarged intercondylar fossa, which may lead to differential overgrowth of one of the femoral condyles. Such deformity may result in posterior subluxation of the tibia and lateral shift of the tibia on the femur.

Treatment

Care of the patient with hemophilia B includes treatment of acute bleeding episodes, rehabilitation and management of the chronic musculoskeletal complications, as well as prophylaxis. Because hemophilia care involves many special requirements, centralization to hemophilia centers is recommended.[425] Such centers should be capable of taking care of the psychological and social problems of the hemophilia family and should provide orthopedic, dental, and surgical treatment. The centers also should provide the laboratory facilities for diagnosis and for monitoring replacement therapy.

Management of Acute Bleeding Episodes and Surgery. The goal for management of acute episodes is to normalize the hemostatic function by replacement of the missing coagulation protein factor IX. Factor IX is relatively stable and the in vivo half-life of about 24 h[426,427] makes it possible to administer factor IX at longer intervals than those used in hemophilia A. Most often, infusion one to two times daily is enough. The in vivo yield, however, is lower than that of factor VIII and is only 20 to 40 percent of the factor IX activity administered as plasma or factor IX concentrate.[426,427] This is ascribed to factor IX being distributed both intra- and extravascularly and to its binding to cellular surfaces.

To achieve hemostasis, the patient's plasma level of factor IX should be increased to 0.6 to 1.0 U/ml (60 U/kg body weight). In minor bleeding situations, it may be enough to reach a plasma level of 0.2 to 0.4 U/ml. Minor bleeding is often managed by treatment for 1 to 3 days. Major hemorrhages, including muscle hematomas, most often require treatment for 7 to 14 days (50 to 60 U/kg the first day, followed by 20 to 30 U/kg on days 2 through 4, and 10 to 20 U/kg for another 4 to 10 days). At major surgery, a plasma level of 0.6 to 1.0 U/ml is desirable during the operation and for the first one to four postoperative days depending on the specific operation. This corresponds to a dose of about 60 U/kg body weight. The dose is then slowly decreased to 30 to 40 U/kg for postoperative days 2 to 4 (a plasma level of 0.3 to 0.4 U/ml) and later to 10 to 20 U/kg (plasma level of 0.1 to 0.2 U/ml) for another 10 to 15 days.[428]

Management of Chronic Musculoskeletal Complications. Surgical correction of chronic musculoskeletal defects in hemophiliacs is possible because of the availability of plasma factor concentrates. Total arthroplasty of the knee and hip joints is successfully performed in hemophiliacs.[429–431] Chronic synovitis is increasingly subject to synovectomy.[432] Although there is some uncertainty regarding joint function deterioration after surgical synovectomy, good long-term results have been reported.[433,434] Arthroscopic synovectomy may reduce the postoperative complication rate.[435,436] Chemical synovectomy, using radioisotopes such as colloid ^{198}Au,[437] ^{90}Y,[438] and ^{32}P,[439] has also been reported to be valuable. In chronic hemophilia, physiotherapy for the arthritis is of major importance.

Prophylaxis. Prophylaxis has been applied in cases of severe hemophilia since the 1960s.[440] The principle involves prevention of the development of heavy bleeding in patients with severe hemophilia by raising the concentration of factor IX in plasma to a level (about 0.04 U/ml) at which spontaneous joint bleeding is rare. This approach was based on earlier observations where substantially less severe musculoskeletal complications were noted in patients with moderate or mild hemophilia. The prophylactic treatment generally consists of regular doses of factor IX concentrate (25 to 30 U/kg) administered twice per week. Such treatment has decreased the chronic musculoskeletal complications substantially. Similar long-term results are reported in patients treated only at times of bleeding.[441] The most important point is an increase in the frequency of treatment, whether given regularly without regard to ongoing bleeding or immediately when symptoms are first noted.[442,443]

Home treatment of hemophilia is now widely accepted. The patients receive greater personal freedom, and the delay in receiving treatment is reduced. Also, financial costs are lowered.[444]

Factor IX Concentrates. Factor IX is largely stable and retains about 80 percent of its activity in plasma stored at 4°C for up to 3 months. Plasma therefore can be used in replacement therapy of mild hemophilia B, but this method does not permit normalization of the plasma level of factor IX in patients with severe hemophilia B.

Crude concentrates of factor IX are prepared by absorption of the vitamin K-dependent coagulation factors (prothrombin and factors VII, IX, and X) on tricalcium phosphate,[445] DEAE-cellulose,[446] or DEAE-Sephadex.[447] The absorbed vitamin K-dependent factors are eluted with phosphate or citrate buffers and the final product is lyophilized. Such concentrates contain approximately equal amounts of prothrombin, factor IX, and factor X. The content of factor VII varies substantially in different preparations. The clinical experience of such factor IX concentrates is documented.[428]

Recombinant factor IX. Factor IX presents unique challenges to recombinant technology because it undergoes extensive posttranslational modification prior to circulating in the blood as a mature proenzyme. The ability to treat patients with recombinant factor IX on a commercial scale has the potential to alleviate the complications of viral transmission and thrombogenicity associated with currently available concentrates of plasma-derived factor IX. A variety of mammalian cell types have been transfected with factor IX cDNA, but secretion of mature, functional factor IX protein is limited by the γ-carboxylation and propeptide processing activities of the transfected cells.[500,501] The recent identification of cDNAs coding for intracellular enzymes capable of γ-carboxylation[79] and propeptide processing,[92] however, facilitated the development of commercially produced recombinant factor IX. Genetics Institute (Cambridge/Andover, MA) currently produces recombinant human factor IX under the trade name Benefix. The full-length cDNA for human factor IX is coexpressed at high levels with the cDNA for the processing protease furin in dihydrofolate-reductase-negative Chinese Hamster Ovary (CHO) cells.[449,452] Recombinant factor IX has procoagulant function indistinguishable from plasma-derived factor IX and has been extensively investigated with respect to posttranslational modifications and clinical characteristics.[450,451] The advantages of recombinant factor IX over that purified from plasma appear to be twofold: The risk of viral transmission is virtually eliminated[453] and the risk of iatrogenic thrombosis is drastically reduced.[450,451] Of particular concern in the clinical setting is the potential for the generation of factor IX inhibitors induced by exposure to the recombinant protein, because recombinant factor IX has slightly different biochemical properties.[454] To date, there are no reports of positive identification of recombinant factor IX-induced antibodies or inhibitors.[450,451] These data suggest that recombinant factor IX is a safe and effective alternative to the traditional plasma-derived preparations.

Side Effects of Factor IX Concentrates

Thrombosis. Venous and arterial thrombotic complications, as well as disseminated intravasculer coagulation (DIC), have been described following the administration of crude concentrates of factor IX.[448,455] The thrombogenic potential varies between different preparations[456] and has been ascribed to either contamination of the concentrates by activated coagulation factors (e.g., factors VIIa, IXa, and Xa),[457,458] the administration of large quantities of the nonactivated vitamin K-dependent factors,[459] and/or by the presence of platelet-derived phospholipids.[460] Patients who are most likely to develop thromboembolic complications or DIC are those with concomitant liver disease and those receiving large doses of factor IX concentrate for support during surgery or as treatment for a factor VIII inhibitor.

Recently, several more highly purified factor IX concentrates were developed.[461–463] These products undergo additional purification steps during the manufacturing process, such as pseudoaffinity chromatography on sulfated proteoglycans (e.g., heparin-sepharose), or monoclonal antibody affinity chromatography. Thus, these newer factor IX concentrates are virtually free of the other, contaminating, vitamin K-dependent clotting factors. Preliminary in vivo studies of these more highly purified concentrates indicate reduced thrombogenicity but similar efficacy compared to the older, cruder concentrates.[464–469] Some of these newer, highly purified factor IX concentrates were recently made available for clinical use, and should ultimately replace the cruder concentrates for treatment of hemophilia B.

Viral Transmission. Concentrates of factor IX are prepared from plasma pooled from several thousand donors. The risk of transmitting blood-borne viral diseases such as hepatitis and AIDS via pooled plasma products, increases substantially with the number of plasma donors involved. In the early to mid-1980s, HIV infection was recognized as one of the most serious hazards of blood transfusion, particularly in recipients of coagulation factor concentrates. Compared to hemophilia A, the HIV seropositivity rate for hemophilia B has been somewhat lower (76 percent vs. 42 percent for severely affected patients).[470] More recently, the introduction of several safety measures has nearly eliminated HIV from currently available blood products. Because the HIV virus is heat labile and is surrounded by a lipid envelope, the introduction of viral inactivation methods such as heat treatment and solvent/detergent treatment successfully eliminated HIV from commercial clotting factor concentrates. Furthermore, screening plasma donors for HIV antibody has nearly eliminated infectious individuals from the donor pool.

The transmission of hepatitis viruses is currently the most significant risk associated with the use of plasma products. Although the current risk of hepatitis B infection is negligible due to the introduction of donor screening assays in the late 1970s and the development of a hepatitis vaccine in the mid-1980s, the risk of transmission of hepatitis C virus (formerly non A-non B hepatitis) remains. The recent isolation of the hepatitis C virus[471] led to the development of a specific immunoassay using recombinant viral antigens.[472] Retrospective serologic studies indicate a prevalence of hepatitis C infection of approximately 70 percent for both hemophilia A and B,[461] although the actual prevalence is even higher when more sensitive assays are used.[473,474] Furthermore, a significant percentage of hemophiliacs infected with hepatitis C virus (HCV) develop chronic progressive liver disease, including cirrhosis.[475,476] Screening blood and plasma donors for anti-HCV should reduce the frequency of hepatitis C transmission via blood products.[477] In addition, several procedures were developed to inactivate viruses present in clotting factor concentrates. These procedures include (a) heat treatment either in the dry state, in solution (i.e., pasteurization), or in the presence of steam or an organic solvent, or (b) combined treatment with an organic solvent together with a detergent to destroy the viral envelope. The most effective methods for inactivation of HCV appear to be dry heat treatment at 80°C for 72 h,[478,479] pasteurization,[480] and solvent/detergent treatment.[481] Dry heat treatment using lower temperatures (60°C) and shorter durations (less than 24 h) and heat treatment in the presence of an organic solvent are less effective.[482,483] The crude factor IX concentrates that are currently available have been heated either in the dry state or in the presence of *n*-Heptane. Most of the newer, more highly purified factor IX concentrates, however, are treated by the solvent/detergent method.

Chronic liver disease secondary to hepatitis C infection is a serious complication of factor IX replacement therapy. Preliminary studies indicate that interferon may be useful in the treatment of hemophiliacs with chronic liver disease.[484,485] Additionally, liver transplantation has been successful in a few selected patients;[486] an additional salutary effect of this procedure is the cure of the patient's hemophilia.

Recently, symptomatic infection with parvovirus B19 has been reported in patients with hemophilia.[487–490] This virus is resistant to current virucidal procedures because it lacks a lipid envelope, and high temperature treatment of lyophilized concentrates contain transmissible parvovirus.[491]

Factor IX Inhibitors. Antibodies against factor IX develop in about 10 percent of patients with severe hemophilia B. In these cases, infused factor IX is rapidly neutralized and does not induce hemostasis until the patient's total amount of antifactor IX is neutralized. Furthermore, an anamnestic response follows administration of any product that contains factor IX. Those hemophilia patients with a substantial anamnestic response following infusion of factor IX are called "high responders."In other patients, the stimulating effect on the antibody formation is not as striking. These patients are called "low responders."Most patients with inhibitors are high responders and develop the antibody at an early age.

Management of patients with factor IX inhibitors includes treatment of acute bleeding episodes as well as attempts to induce tolerance. An acute bleeding episode can be managed by administering factor IX concentrate in amounts high enough to neutralize the inhibitor and also to give a hemostatic effect. This is possible, provided the antibody titer is not too high in relation to the activity of factor IX in the available concentrates. Concomitantly, immunosuppressive treatment can be given to diminish the anamnestic response. Such treatment has been used successfully in a substantial number of patients.[492] In patients with extremely high antibody titers, the inhibitor can be removed by extracorporeal adsorption on protein A-Sepharose[493,494] or by specific immunoadsorption[495] before the administration of factor IX. Recently, recombinant factor VIIa was successfully used to control bleeding in a factor IX-deficient patient with inhibitor.[496]

It has been claimed that tolerance in patients with hemophilia A will develop after long-term administration of high amounts of coagulation factor concentrates. Repeated treatments using the combination of high amounts of factor IX and cyclophosphamide in hemophilia B patients seemed to result in a similar conversion of high responders to low responders.[497] One hemophilia B patient became a low responder after two instances of treatment, including extracorporeal adsorption of his antifactor IX:C on protein A-Sepharose followed by the administration of factor IX, cyclophosphamide, and intravenous IgG.[498] This led to the Malmo treatment protocol comprised of factor IX, cyclophosphamide, and intravenous IgG, that has been successful in inducing immune tolerance in several hemophilia B inhibitor patients.[499]

Future Directions

A "curative"approach to the treatment of inherited metabolic disorders such as hemophilia is the concept of gene transfer therapy.[502] Gene transfer involves the transfection of a target cell with a retroviral vector containing a promoter element, the cDNA for the missing protein, and a selectivity marker. The cells containing the missing cDNA are grown in culture and then transplanted into the deficient host, where, ideally, the missing protein is now able to circulate. This approach has been approved for clinical trials in patients with adenosine deaminase deficiency. In the area of hemophilia, preclinical research has progressed more rapidly for hemophilia B than for hemophilia A[503–505] because the factor IX cDNA and protein are significantly smaller than those of factor VIII. In addition, because of its extravascular distribution, factor IX should not require direct intravascular secretion to achieve adequate circulating levels. Several gene delivery systems have been used to express the factor IX gene in a variety of cell types in vitro and in vivo. These delivery systems include viral vectors derived from retroviruses, adenoviruses, and herpes simplex viruses, as well as nonviral vehicles such as naked DNA, DNA/protein complexes, and liposome-encapsulated DNA.[505] Thus far, several mammalian target cell types (skin fibroblasts,[514] hepatocytes,[506] endothelial cells,[507] keratinocytes,[508] hematopoietic cells,[509] and myoblasts[515]) have been transfected with a variety of retroviral vectors containing human factor IX cDNA. One of the first successful preclinical studies of gene transfer for hemophilia B was accomplished by infusion of an amphotrophic retroviral vector encoding canine factor IX cDNA into the Chapel Hill inbred strain of hemophilia B dogs after partial hepatectomy.[506] In this model, plasma factor IX concentration increased from undetectable amounts to between 1 and 10 ng/ml (about 0.1 percent of normal).[510] Accordingly, the whole-blood clotting time in these animals was decreased from a pretreatment time of 45 to 55 min to 15 to 25 min after viral infusion, and remained at these reduced levels for 11 months. Recently, adeno-associated virus vectors have been used to deliver factor IX cDNA to mouse and dog models with encouraging results.[511–513] Adeno-associated virus vectors contain no viral genes and so do not cause a reactive immune response directed against viral gene products, a phenomenon that results in toxicity and limited gene expression.[511] Additionally, adeno-associated virus vectors, in contrast to adenovirus vectors, have the ability to transduce nondividing cells.[512,513] Investigation into gene therapy for the treatment of hemophilia B is ongoing.

FACTOR X

Factor X ($M_r = 59{,}000$) participates in the middle stage of blood coagulation[122] where it is converted to factor Xa in the intrinsic pathway by the "tenase" complex (factor IXa in the presence of factor VIIIa, phospholipid, and calcium ions) or in the extrinsic pathway by factor VIIa in the presence of tissue factor and calcium ions (Fig. 169-1). Human factor X is a glycoprotein that circulates in blood as a two-chain molecule.[319,516] It contains a light chain ($M_r = 16{,}900$) and a heavy chain ($M_r = 42{,}100$), and these two chains are held together by a disulfide bond. The light chain contains 11 residues of γ-carboxyglutamic acid and two growth factor domains[15–17] (Fig. 169-11). It also contains β-hydroxyaspartic acid at position 63 in the first epidermal growth factor domain.[95–97] Calcium binding occurs through both the Gla and first growth factor domains, and the former is responsible for factor X interaction with membrane surfaces.[40,43,47,61] The total length of the light chain is 139 residues, whereas the heavy chain is composed of 306 residues. The heavy chain also includes the catalytic domain and the active site serine. Human factor X contains 15 percent carbohydrate that includes N-linked chains attached to Asn39 and Asn49 in the activation peptide.

The activation of human factor X by factor IXa results from the cleavage of an Arg52-Ile bond in the N-terminal end of the heavy chain[516] (Fig. 169-11). This releases an activation peptide of 52 amino acids and generates factor Xa, a serine protease. The V_{max} for the activation reaction is accelerated approximately 200,000-fold by the addition of factor VIIIa, while the phospholipid decreases the K_m of the reaction about 3000-fold.[517] The participation of factor VIII as a cofactor in the reaction requires its prior activation by thrombin or factor Xa.[125–128] Present evidence suggests that factor VIIIa forms a complex with the enzyme factor IXa in the presence of phospholipid and calcium ions, and that this complex functions as the activator of factor X.[148,518] This is analogous to the complex formed by factor Xa, factor Va, phospholipid, and calcium ions that carries out the activation of prothrombin. The activation of factor X by factor IXa/factor VIIIa can occur on the membrane surface of platelets,[518] endothelial cells,[156] or monocytes.[519]

Factor X Gene

The gene for human factor X is located on chromosome 13 in the region of q34-qter.[261–263] It contains approximately 25 kb of DNA and includes 7 introns and 8 exons (GenBank M22613).[17] The seven introns in the gene for factor X interrupt the coding sequence at essentially identical locations in the amino acid sequence as do the introns in the genes for human factor VII, factor IX, and protein C.

Recent analysis of the 5′ flanking sequence of the gene for factor X has resulted in the identification of (a) a region upstream of the initiation Met codon 20 bp in length which contains multiple transcription initiation sites;[520] and (b) a region spanning nucleotides (−)457 to (−)1 that contains three distinct elements involved in the regulation of factor X.[521] The first of these, a tissue-specific promoter in the region (−)63 to (−)42 (factor X promoter 1; FXP1), is essential for liver-specific transcription and is homologous to the known liver-specific transcription factor recognition sequences for LF-A1 or HNF-4. An apparent CCAAT-like sequence, present at (−)120 to (−)116 bp, is required for full promoter activity and binds the ubiquitous transcription factor NF-Y.[272] Two additional regulatory sequences encompassing nucleotides (−)215 to (−)149 (FXP2) and (−)457 to (−)351 (FXP3) are also present. Like FXP1, FXP3 is liver-specific, whereas FXP2 is homologous to an SP-1 binding site.

Several polymorphisms have been identified in the gene for factor X. A *Taq*I site with a frequency of 20 percent and less-prevalent *Eco*RI, *Hin*dIII, and *Pst*I RFLPs (frequencies of less common alleles = 5 to 10 percent) have been identified by Southern blotting.[522–524] In addition, a highly polymorphic extragenic *Pvu*II site is present approximately 3 kb downstream of exon VIII.[524] Recently, PCR detected a *Nla*IV polymorphism in exon VII that is due to a C/T dimorphism at codon 817. This polymorphism is silent at the amino acid level and has a frequency of about 25 percent in Caucasians and 50 percent in African-Americans.[525] Because the genes for factor VII and factor X are separated by only 2.8 kb on chromosome 13,[521] these factor X polymorphisms may be useful in studies of families with either congenital factor X or factor VII deficiency.

Factor X Deficiency

In 1955, Duckert and coworkers reported the presence of a serum factor, called factor X, that was depressed by coumarin anticoagulants.[526] Inherited deficiencies were identified shortly thereafter, and the plasma protein was called Prower factor[527] and Stuart factor[528] after the families affected by this disorder. Thus far, more than 50 families have been reported with factor X deficiency. The complete deficiency is inherited as an autosomal recessive disorder, although a subtle bleeding tendency occurs in heterozygotes.[529,530] Clinically, severe factor X deficiency can mimic severe hemophilia A or B, but chronic arthropathy is usually not as prominent. Patients whose levels of factor X clotting activity (factor X:C) are above 15 percent of normal exhibit abnormal bleeding episodes only in connection with major surgery or trauma.

Factor X deficiency is a heterogeneous disorder at both the phenotypic and genotypic levels. The original Stuart plasma demonstrates equally reduced factor X:C levels using PT, APTT, or RVV-based clotting assays. Other variants of factor X, on the other hand, demonstrate different levels of factor X:C, depending on whether factor X activation occurs via the extrinsic system, the intrinsic system, or RVV.[531,532] For example, factor X_{PADUA}[533] and factor $X_{VORARLBERG}$[534] show lower clotting activity as determined by extrinsic activation, whereas factor $X_{MELBOURNE}$[538] and factor X_{ROMA}[539] demonstrate selectively reduced intrinsic activation. Measurement of factor X antigen indicates further heterogeneity as levels may be normal (CRM^+), absent (CRM^-), or reduced (CRM^R).[531]

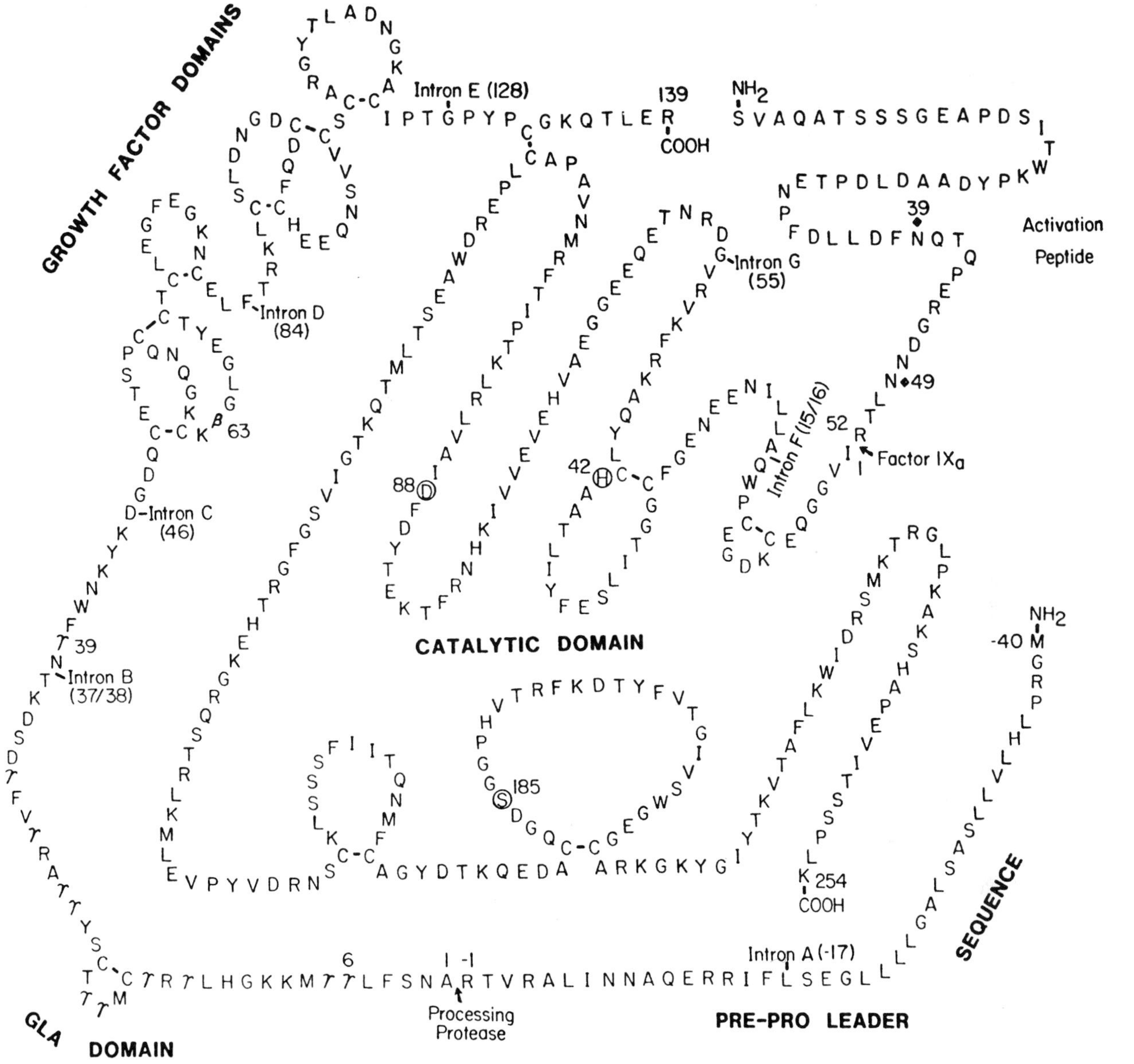

Fig. 169-11 Amino acid sequence and tentative structure of human prepro factor X. The locations of the seven introns (A to G) are shown in the various regions of the protein. The prepro leader sequence (−40 to −1) is cleaved during protein biosynthesis to give rise to the mature protein with an amino-terminal sequence of A-N-S-F- for the light chain. The Arg-Lys-Arg tripeptide that connects the light and heavy chains during the activation reaction is shown with a small arrow. The three amino acids in the catalytic domain (H42, D88, and S185) that participate in catalysis are circled, while the two potential carbohydrate attachment sites in the activation peptide are shown with solid diamonds. The amino acids are numbered as follows, starting with the N-terminal end of the protein: −40 to −1 = prepro leaer sequence; +1 to 139 = light chain; 1 to 52 = activation peptide; 1 to 254 = catalytic chain. The single-letter code for amino acids is shown in the legend to Fig. 169-5. β = β-hydroxyaspartic acid. (*From Leytus et al.*[7] *Used with permission.*)

Several abnormal variants of factor X have been characterized at the molecular level; these range from gross gene deletions to single base substitutions. A patient with severe CRM$^-$ factor X deficiency was found to be heterozygous for two different deletions: a complete gene deletion for which the mother demonstrated germ line mosaicism, and a partial gene deletion of paternal origin, which included exons VII and VIII.[540] A partial deletion encompassing exon VII and the 5′ portion of exon VIII was described in another patient with severe factor X deficiency, who is presumably a compound heterozygote for an as yet unidentified second mutation.[541] Recently, a 3-bp deletion within the polypyrimidine tract of intron D was reported.[542] This deletion is located within an acceptor splicing site where U2 snRNP binds to form spliceosomes, resulting in abnormal splicing and decreased factor X production.

Several point mutations have been identified in patients with factor X deficiency and most of these are transitions within CG dinucleotides. Factor $X_{\text{SANTO DOMINGO}}$ is characterized by a severe CRM$^-$ bleeding disorder due to a homozygous mutation of G to A in exon I. This mutation causes the substitution of Gly with Arg at residue −20 within the signal peptide and prevents factor X secretion from the liver, presumably by disrupting signal peptidase cleavage of the leader sequence.[70] The molecular defect in the original Stuart pedigree[528] is a homozygous mutation of G to A that results in the substitution of Val104 with Met and also appears to impair secretion of the mutant factor X protein from the hepatocyte.[543] Factor $X_{\text{VORARLBERG}}$ is associated with a clinically mild bleeding tendency, preferentially affecting extrinsic factor X activation. This disorder is characterized by diminished calcium affinity caused by a mutation in exon II of Gla_{14} (GAA) to Lys

(AAA).[534] A second transition of G to A in exon V, which changes Glu102 to Lys, was detected in this pedigree, but does not correlate with the factor $X_{VORARLBERG}$ phenotype. Factor $X_{FRANKFURT}$ is caused by Gla25 to Lys[535] and is associated with a mild decrease in both factor X activity and antigen in the heterozygous state. Two other mildly affected variants have been preliminarily described: factor X_{OCKERO} is due to a homozygous mutation of Gly114 to Arg within the second growth factor domain,[544] while an individual with factor $X_{WENATCHEE}$ is heterozygous for a substitution of Arg142 with Cys at the site that is normally cleaved intracellularly to form two-chain factor X.[545] This mutation is analogous to the a activation site mutations in factor $IX_{CHAPEL\ HILL}$ and prothrombins $_{BARCELONA}$ and $_{MADRID}$. Factor $X_{NAGOYA\ 1}$ results in CRM^- deficiency in the homozygous state[536] and is characterized by substitution of Arg306 by Cys in the catalytic domain. Factor $X_{MARSEILLES}$ (Ser334 to Pro)[537] is a CRM^+ variant that results in normal circulating factor X antigen levels with about 20 percent activity when factor $Xa_{MARSEILLES}$ is activated by either the intrinsic, extrinsic or RVV pathways. Factor X_{FRIULI} is a variant found in northern Italian individuals and is characterized by a moderate bleeding tendency in homozygotes with approximately 5 percent factor X:C levels as measured by PT and APTT, although RVV clotting times and factor X:Ag levels remain normal.[531,546,547] The mutation responsible for factor X_{FRIULI} is a substitution of Pro343 (CCC) with Ser (TCC) in a conserved region of the catalytic domain.[548] Factor $X_{SAN\ ANTONIO}$ is a mild CRM^R variant characterized by compound heterozygosity for two mutations in the catalytic domain. The first of these mutations is a single nucleotide deletion at codon 272 in exon VII, which results in the premature termination of translation. The second mutation is a transition of C for T at codon 366 in exon VIII, which results in the substitution of Arg with Cys.[549]

An acquired deficiency of factor X associated with amyloidosis has also been described.[550] Bleeding manifestations in this disorder most commonly involve the skin and gastrointestinal tract.[553] Nine of the ten of these patients described by Fair and Edgington had factor X antigen levels ranging from 15 to 73 percent of normal, while the factor X activity was consistently below normal.[531] Idiopathic, autoantibody acquired factor X deficiency has also been reported,[552] which has been successfully treated with a combination of plasmapheresis, intravenous immunoglobulin, and steroid therapy.[551]

Bleeding episodes in patients with congenital factor X deficiency are generally treated with plasma transfusions to maintain plasma factor X levels above 15 to 20 percent.[554] For major bleeding associated with trauma or surgery, crude factor IX concentrates can be used, because these products contain approximately one unit of factor X per unit of factor IX. More highly purified concentrates of factor X are not currently available, although recombinant factor X has been expressed in mammalian cells.[555]

REFERENCES

1. Stenflo J, Fernlund P, Egan W, Roepstorff P: Vitamin K dependent modifications of glutamic acid residues in prothrombin. *Proc Natl Acad Sci U S A* **71**:2730, 1974.
2. Nelsestuen GL, Zytkovicz TH, Howard JB: The mode of action of vitamin K isolation of a peptide containing the vitamin K-dependent portion of prothrombin. *J Biol Chem* **249**:6347, 1974.
3. Magnusson S, Sottrup-Jensen L, Petersen TE, Morris HR, Dell A: Primary structure of the vitamin K-dependent part of prothrombin. *FEBS Lett* **44**:189, 1974.
4. Esmon CT, Suttie JW, Jackson CM: The functional significance of vitamin K action: Differences in phospholipid binding between normal and abnormal prothrombin. *J Biol Chem* **250**:4095, 1975.
5. Soriano-Garcia M, Padmanabhan K, de Vos AM, Tulinsky A: The Ca^+ ion and membrane binding structure of the Gla domain of Ca-prothrombin fragment 1. *Biochemistry* **31**:2554, 1992.
6. Magnusson S, Petersen TE, Sottrup-Jensen L, Claeys H: Complete primary structure of prothrombin: Isolation, structure and reactivity of ten carboxylated glutamic acid residues and regulation of prothrombin activation by thrombin, in Reich E, Rifkin DB, Shaw E (eds): *Proteases and Biological Control*. Cold Spring Harbor, NY, Cold Spring Harbor Laboratory, 1975, p 123.
7. McMullen BA, Fujikawa K: Amino acid sequence of the heavy chain of human a-factor XIIa. *J Biol Chem* **260**:5328, 1985.
8. Sottrup-Jensen L, Claeys H, Zajdel M, Petersen TE, Magnusson S: The primary structure of human plasminogen: Isolation of two lysine-binding fragments and one "mini"-plasminogen (MW 38,000) by elastase-catalyzed-specific limited proteolysis, in Davidson JF, Rowan RM, Samama MM, Desnoyers PC (eds): *Progress in Chemical Fibrinolysis and Thrombolysis*. New York, Raven, 1978, Vol. 3, p 191.
9. Pennica D, Holmes WE, Kohr WJ, Harkins RN, Vehar GA, Ward CA, Bennett WF, Yelverton E, Seeburg PH, Heyneker HL, Goeddel DV: Cloning and expression of human tissue-type plasminogen activator cDNA in *E. coli*. *Nature* **301**:214, 1983.
10. Gunzler WA, Steffens GJ, Otting F, Kim S-MA, Frankus E, Flohe L: The primary structure of high molecular mass urokinase from human urine: The complete amino acid sequence of the A chain. *Hoppe Seylers Z Physiol Chem* **363**:1155, 1982.
11. Hagen FS, Gray CL, O'Hara P, Grant FJ, Saari GC, Woodbury RG, Hart CE, Insley M, Kisiel W, Kurachi K, Davie EW: Characterization of a cDNA coding for human factor VII. *Proc Natl Acad Sci U S A* **83**:2412, 1986.
12. Kurachi K, Davie EW: Isolation and characterization of a cDNA coding for human factor IX. *Proc Natl Acad Sci U S A* **79**:6461, 1982.
13. Yoshitake S, Schach BG, Foster DC, Davie EW, Kurachi K: Nucleotide sequence of the gene for human factor IX (antihemophilic factor B). *Biochemistry* **24**:3736, 1985.
14. Anson DS, Choo KH, Rees DJG, Giannelli F, Gould K, Huddleston JA, Brownlee GG: The gene structure of human anti-haemophilic factor IX. *EMBO J* **3**:1053, 1984.
15. Leytus SP, Chung DW, Kisiel W, Kurachi K, Davie EW: Characterization of a cDNA coding for human factor X. *Proc Natl Acad Sci U S A* **81**:3699, 1984.
16. Fung MR, Hay CS, MacGillivray RTA: Characterization of an almost full-length cDNA coding for human blood coagulation factor X. *Proc Natl Acad Sci U S A* **82**:3591, 1985.
17. Leytus SP, Foster DC, Kurachi K, Davie EW: Gene for human factor X, a blood coagulation factor whose gene organization is essentially identical to that of factor IX and protein C. *Biochemistry* **25**:5098, 1986.
18. Foster D, Davie EW: Characterization of a cDNA coding for human protein C. *Proc Natl Acad Sci U S A* **81**:4766, 1984.
19. Beckmann RJ, Schmidt RJ, Santerre RF, Plutzky J, Crabtree GR, Long GL: The structure and evolution of a 461 amino acid human protein C precursor and its messenger RNA, based upon the DNA sequence of cloned human liver cDNAs. *Nucleic Acid Res* **13**:5233, 1985.
20. Gray A, Dull TJ, Ullrich A: Nucleotide sequence of epidermal growth factor cDNA predicts a 128,000-molecular weight protein precursor. *Nature* **303**:722, 1983.
21. Doolittle RF, Feng DF, Johnson MS: Computer-based characterization of epidermal growth factor precursor. *Nature* **307**:558, 1984.
22. Carpenter G, Zendegui JG: Epidermal growth factor, its receptor, and related proteins. *Exp Cell Res* **164**:1, 1986.
23. Lundwall A, Dackowski W, Cohen E, Shaffer M, Mahr A, Dahlback B, Stenflo J, Wydro R: Isolation and sequence of the cDNA for human protein S, a regulator of blood coagulation. *Proc Natl Acad Sci U S A* **83**:6716, 1986.
24. Hoskins J, Norman DK, Beckmann RJ, Long GL: Cloning and characterization of human liver cDNA encoding a protein S precursor. *Proc Natl Acad Sci U S A* **84**:349, 1987.
25. Appella E, Weber IT, Blasi F: Structure and function of epidermal growth factor-like regions in proteins. *FEBS Lett* **231**:1, 1988.
26. Stenflo J: Structure-function relationships of epidermal growth factor modules in vitamin K-dependent clotting factors. *Blood* **78**:1637, 1991.
27. Cooke RM, Wilkinson AJ, Baron M, Pastore A, Tappin MJ, Campbell ID, Gregory H, Sheard B: The solution structure of human epidermal growth factor. *Nature* **327**:339, 1987.
28. Campbell ID, Cooke RM, Baron M, Harvey TS, Tappin MJ: The solution structures of epidermal growth factor and transforming growth factor alpha. *Prog Growth Factor Res* **1**:13, 1989.
29. Montelione GT, Wuthrich K, Nice EC, Burgess AW, Scheraga HA: Solution structure of murine epidermal growth factor: Determination of the polypeptide backbone chain-fold by nuclear magnetic resonance and distance geometry. *Proc Natl Acad Sci U S A* **84**:5226, 1987.

30. Mayo KH, Cavalli RC, Peters AR, Boelens R, Kaptein R: Sequence-specific ^{1}H-NMR assignments and peptide backbone conformation in rat epidermal growth factor. *Biochem J* **257**:197, 1989.
31. Montelione GT, Winkler ME, Burton LE, Rinderknecht E, Sporn MB, Wagner G: Sequence-specific ^{1}H-NMR assignments and identification of two small antiparallel β-sheets in the solution structure of recombinant human transforming growth factor a. *Proc Natl Acad Sci U S A* 86:1519, 1989.
32. Kohda D, Shimada I, Miyake T, Fuwa T, Inagaki F: Polypeptide chain fold of human transforming growth factor a analogous to those of mouse and human epidermal growth factors as studied by two-dimensional ^{1}H NMR. *Biochemistry* **28**:953, 1989.
33. Kline TP, Brown FK, Brown SC, Jeffs PW, Kopple KD, Mueller L: Solution structures of human transforming growth factor a derived from ^{1}H-NMR data. *Biochemistry* **29**:7805, 1990.
34. Huang LH, Cheng H, Pardi A, Tam JP, Sweeney WV: Sequence-specific ^{1}H-NMR assignments, secondary structure, and location of the calcium binding site in the first epidermal growth factor like domain of blood coagulation factor IX. *Biochemistry* **30**:7402, 1991.
35. Baron M, Norman DG, Harvey TS, Handford PA, Mayhew M, Tse AGD, Brownlee GG, Campbell ID: The three-dimensional structure of the first EGF-like module of human factor IX: Comparison with EGF and TGF-α. *Protein Sci* **1**:81, 1992.
36. Selander M, Persson E, Stenflo J, Drakenberg T: ^{1}H-NMR assignment and secondary structure of the Ca^{2+}-free form of the amino-terminal epidermal growth factor-like domain in coagulation factor X. *Biochemistry* **29**:8111, 1990.
37. Ullner M, Selander M, Persson E, Stenflo J, Drakenberg T, Teleman O: Three-dimensional structure of the Apo form of the N-terminal EGF-like module of blood coagulation factor X as determined by NMR spectroscopy and simulated folding. *Biochemistry* **31**:5974, 1992.
38. Esmon NL, DeBault LE, Esmon CT: Proteolytic formation and properties of γ-carboxyglutamic acid-domainless protein C. *J Biol Chem* **258**:5548, 1983.
39. Morita T, Isaacs BS, Esmon CT, Johnson AE: Derivatives of blood coagulation factor IX contain a high affinity Ca^{2+}-binding site that lacks γ-carboxyglutamic acid. *J Biol Chem* **259**:5698, 1984.
40. Sugo T, Bjork I, Holmgren A, Stenflo J: Calcium-binding properties of bovine factor X lacking the γ-carboxyglutamic acid-containing region. *J Biol Chem* **259**:5705, 1984.
41. Sugo T, Dahlback B, Holmgren A, Stenflo J: Calcium binding of bovine protein S: Effect of thrombin cleavage and removal of the γ-carboxyglutamic acid-containing region. *J Biol Chem* **261**:5116, 1986.
42. Handford PA, Baron M, Mayhew M, Willis A, Beesley T, Brownlee GG, Campbell ID: The first EGF-like domain from human factor IX contains a high-affinity calcium binding site. *EMBO J* **9**:475, 1990.
43. Persson E, Selander M, Linse S, Drakenberg T, Ohlin A-K, Stenflo J: Calcium binding to the isolated β-hydroxyaspartic acid-containing epidermal growth factor-like domain of bovine factor X. *J Biol Chem* **264**:16897, 1989.
44. Ohlin A-K, Linse S, Stenflo J: Calcium binding to the epidermal growth factor homology region of bovine protein C. *J Biol Chem* **263**:7411, 1988.
45. Dahlback B, Hildebrand B, Linse S: Novel type of very high affinity calcium-binding sites in β-hydroxyasparagine-containing epidermal growth factor-like domains in vitamin K-dependent protein S. *J Biol Chem* **265**:18481, 1990.
46. Handford PA, Mayhew M, Baron M, Winship PR, Campbell ID, Brownlee GG: Key residues invovlved in calcium-binding motifs in EGF-like domains. *Nature* **351**:164, 1991.
47. Selander-Sunnerhagen M, Ullner M, Persson E, Teleman O, Stenflo J, Drakenberg T: How an epidermal growth factor (EGF)-like domain binds calcium: High resolution NMR structure of the calcium form of the NH_2-terminal EGF-like domain in coagulation factor X. *J Biol Chem* **267**:19642, 1992.
48. Sakai T, Lund-Hansen T, Thim L, Kisiel W: The γ-carboxyglutamic acid domain of human factor VIIa is essential for its interaction with cell surface tissue factor. *J Biol Chem* **265**:1890, 1990.
49. Ruf W, Kalnik MW, Lund-Hansen T, Edgington TS: Characterization of factor VII association with tissue factor in solution: High- and low-affinity calcium-binding sites in factor VII contribute to functionally distinct interactions. *J Biol Chem* **266**:15719, 1991.
50. Toomey JR, Smith KJ, Stafford DW: Localization of the human tissue factor recognition determinant of human factor VIIa. *J Biol Chem* **266**:19198, 1991.
51. Clarke BJ, Ofosu FA, Sridhara S, Bona RD, Rickles FR, Blajchman MA: The first epidermal growth factor domain of human coagulation factor VII is essential for binding with tissue factor. *FEBS Lett* **298**:206, 1992.
52. Wildgoose P, Jorgensen T, Komiyama Y, Nakagaki T, Pedersen A, Kisiel W: The role of phospholipids and the factor VII Gla-domain in the interaction of factor VII with tissue factor. *Thromb Haemost* **67**:679, 1992.
53. Ryan J, Wolitzky B, Heimer E, Lambrose T, Felix A, Tam JP, Huang LH, Nawroth P, Wilner G, Kisiel W, Nelsestuen GL, Stern DM: Structural determinants of the factor IX molecule mediating interaction with the endothelial cell binding site are distinct from those involved in phospholipid binding. *J Biol Chem* **264**:20283, 1989.
54. Astermark J, Stenflo J: The epidermal growth factor-like domains of factor IX: Effect on blood clotting and endothelial cell binding of a fragment containing the epidermal growth factor-like domains linked to the γ-carboxyglutamic acid region. *J Biol Chem* **266**:2438, 1991.
55. Rees DJG, Jones IM, Handford PA, Walter SJ, Esnouf MP, Smith KJ, Brownlee GG: The role of β-hydroxyaspartate and adjacent carboxylate residues in the first EGF domain of human factor IX. *EMBO J* **7**:2053, 1988.
56. Lin S-W, Smith KJ, Welsch D, Stafford DW: Expression and characterization of human factor IX and factor IX-factor X chimeras in mouse C127 cells. *J Biol Chem* **265**:144, 1990.
57. Astermark J, Hogg PJ, Bjork I, Stenflo J: Effects of γ-carboxyglutamic acid and epidermal growth factor-like modules of factor IX on factor X activation: Studies using proteolytic fragments of bovine factor IX. *J Biol Chem* **267**:3249, 1992.
58. Cheung W-F, Hamaguchi N, Smith KJ, Stafford D: The binding of human factor IX to endothelial cells is mediated by residues 3-11. *J Biol Chem* **267**:20529, 1992.
59. Toomey JR, Smith KJ, Roberts HR, Stafford DW: The endothelial cell binding determinant of human factor IX resides in the γ-carboxyglutamic acid domain. *Biochemistry* **31**:1806, 1992.
60. Rawala-Sheikh R, Ahmad SS, Monroe DM, Roberts HR, Walsh PN: Role of γ-carboxyglutamic acid residues in the binding of factor IXa to platelets and in factor-X activation. *Blood* **79**:398, 1992.
61. Persson E, Valcarce C, Stenflo J: The γ-carboxyglutamic acid and epidermal growth factor-like domains of factor X: Effect of isolated domains on prothrombin activation and endothelial cell binding of factor X. *J Biol Chem* **266**:2453, 1992.
62. Hertzberg MS, Ben-Tal O, Furie B, Furie BC: Construction, expression, and characterization of a chimera of factor IX and factor X: The role of the second epidermal growth factor domain and serine protease domain in factor Va binding. *J Biol Chem* **267**:14759, 1992.
63. Hogg PJ, Ohlin A-K, Stenflo J: Identification of structural domains in protein C involved in its interaction with thrombin-thrombomodulin on the surface of endothelial cells. *J Biol Chem* **267**:703, 1992.
64. Olsen PH, Esmon NL, Esmon CT, Laue TM: Ca^{2+} dependence of the interactions between protein C, thrombin, and the elastase fragment of thrombomodulin. Analysis by ultracentrifugation. *Biochemistry* **31**:746, 1992.
65. Sunnerhagen M, Olah GA, Stenflo J, Fors'en S, Drakenberg T, Trewhella J: The relative orientation of Gla and EGF domains in coagulation factor X is altered by Ca^{2+} binding to the first EGF domain. A combined NMR-small-angle x-ray scattering study. *Biochemistry* **35**:11547, 1996.
66. Furie B, Bing DH, Feldmann RJ, Robison DJ, Burnier JP, Furie BC: Computer-generated models of blood coagulation factor Xa, factor IXa, and thrombin based upon structural homology with other serine proteases. *J Biol Chem* **257**:3875, 1982.
67. Bode W, Mayr I, Baumann U, Huber R, Stone SR, Hofsteenge J: The refined 1.9 Å crystal structure of human α-thrombin: Interaction with D-Phe-Pro-Arg chloromethylketone and significance of the Tyr-Pro-Pro-Trp insertion segment. *EMBO J* **8**:3467, 1989.
68. Degen SJF, Davie EW: Nucleotide sequence of the gene for human prothrombin. *Biochemistry* **26**:6165, 1987.
69. Jorgensen MJ, Cantor AB, Furie BC, Brown CL, Shoemaker CB, Furie B: Recognition site directing vitamin K-dependent γ-carboxylation residues on the propeptide of factor IX. *Cell* **48**:185, 1987.
70. Watzke HH, Wallmark A, Hamaguchi N, Giardina P, Stafford DW, High KA: Factor $X_{\text{Santo Domingo}}$: Evidence that the severe clinical phenotype arises from a mutation blocking secretion. *J Clin Invest* **88**:1685, 1991.
71. Foster DC, Rudinski MS, Schach BG, Berkner KL, Kumar AA, Hagen FS, Sprecher CA, Insley MY, Davie EW: Propeptide of human protein C is necessary for γ-carboxylation. *Biochemistry* **26**:7003, 1987.

72. Rabiet M-J, Jorgensen MJ, Furie B, Furie BC: Effect of propeptide mutations on post-translational processing of factor IX: Evidence that β-hydroxylation and γ-carboxylation are independent events. *J Biol Chem* **262**:14895, 1987.
73. Ulrich MMW, Furie B, Jacobs MR, Vermeer C, Furie BC: Vitamin K-dependent carboxylation: A synthetic peptide based upon the γ-carboxylation recognition site sequence of the prothrombin propeptide is an active substrate for the carboxylase in vitro. *J Biol Chem* **263**:9697, 1988.
74. Huber P, Schmitz T, Griffin J, Jacobs M, Walsh C, Furie B, Furie BC: Identification of amino acids in the γ-carboxylation recognition site on the propeptide of prothrombin. *J Biol Chem* **265**:12467, 1990.
75. Furie BC, Ratcliffe JV, Tward J, Jorgensen MJ, Blaszkowski LS, DiMichele J, Furie B: The γ-carboxylation recognition site is sufficient to direct vitamin K-dependent carboxylation on an adjacent glutamine-rich region of thrombin in a polypeptide-thrombin chimera. *J Biol Chem* **272**:28258, 1997
76. Stanton C, Taylor R, Wallin R: Processing of prothrombin in the secretory pathway. *Biochem J* **277**:59, 1991.
77. McClure DB, Walls JD, Grinnell BW: Post-translational processing events in the secretion pathway of human protein C, a complex vitamin K-dependent antithrombotic factor. *J Biol Chem* **267**:19710, 1992.
78. Bristol JA, Ratcliffe JV, Roth DA, Jacobs MA, Furie BC, Furie B: Biosynthesis of prothrombin: Intracellular localization of the vitamin K-dependent carboxylase and the sites of γ-carboxylation. *Blood* **88**:2585, 1996.
79. Wu S-M, Cheung W-F, Frazier D, Stafford DW: Cloning and expression of the cDNA for human γ-glutamyl carboxylase. *Science* **254**:1634, 1991.
80. Berkner KL, Harbeck M, Lingenfelter S, Bailey C, Sanders-Hinck CM, Suttie JW: Purification and identification of bovine liver γ-carboxylase. *Proc Natl Acad Sci U S A* **89**:6242, 1992.
81. Suttie JW: Vitamin K-dependent carboxylase. *Ann Rev Biochem* **54**:459, 1985.
82. Furie B, Furie BC: Molecular basis of vitamin K-dependent γ-carboxylation. *Blood* **75**:1753, 1990.
83. Friedman PA, Griep AE: In vitro inhibition of vitamin K-dependent carboxylation by tetrachloropyridinol and the imidazopyridines. *Biochemistry* **19**:3381, 1980.
84. Sugo T, Persson U, Stenflo J: Protein C in bovine plasma after warfarin treatment: Purification, partial characterization, and β-hydroxyaspartic acid content. *J Biol Chem* **260**:10453, 1985.
85. Bentley AK, Rees DJG, Rizza C, Brownlee GG: Defective propeptide processing of blood clotting factor IX caused by mutation of arginine to glutamine at position −4. *Cell* **45**:343, 1986.
86. Diuguid DL, Rabiet MJ, Furie BC, Liebman HA, Furie B: Molecular basis of hemophilia B: A defective enzyme due to an unprocessed propeptide is caused by a point mutation in the factor IX precursor. *Proc Natl Acad Sci U S A* **83**:5803, 1986.
87. Ware J, Diuguid DL, Liebman HA, Rabiet M-J, Kasper CK, Furie BC, Furie B, Stafford DW: Factor $IX_{San\ Dimas}$: Substitution of glutamine for Arg^{-4} in the propeptide leads to incomplete γ-carboxylation and altered phospholipid binding properties. *J Biol Chem* **264**:11401, 1989.
88. Kawabata S, Nakagama K, Muta T, Iwanaga S: Rabbit liver microsomal endopeptidase with substrate specificity for processing proproteins is structurally related to rat testes metalloendopeptidase. *J Biol Chem* **268**:12498, 1993.
89. Wasley LC, Rhemtulla A, Bristol JA, Kaufman RJ: PACE/Furin can process the vitamin K-dependent pro-factor precursor within the secretory pathway. *J Biol Chem* **268**:8458, 1993.
90. Sugimoto M, Miyata T, Kawabata S, Yoshioka A, Fukui H, Iwanaga S: Factor $IX_{Kawachinagano}$: Impaired function of the Gla-domain caused by attached propeptide region due to substitution of arginine by glutamine at position −4. *Br J Haematol* **72**:216, 1989.
91. Thompson AR, Schoof JM, Weinmann AF, Chen S-H: Factor IX mutations: Rapid, direct screening methods for 20 new families with hemophilia B. *Thromb Res* **65**:289, 1992.
92. Barr PJ: Mammalian subtilisins: The long-sought dibasic processing endoproteases. *Cell* **66**:1, 1991.
93. Kawabata S-i, Davie EW: A microsomal endopeptidase from liver with substrate specificity for processing proproteins such as the vitamin K-dependent proteins of plasma. *J Biol Chem* **267**:10331, 1992.
94. Drakenberg T, Fernlund P, Roepstorff P, Stenflo J: β-Hydroxyaspartic acid in vitamin K-dependent proteins. *Proc Natl Acad Sci U S A* **80**:1802, 1983.
95. McMullen BA, Fujikawa K, Kisiel W, Sasagawa T, Howald WN, Kwa EY, Weinstein B: Complete amino acid sequence of the light chain of human blood coagulation factor X: Evidence for identification of residue 63 as β-hydroxyaspartic acid. *Biochemistry* **22**:2875, 1983.
96. McMullen BA, Fujikawa K, Kisiel W: The occurrence of β-hydroxyaspartic acid in the vitamin K-dependent blood coagulation zymogens. *Biochem Biophys Res Commun* **115**:8 1983.
97. Fernlund P, Stenflo J: β-Hydroxyaspartic acid in vitamin K-dependent proteins. *J Biol Chem* **258**:12509, 1983.
98. Stenflo J, Lundwall A, Dahlback B: β-Hydroxyasparagine in domains homologous to the epidermal growth factor precursor in vitamin K-dependent protein S. *Proc Natl Acad Sci U S A* **84**:368, 1987.
99. Gronke RS, VanDusen WJ, Garsky VM, Jacobs JW, Sardana MK, Stern AM, Friedman PA: Aspartyl β-hydroxylase: In vitro hydroxylation of a synthetic peptide based on the structure of the first growth factor-like domain of human factor IX. *Proc Natl Acad Sci U S A* **86**:3609, 1989.
100. Stenflo J, Holme E, Lindstedt S, Chandramouli N, Tsai Huang LH, Tam JP, Merrifield RB: Hydroxylation of aspartic acid in domains homologous to the epidermal growth factor precursor is catalyzed by a 2-oxoglutarate-dependent dioxygenase. *Proc Natl Acad Sci U S A* **86**:444, 1989.
101. Jia S, VanDusen WJ, Diehl RE, Kohl NE, Dixon RAF, Elliston KO, Stern AM, Friedman PA: cDNA cloning and expression of bovine aspartyl (asparaginyl) β-hydroxylase. *J Biol Chem* **267**:14322, 1992.
102. Thim L, Bjoern S, Christensen M, Nicolaisen EM, Lund-Hansen T, Pedersen AH, Hedner U: Amino acid sequence and posttranslational modifications of human factor VIIa from plasma and transfected baby hamster kidney cells. *Biochemistry* **27**:7785, 1988.
103. Nelson RM, VanDusen WJ, Friedman PA, Long GL: β-Hydroxyaspartic acid and β-hydroxyasparagine residues in recombinant human protein S are not required for anticoagulant cofactor activity or for binding to C4b-binding protein. *J Biol Chem* **266**:20586, 1991.
104. Sunnerhagen MS, Persson E, Dahlqvist I, Drakenberg T, Stenflo J, Mayhew M, Robin M, Handford P, Tilley JW, Campbell ID, et al: The effect of apartate hydroxylation on calcium binding to epidermal growth factor-like modules in coagulation factors IX and X. *J Biol Chem* **268**:23339, 1993.
105. Grinnell BW, Walls JD, Gerlitz B: Glycosylation of human protein C affects its secretion, processing, functional activities, and activation by thrombin. *J Biol Chem* **266**:9778, 1991.
106. Sinha U, Wolf DL: Carbohydrate residues modulate the activation of coagulation factor X. *J Biol Chem* **268**:3048, 1993.
107. Hase S, Kawabata S-i, Nishimura H, Takeya H, Sueyoshi T, Miyata T, Iwanaga S, Takao T, Shimonishi Y, Ikenaka T: A new trisaccharide sugar chain linked to a serine residue in bovine blood coagulation factors VII and IX. *J Biochem* **104**:867, 1988.
108. Nishimura H, Kawabata S, Kisiel W, Hase S, Ikenaka T, Takao T, Shimonishi Y, Iwanaga S: Identification of a disaccharide (Xyl-Glc) and a trisaccharide (Xyl_2-Glc) *O*-glycosidically linked to a serine residue in the first epidermal growth factor-like domain of human factors VII and IX and protein Z and bovine protein Z. *J Biol Chem* **264**:20320, 1989.
109. Bjoern S, Foster DC, Thim L, Wiberg FC, Christensen M, Komiyama Y, Pedersen AH, Kisiel W: Human plasma and recombinant factor VII: Characterization of O-glycosylations at serine residues 52 and 60 and effects of site-directed mutagenesis of serine 52 to alanine. *J Biol Chem* **266**:11051, 1991.
110. Nishimura H, Takao T, Hase S, Shimonishi Y, Iwanaga S: Human factor IX has a tetrasaccharide *O*-glycosidically linked to serine 61 through the fucose residue. *J Biol Chem* **267**:17520, 1992.
111. Kentzer EJ, Buko A, Menon G, Sarin VK: Carbohydrate composition and presence of a fucose-protein linkage in recombinant human pro-urokinase. *Biochem Biophys Res Commun* **171**:401, 1990.
112. Harris RJ, Leonard CK, Guzzetta AW, Spellman MW: Tissue plasminogen activator has an *O*-linked fucose attached to threonine-61 in the epidermal growth factor domain. *Biochemistry* **30**:2311, 1991.
113. Harris RJ, Ling VT, Spellman MW: *O*-linked fucose is present in the first epidermal growth factor domain of factor XII but not protein C. *J Biol Chem* **267**:5102, 1992.
114. Bharadwaj D, Harris RJ, Kisiel W, Smith KJ: Enzymatic removal of sialic acid from factor IX and factor X has no effect on their anticoagulant activity. *J Biol Chem* **270**:6537, 1995.
115. Iino M, Foster DC, Kisiel W: Functional consequences of mutations in Ser52 and Ser60 in human blood coagulation factor VII. *Arch Biochem Biophys* **352**:182, 1998.
116. Stanton C, Wallin R: Processing and trafficking of clotting factor X in the secretory pathway. Effects of warfarin. *Biochem J* **284**:25, 1992.

117. Wallin R, Stanton C, Ross RP: Intracellular proteolytic processing of the two-chain vitamin K-dependent coagulation factor X. *Thromb Res* **15**:395, 1994.
118. Miletich JP, Leykam JF, Broze GJ Jr: Detection of single chain protein C in human plasma. *Blood* **62(Suppl 1)**:306a, 1983.
119. Foster DC, Sprecher CA, Holly RD, Gambee JE, Walker KM, Kumar AA: Endoproteolytic processing of the dibasic cleavage site in the human protein C precursor in transfected mammalian cells: Effects of sequence alterations on efficiency of cleavage. *Biochemistry* **29**:347, 1990.
120. Foster DC, Holly RD, Sprecher CA, Walker KM, Kumar AA: Endoproteolytic processing of the human protein C precursor by the yeast Kex2 endopeptidase coexpressed in mammalian cells. *Biochemistry* **30**:367, 1991.
121. Freedman RB: Protein disulfide isomerase: Multiple roles in the modification of nascent secretory proteins. *Cell* **57**:1069, 1989.
122. Davie EW, Fujikawa K, Kisiel W: The coagulation cascade: Initiation, maintenance, and regulation. *Biochemistry* **30**:10363, 1991.
123. Suzuki K, Kahlback B, Stenflo J: Thrombin-catalyzed activation of human coagulation factor V. *J Biol Chem* **257**:6556, 1982.
124. Nesheim ME, Foster WB, Mann KG: Characterization of factor V intermediates. *J Biol Chem* **259**:3187, 1984.
125. Vehar GA, Davie EW: Preparation and properties of bovine factor VIII antihemophilic factor. *Biochemistry* **19**:401, 1980.
126. Fulcher CA, Roberts JR, Zimmerman TS: Thrombin proteolysis of purified factor VIII procoagulant protein: Correlation of activation with generation of specific polypeptide. *Blood* **61**:807, 1983.
127. Fay PJ, Anderson MT, Chavin SI, Marder VJ: The size of human factor VIII heterodimers and the effects produced by thrombin. *Biochim Biophys Acta* **871**:268, 1986.
128. Eaton D, Rodriquez H, Vehar GA: Proteolytic processing of human factor VIII. Correlation of specific cleavages by thrombin, factor Xa and activated protein C with activation and inactivation of factor VIII coagulant activity. *Biochemistry* **25**:505, 1986.
129. Schwartz ML, Pizzo SV, Hill RL, McKee PA: Human factor XIII from plasma and platelets. Molecular weights, subunit structures, proteolytic activation, and cross-linking of fibrinogen and fibrin. *J Biol Chem* **248**:1395, 1973.
130. Takagi T, Doolittle RF: Amino acid sequence studies on factor XIII and the peptide released during its activation by thrombin. *Biochemistry* **13**:750, 1974.
131. Esmon CT, Owen WG: Identification of an endothelial cell cofactor for thrombin-catalyzed activation of protein C. *Proc Natl Acad Sci U S A* **78**:2249, 1981.
132. Owen WG, Esmon CT: Functional properties of an endothelial cell cofactor for thrombin-catalyzed activation of protein C. *J Biol Chem* **256**:5532, 1981.
133. Esmon NL, Owen WG, Esmon CT: Isolation of a membrane-bound cofactor for thrombin-catalyzed activation of protein C. *J Biol Chem* **257**:859, 1982.
134. Gailani D, Broze GJ Jr: Factor XI activation in a revised model of blood coagulation. *Science* **253**:909, 1991.
135. Naito K, Fujikawa K: Activation of human blood coagulation factor XI independent of factor XII. *J Biol Chem* **266**:7353, 1991.
136. Shuman MA: Thrombin-cellular interactions. *Ann N Y Acad Sci* **485**:228, 1986.
137. Vu T-KH, Hung DT, Wheaton VI, Coughlin SR: Molecular cloning of a functional thrombin receptor reveals a novel proteolytic mechanism of receptor activation. *Cell* **64**:1057, 1991.
138. Kahn ML, Zheng YW, Huang W, Bigornia V, Zeng D, Moff S, Farese RV Jr, Tam C, Coughlin SR: A dual thrombin receptor system for platelet activation. *Nature* **394**:690, 1998.
139. Ishihara H, Connolly AJ, Zeng D, Kahn ML, Zheng YW, Timmons C, Tram T, Coughlin SR: Protease-activated receptor 3 is a second thrombin receptor in humans. *Nature* **386**:502, 1997.
140. Coughlin SR: Sol Sherry lecture in thrombosis: how thrombin talks to cells: Molecular mechanisms and roles in vivo. *Arterioscler Thromb Vasc Biol* **18**:514, 1998.
141. Suttie JW, Jackson CM: Prothrombin structure, activation and biosynthesis. *Physiol Rev* **57**:1, 1977.
142. Degen SJF, MacGillivray RTA, Davie EW: Characterization of the cDNA and gene coding for human prothrombin. *Biochemisry* **22**:2087, 1983.
143. Downing MR, Butkowski RJ, Clark MM, Mann KG: Human prothrombin activation. *J Biol Chem* **250**:8897, 1975.
144. Rosing J, Tans G, Grovers-Riemslag JWP, Zwaal RFA, Hemker HC: The role of phospholipids and factor Va in the prothrombinase complex. *J Biol Chem* **255**:274, 1980.
145. Nesheim ME, Taswell JB, Mann KG: The contribution of bovine factor V and factor Va to the activity of prothrombinase. *J Biol Chem* **254**:10952, 1979.
146. Krishnaswamy S, Church WR, Nesheim ME, Mann KG: Activation of human prothrombin by human prothrombinase. *J Biol Chem* **262**:3291, 1987.
147. Rabiet MJ, Blashill A, Furie B, Furie BC: Prothrombin fragment 1.2.3, a major product of prothrombin activation in human plasma. *J Biol Chem* **261**:13210, 1986.
148. Mann KG, Nesheim ME, Church WR, Haley P, Krishnaswamy S: Surface-dependent reactions of the vitamin K-dependent enzyme complexes. *Blood* **76**:1, 1990.
149. Krishnaswamy S: Prothrombinase complex assembly. Contributions of protein-protein and protein-membrane interactions toward complex formation. *J Biol Chem* **265**:3708, 1990.
150. Husten EJ, Esmon CT, Johnson AE: The active site of blood coagulation factor Xa. Its distance from the phospholipid surface and its conformational sensitivity to components of the prothrombinase complex. *J Biol Chem* **262**:12953, 1987.
151. Armstrong SA, Husten EJ, Esmon CT, Johnson AE: The active site of membrane-bound meizothrombin. A fluorescence determination of its distance from the phospholipid surface and its conformational sensitivity to calcium and factor Va. *J Biol Chem* **265**:6210, 1990.
152. Pollock JS, Shepard AJ, Weber DJ, Olson DL, Klapper DG, Pedersen LG, Hiskey RG: Phospholipid binding properties of bovine prothrombin peptide residues 1–45. *J Biol Chem* **263**:14216, 1988.
153. Berkowitz P, Huh N-W, Brostrom KE, Panek MG, Weber DJ, Tulinsky A, Pedersen LG, Hiskey RG: A metal ion-binding site in the kringle region of bovine prothrombin fragment 1. *J Biol Chem* **267**:4570, 1992.
154. Rosing J, van Rijn JLML, Bevers EM, van Dieijen G, Comfurius P, Zwaal FA: The role of activated human platelets in prothrombin and factor X activation. *Blood* **65**:319, 1985.
155. Tracy PB, Eide LL, Mann KG: Human prothrombinase complex assembly and function on isolated peripheral blood cell population. *J Biol Chem* **260**:2119, 1985.
156. Stern D, Nawroth P, Handley D, Kisiel W: An endothelial cell-dependent pathway of coagulation. *Proc Natl Acad Sci U S A* **82**:2523, 1985.
157. Bode W, Turk D, Karshikov A: The refined 1.9 Å x-ray crystal structure of D-Phe-Pro-Arg chloromethylketone-inhibited human α-thrombin: structure analysis, overall structure, electrostatic properties, detailed active site geometry and structure function relationships. *Protein Sci* **1**:426, 1992.
158. Rydel TJ, Tulinsky A, Bode W, Huber R: Refined structure of the hirudin-thrombin complex. *J Mol Biol* **221**:583, 1991.
159. Martin PD, Robertson W, Turk D, Huber R, Bode W, Edwards BFP: The stucture of residues 7–16 of the A-alpha chain of human fibrinogen bound to bovine thrombin at 2.3 A resolution. *J Biol Chem* **267**:7911, 1992.
160. Stubbs MT, Oschkinat H, Mayr I, Huber R, Angliker H, Stone SR, Bode W: The interaction of thrombin with fibrinogen: A structural basis for its specificity. *Eur J Biochem* **206**:187, 1992.
161. Arni RK, Padmanabhan K, Padmanabhan KP, Wu T-P, Tulinsky A: Structures of the non-covalent complexes of human and bovine prothrombin fragment 2 with human PPACK-thrombin. *Biochemistry* **32**:4727, 1993.
162. Mathews II, Padmanabhan KP, Ganesh V, Tulinsky A, Ishii M, Chen J, Turk CW, Coughlin SR, Fenton JW 2nd: Crystallographic structures of thrombin complexed with thrombin receptor peptides: Existence of expected and novel binding modes. *Biochemistry* **33**:3266, 1994.
163. Soriano-Garcia M, Padmanabhan K, de Vos AM, Tulinsky A: The Ca^{2+} ion and membrane-binding structure of the Gla domain of prothrombin fragment 1. *Biochemistry* **31**:2554, 1992.
164. Seshardi TP, Tulinsky A, Skrzypczak-Jankun E, Park CH: Structure of bovine prothrombin fragment 1 refined at 2.25 Å resolution. *J Mol Biol* **220**:481, 1991.
165. Stubbs MT, Bode W: The clot thickens: Clues provided by thrombin structure. *Trends Biochem Sci* **20**:23, 1995.
166. Bourin ML, Lindahl U: Glycosaminoglycans and the regulation of blood coagulation. *Biochem J* **289**:313, 1993.
167. Obst U, Banner DW, Weber L, Diedrich F: Molecular recognition at the thrombin active site: Structure based design and synthesis of potent and selective thrombin inhibitors and the x-ray crystal structures of thwo thrombin-inhibitor complexes. *Chem Biol* **4**:287, 1997.

168. Maikayil JA, Burkhart JP, Schreuder HA, Broersma RJ, tardif C, Kutcher LW 3rd, Mehdi S, Schatzman GL, Neises B, Peet NP: Molecular design and characterization of an alpha-thrombin inhibitor containing a novel P1 moiety. *Biochemistry* **36**:1034, 1997.
169. Royle NJ, Irwin DM, Koschinsky ML, MacGillivray RTA, Hamerton JL: Human genes encoding prothrombin and ceruloplasmin map to 11p11-q12 and 3q21-24, respectively. *Somat Cell Mol Genet* **13**:285, 1987.
170. Breathnach R, Benoist C, O'Hare K, Gannon F, Chambon P: Ovalbumin gene: Evidence for a leader sequence in mRNA and DNA sequences at the exon-intron boundaries. *Proc Natl Acad Sci U S A* **75**:4853, 1978.
171. Mount SM: A catalogue of splice junction sequences. *Nucleic Acids Res* **10**:459, 1982.
172. Rinehart FP, Ritch TG, Deininger PL, Schmid CW: Renaturation rate studies of a single family of interspersed repeated sequences in human deoxyribonucleic acid. *Biochemistry* **20**:3003, 1981.
173. Schmid CW, Jelinek WR: The alu family of dispersed repetitive sequences. *Science* **216**:1065, 1982.
174. Bancroft JD, Schaefer LA, Degen SJF: Characterization of the *Alu*-rich 5′-flanking region of the human prothrombin-encoding gene: Identification of a positive *cis*-acting element that regulates liver-specific expression. *Gene* **95**:253, 1990.
175. Chow BK-C, Ting V, Tufaro F, MacGillivray RTA: Characterization of a novel liver-specific enhancer in the human prothrombin gene. *J Biol Chem* **266**:18927, 1991.
176. de Vetten M, van Amstel HKP, Reitsma PH: RFLP for the human prothrombin (F2) gene. *Nucleic Acids Res* **18**:5917, 1990.
177. McAlpine PJ, Dickson M, Guy C, Wiens A, Irwin DM, MacGillivray RTA: Polymorphism detected by multiple RENS in the human coagulation factor II (F2) gene. *Nucleic Acids Res* **19**:193, 1991.
178. Iwahana H, Yoshimoto K, Itakura M: NcoI RFLP in the human prothrombin (F2) gene. *Nucleic Acids Res* **19**:4309, 1991.
179. Iwahana H, Yoshimoto K, Itakura M: Highly polymorphic region of the human prothrombin (F2) gene. *Hum Genet* **78**:123, 1992.
180. Poort SR, Rosendaal FR, Reitsma PH, Bertina RM: A common genetic variation in the 3′-untranslated region of the prothrombin gene is associated with elevated plasma prothrombin levels and an increase in venous thrombosis. *Blood* **88**:3698, 1996.
181. Rosendaal FR, Doggen CJ, Zivelin A, Arruda VR, Aiach M, Suscovick PS, Hillarp A, Watzke HH, Bernardi F, Cumming AM, Preston FE, Reitsma PH: Geographic distribution of the 20210 G to A prothrombin variant. *Thromb Haemost* **79**:706, 1998.
182. Zivelin A, Rosenberg N, Faier S, Kornbrot N, Peretz H, Mannhalter C, Horellou MH, Seligsohn U: A single genetic origin for the common prothrombotic G20210A polymorphism in the prothrombin gene. *Blood* **92**:1119, 1998.
183. Kattlove HE, Shapiro SS, Spivack M: Hereditary prothrombin deficiency. *N Engl J Med* **282**:57, 1970.
184. Shapiro SS, McCord IS: Prothrombin, in Spaet TH (ed): *Hemostasis and Thrombosis*, Vol. 4. New York, Grune & Stratton, 1978, p 177.
185. Guillin M-C, Bezeaud A, Rabiet M-J, Elion J: Congenitally abnormal prothrombin and thrombin. *Ann N Y Acad Sci* **485**:56, 1986.
186. Rabiet M-J, Furie BC, Furie B: Molecular defect of prothrombin Barcelona. *J Biol Chem* **261**:15045, 1986.
187. Diuguid DL, Rabiet M-J, Furie BC, Furie B: Molecular defects of factor IX Chicago-2 (Arg 145/His) and prothrombin Madrid (Arg 271/Cys): Arginine mutations that preclude zymogen activation. *Blood* **74**:193, 1989.
188. O'Marcaigh AS, Nichols WL, Hassinger NL, Mullins JD, Mallouh AA, Gilchrist GS, Owen WG: Genetic analysis and functional characterization of prothrombins Corpus Christi (Arg382-Cys), Dharhan (Arg271-His) and hypoprothrombinemia. *Blood* **88**:2611, 1996.
189. Henricksen RA, Dunham CK, Miller LD, Casey JT, Menke JB, Knupp CL, Usala SJ: Prothrombin Greenville, Arg517-Gln, identified in an individual heterozygous for dysprothrombinemia. *Blood* **91**:2026, 1998.
190. Degan SJ, McDowell SA, Sparks LM, Scharrer I: Prothrombin Frankfurt: A dysfunctional prothrombin characterized by substitution of Glu-466 by Ala. *Thromb Haemost* **73**:203, 1995.
191. Walz DA, Hewett-Emmett D, Seegers WH: Amino acid sequence of human prothrombin fragments 1 and 2. *Proc Natl Acad Sci U S A* **74**:1969, 1977.
192. Miyata T, Morita T, Inomoto T, Kawuchi S, Shirakami A, Iwanaga S: Prothrombin Tokushima, a replacement of arginine-418 by tryptophan that impairs the fibrinogen clotting activity of derived thrombin Tokushima. *Biochemistry* **26**:1117, 1987.
193. Iwahana H, Yoshimoto K, Shigekiyo T, Shirakami A, Saito S, Itakura M: Detection of a single base substitution of the gene for prothrombin Tokushima. The application of PCR-SSCP for the genetic and molecular analysis of dysprothrombinemia. *Int J Hematol* **55**:93, 1992.
194. Henriksen RA, Owen WG: Characterization of the catalytic defect in the dysthrombin, thrombin Quick. *J Biol Chem* **262**:4664, 1987.
195. Henriksen RA, Mann KG: Identification of the primary structural defect in the dysthrombin thrombin Quick I: Substitution of cysteine for arginine-382. *Biochemistry* **27**:9160, 1988.
196. Leong L, Henriksen RA, Kermode JC, Rittenhouse SE, Tracy PB: The thrombin high-affinity binding site on platelets is a negative regulator of thrombin-induced platelet activation. Structure-function studies using two mutant thrombins, Quick I and Quick II. *Biochemistry* **31**:2567, 1992.
197. Henriksen RA, Mann KG: Substitution of valine for glycine-558 in the congenital dysthrombin thrombin Quick II alters primary substrate specificity. *Biochemistry* **28**:2078, 1989.
198. Bezeaud A, Elion J, Guillin M-C: Functional characterization of thrombin Salakta: An abnormal thrombin derived from a human prothrombin variant. *Blood* **71**:556, 1988.
199. Miyata T, Aruga R, Umeyama H, Bezeaud A, Guillin M-C, Iwanaga S: Prothrombin Salakta: Substitution of glutamic acid-466 by alanine reduces the fibrinogen clotting activity and the esterase activity. *Biochemistry* **31**:7457, 1992.
200. Huisse MG, Dreyfus M, Guillin M-C: Prothrombin Clamart: Prothrombin variant with defective Arg 320-Ile cleavage by factor Xa. *Thromb Res* **44**:11, 1986.
201. Morishita E, Saito M, Asakura H, Jokaji H, Uotani C, Kumabashiri I, Yamazaki M, Hachiya H, Okamura M, Matsuda T: Prothrombin Himi: An abnormal prothrombin characterized by a defective thrombin activity. *Thromb Res* **62**:697, 1991.
202. Rabiet MJ, Jandrot-Perrus M, Boissel JP, Elion J, Josso F: Thrombin Metz: Characterization of the dysfunctional thrombin derived from a variant of human prothrombin. *Blood* **63**:927, 1984.
203. Girolami A, Coccheri S, Palareti G, Poggi M, Burul A, Cappellato G: Prothrombin Molise: A "new" congenital dysprothrombinemia, double heterozygosis with an abnormal prothrombin and true prothrombin deficiency. *Blood* **52**:115, 1978.
204. McMillan CW, Roberts HR: Congenital combined deficiency of coagulation factors II, VII, IX and X. *N Engl J Med* **274**:1313, 1966.
205. Chung K-S, Bezeaud A, Goldsmith JC, McMillan CW, Menache D, Roberts HR: Congenital deficiency of blood clotting factors II, VII, IX and X. *Blood* **53**: 776, 1979.
206. Johnson CA, Chung KS, McGrath KM, Bean PE, Roberts HR: Characterization of a variant prothrombin in a patient congenitally deficient in factors II, VII, IX and X. *Br J Haematol* **44**:461, 1980.
207. Goldsmith GH, Pence RE, Ratnoff OD, Adelstein DJ, Furie B: Studies on a family with combined functional deficiencies of vitamin K-dependent coagulation factor. *J Clin Invest* **69**:1253, 1982.
208. Vicente V, Maia R, Alberca I, Tamagnini GPT, Lopez Borrasca A: Congenital deficiency of vitamin K-dependent coagulation factors and protein C. *Thromb Haemost* **51**:343, 1984.
209. Pauli RM, Lian JB, Mosher DF, Suttie JW: Association of congenital deficiency of multiple vitamin K-dependent coagulation factors and the phenotype of the warfarin embriopathy: Clues to the mechanism of teratogenecity of coumarin derivatives. *Am J Hum Genet* **41**:566, 1987.
210. Brenner B, Tavori S, Zivelin A, Keller CB, Suttie JW, Tatarsky I, Seligsohn U: Hereditary deficiency of all vitamin K-dependent procoagulants and anticoagulants. *Br J Haematol* **75**:537, 1990.
211. Radcliffe R, Nemerson Y: Activation and control of factor VII by activated factor X and thrombin. Isolation and characterization of a single chain form of factor VII. *J Biol Chem* **250**:388, 1975.
212. Kisiel W, Fujikawa K, Davie EW: Activation of bovine factor VII (proconvertin) by factor XIIa (activated Hageman factor). *Biochemistry* **16**:4189, 1977.
213. Seligsohn U, Osterud B, Brown SF, Griffin JH, Rapaport SI: Activation of human factor VII in plasma and in purified systems: Roles of activated factor IX, kallikrein, and activated factor XII. *J Clin Invest* **64**:1056, 1979.
214. Broze GJ Jr, Majerus PW: Purification and properties of human coagulation factor VII. *J Biol Chem* **255**:1242, 1980.
215. Masys DR, Bajaj SP, Rapaport SI: Activation of human factor VII by activated factors IX and X. *Blood* **60**:1143, 1982.
216. Wildgoose P, Kisiel W: Activation of human factor VII by factors IXa and Xa on human bladder carcinoma cells. *Blood* **73**:1888, 1989.

217. Nakagaki T, Foster DC, Berkner KL, Kisiel W: Initiation of the extrinsic pathway of blood coagulation: Evidence for the tissue factor-dependent autoactivation of human coagulation factor VII. *Biochemistry* **30**:10819, 1991.
218. Osterud B, Rapaport SI: Activation of factor IX by the reaction product of tissue factor and factor VII: Additional pathway for initiating blood coagulation. *Proc Natl Acad Sci U S A* **74**:5260, 1977.
219. Nemerson Y: Tissue factor and hemostasis. *Blood* **71**:1, 1988.
220. Drake TA, Morrissey JH, Edgington TS: Selective cellular expression of tissue factor in human tissues. *Am J Pathol* **134**:1087, 1989.
221. Wilcox JN, Smith KM, Schwartz SM, Gordon D: Localization of tissue factor in the normal vessel wall and in the atherosclerotic plaque. *Proc Natl Acad Sci U S A* **86**:2839, 1989.
222. Weiss HJ, Turitto VT, Baumgartner HR, Nemerson Y, Hoffmann T: Evidence for the presence of tissue factor activity of subendothelium. *Blood* **73**:968, 1989.
223. Fair DS, MacDonald MJ: Cooperative interaction between factor VII and cell surface-expressed tissue factor. *J Biol Chem* **262**:11692, 1987.
224. Sakai T, Lund-Hansen T, Paborsky L, Pedersen AH, Kisiel W: Binding of human factors VII and VIIa to a human bladder carcinoma cell line (J82). Implications for the initiation of the extrinsic pathway of blood coagulation. *J Biol Chem* **264**:9980, 1989.
225. Le DT, Rapaport SI, Rao LVM: Relations between factor VIIa binding and expression of factor VII/tissue factor catalytic activity on cell surfaces. *J Biol Chem* **267**:15447, 1992.
226. Bom VJJ, Bertina RM: The contributions of Ca^{2+}, phospholipids and tissue-factor apoprotein to the activation of human blood-coagulation factor X by activated factor VII. *Biochem J* **265**:327, 1990.
227. Komiyama Y, Pedersen AH, Kisiel W: Proteolytic activation of human factors IX and X by recombinant human factor VIIa: Effects of calcium, phospholipids, and tissue factor. *Biochemistry* **29**:9418, 1990.
228. Ruf W, Rehemtulla A, Edgington TS: Phospholipid-independent and -dependent interactions required for tissue factor receptor and cofactor function. *J Biol Chem* **266**:2158, 1991.
229. Nemerson Y, Gentry R: An ordered addition, essential activation model of the tissue factor pathway of coagulation: Evidence for a conformational cage. *Biochemistry* **25**:4020, 1986.
230. Lawson JH, Butenas S, Mann KG: The evaluation of complex-dependent alterations in human factor VIIa. *J Biol Chem* **267**:4834, 1992.
231. Rapaport SI: Inhibition of factor VIIa/tissue factor-induced blood coagulation: With particular emphasis upon a factor Xa-dependent inhibitory mechanism. *Blood* **73**:359, 1989.
232. Broze GJ Jr, Girard TJ, Novotny WF: Regulation of coagulation by a multivalent Kunitz-type inhibitor. *Biochemistry* **29**:7539, 1990.
233. Kisiel W, McMullen BA: Isolation and characterization of human factor VIIa. *Thromb Res* **22**:375, 1981.
234. Wildgoose P, Kazim AL, Kisiel W: The importance of residues 195–206 of human blood clotting factor VII in the interaction of factor VII with tissue factor. *Proc Natl Acad Sci U S A* **87**:7290, 1990.
235. Kumar A, Blumenthal DK, Fair DS: Identification of molecular sites on factor VII which mediate its assembly and function in the extrinsic pathway activation complex. *J Biol Chem* **266**:915, 1991.
236. Higashi S, Nishimura H, Fujii S, Takada K, Iwanaga S: Tissue factor potentiates the factor VIIa-catalyzed hydrolysis of an ester substrate. *J Biol Chem* **267**:17990, 1992.
237. Bazan JF: Structural design and molecular evolution of a cytokine receptor superfamily. *Proc Natl Acad Sci U S A* **87**:6934, 1990.
238. Harlosk K, Martin DMA, O'Brien DP, Jones EY, Stuart DI, Polikarpov DI, Miller A, Tuddenham EGD, Boys CWG: Crystal structure of the extracellular region of human tissue factor. *Nature* **370**:662, 1994.
239. Muller YA, Ultsch MH, Kelly RF, de Vos AM: Structure of the extracellular domain of human tissue factor: Location of factor VIIa binding site. *Biochemistry* **33**:10864, 1994.
240. Walder MR, Windsor WT, Nagabhushan TL, Lundell DJ, Lunn CA, Zauodny PJ, Narula SK: Crystal structure of a complex between interferon-γ and its soluble high-affinity receptor. *Nature* **376**:230, 1995.
241. Rottingen JA, Enden T, Camerer E, Iversen JG, Prydz H: Binding of human factor VIIa to tissue factor induces cytosolic Ca^{2+} signals in J82 cells, transfected COS-1 cells, Madin-Darby canine kidney cells, and human endothelial cells induced to synthesize tissue factor. *J Biol Chem* **270**:4650, 1995.
242. Camerer E, Rottingen JA, Iversen JG, Prydz H: Coagulation factor VII and X induce Ca^{2+} oscillations in Madin-Darby canine kidney cells only when proteolytically active. *J Biol Chem* **271**:29034, 1996.
243. Kirchhofer D, Guha A, Nemerson Y, Konigsberg WH, Vilbois P, Chene C, Banner DW, D'Arcy A: Activation of blood coagulation factor VIIa with cleaved tissue factor extracellular domain and crystallization of the active complex. *Proteins* **22**:419, 1995.
244. Banner DW, D'Arcy AD, Chene C, Winkler FK, Guha A, Konigsberg WH, Nemerson Y, Kirchhofer D: The crystal structure of the complex of blood coagulation factor VIIa with soluble tissue factor. *Nature* **389**:41, 1996.
245. Banner DW: The factor VIIa/tissue factor complex. *Thromb Haemost* **78**:512, 1997.
246. Dickenson CD, Kelly CR, Ruf W: Identification of surface residues mediating tissue factor binding an catalytic function of the serine protease factor VIIa. *Proc Natl Acad Sci U S A* **93**:14379, 1996.
247. Petersen LC, Schiodt J, Christensen U: Involvement of the hydrophobic stack residues 39–44 of factor VIIa in tissue factor interactions. *FEBS Lett* **347**:73, 1994.
248. Ruf W, Schullek JR, Stone MJ, Edgington TS: Mutational mapping of functional residues in tissue factor: Identification of factor VII recognition determinants in both structural modules of the predicted cytokine receptor homology domain. *Biochemistry* **33**:1565, 1994.
249. Gibbs CS, McCurdy SN, Leung LCK, Paborsky LR: Identification of the factor VIIa binding site on tissue factor by homologous loop swap and alanine scanning mutagenesis. *Biochemistry* **33**:14003, 1994.
250. Kelley RF, Costas KE, O'Connell MP, Lazarus RA: Analysis of the factor VIIa binding site on human tissue factor: Effects of tissue factor mutations on the kinetics and thermodynamics of binding. *Biochemistry* **34**:10383, 1995.
251. Ashton AW, Boehm MK, Johnson DJD, Kemball-Cook G, Perkins SJ: The solution structure of human coagulation factor VIIa in its compex with tissue factor is similar to free factor VIIa: A study of heterodimeric receptor-ligand complex by x-ray and neutron scattering and computational modeling. *Biochemistry* **37**:8208, 1998.
252. Scarpati EM, Wen D, Broze GJ Jr, Miletich JP, Flandermeyer RR, Siegel NR, Sadler JE: Human tissue factor: cDNA sequence and chromosome localization of the gene. *Biochemistry* **26**:5234, 1987.
253. Spicer EK, Horton R, Bloem L, Bach R, Williams KR, Guha A, Kraus J, Lin T-C, Nemerson Y, Konigsberg WH: Isolation of cDNA clones coding for human tissue factor: Primary structure of the protein and cDNA. *Proc Natl Acad Sci U S A* **84**:5148, 1987.
254. Morrissey JH, Fakhrai H, Edgington TS: Molecular cloning of the cDNA for tissue factor, the cellular receptor for the initiation of the coagulation protease cascade. *Cell* **50**:129, 1987.
255. Fisher KL, Gorman CM, Vehar GA, O'Brien DP, Lawn RM: Cloning and expression of human tissue factor cDNA. *Thromb Res* **48**:89,1987.
256. Rehemtulla A, Ruf W, Edgington TS: The integrity of the cysteine 186-cysteine 209 bond of the second disulfide loop of tissue factor is required for binding of factor VII. *J Biol Chem* **266**:10294, 1991.
257. Ruf W, Miles DJ, Rehemtulla A, Edgington TS: Cofactor residues lysine 165 and 166 are critical for protein substrate recognition by the tissue factor-factor VIIa protease complex. *J Biol Chem* **267**:6375, 1992.
258. Waxman E, Ross JBA, Lane TM, Guha A, Thiruvikraman SV, Lin TC, Konigsberg WH, Nemerson Y: Tissue factor and its extracellular soluble domain: The relationship between intermolecular association with factor VIIa and enzymatic activity of the complex. *Biochemistry* **31**:3998, 1992.
259. Yamamoto M, Nakagaki T, Kisiel W: Tissue factor-dependent autoactivation of human blood coagulation factor VII. *J Biol Chem* **267**:19089, 1992.
260. Neuenschwander PF, Morrissey JH: Deletion of the membrane-anchoring region of tissue factor abolishes autoactivation of factor VII but not cofactor function. Analysis of a mutant with a selective deficiency in activity. *J Biol Chem* **267**:14477, 1992.
261. de Grouchy J, Dautzenberg MD, Turleau C, Beguin S, Chavin-Colin F: Regional mapping of clotting factors VII and X to 13q34. Expression of factor VII through chromosome 8. *Hum Genet* **66**:230, 1984.
262. Ott R, Pfeiffer RA: Evidence that activities of coagulation factors VII and X are linked to chromosome 13 (q34). *Hum Hered* **34**:123, 1984.
263. Gilgenkrantz S, Briquel ME, Andre E, Alexandre P, Jalbert P, Le Marec B, Pouzol P, Pommereuil M: Structural genes of coagulation factors VII and X located on 13q34. *Ann Genet* **29**:32, 1986.
264. O'Hara PJ, Grant FJ, Haldeman BA, Gray CL, Insley MY, Hagen FS, Murray MJ: Nucleotide sequence of the gene coding for human factor VII, a vitamin K-dependent protein participating in blood coagulation. *Proc Natl Acad Sci U S A* **84**:5158, 1987.
265. O'Hara PJ, Grant FJ: The human factor VII gene is polymorphic due to variation in repeat copy number in a minisatellite. *Gene* **66**:147, 1988.

266. Marchetti G, Gemmati D, Patracchini P, Pinotti M, Bernardi F: PCR detection of a repeat polymorphism within the F7 gene. *Nucleic Acids Res* **19**:4570, 1991.
267. Marchetti G, Patracchini P, Gemmati D, DeRosa V, Pinotti M, Rodorigo G, Casonato A, Girolami A, Bernardi F: Detection of two missense mutations and characterization of a repeat polymorphism in the factor VII gene (F7). *Hum Genet* **89**:497, 1992.
268. Green F, Kelleher C, Wilkes H, Temple A, Meade T, Humphries S: A common genetic polymorphism associated with lower coagulation factor VII levels in healthy individuals. *Arterioscler Thromb* **11**:540, 1991.
269. Greenberg D, Miao CH, Ho WT, Chung DW, Davie EW: Liver-specific expression of the human factor VII gene. *Proc Natl Acad Sci U S A* **92**:12347, 1995.
270. Pollak ES, Hung HL, Godin G, Overton GC, High KA: Functional characterization of the human factor VII 5′-flanking region. *J Biol Chem* **271**:1738, 1996.
271. Salier JP, Hirosawa S, Kurachi K: Functional characterization of the 5′-regulatory region of the human factor IX gene. *J Biol Chem* **265**:7062, 1990.
272. Hung HS, High KA: Liver-enriched transcription factor HNF-4 and ubiquitous factor NF-Y are critical for expression of blood coagulation factor X. *J Biol Chem* **271**:2323, 1996.
273. Arbini A, Pollak ES, Bayleran JK, High KA, Bauer KA: Severe factor VII deficiency due to a mutation disrupting hepatic nuclear factor 4 binding site in the factor VII promoter. *Blood* **89**:176, 1997.
274. Foster DC, Yoshitake S, Davie EW: The nucleotide sequence of the gene for human protein C. *Proc Natl Acad Sci U S A* **82**:4673, 1985.
275. Plutzky J, Hoskins JA, Long GL, Crabtree GR: Evolution and organization of the human protein C gene. *Proc Natl Acad Sci U S A* **83**:546, 1986.
276. Patthy L: Evolutionary assembly of blood coagulation proteins. *Semin Thromb Hemost* **16**:245, 1990.
277. Carson SD, Henry WM, Shows TB: Tissue factor gene localized to human chromosome 1 (1pter/1p21). *Science* **229**:991, 1985.
278. Kao F-T, Hartz J, Horton R, Nemerson Y, Carson SD: Regional assignment of human tissue factor gene (F3) to chromosome 1p21-p22. *Somat Cell Mol Genet* **14**:407, 1988.
279. Mackman N, Morrissey JH, Fowler B, Edgington TS: Complete sequence of the human tissue factor gene, a highly regulated cellular receptor that initiates the coagulation protease cascade. *Biochemistry* **28**:1755, 1989.
280. van der Logt CPE, Reitsma PH, Bertina RM: Alternative splicing is responsible for the presence of two tissue factor mRNA species in LPS-stimulated human monocytes. *Thromb Haemost* **67**:272, 1992.
281. Edgington TS, Mackman N, Brand K, Ruf W: The structural biology of expression and function of tissue factor. *Thromb Haemost* **66**:67, 1991.
282. Dalaker K: Clotting factor VII during pregnancy, delivery and puerperium. *Br J Obstet Gynaecol* **93**:17, 1986.
283. Balleisen L, Bailey J, Epping P-H, Schulte H, van de Loo J: Epidemiological study on factor VII, factor VIII and fibrinogen in an industrial population: I. Baseline data on the relation to age, gender, body-weight, smoking, alcohol, pill-using, and menopause. *Thromb Haemost* **54**:475, 1985.
284. Balleisen L, Assmann G, Bailey J, Epping P-H, Schulte H, van de Loo J: Epidemiological study on factor VII, factor VIII and fibrinogen in an industrial population: II. Baseline data on the relation to blood pressure, blood glucose, uric acid, and lipid fractions. *Thromb Haemost* **54**:721, 1985.
285. Miller GJ, Cruickshank JK, Ellis LJ, Thompson RL, Wilkes HC, Stirling Y, Mitropoulos KA, Allison JV, Fox TE, Walker AO: Fat consumption and factor VII coagulant activity in middle-aged men. *Atherosclerosis* **78**:19, 1989.
286. Miller GJ, Walter SJ, Stirling Y, Thompson SG, Esnouf MP: Assay of factor VII activity by two techniques: Evidence for increased conversion of VII to VIIa in hyperlipidaemia, with possible implications for ischaemic heart disease. *Br J Haematol* **59**:249, 1985.
287. Mitropoulos KA, Miller GJ, Reeves BEA, Wilkes HC, Cruickshank JK: Factor VII coagulant activity is strongly associated with the plasma concentration of large lipoprotein particles in middle-aged men. *Atherosclerosis* **76**:203, 1989.
288. Mitropoulos KA, Martin JC, Reeves BEA, Esnouf MP: The activation of the contact phase of coagulation by physiologic surfaces in plasma: The effect of large negatively charged liposomal vesicles. *Blood* **73**:1525, 1989.
289. Mitropoulos KA, Miller GJ, Watts GF, Durrington PN: Lipolysis of triglyceride-rich lipoproteins activates coagulant factor XII: A study in familial lipoprotein-lipase deficiency. *Atherosclerosis* **95**:119, 1992.
290. Meade TW, Mellows S, Brozovic M, Miller GJ, Chakrabarti RR, North WR, Haines AP, Stirling Y, Imeson JD, Thompson SG: Haemostatic function and ischaemic heart disease: Principal results of the Northwick Park heart study. *Lancet* **2**:533, 1986.
291. Dalaker K, Smith P, Arnesen H, Prydz H: Factor VII-phospholipid complex in male survivors of acute myocardial infarction. *Acta Med Scand* **222**:111, 1987.
292. Broadhurst P, Kelleher C, Hughes L, Imeson JD, Raftery EB: Fibrinogen, factor VII clotting activity and coronary artery disease severity. *Atherosclerosis* **85**:169, 1990.
293. Hall CA, Rapaport SI, Ames SB, DeGroot JA: A clinical and family study of hereditary proconvertin (factor VII deficiency). *Am J Med* **37**:172, 1964.
294. Dische FE, Benfield V: Congenital factor VII deficiency: Haematological and genetic aspects. *Acta Haematol (Basel)* **21**:257, 1959.
295. Kupfer HG, Hanna BL, Kinne DR: Congenital factor VII deficiency with normal Stuart activity: Clinical, genetic and experimental observations. *Blood* **15**:146,1960.
296. Ragni MV, Lewis JH, Spero JA, Hasiba U: Factor VII deficiency. *Am J Haematol* **10**:79, 1981.
297. Gershwin ME, Gude JK: Deep vein thrombosis and pulmonary embolism in congenital factor VII deficiency. *N Engl J Med* **288**:141, 1973.
298. Shifter T, Machtey I, Creter D: Thromboembolism in congenital factor VII deficiency. *Acta Haematol (Basel)* **71**:60, 1984.
299. Godal HC, Madsen K, Nissen-Meyer R: Thromboembolism in a patient with total proconvertin (factor VII) deficiency. *Acta Med Scand* **171**:325, 1962.
300. Mariani G, Mazzucconi MG, Hermans J, Ciavarella N, Faiella A, Hassan HJ, Mannucci PM, Nenci GG, Orlando M, Romoli D, Mandelli F: Factor VII deficiency: Immunological characterization of genetic variants and detection of carriers. *Br J Haematol* **48**:7, 1981.
301. Triplett DA, Brandt JT, McGann Batard MA, Schaeffer Dixon JL, Fair DA: Hereditary factor VII deficiency. Heterogeneity defined by combined functional and immunochemical analysis. *Blood* **66**:1284, 1985.
302. Girolami A, Fabris F, Zanon RDB, Ghiotto G, Burul A: Factor VII Padua: A congenital coagulation disorder due to an abnormal factor VII with a peculiar activation pattern. *J Lab Clin Med* **91**:387, 1978.
303. Tuddenham EGD, Pemberton S, Cooper DN: Inherited factor VII deficiency: Genetics and molecular pathology. *Thromb Haemost* **74**:313, 1995.
304. Bharadwaj D, Iino M, Kontoyianni M, Smith KJ, Foster DC, Kisiel W: Factor VII central. A novel mutation in the catalytic domain that reduces tissue factor binding, impairs activation by factor Xa, and abolishes amidolytic and coagulant activity. *J Biol Chem* **271**:30685, 1996.
305. Kemball-Cook J, Johnson DJD, Takamiya O, Banner DW, McVey JH, Tuddenham EGD: Coagulation factor VII Gln100-Arg. *J Biol Chem* **273**:8516, 1998.
306. Chaing SH, High KA: Severe factor VII deficiency associated with two missense mutations in the factor VII gene. *Thromb Haemost* **65**:1262, 1991.
307. O'Brien DP, Gale KM, Anderson JS, McVey JH, Miller GJ, Meade TW, Tuddenham EGD: Purification and characterization of factor VII 304-Gln: A variant molecule with reduced activity isolated from a clinically unaffected male. *Blood* **78**:132, 1991.
308. Millar DS, Cooper DN, Kakkar VV, Schwartz M, Scheibel E: Prenatal exclusion of severe factor VII deficiency by DNA sequencing. *Lancet* **339**:1359, 1992.
309. Hedner U: Experiences with recombinant factor VIIa in haemophiliacs, in Albertini A, Lenfant CL, Mannucci PM, Sixma JJ (eds): Biotechnology of Plasma Proteins. *Curr Stud Hematol Blood Transfus* **58**:63, 1991.
310. Lusher J, Ingerslev J, Roberts H, Hedner U: Clinical experience with recombinant factor VIIa. *Blood Coagul Fibrinolysis* **9**:119, 1998.
311. Bauer KA: Treatment of factor VII deficiency with recombinant factor VIIa. *Haemostasis* **26(Suppl 1)**:155, 1996.
312. Bernstien DE, Jeffers L, Erhardsten E, Reddy KR, Glazer S, Squiban P, Bech R, Hedner U, Schiff ER: Recombinant factor VIIa corrects prothrombin time in cirrhotic patients: A preliminary study. *Gastroenterology***113**:1930, 1997.
313. Hay CR, Negrier C, Ludlam CA: The treatment of bleeding in acquired hemophilia with recombinant factor VIIa: A mutlicenter study. *Thromb Haemost* **78**:1463, 1997.

314. Kristensen J, Killander A, Hippe E, Helleberg C, Ellegard J, Holm M, Kutti J, Mellqvist UH: Clinical experience with recombiant factor VIIa in patients with thromboscytopenia. *Haemostasis* **26(Suppl 1)**:159, 1996.
315. Arnljots B, Ezban M, Hedner U: Prevention of experimental arterial thrombosis by topical administration of active site-inactivated factor VIIa. *J Vasc Surg* **25**:341, 1997.
316. Aggeler PM, White SG, Glendening MG, Page EW, Leake TB, Bates G: Plasma thromboplastin component (PTC) deficiency: A new disease resembling hemophilia. *Proc Soc Exp Biol Med* **79**:692, 1952.
317. Biggs R, Douglas AS, MacFarlane RG, Dacie JV, Pitney WR, Merskey C, O'Brien JR: Christmas disease: A condition previously mistaken for haemophilia. *BMJ* **2**:1378, 1952.
318. DiScipio RG, Kurachi K, Davie EW: Activation of human factor IX (Christmas factor). *J Clin Invest* **61**:1528, 1978.
319. DiScipio RG, Hermodson MA, Yates SG, Davie EW: A comparison of human prothrombin, factor IX (Christmas factor), factor X (Stuart factor), and protein S. *Biochemistry* **16**:698, 1977.
320. Morita T, Kisiel W: Calcium binding to a human factor IXa derivative lacking γ-carboxyglutamic acid: Evidence for two high-affinity sites that do not involve β-hydroxyaspartic acid. *Biochem Biophys Res Commun* **130**:841, 1985.
321. Derian CK, VanDusen W, Przysiecki CT, Walsh PN, Berkner KL, Kaufman RJ, Friedman PA: Inhibitors of 2-ketoglutarate-dependent dioxygenases block aspartyl β-hydroxylation of recombinant human factor IX in several mammalian expression systems. *J Biol Chem* **264**:6615, 1989.
322. Lindquist PA, Fujikawa K, Davie EW: The activation of bovine factor IX (Christmas factor) by factor XIa (activated plasma thromboplastin antecedent) and a protease from Russell's viper venom. *J Biol Chem* **253**:1902, 1978.
323. Jones ME, Griffith MJ, Monroe DM, Roberts HR, Lentz BR: Comparison of lipid binding and kinetic properties of normal, variant, and γ-carboxyglutamic acid modified human factor IX and factor IXa. *Biochemistry* **24**:8064, 1985.
324. Schwalbe RA, Ryan J, Stern DM, Kisiel W, Dahlback B, Nelsestuen GL: Protein structural requirements and properties of membrane binding by γ-carboxyglutamic acid-containing plasma proteins and peptides. *J Biol Chem* **264**:20288, 1989.
325. Bajaj SP, Sabharwal AK, Gorka J, Birktoft JJ: Antibody-probed conformational transitions in the protease domain of human factor IX upon calcium binding and zymogen activation: Putative high-affinity Ca^2-binding site in the protease domain. *Proc Natl Acad Sci U S A* **89**:152, 1992.
326. Geng JP, Christiansen WT, Plow EF, Castellino FJ: Transfer of specific endothelial cell binding properties from procoagulant protein human factor IX into the anticoagulant protein human protein C. *Biochemistry* **34**:8449, 1995.
327. Prorok M, Geng JP, Warder SE, Castellino FJ: The entire gamma-carboxyglutamic acid and helical stack domains of human coagulation factor IX are required for optimal binding to its endothelial cell receptor. *Int J Pept Protein Res* **48**:281, 1996.
328. Bajaj SP, Rapaport SI, Maki SL: A monoclonal antibody to factor IX that inhibits the factor VIII:Ca potentiation of factor X activation. *J Biol Chem* **260**:11573, 1985.
329. Camerino G, Grzeschik KH, Jaye M, de la Salle H, Tolstoshev P, Lecocq JP, Heilig R, Mandel JL: Regional localization on the human X chromosome and polymorphism of the coagulation factor IX gene (hemophilia B locus). *Proc Natl Acad Sci U S A* **81**:498, 1984.
330. Chance PF, Dyer KA, Kurachi K, Yoshitake S, Ropers H, Wieacker P, Gartler SM: Regional localization of human factor IX gene by molecular hybridization. *Hum Genet* **65**:207, 1983.
331. Crossley M, Ludwig M, Stowell KM, De Vos P, Olek K, Brownlee GG: Recovery from hemophilia B Leyden: An androgen-responsive element in the factor IX promoter. *Science* **257**:377, 1992.
332. Reijnen MJ, Sladek FM, Bertina RM, Reitsma PH: Disruption of a binding site for hepatocyte nuclear factor 4 results in hemophilia B Leyden. *Proc Natl Acad Sci U S A* **89**:6300, 1992.
333. Crossley M, Brownlee GG: Disruption of a C/EBP binding site in the factor IX promoter is associated with haemophilia B. *Nature* **345**:444, 1990.
334. Reijnen MJ, Bertina RM, Reitsma PH: Localization of transcription initiation sites in the human coagulation factor IX gene. *FEBS Lett* **270**:207, 1990.
335. Pang CP, Crossley M, Kent G, Brownlee GG: Comparative sequence analysis of mammalian factor IX promoters. *Nucleic Acids Res* **18**:6731, 1990.
336. Reinjen MJ, Peerlinck K, Massdam D, Bertina RM, Reitsma PH: Hemophilia B Leyden: A substitution of thymine for guanine at position −21 results in a disruption of a hepatocyte nuclear factor 4 binding site in the factor IX promoter. *Blood* **82**:151, 1993.
337. Picketts D, Mueller CR, Lillicrap D: Transcriptional control of the factor IX gene: Analysis of five *cis*-acting elements and the deleterious effects of naturally occurring hemophilia B Leyden mutations. *Blood* **84**:2992, 1994.
338. Picketts D, Lillicrap D, Mueller CR: Synergy between transcription factors DBP and C/EBP compensates for a hemophilia B Leyden factor IX mutation. *Nat Genet* **3**:175, 1993.
339. Sato K, Ito K, Kohara H, Yamaguchi Y, Adachi K, Endo H: Negative regulation of catalase gene expression in hepatoma cells. *Mol Cell Biol* 12:2525, 1992.
340. Brandstetter H, Bauer M, Huber R, Lollar P, Bode W: X-ray structure of clotting factor IXa: Active site and module structure related to Xase activity and hemophilia B. *Proc Natl Acad Sci U S A* **92**:9796, 1995.
341. Brandstetter H, Kuhne A, Bode W, Huber R, von der Saal W, Wirthensohn K, Engh RA: X-ray structure of active site-inhibited clotting factor Xa. Implications for drug design and substrate recognition. *J Biol Chem* **271**:29988, 1996.
342. Thompson AR: Molecular biology of the hemophilias. *Prog Hemost Thromb* **10**:175, 1991.
343. Peake I: Registry of DNA polymorphisms within or close to the human factor VIII and factor IX genes. *Thromb Haemost* **67**:277, 1992.
344. Wiship PR, Nichols CE, Chuansumrit A, Peake IR: An *Mse*I RFLP in the 5′ flanking region of thefactor IX gene: Its use for hemophilia B carrier detection in Caucasians and Thai populations. *Br J Haematol* **84**:101, 1993.
345. McGraw RA, Davis LM, Noyes CM, Lundblad RL, Roberts HR, Graham JB, Stafford DW: Evidence for a prevalent dimorphism in the activation peptide of human coagulation factor IX. *Proc Natl Acad Sci U S A* **82**:2847, 1985.
346. Wallmark A, Ljung R, Nilsson IM, Holmberg L, Hedner U, Lindvall M, Sjögren H-O: Polymorphism of normal factor IX detected by mouse monoclonal antibodies. *Proc Natl Acad Sci U S A* **82**:3839, 1985.
347. Smith KJ, Thompson AR, McMullen BA, Frazier D, Lin SW, Stafford D, Kisiel W, Thibodeau SN, Chen S-H, Smith LF: Carrier testing in hemophilia B with an immunoassay that distinguishes a prevalent factor IX dimorphism. *Blood* **70**:1006, 1987.
348. Fantl P, Sawers RJ, Marr AG: Investigation of a haemorrhagic disease due to beta-prothromboplastin deficiency complicated by a specific inhibitor of thromboplastin formation. *Aust Ann Med* **5**:163, 1956.
349. Roberts HR, Grizzle JE, McLester WD, Penick GO: Genetic variants of hemophilia B. Detection by means of a specific PTC inhibitor. *J Clin Invest* **47**:360, 1968.
350. Thompson AR: Factor IX antigen by radioimmunoassay. Abnormal factor IX protein in patients on warfarin therapy and with hemophilia B. *J Clin Invest* **59**:900, 1977.
351. Giannelli F, Green PM, Sommer S, Poon M, Ludwig M, Schwaab R, Reitsma PH, Goossens M, Yoshioka A, Figueiredo MS, Brownlee GG: Haemophilia B: Database of point mutations and short additions and deletions—Eighth edition, 1998. *Nucleic Acids Res* **26**:265, 1998.
352. Briët E, Bertina RM, Van Tilburg NH, Veltkamp JJ: Hemophilia B Leyden: A sex-linked hereditary disorder that improves after puberty. *N Engl J Med* **306**:788, 1982.
353. Bolton-Maggs PHB, Jones P, Rizza CR, Stowell KM, Figuierido MS, Brownlee GG: Hemophilia B Liverpool: A new British family with mild hemophilia B associated with a G to A mutation at −6 in the factor IX promoter. *Thromb Haemost* **69**:848, 1995.
354. Picketts DJ, D'Souza C, Bridge PJ, Lillicrap DP: An A to T transversion at position −5 of the factor IX promoter results in hemophilia B. *Nature* **345**:444, 1990.
355. Reinjen MJ, Massdam D, Bertina RM, Reitsma PH: Hemophilia B Leyden: The effect of mutations at +13 on the liver-specific transcription of the factor IX gene. *Blood Coagul Fibrinolysis* **5**:341, 1994.
356. Birkenmeier EH, Gwynn B, Howard S, Jerry J, Gordon JI, Lanscholz WH, McKnight SL: Tissue-specific expression, developmenta regulation and genetic mapping of the gene encoding CCAAT/enhancer binding protein. *Genes Dev* **3**:1146, 1989.
357. Mueller CR, Maire P, Schibler U: DBP, a liver-enriched transcriptional activator is expressed late in ontogeny and its tissue specificity is determined post-transcriptionally. *Cell* **61**:279, 1990.

358. Boccia LM, Lillicrap D, Newcombe K, Mueller CR: Binding of Ets factor GA-binding protien to an upstream site in the factor IX promoter is a critical event in transactivation. *Mol Cell Biol* **16**:1929, 1996.
359. Hirosawa S, Fahner JB, Salier J-P, Wu C-T, Lovrien EW, Kurachi K: Structural and functional basis of the developmental regulation of human coagulation factor IX gene: Factor IX Leyden. *Proc Natl Acad Sci U S A* **87**:4421, 1990.
360. Oldenburg J, Quenzel EM, Harbrecht U, Fregin A, Kress W, Muller CR, Hertfelder HJ, Schwaab R, Brackmann HH, Hanfland P: Missense mutations at ALA-10 in the factor IX propeptide: An insignificant variant in normal life but a decisive cause of bellding during oral anticoagulant therapy. *Br J Haematol* **98**:240, 1997.
361. Winship PR, Dragon AC: Identification of haemophilia B patients with mutations in the two calcium binding domains of factor IX: Importance of a β-OH Asp 64-Asn change. *Br J Haematol* **77**:102, 1991.
362. Larson PJ, Stanfield-Oakley SA, VanDusen WJ, Kasper CK, Smith KJ, Monroe DM, High KA: Structural integrity of the gamma-carboxyglutamic acid domain of human blood coagulation IXa is required for its binding to cofactor VIIIa. *J Biol Chem* **271**:3869, 1996.
363. Wojcik EG, van den Berg M, van der Linden IK, Poort SR, Cupers R, Bertina RM: Factor IX Zutphen: A Cys18-Arg mutatin results in the formation of a heterodimer with alpha-1-microglobulin and the inability to form a calcium-induced conformation. *Biochem J* **311**:753, 1995.
364. Nishimura H, Takeya H, Suehiro K, Okamura T, Niho Y, Iwanaga S: Factor IX Fukuoka. Substitution of ASN92 by His in the second epidermal growth factor-like domain results in defective interaction with factors VIIa/X. *J Biol Chem* **268**:24041, 1993.
365. Hamaguchi M, Matsushita T, Tanimoto M, Takahashi I, Yamamoto K, Sugiura I, Takamatsu J, Ogata K, Kamiya T, Saito H: Three distinct point mutations in the factor IX gene of three Japanese CRM$^+$ hemophilia B patients (factor IX B_M Nagoya 2, factor IX Nagoya 3 and 4). *Thromb Haemost* **65**:514, 1991.
366. Chen S-H, Thompson AR, Zhang M, Scott CR: Three point mutations in the factor IX genes of five hemophilia B patients: Identification strategy using localization by altered epitopes in their hemophilic proteins. *J Clin Invest* **84**:113, 1989.
367. Wang NS, Thompson AR, Chen S-H: Factor $IX_{CHONGQING}$: A new mutation in the calcium-binding domain of factor IX resulting in severe hemophilia B. *Thromb Haemost* **63**:24, 1990.
368. Zhang L, Jhingan A, Castellino FJ: Role of individual γ-carboxyglutamic acid residues of activated human protein C in defining its in vitro anticoagulant activity. *Blood* **80**:942, 1992.
369. Davis LM, McGraw RA, Ware JL, Roberts HR, Stafford DW: Factor $IX_{ALABAMA}$: A point mutation in a clotting protein results in hemophilia B. *Blood* **69**:140, 1987.
370. McCord DM, Monroe DM, Smith KJ, Roberts HR: Characterization of the functional defect in factor IX Alabama. *J Biol Chem* **265**:10250, 1990.
371. Lozier JN, Monroe DM, Stanfield-Oakley S, Lin S-W, Smith KJ, Roberts HR, High KA: Factor IX New London: Substitution of proline for glutamine at position 50 causes severe hemophilia B. *Blood* **75**:1097, 1990.
372. Green PM, Bentley DR, Mibashan RS, Nilsson IM, Giannelli F: Molecular pathology of haemophilia B. *EMBO J* **8**:1067, 1989.
373. Chung K-S, Madar DA, Goldsmith JC, Kingdon HS, Roberts HR: Purification and characterization of an abnormal factor IX (Christmas factor) molecule. *J Clin Invest* **62**:1078, 1978.
374. Noyes CM, Griffith MJ, Roberts HR, Lundblad RL: Identification of the molecular defect in factor $IX_{CHAPEL\ HILL}$: Substitution of histidine for arginine at position 145. *Proc Natl Acad Sci U S A* **80**:4200, 1983.
375. Griffith MJ, Breitkreutz L, Trapp H, Briët E, Noyes CM, Lundblad RL, Roberts HR: Characterization of the clotting activities of structurally different forms of activated factor IX. Enzymatic properties of normal human factor IXaa, factor IXab, and activated factor $IX_{CHAPEL\ HILL}$. *J Clin Invest* **75**:4, 1985.
376. Toomey JR, Stafford D, Smith K: Factor IX Albuquerque (arginine 145 to cysteine) is cleaved slowly by factor XIa and has reduced coagulant activity. *Blood* **72**(Suppl 1):312, 1988.
377. Bertina RM, van der Linden IK, Mannucci PM, Reinalda-Poot HH, Cupers R, Poort SR, Reitsma PH: Mutations in hemophilia B_m occur at the Arg180-Val activation site or in the catalytic domain of factor IX. *J Biol Chem* **265**:10876, 1990.
378. Suehiro K, Kawabata S-I, Miyata T, Takeya H, Takamatsu J, Ogata K, Kamiya T, Saito H, Niho Y, Iwanaga S: Blood clotting factor IX B_M Nagoya: Substitution of arginine 180 by tryptophan and its activation by α-chymotrypsin and rat mast cell chymase. *J Biol Chem* **264**:21257, 1989.
379. Monroe DM, McCord DM, Huang M-N, High KA, Lundblad RL: Functional consequences of an arginine-180 to glutamine mutation in factor IX Hilo. *Blood* **73**:1540, 1989.
380. Solera J, Magallén M, Martin-Villar J, Coloma A: Identification of a new haemophilia B_M case produced by a mutation located at the carboxy terminal cleavage site of activation peptide. *Br J Haematol* **78**:385, 1991.
381. Chen S-H, Zhang M, Lovrien EW, Scott CR, Thompson AR: CG dinucleotide transitions in the factor IX gene account for about half of the point mutations in hemophilia B patients: A Seattle series. *Hum Genet* **87**:177, 1991.
382. Ludwig M, Sabharwal AK, Brackmann HH, Olek K, Smith KJ, Birktoft JJ, Bajaj SP: Hemophilia B caused by five different nondeletion mutations in the protease domain of factor IX. *Blood* **79**:1225, 1992.
383. Thompson AR, Chen S-H, Brayer GD: Severe hemophilia B due to a G to T transversion changing GLY 309 to VAL and inhibiting active protease conformation by preventing ion pair formation. *Blood* **74**:134, 1989.
384. Miyata T, Sakai T, Sugimoto M, Naka H, Yamamoto K, Yoshioka A, Fukui H, Mitsui K, Kamiya K, Umeyama H, Iwanaga S: Factor IX Amagasaki: A new mutation in the catalytic domain resulting in the loss of both coagulant and esterase activities. *Biochemistry* **30**:11286, 1991.
385. Miyata T, Kuze K, Matsusue T, Komooka H, Kaniya K, Umeyama H, Matsui A, Kato H, Yoshioka A: Factor IX B_m Kiryu: A Val-313 to Asp substitution in the catalytic domain results in loss of function due to a conformational change of the surface loop: Evidence obtained by chimaeric modeling. *Br J Haematol* **88**:156, 1994.
386. Koeberl DD, Bottema CDK, Ketterling RP, Bridge PJ, Lillicrap DP, Sommer SS: Mutations causing hemophilia B: Direct estimate of the underlying rates of spontaneous germ-line transitions, transversions, and deletions in a human gene. *Am J Hum Genet* **47**:202, 1990.
387. Bajaj SP, Spitzer SG, Welsh WJ, Warn-Cramer BJ, Kasper CK, Birktoft JJ: Experimental and theoretical evidence supporting the role of Gly363 in blood coagulation factor IXa (Gly193 in chymotrypsin) for proper activation of the proenzyme. *J Biol Chem* **265**:2956, 1990.
388. Vidaud M, Attree O, Schaad O, Vidaud D, Edelstein S, Goossens M: Self-inhibition of factor IX by a Gly to Arg mutation at the substrate binding pocket is linked to severe hemophilia B. *Blood* **72**(Suppl 1):313, 1988.
389. Attree O, Vidaud D, Vidaud M, Amselem S, Lavergene J-M, Goossens M: Mutations in the catalytic domain of human coagulation factor IX: Rapid characterization by direct genomic sequencing of DNA fragments displaying an altered melting behavior. *Genomics* **4**:266, 1989.
390. Ware J, Davis L, Frazier D, Bajaj SP, Stafford DW: Genetic defect responsible for the dysfunctional protein: Factor $IX_{LONG\ BEACH}$. *Blood* **72**:820, 1988.
391. Spitzer SG, Warn-Cramer BJ, Kasper CK, Bajaj SP: Replacement of isoleucine-397 by threonine in the clotting proteinase factor IXa (Los Angeles and Long Beach variants) affects macromolecular catalysis but not L-tosylarginine methyl ester hydrolysis. *Biochem J* **265**:219, 1990.
392. Geddes VA, Le Bonniec BF, Louie GV, Brayer GD, Thompson AR, MacGillivray RTA: A moderate form of hemophilia B is caused by a novel mutation in the protease domain of factor $IX_{VANCOUVER}$. *J Biol Chem* **264**:4689, 1989.
393. Hamaguchi N, Charifson PS, Pedersen LG, Brayer GD, Smith KJ, Stafford DW: Expression and characterization of human factor IX: Factor $IX_{thr\text{-}397}$ and factor $IX_{val\text{-}397}$. *J Biol Chem* **266**:15213, 1991.
394. Spitzer SG, Pendurthi UR, Kasper CK, Bajaj SP: Molecular defect in factor IX B_m Lake Elsinore: Substitution of Ala390 by Val in the catalytic domain. *J Biol Chem* **263**:10545, 1988.
395. Sugimoto M, Miyata T, Kawabata S, Yoshioka A, Fukui H, Takahashi H, Iwanaga S: Blood clotting factor IX Niigata: Substitution of alanine-390 by valine in the catalytic domain. *J Biochem* **104**:878, 1988.
396. Hougie C, Twomey JJ: Haemophilia B_M: A new type of factor IX deficiency. *Lancet* **1**:698, 1967.
397. Osterud B, Kasper CK, Lavine KK, Prodanos C, Rapaport SI: Purification and properties of an abnormal coagulation factor IX (factor IX B_m sub): Kinetics of its inhibition of factor X activation by factor VII and bovine tissue factor. *Thromb Haemost* **45**:55, 1981.

398. Sakai T, Yoshioka A, Yamamoto K, Niinomi K, Fujimura Y, Fukui H, Miyata T, Iwanaga S: Blood clotting factor IX Kashihara: Amino acid substitution of valine-182 by phenylalanine. *J Biochem* **105**:756, 1989.
399. Taylor SAM, Liddell MB, Peake IR, Bloom AL, Lillicrap DP: A mutation adjacent to the beta cleavage site of factor IX (valine 182 to leucine) results in mild haemophilia B_M. *Br J Haematol* **75**:217, 1990.
400. Green PM, Montandon AJ, Ljung R, Nilsson IM, Giannelli F: Haplotype analysis of identical factor IX mutants using PCR. *Thromb Haemost* **67**:66, 1992.
401. Thompson AR, Bajaj SP, Chen S-H, MacGillivray RTA: Founder effect in different families with haemophilia B mutation. *Lancet* **335**:418, 1990.
402. Bottema CDK, Koeberl DD, Ketterling RP, Bowie EJW, Taylor SAM, Lillicrap D, Shapiro A, Gilchrist G, Sommer SS: A past mutation at Isoleucine-397 is now a common cause of moderate/mild haemophilia B. *Br J Haematol* **75**:212, 1990.
403. Ketterling RP, Bottema CDK, Koeberl DD, Ii S, Sommer SS: T^{296}-M, a common mutation causing mild hemophilia B in the Amish and others: Founder effect, variability in factor IX activity assays, and rapid carrier detection. *Hum Genet* **87**:333, 1991.
404. Ketterling RP, Bottema CDK, Phillips III JA, Sommer SS: Evidence that descendants of three founders constitute about 25 percent of hemophilia B in the United States. *Genomics* **10**:1093, 1991.
405. Brocker-Vriends AHJT, Bakker E, Kanhai HHH, van Ommen GJB, Reitsma PH, van de Kamp JJP, Briet E: The contribution of DNA analysis to carrier detection and prenatal diagnosis of hemophilia A and B. *Ann Hematol* **64**:2, 1992.
406. Giannelli F, Choo KH, Winship PR, Rizza CR, Anson DS, Rees DJG, Ferrari N, Brownlee GG: Characterization and use of an intragenic polymorphic marker for detection of carriers of haemophilia B (factor IX deficiency). *Lancet* **1**:239, 1984.
407. Winship PR, Anson DS, Rizza CR, Brownlee GG: Carrier detection in haemophilia B using two further intragenic restriction fragment length polymorphisms. *Nucleic Acids Res* **12**:8861, 1984.
408. Camerino G, Oberlé I, Drayna D, Mandel JL: A new *Msp*I restriction fragment length polymorphism in the hemophilia B locus. *Hum Genet* **71**:79, 1985.
409. Hay CW, Robertson KA, Yong S-L, Thompson AR, Growe GH, MacGillivray RTA: Use of a *Bam*HI polymorphism in the factor IX gene for the determination of hemophilia B carrier status: *Blood* **67**:1508, 1986.
410. Tsang TC, Bentley DR, Nilsson IM, Giannelli F: The use of DNA amplification for genetic counselling related diagnosis in haemophilia B. *Thromb Haemost* **61**:343, 1989.
411. Winship PR, Rees DJG, Alkan M: Detection of polymorphisms at cytosine phosphoguanadine dinucleotides and diagnosis of haemophilia B carriers. *Lancet* **1**:631, 1989.
412. Thompson AR, Chen S-H: Characterization of factor IX defects in hemophilia B patients, in Lorand L, Mann KG (eds): *Proteolytic Enzymes in Coagulation, Fibrinolysis and Complement Fixation*. Academic Press, San Diego, 1993. p. 206–237.
413. Green PM, Montandon AJ, Ljung R, Bentley DR, Nilsson IM, Kling S, Giannelli F: Haemophilia B mutations in a complete Swedish population sample: A test of new strategy for the genetic counselling of diseases with high mutational heterogeneity. *Br J Haematol* **78**:390, 1991.
414. Fraser BM, Poon M-C, Hoar DI: Identification of factor IX mutations in haemophilia B: Application of polymerase chain reaction and single strand conformation analysis. *Hum Genet* **88**:426, 1992.
415. Chan V, Yip B, Tong TMF, Chang TPT, Lau K, Yam I, Chan TK: Molecular defects in haemophilia B: Detection by direct restriction enzyme analysis. *Br J Haematol* **79**:63, 1991.
416. Matsushita T, Tanimoto M, Yamamoto K, Sugiura I, Takamatsu J, Kamiya T, Saito H: Direct carrier detection in hemophilia B kindreds: Use of modified primers (mutagenic primers) for enzymatic amplification of the factor IX gene. *Thromb Res* **63**:355, 1991.
417. Forbes CD: Clinical aspects of the hemophilias and their treatment, in Ratnoff OD, Forbes CD (eds): *Disorders of Hemostasis*. Orlando, FL, Grune and Stratton, 1984, p 177.
418. Duthie RB, Matthews JM, Rizza CR, Steel WM, Woods CG: The management of musculo-skeletal problems in the haemophiliacs. Oxford, Blackwell Scientific, 1972.
419. De Valderrama JAF, Matthews JM: The haemophilic pseudotumour of haemophilic subperiosteal haematoma. *J Bone Joint Surg (Br)* **47**:256, 1965.
420. Gilbert MS: The hemophilic pseudotumor. *Prog Clin Biol Res* **324**:257, 1990.
421. Larsson SA, Wiechel B: Deaths in Swedish hemophiliacs, 1957–1980. *Acta Med Scand* **214**:199, 1983.
422. Forbes CD, Prentice CRM: Mortality in haemophilia — A United Kingdom survey, in Fratantoni JC, Aronson DL (eds): *Unsolved Therapeutic Problems in Hemophilia*. Washington, DC, Department of Health, Education, and Welfare, Publication No. (NIH) 77-10899, 1977, p 15.
423. Duthie RB, Rizza CR: Rheumatological manifestations of the haemophiliacs. *Clin Rheum Dis* **1**:53, 1975.
424. Petersson H, Ahlberg A, Nilsson IM: A radiologic classification of hemophilic arthropathy. *Clin Orthop* **149**:153, 1980.
425. Kasper CK, Dietrich SL: Comprehensive management of haemophilia, in Ruggeri ZM (ed): *Clinics in Hematology Coagulation Disorders*, Vol 14/No 2. London, WB Saunders, 1985, p 489.
426. Zauber NP, Levin J: Factor IX levels in patients with hemophilia B (Christmas disease) following transfusion with concentrates of factor IX or fresh frozen plasma. *Medicine (Baltimore)* **56**:213, 1977.
427. Smith KJ, Thompson AR: Labeled factor IX kinetics in patients with hemophilia B. *Blood* **58**:625, 1981.
428. Nilsson IM, Ahlberg A, Bjorlin G: Clinical experience with a Swedish factor IX concentrate. *Acta Med Scand* **19**:257, 1974.
429. Goldberg VM, Heiple KG, Ratnoff OD, Kurczynski E, Arvan G: Total knee arthroplasty in classic hemophilia. *J Bone Joint Surg* **63**:695, 1981.
430. Lachiewicz PF, Inglis AE, Insall JN, Sculco TP, Hilgartner MW, Bussel JB: Total knee arthroplasty in hemophilia. *J Bone Joint Surg* **67A**:1361, 1985.
431. Nelson IW, Sivamurugan S, Latham PD, Matthews J, Bulstrode CJK: Total hip arthroplasty for hemophilic arthropathy. *Clin Orthop* **276**:210, 1992.
432. Storti E, Ascri E: Surgical and chemical synovectomy. *Ann N Y Acad Sci* **240**:316, 1975.
433. Storti E, Ascari E, Gamba G: Postoperative complications and joint function after knee synovectomy in haemophiliacs. *Br J Haematol* **50**:544, 1982.
434. Scarponi R, Silvello L, Landonio G, Baudo F, De Cataldo F: Long-term evaluation of knee-joint function after synovectomy in haemophilia. *Br J Haematol* **52**:337, 1982.
435. Klein K, Aland C, Kim H, Eisele J, Saidi P: Long-term follow-up of arthroscopic synovectomy for chronic hemophilic synovitis. *Arthroscopy* **3**:231, 1987.
436. Wiedel JD: Arthroscopy of the knee in hemophilia. *Prog Clin Biol Res* **324**:231, 1990.
437. Lofqvist T, Pettersson C: Experience with colloid ^{198}Au synoviorthesis in hemophiliacs. *Ric Clin Lab* **16**:97, 1986.
438. Espinosa C, Caballero O, Aznar JA, Querol F: Synoviorthesis with ^{90}Y in hemophilic chronic synovitis. *Ric Clin Lab* **16**:97, 1986.
439. Rivard GE: Synoviorthesis with radioactive colloids in hemophiliacs, in Kasper C (ed): Recent Advances in Hemophilia Care. *Prog Clin Biol Res* **324**:215, 1990.
440. Nilsson IM, Berntorp E, Lofqvist T, Pettersson H: Twenty-five years' experience of prophylactic treatment in severe haemophilia A and B. *J Intern Med* **232**:25, 1992.
441. Brettler DB, Forsberg AD, O'Conell FD, Cederbaum AI, Chaitman AK, Levine PH: A long-term study of hemophilic arthropathy of the knee joint on a program of factor VIII replacement given at time of each hemoarthrosis. *Am J Hematol* **18**:13, 1985.
442. Steven MM, Yogarajah S, Madhok R, Forbes CD, Sturrock RD: Haemophilic arthritis. *QJM* **226**:181, 1986.
443. Guenthner EE, Hilgartner MW, Miller CH, Vienne G: Hemophilic arthropathy: Effect of home care on treatment patterns and joint disease. *J Pediatr* **97**:378, 1980.
444. Ingram GIC, Dykes SR, Creese AL, Mellor P, Swan AV, Karufert J, Rizza CR, Spooner RJD, Biggs R: Home treatment in haemophilia: Clinical, social and economic advantages. *Clin Lab Haematol* **1**:13, 1979.
445. Soulier JP, Blatrix C, Steinbach M: Fractions "coagulants" contenant les facteurs de coagulation absorbables par le phosphate tricalcique. *Presse Med* **72**:1223, 1964.
446. Bidwell E, Booth JM, Dike GWR: The preparation for therapeutic use of a concentrate of factor IX containing also factors II, VII, and X. *Br J Haematol* **13**:568, 1967.
447. Tullis JL, Melin M, Jurgian P: Clinical use of human prothrombin complexes. *N Engl J Med* **273**:667, 1965.

448. Kasper CK: Clinical use of prothrombin complex concentrates: Report on thromboembolic complications. *Thromb Diath Haemorrh* **33**:640, 1975.
449. Wasely LC, Rehemtulla A, Bristol JA, Kaufman RJ: PACE/Furin can process the vitamin K-dependent pro-factor IX precursor within the secretory pathway. *J Biol Chem* **286**:8458, 1993.
450. White GC, Beebe A, Nielsen B: Recombinant factor IX. *Thomb Haemost* **78**:261, 1997.
451. White G, Shapiro A, Ragni M, Garzone P, Goodfellow J, Tubridy K, Courter S: Clinical evaluation of recombinant factor IX. *Semin Hematol* **35(Suppl 2)**:33, 1998.
452. Harrison S, Adamson S, Bonam D, Brodeur T, Charlebois T, Clancy B, Costigan R, Drapeau D, Hamilton M, Hanely K, Kelley B, Knight A, Leonard M, McCarthy M, Oakes P, Sterl K, Switzer M, Walsh R, Foster W: The manufacturing process for recombinant factor IX. *Semin Hematol* **35(Suppl 2)**:4, 1998.
453. Adamson S, Webb C, Bartlett L, Burnett B: Viral safety of recombinant factor IX. *Semin Hematol* **35(Suppl 2)**:22, 1998.
454. Bond M, Janowski M, Patel H, Karnik S, Strang A, Xu B, Rouse J, Koza S, Letwin B, Steckert J, Amphlett G, Scoble H: Biochemical characterization of recombinant factor IX. *Semin Hematol* **35(Suppl 2)**:11, 1998.
455. Lusher JM: Thrombogenicity associated with factor IX complex concentrates. *Semin Hematol* **28(Suppl 6)**:3, 1991.
456. Hedner U, Nilsson IM, Bergentz SE: Various prothrombin complex concentrates and their effect on coagulation and fibrinolysis in vivo. *Thromb Haemost* **35**:386, 1979.
457. White GC II, Roberts HR, Kingdon HS, Lundblad RL: Prothrombin complex concentrates: Potentially thrombogenic materials and clues to the mechanism of thrombosis in vivo. *Blood* **49**:159, 1977.
458. Hultin MB: Activated clotting factors in prothrombin complex concentrates. *Blood* **54**:1028, 1979.
459. Aronson DL, Menache D: Thrombogenicity of factor IX complex: In vivo investigation. *Dev Biol Stand* **67**:149, 1987.
460. Giles AR, Nesheim ME, Hoogendoorn H, Tracy PB, Mann KG: The coagulant-active phospholipid content is a major determinant of in vivo thrombogenicity of prothrombin complex (factor IX) concentrates in rabbits. *Blood* **59**:401, 1982.
461. Smith KJ: Factor IX concentrates: The new products and their properties. *Transfus Med Rev* **6**:124, 1992.
462. Thompson AR: Clinical factor IX concentrates. *Semin Thromb Hemost* **19**:25, 1993.
463. White GC, Shapiro AD, Kurczynski EM, Kim HC, Bergman GE: Variability of in vivo recovery of factor IX after infusion of monoclonal antibody purified factor IX concentrates in patients with hemophilia B. The Mononine study group. *Thromb Haemost* **73**:779, 1995.
464. Menache D, Behre HE, Orthner CL, Nunez H, Anderson HD, Triantaphyllopoulos DC, Kosow DP: Coagulation factor IX concentrate: Method of preparation and assessment of potential in vivo thrombogenicity in animal models. *Blood* **64**:1220, 1984.
465. Mannucci PM, Bauer KA, Gringeri A, Barzegar S, Bottasso B, Simoni L, Rosenberg RD: Thrombin generation is not increased in the blood of hemophilia B patients after the infusion of a purified factor IX concentrate. *Blood* **76**:2540, 1990.
466. Bardin JM, Sultan Y: Factor IX concentrate versus prothrombin complex concentrate for the treatment of hemophilia B during surgery. *Transfusion* **30**:441, 1990.
467. MacGregor IR, Ferguson JM, McLaughlin LF, Burnouf T, Prowse CV: Comparison of high purity factor IX concentrates and a prothrombin complex concentrate in a canine model of thrombogenicity. *Thromb Haemost* **66**:609, 1991.
468. Kim HC, McMillan CW, White GC, Bergman GE, Horton MW, Saidi P: Purified factor IX using monoclonal immunoaffinity technique: Clinical trials in hemophilia B and comparison to prothrombin complex concentrates. *Blood* **79**:568, 1992.
469. Goldsmith JC, Kasper CK, Blatt PM, Gomperts ED, Kessler CM, Thompson AR, Herring SW, Novak PL: Coagulation factor IX: Successful surgical experience with a purified factor IX concentrate. *Am J Hematol* **40**:210, 1992.
470. Goedert JJ, Kessler CM, Aledort LM, Biggar RJ, Andes WA, White GC, Drummond JE, Vaidya K, Mann DL, Eyster ME, Ragni MV, Lederman MM, Cohen AR, Gray GL, Rosenberg PS, Friedman RM, Hilgartner MR, Blattner WA, Kroner B, Gail MH: A prospective study of human immunodeficiency virus type 1 infection and the development of AIDS in subjects with hemophilia. *N Engl J Med* **321**:1141, 1989.
471. Choo QL, Kuo G, Weiner AJ: Isolation of a cDNA clone derived from blood borne non A, non B viral hepatitis genome. *Science* **244**:359, 1989.
472. Kuo G, Choo Q-L, Alter HJ, Gitnick GL, Redeker AG, Purcell RH, Miyamura T, Dienstag JL, Alter MJ, Stevens CE, Tegtmeier GE, Bonino F, Colombo M, Lee W-S, Kuo C, Berger K, Shuster JR, Overby LR, Bradley DW, Houghton M: An assay for circulating antibodies to a major etiologic virus of human non-A, non-B hepatitis. *Science* **244**:362, 1989.
473. Allain J-P, Dailey SH, Laurian Y, Vallari DS, Rafowicz A, Desai SM, Devare SG: Evidence for persistent hepatitis C virus (HCV) infection in hemophiliacs. *J Clin Invest* **88**:1672, 1991.
474. Watson HG, Ludlam CA, Rebus S, Zhang LQ, Peutherer JF, Simmonds P: Use of several second generation serological assays to determine the true prevalence of hepatitis C virus infection in haemophiliacs treated with non-virus inactivated factor VIII and IX concentrates. *Br J Haematol* **80**:514, 1992.
475. Hay CRM, Preston FE, Triger DR: Progressive liver disease in haemophiliacs: An understated problem? *Lancet* **1**:1495, 1985.
476. Makris M, Preston FE, Triger DR, Underwood JCE, Choo Q-L, Kuo G, Moughton M: Hepatitis C antibody and chronic liver disease in haemophilia. *Lancet* **355**:1117, 1990.
477. Esteban JI, Gonzalez G, Hernandez JM, Viladomiu L, Sanchez C, Lopez-Talevera JC, Luccea D, Martin-Vega C, Vidal X, Esteban R, Guardia J: Evaluation of antibodies to hepatitis C virus in a study of transfusion-associated hepatitis. *N Engl J Med* **323**:1107, 1990.
478. Colvin BT, Rizza CR, Hill FGH, Kernoff PBA, Bateman CJT, Bolton-Maggs P, Daly HM, Kenny MW, Taylor PC, Mitchell VE, Wensley RT, Whitmore DN, Lane RS, Smith JK: Effect of dry-heating of coagulation factor concentrates at 80°C for 72 hours on transmission of non-A, non-B hepatitis. *Lancet* **2**:814, 1988.
479. Skidmore SJ, Pasi KJ, Mawson SJ, Williams MD, Hill FGH: Serological evidence that dry heating of clotting factor concentrates prevents transmission of non-A, non-B hepatitis. *J Med Virol* **30**:50, 1990.
480. Kreuz W, Auerswald G, Bruckmann C, Zieger B, Linde R, Funk M, Auberger K, Sutor AH, Rasshofer R, Roggendorf M: Prevention of hepatitis C virus infection in children with haemophilia A and B and von Willebrand's disease. *Thromb Haemost* **67**:184, 1992.
481. Horowitz MS, Rooks C, Horowitz B, Hilgartner MW: Virus safety of solvent/detergent-treated antihaemophilic factor concentrate. *Lancet* **2**:186, 1988.
482. Blanchette VS, Vorstman E, Shore A, Wang E, Petric M, Jett BW, Alter HJ: Hepatitis C infection in children with hemophilia A and B. *Blood* **78**:285, 1991.
483. Carnelli V, Gomperts ED, Friedman A, Aledort L, Hilgartner M, Dietrich S, Fedor EJ: Assessment for evidence of non A-non B hepatitis in patients given *n*-Heptane-suspended heat-treated clotting factor concentrates. *Thromb Res* **47**:827, 1987.
484. Lee CA, Kernoff PBA, Karayiannis P, Thomas HC: Interferon therapy for chronic non-A non-B and chronic delta disease in haemophilia. *Br J Haematol* **72**:235, 1989.
485. Makris M, Preston FE, Triger DR, Adelman MI, Underwood JCE: A prospective randomized controlled liver biopsy study of recombinant alpha interferon in chronic non-A non-B hepatitis in haemophilia. *Br J Haematol* **71(Suppl 1)**:19, 1989.
486. Bontempo FA, Lewis JH, Corenc TJ, Spero JA, Ragni MV, Scott JP, Starzl TE: Liver transplantation in hemophilia A. *Blood* **69**:1721, 1987.
487. Lyon DJ, Chapman CS, Martin C, Brown KE, Clewley JP, Flower AJE, Mitchell VE: Symptomatic parvovirus B19 infection and heat-treated factor IX concentrate. *Lancet* **1**:1085, 1989.
488. Morfini M, Longo G, Rossi Ferrini P, Azzi A, Zakrewska C, Ciappi S, Kolumban P: Hypoplastic anemia in a hemophiliac first infused with a solvent/detergent treated factor VIII concentrate: The role of human B19 parvovirus. *Am J Hematol* **39**:149, 1992.
489. Yee TT, Cohen BJ, Pasi KJ, Lee CA: Transmission of symptomatic parvovirus B19 infection by clotting factor concentrate. *Br J Hematol* **93**:457, 1996.
490. Lefrere JJ, Mariotti M, Thauvin M: B19 parvovirus in slovent/detergent-treated anti-hemophilia concentrates. *Lancet* **343(8891)**:211, 1994.
491. Santagostino E, Mannucci PM, Gringeri A, Azzi A, Morfini M, Musso R, Santoro R, Schiavoni M: Transmission of parvovirus B19 by coagulation factor concentrates exposed to100 degrees C heat after lyholization. *Transfusion* **37**:517, 1997.

492. Hedner U, Sundqvist SB, Nilsson IM: Immunosuppressive treatment in haemophiliacs with inhibitors, in *The State of Art of Managing Hemophilia with FVIII Inhibitors*, Proceedings of the International Meeting on Activated Prothrombin Complex Concentrates. New York, Praeger, 1982. p 68-92.
493. Nilsson IM, Jonsson S, Sundqvist S-B, Ahlberg A, Bergentz S-E: A procedure for removing high-titer antibodies by extracorporeal protein-A-Sepharose adsorption in hemophilia: Substitution therapy and surgery in a patient with hemophilia B and antibodies. *Blood* **58**:38, 1981.
494. Uehlinger J, Button GR, McCarthy J, Forster A, Watt R, Aledort LM: Immunoadsorption for coagulation factor inhibitors. *Transfusion* **31**:265, 1991.
495. Theodorsson B, Hedner U, Nilsson IM, Kisiel W: A technique for specific removal of factor IX alloantibodies from human plasma: Partial characterization of the alloantibodies. *Blood* **61**:973, 1983.
496. Schmidt ML, Smith HE, Gamerman S, DiMichele D, Glazer S, Scott JP: Prolonged recombinant activated factor VII (rFVIIa) treatment for severe bleeding in a factor-IX-deficient patient with an inhibitor. *Br J Haematol* **78**:460, 1991.
497. Hedner U, Nilsson IM: Induced tolerance in hemophilia patients with antibodies against IX:C. *Acta Med Scand* **214**:191, 1983.
498. Nilsson IM, Sundqvist S-B, Ljung R, Holmberg L, Freiburghaus C, Bjorlin G: Suppression of secondary antibody response by intravenous immunoglobulin in a patient with haemophilia B and antibodies. *Scand J Haematol* **30**:458, 1983.
499. Nilsson IM, Berntorp E, Zettervall O: Induction of split tolerance and clinical cure in high-responding hemophiliacs with factor IX antibodies. *Proc Natl Acad Sci U S A* **83**:9169, 1986.
500. Kaufman RJ, Wasley LC, Furie BC, Furie B, Shoemaker CB: Expression, purification, and characterization of recombinant γ-carboxylated factor IX synthesized in Chinese hamster ovary cells. *J Biol Chem* **261**:9622, 1986.
501. Balland A, Faure T, Carvallo D, Cordier P, Ulrich P, Fournet B, de la Salle H, Lecocq J-P: Characterization of two differently processed forms of human recombinant factor IX synthesized in CHO cells transformed with a polycistronic vector. *Eur J Biochem* **172**:565, 1988.
502. Miller AD: Human gene therapy comes of age. *Nature* **357(6378)**:455, 1992.
503. Thompson AR: Progress towards gene therapy for the hemophilias. *Thromb Haemost* **74**:45, 1995.
504. Brinkhous KM: Gene therapy and the hemophilias. *JAMA* **271**:47, 1994.
505. Eisensmith RC, Woo SLC: Viral vector mediated gene therapy for hemophilia B. *Thromb Haemost* **78**:24, 1997.
506. Kay MA, Rothenberg S, landen C, Bellinger D, Leland F, Toman C, Finegold M, Thompson AR, Read MS, Brinkhous KM, Woo SLC: In vivo gene therapy for hemophilia B: Sustained partial correction in factor IX deficient dogs. *Science* **262**:117, 1993.
507. Yao SN, Wilson JM, Nabel EG, Kurachi S, Hachiya HL, Kurachi K: Expression of human factor IX in rat capillary endothelial cells: toward somatic gene threrapy for hemophilia B. *Proc Natl Acad Sci U S A* **88**:8101, 1991.
508. Gerrard AJ, Hudson DL, Brownlee GG, Watt FM: Towards gene therapy for hemophilia B using primary human keratinocytes. *Nat Genet* **3**:180, 1993.
509. Hao QL, Malik P, Slalazar R, Tang H, Gordon EM, Kohn DB: Expression of biologically active human factor IX in human hematopoietic cells after retroviral vector-mediated gene transduction. *Hum Gene Ther* **6**:873, 1995.
510. Kay MA, Landen CN, Rothenberg SR, Taylor LA, Leland F, Wiehle S, Fang B, Bellinger D, Finegold D, Thompson AR, Read M, Brinkhous KM, Woo SLC: In vivo hepatic gene therapy: Complete, albeit transient, correction of factor IX deficiency in hemophilia B dogs. *Proc Natl Acad Sci U S A* **91**:2353, 1994.
511. Koeberl DD, Alexander IE, Halbert CL, Russell DW, Miller AD: Persistent expression of human clotting factor IX from mouse liver after intravenous injection of adeno-associated virus vectors. *Proc Natl Acad Sci U S A* **98**:1426, 1997.
512. Snyder RO, Miao CH, Patijn GA, Spratt SK, Danos O, Nagy D, Gown AM, Winther B, Meuse L, Cohen LK, Thompson AR, Kay MA: Persistent and therapeutic concentrations of human factor IX in mice after hepatic gene transfer of recombinant AAV vectors. *Nat Genet* **16**:270, 1997.
513. Monahan PE, Samulski RJ, Tazelaar J, Xiao X, Nichols TC, Bellinger DA, Read MS, Walsh CE: Direct intramuscular injection with recombinant AAV vectors resustls in sustained expression in a dog model of hemophilia. *Gene Ther* **5**:40, 1998.
514. Palmer TD, Thompson AR, Miller AD: Production of human factor IX in animals by genetically modified skin fibroblasts: Potential therapy for hemophilia B. *Blood* **73**:438, 1989.
515. Dai Y, Roman M, Naviaux RK, Verma IM: Gene therapy via primary myoblasts: Long-term expression of factor IX protein following transplantation in vivo. *Proc Natl Acad Sci U S A* **89**:10892, 1992.
516. DiScipio RG, Hermondson MA, Davie EW: Activation of human factor X (Stuart factor) by a protease from Russell's viper venom. *Biochemistry* **16**:5253, 1977.
517. van Dieijen G, Tans G, Rosing J, Hemker HC: The role of phospholipid and factor VIIIa in the activation of bovine factor X. *J Biol Chem* **256**:3433, 1981.
518. Ahmad SS, Rawala-Sheikh R, Walsh PN: Components and assembly of the factor X activating complex. *Semin Thromb Hemost* **18**:311, 1992.
519. McGee MP, Li LC: Functional difference between intrinsic and extrinsic coagulation pathways. Kinetics of factor X activation on human monocytes and alveolar macrophages. *J Biol Chem* **266**:8079, 1991.
520. Huang M-N, Hung H-L, Stanfield-Oakley SA, High KA: Characterization of the human blood coagulation factor X promoter. *J Biol Chem* **267**:15440, 1992.
521. Miao CH, Leytus SP, Chung DW, Davie EW: Liver-specific expression of the gene coding for human factor X, a blood coagulation factor. *J Biol Chem* **267**:7395, 1992.
522. Jaye M, Ricca G, Kaplan R, Howk R, Mudd R, Ngo KY, Fair DS, Drohan W: Polymorphism associated with the human coagulation factor X (F10) gene. *Nucleic Acids Res* **13**:8286, 1985.
523. Hay CW, Robertson KA, Fung MR, MacGillivray RTA: RFLPs for PstI and EcoRI in the human blood clotting factor X gene. *Nucleic Acids Res* **14**:5118, 1986.
524. Hassan HJ, Guerriero R, Chelucci C, Leonardi A, Mattia G, Leone G, Mariani G, Mannucci PM, Peschle C: Multiple polymorphic sites in factor X locus. *Blood* **71**:1353, 1988.
525. Wallmark A, Rose VL, Ho C, High KA: A NlaIV polymorphism within the human factor X gene. *Nucleic Acids Res* **19**:426, 1991.
526. Duckert F, Fluckiger P, Matter M, Koller F: Clotting factor X: Physiologic and physico-chemical properties. *Proc Soc Exp Biol Med* **90**:17, 1955.
527. Telfer TP, Denson KW, Wright DR: A "new"coagulation defect. *Br J Haematol* **2**:308, 1956.
528. Hougie C, Barrow EM, Graham JB: Stuart clotting defect. I. Segregation of a hereditary hemorrhagic state from the heterogeneous group heretofore called "stable factor"(SPCA, proconvertin, factor VII) deficiency. *J Clin Invest* **36**:485, 1957.
529. Graham JB, Barrow EM, Hougie C: Stuart clotting defect II: Genetic aspects of a "new"hemorrhagic state. *J Clin Invest* **36**:497, 1957.
530. Lechler E, Webster WP, Roberts HR, Penick GD: The inheritance of Stuart disease: Investigation of a family with factor X deficiency. *Am J Med Sci* **249**:191, 1965.
531. Fair DS, Edgington TS: Heterogeneity of hereditary and acquired factor X deficiencies by combined immunochemical and functional analyses. *Br J Haematol* **59**:235, 1985.
532. Girolami A: Tentative and updated classification of factor X variants. *Acta Haematol* **75**:58, 1986.
533. Girolami A, Vicarioto M, Ruzza G, Cappellato G, Vergolani A: Factor X Padua: A "new"congenital factor X abnormality with a defect only in the extrinsic system. *Acta Haematol* **73**:31, 1985.
534. Watzke HH, Lechner K, Roberts HR, Reddy SV, Welsch DJ, Friedman P, Mahr G, Jagadeeswaran P, Monroe DM, High KA: Molecular defect (Gla^{+14}/Lys) and its functional consequences in a hereditary factor X deficiency (factor X "Vorarlberg"). *J Biol Chem* **265**:11982, 1990.
535. Nobauer-Huhmann IM, Holler W, Krinninger B, Turecek PL, Richter G, Scharrer I, Forberg E, Watzkr HH: Factor X Frankfurt I: Molecular and fuctional characterization of a hereditary factor X deficiency (Gly^{+25} to Lys). *Blood Coagul Fibrinolysis* **9**:143, 1998.
536. Miyata T, Kojima T, Suzuki K, Umeyama H, Yamazaki T, Kamiya T, Toyoda H, Kato H: Factor X Nagoya 1 and Nagoya 2; a CRM^- factor deficiency and dysfunctional CRM^+ deficiency characterized by substitiom of Arg306 by Cys and Gly366 by Ser, respectively. *Thromb Haemost* **79**:486, 1998.
537. Bezeaud A, Miyata T, Helley D, Zeng YZ, Kato H, Aillaud MF, Juhan-Vague I, Guillin MC: Functional consequences of the Ser334 to Pro mutation in a human factor X variant (factor X Marseille). *Eur J Biochem* **15**:234, 1995.

538. Parkin JD, Madares F, Sweet B, Castaldi PA: A further inherited variant of coagulation factor X. *Aust N Z J Med* **4**:561, 1974.
539. De Stefano V, Leone G, Ferrelli R, Hassa HJ, Macioce G, Bizzi B: Factor X Roma: A congenital factor X variant defective at different degrees in the intrinsic and the extrinsic activation. *Br J Haematol* **69**:387, 1988.
540. Wieland K, Millar DS, Grundy CB, Mibashan RS, Kakker VV, Cooper DN: Molecular genetic analysis of factor X deficiency: Gene deletion and germline mosaicism. *Hum Genet* **86**:273, 1991.
541. Bernardi F, Marchetti G, Patracchini P, Volinia S, Gemmati D, Simioni P, Girolami A: Partial gene deletion in a family with factor X deficiency. *Blood* **73**:2123, 1989.
542. Hayashi T, Yahagi A, Suzuki K, Sato S, Sasaki H: Molecular abnormality observed in a patient with coagulation factor X deficiency: a novel three base pair (CTT) deletion within the polypyrmidine tract of the factor X intron D. *Br J Haematol* **102**:926, 1998.
543. Asakai R, Roberts HR, Davie EW: unpublished.
544. Wallmark A, Ho C, Monroe DM, Tengborn L, High KA: Molecular defect in F.X "Ockero", a mild congenital F.X deficiency. *Thromb Haemost* **65**:1263, 1991.
545. James HL, Kumar A, Thompson AR, Fair DS: A point mutation destroys a processing site between the light and heavy chains of factor $X_{WENATCHEE}$ [Abstract 7496]. *FASEB J* **5**:A1661, 1991.
546. Girolami A, Molaro G, Lazzarin M, Scarpa R, Brunetti A: A new congenital hemorrhagic condition due to the presence of an abnormal factor X (factor X Fruili): Study of a large kindred. *Br J Haematol* **19**:179, 1970.
547. Fair DS, Revak DJ, Hubbard JG, Girolami A: Isolation and characterization of the factor X Friuli variant. *Blood* **73**:2108, 1989.
548. James HL, Girolami A, Fair DS: Molecular defect in coagulation factor X_{FRIULI} results from a substitution of serine for proline at position 343. *Blood* **77**:317, 1991.
549. Reddy SV, Zhou Z-Q, Rao KJ, Scott JP, Watzke H, High KA, Jagadeeswaran P: Molecular characterization of human factor $X_{SAN\ ANTONIO}$. *Blood* **74**:1486, 1989.
550. Korsan-Bengsten L, Hjort PF, Ygge J: Acquired factor X deficiency in a patient with amyloidosis. *Thromb Diath Haemorrh* **7**:558, 1962.
551. Smith SV, Liles DK, White GC, Brecher ME: Successful treatment of transient acquired factor X deficiency by plasmapheresis with concomitant intravenous immunoglobulin and steroid therapy. *Am J Hematol* **57**:245, 1998.
552. Roa LV, Zivelin A, Iturbe I, Rapaport SI: Antibody-induced acute factor X deficiency: Clinical manifestations and properties of the antibody. *Thromb Haemost* **72**:363, 1994.
553. Greipp PR, Kyle RA, Bowie EJW: Factor-X deficiency in amyloidosis: A critical review. *Am J Hematol* **11**:443, 1981.
554. Knight RD, Barr CF, Alving BM: Replacement therapy for congenital factor X deficiency. *Transfusion* **25**:78, 1985.
555. Messier TL, Pittman DD, Long GL, Kaufman RJ, Church WR: Cloning and expression in COS-1 cells of a full-length cDNA encoding human coagulation factor X. *Gene* **99**:291, 1991.

CHAPTER 170

Anticoagulant Protein C/Thrombomodulin Pathway

Charles T. Esmon

1. **Protein C is converted to an anticoagulant serine protease by a complex between thrombin and thrombomodulin (TM) on the surface of endothelial cells. An endothelial cell protein C/activated protein C receptor (EPCR) augments this process. Activated protein C (APC) binds to protein S on cell surfaces or on negatively charged phospholipid vesicles where the complex inactivates factor Va or factor VIIIa, thereby preventing further thrombin generation.**
2. **Protein C and protein S are vitamin K-dependent proteins. Therefore, their biosynthesis is inhibited by oral anticoagulants that function as vitamin K antagonists. Protein C levels decrease rapidly following initiation of oral anticoagulant therapy with a $t_{\frac{1}{2}} \sim 24$ h.**
3. **Homozygous protein C (MIM 176860) and protein S (MIM 176880) deficiency have been described. When the functional levels of these proteins are extremely low, infants develop purpura fulminans shortly after birth. In the case of protein C deficiency, the purpura can be successfully managed with protein C supplementation. Homozygous or compound heterozygous individuals with low, but detectable, levels of protein C may remain free of thrombosis at least until early adulthood.**
4. **Heterozygous protein C (MIM 176860) and protein S (MIM 176880) deficiency are each associated with approximately 5 percent of familial thrombophilias. Protein C deficiency appears to be relatively prevalent, affecting approximately 0.3 percent of the general population with the majority of these individuals asymptomatic. Patients with TM mutations (MIM 188040) and either arterial or venous thrombosis have been described, but the prevalence of these mutations in the general population and in thrombophilia remains uncertain. EPCR deficiencies have not been described.**
5. **A dimorphism in factor V (MIM 227400) resulting in replacement of Arg 506 with Gln is quite frequent in Caucasians (.5 percent), but much less common in other ethnic groups. Arg 506 is the first bond cleaved during factor Va inactivation and thus the substitution of Arg with Gln results in delayed factor Va inactivation, a situation known as APC resistance or factor V Leiden. Factor V can function as a cofactor for the inactivation of factor VIIIa. The Arg 506 to Gln substitution not only slows factor Va inactivation by APC, but it also appears to eliminate factor V cofactor activity in factor VIIIa inactivation.**
6. **Clinical manifestations of heterozygous protein C or protein S deficiency, and factor V Leiden include venous thrombosis and pulmonary embolism. Arterial thrombosis appears to be a less common complication of these defects in the protein C pathway. Studies have implicated TM mutations in venous thrombosis and in an increased risk of myocardial infarctions, but the epidemiology on TM defects in thrombotic disease is much less developed than for the other factors in the pathway.**

OVERVIEW OF THE PROTEIN C ANTICOAGULANT PATHWAY

The overall function of the protein C pathway is shown schematically in Fig. 170-1. Coagulation is initiated by the factor VIIa-tissue factor complex through the activation of either factor X or factor IX. The factor Xa (Xa) complexes with factor Va (Va) and factor IXa (IXa) complexes with factor VIIIa (VIIIa) to activate prothrombin (pro) or factor X (X), respectively. This process generates thrombin, the enzyme responsible for blood clotting. The protein C pathway serves as an on demand anticoagulant system. The pathway is initiated when thrombin binds to thrombomodulin (TM) on the surface of the endothelium.[1] On large blood vessels,[2] an auxiliary protein, the endothelial cell protein C receptor (EPCR), binds protein C (K_d 0.30 nM)[3] and facilitates protein C activation by the thrombin-TM complex.[4] EPCR is expressed at low levels, if at all, in the capillary circulation. Activated protein C (APC) can also bind to EPCR, but current data based on studies with soluble EPCR suggest that the APC bound to the EPCR cannot inactivate factor Va.[5] APC is bound reversibly to EPCR[3] and hence, when it dissociates, it can interact with protein S. Factor Va or VIIIa are then inactivated by a complex between APC and protein S on the surface of endothelial[6,7] or activated platelet surfaces[8–11] or negatively charged phospholipid liposomes.[12,13] Factor V, but not factor Va, can enhance APC inactivation of factor VIIIa.[14]

Defects in the protein C pathway are the most common hereditary contribution to a propensity for thrombosis. Several reviews are available on the biochemistry,[15–24] physiology, and clinical impact[25–39] of the protein C pathway. For those wishing more information on the basic aspects, a more detailed review of the biochemistry and physiology of the protein C pathway is available.[40]

Of the defects in this pathway that contribute to a propensity for thrombosis, by far the most common is a dimorphism in factor V that replaces the APC target Arg 506 with Gln.[34,37,41] This condition, known as APC resistance[42,43] or factor V Leiden,[36,44] is discussed in a separate section. To appreciate the mechanisms involved in APC resistance, it is useful to describe in considerable detail the biochemical events that are involved in factor Va inactivation.

After protein C activation by the thrombin-TM complex, APC binds to protein S to accelerate factor Va[12] and VIIIa inactivation.[45] In both cases, there is a strong preference for inactivating

A list of standard abbreviations is located immediately preceding the index in each volume. Additional abbreviations used in this chapter include: APC = activated protein C; C4BP = C4b-binding protein; EPCR = endothelial cell protein C receptor; GLA = -carboxyglutamic acid; TAFI = thrombin activatable fibrinolysis inhibitor; TM = thrombomodulin; TNF = tumor necrosis factor .

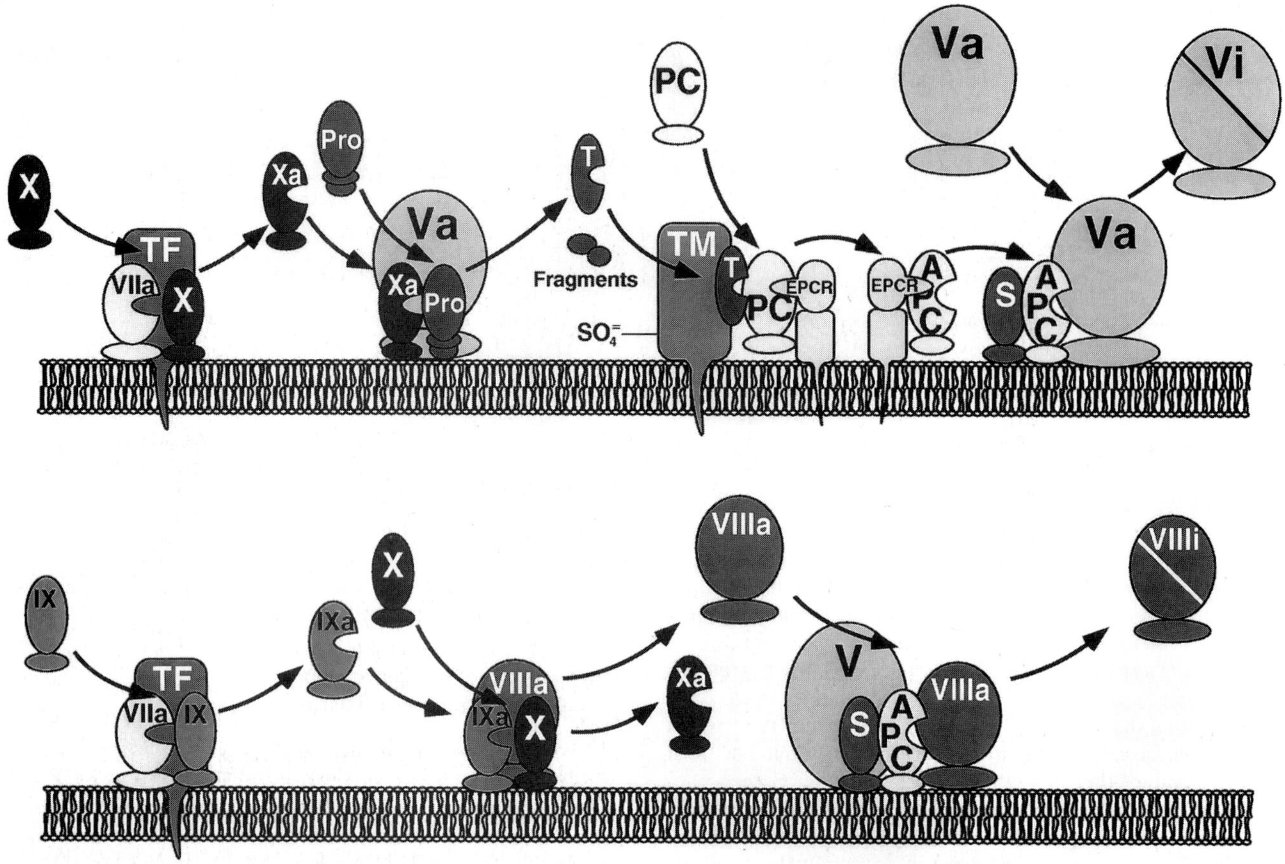

Fig. 170-1 Model of the function of the protein C anticoagulant pathway. All of the reactions of the coagulation and protein C anticoagulation pathway occur at membrane surfaces, depicted below the factors. When tissue factor is exposed to blood, factor VIIa binds and the complex activates either factor IX (IX) or factor X (X). The factor IXa-factor VIIIa complex activates factor X (X) to factor Xa (Xa). The Xa then forms a complex with factor Va to convert prothrombin (pro) to thrombin (T). T then binds to thrombomodulin (TM) to form the protein C activation complex. Protein C (PC) binds to the endothelial cell protein C receptor (EPCR), if present, and this complex is activated by the T-TM complex. In the capillary, where there is no EPCR, the protein C is activated directly by the T-TM complex. Activated protein C (APC) can remain bound to EPCR, but this complex does not seem to be capable of inactivating factor Va, presumably an indication that it is targeted to as yet unidentified alternative substrates. When APC dissociates from EPCR, it can then bind to protein S (PS). This complex inactivates factor Va or factor VIIIa, thus shutting down T formation and preventing blood clot extension. Factor VIIIa inactivation is augmented by factor V in a process that also requires protein S. Factor V Leiden, a factor V mutation that impairs the function of the protein C pathway, cannot serve in this role. See the text for further discussion. (*Modified from Esmon CT: Thrombomodulin as a model of molecular mechanisms that modulate protease specificity and function at the vessel surface.* FASEB *9:946. Used with permission.*)

the activated forms of the cofactors.[46–48] Much more attention has been devoted to the analysis of factor Va inactivation than factor VIIIa. Factor Va is a Ca^{2+}-dependent heterodimer. APC catalyzes three proteolytic cleavages in the heavy chain of factor Va (Fig. 170-2). Cleavage at Arg 306 is sufficient for complete inactivation, but this cleavage is facilitated by cleavage at Arg 506. Cleavage at Arg 672 does not appear to play an important role in factor Va inactivation.[49]

Although protein S is a significant cofactor, it is important to note that unlike the other cofactors involved in blood coagulation, protein S exerts relatively minor influences on factor Va or VIIIa inactivation in purified systems (about twofold under most conditions).[50] In plasma, the protein S dependence is much greater.[51,52] There are several complementary mechanisms that may account for this observation. In the case of factor Va, inactivation involves cleavage at Arg 506 to give a significant reduction of factor Va activity (20 to 80 percent depending on the assay conditions[53]) with subsequent complete inactivation involving cleavage at Arg 306.[49] Protein S enhances cleavage at Arg 306 selectively.[54,55] Thus, depending on how the inactivation is monitored, the protein S effect can vary significantly in vitro. This change in apparent bond specificity is consistent with another set of observations.

Factor Xa can protect factor Va from inactivation by APC.[11,55,56] Protection is selective, however. The Arg 506 cleavage is slowed with little effect on cleavage at Arg 306.[55] Because protein S stimulates the cleavage of factor Va at Arg 306 selectively, the substantial protective effects of factor Xa are largely abolished. How protein S shifts the specificity of bond cleavage is uncertain, but a potential mechanism has emerged.

On the surface of membranes or liposomes, the active site of the enzyme must be able to align with the target cleavage sites in the substrate to effectively cleave the target. Several enzyme cofactor complexes have been observed to undergo a reorientation of the active site of the enzyme relative to the membrane surface following binding of the cofactor. In the case of protein S, the active site of APC is brought approximately 10 Å closer to the membrane surface.[57] If one hypothesizes that the 306 bond is closer to the membrane surface than the 506 bond, then the change in bond specificity can be accounted for based on the change in the height of the APC active site from the membrane surface. Recently, a chimeric form of protein C in which the vitamin K-dependent Gla domain of protein C was exchanged with that of prothrombin was analyzed. This chimera no longer requires protein S for optimal function.[50] Comparison of the distance from

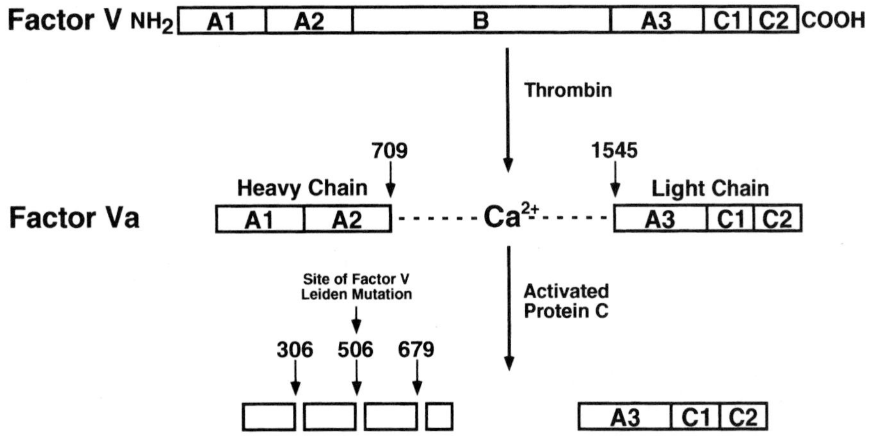

Fig. 170-2 Factor V activation by thrombin and inactivation by APC. Factor V circulates as a single-chain protein. A spanning region, referred to as the B domain, links the heavy and light chains. Thrombin cleaves factor V to release the heavy and light chains, forming factor Va, a heterodimer that requires Ca^{2+} for maintenance of the dimer and function. These chains consist of homologous A and C domains. APC cleaves the heavy chain most rapidly at position Arg 506, and more slowly at Arg 306. Cleavage at 306 leads to complete loss of activity. The heavy chain is also cleaved at Arg 679, but this cleavage does not appear to result in loss of activity. See text for discussion and details.

the membrane surface to the active site of the chimera revealed that the chimera was closer to the distance of the protein S-APC complex than to APC alone.[58]

In vitro, protein S has also been shown to inhibit prothrombin and factor X activation, apparently by binding to factor Xa,[59] factor VIII,[60] and factor Va.[61] Immunodepletion of protein S from plasma has little effect on clotting times or on thrombin generation.[50,62]

The inactivation of factor VIIIa is similar to that of factor Va. Factor IXa protects factor VIIIa from inactivation, and protein S reverses this protection.[45] Unlike factor Va, which is completely inactivated by cleavage at Arg 306 alone, factor VIIIa inactivation appears to require cleavage of at least two bonds (at Arg 336 and Arg 562)[63] with each cleavage leading to partial inactivation. Recently, it was shown that factor V can accelerate the inactivation of factor VIIIa. This process requires protein S, negatively charged phospholipids, and calcium ions.[14,64]

The protein C pathway is controlled, in part, by plasma proteinase inhibitors. Thrombin bound to TM can be inhibited more rapidly by protein C inhibitor[65,66] and antithrombin[67] than free thrombin. APC is neutralized by α_1-antiproteinase inhibitor, protein C inhibitor, and α_2-macroglobulin.[68–76] The estimated half-life for inactivation of the thrombin-TM complex in vivo is about 2 to 3 s[65] compared to 15 min or more for APC.[77] The half-life of protein C is also rather short, approximately 10 h.[78,79]

PROTEIN C STRUCTURE AND FUNCTION

Protein C is a multidomain protein. Mutations influencing protein C activity have been identified in each domain.[32,33] Mature protein C has a mass of approximately 62,000 Daltons and circulates at approximately 65 nM. Protein C is synthesized with a leader peptide followed by a propeptide. The propeptide is involved in recognition by the vitamin K-dependent carboxylase and, hence, mutations in this region could result in incomplete γ-carboxylation of Glu residues with a resultant decrease in biologic activity. Both the leader and propeptide are removed proteolytically during maturation.[80,81] A schematic representation of protein C, protein S, TM and EPCR, in relationship to the membrane surfaces at which they function, is depicted in Fig. 170-3. The sequence of human protein C is shown in Fig. 170-4. The mature protein C molecule consists of an N-terminal Gla domain, a hydrophobic stack region that connects the Gla domain to the two EGF domains, and a protease domain with homology to trypsin. In general, at the gene level, these domains are separated by introns.[82] Human protein C circulates primarily as a two-chain zymogen, but approximately 10 percent of the protein C circulates as a single chain.[83] The thrombin-TM complex is the major physiological activator of human protein C.[84] This activation occurs by cleavage at Arg 169, releasing a 12-residue peptide.[85] In the single chain protein C, no peptide is released during activation.

There are Ca^{2+} binding sites located in the Gla domain,[15] the first EGF domain,[20,86,87] and the protease domain of protein C.[88] The metal-binding sites in the Gla domain are required for binding to phospholipid[15] and to EPCR.[89] Mutational studies of the Gla domain suggest that the N-terminal half of the domain is critical for membrane interaction.[15] Based on site-directed mutagenesis studies, it is clear that mutation of Gla residues 7, 20, 26, and 29 results in nearly complete loss of APC anticoagulant activity, mutation of Gla 25 decreases activity 75 percent, and that Gla 6, 14, and 19 are not critical for any APC functions tested to date[90–93] (reviewed in reference 15). Mutation of the hydrophobic residues near the N-terminus also disrupts phospholipid binding, particularly at Leu 5.[94] In addition to the importance of Gla residues in membrane binding, complete carboxylation is required for protein C binding to EPCR.[89]

APC functions much better on phospholipid vesicles containing phosphatidylethanolamine,[50,95] and protein C activation proceeds more rapidly on these vesicles.[96] In contrast, the prothrombin activation complex demonstrates a lower phosphatidylethanolamine dependence. Chimeric protein C in which the Gla domain (first 46 residues) is replaced with that of prothrombin lacks the phosphatidylethanolamine-dependence characteristic of the normal protein C.[50] Plasma anticoagulant activity of this chimera is also protein S-independent. It is the C-terminal 24 residues of the Gla domain that are responsible for the phosphatidylethanolamine dependence.[50] This same region is necessary for protein S-dependent enhancement of factor Va inactivation and for the participation of protein S as an anticoagulant in plasma. These results suggest that missense mutations in the C-terminal half of the Gla domain could have subtle influences on protein C activity that would require relatively sophisticated assays to detect.

The Ca^{2+} binding site in the first EGF domain aids in stabilizing the functional conformation of the protein C Gla domain.[97,98] This site is not critical for activation by the thrombin-TM complex in solution.[99] Protein C contains a β hydroxy aspartic acid residue[100] in this domain. If this residue is mutated to Glu[101]

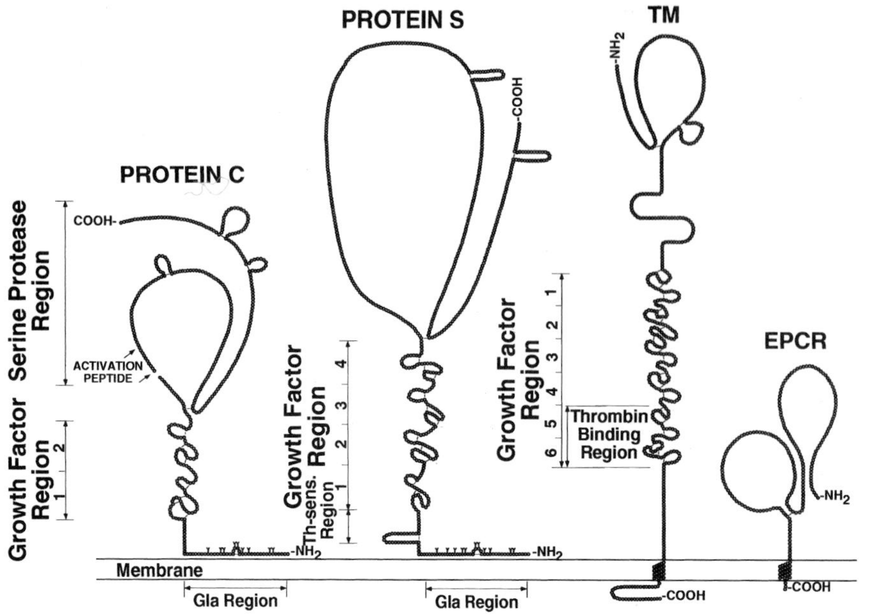

Fig. 170-3 Representation of protein C, protein S, thrombomodulin, and EPCR. The nature and overall domain structure of protein C, protein S, thrombomodulin, and EPCR are illustrated in addition to a representation of the nature of the membrane interactions. Specific domains of each protein are identified. *Gla*, γ-carboxyglutamic acid; *Th-sens.*, thrombin-sensitive. (*Modified from Esmon C: The roles of protein C and thrombomodulin in the regulation of blood coagulation.* J Biol Chem *264:4743, 1989. Used with permission.*)

or Ala,[102] then Ca^{2+} binding to APC is impaired, which results in reduced plasma anticoagulant activity. Therefore, it is likely that other mutations that interfere with Ca^{2+} binding would result in reductions of functional APC activity and probably protein C activation, if the assay system involves any phospholipid- or membrane-dependent steps.

There is a Ca^{2+} binding site in the protease domain[88] that potently modulates protein C activation. With thrombin alone, Ca^{2+} reduces the activation rate more than tenfold primarily by reducing protein C affinity for thrombin.[103] In contrast, activation by the thrombin-TM complex depends on the presence of Ca^{2+}.[104] The Ca^{2+} binding site in the protease domain is similar to that in trypsin.[88,99,105]

The crystal structure of APC lacking the Gla domain has been determined to 2.8 Å (Fig. 170-5),[105] and a molecular model of the protease domain of APC has been published.[106] Regions of APC thought to be functionally important are discussed in the context of the APC structures in these two papers. Several features that are likely to account for the specificity of APC are revealed by the structure. APC has a groove located between the active site and the Ca^{2+} site that is a candidate for engaging the residues on the carboxyl side (P′) of the cleavage site of substrates in a manner analogous to anion binding exosite 1 of thrombin. Both grooves are located in similar regions of the protease domains of their respective molecules. Anion binding exosite 1 in thrombin is the docking site for TM,[107,108] the protease-activated thrombin receptor 1,[109–113] fibrinogen,[114–116] factor V, and factor VIII.[117] Therefore, this groove in APC, when occupied by ligands, is a candidate for eliciting conformational changes and/or interacting with receptors. Of interest, factors V and VIII have highly conserved sequences on the P′ side of Arg 506[118] of factor V and Arg 562 in factor VIII, sites rapidly cleaved by APC in factors Va and VIIIa. These sequences are rich in acidic and hydrophobic residues similar to the corresponding domain in the thrombin receptor.[110]

Highly variable glycosylation of protein C results in a complex pattern when analyzed electrophoretically. Further complicating the pattern, plasma contains both two-chain (90 percent) and single-chain (10 percent) protein C. Both forms exist with 4, 3, and 2 *N*-linked carbohydrate chains.[83] The extent of glycosylation alters the anticoagulant activities of APC and the rate of activation of protein C.[119] Glycosylation at Asn 329 is probably responsible for the highest molecular weight (α) form of protein C. Mutation of the glycosylation sites increases APC anticoagulant activity two- to threefold. Glycosylation at 313 results in a 2.5-fold reduction in activation rate due to a corresponding increase in the K_m. Expression of protein C in human kidney 293 cells leads to decreased sialic acid and increased GalNAc and fucose[120] compared to plasma protein C. A polylactosamine on protein C also has been implicated in inhibiting cell adhesion through E-selectin,[121] a potential anti-inflammatory function of protein C. Thus, alteration of the glycosylation of protein C can significantly influence the biologic activity of the molecule and contribute to discrepancies between the antigen and activity ratios. These ratios are strongly influenced by the nature of the functional assays employed.

Organization of the Protein C Gene

The protein C gene is located in the q13-q14 region of chromosome 2.[122,123] The gene is approximately 11 kb in length and consists of 9 exons and 8 introns (GenBank M11228).[82,124] The first exon codes for the N-terminal portion of the pre-pro leader sequence. The second exon codes for the remainder of this sequence, the basic propeptide involved in recognition by the vitamin K-dependent carboxylase and Gla domain. The third exon codes for the aromatic stack of hydrophobic residues that separates the Gla domain from the EGF domain. The fourth and fifth exons code for the first and second EGF-like domains. The sixth exon encodes for the section between the protease domain and the EGF domain, the activation peptide region and the N-terminal portion of the APC protease domain. The seventh exon codes for the middle portion of the protease domain and contains the active site His, while the eighth exon codes for the C-terminal half of the protease domain and contains the active site Asp and Ser residues. Two major mRNA species are observed that appear to be due to different polyadenylation sites.[125,126] There are several polymorphisms in the protein C gene, none of which result in amino acid changes. The nucleotide polymorphisms are T/A at −1476, C/T at 3204, T/G at 3342, A/G at 6181 and T/C at 7228.[32]

Clinical Manifestations of Protein C Deficiency

The frequency of protein C deficiency (i.e., about a 50 percent reduction in protein C levels) in the general population has been estimated at 1/300[34,127] to 1/500. The majority of heterozygous protein C deficient individuals have no history of thrombosis.[127] However, analysis of patients with thrombosis clearly indicates

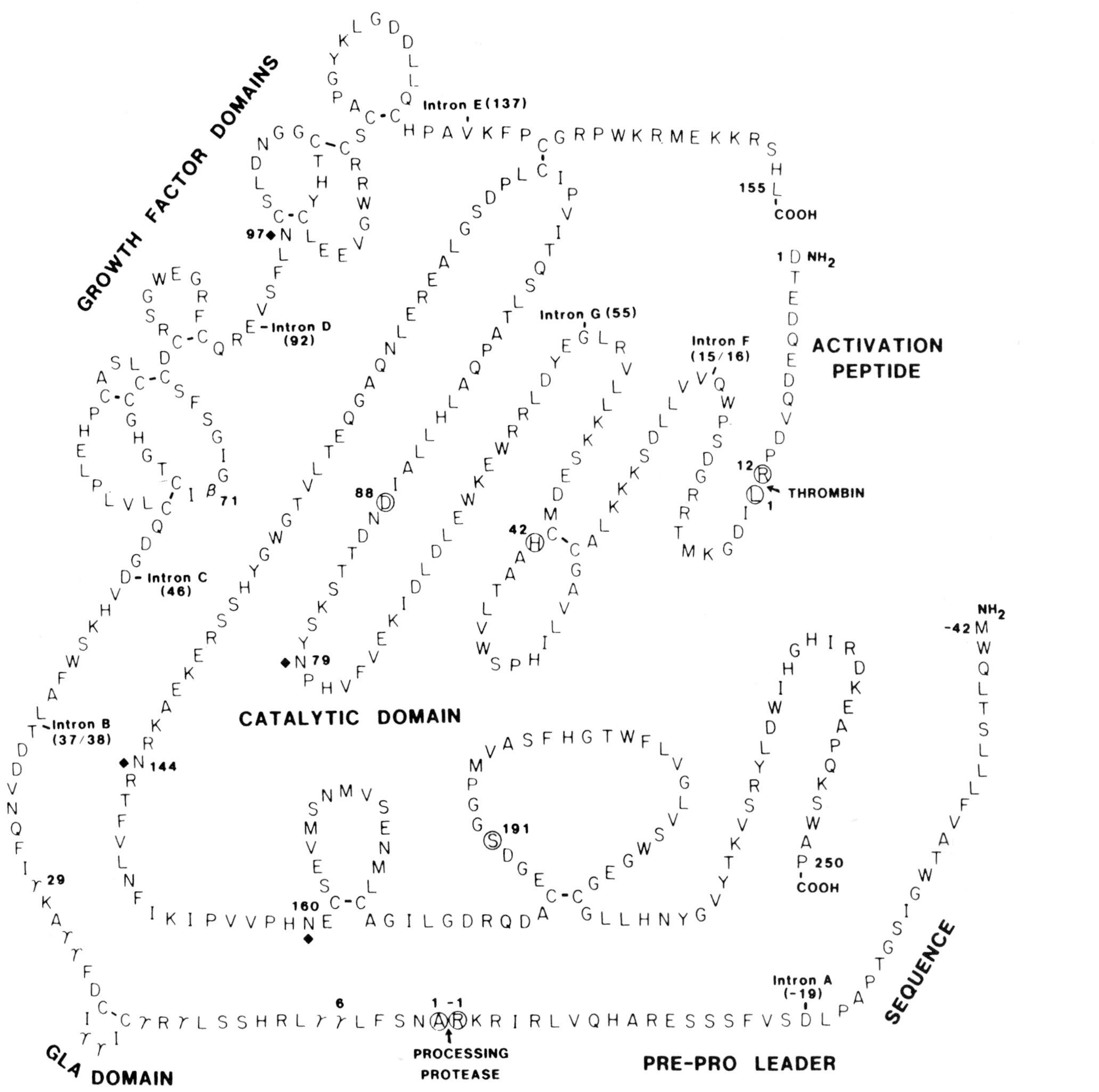

Fig. 170-4 Amino acid sequence of human protein C. Amino acids are numbered from the amino-terminus of the mature protein. Y depicts γ-carboxylation, and an oval depicts hydroxylation of an amino acid. Diamonds represent sites of N-linked glycosylation. Residues within the two EGF-like domains are shaded. The serine, aspartic acid, and histidine residues that constitute the catalytic active site are identified in black. > denotes the location of an intron in the protein C gene, and the roman numeral identifies the following exon. The dipeptide proteolytically removed during the post-translational processing of most protein C molecules is marked by the small arrows. The site of proteolytic cleavage during protein C activation is identified by the large arrow.

that protein C deficiency is a risk factor.[128] Examination of a large family with two mutations in the Gla domain[129] has clearly demonstrated that the protein C deficiency is associated with an increased risk of thrombosis.[130] Clinical manifestations of protein C deficiency include deep vein thrombosis and pulmonary embolism.[32] Although several case reports of protein C deficiency and arterial thrombosis have been published,[129,131,132] protein C deficiency seems to be, at most, a weak risk factor for arterial thrombosis in the general population.[133]

Early studies indicated that patients with protein C deficiency are at an increased risk of developing warfarin-induced skin necrosis.[134–136] Direct involvement of protein C depletion in this process is supported by the observation that the progression of the skin necrosis appears to be prevented by protein C infusion.[27,135] Protein C levels often decrease in patients with septic shock or liver failure, complicating the diagnosis.[78,137]

The Genetic Basis of Protein C Deficiency

The genetic basis of protein C deficiency has been examined in considerable depth.[32,33] The results indicate that the mutations are scattered throughout the gene. Identification of the site of the mutation has yet to aid in the treatment or prediction of future thrombotic complications. In the original review of 142 entries,[32] there were three promoter mutations, 10 splice-site abnormalities, 2 in-frame deletions, 6 frameshift deletions, 1 in-frame insertion, 3 frameshift insertions, 26 nonsense mutations, 93 missense

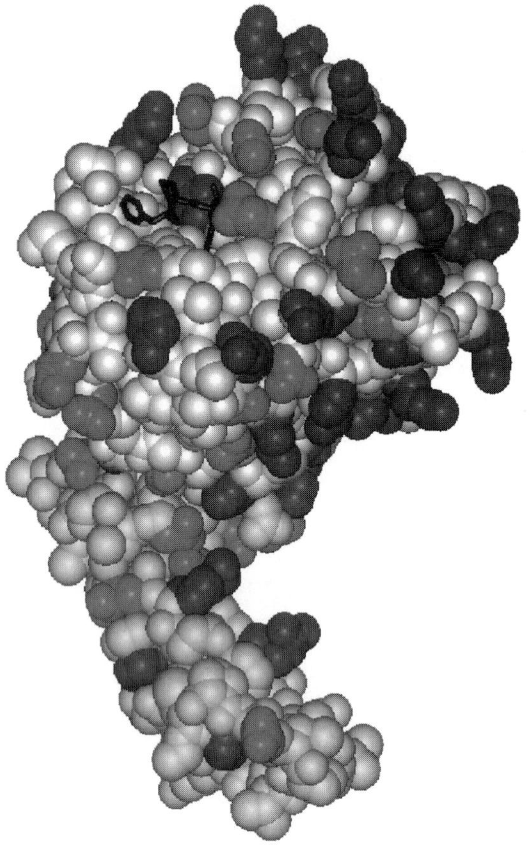

Fig. 170-5 Space-filling model of the activated protein C molecule. The model is based on the crystal structure of activated protein C lacking the Gla domain.[105] The location of a chlormethylketone inhibitor located in the active site is shown in black wire. Basic residues are in black, acidic residues are gray, and other residues are off-white. The protease domain is essentially round and the EGF domains form the "neck" extension at the base of the protease domain. The three basic residues critical for activation by the thrombin-TM complex are at the top of the figure. The exosite runs just underneath these residues. The Ca^{2+} binding site is to the far right of the protease domain near the acidic residue that is almost completely hidden by the basic residues.

mutations, and 1 silent mutation. The protein C gene contains a relatively high percentage (0.60 percent) of guanine plus cytosine. Of the single base-pair substitutions in the protein C gene, 43 percent occurred in CpG dinucleotides that resulted in C6T or G6A transitions, probably indicating a methylation-mediated deamination. Most of the CpG mutations in the protein C gene occur in exon 7.[32] Protein C deficiency is classified as type I (protein C antigen and activity are decreased equivalently) and type II (antigen levels are near normal, but the activity levels are reduced). Characterization of the type II mutations should involve assays of protein C activation and APC anticoagulant activity. A database of protein C mutations can be found at Web site www.xs4all.nl/~reitsma/Prot_C_home.htm.

PROTEIN S STRUCTURE AND FUNCTION

Protein S, like protein C, is synthesized with a leader and propeptide. The propeptide is involved in recognition by the vitamin K-dependent carboxylase and, hence, mutations in this region could result in incomplete γ-carboxylation of Glu residues with a resultant decrease in biologic activity. The leader and propeptide are released proteolytically during protein S secretion from the cell.[138–140] The sequence of protein S is shown in Fig. 170-6. In the mature protein, the vitamin K-dependent Gla domain is followed by an aromatic stack, a unique 29 residue thrombin-sensitive domain encoded by exon 4,[138,140] four EGF-like domains and a terminal domain homologous to the sex hormone-binding globulin and androgen-binding protein.[141,142] Cleavage at Arg 49, 60, or 70 in the thrombin-sensitive region destroys protein S cofactor function.[143–146] Mutation of these three sites generates a form of protein S that is resistant to thrombin inactivation.[143] Physiological levels of Ca^{2+} inhibit thrombin proteolysis of protein S.[147] Activated platelets[148] and neutrophils[149] contain proteases that can cleave protein S in this region and inactivate the protein. The first EGF domain contains a β-hydroxylated aspartic acid residue, while the remaining three EGF domains contain β-hydroxylated asparagine residues. Hydroxylation of these residues is incomplete, however, in human protein S.[150,151] The EGF domains function cooperatively to bind Ca^{2+}.[151] When linked, EGF domains bind Ca^{2+} up to 10,000 times tighter than the isolated domains.[151] The N-terminal EGF domain is critical for the cofactor function.[152] Antibodies directed toward the EGF domains of protein S inhibit cofactor activity.[153] It is likely that mutations in this region of protein S could interfere with the cooperative Ca^{2+} binding and, hence, reduce biologic activity.

The steroid hormone-binding globulin domain is not required for protein S cofactor activity,[154] but is involved in binding to C4b binding protein (C4BP), a regulatory protein of the complement system.[155,156] In plasma, about 60 percent of the protein S is in this complex. The protein S-C4BP complex lacks cofactor activity for APC in plasma anticoagulant assays[52,157] and, hence, it is the free protein S that determines biologic activity. C4BP and protein S interact reversibly and with very high affinity in plasma, an interaction that is tightened substantially by the presence of Ca^{2+}.[158,159] The sex hormone-binding globulin domain appears to be required and sufficient for this binding.[160]

C4BP is a large protein (540 kDa) containing six or seven identical α chains ~70 kDa each[161] and a single β chain.[161] Both subunits are made up of short consensus repeats. Electron microscopy of the complex exhibits a spider-like appearance with arms corresponding to the α chains projecting from a central core that includes the β subunit of C4BP and protein S at its base.[161,162] Consistent with the microscopy, biochemical studies have shown that the β chain is the protein S binding site.[161,163] Most, but not all, circulating C4BP molecules have a covalently linked β chain.[16,164] C4BP is an acute phase reactant, but only the C4BP α chains seem to be elevated in the acute phase response.[165] Truncation studies of the β chain revealed that the protein S binding site is located in the N-terminal repeat.[163] Bovine C4BP, which apparently does not bind to protein S, lacks the N-terminal repeat.[166,167] Mutations that increase C4BP expression are candidates for protein S deficiency because only the free form has cofactor activity (see "Clinical Manifestations of Protein S Deficiency" below).

Organization of the Protein S Gene

There are two protein S genes in the human genome. One is functional (the protein S α gene; GenBank M15036), and the other is a pseudogene (protein S β gene; GenBank M23600).[138,140,168] The β gene has multiple base changes in the coding sequence and lacks exon 1 which contains the initiation Met codon. The genes are located on chromosome 3 at position 3p11.1-q11.2.[169–172] The protein S α gene is 0.80 kb long and contains 15 exons, 14 introns, and 6 repetitive *Alu* sequences. Exon 1 codes for the leader peptide while exon 2 codes for the prepropeptide and Gla domain. Exon 3 codes for the aromatic stack region and exon 4 codes for the thrombin-sensitive region. Exons 5 to 8 code for individual EGF-like domains. The other exons code for the steroid binding-like domain.

Human protein S mRNA is about 4 kb in length, but three mRNA forms have been identified.[139,173] There is one common polymorphism in the coding region of the protein S gene. Pro 626 is encoded by either CCA or CCG at this position with nearly

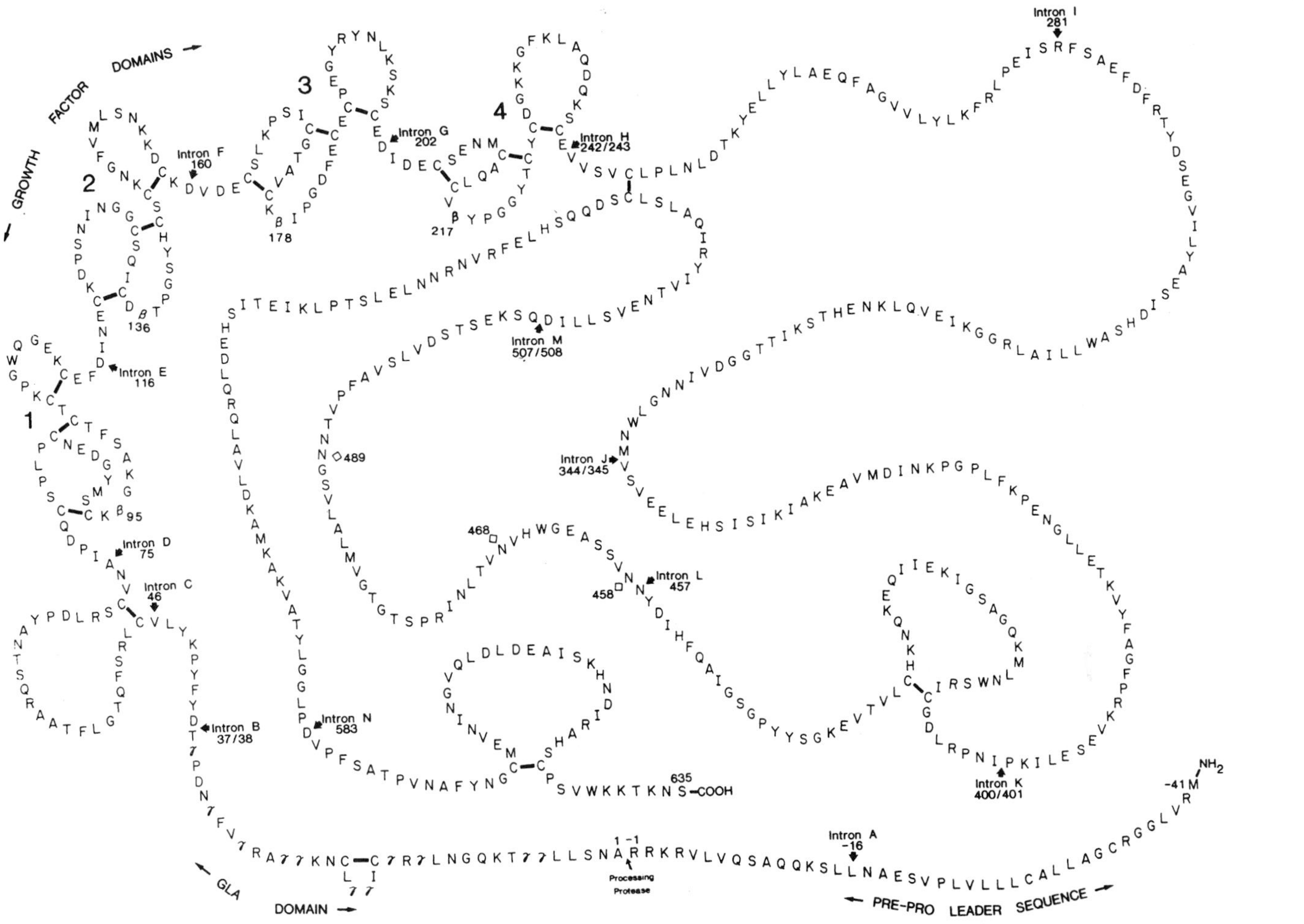

Fig. 170-6 Amino acid sequence of human protein S. Amino acids are numbered from the amino terminus of the mature protein. Y depicts γ-carboxylation, and the oval depicts potential hydroxylation of an amino acid. Diamonds represent potential sites of *N*-linked glycosylation. Residues within the four EGF-like domains are shaded. > denotes the location of an intron in the protein S gene, and the roman numeral identifies the following exon. The amino acid sequence is that reported by Schmidel and colleagues.[140]

equivalent frequency in the Caucasian population that has been studied.[174]

Clinical Manifestation of Protein S Deficiency

Because only free protein S is functional, there are at least three potential mechanisms for protein S deficiency. In all forms, the deficiency is associated with an increased risk of venous thrombosis and pulmonary embolism.[38,52,175–183] Type I is characterized by a reduction in total protein S antigen levels with a corresponding decrease in activity. Antigen reductions have a tendency to decrease functional levels more than the corresponding decrease in antigen because of the high affinity interaction with C4BP, the level of which is not controlled by protein S. Type II deficiency occurs when total and free protein S levels are normal, but functional levels are decreased. Type III deficiency is characterized by normal levels of total protein S but decreased levels of free protein S.[35]

This increased risk is perhaps most evident when analyzed in the context of a large, 122-member family.[184] In this family with a Gly2956Val mutation, the Kaplan Meier plots indicated that the probability of remaining thrombosis free at age 30 for affected members was 0.5 and 0.97 for unaffected family members. This trend continued throughout the life span of the members. Several case reports of protein S deficiency associated with arterial thrombosis have appeared,[176,185–190] but the actual level of increased risk caused by protein S deficiency is uncertain.

Like the situation with protein C, protein S mutations are found throughout the protein S gene (see reference 35 a database summary of the known protein S mutations). Missense mutations account for 53 percent of all mutations in the 125 patients presented in the database. Eighty patients were classified by type using the above criteria; 71 percent were type I, 12.5 percent were type II, and 10 percent were type III. Determination of the type of deficiency is made much more difficult when the patients are on oral anticoagulants. In these patients, protein S antigen levels are reduced but C4BP levels remain stable. Protein S levels can also be decreased in liver disease, with oral contraceptives or pregnancy, in the nephrotic syndrome, and with disseminated intravascular coagulation.[35,191–194]

THROMBOMODULIN STRUCTURE AND FUNCTION

For the overall domain structure of TM, see Fig. 170-3. TM is a type 1 transmembrane protein. The mature human TM molecule is 559 residues in length as deduced from the cDNA sequence.[195–198] The sequence of the mature protein is shown in Fig. 170-7. A model of the thrombin-TM complex, identifying structural and topographic features important in protein C activation, is shown in Fig. 170-8. The N-terminal domain (226 residues) has weak homology (about 20 percent) with lectins, such as the asialoglycoprotein receptor.[199] This region is followed by 6 EGF-like domains (236 residues). EGF domains 5 and 6 are responsible for

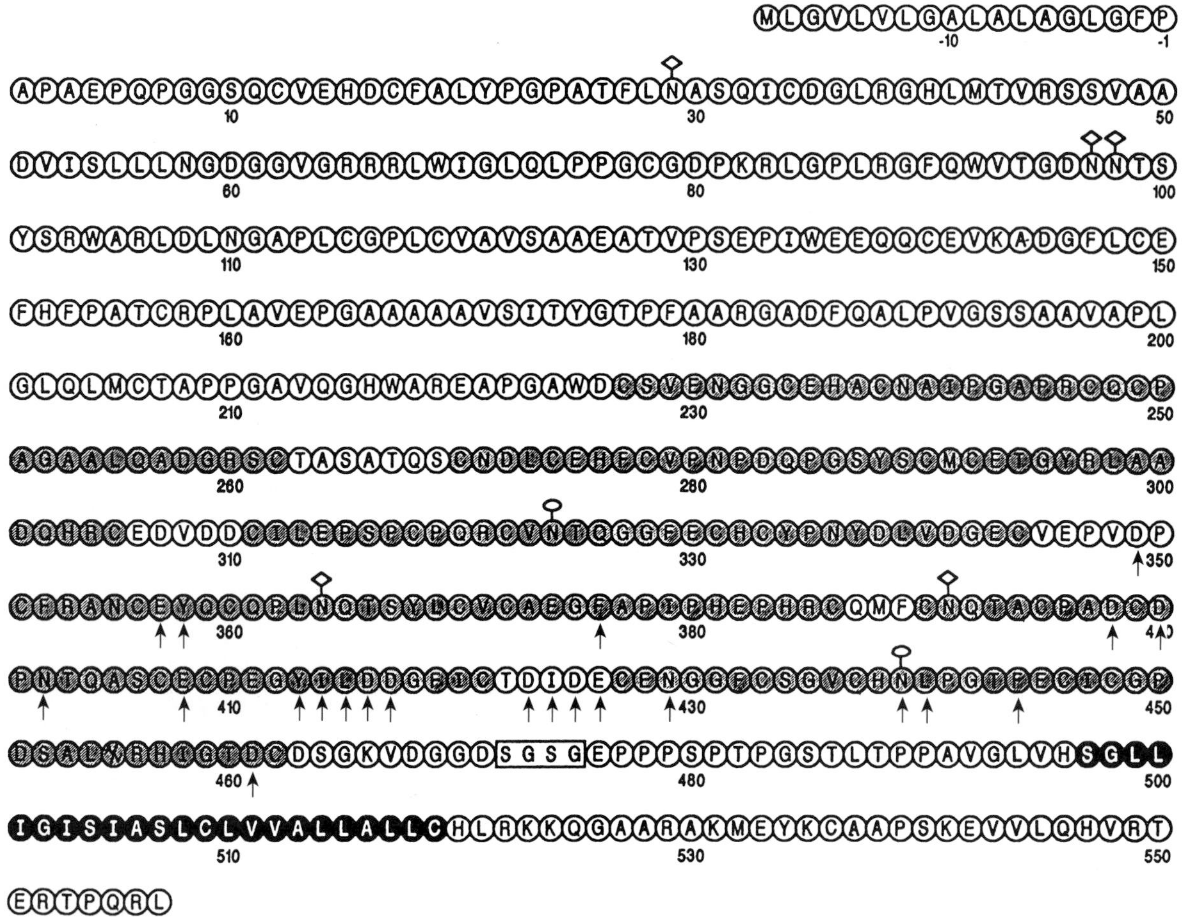

Fig. 170-7 Amino acid sequence of human thrombomodulin. Amino acids are numbered from the amino terminus of the mature protein. Ovals depict sites of potential hydroxylation, and diamonds represent potential sites of *N*-linked glycosylation. Residues within the six EGF-like domains are shaded. Residues in the putative transmembrane domain are shown in black. The consensus sequence for the possible attachment of a glycosaminoglycan is boxed. A/V denotes a genetic polymorphism. Arrows point to the 22 residues thought to be critical for cofactor activity within EGF domains 4 to 6.[207]

the vast majority of the thrombin-binding affinity,[200] but this fragment cannot support protein C activation. Rapid protein C activation requires the linker region between EGF3 and EGF4 and repeats 4 to 6[201–204] or, less effectively, repeats 4 to 5.[205] Many point mutations within EGF 4, 5, and 6 have been identified that reduce thrombin affinity or protein C activation rates.[206,207] Following the EGF domains is a 34-residue region that is rich in Ser and Thr, corresponding to potential O-linked glycosylation sites. The region also contains two sites of potential addition of chondroitin sulfate. Mutational analysis of the proposed sites of chondroitin sulfate attachment, Ser(472)-Gly-Ser(474)-Gly-Glu-Pro, has shown that Ser 474 and 472 are potential sites of chondroitin sulfate addition.[208] Which Ser is modified is cell line-dependent. In the same study, evidence was presented that placental TM can contain chondroitin sulfate(s). Most human TM preparations[209] do not display the characteristic high molecular weight and diffuse electrophoretic pattern observed with rabbit TM.[23,67,210–213] It is unclear whether the human TM has less chondroitin sulfate in vivo or whether the chondroitin-containing material is lost selectively during isolation. Recombinant soluble TM can have chondroitin sulfate attached with relatively high fidelity.[214,215] The presence of chondroitin sulfate (a) tightens thrombin affinity more than tenfold;[216] (b) increases the ability of TM to block fibrinogen clotting and platelet activation;[23,67] (c) stimulates inhibition by antithrombin[23,217] and protein C inhibitor;[65] and (d) modulates the Ca^{2+} dependence of protein C activation.[216,217] Mutations in this chondroitin sulfate attachment site might be expected to increase thrombotic risk. Lack of chondroitin sulfate probably accounts for the relatively ineffective direct anticoagulant activity observed with human TM preparations.[218]

Following the O-linked sugar region is a 23-residue hydrophobic region that corresponds to the transmembrane region. This region is highly conserved among species,[219,220] suggesting a potentially important and selective function for the domain. The cytoplasmic tail is 38 residues in length, contains 1 tyrosine, 1 serine, and 2 threonine residues that are potential sites of phosphorylation. Phosphorylation of serine has been observed following stimulation with phorbol myristate acetate.[219] There is also a Cys residue in this domain. No consensus sequence for internalization via coated pit-mediated endocytosis is present. Nevertheless, coated- and noncoated pit-mediated endocytosis has been observed.[221] The constitutive internalization instead seems to be a property of the N-terminal lectin-like domain.[222] Recently, TM was localized to caveolae,[223] which probably accounts for the constitutive internalization. Whether localization to caveolae is dependent on the lectin domain remains to be determined.

Other Functions of the Thrombin-TM Complex

In addition to activating protein C and catalyzing the inactivation of thrombin, TM in complex with thrombin can promote the activation of a procarboxypeptidase B, often referred to as thrombin activatable fibrinolysis inhibitor or TAFI.[224] The influence of TM on both reactions is comparable.[225] Unlike protein C activation, EGF domain 3, in addition to domains 4 to 6, is required for the TAFI activation.[226] In plasma clots, current

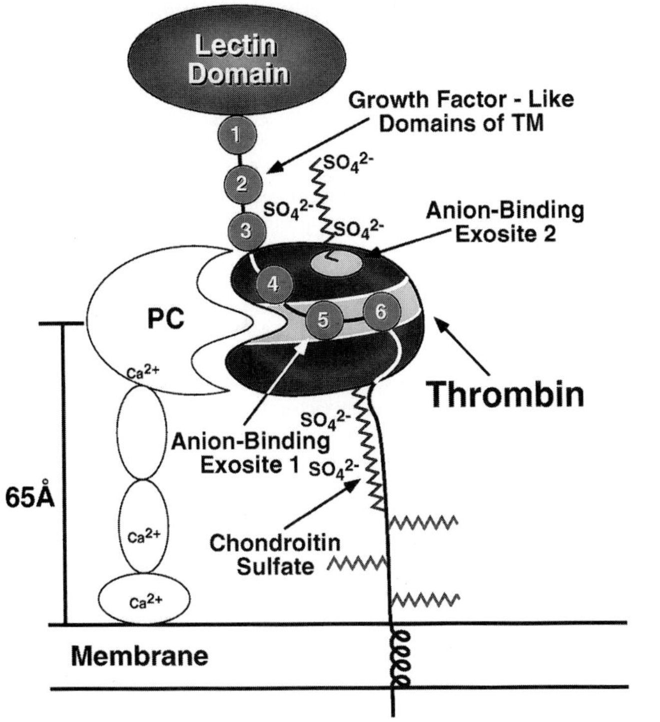

Fig. 170-8 A model of the protein C activation complex. Thrombin binding to thrombomodulin involves anion binding exosite 1 on thrombin (shown as a strip through the middle of thrombin) and EGF domain 4 to 6 on TM. A chondroitin-sulfate moiety on TM increases the affinity for thrombin, but is not required for function. This chondroitin sulfate interacts with anion-binding exosite 2 on thrombin, a second, very basic area near the heparin-binding site. The protein C cleavage site and the thrombin active site are approximately 65 Å from the membrane surface, indicating that TM "lifts" the thrombin off the membrane surface and basically accomplishes the same special functions as those accomplished by the Gla and EGF domains in protein C.

information suggests that the profibrinolytic activity of APC is due to inhibition of thrombin generation with a subsequent decrease in TAFI activation.[224,227] This carboxypeptidase removes C-terminal lysine residues from fibrin, rendering the clot less susceptible to plasmin digestion. This would appear to favor clot stability and would seem to oppose the many anticoagulant functions exhibited by TM. It is possible that this carboxypeptidase has other functions when activated near the vessel surface. In particular, many vasoactive substances, such as complement C5a, are inactivated by removal of their C-terminal Arg. TM also accelerates the proteolytic inactivation of prourokinase by thrombin.[228,229] Urokinase and its receptor have been implicated in cellular remodeling processes, so it is possible that the inhibition of prourokinase may be involved in modulating these processes rather than the fibrinolytic response. These alternative possibilities are in keeping with the many in vivo experiments that have demonstrated that infusion of soluble TM results in a net antithrombotic and/or anti-inflammatory effect.[230–239] Given these in vivo results, the major physiological function of thrombin-TM mediated activation of TAFI or inactivation of prourokinase remains questionable.

Organization of the Thrombomodulin Gene

There is a single copy of the TM gene located at 2p12-cen.[196,240] The TM gene is without introns (GenBank J02973).[195,198] Considerable interest has focused on the regulation of TM expression for two reasons. First, TM expression is regulated by inflammatory cytokines, such as tumor necrosis factor α (TNF α), shear stress, thrombin, heat shock, vascular endothelial cell growth factor, retinoic acid, homocysteine, cyclic AMP, and several other mediators as reviewed elsewhere.[40,241] Second, a recent study by Ireland and associates[242] suggests that mutations in the 5′ region of the TM gene are associated with an increased risk of myocardial infarction. These authors analyzed 104 patients with sustained myocardial infarction (average age 60.5 years). Age-matched control patients were selected from the outpatient clinic who were without a history of thrombosis. Five of the myocardial infarction patients had mutations in the 5′ region of the gene. In three patients, the mutation was a change from GG to AT at nucleotides −9 to −10. No mutations at this site were found in the control patients. A single mutation at −33 from G to A was observed in one myocardial infarction patient and one control patient. A mutation at −133 from C to A was observed in one myocardial infarction patient. These mutations are near putative regulatory elements in the 5′ region of the TM gene, but no direct studies have been reported demonstrating that these mutations cause reduction in TM expression. Nevertheless, that five mutations were observed in the myocardial infarction patient group and only one in the control group suggests that TM deficiency might contribute to myocardial infarction. Given that TM regulates thrombin formation, it is possible that the inability to regulate thrombin functions appropriately near the vessel surface leads to endothelial cell activation and a proinflammatory environment that could contribute to vascular disease.

Clinical Manifestations of Mutations in the TM Gene

Consistent with these findings, Öhlin and colleagues[243] observed that a common dimorphism in the TM gene is associated with an increased risk of myocardial infarction. The C/T dimorphism at nucleotide 1418 results in a substitution of Ala 455 with Val in the sixth EGF domain of TM. The C allele frequency was 0.82 in the patients and 0.72 in the controls ($p = 0.035$). This dimorphism appears to be neutral with respect to deep vein thrombosis.[243,244]

TM mutations leading to arterial thrombosis could be linked to the following observations. Neutrophil elastase can release TM proteolytically from the cell surface.[245,246] TNFα works synergistically to facilitate this release.[245] The neutrophils can also cause oxidative damage to TM by oxidizing a sensitive methionine (Met 388) in TM.[247] Soluble TM degradation products, consisting of the EGF domain repeats, are mitogenic for Swiss 3T3 cells (a fibroblast cell line).[248] This suggests that TM plays a possible role in wound healing or proliferative responses to inflammatory injury, and possibly in atherosclerosis, especially if smooth muscle cell proliferation is also stimulated by these fragments. Mutations that increase susceptibility to oxidation or proteolysis could, therefore, contribute to the development of vascular disease.

TM mutations have also been described as leading to venous thrombosis[249,250] (reviewed in reference 251). In 145 patients with venous thrombosis or pulmonary emboli, 4.8 percent had mutations in the TM gene. To establish the thrombotic risk, future studies need to address the prevalence of these mutations in a larger group of thrombotic patients and in controls. In addition, further interpretation of the mechanism by which these mutations influence arterial or venous thrombotic risk would be advanced substantially by expression and characterization of the mutations in vitro. Even with the limited number of patients characterized to date, it appears likely that TM mutations, like those of protein C and protein S, will be prevalent throughout the gene.

FACTOR V MUTATIONS, APC RESISTANCE, FACTOR V LEIDEN, AND THROMBOSIS

A resistance to the anticoagulant effects of APC is the most common trait observed in patients with thrombosis, particularly familial thrombosis.[28,36,37,41,252,253] It is a further risk factor for patients with heterozygous protein C deficiency.[254] Unlike protein C, protein S, and TM genes, factor V mutations associated with thrombosis are most commonly associated with a single site, a 1691G → A transition resulting in replacement of Arg 506 with Gln (R506Q).[44,255] Patients with this factor V variant (GenBank

M14335) are referred to as APC resistant and the factor V is usually referred to as factor V Leiden. The variant is relatively common in Caucasian populations (about 5 percent), but is very rare in other ethnic groups.[256] This mutation prevents cleavage at the 506 position.

In the original description, Dahlbäck observed that some plasma samples were not anticoagulated effectively by the addition of APC, hence the term APC resistance.[42] This defect could be corrected, however, by the addition of factor V to the plasma.[43] When the nature of the mutation was identified as a substitution of Arg 506 with Gln, first characterized in Leiden,[44,255] the majority of further research focused on the mechanisms by which the mutation would slow inactivation of factor Va.[49,53,257–259] While impaired rates of factor Va inactivation certainly contribute to APC resistance, focusing on factor Va inactivation per se neglects two important observations: factor V can correct the APC resistance defect to some extent and impairment of the APC anticoagulant effect is much greater if assays utilize activation pathways that involve factor VIII.[42,260] Because factor V could partially correct the defect, it appeared that there must be a cofactor effect, but this conclusion seemed inconsistent with the nature of the factor V mutation.

Recent studies have shed light on this apparent contradiction. In purified systems, factor V has now been shown to accelerate factor VIIIa inactivation.[14,64] Enhancement requires protein S, phospholipid, and Ca^{2+} ions. Factor V Leiden cannot stimulate factor VIIIa inactivation under exactly the same in vitro conditions,[64] providing an explanation for the apparent cofactor activity of factor V in APC-resistant plasma.

Given the probable importance of factor V cofactor activity in the anticoagulant response, it became important to identify the region of factor V responsible for the cofactor activity. Because factor V, but not factor Va, possessed cofactor activity, it appeared likely that the region of factor V that is necessary for cofactor activity was lost during the activation process. There is a large region of factor V, the B domain, that serves to link the heavy and light chains of factor Va. This region is released during activation. Deletion mutation analysis indicates that the cofactor activity involves the C-terminal region of this connecting B chain and that this region must remain covalently associated with the light chain of factor V to retain cofactor activity.[261] These authors also demonstrated that replacing the B domain with the corresponding domain of factor VIII resulted in a factor V mutant devoid of cofactor activity. These studies suggest that mutations in this region of the B domain of factor V could lead to a thrombotic tendency.

This cofactor effect is also supported by an unusual clinical condition referred to as pseudohomozygous-activated protein C resistance.[262] In this condition, the patient has a coinheritance of a type I factor V quantitative deficiency and the factor V Leiden mutation. In in vitro assays, plasmas from these patients are as resistant to APC as those of homozygous factor V Leiden patients. Patients with homozygous factor V Leiden appear to exhibit a higher risk for thrombosis than heterozygous patients,[263,264] but not nearly as severe as patients with complete protein C deficiency. It appears likely that the pseudohomozygous-deficient patients may be at greater risk of thrombosis than simple heterozygous patients, but the small number of families screened to date preclude a definitive assessment of the increased risk. The clinical observation that homozygous factor V Leiden patients are at greater thrombotic risk than the heterozygous patients is consistent with the in vitro results suggesting an important cofactor role for factor V.

APC resistance has also been observed in arterial thrombosis.[265–267] In the latter study, the authors found that the factor V Leiden mutation was found in 10 percent of 84 women with their first myocardial infarction compared to 4 percent in the 388 controls. Among nonsmokers, there was very little increased risk, but the risk was significant in the smokers,[267] leading the authors to conclude that smoking and factor V Leiden combined increased the risk of myocardial infarction thirty-twofold as compared to noncarrier nonsmokers. In a larger study population, 373 men and women over the age of 65 with myocardial infarction, stroke, angina, or transient ischemic attacks were compared to 482 controls.[268] This study failed to reveal an association between factor V Leiden and arterial thrombosis. Additional studies are needed to identify which factors, including age, may be associated with increased risk of arterial thrombosis in individuals with factor V Leiden or other defects in the protein C pathway.

Approximately 10 percent of the patients with APC resistance, however, do not have the factor V Leiden dimorphism.[252] A specific factor V haplotype, referred to as HR2, has been described in about 10 percent of the population that leads to APC resistance in the absence of factor V Leiden. The haplotype results in amino acid substitutions at two sites in the B chain of factor V (the linker region) and this may decrease factor V cofactor activity.[269]

Another candidate for APC resistance is Arg 306, which is the second bond in factor V to be cleaved by APC and leads to complete factor Va inactivation. Consistent with this possibility, two patients have been identified with a mutation at this site.[270,271] In addition, a novel form of acquired APC resistance is associated with the use of birth control pills, especially third-generation birth control pills.[272] APC resistance was also observed during pregnancy.[273] How hormonal changes influence the protein C pathway remains to be elucidated.

Epidemiologic studies demonstrate that hereditary defects in the protein C pathway are the most prevalent plasma abnormality associated with venous thrombosis. It is clear that thrombosis in these affected individuals must be associated with other risk factors because families with identical defects can remain thrombosis free. Most of these additional risk factors remain to be identified.

Factor V Leiden, Pregnancy, and Oral Contraceptives

Smoking[274] and oral contraceptives/pregnancy[275,276] are two risk factors that appear to increase the risk of thrombosis synergistically when combined with the factor V Leiden mutation. In addition, factor V Leiden contributes to an increase in risk for pregnancy loss.[277] One possible mechanism for the link between oral contraceptives and factor V Leiden is the observation that protein S levels are reduced by oral contraceptives.[278,279] Protein S plays a critical role in the inactivation of factor V Leiden.[280,281] Therefore, the acquired protein S deficiency would further stabilize the factor V Leiden. In addition, several studies suggest that APC resistance occurs due to some unknown factor that is under the influence of estrogens and possibly other female sex hormones and agents, particularly in the third-generation oral contraceptives.[282,283] This defect does not appear to be due solely to decreased protein S levels because supplementation with protein S does not correct the resistance. It is possible that elevation in other coagulation factors such as the other vitamin K-dependent factors and factor VIII are responsible.[282] Of note, this form of APC resistance is only observed in assays initiated with tissue factor, suggesting that there might be abnormal regulation of the extrinsic pathway of blood coagulation.[283]

Several authors suggest that oral contraceptives are contraindicated in women with the factor V Leiden mutation (heterozygous) in view of the increased risk of thrombosis.[284] Homozygous women would be anticipated to carry still greater risk, but are quite rare, estimated at 1 in 5000.[285] It is estimated that the risk of thrombosis in women taking oral contraceptives who do not carry this trait is approximately 2.2 events/10,000 woman years. The risk of thrombosis in women with factor V Leiden who are not taking oral contraceptives is approximately 4.9/10,000 woman years. The risk when the mutation and oral contraceptives are combined increases to approximately 27.7/10,000 woman years. While the increased risk is readily apparent, it is nevertheless a relatively rare complication leading some to question whether the benefits might balance the risk.[285]

MANAGEMENT OF PATIENTS WITH DEFECTS IN THE PROTEIN C PATHWAY

A consensus view on the management of patients with inherited thrombophilia has been published.[284] The authors conclude that the management of acute venous thrombosis and pulmonary embolism is similar to other patients. In patients with protein C and possibly protein S deficiency, the risk of the rare complication of warfarin skin necrosis following the initial days of therapy is apparently increased. It is recommended that the patients be fully anticoagulated with heparin before oral anticoagulant administration. It may be useful to increase the drug dose slowly. Should skin necrosis occur, protein C has been reported as effective in treating the complication.[286–288]

The risk of recurrence appears greater in patients with hereditary defects in the protein C pathway. If there is a strong family history of recurrent thrombosis in affected members of the family, and the patients thrombotic complications are severe, then longer term oral anticoagulant therapy may be appropriate. Detailed studies on protein S and protein C individuals to validate this view are still preliminary. With factor V Leiden, the risk of recurrent thrombosis appears to be similar or only slightly higher than in other patients following the first thrombotic event.[289]

Thrombosis during pregnancy is often associated with APC resistance,[277,284] with this single defect found in approximately 60 percent of women. With the anticoagulants currently available, the best choice for treating these thrombotic complications is probably subcutaneous heparin administration.[284] The dose, duration, and efficacy of heparin therapy during pregnancy has yet to be established by clinical trials.

ACKNOWLEDGMENTS

I thank Dr. Naomi Esmon for helpful editorial comments and Nici Barnard for final preparation of the manuscript. Dr. Charles Esmon is an investigator for the Howard Hughes Medical Institute.

REFERENCES

1. Esmon CT, Owen WG: Identification of an endothelial cell cofactor for thrombin-catalyzed activation of protein C. *Proc Natl Acad Sci U S A* **78**:2249, 1981.
2. Laszik Z, Mitro A, Taylor FB Jr, Ferrell G, Esmon CT: Human protein C receptor is present primarily on endothelium of large blood vessels: Implications for the control of the protein C pathway. *Circulation* **96**:3633, 1997.
3. Fukudome K, Esmon CT: Identification, cloning and regulation of a novel endothelial cell protein C/activated protein C receptor. *J Biol Chem* **269**:26486, 1994.
4. Stearns-Kurosawa DJ, Kurosawa S, Mollica JS, Ferrell GL, Esmon CT: The endothelial cell protein C receptor augments protein C activation by the thrombin-thrombomodulin complex. *Proc Natl Acad Sci U S A* **93**:10212, 1996.
5. Regan LM, Stearns-Kurosawa DJ, Kurosawa S, Mollica J, Fukudome K, Esmon CT: The endothelial cell protein C receptor: Inhibition of activated protein C anticoagulant function without modulation of reaction with proteinase inhibitors. *J Biol Chem* **271**:17499, 1996.
6. Stern DM, Nawroth PP, Harris K, Esmon CT: Cultured bovine aortic endothelial cells promote activated protein C-protein S-mediated inactivation of Factor Va. *J Biol Chem* **261**:713, 1986.
7. Hackeng TM, Hessing M, van't Veer C, et al.: Protein S binding to human endothelial cells is required for expression of cofactor activity for activated protein C. *J Biol Chem* **268**:3993, 1993.
8. Tans G, Rosing J, Thomassen MCLGD, Heeb MJ, Zwaal RFA, Griffin JH: Comparison of anticoagulant and procoagulant activities of stimulated platelets and platelet-derived microparticles. *Blood* **77**:2641, 1991.
9. Harris KW, Esmon CT: Protein S is required for bovine platelets to support activated protein C binding and activity. *J Biol Chem* **260**:2007, 1985.
10. Dahlbäck B, Wiedmer T, Sims PJ: Binding of anticoagulant vitamin K-dependent protein S to platelet-derived microparticles. *Biochemistry* **31**:12769, 1992.
11. Solymoss S, Tucker MM, Tracy PB: Kinetics of inactivation of membrane-bound factor Va by activated protein C. *J Biol Chem* **263**:14884, 1988.
12. Walker FJ: Regulation of activated protein C by protein S: The role of phospholipid in factor Va inactivation. *J Biol Chem* **256**:11128, 1981.
13. Mann KG, Hockin MF, Begin KJ, Kalafatis M: Activated protein C cleavage of factor Va leads to dissociation of the A2 domain. *J Biol Chem* **272**:20678, 1997.
14. Shen L, Dahlbäck B: Factor V and protein S as synergistic cofactors to activated protein C in degradation of factor VIIIa. *J Biol Chem* **269**:18735, 1994.
15. Castellino FJ: Human protein C and activated protein C. *Trends Cardiovasc Med* **5**:55, 1995.
16. Dahlbäck B: Protein S and C4b-binding protein: Components involved in the regulation of the protein C anticoagulant system. *Thromb Haemost* **66**:49, 1991.
17. Davie EW, Fujikawa K, Kisiel W: The coagulation cascade: Initiation, maintenance and regulation. *Biochemistry* **30**:10363, 1991.
18. Esmon CT: The roles of protein C and thrombomodulin in the regulation of blood coagulation. *J Biol Chem* **264**:4743, 1989.
19. Esmon CT: Thrombomodulin as a model of molecular mechanisms that modulate protease specificity and function at the vessel surface. *FASEB J* **9**:946, 1995.
20. Stenflo J: Structure-function relationships of epidermal growth factor modules in vitamin K-dependent clotting factors. *Blood* **78**:1637, 1991.
21. Preissner KT: Biological relevance of the protein C system and laboratory diagnosis of protein C and protein S deficiencies. *Clin Science* **78**:351, 1990.
22. Walker FJ, Fay PJ: Regulation of blood coagulation by the protein C system. *FASEB J* **6**:2561, 1992.
23. Bourin MC, Lindahl U: Glycosaminoglycans and the regulation of blood coagulation. *Biochem J* **289**:313, 1993.
24. Sadler JE, Lentz SR, Sheehan JP, Tsiang M, Wu Q: Structure-function relationships of the thrombin-thrombomodulin interaction. *Haemostasis* **23**:183, 1993.
25. Aiach M, Borgel D, Gaussem P, Emmerich J, Alhenc-Gelas M, Gandrille S: Protein C and protein S deficiencies. *Semin Hematol* **34**:205, 1997.
26. Alving BM, Comp PC: Recent advances in understanding clotting and evaluating patients with recurrent thrombosis. *Am J Obstet Gynecol* **167**:1184, 1992.
27. Esmon CT, Schwarz HP: An update on clinical and basic aspects of the protein C anticoagulant pathway. *Trends Cardiovasc Med* **5**:141, 1995.
28. Florell SR, Rodgers GM: Inherited thrombotic disorders: An update. *Am J Hematol* **54**:53, 1997.
29. Gladson CL, Groncy P, Griffin JH: Coumarin necrosis, neonatal purpura fulminans, and protein C deficiency. *Arch Dermatol* **123**:1701a, 1987.
30. Lane DA, Mannucci PM, Bauer KA, et al.: Inherited thrombophilia: Part 2. *Thromb Haemost* **76**:824, 1996.
31. Marlar RA, Neumann A: Neonatal purpura fulminans due to homozygous protein C or protein S deficiencies. *Semin Thromb Hemost* **16**:299, 1990.
32. Reitsma PH, Poort SR, Bernardi F, et al.: Protein C deficiency: A database of mutations. For the Protein C & S Subcommittee of the Scientific and Standardization Committee of the International Society on Thrombosis and Haemostasis. *Thromb Haemost* **69**:77, 1993.
33. Reitsma PH, Bernardi F, Doig RG, et al.: Protein C deficiency: A database of mutations, 1995 update. *Thromb Haemost* **73**:876, 1995.
34. Lane DA, Mannucci PM, Bauer KA, et al.: Inherited thrombophilia: Part 1. *Thromb Haemost* **76**:651, 1996.
35. Gandrille S, Borgel D, Ireland H, et al.: Protein S deficiency: A database of mutations. For the plasma coagulation inhibitors subcommittee of the Scientific and Standardization Committee of the International Society on Thrombosis and Haemostasis. *Thromb Haemost* **77**:1201, 1997.
36. Bertina RM: Factor V Leiden and other coagulation factor mutations affecting thrombotic risk. *Clin Chem* **43**:1678, 1997.
37. Dahlbäck B: Physiological anticoagulation. Resistance to activated protein C and venous thromboembolism. *J Clin Invest* **94**:923, 1994.
38. Pabinger I, Brucker S, Kyrle PA, et al.: Hereditary deficiency of antithrombin III, protein C and protein S: Prevalence in patients with a history of venous thrombosis and criteria for rational patient screening. *Blood Coagul Fibrinolysis* **3**:547, 1992.
39. Kemkes-Matthes B: Acquired protein S deficiency. *Clin Invest Med* **70**:529, 1992.

40. Esmon CT: Protein C, protein S, and thrombomodulin, in Colman RW, Hirsh J, Marder VJ, Clowes A, George JN (eds): *Hemostasis and Thrombosis: Basic Principles and Clinical Practice*, 4th ed. Philadelphia, Lippincott-Raven, 1998.
41. Griffin JH, Evatt B, Wideman C, Fernández JA: Anticoagulant protein C pathway defective in majority of thrombophilic patients. *Blood* **82**:1989, 1993.
42. Dahlbäck B, Carlsson M, Svensson PJ: Familial thrombophilia due to a previously unrecognized mechanism characterized by poor anticoagulant response to activated protein C: Prediction of a cofactor to activated protein C. *Proc Natl Acad Sci U S A* **90**:1004, 1993.
43. Dahlbäck B, Hildebrand B: Inherited resistance to activated protein C is corrected by anticoagulant cofactor activity found to be a property of factor V. *Proc Natl Acad Sci U S A* **91**:1396, 1994.
44. Bertina RM, Koeleman BPC, Koster T, et al.: Mutation in blood coagulation factor V associated with resistance to activated protein C. *Nature* **369**:64, 1994.
45. Regan LM, Lamphear BJ, Huggins CF, Walker FJ, Fay PJ: Factor IXa protects factor VIIIa from activated protein C. *J Biol Chem* **269**:9445, 1994.
46. Eaton D, Rodriguez H, Vehar GA: Proteolytic processing of human factor VIII. Correlation of specific cleavages by thrombin, factor Xa, and activated protein C with activation and inactivation of factor VIII coagulant activity. *Biochemistry* **25**:505, 1986.
47. Vehar GA, Davie EW: Preparation and properties of bovine factor VIII (antihemophilic factor). *Biochemistry* **19**:401, 1980.
48. Walker FJ, Sexton PW, Esmon CT: Inhibition of blood coagulation by activated protein C through selective inactivation of activated factor V. *Biochem Biophys Acta* **571**:333, 1979.
49. Egan JO, Kalafatis M, Mann KG: The effect of Arg 306 → Ala and Arg 506 → Gln substitutions in the inactivation of recombinant human factor Va by activated protein C and protein S. *Protein Sci* **6**:2016, 1997.
50. Smirnov MD, Safa O, Regan L, et al.: A chimeric protein C containing the prothrombin Gla domain exhibits increased anticoagulant activity and altered phospholipid specificity. *J Biol Chem* **273**:9031, 1998.
51. Walker FJ: Regulation of activated protein C by a new protein: A role for bovine protein S. *J Biol Chem* **255**:5521, 1980.
52. Comp PC, Nixon RR, Cooper MR, Esmon CT: Familial protein S deficiency is associated with recurrent thrombosis. *J Clin Invest* **74**:2082, 1984.
53. Kalafatis M, Haley PE, Lu D, Bertina RM, Long GL, Mann KG: Proteolytic events that regulate factor V activity in whole plasma from normal and activated protein C (APC)-resistant individuals during clotting: An insight into the APC-resistance assay. *Blood* **87**:4695, 1996.
54. Nicolaes GAF, Tans G, Thomassen MCLGD, et al.: Peptide bond cleavages and loss of functional activity during inactivation of factor Va and Factor Va^{R506Q} by activated protein C. *J Biol Chem* **270**:21158, 1995.
55. Rosing J, Hoekema L, Nicolaes GAF, et al.: Effects of protein S and factor Xa on peptide bond cleavages during inactivation of factor Va and factor Va^{R506Q} by activated protein C. *J Biol Chem* **270**:27852, 1995.
56. Nesheim ME, Canfield WM, Kisiel W, Mann KG: Studies on the capacity of factor Xa to protect factor Va from inactivation by activated protein C. *J Biol Chem* **257**:1443, 1982.
57. Yegneswaran S, Wood GM, Esmon CT, Johnson AE: Protein S alters the active site location of activated protein C above the membrane surface. *J Biol Chem* **272**:25013, 1997.
58. Yegneswaran S, Smirnov MD, Esmon NL, Esmon CT, Johnson AE: Relocation of the active site of activated protein C closer to the membrane surface coincides with an increase in factor Va inactivation activity and an insensitivity to protein S stimulation of activity [Abstract]. *Blood* **90(Suppl 1)**:145a, 1997.
59. Heeb MJ, Rosing J, Bakker HM, Fernandez JA, Tans G, Griffin JH: Protein S binds to and inhibits factor Xa. *Proc Natl Acad Sci U S A* **91**:2728, 1994.
60. Koppelman SJ, Hackeng TM, Sixma JJ, Bouma BN: Inhibition of the intrinsic Factor X activating complex by protein S: Evidence for a specific binding of protein S to factor VIII. *Blood* **86**:1062, 1995.
61. Heeb MJ, Mesters RM, Tans G, Rosing J, Griffin JH: Binding of protein S to Factor Va associated with inhibition of prothrombinase that is independent of activated protein C. *J Biol Chem* **268**:2872, 1993.
62. Duchemin J, Pittet J-L, Tartary M, et al.: A new assay based on thrombin generation inhibition to detect both protein C and protein S deficiencies in plasma. *Thromb Haemost* **71**:331, 1994.
63. Amano K, Michnick DA, Moussalli M, Kaufman RJ: Mutation at either Arg 336 or Arg 562 in factor VIII is insufficient for complete resistance to activated Protein C (APC)-mediated inactivation: Implications for the APC-resistance test. *Thromb Haemost* **79**:557, 1998.
64. Varadi K, Rosing J, Tans G, Pabinger I, Keil B, Schwarz HP: Factor V enhances the cofactor function of protein S in the APC-mediated inactivation of factor VIII: Influence of the factor V^{R506Q} mutation. *Thromb Haemost* **76**:208, 1996.
65. Rezaie AR, Cooper ST, Church FC, Esmon CT: Protein C inhibitor is a potent inhibitor of the thrombin-thrombomodulin complex. *J Biol Chem* **270**:25336, 1995.
66. Elisen MGLM, Borne PAK, Bouma BN, Meijers JCM: Protein C inhibitor acts as a procoagulant by inhibiting the thrombomodulin-induced activation of protein C in human plasma. *Blood* **91**:1542, 1998.
67. Bourin M-C, Öhlin A-K, Lane DA, Stenflo J, Lindahl U: Relationship between anticoagulant activities and polyanionic properties of rabbit thrombomodulin. *J Biol Chem* **263**:8044, 1988.
68. Heeb MJ, Mosher D, Griffin JH: Activation and complexation of protein C and cleavage and decrease of protein S in plasma of patients with intravascular coagulation. *Blood* **73**:455, 1989.
69. Scully MF, Toh CH, Hoogendoorn H, et al.: Activation of protein C and its distribution between its inhibitors, protein C inhibitor, α_1-antitrypsin, and α_2-macroglobulin, in patients with disseminated intravascular coagulation. *Thromb Haemost* **69**:448, 1993.
70. España F, Griffin JH: Determination of functional and antigenic protein C inhibitor and its complexes with activated protein C in plasma by ELISA's. *Thromb Res* **55**:671, 1989.
71. España F, Gilabert J, Aznar J, Estellés A, Kobayashi T, Griffin JH: Complexes of activated protein C with α_1-antitrypsin in normal pregnancy and in severe preeclampsia. *Am J Obstet Gynecol* **164**:1310, 1991.
72. España F, Gruber A, Heeb MJ, Hanson SR, Harker LA, Griffin JH: In vivo and in vitro complexes of activated protein C with two inhibitors in baboons. *Blood* **77**:1754, 1991.
73. Heeb MJ, España F, Geiger M, Collen D, Stump DC, Griffin JH: Immunological identity of heparin-dependent plasma and urinary protein C inhibitor and plasminogen activator inhibitor-3. *J Biol Chem* **262**:15813, 1987.
74. Heeb MJ, Griffin JH: Physiologic inhibition of human activated protein C by α_1-antitrypsin. *J Biol Chem* **263**:11613, 1988.
75. Heeb MJ, España F, Griffin JH: Inhibition and complexation of activated protein C by two major inhibitors in plasma. *Blood* **73**:446, 1989.
76. Heeb MJ, Gruber A, Griffin JH: Identification of divalent metal ion-dependent inhibition of activated protein C by $alpha_2$-macroglobulin and $alpha_2$-antiplasmin in blood and comparisons to inhibition of factor Xa, thrombin, and plasmin. *J Biol Chem* **266**:17606, 1991.
77. Okajima K, Koga S, Kaji M, et al.: Effect of protein C and activated protein C on coagulation and fibrinolysis in normal human subjects. *Thromb Haemost* **63**:48, 1990.
78. D'Angelo SV, Comp PC, Esmon CT, D'Angelo A: Relationship between protein C antigen and anticoagulant activity during oral anticoagulation and in selected disease states. *J Clin Invest* **77**:416, 1986.
79. Dreyfus M, Masterson M, David M, et al.: Replacement therapy with a monoclonal antibody purified protein C concentrate in newborns with severe congenital protein C deficiency. *Semin Thromb Hemost* **21**:371, 1995.
80. Furie B, Furie BC: The molecular basis of blood coagulation. *Cell* **53**:505, 1988.
81. Grinnell BW, Walls JD, Gerlitz B, et al.: Native and modified recombinant human protein C: Function, secretion, and posttranslational modifications, in Bruley DF, Drohan WN (eds): *Protein C and Related Anticoagulants (Advances in Applied Biotechnology Series, vol. 11)*. Houston, TX, Gulf Publishing, 1991, p 29.
82. Plutzky J, Hoskins J, Long GL, Crabtree GR: Evolution and organization of the human protein C gene. *Proc Natl Acad Sci U S A* **83**:546, 1986.
83. Miletich JP, Broze GJ Jr: β Protein C is not glycosylated at asparagine 329: The rate of translation may influence the frequency of usage at asparagine-X-cysteine sites. *J Biol Chem* **265**:11397, 1990.
84. Weiler-Guettler H, Christie PD, Beeler DL, et al.: A targeted point mutation in thrombomodulin generates viable mice with a prethrombotic state. *J Clin Invest* **101**:1983, 1998.
85. Kisiel W: Human plasma protein C: isolation, characterization and mechanism of activation by α-thrombin. *J Clin Invest* **64**:761, 1979.

86. Öhlin A-K, Stenflo J: Calcium-dependent interaction between the EGF region of human protein C and a monoclonal antibody. *J Biol Chem* **262**:13798, 1987.
87. Öhlin A-K, Linse S, Stenflo J: Calcium binding to the epidermal growth factor homology region of bovine protein C. *J Biol Chem* **263**:7411, 1988.
88. Rezaie AR, Mather T, Sussman F, Esmon CT: Mutation of Glu 80 [to] Lys results in a protein C mutant that no longer requires Ca^{2+} for rapid activation by the thrombin-thrombomodulin complex. *J Biol Chem* **269**:3151, 1994.
89. Regan LM, Mollica JS, Rezaie AR, Esmon CT: The interaction between the endothelial cell protein C receptor and protein C is dictated by the Gla domain of protein C. *J Biol Chem* **272**:26279, 1997.
90. Christiansen WT, Tulinsky A, Castellino FJ: Functions of individual gamma-carboxyglutamic acid (Gla) residues of human protein C. Determination of functionally nonessential Gla residues and correlations with their mode of binding of calcium. *Biochemistry* **33**:14993, 1994.
91. Colpitts TL, Prorok M, Castellino FJ: Binding of calcium to individual gamma-carboxyglutamic acid residues of human protein C. *Biochemistry* **34**:2424, 1995.
92. Jhingan A, Zhang L, Christiansen WT, Castellino FJ: The activities of recombinant gamma-carboxyglutamic-acid-deficient mutants of activated human protein C toward human coagulation factor Va and factor VIII in purified systems and in plasma. *Biochemistry* **33**:1869, 1994.
93. Zhang L, Jhingan A, Castellino FJ: Role of individual gamma-carboxyglutamic acid residues of activated human protein C in defining its in vitro anticoagulant activity. *Blood* **80**:942, 1992.
94. Zhang L, Castellino FJ: The binding energy of human coagulation protein C to acidic phospholipid vesicles contains a major contribution from leucine 5 in the gamma-carboxyglutamic acid domain. *J Biol Chem* **269**:3590, 1994.
95. Smirnov MD, Esmon CT: Phosphatidylethanolamine incorporation into vesicles selectively enhances factor Va inactivation by activated protein C. *J Biol Chem* **269**:816, 1994.
96. Horie S, Ishii H, Hara H, Kazama M: Enhancement of thrombin-thrombomodulin-catalysed protein C activation by phosphatidylethanolamine containing unsaturated fatty acids: Possible physiological significance of phosphatidylethanolamine in anticoagulant activity of thrombomodulin. *Biochem J* **301**:683, 1994.
97. Sunnerhagen M, Forsén S, Hoffrén A-M, Drakenberg T, Teleman O, Stenflo J: Structure of the Ca^{2+}-free GLA domain sheds light on membrane binding of blood coagulation proteins. *Nat Struct Biol* **2**:504, 1995.
98. Öhlin A-K, Bjork I, Stenflo J: Proteolytic formation and properties of a fragment of protein C containing the gamma-carboxyglutamic acid rich domain and the EGF-like region. *Biochemistry* **29**:644, 1990.
99. Rezaie AR, Esmon NL, Esmon CT: The high affinity calcium-binding site involved in protein C activation is outside the first epidermal growth factor homology domain. *J Biol Chem* **267**:11701, 1992.
100. Drakenberg T, Fernlund P, Roepstorff P, Stenflo J: β-Hydroxyaspartic acid in vitamin K-dependent protein C. *Proc Natl Acad Sci U S A* **80**:1802, 1983.
101. Öhlin A-K, Landes G, Bourdon P, Oppenheimer C, Wydro R, Stenflo J: β-Hydroxyaspartic acid in the first epidermal growth factor-like domain of protein C: Its role in Ca^{2+} binding and biological activity. *J Biol Chem* **263**:19240, 1988.
102. Cheng C-H, Geng J-P, Castellino FJ: The functions of the first epidermal growth factor homology region of human protein C as revealed by a charge-to-alanine scanning mutagenesis investigation. *Biol Chem* **378**:1491, 1997.
103. Amphlett GW, Kisiel W, Castellino FJ: Interaction of calcium with bovine plasma protein C. *Biochemistry* **20**:2156, 1981.
104. Esmon NL, DeBault LE, Esmon CT: Proteolytic formation and properties of gamma-carboxyglutamic acid-domainless protein C. *J Biol Chem* **258**:5548, 1983.
105. Mather T, Oganessyan V, Hof P, et al.: The 2.8 Å crystal structure of Gla-domainless activated protein C. *EMBO J* **15**:6822, 1996.
106. Fisher CL, Greengard JS, Griffin JH: Models of the serine protease domain of the human antithrombotic plasma factor activated protein C and its zymogen. *Protein Sci* **3**:588, 1994.
107. Ye J, Liu L-W, Esmon CT, Johnson AE: The fifth and sixth growth factor-like domains of thrombomodulin bind to the anion exosite of thrombin and alter its specificity. *J Biol Chem* **267**:11023, 1992.
108. Mathews II, Padmanabhan KP, Tulinsky A, Sadler JE: Structure of a nonadecapeptide of the fifth EGF domain of thrombomodulin complexed with thrombin. *Biochemistry* **33**:13547, 1994.
109. Mathews II, Padmanabhan KP, Ganesh V, et al.: Crystallographic structures of thrombin complexed with thrombin receptor peptides: Existence of expected and novel binding modes. *Biochemistry* **33**:3266, 1994.
110. Coughlin SR: Thrombin receptor function and cardiovascular disease. *Trends Cardiovasc Med* **4**:77, 1994.
111. Liu L-W, Vu T-KH, Esmon CT, Coughlin SR: The region of the thrombin receptor resembling hirudin binds to thrombin and alters enzyme specificity. *J Biol Chem* **266**:16977, 1991.
112. Vu T-KH, Wheaton VI, Hung DT, Charo I, Coughlin SR: Domains specifying thrombin-receptor interaction. *Nature* **353**:674, 1991.
113. Vu T-KH, Hung DT, Wheaton VI, Coughlin SR: Molecular cloning of a functional thrombin receptor reveals a novel proteolytic mechanism of receptor activation. *Cell* **64**:1057, 1991.
114. Stubbs MT, Oschkinat H, Mayr I, et al.: The interaction of thrombin with fibrinogen. A structural basis for its specificity. *Eur J Biochem* **206**:187, 1992.
115. Martin P, Robertson W, Turk D, Huber R, Bode W, Edwards BFP: The structure of residues 7–16 of the A-alpha-chain of human fibrinogen bound to bovine thrombin at 2.3-Å resolution. *J Biol Chem* **267**:7911, 1992.
116. Naski MC, Fenton JW, II, Maraganore JM, Olson ST, Shafer JA: The COOH-terminal domain of hirudin: An exosite-directed competitive inhibitor of the action of alpha-thrombin on fibrinogen. *J Biol Chem* **265**:13484, 1990.
117. Esmon CT, Lollar P: Involvement of thrombin anion-binding exosites 1 and 2 in the activation of factor V and factor VIII. *J Biol Chem* **271**:13882, 1996.
118. Kane WH, Davie EW: Blood coagulation factors V and VIII: Structural and functional similarities and their relationship to hemorrhagic and thrombotic disorders. *Blood* **71**:539, 1988.
119. Grinnell BW, Walls JD, Gerlitz B: Glycosylation of human protein C affects its secretion, processing, functional activities, and activation by thrombin. *J Biol Chem* **226**:9778, 1991.
120. Yan SB, Chao YB, van Halbeek H: Novel Asn-linked oligosaccharides terminating in GalNAcβ(1 to 4)[Fucα(1 to 3)]GlcNAcβ(1 to $) are present in recombinant human protein C expressed in human kidney 293 cells. *Glycobiology* **3**:597, 1993.
121. Grinnell BW, Hermann RB, Yan SB: Human protein C inhibits selectin-mediated cell adhesion: Role of unique fucosylated oligosaccharide. *Glycobiology* **4**:221, 1994.
122. Kato A, Miura O, Sumi Y, Aoki N: Assignment of the human protein C gene (PROC) to chromosome region 2q14-q21 by *in situ* hybridization. *Cytogenet Cell Genet* **47**:46, 1988.
123. Patracchini P, Aiello V, Palazzi P, Calzolari E, Bernardi F: Sublocalization of the human protein C gene on chromosome 2q13-q14. *Hum Genet* **81**:191, 1989.
124. Foster DC, Yoshitake S, Davie EW: The nucleotide sequence of the gene for human protein C. *Proc Natl Acad Sci U S A* **82**:4673, 1985.
125. Tanabe S, Sugo T, Matsuda M: Synthesis of protein C in human umbilical vein endothelial cells. *J Biochem (Tokyo)* **109**:924, 1991.
126. Beckmann RJ, Schmidt RJ, Santerre RF, Plutzky J, Crabtree GR, Long GL: The structure and evolution of a 461 amino acid human protein C precursor and its messenger RNA, based upon the DNA sequence of cloned human liver cDNAs. *Nucleic Acids Res* **13**:5233, 1985.
127. Miletich J, Sherman L, Broze G Jr: Absence of thrombosis in subjects with heterozygous protein C deficiency. *N Engl J Med* **317**:991, 1987.
128. Koster T, Rosendaal FR, Briet E, et al.: Protein C deficiency in a controlled series of unselected outpatients: An infrequent but clear risk factor for venous thrombosis (Leiden Thrombophilia Study). *Blood* **85**:2756, 1995.
129. Bovill EG, Tomczak JA, Grant B, et al.: Protein $C_{Vermont}$: Symptomatic type II protein C deficiency associated with two GLA domain mutations. *Blood* **79**:1456, 1992.
130. Bovill EG, Bauer KA, Dickerman JD, Callas P, West B: The clinical spectrum of heterozygous protein C deficiency in a large New England kindred. *Blood* **73**:712, 1989.
131. Camerlingo M, Finazzi G, Casto L, Laffranchi C, Barbui T, Mamoli A: Inherited protein C deficiency and nonhemorrhagic arterial stroke in young adults. *Neurology* **41**:1371, 1991.
132. Ohwada A, Takahashi H, Uchida K, Nukiwa T, Kira S: Gene analysis of heterozygous protein C deficiency in a patient with pulmonary arterial thromboembolism. *Am Rev Respir Dis* **145**:1491, 1992.
133. Cortellaro M, Boschetti C, Cofrancesco E, et al.: The PLAT Study: Hemostatic function in relation to atherothrombotic ischemic events in vascular disease patients. Principal results. *Arterioscl Thromb Vasc Biol* **12**:1063, 1992.

134. Comp PC, Elrod JP, Karzenski S: Warfarin-induced skin necrosis. *Semin Thromb Hemost* **16**:293, 1990.
135. Schramm W, Spannagl M, Bauer KA, et al.: Treatment of coumarin-induced skin necrosis with a monoclonal antibody purified protein C concentrate. *Arch Dermatol* **129**:753, 1993.
136. Broekmans AW, Bertina RM, Loeliger EA, Hofman V, Klingeman HG: Protein C and the development of skin necrosis during anticoagulant therapy [Letter]. *Thromb Haemost* **49**:251, 1983.
137. Griffin JH, Mosher DF, Zimmerman TS, Kleiss AJ: Protein C, an antithrombotic protein, is reduced in hospitalized patients with intravascular coagulation. *Blood* **60**:261, 1982.
138. Edenbrandt C-M, Lundwall A, Wydro R, Stenflo J: Molecular analysis of the gene for vitamin K-dependent protein S and its pseudogene. Cloning and partial gene organization. *Biochemistry* **29**:7861, 1990.
139. Lundwall A, Dackowski W, Cohen E, et al.: Isolation and sequence of the cDNA for human protein S, a regulator of blood coagulation. *Proc Natl Acad Sci U S A* **83**:6716, 1986.
140. Schmidel DK, Tatro AV, Phelps LG, Tomczak JA, Long GL: Organization of the human protein S genes. *Biochemistry* **29**:7845, 1990.
141. Joseph DR, Baker ME: Sex hormone-binding globulin, androgen-binding protein, and vitamin K-dependent protein S are homologous to laminin A, merosin, and Drosophila crumbs protein. *FASEB J* **6**:2477, 1992.
142. Gershagen S, Fernlund P, Edenbrandt C-M: The genes for SHBG/ABP and the SHBG-like region of vitamin K-dependent protein S have evolved from a common ancestral gene. *J Steroid Biochem Mol Biol* **40**:763, 1991.
143. Chang GTG, Aaldering L, Hackeng TM, Reitsma PH, Bertina RM, Bouma BN: Construction and characterization of thrombin-resistant variants of recombinant human protein S. *Thromb Haemost* **72**:693, 1994.
144. Dahlbäck B: Purification of human vitamin K-dependent protein S and its limited proteolysis by thrombin. *Biochem J* **209**:837, 1983.
145. Walker FJ: Regulation of vitamin K-dependent protein S. Inactivation by thrombin. *J Biol Chem* **259**:10335, 1984.
146. Suzuki K, Nishioka J, Hashimoto S: Regulation of activated protein C by thrombin-modified protein S. *J Biochem (Tokyo)* **94**:699, 1983.
147. Sugo T, Dahlbäck B, Holmgren A, Stenflo J: Calcium binding of bovine protein S. Effect of thrombin cleavage and removal of the gamma-carboxyglutamic acid-containing region. *J Biol Chem* **261**:5116, 1986.
148. Mitchell CA, Salem HH: Cleavage of protein S by a platelet membrane protease. *J Clin Invest* **79**:374, 1987.
149. Oates AM, Salem HH: The binding and regulation of protein S by neutrophils. *Blood Coagul Fibrinolysis* **2**:601, 1991.
150. Stenflo J, Lundwall A, Dahlbäck B: β-Hydroxyasparagine in domains homologous to the epidermal growth factor precursor in vitamin K-dependent protein S. *Proc Natl Acad Sci U S A* **84**:368, 1987.
151. Stenberg Y, Linse S, Drakenberg T, Stenflo J: The high affinity calcium-binding sites in the epidermal growth factor module region of vitamin K-dependent protein S. *J Biol Chem* **272**:23255, 1997.
152. Stenberg Y, Drakenberg T, Dahlbäck B, Stenflo J: Characterization of recombinant epidermal growth factor (EGF)-like modules from vitamin-K-dependent protein S expressed in *Spodoptera* cells. The cofactor activity depends on the N-terminal EGF module in human protein S. *Eur J Biochem* **251**:564, 1998.
153. Dahlbäck B, Hildebrand B, Malm J: Characterization of functionally important domains in human vitamin K-dependent protein S using monoclonal antibodies. *J Biol Chem* **265**:8127, 1990.
154. van Wijnen M, Stam JG, Chang GTG, et al.: Characterization of mini-protein S, a recombinant variant of protein S that lacks the sex hormone binding globulin-like domain. *Biochem J* **330**:389, 1998.
155. Dahlbäck B, Stenflo J: High molecular weight complex in human plasma between vitamin K-dependent protein S and complement component C4b-binding protein. *Proc Natl Acad Sci U S A* **78**:2512, 1981.
156. Chang GTG, Maas BHA, van Amstel HKP, Reitsma PH, Bertina RM, Bouma BN: Studies of the interaction between human protein S and human C4b-binding protein using deletion variants of recombinant human protein S. *Thromb Haemost* **71**:461, 1994.
157. Dahlbäck B: Inhibition of protein Ca cofactor function of human and bovine protein S by C4b-binding protein. *J Biol Chem* **261**:12022, 1986.
158. Dahlbäck B, Frohm B, Nelsestuen G: High affinity interaction between C4b-binding protein and vitamin K-dependent protein S in the presence of calcium. *J Biol Chem* **265**:16082, 1990.
159. Griffin JH, Gruber A, Fernandez JA: Reevaluation of total, free, and bound protein S and C4b-binding protein levels in plasma anti-coagulated with citrate or hirudin. *Blood* **79**:3203, 1992.
160. He X, Shen L, Malmborg A-C, Smith KJ, Dahlbäck B, Linse S: Binding site for C4b-binding protein in vitamin K-dependent protein S fully contained in carboxy-terminal laminin-G-type repeats. A study using recombinant factor IX-protein S chimeras and surface plasmon resonance. *Biochemistry* **36**:3745, 1997.
161. Dahlbäck B, Smith CA, Muller-Eberhard HJ: Visualization of human C4b-binding protein and its complexes with vitamin K-dependent protein S and complement protein C4b. *Proc Natl Acad Sci U S A* **80**:3461, 1983.
162. Dahlbäck B, Muller-Eberhard HJ: Ultrastructure of C4b-binding protein fragments formed by limited proteolysis using chymotrypsin. *J Biol Chem* **259**:11631, 1984.
163. Härdig Y, Dahlbäck B: The amino-terminal module of the C4b-binding protein β-chain contains the protein S-binding site. *J Biol Chem* **271**:20861, 1996.
164. Hillarp A, Dahlbäck B: Novel subunit in C4b-binding protein required for protein S binding. *J Biol Chem* **263**:12759, 1988.
165. Garcia de Frutos P, Alim RIM, Hardig Y, Zoller B, Dahlbäck B: Differential regulation of α and beta chains of C4b-binding protein during acute-phase response resulting in stable plasma levels of free anticoagulant protein S. *Blood* **84**:815, 1994.
166. Hillarp A, Pardo-Manuel F, Ruiz RR, Rodriguez de Cordoba S, Dahlbäck B: The human C4b-binding protein β-chain gene. *J Biol Chem* **268**:15017, 1993.
167. Hillarp A, Thern A, Dahlbäck B: Bovine C4b binding protein. Molecular cloning of the α- and β-chains provides structural background for lack of complex formation with protein S. *J Immunol* **153**:4190, 1994.
168. Ploos van Amstel HK, Reitsma PH, van der Logt CPE, Bertina RM: Intron-exon organization of the active human protein S gene PS alpha and its pseudogene PSβ: Duplication and silencing during primate evolution. *Biochemistry* **29**:7853, 1990.
169. Ploos van Amstel JK, van der Zanden AL, Bakker E, Reitsma PH, Bertina RM: Two genes homologous with human protein S cDNA are located on chromosome 3. *Thromb Haemost* **58**:982, 1987.
170. Watkins P, Eddy R, Fukushima Y, et al.: The gene for protein S maps near the centromere of human chromosome 3. *Blood* **71**:238, 1988.
171. Long GL, Marshall A, Gardner JC, Naylor SL: Genes for human vitamin K-dependent plasma proteins C and S are located on chromosome 2 and 3, respectively. *Somat Cell Mol Genet* **14**:93, 1988.
172. Ploos van Amstel HK, Reitsma PH, Hamulyak K, de Die-Smulders CEM, Mannucci PM, Bertina RM: A mutation in the protein S pseudogene is linked to protein S deficiency in a thrombophilic family. *Thromb Haemost* **62**:897, 1989.
173. Hoskins J, Norman DK, Beckmann RJ, Long GL: Cloning and characterization of human liver cDNA encoding a protein S precursor. *Proc Natl Acad Sci U S A* **84**:349, 1987.
174. Diepstraten CM, Ploos van Amstel JK, Reitsma PH, Bertina RM: A CCA/CCG neutral dimorphism in the codon for Pro 626 of the human protein S gene PSα•*(PROS1)*. *Nucleic Acids Res* **19**:5091, 1991.
175. Faioni EM, Valsecchi C, Palla A, Taioli E, Razzari C, Mannucci PM: Free protein S deficiency is a risk factor for venous thrombosis. *Thromb Haemost* **78**:1343, 1997.
176. Girolami A, Simioni P, Sartori MT, Caenazzo A: Intra-cardial thrombosis with systemic and pulmonary embolism as main symptoms in a patient with protein S deficiency. *Blood Coagul Fibrinolysis* **3**:485, 1992.
177. Kamiya T, Sugihara T, Ogata K, et al.: Inherited deficiency of protein S in a Japanese family with recurrent venous thrombosis: A study of three generations. *Blood* **67**:406, 1986.
178. Lauer CG, Reid TJ, III, Wideman CS, Evatt BL, Alving BM: Free protein S deficiency in a family with venous thrombosis. *J Vasc Surg* **12**:541, 1990.
179. Maccaferri M, Legnani C, Preda L, Palareti G: Protein S activity in patients with heredofamilial protein S deficiency and in patients with juvenile venous thrombosis. Results of a functional method. *Thromb Res* **64**:647, 1991.
180. Mahasandana C, Suvatte V, Chuansumrit A, et al.: Homozygous protein S deficiency in an infant with purpura fulminans. *J Pediatr* **117**:750, 1990.
181. Melissari E, Monte G, Lindo VS, et al.: Congenital thrombophilia among patients with venous thromboembolism. *Blood Coagul Fibrinolysis* **3**:749, 1992.

182. Simmonds RE, Ireland H, Kunz G, Lane DA: The Protein S Study Group: Identification of 19 protein S gene mutations in patients with phenotypic protein S deficiency and thrombosis. *Blood* **88**:4195, 1996.
183. Schwarz HP, Fischer M, Hopmeier P, Batard MA, Griffin JH: Plasma protein S deficiency in familial thrombotic disease. *Blood* **64**:1297, 1984.
184. Simmonds RE, Ireland H, Lane DA, Zöller B, Garcia de Frutos P, Dahlbäck B: Clarification of the risk for venous thrombosis associated with hereditary protein S deficiency by investigation of a large kindred with a characterized gene defect. *Ann Intern Med* **128**:8, 1998.
185. Allaart CF, Aronson DC, Ruys T, et al.: Hereditary protein S deficiency in young adults with arterial occlusive disease. *Thromb Haemost* **64**:206, 1990.
186. Girolami A, Simioni P, Lazzaro AR, Cordiano I: Severe arterial cerebral thrombosis in a patient with protein S deficiency (moderately reduced total and markedly reduced free protein S): A family study. *Thromb Haemost* **61**:144, 1989.
187. Golub BM, Sibony PA, Coller BS: Protein S deficiency associated with central retinal artery occlusion. *Arch Ophthalmol* **108**:918, 1990.
188. Horowitz IN, Galvis AG, Gomperts ED: Arterial thrombosis and protein S deficiency. *J Pediatr* **121**:934, 1992.
189. Sacco RL, Owen J, Mohr JP, Tatemichi TK, Grossman BA: Free protein S deficiency: A possible association with cerebrovascular occlusion. *Stroke* **20**:1657, 1989.
190. Wiesel M-L, Borg J-Y, Grunebaum L, et al.: Influence of protein S deficiency on the risk of arterial thrombosis. *Presse Med* **20**:1023, 1991.
191. Takahashi H, Wada K, Hayashi S, Hanano M, Tatewaki W, Shibata A: Behavior of protein S during long-term oral anticoagulant therapy. *Thromb Res* **51**:241, 1988.
192. Takahashi H, Tatewaki W, Wada K, Shibata A: Plasma protein S in disseminated intravascular coagulation, liver disease, collagen disease, diabetes mellitus, and under oral anticoagulant therapy. *Clinica Chimica Acta* **182**:195, 1989.
193. D'Angelo A, Vigano-D'Angelo S, Esmon CT, Comp PC: Acquired deficiencies of protein S: Protein S activity during oral anticoagulation, in liver disease and in disseminated intravascular coagulation. *J Clin Invest* **81**:1445, 1988.
194. D'Angelo SV, D'Angelo A, Kaufman C, Esmon CT, Comp PC: Acquired functional protein S deficiency occurs in the nephrotic syndrome. *Ann Intern Med* **107**:42, 1987.
195. Jackman RW, Beeler DL, Fritze L, Soff G, Rosenberg RD: Human thrombomodulin gene is intron depleted: Nucleic acid sequences of the cDNA and gene predict protein structure and suggest sites of regulatory control. *Proc Natl Acad Sci U S A* **84**:6425, 1987.
196. Wen D, Dittman WA, Ye RD, Deaven LL, Majerus PW, Sadler JE: Human thrombomodulin: Complete cDNA sequence and chromosome localization of the gene. *Biochemistry* **26**:4350, 1987.
197. Suzuki K, Kusumoto H, Deyashiki Y, et al.: Structure and expression of human thrombomodulin, a thrombin receptor on endothelium acting as a cofactor for protein C activation. *EMBO J* **6**:1891, 1987.
198. Shirai T, Shiojiri S, Ito H, et al.: Gene structure of human thrombomodulin, a cofactor for thrombin-catalyzed activation of protein C. *J Biochem (Tokyo)* **103**:281, 1988.
199. Petersen TE: The amino-terminal domain of thrombomodulin and pancreatic stone protein are homologous with lectins. *FEBS Lett* **231**:51, 1988.
200. Kurosawa S, Stearns DJ, Jackson KW, Esmon CT: A 10-kDa cyanogen bromide fragment from the epidermal growth factor homology domain of rabbit thrombomodulin contains the primary thrombin binding site. *J Biol Chem* **263**:5993, 1988.
201. Stearns DJ, Kurosawa S, Esmon CT: Micro-thrombomodulin: Residues 310–486 from the epidermal growth factor precursor homology domain of thrombomodulin will accelerate protein C activation. *J Biol Chem* **264**:3352, 1989.
202. Suzuki K, Hayashi T, Nishioka J, et al.: A domain composed of epidermal growth factor-like structures of human thrombomodulin is essential for thrombin binding and for protein C activation. *J Biol Chem* **264**:4872, 1989.
203. Zushi M, Gomi K, Yamamoto S, Maruyama I, Hayashi T, Suzuki K: The last three consecutive epidermal growth factor-like structures of human thrombomodulin comprise the minimum functional domain for protein C-activating cofactor activity and anticoagulant activity. *J Biol Chem* **264**:10351, 1989.
204. Zushi M, Gomi K, Honda G, et al.: Aspartic acid 349 in the fourth epidermal growth factor-like structure of human thrombomodulin plays a role in its Ca^{2+}-mediated binding to protein C. *J Biol Chem* **266**:19886, 1991.
205. Vindigni A, White CE, Komives EA, Di Cera E: Energetics of thrombin-thrombomodulin interaction. *Biochemistry* **36**:6674, 1997.
206. Lentz SR, Chen Y, Sadler JE: Sequences required for thrombomodulin cofactor activity within the fourth epidermal growth factor-like domain of human thrombomodulin. *J Biol Chem* **268**:15312, 1993.
207. Nagashima M, Lundh E, Leonard JC, Morser J, Parkinson JF: Alanine-scanning mutagenesis of the epidermal growth factor-like domains of human thrombomodulin identifies critical residues for its cofactor activity. *J Biol Chem* **268**:2888, 1993.
208. Lin J-H, McLean K, Morser J, et al.: Modulation of glycosaminoglycan addition in naturally expressed and recombinant human thrombomodulin. *J Biol Chem* **269**:25021, 1994.
209. Salem HH, Maruyama I, Ishii H, Majerus PW: Isolation and characterization of thrombomodulin from human placenta. *J Biol Chem* **259**:12246, 1984.
210. Esmon NL, Owen WG, Esmon CT: Isolation of a membrane-bound cofactor for thrombin-catalyzed activation of protein C. *J Biol Chem* **257**:859, 1982.
211. Bourin M, Boffa M, Bjork I, Lindahl U: Functional domains of rabbit thrombomodulin. *Proc Natl Acad Sci U S A* **83**:5924, 1986.
212. Bourin MC, Lundgren-Åkerlund E, Lindahl U: Isolation and characterization of the glycosaminoglycan component of rabbit thrombomodulin proteoglycan. *J Biol Chem* **265**:15424, 1990.
213. Bourin M-C: Effect of rabbit thrombomodulin on thrombin inhibition by antithrombin in the presence of heparin. *Thromb Res* **54**:27, 1989.
214. Parkinson JF, Vlahos CJ, Yan SCB, Bang NU: Recombinant human thrombomodulin: Regulation of cofactor activity and anticoagulant function by a glycosaminoglycan side chain. *Biochem J* **283**:151, 1992.
215. Parkinson JF, Koyama T, Bang NU, Preissner KT: Thrombomodulin: An anticoagulant cell surface proteoglycan with physiologically relevant glycosaminoglycan moiety. *Adv Exp Med Biol* **313**:177, 1992.
216. Ye J, Rezaie AR, Esmon CT: Glycosaminoglycan contributions to both protein C activation and thrombin inhibition involve a common arginine-rich site in thrombin that includes residues arginine 93, 97, and 101. *J Biol Chem* **269**:17965, 1994.
217. He X, Ye J, Esmon CT, Rezaie AR: Influence of arginines 93, 97, and 101 of thrombin to its functional specificity. *Biochemistry* **36**:8969, 1997.
218. Maruyama I, Salem HH, Ishii H, Majerus PW: Human thrombomodulin is not an efficient inhibitor of procoagulant activity of thrombin. *J Clin Invest* **75**:987, 1985.
219. Dittman WA, Kumada T, Sadler JE, Majerus PW: The structure and function of mouse thrombomodulin. Phorbol myristate acetate stimulates degradation and synthesis of thrombomodulin without affecting mRNA levels in hemangioma cells. *J Biol Chem* **263**:15815, 1988.
220. Jackman RW, Beeler DL, VanDeWater L, Rosenberg RD: Characterization of a thrombomodulin cDNA reveals structural similarity to the low density lipoprotein receptor. *Proc Natl Acad Sci U S A* **83**:8834, 1986.
221. Conway EM, Boffa M-C, Nowakowski B, Steiner-Mosonyi M: An ultrastructural study of thrombomodulin endocytosis: Internalization occurs via clathrin-coated and non-coated pits. *J Cell Physiol* **151**:604, 1992.
222. Conway EM, Pollefeyt S, Collen D, Steiner-Mosonyi M: The amino terminal lectin-like domain of thrombomodulin is required for constitutive endocytosis. *Blood* **89**:652, 1997.
223. Mulder AB, Smit JW, Bom VJJ, Blom NR, Halie MR, van der Meer J: Association of endothelial tissue factor and thrombomodulin with caveolae. *Blood* **88**:3667, 1996.
224. Bajzar L, Manuel R, Nesheim ME: Purification and characterization of TAFI, a thrombin-activable fibrinolysis inhibitor. *J Biol Chem* **270**:14477, 1995.
225. Bajzar L, Morser J, Nesheim M: TAFI, or plasma procarboxypeptidase B, couples the coagulation and fibrinolytic cascades through the thrombin-thrombomodulin complex. *J Biol Chem* **271**:16603, 1996.
226. Kokami K, Zheng X, Sadler JE: Activation of thrombin-activable fibrinolysis inhibitor requires epidermal growth factor-like domain 3 of thrombomodulin and is inhibited competitively by protein C. *J Biol Chem* **273**:12135, 1998.
227. Bajzar L, Nesheim M: The effect of activated protein C on fibrinolysis in cell-free plasma can be attributed specifically to attenuation of prothrombin activation. *J Biol Chem* **268**:8608, 1993.

228. de Munk GAW, Groeneveld E, Rijken DC: Acceleration of the thrombin inactivation of single chain urokinase-type plasminogen activator (pro-urokinase) by thrombomodulin. *J Clin Invest* **88**:1680, 1991.
229. Molinari A, Giogetti C, Lansen J, et al.: Thrombomodulin is a cofactor for thrombin degradation of recombinant single-chain urokinase plasminogen activator in vitro and in a perfused rabbit heart model. *Thromb Haemost* **67**:226, 1992.
230. Gomi K, Zushi M, Honda G et al.: Antithrombotic effect of recombinant human thrombomodulin on thrombin-induced thromboembolism in mice. *Blood* **75**:1396, 1990.
231. Uchiba M, Okajima K, Murakami K, Nawa K, Okabe H, Takatsuki K: Recombinant human soluble thrombomodulin reduces endotoxin-induced pulmonary vascular injury via protein C activation in rats. *Thromb Haemost* **74**:1265, 1995.
232. Mohri M, Oka M, Aoki Y, et al.: Intravenous extended infusion of recombinant human soluble thrombomodulin prevented tissue factor-induced disseminated intravascular coagulation in rats. *Amer J Hematol* **45**:298, 1994.
233. Ono M, Nawa K, Marumoto Y: Antithrombotic effects of recombinant human soluble thrombomodulin in a rat model of vascular shunt thrombosis. *Thromb Haemost* **72**:421, 1994.
234. Gonda Y, Hirata S, Saitoh K-I, et al.: Antithrombotic effect of recombinant human soluble thrombomodulin on endotoxin-induced disseminated intravascular coagulation in rats. *Thromb Res* **71**:325, 1993.
235. Aoki Y, Takei R, Mohri M, et al.: Antithrombotic effects of recombinant human soluble thrombomodulin (rhs-TM) on arteriovenous shunt thrombosis in rats. *Am J Hematol* **47**:162, 1994.
236. Solis MM, Vitti M, Cook J, et al.: Recombinant soluble human thrombomodulin: A randomized, blinded assessment of prevention of venous thrombosis and effects on hemostatic parameters in a rat model. *Thromb Res* **73**:385, 1994.
237. Hasegawa N, Kandra TG, Husari AW, et al.: The effects of recombinant human thrombomodulin on endotoxin-induced multiple-system organ failure in rats. *Am J Respir Crit Care Med* **153**:1831, 1996.
238. Uchiba M, Okajima K, Murakami K, Johno M, Okabe H, Takatsuki K: Recombinant thrombomodulin prevents endotoxin-induced lung injury in rats by inhibiting leukocyte activation. *Am J Physiol* **271**:L470, 1996.
239. Uchiba M, Okajima K, Murakami K, et al.: rhs-TM prevents ET-induced increase in pulmonary vascular permeability through protein C activation. *Am J Physiol* **273**:L889, 1997.
240. Espinosa RI, Sadler JE, LeBeau MM: Regional localization of the human thrombomodulin gene to 20p12-cen. *Genomics* **5**:649, 1989.
241. Dittman WA: Thrombomodulin: Biology and potential cardiovascular applications. *Trends Cardiovasc Med* **1**:331, 1991.
242. Ireland H, Kunz G, Kyriakoulis K, Stubbs PJ, Lane DA: Thrombomodulin gene mutations in myocardial infarction. *Circulation* **96**:15, 1997.
243. Norlund L, Holm J, Zoller B, Ohlin A-K: A common thrombomodulin amino acid dimorphism is associated with myocardial infarction. *Thromb Haemost* **77**:248, 1997.
244. van der Velden PA, Krommenhoek-Van Es T, Allaart CF, Bertina RM, Reitsma PH: A frequent thrombomodulin amino acid dimorphism is not associated with thrombophilia. *Thromb Haemost* **65**:511, 1991.
245. Boehme MWJ, Deng Y, Raeth U, et al.: Release of thrombomodulin from endothelial cells by concerted action of TNF-α and neutrophils: In vivo and in vitro studies. *Immunology* **87**:134, 1996.
246. Takano S, Kimura S, Ohdama S, Aoki N: Plasma thrombomodulin in health and diseases. *Blood* **76**:2024, 1990.
247. Glaser CB, Morser J, Clarke JH, et al.: Oxidation of a specific methionine in thrombomodulin by activated neutrophil products blocks cofactor activity. *J Clin Invest* **90**:2565, 1992.
248. Hamada H, Ishii H, Sakyo K, Horie S, Nishiki K, Kazama M: The epidermal growth factor-like domain of recombinant human thrombomodulin exhibits mitogenic activity for Swiss 3T3 cells. *Blood* **86**:225, 1995.
249. Norlund L, Zoller B, Öhlin A-K: A novel thrombomodulin gene mutation in a patient suffering from sagittal sinus thrombosis. *Thromb Haemost* **78**:1164, 1997.
250. Ohlin A-K, Marlar RA: The first mutation identified in the thrombomodulin gene in a 45-year-old man presenting with thromboembolic disease. *Blood* **85**:330, 1995.
251. Öhlin A-K, Norlund L, Marlar RA: Thrombomodulin gene variations and thromboembolic disease. *Thromb Haemost* **78**:396, 1997.
252. Zoller B, Svensson PJ, He X, Dahlbäck B: Identification of the same factor V gene mutation in 47 out of 50 thrombosis-prone families with inherited resistance to activated protein C. *J Clin Invest* **94**:2521, 1994.
253. Zoller B, Dahlbäck B: Linkage between inherited resistance to activated protein C and factor V gene mutation in venous thrombosis. *Lancet* **343**:1536, 1994.
254. Koeleman BPC, Reitsma PH, Allaart CF, Bertina RM: Activated protein C resistance as an additional risk factor for thrombosis in protein C-deficient families. *Blood* **84**:1031, 1994.
255. Greengard JS, Sun X, Xu X, Fernandez JA, Griffin JH, Evatt B: Activated protein C resistance caused by Arg506Gln mutation in factor Va. *Lancet* **343**:1361, 1994.
256. Rees DC, Cox M, Clegg JB: World distribution of factor V Leiden. *Lancet* **346**:1133, 1995.
257. Kalafatis M, Rand MD, Mann KG: The mechanism of inactivation of human factor V and human factor Va by activated protein C. *J Biol Chem* **269**:31869, 1994.
258. Kalafatis M, Bertina RM, Rand MD, Mann KG: Characterization of the molecular defect in factor V^{R506Q}. *J Biol Chem* **270**:4053, 1995.
259. Heeb MJ, Kojima Y, Greengard JS, Griffin JH: Activated protein C resistance: Molecular mechanisms based on studies using purified Gln506-factor V. *Blood* **85**:3405, 1995.
260. Sun X, Evatt B, Griffin JH: Blood coagulation factor Va abnormality associated with resistance to activated protein C in venous thrombophilia. *Blood* **83**:3120, 1994.
261. Thorelli E, Kaufman RJ, Dahlbäck B: The C-terminal region of the factor V B-domain is crucial for the anticoagulant activity of factor V. *J Biol Chem* **273**:16140, 1998.
262. Simioni P, Scudeller A, Radossi P, et al.: "Pseudo homozygous" activated protein C resistance due to double heterozygous factor V defects (factor V Leiden mutation and type I quantitative factor V defect) associated with thrombosis: Report of two cases belonging to two unrelated kindreds. *Thromb Haemost* **75**:422, 1996.
263. Rosendaal FR, Koster T, Vandenbroucke JP, Reitsma PH: High risk of thrombosis in patients homozygous for f. V Leiden (activated protein C resistance). *Blood* **85**:1504, 1995.
264. Greengard JS, Eichinger S, Griffin JH, Bauer KA: Brief report: Variability of thrombosis among homozygous siblings with resistance to activated protein C due to an Arg to Gln mutation in the gene for factor V. *N Engl J Med* **331**:1559, 1994.
265. Holm J, Zöller B, Svensson PJ, Berntorp E, Erhardt L, Dahlbäck B: Myocardial infarction associated with homozygous resistance to activated protein C. *Lancet* **344**:952, 1994.
266. Lindblad B, Svensson PJ, Dahlbäck B: Arterial and venous thromboembolism with fatal outcome and resistance to activated protein C. *Lancet* **343**:917, 1994.
267. Rosendaal FR, Siscovick DS, Schwartz SM, et al.: Factor V Leiden (resistance to activated protein C) increases the risk of myocardial infarction in young women. *Blood* **89**:2817, 1997.
268. Cushman M, Rosendaal FR, Psaty BM et al.: Factor V Leiden is not a risk factor for arterial vascular disease in the elderly: Results from the cardiovascular health study. *Thromb Haemost* **79**:912, 1998.
269. Bernardi F, Faioni EM, Castoldi E, et al.: A factor V genetic component differing from factor V R506Q contributes to the activated protein C resistance phenotype. *Blood* **90**:1552, 1997.
270. Chan WP, Lee CK, Kwong YL, Lam CK, Liang R: A novel mutation of Arg 306 of factor V gene in Hong Kong Chinese. *Blood* **91**:1135, 1998.
271. Williamson D, Brown K, Luddington R, Baglin C, Baglin T: Factor V Cambridge: A new mutation (Arg^{306} [to] Thr) associated with resistance to activated protein C. *Blood* **91**:1140, 1998.
272. Rosing J, Tans G, Nicolaes GAF, et al.: Oral contraceptives and venous thrombosis: Different sensitivities to activated protein C in women using second- and third-generation oral contraceptives. *Br J Haematol* **97**:233, 1997.
273. Meinardi JR, Henkens CMA, Heringa MP, van der Meer J: Acquired APC resistance related to oral contraceptives and pregnancy and its possible implications for clinical practice. *Blood Coagul Fibrinolysis* **8**:152, 1997.
274. Rosendaal FR, Siscovick DS, Schwartz SM, et al.: Factor V Leiden (resistance to activated protein C) increases the risk of myocardial infarction in young women. *Blood* **89**:2817, 1997.
275. Danielsson A, Raub E, Lindahl U, Bjork I: Role of ternary complexes, in which heparin binds both antithrombin and proteinase, in the acceleration of the reactions between antithrombin and thrombin or factor Xa. *J Biol Chem* **261**:15467, 1986.

276. Comp PC, Thurnau GR, Welsh J, Esmon CT: Functional and immunologic protein S levels are decreased during pregnancy. *Blood* **68**:881, 1986.
277. Ridker PM, Miletich JP, Buring JE, et al.: Factor V Leiden mutation as a risk factor for recurrent pregnancy loss. *Ann Intern Med* **128**:1000, 1998.
278. Newton JR: Classification and comparison of oral contraceptives containing new generation progestagens. *Hum Reprod Update* **1**:231, 1995.
279. Speroff L, DeCherney A: Evaluation of a new generation of oral contraceptives: The advisory board for the new progestins. *Obstet Gynecol* **81**:1034, 1993.
280. Rosing J, Hoekema L, Nicolaes GAF, et al.: Effects of protein S and factor Xa on peptide bond cleavages during inactivation of factor Va and factor Va^{R506Q} by activated protein C. *J Biol Chem* **270**:27852, 1995.
281. Yegneswaran S, Smirnov MD, Safa O, Esmon NL, Esmon CT, Johnson AE: Relocating the active site of activated protein C eliminates the need for its protein S cofactor. A fluorescence resonance energy transfer study. *J Biol Chem* **274**:5462, 1999.
282. Meinardi JR, Henkens CMA, Heringa MP, van der Meer J: Acquired APC resistance related to oral contraceptives and pregnancy and its possible implications for clinical practice. *Blood Coagul Fibrinolysis* **8**:152, 1997.
283. Rosing J, Tans G, Nicolaes GAF, et al.: Oral contraceptives and venous thrombosis: different sensitivities to activated protein C in women using second- and third-generation oral contraceptives. *Br J Haematol* **97**:233, 1997.
284. Lane DA, Mannucci PM, Bauer KA, et al.: Inherited thrombophilia: Part 2. *Thromb Haemost* **76**:824, 1996.
285. Vandenbroucke JP, Koster T, Briët E, Reitsma PH, Bertina RM, Rosendaal FR: Increased risk of venous thrombosis in oral-contraceptive users who are carriers of factor V Leiden mutation. *Lancet* **344**:1453, 1994.
286. Muntean W, Finding K, Gamillscheg A, Schwarz HP: Multiple thromboses and coumarin-induced skin necrosis in a child with anticardiolipin antibodies: Effects of protein C concentrate administration [Abstract]. *Thromb Haemost* **65**:2017 1991.
287. Schramm W, Spannagl M, Bauer KA, et al.: Treatment of coumarin-induced skin necrosis with a monoclonal antibody purified protein C concentrate. *Arch Dermatol* **129**:753, 1993.
288. Esmon CT, Schwarz HP: An update on clinical and basic aspects of the protein C anticoagulant pathway. *Trends Cardiovasc Med* **5**:141, 1995.
289. Rintelen C, Pabinger I, Lechner K, Mannhalter C: Impact of factor V Leiden mutation on duration of anticoagulation after a single thromboembolic event. *Thromb Haemost* **77**:405, 1997.

CHAPTER 171

Disorders of Fibrinogen and Factor XIII

Dominic W. Chung ▪ Kathleen P. Pratt ▪ Akitada Ichinose

1. Fibrinogen is a dimeric protein consisting of six polypeptide chains $(\alpha\beta\gamma)_2$ (MIM 134820, 134830, 134850) held together by disulfide bonds and folded in a trinodular structure where the globular nodules are connected by coiled coils. Thrombin converts fibrinogen to fibrin, which polymerizes into protofibrils through reciprocal half-staggered interactions. Protofibrils form macroscopic fibers through lateral aggregation and branch point formation. Crystallographic studies show that the polymerization pocket within the C-terminal region of the γ-chain is adjacent to but independent from the calcium-binding site. Fibrinogen is essential for platelet aggregation and wound healing. The genes for the constituent chains of fibrinogen are linked and are located on chromosome 4. Transcription of the fibrinogen genes is mediated by hepatocyte nuclear factor 1 and modulated by interleukin 6.

2. Genetic abnormalities of fibrinogen include afibrinogenemia (MIM 202400), hypofibrinogenemia, dysfibrinogenemia, and hyperfibrinogenemia. Afibrinogenemia is rare and is characterized by neonatal umbilical cord hemorrhage, intracranial and peritoneal bleeding, recurrent abortion, and autosomal recessive inheritance. Hypofibrinogenemia is characterized by fibrinogen levels below 100 mg/dl of plasma (normal 250–320 mg/dl) and can be inherited or acquired. The symptoms of hypofibrinogenemia are similar to but milder than those of afibrinogenemia. Dysfibrinogenemia is highly heterogeneous and may affect any one of the functional properties of fibrinogen, leading to manifestations that include hemorrhage, spontaneous abortion, and thrombosis. Most cases of dysfibrinogenemia are heterozygous for amino acid substitutions; homozygous occurrence is rare but known. Hyperfibrinogenemia is associated with an increased risk for myocardial infarction and stroke.

3. Factor XIII is a proenzyme for a plasma transglutaminase. It is converted to the active form, factor XIIIa, by thrombin in the presence of calcium ions. It catalyzes the formation of γ-glutamyl-ε-lysine bonds between fibrin monomers and between fibrin and α_2-plasmin inhibitor. Factor XIII in plasma is a tetramer (A_2B_2) held together by noncovalent bonds. The A subunit contains the active site, and the B subunit is thought to stabilize the A subunit. The sequence around the active site is identical among all members of the transglutaminase family. The three-dimensional structure of the A subunit of factor XIII determined by x-ray crystallography demonstrated that it is composed of 5 distinct domains. The B subunit contains 10 tandem repeats, which have been designated as Sushi domains or GP-I structures. Homologous Sushi domains have been found in more than 30 other proteins/genes. The A subunit of plasma factor XIII is synthesized, in part, by hemopoietic cells, and is present in many tissues. The B subunit is synthesized in the liver.

4. The genes for the A and B subunits of factor XIII are localized at 6p24-p25 and 1q32-q32.1, respectively. Thus factor XIII deficiency is inherited as an autosomal recessive trait and is caused by the absence of either subunit. Recently, genetic defects have been identified at the DNA level in three patients with B-subunit deficiency (MIM 134580) and in 30 patients with A-subunit deficiency (MIM 134570). Their molecular and cellular bases also were explored in certain cases. This disease is characterized by delayed bleeding ("after bleeding"), though primary hemostasis is normal. Manifestations include neonatal bleeding from the umbilical cord, intracranial hemorrhage, and soft tissue hematomas. In addition, abnormal wound healing and recurrent spontaneous miscarriage are not rare. Infusion of factor XIII concentrates has been successful both for treatment of acute bleeding and for prophylaxis. Recombinant A subunit has been produced in yeast for clinical use.

A list of standard abbreviations is located immediately preceding the index in each volume. Nonstandard abbreviations used in this chapter include: FgBP = fibrinogen-binding protein from *Streptococcus equi*; ICAM-1 = intercellular adhesion molecule 1; NF-IL-6 = nuclear factor for IL-6 expression.

FIBRINOGEN

Fibrinogen participates in two crucial events in hemostasis. It is an adhesive protein essential for platelet aggregation and platelet plug formation at the site of vascular damage. On the surface of the activated platelets, a series of zymogen activations is triggered that culminates in the formation of thrombin. Thrombin catalyzes the conversion of soluble fibrinogen to fibrin, which polymerizes to form a fibrin clot. The fibrin clot is further crosslinked by factor XIIIa (fibrin-stabilizing factor), which introduces covalent bonds between adjacent fibrin monomers, giving rise to a tough, insoluble clot. Congenital fibrinogen deficiency that results in the complete absence of fibrinogen in the circulation, afibrinogenemia, is rare and is usually fatal. Individuals with reduced circulating levels are hypofibrinogenemic and may have a predisposition to bleeding. Inherited structural defects in the fibrinogen molecule cause dysfibrinogenemia, and affected individuals may be asymptomatic or may exhibit a hemorrhagic tendency, abnormal wound healing, or even thrombosis. Individuals with an elevated level of circulating fibrinogen (hyperfibrinogenemia) have an increased risk for cardiovascular disease and stroke.

PRIMARY STRUCTURE OF FIBRINOGEN

Fibrinogen is a plasma glycoprotein of 340 kDa.[1,2] It is a dimeric protein composed of three pairs of nonidentical but homologous polypeptide chains held together by disulfide bonds. The polypeptide chains, designated as the α, β, and γ-chains, are 63, 56, and 47 kDa,[3] and fibrinogen can be represented by the formula $(\alpha\beta\gamma)_2$. The amino acid sequences of the three chains of fibrinogen have been determined.[4–6] Sequence homology indicates that they are derived from a common ancestor. The α-chain is composed of 610 amino acids and does not contain carbohydrate. Fibrinopeptide A, which consists of the N-terminal 16 residues, is removed by thrombin during the conversion of fibrinogen to fibrin. Gly17 thus becomes the new N-terminal residue in fibrin. The region from residues 45 to 165 forms disulfide bonds with the β and γ-chains and participates in coiled coil formation. The region between residues 195 and 239 has a high proline content and is accessible to many proteases, including plasmin.[7,8] The region from residues 240 to 424 is exceptionally rich in glycine, serine, threonine, proline, and tryptophan residues and consists of eight tandem repeats, each 13 residues in length. These tandem repeats and the remaining C-terminal sequence are hydrophilic and vary greatly among species.[9–12] Two Arg-Gly-Asp (RGD) sequences are present in the α-chain. RGD sequences have been shown to bind to integrin receptors and mediate cellular adhesion. The proximal RGD sequence (95–97) occurs in the middle of the coiled-coil region, and the distal RGD sequence (572–574) is present in the C-terminal region and is not conserved among species.

The β-chain of human fibrinogen contains 461 amino acids. Fibrinopeptide B, which consists of the N-terminal 14 residues of the β-chain, is removed by thrombin during clotting, and Gly15 becomes the new N-terminus of the β-chain of fibrin. The region from Cys76 to Cys201 participates in disulfide ring and coiled coil formation. The remainder of the β-chain folds into a globular conformation. Asn364 is the site for an N-linked carbohydrate attachment in the β-chain.

The γ-chain is 411 amino acids in length. The N-terminal region (residues 1–18) that precedes the disulfide ring and the coiled-coil region is significantly shorter than the corresponding regions in the α and β-chains. A single N-linked carbohydrate attachment site is located in the middle of the coiled-coil region at Asn52. The globular C-terminal region (residues 140–411) of the γ-chain is 35 percent identical to the corresponding region of the β-chain, and the conformations are very similar.[13,14] This region contains a polymerization pocket that binds to the thrombin-cleaved α-chain N-terminus, enabling the fibrin monomers to polymerize in linear arrays. The γ-chain has a C-terminal extension of 18 amino acids that contains the factor XIII crosslinking site and the platelet-binding site.

Structure: Function Studies of Fibrinogen

Fibrinogen exhibits properties of both globular and fibrous proteins.[15,16] Electron microscopic studies have shown that fibrinogen forms a trinodular structure.[17] The length of the fibrinogen molecule is approximately 450 Å (Fig. 171-1). The central nodule, also known as the *E domain*, is ~50 Å in diameter and contains the N-termini of all six polypeptide chains.[18] Although a crystal structure of the E region has not yet been reported, a number of structural studies, using both crystallographic and nuclear magnetic resonance (NMR) techniques, have been carried out to characterize the thrombin-fibrinogen interaction. These studies have employed thrombin and peptides corresponding to both native and mutated N-terminal regions of the α- and β-chains of fibrinogen[19–21] and have indicated the structural bases for disrupted thrombin-fibrinogen interactions.

Emerging from opposite sides of the E domain are two coiled coils, which contain stretches of 111 or 112 amino acids from each of the three polypeptide chains.[22] The coiled coils are approximately 150 to 160 Å in length, and the chains in this region are mostly helical. The helical coiled-coil regions impart rigidity to the molecule. The coiled coils are briefly interrupted toward their centers by short nonhelical stretches, and these stretches are sensitive to plasmin digestion. In a structural study on a proteolytic fragment of fibrinogen that contains part of the coiled-coil region,[13] a segment of the α-chain, residues 166 to 195, is also helical and forms a fourth strand of the coiled-coil segment of fibrinogen. A unique arrangement of interchain disulfide bonds among the three chains is termed the *disulfide ring*, and these rings occur both immediately before and immediately after the coiled coils.

The outer nodules, or D domains, are approximately 60 Å in diameter and are composed of the C-terminal two-thirds of the β and γ-chains.[23,24] The C-terminal regions of the α-chains fold into globular domains that appear to bend back and interact with the central "E" nodule.[25]

Several crystal structures of fibrinogen fragments corresponding to the D domain have been reported,[13,14,26,27] and these structures have shed new light on the functional relationships among the various regions of this complex molecule. A recombinant protein corresponding to the C-terminal residues 143 to 411 of the γ-chain (γC-30) was shown to retain functions attributed to this region in intact fibrinogen and in fragment D.[28] The 2.0-Å crystal structure of this molecule shows the overall fold of this region, as well as the precise geometry of the γ-chain calcium-binding site.[14] This fragment is crystallized in a complex with the peptide Gly-Pro-Arg-Pro (GPRP), which mimics the binding of the newly exposed N-terminus of the α-chain of fibrin. Thus the complex reveals the amino acids that comprise the γ-chain polymerization pocket, as well as many of the α:γ-chain (D:E region) interactions that promote protofibril formation in the early stages of fibrin polymerization (Fig 171-2). This region of the molecule is very polar, and the interactions are primarily electrostatic in nature, consistent with the long-established effects of altering salt concentration or pH on the rate of fibrin polymerization. Studies on the γC-30:GPRP complex also show that the calcium-binding site and the polymerization pocket are structurally and functionally distinct.[27,28]

The crystal structures of both fragment D and factor XIII-crosslinked D dimers also have been reported.[13,26] The folding of the C-terminal globular region of the β-chain is similar to that of the γ-chain, as was expected from their strong sequence similarity. The region where the γ-chains abut each other during polymerization was visualized clearly in the D-dimer structures, providing important information on the intermolecular D:D interactions that stabilize and promote protofibril formation. The D dimers are also cocrystallized with the peptides GPRP-amide (mimicking the binding of fibrin α-chain N-terminus) and GHRP-amide (mimicking the binding of the fibrin β-chain N-terminus).[26] The GHRP

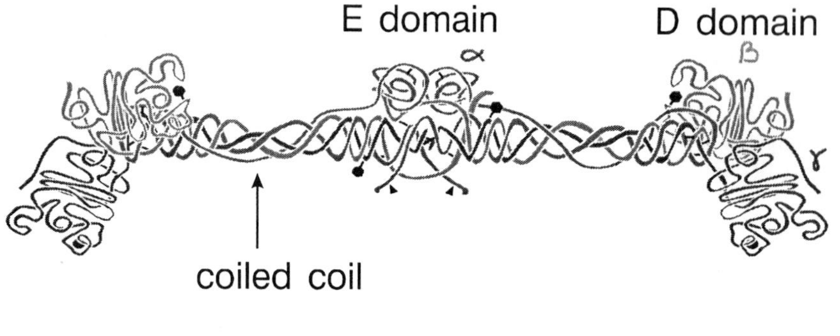

Fig. 171-1 Schematic representation of the trinodular structure of fibrinogen.

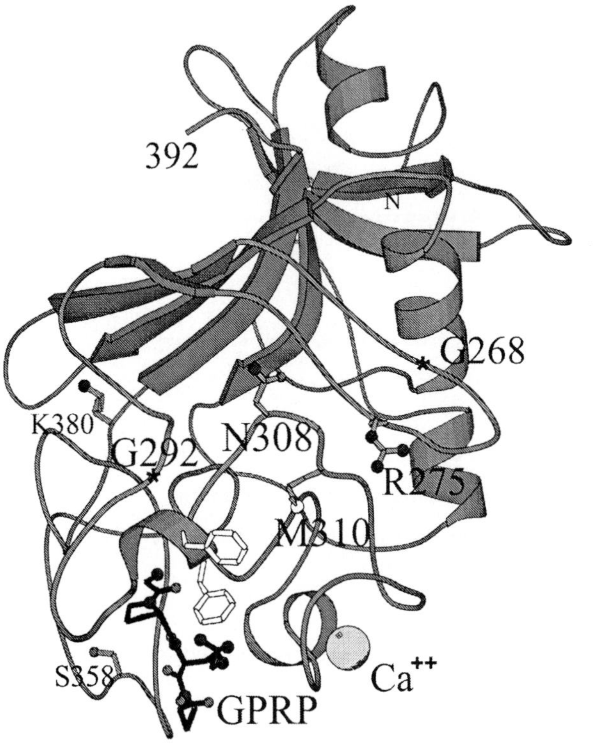

Fig. 171-2 A ribbon model of the γC-30 globular domain showing the calcium-binding site and the polymerization "a" pocket with the GPRP peptide bound to it. *(Modified with permission from Côté et al.[126])*

peptide binds to a second polymerization pocket in the β-chain, and the orientation of the β-chain pockets is consistent with earlier biochemical studies correlating fibrinopeptide B release with lateral aggregation of protofibrils.[29] Finally, an additional low-affinity calcium-binding site is identified in the β-chain, at a position analogous to the γ-chain calcium-binding site.[26] In these studies, the C-terminus of the γ-chain is disordered, and no conformational information is available on the crosslinking site and platelet-binding site.

Heterogeneity

Fibrinogen isolated from plasma is heterogeneous; the heterogeneity is attributed to the presence of variant forms of the constituent chains, polymorphic sequences, different degrees of posttranslational modification, and proteolysis. Polymorphisms in the amino acid sequences of the three chains have been identified by protein and DNA sequencing. These include α47 Ser/Thr, α296 Thr/Ala, α312 Thr/Ala, β162 Pro/Ala, β296 Asn/Asp, β448 Arg/Lys, and γ88 Ile/Lys (summarized in ref. 30). A naturally occurring variant of the γ-chain, designated the γ' or γ_B chain, is translated from a differentially processed form of γ-chain mRNA in which an alternative polyadenylation site in the ninth intron is used. This infrequent processing event enables the immediate 5′ end of the ninth intron to serve as extension of the ninth exon. Translation of this mRNA leads to replacement of residues 408 to 411 (exon X) by a new sequence of 20 amino acids (γ' 408–427).[31,32] In humans, the γ' form comprises ~10 percent of the total γ-chain population.[33] Both the γ and γ' chains are assembled into the dimeric fibrinogen molecule and function normally in fibrin polymerization and in γ-chain crosslinking. The γ' variant, however, does not bind to platelets and does not support platelet aggregation.[34] The γ' variant contains posttranslationally sulfated tyrosines in the C-terminal region.[35] There also exists an extended form of the α-chain, termed *αE*. It contains 236 additional amino acids at the C-terminus that are encoded by the infrequently used exon VI. The extended α-chain has an apparent molecular mass of 110 kDa, and the sequence encoded in exon VI is highly homologous to the C-terminal globular domains of the β and γ-chains.[36] αE chains constitute about 1.3 percent of the α-chain population in adults, whereas levels are about threefold higher in newborns.[37] The structure of the extended domain also has been solved and shows that it has a similar fold as the γC-30 domain and contains a calcium-binding site.[38]

Another source of heterogeneity in fibrinogen is introduced by minor proteolysis in the C-terminus of the α-chain.[39] The level of fibrinogen II, a fraction of 305 kDa, increases in patients with progressive liver diseases and occlusive vascular diseases. This species is composed of two types of α-chains: a normal, homogeneous, intact α-chain population and a second population (α') that has been proteolytically cleaved to terminate at Asn269, Gly297, or Pro309.[40] These cleavage-site sequences bear no resemblance to plasmin-specific recognition sequences. The identity of the proteases responsible for these cleavages remains to be determined.

Another source of heterogeneity in fibrinogen introduced posttranslationally is partial phosphorylation of serines in two locations of the α-chain: Ser3 in the fibrinopeptide A region and Ser345.[41] Fetal fibrinogen has a higher phosphoserine content than adult fibrinogen. The mechanism and regulation of the extent of phosphorylation are not well understood.

The structures of carbohydrates attached to β Asn364 and γ Asn52 have been determined by proton-NMR techniques in conjunction with sequential exoglycosidase digestions.[42] The carbohydrate chains on both polypeptides are identical in structure and contain a core pentasaccharide with biantennary oligosaccharide branch points. Approximately 20 percent of the carbohydrate chains are desialylated. An increased sialic acid content in fibrinogen from patients with inherited dysfibrinogenemia or chronic liver disease[43] causes delayed fibrin polymerization.

Removal of Fibrinopeptides

Fibrinogen is converted to fibrin monomer by thrombin, which cleaves at Arg-Gly bonds near the N-termini of the α and β-chains, releasing two molecules of fibrinopeptide A (α1–16) and two molecules of fibrinopeptide B (β1–14). The release of fibrinopeptide A proceeds more rapidly than that of fibrinopeptide B,[44] generating an intermediate called *des-A fibrin*. The newly exposed N-termini of the α-chains, having the sequence Gly-Pro-Arg, form the polymerization "A" sites in the E domain, which bind to a complementary polymerization pocket or "a" site in the D domain of a second fibrin monomer and thereby initiate fibrin polymerization. (Fig. 171-3). Assembly of des-A fibrin molecules into a polymeric form induces conformational changes in the molecules that enhance the rate of fibrinopeptide B release.[45] In addition to thrombin, several snake venom enzymes have been shown to remove fibrinopeptides from fibrinogen. Ancrod (arvin) from the venom of *Calloselasma rhodostoma* (formerly called *Agkistrodon rhodostoma*) exclusively removes fibrinopeptide A from fibrinogen.[46,47] Batroxobin (reptilase) from *Bothrops atrox moojenim* and crotalase from *Crotalus adamanteus* remove both fibrinopeptides A and B from fibrinogen. An enzyme from the venom of *Agkistrodon contortrix contortrix* preferentially releases fibrinopeptide B but also releases fibrinopeptide A slowly from fibrinogen.[48,49]

Protofibril Assembly

The reciprocal binding of an "A" site to an "a" pocket positions two fibrin molecules in a half-staggered overlapping arrangement.[50] The second "A" site within the E domain is available to bind to the "a" pocket of a third molecule, and subsequent "a-A" associations lead to linear elongation of the two-stranded polymer (see Fig. 171-3). As the D domains of adjacent fibrin monomers come into alignment, additional contacts between the γ-chains stabilize the polymeric structure. This structure is called a *protofibril* and is stabilized by noncovalent interactions entirely.[51,52] A tripeptide with a sequence identical to the

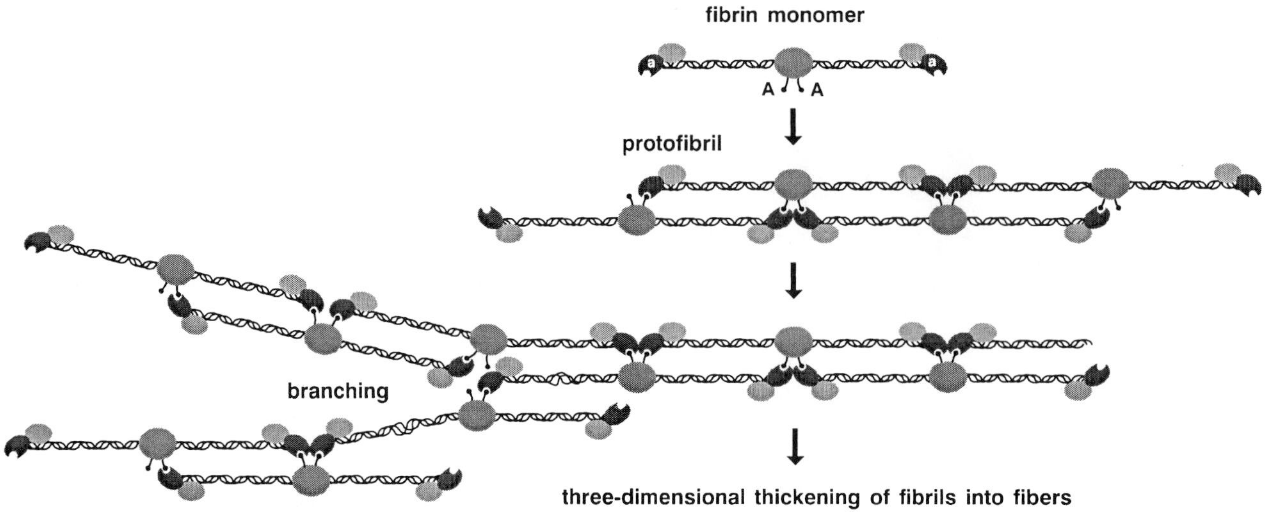

Fig. 171-3 Schematic diagram showing the initial stages of fibrin polymerization. Two stranded protofibrils are formed by "a-A" interactions between fibrin monomers in a half-staggered alignment. (*Modified with permission from Côté et al.*[126])

N-terminus of the fibrin α-chain (Gly-Pro-Arg) can bind to the "a" pockets in the D domains of fibrin(ogen) and inhibit polymerization and protofibril elongation.[53]

Lateral Aggregation

Removal of fibrinopeptides B from des-A fibrin exposes the β-chain N-termini (Gly-His-Arg) of the fibrin molecules, which are called *polymerization "B" sites*. These sites interact with "b" pockets within the C-terminal globular regions of the β-chains of additional fibrin monomers.[54] This promotes lateral aggregation of protofibrils into thick fibers and branching of these fibers to form a fibrin mesh. A tripeptide having the sequence Gly-His-Arg does not inhibit fibrin polymerization.[53,54] The C-terminal region of the α-chain also facilitates lateral aggregation,[55] although the basis for this effect is not fully understood.

Crosslinking

The interactions among fibrin monomers during the polymerization process are noncovalent. The clot is subsequently stabilized by covalent bonds that are introduced by a plasma transglutaminase, factor XIIIa (see below). These covalent links are isopeptide bonds between specific glutamine and lysine residues in aligned fibrin molecules. Initially, Lys406 in the γ-chain of one fibrin molecule is crosslinked to Gln398 or Gln399 in the γ-chain of an adjacent fibrin molecule, and then Lys406 in the γ-chain of the second molecule is reciprocally crosslinked to Gln398 or Gln399 of the first molecule.[56,57] This reciprocal crosslinking results in the formation of covalently linked γ-chain dimers. In a subsequent slower process, multiple crosslinks among α-chains are also introduced,[58–60] leading to the formation of α-chain polymers. In addition to stabilizing the clot, α-chain polymers also protect the coiled-coil regions of fibrin against proteolysis by plasmin.[61] A small proportion of crosslinked γ trimers and tetramers also has been observed. These crosslinked variants arise as a result of trimolecular and tetramolecular branch points in the fibrin clot.[62]

Wound Healing

Wound healing is markedly delayed in individuals with afibrinogenemia.[63] Afibrinogenemic mice were created by targeted disruption of the α-chain gene, and these animals suffered from spontaneous abdominal bleeding and formation of hematomas.[64] These hematomas elicit an unusual wound-healing response, in which fibroblasts form a thick circumscribing capsule without infiltrating the hematomas.[64] This result is consistent with the view that fibrin is important for the adhesion and migration of various cell types to sites of injury and that fibrin(ogen) is necessary for the process of tissue regeneration.

Fibrin Degradation

Fibrin clots deposited at sites of vascular damage are eventually degraded and removed by the protease plasmin. Early studies on the degradation of fibrinogen by plasmin and the identification of protease-susceptible regions have greatly facilitated interpretation of the plasmin digestion patterns of crosslinked fibrin.[65] These early studies showed that plasmin first produces fibrinogen fragment X by cleaving and releasing the C-terminal region of the α-chains. Fragment X is further converted to fragment Y by cleavage within one of the coiled coils. This cleavage releases a fragment D consisting of the globular D domain that is attached to remnants of the coiled coil. A similar cleavage within the second coiled-coil region of fragment Y releases the second D fragment. The remaining fragment E contains the central globular E domain with its attached coiled-coil remnants. The scheme is somewhat simplified, since fragments D and E are not homogeneous, and their masses vary according to the extent of digestion. Plasmin digestion of crosslinked fibrin follows a similar pattern to that of fibrinogen. Crosslinked C-terminal regions of α-chains are released first, exposing the coiled-coil regions of the fibers. Further digestion by plasmin at the coiled coils releases soluble DD-E complexes, each of which contains a crosslinked fragment D-dimer associated with a noncovalently bound fragment E. The D fragments, and to a lesser extent the D-dimers, retain functional "a" polymerization pockets and are effective inhibitors of fibrin polymerization.[66] In some pathologic conditions, e.g., disseminated intravascular coagulation, an excessive amount of plasmin is generated, leading to massive degradation of circulating fibrinogen, accumulation of high levels of fibrinogen degradation products in circulation, and hemorrhage.

Platelet Aggregation

Platelet aggregation is mediated by the binding of fibrinogen and fibrin to the integrin receptor $\alpha_{IIb}\beta_3$ (glycoprotein IIb-IIIa) on the platelet surface.[67] This binding involves the C-terminal 12 amino acids of the γ-chain[68,69] and can be inhibited competitively by peptides containing the sequence RGD. Although the α-chain of human fibrinogen contains two RGD sequences (residues 95–97 and 572–574), mutations abolishing both these sites do not affect platelet aggregation.[70] In addition, electron micrographs have shown that the $\alpha_{IIb}\beta_3$ receptor binds to fragment D, which does not contain the RGD sequences from the α-chain.[71] However, recombinant fibrinogen in which the γ-chain has been truncated, removing the last 5 amino acids, does not support platelet aggregation.[72] These experiments are all consistent with the conclusion that the γ-chain C-terminal residues are the primary site of interaction with $\alpha_{IIb}\ \beta_3$ on the platelet surface.

Interactions with Other Cells

Fibrinogen and fibrin contain additional binding sites that mediate the adhesion of many other types of cells besides platelets. Monocytes, leukocytes, neutrophils, endothelial cells, smooth muscle cells, keratinocytes, and fibroblasts all adhere to fibrin (ogen) and mediate important biologic processes such as clot retraction, angiogenesis, chemotaxis, inflammatory responses, and wound healing. ICAM-1 and several other cell-surface integrins have been implicated in interactions with additional regions of fibrinogen or fibrin. The γ-chain residues 117 to 133 have been shown to mediate the binding of fibrinogen to the ICAM-1 receptor on leukocytes and on endothelial cells,[73] whereas the region γ190–202 is involved in binding to the integrin $\alpha_M\ \beta_2$ on leukocytes.[74] The α-chain residues 17 to 19 mediate binding to the neutrophil integrin $\alpha_X\ \beta_2$.[75] One of the two RGD sequences in the α-chain, α572–574, has been shown to interact with the integrin $\alpha_V\ \beta_3$ on both endothelial cells[76,77] and fibroblasts.[78]

Interactions with Other Molecules

The presence of calcium enhances lateral aggregation of protofibrils and promotes the formation of thick fibers that render the fibrin clot more resistant to lysis. Fibrinogen contains 3 high-affinity calcium-binding sites, 2 of which are within the C-terminal region of the γ-chain.[79] It also contains 10 low-affinity binding sites formed by sialic acids at the ends of carbohydrate chains.[80] Mutations that affect calcium binding result in delayed fibrin polymerization and abnormal patterns of plasmin digestion.[81,82] A lower-affinity calcium-binding site also has been identified recently in the fibrinogen β-chains[26]; its role in the preceding processes remains to be determined.

The conversion of fibrinogen to fibrin is accompanied by a conformational change in the molecule enabling fibrin to interact with tissue plasminogen activator. Fibrin thus serves as a cofactor in the activation of plasminogen to plasmin. The exposure of α148–160 and γ311–379 in fibrin is essential for this cofactor activity.[83]

Besides serving as substrate for factor XIIIa in the crosslinking reactions, fibrin is also a cofactor in the activation of factor XIII to factor XIIIa by thrombin.[84] Saturating levels of the factor XIII zymogen do not affect the binding of active-site-modified factor XIIIa to fibrin. This suggests the presence of a unique nonsubstrate cofactor binding site for factor XIIIa on fibrin.

Fibrin contains two classes of non-substrate-binding sites for thrombin: the high-affinity and the low-affinity sites. Thrombin bound to fibrin is enzymatically active and is protected from inactivation by inhibitors present in the circulation. The low-affinity site is located in the fibrin E domain, and the β-chain residues β15–42 constitute part of this site.[85] The dysfibrinogen$_{\text{NEW YORK I}}$, which has a β-chain deletion of amino acids 9 to 72, lacks the low-affinity binding site and is associated with recurrent thromboembolism.[85] The high-affinity thrombin-binding site is positioned toward the C-terminus of the γ' chain.[86]

A small but significant amount of α_2-plasmin inhibitor is crosslinked to Lys303 of the fibrin(ogen) α-chain and is incorporated into the fibrin clot. Bound α_2-plasmin inhibitor delays the initiation of fibrinolysis. A deficiency in α_2-plasmin inhibitor results in severe hemorrhage characterized by a reduced resistance of fibrin clots to lysis.[87]

Fibrinogen also binds to fibronectin, and this complex can be precipitated from solution at low temperature. Fibronectin is crosslinked to lysine residues within the α-chain of fibrin and is found in fibrin clots in vivo.[88] The presence of fibronectin in fibrin clots enhances the adhesion of cells to fibrin-coated surfaces. This promotes migration and infiltration of fibroblasts and endothelial cells into wound sites and facilitates the healing process.

Bacterial Adhesins

Cell-surface proteins of several bacterial species have been shown to interact specifically with fibrinogen or fibrin. These molecules, called *bacterial adhesins*, increase the ability of the bacteria to invade the host and cause infection.[89] One of the well-characterized adhesins is the *Staphylococcus aureus* clumping factor ClfA, a 130-kDa protein. This protein binds to the C-terminal region of the γ-chain at a site that overlaps with the binding site for the integrin $\alpha_{IIb}\ \beta_3$.[90] By binding to fibrin(ogen)-coated surfaces, this adhesin confers on the bacteria resistance to phagocytosis. This binding also promotes the initial adherence of *Staphylococcus aureus* to wounds, catheters, and endothelium, from which the bacteria then gain access to the bloodstream. *S. aureus* also expresses at least two other fibrinogen-binding proteins, a 19-kDa protein called *Fib*[91] and a 70-kDa protein called *FbpA*.[92] The precise roles played by these proteins in infection remain to be determined. Some strains of *Staphylococcus epidermidis* also express on their surfaces a 119-kDa fibrinogen-binding protein called *Fbe*, which is homologous to the *S. aureus* clumping factor.[93]

Streptococci express several surface proteins that bind to fibrinogen specifically. The M proteins are a group of related proteins containing coiled-coil regions that associate to form M-dimers and multimers. This group of proteins is divided into two classes, A and C. The class A proteins are thermally stable, whereas the class C proteins are heat labile.[94] Fibrinogen and RGD peptides bind to M proteins and enhance the ability of *Streptococcus pyogenes* to invade epithelial cells.[95] A second group of fibrinogen-binding proteins belonging to the protein F family is also expressed on the surface of various strains of *S. pyogenes*. Protein F is a 100-kDa protein that contains a distinct binding site for fibrinogen in its N-terminal region and a fibronectin-binding site in its C-terminal region.[96] A fibrinogen-binding protein called *FgBP* from *Streptococcus equi* also has been characterized.[97] FgBP binds equine fibrinogen, and antibodies to FgBP were found to protect mice against a lethal challenge of *S. equi*. The predicted amino acid sequence of FgBP suggests that it contains a coiled-coil structure as well as a cell wall-anchoring domain.

Fibrin Sealant

Human fibrin can be produced by mixing human fibrinogen with bovine thrombin in the presence of calcium. The resulting fibrin clot can then be used as a tissue adhesive. This material has found widespread application in recent years as an adjunct to sutures in many types of surgeries including cardiothoracic, vascular, urologic, and neurosurgery and is particularly useful in patients with hemostatic disorders.[98,99] The sealant provides an air- and fluid-tight seal to the sutures and is completely absorbed during wound healing. Fibrin sealant has great potential for use in burn patients and for skin grafts. However, exposure to large amounts of sealant and bovine thrombin would elicit an autoimmune response. These risks, together with potential risks of viral infections associated with human fibrinogen from pooled donor plasma, have prevented regulatory approval of fibrin sealant use in the United States. Limited quantities of autologous fibrinogen, which is prepared from the patient's own plasma, have been used successfully.[99] Recombinant human fibrinogen has been purified from the milk of transgenic mice,[100] suggesting a potential for an alternative commercial product in the future.

Gene Structure

The three chains of fibrinogen are encoded by three single-copy genes located at chromosome 4q23-q32.[101,102] The three genes are linked and are arranged in the order of γ-α-β. The gene for the β-chain is oriented in a direction opposite to that of the other two genes.[102] The α-chain gene is 6.5 kb in length and contains 6 exons, whereas the β-chain gene is 8.2 kb and has 8 exons and the γ-chain gene is 8.4 kb and contains 10 exons. The three genes have been completely sequenced (GenBank α = M58569, β = M64983, γ = X02415).[103] The sequences of oligonucleotide primers that can be used to amplify various regions of the three fibrinogen genes by the polymerase chain reaction have been reported.[104] Polymorphic DNA sequences in the genes for the three fibrinogen genes have been identified.[105,106] A *Taq*I restriction fragment length polymorphism (RFLP) and a tetranucleotide repeat polymorphism in the α-chain gene have been identified. In the β-chain gene, four polymorphisms have been identified: a G/A polymorphic site at −455 bp, a C/T polymorphism at 148 bp, a *Hha*I RFLP, and a *Bcl*I RFLP downstream of the gene. In the γ-chain gene, a *Kpn*I/*Sac*I RFLP has been identified.

Assembly

In cultured hepatocytes and in whole animals, only fully assembled fibrinogen molecules are secreted into circulation. Partially assembled intermediates are retained within the cell and are eventually degraded. The intracellular assembly process has been studied in transfected baby hamster kidney cells that can express different combinations of fibrinogen chains.[107] Fibrinogen assembly begins when a γ-chain combines with either a β or an α-chain to form a heterodimeric $\alpha\gamma$ or $\beta\gamma$ intermediate. Subsequently, a β or α-chain is added to the heterodimeric intermediates to form an $\alpha\beta\gamma$ half molecule. Half molecules then dimerize to form the fully assembled six-chain fibrinogen, which is secreted into the circulation.

Regulation

Fibrinogen is synthesized exclusively in the liver by hepatic parenchymal cells, and its level in circulation is maintained at 250 to 320 mg/dl.[108] It has a half-life of 3 to 5 days, and continuous synthesis by the liver is necessary to maintain a relatively constant circulating level. Liver-specific transcription of the α- and β-chain genes is ascribed to the presence of recognition sequences for the liver-specific transcription factor hepatocyte nuclear factor 1 (HNF1).[109–111] Transcription of the γ-chain in the liver is mediated by an upstream stimulatory factor (USF) binding site, which also may be responsible for the extrahepatic transcription of the γ-chain in lung and brain.[112]

Fibrinogen is an acute-phase protein, and its level in circulation rises four- to sevenfold in response to trauma and inflammation.[113] This increase is mediated by a feedback mechanism that involves monocytes and macrophages. After the fibrin clot or fibrinogen is degraded, the degradation product fragment D binds to monocytes and macrophages. This binding stimulates the release of the cytokine interleukin 6 (IL-6) from these cells; IL-6 in turn binds to IL-6 receptors on the surface of hepatocytes. This binding triggers signal transduction in the hepatocytes and leads to, through tyrosine phosphorylation and serine phosphorylation, the activation of the transcription factor NF-IL6.[114] Activated NF-IL6 binds to specific responsive sequences in IL-6-responsive genes and enhances the level of their transcription. The three fibrinogen genes contain single functional type II IL-6-responsive elements (CTGGG/A) in the 5′ flanking regions,[110,111,115] and their transcription is coordinately enhanced by IL-6 stimulation.

GENETIC ABNORMALITIES OF FIBRINOGEN

Afibrinogenemia

Afibrinogenemia is characterized by a complete absence of fibrinogen in the circulation. It is a rare disorder, and over 160 cases have been reported. It is inherited as an autosomal recessive trait of variable penetrance. The cardinal symptom is umbilical cord bleeding at birth and a lifelong predisposition to prolonged bleeding from acute wounds and trauma, delayed wound healing, and spontaneous gastrointestinal bleeding. Intracranial bleeding at birth, caused by pressure of the birth canal on the head, is usually fatal. Laboratory studies have indicated an infinite clotting time, while levels of all other coagulation factors are normal. Afibrinogenemia is usually accompanied by mild thrombocytopenia.[116] Platelets show normal adhesive properties and spreading behavior but are nevertheless defective in aggregation. Because of the early onset and severity of hemorrhages, few afibrinogenemic patients survive beyond age 20 years. Therapy has been focused on the management of acute bleeding by infusion of fibrinogen-containing preparations, which include fresh frozen plasma, fibrinogen concentrate, or cryoprecipitate, to bring the circulating fibrinogen level to 100 mg/dl (~30 percent of normal level). Prophylactic infusion of cryoprecipitate in afibrinogenemic children has been effective.[117] Afibrinogenemic women have complications of recurrent abortions and postpartum hemorrhage. Normal full-term deliveries have been achieved by prophylactic infusion of fibrinogen to maintain a stable level of 100 mg/dl throughout pregnancy. This is consistent with the hypothesis that minute placental separations and hemorrhages occur in a normal pregnancy and are controlled by normal clotting function,[118] which is absent in afibrinogenemic women.

Afibrinogenemic mice with a homozygous deficiency in the α-chain have been constructed.[64] These mice bleed overtly shortly after birth, frequently in the peritoneal cavity, skin, and soft tissues around joints. Adults also exhibit spontaneous abdominal bleeding and delayed wound healing. In females, pregnancy results in fatal uterine bleeding at about the tenth day of gestation. These symptoms are similar to those seen in human afibrinogenemic patients.

Hypofibrinogenemia

Hypofibrinogenemia is characterized by a reduced circulating level of fibrinogen (below 100 mg/dl). There are several causes for this condition. Congenital hypofibrinogenemia may be the heterozygous state of afibrinogenemia. Hypofibrinogenemia also may be acquired as a consequence of disseminated intravascular coagulation, severe liver disease, defibrination by snake venom, and systemic fibrinogenolysis associated with thrombolytic therapy. Defective secretion of fibrinogen from the liver also has been shown to cause inherited hypofibrinogenemia.[118] In one case, a homozygous single nucleotide insertion in the gene for the α-chain, which causes a frameshift and truncation of the α-chain at residue 267, affects the assembly and secretion of fibrinogen and causes severe hypofibrinogenemia.[133] Drug-induced hypofibrinogenemia has been observed following treatments with L-asparaginase and sodium valproate.[119,120] Symptoms of hypofibrinogenemia are similar to those of afibrinogenemia, but they occurr with less frequency and severity. These symptoms include umbilical cord bleeding at birth, cerebral hemorrhage, recurrent abortions, placental separation, and postpartum hemorrhage. Acute bleeding is treated by infusion of fibrinogen.

Dysfibrinogenemia

Dysfibrinogenemia is characterized by the presence of circulating fibrinogen that is functionally impaired. The causes of dysfibrinogenemia are extremely heterogeneous and can be divided into acquired and congenital defects. The most common causes of acquired dysfibrinogenemia are liver diseases, which include cirrhosis, hepatitis, and hepatocarcinoma. These diseases cause an increased branching of the carbohydrate chains in fibrinogen and an increase in sialic acid content, which delays fibrin polymerization. Acquired dysfibrinogenemia also has been attributed to the presence of circulating inhibitors or autoantibodies, which inhibit fibrin polymerization and cause impaired clot retraction.[121,122]

Over 200 cases of dysfibrinogenemias caused by inherited or spontaneous mutations in the fibrinogen genes have been described (summarized in ref. 30). Most dysfibrinogenemias are heterozygous. The resulting heterogeneous mixture of normal and mutated chains accounts for the mild and asymptomatic manifestations of many heterozygous dysfibrinogenemias. However, in some cases the symptoms of dysfibrinogenemic patients are severe and may include a tendency to bleeding, thrombosis, or both. Depending on the locations of the amino acid substitutions, any one of the many functions of fibrinogen may be affected. Thus mutations affecting fibrinopeptide release, fibrin polymerization, factor XIIIa crosslinking, calcium binding, and clot lysis have been described.

Over 40 cases of dysfibrinogenemia with defective fibrinopeptide A release have been reported. These have been attributed to αArg16 to His or αArg16 to Cys mutations. These mutations affect the α-chain thrombin-cleavage site and are associated with either slow release or no detectable release of fibrinopeptide A. Mutations in the neighboring thrombin exosite, namely, αPro18 to Leu and αArg19 to Asn, Gly, or Ser, also affect thrombin binding and cause a delayed release of fibrinopeptide A. The preceding α-chain mutations all affect the conversion of fibrinogen to fibrin and cause bleeding.[123–125]

Mutations at the β-chain thrombin-cleavage site also have been reported.[30] The mutation βArg14 to Cys affected fibrinopeptide B release, but the patient was asymptomatic. This is consistent with the observation that des-A fibrin, which is not cleaved at the β-chain site, can still polymerize to form a clot.

Many mutations between γ275 to 380 in the globular C-terminal region of the γ-chain have been described.[30] The mutations reported to date generally have been detected after routine clinical assays that indicated defective fibrin polymerization or clotting but normal release of fibrinopeptides A and B. The recently reported crystal structures of this region of fibrinogen[13,14,26,27] provide a basis for explaining the functional consequences of many of these mutations. These structure-function correlations have been reviewed and summarized.[126,127] Thus the γAsp318 to Gly substitution and the deletion of residues γAsn319 and Asp320 directly affected calcium binding. The mutations γGly292 to Val and γArg375 to Gly appeared to result in the structural destabilization of the polymerization domain. γGln329 to Arg, γAsp330 to Val/Tyr, γAsn337 to Lys, and γAsp364 to His/Val substitutions affected the integrity of the polymerization pocket and the "a-A" interaction. The mutations γGly268 to Glu, γArg275 to Cys/His, γTyr280 to Cys,[134] and γAsn308 to Ile/Lys altered the D:D (γ:γ) interface between end-to-end aligned fibrin monomers. Some, but not all, patients with mutations at Arg275 and Asn308 suffered from thrombotic disorders. These defects apparently resulted in an abnormal end-to-end alignment of fibrin monomers, leading to formation of clots having altered fiber thickness and branching. These clots were then lysed inefficiently by plasmin. Another dysfibrinogenemia resulted from the insertion of 15 amino acids at γ350. Fibrinogen isolated from this patient was not crosslinked normally by factor XIIIa and did not support platelet aggregation.

Mutations that create novel glycosylation sites in the fibrinogen chains cause polymerization defects, presumably because of steric hindrance as polymerization proceeds or because of the introduction of charged carbohydrate moieties. Thus γMet310 to Thr, which results in glycosylation of Asn308, γLys380 to Asn, which results in glycosylation of Asn 380, and βAla335 to Thr, which results in glycosylation of Asn333, have been shown to affect fibrin polymerization. The molecular structure of the factor XIIIa-crosslinked D-dimer fragment[26] revealed that βAla335 is situated at the entrance of the Gly-His-Arg binding pocket, i.e., at the site where the thrombin-cleaved β-chain of one fibrin molecule binds to the complementary pocket located in the C-terminal region of an adjacent β-chain. The introduction of a bulky carbohydrate at this site would create steric hindrance to this "b-B" interaction and therefore should affect lateral aggregation.

Mutations in the fibrinogen chains that introduce unpaired cysteine residues sometimes result in the linking of the mutant fibrinogen chain to albumin through a disulfide bond. Examples of this type of mutation include αArg554 to Cys, βArg14 to Cys, and γSer358 to Cys. The incorporation of albumin creates a steric hindrance to polymerization and, depending on the site of association, may lead to the formation of clots having abnormal structures, resulting in defective lysis and possibly a tendency to thrombosis in some patients. (*Note:* The γ-mutation patient is asymptomatic.)

Three mutations in the β-chain, βArg44 to Cys, βAla68 to Thr, and deletion of amino acids 9 to 72, are associated with thrombosis. In the cases of the βAla68 to Thr substitution and the Δ9–72 deletion, a thrombin-binding site was eliminated by the substitution.

Hyperfibrinogenemia

The Framingham Study demonstrated that about half the patients who have ischemic heart diseases have high levels of fibrinogen in their plasma ($>$320 mg/dl).[128] After correcting for age, body weight, smoking, and plasma cholesterol levels, elevated fibrinogen levels were still seen to constitute an independent risk factor for myocardial infarction and stroke in men.[128] It was suggested that elevated fibrinogen levels promote platelet hyperaggregation and are correlated with atherogenesis and thrombosis. However, no direct evidence of a causal relationship has been found, and no study has yet suggested that reducing the circulating level of fibrinogen in these individuals may be accompanied by a corresponding decrease in the risk for cardiovascular diseases.

Variations in plasma fibrinogen levels have been attributed to a G/A polymorphism at -453 bp in the promoter region of the gene for the β-chain of human fibrinogen.[129] It was reasoned that in humans, the β-chain is present in a limiting amount in the liver, and therefore, the transcription level for the β-chain gene directly determines the circulating fibrinogen level. The G/A polymorphism, located close to the IL-6 response element in the β-chain gene, may modulate the magnitude of the IL-6 response and hence the transcription level of the β-chain gene. Consistent with this hypothesis, very intensive exercise, which precipitates an acute-phase response, causes a significantly greater increase in circulating fibrinogen levels in individuals carrying the *A* allele. This response is much less marked in individuals carrying the *G* allele.[130] Other studies, however, have not confirmed the correlation of β-chain polymorphism with plasma fibrinogen levels.[131,132] The discrepancy between these studies may be related to population differences and needs to be resolved by future investigations.

COAGULATION FACTOR XIII

Factor XIII (fibrin-stabilizing factor or fibrinoligase) is a plasma glycoprotein that plays an important role in the final stage of blood coagulation, in the regulation of fibrinolysis, and in tissue repair.

Thrombin generated during blood coagulation converts the proenzyme (factor XIII) to an active enzyme (factor XIIIa) in the presence of calcium ions. Factor XIIIa is a transglutaminase that catalyzes the crosslinking of fibrin monomers and the crosslinking of fibrin and α_2-plasmin inhibitor through the formation of intermolecular γ-glutamyl-ε-lysine bonds. These reactions result in a fibrin clot with mechanical strength and increased resistance to proteolytic degradation by plasmin. The crosslinking of fibronectin to fibrin or to collagen is also catalyzed by factor XIIIa, and this reaction appears to be related to wound healing.

A deficiency of factor XIII results in a severe lifelong bleeding tendency and defective wound healing in affected individuals, and spontaneous miscarriage in affected females. Congenital factor XIII deficiency is caused by the absence of either the A or B subunit. This disorder is inherited as an autosomal recessive trait, since the genes coding for the A and B subunits exist on chromosomes 6 and 1, respectively. Disease-causing defects in these two genes have been identified in a number of patients with factor XIII deficiency.

Structure of Factor XIII

Physical Properties. Factor XIII circulates in blood as a tetramer, A_2 B_2 ($\sim$320 kDa) consisting of two A subunits (75 kDa each) and two B subunits (80 kDa each).[135,136] The four polypeptides are held together by noncovalent bonds.[136] The carbohydrate

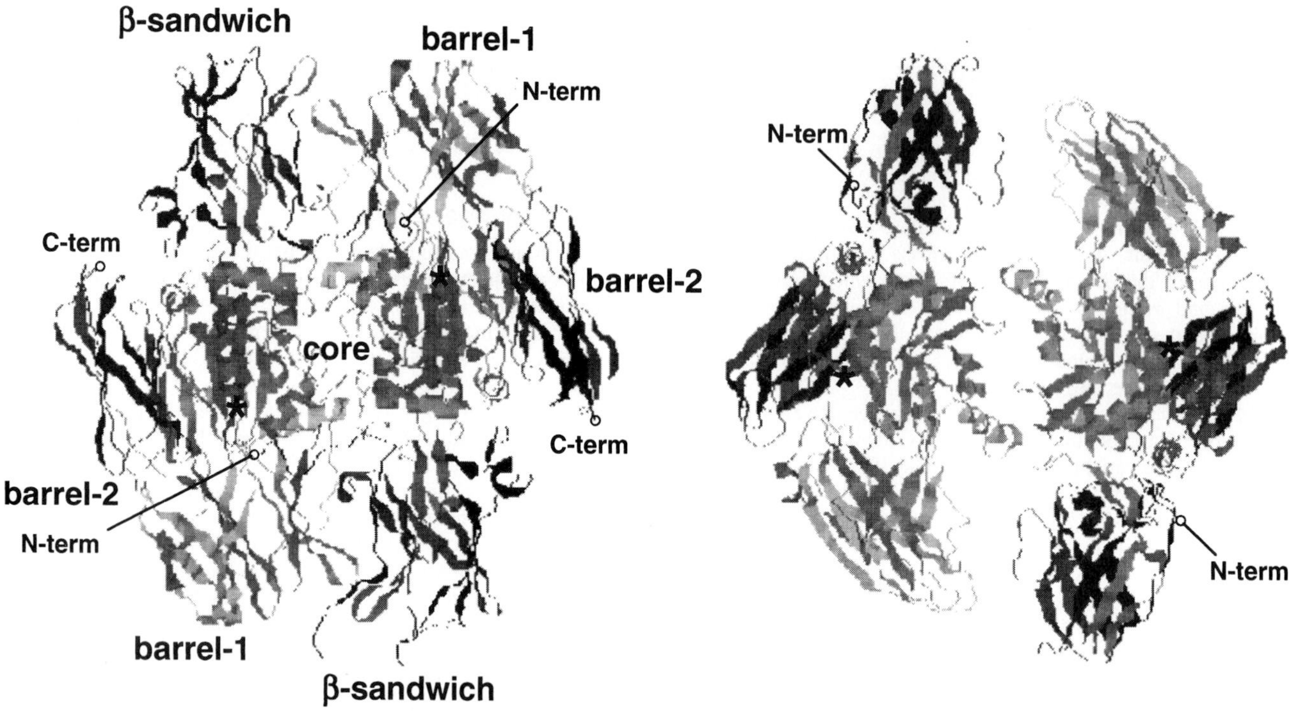

Fig. 171-4 Three-dimensional structure of the A subunit for factor XIII. The A subunit is composed of five distinct domains: from the N-terminus to the C-terminus, an activation peptide (residues 1–37), *β*-sandwich (38-183), central core (first half, 184–332; second half, 333–513), barrel 1 (514–628), and barrel 2 (629–731) domains. The central core domain contains the active site Cys314 and two additional residues (His373 and Asp396) important for enzymatic activity. Both N- and C-termini are identified by small circles. The activation peptide blocks the entrance to the catalytic cavity in the core domain *(left)*. On cleavage by thrombin, the activation peptide remains in the same conformation and occupies the same position with respect to the rest of the molecule, although the catalytic cavity becomes wide open to substrates *(right)*. (*Modified with permission from Yee et al.*[149] *and Yee et al.*[150])

content has been reported to be 1.5 and 8.5 percent for the A and B subunits, respectively.[137,138] The A subunit has more than six free sulfhydryl groups, whereas the B subunit has no free sulfhydryl groups.[136,139] Factor XIII in plasma is complexed with fibrinogen.[139,140] Both the native factor XIII (A_2 B_2) and that potentiated by thrombin, (activated) factor XIIIa′ (A'_2 B_2), bind similarly to calcium ions,[7] although the native factor XIII remains a heterotetramer.[136,142,143] Fibrinogen and factor XIII appear to bind through the B subunit. This observation is based on the fact that placental or platelet factor XIII (A_2), which does not contain B subunits, does not bind fibrinogen.[144] Thus plasma factor XIII (A_2 B_2) circulates in blood in a complex with both fibrinogen and calcium ions.

The three-dimensional structure of factor XIII was demonstrated by an electron microscopic study. The A and B subunits appear to be a globular particle and a filamentous strand, respectively.[145] The A subunit of factor XIII has been purified and characterized,[137,146–148] and crystallized.[146] X-ray crystallography demonstrated that the A subunit is composed of five distinct domains: an activation peptide, *β*-sandwich, central core, barrel 1, and barrel 2 regions[149,150] (Fig. 171-4). The C-terminal portion of the A subunit corresponding to the two *β*-barrels forms thermostable domains, whereas three thermolabile domains are formed by the N-terminal *β*-sandwich and core domains.[151] The core domain is composed of two subdomains where three active-site residues are located as described below. It is of interest that the activation peptide, on cleavage by thrombin, has the same conformation and occupies the same position with respect to the rest of the molecule as it does in the zymogen[152]; moreover, the activation peptide blocks the entrance to the catalytic cavity in the core domain.[149,152]

Primary Structure. The A subunit of factor XIII consists of 731 amino acids.[153,154] The molecular weight of the polypeptide portion of the molecule was calculated to be 83,150. The B subunit is composed of 641 amino acids[155] with a calculated molecular weight of 73,183. The addition of 8.5 percent carbohydrate[138] gives a molecular weight of about 79,700 for each of the B subunits of human factor XIII. These molecular weights are in agreement with those estimated by SDS-polyacrylamide gel electrophoresis.[135,136]

The A Subunit. The N-terminus of the A subunit is acetylated,[156] whereas that of the B subunit is a free Glu residue.[155,156] The A subunit contains several functional regions, including an activation peptide (37 amino acids), an active site (Cys314), putative calcium-binding sites, and a thrombin inactivation site (Fig. 171-5). The amino acid sequence around the active site (Tyr-Gly-Gln-Cys-Trp, YGQCW in Fig. 171-5) is identical to those of other transglutaminases.[157,158] Two additional amino acids, His373 and Asp396, seem to be important for the catalytic activity of factor XIII.[149,159,160] The N-terminal subdomain of the central core domain contains the Cys314, whereas the His373 and Asp396 are located in the C-terminal subdomain.[151] The proposed Cys-His-Asp catalytic triad, which is similar in arrangement to the active site of cysteine proteinases, suggests that the catalytic mechanism of transglutaminases may be similar to the reverse mechanism of the cysteine proteinases.[161] Two nonproline *cis* peptide bonds were identified between Arg310 and Tyr311 close to the active-site Cys314 residue, whereas Gln425 and Phe426 were located at the dimerization interface, indicating their possible importance for factor XIII function.[152]

The A subunit of factor XIII is also present in other tissues and cells such as platelets, megakaryocytes, placenta, uterus, monocytes/macrophages, etc. (see "Synthesis of Factor XIII" below). The A subunits in plasma and in other tissues are identical; the amino acid sequences of the A subunit from plasma,[153,156] platelets,[156] and placenta[153,154,162] are indistinguishable.

The A subunit of factor XIII is highly homologous to other human transglutaminases,[157,163–168] including a novel transgluta-

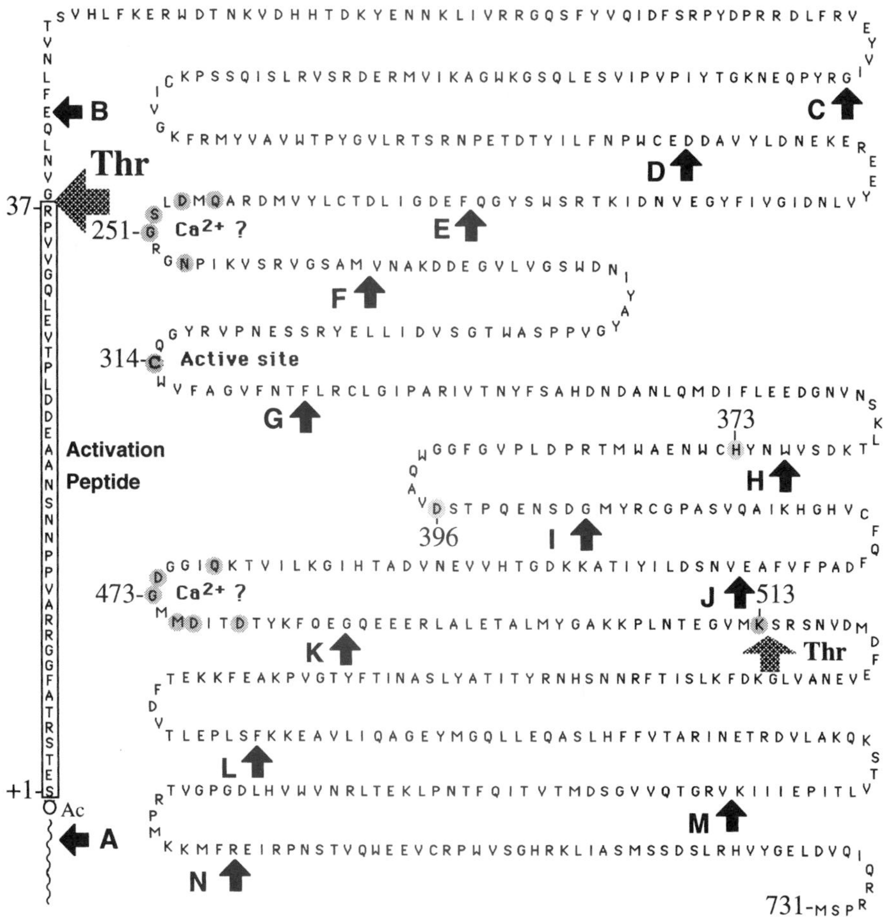

Fig. 171-5 Primary structure of the A subunit and placement of introns. Arrows with capital letters indicate positions of introns. The N- and C-terminal residues are numbered, as are certain other key residues: Arg at an activation cleavage site by thrombin, Cys at an active site, Lys at the second cleavage site by thrombin, etc. The N-terminal Ser residue is acetylated. Wide arrows demonstrate the sites cleaved by thrombin. (*Modified with permission from Ichinose.*[180])

minase identified in keratinocytes.[169] The degree of identity between the A subunit and other transglutaminases ranges from 35 to 45 percent. The middle portion of these proteins contains most of the identical sequences, whereas their N- and C-terminal regions are more diverse. These structural features correspond to the domain organization of the A-subunit molecule; i.e., the middle portion forms a central core homologous with the transglutaminases, and the N- and C-terminal regions form independent domains,[151] which may determine substrate specificity of each transglutaminase. Another transglutaminase has been isolated from horseshoe crab hemocytes, and its primary structure is found to be most homologous to factor XIII.[170] This similarity provides strong evidence that these proteins are derived from a common ancestor. Human erythrocyte membrane band 4.2 protein is also similar to the transglutaminases[171,172]; however, it lacks enzymatic activity because of the substitution of the active site Cys by Ala.

The B Subunit. The B subunit contains 10 tandem repeats (Fig 171-6). These repeats each consist of about 60 amino acids, two disulfide bonds, and highly conserved Pro, Gly, Tyr, and Trp residues.[155] The 10 repeats are subclassified into four groups according to the degree of identity to each other. These repeats have been called *Sushi domains* because of their shape[163] or *GP-I structures*[173] because the disulfide-bond pairing was first established in human β_2-glycoprotein I to be between the first and third and the second and fourth Cys residues in each repeat.[174] This pattern is also found in the bovine counterpart[175] and in the a chain of human C4-binding protein.[176] It is likely, therefore, that a similar pairing occurs with the disulfide bonds in the Sushi domains present in other homologous proteins. Each Sushi domain is independently folded[177] and is predicted to consist of exclusively antiparallel β-sheets,[178] which is consistent with the results obtained experimentally by an NMR study.[179] At least 30 other proteins/genes are found to contain similar Sushi domains.[163,180] Nearly half these 30 proteins are involved in the complement system, and the others are involved in diverse systems such as blood coagulation, lymphocyte regulation, etc. Sushi domains are found even in proteins in invertebrates and viruses, suggesting that the genes for these proteins may have evolved from a common ancestor.

Near the C-terminus of the B subunit of factor XIII within the tenth Sushi domain there is an Arg-Gly-Asp (RGD) sequence that is reported to be responsible for the cell attachment of various proteins.[181] It remains to be determined, however, whether this RGD sequence in the B subunit is related to its function. The amino acid sequence of the mouse B subunit is 78 percent identical to the human counterpart, although the mouse subunit contained 7 amino acid residues at the C-terminus that were not found in the human.[182]

Function of Factor XIII

The A subunit of factor XIII contains the catalytic site, whereas the B subunit is thought to protect or stabilize the A subunit[183–185] or regulate activation of the zymogen.[136,186] The former role is supported by a study using a mammalian expression system demonstrating that recombinant $A_2 B_2$ tetramers are more stable than recombinant A_2 dimers alone.[187] The B subunit also mediates the binding of factor XIII to the C-terminus of the γ' chain of fibrinogen.[144]

Factor XIIIa catalyzes a γ-glutamyl-ε-lysine crosslinking reaction between a number of proteins. Fibrin acts as both an amino donor and an acceptor,[188] whereas α_2-plasmin inhibitor and fibronectin preferentially serve as amino acceptors.[189,190]

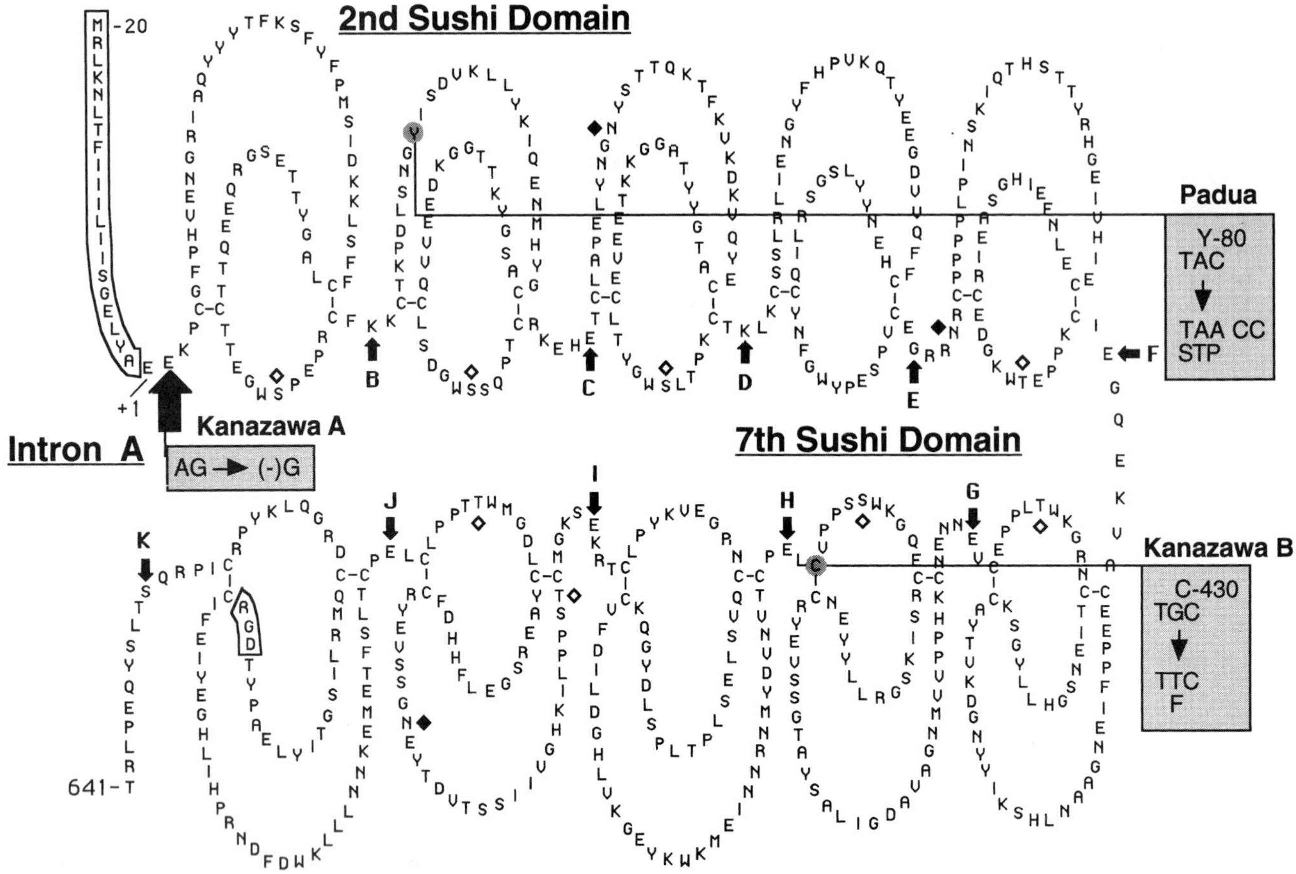

Fig. 171-6 Primary structure of the B subunit and identified mutations. Arrows with capital letters indicate positions of introns. The N- and C-terminal residues of the mature protein are numbered. Residues from (−)1 to (−)20 are enclosed as a signal peptide for secretion. An Arg-Gly-Asp sequence in the tenth Sushi domain is also enclosed. Solid and open diamonds indicate potential carbohydrate attachment sites of the Asn-X-Ser/Thr/Cys and Ser/Thr-X-X-Pro types, respectively. Three mutations identified in patients with the B-subunit deficiency (former type I factor XIII deficiency) are shown in boxes. (*Reprinted with permission from Ichinose et al.*[303])

Crosslinking of Fibrin Monomers. The crosslinking reaction catalyzed by factor XIIIa leads to dimerization of the γ-chains of fibrin, followed by polymerization of the α-chains of fibrin.[135] The crosslinking sites between two γ-chains are Gln398 or Gln399 and Lys406[188] near the C-terminal ends of the polypeptide chain. Gln328 and Gln366[191] and Lys508[192] are involved in the α-chain polymerization. The γ-dimerization and α-polymerization reactions result in a fibrin clot with mechanical strength and elasticity.[193,194] Thus these polymerization reactions aid in hemostasis.

The formation of a γ-trimer, γ-tetramer, and $\alpha\gamma_2$-triad has been demonstrated following the γ-dimerization of both fibrin and fibrinogen.[195,196] These reactions lead to an increase in the resistance of fibrin to fibrinolysis.[197]

Crosslinking of α_2-Plasmin Inhibitor. The crosslinking of α_2-plasmin inhibitor to the α-chain of fibrin[198] or fibrinogen[199] by factor XIIIa occurs at a faster rate than with other proteins. Accordingly, in plasma, α_2-plasmin inhibitor and fibrin are considered the best substrates for factor XIIIa.[200] The crosslinking site in each substrate has been identified as Gln2 in α_2-plasmin inhibitor[190,201] and Lys303 in the α-chain of fibrin(ogen).[202]

The crosslinking of α_2-plasmin inhibitor to fibrin renders the fibrin clot resistant to digestion by plasmin.[203] Consequently, the crosslinked α_2-plasmin inhibitor protects the hemostatic fibrin clot from premature lysis by plasmin.[203,204]

Crosslinking of Fibronectin. Factor XIIIa catalyzes the crosslinking of fibronectin to the α-chain of fibrin[198,205] and to collagen.[206] The crosslinking site of fibronectin is reported to be Gln3 at its N-terminus.[189] The crosslinking of fibronectin to fibrin or collagen may result in anchoring of fibrin clots to cells or to the structural matrix in vessel walls at the site of vascular injury. In a culture system, fibronectin is crosslinked by factor XIIIa and accumulates in fibroblast cell layers. This reaction may be important for a particular assembly process to organize and stabilize the growing extracellular matrix.[207,208] Factor XIII is also reported to enhance fibroblast proliferation.[209] Cultured fibroblasts migrate optimally into gels prepared with fibrinogen at a concentration of about 3 mg/ml (i.e., normal plasma fibrinogen level), and migration is greatly enhanced by extensive crosslinking of the fibrin α-chains by factor XIIIa.[210] In contrast, both the number of migrating macrophages and the distance of migration were reduced when the gel matrix included fibronectin and was crosslinked by factor XIIIa.[211] These reactions appear to be related to wound healing.[212–214]

Other Protein Substrates. The contractile proteins actin and myosin also have been shown to be crosslinked by factor XIIIa.[215–217] Since these proteins exist in platelets, they may be involved in the crosslinking of structural proteins under certain conditions.[216]

Factor XIII is reported to generate a monocyte chemotactic factor by crosslinking of S19 ribosomal protein.[218,219] This reaction may be related to inflammation. Most recently, it has been found that many A-subunit-positive microglia were associated with primitive senile plaques in the brains of patients with Alzheimer disease, whereas few or no microglia containing A subunits were found associated with classic plaques.[220] Factor XIII may play a role(s) in the early phase of Alzheimer disease, since the *tau* protein is reported to be crosslinked by a transglutaminase.[221]

Several other plasma proteins such as von Willebrand factor,[222,223] thrombospondin,[224] factor V,[225] plasminogen, and apolipoprotein(a)[226] have been reported to be crosslinked to themselves or to other substrates by factor XIIIa. The precise functions of these reactions, however, have yet to be established.

Synthesis of Factor XIII

Concentrations of the A and B subunits of factor XIII in normal plasma have been determined by an enzyme-linked immunosorbent assay (ELISA) to be 11 and 21 μg/ml, respectively.[227] Since virtually all the A subunit in plasma is complexed with an equimolar amount of the B subunit, about half the B subunit (10 μg/ml) exists in the "free" form in plasma.[184,228,229] The free B subunit may act as a reserve by binding and stabilizing the A subunit immediately on its release from cells into circulation.

Site of Synthesis for Factor XIII. The liver has long been thought to be the major site of synthesis for both the A and B subunits of plasma factor XIII.[230,231] In addition, the biosynthesis and secretion of both subunits by the human hepatoma cell line HepG-2 have been reported.[232] No cDNA clone for the A subunit, however, was obtained from liver libraries, despite extensive screening.[153,233] Northern blot analyses of mRNA samples from normal liver, HepG-2 cells, and fibroblasts also showed little or no detectable hybridization signal, whereas a single mRNA species (about 4.0 kb) for the A subunit was obtained from mRNA samples from placenta,[154] macrophages,[234,235] and megakaryoblastoid cells (Kida and Ichinose, unpublished data). These results suggest that placenta, macrophages, and megakaryocytes do synthesize the A subunit, whereas liver does not.

Free A subunits are also present in a number of organs, tissues, and cells, such as placenta, uterus, prostate, platelets, megakaryocytes, and monocytes/macrophages.[236–241] The A subunit in these cells, however, is localized in the cytoplasm by immunohistochemical and immunobiochemical methods. In particular, the amount of A subunit in platelets is equal to that in plasma,[242,243] but the A subunit in platelets is present in the cytoplasm[241,243] and is not secreted.[242,243] An acetylated N-terminus and the absence of glycosylation and disulfide bonds are also consistent with the fact that the A subunit is a typical cytoplasmic protein. At present, the function of these intracellular forms of the A subunit is not known, although other cytosolic transglutaminases are thought to be related to apoptosis[244,245] and the synthesis of a cornified envelope in the skin.[246] Dermis-peculiar cells named *dendrocytes* were found to contain the A subunit of factor XIII.[247] Since dendrocytes share several common surface epitopes with monocytes/macrophages, they are considered to be derived from bone marrow and become perivascular resident macrophages.

After bone marrow transplantation, the phenotype of the A subunit in the plasma of the recipient was replaced by that of the donor, whereas the phenotype of the B subunit remained unchanged.[248] In addition, complete or partial conversion of the phenotype of the A subunit in monocytes and platelets as well as in plasma was detected in patients after bone marrow transplantation.[249] Therefore, it is likely that the A subunit of plasma factor XIII is produced at least in part by hemopoietic cells.

The site of synthesis for the B subunit has been suggested to be the liver.[230,231] HepG-2 and PLC/PRF/5 hepatoma cells secrete the B subunit,[232] and cDNA clones coding for the B subunit have been obtained from a normal human liver library.[155,233] In addition, the phenotype of a recipient's B subunit changed to the donor's phenotype after liver transplantation, whereas that of the A subunit remained unchanged.[248] Therefore, it is clear that the liver is the major site of synthesis for the B subunit.

Mechanism of Release of the A Subunit of Factor XIII. Like those of other transglutaminases, the 5′ end of the cDNA for the placental A subunit does not encode a typical hydrophobic leader sequence for secretion.[153,154] A search for a possible preproleader sequence or internal signal has been unsuccessful, although the corresponding portions of the A-subunit gene have been examined extensively.[233,250] Because the A subunit of factor XIII is known to remain in the cytoplasm of placenta,[236] macrophages,[239,240] megakaryocytes,[238] platelets,[241,243] and skin dendrocytes,[247] it is very likely that the Met at position (−)1 functions as the initiator for biosynthesis. The removal of the Met by an aminopeptidase(s) would then be followed by acetylation of the N-terminal Ser residue.[156]

If any of the cells mentioned earlier is the major source of the A subunit of "plasma" factor XIII, there should be a unique mechanism(s) for its release into circulation, where the free B subunit can readily bind to and form an $A_2 B_2$ tetramer. Results of the expression of the A and/or B subunits in a mammalian cell system suggest that the A subunit is not secreted through the conventional secretory pathway but is released from cells after cell damage.[187] There are more than 20 proteins that lack typical hydrophobic leader sequences and distinct internal hydrophobic signals but are present and function in extracellular spaces.[251–255] In the case of IL-1b, two different mechanisms, a novel pathway and apoptosis, are proposed for its release from cells.[256,257]

The 5′ end of the cDNA and the corresponding exon in the gene for the B subunit code for a typical hydrophobic leader sequence that aids in its secretion from hepatocytes into the circulation.[155,258] This is supported by the fact that the HepG-2 and PLC/PRF/5 hepatoma cells secrete the B subunit[232] and by the results that the recombinant B subunit is secreted through the conventional secretory pathway in a mammalian cell system.[187]

Regulation of B-Subunit Levels. Patients with congenital factor XIII deficiency lack an immunologically detectable A subunit (<1 percent of normal) and have a reduced amount (about 50 percent of normal) of the B subunit.[184,259] Heterozygotes have about 50 and 80 percent of the A and B subunits, respectively.[260] Furthermore, administration of the A subunit obtained from placenta increased not only the A-subunit level in plasma but also the level of the B subunit, which reached a maximum after several days and was maintained at that level for a prolonged period.[231,261] An ELISA assay revealed that the plasma concentration of the complexed form of the B subunit is decreased to almost 0 percent of normal in homozygotes and about 50 percent in heterozygotes of the A-subunit deficiency, whereas that of the free B subunit is essentially the same among normal individuals, homozygotes, and heterozygotes.[227] Therefore, it is likely that the concentration of the complex form of the B subunit ($A_2 B_2$) depends on the amount of the A subunit in plasma and that the concentration of the free B subunit is regulated to be constant. The increase in the A subunit caused by the infusion of exogenous A subunit may induce the synthesis of the B subunit as a response to the increased A subunit or decreased free B subunit. This response was absent in a patient whose complete B-subunit deficiency was genetic in origin.[262,263]

Metabolism of Factor XIII

The half-life of the A subunit of factor XIII in circulation is about 10 days.[214,231,264,265] It is of interest that the half-life of placental concentrates (A_2) infused into a patient with complete B-subunit deficiency was shorter than those in patients with A-subunit deficiency,[262] probably because the placental A_2 dimer is stabilized by immediate formation of an $A_2 B_2$ tetramer with the free B_2 dimer in the plasma of patients with A-subunit deficiency.

In rabbit, factor XIIIa (the activated form) is removed from circulation faster than factor XIII (the zymogen form), probably through the reticuloendothelial system in liver.[230] The retention of factor XIIIa in fibrin clots[266] could be an additional mechanism for its clearance from plasma.

Activation of the Zymogen. During the final stage of blood coagulation, thrombin converts the proenzyme (factor XIII) to a potentiated form (factor XIIIa′) by releasing an activation peptide

(4 kDa) from the N-terminus of each of the A subunits [135,156] (Fig 171-5). The site of cleavage by thrombin is between Arg37 and Gly38. This reaction is stimulated by fibrin monomers.[267,268] The cofactor activity of fibrin I (polymerized des-A fibrinogen) has been attributed to formation of a fibrin I-factor XIII complex (K_d = 65 nM), which is potentiated by α-thrombin 80-fold more efficiently than free, uncomplexed factor XIII.[269] In contrast, fibrin crosslinked by factor XIIIa in the presence of calcium ions loses its cofactor activity as γ-dimers appear.[268] Thus crosslinked fibrin may function as a negative feedback to prevent further generation of factor XIIIa.

In the presence of calcium ions, the potentiated A'_2 dimer dissociates from the B_2 dimer[136,183,186] and binds to fibrin more tightly,[270] whereas the B_2 dimer remains in liquid phase.[266] Calcium ions bind to the A′ subunit and unmask the active site.[141,183,186,271] Fibrin(ogen) lowers the calcium concentration required both for the dissociation of the A'_2 and B_2 dimers and for the exposure of the active site to the physiologic level (1.5 mM).[270,272]

Several other enzymes, including trypsin, factor Xa, elastase, and cathepsin C, have been reported to activate (or potentiate) factor XIII.[135,239,273–275] Factor XIII also can be activated by high concentrations of calcium and salt.[276] This reaction may be specific for the intracellular form of factor XIII, since nonproteolytic activation of the A subunit in platelets is abolished by the addition of the B subunit in a stoichiometric amount.[276] Thrombin-independent activation actually may play an important role(s) in the activation of intracellular factor XIII (A_2 alone), since thrombin does not exist in the cytoplasm.

Degradation of the Enzyme. The loss of biologic activity of factor XIIIa during prolonged incubation with thrombin occurs in parallel with the generation of fragments of 56 and 24 kDa from the A subunit, whereas the molecular weight of the B subunit remains unchanged.[135,277] The cleavage site for thrombin is reported to be between Lys513 and Ser514[162]; however, Hornyak et al. have claimed that the loss of activity does not correlate with the appearance of the cleaved fragments.[278] An expression study of mutant A subunits suggests that removal of the C-terminal portion makes the molecule unstable (Ichinose, unpublished data),[279,280] which is consistent with the idea that the C-terminal domains are involved in the interaction of the two A subunits.[151] Degradation of factor XIII or factor XIIIa also has been reported to occur by digestion with elastase and trypsin.[135,151,274]

Acquired deficiencies in factor XIII and its elevated plasma levels are seen in various disease states.[214,281]

Genetics of Factor XIII

Chromosomal Localization and Gene Structures. The gene for the A subunit of factor XIII is located on chromosome 6p24-p25.[282] The gene encoding the keratinocyte (epidermal) transglutaminase is localized to chromosome 14q11.2–q13,[283–285] whereas the gene for tissue transglutaminase is located on chromosome 20q12[167] and that for prostate transglutaminase (type IV, TGM4) on chromosome 3p21.33-p22.[286] Thus gene loci for the various transglutaminases are not clustered but rather are dispersed throughout the genome. The gene for the B subunit of factor XIII is localized to chromosome 1q32-q32.1.[287] In contrast, the genes for several proteins containing multiple Sushi domains, such as factor H, the a and b chains of C4b-binding protein, complement receptors type I and II, membrane cofactor protein, and decay accelerating factor, are clustered at the same locus.[288,289] Because of the presence of a number of genes that are homologous to either the A or B subunit of factor XIII, their chromosomal localization was reexamined and confirmed by in vitro amplification of genomic DNAs from human-hamster hybrid cell lines employing gene-specific primers.[233]

The genes for both the A and B subunits of factor XIII have been characterized.[250,258] The gene for the A subunit spans more than 160 kb (GenBank M21987, J03834). It consists of 15 exons interrupted by 14 introns, and each functional region is encoded by a separate exon. The genomic organizations of keratinocyte, tissue, and hair follicle transglutaminases and erythrocyte membrane band 4.2 protein are nearly identical to that of the A subunit.[158,284,285,290–292]

The gene for the B subunit is about 28 kb in length (GenBank M64554).[258] It is composed of 12 exons interrupted by 11 introns, and each of the 10 Sushi domains is encoded by a single exon. This is also true of the genes for other Sushi domain-containing proteins, with few exceptions.

Gene Regulation of the A subunit. Recently, the cell type-specific transcriptional regulation of the A-subunit gene has been characterized.[293] Although the A subunit and other transglutaminases share significant similarity in their gene organization, their 5′-flanking nucleotide sequences differ from each other, and the mechanisms for their gene regulation seem to be diverse as well.[294–297]

It has been reported that the conditioned medium from type II human T-cell leukemia virus-infected T cells induces the conversion of endothelial cells to a Kaposi sarcoma cell-like phenotype and that the endothelial cells cultured in the presence of hepatocyte growth factor acquired the ability to express the A subunit of factor XIII.[298,299] These findings suggest that hepatocyte growth factor and factor XIII play a role in the initiation and maintenance of Kaposi sarcoma lesions. The expression of the A subunit may be induced by other cytokines and growth factors as well.

Genetic Polymorphism. By use of agarose gel electrophoresis, several different allelic forms of the A subunit of factor XIII were identified in the normal population.[300,301] Heterogeneity in these A subunits was confirmed by both amino acid and DNA sequencing.[153,154,162,250,302] All amino acid substitutions can be explained by point mutations; these include Val34/Leu, Phe204/Tyr, Leu564/Pro, Val650/Ile, and Glu651/Gln.[303] Although Arg77/Gly, Arg78/Lys, and Phe88/Leu polymorphisms have been described in the literature,[154,162] genetic studies failed to identify the corresponding nucleotide changes. It has been reported that the Val34/Leu polymorphism is associated with myocardial infarction.[304] A mechanism whereby Leu34 is protective against myocardial infarction remains to be determined. It also has been shown by restriction fragments length polymorphism (RFLP) that extensive DNA polymorphism exists in the A-subunit gene.[250,307,308] Furthermore, a short tandem repeat polymorphism exists in the 5′-flanking region in the A-subunit gene.[250,307,308]

Microheterogeneity of the B subunit[271] has been observed in several alleles.[309] Differences in amino acid sequences or DNA sequences, however, were not detected.[155,258] Several nucleotide substitutions were found in the noncoding and flanking regions of the B-subunit gene.[263,310,311] A short tandem repeat polymorphism also was found in the 3′-flanking region of the B-subunit gene.[258,312] Most recently, several nucleotide substitutions in the B-subunit gene corresponding to the heterogeneity described earlier have been identified (Umetsu and Ichinose, unpublished data).

Hereditary Disorders of Factor XIII

Congenital Deficiency and Molecular Abnormality. The incidence of congenital factor XIII deficiency (<1 percent of the normal activity level) is about 1 in 5 million in the United Kingdom[214] and in Japan. Most patients appear to be deficient in the A subunit in plasma. The mode of inheritance is autosomal recessive,[214,260] which is consistent with the A-subunit gene being on chromosome 6.

In affected individuals, the first manifestation of bleeding is usually from the umbilical cord after birth, and this occurs in approximately 90 percent of the patients.[212] Intracranial hemorrhage occurs in one-fourth of patients and is the leading cause of death. Superficial bruising and hematomas in subcutaneous tissue and muscle are common, and the bleeding at these sites may recur if not treated. Patients may bleed around the joint after trauma but have much less spontaneous hemarthrosis than hemophiliacs.

Deficiency of either factor XIII[212,214] or α_2-plasmin inhibitor[313] results in "delayed bleeding" after trauma, whereas primary hemostasis in individuals with these traits is normal. The delayed bleeding is caused by premature lysis of hemostatic clots. Because of the absence of crosslinking between α_2-plasmin inhibitor and fibrin, these clots have decreased resistance to proteolytic degradation by plasmin.[203,204]

In addition to a lifelong bleeding tendency, abnormal wound healing in affected individuals and habitual spontaneous abortion in affected females are not rare.[212,214] It is noteworthy that recurrent miscarriage also has been described in patients with congenital hypofibrinogenemia or afibrinogenemia.[314,315] Moreover, abnormal wound healing and repetitive spontaneous miscarriage are reported in patients with congenital dysfibrinogenemia (reviewed in ref. 316). These symptoms underscore the importance of the function of factor XIII and fibrin in vivo.

Molecular and Cellular Bases. Factor XIII deficiency has been classified previously into two categories: type I deficiency, characterized by the lack of both the A and B subunits, and type II deficiency, characterized by the lack of the A subunit alone.[317] Based on genetic analyses, a new classification for factor XIII deficiency has been proposed: a deficiency of the A subunit (former type II), a deficiency of the B subunit (former type I), and a possible combined deficiency of both A and B subunits.[303]

Deficiency of the A Subunit. Mutations in the gene for the A subunit have been detected by in vitro amplification of DNA samples obtained from patients with A-subunit deficiency.[233] These include a variety of missense and nonsense mutations, small deletions and insertions with or without frameshift/premature termination, splicing abnormalities, and a large deletion[280,318–333] (Fig 171-7). Effects of these mutations on A-subunit biosynthesis have been confirmed in several cases. For example, in one case a deletion of 4 bp was observed in exon XI, whereas in another case Gly562 was found to have been replaced by Arg.[280] The deletion in the former case leads to a premature termination at codon 464. Reverse transcription (RT) polymerase chain reaction (PCR) analysis demonstrated that the level of mRNA was greatly reduced in the former case, whereas the level of mutant mRNA expressed in the latter case was normal. To determine how these mutations impaired synthesis of the A subunit, recombinant A subunits bearing the mutations were expressed in mammalian cells, showing that the mutants were synthesized normally but disappeared rapidly, whereas the wild type remained for a

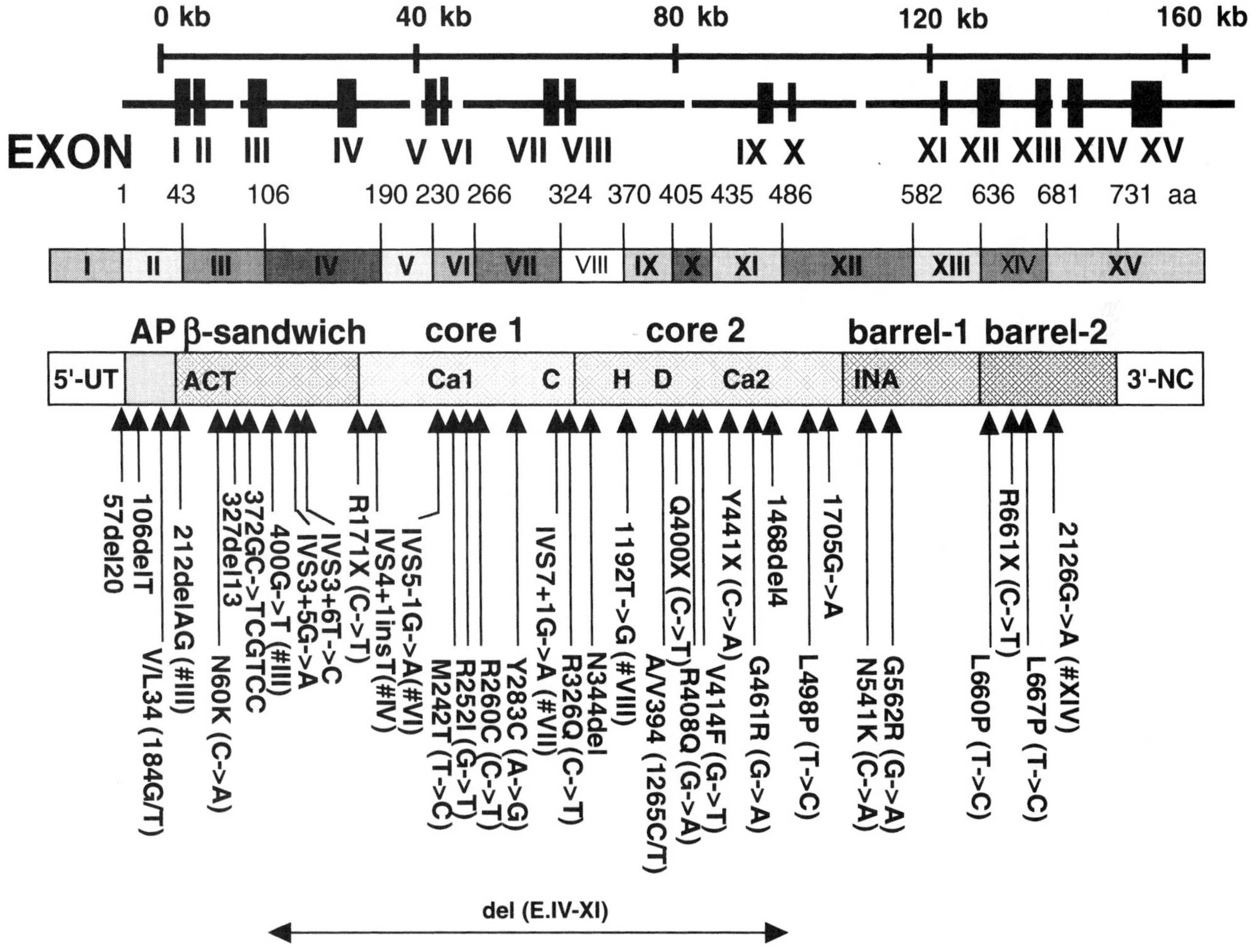

Fig. 171-7 Structure of the A-subunit gene and identified mutations. ***(Above)*** **Exons are indicated by wide vertical bars and Roman numerals.** ***(Center)*** **The 5′-untranslated region (5′-UT), region coding each exon (with Roman numeral), and the 3′-noncoding region (3′-NC) of the cDNA are shown by boxes. ACT, Ca1, C, H, D, Ca2, and INA stand for the activation cleavage site, a candidate for a calcium binding site, the active site Cys314, His373, and Asp396, another candidate for a calcium-binding site, and the inactivation cleavage site, respectively.** ***(Below)*** **The mutations were identified in various patients with the A-subunit deficiency (former type II deficiency). Short, medium, and long vertical arrows indicate mutations with premature termination, mutations resulting in exon skipping, and missense mutations, respectively. A large deletion is depicted by a long horizontal arrow at the bottom. The mutations discussed in the text are boxed. *, premature termination; #, exon skipping; −, deletion; +, insertion; =, substitution.**

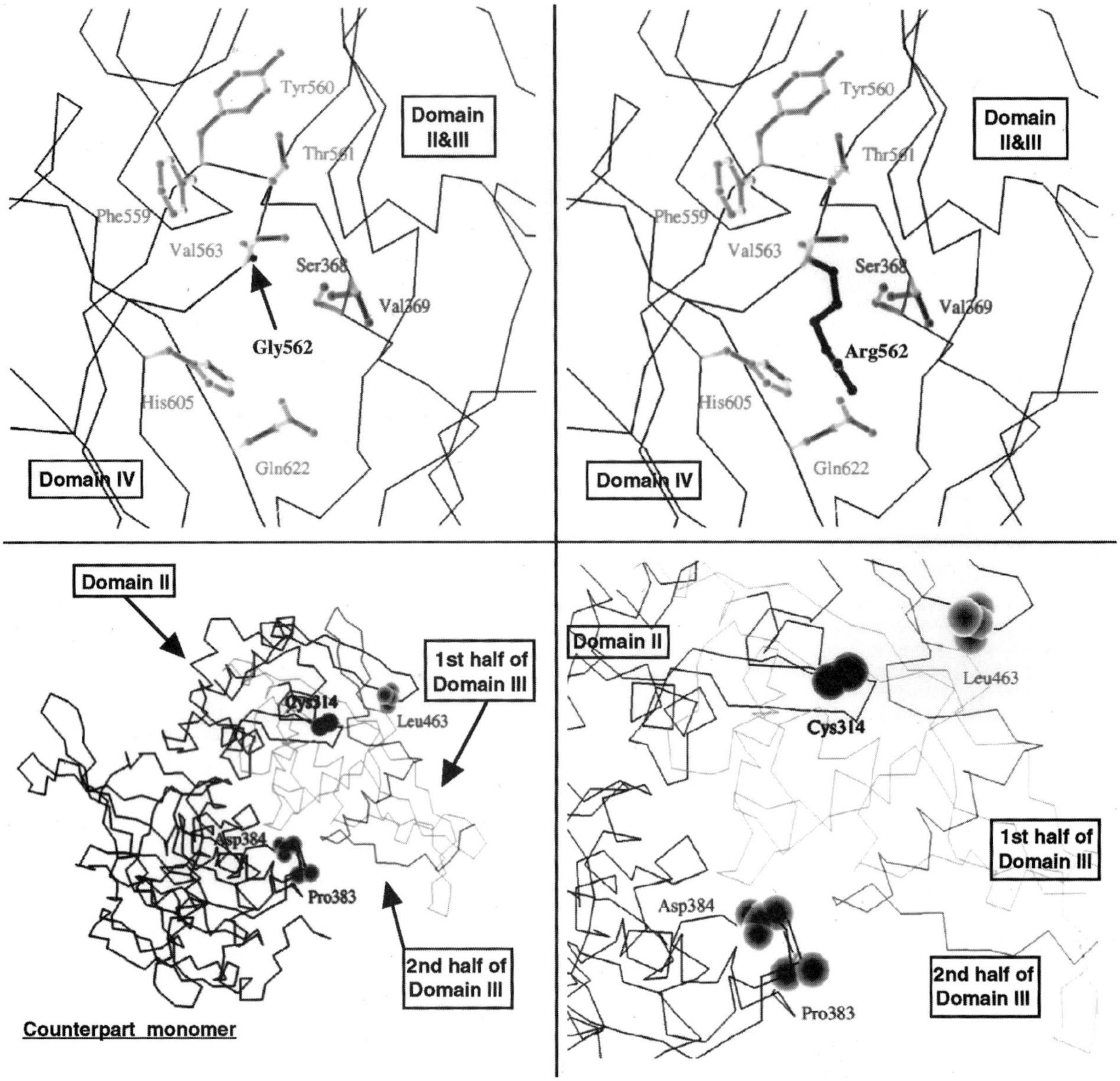

Fig. 171-8 ***(Above)*** **Close-up model view of the native (*left*, Gly562) or mutant (*right*, Arg562) A subunit. The tertiary structure of the normal A subunit is based on x-ray diffraction analysis. The main chain of the protein is drawn as a carbon trace; domains II and III are shown by light lines and domain IV by dark lines. Side-chain groups of labeled residues are shown as ball-and-stick structures; residues belonging to domains II and III are drawn in a light color and those in domain IV in a faint color. Although the mutant Arg562 residue can be accommodated by the chemical structure, it generates unfavorable short contacts with neighboring residues. Accordingly, the substitution of a small residue by a large charged amino acid is expected to yield an unstable, misfolded structure. (*Below, left*) Model view for the A-subunit dimer including the normal domain II (dark line), the first half of domain III (faint line), the second half of domain III (light line) in a monomer, and the same domains II and III in the counterpart monomer. Domains IV and V are not shown in this figure. A total of 268 residues consisting of the second half of domain III and domains IV and V are removed from the molecule in the deletion mutant. The C-terminal Leu463 residue of the truncated molecule is shown in a light color. Pro383 and Asp384 residues contact with the second part of domain III, which is absent in the mutant. (*Below, right*) Closer view of the environment around domains II and III. Since premature termination at position 464 would lead to the loss of a C-terminal part of the core domain and the entire domains IV and V (barrel 1 and 2), the protein is expected to misfold and/or be incapable of dimer formation. (*Reprinted with permission from Takahashi et al.*[280])**

prolonged period of time.[280] Molecular modeling also showed that the Arg562 substitution changed the conformation of the A subunit, causing misfolding and/or destabilization of the molecule (Fig. 171-8).

An amino acid substitution of Arg260 by Cys has been predicted by molecular modeling and mechanics to result in instability of the A-subunit molecule.[334] Rapid degradation of this mutant has been confirmed by an expression study in yeast (Maeda and Ichinose, unpublished data). Rapid degradation of a novel Tyr283 to Cys mutant also has been ascribed to its instability by characterization in an expression system employing megakaryoblastoid MEG01 cells that endogeneously synthesize the A subunit (Souri and Ichinose, unpublished data). In contrast, a previously described Ala394 to Val mutation[233] appears to be a rare polymorphism, since this mutation also was detected in a normal allele of the patient's father. Moreover, molecular modeling and mechanics predicted no significant alteration in its conformation.[334]

A 20-bp deletion at the boundary of exon I/intron A and an insertion of T in the invariant GT dinucleotide at the splicing donor site of exon IV/intron D also were found in a patient.[335] RT-PCR analysis demonstrated that only one kind of mRNA without exon

IV was detected, although its level was reduced to less than 5 percent of normal. Transcript of the other defective allele of the A-subunit gene containing the 20-bp deletion was not detected. Thus both mutations impaired normal processing of mRNA for the A subunit.

Deficiency of the B Subunit. A rare case of complete deficiency of the B subunit of factor XIII was found in Japan and has been characterized.[262] The patient, who manifests a mild bleeding tendency, has no B subunit and a significantly reduced level of the A subunit in plasma. The half-life of an infused placental concentrate (A_2) in the patient was shorter than that in the plasma of patients with A-subunit deficiency; therefore, the lack of the B subunit most likely causes instability of the A subunit. Nucleotide sequence analysis of the B-subunit gene of this patient revealed that the patient is a compound heterozygote for two separate defects in the B-subunit genes. The deletion of an A at the splicing acceptor junction of the intron A/exon II boundary and the amino acid substitution of Cys430 by Phe in exon VIII (see Fig 171-6) result in abnormal splicing of pre-mRNA and the breakup of a disulfide bond in the seventh Sushi domain, respectively.[263] The Cys430 to Phe mutation does not prevent the *de novo* synthesis of the B subunit but alters the conformation of the mutant protein sufficiently to impair its intracellular transport, resulting in its deficiency in this patient.[336]

Additionally, two unrelated Italian families were found to be deficient in the B subunit.[265,317,337] Surprisingly, these families share the same AAC insertion mutation in exon III and identical polymorphisms in the 3′-noncoding and 3′-flanking regions of the B-subunit gene.[310,311] These results suggest that this mutation reflects a founder effect, at least among Italians.

Diagnosis for Factor XIII Deficiency. The diagnosis of a homozygote with congenital deficiency of factor XIII is based on the pattern of inheritance, clinical symptoms, and laboratory tests. In addition to the typical umbilical cord bleeding after birth, the characteristic delayed bleeding after trauma strongly suggests this disorder. Deficiencies and molecular abnormalities of α_2-plasmin inhibitor and fibrinogen should be ruled out before the final diagnosis, since these disorders show symptoms similar to those described earlier.

Tests for factor XIII deficiency are based on transglutaminase activity. These include thromboelastography and, more specifically, a solubility test of the recalcified plasma clot in 5 M urea or 1% monochloroacetic acid. Visualization of a γ-dimer or α-polymers of fibrin by SDS-polyacrylamide gel electrophoresis is useful to obtain a rough estimate of the functional level of factor XIII in plasma. The transglutaminase activity of factor XIII is quantitatively measured by amine incorporation assays.[338,339] A standardized method for screening of factor XIII deficiency, however, needs to be established so that patients with this disease will not be misdiagnosed or completely overlooked.

Immunologic quantitation of the A and B subunits in plasma is essential in determining which subunit is primarily deficient, although the incidence of B-subunit deficiency appears to be rather rare. Although concentrations of the A and B subunits were measured routinely by the Laurell rocket electrophoresis method,[184,259] these measurements can now be determined more precisely by an ELISA.[227] Laboratory coagulation tests other than factor XIII are within the normal range.

Diagnosis of a heterozygote, who usually lacks symptoms of factor XIII deficiency, can be made only by specific quantitative measurements of both the A and B subunits. Genetic diagnosis at the DNA level will help both in prenatal detection of affected patients and in determination of carrier states. It would be difficult, however, to perform genetic diagnosis for a new subject unless the type of mutation is known in at least one member of the subject's family. This is so because mutations causing factor XIII deficiency are highly heterogeneous, as discussed earlier.

Therapy for Factor XIII Deficiency. Both congenital and acquired factor XIII deficiencies have been treated successfully with fresh frozen plasma, cryoprecipitate, and crude factor XIII concentrates from placenta.[340,341] Maintaining the level of plasma factor XIII at 10 to 20 percent of the normal level is sufficient to alleviate symptoms, since bleeding occurs frequently in patients with less than 1 percent of the normal level, and levels of 1 and 10 percent of normal are adequate for the in vitro γ-dimerization and α-polymerization of fibrin, respectively. The long half-life of factor XIII in plasma and its minimal requirement for hemostasis are beneficial both for the treatment of acute bleeding and for prophylaxis. Prophylactic infusion of factor XIII concentrates would be desirable for severe deficiency patients, who otherwise may bleed frequently. Although development of inhibitors to factor XIII following multiple infusions is rare, it must be considered when bleeding is uncontrollable by a therapeutic dosage of factor XIII. In such a case, immunosuppressive therapy may be required as well.

The cloning of human factor XIII[153,154] made it possible to prepare recombinant A subunit as a therapeutic material that is free of viral contamination. The recombinant A subunit is comparable with the native A-subunit protein with respect to structural and functional properties.[148,187] Thus it is a safe substitute for the placental and plasma factor XIII concentrates currently used in transfusion therapy. It also has been introduced as an essential component in fibrin sealant, which has been used widely for many types of surgery and for the treatment of trauma.

REFERENCES

1. Scheraga HA, Laskowski M Jr: The fibrinogen-fibrin conversion. *Adv Protein Chem* **12**:1, 1957.
2. Doolittle RF: Structural aspects of the fibrinogen-fibrin conversion. *Adv Protein Chem* **27**:1, 1973.
3. McKee PA, Rogers LA, Marler E, Hill RL: The subunit polypeptides of human fibrinogen. *Arch Biochem Biophys* **116**:271, 1966.
4. Doolittle RF, Watt KWK, Cottrell BA, Strong DD, Riley M: The amino acid sequence of the α-chain of human fibrinogen. *Nature* **280**:464, 1979.
5. Henschen A, Lottspeich F: Amino acid sequence of human fibrin: Preliminary note on the completion of the β-chain sequence. *Hoppe-Seylers Z Physiol Chem* **358**:1643, 1977.
6. Henschen A, Lottspeich F: Amino acid sequence of human fibrin: Preliminary note on the γ-chain sequence. *Hoppe-Seylers Z Physiol Chem* **358**:935, 1977.
7. Tagaki T, Doolittle RF: Amino acid sequence studies on the α-chain of human fibrinogen: Location of four plasmin attack points and a covalent cross-linking site. *Biochemistry* **14**:5149, 1975.
8. Takagi T, Doolittle, RF: The amino acid sequences of those portions of human fibrinogen fragment E which are not included in the amino-terminal disulfide knot. *Thromb Res* **7**:813, 1975.
9. Chung DW, Rixon MW, Davie EW: The biosynthesis of fibrinogen and the cloning of its cDNA, in Bradshaw RA, Hill RL, Tang J, Liang CC, Tsao TC, Tsou CL (eds): *Proteins in Biology and Medicine*. New York, Academic Press, 1982, p 309.
10. Crabtree GR, Comeau CM, Fowlkes DM, Fornace AJ, Malley JD, Kant JA: Evolution and structure of the fibrinogen genes: Random insertion of introns or selective loss? *J Mol Biol* **185**:1, 1985.
11. Weissbach L, Grieninger G: Bipartite mRNA for chicken alpha-fibrinogen potentially encodes an amino acid sequence homologous to beta- and gamma-fibrinogens. *Proc Natl Acad Sci USA* **87**:5198, 1990
12. Pan Y, Doolittle RF: cDNA sequence of a second fibrinogen alpha chain in lamprey: An archetypal version alignable with full-length beta and gamma chains. *Proc Natl Acad Sci USA* **89**:2066, 1992.
13. Spraggon G, Everse SJ, Doolittle RF: Crystal structures of fragment D from human fibrinogen and its crosslinked counterpart from fibrin. *Nature* **389**:455, 1997.
14. Yee VC, Pratt KP, Cote HC, Trong IL, Chung DW, Davie EW, Stenkamp RE, Teller DC: Crystal structure of a 30 kDa C-terminal fragment from the gamma chain of human fibrinogen. *Structure* **5**:125, 1997.
15. Bailey K, Astbury WT, Rudall KM: Fibrinogen and fibrin as members of the keratin-myosin group. *Nature* **151**:716, 1943.

16. Hall CE, Slayter HS: The fibrinogen molecule: Its size, shape and mode of polymerization. *J Biophys Biochem Cytol* **5**:11, 1959.
17. Williams RC: Morphology of fibrinogen monomers and of fibrin protofibrils. *Ann NY Acad Sci* **408**:180, 1983.
18. Blomback B, Blomback M, Hanschen A, Hessel B, Iwanaga S, Woods KR: N-terminal disulfide knot of human fibrinogen. *Nature* **218**:130, 1968.
19. Marsh HC, Meinwald YC, Lee S, Martinelli RA, Scheraga HA: Mechanism of action of thrombin on fibrinogen: NMR evidence for a beta-bend at or near fibrinogen A alpha Gly(P5)-Gly(P4). *Biochemistry* **24**:2806, 1985.
20. Marti PD, Robertson W, Turk D, Huber R, Bode W, Edwards BF: The structure of residues 7-16 of the A alpha-chain of human fibrinogen bound to bovine thrombin at 2.3-Å resolution. *J Biol Chem* **267**:7911, 1992.
21. Ni F, Zhu Y, Scheraga HA: Thrombin-bound structures of designed analogues of human fibrinopeptide A determined by quantitative transferred NOE spectroscopy: A new structural basis for thrombin specificity. *J Mol Biol* **252**:656, 1995.
22. Doolittle RF, Goldbaum DM, Doolittle LR: Designation of sequences involved in the "coiled coil" interdomainal connector in fibrinogen: Construction of an atomic scale model. *J Mol Biol* **120**:311, 1978.
23. Weisel JW, Stauffacher CV, Bullit E, Cohen C: A model for fibrinogen: Domains and sequence. *Science* **230**:1388, 1985.
24. Medved LV, Litvinovich SV, Privalov PL: Domain organization of the terminal parts in the fibrinogen molecule. *FEBS Lett* **202**:298, 1986.
25. Beklich YL, Gorkun OV, Medved LV, Nieuwenhuizen W, Weisel JW: Carboxyl-terminal portions of the alpha chains of fibrinogen and fibrin: Localization by electron microscopy and the effects of isolated alpha C fragments on polymerization. *J Biol Chem* **268**:13577, 1993.
26. Everse SJ, Spraggon G, Veerapandian L, Riley M, Doolittle RF: Crystal structure of fragment double-D from human fibrin with two different bound ligands. *Biochemistry* **37**:8637, 1998.
27. Pratt KP, Cote HC, Chung DW, Stenkamp RE, Davie EW: The primary fibrin polymerization pocket: Three-dimensional structure of a 30-kDa C-terminal gamma chain fragment complexed with the peptide Gly-Pro-Arg-Pro. *Proc Natl Acad Sci USA* **94**:7176, 1997.
28. Cote HC, Pratt KP, Davie EW, Chung DW: The polymerization pocket "a" within the carboxyl-terminal region of the gamma chain of human fibrinogen is adjacent to but independent from the calcium-binding site. *J Biol Chem* **272**:23792, 1997.
29. Hantgan R, McDonagh J, Hermans J: Fibrin assembly. *Ann NY Acad Sci* **408**:344, 1983.
30. Ebert RF: *Index of Variant Human Fibrinogens*. Boca Raton, FL, CRC Press, 1994.
31. Chung DW, Davie EW: γ and γ' chains of human fibrinogen are produced by alternative mRNA processing. *Biochemistry* **23**:4232, 1984.
32. Fornace AJ, Cummings D, Comeau CM, Kant JA, Crabtree GR: The γ_B chain of human fibrinogen is produced by alternate splice patterns of mRNA from a single gene. *J Biol Chem* **259**:12826, 1984.
33. Mosesso MW, Finlayson JS, Umfleet RA: Human fibrinogen heterogeneities: III. Identification of chain variants. *J Biol Chem* **247**:5223, 1972.
34. Farrell DH, Thiagarajan P, Chung DW, Davie EW: Role of fibrinogen alpha and gamma chain sites in platelet aggregation. *Proc Natl Acad Sci USA* **89**:10729, 1992.
35. Farrell DH, Mulvihill ER, Huang SM, Chung DW, Davie EW: Recombinant human fibrinogen and sulfation of the gamma′ chain. *Biochemistry* **30**:9414, 1991.
36. Fu Y, Grieninger G: Fib420: A normal human variant of fibrinogen with two extended alpha chains. *Proc Natl Acad Sci USA* **91**:2625, 1994.
37. Grieninger G, Lu X, Cao Y, Fu Y, Kudryk BJ, Galanakis DK, Hertzberg KM: Fib420, the novel fibrinogen subclass: newborn levels are higher than adult. *Blood* **90**:2609, 1997.
38. Spraggon G, Applegate D, Everse SJ, Zhang JZ, Veerapandian L, Redman C, Doolittle RF, Grieninger G: Crystal structure of a recombinant alphaEC domain from human fibrinogen-420. *Proc Natl Acad Sci USA* **95**:9099, 1998.
39. Mosesson MW: Fibrinogen heterogeneity. *Ann NY Acad Sci* **408**:97, 1083.
40. Nakashima A, Sasaki S, Miyazaki K, Miyata T, Iwanaga S: Human fibrinogen heterogeneity: the COOH-terminal residues of defective Aα-chains of fibrinogen II. *Blood Coagul Fibrinol* **3**:361, 1992.
41. Seydewitz HH, Kaiser C, Rothweiler H, Witt I: The location of a second in vivo phosphorylation site in the A alpha chain of human fibrinogen. *Thromb Res* **33**:487, 1983.
42. Townsend RR, Hilliker E, Li YT, Laine RA, Bell WR, Lee YC: Carbohydrate structure of human fibrinogen: Use of 300-MHz ^{1}H-NMR to characterize glycosidase-treated glycopeptides. *J Biol Chem* **257**:9704, 1982.
43. Martinez J, Palascak JE, Dwasniak D: Abnormal sialic acid content of the dysfibrinogenemia associated with liver disease. *J Clin Invest* **61**:535, 1978.
44. Blomback B, Vestermark A: Isolation of fibrinopeptides by chromatography. *Arkiv Kemi* **12**:173, 1958.
45. Lewis SD, Shields PP, Shafer JA: Characterization of the kinetic pathway for liberation of fibrinopeptides during assembly of fibrin. *J Biol Chem* **260**:10192, 1985.
46. Stocker K, Fischer H, Meier J: Thrombin-like snake venom proteinases. *Toxicon* **20**:265, 1982.
47. Bell WR Jr: Defibrinogenating enzymes. *Drugs* **54**(suppl 3)18, 1997.
48. Shainoff JR, Dardik BN: Fibrinopeptide B and aggregation of fibrinogen. *Science*: **204**:200, 1979.
49. Dyr JE, Blomback B, Kornalik F: The fibrinogenolytic and procoagulant activity of southern copperhead venom enzymes. *Thromb Res* **30**:185, 1983.
50. Fowler WE, Hantgan RR, Hermans J, Erickson HP: Structure of the fibrin protofibril. *Proc Natl Acad Sci USA* **78**:4872, 1981.
51. Hantgan RR, Hermans J: Assembly of fibrin: A light scattering study. *J Biol Chem* **254**:11272, 1979.
52. Hantgan RR, Fowler RW, Erickson HP, Hermans J: Fibrin assembly: A comparison of electron microscopic and light scattering results. *Thromb Haemost* **44**:119, 1980.
53. Laudano AP, Doolittle RF: Studies on synthetic peptides that bind to fibrinogen and prevent fibrin polymerization. *Proc Natl Acad Sci USA* **75**:3085, 1978.
54. Laudano AP, Doolittle RF: Studies on synthetic peptides that bind to fibrinogen and prevent fibrin polymerization: Structural requirements, number of binding sites, and species differences. *Biochemistry* **19**:1013, 1980
55. Gorkun OV, Bveklich YI, Medved LV, Henschen AH, Weisel JW: Role of the alpha C domains of fibrin in clot formation. *Biochemistry* **33**:6986, 1994.
56. Chen R, Doolittle RF: Identification of the polypeptide chains involved in the crosslinking of fibrin. *Proc Natl Acad Sci USA* **63**:420, 1969.
57. Chen R, Doolittle RF: γ cross-linking sites in human and bovine fibrin. *Biochemistry* **10**:4486, 1971.
58. Cottrell BA, Strong DD, Watt KWK, Doolittle RF: Amino acid sequence studies on the α-chain of human fibrinogen: Exact location of crosslinking acceptor sites. *Biochemistry* **18**:5405, 1979.
59. Fretto LJ, Ferguson EW, Steinman HM, McKee PA: Localization of the α-chain crosslink acceptor sites of human fibrin. *J Biol Chem* **253**:2184, 1978.
60. Corcoran DH, Ferguson EW, Fretto LJ, McKee PA: Localization of a cross-link donor site in the alpha-chain of human fibrin. *Thromb Res* **19**:883, 1980.
61. Gaffney PJ, Whitaker AN: Fibrin crosslinks and lysis rates. *Thromb Res* **14**:85, 1979.
62. Mosesson MW, Siebenlist KR, Amrani DL, DiOrio JP: Identification of covalently linked trimeric and tetrameric D domains in crosslinked fibrin. *Proc Natl Acad Sci USA* **86**:1113, 1989.
63. Al-Mondhiry H, Ehmann WC: Congenital afibrinogenemia. *Am J Hematol* **46**:343, 1994.
64. Suh TT, Holmback K, Jensen NJ, Daugherty CC, Small K, Simon DI, Potter S, Degen JL: Resolution of spontaneous bleeding events but failure of pregnancy in fibrinogen-deficient mice. *Genes Dev* **9**:2020, 1995.
65. Marder VJ, Shulman NR, Carroll WR: High molecular weight derivatives of human fibrinogen produced by plasmin: I. Physicochemical and immunological characterization. *J Biol Chem* **244**:2111, 1969.
66. Haverkate F, Tman G, Nieuwenhuizen W: Anticlotting properties of fragments D from human fibrinogen and fibrin. *Eur J Clin Invest* **9**:253, 1979.
67. Bennett JS: Integrin structure and function in hemostasis and thrombosis. *Ann NY Acad Sci* **614**:214, 1991.
68. Kloczewiak M, Timmons S, Hawiger J: Recognition site for the platelet receptor is present on the 15-residue carboxy-terminal fragment of the gamma chain of human fibrinogen and is not involved in the fibrin polymerization reaction. *Thromb Res* **29**:249, 1983.

69. Kloczewiak M, Timmons S, Lukas TJ, Hawiger J: Platelet receptor recognition site on human fibrinogen: Synthesis and structure-function relationship of peptides corresponding to the carboxy-terminal segment of the gamma chain. *Biochemistry* **23**:1767, 1984.
70. Farrell DH, Thiagarajan P, Chung DW, Davie EW: Role of dfibrinogen alpha and gamma chain sites in platelet aggregation. *Proc Natl Acad Sci USA* **89**:10729, 1992.
71. Weisel JW, Nagaswami C, Vilaire G, Bennett JS: Examination of the platelet membrane glycoprotein IIb-IIIa complex and its interaction with fibrinogen and other ligands by electron microscopy. *J Biol Chem* **267**:16637, 1992.
72. Holmback K, Danton MJ, Suh TT, Daugherty CC, Degen JL: Impaired platelet aggregation and sustained bleeding in mice lacking the fibrinogen motif bound by integrin alpha IIb beta 3. *EMBO J* **15**:5760, 1996.
73. Altieri DC, Duperray A, Plescia J, Thornton GB, Languino LR: Structural recognition of a novel fibrinogen gamma chain sequence (117–133) by intercellular adhesion molecule-1 mediates leukocyte-endothelium interaction. *J Biol Chem* **270**:696, 1995.
74. Altieri DC, Plescia J, Plow EF: The structural motif glycine 190-valine 202 of the fibrinogen gamma chain interacts with CD11b/CD18 integrin (alpha M beta 2, Mac-1) and promotes leukocyte adhesion. *J Biol Chem* **268**:1847, 1993.
75. Loike JD, Sodeik B, Cao L, Leucona S, Weitz JI, Detmers PA, Wright SD, Silverstein SC: CD11c/CD18 on neutrophils recognizes a domain at the N terminus of the A alpha chain of fibrinogen. *Proc Natl Acad Sci USA* **88**:1044, 1991.
76. Cheresh DA, Berliner SA, Vicente V, Ruggeri ZM: Recognition of distinct adhesive sites on fibrinogen by related integrins on platelets and endothelial cells. *Cell* **58**:945, 1989.
77. Thiagarajan P, Rippon AJ, Farrell DH: Alternative adhesion sites in human fibrinogen for vascular endothelial cells. *Biochemistry* **35**:4169, 1996.
78. Farrell DH, Al-Mondhiry HA: Human fibroblast adhesion to fibrinogen. *Biochemistry* **36**:1123, 1997.
79. Nieuwenhuizen W, Haverkate F: Calcium binding regions in fibrinogen. *Ann NY Acad Sci* **408**:92, 1983.
80. Dang CV, Shin CK, Bell WR, Nagaswami C, Weisel JW: Fibrinogen sialic acid residues are low affinity calcium-binding sites that influence fibrin assembly. *J Biol Chem* **264**:15104, 1989.
81. Yoshida N, Hirata H, Morigami Y, Imaoka S, Matsuda M, Yamazumi K, Asakura S: Characterization of an abnormal $fibrinogen_{OSAKA\ V}$ with the replacement of γ-arginine 375 by glycine: The lack of high affinity calcium binding to D-domains and the lack of protective effect of calcium on fibrinolysis. *J Biol Chem* **267**:2753, 1992.
82. Koopman J, Haverkate F, Brieet E, Lord ST: A congenitally abnormal fibrinogen (Vlissingen) with a 6-base deletion in the gamma-chain gene, causing defective calcium binding and impaired fibrin polymerization. *J Biol Chem* **266**:13456, 1991.
83. Yonekawa O, Voskuilen M, Nieuwenhuizen W: Localization in the fibrinogen gamma chain of a new site that is involved in the acceleration of the tissue-type plasminogen activator-catalysed activation of plasminogen. *Biochem J* **283**:187, 1992.
84. Hornyak TJ, Shafer JA: Interactions of factor XIII with fibrin as substrate and cofactor. *Biochemistry* **31**:423, 1992.
85. Liu CY, Koehn JA, Morgan FJ: Characterization of $fibrinogen_{NEW\ YORK\ I}$: A dysfunctional fibrinogen with a deletion of Bb(9–72) corresponding exactly to exon 2 of the gene. *J Biol Chem* **260**:4390, 1985.
86. Meh DA, Siebenlist KR, Mosesson MW: Identification and characterization of the thrombin binding sites on fibrin. *J Biol Chem* **271**:23121, 1996.
87. Aoki N, Saito H, Kamiya T, Koie K, Dakata Y, Kobokura M: Congenital deficiency of α_2-plasmin inhibitor associated with severe hemorrhagic tendency. *J Clin Invest* **63**:877, 1979.
88. Mosher DF: Crosslinking of cold-insoluble globulin by fibrin-stabilizing factor. *J Biol Chem* **250**:6614, 1975.
89. Francois P, Vaudaux P, Foster TJ, Lew DP: Host-bacteria interactions in foreign body infections. *Infect Control Hosp Epidemiol* **17**:514, 1996.
90. McDevitt D, Nanavaty T, House-Pompeo K, Bell E, Turner N, McIntire L, Foster T, Hook M: Characterization of the interaction between the *Staphylococcus aureus* clumping factor (ClfA) and fibrinogen. *Eur J Biochem* **247**:416, 1997.
91. Boden MK, Flock JI: Cloning and characterization of a gene for a 19-kDa fibrinogen-binding protein from *Staphylococcus aureus*. *Mol Microbiol* **12**:599, 1994.
92. Cheung AI, Projan SJ, Edelstein RE, Rischetti VA: Cloning, expression, and nucleotide sequence of a *Staphylococcus aureus* gene (*flpA*) encoding a fibrinogen-binding protein. *Infect Immun* **63**:1914, 1995.
93. Nilsson M, Frykberg L, Flock JI, Pei L, Lindberg M, Guss B: A fibrinogen-binding protein of *Staphylococcus epidermidis*. *Infect Immun* **66**:2666, 1998.
94. Cedervall T, Johansson MU, Akerstrom B: Coiled-coil structure of group A streptococcal M proteins: Different temperature stability of class A and C proteins by hydrophobic-nonhydrophobic amino acid substitutions at heptad positions a and d. *Biochemistry* **36**:4987, 1997.
95. Cue DR, Cleary PP: High-frequency invasion of epithelial cells by *Streptococcus pyogenes* can be activated by fibrinogen and peptides containing the sequence RGD. *Infect Immun* **65**:2759, 1997.
96. Katerov V, Andreev A, Schalen C, Totolian AA: Protein F, a fibronectin-binding protein of *Streptococcus pyogenes*, also binds human fibrinogen: isolation of the protein and mapping of the binding region. *Microbiology* **144**:119, 1998.
97. Meehan M, Nowlan P, Owen P: Affinity purification and characterization of a fibrinogen-binding protein complex which protects mice against lethal challenge with *Streptococcus equi* subsp. *equi*. *Microbiology* **144**:993, 1998.
98. Brennan M: Fibrin glue. *Blood Rev* **5**:240, 1991.
99. Spotnitz WD: Fibrin sealant in the United States: Clinical use at the University of Virginia. *Thromb Haemost* **74**:482, 1995.
100. Prunkard D, Cottingham I, Garner I, Bruce S, Dalrymple M, Lasser G, Bishop P, Foster D: High-level expression of recombinant human fibrinogen in the milk of transgenic mice. *Nature Biotechnol* **14**:867, 1996.
101. Henry I, Uzan G, Weil D, Nicolas H, Kaplan JC, Marguerie C, Kahn A, Junien C: The genes coding for A alpha-, B beta-, and gamma-chains of fibrinogen map to 4q2. *Am J Hum Genet* **36**:760, 1984.
102. Kant JA, Fornace AJ Jr, Saxe D, Simon ML, McBride OW, Crabtree GR: Organization and evolution of the human fibrinogen locus on chromosome four. *Proc Natl Acad Sci USA* **82**:2344, 1985.
103. Chung DW, Harris JE, Davie EW: Nucleotide sequences of the three genes coding for human fibrinogen. *Adv Exp Med Biol* **281**:39, 1990.
104. Lord ST: Fibrinogen oligonucleotide primers, in Ebert RF (ed): *Index of Variant Human Fibrinogens*. Boca Raton, FL, CRC Press, 1994, pp 25–29.
105. Connor JM, Fowkes FG, Wood J, Smith FB, Donnan PT, Lowe GD: Genetic variation at fibrinogen loci and plasma fibrinogen levels. *J Med Genet* **29**:480, 1992.
106. Mills KA, Even D, Murray JC: Tetranucleotide repeat polymorphism at the human alpha fibrinogen locus (FGA). *Hum Mol Genet* **1**:779, 1992.
107. Huang S, Cao Z, Chung DW, Davie EW: The role of betagamma and alphagamma complexes in the assembly of human fibrinogen. *J Biol Chem* **271**:27942, 1996.
108. Straub PW: A study of fibrinogen production by human liver slices in vitro by immunoprecipitin method. *J Clin Invest* **42**:130, 1963.
109. Courtois G, Morgan JG, Campbell LA, Fourel G, Crabtree GR: Interaction of a liver-specific nuclear factor with the fibrinogen and α_1-antitrypsin promoter. *Science* **238**:688, 1987.
110. Hu CH, Harris JE, Davie EW, Chung DW: Characterization of the 5′-flanking region of the gene for the alpha chain of human fibrinogen. *J Biol Chem* **270**:28342, 1995.
111. Dalmon J, Laurent M, Courtois G: The human beta fibrinogen promoter contains a hepatocyte nuclear factor 1-dependent interleukin-6-responsive element. *Mol Cell Biol* **13**:1183, 1993.
112. Haidaris PJ, Courtney MA: Tissue-specific and ubiquitous expression of fibrinogen gamma-chain mRNA. *Blood Coagul Fibrinol* **1**:433, 1990.
113. Ritchie DG, Fuller GM: Hepatocyte-stimulating factor: A monocyte-derived acute-phase regulatory protein. *Ann NY Acad Sci* **408**:490, 1983.
114. Akira S, Isshiki H, Sugita T, Tanabe O, Kinoshita S, Nishio Y, Nakajima T, Hirano T, Kishimoto T: A nuclear factor for IL-6 expression (NF-IL6) is a member of a C/EBP family. *EMBO J* **9**:1897, 1990.
115. Mizuguchi J, Hu CH, Cao Z, Loeb KR, Chung DW, Davie EW: Characterization of the 5′-flanking region of the gene for the gamma chain of human fibrinogen. *J Biol Chem* **270**:28305, 1995.
116. Flute PT: Disorders of plasma fibrinogen synthesis. *Br Med Bull* **33**:253, 1977.
117. Rodriguez RC, Buchanan GR, Clanton MS: Prophylactic cryoprecipitate in congenital afibrinogenemia. *Clin Pediatr* **27**:543, 1988.
118. Pfeifer U, Ormanns W, Klinge O: Hepatocellular fibrinogen storage in familial hypofibrinogenemia. *Virchows Arch* **36**:247, 1981.

119. Gralnick HR, Henderson E: Hypofibrinogenemia and coagulation factor deficiencies with L-asparaginase treatment. *Cancer* **27**:1313, 1971.
120. Majer RV, Green PJ: Neonatal afibrinogenemia due to sodium valproate. *Lancet* **11**:740, 1987.
121. Coleman M, Bigliano EM, Weksler ME, Nachman RL: Inhibition of fibrin monomer polymerization by lambda myeloma globulins. *Blood* **39**:210, 1972.
122. Davey F: Immunoglobulin inhibition of fibrin clot formation. *Ann Clin Lab Sci* **6**:72, 1976.
123. Henschen A, Southan C, Kehl M, Lottspeich F: The structural error and its relation to the malfunction in some abnormal fibrinogens. *Thromb Haemost* **46**:181, 1981.
124. Hessel B, Stenbjerg S, Dyr J, Kudryk B, Therkildsen L, Blomback B: Fibrinogen$_{\mathrm{AARHUS}}$: A new case of dysfibrinogenemia. *Thromb Res* **42**:21, 1986.
125. Kudryk B, Blamback B, Blomback M: Fibrinogen$_{\mathrm{DETROIT}}$: An abnormal fibrinogen with nonfunctional NH_2 -terminal polymerization domain. *Thromb Res* **9**:25, 1976.
126. Cote HC, Lord ST, Pratt KP: Gamma chain dysfibrinogenemias: Molecular structure-function relationships of naturally occurring mutations in the gamma chain of human fibrinogen. *Blood* **92**:2195, 1998.
127. Everse SJ, Spraggon G, Doolittle RF: A three-dimensional consideration of variant human fibrinogens. *Thromb Haemost* **80**:1, 1998.
128. Kannel WB, D'Agostino RB, Belanger AJ: Fibrinogen, cigarette smoking, and risk of cardiovascular disease: Insights from the Framingham Study. *Am Heart J* **113**:1006, 1987.
129. Thomas AE, Green FR, Kelleher CH, Wilkes HC, Brennan PJ, Meade TW, Humphries SE: Variation in the promoter region of the b fibrinogen gene is associated with plasma fibrinogen levels in smokers and nonsmokers. *Thromb Haemost* **65**:487, 1991.
130. Montgomery HE, Clarkson P, Nwose OM, Mikailidis DP, Jagroop IA, Dollery C, Moult J, Benhizia F, Deanfield J, Jubb M, World M, McEwan JR, Winder A, Humphries S: The acute rise in plasma fibrinogen concentration with exercise is influenced by the G453-A polymorphism of the beta-fibrinogen gene. *Arterioscler Thromb Vasc Biol* **16**:386, 1996.
131. Berg K, Kierulf P: DNA polymorphisms at fibrinogen loci and plasma fibrinogen concentration. *Clin Genet* **36**:229, 1989.
132. Vaisanen S, Rauramaa R, Penttila I, Rankinen T, Gagnnon J, Perusse L, Chagnon M, Bouchard C: Variation in plasma fibrinogen over one year: Relationships with genetic polymorphisms and nongenetic factors. *Thromb Haemost* **77**:884, 1997.
133. Ridgway HJ, Brannan SO, Faed JM, George PM: Fibrinogen$_{\mathrm{OTAGO}}$: A major alpha chain truncation associated with severe hypofibrinogenemia and recurrent miscarriage. *Br J Haematol* **98**:632, 1997.
134. Fellowe AP, Brannan SQ, Ridgway HJ, Heaton DC, George PM: Electrospray ionization mass spectrometry identification of fibrinogen$_{\mathrm{BANKS\ PENINSULA}}$ (gamma280Tyr → Cys): A new variant with defective polymerization. *Br J Haematol* **101**:24, 1998.
135. Schwartz ML, Pizzo SV, Hill RL, McKee PA: Human factor XIII from plasma and platelets. Molecular weights, subunit structures, proteolytic activation, and crosslinking of fibrinogen and fibrin. *J Biol Chem* **248**:1395, 1973.
136. Chung SI, Lewis MS, Folk JE: Relationships of the catalytic properties of human plasma and platelet transglutaminases (activated blood coagulation factor XIII) to their subunit structures. *J Biol Chem* **249**:940, 1974.
137. Bohn H: Isolation and characterization of the fibrin stabilizing factor from human thrombocytes. *Thromb Diath Haemorrh* **23**:455, 1970.
138. Bohn H, Haupt H, Kranz T: Molecular structure of human fibrin stabilizing factors. *Blut* **25**:235, 1972.
139. Loewy A, Dahlberg A, Dunathan K, Kriel R, Wolfinger H: Fibrinase: Some physical properties. *J Biol Chem* **236**:2634, 1961.
140. Greenberg CS, Shuman MA: The zymogen forms of blood coagulation factor XIII bind specifically to fibrinogen. *J Biol Chem* **257**:6096, 1982.
141. Lewis BA, Freyssinet JM, Holbrook JJ: An equilibrium study of metal ion binding to human plasma coagulation factor XIII. *Biochem J* **169**:397, 1978.
142. Freyssinet JM, Lewis BA, Holbrook JJ, Shore JD: Protein-protein interactions in blood clotting: The use of polarization of fluorescence to measure the dissociation of plasma factor XIIIa. *Biochem J* **169**:403, 1978.
143. Achyuthan KE, Rowland TC, Birckbichler PJ, Lee KN, Bishop PD, Achyuthan AM: Hierarchies in the binding of human factor XIII, factor XIIIa, and endothelial cell transglutaminase to human plasma fibrinogen, fibrin, and fibronectin. *Mol Cell Biochem* **162**:43, 1996.
144. Siebenlist KR, Meh DA, Mosesson MW: Plasma factor XIII binds specifically to fibrinogen molecules containing gamma chains. *Biochemistry* **35**:10448, 1996.
145. Carrell NA, Erickson HP, McDonagh J: Electron microscopy and hydrodynamic properties of factor XIII subunits. *J Biol Chem* **264**:551, 1989.
146. Bohn H, Schwick HG: Isolation and characterization of a fibrin-stabilizing factor from human placenta. *Arzneimittel-Forschung* **21**:1432, 1971.
147. Hilgenfeld R, Liesum A, Storm R, Metzner HJ, Karges HE: Crystallization of blood coagulation factor XIII by an automated procedure. *FEBS Lett* **265**:110, 1990.
148. Bishop PD, Teller DC, Smith RA, Lasser GW, Gilbert T, Seale RL: Expression, purification, and characterization of human factor XIII in *Saccharomyces cerevisiae*. *Biochemistry* **29**:1861, 1990.
149. Yee VC, Pedersen LC, Le Trong I, Bishop PD, Stenkamp RE, Teller DC: Three-dimensional structure of a transglutaminase: Human blood coagulation factor XIII. *Proc Natl Acad Sci USA* **91**:7296, 1994.
150. Yee VC, Pedersen LC, Bishop PD, Stenkamp RE, Teller DC: Structural evidence that the activation peptide is not released upon thrombin cleavage of factor XIII. *Thromb Res* **78**:389, 1995.
151. Kurochkin IV, Procyk R, Bishop PD, et al: Domain structure, stability and domain-domain interactions in recombinant factor XIII. *J Mol Biol* **248**:414, 1995.
152. Weiss MS, Metzner HJ, Hilgenfeld R: Two nonproline cis peptide bonds may be important for factor XIII function. *FEBS Lett* **423**:291, 1998.
153. Ichinose A, Hendrickson LE, Fujikawa K, Davie EW: Amino acid sequence of the a subunit of human factor XIII. *Biochemistry* **25**:6900, 1986.
154. Grundmann U, Amann E, Zettlmeissl G, Kupper HA: Characterization of cDNA coding for human factor XIIIa. *Proc Natl Acad Sci USA* **83**:8024, 1986.
155. Ichinose A, McMullen BA, Fujikawa K, Davie EW: Amino acid sequence of the b subunit of human factor XIII, a protein composed of ten repetitive segments. *Biochemistry* **25**:4633, 1986.
156. Takagi T, Doolittle RF: Amino acid sequence studies on factor XIII and the peptide released during its activation by thrombin. *Biochemistry* **13**:750, 1974.
157. Gentile V, Saydak M, Chiocca EA, et al: Isolation and characterization of cDNA clones to mouse macrophage and human endothelial cell tissue transglutaminases. *J Biol Chem* **266**:478, 1991.
158. Phillips MA, Stewart BE, Rice RH: Genomic structure of keratinocyte transglutaminase: Recruitment of new exon for modified function. *J Biol Chem* **267**:2282, 1992.
159. Micanovic R, Procyk R, Lin W, Matsueda GR: Role of histidine 373 in the catalytic activity of coagulation factor XIII. *J Biol Chem* **269**:9190, 1994.
160. Hettasch JM, Greenberg CS: Analysis of the catalytic activity of human factor XIIIa by site-directed mutagenesis. *J Biol Chem* **269**:28309, 1994.
161. Pedersen LC, Yee VC, Bishop PD, Le Trong I, Teller DC, Stenkamp RE: Transglutaminase factor XIII uses proteinase-like catalytic triad to crosslink macromolecules. *Protein Sci* **3**:1131, 1994.
162. Takahashi N, Takahashi Y, Putnam FW: Primary structure of blood coagulation factor XIIIa (fibrinoligase, transglutaminase) from human placenta. *Proc Natl Acad Sci USA* **83**:8019, 1986.
163. Ichinose A, Bottenus RE, Davie EW: Structure of transglutaminases. *J Biol Chem* **265**:13411, 1990.
164. Phillips MA, Stewart BE, Qin Q, et al: Primary structure of keratinocyte transglutaminase. *Proc Natl Acad Sci USA* **87**:9333, 1990.
165. Kim HC, Idler WW, Kim IG, Han JH, Chung SI, Steinert PM: The complete amino acid sequence of the human transglutaminase K enzyme deduced from the nucleic acid sequences of cDNA clones. *J Biol Chem* **266**:536, 1991.
166. Yamanishi K, Liew FM, Konishi K, et al: Molecular cloning of human epidermal transglutaminase cDNA from keratinocytes in culture. *Biochem Biophys Res Commun* **175**:906, 1991.
167. Gentile V, Davies PJ, Baldini A: The human tissue transglutaminase gene maps on chromosome 20q12 by *in situ* fluorescence hybridization. *Genomics* **20**:295, 1994.
168. Grant FJ, Taylor DA, Sheppard PO, et al: Molecular cloning and characterization of a novel transglutaminase cDNA from a human prostate cDNA library. *Biochem Biophys Res Commun* **203**:1117, 1994.

169. Aeschlimann D, Koeller MK, Allen-Hoffmann BL, Mosher DF: Isolation of a cDNA encoding a novel member of the transglutaminase gene family from human keratinocytes: Detection and identification of transglutaminase gene products based on reverse transcription-polymerase chain reaction with degenerate primers. *J Biol Chem* **273**:3452, 1998.
170. Tokunaga F, Muta T, Iwanaga S, et al: Limulus hemocyte transglutaminase: cDNA cloning, amino acid sequence, and tissue localization. *J Biol Chem* **268**:262, 1993.
171. Sung LA, Chien S, Chang LS, et al: Molecular cloning of human protein 4.2: A major component of the erythrocyte membrane. *Proc Natl Acad Sci USA* **87**:955, 1990.
172. Korsgren C, Lawler J, Lambert S, Speicher D, Cohen CM: Complete amino acid sequence and homologies of human erythrocyte membrane protein band 4.2. *Proc Natl Acad Sci USA* **87**:613, 1990.
173. Davie EW, Ichinose A, Leytus SP: Structural features of the proteins participating in blood coagulation and fibrinolysis. *Cold Spring Harbor Symp Quant Biol* **51**:509, 1986.
174. Lozier J, Takahashi N, Putnam FW: Complete amino acid sequence of human plasma beta 2-glycoprotein I. *Proc Natl Acad Sci USA* **81**:3640, 1984.
175. Kato H, Enjyoji K: Amino acid sequence and location of the disulfide bonds in bovine beta 2 glycoprotein I: The presence of five Sushi domains. *Biochemistry* **30**:11687, 1991.
176. Janatova J, Reid KB, Willis AC: Disulfide bonds are localized within the short consensus repeat units of complement regulatory proteins: C4b-binding protein. *Biochemistry* **28**:4754, 1989.
177. Medved LV, Busby TF, Ingham KC: Calorimetric investigation of the domain structure of human complement Cl-s: Reversible unfolding of the short consensus repeat units. *Biochemistry* **28**:5408, 1989.
178. Perkins SJ, Haris PI, Sim RB, Chapman D: A study of the structure of human complement component factor H by Fourier transform infrared spectroscopy and secondary structure averaging methods. *Biochemistry* **27**:4004, 1988.
179. Barlow PN, Baron M, Norman DG, et al.: Secondary structure of a complement control protein module by two-dimensional ^{1}H NMR. *Biochemistry* **30**:997, 1991.
180. Ichinose A: The physiology and biochemistry of factor XIII, in Bloom AL, Forbes CD, Thomas DP, Tuddenham EGD (eds): *Haemostasis and Thrombosis,* vol 1, 3d ed. Edinburgh, Churchill-Livingstone, 1994, p 531.
181. Pierschbacher MD, Ruoslahti E: Cell attachment activity of fibronectin can be duplicated by small synthetic fragments of the molecule. *Nature* **309**:30, 1984.
182. Nonaka M, Matsuda Y, Shiroishi T, Moriwaki K, Nonaka M, Natsuume-Sakai S: Molecular cloning of the b subunit of mouse coagulation factor XIII and assignment of the gene to chromosome 1: Close evolutionary relationship to complement factor H. *Genomics* **15**:535, 1993.
183. Cooke RD: Calcium-induced dissociation of human plasma factor XIII and the appearance of catalytic activity. *Biochem J* **141**:683, 1974.
184. Bohn H, Becker W, Trobisch H: Molecular structure of fibrin stabilizing factors in man: II. Comparative immunologic studies on factor XIII deficient plasma and normal plasma. *Blut* **26**:303, 1973.
185. Lorand L, Murthy SN, Velasco PT, Karush F: Identification of transglutaminase substrates in inside-out vesicles from human erythrocytes: immunoblotting with anti-dansyl antibody. *Biochem Biophys Res Commun* **134**:685, 1986.
186. Lorand L, Gray AJ, Brown K, et al: Dissociation of the subunit structure of fibrin stabilizing factor during activation of the zymogen. *Biochem Biophys Res Commun* **56**:914, 1974.
187. Kaetsu H, Hashiguchi T, Foster D, Ichinose A: Expression and release of the a and b subunits for human coagulation factor XIII in baby hamster kidney (BHK) cells. *J Biochem* **119**:961, 1996.
188. Chen R, Doolittle RF: γ-Crosslinking sites in human and bovine fibrin. *Biochemistry* **10**:4487, 1971.
189. McDonagh RP, McDonagh J, Petersen TE, et al: Amino acid sequence of the factor XIIIa acceptor site in bovine plasma fibronectin. *FEBS Lett* **127**:174, 1981.
190. Tamaki T, Aoki N: Crosslinking of alpha 2-plasmin inhibitor to fibrin catalyzed by activated fibrin-stabilizing factor. *J Biol Chem* **257**:14767, 1982.
191. Cottrell BA, Strong DD, Watt KW, Doolittle RF: Amino acid sequence studies on the alpha chain of human fibrinogen: Exact location of crosslinking acceptor sites. *Biochemistry* **18**:5405, 1979.
192. Corcoran DH, Ferguson EW, Fretto LJ, McKee PA: Localization of a crosslink donor site in the alpha-chain of human fibrin. *Thromb Res* **19**:883, 1980.
193. Lorand L: Fibrinoligase: the fibrin-stabilizing factor system of blood plasma. *Ann NY Acad Sci* **202**:6, 1972.
194. Shen L, Lorand L: Contribution of fibrin stabilization to clot strength: Supplementation of factor XIII-deficient plasma with the purified zymogen. *J Clin Invest* **71**:1336, 1983.
195. Mosesson MW, Siebenlist KR, Amrani DL, Diorio JP: Identification of covalently linked trimeric and tetrameric D domains in crosslinked fibrin. *Proc Natl Acad Sci USA* **86**:1113, 1989.
196. Shainoff JR, Urbanic DA, Dibello PM: Immunoelectrophoretic characterizations of the crosslinking of fibrinogen and fibrin by factor XIIIa and tissue transglutaminase: Identification of a rapid mode of hybrid alpha-/gamma-chain crosslinking that is promoted by the gamma-chain crosslinking. *J Biol Chem* **266**:6429, 1991.
197. Siebenlist KR, Mosesson MW: Progressive crosslinking of fibrin gamma chains increases resistance to fibrinolysis. *J Biol Chem* **269**:28414, 1994.
198. Tamaki T, Aoki N: Crosslinking of alpha 2-plasmin inhibitor and fibronectin to fibrin by fibrin-stabilizing factor. *Biochem Biophys Acta* **661**:280, 1981.
199. Ichinose A, Aoki N: Reversible crosslinking of alpha 2-plasmin inhibitor to fibrinogen by fibrin-stabilizing factor. *Biochemistry* **706**:158, 1982.
200. Carmassi F, Chung SI: Regulation of fibrinolysis by factor XIII. *Prog Fibrinol* **6**:281, 1983.
201. Ichinose A, Tamaki T, Aoki N: Factor XIII-mediated crosslinking of NH_2 -terminal peptide of alpha 2-plasmin inhibitor to fibrin. *FEBS Lett* **153**:369, 1983.
202. Kimura S, Aoki N: Crosslinking site in fibrinogen for alpha 2-plasmin inhibitor. *J Biol Chem* **261**:15591, 1986.
203. Sakata Y, Aoki N: Significance of crosslinking of alpha 2-plasmin inhibitor to fibrin in inhibition of fibrinolysis and in hemostasis. *J Clin Invest* **69**:536, 1982.
204. Sakata Y, Aoki N: Crosslinking of alpha 2-plasmin inhibitor to fibrin by fibrin-stabilizing factor. *J Clin Invest* **65**:290, 1980.
205. Mosher DF: Crosslinking of cold-insoluble globulin by fibrin-stabilizing factor. *J Biol Chem* **250**:6614, 1975.
206. Mosher DF, Schad PE: Crosslinking of fibronectin to collagen by blood coagulation factor XIIIa. *J Clin Invest* **64**:781, 1979.
207. Barry EL, Mosher DF: Factor XIII crosslinking of fibronectin at cellular matrix assembly sites. *J Biol Chem* **263**:10464, 1988.
208. Barry EL, Mosher DF: Factor XIIIa-mediated crosslinking of fibronectin in fibroblast cell layers: Crosslinking of cellular and plasma fibronectin and of amino-terminal fibronectin fragments. *J Biol Chem* **264**:4179, 1989.
209. Grinnell F, Feld M, Minter D: Fibroblast adhesion to fibrinogen and fibrin substrata: requirement for cold-insoluble globulin (plasma fibronectin). *Cell* **19**:517, 1980.
210. Brown LF, Lanir N, McDonagh J, Tognazzi K, Dvorak AM, Dvorak HF: Fibroblast migration in fibrin gel matrices. *Am J Pathol* **142**:273, 1993.
211. Lanir N, Ciano PS, Van de Water L, McDonagh J, Dvorak AM, Dvorak HF: Macrophage migration in fibrin gel matrices: II. Effects of clotting factor XIII, fibronectin, and glycosaminoglycan content on cell migration. *J Immunol* **140**:2340, 1988.
212. Duckert F: Documentation of the plasma factor XIII deficiency in man. *Ann NY Acad Sci* **202**:190, 1972.
213. Folk JE, Finlayson JS: The epsilon-(gamma-glutamyl)lysine crosslink and the catalytic role of transglutaminases. *Adv Protein Chem* **31**:1, 1977.
214. Lorand L, Losowsky MS, Miloszewski KJ: Human factor XIII: Fibrin-stabilizing factor. *Prog Hemost Thromb* **5**:245, 1980.
215. Mui PT, Ganguly P: Crosslinking of actin and fibrin by fibrin-stabilizing factor. *Am J Physiol* **233**:H346, 1977.
216. Cohen I, Glaser T, Veis A, Bruner-Lorand J: Ca^{2+}-dependent crosslinking processes in human platelets. *Biochem Biophys Acta* **676**:137, 1981.
217. Cohen I, Young-Bandala L, Blankenberg TA, Siefring GE Jr, Bruner-Lorand J: Fibrinoligase-catalyzed crosslinking of myosin from platelet and skeletal muscle. *Arch Biochem Biophys* **192**:100, 1979.
218. Okamoto M, Yamamoto T, Matsubara S, et al: Factor XIII-dependent generation of 5th complement component (C5)-derived monocyte chemotactic factor coinciding with plasma clotting. *Biochem Biophys Acta* **1138**:53, 1992.
219. Nishiura H, Shibuya Y, Matsubara S, Tanase S, Kambara T, Yamamoto T: Monocyte chemotactic factor in rheumatoid arthritis synovial tissue:

Probably a crosslinked derivative of S19 ribosomal protein. *J Biol Chem* **271**:878, 1996.
220. Yamada T, Yoshiyama Y, Kawaguchi N, et al: Possible roles of transglutaminases in Alzheimer's disease. *Dement Geriatr Cogn Dis* **9**:103, 1998.
221. Miller ML, Johnson GV: Transglutaminase crosslinking of the tau protein. *J Neurochem* **65**:1760, 1995.
222. Hada M, Kaminski M, Bockenstedt P, McDonagh J: Covalent crosslinking of von Willebrand factor to fibrin. *Blood* **68**:95, 1986.
223. Bockenstedt P, McDonagh J, Handin RI: Binding and covalent crosslinking of purified von Willebrand factor to native monomeric collagen. *J Clin Invest* **78**:551, 1986.
224. Bale MD, Mosher DF: Thrombospondin is a substrate for blood coagulation factor XIIIa. *Biochemistry* **25**:5667, 1986.
225. Francis RT, McDonagh J, Mann KG: Factor V is a substrate for the transamidase factor XIIIa. *J Biol Chem* **261**:9787, 1986.
226. Borth W, Chang V, Bishop P, Harpel PC: Lipoprotein (a) is a substrate for factor XIIIa and tissue transglutaminase. *J Biol Chem* **266**:18149, 1991.
227. Yorifuji H, Anderson K, Lynch GW, Van de Water L, McDonagh J: B protein of factor XIII: Differentiation between free B and complexed B. *Blood* **72**:1645, 1988.
228. Cooke RD, Holbrook JJ: The calcium-induced dissociation of human plasma clotting factor XIII. *Biochem J* **141**:79, 1974.
229. Bannerjee D, Mosesson MW: Characteristics of platelet protransglutaminase (factor XIII)-binding activity in human plasma. *Thromb Res* **7**:323, 1975.
230. Lee SY, Chung SI: Biosynthesis and degradation of plasma protransglutaminase (factor XIII). *Fed Proc* **35**:1486, 1976.
231. Ikematsu S: An approach to the metabolism of factor XIII. *Acta Haematol Jpn* **44**:1499, 1981.
232. Nagy JA, Henriksson P, McDonagh J: Biosynthesis of factor XIII B subunit by human hepatoma cell lines. *Blood* **68**:1272, 1986.
233. Ichinose A, Kaetsu H: Molecular approach to structure-function relationship of human coagulation factor XIII. *Methods Enzymol* **222**:36, 1993.
234. Weisberg LJ, Shiu DT, Greenberg CS, Kan YW, Shuman MA: Localization of the gene for coagulation factor XIII a-chain to chromosome 6 and identification of sites of synthesis. *J Clin Invest* **79**:649, 1987.
235. Weisberg LJ, Shiu DT, Conkling PR, Shuman MA: Identification of normal human peripheral blood monocytes and liver as sites of synthesis of coagulation factor XIII a-chain. *Blood* **70**:579, 1987.
236. Fear JD, Jackson P, Gray C, Miloszewski KJ, Losowsky MS: Localisation of factor XIII in human tissues using an immunoperoxidase technique. *J Clin Pathol* **37**:560, 1984.
237. Chung SI: Comparative studies on tissue transglutaminase and factor XIII. *Ann NY Acad Sci* **202**:240, 1972.
238. Kiesselbach TH, Wagner RH: Demonstration of factor XIII in human megakaryocytes by a fluorescent antibody technique. *Ann NY Acad Sci* **202**:318, 1972.
239. Henriksson P, Becker S, Lynch G, McDonagh J: Identification of intracellular factor XIII in human monocytes and macrophages. *J Clin Invest* **76**:528, 1985.
240. Muszbek L, Adany R, Szegedi G, Polgar J, Kavai M: Factor XIII of blood coagulation in human monocytes. *Thromb Res* **37**:401, 1985.
241. Sixma JJ, Van den Berg A, Schiphorst M, Geuze HJ, McDonagh J: Immunocytochemical localization of albumin and factor XIII in thin cryosections of human blood platelets. *Thromb Haemost* **51**:388, 1984.
242. McDonagh J, McDonagh RP Jr, Delage JM, Wagner RH: Factor XIII in human plasma and platelets. *J Clin Invest* **48**:940, 1969.
243. Lopaciuk S, Lovette KM, McDonagh J, Chuang HY, McDonagh J: Subcellular distribution of fibrinogen and factor XIII in human blood platelets. *Thromb Res* **8**:453, 1976.
244. Fesus L, Thomazy V, Autuori F, Ceru MP, Tarcsa E, Piacentini M: Apoptotic hepatocytes become insoluble in detergents and chaotropic agents as a result of transglutaminase action. *FEBS Lett* **245**:150, 1989.
245. Knight CR, Rees RC, Griffin M: Apoptosis: A potential role for cytosolic transglutaminase and its importance in tumour progression. *Biochem Biophys Acta* **1096**:312, 1991.
246. Baden HP: Common transglutaminase substrates shared by hair, epidermis and nail and their function. *J Dermatol Sci* **7**:S20, 1994.
247. Cerio R, Spaull J, Jones EW: Histiocytoma cutis: A tumour of dermal dendrocytes (dermal dendrocytoma). *Br J Dermatol* **120**:197, 1989.
248. Wolpl A, Lattke H, Board PG, et al: Coagulation factor XIII A and B subunits in bone marrow and liver transplantation. *Transplantation* **43**:151, 1987.
249. Poon MC, Russell JA, Low S, et al: Hemopoietic origin of factor XIII A subunits in platelets, monocytes, and plasma: Evidence from bone marrow transplantation studies. *J Clin Invest* **84**:787, 1989.
250. Ichinose A, Davie EW: Characterization of the gene for the a subunit of human factor XIII (plasma transglutaminase), a blood coagulation factor. *Proc Natl Acad Sci USA* **85**:5829, 1988.
251. Auron PE, Webb AC, Rosenwasser LJ, et al: Nucleotide sequence of human monocyte interleukin 1 precursor cDNA. *Proc Natl Acad Sci USA* **81**:7907, 1984.
252. Wallner BP, Mattaliano RJ, Hession C, et al: Cloning and expression of human lipocortin, a phospholipase A2 inhibitor with potential anti-inflammatory activity. *Nature* **320**:77, 1986.
253. Jaye M, Howk R, Burgess W, et al: Human endothelial cell growth factor: Cloning, nucleotide sequence, and chromosome localization. *Science* **233**:541, 1986.
254. Kurokawa T, Sasada R, Iwane M, Igarashi K: Cloning and expression of cDNA encoding human basic fibroblast growth factor. *FEBS Lett* **213**:189, 1987.
255. Ye RD, Wun TC, Sadler JE: cDNA cloning and expression in *Escherichia coli* of a plasminogen activator inhibitor from human placenta. *J Biol Chem* **262**:3718, 1987.
256. Hogquist KA, Nett MA, Unanue ER, Chaplin DD: Interleukin 1 is processed and released during apoptosis. *Proc Natl Acad Sci USA* **88**:8485, 1991.
257. Rubartelli A, Cozzolino F, Talio M, Sitia R: A novel secretory pathway for interleukin-1 beta, a protein lacking a signal sequence. *EMBO J* **9**:1503, 1990.
258. Bottenus RE, Ichinose A, Davie EW: Nucleotide sequence of the gene for the b subunit of human factor XIII. *Biochemistry* **29**:11195, 1990.
259. Barbui T, Cartei G, Chisesi T, Dini E: Electroimmunoassay of plasma subunits-a and -s in a case of congenital fibrin stabilizing factor deficiency. *Thromb Diathes Haemorrh* **32**:124, 1974.
260. Barbui T, Rodeghiero F, Dini E, et al: Subunits A and S inheritance in four families with congenital factor XIII deficiency. *Br J Haematol* **38**:267, 1978.
261. Rodeghiero F, Morbin M, Barbui T: Subunit A of factor XIII regulates subunit B plasma concentration. *Thromb Haemost* **46**:621, 1981.
262. Saito M, Asakura H, Yoshida T, et al: A familial factor XIII subunit B deficiency (see comments). *Br J Haematol* **74**:290, 1990.
263. Hashiguchi T, Saito M, Morishita E, Matsuda T, Ichinose A: Two genetic defects in a patient with complete deficiency of the b-subunit for coagulation factor XIII. *Blood* **82**:145, 1993.
264. Fear JD, Miloszewski KJ, Losowsky MS: The half life of factor XIII in the management of inherited deficiency. *Thromb Haemost* **49**:102, 1983.
265. Rodeghiero F, Tosetto A, Di Bona E, Castaman G: Clinical pharmacokinetics of a placenta-derived factor XIII concentrate in type I and type II factor XIII deficiency. *Am J Hematol* **36**:30, 1991.
266. Folk JE, Chung SI: Blood coagulation factor XIII: Relationship of some biological properties to subunit structure, in Reich E, et al (eds): *Proteases and Biological Control,* vol 2. Cold Spring Harbor, NY, Cold Spring Harbor Laboratory, 1975, pp 157–170.
267. Janus TJ, Lewis SD, Lorand L, Shafer JA: Promotion of thrombin-catalyzed activation of factor XIII by fibrinogen. *Biochemistry* **22**:6269, 1983.
268. Lewis SD, Janus TJ, Lorand L, Shafer JA: Regulation of formation of factor XIIIa by its fibrin substrates. *Biochemistry* **24**:6772, 1985.
269. Naski MC, Lorand L, Shafer JA: Characterization of the kinetic pathway for fibrin promotion of alpha-thrombin-catalyzed activation of plasma factor XIII. *Biochemistry* **30**:934, 1991.
270. Hornyak TJ, Shafer JA: Role of calcium ion in the generation of factor XIII activity. *Biochemistry* **30**:6175, 1991.
271. Curtis CG, Brown KL, Credo RB, et al: Calcium-dependent unmasking of active center cysteine during activation of fibrin stabilizing factor. *Biochemistry* **13**:3774, 1974.
272. Credo RB, Curtis CG, Lorand L: Alpha-chain domain of fibrinogen controls generation of fibrinoligase (coagulation factor XIIIa): Calcium ion regulatory aspects. *Biochemistry* **20**:3770, 1981.
273. McDonagh J, McDonagh RP: Alternative pathways for the activation of factor XIII. *Br J Haematol* **30**:465, 1975.
274. Henriksson P, Nilsson IM, Ohlsson K, Stenberg P: Granulocyte elastase activation and degradation of factor XIII. *Thromb Res* **18**:343, 1980.
275. Lynch GW, Pfueller SL: Thrombin-independent activation of platelet factor XIII by endogenous platelet acid protease. *Thromb Haemost* **59**:372, 1988.

276. Credo RB, Curtis CG, Lorand L: Ca^{2+}-related regulatory function of fibrinogen. *Proc Natl Acad Sci USA* **75**:4234, 1978.
277. Shrode J, Chung SI, Folk JE: Thrombin cleavage products of human placental transglutaminase. *Fed Proc* **35**:1487, 1976.
278. Hornyak TJ, Bishop PD, Shafer JA: Alpha-thrombin-catalyzed activation of human platelet factor XIII: relationship between proteolysis and factor XIIIa activity. *Biochemistry* **28**:7326, 1989.
279. Lai TS, Achyuthan KE, Santiago MA, Greenberg GS: Carboxy-terminal truncation of recombinant factor XIII A-chains: Characterization of minimum structural requirement for transglutaminase activity. *J Biol Chem* **269**:24596, 1994.
280. Takahashi N, Tsukamoto H, Umeyama H, Castaman G, Rodeghiero F, Ichinose A: Molecular mechanisms of type II factor XIII deficiency: Novel Gly562-Arg mutation and C-terminal truncation of the A subunit cause factor XIII deficiency as characterized in a mammalian expression system. *Blood* **91**:2830, 1998.
281. Chung D, Ichinose A: Hereditary disorders related to fibrinogen and factor XIII, in Scriver CR, Beaudet AL, Sly WS, Valle D (eds): *The Metabolic Basis of Inherited Disease,* vol 2, 6th ed. New York, McGraw-Hill, 1989, p 2135.
282. Board PG, Webb GC, McKee J, Ichinose A: Localization of the coagulation factor XIII A subunit gene (F13A) to chromosome bands 6p24-p25. *Cytogenet Cell Genet* **48**:25, 1988.
283. Polakowska RR, Eddy RL, Shows TB, Goldsmith LA: Epidermal type I transglutaminase (TGM1) is assigned to human chromosome 14. *Cytogenet Cell Genet* **56**:105, 1991.
284. Kim IG, Mcbride OW, Wang M, Kim SY, Idler WW, Steinert PM: Structure and organization of the human transglutaminase 1 gene. *J Biol Chem* **267**:7710, 1992.
285. Yamanishi K, Inazawa J, Liew FM, et al: Structure of the gene for human transglutaminase 1. *J Biol Chem* **267**:17858, 1992.
286. Gentile V, Grant FJ, Porta R, Baldini A: Localization of the human prostate transglutaminase (type IV) gene (TGM4) to chromosome 3p21.33-p22 by fluorescence in situ hybridization. *Genomics* **27**:219, 1995.
287. Webb GC, Coggan M, Ichinose A, Board PG: Localization of the coagulation factor XIII B subunit gene (F13B) to chromosome bands 1q31-32.1 and restriction fragment length polymorphism at the locus. *Hum Genet* **81**:157, 1989.
288. Rodriguez de Cordoba S, Rey-Campos J, Dykes DD, McAlpine PJ, Wong P, Rubinstein P: Coagulation factor XIII B subunit is encoded by a gene linked to the regulator of complement activation (*RCA*) gene cluster in man. *Immunogenetics* **28**:452, 1988.
289. Pardo-Manuel F, Rey-Campos J, Hillarp A, Dahlback B, Rodriguez de Cordoba S: Human genes for the alpha and beta chains of complement C4b-binding protein are closely linked in a head-to-tail arrangement. *Proc Natl Acad Sci USA* **87**:4529, 1990.
290. Fraij BM, Gonzales RA: Organization and structure of the human tissue transglutaminase gene. *Biochem Biophys Acta* **1354**:65, 1997.
291. Kim IG, Lee SC, Lee JH, Yang JM, Chung SI, Steinert PM: Structure and organization of the human transglutaminase 3 gene: Evolutionary relationship to the transglutaminase family. *J Invest Dermatol* **103**:137, 1994.
292. Korsgren C, Cohen CM: Organization of the gene for human erythrocyte membrane protein 4.2: Structural similarities with the gene for the a subunit of factor XIII. *Proc Natl Acad Sci USA* **88**:4840, 1991.
293. Kida M, Souri M, Izumi T, Ichinose A: Gene regulation of cell type-specific expression of the A subunit for factor XIII. *Blood* **90**:31a, 1998.
294. Lee JH, Jang SI, Yang JM, Markova NG, Steinert PM: The proximal promoter of the human transglutaminase 3 gene: Stratified squamous epithelial-specific expression in cultured cells is mediated by binding of Sp1 and its transcription factors to a proximal promoter element. *J Biol Chem* **271**:4561, 1996.
295. Mariniello L, Qin Q, Jessen BA, Rice RH: Keratinocyte transglutaminase promoter analysis. Identification of a functional response element. *J Biol Chem* **270**:31358, 1995.
296. Lu S, Saydak M, Gentile V, Stein JP, Davies PJ: Isolation and characterization of the human tissue transglutaminase gene promoter. *J Biol Chem* **270**:9748, 1995.
297. Yamada K, Matsuki M, Morishima Y, et al: Activation of the human transglutaminase 1 promoter in transgenic mice: Terminal differentiation-specific expression of the *TGM*1-*lacZ* transgene in keratinized stratified squamous epithelia. *Hum Mol Genet* **6**:2223, 1997.
298. Nickoloff BJ, Griffiths CE: Factor XIIIa-expressing dermal dendrocytes in AIDS-associated cutaneous Kaposi's sarcomas. *Science* **243**:1736, 1989.
299. Naidu YM, Rosen EM, Zitnick R, et al: Role of scatter factor in the pathogenesis of AIDS-related Kaposi sarcoma. *Proc Natl Acad Sci USA* **91**:5281, 1994.
300. Board PG: Genetic polymorphism of the A subunit of human coagulation factor XIII. *Am J Hum Genet* **31**:116, 1979.
301. Castle SL, Board PG: An extended survey of the genetic polymorphism at the human coagulation factor XIII: A subunit structural locus. *Hum Hered* **35**:101, 1985.
302. Suzuki K, Henke J, Iwata M, et al: Novel polymorphisms and haplotypes in the human coagulation factor XIII A-subunit gene. *Hum Genet* **98**:393, 1996.
303. Ichinose A, Izumi T, Hashiguchi T: The normal and abnormal genes of the a and b subunits in coagulation factor XIII. *Semin Thromb Hemost* **22**:385, 1996.
304. Kohler HP, Stickland MH, Ossei-Gerning N, Carter A, Mikkola H, Grant PJ: Association of a common polymorphism in the factor XIII gene with myocardial infarction. *Thromb Haemost* **79**:8, 1998.
305. Zoghbi HY, Daiger SP, McCall A, O'Brien WE, Beaudet AL: Extensive DNA polymorphism at the factor XIIIa (F13A) locus and linkage to HLA. *Am J Hum Genet* **42**:877, 1988.
306. Board PG, Chapple R, Coggan M: Haplotypes of the coagulation factor XIII A subunit locus in normal and deficient subjects. *Am J Hum Genet* **42**:712, 1988.
307. Polymeropoulos MH, Rath DS, Xiao H, Merril CR: Tetranucleotide repeat polymorphism at the human coagulation factor XIII A subunit gene (F13A1). *Nucl Acids Res* **19**:4306, 1991.
308. Puers C, Hammond HA, Caskey CT, et al: Allelic ladder characterization of the short tandem repeat polymorphism located in the 5′ flanking region to the human coagulation factor XIII A subunit gene. *Genomics* **23**:260, 1994.
309. Board PG: Genetic polymorphism of the B subunit of human coagulation factor XIII. *Am J Hum Genet* **32**:348, 1980.
310. Izumi T, Hashiguchi T, Castaman G, et al: Type I factor XIII deficiency is caused by a genetic defect of its b subunit: Insertion of triplet AAC in exon III leads to premature termination in the second Sushi domain. *Blood* **87**:2769, 1996.
311. Souri M, Izumi T, Higashi Y, Girolami A, Ichinose A: A founder effect is proposed for factor XIII B subunit deficiency caused by the insertion of triplet AAC in exon III encoding the second sushi domain. *Thromb Haemost* **80**:211, 1998.
312. Nishimura DY, Murray JC: A tetranucleotide repeat for the F13B locus. *Nucl Acids Res* **20**:1167, 1992.
313. Aoki N, Saito H, Kamiya T, Koie K, Sakata Y, Kobakura M: Congenital deficiency of alpha 2-plasmin inhibitor associated with severe hemorrhagic tendency. *J Clin Invest* **63**:877, 1979.
314. Evron S, Anteby SO, Brzezinsky A, Samueloff A, Eldor A: Congenital afibrinogenemia and recurrent early abortion: a case report. *Eur J Obstet Gynecol Reprod Biol* **19**:307, 1985.
315. Hahn L, Lundberg PA: Congenital hypofibrinogenaemia and recurrent abortion: Case report. *Br J Obstet Gynaecol* **85**:790, 1978.
316. McDonagh J, Carrell N: Dysfibrinogenemia and other disorders of fibrinogen structure and function, in Colman RW, Hirsh J, Marder VJ, Salzman EW (eds): *Hemostasis and Thrombosis: Basic Principles and Clinical Practice,* 3d ed. Philadelphia, Lippincott, 1994, p 314.
317. Girolami A, Burul A, Fabris F, Cappellato G, Betterle C: Studies on factor XIII antigen in congenital factor XIII deficiency: A tentative classification of the disease in two groups. *F Haematol Int Mag Klin Morphol Blut* **105**:131, 1978.
318. Anwar R, Stewart AD, Miloszewski KJ, Losowsky MS, Markham AF: Molecular basis of inherited factor XIII deficiency: identification of multiple mutations provides insights into protein function. *Br J Haematol* **91**:728, 1995.
319. Mikkola H, Syrjala M, Rasi V, et al: Deficiency in the A-subunit of coagulation factor XIII: Two novel point mutations demonstrate different effects on transcript levels. *Blood* **84**:517, 1994.
320. Coggan M, Baker R, Miloszewski K, Woodfield G, Board P: Mutations causing coagulation factor XIII subunit A deficiency: Characterization of the mutant proteins after expression in yeast. *Blood* **85**:2455, 1995.
321. Mikkola H, Yee VC, Syrjala M, et al: Four novel mutations in deficiency of coagulation factor XIII: Consequences to expression and structure of the A-subunit. *Blood* **87**:141, 1996.
322. Inbal A, Yee VC, Kornbrot N, Zivelin A, Brenner B, Seligsohn U: Factor XIII deficiency due to a Leu660Pro mutation in the factor XIII subunit-a gene in three unrelated Palestinian Arab families. *Thromb Haemost* **77**:1062, 1997.
323. Mikkola H, Muszbek L, Haramura G, Hamalainen E, Jalanko A, Palotie A: Molecular mechanisms of mutations in factor XIII A-subunit

deficiency: In vitro expression in COS-cells demonstrates intracellular degradation of the mutant proteins. *Thromb Haemost* **77**:1068, 1997.

324. Aslam S, Poon MC, Yee VC, Bowen DJ, Standen GR: Factor $XIIIA_{CALGARY}$: A candidate missense mutation (Leu667Pro) in the beta barrel 2 domain of the factor XIIIA subunit. *Br J Haematol* **91**:452, 1995.
325. Aslam S, Yee VC, Narayanan S, Duraisamy G, Standen GR: Structural analysis of a missense mutation (Val414Phe) in the catalytic core domain of the factor XIII(A) subunit. *Br J Haematol* **98**:346, 1997.
326. Standen GR, Bowen DJ: Factor $XIIIA_{BRISTOL\ 1}$: Detection of a nonsense mutation (Arg171 → stop codon) in factor XIII A subunit deficiency. *Br J Haematol* **85**:769, 1993.
327. Kamura T, Okamura T, Murakawa M, et al: Deficiency of coagulation factor XIII A subunit caused by the dinucleotide deletion at the 5′ end of exon III. *J Clin Invest* **90**:315, 1992.
328. Aslam S, Bowen DJ, Mandalaki T, Gialeraki R, Standen GR: Factor XIII(A) subunit deficiency due to a homozygous 13-base pair deletion in exon 3 of the A subunit gene. *Am J Hematol* **53**:77, 1996.
329. Kangsadalampai S, Farges-Berth A, Caglayan SH, Board PG: New mutations causing the premature termination of translation in the A subunit gene of coagulation factor XIII. *Thromb Haemost* **76**:139, 1996.
330. Mikkola H, Muszbek L, Laiho E, et al: Molecular mechanism of a mild phenotype in coagulation factor XIII (FXIII) deficiency: A splicing mutation permitting partial correct splicing of FXIII A-subunit mRNA. *Blood* **89**:1279, 1997.
331. Board P, Coggan M, Miloszewski K: Identification of a point mutation in factor XIII A subunit deficiency. *Blood* **80**:937, 1992.
332. Vreken P, Niessen RW, Peters M, Schaap MC, Zuithoff-Rijntjes JG, Sturk A: A point mutation in an invariant splice acceptor site results in a decreased mRNA level in a patient with severe coagulation factor XIII subunit A deficiency. *Thromb Haemost* **74**:584, 1995.
333. Anwar R, Miloszewski KJ, Markham AF: Identification of a large deletion, spanning exons 4 to 11 of the human factor XIIIA gene, in a factor XIII-deficient family. *Blood* **91**:149, 1998.
334. Ichinose A, Tsukamoto H, Izumi T, et al: Arg260-Cys mutation in severe factor XIII deficiency: Conformational change of the A subunit is predicted by molecular modeling and mechanics. *Br J Haematol* **101**:264, 1998.
335. Izumi T, Nagaoka U, Saito T, Takamatsu J, Saito H, Ichinose A: Novel deletion and insertion mutations cause splicing defects, leading to severe reduction in mRNA levels of the A subunit in severe factor XIII deficiency. *Thromb Haemost* **79**:479, 1998.
336. Hashiguchi T, Ichinose A: Molecular and cellular basis of deficiency of the b subunit for factor XIII secondary to a Cys430-Phe mutation in the seventh Sushi domain. *J Clin Invest* **95**:1002, 1995.
337. Capellato MG, Lazzaro AR, Marafioti F, Polato G, Girolami A: A new family with congenital factor XIII deficiency showing a deficit of both subunit A and B: Type I factor XIII deficiency. *Haematologia* **20**:179, 1987.
338. Lorand L, Campbell-Wilkes LK, Cooperstein L: A filter paper assay for transamidating enzymes using radioactive amine substrates. *Anal Biochem* **50**:623, 1972.
339. Nishida Y, Ikematsu S, Fukutake K, Fujimaki M, Fukutake K, Kakishita E: A new rapid and simple assay for factor XIII activity using dansylcadaverine incorporation and gel filtration. *Thromb Res* **36**:123, 1984.
340. Trobisch H, Egbring R: Substitution treatment of factor XIII deficiency with a new factor XIII concentrate. *Dtsch Med Wochenschr* **97**:499, 1972.
341. Kuratsuji T, Oikawa T, Fukumoto T, et al: Factor XIII deficiency in antibiotic-associated pseudomembranous colitis and its treatment with factor XIII concentrate. *Thromb Haemost* **11**:229, 1982.

CHAPTER 172

Hemophilia A: Deficiency of Coagulation Factor VIII

Haig H. Kazazian, Jr. ▪ Edward G. D. Tuddenham
Stylianos E. Antonarakis

1. Hemophilia A (MIM 206700; classic hemophilia) is an X-linked bleeding disorder characterized by a deficiency in the activity of factor VIII, a key component of the coagulation cascade. Approximately 1 in 5000 to 10,000 males are affected in all populations.

2. Affected individuals suffer joint and muscle hemorrhage, easy bruising, and prolonged bleeding from wounds. Because platelet function is not affected, blood loss from minor cuts and abrasions is not excessive. Of hemophilia A patients, 50 to 60 percent have severe hemophilia with factor VIII activity <1 percent, while the remainder have mild to moderate disease with factor VIII levels of 1 to 20 percent. Nearly all patients with severe disease have no factor VIII protein in their plasma (cross-reacting material negative or [CRM−]), but a small proportion of these patients (about 5 percent) have inactive factor VIII protein circulating in their plasma (CRM+).

3. Factor VIII functions as a cofactor in the activation of factor X to factor Xa in a reaction catalyzed by factor IXa on a phospholipid surface. Factor VIII is activated following specific proteolytic cleavages by thrombin and factor Xa, which results in an effective amplification of the signal through this step of the cascade. Factor VIII is inactivated by limited proteolysis by factor Xa or by activated protein C (APC).

4. Hemophilia A arises from a variety of mutations within the factor VIII gene, which is located near the telomere of the long arm of the X chromosome. The gene comprises 26 exons and spans 186 kb. The cDNA sequence reveals that factor VIII is synthesized as a large precursor molecule (2332 amino acids). The amino acid sequence of the protein has considerable sequence similarity to that of ceruloplasmin and coagulation factor V.

5. Approximately 43 percent of patients with severe disease and approximately 25 percent of all patients have an inversion at the tip of the X chromosome that disrupts the factor VIII gene. This mutation almost always has its origin in male meiosis. Of the remaining 75 percent of patients, approximately 95 percent have one of a large variety of point mutations. Although the functional consequences of some of the 400-odd point mutations producing the disease are known (for example, some alter a thrombin cleavage site, a factor IX binding site, or a von Willebrand factor binding site), the structure-function relationships of most mutations remain unknown.

6. Combined deficiency of factors V and VIII is an uncommon autosomal recessive disease with factor levels in the 5 to 30 percent range and symptoms similar to mild factor VIII deficiency. Recently, mutations in the ERGIC-53 gene were shown to cause this combined deficiency. The ERGIC-53 gene encodes a protein that likely transports proteins from the endoplasmic reticulum to the Golgi compartment. Deficiency of this protein in combined factor V and factor VIII deficiency suggests that it may act uniquely to facilitate the intracellular transport and secretion of these two coagulation factors.

7. Treatment of hemophilia A is accomplished by infusions of factor VIII, usually prepared by recombinant DNA technology, or sometimes prepared as concentrates from human plasma. The *in vivo* half-life of such preparations is approximately 12 h. Although such therapy is effective in most cases, approximately 15 percent of affected individuals eventually develop neutralizing antibodies (inhibitors) that complicate further therapy.

8. Gene therapy for hemophilia A is likely in the future. Animal model systems (affected dogs and mice) are greatly aiding experimentation in this rapidly advancing field. As of early 2000, there is substantial hope that clinical trials with an effective vector will be successful in the next few years.

HISTORICAL PERSPECTIVE

Sex-linked hemophilia, of which factor VIII deficiency is the leading cause, was first recognized by Rabbi Simon ben Gamaliel in the second century AD. He gave dispensation from circumcision to an infant whose three maternal cousins had died after the operation (Babylonian Talmud).[1,2] The first reference to a male-specific bleeding disorder in the medical literature appeared eight centuries later. Khalif ibn Abbas, a great surgical writer of the Moorish period in Spain, described a village in which men, when wounded, suffered uncontrollable, lethal hemorrhage.[3] The first modern report of hemophilia was by John Otto (reference 4, reprinted in reference 5). He particularly noted the familial pattern of transmission of severe bleeding after trivial injury.

In 1813, another North American family of bleeders — the Appleton-Swain kindred — was reported.[6] Oliver Appleton, its founder, an English immigrant, was himself a bleeder; Appleton had three daughters (Fig. 172-1). Both daughters who married had "bleeder" sons who themselves had daughters who bore bleeder sons — the great-great-grandsons of Oliver Appleton. This family was later studied by Osler.[7]

The first recorded usage of the term hemophilia was by Hopff in 1828.[8] His cases were four brothers who bled to death either

A list of standard abbreviations is located immediately preceding the index in each volume. Additional abbreviations used in this chapter include: AHG = antihemophilic globulin; APC = activated protein C; DDAVP = 1-desamino-8-D-arginine vasopressin; FVIII = factor VIII; vWF = von Willebrand factor.

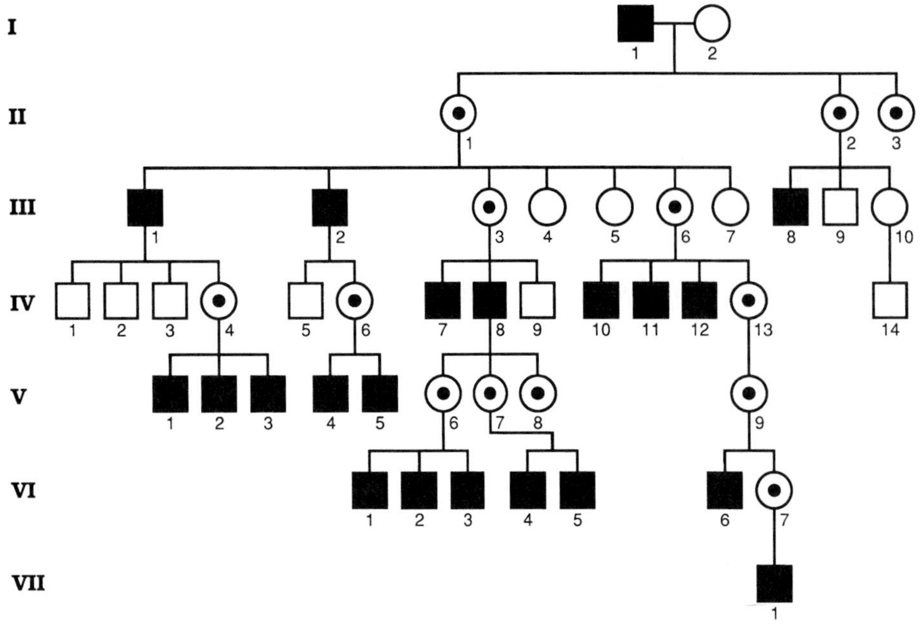

Fig. 172-1 The Appleton-Swain kindred, the first kindred and which was published in 1813, shows all the characteristics of a sex-linked bleeding disorder.[6] Solid squares = bleeder males; open squares = normal males; circles with dot = obligatory carrier females.

from a trivial injury or, in one case, from a ruptured hemophilic pseudotumor of the thigh.

In a monumental compilation in 1911, Bulloch and Fildes critically reviewed almost 1000 publications on hemophilia and related conditions, extracting from them 224 pedigrees.[1] Almost all of the clinical features of untreated hemophilia recognized today were described in this publication. A satisfactory theory of the genetics of sex-linked disorders had just become available. Bateson's 1909 book, *Mendel's Principles of Heredity,* contains an account of sex-linked recessive color blindness.[9] He made the correct interpretation that female carriers are heterozygous, and therefore are unaffected. Bateson realized the importance of the normality of affected men's sons and the carrier status of their daughters, and rightly concluded that this implied dimorphism of spermatozoa (X or Y). It was soon realized that hemophilia, as classically defined, fit perfectly the prediction of an X-linked recessive disorder. The occurrence of homozygous affected females was also predicted and correctly explained by Bateson.[9]

The most famous hemophilic kindred is that descended from Queen Victoria (Fig. 172-2). None of Victoria's ancestors suffered from a bleeding tendency, but she was clearly a carrier of X-linked hemophilia because one of her sons (Leopold) was affected and two of her daughters (Alice and Beatrice) were carriers, transmitting the disease to their descendants.[10] Through dynastic marriage and intermarriage, the gene was passed to three other royal families in Europe, with particularly tragic consequences for the Russian royal family. Among the affected males in this kindred, only Leopold lived to have children, and he died at the age of 31. All the other hemophilic males had died of bleeding without issue by 1945, demonstrating the short life expectancy and low reproductive fitness of hemophiliacs before replacement therapy. Because their death predated the discovery that X-linked hemophilia can be due to either factor VIII or factor IX deficiency, we do not know to which type the royal hemophilia belonged. A plausible origin for the royal hemophilia gene is the gamete supplied by Victoria's father, Edward, Duke of Kent, who was 54 at the time of Victoria's birth.

Research into the defect in the blood of hemophiliacs began in the late nineteenth century. Wright[11] showed that whereas normal blood clotted in a capillary tube in 6 min, blood from a boy with severe hemophilia took over 10 min to clot. Addis[12,13] showed that the prolonged clotting time of hemophilic blood could be corrected by a fraction from normal blood. He also demonstrated a delay in the conversion of prothrombin to thrombin and concluded that this was sufficient to completely explain the hemostatic failure. The fraction of plasma that Addis used to study prothrombin content was a euglobulin fraction that contains both prothrombin and factor VIII among many other proteins. Therefore, Addis concluded that hemophilia is due to prothrombin deficiency, an inescapable conclusion in terms of the theory of blood coagulation proposed by Morawitz,[14] which prevailed then and for 30 years thereafter. Based on this theory, the coagulation defect of hemophilia could only be due to a deficiency of prothrombin, calcium, thrombokinase, or fibrinogen. The last option was excluded by the finding that hemophilic blood could form a firm clot if "thrombokinase" or tissue extract was added to it.[11] Although Addis' experiment pointed to a prothrombin defect, Govaerts and Gratia[15] demonstrated that the correcting fraction in normal plasma was not absorbed by tricalcium phosphate and therefore could not be prothrombin. Subsequently, Quick,[16] using his newly devised prothrombin time, showed that prothrombin was normal in hemophilic blood. Addis had shown that hemophilic blood clotted more slowly than normal in response to diluted tissue extract, but the explanation for this correct observation has only recently come to light.[17]

Morawitz and Lossen had studied the blood of a hemophilic boy in 1908 and concluded that there was a deficiency of thrombokinase production by the corpuscles.[18] Sahli drew the similar conclusion that the tissues were deficient in thrombokinase.[19] Neither hypothesis was supported by later experiments. Thus, an intellectual impasse was reached that could only be surmounted by a new attack on theory. This came in 1937, when Patek and Taylor reexamined a plasma fraction similar to Addis' and confirmed that it would correct the prolonged clotting time of hemophilic blood.[20] They called this fraction "globulin" and, later, "antihemophilic globulin" (AHG).[21]

A further advance came when quantitative assays were devised for measuring the correcting fraction.[22,23] Hemophilia became defined as the condition that results from AHG deficiency and that is inherited in an X-linked recessive fashion, with sporadic cases due to new mutation. In 1952, three groups[24–26] simultaneously reported that one hemophiliac's blood could cross-correct that of other clinically identical cases, and that hemophilia, therefore, could be caused by deficiency of more than one factor. The new

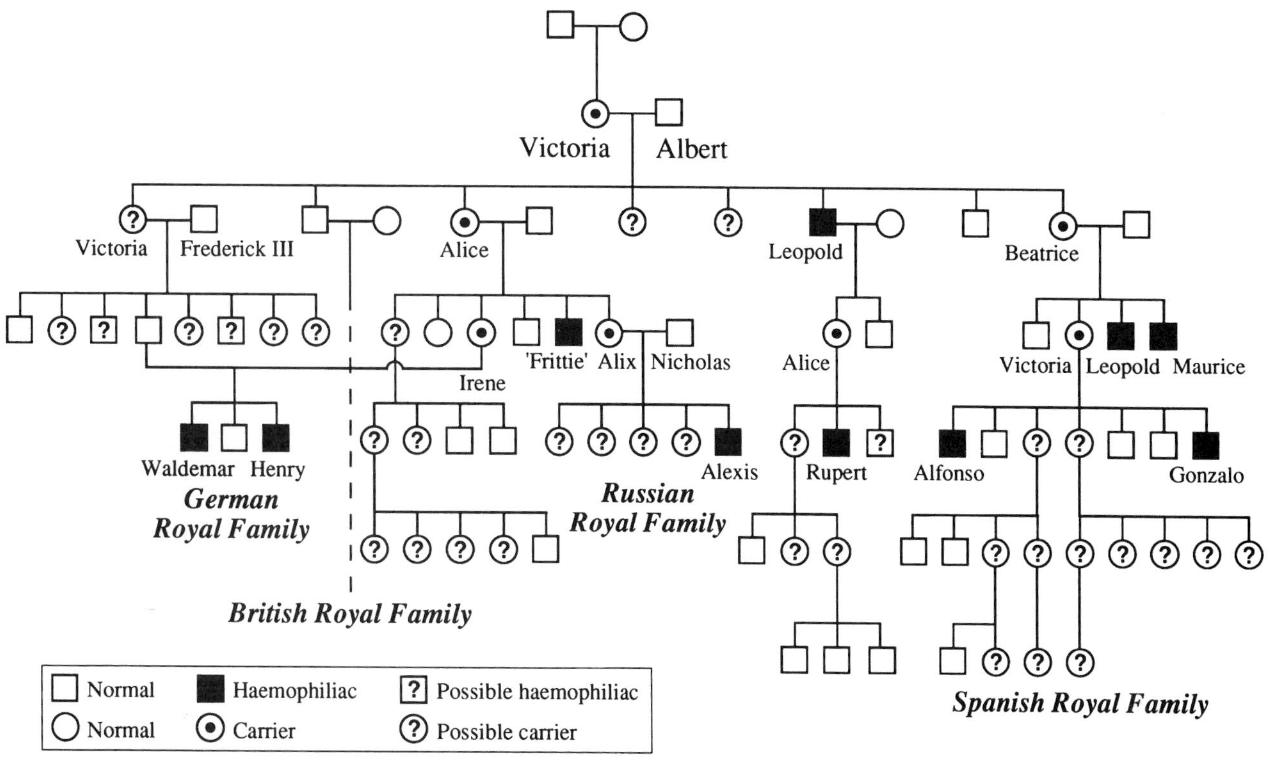

Fig. 172-2 The royal hemophilia pedigree of Queen Victoria's descendants, emphasizing the lines affected by bleeding. The present British royal family is unaffected, being descended through a normal male. The defective gene almost certainly died out with Leopold's daughter Alice in 1980.

factor was factor IX, and its deficiency is responsible for about one-sixth of the cases of X-linked hemophilia. By international convention, AHG was assigned the Roman number VIII.[27] The two disorders are now called hemophilia A and B (factor VIII and factor IX deficiency, respectively). Attempts to purify factor VIII began in the 1950s as soon as an assay became available. In retrospect, the early work failed because (a) factor VIII copurifies with its carrier protein, von Willebrand factor (vWF), and (b) factor VIII is unstable and is present in a very low concentration in blood. In 1972, Owen and Wagner used gel filtration[28] to establish that 0.25 M $CaCl_2$ was highly effective at lowering the molecular weight of factor VIII.

In 1971, Zimmerman and colleagues showed that the concentration of an antigen detected by antisera raised in rabbits against partially purified factor VIII was reduced in the blood of patients with von Willebrand disease[29] (see Chap. 174), but present in normal quantities in the blood of hemophilia A patients. This antigen was first called factor VIII-related antigen (VIIIR:Ag), but is now designated von Willebrand antigen (vW:Ag).

In 1973, Zimmerman and Edgington used immobilized antibodies to obtain differential absorption of VIII:C and vWF.[30] They concluded that "Factor VIII coagulant activity resides on a molecule distinct from that expressing the von Willebrand's antigen."

In 1979, factor VIII was separated from vWF by immunoaffinity purification.[31] In 1982, Fass and colleagues succeeded in isolating porcine factor VIII using a monoclonal antibody.[32] These techniques were used by several groups to isolate sufficient factor VIII for partial sequence determination, and the availability of a partial protein sequence made possible the cloning of factor VIII cDNA and its gene.[33–35] This chapter describes the clinical features of hemophilia A; the structure and physiology of factor VIII in blood coagulation; the molecular pathology of the disease and the general biologic lessons learned from studies of its mutational basis; the molecular basis of combined factor VIII and factor V deficiency; carrier and antenatal diagnosis of hemophilia A; and treatment of the disease.

CLINICAL FEATURES OF HEMOPHILIA A (MIM 306700)

Incidence

The frequency of this disorder is often stated to be 1 in 10,000 male births. This is certainly an underestimate, because countries that compile central records (e.g., the UK and Sweden) have a much higher frequency in the general population. Currently, the UK has 5000 cases of hemophilia A known to the Haemophilia Centre Directors, which approaches 1:5000 male births (allowing for a shorter than normal life expectancy), or 1:10,000 in the general population.[36] A possible cause of the lower estimates could be underreporting of moderate and mild hemophilia A; these forms of the disease account for up to half of all cases and present later in life than does severe hemophilia.

Clinical Features

Almost all patients are male (see "Hemophilia A in Females" below). The severity and frequency of bleeding in X-linked factor VIII deficiency is inversely correlated with the residual factor VIII level. Table 172-1 summarizes this relationship and gives the relative frequencies of categories, based on UK national data.[36] The joints most affected are the main weight-bearing articulations — ankles, knees, hips, and elbows — but any joint can be the site of bleeding. If untreated, this intracapsular bleeding causes severe swelling, pain, stiffness, and inflammation, which gradually resolve over days or weeks (for a vivid account of a classical case, see reference 37). Blood is highly irritating to the synovium and causes synovial overgrowth, with a tendency to rebleed from friable vascular tissue, thus establishing a vicious cycle. Probably through accumulation of iron in chondrocytes, a rapid

Table 172-1 Relationship of Factor VIII Activity to Severity of Hemophilia A

Factor VIII (U/dl)	Bleeding Tendency	Relative Incidence of Cases (percent)
<2	Severe; frequent spontaneous* bleeding into joints, muscles, and internal organs	50
2–10	Moderately severe; some spontaneous bleeds; bleeding after minor trauma	30
>10–30	Mild; bleeding only after significant trauma or surgery	20

* "Spontaneous bleeding" refers to episodes where no obvious precipitating event precedes the bleed. Presumably, minor tissue damage caused by everyday activities actually initiates bleeding.

degenerative arthritis occurs, leading to irregularity of the articular contour, then to thinning of the cartilage and bony overgrowth, and finally to ankylosis (Figs. 172-3, 172-4, and 172-5). A particular joint or joints tend to be the target for this destructive process in a given patient, while other joints may be relatively spared.

Muscle bleeding occurs most often in the large, load-bearing groups of the thigh, calf, posterior abdominal wall, and buttocks. Local pressure effects often cause entrapment neuropathy, particularly of the femoral nerve with iliopsoas bleeding. The latter causes a common symptom triad of groin pain, hip flexure, and cutaneous sensory loss over the femoral nerve distribution. Bleeding into the calf, forearm, or peroneal muscles can lead to ischemic necrosis and contracture (Fig. 172-6).

Hematuria is less common than joint or muscle bleeding in hemophiliacs, but most severely affected patients have one or two episodes per decade. These may be painless and resolve spontaneously, but if bleeding is heavy, they can produce severe pain owing to obstruction by a large blood clot. Usually, no anatomic abnormality is found on radiologic investigation to account for the hematuria.

Central nervous system bleeding is uncommon, but can occur after slight head injury and was formerly the most common cause of death in hemophilia A. Intestinal tract bleeding usually presents as obstruction due to intramural hemorrhage, but hematemesis and melena occur occasionally and should be routinely investigated because they may be due to peptic ulcer or malignancy.

Oropharyngeal bleeding, although uncommon, is clinically dangerous because extension through the soft tissue of the floor of the mouth can lead to respiratory obstruction (Fig. 172-7). Bleeding from the tongue after laceration can be very persistent and troublesome because of the fibrinolytic substances in saliva and the impossibility of immobilizing the tongue.

Surgery and open trauma invariably lead to dangerous hemorrhage in the untreated hemophiliac. The most impressive feature is not the rate of hemorrhage but its persistence, often after an initial short-lived period of hemostasis. Clots, if formed, are bulky and friable and break off, with renewed hemorrhage occurring intermittently over days and weeks. Occasionally, a hemorrhage into a large muscle, such as the gluteus, fails to resolve, instead becoming encysted and enlarging slowly as a result of repeated bleeding, forming a hemophilic pseudotumor (Fig. 172-8). This development is only seen today in patients who are resistant to conventional replacement therapy owing to the presence of inhibitors (see below) or who live where little treatment is available; that is, in most developing countries.

Bruising is a feature of hemophilia A, but usually is of only cosmetic significance because it remains superficial and self-limited. Large, extending ecchymoses may occasionally require treatment.

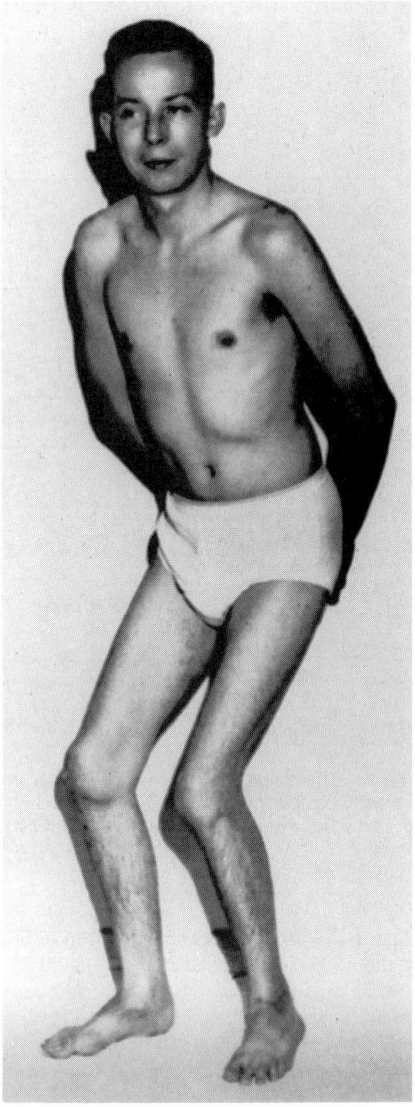

Fig. 172-3 Patient with hemophilia A who grew to maturity before the availability of factor VIII concentrate. He has fixed flexion deformities of both knees and both elbows owing to hemarthroses.

When a pregnant woman is known to be a carrier or at high risk, a cord blood factor VIII level will establish the diagnosis in her infant. Up to one-third of cases are sporadic, however, and in these the hemophilic condition may become known in the neonatal period as a result of cephalohematoma or as a result of prolonged bleeding from the cord or penis following circumcision. Often the diagnosis is not made until the infant is noticed to have many large bruises caused by the pressure of being lifted or by minor bumps on the crib (Fig. 172-9). These sometimes cause diagnostic confusion and the erroneous label of "battered baby syndrome," with needless psychologic trauma to the parents. As soon as the infant starts to crawl actively, joint bleeding begins to appear. In other children, excessive bleeding from eruption of primary dentition or from lacerations leads to the performance of diagnostic tests. Patients with mild disease present in later life when severe trauma or surgery provokes unusual bleeding.

Pathophysiology

All the clinical features of hemophilia A are due directly or indirectly to lack of clotting factor VIII. Affected males are unable to produce normal levels of factor VIII because of various mutations (see below) at the factor VIII locus. Lack of the cofactor drastically slows the rate of generation of factor Xa, even though all other coagulation factors and platelets are present in normal

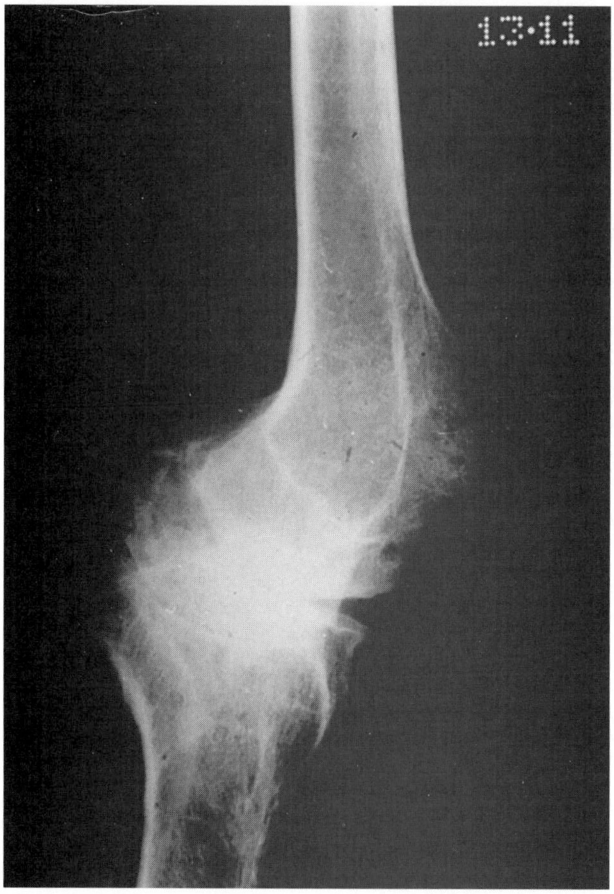

Fig. 172-4 X-ray of the right knee of a hemophiliac showing end-stage hemophilic osteoarthropathy. Note loss of cartilage, osteoporosis, cysts in bone near joint surface, anterior subluxation, deformity, and ankylosis.

amounts. Conversely, replacement of factor VIII by intravenous infusion completely normalizes the hemophiliac's hemostatic mechanism for as long as the infused factor remains in the circulation at physiological concentration (see "Treatment of Hemophilia A" below).

Laboratory Diagnosis

Screening tests show a prolonged partial thromboplastin time (PTT), normal prothrombin time (PT), normal thrombin clotting time (TCT), normal bleeding time, and normal platelet count. Specific assays show factor VIII clotting activity below 35 U/dl with all other factors normal, including vWF antigen and ristocetin cofactor. A test for antibodies to factor VIII should also be performed.

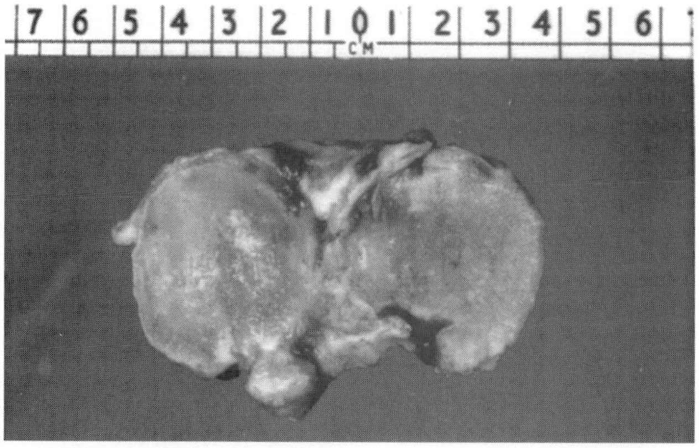

Fig. 172-5 Tibial condyles removed from the knee of a hemophiliac undergoing total knee replacement for advanced arthropathy. Note severe roughening of joint surface with aberrant vascular tissue in the normally avascular area and brown hemosiderin deposition in synovial tissues, the residue of repeated bleeding episodes.

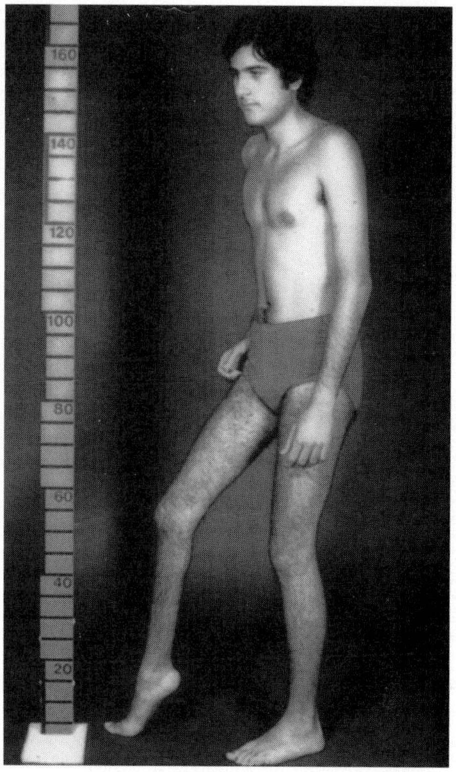

Fig. 172-6 Joint contractures in a patient with hemophilia A. Talipes equinovarus of right foot secondary to untreated bleeding into the calf muscles with ischemic necrosis, followed by contraction and fibrosis causing fixed extension of the ankle. The patient's right elbow is held in fixed flexion owing to hemarthrosis leading to osteoarthropathy.

A normal bleeding time and ristocetin cofactor assay help to distinguish mild hemophilia A from von Willebrand disease, the only condition with which it is likely to be confused on laboratory test results. Recently, a number of individuals were described with apparently autosomal recessive hemophilia A due to defects in the region of vWF involved in binding to factor VIII.[38] Specific assays for the interaction of vWF with factor VIII are required to identify these rare cases.

THE STRUCTURE AND PHYSIOLOGY OF FACTOR VIII

The Factor VIII Gene and Its Deduced Protein Structure

The gene for factor VIII was first cloned in 1984.[33–35,39] The cloning was accomplished by screening bacteriophage λ genomic libraries with oligonucleotide probes synthesized to correspond to sequenced tryptic peptides from purified human[39] or porcine factor VIII.[35]

The factor VIII gene is 186 kb long (approximately 0.1 percent of the DNA of the X chromosome) and has 26 exons. The nucleotide sequence of the exons, intron-exon boundaries, and 5′ flanking region has been determined.[33–35,39] The exon length varies from 69 to 262 bp except for exon 14, which is 3106 bp long, and the last exon (exon 26), which is 1958 bp long (Fig. 172-10). Some of the intervening sequences are quite large; intron 22 is 32 kb, and introns 1, 6, 13, 14, and 25 are 14 to 23 kb.

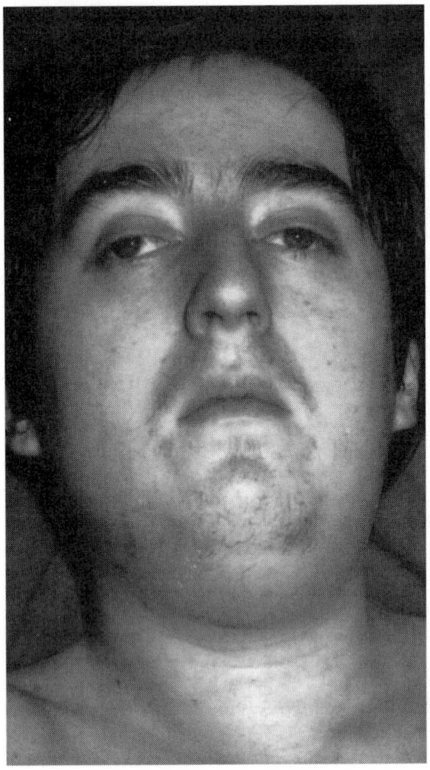

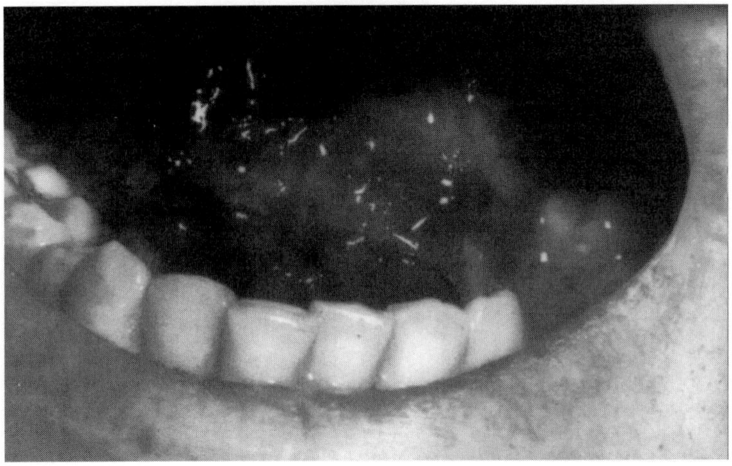

Fig. 172-7 Hemophilia A patient with a factor VIII inhibitor. ***A,*** **Sublingual bleeding with extension to oropharyngeal region. The patient developed respiratory distress before the bleeding could be controlled by porcine factor VIII.** ***B,*** **Intralingual soft tissues distended with blood.**

Normal factor VIII mRNA consists of approximately 9 kb, of which the coding sequence is 7053 nucleotides. There is a CpG island in intron 22, which is associated with two additional transcripts. One transcript of 1.8 kb is produced abundantly in a wide variety of cells. The orientation of this transcript is opposite to that of factor VIII and contains no intervening sequence.[40] This 1739-nucleotide-long cDNA is termed *factor VIII-associated gene A* (F8A) and is conserved in the mouse.[41] The F8A sequence, along with roughly 8 kb of flanking sequence, is repeated twice more at some distance 5′ to the FVIII gene and close to the tip of the X chromosome. These three repeated sequences, which are 99.9 percent identical in sequence,[39a] are involved in a frequent rearrangement of the FVIII gene, which causes severe hemophilia A (see below). The second transcript of 2.5 kb is transcribed in the same direction as factor VIII. After a short exon that may encode eight amino acids, it uses exons 23 to 26 of the factor VIII gene.[42] This gene has been termed *factor VIII-associated gene B* (F8B). The two transcripts, F8A and F8B, originate within 122 bases of each other. The function of these transcripts and their potential protein products are unknown.

Factor VIII is expressed in the liver, spleen, lymph nodes, and a variety of other human tissues but not in bone marrow, peripheral blood lymphocytes, or endothelial cells.[43] In the liver, the hepatocyte is the predominant cell that synthesizes factor VIII mRNA.[43,44]

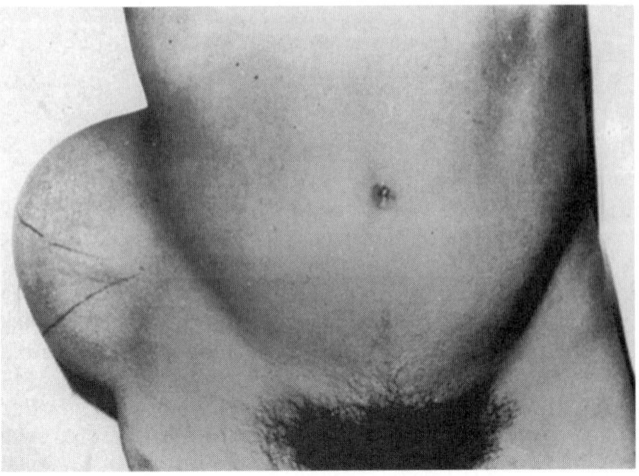

Fig. 172-8 Hemophilic pseudotumor arising in the gluteus muscle. Surgical excision of the entire pseudotumor is mandatory, since rupture and infection of such lesions is invariably fatal.

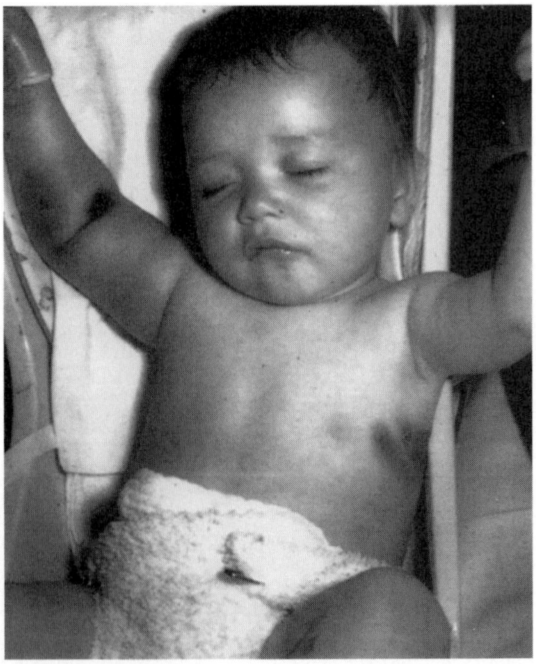

Fig. 172-9 Hemophilia A presentation in infancy with bruising on left chest wall. This led to unsuccessful attempts to obtain a blood sample via the right antecubital fossa, resulting in further bruising.

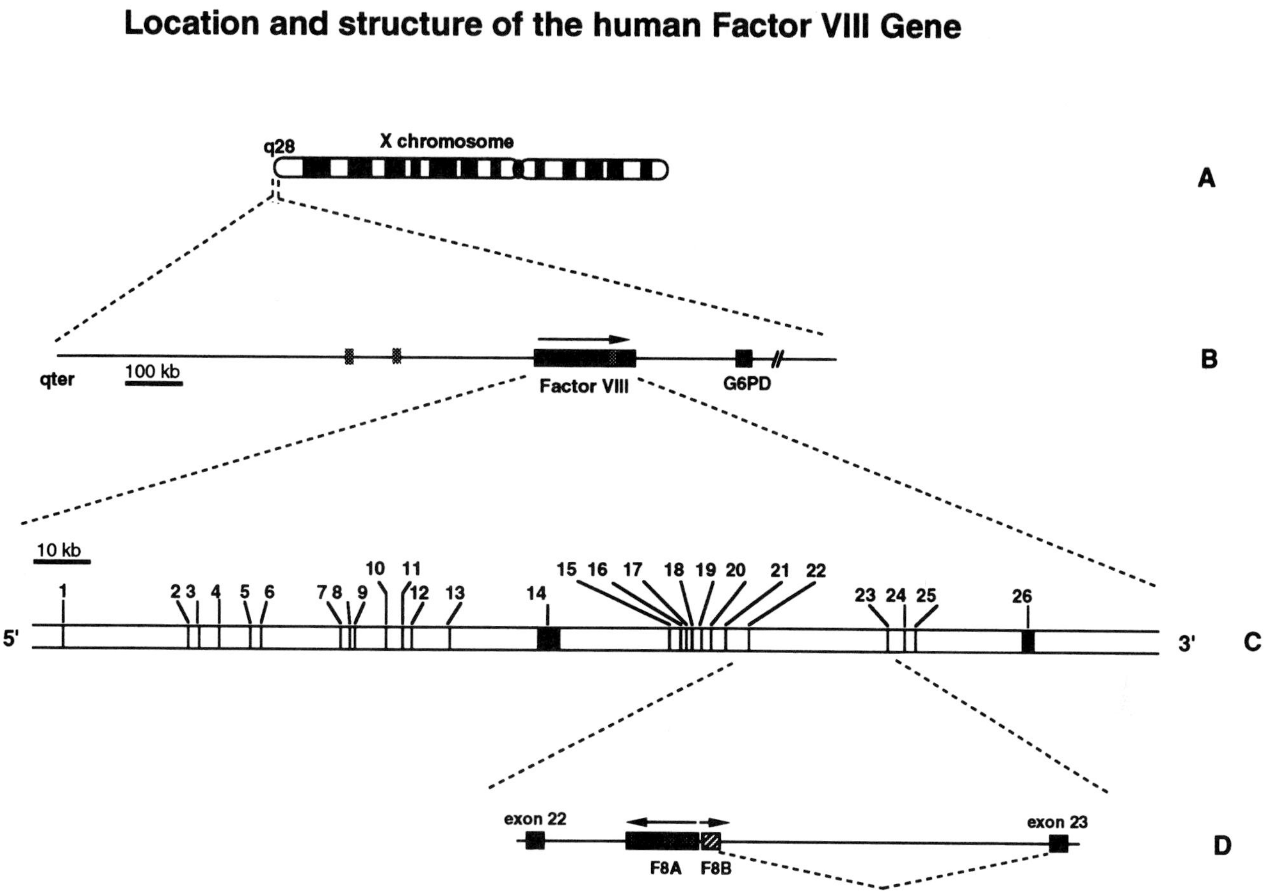

Fig. 172-10 Chromosomal location and structure of the factor VIII genes. *A,* The 186-kb gene is located near the tip of Xq. It contains 26 exons and an unusual bifunctional promoter in intron 22. *B,* Enlargement. The G-6-PD rectangle represents the G-6-PD gene, and the two small rectangles to the right of the factor VIII gene are copies of the F8A gene, which is seen in *C* in intron 22. *D,* Within intron 22 are the two nonfactor-VIII coding sequences, F8A and F8B, which can be transcribed from the bifunctional promoter mentioned above in opposite directions, as shown by the arrows.

The promoter region of the factor VIII gene appears to be located in the 300 nucleotides 5′ to the gene.[44a,44b] Site-directed metagenesis in this region indicates that a putative TATA box is not essential for transcription, but liver-enriched transcription factors, such as HNF1, NFkB, C/EBPa, and C/EBPb, interact with the factor VIII promoter region.[44a] Interestingly, no natural mutations producing hemophilia A have been found in this promoter region.

The gene for factor VIII encodes a precursor protein of 2351 amino acid residues (Fig. 172-11). The first 19 amino acids constitute the leader peptide.[33] This peptide contains 10 hydrophobic amino acids flanked by two charged residues, a structure that is observed in the leader sequences of most proteins. The mature protein contains 2332 amino acids with a calculated molecular weight of 264,763. There are 25 potential asparagine-linked glycosylation sites and 23 cysteine residues.

Factor VIII has several domains with internal homology. The first three are the A1 (amino acid residues 1 to 329), A2 (residues 380 to 711), and A3 (residues 1649 to 2019) domains. These domains have an amino acid sequence homology of approximately 30 percent. The A1 domain is encoded by exons 1 through 8, A2 by exons 9 through 13 and a small region of exon 14, and A3 by the 3′ end of exon 14 and exons 15 through 18. These A domains are homologous to the A domains of ceruloplasmin and factor V.[33,45,46,48a] The A2 and A3 domains are separated by a region of 983 amino acids, the B domain, which contains 19 of the 25 potential N-glycosylation sites. The B domain has no known function; it is encoded by nearly all of the large exon 14, and it is not conserved between factor VIII and factor V.[47] The B domain is discussed further in "The Mystery of the B Domain" below.

At the C-terminus of the mature factor VIII protein, there are two homologous domains, C1 and C2. These domains are also homologous to the A, C, and D chains of discoidin I, the C domains of factor V, integrin binding protein Del-1, mouse protein mP47, and mouse milkfat globule protein.[33,48,48a,48b,48c] Domain C1 is encoded by exons 20 to 23 and includes amino acid residues 2020 to 2172; domain C2 includes amino acids 2173 to 2332 and is encoded by exons 24 to 26 of the factor VIII gene. The order of the six domains described above from the N-terminus to the C-terminus is A1-A2-B-A3-C1-C2 (Fig. 172-11).

In addition, there are two acidic regions in the factor VIII protein. One lies between the A1 and A2 domains, includes amino acid residues 331 to 379, and contains 15 aspartic acid and glutamic acid residues. The second consists of amino acid residues 1649 to 1689 and also contains 15 aspartic acid and glutamic acid residues. Of the 23 cysteine residues in factor VIII, 14 are conserved between factors V and VIII, suggesting that these proteins may be folded in a similar manner. The murine factor VIII cDNA has been cloned and sequenced.[49] The mouse cDNA encodes a protein of 2319 amino acids with an overall identity of 74 percent with the human sequence. The amino acid identity in the A and C domains is 84 to 93 percent, whereas the B domain and the two acidic regions are more divergent, with identities of 42 to 70 percent. All thrombin cleavage sites and sulfated tyrosine residues are conserved. Five of six potential N-glycosylation sites in the non-B domain regions of factor VIII are conserved. The B domain of the murine-deduced protein sequence contains 19 potential N-glycosylation sites in positions different from the human sequence. The human sequence contains the same number of potential N-glycosylation sites, suggesting that

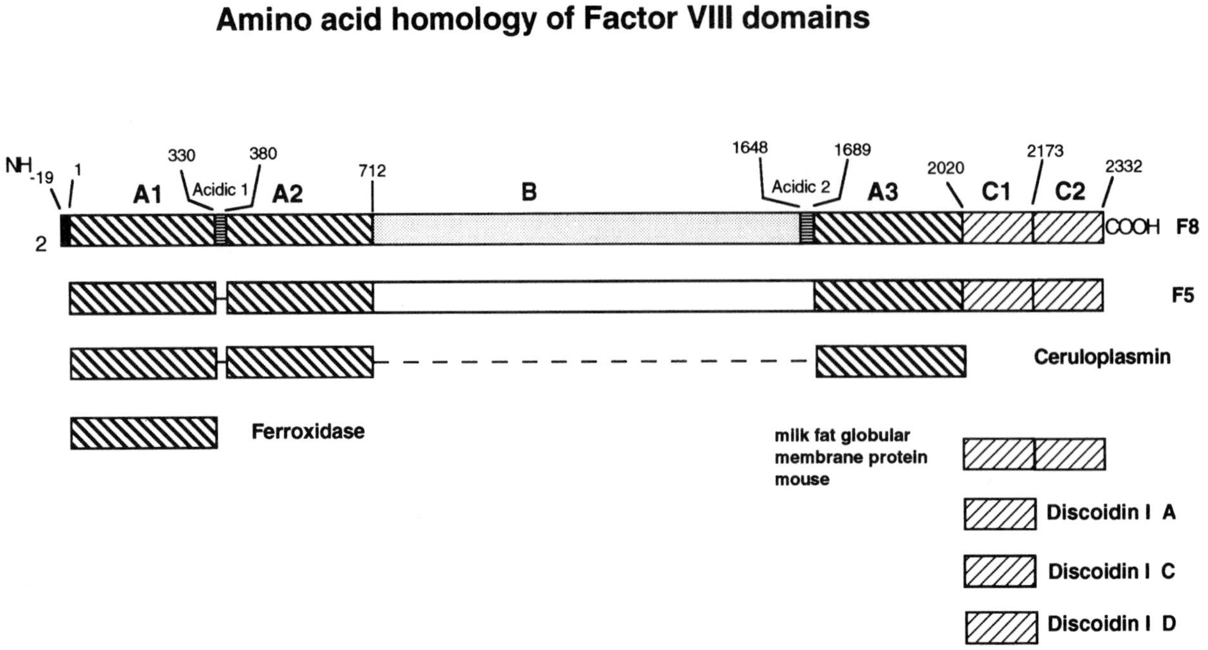

Fig. 172-11 Amino acid homologies of factor VIII domains. The A and C domains have significant homology with factor V. All three A domains have homology with ceruloplasmin and ferroxidase. The C domains also have homology with the milkfat globule membrane protein of mouse and the discoidins of Dictyostelium.

glycosylation of the B domain is important for the biosynthesis of factor VIII.

Genomic Mapping of Factor VIII

The factor VIII gene is located on the long arm of the X chromosome, in the most distal band Xq28. Haldane and Smith[50] reported linkage of hemophilia A with color blindness and Boyer and Graham[51] demonstrated close linkage of hemophilia A with polymorphisms at the G-6-PD locus. Additional studies confirmed the close linkage of factor VIII with G-6-PD.[52] Patterson *et al.*[53] showed that the G-6-PD and factor VIII genes lie within 500 kb of each other. Pulsed field gel electrophoresis and physical mapping of Xq28 using yeast artificial chromosomes suggested that the factor VIII gene maps distal to G-6-PD.[54,55] The order of these loci and the direction of transcription is Xcen-G-6-PD-3′F8-5′F8-Xqter.[55,56] The distance from the factor VIII gene to the Xq telomere is approximately 1 Mb.

Biosynthesis and Activation of Factor VIII

Several excellent reviews describe the biosynthesis, proteolytic cleavages, activation, and inactivation of factor VIII.[57,58]

Activated factor VIII is a critical participant in the intrinsic pathway of blood coagulation (see Chap. 169 for an overview of hemostasis). It is essential for the activation of factor X by factor IXa. Factor IXa is a serine protease; in the presence of active factor VIII, negatively charged phospholipids, and calcium ions, it cleaves an approximately 11-kDa N-terminal activation peptide from factor X to produce factor Xa. The catalytic activity of factor IXa is increased by approximately 10^4 when factor VIIIa is added to IXa, Ca^{2+}, and phospholipids.[59] This increased activity is believed to result from a direct association of factor VIIIa with factor IXa on the phospholipid surface.

In plasma, factor VIII exists as a heavy chain of 90 to 200 kDa (multiple partially processed polypeptides) in a metal-ion association with a light chain of 80 kDa[33,35] (Fig. 172-12). The complex is stabilized by association with vWF.[60,61] The concentration of factor VIII in plasma is about 100 to 200 ng/ml,[62] and the protein is extremely sensitive to proteolysis. The cloning of factor VIII and its heterologous expression in mammalian cells have made possible the analysis of some aspects of its biosynthesis, processing, and function. Liver transplantation and *in situ* hybridization of factor VIII mRNA suggest that the liver is the major site of its synthesis;[63,64] however, factor VIII mRNA has been detected in many other tissues.[43] There are no known natural cell lines that synthesize factor VIII. The experiments of Kaufman using factor VIII cDNA cloned in expression vectors and introduced into mammalian cells (either Chinese hamster ovary cells or COS-1 monkey kidney cells) showed that factor VIII is synthesized as a single polypeptide chain precursor of 2351 amino acid residues, from which the 19-amino acid signal peptide is cleaved on translocation into the endoplasmic reticulum (ER).[60] In the ER, high-mannose oligosaccharide is added to asparagine residues. A significant portion of factor VIII in the ER is bound to a protein called GRP78 (glucose-regulated protein 78 kDa or BiP).[64,65] It is not known if the GRP78-associated factor VIII is secreted or degraded, but binding of factor VIII to BiP reduces the secretion of factor VIII into the circulation. BiP binding is completely abolished by a single amino acid substitution F309S in the A1 domain of the factor VIII protein.[65a] Interestingly, factor VIII binds one molecule of the copper ion Cu(I) with a binding site at C310, one amino acid removed from the BiP binding site. Mutation of C310 to serine destroys copper binding in the A1 domain, eliminates FVIII activity, and yields heavy and light chains that are not associated.[65b] These data suggest that the BiP may play a role in copper binding to factor VIII.

A significant fraction of factor VIII from the ER never transits the Golgi, but is instead degraded within the cell. The portion of the protein that is destined for secretion moves through the Golgi apparatus, where it is cleaved at sites R1313/A1314 and R1648/E1649 in the B domain to generate the 90- to 200-kDa N-terminal heavy chain(s) and the 80-kDa C-terminal light chain[60] (Fig. 172-13). Within the Golgi apparatus, factor VIII is modified by addition of carbohydrate to serine and threonine residues, modification of asparagine-linked high-mannose oligosaccharides, and sulfation of six specific tyrosine residues in the heavy and light chains.[60,66] In cultured cells, factor VIII synthesized without vWF in the medium is secreted as separate chains and degraded. Addition of vWF results in stable association of the two chains.[60,67] Factor VIII and vWF have a half-life of about 12 h

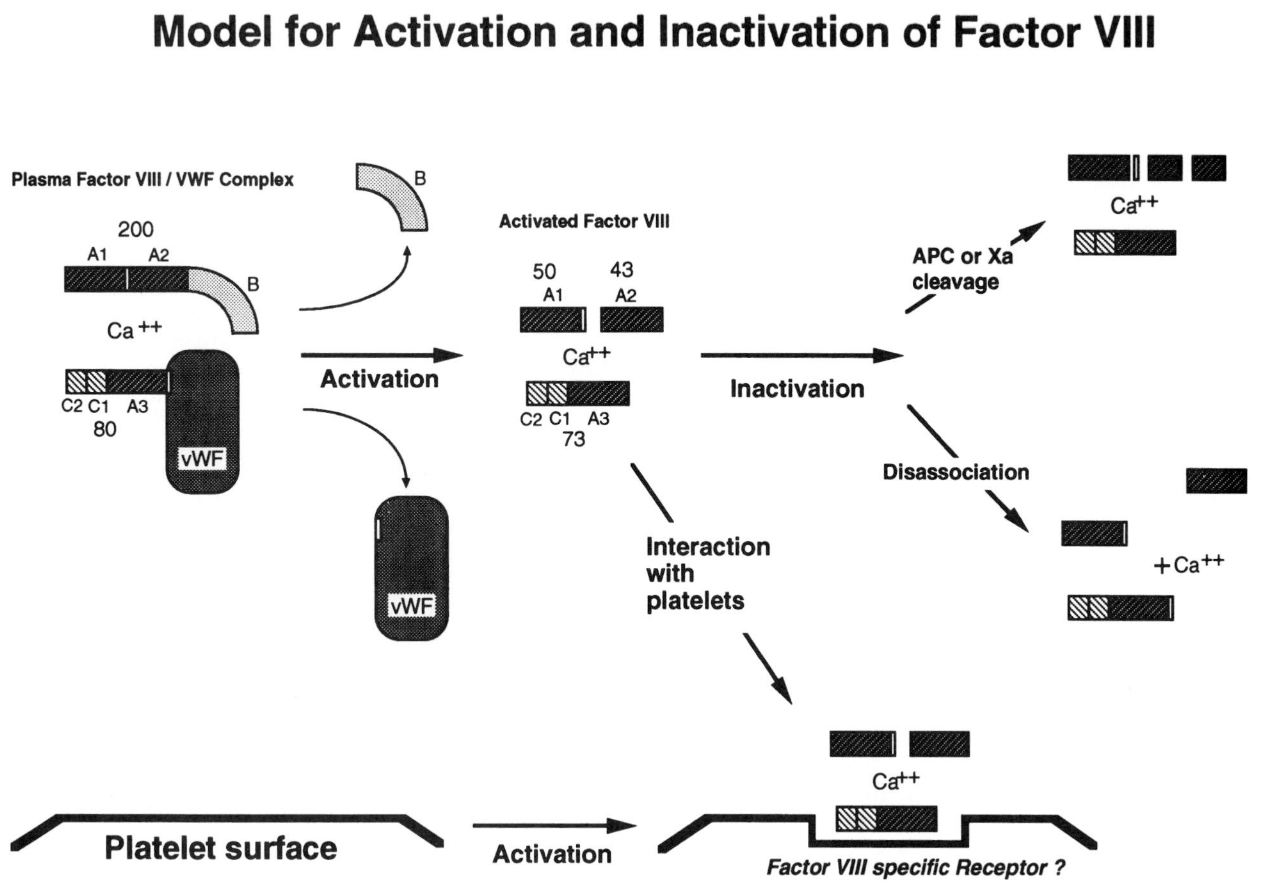

Fig. 172-12 A model for activation and inactivation of factor VIII. Activation involves protease cleavages and interaction with Ca^{2+} ions and platelet surfaces. Inactivation requires proteolysis or dissociation of the subunits. (Modified from Kaufman.[58] Used with permission.)

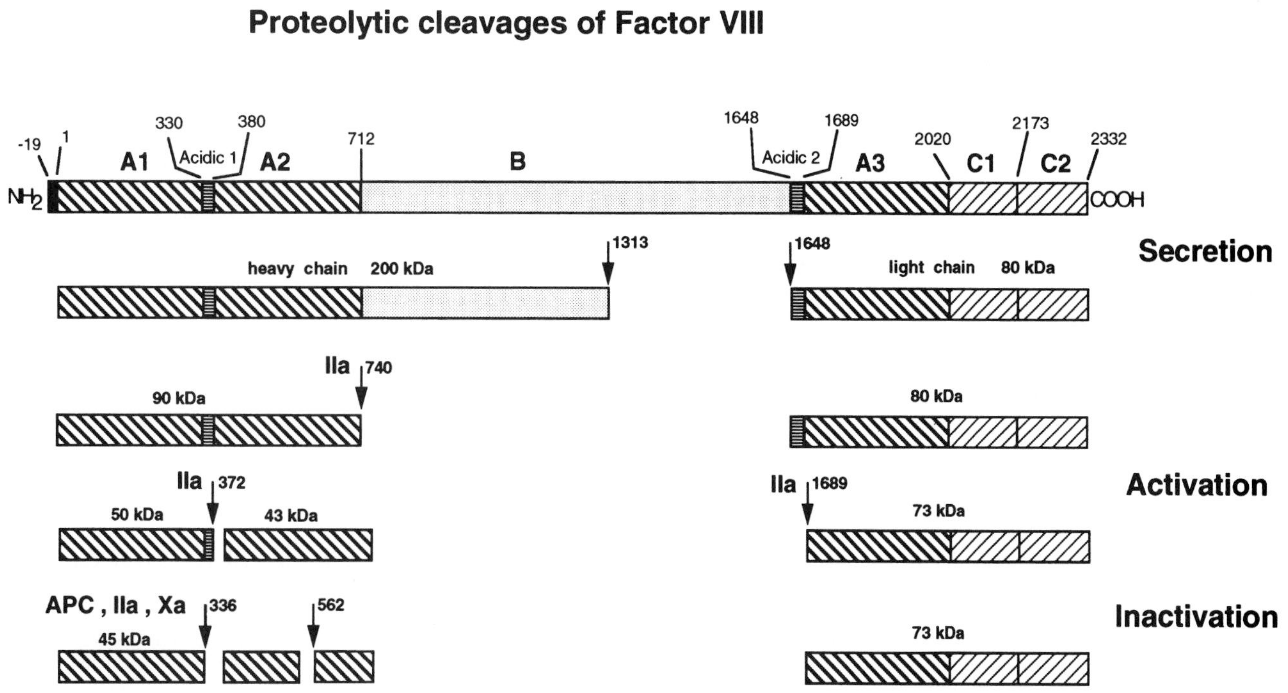

Fig. 172-13 Relationship of proteolytic cleavages of factor VIII to its secretion, activation, and inactivation. (Modified from Kaufman.[58] Used by permission.)

when the factor VIII/vWF complex is infused into hemophilia A patients. In contrast, infused factor VIII is cleared from the plasma of vWF patients with a half-life of 2.4 h.[67a,67b]

Proteolytic Activation of Factor VIII

Factor VIII is activated by proteolytic cleavages by proteases such as thrombin (factor IIa) or factor Xa in the presence of phospholipid surfaces. The following cleavages by thrombin occur in factor VIII after secretion (Figs. 172-12 and 172-13).[68,69] Cleavage of the heavy chain at R740/S741 generates a 90kDa polypeptide, which is subsequently cleaved at R372/S373 to generate polypeptides of 50 kDa and 43 kDa. The light chain is cleaved at R1689/S1690 to produce a 73kDa polypeptide. Factor Xa cleaves at the same sites and at R1721/A1722. Transfection of COS-1 cells with factor VIII cDNA mutated to alter the Arg residues at these cleavage sites to Ile or Leu suggests that the cleavages at R740 or R1721 have no effect on coagulation activity.[70,71] However, the cleavages at R372 or R1689 are important for the procoagulant activity of factor VIII. The cleavage at R1689 releases factor VIII from vWF and permits factor VIII to interact with phospholipids and platelets.[71,72] The Arg residues at positions 372, 740, 1689, and 1721 are conserved in murine and porcine factor VIII.[49]

Missense mutations have been described in factor VIII at R372 and R1689 residues in patients with hemophilia A. The mutations R372C and R372H at the first cleavage site, and R1689C and R1689H at the second site, have been found in more than a dozen unrelated patients.[73–80] All of these patients have CRM+ hemophilia A with normal levels of circulating factor VIII protein but very low activity (1 to 7 percent). The circulating dysfunctional plasma factor VIII from these patients, isolated by immunopurification, cannot be cleaved *in vitro* by thrombin at the site of the amino acid substitution.[78–80a]

After cleavage with thrombin and activation, factor VIII exists as a heterotrimer consisting of the 50kDa A1 subunit, 43kDa A2 subunit, and 73kDa A3-C1-C2 subunit.[66,81,82] Dissociation or deletion of the A2 subunit results in loss of activity, and addition of the A2 subunit restores the procoagulant activity.[81–85] It is clear that the A2 subunit is required for the activity of factor VIII; however, its function is not yet known. Over 50 missense mutations have been identified in the A2 subunit in patients with hemophilia A, underscoring its importance.

The Mystery of the B Domain

The B domain (amino acid residues 740 to 1648) is cleaved during proteolytic activation.[60] Deletions of the B domain by mutagenesis (amino acid residues 797 to 1652) in one experiment[86] and 759 to 1639 in another[87] resulted in normal cofactor activity. In addition, B-domainless factor VIII was activated by thrombin to the same extent as native factor VIII. Furthermore, the derived factor VIII interacted normally with vWF with a half-life of about 13 h, similar to that of factor VIII encoded by the full-length cDNA. The function of the B domain is unknown. It is possible that it may regulate the intracellular processing and/or secretion of factor VIII, as B-domain-deleted molecules are expressed at five- to tenfold higher levels than non-B-deleted factor VIII, and have decreased association with GRP78 (BiP) in the ER.[64,87]

Surprisingly, the B domain is not well conserved during evolution. The murine B domain of factor VIII is only 55 percent identical to the human domain in amino acid sequence[49] (the other domains have identities of 84 to 93 percent between the two species). The murine B domain contains 19 potential N-glycosylation sites, most in positions different from the 19 potential N-glycosylation sites in the human B domain.[49] Thus, the number of N-glycosylation sites may be of functional importance. The B domains of human and bovine factor V contain 26 and 18 potential N-glycosylation sites, respectively, and otherwise have no similarity with the human factor VIII B domain.[47,88,89]

Finally, the B domain may have coagulant, anticoagulant, vasoactive, or other properties at present unknown and unsuspected. No clearcut disease-producing missense mutations have been reported in this region in patients with hemophilia A.

Inactivation of Factor VIII

The activity of activated factor VIII requires all three heterotrimer polypeptides, the 50 kDa A1 subunit, the 43 kDa A2 subunit, and the 73 kDa A3 subunit. The A1 subunit is in a copper ion-dependent association with the A3 subunit or light chain. The A2 subunit associates with the A1 subunit by electrostatic interactions that probably involve amino acids 336 to 372 of the A1 fragment.[90b,90c] After it is activated by thrombin, the factor VIII heterotrimer is stabilized by factor X and phospholipid.[90] Covalent attachment of the A2 subunit to the A3 light chain produced a factor VIII moiety that was stable after thrombin activation.[90e] These results indicate the significance of A2 subunit dissociation in the inactivation of factor VIII.

Although physiological inactivation of factor VIII activity may not require a proteolytic event, inactivation can be mediated by proteolytic cleavage.[68] Activated protein C (APC) cleaves and inactivates factor VIII.[91–93] Two APC cleavage sites, at R336/M337 and R562/G563, have been identified in factor VIII.[64,87] The cleavage at R562 correlates most significantly with inactivation.[94] R336 is not conserved in the murine factor VIII sequence;[49] however, site-directed mutagenesis of residue 336 from R to I resulted in a factor VIII molecule with increased activity, possibly because of resistance to proteolytic inactivation.[70] Factor Xa and thrombin also cleave at R336.[68,70] Factor IXa has been shown to inactivate factor VIII by specific cleavages at R336/M337 and R1719/N1720.[94a] No natural missense mutations have been identified in the inactivation cleavage sites. An inherited increased ability to form blood clots, called "hereditary thrombophilia," which is due to resistance of factor VIII to APC, has been reported.[95] The molecular defect behind this condition is a mutation in factor V which renders it more sensitive to APC (see Chap. 170). Other studies indicate that a single mutation in an APC cleavage site of factor VIII, which rendered the site cleavage resistant, is insufficient to produce a thrombophilia state, and no thrombophilia-generating mutations have been observed in the factor VIII gene.[95]

Interactions of Factor VIII with Other Molecules

Binding to von Willebrand Factor. Von Willebrand factor is required for normal stability of factor VIII in plasma and is encoded by a gene on chromosome 12p. It is synthesized by endothelial cells and megakaryocytes[96,97] and binds to factor VIII in the extracellular fluid.[60] Infused factor VIII-vWF complex in hemophilia A patients has a half-life of 12 h.[98,99] Infused factor VIII is cleared at a rate similar to the factor VIII-vWF complex, probably because factor VIII binds immediately to vWF. However, infused factor VIII in patients with vWF disease or in vWF-deficient dogs has a half-life of only 2.4 h.[99,100] Infusion of vWF in patients with vWF deficiency also elevates factor VIII levels.[98,99] vWF plays an important role in the regulation of factor VIII activity in a four ways:

1. In addition to its stabilizing effect, it promotes the association of light and heavy chains of factor VIII;[67,101]
2. It protects factor VIII from inactivation by activated protein C;[93,102]
3. It facilitates cleavage of the light chain (or A3 subunit) of factor VIII by thrombin[103] and does not interfere with the other thrombin cleavages;[104] and
4. It inhibits the binding of factor VIII to phospholipids and activated platelets.[105–107]

Several investigators have localized the portion of vWF protein that interacts with factor VIII to the first 272 amino acids of the secreted vWF.[108–110] In fact, missense mutations, such as T28M,[111] R53W, and R91Q,[112,113] in this portion of vWF, result in defective binding to factor VIII and a clinical phenotype that mimics hemophilia A (autosomal recessive hemophilia or Type N von Willebrand's disease).[114]

The N-terminus of the light chain of factor VIII has also been shown to interact with vWF.[104,115] After thrombin cleavage at residue R1689 of the factor VIII light chain, vWF no longer binds to factor VIII, suggesting that the peptide from E1649 to R1689 contains the vWF binding capacity of factor VIII.[116] This region, E1649 to R1689, corresponds to the second acidic region, which contains 15 aspartic and glutamic acid residues. The use of monoclonal antibodies against specific residues of factor VIII further localized the vWF binding site of factor VIII to amino acids K1673 to E1684.[116,117]

Deletion of the acidic region of the light chain results in a factor VIII molecule that does not bind vWF but has normal specific activity when compared to normal factor VIII.[118] In addition, the second acidic region contains two tyrosine residues, Y1664 and Y1680, which are sulfated.[66] Site-directed mutagenesis of Y1680 to F, which cannot be sulfated, results in a molecule that lacks high-affinity binding to vWF.[119] Patients with the naturally occurring Y1680F mutation[76] have moderately severe, CRM-reduced hemophilia (10 percent factor VIII activity and about 20 percent factor VIII antigen). Therefore, the sulfation of Y1680 is an important posttranslational modification required for proper binding of factor VIII to vWF. Not only is the N-terminus of the light chain required for vWF binding, but the C-terminus from residues 2248 to 2312 in the C2 domain was recently shown to be crucial for high-affinity binding of vWF to factor VIII.[119a]

Tyrosine Sulfation. Using ^{35}S metabolic-labeling in cultured Chinese hamster ovary cells expressing human recombinant factor VIII, Pittman and Kaufman[66] identified six sulfated tyrosine residues. Of these residues, Y346, Y718, Y719, and Y723 are in the heavy chain, and Y1664 and Y1680 are in the light chain.

Tyrosine sulfation is a posttranslational modification that occurs on a number of secretory proteins as they traverse the Golgi apparatus,[120] and it is required for full factor VIII activity. It may also affect the interaction of factor VIII with other components of the coagulation cascade. However, inhibition of tyrosine sulfation does not alter the synthesis or secretion of factor VIII. The sulfated tyrosine residues of human factor VIII are conserved in murine and porcine factor VIII.[49] Y1680 has been shown to be important for interaction with vWF,[117,119] and, as mentioned earlier, site-directed mutagenesis of Y1680 to F resulted in a factor VIII molecule with defective binding to vWF.[71,119]

Binding to Factors IXa and X. Data on the location of contact sites of factor VIII with factor IXa was recently published. Studies of the binding of factor VIII to fluorescently labeled factor IXa demonstrated that the A2 domain is required to induce a maximal conformational change in factor IXa.[120a,120b] Peptide-inhibition studies showed that a factor IXa binding site is present at residues 558 to 565 within the A2 domain of factor VIII.[120c,120d] However, monoclonal antibody inhibition experiments indicate that a factor IXa binding site exists between residues 1770 and 1840, and other studies have narrowed this site to 1811 to 1818 of the factor VIII light chain.[120e]

The binding of substrate factor X to factor VIII has also been studied.[120f] The data suggest that a factor X binding site exists within the acidic region at the C-terminus of the A1 domain.[120f] Factor X binding at this site likely occurs whether factor VIII is activated or not.

Binding to Phospholipids. The C1 and C2 domains of factor VIII are thought to interact with phospholipids. These domains have amino acid homology with discoidins, which are Dictyostelium lectins that are capable of binding negatively charged phospholipids.[121] Phospholipids are important components in the activation of factor X by activated factor IX and the factor-VIII cofactor activity.[59,121] The light chain of factor VIII contains a phospholipid binding site,[122,123] which is not abolished after thrombin cleavage and elimination of the vWF-binding domain.[106]

A subset of human factor VIII inhibitor antibodies that have epitopes contained in the C2 domain inhibit the binding of factor VIII to immobilized phosphatidylserine.[124] Furthermore, a study of the capability of synthetic peptides to inhibit the binding of purified factor VIII to immobilized phosphatidylserine indicated that the region between residues T2303 and Y2332—that is, the C-terminal portion of the C2 domain—is an important phospholipid-binding domain of factor VIII.[125]

The surface of thrombin-activated platelets binds factor VIII, and vWF inhibits this binding.[107] As platelets are activated by thrombin, their phosphatidylserine levels rise from 2 percent to 13 percent.[126] Because factor VIII has specific binding to this phospholipid by both hydrophobic and electrostatic interactions,[127] the increase in phosphatidylserine content likely accounts for the specific binding of factor VIII to the surface of activated platelets. Alternatively, factor VIII may bind to a specific, unidentified receptor that appears in the platelet membrane after activation. There are approximately 400 factor VIII sites per activated platelet.[128,129] Although factor V has a C2 domain similar to that of factor VIII, it cannot compete with factor VIII for platelet binding.

Several natural mutations have been identified in the last 30 amino acid residues of factor VIII in patients with hemophilia A, including R2304C, R2307Q, and R2307L, which result in both mild and severe forms of the disease. However, the role of these residues in phospholipid binding is not known.[130–133] Endothelial cells are important components of the coagulation mechanism; however, it is not known if these cells have specific binding sites for factor VIII.

The Structural Mechanism of Factor VIII Action

Although little is known about how the complex factor VIII molecule induces a specific conformational change in the active site of factor IXa, this information remains a major future goal. The three-dimensional structure of factor IXa is now available.[133] In addition, a molecular model of the A domain of factor VIII based on the structure of the homologous ceruloplasmin protein has been proposed.[133b] The model suggests that factor IXa binding sites in the A2 and A3 domains are in close proximity and exposed to the surface. Greater understanding of the conformational change that factor VIII mediates in factor IXa may allow production of a small peptide (peptidomimetic) that carries out the same change. If such a peptide could be effective following oral administration, it would be a major advance in the treatment of hemophilia A.

MOLECULAR PATHOLOGY OF HEMOPHILIA A

Until recent times, hemophilia A was a lethal genetic disease, and affected males had little chance of reproduction. Therefore, the observed gene frequency for the disorder indicates that a large fraction of cases must arise by new mutation. In fact, in the 1930s, Haldane predicted that one-third of all isolated cases would arise by new mutation in noncarrier females, and that another one-third of the remaining cases would have arisen by new mutation in the grandparental generation.[134] This prediction has now been largely verified in studies of the molecular basis of the disease.[135] An important exception is mothers of severe hemophiliacs with an inversion mutation (see below), nearly all of whom are carriers.[136] A corollary of the Haldane hypothesis is that if a number of potential molecular defects can give rise to hemophilia A, multiple new mutations will be significantly heterogeneous. One could predict that, in the absence of a "common mutation" or "mutation hotspot" in the factor VIII gene, the great majority of unrelated hemophilic males carry a different mutation in the factor VIII gene. As it turns out, a large number of mutations can produce the disease, and over 50 percent of unrelated patients have a different mutation. A database of nucleotide substitutions, deletions, insertions, and rearrangements of the factor VIII gene in hemophilia A

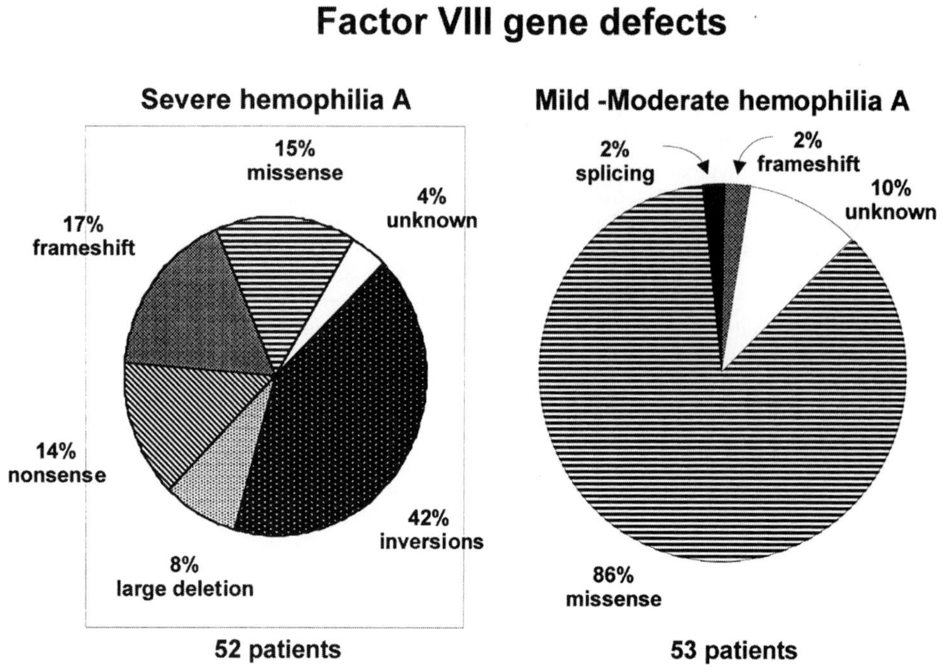

Fig. 172-14 Factor VIII gene defects in patients with severe and mild-to-moderate hemophilia A. Data are from references 90, 137a, and 166, and updated after the identification of the common inversions.[139]

was compiled in late 1991.[137] (See the Web site at http://146.179.66.63/usr/www/WebPages/main.dir/main.htm). Figure 172-14 depicts the mutation types found in patients with hemophilia A.

Gross Rearrangements of the Factor VIII Gene

Common Inversions Involving the Factor VIII Gene. Efforts to characterize all mutations in the factor VIII gene in a defined group of hemophilia A patients revealed an unexpected finding. After scanning all the exons of the factor VIII gene using denaturing gradient gel electrophoresis, Higuchi *et al.* found the causative mutation in about 90 percent of patients with mild to moderate hemophilia A.[90] However, when severely affected patients were similarly extensively studied, the causative mutation was found in only about 50 percent of patients.[137a] The etiology of the remaining 50 percent of severe patients was unknown.

Naylor *et al.* used RT-PCR of illegitimate transcripts of the factor VIII gene to provide the beginnings of an answer to the mystery.[138] They found that transcripts were interrupted between exons 22 and 23 in 40 percent of patients with severe hemophilia A. These patients must all have one or more different mutations at a hotspot in the large intron 22. Because an unusual duplicated gene (gene A) was located in this intron (see Fig. 172-10), along with a promoter that can result in a transcript containing 8 codons from the intron-22 sequence connected to exons 23 through 26, this region had interesting possibilities for an unusual mutation hotspot. Lakich *et al.*[139] and Naylor *et al.*[140] found that the region encompassing gene A in intron 22 inappropriately pairs with one of the two homologous regions 5′ (telomeric) to the factor VIII gene on the same X chromosome (Figs. 172-10 and 172-15). This unusual pairing is sometimes followed by homologous recombination, resulting in one of two potential large inversions (depending on which extragenic gene A is involved) that disrupt the factor VIII gene (Fig. 172-15). These inversions place exons 1 to 22 some 400 kb upstream of exons 23 to 26 and oriented in the opposite direction. Because these mutations involve the tip of the X chromosome, they have been dubbed the "flip tip" mutations. It is interesting to note that the three gene A regions are each 9.5kb long and that there is greater than 99.5 percent nucleotide sequence identity among them.[39a] Depending on which extragenic copy of gene A is involved in the recombination event, two main inversion types are seen. Type 1 affects the distal gene A copy, while type 2 affects the proximal copy. A rare third type is thought to arise from inversion in individuals carrying three extragenic copies of gene A. A consortium analysis of about 2100 patients with severe hemophilia A demonstrated inversions in 43 percent of cases.[141] Thus, these recurring mutations account for about 25–30 percent of all hemophilia A patients. Because nearly all inversions originate in male meiosis,[39a] almost all mothers of inversion patients are carriers of factor VIII deficiency. This means that slightly over 80 percent of mothers of an isolated case of severe hemophilia A are carriers of a mutant factor VIII gene.

Deletions in the Factor VIII Gene. Large deletions account for about 5 percent of characterized mutations in the disease. The mutation database contains[92] deletions as of May 1999. Deletions usually produce severe hemophilia A with no factor VIII activity. Two exceptions are deletions that eliminate only the 156-bp exon 22 or the 294-bp of exons 23 and 24 from the coding region of the gene. These deletions are associated with moderate disease, probably because of in-frame splicing of exon 21 to exon 23 or exon 22 to exon 25.[142,143] Large deletions are often associated with inhibitor formation (27 of 73 patients [37 percent] with deletions for whom data are available on inhibitor formation), and they show no particular predilection for one or another region of the factor VIII gene. They nearly all result from non-homologous loss of a region of the gene[144]—that is, they generally are not caused by mispairing of homologous DNA, such as Alu sequences, followed by unequal crossing over. That said, there is often a 2 to 4 nucleotide homology at the junctions flanking the deletion.

Retrotransposon Insertions. The first insertions of a transposable element in humans were observed in the factor VIII gene in 1987. Although transposable elements are present in a large variety of organisms, including yeast, maize, *Drosophila*, and mouse, they had not been seen in humans until hemophilia A—a disorder with a wide spectrum of mutations—was studied. Two patients were found with truncated L1 elements inserted into exon 14 of the factor VIII gene.[145]

L1 elements make up about 15 percent of the human genome and are present in about 500,000 copies, but only 3000 are full length and approximately 40 are active transposons.[146] These active elements are retrotransposable in that they produce a new

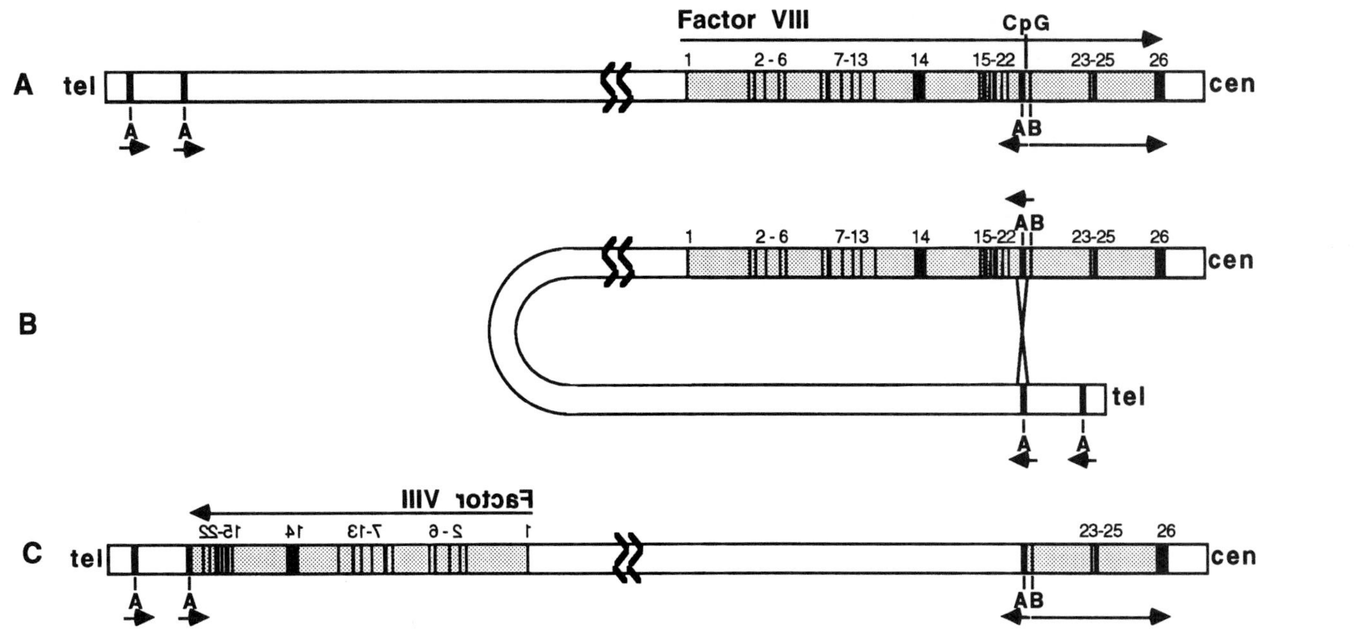

Fig. 172-15 **Inversions involving the factor VIII gene. *A,* The region of Xq28 that includes the factor VIII gene, oriented with the telomere at the left. Three copies of gene A are indicated, two lying upstream of factor VIII and one inside intron 22 of factor VIII. The location of the B transcript is also shown. The arrows indicate the direction of transcription of the factor VIII and internal A and B genes. The direction of the upstream A genes is hypothesized to be as shown. *B,* The proposed homologous recombination between the intron-22 copy of gene A and one of the two upstream copies. A crossover between these two identical regions, oriented in the manner illustrated, results in an inversion of sequence between the two recombined A genes, as shown in *C.* A recombination could involve either of the upstream A genes, but only one is presented. The crossover could occur anywhere in the region of homology that includes the A genes.**

insertion through an RNA intermediate. They are transcribed into RNA, the RNA is translated into two proteins in the cytoplasm, and somehow makes its way back into the nucleus with at least one of its encoded proteins. That protein then makes a nick in a single strand of the DNA using its endonuclease activity and reverse transcribes the RNA into DNA using its reverse transcriptase activity and the 3′-OH at the DNA nick as a primer. By other unknown mechanisms the first-strand DNA is ligated to genomic DNA, the second strand is nicked, and a second strand DNA is made and ligated to complete the retrotransposition event.[147] Thus, L1s are "copy and paste" mobile elements.[147] In the case of the *de novo* L1 insertions into exon 14 of the factor VIII gene, one insertion that contained the 3′ two-thirds of an L1 element was shown to result from retrotransposition of an active element located on chromosome 22. As of February 2000, 14 new insertions of different L1 elements into the factor VIII gene,[145] the adenomatosis polyposis coli gene,[148] the dystrophin gene,[149–151] the β-globin gene,[152] a retinitis pigmentosa gene,[153] and a chronic granulomatous disease gene[154] were known. In addition, 17 insertions of Alu elements have been reported.[155–159]

Duplications. Duplications are rarely seen in human genes. In the factor VIII gene, two such events have been described. One was a duplication of 23 kb of intron 22 inserted between exons 23 and 25.[160] This rearrangement was found in two females, was unstable, and led to deletion of exons 23 to 25 in a male offspring of one female. The second case was an in-frame duplication of exon 13 in a patient with mild disease.[161]

Chromosomal Rearrangement Disrupting the Factor VIII Gene

A single chromosomal X-autosome translocation with a breakpoint in the factor VIII gene has been reported.[162] A complex *de novo* translocation of chromosomes X and 17 in a female resulted in severe hemophilia A. The der(17) contained a deleted factor VIII gene lacking exons 1 to 15; exons 16 to 26 were present on another autosome. Thus, one breakpoint of this complex rearrangement occurred between exons 15 and 16 of the factor VIII gene. The normal X contained a normal factor VIII gene that was inactivated by X-inactivation in all cells.

Point Mutations in the Factor VIII Gene

Small Deletions/Insertions (Frameshift Mutations). Frameshift mutations that cause severe hemophilia A have been reported in 86 unrelated patients.[163–165] In the database, 63 of 572 point mutations(11 percent) are frameshifts. Most small deletions/insertions occur in DNA regions of short repeat sequences. Although all frameshifts would be expected to result in severe hemophilia A, there is one exception. In this family, a single nucleotide deletion in exon 14 within an A_8TA_2 sequence resulted in moderately severe hemophilia A (factor VIII activity = 2 percent). Analysis of DNA and RNA from normal and affected individuals suggested a partial correction of the molecular defect *in vivo* due to DNA replication/RNA transcription errors resulting in restoration of the reading frame, and/or ribosomal frameshifting during translation resulting in production of some normal factor VIII. Either of these mechanisms could have been promoted by the longer stretch of adenines, A_{10} instead of A_8TA_2, which followed the delT mutation.[90]

Nonsense Mutations. According to the database, 115 nonsense mutations in 48 different codons account for about 20 percent of the total point mutations in the disease. Indeed, in two samples of severe hemophilia A patients in which all point mutations were characterized, the frequency of nonsense mutations was 18 percent.

Exon Skipping Due to Nonsense Mutations. An important observation concerning the pathophysiology of nonsense mutations has been made in the factor VIII gene.[166] This observation, independently made in the fibrillin and ornithine aminotransferase genes,[167] indicates that a nonsense mutation can, on occasion, lead to aberrant RNA processing in which the exon harboring the mutation is skipped. The mechanism for this unusual RNA

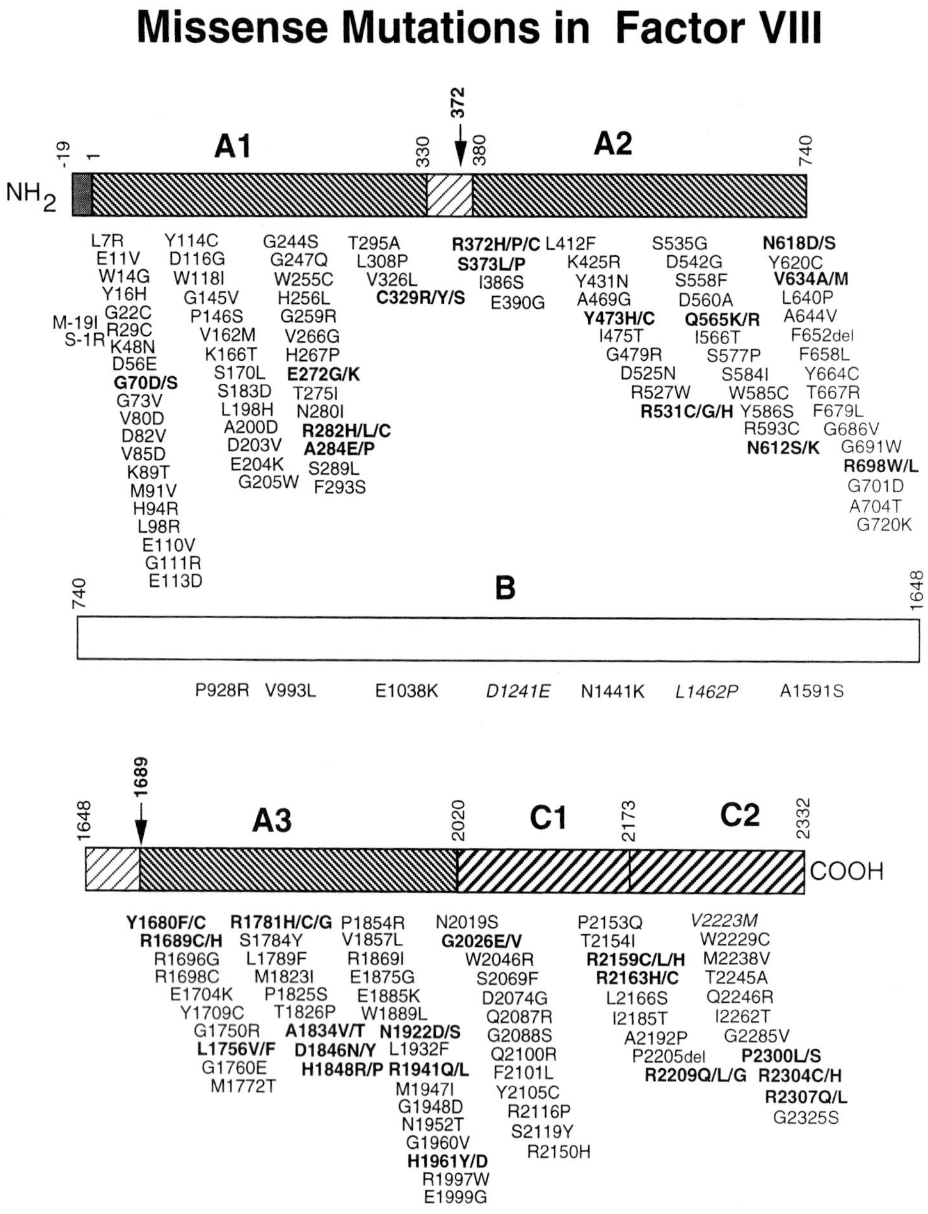

Fig. 172-16 Missense mutations in the factor VIII protein. The structural domains of the protein are shown and amino acid substitutions use the one-letter code for amino acids. For example, L7R is a leucine to arginine substitution at amino acid 7. When two or more substitutions are observed at the same residue, bold type is used (R372H/P/C indicates substitutions at arginine372 to histidine, proline, or cysteine.) Substitutions in the B domain are neutral variants, and are not disease producing.

processing is unknown. At least two instances of the skipping of an exon containing a nonsense codon have been discovered in the factor VIII gene.[166] The fraction of factor VIII mRNA missing the exon of interest was nearly 100 percent in one case and about 50 percent in the other, and in both cases the skipping of an in-frame exon would lead to an otherwise normal factor VIII protein missing the amino acids encoded by the skipped exon. In both cases, the phenomenon explains the lack of inhibitor formation by the patient (see "Etiology of Inhibitors in Hemophilia A" below). Presumably, a small amount of near-normal protein protects the patient from producing factor VIII antibodies.

Exon skipping in factor VIII gene mutants was demonstrated by taking advantage of the low level of factor VIII transcripts, so-called illegitimate transcripts, present in lymphocytes.[170] As mentioned earlier, the major site of factor VIII transcription is the liver, but transcript levels of about one factor VIII mRNA per 10 cells can be detected in lymphocytes using reverse transcriptase followed by PCR. In a number of gene systems, these transcripts have been shown to accurately reflect the transcription and splicing of the gene of interest at its major site of expression. Thus, illegitimate transcripts can be used to characterize mutations in genomic DNA.[168]

Missense Mutations. Missense mutations, nucleotide substitutions that lead to amino acid substitutions, account for 191 mutations in 457 unrelated patients in the database (Fig. 172-16). These nucleotide substitutions are spread throughout the factor VIII gene, except for the bulk of exon 14 that encodes the B domain and is devoid of missense mutations. However, there are regions, such as the A2 domain, in which they concentrate.[90,169] For most of the missense mutations, the antigen level is commensurate with the factor VIII activity, that is, very low. Indeed, for most of these mutations, the mechanism that produces reduced factor VIII in plasma is unknown and is very difficult to study. The structure-function relationship is known for only approximately 10 of these mutations. Mutations at the thrombin cleavage sites — arginine residues 372 and 1689 — are known to block activation of factor VIII by thrombin, producing CRM+ hemophilia in which FVIII:Ag levels are normal.[73–80] The mutation Y1680F produces a mild CRM-reduced phenotype owing to a block in tyrosine sulfation and concomitant vWF binding to factor VIII.[76,137a] A nearby tyrosine substitution, Y1709C, causes a severe hemophilia A.[170]

Two other CRM+ mutations, I566T and M1772T, produce severe hemophilia A phenotypes by creating new N-glycosylation sites in the protein.[171] The consensus amino acid sequence for N-glycosylation is Asn-X-Ser/Thr. One site created by the I566T mutation is in the A2 domain, producing glycosylation at N564 (Asn-X-Ile to Asn-X-Thr). The second new glycosylation is in the A3 domain of the light chain at residue 1770. In both cases, factor VIII is present at normal levels in the plasma but is completely inactive. In either case, deglycosylation of the plasma restores factor VIII activity to a significant degree.[171] Position 564 is in the putative interaction site with activated factor IX, and abnormal glycosylation produced at this site sterically hinders interaction of factor IXa with factor VIII.[172]

Other CRM+ mutations that greatly reduce factor VIII activity while leaving factor VIII antigen levels intact or only modestly reduced should provide clues to important sites of interaction of factor VIII with other molecules, such as factor Xa, APC, phospholipid surfaces, and calcium ions. Sites of CRM+ mutations include S289, R527, and S558, defects of which produce mild factor VIII deficiency, and V634.[137a,169] A V634A substitution produces moderate hemophilia A, whereas a V634M substitution leads to severe hemophilia A.[169] An R282H substitution in domain A1 leads to a severe hemophilia with 18 percent of normal antigen.[90]

In general, studies of the small numbers of CRM+ and CRM-reduced patients point to potentially important residues in the protein. Because 11 of 26 of the known CRM+ mutations occur in the A2 domain, which consists of 228 amino acids, or about 10 percent of the coding region of factor VIII, this region must be important in procoagulant activity.[169] The great majority of mutations are CRM−, and these probably affect protein folding and stability. Because these mutations result in an absence of secreted factor VIII, and *in vitro* functional studies depend on analysis of the protein produced in eukaryotic cells after transfection with factor VIII cDNA, the mechanisms of action of these mutations are difficult to elucidate.

CpG Dinucleotide Hypermutability. A general mutation hotspot exists in human genomic DNA at CpG dinucleotides in which the canonical mutation is either a CG-to-TG, or, if the C-T substitution occurs in the antisense strand, a CG-to-CA substitution.[173–175] These CG dinucleotides are the only general hotspot known, and the mutations occur because cytosine residues 5′ to guanine are the only methylation site in mammalian DNA. These cytosines are methylated by a methyltransferase to produce 5-methylcytosine. When 5-methylcytosine is spontaneously deaminated in a nonenzymatic reaction, thymine is produced. Canonical CG-to-TG or CG-to-CA substitutions account for 38 percent of the point mutations observed in the factor VIII gene after unbiased scanning of the exons for mutations in patients (32/84).[90,137a] They account for 25 to 40 percent of the mutations observed in a wide variety of other human genes (see reference 176 and Chap. 13), and are estimated to be 10 to 20 times more frequent than mutations at other dinucleotides.[177]

Splicing Errors. Despite the factor VIII gene containing 50 splice junctions (25 donor sites and 25 acceptor sites), mutations leading to splicing errors are uncommon. Only 25 of 572 point mutations (4 percent) are present in splice junctions or consensus sequences, and are likely to cause splicing defects.

General Lessons from the Study of Factor VIII Mutations

The factor VIII gene was one of the first large genes with a high rate of new mutation studied at the molecular level. Some general lessons concerning human mutation have been learned from this experience. These lessons regarding our genome include:

1. It supports long-range rearrangements after mispairing of homologous sequences and recombination;
2. It contains a hypermutable dinucleotide, CpG;
3. It supports retrotransposition of DNA sequences by a "copy and paste" mechanism; and
4. Some mechanism recognizes nonsense mutations in exons, sometimes resulting in exon skipping.

FACTOR VIII INHIBITORS

Development of inhibitors to factor VIII occurs predominantly, but not exclusively, in severely affected patients (factor VIII:C and factor VIII:Ag undetectable) after treatment with factor VIII. The phenomenon is a fairly typical immune response to foreign protein, in that several doses are required to produce a maximum response. Most such antibodies are IgG subtype 4.[178] Epitope mapping shows that specificities against the heavy chain, or light chain, or both, can be detected in different patients.[179] The most common factor VIII epitopes that induce inhibitors are localized to the A2 domain (residues 373 to 740), the C2 domain (2173 to 2332) and possibly the A3 domain.[180–185] Because only a few regions of factor VIII appear to be antigenic, attempts have been made to engineer less-immunogenic factor VIII by recombinant DNA technology. Lollar *et al.* found that a human factor VIII with residues 484 to 508 replaced by porcine residues was less reactive to antifactor VIII inhibitors.[186] Other than neutralization of infused factor VIII, no additional immune-complex-type pathology occurs. A relationship to HLA subtype BFF, C4A4, and C4B2 was detected in one survey.[187] Recently, Lippert and colleagues[188] found a highly significant association between inhibitor formation and HLA class II genes but no association with HLA-DR. Likewise, Aly *et al.*[189] found a strong association between HLA-Cw5 and inhibitors (16 of 16) in their survey of 44 patients, but no linkage to HLA-DR. Conversely, Simmoney *et al.*[190] detected an association between inhibitors and HLA-DR4. All these surveys involved rather small numbers of patients, but an association with the HLA class II locus seems likely.

Familial incidence of antibodies was noted before the recent molecular genetic analysis of hemophilia A. From the published database of mutations, it is now possible to draw some inferences about mutational associations with inhibitor development. In the recent consortium analysis of more than 900 patients with factor VIII inversions, 130 of 642 studied (20 percent) had developed inhibitors. In severe hemophilia A patients without inhibitors, 131 of 821 (16 percent) developed inhibitors. This result suggests that inversions are not a specific predisposing factor for inhibitor production.

Nearly all other reported patients with inhibitors have nonsense mutations or deletions in their factor VIII gene. The incidence varies for different sites; R336X is associated with inhibitors in 0 of 8 cases, R2116X in 0 of 9, R1941X in 8 of 11, R2147X in 3 of 8, and R2209X in 6 of 16. The low incidence for R336X and R2116X may be explained by exon skipping, which has been observed specifically in the processed mRNA for these mutations,[166] giving rise to factor VIII merely lacking 20 to 50 amino acids in sufficient quantity to induce tolerance to most of the factor VIII sequence (see above).

Patients with gross deletions (>2 kb) in the factor VIII gene, have two to three times the incidence of inhibitors as patients without detectable deletions.[137,191]

Mild hemophilia A is almost always associated with missense mutations and a very low incidence of inhibitors (only 10 cases have been reported with low levels of inhibitor). Perhaps the missense mutations in these cases create local structural variations such that the wild-type sequence presents an immunogenic epitope.

CARRIER AND ANTENATAL DIAGNOSIS

At present, the two inversions mentioned above are easily detectable by Southern blotting and account for approximately 40 percent of factor VIII mutations in families seeking genetic counseling. Recently, a technique to detect the inversions by PCR analysis of genomic DNA was reported that could have a significant impact on the speed of carrier diagnosis.[192] In early

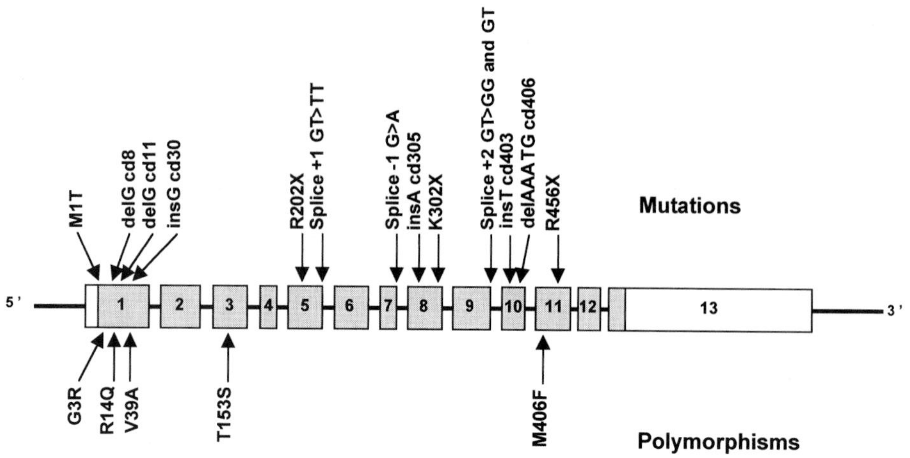

Fig. 172-17 Mutations and polymorphisms of the ERG1C-53 gene in combined deficiency of factor V and factor VIII. The location and the type of 13 disease-producing mutations is shown above the gene structure. Five polymorphisms are depicted below the genes.

1998, the DNA diagnostic lab at the University of Pennsylvania began offering analysis of point mutations in the factor VIII gene. The lab uses PCR amplification of all exons and conformation-sensitive gel electrophoresis,[193] a form of heteroduplex analysis, to screen for mutations. Among the first 45 inversion-negative-affected males studied, a mutation was identified in 42 (93 percent). Inversion testing and direct mutation analysis have greatly altered our ability to provide exact counseling for nearly all families that have one or more cases of hemophilia A. However, the cost of direct mutation analysis is still high and its availability is limited to a small number of labs. It is hoped that the use of high-density oligonucleotide arrays[194] ("chips") will soon permit more rapid and less expensive detection of factor VIII mutations.

Meanwhile, carrier and antenatal diagnosis by DNA analysis can still be carried out using indirect detection via linked DNA polymorphisms. The affected factor VIII gene is tracked in these families using DNA polymorphisms both within the gene (BclI, XbaI, BglI restriction site polymorphisms)[195,196] and outside the gene.[197,198] Simple sequence repeats (CAn repeats) present in two introns of the gene are also valuable in this process.[199,200] Nearly all families are informative with one or more DNA polymorphism, but 20 to 30 percent of families are informative for extragenic polymorphisms only. In these families, the chance of error in the diagnosis is 2 to 3 percent in some, and 4 to 6 percent in others, depending on the number of meioses in question. When an intragenic polymorphism is used for the diagnosis of carrier or affected status, the chance of an error is < 1 percent.

In families with only one affected male who does not carry an inversion, however, there is often further uncertainty in determining carrier status by linkage analysis, and one must often rely heavily on biochemical determinations of factor VIII levels for determination of carrier status. Because of uncertainty of carrier status in those females whose tests fall into an inconclusive range, this approach is unsatisfactory and often leads to an uncertain status for potential carriers. This problem further highlights the usefulness of direct mutation analysis. When the mutation causing hemophilia A is characterized in the affected male, its presence or absence in a female relative of the patient can easily be determined.

As of 1999, hundreds of families have undergone carrier and antenatal diagnosis for factor VIII deficiency by DNA analysis, with generally satisfactory results and a minimum of error. Although exact numbers of pregnancy terminations for affected fetuses are hard to obtain, a sizable percentage of couples (perhaps 50 percent) who underwent antenatal diagnosis and were informed that their fetus was affected, decided to carry the pregnancy to term. Now that one can determine the causative mutation in essentially all patients within 4 weeks, the ability to analyze any family member for that mutation should have a major effect on the genetic counseling for this important condition.

COMBINED DEFICIENCIES OF FACTORS V and VIII

Combined deficiencies of factors V and VIII (F5F8D) is an autosomal recessive disorder described in 1954.[201] A total of 89 patients in 58 families, 24 of whom originate from the Mediterranean Basin, have been reported. Patients have excessive blood loss after dental extraction or other surgery, epistaxes, and large bruises. A few cases have had hemarthroses or muscle hematomas. Treatment with fresh frozen plasma is effective. Factor VIII concentrates contain insufficient factor V to be effective. The patients have factor V and factor VIII activity and antigen levels in the range of 5 to 30 percent. All other plasma protein concentrations are normal. Recently, homozygosity mapping, a method proposed by Lander and Botstein,[202] and positional cloning were successful in identifying the location of the defective gene.[203,204] Analysis of 14 patients from nine unrelated families mapped the gene to the long arm of chromosome 18. Positional cloning identified the responsible gene as ERGIC-53.[205] In the original nine families, only two mutations were found. However, subsequent studies identified 13 mutant alleles accounting for 52 (74 percent) of 70 mutant ERGIC-53 genes examined (Fig. 172-17). Interestingly, all the mutations identified produce null alleles; they are nonsense, frameshift, splice site, and initiation codon mutants.[205,206] In some families with combined deficiency of factors V and VIII, ERGIC-53 levels are normal and no mutations were detected. Thus, it is likely that mutations in at least one additional gene produce the combined factor V and VIII deficiency phenotype.

ERGIC-53 encodes a 53-kDa transmembrane protein in the ER-Golgi intermediate compartment (hence, ERGIC-53) with mannose-binding capability and the capability to cycle between the ER and Golgi.[207,208] Lymphocytes of patients with combined factor V and VIII deficiency lack the ERGIC-53 protein.[205] ERGIC-53 has the properties of a protein chaperone between the ER and Golgi, but it appears that the protein acts selectively on the intracellular transport and secretion of factors V and VIII. Both of these coagulation factors contain the heavily glycosylated B domain, suggesting the ERGIC-53 may interact with the B domain of these factors.

TREATMENT OF HEMOPHILIA A

The mainstay of treatment is replacement therapy by means of intravenous infusion with factor VIII. Until 7 years ago, all factor VIII used was blood-derived (Table 172-2). Now two recombinant products are licensed. Ideally, all severely affected patients are maintained on long-term prophylaxis with daily or alternate-day infusions to keep spontaneous hemorrhages to a minimum. This is impossible for most patients owing to limitations of supply and

Table 172-2 Therapeutic Materials for Treatment of Hemophilia A

Material	Factor VIII (U/ml)	vWF (U/ml)	Donors per Unit	Advantages	Disadvantages
Cryoprecipitate	5–10	5–10	1	Low infection hazard (unless many units used); simple to prepare.	Storage at −20°C. Allergic reactions. Not virus-inactivated. Potency not assayed.
Heat or solvent detergent treated factor VIII concentrate	20–50	20–50	3,000–15,000	Assayed higher potency, HIV and hepatitis B and C infectivity. Store at 4°C. Few allergic reactions.	Heavy load of non-factor-VIII proteins, including B_2-microglobulin iso-anti-A, anti-B, β-microglobulin, fibrinogen, etc. Falling CD4 count in HIV-positive patients.
DDAVP	—	—	0	No infection risk as totally synthetic.	Only effective in mild cases.
High-purity plasma-derived factor VIII	~5000 U/mg*	0	3000–15,000	Convenience. Preserves CD4 count in HIV-positive cases.	High cost;? increased incidence of inhibitors.
Recombinant factor VIII	~5000 U/mg*	0	0	No infectious risk. Totally pure.	High cost;? increased incidence of inhibitors.

* Before addition of albumen carrier.

finance. Because the half-life of factor VIII is 8 to 12 h, twice-daily infusions are needed to maintain a normal level at all times. However, for prophylactic purposes, a fairly wide fluctuation is still very effective. In practice, most patients are treated on demand, which means that they receive an infusion of factor at the first symptom of bleeding. Patients become skilled at recognizing very early joint bleeding and, provided that an infusion of factor VIII is given within a few minutes to 1 h of onset, the bleeding can be halted before a significant amount of blood has leaked into a joint. Normal activities can then be resumed almost immediately.

It was realized in the 1960s that such prompt treatment could only be achieved if the patient or the patient's relatives gave the injection. Therefore, home therapy programs were instituted, leading to a dramatic reduction in time lost from school or work, as well as a dramatic reduction in the onset of new joint damage and the progression of old joint damage. Severely affected patients who have grown up under this regimen are now reaching their twenties with little arthritis. This result is in sharp contrast to the situation in older patients or patients from developing countries, nearly all of whom have severe damage in several joints. However, it is becoming clear that to completely prevent joint damage a high-dose prophylactic regimen is necessary (L. Aledort, personal communication).

The dosage of factor VIII is adjusted to obtain a desired level in the circulation (Table 172-3). Formulas based on plasma volume and expected recovery give a rough guide to dosage, but where the level is critical, as for surgery or in case of serious bleeding, it should always be checked by assay after infusion. On average, factor VIII infusion produces a plasma increment of 2 U/dl per unit infused per kilogram body weight. From this a simple formula can be derived:

$$\text{Dose to be infused (units)} = \text{weight(kg)} \times \text{increment needed (U/dl)}/2.0.$$

Assessing the period of treatment required is a matter of clinical judgment with respect to the individual episode or lesion. An early joint bleed often resolves with a single infusion. For surgery other than very minor procedures, treatment needs to be continued at full dosage twice daily, adjusted according to pre- and posttreatment assays, for a week or more, followed by a period of treatment at reduced dosage during convalescence.

Detailed discussion of the orthopedic management of hemophilic arthropathy is beyond the scope of this chapter; the reader is referred to the texts on comprehensive care.[209–211] Suffice it to say, a large number of patients have had total hip or knee joint replacements with good results and arthrodesis of the knee or

Table 172-3 Plasma Levels of Factor VIII Required for Hemostasis

Clinical Indication	Plasma Factor VIII (U/dl)	Dosage (U/kg)
Early hemarthrosis or muscle bleeding	15–20	8–10
More severe bleeding, minor trauma	30–50	15–25
Surgery, major trauma, head injury	80–120	40–60

ankle can provide pain relief and improved locomotion where arthroplasty is impractical.

Physical therapy plays a very important role in maintaining and improving the function of joints and muscles damaged or weakened by bleeding and enforced periods of immobilization.

Factor VIII concentrate, with its advantages of storage, convenience, and assayed potency, is the material of choice in severe hemophilia and in the treatment of major bleeding where it is essential to maintain high levels. The realization that it carries a risk of infection (see "Complications of Therapy" below) has given rise to intensive and by now successful efforts to use inactive viruses in concentrate, use recombinant factor VIII, and use a non-blood-derived alternative, DDAVP (desamino-D-arginine vasopressin). This synthetic analogue of vasopressin was noted to cause a rise in factor VIII and vWF levels without pressor effects. DDAVP retains the antidiuretic action of natural vasopressin and also stimulates the release of vascular plasminogen activator. In practice, these effects can be used to elevate the plasma factor VIII level to two to four times baseline, presumably by inducing release from a storage site(s).

Given together with a fibrinolytic inhibitor such as tranexamic acid (to neutralize the fibrinolytic stimulus), DDAVP can correct the hemostatic defect in mild hemophilia A or von Willebrand disease well enough to cover minor surgery or treat a minor bleeding episode. A typical regimen is to give 0.3 mg per kilogram body weight by slow intravenous infusion over 20 min together with 1 g of tranexamic acid. The effect reaches a maximum at 1 h, at which point, for example, the factor VIII level in a mild hemophiliac may have risen from 10 to 40 U/dl. The half-life of the endogenously released factor VIII is about 8 h, and repeat doses can be given, but with progressively diminishing response. The maximum useful number of doses is 3 doses in 24 h, after which a rest period is needed to enable stores to reaccumulate. Fibrinolytic inhibition is also useful for management of oral and intestinal tract bleeding. It must be strictly avoided when there is upper urinary tract bleeding, because it can cause obstructive nephropathy and acute renal failure owing to mechanical outflow occlusion by blood clots.

Complications of Therapy

Management of Inhibitors. Routine testing for factor VIII inhibitors is always performed before elective surgery and regularly at follow-up in severe cases. Laboratory tests for antibody rely on neutralization of clotting activity in mixtures of normal and patient plasma. Because the plasma concentration of factor VIII is very low (200 ng/ml, or 0.5 nM), it is necessary to prolong the incubation of the mixture to attain equilibrium binding of antibody to antigen. This test is standardized to Bethesda units,[212] 1 unit being the amount of antibody that neutralizes 50 percent of the factor VIII in 1 ml of normal plasma after 2 h incubation at 37°C. Three aspects of an individual patient's antibody are of clinical importance: the level in units at the time of treatment, the type of immune response to infusion of factor VIII (low or high), and whether there is cross-reaction with porcine factor VIII. When the antibody titer is low (Table 172-4), treatment can consist of an increased dose of factor, so that enough factor remains after the circulating inhibitor is neutralized to give a hemostatic level. In some patients, the level of antibody remains low to moderate (low responders), but in others, treatment with factor VIII elicits a sharp "anamnestic" response (high

Table 172-4 Guidelines for Treatment of Patients with Factor VIII Inhibitors

Inhibitor Level (BU/ml)*			
Antihuman	Antiorcina	Type of Therapeutic Responder	Strategies
1–5	1–5	Low	Human factor VIII at increased dosage
		High	1. Institute immune-tolerance-inducing regimen 2. Human factor VIII at high dose first, then as below
5–13	1–5	Low	Porcine factor VIII for all bleeds
		High, developing antiporcine antibodies	1. Factor VIIa or activated factor complex for minor bleeds 2. Attempt to induce tolerance
>13	>13	High	1. Treat bleeds with factor VIIa or activated factor complex 2. Plasmapheresis with extracorporeal antibody binding column for severe bleeds, then high-dose human or porcine factor VIII 3. Attempt to induce tolerance

* BU = Bethesda units.

responders). The low responders can be treated repeatedly with human or porcine factor VIII, but high responders become refractory; thus, alternative therapies were developed. Most often, the antibody is species-specific to human factor VIII and has little or no cross-reactivity with porcine factor VIII.

When the factor VIII inhibitor titer rises sharply to hundreds or even thousands of units per milliliter, factor VIII therapy is ineffective. In this situation, an alternative strategy is to attempt to bypass factor VIII with partly activated mixtures of the vitamin K-dependent factors. Conventional factor IX concentrate contains activated species (and is, in fact, liable to produce thrombosis, particularly in patients with liver damage). Controlled trials have shown it to be more effective than albumin solution in hastening recovery from a hemarthrosis. More effective are the deliberately activated coagulation factor mixtures FEIBA and AUTOPLEX. It is not clear what the active principle in these products consists of, nor how to monitor the response by blood tests. Empirical dosage regimens are established and these products are strikingly effective on some occasions but they do fail to control bleeding on other occasions. Elective surgical procedures should not be attempted based on treatment with these products. Recently, recombinant factor VIIa was used for these patients, with excellent results in most cases, along with a few failures. Doses are high, and there is a risk of inducing generalized coagulation activation in the presence of infection.[213]

Induction of immune tolerance has been attempted on many occasions. Immunosuppressive agents, such as glucocorticoids and alkylating agents, are of no benefit (although probably valuable for treatment of spontaneous acquired autoantibodies to factor VIII). Brackman[214] demonstrated that a megadose regimen of factor VIII infusion continued over many months is effective in abolishing inhibitory antibodies in over 90 percent of cases. In the long-term, a medium intermittent dose regimen is also fairly effective in blunting or abolishing immune response to factor VIII.[215] Various schemes have been proposed for inducing specific immune tolerance, but no consistently successful protocol has been reported. Infusion of intravenous gamma-globulin has been successful in temporarily lowering inhibitor titers,[216] presumably through the action of anti-idiotypic antibodies.

Recently, intensive observation of previously untreated patients after exposure to new, high-purity (recombinant or plasma-derived) factor VIII revealed a disturbingly high incidence of inhibitors (up to 30 percent).[217] The implications of this observation are debatable, but inhibitor development after recombinant factor VIII treatment is presently the subject of well-controlled studies.

The multiplicity of therapies proposed and the space devoted to this topic reflect the lack of any universally successful regimen and the large amount of time, expense, and effort required for the management of these unfortunate patients. For further details, the reviews of Kasper[218] and Bloom[178] should be consulted.

Viruses Transmitted by Factor VIII Concentrates. Multiple-donor concentrates were introduced in the late 1960s. Very soon thereafter, it was noted that a high incidence of hepatitis occurred in patients treated with them, and that the newly discovered Australia antigen was present in most attacks. Most older patients now test positive for hepatitis B antibody or are chronically antigen-positive. During the 1970s, despite screening of blood for hepatitis B antigen, both acute and chronic hepatitis continued to appear in hemophiliacs, and it was realized that this was mainly due to another virus, now known to be hepatitis C. Up to half of hemophiliacs have chronically or intermittently elevated liver enzymes[219] that developed after a first attack of hepatitis C; this disease may cause a very severe acute episode before converting to chronicity. Liver biopsies show characteristic histologic features[220] and chronic active or chronic persistent hepatitis in a high proportion of cases.[219] The long-term effect of this process is eventual liver failure.[220] Prevention of hepatitis B is now assured by vaccinating all nonimmune patients. The management of chronic viral hepatitis, especially when there is coexisting delta agent, includes interferon, which is effective in suppressing biochemical signs of hepatitis in approximately 25 percent of cases. Whether this treatment will prevent eventual liver failure or hepatocarcinoma remains to be seen.

The first hemophilic patient to develop AIDS was reported from the United States in 1983. Retrospective surveys of stored blood serum of hemophiliacs in the UK and in the United States show that seroconversion to HIV-antibody-positive began in 1978. Currently, all factor concentrates are from HIV-antibody-negative plasma and are treated with heat or solvent detergent, which successfully prevents transmission. Tragically, 30 to 90 percent of hemophiliacs (the rate varies in different countries) were infected by HIV before the cause of AIDS and the means of avoiding it were discovered. The conversion rate of HIV-antibody-positive patients to clinical AIDS is similar for hemophiliacs and other high risk groups (70 percent conversion rate at 11 years).[221]

AIDS has now become the most common cause of death in hemophilia A. The only clinical point of difference between AIDS in hemophiliacs and in other high-risk groups is that Kaposi's sarcoma is very uncommon in hemophiliacs. Surveys of the families of HIV-antibody-positive hemophiliacs show that up to 5 percent of wives and sexual partners test positive, but that no other household contacts do. Several wives of hemophiliacs have died of AIDS. This devastating situation has thrown a great strain on patients, their families, and those who care for them. Intensive counseling and treatment of the condition, once it develops, with AZT, protease inhibitors, and appropriate antimicrobials for infections, are all that can be offered at present. Patients have been strongly advised to use barrier contraception if they test positive.

PROSPECTS FOR GENE THERAPY

Hemophilia A is considered a suitable condition for gene therapy for several reasons. Because the protein acts in the circulation, any convenient tissue or site can be targeted for expression, provided the protein is exported to plasma. *In vitro* studies show that a wide variety of cell types will make functional factor VIII, including fibroblasts, endothelial cells, hepatocytes, and kidney-derived cell lines. Tight control of expression levels is not essential, and a partial correction, for example, from 0 to 5 percent, will bring substantial relief to the clinical phenotype. Present treatments, although effective, are inconvenient to administer and expensive.

The argument against gene therapy for hemophilia A is that the disease is not usually lethal and that replacement therapy is effective, with a long history of success. Therefore, gene therapy will need to be completely free of harmful side effects, a stricture that few therapies of any kind can meet.

The most worrisome aspects of current approaches to gene therapy based on retroviral or adenovirus-associated vectors (AAV) are the potentials for insertional mutagenesis and for reversion of the virus to replication competence. Furthermore, studies in mice, where retroviral vectors have been used to transfer a factor VIII cDNA to fibroblasts and to hematopoietic progenitor cells, have shown either no expression or short-lived expression of factor VIII.[200] Nevertheless, the field of gene therapy is extremely active, new strategies are being devised almost weekly, and advances are being made.

Animal models have been developed to evaluate therapeutic regimens and to study factor VIII *in vivo*. Several natural dog colonies with hemophilia A have been propagated, and targeted disruption of the factor VIII gene has been used to produce a mouse model with severe factor VIII deficiency.[222] Two mice strains, carrying disruptions of either exon 16 or exon 17, have < 1 percent factor VIII activity and do not survive the minor trauma of tail snipping. However, affected mice usually do not bleed spontaneously, and affected females have been bred with affected males to produce a strain in which every animal is affected.[223] Assay of cryoprecipitate from the plasma of affected mice using a monoclonal antibody failed to detect factor VIII light chain.[223] These mice provide an excellent small-animal model of the disease, and have been used in a number of labs studying potential gene-therapy protocols.

A number of different vector backbones and delivery systems have been contemplated for gene therapy of hemophilia A. For factor IX delivery, AAV vectors have been particularly successful in affected mice and dogs. The factor IX gene is sufficiently small to fit the capacity of the AAV backbone (4.7 kb), and intramuscular injection of the gene in an AAV backbone has not led to immunogenic response.[224] Although the long-term levels achieved by this approach are low, they are still corrective of the bleeding phenotype in the animals. Gene therapy in humans with factor IX deficiency was initiated using this vector system in 1999. Gene therapy for factor VIII deficiency using AAV vectors has not advanced so swiftly. Because of the large size of the factor VIII cDNA, it has been difficult to effectively insert an active factor VIII gene (the B domainless cDNA) in the AAV backbone. Intramuscular injection of separate AAV vectors containing portions of the factor VIII B domainless cDNA (heavy chain and light chain segments) has not been very successful, but has shown promise when the vectors are delivered to the liver by portal vein injection. In one study, adenoviral delivery to liver of human factor VIII B domainless cDNA under the control of a liver specific promoter led to long-term correction of the factor VIII-deficient mice.[225] In other work, adenoviral delivery to liver, especially after immune suppression with antibodies to block the T-cell response to both vector and foreign antigen (factor VIII) has led to long-term, low-level correction.[226] Transgenic experiments using affected mice demonstrate that the epidermis is also a potential site for factor VIII gene delivery. In these experiments, factor VIII deficiency was corrected by transplanted skin expressing factor VIII protein.[226a] In summary, although many problems still require overcoming, the future of gene therapy for factor VIII deficiency appears brighter than ever, leading to the prediction of successful clinical trials in the near-term.

HEMOPHILIA A IN FEMALES

Hemophilia A is very rare in females; yet a number of biologic bases exist for the observation. If the frequency of affected males in the population is 1 in 5000, and up to one-third of affected males result from new mutations occurring in females who are not carriers of the disease, then about 1 in 7000 males inherit the disease from a carrier female. Because carrier females have a 1 in 2 chance of having an affected male with each pregnancy, the incidence of carrier females is approximately 1 in 3500. A true homozygous female will result from matings of affected males and carrier females, with an incidence of 1 in every 2 female offspring. Thus, the general population frequency of homozygous affected females is approximately $(1/7000) \times (1/3500) \times (1/2)$, or about 1 in 50 million females. Such cases have been described.[227–229]

Another cause of hemophilia in a phenotypic female is a defective factor VIII gene in an XO, or Turner syndrome, female.[230] In such females, Turner syndrome should be suspected on the basis of the typical dysmorphic features, including short stature, webbed neck, and shield chest.

A potentially more frequent cause of hemophilia A in a female is inappropriate lyonization such that by chance, the X chromosome bearing the mutant factor VIII gene in a female heterozygote is the active X chromosome in the vast majority of factor VIII-producing cells in the liver.

A fourth cause of hemophilia A in a female is an X-autosome translocation involving a breakpoint within the factor VIII gene.[162] Because cells with one or three copies of autosomal genes are at a survival disadvantage to those with two copies of all autosomal genes, the normal X chromosome is the inactive X in all cells in females carrying such an X-autosome translocation. Because the factor VIII gene is very close to the telomere of the long arm of the X chromosome, translocations involving the factor VIII gene and the tip of an autosomal arm are cryptic and impossible to detect by conventional cytogenetic analysis. This type of translocation, although rarely reported to date, could be a significant contributor to the incidence of females with hemophilia A.

A fifth possible cause of hemophilia A in a female is uniparental isodisomy, the inheritance of two copies of one chromosomal homologue of a pair from one parent and no copies of that chromosome from the other parent. In this instance, uniparental isodisomy requires inheritance in an affected female of two copies of the X chromosome bearing a factor VIII mutation from her carrier mother. Such a female, who is homozygous for all genes on the X chromosome, may not be viable. Isodisomy has been observed in one case of male-to-male transmission of hemophilia A; an affected male passed both his X chromosome and his Y chromosome to his affected son, who received no sex chromosome from his mother.[231]

REFERENCES

1. Bulloch W, Fildes P: *Haemophilia*, in *Treasury of Human Inheritance Parts V and VI, Eugenics Laboratory Memoirs*, Vol 12. London, Dulau, 1911, p 173.
2. Rosner F: Hemophilia in the Talmud and Rabbinic writings. *Ann Intern Med* **70**:833, 1969.
3. Alsaharavius: Liber Theoricae Necnon Practicae Alsaharavii ... qui Vulgo caravius Dicitur; Jam....Deprompttus in Lucem. tractatus XXXI, sectio II, capitulum XV, folio CXLV. Augsburg, published by S. Grim and M. Vuirsung, 1519. Translated from the original Arabic into Latin by Paul Ricius.
4. Otto JC: *An Account of an Haemorrhagic Disposition Existing in Certain Families* vol. 6, no. 1. New York, The Medical Repository, 1803, p 1.
5. Major M: *Classic Descriptions of Disease* 3rd ed. Springfield, IL, Charles C Thomas, 1945, p 521. (Reproduction of J. C. Otto's classic paper, with a short biographical note on Otto.)
6. Hay J: An account of a remarkable haemorrhagic disposition existing in many individuals of the same family. *N Engl J Med Surg* (Boston) **2**:221, 1813.
7. Osler W: Haemophilia, in *Pepper's System of Medicine* vol. 3. London, Lea Brothers & Co., 1885, p 933.
8. Hopff F: *Ueber die Haemophilie oder die erbliche Anlage zu todtlichen Blutungen* [Inaugural Dissertation]. Wurzburg, Germany, Wurzburg University, 1828.
9. Bateson W: *Mendel's Principles of Heredity.* Cambridge, Cambridge University Press, 1909, p 222.
10. McKusick VA: The Royal hemophilia. *Sci Am* **213**:88, 1965.
11. Wright AE: On a method of determining the condition of blood coagulability for clinical and experimental purposes and on the effect of the administration of calcium salts in haemophilia and actual or threatened haemorrhage. *BMJ* **2**:223, 1893.
12. Addis T: Hereditary haemophilia: Deficiency in the coagulability of the blood the only immediate cause of the condition. *QJM* **4**:14, 1910.
13. Addis T: The pathogenesis of hereditary haemophilia. *J Pathol Bacteriol* **15**:427, 1911.
14. Morawitz P: Die Chemie der Blutgerinnung. *Adv Anat Embryol Cell Biol* **4**:307, 1905.
15. Govaerts P, Gratia A: Contribution a l'etude de l'hemophilie. *Rev Belg Sci Med* **3**:689, 1931.
16. Quick AJ, Stanley-Brown M, Bancroft FW: A study of the coagulation defect in hemophilia and in jaundice. *Am J Med Sci* **190**:501, 1935.
17. Repke K, Gemmell CH, Guha A, Turitto VT, Broze GJ, Nemerson Y: Hemophilia as a defect of the tissue factor pathway of blood coagulation. Effect of factors VIII and IX on factor X activation in a continuous flow reactor. *Proc Natl Acad Sci U S A* **87**:7623, 1990.
18. Morawitz P, Lossen J: Ueber Hamophilie. *Deutsch Arch Klin Med* (Leipzig) Bd. **XCIV**:S.110, 1908.
19. Sahli H: Ueber das Wesen der Haemophilie. *Z Klin Med* (Berlin) Bd. **LVI**:S.264, 1904.
20. Patek AJJ, Taylor FHL: Hemophilia II. Some properties of a substance obtained from normal human plasma effective in accelerating the coagulation of hemophilic blood. *J Clin Invest* **16**:113, 1937.
21. Lewis JH, Tagnon HJ, Davidson CS, Minot GR, Taylor FHL: The relation of certain fractions of the plasma globulins to the coagulation defect in hemophilia. *Blood* **1**:166, 1946.

22. Merskey C: The laboratory diagnosis of haemophilia. *J Clin Pathol* **3**:301, 1950.
23. Merskey C, MacFarlane RG: The female carrier of haemophilia: A clinical and laboratory study. *Lancet* **1**:487, 1951.
24. Aggeler PM, White SG, Glendening MB, Page EW, Leake TB, Bates B: Plasma thromboplastin component (PTC) deficiency: A new disease resembling haemophilia. *Proc Soc Exp Biol Med* **79**:692, 1952.
25. Biggs R, Douglas AS, Macfarlane RG, Dacie JV, Pitney WR, Merskey C, O'Brien JR: Christmas disease: A condition previously mistaken for haemophilia. *BMJ* **2**:1378, 1952.
26. Schulman I, Smith CH: Hemorrhagic disease in an infant due to deficiency of a previously undescribed clotting factor. *Blood* **7**:794, 1952.
27. Wright IS: The nomenclature of blood clotting factors. *Thromb Diath Haemorrh* **7**:381, 1962.
28. Owen WG, Wagner RH: Antihemophilic factor: Separation of an active fragment following dissociation by salts or detergents. *Thromb Diath Haemorrh* **27**:502, 1972.
29. Zimmerman TS, Ratnoff OD, Powell AE: Immunologic differentiation of classic haemophilia (factor VIII deficiency) and von Willebrand's disease. *J Clin Invest* **50**:244, 1971.
30. Zimmerman TS, Edgington TS: Factor VIII coagulant activity and factor VIII like antigen: Independent molecular entities. *J Exp Med* **138**:1015, 1973.
31. Tuddenham EGD, Trabold NS, Collins JA, Hoyer LW: The properties of factor VIII coagulant activity prepared by immunoadsorbent chromatography. *J Lab Clin Med* **93**:40, 1979.
32. Fass DN, Knutson GJ, Katzmann JA: Monoclonal antibodies to porcine factor VIII coagulant and their use in the isolation of active coagulant protein. *Blood* **59**:594, 1982.
33. Vehar GA, Keyt B, Eaton D, Rodriguez H, O'Brien DP, Rotblat F, Oppermann H, Keck R, Wood WI, Harkins RN, Tuddenham EGD, Lawn RM, Capon DJ: Structure of human factor VIII. *Nature* **312**:337, 1984.
34. Wood WI, Capon DJ, Simonsen CC, Eaton DL, Gitschier J, Keyt B, Seeburg PH, Smith DL, Hollingshead P, Wion KL, Delwart E, Tuddenham EGD, Vehar GA, Lawn RM: Expression of active human factor VIII from recombinant DNA clones. *Nature* **312**:330, 1984.
35. Toole JJ, Knopf JL, Wozney JM, Sultzman LA, Buecker JL, Pittman DD, Kaufman RJ, Brown E, Shoemaker C, Orr EC, Amphlett GW, Foster WB, Coe ML, Knutson GJ, Fass DN, Hewick RM: Molecular cloning of a cDNA encoding human antihaemophilic factor. *Nature* **312**:342, 1984.
36. Rizza CR, Spooner RJD: Treatment of haemophilia and related disorders in Britain and Northern Ireland during 1976-80: Report on behalf of the directors of Haemophilia Centres in the United Kingdom. *BMJ* **286**:929, 1983.
37. Massie R, Massie S: *Journey.* New York, Knopf, 1973.
38. Mazurier C: von Willebrand's disease masquerading as haemophilia A. *Thromb Haemost* **67**:391, 1992.
39. Gitschier J, Wood WI, Goralka TM, Wion KL, Chen EY, Eaton DE, Vehar GA, Capon DJ, Lawn RM: Characterization of the human factor VIII gene. *Nature* **312**:326, 1984.
39a. Naylor JA, Buck D, Green P, Williamson H, Bentley D, Giannelli F: Investigation of the factor VIII intron 22 repeated region (int22h) and the associated inversion junctions. *Hum Mol Genet* **4**:1217, 1995.
40. Levinson B, Kenwrick S, Lakich D, Hammonds G, Gitschier J: A transcribed gene in an intron of the human factor VIII gene. *Genomics* **7**:1, 1990.
41. Levinson B, Bermingham JR, Metzenberg A, Kenwrick S, Chapman V, Gitschier J: Sequence of the human factor VIII-associated gene is conserved in mouse. *Genomics* **13**:862, 1992.
42. Levinson B, Kenwrick S, Gamel P, Fisher K, Gitschier J: Evidence for a third transcript from the human factor VIII gene. *Genomics* **14**:585, 1992.
43. Wion KL, Kelly D, Summerfield JA, Tuddenham EGD, Lawn RM: Distribution of factor VIII mRNA and antigen in human liver and other tissues. *Nature* **317**:726, 1985.
44. Zelechowska MG, van Mourik JA, Brodniewicz-Proba T: Ultrastructural localization of factor VIII procoagulant antigen in human liver hepatocytes. *Nature* **317**:729, 1985.
44a. Figueiredo MS, Brownlee GG: cis-Acting elements and transcription factors involved in the promoter activity of the human factor VIII gene. *J Biol Chem* **270**:11828, 1995.
44b. McGlynn LK, Mueller CR, Begbie M, Notley CR, Lillicrap D: Role of the liver-enriched transcription factor hepatocyte nuclear factor 1 in transcriptional regulation of the factor V111 gene. *Mol Cell Biol* **16**:1936, 1996.
45. Koschinsky ML, Funk WD, van Ooar BA, MacGillivray TRA: Complete cDNA sequence of human preceruloplasmin. *Proc Natl Acad Sci U S A* **83**:5086, 1986.
46. Kane WH, Davie EW: Cloning of a cDNA coding for human factor V, a blood coagulation factor homologous to factor VIII and ceruloplasmin. *Proc Natl Acad Sci U S A* **83**:800, 1986.
47. Kane WH, Ichinose A, Hagen FS, Davie EW: Cloning of cDNAs coding for the heavy chain region and connecting region of human factor V, a blood coagulation factor with four types of repeats. *Biochemistry* **26**:6508, 1987.
48. Stubbs JD, Lekutis C, Singer KL, Bui A, Yuzuki D, Srinivasan U, Parry G: cDNA cloning of a mouse mammary epithelial cell surface protein reveals the existence of epidermal growth factor-like sequences. *Proc Natl Acad Sci U S A* **87**:8417, 1990.
48a. Larocca D, Paterson JA, Urrea R, Kuniyoshi J, Bistrain AM, Cerioni RL: A Mr 46,000 human milk globule protein that is highly expressed in human breast tumours contains factor VIII-like domains. *Cancer Res* **51**:4994, 1991.
48b. Hidai C, Zupancic TJ, Penta K, Mikhail A, Kawana M, Quertermous EE, Aoka Y, Fukagawa M, Matsui Y, Platika DJ, Auerbach R, Hogan BZM, Snodgrass R, Quertermous T: Cloning and characterization of developmental endothelial locus-1; an embryonic endothelial cell protein that binds an $\alpha v\beta 3$ integrin receptor. *Genes Dev* **12**:21, 1998.
48c. Ensslin H, Vogel T, Calvete JJ, Thole HH, Schmidtke J, Matsuda T, Topfer-Petersen E: Molecular cloning and characterization of P47, a novel boar sperm-associated zone pellucida-binding protein homologous to a family of mammalian secretory proteins. *Biol Reprod* **58**:1057, 1998.
49. Elder B, Lakich D, Gitschier J: Sequence of the murine Factor VIII cDNA. *Genomics* **16**:374, 1993.
50. Haldane JBS, Smith CAB: A new estimate of the linkage between the genes for colour-blindness and haemophilia in man. *Ann Eugen* **14**:10, 1947.
51. Boyer SH, Graham JB: Linkage between the X chromosome loci for G6PD electrophoretic variation and hemophilia A. *Am J Hum Genet* **17**:320, 1965.
52. Filippi G, Mannucci PM, Coppola R, Farris A, Rinaldi A, Siniscalco M: Studies on hemophilia A in Sardinia bearing on the problems of multiple allelism, carrier detection and differential mutation rate in the two sexes. *Am J Hum Genet* **36**:44, 1984.
53. Patterson M, Schwartz C, Bell M, Sauer S, Hofker M, Trask B, van den Engh G, Davies KE: Physical mapping studies on the human X chromosome in the region Xq27-Xqter. *Genomics* **1**:297, 1987.
54. Poustka A, Detrich A, Langenstein G, Toniolo D, Warren ST, Lehrach H: Physical map of Xq27-Xqter: Localizing the region of the fragile X mutation. *Proc Natl Acad Sci U S A* **88**:8302, 1991.
55. Freije D, Schlessinger D: A 1.6 mb contig of yeast artificial chromosomes around the human factor VIII gene reveals three regions homologous to probes for the DXS115 locus and two for the DXYS64 locus. *Am J Hum Genet* **51**:66, 1992.
56. Migeon BR, McGinnis MJ, Antonarakis SE, Axelman J, Stasiowski B, Youssoufian H, Keams WG, Chung A, Pearson PL, Kazazian HH Jr, Muneer RS: Severe hemophilia A in a female by cryptic translocation: Order and orientation of factor VIII within Xq28. *Genomics* **16**:20, 1993.
57. Kaufman RJ: Structure and biology of factor VIII, in Hoffman R, Benz EJ, Shattil SJ, Furie B, Cohen HJ (eds): *Hematology: Basic Principles and Practice.* New York, Churchill Livingstone, 1991, p 1276.
58. Kaufman RJ: Biological regulation of Factor VIII activity. *Annu Rev Med* **43**:325, 1992.
58a. Kaufman RJ, Antonarakis SE: Structure, biology and genetics of factor VIII, in Hoffman R, Benz EJ, Shattil SJ, Furie B, Cohen HJ, Silberstein LE (eds). *Hematology; Basic Principles and Practice* 3rd ed. Philadelphia, Churchill Livingstone, 1999, p 1850.
59. van Dieijen G, Tans G, Rosing J, Hemker HC: The role of phospholipid and factor VIIIa in the activation of bovine factor X. *J Biol Chem* **256**:3433, 1981.
60. Kaufman RJ, Wasley LC, Dorner AJ: Synthesis, processing and secretion of recombinant human factor VIII expressed in mammalian cells. *J Biol Chem* **263**:6352, 1988.
61. Weiss HJ, Sussman I, Hoyer LW: Stabilization of factor VIII in plasma by the von Willebrand factor. Studies on posttransfusion and dissociated factor VIII and in patients with von Willebrand disease. *J Clin Invest* **60**:390, 1977.

62. Fulcher CA, Zimmerman TS: Characterization of the human factor VIII procoagulant protein with a heterologous precipitating antibody. *Proc Natl Acad Sci U S A* **79**:1648, 1982.
63. Bontempo FA, Lewis JH, Gorenc TJ, Spero JA, Ragni MV, Scott JP, Starzl TE: Liver transplantation in hemophilia A. *Blood* **68**:1721, 1986.
64. Dorner AJ, Bole DG, Kaufman RJ: The relationship of N-linked glycosylation and heavy chain binding protein association with the secretion of glycoproteins. *J Cell Biol* **105**:2665, 1987.
65. Munro S, Pelham HRB: An Hsp70-like protein in the ER: Identity with the 78-kD glucose-regulated protein and immunoglobulin heavy chain binding protein. *Cell* **46**:291, 1986.
65a. Swaroop M, Moussalli M, Pipe SW, Kaufman RJ: Mutagenesis of a potential BiP binding site enhances secretion of coagulation factor VIII. *J Biol Chem* **272 (39)**:24121, 1997.
65b. Tagliavacca L, Moon N, Dunham WR, Kaufman RJ: Identification and functional requirement of Cu(II) and its ligands within coagulation factor VIII. *J Biol Chem* **272**:27428, 1997.
66. Pittman DD, Wang JH, Kaufman RJ: Identification and functional importance of tyrosine sulfate residues within recombinant factor VIII. *Biochemistry* **31**:3315, 1992.
67. Wise RJ, Dorner AJ, Krane M, Pittman DD, Kaufman RJ: The role of von Willebrand factor multimers and propeptide cleavage in binding and stabilization of factor VIII. *J Biol Chem* **266**:21948, 1991.
67a. Tuddenham EGD, Lane RS, Rotblat F, Johnson AJ, Snape TJ, Middleton S, Kernoff PB: Response to infusions of polyelectrolyte fractionated human factor VIII concentrate in human hemophilia A and von Willebrand's disease. *Br J Haematol* **52**:259, 1982.
67b. Brinkhous KM, Sandberg H, Garris JB, Mattsson C, Palm M, Griggs T, Read MS: Purified human factor VIII procoagulant protein: Comparative hemostatic response after infusions into hemophilic and von Willebrand disease dogs. *Proc Natl Acad Sci U S A* **82**:8752, 1985.
68. Eaton D, Rodriguez H, Vehar GA: Proteolytic processing of human factor VIII. Correlation of specific cleavages by thrombin, factor Xa, and activated protein C with activation and inactivation of factor VIII coagulant activity. *Biochemistry* **25**:505, 1986.
69. Fulcher CA, Roberts JR, Zimmerman TS: Thrombin proteolysis of purified factor VIII. Correlation of activation with generation of a specific polypeptide. *Blood* **61**:807, 1983.
70. Pittman DD, Kaufman RJ: Proteolytic requirements for thrombin activation of antihemophilic factor (factor VIII). *Proc Natl Acad Sci U S A* **85**:2429, 1988.
71. Pittman DD, Kaufman RJ: Structure-function relationships of factor VIII elucidated through recombinant DNA technology. *Thromb Haemost* **61**:161, 1989.
72. Hill-Eubanks DC, Parker CG, Lollar P: Differential proteolytic activation of factor VIII-von Willebrand factor complex by thrombin. *Proc Natl Acad Sci U S A* **86**:6508, 1989.
73. Shima M, Ware J, Yoshioka A, Fukui H, Fulcher CA: An arginine to cysteine amino acid substitution at a critical thrombin cleavage site in a dysfunctional factor VIII molecule. *Blood* **74**:1612, 1989.
74. Gitschier J, Kogan S, Levinson B, Tuddenham EGD: Mutations of factor VIII cleavage sites in hemophilia A. *Blood* **72**:1022, 1988.
75. Pattinson J, Millar DS, McVey J, Grundy CB, Wieland K, Mibashsan RS, Martinowitz U, Tan-Un K, Vidaud M, Goossens M, Sampietro M, Manucci PM, Krawczak M, Reiss J, Zoll B, Whitmore D, Bowcock S, Wensley R, Ajani A, Mitchell V, Rizza C, Maia R, Winter P, Mayne EE, Schwartz M, Green PJ, Kakker VV, Tuddenham EGD, Cooper DN: The molecular genetic analysis of hemophilia A: A directed search strategy for the detection of point mutations in the human factor VIII gene. *Blood* **76**:2242, 1990.
76. Higuchi M, Wong C, Kochhan L, Olek K, Aronis S, Kasper CK, Kazazian HH, Antonarakis SE: Characterization of mutations in the factor VIII gene by direct sequencing of amplified genomic DNA. *Genomics* **6**:65, 1990.
77. Schwaab R, Ludwig M, Kochhan L, Oldenburg J, McVey JH, Egli H, Brackmann HH, Olek K: Detection and characterisation of two missense mutations at a cleavage site in the factor VIII light chain. *Thromb Res* **61**:225, 1991.
78. Arai M, Inaa H, Higuchi M, Antonarakis SE, Kazazian HH, Fujimaki M, Hoyer LW: Detection of a mutation altering a thrombin cleavage site (arginine-372-histidine). *Proc Natl Acad Sci U S A* **86**:4277, 1989.
79. O'Brien D, Pattinson JK, Tuddenham EGD: Purification and characterization of factor VIII 372-cys: A hypofunctional cofactor from a patient with moderately severe hemophilia A. *Blood* **75**:1664, 1990.
80. Arai M, Higuchi M, Antonarakis SE, Kazazian HH, Phillips JA, Janco RL, Hoyer LW: Characterization of a thrombin cleavage site mutation (arg 1689 to cys) in the factor VIII gene of two unrelated patients with cross-reacting material positive hemophilia A. *Blood* **75**:384, 1990.
80a. O'Brien DP, Tuddenham EGD: Purification and characterization of factor VIII 1689Cys: A non-functional cofactor occurring in a patient with severe haemophilia A. *Blood* **73**:2117, 1989.
81. Lollar C, Parker CG: Subunit structure of thrombin-activated porcine factor VIII. *Biochemistry* **28**:666, 1989.
82. Fay PJ, Haidaris PJ, Smudzin TM: Human factor VIIIa subunit structure: Reconstitution of factor VIIIa from the isolated A1/A3-C1-C2 dimer and A2 subunit. *J Biol Chem* **266**:8957, 1991.
83. Lollar P, Parker CG: pH-dependent denaturation of thrombin-activated porcine factor VIII. *J Biol Chem* **265**:1688, 1990.
84. Lollar P, Parker ET: Structural basis for the decreased procoagulant activity of human factor VIII compared to the porcine homolog. *J Biol Chem* **266**:12481, 1991.
85. Pittman DD, Millenson M, Marquette K, Bauer K, Kaufman RJ: The A2 domain of human recombinant derived factor VIII is required for procoagulant activity but not for thrombin cleavage. *Blood* **79**:389, 1992.
86. Eaton DL, Wood WI, Eaton D, Hass PE, Hollingshead P, Wion K, Mather J, Lawn RM, Vehar GA, Gorman C: Construction and characterization of an active factor VIII variant lacking the central one-third of the molecule. *Biochemistry* **25**:8343, 1987.
87. Toole JJ, Pittman DD, Orr EC, Murtha P, Wasley LC, Kaufman RJ: A large region (= 95 kDa) of human factor VIII is dispensable for in vitro procoagulant activity. *Proc Natl Acad Sci U S A* **83**:5939, 1986.
88. Jenny RJ, Pittman DD, Toole JJ, Kriz RW, Aldape RA, Hewick RM, Kaufman RJ, Mann KG: Complete cDNA and amino acid sequence of human factor V. *Proc Natl Acad Sci U S A* **84**:4846, 1986.
89. Guinto ER, Esmon CT: Loss of prothrombin and of factor Xa-factor Va interactions upon inactivation of factor Va by activated protein C. *J Biol Chem* **259**:13986, 1983.
90. Higuchi M, Antonarakis SE, Kasch L, Oldenburg J, Economou-Petersen E, Olek K, Inaba H, Kazazian HH: Towards a complete characterization of mild to moderate hemophilia A: Detection of the molecular defect in 25 of 29 patients by denaturing gradient gel electrophoresis. *Proc Natl Aca Sci U S A* **88**:8307, 1991.
90a. Young M, Inaba H, Hoyer LW, Higuchi M, Kazazian HH Jr, Antonarakis SE: Partial correction of a severe molecular defect in hemophilia A, because of errors during expression of the factor VIII gene. *Am J Hum Genet* **60**:565, 1997
90b. Fay PJ, Smudzin TM: Characterization of the interaction between the A2 subunit and A1/A3-C1-C2 dimer in human factor VIIIa. *J Biol Chem* **267**:13246, 1992
90c. Fay PJ, Haidaris PJ, Huggins CF: Role of the COOH-terminal acidic region of A1 subunit in A2 subunit retention in human factor VIIIa. *J Biol Chem* **268(24)**:17861, 1993.
90d. Lollar P, Parker CG: pH-dependent denaturation of thrombin-activated porcne factor VIII. *J Biol Chem* **265**(3):1688, 1990.
90e. Lollar P, Knutson GJ, Fass DN: Stabilization of thrombin-activated porcine factor VIII:C by factor IXa and phospholipid. *Blood* **63**:1303, 1984.
91. Walker FJ, Scandella D, Fay PJ: Identification of the binding site for activated protein C on the light chain of factors V and VIII. *J Biol Chem* **265**:1484, 1990.
92. Fulcher CA, Gardiner JE, Griffin JH, Zimmerman TS: Proteolytic inactivation of human factor VIII procoagulant protein by activated protein C and its analogy with factor V. *Blood* **63**:486, 1984.
93. Fay PJ, Walker FJ: Inactivation of human factor VIII by inactivated protein C: Evidence that the factor VIII light chain contains the activated protein C binding site. *Biochim Biophys Acta* **994**:142, 1989.
94. Fay PJ, Smudzin TM, Walker FJ: Activated protein C-catalyzed inactivation of human factor VIII and factor VIIIa. Identification of cleavage sites and correlation of proteolysis with cofactor activity. *J Biol Chem* **266**:20139, 1991.
94a. O'Brien DP, Johnson D, Byfield P, Tuddenham EGD: Inactivation of factor VIII by factor IXa. *Biochemistry* **31**:2805, 1992.
95. Dahlback B, Carlsson M: Factor VIII defect associated with familial thrombophilia [Abstract 39]. *Thromb Haemost* **65**:658, 1991.
95a. Amano K, Michnick DA, Moussalli M, Kaufman RJ: Mutation at either Arg336 or Arg562 in Factor VIII is insufficient for complete resistance to activated protein C (APC)-mediated inactivation:

Implications for the APC resistance test. *Thromb Haemost* **79**:557, 1998.

96. Bonthron DT, Hardin R, Kaufman RJ, Wasley LC, Orr EC, Mitsork LM, Ewenstein B, Loscalzo J, Ginsburg D, Orkin SH: Structure of pre-pro-von Willebrand factor and its expression in heterologous cells. *Nature* **324**:270, 1986.
97. Marcuso DJ, Tuley EA, Westfield LA, Worval NK, Shelton-Inloes BB, Sorace JM, Alevy YG, Sadler JE: Structure of the gene for human von Willebrand factor. *J Biol Chem* **264**:19514, 1989.
98. Pver K. Sixma JJ, Bruine MH, Trieschnigg AM, Vlooswijk RA, Beeser-Visser NH, Bonnon B: Survival of 125iodine-labeled factor VIII in normals and patients with classic hemophilia. Observations on the heterogeneity of human factor VIII. *J Clin Invest* **62**:233, 1978.
99. Tuddenham EGD, Lane RS, Rotblat F, Johnson AJ, Snapp TJ, Middleton S, Kernoff PB: Response to infusions of polyelectrolyte fractionated human factor VIII concentrate in human hemophilia A and von Willebrand's disease. *Br J Haematol* **52**:259, 1982.
100. Brinkhous KM, Sandberg H, Garris JB, Mattsson C, Palm M, Griggs T, Read MS: Purified human factor VIII procoagulant protein: Comparative hemostasis response after infusions into hemophilic and von Willebrand disease dogs. *Proc Natl Acad Sci U S A* **82**:8752, 1985.
101. Fay PJ, Coumans J-V, Walker FJ: Von Willebrand factor mediates protection of factor VIII from activated protein C-catalyzed inactivation. *J Biol Chem* **266**:2172, 1991.
102. Koedam JAS, Meijers JCM, Sixma JJ, Bouma BN: Inactivation of human factor VIII by activated protein C cofactor activity of protein S and protective effect of von Willebrand factor. *J Clin Invest* **82**:12336, 1988.
103. Hill-Eubanks DC, Lollar P: Von Willebrand factor is a cofactor for thrombin-catalyzed cleavage of the factor VIII light chain. *J Biol Chem* **265**:17854, 1990.
104. Hamer RJ, Koedam JA, Beeser-Visser NH, Bertina RM, van Mourik JA, Sixma JJ: Factor VIII binds to von Willebrand factor via its Mr-80,000 light chain. *Eur J Biochem* **166**:37, 1987.
105. Andersson L-O, Brown JE: Interaction of factor VIII-von Willebrand factor with phospholipid vesicles. *Biochem J* **200**:161, 1981.
106. Lajmonovich A, Hudry-Clergeon G, Freyssinet JM, Marguerie G: Human factor VIII procoagulant activity and phospholipid interaction. *Biochim Biophys Acta* **678**:123, 1991.
107. Nesheim M, Pittman DD, Giles AR, Fass DN, Wang JH, Slonosky D, Kaufman RJ: The effect of von Willebrand factor on the binding of factor VIII to thrombin activated platelets. *J Biol Chem* **266**:17815, 1991.
108. Foster PA, Fulcher CA, Marti T, Titani K, Zimmerman TS: A major factor VIII binding domain resides within the amino-terminal 272 amino acid residues of von Willebrand factor. *J Biol Chem* **262**:8443, 1987.
109. Takahashi Y, Kalafatis M, Girma J-P, Sewerin K, Andersson L-O, Meyer D: Localization of factor VIII binding domain on a 34-kilodalton fragment of the N-terminal portion of von Willebrand factor. *Blood* **70**:1679, 1987.
110. Bahou WF, Ginsburg D, Sikkink R, Litwiller R, Fass DN: A monoclonal antibody to von Willebrand factor (vWF) inhibits factor VIII binding. *J Clin Invest* **84**:56, 1989.
111. Tuley EA, Gaucher C, Jorieux S, Worrall NK, Sadler JE, Mazurier C: Expression of von Willebrand factor "Normandy": An autosomal mutation that mimics hemophilia A. *Proc Natl Acad Sci U S A* **88**:6377, 1991.
112. Gaucher C, Mercier B, Jorieux S, Oufkir D, Mazurier C: Identification of two point mutations in the von Willebrand factor gene of three families with the "Normandy" variant of van Willebrand disease. *Br J Haematol* **78**:506, 1991.
113. Cacheris PM, Nichols WC, Ginsburg D: Molecular characterization of a unique von Willebrand disease variant. *J Biol Chem* **266**:13499, 1991.
114. Nishino M, Girma J-P, Rothschild C, Fressinaud E, Meyer D: New variant of von Willebrand disease with defective binding to factor VIII. *Blood* **74**:1591, 1989.
115. Leyte A, Verbeet MP, Brodniewicz-Proba T, Van Mourik JA, Mertens K: The interaction between human blood-coagulation factor VIII and von Willebrand factor: Characterization of a high-affinity binding site on factor VIII. *Biochem J* **257**:679, 1989.
116. Lollar P, Hill-Eubanks DC, Parker CG: Association of the factor VIII light chain with von Willebrand factor. *J Biol Chem* **263**:10451, 1988.
117. Foster PA, Fulcher CA, Houghten RA, Zimmerman TS: An immunogenic region within amino acid residues Val1670-Glu1684 of the factor VIII chain induces antibodies which inhibit binding of factor VIII to von Willebrand factor. *J Biol Chem* **264**:5230, 1988.
118. Pittman DD, Kaufman RJ: Internal deletions of factor VIII identify potentially important peptide sequences for binding to von Willebrand factor. *Blood* **70**:392, 1987.
119. Leyte A, van Schijndel HB, Niehrs C, Huttner WB, Verbeet MPH, et al: Sulfation of Tyr1680 of human blood coagulation factor VIII is essential for the interaction of factor VIII with von Willebrand factor. *J Biol Chem* **266**:17572, 1991.

119a. Saenko EL, Scandella D: The acidic region of the factor VIII light chain and the C2 domain together form the high affinity binding site for von Willebrand factor. *J Biol Chem* **272**:18007, 1997.

120. Baeuerle PA, Huttner WB: Tyrosine sulfation is a trans-Golgi-specific protein modification. *Mol Cell Biol* **6**:97, 1988.

120a. Mutucumarana VP, Duffy EJ, Lollar P, Johnson AE: The active site of factor IXa is located far above the membrane surface and its conformation is altered upon association with factor VIIIa: A fluorescence study. *J Biol Chem* **267**:17012, 1992.

120b. Lamphear BJ, Fay PJ: Factor IXa enhances reconstitution of factor VIIIa from isolated A2 subunit and Al/A3-C1-C2 dimer. *J Biol Chem* **267**:3725, 1992.

120c. Fay PJ, Beattie T, Huggins CF, Regan LM: Factor VIIIa A2 subunit residues 558–565 represent a factor IXa interactive site. *J Biol Chem* **269(12)**:20522, 1994.

120d. O'Brien LM, Medved LV, Fay PJ: Localization of factor IXa and factor VIIIa interactive sites. *J Biol Chem* **270**:27087, 1995.

120e. Lenting PJ, van de Loo JW, Donath MJ, van Mourik JA, Mertens K: The sequence Glu1811-Lys1818 of human blood coagulation factor VIII comprises a binding site for activated factor IX. *J Biol Chem* **271**:1935, 1996.

120f. Lapan KA, Fay PJ: Localization of a factor X interactive site in the A1 subunit of factor VIIIa. *J Biol Chem* **272**:2082, 1997.

121. Poole S, Firtel RA, Lamar E, Rowekamp W: Structure and expression of the discoidin I gene family in Dictyostelium discoideum. *J Mol Biol* **153**:273, 1981.
122. Brown JE, Baugh RF, Hougie C: Effect of exercise on the factor VIII complex: A correlation of the von Willebrand antigen and factor VIII coagulant antigen increase. *Thromb Res* **15**:61, 1979.
123. Bloom JW: The interaction of rDNA, factor VIII, factor VIIIdes-797-1562 and factor VIIIdes-797–1562-derived peptides with phospholipid. *Thromb Res* **48**:439, 1987.
124. Kemball-Cook G, Edwards SJ, Sewerin K, Andersson L-O, Barrowcliffe TW: The phospholipid-binding site of factor VIII is located on the 80-kD light chain. *Thromb Haemost* **58**:222, 1987.
125. Arai M, Scandella D, Hoyer LW: Molecular basis of factor VIII inhibition by human antibodies. *J Clin Invest* **83**:1978, 1989.
126. Foster PA, Fulcher CA, Houghten RA, Zimmerman TS: Synthetic factor VIII peptides with amino acid sequences contained within the C2 domain of factor VIII inhibit factor VIII binding to phosphatidylserine. *Blood* **75**:1999, 1990.
127. Bevers EM, Comfurius P, Zwaal RF: Changes in membrane phospholipid distribution during platelet activation. *Biochim Biophys Acta* **736**:57, 1983.
128. Gilbert GE, Furie BC, Furie B: Binding of human factor VIII to phospholipid. *J Biol Chem* **265**:815, 1990.
129. Nesheim ME, Pittman DD, Wang JH, Slonosky D, Giles AR, Kaufman RJ: The binding of 35_S-labeled recombinant factor VIII to activated and unactivated human platelets. *J Biol Chem* **263**:16467, 1988.
130. Muntean W, Leschnik B, Haas J: Factor VIII coagulant moiety binds to platelets by binding to phospholipids of the platelet membrane. *Thromb Res* **45**:345, 1987.
131. Inaba H, Fujimaki M, Kazazian HH, Antonarakis SE: Mild hemophilia A resulting from Arg to Leu substitution in exon 26 of the factor VIII gene. *Hum Genet* **81**:335, 1989.
132. Gitschier J, Wood WI, Shuman MA, Lawn RM: Identification of a missense mutation in the factor VIII gene of a mild hemophiliac. *Science* **232**:1415, 1986.
133. Casula L, Murru S, Pecorara M, Ristaldi MS, Restagno G, Mancuso G, Morfini M, DeBiasi R, Baudo F, Carbonara A, Mori PG, Cao A, Pirastu M: Recurrent mutations and three novel deletions in the factor VIII gene of hemophilia A patients of Italian descent. *Blood* **75**:662, 1990.

133a. Brandstetter H, Bauer M, Huber R, Lollar P, Bode W: X-ray structure of clotting factor IXa: Active site and module structure related to Xase activity and hemophilia B. *Proc Natl Acad Sci U S A* **92**:9796, 1995.

133b. Pemberton S, Lindley P, Zaitsev V, Card G, Tuddenham EGD, Kemball-Cook G: A molecular model for the triplicated A domains of human factor VIII based on the crystal structure of human ceruloplasmin. *Blood* **89**:2413, 1997.
134. Haldane JBS: The rate of spontaneous mutation of a human gene. *J Genet* **31**:317, 1935.
135. Antonarakis SE, Kazazian HH Jr: The molecular basis of hemophilia A in man. *Trends Genet* **4**:233, 1988.
136. Rossiter JP, Young M, Kimberland ML, Hutter P, Ketterling RP, Gitschier J, Horst J, Morris MA, Schaid DJ, de Moerloose P, Sommer SS, Kazazian HH Jr, Antonarakis SE: Factor VIII gene inversions causing severe hemophilia A originate almost exclusively in male germ cells. *Hum Mol Genet* **3**:1035, 1994.
137. Tuddenham EGD, Cooper DN, Gitschier J, Higuchi M, Hoyer L, Yoshioka A, Peake I, Schwaab R, Olek K, Kazazian H, Lavergne J-M, Giannelli F, Antonarakis S: Haemophilia A: Database of nucleotide substitutions, deletions, insertions and rearrangements of the factor VIII gene. *Nucleic Acids Res* **19**:4821, 1991.
137a. Higuchi M, Kazazian HH, Kasch L, Warren TC, McGinniss MJ, Phillips JA, Kasper C, Janco R, Antonarakis SE: Molecular characterization of severe hemophilia A suggests that about half the mutations are not within the coding region and splice junctions of the factor VIII gene. *Proc Natl Acad Sci U S A* **88**:7405, 1991.
138. Naylor JA, Green PM, Rizza CR, Giannelli F: Factor VIII gene explains all cases of haemophilia A. *Lancet* **340**:1066, 1992.
139. Lakich D, Kazazian HH, Antonarakis SE, Gitschier J: Inversions disrupting the factor VIII gene as a common cause of severe hemophilia A. *Nat Genet* **5**:236, 1993.
140. Naylor J, Brinke A, Hassock S, Green PM, Giannelli F: Characteristic mRNA abnormality found in half the patients with severe haemophilia A is due to large DNA inversions. *Hum Mol Genet* **2**:1773, 1993.
141. Antonarakis SE, Rossiter JP, Young M, Horst J, de Moerloose P, Sommer SS, Ketterling RP, Kazazian HH Jr, Negrier C, Vinciguerra C: Factor VIII gene inversions in severe hemophilia A: Results of an international consortium study. *Blood* **86**:2206, 1995.
142. Youssoufian H, Antonarakis SE, Aronis S, Triftis G, Phillips DG, Kazazian HH Jr: Characterization of five partial deletions of the factor VIII gene. *Proc Natl Acad Sci U S A* **84**:3772, 1987.
143. Lavergne JM, Bahnak BR, Vidaud M, Laurian Y, Meyer D: A directed search for mutations in hemophilia A using restriction enzyme analysis and denaturing gradient gel electrophoresis. A study of seven exons in the factor VIII gene of 170 cases. *Nouv Rev Fr Hematol* **34**:85, 1992.
144. Woods Samuels P, Kazazian HH Jr, Antonarakis SE: Nonhomologous recombination in the human genome: Deletions in the human factor VIII gene. *Genomics* **10**:94, 1991.
145. Kazazian HH Jr, Wong C, Youssoufian HG, Scott AF, Phillips D, Antonarakis SE: A novel mechanism of mutation in man: Hemophilia A due to de novo insertion of L1 sequences. *Nature* **332**:164, 1988.
146. Sassaman DM, Dombroski BA, Moran JV, Kimberland ML, Naas TP, DeBerardinis RJ, Gabriel A, Swergold GD, Kazazian HH Jr: Many human L1 elements are capable of retrotransposition. *Nat Genet* **16**:37, 1997.
147. Kazazian HH, Jr., Moran JV: The impact of L1 retrotransposons on the human genome. *Nat Genet* **19**:19, 1998.
148. Miki Y, Nishisho I, Horii A, Miyoshi Y, Utsunomiya J, Kinzler KW, Vogelstein B, Nakamura Y: Disruption of the APC gene by a retrotransposal insertion of L1 sequence in a colon cancer. *Cancer Res* **52**:643, 1992.
149. Narita N, Nishio H, Kitoh Y, Ishikawa Y, Ishikawa Y, Minami R, Nakamura H, Matsuo M: Insertion of a 5′ truncated L1 element into the 3′ end of exon 44 of the dystrophin gene resulted in skipping of the exon during splicing in a case of Duchenne muscular dystrophy. *J Clin Invest* **91**:1862, 1993.
150. Bakker E, van Omenn GM, personal communication.
151. Holmes SH, Dombroski BA, Boehm CD, Krebs C, Kazazian HH Jr: A new retrotransposable human L1 element from the LRE2 locus on chromosome 1q produces a chimaeric insertion. *Nat Genet* **7**:143, 1994.
152. Divoky V, Indrak K, Mrug, M, Brabec V, Huisman THJ, Prchal JT: A novel mechanism of β-thalassemia. The insertion of L1 retrotransposable element into β globin IVSII. *Blood* **88**:148a, 1996.
153. Schwahn U, Lenzner S, Dong J, Feil S, Hinzmann B, van Duijnhoven G, Kirschner R, Hemberger M, Bergen AAB, Rosenberg T, Pinckers AJLG, Fundele R, Rosenthal A, Cremers FPM, Ropers H-H, Berger W: Positional cloning of the gene for X-linked retinitis pigmentosa 2. *Nat Genet* **19**:327, 1998.
154. Meischl C, de Boer M, Roos D: Chronic granulomatous disease caused by LINE-1 retrotransposons. *Eur J Haematol* **60**:349, 1998.
155. Wallace MR, Andersen LB, Saulino AM, Gregory TW, Collins FS: A de novo Alu insertion results in neurofibromatosis type 1. *Nature* **353**:864, 1991.
156. Muratani K, Hada T, Yamamoto Y, Kaneko T, Shigeto Y, Ohue T, Furuyama J, Higashino K: Inactivation of the cholinesterase gene by Alu insertion: Possible mechanism for human gene transposition. *Proc Natl Acad Sci U S A* **88**:11315, 1991.
157. Vidaud D, Vidaud M, Bahnak BR, Siguret V, Sanchez SG, Laurian Y, Meyer D, Goossens M, Lavergne JM: Haemophilia B due to a de novo insertion of a human-specific Alu subfamily member within the coding region of the factor IX gene. *Eur J Hum Genet* **1**:30, 1993.
158. Goldberg YP, Rommens JM, Andrew SE, Hutchinson GB, Lin B, Theilmann J, Graham R, Glaves ML, Starr E, McDonald H, Nasir J, Schappert K, Kalchman MA, Clarke LA, Hayden MR: Identification of an Alu retrotransposition event in close proximity to a strong candidate gene for Huntington's disease. *Nature* **362**:370, 1993.
159. Kazazian HH Jr: Mobile elements and disease. *Curr Opin Genet Dev* **81**:343, 1998.
160. Gitschier J: Maternal duplication associated with gene deletion in sporadic hemophilia. *Am J Hum Genet* **43**:274, 1988.
161. Murru S, Casula L, Pecorara M, Mori P, Cao A, Pirastu M: Illegitimate recombination produced a duplication within the factor VIII gene in a patient with mild hemophilia A. *Genomics* **7**:115, 1990.
162. Migeon BR, McGinnis MJ, Antonarakis SE, Stasiowski B, Youssoufian H, Keams WG, Chung A, Pearson PL, Kazazian HH Jr, Muneer RS: Severe hemophilia A in a female by cryptic translocation: Order and orientation of factor VIII within Xq28. *Genomics* **16**:20, 1993.
163. Tuddenham EGD, Cooper DN, Gitscher J, Higuchi M, Hoyer L, Yoshioka A, Peaker I, Schwaab R, Olek K, Kazazian H, Lavergne J-M, Giannelli F, Antonarakis S: Haemophilia A: Database of nucleotide substitutions, deletions, insertions and rearrangements of the factor VIII gene. *Nucleic Acids Res* **19**:4821, 1991.
164. Antonarakis SE, Kazazian HH, Tuddenham EG: Molecular etiology of factor VIII deficiency in hemophilia A. *Hum Mutat* **5**:1, 1995.
165. Wacey AI, Kemball-Cook G, Kazazian HH, Antonarakis SE, Schwaab R, Lindley P, Tuddenham EG: The haemophilia A mutation search test and resource site, home page of the factor VIII mutation database: HAMSTeRS. *Nucleic Acids Res* **24**:100, 1996.
166. Naylor JA, Green PM, Rizza CR, Ginnelli F: Analysis of factor VIII mRNA reveals defects in every one of 28 haemophilia A patients. *Hum Mol Genet* **2**:11, 1993.
167. Dietz HC, Valle D, Francomano CA, Kendzior RJ Jr, Pyeritz RE, Cutting GR: The skipping of constitutive exons in vivo induced by nonsense mutations. *Science* **259**:680, 1993.
168. Kaplan J-C, Kahn A, Chelly J: Illegitimate transcription: Its use in the study of inherited disease. *Hum Mutat* **1**:357, 1992.
169. McGinniss MJ, Kazazian HH Jr, Hoyer LW, Bi L, Inaba H, Antonarakis SE: Spectrum of mutations in CRM-positive and CRM-reduced hemophilia A. *Genomics* **15**:392, 1993.
170. Traystman MD, Higuchi M, Antonarakis SE, Kazazian HH Jr: Use of denaturing gradient gel electrophoresis to detect point mutations in the factor VIII gene. *Genomics* **6**:293, 1990.
171. Aly AM, Higuchi M, Kasper CK, Kazazian HH Jr, Antonarakis SE, Hoyer LW: Hemophilia A due to mutations that create new N-glycosylation sites. *Proc Natl Acad Sci U S A* **89**:4933, 1992.
172. Amano K, Sarkar R, Pemberton S, Kemball-Cook G, Kazazian HH Jr, Kaufman RJ: The molecular basis for cross-reacting material-positive hemophilia A due to missense mutations within the A2-domain of factor VIII. *Blood* **91**:538, 1998.
173. Barker D, Schafer M, White R: Restriction sites containing CpG show a higher frequency of polymorphism in human DNA. *Cell* **36**:343, 1984.
174. Gitschier J, Wood WI, Tuddenham EGD, Shuman MA, Goralka TM, Chen EY, Lawn RM: Detection and sequence of mutations in the factor VIII gene of haemophiliacs. *Nature* **315**:427, 1985.
175. Youssoufian H, Kazazian HH Jr, Phillips DG, Aronis S, Tsiftis G, Brown VA, Antonarakis SE: Recurrent mutations in haemophilia A give evidence for CpG mutations hotspots. *Nature* **324**:380, 1986.
176. Sommer S: Assessing the underlying pattern of human germline mutations: Lessons from the factor IX gene. *FASEB* J **6**:2767, 1992.
177. Youssoufian H, Antonarakis SE, Bell W, Griffin AM, Kazazian HH Jr: Nonsense and missense mutation in hemophilia A: Estimate of the relative mutation rate at CpG dinucleotides. *Am J Hum Genet* **42**:718, 1988.

178. Bloom AL: The treatment of factor VIII inhibitors, in Verstraete M, Vermylen J, Lijnene R, Arnout J (eds): *Thrombosis and Haemostasis 1987*. Leuven, Leuven University Press, 1987, p 447.
179. Fulcher CA, de Graaf S, Mahoney S, Zimmerman TS: FVIII inhibitor IgG subsclass and FVIII polypeptide specificity determined by immunoblotting. *Blood* **69**:1475, 1987.
180. Gilles JG, Arnout J, Vermylen J, Saint-Remy JM: Anti-factor VIII antibodies of hemophiliac patients are frequently directed towards nonfunctional determinants and do not exhibit isotypic restriction. *Blood* **82**:2452, 1993.
181. Scandella D, Mattingly M, de Graaf S, Fulcher CA: Localization of epitopes for human factor VIII inhibitor antibodies by immunoblotting and antibody neutralization. *Blood* **74**:1618, 1989.
182. Scandella D, DeGraaf Mahoney S, Mattingly M, Roeder D, Timmons L, Fulcher CA: Epitope mapping of human factor VIII inhibitor antibodies by deletion analysis of factor VIII fragments expressed in Escherichia coli [published erratum appears in *Proc Natl Acad Sci U S A* 86(4):1387, 1989]. *Proc Natl Acad Sci U S A* **85**:6152, 1988.
183. Scandella D, Mattingly M, de Graaf S, Fulcher CA: Localization of epitopes for human factor VIII inhibitor antibodies by immunoblotting and antibody neutralization. *Blood* **74**:1618, 1989.
184. Fulcher CA, de Graaf Mahoney S, Roberts JR, Kasper CK, Zimmerman TS: Localization of human factor FVIII inhibitor epitopes to two polypeptide fragments. *Proc Natl Acad Sci U S A* **82**:7728, 1985.
185. Zhong D, Scandella D: Epitope of a hemophilia A inhibitor antibody overlaps the factor VIII binding site for factor IX. *Blood* **88**:324a, 1996.
186. Healey JF, Lubin IM, Nakai H, Saenko EL, Hoyer LW, Scandella D, Lollar P: Residues 484-508 contain a major determinant of the inhibitory epitope in the A2 domain of human factor VIII. *J Biol Chem* **270**:14505, 1995.
187. Alper CA, Raum DD, Awdeh ZL, Sahpiro SS, Yunis EJ: Major histocompatibility complex (MHC)-linked complement alleles as markers for the development of anti-factor VIII in hemophiliacs, in Hyouer L (ed): *Factor VIII Inhibitors*. New York, Alan R Liss, 1984, p 141.
188. Lippert LE, Fisher LM, Schook LB: Relationship of major histocompatibility complex class II genes to inhibitor antibody formation in hemophilia A. *Thromb Haemost* **64**:564, 1990.
189. Aly AM, Aledort LM, Lee TD, Hoyer LW: Histocompatibility antigen patterns in patients with factor VIII antibodies. *Br J Haematol* **76**:238, 1990.
190. Simmoney N, DeBosch N, Argueyo A, Garcia E. Layrise Z: HLA antigens in hemophiliacs A with or without factor VIII antibodies in a Venezuelan Mestizo population. *Tissue Antigens* **25**:216, 1985.
191. Millar DS, Steinbrecher RA, Wieland K, Grundy CB, Martinowitz U, Krawczak M, Zoll B, Whitmore D, Stephenson I, Mibashan RS, Kakkar VV, Cooper DN: The molecular genetic analysis of haemophilia A: Characterization of six partial deletions in the factor VIII gene. *Hum Genet* **86**:219, 1990.
192. Qiang L, Sommer S: Subcycling-PCR for multiplex long-distance amplification of regions with high and low GC content: Application to the inversion hotspot in the factor VIII gene. *Biotechniques* **25**:140, 1998.
193. Ganguly A, Rock MJ, Prockop DJ: Conformation sensitive gel electrophoresis for rapid detection of single-base differences in double-stranded PCR products and DNA fragments: Evidence for solvent-induced bends in DNA heteroduplexes. *Proc Natl Acad Sci U S A* **90**:10325, 1993.
194. Chee M, Yang R, Hubbell E, Berno A, Huang XC, Stern D, Winkler J, Lockhart DJ, Morris MS, Fodor SP: Accessing genetic information with high-density DNA arrays. *Science* **274**:610, 1996.
195. Gitschier J, Drayne D, Tuddenham EGD, White RL, Lawn RM: Genetic mapping and diagnosis of haemophilia A achieved through a BclI polymorphism in the factor VIII gene. *Nature* **314**:738, 1985.
196. Wion KL, Tuddenham EGD, Lawn RM: A new polymorphism in the factor VIII gene for prenatal diagnosis of hemophilia A. *Nucleic Acids Res* **14**:4535, 1986.
197. Antonarakis SE, Waber PG, Kittur SD, Patel AS, Kazazian HH Jr, Mellis MA, Stamatoyannopoulos G, Counts RB, Bowie EJW, Fass DN, Pittman DD, Wozney JM, Toole JJ: Hemophilia A: Molecular defects and carrier detection by DNA analysis. *N Engl J Med* **313**:843, 1985.
198. Harper K, Winter RM, Pembrey ME, Hartley D, Davies KE, Tuddenham EGD: A clinically useful DNA probe linked to haemophilia A. *Lancet* **2**:6, 1984.
199. Oberle I, Camerino G, Heilig R, Grunebaum L, Cazenave J-P, Crapanzano C, Manucci P, Mandel JL: Genetic screening for hemophilia A (classic hemophilia) with a polymorphic DNA probe. *N Engl J Med* **312**:682, 1985.
200. Lalloz MR, McVey JH, Pattinson JK, Tuddenham EGD: Haemophilia A diagnosis by analysis of a hypervariable dinucleotide repeat within the factor VIII gene. *Lancet* **338**:207, 1991.
201. Oeri J, Matter M, Isenschmid H, Hauser F, Koller F: Angeborener mangel an faktor V (parahaemophilie) verbunden mit echter haemophilie A bein zwei brudern. *Med Probl Paediatr* **1**:575, 1954.
202. Lander ES, Botstein D: Homozygosity mapping: A way to map human recessive traits with the DNA of inbred children. *Science* **236**:1567, 1987.
203. Nichols WC, Seligsohn U, Zivelin A, Terry VH, Arnold ND, Siemieniak DR, Kaufman RJ, Ginsburg D: Linkage of combined factors V and VIII deficiency to chromosome 18q by homozygosity mapping. *J Clin Invest* **99**:596, 1997.
204. Neerman-Arbez M, Antonarakis SE, Blouin J-L, Akhtari M, Afshar Y, Tuddenham EGD: The locus for combined factor V-factor VIII deficiency (F5F8D) maps to 18q21, between D18S849 and D18S1103. *Am J Hum Genet* **61**:143, 1997.
205. Nichols WC, Seligsohn U, Zivelin A, Terry VH, Hertel CE, Wheatley MA, Moussalli MJ, Hauri H-P, Ciavarella N, Kaufman RJ, Ginsburg D: Mutations in an endoplasmic reticulum-Golgi intermediate compartment protein cause combined deficiency of coagulation factors V and VIII. *Cell* **93**: 61, 1998.
206. Neerman-Arbez M, Johnson KM, Morris MA, McVey JH, Peyvandi F, Nichols WC, Ginsburg D, Rossier C, Antonarakis SE, Tuddenham EGD. Molecular analysis of the ERGIC-53 gene in 35 families with combined factor V-factor VIII deficiency (F5F8D). *Blood* **93**:2253, 1999.
207. Schweizer A, Fransen JA, Bachi T, Ginsel L, Hauri HP: Identification, by a monoclonal antibody, of a 53-kD protein associated with a tubulovesicular compartment at the *cis*-side of the Golgi apparatus. *J Cell Biol* **107**:1643, 1988.
208. Arar C, Carpentier V, Le Caer JP, Monsigny M, Legrand A, Roche AC: ERGIC-53, a membrane protein of the endoplasmic reticulum-Golgi intermediate compartment, is identical to MR60, an intracellular mannose-specific lectin of myelomonocytic cells. *J Biol Chem* **270**:3551, 1995.
209. Biggs R: *The Treatment of Haemophilia A and B and von Willebrand's Disease*. Oxford, Blackwell, 1978.
210. Boone DC: *Comprehensive Management of Haemophilia*. Philadelphia, FA Davis, 1976.
211. Gilbert MS, Aledort L: Comprehensive care in hemophilia: A team approach. *Mount Sinai Med* **44**:3, 1977.
212. Kasper CK, Aledort LM, Counts RB, Edson JR, Fratantoni J, Green D, Hampton JW, Hilgartner MW, Lazerson J, Levine PH, McMillan CW, Pool JG, Shapiro SS, Shulman NR, van Eys J: A more uniform measurement of factor VIII inhibitors. *Thromb Diath Haemorrh* **34**:869, 1975.
213. Hedner U, Glazer S, Pingel K, Alberta KA, Blombaeck M, Schulman S, Johnson M: Successful use of recombinant factor VIIa in patients with severe haemophilia A during synovectomy. *Lancet* **2**:1193, 1988.
214. Brackman HH: The treatment of inhibitor against factor VIII by continuous treatment with factor VIII and activated prothrombin complex concentrate, in Mariani G, Russo MA, Mandelli F (eds): *Activated Prothrombin Complex Concentrates*. New York, Praeger Publishers, 1982.
215. Rizza CR, Mathews JM: Effect of frequent factor VIII replacement on the level of factor VIII antibodies in haemophiliacs. *Br J Haematol* **52**:13, 1982.
216. Sultan U, Maisonneuve D, Kazatchkine MD, Nydegger UE: Anti-idiotypic suppression of autoantibodies to factor VIII (antihaemophilic factor) by high dose intravenous gamma-globulin. *Lancet* **2**:765, 1984.
217. Lusher JM, Arkin S, Abildgaard CF, Schwartz RS, Kogenate Previously Untreated Patient Study Group: Recombinant factor VIII for the treatment of previously untreated patients with hemophilia A. *N Engl J Med* **328**:453, 1993.
218. Kasper CK: Treatment of factor VIII inhibitors. *Prog Hemost Thromb* **9**:57, 1989.
219. Aledort LM, Levine PH, Hilgartner M, Blatt P, Spero JA, Goldberg JD, Bianchi L, Desmet V, Scheuer P, Popper H, Berk PD: A study of liver biopsies and liver disease among haemophiliacs. *Blood* **66**:367, 1985.
220. Triger DR, Preston FE: Chronic liver disease in haemophiliacs [Annotation]. *BMJ* **74**:241, 1990.

221. Lee CA, Phillips AN, Elford J, Janossy G, Griffiths P, Kernoff PBA: Progression of HIV disease in a haemophiliac cohort followed for 11 years and the effect of treatment. *BMJ* **303**:1093, 1991.
222. Bi L, Lawler AM, Antonarakis SE, High KA, Gearhart JD, Kazazian HH Jr: Targeted disruption of the mouse factor VIII gene produces a model of haemophilia A [Letter]. *Nat Genet* **10**:119, 1995.
223. Bi L, Sarkar R, Naas T, Lawler AM, Pain J, Shumaker SL, Bedian V, Kazazian HH Jr: Further characterization of factor VIII-deficient mice created by gene targeting: RNA and protein studies. *Blood* **88**:3446, 1996.
224. Herzog RW, Yang EY, Cuoto LB, Hagstrom JN, Elwell D, Fields PA, Burton M, Bellinger DA, Read MS, Brinkhous KM, Nichols T, Kurtzman GJ, High KA: Long-term correction of canine hemophilia B by AAV-mediated gene transfer of blood coagulation factor IX. *Nat Med* **5**:56, 1999.
225. Connelly S, Andrews JL, Gallo AM, Kayda DB, Qian J, Hoyer L, Kadan MJ, Gorziglia MI, Trapnell BC, McClelland A, Kaleko M: Sustained phenotypic correction of murine hemophilia A by *in vivo* gene therapy. *Blood* **91**:3273, 1998.
226. Sarkar R, Gao G-P, Chirmule N, Tazelaar J, Kazazian HH Jr: Partial correction of hemophilia A with neo-antigenic murine factor VIII. *Hum Gene Ther*, in press.
226a. Fakharzadeh SS, Zhang Y, Sarkar R, Kazazian HH Jr: Further progress towards examining the epidermis as a target tissue for factor VIII gene therapy. *Blood*, in press.
227. Merskey C: The occurrence of haemophilia in the human female. *QJM* **3**:301, 1951.
228. Lusher JM, Zuelaer WW, Evans RK: Hemophilia A in chromosomal female subjects. *J Pediatr* **74**:265, 1969.
229. Morita H: The occurrence of homozygous hemophilia in the female. *Acta Haematol* **45**:112, 1971.
230. Panarello C, Acquila M, Caprino D, Gimelli G, Pecorara M, Mori PG: Concomitant Turner syndrome and hemophilia A in a female with an idic (X) (p11) heterozygous at locus DXS52. *Cytogenet Cell Genet* **59**:241, 1992.
231. Vidaud D, Vidaud M, Plassa F, Gazengel C, Noel B, Goossens M: Father-to-son transmission of hemophilia A due to uniparental disomy. *Am J Hum Genet* **45**:A226, 1989.

CHAPTER 173

Hemophilia B: Factor IX Deficiency

Eleanor S. Pollak ▪ Katherine A. High

1. **The activated form of factor IX (F.IXa), a vitamin K-dependent protein made exclusively in the liver, is an enzyme required for amplification in the series of reactions leading to blood clot formation. Factor IX deficiency (hemophilia B or Christmas disease) results in a bleeding disorder, phenotypically identical to the more common Hemophilia A, which results from a deficiency of factor VIII.**
2. **Clinically, the disease exists in severe (F.IX levels < 1 percent normal), moderate (1 to 5 percent), and mild (6 to 30 percent) forms. The major symptom of the disease is spontaneous bleeding into joints and soft tissues. Bleeding at others sites is less common but can be life or limb threatening; for example, intracranial or compartmental syndrome bleeding.**
3. **A detailed and extensive database of mutations resulting in hemophilia B that includes more than 1918 patient entries as of mid 2000 (www.umds.ac.uk/molgen/) provides information about all known mutations.**
4. **Treatment options include replacement of the missing protein with purified or recombinant F.IX protein and most recently gene therapy. Complications of treatment include thrombogenicity, blood-borne viral diseases, and the development of an inhibitory F.IX antibody. The presence of an anti-F.IX inhibitory antibody is clinically problematic and treated acutely by delivery of proteins (recombinant Factor VIIa) that bypass the requirement for F.IX. In addition, initiation of immune tolerance regimens (daily injection of high doses of F.IX) is designed to eradicate the inhibitory antibody.**
5. **Murine and canine models of hemophilia B facilitate testing of novel therapies such as gene therapy.**

HISTORICAL PERSPECTIVE

Hemophilia B, also called factor IX deficiency or Christmas disease, is an X-linked blood clotting disorder caused by a deficiency of the vitamin K-dependent blood procoagulant protein factor IX (F.IX). Hemophilia B occurs in approximately 1 in 30,000 live male births and is clinically indistinguishable from the more common hemophilia A, which is caused by a deficiency of factor VIII (F.VIII), which in the activated state, serves as the catalytic cofactor for the activated factor F.IX (F.IXa).

Hemophilia is thought to be the first X-linked genetic disease described; the Talmud vindicates abstention from circumcision, a mandated Jewish ritual in the newborn male, when the mother had a history of two sons who had died at circumcision.[1] John Conrad Otto from the Philadelphia Dispensary is said to have given the first description of hemophilia in the modern day literature in 1813 and the name "hemophilia" is attributed to Hopff in 1828,[6] and Schönlein in 1839.[1] The distinction between the two hemophilia disorders, later shown to be F.VIII and F.IX deficiencies, was discovered in 1952 when Aggeler et al. in San Francisco,[2] Biggs, MacFarlane et al. in Oxford,[3] and Schulman and Smith in New York[4] noted the difference between samples from patients with classic hemophilia, deficient in antihemophiliac factor (F.VIII), and a subset of other hemophilia patients.[5,6] The term "Christmas disease" refers to one of the initial reports of F.IX deficiency in a family with the surname Christmas; the report appeared in the 1952 Christmas number of the British Medical Journal.[3] Detailed study of procoagulant protein functions later revealed that the activated form of F.VIII (F.VIIIa) is a cofactor for the activated form of F.IX (F.IXa) in catalyzing the activation of factor X (F.X), which ultimately leads to fibrin clot formation and physiologic hemostasis (Fig. 173-1).

Medical remedies for treating hemophilia were plentiful in the early 1900s, including local application of diluted Russell viper venom, a reagent still used today as a diagnostic tool in the clinical coagulation laboratory. However, the first effective treatment of hemophilia with blood transfusions occurred in the 1930s when MacFarlane recognized the need to replace a missing essential component with blood from a nonhemophiliac.[6] This understanding of the need to replace a deficient factor led to increasingly specific transfusions of the normal protein from whole blood, to plasma, to purified vitamin K-dependent coagulation protein concentrate, to purified F.IX, and most recently to recombinant F.IX (rFIX). With this understanding, the life expectancy of people with severe hemophilia has increased from 11 years at the beginning of the century to within several years of the average male expectancy in the early 1980s, before the devastating effects of blood-borne viral disease again shortened average life expectancy.[7,8]

Health and therapeutic intervention issues concerning patients with deficiencies of F.VIII and F.IX underwent intense scrutiny during the 1980s and 1990s due to complications associated with viral contamination of purified blood product components with HIV and hepatitis viruses. The complications of treatment with plasma-derived clotting factors have fueled an interest in exploring new treatment strategies, including the use of recombinant proteins and of gene therapy approaches. Professional

A list of standard abbreviations is located immediately preceding the index in each volume. Additional abbreviations used in this chapter include: a = activated as in factor IXa (F.IXa); AAV = adeno-associated virus; aPTT = activated partial thromboplastin time; ARE = androgen response element; BSE = bovine spongiform encephalopathy; BU = Bethesda unit; C/EBP- = CAAT/enhancer-binding protein; CJD = Creutzfeldt-Jakob disease; DBP = albumin D-site-binding protein; DIC = disseminated intravascular coagulation; F.II = factor II (prothrombin); F.VII, F.VIII, F.IX, F.X, F.XI = factor VII, VIII, IX, X, XI, respectively; FDA = Food and Drug Administration; FFP = fresh frozen plasma; GABP- = Ets transcription factor GA-binding protein; Gla = -carboxyglutamic acid; HAV, HBV, HCV, HDV, HEV, HGV = hepatitis A, B, C, D, E, and G virus, respectively; HLF = hepatic leukemia factor; HNF-4 = hepatocyte nuclear factor 4; ICH = intracranial hemorrhage; IU = International unit; PCC = prothrombin complex concentrate; PT = prothrombin time; rFVIIa = recombinant activated factor VII; rFIX = recombinant factor IX; RVV = Russell viper venom; TF = tissue factor; TTV = transfusion-transmitted virus; Xase = factor X enzymatic complex.

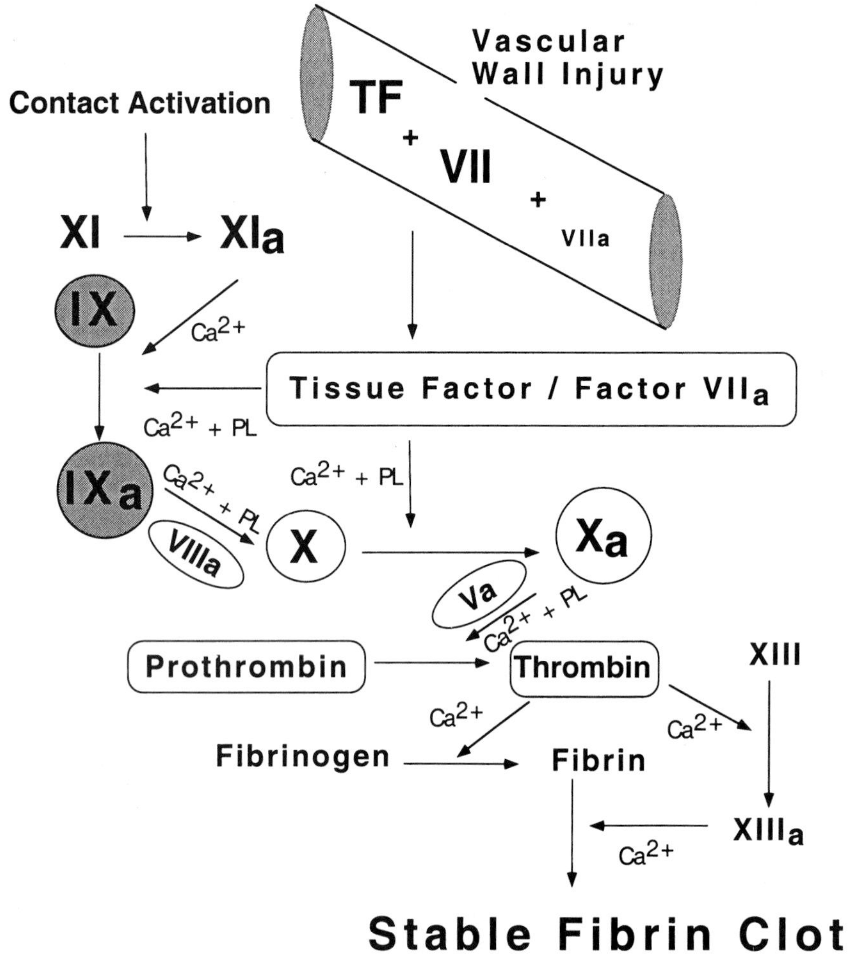

Fig. 173-1 A simplified diagram of the sequence of coagulant protein activation reactions leading to the formation of a stable fibrin clot. F.IX is activated to F.IXa by either the complex of tissue factor (TF) and F.VIIa, primarily generated at sites of vascular injury, or by F.XIa activated through the contact activation system. Activated F.IXa activates F.X in combination with its cofactor F.VIIIa along with calcium and phospholipid (PL).

and patient-oriented organizations provide a network of information and support for both patients and physicians confronting medical, economic, and social issues related to hemophilia B, including the Coalition for Hemophilia B, the National Hemophilia Foundation and subcommittees of the American Society of Hematology and the International Society for Thrombosis and Haemostasis.

CLINICAL FEATURES

Hemophilia B, occurring in 1 in 30,000 male births, is clinically indistinguishable from hemophilia A, which occurs at 4 to 5 times the frequency in most populations.[7,9,10] *De novo* cases occur quite commonly. Approximately one-fourth to one-third of cases arise without a previous family history. Clinically, the severity of disease is correlated with in vitro functional clotting assay levels compared with 100 percent normal levels. Normal levels are based on studies of a pool of at least 20 nonsmoking, nonpregnant, nonhemophiliac donors aged 18 to 65. Disease is classified as severe (<1 percent of normal F.IX levels), moderate (1 to 5 percent), or mild (6 to 30 percent) (see Fig. 173-2A).

The most common clinical problems requiring therapy include hemarthroses and soft tissue hemorrhage. Intracranial hemorrhage is a leading cause of death in hemophilia.[11] Centuries of documentation of excessive bleeding at circumcision might lead one to suspect that this is always the initial manifestation of disease, but in fact the first symptom is more commonly the presence of easy bruising, hematoma formation, and bleeding associated with venipuncture.[12,13] Severely affected patients are usually diagnosed before 1 year of age, although moderate and mild cases may present later.[9,12,14] Bleeding is often delayed and may occur several days after trauma. During the past decade, morbidity in hemophilia has been largely related to complications of disease due to blood-borne viruses transmitted by plasma-derived clotting factor.[8,15] Now, with increased safety of products and better understanding of treatment options, patients may even involve themselves in sports activities with appropriate self-administered F.IX prophylaxis when necessary.

Hemarthroses

Hemophilic arthropathy and joint deformity, resulting from acute and chronic hemarthroses, are inevitable clinical complications in the untreated patient with severe hemophilia. Joint problems begin in infancy with minor trauma or occur spontaneously.[16] Affected joints in decreasing order of involvement include the knee, elbow, ankle, shoulder, wrist, and hip. Patients may develop a "target joint" more prone to recurrent bleeding episodes due to chronic inflammation and a hypertrophic synovial lining. The intra-articular synovial lining limits the extent of hemorrhage but may become chronically inflamed resulting in increased vascularization. Ideally, treatment of the synovitis should begin before subsequent episodes become a pattern. High-dose concentrate therapy to minimize bleeding is recommended. In one study of patients with hemophilia A and B, hemarthroses accounted for 70 percent of bleeding episodes requiring treatment and 40 percent of concentrate usage.[17]

There is a growing consensus that factor concentrate should be recommended for acute joint hemorrhage, as well as for prophylactic therapy that will prevent damage to articular cartilage and that may reduce hemophilic arthropathy when started in young patients (<5 years) with severe hemophilia.[18] Prophylaxis is probably most valuable when instituted at 1 to 2 years of age; in large series in the U.S., however, this has been associated with a high rate of sepsis related to the intravenous access devices that are generally required for prophylactic therapy in very young children. For this reason, many pediatric centers in the U.S. defer

Factor IX level	% F.IX activity *
Normal reference range	75-125%
Severe hemophilia	<1%
Moderate hemophilia	1-5%
Mild hemophilia	6-30%

* F.IX activity based on an in vitro aPTT-based F.IX assay

A

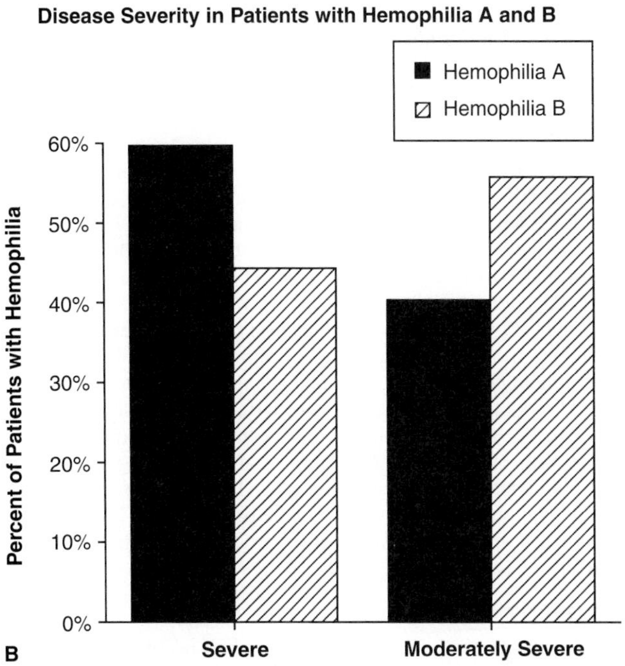

B

Fig. 173-2 ***A*****, Diagnosis of clinical severity (mild, moderate, severe) of hemophilia is based on in vitro coagulant activity as shown.** ***B*****, Distribution of severe and moderately severe disease in hemophilia A and hemophilia B. Data based on a survey of hemophilia treaters in the United States in the early 1970s and included 20,297 patients with hemophilia A and 5202 patients with hemophilia B. Estimates were made from the number of patients requiring blood products during the year prior to survey: Patients with mild disease were excluded. (*****From Department of Health and Human Services, 1972*****[285]).**

prophylactic therapy until children are 4 to 5 years of age, at which point intravenous therapy may not require an indwelling line. If joint preservation by the use of prophylactic or aggressive episode-based factor infusion fails, treatment options for individuals with severe joint disease are limited. In small joints or, in patients with inhibitor when high-dose prophylaxis is not successful, chemical or radioactive synoviorthosis (injection into a joint of a synovium-ablating drug such as rifampicin or a radioactive gold compound can be helpful.[19,20] Surgical management and correction of articular problems is often highly successful.[16,21–23]

Hematoma

Soft-tissue hemorrhage is a frequent complication of hemophilia B. Hemorrhage can arise spontaneously, in association with trauma, or as a complication of surgery. Seemingly, confined soft-tissue hemorrhages in the retroperitoneal space have the potential to dissect. Appropriate control of soft-tissue hemorrhage is necessary to prevent major blood loss, compartment syndromes, and subsequent neurologic compromise. In addition to factor replacement, recommendations for treatment of compartment syndrome in patients with coagulation deficiencies include obtaining mean arterial blood pressure and the compartment pressure to determine the pressure difference for assessing the potential for tissue damage and the necessity of fasciotomy.[24]

Neurologic Complications

Intracranial hemorrhage (ICH) is a life threatening and potentially fatal complication of bleeding associated with hemophilia B and occurs in approximately 2 to 8 percent of patients.[25,26] Although the mortality from intracranial bleeding has dramatically decreased since the availability of concentrated factor, the mortality from ICH remains a leading cause of death in this patient population.[11] Immediate evaluation and treatment of potential bleeds is critical, especially during the first 6 to 8 h after injury, to prevent devastating consequences.[27] ICH can arise either spontaneously, primarily in adult patients and patients with severe hemophilia,[28] or after head trauma.[25] Although a large proportion of pediatric patients with hemophilia presents with recent head trauma, only a small fraction of these is associated with ICH. The majority of central nervous system bleeds are seen in patients under the age of 20 years (72 percent),[25] with the median age of incidence being 9 years. Common clinical signs and symptoms associated with ICH in this setting include an impaired mental status (Glasgow scale ≤ 14), vomiting, and a neurologic deficit.[11] Although a delayed presentation has been noted in the past, Dietrich et al.[11] found presentation within 24 h of an incident to be most common.

The prevalence of neonatal ICH in infants with hemophilia B is unknown. There are many case reports in the literature,[29] and some have proposed that a prospective study be carried out in which infants with hemophilia undergo an imaging procedure before leaving the hospital. Recommendations for management of known carriers at the time of delivery are summarized (see "Hemophilia B in Females" below). Cervical spine involvement is common as well and may be associated with vague complaints of neck discomfort.[30] Compartment syndromes due to bleeding episodes may also result in entrapment neuropathies.[31]

Renal Problems and Hematuria

Hematuria is seen frequently in patients with hemophilia.[32] The severity can range from minor self-limited episodes lasting only several days to gross hematuria leading to significant blood loss. Although structural lesions are not commonly found even when patients present with gross hematuria, appropriate workup is recommended as patients may experience renal complications unrelated to hemophilia. Additional renal complications may include hematuria associated with flank pain and/or renal stones in hemophilia B patients taking protease inhibitors, particularly indinavir, for treatment of HIV;[33] nephrotic syndrome may occur in patients placed on immune tolerance regimens.[34]

Dental Procedures

Routine dental procedures, including tooth extraction, warrant involvement by a specialist in the treatment of hemophilia. Optimal levels for dental extractions have been suggested as 25 to

50 percent F.IX and 70 to 100 percent for more complicated dental procedures. Antifibrinolytic agents, ε-aminocaproic acid or tranexamic acid, and fibrin sealants are often recommended as adjuncts to minimize mucosal bleeding.[35–39]

Pseudotumor

A very rare but extremely serious complication seen in patients with hemophilia is the development of an encapsulated collection of blood known as a pseudotumor. Pseudotumors, found in bone or soft tissues, arise from extraarticular hemorrhage. Although the muscles and bones of the limbs are most commonly affected,[40] reports also document other locations including the jaw.[41] A multicenter, 25-year retrospective analysis of 1831 patients with a bleeding diathesis revealed a frequency of 2.32 percent (4 cases) of this complication in the 172 hemophilia B patients included in this study.[40] Pseudotumor was seen in mild and moderate cases, as well as in severely affected patients, and occurs most frequently in patients with an inhibitor. No definitive treatment regimen has been established for pseudotumors. Although the reported mortality for surgical intervention with pseudotumor is high, it may represent the best option; such surgery, however, should only be performed at specialized centers.[40]

Emergency Room Visits

In 1993, Morgan et al. reported a 10-year chart review of patients with hemophilia presenting to a pediatric emergency department.[42] Twenty-eight percent of the patients (10/36) were F.IX deficient, 7 mildly deficient and 3 severely deficient. This distribution is common because most patients with mild disease bleed so infrequently that they are not on home infusion regimens; instead, they seek medical care when a bleed occurs. Seventy-eight percent of visits were by children between 1 and 5 years of age, 48 percent for soft tissue hemorrhages, 24 percent for hemarthroses, and 12 percent for head injuries. Watchful assessment and treatment of head injuries is essential. A rare but life-threatening complication is bleeding into the upper airway, primarily in the pediatric population. Even patients presenting with nonspecific symptomatology of a sore throat can have retropharyngeal bleeds requiring emergency treatment.[43] An emergency in a patient with a F.IX inhibitor can present a serious challenge in the acute care setting due to management difficulties in addressing appropriate laboratory assessment and treatment options. Blood volume replacement with saline and packed RBCs is necessary to maintain appropriate volume and oxygen carrying capacity. In patients with low titer inhibitors, high-dose treatment with a F.IX concentrate may be used. In patients with high titer inhibitors, either preparations of activated factors (Autoplex) or recombinant F.VIIa (rFVIIa) can be life-saving.

Hemophilia B in Females

Because hemophilia B is an X-linked disease, symptoms of hemophilia B in heterozygous females are rare except immediately postpartum. Recognition of affected females was noted soon after the initial report of Christmas disease.[44] Hemophilia B in female patients is most often associated with extreme lyonization.[45,46] Other rare causes for X-linked disease manifestation in females are possible. Heterozygote females are rarely affected by problems faced by patients with hemophilia. However, a recent review of 55 patients with mild hemophilia (levels >5 percent) revealed that 5 of the patients were female and the authors suggest that mild disease may affect females more commonly than appreciated.[14]

The management of heterozygous women in the antepartum period warrants special obstetric care; a high percentage of pregnancies is associated with either primary or secondary hemorrhage in the mother.[47] Knowledge of the gender of the fetus is recommended. Neonatal problems in affected infants include subgaleal or cephalic hematoma, intracranial hemorrhage, umbilical bleeding, or bleeding after injection or venipuncture.[48] In reviewing other cases in carriers of hemophilia, Guy et al. recommend periodic monitoring of F.IX levels during pregnancy in addition to measurement of fibrin degradation products, platelet studies, and ultrasound to look for occult hemorrhage.[49] Unlike the rise of the acute phase reactant F.VIII, F.IX does not rise significantly in pregnancy. Prolonged labor, traumatic delivery, and invasive fetal monitoring should be avoided,[47,50] and some authors have recommended caesarian delivery.[13] Vaginal delivery does not appear to cause an increased risk of intracranial hemorrhage in the newborn with hemophilia, although vacuum extraction deliveries and mid-cavity forceps deliveries are not recommended.[48] In affected neonates, intramuscular injections of vitamin K and vaccine should be avoided if possible, and venipuncture should be minimized.[47]

BIOLOGY OF FACTOR IX

F.IX is a zymogen of the vitamin K-dependent serine protease, F.IXa (see Chap. 169). The activation of F.IX is achieved through the cleavage of two bonds within the 415 amino acid F.IX, at Arg 145 to Ala 146 and Arg 180 to Val 181. The catalysts for this reaction are factor VIIa (F.VIIa)-tissue factor (TF)-Ca^{2+}, generated at sites of vascular injury, and activated factor XI (F.XIa)-Ca^{2+} (Fig. 173-1). Cleavage at these two bonds generates a 35-amino acid, 10-kDa activation peptide and a 45-kDa, 380-amino acid-activated F.IX (F.IXa) consisting of a light chain (amino acids 1 to 145) and a heavy chain (amino acids 181 to 415) connected by the disulfide bond between Cys 132 and Cys 289.[51] F.IX has a molecular weight of 57 kDa with a carbohydrate content of about 17 percent.[52] Numerous posttranslational modifications are present on the activation peptide of F.IX, including tyrosine sulfation at Tyr 155, serine phosphorylation at Ser 158, *O*-glycosylation at Thr 159, Thr 169, and Thr 172, and *N*-glycosylation at Asn 157 and Asn 167.[53] For a more in-depth discussion of the structural properties of the group of vitamin K-dependent proteins, including F.IX, see Chap. 169.

Under some conditions, an inactive intermediate, F.IXaα, is generated after the Arg 145-Ala 146 bond is first cleaved and before cleavage of the Arg 180 to Val 181 bond; however, a recent study suggests that F.XIa-catalyzed activation of F.IX proceeds without release of a free intermediate.[54] The activation by XIa and F.VIIa-TF are thought to be similar; however, Larson et al. showed that a mutant F.IX (F.IX LA4) prevented activation by F.VIIa-TF, whereas the mutant F.IXLA4 can still be activated normally by F.XIa.[55] Venom from the Russell viper (RVV), which is used in the clinical laboratory, cleaves F.IX, primarily resulting in F.IXaα; however, the 10 to 20 times faster rate of F.X activation by RVV indicates that F.X activation is the primary means by which RVV activates clot formation.[52] F.IXa is inhibited by formation of a 1:1 complex with antithrombin[52] and heparin.

Structurally, the F.IX protein (Fig. 173-3) consists of a prepropeptide region (approximately residues -39 to -1; see "Synthesis" below), a modified glutamic acid-rich region referred to as the Gla domain (residues 1 to 40), a short aromatic stack (residues 41 to 46), two epidermal growth factor regions (EGF1, residues 47 to 84; and EGF2, residues 85 to 127), an activation peptide (residues 146 to 180), and a catalytic region (residues 181 to 415).[56] F.IXa amplifies clot formation through its direct activation of F.X by cleavage of the Arg 52 to Ile 53 bond within the F.X heavy chain. F.Xa then activates prothrombin to thrombin, a molecule with diverse and potent hemostatic activities (Fig. 173-1). The F.IX interacts with calcium ions needed to induce a conformational change while the phospholipid surface enables assembly of the F.X activating complex. Calcium and phospholipid lower the K_m of F.IXa for F.X by over 5000-fold; F.VIIIa increases the catalytic efficiency of F.X cleavage by F.IXa by 200,000-fold but affects the K_m only slightly.[57]

Brandstetter et al. reported the 3.0 Å-resolution structure of porcine F.IXa that clearly shows the structures of the serine proteinase module and the two preceding epidermal growth factor (EGF)-like domains.[58] The structural data show that mutations that cause hemophilia B often occur at surface site residues on the

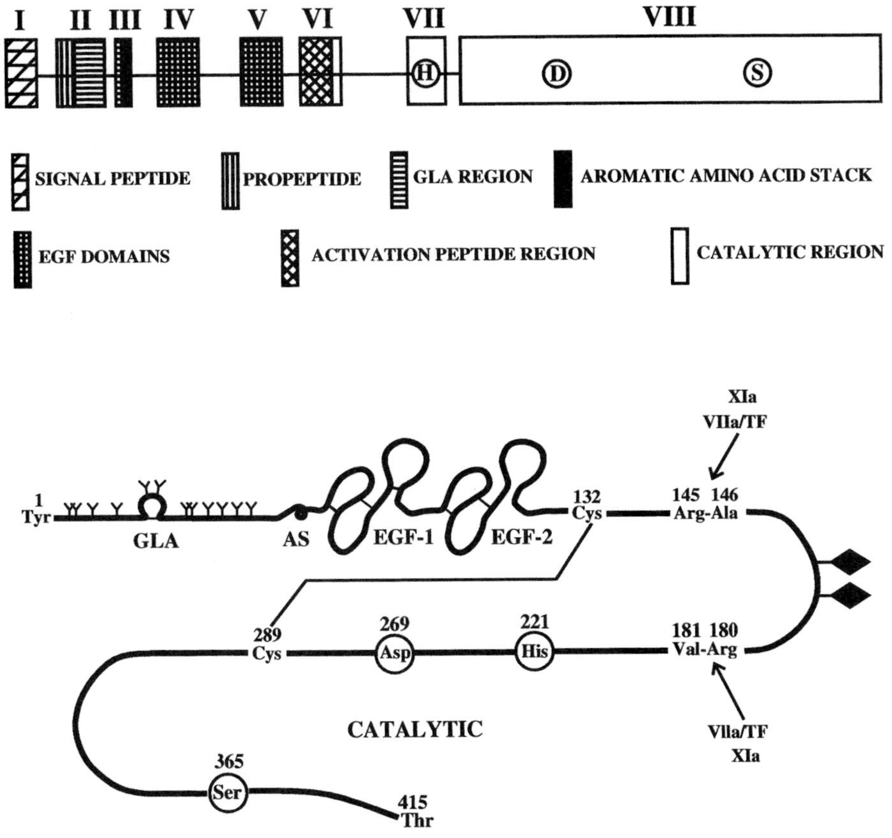

Fig. 173-3 *Top,* Exon-intron locations of the human F.IX gene and regions of the protein encoded by exons. *Bottom,* View of human F.IX protein domains: Gla (γ-glutamic acid); AS (aromatic stack); EGF1 (epidermal growth factor-like domain-1); EGF2 (epidermal growth factor-like domain-2); AP (activation peptide); and catalytic. TF = tissue factor. The diamond-shaped structures represent potential *N*-linked carbohydrate side chains in the activation peptide. (*From Bajaj, SP and Birktoft JJ. Human Factor IX and Factor IXa. Methods Enzymol, 222:97, 1993. Used with permission.*)

concave surface of F.IX. The hypothesized model of F.IXa/F.VIIIa/F.X interactions (Fig. 173-4) illustrates how F.VIIIa stabilizes the F.IXa catalytic active site to position it for activating F.X.[58] Mutations of specific regions as detailed below help define the functions and physiological contacts of the F.IX protein.

SYNTHESIS

The F.IX gene is 34 kb in length and located on chromosome Xq27.1, centromeric to the fragile X locus and the F.VIII gene.[59,60] The F.IX gene includes 8 exons ranging in size from 25 to 1935 nucleotides with a high degree of homology to members of the vitamin K-dependent protein family, particularly F.VII, F.X, and Protein C.[61] Repetitive *Alu* sequences are present in intron 1, intron 6, and the 3′ untranslated region. *Kpn* repeats are found in the 5′ flanking region and in intron 4.[62]

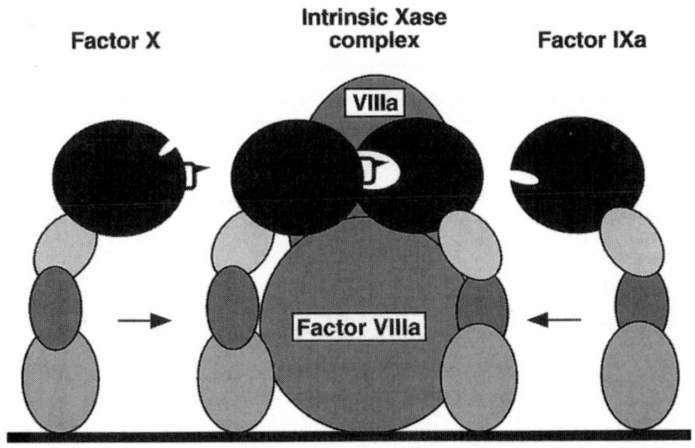

Fig. 173-4 Drawing of the intrinsic Xase complex, the interaction between F.IXa with F.VIIIa leading to the activation of F.X. (*From Bode et al: Comparative analysis of hemostatic proteinases: Structural aspects of thrombin factor Xa, factor IXa, and protein O. Thromb Haemost 78(1):507, 1997. Used with permission.*)

Levels of F.IX are 50 percent of adult values in the healthy full-term infant and are even further reduced in preterm infants. Levels gradually rise toward full-term infant values as a function of gestational age; levels reach approximately 80 percent of adult levels by day 180 of life.[13] Levels in healthy children (average age 7.5 years) remain only 83 percent of adult values.[63] This is in contradistinction to the normal F.VIII levels seen during the neonatal period. Regulation of the expression of F.IX reveals several interesting characteristics, particularly with respect to the clinical entity known as hemophilia B Leyden, an unusual condition that results in hemophilia until puberty, at which time F.IX levels climb to near normal (see "Hemophilia B Leyden" below and Fig. 173-5).[64]

Human F.IX is synthesized in the liver as a precursor, an approximately 454-amino acid compound that contains an amino acid hydrophobic signal peptide that is followed by an 18-amino acid propeptide, both of which are removed proteolytically to produce the mature F.IX zymogen.[62] The physiologically precise start of translation of the proenzyme is unknown; however, homology with dog, rat, and mouse genes, and similarity to the Kozak consensus sequence favors the −39 methionine as the start site, although methionines at −46 and −41 may also be used.[65,66] The organization of the human F.IX gene and a diagram of the protein structure are shown in Fig. 173-3.[56]

As a member of the family of vitamin K-dependent proteins, F.IX requires posttranslational carboxylation for functional coagulant activity. This posttranslational modification, carboxylation of 12 specific glutamic acid residues at the N-terminus of the mature protein, is catalyzed by γ-glutamyl carboxylase, and requires as a cofactor the reduced form of vitamin K (KH_2), which is converted to vitamin K epoxide (KO) in the course of the reaction. The clinically important anticoagulant medication warfarin inhibits the regeneration of reduced vitamin K (KH_2) from the vitamin K epoxide.[67] F.IX undergoes several other

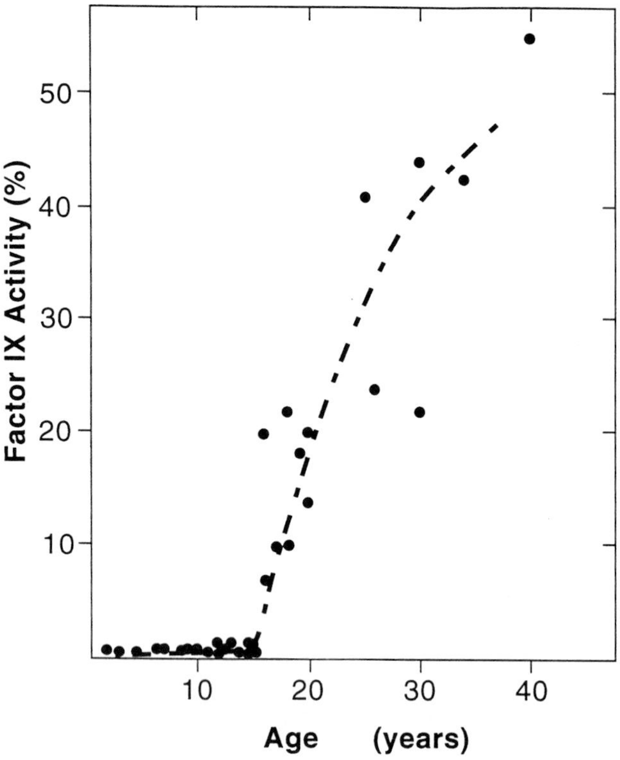

Fig. 173-5 Graph showing the postpuberty age-related increase in F.IX activity levels in patients with Hemophilia B Leyden. (*From Briet et al.: Hemophilia B Leyden—A sex-linked hereditary disorder that improves after puberty. N Engl J Med 306:788, 1982. Used with permssion.*)

posttranslational modifications, most prominently glycosylation and tyrosine sulfation and serine phosphorylation of the activation peptide. Analysis of these modifications assumed special importance with the advent of recombinant protein and gene-based therapeutic approaches. Both choice of cell lines for production, in the case of recombinant proteins, and choice of target cell, in the case of gene therapy, must be designed with a view toward ensuring that the posttranslational modifications required for stability and coagulant activity are carried out efficiently.

Polymorphisms and Normal Variants in the F.IX Gene

Eight common polymorphisms have been described in populations of European and African descent at different frequencies in these populations (Table 173-1) such that linkage analysis can provide a variable certainty (between 50 and 100 percent) of carrier status in the heterozygous female. These polymorphisms, however, are much less common in Asian and other populations. The most informative polymorphism documented in the Asian population is *Hha*I (allele frequency = 0.17);[68,69] several recent reports have described additional polymorphic loci in these populations facilitating molecular diagnosis of non-Caucasian carriers and patients with hemophilia B.[69–73] With increasing laboratory familiarity with PCR amplification, definitive diagnosis of point mutations leading to hemophilia B is becoming more commonplace.[74–76] The laboratory of Dr. Arthur Thompson describes 19 common mutations for which they commonly screen.[77] This facilitates genetic counseling and provides information concerning the molecular basis of the disease. Characterization of mutations in kindreds provides more definitive information than activity testing, particularly in pregnant carriers.

One polymorphism exists within the F.IX *coding* region, resulting in an Ala/Thr variation at residue 148 within the activation peptide. Unlike amino acid polymorphisms associated with other clotting factors such as F.VII and fibrinogen,[78,79] the F.IX 148 polymorphism is not correlated with any change in either F.IX activity or antigen levels. The polymorphism occurs at high frequency in the Caucasian population (frequency of the Thr allele is 0.3), however, the Thr allele occurs much less frequently in the African-American population (0.053 to 0.15) and Asian[FES3] populations (< 0.01).

MUTATIONS RESULTING IN F.IX DEFICIENCY

A detailed and extensive database of mutations resulting in F.IX deficiency is available as a Web site supplement to the January 1998 Nucleic Acids Research article at www.umds.ac.uk/molgen/haemBdatabase.htm. This ninth edition of the hemophilia B published database (www.umds.ac.uk/molgen/),[80] updated annually since the original compilation in 1990,[81] includes a description of all known F.IX mutations due to base substitutions and short additions and/or deletions of <30 base pairs. The database includes 1918 patient entries entered in ascending order by nucleotide position using the Yoshitake nucleotide numbering system[62] and details the following: (a) nucleotide mutation and position; (b) the amino acid change and location using the Anson amino acid numbering system; (c) the resultant coagulant activity and antigen levels; (d) the mechanism responsible for the mutation, if known; (e) whether or not the mutation occurs at a CpG dinucleotide; (f) the initial publication reference describing the mutation; and (g) additional information such as the occurrence of a *de novo* mutation, the occurrence in a female, and the presence of an inhibitor antibody when known. The

Table 173-1 Frequency of Rare Allelle

Polymorphic site	Location	Caucasian*	U.S. African-American	Asian†	References
−793 promoter	5′ flanking sequence	0.44		0.48	69, 73
*Mse*I	5′ flanking sequence (−698)	0.33		0.32 (Thai)	71
5′ *Bam*HI	5′ flanking sequence	<0.01–0.06	0.30–0.48	<0.01	276, 281, 286
*Hin*fI/*Dde*I	Intron 1	0.24	0.17–0.36	<0.01–0.07	71, 276, 278, 281, 286
FIX192	Intron 1			0.26	69
*Bam*HI	Intron 2	0.02–0.07	0.13–0.36	<0.01–0.02	277–279, 286
*Xmn*I	Intron 3	0.15–0.30	0.05–0.12	0.01–0.02	276–279
*Taq*I	Intron 4	0.29–0.35	0.10–0.14	0.01–0.04	59, 277, 279, 280, 286
*Msp*I	Intron 4	0.22	0.39–0.45	<0.01	59, 279, 281
Ala/Thr	Exon 6 (Ala148 in the activation peptide of the FIX zymogen)	0.33	0.03–0.15	0.01–0.04	277, 282, 283, 286
*Hha*I	8 kb 3′ of exon 8	0.40–0.51	0.33–0.57	0.17–0.18	68, 277

*Numbers are frequency of rare allele.
†Asian includes individuals of East Asian decent including individuals from China, Japan, and Thailand.

database is the largest compilation of naturally occurring mutations associated with a human disease; a description of these mutations is far beyond the scope of this chapter.

Mutations are often described based on the presence of F.IX antigen when compared to in vitro coagulant activity. Plasma from patients with CRM^- mutations (cross-reactive material negative), is F.IX antigen-negative. CRM^R mutations have a reduced F.IX antigen level compared to coagulant activity and CRM^+ mutations have normal F.IX antigen levels but a dysfunctional protein (i.e., F.IX B_M). Several representative abnormal variants of historic, biologic, and clinical interest are described below.

Analysis of mutations responsible for hemophilia B reveals that vital amino acids in the F.IX protein can be divided into two main classes: those in which the nature of the specific amino acid is critical such that a change results in a dysfunctional protein, and those that are necessary as "spacers" to provide appropriate conformation.[82] Approximately half of point mutations in the F.IX gene are related to mutations arising due to gene methylation at CpG dinucleotides; approximately 40 percent arise at 11 mutation hot spots.[83] Because of the lack of geographic regional variation in the mutation pattern as expected with environmental mutagens, the lack of characteristic mutagen-induced patterns of mutations, and the frequency of the deamination, depurination, and replication errors, the F.IX mutation pattern reveals that the majority of germ line mutations arose from an endogenous process rather than from environmental mutagens. Extensive documentation of mutations leading to hemophilia B provides a useful model for understanding principles related to inheritance of monogenic disorders.[82] Sommer points out the following inherited pattern of germ line mutations in the United States:

1. Mild disease arose from transmission by three founders in the majority of individuals (two-thirds of the cases);
2. Moderate to severe disease arose within the last 150 years, almost entirely from independent mutations;
3. Mutations occur in the following order: transitions > transversions > deletions and insertions;
4. Transitions at CpG dinucleotides are elevated approximately twenty-fourfold relative to transitions at non-CpG dinucleotides; transversions at CpG are elevated approximately eightfold relative to transversions at non-CpG dinucleotides;
5. The evolutionarily conserved GC content of the F.IX gene (40 percent) is consistent with the bias against G + C bases due to the sum total of the GC dinucleotide mutation rates;
6. In Caucasian U.S. inhabitants, the mutation pattern is similar to that in Asians residing in Asia.

Mutations Affecting Regulatory Sequences of the F.IX Gene

Hemophilia B Leyden. A number of functional mutations have been described within the well-characterized promoter region of the F.IX gene. The majority of these mutations result in the lack of coagulant activity due to the absence of antigen. A unique group of mutations exist within the promoter region between bases −20 and +13, which result in the phenotype of hemophilia B Leyden, a severe form of hemophilia B that largely resolves after puberty.[64,84] This unique phenotype is characterized by prepubertal low levels of F.IX (usually <1 percent) which rise approximately 5 percent a year postpuberty and reach near normal levels at around 20 years of age (Fig. 173-5).[64,85] Five distinct protein-binding regions are present in the approximately 40-bp Leyden region of the F.IX promoter.[86,87] A number of point mutations at bases −21, −20, −6, −5, +8, +13[88–94] in proximity to the major transcription start sites (+1, +4, +30)[95,96] are associated with the Leyden phenotype.

The molecular mechanism responsible for the phenotype resulting from this group of mutations is under scrutiny. Surprisingly, the HepG2 hepatoblastoma cell line, used for many studies of liver specific protein synthesis, does not naturally synthesize F.IX,[97] which makes the in vitro study of F.IX transcriptional regulation more difficult. One hypothesis advanced to explain the phenotype of hemophilia B Leyden involves a putative androgen response element (ARE) which overlaps the binding site of hepatocyte nuclear factor-4 (HNF-4), a liver-enriched transcription factor essential for the synthesis of F.IX and many other liver-specific proteins.[98] According to this hypothesis, the increase in androgens at puberty compensates for the lack of binding of HNF-4 thus allowing synthesis of near normal concentrations of F.IX. The original description of this mechanism distinguishes the hemophilia B Leyden phenotype from that seen in the Brandenburg mutation at −26 in the F.IX promoter, resulting in a life-long disease state.[98] Mutations at −26 are associated not only with loss of binding of HNF-4 but also with disruption of the consensus ARE.[98,99] However, this hypothesis does not fully explain the similar phenotype seen with mutations further downstream, which inhibit binding of distinct proteins that are not HNF-4. Moreover, footprinting studies have never convincingly demonstrated binding of purified androgen receptor to the putative ARE.

Other hypotheses include indirect effects through the binding of nonandrogen response element proteins such as the albumin D-site-binding protein (DBP), which also increases postpuberty. Transactivation of the F.IX promoter by the PAR (proline and acidic amino acid rich) domain proteins DBP or HLF (hepatic leukemia factor) is also dependent on the binding of the Ets transcription factor GA-binding protein (GABP-α) and enhanced by the CAAT/enhancer-binding protein (C/EBP-α).[100–102] Thus, while the current understanding of the F.IX promoter provides a reasonable explanation for the low levels of protein during childhood, the molecular basis of the recovery remains a mystery.

Mutations Affecting the Signal Sequence and Propeptide Region

The F.IX protein contains an amino acid prepropeptide region containing a leader sequence, followed by an 18-amino acid propeptide, which is cleaved to produce the mature F.IX zymogen.[103] In addition to several frameshift and stop mutations in the signal peptide sequence, missense mutations have been reported at two residues (− 30 and − 19).[80] The − 30 mutation (Ile − 30 → Asp − 30) results in severe, CRM^- disease attributed to lack of hepatic secretion of F.IX due to a disruption of the hydrophobic signal sequence core.[104]

Naturally occurring single amino acid substitutions in the F.IX propeptide at Arg −4 (F.IX Kawachinagano, F.IX Bostexl, F.IX Bendorf, and F.IX Seattle C) produce dysfunctional F.IX molecules; the propeptide is retained in the circulating protein. The mutant F.IX has normal total γ-Gla content,[105,106] but the mutation is thought to interfere with the N-terminus, preventing necessary metal-induced conformational changes for functional F.IX activity.[105] Further studies have confirmed these results and suggest that mutations in F.IX that interfere with propeptide cleavage principally decrease its activity by destabilizing the calcium-induced conformation.[107] Other mutations in the propeptide of F.IX (F.IX Cambridge) that result in retention of the 18-residue propeptide (Arg −1 → Ser −1) also result in decreased functional activity.[108]

Mutations Affecting the Glutamic Acid and Aromatic Stack Regions

The vitamin K-dependent coagulant proteins (F.II, F.VII, F.IX, F.X, protein C, protein S, and protein Z) require γ-carboxylation of between 9 and 13 glutamic acid residues near the amino terminus (Fig. 173-3; see Chap. 169). Vitamin K serves as a cofactor for the γ-glutamyl carboxylase that catalyzes this reaction (see "Synthesis" above). An intact Gla domain is essential for functional activity; however, the additional eleventh and twelfth Gla residues of F.IX (residues 36 and 40), which are not conserved in other vitamin K-dependent proteins, are not required for functional activity.[109]

A number of naturally occurring missense Gla mutations have been described which result in CRM^-, CRM^R, or CRM^+ mutations, depending on both the amino acid position of the change and the amino acid substitution.[80] A naturally occurring CRM^R mutant at Gla 12 (F.IXLA4) does not affect activation of F.IX by XIa, but does preclude activation by the F.VIIa-TF complex.[55] Analysis of this F.IXLA4 also showed that structural integrity of the F.IX Gla domain is necessary for F.IXa/F.VIIIa binding enabling formation of the active enzymatic Xase complex.[55]

The F.IXa Gla domain facilitates F.IX/IXa cellular binding; residues 3 to 11 bind collagen IV[110] and residues 4 to 11 mediate binding to a site on activated human platelets distinct from the site used for assembly of the Xase complex.[111] Residues 6 and 9 in the Gla domain are thought to be particularly important in interacting with phospholipids.[112] Full binding activity to endothelial cells is additionally thought to require proper folding with the entire Gla domain and aromatic stack.[113]

In the short hydrophobic region (the aromatic stack), located at residues 41 through 46, several missense mutations, resulting in mild CRM^+ or CRM^R disease, have been reported. However, these reports are not accompanied by structure-function analysis.[80]

Mutations Affecting EGF Domains

The EGF modules of the vitamin K-dependent proteins do not retain growth factor activity, but rather serve as Ca^{2+} binding modules, and also serve as spacers between the Gla and catalytic domains.[114] F.IX has two EGF modules at residues 47 to 84 (EGF1) and residues 85 to 127 (EGF2). Posttranslational modifications in EGF1 include partial γ-hydroxylation (30 percent) of Asp 64[115] and glycosylation of Ser 53. Site-directed mutagenesis studies confirm the necessity of Asp residues 47, 49, and Asp/Hya 64 in F.IXa. (Hya is erythro-β-hydroxyaspartic acid, which is a posttranslational hydroxylation of aspartic acid.[114,115]) Mutations affecting the Asp 64 site result in reduced F.VIIIa binding by F.IXa in the presence of Ca^{2+}.[116] Replacement of the EGF1-F.IX by that from F.VII increases the affinity of the chimeric molecule for F.VIIIa.[117]

Naturally occurring mutations have been described in EGF2;[80] however, the role of this EGF module is less clear. Studies examining the EGF2 domain suggest its importance in specific high-affinity F.IXa binding to platelets in the presence of F.VIIIa and F.X.[118] Opposite charges on EGF1 and EGF2 domains at residues Glu 78 and Arg 94 are thought necessary for linking the domains to maintain the F.VIII light chain binding site.[119]

Mutations Affecting the Catalytic Region

The catalytic region of F.IX encoded by part of the sixth, and the seventh, and eighth exons of the F.IX gene, contains the enzymatic serine protease-like portion of F.IXa, with residues His 221, Asp 269, and Ser 365 forming the classic catalytic triad characteristic of serine-like proteases. Of the coagulant proteins, the catalytic domain of F.IXa most closely resembles that of F.Xa.[120] Numerous mutations have been described which alter the functional F.IX protein by either disrupting necessary conformational elements or ionic charges. Mutations also occur at donor and acceptor splice sites and within introns to create new cryptic splice sites. As noted earlier, a number of the most frequently reported mutations occur at CG dinucleotides and involve a CG→TG or CA change (hot spots for mutations). Other frequently observed mutations seem to be caused by a "founder" effect; based on haplotype analysis, these mutations, described from distinct geographic locations, appear to have arisen from a single common ancestor.[121,122] Additionally, one study suggests that the C-terminal region is critical for cellular secretion of F.IX such that mutations in this region can make the mutant protein subject to proteasomal degradation.[123]

Hemophilia B_M. Hemophilia B_M presents an interesting phenotype caused by a heterogeneous group of mutations in the catalytic domain or the activation peptide of F.IX. The phenotype was named after the first patient (surname Martin) described in 1967 by Hougie.[124] The phenotype is defined by a CRM^+ F.IX deficiency[125] with coagulant activity usually <1 percent with normal F.IX antigen levels, with the unique feature that not only the aPTT (activated partial thromboplastin time) is prolonged, but the PT (prothrombin time) is prolonged when ox-brain (also called bovine brain) thromboplastin reagent, but not rabbit or human thromboplastin reagent, is used.[126] This ox-brain prothrombin time prolongation is not corrected after the addition of a quantity of normal plasma sufficient to produce a full correction of the aPTT. Additional studies reveal that the concentrations of reagents (thromboplastin, and F.IX and F.X levels) are important and that high concentrations of either normal F.IX or rabbit or human thromboplastins can inhibit PT assays.[126]

At least nine naturally occurring single amino acid substitutions have been described that result in this phenotype, including mutations at residue 180 at the C-terminus of the activation peptide, at residues 181 and 182 near the N-terminus of the heavy chain, and at residues 311, 364, 368, 390, 396, and 397 near the F.IX activation site.[81] In vitro mutagenesis reveals that not only the location but the identity of the amino acid substitution is important in causing the F.IX B_M phenotype.[127] The mutations result in variable effects with respect to F.XI activation, but they share the common property that the molecule interacts with components of the tissue factor pathway as a competitive inhibitor of F.X activation, thus prolonging the ox-brain PT,[128] even in the presence of normal F.IX. Removal of F.IXB_M from patient plasma by immunoadsorption corrects the prolonged ox-brain prothrombin time while addition of F.IXB_M to normal plasma prolongs the time.[128,129]

MUTATIONS LEADING TO DISEASE STATES OTHER THAN HEMOPHILIA B

Warfarin Sensitivity

Recently, two mutations in the propeptide of F.IX were reported in association with a unique phenotype, warfarin sensitivity.[130,131] Patients with mutations at Ala −10 (Ala −10 → Thr −10, Ala −10 → Val−10) have a normal hemostatic profile with aPTTs and F.IX levels within the normal range. However, upon treatment with warfarin, the F.IX level drops precipitously to <1 percent in the setting of therapeutically acceptable levels (15 to 30 percent) of the other vitamin K-dependent clotting enzymes (F.II, F.VII and F.X). In vitro biochemical analysis of the Ala −10 → Thr −10 defect revealed a direct effect on the efficiency of carboxylation due to a thirtyfold reduced affinity for the carboxylase enzyme with unchanged affinity for vitamin K.[130] The question of prophylactic screening of male patients being placed on warfarin has been addressed by Peters et al. who conclude that the incidence of this mutation is too low to warrant screening.[132] However, in patients taking warfarin who exhibit recurrent hemorrhage, evaluation and documentation of a disproportionately prolonged aPTT should warrant examination of F.IX levels in proportion to F.VII levels to address the possibility of warfarin sensitivity.

Hypercoagulability

Using alanine scanning mutagenesis to identify residues critical for the interaction between F.IXa and F.VIIIa, Stafford et al. identified a residue (Arg 338), which, when changed to alanine, resulted in coagulant activity three times higher than that of wild-type or plasma-derived F.IX.[133] Although the exact mechanism for this enhanced activity is not known, Stafford et al. suggest that Arg 338 is part of an extended macromolecular binding site which, when changed to the uncharged and less sterically constricting Ala 338, enables F.IXa to interact more favorably with its cofactor F.VIIIa and increases the enzymatic efficiency resulting in enhanced ability to activate F.X. Studies also show an enhanced interaction with the anticoagulant heparin. Interestingly, the codon for Arg 338 contains a CpG dinucleotide that had been predicted to be a mutation "hotspot." Sommer and colleagues pointed out several years ago the absence of mutations at Arg 338 from the hemophilia B database and raised the question of whether a mutation at this site resulted in a nonhemophilic phenotype.[133]

LABORATORY DIAGNOSIS

The principal tests performed by a routine clinical laboratory for screening patients for potential bleeding problems due to coagulation factor defects are the PT (prothrombin time) and the aPTT (activated partial thromboplastin time).

Hemophilia most commonly presents during infancy or early childhood. When a long aPTT is found in the presence of a normal PT, particularly in a symptomatic male child, subsequent analyses for F.VIII and F.IX levels are performed to diagnose hemophilia A or B. Analyses are performed by measuring the time to clot formation after diluting the patient's plasma with reagent plasma, deficient in the coagulation protein being assayed. When a long aPTT is found in an adult male in the absence of anticoagulant therapy, the subsequent diagnostic test, an inhibitor screen, distinguishes between a prolongation due to a clotting protein deficiency state versus prolongation due to an inhibitory antibody. Liver disease and/or vitamin K deficiency may result in low F.IX levels in either the adult or pediatric patient, but the PT is usually prolonged in this setting. Thus, it may be necessary to assay other coagulant protein levels for appropriate diagnosis. Acquired inhibitory F.VIII antibodies are seen occasionally in individuals without hemophilia A; only rare case reports exist that describe such antibody formation to F.IX in patients who do not have hemophilia B.[134]

Patients with F.IX deficiency can often be misdiagnosed historically and from a laboratory perspective. Although F.VIII is a heat-labile protein that is easily degraded during prolonged specimen retrieval, F.IX can better withstand prolonged exposure to room temperature, which means that fewer false positive F.IX-deficiency results will be seen from inappropriately stored specimens. The sensitivity of partial thromboplastin reagents to deficiencies of various clotting proteins varies widely. With currently available partial thromboplastin reagents in the setting of other normal clotting factor levels, F.IX levels associated with a prolonged aPTT are less than 50 percent. Marked prolongation of the aPTT is seen below F.IX levels of 10 percent (Fig. 173-6). In the early 1980s, there was an increase in the number of patients diagnosed with mild hemophilia (from 35 percent of cases in 1960 to 54 percent of cases in 1980), as a comprehensive Swedish survey in 1980 of the hemophilia A and B population showed. This increase was attributed to improved ability of laboratories to diagnose mild disease.[135] It has also been recognized that approximately 50 percent of healthy children have aPTT values over the 95th percentile of the healthy adult aPTT values.[63]

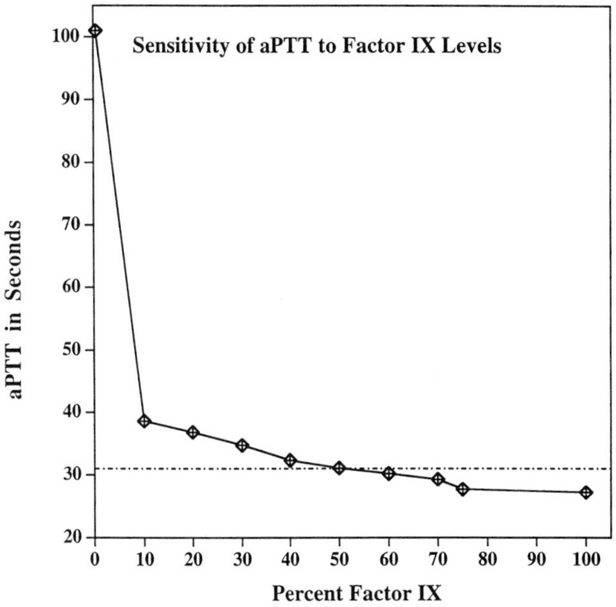

Fig. 173-6 Sensitivity of activated partial thromboplastin (aPTT) to levels of F.IX activity. The curve is generated by dilution of pooled plasma with F.IX-deficient plasma from a patient with severe hemophilia (<1 percent activity). The upper range of normal is 31 seconds (horizontal dotted line). aPTT values are beyond the reference range at levels <50 percent. The curve is based on values generated at the Hospital of the University of Pennsylvania using a standard 1998 lot of a commercially available partial thromboplastin reagent (Organon-Technika) and performed on an automated coagulation instrument.

TREATMENT

Acute Bleeding Episodes

A number of treatment options are currently available for the management of acute bleeding episodes for patients with hemophilia B. Available products containing F.IX include fresh frozen plasma (FFP), prothrombin complex concentrates (PCCs), activated prothrombin complex concentrates, monoclonal-antibody purified F.IX, and recombinant F.IX. Recombinant F.VIIa (rFVIIa) has recently been approved by the FDA and may be used for hemophilia B patients with inhibitors during acute bleeds. In addition, gene therapy approaches are currently undergoing clinical investigation. When possible, it is most advantageous to treat patients with hemophilia B with either highly purified F.IX concentrates or recombinant F.IX. Issues dictating the choice of F.IX product include availability, ease of administration, cost, viral safety, and thrombotic risk, particularly in patients undergoing high-dose therapy or procedures with a high risk of thrombotic complications. In scenarios in which coadministration of additional clotting proteins is advantageous, FFP and PCCs provide a complement of other clotting proteins. Cryoprecipitate, containing approximately 80 units of F.VIII/unit, does not contain F.IX.[136] Available F.IX concentrates in the U.S. and Europe are shown in Table 173-2.

FFP is readily available in most emergency settings. Methods for viral inactivating have not been previously applied to FFP production in the past; however, solvent-detergent treated plasma is now available, and as each unit is from only one screened donor, the risk of viral transmission is low.[137] Concentrated F.IX preparations have been available since the 1960s.[138] From the standpoint of both viral transmission and thrombogenicity, these products have dramatically improved over the past 15 years. Several immunoaffinity-purified plasma-derived F.IX products are available in the United States and Europe, and have excellent records of viral safety, efficacy, and lack of thrombogenicity. These products have two orders of magnitude higher F.IX-specific activities in IU/mg protein as compared to PCCs. A safety and efficacy study in previously untreated hemophilia B patients using a monoclonal antibody purified F.IX product yielded excellent results.[139] Such high-purity concentrates are recommended in settings in which thrombosis is more likely such as surgery; trauma involving the central nervous system or massive injury in which release of natural tissue thromboplastin is suspected; high and/or long-term use of F.IX concentrate; a history of thrombosis; reduced clearance of active complexes; liver disease; and immature newborns.[140]

rFIX was licensed in 1997. It is produced from cultured Chinese hamster ovary cells containing an expression construct for F.IX, purified from conditioned medium through a process of seven steps of chromatographic, chemical, and filtration techniques,[141]

Table 173-2 Preparations for Treatment of Hemophilia B

Product	Viral inactivation procedure(s)	Specific activity (IU/mg protein) final product
Prothrombin Complex Concentrates:		
Bebulin VH (Immuno distributed by Baxter)	Vapor heat (10 h, 60°C, 1190 mbar pressure plus 1 h, 80°C, 1375 mbar pressure)	2.0
Proplex T (Baxter)	Dry heat (68°C, 144 h)	3.9
Profilinine SD (Alpha)	Solvent detergent (TNBP and polysorbate 80)	4.5
Konyne 80 (Bayer)	Dry heat (80°C, 72 h)	1.25
Highly Purified Factor IX Concentrates:		
AlphaNine SD (Alpha)	(1) Dual affinity chromatography (2) Solvent detergent (TNBP and polysorbate 80) (3) Nanofiltration	230
Mononine (Centeon)	(1) Immunoaffinity chromatography (2) Sodium thiocyanate (3) Ultrafiltration	>160
Recombinant Factor IX Concentrates:		
Benefix (Genetic Institute)	(1) Affinity chromatography (2) Ultrafiltration	>200
Bypassing Agents:		
Activated Prothrombin Complex Concentrates:		
Autoplex T (Baxter distributed by Nabi)	Dry heat (68°C, 144 h)	5
FEIBA (Immuno distributed by Baxter)	Vapor heat 10 h, 60°C, 1190 mbar Plus 1 h, 80°, 1375 mbar)	0.8

and processed in a form devoid of human plasma proteins that is optimal for storage and administration.[142] Empirically, it has been shown that rFIX has a similar half-life to plasma-derived products. However, the recovered in vivo coagulant activity is 80 percent of in vitro estimates used for labeling of product in IU/mg. Thus, it is recommended to multiply the calculated F.IX administration dosage by a factor of 1.2 for dosage calculation when using rFIX. A plausible explanation for this discrepancy is a difference in posttranslational modifications.[53]

rF.VIIa is used with great efficacy with few serious adverse side effects in F.VIII or F.IX inhibitor patients, patients whose management can be extremely difficult. Treatment in over 400 hemophilia patients with over 1900 treatments was rated as excellent and efficacious in 92 percent, 88 percent, 80 percent, 76 percent, 75 percent, or 62 percent of dental, central nervous system, ear/nose/throat, joint, retroperitoneal or internal, or muscle bleeds, respectively.[143] This product, was approved for use by the FDA in 1999.

During severe and critical bleeds it is optimal to achieve 50 to 100 percent F.IX activity levels for 7 to 10 days (e.g. for pharyngeal, retropharyngeal, retroperitoneal, and central nervous system bleeds). More modest levels of 20 to 50 percent for 2 to 7 days are generally adequate for dental extractions, hematuria, intramuscular or soft tissue bleeds with dissection, or bleeds of the mucous membranes. Levels of 20 to 30 percent for 1 to 2 days are recommended for uncomplicated hemarthroses, superficial muscle or soft tissue bleeds. The frequency of dosing is every 12 to 24 h.[144] At 24 h, the calculated amount to infuse is one-half the initial amount of F.IX, required as the half-life of F.IX is approximately 24 h.[38] Due to the variable response in patient F.IX levels to F.IX concentrate administration, a trial should be performed in a nonemergency setting to assess a patient's response to a given product before needing to urgently administer the F.IX concentrate during a life-threatening bleed.

The following formula calculates the optimal F.IX concentration for administration:

$$\text{Number of F.IX IU (International Units) required}^{*} = (\text{kg body weight}) \times (\text{desired percent increase in factor IX level}) \times (1.2)\dagger$$

The timing of F.IX level determination is suggested as 15 min after the loading dose and immediately before subsequent doses for appropriate dosing adjustments.[144] When F.IX concentrate is used for a patient with an inhibitor, higher doses are likely to be required. Additionally, some authors have reported good success and reduced cost with constant infusion regimens.[147–149]

Surgery in Patients with Hemophilia

Institution of treatment by caregivers aware of major and minor adverse reactions and complications that occur in this patient population is one of the most important measures to minimize complications in the surgical management of patients with hemophilia. It is also essential that care be given in association with an experienced reference laboratory able to provide timely evaluation of a patient's response to treatment. A therapeutic level of F.IX should be obtained before surgery. Depending on the type of surgery, the F.IX level should reach 50 to 100 percent of normal levels and should be maintained for 2 to 7 days postprocedure. Complications from high-dose prophylactic therapy have greatly decreased with the availability of higher purity factors.[150] In

* Because F.IX is not confined to the intravascular space, in part due to binding of F.IX to endothelial cells, twice as much F.IX concentrate is administered compared to the dosage of F.VIII that would be administered under similar conditions.

†When using the only available recombinant protein (BeneFix), it has empirically been shown that it is necessary to multiply this dosage by a factor of 1.2 IU/kg to achieve the projected desired level[145,146]

addition to factor concentrates, fibrin glue has been recommended with circumcision,[151] antifibrinolytics with dental procedures,[37,152] aprotinin with cardiac procedures,[153] and rFVIIa and/or apheresis in patients with high titer inhibitors (in whom surgery should be avoided if at all possible (see "Complications of Treatment" below).[154–157] The use of aprotinin, however, has been proposed to increase the risk of thrombogenicity.[158,159] Brain or prostate surgery, in particular, present a higher risk of bleeding; a level approaching 100 percent is appropriate in these cases. The administration of DDAVP, helpful in the treatment of von Willebrand disease and hemophilia A, does not cause a rise in F.IX levels.

COMPLICATIONS OF THERAPY

The main adverse outcomes related to treatment with F.IX concentrates include viral transmission, thrombosis, and development of inhibitory F.IX antibodies. The incidence of viral contamination has markedly decreased since the recognition of the problem and development of purification schemes that eradicate viruses or prevent exposure through recombinant synthesis of F.IX. Thrombotic complications were principally, although not exclusively, a problem with early preparations of PCCs, which now have additional purification steps to eliminate activated phospholipid constituents. Inhibitor development, although uncommon in the setting of F.IX deficiency, remains problematic, especially in light of the recent recognition of anaphylactoid reactions in inhibitor patients.[160]

Viral Diseases

Viral infection due to contamination of plasma-derived products pooled from thousands of donors is a major cause of morbidity and mortality in the hemophilia population. This is most problematic in severely affected patients requiring multiple doses of products, especially in those treated before 1985.[161] Over the course of a 70-year life span, a patient with severe hemophilia may be exposed to donations from 70 million individuals due to the pooling of thousands of donor units for concentrate production.[162] There are ongoing efforts to reduce the size of the donor pool to 15,000 donors for each lot of concentrate. Now, better screening procedures for donors, including a detailed donor history of risk factors for hepatitides and HIV, testing for increased levels of liver enzymes, and specific laboratory tests to screen for HIV, HCV, and HBV have dramatically limited the number of donations from individuals carrying viral diseases.

Inactivation procedures for both the enveloped viruses (HIV and hepatitis viruses B, C, D, and G) susceptible to many solvent decontamination procedures, and nonenveloped viruses (hepatitis A and E viruses and parvovirus B19) largely inactivated by heat treatment, has decreased the risk of viral infection from plasma-derived products. Currently used viral inactivation procedures include pasteurization, vapor heating, high-dry heating, and nanofiltration.[163] Regulations instituted in the mid-1980s mandating virucidal steps in the manufacturing process drastically reduced the incidence of virally contaminated concentrates.[164,165] Recent contamination of concentrates with HIV have been due to ineffective virucidal techniques such as beta-propiolactone UV inactivation.[163,166] The recent availability of recombinant product devoid of any plasma-derived product has changed the expected morbidity associated with administration of F.IX concentrates.[167]

HIV. The appearance of HIV in the blood supply in the late 1970s and early 1980s predated the routine laboratory testing for contamination. In 1982, hemorrhage was still the leading cause of death in U.S. hemophilia patients; however, the incidence of viral disease began rising sharply in 1984,[168] after seroconversion, principally during the period between 1979 to 1983. A large proportion of hemophilia patients became infected with HIV and subsequently died from AIDS.[8,169] The proportion of patients infected was largely associated with the specific concentrate used (F.VIII vs. F.IX concentrate),[170] the viral inactivation procedures, the severity of the disease (severely affected patients much more commonly affected than those with moderate or mild disease),[161] and the geographic location of the patient with regard to percentage of blood products contaminated.[15,161] A U.S. study of patients treated with plasma-derived concentrates between 1979 and 1984 showed a much lower incidence of HIV infection (55 percent) in patients receiving F.IX complex concentrates than in those receiving F.VIII concentrates (approximately 90 percent infection with F.VIII).[161,171] Although the proportion of patients infected with HIV was extremely high and was devastating for the individuals affected, the projected impact on births over the next two centuries of patients with hemophilia is minimal (1.79 percent).[172]

Hepatitides. In addition to the tragic effects of HIV on the hemophilia population, significant morbidity and mortality is associated with hepatitis viruses transmitted through the administration of plasma-derived concentrates. The availability of effective virucidal techniques has greatly reduced the incidence of hepatitic viral disease in this population. A lag in technology of virus attenuation of F.IX concentrates compared to that of F.VIII was thought to contribute to higher incidences of hepatitis in hemophilia B patients in the late 1980s.[173] Troisi et al. documented the severity of hepatitis in the hemophilia A and B population at this time; 87 percent of the 345 HIV-negative, and >99 percent of the HIV-positive patients showed evidence of prior infection with hepatitis B, hepatitis C, or hepatitis D viruses.[173] Infection due to hepatitis A virus (HAV) has rarely been reported in patients with hemophilia B in the United States. The association with a high prevalence of HAV antibodies and reports of outbreaks in Europe were thought to be associated with solvent/detergent inactivation.[162,174] Recently, there has been evidence of HAV in F.IX concentrates[175] and a report of HAV in patients receiving F.IX has been documented.[176]

Hepatitis B was commonly seen in patients with hemophilia B until routine screening of liver enzymes and subsequently hepatitis specific antibody and antigen tests became available in the 1980s.[173,177,178] A study in 1987 to 1988 showed a high incidence of positivity for hepatitis B markers in hemophilia patients and a small but notable proportion of patients (8 percent) manifesting markers of an active state (HBsAg).[173] Most patients are now vaccinated against hepatitis B, making it difficult to estimate hepatitis B infection from concentrate administration. However, there still are rare reports of hepatitis B outbreak.[158,179] The hepatitis delta virus, dependent on coinfection with hepatitis B virus (HBV), has also been a significant cause of morbidity in the hemophilia B population. After controlling for disease severity, Troisi et al. found that HDV markers were prevalent in patients with hemophilia B and attributed this finding to administration of PCCs.[173]

Although specific testing has reduced infection with hepatitis B, non-A, non-B hepatitis, primarily due to hepatitis C virus (HCV), remains a problem. In hepatitis B-negative patients in the late 1980s, the prevalence of HCV in patients with hemophilia was 67 to 97 percent.[173] Routine testing for hepatitis C, instituted in the early 1990s, has reduced but not eliminated the hepatitis C contamination in the donor pool. A variable susceptibility and morbidity is seen in response to hepatitis infection; cirrhosis was estimated at approximately 20 percent[180] and liver failure 20 years after infection at 10 to 20 percent.[181] Concurrent infection with HIV accelerates complications of HCV.[182] Another long-term complication of infection with viral hepatitis is the increased likelihood of development of hepatocellular carcinoma.[183–186]

Although an increased incidence of antibodies to hepatitis E virus (HEV) is found in some, but not all, studies, an association has not been seen between hepatitis E disease and patients with hemophilia transfused with factor concentrates, even in patients positive for other hepatitis viruses.[187–189] Another recently identified virus, hepatitis G virus (HGV), has been seen in patients with hemophilia,[190] and stored serum samples have documented long periods of HGV viremia. The classification of HGV as a "hepatitis" virus occurred mainly because of its similarity to HCV; HGV viremia is not thought to be associated with the severity of or persistence of liver disease or the presence of liver pathology.[190–192] Additionally, coinfection with HGV does not appear to affect the course of HIV.[193]

Other Infectious Agents. Parvovirus B19 is a small, nonlipid enveloped, highly heat-resistant virus that contaminates plasma-derived products.[194,195] The vast majority of patients with hemophilia have antibodies to parvovirus B19 and methods to decontaminate other nonlipid enveloped viruses in products are not routinely effective against this virus.[194–196] Although parvovirus B19 infection is often mild and self-limited, in the immune deficiency state, infection with parvovirus B19 has the potential to severely compromise the infected patient's health.[197]

Blood donor screening for risk of prion diseases such as Creutzfeldt-Jakob disease (CJD) is currently performed through a questionnaire administered by the American Red Cross. There is experimental evidence in animal models that cellular blood components, plasma, and plasma components have a potential, although minimal, risk of transmitting CJD.[198] To date, transmission through cadaveric pituitary hormones, and corneal and dura mater grafts have been reported, but no definitive direct infection of a blood product recipient or blood product concentrate has been documented.[199,200] A new variant of CJD (nvCJD) has been described in geographic proximity to outbreaks of bovine spongiform encephalopathy (BSE), potentially from dietary exposure.[201] Thus there is concern that transmission of nvCJD may differ from classical CJD and could potentially be transmitted through plasma-derived concentrates. This increased concern is further fueled by experimental evidence that BSE and nvCJD are caused by the same infectious agent, as well as findings of prion-related protein in lymphoid tissue of patients with nvCJD.[202,203] In Europe, particular lots of concentrate have been removed from the market due to the development of a nvCJD in product donors.[204–206]

Recently, a novel single-stranded DNA virus, transfusion-transmitted virus (TTV), was identified in a Japanese patient with posttransfusion hepatitis not due to HAV, HBV, or HCV.[207] Since then, TTV viremia has been detected in approximately 2 percent of 1000 volunteer blood donors in the United Kingdom. Virucidal treatment of factor concentrates is thought to eliminate infectivity; however, PCR detection reveals approximately 50 percent TTV contamination of concentrate inactivated with solvent detergent treatment.[208] Further studies are needed to investigate an association between TTV and hepatic failure.

Treatment of Patients Infected with Hepatitis Virus and/or HIV. Vaccination of patients who receive concentrates and lack viral antibodies indicative of past infection is highly recommended despite the current low incidence of viral contamination in such products. Vaccines have now been licensed against hepatitis A and B.[176] In patients with hemophilia who are candidates for a surgical procedure, the presence of viral disease in and of itself has not been shown to significantly impact the success and benefits of the procedure or the course of HIV.[170,209] Although some studies have not reported explicit interactions between coinfection with HIV and HCV, other studies have indicated more accelerated hepatic disease.[169,182] Treatment of hepatitis C with interferon-α is associated with significant improvement in approximately half of the patients in most, but not all, studies.[210–213] In patients with liver failure who are unresponsive to treatment, liver transplant has been successful in many cases. Liver transplantation, most commonly performed subsequent to hepatitis C-associated liver disease, fortuitously corrects the clotting protein deficiency due to synthesis of F.IX in the orthotopic liver.[183,214] The possibility of reinfection, however, is significant and must be included in management decisions.

Complications of treatment of HIV in patients with hemophilia have been documented and include the development of drug-related hepatitis,[215] particularly in response to indinavir.[33] Additionally, complications in HIV-positive hemophiliacs taking protease inhibitors include hematuria (see "Renal Problems and Hematuria" above), intracranial bleeds, and excessive bleeding that often requires hospitalization and higher than expected doses of factor concentrate to correct the bleeding.[216] A 6-month prospective study of 20 hemophilia patients receiving protease inhibitors revealed one unusual bleed corrected by factor infusion, which led the authors to conclude that further prospective studies are needed, but that protease inhibitor therapy should not be withheld from HIV-positive hemophiliacs.[217]

Thrombosis

With early preparations of PCCs containing F.IX, thrombosis was a major, well-recognized, potentially life-threatening complication of therapy occurring in 11 to 50 percent of cases.[218–221] In 1973, Dr. Kasper reported 6 episodes of thrombosis, including 3 episodes of pulmonary emboli, in 13 operations in which PCCs were administered; during the same time period none of 72 patients receiving lyophilized F.VIII concentrates had thrombotic complications.[222] Major risk factors contributing to thrombogenicity include the underlying diagnosis, the quality of the PCC used, and the dose of concentrate.[223] Although thrombotic complications due to PCC administration are now rare, particular preparations and/or lots have been recently associated with fatal thromboses leading to withdrawal of the license for this brand.[158] Current preparations of high purity F.IX and recombinant F.IX have not been reported to cause such complications.

Hypotheses presented to explain PCC-associated thromboses include depletion of the anticoagulant protein antithrombin III, which forms complexes with many of the procoagulant proteins found in these earlier preparations; presence of activated procoagulant proteins thrombin, F.VIIa, F.IXa, or F.Xa; cumulative prolonged presence of numerous zymogen procoagulant proteins; and the presence of activated coagulant phospholipid complexes. The occurrence of thrombotic complications was not limited to hemophilia B patients but was also reported in patients receiving PCC for liver disease or as a bypass treatment in hemophilia A patients with inhibitors.[220] In addition to venous thrombosis and DIC, many reports also include arterial thrombotic complications.[220,224] A number of animal models have been used to study this complication, including mice, cats, dogs, and rabbits. There are no reports of thrombosis with the newly available rFIX. Phlebitis at the site of infusion is the only complication noted with a highly purified F.IX concentrate.[225,226]

Inhibitors

One complication of treatment in hemophilia is the development of inhibitors stimulated by the immune system's reaction to the F.IX protein. For unclear reasons, the frequency of inhibitor development in hemophilia B, 1 to 3 percent, is much less than that in hemophilia A, 7 to 52 percent.[227–229] Potential explanations for the difference between the two disorders include the lower number of hemophilia B patients with severe disease (see Fig. 173-2B), the presence of higher plasma F.IX levels (5 μg/ml versus 100 ng/ml for F.VIII allowing, in the case of F.IX, tolerance to develop even though circulating levels are <1 percent), the structural similarities between F.IX and the other vitamin K-dependent proteins, and the inherent F.VIII immunogenicity as illustrated by nonhemophiliacs who acquire a hemophilia A phenotype from autoantibody development. The inhibitors that develop in hemophilia B, like those in hemophilia A, are principally IgG subclass 4,[230,231] the least common of the immunoglobulin subtypes and one not normally associated with complement binding. Additional IgG2 and IgG1 subtypes are occasionally seen along with the IgG4. IgG3 does not appear to develop. An IgA inhibitor has been reported,[232] and red blood cell incompatibility testing due to F.IX inhibitors has also been described.[233]

Although standard assays for measurement of a F.VIII inhibitor are established, the testing of F.IX inhibitors is less routine. In 1988, Gadarowski modified the F.VIII Bethesda inhibitor assay for use with F.IX.[234] The Bethesda inhibitor titer (BU) is equal to the reciprocal of the dilution of test plasma (expressed as a percentage) that gives a residual F.IX activity of 50 percent.[235] Clinically, patients with inhibitors are divided into high and low responders; low responders are those whose inhibitor titers never rise above 10 BU, whereas high responders are those who can manifest peaks > 10 BU on reexposure to antigen. ELISA assays also exist that measure absorbance and can be converted into the F.IX inhibitor titer.[236]

Deletions account for only 5 percent of hemophilia B mutations overall, but they account for approximately 50 percent of hemophilia B patients who develop inhibitors.[237] Mutations leading to the loss of coding information, CRM(−), account for approximately 20 to 30 percent of patients, whereas inhibitor development in patients with missense mutations is almost zero.[129,238] It should be noted that the nature of the specific mutation contributes, but is not the only factor, to inhibitor development as only some patients with a given mutation develop inhibitors. The purity of the factor concentrate has also been suggested to play an important role; the different intensities of follow-up for inhibitor development, however, make such studies difficult to compare. Studies of inhibitor development with recombinant F.VIII reveal a cumulative incidence of inhibitor development of between 30 and 40 percent after the first 10 to 20 exposure days, although some of these prove to be transient and low titer.[239]

In 1997, Warrier et al. reported a potentially life-threatening anaphylactic complication to F.IX treatment in 18 very young children with severe hemophilia B from 12 hemophilia treatment centers in the United States, Canada, and Europe.[160] This complication tended to occur in very young patients (median age of 16 months) with a median of only 11 exposure days and occurred simultaneously with the development of the F.IX inhibitor in 12 of the patients. The IgG1 subclass appears to arise in association with the development of an allergic reaction to F.IX administration; the development of IgG1 is not necessarily pathologic, but it could be a marker for the simultaneous development of IgA or IgE antibodies. Shapiro et al. also documented an anaphylactic reaction in a patient with a F.IX gene deletion concurrent with the development of a F.IX inhibitor.[139] Although immune tolerance induction in these patients elicited a poor response, with 2 patients developing nephrotic syndrome, rFVIIa was successfully used in 11 patients to manage acute bleeding episodes. Other reports of patients with allergic reactions to F.IX have also documented nephrotic syndrome as a complication of immune tolerance regimens with F.IX.[34] The authors suggest that patients with major F.IX gene deletions, identified to be at higher risk for inhibitor development, should be monitored closely during their initial 10 to 20 treatments.

The treatment of inhibitors requires the management of acute bleeding episodes and ongoing efforts to eradicate the inhibitor. The most successful strategy for eradication of inhibitors is based on daily infusion of high doses of factor.[240,241] Referred to as immune tolerance induction, this treatment has a high rate of success (approximately 70 to 90 percent of patients achieve long-lasting remission of inhibitor) among patients who are able to persist with treatment.[242] The two best predictors of outcome for patients treated on this regimen are (a) a low Bethesda titer at the time of initiation of treatment and (b) the use of high-dose (> 100 IU/kg/day) regimens. In addition to high doses of F.IX over an extended period of time, a newer regimen, referred to as the Malmö protocol, includes immune modulation through the use of intravenous immune globulin, cyclophosphamide, and plasmapheresis of high titer antibodies with a Staphylococcal protein A column. The overall success rate of the Malmö protocol is estimated at 80 percent, with a mean time to developing tolerance of 28 days at a cost of $125,000.[243]

The immunologic mechanism by which high-dose infusion of clotting factor brings about disappearance of the inhibitor is unclear. Earlier theories proposed that immune tolerance for hemophilia A resulted in a decrease in affinity of the antibodies for F.VIII and/or an epitope switch to epitopes not required for functional activity.[244] Gilles et al. recently presented evidence for the development of anti-idiotype antibodies (secondary antibodies specific for the antigen-binding site for the original or primary antibody — anti-idiotype antibodies thus mimic the epitope of the original antigen) as the mechanism for "disappearance" of the inhibitor (i.e., the titer of the inhibitory antibodies does not decrease but their activity is neutralized by the presence of the anti-idiotype antibodies).[245] Other possibilities, such as induction of anti-idiotypic T cells, induction of T-cell tolerance by inappropriate antigen presentation in the absence of costimulatory determinants (unlikely for a memory response), or induction of immunologic exhaustion by recruiting all the memory T cells into the effector cell pool, have not been aggressively pursued. It is entirely possible that immune tolerance induction owes success to some combination of these mechanisms.

ANIMAL MODELS OF HEMOPHILIA B

Development of novel therapies for hemophilia B, including rF.IX and gene therapy approaches, has been facilitated by the existence of both large and small animal models of hemophilia B.[246–248] These include a naturally occurring dog model, and genetically engineered mouse models. Canine hemophilia B was first described in 1960;[249] it occurs naturally in a number of strains and closely mimics the human disease with frequent spontaneous joint and soft tissue bleeds. The canine F.IX cDNA was isolated in 1989 by screening a canine liver cDNA library with a human F.IX cDNA.[250] The F.IX cDNA sequence shows extensive conservation when compared with the human sequence and the predicted canine amino acid sequence is 86 percent conserved compared to the human amino acid sequence. As is the case generally for F.IX sequences from a number of species, conservation of amino acid sequence is very high in some portions of the sequence (the Gla domain and the catalytic domain, for example, where conservation of sequence at the amino acid level is > 90 percent), and much less so in other portions (<33 percent in the activation peptide).

A large number of mutations resulting in human hemophilia B have been described (see "Mutations Resulting in Hemophilia" above). Similarly, a number of different mutations have also been described for canine hemophilia B, although the canine disease has not been studied nearly as extensively. The first canine mutation described was that associated with severe hemophilia B in the Chapel Hill dog colony.[251] The causative mutation is a G $\rightarrow$ A transition in the triplet encoding amino acid 379 in the catalytic domain of canine F.IX. The nucleotide change results in the substitution of a glutamic acid residue for a glycine that is highly conserved in serine proteases from bacteria to man. Modeling studies indicate that the glycine normally present at 379 occupies a hydrophobic pocket in a closely packed internal region of the molecule. Substitution of a glutamic acid residue with a large, charged side chain is likely to result in steric hindrance to proper folding, and structural instability on that basis. This prediction is consistent with the fact that no F.IX protein (antigen or activity) is detectable in the plasma of these dogs. In another study, Mauser and colleagues described a mutation in Lhasa Apso dogs with hemophilia B.[252] These dogs also had <1 percent F.IX antigen and activity, but in contrast to the Chapel Hill dogs, which have normal levels of F.IX transcript on northern analysis, the Lhasa Apso mutation is associated with a marked decrease in F.IX mRNA levels. Nucleotide sequence analysis reveals a 5-bp deletion at nucleotides 772 to 776 of the canine cDNA and a C $\rightarrow$ T transition at nucleotide 777. These changes result in a termination codon at amino acid 146 (at the start of the activation peptide) and account for the absence of detectable antigen or activity in these dogs. Brooks et al.[253] have described a large gene deletion in a

Labrador retriever with severe hemophilia B. PCR and Southern analysis indicate that there is no evidence of F.IX coding sequence in this animal. Interestingly, this dog with a large gene deletion was reported to develop an inhibitor in response to canine plasma, whereas the Chapel Hill dogs, with a missense mutation, have not been reported to develop inhibitors. In this sense, too, then, the hemophilic dogs exhibit a response similar to that seen in human hemophilia B.

The availability of a large animal model that faithfully mirrors the human disease has been a considerable asset in the assessment of novel therapies for hemophilia. The pharmacokinetics of recombinant F.IX were extensively investigated in these dogs prior to initiation of human trials,[246] and the dogs have also proven useful in the investigation of gene therapy approaches, particularly in determining whether an approach that appears successful in rodents can be extended to large animals (and thus, presumably, to humans).[254] However, certain disadvantages of a large animal model, including the expense of maintaining a colony and the long breeding times, have made the generation of a small animal model of the disease desirable. In recent work, several groups have used gene-targeting techniques to develop genetically engineered models of hemophilia B in mice. Lin et al.,[255] using a plug-socket targeting strategy developed by Smithies and colleagues,[256] produced a mouse with a deletion of exons 1, 2, and 3. These mice have an absence of F.IX transcript by RT-PCR. Phenotypically, they exhibit the phenomenon first described in mice with hemophilia A,[257] hemorrhage and death following tail transection if the tail is not cauterized. They also experience spontaneous soft-tissue hemorrhage and hemorrhage into the intracranial space. A similar phenotype was described by Wang et al., who generated a mouse with a deletion of the coding sequence corresponding to exon 8 in the human gene (encoding the catalytic domain),[258] and by Kundu et al., who engineered a mouse with deletions of exons 7 and 8.[259]

Kung et al.[260] showed that human F.IX corrects the bleeding diathesis of mice with hemophilia B, as measured both by plasma-based clotting assays and tail bleeding times. This is an important observation because it means that gene transfer vehicles expressing *human* F.IX can be assessed for efficacy in the hemophilic mice, and that the function of mutant human F.IX proteins can be assessed in vivo in the mice. The mouse generated by Lin et al. should prove especially useful in this regard because the plug-socket-targeting construct used to install the deletion makes the generation of a "knock-in" construct a straightforward matter.

NOVEL APPROACHES TO THE TREATMENT OF HEMOPHILIA

Hemophilia has been the focus of a number of studies aimed at developing gene therapy approaches for the treatment of inherited disease. After a long period of development, some of these studies have now been translated into clinical protocols that will allow investigators to determine whether these approaches will be successful in treating patients with hemophilia. A detailed discussion of the preclinical data supporting various viral and nonviral approaches is beyond the scope of this chapter, but strategies that are currently in clinical trials or are being proposed for clinical trials are reviewed briefly. For a more comprehensive analysis of these novel therapeutics, the reader is referred to recent reviews (references 261 and 262) and to papers referenced in the text.

As noted earlier, the availability of clotting factor concentrates has resulted in a marked increase in life expectancy for people with hemophilia, but protein-based therapy, whether recombinant or plasma-derived, has a number of disadvantages. First, the short half-life of these proteins in the circulation requires that factor be infused on a daily or twice daily basis to achieve hemostasis. Second, plasma-derived concentrates have caused extensive transmission of blood-borne diseases in the hemophilia population (see "Complications of Treatment" above). Current methods of viral inactivation have greatly reduced, but not eliminated this risk, a fact attested to by recent product recalls due to possible contamination with the agent responsible for Creutzfeldt-Jakob disease, and by recent reports of a novel blood-borne DNA virus associated with posttransfusion hepatitis.[208,263] Even recombinant clotting factor concentrates carry some risk of transmission of viral disease, because most are stabilized with human plasma-derived albumin. A third disadvantage is that protein-based therapy is mostly given in response to bleeds (episode-based treatment) rather than prophylactically, so that bleeds are simply treated rather than prevented altogether. The reliance on treatment rather than prophylaxis is due partly to the expense and partly to the inconvenience associated with prophylactic factor infusion (in young children prophylaxis generally requires the placement of an intravenous access device, with attendant risks of infection). At any rate, it is very difficult to prevent long-term joint damage using episode-based therapy, which leads to the most common complication of the disease, hemophilic arthropathy. Finally, protein-based therapy is very expensive. Factor costs alone are ~\$100,000/year for an adult with severe hemophilia on an episode-based treatment regimen, and can be three times higher for a prophylactic regimen. Thus, the motivation to develop a gene-based treatment is strong.

Hemophilia has been a particularly appealing model for those interested in gene therapy approaches to inherited disease because, as a disease model, it has a number of features that facilitate a gene therapy strategy. First, in contrast to many other inherited diseases, the transgene product can be expressed in any of a number of different target tissues and still produce a therapeutic effect. Work by a number of investigators has established that biologically active clotting factors can be synthesized in muscle cells, endothelial cells, kidney cells, and fibroblasts in addition to hepatocytes, the normal site of synthesis. Thus, there is considerable latitude in choice of target cell, which expands the therapeutic options available. Second, the level of protein production required for therapeutic efficacy is well established based on two decades of experience with clotting factor concentrates. The Swedish prophylaxis studies[18] clearly demonstrate that maintenance of trough clotting factor levels of >1 percent result in radiographically and orthopedically normal joints. Moreover, studies on the natural history of central nervous system bleeding in hemophilia[264] document that this serious complication is overwhelmingly limited to patients with severe disease (<1 percent). Thus, there is strong evidence to suggest that even modest elevations in the levels of clotting factors will be adequate to correct the spontaneous bleeding episodes that are the major manifestation of the disease. A third advantage of hemophilia as a disease model for gene therapy is the existence of both large and small animal models of the disease (see "Animal Models" above). Both genetically engineered mice[255] and naturally occurring dog models[251] manifest a phenotype that closely mimics the disease in humans. Finally, determination of a clinically relevant endpoint is straightforward and unequivocal in the case of hemophilia, where phenotypic correction can be accurately measured by a number of well-characterized clotting assays.

From a gene transfer standpoint, there are a number of important differences between F.IX and F.VIII, so that, despite the clinical similarities of these two deficiency states, the optimal choice of vector and target cell may ultimately be different for the two genes. The F.IX cDNA is relatively small, ~3 kb, and thus fits well into most viral vectors, while the F.VIII cDNA, at 7 kb (or even at 4.4 kb for the B-domain deleted construct) is less well-accommodated by some vectors. In protein-based therapy, neutralizing antibodies occur much more frequently in the case of F.VIII deficiency than in the case of F.IX deficiency.[229] If the same holds true for gene-based therapies, this will favor hemophilia B as a model because the development of neutralizing antibodies confounds analysis of transgene expression. On the other hand, normal circulating levels of F.VIII (100 to 200 ng/ml) are much lower than plasma levels of F.IX (5 μg/ml), so levels of protein expression required are much less for F.VIII.

In addition to the differences between the transgenes, the recipient patient population is a heterogeneous one. For example, many of the older patients are hepatitis B and/or C positive, with varying degrees of liver disease, while most of the younger patients have not been infected with hepatitis viruses. Thus, a liver-directed treatment strategy may be more suitable for younger patients who are free of liver disease. Similarly, many of the patients treated before 1983 are already infected with HIV and have a decreased life expectancy on that basis, while most of those treated since are HIV-negative. Thus, older patients may be less concerned about the potential for late-appearing complications following treatment with integrating vectors, while younger patients, with nearly normal life expectancy, would be more concerned about this possibility.

Several gene therapy strategies are either already approved for clinical trials in hemophilia or are currently being proposed for clinical trials. In the only FDA-approved protocol to date, gene transfer is effected by a plasmid that is introduced into autologous fibroblasts. The plasmid contains the clotting factor cDNA sequence under the control of an eukaryotic promoter, and a *neo* gene to allow selection of transfected fibroblasts in G418. In the planned phase I trial, patient fibroblasts will be obtained from a skin biopsy, cultured in vitro, and transfected with the plasmid expressing the clotting factor. A small number of stably transfected clones are isolated in selective (G418-containing) media, and a single clone is selected for production. This clone is then grown in nonselective media and implanted onto the patient's omentum in a laparoscopic procedure.[265] Preclinical studies supporting this approach have been carried out using stably transfected rabbit fibroblasts implanted into the omenta of nude mice.[265]

The majority of the experience with human gene therapy trials has been with retroviral vectors, but earlier preclinical studies with retroviral vectors for F.IX gene delivery to the liver were disappointing in that the level of F.IX expression was too low to be therapeutic, and even this level of hepatocyte transduction required preparative partial hepatectomy.[248] However, Greengard and colleagues[266] recently presented preliminary findings suggesting that a retroviral approach may be feasible. A key to their studies is the preparation of high-titer retroviral vector, which results in much improved transduction efficiency. In experiments in which juvenile rabbits or dogs were infused intravenously with high-titer retrovirus expressing human F.VIII, $\sim$50 percent of animals expressed F.VIII in a therapeutic range. These immunocompetent animals rapidly develop antibodies to the human transgene product, but results suggest that expression is present for periods of >1 year. PCR data show that the donated gene is found in liver and spleen. Definitive proof-of-principle for this strategy will require the use of a species-specific transgene such as canine F.VIII in canine hemophilia A. Whether this approach can be extended to hemophilia B is unclear; the higher levels of expression required for hemophilia B may prevent successful application of this strategy to F.IX deficiency.

In another approach, High and coworkers have shown in mice and in hemophilic dogs that intramuscular injection of an AAV vector expressing factor IX can result in long-term expression of F.IX (>1 year) at levels that would be therapeutic in humans (70 to 300 ng/ml; 1.4 to 6 percent normal human F.IX levels).[267,268] The studies in hemophilic dogs were carried out with an AAV vector-expressing canine F.IX. The use of a species-specific transgene in a hemophilic animal model permits not only demonstration of proof-of-principle, but also allows assessment of the immune response to the transgene product in an immunocompetent animal. This is a matter of concern in any novel approach to the treatment of hemophilia, because the possibility of development of neutralizing antibodies to the clotting factor is always a risk. Studies to date have shown that neutralizing antibodies are either absent or present only transiently in hemophilic dogs treated by this approach. A clinical trial based on these findings is currently underway.[268a]

In a similar approach, two groups, Kay and coworkers and Nakai et al., demonstrated that injection of an AAV vector-expressing F.IX into the portal circulation results in high levels of liver-derived F.IX expression in mice.[269,270] Direct comparisons of similar AAV vectors (differing only in promoter) injected into either muscle or portal vein by one group suggest that the vector may be approximately five times more efficient in liver. This likely reflects the ready access of hepatocyte-synthesized material to the circulation, although other factors, including transduction efficiency, promoter strength, and mRNA stability, and cellular synthetic capacity may also be involved. Kay and coworkers extended this approach to hemophilic dogs and obtained levels of F.IX expression in the range of 1 to 2 percent of normal human plasma levels (M. Kay, personal communication). Again, a clinical trial is being designed based on these findings.

There are two other gene transfer strategies for which intriguing preclinical data exist. The first involves the use of the so-called gutted adenoviral vector, an adenoviral vector from which all viral coding sequences have been deleted.[271] Compared to earlier-generation adenoviral vectors, these gutted vectors result in decreased host immune response to the vector, longer duration of expression, and increased capacity to accommodate large DNA inserts. These features are particularly attractive in the case of F.VIII gene transfer. That adenoviral vectors do not integrate into the host cell genome provides an additional measure of safety over vectors, such as retrovirus, that do integrate and thus carry a risk of insertional mutagenesis. In another novel strategy, Kren et al.[272] showed that chimeric RNA/DNA oligonucleotides could be used to induce a site-specific mutation in rat hepatocyte DNA. The utility of this modality for gene correction will depend on the efficiency with which site-specific correction occurs; current studies suggest that the efficiency is sequence-dependent, so that this strategy may be more effective for some mutations than for others. In addition, of course, this treatment strategy will require that the patient's mutation be known at the nucleotide level (a requirement that can be met), and that the mutation be a point mutation (a requirement that will impede application to F.VIII deficiency because 40 percent of patients with severe hemophilia A have a gene inversion mutation).[273]

REFERENCES

1. Rosner F: Hemophilia in the Talmud and rabbinic writings. *Ann Intern Med* **70**:833, 1969.
2. Aggeler PM, White SG, Glendening MG, Page EW, Leake TB, Bates G: Plasma thromboplastin component (PTC) deficiency: A new disease resembling hemophilia. *Proc Soc Exp Biol* **79**:602, 1952.
3. Biggs R, Douglas AS, MacFarlane RG, Dacie JV, Pitney WR, Merskey C, O'Brien JR: Christmas disease: A condition previously mistaken for haemophilia. *BMJ* **ii**:1378, 1952.
4. Schulman I, Smith CH: Hemorrhagic disease in an infant due to deficiency of a previously undescribed clotting factor. *Blood* **7**:794, 1952.
5. Simpson NE, Biggs R: The inheritance of Christmas factor. *B J Haematol* **8**:191, 1962.
6. Ingram GI: The history of haemophilia. *J Clin Pathol* **2**:469, 1976.
7. Larsson SA: Hemophilia in Sweden. Studies on demography of hemophilia and surgery in hemophilia and von Willebrand's disease. *Acta Med Scand Suppl* **684**:1, 1984.
8. Eyster ME, Schaefer JH, Ragni MV, Gorenc TJ, Shapiro S, Cutter S, Kajani MK, et al.: Changing causes of death in Pennsylvania's hemophiliacs 1976 to 1991: Impact of liver disease and acquired immunodeficiency syndrome. *Blood* **79**:2494, 1992.
9. Kim KY, Yang CH, Cho MJ, Lee M: Comprehensive clinical and statistical analysis of hemophilia in Korea. *J Korean Med Sci* **3**:107, 1988.
10. Walker I, Pai M, Akabutu J, Ritchie B, Growe G, Poon MC, Card R, et al.: The Canadian Hemophilia Registry as the basis for a national system for monitoring the use of factor concentrates. *Transfusion* **35**:548, 1995.
11. Dietrich AM, James CD, King DR, Ginn-Pease ME, Cecalupo AJ: Head trauma in children with congenital coagulation disorders. *J Pediatri Surg* **29**:28, 1994.

12. Ljung R, Petrini P, Nilsson IM: Diagnostic symptoms of severe and moderate haemophilia A and B. A survey of 140 cases. *Acta Paediatr Scand* **79**:196, 1990.
13. Smith PS: Congenital coagulation protein deficiencies in the perinatal period. *Semin Perinatol* **14**:384, 1990.
14. Venkateswaran L, Wilimas JA, Jones DJ, Nuss R: Mild hemophilia in children: Prevalence, complications, and treatment. *J Pediatri Hematol Oncol* **20**:32, 1998.
15. Triemstra M, Rosendaal FR, Smit C, Van der Ploeg HM, Briet E: Mortality in patients with hemophilia. Changes in a Dutch population from 1986 to 1992 and 1973 to 1986. *Ann Intern Med* **123**:823, 1995.
16. Rodriguez-Merchan EC: Management of the orthopaedic complications of haemophilia. *J Bone Joint Surg Br* **80**:191, 1998.
17. Eyster ME, Lewis JH, Shapiro SS, Gill F, Kajani M, Prager D, Djerassi I, et al.: The Pennsylvania hemophilia program 1973–1978. *Am J Hematol* **9**:277, 1980.
18. Lofqvist T, Nilsson IM, Berntorp E, Pettersson H: Haemophilia prophylaxis in young patients — A long-term follow-up. *J Intern Med* **241**:395, 1997.
19. Caviglia HA, Fernandez-Palazzi F, Maffei E, Galatro G, Barrionuevo A: Chemical synoviorthosis for hemophilic synovitis. *Clin Orthop Rel Res* **343**:30, 1997.
20. Lofqvist T, Petersson C, Nilsson IM: Radioactive synoviorthosis in patients with hemophilia with factor inhibitor. *Clin Orthop Rel Res* **343**:37, 1997.
21. Eickhoff HH, Koch W, Raderschadt G, Brackmann HH: Arthroscopy for chronic hemophilic synovitis of the knee. *Clin Orthop Rel Res* **343**:58, 1997.
22. Esposito C, Melanotte PL, Olmeda A, Traldi A, Bonaga R: Early synovectomy in haemophilia. *Ital J Orthop Traumatol* **8**:309, 1982.
23. Wiedel JD: Arthroscopy of the knee in hemophilia. *Prog Clin Biol Res* **324**:231, 1990.
24. Naranja RJ Jr, Chan PS, High K, Esterhai JL Jr, Heppenstall RB: Treatment of considerations in patients with compartment syndrome and an inherited bleeding disorder. *Orthopedics* **20**:706, 1997.
25. de Tezanos Pinto M, Fernandez J, Perez Bianco PR: Update of 156 episodes of central nervous system bleeding in hemophiliacs. *Haemostasis* **22**:259, 1992.
26. Silverstein A: Intracranial bleeding in hemophilia. *Arch Neurol* **3**:141, 1960.
27. Andes WA, Wulff K, Smith WB: Head trauma in hemophilia: A prospective study. *Arch Intern Med* **144**:1981, 1984.
28. Bray GL, Luban NL: Hemophilia presenting with intracranial hemorrhage. *Am J Dis Child* **141**:1215, 1987.
29. Yoffe G, Buchanan GR: Intracranial hemorrhage in newborn and young infants with hemophilia. *J Pediatr* **113**:333, 1988.
30. Romeyn RL, Herkowitz HN: The cervical spine in hemophilia. *Clin Orthop Rel Res* 210:113, 1986.
31. Dumontier C, Sautet A, Man M, Bennani M, Apoil A: Entrapment and compartment syndromes of the upper limb in haemophilia. *J Hand Surg [Br]* **19**:427, 1994.
32. Forbes CD, Prentice CR: Renal disorders in haemophilia A and B. *Scand J Haematol Suppl* **30**:43, 1977.
33. Matsuda J, Gohchi K: Severe hepatitis in patients with AIDS and haemophilia B treated with indinavir. *Lancet* **350**:364, 1997.
34. Ewenstein BM, Takemoto C, Warrier I, Lusher J, Saidi P, Eisele J, Ettinger LJ, et al.: Nephrotic syndrome as a complication of immune tolerance in hemophilia B. *Blood* **89**:1115, 1997.
35. Needleman HL, Kaban LB, Kevy SV: The use of epsilon-aminocaproic acid for the management of hemophilia in dental and oral surgery patients. *J Am Dental Assoc* **93**:586, 1976.
36. Djulbegovic B, Marasa M, Pesto A, Kushner GM, Hadley T, Joseph G, Goldsmith G: Safety and efficacy of purified factor IX concentrate and antifibrinolytic agents for dental extractions in hemophilia B. *Am J Hematol* **51**:168, 1996.
37. Djulbegovic B, Hannan MM, Bergman GE: Concomitant treatment with factor IX concentrates and antifibrinolytics in hemophilia B. *Acta Haematol* **94(Suppl 1)**:43, 1995.
38. Furie B, Limentani SA, Rosenfield CG: A practical guide to the evaluation and treatment of hemophilia. *Blood* **84**:3, 1994.
39. Martinowitz U, Schulman S, Horoszowski H, Heim M: Role of fibrin sealants in surgical procedures on patients with hemostatic disorders. *Clin Orthop Rel Res* **328**:65, 1996.
40. Magallon M, Monteagudo J, Altisent C, Ibanez A, Rodriguez-Perez A, Riba J, Tusell J, et al.: Hemophilic pseudotumor: Multicenter experience over a 25-year period. *Am J Hematol* **45**:103, 1994.
41. de Sousa SO, de Piratininga J, Pinto Junior DS, de Araujo N: Hemophilic pseudotumor of the jaws: Report of two cases. *Oral Surg Oral Med Oral Pathol Oral Radiol Endod* **216(9)**:216, 1995.
42. Morgan LM, Kissoon N, de Vebber BL: Experience with the hemophiliac child in a pediatric emergency department. *J Emerg Med* **11**:519, 1993.
43. Bray G, Nugent D: Hemorrhage involving the upper airway in hemophilia. *Clin Pediatr* **25**:436, 1986.
44. Hardisty RM: Christmas disease in a woman. *BMJ* **i**:1039, 1957.
45. Orstavik KH, Stormorken H, Sparr T: Hemophilia B_M in a female. *Thromb Res* **37**:561, 1985.
46. Schroder W, Wulff K, Wollina K, Herrmann FH: Haemophilia B in female twins caused by a point mutation in one factor IX gene and nonrandom inactivation patterns of the X-chromosomes. *Thromb Haemost* **78**:1347, 1997.
47. Kadir RA, Economides DL, Braithwaite J, Goldman E, Lee CA: The obstetric experience of carriers of haemophilia. *Br J Obstet Gynaecol* **104**:803, 1997.
48. Ljung R, Lindgren AC, Petrini P, Tengborn L: Normal vaginal delivery is to be recommended for haemophilia carrier gravidae. *Acta Paediatr* **83**:609, 1994.
49. Guy GP, Baxi LV, Hurlet-Jensen A, Chao CR: An unusual complication in a gravida with factor IX deficiency: Case report with review of the literature. *Obstet Gynecol* **80**:502, 1992.
50. National Hemophilia Foundation: Medical and scientific advisory council (MASAC) recommendations. New YorkNational Hemophilia Foundation, 1998.
51. Bajaj SP, Rapaport SI, Russell WA: Redetermination of the rate-limiting step in the activation of factor IX by factor XIa and by factor VIIa/tissue factor. Explanation for different electrophoretic radio-activity profiles obtained on activation of ^{3}H- and ^{125}I-labeled factor IX. *Biochemistry* **22**:4047, 1983.
52. Di Scipio RG, Kurachi K, Davie EW: Activation of human factor IX (Christmas factor). *J Clin Invest* **61**:1528, 1978.
53. Bond M, Jankowski M, Patel H, Karnik S, Strang A, Xu B, Rouse J, et al.: Biochemical characterization of recombinant factor IX. *Semin Hematol* **35**:11, 1998.
54. Wolberg AS, Morris DP: Factor IX activation by factor XIa proceeds without release of a free intermediate. *Biochemistry* **36**:4074, 1997.
55. Larson PJ, Stanfield-Oakley SA, VanDusen WJ, Kasper CK, Smith KJ, Monroe DM, High KA: Structural integrity of the gamma-carboxyglutamic acid domain of human blood coagulation factor IXa is required for its binding to cofactor VIIIa. *J Biol Chem* **271**:3869, 1996.
56. Bajaj SP, Birktoft JJ: Human Factor IX and IXa. *Methods Enzymol* **222**:96, 1993.
57. Van Dieijen G, Tans G, Rosing J, Hemker HC: The role of phospholipid and factor VIIIa in the activation of bovine factor X. *J Biol Chem* **256**:3433, 1981.
58. Brandstetter H, Bauer M, Huber R, Lollar P, Bode W: X-ray structure of clotting factor IXa: Active site and module structure related to Xase activity and hemophilia B. *Proc Natl Acad Sci U S A* **92**:9796, 1995.
59. Camerino G, Grezschik KH, Jaye M, De La Salle H, Tolstoshev P, Lecocq JP, Heilig R, et al.: Regional localization on the human X chromosome and polymorphism of the coagulation factor IX gene (hemophilia B locus). *Proc Natl Acad Sci U S A* **81**:498, 1984.
60. Purrello M, Alhadeff B, Esposito D, Szabo P, Rocchi M, Truett M, Masiarz F, et al.: The human genes for hemophilia A and hemophilia B flank the X chromosome fragile X site at Xq27.3. *EMBO J* **4**:725, 1985.
61. Furie B, Furie BC: The molecular basis of blood coagulation. *Cell* **53**:505, 1988.
62. Yoshitake S, Schach BF, Foster DC, Davie EW, Kurachi K: Nucleotide sequence of the gene for human factor IX (antihemophilic factor B). *Biochemistry* **24**:3736, 1985.
63. Gallistl S, Muntean W, Leschnik B, Meyers W: Longer aPTT values in healthy children than in adults: No single cause. *Thromb Res* **88**:355, 1997.
64. Briet E, Bertina RM, van Tilburg NH, JJ V: Hemophilia B Leyden: A sex-linked hereditary disorder that improves after puberty. *N Engl J Med* **306**:788, 1982.
65. Pang CP, Crossley M, Kent G, Brownlee GG: Comparative sequence analysis of mammalian factor IX promoters. *Nucleic Acids Res* **12**:6731, 1984.

66. Kozak M: Compilation and analysis of sequences upstream from the translation start site in eukaryotic mRNAs. *Nucleic Acids Res* **12**:857, 1984.
67. Whitlon DS, Sadowski JA, Suttie JW: Mechanism of coumarin action: Significance of vitamin K epoxide reductase inhibition. *Biochemistry* **17**:1371, 1978.
68. Reiner AP, Thompson AR: An *Hha*I polymorphism is present in factor IX genes of Asian subjects. *Hum Genet* **86**:87, 1990.
69. Toyozumi H, Kojima T, Matsushita T, Hamaguchi M, Tanimoto M, Saito H: Diagnosis of hemophilia B carriers using two novel dinucleotide polymorphisms and *Hha*I RFLP of the factor IX gene in Japanese subjects. *Thromb Haemost* **74**:1009, 1995.
70. Bao Y, Lu D, Shi Q, Xu H, Qiu X, Xue J: Determination of the polymorphism of DXS102 locus and its application in gene diagnosis. *Chung-Hua I Hsueh Tsa Chih* **15**:27, 1998.
71. Goodeve AC, Chuansumrit A, Sasanakul W, Isarangkura P, Preston FE, Peake IR: A comparison of the allelic frequencies of ten DNA polymorphisms associated with factor VIII and factor IX genes in Thai and Western European populations. *Blood Coagul Fibrinol* **5(1)**:29, 1994.
72. Chuansumrit A, Goodeve A, Sasanakul W, Peake IR, Pintadit P, Hathirat P, Preston FE, et al.: DNA polymorphisms for carrier detection of hemophilia in Thailand. *Southeast Asian J Trop Med Public Health* **26(Suppl 1)**:201, 1995.
73. Rai HK, Winship PR: A −793 G to A transition in the factor IX gene promoter is polymorphic in the Caucasian population. *Br J Haematol* **92**:501, 1996.
74. Young JH, Wang JC, Gau JP, Hu HT: Prenatal and molecular diagnosis of hemophilia B. *Am J Hematol* **52**:243, 1996.
75. Rowley G, Saad S, Giannelli F, Green PM: Ultrarapid mutation detection by multiplex, solid-phase chemical cleavage. *Genomics* **30**:574, 1995.
76. Martinez PA, Romey MC, Schved JF, Gris JC, Demaille J, Claustres M: Direct carrier testing of haemophilia B by SSCP. *Clin Lab Haematol* **16(1)**:15, 1994.
77. Thompson AR, Chen SH: Characterization of factor IX defects in hemophilia B patients. *Methods Enzymol* **222**:143, 1993.
78. Thomas AE, Green FR, Kelleher CH, Wilkes HC, Brennan PJ, Meade TW, Humphries SE: Variation in the promoter region of the beta fibrinogen gene is associated with plasma fibrinogen levels in smokers and non-smokers. *Thromb Haemost* **65**:487, 1991.
79. Bernardi F, Marchetti G, Pinotti M, Arcieri P, Baroncini C, Papacchini M, Zepponi E, et al.: Factor VII gene polymorphisms contribute about one-third of the factor VII level variation in plasma. *Arterioscler Thromb Vasc Biol* **16**:72, 1996.
80. Giannelli F, Green PM, Sommer SS, Poon M, Ludwig M, Schwaab R, Reitsma PH, et al.: Haemophilia B: database of point mutations and short additions and deletions — Eighth edition. *Nucleic Acids Res* **26**:265, 1998.
81. Giannelli F, Green PM, High KA, Lozier JN, Lillicrap DP, Ludwig M, Olek K, et al.: Haemophilia B: Database of point mutations and short additions and deletions. *Nucleic Acids Res* **18**:4053, 1990.
82. Sommer SS: Assessing the underlying pattern of human germline mutations: Lessons from the factor IX gene. *FASEB J* **6**:2767, 1992.
83. Mazin AL: Methylation of the factor IX gene — A basic reason for the mutation causing hemophilia B. *Molekuliarnaia Biologiia* **29**:71, 1995.
84. Veltkamp JJ, Meilof J, Remmelts HG, van der Vlerk D, Loeliger EA: Another genetic variant of haemophilia B: Haemophilia B Leyden. *Scand J Haematol* **7**:82, 1970.
85. Reitsma PH, Bertina RM, Ploos van Amstel JK, Riemens A, Briet E: The putative factor IX gene promoter in hemophilia B Leyden. *Blood* **72**:1074, 1988.
86. Kurachi S, Furukawa M, Salier JP, Wu CT, Wilson EJ, French FS, Kurachi K: Regulatory mechanism of human factor IX gene: Protein binding at the Leyden-specific region. *Biochemistry* **33**:1580, 1994.
87. Picketts DJ, Mueller CR, Lillicrap D: Transcriptional control of the factor IX gene: Analysis of five *cis*-acting elements and the deleterious effects of naturally occurring hemophilia B Leyden mutations. *Blood* **84**:2992, 1994.
88. Reijnen MJ, Peerlinck K, Maasdam D, Bertina RM, Reitsma PH: Hemophilia B Leyden: Substitution of thymine for guanine at position −21 results in a disruption of a hepatocyte nuclear factor 4 binding site in the factor IX promoter. *Blood* **82**:151, 1993.
89. Reijnen MJ, Maasdam D, Bertina RM, Reitsma PH: Haemophilia B Leyden: The effect of mutations at position +13 on the liver-specific transcription of the factor IX gene. *Blood Coagul Fibrinol* **5**:341, 1994.
90. Reijnen MJ, Sladek FM, Bertina RM, Reitsma PH: Disruption of a binding site for hepatocyte nuclear factor 4 results in hemophilia B Leyden. *Proc Natl Acad Sci U S A* **89**:6300, 1992.
91. Picketts DJ, D'Souza C, Bridge PJ, Lillicrap D: An A to T transversion at position −5 of the factor IX promoter results in hemophilia B. *Genomics* **12**:161, 1992.
92. Vidaud D, Tartary M, Costa JM, Bahnak BR, Gispert-Sanchez S, Fressinaud E, Gazengel C, et al.: Nucleotide substitutions at the −6 position in the promoter region of the factor IX gene result in different severity of hemophilia B Leyden: Consequences for genetic counseling. *Hum Genet* **91**:241, 1993.
93. Reitsma PH, Mandalaki T, Kasper CK, Bertina RM, Briet E: Two novel point mutations correlate with an altered developmental expression of blood coagulation factor IX (hemophilia B Leyden phenotype). *Blood* **73**:743, 1989.
94. Royle G, Van de Water NS, Berry E, Ockelford PA, Browett PJ: Haemophilia B Leyden arising *de novo* by point mutation in the putative factor IX promoter region. *Br J Haematol* **77**:191, 1991.
95. Reijnen MJ, Bertina RM, Reitsma PH: Localization of transcription initiation sites in the human coagulation factor IX gene. *FEBS Lett* **270**:207, 1990.
96. Anson DS, Choo KH, Rees DJ, Giannelli F, Gould K, Huddleston JA, Brownlee GG: The gene structure of human anti-haemophilic factor IX. *EMBO J* **3**:1053, 1984.
97. Fair DS, Bahnak BR: Human hepatoma cells secrete single chain factor X, prothrombin, and antithrombin III. *Blood* **64**:194, 1984.
98. Crossley M, Ludwig M, Stowell KM, De Vos P, Olek K, Brownlee GG: Recovery from hemophilia B Leyden: An androgen-responsive element in the factor IX promoter. *Science* **257**:377, 1992.
99. Morgan GE, Rowley G, Green PM, Chisholm M, Giannelli F, Brownlee GG: Further evidence for the importance of an androgen response element in the factor IX promoter. *Br J Haematol* **98**:79, 1997.
100. Crossley M, Brownlee GG: Disruption of a C/EBP binding site in the factor IX promoter is associated with haemophilia B. *Nature* **345**:444, 1990.
101. Picketts DJ, Lillicrap DP, Mueller CR: Synergy between transcription factors DBP and C/EBP compensates for a haemophilia B Leyden factor IX mutation. *Nat Genet* **3**:175, 1993.
102. Boccia LM, Lillicrap D, Newcombe K, Mueller CR: Binding of the Ets factor GA-binding protein to an upstream site in the factor IX promoter is a critical event in transactivation. *Mol Cell Biol* **16**:1929, 1996.
103. Bentley AK, Rees DJ, Rizza C, Brownlee GG: Defective propeptide processing of blood clotting factor IX caused by mutation of arginine to glutamine at position −4. *Cell* **45**:343, 1986.
104. Green PM, Mitchell VE, McGraw A, Goldman E, Giannelli F: Haemophilia B caused by a missense mutation in the prepeptide sequence of factor IX. *Hum Mutat* **2**:103, 1993.
105. Sugimoto M, Miyata T, Kawabata S, Yoshioka A, Fukui H, Iwanaga S: Factor IX Kawachinagano: Impaired function of the Gla-domain caused by attached propeptide region due to substitution of arginine by glutamine at position −4. *Br J Haematol* **72**:216, 1989.
106. Wojcik EG, Cheung WF, van den Berg M, van der Linden IK, Stafford DW, Bertina RM: Identification of residues in the Gla-domain of human factor IX involved in the binding to conformation specific antibodies. *Biochim Biophys Acta* **13821**:91, 1998.
107. Wojcik EG, Van Den Berg M, Poort SR, Bertina RM: Modification of the N-terminus of human factor IX by defective propeptide cleavage or acetylation results in a destabilized calcium-induced conformation: Effects on phospholipid binding and activation by factor XIa. *Biochem J* **323**:629, 1997.
108. Diuguid DL, Rabiet MJ, Furie BC, Liebman HA, Furie B: Molecular basis of hemophilia B: A defective enzyme due to an unprocessed propeptide is caused by a point mutation in the factor IX precursor. *Proc Natl Acad Sci U S A* **83**:5803, 1986.
109. Gillis S, Furie BC, Furie B, Patel H, Huberty MC, Switzer M, Foster WB, et al.: Gamma-carboxyglutamic acids 36 and 40 do not contribute to human factor IX function. *Protein Sci* **6**:185, 1997.
110. Cheung WF, van den Born J, Kuhn K, Kjellen L, Hudson BG, Stafford DW: Identification of the endothelial cell binding site for factor IX. *Proc Natl Acad Sci U S A* **93**:11068, 1996.
111. Ahmad SS, Wong MY, Rawala R, Jameson BA, Walsh PN: Coagulation factor IX residues G4-Q11 mediate its interaction with a shared factor IX/IXa binding site on activated platelets but not the

assembly of the functional factor X activating complex. *Biochemistry* **37**:1671, 1998.
112. Freedman SJ, Blostein MD, Baleja JD, Jacobs M, Furie BC, Furie B: Identification of the phospholipid binding site in the vitamin K-dependent blood coagulation protein factor IX. *J Biol Chem* **271**:16227, 1996.
113. Prorok M, Geng JP, Warder SE, Castellino FJ: The entire gamma-carboxyglutamic acid- and helical stack-domains of human coagulation factor IX are required for optimal binding to its endothelial cell receptor. *Int J Pept Protein Res* **48**:281, 1996.
114. Stenflo J: Structure-function relationships of epidermal growth factor modules in vitamin K-dependent clotting factors. *Blood* **78**:1637, 1991.
115. Fernlund P, Stenflo J: Beta-hydroxyaspartic acid in vitamin K-dependent proteins. *J Biol Chem* **258**:12509, 1983.
116. Lenting PJ, Christophe OD, Maat H, Rees DJG, Mertens K: Ca^{2+} binding to the first epidermal growth factor-like domain of human blood coagulation factor IX promotes enzyme activity and factor VIII light chain binding. *J Biol Chem* **271**:25332, 1996.
117. Chang JY, Monroe DM, Stafford DW, Brinkhous KM, Roberts HR: Replacing the first epidermal growth factor-like domain of factor IX with that of factor VII enhances activity in vitro and in canine hemophilia B. *J Clin Invest* **100**:886, 1997.
118. Ahmad SS, Rawala R, Cheung WF, Stafford DW, PN W: The role of the second growth-factor domain of human factor IXa in binding to platelets and in factor-X activation. *Biochem J* **310**:427, 1995.
119. Christophe OD, Lenting PJ, Kolkman JA, Brownlee GG, Mertens K: Blood coagulation factor IX residues Glu78 and Arg94 provide a link between both epidermal growth factor-like domains that is crucial in the interaction with factor VIII light chain. *J Biol Chem* **273**:222, 1998.
120. Bode W, Brandstetter H, Mather T, Stubbs MT: Comparative analysis of haemostatis proteinases: Structural aspects of thrombin, factor Xa, factor IXa, and Protein C. *Thromb Haemost* **78**:501, 1997.
121. Ketterling RP, Bottema CDK, Phillips JA III, Sommer SS: Evidence that descendants of three founders constitute about 25% of hemophilia B in the United States. *Genomics* **10**:1093, 1991.
122. Thompson AR, Bajaj SP, Chen SH, MacGillivray RTA: "Founder" effect in different families with haemophilia B mutation. *Lancet* **335**:418, 1990.
123. Kurachi S, Pantazatos DP, Kurachi K: The carboxyl-terminal region of factor IX is essential for its secretion. *Biochemistry* **36**:4337, 1997.
124. Hougie C, Twomey JJ: Haemophilia B_M: A new type of factor-IX deficiency. *Lancet* **1**:698, 1967.
125. Miyata T, Kuze K, Matsusue T, Komooka H, Kamiya K, Umeyama H, Matsui A, et al.: Factor IX Bm Kiryu: A Val-313-to-Asp substitution in the catalytic domain results in loss of function due to a conformational change of the surface loop: Evidence obtained by chimaeric modelling. *Br J Haematol* **88**:156, 1994.
126. Lefkowitz JB, Monroe DM, Kasper CK, Roberts HR: Comparison of the behavior of normal factor IX and the factor IX B_M variant Hilo in the prothrombin time test using tissue factors from bovine, human, and rabbit sources. *Am J Hematol* **43**:177, 1993.
127. Hamaguchi N, Roberts H, Stafford DW: Mutations in the catalytic domain of factor IX that are related to the subclass hemophilia B_M. *Biochemistry* **32**:6324, 1993.
128. Monroe DM, McCord DM, Huang MN, High KA, Lundblad RL, Kasper CK, Roberts HR: Functional consequences of an arginine180 to glutamine mutation in factor IX Hilo. *Blood* **73**:1540, 1989.
129. High KA, Roberts HR: Factor IX, in High KA RH (ed): *Molecular Basis of Thrombosis and Hemostasis*. New York, Marcel Dekker, 1995, p 215.
130. Chu K, Wu SM, Stanley T, Stafford DW, High KA: A mutation in the propeptide of factor IX leads to warfarin sensitivity by a novel mechanism. *J Clin Invest* **98**:1619, 1996.
131. Oldenburg J, Quenzel EM, Harbrecht U, Fregin A, Kress W, Muller CR, Hertfelder HJ, et al.: Missense mutations at ALA-10 in the factor IX propeptide: An insignificant variant in normal life but a decisive cause of bleeding during oral anticoagulant therapy. *Br J Haematol* **98**:240, 1997.
132. Peters J, Luddington R, Brown K, Baglin C, Baglin T: Should patients starting anticoagulant therapy be screened for missense mutations at Ala-10 in the factor IX propeptide? *Br J Haematol* **99**:467, 1997.
133. Chang J, Jin J, Lollar P, Bode W, Brandstetter H, Hamaguchi N, Straight DL, et al.: Changing residue 338 in human factor IX from arginine to alanine causes an increase in catalytic activity. *J Biol Chem* **273**:12089, 1998.
134. Miller K, Neely JE, Krivit W, Edson JR: Spontaneously acquired factor IX inhibitor in a nonhemophiliac child. *J Pediatr* **93**:232, 1978.
135. Larsson SA, Nilsson IM, Blomback M: Current status of Swedish hemophiliacs. I. A demographic survey. *Acta Med Scand* **212**:195, 1982.
136. Vengelen-Tyler V (ed): *Technical Manual*. Bethesda, MD, American Association of Blood Banks, 1996, p 144.
137. Schreiber GB, Busch MP, Kleinman SH, Korelitz JJ: The risk of transfusion-transmitted viral infections. The retrovirus epidemiology donor study. *N Engl J Med* **334**:1685, 1996.
138. Larrieu MJ, Caen J, Soulier JP, Bernard J: Treatment of hemophilia B with plasma fraction rich in the antihemophilic B factor (PPSB). *Pathol Biol (Paris)* **7**:2507, 1959.
139. Shapiro AD, Ragni MV, Lusher JM, Culbert S, Koerper MA, Bergman GE, Hannan MM: Safety and efficacy of monoclonal antibody purified factor IX concentrate in previously untreated patients with hemophilia B. *Thromb Haemost* **75**:30, 1996.
140. Kasper CK: Clotting factor concentrates in 1997. XVIth National Meeting of the Brazilian College of Hematology in Belo Horizonte, MG, Brazil, 1997.
141. Harrison S, Adamson S, Bonam D, Brodeur S, Charlebois T, Clancy B, Costigan R, et al.: The manufacturing process for recombinant factor IX. *Semin Hematol* **35**:4, 1998.
142. Bush L, Webb C, Bartlett L, Burnett B: The formulation of recombinant factor IX: Stability, robustness, and convenience. *Semin Hematol* **35**:18, 1998.
143. Lusher J, Ingerslev J, Roberts H, Hedner U: Clinical experience with recombinant factor VIIa. *Blood Coagul Fibrinol* **9**:119, 1998.
144. Roberts HR, Eberst ME: Current management of hemophilia B. *Hematol Oncol Clin North Am* **7**:1269, 1993.
145. Schaub R, Garzone P, Bouchard P, Rup B, Keith J, Brinkhous K, Larsen G: Preclinical studies of recombinant factor IX. *Semin Hematol* **35**:28, 1998.
146. White G, Shapiro A, Ragni M, Garzone P, Goodfellow J, Tubridy K, Courter S: Clinical evaluation of recombinant factor IX. *Semin Hematol* **35**:33, 1998.
147. Berntorp E: The treatment of haemophilia, including prophylaxis, constant infusion and DDAVP. *Baillieres Clin Haematol* **9**:259, 1996.
148. Bona RD, Weinstein RA, Weisman SJ, Bartolomeo A, Rickles FR: The use of continuous infusion of factor concentrates in the treatment of hemophilia. *Am J Hematol* **32**:8, 1989.
149. Martinowitz UP, Schulman S: Continuous infusion of factor concentrates: review of use in hemophilia A and demonstration of safety and efficacy in hemophilia B. *Acta Haematol* **94(Suppl 1)**:35, 1995.
150. Conlan MG, Hoots WK: Disseminated intravascular coagulation and hemorrhage in hemophilia B following elective surgery. *Am J Hematol* **35**:203, 1990.
151. Martinowitz U, Varon D, Jonas P, Bar-Maor A, Brenner B, Leibovitch I, Heim M: Circumcision in hemophilia: The use of fibrin glue for local hemostasis. *J Urol* **148**:855, 1992.
152. Sindet-Pedersen S, Stenbjerg S: Effect of local antifibrinolytic treatment with tranexamic acid in hemophiliacs undergoing oral surgery. *J Oral Maxillofac Surg* **44**:703, 1986.
153. Palanzo DA, Sadr FS: Coronary artery bypass grafting in a patient with haemophilia B. *Perfusion* **10**:265, 1995.
154. Theodorsson B, Hedner U, Nilsson IM, Kisiel W: A technique for specific removal of factor IX alloantibodies from human plasma: Partial characterization of the alloantibodies. *Blood* **61**:973, 1983.
155. Nilsson IM, Freiburghaus C: Apheresis. *Adv Exp Med Biol* **386**:175, 1995.
156. Lusher JM: Recombinant factor VIIa (NovoSeven) in the treatment of internal bleeding in patients with factor VIII and IX inhibitors. *Haemostasis* **26(Suppl 1)**:124, 1996.
157. Ingerslev J, Freidman D, Gastineau D, Gilchrist G, Johnsson H, Lucas G, McPherson J, et al.: Major surgery in haemophilic patients with inhibitors using recombinant factor VIIa. *Haemostasis* **26**:118, 1996.
158. Köhler M, Lellstern P, Lechler E, Überhfuhr P, Müller-Berghaus G: Thromboembolic complications associated with the use of prothrombin complex and factor IX concentrates. *Thromb Haemost* **80**:399, 1998.
159. van der Meer J, Hillege HL, Ascop CAPL, Dunselman JM, Mulder BJM, van Omnen GVA, Pfisterer M, et al.: Aprotinin in aortocoronary bypass surgery: Increased risk of vein-graft occlusion and myocardial infarction? Supportive evidence from a retrospective study. *Thromb Haemost* **75**:1, 1996.

160. Warrier I, Ewenstein BM, Koerper MA, Shapiro A, Key N, DiMichele D, Miller RT, et al.: Factor IX inhibitors and anaphylaxis in hemophilia B. *J Pediatr Hematol Oncol* **19**:23, 1997.
161. Ragni MV, Winkelstein A, Kingsley L, Spero JA, Lewis JH: 1986 update of HIV seroprevalence, seroconversion, AIDS incidence, and immunologic correlates of HIV infection in patients with hemophilia A and B. *Blood* **70**:786, 1987.
162. Ludlam CA: Viral safety of plasma-derived factor VIII and IX concentrates. *Blood Coagul Fibrinol* **8**:S19, 1997.
163. Mannucci PM: Clinical evaluation of viral safety of coagulation factor VIII and IX concentrates. *Vox Sang* **64**:197, 1993.
164. Aronson DL: Regulation and licensing of U.S. plasma products: Response to AIDS. *Dev Biol Stand* **67**:215, 1986.
165. Craven BM, Stewart GT, Khan M: AIDS: Safety, regulation and the law in procedures using blood and blood products. *Med Sci Law* **37**:215, 1997.
166. Kupfer B, Oldenburg J, Brackmann HH, Matz B, Schneweis KE, Kaiser R: Beta-propiolactone UV inactivated clotting factor concentrate is the source of HIV-infection of 8 hemophilia B patients: Confirmed. *Thromb Haemost* **74**:1386, 1995.
167. Adamson S, Charlebois T, O'Connell B, Foster W: Viral safety of recombinant factor IX. *Semin Hematol* **35**:22, 1998.
168. Johnson RE, Lawrence DN, Evatt BL, Bregman DJ, Zyla LD, Curran JW, Aledort LM, et al.: Acquired immunodeficiency syndrome among patients attending hemophilia treatment centers and mortality experience of hemophiliacs in the United States. *J Epidemiol* **121**:797, 1985.
169. Diamondstone LS, Blakley SA, Rice JC, Clark RA, Goedert JJ: Prognostic factors for all-cause mortality among hemophiliacs infected with human immunodeficiency virus. *Am J Epidemiol* **142**:304, 1995.
170. Hardy AM, Allen JR, Morgan WM, Curran JW: The incidence rate of acquired immunodeficiency syndrome in selected populations. *JAMA* **253**:215, 1985.
171. Lusher JM: Factor IX concentrates, in Forbes CD AL, Madhok R (ed): *Hemophilia*. London, Chapman and Hall, 1997, p 203.
172. Ragni MV, Weissfeld JL: Model of the impact of HIV infection on the size of future hemophilia and carrier birth cohorts. *J Acquir Immune Defic Syndr Hum Retrovirol* **13**:160, 1996.
173. Troisi CL, Hollinger FB, Hoots WK, Contant C, Gill J, Ragni M, Parmley R, et al.: A multicenter study of viral hepatitis in a United States hemophilic population. *Blood* **81**:412, 1993.
174. Vermylen J, Peerlinck K: Review of the hepatitis A epidemics in hemophiliacs in Europe. *Vox Sang* **67**:8, 1994.
175. Lawlor E, Graham S, Davidson E, Yap PL, Cunningham C, Daly H, Temperley IJ: Hepatitis A transmission by factor IX concentrates. *Vox Sang* **71**:126, 1996.
176. Centers for Disease Control and Prevention: Hepatitis A among persons with hemophilia who received clotting factor concentrate—United States, September-December 1995. *JAMA* **275**:427, 1996.
177. Rollag H, Evensen SA, Froland SS, Glomstein A: Serological markers of hepatitis B virus and cytomegalovirus infections in Norwegians with coagulation factor defects. *Blut* **60**:93, 1990.
178. Kumar A, Kulkarni R, Murray DL, Gera R, Scott-Emuakpor AB, Bosma K, Penner JA: Serologic markers of viral hepatitis A, B, C, and D in patients with hemophilia. *J Med Virol* **41**:205, 1993.
179. Jantsch-Plunger V, Beck G, Maurer W: PCR detection of a low viral load in a prothrombin complex concentrate that transmitted hepatitis B virus. *Vox Sang* **69**:352, 1995.
180. Preston FE, Jarvis LM, Makris M, Philp L, Underwood JC, Ludlam CA, Simmonds P: Heterogeneity of hepatitis C virus genotypes in hemophilia: Relationship with chronic liver disease. *Blood* **85**:1259, 1995.
181. Telfer P, Sabin C, Devereux H, Scott F, Dusheiko G, Lee C: The progression of HCV-associated liver disease in a cohort of haemophilic patients. *Br J Haematol* **87**:555, 1994.
182. Sabin CA, Telfer P, Phillips AN, Bhagani S, Lee CA: The association between hepatitis C virus genotype and human immunodeficiency virus disease progression in a cohort of hemophilic men. *J Infect Dis* **175**:164, 1997.
183. Gordon FH, Mistry PK, Sabin CA, Lee CA: Outcome of orthotopic liver transplantation in patients with haemophilia. *Gut* **42**:744, 1998.
184. Makris M, Preston FE, Rosendaal FR, Underwood JC, Rice KM, Triger DR: The natural history of chronic hepatitis C in haemophiliacs. *Br J Haematol* **94**:746, 1996.
185. Tatsunami S, Mimaya J, Nakamura I, Yago N, Meguro T, Yamada K: Life time expectancy of hemophilia patients infected with HIV-1 with the risk of hepatocellular carcinoma after HCV infection. *Medinfo* **8**:912, 1995.
186. Tradati F, Colombo M, Mannucci PM, Rumi MG, De Fazio C, Gamba G, Ciavarella N, et al.: A prospective multicenter study of hepatocellular carcinoma in Italian hemophiliacs with chronic hepatitis C. The Study Group of the Association of Italian Hemophilia Centers. *Blood* **91**:1173, 1998.
187. Zaaijer HL, Mauser-Bunschoten EP, ten Veen JH, Kapprell HP, Kok M, van den Berg HM, Lelie PN: Hepatitis E virus antibodies among patients with hemophilia, blood donors, and hepatitis patients. *J Med Virol* **46**:244, 1995.
188. Mannucci PM, Gringeri A, Santagostino E, Romano L, Zanetti A: Low risk of transmission of hepatitis E virus by large-pool coagulation factor concentrates. *Lancet* **343**:597, 1994.
189. Barzilai A, Schulman S, Karetnyi YV, Favorov MO, Levin E, Mendelson E, Weiss P, et al.: Hepatitis E virus infection in hemophiliacs. *J Med Virol* **46**:153, 1995.
190. De Filippi F, Colombo M, Rumi MG, Tradati F, Prati D, Zanella A, Mannucci PM: High rates of hepatitis G virus infection in multitransfused patients with hemophilia. *Blood* **90**:4634, 1997.
191. Wilde JT, Ahmed MM, Collingham KE, Skidmore SJ, Pillay D, Mutimer D: Hepatitis G virus infection in patients with bleeding disorders. *Br J Haematol* **99**:285, 1997.
192. Hanley JP, Jarvis LM, Hayes PC, Lee AJ, Simmonds P, Ludlam CA: Patterns of hepatitis G viraemia and liver disease in haemophiliacs previously exposed to non-virus inactivated coagulation factor concentrates. *Thromb Haemost* **79**:291, 1998.
193. Toyoda H, Fukuda Y, Hayakawa T, Takamatsu J, Saito H: Effect of GB virus C/hepatitis G virus coinfection on the course of HIV infection in hemophilia patients in Japan. *J Acquir Immune Defic Syndr Hum Retrovirol* **17**:209, 1998.
194. Santagostino E, Mannucci PM, Gringeri A, Azzi A, Morfini M, Musso R, Santoro R, et al.: Transmission of parvovirus B19 by coagulation factor concentrates exposed to 100 degrees C heat after lyophilization. *Transfusion* **37**:517, 1997.
195. Remafedi G, Parsons JT, Schultz JR, Schulz SL: Sexual behavior of HIV-seropositive young men with congenital coagulopathies. Hemophilia Behavioral Intervention Projects (HBIEP) Study Group. *J Adolesc Health* **21**:232, 1997.
196. Eis-Hubinger AM, Oldenburg J, Brackmann HH, Matz B, Schneweis KE: The prevalence of antibody to parvovirus B19 in hemophiliacs and in the general population. *Zentralbl Bakteriol* **284**:232, 1996.
197. Yee TT, Lee CA, Pasi KJ: Life-threatening human parvovirus B19 infection in immunocompetent haemophilia. *Lancet* **345**:794, 1995.
198. Brown P, Rohwer RG, Dunstan BC, MacAuley C, Gadjusek DC, Drohan WN: The distribution of infectivity in blood components and plasma derivatives in experimental models of transmissible spongiform encephalopathy. *Transfusion* **38**:810, 1998.
199. Dodd RY, Sullivan MT: Creutzfeldt-Jakob disease and transfusion safety: Tilting at icebergs? *Transfusion* **38**:221, 1998.
200. Evatt B, Autstin H, Barnhart E, Schonberger L, Sharer L, Jones R, DeArmond S: Surveillance for Creutzfeldt-Jakob disease among persons with hemophilia. *Transfusion* **38**:817, 1998.
201. Will RG, Ironside JW, Zeidler M, Cousens SN, Estibeiro K, Alperovitch A, Poser S, et al.: A new variant of Creutzfeldt-Jakob disease in the UK. *Lancet* **347**:921, 1996.
202. Bruce ME, Will RG, Ironside JW, McConnell I, Drummond D, Suttie A, McCardle L, et al.: Transmissions to mice indicate that "new variant" CJD is caused by the BSE agent. *Nature* **389**:498, 1997.
203. Kawashima T, Furukawa H, Doh-ura K, Iwaki T: Diagnosis of new variant Creutzfeldt-Jakob disease by tonsil biopsy. *Lancet* **350**:68, 1997.
204. Baxter T, Black D, Birks D: New-variant Creutzfeldt-Jakob disease and treatment of haemophilia. *Lancet* **351**:600, 1998.
205. Ludlam CA: New-variant Creutzfeldt-Jakob disease and treatment of haemophilia. Executive Committee UK Haemophilia Directors' Organisation. *Lancet* **351**:1289, 1998.
206. Saegusa A: UK plays safe on risks from blood products. *Nature* **392**:3, 1998.
207. Nishizawa T, Okamoto H, Konishi K, Yoshizawa H, Miyakawa Y, Mayumi M: A novel DNA virus (TTV) associated with elevated transaminase levels in posttransfusion hepatitis of unknown aetiology. *Biochem Biophys Res Commun* **241**:92, 1997.
208. Simmonds P, Davidson F, Lycett C, Prescott LE, MacDonald DM, Ellender J, Yap PL, et al.: Detection of a novel DNA virus (TTV) in blood donors and blood products. *Lancet* **352**:191, 1998.

209. Unger AS, Kessler CM, Lewis RJ: Total knee arthroplasty in human immunodeficiency virus-infected hemophiliacs. *J Arthroplasty* **10**:448, 1995.
210. Yamada M, Fukuda Y, Koyama Y, Nakano I, Urano F, Isobe K, Takamatsu J, et al.: A long-term follow-up study of interferon treatment for chronic hepatitis C in Japanese patients with congenital bleeding disorders. *Eur J Haematol* **57**:165, 1996.
211. Makris M, Preston FE, Triger DR, Underwood JC, Westlake L, Adelman MI: Interferon alfa for chronic hepatitis C in haemophiliacs. *Gut* **34**:S121, 1993.
212. Pinilla J, Quintana M, Magallon M: High-dose and long-term therapy of alpha interferon in hemophiliac patients with chronic C virus hepatitis. *Blood* **91**:727, 1998.
213. Rumi MG, Santagostino E, Morfini M, Gringeri A, Tagariello G, Chistolini A, Pontisso P, et al.: A multicenter controlled, randomized, open trial of interferon alpha2b treatment of anti-human immunodeficiency virus-negative hemophilic patients with chronic hepatitis C. Hepatitis Study Group of the Association of Italian Hemophilia Centers. *Blood* **89**:3529, 1997.
214. McCarthy M, Gane E, Pereira S, Tibbs CJ, Heaton N, Rela M, Hambley H, et al.: Liver transplantation for haemophiliacs with hepatitis C cirrhosis. *Gut* **39**:870, 1996.
215. Ragni MV, Amato DA, LoFaro ML, DeGruttola V, Van Der Horst C, Eyster ME KC, Gjerset GF, et al.: Randomized study of didanosine monotherapy and combination therapy with zidovudine in hemophilic and nonhemophilic subjects with asymptomatic human immunodeficiency virus-1 infection. AIDS Clinical Trial Groups. *Blood* **85**:2337, 1995.
216. Racoosin JA, Kessler C: A series of bleeding episodes in HIV-positive hemophiliacs (HEM) taking protease inhibitors. *Blood* **40**:34a, 1997.
217. Merry C, McMahon C, Ryan M, O'Shea E, Mulcahy F, Smith OP: Successful use of protease inhibitors in HIV-infected haemophilia patients. *Br J Haematol* **101**:475, 1998.
218. Aledort LM: Factor IX and thrombosis. *Scand J Haematol Suppl* **30**:40, 1977.
219. Anonymous: Prothrombin-complex concentrates and thrombosis. *N Engl J Med* **290**:403, 1974.
220. Aronson DL, Menache D: Thrombogenicity of factor IX complex: In vivo investigation. *Dev Biol Stand* **67**:149, 1987.
221. Chandra S, Brummelhuis HG: Prothrombin complex concentrates for clinical use. *Vox Sang* **41**:257, 1981.
222. Kasper CK: Postoperative thromboses in hemophilia B. *N Engl J Med* **289**:160, 1973.
223. Lusher JM: Thrombogenicity associated with factor IX complex concentrates. *Semin Hematol* **28(3 Suppl 6)**:3, 1991.
224. Lusher JM: Use of prothrombin complex concentrates in management of bleeding in hemophiliacs with inhibitors—Benefits and limitations. *Semin Hematol* **31(Suppl 4)**:49, 1994.
225. White GC 2nd, Shapiro AD, Kurczynski EM, Kim HC, Bergman GE: Variability of in vivo recovery of factor IX after infusion of monoclonal antibody purified factor IX concentrates in patients with hemophilia B. The Mononine Study Group. *Thromb Haemost* **73**:779, 1995.
226. White GC 2nd: Safety and recovery of mononine in multiple-dose, high-dose regimens. *Acta Haematol* **94(Suppl 1)**:53, 1995.
227. Brettler DB: Inhibitors in congenital haemophilia. *Baillieres Clin Haematol* **9**:319, 1996.
228. Sultan Y: Prevalence of inhibitors in a population of 3435 hemophilia patients in France. French Hemophilia Study Group. *Thromb Haemost* **67**:600, 1992.
229. High KA: Factor IX: Molecular structure, epitopes and mutations associated with inhibitor formation, in Aledort LM (ed): *Inhibitors to Coagulation Factors*. New York, Plenum Press, 1995, p 79.
230. Sawamoto Y, Shima M, Yamamoto M, Kamisue S, Nakai H, Tanaka I, Hayashi K, et al.: Measurement of anti-factor IX IgG subclasses in haemophilia B patients who developed inhibitors with episodes of allergic reactions to factor IX concentrates. *Thromb Res* **83**:279, 1996.
231. Orstavik KH, Miller CH: IgG subclass identification of inhibitors to factor IX in haemophilia B patients. *Br J Haematol* **68**:451, 1988.
232. Carroll RR, Panush RS, Kitchens CS: Spontaneous disappearance of an IgA anti-factor IX inhibitor in a child with Christmas disease. *Am J Hematol* **17**:321, 1984.
233. Swanson JL, Moertel CL, Stroncek DF, Key NS: Serologic evidence that factor IX inhibitor in the plasma of hemophilia B patients detects factor IX on normal red cells. *Transfusion* **36**:467, 1996.
234. Gadarowski JJ Jr, Czapek EE, Ontiveros JD, Pedraza JL: Modification of the Bethesda assay for factor VIII or IX. *Acta Haematol* **80**:134, 1988.
235. Kasper CK, Aledort LW, Counts RB, et al.: A more uniform measurement of factor VIII inhibitors. *Thromb Diath Haemorrhag* **34**:869, 1975.
236. Takamiya O, Kinoshita S: A simple method for detection of human factor IX inhibitor using ELISA. *Scand J Clin Lab Invest* **57**:683, 1997.
237. Sommer SS, Ketterling RP: The factor IX gene as a model for analysis of human germline mutations: An update. *Hum Mol Genet* **5**:1505, 1996.
238. Ljung RC: Gene mutations and inhibitor formation in patients with hemophilia B. *Acta Haematol* **94**:49, 1995.
239. Hoyer LW: Why do so many haemophilia A patients develop an inhibitor? *Br J Haematol* **90**:498, 1995.
240. Brackmann H, Gormsen J: Massive factor-VIII infusion in hemophiliac with factor VIII-inhibitor, high responder. *Lancet* **2**:933, 1977.
241. Brackmann HH, Oldenburg J, Schwaab R: Immune tolerance for the treatment of factor VIII inhibitors—Twenty years' "Bonn Protocol." *Vox Sang* **70**:30, 1996.
242. DiMichele D (ed.): *Pediatric Issues in Hemophilia: III. Pathophysiology and Management of Inhibitors*, San Diego, CA, Education Program of the American Society of Hematology, in 1997.
243. Berntorp E, Nilsson IM: Immune tolerance and the immune modulation protocol. *Vox Sang* **70(Suppl 1)**:36, 1996.
244. Nilsson IM, Berntorp E: Induction of immune tolerance in hemophiliacs with inhibitors by combined treatment with i.v. IgG, cyclophosphamide and factor VIII or IX. *Prog Clin Biol Res* **324**:69, 1990.
245. Gilles JG, Desqueper B, Lenk H, Vermylen J, Saint-Remy JM: Neutralizing anti-idiotypic antibodies to factor VIII inhibitors after desensitization in patients with hemophilia A. *J Clin Invest* **97**:1382, 1996.
246. Brinkhous KM, Sigman JL, Read MS, Stewart PF, McCarthy KP, Timony GA, Leppanen SD, et al.: Recombinant human factor IX: Replacement therapy, prophylaxis, and pharmacokinetics in canine hemophilia B. *Blood* **88**:2603, 1996.
247. Kay MA, Landen CN, Rothenberg SR, Taylor LA, Leland F, Wiehle S, Fang B, et al.: In vivo hepatic gene therapy: Complete albeit transient correction of factor IX deficiency in hemophilia B dogs. *Proc Natl Acad Sci U S A* **91**:2353, 1994.
248. Kay MA, Rothenberg S, Landen CN, Bellinger DA, Leland F, Toman C, Finegold M, et al.: In vivo gene therapy of hemophilia B: Sustained partial correction in factor IX-deficient dogs. *Sci* **262**:117, 1993.
249. Mustard JF, Rowsell HC, Robinson GA, Hoeksema TC, Downie HG: Canine hemophilia B (Christmas disease). *Br J Haematol* **6**:259, 1960.
250. Evans JP, Watzke HH, Ware JL, Stafford DW, High KA: Molecular cloning of a cDNA encoding canine factor IX. *Blood* **74**:207, 1989.
251. Evans JP, Brinkhous KM, Brayer GD, Reisner HM, High KA: Canine hemophilia B resulting from a point mutation with unusual consequences. *Proc Natl Acad Sci U S A* **86**:10095, 1989b.
252. Mauser AE, Whitlark J, Whitney KM, Lothrop CD Jr: A deletion mutation causes hemophilia B in Lhasa Apso dogs. *Blood* **88**:3451, 1996.
253. Brooks MB, Gu W, Ray K: Complete deletion of factor IX gene and inhibition of factor IX activity in a Labrador retriever with hemophilia B. *J Am Vet Med Assoc* **211**:1418, 1997.
254. Cristiano RJ, Smith LC, Kay MA, Brinkley BR, Woo SL: Hepatic gene therapy: efficient gene delivery and expression in primary hepatocytes utilizing a conjugated adenovirus-DNA complex. *Proc Natl Acad Sci U S A* **90**:11548, 1993.
255. Lin HF, Maeda N, Smithies O, Straight DL, Stafford DW: A coagulation factor IX-deficient mouse model for human hemophilia B. *Blood* **90**:3962, 1997.
256. Detloff PJ, Lewis J, John SW, Shehee WR, Langenbach R, Maeda N, Smithies O: Deletion and replacement of the mouse adult beta-globin genes by a "plug and socket" repeated targeting strategy. *Mol Cell Biol* **14**:6936, 1994.
257. Li B, Lawler AM, Antonarkis SE, High KA, Gearhart JD, Kazazian HH: Targeted disruption of the mouse factor VIII gene: A model for hemophilia A. *Nat Genet* **10**:119, 1995.
258. Wang L, Zoppe M, Hackeng TM, Griffin JH, Lee KF, Verma IM: A factor IX-deficient mouse model for hemophilia B gene therapy. *Proc Natl Acad Sci U S A* **94**:11563, 1997.

259. Kundu RK, Sangiorgi F, Wu L-Y, Kurachi K, Anderson WF, Maxson R, Gordon EM: Targeted inactivation of the coagulation factor IX gene causes hemophilia B in mice. *Blood* **92**:168, 1998.
260. Kung SH, Hagstrom JN, Cass D, Tai SJ, Lin HF, Stafford DW, High KA: Human factor IX corrects the bleeding diathesis of mice with hemophilia B. *Blood* **91**:784, 1998.
261. Verma IM, Somia N: Gene therapy-promises, problems and prospects. *Nature* **389**:239, 1997.
262. Herzog RW, High KA: Problems and prospects in gene therapy for hemophilia. *Curr Opin Hematol* **5**:321, 1998.
263. Naoumov NV, Petrova EP, Thomas MG, Williams R: Presence of a newly described human DNA virus (TTV) in patients with liver disease. *Lancet* **352**:195, 1998.
264. Eyster ME, Gill FM, Blatt PM, Hilgartner MW, Ballard JO, Kinney TR: Central nervous system bleeding in hemophiliacs. *Blood* **51**:1179, 1978.
265. Roth Protocol #9804-247, Office of Recombinant DNA Activities NIH, *Recombinant DNA Advisory Committee Meeting*, Bethesda, MD, 1998.
266. Greengard JS, Jolly DJ:Animal testing of retroviral-mediated gene therapy for factor VIII deficiency. Thromb Haemost **82**:555, 1999.
267. Herzog RW, Hagstrom JN, Kung SH, Tai SJ, Wilson JM, Fisher KJ, High KA: Stable gene transfer and expression of human blood coagulation factor IX after intramuscular injection of recombinant adeno-associated virus. *Proc Natl Acad Sci U S A* **94**:5804, 1997.
268. Herzog RW, Yang EY, Couto LB, Hagstrom JN, Elwell D, Tai SJ, Colosi P, et al.: *AAV-mediated transfer in dogs with hemophilia B*. Seattle, WA, American Society of Gene Therapy, 1998, p 116a.
268a. Kay MA, Manno CS, Ragni MV, Larson PJ, Couto LB, McClelland A, Glader B, Chew AJ, Tai SJ, Herzog RW, Arruda V, Johnson F, Scallan C, Skarsgard E, Flake AW, High KA: Evidence for gene transfer and expression of factor IX in haemophilia B patients treated with an AAV vector. *Nat Genet* **24**:257, 2000.
269. Snyder RO, Miao CH, Patijn GA, Spratt SK, Danos O, Nagy D, Gown AM, et al.: Persistent and therapeutic concentrations of human factor IX in mice after hepatic gene transfer of recombinant AAV vectors. *Nat Genet* **16**:270, 1997.
270. Nakai H, Herzog R, Hagstrom JN, Kung J, Walter JTai SJ, Iwaki Y, et al.: AAV-mediated gene transfer of human blood coagulation factor IX into mouse liver. *Blood* **91**:4600, 1998.
271. Kochanek S, Clemens PR, Mitani K, Chen HH, Chan S, Caskey CT: A new adenoviral vector: replacement of all viral coding sequences with 28kb of DNA independently expressing both full length dystrophin and β-galactosidase. *Proc Natl Acad Sci U S A* **93**:5731, 1996.
272. Kren BT, Bandyopadhyay P, Steer CJ: In vivo site-directed mutagenesis of the factor IX gene by chimeric RNA/DNA oligonucleotides. *Nat Med* **4**:285, 1998.
273. Lakich D, Kazazian HH, Antonarakis SE, Gitschier J: Inversions disrupting the factor VIII gene as a common cause of severe haemophilia A. *Nat Genet* **5**:236, 1993.
274. Hay CW, Robertson KA, Yong SL, Thompson AR, Growe GH, MacGillivray RTA: Use of a *Bam*HI polymorphism in the factor IX gene for the determination of hemophilia B carrier status. *Blood* **67**:1508, 1986.
275. Zhang M, Chen S-H, Thompson AR, Scott CR: *Bam*HI polymorphism of factor IX (T $\rightarrow$ G) transversion at nucleotide sequence −561, and high polymorphic frequency in black population. *Hum Genet* **82**:283, 1989.
276. Winship PR, Anson DS, Rizza CR, Brownlee GG: Carrier detection in haemophilia B using two further intragenic restriction fragment length polymorphisms. *Nucleic Acids Res* **12**:8861, 1984.
277. Graham JB, Kunkel GR, Egilmez NK, Wallmark A, Fowlkes DM, Lord ST: The varying frequencies of five DNA polymorphisms of X-linked coagulant factor IX in eight ethnic groups. *Am J Hum Genet* **49**:537, 1991.
278. Driscoll MC, Dispenzieri A, Tobias E, Miller CH, Aledort LM: A second *Bam*HI DNA polymorphism and haplotype association in the factor IX gene. *Blood* **72**:61, 1988.
279. Scott CR, Chen S-H, Schoof J, Kurachi K: Hemophilia B: Population differences in RFLP frequencies useful for carrier detection. *Am J Hum Genet* **41**:A262, 1987.
280. Giannelli F, Anson DS, Choo KH, Rees DJ, Winship PR, Ferrari N, Rizza CR, et al.: Characterisation and use of an intragenic polymorphic marker for detection of carriers of haemophilia B (factor IX deficiency). *Lancet* **1**:239, 1984.
281. Freedenburg DL, Chen SH, Kurachi K, Scott CR: *Msp*I polymorphic site within the factor IX gene. *Hum Genet* **76**:262, 1987.
282. Wallmark A, Kunkel G, Mouhli H, Bosco J, Ljung R, Nilsson IM, Graham JB: Population genetics of the Malmö polymorphism of coagulation factor IX. *Hum Hered* **41**:391, 1991.
283. Thompson AR, Chen SH, Smith KJ: Diagnostic role of an immunoassay-detected polymorphism of factor IX for potential carriers of hemophilia B. *Blood* **72**:1633, 1988.
284. Winship PR, Rees DJ, Alkan M: Detection of polymorphisms at cytosine phosphoguanidine dinucleotides and diagnosis of haemophilia B carriers. *Lancet* **1**:631, 1989.
285. Department of Health and Human Services: National Heart and Lung Institute Blood Resource Studies. *Pilot Study of Hemophilia Treatment in the U.S.*, vol. 3. Washington, DC, U.S. Government Printing Office, 1972.
286. Goodeve AC, Chuansumrit A, Sasanakul W, Isarangkura P, Preston FE, Peake IR: A comparison of the allelic frequencies of ten DNA polymorphisms associated with factor VII and factor IX genes in Thai and Western European populations. *Blood Coagul Fibrinolysis* **5**:29, 1994.

CHAPTER 174

Von Willebrand Disease

J. Evan Sadler

1. **von Willebrand factor (VWF) is a complex multimeric glycoprotein that is found in plasma, in platelet α granules, and in subendothelial connective tissue. VWF performs two biologic functions that are required for normal hemostasis: it binds to specific receptors on the platelet surface and in subendothelial connective tissue to form a bridge between the platelet and areas of vascular damage, and it binds to and stabilizes blood coagulation factor VIII. This interaction between VWF and factor VIII is necessary for normal factor VIII survival in the circulation. Deficiency of VWF results in defective platelet adhesion and also causes a secondary deficiency of factor VIII. Consequently, deficiency of VWF may cause bleeding that mimics either platelet dysfunction or hemophilia.**
2. **Inherited deficiency of VWF causes von Willebrand disease (VWD). Clinically significant VWD affects approximately 125 people per million population, a prevalence approximately twice that of hemophilia A. The prevalence of severely affected homozygous or compound heterozygous patients suggests that between 1500 and 3500 people per million population are heterozygous for a defective VWF allele; therefore, a relatively small fraction of persons harboring VWF mutations are symptomatic.**
3. **VWD is a heterogeneous disorder that has been classified into several major subtypes (dominant, MIM 193400; recessive, MIM 277480). The most common form (type 1) is transmitted as an autosomal dominant trait and appears to be due to simple quantitative deficiency of all VWF multimers. Recessive inheritance and virtual absence of VWF characterize a clinically severe variant (type 3). Variants that are characterized by a dysfunctional protein are classified as type 2. Type 2 VWD is further subdivided into four variants (2A, 2B, 2M, and 2N) based on the functional characteristics of the mutant protein.**
4. **Bleeding in severe VWD is treated with blood products containing factor VIII-VWF complex; these include certain factor VIII concentrates and plasma cryoprecipitate. Clinically milder variants can often be treated without exposure to blood products through pharmacologic manipulation of plasma VWF levels. For many patients with VWD the intravenous or intranasal administration of the vasopressin analogue DDAVP causes a rise in plasma VWF that is sufficient either to treat spontaneous and traumatic bleeding or to sustain normal hemostasis during surgery.**
5. **Molecular defects have been characterized in many types of VWD. Nonsense mutations and gene deletions are causes of severe VWD (type 3). Gene deletions predispose to the development of alloantibody inhibitors to transfused VWF, a rare complication of therapy. Missense mutations have been characterized that cause specific gain-of-function and loss-of-function variants of type 2 VWD. Many polymorphisms have been described for the VWF gene that can augment the use of biochemical testing for genetic counseling.**

A list of standard abbreviations is located immediately preceding the index in each volume. Additional abbreviations used in this chapter include: CK = cysteine knot; DDAVP = 1-desamino-8-D-arginine vasopressin; GPIb (GPIIb, GPIIIa) = platelet glycoprotein Ib (IIb, IIIa); GPIIb-IIIa = platelet glycoprotein IIb-IIIa complex; RIPA = ristocetin-induced platelet aggregation; RGD = Arg-Gly-Asp sequences; VWAgII = von Willebrand antigen II; VWD = von Willebrand disease; VWF = von Willebrand factor.

HISTORICAL ASPECTS

von Willebrand factor (VWF) and the corresponding inherited deficiency state take their name from Erik von Willebrand, who, in 1926, described a bleeding disease that affected several branches of a large family from the Åland islands in the Gulf of Bothnia, Finland.[1,2] In contrast to classic hemophilia, the mode of inheritance was autosomal rather than X-linked, and the bleeding was usually from mucocutaneous sites rather than joints and deep tissues. The disorder was characterized by a prolonged bleeding time, with normal coagulation time, clot retraction, and platelet count. von Willebrand named the condition hereditary pseudohemophilia, distinguishing it from thrombocytopenic purpura and Glanzmann thrombasthenia.

The pathogenesis of von Willebrand disease (VWD) remained controversial for more than 30 years. von Willebrand and subsequent investigators thought that the bleeding disorder was caused either by platelet dysfunction or by a lesion of the vasculature.[3,4] In 1953, several reports described patients with prolonged bleeding times who also had decreased plasma factor VIII activity, suggesting that an abnormality of the blood might be responsible for their apparent platelet or vascular dysfunction.[4–6] These patients were not immediately recognized to have VWD, but later studies showed that the original patients described by von Willebrand were indistinguishable and also had reduced factor VIII activity.[7,8]

The concept of a plasma deficiency was confirmed when the prolonged bleeding time and factor VIII deficiency in VWD were shown to be corrected by transfusion of a plasma factor VIII concentrate.[7,8] The same plasma fraction prepared from patients with severe hemophilia A was also effective,[9] indicating that the hemostatic defect in VWD could be corrected by a "von Willebrand factor" (VWF) that was found in normal or hemophilia A plasma. This VWF clearly was not identical to factor VIII.

Despite this clinical evidence that VWF and factor VIII were different, recognition that they were distinct proteins was obscured by the fact that factor VIII is usually deficient in VWD. Furthermore, the transfusion of VWF into patients with

VWD produces a sustained rise in plasma factor VIII levels that cannot be explained by the content of factor VIII transfused. Factor VIII may remain elevated for several days, and decays with a half-life much longer than that of exogenous factor VIII in normal subjects.[9–12]

The relationship between factor VIII and VWF was further confused because early partial purifications of factor VIII activity yielded a protein that by immunochemical assays was clearly deficient in VWD plasma, but that was present in normal antigenic amounts in hemophilia A plasma.[13–15] Conversely, the antibodies to factor VIII that developed in some patients with hemophilia A did not recognize this "factor VIII-related antigen."[16–18] To reconcile these data, some investigators proposed that VWF was a protein specified by an autosomal gene that served as a precursor to factor VIII, which was produced when a protein specified by an X-linked gene acted on VWF.[19–21] These observations gave rise to one of the most persistent confusions in the study of hemostasis, in which the term factor VIII referred either to (antihemophilic) factor VIII or to VWF, depending on the context.

The first evidence that VWF was specifically required for platelet adhesion in vivo was obtained in 1960 by Borchgrevink, who found that patients with VWD had higher platelet counts in blood from capillary lesions than did normal controls.[22] Subsequently, decreased platelet adhesion in vitro was demonstrated by the perfusion of blood from patients with VWD through a column of glass beads.[23,24] Transfusion of either normal plasma, hemophilia A plasma, or factor VIII concentrate was shown to correct both the bleeding time and the in vitro platelet adhesion defect in VWD.[7,8,23,25] This glass bead retention assay was used for the first documented purification of VWF.[26]

A more convenient assay for human VWF was developed in 1971 by Howard and Firkin, who discovered that the antibiotic ristocetin induced platelet aggregation in normal platelet-rich plasma, but not in plasma from patients with VWD.[27] The defect was corrected by normal plasma, hemophilia A plasma, or partially purified VWF. A similar defect could be induced in normal plasma by heteroantiserums to VWF.

Factor VIII was known to behave as a very large macromolecule that could be dissociated into a smaller active species by buffers of high ionic strength.[28] This salt-induced transition resolved factor VIII from the ristocetin-dependent platelet aggregating activity of VWF, which did not decrease in apparent size.[29] Bovine plasma aggregates human platelets in the absence of ristocetin, and similar experiments demonstrated that bovine platelet aggregating activity, or VWF, could also be resolved from factor VIII.[30]

Protein sequencing and cDNA cloning subsequently provided conclusive proof that factor VIII and VWF were independent proteins, as discussed below for VWF and in Chap. 172 for factor VIII. Together, these methods demonstrated that the two proteins have unique primary sequences that are encoded by distinct genes. Furthermore, the product of each gene has the appropriate biologic activity in the absence of the other.

At one time, VWD was thought to be a single entity that was characterized in part by deficiency of both VWF activity and the corresponding protein antigen. In 1972, Holmberg and Nilsson showed that a subgroup of patients with VWD have a normal plasma concentration of VWF antigen.[31] By crossed immunoelectrophoresis, the VWF antigen in these patients was shown to have excessively rapid mobility, consistent with a structural abnormality.[32,33] Subsequent studies revealed considerable additional phenotypic heterogeneity in VWD.

BIOCHEMISTRY OF VON WILLEBRAND FACTOR

Knowledge of the biochemistry of VWF provides a necessary framework for organizing and understanding the pathogenesis of the many variants of VWD. VWF has a particularly complex structure that requires a correspondingly complicated biosynthesis. Accordingly, VWF deficiency could result from defects in biosynthetic processing or from the structural alteration of specific functional domains.

Biosynthesis and Localization of von Willebrand Factor

VWF is synthesized by endothelial cells,[34] megakaryocytes,[35] and perhaps by the syncytiotrophoblast of placenta.[36] The structure of VWF was determined by a combination of protein chemistry methods and cDNA cloning. The ≈9-kb VWF mRNA encodes a primary translation product of 2813 amino acids (Fig. 174-1) that includes a conventional signal peptide of 22 residues, an unusually large propeptide of 741 residues or ≈100 kDa, and the mature subunit of 2050 residues or ≈270 kDa.[37–44] The proVWF contains five distinct types of repeated domains, or motifs shared with other proteins, that together make up over 95 percent of the protein and are arranged in the sequence D1-D2-D′-D3-A1-A2-A3-D4-B1-B2-B3-C1-C2-CK as reviewed elsewhere.[45]

VWF contains a remarkable amount of cysteine. In fact, cysteine is the most abundant amino acid in the protein, comprising 234 of the 2813 residues (8.3 percent). The cysteines are clustered at the N-terminal and C-terminal ends of the sequence, and the triplicated A domains correspond to a cysteine-poor region in the middle of the protein.

Shortly after removal of the signal peptide, the ≈370 kDa proVWF dimerizes by disulfide bond formation between the CK domains at the C-terminal ends of the subunits (Fig. 174-2) to yield the basic repeating unit of VWF.[46–50] The dimers undergo further polymerization by forming disulfide bonds between the N-terminal ends of subunits to yield a series of oligomers. This polymerization appears to occur at about the same time that the pro-VWF dimers arrive in the Golgi apparatus, and is associated with removal of the propeptide from all but ≈1 percent of the subunits.[49] The oligomers in plasma range in size from ≈500 kDa dimers to species of over 10 million daltons and 20 subunits.[51–54] Subunits that retain the propeptide are found in all of the multimers.[49]

The propeptide of VWF is identical to von Willebrand antigen II (VWAgII),[55] a ≈100 kDa protein that is found in blood plasma and platelet α granules.[56,57] The free propeptide spontaneously forms noncovalent dimers.[58] Many deletions or insertions within the propeptide lead to the formation of VWF dimers but not to the formation of higher multimers,[59–61] although missense mutations that abolish propeptide cleavage are compatible with normal multimer assembly.[60,62] These observations suggest that the propeptide is needed for VWF multimer assembly; whether it has another independent biologic function is not known.

In addition to proteolytic processing and disulfide bond formation, VWF is subject to several other posttranslational modifications that may affect its function. There are a total of 17 potential *N*-linked glycosylation sites in preproVWF with the sequence Asn-X-Thr/Ser (Fig. 174-1). Plasma VWF contains ≈19 percent carbohydrate by weight,[63] distributed among 12 asparagine-linked and 10 serine/threonine-linked oligosaccharides.[43] Eleven of the 13 potential *N*-linked sites in the mature subunit are glycosylated, and one glycosylated asparagine residue occurs in the unusual sequence Asn-Ser-Cys. Additional carbohydrate is attached to the von Willebrand antigen II propeptide. The antibiotic tunicamycin inhibits the asparagine-linked glycosylation of nascent VWF. The resultant carbohydrate-deficient proVWF monomers do not dimerize and the propeptide is not removed, suggesting that this glycosylation is required for the normal assembly of VWF structure.[64] Also, cultured endothelial cells incorporate sulfate into one or both of the *N*-linked oligosaccharides at Asn384 and Asn468 of the mature subunit.[65] The *N*-linked oligosaccharides of VWF are unusual compared to those of other plasma glycoproteins because they contain ABO blood group structures.[66]

Mature VWF and VWAgII both are stored in endothelial cells in a unique membrane enclosed organelle, the Weibel-Palade body.[67] These are 0.1 to 0.2 μM wide and up to 4 μM long, and

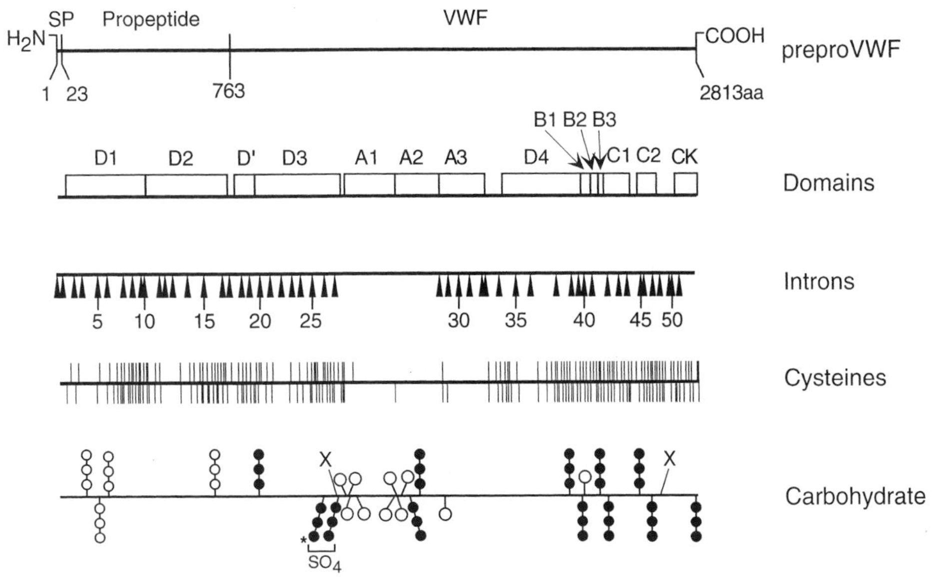

Fig. 174-1 Structural features of the human VWF precursor. PreproVWF: The signal peptide, or prepeptide, consists of amino acid residues (aa) 1 to 22, the propeptide consists of aa 23 to 763, and the mature subunit consists of aa 764-2813. Domains: The repeated domains are labeled A, B, C, D, and CK. "CK" stands for "cysteine knot" domain. Introns: The locations within the amino acid sequence of the 51 VWF introns are indicated by arrowheads, and every fifth intron is numbered. Cysteines: The sites of cysteine residues are indicated by vertical marks. In regions with a very high density of cysteine residues, one mark may represent several cysteines. Carbohydrate: The sites of potential *N*-linked glycosylation sites are indicated by the open symbols, O-O-O. The similar filled symbols, ●-●-●, indicate sites shown to be glycosylated by protein sequencing. The asterisk (*) marks a glycosylated asparagine residue in the unusual sequence Asn-Ser-Cys. Oligosaccharides that are sulfated (SO_4) are indicated by the bracket. The symbol X indicates two potential *N*-linked glycosylation sites that are not glycosylated in mature VWF. The slightly larger open circles (O) mark sites of *O*-linked glycosylation. (*Adapted from Sadler.[288] Used by permission.*)

contain regularly spaced longitudinal tubular structures[68] that appear to represent closely packed VWF molecules. VWF is also found at the periphery of the α granules of platelets in tubular structures that resemble those of Weibel-Palade bodies,[69] as well as in subendothelial connective tissue,[70,71] and the syncytiotrophoblast of placenta.[36]

Metabolism

The plasma concentration of VWF is ≈10 mg/ml,[72] with a wide range of normal concentration from 40 to 200 percent of the mean.[73] Some of this variability may be due to an effect of blood type. Both VWF antigen levels[74,75] and ristocetin-cofactor activity[76] are lower in individuals of blood type O. Plasma VWF levels increase slightly with increasing age.[75,76] Approximately 15 percent of circulating VWF is found in platelets.[77]

The plasma concentration of VWF increases in response to many physiological stimuli including adrenergic stress, vasopressin, growth hormone, and estrogens as reviewed elsewhere.[78] Adrenergic agents and vasopressin appear to act through independent pathways to induce the secretion of VWF stored in Weibel-Palade bodies. The effect of adrenergic agonists is blocked by propranolol and is probably mediated by β-adrenoreceptors.

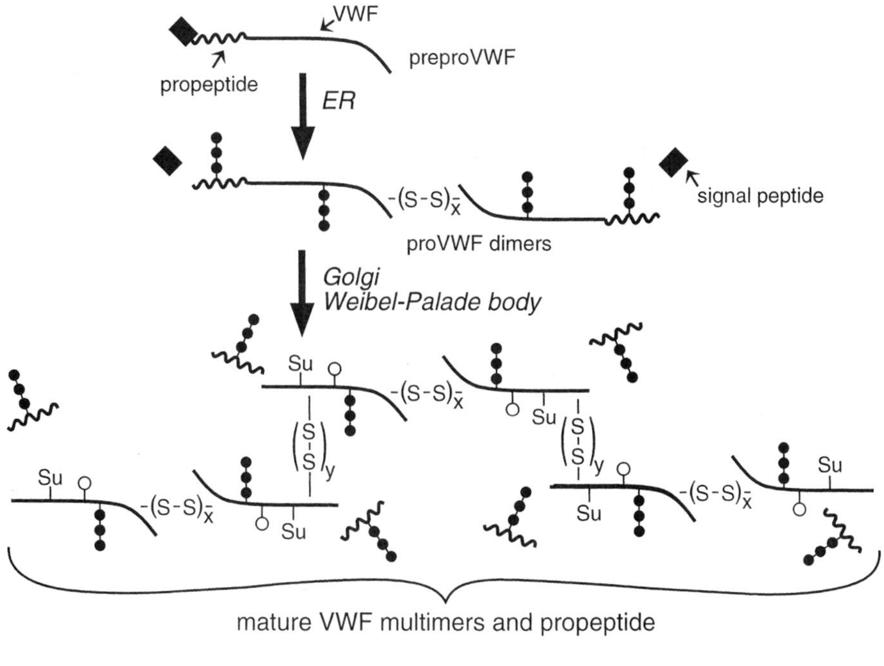

Fig. 174-2 Biosynthesis of VWF. The primary translation product of the mRNA for VWF is translocated into the lumen of the rough endoplasmic reticulum (ER), where the signal peptide is removed and *N*-linked glycosylation begins. The resultant proVWF rapidly dimerizes by the formation of a number (*x*) of disulfide bonds in the C-terminal region of the protein sequence. ProVWF dimers are transported to the Golgi apparatus and then to Weibel-Palade bodies. In the Golgi apparatus, *O*-linked and *N*-linked glycosylation is completed, inorganic sulfate (Su) is incorporated into some *N*-linked oligosaccharides, the propeptide is cleaved from almost all of the subunits, and multimers are created by the formation of a number (*y*) of intersubunit disulfide bonds near the N-terminal end of the subunits. The symbols for *N*-linked and *O*-linked oligosaccharides are as in Fig. 174-1.

Propranolol has no effect on the response to the vasopressin analogue, 1-desamino-8-D-arginine vasopressin (DDAVP). DDAVP does not stimulate the secretion of VWF by cultured vascular endothelial cells, so its mechanism of action in vivo appears to be indirect.[79,80]

Certain products of blood coagulation act directly on endothelial cells to stimulate the secretion of VWF. Human α-thrombin induces the rapid release of VWF that appears to be complete after 10 min of exposure to thrombin and does not require continued protein synthesis.[81,82] Release requires the presence of extracellular calcium, is associated with depletion of the Weibel-Palade bodies,[82] and requires the thrombin active site.[81] Fibrin also induces the release of VWF, and this effect is not duplicated by fibrinogen, fibrinopeptides A and B, factor XIII, or tissue plasminogen activator. The specific fibrin structure that is required includes the N-terminus of the β-chain.[83] Thus, products of thrombosis may have localized effects on the adjacent vascular endothelium to recruit additional VWF to the clot environment. In addition, the VWF secreted by endothelial cells in response to such stimuli appears to contain especially large and biologically potent VWF multimers.[84]

The metabolic fate of VWF is not known in much detail. Clearance from the circulation of ^{125}I-labeled VWF occurs in two phases. In both normal persons and patients with hemophilia A, an initial rapid phase with a disappearance half-life of 4.5 h is followed by a slower phase with a disappearance half time of 20 h. Larger multimers seem to clear more rapidly than smaller multimers.[11] The catabolism of VWF probably involves proteolysis within the circulation. Specific proteolytic fragments of the basic subunit are present in plasma VWF.[63,85] These fragments are reduced or absent in the larger VWF multimers that are released into the circulation by the administration of DDAVP, and with time, both the multimer pattern and subunit fragmentation pattern return to those present before DDAVP.[86] This proteolysis may contribute to the relatively rapid disappearance of larger multimers from the circulation, whether transfused or endogenous.

Biologic Activities and Structure-Function Relationships of von Willebrand Factor

VWF has two well-characterized biologic functions. It is necessary for the adhesion of platelets to regions of vascular damage, and it is necessary for the normal survival of factor VIII in circulation. These functions have been dissected in vitro into several distinct binding interactions that depend on specific domains of the protein sequence and on higher orders of structure that include organization into multimers (Table 174-1). Abnormalities in any of these interactions might contribute to the phenotype of von Willebrand disease.

Table 174-1 Binding Activities of VWF

Ligand	Biologic Function
Collagens	May mediate platelet adhesion to subendothelium
Other connective tissue elements	May mediate platelet adhesion to subendothelium
Platelet glycoprotein Ib	Required for platelet adhesion to subendothelium
Platelet glycoprotein IIb-IIIa	May mediate platelet adhesion to subendothelium and VWF-dependent platelet aggregation
Factor VIII	Stabilizers factor VIII in the circulation
Heparin	Unknown
Sulfated glycolipids	Unknown

NOTE: References can be found in the text

The Role of von Willebrand Factor in Platelet Adhesion to Subendothelial Connective Tissue. Several in vitro perfusion systems have been described for the study of VWF function in promoting platelet adhesion to damaged blood vessels and connective tissue constituents. When whole blood is perfused over everted blood-vessel segments, platelets adhere to the surface, if the endothelium was removed.[87] Platelet adherence to the subendothelium is decreased in blood from patients with VWD,[88–90] but can be corrected by the addition of purified VWF.[90,91] Conversely, platelet adherence using blood from patients with hemophilia A is normal[89,90], and that observed with normal blood is inhibited by antibodies to VWF.[92,93] This dependence on VWF is most apparent at high wall-shear rates that may occur in the microcirculation.[89,92] The platelet adhesion that is observed at low shear rates is not increased by VWF and may depend on other proteins in the blood or subendothelium.

There are three principal sites of VWF localization that might contribute to VWF-dependent platelet adhesion: plasma, platelet α granule, and subendothelial connective tissue. The importance of plasma VWF for platelet adhesion is readily demonstrated in the perfusion systems just discussed. An independent contribution by the VWF already localized in the subendothelium is strongly supported by perfusion studies using rabbit[94] and human vessel segments.[95] The activation of platelets induces the release of additional VWF from platelet α granules that could augment VWF-dependent processes. Platelet VWF promotes adhesion to collagen in perfusates that lack VWF[96] and correlates inversely with the bleeding time in some patients with VWD type 1.[97] The relative role of VWF in these three locations in normal hemostasis is difficult to assess, but all of these pools may participate in VWF-mediated platelet adhesion in vivo.

Binding of von Willebrand Factor to Subendothelial Connective Tissue. The substances in subendothelial connective tissue that support VWF-dependent platelet adhesion have not been completely characterized, and more than one may be important. Among connective tissue constituents, VWF binds to fibrillar collagens, collagen type VI (a nonfibrillar collagen), and heparin; furthermore, VWF mediates platelet adhesion to native collagen types I and III,[98,99] but not to denatured collagens.[100–102] VWF binds to extracellular matrix that is depleted of fibrillar collagens with collagenase or α,α′-dipyridyl.[103] Also, a monoclonal anti-VWF antibody that inhibits VWF binding to collagen types I and III does not inhibit binding to extracellular matrix; conversely, another monoclonal antibody that inhibits VWF binding to extracellular matrix does not inhibit binding to the same collagens.[104] These results suggest that interaction of VWF with fibrillar collagens might not be required for platelet adhesion. Collagen type VI consists mostly of large noncollagenous domains, as reviewed elsewhere,[105] and binds VWF.[106] Because this collagen is abundant in subendothelium[106] and is resistant to both collagenase[107] and α,α′-dipyridyl,[108] collagen type VI may be a physiologically significant VWF binding site in the subendothelium.

The VWF propeptide has at least one binding site for collagen.[109] The physiological significance of this interaction is not known.

Interaction of von Willebrand Factor with Specific Platelet Receptors. Two distinct receptors for VWF have been identified in the platelet plasma membrane. Platelet glycoprotein Ib (GPIb) appears to be the principal receptor responsible for VWF-dependent platelet adhesion to vascular subendothelium. Patients afflicted with the Bernard-Soulier syndrome, which is characterized by deficiency of platelet membrane GPIb,[110,111] have a severe bleeding disorder associated with defective VWF-dependent platelet adhesion to subendothelium in vitro (see Chap. 177).[89,112] This phenomenon is mimicked by treatment of normal platelets with antibodies to GPIb.[113] This same receptor also mediates the ristocetin-dependent platelet aggregating activity of

VWF.[114,115] This interaction does not require platelet activation and can be demonstrated with formalin-fixed normal platelets.[116,117] Ristocetin-induced binding of VWF to platelets is deficient in the Bernard-Soulier syndrome,[118] and binding to normal platelets is inhibited by monoclonal antibodies to GPIb.[119,120]

A second receptor for VWF is present on activated platelets. The platelet glycoprotein IIb-IIIa complex (GPIIb-IIIa) does not bind VWF in resting platelets. Upon activation with thrombin or other agonists, GPIIb-IIIa acquires the capability to bind several plasma proteins, including fibrinogen,[121–123] fibronectin,[124] and VWF.[125] Thus, ligand binding to GPIIb-IIIa may contribute to platelet adhesion that is initiated by GPIb binding to VWF. These proteins appear to interact competitively with a common site on GPIIb-IIIa through similar short Arg-Gly-Asp-containing recognition sequences in all three proteins.[126] Additional sequences may contribute to the binding of certain proteins to GPIIb-IIIa, particularly the C-terminal 12 amino acids of the γ chain of fibrinogen.[127] Binding of VWF to normal activated platelets is inhibited by antibodies to GPIIb-IIIa,[120] and does not occur at all in Glanzmann thrombasthenia, which is characterized by deficiency of GPIIb-IIIa (see Chap. 177).[128] The binding of VWF to GPIIb-IIIa requires calcium ions,[125] in contrast to the ristocetin-induced binding of VWF to GPIb, which is calcium-independent.[129]

Stabilization of Factor VIII by von Willebrand Factor. Factor VIII is noncovalently bound to VWF in the blood and the two proteins can be resolved by chromatography in buffers of high ionic strength.[28,29] Activation of factor VIII by thrombin also appears to cause dissociation from VWF.[130] The VWF binding site is on the light chain of factor VIII.[131] Factor VIII is a minor constituent of this factor VIII-VWF complex, comprising ≈1 percent of the mass of circulating VWF. This interaction is necessary for the normal survival of factor VIII in the circulation. Pure factor VIII transfused into patients with hemophilia A or normal volunteers disappears from the circulation with a half-life of about 12 h, and this is similar to the half-life of the factor VIII-VWF complex.[11,12] In contrast, pure factor VIII transfused into patients with severe VWD has a half-life of ≈2.4 h.[12] As discussed under "Historical Aspects," above, the transfusion of VWF in severe VWD produces a rise in plasma factor VIII that may persist for several days, while the bleeding time and ristocetin cofactor activity are only corrected for several hours.[9,10,12] This response to transfusion is adequately explained by a model in which endogenously synthesized factor VIII binds to and is stabilized by the infused VWF. The larger multimers that can correct the bleeding time and ristocetin cofactor levels are more rapidly metabolized,[11] and the remaining smaller multimers continue to protect factor VIII. Thus, severe deficiency of VWF causes a secondary deficiency of factor VIII. Defective interaction between VWF and factor VIII gives rise to a phenotype of apparent autosomal dominant hemophilia A with normal VWF function, as described below under "Type 2N von Willebrand Disease."

Other Binding Activities of von Willebrand Factor. Additional binding activities of VWF have been described that have no known physiological function at this time. VWF binds to immobilized heparin, and this interaction was used for the purification of VWF by affinity chromatography on heparin agarose.[132] It is possible that binding to heparin-like glycosaminoglycans contributes to the interaction of VWF with the vascular subendothelium. VWF also binds specifically and with high affinity to certain sulfated glycolipids. This interaction is only weakly inhibited by heparin and may be mediated by an independent binding site.[133,134] Whether appropriate sulfated glycolipids are accessible to VWF in vivo is not known.

Structure-Function Relationships of von Willebrand Factor. The multimeric structure of VWF is important for its function in promoting platelet adhesion. Larger multimers in plasma adhere selectively to resting platelets in the presence of ristocetin[135] and to collagen,[136] whereas the smaller multimers (e.g., <4 million Da) do not. Large multimers support platelet adhesion to subendothelium in perfusion systems, whereas the smaller multimers found in plasma do not.[137] Accordingly, some degree of polymerization appears to be necessary for optimal VWF function.

Binding sites for several ligands have been localized to the A domains of the VWF subunit (Fig. 174-3). The VWF A1 domain contains the site of interaction for platelet GPIb,[138] the snake-venom protein botrocetin,[139] heparin,[140] and sulfatides,[134] as well as a minor binding site for collagen.[141,142] The major collagen-binding site is within VWF domain A3.[141–144] Amino acids that participate in several of these binding interactions have been identified by scanning mutagenesis.[145,146] The crystallographic structures of the VWF A1 and A3 domains have been determined and provide a framework for interpreting the effects of mutations on VWF function.[147–150]

The factor VIII binding site is located within the first 273 amino acid residues of the mature VWF subunit, corresponding to domains D′ and part of D3.[151] A second heparin-binding site has been reported in this region, although this site appears not to be accessible in the intact protein.[152]

The tetrapeptide sequence, Arg-Gly-Asp-Ser, occurs near the C-terminus of domain C1[37] and appears to mediate the binding of VWF to the platelet GPIIb-IIIa complex of activated platelets.[153–155] Several other adhesive glycoproteins appear to interact with receptors through sites that contain Arg-Gly-Asp sequences (also known as RGD sequences in single letter code), including fibronectin, vitronectin, and fibrinogen as reviewed elsewhere.[156] None of these proteins are known to be homologous, and the presence of similar functional binding sites may represent convergent evolution. A second Arg-Gly-Asp sequence occurs in the VWF propeptide;[44] whether it has any function is not known.

The glycosidically bound oligosaccharides of VWF have nonspecific but nevertheless essential functions. The sialic acid and galactose residues appear to protect the native protein from degradation by proteases.[157] The sialic acid residues are necessary to prevent clearance of VWF from the circulation by the liver.[158]

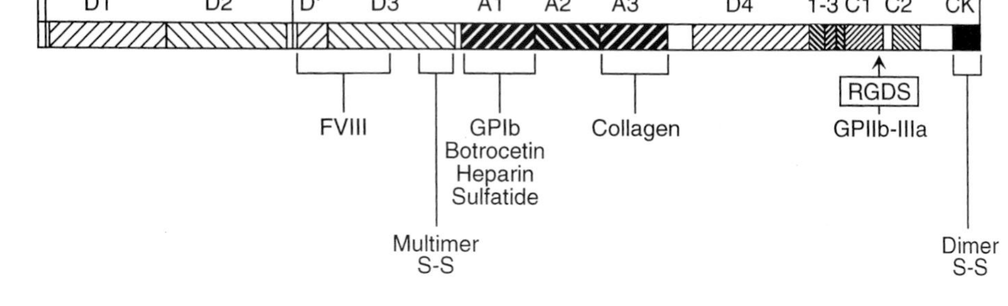

Fig. 174-3 Structure-function relationships of VWF. The repeated domains are shaded and labeled, and the positions of the signal peptide, propeptide, and mature subunit sequences are indicated. The locations of intersubunit disulfide bonds, an Arg-Gly-Asp-Ser (RGDS) sequence, and various ligand binding sites are shown.

They also prevent spontaneous interaction of VWF with platelet GPIb in the absence of ristocetin, as discussed above under "Interaction of VWF with Specific Platelet Receptors."

MOLECULAR BIOLOGY OF VON WILLEBRAND FACTOR

Chromosome Localization and Structure of the von Willebrand Factor Gene and Pseudogene

The gene for VWF is located near the tip of the short arm of human chromosome 12.[39,40] It spans ≈180 kb of DNA and consists of 52 exons.[159,160] There is a rough correlation between the placement of certain intron-exon boundaries and the repeated domains defined-by examination of the protein sequence, which lends support to the hypothesis that these domains evolved by gene segment duplication (GenBank pre-pro-VWF cDNA X04385). VWF lies within a region for which recombination is more frequent in males than in females, in contrast to the rest of chromosome 12 for which recombination is more frequent in females.[161]

A partial, unprocessed VWF pseudogene is located on chromosome 22q11.2.[162–164] The VWF pseudogene spans ≈21 to 29 kb of DNA and corresponds to exons 23 through 34 of the VWF gene. These exons encode mainly the triplicated A domains of VWF. The VWF gene and pseudogene diverged ≈3.1 percent in nucleotide sequence; this is consistent with a relatively recent origin of the pseudogene, perhaps < 10 million years ago.

Evolution of von Willebrand Factor and Homology to Other Proteins

The highly repeated structure of VWF indicates that the VWF gene has a complex evolutionary history including several gene segment duplications. Comparison of the VWF amino acid sequence to other protein sequences further indicates that VWF shares domains with a variety of proteins that otherwise do not appear to be homologous; thus, VWF also is a mosaic protein that has evolved in part by exon shuffling as reviewed elsewhere.[45] Vertebrate homologues of the VWF A domains are present in at least 22 proteins from at least 6 other protein "superfamilies": (a) the complement protease zymogens factor B and component C2; (b) the α subunits of a subset of heterodimeric cell surface integrins, the leukocyte adhesion molecules (Mac-1, LFA-1, p150,95, $\alpha d\beta 2$ and $\alpha E\beta 7$) and collagen receptors ($\alpha 1\beta 1$ and $\alpha 2\beta 2$); (c) cartilage matrix protein and the related matrilin-2 and matrilin-3; (d) unusual collagens with large noncollagenous domains, including the homotrimeric collagens type VII, XII, and XIV, and the three chains of collagen type VI; (e) the noninhibitory $\alpha 2$ and $\alpha 3$ subunits of inter-α-trypsin inhibitor; and (f) the $\alpha 2$ subunit of a dihydropyridine-sensitive calcium channel. As in VWF, the A domains in several of these other proteins bind macromolecular ligands. Homologues of VWF A domains also are found in proteins from several invertebrates, including *Caenorhabditis elegans* and *Plasmodium falciparum*.

VWF C and CK domains are shared with certain epithelial mucins, often in association with D domains and, sometimes, B domains.[165,166] These proteins form disulfide-linked dimers or larger oligomers through their CK or "cystine knot" domains. These CK domains are homologous to the transforming growth factor-β family.[167] Growth factors in this family usually are dimeric,[168] suggesting that CK domains function as dimerization motifs in several contexts.

CLINICAL ASPECTS OF VON WILLEBRAND DISEASE

Diagnosis

von Willebrand disease should be suspected in any patient with mucocutaneous bleeding despite a normal platelet count. The symptoms may be highly variable with time in a single patient, and all affected members of a given pedigree may not have the same difficulty with bleeding.[73,169–171] Even for severely affected patients with symptoms since birth and a clear family history, the pattern of bleeding is not specific for von Willebrand disease. Thus, final diagnosis depends on laboratory testing and may require repeated examinations of patients and family members.

Detailed reviews of the laboratory assessment of VWD can be found elsewhere.[172,173] Tests commonly applied to the diagnosis of VWD fall into four general categories:

1. *The template bleeding time.* This test assesses the formation of the platelet plug in vivo by determining the time required to stop bleeding from a standard skin laceration. It is difficult to standardize, and consistent results depend strongly upon the skill of the tester. A prolonged bleeding time is not at all specific for VWD because connective tissue and platelet disorders may also exhibit this abnormality. Patients with mild VWD intermittently may have normal bleeding times.[73]
2. *Platelet aggregation stimulated by the antibiotic ristocetin.* This test measures VWF binding to platelet GPIb. Two variations are used. One (ristocetin-induced platelet aggregation, or RIPA) employs patient platelets suspended in autologous plasma. The second (ristocetin cofactor activity) employs patient plasma with washed and fixed allogeneic platelets. In each assay, platelet aggregation as a function of ristocetin concentration is compared to normal controls, and the concentration required to achieve a specific degree or rate of aggregation is noted. The snake-venom factor botrocetin has effects similar, but not identical, to those of ristocetin, and can also be used to measure the ability of VWF to bind to resting platelets.[174,175]
3. *Measurement of factor VIII antigen or activity in patient plasma.* Factor VIII binds to plasma VWF, so that factor VIII levels usually reflect VWF antigen concentration. Comparison of ristocetin cofactor activity with factor VIII level provides an estimate of the specific activity of the residual VWF protein in patient plasma. This ratio of ristocetin cofactor activity to factor VIII level is expected to be normal for quantitative deficiencies of VWF and reduced for variants of VWD with a qualitatively abnormal protein.
4. *Physical characterization of patient VWF.* Gel electrophoresis and immunochemical assays measure VWF concentration, as well as multimer distribution. This category of assays includes the quantitative immunoassay of VWF antigen and the qualitative assessment of multimer distribution by counterimmunoelectrophoresis. More precise assessment of multimer distribution is obtained by electrophoresis of plasma on agarose or agarose/acrylamide copolymer gels in the presence of sodium dodecyl sulfate (Fig. 174-4). In such systems, the VWF multimers are separated according to size and can be visualized by reaction with ^{125}I-labeled antihuman VWF antibody and autoradiography[53,54] or by immunoenzymatic methods.

Comparison of platelet and plasma VWF with these assays may be useful in the further characterization of specific variants of VWD.[176,177] In addition, the time course of response of plasma factor VIII, VWF antigen, ristocetin cofactor activity, and VWF multimer structure to a trial infusion of the vasopressin analogue DDAVP can distinguish still more phenotypic heterogeneity.[177–179] Assays of VWF binding to collagen, heparin, or factor VIII also have been described, but are less widely available. Finally, the detailed investigation of family members to show inheritance of VWD is useful to firmly exclude acquired conditions that may mimic VWD.

Prevalence

von Willebrand disease appears to be the most common inherited bleeding disorder of human beings, but the prevalence is difficult to determine precisely because of substantial variation in the severity of disease. If all cases that come to the attention of specialized referral centers are included, the prevalence of

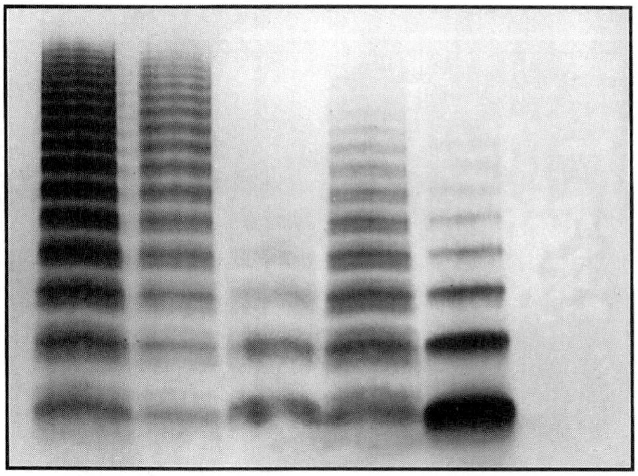

Fig. 174-4 Multimer patterns in variants of von Willebrand disease. Plasma VWF multimers in type 1 VWD have mobility similar to those from normal controls (N). Larger multimers are missing in VWD type 2A (lanes 3 and 5) and type 2B (lane 4). No multimers are visualized in VWD type 3 (lane 6). (*Adapted from Sadler.*[289] *Used by permission.*)

symptomatic VWD in Sweden is approximately 125 per million population.[180] However, the screening of an unselected population of schoolchildren in Italy suggests that the prevalence of inherited VWF abnormalities is much higher, ≈8000 per million population.[76] Severe VWD with essentially no detectable circulating VWF antigen is quite rare and affects 0.5 to 3 per million population in Western Europe and Scandinavia,[181] and perhaps as many as 5.3 per million population among selected Arab populations in the Middle East.[182]

The genetics of VWD illustrate some of the problems in the use of the terms dominant and recessive to describe human phenotypes (see Chap. 1). In many families, heterozygosity is consistently associated with obvious phenotypic effects and the dominant description is satisfactory. In other instances, heterozygosity is relatively or totally asymptomatic and may be associated with subtle laboratory abnormalities, thus blurring the separation of dominant and recessive phenotypes. In addition, it is likely that the genotype at other loci and nongenetic factors influence the phenotype, particularly in individuals heterozygous for VWD. Recognizing these limitations, it is still useful to separate phenotypes generally as dominant or recessive disorders.

In most pedigrees, VWD is transmitted as an autosomal dominant trait. By contrast, many patients with severe VWD who appear to be homozygotes or compound heterozygotes for a mutant allele at the VWF locus are born to clinically normal parents. Sensitive testing may disclose mild functional abnormalities in such parents who are obligate heterozygotes, but these families are usually considered affected by a recessive disease. Selected pedigrees may exhibit both dominant and recessive patterns of inheritance.[1,170,171] This variability suggests that some interplay between specific mutant alleles and the genetic background of the host determines whether clinically significant bleeding may occur. Certain variants of type 2 VWD consistently exhibit recessive inheritance although most are dominant.

One unlinked modifier of plasma VWF levels appears to be related to ABO blood type. Both VWF antigen[74,75] and ristocetin cofactor activity[76] are lower in persons of blood type O compared to blood types A and B.

Classification and Molecular Defect

The current classification of VWD is based on pathophysiological mechanism.[183] The correspondence with previous classifications is straightforward.[183] VWD is divided into three broad categories based on whether the VWF in blood plasma is qualitatively normal (type 1), abnormal (type 2), or absent (type 3). These categories correlate fairly well with the VWF multimer pattern observed in plasma. In type 1 VWD, all normal multimer species are present but reduced proportionally; assays of VWF antigen and function also are reduced proportionally. This pattern suggests a simple quantitative deficiency of VWF. In type 2 VWD, the plasma VWF exhibits defective structure or function, indicating a qualitative abnormality of the protein. In some such variants, the larger VWF multimers are absent (Fig. 174-4). Further subdivision of type 2 VWD is made based on the response of patient VWF to ristocetin, on the VWF multimer structure, and on the affinity of VWF for factor VIII. A third category, type 3 VWD, is distinguished by the virtual absence of VWF antigen and activity from plasma, and by clinically recessive inheritance. This scheme has the advantage that the major subdivisions identify patient groups having distinctive biochemical and clinical characteristics.

In principle, deficiency of VWF activity could result from lesions within the VWF gene or indirectly as a consequence of mutations that affect biosynthesis or metabolism. No cause of human VWD that is unlinked to the VWF locus has been described to date.

This chapter emphasizes the properties of VWD types for which molecular defects are defined (Table 174-2). A database of VWD mutations with comprehensive references has been published.[184] An updated version is maintained by David Ginsburg at the University of Michigan and is accessible online at http://mmg2.im.med.umich.edu/vWF. A catalogue of most known variants of VWD was compiled by Zaverio Ruggeri;[185] that review and selected more recent publications[186,187] can be consulted for references to case reports for rare or unclassified variants.

Type 1 von Willebrand Disease. VWD type 1 is the most common form of VWD and accounts for approximately 70 percent of cases seen in specialized treatment centers.[180,188] Plasma VWF is reduced; ristocetin cofactor activity and factor VIII usually are reduced proportionately, and the multimer distribution is normal. This is compatible with a simple quantitative deficiency of VWF with no intrinsic functional abnormality. Inheritance is usually autosomal dominant.

VWD type 1 is a heterogeneous disorder. Patients in some pedigrees have a normal content of platelet VWF, while in other families the patients have similar deficiencies of both plasma and platelet VWF.[176,177] These distinctions may correlate with the efficacy of therapy with DDAVP.[177] The mutations in VWD type 1 that have been characterized so far mainly consist of nonsense mutations, frameshifts, and deletions that also are found in VWD type 3.[189–191]

A few families are affected by VWD type 1 that is inherited with high penetrance and characterized by exceptionally low VWF levels. VWF is multimeric, and mutations that interfered with multimer synthesis or secretion could explain such a strongly dominant phenotype. In one family, the missense mutation $C386_{m}R$ (see mutation nomenclature note under "Type 2 von Willebrand disease" below) was shown to reduce the secretion of coexpressed normal VWF subunits, probably by causing the retention of heterodimers in the endoplasmic reticulum. This dominant-negative mechanism may explain some unexpectedly severe VWD type 1 phenotypes.[192]

A normal-appearing multimer distribution does not correlate perfectly with normal function. Because type 1 VWD is constrained to include only quantitative disorders, some variants previously designated as type 1 were reclassified under type 2, mainly as type 2M.

Type 2 von Willebrand Disease. Type 2 VWD includes all variants in which the circulating protein is qualitatively abnormal, with a defect in stability, function, or multimer distribution. Additional subdivision of type 2 VWD is made on the nature of

Table 174-2 Classification of von Willebrand Disease

Von Willebrand Disease	Genetics	Factor VIII	VWF Antigen	Ristocetin Cofactor Activity	RIPA	Multimer Structure
Type 1	Dominant	Decreased	Decreased	Decreased	Decreased	Normal in plasma and platelets
Type2A	Dominant (usually)	Decreased or normal	Decreased or normal	Decreased relative to antigen	Decreased relative to antigen	Large and intermediate multimers absent from plasma; variable in platelets
Type 2B	Dominant	Decreased or normal	Decreased or normal	Decreased or normal	Increased	Large and intermediate multimers absent from plasma; normal in platelets
Type 2M	Dominant (usually)	Decreased or normal	Decreased or normal	Decreased relative to antigen	Decreased relative to antigen	Large and intermediate multimers present in plasma and platelets
Type 2N	Recessive	Moderately to markedly decreased	Normal	Normal	Normal	Normal in plasma and platelets
Type 3	Recessive	Moderately to markedly decresed	Absent or trace	Absent	Absent	None or trace in plasma or platelets

RIPA = Ristocetin-induced platelet aggregation in platelet-rich plasma

the functional defect and analysis of VWF multimer patterns (Fig. 174-4).

Type 2A von Willebrand Disease. In type 2A VWD, both ristocetin-induced platelet aggregation and ristocetin cofactor activity are disproportionately decreased relative to VWF antigen, indicating that the residual plasma VWF has reduced function.[54] Large and intermediate plasma VWF multimers are absent, and the smallest multimer may be relatively increased. This subgroup is heterogeneous: the plasma VWF levels may be normal or decreased, and the distribution of platelet VWF multimers is variable.[54,176] In some patients, the plasma and platelet multimers exhibit similar decreases in large multimers that suggest a defect in polymerization. In other patients, the platelet multimer distribution appears normal, and increased sensitivity to proteolysis may contribute to the abnormal plasma VWF multimer distribution.[193,194] This heterogeneity is supported by the variable response to DDAVP in VWD type 2A. Some patients show at least a partial correction of both bleeding time and multimer distribution after treatment with DDAVP; others consistently fail to respond.[179,194,195] The mode of inheritance usually is dominant, and this variant accounts for approximately three-fourths of all type 2 VWD.

Several missense mutations that cause dominant type 2A VWD have been characterized, most of which are within VWF domain A2 (Fig. 174-5).[184] As was predicted from the phenotypic variability of type 2A VWD, these mutations can be divided into two groups that appear to cause similarly abnormal plasma VWF multimer patterns by distinct mechanisms.[196] One group includes the mutations $V844_mD$, $S743_mL$, and $G742_mR$. (Missense mutations are designated in single-letter code with the normal amino acid followed by the number of the position, which is followed by the mutant amino acid. Positions in the prepro region are numbered by codon number and are indicated by subscript p. Positions in the mature subunit are numbered from the first residue of the mature subunit, which corresponds to codon 764, and are indicated by subscript m (e.g. $V844_mD$ is Val at position 844 in the mature subunit mutated to Asp).) These particular mutations were shown to impair the assembly and secretion of normal VWF multimers, and patients with these mutations have decreased large VWF multimers in both plasma and platelets. The second group includes the mutations $R834_mW$ and $G742_mE$, which are compatible with the synthesis and secretion of normal appearing VWF multimers. Patients with these mutations have normal platelet VWF multimer patterns, and the deficiency of plasma VWF multimers apparently is caused by increased proteolytic

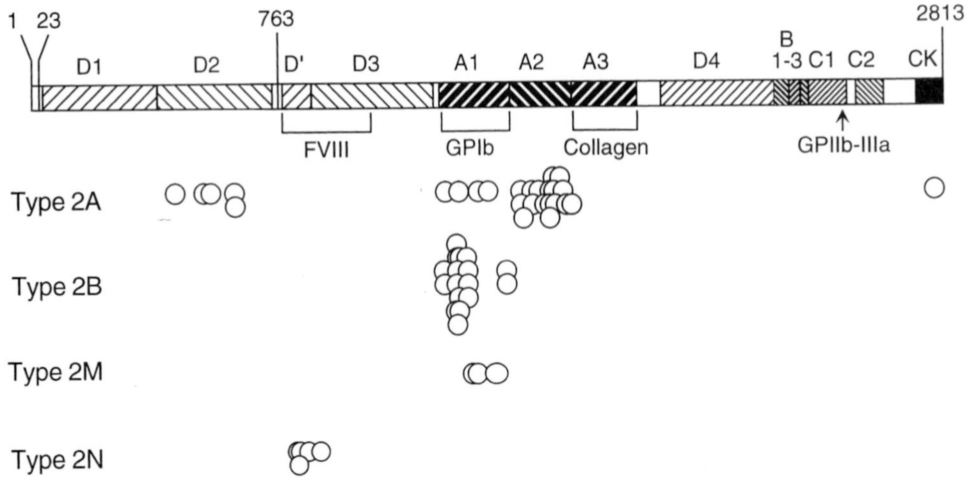

FIG. 174-5 Mutations in VWD type 2. References to the individual mutations can be found in the database of VWD mutations[184] maintained at the University of Michigan and accessible at http://mmg2.im.med.umich.edu/vWF.

degradation in the circulation.[196] For some patients with type 2A VWD, a major site of proteolytic cleavage in the VWF subunit was shown to be the $Tyr842_m$-$Met843_m$ bond.[197] A metalloprotease recently was partially purified from plasma that can cleave this bond.[198,199] The dominant variant originally described as type IID[206,207] is caused by mutations in the CK domain that prevent the formation of proVWF dimers within the endoplasmic reticulum. The mutant proVWF monomers are transported to the Golgi where they form nonfunctional "head-to-head" dimers.[208]

Recessive forms of VWD type 2A have been described. The variant originally designated VWD type IIC[200–204] is caused by mutations in the propeptide that impair multimer assembly in the Golgi apparatus, probably by interfering with the normal function of the propeptide in promoting intersubunit disulfide bond formation.[205] The recessive and dominant type 2A variants share a common pathophysiologic mechanism in which the lack of large VWF multimers prevents effective VWF-dependent platelet adhesion.

Several other rare type 2 variants are included under VWD type 2A. In general, these loss of function variants were defined initially by unique features of individual multimers upon high-resolution gel electrophoresis. These include the former type IIE,[85] type IIF,[209] type IIG,[210] type IIH,[211] and type II-I.[187] The latter four types represent single case reports.

Type 2B von Willebrand Disease. Type 2B VWD includes variants in which the mutant VWF has increased affinity for platelet GPIb. Laboratory testing shows hyperresponsiveness of platelet-rich plasma to ristocetin in the RIPA assay,[212] although ristocetin cofactor activity may be decreased or normal. Plasma VWF multimers usually show a decrease in large multimers, but platelets contain a normal multimer distribution.[54] Administration of DDAVP to patients with type 2B VWD causes the release of large multimers into the circulation, but the larger species are rapidly cleared, apparently through spontaneous binding to platelet GPIb. The binding of mutant VWF to platelets is accompanied by transient thrombocytopenia that can be severe.[213] Thus, the small multimer pattern in this variant is at least partly due to enhanced clearance of large multimers rather than to a polymerization defect. The increased RIPA is due to the presence of large, abnormal, hyperresponsive VWF multimers adsorbed to patient platelets in platelet-rich plasma. The normal or decreased ristocetin cofactor activity is due to the absence of these same multimers from (platelet-poor) patient plasma, so that added allogeneic platelets are not agglutinated by them. Variants of this subtype have been reported with chronic thrombocytopenia, circulating platelet aggregates, and spontaneous platelet aggregation in vitro.[214,215] The disorder is transmitted as a dominant trait; a few families with de novo mutations have been reported.[184,216,217] The few cases described of normal multimer distribution with hyperresponsiveness to ristocetin[218,219] appear to represent a mild form of type 2B defect. Type 2B VWD appears to account for less than 20 percent of all type 2 VWD.

Mutations that cause VWD type 2B (Fig. 174-5)[184] cluster within a spatially restricted region of VWF domain A.[149,150] This cluster may mark the location of a regulatory site that normally inhibits the binding of domain A1 to platelet GPIb. Mutations within this region appear to relieve this inhibition and cause the observed dominant gain-of-function phenotype.

Type 2M von Willebrand Disease. Type 2M (for "multimer") refers to variants with decreased platelet-dependent function that is not caused by the absence of large VWF multimers.[183] Despite the normal sized multimers, the presence of a functional defect indicates that the multimers must contain qualitatively abnormal VWF subunits. Type 2M includes variants with normal multimer distribution but decreased ristocetin cofactor activity,[220,221] the presence of large amounts of uncleaved proVWF in the multimers,[222] or larger than normal plasma multimers.[223] Such variants often were classified previously as distinct forms of VWD "type I."

One mechanism that causes VWD type 2M is decreased binding affinity for platelet GPIb due to mutations in VWF domain A1, and several patients with normal VWF multimer distributions have had mutations in the $Cys509_m$-$Cys695_m$ disulfide loop of domain A1 that prevented binding to GPIb. These mutations include deletion of the segment $R629_m$-$Q639_m$,[224] and the missense mutations $F606_mI$,[225] $I662_mF$,[225] and $G561_mS$[226].

Type 2N Von Willebrand Disease. An interesting variant of type 2 VWD is characterized by factor VIII deficiency that is caused indirectly by mutations in VWF.[227,228] The abnormal VWF does not bind to factor VIII and consequently does not stabilize it in the circulation; otherwise it apparently is normal, with normal levels of VWF antigen, normal indices of platelet-dependent VWF function such as bleeding time and ristocetin cofactor activity, and normal VWF multimer distribution. Thus, this type 2 VWD variant mimics hemophilia A except that the pattern of inheritance is autosomal recessive rather than X-linked recessive. This phenotype was named VWD type 2N after Normandy, the birth province of one proband.[228]

In one affected family, a male patient with VWD type 2N was misdiagnosed with hemophilia A, and moderate factor VIII deficiency in a sister was incorrectly attributed to extreme lyonization in a carrier of hemophilia A.[229] The prevalence of VWD type 2N is not known precisely, but screening of clinic patients suggests that a few percent of patients with apparent mild hemophilia A actually have VWD type 2N.[230] This diagnosis should be considered in patients with congenital factor VIII deficiency in whom the disorder is not clearly X-linked, because correct diagnosis has important implications for therapy and genetic counseling.[229]

Several mutations causing VWD type 2N have been identified within the factor VIII binding domain of VWF (Fig. 174-5).[184] In some patients, defects in factor VIII binding are associated with symptomatic decreases in platelet-dependent VWF functions. Such intermediate phenotypes can be caused by coinheritance of VWD type 1 and type 2N alleles,[231] and indicate that compound heterozygosity can strongly influence the clinical presentation of VWD variants.

Type 3 von Willebrand Disease. Patients with type 3 VWD have essentially no detectable VWF antigen or activity in blood plasma, and usually have factor VIII levels <10 percent of normal.[25,232,233] These patients appear to have received two defective VWF alleles, and many have clinically unaffected parents.

Because the prevalence of recessive type 3 VWD (q^2) is ≈ 0.5 to 3 per million population, heterozygotes (2pq) should comprise at least 1400 to 3500 per million population; however, the prevalence of symptomatic type 1 VWD appears to be at least tenfold lower. Clearly, most heterozygous relatives of patients with type 3 VWD are not symptomatic. There is variability in expression among heterozygotes within families that contain type 3 VWD patients, and deficiencies of VWF antigen and ristocetin cofactor activity can often be detected in clinically normal relatives.[170,171]

Patients with VWD type 3 usually are compound heterozygous for VWF alleles with frameshifts, large deletions, or nonsense mutations; homozygosity has been demonstrated in a few consanguineous families.[184,189,190,191] The mutation in the original von Willebrand family is a single nucleotide insertion in exon 18 that causes a frameshift and premature termination within the propeptide.[234] Large deletions in the VWF gene predispose patients with VWD type 3 to the development of inhibitors during therapy. A similar correlation has been noted for hemophilia B and deletions of the factor IX gene[235] (see Chap. 173).

Clinical Course

For patients with a quantitative deficiency of VWF (VWD types 1 and 3) the severity of disease generally correlates with the degree of VWF functional deficiency, and may vary from clinically insignificant to life threatening. The severity of the disease in patients with qualitative disorders of VWF (VWD type 2) may exceed what might be expected based on the functional deficiency ascertained by laboratory tests.[201,203,206,209] Symptoms are usually present from childhood, and often from birth.[7,8,10,25] These commonly include easy bruising, cutaneous hematomas, epistaxis, bleeding from gums, and prolonged bleeding from cuts. Persistent severe bleeding after minor oral trauma and after dental extraction is common. Most affected women have menorrhagia that may require blood transfusion.[169] Bleeding from a ruptured ovarian follicle or corpus luteum may also be severe.[180,203] Gastrointestinal bleeding seems to be relatively rare but may be life threatening. Patients with VWD type 3 and essentially undetectable VWF can have factor VIII levels low enough to predispose to spontaneous hemarthrosis, joint deformities, and soft tissue bleeding.[7,8,25] Milder forms of VWD are almost never associated with hemarthrosis. The bleeding tendency of VWD has been reported to decrease with advancing age,[7,25] although this is not a uniform feature of the disease.

During pregnancy the plasma VWF levels are increased in normal individuals and in patients with most forms of VWD other than VWD type 3.[236–239] This increase is most marked in the third trimester. If the increase represents functional VWF, then labor and delivery are usually uncomplicated. Patients with dysfunctional VWF (VWD type 2) frequently have difficulty with hemorrhage during labor and delivery.[201,206,219] Plasma VWF levels return to baseline within a few days, and patients with VWD should be watched closely during at least the first week after delivery for postpartum bleeding.

Type 2B VWD can present special problems during pregnancy. The increased plasma concentration of abnormal VWF that is a consequence of the physiological stimulus of pregnancy can cause severe and prolonged thrombocytopenia, rarely with marked blood loss during delivery.[240] Children born with VWD type 2B may present with congenital thrombocytopenia.[217]

The development of alloantibodies to VWF is distinctly uncommon in VWD as reviewed elsewhere.[241] All of the reported cases have occurred in patients with VWD type 3 with no detectable VWF-like protein. Among patients with VWD type 3, the prevalence of alloantibodies to VWF is about 7.5 percent. Not all severely affected patients develop antibodies, and there may be a familial predisposition to this complication of therapy. The apparent association between deletions within the VWF gene and the development of such antibodies was discussed above.

Differential Diagnosis

The symptoms that occur in VWD are not specific, and many conditions of quite different pathogenesis may be associated with a similar bleeding diathesis. These include primary platelet disorders, such as Bernard-Soulier syndrome, and the ingestion of antiplatelet drugs. In particular, the use of aspirin by patients with hemophilia A can produce a clinical picture quite similar to severe VWD.[242] In most cases, VWD can be excluded easily by appropriate laboratory testing.

VWD type 2B can cause thrombocytopenia that may be confused with idiopathic thrombocytopenic purpura. Such patients who present during pregnancy have received unnecessary therapy with prednisone[240,243] or intravenous γ-globulin,[244,245] while appropriate therapy with factor VIII concentrates was withheld. Two men, who were ultimately found to have VWD type 2B, underwent splenectomy for presumed idiopathic thrombocytopenic purpura unresponsive to prednisone.[214,246] This subtype of VWD also is associated with postoperative thrombocytopenia,[247] and has presented as congenital thrombocytopenia.[217]

Two conditions are especially difficult to distinguish from VWD because they may cause low VWF levels and abnormal VWF multimer distributions. These are the acquired von Willebrand syndrome and "platelet-type," or "pseudo," VWD. The *acquired von Willebrand syndrome* refers to a condition of spontaneous bleeding associated with decreased VWF occurring in adults without a prior personal or family history of VWD as reviewed elsewhere.[241] Most have been associated with a recognized autoimmune or lymphoproliferative disorder that suggests an immunologic cause. Some patients have lacked such underlying diseases, and fewer than half of the afflicted patients were shown to possess autoantibodies to VWF. The multimer distribution in plasma may be normal, or the largest multimers may be absent. In the latter case, discrimination between VWD type 2A and the acquired von Willebrand syndrome may be difficult. Both conditions may be characterized by relatively normal platelet VWF structure and concentration, and by shortened survival in the circulation of the endogenous VWF released by DDAVP. In contrast to VWD type 2A, the ristocetin sensitivity of platelet VWF is normal in the acquired von Willebrand syndrome, and exogenous VWF administered by transfusion has shortened survival.

Platelet-type or pseudo-VWD is clinically very similar to VWD type 2B, but the abnormality lies with the platelet rather than with the VWF.[248–250] The condition is inherited as an autosomal dominant trait. Symptoms resemble those of moderately severe VWD, and laboratory abnormalities include a prolonged bleeding time, decreased plasma VWF and factor VIII levels, increased ristocetin-induced platelet aggregation, absence of larger multimers from plasma, and presence of all multimers in platelets. The effect of DDAVP is like that in VWD type 2B, with transient thrombocytopenia and spontaneous platelet aggregation.[251] In contrast to VWD type 2B, the addition of normal plasma, hemophilic plasma, cryoprecipitate, or purified VWF to platelet-rich plasma in this disorder causes platelet aggregation without the addition of ristocetin.[249,250,252] Mutations within the gene for platelet GPIba were found in two patients with this disorder: G233V[253] and M239V (see Chap. 177).[254]

Therapy

Patients with severe VWD may bleed either because they lack sufficient VWF to support normal platelet function or because they are factor VIII-deficient, and the response to therapy in VWD emphasizes the distinct functions of these molecules in hemostasis. Hemarthroses, soft tissue hematomas, and postoperative bleeding usually respond to raising the level of factor VIII, whereas mucocutaneous bleeding responds to infusions of functional VWF.

Factor VIII levels are usually easy to support because even limited amounts of small VWF multimers can stabilize and cause a prolonged elevation of plasma factor VIII level. Correction of the platelet adhesion abnormality is more difficult. Fresh frozen plasma and cryoprecipitate consistently contain functional VWF multimers. The large volume of fresh frozen plasma that is needed to infuse sufficient VWF limits its utility. Cryoprecipitate may shorten the bleeding time in VWD, but the possible transmission of disease by cryoprecipitate makes it less than an ideal therapy. Several virucidally treated factor VIII concentrates that are used for the treatment of hemophilia A contain functional VWF multimers and appear to be effective.[255–257] These currently are the products of choice for the treatment or prevention of serious bleeding in VWD.

A very high purity VWF concentrate that contains little factor VIII was effective in several types of VWD.[258–260] The infused pure VWF binds and stabilizes endogenously synthesized factor VIII, so that factor VIII levels rise in a delayed fashion and peak levels are achieved only after many hours. Recombinant VWF has undergone therapeutic testing in animal models including VWF-deficient dogs.[261]

The highly purified "monoclonal" or recombinant factor VIII preparations commonly used for the treatment of hemophilia A are inappropriate for almost all patients with VWD because they do not treat the deficiency of functional VWF. In addition, the factor VIII in these products cannot be stabilized effectively by endogenous VWF in patients with VWD type 3 or type 2N.[256,262]

Platelet transfusions shorten the bleeding time in some VWD patients who are refractory to treatment with factor VIII-VWF concentrates. This effect may reflect the participation of both platelet and plasma VWF in hemostasis.[263–265]

Many patients with mild VWD can avoid exposure to blood products through the pharmacologic manipulation of plasma VWF levels. In many patients, the vasopressin analogue DDAVP administered intravenously, subcutaneously, or intranasally causes a three- to sixfold elevation of VWF and factor VIII levels that is maximal in 30 to 90 min.[266,267] Levels decrease to baseline over several hours to several days. Repeated doses often elicit a diminished response, but tachyphylaxis is not consistently observed and the efficacy of repeated doses should be evaluated in individual patients as indicated.[268,269] For therapy with DDAVP to be effective, the patient must be able to synthesize at least a partially functional VWF. Consequently, DDAVP is expected to be most useful in VWD type 1 with a simple quantitative deficiency of VWF. Patients with VWD type 3 generally do not have a useful response to DDAVP.[267,270]

The response to DDAVP in VWD type 2 variants is variable and frequently is unsatisfactory.[179,270–273] However, patients who will respond favorably are identifiable with a test infusion, which should be considered for all variants with low ristocetin cofactor activity.[269] In VWD type 2N, DDAVP increases plasma VWF levels but often does not significantly increase factor VIII levels; this pattern is consistent with the inability of VWF type 2N to bind and stabilize factor VIII.[272,273]

In patients with VWD type 2B, DDAVP causes transient thrombocytopenia and spontaneous platelet aggregation,[213] and the bleeding time usually is not shortened.[195,213,274] Concerns over the potential for promoting thrombosis have led to the recommendation that DDAVP should not be used in type 2B VWD.[213,271] Experience with DDAVP in this VWD subtype is very limited and the risk of thrombosis is not known, but no thrombotic complications have been described to date. In a few patients with VWD type 2B, DDAVP was therapeutically effective and did not cause a significant decrease in platelet count.[275–279] Thus, DDAVP may be acceptable therapy for a subset of patients with type 2B VWD.

Fibrinolytic inhibitors may be useful adjuncts for the control of nasopharyngeal and oral bleeding. Menorrhagia in women with VWD can be treated successfully with oral contraceptives.

Genetic Counseling

Assessment of the risk of VWD is usually straightforward and requires only the determination of whether a family is affected by a dominant or recessive variant. For families affected with severe forms of VWD (type 3 and some type 2 variants), genetic counseling is the same as for any severe recessive disorder. Prenatal diagnosis has been accomplished for VWD type 3 by assays of factor VIII and VWF in fetal blood samples.[280,281] The VWF multimer distribution in fetal blood may be diagnostic of type 2 VWD even if the levels of antigen are not depressed, provided there is no intercurrent disease that might consume large VWF multimers.[282] The VWF gene is highly polymorphic; at least 32 marker systems are available for genetic studies in VWD.[283] The most informative of these is a tetranucleotide repeat polymorphism in intron 40, with >98 alleles,[284] and this system was used for prenatal diagnosis of severe VWD.[285] DNA sequence polymorphisms also have been used to confirm the neonatal diagnosis of VWD.[286,287]

Carriers of the defective allele in mildly affected pedigrees could be identified with greater certainty by combining the currently employed VWF and factor VIII assays with analysis of DNA sequence polymorphisms. Such families should receive counseling, but most families do not choose to alter reproductive plans because of the mild phenotype.

REFERENCES

1. von Willebrand EA: Hereditär pseudohemofili. *Fin Laekaresaellsk Hand* **68**:87, 1926.
2. von Willebrand EA: Über hereditäre pseudohæmophilie. *Acta Med Scand* **76**:521, 1931.
3. von Willebrand EA, Jürgens R: Über eine neues vererbbares Blutungsübel: Kie konstitutionelle Thrombopathie. *Dtsch Arch Klin Med* **175**:453, 1933.
4. Alexander B, Goldstein B: Dual hemostatic defect in pseudohemophilia. *J Clin Invest* **32**:551, 1953.
5. Larrieu MJ, Soulier JP: Déficit en facteur antihémophilique A chez une fille associé à un trouble saignement. *Rev Hematol* **8**:361, 1953.
6. Quick AJ, Hussey CV: Hemophilic condition in the female. *J Lab Clin Med* **42**:929, 1953.
7. Nilsson IM, Blombäck M, Jorpes E, Blombäck B, Johansson S-A: v. Willebrand's disease and its correction with human plasma fraction 1-0. *Acta Med Scand* **159**:179, 1957.
8. Nilsson IM, Blombäck M, von Francken I: On an inherited autosomal hemorrhagic diathesis with antihemophilic globulin (AHG) deficiency and prolonged bleeding time. *Acta Med Scand* **159**:35, 1957.
9. Nilsson IM, Blombäck M, Blombäck B: von Willebrand's disease in Sweden. Its pathogenesis and treatment. *Acta Med Scand* **164**:263, 1959.
10. Cornu P, Larrieu MJ, Caen J, Bernard J: Transfusion studies in von Willebrand's disease: Effect on bleeding time and factor VIII. *Br J Haematol* **9**:189, 1963.
11. Over J, Sixma JJ, Bouma BN, Bolhuis PA, Vlooswijk RA, Beeser-Visser NH: Survival of ^{125}Iodine-labeled factor VIII in patients with von Willebrand's disease. *J Lab Clin Med* **97**:332, 1981.
12. Tuddenham EG, Lane RS, Rotblat F, Johnson AJ, Snape TJ, Middleton S, and Kernoff PB: Response to infusions of polyelectrolyte fractionated human factor VIII concentrate in human haemophilia A and von Willebrand's disease. *Br J Haematol* **52**:259, 1982.
13. Stites DP, Hershgold EJ, Perlman JD, and Fudenberg HH: Factor VIII detection by hemagglutination inhibition: Hemophilia A and von Willebrand's disease. *Science* **171**:196, 1971.
14. Zimmerman TS, Ratnoff OD, Powell AE: Immunologic differentiation of classic hemophilia (factor VIII deficiency) and von Willebrand's disease, with observations on combined deficiencies of antihemophilic factor and proaccelerin (factor V) and on an acquired circulating anticoagulant against antihemophilic factor. *J Clin Invest* **50**:244, 1971.
15. Shapiro GA, Andersen JC, Pizzo SV, McKee PA: The subunit structure of normal and hemophilic factor VIII. *J Clin Invest* **52**:2198, 1973.
16. Zimmerman TS, Edgington TS: Factor VIII coagulant activity and factor VIII-like antigen: Independent molecular entities. *J Exp Med* **138**:1015, 1973.
17. Lazarchick J, Hoyer LW: Immunoradiometric measurement of the factor VIII procoagulant antigen. *J Clin Invest* **62**:1048, 1978.
18. Peake IR, Bloom AL: Immunoradiometric assay of procoagulant factor-VIII antigen in plasma and serum and its reduction in haemophilia. Preliminary studies on adult and fetal blood. *Lancet* **1**:473, 1978.
19. Bennett B, Ratnoff OD, Levin J: Immunologic studies in von Willebrand's disease. Evidence that the antihemophilic factor (AHF) produced after transfusions lacks an antigen associated with normal AHF and the inactive material produced by patients with classic hemophilia. *J Clin Invest* **51**:2597, 1972.
20. Gralnick HR, and Coller BS: Molecular defects in haemophilia A and von Willebrand's disease. *Lancet* **1**:837, 1976.
21. Graham JB: Genetic control of factor VIII. *Lancet* **1**:340, 1980.
22. Borchgrevink CF: A method for measuring platelet adhesiveness in vivo. *Acta Med Scand* **162**:361, 1960.
23. Salzman EW: Measurement of platelet adhesiveness: A simple in vitro technique demonstrating an abnormality in von Willebrand's disease. *J Lab Clin Med* **62**:724, 1963.
24. Zucker MB: In vitro abnormality of the blood in von Willebrand's disease correctable by normal plasma. *Nature* **197**:601, 1963.
25. Larrieu MJ, Caen JP, Meyer DO, Vainer H, Sultan Y, Bernard J: Congenital bleeding disorders with long bleeding time and normal platelet count. II. Von Willebrand's disease (report of thirty-seven patients). *Am J Med* **45**:354, 1968.
26. Bouma BN, Wiegerinck Y, Sixma JJ, van Mourik JA, Mochtar IA: Immunological characterization of purified anti-haemophilic factor A (factor VIII) which corrects abnormal platelet retention in von Willebrand's disease. *Nature New Biol* **236**:104, 1972.
27. Howard MA, Firkin BG: Ristocetin—A new tool in the investigation of platelet aggregation. *Thromb Diath Haemorrh* **26**:362, 1971.

28. Thelin GM, Wagner RH: Sedimentation of plasma antihemophilic factor. *Arch Biochem Biophys* **95**:70, 1960.
29. Weiss HJ, Hoyer LW: Von Willebrand factor: Dissociation from antihemophilic factor procoagulant activity. *Science* **182**:1149, 1973.
30. Griggs TR, Cooper HA, Webster WP, Wagner RH, Brinkhous KM: Plasma aggregating factor (bovine) for human platelets: A marker for study of antihemophilic and von Willebrand factors. *Proc Natl Acad Sci U S A* **70**:2814, 1973.
31. Holmberg L, Nilsson IM: Genetic variants of von Willebrand's disease. *Br Med J* **3**:317, 1972.
32. Kernoff PBA, Gruson R, Rizza CR: A variant of factor VIII related antigen. *Br J Haematol* **26**:435, 1974.
33. Peake IR, Bloom AL, Giddings JC: Inherited variants of factor VIII-related protein in von Willebrand's disease. *N Engl J Med* **291**:113, 1974.
34. Jaffe EA, Hoyer LW, Nachman RL: Synthesis of von Willebrand factor by cultured human endothelial cells. *Proc Natl Acad Sci U S A* **71**:1906, 1974.
35. Nachman R, Levine R, Jaffe EA: Synthesis of factor VIII antigen by cultured guinea pig megakaryocytes. *J Clin Invest* **60**:914, 1977.
36. Maruyama I, Bell CE, Majerus PW: Thrombomodulin is found on endothelium of arteries, veins, capillaries, and lymphatics, and on syncytiotrophoblast of human placenta. *J Cell Biol* **101**:363, 1985.
37. Sadler JE, Shelton-Inloes BB, Sorace JM, Harlan JM, Titani K, Davie EW: Cloning and characterization of two cDNAs coding for human von Willebrand factor. *Proc Natl Acad Sci U S A* **82**:6394, 1985.
38. Lynch DC, Zimmerman TS, Collins CJ, Brown M, Morin MJ, Ling EH, Livingston DM: Molecular cloning of cDNA for human von Willebrand factor: Authentication by a new method. *Cell* **41**:49, 1985.
39. Verweij CL, de Vries CJ, Distel B, van Zonneveld AJ, van Kessel AG, van Mourik JA, Pannekoek H: Construction of cDNA coding for human von Willebrand factor using antibody probes for colony-screening and mapping of the chromosomal gene. *Nucleic Acids Res* **13**:4699, 1985.
40. Ginsburg D, Handin RI, Bonthron DT, Donlon TA, Bruns GAP, Latt SA, Orkin SH: Human von Willebrand factor (vWF): Isolation of complementary DNA (cDNA) clones and chromosomal localization. *Science* **228**:1401, 1985.
41. Bonthron DT, Orr EC, Mitsock LM, Ginsburg D, Handin RI, Orkin SH: Nucleotide sequence of pre-pro-von Willebrand factor cDNA. *Nucleic Acids Res* **14**:7125, 1986.
42. Shelton-Inloes BB, Titani K, Sadler JE: cDNA sequences for human von Willebrand factor reveal five types of repeated domains and five possible protein sequence polymorphisms. *Biochemistry* **25**:3164, 1986.
43. Titani K, Kumar S, Takio K, Ericsson LH, Wade RD, Ashida K, Walsh KA, et al: Amino acid sequence of human von Willebrand factor. *Biochemistry* **25**:3171, 1986.
44. Verweij CL, Diergaarde PJ, Hart M, Pannekoek H: Full-length von Willebrand factor (vWF) cDNA encodes a highly repetitive protein considerably larger than the mature vWF subunit. *EMBO J* **5**:1839, 1986.
45. Sadler JE: Biochemistry and genetics of von Willebrand factor. *Annu Rev Biochem* **67**:395, 1998.
46. Wagner DD, Marder VJ: Biosynthesis of von Willebrand protein by human endothelial cells. Identification of a large precursor polypeptide chain. *J Biol Chem* **258**:2065, 1983.
47. Lynch DC, Williams R, Zimmerman TS, Kirby EP, Livingston DM: Biosynthesis of the subunits of factor VIIIR by bovine aortic endothelial cells. *Proc Natl Acad Sci U S A* **80**:2738, 1983.
48. Lynch DC, Zimmerman TS, Kirby EP, Livingston DM: Subunit composition of oligomeric human von Willebrand factor. *J Biol Chem* **258**:12757, 1983.
49. Wagner DD, Marder VJ: Biosynthesis of von Willebrand protein by human endothelial cells: processing steps and their intracellular localization. *J Cell Biol* **99**:2123, 1984.
50. Wagner DD, Lawrence SO, Ohlsson-Wihelm BM, Fay PJ, Marder VJ: Topology and order of formation of interchain disulfide bonds in von Willebrand factor. *Blood* **69**:27, 1987.
51. van Mourik JA, Bouma BN, LaBruyére WT, de Graaf S, Mochtar IA: Factor VIII, a series of homologous oligomers and a complex of two proteins. *Thromb Res* **4**:155, 1974.
52. Counts RB, Paskell SL, Elgee SK: Disulfide bonds and the quaternary structure of factor VIII/von Willebrand factor. *J Clin Invest* **62**:702, 1978.
53. Hoyer LW, Shainoff JR: Factor VIII-related protein circulates in normal human plasma as high molecular weight multimers. *Blood* **55**:1056, 1980.
54. Ruggeri ZM, Zimmerman TS: Variant von Willebrand's disease. Characterization of two subtypes by analysis of multimeric composition of factor VIII/von Willebrand factor in plasma and platelets. *J Clin Invest* **65**:1318, 1980.
55. Fay PJ, Kawai Y, Wagner DD, Ginsburg D, Bonthron D, Ohlsson-Wilhelm BM, Chavin SI, et al: Propolypeptide of von Willebrand factor circulates in blood and is identical to von Willebrand antigen II. *Science* **232**:995, 1986.
56. Montgomery RR, Zimmerman TS: von Willebrand's disease antigen II. A new plasma and platelet antigen deficient in severe von Willebrand's disease. *J Clin Invest* **61**:1498, 1978.
57. Scott JP, Montgomery RR: Platelet von Willebrand's antigen II: Active release by aggregating agents and a marker of platelet release reaction in vivo. *Blood* **58**:1075, 1981.
58. Wagner DD, Fay PJ, Sporn LA, Sinha S, Lawrence SO, Marder VJ: Divergent fates of von Willebrand factor and its propolypeptide (von Willebrand antigen II) after secretion from endothelial cells. *Proc Natl Acad Sci U S A* **84**:1955, 1987.
59. Verweij CL, Hart M, Pannekoek H: Expression of variant von Willebrand factor (vWF) cDNA in heterologous cells: Requirement of the pro-polypeptide in vWF multimer formation. *EMBO J* **6**:2885, 1987.
60. Wise RJ, Pittman DD, Handin RI, Kaufman RJ, Orkin SH: The propeptide of von Willebrand factor independently mediates the assembly of von Willebrand multimers. *Cell* **52**:229, 1988.
61. Mayadas TN, Wagner DD: Vicinal cysteines in the prosequence play a role in von Willebrand factor multimer assembly. *Proc Natl Acad Sci U S A* **89**:3531, 1992.
62. Verweij CL, Hart M, Pannekoek H: Proteolytic cleavage of the precursor of von Willebrand factor is not essential for multimer formation. *J Biol Chem* **263**:7921, 1988.
63. Chopek MW, Girma JP, Fujikawa K, Davie EW, Titani K: Human von Willebrand factor: A multivalent protein composed of identical subunits. *Biochemistry* **25**:3146, 1986.
64. Wagner DD, Mayadas T, Marder VJ: Initial glycosylation and acidic pH in the Golgi apparatus are required for multimerization of von Willebrand factor. *J Cell Biol* **102**:1320, 1986.
65. Carew JA, Browning PJ, Lynch DC: Sulfation of von Willebrand factor. *Blood* **76**:2530, 1990.
66. Matsui T, Titani K, Mizuochi T: Structures of the asparagine-linked oligosaccharide chains of human von Willebrand factor. Occurrence of blood group A, B, and H(O) structures. *J Biol Chem* **267**:8723, 1992.
67. Wagner DD, Olmsted JB, Marder VJ: Immunolocalization of von Willebrand protein in Weibel-Palade bodies of human endothelial cells. *J Cell Biol* **95**:355, 1982.
68. Weibel ER, Palade GE: New cytoplasmic components in arterial endothelia. *J Cell Biol* **23**:101, 1964.
69. Cramer EM, Meyer D, le Menn R, Breton-Gorius J: Eccentric localization of von Willebrand factor in an internal structure of platelet α-granule resembling that of Weibel-Palade bodies. *Blood* **66**:710, 1985.
70. Bloom AL, Giddings JC, Wilks CJ: Factor VIII on the vascular intima: Possible importance in haemostasis and thrombosis. *Nature New Biol* **241**:217, 1973.
71. Hoyer LW, De los Santos RP, Hoyer JR: Antihemophilic factor antigen. Localization in endothelial cells by immunofluorescent microscopy. *J Clin Invest* **52**:2737, 1973.
72. Borchiellini A, Fijnvandraat K, ten Cate JW, Pajkrt D, van Deventer SJ, Pasterkamp G, Meijer-Huizinga F, et al: Quantitative analysis of von Willebrand factor propeptide release in vivo: Effect of experimental endotoxemia and administration of 1-deamino-8-D-arginine vasopressin in humans. *Blood* **88**:2951, 1996.
73. Abildgaard CF, Suzuki Z, Harrison J, Jefcoat K, Zimmerman TS: Serial studies in von Willebrand's disease: Variability versus "variants." *Blood* **56**:712, 1980.
74. Wahlberg TB, Blomback M, Magnusson D: Influence of sex, blood group, secretor character, smoking habits, acetylsalicylic acid, oral contraceptives, fasting and general health state on blood coagulation variables in randomly selected young adults. *Haemostasis* **14**:312, 1984.
75. Gill JC, Endres-Brooks J, Bauer PJ, Marks WJ, Montgomery RR: The effect of ABO blood group on the diagnosis of von Willebrand disease. *Blood* **69**:1691, 1987.
76. Rodeghiero F, Castaman G, Dini E: Epidemiological investigation of the prevalence of von Willebrand's disease. *Blood* **69**:454, 1987.
77. Nachman RL, Jaffe EA: Subcellular platelet factor VIII antigen and von Willebrand factor. *J Exp Med* **141**:1101, 1975.

78. Wagner DD: Cell biology of von Willebrand factor. *Annu Rev Cell Biol* **6**:217, 1990.
79. Moffat EH, Giddings JC, Bloom AL: The effect of desamino-D-arginine vasopressin (DDAVP) and naloxone infusions on factor VIII and possible endothelial cell (EC) related activities. *Br J Haematol* **57**:651, 1984.
80. Booth F, Allington MJ, Cederholm-Williams SA: An in vitro model for the study of acute release of von Willebrand factor from human endothelial cells. *Br J Haematol* **67**:71, 1987.
81. Levine JD, Harlan JM, Harker LA, Joseph ML, Counts RB: Thrombin-mediated release of factor VIII antigen from human umbilical vein endothelial cells in culture. *Blood* **60**:531, 1982.
82. Loesberg C, Gonsalves MD, Zandbergen J, Willems C, van Aken WG, Stel HV, Van Mourik JA, et al: The effect of calcium on the secretion of factor VIII-related antigen by cultured human endothelial cells. *Biochim Biophys Acta* **763**:160, 1983.
83. Ribes JA, Ni F, Wagner DD, Francis CW: Mediation of fibrin-induced release of von Willebrand factor from cultured endothelial cells by the fibrin β-chain. *J Clin Invest* **84**:435, 1989.
84. Sporn LA, Marder VJ, Wagner DD: Inducible secretion of large, biologically potent von Willebrand factor multimers. *Cell* **46**:185, 1986.
85. Zimmerman TS, Dent JA, Ruggeri ZM, Nannini LH: Subunit composition of plasma von Willebrand factor. Cleavage is present in normal individuals, increased in IIA and IIB von Willebrand disease, but minimal in variants with aberrant structure of individual oligomers (types IIC, IID, and IIE). *J Clin Invest* **77**:947, 1986.
86. Batlle J, Lopez-Fernandez MF, Lopez-Borrasca A, Lopez-Berges C, Dent JA, Berkowitz SD, Ruggeri ZM, et al: Proteolytic degradation of von Willebrand factor after DDAVP administration in normal individuals. *Blood* **70**:173, 1987.
87. Baumgartner HR: The role of blood flow in platelet adhesion, fibrin deposition, and formation of mural thrombi. *Microvasc Res* **5**:167, 1973.
88. Tschopp TB, Weiss HJ, Baumgartner HR: Decreased adhesion of platelets to subendothelium in von Willebrand's disease. *J Lab Clin Med* **83**:296, 1974.
89. Weiss HJ, Turitto VT, Baumgartner HR: Effect of shear rate on platelet interaction with subendothelium in citrated and native blood. I. Shear rate-dependent decrease of adhesion in von Willebrand's disease and the Bernard-Soulier syndrome. *J Lab Clin Med* **92**:750, 1978.
90. Sakariassen KS, Bolhuis PA, Sixma JJ: Human blood platelet adhesion to artery subendothelium is mediated by factor VIII-von Willebrand factor bound to the subendothelium. *Nature* **279**:636, 1979.
91. Weiss HJ, Baumgartner HR, Tschopp TB, Turitto VT, Cohen D: Correction by factor VIII of the impaired platelet adhesion to subendothelium in von Willebrand disease. *Blood* **51**:267, 1978.
92. Baumgartner HR, Tschopp TB, Meyer D: Shear rate dependent inhibition of platelet adhesion and aggregation on collagenous surfaces by antibodies to human factor VIII/von Willebrand factor. *Br J Haematol* **44**:127, 1980.
93. Meyer D, Baumgartner HR, Edginton TS: Hybridoma antibodies to human von Willebrand factor. II. Relative role of intramolecular loci in mediation of platelet adhesion to the subendothelium. *Br J Haematol* **57**:609, 1984.
94. Turitto VT, Weiss HJ, Zimmerman TS, Sussman II: Factor VIII/von Willebrand factor in subendothelium mediates platelet adhesion. *Blood* **65**:823, 1985.
95. Stel HV, Sakariassen KS, de Groot PG, van Mourik JA, Sixma JJ: Von Willebrand factor in the vessel wall mediates platelet adherence. *Blood* **65**:85, 1985.
96. Fressinaud E, Baruch D, Rothschild C, Baumgartner HR, Meyer D: Platelet von Willebrand factor: Evidence for its involvement in platelet adhesion to collagen. *Blood* **70**:1214, 1987.
97. Gralnick HR, Rick ME, McKeown LP, Williams SB, Parker RI, Maisonneuve P, Jenneau C, et al: Platelet von Willebrand factor: An important determinant of the bleeding time in type I von Willebrand's disease. *Blood* **68**:58, 1986.
98. Muggli R, Baumgartner HR, Tschopp TB, Keller H: Automated microdensitometry and protein assays as a measure for platelet adhesion and aggregation on collagen-coated slides under controlled flow conditions. *J Lab Clin Med* **95**:195, 1980.
99. Sakariassen KS, Aarts PAMM, de Groot PG, Houdijk WPM, Sixma JJ: A perfusion chamber developed to investigate platelet interaction in flowing blood with human vessel wall cells, their extracellular matrix, and purified components. *J Lab Clin Med* **102**:522, 1983.
100. Santoro SA: Adsorption of von Willebrand factor/factor VIII by the genetically distinct interstitial collagens. *Thromb Res* **21**:689, 1981.
101. Santoro SA, Cowan JF: Adsorption of von Willebrand factor by fibrillar collagen — Implications concerning the adhesion of platelets to collagen. *Coll Rel Res* **2**:31, 1982.
102. Morton LF, Griffin B, Pepper DS, Barnes MJ: The interaction between collagens and factor VIII/von Willebrand factor: Investigation of the structural requirements for interaction. *Thromb Res* **32**:545, 1983.
103. Wagner DD, Urban-Pickering M, Marder VJ: Von Willebrand protein binds to extracellular matrices independently of collagen. *Proc Natl Acad Sci U S A* **81**:471, 1984.
104. de Groot PG, Ottenhof-Rovers M, van Mourik JA, Sixma JJ: Evidence that the primary binding site of von Willebrand factor that mediates platelet adhesion on subendothelium is not collagen. *J Clin Invest* **82**:65, 1988.
105. Colombatti A, Bonaldo P: The superfamily of proteins with von Willebrand factor type A-like domains: One theme common to components of extracellular matrix, hemostasis, cellular adhesion, and defense mechanisms. *Blood* **77**:2305, 1991.
106. Rand JH, Patel ND, Schwartz E, Zhou SL, Potter BJ: 150-kD von Willebrand factor binding protein extracted from human vascular subendothelium is type VI collagen. *J Clin Invest* **88**:253, 1991.
107. von der Mark H, Aumailley M, Wick G, Fleischmajer R, Timpl R: Immunochemistry, genuine size and tissue localization of collagen VI. *Eur J Biochem* **142**:493, 1984.
108. Colombatti A, Bonaldo P: Biosynthesis of chick type VI collagen. II. Processing and secretion in fibroblasts and smooth muscle cells. *J Biol Chem* **262**:14461, 1987.
109. Takagi J, Fujisawa T, Sekiya F, Saito Y: Collagen-binding domain within bovine propolypeptide of von Willebrand factor. *J Biol Chem* **266**:5575, 1991.
110. Nurden AT, Caen JP: Specific roles for platelet surface glycoproteins in platelet function. *Nature* **255**:720, 1975.
111. Nurden AT, Dupuis D, Kunicki TJ, Caen JP: Analysis of the glycoprotein and protein composition of Bernard-Soulier platelets by single and two-dimensional sodium dodecyl sulfate-polyacrylamide gel electrophoresis. *J Clin Invest* **67**:1431, 1981.
112. Weiss HJ, Tschopp TB, Baumgartner HR, Sussman II, Johnson MM, Egan JJ: Decreased adhesion of giant (Bernard-Soulier) platelets to subendothelium. Further implications on the role of the von Willebrand factor in hemostasis. *Am J Med* **57**:920, 1974.
113. Sakariassen KS, Nievelstein PF, Coller BS, Sixma JJ: The role of platelet membrane glycoproteins Ib and IIb-IIIa in platelet adherence to human artery subendothelium. *Br J Haematol* **63**:681, 1986.
114. Caen JP, Nurden AT, Jeanneau C, Michel H, Tobelem G, Levy-Toledano S, Sultan Y, et al: Bernard-Soulier syndrome: A new platelet glycoprotein abnormality. Its relationship with platelet adhesion to subendothelium and with the factor VIII von Willebrand protein. *J Lab Clin Med* **87**:586, 1976.
115. Jenkins CSP, Phillips DR, Clemetson KJ, Meyer D, Larrieu MJ, Luscher EF: Platelet membrane glycoproteins implicated in ristocetin-induced aggregation. Studies of the proteins on platelets from patients with Bernard-Soulier syndrome and von Willebrand's disease. *J Clin Invest* **57**:112, 1976.
116. Macfarlane DE, Stibbe J, Kirby EP, Zucker MB, Grant RA, and McPherson J: A method for assaying von Willebrand factor (ristocetin cofactor). *Thromb Diath Haemorrh* **34**:306, 1975.
117. Allain JP, Cooper HA, Wagner RH, Brinkhous KM: Platelets fixed with paraformaldehyde: A new reagent for assay of von Willebrand factor and platelet-aggregating factor. *J Lab Clin Med* **85**:318, 1975.
118. Moake JL, Olson JD, Troll JH, Tang SS, Funicella T, Peterson DM: Binding of radioiodinated human von Willebrand factor to Bernard-Soulier, thrombasthenic and von Willebrand's disease platelets. *Thromb Res* **19**:21, 1980.
119. Coller BS, Peerschke EI, Scudder LE, Sullivan CA: Studies with a murine monoclonal antibody that abolishes ristocetin-induced binding of von Willebrand factor to platelets: Additional evidence in support of GPIb as a platelet receptor for von Willebrand factor. *Blood* **61**:99, 1983.
120. Ruggeri ZM, De Marco L, Gatti L, Bader R, Montgomery RR: Platelets have more than one binding site for von Willebrand factor. *J Clin Invest* **72**:1, 1983.
121. Marguerie GA, Plow EF, Edgington TS: Human platelets possess an inducible and saturable receptor specific for fibrinogen. *J Biol Chem* **254**:5357, 1979.
122. Coller BS, Peerschke EI, Scudder LE, Sullivan CA: A murine monoclonal antibody that completely blocks the binding of fibrinogen to platelets produces a thrombasthenic-like state in normal platelets and binds to glycoproteins IIb and/or IIIa. *J Clin Invest* **72**:325, 1983.

123. Bennett JS, Hoxie JA, Leitman SF, Vilaire G, Cines DB: Inhibition of fibrinogen binding to stimulated human platelets by a monoclonal antibody. *Proc Natl Acad Sci U S A* **80**:2417, 1983.
124. Plow EF, Ginsberg MH: Specific and saturable binding of plasma fibronectin to thrombin-stimulated human platelets. *J Biol Chem* **256**:9477, 1981.
125. Fujimoto T, Ohara S, Hawiger J: Thrombin-induced exposure and prostacyclin inhibition of the receptor for factor VIII/von Willebrand factor on human platelets. *J Clin Invest* **69**:1212, 1982.
126. Plow EF, Srouji AH, Meyer D, Marguerie G, Ginsberg MH: Evidence that three adhesive proteins interact with a common recognition site on activated platelets. *J Biol Chem* **259**:5388, 1984.
127. Kloczewiak M, Timmons S, Lukas TJ, Hawiger J: Platelet receptor recognition site on human fibrinogen. Synthesis and structure-function relationship of peptides corresponding to the carboxy-terminal segment of the γ chain. *Biochemistry* **23**:1767, 1984.
128. Ruggeri ZM, Bader R, De Marco L: Glanzmann thrombasthenia: Deficient binding of von Willebrand factor to thrombin-stimulated platelets. *Proc Natl Acad Sci U S A* **79**:6038, 1982.
129. Kao K-J, Pizzo SV, McKee PA: Demonstration and characterization of specific binding sites for factor VIII/von Willebrand factor on human platelets. *J Clin Invest* **63**:656, 1979.
130. Cooper HA, Reisner FF, Hall M, Wagner RH: Effects of thrombin treatment of preparations of factor VIII and the Ca^{2+}-dissociated small active fragment. *J Clin Invest* **56**:751, 1975.
131. Hamer RJ, Koedam JA, Beeser-Visser NH, Bertina RM, Van Mourik JA, Sixma JJ: Factor VIII binds to von Willebrand factor via its M_r-80,000 light chain. *Eur J Biochem* **166**:37, 1987.
132. Fowler WE, Fretto LJ, Hamilton KK, Erickson HP, McKee PA: Substructure of human von Willebrand factor. *J Clin Invest* **76**:1491, 1985.
133. Roberts DD, Williams SB, Gralnick HR, Ginsburg V: von Willebrand factor binds specifically to sulfated glycolipids. *J Biol Chem* **261**:3306, 1986.
134. Christophe O, Obert B, Meyer D, Girma JP: The binding domain of von Willebrand factor to sulfatides is distinct from those interacting with glycoprotein Ib, heparin, and collagen and resides between amino acid residues Leu 512 and Lys 673. *Blood* **78**:2310, 1991.
135. Martin SE, Marder VJ, Francis CW, Barlow GH: Structural studies of the functional heterogeneity of von Willebrand protein polymers. *Blood* **57**:313, 1981.
136. Aihara M, Kimura A, Chiba Y, Yoshida Y: Plasma collagen cofactor correlates with von Willebrand factor antigen and ristocetin cofactor but not with bleeding time. *Thromb Haemost* **59**:485, 1988.
137. Sixma JJ, Sakariassen KS, Beeser-Visser NH, Ottenhof-Rovers M, and Bolhuis PA: Adhesion of platelets to human artery subendothelium: Effect of factor VIII-von Willebrand factor of various multimeric composition. *Blood* **63**:128, 1984.
138. Fujimura Y, Titani K, Holland LZ, Russell SR, Roberts JR, Elder JH, Ruggeri ZM, et al: von Willebrand factor. A reduced and alkylated 52/48-kDa fragment beginning at amino acid residue 449 contains the domain interacting with platelet glycoprotein Ib. *J Biol Chem* **261**:381, 1986.
139. Andrews RK, Gorman JJ, Booth WJ, Corino GL, Castaldi PA, Berndt MC: Cross-linking of a monomeric 39/34-kDa dispase fragment of von Willebrand factor (Leu-480/Val-481-Gly-718) to the N-terminal region of the alpha-chain of membrane glycoprotein Ib on intact platelets with bis(sulfosuccinimidyl) suberate. *Biochemistry* **28**:8326, 1989.
140. Fujimura Y, Titani K, Holland LZ, Roberts JR, Kostel P, Ruggeri ZM, Zimmerman TS: A heparin-binding domain of human von Willebrand factor. Characterization and localization to a tryptic fragment extending from amino acid residue Val-449 to Lys-728. *J Biol Chem* **262**:1734, 1987.
141. Roth GJ, Titani K, Hoyer LW, Hickey MJ: Localization of binding sites within human von Willebrand factor for monomeric type III collagen. *Biochemistry* **25**:8357, 1986.
142. Pareti FI, Niiya K, McPherson JM, Ruggeri ZM: Isolation and characterization of two domains of human von Willebrand factor that interact with fibrillar collagen types I and III. *J Biol Chem* **262**:13835, 1987.
143. Kalafatis M, Takahashi Y, Girma JP, Meyer D: Localization of a collagen-interactive domain of human von Willebrand factor between amino acid residues Gly 911 and Glu 1,365. *Blood* **70**:1577, 1987.
144. Lankhof H, van Hoeij M, Schiphorst ME, Bracke M, Wu YP, Ijsseldijk MJ, Vink T, et al: A3 domain is essential for interaction of von Willebrand factor with collagen type III. *Thromb Haemost* **75**:950, 1996.
145. Matsushita T, Sadler JE: Identification of amino acid residues essential for von Willebrand factor binding to platelet glycoprotein Ib. Charged-to-alanine scanning mutagenesis of the A1 domain of human von Willebrand factor. *J Biol Chem* **270**:13406, 1995.
146. Kroner PA, Frey AB: Analysis of the structure and function of the von Willebrand factor A1 domain using targeted deletions and alanine-scanning mutagenesis. *Biochemistry* **35**:13460, 1996.
147. Huizinga EG, van der Plas RM, Kroon J, Sixma JJ, Gros P: Crystal structure of the A3 domain of human von Willebrand factor: Implications for collagen binding. *Structure* **5**:1147, 1997.
148. Bienkowska J, Cruz M, Atiemo A, Handin R, Liddington R: The von Willebrand factor A3 domain does not contain a metal ion-dependent adhesion site motif. *J Biol Chem* **272**:25162, 1997.
149. Celikel R, Varughese KI, Madhusudan, Yoshioka A, Ware J, Ruggeri ZM: Crystal structure of the von Willebrand factor A1 domain in complex with the function blocking NMC-4 Fab. *Nat Struct Biol* **5**:189, 1998.
150. Emsley J, Cruz M, Handin R, Liddington R: Crystal structure of the von Willebrand Factor A1 domain and implications for the binding of platelet glycoprotein Ib. *J Biol Chem* **273**:10396, 1998.
151. Foster PA, Fulcher CA, Marti T, Titani K, Zimmerman TS: A major factor VIII binding domain resides within the amino-terminal 272 amino acid residues of von Willebrand factor. *J Biol Chem* **262**:8443, 1987.
152. Fretto LJ, Fowler WE, McCaslin DR, Erickson HP, McKee PA: Substructure of human von Willebrand factor. Proteolysis by V8 and characterization of two functional domains. *J Biol Chem* **261**:15679, 1986.
153. Plow EF, Pierschbacher MD, Ruoslahti E, Marguerie GA, Ginsberg MH: The effect of Arg-Gly-Asp-containing peptides on fibrinogen and von Willebrand factor binding to platelets. *Proc Natl Acad Sci U S A* **82**:8057, 1985.
154. Berliner S, Niiya K, Roberts JR, Houghten RA, Ruggeri ZM: Generation and characterization of peptide-specific antibodies that inhibit von Willebrand factor binding to glycoprotein IIb-IIIa without interacting with other adhesive molecules. Selectivity is conferred by Pro1743 and other amino acid residues adjacent to the sequence Arg1744-Gly1745-Asp1746. *J Biol Chem* **263**:7500, 1988.
155. Beacham DA, Wise RJ, Turci SM, Handin RI: Selective inactivation of the Arg-Gly-Asp-Ser (RGDS) binding site in von Willebrand factor by site-directed mutagenesis. *J Biol Chem* **267**:3409, 1992.
156. Ruoslahti E: RGD and other recognition sequences for integrins. *Annu Rev Cell Dev Biol* **12**:697, 1996.
157. Federici AB, Elder JH, De Marco L, Ruggeri ZM, Zimmerman TS: Carbohydrate moiety of von Willebrand factor is not necessary for maintaining multimeric structure and ristocetin cofactor activity but protects from proteolytic degradation. *J Clin Invest* **74**:2049, 1984.
158. Sodetz JM, Pizzo SV, McKee PA: Relationship of sialic acid to function and in vivo survival of human factor VIII/von Willebrand factor protein. *J Biol Chem* **252**:5538, 1977.
159. Collins CJ, Underdahl JP, Levene RB, Ravera CP, Morin MJ, Dombalagian MJ, Ricca G, et al: Molecular cloning of the human gene for von Willebrand factor and identification of the transcription initiation site. *Proc Natl Acad Sci U S A* **84**:4393, 1987.
160. Mancuso DJ, Tuley EA, Westfield LA, Worrall NK, Shelton-Inloes BB, Sorace JM, Alevy YG, et al: Structure of the gene for human von Willebrand factor. *J Biol Chem* **264**:19514, 1989.
161. O'Connell P, Lathrop GM, Law M, Leppert M, Nakamura Y, Hoff M, Kumlin E, et al: A primary genetic linkage map for human chromosome 12. *Genomics* **1**:93, 1987.
162. Shelton-Inloes BB, Chehab FF, Mannucci PM, Federici AB, Sadler JE: Gene deletions correlate with the development of alloantibodies in von Willebrand disease. *J Clin Invest* **79**:1459, 1987.
163. Patracchini P, Calzolari E, Aiello V, Palazzi P, Banin P, Marchetti G, Bernardi F: Sublocalization of von Willebrand factor pseudogene to 22q11.22-q11.23 by in situ hybridization in a 46,X,t(X;22)(pter;q11.21) translocation. *Hum Genet* **83**:264, 1989.
164. Mancuso DJ, Tuley EA, Westfield LA, Lester-Mancuso TL, Le Beau MM, Sorace JM, Sadler JE: Human von Willebrand factor gene and pseudogene: Structural analysis and differentiation by polymerase chain reaction. *Biochemistry* **30**:253, 1991.
165. Desseyn J-L, Aubert JP, Van Seuningen I, Porchet N, Laine A: Genomic organization of the 3′ region of the human mucin gene *MUC5B*. *J Biol Chem* **272**:16873, 1997.
166. Toribara NW, Ho SB, Gum E, Gum JR Jr, Lau P, Kim YS: The carboxyl-terminal sequence of the human secretory mucin, MUC6.

Analysis of the primary amino acid sequence. *J Biol Chem* **272**:16398, 1997.
167. Meitinger T, Meindl A, Bork P, Rost B, Sander C, Haasemann M, Murken J: Molecular modelling of the Norrie disease protein predicts a cystine knot growth factor tertiary structure. *Nat Genet* **5**:376, 1993.
168. McDonald NQ, Hendrickson WA: A structural superfamily of growth factors containing a cystine knot motif. *Cell* **73**:421, 1993.
169. Silwer J: von Willebrand's disease in Sweden. *Acta Paediatr Scand* **238**(Suppl):1, 1973.
170. Bloom AL, Peake IR: Apparent "dominant" and "recessive" inheritance of von Willebrand's disease within the same kindreds. Possible biochemical mechanisms. *Thromb Res* **15**:505, 1979.
171. Miller CH, Graham JB, Goldin LR, Elston RC: Genetics of classic von Willebrand's disease. I. Phenotypic variation within families. *Blood* **54**:117, 1979.
172. Hoyer LW: The assessment of von Willebrand's disease, in Bloom AL (ed): *The Hemophilias*. Edinburgh, Churchill Livingstone, 1982, p 106.
173. Zimmerman TS, Roberts JR, Ruggeri ZM: Factor VIII-related antigen: Characterization by electrophoretic techniques, in Bloom AL (ed): *The Hemophilias*. Edinburgh, Churchill Livingstone, 1982, p 81.
174. Read MS, Shermer RW, Brinkhous KM: Venom coagglutinin: An activator of platelet aggregation dependent on von Willebrand factor. *Proc Natl Acad Sci U S A* **75**:4514, 1978.
175. Brinkhous KM, Read MS: Use of venom coagglutinin and lyophilized platelets in testing for platelet-aggregating von Willebrand factor. *Blood* **55**:517, 1980.
176. Weiss HJ, Piétu G, Rabinowitz R, Girma JP, Rogers J, Meyer D: Heterogeneous abnormalities in the multimeric structure, antigenic properties, and plasma-platelet content of factor VIII/von Willebrand factor in subtypes of classic (type I) and variant (type IIA) von Willebrand's disease. *J Lab Clin Med* **101**:411, 1983.
177. Mannucci PM, Lombardi R, Bader R, Vianello L, Federici AB, Solinas S, Mazzucconi MG, et al: Heterogeneity of type I von Willebrand disease: Evidence for a subgroup with an abnormal von Willebrand factor. *Blood* **66**:796, 1985.
178. Hanna WT, Slywka J, Dent J, Ruggeri ZM, Zimmerman TS: 1-Deamino-8-D-arginine vasopressin and cryoprecipitate in variant von Willebrand disease. *Am J Hematol* **20**:169, 1985.
179. Gralnick HR, Williams SB, McKeown LP, Rick ME, Maisonneuve P, Jenneau C, Sultan Y: DDAVP in type IIA von Willebrand's disease. *Blood* **67**:465, 1986.
180. Holmberg L, Nilsson IM: von Willebrand's disease. *Eur J Haematol* **48**:127, 1992.
181. Mannucci PM, Bloom AL, Larrieu MJ, Nilsson IM, West RR: Atherosclerosis and von Willebrand factor. I. Prevalence of severe von Willebrand's disease in Western Europe and Israel. *Br J Haematol* **57**:163, 1984.
182. Berliner SA, Seligsohn U, Zivelin A, Zwang E, Sofferman G: A relatively high frequency of severe (type III) von Willebrand's disease in Israel. *Br J Haematol* **62**:535, 1986.
183. Sadler JE: A revised classification of von Willebrand disease. *Thromb Haemost* **71**:520, 1994.
184. Ginsburg D, Sadler JE: von Willebrand disease: A database of point mutations, insertions, and deletions. *Thromb Haemost* **69**:177, 1993.
185. Ruggeri ZM: Structure and function of von Willebrand factor: Relationship to von Willebrand's disease. *Mayo Clin Proc* **66**:847, 1991.
186. Lopez-Fernandez MF, Gonzalez-Boullosa R, Blanco-Lopez MJ, Perez M, Batlle J: Abnormal proteolytic degradation of von Willebrand factor after desmopressin infusion in a new subtype of von Willebrand disease (ID). *Am J Hematol* **36**:163, 1991.
187. Castaman G, Rodeghiero F, Lattuada A, Mannucci PM: A new variant of von Willebrand disease (type II-I) with a normal degree of proteolytic cleavage of von Willebrand factor. *Thromb Res* **65**:343, 1992.
188. Hoyer LW, Rizza CR, Tuddenham EG, Carta CA, Armitage H, Rotblat F: Von Willebrand factor multimer patterns in von Willebrand's disease. *Br J Haematol* **55**:493, 1983.
189. Zhang ZP, Lindstedt M, Falk G, Blombäck M, Egberg N, Anvret M: Nonsense mutations of the von Willebrand factor gene in patients with von Willebrand disease type III and type I. *Am J Hum Genet* **51**:850, 1992.
190. Zhang ZP, Blombäck M, Egberg N, Falk G, Anvret M: Characterization of the von Willebrand factor gene (VWF) in von Willebrand disease type III patients from 24 families of Swedish and Finnish origin. *Genomics* **21**:188, 1994.
191. Schneppenheim R, Krey S, Bergmann F, Bock D, Budde U, Lange M, Linde R, et al: Genetic heterogeneity of severe von Willebrand disease type III in the German population. *Hum Genet* **94**:640, 1994.
192. Eikenboom JCJ, Matsushita T, Reitsma PH, Tuley EA, Castaman G, Briët E, Sadler JE: Dominant type 1 von Willebrand disease caused by mutated cysteine residues in the D3 domain of von Willebrand factor. *Blood* **88**:2433, 1996.
193. Gralnick HR, Williams SB, McKeown LP, Maisonneuve P, Jenneau C, Sultan Y, Rick ME: In vitro correction of the abnormal multimeric structure of von Willebrand factor in type IIA von Willebrand's disease. *Proc Natl Acad Sci U S A* **82**:5968, 1985.
194. Batlle J, Lopez Fernandez MF, Campos M, Justica B, Berges C, Navarro JL, Diaz Cremades JM, et al: The heterogeneity of type IIA von Willebrand's disease: Studies with protease inhibitors. *Blood* **68**:1207, 1986.
195. Ruggeri ZM, Mannucci PM, Lombardi R, Federici AB, Zimmerman TS: Multimeric composition of factor VIII/von Willebrand factor following administration of DDAVP: Implications for pathophysiology and therapy of von Willebrand's disease subtypes. *Blood* **59**:1272, 1982.
196. Lyons SE, Bruck ME, Bowie EJW, Ginsburg D: Impaired intracellular transport produced by a subset of type IIA von Willebrand disease mutations. *J Biol Chem* **267**:4424, 1992.
197. Dent JA, Berkowitz SD, Ware J, Kasper CK, Ruggeri ZM: Identification of a cleavage site directing the immunochemical detection of molecular abnormalities in type IIA von Willebrand factor. *Proc Natl Acad Sci U S A* **87**:6306, 1990.
198. Furlan M, Robles R, Lämmle B: Partial purification and characterization of a protease from human plasma cleaving von Willebrand factor to fragments produced by in vivo proteolysis. *Blood* **87**:4223, 1996.
199. Tsai H-M: Physiologic cleavage of von Willebrand factor by a plasma protease is dependent on its conformation and requires calcium ion. *Blood* **87**:4235, 1996.
200. Ruggeri ZM, Nilsson IM, Lombardi R, Holmberg L, Zimmerman TS: Aberrant multimeric structure of von Willebrand factor in a new variant of von Willebrand's disease (type IIC). *J Clin Invest* **70**:1124, 1982.
201. Mannucci PM, Lombardi R, Pareti FI, Solinas S, Mazzucconi MG, Mariani G: A variant of von Willebrand's disease characterized by recessive inheritance and missing triplet structure of von Willebrand factor multimers. *Blood* **62**:1000, 1983.
202. Batlle J, Lopez Fernandez MF, Lasierra J, Fernandez Villamor A, Lopez Berges C, Lopez Borrasca A, Ruggeri ZM, et al: von Willebrand disease type IIC with different abnormalities of von Willebrand factor in the same sibship. *Am J Hematol* **21**:177, 1986.
203. Mazurier C, Mannucci PM, Parquet-Gernez A, Goudemand M, Meyer D: Investigation of a case of subtype IIC von Willebrand disease: Characterization of the variability of this subtype. *Am J Hematol* **22**:301, 1986.
204. Batlle J, Lopez Fernandez MF, Fernandez Villamor A, Lopez Berges C, Zimmerman TS: Multimeric pattern discrepancy between platelet and plasma von Willebrand factor in type IIC von Willebrand disease. *Am J Hematol* **22**:87, 1986.
205. Gaucher C, Diéval J, Mazurier C: Characterization of von Willebrand factor gene defects in two unrelated patients with type IIC von Willebrand disease. *Blood* **84**:1024, 1994.
206. Kinoshita S, Harrison J, Lazerson J, Abildgaard CF: A new variant of dominant type II von Willebrand's disease with aberrant multimeric pattern of factor VIII-related antigen (type IID). *Blood* **63**:1369, 1984.
207. Hill FG, Enayat MS, George AJ: Investigation of a kindred with a new autosomal dominantly inherited variant type von Willebrand's disease (possible type IID). *J Clin Pathol* **38**:665, 1985.
208. Schneppenheim R, Brassard J, Krey S, Budde U, Kunicki TJ, Holmberg L, Ware J, et al: Defective dimerization of von Willebrand factor subunits due to a Cys Ø Arg mutation in type IID von Willebrand disease. *Proc Natl Acad Sci U S A* **93**:3581, 1996.
209. Mannucci PM, Lombardi R, Federici AB, Dent JA, Zimmerman TS, Ruggeri ZM: A new variant of type II von Willebrand disease with aberrant multimeric structure of plasma but not platelet von Willebrand factor (type IIF). *Blood* **68**:269, 1986.
210. Gralnick HR, Williams SB, McKeown LP, Maisonneuve P, Jenneau C, Sultan Y: A variant of type II von Willebrand disease with an abnormal triplet structure and discordant effects of protease inhibitors on plasma and platelet von Willebrand factor structure. *Am J Hematol* **24**:259, 1987.
211. Federici AB, Mannucci PM, Lombardi R, Lattuada A, Colibretti ML, Dent JA, Zimmerman TS: Type II H von Willebrand disease: New

structural abnormality of plasma and platelet von Willebrand factor in a patient with prolonged bleeding time and borderline levels of ristocetin cofactor activity. *Am J Hematol* **32**:287, 1989.
212. Ruggeri ZM, Pareti FI, Mannucci PM, Ciavarella N, Zimmerman TS: Heightened interaction between platelets and factor VIII/von Willebrand factor in a new subtype of von Willebrand's disease. *N Engl J Med* **302**:1047, 1980.
213. Holmberg L, Nilsson IM, Borge L, Gunnarsson M, Sjorin E: Platelet aggregation induced by 1-desamino-8-D-arginine vasopressin (DDAVP) in Type IIB von Willebrand's disease. *N Engl J Med* **309**:816, 1983.
214. Saba HI, Saba SR, Dent J, Ruggeri ZM, Zimmerman TS: Type IIB Tampa: A variant of von Willebrand disease with chronic thrombocytopenia, circulating platelet aggregates, and spontaneous platelet aggregation. *Blood* **66**:282, 1985.
215. Gralnick HR, Williams SB, McKeown LP, Rick ME, Maisonneuve P, Jenneau C, Sultan Y: Von Willebrand's disease with spontaneous platelet aggregation induced by an abnormal plasma von Willebrand factor. *J Clin Invest* **76**:1522, 1985.
216. Federici AB, Mannucci PM, Bader R, Lombardi R, Lattuada A: Heterogeneity in type IIB von Willebrand disease: Two unrelated cases with no family history and mild abnormalities of ristocetin-induced interaction between von Willebrand factor and platelets. *Am J Hematol* **23**:381, 1986.
217. Donnér M, Holmberg L, Nilsson IM: Type IIB von Willebrand's disease with probable autosomal recessive inheritance and presenting as thrombocytopenia in infancy. *Br J Haematol* **66**:349, 1987.
218. Holmberg L, Berntorp E, Donnér M, Nilsson IM: von Willebrand's disease characterized by increased ristocetin sensitivity and the presence of all von Willebrand factor multimers in plasma. *Blood* **68**:668, 1986.
219. Weiss HJ, Sussman II: A new von Willebrand variant (type I, New York): Increased ristocetin-induced platelet aggregation and plasma von Willebrand factor containing the full range of multimers. *Blood* **68**:149, 1986.
220. Ciavarella G, Ciavarella N, Antoncecchi S, De Mattia D, Ranieri P, Dent J, Zimmerman TS, et al: High-resolution analysis of von Willebrand factor multimeric composition defines a new variant of type I von Willebrand disease with aberrant structure but presence of all size multimers (type IC). *Blood* **66**:1423, 1985.
221. Tavori S, Tatarsky I: Additional variant of type I von Willebrand disease. *Am J Hematol* **24**:189, 1987.
222. Montgomery RR, Dent J, Schmidt W, Kyrle P, Hiessner H, Ruggeri ZM, Zimmerman TS: Hereditary persistence of circulating pro von Willebrand factor (pro-vWF). *Circulation* 74(Suppl II): 406, 1986.
223. Mannucci PM, Lombardi R, Castaman G, Dent JA, Lattuada A, Rodeghiero F, Zimmerman TS: von Willebrand disease "Vicenza" with larger-than-normal (supranormal) von Willebrand factor multimers. *Blood* **71**:65, 1988.
224. Mancuso DJ, Kroner PA, Christopherson PA, Vokac EA, Gill JC, Montgomery RR: Type 2M:Milwaukee-1 von Willebrand disease: An in-frame deletion in the Cys509-Cys695 loop of the von Willebrand factor A1 domain causes deficient binding of von Willebrand factor to platelets. *Blood* **88**:2559, 1996.
225. Hillery CA, Mancuso DJ, Sadler JE, Ponder JW, Jozwiak MA, Christopherson PA, Gill JC, et al: Type 2M von Willebrand disease: F606I and I662F mutations in the glycoprotein Ib binding domain selectively impair ristocetin- but not botrocetin-mediated binding of von Willebrand factor to platelets. *Blood* **91**:1572, 1998.
226. Rabinowitz I, Tuley EA, Mancuso DJ, Randi AM, Firkin BG, Howard MA, Sadler JE: von Willebrand disease type B: A missense mutation selectively abolishes ristocetin-induced von Willebrand factor binding to platelet glycoprotein Ib. *Proc Natl Acad Sci U S A* **89**:9846, 1992.
227. Nishino M, Girma J-P, Rothschild C, Fressinaud E, Meyer D: New variant of von Willebrand disease with defective binding to factor VIII. *Blood* **74**:1591, 1989.
228. Mazurier C, Dieval J, Jorieux S, Delobel J, Goudemand M: A new von Willebrand factor (vWF) defect in a patient with factor VIII (FVIII) deficiency but with normal levels and multimeric patterns of both plasma and platelet vWF. Characterization of abnormal vWF/FVIII interaction. *Blood* **75**:20, 1990.
229. Mazurier C, Gaucher C, Jorieux S, Parquet GA, Goudemand M: Evidence for a von Willebrand factor defect in factor VIII binding in three members of a family previously misdiagnosed mild haemophilia A and haemophilia A carriers: Consequences for therapy and genetic counselling. *Br J Haematol* **76**:372, 1990.
230. Schneppenheim R, Budde U, Krey S, Drewke E, Bergmann F, Lechler E, Oldenburg J, et al: Results of a screening for von Willebrand disease type 2N in patients with suspected haemophilia A or von Willebrand disease type 1. *Thromb Haemost* **76**:598, 1996.
231. Eikenboom JC, Reitsma PH, Peerlinck KMJ, Briët E: Recessive inheritance of von Willebrand's disease type I. *Lancet* **341**:982, 1993.
232. Italian Working Group: Spectrum of von Willebrand's disease: A study of 100 cases. *Br J Haematol* **35**:101, 1977.
233. Zimmerman TS, Abildgaard CF, Meyer D: The factor VIII abnormality in severe von Willebrand's disease. *N Engl J Med* **301**:1307, 1979.
234. Zhang ZP, Blömback M, Nyman D, Anvret M: Mutations of von Willebrand factor gene in families with von Willebrand disease in the Aland Islands. *Proc Natl Acad Sci U S A* **90**:7937, 1993.
235. Giannelli F, Choo KH, Rees DJ, Boyd Y, Rizza CR, Brownlee GG: Gene deletions in patients with haemophilia B and anti-factor IX antibodies. *Nature* **303**:181, 1983.
236. Straus HD, Diamond LK: Elevation of factor VIII (antihemophilic factor) during pregnancy in normal persons and in a patient with von Willebrand's disease. *N Engl J Med* **269**:1251, 1963.
237. Noller KL, Bowie EJ, Kempers RD, Owen CA Jr: Von Willebrand's disease in pregnancy. *Obstet Gynecol* **41**:865, 1973.
238. Bennett G, Oxnard SC, Douglas AS, Ratnoff OD: Studies on antihemophilic factor (AHF, factor VIII) during labor in normal women, in patients with premature separation of the placenta, and in a patient with von Willebrand's disease. *J Lab Clin Med* **84**:851, 1974.
239. Telfer MC, Chediak J: Factor-VIII-related disorders and their relationship to pregnancy. *J Reprod Med* **19**:211, 1977.
240. Rick ME, Williams SB, Sacher RA, McKeown LP: Thrombocytopenia associated with pregnancy in a patient with type IIB von Willebrand's disease. *Blood* **69**:786, 1987.
241. Mannucci PM, Mari D: Antibodies to factor VIII-von Willebrand factor in congenital and acquired von Willebrand's disease, in Hoyer LW (ed): *Factor VIII Inhibitors*. New York, Alan R. Liss, 1984, p 109.
242. Kaneshiro MM, Mielke CH Jr, Kasper CK, Rapaport SI: Bleeding time after aspirin in disorders of intrinsic clotting. *N Engl J Med* **281**:1039, 1969.
243. Giles AR, Hoogendoorn H, Benford K: Type IIB von Willebrand's disease presenting as thrombocytopenia during pregnancy. *Br J Haematol* **67**:349, 1987.
244. Valster FAA, Feijen HL, Hutten JW: Severe thrombocytopenia in a pregnant patient with platelet-associated IgM, and known von Willebrand's disease: A case report. *Eur J Obstet Gynecol Reprod Biol* **36**:197, 1990.
245. Ieko M, Sakurama S, Sagawa A, Yoshikawa M, Satoh M, Yasukouchi T, Nakagawa S: Effect of a factor VIII concentrate on type IIB von Willebrand's disease-associated thrombocytopenia presenting during pregnancy in identical twin mothers. *Am J Hematol* **35**:26, 1990.
246. Sakariassen KS, Nieuwenhuis HK, Sixma JJ: Differentiation of patients with subtype IIb-like von Willebrand's disease by means of perfusion experiments with reconstituted blood. *Br J Haematol* **59**: 459, 1985.
247. Hultin MB, Sussman II: Postoperative thrombocytopenia in type IIB von Willebrand disease. *Am J Hematol* **33**:64, 1990.
248. Takahashi H: Studies on the pathophysiology and treatment of von Willebrand's disease. IV. Mechanism of increased ristocetin-induced platelet aggregation in von Willebrand's disease. *Thromb Res* **19**:857, 1980.
249. Miller JL, Castella A: Platelet-type von Willebrand's disease: Characterization of a new bleeding disorder. *Blood* **60**:790, 1982.
250. Weiss HJ, Meyer D, Rabinowitz R, Pietu G, Girma JP, Vicic WJ, Rogers J: Pseudo-von Willebrand's disease. An intrinsic platelet defect with aggregation by unmodified human factor VIII/von Willebrand factor and enhanced adsorption of its high-molecular-weight multimers. *N Engl J Med* **306**:326, 1982.
251. Takahashi H, Nagayama R, Hattori A, Shibata A: Platelet aggregation induced by DDAVP in platelet-type von Willebrand's disease. *N Engl J Med* **310**:722, 1984.
252. Miller JL, Kupinski JM, Castella A, Ruggeri ZM: von Willebrand factor binds to platelets and induces aggregation in platelet-type but not type IIB von Willebrand disease. *J Clin Invest* **72**:1532, 1983.
253. Miller JL, Cunningham D, Lyle VA, Finch CN: Mutation in the gene encoding the α chain of platelet glycoprotein Ib in platelet-type von Willebrand disease. *Proc Natl Acad Sci U S A* **88**:4761, 1991.
254. Russell SD, Roth GJ: Pseudo-von Willebrand disease: A mutation in the platelet glycoprotein Ib alpha gene associated with a hyperactive surface receptor. *Blood* **81**:1787, 1993.

255. Rodeghiero F, Castaman G, Meyer D, Mannucci PM: Replacement therapy with virus-inactivated plasma concentrates in von Willebrand disease. *Vox Sang* **62**:193, 1992.
256. Berntorp E: Plasma product treatment in various types of von Willebrand's disease. *Haemostasis* **24**:289, 1994.
257. Scharrer I, Vigh T, Aygoren-Pursun E: Experience with haemate P in von Willebrand's disease in adults. *Haemostasis* **24**:298, 1994.
258. Goudemand J, Mazurier C, Marey A, Caron C, Coupez B, Mizon P, Goudemand M: Clinical and biological evaluation in von Willebrand's disease of a von Willebrand factor concentrate with low factor VIII activity. *Br J Haematol* **80**:214, 1992.
259. Meriane F, Zerhouni L, Djeha N, Goudemand M, Mazurier C: Biological effects of a S/D-treated, very high purity, von Willebrand factor concentrate in five patients with severe von Willebrand disease. *Blood Coag Fibrinol* **4**:1023, 1993.
260. Smith MP, Rice KM, Bromidge ES, Lawn M, Beresford-Webb R, Spence K, Khair K, et al: Continuous infusion therapy with very high purity von Willebrand factor concentrate in patients with severe von Willebrand disease. *Blood Coag Fibrinol* **8**:6, 1997.
261. Turecek PL, Gritsch H, Pichler L, Auer W, Fischer B, Mitterer A, Mundt W, et al: In vivo characterization of recombinant von Willebrand factor in dogs with von Willebrand disease. *Blood* **90**:3555, 1997.
262. Morfini M, Mannucci PM, Tenconi PM, Longo G, Mazzucconi MG, Rodeghiero F, Ciavarella N, et al: Pharmacokinetics of monoclonally-purified and recombinant factor VIII in patients with severe von Willebrand disease. *Thromb Haemost* **70**:270, 1993.
263. Castillo R, Monteagudo J, Escolar G, Ordinas A, Magallon M, Martin Villar J: Hemostatic effect of normal platelet transfusion in severe von Willebrand disease patients. *Blood* **77**:1901, 1991.
264. Mannucci PM: Platelet von Willebrand factor in inherited and acquired bleeding disorders. *Proc Natl Acad Sci U S A* **92**:2428, 1995.
265. Castillo R, Escolar G, Monteagudo J, Aznar-Salatti J, Reverter JC, Ordinas A: Hemostasis in patients with severe von Willebrand disease improves after normal platelet transfusion and normalizes with further correction of the plasma defect. *Transfusion* **37**:785, 1997.
266. Mannucci PM, Ruggeri ZM, Pareti FI, Capitanio A: 1-Deamino-8-D-arginine vasopressin: A new pharmacological approach to the management of haemophilia and von Willebrands' diseases. *Lancet* **1**:869, 1977.
267. Mannucci PM: Desmopressin (DDAVP) in the treatment of bleeding disorders: The first 20 years. *Blood* **90**:2515, 1997.
268. Mannucci PM, Bettega D, Cattaneo M: Patterns of development of tachyphylaxis in patients with haemophilia and von Willebrand disease after repeated doses of desmopressin (DDAVP). *Br J Haematol* **82**:87, 1992.
269. Rodeghiero F, Castaman G, Di Bona E, Ruggeri M: Consistency of responses to repeated DDAVP infusions in patients with von Willebrand's disease and hemophilia A. *Blood* **74**:1997, 1989.
270. Rodeghiero F, Castaman G, Mannucci PM: Clinical indications for desmopressin (DDAVP) in congenital and acquired von Willebrand disease. *Blood Rev* **5**:155, 1991.
271. de la Fuente B, Kasper CK, Rickles FR, Hoyer LW: Response of patients with mild and moderate hemophilia A and von Willebrand's disease to treatment with desmopressin. *Ann Int Med* **103**:6, 1985.
272. Lopez-Fernandez MF, Blanco-Lopez MJ, Castiñeira MP, Batlle J: Further evidence for recessive inheritance of von Willebrand disease with abnormal binding of von Willebrand factor to factor VIII. *Am J Hematol* **40**:20, 1992.
273. Mazurier C, Gaucher C, Jorieux S, Goudemand M, and the Collaborative Group: Biological effect of desmopressin in eight patients with type 2N ("Normandy") von Willebrand disease. *Br J Haematol* **88**:849, 1994.
274. Ruggeri ZM, Lombardi R, Gatti L, Bader R, Valsecchi C, and Zimmerman TS: Type IIB von Willebrand's disease: Differential clearance of endogenous versus transfused large multimer von Willebrand factor. *Blood* **60**:1453, 1982.
275. Kyrle PA, Niessner H, Dent J, Panzer S, Brenner B, Zimmerman TS, Lechner K: IIB von Willebrand's disease: Pathogenetic and therapeutic studies. *Br J Haematol* **69**:55, 1988.
276. Fowler WE, Berkowitz LR, Roberts HR: DDAVP for type IIB von Willebrand disease. *Blood* **74**:1859, 1989.
277. Casonato A, Pontara E, Dannhaeuser D, Bertomoro A, Sartori MT, Zerbinati P, Girolami A: Re-evaluation of the therapeutic efficacy of DDAVP in type IIB von Willebrand's disease. *Blood Coag Fibrinol* **5**:959, 1994.
278. McKeown LP, Connaghan G, Wilson O, Hansmann K, Merryman P, Gralnick HR: 1-Desamino-8-arginine-vasopressin corrects the hemostatic defects in type 2B von Willebrand's disease. *Am J Hematol* **51**:158, 1996.
279. Mauz-Korholz C, Budde U, Kruck H, Korholz D, Gobel U: Management of severe chronic thrombocytopenia in von Willebrand's disease type 2B. *Arch Dis Child* **78**:257, 1998.
280. Hoyer LW, Lindsten J, Blomback M, Hagenfeldt L, Cordesius E, Stromberg P, Gustavii B: Prenatal evaluation of fetus at risk for severe von Willebrand's disease. *Lancet* **2**:191, 1979.
281. Mibashan RS, Millar DS: Fetal haemophilia and allied bleeding disorders. *Br Med Bull* **39**:392, 1983.
282. Montgomery RR, Marlar RA, Gill JC: Newborn haemostasis. *Clin Haematol* **14**:443, 1985.
283. Sadler JE, Ginsburg D: A database of polymorphisms in the von Willebrand factor gene and pseudogene. *Thromb Haemost* **69**:185, 1993.
284. Gaucher C, Mercier B, Mazurier C: von Willebrand disease family studies: Comparison of three methods of analysis of the von Willebrand factor gene polymorphism related to a variable number tandem repeat sequence in intron 40. *Br J Haematol* **82**:73, 1992.
285. Peake IR, Bowen D, Bignell P, Liddell MB, Sadler JE, Standen G, Bloom AL: Family studies and prenatal diagnosis in severe von Willebrand disease by polymerase chain reaction amplification of a variable number tandem repeat region of the von Willebrand factor gene. *Blood* **76**:555, 1990.
286. Bignell P, Standen GR, Bowen DJ, Peake IR, Bloom AL: Rapid neonatal diagnosis of von Willebrand's disease by use of the polymerase chain reaction. *Lancet* **336**:638, 1990.
287. Mannhalter C, Kyrle PA, Brenner B, Lechner K: Rapid neonatal diagnosis of type IIB von Willebrand disease using the polymerase chain reaction. *Blood* **77**:2539, 1991.
288. Sadler JE: von Willebrand factor. *J Biol Chem* **266**:22777, 1991.
289. Sadler JE: von Willebrand disease, in Bloom AL, Forbes CD, Thomas DP, Tuddenham EGD (eds): *Haemostasis and Thrombosis*, 3rd ed. Edinburgh, Churchill-Livingstone, 1994, p 843.

CHAPTER 175

Factor XI and the Contact System

David Gailani ▪ George J. Broze, Jr.

1. **Exposure of blood or plasma to negatively charged surfaces results in activation of the plasma proteins factor XII and prekallikrein (PK) by a process termed *contact activation*. These reactions require the cofactor high-molecular-weight-kininogen (HK). Contact activation triggers fibrinolysis, kinin formation, and blood coagulation through activation of factor XI.**
2. **The cDNAs for human factor XI, factor XII, PK, and HK have been cloned, and the amino acid sequences and domain structures of the proteins have been determined. Factor XI, factor XII, and PK are zymogens of serine proteases containing C-terminal trypsin-like catalytic domains and N-terminal domains that bind other macromolecules. Factor XI is a homodimer of 80-kDa polypeptides structurally similar to PK. Factor XI and PK circulate as noncovalent complexes with HK. HK is a multifunctional 110-kDa protein with domains for binding to cells, factor XI, PK, and negatively charged surfaces, and two domains that inhibit cysteine proteases. HK is a source of the potent vasodilatory nanopeptide bradykinin.**
3. **Genes for factor XI, factor XII, PK, and HK have been characterized and their chromosomal locations determined. Mutations causing hereditary deficiency states have been identified for each protein except PK. The genes, cDNAs, and amino acid sequence for factor XI and PK are very similar, which suggests that they are the products of a duplication event involving a common ancestral gene.**
4. **Deficiency of factor XI (mim 264900) results in excessive bleeding following trauma or surgery indicating that this protein is essential for normal coagulation. In contrast, deficiencies of factor XII (mim 234000), PK (mim 229000), HK (mim 228960) are not associated with clinical abnormalities. These observations suggest that factor XI is activated in vivo by processes other than contact activation.**
5. **Factor XI deficiency is common in Ashkenazi Jews, in whom the carrier frequency has been estimated to be 5 to 13 percent. Two distinct point mutations account for the majority of abnormal alleles in this group. The type II mutation results in early termination of the protein, while the type III mutation causes greatly reduced protein secretion from the liver.**
6. **While deficiencies of factor XII, PK, or HK are not associated with an abnormal phenotype, inappropriate activation of these proteins may contribute to pathologic processes in several clinical conditions such as sepsis, inflammation, and hereditary angioedema.**

INTRODUCTION

When blood is exposed to a variety of negatively charged surfaces, a series of reactions are initiated that activate the plasma proteins factor XII, prekallikrein (PK), and factor XI in the presence of the cofactor high-molecular-weight-kininogen (HK).[1–5] These processes, collectively referred to as contact activation reactions, trigger a number of plasma host-defense systems including blood coagulation,[6,7] fibrinolysis,[8] and the liberation of vasoactive kinins[9,10] (Fig. 175-1). Factor XII, PK, HK, and factor XI have now been purified from the plasma of several species including humans, the amino acid sequence and structural features of each protein have been determined, and detailed data concerning the protein-protein interactions in contact activation are available. The genes for these proteins have been cloned, and mutations causing hereditary deficiency states have been described. Despite these advances, the physiological role of contact activation remains unclear.

The four proteins involved in contact activation are required for normal blood coagulation in in vitro assays such as the activated partial thromboplastin time (aPTT).[11] Indeed, factor XII and factor XI were first recognized as plasma factors missing in patients with abnormal in vitro blood coagulation.[12–18] However, the clinical symptoms of patients deficient in components of this system are difficult to reconcile with the profoundly abnormal results of these tests. Factor XI is required for normal hemostasis, as patients lacking this protein have a bleeding diathesis that is characterized by excessive postoperative and trauma-induced hemorrhage.[19] In contrast, deficiencies of factor XII, PK, or HK are not associated with either abnormal bleeding or any clear-cut clinical abnormalities. While these observations demonstrate the importance of factor XI to normal hemostasis, they bring into question the physiological relevance of contact activation. It is possible that abnormalities associated with deficiency of factor XII, PK, or HK are subtle, or are compensated for by other proteins. Alternatively, these proteins may not be as important to human physiology as for other species. Plasmas of marine mammals of the order *cetacea* (whales and porpoises) do not undergo contact activation mediated coagulation due to a lack of factor XII activity, consistent with a variable requirement for contact activation between species.[20,21]

Recent clinical and biochemical data provide new insights into the roles of factor XI and the contact proteins in normal and pathologic conditions. Factor XI is no longer considered to be a component of a mechanism for initiating clot formation (contact activation) but, instead, is required to sustain coagulation after

A list of standard abbreviations is located immediately preceding the index in each volume. Additional abbreviations used in this chapter include: A1–A4 = apple domains of factor XI or prekallikrein; aPTT = activated partial thromboplastin time; AT III = antithrombin III; C1, C3 = complement factors 1, 3; C1–INH = C1-inhibitor; Clq = subcomponent of C1; D1–D6, D5L, D6H, etc. = domains of high and low molecular weight kininogen; α-factor XIIa = activated factor XII, 80-kDa form; β-factor XIIa = activated factor XII, 28-kDa form; FFP = fresh frozen plasma; gClqR = receptor for the globular "head" region of Clq; HAE = hereditary angioedema; HepG2 = hepatocyte cell line; HK = high molecular weight kininogen; HKa = kinin-free HK; LK = low molecular weight kininogen; PK = prekallikrein; PAI-1 = plasminogen activator inhibitor-1; proUK = prourokinase; TAFI = thrombin activatable fibrinolysis inhibitor; TF = tissue factor; TFPI = tissue factor pathway inhibitor; TNFα = tumor necrosis factor-α; tPA = tissue plasminogen activator; UK = urokinase.

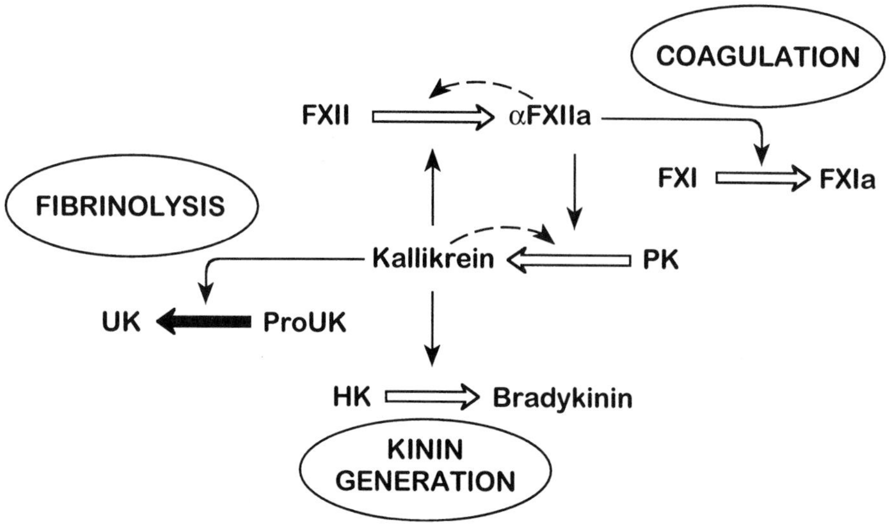

Fig. 175-1 Contact activation reactions. Large open arrows signify the conversion of a protease zymogen or uncleaved protein to the activated or cleaved form on a negatively charged surface; the large closed arrow indicates the activation of pro-urokinase in solution; small arrows designate the enzyme responsible for cleaving a protein; interrupted arrows signify autoactivation. Contact activation is initiated by the activation of factor XII (FXII) to factor XIIa (FXIIa) when plasma is exposed to a negatively charged surface. Reciprocal activation of prekallikrein (PK) by FXIIa, and FXII by kallikrein amplifies the process. FXIIa promotes coagulation through the activation of factor XI (FXI), while kallikrein cleaves high molecular weight kininogen to liberate bradykinin and activates the fibrinolytic system through the activation of the plasminogen activator pro-urokinase (pro-UK) to urokinase (UK).

initial fibrin formation to consolidate the clotting process.[22–25] Furthermore, alternative factor XII-independent reactions for the activation of factor XI have been described.[23,25] The key coagulation protease thrombin has been shown to activate factor XI in a number of experimental systems, possibly explaining the lack of bleeding seen in factor XII deficiency.[23,26] While an abnormal phenotype has yet to be assigned to deficiencies of factor XII, PK or HK, these proteins may play important roles in a number of pathologic processes.[5,27] In addition, a physiological replacement for the artificial surfaces required for contact activation, the surface of endothelial cells, has been identified.[28,29] This chapter discusses new biochemical and clinical data related to factor XI and the contact system, with an emphasis on factor XI and its deficiency state because of the clear physiological importance of this protein. The reader may wish to consult several excellent reviews for further information.[1–5,30]

Contact Activation

Contact activation in plasma is initiated when factor XII binds to and is activated on a negatively charged surface by limited proteolysis (Fig. 175-1). Activated factor XII (α-factor XIIa), then activates PK to kallikrein, and kallikrein, in turn, amplifies the process by activating additional factor XII.[31] The process that triggers contact activation is not known. It is clear, however, that alternatives to kallikrein for factor XII activation exist, because the abnormal coagulation associated with PK deficiency is corrected by prolonged incubation with the contact surface.[32] Factor XII undergoes autoactivation by α-factor XIIa when bound to a surface.[33,34] It is conceivable that α-factor XIIa, kallikrein, or other proteases from plasma or tissue are continuously present in plasma in sufficient amounts to initiate factor XII activation. Alternatively, surface bound factor XII zymogen may undergo conformational changes that result in a weakly active zymogen[35] similar to the phenomena noted for trypsinogen and chymotrypsinogen.[36] Along similar lines, conformational changes in factor XII when bound to surface could allow substrate-induced activation by PK or factor XI.[37,38] Regardless of the initiating event, the activation of factor XII by kallikrein and PK by α-factor XIIa are orders of magnitude more efficient than factor XII "autoactivation."[39] Optimal activation of PK by α-factor XIIa on a surface requires the nonenzymatic cofactor HK.[15,16,18,40–44] PK circulates in a noncovalent complex with HK.[44–47] Binding of HK to the contact surface brings PK to the surface, where it is activated to kallikrein by surface bound α-factor XIIa.[41] Kallikrein remains bound to the surface by HK, where it is available to amplify the contact process by activation of surface-bound factor XII.

The α-factor XIIa and kallikrein produced during contact activation can activate a number of host defense systems in plasma. The physiological importance of these reactions is not clear. Each system activated by contact activation proteases is also activated by alternative, and in most instances more potent, mechanisms. This fact, in conjunction with the apparent lack of abnormal phenotypes associated with factor XII, PK, or HK deficiency, suggests that the contact activation process is an in vitro phenomena distinct from the true physiological roles of these proteins. α-Factor XIIa promotes the coagulation of blood by activating factor XI.[6,7,48,49] Analogous to the situation with PK, factor XI circulates in a complex with HK, and is bound to negatively charged surfaces by HK where it is activated by surface bound α-factor XIIa.[37,41] Activated factor XI (factor XIa) then activates factor IX, which, in turn, activates factor X. Activated factor X converts prothrombin to thrombin which cleaves soluble fibrinogen into fibrin to form a clot.[6,7,22,30] This cascade or waterfall hypothesis of blood coagulation is the basis for the aPTT assay used for more than 30 years in hospital coagulation laboratories. Kallikrein is a kininogenase which cleaves HK to liberate the potent vasoactive nonapeptide bradykinin.[50,51] Kallikrein also activates the fibrinolytic system by converting prourokinase plasminogen activator (proUK) to its active form urokinase (UK).[52–55] Factor XIIa may directly activate plasminogen to the fibrinolytic enzyme plasmin, but the physiological significance of this reaction is not known.[56–58]

Contact activation reactions on negatively charged surfaces may be propagated into the fluid phase of plasma by several mechanisms. Kallikrein can dissociate from HK and liberate bradykinin from HK in the fluid phase,[43,59] and activate the renin-angiotensin system of blood pressure regulation by proteolytically converting prorenin to renin.[60–62] In addition, kallikrein triggers the alternative pathway of the complement system by activation of plasma C3.[63] Surface-bound α-factor XIIa, an 80-kDa protein, can undergo further cleavage in the heavy chain to produce β-factor XIIa, a 28-kDa protease that does not bind to surface.[31,64–66] β-factor XIIa does not activate factor XI well, but it is a potent activator of PK in fluid phase and can initiate the classic pathway of the complement system through activation of C1.[67]

Many different types of materials initiate contact activation in plasma. Highly purified nonphysiological substances such as kaolin (aluminum silicate), celite (diatomaceous earth), and ellagic acid are often used in clinical in vitro assays such as the aPTT.[11] Glycosaminoglycans, such as heparin and chondroitin sulfate, articular cartilage, sulfatide, cholesterol sulfate, acid phospholipids and several proteoglycans, all induce contact activation, although under conditions that are not likely to be physiological.[34,68–71] Sulfatides[34] and dextran sulfate[39,72] are particularly popular compounds for studying contact activation because they are potent and are available in highly purified forms. An in vivo counterpart for the materials used to induce contact activation in vitro has not been identified. Indeed, recent data suggest that factor XII and PK may be activated by mechanisms distinct from contact activation. Factor XII binds to endothelial cells in a zinc-dependent manner, where it undergoes slow activation to α-factor XIIa.[73] The endothelial cell membrane protein involved in this interaction is called gC1qR, a receptor for the globular "head" regions of the C1q component of complement. PK also binds to endothelial cells in a process requiring zinc and HK, and undergoes activation by a factor XIIa-independent process that may involve an endothelial cell thiol protease.[29] gC1qR appears to be required for this process as a binding site for HK.[74,75] The long sought "physiological" surface for the activation of the contact proteases may, therefore, be the endothelial cell surface, and activation may proceed by processes unlike those involved in classic contact activation.

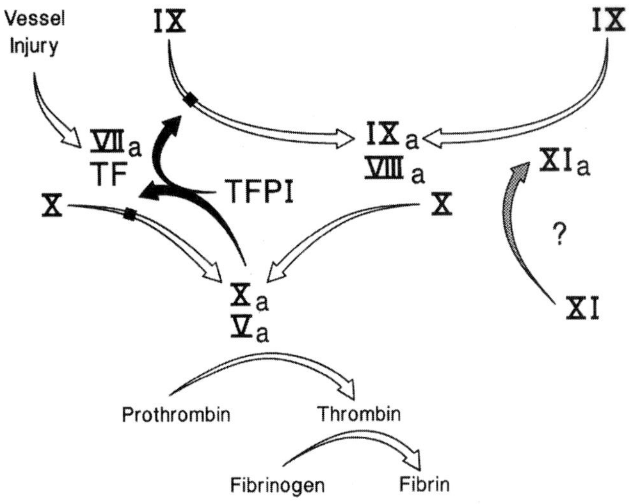

Fig. 175-2 The role of factor XI in blood coagulation. The lowercase "a" next to the Roman numerals indicates the activated form of the proteins. Coagulation is initiated when factor VIIa in plasma is exposed to tissue factor (TF) at a wound site. Factor VIIa/TF activates some factor IX and factor X to start the process of thrombin generation and fibrin production. The activity of factor VIIa/TF is limited through feedback inhibition by tissue factor pathway inhibitor (TFPI). To sustain thrombin production to complete coagulation, factor X activation by factor IXa is necessary. Factor XIa appears to contribute to coagulation by activating additional factor IX to supplement the factor IXa initially produced by factor VIIa/TF. The protease responsible for factor XI activation in vivo is not certain, however, thrombin is a candidate.

Factor XI and Coagulation

Congenital deficiency of factor XI is associated with a variable bleeding abnormality that presents as excessive hemorrhage after trauma or surgery.[76–80] Bleeding is usually mild to moderate and the severe spontaneous bleeding symptoms seen in patients with hemophilia (factor VIII or factor IX deficiency, see Chap. 172 and 173) are rare in factor XI deficiency. These clinical observations indicate that factor XI is required for normal hemostasis. The nature of the bleeding suggests, however, that factor XI is unlikely to be part of a major mechanism for initiating clot formation, as the contact activation model proposes. In current models of hemostasis, coagulation is initiated when factor VIIa in plasma is exposed to the integral membrane protein tissue factor (TF) at a wound site (Fig. 175-2).[22,24,30,81,82] The factor VIIa/TF complex activates some factors X and IX to generate thrombin for initial fibrin formation. This process is limited by the tissue factor pathway inhibitor (TFPI), which binds factor Xa and causes feedback inhibition of factor VIIa/TF.[22,24] Further activation of factor X to continue the clotting process must proceed through factors VIII and IX. Factor XIa activates additional factor IX to supplement the factor IXa produced initially by factor VIIa/TF. The reader is referred to Chap. 169 and several outstanding review articles[24,30,81,83,84] for additional information on blood coagulation.

In the model proposed above, factor XI is not required for initiating fibrin formation, but instead sustains thrombin production after the inhibition of factor VIIa/TF by TFPI. In situations where blood vessel integrity is severely challenged (trauma or surgery) or processes opposing coagulation are particularly active (fibrinolysis), the factor IXa produced by factor VIIa/TF may be insufficient for adequate hemostasis and must be supplemented through factor XIa. This premise fits well with the excessive posttraumatic and surgical bleeding seen in factor XI deficiency, which is most severe when involving tissues rich in fibrinolytic activity, such as the oral cavity and urinary tract.[19,85] The mechanism by which factor XI is activated in vivo is not certain, however, the model predicts that it would be activated relatively late in the course of coagulation, after initial thrombin and fibrin formation.[22] Furthermore, the lack of excessive bleeding seen in factor XII deficiency suggests a factor XII-independent process for factor XI activation. Thrombin activates factor XI in a number of experimental systems, including on the surface of platelets,[23,26,86–90] and may be more important than factor XIIa for factor XI activation in vivo.

The requirement for sustained thrombin production through factor XIa may be due, in part, to a need for additional fibrin formation over time, however, recent data suggest that it also leads to modifications of the fibrin clot that retard fibrinolysis.[89] A recent study in which inhibition of factor XI in rabbits by infusion of a monoclonal antibody renders artificially induced jugular vein clots more susceptible to degradation after tissue plasminogen activator infusion supports this observation.[91] This process may ultimately involve a thrombin-activated plasma carboxypeptidase termed TAFI (thrombin activatable fibrinolysis inhibitor), which proteolytically alters fibrin, removing binding sites for plasminogen and plasminogen activators.[92–94] The current hypothesis, therefore, is that factor XI is required to sustain activation of factor IX, and, ultimately, generation of thrombin to counteract fibrinolytic degradation of the fibrin clot. Bleeding in factor XI deficiency, then, is due to the inability of plasma to counter fibrinolysis adequately, rather than a failure to form the fibrin clot.

PROTEINS AND GENES

Factor XI (Plasma thromboplastin antecedent)

Factor XI is the zymogen of a serine protease present in plasma at a concentration of 20 to 45 nM (3 to 7 μg/ml),[48,49,95] almost all of which circulates in a complex with HK.[96] Factor XI has been purified from bovine,[97] human,[49] porcine,[98] and rabbit[99] plasma; additionally, recombinant mouse factor XI[100] has been expressed. Except for the rabbit molecule, the protein is a 160-kDa disulfide-linked dimer of identical 80-kDa polypeptides.[49] Rabbit factor XI, also an 80-kDa polypeptide, lacks the disulfide bond, but may circulate as a noncovalently associated homodimer.[99] Factor XI is the only coagulation protease that is polymeric, a feature that has

Table 175-1 Factor XI and the Contact Activation Factors—Proteins and Genes

	Factor XI	PK	Factor XII	HMWK
Protein				
Molecular mass (kDa)	160	86–88	80	110
Carbohydrate (w/w %)	5	15	17	40
Isoelectric point	8.6	8.7	6.3	4.7
Plasma concentration				
μg/ml	5	50	30	70
n*M*	30	580	375	670
In vivo half-life (hours)	52	35	60	150
mRNA				
Size (kb)	2.1 & 4.2	2.4	2.4	3.5
Amino acids	1214	619	596	626
Gene				
Chromosomal location	4q35	4q35	5q33-qter	3q27
Size (kilobases)	23	22*	12	27
Number of exons	15	15*	14	11

*Values are for the rat gene.

implications for the genetics of its deficiency state (see "Genetics" under "Factor XI Deficiency" below). The mRNA for human factor XI has been detected in liver, pancreas, kidney, and platelets.[100–102] The primary source of plasma factor XI is the liver, as factor XI levels decrease during liver failure; two patients acquired factor XI deficiency after liver transplantation from factor XI-deficient donors.[103,104] The gene (GenBank M18295)[105] and cDNA (GenBank M13142)[106] for human factor XI have been cloned (Table 175-1), and the primary amino acid sequence and disulfide bond configuration has been determined (Fig. 175-3).[107] The structure of factor XI monomer is similar to that of plasma PK with which it shares 58 percent identity in amino acid sequence (Fig. 175-4).[106–109] The genes for the two proteins have the same number of exons,[105,110] identical intron/exon boundaries,[105,110,111] and are located on the same area of chromosome 4 (4q34-35)[112] in humans and of chromosome 8 in mice.[113] These data indicate that the two genes are products of a duplication event involving a common ancestral gene. Mature factor XI monomer contains 607 amino acids and is divided into a C-terminal catalytic trypsin-like serine protease (light chain) domain and an N-terminal heavy chain required for binding interactions with other macromolecules.[114] The heavy chain, in turn, is comprised of four in tandem 90 to 91-amino acid repeats called apple domains (designated A1 to A4, Fig. 175-3).[106,109]

Zymogen factor XI is converted to active factor XI (factor XIa) by proteolytic cleavage of the bond between Arg369 and Ile370, resulting in a heavy chain of 47 kDa and a light chain of 33 kDa.[48,49] Factor XIIa,[48,49] thrombin,[23,26] trypsin,[115,116] and

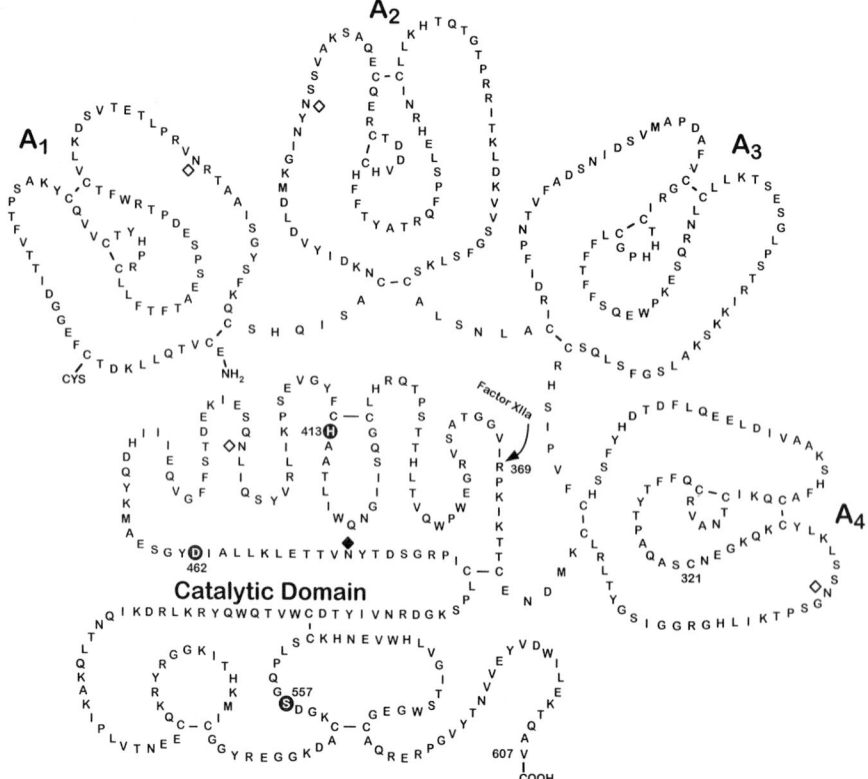

Fig. 175-3 The amino acid sequence and disulfide bond structure of human factor XI monomer. The four apple domains of the noncatalytic heavy chain are designated A1 to A4. Binding sites for HK and factor XIIa have been identified on the A1 and A4 domains, respectively. The factor IX binding site involves sequences in the A3 domain and possibly the C-terminal portion of the A2 domain. Cys321 (designated by the asterisk) in the A4 domain is involved in the disulfide bond between the two polypeptides of the factor XI homodimer. The Arg369-Ile370 bond cleaved by factor XIIa, thrombin, or factor XIa during factor XI activation is designated by the curved arrow. The circled residues comprise the catalytic triad typical of serine proteases. A carbohydrate attachment site at Asn473 is designated by a closed diamond. Four additional potential carbohydrate attachment sites at Asn72, 108, 335, and 432 are marked with open diamonds. (*Reprinted with permission from McMullen et al.*[107] *Copyright 1991 American Chemical Society.*)

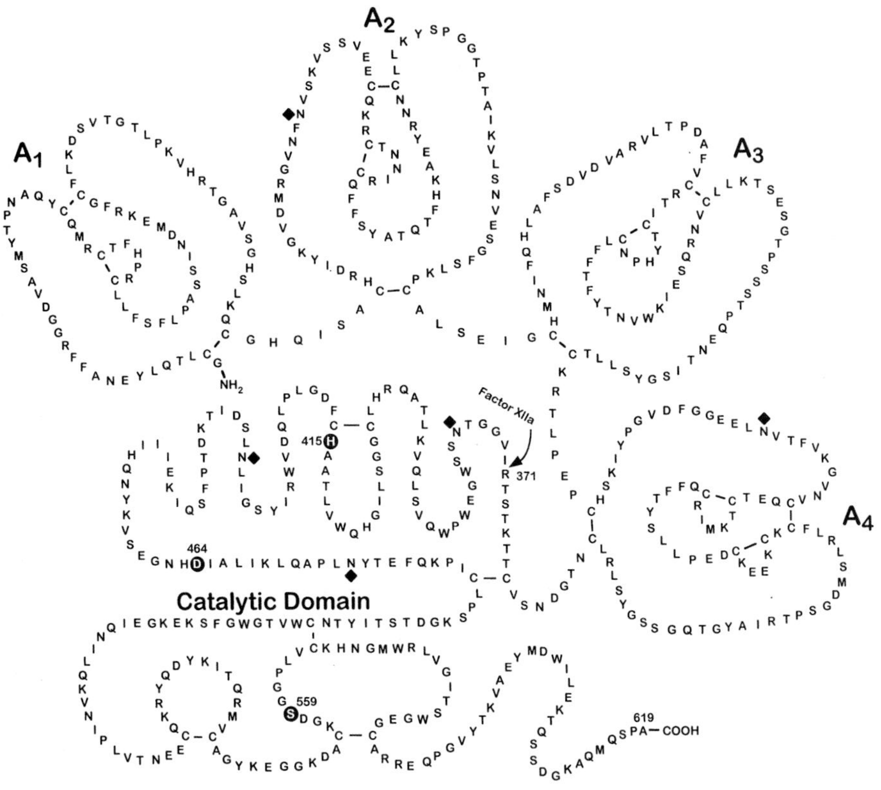

Fig. 175-4 The amino acid sequence and disulfide bond structure of human plasma prekallikrein. The four apple domains of the noncatalytic heavy chain are designated A1 to A4. Amino acid sequences involved in HK binding are present in the C-terminal portion of the A1 and N-terminal portion of the A4 domains. The Arg371-Ile372 bond cleaved by factor XIIa during activation of prekallikrein is designated by the curved arrow. The amino acids of the serine protease catalytic triad are circled. Asn residues at positions 108, 289, 377, 434, and 475 that are attachment sites for carbohydrates are designated by the closed diamonds. (Reprinted with permission from McMullen et al.[109] Copyright 1991 American Chemical Society.)

factor XIa[23,26,86] activate factor XI, and there is evidence that the thrombin precursor meizothrombin activates factor XI on phospholipid vesicles.[117] Recent studies by Baglia and coworkers indicate that the platelet surface may be a physiological site for factor XI binding and activation by thrombin.[90,118–120] The primary function of factor XIa in blood coagulation is the activation of factor IX by limited, calcium-dependent proteolysis.[121–124] Factor XIa cleaves factor IX first at the Arg145-Ala146 bond producing an intermediate factor IXaα. A second cleavage between Arg180 and Val181 releases a 10-kDa activation peptide and the fully activated factor IX molecule, factor IXaβ.[121,125,126] The activation of factor IX by factor XIa does not require negatively charged surfaces, phospholipids, or HK; magnesium ions, however, enhance this reaction, probably through conformational effects on factor IX.[127] Factor XIa also proteolytically activates or cleaves several other plasma protein, although the physiological importance of these reactions is not clear. Factor XII,[128] plasminogen,[58,129,130] and factor XI[23,26] may be activated by factor XIa. In addition, factor XIa will cleave HK to liberate bradykinin, although at a substantially slower rate than kallikrein.[131]

A series of recent reports has expanded our understanding of the roles of the factor XI domains in interactions with other macromolecules. Studies in which the heavy and light chains of factor XIa were separated by mild reduction and alkylation, demonstrate that catalytic activity resides in the light chain, while the heavy chain is required for optimal calcium-dependent activation of factor IX.[114] The A1 domain has been implicated in binding interactions with HK[132] and thrombin,[133] while the A4 domain binds factor XIIa.[134] A4 is also involved in factor XI dimer formation, with Cys321 forming the disulfide bond between the two polypeptides.[135,136] There are conflicting data regarding the location of the factor IX binding site. Studies using peptide inhibition techniques suggest the binding site is on the A2 domain.[137] However, work with recombinant factor XI mutants favors sequences in the N- and C-terminal areas of the A3 domain.[138,139] The A3 domain also contains distinct binding sites for platelets[140,141] and heparin.[142,143]

The regulation of factor XIa involves several plasma serine protease inhibitors (serpins). Initial work suggested that α_1-antitrypsin[144,145] is the major inhibitor with some contribution from antithrombin III (ATIII).[146–148] C1-inhibitor (C1-INH),[149,150] α_2-antiplasmin,[151] and protein C inhibitor[152] also inhibit factor XIa. In addition, platelets release a form of the amyloid precursor protein from α-granules called protease nexin II,[153,154] which is a potent inhibitor of factor XIa. More recent work using enzyme-serpin capture techniques indicate that C1-INH may be the predominant regulator of factor XIa.[155,156] Heparin enhances inhibition of factor XIa by ATIII[147,148,157] and C1-INH.[156] At therapeutic concentrations of heparin the effect on inhibition by ATIII appears to be greater than on C1-INH.[143] Heparin will also enhance factor XIa inhibition by protease nexin II.[153]

Although liver is the primary source of plasma factor XI, there is evidence that platelets contain factor XI-like activity. Well-washed platelets are reported to contain small amounts of factor XI activity (0.67 units/10^{11} platelets),[158] although this finding has been challenged.[159,160] Three groups have reported on the immunoprecipitation of a 220-kDa protein from platelets using polyclonal antifactor XI antibodies.[158,160a,161] It is proposed that this protein is a tetramer of a 50- to 55-kDa product of the factor XI gene lacking the amino acids encoded by exon 5. In support of this is a report of a truncated factor XI mRNA lacking exon 5, isolated from a leukemia cell line cDNA library.[101] It is not clear if normal platelets express this message. Hu and coworkers reported on immunofluorescence studies of human platelets indicating the presence of factor XI-like protein in both normal individuals and patients with deficiency of plasma factor XI.[162] Recently, Martincic and colleagues identified full-length factor XI mRNA in platelets and bone marrow, but did not find truncated messages representing alternatively spliced mRNAs.[102]

Prekallikrein (Fletcher Factor)

Plasma PK is the zymogen of the serine protease plasma kallikrein, a protein with similar structure to factor XI with which it shares 58 percent amino acid homology (Fig. 175-4).[106–109] PK is distinct from a group of kininogenases called tissue-type (glandular) kallikreins.[163] It is an 86- to 88-kDa monomeric glycoprotein that circulates at a concentration of 580 nM (50 μg/ml),[129,164,165] 75 to 90 percent of which is in a noncovalent complex with HK.[45–47] Plasma PK mRNA has been reported only in liver.[100,108] The gene for human PK is located on chromosome 4q34-35 near the factor XI gene;[110] however, it has not been completely characterized (GenBank M62345).[166] Data is available for the rat PK gene which contains 15 exons with identical intron/exon boundaries to the human factor XI gene.[110] The complementary cDNA for human[108] and mouse[167] PK have been cloned, and amino acid sequence and disulfide bond structures determined.[109] The human protein is 619 amino acids long with a trypsin-like serine protease domain at the C-terminus, and an N-terminal heavy chain comprised of four in tandem 90- to 91-amino acid apple domain repeats (Fig. 175-4).[108,109] The heavy chain of PK is required for binding to HK and for surface-dependent activation of factor XII.[168] Key residues for HK binding are located in the A1 (Phe56-Gly86) and A4 domains (Gly284-Arg331).[74] In the absence of HK, the heavy chain can bind directly to negatively charged surfaces.[168,169]

PK is converted to its active form α-kallikrein by proteolytic cleavage between Arg371 and Ile372, generating a 50-kDa heavy chain and a 35-kDa light chain connected by a disulfide bond.[108,129,164,170] α-Factor XIIa, β-factor XIIa, kallikrein, and trypsin will activate plasma PK.[129,164,170] Surface-dependent autoactivation of PK has also been demonstrated.[171] With the exception of β-factor XIIa, all these reactions are promoted by negatively charged artificial surfaces. A study by Motta and coworkers indicates that PK may be activated on endothelial cells by a cell-associated thiol protease in a reaction that is independent of factor XIIa.[29] Autocatalytic cleavage of α-kallikrein at Lys140-Ala141 generates β-kallikrein, a 65-kDa protein.[172,173] Plasma kallikrein is a kininogenase, releasing bradykinin from HK and low-molecular-weight-kininogen by limited proteolysis.[51,174–176] Kallikrein also activates surface-bound factor XII to α- and β-XIIa,[31,41,128] prourokinase to urokinase,[55] plasminogen to plasmin,[58,152,170] and the renin-angiotensin system through conversion of prorenin to renin.[60–62] In the absence of calcium, kallikrein and factor XIa activate factor IX with similar efficiency.[122] Addition of physiological concentrations of calcium reduces the K_m two-orders of magnitude for the reaction with factor XIa but has no effect on activation by kallikrein.[138,122] While the activation of factor IX by kallikrein is probably not significant in hemostasis, it is required for activation of factor VII during "cold activation" of citrated plasma at 4°C.[177,178] Kallikrein has potent in vitro effects on neutrophils, inducing aggregation, chemotaxis, and elastase release.[2,3,179] Monocytes are also stimulated by kallikrein.[180]

Plasma kallikrein is inhibited primarily by C1-INH[181] and α_2-macroglobulin,[182,183] with some contribution from ATIII.[181] Heparin appears to have little effect on C1-INH inhibition of kallikrein.[156] Plasminogen activator inhibitor-1 (PAI-1)[184] and protein C inhibitor[152,185] have also been shown to inhibit plasma kallikrein.

Factor XII (Hageman Factor)

Factor XII is the zymogen of a plasma serine protease, and is an 80-kDa single-chain glycoprotein that circulates in plasma at 375 nM (30 μg/ml).[186] The ~12-kb factor XII gene has 14 exons and maps to human chromosome 5q33-qter (GenBank cDNA M11723 and gDNA M17464).[187,188] The organization of the gene is similar to those of the plasminogen activators tissue plasminogen activator (tPA) and prourokinase (pro UK) and differs from that of most other coagulation factors.[187] Based on homology to known structural motifs, a variety of domains have been identified within the factor XII molecule (Fig. 175-5). An N-terminal fibronectin type II domain (encoded by exons 3 and 4) is followed by an epidermal growth factor (EGF) domain (exon 5), a fibronectin type 1 domain (exon 6), a second EGF domain (exon 7), a kringle domain (exons 8 and 9), a unique 55-amino acid "proline-rich" domain (exon 9), and the trypsin-like serine protease domain (exons 10–14). Three regions within the molecule appear to mediate its binding to negatively charged surfaces: one at the proximal N-terminus (residues 1–28), a second within the fibronectin type 1 domain (residues 134–153), and a third in the second EGF-like or kringle domain.[189–191] Two zinc binding sites in factor XII have been identified (residues 40–44 and 78–82).[192] The major site of synthesis of factor XII is thought to be the liver.[193,194] The promoter of the factor XII gene contains an estrogen response element (at −43 to −31) and the plasma level of factor XII is increased by the administration of estrogen and during pregnancy.[189,195–197] Interleukin-6 down-regulates factor XII expression in cultured hepatoma cells (HepG2) and factor XII appears to behave as a negative acute-phase protein.[198]

Factor XII is activated by proteolytic cleavage after Arg353 producing α-factor XIIa, a two-chain disulfide-linked molecule with an N-terminal heavy chain (52 kDa) and C-terminal light chain (28 kDa) that contains the catalytic site.[199,200] Cleavage at this site is dramatically enhanced when factor XII is bound to a negatively charged surface[128] and by the presence of zinc ions.[201–204] Kallikrein, factor XIa, factor XIIa, plasmin, or trypsin can activate factor XII. Kallikrein is the most potent endogenous activator of factor XII. Plasmin-mediated factor XII activation has been documented in patients receiving thrombolytic therapy.[205] β-Factor XIIa (Hageman factor fragment) is generated by additional cleavages at Arg334 and Arg343.[199,200] Because it lacks the bulk of the heavy chain that is responsible for the interaction of factor XII(a) with negatively charged surfaces, β-factor XIIa does not produce contact-mediated activation of PK or factor XI.[66] Nevertheless, β-factor XIIa retains the ability to activate PK in the fluid phase and can also activate the complement factor C1.[31,66,206,207] Factor XII can bind to endothelial cells in a zinc-dependent manner; it undergoes slow activation in this environment.[5] Factor XII binds to gC1qR on endothelial cells, a protein that binds the globular "heads" of the C1q component of the complement system.[73] Besides PK and factor XI, factor XIIa activates plasminogen and factor VII, and cleaves bradykinin from HK.[56,208–210] The importance of the latter reactions is not clear. Factor XII and factor XIIa also possess mitogenic activity that may reside in their EGF-like domains and stimulate the proliferation of cultured human hepatoma cells (HepG2).[211,212] Indeed, the structure of factor XII is highly homologous to hepatocyte growth factor activator,[213] a serine protease that activates hepatocyte growth factor, itself a serine protease with homology to plasminogen.[214]

The predominant plasma inhibitor of α-factor XIIa and β-factor XIIa is C1-INH, although ATIII and PAI-1 have also been shown to inhibit factor XIIa.[184,215,216] Endothelial cells reportedly produce a substance that interferes with contact-mediated factor XII activation, but not factor XIIa proteolytic activity.[217] Likewise, certain plasma proteins, such as fibrinogen, β_2-glycoprotein I, and C1q, compete with factor XII for surface binding and inhibit contact activation.[218,219]

High Molecular Weight Kininogen

HK is a 110-kDa glycoprotein with a plasma concentration of 670 nM (70 μg/ml). The protein migrates anomalously on gel filtration (~220,000), indicating a large, partial, specific volume, and electron microscopy studies show that HK is a complex of linked globular units.[220] Low molecular weight kininogen (LK), also known as α_1-cysteine protease inhibitor, is a 66-kDa glycoprotein that circulates at a plasma concentration of 2.4 μM (160 μg/ml).[221] The ~27-kb kininogen gene contains 11 exons and maps to 3q27, close to two other members of the cystatin gene family, α_2HS-glycoprotein and histidine-rich glycoprotein.[222–225] Through alternative mRNA processing and the use of different polyadenylation signals, the single kininogen gene (GenBank M11438, M11260) produces transcripts for both HK (3.5 kb) and LK (1.7 kb) (Fig. 175-6).[223] Exons 1–9 and a portion

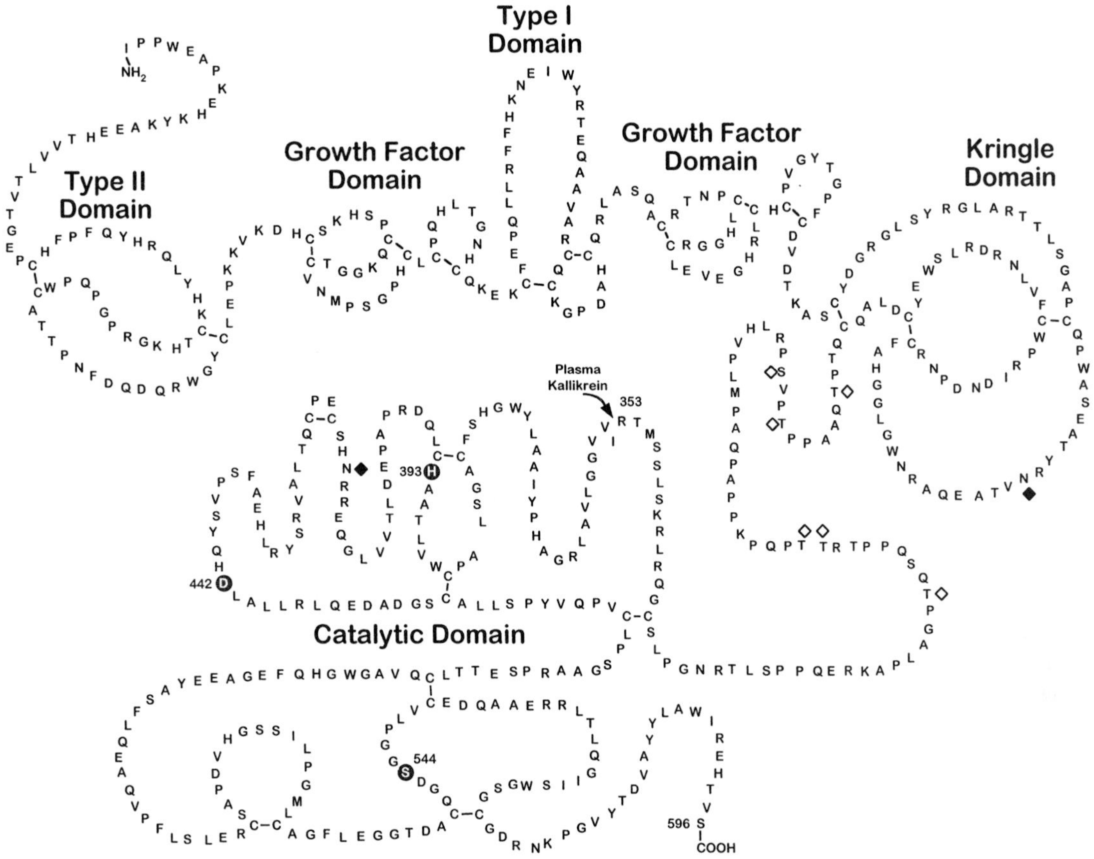

Fig. 175-5 The amino acid sequence and disulfide bond structure of human factor XII. Portions of the noncatalytic heavy chain with homology to fibronectin types I and II domains, growth factor-like domains, and a kringle domain are indicated. The Arg353-Val354 bond cleaved during activation of factor XII by plasma kallikrein is designated by the curved arrow. The amino acids of the serine protease catalytic triad are circled. The closed diamonds designate N-glycosylation sites, while opened diamonds signify possible O-glycosylation sites. (From Fujikawa, and based on available sequence data.[193,199,200] Reprinted by permission.)

of exon 10, encoding bradykinin and the following 12 amino acids, are shared in the mRNAs of HK and LK. HK mRNA contains the remainder of exon 10 encoding the unique 56-kDa C-terminus of HK, whereas in LK mRNA this part of exon 10 and its flanking 90-nucleotide sequence is spliced out and exon 11 is used to encode the unique 4-kDa C-terminus of LK. Liver contains mRNA for both HK and LK.[222,223] Cultured umbilical vein endothelial cells express HK, and kininogen antigen has been detected in

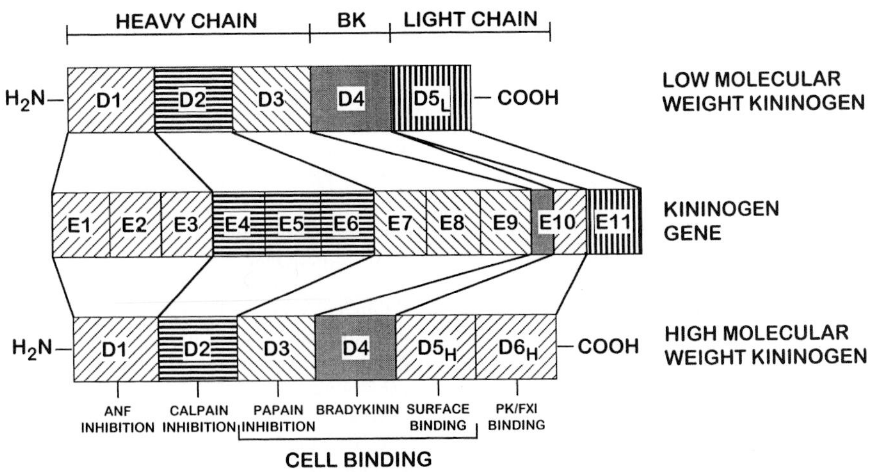

Fig. 175-6 The exons of the kininogen gene and corresponding domain structures of the kininogen proteins. Both high (HK) and low (LK) molecular weight kininogen are products of a single gene containing 11 exons (designated E1 to E11 in the center of the figure). Parts of domain 1 (D1, encoded by exons 1-3) on HK and LK inhibit atrial naturetic factor (ANF). Domain 2 (D2, encoded by E4-6) contains unique papain and calpain inhibitory sequences. Domain 3 (D3, E7-9) has papain inhibitory sequences. Domain 4 (D4), encoded by part of exon 10, contains the nonapeptide bradykinin and the first 12 amino acids of the HK and LK light chains. The remainder of E10 encodes HK's light chain, which consists of a domain for binding to negatively charged surfaces ($D5_H$), and a domain for binding to factor XI or PK ($D6_H$). Domains 3 to 5 on HK are also required for HK binding to cells. The remainder of the light chain of LK ($D5_L$) is encoded by exon 11. (From Colman and Schmaier.[27] Reprinted with permission.)

granulocytes, renal tubular cells, skin, and platelets.[226–232] The quantity of HK contained by platelets is very low in comparison to the plasma HK concentration (0.23 percent).[232] Platelets secrete HK from their α granules following activation, however, and platelet HK may contribute significantly to local HK concentrations at sites where platelets aggregate.[231,233] Kininogen gene transcription is affected by estrogen and plasma concentrations of HK increase in pregnancy.[234,235] Cyclic AMP, forskolin, prostaglandin E2, and TNF-α enhance the expression of kininogens by cultured murine fibroblasts and TNF-α increases kininogen expression in a hepatoma cell line (HepG2).[236,237]

Based on limited proteolysis, the structures of the kininogens have been separated into domains (Fig. 175-6). HK and LK share an identical heavy chain (D1-D3) and a bradykinin-containing domain (D4). The unique light chain of LK is designated D5L, whereas the light chain of HK contains two domains (D5H and D6H). Domains D1, D2, and D3 are homologous to cystatin and domains D2 and D3 retain cysteine protease inhibitory activity.[238] A peptide derived from D1 reportedly inhibits atrial naturetic peptide.[239,240] The role of a low-affinity calcium binding site in D1 is not known.[241] Platelet calpain is inhibited by D2, and papain and cathepsins are inhibited by D2 and D3.[238,242,243] Regions within D3 and D4 inhibit thrombin-induced platelet aggregation by interfering with the binding of thrombin to platelet glycoprotein Ib_a and by interacting with protease-activated receptor-1 (PAR-1), inhibiting its proteolytic activation by thrombin.[244–246]

Regions within D3 and D4 in LK, and in D3, D4, and D5H in HK, are responsible for the zinc-dependent binding of the kininogens to the surface of cells, including granulocytes, platelets, and endothelial cells.[247–251] The cellular binding of kininogen is of high affinity (K_d 10 to 50 nM). HK serves as an intermediary in the binding of factor XI and PK to platelets, endothelial cells, and granulocytes.[29,119,120,252–257] Identification of the cell surface receptor(s) mediating kininogen binding is an area of active investigation. Candidate proteins include Mac-1 (CD11b/18),[248,258] gC1qR,[73,75,259] urokinase plasminogen activator receptor,[27] thrombospondin − 1,[260] and cytokeratin-1.[261] The kininogen receptor(s) may differ between cells and perhaps comprise a multiprotein complex. Several in vitro studies suggest that HK and/or kinin-free HK may function as antiadhesive proteins by interfering with the binding of fibrinogen to artificial surfaces, neutrophils, and platelets, and by inhibiting the attachment and spreading of platelets, monocytes, and other cells on fibrinogen, vitronectin, and matrix protein-coated surfaces.[252,262,263]

The D4 domain of the kininogens contains the biologically active peptide bradykinin that is released by plasma and tissue kallikreins by limited proteolysis. HK is the preferred substrate for plasma kallikrein and LK is the preferred substrate for tissue kallikrein. Cleavage of kininogen by plasma kallikrein at Lys362 and Arg371 produces bradykinin (ArgProProGlyPheSerProPheArg), whereas cleavage by tissue kallikrein produces Lys-bradykinin (kallidin) that is subsequently converted to bradykinin by a plasma aminopeptidase.[264] Kinin-free HK (HKa) initially consists of a 64-kDa heavy chain and a 56-kDa light chain that are linked by a disulfide bridge. Subsequent cleavage in the light chain produces a stable form of HKa with a 64-kDa heavy chain and 45-kDa light chain. Kininogen is also cleaved by factor XIIa, factor XIa, and plasmin, but the physiological relevance of these reactions is not clear.[131,208,265] Bradykinin produces a multitude of effects including vasodilatation, increased vascular permeability, hypotension, pain, smooth-muscle cell contraction, and the stimulation of prostacyclin synthesis, PA release, superoxide formation, and nitric oxide formation in endothelial cells.[266–270] These effects of bradykinin are mediated through its interaction with two seven-transmembrane, G-protein-linked cellular receptors termed B1 and B2.[271–273] The degradation of bradykinin initially proceeds through the actions of carboxypeptidase-N (and perhaps other carboxypeptidase B-like enzymes) and angiotensin converting enzyme (ACE).[274–276]

Two histidine/glycine-rich regions in the D5H domain in the light chain of HK bind zinc and mediate the binding of HK to anionic artificial surfaces and heparin.[277–280] This surface-binding subdomain overlaps with the region in D5H involved in HK interactions with cells.[251] The binding of HK to anionic surfaces is dramatically increased following the proteolytic release of bradykinin.[281] The D6H domain in the light chain of HK contains binding sites for factor XI and PK and a substantial proportion of these proteins circulate in plasma bound to HK.[282,283] The factor XI and PK binding sites on HK overlap, therefore one molecule of HK can bind either a molecule of factor XI or a molecule of PK. The coagulant activity of HK as measured in the aPTT assay requires the D5H-mediated association of HK with artificial surfaces and the D6H-mediated binding of factor XI and PK to HK.[284–286] Granulocyte elastase cleavage of HK destroys its coagulant activity.[287] The domains present in the HK light chain are lacking in LK, which does not possess procoagulant activity. The function of the light chain of LK (D5L) is not known.

CONGENITAL DEFICIENCY STATES AND CLINICAL DISORDERS

Factor XI Deficiency

Factor XI deficiency was first identified in two sisters and their uncle in 1953 by Rosenthal and coworkers, and was initially called hemophilia C.[12] The bleeding tendency was milder and more variable than in hemophilias A or B (factor VIII or IX deficiency, respectively), and was inherited as an autosomal trait.[288] The plasma factor missing in these individuals was originally termed plasma thromboplastin antecedent, and subsequently was designated factor XI. While the mode of inheritance was initially thought to be autosomal dominant, the preponderance of data suggested that factor XI deficiency was an autosomal recessive condition,[76] with a particularly high incidence in Ashkenazi Jews.[76,77,289–291]

Genetics. Factor XI deficiency is an autosomal condition, presenting in the homozygous or compound heterozygous state with factor XI activity levels of < 15 percent of that of normal plasma (< 0.15 units/ml).[76,79,80,292] Heterozygotes have partial deficiency or low normal levels (30 to 70 percent of normal). Circulating dysfunctional (cross-reactive material +, or CRM^+) factor XI molecules appear to be rare. Reports of 122 individuals of various ethnic background with severe factor XI deficiency in whom activity and antigen levels were measured[79,293–298] identify only two patients, one German[296] and one Japanese,[298] with significant factor XI antigen. Two German patients with modest decreases in activity and discordantly high antigen levels have also been reported.[79] Therefore, unlike the situation for deficiency of factors VIII and IX in which large numbers of dysfunctional variants occur, little information regarding protein structure/function relationships have been obtained by studying factor XI deficient patients.

Three distinct mutations in the human factor XI gene, designated types I through III were first reported in six patients of Ashkenazi Jewish descent by Asakai et al. (Table 175-2).[299] Subsequent work demonstrated that the types II and III mutations were common in the Jewish population accounting for > 90 percent of the abnormal factor XI alleles in this group.[85,300] The type II mutation introduces a premature termination codon in the A2 domain.[299] The type III mutation substitutes leucine for phenylalanine at amino acid 283 (F283L) within A4.[299] The A4 domain is involved in interactions between the two polypeptides of the factor XI dimer.[136] Work by Meijers and coworkers suggests that the type III mutation interferes with intracellular dimer formation, resulting in greatly reduced protein secretion.[135] Consistent with this is a report of three patients from England with factor XI deficiency associated with mutations in the A4

Table 175-2 Reported Mutations in the Human Factor XI Gene

DNA change*	Result of DNA change	Reference
Exon 3 143G → C	D16H	301
Exon 4 352ins7	frameshift	315
Exon 5 446G → T	E117X (type II mutation)	299
Exon 5 481C → A	C128X	426
Intron E +5G → C	Splicing	301
Exon 7 774A → G	Q226R	302
Exon 7 781G → C	W228C	427
Exon 8 840G → A	S248N	302
Exon 9 944T → C	F283Leu (type III mutations)	299
Exon 9 1002T → C	L302P	301
Exon 9 1008C → T	T304I	301
Exon 9 1064G → A	E323K	301
Intron I -2A → G	splicing	301
Exon 10 1115delA	frameshift	315
Intron J +1G → A	splicing	298
Exon 11 1254C → A	T386N	310
Intron K T to A	splicing	315
Exon 12 1421T → G	F442V	426
Exon 14/Intron 1757del14	splicing (type IV mutation)	428
Intron N + 1G → A	splicing (type I mutations)	299

*Base pair numbering system refers to position in the human factor XI cDNA.[106]

domain that interfere with protein secretion in in vitro expression systems.[301]

Twenty distinct mutations and deletions have now been reported in the human factor XI gene (Table 175-2), the majority of which are associated with low levels of both antigen and activity in plasma. Recently, two amino acid substitutions, one on each allele, were found in a 9-year-old African-American male with mild factor XI deficiency and a life-long history of excessive bleeding.[302] These mutations are associated with significant amounts of circulating factor XI antigen; however, the effects of the individual mutations on protein function have yet to be determined. Hayashi and colleagues reported a CRM^{+} variant causing severe factor XI deficiency (Factor XI Yamagata) associated with a mutation in an intron J splice acceptor site.[298] As this type of change would be expected to result in CRM^{-} deficiency, it is not yet clear if the reported mutation is responsible for this variant. Eight neutral polymorphisms (unassociated with amino acid substitutions) have been identified in the human factor XI gene (Table 175-3), four of which are in the coding sequence. These substitutions should prove useful in population analyses.

Frequency. Factor XI deficiency is prevalent in individuals of Ashkenazi Jewish heritage, in whom surveys involving 1141 persons determined a frequency for severe deficiency of 1 in 190.[303] This impressive result implies a carrier frequency of 13.5 percent. The majority (>90 percent) of abnormal alleles in severe factor XI deficiency in Jews are of types II or III, and the two mutations are equally prevalent.[85,300,304] A recent study of 531 Ashkenazi Jews determined allele frequencies of 0.0217 and 0.0254 for the types II and III mutations, respectively.[304] A frequency for the type II mutation of 0.0167 was seen in Iraqi Jews.[304] The type II allele was subsequently detected at significant frequencies in Arabs (0.0065), Sephardic/North African Jews (0.0027), and Middle Eastern Jews of non-Iraqi origin (0.0026), consistent with an ancient origin for this allele.[305] The type III mutation, found predominantly in Ashkenazi Jews, appears to be of more recent European origin.[305] The reason for the high frequency of factor XI deficiency in this population is not clear. A founder effect coupled with migration and significant fluctuations in population size would appear to be most likely,[306–308] as no selective advantage for deficient patients or carriers of abnormal alleles has been detected.

Factor XI deficiency is rare among individuals not of Jewish heritage, with one study estimating occurrence at 1 in 10^5 to 10^6 individuals,[309] although deficient persons are undoubtedly missed due to the relatively mild nature of the bleeding disorder. Factor XI deficiency has been reported sporadically in patients of Arab,[295,310] African-American,[295,302,311] Chinese,[312] Czechoslovakian,[313] Dutch,[79] English,[295,301,314] German,[79,296] Indian,[295] Italian,[79,313] Korean,[295] Japanese,[295,298] Portuguese,[315] Swedish,[300] and Yugoslav[79] origin. The types II and III mutations are relatively infrequent in this heterogeneous population (probably <15 percent of abnormal alleles).[300] While no single mutation appears to predominate in this group, Bolton-Maggs and coworkers recently identified the C128X mutation in six unrelated patients in north west England.[315a]

Clinical Presentation. Bleeding in factor XI deficient patients is usually triggered by trauma or surgery, and "spontaneous" bleeding such as occurs in patients with hemophilia A or B is very uncommon.[76–80,292] Excessive bleeding may start at the time of injury and persist over hours to days, or may be delayed for several hours. Oozing from wounds, such as a site of tooth extraction, may persist for several days. In contrast to hemophilia A or B, the bleeding in factor XI deficiency correlates poorly with factor XI activity levels.[79,80] Indeed, there are patients with <1 percent of normal levels that do not bleed excessively despite surgery or trauma.[76,316,317] As puzzling is the tendency for bleeding to vary in the same patient over time.[80,85] A seminal study by Asakai and colleagues shed light on this conundrum,

Table 175-3 Neutral Polymorphisms in the Human Factor XI Gene

Location	Polymorphism*	Population†	Allele Frequency	Reference
Intron A	139A/C	C	Unreported	305‡, 315
Intron B	CA repeats	C	Four different alleles	305, 429
Exon 5	472 C/T	C, B	C = 0.93 T = 0.07	302, 315
Intron E	RFLP (*Hha* I)	C	A1 = 0.4, A2 = 0.6	305, 430
Exon 8	844A/G	C, B	A = 0.81 G = 0.19	302, 315
Exon 11	1234C/T	C, B	C = 0.82 T = 0.18	302
Intron M	AT repeats	C	Four different alleles	305
Exon 14	1750C/T	B	C = 0.85 T = 0.15	§

*Base pair numbering system refers to position in the human factor XI cDNA[106] for changes in exons, and to the position in the individual introns of the factor XI gene.[105]
‡This study identified an abnormality in intron A which may be the specific nucleotide change identified in reference 315.
†C = Caucasian, B = Black
§Martincic and Gailani, 1998, unpublished observation.

demonstrating that both genotype (factor XI level) and the site of injury influence bleeding tendency.[85] Surgical procedures on tissues with high fibrinolytic activity, such as the oral cavity and the urinary tract, were associated with excessive bleeding in two-thirds of cases, independent of genotype. Bleeding with surgery at other locations and injury-related bleeding were genotype dependent with patients homozygous for the type III mutation experiencing significantly fewer bleeding problems than those homozygous for the type II mutation or compound heterozygosity for both mutations. This probably relates to the slightly higher factor XI level in the type III homozygotes compared to the other genotypes.

Bleeding variability in this disorder may be due to the coexistence of other hemostatic problems. von Willebrand disease was found in one study to be more prevalent in factor XI-deficient patients who bleed, than in those who do not,[318] although subsequent reports did not confirm this.[319] It has been proposed that platelets contain factor XI activity in the form of an alternatively spliced product of the factor XI gene, and that the presence of this protein in some individuals may ameliorate bleeding symptoms in factor XI deficiency.[101,162,320] It is not clear if this protein is present in factor XI-deficient nonbleeders and absent in bleeders, and if so, why the protein expression would vary to such a large degree between individuals.

There is controversy regarding the issue of abnormal hemostasis in mild (heterozygous) factor XI deficiency. Several studies have reported minimal bleeding problems following a variety of surgical procedures including tooth extraction, tonsillectomy, nasal surgery, and urologic surgery.[76,321] However, several groups have found poor correlation between factor XI levels and bleeding,[80,300] and some studies report an inability to distinguish severe (homozygous) from mild (heterozygous) factor XI deficiency based on bleeding symptoms.[77,79,322] While interpretation of these results is difficult due to different criteria for excessive bleeding and the wide range of hemostatic challenges involved, it is possible that some factor XI deficiency genotypes could present with abnormal bleeding in the heterozygous form. As factor XI is a homodimer, heterozygotes could have normal factor XI, heterodimers of normal and abnormal polypeptides, and homodimers of abnormal polypeptides in a 1:2:1 ratio, assuming the two alleles are expressed equally. In this case, three-fourths of circulating factor XI would have at least one abnormal chain, and may be associated with abnormal hemostasis despite modest abnormalities on in vitro clotting assays. A similar autosomal "dominant" mechanism appears to be involved in some forms of type II deficiency of von Willebrand factor, another multimeric protein.[323] This scenario does not appear to apply to the majority of known factor XI mutations, which cause severely decreased expression of the abnormal allele. Indeed, only one report of mutations that may be consistent with an autosomal dominant mode of transmission is available.[302] The general consensus is that, with rare exception, most persons with mild heterozygous factor XI deficiency are not at greater risk for trauma-or surgery-related bleeding than are normal individuals.

Diagnosis. Factor XI deficiency is suspected following excessive trauma-related bleeding or as an incidental finding of a prolonged aPTT.[19,79,322] A history of mild to moderate bleeding after tooth extraction, tonsillectomy, nasal surgery, or urologic surgery, particularly in a Jewish individual, suggests the diagnosis. Diagnosis is established by a modified aPTT assay that assesses the capacity of patient plasma to correct the defect in a factor XI-deficient test plasma.[76] This assay requires careful standardization, as the intra- and interlaboratory coefficient of variation is substantial.[324] Amydolytic[325,326] and immunoassays[295,325,327] for factor XI are available, but are not routinely used for diagnosis. Almost all individuals with severe deficiency have factor XI coagulant and antigen levels < 15 percent of normal and an aPTT greater than two SD above the mean.[295,328] Patients homozygous for the type II mutation have the lowest level (1.2 ± 0.5 percent), while higher levels are noted in homozygotes for the type III mutation (9.7 ± 1.2 percent) and in compound typeII/type III heterozygotes (3.3 ± 1.6 percent).[85] While the mean factor XI level in heterozygotes is significantly lower than the normal mean, a significant number of obligate carriers have factor XI levels within normal range, making diagnosis difficult.[292] The aPTT assay is frequently normal in heterozygous patients and is not useful for identifying these individuals.[85,328] If detection of the carrier state is required, genotypic analysis for the types II and III mutation may be done by restriction endonulease digestion of PCR fragments.

Association with Other Disorders. Factor XI deficiency has been detected in patients with a variety of other coagulation disorders including von Willebrand disease,[318,329] factor VII deficiency,[330] factor VIII deficiency,[80,331] factor IX deficiency (familial multiple factor deficiency type VI),[332] combined factor VIII and IX deficiency (familial multiple factor deficiency type V),[332,333] factor XII deficiency,[334] and abnormal platelet function.[335] Most of these cases likely represent chance occurrence of two disorders in the same patient. A possible exception is combined factor XI and factor IX deficiency (reported in two families) and combined factors VII, IX, and XI deficiency (reported in five families). Studies in some of these cases suggest a single genetic abnormality, possibly in a protein synthesis or secretion pathway, although thorough molecular analysis of the genes of the factors in question have not been reported.[332] Noonan syndrome, an autosomal dominant disorder characterized by face and neck abnormalities, short stature, and heart defects, is associated with a bleeding diathesis in 20 to 65 percent of cases.[336] Several coagulation abnormalities have been reported in these patients, the most common of which is factor XI deficiency.[322,336] Factor XI deficiency has been reported in Jewish patients with Gaucher disease.[337,338] Given the high frequency for the types II and III alleles in the Jewish population, it is not surprising that factor XI deficiency occurs in conjunction with other inherited disorders that are common to this group. Factor XI deficiency has been noted, along with deficiencies of other plasma proteins, in the carbohydrate-deficient glycoprotein syndrome, a group of recently recognized genetic diseases involving multiple organ systems (see Chap. 74).[339] The hallmark of the disorder is deficiency of the three terminal sugar residues (sialic acid, galactose, and *N*-acetylglucosamine) on secretory glycoproteins. Factor XI may contain up to five N-linked sugar moieties,[107] which may explain why it is affected in this syndrome.

Treatment. The highly variable bleeding tendency in patients with factor XI deficiency makes planning perioperative therapy particularly challenging. While some practitioners wait for a surgical patient to bleed before giving replacement therapy, several authorities strongly discourage this strategy.[312] Surgery in these patients, particularly urologic procedures, may be associated with significant and prolonged bleeding, and stopping hemorrhage once it has started is considerably more difficult than preventing it.[78,321,340–342] In the seventh edition of this book, Seligsohn and Griffin presented a list of recommendations for handling surgery patients with factor XI deficiency[312] that remains the standard of care: (a) the procedure should be absolutely indicated; (b) avoid ingestion of antiplatelet drugs, such as aspirin, for one week prior to surgery; (c) the platelet count and prothrombin time (PT) should be normal and a factor XI inhibitor should be ruled out, particularly in patients with prior exposure to plasma infusions; (d) bleeding vessels should be ligated rather than cauterized to avoid postsurgical oozing from damaged vessels; (e) consider the use of antifibrinolytic agents such as ε-amino caproic acid when surgery involves the oral cavity, nasal passages, or urinary tract; and (f) replacement therapy should be initiated prior to surgery and monitored with factor XI activity assays. Replacement therapy for major surgical procedures should continue for 10 to 14 days, while 5 days of therapy is sufficient for minor procedures.[321,322,342]

Replacement therapy for factor XI deficiency is with fresh frozen plasma (FFP). Factor XI concentrates have been prepared and are currently under investigation.[343,344] Factor XI recovery following infusion of either FFP[345] or concentrate[343] is >90 percent and the half-life is relatively long (52 ± 22 h) facilitating treatment. There is no consensus regarding appropriate plasma concentrations of factor XI for surgical procedures, with levels from 20 to 100 percent of normal activity being advocated.[76,291,321,322,343] Excessive postoperative bleeding in some patients with modest reductions in factor XI level (50 to 60 percent of normal) are used in support of higher levels,[79,80,322] while reports of prostatectomy patients doing well with 30 to 35 percent of normal levels suggests lower levels may be adequate.[321,342] It seems prudent to keep the nadir factor XI level above 45 U/dl for major surgery and 30 U/dl for minor surgery.[312] These guidelines may be applied to patients with severe (< 15 percent) and mild (20 to 60 percent) deficiency.

Oral surgery is frequently accompanied by excessive bleeding in untreated factor XI-deficient patients, probably because of brisk fibrinolytic activity in the mouth.[19,76,78] Plasma infusion, with or without fibrinolytic inhibitors, has been used to successfully manage these patients.[345,346] Patients undergoing dental surgery have been successfully treated with the antifibrinolytic agent tranexamic acid without plasma infusion,[347] therefore, FFP is not required for dental procedures in severe factor XI deficiency. Tranexamic acid is administered 12 h before the procedure and continued for 7 days. Spontaneous bleeding is rarely noted in factor XI deficiency. Kitchens observed that these episodes are often associated with aspirin ingestion and resolved after discontinuing aspirin.[322] Factor XI deficiency rarely causes problems with pregnancy or delivery, therefore, prophylactic FFP infusions are not recommended.[322,348]

Factor XII (Hageman Factor) Deficiency

In 1955, Ratnoff and Colopy described three asymptomatic individuals with markedly prolonged clotting times.[13] The missing plasma component was initially termed Hageman factor after the index case and was later assigned the designation factor XII. The incidence of factor XII deficiency is not known, although the condition appears to be more common than deficiencies of PK or HK. Undoubtedly, deficient persons go undiagnosed due to the lack of associated symptoms.

Genetics. Factor XII deficiency is inherited as an autosomal recessive trait. Autosomal dominant inheritance of factor XII deficiency has been reported in a single nonconsanguineous family.[349] Perhaps due to an effect on mRNA translation, a polymorphism (46C/T, detected by *Hga*I restriction digestion) in the 5′-untranslated region of the factor XII gene modifies the plasma level of factor XII.[350] Expression of factor XII by the 46T allele appears to be ~40 percent that of the 46C allele. The estimated 46T allele frequency is 0.73 in Orientals and 0.20 in Caucasians, and Orientals have lower levels of factor XII in plasma.[350,351]

Plasma levels of factor XII activity and antigen are reduced in parallel in most individuals with factor XII deficiency (CRM$^-$), and dysfunctional factor XII (CRM$^+$) has been detected in only a limited number of subjects. Reported genetic abnormalities associated with factor XII deficiency are listed in Table 175-4. In many CRM$^-$ patients, an additional *Taq*I restriction site is present in intron B of the factor XII gene due to a T to C transition 224 nucleotides upstream of exon 3.[352–354] The majority of alleles with the anomalous *Taq*I site contain an additional mutation in the 5′-flanking region of the factor XII gene, −8 G to C.[353,354] The mechanism by which this combination of mutations reduces factor XII gene expression is not known. The *Taq*I abnormality has also been reported in combination with the single base pair deletion (10590 delC) that produces a frame shift in exon 12, and in another CRM$^-$ subject in whom additional mutations in the factor XII gene were not detected.[354] Isolated mutations leading to frameshifts within exon 12 and exon 14 and amino acid substitutions in exon 10 have also been detected in CRM$^-$ individuals (Table 175-4).[354–356] The mechanism by which missense mutations producing Lys395 to Met, or Arg398 to Gln substitutions leads to a CRM$^-$ phenotype is not clear.

Table 175-4 Genetic Abnormalities Associated with Factor XII Deficiency

DNA change*	CRM	Result of DNA change	Reference
-8G → C†	−	not determined	353
Exon 10§	+	R353P	358
Exon 10 9988C → A	−	K395M	354
Exon 10 9998G → A	−	R398Q	354
Exon 11 10372G → A	+	D442N	354
Exon 12 10586delG	−	frameshift	355
Exon 12 10590delC†	−	frameshift	354
Exon 14 11397G → A	−	splice/frameshift	356
Exon 14 11482G → C	+	G570R	354
Exon 14§	+	C571S	359, 360

* Basepair numbering system refers to position in the human factor XII gene.[187]
† TaqI—alterations.
§ Abnormality determined by amino acid sequencing; DNA change not known.

The abnormalities associated with factor XII deficiency in four CRM$^+$ patients have been identified (Table 175-4). In factor XII Locarno, the dysfunctional molecule is produced by an Arg353 to Pro substitution that destroys the cleavage site required for factor XII activation.[357,358] The 10372(G to A) mutation in exon 11 changes Asp442 of the protease catalytic triad to Asn.[354] In factor XII Washington D.C., Cys571 is replaced by Ser in the catalytic domain.[359,360] This amino acid substitution prevents the formation of a disulfide bond between Cys540 and Cys571 and presumably abrogates enzymatic activity by altering the conformation of the catalytic site. A similar mechanism may explain the loss of function associated with an amino acid substitution (Gly570 to Arg) at the residue immediately preceding Cys571.[354]

Clinical Presentation. Factor XII deficiency is not associated with spontaneous or postsurgical bleeding. It is identified most frequently when an incidental aPTT is markedly prolonged in an asymptomatic subject. Occasional factor XII-deficient patients with excessive bleeding have been reported; however, other causes for the hemorrhage were present or not rigorously excluded.[361–363] Some reports suggest a potential association between severe, and even heterozygous, factor XII deficiency and thromboembolic disease.[364–372] Presumably, the loss of factor XIIa-induced fibrinolytic activity plays a role in this phenomena.[373] Although this hypothesis is intriguing, additional carefully controlled and prospective investigations are necessary before it can be concluded that factor XII deficiency is a prothrombotic risk factor.

Diagnosis. Factor XII deficiency is characterized by a prolonged aPTT. Definitive diagnosis is established by modified aPTT using factor XII-deficient plasma. Immunoassays are available.[374] Certain antiphospholipid antibodies in patients with lupus anticoagulants can affect the measurement of factor XII by coagulation assay.[375]

Prekallikrein Deficiency (Fletcher Trait)

In 1963, an 11-year-old African-American girl, who was hospitalized after a house fire in eastern Kentucky, was noted to have a prolonged aPTT. Evaluation at the University of Kentucky confirmed that this child and three of her ten siblings had prolonged aPTTs, which corrected when the plasma underwent prolonged incubation with glass.[14] There was no history of excessive bleeding and other parameters of blood coagulation were normal. It was proposed that this abnormality was due to deficiency of an unrecognized coagulation factor, which was named Fletcher factor after the family in which the disorder was discovered. Wuepper and colleagues subsequently demonstrated that Fletcher factor was identical to plasma PK.[376] Severe PK deficiency (Fletcher trait), an apparently rare disorder, has now been reported in more than 50 individuals from at least 37 unrelated families.[14,32,377–398] Many milder cases may be missed because 2 to 5 percent of normal PK activity in plasma is sufficient to bring the aPTT into normal range.[376]

Genetics. PK deficiency is an autosomal trait, presenting in the homozygous or compound heterozygous condition with levels of < 1 percent of normal. Data on obligate carriers for PK deficiency (parents and children of severely deficient persons), show that 15 of 27 have PK activity levels less than 2 SD below the normal mean, while the remainder fall within the normal range.[32,378,380,382,386–388,390,391,393,399] Circulating dysfunctional PK variants are relatively common. The antigen status of 38 severely PK-deficient patients from 29 separate families was reported by Seligsohn and Griffin in the seventh edition of this book.[312] Nineteen of those individuals had PK antigen levels of 10 to 54 percent of normal and were considered CRM+, while 19 were CRM – . The Black patients in this group, representing 15 families, were all CRM – , accounting for all but three of the CRM – families. The 11 CRM+ families were Caucasian or Japanese. Other published studies contain data on 27 individuals, with all 12 Caucasian patients being CRM+[385,388,391,392,396] and 14 of 15 Black patients being CRM – .[385,387,400] There is a single report of a Black patient with CRM+PK deficiency.[400] Two dysfunctional PK molecules have been studied in detail: PK Long Beach[391] and PK Zurich.[396] These variants are immunologically similar to wild-type PK and bind HK; however, both show reduced activation by β-factor XIIa and have no enzymatic activity. No gene mutation responsible for PK deficiency has been reported.

Clinical Presentation. Despite being associated with pronounced abnormalities in in vitro coagulation assays such as the aPTT, PK deficiency is not associated with excessive bleeding. Anecdotal reports of easy bruising and epsitaxis in patients who have no other bleeding problems are difficult to evaluate and are probably not related to PK deficiency. A 5-month-old boy with severe PK deficiency developed hemarthroses during an infectious illness; however, he had no subsequent problems, which indicate that PK deficiency was not responsible for the bleeding episode.[379] An 11-year-old boy required plasma transfusions after prolonged bleeding posttonsillectomy,[386] and a 3-year-old girl required 1 U of packed red blood cells after an amygdaloidectomy.[380] In only three reported cases, therefore, is it possible that bleeding may be related to PK deficiency. Arterial[364,378,390,395] and venous[377,385] thrombotic events were reported in several patients less than 45 years of age with severe PK deficiency. Some of these individuals had other obvious risk factors for vascular disease. While PK deficiency did not protect these individuals from thrombotic episodes, insufficient data are available to determine that PK deficiency could have contributed to pathologic clot formation.

Diagnosis. Severe PK deficiency presents as an incidental prolongation of the aPTT in an individual without a history of excessive bleeding. Current automated coagulation analyzers often utilize an aPTT reagents containing ellagic acid as the contact activation initiator. As ellagic acid appears to be relatively insensitive to deficiency of PK, it is conceivable that a significant number of PK deficient patients are missed.[399] The abnormal aPTT in PK deficiency may be corrected by prolonging the incubation time with the contact activation-inducing reagent,[32] distinguishing PK deficiency from those of other intrinsic pathway proteins, which do not correct on prolonged incubation. The diagnosis may be confirmed by a specific PK assay that measures the ability of patient plasma to correct the clotting defect in PK deficient test plasma in an aPTT-based assay.[399] Specific monoclonal antibody based immunoassays[385,391] and chromogenic substrate based amydolitic assays[326,391] have also been developed.

HK Deficiency

In 1974, Schiffman and Lee reported that a previously unrecognized plasma factor, separate from PK, was involved in the activation of factor XI by factor XIIa.[401] Shortly thereafter, three asymptomatic patients (Fitzgerald, Williams, and Flaujeac) were described with an inherited deficiency of a clotting factor, later identified as HK, that was required for the contact phase of coagulation in plasma.[15–18] Reports of HK deficiency are infrequent, the disorder having been described in 18 patients from 16 separate families of African-American, Caucasian, Japanese, Pakistani, and Australian Aboriginal origins.[15,17,18,40,402–411]

Genetics. HK deficiency is inherited as an autosomal recessive trait. Depending on the genetic abnormality, patients may have isolated HK deficiency[405,408,411] or combined HK and LK deficiency.[40,402,410,411] A point mutation in exon 5 of the kininogen gene, CGA (Arg) to TGA (stop), has been reported in an individual with total kininogen deficiency (Williams trait).[412] In another subject with isolated HK deficiency, a partial deletion in intron 7 was detected by Southern analysis, but was not further characterized.[411]

Clinical Presentation and Diagnosis. Diagnostic evaluation for HK deficiency is typically prompted by the presence of a very prolonged aPTT in an asymptomatic individual. A convincing association between severe HK deficiency and hemorrhage, thrombosis, or other clinical abnormality has not been documented. Thus, there does not appear to be any in vivo function for which HK is absolutely essential. Partial PK deficiency (10 to 50 percent of normal) is common in patients with severe HK deficiency and may stem from increased catabolism of PK when it is not complexed with HK in plasma.[18,40,408,410]

Clinical Conditions Associated with Activation of Contact System Proteases

Hereditary Angioedema (HAE). HAE is an inherited condition caused by a deficiency or defect in C1-INH, the plasma inhibitor of the first (C1) component of the complement system (see Chap. 186).[413] Activation of the contact system is a consistent finding during acute attacks of HAE, and is probably directly due to the deficiency of C1-INH, which is a major inhibitor of factor XIIa and plasma kallikrein.[414–416] Generation of increased amounts of bradykinin is thought to be an important mediator of the edema that occurs in this condition.[415,417] In addition, β-factor XIIa may directly activate complement components C1r and C1s, perpetuating the process.[207]

Sepsis. Activation of the contact system proteases appears to accompany sepsis syndromes related to Gram-negative bacteria, viruses, fungi, and Rickettsia.[418,419] Significant increases in plasma kallikrein-α_2 macroglobulin complexes in conjunction with a hyperdynamic cardiovascular state were measured in healthy volunteers injected with *E. coli* endotoxin.[420] Injection of a lethal dose of endotoxin in baboons was associated with a decline in functional HK levels and a significant increase in kallikrein-α_2 macroglobulin complexes in conjunction with severe hypotension, while less striking abnormalities were associated with nonlethal doses of endotoxin.[421,422] In this model, infusion of a monoclonal antibody that inhibits factor XIIa prior to administration of endotoxin blocked these abnormalities and prolonged the survival of the animals, although all eventually died.[422] The antifactor XII antibody did not prevent the consumptive coagulopathy that accompanied endotoxin infusion. This is consistent with the premise that tissue factor is probably more important than contact activation for triggering coagulation during sepsis.

Other Conditions Associated with Activation of the Contact System. Activation of contact system proteins have been observed in a number of inflammatory conditions. The synovial fluid of rheumatoid arthritis patients contains plasma kallikrein, which may contribute to joint destruction through the activation of procollagenase.[423] Contact activation can occur on the surface of uric acid or pyrophosphate crystals and may contribute to inflammation in the crystal-induced arthropathies, gout, and pseudogout.[424,425] Pancreatitis is associated with release of tissue-type kallikreins and the generation of bradykinin, which may contribute to formation of ascites and hypotension.[5]

ACKNOWLEDGMENTS

The authors are grateful to Drs. K. Fujikawa, E.W. Davie, D.W. Chung, and B.A. McMullen for permission to use figures displaying the structures of factor XI, factor XII, and PK; and to Drs. A. H. Schmaier and R.W. Colman for permission to use the diagram of the kininogen gene and proteins. We wish to thank Jean McClure for art work and Terri Lewis for preparation of portions of the manuscript.

REFERENCES

1. Saito H: Contact factors in health and disease. *Sem Thromb Hemost* **13**:35, 1987.
2. Kaplan A, Silberberg M: The coagulation-kinin pathway of human plasma. *Blood* **70**:1, 1987.
3. Colman R: Contact system in infectious disease. *Rev Infect Dis* **11(Supp 4)**:S689, 1989.
4. DeLa Cadena R, Wachtfogel Y, Colman R. Contact activation pathway: Inflammation and coagulation, in: Colman R, Hirsh J, Marder V, Salzman E (eds): *Hemostasis and Thrombosis: Basic Principles and Clinical Practice 3rd ed.* Philadelphia: J.B. Lippincott, 1994, p 219.
5. Kaplan A, Joseph K, Shibayama Y, Reddigari S, Ghebrehiwet B, Silverberg M: The intrinsic coagulation/kinin-forming cascade: Assembly in plasma and cell surfaces in inflammation. *Adv Immunol* **66**:225, 1997.
6. Macfarlane R: An enzyme cascade in the blood clotting mechanism, and its function as a biochemical amplifier. *Nature* **202**:498, 1964.
7. Davie E, Ratnoff O: Waterfall sequence for intrinsic clotting. *Science* **145**:1310, 1964.
8. Niewiarowski S, Prou-Wartelle O: Role du facteur contact (facteur Hageman) dans La fibrinolyse. *Thromb Diath Haemorrh* **3**:593, 1959.
9. Armstrong D, Keele C, Jepson J, Stewart J: Development of pain-producing substance in human plasma. *Nature* **174**:791, 1954.
10. Margolis J: Activation of plasma by contact with glass: Evidence of a common reaction which releases plasma kinin and initiates coagulation. *J Physiol (Lond)* **144**:1, 1958.
11. Santoro S, Eby C: Laboratory evaluation of hemostatic disorders, in: Hoffman R, Benz E, Shattil S, Furie B, Cohen H, Silberstein L (eds): *Hematology: Basic Principles and Practice 2nd ed.* New York: Churchill Livingstone, 1995, p 1622.
12. Rosenthal R, Dreskin O, Rosenthal N: New hemophilia-like disease caused by deficiency of a third plasma thromboplastin factor. *Proc Soc Exp Biol Med* **82**:171, 1953.
13. Ratnoff O, Colopy J: A familial hemorrhagic trait associated with a deficiency of a clotpromoting fraction of plasma. *J Clin Invest* **34**:602, 1955.
14. Hathaway W, Belhasen L, Hathaway H: Evidence for a new plasma thromboplastin factor. I. Case report, coagulation studies and physiochemical properties. *Blood* **26**:521, 1965.
15. Saito H, Ratnoff O, Waldmann R, Abraham J: Deficiency of a hitherto unrecognized agent, Fitzgerald factor, participating in surface-mediated reactions of clotting, fibrinolysis, generation of kinins, and the property of diluted plasma enhancing vascular permeability. *J Clin Invest* **55**:1082, 1975.
16. Wuepper K, Miller D, Lacombe M: Flaujeac trait. Deficiency of human plasma kininogen. *J Clin Invest* **56**:1663, 1975.
17. Waldmann R, Abraham J, Rebick J, Caldwell J, Saito H, Ratnoff O: Fitzgerald factor: A hitherto unrecognized coagulation factor. *Lancet* **1**:949, 1975.
18. Colman R, Bagdasarian A, Talamo R, Scott C, Seavey M, Guimaraes J, Pierce J, et al: Williams trait: Human kininogen deficiency with diminished levels of plasminogen proactivator and prekallikrein associated with abnormalities of the Hageman factor-dependent pathways. *J Clin Invest* **56**:1650, 1975.
19. Seligsohn U: Factor XI deficiency. *Thromb Haemost* **70**:68, 1993a.
20. Robinson A, Kropatkin M, Aggeler P: Hageman factor (factor XII) deficiency in marine mammals. *Science* **166**:1420, 1969.
21. Lewis J, Bayer W, Szeto I: Coagulation factor XII deficiency in the porpoise, *Tursiops truncatus*. *Comp Biochem Physiol* **31**:667, 1969.
22. Broze G, Girard T, Novotny W: Regulation of coagulation by a multivalent Kunitz-type inhibitor. *Biochemistry* **29**:7539, 1990.
23. Gailani D, Broze G: Factor XI activation in a revised model of blood coagulation. *Science* **253**:909, 1991.
24. Broze G: The role of tissue factor pathway inhibitor in a revised coagulation cascade. *Semin Hematol* **29**:159, 1992.
25. Broze G, Gailani D: The role of factor XI in coagulation. *Thromb Haemost* **70**:72, 1993.
26. Naito K, Fujikawa K: Activation of human blood coagulation factor XI independent of factor XII: Factor XI is activated by thrombin and factor XIa in the presence of negatively charged surfaces. *J Biol Chem* **266**:7353, 1991.
27. Colman R, Schmaier A: Contact system: A vascular biology modulator with anticoagulant, profibrinolytic, antiadhesive, and proinflammatory attributes. *Blood* **90**:3819, 1997.
28. Reddigari S, Shibayama Y, Brunnee T, Kaplan A: Human Hageman factor (FXII) and high molecular weight kininogen compete for the same binding site on human umbilical vein endothelial cells. *J Biol Chem* **268**:11982, 1993.
29. Motta G, Rojkjaer R, Hasan AAK, Cines DB, Schmaier AH: High molecular weight kininogen regulates prekallikrein assembly and activation on endothelial cells: A novel mechanism for contact activation. *Blood* **91**:516, 1998.
30. Davie E, Fujikawa K, Kisiel W: The coagulation cascade: Initiation, maintenance and regulation. *Biochemistry* **30**:10363, 1991.
31. Cochrane C, Revak S, Wuepper K: Activation of Hageman factor in solid and fluid phases: A critical role for prekallikrein. *J Exp Med* **138**:1564, 1973.
32. Hattersley P, Hayse D: Fletcher factor deficiency: A report of three unrelated cases. *Brit J Haematol* **18**:411, 1970.
33. Silverberg M, Dunn JT, Garen L, Kaplan AP: Autoactivation of human Hageman factor: Demonstration utilizing a synthetic substrate. *J Biol Chem* **255**:7281, 1980.
34. Tans G, J R, Griffin J: Sulfatide-dependent autoactivation of human blood coagulation factor XII (Hageman factor). *J Biol Chem* **258**:8215, 1983.
35. Ratnoff O, Saito H: Amidolytic properties of a single chain activated Hageman factor. *Proc Natl Acad Sci U S A* **76**:1411, 1979.
36. Morgan P, Robinson N, Walsh K, Neurath H: Inactivation of bovine trypsinogen and chymotrypsinogen by diisopropyl phosphofluoridate. *Proc Natl Acad Sci U S A* **69**:3312, 1972.
37. Heimark R, Kurachi K, Fujikawa K, Davie E: Surface activation of blood coagulation, fibrinolysis and kinin formation. *Nature* **286**:456, 1980.
38. Kurachi K, Fujikawa K, Davie E: Mechanism of activation of bovine factor XI by factor XII and factor XIIa. *Biochemistry* **19**:1330, 1980.
39. Tankersley DL, Finlayson JS: Kinetics of activation and autoactivation of human factor XII. *Biochemistry* **23**:273, 1984.
40. Donaldson V, Glueck H, Miller M, Movat H, Habal F: Kininogen deficiency in Fitzgerald trait: Role of high molecular weight kininogen in clotting and fibrinolysis. *J Lab Clin Med* **87**:327, 1976.
41. Griffin J, Cochrane C: Mechanism for the involvement of high molecular weight kininogen in surface-dependent reactions of Hageman factor. *Proc Natl Acad Sci U S A* **73**:2554, 1976.
42. Saito H: Purification of high molecular weight kininogen and the role of this agent in blood coagulation. *J Clin Invest* **60**:584, 1977.
43. Wiggins R, Bouma B, Cochrane C, Griffin J: Role of high molecular weight kininogen in surface-binding and activation of coagulation factor XI and prekallikrein. *Proc Natl Acad Sci U S A* **74**:4636, 1977.
44. Thompson R, Mandle R, Kaplan A: Studies of binding of prekallikrein and factor XI to high molecular weight kininogen and its light chain. *Proc Natl Acad Sci U S A* **76**:4862, 1979.

45. Mandle R, Colman R, Kaplan A: Identification of prekallikrein and high molecular weight kininogen as a complex in human plasma. *Proc Natl Acad Sci U S A* **73**:4179, 1976.
46. Kerbiriou D, Bouma B, Griffin J: Immunochemical studies of human high molecular weight kininogen and of its complexes with plasma prekallikrein or kallikrein. *J Biol Chem* **255**:3952, 1980.
47. Reddigari S, Kaplan A: Quantification of human high molecular weight kininogen by immunoblotting with a monoclonal anti-light chain antibody. *J Immunol Methods* **119**:19, 1989.
48. Kurachi K, Davie E: Activation of human factor XI (plasma thromboplastin antecedent) by factor XIIa (activated Hageman factor). *Biochemistry* **16**:5831, 1977.
49. Bouma B, Griffin J: Human blood coagulation factor XI, purification, properties, and mechanism of activation by activated factor XII. *J Biol Chem* **252**:6432, 1977.
50. Cochrane C, Griffin J: The biochemistry and pathophysiology of the contact system of plasma. *Adv Immunol* **33**:241, 1982.
51. Muller-Esterl W, Iwanaga S, Nakanishi S: Kininogens revisited. *TIBS* **11**:336, 1986.
52. Miles LA, Rothschild Z, Griffin J: Dextran sulfate stimulated fibrinolytic activity in whole human plasma. Dependence on the contact activation system and a urokinase-related antigen. *Thromb Haemost* **46**:211, 1981.
53. Kluft C, Wijngaards G, Jie A: Intrinsic plasma fibrinolysis: Involvement of urokinase-related activity in the factor XII-independent plasminogen proactivator pathway. *J Lab Clin Med* **103**:408, 1984.
54. Hauert J, Bachmann F: Prourokinase activation in euglobulin fractions. *Thromb Haemost* **54**:122, 1985.
55. Ichinose A, Fujikawa K, Suyama T: The activation of pro-urokinase by plasma kallikrein and its inactivation by thrombin. *J Biol Chem* **261**:3486, 1986.
56. Goldsmith G, Saito H, Ratnoff OD: The activation of plasminogen by Hageman FXII (factor XII) and Hageman factor fragments. *J Clin Invest* **62**:54, 1978.
57. Mandle R, Kaplan A: Hageman factor dependent fibrinolysis. Generation of fibrinolytic activity by the interaction of human activated factor XI and plasminogen. *Blood* **54**:850, 1979.
58. Miles L, Greengard J, Griffin J: A comparison of the abilities of plasma kallikrein, b-factor XIIa, factor XIa and urokinase to activate plasminogen. *Thromb Res* **29**:407, 1983.
59. Cochrane C, Revak S: Dissemination of contact activation in plasma by plasma kallikrein. *J Exp Med* **152**:608, 1985.
60. Sealey J, Atlas S, Laragh J, Silverberg M, Kaplan A: Initiation of plasma prorenin activation by Hageman factor-dependent conversion of prekallikrein to kallikrein. *Proc Natl Acad Sci U S A* **76**:5914, 1979.
61. Derkx F, Bouma B, Schalekamp M, Schalekamp M: An intrinsic factor XII-prekallikrein-dependent pathway activates the human plasma renin-angiotensin system. *Nature* **280**:315, 1979.
62. Blumberg A, Sealey J, Atlas S, Laragh J, Dharmgrongartama B, Kaplan A: Contact activation of plasma prorenin in vitro. *J Lab Clin Med* **97**:771, 1981.
63. DiScipio R: The activation of the alternative pathway C3 convertase by human plasma kallikrein. *Immunology* **45**:587, 1982.
64. Revak S, Cochrane C, Griffin J: Structural changes accompanying enzymatic activation of Hageman factor. *J Clin Invest* **54**:619, 1974.
65. Revak S, Cochrane C, Griffin J: The binding and cleavage characteristics of human Hageman factor during contact activation: A comparison of normal plasma with plasmas deficient in factor XI, prekallikrein, or high molecular weight kininogen. *J Clin Invest* **59**:1167, 1977.
66. Revak SD, Cochrane CG, Bouma BN, Griffin JH: Surface and fluid phase activities of two forms of activated Hageman factor produced during contact activation of plasma. *J Exp Med* **147**:719, 1978.
67. Ghebrehiwet B, Randazzo B, Dunn J, Silverberg M, Kaplan A: Mechanisms of activation of the classical pathway of complement by Hageman factor fragment. *J Clin Invest* **71**:1450, 1983.
68. Moskowitz R, Schwartz H, Michel B, Ratnoff O: Generation of kinin-like agents by chondroitin sulfate, heparin, chitin sulfate, and human articular cartilage: Possible pathophysiologic implications. *J Lab Clin Med* **76**:790, 1970.
69. Hojima Y, Cochrane C, Wiggins R, Austen K, Stevens R: *In vitro* activation of the contact (Hageman factor) system of plasma by heparin and chondroitin sulfate. *Blood* **63**:1453, 1984.
70. Shimada T, Kato H, Iwanaga S, Iwamori M, Nagai Y: Activation of factor XII and prekallikrein with cholesterol sulfate. *Thromb Res* **38**:21, 1985.
71. Griep M, Fujikawa K, Nelsestuen G: Binding and activation properties of human factor XII, prekallikrein, and derived peptides with acidic lipid vesicles. *Biochemistry* **24**:4124, 1985.
72. van der Graaf F, Keus F, Vlooswijk R, Bouma B: The contact activation mechanism of human plasma: Activation induced by dextran sulfate. *Blood* **59**:1225, 1982.
73. Joseph K, Ghebrehiwet B, Peerschke EIB, Reid KBM, Kaplan AP: Identification of the zinc-dependent endothelial cell binding protein for high molecular weight kininogen and factor XII. Identity with the receptor that binds to the globular "heads" of C1q (gC1qR). *Proc Natl Acad Sci U S A* **93**:8552, 1996.
74. Herwald H, Renne T, Meijers J, Chung D, Page J, Colman R: Mapping of the discontinuous kininogen binding site of prekallikrein. *J Biol Chem* **271**:13061, 1996.
75. Dedio J, Mueller-Esterl W: Kininogen binding protein p33/gC1qR is localized in the vesicular fraction of endothelial cells. *FEBS Lett* **399**:255, 1996.
76. Rapaport S, Proctor R, Patch M, Yettra M: The mode of inheritance of PTA deficiency: Evidence for the existence of major PTA deficiency and minor PTA deficiency. *Blood* **18**:149, 1961.
77. Leiba H, Ramot B, Many R: Heredity and coagulation studies in ten families with factor XI (plasma thromboplastin antecedent) deficiency. *Br J Haematol* **11**:654, 1965.
78. Britten A, Salzman E: Surgery in congenital disorders of blood coagulation. *Surg Gynecol Obstet* **123**:1333, 1966.
79. Ragni M, Sinha D, Seaman F, Lewis J, Spero J, Walsh P: Comparison of bleeding tendency, factor XI coagulant activity, and factor XI antigen in 25 factor XI-deficient kindreds. *Blood* **65**:719, 1985.
80. Bolton-Maggs P, Wan-Yin B, McGraw A, Slack J, Kernoff P: Inheritance and bleeding in factor XI deficiency. *Br J Haematol* **69**:521, 1988.
81. Rapaport S, Rao L: Initiation and regulation of tissue factor-dependent blood coagulation. *Arterioscler Thromb Vasc Biol* **12**:1111, 1992.
82. Nemerson Y: The tissue factor pathway of blood coagulation. *Semin Hematol* **29**:170, 1992.
83. Furie B, Furie B: The molecular basis of blood coagulation. *Cell* **53**:505, 1988.
84. Furie B, Furie B: Molecular and cellular biology of blood coagulation. *N Engl J Med* **326**:800, 1992.
85. Asakai R, Chung D, Davie E, Seligsohn U: Factor XI deficiency in Ashkenazi Jews in Israel. *N Eng J Med* **325**:153, 1991.
86. Gailani D, Broze G: Effects of glycosaminoglycans on factor XI activation by thrombin. *Blood Coagul Fibrinolysis* **4**:15, 1993.
87. Gailani D, Broze G: Factor XI activation by thrombin and factor XIa. *Semin Thromb Hemost* **19**:396, 1993.
88. Gailani D, Broze G: Factor XII-independent activation of factor XI in plasma: Effects of sulfatides on tissue factor-induced coagulation. *Blood* **82**:813, 1993.
89. von dem Borne P, Meijers J, Bouma, BN: Feedback activation of factor XI by thrombin in plasma results in additional formation of thrombin that protects fibrin clots from fibrinolysis. *Blood* **86**:3035, 1995.
90. Baglia F, Walsh P: Prothrombin is a cofactor for binding of factor XI to the platelet surface and for platelet-mediated factor XI activation by thrombin. *Biochemistry* **37**:2271, 1998.
91. Minnema M, Friederick P, Levi M, von dem Borne P, Mosnier L, Meijers J, Briemond B, et al: Enhancement of rabbit jugular vein thrombolysis by neutralization of factor XI. *In vivo* evidence for a role of factor XI as an anti-fibrinolytic factor. *J Clin Invest* **101**:10, 1998.
92. Bajzar L, Manuci R, Nesheim M: Purification and characterization of TAFI, a thrombin-activatable fibrinolysis inhibitor. *J Biol Chem* **270**:14477, 1995.
93. Redlitz A, Tan A, Eaton D, Plow E: Plasma carboxypeptidases as regulators of the plasminogen system. *J Clin Invest* **96**:2534, 1995.
94. Broze G, Higuchi D: Coagulation-dependent inhibition of fibrinolysis: Role of carboxypeptidase-U and the premature lysis of clots from hemophilic plasma. *Blood* **88**:3815, 1996.
95. Saito H, Goldsmith G: Plasma thromboplastin antecedent (factor XI): A specific and sensitive radioimmunoassay. *Blood* **50**:377, 1977.
96. Thompson R, Mandle R, Kaplan A: Association of factor XI and high molecular weight kininogen in human plasma. *J Clin Invest* **60**:1376, 1977.
97. Fujikawa K, Lagaz M, Kato H, Davie E: The mechanism of activation of bovine factor IX (Christmas factor) by bovine factor XIa (activated plasma thromboplastin antecedent). *Biochemistry* **13**:4508, 1974.

98. Mashiko H: Factor XI: Purification from porcine plasma by affinity chromatography and some properties of factor XI and activated factor XI. *Biol Chem Hoppe Seyler* **375**:481, 1994.
99. Wiggins R, Cochrane C, Griffin J: Rabbit blood coagulation factor XI: Purification and properties. *Thromb Res* **15**:475, 1979.
100. Gailani D, Sun M, Sun Y: A comparison of murine and human factor XI. *Blood* **90**:1055, 1997.
101. Hsu T, Shore S, Seshsmma T, Bagasra O, Walsh P: Molecular cloning of platelet factor XI, an alternative splicing product of the plasma factor XI gene. *J Biol Chem* **273**:13787, 1998.
102. Martincic D, Kravtsov V, Gailani D: Factor XI messenger RNA in human platelets. *Blood* **94**:3397, 1999.
103. Dzik W, Arkin C, Jenkins R: Transfer of congenital factor XI deficiency from a donor to a recipient by liver transplantation. *N Engl J Med* **316**:1217, 1987.
104. Clarkson K, Rosenfeld B, Fair J, a K, Bell W: Factor XI deficiency acquired by liver transplantation. *Ann Int Med* **115**:877, 1991.
105. Asakai R, Davie E, Chung D: Organization of the gene for human factor XI. *Biochemistry* **26**:7221, 1987.
106. Fujikawa K, Chung D, Hendrickson L, Davie E: Amino acid sequence of human factor XI, a blood coagulation factor with four tandem repeats that are highly homologous with plasma prekallikrein. *Biochemistry* **25**:2417, 1986.
107. McMullen B, Fujikawa K, Davie E: Location of the disulfide bonds in human coagulation factor XI: The presence of tandem apple domains. *Biochemistry* **30**:2056, 1991.
108. Chung D, Fujikawa K, McMullen B, Davie E: Human plasma prekallikrein, a zymogen to a serine protease that contains four tandem repeats. *Biochemistry* **25**:2410, 1986.
109. McMullen B, Fujikawa K, Davie E: Location of the disulfide bonds in human plasma prekallikrein: Presence of four novel apple domains in the amino-terminal portion of the molecule. *Biochemistry* **30**:2050, 1991.
110. Beaubien G, Rosinski-Chupin I, Mattei M, Mbikay M, Chretien M, Seidah N: Gene structure and chromosomal localization of plasma prekallikrein. *Biochemistry* **30**:1628, 1991.
111. Kunapuli S, Stark P, Rick L, Colman R: Determination of gene structure by intron trapping using polymerase chain reaction: Application to the plasma prekallikrein gene. *DNA Cell Biol* **14**:343, 1995.
112. Kato A, Asakai R, Davie E, Aoki N: Factor XI gene (F11) is located on the distal end of the long arm of human chromosome 4. *Cytogenet Cell Genet* **52**:77, 1989.
113. Mills K, Mathews K, Scherpbier-Heddema T, Schelper R, Schmalzel R, Bailey H, Nadeau J, et al: Genetic mapping near the myd locus on mouse chromsome 8. *Mamm Genome* **6**:278, 1995.
114. van der Graaf F, Greengard J, Bouma B, Kerbiriou D, Griffin J: Isolation and functional characterization of the active light chain of activated human blood coagulation factor XI. *J Biol Chem* **258**:9669, 1983.
115. Saito H, Ratnoff O, Marshall J, Pensky J: Partial purification of plasma thromboplastin antecedent (factor XI) and activation by trypsin. *J Clin Invest* **52**:850, 1973.
116. Mannhalter C, Schiffman S, Jacobs A: Trypsin activation of human factor XI. *J Biol Chem* **255**:2667, 1980.
117. von dem Borne P, Mosnier L, Tans G, Meijers J, Bouma B: Factor XI activation by meizothrombin: Stimulation by phospholipid vesicles containing both phosphotidylserine and phosphotidylethanolamine. *Thromb Haemost* **78**:834, 1997.
118. Sinha D, Seaman F, Koshy A, Walsh P: Blood coagulation factor XIa binds specifically to a site on activated human platelets distinct from that of factor XI. *J Clin Invest* **73**:1559, 1984.
119. Greengard J, Heeb M, McGann M, Ersdal E, Griffin J: Coordinate Zn++ and Ca++ ion-dependent binding of high molecular weight kininogen and factor XI to platelets. *Circulation* **70**(Supp II):1409(abstract), 1984.
120. Greengard J, Heeb M, Ersdal E, Walsh P, Griffin J: Binding of coagulation factor XI to washed human platelets. *Biochemistry* **25**:3884, 1986.
121. DiScipio R, Kurachi K, Davie E: Activation of human factor IX (Christmas factor). *J Clin Invest* **61**:1528, 1978.
122. Osterud B, Bouma B, Griffin G: Human blood coagulation factor IX: Purification, properties, and mechanism of activation by activated factor XI. *J Biol Chem* **253**:5946, 1978.
123. Bajaj S: Cooperative calcium binding to human factor IX: Effects of calcium on the kinetic parameters of the activation of factor IX by factor XIa. *J Biol Chem* **257**:4127, 1982.
124. Walsh B, Bradford H, Sinha D, Piperno J, Tuszynzki G: Kinetics of the factor XIa catalyzed activation of human coagulation factor IX. *J Clin Invest* **73**:1392, 1984.
125. Lindquist P, Fujikawa K, Davie E: Activation of bovine factor IX (Christmas factor) by factor XIa (activated plasma thromboplastin antecedent) and a protease from Russel's viper venom. *J Biol Chem* **253**:1902, 1978.
126. Kurachi K, Davie E: Isolation and characterization of a cDNA coding for human factor IX. *Proc Natl Acad Sci U S A* **79**:6461, 1982.
127. Seikiya F, Yamashita T, Atoda H, Komiyama Y, Morita T: Regulation of the tertiary structure and function of coagulation factor IX by magnesium (II) ions. *J Biol Chem* **270**:14325, 1995.
128. Griffin JH: Role of surface-dependent activation of Hageman factor (blood coagulation factor XII). *Proc Natl Acad Sci U S A* **75**:1997, 1978.
129. Mandle R, Kaplan A: Hageman factor substrates. Human prekallikrein: Mechanism of activation by Hageman factor and participation in Hageman factor-dependent fibrinolysis. *J Biol Chem* **252**:6097, 1977.
130. Saito H: The participation of plasma thromboplastin antecedent (factor XI) in contact-activated fibrinolysis. *Proc Soc Exp Biol Med* **164**:153, 1980.
131. Scott C, Silver L, Purdon D, Colman R: Cleavage of human high molecular weight kininogen by factor XIa in vitro. *J Biol Chem* **260**:10856, 1985.
132. Baglia F, Jameson B, Walsh P: Fine mapping of the high molecular weight kininogen binding site on blood coagulation factor XI through the use of rationally designed synthetic analogs. *J Biol Chem* **267**:4247, 1992.
133. Baglia F, Walsh P: A binding site for thrombin in the apple 1 domain of factor XI. *J Biol Chem* **271**:3652, 1996.
134. Baglia F, Jameson B, Walsh P: Identification and characterization for a binding site for factor XIIa in the apple 4 domain of coagulation factor XI. *J Biol Chem* **268**:3838, 1993.
135. Meijers J, Davie E, Chung D: Expression of human blood coagulation factor XI: Characterization of the defect in factor XI type III deficiency. *Blood* **79**:1435, 1992.
136. Meijers J, Mulvihill E, Davie E, Chung D: Apple 4 in human blood coagulation factor XI mediates dimer formation. *Biochemistry* **31**:4680, 1992.
137. Baglia F, Jameson B, Walsh P: Identification and chemical synthesis of a substrate binding site for factor IX on coagulation factor XIa. *J Biol Chem* **266**, 1991.
138. Sun Y, Gailani D: Identification of a factor IX binding site on the third apple domain of activated factor XI. *J Biol Chem* **271**:29023, 1996.
139. Sun M-F, Zhao M, Gailani D: Identification of amino acids in the factor XI apple 3 domain required for activation of factor IX. *J Biol Chem* **274**:36373, 1999.
140. Baglia F, Jameson B, Walsh P: Identification and characterization of a binding site for platelets in the apple 3 domain of coagulation factor XI. *J Biol Chem* **270**:6734, 1995.
141. Ho D, Baglia F, Zhao M, Gailani D, Walsh P: Fine mapping of a platelet binding site in the apple 3 domain of factor XI. *Blood* **92**:708a-709a(Abstract), 1998.
142. Ho D, Baglia F, Walsh P: Identification of contiguous and distinct binding sites for platelets and heparin in the apple 3 domain of coagulation factor XI. *Blood* **88**:282a(Abstract), 1996.
143. Zhao M, Abdel-Razek T, Sun M, Gailani D: Characterization of a heparin binding site on the heavy chain of factor XI. *J Biol Chem* **273**:31153, 1998.
144. Heck L, Kaplan A: Substrates of Hageman factor: I. Isolation and characterization of human factor XI (PTA) and inhibition of the activated enzyme by alpha-1-antitrypsin. *J Exp Med* **140**:1615, 1974.
145. Scott C, Schapira M, James H, Cohen A, Colman R: Inactivation of factor XIa by plasma protease inhibitors: Predominant role of alpha-1-protease inhibitor and protective effect of high molecular weight kininogen. *J Clin Invest* **69**:844, 1982.
146. Damus P, Hick M, Rosenberg R: Anticoagulant action of heparin. *Nature* **240**:355, 1973.
147. Scott C, Colman R: Factors influencing the acceleration of human factor XIa inactivation by antithrombin III. *Blood* **73**:1873, 1989.
148. Soons H, Janssen-Claesson T, Tans G, Hemker H: Inhibition of factor XIa by antithrombin III. *Biochemistry* **26**:4624, 1989.
149. Forbes C, Pensky J, Ratnoff O: Inactivation of activated Hageman factor and activated partial thromboplastin antecedent by purified serum C1 inactivator. *J Lab Clin Med* **76**:809, 1970.
150. Meijers J, Vlooswijk R, Bouma B: Inhibition of human blood coagulation factor XIa by C1 inhibitor. *Biochemistry* **27**:959, 1988.

151. Saito H, Goldsmith G, Moroi M, Aoki N: Inhibitory spectrum of alpha-2-antiplasmin inhibitor. *Proc Natl Acad Sci U S A* **76**:2103, 1979.
152. Meijers J, Kanters D, Vlooswijk R, van Erp H, Hessing M, Bouma B: Inactivation of human plasma kallikrein and factor XIa by protein C inhibitor. *Biochemistry* **27**:4231, 1988.
153. Smith R, Higuchi D, Broze G: Platelet coagulation factor XIa-inhibitor, a form of Alzheimer Amyloid Precursor Protein. *Science* **248**:1126, 1990.
154. Smith R, Broze G: Characterization of platelet-releasable forms of beta-amyloid precursor protein: The effect of thrombin. *Blood* **80**:2252, 1992.
155. Wuillemin W, Minnema M, Meijers J, Roem D, Eerenberg A, Niujens J, ten Cate H, et al: Inactivation of factor XIa in human plasma assessed by measuring factor XIa-protease inhibitor complexes: Major role for C1-Inhibitor. *Blood* **85**:1517, 1995.
156. Wuillemin W, Eldering E, Citarell F, de Ruig C, ten Cate H, Hack C: Modulation of contact system proteases by Glycosaminoglycans: Selective enhancement of the inhibition of factor XIa. *J Biol Chem* **271**:12913, 1996.
157. Beeler D, Marcum J, Schiffman S, Rosenberg R: Interaction of factor XIa and antithrombin in the presence and absence of heparin. *Blood* **67**:1488, 1986.
158. Tuszynski G, Bevacqua S, Schmaier A, Colman R, Walsh P: Factor XI antigen and activity in human platelets. *Blood* **59**:1148, 1982.
159. Schiffman S, Rimon A, Rapaport S: Factor XI and platelets: Evidence that platelets contain only minimal factor XI activity and antigen. *Br J Haematol* **35**:429, 1977.
160. Osterud B, Harper E, Rapaport S, Lavine K: Evidence against collagen activation of platelet-associated factor XI as a mechanism for initiating intrinsic clotting. *Scand J Haematol* **22**:205, 1979.
160a. Schiffman S, Yeh C-H: Purification and characterization of platelet factor XI. *Thromb Res* **60**:87, 1990.
161. Komiyama Y, Nomura S, Murakami T, Masuda M, Egawa H, Murata L, Okubo S, et al: Purification and characterization of platelet-type factor XI from human platelets. *Thromb Haemost* **69**:1238(Abstract), 1993.
162. Hu C, Baglia F, Mills D, Konkle B, Walsh P: Tissue-specific expression of functional platelet factor XI is independent of plasma factor XI expression. *Blood* **91**:3800, 1998.
163. Drinkwater C, Evans B, Richards R: Kallikreins, kinins and growth factor biosynthesis. *TIBS* **13**:169, 1988.
164. Wuepper K, Cochrane C: Plasma prekallikrein: Isolation, characterization and mechanism of activation. *J Exp Med* **135**:1, 1972.
165. Bouma B, Keribiriou D, Vlooswijk R, Griffin J: Immunological studies of prekallikrein, kallikrein and high molecular weight kininogen in normal and deficient plasmas and in normal plasma after cold-dependent activation. *J Lab Clin Med* **96**:693, 1980.
166. Kanapuli S, Stark P, Rick L, Colman R: Determination of gene structure by intron trapping using polymerase chain reaction: Application to the human plasma prekallikrein gene. *DNA Cell Biol* **14**:343, 1995.
167. Seidah N, Sawyer N, Hamelin J, Mion P, Beaubien G, Brachpapa L, Rochemont J, et al: Mouse plasma kallikrein: cDNA structure, enzyme characterization, and comparison of protein and mRNA levels among species. *DNA Cell Biol* **9**:737, 1990.
168. van der Graaf F, Tans G, Bouma B, Griffin J: Isolation and functional properties of the heavy and light chains of human plasma kallikrein. *J Biol Chem* **257**:14300, 1982.
169. Rosing J, Tans G, Griffin J: Surface-dependent activation of human factor XII (Hageman factor) by kallikrein and its light chain. *Eur J Biochem* **151**:531, 1985.
170. Bouma B, Miles L, Beretta G, Griffin J: Human plasma prekallikrein: Studies of its activation by activated factor XII and of its inactivation by diisopropyl phosphofluoridate. *Biochemistry* **19**:1151, 1980.
171. Tans G, Rosing J, Berrettini M, Lammle B, Griffin J: Autoactivation of plasma prekallikrein. *J Biol Chem* **262**:11308, 1987.
172. Colman R, Wachtfogel Y, Kucich U, Weinbaum G, Hahn S, Pixley R, Scott C, et al: Effects of cleavage of the heavy chain of human plasma kallikrein on its functional properties. *Blood* **65**:311, 1985.
173. Burger D, Schleuning W, Scahpira M: Human plasma prekallikrein: Immunoaffinity purification and activation to a- and b-kallikrein. *J Biol Chem* **262**:324, 1986.
174. Keribiriou D, Griffin J: High molecular weight kininogen. Studies of structure-function relationships and of proteolysis of the molecule during contact activation of plasma. *J Biol Chem* **254**:12020, 1979.
175. Nakayasa T, Nagasawa S: Studies on human kininogen I. Isolation, characterization, and cleavage by plasma kallikrein of high molecular weight (HMW) kininogen. *J Biochem* **85**:249, 1979.
176. Mori K, Nagasawa S: Studies on human high molecular weight (HMW) kininogen II. Structural change of HMW-kininogen by the action of human plasma kallikrein. *J Biochem* **84**:1465, 1981.
177. Seligsohn U, Osterud B, Griffin J, Rapaport S: Evidence for the participation of both activated factor XII and activated factor IX in cold-promoted activation of factor VII. *Thromb Res* **13**:1049, 1978.
178. Seligsohn U, Osterud B, Brown J, Griffin J, Rapaport S: Activation of factor VII in plasma and purified systems. *J Clin Invest* **64**:1056, 1979.
179. Gustafson E, Colman R: Interaction of polymorphonuclear cells with contact activation factors. *Semin Thromb Hemost* **13**:95, 1987.
180. Gallin JI, Kaplan A: Mononuclear cell chemotactic activity of kallikrein and plasminogen activator and its inhibition by C1-INH and α_2-macroglobulin. *J Immunol* **113**:1928, 1974.
181. van der Graaf F, Koedam J, Bouma B: Inactivation of kallikrein in human plasma. *J Clin Invest* **71**:149, 1983.
182. van der Graaf F, Rietveld A, Keus F, Bouma B: Interaction of human plasma kallikrein and its light chain with α_2-macroglobulin. *Biochemistry* **23**:1760, 1984.
183. Harpel P, Lewin M, Kaplan A: Distribution of plasma kallikrein between C1-inhibitor and α_2-macroglobulin in plasma utilizing a new assay for α_2-macroglobulin-kallikrein complexes. *J Biol Chem* **260**:4257, 1985.
184. Berrettini M, Schleef R, Espana F, Loskutoff D, Griffin J: Interaction of type 1 plasminogen activator inhibitor with the enzymes of the contact activation system. *J Biol Chem* **264**:11738, 1989.
185. Espana F, Berrettini M, Griffin J: Purification of characterization of plasma protein C inhibitor. *Thromb Res* **55**:369, 1989.
186. Fujikawa K, Davie EW: Human factor XII (Hageman factor). *Methods Enzymol* **80**:10924, 1981.
187. Cool DE, MacGillivray RTA: Characterization of the human blood coagulation factor XII gene. *J Biol Chem* **262**:13662, 1987.
188. Rolye NJ, Nigli M, Cool D, MacGilivray RTA, Hamerton JL: Structural gene encoding human factor XII is located at 5q33-qter. *Somat Cell Mol Genet* **14**:217, 1988.
189. Citarella F, Misiti S, Felici A, Aiuti A, La Porta C, Fantoni A: The 5′ sequence of human factor XII gene contains transcription regulatory elements typical of liver specific, estrogen-modulated genes. *Biochim Biophys Acta* **1172**:197, 1993.
190. Pixley RA, Stumpo LG, Birkmeyer K, Silver L, Colman RW: A monoclonal antibody recognizing an icosapeptide sequence in the heavy chain of human factor XII inhibits surface-catalyzed activation. *J Biol Chem* **262**:10140, 1987.
191. Clarke BJ, Cote HCF, Cool DE, Clark-Lewis I, Saito H, Pixley RA, Colman RW, et al: Mapping of a putative surface-binding site of human coagulation factor XII. *J Biol Chem* **264**:11497, 1989.
192. Rojkjaer R, Schousboe I: Identification of the Zn^{2+} binding sites in factor XII and its activation derivatives. *Eur J Biochem* **247**:491, 1997.
193. Cool D, Edgell C, Louie G, Zoller M, Brayer G, MacGillivray R: Characterization of human blood coagulation factor XII cDNA. *J Biol Chem* **260**:13666, 1985.
194. Gordon EM, Gallagher CA, Johnson TR, Blossey BK, Ilan J: Hepatocytes express blood coagulation factor XII (Hageman factor). *J Lab Clin Med* **115**:463, 1990.
195. Citarella F, Ravon DM, Pascucci B, Felici A, Fantoni A, Hack CE: Structure/function analysis of human factor XII using recombinant deletion mutants. Evidence for an additional region involved in the binding to negatively charged surfaces. *Eur J Biochem* **238**:240, 1996.
196. Gordon EM, Williams SR, Frenchek B, Mazur CA, Speroff L: Dose-dependent effects of postmenopausal estrogen and progestin on antithrombin III and factor XII. *J Lab Clin Med* **111**:52, 1988.
197. Gordon EM, Johnson TR, Ramos LP, Schmeidler-Sapiro KT: Enhanced expression of factor XII (Hageman factor) in isolated livers of estrogen- and prolactin-treated rats. *J Lab Clin Med* **117**:353, 1991.
198. Citarella F, Felici A, Brouwer M, Wagstaff J, Fantoni A, Hack CE: Interleukin-6 downregulates factor XII production by human hepatoma cell line (HepG2). *Blood* **90**:1501, 1997.
199. Fujikawa K, McMullen BA: Amino acid sequence of human β-factor XIIa. *J Biol Chem* **258**:10924, 1983.
200. McMullen BA, Fujikawa K: Amino acid sequence of the heavy chain of human α-factor XIIa (activated Hageman factor). *J Biol Chem* **260**:5328, 1985.

201. Shore JD, Day DE, Bock PE, Olson ST: Acceleration of surface-dependent autocatalytic activation of blood coagulation factor XII by divalent metal ions. *Biochemistry* **26**:2250, 1987.
202. Schousboe I: Contact activation in human plasma is triggered by zinc ion modulation of factor XII (Hageman factor). *Blood Coagul Fibrinolysis* **4**:671, 1993.
203. Bernardo MM, Day DE, Olson ST, Shore JD: Surface-independent acceleration of factor XII activation by zinc ions. II. Direct binding and fluorescence studies. *J Biol Chem* **268**:12477, 1993.
204. Bernardo MM, Day DE, Halvorson HR, Olson ST, Shore JD: Surface-independent acceleration of factor XII activation by zinc ions. II. Direct binding and fluorescence studies. *J Biol Chem* **268**:12477, 1993.
205. Ewald GA, Eisenberg PR: Plasmin-mediated activation of contact system in response to pharmacological thrombolysis. *Circulation* **91**:28, 1995.
206. Dunn JT, Silverberg M, Kaplan AP: The cleavage and formation of activated human Hageman factor by autodigestion and by kallikrein. *J Biol Chem* **257**:1779, 1982.
207. Ghebrehiwet B, Randazzo BP, Dunn JT, Silverberg M, Kaplan AP: Mechanism of activation of the classical pathway of complement by Hageman factor fragment. *J Clin Invest* **71**:1450, 1983.
208. Wiggins RC: Kinin release from high molecular weight kininogen by the action of Hageman factor in the absence of kallikrein. *J Biol Chem* **258**:8963, 1983.
209. Schousboe I: Factor XIIa activation of plasminogen is enhanced by contact activating surfaces and Zn^2. *Blood Coagul Fibrinolysis* **8**:97, 1997.
210. Kisiel W, Fujikawa K, Davie E: Activation of bovine factor VII (proconvertin) by factor XIIa (activated Hageman factor). *Biochemistry* **16**:4189, 1977.
211. Schmedler-Sapiro KT, Ratnoff OD, Gordon EM: Mitogenic effect of coagulation factor XII and factor XIIa on HepG2 cells. *Proc Natl Acad Sci U S A* **88**:4382, 1991.
212. Gordon EM, Venkatesan N, Salazar R, Tang H, Schmeidler K, Buckley S, Warburton D, et al: Factor XII-induced mitogenesis is mediated via a distinct signal transduction pathway that activates a mitogen-activated protein kinase. *Proc Natl Acad Sci U S A* **93**:2174, 1996.
213. Miyazawa K, Shimomura T, Kitamura A, Kondo J, Morimoto Y, Kitamura N: Molecular cloning and sequence analysis of the cDNA for a human serine protease responsible for activation of hepatocyte growth factor. *J Biol Chem* **269**:10024, 1993.
214. Nakamura T, Nishizawa T, Hagiya M, Seki T, Shimonishi M, Sugimura A, Tashiro K, et al: Molecular cloning and expression of human hepatocyte growth factor. *Nature* **342**:440, 1989.
215. Pixley RA, Schapira M, Colman RW: The regulation of human factor XIIa by plasma protease inhibitors. *J Biol Chem* **260**:1723, 1985.
216. Pixley RA, Colman RW: Effect of heparin on the inactivation rate of human activated factor XII by antithrombin III. *Blood* **66**:198, 1985.
217. Kleniewski J, Donaldson VH: Endothelial cells produce a substance that inhibits contact activation of coagulation by blocking the activation of Hageman factor. *Proc Natl Acad Sci U S A* **90**:198, 1993.
218. Henry ML, Everson B, Ratnoff OD: Inhibition of the activation of Hageman factor (Factor XII) by β_2-glycoprotein I. *J Lab Clin Med* **111**:519, 1988.
219. Rehmus EH, Greene BM, Everson BA, Ratnoff OD: Inhibition of the activation of Hageman factor (factor XII) by complement subcomponent Clq. *J Clin Invest* **80**:516, 1987.
220. Weisel JW, Nagaswami C, Woodhead JL, DeLa Cadena RA, Page JD, Colman RW: The shape of high molecular weight kininogen: Organization into structural domains, changes with activation, and interactions with prekallikrein, as determined by electron microscopy. *J Biol Chem* **269**:10100, 1994.
221. Ohkubo I, Kurachi K, Takasawa T, Shiokawa H, Sasaki M: Isolation of a human cDNA for alpha 2-thiol proteinase inhibitor and its identity with low molecular weight kininogen. *Biochemistry* **23**:5691, 1984.
222. Takagaki Y, Kitamura N, Nakanishi S: Cloning and sequence analysis of cDNAs for human high molecular weight and low molecular weight prekininogens. Primary structures of two human prekininogens. *J Biol Chem* **260**:8601, 1985.
223. Kitamura N, Kitagawa H, Fukushima D, Takagaki Y, Miyata T, Nakanishi S: Structural organization of the human kininogen gene and a model for its evolution. *J Biol Chem* **260**:8610, 1985.
224. Cheung PP, Cannizzaro LA, Colman RW: Chromosomal mapping of human kininogen gene (KNG) to 3q26-qter. *Cytogenet Cell Genet* **59**:24, 1992.
225. Rizzu P, Baldini A: Three members of the human cystatin gene superfamily, AHSG, HRG, and KNG, map within one megabase of genomic DNA at 3q27. *Cytogenet Cell Genet* **70**:26, 1995.
226. Schmaier AH, Kuo A, Lundberg D, Murray S, Cines DB: The expression of high molecular weight kininogen on human umbilical vein endothelial cells. *J Biol Chem* **263**:16327, 1988.
227. Gustafson EJ, Schmaier AH, Wachtfogel YT, Kaufman N, Kucich U, Colman RW: Human neutrophils contain and bind high molecular weight kininogen. *J Clin Invest* **84**:28, 1989.
228. Proud D, Perkins M, Pierce JV, Yates KN, Highet PF, Herring PL, Mangkornkano M, et al: Characterization and localization of human renal kininogen. *J Biol Chem* **256**:10634, 1981.
229. Hallbach J, Adams G, Wirthensohn G, Guder WG: Quantification of kininogen in human renal medulla. *Biol Chem Hoppe Seyler* **368**:1151, 1987.
230. Yamamoto T, Tsuruta J, Kambara T: Interstitial-tissue localization of high molecular weight kininogen in guinea-pig skin. *Biochim Biophys Acta* **916**:332, 1987.
231. Schmaier AH, Zuckerberg A, Silverman C, Kuchibhotla J, Tuszynski GP, Colman RW: High molecular weight kininogen. A secreted platelet protein. *J Clin Invest* **71**:1477, 1983.
232. Kerbiriou-Nabias DM, Garcia FO, Larrieu MJ: Radioimmunoassays of human high and low molecular weight kininogens in plasmas and platelets. *Br J Haematol* **56**:273, 1984.
233. Schmaier AH, Smith PM, Purdon AD, White JG, Colman RW: High molecular weight kininogen: Localization in the unstimulated and activated platelet and activation by a platelet calpain(s). *Blood* **67**:119, 1986.
234. Chen LM, Chung P, Chao S, Chao L, Chao J: Differential regulation of kininogen gene expression by estrogen and progesterone in vivo. *Biochim Biophys Acta* **1131**:145, 1992.
235. Chibber G, Cohen A, Lane S, Farber A, Meloni FJ, Schmaier AH: Immunoblotting of plasma in a pregnant patient with hereditary angioedema. *J Lab Clin Med* **115**:112, 1990.
236. Takano M, Yokoyama K, Yayama K, Okamoto H: Murine fibroblasts synthesize and secrete kininogen in response to cyclic-AMP, prostaglandin E_2 and tumor necrosis factor. *Biochim Biophys Acta* **1265**:189, 1995.
237. Scott C, Colman R: Fibrinogen blocks the autoactivation and thrombin-mediated activation of factor XI on dextran sulfate. *Proc Natl Acad Sci U S A* **89**:11189, 1992.
238. Salvesen G, Parkes C, Abrahamson M, Grubb A, Barrett AJ: Human low-Mr kininogen contains three copies of a cystatin sequence that are divergent in structure and in inhibitory activity for cysteine proteinases. *Biochem J* **234**:429, 1986.
239. Croxatto HR, Boric MP, Roblero J, Albertini R, Silva R: Digestive process and regulation of renal excretory function. Pepsanurin and prokinin inhibitors of diuresis mediated by atrial natriuretic peptide. *Rev Med Chile* **122**:1162, 1995.
240. Croxatto HR, Silva R, Figueroa X, Albertini R, Roblero J, Boric MP: A peptide released by pepsin from kininogen domain 1 is a potent blocker of ANP-mediated diuresis-natriuresis in the rat. *Hypertension* **30**:897, 1997.
241. Ishiguro H, Higashiyama S, Ohkubo I, Sasaki M: Heavy chain of human high molecular weight and low molecular weight kininogen binds calcium ion. *Biochemistry* **26**:7021, 1987.
242. Bradford HN, Jameson BA, Adam AA, Wassell RP, Colman RW: Contiguous binding and inhibitory sites on kininogens required for the inhibition of platelet calpain. *J Biol Chem* **268**:26546, 1993.
243. Bano B, Kanapuli S, Bradford H, Colman R: Structural requirements for cathepsin B and cathepsin h inhibition by kininogens. *J Protein Chem* **15**:519, 1996.
244. Kunapuli SP, Bradford HN, Hameson BA, DeLa Cadena RA, Rick L, Wassell RP, Colman RW: Thrombin-induced platelet aggregation is inhibited by the heptapeptide Leu271-Ala277 of domain 3 in the heavy chain of high molecular weight kininogen. *J Biol Chem* **271**:11228, 1996.
245. Bradford HN, Dela Cadena RA, Kunapuli SP, Dong J-F, Lopez JA, Colman RW: Human kininogens regulate thrombin binding to platelets through the glycoprotein Ib-IX-V complex. *Blood* **90**:1508, 1997.
246. Hasan AAK, Amenta S, Schmaier AH: Bradykinin and its metabolite, Arg-Pro-Pro-Gly-Phe, are selective inhibitors of α-thrombin-induced platelet activation. *Circulation* **94**:517, 1996.

247. Reddigari SR, Kuna P, Miragliotta G, Shibayama Y, Nishikawa K, Kaplan AP: Human high molecular weight kininogen binds to human umbilical vein endothelial cells via its heavy and light chains. *Blood* **81**:1306, 1993.
248. Wachtfogel YT, DeLa Cadena RA, Kunapuli SP, Rick L, Miller M, Schultze RL, Altieri DC, et al: High molecular weight kininogen binds to Mac-1 on neutrophils by its heavy chain (domain 3) and its light chain (domain 5). *J Biol Chem* **269**:19307, 1994.
249. Hasan AAK, Cines DB, Zhang J, Schmaier AH: The carboxyl terminus of bradykinin and amino terminus of the light chain of kininogens comprise an endothelial cell binding domain. *J Biol Chem* **269**:31822, 1994.
250. Herwald H, Hasan AAK, Godovac-Zimmermann J, Schmaier AH, Muller-Esterl W: Identification of an endothelial cell binding site on kininogen domain D3. *J Biol Chem* **270**:14634, 1995.
251. Hasan AAK, Cines DB, Herwald H, Schmaier AH, Muller-Esterl W: Mapping the cell binding site on high molecular weight kininogen domain 5. *J Biol Chem* **270**:19256, 1995.
252. Gustafson EJ, Lukasiewica H, Wachtfogel YT, Norton KJ, Schmaier AH, Niewiarowski S, Colman RW: High molecular weight kininogen inhibits fibrinogen binding to cytoadhesins of neutrophils and platelets. *J Cell Biol* **109**:377, 1989.
253. van Iwaarden F, deGroot PG, Bouma BN: The binding of high molecular weight kininogen to cultured human endothelial cells. *J Biol Chem* **263**:4698, 1988.
254. van Iwaarden F, de Groot PG, Sixma JJ, Berrettini M, Bouma BN: High molecular weight kininogen is present in cultured human endothelial cells. Localization, isolation and characterization. *Blood* **71**:1268, 1988.
255. Greengard J, Griffin J: Receptors for high molecular weight kininogen on stimulated washed human platelets. *Biochemistry* **23**:6863, 1984.
256. Berrettini M, Schleef R, Heeb M, Hopmeier P, Griffin J: Assembly and expression of an intrinsic factor IX activator complex on the surface of cultured human endothelial cells. *J Biol Chem* **267**:19833, 1992.
257. Lenich C, Pannell R, Gurewich V: Assembly and activation of the intrinsic fibrinolytic pathway on the surface of human endothelial cells in culture. *Thromb Haemost* **74**:698, 1995.
258. Sheng N, Fairbanks M, Henrikson R, Canziani G, Chaiken I, Moser D, Colman RW: The integrin, CD11b/18 (Mac-1) is a major cell receptor for high molecular weight kininogen (HK). *FASEB* **11**:19920, 1997.
259. Herwald H, Dedio J, Kellner R, Loos M, Mueller-Esterl W: Isolation and characterization of the kininogen-binding protein p33 from endothelial cells: Identity with the gC1q receptor. *J Biol Chem* **271**:13040, 1996.
260. DeLa Cadena RA, Kunapuli SP, Walz DA, Colman RW: Expression of thrombospondin 1 on the surface of activated platelets mediates their interaction with the heavy chains of human kininogens through Lys244-Pro254. *Thromb Haemost* **79**:186, 1998.
261. Hasan AAK, Zisman T, Schmaier AH: Cytokeratin 1 is the major cell receptor for kininogens. *Thromb Haemost* **77**:141, 1997.
262. Asakura S, Hurley RW, Skorstengaard K, Ohkubo I, Mosher DF: Inhibition of cell adhesion by high molecular weight kininogen. *J Cell Biol* **116**:465, 1992.
263. Brash JL, Scott CRF, ten Hove P, Wojciechowski P, Colman RW: Mechanism of transient adsorption of fibrinogen from plasma to solid surfaces: Role of the contact and fibrinolytic systems. *Blood* **71**:932, 1988.
264. Guimaraes JA, Borges DR, Prado ES, Prado JL: Kinin converting aminopeptidase from human serum. *Biochem Pharmacol* **22**:403, 1973.
265. Kleniewski J, Donaldson VH: Comparison of human HMW kininogen digestion by plasma kallikrein and by plasmin. A revised method of purification of HMW-kininogen. *J Lab Clin Med* **110**:469, 1987.
266. Regoli D, Barabe J: Pharmacology of bradykinin and related kinins. *Pharmacol Rev* **32**:1, 1980.
267. Hong SL: Effect of bradykinin and thrombin on prostacyclin synthesis in endothelial cells from calf and pig aorta and human umbilical cord vein. *Thromb Res* **18**:787, 1980.
268. Brown NJ, Nadeau JH, Vaughan DE: Selective stimulation of tissue-type plasminogen activator (t-PA) in vivo by infusion of bradykinin. *Thromb Haemost* **77**:522, 1997.
269. Holland JA, Pritchard KA, Pappolla MA, Wolin MS, Rogers NJ, Stemermen MB: Bradykinin induces superoxide anion release from human endothelial cells. *J Cell Physiol* **143**:21, 1990.
270. Palmer R, Ferrige A, Moncada S: Nitric oxide release accounts for biologic activity of endothelium-derived relaxing factor. *Nature* **327**:524, 1987.
271. Hall JM: Bradykinin receptors: Pharmacological properties and biological roles. *Pharmacol Ther* **56**:131, 1992.
272. McEachern AE, Shelton ER, Bhakta S, Obernolte R, Bach C, Zuppan P, Fujisaki J, et al: Expression cloning of a rat B2 bradykinin receptor. *Proc Natl Acad Sci U S A* **88**:7724, 1991.
273. Menke JG, Borkowski JA, Bierilo K, MacNeil T, Derrick A, Schneck KA, Ransom RW, et al: Expression cloning of a human B1 bradykinin receptor. *J Biol Chem* **269**:21583, 1994.
274. Erdos EG, Sloane GM: An enzyme in human plasma that inactivates bradykinin and kallidins. *Biochem Pharmacol* **11**:585, 1962.
275. Sheikh IA, Kaplan AP: Studies of the digestion of bradykinin, lysyl-bradykinin and kinin degradation products by carboxypeptidases A, B and N. *Biochem Pharmacol* **35**:1957, 1986.
276. Sheikh IA, Kaplan AP: Studies of the digestion of bradykinin, Lys-bradykinin and des-arg9 bradykinin by angiotensin converting enzyme. *Biochem Pharmacol* **35**:1951, 1986.
277. DeLa Cadena RA, Colman RW: The sequence HGLGHGHEQQH-GLIGHGH in the light chain of high molecular weight kininogen serves as a primary structural feature for zinc-dependent binding to an anionic surface. *Protein Sci* **1**:151, 1992.
278. Retzios AD, Rosenfeld R, Schiffman S: Effects of chemical modifications on the surface- and protein-binding properties of the light chain of human high molecular weight kininogen. *J Biol Chem* **262**:3074, 1987.
279. Kunapuli SP, DeLa Cadena RA, Colman RW: Deletion mutagenesis of high molecular weight kininogen light chain: Identification of two anionic surface binding subdomains. *J Biol Chem* **268**:2486, 1993.
280. Bjork I, Olson ST, Sheffer RG, Shore JD: Binding of heparin to human high molecular weight kininogen. *Biochemistry* **28**:1213, 1989.
281. Scott C, Silver L, Schapira M, Colman R: Cleavage of high molecular weight kininogen markedly enhances its coagulant activity: Evidence that this molecule exists as a procofactor. *J Clin Invest* **73**:954, 1984.
282. Tait J, Fujikawa K: Primary structure requirements for the binding of human high molecular weight kininogen to plasma prekallikrein and factor XI. *J Biol Chem* **262**:11651, 1987.
283. You JL, Page JD, Scarsdale JN, Colman RW, Harris RB: Conformational analysis of synthetic peptides encompassing the factor XI and prekallikrein overlapping binding domains of high molecular weight kininogen. *Peptides* **14**:867, 1993.
284. Schmaier AH, Schutsky D, Farber A, Silver LD, Bradford HN, Colman RW: Determination of the bifunctional properties of high molecular weight kininogen by studies with monoclonal antibodies directed to each of its chains. *J Biol Chem* **262**:1405, 1987.
285. Reddigari S, Kaplan AP: Monoclonal antibody to human high molecular weight kininogen recognizes its prekallikrein binding site and inhibits coagulant activity. *Blood* **74**:695, 1989.
286. Kaufmann J, Haasemann M, Modrow S, Muller-Esterl W: Structural dissection of the multidomain kininogens. Fine mapping of the target epitopes of antibodies interfering with their functional properties. *J Biol Chem* **268**:9079, 1993.
287. Kleniewski J, Donaldson V: Granulocyte elastase cleaves human high molecular weight kininogen and destroys its clot-promoting activity. *J Exp Med* **167**:1895, 1988.
288. Rosenthal R, Dreskin O, Rosenthal N: Plasma thromboplastin antecedent (PTA) deficiency: Clinical, coagulation, therapeutic and hereditary aspects of a new hemophilia-like disease. *Blood* **10**:120, 1955.
289. Biggs R, Sharp A, Margolis J, Hardisty R, J S, Davidson W: Defects in the early stages of blood coagulation: A report of four cases. *Br J Haematol* **4**:177, 1958.
290. Kurtides E: Plasma thromboplastin antecedent deficiency. *Quarterly Bulletin, Northwestern University Medical School* **36**:329, 1962.
291. Nossel H, Niemetz J, Mibasgan R, Schulze W: The measurement of factor XI (plasma thromboplastin antecedent). *Br J Haematol* **12**:133, 1966.
292. Seligsohn U: High gene frequency of factor XI (PTA) deficiency in Ashkenazi Jews. *Blood* **51**:1223, 1978.
293. Forbes C, Ratnoff O: Studies on plasma thromboplastin antecedent (factor XI), PTA deficiency and inhibition of PTA by plasma: Pharmacologic inhibitors and specific antiserum. *J Lab Clin Med* **79**:113, 1972.
294. Rimon A, Schiffman S, Feinstein D, Rapaport S: Factor XI activity and factor XI antigen in homozygous and heterozygous factor XI deficiency. *Blood* **48**:165, 1976.

295. Saito H, Ratnoff O, Bouma B, Seligsohn U: Failure to detect variant (CRM+) plasma thromboplastin antecedent (factor XI) molecules in hereditary plasma thromboplastin antecedent deficiency: A study of 125 patients of several ethnic backgrounds. *J Lab Clin Med* **106**:718, 1985.
296. Mannhalter C, Hellstern P, Deutsch E: Identification of a defective factor XI cross-reacting material in a factor XI-deficient patient. *Blood* **70**:31, 1987.
297. Ohkubo Y, O'Brien D, Kanehiro T, Fukui H, Tuddenham E: Characterization of a panel of monoclonal antibodies to human coagulation factor XI and detection of factor XI in HepG2 cell conditioned medium. *Thromb Haemost* **63**:417, 1990.
298. Hayashi T, Satoh S, Suzuki S, Yahagi A, Yoshino M, Saski, H: Cross-reacting material positive (CRM+) factor XI deficiency, factor XI Yamagata, with a GT to AT transition at donor splicing site in intron J of the factor XI gene. *Thromb Haemost* **78**:PS1883(Abstract), 1997.
299. Asakai R, Chung D, Ratnoff O, Davie E: Factor XI (plasma thromboplastin antecedent) deficiency in Ashkenazi Jews is a bleeding disorder that can result from three types of point mutations. *Proc Natl Acad Sci U S A* **86**:7667, 1989.
300. Hancock J, Wieland K, Pugh R, Martinowitz U, Kakkar V, Kernoff P, Cooper D: A molecular genetic study of factor XI deficiency. *Blood* **77**:1942, 1991.
301. Pugh R, McVey J, Tuddenham E, Hancock J: Six point mutations that cause factor XI deficiency. *Blood* **85**:1509, 1995.
302. Martincic D, Zimmerman S, Ware R, Sun M, Whitlock J, Gailani D: Identification of mutations and polymorphisms in the factor XI genes of an African-American family by dideoxyfingerprinting. *Blood* **92**:3309, 1998.
303. Seligsohn U. *Factor XI (PTA) deficiency.* New York: Raven, 1979.
304. Shpilberg O, Peretz H, Zivelin A, Yatuv R, Chetrit A, Kulka T, Stern C, et al: One of the two common mutations causing factor XI deficiency in Ashkenazi Jews (type II) is also prevalent in Iraqi Jews, who represent the ancient gene pool of Jews. *Blood* **85**:429, 1995.
305. Peretz H, Mulai A, Usher S, Zivelin A, Segal A, Weisman Z, Mittleman M, et al: The two common mutations causing factor XI deficiency in Jews stem from distinct founders: One of ancient Middle Eastern origin and another of more recent European Origin. *Blood* **90**:2654, 1997.
306. Meals R: Paradoxical frequencies of recessive disorders in Ashkenazic Jews. *J Chron Dis* **23**:547, 1971.
307. Goodman R. A perspective on genetic disease among the Jewish people. New York: Raven, 1979.
308. Motulsky A: Jewish diseases and origins. *Nature Genet* **9**:99, 1995.
309. Frick P: The relative incidence of anti-hemophilic globulin (AHG), plasma thromboplastin component (PTC), plasma thromboplastin antecedent (PTA) deficiency: A study of 55 cases. *J Lab Clin Med* **43**:860, 1955.
310. Wistinghausen B, Reischer A, Nardi M, Karpatkin M: Severe factor XI deficiency in an Arab family associated with a novel mutation in exon 11. *Thromb Haemost* **78**:PS857(Abstract), 1997.
311. Niskanen E, Saito S, Cline M: Plasma thromboplastin antecedent (factor XI) deficiency in a Black family. *Arch Intern Med* **141**:936, 1981.
312. Seligsohn U, Griffin J. Contact activation and factor XI, in Scriver CR, Beaudet AL, Sly WS, Valle D, (eds): *The Metabolic and Molecular Bases of Inherited Diesease. 7th ed.* New York: McGraw-Hill, 1995.
313. Litz C, Swaim W, Dalmasso A: Factor XI deficiency: Genetic and clinical studies of a single kindred. *Am J Hematol* **28**:8, 1988.
314. Zacharski L, French E: Factor XI (PTA) deficiency in an English-American kindred. *Thromb Haemost* **39**:215, 1978.
315. Ventura C, Santos A, Tavares A, de Deus G, Gago T, David D: Molecular pathology of factor XI deficiency in the Portuguese population. *Thromb Haemost* **78**:PS859(Abstract), 1997.
315a. Bolton-Maggs PHB, Butler R, Harding I, Mountford R: Six non-Jewish families with factor XI deficiency in north west England share a common mutation. *Blood* **92**:355a(Abstract), 1998.
316. Egeberg O: A family with antihemophilic factor (AHC-plasma thromboplastin antecedent) deficiency without bleeding tendency. *Scand J Clin Invest* **14**:478, 1962.
317. Edson J, White J, Krivit W: The enigma of severe factor XI deficiency without hemorrhagic symptoms. *Thromb Diath Haemorrh* **18**:342, 1967.
318. Tavori S, Brenner B, Tirski I: The effect of combined factor XI deficiency with von Willebrand factor abnormalities on hemorrhagic diathesis. *Thromb Haemost* **63**:36, 1990.
319. Brenner B, Laor A, Lupo H, Zivelin A, Lanir N, Seligsohn U: Bleeding predictors in factor XI-deficient patients. *Blood Coagul Fibrinolysis* **8**:511, 1997.
320. Lipscomb M, Walsh R: Human platelets and factor XI: Localization in platelet membranes of factor XI-like activity and its functional distinction from plasma factor XI. *J Clin Invest* **63**:1006, 1979.
321. Sidi A, Seligsohn U, Jonas P, Many M: Factor XI deficiency: Detection and management during urologic surgery. *J Urol* **119**:528, 1978.
322. Kitchens C: Factor XI: A review of its biochemistry and deficiency. *Semin Thromb Hemost* **17**:55, 1991.
323. Ginsburg D, Sadler J: von Willebrand disease: A database of point mutation, insertions, and deletions. *Thromb Haemost* **69**:177, 1993.
324. Pearson R, Tripplet D: Factor XI assay results in the CAP survey. *Am J Clin Pathol* **78**(Supp):615, 1982.
325. Scott C, Sinha D, Seaman F, Walsh P, Colman R: Amidolytic assay of human factor XI in plasma: Comparison with a coagulant assay and a new rapid immunoassay. *Blood* **63**:42, 1984.
326. Retzios A, Rosenfeld R, Schiffman S: Enzymes of the contact phase of blood coagulation: Kinetics with various chromogenic substrates and a two-substrate assay for the joint estimation of plasma prekallikrein and factor XI. *J Lab Clin Med* **112**:560, 1988.
327. Bouma B, Vlooswijk R, Davie E: Immunologic studies of human coagulation factor XI and its complex with high molecular weight kininogen. *Blood* **62**:1123, 1983.
328. Seligsohn U, Modan M: Definition of the population at risk of bleeding due to factor XI deficiency in Ashkenazic Jews and the value of the activated thromboplastin time in its detection. *Isr J Med Sci* **17**:413, 1981.
329. Chediak J, Lambert E, Johnson E, Telfer M: Combined severe factor XI deficiency and von Willebrand disease. *Am J Clin Path* **74**:108, 1980.
330. Berube C, Ofosu F, Kelton J, Blajchman M: A novel congenital haemostatic defect: Combined factor VII and factor XI deficiency. *Blood Coagul Fibrinolysis* **3**:357, 1992.
331. Lian E, Deykin D, Harkness D: Combined deficiency of factor VIII (AHF) and factor XI (PTA). *Am J Hematol* **1**:319, 1976.
332. Soff G, Levin J, Bell W: Familial multiple coagulation deficiency and combined factor IX and XI deficiency: Two previously uncharacterized familial multiple factor deficiency syndromes. *Semin Thromb Hemost* **7**:149, 1981.
333. Angelopoulos B, Kourepi M, Vicatou M, Mourdjinis A: Hamophilia due to combined AHG, PTC and PTA factors. *Acta Haematol* **31**:36, 1964.
334. Hollstern P, Mannhalter C, Kohler M, Kiehl R, von Blohn G, Wenzel E, Deutsch E: Combined dys-form of homozygous factor XI deficiency and heterozygous factor XII deficiency. *Haemostasis* **15**:215, 1985.
335. Winter M, Needham J, Barkhan P: Factor XI deficiency and a platelet defect. *Haemostasis* **13**:83, 1983.
336. Singer S, Hurst D, Addiego J: Bleeding disorders in Noonan Syndrome: Three case reports and review of the literature. *J Pediatr Hematol Oncol* **19**:130, 1997.
337. Seligsohn U, Zitman D, Many A, Klibansky C: Coexistence of factor XI (plasma thromboplastin antecedent) deficiency and Gaucher's disease. *Isr J Med Sci* **12**:1448, 1976.
338. Berrebi A, Malnick S, Vorst E, Stein D: High incidence of factor XI deficiency in Gaucher's disease. *Am J Hematol* **40**:153, 1992.
339. van Geet C, Jaeken J: A unique pattern of coagulation abnormalities in Carbohydrate-deficient glycoprotein syndrome. *Pediatr Res* **33**:540, 1993.
340. Kaufman J: Prostatectomy in factor XI deficiency. *J Urol* **117**:75, 1977.
341. Bashevkin M, Nawabi I: Factor XI deficiency in surgical patients. *NY State J Med* **79**:1360, 1979.
342. Jonas P, Sidi A, Goldwasser B, Many M: Prostatectomy in factor XI (plasma thromboplastin antecedent) deficiency. *J Urol* **128**:1209, 1982.
343. Bolton-Maggs P, Wensley R, Kernoff P, Kasper C, Winkelman L, Lane R, Smith J: Production and therapeutic use of a factor XI concentrate from plasma. *Thromb Haemost* **67**:314, 1992.
344. Burnouf-Radosevich M, Burnouf T: A therapeutic, highly purified factor XI concentrate from human plasma. *Transfusion* **32**:861, 1992.
345. Nossel H, Niemetz J, Sawitsky A: Blood PTA (factor XI) levels following plasma infusion. *Proc Soc Exp Biol Med* **115**:896, 1964.
346. Williams J: Plasma thromboplastin antecedent deficiency. *Br J Oral Surg* **10**:126, 1972.

347. Berliner S, Horowitz I, Martinowitz U, Brenner B, Seligsohn U: Dental surgery in patients with severe factor XI deficiency without plasma replacement. *Blood Coagul Fibrinolysis* **3**:465, 1992.
348. Steinberg M, Saletan S, Funt M, Baker D, Coller B: Management of factor XI deficiency in gynecologic and obstetric patients. *Obstet Gynecol* **68**:130, 1986.
349. Bennett B, Ratnoff OD, Holt JB, Roberts HR: Hageman trait (factor XII deficiency): A probable second genotype inherited as an autosomal dominant characteristic. *Blood* **40**:412, 1972.
350. Kanaji T, Okamura T, Osaki K, Kuroiwa M, Shimoda K, Hamasaki N, Niho Y: A common gene polymorphism (46 C to T substitution) in the 5′-untranslated region of the coagulation factor XII gene is associated with low translation efficiency and decrease in plasma factor XII level. *Blood* **91**:2010, 1998.
351. Gordon EM, Donaldson VH, Saito H, Su E, Ratnoff OD: Reduced titers of Hageman factor (Factor XII) in Orientals. *Ann Intern Med* **95**:697, 1981.
352. Bernardi F, Marchetti G, Patracchini P, del Senno L, Tripodi N, Fantoni A, Bartolai S, et al: Factor XII gene alteration in Hageman trait detected by Taq1 restriction enzyme. *Blood* **69**:1421, 1987.
353. Hofferbert S, Muller J, Kostering H, von Ohlen WD, Schloesser M: A novel 5′ upstream mutation in the factor XII gene is associated with a Taq I restriction site in an Alu repeat in factor XII-deficient patients. *Hum Genet* **97**:838, 1996.
354. Schloesser M, Zeerleder S, Lutze G, Halbmayer W, Hofferbert S, Hinney B, Koestering H, et al: Mutations in the human factor XII gene. *Blood* **90**:3967, 1997.
355. Kemptner B, Reuth S, Epple I, Lohse P: Untersuchungen zur Genetik des Faktor-XII-Mangels, in Kretschmer V, Stangel W, Eckstein R (eds).*Beitr Infusionsther: 31*. Germany: Karger, Freiburg, 1993, p 174.
356. Schloesser M, Hofferbert S, Bartz U, Lutze G, Lammle B, Engel W: The novel acceptor splice site mutation 11396(G- > A) in the factor XII gene causes a truncated transcript in cross-reacting material negative patients. *Hum Mol Genet* **4**:1235, 1995.
357. Wuillemin WA, Furlan M, Stricker H, Lammle B: Functional characterization of a variant factor XII (F XII Locarno) in a cross reacting material positive F XII deficient plasma. *Thromb Haemost* **67**:219, 1992.
358. Kremer-Hovinga J, Schaller J, Stricker H, Wuillemin WA, Furlan M, Lammle B: Coagulation factor XII Locarno: The functional defect is caused by the amino acid substitution Arg 353- > Pro leading to loss of a kallikrein cleavage site. *Blood* **84**:1173, 1994.
359. Saito H, Scialla SJ: Isolation and properties of an abnormal Hageman factor (factor XII) molecule in a cross-reacting material-positive Hageman trait plasma. *J Clin Invest* **68**:1028, 1981.
360. Miyata T, Kawabata SI, Iwanaga S, Takahashi I, Alving B, Saito H: Coagulation factor XII (Hageman factor) Washington D.C.: Inactive factor XIIa results from Cys-571-Ser substitution. *Proc Natl Acad Sci U S A* **86**:8319, 1989.
361. Didisheim P: Hageman Factor deficiency (Hageman Trait): Case report and review of the literature. *Arch Intern Med* **110**:170, 1962.
362. Ikkala E, Myllyla G, Nevablinna H: Rare congenital coagulation factor defects in Finland. *Scand J Haematol* **8**:210, 1971.
363. Nicholls J, Chan L, Koo Y, Kwong Y, Tsoi N: Subdural haematoma and factor XII deficiency in a Chinese infant. *Br J Accident Surg* **24**:202, 1993.
364. Goodnough L, Saito H, Ratnoff O: Thrombosis or myocardial infarction in congenital clotting factor abnormalities and chronic thrombocytopenias: A report of 21 patients and a review of 50 previously reported cases. *Medicine (Baltimore)* **62**:248, 1983.
365. Hellstern P, Kohler M, Schmengler K, Doenecke P, Wenzel E: Arterial and venous thrombosis and normal response to streptokinase treatment in a young patient with severe Hageman factor deficiency. *Acta Haematol* **69**:123, 1983.
366. Lodi S, Isa L, Pollini E, Bravo AF, Scalvini A: Defective intrinsic fibrinolytic activity in a patient with severe factor XII-deficiency and myocardial infarction. *Scand J Haematol* **33**:80, 1984.
367. Mannhalter C, Fisher M, Hopmeier P, Deutch E: Factor XII activity and antigen concentrations in patients suffering from recurrent thrombosis. *Fibrinolysis* **1**:259, 1987.
368. Lammle B, Wuillemin W, Huber I, Krauskopf M, Zurcher C, Plugshaupt R, Furlan M: Thrombo-embolism and bleeding tendency in congenital factor XII deficiency: A study of 74 subjects from 14 Swiss families. *Thromb Haemost* **65**:117, 1991.
369. Halbmayer WM, Mannhaltaer C, Feichtinger C, Rubi K, Fischer M: The prevalence of factor XII deficiency in 103 orally anticoagulated outpatients suffering from recurrent venous and/or arterial thromboembolism. *Thromb Haemost* **68**:285, 1992.
370. von Kanel R, Wuillemin W, Furlan M, Lammle B: Factor XII clotting activity and antigen levels in patients with thromboembolic disease. *Blood Coagul Fibrinolysis* **3**:555, 1992.
371. Jespersen J, Munkvad S, Pedersen OD, Gram J, Kluft C: Evidence for a role of factor XII-dependent fibrinolysis in cardiovascular diseases. *Ann NY Acad Sci* **667**:454, 1992.
372. Winter M, Gallimore M, Jones DW: Should factor XII assays be included in thrombophilia screenings? *Lancet* **346**:52, 1995.
373. Levi M, Hack C, de Boer J, Brandjes D, Buller H, ten Cate J: Reduction of contact activation related fibrinolytic activity in factor XII deficient patients. *J Clin Invest* **88**:1155, 1991.
374. Saito H, Scott JG, Movat HZ, Scialla SJ: Molecular heterogeneity of Hageman trait (factor XII deficiency). Evidence that two of 49 subjects are cross-reacting material positive (CRM+). *J Lab Clin Med* **94**:256, 1979.
375. Gallimore MJ, Jones DW, Winter M: Factor XII determinations in the presence and absence of phospholipid antibodies. *Thromb Haemost* **79**: 87, 1998.
376. Wuepper K: Prekallikrein deficiency in man. *J Exp Med* **138**: 1345, 1973.
377. Hathaway W: Fletcher factor. *Blood* **46**: 817, 1975.
378. Currimbhoy Z, Vinciguerra V, Palakavongs P, Kuslansky P, Degnan T: Fletcher factor deficiency and myocardial infarction. *Am J Clin Pathol* **65**: 970, 1976.
379. Essien E, Ebhota M: Fletcher factor deficiency: Detection of a severe case in a population survey. *Acta Haematol* **58**: 353, 1977.
380. Aznar J, Espana F, Aznar J, Tascon A, Jimenez C: Fletcher factor deficiency: Report of a new family. *Scand J Haematol* **21**:94, 1978.
381. Ragni M, Lewis J, Hasiba U, Spero J: Prekallikrein (Fletcher factor) deficiency in clinical disease states. *Thromb Res* **18**:45, 1980.
382. Saade M: Fletcher factor deficiency with a mildly prolonged activated PTT. *South Med J* **73**:958, 1980.
383. Waddell C, Brown J, Udden M: Plasma prekallikrein (Fletcher factor) deficiency in a patient with chronic lymphocytic leukemia. *South Med J* **73**:1653, 1980.
384. Entes K, LaDuca F, Tourbaf K: Fletcher factor deficiency, source of variation of the partial thromboplastin time. *Am J Clin Pathol* **75**:626, 1981.
385. Saito H, Goodnough L, Soria J, Soria C, Aznar J, Espana F: Heterogenity of human prekallikrein deficiency (Fletcher trait). Evidence that five of 18 cases are positive for cross-reacting material. *N Eng J Med* **305**:910, 1981.
386. Raffoux C, Alexandre P, Perrier P, Briquel M, Streiff H: HLA typing in a new family with Fletcher factor deficiency. *Hum Genet* **60**:71, 1982.
387. Poon M, Moore M, Castleberry R, Lurie A, Huang S, Lehmeyer J: Combined deficiencies of Fletcher factor (plasma prekallikrein) and Hageman factor (factor XII). Report of a case with observation on in vivo and in vitro leukocyte chemotaxis. *Am J Hematol* **12**:261, 1982.
388. Kyrle P, Neissner H, Deutsch E, Lechner K, Korninger C, Manhalter C: CRM + severe Fletcher factor deficiency associated with Graves' disease. *Haemostasis* **14**:302, 1984.
389. Sollo D, Saleem A: Prekallikrein (Fletcher factor) deficiency. *Ann Clin Lab Sci* **15**:279, 1985.
390. Harris M, Exner T, Rickard K, Kronenberg H: Multiple cerebral thrombosis in Fletcher factor (prekallikrein) deficiency: A case report. *Am J Haematol* **19**:387, 1985.
391. Bouma B, Keribiriou D, Baker J, Griffin J: Characterization of a variant prekallikrein, prekallikrein Long Beach, from a family with mixed cross-reacting material-positive and cross-reacting material negative prekallikrein deficiency. *J Clin Invest* **78**:170, 1986.
392. De Stefano V, Leone G, Teofili L, De Marinis L, Micalizzi P, Fiumara C, Bizzi B: Association of Graves' disease and prekallikrein congenital deficiency in a patient belonging to the first CRM+ prekallikrein-deficient Italian family. *Thromb Res* **60**:397, 1990.
393. Castaman R, Ruggeri M, Rodeghiero F: A new Italian family with severe prekallikrein deficiency. Desmopression-induced fibrinolysis and coagulation changes in homozygous and heterozygous members. *Res Clin Lab* **20**:239, 1990.
394. Joggi J, Stalder M, Knecht H, Hauert J, Bacjmann F: Deficience en prekallicreine: A propos de 2 cas. *Schweiz Med Wochenschr* **120**:1942, 1990.
395. Hess D, Krauss J, Rardin D: Stroke in a young adult with Fletcher trait. *South Med J* **84**:507, 1991.

396. Wuillemin W, Furlan M, von Felten A, Lammle B: Functional characterization of a variant prekallikrein (PK Zurich). *Thromb Haemost* **70**:427, 1993.
397. DeLa Cadena R, Stadnicki A, Uknis A, Sartor R, Kettner C, Ada A, Colman R: Inhibition of plasma kallikrein prevents peptidoglycan-induced arthritis in the Lewis rat. *FASEB J* **9**:446, 1995.
398. Sanfelippo M, Cafaro A, Winston W: aPTT prolonged by prekallikrein deficiency. *Lab Med* **29**:274, 1998.
399. Abildgaard C, Harrison J: Fletcher factor deficiency: Family study and detection. *Blood* **43**:641, 1974.
400. DeLa Cadena R: Fletcher factor deficiency in a 9-year-old girl: Mechanisms of the contact pathway of blood coagulation. *Am J Hematol* **48**:273, 1995.
401. Schiffman S, Lee P: Preparation, characterization, and activation of a highly purified factor XI. Evidence that a hitherto unrecognized plasma activating factor participates in the interaction of factors XI and XII. *Br J Haematol* **27**:101, 1974.
402. Lacombe M, Varet B, Levy J: A hitherto undescribed plasma factor acting at the contact phase of blood coagulation (Flaukeac factor): Case report and coagulation studies. *Blood* **46**:761, 1975.
403. Donaldson V, Kleniewski J, Saito H, Sayed J: Prekallikrein deficiency in a kindred with kininogen deficiency and Fitzgerald trait clotting defect. *J Clin Invest* **60**:571, 1977.
404. Lutcher C: A new expression of high molecular weight kininogen (HMW-kininogen) deficiency. *Clin Res* **34**:440, 1979.
405. Proud D, Pierce JV, Pisano JJ: Radioimmunoassay of human high molecular weight kininogen in normal and deficient plasma. *J Lab Clin Med* **95**:563, 1980.
406. Nakamura K, Iijima K, Fukuda C, Kadowaki H, Ikoma H, Oh-ishi S, Uchida Y, et al: Tachibana Trait: Human high molecular weight kininogen deficiency with diminished levels of prekallikrein and low molecular weight kininogen. *Acta Haematol Jpn* **48**:1473, 1985.
407. Lefrere J, Horellou M, Gozin D, Conrad J, Muller J, Clark M, Soulier J, et al: A new case of high molecular weight kininogen inherited deficiency. *Am J Hematol* **22**:415, 1986.
408. Vicente V, Alberca I, Gonzalez R, Alegre A, Redondo C, Moro J: New congenital deficiency of high molecular weight kininogen and prekallikrein (Fitzgerald trait). Study of response to DDAVP and venous occlusion. *Haematologic* **19**:41, 1986.
409. Exner T, Barber S, Naujalis J: Fitzgerald factor deficiency in an Australian Aborigine. *Med J Aust* **146**:545, 1987.
410. Stormorken H, Briseid K, Hellum B, Hoem NO, Johansen HT, Ly B: A new case of total kininogen deficiency. *Thromb Res* **60**:457, 1990.
411. Hayashi H, Ishimaru F, Fujita T, Tsurumi N, Tsuda T, Kimura I: Molecular genetic survey of five Japanese families with high molecular weight kininogen deficiency. *Blood* **75**:1296, 1990.
412. Cheung PP, Kunapuli SP, Scott CF, Wachfogel YT, Colman RT: Genetic basis of total kininogen deficiency in Williams' trait. *J Biol Chem* **268**:23361, 1993.
413. Donaldson V, Evans R: Biochemical abnormality in hereditary angioneurotic edema. *Am J Med* **35**:37, 1963.
414. Curd J, Prograis L, Cochrane C: Detection of active kallikrein in induced blister fluids of hereditary angioedema. *J Exp Med* **152**:742, 1980.
415. Schapira M, Silver L, Scott C, Schmaier A, Prograis L, Curd J, Colman R: Prekallikrein activation and high molecular weight kininogen consumption in hereditary angioedema. *N Engl J Med* **308**:1050, 1983.
416. Cugno M, Hack C, de Boer J, Eerenberg A, Agostini A, Cicardi M: Generation of plasmin during acute attacks of hereditary angioedema. *J Lab Clin Med* **121**:38, 1993.
417. Fields A, Ghebrehiwet B, Kaplan A: Kinin formation in hereditary angioedema plasma: Evidence against kinin derivation from C2 and in support of "spontaneous" formation of bradykinin. *J Allergy Clin Immunol* **72**:54, 1983.
418. Kalter E, Daha M, Verhoef J, Bouma B: Activation and inhibition of Hageman-factor dependent pathways and the complement system in uncomplicated bacteremia and bacterial shock. *J Infect Dis* **151**:1019, 1985.
419. Colman R: The role of plasma proteases in septic shock. *N Engl J Med* **320**:1207, 1989b.
420. DeLa Cadena R, Suffredini A, Page J, Pixley R, Kauffman N, Perilo J, Colman R: Activation of the kallikrein-kinin system after endotoxin administration to normal human volunteers. *Blood* **81**:3313, 1993.
421. Pixley R, DeLa Cadena R, Page J, Kauffman N, Wyshock E, Chang A, Taylor F, et al: Activation of the contact system in lethal hypotensive bacteremia in a baboon model. *Am J Pathol* **140**:1, 1992.
422. Pixley R, DeLa Cadena R, Page J, Kauffman N, Wyshock E, Change A, Taylor F, et al: The contact system contributes to hypotension but not disseminated intravascular coagulation in lethal bacteremia: In vivo use of a monoclonal anti-factor XII antibody to block contact activation in baboons. *J Clin Invest* **91**:61, 1993.
423. Nagase H, Cawston J, DeSilva M, Barrett A: Identification of plasma kallikrein an activator of latent collagenase in rheumatoid synovial fluid. *Biochim Biophys Acta* **707**:133, 1982.
424. Ginsberg M, Jaques B, Cochrane C, Griffin J: Urate crystal dependent cleavage of Hageman factor in human plasma and synovial fluid. *J Lab Clin Med* **95**:497, 1980.
425. Kellermeyer R, Breckenridge R: The inflammatory process in acute gouty arthritis. I. Activation of Hageman factor by sodium urate crystals. *J Lab Clin Med* **63**:307, 1965.
426. Imanaka Y, Lala K, Nishimura T, Bolton-Maggs P, Tuddenham E, McVey J: Identification of two novel mutations in non-Jewish factor XI deficiency. *Brit J Haematol* **90**:916, 1995.
427. Alhaq A, Mitchell M, Sethi M, Boulton G, Caenaro G, Smith M, Savidge G: Identification of a novel mutation in a non-Jewish factor XI deficient kindred. *Blood* **90**:467A(Abstract), 1997.
428. Peretz H, Zivelin A, Usher S, Seligsohn U: A 14-base pair deletion (codon 554 del AAGgtaacagagtg) at exon 14/intron N junction of the coagulation factor XI gene disrupts splicing and causes severe factor XI deficiency. *Human Mutat* **8**:77, 1996.
429. Bodfish P, Warne D, Watkins C, Nyberg K, Spurr N: Dinucleotide repeat polymorphism in the human coagulation factor XI gene, intron B (F11), detected using the polymerase chain reaction. *Nucleic Acids Res* **19**:6979, 1991.
430. Butler M, Parsons A: RFLP for intron E of factor XI gene. *Nucleic Acids Res* **18**:5327, 1990.

CHAPTER 176

Antithrombin Deficiency

Douglas M. Tollefsen

1. **Antithrombin is a 58-kDa glycoprotein that is present in human plasma at a concentration of ~2.6 μM. It inhibits several activated coagulation factors, including thrombin, factor IXa, and factor Xa. Inhibition occurs by formation of a stable 1 : 1 complex between antithrombin and the protease.**
2. **Heparin and heparan sulfate increase the rate of the antithrombin-protease reaction at least 1000 times by a catalytic mechanism that requires binding of the glycosaminoglycan chain to antithrombin. The binding site for antithrombin is a specific pentasaccharide sequence that contains an unusual 3-O-sulfated glucosamine residue. This structure occurs in ~30 percent of heparin molecules isolated from mast cells and in 1 to 10 percent of heparan sulfate molecules synthesized by vascular endothelial cells. Current evidence suggests that heparan sulfate proteoglycans anchored in the vessel wall interact with circulating antithrombin to inhibit thrombus formation.**
3. **Antithrombin deficiency (MIM 107300) is present in ~2 percent of patients with venous thromboembolic disease, in whom it is generally inherited as an autosomal dominant trait. The prevalence of symptomatic antithrombin deficiency is estimated to range from 1 per 2000 to 1 per 5000 in the general population. Affected heterozygous individuals have ~50 percent of the normal plasma antithrombin activity. Deficiency results from mutations that affect the biosynthesis or stability of antithrombin and hence lower the amount of antithrombin antigen detectable in plasma, or from mutations that affect the protease and/or heparin-binding sites and are associated with essentially normal levels of antithrombin antigen. Mutations confined to the heparin binding site appear to be more common than the other types of mutations and are usually asymptomatic unless present in a homozygous state.**
4. **Clinical manifestations of antithrombin deficiency include deep vein thrombosis and pulmonary embolism. Thrombosis may occur spontaneously or in association with pregnancy, trauma, or surgery. Arterial thrombosis is rare. Many patients experience recurrent thromboembolic disease beginning in early adulthood. It has been estimated that by 30 years of age ~60 percent of patients with antithrombin deficiency will have had at least one thrombotic episode. Acute episodes are generally treated with a 5- to 7-day infusion of heparin followed by oral anticoagulant therapy for an indefinite period of time. Prophylactic therapy of asymptomatic patients remains controversial.**
5. **Heparin cofactor II, which is homologous to antithrombin, inhibits thrombin in the presence of heparin or dermatan sulfate but does not inhibit other coagulation proteases. The concentration of heparin cofactor II in plasma is normal (~1.2 μM) in patients with inherited antithrombin deficiency. Several patients with thrombosis and inherited deficiency of heparin cofactor II have been reported (MIM 142360), but a causal relationship between these phenomena has not been established.**

A list of standard abbreviations is located immediately preceding the index in each volume. Additional abbreviations used in this chapter include: HBS = heparin binding site; PE = pleiotropic effect; and RS = reactive site.

FUNCTIONS OF THROMBIN

Blood coagulation results from activation of a series of protease zymogens in the presence of nonenzymatic protein cofactors, calcium, and platelets (Fig. 176-1) (see Chap. 169). The initial event in coagulation is exposure of plasma to tissue factor, a protein expressed on the surface of many cells not normally in contact with the bloodstream, which leads to the activation of factors IX and X by the factor VIIa-tissue factor complex. This triggering mechanism is inactivated rapidly by tissue factor pathway inhibitor,[1] but additional factor Xa can be generated by the factor IXa-VIIIa complex. Factor Xa in a complex with factor Va then converts prothrombin to thrombin, the final protease in the coagulation cascade. This conversion occurs in two steps: factor Xa first cleaves prothrombin at Arg 320 to produce the intermediate meizothrombin; subsequent cleavage at Arg 271 in meizothrombin yields thrombin.[2] Thrombin cleaves fibrinogen near the N-terminal ends of the Aα and Bβ chains, yielding fibrin monomers that polymerize to form the clot.

Thrombin promotes hemostasis by several mechanisms in addition to the clotting of fibrinogen. Thrombin cleaves the platelet thrombin receptor to generate a tethered peptide ligand that stimulates platelet aggregation and secretion.[3] The aggregated platelets serve as the primary hemostatic plug and provide a surface on which the factor IXa-VIIIa and Xa-Va complexes are localized. Thrombin directly activates factors V and VIII, which serve as the nonenzymatic cofactors in these complexes. In addition, thrombin converts factor XI to XIa, which activates factor IX.[4,5] The reactions of thrombin with platelets and factors V, VIII, and XI provide positive feedback to accelerate thrombin generation at the site of a wound. Two other enzymes are also activated by thrombin: a transglutaminase (factor XIII) that covalently crosslinks polymerized fibrin and a plasma carboxypeptidase that inhibits fibrinolysis.[6]

If thrombin is generated within a normal blood vessel, it binds to the endothelial membrane protein thrombomodulin and activates protein C. Activated protein C produces a local anticoagulant effect by proteolytic inactivation of factors Va and VIIIa (see Chap. 170). Although meizothrombin is much less active than thrombin with respect to fibrinogen, platelets, and the plasma carboxypeptidase, meizothrombin activates protein C faster than thrombin does in the presence of thrombomodulin.[7,8] Thus, meizothrombin may function as an anticoagulant protease.

Thrombin has a number of activities that are not directly related to coagulation (reviewed in Coughlin et al.[9]). It is mitogenic for lymphocytes and vascular smooth muscle cells, induces chemotaxis in monocytes, promotes adhesion of neutrophils to endothelial cells, and stimulates endothelial cells to produce prostacyclin, platelet-activating factor, plasminogen activator inhibitor-1, and platelet-derived growth factor. These activities may be important in wound healing and inflammation. Thrombin also inhibits neurite outgrowth in neuroblastoma cells and

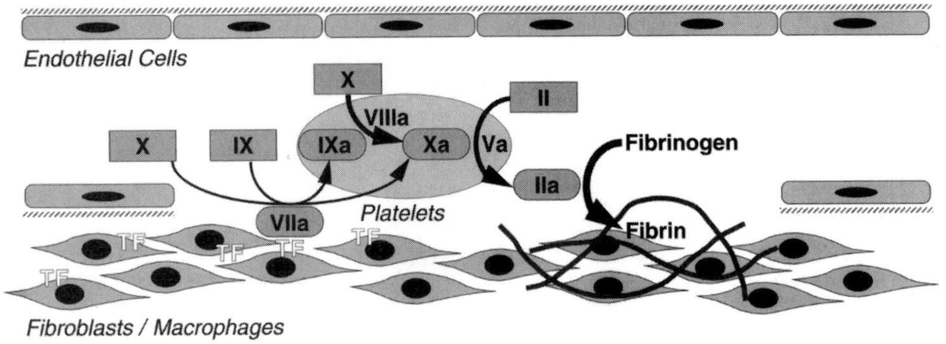

Fig. 176-1 Major reactions in blood coagulation. Rectangles indicate protease zymogens; ovals indicate active proteases. The activated forms of the nonenzymatic protein cofactors V and VIII are designated Va and VIIIa, respectively. TF, tissue factor; II, prothrombin; IIa, thrombin.

sympathetic neurons, a process that appears to be regulated by glial-derived nexin (protease nexin-I) in the brain.[10]

Regulation of Thrombin by Protease Inhibitors in Plasma

Antithrombin, heparin cofactor II, and protein C inhibitor inhibit thrombin, whereas heparin cofactor II preferentially inhibits meizothrombin.[11] Antithrombin and heparin cofactor II require the presence of a glycosaminoglycan, such as heparin, for maximal activity. Protein C inhibitor rapidly inactivates thrombin bound to thrombomodulin.[12] The association between antithrombin deficiency and recurrent venous thromboembolism, first reported by Egeberg in 1965,[13] established the idea that antithrombin plays a critical role in regulating hemostasis. Heparan sulfate synthesized by vascular endothelial cells appears to activate antithrombin and thereby prevent thrombosis within normal blood vessels.[14] The physiologic roles of heparin cofactor II and protein C inhibitor are unknown.

BIOCHEMISTRY AND MOLECULAR BIOLOGY OF ANTITHROMBIN

In 1939, Brinkhous and coworkers discovered that the anticoagulant activity of heparin is mediated by an endogenous plasma component termed heparin cofactor.[15] The nature of this component was obscure until 1968, when Abildgaard purified antithrombin (formerly called antithrombin III) from plasma and showed that this protein has heparin cofactor activity.[16] Rosenberg and Damus later purified a sufficient amount of antithrombin for biochemical characterization.[17]

Structure and Biosynthesis

Structure. Antithrombin is a single-chain, 58-kDa glycoprotein that belongs to the serpin superfamily.[18] The cDNA for antithrombin encodes a polypeptide that is 432 amino acids in length and that is preceded by a 32-residue signal peptide.[19–21] Antithrombin contains three disulfide bonds, one of which is required for heparin cofactor activity.[22,23] It also contains four biantennary asparagine-linked oligosaccharides in its fully glycosylated form.[24] No other biosynthetic modifications have been reported.

Two forms of antithrombin that differ in their carbohydrate content were isolated from normal human plasma by heparin-agarose affinity chromatography.[25] The major form (α-antithrombin), which comprises ~90 percent of the total antithrombin, is eluted from the affinity matrix with 1 M NaCl and is fully glycosylated. The minor form (β-antithrombin) is eluted at a higher salt concentration and lacks the oligosaccharide unit linked to Asn 135, which is near the heparin binding site.[26] Both α- and β-antithrombin inhibit thrombin rapidly in the presence of heparin, but β-antithrombin requires a lower concentration of heparin for maximal activity, consistent with its higher affinity for heparin.

Nonenzymatic glycation of one or two lysine residues of antithrombin occurs in vitro in the presence of high concentrations of glucose. This modification, which may occur in some patients with diabetes mellitus, has been reported to decrease the heparin-dependent thrombin inhibitory activity ~10 to 20 percent.[27]

Gene. The antithrombin gene on human chromosome 1q23-25[28] contains seven exons distributed over ~13.5 kb of DNA (GenBank X68793).[29] The introns contain 10 *Alu* repeats, which are present at a greater density than average for the human genome. Homologous recombination among these repetitive elements appears to have been an important mechanism by which deletions producing type I deficiency occurred.[29] Antithrombin mRNA is expressed in the liver, and synthesis of antithrombin has been demonstrated in cultured human hepatoma cells.[30] Alternative splicing of the antithrombin mRNA has been demonstrated.[31] The alternative splicing event introduces a 42-base segment between codons -19 and -18 of the signal peptide. This segment of mRNA contains an in-frame termination codon such that the predicted protein product encoded by the alternatively spliced mRNA is only 19 amino acids long. Although the alternatively spliced mRNA accounts for 20 to 40 percent of the antithrombin mRNA in human liver, it is not known whether translation of this mRNA occurs. In the adult rat, antithrombin mRNA was detected in the kidney at a level ~20 percent of that found in the liver.[32]

Biosynthesis. The 5′ flanking sequence of the antithrombin gene lacks a TATA-like sequence at the expected location 25 to 30 bases upstream from the transcription initiation site,[31] but contains short sequences that are similar to an enhancer element found in the immunoglobulin Jκ-Cκ gene.[33] When the antithrombin enhancer element was ligated to the chloramphenicol acetyltransferase gene and transfected into cells, expression of chloramphenicol acetyltransferase activity was increased preferentially in Alexander hepatoma (liver) and Cos-1 (kidney) cells. Thus, the enhancer may be involved in tissue-specific expression of the antithrombin gene. More recently, a 700-bp fragment of the human antithrombin promoter was shown to confer a high level of tissue-specific expression in the liver and kidney of transgenic mice,[34] and several transcription factors that bind to regions flanking exon 1 of the antithrombin gene were identified.[35] A DNA length polymorphism has been identified, resulting from insertion of either 32 or 108 bp of DNA at the position 345 bases upstream from the translation initiation codon.[36] This polymorphism does not appear to affect the level of expression of antithrombin in human plasma.[37]

Little is known about the regulation of antithrombin biosynthesis. Biosynthesis of antithrombin by isolated rat hepatocytes is unaffected by the presence of protease-antithrombin complexes or by the supernatant medium of macrophages incubated with these complexes.[38] However, antithrombin biosynthesis is stimulated by the supernatant medium of macrophages incubated with endotoxin or fibrinogen fragment D. Under these conditions, fibrinogen and α_1-antitrypsin biosynthesis are also stimulated.

Protease Inhibition by Antithrombin

Specificity. Antithrombin inhibits several of the proteases involved in blood coagulation, including thrombin, factor Xa, factor IXa, and factor XIa.[39] Antithrombin also inhibits factor VIIa

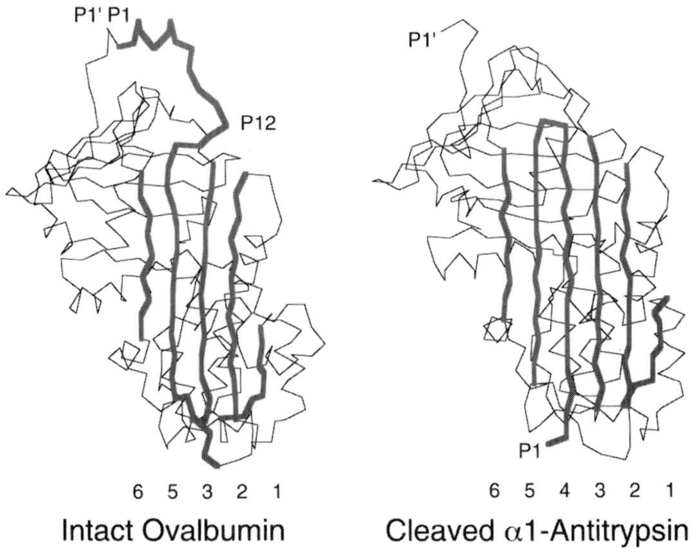

Fig. 176-2 Typical structures and native and cleaved serpins. The structures of native ovalbumin[62] and cleaved α_1-antitrypsin[309] determined by x-ray crystallography are shown. The α-carbon tracing of the polypeptide backbone is indicated for each protein. The P1 to P12 residues of ovalbumin form an exposed loop on the surface of the protein that is susceptible to proteolytic attack. After cleavage of the reactive site peptide bond (P1-P1′) of α_1-antitrypsin, residues P1 to P12 become incorporated into a β-sheet structure (thick lines; strands numbered according to α_1-antitrypsin), and the P1 and P1′ amino acid residues are separated by 69Å.

bound to tissue factor.[40,41] In vitro experiments in which ^{125}I-labeled proteases were incubated with plasma in the absence of heparin suggest that antithrombin is the major inhibitor of factor IXa, factor Xa, and thrombin, although α_1-antitrypsin and α_2-macroglobulin also contribute to inhibition of the latter two proteases.[42–44] In the presence of heparin at concentrations likely to be achieved therapeutically, factor IXa, factor Xa, and thrombin are inhibited almost exclusively by antithrombin. In the presence of higher concentrations of heparin or dermatan sulfate, thrombin is inhibited primarily by heparin cofactor II.[45,46] Factor Xa is also inhibited by tissue factor pathway inhibitor, which is present in plasma bound to lipoproteins at about one-thousandth the concentration of antithrombin,[47] and it is the factor Xa-tissue factor pathway inhibitor complex that inhibits factor VIIa-tissue factor.[48] Factor XIa is inhibited primarily by α_1-antitrypsin in plasma[49] or by protease nexin-2, a form of the amyloid precursor protein released from platelets.[50,51] Antithrombin does not inhibit activated protein C.[52]

Antithrombin may regulate several proteases in addition to those involved in blood coagulation. In the presence of heparin, the streptokinase-plasminogen complex (which has plasmin-like activity) is inhibited more rapidly by antithrombin than by α_2-antiplasmin,[53] whereas plasmin itself is inhibited more rapidly by α_2-antiplasmin.[54,55] Antithrombin also inhibits granzyme A (tryptase), a protease from cytotoxic T lymphocytes,[56,57] and inhibits one or more of the steps in complement activation.[58]

Mechanism. Antithrombin forms an essentially irreversible, equimolar complex with each of its target proteases.[17] The serine residue at the active site of the protease is required for complex formation but thereafter becomes inaccessible to substrates. Furthermore, a small peptide is cleaved from the C-terminus of antithrombin during complex formation.[59] Thrombin, factor Xa, and factor IXa cleave the same peptide bond in antithrombin (Arg 393 to Ser 394)*, which is termed the reactive site.[60] The antithrombin-protease complex resists dissociation in denaturing agents, suggesting that a covalent bond is formed between the two proteins. The complex can be dissociated by treatment with nucleophiles, which release the protease along with the cleaved form of antithrombin from the complex.[59,61] These properties are consistent with the presence of an ester linkage between the active center serine hydroxyl group of thrombin and the α-carbonyl group of Arg 393 in the reactive site of antithrombin. Currently, it is unknown whether the reactive site peptide bond is cleaved in the native antithrombin-protease complex or whether cleavage occurs on exposure to a denaturing agent.

Antithrombin and other serpins undergo a striking conformational change after proteolytic cleavage at the reactive site (Fig. 176-2). X-ray crystallography of intact serpins, such as ovalbumin, suggests that the P1 to P12 residues N-terminal to the cleavage site form an exposed loop on the surface of the molecule.[62] This structure is consistent with the finding that the region immediately upstream from the reactive site in many serpins is susceptible to proteolytic cleavage by enzymes other than the target protease, resulting in loss of the serpin's inhibitory activity.[63,64] In α_1-antitrypsin cleaved at P1-P1′, movement of the exposed loop about a "hinge" located near P12 allows residues P1 to P12 to become the fourth strand of a six-membered β-sheet (termed β-sheet A), separating the P1 and P1′ amino acids by 69Å.[18] This conformational change results in greater thermal stability of the cleaved ("relaxed") form in comparison with the intact ("stressed") form of the serpin. Mutations of the "hinge" region of antithrombin (e.g., P10 Ala $\rightarrow$ Pro or P12 Ala $\rightarrow$ Thr) appear to interfere with insertion of the exposed reactive site loop into β-sheet A, prevent the "stressed" to "relaxed" conformational change, and convert antithrombin from an inhibitor to a substrate for thrombin and factor Xa.[65,66] Antithrombin is also converted from an inhibitor to a substrate by a monoclonal antibody that recognizes the P8–P12 sequence[67] or by a synthetic peptide that corresponds to P1–P14;[68,69] these reagents are assumed to prevent insertion of the reactive site loop into β-sheet A. Thus, the ability of the reactive site loop to become inserted into β-sheet A appears to be critical for the inhibitory activity of a serpin. Recent x-ray crystallographic studies demonstrate partial insertion of the reactive site loop into β-sheet A of the uncleaved, inhibitory form of antithrombin.[70–73]

Proteolytic Inactivation. Neutrophil elastase inactivates antithrombin by proteolytic cleavage in the reactive site loop to yield the "relaxed" conformation of the inhibitor.[74] Inactivation by this protease may explain the decreased antithrombin activity observed in patients with sepsis.[75] Other proteases involved in inflammation, including matrix metalloproteinases-1, -2, and -3, inactivate antithrombin very slowly or not at all.[76] Antithrombin is also inactivated by certain snake venom proteases.[77]

Proteolytic inactivation of antithrombin by target proteases such as thrombin and factor Xa occurs in the presence of heparin at low ionic strength.[78,79] Thus, the stoichiometry of inhibition of thrombin in the presence of heparin decreases from ~0.9 to

*Residues that extend in the N-terminal direction from the reactive site are numbered P1, P2, P3, ... beginning with Arg 393, whereas those extending in the C-terminal direction are numbered P1′, P2′, P3′, ... beginning with Ser 394.

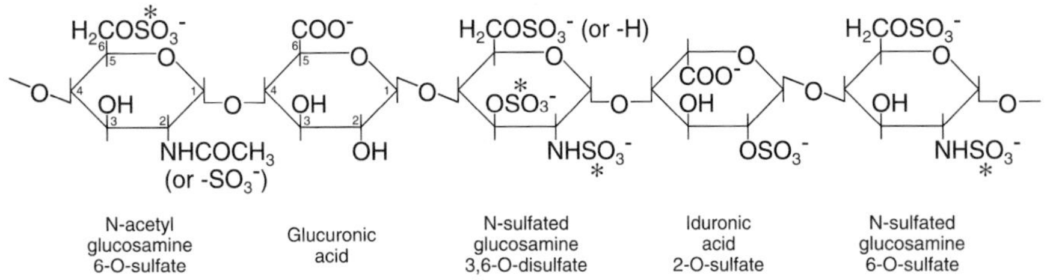

Fig. 176-3 Structure of the antithrombin binding pentasaccharide of heparin. Sulfate groups marked with asterisks are essential for high-affinity binding to antithrombin. The first residue may be either N-sulfated or N-acetylated, and the C6 position of the third residue may or may not be sulfated.

~0.1 mol of thrombin per mol of antithrombin as the ionic strength is lowered from 0.3 to 0.01.[78] The mechanism by which heparin at low ionic strength favors cleavage of the reactive site rather than stable complex formation is unclear.

Stimulation of Antithrombin by Heparin

Kinetics. The concentration of antithrombin in plasma (2 to 3 μM) greatly exceeds that of any of the target proteases generated during coagulation. Under these conditions, protease inhibition follows pseudo-first-order kinetics. In the absence of heparin, thrombin and factor Xa are inhibited by antithrombin in plasma with $t_{\frac{1}{2}}$'s of 0.5 to 1.5 min, while factor IXa is inhibited about 10 times more slowly.[80] Addition of heparin to plasma increases the rate of inhibition of all three proteases ~1000 times. As a result, inhibition of thrombin, factor Xa, and factor IXa by antithrombin becomes essentially instantaneous ($t_{\frac{1}{2}}$ = 10 to 60 ms).[80] Heparin also stimulates inhibition of XIa, XIIa, kallikrein, and plasmin, but the magnitude of the effect is much less.

The anticoagulant effect produced by an IV infusion of heparin is thought to be caused mainly by stimulation of antithrombin-protease reactions, although inhibition of thrombin by heparin cofactor II[45] and factor Xa by tissue factor pathway inhibitor may also contribute.[81] The major effect of heparin is apparently to blunt the positive feedback reactions of thrombin on activation of factors V and VIII, thus decreasing the rate of generation of thrombin.[82–84]

Structure of Heparin and Heparan Sulfate. Heparin occurs in the secretory granules of mast cells. A closely related glycosaminoglycan, heparan sulfate, is found on the surface of most eukaryotic cells and in the extracellular matrix. Heparin and heparan sulfate are synthesized from UDP-sugar precursors as linear polymers of alternating D-glucuronic acid and *N*-acetyl-D-glucosamine.[14,85,86] Each glycosaminoglycan chain is built on a core structure consisting of one xylose and two galactose residues covalently attached to serine in a polypeptide backbone. About 10 to 15 glycosaminoglycan chains, each containing 200 to 300 monosaccharide units, are attached to the core protein serglycin to yield the heparin proteoglycan, which has a molecular mass of 750 to 1000 kDa. By contrast, heparan sulfate proteoglycans vary considerably in structure. They are generally smaller than the heparin proteoglycan and contain fewer glycosaminoglycan chains linked to one of several core proteins (e.g., syndecan, glypican, perlecan). In some cases, the core protein has a hydrophobic domain that anchors the proteoglycan to a cell membrane.

As the glycosaminoglycan chains are being synthesized, they undergo a series of modification reactions that include:[14,85,86] (a) N-deacetylation of glucosamine residues, followed by sulfation of the free amino groups to yield N-sulfated glucosamine; (b) epimerization at the C5 position of D-glucuronic acid to yield L-iduronic acid; (c) O-sulfation of iduronic acid residues at the C2 position; and (d) O-sulfation of glucosamine residues at the C6 position. In addition, several minor but important reactions occur, including O-sulfation of glucuronic acid at C2 and C3 and glucosamine at C3. The reactions that modify the glycosaminoglycan chain appear to be catalyzed by membrane-bound enzymes in the Golgi apparatus and are completed within minutes of synthesis of the core protein. Many of these reactions are regulated by modifications that have occurred on neighboring sugar residues. Furthermore, all the reactions, with the exception of N-sulfation, are incomplete, yielding heterogeneous oligosaccharide structures within the glycosaminoglycan chain. Heparan sulfate generally undergoes less polymer modification than heparin and, therefore, contains higher proportions of glucuronic acid and N-acetylglucosamine and fewer sulfate groups.

Binding Site in Heparin for Antithrombin. Heparin can be fractionated according to its ability to bind to antithrombin.[87–89] The high affinity molecules account for virtually all the anticoagulant activity of the starting material, while the low affinity molecules are inactive. Heparin binds to antithrombin with a dissociation constant of ~20 nM.[90,91] Binding is disrupted at high ionic strength, and therefore appears to result primarily from electrostatic interactions between sulfate or carboxylate groups in heparin and basic amino acid residues in antithrombin. The smallest fragment of heparin that binds to antithrombin with high affinity is the pentasaccharide shown in Fig. 176-3.[92–94] This structure contains a 3-O-sulfate group that occurs predominantly in the high affinity binding site. Several of the sulfate groups within the pentasaccharide are essential for binding to antithrombin, while others do not appear to be required. In commercial heparin preparations, ~30 percent of the molecules contain this structure and bind to antithrombin with high affinity. A similar pentasaccharide structure can arise during the biosynthesis of heparan sulfate, although usually at a much lower frequency in comparison with mast cell heparin. Other types of glycosaminoglycans (e.g., dermatan sulfate, chondroitin 4-sulfate, and chondroitin 6-sulfate) do not interact with antithrombin.[46]

About 1 to 10 percent of the heparan sulfate chains synthesized by vascular endothelial cells contain antithrombin binding sites and stimulate protease inhibition by antithrombin.[95] The high affinity heparan sulfate chains appear to be segregated from the low affinity chains on different subpopulations of endothelial cell core proteins.[96] A variety of other cells, including fibroblasts and melanoma cells, also synthesize high affinity heparan sulfate chains.[97] Antithrombin binding sites are particularly abundant in heparan sulfate isolated from mouse Reichert's membrane (an extraembryonic uterine basement membrane)[98] and the basement membrane of mouse mammary epithelial cells.[99] There is good evidence that antithrombin interacts with endothelial heparan sulfate (see "Activation of Antithrombin by Vascular Heparan Sulfate" below), but the physiological significance of antithrombin binding sites in other tissues is unknown.

Binding Site in Antithrombin for Heparin. The heparin binding site in antithrombin has been studied by chemical modification, analysis of natural and site-directed mutants, and x-ray crystallography. The following observations suggest that amino acid residues between positions 107 and 145 are involved in binding to heparin: (a) Heparin blocks the chemical modification of Lys 107, Lys 114, Lys 125, Arg 129, Lys 136, and Arg 145, and these modifications decrease the heparin cofactor activity of antithrombin without affecting its ability to inhibit thrombin in the absence of heparin.[100–103] (b) An antibody against residues 124 to 145 blocks heparin binding and partially mimics the ability of heparin to stimulate formation of the thrombin-antithrombin complex.[104] (c) The synthetic peptide corresponding to residues 123 to 139, but not a random peptide of the same composition, competes with

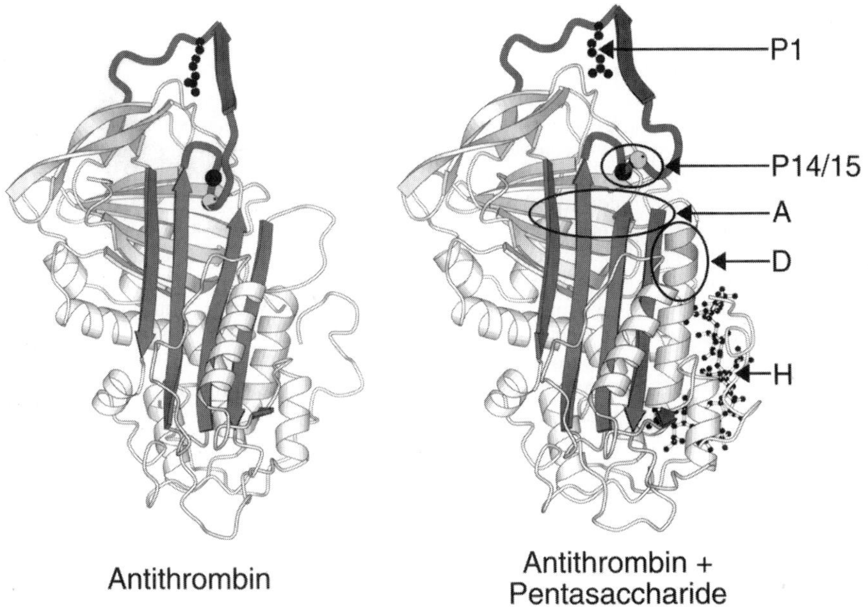

Fig. 176-4 Conformational changes in antithrombin induced by heparin. Shown are the structures of native inhibitory antithrombin[73] and the antithrombin-pentasaccharide complex[72] determined by x-ray crystallography. Binding of heparin (H) is associated with elongation of α-helix D (D), closure of the upper portion of β-sheet A (A), and expulsion of residues P14 and P15 of the reactive site loop (P14/15). As a result of heparin binding, the orientation of the P1 arginine residue (P1) may change so that it becomes accessible to attack by a target protease. However, this change is not apparent on comparison of the two structures, because the P1 residue in both crystals was constrained by contact with an adjacent antithrombin molecule.

antithrombin for binding to heparin.[105] (d) The presence of an oligosaccharide linked to Asn 135 decreases the affinity of α-antithrombin for heparin relative to that of β-antithrombin.[26] (e) The disulfide bond between Cys 8 and Cys 128 is required for the integrity of the heparin binding site.[22]

Other studies suggest that the heparin-binding site includes residues in the N-terminal portion of antithrombin. For example, natural mutations of Ile 7, Arg 24, Pro 41, and Arg 47,[106–110] as well as chemical modification of Trp 49,[111] decrease the affinity of antithrombin for heparin. In addition, proton NMR experiments implicate His 1 and possibly His 65 in heparin binding.[112] Based on molecular modeling, the suggestion was made that Arg 47 and the basic amino acid residues near Lys 125 are clustered on the surface of antithrombin to form a single heparin-binding site.[18]

Estimates of the number of ion pairs (four or five) that exist in the antithrombin-heparin complex imply that not all of the basic amino acid residues identified in the experiments mentioned above participate directly in heparin binding.[79] Recently, Carrell and coworkers crystallized antithrombin complexed with a synthetic analog of the high affinity heparin pentasaccharide.[72] X-ray diffraction analysis suggested that hydrogen bonds occur between sulfate and carboxylate groups on the pentasaccharide and the side chains of Arg 46, Arg 47, Lys 114, Lys 125, and Arg 129, in general agreement with the previous studies.

Allosteric and Template Effects of Heparin. Rapid kinetic analyses indicate that heparin binding induces a conformational change in antithrombin that locks the glycosaminoglycan into place on the surface of the inhibitor.[91] The heparin-antithrombin complex then reacts rapidly with a target protease. Formation of the antithrombin-protease complex reduces the affinity of antithrombin for heparin, allowing the complex to dissociate from the heparin molecule.[113] Thus a single heparin molecule can catalyze the formation of many antithrombin-protease complexes.

The mechanism by which heparin catalyzes the inhibition of proteases by antithrombin involves both allosteric and template effects. Heparin binding induces a conformational change that affects the reactive site of antithrombin, which permits target proteases to interact more rapidly with this site. This model is supported by the fact that changes in antithrombin as a consequence of heparin binding can be detected by UV absorbance,[114] fluorescence,[115,116] circular dichroism,[114,117] and proton NMR.[118] Additional evidence for a conformational linkage between the heparin-binding site and the reactive site was obtained using a fluorescence probe covalently attached to the reactive site P1 residue[119] and a monoclonal antibody that binds to the 1C/4B region adjacent to the reactive site loop.[120] Comparison of the structures of antithrombin crystallized with and without the heparin pentasaccharide suggests that binding of heparin induces elongation of α-helix D, which, in turn, causes closure of β-sheet A with expulsion of the partially inserted reactive site loop (Fig. 176-4).[72,121] As a result, the orientation of the P1 arginine residue may change so that it becomes accessible to attack by a proteolytic enzyme.[122]

Heparin can also function as a template to which both antithrombin and the target protease bind. Thus, catalysis occurs by an approximation effect. This model is supported by the fact that heparin molecules containing ≥ 18 sugar residues are required to catalyze the reaction of antithrombin with thrombin, even though smaller molecules bind with high affinity and induce a conformational change.[93,123] Physical evidence also indicates formation of ternary complexes containing antithrombin, heparin, and thrombin.[124,125]

The balance between the allosteric and template effects appears to explain differences in the rate enhancement for inhibition of thrombin and factor Xa produced by heparin chains of varying length (Table 176-1). For example, the synthetic pentasaccharide that contains only the antithrombin binding site of heparin increases the rate of inhibition of factor Xa ~270 times, but has relatively little effect on the rate of inhibition of thrombin.[79] Because an oligosaccharide of this size is unlikely to function as a template, induction of a conformational change in the reactive site of antithrombin may be sufficient to promote inhibition of factor Xa. Longer heparin chains produce only an additional twofold increase in the rate of factor Xa inhibition. Stimulation of the thrombin-antithrombin reaction requires heparin molecules that

Table 176-1 Second-Order Rate Constants for Inhibition of Proteases by Antithrombin-Heparin Complexes

	Thrombin	Factor Xa
	$\times 10^6\ M^{-1}s^{-1}$ (increase)	
Antithrombin	0.0087	0.0023
Antithrombin + pentasaccharide	0.0146 (1.7)	0.61 (270)
Antithrombin + full-length heparin*	37 (4300)	1.3 (570)

*24 to 28 monosaccharide units in length.
Data from Olson et al.[79]

contain at least 18 sugar residues, which are the smallest chains capable of forming a ternary complex with antithrombin and active site-blocked thrombin.[125] The factor IXa-antithrombin reaction has a similar requirement for longer heparin chains. Therefore, inhibition of thrombin and factor IXa appear to depend primarily on the template effect.

At low heparin concentrations, the rate of inhibition of thrombin or factor Xa is proportional to the concentration of heparin-antithrombin complexes present in the incubation.[80,90] The rate of inhibition plateaus at a concentration of heparin that is sufficient to saturate the antithrombin. Higher concentrations of heparin decrease the rate of inhibition of thrombin, presumably by favoring the binding of thrombin and antithrombin to separate heparin chains, but do not decrease the rate of inhibition of factor Xa.[80,90] These observations are consistent with predominance of the template effect in catalysis of the thrombin-antithrombin reaction.[126]

Thrombin binds to heparin with a dissociation constant of 6 to 10 μM under physiologic conditions.[127] An increase in the NaCl concentration from 0.15 to 0.30 M causes parallel reductions of 20 to 30 times in the affinity of thrombin for heparin and in the rate of inhibition of thrombin by antithrombin in the presence of full-length heparin.[79,126] By contrast, the thrombin-antithrombin reaction in the absence of heparin is much less dependent on the ionic strength. Chemical modifications of thrombin that decrease its affinity for heparin greatly reduce the ability of heparin to stimulate the thrombin-antithrombin reaction.[124] Factor Xa also binds to heparin, but apparently with a much lower affinity in comparison to thrombin. Inhibition of factor Xa by antithrombin in the presence or absence of heparin is essentially unaffected by changes in ionic strength or by chemical modification of factor Xa to reduce its affinity for heparin.[79,128] These observations suggest that binding of thrombin, but not factor Xa, to heparin is required for catalysis of the antithrombin-protease reaction.

Modulators of Heparin Catalysis. Several proteins competitively inhibit binding of antithrombin to heparin. They include histidine-rich glycoprotein[129] and vitronectin (complement S protein),[130] both of which are present in plasma at micromolar concentrations. Whether these proteins regulate hemostasis remains to be determined. In this regard, histidine-rich glycoprotein does not inhibit the interaction of antithrombin with heparan sulfate on the surface of cultured aortic endothelial cells.[131] Platelet factor 4 is released from the α-granules during platelet aggregation and binds tightly to heparin.[129] It may promote local clot formation at the site of hemostasis by blocking the binding of antithrombin to heparan sulfate. Soluble fibrin monomers decrease the rate of inhibition of thrombin by antithrombin in the presence or absence of heparin,[132] and thrombin bound to a fibrin clot is protected from inhibition by antithrombin in the presence of heparin.[133]

Activity of Antithrombin in Vivo

Protease Inhibition. Radiolabeled thrombin rapidly forms complexes with antithrombin after IV injection in rabbits.[134] Furthermore, low concentrations of thrombin-antithrombin complex (20 to 100 pM) can be detected in plasma from healthy human subjects and may reflect the basal rate of generation of thrombin under normal circumstances.[135] The concentration of the thrombin-antithrombin complex is increased in certain pathological conditions such as disseminated intravascular coagulation.[135,136]

Formation of factor IXa-antithrombin complexes also occurs rapidly in vivo.[42] By contrast, factor Xa mainly forms complexes with α_2-macroglobulin after IV injection in the mouse, although the major inhibitors of factor Xa incubated with murine plasma in vitro are α_1-antitrypsin and antithrombin.[137] Factor Xa is protected from inhibition by antithrombin in vitro when the protease is bound to platelets[138] or to the prothrombinase complex which contains factor Va, prothrombin, and phospholipids.[139] It is uncertain whether these mechanisms also protect factor Xa from inhibition by antithrombin in vivo. The factor Xa-antithrombin complex can be detected at low concentrations (20 to 50 pM) in normal subjects.[140]

Clearance of Antithrombin-Protease Complexes. Antithrombin-protease complexes are cleared from the circulation by hepatocytes with a half-life of 2 to 3 min,[42,141] which is considerably more rapid than the rate of clearance of free antithrombin ($t_{\frac{1}{2}}$ ~3 days).[142] The hepatocyte uptake mechanism is saturable both in vivo and in vitro.[143] Cross-competition experiments suggest that the receptor for hepatic uptake also recognizes complexes of proteases with α_1-antitrypsin, α_1-antichymotrypsin, and heparin cofactor II.[144] The low density lipoprotein receptor-related protein (LRP) is responsible for endocytosis and degradation of thrombin-antithrombin, thrombin-heparin cofactor II, and trypsin-α_1-antitrypsin complexes by human hepatoma (HepG2) cells and for the in vivo clearance of ^{125}I-thrombin-antithrombin complexes in rats.[145] In human serum, the thrombin-antithrombin complex is associated with vitronectin.[146] Vitronectin mediates binding of the thrombin-antithrombin complex to endothelial cells in vitro,[147] and internalization of the thrombin-antithrombin complex by cultured human umbilical vein endothelial cells has been demonstrated.[148] Whether these processes contribute to the clearance of thrombin-antithrombin complexes from the circulation or serve some other function remains to be determined.

Activation of Antithrombin by Vascular Heparan Sulfate

Because of the dramatic effect of heparin on the activity of antithrombin in vitro, it has long been assumed that an endogenous heparin-like substance must stimulate antithrombin in vivo. Under normal circumstances, heparin is not released from mast cells into the circulation and cannot be detected in plasma. However, a small amount of heparin may appear in the circulation of patients with systemic mastocytosis and produce a mild prolongation of the activated partial thromboplastin time.[149] Circulating heparan sulfate, apparently released from damaged tissues, has been reported to cause marked prolongation of the activated partial thromboplastin time and bleeding in a few severely ill patients.[150–153]

Interaction of Antithrombin with Endothelial Cells. Current evidence suggests that heparan sulfate proteoglycans anchored in the vessel wall interact with circulating antithrombin to produce an antithrombotic effect. Glycosaminoglycans extracted from cloned endothelial cells possess anticoagulant activity.[154] Treatment of the extracts with heparinase abolishes the activity, indicating that the active moiety is heparin-like. De novo biosynthesis of heparan sulfate proteoglycans has been demonstrated by culturing endothelial cells in the presence of [^{35}S]sulfate.[95] Approximately 1 to 10 percent of the labeled heparan sulfate from endothelial cells binds to immobilized antithrombin with high affinity, and this fraction possesses essentially all the anticoagulant activity of the cell extract. Structural analysis of the high-affinity heparan sulfate has revealed the presence of the 3-O-sulfated glucosamine residue that is characteristic of the antithrombin-binding structure of heparin.[95]

Direct binding of antithrombin to endothelial cells cloned from bovine aorta has been demonstrated. The inhibitor binds to approximately 60,000 sites per cell with a dissociation constant of 12 nM.[95] Binding is diminished by pretreatment of the cells with heparinase. Similar results were obtained with intact segments of bovine aorta.[155] However, the binding of antithrombin to intact rabbit aortic endothelium is weak, whereas antithrombin appears to bind more avidly to heparinase-sensitive components beneath the endothelial cell layer.[156] Electron microscopic autoradiography of ^{125}I-labeled antithrombin bound to endothelial cells in culture or after perfusion of segments of rat aorta ex vivo indicates that >90 percent of the antithrombin is associated with the extracellular matrix located in the subendothelium.[157] Binding to the subendothelial matrix is greatly increased after crush injury of the aorta, which removes most of the endothelial cells. Because the intact endothelium appears to be permeable to proteins, coagulation proteases may interact with antithrombin bound to subendothelial heparan sulfate proteoglycans.[157] Inhibition of thrombin in the subendothelium appears to be mediated primarily by β-antithrombin.[158]

Interleukin-1 and tumor necrosis factor decrease heparan sulfate biosynthesis in cultured endothelial cells and reduce the amount of antithrombin that can be bound per cell by ~50 percent.[159] This mechanism could contribute to the increased thrombogenicity of the endothelium induced by cytokines.

Stimulation of Antithrombin Activity In Vivo. Evidence for the stimulation of antithrombin by vascular heparan sulfate in vivo was obtained using a rodent hind limb preparation.[160] The hind limb was first perfused with thrombin to saturate thrombin binding sites (most likely thrombomodulin) present in the microvasculature. When the concentration of thrombin present in the venous effluent had reached a steady state, antithrombin was perfused through the preparation, and the amount of thrombin-antithrombin complex recovered in the effluent was determined. Complex formation occurred fifteenfold to nineteenfold more rapidly within the microvasculature as compared with in vitro incubations in the absence of heparin. The rate enhancement was diminished by prior perfusion of the hind limb preparation with heparinase or by chemical modification of the antithrombin at Trp 49 to decrease the affinity for heparin, suggesting that interaction of antithrombin with microvascular heparan sulfate was responsible for the enhanced rate of inhibition.

Role of Thrombomodulin. When a trace amount of thrombin is injected into the circulation, the thrombin appears to become bound initially to thrombomodulin on the endothelial cell surface.[134] Thrombomodulin mediates internalization of thrombin by endothelial cells in vitro, but the importance of this pathway for the clearance of thrombin in vivo is uncertain.[161] In comparison with free thrombin, thrombin bound to bovine lung thrombomodulin reacts less rapidly with fibrinogen and heparin cofactor II, more rapidly with protein C, and at about the same rate with antithrombin.[162] The net effect of these changes in substrate specificity may be a small increase (approximately threefold) in the rate of the thrombin-antithrombin reaction because of diminished competition from other substrates. Accordingly, only when thrombomodulin becomes saturated with thrombin is the excess thrombin inhibited rapidly by antithrombin bound to heparan sulfate proteoglycans.

Thrombomodulin may have different effects on the thrombin-antithrombin reaction depending on the tissue or species of origin. Rabbit lung thrombomodulin is a proteoglycan that bears a single chondroitin sulfate chain. It accelerates the thrombin-antithrombin reaction fourfold to eightfold by a mechanism that depends on the presence of both the protein and glycosaminoglycan components.[163,164] Expression of recombinant human thrombomodulin in human embryonal kidney cells yields two forms of the protein; the higher molecular weight form contains a chondroitin sulfate chain and stimulates the thrombin-antithrombin reaction.[165] By contrast, thrombomodulin purified from human placenta or bovine lung does not have these properties.[162,166]

ANTITHROMBIN DEFICIENCY

Antithrombin deficiency was the first inherited abnormality to be associated with a thrombotic tendency.[13] The diagnosis is usually made in patients who experiences the onset of recurrent thromboembolic disease at an early age or in whom a positive family history of thromboembolic disease is obtained. The diagnosis is established by determination of the antithrombin activity in the patient's plasma.

Assay Methods

The antithrombin concentration in plasma is determined with a functional assay that measures the capacity of a sample to inhibit exogenous thrombin or factor Xa over a short period of time in the presence of heparin (heparin cofactor assay). Such assays are conveniently performed with a chromogenic substrate to detect the residual protease activity at the end of the incubation. Heparin cofactor assays that use thrombin as the target protease may overestimate the concentration of antithrombin to a modest degree due to the presence of heparin cofactor II in the sample.[45,167,168] The use of factor Xa allows greater specificity because heparin cofactor II does not react with this protease.[169] An assay that measures the inhibition of thrombin over a longer time in the absence of heparin (so-called "progressive" antithrombin assay) gives a rough indication of the antithrombin concentration but may also be influenced by α_1-antitrypsin and α_2-macroglobulin.[170] Immunologic assays are used in conjunction with functional assays to detect inactive variants of antithrombin. Crossed immunoelectrophoresis in the presence and absence of heparin is commonly used to detect variants with altered heparin binding properties.

Normal Levels

The mean concentration of antithrombin in plasma from adults is ~2.6 μM (150 μg/ml).[171] The range of antithrombin activity determined in 9669 healthy individuals 17 to 65 years of age was 105.6 ± 11.2 IU/dl (mean ± SD).[172] Small differences in antithrombin levels have been noted depending on age, sex, hormonal status, and cardiovascular risk factors.[172,173] Healthy, full-term newborn infants have antithrombin antigen concentrations 39 to 87 percent of the mean adult value.[174] The level gradually increases into the normal adult range by 3 months of age.

Classification of Inherited Deficiencies

There is no universally accepted nomenclature for the various types of antithrombin deficiency. The classification described below is that proposed by Lane et al. for the Antithrombin Mutation Database: 2nd (1997) Update (http://www.med.ic.ac.uk/dd/ddhc/default.htm).

Type I. Classical (type I) antithrombin deficiency is inherited as an autosomal dominant trait. Affected heterozygous individuals have ~50 percent of the normal plasma levels of both antithrombin activity and antigen.[176] Total absence of antithrombin has not been reported and may be lethal in utero. Type I antithrombin deficiency can result from deletion of one of the two antithrombin alleles, from a dysfunctional allele, or from missense, nonsense, or frameshift mutations in the coding sequence. Approximately 80 point mutations and 12 large deletions have been reported to cause type I deficiency.[175] The catabolic rate of infused radiolabeled antithrombin is normal in patients with inherited antithrombin deficiency, suggesting that the deficiency is not exacerbated by accelerated clearance of antithrombin produced by the normal allele.[177,178]

Type II. Patients who have a low level of antithrombin activity but approximately normal antithrombin antigen have type II deficiencies. The occurrence of variant forms of the inhibitor with impaired activity has provided important insights into the mechanism of action of antithrombin.[179,180] Approximately 35 such variants are identified and are grouped into several categories:[175] (a) Type II RS (reactive site) mutations interfere with the ability of antithrombin to inhibit proteases. These mutations generally have been found at the P2, P1, or P1′ residue of the reactive site or at the "hinge" region (P10 or P12). Another type II RS mutation (Asn-187 → Asp) is associated with formation of inactive polymers of antithrombin at 41°C, which may explain the occurrence of thrombosis during febrile episodes in patients with this abnormality.[181] (b) Type II HBS (heparin binding site) mutations occur in residues that appear to bind directly to heparin (e.g., Arg 47 or Arg 129) or at nearby locations where mutations may distort the structure of the heparin binding site (e.g., Pro 41 and Leu 99). The Ile-7 → Asn mutation creates a new glycosylation site, and the presence of an oligosaccharide at this site may sterically interfere with heparin binding.[106] (c) Type II PE (pleiotropic effect) mutations affect both the reactive site and the heparin binding site. Most of these mutations occur in the region P9′ to P14′, which is thought to be involved in the conformational linkage between the reactive site and the heparin binding site. Although some type II mutations may impair the intracellular processing and secretion of antithrombin,[182] type II variants generally appear to be synthesized at a normal rate and have a normal half-life in the circulation. Therefore, in most instances the plasma of an affected heterozygote has approximately equimolar amounts of normal and variant antithrombin. In contrast to type I antithrombin deficiency, several homozygous patients with type II HBS deficiency have been identified,[109,183,184] and individuals with heterozygous type II HBS deficiency are generally asymptomatic.[185]

Prevalence

The prevalence of inherited antithrombin deficiency in the general population has been estimated to range from 1 per 2000 to 1 per 5000, based on the number of symptomatic patients identified in large referral populations.[186,187] However, a more recent study of 4189 healthy blood donors 18 to 65 years of age in Scotland identified 16 unrelated individuals with antithrombin deficiency (1 type I, 2 type II RS, and 13 type II HBS), suggesting that the prevalence may be closer to 1 per 250.[188] Only one of the deficient individuals in this series had a history of thrombosis, which is consistent with the earlier estimates for the prevalence of symptomatic antithrombin deficiency.

The prevalence of antithrombin deficiency in patients with thrombosis has been estimated to range from 2 to 6 percent,[185] although a recent Spanish study found a prevalence of only 0.5 percent.[189] In a series of 752 patients with thromboembolic disease, inherited antithrombin deficiency was established in 13 (1.7 percent) by family studies.[190] Only 1 of the 13 deficient patients in this series had a type II abnormality, in contrast to the much more frequent occurrence of type II abnormalities in asymptomatic individuals.[188] The observation that type I antithrombin deficiency appears to be more common in patients with thromboembolism than in asymptomatic individuals suggests that this type of antithrombin deficiency increases the risk for development of the disease.

Clinical Manifestations

The prevalence of thromboembolic complications in patients with inherited antithrombin deficiency has been estimated from retrospective reviews of published case reports and medical records.[185,191–193] Clinical data from 62 families with antithrombin deficiency, excluding 14 families with type II HBS deficiency, are summarized in Table 176-2.[194] About half of the 964 individuals studied had low plasma antithrombin activities and were apparently heterozygous. The mean prevalence of venous thromboembolism was 50.8 percent in the deficient subjects in comparison with 1.5 percent in the nondeficient subjects. However, the prevalence of venous thromboembolism in the deficient members of different families ranged from 15 to 100 percent. Thrombosis occurred with approximately equal frequency in male and female patients and included deep vein thrombosis of the lower extremities or pulmonary embolism (89.9 percent), mesenteric vein thrombosis (3.1 percent), and cerebral vein thrombosis (0.9 percent). Arterial occlusion was rare. Risk factors such as pregnancy or surgery were associated with 32 percent of the thrombotic episodes and were noted to be absent in 16 percent; however, information about risk factors was not included in the majority of case reports. In some families, coinheritance of antithrombin deficiency and factor V Leiden (see Chap. 170) (which maps to chromosome 1q21-25 and is 3 to 11 cM from the antithrombin gene) appears to result in a more severe thromboembolic phenotype in comparison with individuals who have only one or the other of these molecular abnormalities.[195–197]

Thrombosis has been reported rarely in antithrombin-deficient patients before 15 years of age. It has been suggested that the high levels of α_2-macroglobulin present during childhood (two to three times the adult level) protect antithrombin-deficient children from thrombosis.[198] The incidence of thrombosis in the reported cases was greatest between 15 and 35 years of age and decreased thereafter, presumably because the majority of individuals who became symptomatic were given long-term oral anticoagulant therapy. By 30 years of age, ~60 percent of the antithrombin-deficient subjects had experienced at least one thromboembolic episode.[194] Despite the high incidence of thrombosis, the mortality of patients with antithrombin deficiency, many of whom are anticoagulated indefinitely after their first thromboembolic episode, appears to be no different from that of the general population.[199–201] It is uncertain whether less aggressive treatment of patients with antithrombin deficiency would result in increased mortality.

Most reported cases of antithrombin deficiency were discovered by laboratory investigation of patients with recurrent thromboembolic disease. The bias of ascertainment inherent in such reports may lead to overestimation of the frequency of complications in patients with antithrombin deficiency. Furthermore, the diagnosis of thromboembolism was established by objective tests in a minority of the reported episodes (Table 176-2).

Table 176-2 Summary of Clinical Data from 62 Families with Antithrombin Deficiency

	Number of Subjects	Percent
Prevalence of antithrombin deficiency	449/964	46.6
Prevalence of venous thromboembolism in nondeficient subjects	6/400*	1.5
Prevalence of venous thromboembolism in deficient subjects	228/449	50.8
Site of venous thromboembolism		
Deep vein thrombosis/pulmonary embolism	205	89.9
Mesenteric vein thrombosis	7	3.1
Cerebral vein thrombosis	2	0.9
No information provided	14	6.1
Subtotals	228	100.0
Diagnostic tests		
Venogram	27	11.8
Surgery	3	1.3
Autopsy	3	1.3
Lung scan	2	0.9
Angiogram	2	0.9
CT scan	1	0.4
No information provided	190	83.3
Subtotals	228	100.0
Risk factors		
None identified	36	15.8
Postpartum	22	9.6
Surgery	19	8.3
Pregnancy	18	7.9
Oral contraceptives	5	2.2
Trauma	4	1.8
Immobilization	4	1.8
No information provided	120	52.6
Subtotals	228	100.0

*Includes only studies that provided prevalence of venous thrombosis for nondeficient subjects.
Data from Demers et al.[194]

Because the clinical manifestations of deep vein thrombosis and pulmonary embolism are nonspecific, thromboembolism has probably been misdiagnosed in at least some individuals with antithrombin deficiency. In a large Canadian family, type II RS antithrombin deficiency was established in 31 of 67 individuals by analysis of genomic DNA.[194] Only 6 episodes of venous thromboembolism, 5 of which were associated with known risk factors, were documented by objective tests in the 31 deficient subjects (mean age 36 years), whereas none occurred in the 36 nondeficient subjects. This study suggests that idiopathic thrombosis may occur less frequently than previously estimated in antithrombin-deficient patients.

The clinical manifestations of patients with type II HBS antithrombin deficiency, in which abnormalities are limited to the heparin-binding site, are distinct from those of patients with the other types of deficiencies. Only 3 episodes of thrombosis have been reported among 51 individuals with inherited type II HBS antithrombin deficiency;[185] all 3 episodes occurred in homozygous patients. For example, one family included a child born to consanguineous parents, both of whom had asymptomatic antithrombin deficiency.[184] The child had undetectable heparin cofactor activity and died at 3 years of age of massive intracardiac thrombosis while receiving oral anticoagulant therapy.

Laboratory Abnormalities

With the exception of decreased plasma antithrombin activity, no laboratory abnormalities are associated consistently with antithrombin deficiency. Immunoassays of plasma for prothrombin activation fragment 1·2 and fibrinopeptide A, which are indicative of factor Xa and thrombin activity, respectively, have been used to assess the degree of activation of the coagulation system in vivo. A report that fragment 1·2 levels are elevated two- to threefold in patients with antithrombin deficiency was later found to be incorrect due to an artifact of sample collection.[202,203] A more recent study found a small but statistically significant increase in mean plasma fragment 1·2 concentration in deficient adults not receiving warfarin (0.87 ± 0.26 nM) in comparison with nondeficient adults (0.70 ± 0.21 nM, $p = 0.03$).[204] However, most of the fragment 1·2 values in the deficient adults were within the normal range. No increase in fibrinopeptide A has been found in antithrombin-deficient subjects.[202,204]

Oral anticoagulant therapy is reported to increase the antithrombin level into the normal range in some deficient patients.[205]

Treatment

Anticoagulant therapy is indicated for patients with antithrombin deficiency following acute episodes of deep vein thrombosis or pulmonary embolism. The treatment is similar to that used for patients with normal antithrombin and routinely consists of an initial 5- to 7-day course of heparin administered by continuous IV infusion followed by oral anticoagulation with warfarin.[206] Warfarin is initiated on the first hospital day to allow time for depletion of the vitamin K dependent coagulation factors before the heparin is discontinued. Patients with antithrombin deficiency generally respond to standard doses of IV heparin as indicated by an increase in the activated partial thromboplastin time.[207] However, an occasional patient with inherited antithrombin deficiency, as well as patients with severe acquired antithrombin deficiency (< 10 percent of normal), may be resistant to heparin.[208] In theory, treatment with a concentrate of purified antithrombin in combination with IV heparin might benefit patients with heparin resistance. Heparin itself can cause a modest ($\sim$15 percent) decrease in the circulating antithrombin concentration, but this effect is unlikely to have clinical significance.[209]

The duration of therapy with warfarin remains controversial. Most authors recommend lifelong treatment of antithrombin-deficient patients after the first thromboembolic episode. Some advocate treatment of asymptomatic family members with documented antithrombin deficiency who have never had a thromboembolic episode. These recommendations are based on anecdotal experience and may not be warranted in view of the morbidity due to hemorrhage associated with long-term anticoagulant therapy.[210] However, patients with recurrent thromboembolism may be candidates for indefinite oral anticoagulant therapy, regardless of whether they have antithrombin deficiency.[211]

The incidence of thrombotic complications in women with antithrombin deficiency during pregnancy and postpartum is estimated to range from 37 to 68 percent.[212–214] A recent study, however, identified only one episode of venous thromboembolism during 33 pregnancies (3 percent) in antithrombin-deficient women who were previously asymptomatic.[215] Nevertheless, antithrombin-deficient patients, especially those with a history venous thromboembolism, should be considered for prophylactic anticoagulation during pregnancy and postpartum. Because warfarin is associated with an increase in the incidence of fetal hemorrhage, stillbirth, and developmental abnormalities, subcutaneous heparin regimens that appear to be effective in preventing thrombosis in these patients have been developed.[216] Some physicians have used antithrombin concentrates and a lower dose of heparin in the peripartum period to minimize the risk of bleeding.[217] However, delivery has been managed successfully without the use of antithrombin concentrates in some antithrombin-deficient patients.[207,218]

Approximately 30 percent of pregnancies in women with antithrombin deficiency end with fetal death in utero.[219,220] It is unknown whether prophylactic anticoagulation would reduce the incidence of this complication.

Antithrombin concentrates[221,222] and androgens[223–225] have been used to treat deep vein thrombosis and to prevent thrombosis at the time of surgery in antithrombin-deficient patients. Although these agents increase the plasma concentration of antithrombin, their clinical efficacy is unproven.

Acquired Deficiencies

Acquired antithrombin deficiency with very low plasma concentrations (10 to 30 percent of normal) can occur in liver disease,[226] in the nephrotic syndrome,[227] and during disseminated intravascular coagulation.[228] Whether antithrombin deficiency contributes to the thrombotic complications associated with these conditions is unclear. Less severe acquired deficiencies have been reported in preeclampsia[229] and diabetes mellitus.[230] Antithrombin is mildly decreased in patients taking estrogens[231] or diethylstilbesterol,[232] and these medications should probably be avoided in patients with inherited antithrombin deficiency. A more profound decrease in antithrombin occurs in patients receiving L-asparaginase.[233] The levels of procoagulant factors such as prothrombin are decreased concomitantly by L-asparaginase, and there is uncertainty about the existence of a hypercoagulable state attributable to antithrombin deficiency in these patients.[234,235]

HEPARIN COFACTOR II

Antithrombin was initially thought to be the only heparin-dependent inhibitor of thrombin in plasma.[17,236] However, experiments suggesting the presence of a second heparin cofactor activity[45,237] were confirmed by the isolation of heparin cofactor II from human plasma.[238] Heparin cofactor II has a more restricted protease specificity than antithrombin,[239] and its activity is stimulated by dermatan sulfate as well as by heparin.[46] These properties suggest that the physiological function of heparin cofactor II is distinct from that of antithrombin.

Structure and Biosynthesis

Heparin cofactor II is a single-chain, 66-kDa glycoprotein.[238] The cDNA for heparin cofactor II encodes a polypeptide 480 amino acids in length preceded by a 19-residue signal peptide (GenBank M12849).[240,241] Heparin cofactor II is $\sim$30 percent identical in sequence to antithrombin and other serpins, the greatest similarity occurring in the C-terminal two-thirds of the protein. By contrast, the first 80 amino acid residues at the N-terminal end of heparin cofactor II share no homology with other serpins and include two tyrosine residues that become O-sulfated during biosynthesis.[242] Peptides cleaved from this portion of heparin cofactor II by neutrophil proteases have potent chemotactic activity.[243] Heparin cofactor II contains three asparagine-linked glycosylation sites and three cysteine residues that apparently do not form disulfide bonds.[244]

The gene for heparin cofactor II is located on human chromosome 22q11.[245] It contains five exons distributed over ~16 kb of DNA (GenBank M58600).[245,246] No TATA or CAAT sequence is present in the 5′ flanking region of the heparin cofactor II gene, and transcription may initiate at several positions.[246] Human liver contains a 2200-nucleotide mRNA for heparin cofactor II,[240] and biosynthesis has been demonstrated in cultured human hepatoma cells.[242,247]

Protease Specificity

Heparin cofactor II differs from antithrombin with respect to its protease specificity. Among the proteases involved in coagulation and fibrinolysis, heparin cofactor II inhibits only thrombin.[239] The reactive site peptide bond attacked by thrombin contains a leucine residue in the P1 position, which is atypical of thrombin substrates.[248] In fact, heparin cofactor II inhibits chymotrypsin more rapidly than it inhibits thrombin in the absence of a glycosaminoglycan.[249] Mutation of the P1 leucine to arginine increases the basal rate of inhibition of thrombin in the absence of a glycosaminoglycan ~100 times and eliminates the ability of heparin cofactor II to inhibit chymotrypsin.[250] These results emphasize the importance of the P1 residue as a determinant of protease specificity and suggest that heparin cofactor II has evolved to be essentially inactive toward thrombin in the absence of a glycosaminoglycan.

Stimulation by Glycosaminoglycans

The rate of inhibition of thrombin by heparin cofactor II is increased ~1000 times by heparin, heparan sulfate, or dermatan sulfate.[46] The affinity of heparin cofactor II for heparin is lower than that of antithrombin, and a tenfold higher concentration of heparin is required to accelerate thrombin inhibition by heparin cofactor II.[46,238] Heparin cofactor II does not require the specific pentasaccharide structure shown in Fig. 176-3 for stimulation by heparin.[251,252] Moreover, heparin cofactor II appears to bind nonspecifically to heparin oligosaccharides that contain ≥ 4 monosaccharide units regardless of their composition.[253] Heparin chains containing ≥ 26 monosaccharide units stimulate thrombin inhibition by heparin cofactor II, although shorter oligosaccharides also possess weak activity.[254,255]

Heparin cofactor II is unique with regard to its capability to be stimulated by dermatan sulfate. Dermatan sulfate is a repeating polymer of D-glucuronic or L-iduronic acid and *N*-acetyl-D-galactosamine.[256] O-Sulfation of iduronic acid residues at the C2 position and of galactosamine residues at the C4 and C6 positions occurs to a variable extent, yielding heterogeneous structures within the polymer. Like heparan sulfate, dermatan sulfate is a component of proteoglycans on the cell surface and in the extracellular matrix. Heparin cofactor II binds preferentially to a minor subpopulation of dermatan sulfate oligosaccharides, in contrast to the nonspecific binding observed with heparin oligosaccharides. The high affinity binding site for heparin cofactor II in dermatan sulfate is a tandem repeat of three iduronic acid 2-sulfate → N-acetylgalactosamine 4-sulfate disaccharide subunits, which appear to be clustered within the polymer.[257] The high affinity hexasaccharide increases the rate of inhibition of thrombin by heparin cofactor II ~50 times,[257] although dermatan sulfate chains containing ≥ 14 monosaccharide units are required for maximal stimulation.[258] An invertebrate dermatan sulfate composed predominantly of iduronic acid 2-sulfate → N-acetylgalactosamine 6-sulfate disaccharide subunits is 100 times less active than mammalian dermatan sulfate, indicating that 4-O-sulfation of galactosamine is essential for activity with heparin cofactor II.[259] Addition of dermatan sulfate to plasma in vitro causes prolongation of the thrombin time and the activated partial thromboplastin time,[260] and IV infusion of dermatan sulfate produces an antithrombotic effect in experimental animals[261–264] and humans.[265–267] These effects appear to be mediated primarily by heparin cofactor II.[46,268,269]

Glycosaminoglycan Binding Site

Analysis of the natural variant heparin cofactor II Oslo (Arg 189 → His) established that heparin and dermatan sulfate interact with different amino acid residues on the surface of the inhibitor.[270,271] This mutation results in a large decrease (~60 times) in the affinity of heparin cofactor II for dermatan sulfate, but does not affect the affinity of the inhibitor for heparin. Arg 189 occurs within a cluster of basic amino acid residues that can be aligned with basic residues in the heparin-binding site of antithrombin but are poorly conserved in other serpins. Mutations of Lys 173, Arg 184, and Arg 185 in recombinant heparin cofactor II affect heparin binding, whereas mutations of Arg 184, Arg 185, Arg 189, Arg 192, and Arg 193 affect dermatan sulfate binding.[271–275] These results indicate that, although the binding sites for heparin and dermatan sulfate overlap, they are not identical.

Mechanism of Stimulation by Glycosaminoglycans

The stimulatory effect of heparin and dermatan sulfate depends on the presence of an acidic polypeptide domain near the N-terminus of heparin cofactor II.[276] The acidic domain contains a tandem repeat of two nearly identical sequences (-Glu-Asp-Asp-Asp-Tyr(SO_4)-Leu/Ile-Asp-), each of which is similar to the C-terminal sequence of hirudin, a potent thrombin inhibitor in the saliva of the medicinal leech. The C-terminal portion of hirudin binds with high affinity to anion-binding exosite I of thrombin, while the N-terminal domain of hirudin occupies the catalytic site.[277,278] A synthetic peptide that corresponds to the acidic domain of heparin cofactor II competes with hirudin for binding to thrombin but does not affect the ability of thrombin to hydrolyze a tripeptide *p*-nitroanilide substrate.[279] Thus, binding of thrombin to the acidic domain of heparin cofactor II could facilitate inhibition by bringing the active site of thrombin into approximation with the reactive site of heparin cofactor II.

Experiments with recombinant heparin cofactor II established the importance of the N-terminal acidic domain.[273,274,276] Although deletion of both acidic repeats does not affect the rate of inhibition of thrombin or chymotrypsin in the absence of a glycosaminoglycan, deletion of the first acidic repeat greatly diminishes the ability of dermatan sulfate or heparin to stimulate the inhibition of thrombin.[276] The deletion mutants bind heparin more tightly, which suggests that the acidic domain occupies the glycosaminoglycan binding site in native heparin cofactor II. These findings are consistent with a model in which heparin or dermatan sulfate displaces the N-terminal acidic domain from the glycosaminoglycan binding site of heparin cofactor II, thus enabling the acidic domain to interact with exosite I of thrombin (Fig. 176-5).

In addition to anion-binding exosite I, thrombin contains a distinct site termed anion-binding exosite II. Exosite II binds glycosaminoglycans, including heparin and dermatan sulfate. Studies with thrombin variants have clarified the roles these exosites play in inhibition by heparin cofactor II and antithrombin.[280–285] Mutations in exosite I do not affect the rate of inhibition of thrombin by antithrombin in the presence of heparin, whereas exosite II mutations markedly decrease the rate. Conversely, mutations in exosite I greatly decrease the rate of inhibition of thrombin by heparin cofactor II in the presence of heparin or dermatan sulfate, whereas exosite II mutations have little or no effect. These observations suggest that antithrombin and heparin cofactor II inhibit thrombin by different mechanisms

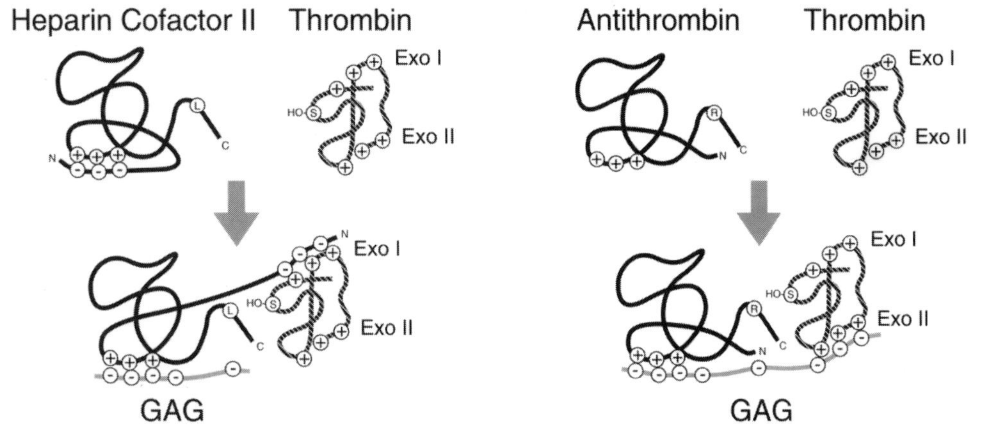

Fig. 176-5 Comparison of the proposed mechanisms for inhibition of thrombin by antithrombin and heparin cofactor II. Heparin stimulates the thrombin-antithrombin reaction primarily by a template effect, involving interactions with the heparin-binding site of antithrombin and exosite II of thrombin. Dermatan sulfate or heparin stimulates the thrombin-heparin cofactor II reaction primarily by an allosteric mechanism that involves displacement of the N-terminal acidic domain from the glycosaminoglycan-binding site of heparin cofactor II. The N-terminal acidic domain then interacts with exosite I of thrombin. Exo I, exosite I; Exo II, exosite II; GAG, glycosaminoglycan.

as shown schematically in Fig. 176-5. In meizothrombin, exosite II is blocked by the fragment 2 domain of prothrombin.[286] Because of this, meizothrombin is preferentially inhibited by heparin cofactor II.[7,11]

Physiology of Heparin Cofactor II

The function of heparin cofactor II in vivo remains obscure. Heparin cofactor II is present in normal human plasma at a concentration of 1.2 ± 0.4 μM (mean $\pm$ 2 SD),[287] and individuals with inherited partial deficiency of heparin cofactor II ($\sim$50 percent of normal) have been reported in association with histories of thrombotic disease.[288–295] In one study, however, 4 of 379 apparently healthy individuals had heparin cofactor II levels < 60 percent of normal.[296] Thus, heterozygous deficiency of heparin cofactor II may be a coincidental finding in $\sim$1 percent of patients with thrombosis, and it is premature to conclude that heparin cofactor II deficiency is a risk factor for development of the disease.[297] No patients with homozygous heparin cofactor II deficiency have been identified.

The concentration of heparin cofactor II is markedly decreased in some patients with liver disease, disseminated intravascular coagulation, and obstetric complications.[287,298–300] In these situations, the heparin cofactor II and antithrombin levels are usually decreased to a similar degree. A moderately elevated concentration of heparin cofactor II is present in women who are pregnant or use oral contraceptives.[301,302] Normal levels are present in patients taking oral anticoagulants, in the vast majority of patients with venous thromboembolic disease,[297,299,300] and in symptomatic patients with inherited antithrombin deficiency.[298,299,303]

Cultured fibroblasts and vascular smooth muscle cells accelerate inhibition of thrombin by heparin cofactor II, whereas endothelial cells do not.[304] In the case of fibroblasts, a dermatan sulfate proteoglycan was demonstrated to be responsible for the stimulatory effect. By contrast, a heparan sulfate proteoglycan has been implicated in the case of arterial smooth muscle cells.[305] These results suggest that heparin cofactor II may inhibit thrombin in the connective tissues rather than within the blood vessels and perhaps modulate wound healing or inflammation. Theoretically, heparin cofactor II could promote coagulation by inhibiting the activation of protein C by meizothrombin.[11]

During pregnancy, both the maternal and fetal plasma contain a dermatan sulfate proteoglycan that stimulates inhibition of thrombin by heparin cofactor II approximately twofold,[306] and elevated levels of the thrombin-heparin cofactor II complex are present.[307] The placenta is rich in dermatan sulfate and may be the source of this proteoglycan.[308] Thus, heparin cofactor II could inhibit coagulation locally within the placenta.

REFERENCES

1. Broze GJ Jr: Tissue factor pathway inhibitor. *Thromb Haemost* **74**:90, 1995.
2. Krishnaswamy S, Church WR, Nesheim ME, Mann KG: Activation of human prothrombin by human prothrombinase. Influence of factor Va on the reaction mechanism. *J Biol Chem* **262**:3291, 1987.
3. Coughlin SR: How thrombin "talks" to cells: Molecular mechanisms and roles in vivo. *Arterioscler Thromb Vasc Biol* **18**:514, 1998.
4. Naito K, Fujikawa K: Activation of human blood coagulation factor XI independent of factor XII. Factor XI is activated by thrombin and factor XIa in the presence of negatively charged surfaces. *J Biol Chem* **266**:7353, 1991.
5. Gailani D, Broze GJ Jr: Factor XI activation in a revised model of blood coagulation. *Science* **253**:909, 1991.
6. Bajzar L, Manuel R, Nesheim ME: Purification and characterization of TAFI, a thrombin-activable fibrinolysis inhibitor. *J Biol Chem* **270**:14477, 1995.
7. Côté HCF, Bajzar L, Stevens WK, Samis JA, Morser J, MacGillivray RTA, Nesheim ME: Functional characterization of recombinant human meizothrombin and meizothrombin(desF1). Thrombomodulin-dependent activation of protein C and thrombin-activatable fibrinolysis inhibitor (TAFI), platelet aggregation, antithrombin-III inhibition. *J Biol Chem* **272**:6194, 1997.
8. Hackeng TM, Tans G, Koppelman SJ, de Groot PG, Rosing J, Bouma BN: Protein C activation on endothelial cells by prothrombin activation products generated *in situ*: Meizothrombin is a better protein C activator than α-thrombin. *Biochem J* **319**:399, 1996.
9. Coughlin SR, Vu T-KH, Hung DT, Wheaton VI: Characterization of a functional thrombin receptor. Issues and opportunities. *J Clin Invest* **89**:351, 1992.
10. Cunningham DD, Donovan FM: Regulation of neurons and astrocytes by thrombin and protease nexin-1. Relationship to brain injury. *Adv Exp Med Biol* **425**:67, 1997.
11. Han J-H, Côté HCF, Tollefsen DM: Inhibition of meizothrombin and meizothrombin(desF1) by heparin cofactor II. *J Biol Chem* **272**:28660, 1997.
12. Rezaie AR, Cooper ST, Church FC, Esmon CT: Protein C inhibitor is a potent inhibitor of the thrombin-thrombomodulin complex. *J Biol Chem* **270**:25336, 1995.
13. Egeberg O: Inherited antithrombin deficiency causing thrombophilia. *Thromb Diath Haemorrh* **13**:516, 1965.
14. Rosenberg RD, Shworak NW, Liu J, Schwartz JJ, Zhang L: Heparan sulfate proteoglycans of the cardiovascular system. Specific structures emerge but how is synthesis regulated? *J Clin Invest* **99**:2062, 1997.
15. Brinkhous KM, Smith HP, Warner ED, Seegers WH: The inhibition of blood clotting: An unidentified substance which acts in conjunction

with heparin to prevent the conversion of prothrombin into thrombin. *Am J Physiol* **125**:683, 1939.
16. Abildgaard U: Highly purified antithrombin III with heparin cofactor activity prepared by disc electrophoresis. *Scand J Clin Lab Invest* **21**:89, 1968.
17. Rosenberg RD, Damus PS: The purification and mechanism of action of human antithrombin-heparin cofactor. *J Biol Chem* **248**:6490, 1973.
18. Huber R, Carrell RW: Implications of the three-dimensional structure of α_1-antitrypsin for structure and function of serpins. *Biochemistry* **28**:8951, 1989.
19. Bock SC, Wion KL, Vehar GA, Lawn RM: Cloning and expression of the cDNA for human antithrombin III. *Nucleic Acids Res* **10**:8113, 1982.
20. Prochownik EV, Markham AF, Orkin SH: Isolation of a cDNA clone for human antithrombin III. *J Biol Chem* **258**:8389, 1983.
21. Stackhouse R, Chandra T, Robson KJ, Woo SL: Purification of antithrombin III mRNA and cloning of its cDNA. *J Biol Chem* **258**:703, 1983.
22. Sun XJ, Chang JY: Heparin binding domain of human antithrombin III inferred from the sequential reduction of its three disulfide linkages. An efficient method for structural analysis of partially reduced proteins. *J Biol Chem* **264**:11288, 1989.
23. Zhou ZR, Smith DL: Location of disulfide bonds in antithrombin III. *Biomed Environ Mass Spectrom* **19**:782, 1990.
24. Franzén L-E, Svensson S, Larm O: Structural studies on the carbohydrate portion of human antithrombin III. *J Biol Chem* **255**:5090, 1980.
25. Peterson CB, Blackburn MN: Isolation and characterization of an antithrombin III variant with reduced carbohydrate content and enhanced heparin binding. *J Biol Chem* **260**:610, 1985.
26. Brennan SO, George PM, Jordan RE: Physiological variant of antithrombin-III lacks carbohydrate side chain at Asn 135. *FEBS Lett* **219**:431, 1987.
27. Hall PK, Roberts RC: Phosphate promotes glycation of antithrombin III which interferes with heparin binding. *Biochim Biophys Acta* **993**:217, 1989.
28. Bock SC, Harris JF, Balazs I, Trent JM: Assignment of the human antithrombin III structural gene to chromosome 1q23-25. *Cytogenet Cell Genet* **39**:67, 1985.
29. Olds RJ, Lane DA, Chowdury V, De Stefano V, Leone G, Thein SL: Complete nucleotide sequence of the antithrombin gene. Evidence for homologous recombination causing thrombophilia. *Biochemistry* **32**:4216, 1993.
30. Fair DS, Bahnak BR: Human hepatoma cells secrete single chain factor X, prothrombin, and antithrombin III. *Blood* **64**:194, 1984.
31. Prochownik EV, Orkin SH: In vivo transcription of a human antithrombin III "minigene." *J Biol Chem* **259**:15386, 1984.
32. D'Souza SE, Mercer JF: Antithrombin III mRNA in adult rat liver and kidney and in rat liver during development. *Biochem Biophys Res Commun* **142**:417, 1987.
33. Prochownik EV: Relationship between an enhancer element in the human antithrombin III gene and an immunoglobulin light-chain gene enhancer. *Nature* **316**:845, 1985.
34. Tremp GL, Duchange N, Branellec D, Cereghini S, Tailleux A, Berthou L, Fievet C, et al.: A 700-bp fragment of the human antithrombin III promoter is sufficient to confer high, tissue-specific expression on human apolipoprotein A-II in transgenic mice. *Gene* **156**:199, 1995.
35. Fernandez-Rachubinski FA, Weiner JH, Blajchman MA: Regions flanking exon 1 regulate constitutive expression of the human antithrombin gene. *J Biol Chem* **271**:29502, 1996.
36. Bock SC, Levitan DJ: Characterization of an unusual DNA length polymorphism 5′ to the human antithrombin III gene. *Nucleic Acids Res* **11**:8569, 1983.
37. Winter PC, Scopes DA, Berg L-P, Millar DS, Kakkar VV, Mayne EE, Krawczak M, et al.: Functional analysis of an unusual length polymorphism in the human antithrombin III (AT3) gene promoter. *Blood Coagul Fibrinolysis* **6**:659, 1995.
38. Hoffman M, Fuchs HE, Pizzo SV: The macrophage-mediated regulation of hepatocyte synthesis of antithrombin III and α1-proteinase inhibitor. *Thromb Res* **41**:707, 1986.
39. Rosenberg RD: Regulation of the hemostatic mechanism, in Stamatoyannopoulos G, Nienhuis AW, Leder P, Majerus PW (eds): *The Molecular Basis of Blood Diseases*. Philadelphia, WB Saunders Company, 1987, p 534.
40. Rao LVM, Rapaport SI, Hoang AD: Binding of factor VIIa to tissue factor permits rapid antithrombin III/heparin inhibition of factor VIIa. *Blood* **81**:2600, 1993.
41. Rao LVM, Nordfang O, Hoang AD, Pendurthi UR: Mechanism of antithrombin III inhibition of factor Xa/tissue factor activity on cell surfaces. Comparison with tissue factor pathway inhibitor/factor Xa-induced inhibition of factor VIIa/tissue factor activity. *Blood* **85**:121, 1995.
42. Fuchs HE, Trapp HG, Griffith MJ, Roberts HR, Pizzo SV: Regulation of factor IXa in vitro in human and mouse plasma and in vivo in the mouse. Role of the endothelium and the plasma proteinase inhibitors. *J Clin Invest* **73**:1696, 1984.
43. Gitel SN, Medina VM, Wessler S: Inhibition of human activated Factor X by antithrombin III and α1-proteinase inhibitor in human plasma. *J Biol Chem* **259**:6890, 1984.
44. Vogel CN, Kingdon HS, Lundblad RL: Correlation of in vivo and in vitro inhibition of thrombin by plasma inhibitors. *J Lab Clin Med* **93**:661, 1979.
45. Tollefsen DM, Blank MK: Detection of a new heparin-dependent inhibitor of thrombin in human plasma. *J Clin Invest* **68**:589, 1981.
46. Tollefsen DM, Pestka CA, Monafo WJ: Activation of heparin cofactor II by dermatan sulfate. *J Biol Chem* **258**:6713, 1983.
47. Novotny WF, Brown SG, Miletich JP, Rader DJ, Broze GJ Jr: Plasma antigen levels of the lipoprotein-associated coagulation inhibitor in patient samples. *Blood* **78**:387, 1991.
48. Broze GJ Jr, Warren LA, Novotny WF, Higuchi DA, Girard JJ, Miletich JP: The lipoprotein-associated coagulation inhibitor that inhibits the factor VII-tissue factor complex also inhibits factor Xa: Insight into its possible mechanism of action. *Blood* **71**:335, 1988.
49. Scott CF, Colman RW: Factors influencing the acceleration of human factor XIa inactivation by antithrombin III. *Blood* **73**:1873, 1989.
50. Smith RP, Higuchi DA, Broze GJ Jr: Platelet coagulation factor XIa-inhibitor, a form of Alzheimer amyloid precursor protein. *Science* **248**:1126, 1990.
51. Van Nostrand WE, Wagner SL, Farrow JS, Cunningham DD: Immunopurification and protease inhibitory properties of protease nexin-2/amyloid beta-protein precursor. *J Biol Chem* **265**:9591, 1990.
52. Suzuki K, Nishioka J, Hashimoto S: Protein C inhibitor: purification from human plasma and characterization. *J Biol Chem* **258**:163, 1983.
53. Anonick PK, Wolf B, Gonias SL: Regulation of plasmin, miniplasmin, and streptokinase-plasmin complex by α2-antiplasmin, α2-macroglobulin, and antithrombin III in the presence of heparin. *Thromb Res* **59**:449, 1990.
54. Highsmith RF, Rosenberg RD: The inhibition of human plasmin by human antithrombin-heparin cofactor. *J Biol Chem* **249**:4335, 1974.
55. Wiman B, Collen D: On the kinetics of the reaction between human antiplasmin and plasmin. *Eur J Biochem* **84**:573, 1978.
56. Masson D, Tschopp J: Inhibition of lymphocyte protease granzyme A by antithrombin III. *Mol Immunol* **25**:1283, 1988.
57. Poe M, Bennett CD, Biddison WE, Blake JT, Norton GP, Rodkey JA, Sigal NH, et al.: Human cytotoxic lymphocyte tryptase. Its purification from granules and the characterization of inhibitor and substrate specificity. *J Biol Chem* **263**:13215, 1988.
58. Weiler JM, Linhardt RJ: Antithrombin III regulates complement activity in vitro. *J Immunol* **146**:3889, 1991.
59. Fish WW, Björk I: Release of a two-chain form of antithrombin from the antithombin-thrombin complex. *Eur J Biochem* **101**:31, 1979.
60. Björk I, Jackson CM, Jörnvall H, Lavine KK, Nordling K, Salsgiver WJ: The active site of antithrombin. Release of the same proteolytically cleaved form of the inhibitor from complexes with factor IXa, factor Xa, and thrombin. *J Biol Chem* **257**:2406, 1982.
61. Owen WG: Evidence for the formation of an ester between thrombin and heparin cofactor. *Biochim Biophys Acta* **405**:380, 1975.
62. Stein PE, Leslie AGW, Finch JT, Turnell WG, McLaughlin PJ, Carrell RW: Crystal structure of ovalbumin as a model for the reactive centre of serpins. *Nature* **347**:99, 1990.
63. Carrell RW, Owen MC: Plakalbumin, α1-antitrypsin, antithrombin and the mechanism of inflammatory thrombosis. *Nature* **317**:730, 1985.
64. Mast AE, Enghild JJ, Salvesen G: Conformation of the reactive site loop of α1-proteinase inhibitor probed by limited proteolysis. *Biochemistry* **31**:2720, 1992.
65. Perry DJ, Harper PL, Fairham S, Daly M, Carrell RW: Antithrombin Cambridge, 384 Ala to Pro: A new variant identified using the polymerase chain reaction. *FEBS Lett* **254**:174, 1989.
66. Austin RC, Rachubinski RA, Ofosu FA, Blajchman MA: Antithrombin-III-Hamilton, Ala 382 to Thr: An antithrombin-III variant that acts as a substrate but not an inhibitor of α-thrombin and factor Xa. *Blood* **77**:2185, 1991.
67. Asakura S, Hirata H, Okazaki H, Hashimoto-Gotoh T, Matsuda M: Hydrophobic residues 382-386 of antithrombin III, Ala-Ala-Ala-Ser-

Thr, serve as the epitope for an antibody which facilitates hydrolysis of the inhibitor by thrombin. *J Biol Chem* **265**:5135, 1990.
68. Carrell RW, Evans DL, Stein PE: Mobile reactive centre of serpins and the control of thrombosis. *Nature* **353**:576, 1991.
69. Björk I, Ylinenjärvi K, Olson ST, Bock PE: Conversion of antithrombin from an inhibitor of thrombin to a substrate with reduced heparin affinity and enhanced conformational stability by binding of a tetradecapeptide corresponding to the P1 to P14 region of the putative reactive bond loop of the inhibitor. *J Biol Chem* **267**:1976, 1992.
70. Carrell RW, Stein PE, Fermi G, Wardell MR: Biological implications of a 3 Å structure of dimeric antithrombin. *Structure* **2**:257, 1994.
71. Schreuder HA, de Boer B, Dijkema R, Mulders J, Theunissen HJ, Grootenhuis PD, Hol WG: The intact and cleaved human antithrombin III complex as a model for serpin-proteinase interactions. *Nat Struct Biol* **1**:48, 1994.
72. Jin L, Abrahams JP, Skinner R, Petitou M, Pike RN, Carrell RW: The anticoagulant activation of antithrombin by heparin. *Proc Natl Acad Sci U S A* **94**:14683, 1997.
73. Skinner R, Abrahams J-P, Whisstock JC, Lesk AM, Carrell RW, Wardell MR: The 2.6 Å structure of antithrombin indicates a conformational change at the heparin binding site. *J Mol Biol* **266**:601, 1997.
74. Jordan RE, Nelson RM, Kilpatrick J, Newgren JO, Esmon PC, Fournel MA: Inactivation of human antithrombin by neutrophil elastase. Kinetics of the heparin-dependent reaction. *J Biol Chem* **264**:10493, 1989.
75. Duswald K-H, Jochum M, Schramm W, Fritz H: Released granulocytic elastase: an indicator of pathobiochemical alterations in septicemia after abdominal surgery. *Surgery* **98**:892, 1985.
76. Mast AE, Enghild JJ, Nagase H, Suzuki K, Pizzo SV, Salvesen G: Kinetics and physiologic relevance of the inactivation of α1-proteinase inhibitor, α1-antichymotrypsin, and antithrombin III by matrix metalloproteinases-1 (tissue collagenase), -2 (72-kDa gelatinase/type IV collagenase), and -3 (stromelysin). *J Biol Chem* **266**:15810, 1991.
77. Kress LF, Catanese JJ: Identification of the cleavage sites resulting from enzymatic inactivation of human antithrombin III by Crotalus adamanteus proteinase II in the presence and absence of heparin. *Biochemistry* **20**:7432, 1981.
78. Olson ST: Heparin and ionic strength-dependent conversion of antithrombin III from an inhibitor to a substrate of α-thrombin. *J Biol Chem* **260**:10153, 1985.
79. Olson ST, Björk I, Sheffer R, Craig PA, Shore JD, Choay J: Role of the antithrombin-binding pentasaccharide in heparin acceleration of antithrombin-proteinase reactions. Resolution of the antithrombin conformational change contribution to heparin rate enhancement. *J Biol Chem* **267**:12528, 1992.
80. Jordan RE, Oosta GM, Gardner WT, Rosenberg RD: The kinetics of hemostatic enzyme-antithrombin interactions in the presence of low molecular weight heparin. *J Biol Chem* **255**:10081, 1980.
81. Abildgaard U, Lindahl AK, Sandset PM: Heparin requires both antithrombin and extrinsic pathway inhibitor for its anticoagulant effect in human blood. *Haemostasis* **21**:254, 1991.
82. Ofosu FA, Sié P, Modi GJ, Fernandez F, Buchanan MR, Blajchman MA, Boneu B, et al.: The inhibition of thrombin-dependent positive-feedback reactions is critical to the expression of the anticoagulant effect of heparin. *Biochem J* **243**:579, 1987.
83. Béguin S, Lindhout T, Hemker HC: The mode of action of heparin in plasma. *Thromb Haemost* **60**:457, 1988.
84. Ofosu FA, Hirsh J, Esmon CT, Modi GJ, Smith LM, Anvari N, Buchanan MR, et al.: Unfractionated heparin inhibits thrombin-catalysed amplification reactions of coagulation more efficiently than those catalysed by factor Xa. *Biochem J* **257**:143, 1989.
85. Salmivirta M, Lidholt K, Lindahl U: Heparan sulfate: A piece of information. *FASEB J* **10**:1270, 1996.
86. Conrad HE: *Heparin-Binding Proteins*. San Diego, Academic Press, 1998.
87. Höök M, Björk I, Hopwood J, Lindahl U: Anticoagulant activity of heparin: Separation of high-activity and low-activity species by affinity chromatography on immobilized antithrombin. *FEBS Lett* **66**:90, 1976.
88. Andersson L-O, Barrowcliffe TW, Holmer E, Johnson EA, Sims GEC: Anticoagulant properties of heparin fractionated by affinity chromatography on matrix-bound antithrombin III and by gel filtration. *Thromb Res* **9**:575, 1976.
89. Lam LH, Silbert JE, Rosenberg RD: The separation of active and inactive forms of heparin. *Biochem Biophys Res Commun* **69**:570, 1976.
90. Jordan R, Beeler D, Rosenberg R: Fractionation of low molecular weight heparin species and their interaction with antithrombin. *J Biol Chem* **254**:2902, 1979.
91. Olson ST, Srinivasan KR, Björk I, Shore JD: Binding of high affinity heparin to antithrombin III. Stopped flow kinetic studies of the binding interaction. *J Biol Chem* **256**:11073, 1981.
92. Choay J, Petitou M, Lormeau JC, Sinay P, Casu B, Gatti G: Structure-activity relationship in heparin: A synthetic pentasaccharide with high affinity for antithrombin III and eliciting high anti-factor Xa activity. *Biochem Biophys Res Commun* **116**:492, 1983.
93. Lindahl U, Thunberg L, Bäckström G, Riesenfeld J, Nordling K, Björk I: Extension and structural variability of the antithrombin-binding sequence in heparin. *J Biol Chem* **259**:12368, 1984.
94. Atha DH, Lormeau JC, Petitou M, Rosenberg RD, Choay J: Contribution of monosaccharide residues in heparin binding to antithrombin III. *Biochemistry* **24**:6723, 1985.
95. Marcum JA, Atha DH, Fritze LM, Nawroth P, Stern D, Rosenberg RD: Cloned bovine aortic endothelial cells synthesize anticoagulantly active heparan sulfate proteoglycan. *J Biol Chem* **261**:7507, 1986.
96. Kojima T, Leone CW, Marchildon GA, Marcum JA, Rosenberg RD: Isolation and characterization of heparan sulfate proteoglycans produced by cloned rat microvascular endothelial cells. *J Biol Chem* **267**:4859, 1992.
97. Piepkorn M, Hovingh P, Hentschel WM: Isolation of heparan sulfates with antithrombin III affinity and anticoagulant potency from BALB/c 3T3, B16.F10 melanoma, and cutaneous fibrosarcoma cell lines. *Biochem Biophys Res Commun* **151**:327, 1988.
98. Pejler G, Bäckström G, Lindahl U, Paulsson M, Dziadek M, Fujiwara S, Timpl R: Structure and affinity for antithrombin of heparan sulfate chains derived from basement membrane proteoglycans. *J Biol Chem* **262**:5036, 1987.
99. Pejler G, David G: Basement-membrane heparan sulphate with high affinity for antithrombin synthesized by normal and transformed mouse mammary epithelial cells. *Biochem J* **248**:69, 1987.
100. Pecon JM, Blackburn MN: Pyridoxylation of essential lysines in the heparin-binding site of antithrombin III. *J Biol Chem* **259**:935, 1984.
101. Peterson CB, Noyes CM, Pecon JM, Church FC, Blackburn MN: Identification of a lysyl residue in antithrombin which is essential for heparin binding. *J Biol Chem* **262**:8061, 1987.
102. Chang J-Y: Binding of heparin to human antithrombin III activates selective chemical modification at lysine 236. Lys-107, Lys-125, and Lys-136 are situated within the heparin-binding site of antithrombin III. *J Biol Chem* **264**:3111, 1989.
103. Sun X-J, Chang J-Y: Evidence that arginine-129 and arginine-145 are located within the heparin binding site of human antithrombin III. *Biochemistry* **29**:8957, 1990.
104. Smith JW, Dey N, Knauer DJ: Heparin binding domain of antithrombin III: Characterization using a synthetic peptide directed polyclonal antibody. *Biochemistry* **29**:8950, 1990.
105. Lellouch AC, Lansbury PT Jr: A peptide model for the heparin binding site of antithrombin III. *Biochemistry* **31**:2279, 1992.
106. Brennan SO, Borg J-Y, George PM, Soria C, Soria J, Caen J, Carrell RW: New carbohydrate site in mutant antithrombin (7Ile → Asn) with decreased heparin affinity. *FEBS Lett* **237**:118, 1988.
107. Borg JY, Brennan SO, Carrell RW, George P, Perry DJ, Shaw J: Antithrombin Rouen IV 24 Arg to Cys. The amino terminal contribution to heparin binding. *FEBS Lett* **266**:163, 1990.
108. Chang JY, Tran TH: Antithrombin III Basel. Identification of a Pro-Leu substitution in a hereditary abnormal antithrombin with impaired heparin cofactor activity. *J Biol Chem* **261**:1174, 1986.
109. Koide T, Odani S, Takahashi K, Ono T, Sakuragawa N: Antithrombin III Toyama: Replacement of arginine-47 by cysteine in hereditary abnormal antithrombin III that lacks heparin-binding ability. *Proc Natl Acad Sci U S A* **81**:289, 1984.
110. Owen MC, Borg JY, Soria C, Soria J, Caen J, Carrell RW: Heparin binding defect in a new antithrombin III variant: Rouen, 47 Arg to His. *Blood* **69**:1275, 1987.
111. Blackburn MN, Smith RL, Carson J, Sibley CC: The heparin-binding site of antithrombin III. Identification of a critical tryptophan in the amino acid sequence. *J Biol Chem* **259**:939, 1984.
112. Gettins P, Wooten EW: On the domain structure of antithrombin III. Tentative localization of the heparin binding region using ^{1}H NMR spectroscopy. *Biochemistry* **26**:4403, 1987.
113. Olson ST, Shore JD: Transient kinetics of heparin-catalyzed protease inactivation by antithrombin III. The reaction step limiting heparin turnover in thrombin neutralization. *J Biol Chem* **261**:13151, 1986.

114. Nordenman B, Björk I: Binding of low-affinity and high-affinity heparin to antithrombin. Ultraviolet difference spectroscopy and circular dichroism studies. *Biochemistry* **17**:3339, 1978.
115. Einarsson R, Andersson L-O: Binding of heparin to human antithrombin III as studied by measurements of tryptophan fluorescence. *Biochim Biophys Acta* **490**:104, 1977.
116. Olson ST, Shore JD: Binding of high affinity heparin to antithrombin III. Characterization of the protein fluorescence enhancement. *J Biol Chem* **256**:11065, 1981.
117. Stone AL, Beeler D, Oosta G, Rosenberg RD: Circular dichroism spectroscopy of heparin-antithrombin interactions. *Proc Natl Acad Sci U S A* **79**:7190, 1982.
118. Horne AP, Gettins P: ^{1}H NMR spectroscopic studies on the interactions between human plasma antithrombin III and defined low molecular weight heparin fragments. *Biochemistry* **31**:2286, 1992.
119. Gettins PGW, Fan B, Crews BC, Turko IV, Olson ST, Streusand VJ: Transmission of conformational change from the heparin binding site to the reactive center of antithrombin. *Biochemistry* **32**:8385, 1993.
120. Dawes J, James K, Lane DA: Conformational change in antithrombin induced by heparin, probed with a monoclonal antibody against the 1C/4B region. *Biochemistry* **33**:4375, 1994.
121. Huntington JA, Olson ST, Fan B, Gettins PG: Mechanism of heparin activation of antithrombin. Evidence for reactive center loop preinsertion with expulsion upon heparin binding. *Biochemistry* **35**:8495, 1996.
122. Pike RN, Potempa J, Skinner R, Fitton HL, McGraw WT, Travis J, Owen M, et al.: Heparin-dependent modification of the reactive center arginine of antithrombin and consequent increase in heparin binding affinity. *J Biol Chem* **272**:19652, 1997.
123. Oosta GM, Gardner WT, Beeler DL, Rosenberg RD: Multiple functional domains of the heparin molecule. *Proc Natl Acad Sci U S A* **78**:829, 1981.
124. Pomerantz MW, Owen WG: A catalytic role for heparin. Evidence for a ternary complex of heparin cofactor, thrombin and heparin. *Biochim Biophys Acta* **535**:66, 1978.
125. Danielsson Å, Raub E, Lindahl U, Björk I: Role of ternary complexes, in which heparin binds both antithrombin and proteinase, in the acceleration of the reactions between antithrombin and thrombin or factor Xa. *J Biol Chem* **261**:15467, 1986.
126. Olson ST, Björk I: Predominant contribution of surface approximation to the mechanism of heparin acceleration of the antithrombin-thrombin reaction. Elucidation from salt concentration effects. *J Biol Chem* **266**:6353, 1991.
127. Olson ST, Halvorson HR, Björk I: Quantitative characterization of the thrombin-heparin interaction. Discrimination between specific and nonspecific binding models. *J Biol Chem* **266**:6342, 1991.
128. Owen BA, Owen WG: Interaction of factor Xa with heparin does not contribute to the inhibition of factor Xa by antithrombin III-heparin. *Biochemistry* **29**:9412, 1990.
129. Lane DA, Pejler G, Flynn AM, Thompson EA, Lindahl U: Neutralization of heparin-related saccharides by histidine-rich glycoprotein and platelet factor 4. *J Biol Chem* **261**:3980, 1986.
130. Preissner KT, Müller-Berghaus G: S protein modulates the heparin-catalyzed inhibition of thrombin by antithrombin III. Evidence for a direct interaction of S protein with heparin. *Eur J Biochem* **156**:645, 1986.
131. Shimada K, Kawamoto A, Matsubayashi K, Ozawa T: Histidine-rich glycoprotein does not interfere with interactions between antithrombin III and heparin-like compounds on vascular endothelial cells. *Blood* **73**:191, 1989.
132. Hogg PJ, Jackson CM: Fibrin monomer protects thrombin from inactivation by heparin-antithrombin III: implications for heparin efficacy. *Proc Natl Acad Sci U S A* **86**:3619, 1989.
133. Weitz JI, Hudoba M, Massel D, Maraganore J, Hirsh J: Clot-bound thrombin is protected from inhibition by heparin-antithrombin III but is susceptible to inactivation by antithrombin III-independent inhibitors. *J Clin Invest* **86**:385, 1990.
134. Lollar P, Owen WG: Clearance of thrombin from the circulation in rabbits by high-affinity binding sites on the endothelium. Possible role in the inactivation of thrombin by antithrombin III. *J Clin Invest* **66**:1222, 1980.
135. Boisclair MD, Lane DA, Wilde JT, Ireland H, Preston FE, Ofosu FA: A comparative evaluation of assays for markers of activated coagulation and/or fibrinolysis: Thrombin-antithrombin complex, D-dimer and fibrinogen/fibrin fragment E antigen. *Br J Haematol* **74**:471, 1990.
136. Deguchi K, Noguchi M, Yuwasaki E, Endou T, Deguchi A, Wada H, Murashima S, et al.: Dynamic fluctuations in blood of thrombin/antithrombin III complex (TAT). *Am J Hematol* **38**:86, 1991.
137. Fuchs HE, Pizzo SV: Regulation of factor Xa in vitro in human and mouse plasma and in vivo in mouse. Role of the endothelium and plasma proteinase inhibitors. *J Clin Invest* **72**:2041, 1983.
138. Miletich JP, Jackson CM, Majerus PW: Properties of the factor Xa binding site on human platelets. *J Biol Chem* **253**:6908, 1978.
139. Lindhout T, Baruch D, Schoen P, Franssen J, Hemker HC: Thrombin generation and inactivation in the presence of antithrombin III and heparin. *Biochemistry* **25**:5962, 1986.
140. Gouin-Thibault I, Dewar L, Kulczycky M, Sternbach M, Ofosu FA: Measurement of factor Xa-antithrombin III in plasma: Relationship to prothrombin activation in vivo. *Br J Haematol* **90**:669, 1995.
141. Shifman MA, Pizzo SV: The in vivo metabolism of antithrombin III and antithrombin III complexes. *J Biol Chem* **257**:3243, 1982.
142. Collen D, de Cock F, Verstraete M: Quantitation of thrombin-antithrombin III complexes in human blood. *Eur J Clin Invest* **7**:407, 1977.
143. Fuchs HE, Shifman MA, Michalopoulos G, Pizzo SV: Hepatocyte receptors for antithrombin III-proteinase complexes. *J Cell Biochem* **24**:197, 1984.
144. Pizzo SV, Mast AE, Feldman SR, Salvesen G: In vivo catabolism of α1-antichymotrypsin is mediated by the serpin receptor which binds α1-proteinase inhibitor, antithrombin III and heparin cofactor II. *Biochim Biophys Acta* **967**:158, 1988.
145. Kounnas MZ, Church FC, Argraves WS, Strickland DK: Cellular internalization and degradation of antithrombin III-thrombin, heparin cofactor II-thrombin, and α1-antitrypsin-trypsin complexes is mediated by the low density lipoprotein receptor-related protein. *J Biol Chem* **271**:6523, 1996.
146. Ill CR, Ruoslahti E: Association of thrombin-antithrombin III complex with vitronectin in serum. *J Biol Chem* **260**:15610, 1985.
147. de Boer HC, Preissner KT, Bouma BN, de Groot PG: Binding of vitronectin-thrombin-antithrombin III complex to human endothelial cells is mediated by the heparin binding site of vitronectin. *J Biol Chem* **267**:2264, 1992.
148. van Iwaarden F, Acton DS, Sixma JJ, Meijers JCM, de Groot PG, Bouma BN: Internalization of antithrombin III by cultured human endothelial cells and its subcellular localization. *J Lab Clin Med* **113**:717, 1989.
149. Nenci GG, Berrettini M, Parise P, Agnelli G: Persistent spontaneous heparinaemia in systemic mastocytosis. *Folia Haematol (Leipz)* **109**:453, 1982.
150. Khoory MS, Nesheim ME, Bowie EJW, Mann KG: Circulating heparan sulfate proteoglycan anticoagulant from a patient with a plasma cell disorder. *J Clin Invest* **65**:666, 1980.
151. Bussel JB, Steinherz PG, Miller DR, Hilgartner MW: A heparin-like anticoagulant in an 8-month-old boy with acute monoblastic leukemia. *Am J Hematol* **16**:83, 1984.
152. Palmer RN, Rick ME, Rick PD, Zeller JA, Gralnick HR: Circulating heparan sulfate anticoagulant in a patient with a fatal bleeding disorder. *N Engl J Med* **310**:1696, 1984.
153. Tefferi A, Nichols WL, Bowie EJW: Circulating heparin-like anticoagulants: report of five consecutive cases and a review. *Am J Med* **88**:184, 1990.
154. Marcum JA, Rosenberg RD: Heparin-like molecules with anticoagulant activity are synthesized by cultured endothelial cells. *Biochem Biophys Res Commun* **126**:365, 1985.
155. Stern D, Nawroth P, Marcum J, Handley D, Kisiel W, Rosenberg R, Stern K: Interaction of antithrombin III with bovine aortic segments. Role of heparin in binding and enhanced anticoagulant activity. *J Clin Invest* **75**:272, 1985.
156. Hatton MW, Moar SL, Richardson M: On the interaction of rabbit antithrombin III with the luminal surface of the normal and de-endothelialized rabbit thoracic aorta in vitro. *Blood* **67**:878, 1986.
157. de Agostini AI, Watkins SC, Slayter HS, Youssoufian H, Rosenberg RD: Localization of anticoagulantly active heparan sulfate proteoglycans in vascular endothelium: antithrombin binding on cultured endothelial cells and perfused rat aorta. *J Cell Biol* **111**:1293, 1990.
158. Frebelius S, Isaksson S, Swedenborg J: Thrombin inhibition by antithrombin III on the subendothelium is explained by the isoform AT beta. *Arterioscler Thromb Vasc Biol* **16**:1292, 1996.
159. Kobayashi M, Shimada K, Ozawa T: Human recombinant interleukin-1β- and tumor necrosis factor α-mediated suppression of heparin-like compounds on cultured porcine aortic endothelial cells. *J Cell Physiol* **144**:383, 1990.

160. Marcum JA, McKenney JB, Rosenberg RD: Acceleration of thrombin-antithrombin complex formation in rat hindquarters via heparinlike molecules bound to the endothelium. *J Clin Invest* **74**:341, 1984.
161. Maruyama I, Majerus PW: The turnover of thrombin-thrombomodulin complex in cultured human umbilical vein endothelial cells and A549 lung cancer cells. Endocytosis and degradation of thrombin. *J Biol Chem* **260**:15432, 1985.
162. Jakubowski HV, Kline MD, Owen WG: The effect of bovine thrombomodulin on the specificity of bovine thrombin. *J Biol Chem* **261**:3876, 1986.
163. Bourin M-C, Lundgren-Åkerlund E, Lindahl U: Isolation and characterization of the glycosaminoglycan component of rabbit thrombomodulin proteoglycan. *J Biol Chem* **265**:15424, 1990.
164. He X, Ye J, Esmon CT, Rezaie AR: Influence of arginines 93, 97, and 101 of thrombin to its functional specificity. *Biochemistry* **36**:8969, 1997.
165. Koyama T, Parkinson JF, Sié P, Bang NU, Müller-Berghaus G, Preissner KT: Different glycoforms of human thrombomodulin. Their glycosaminoglycan-dependent modulatory effects on thrombin inactivation by heparin cofactor II and antithrombin III. *Eur J Biochem* **198**:563, 1991.
166. Preissner KT, Koyama T, Müller D, Tschopp J, Müller-Berghaus G: Domain structure of the endothelial cell receptor thrombomodulin as deduced from modulation of its anticoagulant functions. Evidence for a glycosaminoglycan-dependent secondary binding site for thrombin. *J Biol Chem* **265**:4915, 1990.
167. Tran TH, Duckert F: Influence of heparin cofactor II (HCII) on the determination of antithrombin III (AT). *Thromb Res* **40**:571, 1985.
168. Conard J, Bara L, Horellou MH, Samama MM: Bovine or human thrombin in amidolytic AT III assays. Influence of heparin cofactor II. *Thromb Res* **41**:873, 1986.
169. Andersson N-E, Menschik M, van Voorthuizen H: New chromogenic ATIII activity kit which is insensitive to heparin cofactor II and designed for use on automated instruments. *Thromb Haemost* **65**:912, 1991.
170. Downing MR, Bloom JW, Mann KG: Comparison of the inhibition of thrombin by three plasma protease inhibitors. *Biochemistry* **17**:2649, 1978.
171. Conard J, Brosstad F, Lie-Larsen M, Samama M, Abildgaard U: Molar antithrombin concentration in normal human plasma. *Haemostasis* **13**:363, 1983.
172. Tait RC, Walker ID, Islam SIAM, McCall F, Conkie JA, Mitchell R, Davidson JF: Influence of demographic factors on antithrombin III activity in a healthy population. *Br J Haematol* **84**:476, 1993.
173. Conlan MG, Folsom AR, Finch A, Davis CE, Marcucci G, Sorlie P, Wu KK: Antithrombin III: Associations with age, race, sex and cardiovascular risk factors. *Thromb Haemost* **72**:551, 1994.
174. Andrew M, Paes B, Milner R, Johnston M, Mitchell L, Tollefsen DM, Powers P: Development of the human coagulation system in the full-term infant. *Blood* **70**:165, 1987.
175. Lane DA, Bayston T, Olds RJ, Fitches AC, Cooper DN, Millar DS, Jochmans K, et al.: Antithrombin mutation database: 2nd (1997) update. *Thromb Haemost* **77**:197, 1997.
176. van Boven HH, Lane DA: Antithrombin and its inherited deficiency states. *Semin Hematol* **34**:188, 1997.
177. Ambruso DR, Leonard BD, Bies RD, Jacobson L, Hathaway WE, Reeve EB: Antithrombin III deficiency: Decreased synthesis of a biochemically normal molecule. *Blood* **60**:78, 1982.
178. Knot EA, de Jong E, ten Cate JW, Iburg AH, Henny CP, Bruin T, Stibbe J: Purified radiolabeled antithrombin III metabolism in three families with hereditary AT III deficiency: Application of a three-compartment model. *Blood* **67**:93, 1986.
179. Perry DJ, Carrell RW: Molecular genetics of human antithrombin deficiency. *Hum Mutat* **7**:7, 1996.
180. Bayston TA, Lane DA: Antithrombin: molecular basis of deficiency. *Thromb Haemost* **78**:339, 1997.
181. Bruce D, Perry DJ, Borg JY, Carrell RW, Wardell MR: Thromboembolic disease due to thermolabile conformational changes of antithrombin Rouen-VI (187 Asn → Asp). *J Clin Invest* **94**:2265, 1994.
182. Sheffield WP, Castillo JE, Blajchman MA: Intracellular events determine the fate of antithrombin Utah. *Blood* **86**:3461, 1995.
183. Fischer AM, Cornu P, Sternberg C, Meriane F, Dautzenberg MD, Chafa O, Beguin S, et al.: Antithrombin III Alger: a new homozygous AT III variant. *Thromb Haemost* **55**:218, 1986.
184. Boyer C, Wolf M, Vedrenne J, Meyer D, Larrieu MJ: Homozygous variant of antithrombin III: AT III Fontainebleau. *Thromb Haemost* **56**:18, 1986.
185. Hirsh J, Piovella F, Pini M: Congenital antithrombin III deficiency. Incidence and clinical features. *Am J Med* **87**:34S, 1989.
186. Ødegård OR, Abildgaard U: Antithrombin III: Critical review of assay methods. Significance of variations in health and disease. *Haemostasis* **7**:127, 1978.
187. Rosenberg RD: Actions and interactions of antithrombin and heparin. *N Engl J Med* **292**:146, 1975.
188. Tait RC, Walker ID, Perry DJ, Carrell RW, Islam SIA, McCall F, Mitchell R, et al.: Prevalence of antithrombin III deficiency subtypes in 4000 healthy blood donors. *Thromb Haemost* **65**:839, 1991.
189. Mateo J, Oliver A, Borrell M, Sala N, Fontcuberta J: Laboratory evaluation and clinical characteristics of 2,132 consecutive unselected patients with venous thromboembolism—results of the Spanish Multicentric Study on Thrombophilia (EMET-Study). *Thromb Haemost* **77**:444, 1997.
190. Vikydal R, Korninger C, Kyrle PA, Niessner H, Pabinger I, Thaler E, Lechner K: The prevalence of hereditary antithrombin-III deficiency in patients with a history of venous thromboembolism. *Thromb Haemost* **54**:744, 1985.
191. Thaler E, Lechner K: Antithrombin III deficiency and thromboembolism. *Clin Haematol* **10**:369, 1981.
192. Cosgriff TM, Bishop DT, Hershgold EJ, Skolnick MH, Martin BA, Baty BJ, Carlson KS: Familial antithrombin III deficiency: Its natural history, genetics, diagnosis and treatment. *Medicine (Baltimore)* **62**:209, 1983.
193. Pabinger I, Schneider B: Thrombotic risk in hereditary antithrombin III, protein C, or protein S deficiency. A cooperative, retrospective study. *Arterioscler Thromb Vasc Biol* **16**:742, 1996.
194. Demers C, Ginsberg JS, Hirsh J, Henderson P, Blajchman MA: Thrombosis in antithrombin-III-deficient persons. Report of a large kindred and literature review. *Ann Intern Med* **116**:754, 1992.
195. McColl M, Tait RC, Walker ID, Perry DJ, McCall F, Conkie JA: Low thrombosis rate seen in blood donors and their relatives with inherited deficiencies of antithrombin and protein C: Correlation with type of defect, family history, and absence of the factor V Leiden mutation. *Blood Coagul Fibrinolysis* **7**:689, 1996.
196. van Boven HH, Reitsma PH, Rosendaal FR, Bayston TA, Chowdhury V, Bauer KA, Scharrer I, et al.: Factor V Leiden (FV R506Q) in families with inherited antithrombin deficiency. *Thromb Haemost* **75**:417, 1996.
197. Martinelli I, Magatelli R, Cattaneo M, Mannucci PM: Prevalence of mutant factor V in Italian patients with hereditary deficiencies of antithrombin, protein C or protein S. *Thromb Haemost* **75**:694, 1996.
198. Mitchell L, Piovella F, Ofosu F, Andrew M: α-2-Macroglobulin may provide protection from thromboembolic events in antithrombin III-deficient children. *Blood* **78**:2299, 1991.
199. Rosendaal FR, Heijboer H, Briët E, Büller HR, Brandjes DPM, de Bruin K, Hommes DW, et al.: Mortality in hereditary antithrombin-III deficiency—1830 to 1989. *Lancet* **337**:260, 1991.
200. Rosendaal FR, Heijboer H: Mortality related to thrombosis in congenital antithrombin III deficiency. *Lancet* **337**:1545, 1991.
201. van Boven HH, Vandenbroucke JP, Westendorp RG, Rosendaal FR: Mortality and causes of death in inherited antithrombin deficiency. *Thromb Haemost* **77**:452, 1997.
202. Bauer KA, Goodman TL, Kass BL, Rosenberg RD: Elevated factor Xa activity in the blood of asymptomatic patients with congenital antithrombin deficiency. *J Clin Invest* **76**:826, 1985.
203. Bauer KA, Barzegar S, Rosenberg RD: Influence of anticoagulants used for blood collection on plasma prothrombin fragment F1 + 2 measurements. *Thromb Res* **63**:617, 1991.
204. Demers C, Ginsberg JS, Henderson P, Ofosu FA, Weitz JI, Blajchman MA: Measurement of markers of activated coagulation in antithrombin III deficient subjects. *Thromb Haemost* **67**:542, 1992.
205. Marciniak E, Farley CH, DeSimone PA: Familial thrombosis due to antithrombin III deficiency. *Blood* **43**:219, 1974.
206. Ginsberg JS: Management of venous thromboembolism. *N Engl J Med* **335**:1816, 1996.
207. Leclerc JR, Geerts W, Panju A, Nguyen P, Hirsh J: Management of anti-thrombin III deficiency during pregnancy without administration of anti-thrombin III. *Thromb Res* **41**:567, 1986.
208. Nielsen LE, Bell WR, Borkon AM, Neill CA: Extensive thrombus formation with heparin resistance during extracorporeal circulation. A new presentation of familial antithrombin III deficiency. *Arch Intern Med* **147**:149, 1987.
209. Holm HA, Kalvenes S, Abildgaard U: Changes in plasma antithrombin (heparin cofactor activity) during intravenous heparin therapy: observations in 198 patients with deep venous thrombosis. *Scand J Haematol* **35**:564, 1985.

210. Petitti DB, Strom BL, Melmon KL: Duration of warfarin anticoagulant therapy and the probabilities of recurrent thromboembolism and hemorrhage. *Am J Med* **81**:255, 1986.
211. Schulman S, Granqvist S, Holmström M, Carlsson A, Lindmarker P, Nicol P, Eklund S-G, et al.: The duration of oral anticoagulant therapy after a second episode of venous thromboembolism. *N Engl J Med* **336**:393, 1997.
212. Hellgren M, Tengborn L, Abildgaard U: Pregnancy in women with congenital antithrombin III deficiency: Experience of treatment with heparin and antithrombin. *Gynecol Obstet Invest* **14**:127, 1982.
213. Conard J, Horellou MH, Van Dreden P, Lecompte T, Samama M: Thrombosis and pregnancy in congenital deficiencies in AT III, protein C or protein S: Study of 78 women. *Thromb Haemost* **63**:319, 1990.
214. De Stefano V, Leone G, Mastrangelo S, Tripodi A, Rodeghiero F, Castaman G, Barbui T, et al.: Thrombosis during pregnancy and surgery in patients with congenital deficiency of antithrombin III, protein C, protein S. *Thromb Haemost* **71**:799, 1994.
215. Friederich PW, Sanson B-J, Simioni P, Zanardi S, Huisman MV, Kindt I, Prandoni P, et al.: Frequency of pregnancy-related venous thromboembolism in anticoagulant factor-deficient women: implications for prophylaxis. *Ann Intern Med* **125**:955, 1996.
216. Ginsburg JS, Hirsh J: Use of antithrombotic agents during pregnancy. *Chest* **108(Suppl)**:305S, 1995.
217. Owen J: Antithrombin III replacement therapy in pregnancy. *Semin Hematol* **28**:46, 1991.
218. Blondel-Hill E, Mant MJ: The pregnant antithrombin III deficient patient: Management without antithrombin III concentrate. *Thromb Res* **65**:193, 1992.
219. Sanson B-J, Friederich PW, Simioni P, Zanardi S, Hilsman MV, Girolami A, ten Cate J-W, et al.: The risk of abortion and stillbirth in antithrombin-, protein C-, and protein S-deficient women. *Thromb Haemost* **75**:387, 1996.
220. Preston FE, Rosendaal FR, Walker ID, Briët E, Berntorp E, Conard J, Fontcuberta J, et al.: Increased fetal loss in women with heritable thrombophilia. *Lancet* **348**:913, 1996.
221. Menache D, O'Malley JP, Schorr JB, Wagner B, Williams C, Alving BM, Ballard JO, et al.: Evaluation of the safety, recovery, half-life, and clinical efficacy of antithrombin III (human) in patients with hereditary antithrombin III deficiency. *Blood* **75**:33, 1990.
222. Menache D: Replacement therapy in patients with hereditary antithrombin III deficiency. *Semin Hematol* **28**:31, 1991.
223. Winter JH, Fenech A, Bennett B, Douglas AS: Prophylactic antithrombotic therapy with stanozolol in patients with familial antithrombin III deficiency. *Br J Haematol* **57**:527, 1984.
224. Fairfax AJ, Ibbotson RM: Effect of danazol on the biochemical abnormality of inherited antithrombin III deficiency. *Thorax* **40**:646, 1985.
225. Eyster ME, Parker ME: Treatment of familial antithrombin-III deficiency with danazol. *Haemostasis* **15**:119, 1985.
226. Knot E, ten Cate JW, Drijfhout HR, Kahle LH, Tytgat GN: Antithrombin III metabolism in patients with liver disease. *J Clin Pathol* **37**:523, 1984.
227. Kauffmann RH, Veltkamp JJ, van Tilburg NH, van Es LA: Acquired antithrombin III deficiency and thrombosis in the nephrotic syndrome. *Am J Med* **65**:607, 1978.
228. Spero JA, Lewis JH, Hasiba U: Disseminated intravascular coagulation. Findings in 346 patients. *Thromb Haemost* **43**:28, 1980.
229. Brenner B: Antithrombin III and preeclampsia. *Isr J Med Sci* **26**:121, 1990.
230. Ceriello A, Quatraro A, Marchi E, Barbanti M, Dello Russo P, Lefebvre P, Giugliano D: The role of hyperglycaemia-induced alterations of antithrombin III and factor X activation in the thrombin hyperactivity of diabetes mellitus. *Diabetic Med* **7**:343, 1990.
231. Fagerhol MK, Abildgaard U, Bergsjø P, Jacobsen JH: Oral contraceptives and low antithrombin III concentration. *Lancet* **1**:1175, 1970.
232. Henny CP, ten Cate H, Dabhoiwala NF, Büller HR, ten Cate JW: The effect of different hormonal approaches in treatment of prostatic cancer on the plasma antithrombin III activity. *Thromb Haemost* **50**:50, 1983.
233. Conard J, Cazenave B, Maury J, Horellou MH, Samama M: L-Asparaginase, antithrombin III, and thrombosis. *Lancet* **1**:1091, 1980.
234. Bauer KA, Teitel JM, Rosenberg RD: L-Asparaginase induced antithrombin III deficiency: Evidence against the production of a hypercoagulable state. *Thromb Res* **29**:437, 1983.
235. Gugliotta L, D'Angelo A, Mattioli Belmonte M, Viganò-D'Angelo S, Colombo G, Catani L, Gianni L, et al.: Hypercoagulability during L-asparaginase treatment: The effect of antithrombin III supplementation in vivo. *Br J Haematol* **74**:465, 1990.
236. Holmer E, Soderstrom G, Andersson L-O: Properties of antithrombin III depleted plasma. I. Effect of heparin. *Thromb Res* **17**:113, 1980.
237. Briginshaw GF, Shanberge JN: Identification of two distinct heparin cofactors in human plasma. Separation and partial purification. *Arch Biochem Biophys* **161**:683, 1974.
238. Tollefsen DM, Majerus DW, Blank MK: Heparin cofactor II. Purification and properties of a heparin-dependent inhibitor of thrombin in human plasma. *J Biol Chem* **257**:2162, 1982.
239. Parker KA, Tollefsen DM: The protease specificity of heparin cofactor II. Inhibition of thrombin generated during coagulation. *J Biol Chem* **260**:3501, 1985.
240. Ragg H: A new member of the plasma protease inhibitor gene family. *Nucleic Acids Res* **14**:1073, 1986.
241. Blinder MA, Marasa JC, Reynolds CH, Deaven LL, Tollefsen DM: Heparin cofactor II: cDNA sequence, chromosome localization, restriction fragment length polymorphism, and expression in *Escherichia coli*. *Biochemistry* **27**:752, 1988.
242. Hortin G, Tollefsen DM, Strauss AW: Identification of two sites of sulfation of human heparin cofactor II. *J Biol Chem* **261**:15827, 1986.
243. Church FC, Pratt CW, Hoffman M: Leukocyte chemoattractant peptides from the serpin heparin cofactor II. *J Biol Chem* **266**:704, 1991.
244. Church FC, Meade JB, Pratt CW: Structure-function relationships in heparin cofactor II: Spectral analysis of aromatic residues and absence of a role for sulfhydryl groups in thrombin inhibition. *Arch Biochem Biophys* **259**:331, 1987.
245. Herzog R, Lutz S, Blin N, Marasa JC, Blinder MA, Tollefsen DM: Complete nucleotide sequence of the gene for human heparin cofactor II and mapping to chromosomal band 22q11. *Biochemistry* **30**:1350, 1991.
246. Ragg H, Preibisch G: Structure and expression of the gene coding for the human serpin hLS2. *J Biol Chem* **263**:12129, 1988.
247. Jaffe EA, Armellino D, Tollefsen DM: Biosynthesis of functionally active heparin cofactor II by a human hepatoma-derived cell line. *Biochem Biophys Res Commun* **132**:368, 1985.
248. Griffith MJ, Noyes CM, Tyndall JA, Church FC: Structural evidence for leucine at the reactive site of heparin cofactor II. *Biochemistry* **24**:6777, 1985.
249. Church FC, Noyes CM, Griffith MJ: Inhibition of chymotrypsin by heparin cofactor II. *Proc Natl Acad Sci U S A* **82**:6431, 1985.
250. Derechin VM, Blinder MA, Tollefsen DM: Substitution of arginine for Leu444 in the reactive site of heparin cofactor II enhances the rate of thrombin inhibition. *J Biol Chem* **265**:5623, 1990.
251. Hurst RE, Poon M-C, Griffith MJ: Structure-activity relationships of heparin. Independence of heparin charge density and antithrombin-binding domains in thrombin inhibition by antithrombin and heparin cofactor II. *J Clin Invest* **72**:1042, 1983.
252. Maimone MM, Tollefsen DM: Activation of heparin cofactor II by heparin oligosaccharides. *Biochem Biophys Res Commun* **152**:1056, 1988.
253. Maimone MM: Characterization of heparin and dermatan sulfate molecules that bind and activate heparin cofactor II. PhD thesis. St. Louis, Washington University, 1990.
254. Sié P, Petitou M, Lormeau J-C, Dupouy D, Boneu B, Choay J: Studies on the structural requirements of heparin for the catalysis of thrombin inhibition by heparin cofactor II. *Biochim Biophys Acta* **966**:188, 1988.
255. Bray B, Lane DA, Freyssinet J-M, Pejler G, Lindahl U: Anti-thrombin activities of heparin. Effect of saccharide chain length on thrombin inhibition by heparin cofactor II and by antithrombin. *Biochem J* **262**:225, 1989.
256. Conrad HE: Structure of heparan sulfate and dermatan sulfate. *Ann N Y Acad Sci* **556**:18, 1989.
257. Maimone MM, Tollefsen DM: Structure of a dermatan sulfate hexasaccharide that binds to heparin cofactor II with high affinity. *J Biol Chem* **265**:18263, 1990.
258. Tollefsen DM, Peacock ME, Monafo WJ: Molecular size of dermatan sulfate oligosaccharides required to bind and activate heparin cofactor II. *J Biol Chem* **261**:8854, 1986.
259. Pavão MSG, Mourão PAS, Mulloy B, Tollefsen DM: A unique dermatan sulfate-like glycosaminoglycan from ascidian: Its structure and the effect of its unusual sulfation pattern on anticoagulant activity. *J Biol Chem* **270**:31027, 1995.
260. Teien AN, Abildgaard U, Höök M: The anticoagulant effect of heparan sulfate and dermatan sulfate. *Thromb Res* **8**:859, 1976.
261. Fernandez F, van Ryn J, Ofosu FA, Hirsh J, Buchanan MR: The haemorrhagic and antithrombotic effects of dermatan sulfate. *Br J Haematol* **64**:309, 1986.

262. Maggi A, Abbadini M, Pagella PG, Borowska A, Pangrazzi J, Donati MB: Antithrombotic properties of dermatan sulphate in a rat venous thrombosis model. *Haemostasis* **17**:329, 1987.
263. Merton RE, Thomas DP: Experimental studies on the relative efficacy of dermatan sulphate and heparin as antithrombotic agents. *Thromb Haemost* **58**:839, 1987.
264. Van Ryn-McKenna J, Gray E, Weber E, Ofosu FA, Buchanan MR: Effects of sulfated polysaccharides on inhibition of thrombus formation initiated by different stimuli. *Thromb Haemost* **61**:7, 1989.
265. Agnelli G, Cosmi B, Di Filippo P, Ranucci V, Veschi F, Longetti M, Renga C, et al.: A randomised, double-blind, placebo-controlled trial of dermatan sulphate for prevention of deep vein thrombosis in hip fracture. *Thromb Haemost* **67**:203, 1992.
266. Cofrancesco E, Boschetti C, Leonardi P, Cortellaro M: Dermatan sulphate in acute leukaemia. *Lancet* **339**:1177, 1992.
267. Lane DA, Ryan K, Ireland H, Curtis JR, Nurmohamed MT, Krediet RT, Roggekamp MC, et al.: Dermatan sulphate in haemodialysis. *Lancet* **339**:334, 1992.
268. Ofosu FA, Modi GJ, Smith LM, Cerskus AL, Hirsh J, Blajchman MA: Heparan sulfate and dermatan sulfate inhibit the generation of thrombin activity in plasma by complementary pathways. *Blood* **64**:742, 1984.
269. Sié P, Ofosu F, Fernandez F, Buchanan MR, Petitou M, Boneu B: Respective role of antithrombin III and heparin cofactor II in the in vitro anticoagulant effect of heparin and of various sulphated polysaccharides. *Br J Haematol* **64**:707, 1986.
270. Andersson TR, Larsen ML, Abildgaard U: Low heparin cofactor II associated with abnormal crossed immunoelectrophoresis pattern in two Norwegian families. *Thromb Res* **47**:243, 1987.
271. Blinder MA, Andersson TR, Abildgaard U, Tollefsen DM: Heparin cofactor II Oslo. Mutation of Arg-189 to His decreases the affinity for dermatan sulfate. *J Biol Chem* **264**:5128, 1989.
272. Blinder MA, Tollefsen DM: Site-directed mutagenesis of arginine 103 and lysine 185 in the proposed glycosaminoglycan-binding site of heparin cofactor II. *J Biol Chem* **265**:286, 1990.
273. Ragg H, Ulshöfer T, Gerewitz J: On the activation of human leuserpin-2, a thrombin inhibitor, by glycosaminoglycans. *J Biol Chem* **265**: 5211, 1990.
274. Ragg H, Ulshöfer T, Gerewitz J: Glycosaminoglycan-mediated leuserpin-2/thrombin interaction. Structure-function relationships. *J Biol Chem* **265**:22386, 1990.
275. Whinna HC, Blinder MA, Szewczyk M, Tollefsen DM, Church FC: Role of lysine 173 in heparin binding to heparin cofactor II. *J Biol Chem* **266**:8129, 1991.
276. Van Deerlin VMD, Tollefsen DM: The N-terminal acidic domain of heparin cofactor II mediates the inhibition of α-thrombin in the presence of glycosaminoglycans. *J Biol Chem* **266**:20223, 1991.
277. Grutter MG, Priestle JP, Rahuel J, Grossenbacher H, Bode W, Hofsteenge J, Stone SR: Crystal structure of the thrombin-hirudin complex: A novel mode of serine protease inhibition. *EMBO J* **9**:2361, 1990.
278. Rydel TJ, Ravichandran KG, Tulinsky A, Bode W, Huber R, Roitsch C, Fenton JW II: The structure of a complex of recombinant hirudin and human α-thrombin. *Science* **249**:277, 1990.
279. Hortin GL, Tollefsen DM, Benutto BM: Antithrombin activity of a peptide corresponding to residues 54-75 of heparin cofactor II. *J Biol Chem* **264**:13979, 1989.
280. Rogers SJ, Pratt CW, Whinna HC, Church FC: Role of thrombin exosites in inhibition by heparin cofactor II. *J Biol Chem* **267**:3613, 1992.
281. Phillips JE, Shirk RA, Whinna HC, Henriksen RA, Church FC: Inhibition of dysthrombins Quick I and II by heparin cofactor II and antithrombin. *J Biol Chem* **268**:3321, 1993.
282. Sheehan JP, Wu Q, Tollefsen DM, Sadler JE: Mutagenesis of thrombin selectively modulates inhibition by serpins heparin cofactor II and antithrombin III. Interaction with the anion-binding exosite determines heparin cofactor II specificity. *J Biol Chem* **268**:3639, 1993.
283. Sheehan JP, Tollefsen DM, Sadler JE: Heparin cofactor II is regulated allosterically and not primarily by template effects. Studies with mutant thrombins and glycosaminoglycans. *J Biol Chem* **269**:32747, 1994.
284. Sheehan JP, Sadler JE: Molecular mapping of the heparin-binding exosite of thrombin. *Proc Natl Acad Sci U S A* **91**:5518, 1994.
285. Tsiang M, Jain AK, Gibbs CS: Functional requirements for inhibition of thrombin by antithrombin III in the presence and absence of heparin. *J Biol Chem* **272**:12024, 1997.
286. Arni RK, Padmanabhan K, Padmanabhan KP, Wu T-P, Tulinsky A: Structures of the noncovalent complexes of human and bovine prothrombin fragment 2 with human PPACK-thrombin. *Biochemistry* **32**:4727, 1993.
287. Tollefsen DM, Pestka CA: Heparin cofactor II activity in patients with disseminated intravascular coagulation and hepatic failure. *Blood* **66**:769, 1985.
288. Sié P, Dupouy D, Pichon J, Boneu B: Constitutional heparin co-factor II deficiency associated with recurrent thrombosis. *Lancet* **2**:414, 1985.
289. Tran TH, Marbet GA, Duckert F: Association of hereditary heparin co-factor II deficiency with thrombosis. *Lancet* **2**:413, 1985.
290. Simioni P, Lazzaro AR, Coser E, Salmistraro G, Girolami A: Hereditary heparin cofactor II deficiency and thrombosis: Report of six patients belonging to two separate kindreds. *Blood Coagul Fibrinolysis* **1**:351, 1990.
291. Jobin F, Vu L, Lessard M: Two cases of inherited triple deficiency in a large kindred with thrombotic diathesis and deficiencies of antithrombin III, heparin cofactor II, protein C and protein S. *Thromb Haemost* **66**:295, 1991.
292. Weisdorf DJ, Edson JR: Recurrent venous thrombosis associated with inherited deficiency of heparin cofactor II [published erratum appears in *Br J Haematol* **77(3)**:446, 1991]. *Br J Haematol* **77**:125, 1991.
293. Simioni P, Zanardi S, Prandoni P, Girolami A: Combined inherited protein S and heparin co-factor II deficiency in a patient with upper limb thrombosis: A family study. *Thromb Res* **67**:23, 1992.
294. Bernardi F, Legnani C, Micheletti F, Lunghi B, Ferraresi P, Palareti G, Biagi R, et al.: A heparin cofactor II mutation (HCII Rimini) combined with factor V Leiden or type I protein C deficiency in two unrelated thrombophilic subjects. *Thromb Haemost* **76**:505, 1996.
295. Kondo S, Tokunaga F, Kario K, Matsuo T, Koide T: Molecular and cellular basis for type I heparin cofactor II deficiency (heparin cofactor II Awaji). *Blood* **87**:1006, 1996.
296. Andersson TR, Larsen ML, Handeland GF, Abildgaard U: Heparin cofactor II activity in plasma: Application of an automated assay method to the study of a normal adult population. *Scand J Haematol* **36**:96, 1986.
297. Bertina RM, van der Linden IK, Engesser L, Muller HP, Brommer EJP: Hereditary heparin cofactor II deficiency and the risk of development of thrombosis. *Thromb Haemost* **57**:196, 1987.
298. Tran TH, Duckert F: Heparin cofactor II determination — levels in normals and patients with hereditary antithrombin III deficiency and disseminated intravascular coagulation. *Thromb Haemost* **52**:112, 1984.
299. Abildgaard U, Larsen ML: Assay of dermatan sulfate cofactor (heparin cofactor II) activity in human plasma. *Thromb Res* **35**:257, 1984.
300. Ezenagu LC, Brandt JT: Laboratory determination of heparin cofactor II. *Arch Pathol Lab Med* **110**:1149, 1986.
301. Massouh M, Jatoi A, Gordon EM, Ratnoff OD: Heparin cofactor II activity in plasma during pregnancy and oral contraceptive use. *J Lab Clin Med* **114**:697, 1989.
302. Toulon P, Bardin JM, Blumenfeld N: Increased heparin cofactor II levels in women taking oral contraceptives. *Thromb Haemost* **64**:365, 1990.
303. Griffith MJ, Carraway T, White GC, Dombrose FA: Heparin cofactor activities in a family with hereditary antithrombin III deficiency: evidence for a second heparin cofactor in human plasma. *Blood* **61**:111, 1983.
304. McGuire EA, Tollefsen DM: Activation of heparin cofactor II by fibroblasts and vascular smooth muscle cells. *J Biol Chem* **262**:169, 1987.
305. Shirk RA, Church FC, Wagner WD: Arterial smooth muscle cell heparan sulfate proteoglycans accelerate thrombin inhibition by heparin cofactor II. *Arterioscler Thromb Vasc Biol* **16**:1138, 1996.
306. Andrew M, Mitchell L, Berry L, Paes B, Delorme M, Ofosu F, Burrows R, et al.: An anticoagulant dermatan sulfate proteoglycan circulates in the pregnant woman and her fetus. *J Clin Invest* **89**:321, 1992.
307. Liu L, Dewar L, Song Y, Kulczycky M, Blajchman MA, Fenton JW, II, Andrew M, et al.: Inhibition of thrombin by antithrombin III and heparin cofactor II in vivo. *Thromb Haemost* **73**:405, 1995.
308. Brennan MJ, Oldberg A, Pierschbacher MD, Ruoslahti E: Chondroitin/dermatan sulfate proteoglycan in human fetal membranes: demonstration of an antigenically similar proteoglycan in fibroblasts. *J Biol Chem* **259**:13742, 1984.
309. Loebermann H, Tokuoka R, Deisenhofer J, Huber R: Human α1-proteinase inhibitor. Crystal structure analysis of two crystal modifications, molecular model and preliminary analysis of the implications for function. *J Mol Biol* **177**:531, 1984.

CHAPTER 177

Inherited Disorders of Platelets

Deborah L. French ▪ Peter J. Newman ▪ Mortimer Poncz

1. **Human platelets participate in a number of adhesive events that are crucial for repair of the vasculature. Although lacking in protein synthetic capability, platelets come equipped with a variety of membrane receptors and intracellular organelles that make them highly efficient "adhesion machines" for mediating the primary hemostatic process. Adhesion itself is an activating event, and it results in the transmission of signals to the cell interior by virtue of cell-surface receptors that form cytoplasmic connections with intracellular kinases, G proteins, and cytoskeletal components. Platelet activation, in turn, elicits the secretion of several types of intracellular granules, the contents of which serve to embellish further the formation of the platelet plug by providing additional adhesive ligands that can add to the local concentration of intercellular glue molecules.**
2. **The αIIbβ3 integrin receptor (also called glycoprotein [GP] IIb-IIIa) is the most abundant receptor on the platelet surface, representing nearly 15 percent of total surface protein. Glanzmann thrombasthenia is a rare, inherited, autosomal recessive bleeding disorder, the hallmark of which is the failure of platelets to bind fibrinogen and aggregate following stimulation by physiological agonists such as ADP, thrombin, epinephrine, or collagen. Underlying this disorder are abnormalities of either the αIIb or β3 gene. Glanzmann thrombasthenia is characterized by significant mucocutaneous bleeding beginning at an early age. Nearly 200 individuals with Glanzmann thrombasthenia have been described in the literature and 75 molecular defects have been identified in 61 kindreds. The molecular abnormalities have ranged from major deletions and inversions easily detectable by Southern blot analysis to single point mutations identified only by nucleotide sequence analysis of the genome or platelet mRNA-derived PCR products.**
3. **The GPIb complex is crucial for initial attachment and proper adhesion to the extracellular matrix of a damaged vessel. Bernard-Soulier syndrome represents the second most recognized inherited platelet disorder, and is characterized by a prolonged bleeding time, giant platelets, normal platelet aggregation with ADP, collagen, and epinephrine, but absent platelet agglutination in the presence of ristocetin. The Bernard-Soulier syndrome is an autosomal recessive disorder in which most patients have a decrease to absence of all four members of the GPIb complex, each encoded by a separate gene: GPIbα, GPIbβ, GPIX, and GPV. These genes have been cloned and characterized, and a growing number of patients have had the responsible defect defined on a molecular level. Defects in the GPIb complex are also responsible for another bleeding disorder—platelet-type (or pseudo-) von Willebrand disease—in which the platelet receptor exhibits increased affinity for von Willebrand factor (VWF).**
4. **In addition to amino acid changes that disrupt function and result in bleeding diatheses, several platelet membrane glycoproteins have naturally occurring allelic forms within the human gene pool. Two clinically recognized immunologic syndromes are attributable to "platelet-specific" polymorphisms. Neonatal alloimmune thrombocytopenia is characterized by neonatal thrombocytopenia due to passively transmitted maternal antibodies directed against a platelet antigen inherited from the father and lacking on maternal platelets. Posttransfusion purpura is quite rare, and is characterized by acute, usually severe, thrombocytopenia 7 to 10 days after a blood transfusion. As the precise nucleotide sequence polymorphisms associated with the major human platelet alloantigen systems have become defined, it has become possible to develop and apply DNA-based diagnostic tests.**
5. **Human platelets contain several different types of intracytoplasmic granules that can be distinguished by electron microscopy, including α-granules, dense (or δ-) granules, and lysosomes. These granules play a major role in platelet plug formation following platelet activation. Patients with defects in the platelet-dense granules have a storage pool deficiency. The two most common platelet storage pool disorders are known as Hermansky-Pudlak syndrome and Chediak-Higashi syndrome, and the genes involved in these diseases have been cloned. A number of patients have been described who have a deficiency in α-granules, a disorder known as the gray platelet syndrome. These platelets are markedly deficient in α-granule-specific proteins such as platelet factor 4, β-thromboglobulin, VWF, factor V, fibronectin, and platelet-derived growth factor.**
6. **Following the binding of an agonist to its platelet receptor, a signal is transferred across the cell membrane into the cell either directly by the membrane receptor or through intervening $G_{\alpha\beta\delta}$ heterotrimeric proteins. Signal transduction results in secondary changes within the platelet that include ionic calcium fluxes, cAMP formation, phospholipase A2 and C activation, changes in arachidonate pathway metabolism, protein kinase C activation, and protein phosphorylation. Patients with inherited disorders of platelet signal transduction have been described. The most prominent of these has been the Wiskott-Aldrich syndrome (WAS) that affects both platelets and lymphocytes.**
7. **Activated platelets play a role in accelerating the proteolytic events that take place as part of the coagulation cascade, and this property has been termed "platelet factor 3 activity." The procoagulant properties have been attributed to a number of characteristics unique to the surface of activated platelets, including exposure of phosphatidylserine moieties, redistribution of specific receptors for factors V and X, and development of platelet microvesicles. One of the best-characterized inherited disorders of platelet factor**

3 activity is known as Scott syndrome. The defect in this disorder is not limited to platelet membranes, as erythrocytes from patients with Scott syndrome also have decreased microvesiculation and fewer factor Va binding sites than normal following A23187 ionophore stimulation. The molecular basis of any of these disorders has yet to be determined.

8. The process by which platelet formation occurs is a fascinating one. Megakaryocytopoiesis begins with the self-renewing hematopoietic stem cell in the bone marrow that becomes progressively committed to the megakaryoblast lineage, eventually resulting in the production of a mature megakaryocyte that "terminally differentiates" by releasing a shower of $\sim 10^4$ platelets. The size variation and heterogeneity in platelets seen in various disease states may be related to cytoskeletal problems or to the site and mechanism of formation. A number of the inherited platelet disorders involve abnormal platelet size, including the macrothrombocytopenic states seen in Bernard-Soulier syndrome and the May-Hegglin anomaly, as well as the microthrombocytopenia seen in WAS. Decreased platelet counts also occur and involve the above three disorders as well as the recently recognized family platelet deficiency/acute myelogenous leukemia (FPD/AML) syndrome.

THE ROLE OF PLATELETS IN HEMOSTASIS AND THROMBOSIS

Human platelets are anucleate cellular derivatives of bone marrow megakaryocytes that circulate throughout the bloodstream at a concentration of 1.5 to 4.0 × $10^5/\text{mm}^3$. With a life span of only ~10 days, resting platelets maintain a disk-like shape unless activated, usually by exposure to a damaged vessel wall. Following activation, platelets undergo a rapid metamorphosis from nonadherent plate-shaped cells into highly adherent, pseudopod-containing, ameba-like entities, and participate in the formation of the so-called platelet plug at a site of vascular injury.

Platelet Adhesion and Aggregation

Platelets come equipped with a variety of membrane receptors and intracellular organelles that make them highly efficient "adhesion machines" for mediating the primary hemostatic process. The mechanisms by which platelets become activated are multiple and complex, and have a great deal of built-in redundancy to ensure rapid, efficient sealing of the wound. As illustrated in Fig. 177-1, platelets can be activated by numerous agonists, both soluble and insoluble. Damage to a vessel wall leads to disruption of the normal endothelial cell barrier, with exposure of extracellular matrix components, including fibronectin, collagen, and VWF. Platelets have receptors for these ligands, and rapidly initiate an adhesive cascade at the site of injury. Membrane-receptor complexes GPIb and $\alpha 2\beta 1$ bind VWF and collagen, respectively, and mediate the primary adhesion of an initial layer of platelets that applies a thin bandage to the injury. Nearby platelets become secondarily exposed to extracellular agonists, such as thrombin, epinephrine, ADP, and various thromboxane metabolites that are released as a result of local tissue injury. Platelets become activated by one or more of these agonists, and mobilize still another adhesive receptor, the $\alpha\text{IIb}\beta 3$ complex. On activation, this receptor complex undergoes conformational changes and binds fibrinogen, which, due to its symmetric structure, serves to crosslink platelets to each other, that is, platelet aggregation. The membrane receptors and their ligands that mediate these important adhesive interactions are summarized in Fig. 177-2.

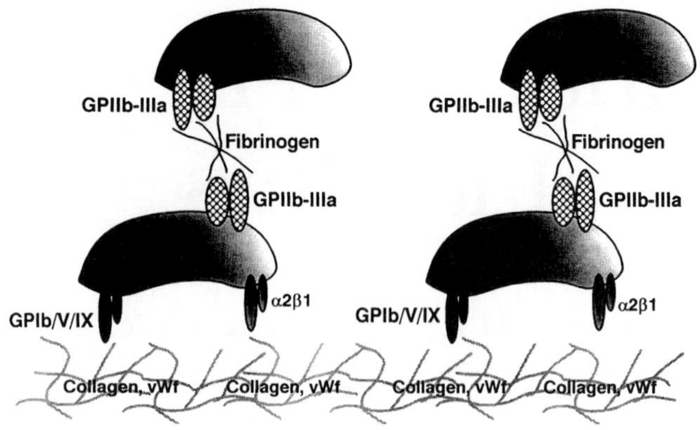

Fig. 177-2 Platelet adhesive interactions. Platelet receptors involved in platelet-platelet interactions are shown, together with the adhesive ligands with which they interact.

Platelet Granules

Adhesion is an activating event; it causes the secretion of several types of intracellular granules, the contents of which serve to embellish further the formation of the platelet plug by providing additional adhesive ligands that add to the local intercellular glue molecules. A number of soluble agonists that aid in recruiting other platelets to the site of injury are also secreted. The three major types of platelet granules, and some of their more interesting components, are listed in Table 177-1. The α-granules contain a large number of adhesive protein ligands, some of which, on secretion, bind to specific platelet plasma membrane receptors and help to crosslink platelets to each other during platelet aggregation. Dense, or δ-granules, contain most of the platelet calcium and stored ADP and serotonin. Although the function of serotonin in platelet function is not well understood, released calcium and ADP play important roles in mediating the platelet aggregation process. Lysosomal granules, as in other cell types, probably function in

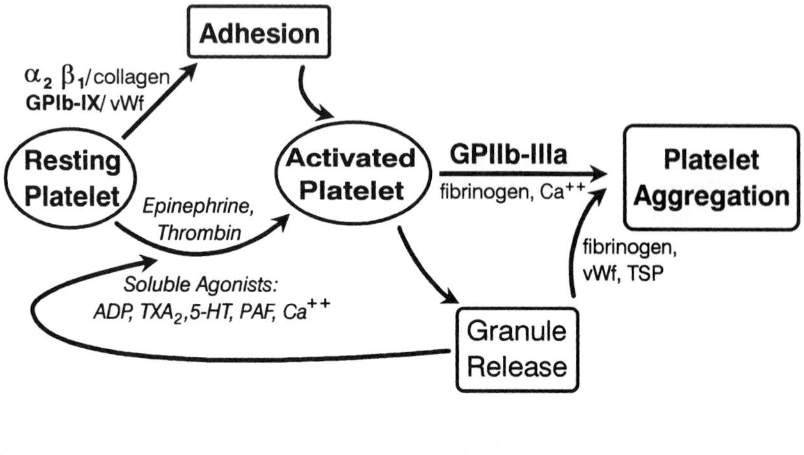

Fig. 177-1 Role of platelets in hemostasis. The transformation of platelets from a resting to an adherent state is depicted, together with several of the known soluble and insoluble agonists that can trigger the event. Adhesion to extracellular matrix components, exposed as a result of endothelial cell damage, is an activating event, and leads to granule release and the conversion of cell-surface receptors into an adhesive conformation. Additional soluble agonists, including thrombin, ADP, and epinephrine, generated at the site of the injury, serve to enhance the activation process, and recruit additional platelets into the developing platelet aggregate. TSP = thrombospondin.

Table 177-1 Platelet Granules and Their Contents

α-Granules	δ-Granules	Lysosomes
Fibrinogen	Serotonin	β-*N*-acetylglucosaminidase
VWF	Calcium	β-Glucuronidase
Fibronectin	ADP	β-Galactosidase
Thrombospondin	Guanine nucleotides	Other acid hydrolases
Factor V		
Platelet factor 4	ATP, AMP	
β-Thromboglobulin	Inorganic pyrophosphate	

degrading various endocytosed plasma constituents, and may also play a role in receptor recycling.

Platelet Adhesion Receptors

Central to the role of platelets to adhere to both extracellular matrix components and to aggregation is an abundant supply of cell-surface adhesion molecules that exist in multiple states of activation. These cell adhesion receptors, in turn, are capable of transmitting signals to the cell interior by virtue of their ability to form cytoplasmic connections with G proteins, kinases, and cytoskeletal components. Many platelet cell-surface receptors have now been cloned and characterized, and while >50 platelet plasma membrane proteins are recognizable by two-dimensional electrophoresis, many of them fall into a limited number of well-recognized families. Five gene families, the integrins, the leucine-rich glycoproteins, the immunoglobulin superfamily, and the selectins, as well as their members that are present in human platelets, are summarized in Table 177-2. A brief description of the major distinguishing characteristics of each family follows.

The Leucine-Rich Glycoprotein Family. Platelets contain four members of the leucine-rich glycoprotein family[1,2] and, interestingly enough, these proteins (GPIbα, GPIbβ, GPIX, and GPV) exist on the platelet surface in a 2:2:2:1 stoichiometric complex,[3,4] and are referred to in the remainder of this chapter as the GPIb complex. Each member of this receptor complex has been cloned.[1,2,5] Each platelet expresses 2 to 3 × 10^4 copies of the GPIb complex on its surface, and all four components of the complex are missing from the platelet surface in patients with the Bernard-Soulier syndrome,[2,6] a defect that is discussed in greater detail below.

Table 177-2 Cell Adhesion Molecule Families in Human Platelets

Gene family	Members on human platelets	Functions
Integrins	αIIbβ3, αvβ3, α2β1, α5β1, α6β1	Cell-cell and cell-matrix interactions
Leucine-rich	GPIbα, GPIbβ, GPV, GPIX	Adhesion to subendothelium glycoprotein
Immunoglobulin	FcγRIIA, Class I GMP, PECAM-1	Immunoregulation, adhesion gene (ITAM/ITIM) superfamily
Selectins	P-selectin (HLA-140, PADGEM)	Platelet-endothelial cell and platelet-leukocyte interactions

The Immunoglobulin Superfamily. The distinguishing feature of the immunoglobulin gene (Ig) superfamily is the presence of one or more immunoglobulin-like homology domains. Structurally, these homology domains resemble antibodies, containing 7 β-strands folded into 2 β-pleated sheets held together by 2 cysteines spaced approximately 50 residues apart. Human platelets are known to express three members of the Ig superfamily: class I histocompatibility antigens (HLA), FcγRIIA, and PECAM-1. Of these, the HLA molecules are extremely polymorphic, and probably account for the majority of cases of platelet transfusion refractoriness.

Seven Transmembrane Receptors. There is a series of two transmembrane receptors present on platelets that bind to platelet agonists. For example, P242, P2X, and P2YAC are three such receptors for ADP binding and platelet activation. For thrombin, PAR1 and PAR4 are present on platelets. Epinephrine and thromboxane AZ also stimulate platelets through such receptors. The seven transmembrane receptors signal to the platelet via $G_{\alpha\beta\gamma}$ heterotrimers.

Selectins. This family contains only three members, each named for the cell type in which it was first discovered: P-selectin, originally described in human platelets;[7,8] E-selectin, which is present only on endothelium;[9,10] and L-selectin, found on lymphocytes. Selectins share a common N-terminal lectin-like domain that is capable of interacting with carbohydrate moieties on nearby cellular receptors, and it is this structural motif that gives the family its name.[10] P-selectin (previously called GMP-140 or PADGEM) is the only platelet selectin, and resides within the membrane of α-granules of resting platelets. On platelet activation, the α-granule membranes fuse with the plasma membrane, exposing 1.0 to 1.5 × 10^4 P-selectin molecules per platelet, where they participate in recruiting monocytes and neutrophils to the site of vascular injury.[11]

Integrins. The integrins are composed of an αβ heterodimeric membrane complex that mediates cell-cell and cell-extracellular matrix adhesive interactions.[12,13] At least 8 different β subunits and 11 different α-chains have been cloned and sequenced. It is now recognized that distinct α and β subunits can cross-pair in different cell types to form multiple, distinct functional entities. More than 15 members of this heterodimer family have been identified in species ranging from *Drosophila* to humans,[12,13] with at least 5 members (α2β1, α5β1, α6β1, αIIbβ3, and αvβ3) expressed on the platelet surface. Of these, αIIbβ3 is uniquely expressed on platelets, and is by far the most abundant member of the integrin family to be found on the platelet surface, with 8 × 10^4 molecules/platelet.[14] Other platelet integrins, although not as extensively studied as αIIbβ3, are thought to share similar overall structure due to the presence of multiple highly conserved cysteine residues.[15,16] The integrin most closely related to αIIbβ3 is the receptor for vitronectin, αvβ3. This integrin uses the same β3 subunit, but forms the vitronectin receptor (VNR) by complexing with the αv subunit that shares 74 percent sequence similarity with αIIb.[15] Although there are at most 50 to 100 αvβ3 molecules per platelet,[17] there are nearly 10^5 VNR per endothelial cell,[18] and they probably play an important adhesive function in this and other cell types. The other three platelet integrins share a different common β subunit (β1), which forms a complex with either an α2, α5, or α6 chain to form receptors for collagen, fibronectin, or laminin, respectively.[19–22] Interestingly, of the three β1 integrin α-subunits that are present on platelets, only α2 is known to be naturally polymorphic in humans (see below). Of the β1 integrin α-chain subunits present on the platelet surface, α2 is unique in that it contains an inserted "I" domain of approximately 200 amino acids, which is also present in the α-chain subunits that pair with leukocyte β2 integrin subunits (LFA-1, p150,95, and MAC-1). High-resolution crystal structures of isolated I domains have established this motif as part of a unique metal coordination site designated the metal ion-dependent adhesion site or MIDAS domain.[23] Interestingly, this motif has also been identified in integrin β-chain subunits and has been predicted to play a direct role in ligand binding function.[24–26]

Diseases Associated with the αIIbβ3 Complex

The αIIbβ3 receptor is one of the most abundant receptors on the platelet surface, representing nearly 15 percent of total surface protein. This receptor is a key component in the pathway to platelet aggregation and consequently has become a target for therapeutic intervention.[27] Platelet aggregation and fibrin formation are essential for the maintenance of normal hemostasis, but these processes can also be triggered by pathogenic events such as the rupture of an atherosclerotic plaque. A paradigm of antiplatelet therapy is found in the inherited bleeding disorder Glanzmann thrombasthenia. A key feature of this disease is that patients present with mucocutaneous bleeding and rarely demonstrate spontaneous central nervous system hemorrhage,[28] a feared complication of anticoagulant and antiplatelet therapy. All of the mutations that have been identified in patients with Glanzmann thrombasthenia result in a functional deficiency of platelet αIIbβ3 receptors,[29] and a hallmark of this disease is the absence of agonist-induced platelet aggregation. In addition to its role as the major receptor for adhesive ligands, αIIbβ3 is also highly immunogenic and is the target molecule for human auto-, allo-, and drug-dependent antibodies in immune-mediated platelet disorders. Because of its clinical significance in both immunologic, hemostatic, and thrombotic platelet disorders, αIIbβ3 is one of the most completely characterized membrane glycoproteins, and an abundant literature exists describing its biochemical, immunologic, and cell and molecular biologic properties (for reviews, see references 29 to 32).

Biology of αIIbβ3. The αIIb and β3 subunits are derived from separate mRNA transcripts,[33,34] although the genes encoding them are closely linked,[35] on chromosome 17.[36,37] The amino acid sequences of both these membrane glycoproteins have been determined in full from cloned cDNA, and a diagram of the complex is shown in Fig. 177-3. αIIb is ~145 kDa in size and

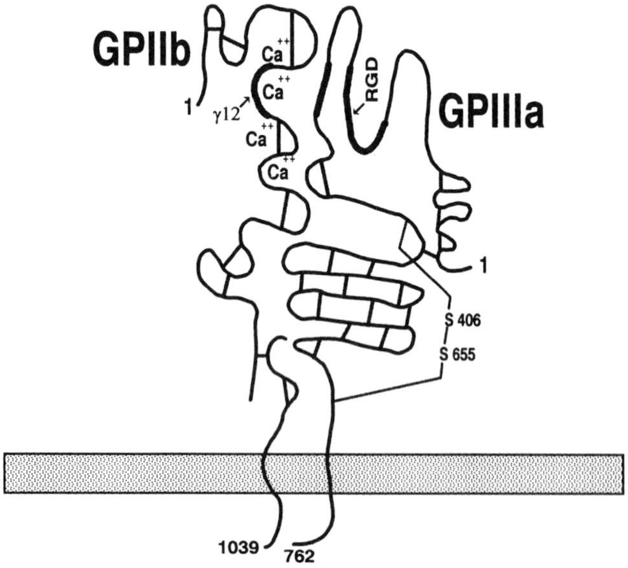

Fig. 177-3 Representation of the major platelet integrin receptor αIIbβ3. The major features of β3 include the presence of five cysteine-rich regions, including one at the N-terminus, and four cysteine-rich repeats positioned closed to the membrane. Two long-range disulfide bonds (5 to 435, and 406 to 655) are depicted, as well as putative sites of interaction with fibrinogen (stippled areas). The four calcium-binding domains of αIIb are shown, as well as the site on this integrin α-subunit that was shown biochemically to bind the γ chain of fibrinogen (H12).

contains 18 cysteine residues arranged in 9 disulfide bonds that are rather evenly spaced throughout its length.[37] Like most other integrin α chains, αIIb contains four calcium-binding domains, similar in sequence to those found in calcium-binding proteins such as troponin C, tropomyosin, and calmodulin.[37] Marguerie and coworkers have shown that all four sites must be occupied by divalent cations for proper functioning,[38] and several groups have demonstrated that the ability of αIIb to associate with β3 depends on the continuous presence of at least micromolar levels of calcium.[39–41] The four calcium-binding sites are located within the amino-terminal 450 amino acids of αIIb that have been identified as the minimal sequence required for ligand-binding.[42] This region in all α-subunits contains seven homologous repeats that are comprised predominantly of β-strands[43] predicted to fold into a β-propeller structure[44] (Fig. 177-4). The β-propeller is highly conserved and contains seven repeats of β-sheets that are arranged similar to propeller blades around a central axis.[44] Ligand binding has been proposed to occur on the face opposite the cation-binding sites that lie on the bottom of the structure.[44] The biologic importance of the β-propeller domain of αIIb is illustrated below by examination of specific mutations that lead to dysfunctional platelet aggregation responses.

Similar to other integrin β chains, β3 is ~90 kDa, and contains 762 amino acid residues in its mature form.[45–47] β3 contains five cysteine-rich regions — one at the N-terminus and four located proximal to the transmembrane domain.[46] β3 contains 56 cysteine residues in locations that are highly conserved in other human integrin β subunits. Each cysteine is involved in the formation of a disulfide bond that stabilizes the overall structure of the mature glycoprotein. Another distinguishing feature of β3 and other integrin β subunits is the presence of a large disulfide-bonded loop that extends from amino acids Cys^5 to Cys^{435}.[48] At least one critical fibrinogen-binding functional domain of β3 has been localized within this loop[49] (see below). Treatment of intact platelets with the proteolytic enzyme chymotrypsin results in cleavage of β3 at residues 121 and 348,[50] effectively removing half the loop and leaving a nonfunctional 66-kDa fragment associated with the plasma membrane. The 66-kDa remnant is composed of two disulfide-linked chains — an N-terminal 17-kDa chain containing amino acids 1 to 120 and a larger fragment extending from residues 349 to 762. Immunochemical analyses of such proteolytic fragments have been useful in determining the antigenic epitopes that form the targets of alloimmune antibodies.

To understand the molecular nature of inherited disorders associated with αIIb and β3, it is necessary first to understand the mechanism by which these two glycoproteins are synthesized, associate in a complex, and are transported through the intercellular organelles of the megakaryocyte to reach the cell surface. The biosynthetic pathway for the formation of the αIIbβ3 complex is illustrated in Fig. 177-5. As shown, both αIIb and β3 are synthesized in the RER as single-chain precursors that associate to form a pre-αIIbβ3 complex. Both proteins are cotranslationally modified with high-mannose carbohydrate moieties that represent ~15 percent of each subunit's molecular mass.[51–53] Following subunit association, pre-αIIbβ3 moves to the Golgi apparatus, where the pre-αIIb (1039 amino acids in length) is cleaved at amino acid 859 into a heavy and a light chain[54] that remain linked by a disulfide bridge formed by residues Cys^{826} to Cys^{880}. The high-mannose carbohydrate residues of αIIb, but not β3, are converted to complex sugars, as indicated by a change in the susceptibility of αIIb to endoglycosidase H. There is evidence from endoglycosidase studies that *O*-linked sugars may be added to the protein backbone of αIIb as well.[53] Following posttranslational processing, the mature αIIbβ3 complex is rapidly transported to the cell surface, where it is maintained in a resting conformation.

There are $\sim 8 \times 10^4$ αIIbβ3 receptors per platelet.[14,56] Although >70 percent of these receptors are present on the platelet surface,[14,57,58] the complex exists in a resting, nonadhesive state, and does not normally interact with its ligand fibrinogen,

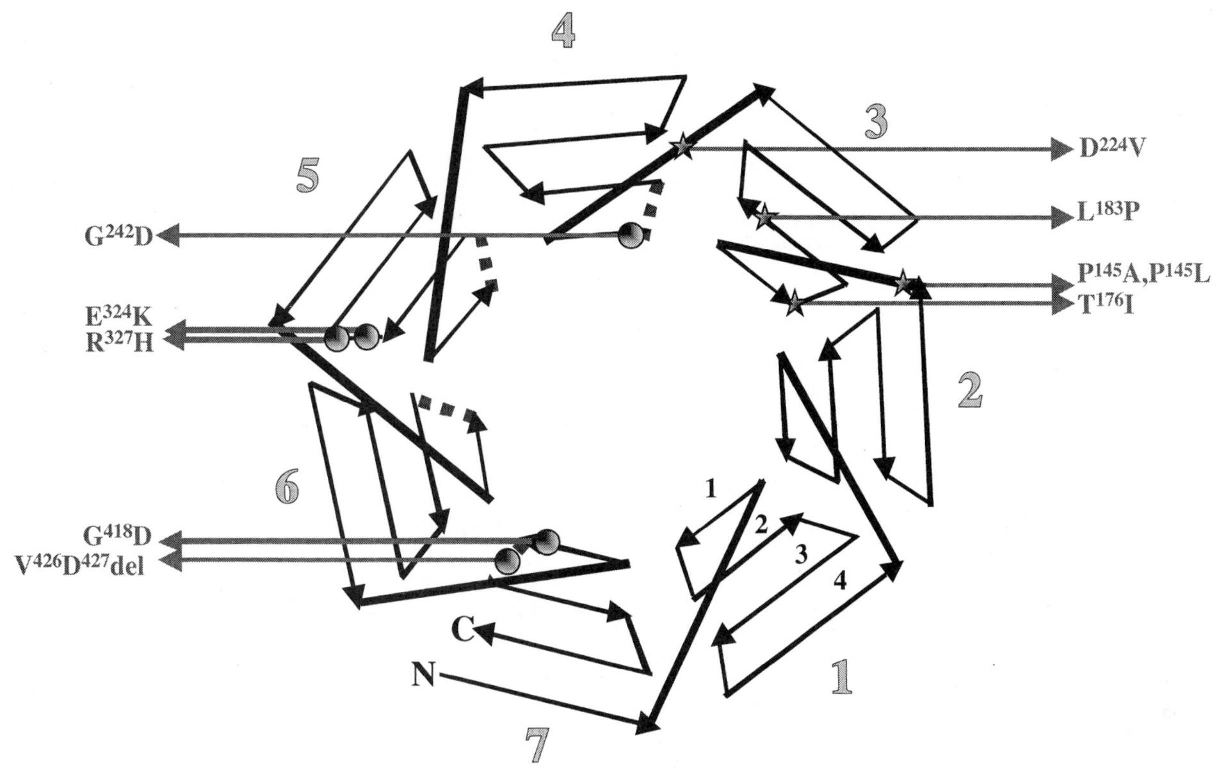

Fig. 177-4 **β-Propeller model of the N-terminus of αIIb. This representation of the β-propeller model of the N-terminus of αIIb depicts the known thrombasthenic mutations in this region of αIIb. The N- and C-termini of this region are shown, as are the seven propeller blades, each of which has four β-strands (depicted as arrows) and which are numbered 1 to 4 for the first propeller only. Those mutations that decrease surface expression and interfere with ligand binding are shown as stars, while the mutations that prevent intracellular processing of the αIIbβ3 receptor with no surface expression of the receptor are shown as circles.**

despite being bathed in 3 to 4 mg/ml concentrations of this abundant plasma protein. If, however, the platelet becomes activated by thrombin, ADP, thromboxane A2, or some other agonist, an inside-out signaling event takes place (for review see reference 59) that results in the conversion of the complex into an active receptor that can bind ligand, resulting in platelet aggregation. Following ligand binding, "outside-in" signal transduction mechanisms[59] mediate integrin-cytoskeleton interactions and receptor clustering. These are requirements for post-ligand occupancy events such as cell spreading and formation of focal adhesion sites (for review see reference 60).

Ligands for many integrins contain the tripeptide sequence Arg-Gly-Asp (RGD).[61] Thus, fibrinogen, fibronectin, VWF, and collagen contain one or more RGD sequences.[61–64] Fibrinogen, which is an elongated, cigar-shaped, six-chain molecule composed of two Aα, two Bβ, and two γ chains held together in symmetrical fashion by a centrally located disulfide-dependent knot, contains four such RGD sequences, two on each Aα chain. On conversion of αIIbβ3 into the active state, one fibrinogen Aα chain binds,[65] presumably through the RGD, at residues 572 to 575.[66] Due to its symmetric nature, the other fibrinogen Aα chain is free to interact with an αIIbβ3 on a nearby platelet, thus serving to bridge the two cells and mediate platelet-platelet cohesion (see Fig. 177-2). Synthetic RGD peptides block fibrinogen binding and platelet aggregation,[62,67,68] and photoaffinity-labeled RGD peptides interact directly with residues 109 to 171 of the β3 subunit.[49] Another region on β3 also contributes to the interaction with fibrinogen, as a small linear synthetic peptide corresponding to amino acids 211 to 222 blocks fibrinogen binding to platelets and the subsequent platelet aggregation response.[69] These findings are supported by mutations in patients with Glanzmann thrombasthenia (see below) and by mutagenesis studies,[70–72] and define molecularly one mechanism of receptor-ligand interaction within the β3 MIDAS domain.[25,26,42]

The binding of fibrinogen to αIIbβ3 on the platelet surface, however, seems to be multivalent,[65] as fibrinogen is also known to interact with its receptor via a dodecapeptide sequence (labeled γ12 in Fig. 177-3) located at residues 400 to 411 in a KGD recognition motif of the γ chain.[73–76] As defined biochemically, the γ12 binds to amino acids 296 to 313 of the αIIb subunit, located

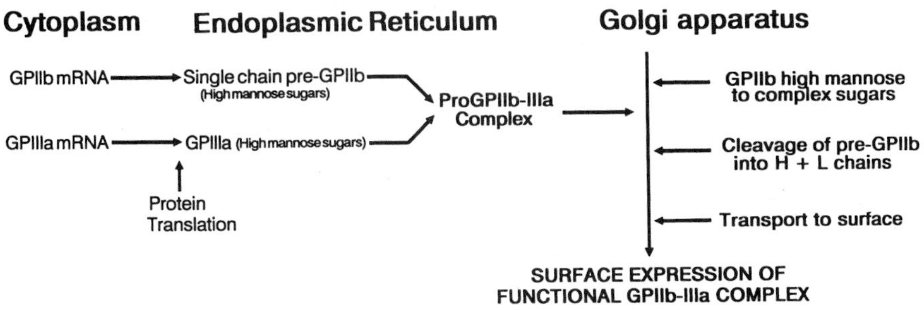

Fig. 177-5 **Flow chart of the biosynthetic pathway of the αIIbβ3 complex. Each subunit is translated from separate mRNA transcripts into single-chain precursors within the ER of the megakaryocyte, and assembled into a pre-αIIbβ3 complex before transport to the Golgi. Modification of αIIb carbohydrate chains and cleavage of αIIb into heavy and light chains takes place before eventual transport of the now mature complex to the cell surface.**

Table 177-3 Sites of Interaction between αIIbβ3 and Fibrinogen

Region of the αIIbβ complex	Region on fibrinogen
β3 109–171	Aα Chain RGD residues 572 to 575
β3 211–222	Unknown
αIIb 296–313	γ-Chain residues 400 to 411

in the fifth blade of the β-propeller model (Fig. 177-4).[77,78] Due to the absence of a crystal structure of the αIIbβ3 receptor complex, precise information concerning the sites within integrin receptors that recognize ligands is not available, but the three putative regions on αIIbβ3 that interact with fibrinogen, as well as the corresponding site on the fibrinogen molecule, are summarized in Table 177-3.

Molecular Genetic Characterization of Platelet-Specific Defects

PCR technology[79] combined with the discovery that human platelets contain enough RNA to generate cDNA fragments by reverse transcriptase (RT)-PCR[80] revolutionized the field of platelet molecular biology. The αIIb and β3 Glanzmann thrombasthenia mutations are now routinely determined by sequence analysis of genomic DNA and platelet RNA using specific oligonucleotide primers and PCR.[81] Briefly, the methodologies used include RT-PCR of platelet RNA, PCR of genomic DNA, and single-stranded conformational polymorphism (SSCP) analysis of PCR fragments containing intron and exon boundaries. PCR fragments are sequenced either directly, which provides the advantage of immediately determining homozygosity versus heterozygosity of the mutation, or from a cloned product. The mutations that affect RNA splicing are usually identified by sequence analysis of the patients' genomic DNA followed by analysis of the patients' platelet RNA. Using these methodologies, the molecular genetic defects responsible for the diseases Glanzmann thrombasthenia, Bernard-Soulier syndrome, von Willebrand disease, and the alloimmune thrombocytopenias have been identified, and our ability to diagnose these disorders, both prenatally and postnatally, is a reality. Much of the remainder of this chapter describes our current understanding of the molecular biologic basis of inherited platelet defects, and describes lessons learned from these findings.

Glanzmann Thrombasthenia

In 1918, Glanzmann, a Swiss pediatrician, described a somewhat heterogeneous group of disorders that he termed "thrombasthenie" ("weak platelets"), that were characterized by normal platelet counts but abnormal clot retraction.[82] Braunsteiner and Pakesch added to our understanding of what is now termed Glanzmann thrombasthenia (GT) by noting, in 1956, that platelets from these patients failed to spread onto a surface,[83] while the laboratories of Hardisty[84] and Zucker[85] first described the failure of thrombasthenic platelets to stick to each other (aggregate). Glanzmann thrombasthenia is known to be a rare, inherited, autosomal recessive bleeding disorder, the hallmark of which is the failure of platelets to bind fibrinogen and aggregate following stimulation by physiological agonists such as ADP, thrombin, epinephrine, or collagen. In all patients with this disorder described to date, the underlying defect is an abnormality of the genes encoding either αIIb or β3, although it is theoretically possible that molecules involved in transmitting the signal to or from the αIIbβ3 receptor could also be affected.

Clinical Features. GT is a lifelong disease characterized by repeat mucocutaneous bleeding beginning at an early age. Thus, epistaxis, gingival bleeding, and purpura or petechiae at sites of minor trauma are the most common features. Menorrhagia is a critical problem in teenage girls and younger women, when heavy bleeding during menstruation may need medical intervention.[28] Bleeding that normally accompanies pregnancy, surgical procedures, tooth extractions, or physical trauma can be excessive in GT patients, although the severity of hemorrhage is not predictable, even in defined subtypes of the disease (see below). Severe unprovoked intracranial or gastrointestinal hemorrhages occur and account for a significant portion of the observed mortality in 5 to 10 percent of the patients. In addition, some patients experience joint bleeding or visceral hematomas more characteristic of coagulation protein disorders (the hemophilias).[28] Treatment is limited to local measures although platelet transfusions may be useful until resistance to platelet infusions develop. Recent evidence suggests that recombinant activated Factor VII may be a useful addition in such a circumstance.[86] An animal model for Glanzmann thrombasthenia was created by knocking out the β3 gene.[87] The platelets from these animals do not express surface β3 as determined by flow cytometry and immunoblot of whole platelet lysates. Due to the absence of β3, αIIb is degraded and undetectable by immunoblot. Platelet aggregation in response to ADP is absent, but shape change is present. Platelet fibrinogen is markedly decreased. The mice have greatly prolonged bleeding times and suffer various degrees of anemia. Tests for occult blood show that more than 60 percent of null animals have blood in their stools. The mice are viable and fertile and some animals do die, either preweaning or later. Necropsies reveal a variety of abnormalities, including ulcerative dermatitis, enlarged spleens, and blood in the gastrointestinal tract.

Incidence. Like many other rare disorders, GT is found at an unusually high incidence among certain isolated population clusters and/or those in which consanguinity is commonplace. Thus, in spite of its infrequent occurrence worldwide, a high carrier rate for thrombasthenia exists among Iraqi Jews,[88–90] selected Arab populations,[89–91] French gypsies,[92–94] and individuals from southern India.[95] Carriers or obligate heterozygotes of this disease have ~50 percent the normal number of αIIbβ3 receptors and these individuals do not have abnormalities of platelet function or clinically significant bleeding.[28,90] The occurrence of abnormal αIIb and β3 genes in the human gene pool is low, but to date, ~40% of the patients with identified mutations are compound heterozygotes. Due to the autosomal recessive nature of this disorder, all of the identified homozygous mutations result from consanguinity (except one due to uniparental disomy[96]) and a putative founder effect has been described for two of the mutant genes identified in the Iraqi-Jewish population in Israel.[97]

Classification and Laboratory Diagnosis. Despite several attempts to categorize Glanzmann thrombasthenia into subtypes, it will become apparent from the studies discussed below that there are almost as many molecular biologic etiologies of thrombasthenia as there are patient populations. In 1972, Caen proposed the first classification of this disease based on platelet intracellular fibrinogen content and the ability of platelets to retract a fibrin clot.[98] Type I patients, representing 80 percent of those studied, lacked platelet fibrinogen and had absent clot retraction, whereas type II thrombasthenic platelets contained appreciable levels of platelet fibrinogen and maintained some clot retraction capability. Soon thereafter, the technique of SDS-PAGE became widespread, and Nurden and Caen used this method to detect an abnormal "glycoprotein II" pattern in three cases of GT.[99,100] Phillips and Agin used two-dimensional SDS-PAGE analysis of radiolabeled platelets to show convincingly that both αIIb and β3 were specifically decreased in GT versus normal platelets.[101] Several laboratories made the observation that whereas type I patients lacked detectable levels of αIIbβ3, type II GT platelets expressed moderate (15 to 25 percent) levels of this glycoprotein, as measured using immunochemical[102–104] and electrophoretic[105]

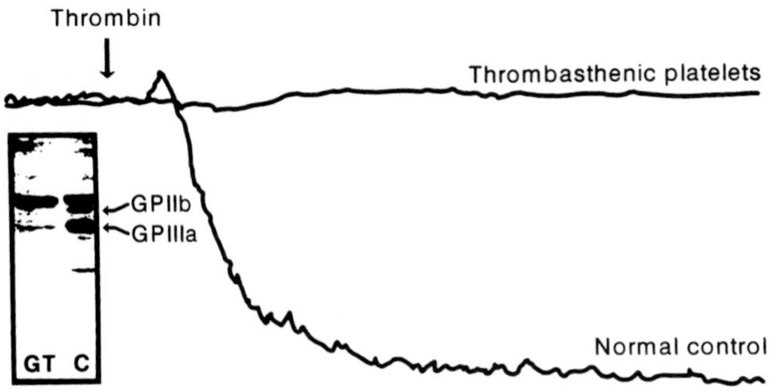

Fig. 177-6 Typical platelet aggregation profiles of normal versus GT individuals. Whereas normal platelets aggregate readily when exposed to thrombin or other agonists, platelets from a patient with thrombasthenia fail to respond. *Inset*: Immunoblot of detergent lysates from normal control (C) and GT platelets. Rabbit polyclonal antibodies specific for αIIb, β3, and PECAM-1 (top band) were exposed to Immobilon strips containing 100 mg each of a platelet lysate, and developed with an alkaline phosphatase-conjugated second antibody. Platelets from the GT patient shown express less than 5 percent of normal β3 levels, and no αIIb can be detected, typical of an αIIb genetic defect.

techniques. Adding to the complexity of this classification was the identification of variant forms of thrombasthenia which are characterized by normal to near-normal levels of a dysfunctional form of αIIbβ3 present on the cell surface.[106–109] It is important to note that platelets from these patients are functionally indistinguishable from type I and II platelets in that laboratory diagnosis for all three GT subgroups have in common the complete failure to aggregate in response to physiological agonists such as ADP, thrombin, or epinephrine, as illustrated in Fig. 177-6. The functional deficiency of platelet surface αIIbβ3 receptors and the failure to bind fibrinogen,[110] VWF,[111] and other adhesive ligands is the reason for the inability of platelets to cohere.

As the genetic defects underlying the thrombasthenic phenotype have become defined, the rationale for maintaining these three traditional categories of GT becomes less convincing. Alternatively, more complicated classifications based on surface expression or on the fate of αIIb and β3 subunits as they traffic through the cell to reach the plasma membrane[112] have been proposed. None of these are entirely satisfying, as biologic exceptions to each appear as readily as classification schemes are devised. Furthermore, no correlation exists between any of the proposed subtypes of GT and the severity of bleeding symptoms in patients.[28] Some patients with absolutely no αIIbβ3 have relatively mild clinical symptoms, while others with a full complement of αIIbβ3, albeit dysfunctional, can have frequent bleeding episodes requiring multiple platelet transfusions. Nonetheless, even in the absence of predictive value, it remains instructive for both clinical diagnosis and research purposes to determine the level of αIIbβ3 complex surface expression in GT patients.

Currently, the most common method used for determining the levels of αIIbβ3 on thrombasthenic platelets involves flow cytometry,[113] radiolabeled monoclonal antibody binding,[56,115,116] and western blot (immunoblot) analysis,[114] each of which offers the advantage of increased sensitivity over the previously used crossed immunoelectrophoretic technique.[92,93] An immunoblot illustrating αIIbβ3 content of both a normal control and a GT patient platelet lysate is shown in the inset to Fig. 177-6, and demonstrates the severe deficiency of αIIbβ3 in this patient. In patients with <5 percent of the normal αIIbβ3 content, a trace of even one of the two integrin subunits can be instructive as to the nature of the molecular defect.[117] In the example shown, a trace amount of β3 is apparent, while there is no detectable αIIb. This patient was later found to have a large deletion in the αIIb gene (see below), consistent with the immunoblot analysis. Because it is known that β3 does not survive intracellular trafficking in the absence of an integrin α-chain subunit, it is presumed that a small number of β3 molecules expressed on the platelet surface were "rescued" by their ability to form a complex with the VNR αv subunit (see "Biology of αIIbβ3" above). Analysis of surface expression of αvβ3 on either patient platelets[118] or lymphocytes[119] is a reliable indicator of αIIb and β3 defects. The decreased or undetectable binding of both αIIbβ3 and αvβ3-specific monoclonal antibodies indicates a defect in β3, whereas decreased or undetectable binding of αIIbβ3-specific, but not αvβ3-specific monoclonal antibody, indicates a defect in αIIb. This analysis has been utilized to identify defective αIIb or β3 subunits in numerous patients with GT and subsequent identification of the mutation in either gene has confirmed the reliability and usefulness of this assay.[120–124]

Molecular Abnormalities of αIIb and β3 Genes Resulting in Glanzmann Thrombasthenia. Nearly 200 individuals with GT have been described in the literature. More than 61 of these have been solved at the molecular level. As in most genetic disorders, the molecular abnormalities have been found to range from major deletions and inversions to single-point mutations identified by nucleotide sequence analysis of genomic DNA or platelet mRNA-derived PCR products (for review see reference 125). Forty-five of these mutations are in αIIb gene and 30 are in β3. In vitro studies indicate that production of both protein subunits is required for proper surface expression and function,[125] and this concept has been nicely corroborated at the level of human biology through the molecular biologic analysis of GT defects. The mutations that have been identified in the αIIb and β3 genes result in qualitative and/or quantitative abnormalities of the platelet membrane proteins[28–30,125] and the molecular characterization of GT in patients and their families has permitted DNA-based carrier detection and prenatal diagnoses to be performed.[126,127] A worldwide interactive Internet database (http://med.mssm.edu/glanzmanndb) that includes all reported clinical, biochemical, and molecular information on patients with GT has been created from a published database[125] in which the GT mutations are identified by amino acid number beginning with methionine of the ATG start codons and by nucleotide number beginning with the A of the ATG start codons in the reported cDNA sequences of αIIb[37] and β3.[46]

Of the propositi kindreds with affected individuals described in the literature, ~40% were identified as compound heterozygotes and ~60% as homozygotes, in which one of the latter may have arisen from a rare uniparental disomy event.[96] With an increasing number of mutations identified and characterized at the molecular level, the Glanzmann thrombasthenia subtypes can be categorized according to the biochemical consequences of their molecular genetic abnormality (Table 177-4). The αIIb and β3 mutations can be divided into two broad subsets of those that affect biosynthesis and those that affect function of the receptor complex, with some mutations resulting in both quantitative and qualitative defects.[124,127,128] Mutations that result in biosynthetic defects of the receptor can be further divided into those that affect (a) RNA transcription, (b) subunit assembly or stability, and (c) complex maturation. A number of patients with point mutations or small deletions in αIIb or β3 genes leading to defects in the maturation of complex will be described below. Depending on the location of the mutation, the blockade can take place at the level of subunit association in the ER (complex formation), sorting to the Golgi apparatus, or trafficking to the cell surface (Fig. 177-5). Examples for each have been found, and each is characterized by absent to reduced levels of αIIbβ3 on the cell surface, although significant intracellular pools of the affected subunit can be recovered in transfection/immunoprecipitation studies of recombinant forms of the mutated subunit. Mutations that result in functional defects of the receptor complex can be further divided into those that affect (a) stability of the receptor complex and (b) the ability of the receptor complex to be activated.

Table 177-4 Classification of Glanzmann Thrombasthenia Subtypes by Biochemical Consequence of the Molecular Genetic Abnormality

Defect (examples)	Characteristics	mRNA	Subunit synthesis	Surface expressions
Transcriptional				
(KW, GT3*)	Major gene deletions, insertions, or rearrangements	−/+	—	—
Subunit stability				
(I-J, Arab)	Small deletions or insertions leading to a change in the number of amino acids, or substitution to a destabilizing amino acid. Binding of GPIIb-IIIa complex-specific antibodies and at least one subunit-specific antibody, even to intracellular pools are absent.	+	Absent to reduced	—
Complex maturation				
(LM, FLD, KJ, SH)	Point mutations affecting Ca^{2+}-binding, subunit association, etc. that affect intracellular trafficking and surface expression. Binding of complex-specific antibodies is often affected, though subunit-specific antibodies bind to intracellular forms.	+	Near normal	Absent to reduced
Ligand binding				
A. Complex stability (CAM, ET, Stras I) B. Activatability (Paris I)	Normal to somewhat reduced levels of GPIIb-IIIa complex on the platelet surface. Often easily dissociable with EDTA. Binding of many subunit- and complex-specific antibodies is normal.	+	Normal to mildly reduced	Normal to mildly reduced

*For references see http://med.mssm.edu/glanzmanndb

Patients with mutations resulting in defects affecting complex maturation, complex stability, ligand binding, and activation of the receptor complex are described below. These mutations are located within the α-chain β-propeller domain, the MIDAS domain of β3, and the cytoplasmic domain of β3 (Table 177-5). To view all of the mutations as well as clinical and biochemical information on the reported patients with Glanzmann thrombasthenia, the reader is referred to the Internet database (http://med.mssm.edu/glanzmanndb).

Mutations Within the α-Chain β-Propeller Domain. Different groups of Glanzmann thrombasthenia mutations located within the α-chain β-propeller are beginning to emerge. One group of mutations is located within and surrounding the calcium-binding domains, and another group is located within the vicinity of the third blade of the β-propeller structure. The mutations that are located within and surrounding the calcium-binding domains affect transport of the receptor complex to the cell surface. Six missense mutations and one in-frame deletion mutation in nine kindreds have been identified and their locations within the β-propeller model are shown in Fig. 177-4. These mutations include a $G^{242}D$ substitution (patient FLD)[122] that precedes the first calcium-binding domain, an $F^{289}S$ substitution (Japanese-1) that precedes the second calcium-binding domain, an $E^{324}K$ (patients FL, Swiss, and Japanese-2)[129,130] substitution located between the second and third calcium-binding domains, an $R^{327}H$ (patients KJ and Mila-1)[131,132] substitution also located between the second and third calcium-binding domains, a $G^{418}D$ (patient LM)[133] substitution that precedes the fourth calcium-binding domain, and a $V^{425}D^{426}$ (patient LeM)[134] deletion at the beginning of the fourth calcium-binding domain. In patients FLD, LM, and LeM, the mutations lead to improperly folded pre-αIIb subunits that are stable but unable to assemble with β3 properly. In the cases of LM and LeM, the abnormal complexes accumulate within the ER. Thus, these patients' platelets do not express αIIbβ3 on their surface, as illustrated in the representative flow cytometric profile of patient LM shown in Fig. 177-7. The defects in patients KJ and Mila-1 differ somewhat from the others in that moderate amounts of their abnormal αIIbβ3 complex reach the cell surface (see Fig. 177-7). This group of GT patients can best be categorized as having maturational defects in the αIIbβ3 complex, as suggested by the decreased to absent levels that reach the cell surface, and by the inability of the residual surface receptor to bind fibrinogen or fibrinogen mimetics. Failure of complex, but not subunit-specific, monoclonal antibodies to bind to residual pools of abnormal subunits that accumulate intracellularly may also be a common feature.

Another group of mutations has been localized to the vicinity of the third blade (W3) of the β-propeller. These mutations are located close to a predicted β-turn structure that has been implicated in ligand-binding of αIIbβ3 and other integrin receptors.[135,136] Four missense mutations and one in-frame insertion mutation in five kindreds have been identified and their locations within the β-propeller model are shown in Fig. 177-4. These mutations include an RTins (patient KO) located in the connecting strand between W2 β-strand 4 and W3 β-strand 1, a $T^{176}I$ (Frankfurt I)[137] located in the connecting strand between W3 β-strands 1 and 2, an $L^{183}P$ (patient LW)[124] located at the end of the second β-strand in W3 near the 2-3 connecting strand, and a $P^{145}A$ (Mennonite and JF) and a $P^{145}L$ (Chinese-14)[128] located within the 4-1 connecting strand between the second and third blades of the propeller. The $L^{183}P$ and $P^{145}A$ mutations both result in quantitative and qualitative defects of the receptor complex. The RTins mutation results in a quantitatively normal surface expressed receptor that is qualitatively defective. Independent support for the functional importance of this region has been shown by the $D^{224}V$ mutation,[138] located within the 4-1 connecting strand between the third and fourth blades of the propeller. This mutation was identified from in vitro generated mutant αIIbβ3 receptors expressed in CHO cells[72] and disrupts ligand-binding function of the receptor.

Mutations Within the β3 MIDAS Domain. This group of thrombasthenic defects is characterized by significant levels of αIIbβ3 surface expression, although the complex is not able to interact with its natural ligands. In contrast to the platelets of

Table 177-5 Glanzmann Thrombasthenia Mutations*

Mutations within the αIIb β-Propeller Domain

Patient	Genotype	Mutation†	Mutation phenotype	Amino acid substitution‡	Biochemical defect
FLD	Homozygote	818G → A	Missense	$G^{242}D$	Complex maturation
Japanese-1	Compound	959T → C	Missense	$F^{289}S$	Subunit assembly
	heterozygote	unknown	Unknown	Unknown	or complex maturation?
FL	Homozygote	1063G → A	Missense	$E^{324}K$	Subunit assembly?
Swiss	Compound	1063G → A	Missense	$E^{324}K$	Subunit assembly?
	heterozygote	1787T → C	Missense	$I^{565}T$	
Japanese-2	Compound	1063G → A	Missense	$E^{324}K$	Subunit assembly?
	heterozygote	Unknown	Unknown	Unknown	
KJ	Homozygote	1073G → A	Missense	$R^{327}H$	Complex maturation ligand binding?
Mila-1	Homozygote	1073G → A	Missense	$R^{327}H$	Complex maturation ligand binding?
LM	Homozygote	1346G → A	Missense	$G^{418}D$	Complex maturation
LeM	Compound	1366-1371del	Del: In frame	$V^{425}D^{426}del$	Complex maturation
	heterozygote	Unknown	Unknown	Unknown	
Frankfurt I	Homozygote	620C → T	Missense	$T^{176}I$	Complex maturation ligand binding
LW	Homozygote	641T → C	Missense	$L^{183}P$	Complex maturation ligand binding
Mennonite	Homozygote	526C → G	Missense	$P^{145}A$	Complex maturation ligand binding
JF	Compound	526C → G	Missense	$P^{145}A$	Complex maturation
	heterozygote	2929C → T	Nonsense	$R^{946}X$	Premature termination
Chinese-14	Compound	527C → T	Missense	$P^{145}L$	Complex maturation ligand binding?
	heterozygote	IVS15(−1)Gdel	Unknown	Unknown	

Mutations within the β3 MIDAS Domain

Patient	Genotype	Mutation†	Mutation phenotype	Amino acid substitution‡	Biochemical defect
Cam	Homozygote	433G → T	Missense	$D^{119}Y$	Ligand binding
NR	Homozygote	433G → A	Missense	$D^{119}N$	Ligand binding
Strasbourg I	Homozygote	718C → T	Missense	$R^{214}W$	Ligand binding complex stability
CM	Homozygote	718C → T	Missense	$R^{214}W$	Ligand binding complex stability
ET	Homozygote	719G → A	Missense	$R^{214}Q$	Ligand binding complex stability
SH	Homozygote	725G → A	Missense	$R^{216}Q$	Complex maturation ligand binding
MK	Homozygote	428T → G	Missense	$L^{177}W$	Complex maturation
BL	Homozygote	563C → T	Missense	$S^{162}L$	Ligand binding complex stability
LD	Compound	847delGC	Del: Out of	Premature	Ligand binding complex stability
	heterozygote	863T → C	frame missense	termination $L^{262}P$	

Mutations within the β3 Cytoplasmic Domain

Patient	Genotype	Mutation†	Mutation phenotype	Amino acid substitution‡	Biochemical defect
RM	Compound	1791delT	Del: Out of	Premature	Receptor activation inside-out signaling
	heterozygote	2248C → T	frame missense	termination $R^{724}X$	
Paris I	Compound	2332T → C	Missense	$S^{752}P$	Receptor activation
	heterozygote	Unknown	Unknown	No transcript	

*For references see reference 125 and http://med.mssm.edu/glanzmanndb
†Nomenclature is based on recommendations by Beaudet et al. *Hum Mutat* 8:197–202, 1996; *ibid.* 203–206. The cDNA nucleotide numbering begins with the A nucleotide of the ATG start codon as +1.[49] Nucleotide substitutions: cDNA nucleotide number followed by nucleotide → nucleotide substitution. Abbreviations: del-deletion, ins-insertion, inv-inversion, IVS-intervening sequence.
‡Amino acid numbering begins with methionine of the ATG start codon[49] and the amino acid codon number excluding the leader sequence is in parentheses. Amino acid substitutions are designated by amino acid-codon number-amino acid. Single letter amino acid code: C = cysteine, D = aspartate, E = glutamate, K = lysine, L = leucine, M = methionine, N = asparagine, P = proline, Q = glutamine, R = arginine, S = serine, V = valine, W = tryptophan, Y = tyrosine, X = nonsense mutation.

patients having integrin maturational defects, such as those described in the previous section, the binding of many αIIbβ3 complex-specific antibodies are normal in this group, indicating that subunit association and intracellular trafficking are largely unaffected by the nature of the mutation. That the αIIbβ3 complex is not normal is indicated by the fact that divalent-cation dependent regulation of its conformation can be affected and the complex may be easily dissociable by chelation of external calcium ions with EDTA (patient Cam, $D^{119}Y$ mutation).[139] Nine missense mutations in twelve patients with Glanzmann thrombasthenia have been identified within the cation-binding sphere of the MIDAS domain (Fig. 177-8). Two mutations, the Cam variant and $D^{119}N$ (patient NR),[140] are located within the conserved DXSXS amino acid motif; three mutations, $R^{214}W$ (Strasbourg I variant and patient CM),[141,142] $R^{214}Q$ (patient ET),[70] and $R^{216}Q$ (patient SH),[143] are located within the putative coordinating sites;[43] and four mutations, $D^{117}W$ (patient MK),[144] $S^{162}L$ (patient BL),[145] $L^{262}P$ (patient LD),[146] and $H^{280}P$ (patients HJ, NT, TK) are

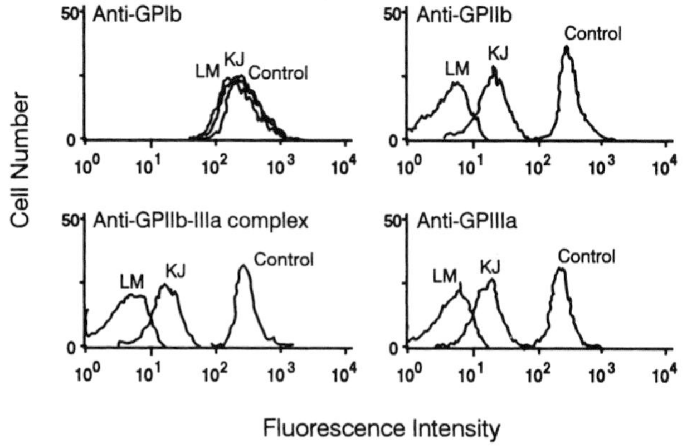

Fig. 177-7 Flow cytometric profile of two patients with GT as compared with a normal control individual. Both patients KJ and LM have mutations that affect the maturation of the αIIbβ3 complex, but differ in that the mutation in patient LM is within the calcium-binding domain of αIIb and perturbs maturation such that no part of the complex is able to traffic to the cell surface. The nature of the mutation in KJ is such that 20 to 30 percent levels of αIIbβ3 are expressed, but fail to function normally.

located within the vicinity of the MIDAS domain. The mutations at residue D^{119} result in abnormalities of platelet αIIbβ3 function, but do not affect surface expression, while the mutation at D^{117} results in the intracellular retention of misfolded receptor complexes. The mutations at residue R^{214} result in surface expressed αIIbβ3 receptors that are abnormally sensitive to dissociation by calcium chelation, the mutation at R^{216} results in surface expressed αIIbβ3 that are unreactive with complex-dependent antibodies and cannot bind ligand, the mutations at residues S^{162} and L^{262} result in surface expression levels of ~30 percent of normal, but also show sensitivity to dissociation by calcium, and the mutation at residue $H^{280}P$ results in surface expression levels of ~17% of normal but does not appear to affect the function of the receptor complex. The importance of these sites is reinforced by the identification of a group of in vitro-generated mutant αIIbβ3 receptors expressed in CHO cells.[72] The mutations $D^{119}N$, $R^{214}W$, $D^{198}N$, $E^{220}Q$, and $E^{220}K$ were identified as functional defects providing independent support for the importance of the MIDAS domain in ligand binding.

Mutations that Affect Receptor Activation. The cytoplasmic domain of β3 is important for integrin activation and regulation of ligand binding.[147–149] Two Glanzmann thrombasthenia mutations in two kindreds have been identified in this region. One is an $R^{724}X$ nonsense mutation (patient RM)[150] that deletes the C-terminal 39 residues of β3, and the other is an $S^{752}P$ missense mutation (patient P or Paris I).[147,148,151] These mutations do not affect surface expression of platelet αIIbβ3 complexes, but mutant receptors are unresponsive to agonist stimulation. Mammalian cell expression studies show normal adhesion to immobilized fibrinogen, but abnormal cell spreading. Cells expressing the $S^{752}P$ mutant receptors have reduced focal adhesion plaque formation and cells expressing the $R^{724}X$ mutant receptors have undetectable tyrosine phosphorylation of focal adhesion kinase $pp125^{FAK}$. These mutations provide compelling evidence for the role of the β3 cytoplasmic tail in the function of the αIIbβ3 receptor complex.

INHERITED DISORDERS OF THE PLATELET GPIb COMPLEX

Biology of the GPIb Complex

An initial event that occurs when circulating platelets come into contact with the arterial subendothelium at a site of injury is adhesion to VWF molecules that have themselves adhered to the subendothelial matrix.[1,152] This process is especially important in arterioles and in the microcirculation, where high shear rates are present.[1,153–155] Following this initial adhesion event, additional platelets aggregate to the site of injury, forming the platelet plug.[156–158]

Platelet membranes contain two binding sites for VWF.[159] One of these sites requires prior platelet activation, and is located on the platelet membrane αIIbβ3 complex.[159] The second binding site involves the GPIb-IX-V complex, and it is this membrane

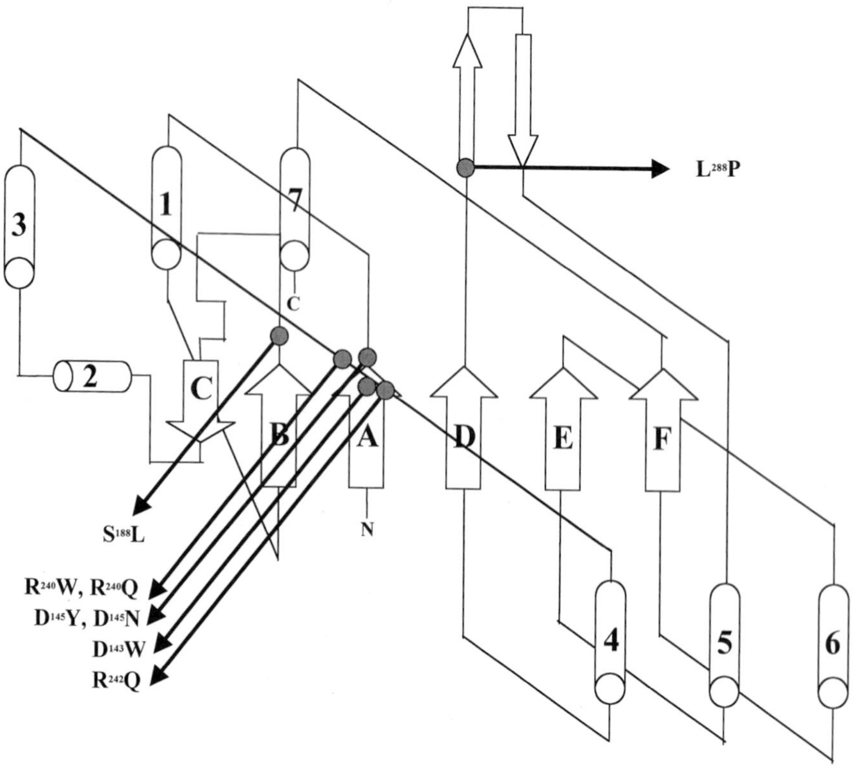

Fig. 177-8 MIDAS model of the β3. This representation of the MIDAS model of the N-terminus of β3 depicts the known thrombasthenic mutations in this region of β3. The N- and C-termini of this region are shown. Thrombasthenic mutations are shown as circles; β-sheets are depicted as arrows; and α-helical regions are depicted as cylinders.

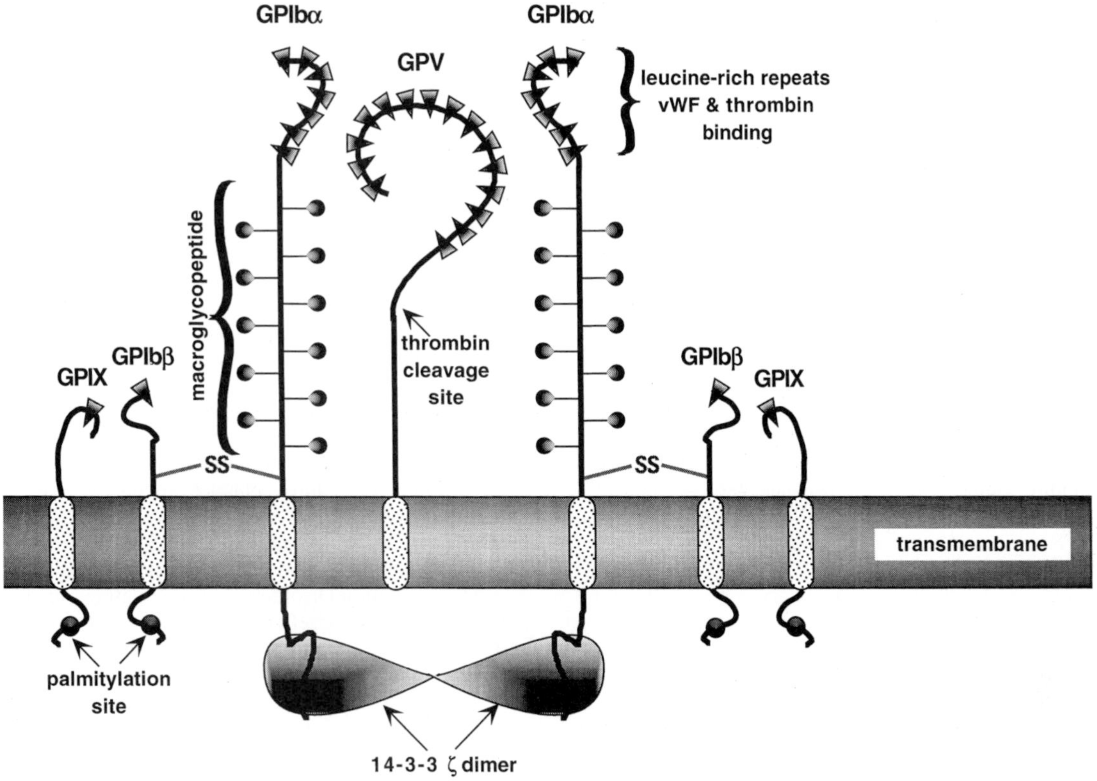

Fig. 177-9 The GPIb complex on platelets. This receptor consist of four separately encoded proteins: GPIbα, GPIbβ, GPIX, and GPV in a 2:2:2:1 stoichiometric ratio.[3,4] Some of the structural features found in this receptor complex are depicted, including the leucine-rich repeats found in each protein, the *O*-linked carbohydrate-rich region of GPIbα, the thrombin cleavage site in GPIbα, the disulfide bond linking GPIbα and GPIbβ, the thrombin- and VWF-binding domain of GPIbα, and some of the intracellular interaction sites, as well as the 14-3-3 ζ intracytoplasmic dimer.

complex that is crucial for initial attachment and proper adhesion to the extracellular matrix of a damaged vessel wall[160,161] (see Fig. 177-2). The GPIb-IX-V complex represents the second most common receptor on the platelet membrane surface, with ~25,000 copies per platelet.[162] As shown in Fig. 177-9, the GPIb complex actually consists of four different proteins. All of these proteins have an N-terminal signal peptide and a hydrophobic transmembrane domain near the C-terminus. The four proteins also share an interesting structural element known as the leucine-rich repeat, which is comprised of a 24-amino-acid motif that contains 7 conserved leucine positions. Other proteins have been described with this leucine-rich repeat, but the biologic significance of this structure is unknown, as the proteins have disparate functions such as a photoreceptor (chaoptin),[162] a hormone receptor (lutropin-choriogonadotropin receptor),[163] and adenylate cyclase.[164] In addition, these repeats have some similarity with the DNA-binding leucine-zipper proteins.[165–167] These repeats may function in binding to the VWF ligand and there is some suggestion that they are important in subunit interaction (see below).

GPIbα is the largest subunit (135 kDa, 610 amino acids) with 7 leucine repeats. It is susceptible to cleavage by trypsin or by the calcium-dependent platelet protease calpain, giving rise to a water-soluble, heavily glycosylated 135-kDa N-terminal fragment known as "glycocalicin."[168,169] In addition to containing the binding site for VWF, the glycocalicin portion of GPIbα may also contain a binding site for thrombin.[170–172] The biologic role of the thrombin-binding site is unclear, because enzymatic cleavage of the GPIb complex, while leading to a loss of VWF-mediated platelet agglutination, does not significantly affect the ability of human platelets to respond to thrombin.[173] These data may be explained by the cloning of a family of seven membrane-spanning functional thrombin receptors found on several cells of the vasculature, including the platelet surface, that are activated following proteolysis by thrombin and are now termed protease-activated receptors.[174]

In between the leucine-rich domains and the *O*-linked glycosylation sites of GPIbα is a region from amino acid residues 220 to 310 that contains the VWF and thrombin-binding regions. Studies with peptide inhibitors suggest that amino acids 269 to 301 contain two charged domains that represent the major binding site for VWF.[175,176] In vivo, plasma VWF does not bind to the GPIb complex, and it is likely that changes in VWF conformation occur once it has bound to components of the subendothelium that enable it to then interact with its platelet receptor. In vitro, the antibiotic ristocetin is used to mimic this effect, and similarly induces conformational changes in VWF that promote binding to GPIb in stirred platelet-rich plasma.[177]

All four chains of the GPIb complex are glycosylated. GPIbα has four *N*-glycosylation sites, while GPIbβ and GPIX each have a single *N*-glycosylation site. In GPIbα, *O*-linked carbohydrates are associated with a series of five 9-amino-acid repeats in a region of glycocalicin that is heavily glycosylated.[178] Thus, members of the GPIb complex contain carbohydrate moieties ending with sialic acid residues, contributing significantly to the negative charge of the platelet surface.[170] This *O*-linked sugar-rich domain is highly polymorphic with 1 to 4 repeats in various individuals.[179] Each repeat extends the N-terminal globular region out ~45 nM from the cell surface. The thrombophilic implications of this polymorphism are not clear.

GPIbα is disulfide-bonded to GPIbβ (25 kDa, 181 amino acids)[3,180] through a single cysteine residue located in each subunit near the transmembrane domains of GPIbα and GPIbβ. This peptide has only one leucine repeat. The cytoplasmic tail of GPIbβ contains a potential serine phosphorylation site that may be important in tethering the receptor to the cytoskeleton following agonist stimulation.[181]

These two proteins are, in turn, noncovalently associated with platelet GPIX and V.[4,182] GPIX is the smallest member of the GPIb complex (22 kDa, 160 amino acids) and has only one leucine repeat.[183,184] Both the cytoplasmic tails of GPIbβ and GPIX have potential palmitylation sites that may anchor the entire complex into the membrane.[185] GPV (82 kDa, 344 amino acids) is a transmembrane protein with 15 leucine repeats. This protein is susceptible to digestion by calpain, and in addition is the only known proteolytic substrate for thrombin on the platelet surface, releasing a 69-kDa soluble fragment.[2,186]

The genes encoding the subunits of the GPIb-IX-V complex are dispersed in the human genome. GPIbα is on the short arm of chromosome 17,[5] and GPIbβ is on the long arm of chromosome 22, while the genes for GPV and GPIX are all on chromosome 3, but at distinct chromosomal sites.[187] All four genes are intronless, but appear to share GATA, Ets, and Sp1 binding sites in the 5′-flanking region, like other megakaryocyte-specific genes.

Studies utilizing proteolytic fragments of VWF have localized the GPIb binding domain to VWF residues 480 to 718.[188,189] Studies of patients with type IIB von Willebrand disease (vWD), in which VWF multimers have increased affinity for nonactivated platelets, have further defined a small disulfide loop in VWF between Cys^{509} and Cys^{695} that is necessary for GPIb binding. Multiple mutations in this loop in patients with type IIB vWD have been defined at the molecular level, and each appears to be capable of increasing the affinity of VWF for the platelet surface.[189–196] It is important to distinguish the increased VWF-GPIb interactions seen in this disorder from an inherited disorder of GPIbα known as platelet-type or pseudo-vWD, which is discussed below.

Even in resting platelets, the GPIb complex is associated with the cytoskeleton. A small deletion in the cytoplasmic tail of GPIbα results in increased mobility of the complex in the platelet membrane.[197] Binding of VWF/ristocetin or VWF/collagen to the GPIb complex is itself an activating event (see Fig. 177-1), and operates through an arachidonic acid metabolite-dependent activation of phospholipase C. This signal results in the mobilization of protein kinase C, which together with increases in $(Ca^{2+})_i$ promotes platelet secretion and potentiates platelet aggregation.[198] The GPIb-IX-V complex also appears to activate the cell through the cytoskeleton protein 14-3-3ζ[199] that, in turn, binds Raf-1.[200]

Bernard-Soulier Syndrome

Bernard-Soulier syndrome (BSS) was first described in 1948 in a 5-month-old infant with a prolonged bleeding time, giant platelets on blood smear, and a sibling who had died from hemorrhage at the age of 3 years.[201] Over the following years, additional patients with the combination of mucocutaneous bleeding; enlarged platelets; normal platelet aggregation with ADP, collagen, and epinephrine with a delayed response to thrombin; and absent platelet aggregation with human VWF and ristocetin or with bovine VWF alone were described as having Bernard-Soulier syndrome (for review see reference 2). This syndrome represents the second most recognized inherited platelet disorder.

Clinical Features. The bleeding manifestations of these patients are similar to other patients with platelet dysfunctions and center on mucocutaneous bleeding with purpuric skin bleeding epistaxis, gastrointestinal hemorrhage, and menorrhagia.[2,202] Alloantibodies to components of the GPIb-IX-V complex can develop following platelet transfusions, and thereby secondary complications from their refractoriness to platelet therapy develop.[2,202–204] In addition to local forms of therapy such as proper pressure and topical thrombin, platelet transfusion therapy, and hormonal management of menses, there have been several reports that have suggested that the synthetic vasopressin homologue DDAVP (1-deamino-8-D-arginine vasopressin) may be useful in the treatment of a number of inherited bleeding disorders such as BSS.[205,206] These studies demonstrate improved bleeding times in these patients following DDAVP therapy, although the improvement did not correlate with the ability of the DDAVP to increase the levels of circulating VWF.

Incidence. BSS is an autosomal recessive disorder in which most patients have a decrease to absence of all four members of the GPIb complex — GPIbα, GPIbβ, GPIX, and GPV.[2,207] In 1969, platelets from these patients were shown to have an altered electrophoretic mobility and sialic acid content,[208] and in 1975, membrane protein fractionation of platelets by SDS-PAGE demonstrated a marked decrease in a major 155-kDa glycoprotein, then termed GPI, in these patients.[100] Since that time, further refinements in protein analysis demonstrated a variable decrease, ranging from the GPIb complex being almost fully present to being virtually absent in homozygous patients.[209]

Classification and Laboratory Diagnosis. Laboratory evaluation of BSS patients demonstrates a variable degree of thrombocytopenia. Most patients are thrombocytopenic to some degree, but some patients may have platelet counts as low as 20,000/ml.[2,210,211] The platelets tend to be increased in size, with a mean diameter ranging from 3 to 20 times normal[211] (Fig. 177-10). Other cell types appear normal. As mentioned below in "Platelet Size and Production Disorders," the circulating total platelet mass in people is more precisely conserved than is platelet count,[212] and part of the decrease in platelet count in this disease may well reflect this compensation mechanism. Megakaryocytes in this disorder appear normal in size and appearance by light microscopic examination. However, on electron microscopy, a striking feature in these cells is the variable and intermittent nature of the demarcation system, which is often vacuolar.[213] The relationship between this structural feature in the megakaryocyte and the giant platelet is not understood. It is believed that the absence of interactions between the GPIb-IX-V complex and the platelet cytoskeleton underlies both the morphologic abnormality seen in the megakaryocyte and the size of the platelets.

Bleeding times are prolonged in these patients, but the distinctive abnormality of BSS platelets is the failure of agglutination in the presence of ristocetin, an abnormality that cannot be corrected by the addition of normal plasma.[214] Aggregation by other agonists such as ADP, collagen, and epinephrine is normal, though the response to low-dose thrombin may be delayed.[211,214,215]

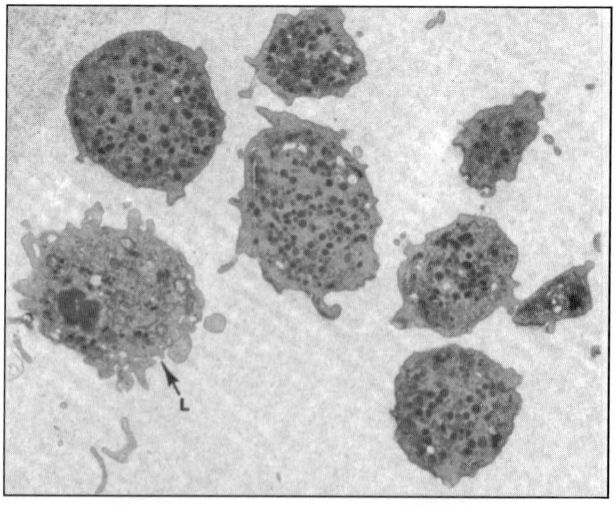

Fig. 177-10 Thin-section electron micrograph of platelets from a patient with BSS. Whereas normal platelets are 1 to 2 mm in diameter, several of the BSS platelets in this section are the same size as a lymphocyte (L) (8 to 10 mm). Aside from their increased size, the morphology of BSS platelets is comparable to that of normal platelets. Magnification: ×5000. (*Electron micrographs generously provided by Dr. James G. White, University of Minnesota.*)

Table 177-6 Summary of Molecular Abnormalities Causing Bernard-Soulier Syndrome

Patient	Molecular defect	Clinical features	Platelet count (/mm^3)	Reference
GP1bα				
1.	TGG → TGA(hetero) $W^{343}X$	Male with spontaneous epistaxis.	32,000	216
2.	GCT → GTT(homo) $A^{156}V$	Bolzano variant. Affected child died with intracranial hemorrhage.	81,000	231
3.	CTC → TTC(hetero) $L^{57}F$	Autosomal dominant. Recurrent mucosal bleeds.	80,000	219
4.	TGC → AGC(homo) $C^{209}S$	Spanish male, splenectomized secondary to thrombocytopenia.	25,000	232
5.	CTC → CCC(homo) $L^{129}P$	African-American, mucosal, menstrual hemorrhage.	75,000	233
6.	TGG → TGA(homo) $W^{498}X$	Karlstad variant. Swedish with severe recurrent mucosal bleeds.	10,000	234
7.	2 base deletion(homo) at AA^{654}	German siblings required transfusion.	66,000	235
8.	TCA → TAA(homo) $S^{444}X$	Japanese female.	24,000	236
9.	1 base deletion (homo) at AA 76	Caucasian with splenectomy and multiple transfusions.	35,000	237
10.	2 base deletion (homo) at AA 294	Japanese female with recurrent mucosal hemorrhages.	60,000	238
11.	T insertion (hetero) at 1418 A deletion (hetero) at 1438	Japanese male with recurrent mucosal hemorrhages.	25,000	238
GP1bβ:				
1.	GATA site (hetero) deletion gene deletion (hetero)	Male with velo-facial-cranial defects and with mucosal hemorrhage.	80,000	220
2.	TAC → TCC(hetero) $Y^{88}C$ GCC → CCC(hetero) $A^{108}P$	Japanese female variant with decreased bleeding in adulthood.	180,000	221
GP1X:				
1.	GAC → GGC(hetero) $D^{21}G$ AAC → AGC(hetero) $N^{45}S$	Caucasian female with recurrent mucosal hemorrhages.	???	221
2.	ACC → AGC(homo) $N^{45}S$	Caucasian male with mild mucosal hemorrhage.	60,000	222
3.	TGG → TGA $W^{126}X$	Japanese female with moderate mucosal bleeding.	75,000	239
4.	TGT → TAT $C^{73}Y$	Japanese patients with recurrent mucosal hemorrhages. One patient died from blood loss.	???	240
5.	TTT → TCT(homo) $F^{55}S$	Male with moderate mucosal hemorrhages.	50,000	241

Molecular Abnormalities. There are over 55 cases of BSS published, and 18 molecular defects have been defined.[2] In general, these disorders can be classified by whether any complex reaches the platelet membrane and by the specific subunit that is affected (Table 177-6). The first described mutation was found within the coding sequence of the GPIbα gene,[216] in which a TGG → TGA mutation resulted in the conversion of $W^{343}X$ (GPIbα; 1 in Table 177-6). The resulting GPIbα chain lacks a portion of the extracellular domain and the entire transmembrane and cytoplasmic domains, providing a likely explanation for the absence of GPIb complex expression on the platelet surface.

Several dominant variants of BSS have been defined in which surface expression of the GPIb complex is approximately 50 percent of normal.[217–219] In two cases, point mutations within the leucine-rich repeat region of GPIba were found to be associated with the defect.[211] In the Balzano variant (GPIbα; 2 in Table 177-6), an $A^{156}V$ substitution within the leucine-rich repeat domain of GPIbα was identified and was shown to be responsible for the defect in that a recombinant GPIbα protein containing this substitution, when reconstituted into an otherwise normal GPIb complex, was shown to have impaired binding to VWF, but normal thrombin binding. In an American variant (GPIbα; 3 in Table 177-6), an $L^{57}F$ mutation was found.[219] It is of interest that the American variant mutation occurs in one of the highly conserved leucine residues, whereas the Balzano mutation is positioned within a nonconserved position. Both variants have in common an abnormally small GPIbα protein, and the mutations may lead to increased susceptibility of the N-terminus of the GPIbα chain to cleavage. A monoclonal antibody AS-7, which is directed to the N-terminus of GPIbα, binds to GPIbα of normal platelets but does not bind to the faster-migrating band in the American variant.

It is clear that BSS can also be due to mutations of the GPIbβ and GPIX genes (see Table 177-6). Because these two genes and GPV have been more recently cloned than GPIbα, it is unclear what the relative importance of each is to the appearance of the BSS phenotype. There are two described GPIbβ forms of BSS. In one, the patient is heterozygous for a large deletion on one chromosome resulting in the velo-cranial-facial syndrome as well as BSS (GPIbβ; 1 in Table 177-6).[220] This patient is also of interest in that her remaining GPIbβ gene has the first demonstrated naturally occurring mutation in a GATA-binding site, providing important evidence for the role of the GATA-1 transcription factor in the regulated expression of a megakaryocyte-specific gene. The other GPIbβ mutation occurred in a Japanese patient and resulted in a mild bleeding diathesis (GPIbβ; 2 in Table 177-6).[221] The platelets were not defective to activation by either botrocetin- or ristocetin-activated VWF in vitro, nor was there a significant decrease in surface GPIb-IX-V complex. The patient had large platelets and it was proposed that the defect was in GPIbα-GPIbβ disulfide linkage and intracellular signaling.

Mutations in the gene for GPIX also occur, demonstrating that this chain is important for normal receptor expression and function. The first described defects were missense mutations in the leucine-rich repeats (GPIX 1 and 2 in Table 177-6).[222,223] Expression studies in culture demonstrated that these mutations prevented complex formation with GPIbα and GPIbβ, suggesting that the leucine-rich repeats may have a role in subunit interactions.

Platelet-Type (Pseudo-) von Willebrand Disease

Platelet-type vWD is an autosomal dominant bleeding disorder often associated with a prolonged bleeding time, mild thrombocytopenia, and decreased circulating levels of high-molecular-weight VWF multimers.[224–226] Patients with this disorder have a mild-to-moderate bleeding diathesis. Platelet-type vWD is very similar to type IIB vWD in that both are characterized by platelet agglutination in the presence of lower than normal concentrations of ristocetin, and by decreased circulating levels of high-molecular-weight VWF. Binding of VWF to the circulating platelet pool results in the reduced levels of circulating levels of VWF seen in these patients, as well as some degree of platelet activation and mild thrombocytopenia.

Unlike type IIB vWD, in which mutations in VWF result in increased affinity for normal platelet GPIb, pseudo-vWD is caused by an alteration in the platelet GPIb receptor that leads to increased affinity for normal VWF multimers. Platelet-type vWD can be distinguished from type IIB vWD by addition of normal VWF to patient platelet-rich plasma, which results in spontaneous aggregation of pseudo-vWD, but not type IIB vWD, platelets.[226,227] It is important to distinguish patients with platelet-type vWD from other vWD patients, as the standard form of therapy for vWD involves infusion of cryoprecipitate or DDAVP and can lead to severe thrombocytopenia in these patients.[227] A patient with mild thrombocytopenia and a prolonged bleeding time should be evaluated for this disorder as described above, and if it is found, treatment should be more carefully monitored.[228]

The molecular basis of platelet-type vWD has been defined in two patients.[229,230] Both mutations occur in the region of GPIbα that was previously shown to be important in VWF binding.[176] These mutations are a Gly^{233}Val and Met^{239}Val. It has been hypothesized that these mutations alter GPIbα such that it is maintained in an adhesive conformation. Further examination of mutations in this region of GPIb may provide important insights into how this receptor becomes activated on exposure to components of the extracellular matrix at sites of vascular injury.

OTHER PLATELET MEMBRANE GLYCOPROTEIN DEFECTS

The integrin $\alpha2\beta1$ (platelet GPIa-IIa) is a heterodimer complex that, like αIIb$\beta3$, is held together by noncovalent, divalent cation-dependent interactions.[242] In platelets and other cell types, $\alpha2\beta1$ serves as a receptor for collagen[20,21] and functions in mediating platelet-extracellular matrix interactions as well as cellular activation events, because adherence to fibrillar collagen causes platelets to change their shape rapidly, secrete the contents of their granules, and transform surface receptors into an adhesive phenotype (see Fig. 177-1). The physiological and clinical significance of $\alpha2\beta1$ was underscored by the discovery that human platelets from a patient with a long bleeding time, normal platelet count, and normal aggregation response to thrombin, ADP, and epinephrine fail to aggregate in response to collagen, and have a parallel absence of $\alpha2$ on the platelet surface.[243] A defect in platelet spreading on collagen-coated surfaces has also been associated with $\alpha2$ defects.[243,244]

Platelet GPIV, also known as the CD36 differentiation antigen, is an 88-kDa transmembrane glycoprotein found in a wide variety of cells types, including platelets, endothelial cells, erythrocytes, and melanoma cells.[245] GPIV is a multifunctional protein that has been implicated in mediating platelet adherence to collagen[246] and thrombospondin,[207] and also serves as a receptor on endothelial cells, monocytes, and platelets for the binding of *Plasmodium falciparum*-infected erythrocytes.[246–248] Several years ago, a population of healthy Japanese individuals, known as Naka-negative,[249] was identified, and its members were shown to lack expression of GPIV on their platelets.[250] Interestingly, platelets from these individuals displayed normal platelet function, in that thrombospondin binding and platelet aggregation in response to collagen were normal,[251] although platelet adhesion to collagen under conditions of minimal shear flow was mildly diminished.[251] Because up to 3 percent of the Japanese population do not express GPIV on the platelet surface and are, at the same time, free of any overt bleeding abnormality,[250] it would appear that the adhesive functions mediated by this major platelet membrane glycoprotein are adequately compensated for by other adhesive receptors.

ALLOIMMUNE DISORDERS

In addition to amino acid changes that disrupt function and result in bleeding diatheses, several platelet-membrane glycoproteins have naturally occurring allelic forms within the human gene pool. Although the molecular variants of these platelet-surface glycoproteins are thought to function identically, their presence has important clinical consequences not unlike those found in other cellular and organ systems, in that the polymorphisms can be and are recognized as immunologic targets in settings that include organ transplantation, blood transfusion, and pregnancy. A detailed understanding of the molecular basis of these naturally occurring variations, therefore, is crucial to our ability to design rational therapeutic and diagnostic approaches for the management of platelet immunologic disorders.

Two clinically recognized immunologic syndromes are attributable to "platelet-specific" polymorphisms. The first such syndrome, posttransfusion purpura, or PTP, is quite rare, with less than 200 cases reported to date.[252] PTP is characterized by acute, usually severe, thrombocytopenia occurring 7 to 10 days following a blood transfusion, and it is thought to be induced by platelets or platelet fragments bearing an incompatible allelic form of one or more platelet membrane glycoproteins, usually $\beta3$. Neonatal alloimmune thrombocytopenia (NAT) is the second immunologically related bleeding disorder due to platelet-antigen incompatibility and is characterized by thrombocytopenia in the neonate due to passively transmitted maternal antibody directed against a fetal platelet antigen inherited from the father and lacking on the mother's platelets. The incidence of NAT is about 1 in 2500 live births,[253] and like PTP, it is usually caused by an alloimmune response to an incompatible allelic form of $\beta3$.

There are currently six known molecular variants of $\beta3$ in the human gene pool; these are shown in Table 177-7. The PlA1 allele of $\beta3$, as defined serologically, is by far the most common, with a gene frequency in Caucasians of about 85 percent, and it is this allelic form of $\beta3$ that is most often responsible for inducing the alloimmune response causing both PTP and NAT in individuals that have inherited one of the other, less common, $\beta3$ isoforms. The molecular basis of the polymorphisms underlying NAT and PTP is now known to involve, almost exclusively, single amino acid substitutions along the length of the polypeptide chain. Thus, an L^{33}F substitution controls the formation of the PlA1/PlA2 alloantigen system,[254,255] while an R^{143}Q polymorphism is

Table 177-7 Naturally Occuring Allelic Forms of Platelet Membrane Glycoproteins That Can Induce Immune Thrombocytopenias

Allelic form	*Gene frequency (%)	Serologic designation
$\alpha2$: D^{505}	89	Brb
$\alpha2$: K^{505}	11	Bra
GPIb: T^{145}	93	Kob
GPIb: M^{145}	7	Koa
αIIb: I^{843}	61	Baka
αIIb: S^{843}	39	Bakb
$\beta3$: $\underline{L^{33}}$, R^{143}, P^{407}, R^{489}, R^{636}	85	P1A1
$\beta3$: $\underline{P^{33}}$, R^{143}, P^{407}, R^{489}, R^{636}	15	P1A2
$\beta3$: L^{33}, $\underline{E^{143}}$, P^{407}, R^{489}, R^{636}	$\ll1$	Penb
$\beta3$: L^{33}, R^{143}, $\underline{A^{407}}$, R^{489}, R^{636}	$\ll1$	Mo
$\beta3$: L^{33}, R^{143}, P^{407}, $\underline{Q^{489}}$, R^{636}	$\ll1$	CA
$\beta3$: L^{33}, R^{143}, P^{407}, R^{489}, $\underline{C^{636}}$	$\ll1$	Sr

*In the Caucasian population. Gene frequencies in African and Asian populations differ. The amino acid substitutions in allelic forms of $\beta3$ are underlined.

responsible for the Pen^a/Pen^b alloantigens.[256] Other, rare allelic forms of $\beta 3$ that can elicit an alloimmune response have also been reported,[257–261] and are summarized in Table 177-7.

In addition to $\beta 3$, more than one allele each is known to exist for $\alpha 2$, GPIb, and αIIb; they, too, have been defined at the molecular biologic level and shown to be caused by single-amino-acid substitutions. As shown in Table 177-7, these include an Asp^{505}Lys polymorphism of $\alpha 2$ associated with the Bra/Brb alloantigen system,[262] a T^{145}M substitution in GPIbα,[263] and an I^{843}S allelic form of αIIb that controls the formation of the Bak^a and Bak^b alloantigens.[255] As the precise nucleotide sequence polymorphisms associated with the major human platelet alloantigen systems have become defined, our ability to design novel diagnostic and therapeutic approaches for the treatment of patients with NAT and PTP has improved, and it has now become a routine matter to develop and apply DNA-based diagnostic tests for the molecular analysis of these clinically important molecular variations.[81]

More recently, there has been growing interest in these polymorphisms to see if they are associated with a prothrombotic risk. The issue is not completely settled. The greatest controversy concerns the role of PLA2 in thrombosis.[264,265] More recently, it was suggested that PLA2 may be a risk factor for early stroke in females.[266]

PLATELET STORAGE GRANULE DEFECTS

Biology of the Platelet Granules

As mentioned in the introduction, human platelets contain several different types of intracytoplasmic granules that can be distinguished by electron microscopy, including α-granules, dense (δ-) granules, and lysosomes[253] (see Table 177-1). These granules play a major role in platelet plug formation following platelet activation. This is especially true for the α- and δ-granules, which are uniquely designed to participate in the clotting process.

δ-Granules are the most rapidly secreted granules following platelet activation; they contain ADP, ATP, serotonin, and calcium.[267] Released ADP serves as a potent agonist for recruiting other platelets,[268] and ATP is an agonist for other cells.[269] Two-thirds of platelet adenine nucleotides are stored in these granules, with an ADP:ATP ratio of 3:2, as opposed to the 1:8 ratio in the cytoplasmic pool.[270] Serotonin is a biogenic amine that can influence vascular tone, while secreted calcium ions mediate adhesive interactions and serve in addition as an intracellular second messenger for signal transduction within the activated platelet (discussed below).

Platelet α-granules contribute a vast array of proteins uniquely involved in platelet plug formation. Following platelet activation, the α-granules move to the center of the platelet and release their contents into the bloodstream via membrane fusion with the open canalicular system.[271] Interestingly, not all proteins present in α-granules have the same origin. Some, like VWF, thrombospondin, and platelet factor 4 (PF4), are synthesized in and packaged by the megakaryocyte during maturation,[272,273] while others, such as albumin, IgG, and fibrinogen, are acquired by endocytosis of plasma components.[274,275] Secreted α-granule products participate in important ways in hemostasis: fibrinogen, fibronectin, vitronectin, VWF, and thrombospondin serve as adhesive ligands; platelet derived-growth factor (PDGF), β-thromboglobulin (βTG), PF4, tissue-growth factor-β, and thrombospondin modulate cell growth; and factors V and XI, high-molecular-weight kininogen, C1 inhibitor, fibrinogen, plasminogen activator inhibitor-1, and protein S each participate in the coagulation process.[272–278] The membrane of the α-granule itself also contributes to platelet adhesiveness in that it harbors P-selectin (formerly called PADGEM or GMP-140),[279,280] which becomes expressed on the surface of activated platelets and endothelial cells following granule fusion, and mediates the subsequent binding of neutrophils and monocytes during the inflammatory process.[11]

Dense Granule Defects

Storage Pool Diseases. Patients with defects in the platelet-dense granules have a storage pool deficiency (for review see references 270 and 281). These patients present with mild-to-moderate bleeding diatheses, as well as abnormalities in their platelet aggregation patterns. The second wave of aggregation is absent in response to ADP and epinephrine, and virtually absent in response to collagen. Bleeding times in these patients are often prolonged. In 1969, it was shown that these patients have a deficiency in total platelet ADP,[282] and this deficit was subsequently localized to the ADP pool of the δ-granule (known as the nonmetabolic pool).[283] Direct measurements of other platelet-dense granular components also confirm their absence.[284] Platelets from these patients have a defect in their ability to take up serotonin from their environment,[285] and electron microscopic examination revealed an absence of characteristic dense granules.[281] In addition to the δ-granule storage-pool deficit seen in all of these patients, a subset of individuals have other associated defects. The two most common platelet storage pool disorders are known as Hermansky-Pudlak syndrome (HPS)[286,287] and Chediak-Higashi syndrome (CHS),[288–291] and are discussed below. For both of these disorders, some of the genes affected and a series of mutations resulting in the observed phenotype were recently defined.

Hermansky-Pudlak Syndrome. This disorder is characterized by tyrosinase-positive severe oculocutaneous albinism that is associated with photophobia rotatory nystagmus and loss of visual acuity, excessive accumulation of ceroid-like material in reticuloendothelial cells in the bone marrow and other tissues, and a mild-to-moderate hemorrhagic diathesis (see Table 177-8). This disease is inherited as an autosomal recessive disorder, and while it occurs in many populations, it occurs with higher frequency in the Puerto Rican population.[292] Although their platelets completely lack δ-granules, these patients often have no significant bleeding diathesis unless complicated by aspirin exposure or by pregnancy.[270,293] In one study, however, deaths from bleeding were second only to deaths from pulmonary fibrosis, a complication that probably is secondary to the serotonin released from failure to package the serotonin into δ-granules.[281] HPS is also associated with a higher incidence of granulomatous colitis,[294] although the connection of this gastrointestinal disorder and the granule defect is unclear.

The gene involved in the common form of HPS was positionally cloned on the long arm of chromosome 10.[295] The 700-amino-acid protein has one transmembrane domain, but has little homology with other known proteins, although the transcript appears to be present in multiple tested tissues. The HPS protein is homologous to the pale ear (ep) mutation in mice.[296] The Puerto Rican form of HPS appears to be due to a 16-base pair insert at codon Pro^{496} that results in a frameshift. Similar frameshifts were detected in other ethnic forms of HPS, including at Ala^{441} (Japanese) and Pro^{324} (Swiss and Irish).

Chediak-Higashi Syndrome. CHS involves only partial albinism, with patients often having a white forelock or ashen hair, secondary to abnormally large melanosomes.[281–285] Platelets from these patients are characterized by the presence of large intracytoplasmic granules (Fig. 177-11*A*). In addition, these patients have an associated immune defect, as characterized by the presence of large intracellular granules in their leukocytes (Fig. 177-12*A*), with a concurrent immune dysfunction involving poor mobilization of the marrow leukocyte pool,[297] defective chemotaxis,[298,299] and decreased bactericidal activity[300] (Table 177-8). Many other tissues also contain abnormal granules, including renal tubular cells, pneumocytes, chief and parietal gastric cells, hepatocytes, neuronal cells, and fibroblasts.[301] Chediak-Higashi patients often die in the first two decades of life from either overwhelming infections or lymphoproliferative disorders, especially in what is termed the "accelerated phase" of the disease.[302] These patients are particularly susceptible to Epstein-Barr viral infections.[297]

Table 177-8 Inherited Platelet Defects Associated with Morphologic Abnormalities

Category	Disease	Major feature
δ-Granule defect	Storage pool disease	Absence of dense granules in plates associated with a mild-to-moderate bleeding diathesis. Decreased level of platelet serotonin and ADP:ATP ratio. Absent second wave on platelet aggregation.
	Chediak-Higashi syndrome	Same as storage pool deficiency, but also associated with partial albinism and large cytoplasmic granules in white cells with a mild bleeding diathesis and an immune dysfunction.
	Hermansky-Pudlak syndrome	Same as storage pool deficiency, but also associated with severe albinism and a very mild bleeding diathesis.
α-Granule defect	Gray platelet syndrome	Absence of α granules in platelets, associated with very mild bleeding diathesis and decreased α-granular content.
Large platelets	Bernard-Soulier syndrome	Deficiency of the platelet GPIIb-IX-V complex associated with moderate bleeding. Associated with large platelets and often a mild thrombocytopenia.
	May-Hegglin anomaly	Large platelets without a bleeding diathesis, associated with mild thrombocytopenia, no bleeding diathesis, but Dohle body inclusions in white cells.
	Fechtner syndrome	Same as May-Hegglin, but with associated deafness, nephritis, and ocular abnormalities.
	Montreal platelet syndrome	Large platelets and a mild bleeding diathesis. Spontaneous platelet aggregation at pH 7.4.
Small platelets	Familial platelet deficiency/acute myelogenous leukemia (FPD/AML)	Mild thrombocytopenia and out-of-proportion bleeding tendency. ~30% life-risk of AML.
	Wiskott-Aldrich syndrome (WAS)	Presplenectomy has small platelets, severe thrombocytopenia. Has eczema and immune dysfunction ultimately resulting in severe infections, immune complex diseases, and lymphomas/leukemias.

The gene involved in the common form of CHS has been identified on the long arm of chromosome 1, and this gene encodes a large protein of 3801 amino acids.[303] This complex protein has several repeated motifs that contain a series of hydrophobic helices interspersed with hydrophobic membrane association domains. The helical regions resemble previously defined HEAT elements that appear to be involved in vesicular transportation.[304] It is highly homologous to the yeast proteins whose mutations result in defective protein sorting called Vps.[305] The murine equivalent of the CHS gene is the gene defective in beige (bg) mice. Mutations have been defined in four patients with CHS. All involved truncated products. Two were frameshifts (nucleotide 489 in one patient and nucleotides 3073 and 3074 in another) and three were nonsense mutations leading to a stop codon ($R^{1103}X$, $R^{50}X$, and $Q^{1029}X$). It appears that full-length CHS is needed for proper function.[306]

α-Granule Defects: The Gray Platelet Syndrome

A number of patients who have a deficiency in α-granules have been described (for review, see reference 270). These patients have a bleeding history similar to δ-granule storage pool defective patients, with mild to moderate bleeding, mild thrombocytopenia, and a prolonged bleeding time (see Table 177-8). Because of the initial light microscopic observation of gray platelets in the peripheral blood smear of these patients following Romanovsky stain,[307] this disorder was termed gray platelet syndrome. On electron microscopy, these platelets appear somewhat enlarged, but are most notable for the absence or marked reduction of α-granules, as shown in Fig. 177-11*B*.[281] These platelets are also deficient in α-granule-specific proteins such as PF4, βTG, VWF, factor V, fibronectin, and PDGF.[308] Gray platelet aggregation to various agonists, especially to thrombin, appears to be impaired. There have been many mild alterations noted in platelet aggregation, such as a delayed and blunted Ca^{2+} mobilization response in these platelets.[309] The observed platelet aggregation abnormalities may be secondary effects of the absence of any of the many different α-granule components.

The vacuolar structures seen in gray platelets appear to be aborted α-granules.[310] Immunocytochemical studies show that these structures contain both P-selectin and αIIbβ3 in their membranes, and that these proteins are transferred to and, via granule fusion with the plasma membrane, expressed normally on the cell surface following platelet activation.[311] The vacuolar structures appear to become centralized like normal α-granules following platelet activation. They also appear to contain significant amounts of proteins, including immunoglobulin and albumin,[311] that are normally incorporated into α-granules by passive endocytosis (see above). Further, endogenously synthesized α-granule-specific proteins such as PDGF, PF4, and βTG do not seem to be retained within the platelet, leaking out of the cell instead.[312] This latter phenomenon may account for several reports of myelofibrosis and pulmonary fibrosis associated with gray platelet syndrome.[312]

The biologic basis of how proteins are processed intracellularly and targeted to particular organelles is just now beginning to be understood.[313] Because multiple α-granule proteins normally synthesized in the megakaryocyte are affected, while granule proteins derived by endocytosis are present at near-normal levels, and because this disease is limited to megakaryocytes and platelets, it appears that a platelet-specific chaperon-like protein necessary to transport proteins to, or retain them in, the α-granules may be missing or defective.

Patients with gray platelet syndrome have a mild bleeding diathesis that may be treated by administration of DDAVP or local care of a bleeding site through the use of ε-amino caproic acid, an inhibitor of plasminogen activation.[270,314] Platelet transfusions are not often necessary, but may be lifesaving. There is one report of az 68-year-old man in whom the diagnosis of gray platelet syndrome was made while he was being evaluated for thrombocytopenia.[315] Bone marrow analysis demonstrated mild reticular

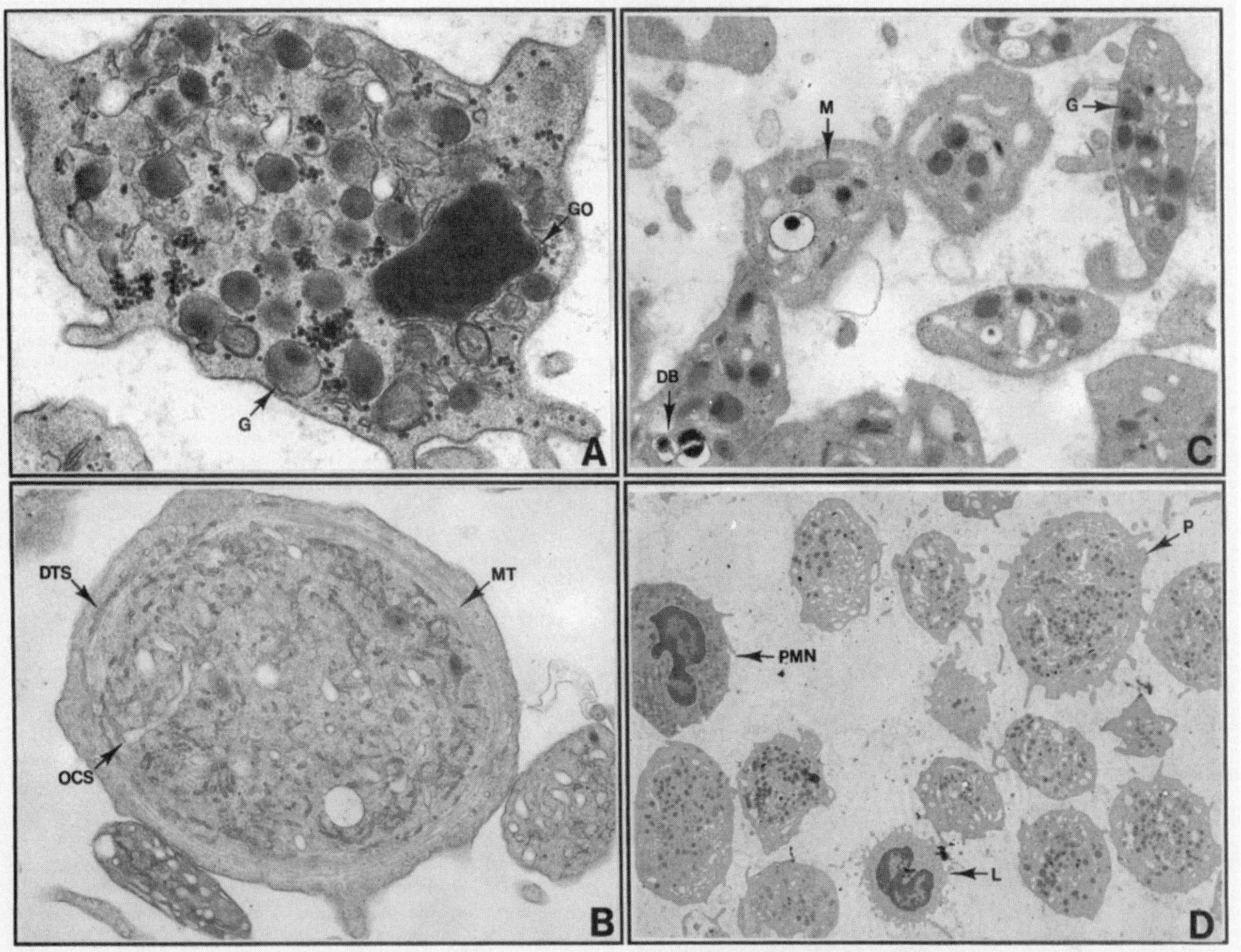

Fig. 177-11 Thin-section electron micrographs of platelets. *A*, Chediak-Higashi platelet demonstrating a giant organelle (GO) present among many normal sized granules (G). Magnification: ×32,000. *B*, A platelet from a patient with gray platelet syndrome reveals the presence of the normal circumferential band of microtubules (MT), elements of the open canalicular system (OCS), and dense tubular system (DTS), and the absence of other organelles. Magnification: ×23,000. *C*, Wiskott-Aldrich platelets are about half normal size, but contain normal-appearing α-granules (G), dense bodies (DB), and mitochondria (M), all of which appear large by comparison. Magnification: ×22,000. *D*, Platelets from patients with May-Hegglin anomaly are as large as lymphocytes (L), and a few platelets (P) are larger than polymorphonuclear leukocytes (PMN). Occasional large α-granules are present, and channels of both the OCS and the DTS are prominent in the cytoplasm. Magnification: ×3500. (*Courtesy of Dr. James G. White, University of Minnesota.*)

fibrosis that may have resulted from the unregulated secretion of α-granule constituents from megakaryocytes and platelets. The clinical importance of the marrow myelofibrosis in this disorder is as yet unclear.

A variant of the gray platelet syndrome has been described in the Wistar-Furth rat, in which there is thrombocytopenia and platelet size heterogeneity with small α-granules and a canalicular system containing α-granular material.[316] The defect in this disorder may be different than in the human disorder and may involve a protein important in the division of the megakaryocyte into platelets as well as in the formation of α-granules.

A small number of patients have been described with a combined α/δ-granule deficiency.[271,284] The δ-granule deficiency was often much more severe than the α-granule deficiency. These patients also have mild to moderate bleeding histories, and the laboratory evaluation is similar to that of the δ-granule-deficient patient, with a decreased platelet ADP:ATP ratio in the cells and low levels of serotonin. In one patient with a severe deficiency of both α- and δ-granules, there was a deficiency in total platelet P-selectin,[317] suggesting that, unlike the gray platelet syndrome in which there may be α-granule-targeting defect, platelet granule formation itself may underlie this disorder.

Quebec Platelet Syndrome. This rare disease has been associated with a deficiency of Factor V levels.[318] Initially, the disorder was thought to be due to an absence of a carrier protein for Factor V,[319] but more recent studies suggest that there is a generalized autolysis of many α-granule proteins in this disease.[320]

Therapeutic treatment of these patients is the same as other storage-pool-deficient patients. It is not known whether there are concomitant, related syndromes, such as pulmonary fibrosis, myelofibrosis, or granular defects in other tissues.

DEFECTS IN SIGNAL TRANSDUCTION

Following the binding of an agonist to its platelet receptor, a signal is transferred across the cell membrane into the cell either directly by the membrane receptor or, for the 7 transmembrane family of receptors, through intervening $G_{\alpha\beta\delta}$ heterotrimeric proteins.[321] The following G_α proteins have been described in platelets: G_s, $G_{\alpha i1}$, $G_{\alpha i2}$, $G_{\alpha i3}$, G_z, and G_q.[321] These different G proteins have separate roles in the biology of signal transduction and may modulate the response of a particular receptor to a given agonist. Signal transduction results in secondary changes within the platelet that include ionic calcium fluxes, cAMP formation,

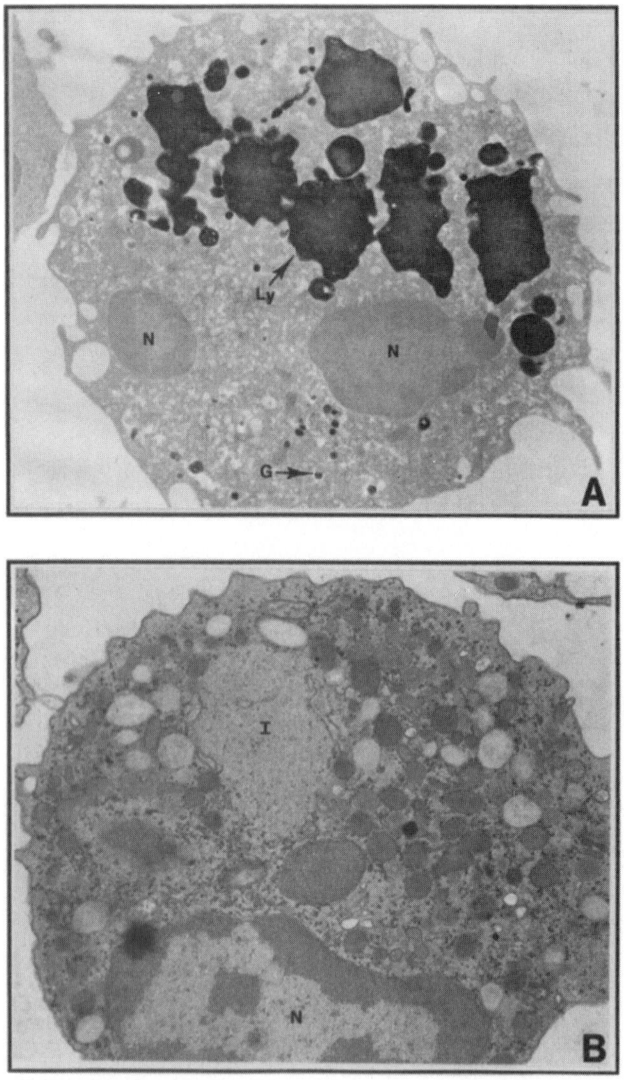

Fig. 177-12 Thin-section electron micrographs of neutrophils. *A*, Thin-section electron micrographs of a typical neutrophil from a patient with CHS stained for myeloperoxidase. Osmium black reaction product identifies a few normal size granules (G) and numerous huge lysosomes (Ly) characteristic of this disorder. Nuclear lobes (N) are not stained. Magnification: ×14,500. *B*, Neutrophil from a patient with May-Hegglin anomaly (MHA), containing a characteristic spindle-shaped inclusion (I) present in nearly all granulocytes from these patients. Fibers resembling intermediate filaments are oriented in the long axis of the inclusions, and are probably responsible for their shape. Clusters of ribosomes are present on the filaments and produce the basophilia of the occlusions on smears stained with Wright-Giemsa. Membrane segments are close by but do not enclose MHA inclusions. Magnification: ×25,000. (*Courtesy of Dr. James G. White, University of Minnesota.*)

phospholipase A2 and C activation, changes in arachidonate pathway metabolism, protein kinase C activation, and protein phosphorylation. These diverse pathways interact with each other in multiple complex ways that are still being defined. For example, phospholipase C releases diacylglycerol,[322,323] which, in turn, activates protein kinase C[324] and, consequently, phosphorylation of numerous intracellular proteins, including cytoskeletal elements.[325]

With multiple overlapping pathways of activation, as well as overlapping phenotypes, it has been difficult to define specific defects in patients with inherited disorders of platelet signal transduction. Nonetheless, a small number of patients have been described, many of whom have a mild bleeding diathesis with moderate prolongation of the bleeding time. Most studies have demonstrated abnormal platelet aggregation patterns, with only partial response to certain agonists, which resemble those in patients with storage pool disorders (see above). One such group of patients lack the ability to liberate arachidonic acid.[326] This may be due to a phospholipase A2 deficiency in at least one of the described patients.[327] In others, the failure of phospholipase A2 to release arachidonic acid may be due to decreased thrombin mobilization of Ca^{2+}. Another patient appears to have difficulty with tyrosine phosphorylation through the ADP receptor system.[328]

Other patients have diminished cyclooxygenase enzyme activity that mimics an aspirin-like defect.[329–332] These patients have abnormal platelet aggregation in response to ADP, epinephrine, collagen, and arachidonic acid, while responding normally to prostaglandin G2, suggesting a defect in cyclooxygenase and subsequent thromboxane A2 synthesis. In one study, radioimmunoassay using an anticyclooxygenase antibody showed that five of six patients with this disorder had normal antigen levels of an apparently functionally abnormal protein.[333] Additionally, two affected patients have been described who appear to lack thromboxane synthetase that converts prostaglandin H2 to thromboxane A2.[334,335] Bassett hound hereditary thrombopathy represents a possible animal model of a signal transduction defect in platelets.[336] Originally thought to be an animal model of Glanzmann thrombasthenia, it appears that fibrinogen binding is normal in these animals, but that there is a delay in platelet activation following fibrinogen binding.[337]

Over the past few years, two additional models of platelet dysfunction secondary to a signaling defect have been recognized. These are the Wiskott-Aldrich syndrome (WAS) and a deficiency of G_q protein. WAS is described below under disorders of platelet size and numbers, but clearly also involves a defect in signaling within the developing megakaryocyte.

A mouse model for G_q targeted disruption has recently been published.[338] G_q is expressed in multiple tissues, such as the cerebellum, as well as in platelets. This may explain the observed phenotype of cerebellar ataxia plus a bleeding diathesis most noted for many of the newborn pups bleeding to death. Platelets from affected animals did not aggregate in response to low-dose ADP, collagen, thrombin, or the thromboxane A-mimetic U46619; however, G_q-deficient platelets underwent a pronounced shape change to thrombin, collagen, or U46619, as indicated by an immediate decrease in light transmission upon addition of platelet agonists. They did respond well to the calcium ionophore A23187 and to PMS stimulation. This animal model shows that in platelets, a number of G-protein-coupled receptor outside-in signals appear to rely heavily on G_q-coupled pathways.

DISORDERS OF PLATELET PROCOAGULANT ACTIVITY

Activated platelets play a role in accelerating the proteolytic events that take place as part of the coagulation cascade, and this property has been termed platelet factor 3 activity.[339] The procoagulant properties have been attributed to a number of characteristics unique to the surface of activated platelets, including exposure of phosphatidylserine moieties, the redistribution of specific receptors for Factors V and X, and the development of platelet microvesicles.

One of the best-characterized inherited disorders of platelet factor 3 activity is known as Scott syndrome.[340,341] In the first case studies of this bleeding disorder, the patient presented with prolonged bleeding after dental extractions, excessive postoperative bleeding, and a spontaneous retroperitoneal hemorrhage.[340] Serum prothrombin time was short, with normal prothrombin and partial thromboplastin times, normal bleeding times, and normal platelet aggregation and secretion. Measurement of prothrombinase activity of the patient's activated platelets demonstrated a 75 percent reduction in Factor Xa binding even in the presence of added factor Va, implying a defect in a membrane component necessary for Factor Va-Xa assembly. These platelets are ineffective at moderate shear rates in promoting fibrinopeptide A formation and in fibrin deposition on subendothelium.[342] The molecular basis of this disease may be related to a defect in a protein called scrambalase, with a failure to move phosphatidylserine onto the activated platelet surfaces[343,344] and decreased microvesicle formation.[345] The defect in this disorder is not limited to platelet membranes, as erythrocytes from patients with Scott syndrome also have decreased microvesiculation and fewer Factor Va binding sites than normal following A23187 ionophore stimulation.[346]

PLATELET SIZE AND PRODUCTION DISORDERS: THE INHERITED THROMBOCYTOPENIAS

General Comments

The process by which platelet formation occurs is a fascinating one that is only now beginning to be understood. Megakaryocytopoiesis begins with the self-renewing hematopoietic stem cell in the bone marrow that becomes progressively committed to the megakaryoblast lineage, eventually resulting in the diploid megakaryoblast, a cell that is indistinguishable from other lymphocytic-like cells by routine staining techniques. Over an $\sim$4-day period, this precursor cell undergoes an explosive series of changes, with endoreduplication of the nucleus, an increase in cytoplasmic content to an average volume of $\sim 10^4$ μm^3, and an accumulation of proteins and morphologic features characteristic of platelets. Eventually, either in the bone marrow or in the pulmonary vascular bed, each megakaryocyte sheds several thousand platelets.[347]

The study of the process of platelet formation is of considerable clinical interest. Regulating this process may be valuable in altering thrombotic tendency and in limiting the incidence of clinically significant thrombocytopenia during chemotherapeutic treatment of tumors. In addition, there are a large number of inherited disorders and murine-targeting gene-disruption models, resulting in decreased platelet production. A number of these are well-defined clinical syndromes, such as thrombocytopenia and absent radii (TAR) syndrome, in which skeletal abnormalities occur in association with clinically significant thrombocytopenia (also see below).[348] Interestingly, in most of these patients, the thrombocytopenia disappears with time. Other inherited thrombocytopenic states occur in conjunction with more recognized platelet disorders such as platelet-type vWD (discussed above), the storage pool platelet defects, and May-Hegglin syndrome, in which there are large, often bizarre-shaped platelets associated with the thrombocytopenia and inclusion bodies in the lymphocytes and neutrophils (see below). In many of these states, decreased production may be inversely related to increased platelet size, so that total platelet mass is conserved.

Some of the above described disorders may involve a defect in hematopoietic stem cell commitment to the megakaryocyte lineage, while others may involve defects in the final process of differentiation into mature megakaryocytes and the subsequent shedding of platelets. Below we discuss the state of knowledge of these two interrelated processes — megakaryocytopoiesis and platelet formation.

Megakaryocytopoiesis

Megakaryocytes are large, polyploid, terminally differentiated hematopoietic cells that release platelets into the peripheral bloodstream.[349] As shown in Fig. 177-13, these cells arise from self-regenerating pluripotent stem cells that also give rise to all other hematopoietic lineages. Megakaryocyte lineage commitment involves a number of precursor stages that are distinguishable by the final differentiated cells to which they can give rise. The

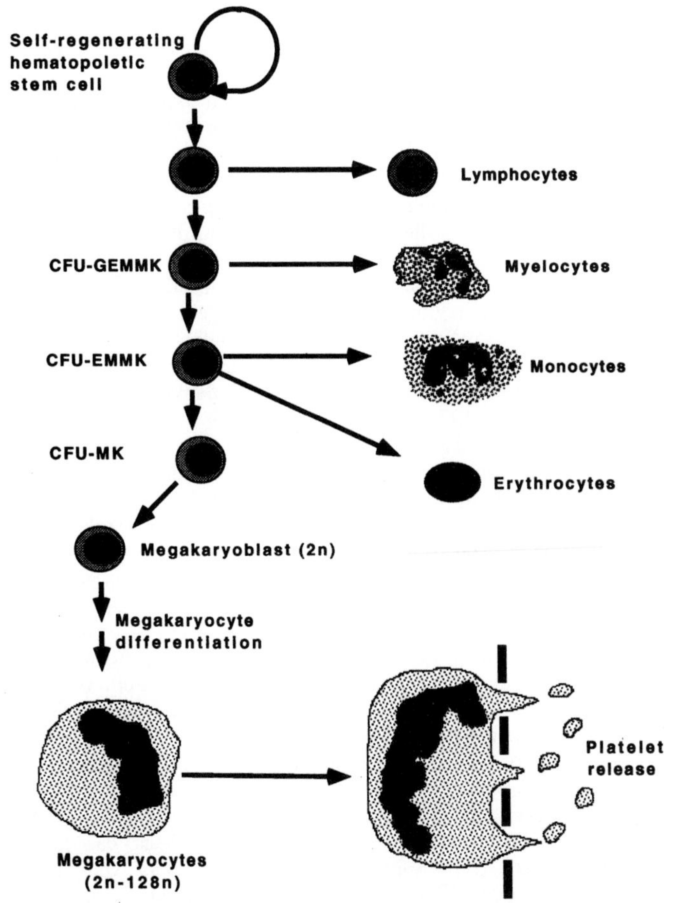

Fig. 177-13 Megakaryocyte development from the pluripotent hematopoietic stem cell involves two steps. In the first, the mononuclear stem cell undergoes increasing commitment toward the megakaryocyte cell lineage. These cells undergo proliferation. In the second, the mononuclear megakaryoblast undergoes nuclear endoreduplication, increases in cell size, and develops special structures and organization. This terminally differentiated cell eventually releases a shower of platelets.

earliest precursor after the pluripotent stem cell appears to be the CFU-GEMMK (colony-forming unit — granulocyte, erythrocyte, monocyte, megakaryocyte) that in culture results in a mix of granulocytes, erythrocytes, monocytes, and megakaryocytes. The next apparent stage of commitment appears to be the CFU-EMM that gives rise to mixed colonies of erythrocytes, monocytes, and megakaryocytes. The BFU-MK (burst-forming unit — megakaryocyte) gives rise to a burst of approximately 10 to 20 megakaryocytes after 3 weeks in culture, and the CFU-MK gives rise to a smaller megakaryocyte colony after 10 days in culture (for review, see reference 349). Various growth factors regulate megakaryocyte differentiation at different points of their development. Certain cytokines stimulate proliferation of megakaryocytic progenitors such as interleukin-3 (IL-3), IL-6, IL-11, IL-12, granulocyte-macrophage colony stimulating factor (GM-CSF), and erythropoietin (EPO).[350] Others have been reported to modulate megakaryocyte maturation and platelet development, including IL-1α and leukemia inhibitory factor (LIF).[349,350] However, all of the above mentioned growth factors and cytokines have very broad effects on all hematopoietic cell lines. The discovery and cloning of thrombopoietin (TPO), the ligand of the orphan c-Mpl receptor,[351] opened a new avenue in megakaryocyte differentiation studies. TPO was found to be a specific factor that controls megakaryocytic cell proliferation as well as maturation, and that can enhance platelet reactivity.[352–355]

This 353-amino-acid protein is highly homologous at its N-terminus with erythropoietin. The full-length protein, a truncated N-terminal TPO and even mimetic peptides can dimerize the myeloproliferative ligand receptor (Mpl) that is present on multiple hematopoietic precursor cells and on maturing megakaryocytes.[356] On immature cells, this activated receptor stimulates general proliferation, much like IL-11 or *c*-kit ligand. On megakaryocyte precursors and megakaryocytes, it leads to increased megakaryocyte differentiation and platelet formation. Targeted disruption murine models of the Mpl and TPO genes both result in a decrease in platelet count to ~5 percent of normal with normal appearing megakaryocytes;[357–359] however, the Mpl-deficient mice also have a proliferative deficiency in their hematopoietic stem cells in vitro.[360,361] Thus, this cytokine pathway appears to be permissive for megakaryocytopoiesis, but not absolutely required for this differentiation process. Certainly, a defect in the ability to produce TPO or its receptor may be the basis of the thrombocytopenia seen in an inherited disorder such as the TAR syndrome (see below) or Fanconi anemia. The relationship between the marrow dysfunction in these disorders and the inherited skeletal abnormality is intriguing.

Cell and Molecular Biology of Platelet Formation

The end product of this lineage commitment is the megakaryoblast, a small lymphocyte-like cell that undergoes the process of nuclear endoreduplication,[349] cytoplasmic enlargement, and differentiation to form the mature megakaryocyte (see Fig. 177-13). Each of these huge cells eventually results in the formation of approximately 10^3 to 10^4 platelets. Because erythrocytes and white cells are directly released from the bone, it has been assumed that platelets are released from there as well. The findings of naked megakaryocyte nuclei[362] in the marrow and the presence of proplatelets in the central venous blood[363] support the hypothesis that platelets are formed in the marrow. It is possible, however, that platelets are, at least in part, released from megakaryocytes that have migrated to the pulmonary bed.[364–367] Studies demonstrate that there are more circulating megakaryocytes in the pulmonary artery than in the pulmonary venous system and that the opposite is true for platelet numbers.[366,367]

The process by which platelets actually derive from megakaryocytes is not well understood. The mature megakaryocyte contains an extensive membrane system termed the demarcation membrane system (DMS) that may represent inverted membranes. Two hypotheses for the mechanism of platelet production have been proposed: that the DMS fuses and the megakaryocyte cytoplasm fractures to release a shower of platelets, or that the DMS represents reserve plasma membrane that allows the formation of projections from the megakaryocyte surface that then break off to form proplatelets and platelets.[368,369] A great deal of effort has been directed at establishing an in vitro megakaryocyte system that sheds platelets. In some cases, cultured cells have been shown to form spindles, while in others, cellular processes take on a beaded appearance and fragment to form particles with the size and ultrastructural appearance of platelets.[369] This process can be inhibited by agents that disrupt microtubules[370,371] and promoted by actin filament depolymerizing agents,[371,372] suggesting involvement of the cytoskeleton in this process. A targeted disruption of the hematopoietic transcription factor NF-E2 results in severe thrombocytopenia and very large, bizarre megakaryocytes.[373] The defect may involve loss of β-tubulin expression in these cells and an inability of normal demarcation and release of platelets, and thus may represent the first model of a specific defect that inhibits platelet release from megakaryocytes.[374] The size variation and heterogeneity in platelets seen in various disease states may be related to the site and mechanism of formation, and a number of the inherited platelet disorders to be discussed below appear to involve abnormal platelet size, including the macrothrombocytopenic states seen in Bernard-Soulier syndrome, May-Hegglin anomaly, and the Wistar-Furth rat, and the microthrombocytopenia seen in Wiskott-Aldrich syndrome.

The normal range of platelet counts is 150 to 400 $\times$ 10^3/ml.[375] Even more constant than the circulating platelet count, however, is the circulating platelet mass in which the platelet count is multiplied by the mean platelet volume, so that there is an inverse relationship between platelet count and platelet size.[212] Because platelets also express Mpl, it has been suggested that TPO regulation has to do not with a constant production of TPO, but with a variable circulating absorption of TPO to platelets.[376] As platelet mass rises, the amount of the constant TPO bound increases and less is available for marrow megakaryocyte stimulation. The converse situation would also be true: as platelet mass falls, there is more free TPO to stimulate marrow megakaryocyte development.

The molecular biology of the regulated expression of genes during megakaryocytopoiesis is only now beginning to be understood. Several platelet-specific genes have had regulatory studies on their 5′-flanking region. The best studied have been the PF4 and αIIb promoters. Transgenic mice containing a 1.1-kb segment from the 5′-flanking region of the rat PF4 gene linked to the prokaryote β-galactosidase gene drove expression in a virtually megakaryocyte-specific fashion.[377] Further deletional studies with the 5′-flanking region of the rat PF4 gene and a transient expression assay utilizing rat marrow and a growth hormone expression vector demonstrated the presence of three enhancer regions and one silencer region in the 5′-flanking region.[378] As shown in Fig. 177-14, these regions define the elements that partially control tissue specificity, and include a GATA consensus sequence 31 bp upstream from the transcriptional start site that may contribute to tissue-specific expression.

Two GATA boxes may also play an important role in the regulation of expression of the αIIb gene. DNase I protection sites have been defined within the 5′-flanking region of this gene (see Fig. 177-14),[379] with two of them shown to be megakaryocyte-specific. Transient expression assays using constructs in which these two regions, beginning 456 and 502 bp upstream of the transcriptional start site, have been deleted resulted in a threefold decrease in expression. The −456-bp site contains a GATA consensus sequence, and a second GATA site at −55 has also been defined, and may be an important regulator of megakaryocyte-specific expression.[380]

GATA-binding proteins are nuclear transcription factors that were first defined in erythroid cells.[381] At least one family member, GATA-1, was thought to be restricted in its expression to erythroid tissues.[382] More recently, this transcription factor was

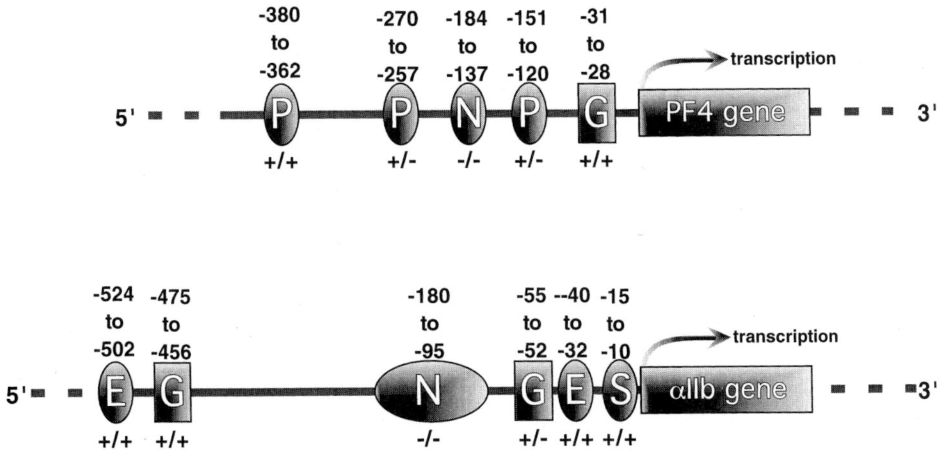

Fig. 177-14 Promoter, enhancer, and silencer elements in the 5′-flanking regions of the rat PF4 and human GPIIb genes that influence megakaryocyte-specific gene expression. Both genes are numbered from the transcriptional start site. P = promoter element; N = silencer element; G = GATA consensus sequence; E = Ets promoter element; and S = Sp1 promoter element. The three different P regions do not share significant sequence similarity. The first + or − refers to whether the element enhances or silences transcriptional activity, while the second + or − refers to whether the element is megakaryocyte specific (+) or not (−).

also shown to be present in megakaryocytes, megakaryocyte cell lines, and monocytes.[383,384] As these three cell lines share a common progenitor, it is not surprising that there is a common nuclear regulatory factor like GATA-1. The role of GATA-1 in megakaryocyte-specific expression became clear with the creation of a "knockdown" transgenic mouse in which a deletion was introduced upstream of the GATA-1 gene.[385] As opposed to the targeted disruption of the GATA-1 gene that was embryonically lethal because of a block in erythroid development,[386] these animals were born, but had a severe thrombocytopenia, with an abundance of dysmorphic marrow megakaryocytes.

In addition to the role of GATA-1 and NF-E2 in megakaryocyte-specific expression, a number of transcription factors belonging to the Ets family have been implicated in megakaryocyte-specific expression (see Fig. 177-14).[387,388] Furthermore, two mice with targeted gene disruptions of erythroid-specific nuclear factors also have the surprising absence of megakaryocytopoiesis. The first is FOG, a transcription factor first recognized by its ability to bind to GATA-1.[389] Targeted disruption of this is embryonically lethal with an absence of mature erythroid cells and a severe deficit of normal-appearing megakaryocytes.[390] Targeted disruption of another erythroid transcription factor NF-E2 also resulted in a defect in megakaryopoiesis, and this was discussed above. Thus, in all of these transcription factor knockouts, megakaryopoiesis goes on, but there is a disruption of different subsets of genes involved in the full development of mature megakaryocytes giving rise to the different morphologies of the megakaryocytes and the difference in the released platelet numbers and sizes.

Defects in Platelet Size and Production

Until very recently, none of the above targeted disruptions of megakaryocyte transcription factors had a homologous human disease. A recent report of a family with X-linked severe thrombocytopenia and anemia due to a mutation in the FOG-binding domain of GATA-1 has been described.[391] In addition, several platelet abnormalities have been described that are associated with altered numbers and size of platelets. Some of these are associated with large platelets and thrombocytopenia. The most common of these is the May-Hegglin anomaly, in which macrothrombocytes (see Fig. 177-11*D*) are associated with thrombocytopenia and normal coagulation studies.[392] In addition, leukocytes appear to contain large spindle-shaped inclusions known as Dohle bodies (Fig. 177-12*B*). A similar disorder, but with inclusions that look different, is Sebastian syndrome.[393] Again, no intrinsic platelet defect has been described. The association of the morphologic finding of May-Hegglin anomaly with sensorineural deafness, nephritis, and ocular abnormalities has been called Fechtner syndrome.[394] In Montreal platelet syndrome, there are macrothrombocytes, a prolonged bleeding time, and spontaneous aggregation of platelets at pH 7.4.[395,396] The molecular bases of these abnormalities are unknown.

Inherited disorders in platelet production alone without defects in other hematopoietic cell lines are rare. The most common ones are the TAR syndrome,[348,397,398] X-linked thrombocytopenia,[399,400] and familial platelet deficiency/acute myelogenous anemia (FPD/AML).[401,402] TAR syndrome was first described in 1951,[397] and is a relatively common disorder involving hypomegakaryocytic thrombocytopenia and bilateral absence of the radii.[348,397,398] These patients are born with a low platelet count in the approximately 10,000/mm^3 range, which improves slowly, reaching normal levels after the first year. During infancy, environmental stress such as viral illness can precipitate episodes of severe thrombocytopenia. Several TAR patients have an associated storage-pool defect.[403] In addition, these patients have other hematologic changes, including leukemoid reactions to the 30,000 to 40,000/mm^3 range and anemia, at least in part due to blood loss.[398] The skeletal manifestations include complete absence of the radii, but presence of functional thumbs. Other orthopedic abnormalities are seen in 50 percent of cases, and the more severe the upper limb deformity, the more likely the patient is to have a lower limb deformity. In about 30 percent of the patients, there are cardiac anomalies, including tetralogy of Fallot and atrial septal defects.

The etiology of this disorder is unknown. Megakaryocytes are present in the bone marrow, although there may be some decrease as compared with what one would see in thrombocytopenia secondary to increased peripheral destruction.[404] Recently, it was reported that the level of TPO in patients with TAR is elevated despite the presence of Mpl on hematopoietic cells.[405] Whether there is a block in signaling through the Mpl receptor remains to be determined. Certainly other disorders, such as Fanconi anemia and Schwachman syndrome, also have a similar relationship in which skeletal abnormalities occur in conjunction with hematopoietic defects.[406,407] Whether a common growth factor or shared environmental factors underlie these disorders remains to be established.

Familial Platelet Deficiency/Acute Myelogenous Anemia. FPD/AML is a syndrome being recognized with increasing frequency. The initial descriptions of this disorder were based on extended families in which there were enough family members to make a clear diagnosis.[401,402] These families have a dominantly inherited platelet count of ~100,000/mm^3, often associated with a bleeding diathesis out of proportion to the decreased platelet count. Platelet studies in some families show a classic and profound storage-pool defect,[401] but this defect can vary between families and initially suggested that these families have similar phenotypes with different underlying defects. Affected platelets may also be microthrombocytes. There is an ~30 percent lifetime risk of any affected family member developing acute myelogenous leukemia. There is also an increased risk of developing other cancers as well.

In two extended families with dominantly inherited thrombocytopenia, recent studies show the defect localized to a single locus on chromosome 21 near the AML-1 gene.[402,408] AML-1 is a nuclear transcription factor often involved in translocations that result in AML or related cancers. In a recent report, six affected families clearly show that in each, a disrupting mutation is inherited by the affected family members and causes disease by haploinsufficiency.[409] The AML-1 homozygous targeted knockout mice are embryonically lethal, and the heterozygotes have decreased myeloid and erythroid colonies, although no one has determined their megakaryocytic marrow potential or the presence of thrombocytopenia.

Wiskott-Aldrich Syndrome. WAS is associated with platelet size abnormalities, but certainly the phenotype seen is much wider, affecting multiple aspects of platelet and lymphocyte biology. Now that the affected protein has been cloned and termed WAS protein or WASP, it is becoming clear that it is much more appropriate to discuss it under signal transduction, perhaps linked to cytoskeletal rearrangement. WAS was first recognized in two case reports, one in 1954 and one in 1973, as a sex-linked disorder of thrombocytopenia and eczema.[410,411] Platelets are small (Fig. 177-11*C*), usually half-normal volume, and the platelet mass is decreased.[411,412] There appears to be an associated platelet storage-pool defect.[411,412] The thrombocytopenia seen is severe, and can be less than 10,000 platelets/mm^3. These patients have a severe immune defect, in addition to the platelet disorder and eczema. Many die during the first decade from overwhelming infections or immune-based disorders, such as immune thrombocytopenia or hemolytic anemia, and from lymphoma-like illnesses during the second decade of life.[413,414] These patients have an impaired ability to form antibodies to carbohydrate antigens[415] and appear to have a defect in both B and T lymphocytes, but primarily in the latter.[416–419] In fact, the defect in T-lymphocyte function has been used clinically to confirm carrier status, because female carriers for this condition have selective inactivation of their X chromosome in their T lymphocytes.[417–419]

Splenectomy, although it increases the risk of opportunistic infection, often alleviates the thrombocytopenia and bleeding diathesis in this disorder[420] and should be undertaken in spite of the increased risk of bleeding. Immune-related complications respond variably to steroids, IV immunoglobulin, vincristine, or plasmapheresis. Bone marrow transplantation has been efficacious in treating this disorder,[421,422] although the success rate with nonrelated marrow donors is poor.[423]

In addition, there are variations on the classical Wiskott-Aldrich presentation, in which initially the thrombocytopenia is the predominant feature, or in which X-linked thrombocytopenia occurs alone.[399,400] Linkage analysis studies have shown that both the X-linked thrombocytopenia and Wiskott-Aldrich syndrome are localized to the same pericentric region of the X chromosome.[399] In fact, maternal X-chromosome inactivation studies in one of these families demonstrated nonrandom X-inactivation limited to T and B cells and granulocytes, similar to that seen in Wiskott-Aldrich syndrome.[419]

The gene involved in WAS and X-linked thrombocytopenia has been localized on the short arm of the X chromosome and has been cloned.[424] WASP is 501 amino acids long and has no transmembrane domain, but it does have two highly charged C-terminal domains, HHHRHHRHRR (amino acids 394 to 403) and DEGEDQAGDEDEDDEWDD (amino acids 484 to 501).[424] In addition, there is a potential nuclear localization signal (PADKKRSGKKKISK) (amino acids 222 to 235). There is a pleckstrin homology domain and a cofilin domain by which WASP can depolymerize actin. The gene involves 11 exons spanning ~9 kb. WASP expression is limited to lymphocytes and platelets, consistent with the known phenotype of WAS. WASP binds to a number of intracellular signaling proteins such as the Rho family member GTPase Cdc42.[425,426] Tyrosine phosphorylation signaling in the cell appears to cause WASP to become bound to the cytoskeleton through PSTPIP, a cytoskeletal-associated protein,[427] and to be involved in megakaryocytopoiesis.[428,429] A homologous protein has been isolated from neural tissue and termed N-WASP.[430] This protein is involved as a novel actin-depolymerizing protein regulated in a PIP2-dependent manner downstream of tyrosine kinases.

Additional proof that WASP was involved in WAS came in the original description of the gene by the analysis of three affected patients. One had a single nucleotide deletion, the second had a G to T transversion that led to an Arg^{86}Leu substitution, and the third had a G to A transition of the same Arg leading to a His substitution.[424] Since then, more than 20 mutations have been defined.[431,432] Several insights have come from these studies. Aside from the hotspot at codon 86, there is no consistent pattern seen with the defined mutations in the WAS gene, which include deletions and missense, nonsense, and splice junction mutations. Within an individual family with WAS, some patients with WAS may have a milder phenotype than other affected family members with the same mutations. Patients with the X-linked thrombocytopenia phenotype all have missense mutations of the WASP, some of which overlap with mutations seen in WAS. It should be noted that the GATA-1 gene is closely linked to the WAS gene locus.[391] It is therefore possible that X-linked cases of thrombocytopenia may be due to GATA-1 gene mutations when the WAS gene is sequenced and is normal.

ACKNOWLEDGMENTS

We are grateful to Dr. James G. White (University of Minnesota) for providing the electron micrographs used in this chapter. This research was supported by grants HL44612 (to P.J.N.) and HL40387 (to M.P.) from the National Institutes of Health, and by a grant (9750841A, D.L.F.) from the American Heart Association Heritage Affiliate, Inc. P.J.N. is an established investigator (92001390) of the American Heart Association.

REFERENCES

1. Roth GJ: Developing relationships: Arterial platelet adhesion, glycoprotein Ib, and leucine-rich glycoproteins. *Blood* **77**:5, 1991.
2. Lopez JA, Andrews RK, Afshar-Kharghan V, Berndt MC: Bernard-Soulier Syndrome. *Blood* **91**:4397, 1998.
3. Du X, Beutler L, Ruan C, Castaldi PA, Berndt MC: Glycoprotein Ib and glycoprotein IX are fully complexed in the intact platelet membrane. *Blood* **69**:1524, 1987.
4. Modderman PW, Admiraal LG, Sonnenberg A, von dem Borne AEGK: Glycoprotein-V and glycoprotein-Ib-IX form a noncovalent complex in the platelet membrane. *J Biol Chem* **267**:364, 1992.
5. Lanz F, Morales M, de La Salle C, Cazenave J-P, Clemetson KJ, Shimomura T, Phillips DR: Cloning and characterization of the gene encoding the human platelet glycoprotein V. A member of the leucine-rich glycoprotein family cleaved during thrombin-induced platelet activation. *J Biol Chem* **268**:20801, 1993.
6. Caen JP, Levy-Toledano: Interaction between platelets and von Willebrand factor provides a new scheme for primary hemostasis. *Nature* **244**:159, 1971.
7. McEver RP, Martin MN: A monoclonal antibody to a membrane glycoprotein binds only to activated platelets. *J Biol Chem* **259**:9799, 1984.
8. Hsu-Lin S, Berman CL, Furie BC, August D, Furie B: A platelet membrane protein expressed during platelet activation and secretion. Studies using a monoclonal antibody specific for thrombin-activated platelets. *J Biol Chem* **259**:9121, 1984.
9. Bevilacqua M, Butcher E, Furie B, Furie B, Gallatin M, Gimbrone M, Harlan J, Kishimoto K, Lasky L, McEver R, Paulson J, Rosen S, Seed B, Siegelman M, Springer T, Stoolman L, Tedder T, Varki A, Wagner D, Weissman I, Zimmerman G: Selectins: A family of adhesion receptors. *Cell* **67**:233, 1991.
10. McEver RP: Selectins: Novel receptors that mediate leukocyte adhesion during inflammation. *Thromb Haemost* **65**:223, 1991.
11. Larsen E, Celi A, Gilbert GE, Furie BC, Erban JK, Bonfanti R, Wagner DD, Furie B: PADGEM protein: A receptor that mediates the interaction of activated platelets with neutrophils and monocytes. *Cell* **59**:305, 1989.

12. Albelda SM, Buck CA: Integrins and other cell adhesion molecules. *FASEB J* **4**:2868, 1990.
13. Hynes RO: Integrins, a family of cell surface receptors. *Cell* **48**:549, 1987.
14. Wagner CL, Mascelli MA, Neblock DS, Weisman HF, Coller BS, Jordan RE: Analysis of GPIIb/IIIa receptor number by quantitation of 7E3 binding to human platelets. *Blood* **88**:907, 1996.
15. Fitzgerald LA, Poncz M, Steiner B, Rall SC Jr, Bennett JS, Phillips DR: Comparison of cDNA-derived protein sequences of the human fibronectin and vitronectin receptor alpha-subunits and platelet glycoprotein IIb. *Biochemistry* **26**:8158, 1987.
16. Poncz M, Newman PJ: Analysis of rodent platelet glycoprotein IIb: Evidence for evolutionarily conserved domains and alternative proteolytic processing. *Blood* **75**:1282, 1990.
17. Coller BS, Cheresh DA, Asch E, Seligsohn U: Platelet vitronectin receptor expression differentiates Iraqi-Jewish from Arab patients with Glanzmann thrombasthenia in Israel. *Blood* **77**:75, 1991.
18. Thiagarajan P, Shapiro SS, Levine E, DeMarco L, Yalcin A: A monoclonal antibody to human platelet Glycoprotein IIIa detects a related protein in cultured human endothelial cells. *J Clin Invest* **75**:896, 1985.
19. Santoro SA: Identification of a 160,000-dalton platelet membrane protein that mediates the initial divalent cation-dependent adhesion of platelets to collagen. *Cell* **46**:913, 1986.
20. Kunicki TJ, Nugent DJ, Staats SJ, Orchekowski RP, Wayner EA, Carter WG: The human fibroblast class II extracellular matrix receptor mediates platelet adhesion to collagen and is identical to the platelet glycoprotein Ia-IIa complex. *J Biol Chem* **263**:4516, 1988.
21. Piotrowicz RS, Orchekowski RP, Nugent DJ, Yamada KY, Kunicki TJ: Glycoprotein Ic-IIa functions as an activation-independent fibronectin receptor on human platelets. *J Cell Biol* **106**:1359, 1988.
22. Sonnenberg A, Modderman PW, Hogervorst F: Laminin receptor on platelets in the integrin VLA-6. *Nature* **336**:487, 1988.
23. Lee J-O, Rieu P, Arnaout MA, Liddington R: Crystal structure of the A domain from the α subunit of integrin CR3 (CD11b/CD18). *Cell* **80**:631, 1995.
24. Tozer EC, Liddington RC, Sutcliffe MJ, Smeeton AH, Loftus JC: Ligand binding to integrin αIIbβ3 is dependent on a MIDAS-like domain in the β3 subunit. *J Biol Chem* **271**:21978, 1996.
25. Tuckwell DS, Humphries MJ: A structure prediction for the ligand-binding region of the integrin β subunit: Evidence for the presence of a von Willebrand factor A domain. *FEBS Lett* **400**:297, 1997.
26. Takagi J, Kamata T, Meredith J, Puzon-McLaughlin W, Takada Y: Changing ligand specificities of αvβ1 and αvβ3 integrins by swapping a short diverse sequence of the β subunit. *J Biol Chem* **272**:19794, 1997.
27. Coller BS: Blockade of platelet GPIIb/IIIa receptors as an antithrombotic strategy. *Circulation* **92**:2373, 1995.
28. George JN, Caen JP, Nurden AT: Glanzmann's thrombasthenia: The spectrum of clinical disease. *Blood* **75**:1383, 1990.
29. French DL: The molecular genetics of Glanzmann's thrombasthenia. *Platelets* **9**:5, 1998.
30. Newman PJ: Platelet GPIIb-IIIa: Molecular variations and alloantigens. *Thromb Haemost* **66**:111, 1991.
31. Calvete JJ: On the structure and function of platelet integrin αIIbβ3, the fibrinogen receptor. *Proc Soc Exp Biol Med* **208**:346, 1995.
32. Shattil SJ, Kashiwagi H, Pampori N: Integrin signaling: The platelet paradigm. *Blood* **91**:2645, 1998.
33. Bray PF, Rosa JP, Lingappa VR, Kan YW, McEver RP, Shuman MA: Biogenesis of the platelet receptor for fibrinogen: Evidence for separate precursors for glycoproteins IIb and IIIa. *Proc Natl Acad Sci U S A* **83**:1480, 1986.
34. Silver SM, McDonough MM, Vilaire G, Bennett JS: The in vitro synthesis of polypeptides for the platelet membrane glycoproteins IIb and IIIa. *Blood* **69**:1031, 1987.
35. Thornton MA, Poncz M, Korostishevsky M, Yakobson E, Usher S, Seligsohn U, Peretz H: The human platelet αIIb gene is not closely linked to its integrin partner β3. *Blood* **44**:2039, 1999.
36. Bray PF, Rosa JP, Johnston GI, Shiu DT, Cook RG, Lau C, Kan YW, McEver RP, Shuman MA: Platelet glycoprotein IIb. Chromosomal localization and tissue expression. *J Clin Invest* **80**:1812, 1987.
37. Poncz M, Eisman R, Heidenreich R, Silver SM, Vilaire G, Surrey S, Schwartz E, Bennett JS: Structure of the platelet membrane glycoprotein IIb. Homology to the alpha subunits of the vitronectin and fibronectin membrane receptors. *J Biol Chem* **262**:8476, 1987.
38. Gulino D, Boudignon C, Zhang LY, Concord E, Rabiet MJ, Marguerie G: Ca(2+)-binding properties of the platelet glycoprotein IIb ligand-interacting domain. *J Biol Chem* **267**:1001, 1992.
39. Brass LF, Shattil SJ, Kunicki TJ, Bennett JS: Effect of calcium on the stability of the platelet membrane glycoprotein IIb-IIIa complex. *J Biol Chem* **260**:7875, 1985.
40. Kunicki TJ, Pidard D, Rosa J-P, Nurden AT: The formation of Ca++-dependent complexes of platelet membrane glycoproteins IIb and IIIa in solution as determined by crossed immunoelectrophoresis. *Blood* **58**:268, 1981.
41. Fitzgerald LA, Phillips DR: Calcium regulation of the platelet membrane glycoprotein IIb-IIIa complex. *J Biol Chem* **260**:11366, 1985.
42. Loftus JC, Halloran CE, Ginsberg MH, Feigen LP, Zablocki JA, Smith JW: The amino-terminal one-third of αIIb defines the ligand recognition specificity of integrin αIIbβ3. *J Biol Chem* **271**:2033, 1996.
43. Tuckwell DS, Humphries MJ, Brass A: A secondary structure model of the integrin α subunit N-terminal domain based on analysis of multiple alignments. *Cell Adhes Commun* **2**:385, 1994.
44. Springer TA: Folding of the N-terminal, ligand-binding region of integrin α-subunits into a β-propeller domain. *Proc Natl Acad Sci U S A* **94**:65, 1997.
45. Zimrin AB, Eisman R, Vilaire G, Schwartz E, Bennett JS, Poncz M: Structure of platelet glycoprotein IIIa. A common subunit for two different membrane receptors. *J Clin Invest* **81**:1470, 1988.
46. Fitzgerald LA, Steiner B, Rall SC Jr, Lo SS, Phillips DR: Protein sequence of endothelial glycoprotein IIIa derived from a cDNA clone. Identity with platelet glycoprotein IIIa and similarity to "integrin." *J Biol Chem* **262**:3936, 1987.
47. Rosa JP, Bray PF, Gayet O, Johnston GI, Cook RG, Jackson KW, Shuman MA, McEver RP: Cloning of glycoprotein IIIa cDNA from human erythroleukemia cells and localization of the gene to chromosome 17. *Blood* **72**:593, 1988.
48. Calvete JJ, Henschen A, Gonzalez-Rodriguez J: Assignment of disulphide bonds in human platelet GPIIIa. A disulphide pattern for the beta-subunits of the integrin family. *Biochem J* **274**:63, 1991.
49. D'Souza SE, Ginsberg MH, Lam SC, Plow EF: Chemical cross-linking of arginyl-glycyl-aspartic acid peptides to an adhesion receptor on platelets. *J Biol Chem* **263**:3943, 1988.
50. Beer J, Coller BS: Evidence that platelet glycoprotein IIIa has a large disulfide-bonded loop that is susceptible to proteolytic cleavage. *J Biol Chem* **264**:17564, 1989.
51. McEver RP, Baenziger JU, Majerus PW: Isolation and structural characterization of the polypeptide subunits of membrane glycoprotein IIb-IIIa from human platelets. *Blood* **59**:80, 1982.
52. Newman PJ, Martin LS, Knipp MA, Kahn RA: Studies on the nature of the human platelet alloantigen, PlA1: Localization to a 17,000-dalton polypeptide. *Mol Immunol* **22**:719, 1985.
53. Tsuji T, Osawa T: Structures of the carbohydrate chains of membrane glycoproteins IIb and IIIa of human platelets. *Biochem J* **100**:1387, 1986.
54. Duperray A, Berthier R, Chagnon E, Ryckewaert JJ, Ginsberg M, Plow E, Marguerie G: Biosynthesis and processing of platelet GPIIb-IIIa in human megakaryocytes. *J Cell Biol* **104**:1665,1987.
55. Calvete JJ, Henschen A, Gonzalez-Rodriguez J: Complete localization of the intrachain disulphide bonds and the *N*-glycosylation points in the alpha-subunit of human platelet glycoprotein IIb. *Biochem J* **261**:561, 1989.
56. Newman PJ, Allen RW, Kahn RA, Kunicki TJ: Quantitation of membrane glycoprotein IIIa on intact human platelets using the monoclonal antibody, AP-3. *Blood* **65**:227, 1985.
57. Woods VL Jr, Wolff LE, Keller DM: Resting platelets contain a substantial centrally located pool of glycoprotein IIb-IIIa complex which may be accessible to some but not other extracellular proteins. *J Biol Chem* **261**:15242, 1986.
58. Wencel-Drake JD, Plow EF, Kunicki TJ, Woods VL, Keller DM, Ginsberg MH: Localization of internal pools of membrane glycoproteins involved in platelet adhesive responses. *Am J Pathol* **124**:324, 1986.
59. Shattil SJ, Kashiwagi H, Pampori N: Integrin signaling: The platelet paradigm. *Blood* **91**:2645, 1998.
60. Yamada KM, Geiger B: Molecular interactions in cell adhesion complexes. *Curr Biol* **9**:76, 1997.
61. Pierschbacher MD, Ruoslahti E: Cell attachment activity of fibronectin can be duplicated by small synthetic fragments of the molecule. *Nature* **309**:30, 1984.

62. Haverstick DM, Cowan JF, Yamada KM, Santoro SA: Inhibition of platelet adhesion to fibronectin, fibrinogen, and von Willebrand factor by a synthetic tetrapeptide derived from the cell-binding domain of fibronectin. *Blood* **66**:946, 1985.
63. Pytela R, Pierschbacher MD, Ginsberg MH, Plow EF, Ruoslahti E: Platelet membrane glycoprotein IIb/IIIa: Member of a family of Arg-Gly-Asp-specific adhesion receptors. *Science* **231**:1559, 1986.
64. Ginsberg MH, Pierschbacher MD, Ruoslahti E, Marguerie G, Plow EF: Inhibition of fibronectin binding to platelets by proteolytic fragments and synthetic peptides which support fibroblast adhesion. *J Biol Chem* **260**:3931, 1985.
65. Hawiger J, Timmons S, Kloczewiak M, Strong DD, Doolittle RF: Gamma and alpha chains of human fibrinogen possess sites reactive with human platelet receptors. *Proc Natl Acad Sci U S A* **79**:2068, 1982.
66. Amrani DL, Newman PJ, Meh D, Mosesson MW: The role of fibrinogen A alpha chains in ADP-induced platelet aggregation in the presence of fibrinogen molecules containing gamma chains. *Blood* **72**:919, 1988.
67. Gartner TK, Bennett JS: The tetrapeptide analogue of the cell attachment site of fibronectin inhibits platelet aggregation and fibrinogen binding to activated platelets. *J Biol Chem* **260**:11891, 1985.
68. Plow EF, Pierschbacher MD, Ruoslahti E, Marguerie G, Ginsberg MH: The effect of Arg-Gly-Asp-containing peptides on fibrinogen and von Willebrand factor binding to platelets. *Proc Natl Acad Sci U S A* **82**:8057, 1985.
69. Charo IF, Nannizzi L, Phillips DR, Hsu MA, Scarborough RM: Inhibition of fibrinogen binding to GP IIb-IIIa by a GP IIIa peptide. *J Biol Chem* **266**:1415, 1991.
70. Bajt ML, Ginsberg MH, Frelinger AL, III, Berndt MC, Loftus JC: A spontaneous mutation of integrin αIIbβ3 (platelet glycoprotein IIb-IIIa) helps define a ligand binding site. *J Biol Chem* **267**:3789, 1992.
71. Bajt ML, Loftus JC: Mutation of a ligand binding domain of β3 integrin. Integral role of oxygenated residues in αIIbβ3 (GPIIb/IIIa) receptor function. *J Biol Chem* **269**:20913, 1994.
72. Baker EK, Tozer EC, Pfaff M, Shattil SJ, Loftus JC, Ginsberg MH: A genetic analysis of integrin function: Glanzmann thrombasthenia in vitro. *Proc Natl Acad Sci U S A* **94**:1973, 1997.
73. Kloczewiak M, Timmons S, Lukas TJ, Hawiger J: Platelet receptor recognition site on human fibrinogen. Synthesis and structure-function relationships of peptides corresponding to the carboxy-terminal segment of the gamma chain. *Biochemistry* **23**:1767, 1984.
74. Timmons S, Bednarek MA, Kloczewiak M, Hawiger J: Antiplatelet "hybrid" peptides analogous to receptor recognition domains on gamma and alpha chains of human fibrinogen. *Biochemistry* **28**:2929, 1989.
75. Hawiger J, Timmons S: Binding of fibrinogen and von Willebrand factor to platelet glycoprotein IIb-IIIa complex. *Methods Enzymol* **215**:228, 1982.
76. Farrell DH, Thiagarajan P, Chung DW, Davie EW: Role of fibrinogen α and γ chain sites in platelet aggregation. *Proc Natl Acad Sci U S A* **89**:10729, 1992.
77. D'Souza SE, Ginsberg MH, Burke TA, Plow EF: The ligand binding site of the platelet integrin receptor GPIIb-IIIa is proximal to the second calcium binding domain of its alpha subunit. *J Biol Chem* **265**:2440, 1990.
78. D'Souza SE, Ginsberg MH, Matsueda GR, Plow EF: A discrete sequence in a platelet integrin is involved in ligand recognition. *Nature* **350**:66, 1991.
79. Saiki RK, Gelfand DH, Stoffel S, Scharf SJ, Higuchi RG, Horn GT, Mullis KB, Erlich HA: Primer-directed enzymatic amplification of DNA with a thermostable DNA polymerase. *Science* **239**:487, 1988.
80. Newman PJ, Gorski J, White GCI, Gidwitz S, Cretney CJ, Aster RH: Enzymatic amplification of platelet-specific messenger RNA using the polymerase chain reaction. *J Clin Invest* **82**:739, 1988.
81. Bray PF: Inherited diseases of platelet glycoproteins: Considerations for rapid molecular characterization. *Thromb Haemost* **72**:492, 1994.
82. Glanzmann E: Hereditare hamorrhagische thrombasthenie: ein beitrag zur pathologie der blut plattchen. *J Kinderkr* **88**:113, 1918.
83. Braunsteiner H, Pakesch F: Thrombocytasthenia and thrombocytopathia. Old names and new diseases. *Blood* **2**:965, 1956.
84. Hardisty RM, Dormandy KM, Hutton RA: Thrombasthenia: Studies on three cases. *Br J Haematol* **10**:371, 1964.
85. Zucker MB, Pert JH, Hilgartner HR: Platelet function in a patient with thrombasthenia. *Blood* **28**:524, 1966.
86. Tengborn L, Petruson B: A patient with Glanzmann thrombasthenia and epistaxis successfully treated with recombinant factor VIIa. *Thromb Haemost* **75**:981, 1996.
87. Hodivala-Dilke KM, McHugh KP, Tsakiris DA, Rayburn H, D C, M U-C, Ross FP, Coller BS, Teitelbaum S, Hynes RO: Beta3-integrin-deficient mice are a model for Glanzmann thrombasthenia showing placental defects and reduced survival. *J Clin Invest* **103**:229, 1999.
88. Reichert N, Seligsohn U, Ramot B: Thrombasthenia in Iraqi Jews. *Isr J Med Sci* **9**:1406, 1973.
89. Reichert N, Seligsohn U, Ramot B: Clinical and genetic aspects of Glanzmann's thrombasthenia in Israel. Report of 22 cases. *Thromb Diath Haemorrh* **34**:806, 1975.
90. Seligsohn U, Rososhansky S: A Glanzmann's thrombasthenia cluster among Iraqi Jews in Israel. *Thromb Haemost* **52**:230, 1984.
91. Awidi AS: Increased incidence of Glanzmann's thrombasthenia in Jordan as compared with Scandinavia. *Scand J Haematol* **30**:218, 1983.
92. Caen JP, Castaldi PA, Leclerc JC, Inceman S, Larrieu M-J, Probst M, Bernard J: Congenital bleeding disorders with long bleeding time and normal platelet count. I. Glanzmann's thrombasthenia (report of fifteen patients). *Am J Med* **41**:4, 1966.
93. Bentegeat J, Verger P, Boisseau M, De Ioigny C, Guiliard JM, Le Menn R: Considerations cliniques, genetiques, biologiques et physiologiques sur la thrombasthenie de Glanzmann (a propos de 5 cas). *Coagulation* **1**:237, 1968.
94. Levy JM, Mayer G, Sacrez R, Ruff R, Francfort JJ, Rodier L: Glanzmann thrombasthenia-Naegeli. Study of a strongly endogamous ethnic group. *Semin Hosp Paris* **47**:129, 1971.
95. Khanduri U, Pulimood R, Sudarsanam A, Carman RH, Jadhav M, Pereira S: Glanzmann's thrombasthenia. A review and report of 42 cases from South India. *Thromb Haemost* **46**:717, 1981.
96. Jin Y, Dietz HC, Montgomery RA, Bell WR, McIntosh I, Coller B, Bray PF: Glanzmann thrombasthenia. Cooperation between sequence variants in *cis* during splice site selection. *J Clin Invest* **98**:1745, 1996.
97. Rosenberg N, Yatuv R, Orion Y, Zivelin A, Dardik R, Peretz H, Seligsohn U: Glanzmann thrombasthenia caused by an 11.2-kb deletion in the glycoprotein IIIa (β_3) is a second mutation in Iraqi Jews that stemmed from a distinct founder. *Blood* **89**:3654, 1997.
98. Caen JP: Glanzmann's thrombasthenia. *Clin Haematol* **1**:383, 1972.
99. Nurden AT, Caen JP: An abnormal platelet glycoprotein pattern in three cases of Glanzmann's thrombasthenia. *Br J Haematol* **28**:253, 1974.
100. Nurden AT, Caen JP: Specific roles for platelet surface glycoproteins in platelet function. *Nature* **255**:720, 1975.
101. Phillips DR, Agin PP: Platelet membrane defects in Glanzmann's thrombasthenia. Evidence for decreased amounts of two major glycoproteins. *J Clin Invest* **60**:535, 1977.
102. Kunicki TJ, Aster RH: Deletion of the platelet-specific alloantigen PlA1 from platelets in Glanzmann's thrombasthenia. *J Clin Invest* **61**:1225, 1978.
103. Hagen I, Nurden AT, Bjerrum OJ, Solum NO, Caen JP: Immunochemical evidence for protein abnormalities in platelets from patients with Glanzmann's thrombasthenia and Bernard Soulier syndrome. *J Clin Invest* **65**:722, 1980.
104. Kunicki TJ, Nurden AT, Pidard D, Russell NR, Caen JP: Characterization of human platelet glycoprotein antigens giving rise to individual immunoprecipitates in crossed-immunoelectrophoresis. *Blood* **58**:1190, 1981.
105. Holahan JR, White GC: Heterogeneity of membrane surface proteins in Glanzmann's thrombasthenia. *Blood* **57**:174, 1981.
106. Ginsberg MH, Lightsey A, Kunicki TJ, Kaufmann A, Marguerie G, Plow EF: Divalent cation regulation of the surface orientation of platelet membrane glycoprotein IIb. Correlation with fibrinogen binding function and definition of a novel variant of Glanzmann's thrombasthenia. *J Clin Invest* **78**:1103, 1986.
107. Caen JP, Rosa JP, Boizard B, Nurden AT: Thrombasthenia Paris I Lariboisiere variant, a model for the study of the platelet glycoprotein (GP) IIb-IIIa complex. *Blood* **62**:951a, 1983.
108. Nurden AT, Rosa JP, Fournier D, Legrand C, Didry D, Parquet A, Pidard D: A variant of Glanzmann's thrombasthenia with abnormal glycoprotein IIb-IIIa complexes in the platelet membrane. *J Clin Invest* **79**:962, 1987.
109. Fournier DJ, Kabral A, Castaldi PA, Berndt MC: A variant of Glanzmann's thrombasthenia characterized by abnormal glycoprotein IIb/IIIa complex formation. *Thromb Haemost* **62**:977, 1989.

110. Bennett JS, Vilaire G: Exposure of platelet fibrinogen receptors by ADP and epinephrine. *J Clin Invest* **64**:1393, 1979.
111. Ruggeri ZM, Bader R, De Marco L: Glanzmann thrombasthenia: Deficient binding of von Willebrand factor to thrombin-stimulated platelets. *Proc Natl Acad Sci U S A* **79**:6038, 1982.
112. Kato A, Yamamoto K, Aoki N: Classification of Glanzmann's thrombasthenia based on the intracellular transport pathway of GPIIb-IIIa. *Thromb Haemost* **68**:615, 1992.
113. Jennings LK, Ashmun RA, Wang WC, Docker ME: Analysis of human platelet glycoproteins IIb-IIIa and Glanzmann's thrombasthenia in whole blood by flow cytometry. *Blood* **68**:173, 1986.
114. Nurden AT, Didry D, Kieffer N, McEver RP: Residual amounts of glycoproteins IIb and IIIa may be present in the platelets of most patients with Glanzmann's thrombasthenia. *Blood* **65**:1021, 1985.
115. McEver RP, Baenziger NL, Majerus PW: Isolation and quantitation of the platelet membrane glycoprotein deficient in thrombasthenia using a monoclonal hybridoma antibody. *J Clin Invest* **66**:1311, 1980.
116. Montgomery RR, Kunicki TJ, Taves C, Pidard D, Corcoran M: Diagnosis of Bernard-Soulier syndrome and Glanzmann's thrombasthenia with a monoclonal assay on whole blood. *J Clin Invest* **71**:385, 1983.
117. Coller BS, Seligsohn U, Little PA: Type I Glanzmann thrombasthenia patients from the Iraqi-Jewish and Arab populations in Israel can be differentiated by platelet glycoprotein IIIa immunoblot analysis. *Blood* **69**:1696, 1987.
118. Coller BS, Cheresh DA, Asch E, Seligsohn U: Platelet vitronectin receptor expression differentiates Iraqi-Jewish from Arab patients with Glanzmann thrombasthenia in Israel. *Blood* **77**:75, 1991.
119. Rosenberg N, Dardik R, Rosenthal E, Zivelin A, Seligsohn U: Mutations in the alphaIIb and beta3 genes that cause Glanzmann thrombasthenia can be distinguished by a simple procedure using transformed B-lymphocytes. *Thromb Haemost* **79**:244, 1998.
120. Newman PJ, Seligsohn U, Lyman S, Coller BS: The molecular genetic basis of Glanzmann thrombasthenia in the Iraqi-Jewish and Arab populations in Israel. *Proc Natl Acad Sci U S A* **88**:3160, 1991.
121. Burk CD, Newman PJ, Lyman S, Gill J, Coller BS, Poncz M: A deletion in the gene for glycoprotein IIb associated with Glanzmann's thrombasthenia. *J Clin Invest* **87**:270, 1991.
122. Poncz M, Rifat S, Coller BS, Newman PJ, Shattil SJ, Parrella T, Fortina P, Bennett JS: Glanzmann thrombasthenia secondary to a Gly^{273}Asp mutation adjacent to the first calcium-binding domain of platelet glycoprotein IIb. *J Clin Invest* **93**:172, 1994.
123. Grimaldi CM, Chen FP, Scudder LE, Coller BS, French DL: A Cys^{374}Tyr homozygous mutation of platelet glycoprotein IIIa ($\beta 3$) in a Chinese patient with Glanzmann's thrombasthenia. *Blood* **88**:1666, 1996.
124. Grimaldi CM, Chen FP, Wu CH, Weiss HJ, Coller BS, French DL: Glycoprotein IIb Leu^{214}Pro mutation produces Glanzmann thrombasthenia with both quantitative and qualitative abnormalities in GPIIb/IIIa. *Blood* **91**:1562, 1998.
125. French DL, Coller BS: Hematologically important mutations: Glanzmann thrombasthenia. *Blood Cells Mol Dis* **23**:39, 1996.
126. Seligsohn U, Mibashan RS, Rodeck CH, Nicolaides KH, Millar DS, Coller BS: Prenatal diagnosis of Glanzmann's thrombasthenia. *Lancet* **II**:1419, 1985.
127. French DL, Coller BS, Usher S, Berkowitz R, Eng C, Seligsohn U, Peretz H: Prenatal diagnosis of Glanzmann thrombasthenia using the polymorphic markers BRCA1 and THRA1 on chromosome 17. *Br J Haematol* **102**:582,1998.
128. Basani RB, French DL, Vilaire G, Brown DL, Chen FP, Coller BS, Derrick JM, Gartner TK, Bennett JS, Poncz M: A naturally occurring mutation near the amino terminus of αIIb defines a new region involved in ligand binding to αIIbβ3. *Blood* **95**:180, 2000.
129. Ruan J, Peyruchaud O, Alberio L, Valles G, Clemetson K, Bourre F, Nurden AT: Double heterozygosity of the GPIIb gene in a Swiss patient with Glanzmann's thrombasthenia. *Br J Haematol* **102**:918, 1998.
130. Bourre R, Peyruchaud O, Bray P, Combrie R, Nurden P, Nurden AT: A point mutation in the gene for platelet GPIIb leads to a substitution in a highly conserved amino acid located between the second and the third Ca^{++}-binding domain. *Blood* **86**:452a, 1995.
131. Wilcox DA, Paddock CM, Lyman S, Gill JC, Newman PJ: Glanzmann thrombasthenia resulting from a single amino acid substitution between the second and third calcium-binding domains of GPIIb. *J Clin Invest* **95**:1553, 1995.
132. Ferrer M, Fernandez-Pinel M, Gonzalez-Manchon C, Gonzalez J, Ayuso MS, Parrilla R: A mutant (Arg327His) GPIIb associated to thrombasthenia exerts a dominant negative effect in stably transfected CHO cells. *Thromb Haemost* **76**:292, 1996.
133. Wilcox DA, Wautier JL, Pidard D, Newman PJ: A single amino acid substitution flanking the fourth calcium binding domain of αIIb prevents maturation of the integrin αIIbβ3 complex. *J Biol Chem* **269**:4450, 1994.
134. Basani RB, Vilaire G, Shattil SJ, Kolodziej MA, Bennett JS, Poncz M: Glanzmann thrombasthenia due to a two amino acid deletion in the fourth calcium-binding domain of αIIb: Demonstration of the importance of calcium-binding domains in the conformation of αIIbβ. *Blood* **88**:167, 1996.
135. Irie A, Kamata T, Puzon-McLaughlin W, Takada Y: Critical amino acid residues for ligand binding are clustered in a predicted β-turn of the third N-terminal repeat in the integrin α4 and α5 subunits. *EMBO J* **14**:5550, 1995.
136. Kamata T, Irie A, Tokuhira M, Takada Y: Critical residues of integrin αIIb subunit for binding of αIIbβ3 (glycoprotein IIb-IIIa) to fibrinogen and ligand-mimetic antibodies (PAC-1, OP-G2, and LJ-CP3). *J Biol Chem* **271**:18610, 1996.
137. Westrup D, Santoso S, Becker-Hagendorff K, Just M, Jablonka B, Siefried E, Kirchmaier CM: Transfection of GPIIbIle176/IIIa (Frankfurt I) in mammalian cells. *Thromb Haemost* **77**:671, 1997.
138. Tozer EC, Baker E, Ginsberg MH, Loftus JC: A mutation in the α subunit of the platelet integrin αIIbβ3 identifies a novel region important for ligand binding. *Blood* **93**:918, 1999.
139. Loftus JC, O'Toole TE, Plow EF, Glass A, Frelinger AL, III, Ginsberg MH: A β3 integrin mutation abolishes ligand binding and alters divalent cation-dependent conformation. *Science* **249**:915, 1990.
140. Ward CM, Chao YL, Kato GJ, Casella J, Bray PF, Newman PJ: Substitution of Asn, but not Tyr, for Asp119 of the β3 integrin subunit preserves fibrin binding and clot retraction. *Blood* **90**:26a, 1997.
141. Lanza F, Stierle A, Fournier D, Morales M, Andre G, Nurden AT, Cazenave J-P: A new variant of Glanzmann's thrombasthenia (Strasbourg I). Platelets with functionally defective glycoprotein IIb-IIIa complexes and a glycoprotein IIIa Arg^{214}Trp mutation. *J Clin Invest* **89**:1995, 1992.
142. Djaffer I, Rosa J-P: A second case of variant of Glanzmann's thrombasthenia due to substitution of platelet GPIIIa (integrin β_3) Arg^{214} by Trp. *Hum Mol Genet* **2**:2179, 1993.
143. Newman PJ, Weyerbusch-Bottum S, Visentin GP, Gidwitz S, White GCI: Type II Glanzmann thrombasthenia due to a destabilizing amino acid substitution in platelet membrane glycoprotein IIIa. *Thromb Haemost* **69**:1017, 1993.
144. Basani RB, Brown DL, Vilaire G, Bennett JS, Poncz M: A Leu^{117}Trp mutation within the RGD-peptide cross-linking region of β3 results in Glanzmann thrombasthenia by preventing αIIbβ3 export to the platelet surface. *Blood* **90**:3082, 1997.
145. Jackson DE, White MM, Jennings LK, Newman PJ: A Ser^{162}Leu mutation within glycoprotein (GP) IIIa (integrin β3) results in an unstable αIIbβ3 complex that retains partial function in a novel form of type II Glanzmann thrombasthenia. *Thromb Haemost* **80**:42, 1998.
146. Ward CM, Kestin AS, Newman PJ: A Leu^{262}Pro mutation in the integrin β3 subunit results in an αIIbβ3 complex that binds fibrin but not fibrinogen. *Blood* **96**:161, 2000.
147. Chen Y-P, I, Pidard D, Steiner B, Cieutat A-M, Caen JP, Rosa J-P: Ser^{752}Pro mutation in the cytoplasmic domain of integrin β3 subunit and defective activation of platelet integrin αIIbβ3(glycoprotein IIb-IIIa) in a variant of Glanzmann thrombasthenia. *Proc Natl Acad Sci U S A* **89**:10169, 1992.
148. Ylanne J, Chen Y, O'Toole TE, Loftus JC, Takada Y, Ginsberg MH: Distinct functions of integrin α and β subunit cytoplasmic domains in cell spreading and formation of focal adhesions. *J Cell Biol* **122**:223, 1993.
149. Ylanne J, Huuskonen J, O'Toole TE, Ginsberg MH, Virtanen I, Gahmberg CG: Mutation of the cytoplasmic domain of the integrin β_3 subunit. *J Biol Chem* **270**:9550, 1995.
150. Wang R, Shattil SJ, Ambruso DR, Newman PJ: Truncation of the cytoplasmic domain of β3 in a variant form of Glanzmann thrombasthenia abrogates signaling through the integrin αIIbβ3 complex. *J Clin Invest* **100**:2393, 1997.
151. Chen Y-P, O'Toole TE, Ylanne J, Rosa J-P, Ginsberg MH: A point mutation in the integrin β3 cytoplasmic domain (S752P) impairs bidirectional signaling through αIIbβ3 (platelet glycoprotein IIb-IIIa). *Blood* **84**:1857, 1994.

152. Baumgartner HR, Muggli R: Adhesion and aggregation: Morphological demonstration and quantitation in vivo and in vitro, in Gordon JL (ed): *Platelets in Biology and Pathology.* New York, Elsevier, 1976, p 23.
153. Baumgartner HR, Tschopp TB, Meyer D: Shear rate dependent inhibition of platelet adhesion and aggregation on collagenous surfaces by antibodies to Factor VIII/von Willebrand factor. *Br J Haematol* **44**:127, 1980.
154. Turritto VT, Weiss HJ, Zimmerman TS, Sussman II: Factor VIII/von Willebrand factor in subendothelium mediates platelets adhesion. *Blood* **65**:823, 1985.
155. Turritto VT, Weiss HJ, Baumgartner HS: Decreased platelet adhesion on vessel segment in von Willebrand's disease: A defect in initial platelet attachment. *J Lab Clin Med* **102**:551, 1983.
156. Jorgensen L, Borchgrevink CF: The hemostatic mechanism in patients with haemorrhagic diseases: A histological study of wounds made for primary and secondary bleeding time tests. *Acta Pathol Microbiol Scand* **60**:55, 1964.
157. Hovig T, Stormorken H: Ultrastructural studies on the platelet plug in bleeding time wounds from normal individuals and patients with von Willebrand's Disease. *Acta Pathol Microbiol Immunol Scand* **248**:105, 1974.
158. Sixma JJ, Wester J: The hemostatic plug. *Semin Hematol* **14**:265, 1977.
159. Ruggeri ZM, De Marco L, Gatti L, Bader R, Montgomery RR: Platelets have more than one binding site for von Willebrand factor. *J Clin Invest* **72**:1, 1983.
160. Sixma JJ, Sakariassen KS, Besser-Visser NH, Ottenhof-Rovers M, Bolhuis PA: Adhesion of platelets to human artery subendothelium: Effect of factor VIII-von Willebrand factor of various multimeric composition. *Blood* **63**:128, 1984.
161. Chopek MW, Gilma J-P, Fujikawa K, Davis EW, Titani K: Human von Willebrand factor: A multivalent protein composed of identical subunits. *Biochemistry* **25**:3146, 1986.
162. Coller BS, Peerschke EL, Scudder IE, Sullivan CA: Studies with a murine monoclonal antibody that abolishes ristocetin-induced binding of von Willebrand factor to platelets: Additional evidence in support of GPIb as a platelet receptor for von Willebrand factor. *Blood* **61**:99, 1983.
162a. Reinke R, Krantz DE, Yen D, Zipursky SL: Chaoptin, a cell-surface glycoprotein required for *Drosophila* photoreceptor cell morphogenesis, contains a repeat motif found in yeast and human. *Cell* **52**:291, 1988.
163. McFarland KC, Sprengel R, Phillips HS, Kohler M, Rosemblit N, Nikolics K, Segaloff DL, Seeburg PH: Lutropin-choriogonadotropin receptor: An unusual member of the G protein-coupled receptor family. *Science* **245**:494, 1989.
164. Kataoka T, Broek D, Wigler M: DNA sequence and characterization of the *S. cerevisiae* gene encoding adenylate cyclase. *Cell* **43**:493, 1985.
165. Landschultz WH, Johnson OF, McKnight SL: The leucine zipper: A hypothetical structure common to a new class of DNA binding proteins. *Science* **240**:1759, 1990.
166. Bohmann D, Bos TJ, Admon A, Nishimura T, Vogt PK, Tjian R: Human proto-oncogene *c*-jun encodes a DNA binding protein with structural and functional properties of transcription factor AP-1. *Science* **238**:1386, 1987.
167. Setoyama C, Frunzio R, Liau G, Mudryj M, de Crombrugghe B: Transcription activation encoded by the *v*-fos gene. *Proc Natl Acad Sci U S A* **83**:3213, 1986.
168. Phillips DR, Jakabova M: Ca2+-dependent protease in human platelets. Specific cleavage of platelet polypeptides in the presence of added Ca2+. *J Biol Chem* **252**:5602, 1977.
169. Okumura T, Lombart C, Jamieson GA: Platelet glycocalicin II. Purification and characterization. *J Biol Chem* **251**:5950, 1976.
170. Handa M, Titani K, Holland LZ, Roberts JR, Ruggeri Z: The von Willebrand factor-binding domain of platelet membrane glycoprotein Ib. *J Biol Chem* **261**:12579, 1986.
171. Wicki AN, Clemetson KJ: Structure and function of platelet membrane glycoprotein Ib and V. Effects of leucocyte elastase and other proteases on platelet response to von Willebrand factor and thrombin. *Eur J Biochem* **153**:1, 1985.
172. Yamamoto K, Yamamoto N, Kitagawa H, Tanoue K, Kosaki G, Yamazaki H: Localization of a thrombin-binding site on human platelet membrane Ib determined by a monoclonal antibody. *Thromb Haemost* **55**:162, 1986.
173. Berndt MC, Gregory C, Dowden G, Castaldi PA: Thrombin interactions with platelet membrane proteins. *Ann N Y Acad Sci* **485**:374, 1986.
174. Coughlin SR: Sol Sherry lecture in thrombosis: How thrombin "talks" to cells: Molecular mechanisms and roles in vivo. *Arterioscler Thromb Vasc Biol* **18**:514, 1998.
175. Vicente V, Houghten RA, Ruggeri ZM: Identification of a site in the alpha chain of platelet glycoprotein Ib that participates in von Willebrand factor binding. *J Biol Chem* **265**:274, 1990.
176. Handin RI, Peterson E: Production of recombinant glycoprotein Ibalpha fragments and delineation of the von Willebrand factor binding site. *Blood* **74**:4777, 1989.
177. Howard MA, Firkin BG: Ristocetin — A new tool in the investigation of platelet aggregation. *Thromb Diath Haemorrh* **26**:362, 1971.
178. Pepper DS, Jamieson GA: Isolation of a macroglycopeptide from human platelets. *Biochemistry* **9**:3706, 1970.
179. Lopez JA, Ludwig EH, McCarthy BJ: Polymorphism of human glycoprotein Ibα results from a variable number of tandem repeats of a 13-amino acid sequence in the mucin-like macroglycopeptide region. Structure/function implications. *J Biol Chem* **267**:10055, 1992.
180. Fox JEB, Aggerbeck LP, Berndt MC: Structure of the glycoprotein Ib-IX complex from platelet membranes. *J Biol Chem* **263**:4882, 1988.
181. Fox JE, Berdnt MC: Cyclic AMP-dependent phosphorylation of glycoprotein GPIb inhibits collagen-induced polymerization on platelets. *J Biol Chem* **264**:9520, 1989.
182. Phillips DR, Agin PP: Platelet plasma membrane glycoproteins. Evidence for the presence of nonequivalent disulfide bonds using nonreduced-reduced two-dimensional gel electrophoresis. *J Biol Chem* **252**:2121, 1977.
183. Hickey MJ, Williams SA, Roth GJ: Human platelet glycoprotein IX: An adhesive prototype of leucine-rich glycoproteins with flank-center-flank structures. *Proc Natl Acad Sci U S A* **86**:6773, 1989.
184. Roth GJ, Ozols J, Nugent DJ, Williams SA: Isolation and characterization of human platelet glycoprotein IX. *Biochem Biophys Res Commun* **156**:931, 1988.
185. Muszbek L, Laposata M: Glycoprotein Ib and glycoprotein IX in human platelets are acetylated with palmitic acid through thioester linkages. *J Biol Chem* **264**:9716, 1989.
186. Zafar RS, Walz DA: Platelet membrane glycoprotein V: Characterization of the thrombin-sensitive glycoprotein from human platelets. *Thromb Res* **53**:31, 1989.
187. Yagi M, Edelhoff S, Disteche CM, Roth GJ: Human platelet glycoproteins V and IX: mapping of two leucine-rich glycoprotein genes to chromosome 3 and analysis of structures. *Biochemistry* **34**:16132, 1995.
188. Andrews RK, Gorman JJ, Booth WJ, Corino GL, Castaldi PA, Berndt MC: Cross-linking of a monomeric 39/34-kDa dispase fragment of von Willebrand factor (Leu-480/Val-481-Gly-718) to the N-terminal region of the a-chain of membrane glycoprotein Ib on intact platelets with *bis*(sulfosuccinimidyl)suberate. *Biochemistry* **28**:8326, 1989.
189. Mohri H, Yoshioka A, Zimmerman TS, Ruggeri ZM: Isolation of the von Willebrand factor domain interacting with platelet glycoprotein Ib, heparin, and collagen and characterization of its three distinct functional sites. *J Biol Chem* **264**:17361, 1989.
190. Randi AM, Rabinowitz I, Mancuso DJ, Mannucci PM, Sadler JE: Molecular basis of von Willebrand disease type IIB. Candidate mutations cluster in one disulfide loop between proposed platelet glycoprotein Ib binding sequences. *J Clin Invest* **87**:1220, 1991.
191. Cooney KA, Nichols WC, Bruck ME, Bahou WF, Shapiro AD, Bowie EJW, Gralnick HR, Ginsberg D: The molecular defect in type IIB von Willebrand disease. *J Clin Invest* **87**:1227, 1991.
192. Ribba AS, Lavergne JM, Bahnak BR, Derion A, Pietu G, Meyer D: Duplication of a methionine within the glycoprotein Ib binding domain of von Willebrand factor detected by denaturing gradient gel electrophoresis in a patient with type IIB von Willebrand disease. *Blood* **78**:1738, 1991.
193. Lillicrap D, Murray EW, Benford K, Blanchette VS, Rivard GE, Wensley R, Giles AR: Recurring mutations at CpG dinucleotides in the region of the von Willebrand factor gene encoding the glycoprotein Ib binding domain, in patients with type IIB von Willebrand's disease. *Br J Haematol* **79**:612, 1991.
194. Holmberg L, Donner M, Dahlback B, Nilsson IB: Apparently recessive IIB von Willebrand disease (vWD) is caused by de novo mutations (Arg543 → Trp; Val551 → Leu). *Blood* **78**:150, 1991.

195. Randi AM, Tuley EA, Jorieux S, Rabinowitz I, Sadler JE: A missense mutation (R578Q) in von Willebrand disease (vWD) affects von Willebrand factor (vWF) binding to GPIb but not to collagen or heparin: Studies with recombinant vWF. *Blood* **78**:179, 1991.
196. Rabinowitz I, Mancuso DJ, Tuley EA, Randi AM, Firkin BG, Howard MA, Sadler JE: von Willebrand disease (vWD) type B, a variant with absent ristocetin—But normal ristocetin cofactor activity is caused by a missense mutation in the GPIb binding domain of von Willebrand factor (vWf). *Blood* **78**:179, 1991.
197. Dong J-F, Li CQ, Sae-Tung G, Hyun W, Afshar-Kharghan V, Lopez JA: The cytoplasmic domain of glycoprotein (GP) Ibα constrains the lateral mobility of the GPIb-IX complex and modulates von Willebrand factor binding. *Biochemistry* **36**:12421, 1997.
198. Krolls MH, Harris TS, Moake JL, Handin RI, Schafer AI: von Willebrand factor binding to platelet GPIb initiates signals for platelet activation. *J Clin Invest* **88**:1568, 1991.
199. Du X, Harris SJ, Tetaz TJ, Ginsberg MH, Berndt: Association of the phospholipase A_2 (14-3-3ζ) with the platelet glycoprotein Ib-IX complex. *J Biol Chem* **269**:18287, 1994.
200. Muslin AJ, Tanner JW, Allen PM, Shaw AS: Interaction of 14-3-3 with signaling proteins is mediated by the recognition of phosphoserine. *Cell* **84**:889, 1996.
201. Bernard J, Soulier JP: Sur une nouvele variete de dystrophie thrombocytaire haemoragipare congenitale. *Semin Hosp Paris* **24**:3217, 1948.
202. Blanchette VS, Sparling C, Turner C: Inherited bleeding disorders. *Baillieres Clin Haematol* **4**:291, 1991.
203. Peng TC, Kickler TS, Bell WR, Haller E: Obstetric complications in a patient with Bernard-Soulier syndrome. *Am J Obstet Gynecol* **165**:425, 1991.
204. Saade G, Homsi R, Seoud M: Bernard-Soulier syndrome in pregnancy: A report of four pregnancies in one patient and review of the literature. *Eur J Obstet Gynecol Reprod Biol* **40**:149, 1991.
205. Cuthbert RJG, Watson HH, Handa SI, Abbott I, Ludlam CA: DDAVP shortens the bleeding time in Bernard-Soulier syndrome. *Thromb Res* **49**:649, 1988.
206. Mant MJ: DDAVP in Bernard-Soulier syndrome. *Thromb Res* **52**:77, 1988.
207. Clemetson KJ, McGregor JL, James E, Dechavanne M, Luscher EF: Characterization of the platelet membrane glycoprotein abnormalities in Bernard-Soulier syndrome and comparison with normal by surface labeling techniques and high resolution two-dimensional electrophoresis. *J Clin Invest* **70**:304, 1982.
208. Grottum KA, Solum NO: Congenital thrombocytopenia with giant platelets: A defect in the platelet membrane. *Br J Haematol* **16**:277, 1969.
209. Poulsen LO, Taaning E: Variation in surface platelet glycoprotein Ib expression in Bernard-Soulier syndrome. *Haemostasis* **20**:155, 1990.
210. Bithell TC, Parekh SJ, Strong RR: Platelet-function studies in the Bernard-Soulier syndrome. *Ann N Y Acad Sci* **201**:145, 1972.
211. George JN, Reimann TA, Moake JL, Morgan RK, Cimo PL, Sears DA: Bernard-Soulier disease: A study of four patients and their parents. *Br J Haematol* **48**:459, 1981.
212. Bessman JD, Williams LJ, Gilmer PR Jr: Mean platelet volume. The inverse relation between platelet size and count in normal subjects and an artifact of other particles. *Am J Clin Pathol* **76**:289, 1981.
213. Hourdille P, Pico M, Jandrot-Perrus M, Lacaze D, Lozano M, Nurden AT: Studies on the megakaryocytes of a patient with the Bernard-Soulier syndrome. *Br J Haematol* **76**:521, 1990.
214. Howard MA, Hutton RA, Hardisty RM: Hereditary giant platelet syndrome: A disorder of a new aspect of platelet function. *BMJ* **2**:586, 1973.
215. Weiss HJ, Tschopp TB, Baumgartner HR, Sussman II, Johnson MM, Egan JJ: Decreased adhesion of giant (Bernard-Soulier) platelets to subendothelium. Further implications on the role of the von Willebrand factor in hemostasis. *Am J Med* **57**:920, 1974.
216. Ware J, Russell SR, Vicente V, Scharf RE, Tomer A, McMillan R, Ruggeri ZM: Nonsense mutation in the glycoprotein Ib alpha coding sequence associated with Bernard-Soulier syndrome. *Proc Natl Acad Sci U S A* **87**:2026, 1990.
217. De Marco L, Mazzucato M, Fabris F, De Roia D, Coser P, Girolami A, Vicente V, Ruggeri ZM: Variant Bernard-Soulier syndrome type Bolzano. A congenital bleeding disorder due to a structural and functional abnormality of the platelet glycoprotein Ib-IX complex. *J Clin Invest* **86**:25, 1990.
218. Aakhus AM, Stavem P, Hovig T, Pedersen TM, Solum NO: Studies on a patient with thrombocytopenia, giant platelets and a platelet membrane Ib with reduced sialic acid. *Br J Haematol* **74**:320, 1987.
219. Miller JL, Lyle VA, Cunningham D: Mutation of leucine-57 to phenylamine in a platelet glycoprotein Ibα leucine tandem repeat occurring in patients with an autosomal dominant variant of Bernard-Soulier disease. *Blood* **79**:439, 1992.
220. Budarf ML, Konkle BA, Ludlow LB, Michaud D, Li M, Yamashiro DJ, McDonald D, Zackai EH, Driscoll DA: Identification of a patient with Bernard-Soulier syndrome and a deletion in the DiGeorge/velo-cardio-facial chromosomal region in 22q11.2. *Hum Mol Genet* **4**:763, 1995.
221. Kunishima S, Lopez JA, Kobayashi S, Imai N, Kamiya T, Saito H, Naoe T: Missense mutations of the glycoprotein (GP) Ibβ gene impairing the GPIbαβ disulfide linkage in a family with giant platelet disorder. *Blood* **89**:2404, 1997.
222. Wright SD, Michaelides K, Johnson DJ, West NC, Tuddenham EG: Double heterozygosity for mutations in the platelet glycoprotein IX gene in three siblings with Bernard-Soulier Syndrome. *Blood* **81**:2339, 1993.
223. Clemetson JM, Kyrle PA, Brenner B, Clemetson KJ: Variant Bernard-Soulier syndrome associated with a homozygous mutation in the leucine-rich domain of glycoprotein IX. *Blood* **84**:1124, 1994.
224. Takahashi H: Studies of the pathophysiology and treatment of von Willebrand's disease. IV. Mechanism of increased ristocetin-induced platelet aggregation in von Willebrand's disease. *Thromb Res* **19**:857, 1980.
225. Weiss HJ, Meyer D, Rabinowitz R, Grima J-P, Vicic WJ, Rogers J: Pseudo-von Willebrand's disease. An intrinsic platelet defect with aggregation by unmodified human factor VIII/von Willebrand factor and enhanced absorption of its high-molecular-weight multimers. *N Engl J Med* **306**:326, 1982.
226. Miller JL, Castella A: Platelet-type von Willebrand's disease: Characterization of a new bleeding disorder. *Blood* **60**:790, 1982.
227. Miller JL, Kupinski JM, Castella A, Ruggeri ZM: Von Willebrand factor binds to platelets and induces aggregation in platelet-type but not type IIb von Willebrand disease. *J Clin Invest* **72**:1532, 1983.
228. Takahashi H, Handa M, Watanabe K, Ando Y, Nagayama R, Hattori A, Shibata A, Federici A, Ruggeri ZM, Zimmerman TS: Further characterization of platelet-type von Willebrand's disease in Japan. *Blood* **64**:1254, 1984.
229. Miller JL, Cunningham D, Lyle VA, Finch CN: Mutation in the gene encoding the alpha chain of platelet glycoprotein Ib in platelet-type von Willebrand disease. *Proc Natl Acad Sci U S A* **88**:4761, 1991.
230. Russell SD, Roth GJ: A mutation in the platelet glycoprotein (GP) Iba gene associated with pseudo-von Willebrand disease [Abstract]. *Blood* **78**:131a, 1991.
231. Ware J, Russell SR, Marchese P, Murata M, Mazzucato M, De Marco L, Ruggeri ZM: Point mutation in a leucine-rich repeat of platelet glycoprotein Iba resulting in the Bernard-Soulier syndrome. *J Clin Invest* **92**:1213, 1993.
232. Simesk S, Noris P, Lozano M, Pico M, von dem Borne AEGK, Ribera A, Gallardo D: Cys209Ser mutation in the platelet membrane glycoprotein Ibα gene is associated with Bernard-Soulier syndrome. *Br J Haematol* **88**:839, 1994.
233. Li C, Martin S, Roth G: The genetic defect in two well-studied cases of Bernard-Soulier syndrome: A point mutation in the fifth leucine-rich repeat of platelet glycoprotein Ibα. *Blood* **86**:3805, 1996.
234. Holmberg L, Karpman D, Nilsson I, Olofsson T: Bernard-Soulier Karlstad: Trp498 → Stop mutation resulting in a truncated glycoprotein Ibα that contains part of the transmembrane domain. *Br J Haematol* **98**:57, 1997.
235. Afshar-Kharghan V, Lopez JA: Bernard-Soulier syndrome caused by a dinucleotide deletion and frameshift in the region encoding the glycoprotein Ibα transmembrane domain. *Blood* **90**:2634, 1997.
236. E. Kunishima S, Miura H, Fukutani H, Yoshida H, Osumi K, Kobayashi S, Ohno R, Naoe T: Bernard-Soulier syndrome Kagoshima: Ser444 → Stop mutation of glycoprotein (GP) Ibα resulting in circulating truncated GPIbα and surface expression of GPIbβ and GPIX. *Blood* **84**:3356, 1994.
237. F. Simesk S, Admiraal LG, Modderman PW, van der Schoot CE, von dem Borne AEGK: Identification of a homozygous single base pair deletion in the gene coding for the human platelet glycoprotein Ibα causing Bernard-Soulier syndrome. *Thromb Haemost* **72**:444, 1994.
238. Kanaji T, Okamura T, Kuroiwa M, Noda M, Fujimura K, Kuramoto A, Sano M, Nakano Y: Molecular and genetic analysis of two patients with Bernard-Soulier syndrome: Identification of new mutations in glycoprotein Ibα gene. *Thromb Haemost* **77**:1055, 1997.

239. Noda M, Fujimura K, Takafuta T, Shimomura T, Fujimoto T, Yamamoto N, Tanoue K, Arai M, Suehiro A Kakishita E, Shimasaki A, Kuramoto A: Heterogeneous expression of glycoprotein Ib, IX and V in platelets from two patients with Bernard-Soulier syndrome caused by different genetic abnormalities. *Thromb Haemost* **74**:1411, 1995.
240. Noda M, Fujimura K, Takafuta T, Shimomura T, Fujii T, Katsutani S, Fujimoto T, Kuramoto A, Yamazaki T, Mochizuki T, Matsuzaki M, Sano M: A point mutation in glycoprotein IX coding sequence (Cys73(TGT) to Tyr(TAT) causes impaired surface expression of GPIb-IX-V complex in two families with Bernard-Soulier syndrome. *Thromb Haemost* **74**:874, 1996.
241. Noris P, Simesk S, Stibbe J, von dem Borne AEGK: A phenylalanine-55 to serine amino acid substitution in the human glycoprotein IX leucine-rich repeat is associated with Bernard-Soulier syndrome. *Br J Haematol* **97**:312, 1997.
242. Santoro SA, Rajpara SM, Staatz WD, Woods VL: Isolation and characterization of a platelet surface collagen binding complex related to VLA-2. *Biochem Biophys Res Commun* **153**:217, 1988.
243. Nieuwenhuis HK, Akkerman JWN, Houdijk WPM, Sixma JJ: Human blood platelets showing no response to collagen fail to express surface glycoprotein Ia. *Nature* **318**:470, 1985.
244. Kehrel B, Balleisen L, Kokott R, Mesters R, Stenzinger W, Clemetson KJ, van de Loo J: Deficiency of intact thrombospondin and membrane glycoprotein Ia in platelets with defective collagen-induced aggregation and spontaneous loss of disorder. *Blood* **71**:1074, 1988.
245. Greenwalt DE, Lipsky RH, Ockenhouse CF, Ikeda H, Tandon NN, Jamieson GA: Membrane glycoprotein CD36: A review of its roles in adherence, signal transduction, and transfusion medicine. *Blood* **80**:1105, 1992.
246. Ockenhouse CF, Tandon NN, Magowan C, Jamieson GA, Chulay JD: Identification of a platelet membrane glycoprotein as a falciparum malaria sequestration receptor [see comments]. *Science* **243**:1469, 1989.
247. Oquendo P, Hundt E, Lawler J, Seed B: CD36 directly mediates cytoadherence of *Plasmodium falciparum* parasitized erythrocytes. *Cell* **58**:95, 1989.
248. Barnwell JW, Asch AS, Nachman RL, Yamaya M, Aikawa M, Ingravallo P: A human 88-kD membrane glycoprotein (CD36) functions in vitro as a receptor for a cytoadherence ligand on Plasmodium falciparum-infected erythrocytes. *J Clin Invest* **84**:765, 1989.
249. Tomiyama Y, Take H, Ikeda H, Mitani T, Furubayashi T, Mizutani H, Yamamoto N, Tandon NN, Sekiguchi S, Jamieson GA, Kurata Y, Yonezawa T, Tarui S: Identification of the platelet-specific alloantigen, Naka, on platelet membrane glycoprotein IV. *Blood* **75**:684, 1990.
250. Yamamoto N, Ikeda H, Tandon NN, Herman J, Tomiyama Y, Mitani T, Sekiguchi S, Lipsky R, Kralisz U, Jamieson GA: A platelet membrane glycoprotein (GP) deficiency in healthy blood donors: Naka-platelets lack detectable GPIV (CD36). *Blood* **76**:1698, 1990.
251. Tandon NN, Ockenhouse CF, Greco NJ, Jamieson GA: Adhesive functions of platelets lacking glycoprotein-IV (CD36). *Blood* **78**:2809, 1991.
252. Aster RH: The immunologic thrombocytopenias, in Kunicki TJ, George JN (eds): *Platelet Immunobiology*. Philadelphia, JB Lippincott, 1989, p 387.
253. Blanchette VS, Peters MA, Pegg-Feige K: Alloimmune thrombocytopenia: Review from a neonatal intensive care unit. *Curr Stud Hematol Blood Transfus* **52**:87, 1986.
254. Newman PJ, Derbes RS, Aster RH: The human platelet alloantigens, PlA1 and PlA2, are associated with a leucine33/proline33 amino acid polymorphism in membrane glycoprotein IIIa, and are distinguishable by DNA typing. *J Clin Invest* **83**:1778, 1989.
255. Goldberger A, Kolodziej M, Poncz M, Bennett JS, Newman PJ: Effect of single amino acid substitutions on the formation of the PlA and Bak alloantigenic epitopes. *Blood* **78**:681, 1991.
256. Wang R, Furihata K, McFarland JG, Friedman K, Aster RH, Newman PJ: An amino acid polymorphism within the RGD binding domain of platelet membrane glycoprotein IIIa is responsible for the formation of the Pena/Penb alloantigen system. *J Clin Invest* **90**:2038, 1992.
257. Kroll H, Kiefel V, Santoso S, Mueller-Eckhardt C: Sra, a private platelet antigen on glycoprotein IIIa associated with neonatal alloimmune thrombocytopenia. *Blood* **76**:2296, 1990.
258. Santoso S, Newman PJ, Kalb R, Kroll H, Walka M, Kiefel V, Mueller-Eckhardt C: An unpaired cysteine residue is involved in epitope formation but has no influence on platelet GPIIIa expression and function. *Blood* **80**:128a, 1992.
259. Kuijpers RWAM, Simsek S, Faber NM, Goldschmeding R, van Wermerkerken RKV, von dem Borne AEGK: Single point mutation in human glycoprotein IIa is associated with a new platelet-specific alloantigen (Mo) involved in neonatal alloimmune thrombocytopenia. *Blood* **81**:70, 1993.
260. McFarland JG, Blanchette V, Collins J, Wang R, Newman PJ, Aster RH: Neonatal alloimmune thrombocytopenia due to a new platelet-specific alloantibody. *Blood* **81**:3318, 1993.
261. Wang R, McFarland JG, Kekomaki R, Newman PJ: Amino acid 489 is a mutational "hot spot" on the $\beta3$ integrin chain. The CA/Tu human platelet alloantigen system. *Blood* **82**:3386, 1993.
262. Santoso S, Kalb R, Walka M, Kiefel V, Mueller-Eckhardt C, Newman PJ: The human platelet alloantigens Bra and Brb are associated with a single amino acid polymorphism on glycoprotein Iα (integrin subunit $\alpha2$). *J Clin Invest* **92**:2427, 1993.
263. Kuijpers RW, Faber NM, Cuypers HT, Ouwehand WH, von dem Borne AE: The N-terminal globular domain of human platelet glycoprotein Ibα has a methionine145/threonine145 amino acid polymorphism which is associated with the HPA-2 (Ko) alloantigens. *J Clin Invest* **89**:381, 1992.
264. Weiss EJ, Bray PF, Tayback M, Schulman SP, Kickler TS, Becker LC, Weiss JL, Gerstenblith G, Goldschmidt-Clermont PJ: A polymorphism of a platelet glycoprotein receptor as an inherited risk factor for coronary thrombosis. *N Engl J Med* **334**:1090. 1996.
265. Ridker PM, Hennekens CH, Schmitz C, Stampfer MJ, Lindpainter K: P1A1/A2 polymorphism of platelet glycoprotein IIIa and risks of myocardial infarction, stroke, and venous thrombosis. *Lancet* **349**:385, 1997.
266. Wagner KR, Giles WH, Johnson CJ, Ou CY, Bray PF, Goldschmidt-Clermont PJ, Croft JB, Brown VK, Stern BJ, Feeser BR, Buchholz DW, Earley CJ, Macko RF, McCarter RJ, Sloan MA, Stolley PD, Wityk RJ, Wozniak MA, Price TR, Kittner SJ: Platelet glycoprotein receptor IIIa polymorphism P1A2 and ischemic stroke risk: the Stroke Prevention in Young Women Study. *Stroke* **29**:581, 1998.
267. Ginsberg MH, Taylor L, Painter RG: The mechanism of thrombin-induced platelet factor 4 secretion. *Blood* **55**:661, 1980.
268. Grant JA, Scrutton MC: Positive interaction between agonists in the aggregation response of human blood platelet: Interaction between ADP, adrenaline and vasopressin. *Br J Haematol* **44**:109, 1980.
269. Sung SS, Young JD, Origlio AM, Heiple JM, Kaback HR, Silverstein SC: Extracellular ATP perturbs transmembrane ion fluxes, elevates cytosolic (Ca2+), and inhibits phagocytosis in mouse macrophages. *J Biol Chem* **260**:13442, 1985.
270. Rao AK: Congenital disorders of platelet function. *Hematol Oncol Clin North Am* **4**:65, 1990.
271. White JG, Krumwiede M: Further studies on the secretory pathway in thrombin-stimulated human platelets. *Blood* **69**:1196, 1987.
272. Cramer EM, Debili N, Martin JF, Gladwin A-M, Breton-Gorius J, Harrison P, Savidge GF, Vainchecker W: Uncoordinated expression of fibrinogen compared with thrombospondin and von Willebrand factor in maturing megakaryocytes. *Blood* **73**:1123, 1989.
273. Nachman R, Levine R, Jaffe EA: Synthesis of factor VIII antigen by cultured guinea pig megakaryocytes. *J Clin Invest* **60**:914, 1977.
274. Handagama P, Rappolee DA, Werb Z, Levin J, Bainton DF: Platelet α-granule fibrinogen, albumin and immunoglobulin G are not synthesized by rat and mouse megakaryocytes. *J Clin Invest* **86**:1364, 1990.
275. Handagama PJ, George JN, Shuman MA, McEver RP, Bainton DF: Incorporation of a circulating protein into megakaryocyte and platelet granules. *Proc Natl Acad Sci U S A* **84**:861, 1987.
276. Gewirtz AM, Keefer M, Doshi K, Annamalai AE, Chiu HC, Colman RW: Biology of human megakaryocyte Factor V. *Blood* **67**:1639, 1986.
277. Stenberg PE, Beckstead JH, McEver RP, Levin J: Immunohistochemical localization of membrane and alpha-granule proteins in plastic-embedded mouse bone marrow megakaryocytes and murine megakaryocyte colonies. *Blood* **68**:696, 1986.
278. Ross R: Platelet-derived growth factor. *Lancet* **1**:1179, 1989.
279. Berman CL, Yeo EL, Wencel-Drake JD, Furie BC, Ginsberg MH, Furie B: A platelet alpha granule membrane protein that is associated with the plasma membrane after activation. *J Clin Invest* **78**:130, 1986.
280. Stenberg PE, McEver RP, Shuman MA, Jacques YV, Bainton DF: A platelet alpha-granule membrane protein (GMP-140) is expressed on the plasma membrane after activation. *J Cell Biol* **101**:880, 1985.

281. White JG: Inherited abnormalities of the platelet membrane and secretory granules. *Hum Pathol* **18**:123, 1987.
282. Weiss HJ, Chervenick PA, Zalusky R, Factor A: A familial defect in platelet function associated with impaired release of adenosine diphosphate. *N Engl J Med* **281**:1264, 1969.
283. Holmsen H, Weiss HJ: Hereditary defect in the release reaction caused by a deficiency in the storage pool of platelet adenine nucleotides. *Br J Haematol* **19**:643, 1970.
284. Weiss HJ, Witte LD, Kaplan KL, Lages BA, Chernoff A, Nossel HL, Goodman DS, Baumgartner HR: Heterogeneity in storage pool deficiency: Studies on granule-bound substances in 18 patients including variants deficient in alpha-granules, platelet factor 4, β-thromboglobulin and platelet-derived growth factor. *Blood* **54**:1296, 1979.
285. Weiss HJ, Tschopp TB, Rogers J, Brand H: Studies on platelet 5-hydroxytryptamine (serotonin) in patients with storage-pool disease and albinism. *J Clin Invest* **54**:421, 1974.
286. White JG, Gerrard JM: Ultrastructural features of abnormal blood platelets. *Am J Pathol* **83**:590, 1976.
287. DePinho RA, Kaplan KL: The Hermansky-Pudlak syndrome. Report of three cases and review of the pathophysiology and management considerations. *Medicine (Baltimore)* **64**:192, 1985.
288. Barak Y, Nir E: Chediak-Higashi syndrome. *Am J Pediatr Hematol Oncol* **9**:42, 1987.
289. Bequez-Cesar A: Neutropenia cronica maligna familiar con granulaciones atipicas de los leucocitos. *Soc Cubana Pediatr Biol* **15**:900, 1943.
289a. Steinbrink W: Uber eine neue Granulationsanomalie der keukocyten. *Dtsch Arciv Klin Med* **193**:577, 1948.
290. Chediak MM: Nouvelle anomalie leucocytaire de caractere constitutionnel et familial. *Rev Hematol* **7**:362, 1952.
291. Higashi O: Congenital gigantism of peroxidase granules. *Tohoku J Exp Med* **59**:315, 1959.
292. Witkop CJ, Almadovar C, Pineeiro B, Nunez-Babcock M: Hermansky-Pudlak syndrome (HPS). An epidemiological study. *Ophthalmic Paediatr Genet* **11**:245, 1990.
293. Witkop CJ Jr, White JG, King RA: Oculocutaneous albinism, in Nyhan WL (ed): *Heritable Disorders of Amino Acid Metabolism. Pattern of Clinical Expression and Genetic Variation*. New York, John Wiley, 1974, p 177.
294. Mahadeo R, Markowitz J, Fisher S, Daum F: Hermansky-Pudlak syndrome with granulomatous colitis in children. *J Pediatr* **118**:904, 1991.
295. Oh J, Bailin T, Fukai K, Feng GH, Ho L, Mao J, Frenk E, Tamura N, Spritz RA: Positional cloning of a gene for Hermansky-Pudlak syndrome, a disorder of cytoplasmic organelles. *Nat Genet* **14**:300, 1998.
296. Gardner JM, Wildenberg SC, Keiper NM, Novak EK, Rusiniak ME, Swank RT, Puri N, Finger JN, Hagiwara N, Lehman AL, Gales TL, Bayer ME, King RA, Brilliant MH: The mouse pale ear (ep) mutation is the homologue of human Hermansky-Pudlak syndrome. *Proc Natl Acad Sci U S A* **94**:9283, 1997.
297. Blume RS, Bennet JM, Yankee RA, Wolff SM: Defective granulocyte regulation in the Chediak-Higashi syndrome. *N Engl J Med* **279**:1009, 1969.
298. Clark R, Kimball H: Defective granulocyte chemotaxis in the Chediak-Higashi syndrome. *J Clin Invest* **50**:2645, 1971.
299. Barak Y, Karov Y, Nir E, Wagner Y, Kristal H, Levin S: Chediak-Higashi syndrome: Expression of the cytoplasmic defect by in vitro cultures of bone marrow progenitors. *Am J Pediatr Hematol Oncol* **8**:128, 1981.
300. Root RK, Rosenthal AS, Balestra DJ: Abnormal bactericidal metabolic and lysosomal functions of Chediak-Higashi syndrome. *J Clin Invest* **51**:649, 1979.
301. Spicer SS, Sato A, Vincent R, Eguchhi M, Poon KC: Lysosomal enlargement in the Chediak-Higashi syndrome. *Fed Proc* **40**:1451, 1981.
302. Blume RS, Wolff SM: The Chediak Higashi syndrome: Studies in four patients and a review of the literature. *Medicine (Baltimore)* **51**:247, 1972.
303. Nagle DL, Karim MA, Woolf EA, Holmgren L, Bork P, Misumi DJ, McGrail SH, Dussault BJ Jr, Perou CM, Boissy RE, Duyk GM, Spritz RA, Moore KJM: Identification and mutation analysis of the complete gene for Chediak-Higashi syndrome. *Nat Genet* **14**:307, 1996.
304. Andrade MA, Bork P: HEAT repeats in the Huntington's disease protein. *Nat Genet* **11**:115, 1995.
305. Kilonsky DJ, Emr, SD: A new class of lysosomal/vacuolar protein sorting signals. *J Biol Chem* **265**:5349, 1990.
306. Barbosa MD, Barrat FJ, Tchernev VT, Nguyen QA, Mishra VS, Colman SD, Pastural E, Dufourcq-Lagelouse R, Fischer A, Holcombe RF, Wallace MR, Brandt SJ, de Saint Basile G, Kingmore SF: Identification of mutations in two major isoforms of the Chediak-Higashi syndrome gene in human and mouse. *Hum Mol Genet* **6**:1091, 1997.
307. Raccuglio G: Grey platelet syndrome: A variety of qualitative platelet disorder. *Am J Med* **51**:818, 1971.
308. Nurden AT, Kunicki TJ, Dupuis D, Soria C, Caen JP: Specific protein and glycoprotein deficiencies in platelets isolated from two patients with the gray platelet syndrome. *Blood* **59**:709, 1982.
309. Srivastava PC, Powling MJ, Nokes TJ, Patrick AD, Dawes J, Hardisty RM: Grey platelet syndrome: Studies on platelet alpha granules, lysosomes and defective response to thrombin. *Br J Haematol* **65**:441, 1987.
310. Breton-Gorius J, Vainchecker W, Nurden A, Levy-Toledano S, Caen J: Defective α-granule production in megakaryocytes from platelet gray syndrome: Ultrastructural studies of bone marrow cells and megakaryocytes growing in culture from blood precursors. *Am J Pathol* **102**:10, 1981.
311. Rosa JP, George JN, Bainton DF, Nurden AT, Caen JP, McEver RP: Gray platelet syndrome. Demonstration of alpha granule membranes that can fuse with the cell surface. *J Clin Invest* **80**:1138, 1987.
312. Caen JP, Deschamps JF, Bodevin E, Byckaerrt MC, Dupuy E, Wasteson A: Megakaryocytes and myelofibrosis in gray platelet syndrome. *Nouv Rev Fr Hematol* **29**:109, 1987.
313. Rothman JE, Orci L: Molecular dissection of the secretory pathway. *Nature* **355**:409, 1992.
314. Pfueller SL, Howard MA, White JG, Menon C, Berry EW: Shortening of bleeding time by 1-deamino-8-arginine vasopressin (DDAVP) in the absence of platelet von Willebrand factor in gray platelet syndrome. *Thromb Haemost* **18**:1060, 1987.
315. Berrebi A, Klepfish A, Varon D, Shtalrid M, Vorst E, Nir E, Lahav J: Gray platelet syndrome in the elderly. *Am J Hematol* **28**:270, 1988.
316. Jackson CW, Hutson NK, Steward SA, Saito N, Cramer EM: Platelets of the Wistar Furth rat have reduced levels of alpha-granule proteins. An animal model resembling gray platelet syndrome. *J Clin Invest* **87**:1985, 1991.
317. Lages B, Shattil SJ, Bainton DF, Weiss HJ: Decreased content and surface expression of alpha-granule membrane protein GMP-140 in one of two types of platelet alpha delta storage pool deficiency. *J Clin Invest* **87**:919, 1991.
318. Janeway CM, Rivard GE, Tracy PB, Mann KG: Factor V Quebec revisited. *Blood* **87**:3571,1996.
319. Hayward CP, Rivard GE, Kane WH, Drouin J, Zheng S, Moore JC, Kelton JG: An autosomal dominant, qualitative platelet disorder associated with multimeric deficiency, abnormalities in platelet factor V, thrombospondin, von Willebrand factor, and fibrinogen and an epinephrine aggregation defect. *Blood* **87**:4967, 1996.
320. Hayward CP, Cramer EM, Kane WH, Zheng S, Bouchard M, Masse JM, Rivard GE: Studies of a second family with the Quebec platelet disorder: evidence that the degradation of the alpha-granule membrane and its soluble contents are not secondary to a defect in targeting proteins to alpha-granules. *Blood* **89**:1243, 1997.
321. Brass LF: The biochemistry of platelet activation, in Hoffman R, Benz EJ Jr, Shattil SJ, Furie B, Cohen JJ (eds): *Hematology: Basic Principles and Practice*. New York, Churchill Livingstone, 1991, p 1176.
322. Rittenhouse SE, Sasson JP: Mass changes in myoinositoltrisphosphate in human platelet stimulated by thrombin. Inhibitory effects of phorbol esters. *J Biol Chem* **260**:8657, 1985.
323. Lapetina EG: Inositol phospholipids and GTP-binding in signal transduction in stimulated platelets. *Adv Prostaglandin Thromboxane Leukot Res* **16**:217, 1986.
324. Irvine RF: Metabolism and function of inositol phosphates: Synthesis and degradation. *ISI Atlas Sci Biochem* **1**:337, 1988.
325. Litchfield DW, Ball EH: Phosphorylation of caldesmon 77 by protein kinase C in vitro and in intact platelets. *J Biol Chem* **262**:8056, 1987.
326. Rao AK, Koike K, Willis J, Daniel JL, Beckett C, Hassel B, Day HJ, Smith JB: Platelet secretion defect associated with impaired liberation of arachidonate metabolism and normal myosin light chain phosphorylation. *Blood* **64**:914, 1984.
327. Rendu F, Breton-Gorius J, Trugnan G, Malaspina HC, Andrieu JM, Bereziat G, Lebret M, Caen JP: Studies on a new variant of the Hermansky-Pudlak syndrome: Qualitative, ultrastructural, and functional abnormalities of the platelet-dense bodies associated with a phospholipase A defect. *Am J Hematol* **4**:387, 1978.

328. Levy-Toledano S, Maclouf J, Rosa JP, Gallet C, Valles G, Nurden P, Nurden AT: Abnormal tyrosine phosphorylation linked to a defective interaction between ADP and its receptor on platelets. *Thromb Haemost* **80**:463, 1998.
329. Malmsten C, Hamberg M, Samuelsson B: Physiological role of an endoperoxide in human platelets: Hemostatic defect due to platelet cyclooxygenase deficiency. *Proc Natl Acad Sci U S A* **72**:1446, 1975.
330. Horellou MH, Lecompte T, Lecrubier C, Fouque F, Chignard M, Conard J, Vargaftig BB, Dray F, Samama M: Familial and constitutional bleeding disorder due to platelet cyclo-oxygenase deficiency. *Am J Hematol* **14**:1, 1983.
331. Lagarde M, Byron PA, Vargaftig BB, Dechavanne M: Impairment of platelet thromboxane A2 generation and of the platelet release reaction in two patients with congenital deficiency of platelet cyclooxygenase. *Br J Haematol* **38**:251, 1978.
332. Pareti FI, Manucci PM, D'Angelo A, Smith JB, Sautebini L, Galli G: Congenital deficiency of thromboxane and prostacyclin. *Lancet* **1**:898, 1980.
333. Roth GJ, Machuga R: Radioimmune assay of human platelet prostaglandin synthetase. *J Lab Clin Med* **99**:187, 1982.
334. Defryn G, Machin SJ, Carreras LO, Dauden M, Chamone AF, Vermylen J: Familial bleeding tendency with partial platelet thromboxane synthetase deficiency: Reorientation of cyclic endoperoxide metabolism. *Br J Haematol* **49**:29, 1981.
335. Mestel F, Oetliker O, Beck E, Felix R, Imbach P, Wagner H-P: Severe bleeding associated with defective thromboxane synthetase. *Lancet* **1**:157, 1980.
336. Bell TG, Leader RW, Olsen PM, Padgett GA, Penner JA, Patterson WR: Basset hound hereditary thrombopathy: An autosomally recessively inherited platelet dysfunction with 11 cases in a kindred of 56 dogs, in Ryder OA, Byrd ML (eds): *One Medicine*. New York, Springer-Verlag, 1984, p 335.
337. Patterson WR, Estry DW, Schwartz KA, Borchert RD, Bell TG: Absent platelet aggregation with normal fibrinogen binding in Basset hound hereditary thrombopathy. *Thromb Haemost* **62**:1011, 1989.
338. Offermanns S, Toombs CF, Hu YH, Simon MI: Defective platelet activation in G alpha(q)-deficient mice. *Nature* **389**:183, 1997.
339. Walsh PN, Schmaier AH: Platelet-coagulation protein interactions, in Colman RW, Hirsh J, Marder VJ, Salzman EW (eds): *Hemostasis and Thrombosis: Basic Principles and Clinical Practice*. Philadelphia, JB Lippincott, 1992, p 689.
340. Weiss HJ, Vicic WJ, Lages BA, Rogers J: Isolated deficiency of platelet procoagulant activity. *Am J Med* **67**:206, 1979.
341. Miletich JP, Kane WH, Hofmann SL, Stanford N, Majerus PW: Deficiency of factor Xa-factor Va binding sites on the platelets of a patient with a bleeding disorder. *Blood* **54**:1015, 1979.
342. Stout JG, Basse F, Luhm RA, Weiss HJ, Wiedmer T, Sims PJ: Scott syndrome erythrocytes contain a membrane protein capable of mediating Ca^{2+}-dependent transbilayer migration of membrane phospholipids. *J Clin Invest* **99**:2232, 1997.
343. Dekkers DW, Comfurius P, Vuist WM, Billheimer JT, Dicker I, Weiss HJ, Zwaal RF, Bevers EM: Impaired Ca^{2+}-induced tyrosine phosphorylation and defective lipid scrambling in erythrocytes from a patient with Scott syndrome: a study using an inhibitor for scramblase that mimics the defect in Scott syndrome. *Blood* **91**:2133, 1998.
344. Rosing EM, Bevers P, Comfurius P, Hemker HC, van Diejan G, Weiss HJ, Zwaal RFA: Impaired factor X- and prothrombin activation associated with decreased phospholipid exposure in platelets from a patient with a bleeding disorder. *Blood* **65**:1557, 1985.
345. Sims PJ, Wiedmer T, Esmon CT, Weiss HJ, Shattil SJ: Assembly of the platelet prothrombinase complex is linked to vesiculation of the platelet plasma membrane: Studies in Scott syndrome: An isolated defect in platelet procoagulant activity. *J Biol Chem* **264**:17049, 1989.
346. Bevers EM, Wiedmer T, Comfurius P, Shattil SJ, Weiss HJ, Zwaal RFA, Sims PJ: Defective $Ca2^{+}$-induced microvesiculation and deficient expression of procoagulant activity in erythrocytes from a patient with a bleeding disorder: A study of the red blood cells of Scott syndrome. *Blood* **79**:380, 1992.
347. Gewirtz AM, Poncz M: Megakaryocytopoiesis and platelet production, in Hoffman R, Benz EJ Jr, Shattil SJ, Furie B, Cohen HJ (eds): *Hematology: Basic Principles and Practice*. New York, Churchill Livingstone, 1991, p 1148.
348. Hall JG: Thrombocytopenia and absent radius (TAR) syndrome. *J Med Genet* **24**:79, 1987.
349. Vainchenker W, Debili N, Mouthon MA, Wendling F: Megakaryocytopoiesis: Cellular aspects and regulation. *Crit Rev Oncol Hematol* **20**:165, 1995.
350. Gordon M, Hoffman R: Growth factors affecting human thrombocytopoiesis: Potential agents for the treatment of thrombocytopenia. *Blood* **80**:302 1992.
351. Souyri M, Vigon I, Penciolelli JF, Heard JM, Tambourin P, Wendling F: A putative truncated cytokine receptor gene transduced by the myeloproliferative leukemia virus immortalizes hematopoietic progenitors. *Cell* **63**:1137, 1990.
352. Bartley TD, Bogenberger J, Hunt P, Li YS, Lu HS, Martin F, Chang MS, Samal B, Nichol JL, Swift S: Identification and cloning of a megakaryocyte growth and development factor that is a ligand for the cytokine receptor Mpl. *Cell* **77**:1117, 1994.
353. Kaushansky K, Lok S, Holly RD, Broudy VC, Lin N, Bailey MC, Forstrom JW, Buddle MM, Oort PJ, Hagen FS: Promotion of megakaryocyte progenitor expansion and differentiation by the c-Mpl ligand thrombopoietin. *Nature* **369**:568, 1994.
354. Lok S, Kaushansky K, Holly RD, Kuijper JL, Lofton-Day CE, Oort PJ, Grant FJ, Heipel MD, Burkhead SK, Kramer JM: Cloning and expression of murine thrombopoietin cDNA and stimulation of platelet production in vivo. *Nature* **369**:565, 1994.
355. de Sauvage FJ, Hass PE, Spencer SD, Malloy BE, Gurney AL, Spencer SA, Darbonne WC, Henzel WJ, Wong SC, Kuang WJ: Stimulation of megakaryocytopoiesis and thrombopoiesis by the c-Mpl ligand. *Nature* **369**:533, 1994.
356. Cwirla SE, Balasubramanian P, Duffin DJ, Wagstrom CR, Gates CM, Singer SC, Davis AM, Tansik RL, Mattheakis LC, Boytos CM, Schatz PJ. Baccanari DP, Wrighton NC, Barrett RW, Dower WJ: Peptide agonist of the thrombopoietin receptor as potent as the natural cytokine. *Science* **276**:1696, 1997.
357. Gurney AL, Carver-Moore K, de Sauvage FJ, Moore MW: Thrombocytopenia in c-mpl-deficient mice. *Science* **265**:1445, 1994.
358. Carver-Moore K, Broxmeyer HE, Luoh SM, Cooper S, Peng J, Burstein SA, Moore MW, de Sauvage FJ: Low levels of erythroid and myeloid progenitors in thrombopoietin- and c-mpl-deficient mice. *Blood* **88**:803, 1996.
359. Bunting S, Widmer R, Lipari T, Rangell L, Steinmetz H, Carver-Moore K, Moore MW, Keller GA, de Sauvage FJ: Normal platelets and megakaryocytes are produced in vivo in the absence of thrombopoietin. *Blood* **90**:3423, 1997.
360. Kimura S, Roberts AW, Metcalf D, Alexander WS: Hematopoietic stem cell deficiencies in mice lacking c-Mpl, the receptor for thrombopoietin. *Proc Natl Acad Sci U S A* **95**:1195, 1998.
361. Alexander WS, Roberts AW, Nicola NA, Li R, Metcalf D: Deficiencies in progenitor cells of multiple hematopoietic lineages and defective megakaryocytopoiesis in mice lacking the thrombopoietic receptor c-Mpl. *Blood* **87**:2162, 1996.
362. Radley JM, Haller CJ: Fate of senescent megakaryocytes in the bone marrow. *Br J Haematol* **53**:277, 1983.
363. Tong M, Seth P, Pennington DG: Proplatelets and stress platelets. *Blood* **69**:522, 1987.
364. Kaufman RM, Airo R, Pollack S, Crosby WH: Circulating megakaryocytes and platelet release in the lung. *Blood* **26**:720, 1985.
365. Pederson NT: Occurrence of megakaryocytes in various vessels and their retention in the pulmonary capillaries in man. *Scand J Haematol* **21**:369, 1978.
366. Scheinen TM, Koivuiniemi AP: Megakaryocytes in the pulmonary circulation. *Blood* **22**:82, 1963.
367. Kallinikos-Maniatis A: Megakaryocytes and platelets in central venous and arterial blood. *Acta Haematol (Basel)* **42**:330, 1969.
368. Radley JM, Haller CJ: The demarcation membrane system of the megakaryocyte: A misnomer? *Blood* **60**:213, 1982.
369. White JG: Interaction of membrane systems in blood platelet. *Am J Pathol* **66**:295, 1972.
370. Handagama PJ, Feldman BF, Jain NC, Farver TB, Kono CS: In vitro platelet release by rat megakaryocytes: Effects of metabolic inhibitors and cytoskeletal disrupting agents. *Am J Vet Res* **48**:1142, 1987.
371. Tablin F, Gastro M, Leven RM: Blood platelet formation in vitro. The role of the cytoskeleton in megakaryocyte fragmentation. *J Cell Sci* **97**:59, 1990.
372. Radley JM, Scurfield G: The mechanism of platelet release. *Blood* **56**:996, 1980.
373. Lecine P, Villeval JL, Vyas P, Swencki B, Xu Y, Shivdasani RA: Mice lacking transcription factor NF-E2 provide in vivo validation of the proplatelet model of thrombocytopoiesis and show a platelet production defect that is intrinsic to megakaryocytes. *Blood* **92**:1608, 1998.

374. Italiano JE, Lecine P, Shivdasani RA: Ultrastructure and dynamics of proplatelet formation by mouse megakaryocytes [Abstract]. *Blood* **92**:376a, 1998.
375. Williams WJ: Clinical evaluation of the patient, in Williams WJ, Beutler E, Erslev AJ, Lichtman MA (eds): *Hematology*. New York, McGraw-Hill, 1983, p 9.
376. Sheridan WP, Kuter DJ: Mechanism of action and clinical trials of Mpl ligand. *Curr Opin Hematol* **4**:312, 1997.
377. Ravid K, Beeler DL, Rabin MS, Ruley HE, Rosenberg RD: Selective targeting of gene products with the megakaryocyte platelet factor 4 gene. *Proc Natl Acad Sci U S A* **88**:1521, 1991.
378. Ravid K, Doi T, Beeler DL, Kuter DJ, Rosenberg RD: Transcriptional regulation of the rat platelet factor 4 gene: Interaction between an enhancer/silencer domain and the GATA site. *Mol Cell Biol* **11**:6116, 1991.
379. Uzan G, Prenant M, Prandini MH, Martin F, Marguerie G: Tissue-specific expression of the platelet GPIIb gene. *J Biol Chem* **266**:8932, 1991.
380. 404. Lemarchandel V, Ghysdael J, Mignotte V, Rahuel C, Romeo P-H: GATA and Ets *cis*-acting sequences mediate megakaryocyte-specific expression. *Mol Cell Biol* **13**:668, 1993.
381. Martin DIK, Tsai S-F, Orkin SH: Increased gamma-globin expression in a nondeletional HPFH mediated by an erythroid-specific DNA-binding factor. *Nature* **338**:435, 1989.
382. Tsai S-F, Martin DIK, Zon L, D'Andrea A, Wong G, Orkin SH: Cloning of the cDNA for the major DNA-binding protein of the erythroid lineage through expression in mammalian cells. *Nature* **339**:446, 1989.
383. Martin DIK, Zon LI, Mutter G, Orkin SH: Expression of the erythroid transcription factor in megakaryocytic and mast cell lineages. *Nature* **344**:444, 1990.
384. Romeo P-H, Prandini M-H, Joulin V, Mignotte V, Prenant M, Vainchenker W, Marguerie G, Uzan G: Megakaryocytic and erythrocytic lineages share specific transcription factors. *Nature* **344**:447, 1990.
385. Shivdasani RA, Fujiwara Y, McDevitt MA, Orkin SH: A lineage-selective knockout establishes the critical role of transcription factor GATA-1 in megakaryocyte growth and platelet development. *EMBO J* **16**:3965, 1997.
386. Pevny L, Simon CS, Robertson E, Klein WH, Tsai S-F, D'Agati V, Orkin SH, Constantini F: Erythroid differentiation in chimaeric mice blocked by a targeted mutation in the gene for transcription factor GATA-1. *Nature* **349**:257, 1991.
387. Minami T, Tachibana K, Imanishi T, Doi T: Both Ets-1 and GATA-1 are essential for positive regulation of platelet factor 4 gene expression. *Eur J Biochem* **258**:879, 1998.
388. Zhang C, Gadue P, Scott E, Atchison M, Poncz M: Activation of the megakaryocyte-specific gene platelet basic protein (PBP) by the Ets family factor PU.1. *J Biol Chem* **272**:26236, 1997.
389. Tsang AP, Visvader JE, Turner CA, Fujiwara Y, Yu C, Weiss MJ, Crossley M, Orkin SH: FOG, a multitype zinc finger protein, acts as a cofactor for transcription factor GATA-1 in erythroid and megakaryocytic differentiation. *Cell* **90**:109, 1997.
390. Tsang AP, Fujiwara Y, Hom DB, Orkin SH: Failure of megakaryopoiesis and arrested erythropoiesis in mice lacking the GATA-1 transcriptional cofactor FOG. *Genes Dev* **12**:1176, 1998.
391. Song W-J, Sullivan MG, Legare RD, Hutchings S, Tan X, Kufrin D, Ratajczak J: Haploinsufficiency of *CBFA2* causes familial thrombocytopenia with propensity to develop acute myelogenous leukaemia. *Nat Genet* **23**:166, 1999.
392. Coller BS, Zarrabi MH: Platelet membrane studies in the May-Hegglin anomaly. *Blood* **58**:279, 1981.
393. Greinacher A, Mueller-Eckhardt C: Hereditary types of thrombocytopenia with giant platelets and inclusion bodies in the leukocytes. *Blut* **60**:53, 1990.
394. Greinacher A, Nieuwenhuis HK, White JG: Sebastian platelet syndrome: A new variant of hereditary macrothrombocytopenia with leukocyte inclusions. *Blut* **61**:282, 1990.
395. Milton JG, Frojmovic MM: Shape-change agent produce abnormally large platelets in hereditary "giant platelet syndrome (MPS)." *J Lab Clin Med* **93**:154, 1979.
396. Milton JG, Frojmovic MM, Tang SS, White JG: Spontaneous platelet aggregation in a hereditary giant platelet syndrome (MPS). *Am J Pathol* **114**:336, 1984.
397. Bernhardt SG, Gore I, Kelby RA: Congenital leukemia. *Blood* **6**:990, 1951.
398. Hall JG, Levin J, Kuhn JP, Ottenheimer EJ, van Berkum KAP, McKusick VA: Thrombocytopenia with absent radius (TAR). *Medicine (Baltimore)* **48**:411, 1969.
399. Donner M, Schwartz M, Carlsson KU, Holmberg L: Hereditary X-linked thrombocytopenia maps to the same chromosomal region as the Wiskott-Aldrich syndrome. *Blood* **72**:1849, 1988.
400. Notarangelo LD, Parolini O, Faustini R, Porteri V, Albertini A, Ugazio AG: Presentation of Wiskott Aldrich syndrome as isolated thrombocytopenia. *Blood* **77**:1125, 1991.
401. Gerrard JM, Israels ED, Bishop AJ, Schroeder ML, Beattie LL, McNicol A, Israels SJ, Walz D, Greenberg AH, Ray M, Israels LG: Inherited platelet-storage pool deficiency associated with a high incidence of acute myeloid leukaemia. *Br J Haematol* **79**:246, 1991.
402. Ho CY, Otterud B, Legare RD, Varvil T, Saxena R, DeHart DB, SE, Aster JC, Dowton SB, Li FP, Leppert M, Gilliland DG: Linkage of a familial platelet disorder with a propensity to develop myeloid malignancies to human chromosome 21q22.1-22.2. *Blood* **87**:5218, 1996.
403. Day HJ, Holmsen H: Platelet adenine nucleotide "storage pool deficiency" in thrombocytopenic absent radii syndrome. *JAMA* **221**:1053, 1972.
404. de Alarcon PA, Graeve JA, Levine RF, McDonald TP, Beal DW: Thrombocytopenia and absent radii syndrome: Defective megakaryocytopoiesis-thrombocytopoiesis. *Am J Pediatr Hematol Oncol* **13**:77, 1991.
405. Ballmaier M, Schulze H, Strauss G, Cherkaoui K, Wittner N, Lynen S, Wolters S, Bogenberger J, Welte K: Thrombopoietin in patients with congenital thrombocytopenia and absent radii: Elevated serum levels, normal receptor expression, but defective reactivity to thrombopoietin. *Blood* **90**:612, 1997.
406. Alter BP: The bone marrow failure syndrome, in Nathan DG, Oski F (eds): *Hematology of Infancy and Childhood*. Philadelphia, WB Saunders, 1981, p 159.
407. Aggett PJ, Cavanagh NP, Matthew DJ, Pincott JR, Sutcliffe J, Harries JT: Schwachman's syndrome: A review of 21 cases. *Arch Dis Child* **55**:331, 1980.
408. Arepally G, Rebbeck TR, Song W, Gilliland G, Maris JM, Poncz M: Evidence for genetic homogeneity in a familial platelet disorder with predisposition to acute myelogenous leukemia (FPD/AML). *Blood* **92**:2600, 1998.
409. Nichols KE, Crispino JD, Poncz M, White JG, Orkin SH, Maris JM, Weiss MJ: Familial dyserythropoietic anaemia and thrombocytopenia due to an inherited mutation in *GATA1*. *Nat Genet* **24**:266, 2000.
410. Wiskott A: Familiarer angeborener Morbus Werlhofi? *Monatsschr Kinderheilkd* **68**:212, 1937.
411. Aldrich RA, Steinberg AG, Campbell DC: Pedigree demonstrating a sex-linked recessive condition characterized by draining ears, eczematoid dermatitis and bloody diarrhea. *Pediatrics* **13**:133, 1954.
412. Grottum KA, Hovig T, Holmsen H, Abramsen AF, Jeremic M, Seip M: Wiscott-Aldrich syndrome: Qualitative platelet defects and short platelet survival. *Br J Haematol* **17**:373, 1969.
413. Perry GS, Spector BD, Schuman LM, Mandel JS, Anderson E, McHugh RB, Hanson MR, Fahlstrom SM Krivitz W, Kersey JH: The Wiskott-Aldrich syndrome in the United States and Canada (1892-1979). *J Pediatr* **97**:72, 1980.
414. Cotelingam JD, Witebsky FG, Hsu SM, Blaese RM, Jaffe ES: Malignant lymphoma in patients with the Wiskott-Aldrich syndrome. *Cancer Invest* **3**:515, 1985.
415. Cooper MD, Chase HP, Lowman JT, Krivit W, Good RA: Wiskott-Aldrich Syndrome. An immunologic deficiency disease involving the afferent limb of immunity. *Am J Med* **44**:499, 1968.
416. Gahmberg CG, Autero M, Mermonen J: Major O-glycosylated sialoglycoproteins of human hematopoietic cells: Differentiation antigens with poorly understood functions. *J Cell Biochem* **37**:91, 1988.
417. Gealy WJ, Dwyer JM, Harley JB: Allelic exclusion of glucose-6-phosphate dehydrogenase in platelet and T lymphocytes from a Wiskott-Aldrich syndrome carrier. *Lancet* **1**:63, 1980.
418. Prchal JT, Carroll AJ, Prchal JF, Crist WM, Skalka HW, Gealy WJ, Harley J, Malluh A: Wiskott-Aldrich syndrome: Cellular impairments and their implications for carrier detection. *Blood* **56**:1048, 1980.
419. Puck JM, Siminovitch KA, Poncz M, Greenberg CR, Rottem M, Conley ME: Atypical presentation of Wiskott-Aldrich syndrome: Diagnosis in two unrelated males based on studies of maternal T cell X-chromosome inactivation. *Blood* **75**:2369, 1990.

420. Stormoken H, Hellum B, Egeland T, Abrahamsen TG, Hovig T: X-linked thrombocytopenia and thrombocytopathia: Attenuated Wiskott-Aldrich syndrome. Functional and morphological studies of platelet and lymphocytes. *Thromb Haemost* **65**:300, 1991.
421. Brochstein JA, Gillio AP, Ruggerio M, Kernan N, Emanuel D, Laver J, Small T, O'Reilly RJ: Marrow transplantation from human leucocyte antigen-identical or haploidentical donors for correction of Wiskott-Aldrich syndrome year follow-up of a patient with Wiskott-Aldrich syndrome. *J Pediatr* **119**:907, 1991.
422. Rimm IJ, Rappeport JM: Bone marrow transplantation for the Wiskott-Aldrich syndrome: Long-term follow-up. *Transplantation* **50**:617, 1990.
423. Brochstein JA, Gillio AP, Ruggiero M, Kernan NA, Emanuel M, Small T, O'Reilly RJ: Marrow transplantation from human leukocyte antigen-identical or haploidentical donors for correction of Wiskott-Aldrich syndrome. *J Pediatr* **119**:907, 1991.
424. Derry JM, Ochs HD, Francke U: Isolation of a novel gene mutated in Wiskott-Aldrich syndrome. *Cell* **78**:635, 1994.
425. Kolluri R, Tolias KF, Carpenter CL, Rosen FS, Kirchhausen T: Direct interaction of the Wiskott-Aldrich syndrome protein with the GTPase Cdc42. *Proc Nat Acad Sci U S A* **93**:5615, 1996.
426. Symons M, Derry JM, Karlak B, Jiang S, Lemahieu V, McCormick F, Francke U, Abo A: Wiskott-Aldrich syndrome protein, a novel effector for the GTPase CDC42Hs, is implicated in actin polymerization. *Cell* **84**:723, 1996.
427. Wu Y, Spencer SD, Lasky LA: Tyrosine phosphorylation regulates the SH3-mediated binding of the Wiskott-Aldrich syndrome protein to PSTPIP, a cytoskeletal-associated protein. *J Biol Chem* **273**:5765, 1998.
428. Miki H, Nonoyama S, Zhu Q, Aruffo A, Ochs HD, Takenawa T: Tyrosine kinase signaling regulates Wiskott-Aldrich syndrome protein function, which is essential for megakaryocyte differentiation. *Cell Growth Diff* **8**:195, 1997.
429. Miki H, Miura K, Takenawa T: N-WASP, a novel actin-depolymerizing protein regulates the cortical cytoskeletal rearrangement in a PIP2-dependent manner downstream of tyrosine kinases. *EMBO J* **15**:5326, 1996.
430. Fukuoka M, Miki H, Takenawa T: Identification of N-WASP homologues in human and rat brains. *Gene* **196**:43, 1997.
431. Zhu Q, Watanabe C, Liu T, Hollenbaugh D, Blaese RM, Kanner SB, Aruffo A, Ochs HD: Wiskott-Aldrich syndrome/X-linked thrombocytopenia: WASP gene mutations, protein expression, and phenotype. *Blood* **90**:2680, 1997.
432. Greer WL, Shehabeldin A, Schulman J, Junker A, Siminovitch KA: Identification of WASP mutations, mutation hotspots and genotype-phenotype disparities in 24 patients with the Wiskott-Aldrich syndrome. *Hum Genet* **98**:685, 1996.
433. Zhu Q, Zhang M, Blaese RM, Derry JM, Junker A, Francke U, Chen SH, Ochs HD: The Wiskott-Aldrich syndrome and X-linked congenital thrombocytopenia are caused by mutations of the same gene. *Blood* **86**:3797, 1995.

CHAPTER 178

Disorders of the Fibrinolytic System

David Ginsburg

1. **The fibrinolytic system plays a central role in hemostasis through the controlled dissolution of the fibrin blood clot. Clot lysis is achieved by the direct action of the protease plasmin, which is, in turn, activated through proteolytic cleavage of its inactive zymogen, plasminogen. The known physiologic activators of plasminogen are tissue plasminogen activator (tPA) and urokinase-type plasminogen activator (uPA). In addition, a number of nonphysiologic plasminogen activators have been identified, including several bacterial gene products that may play important roles in microbial pathogenesis. The fibrinolytic system constitutes a primary mechanism for the defense against extensive intravascular thrombosis and is tightly regulated at many levels. The specific serine protease inhibitors α_2-antiplasmin (α2AP) and plasminogen activator inhibitors (PAIs) target plasmin and the PAs, respectively. In addition, cellular receptors for uPA (the uPA receptor [uPAR]), tPA, and plasmin, together with specific interactions of fibrinolytic system components with fibrin, serve to localize and fine-tune the process of clot lysis.**
2. **Acquired or inherited disorders of fibrinolytic system components can result in pathologic bleeding or thrombosis. The proteases of the fibrinolytic system are all homologous members of the serine protease family with similar structures. Plasminogen is activated to plasmin by specific cleavage at the Arg560-Val561 peptide bond. Plasminogen is synthesized primarily in the liver and circulates at high concentrations in plasma. Plasminogen binds to its substrate, fibrin, through "lysine-binding" sites in kringle domains 1 and 4. tPA also has a high affinity for fibrin, with the presence of fibrin markedly enhancing the rate of plasminogen activation. tPA appears to be the primary physiologic activator of plasminogen within the vascular space, whereas uPA activity may be required primarily at extracellular sites. α2AP efficiently inhibits plasmin in the circulation, whereas clot-bound plasmin is relatively resistant. The combined effect of these interactions is to localize plasmin activity to the fibrin clot and to protect circulating fibrinogen from degradation.**
3. **Though partial deficiency of plasminogen has been described as predisposing to thrombosis, this has not been consistently observed. However, complete deficiency of plasminogen was recently shown to explain a distinct clinical syndrome previously known as ligneous conjunctivitis. The predominant manifestations of this disorder are ocular. Surprisingly, widespread vascular thrombosis has not been observed in these patients. Several mutations leading to complete loss of plasminogen antigen and activity have been identified in patients with ligneous conjunctivitis. The absence of clinically evident vascular thrombosis in these patients, in contrast to observations in plasminogen-deficient mice, suggests that alternative mechanisms for clot lysis and the clearance of fibrin may exist in humans.**
4. **Deficiency states for α2AP and PAI-1 have been described in a limited number of patients. Both of these disorders are autosomal recessive and associated with inactivating mutations in the corresponding genes. Clinical manifestations are mild to moderate bleeding, particularly after trauma. Patients can be successfully treated with inhibitors of plasmin activity, including ε-aminocaproic acid (EACA) and tranexamic acid.**

HISTORICAL PERSPECTIVE

The observation that blood clots often spontaneously liquefy after death has been know since at least the early part of the nineteenth century. In the early part of the twentieth century, this process was linked to proteolysis and cells growing in plasma clots were shown to promote dissolution, suggesting that they contained an activator of clot lysis.[1] In 1933, Tillett and Garner[2,3] isolated a fraction from beta hemolytic streptococci that was capable of rapidly dissolving human plasma clots and termed the substance "streptococcal fibrinolysin." In the early 1940s, Christensen showed that the streptococcal fibrinolysin required another component of plasma referred to as plasminogen and renamed the bacterial fibrinolysin "streptokinase."[4] Sol Sherry and his collaborators first pioneered the use of streptokinase to treat pathologic vascular thromboses in the 1950s.[5] However, it was not until the introduction of recombinant tissue plasminogen activator (tPA) in the 1980s that this approach received widespread application, rapidly becoming a mainstay of modern medical therapy for myocardial infarction and other thrombotic disorders. Spurred by the pharmaceutical potential of this therapeutic approach, as well as the proposed role of plasmin proteolysis in tissue remodeling and tumor invasion, extensive investigation by many laboratories led to the identification of the array of protease activators and their receptors and inhibitors that constitute our current model of fibrinolytic system function today. (For additional historical background see references 1 and 3.)

OVERVIEW OF PLASMINOGEN ACTIVATION

Our current concept of fibrinolytic system function is shown schematically in Fig. 178-1. Fibrinolysis serves as a counterbalance to the vascular occlusion produced by platelet deposition and fibrin clot formation at sites of vascular injury. An intricate control mechanism interconnecting all of these processes has evolved to minimize blood loss following injury, but at the same time to limit the tissue damage resulting from vascular occlusion. Similar to the coagulation cascade (see Chap. 169), the fibrinolytic system is composed of a series of proteases regulated by their corresponding specific inhibitors. The final effector protease of this cascade is plasmin, which efficiently degrades fibrin but also exhibits a range of protease activity against other proteins. In

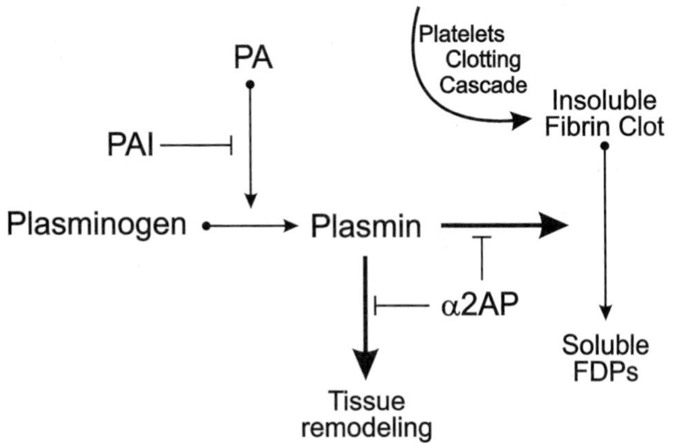

Fig. 178-1 Hemostasis is the balance of platelet and fibrin deposition by the coagulation cascade with fibrin dissolution by the fibrinolytic system. Plasminogen activators (PAs) cleave plasminogen to generate the active enzyme plasmin, which degrades the fibrin clot to soluble fibrin degradation products (FDPs). The PAs are inhibited by plasminogen activator inhibitors (PAIs) and plasmin is directly inhibited by α2AP.

addition to its central role in hemostasis, plasmin is thought to contribute to a variety of other biologic processes including tissue remodeling and wound healing, as well as a number of disease processes including atherosclerosis, tumor invasion, and metastasis.

A more detailed view of the fibrinolytic system and its components is shown in Fig. 178-2. Plasminogen is present in high concentrations in plasma where it circulates as an inactive zymogen. Specific cleavage at the Arg560-Val561 peptide bond by one of several serine proteases termed plasminogen activators (PAs) converts plasminogen to the active proteolytic enzyme, plasmin. Plasmin clips multiple bonds within fibrin to produce soluble fibrin degradation products (FDPs). Plasmin is also capable of degrading circulating fibrinogen, and thus, unregulated, could deplete the plasma pool of the fibrinogen required for subsequent clot formation. However, free plasmin in the circulation is rapidly inactivated through the action of its specific inhibitor, α2AP.

There are two major physiologic PAs, tissue plasminogen activator (tPA) and urokinase-like plasminogen activator (uPA). tPA is the predominant PA in the intravascular compartment, whereas uPA plays an important role in the genitourinary tract (hence its name), as well as at extravascular sites. Plasminogen and tPA both bind to fibrin with high affinity, leading to the concentration of plasmin activity at the site of the fibrin clot, where it is needed. Although tPA exhibits some activity in its uncleaved, native form, it is fully activated through cleavage by plasmin, providing an amplification loop for further plasmin activation. Cellular receptors for tPA and plasminogen also serve to assemble these components on the endothelial cell surface, potentially contributing to maintaining the integrity of the healthy blood vessel wall. uPA is also localized to specific sites on the cell surface through interactions with its high affinity receptor (uPAR). uPA and tPA are further regulated by interactions with their specific inhibitor, plasminogen activator inhibitor-1 (PAI-1). The functional role of a second PA inhibitor, PAI-2, is unknown.

Figure 178-2 also illustrates several connections between the fibrinolytic system and other components of hemostasis. PAI-1 may inhibit thrombin under some circumstances.[6] In addition, thrombin activates carboxypeptidase B (TAFI, see below), which removes free lysines from fibrin, inhibiting plasminogen binding.

GENES AND PROTEINS OF THE FIBRINOLYTIC SYSTEMS

Plasminogen

The plasminogen coding sequence is interrupted by 18 introns, as shown schematically in Fig. 178-3. The plasminogen gene (*PLG*) spans a total of 52.5 kb on human chromosome 6q26-27.[7–9] Plasminogen is a member of a gene family of closely related serine proteases that also includes the plasminogen activators tPA and uPA (see below[10]). This gene family also includes the highly homologous nonprotease, apolipoprotein (a) (Lp(a)), which may contribute to thrombosis and atherosclerosis by interfering with plasminogen function (Chaps. 116 and 169).

The gene for Lp(a) is located ≈50 kb from the *PLG* gene on 6q. Plasminogen is an abundant plasma protein and a number of variant alleles have been identified based on pI. The most common variants are PLGA and PLGB, with rarer variants designated as PLGM1, M2, and so forth.[11] Plasminogen is first synthesized as a single-chain proenzyme with molecular mass of 92 kDa. It circulates in plasma at a concentration of 1.5 μM and is thought to be derived primarily from synthesis within the liver.[12] The

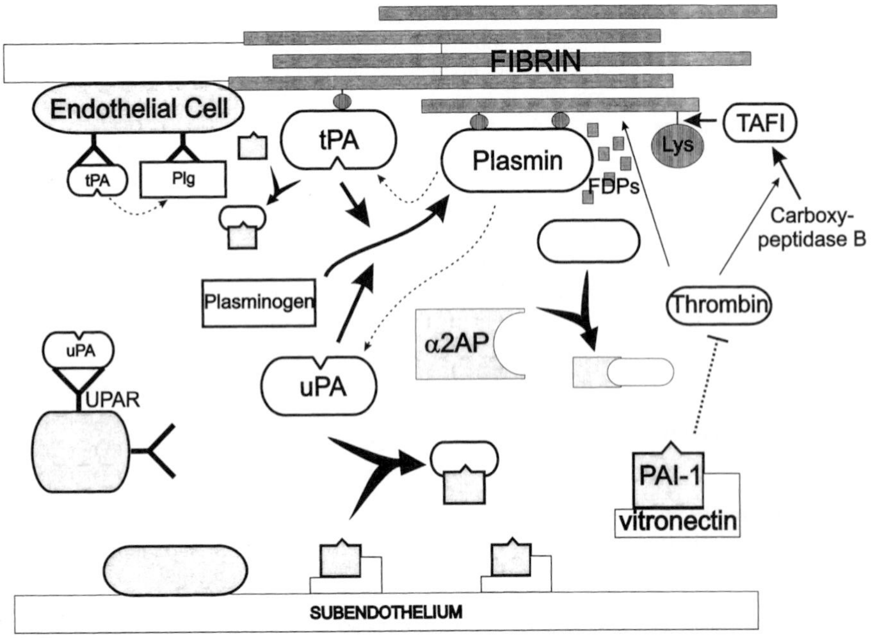

Fig. 178-2 More detailed view of the process shown in Fig. 178-1. Both plasminogen activators, tPA and uPA, are shown. Plasmin also activated tPA and uPA to form an amplification loop. PAI-1 binds to vitronectin, which stabilizes PAI-1 in the active form and localizes PAI-1 to the subendothelial matrix. Specific cellular receptors for uPA (uPAR), tPA, and plasminogen are indicated. Plasmin binds to fibrin, where it is protected from inhibition by α2AP. Fibrin also accelerates the activation of plasminogen by tPA. TAFI is activated by thrombin and inhibits fibrinolysis by removing lysine-binding sites for tPA and plasminogen. PAI-1 may form another link between hemostasis and fibrinolysis by inhibiting thrombin.

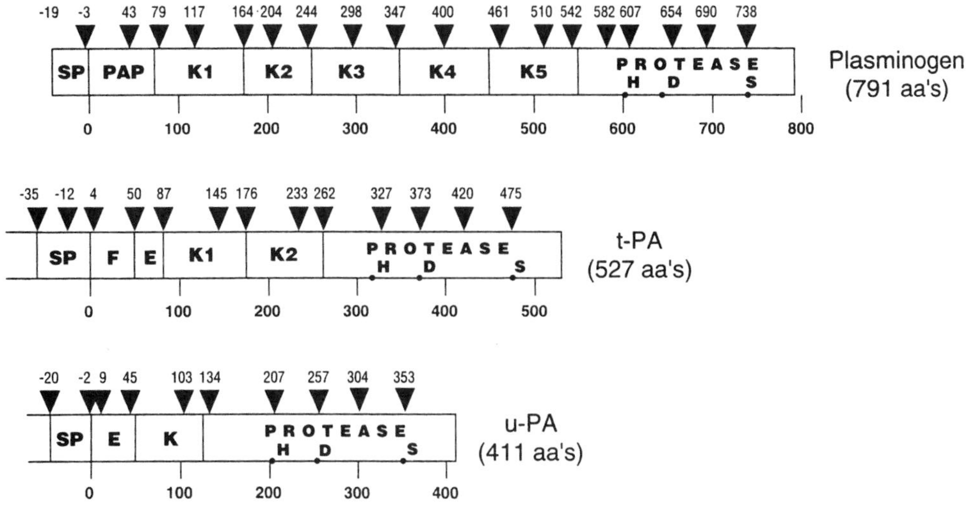

Fig. 178-3 An alignment of the intron/exon structures for plasminogen, tPA, and uPA is shown. Intron positions are indicated by triangles, with the preceding codon number given above the triangle. Labeled protein domains are the signal peptide (SP), preactivation peptide (PAP), "kringle" domains (K1-5), fibronectin-like "finger" domain (F), epidermal growth factor-like domain (E), and the protease domain. The catalytic triad amino acid residues in the latter domain are also indicated (H, D, and S). (*Adapted from Hajjar.*[45] *Used with permission.*)

791-amino-acid protein contains 24 disulfide bonds (Fig. 178-4). Most of these disulfides (16) are contained within the five repeated homologous loop structures referred to as "kringles," because of a fanciful resemblance to a Danish pastry of that name.[9] Each kringle domain contains approximately 80 amino acids, with a molecular mass of about 10,000 daltons and is held in its unique loop conformation by 3 disulfide bonds present in homologous locations within the structure (Fig. 178-5). Plasminogen interacts with free lysines on fibrin and α2AP. A high-affinity lysine-binding site appears to be localized to the first kringle domain and a lower affinity site to the fourth kringle.[13] Binding to surface receptors for plasminogen is also dependent on lysine interactions. All of these lysine-binding interactions can be inhibited by lysine analogues such as ε-aminocaproic acid and tranexamic acid, both of which are used effectively as pharmacologic inhibitors of fibrinolysis.[14]

Two circulating isoforms of plasminogen can be biochemically identified containing different amino termini.[15,16] Glu-plasminogen contains the full-length molecule formed following cleavage of the signal peptide. Limited proteolysis of the peptide bond between lysines 77 and lysine 78 generates Lys-plasminogen (Fig. 178-4), which is missing the first 77 amino acids of Glu-plasminogen. Limited proteolysis is also seen after Arg68 and Lys78. All three of these variant molecules are referred to together as Lys-plasminogen. All of these forms of Lys-plasminogen show enhanced binding to both fibrin and cellular receptors and can be activated to plasmin by plasminogen activators at a 10 to 20 times more rapid rate than Glu-plasminogen.[17] Small amounts of Lys-plasminogen can be detected in plasma. Both Lys- and Glu-plasminogen are activated to plasmin by specific cleavage of the peptide bond between Arg560 and Val561, yielding the two-chain active serine protease.[18] Most of the plasminogen activated at the cell surface is of the Lys-form whereas the majority of circulating plasminogen is in the Glu-form.[19] Plasminogen contains a typical serine protease active site triad formed by His602, Asp645, and Ser740.

Recently, an internal fragment of plasminogen containing the first four kringle domains was shown to be a potent inhibitor of angiogenesis termed angiostatin.[20,21] Angiostatin is currently under study as a potential therapeutic agent for the treatment of human malignancies.

Tissue Plasminogen Activator (tPA)

tPA appears to be the primary physiological activator of plasminogen within the vascular space. tPA is a serine protease with significant homology to plasminogen (Figs. 178-3 and 178-5). The human tPA gene (*PLAT*) is localized to chromosome 8[22] and is composed of 14 exons spanning approximately 36 kb.[23,24] The mature protein contains 527 amino acids with a molecular mass of 72 kDa. tPA was originally assumed to begin with a serine designated as amino acid 1.[25] Although the N-terminus was subsequently shown to include three additional proximal amino acids,[26] the original numbering scheme is still generally used. As in plasminogen, the serine protease domain is at the C-terminus and is preceded by two kringle domains (compared to the five in plasminogen, Fig. 178-5). At the immediate amino terminus following the signal peptide is a 47-residue domain referred to as the finger domain, which is homologous to a similar segment in fibronectin. The next 38 amino acids following the finger domain are homologous to epidermal growth factor and are referred to as the EGF or growth factor domain (Fig. 178-5). The finger and kringle 2 domains appear to be most important for fibrin binding.[27] Note that the finger, EGF, and kringle domains are all encoded by single exons or two adjacent exons (Fig. 178-3). A comparison of the domain and intron/exon structures of plasminogen, tPA, and uPA, along with the homologous serine proteases of the coagulation cascade, suggests that these genes arose by assembly of common modules, and is one of the original observations supporting the notion of exon shuffling.[10]

tPA is cleaved by plasmin at the bond between Arg275 and Ile276 to generate the two-chain, disulfide-linked form of tPA.[28] Although single-chain tPA has less activity than the two-chain form in solution, both molecules show similar activity toward plasminogen when bound to fibrin. Fibrin binding increases the activity of both forms of tPA toward plasminogen by at least two orders of magnitude, primarily by lowering the K_m,[29] presumably through the colocalization of both molecules on the fibrin surface. The significant functional activity of the single-chain, uncleaved form of tPA is unique among serine proteases, with other members of this family exhibiting more typical zymogen behavior.[30,31] tPA exists in at least two variants, referred to as type 1 and type 2, defined by differences in glycosylation. The carbohydrate structures of tPA are thought to play an important role in clearance and may also modulate binding to cell-surface receptors.[32]

tPA is thought to be derived primarily from synthesis in the endothelial cell. Its secretion from the endothelial cell is regulated by a variety of agonists including thrombin, histamine, epinephrine, and DDAVP and is also induced by exercise or venous occlusion, as well as shear stress. All of these responses may be important in maintaining the integrity of the vascular space under a variety of physiological and pathologic conditions.[33–35]

Urokinase-Type Plasminogen Activator (uPA)

The mature uPA molecule contains 411 amino acids with a molecular mass of approximately 54 kDa.[36,37] Similar to tPA, uPA exists in a single-chain, uncleaved form referred to as prourokinase or single-chain uPA (abbreviated scu-PA). Though prourokinase

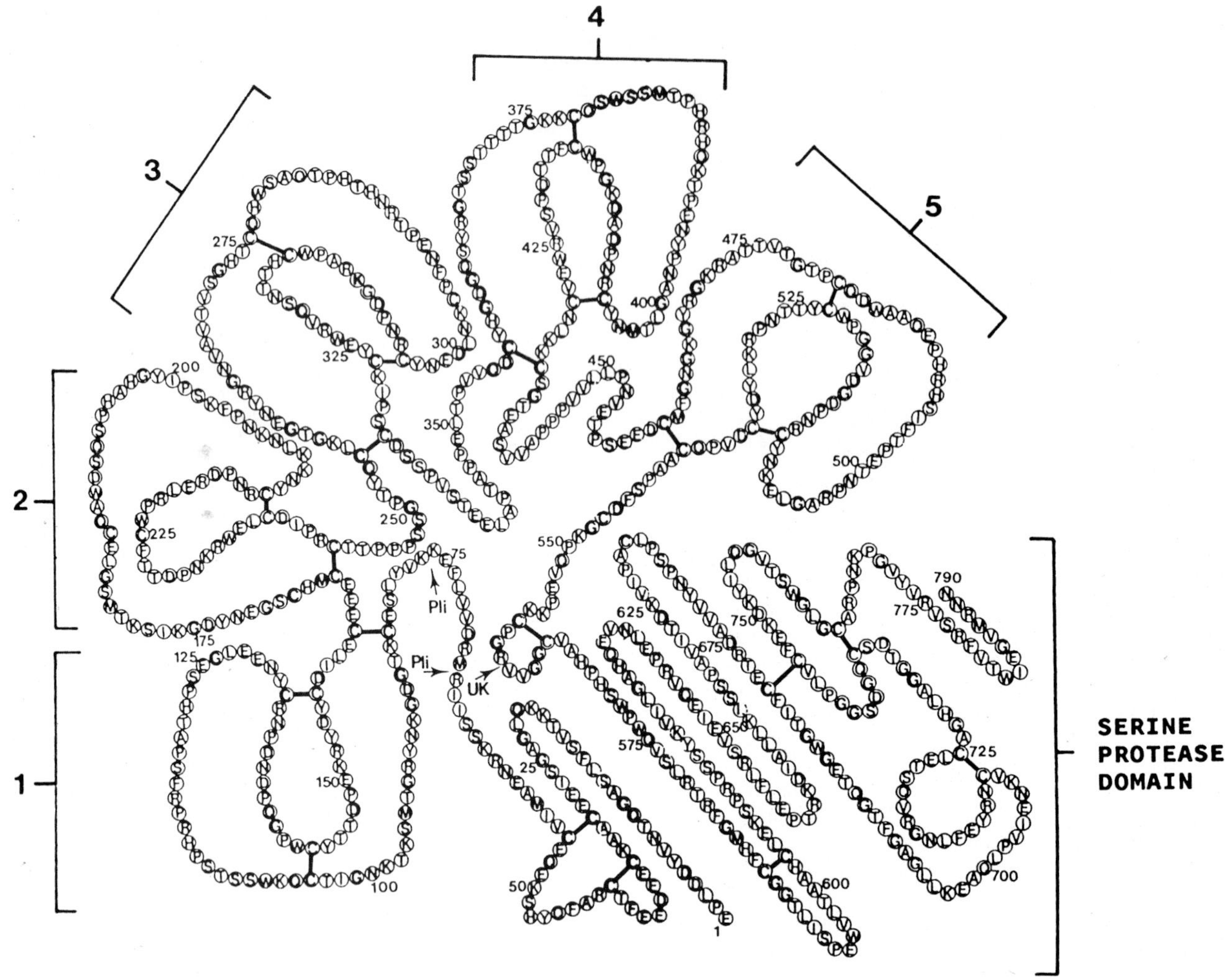

Figure 4

Fig. 178-4 The primary structure of plasminogen is depicted in single letter amino acid code. "Pli" indicates the site of cleavage to generate Lys-plasminogen from Glu-plasminogen. UK indicates the Arg560-Val561 bond that is cleaved by both uPA and tPA to activate plasminogen to plasmin. Black bars indicate disulfide bonds. Kringles 1 to 5 are indicated by the numbered brackets. (*Adapted from Collen and Lijnen.*[149] *Used with permission.*)

has been reported to exhibit a small amount of intrinsic PA activity,[38–40] the significance of this observation is controversial.[41] uPA is cleaved by plasmin or kallikrein at the peptide bond between Lys158 and Ile159 to generate the two-chain form.[42] The uPA domain structure (Fig. 178-5) consists of an N-terminal EGF domain, followed by a single kringle, and, finally, by the C-terminal protease domain.

The human uPA gene *(PLAU)* contains 11 exons and spans 6.4 kb on chromosome 10,[22,37,43] again, with considerable homology to the gene structures of other members of the serine protease gene family (Fig. 178-3). Two-chain uPA can be cleaved between Lys135 and Lys136 by plasmin to remove the N-terminal 135 residues, generating a low-molecular-weight form (33 kDa).[44] Both the high- and low-molecular-weight forms of uPA activate plasminogen with similar efficiency, although only the high-molecular-weight form of uPA can bind to its specific cellular receptor, the uPA receptor (uPAR see below). In contrast to tPA, uPA has a low affinity for fibrin and appears to function primarily in the extravascular space.

Other Plasminogen Activators

In addition to the specific plasminogen activators tPA and uPA, proteases of the intrinsic coagulation system, including kallikrein, factor XIa, and factor XIIa, can also activate plasminogen under some conditions, although this is thought to account for <15 percent of the total plasmin-generating activity of plasma.[45] The observation that knockout mice deficient for both tPA and uPA[46] have a phenotype quite similar to plasminogen knockout mice[47,48] suggests that the physiologic contribution of these additional pathways for plasminogen activation is minimal.

A number of pathogenic bacteria produce their own plasminogen activators, which are sometimes referred to as exogenous plasminogen activators, in contrast to the endogenous PAs discussed above. In several examples, these exogenous activators have been shown to play an important role in microbial pathogenesis.[49,50] Streptokinase is a 414-amino-acid polypeptide produced by streptococci that does not exhibit direct protease activity. However, when bound to plasminogen, the complex induces a conformational change, exposing the active site of the enzyme, which is then capable of activating a second plasminogen molecule to plasmin.[51–53] Plasminogen in complex with streptokinase is also converted to plasmin and the plasmin/streptokinase complex is resistant to inhibition by α2AP, in contrast to free plasmin, which is rapidly inhibited by this serpin (see below). A 36-amino-acid protein produced by *S. aureus*, a staphylokinase-like streptokinase, forms a 1:1 complex with plasminogen that is also capable of activating additional plasminogen molecules.[54] However, the staphylokinase/plasmin complex is inhibited by α2AP. Both staphylokinase and streptokinase are used as pharmacologic agents to induce clot lysis by activating plasminogen.

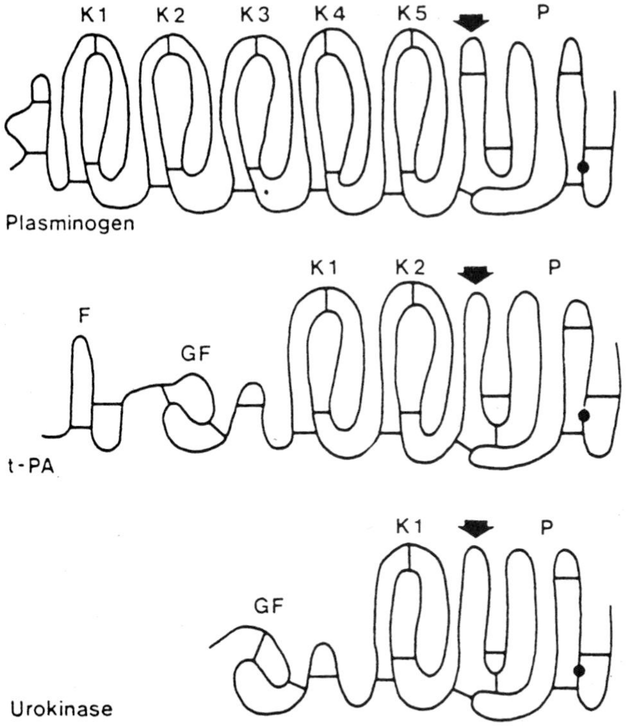

Fig. 178-5 The domain structures of plasminogen, tPA, and uPA. P = protease domain and GF = epidermal growth factor-like domain; other domain abbreviations are as in Fig. 178-3. Arrows indicate the cleavage sites that yield the two-chain activated form of each protease. The active sites are depicted by dots. (*Adapted from Wiman and Hamsten.*[150] *Used with permission.*)

Inhibitors of Plasmin

α2AP has a molecular mass of 70,000 and contains 452 amino acids.[55] α2AP is a member of the serpin gene family, with its P1 and P1′ residues corresponding to Arg364 and Met365. α2AP circulates in plasma at concentrations of approximately 1 μm and has a half-life of approximately 2.5 days. The human α2AP gene (*PLI*) is located on chromosome 17 and contains 10 exons, spanning approximately 16 kb.[56] The primary site of synthesis of α2AP is in the liver, although the protein is also found in the platelet α-granule. Free plasmin in the circulation is promptly neutralized through the formation of a 1:1 complex with α2AP via the standard serpin inhibitory mechanism and the α2AP/plasmin complex is rapidly cleared from plasma.[57] A modified form of α2AP lacking the 26 carboxy-terminal residues constitutes a small portion of circulating α2AP, but is inactive. α2AP is efficiently cross-linked to the fibrin α-chain in the blood clot by the action of factor XIII. This localization serves to stabilize the fibrin clot against plasmin degradation.[58]

α2-Macroglobulin, a large 725-kDa dimeric protein, can also inhibit plasmin, although only with ≈10 percent of the efficiency of α2AP. Unlike other protease inhibitors of the fibrinolytic system, α2-macroglobulin is not a serpin and its complex with plasmin is noncovalent. α2-Macroglobulin is synthesized in endothelial cells and macrophages, and is also found in the platelet α-granule.[45]

Plasminogen Activator Inhibitors

There are two major plasminogen activator inhibitors (PAIs), PAI-1 and PAI-2. PAI-1 is the major inhibitor found in normal plasma. It is a single-chain, 52-kDa molecule that is devoid of cysteines, and thus of disulfide bonds.[59–61] PAI-1 is synthesized in many cell types in tissue culture, although in vivo its primary sites of synthesis appear to be megakaryocytes (leading to storage in the platelet α-granule), smooth muscle cells, and adipocytes.[62–64] In response to inflammation, PAI-1 expression is markedly induced in endothelial cells and several other cell types, including hepatocytes. The synthesis of PAI-1 is regulated by a broad range of inflammatory mediators and cytokines, and its transcriptional regulation has been extensively studied.[65,66]

The PAI-1 gene spans approximately 12 kb on human chromosome 7q and consists of 9 exons.[67,68] PAI-1 is unique among serpins in its propensity to decay to an inactive, latent form as a result of a conformational change with a half-life of approximately 2 h.[69–71] PAI-1 forms a complex with the adhesive glycoprotein vitronectin that serves to stabilize PAI-1 in the active form and also to localize it to specific regions within the extracellular matrix.[72] PAI-1 is an efficient inhibitor of both tPA and uPA and appears to be the major physiological inhibitor of these proteases.[73,74]

PAI-2 is a 393-amino-acid member of the serpin family with an 8-exon, approximately 16-kb gene localized to human chromosome 18q. PAI-2 was originally purified from human placenta and is only found in the circulation at significant concentrations during pregnancy. PAI-2 is a poor inhibitor of single-chain tPA, but efficiently inhibits both two-chain tPA and two-chain uPA.[75] PAI-2 does not contain a typical signal peptide, similar to other members of the ovalbumin subgroup of serine protease inhibitors. Approximately 70 percent of PAI-2 remains intracellular, where its function is unknown, although it has been proposed to play a role in regulating apoptosis.[76] Approximately 20 percent of PAI-2 is secreted via a unique mechanism not involving a signal peptide.[77,78] The transcriptional regulation of PAI-2 has been extensively studied and, as for PAI-1, this gene also appears to be regulated by a broad range of inflammatory mediators.[75,79]

Other Inhibitors of Fibrinolysis

Another serpin, the protein C inhibitor, is also capable of inhibiting uPA and is sometimes referred to as PAI-3.[80] Protease nexin, designated as PAI-4, can also inhibit a broad range of proteases including the PAs. Protease nexin is a much more efficient inhibitor of uPA than tPA, and also inhibits plasmin, thrombin, trypsin, and factor Xa.[81] Finally, another inhibitor of fibrinolysis termed TAFI (*t*hrombin *a*ctivated *f*ibrinolysis *i*nhibitor) is produced by the coagulation cascade[82] and serves as a connection between these two limbs of hemostasis. TAFI has been shown to be identical to carboxypeptidase B and functions by removing free lysines (the binding sites for plasminogen) from the fibrin clot.[83] Carboxypeptidase B is activated by thrombin. Thus, coincident with the formation of the fibrin clot by thrombin, TAFI generation also serves to protect the clot from rapid degradation by plasmin.[84]

Cellular Receptors for the Fibrinolytic System

Specific cellular receptors have been proposed for plasminogen as well as for the natural PAs, uPA and tPA.[85] The best characterized of these is the uPA receptor or uPAR. This protein is widely expressed on monocytes, macrophages, fibroblasts, endothelial cells, platelets, and many tumor cells.[85] uPAR has a molecular mass of 55 to 60 kDa and binds single-chain uPA as well as the high-molecular-weight form of two-chain uPA. The uPAR protein contains 313 amino acids with a 21-residue signal peptide.[86] uPAR does not have a typical transmembrane domain and belongs to the family of glycosylphosphatidyl-inositol-linked surface proteins.[87] uPAR may serve to localize uPA activity to specific sites on the cell surface and has been proposed to play a role in cell migration and possibly also in uPA clearance.[88]

Annexin II has been proposed as a specific receptor for tPA on the cell surface and may also bind plasminogen, potentially coordinating their interaction.[89] α-Enolase has been proposed as a receptor for plasminogen.[90] Plasminogen has also been shown to bind to the glycoprotein IIb/IIIa receptor on the platelet surface.[91] Finally, complexes formed between the uPA and tPA proteases and PAI-1 or PAI-2 are cleared through the low-density lipoprotein receptor-related protein, LRP.[92,93]

Fibrin Degradation by Plasmin

Plasmin is capable of degrading both intact fibrinogen in the circulation as well as fibrin deposited in a blood clot. Fibrinogen thus serves as a substrate for both plasmin and thrombin. Thrombin cleaves at the C-termini of fibrinogen α-chains to liberate fibrinopeptide A and expose the Gly-Pro-Arg tripeptide facilitating polymerization to form insoluble fibrin (see Chap. 169). Plasmin first cleaves fibrinogen to release the C-terminal fragments of the α-chain and simultaneously, but more slowly, liberates fibrinopeptide B from the β-chain. Alhough plasmin can cleave fibrinogen in the circulation, its primary physiological role is the degradation of insoluble fibrin. Fibrin degradation by plasmin liberates a number of soluble fragments, including dimers of the central "coiled coil" D domains of fibrin. The latter fragments, termed D-dimers, are measured clinically as a marker of disseminated intravascular coagulation. These fragments can inhibit platelet function and also may contribute to the inflammatory response through effects on blood pressure regulation, chemotaxis, and immune modulation.[45]

As noted above, both tPA and plasminogen bind to fibrin, resulting in an increase in the rate of plasminogen activation by at least two orders of magnitude in the presence of fibrin.[29] Plasmin molecules on the fibrin surface have their lysine binding sites and active sites occupied, interfering with their interaction with α2AP.[94] Thus, fibrin both enhances the catalytic efficiency of tPA for plasminogen activation and also protects active plasmin from inhibition by α2AP.

Table 178-1 Plasminogen Gene Mutations

Mutation	Clinical disorder	Reference
Val355Phe	Dysplasminogenemia	100
Ser572Pro	Dysplasminogenemia	102
Ala600Thr	Dysplasminogenemia (asymptomatic in homozygote)	100
Trp597Ter	Ligneous conjunctivitis in homozygote	110
Arg216Cys	Ligneous conjunctivitis in homozygote and compound heterozygote	110;112
Trp597Cys	Asymptomatic in compound heterozygote with Trp597Ter	110
Lys19Glu	Ligneous conjunctivitis in compound heterozygote	112
Arg513His	Ligneous conjunctivitis in compound heterozygote	112
Leu128Pro	Ligneous conjunctivitis in compound heterozygote	112
Lys212Del	Ligneous conjunctivitis in compound heterozygote	112
IVS17,1-bp Del, G+1	Ligneous conjunctivitis in compound heterozygote	112
Glu460Ter	Ligneous conjunctivitis in homozygote	111

GENETIC DISORDERS OF PROTEASE FUNCTION

Partial Deficiency of Plasminogen

Plasminogen deficiency has been classified in the past as either (a) hypoplasminogenemia, or type I deficiency, in which both antigen level and functional activity are coordinately decreased, or (b) dysplasminogenemia, or type II deficiency, in which antigen levels are normal and functional activity is disproportionately decreased. Only a few cases of hypoplasminogenemia have been reported, generally in association with thromboembolic disease.[95–97] Alhough the low plasminogen level could be shown to be inherited in an autosomal dominant pattern in some of these families, individuals other than the proband were generally found to be asymptomatic.

Dysplasminogenemia (type II plasminogen deficiency) was first described by Aoki et al. in 1978.[98] Although the propositus had a history of recurrent thrombosis, none of the other family members inheriting the same biochemical defect demonstrated thrombosis. The mutation in this pedigree was later shown to be a single nucleotide substitution resulting in Ala600Thr.[99] This mutation was subsequently identified in additional patients, including a homozygous patient who was asymptomatic, despite plasma plasminogen activity decreased to 8 percent of normal.[100] Ala600Thr is now known to be a common mutation in the Japanese population with an allele frequency of about 1 percent.[101] Despite this high allele frequency, no other homozygous Ala600Thr patients have been identified, suggesting that most such individuals are asymptomatic, similar to the single previously reported case.

Several examples of dysplasminogenemia due to other substitutions have also been reported, including Val355Phe[100] and Ser572Pro[102] (Table 178-1). In a recent analysis of a large cohort of patients with thrombophilia, approximately 2 percent (23/1192) had low plasma plasminogen levels, with similar levels found among approximately half of the available family members. However, the incidence of thrombosis was no greater in plasminogen-deficient family members than in the nondeficient group, indicating that partial plasminogen deficiency of this type is not, by itself, a significant risk factor for thrombosis.[103] In another study of 9611 normal Scottish blood donors, 66 individuals with decreased plasminogen activity were identified, with this reduction shown to be familial in 28 cases. The prevalence of plasminogen deficiency in these unselected healthy blood donors was not found to be significantly different than that calculated from published reports of plasminogen deficiency in thrombotic cohorts, again suggesting that heterozygous plasminogen deficiency does not constitute a significant thrombotic risk factor.[104] Taking all of this evidence together, along with the recent finding of autosomal recessive inheritance in families with ligneous conjunctivitis (due to severe plasminogen deficiency, see below), mild to moderate reduction in plasma plasminogen activity does not appear to confer a significant predisposition to thrombosis.

Targeted inactivation of the plasminogen gene in mice provided important new insight into the biologic function of this protease.[47,48] Although plasminogen-deficient mice develop normally and are fertile, they exhibit widespread thrombosis and shortened survival. Fibrin deposition is observed in vessels of multiple tissues and rectal prolapse is nearly uniform in older animals, presumably due to thromboses in surrounding vessels. Plasminogen-deficient animals also demonstrate impaired wound healing,[105] abnormalities in response to vascular injury,[106] and accelerated progression of atherosclerosis.[107] Failure to identify a similar syndrome in humans initially suggested either that this disorder is quite rare or that it has been missed because of early fatality. Introduction of concurrent genetic deficiency for fibrinogen rescues plasminogen-null mice from nearly all of the pleiotropic abnormalities associated with complete plasminogen deficiency,[108] except for a recently reported abnormality in tissue remodeling following toxic injury to the liver.[109]

Ligneous Conjunctivitis

In the context of these preceding observations, it was thus quite surprising and unexpected when homozygosity for a null mutation in plasminogen was identified as the molecular basis for a rare ophthalmologic disorder, ligneous conjunctivitis.[110] This disease was first described in 1847 and more than 100 cases have been reported.[110–112] Ligneous conjunctivitis usually first presents in early infancy as a chronic pseudomembranous conjunctivitis, although in some patients, onset is delayed even into adulthood. These lesions have a wood-like consistency, giving rise to the term "ligneous," and may be initiated by minor trauma or infection (Fig. 178-6). Similar pseudomembranes can occur on other mucosal

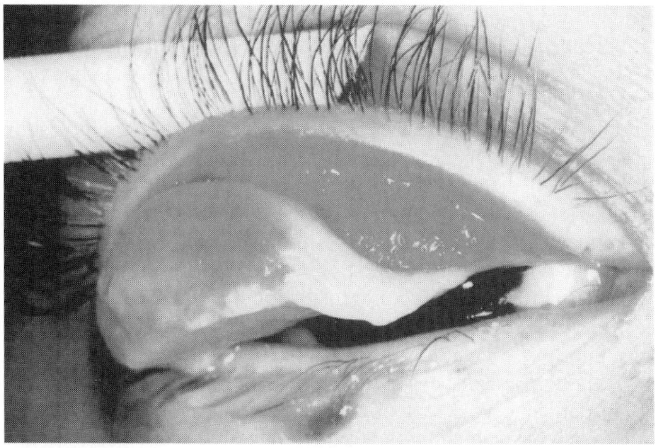

A

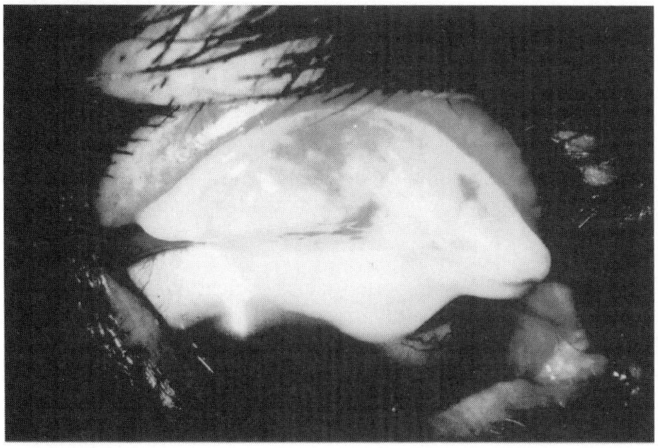

B

Fig. 178-6 Ligneous conjunctivitis in the two patients reported by Schuster and coworkers.[110] (*Adapted from Schuster et al.[110] Used with permission.*)

surfaces including the oropharynx, tracheobronchial tree, and female genital tract. A significant minority of patients is noted to have congenital occlusive hydrocephalus. Most cases appear to be sporadic and an inheritance pattern consistent with an autosomal recessive disorder was first noted in 1986.[113] Histologic examination of the pseudomembranes reveals disrupted epithelium and massive deposits of fibrin along with an inflammatory infiltrate.

In 1997, Schuster, et al.[110] studied two patients with ligneous conjunctivitis and documented undetectable plasma plasminogen activity and antigen (Fig. 178-6). One patient was homozygous for Arg216Cys and the other for Trp597Ter. The father of the latter child was compound heterozygous for this nonsense mutation and a second mutation in the same codon on the other allele, Trp597Cys, resulting in plasma plasminogen activity of 15 percent. Plasminogen levels in the other parents were about half-normal. The same investigators subsequently reported five additional patients, ranging in age from 5 years to 71 years, who were all found to be compound heterozygotes for mutations in the plasminogen gene (Table 178-1). There appears to be a correlation between the type of mutation, residual plasminogen activity, and severity of disease.[112]

In a recent report,[111] a patient with severe ligneous conjunctivitis (homozygous for Glu460Ter), was successfully treated with a Lys-plasminogen concentrate prepared from human plasma. This treatment resulted in a rapid decline in thrombin/antithrombin complexes and D-dimer levels and a dramatic clinical response (Fig. 178-7).

The complete absence of thromboembolic complications in ligneous conjunctivitis patients or their families is in striking contrast to the findings in plasminogen-deficient mice. These observations suggest that the primary role of plasminogen in humans is in extravascular fibrin clearance, implying the existence of an alternative or overlapping system for intravascular fibrinolysis.

A recent careful reexamination of plasminogen-deficient mice[114] revealed that ocular lesions highly reminiscent of human ligneous conjunctivitis do indeed occur in these animals, but were missed in the initial analysis. In addition, it was also noted that hydrocephalus is occasionally observed among these mice, again

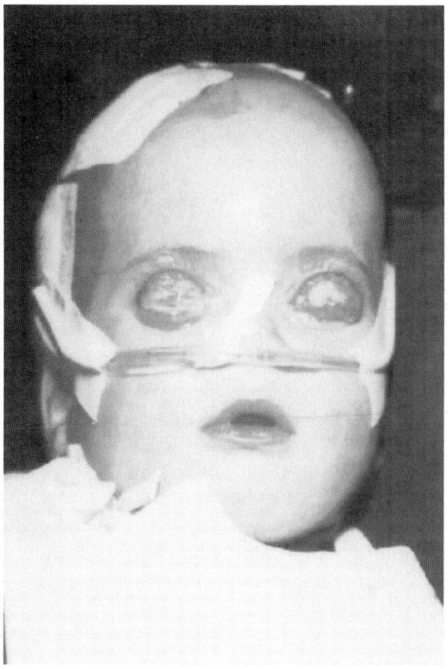

A

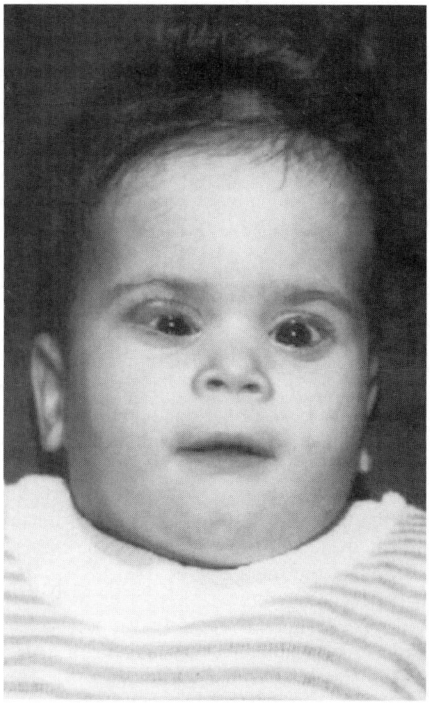

B

Fig. 178-7 Panel *A* is the initial appearance of a child with homozygous plasminogen deficiency resulting in ligneous conjunctivitis. Panel *B* shows the same child after 7 months of replacement with Lys-plasminogen. See Color Plate 8. (*Adapted from Schott et al.[111] Used with permission.*)

similar to the human disease. Thus, in retrospect, the mouse and human phenotypes more closely resemble each other than was originally appreciated. These results highlight the difficulty of accurately characterizing subtle phenotypes in the mouse and the extent to which the diagnostic evaluation of humans is often considerably more sophisticated. Ligneous conjunctivitis has also been reported in Doberman pinschers.[115] It will be interesting to learn whether this latter disorder is also due to plasminogen gene mutations and whether there are associated thrombotic abnormalities.

tPA and uPA

No genetic deficiencies of tPA or uPA have yet been identified in humans. A few case reports have described patients with low tPA in plasma or defective release of tPA from the vessel wall during venous occlusion. However, none have convincingly demonstrated an inherited protein abnormality or tPA gene mutation.

Gene-targeting experiments in mice have generated mouse models for complete deficiency of both proteins.[46] Mice deficient in either tPA or uPA demonstrate normal development and survival and do not exhibit an overt thrombotic phenotype. Although no spontaneous fibrin deposits are observed in tPA-deficient mice, uPA null animals develop occasional small fibrin deposits in the liver and intestines, as well as chronic nonhealing skin ulcerations. However, a genetic cross to generate doubly deficient mice lacking both tPA and uPA results in widespread thrombosis and shortened life span, very similar to the phenotype observed in plasminogen-null mice. These results indicate that tPA and uPA are the primary activators of plasminogen in vivo, with at least partial overlap in function resulting in compensation for deficiency of a single PA. If similar overlapping functions also occur in humans with single uPA or tPA deficiency, this could explain the failure to identify symptomatic patients with either of these disorders.

INHERITED ABNORMALITIES OF FIBRINOLYSIS INHIBITORS

α2AP

Deficiency of α2AP results in a rare autosomal recessive bleeding disorder due to unopposed plasmin activity. The first patient was reported in 1978.[116,117] The proband had lifelong severe bleeding, including the occurrence of hemarthroses and excessive bleeding after trauma. An extensive evaluation with the coagulation tests available at the time was entirely normal, except for a rapid whole-blood clot-lysis time. This led to the evaluation of α2AP levels in the patient's plasma, which were undetectable by either immunologic or functional assay. The accelerated fibrinolysis of the patient's whole-blood in vitro was corrected by the addition of purified α2AP. All other family members were asymptomatic, although the parents and several siblings had approximately 50 percent levels of α2AP.[117]

Molecular analysis in the same family performed 10 years later identified a trinucleotide deletion in exon 7 that results in the deletion of Glu137. In vitro analysis of transfected COS-7 cells revealed that the mutant protein was largely retained within the ER and only a small fraction secreted. However, plasma α2AP levels in the patient were even lower (<1 percent) probably due to additional acceleration of clearance of this secreted mutant protein in vivo.[118] Analysis of another α2AP-deficient family identified a single nucleotide insertion in the last coding exon resulting in a frame-shift, which leads to the replacement of the C-terminal 12 amino acid residues with a 178-amino-acid unrelated extension.[119] Transfection of tissue culture cells demonstrated that the mutant protein is also poorly secreted, accumulating in the cell culture media at approximately 4 percent of wild-type levels. The undetectable α2AP level in the patient's plasma was presumably also due to accelerated clearance.[119]

A particularly interesting mutation in α2AP was identified in another family from Holland, first reported in 1979.[120] The proband was a 17-year-old boy with severe bleeding. Analysis of an extended pedigree identified a homozygous younger sister, as well as eight heterozygotes.[121] Both affected individuals had very low α2AP activity (≤ 4 percent of normal), although α2AP antigen levels were normal. Heterozygotes were asymptomatic, with approximately 50 percent activity levels. This variant was termed α2AP Enschede, and the molecular defect was shown to be a 3-nucleotide insertion resulting in an additional alanine in a run of 4 alanines between amino acid positions 354 and 357. This single amino acid insertion within the reactive center loop of α2AP appears to produce a structural distortion that alters the interaction between this serpin and its target protease and converts α2AP from an inhibitor of plasmin to a substrate.[122]

Although it has been suggested that some heterozygotes for α2AP deficiency may experience mild bleeding,[123] this observation may be explained by the frequent history of mild bleeding and bruising that can be obtained in the general population. The vast majority of heterozygotes in the reported families with α2AP deficiency are asymptomatic.[118,119,123] α2AP-deficient patients have been successfully treated with orally available inhibitors of the fibrinolytic system, such as ε-aminocaproic acid or tranexamic acid, particularly at the time of surgery or trauma.

A knockout mouse completely deficient in α2AP was recently reported.[124] These animals demonstrate accelerated fibrinolysis after thrombotic challenge, but do not suffer from overt bleeding.

Elevated PAI-1

In 1978, a family was reported with deficient fibrinolytic activity in the vessel wall thought to be due to tPA deficiency.[125] This family was subsequently shown to have increased PAI-1 rather than decreased tPA,[126] and this abnormality was proposed as a potential general mechanism for increased risk of venous thrombosis.[127] The report in 1985 by Hamsten and coworkers[128] of elevated plasma PAI-1 levels in young myocardial infarction victims stimulated considerable interest in PAI-1 as a potential genetic risk factor for cardiovascular disease.

Recent attention has focused on a common single base pair insertion/deletion polymorphism resulting in a run of either 4 or 5 G residues, located 675 base pairs upstream from the start site of transcription for the PAI-1 gene. The two alleles of the 4G/5G polymorphism are found with approximately equal frequencies and in vitro studies suggest a difference in transcription factor binding, with significantly greater transcriptional activity associated with the 4G allele. Individuals homozygous for the 4G allele exhibited significantly higher plasma PAI-1 levels than those with other genotypes, both among control and young MI patients.[129,130] However, several large-scale epidemiologic studies have failed to confirm the association of this polymorphism with either arterial or venous thrombosis, most notably the U.S. Physicians' Health Study, a prospective analysis of approximately 15,000 males.[131] A large European study confirmed the correlation of the 4G allele with elevated plasma PAI-1, but not with the risk of myocardial infarction.[132] A recent twin study[133] failed to identify significant differences in PAI-1 level between dizygotic twins either concordant or discordant for the PAI-1 4G/5G polymorphism, suggesting that these alleles are not a major determinant. However, the strong concordance in PAI-1 levels among monozygotic twins indicated the contribution of other genetic factors to the determination of plasma PAI-1 level.

Elevated PAI-1 levels were recently reported in several pedigrees in association with osteonecrosis.[134,135] The mechanism responsible for this potential association, or the candidate molecular defect(s) in the PAI-1 gene, have not yet been identified.

PAI-1 Deficiency

Two reports of sporadic patients with decreased levels of PAI-1 and clinically significant bleeding have appeared in the literature.[136,137] The first reported case of complete PAI-1 deficiency was that of a 9-year-old Amish girl who presented with several episodes of life-threatening hemorrhage following minor trauma or surgery.[138] This patient was found to be homozygous for a two-base pair insertion at the end of PAI-1 exon 4 resulting in a frameshift that removes the C-terminal half of the protein, including the reactive center. The mRNA resulting from this mutation was shown to be unstable, as was the truncated protein. The patient had undetectable levels of both PAI-1 antigen and activity in platelets and in plasma and the heterozygous parents and four heterozygous siblings all showed intermediate PAI-1 levels. This observation was surprising at the time, given the extensive prior evidence for PAI-1 function in a wide range of biologic processes and suggested that the primary role of PAI-1 in vivo is restricted to the regulation of hemostasis.[138]

Subsequent analysis in an extended Amish pedigree identified an additional 19 heterozygous and 7 homozygous null patients. Clinical manifestations were restricted to abnormal bleeding, which was observed only after trauma or surgery in the homozygous individuals. The clinical spectrum included intracranial and joint hemorrhage after mild trauma, delayed surgical bleeding, severe menstrual bleeding, and frequent bruising. Fibrinolytic inhibitors including ε-aminocaproic acid and tranexamic acid were effective in treatment and prevention of bleeding episodes.[139]

Knockout mice deficient in PAI-1 have also been generated.[140,141] Homozygous PAI-1-deficient animals appear normal, but they are resistant to prothrombic challenge due to enhanced endogenous fibrinolysis. Although the phenotype in the deficient mice is frequently characterized as "milder" than the human phenotype, as for plasminogen (see above) this may be due to a bias in the observation of mouse models compared to human patients. Of note: although the initial human patient did suffer life-threatening hemorrhage, her first episode was at age 3 following minor head trauma. It is likely that a phenotype of this type could easily be missed when observing mice in the protected environment of the research laboratory.[142]

DEFICIENCIES OF OTHER COMPONENTS OF THE FIBRINOLYTIC SYSTEM

Human deficiencies of PAI-2, vitronectin, and TAFI have not yet been reported. PAI-2-deficient mice exhibit no obvious disease phenotype and enjoy normal survival and fertility, excluding an essential role in placental function.[143] PAI-2 deficiency did not result in significant bleeding, even after surgical challenge. In addition, mice crossed to be doubly deficient for both PAI-1 and PAI-2 also appeared normal and exhibited normal wound healing.[143]

As noted above, vitronectin is an abundant plasma glycoprotein that serves as a carrier for PAI-1 and stabilizes it in the active conformation. Consistent with this function, vitronectin-deficient mice have reduced levels of PAI-1. Vitronectin contains an RGDS sequence which can serve as a ligand for the integrin referred to as the vitronectin receptor ($\alpha V\beta 3$) and is responsible for the "spreading factor" activity of serum for tissue culture cells.[72] Although this interaction has been proposed to be critical for vascular development,[144] vitronectin null animals develop normally and exhibit no gross abnormality in the vascular tree or the response to injury.[145] Vitronectin null mice have recently been reported to exhibit an exaggerated thrombotic response to vascular injury, suggesting that vitronectin may play an anticoagulant role that has previously been unappreciated.[146]

Therapeutic Modulation of Fibrinolysis

The fibrinolytic system plays a central role in regulating the thrombotic response to vascular injury. It is perturbed in a number of disease states and offers a valuable therapeutic target for a number of human diseases. The inhibition of natural fibrinolysis can enhance clot stability in patients with bleeding disorders due to poor thrombin generation, such as hemophilia.[147] Indeed, ε-aminocaproic acid and related drugs that inhibit plasmin activity have been used successfully to treat patients with a variety of hemorrhagic disorders. Pharmacologic activation of the fibrinolytic system has been exploited as a therapeutic approach to pathologic thrombosis, particularly in the setting of myocardial infarction and stroke. In these disorders, prompt activation of fibrinolysis can result in dissolution of an acute thrombus occluding a coronary or cerebral artery, leading to rescue of the endangered tissue and significantly improved outcome. Therapeutic agents currently in use include tPA, streptokinase, uPA, and staphylokinase.[54,148]

REFERENCES

1. Ratnoff OD: Evolution of knowledge about hemostasis, in Ratnoff OD, Forbes CD (eds): *Disorders of Hemostasis*. Philadelphia, WB Saunders, 1991, p 1.
2. Tillett WS, Garner RL: The fibrinolytic activity of hemolytic streptococci. *J Exp Med* **58**:485, 1933.
3. Sherry S: Basic Concepts of fibrinolysis, in Bussy RK, Stead L (eds): *Fibrinolysis, Thrombosis, and Hemostasis Concepts, Perspectives, and Clinical Applications*. Philadelphia, Lea & Febiger, 1992, p 3.
4. Christensen LR: Streptococcal fibrinolysis: A proteolytic reaction due to a serum enzyme activated by streptococcal fibrinolysis. *J Gen Physiol* **28**:363, 1945.
5. Sherry S, Fletcher A, Alkjaersig N: Fibrinolysis and fibrinolytic activity in man. *Physiol Rev* **39**:343, 1959.
6. Stoop A, Van Meijer M, Horrevoets AJG, Pannekoek H: Molecular advances in plasminogen activator inhibitor 1 interaction with thrombin and tissue-type plasminogen activator. *Trends Cardiovasc Med* **7**:47, 1997.
7. Edlund T, Ny T, Ranby M, Heden L-O, Palm G, Holmgren E, Josephson S: Isolation of cDNA sequences coding for a part of human tissue plasminogen activator. *Proc Natl Acad Sci U S A* **80**:349, 1983.
8. Petersen TE, Martzen MR, Ichinose A, Davie EW: Characterization of the gene for human plasminogen, a key proenzyme in the fibrinolytic system. *J Biol Chem* **265**:6104, 1990.
9. Forsgren M, Raden B, Israelsson M, Larsson K, Heden LO: Molecular cloning and characterization of a full-length cDNA clone for human plasminogen. *FEBS Lett* **213**:254, 1987.
10. Patthy L: Evolution of the proteases of blood coagulation and fibrinolysis by assembly from modules. *Cell* **41**:657, 1985.
11. Skoda U, Bertrams J, Dykes D, Eiberg H, Hobart M, Hummel K, Kuhnl P, Mauff G, Nakamura S, Nishimukai H: Proposal for the nomenclature of human plasminogen (PLG) polymorphism. *Vox Sang* **51**:244, 1986.
12. Raum D, Marcus D, Alper CA, Levey R, Taylor PD, Starzl TE: Synthesis of human plasminogen by the liver. *Science* **208**:1036, 1980.
13. Miles LA, Dahlberg CM, Plow EF: The cell-binding domains of plasminogen and their function in plasma. *J Biol Chem* **263**:11928, 1988.
14. Plow EF, Felez J, Miles LA: Cellular regulation of fibrinolysis. *Thromb Haemost* **66**:32, 1991.
15. Wallen P, Wiman B: Characterization of human plasminogen. II. Separation and partial characterization of different molecular forms of human plasminogen. *Biochim Biophys Acta* **257**:122, 1972.
16. Wallen P, Wiman B: Characterization of human plasminogen. I. On the relationship between different molecular forms of plasminogen demonstrated in plasma and found in purified preparations. *Biochim Biophys Acta* **221**:20, 1970.
17. Holvoet P, Lijnen HR, Collen D: A monoclonal antibody specific for Lys-plasminogen. Application to the study of the activation pathways of plasminogen in vivo. *J Biol Chem* **260**:12106, 1985.
18. Robbins KC, Summaria L, Hsieh B, Shah RJ: The peptide chains of human plasmin. Mechanism of activation of human plasminogen to plasmin. *J Biol Chem* **242**:2333, 1967.
19. Hajjar KA, Nachman RL: Endothelial cell-mediated conversion of Glu-plasminogen to Lys- plasminogen. Further evidence for assembly of the fibrinolytic system on the endothelial cell surface. *J Clin Invest* **82**:1769, 1988.
20. O'Reilly MS, Holmgren L, Shing Y, Chen C, Rosenthal RA, Moses M, Lane WS, Cao Y, Sage EH, Folkman J: Angiostatin: A novel angiogenesis inhibitor that mediates the suppression of metastases by a Lewis lung carcinoma. *Cell* **79**:315, 1994.
21. Cao Y, Ji RW, Davidson D, Schaller J, Marti D, Sohndel S, McCance SG, O'Reilly MS, Llinas M, Folkman J: Kringle domains of human angiostatin. Characterization of the anti- proliferative activity on endothelial cells. *J Biol Chem* **271**:29461, 1996.
22. Rajput B, Degen SF, Reich E, Waller EK, Axelrod J, Eddy RL, Shows TB: Chromosomal locations of human tissue plasminogen activator and urokinase genes. *Science* **230**:672, 1985.

23. Ny T, Elgh F, Lund B: The structure of the human tissue-type plasminogen activator gene: Correlation of intron and exon structures to functional and structural domains. *Proc Natl Acad Sci U S A* **81:**5355, 1984.
24. Degen SJ, Rajput B, Reich E: The human tissue plasminogen activator gene. *J Biol Chem* **261:**6972, 1986.
25. Pennica D, Holmes WE, Kohr WJ, Harkins RN, Vehar GA, Ward CA, Bennett WF, Yelverton E, Seeburg PH, Heyneker HL, Goeddel DV, Collen DV: Cloning and expression of human tissue-type plasminogen activator cDNA in *E. coli*. *Nature* **301:**214, 1983.
26. Jornvall H, Pohl G, Bergsdorf N, Wallen P: Differential proteolysis and evidence for a residue exchange in tissue plasminogen activator suggest possible association between two types of protein microheterogeneity. *FEBS Lett* **156:**47, 1983.
27. van Zonneveld A-J, Veerman H, Pannekoek H: Autonomous functions of structural domains on human tissue-type plasminogen activator. *Proc Natl Acad Sci U S A* **83:**4670, 1986.
28. Tate KM, Higgins DL, Holmes WE, Winkler ME, Heyneker HL, Vehar GA: Functional role of proteolytic cleavage at arginine-275 of human tissue plasminogen activator as assessed by site-directed mutagenesis. *Biochemistry* **26:**338, 1987.
29. Hoylaerts M, Rijken DC, Lijnen HR, Collen D: Kinetics of the activation of plasminogen by human tissue plasminogen activator. *J Biol Chem* **257:**2912, 1982.
30. Madison EL, Kobe A, Gething M-J, Sambrook JF, Goldsmith EJ: Converting tissue plasminogen activator to a zymogen: A regulatory triad of Asp-His-Ser. *Science* **262:**419, 1993.
31. Tachias K, Madison EL: Converting tissue type plasminogen activator into a zymogen. *J Biol Chem* **272:**28, 1997.
32. Hajjar KA, Reynolds CM: α-Fucose-mediated binding and degradation of tissue-type plasminogen activator by HepG2 cells. *J Clin Invest* **93:**703, 1994.
33. Diamond SL, Eskin SG, McIntire LV: Fluid flow stimulates tissue plasminogen activator secretion by cultured human endothelial cells. *Science* **243:**1483, 1989.
34. Hanss M, Collen D: Secretion of tissue-type plasminogen activator and plasminogen activator inhibitor by cultured human endothelial cells: Modulation by thrombin, endotoxin, and histamine. *J Lab Clin Med* **109:**97, 1987.
35. Shi G-Y, Hau J-S, Wang S-J, Wu I-S, Chang B-I, Lin MT, Chow Y-H, Chang W-C, Wing L-YC, Jen CJ, Wu H-L: Plasmin and the regulation of tissue-type plasminogen activator biosynthesis in human endothelial cells. *J Biol Chem* **267:**19363, 1992.
36. Kasai S, Arimura H, Nishida M, Suyama T: Primary structure of single-chain pro-urokinase. *J Biol Chem* **260:**12382, 1985.
37. Holmes WE, Pennica D, Blaber M, Rey MW, Guenzler WA, Steffens GJ, Heyneker HL: Cloning and expression of the gene for pro-urokinase in *Esherichia coli*. *Biotechnology* **3:**923, 1985.
38. Higazi AA, Cohen R, Henkin J, Kniss D, Schwartz BS, Cines D: Enchancement of the enzymatic activity of single-chain urokinase plasminogen activator by soluble urokinase receptor. *J Biol Chem* **270:**17375, 1995.
39. Manchanda N, Schwartz BS: Single chain urokinase. Augmentation of enzymatic activity upon binding to monocytes. *J Biol Chem* **266:**14580, 1991.
40. Lijnen HR, Van Hoef B, De Cock F, Collen D: The mechanism of plasminogen activation and fibrin dissolution by single chain urokinase-type plasminogen activator in a plasma milieu in vitro. *Blood* **73:**1864, 1989.
41. Petersen LC, Lund LR, Nielsen LS, Dano K, Skriver L: One-chain urokinase-type plasminogen activator from human sarcoma cells is a proenzyme with little or no intrinsic activity. *J Biol Chem* **263:**11189, 1988.
42. Gunzler WA, Steffens GJ, Otting F, Buse G, Flohe L: Structural relationship between human high and low molecular mass urokinase. *Hoppe Seylers Z Physiol Chem* **363:**133, 1982.
43. Riccio A, Grimaldi G, Verde P, Sebastio G, Boast S, Blasi F: The human urokinase-plasminogen activator gene and its promoter. *Nucleic Acids Res* **13:**2759, 1985.
44. Stump DC, Lijnen HR, Collen D: Purification and characterization of a novel low-molecular-weight form of single-chain urokinase-type plasminogen activator. *J Biol Chem* **261:**17120, 1986.
45. Hajjar KA: The molecular basis of fibrinolysis, in Nathan DG, Orkin SH (eds): *Hematology of Infancy and Childhood*. Philadelphia, WB Saunders, 1998, p 1557.
46. Carmeliet P, Schoonjans L, Kieckens L, Ream B, Degen JL, Bronson R, De Vos R, van den Oord JJ, Collen D, Mulligan RC: Physiological consequences of loss of plasminogen activator gene function in mice. *Nature* **368:**419, 1994.
47. Bugge TH, Flick MJ, Daugherty CC, Degen JL: Plasminogen deficiency causes severe thrombosis but is compatible with development and reproduction. *Genes Dev* **9:**794, 1995.
48. Ploplis VA, Carmeliet P, Vazirzadeh S, Van Vlaenderen I, Moons L, Plow EF, Colleen D: Effects of disruption of the plasminogen gene on thrombosis, growth, and health in mice. *Circulation* **92:**2585, 1995.
49. Boyle MD, Lottenberg R: Plasminogen activation by invasive human pathogens. *Thromb Haemost* **77:**1, 1997.
50. Sodeinde OA, Subrahmanyam YVBK, Stark K, Quan T, Bao Y, Goguen JD: A surface protease and the invasive character of plague. *Science* **258:**1004, 1992.
51. Wang X, Lin X, Loy JA, Tang J, Zhang XC: Crystal structure of the catalytic domain of human plasmin complexed with streptokinase. *Science* **281:**1662, 1998.
52. Collen D: Coronary thrombolysis: Streptokinase or recombinant tissue-type plasminogen activator? *Ann Intern Med* **112:**529, 1990.
53. Collen D, Lijnen HR: Basic and clinical aspects of fibrinolysis and thrombolysis. *Blood* **78:**3114, 1991.
54. Collen D: Staphylokinase: A potent, uniquely fibrin-selective thrombolytic agent. *Nat Med* **4:**279, 1998.
55. Holmes WE, Nelles L, Lijnen HR, Collen D: Primary structure of human alpha 2-antiplasmin, a serine protease inhibitor (serpin). *J Biol Chem* **262:**1659, 1987.
56. Hirosawa S, Nakamura Y, Miura O, Sumi Y, Aoki N: Organization of the human α-2-plasmin inhibitor gene. *Proc Natl Acad Sci U S A* **85:**6836, 1988.
57. Wiman B, Collen D: On the mechanism of the reaction between human alpha 2-antiplasmin and plasmin. *J Biol Chem* **254:**9291, 1979.
58. Sakata Y, Aoki N: Significance of cross-linking of alpha 2-plasmin inhibitor to fibrin in inhibition of fibrinolysis and in hemostasis. *J Clin Invest* **69:**536, 1982.
59. Pannekoek H, Veerman H, Lambers H, Diergaarde P, Verweij CL, van Zonneveld A-J, van Mourik JA: Endothelial plasminogen activator inhibitor (PAI): a new member of the Serpin gene family. *EMBO J* **5:**2539, 1986.
60. Ny T, Sawdey M, Lawrence D, Millan JL, Loskutoff DJ: Cloning and sequence of a cDNA coding for the human beta-migrating endothelial-cell-type plasminogen activator inhibitor. *Proc Natl Acad Sci U S A* **83:**6776, 1986.
61. Ginsburg D, Zeheb R, Yang AY, Rafferty UM, Andreasen PA, Nielsen L, Dano K, Lebo RV, Gelehrter TD: cDNA cloning of human plasminogen activator-inhibitor from endothelial cells. *J Clin Invest* **78:**1673, 1986.
62. Fay WP, Owen WG: Platelet plasminogen activator inhibitor: Purification and characterization of interaction with plasminogen activators and activated protein C. *Biochemistry* **28:**5773, 1989.
63. Samad F, Yamamoto K, Loskutoff DJ: Distribution and regulation of plasminogen activator inhibitor-1 in murine adipose tissue *in vivo*. Induction by tumor necrosis factor-α and lipopolysaccharide. *J Clin Invest* **97:**37, 1996.
64. Loskutoff DJ, Sawdey M, Keeton M, Schneiderman J: Regulation of PAI-1 gene expression in vivo. *Thromb Haemost* **70:**135, 1993.
65. Sawdey MS, Loskutoff DJ: Regulation of murine type 1 plasminogen activator inhibitor gene expression in vivo. Tissue specificity and induction by lipopolysaccharide, tumor necrosis factor-α, and transforming growth factor-β. *J Clin Invest* **88:**1346, 1991.
66. Fearns C, Loskutoff DJ: Induction of plasminogen activator inhibitor 1 gene expression in murine liver by lipopolysaccharide: Cellular localization and role of endogenous tumor necrosis factor-α. *Am J Pathol* **150:**579, 1997.
67. Loskutoff DJ, Linders M, Keijer J, Veerman H, van Heerikhuizen H, Pannekoek H: Structure of the human plasminogen activator inhibitor 1 gene: Nonrandom distribution of introns. *Biochemistry* **26:**3763, 1987.
68. Follo M, Ginsburg D: Structure and expression of the human gene encoding plasminogen activator inhibitor, PAI-1. *Gene* **84:**447, 1989.
69. Carrell RW, Gooptu B: Conformational changes and disease - serpins, prions and Alzheimer's. *Curr Opin Struct Biol* **8:**799, 1998.
70. Berkenpas MB, Lawrence DA, Ginsburg D: Molecular evolution of plasminogen activator inhibitor-1 functional stability. *EMBO J* **14:**2969, 1995.
71. Sharp AM, Stein PE, Pannu NS, Carrell RW, Berkenpas MB, Ginsburg D, Lawrence DA, Read RJ: The active conformation of plasminogen

activator inhibitor 1, a target for drugs to control fibrinolysis and cell adhesion. *Structure* **7:**111, 1999.
72. Preissner KT: Structure and biological role of vitronectin. *Annu Rev Cell Biol* **7:**275, 1991.
73. Kruithof EKO, Tran-Thang C, Ransijn A, Bachmann F: Demonstration of a fast-acting inhibitor of plasminogen activators in human plasma. *Blood* **64:**907, 1984.
74. Lawrence DA, Ginsburg D: Plasminogen Activator Inhibitors, in High KA, Roberts HR (eds): *Molecular Basis of Thrombosis and Hemostasis*. New York, Marcel Dekker, 1995, p 517.
75. Kruithof EKO, Baker MS, Bunn CL: Biological and clinical aspects of plasminogen activator inhibitor type 2 (PAI-2). *Blood* **86:**4007, 1995.
76. Dickinson JL, Bates EJ, Ferrante A, Antalis TM: Plasminogen activator inhibitor type 2 inhibits tumor necrosis factor α-induced apoptosis. Evidence for an alternate biological function. *J Biol Chem* **270:**27894, 1995.
77. von Heijne G, Liljestrom P, Mikus P, Andersson H, Ny T: The efficiency of the uncleaved secretion signal in the plasminogen activator inhibitor type 2 protein can be enhanced by point mutations that increase its hydrophobicity. *J Biol Chem* **266:**15240, 1991.
78. Mikus P, Ny T: Intracellular polymerization of the serpin plasminogen activator inhibitor type 2. *J Biol Chem* **271:**10048, 1996.
79. Maurer F, Medcalf RL: Plasminogen activator inhibitor type 2 gene induction by tumor necrosis factor and phorbol ester involves transcriptional and post-transcriptional events: Identification of a functional nonameric AU-rich motif in the 3′-untranslated region. *J Biol Chem* **271:**26074, 1996.
80. Suzuki K, Deyashiki Y, Nishioka J, Toma K: Protein C inhibitor: Structure and function. *Thromb Haemost* **61:**337, 1989.
81. Festoff BW, Rao JS, Hantai D: Plasminogen activators and inhibitors in the neuromuscular system: III. The serpin protease nexin I is synthesized by muscle and localized at neuromuscular synapses. *J Cell Physiol* **147:**76, 1991.
82. Bajzar L, Manuel R, Nesheim ME: Purification and characterization of TAFI, a thrombin-activable fibrinolysis inhibitor. *J Biol Chem* **270:**14477, 1995.
83. Bajzar L, Morser J, Nesheim M: TAFI, or plasma procarboxypeptidase B, couples the coagulation and fibrinolytic cascades through the thrombin-thrombomodulin complex. *J Biol Chem* **271:**16603, 1996.
84. Loskutoff DJ: Carboxypeptidases: New regulators of plasminogen activation in vivo? *J Clin Invest* **96:**2104, 1995.
85. Hajjar KA: Cellular receptors in the regulation of plasmin generation. *Thromb Haemost* **74:**294, 1995.
86. Roldan AL, Cubellis MV, Masucci MT, Behrendt N, Lund LR, Dane K, Appella E, Blasi F: Cloning and expression of the receptor for human urokinase plasminogen activator, a central molecule in cell surface, plasmin dependent proteolysis. *EMBO J* **9:**467, 1990.
87. Ploug M, Ronne E, Behrendt N, Jensen AL, Blasi F, Dano K: Cellular receptor for urokinase plasminogen activator. Carboxyl-terminal processing and membrane anchoring by glycosyl-phosphatidylinositol. *J Biol Chem* **266:**1926, 1991.
88. Cubellis MV, Wun T-C, Blasi F: Receptor-mediated internalization and degradation of urokinase is caused by its specific inhibitor PAI-1. *EMBO J* **9:**1079, 1990.
89. Hajjar KA, Jacovina AT, Chacko J: An endothelial cell receptor for plasminogen/tissue plasminogen activator. I. Identity with Annexin II. *J Biol Chem* **269:**21191, 1994.
90. Miles LA, Dahlberg CM, Plescia J, Felez J, Kato K, Plow EF: Role of cell-surface lysines in plasminogen binding to cells: identification of alpha-enolase as a candidate plasminogen receptor. *Biochemistry* **30:**1682, 1991.
91. Miles LA, Ginsberg MH, White JG, Plow EF: Plasminogen interacts with human platelets through two distinct mechanisms. *J Clin Invest* **77:**2001, 1986.
92. Herz J, Clouthier DE, Hammer RE: LDL receptor-related protein internalizes and degrades uPA-PAI-1 complexes and is essential for embryo implantation. *Cell* **71:**411, 1992.
93. Orth K, Madison EL, Gething MJ, Sambrook JF, Herz J: Complexes of tissue-type plasminogen activator inhibitor and its serpin inhibitor plasminogen-activator inhibitor type 1 are internalized by means of the low-density lipoprotein receptor-related protein/α_2-macroglobulin receptor. *Proc Natl Acad Sci U S A* **89:**7422, 1992.
94. Wiman B, Collen D: On the kinetics of the reaction between human antiplasmin and plasmin. *Eur J Biochem* **84:**573, 1978.
95. Hach-Wunderle V, Scharrer I, Lottenberg R: Congenital deficiency of plasminogen and its relationship to venous thrombosis. *Thromb Haemost* **59:**277, 1988.
96. Mannucci PM, Kluft C, Traas DW, Seveso P, D'Angelo A: Congenital plasminogen deficiency associated with venous thromboembolism: therapeutic trial with stanozolol. *Br J Haematol* **63:**753, 1986.
97. Dolan G, Greaves M, Cooper P, Preston FE: Thrombovascular disease and familial plasminogen deficiency: A report of three kindreds. *Br J Haematol* **70:**417, 1988.
98. Aoki N, Moroi M, Sakata Y, Yoshida N, Matsuda M: Abnormal plasminogen. A hereditary molecular abnormality found in a patient with recurrent thrombosis. *J Clin Invest* **61:**1186, 1978.
99. Miyata T, Iwanaga S, Sakata Y, Aoki N: Plasminogen Tochigi: Inactive plasmin resulting from replacement of alanine-600 by threonine in the active site. *Proc Natl Acad Sci U S A* **79:**6132, 1982.
100. Ichinose A, Espling ES, Takamatsu J, Saito H, Shinmyozu K, Maruyama I, Petersen TE, Davie EW: Two types of abnormal genes for plasminogen in families with a predisposition for thrombosis. *Proc Natl Acad Sci U S A* **88:**115, 1991.
101. Kikuchi S, Yamanouchi Y, Li L, Kobayashi K, Ijima H, Miyazaki R, Tsuchiya S, Hamaguchi H: Plasminogen with type-I mutation is polymorphic in the Japanese population. *Hum Genet* **90:**7, 1992.
102. Azuma H, Uno Y, Shigekiyo T, Saito S: Congenital plasminogen deficiency caused by a Ser^{572} to Pro mutation. *Blood* **82:**475, 1993.
103. Demarmels BF, Sulzer I, Stucki B, Wuillemin WA, Furlan M, Lammle B: Is plasminogen deficiency a thrombotic risk factor? A study on 23 thrombophilic patients and their family members. *Thromb Haemost* **80:**167, 1998.
104. Tait RC, Walker ID, Conkie JA, Islam SIAM, McCall F: Isolated familial plasminogen deficiency may not be a risk factor for thrombosis. *Thromb Haemost* **76:**1004, 1996.
105. Romer J, Bugge TH, Pyke C, Lund LR, Flick MJ, Degen JL, Dano K: Impaired wound healing in mice with a disrupted plasminogen gene. *Nat Med* **2:**287, 1996.
106. Carmeliet P, Moons L, Ploplis V, Plow EF, Collen D: Impaired arterial neointima formation in mice with disruption of the *plasminogen* gene. *J Clin Invest* **99:**200, 1997.
107. Xiao Q, Danton MJS, Witte DP, Kowala MC, Valentine MT, Bugge TH, Degen JL: Plasminogen deficiency accelerates vessel wall disease in mice predisposed to atherosclerosis. *Proc Natl Acad Sci U S A* **94:**10335, 1997.
108. Bugge TH, Kombrinck KW, Flick MJ, Daugherty CC, Danton MJS, Degen JL: Loss of fibrinogen rescues mice from the pleiotropic effects of plasminogen deficiency. *Cell* **87:**709, 1996.
109. Bezerra JA, Bugge TH, Melin-Aldana H, Sabla G, Kombrinck KW, Witte DP, Degen JL: Plasminogen deficiency leads to impaired remodeling after a toxic injury to the liver. *Proc Natl Acad Sci U S A* **96:**15143, 1999.
110. Schuster V, Mingers A-M, Seidenspinner S, Nüssgens Z, Pukrop T, Kreth HW: Homozygous mutations in the plasminogen gene of two unrelated girls with ligneous conjunctivitis. *Blood* **90:**958, 1997.
111. Schott D, Dempfle C-E, Beck P, Liermann A, Mohr-Pennert A, Goldner M, Mehlem P, Azuma H, Schuster V, Mingers A-M, Schwarz HP, Kramer MD: Therapy with a purified plasminogen concentrate in an infant with ligneous conjunctivitis and homozygous plasminogen deficiency. *N Engl J Med* **339:**1679, 1998.
112. Schuster V, Seidenspinner S, Zeitler P, Escher C, Pleyer U, Bernauer W, Stiehm ER, Isenberg S, Seregard S, Olsson T, Mingers A-M, Schambeck C, Kreth HW: Compound-heterozygous mutations in the plasminogen gene predispose to the development of ligneous conjunctivitis. *Blood* **93:**3457, 1999.
113. Bateman JB, Pettit TH, Isenberg SJ, Simons KB: Ligneous conjunctivitis: an autosomal recessive disorder. *J Pediatr Ophthalmol Strabismus* **23:**137, 1986.
114. Drew AF, Kaufman AH, Kombrinck KW, Danton MJS, Daugherty CC, Degen JL, Bugge TH: Ligneous conjunctivitis in plasminogen-deficient mice. *Blood* **91:**1616, 1998.
115. Ramsey DT, Ketring KL, Glaze MB, Knight B, Render JA: Ligneous conjunctivitis in four Doberman pinschers. *J Am Anim Hosp Assoc* **32:**439, 1996.
116. Koie K, Kamiya T, Ogata K, Takamatsu J: Alpha2-plasmin-inhibitor deficiency (Miyasato disease). *Lancet* **2:**1334, 1978.
117. Aoki N, Saito H, Kamiya T, Koie K, Sakata Y, Kobakura M: Congenital deficiency of α_2-plasmin inhibitor associated with severe hemorrhagic tendency. *J Clin Invest* **63:**877, 1979.
118. Miura O, Sugahara Y, Aoki N: Hereditary α_2-plasmin inhibitor deficiency caused by a transport-deficient mutation(a_2-PI-Okinawa). *J Biol Chem* **264:**18213, 1989.
119. Miura O, Hirosawa S, Kato A, Aoki N: Molecular basis for congenital deficiency of α_2-plasmin inhibitor. A frameshift mutation leading to

elongation of the deduced amino acid sequence. *J Clin Invest* **83:**1598, 1989.
120. Kluft C, Vellenga E, Brommer EJ: Homozygous alpha 2-antiplasmin deficiency [Letter]. *Lancet* **2:**206, 1979.
121. Kluft C, Nieuwenhuis HK, Rijken DC, Groeneveld E, Wijngaards G, van Berkel W, Dooijewaard G, Sixma JJ: alpha 2-Antiplasmin Enschede: Dysfunctional alpha 2-antiplasmin molecule associated with an autosomal recessive hemorrhagic disorder. *J Clin Invest* **80:**1391, 1987.
122. Holmes WE, Lijnen HR, Nelles L, Kluft C, Nieuwenhuis HK, Rijken DC, Collen D: α_2-Antiplasmin Enschede: Alanine insertion and abolition of plasmin inhibitory activity. *Science* **238:**209, 1987.
123. Leebeek FW, Stibbe J, Knot EA, Kluft C, Gomes MJ, Beudeker M: Mild haemostatic problems associated with congenital heterozygous alpha 2-antiplasmin deficiency. *Thromb Haemost* **59:**96, 1988.
124. Lijnen HR, Okada K, Matsuo O, Collen D, Dewerchin M: α_2-Antiplasmin gene deficiency in mice is associated with enhanced fibrinolytic potential without overt bleeding. *Blood* **93:**2274, 1999.
125. Johansson L, Hedner U, Nilsson IM: A family with thromboembolic disease associated with deficient fibrinolytic activity in vessel wall. *Acta Med Scand* **203:**477, 1978.
126. Nilsson IM, Tengborn L: Impaired fibrinolysis: New evidence in relation to thrombosis, in Jespersen J, Kluft C, Korsgaard O (eds): *Clinical Aspects of Fibrinolysis and Thrombolysis*. Esbjerg, Sweden, South Jutland University Press, 1983, p 273.
127. Nilsson IM, Ljungner H, Tengborn L: Two different mechanisms in patients with venous thrombosis and defective fibrinolysis low concentration of plasminogen activator or increased concentration of plasminogen activator inhibitor. *BMJ* **290:**1453, 1985.
128. Hamsten A, Wiman B, de Faire U, Blombäck M: Increased plasma levels of a rapid inhibitor of tissue plasminogen activator in young survivors of myocardial infarction. *N Engl J Med* **313:**1557, 1985.
129. Dawson SJ, Wiman B, Hamsten A, Green F, Humphries S, Henney AM: The two allele sequences of a common polymorphism in the promoter of the plasminogen activator inhibitor-1 (PAI-1) gene respond differently to interleukin-1 in HepG2 cells. *J Biol Chem* **268:**10739, 1993.
130. Eriksson P, Kallin B, Van't Hooft FM, Båvenholm P, Hamsten A: Allele-specific increase in basal transcription of the plasminogen-activator inhibitor 1 gene is associated with myocardial infarction. *Proc Natl Acad Sci U S A* **92:**1851, 1995.
131. Ridker PM, Hennekens CH, Lindpaintner K, Stampfer MJ, Miletich JP: Arterial and venous thrombosis is not associated with the 4G/5G polymorphism in the promoter of the plasminogen activator inhibitor gene in a large cohort of US men. *Circulation* **95:**59, 1997.
132. Ye S, Green FR, Scarabin PY, Nicaud V, Bara L, Dawson SJ, Humphries SE, Evans A, Luc G, Cambou JP, Arveiler D, Henney AM, Cambien F: The 4G/5G genetic polymorphism in the promoter of the plasminogen activator inhibitor-1 (PAI-1) gene is associated with differences in plasma PAI-1 activity but not with risk of myocardial infarction in the ECTIM study. *Thromb Haemost* **74:**837, 1995.
133. Cesari M, Sartori MT, Patrassi GM, Vettore S, Rossi GP: Determinants of plasma levels of plasminogen activator inhibitor-1: A study of normotensive twins. *Arterioscler Thromb Vasc Biol* **19:**316, 1999.
134. Glueck CJ, Glueck HI, Mieczkowski L, Tracy T, Speirs J, Stroop D: Familial high plasminogen activator inhibitor with hypofibrinolysis, a new pathophysiologic cause of osteonecrosis? *Thromb Haemost* **69:**460, 1993.
135. Glueck CJ, Glueck HI, Welch M, Freiberg R, Tracy T, Hamer T, Stroop D: Familial idiopathic osteonecrosis mediated by familial hypofibrinolysis with high levels of plasminogen activator inhibitor. *Thromb Haemost* **71:**195, 1994.
136. Schleef RR, Higgins DL, Pillemer E, Levitt LJ: Bleeding diathesis due to decreased functional activity of Type 1 plasminogen activator inhibitor. *J Clin Invest* **83:**1747, 1989.
137. Diéval J, Nguyen G, Gross S, Delobel J, Kruithof EKO: A lifelong bleeding disorder associated with a deficiency of plasminogen activator inhibitor type I. *Blood* **77:**528, 1991.
138. Fay WP, Shapiro AD, Shih JL, Schleef RR, Ginsburg D: Complete deficiency of plasminogen-activator inhibitor type 1 due to a frame-shift mutation. *N Engl J Med* **327:**1729, 1992.
139. Fay WP, Parker AC, Condrey LR, Shapiro AD: Human plasminogen activator inhibitor-1 (PAI-1) deficiency: Characterization of a large kindred with a null mutation in the PAI-1 gene. *Blood* **90:**204, 1997.
140. Carmeliet P, Stassen JM, Schoonjans L, Ream B, van den Oord JJ, De Mol M, Mulligan RC, Collen D: Plasminogen activator inhibitor-1 gene-deficient mice. II. Effects on hemostasis, thrombosis, and thrombolysis. *J Clin Invest* **92:**2756, 1993.
141. Carmeliet P, Kieckens L, Schoonjans L, Ream B, Van Nuffelen A, Prendergast GC, Cole MD, Bronson R, Collen D, Mulligan RC: Plasminogen activator inhibitor-1 gene-deficient mice. I. Generation by homologous recombination and characterization. *J Clin Invest* **92:**2746, 1993.
142. Eitzman DT, Ginsburg D: Of mice and men: The function of plasminogen activator inhibitors (PAIs) in vivo. *Adv Exp Med Biol* **425:**131, 1997.
143. Dougherty KM, Pearson JM, Yang AY, Westrick RJ, Baker MS, Ginsburg D: The plasminogen activator inhibitor-2 gene is not required for normal murine development or survival. *Proc Natl Acad Sci U S A* **96:**686, 1999.
144. Stefansson S, Lawrence DA: The serpin PAI-1 inhibits cell migration by blocking integrin $\alpha_v\beta_3$ binding to vitronectin. *Nature* **383:**441, 1996.
145. Zheng X, Saunders TL, Camper SA, Samuelson LC, Ginsburg D: Vitronectin is not essential for normal mammalian development and fertility. *Proc Natl Acad Sci U S A* **92:**12426, 1995.
146. Fay WP, Parker AC, Ansari MN, Zheng X, Ginsburg D: Vitronectin inhibits the thrombotic response to arterial injury in mice. *Blood* **93:**1825, 1998.
147. Ginsburg D: Hemophilia and other inherited disorders of hemostasis and thrombosis, in Rimoin DL, Connor JM, Pyeritz RE, Emery AEH (eds): *Emery and Rimoin's Principles and Practice of Medical Genetics*, vol II. New York, Churchill-Livingstone, 1997, p 1651.
148. Anderson HV, Willerson JT: Thrombolysis in acute myocardial infarction. *N Engl J Med* **329:**703, 1993.
149. Collen D, Lijnen HR: Fibrinolysis and the control of hemostasis, in Stamatoyannopoulos G (ed): *The Molecular Basis of Blood Diseases*. Philadelphia, WB Saunders, 1994, p 725.
150. Wiman B, Hamsten A: The fibrinolytic enzyme system and its role in the etiology of thromboembolic disease. *Semin Thromb Hemost* **16:**207, 1990.

CHAPTER 179

Glucose 6-Phosphate Dehydrogenase Deficiency

Lucio Luzzatto ▪ Atul Mehta ▪ Tom Vulliamy

Quod aliis cibus est, aliis fuat acre venenum
What is food to some men may be fierce poison to others
Lucretius Caro
De Rerum Natura 4641, 65 BC

1. Glucose-6-phosphate dehydrogenase (G6PD) is a cytoplasmic enzyme that is distributed in all cells. G6PD catalyzes the first step in the hexose monophosphate pathway, and it produces NADPH, which is required for reactions of various biosynthetic pathways as well as for the stability of catalase and the preservation and regeneration of the reduced form of glutathione (GSH). Because catalase and glutathione (via glutathione peroxidase) are essential for the detoxification of hydrogen peroxide, the defense of cells against this compound depends ultimately and heavily on G6PD. This is especially true in red cells, which are exquisitely sensitive to oxidative damage and in which other NADPH-producing enzymes are lacking.
2. G6PD in its active enzyme form is made up of either two or four identical subunits, each having a molecular mass of about 59 kDa. The primary sequence of 515 amino acids has been determined from the cDNA sequence, and it shows more than 90 percent identity with the protein sequence of rat liver G6PD. The gene encoding G6PD maps to band Xq28 on the long arm of the X chromosome (just over 1 Mb from the telomere, between the GD1 mental retardation locus and the dyskeratosis congenita locus). Therefore, one of the two G6PD alleles is subject to inactivation in females. As determined from overlapping genomic phage clones, the gene spans 18 kb and consists of 13 exons (the first of which is noncoding). The sequence of the DNA region upstream from the major transcription initiation site has features similar to those found in other housekeeping gene promoters.
3. G6PD deficiency is the most common known enzymopathy; it is estimated to affect 400 million people worldwide. The highest prevalence rates (with gene frequencies in the range of 5 to 25 percent) are found in tropical Africa, in the Middle East, in tropical and subtropical Asia, in some areas of the Mediterranean, and in Papua New Guinea. The most common clinical manifestations are neonatal jaundice and acute hemolytic anemia. In some cases, the neonatal jaundice is severe enough to cause death or permanent neurologic damage. The acute hemolytic anemia can be triggered by a number of drugs, by infections, or by the ingestion of fava beans. These manifestations may be life threatening, especially favism in children. The detailed mechanism of hemolysis is not fully known, but it results undoubtedly from the inability of G6PD-deficient red cells to withstand the oxidative damage produced, directly or indirectly, by the triggering agents mentioned above. Red cell destruction in these acute hemolytic events is largely intravascular and therefore is associated with hemoglobinuria. Fortunately, apart from these episodes of hemolytic anemia, most G6PD-deficient individuals are entirely asymptomatic. However, a rare subset of G6PD-deficient patients has, instead, a chronic hemolytic disorder, which may be severe.
4. G6PD deficiency is genetically heterogeneous. About 400 different variants have been reported on the basis of diverse biochemical characteristics; this diversity suggests that these variants result from many allelic mutations in the G6PD gene. In addition, several structural mutants without enzyme deficiency have been characterized. Molecular analysis has confirmed that the basis for G6PD deficiency is widely heterogeneous. In some cases, variants that had been assigned different names turned out to be identical; conversely, however, some variants that had been thought to be homogeneous have turned out to be heterogeneous on the molecular level. Thus far, some 130 different point mutations have been identified, but only five in-frame deletions of one to eight codons and no larger deletions have been observed. Different mutants, each one having a polymorphic frequency, underlie G6PD deficiency in the various parts of the world where this abnormality is prevalent. Genetic heterogeneity also explains to a large extent the diversity of clinical manifestations. Different mutations are responsible for the less common patients who have chronic hemolytic anemia and for the frequent patients who are only at risk of developing episodic hemolysis.
5. The remarkable geographic correlation between the prevalence of G6PD deficiency and the past and present endemicity of *Plasmodium falciparum* malaria strongly suggests that the former confers resistance against the latter. The high prevalence in malaria-endemic areas of G6PD mutants that have arisen independently corroborates this notion; indeed, it constitutes an example of convergent evolution through balanced polymorphism. Clinical data further support this notion, although it is not certain whether malaria resistance is a feature of heterozygous females only, or also of hemizygous males. In vitro culture studies have shown that the growth of malaria parasites is impaired in G6PD-deficient red cells, and that G6PD-deficient parasitized red cells are phagocytosed by macrophages more effectively than G6PD normal parasitized red cells.

A list of standard abbreviations is located immediately preceding the index in each volume. Additional abbreviations used in this chapter include: CNSHA = chronic nonspherocytic hemolytic anemia; GSHPX = glutathione peroxidase; NNJ = neonatal jaundice.

The recognition of human pathology associated with deficiency of glucose-6-phosphate dehydrogenase (G6PD) in red blood cells is quite ancient. It has gone through several stages.[1] First came the anecdotal observation by the Greek philosopher and mathematician Pythagoras, who is said to have warned his disciples against the dangers of eating fava beans (or broad beans, *Vicia faba*). Second was the clinical picture of favism drawn at the turn of the century by a number of physicians in Southern Italy and in Sardinia.[2–4] In contrast to some other inborn errors of metabolism, the mode of inheritance was not easy to establish, because exposure and response to fava beans is erratic; thus both a "toxic theory" and an "allergic theory" of the pathogenesis of favism were popular.[5] However, observant general practitioners had noticed that the condition did "run in families."[2] The third stage was the recognition of hemolytic anemia caused by drugs. Again, it soon became clear that with certain drugs only some individuals were susceptible, and the term "primaquine sensitivity" was appropriately coined.[6] For hematology, this syndrome was important because hemolytic anemia had been traditionally classified as being due to either intracorpuscular or extracorpuscular causes. Here was one that was caused by an exogenous agent, but only in people who presumably already had abnormal red cells.[7] The final stage was the discovery by Carson et al.[8] in Chicago that, indeed, primaquine-sensitive people had a very low level of G6PD activity in their red cells. Soon thereafter, similar observations were made in Germany[9] and in Italy on the red cells of people with a past history of favism.[10] The genetic heterogeneity of this abnormality then became quickly apparent,[11,12] and the question arose as to whether G6PD deficiency was due mainly to qualitative or to quantitative changes in the enzyme. In other words, it was not clear whether it was more similar to a structural hemoglobinopathy or to a thalassemia-like disorder.

Over the last 30 years, the biochemical basis and the clinical implications of G6PD deficiency have been largely established, and we now know that G6PD deficiency is caused by a multitude of different structural allelic mutants. The molecular structures of the normal gene and of many mutants have been elucidated, and very recently, the three-dimensional structure of G6PD was solved. Since the previous edition of this book, some new reviews dealing with G6PD have appeared.[13–15] The hematologic aspects of G6PD deficiency have also been covered in textbooks and monographs.[16–18]

STRUCTURE AND FUNCTION OF G6PD

G6PD in its active form is either a dimer or a tetramer consisting of identical subunits.[18,19] Both the dimer and the tetramer are active, and the two forms are in a pH-dependent equilibrium with each other, with about equal proportions present at neutral pH.[20,21] There are two molecules of tightly bound NADP per molecule of dimer.[22] The primary structure of the single subunit polypeptide chain was determined from the cDNA sequence (see "The G6PD Gene," below). It consists of 515 amino acids (Fig. 179-1), with a molecular weight of 59,265 daltons. The rat liver G6PD amino acid sequence, obtained by protein analysis,[23] shows 94 percent identity with the human sequence and provides evidence that the N-terminal amino acid is *N*-acetylalanine, which must result from posttranslational cleavage of the N-terminal methionine followed by acetylation. This was confirmed by tryptic peptide analysis of human red cell G6PD.[24] There are 11 cysteine residues per subunit, and one or more of them must be important for enzyme activity, because sulfhydryl group inhibitors, such as hydroxymercuribenzoate and *N*-ethylmaleimide, cause marked inhibition.[25] Recent data revealed one intra-chain disulfide bridge.[26] A recent analysis[27] retrieved from available databases 57 G6PD sequences from 54 organisms, including bacteria, yeast, fungi, plants, and numerous metazoa. The predicted amino acid sequences from these organisms show from 29 to 94 percent homology to human G6PD. Not surprisingly, the homology regions are not randomly distributed; indeed, one can identify several stretches of conserved residues, which generally correspond to important functional domains and/or to the hydrophobic core (see Fig. 179-1 and reference 27). An NADP-binding protein previously reported to be increased in G6PD-deficient subjects[28] was found to be the human homologue of the mouse "tum"-transplantation antigen p35B.[29]

The Three-Dimensional Structure and the Mechanism of Catalysis

The crystal structure of the G6PD from *Leuconostoc mesenteroides* has been solved at a resolution of 2.8 Å[30] and, based on this structure, a model of the human G6PD dimer has been obtained[31] (see Fig. 179-2). Each subunit has a smaller, N-terminal coenzyme domain and a larger C-terminal domain that includes the substrate-binding site; this arrangement is clearly conserved in the human enzyme. There are a total of 15 α-helical regions and 15 β-sheets. The boundary between the coenzyme domain and the substrate domain is at the end of sheet strand βF. The active site can be identified at the domain boundary and it includes the nonapeptide 198–206, which is highly conserved in evolution, and which, in turn, includes the lysine residue 205, already known to be part of the G6P binding site.[32] Mutating this residue to either arginine or threonine showed that lysine 205 is not indispensable for binding of the substrate G6P, but that it is essential for the catalytic action of the enzyme.[33] Work on the *Leuconostoc* enzyme has identified a histidine residue, corresponding to His263 in the human enzyme, as the base that mobilizes the proton from the C1 position of G6PD;[34] this had been in fact hypothesized from the pH-dependence of G6P binding.[20] The NADP binding site is a fan of β-sheet structures, with a critical G-X-X-G-X-X peptide motif that corresponds to amino acids 38 to 43 in exon 3. There are no known mutations in these amino acids in human G6PD variants, but an Ala → Gly replacement at amino acid 44 has been reported in G6PD Orissa, and this has a markedly decreased affinity for NADP.[35] Site-directed mutagenesis experiments on the *L. mesenteroides* G6PD, which can use either NAD or NADP as coenzyme, have identified an arginine residue in position 46 that is critical for NADP, but not for NAD binding.[36] This residue is highly conserved throughout evolution and it corresponds in the human enzyme to arginine 72, which so far has never been found mutated in human G6PD variants. The dimer interface of human G6PD is formed by association of the sheets and two helices in the C-terminal domain of each subunit to form a barrel. The two active sites in the dimer are more than 50 Å apart, separated by the large, predominantly antiparallel sheets of the dimer interface that together form a half-barrel. The structure of the human G6PD model as described has been recently essentially confirmed by direct crystallographic analysis.[26] The mechanism of catalysis has been discussed in greater detail elsewhere.[15]

METABOLIC ROLE OF G6PD

G6PD is depicted classically in intermediary metabolism as a step in the conversion of glucose-6-phosphate to pentose phosphate. Indeed, it is the first enzyme in the so-called pentose phosphate pathway, also referred to as the oxidative "shunt" (by contrast to the "mainstream" glycolytic Embden-Meyerhof pathway). However, pentose can be produced alternatively by the concerted action of transketolase and transaldolase, thus bypassing G6PD. There are limited data on what fraction of pentose is normally produced via G6PD as opposed to the transketolase-transaldolase route, and the ratio may vary in different cells and under different circumstances. However, Chinese hamster ovary cells[37] and human fibroblasts[38] with less than 5 percent of normal G6PD activity can grow normally, suggesting that G6PD does not need to contribute much to the large amount of pentose that is needed for nucleic acid synthesis. On the other hand, G6PD produces NADPH, the coenzyme that is the main hydrogen donor for numerous other enzymatic reactions. Some of these reactions are essential steps in biosynthetic pathways; another, catalyzed by

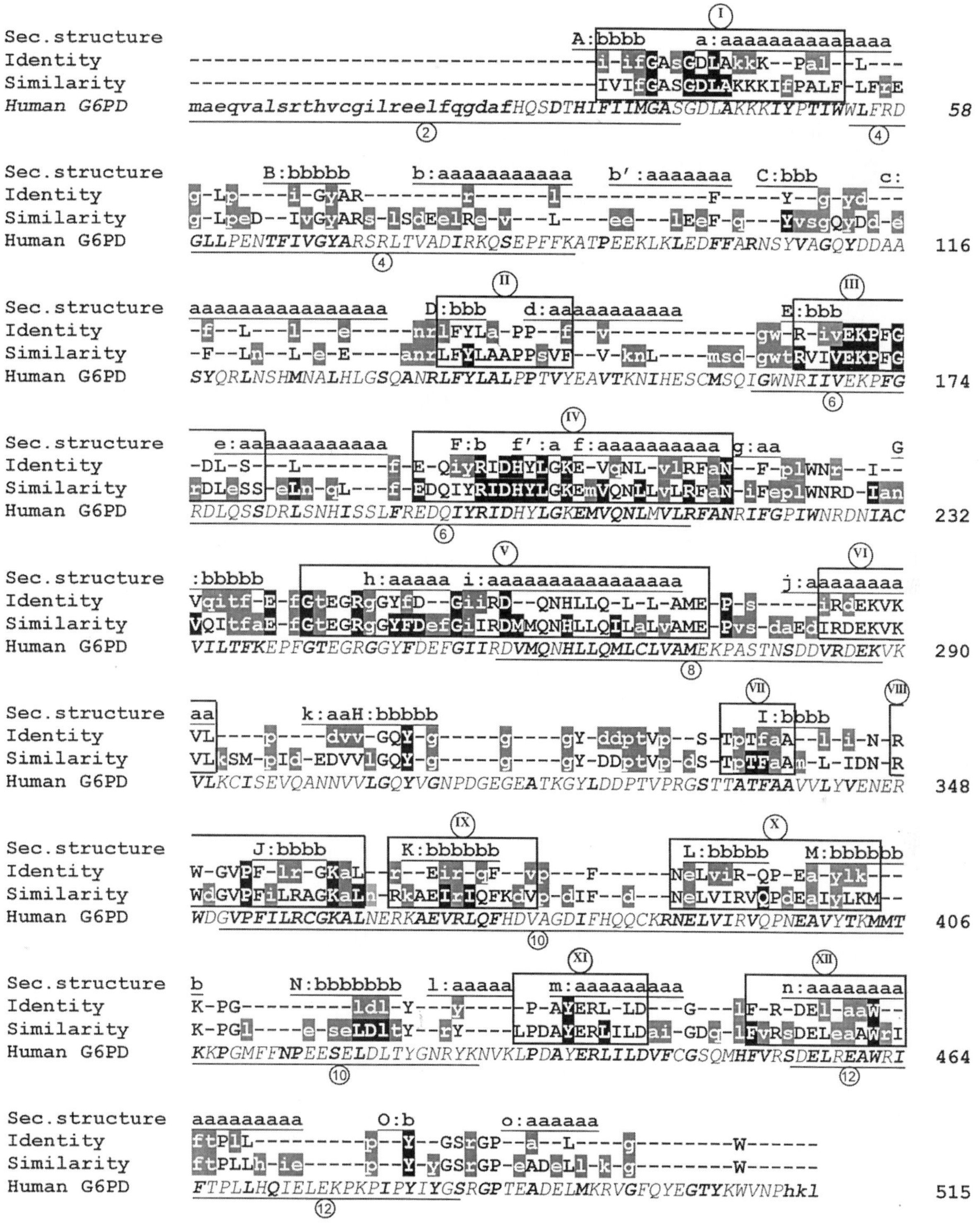

Fig. 179-1 Macro-evolution of the G6PD molecule. This diagram reflects a synoptic analysis of 52 different G6PD sequences. Human G6PD is used as the reference sequence and the even exons are underlined and numbered: the coding sequence starts in exon 2. In the lettering of human G6PD aa solvent accessibility (SA) is reported with the following code: bold uppercase, buried aa (SA <10%), non-bolded uppercase, exposed aa (SA ≥10%). Immediately above the human sequence we show the similarity consensus for the 52 sequences analyzed (Similarity), and above that the identity consensus sequence (Identity). At each position the most frequent aa is shown, with a coding for its frequency (white uppercase in black field: 100%; black uppercase: 76–99%; white lowercase in medium gray field: 51–75%); hyphens are entered in the two consensus lines for aa with <50% conservation. For aa similarity we have adopted the criteria of the Dayhoff PAM 250 matrix, *i.e.:* (a) DEQHN, (b) FY, (c) KR, (d) SAT, and (e) LIVM. Conserved blocks described in the text are boxed and identified with Roman numerals. Above the identity consensus sequence, runs of underlined *a* and *b* indicate α-helices and β-strands, respectively, as found in the *Leuconostoc mesenteroides* molecule[30] (Sec. structure).

The N-terminal methionine is not present in the mature protein and the N-terminal alanine is acetylated. It is seen that the lysine 205 lies within a highly conserved stretch of amino acids. This residue is part of the G6P-binding site. Also highly conserved is the NADP binding site at amino acids 38–44. Above the amino acid sequence the secondary structure is indicated by lettered stretches of a's and b's indicating the α-helices and β-sheets, respectively.

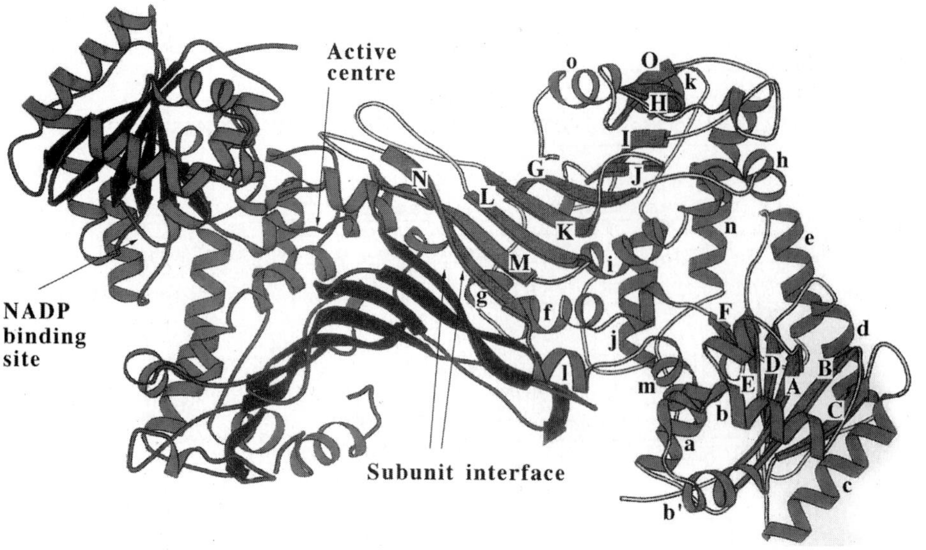

Fig. 179-2 The 3-D structure of human G6PD.[31] This model of the active dimer is derived from the structure of *Leuconostoc mesenteroides* G6PD. α-Helices are shown by medium gray helicoidal ribbons; β-sheets are shown by dark gray flat arrowheaded ribbons; coils are shown by either dark or light gray strings. In one subunit the sheets and helices are labeled in sequence order by capital and small letters, respectively.

glutathione reductase, is essential in protecting cells against oxidative damage (Fig. 179-3). Glutathione (GSH) converts H_2O_2 to H_2O stoichiometrically via glutathione peroxidase (GSHPX). Thus, the detoxification of each molecule of hydrogen peroxide requires one molecule of NADPH, ultimately provided by G6PD. That maintaining the level of intracellular GSH is a crucial function of G6PD in red cells has been obvious since the glutathione stability test was developed.[39] Recent data suggest that this notion has a much more general validity. Thus, HeLa cell clones[40] and fibroblast clones[41] overexpressing G6PD have an increased resistance to oxidative stress and an increased capacity to regenerate GSH under stress. Overexpression of G6PD in other cell types can protect against the lethal effect of peroxides,[42] and the similar effect of small stress proteins may be mediated by increased G6PD activity.[43]

An alternative pathway of H_2O_2 detoxification is via catalase. This route has been regarded as ineffective under normal circumstances,[44] because the affinity of catalase for H_2O_2 is much lower than that of GSHPX. In addition, the rare genetic defect acatalasemia is not associated with hemolytic anemia.[45] However, Kirkman and Gaetani[46,47] have discovered that catalase has four moles of tightly bound NADPH per mole of enzyme dimer, thereby bringing to light a further unexpected link between the G6PD coenzyme and H_2O_2 detoxification. From a comparison of normal and catalase-deficient red cells, they further inferred that catalase accounts for more than half of the destruction of H_2O_2

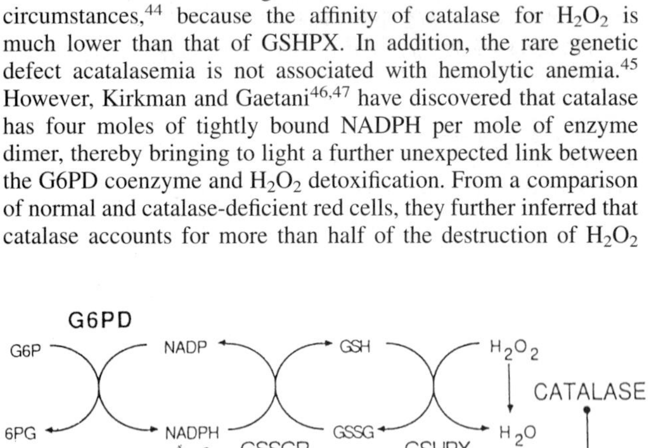

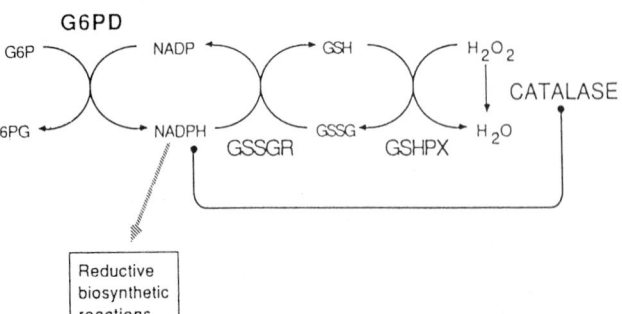

Fig. 179-3 The main metabolic role of G6PD in red cells is the defense against oxidizing agents, epitomized by hydrogen peroxide. NADPH, a product of the reaction, is both the hydrogen donor for regeneration of reduced glutathione and a ligand for catalase (see text). GSSGR = glutathione reductase; GSHPX = glutathione peroxidase; G-6-P = glucose-6-phosphate; 6PG = phosphogluconate.

when the latter is generated at a rate comparable to that which leads to hemolysis in G6PD-deficient erythrocytes.[48] Thus, we must now regard NADPH as essential for both pathways of H_2O_2 detoxification. Its role is stoichiometric when GSHPX is used, whereas it is catalytic when catalase is used. It has been postulated that when NADPH is in short supply owing to a G6PD deficiency, the role of the latter may become more important.[49] Amongst the NADPH-dependent biosynthetic reactions nitric oxide synthesis is prominent in many cell types; recently, it was shown to be impaired in G6PD-deficient granulocytes.[50]

Evidence from Model Systems

The notion that the primary role of G6PD consists in providing reductive power rather than in pentose synthesis is firmly based in evolution. In microbial organisms, G6PD is absent only from Archaea that are strict anaerobes and from intracellular bacteria.[27] G6PD null *E. coli*[51] and yeast[52] are viable, but unable to adapt to oxidative stress.[53] G6PD null mouse embryonic stem (ES) cells are also viable, but exquisitely sensitive to oxidative stress.[54] When injected into blastocysts, G6PD null ES cells yield chimeras and normal heterozygotes, but no hemizygous mice progeny,[55] confirming that G6PD null mutations are lethal. A mouse G6PD-deficient mutant with a red cell G6PD activity of about 15 percent of normal was obtained by chemical mutagenesis and was reported to have a normal phenotype.[56] However, it was recently shown that hemizygous mice with this mutation (identified as a splicing mutation[57]) have a significant rate of embryonic and postnatal death; that they have a marked reduction of G6PD activity also in non-hematopoietic tissues, particularly lung and brain; and that a high rate of teratogenesis is produced by administration of phenytoin during pregnancy.[58] Phenytoin is known to cause damage to embryos through oxidative stress,[59,60] providing a direct explanation as to why severe G6PD deficiency may be an embryonic lethal. By contrast, cells made to overexpress G6PD by introduction of a G6PD transgene have an increased growth rate.[61]

REGULATION OF G6PD ACTIVITY

As for all enzymes, the activity of G6PD in a cell could theoretically be changed by two general mechanisms, which are discussed in turn.

Variation in the Number of G6PD Molecules

Enzyme activity measured in cell extracts under optimal conditions and with saturating substrate concentrations is assumed to be proportional to the number of molecules present. While G6PD is

Table 179-1 G-6PD Activity in Selected Tissues*

	In normal subjects milliunits/mg protein	In G6PD-deficient subjects, % of normal*
Erythrocytes	8.5	1–50
Granulocytes	851	1–90
Fibroblasts	174	2–90
Muscle	3.2	—
Liver	7.2	15–50
Brain (fetal)	85	—

*From Battistuzzi et al.,[66] from Luzzatto and Battistuzzi[386] and unpublished results. The range is very wide because the expression of G-6-PD deficiency, defined by assaying erythrocytes, varies widely with different Gd-alleles.

found in all cells, its level varies over a range of about two orders of magnitude in different tissues (Table 179-1), regardless of whether the activity is expressed per cell or per milligram of protein. This has been studied particularly in the liver in relation to diet,[62] where regulation may be posttranscriptional.[63] These tissue-specific differences may result from variations in the rate of transcription, in posttranscriptional processing, in mRNA stability, in the rate of translation, or in posttranslational changes, especially the rate of proteolytic degradation. Each of these possibilities is likely to be important in specific circumstances. For instance, an increase in G6PD-specific mRNA has been observed in the liver of rats in which fatty acid synthesis is stimulated by a high-carbohydrate diet after starvation,[64,65] and variation of mRNA is seen in various fetal and adult human organs.[66] Different rates of proteolysis are suggested by the wide difference between the half-life of normal G6PD in fibroblasts (about 2 days[67]) and in red cells (about 60 days[68]). Variation in the rate of transcription was suggested by an empirical correlation between the extent of methylation of cytosine residues in a DNA region located 3′ to the G6PD gene and the level of G6PD activity in a variety of fetal and adult organs.[66] Recently, it was shown that oxidative stress produces increased G6PD activity in a variety of human cell lines and in primary rat hapatocytes,[69] and that this is due mainly to an increased rate of transcription.[70]

Variation in the Enzyme Activity of Existing G6PD Molecules

The actual intracellular activity of G6PD, like that of any other enzyme, may be very different from what is measured under optimal conditions in cell-free extracts. Many effectors, including pH,[20,21] divalent cations,[71] inorganic phosphate, phosphorylated intermediates, and other compounds,[72,73] have been found to affect G6PD activity. Among known metabolites, at least three must be major determinants of the intracellular G6PD activity: the two substrates, G-6-P and NADP, and one of the reaction products, NADPH, which is a potent, partially competitive inhibitor of G6PD.[74,75] In red cells, the estimated concentration of G-6-P is about 32 μM (well below the K_m of G-6-P of 72 μM) and the concentration of NADP is extremely low (probably less than 1 μM[76]), whereas the concentration of NADPH is high. (Estimating the concentrations of NADP and NADPH is complicated by the fact that substantial fractions of these compounds are bound to catalase and NADPH diaphorase, respectively[47]). Thus, it can be predicted that the intracellular G6PD activity is only a small fraction of the maximum activity that would be available if substrate concentrations were saturating.[73] It is practically impossible to faithfully simulate intracellular conditions, but in the case of G6PD the intracellular activity can be measured experimentally by the rate of production of $^{14}CO_2$ from (1-^{14}C)glucose. Using this technique,[77] the above predictions were validated. In normal red cells, G6PD operates at only about 1 to 2 percent of its maximal potential, even under the stimulatory action of methylene blue (which tends to continuously reoxidize the NADPH produced by G6PD). This finding quantifies the vast reserve of reductive potential that is available to normal red cells, and which is substantially decreased in G6PD-deficient red cells, thus determining their pathophysiological features (see "Mechanism of Hemolysis," below). It has long been known[78,79] that certain steroid compounds, particularly dehydroepiandrosterone (DHEA), are potent inhibitors of G6PD, by a noncompetitive mechanism that probably involves an unusual binding of the inhibitor to the G6PD-G6P-NADP ternary complex.[80] It has been suggested that DHEA might help to prevent breast cancer through inhibition of G6PD,[81] but recent biochemical analysis does not support this claim.[82]

GENETICS

Inheritance of G6PD shows a characteristic X-linked pattern, and the much higher incidence of favism in males than in females was recognized even before G6PD deficiency was discovered.[83] In contrast to several other X-linked conditions, however, there are many populations in which the frequency of G6PD deficiency is so high that homozygous females are not rare (see reference 84). In biochemical terms, the inheritance of G6PD is typically co-dominant, as can be seen easily when electrophoretic variants segregate in a pedigree (Fig. 179-4). In terms of clinical expression, G6PD deficiency is sometimes classified as X-linked recessive.[85] Although X-linked, it is not truly recessive because heterozygous females can develop hemolytic attacks, even severe ones. This is explained by the coexistence in heterozygotes of two cell populations, G6PD(+) and G6PD(−), as a result of X-chromosome inactivation (see Fig. 179-12 later in this chapter). Beutler et al.[86] first demonstrated this physiological mosaicism in human red cells using G6PD as a marker. Soon afterward, Davidson et al.[87] obtained cellular clones expressing different G6PD alleles (GdB and GdA) from skin fibroblasts of heterozygotes, which proved conclusively that mosaicism was

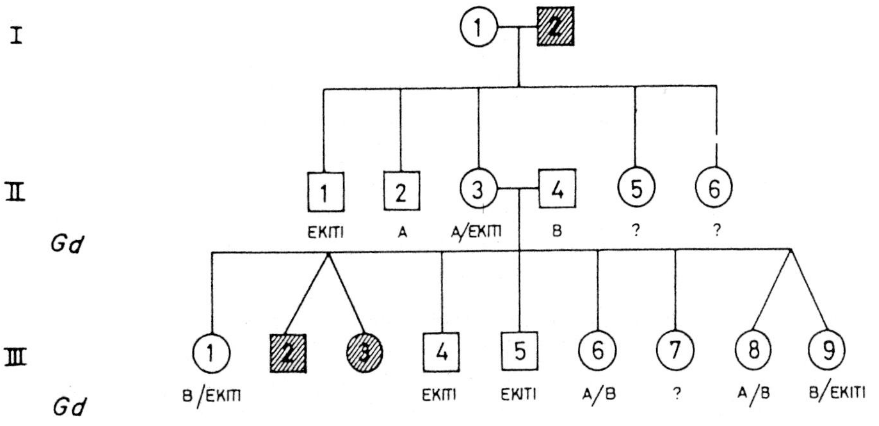

Fig. 179-4 X-linked inheritance of G6PD in a family segregating three different alleles (A, B, and Ekiti) at the locus Gd. Shaded symbols denote decreased subjects. (*From Usanga et al.*[594] *Reproduced with permission.*)

genetically determined in somatic cells by faithful maintenance of the active state of one or the other X chromosome in each cell and its progeny. Formal genetic analysis has already established that Gd was closely linked to several other X-linked genes,[88,89] including those for hemophilia A, color blindness, and adrenoleukodystrophy. The use of somatic cell hybrids[90] and of *in situ* hybridization with G6PD-specific probes[91,92] firmly mapped Gd as being distal to the fragile site Xq27.3. Subsequently, physical linkage between Gd and the factor VIII gene was established, within a length of about 400 kb, through analysis by pulsed-field gel electrophoresis of large DNA restriction fragments.[93] Yeast artificial chromosome (YAC) contigs established the physical relationship between Gd, factor VIII, and the color vision genes.[94] From an extended genomic sequence of Xq28 we now know that G6PD is embedded in a gene-rich region,[95] with a transcriptional map that is highly conserved between mouse and human.[96] The DNA replication origins have been also mapped in this region.

The G6PD Gene

Comparison of cDNA clones with genomic clones revealed thattheG6PD gene consists of 13 exons and 12 introns[97] (Fig. 179-5*A*). The coding exons vary in size from 38 to 236 bp. All introns are small (less than 1 kb), except for intron II, which is about 11 kb long. The 5′ untranslated portion of the mRNA corresponds to exon I and part of exon II; the initiation codon is in exon II, and the large intron (the significance of which is unknown, but which in the mouse includes a DNAse hypersensitive site[98]) interrupts the coding sequence at codon 36. The size of the G6PD mRNA expected from the sequence is 2269 nucleotides. This is in good agreement with the size of about 2.4 kb (including the poly(A) tail) measured on northern blots.[99]

The G6PD mRNA, like that of most genes, has a relatively short 5′ untranslated region of 69 bp and a longer 3′ untranslated region of 655 bp (Table 179-2). The entire genomic gene has been sequenced,[100] including about 2 kb of sequence upstream of the transcription initiation site. The mouse genomic gene has also been characterized and has considerable similarity to the human gene, not only in the coding region, but also in its overall organization.[101] The G6PD promoter[97] is very GC-rich (more than 70 percent), and it contains many unmethylated CG dinucleotides, constituting an island of HTF (*Hpa*II tiny fragments), regarded as characteristic of DNA flanking a gene.[102] As in other housekeeping-gene promoters,[103,104] there are several SP1-binding elements (see Fig. 179-6), GGCGGG and CCGCCC, which are reminiscent of the 21-bp repeats of the SV40 early promoter.[105] There is also an ATTAAA element at position −30 to −25, which may play the role of a "TATA box" (present in some housekeeping genes but not in others).[97] The size of the G6PD "minimal promoter" has been narrowed down to about 160 bp by deletion analysis.[106] The promoter region has been further characterized by band shift assays and systematic mutagenesis.[107,108] From this work it appears that only two of seven GC boxes are essential for basal transcriptional activity, and that different regions may influence transcription rate in different cell types.[108] This work also shows that point mutations in the promoter can markedly affect transcriptional activity. Thus, it is possible that in some cases, human G6PD deficiency is due to such mutations, although this has not yet been reported. The HIV-1-encoded Tat protein increases the rate of G6PD transcription in HeLa cells; this may be mediated by a short sequence element near the transcription start site, which has some features in common with the NFκB motif.[109] We do not yet know what precise structural elements determine the rate of transcription in different cells, under different physiological conditions (e.g., in response to changes in diet[98,110] or to hormones[111]), or in tissues with markedly increased G6PD activity, such as the lactating mammary gland[112] or certain tumors.[113] However, extensive work in transgenic mice has shown that, with a 630-bp promoter, the levels of enzyme activity produced by a human G6PD transgene parallel closely those of the endogenous mouse G6PD gene in all tissues that were tested,[114] suggesting that this promoter is sufficient for the physiology of G6PD expression. Overexpression of G6PD in erythroid cells was obtained in a transgenic mouse in which the G6PD gene was driven by an SV40 promoter placed downstream of the human beta-globin locus control region.[115]

An intronless, presumably retroposed autosomal G6PD gene has been discovered in the mouse.[116] Its predicted amino acid sequence has 92 percent identity to the X-linked G6PD, and its expression is strictly confined to postmeiotic spermatogenic cells, suggesting that it is required at the time when the X chromosome is inactivated in these cells. This situation is highly reminiscent of that already known for another X-linked housekeeping gene, phosphoglycerate kinase[117] (see Chap. 182). This autosomal G6PD has not yet been demonstrated in humans, but one wonders

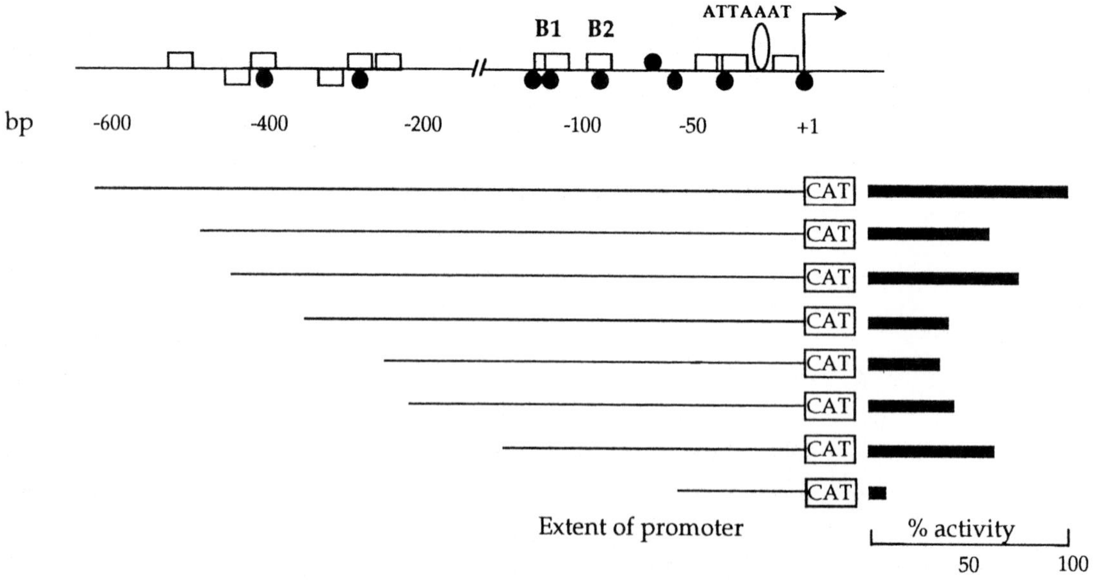

Fig. 179-5 The promoter.[108] On the top line, the location of consensus sequences for Sp1 and AP2 binding (filled circles and open squares, respectively) are shown in the region upstream of the G6PD transcription initiation site (+1). Note the change in scale at −150. The B1 and B2 boxes are both essential for transcription. The horizontal lines below show the extent of the promoter left intact after serial deletions, starting from −613 bp. The horizontal bars to the right show the extent of transcriptional activity of these deletions relative to the −613 bp promoter, as determined by CAT expression in HeLa cells.

Table 179-2 Molecular Numerology of Human G6PD

DNA	
Size of gene, kb	18.5
Total number of exons	13
Coding exons	12
mRNA	
Size of nucleotides	2269
5′ untranslated region	69
Coding region	1545
3′ untranslated region	655
Protein	
Amino acids, number	515
Molecular weight	59,265
Subunits per molecule of active enzyme	2 or 4
Molecules of tightly bound NADP per subunit	1
Molecular specific activity, IU/nmole	13

whether it may correspond to a chromosome 17 sequence previously identified by cross-hybridization to G6PD on Southern blots.[118]

Genetic Variation of G6PD

It became apparent almost immediately after the discovery of G6PD deficiency that the condition was caused not by a single mutation but by a variety of genetic changes. The initial criteria for this inference were the level of residual activity and the electrophoretic mobility. Subsequently, the study of other physicochemical properties (thermostability, chromatographic behavior) and of kinetic properties (K_m for G6P, K_m for NADP, pH dependence, utilization of substrate analogues) revealed that numerous variants must exist, even within a set having the same or very similar residual activity and electrophoretic mobility. In 1967, a WHO study group made recommendations on standardized methods of analysis,[119] which have been followed by most investigators and subsequently updated.[120] For taxonomic purposes, it is convenient to classify G6PD variants according to the level of enzyme activity and to the clinical manifestations (classes I to V; see Table 179-3) or according to whether they are sporadic or polymorphic. Not surprisingly, these classification criteria are not unrelated to each other. For instance, variants in class I (chronic nonspherocytic hemolytic anemia, CNSHA) are never polymorphic, presumably because their clinical expression is too severe to become balanced by malaria selection. All variants in class IV (normal activity) are electrophoretically different from the wild-type (B), because otherwise they would not have been detected. Some 400 different variants reported before 1994 were listed in Table 111-4*B* in the previous edition of this book.[121] It was not always easy to be sure whether the claim of a "new" variant was valid; multivariate analysis had been proposed for testing the identity of G6PD variants and the relationships among them.[122] Now molecular analysis is the definitive criterion, and in several cases, variants that had been claimed to be different turned out to be the same (see, for example, footnotes to Table 179-4). In the case of G6PD Cagliari and G6PD Sassari, which have the same mutation as G6PD Mediterranean, painstaking biochemical work still finds some different properties,[123,124] the structural basis for which is unknown.

Although there were reports in the earlier literature of "complete" absence of G6PD,[125,126] complete G6PD deficiency has yet to be identified; all the human mutants are, in the language of classic microbial genetics, "leaky." Therefore, we must understand the pathophysiology of G6PD deficiency in terms of the quantity and quality of the residual mutant enzyme. As for any other genetically determined enzymopathy, deficiency of G6PD might be due to a quantitative reduction in the number of enzyme molecules, to a qualitative change in the structure of the enzyme molecule, or to both. The findings reviewed in the previous section strongly supported the notion that most subjects with G6PD deficiency have a qualitatively abnormal enzyme, and that a wide

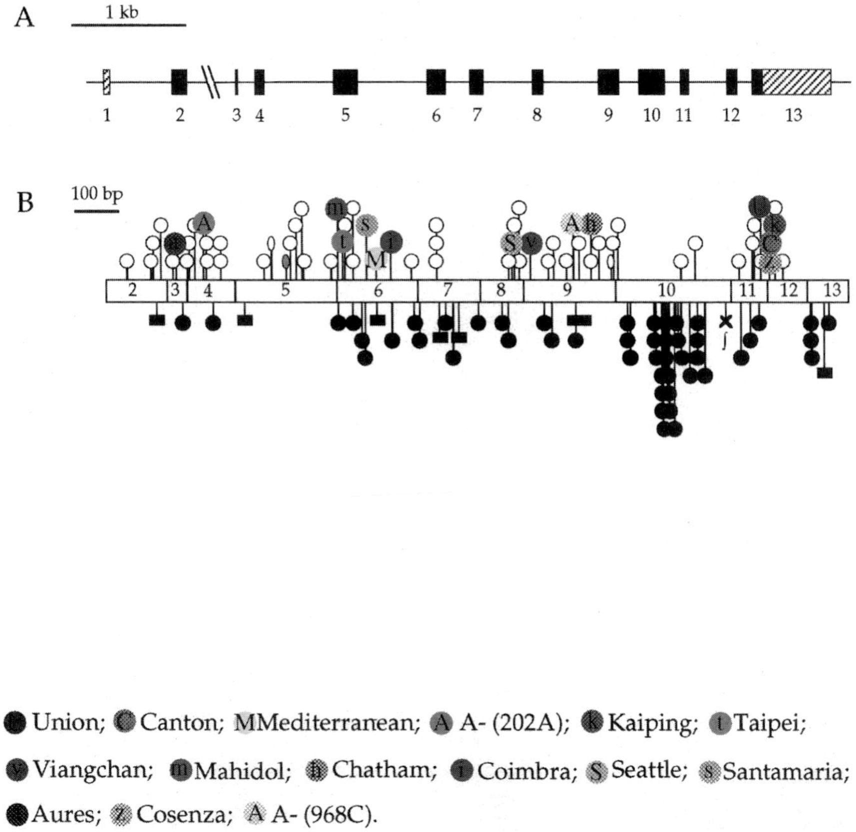

Fig. 179-6 Distribution of mutations along the structure of the human G6PD gene. *A*, Coding exons are shown as numbered black rectangles. Noncoding sequences of the mRNA are shown as shaded rectangles. *B*, The locations of amino acid substitutions are shown along the coding sequence of the gene, in which the exons are shown as open boxes. Those giving rise to the more severe (Class I) variants are shown as filled circles below. Small deletions, a nonsense mutation, and a splice site mutation are shown as filled rectangles, a cross, and a ∫, respectively. The milder class II and III variants are shown as open circles above, while class IV variants are shown as open ellipses.

Table 179-3 **Summary of Biochemically Defined G6PD Variants**

Polymorphic			Electrophoretic mobility			Altered electrophoretic mobility, %
Class	Number	%	Fast	Normal	Slow	
I	1	1	—	34	39	64
II	37	30	—	37	54	70
III	22	21	41	16	46	84
IV	12	23	—	3	29	94
V	0		—			100
Total	**72**	**19**	**—**	**90**	**168**	**76**
With known mutation*	35	28	16	27	27	60

* For comparative purposes, this line shows the eletrophoretic data on those 70 variants from Table 179-4 for which this information is available.

range of different mutational changes have taken place in human populations. As soon as it became possible to sequence variants, these expectations were verified in broad outline.

An analysis of 130 variants fully characterized at the DNA level (Table 179-4) provides a reasonably clear picture of the molecular basis of G6PD deficiency. (a) In nearly all the G6PD variants, we find a single amino acid replacement, caused by a single missense point mutation; these point mutations are spread throughout the entire coding region. Because in most cases G6PD deficiency is due to instability, this must mean that many different amino acid (aa) replacements in many different locations can destabilize the enzyme molecule. (b) Conspicuous by their absence are large deletions, major rearrangements, and nonsense point mutations; in other words, *null* mutations have never been observed, suggesting that they are lethal, in keeping with the mouse evidence cited above. (c) Mutations that drastically compromise the binding of either substrate or the catalytic mechanism would be expected to affect G6PD function to approximately the same extent in all cells (rather than just in red cells), and ought to cluster in the respective regions of the sequence. We do not see these clusters, presumably because such mutations again may be frequently lethal. (d) Mutations that cause instability of the G6PD protein molecule would be expected to produce marked deficiency of G6PD in red cells (much more than in other cells), because these cells have a long life span after they have lost their capacity for protein synthesis. The majority of the G6PD variants associated with G6PD deficiency fall into this category. (e) The most conspicuous cluster of mutations emerges between aa 380 and aa 410, a region that corresponds to the subunit interface in the enzymatically active G6PD dimer. Moreover, nearly all of the mutations in this cluster cause a severe phenotype (class I); indeed, 34 percent of all class I mutations fall within this 6 percent of the entire sequence. This highlights the critical role of precisely fitting noncovalent interactions for the formation and stability of the dimeric molecule.

The distribution of mutations found in human patients seems to bear some relationship to the evolutionary history of G6PD. Indeed, over two-thirds of the amino acid replacements that cause G6PD deficiency are in residues that we could score as intermediate in terms of evolutionary conservation (see reference 27). In contrast, fully conserved amino acids are underrepresented in G6PD-deficient mutants, presumably because of a higher probability that their replacement may be lethal; and poorly conserved amino acids are also underrepresented, presumably because in many cases, their replacement may not cause G6PD deficiency and therefore such mutations may go undetected.

Sporadic Mutations

Databases comprising 100 or more mutations are now available for many human disease genes. However, G6PD is the only case of a housekeeping gene in which at least one-third of the known mutations are both potentially pathogenic and polymorphic (as a result of malaria selection; see below). Each of the polymorphic alleles must be an example of a fine equipoise, whereby the deleterious phenotypic consequences of the mutation are balanced by the resistance that it confers against *Plasmodium falciparum*. By contrast, we can presume — in first approximation — that each of the sporadic G6PD mutants has remained sporadic because its phenotypic consequences are *too* deleterious to be balanced by the resistance that it might confer against *P. falciparum*. On the one hand, they cannot cause complete loss of G6PD activity; otherwise they would fall into the same category as deletions (see above). On the other hand, they must cause sufficient loss of activity in red cells to become limiting for their in vivo survival. This in turn may result, in principle, from two (nonmutually-exclusive) mechanisms: (a) severe alterations in the interaction with the substrates, particularly G-6-P (see above under regulation); and (b) marked intracellular instability. With both mechanisms, the changes must be relatively subtle, as they seem to affect red cells more than other somatic cells. Although we do not yet know exactly how this is brought about, it is not too difficult to imagine that intracellular stability, for instance, has very different consequences in red cells, which have a long life span after they have lost the ability to synthesize proteins, compared to other somatic cells, which are capable of regenerating continuously effete protein molecules. There is also evidence that protease activity is different in red cells.[67,127]

We have already seen that severe instability of the G6PD molecule, causing severe G6PD deficiency, is usually brought about by single aa replacements, many of which cluster in exon 10 (see Fig. 179-5). This cluster, as well as several mutations in exons 7 and 8, affect the subunit interface. We do not yet have a precise explanation as to why each sporadic mutation gives a severe phenotype. Seven variants are in-frame deletions with loss of 1 aa (G6PD Sunderland, G6PD Urayasu, G6PD Tsukui, G6PD North Dallas, G6PD Brighton), or 2 aa (G6PD Stonybrook), or 8 aa (G6PD Nara). One variant has a splice-site mutation (G6PD Varnsdorf). In the G6PD Vancouver variant, three separate amino acid replacements have been reported (one of which is the same as in the polymorphic variant G6PD Coimbra).

Sporadic variants associated with CNSHA are not likely to spread by genetic drift. Nevertheless, from molecular analysis of G6PD-deficient patients who present with CNSHA, it is increasingly common that one finds a mutation already previously seen in other patients who are almost certainly not ancestrally related.[128–130] It is a safe prediction that more G6PD mutations will be discovered. However, the finding that patients with CNSHA keep turning up with the same mutation in disparate parts of the world is not trivial. It can be presumed that these are independently arisen mutations: indeed, in several cases, these mutations were proven to be *de novo* by demonstrating their absence in the patient's mother. In some cases, these may be

Table 179-4 Genetic Variants of G6PD Characterized at the Molecular Level

Name	Nucleotide substitution	Restriction enzyme site change	Amino acid replacement	Protein location	Class	Electro-phoretic mobility	K_mG6P, µM	Population (*: polymorphic)	References
Sinnai	34 G → T	−*Afl*III	12 Val → Leu	pre βA	III			Sardinian	478
Lages	40 G → A	+*Bsg*I	14 Gly → Arg	pre βA	II or III			Brazilian	138
Gaohe[1]	95 A → G		32 His → Arg	βA	III	96	31	Chinese*	479
Honiara	99 A → G	+*Nla*III	33 Ile → Met	βA inter αm/αn	II			Solomon Is*	480
	1360 C → T	*Hha*I	454 Arg → Cys						
Sunderland	Δ105–107		35 or 36 Δ Ile	βA	I	95		English	481
Gidra	110 T → C	−*Nla*III	37 Met → Thr	βA					See Vulliamy et al.[482]
Orissa	131 C → G	−*Hae*III	44 Ala → Gly	αa	III	100	69		35
Aures	143 T → C	−*Bgl*II	48 Ile → Thr	αa	II	100	59	Algerian*, Middle Eastern, Spanish	483
Kozukata	159 G → C	+*Pvu*II	53 Trp → Cys	αa	I			Japanese	See Vulliamy et al.[482]
Kamogawa	169 C → T	−*Msp*I	57 Arg → Trp	αa	II			Japanese	See Vulliamy et al.[482]
Metaponto	172 G → A	−*Fok*I	58 Asp → Asn	inter αa/βB	III	90	47	Italian*	132
Musashino	185 C → T	+*Taq*I	62 Pro → Leu	inter αa/βB	III	90	32	Japanese	129
A^{-}[2]	202 G → A	+*Nla*III	68 Val → Met	βB	III	110	60	African*, European, Middle Eastern, Brazilian, Central American	132, 134, 139, 484–486
	376 A → G	+*Fok*I	126 Asn → Asp	αc					
Namouru	208 T → C	+*Nla*III	70 Tyr → His	βB	II	92		S Pacific*	151
Murcia	209 A → G	+*Bsp*1286 I	70 Tyr → Cys	βB	II	98	54	Spanish	487
Swansea	224 T → C	−*Mnl*I	75 Leu → Pro	inter βB/αb	I			Welsh	128
Ube[3]	241 C → T	−*Fok*I	81 Arg → Cys	αb	III	108	52	Japanese*	488
Lagosanto	242 G → A		81 Arg → His	αb	III	105	65	Italian	489
Urayasu	Δ 281–283	+*Sac*I	95 Δ Lys	αb′	I	109	40	Japanese	490
Vancouver	317 C → G	−*Msp*I	106 Ser → Cys	βC	I			Canadian	491
	544 C → T		182 Arg → Trp	αe					
	592 C → T		198 Arg → Cys	βf					
Hammersmith	323 T → A	+*Mnl*I	108 Val → Glu	βC	III	108		Indian	143
Sao Borja	337 G → A		113 Asp → Asn	inter βC/αc	IV	83	96	Brazilian, Cuban, Italian	138
A	376 A → G	+*Fok*I	126 Asn → Asp	αc	IV	110	60	African*	492
Vanua Lava	383 T → C	−*Mnl*I	128 Leu → Pro	αc	II	96		S Pacific*	151
Quing Yan	392 G → T	+*Dra*III	131 Gly → Val	inter αc/βD	III	100	56	Chinese*	162
Cairo	404 A → C	+*Fau*I	135 Asn → Thr	βD	II			Egyptian	See Vulliamy et al.[482]
Valladolid	406 C → T		136 Arg → Cys	βD	II	112	41	Spanish	493
Acrokorinthos	463 C → A	*Fok*I	155 His → Asn	αd	II			Greek	494
	376 A → G		126 Asn → Asp	αc					
Ilesha	466 G → A	−*Hinf*I	156 Glu → Lys	αd	III	75	83	Nigerian, Algerian	132
Mahidol	487 G → A	+*Alu*I	163 Gly → Ser	inter αd/βE	III	100	40	SE Asian*	495
Plymouth	488 G → A		163 Gly → Asp	inter αd/βE	I	103	48	English	128
Taipei	493 A → G	+*Ava*II	165 Asn → Asp	βE	II		54	Chinese*, Filipino*	496
Naone	497 G → A	−*Sfa*NI	166 Arg → His	βE	II	103		S Pacific*	151
Volendam	514 C → T		172 Pro → Ser	interβE/αe	I			Dutch	497
Nankang	517 T → C	+*Ava*I	173 Phe → Leu	inter βE/αe	II			Chinese	498
Miaoli	519 C → G	−*Xmn*I	173 Phe → Leu	inter βE/αe				Chinese*	499
Shinshu	527 A → G	+*Hae*III	176 Asp → Gly	inter βE/αe	I		85	Japanese, English	500

(Continued on next page)

Table 179-4 Genetic Variants of G6PD Characterized at the Molecular Level (*Continued*)

Name	Nucleotide substitution	Restriction enzyme site change	Amino acid replacement	Protein location	Class	Electro-phoretic mobility	K_mG6P, μM	Population (*: polymorphic)	References
Chikugo	535 A → T	+*Sac*I	179 Ser → Cys	αe	I			Japanese	See Vulliamy et al.[482]
Malaga	542 A → T	−*Cfr*10 I	181 Asp → Val	αe	II	81	26	Spanish*	501
Santamaria	542 A → T	−*Cfr*10 I	181 Asp → Val	αe	II	98	16	Algerian*, Costa Rican, Canary Is, Spanish, Italian	502
	376 A → G	+*Fok*I	126 Asn → Asp	αc					
Tsukui	Δ 561–563	−*Mnl*I	188 or 189_Ser	αe	I	89	100	Japanese	490
Mediterranean[4]	563 C → T	+*Mbo* II	188 Ser Δ Phe	αe	II	100	23	Mediterranean*, Middle Eastern, Indian, SE Asian	132,145,503
Coimbra[5]	592 C → T		198 Arg → Cys	βF	II	100	7	Mediterranean*, Taiwanese	152
Santiago	593 G → C	−*Sfa*N I	198 Arg → Pro	βF	I			Chilean	504
Sibari	634 A → G	−*Nla* III	212 Met → Val	αf	III	100	31	Italian*	133
Minnesota[6]	637 G → T		213 Val → Leu	αf	I	95	88	USA (white)	506,507
Harilaou	648 T → G	+*Hae* III	216 Phe → Leu	αf	I	100		Greek	508
Radlowo	679 C → T	−*Msp*I	227 Arg → Trp	inter αg/βG					509
Mexico City	680 G → A	+*Bst*N I	227 Arg → Gln	inter αg/βG	III	110		Mexican	504
A⁻	680 G → T	+*Bst*N I +*Fok*I	227 Arg → Leu	inter αg/βG	III	110		USA (black)	134
	376 A → G		126 Asn → Asp	αc					
North Dallas	Δ 683–685		229 Δ Asn	inter αg/βG	I			USA	See Vulliamy et al.[482]
Asahikawa	695 G → A	+*Mae* II	232 Cys → Tyr	βG	I	98	30	Japanese	129
Durham	713 A → G	+*Eco*57 I	238 Lys → Arg	βG	I	100		USA (white)	510
Stonybrook	Δ 724–729	−*Dde*I	242–243 Δ Gly, Thr	inter βG/αh	I			USA (white)	511
Wayne	769 C → G	−*Fok*I	257 Arg → Gly	αh	I	107	78	USA (white)	507
Aveiro	806 G → A		269 Cys → Tyr	αh	I			Brazilian	512
Corum[7]	820 G → A	+*Mbo*II	274 Glu → Lys	inter αi/αj	I	85	35	Turkish, USA (white)	511
Wexham	833 C → T	−*Mnl*I	278 Ser → Phe	inter αi/αj	I	96		English	128
Chinese-1	835 A → T	+*Mme*I	279 Thr → Ser	inter αi/αj	II			Chinese	513
Seattle[8]	844 G → C	−*Dde*I	282 Asp → His	αj	III	80	20	European*, Algerian, Mexican, Brazilian, Canaries	145, 514–516
Papua	849 C → A	−*Aat*II	283 Asp → Glu	αj					Unpublished
Osaka	853 C → T		285 Arg → Cys	αj	II			Japanese	See Vulliamy et al.[482]
Montalbano	854 G → A	+*Nla*III	285 Arg → His	αj	III	93	49	Italian *	517
Viangchan[9]	871 G → A		291 Val → Met	αj	III	100	105	Laotian*, Filipino, Chinese	507
West Virginia	910 G → T	−*Ava*II	303 Val → Phe	αk	I			USA (white)	511
Seoul	916 G → A	+*Dde*I	306 Gly → Ser	βH	II				See Vulliamy et al.[482]
Omiya	921 G → C	−*Rsa*I	307 Gln → His	βH	I				See Vulliamy et al.[482]
Ludhiana	929 G → A	−*Nla*IV	310 Gly → Glu	βH	II or III			Indian	See Vulliamy et al.[482]
Kalyan[10]	949 G → A		317 Glu → Lys	inter βH/βI	III	75	105	Indian*	156
Nara	Δ 953–976	−*Kpn*I	319–236 Δ TKGYLDDP	inter βH/βI	I			Japanese, Portuguese	289
Manhattan	962 G → A	−*Kpn*I	321 Gly → Glu	inter βH/βI	I				See Vulliamy et al.[482]
A⁻[11]	968 T → C	+*Nci*I	323 Leu → Pro	inter βH/βI	III	110		USA (black), Mexican Spanish*, Canaries, Portuguese	134
	376 A → G	+*Fok*I	126 Asn → Asp	αc					
Farroupilha	977 C → A	+*Dra*III	326 Pro → His	inter βH/βI	II or III			Brazilian	138
Chatham	1003 G → A	−*Bsp*W I	335 Ala → Thr	inter βH/βI	III	100	60	Filipino*, Indian, Middle Eastern, Mediterranean, Brazilian, Japanese	132

Table 179-4 Genetic Variants of G6PD Characterized at the Molecular Level (*Continued*)

Name	Nucleotide substitution	Restriction enzyme site change	Amino acid replacement	Protein location	Class	Electro-phoretic mobility	K_mG6P, μM	Population (*: polymorphic)	References
Fushan	1004 C → A	+*Alu* I	335 Ala → Asp	inter βH/βI	II			Chinese	511
Torun	1006 A → G		336 Thr → Ala	βI	I			Polish	509
Chinese-5	1024 C → T	+*Mbo* II	342 Leu → Phe	βI	III	91	65	Chinese*	162
Mira d'Aire	1048 G → C	+*Nla* III	350 Asp → His	inter βI/βJ	IV			Portuguese	See Vulliamy et al.[482]
Partenope	1052 G → T		351 Gly → Val	inter βI/βJ	II	100	19	Italian	124
Ierapetra	1057 C → T	−*Nla* IV	353 Pro → Ser	inter βI/βJ	II			Greek*	504
Iwatsuki	1081 G → A	−*Hae* III	361 Ala → Thr	inter βJ/βK	I			Japanese	See Vulliamy et al.[482]
Serres	1082 C → T	+*Ava* II	361 Ala → Val	inter βJ/βK	I			Greek	130
Loma Linda	1089 C → A		363 Asn → Lys	inter βJ/βK	I	98	70	USA (Mexican)	506
Calvo Mackenna	1138 A → G	+*Mae* II	380 Ile → Val	inter βK/βL	I				518
Riley	1139 T → C	−*Mbo* II	380 Ile → Thr	inter βK/βL	I				518
Olomouc	1141 T → C	+*Fok* I	381 Phe → Leu	inter βK/βL	I			Czech	511
Tomah	1153 T → C	+*Fnu*4H I	385 Cys → Arg	inter βK/βL	I	92	42	USA, Spanish, Portuguese	519
Lynwood	1154 G → T		385 Cys → Phe	inter βK/βL	I				See Vulliamy et al.[482]
Madrid	1155 C → G		385 Cys → Trp	inter βK/βL	I	91	76	Spanish	493
Iowa[12]	1156 A → G		386 Lys → Glu	inter βK/βL	I	100	65	USA (white), English	519
Guadalajara	1159 C → T	−*Hha* I	387 Arg → Cys	inter βK/βL	I	100	36	Mexican, Irish, USA (white), Danish, Indian, Japanese	128, 504, 520, 521
Mount Sinai	1159 C → T 376 A → G	−*Hha* I *Fok* I	387 Arg → Cys 126 Asn → Asp	inter βK/βL αc	I				131
Beverly Hills[13]	1160 G → A	−*Hla* I	387 Arg → His	inter βK/βL	I	95	41	USA (white), Italian, Scottish, Japanese	129, 519, 522
Hartford	1162 A → G	+*BstU* I	388 Asn → Asp	βL	I				See Vulliamy et al.[482]
Praha	1166 A → G	−*Alu* I	389 Glu → Gly	βL	I			Czech	511
Wisconsin	1177 C → G	−*BstU* I	393 Arg → Gly	βL	I				518
Nashville[14]	1178 G → A	−*BstU* I	393 Arg → His	βL	I	100	87	USA, Italian, Portuguese, Israeli	506,524
Alhambra	1180 G → C	+*Pst* I	394 Val → Leu	βL	I	96	55	Finnish/Swedish	504
Bari	1187 C → T	+*Alu* I	396 Pro → Leu	inter βL/βM	I			Italian	
Puerto Limon	1192 G → A	−*Mnl* I	398 Glu → Lys	inter βL/βM	I	98	32	Costa Rican	502
Anadia	1193 A → G	+*Sau*96 I	398 Glu → Gly	inter βL/βM	II	90		Portuguese	See Vulliamy et al.[482]
Clinic	1215 G → A		405 Met → Ile	βM	I	100	52	Spanish, French	487
Abeno	1220 A → C		407 Lys → Thr	βM	II				See Vulliamy et al.[482]
Riverside	1228 G → T	−*Msp* I	410 Gly → Cys	inter βM/βN	I	100	326	German/English	519
Kawasaki	1229 G → C	+*Hae* III	410 Gly → Ala	inter βM/βN	I			Japanese	See Vulliamy et al.[482]
Shinagawa	1229 G → A	−*Nci* I	410 Gly → Asp	inter βM/βN	I		242	Japanese	500, 504
Tokyo[15]	1246 G → A	+*Sty* I	416 Glu → Lys	βN	I	90	65	Japanese, Scottish, Italian	128,129,525
Georgia	1284 C → A		428 Try → STOP	αl	I			Filipino female	511
Varnsdorf	Δ−2,−1	+*Dra* III	3′*splice* Δ AG		I			Czech	511
Sumare	1292 T → G	−*Mae* II	431 Val → Gly	αl	I			Brazilian	526
Pawnee	1316 G → C	−*Hinp* I	439 Arg → Pro	αm	i	103	50	USA (white)	504
Kobe[16]	1318 C → T	−*Mnl* I	440 Leu → Phe	αm	I	89	143	Japanese, Italian	
Santiago de Cuba[17]	1339 G → A	+*Pst* I	447 Gly → Arg	inter αm/αn	I	80	50	Cuban, Japanese	132
San Antioco	1342 A → G	+*Hae* III	448 Ser → Gly	inter αm/αn	II			Italian*	124

Table 179-4 Genetic Variants of G6PD Characterized at the Molecular Level (*Continued*)

Name	Nucleotide substitution	Restriction enzyme site change	Amino acid replacement	Protein location	Class	Electro-phoretic mobility	K_mG6P, μM	Population (*: polymorphic)	References
Cassano	1347 G → C	+*Nla* III	449 Gln → His	inter αm/αn	II	93	14	Italian*	133
Hermoupolis	1347 G → C 1360 C → T	+*Nla* III −*Hha* I	449 Gln → His 454 Arg → Cys	inter αm/αn inter αm/αn	II				494
Harima	1358 T → A	+*Taq* I	453 Val → Glu	inter αm/αn	I				See Vulliamy et al.[482]
Union[18]	1360 C → T	−*Hha* I	454 Arg → Cys	inter αm/αn	II	105	8	Polynesian*, SE Asian, Chinese, Mediterranean	149, 150, 133, 513, 527, 528
Andalus	1361 G → A	−*Hha* I	454 Arg → His	inter αm/αn	II	100	14	Spanish, Japanese	529
Figuera da Foz	1366 G → C		456 Asp → His	αn	II			Portuguese	Unpublished
Canton[19]	1376 G → T		459 Arg → Leu	αn	II	105	28	Chinese *, SE Asian	530
Cosenza	1376 G → C	+*Dde* I	459 Arg → Pro	αn	II	100	27	Mediterranean*	133
Kamiube[20]	1387 C → T		463 Arg → Cys	αn	III	100	57	Japanese*	129
Kaiping[21]	1388 G → A		463 Arg → His	αn	II	100	40	Chinese*	163
Neapolis	1400 C → G		467 Pro → Arg	αn	III	85	55	Italian	169
Fukaya	1462 G → A	−*Hae* III	488 Gly → Ser	inter βO/αo	I			Japanese	See Vulliamy et al.[482]
Campinas	1463 G → T	+*Hinf* I	488 Gly → Val	inter βO/αo	I			Brazilian	531
Arakawa	1466 C → T	−*Sau*96 I	489 Pro → Leu	inter βO/αo	I			Japanese	See Vulliamy et al.[482]
Brighton	Δ1488-1490	−*Mbo* II	497 Δ Lys	αo	I	100	50	English	Unpublished
Bangkok Noi	1502 T → G 1376 G → T		501 Phe → Cys 459 Arg → Leu	post αo αn	I			Japanese	See Vulliamy et al.[482]

*Other named variants share some of the listed mutations as follows: [1]Gaozhou. [2]Distrito Federal, Matera, Castilla, Alabama, Betica, Tepic, Ferrara I, Laghouat, Kabyle. [3]Konan. [4]Dallas, Birmingham, Sassari, Caliari, Panama. [5]Shunde. [6]Marion, Gastonia, Le Jeune. [7]Cleveland. [8]Lodi, Modena Ferrara II, Athens-like, Mexico. [9]Jammu. [10]Kerala. [11]Betica, Selma, Guantanemo. [12]Iowa City, Walter Reed, Springfield. [13]Genova, Worcester, Yamaguchi, Iwate, Niigata. [14]Anaheim, Caligari, Portici. [15]Fukushima. [16]Telti. [17]Morioka. [18]Maewo, Chinese-2. [19]Taiwan-Hakka, Gifu-like, Agrigento-like. [20]Keelung. [21]Anant, Dhon, Petrich, Sapporo, Wosera.

mutational hot spots, particularly when the mutation is a C → T transition (which may result from methyl-C deamination) in a CpG pair, as in G6PD Guadalajara, G6PD Nashville, and others, all of which have been found recurrently.[130] (In one case, the G6PD Guadalajara mutation must have taken place in a G6PD A background, yielding G6PD Mount Sinai.[131]) However, perhaps the most interesting inference is that there is a limited set of mutations that give G6PD deficiency; thus, we have a kind of ascertainment bias in collecting mutations mostly from patients who present with clinical disease (see Table 179-4). In summary, there is a limited number of ways in which the G6PD molecule can be altered so that it will cause a distinctly severe clinical expression while remaining compatible with life.

Polymorphic Mutations

Most known mutations in this category are again associated with G6PD deficiency (see Table 179-4), and there is overwhelming evidence that they have become polymorphic as a result of malaria selection. For these mutations, we can visualize more stringent constraints. While they cause deficiency in red cells probably by similar mechanisms, they must not affect the red cells so severely as to outweigh the advantage with respect to malaria. Thus, it is not surprising that nearly all the polymorphic variants fall in classes II or III, and none of them causes CNSHA (class I).

If we analyze separately the severe sporadic mutations and the mild polymorphic mutations against the backdrop of macro-evolution (see reference 27), we find that the former are slightly more frequent in the 76 to 99 percent conservation bracket, whereas the latter are more frequent in the 50 to 75 percent conservation bracket (difference not yet statistically validated).

Two of the three known mutations that give rise to class IV variants (i.e., with normal activity), G6PD A and G6PD São Boria, are quite close to each other in the α helix c. G6PD A was one of the first G6PD variants to be extensively investigated, and it is probably also quite ancient in human evolution, based on the fact that the respective mutation has been found in three different haplotypes. G6PD became so widespread, originally in Africa, that we know of at least five G6PD double-mutants that must be derivatives of G6PD A through a second mutation (see Fig. 179-9). Finally, we must remember that, as in the case of other protein polymorphisms, electrophoretically silent G6PD variants—hitherto undetected—are likely to exist as well.

Spread of Polymorphic Variants of G6PD

The world distribution of G6PD deficiency (Fig. 179-7) has not changed much since previous editions. However, it is gradually becoming possible to supplement this phenotypic map (i.e., one that reflects the prevalence of G6PD deficiency as a whole), with a genetic map, showing the distribution of individual polymorphic alleles. Ideally, we would like to know for any given population the quantitative contribution of each of these to the overall prevalence of G6PD deficiency. A first attempt has been made here (Fig. 179-8): although the information is sketchy and often not quantitative, some pattern is emerging. G6PD A− is widespread in Africa, in the Americas, in the West Indies, and wherever there are immigrant populations of African origin. In addition, G6PD A− is present with significant frequency in southern Europe (for instance in southern Italy,[132,133] Spain,[134] the Canary Islands,[135] and Portugal), and in the Arabian peninsula.[134] G6PD A− has also been reported in white Brazilians,[136–138] and we have seen it in a white American from South Carolina, and in Corsica. The population distribution of the nondeficient variant, G6PD A, is practically the same as that of G6PD A−. G6PD Mediterranean was very appropriately named because it is polymorphic in all countries surrounding the Mediterranean sea, including North African countries.[139] But it is also widespread in the Middle East, including the Arab countries and Israel, and it accounts for almost all the G6PD deficiency in Kurdish Jews,[140] the population that has the highest known frequency of this trait (estimated gene frequency = 0.65). In addition, G6PD Mediterranean is one of the

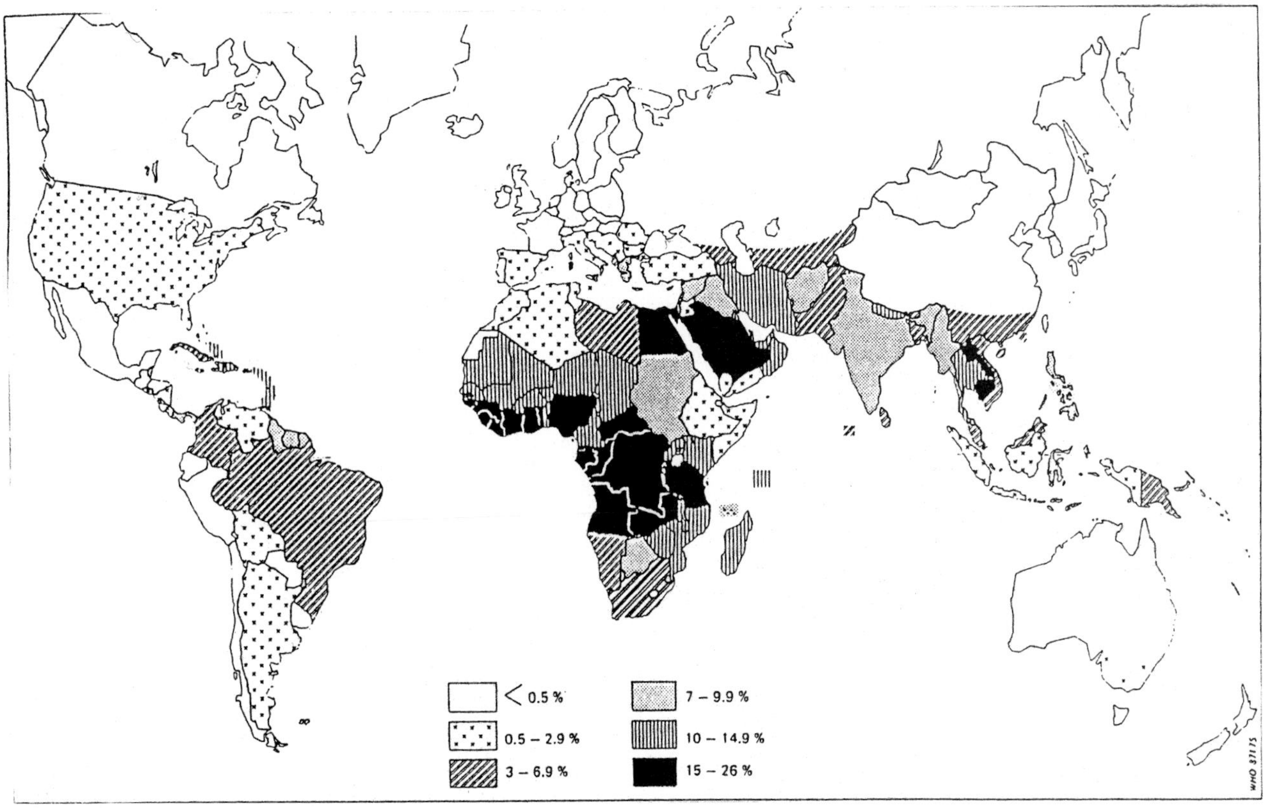

Fig. 179-7 World distribution of G6PD deficiency (from reference 120). The values shown by the different shadings are frequencies in the populations of the various countries of G6PD-deficient males (which are also gene frequencies, because the gene is X-linked).

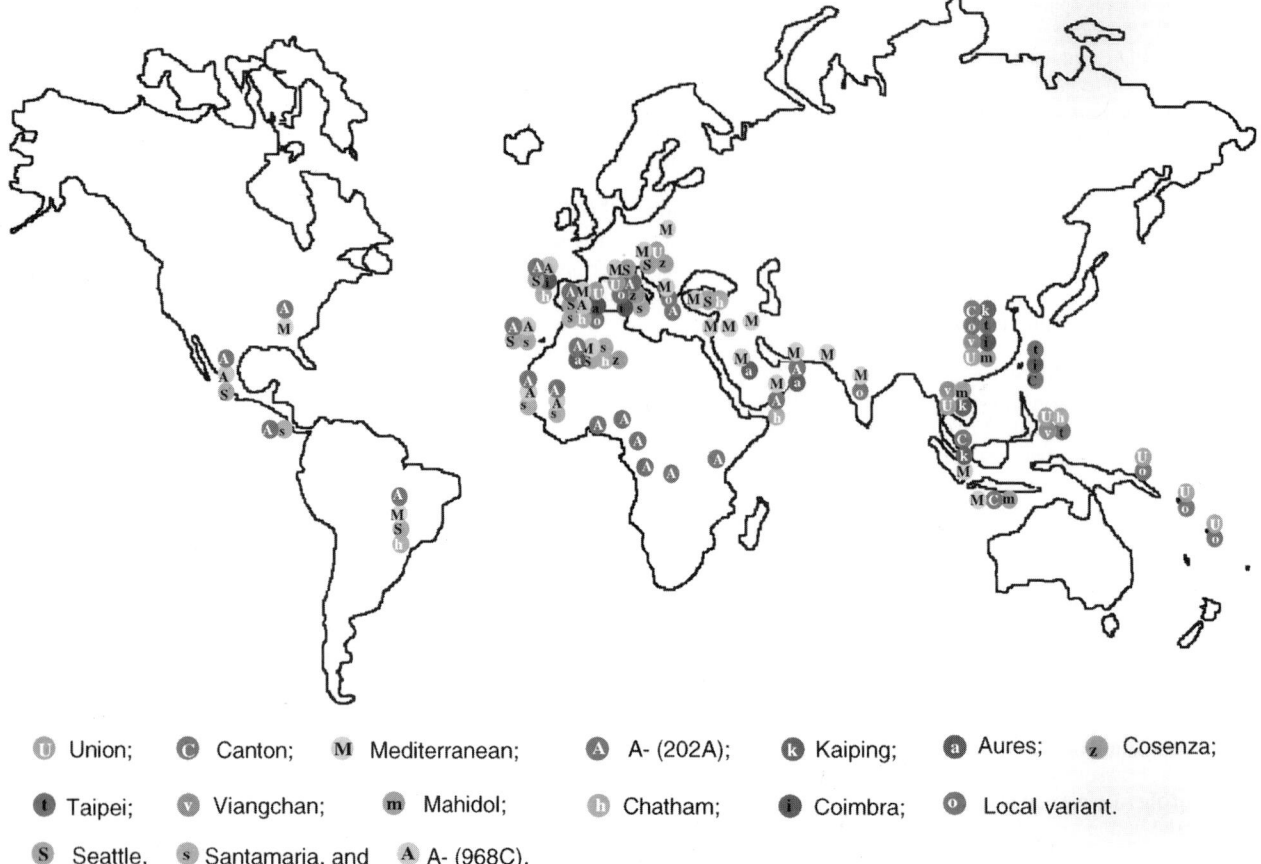

Fig. 179-8 Worldwide distribution of polymorphic variants of G6PD. The variants in each country are shown in order of prevalence according to these symbols: U = Union; C = Canton; M = Mediterranean; A = A− (202A); k = Kaiping; t = Taipei; v = Viangchan; m = Mahidol; h = Chatham; i = Coimbra; S = Seattle; s = Santamaria; a = Aures; z = Cosenza; A = A− (968C). See Color Plate 9.

most common G6PD-deficient variants in the Indian subcontinent, and it has spread as far as Indonesia. G6PD A− and G6PD Mediterranean coexist at polymorphic frequencies in several populations, for instance in the Persian Gulf,[141,142] and in the island of Mauritius.[143] G6PD Seattle was first reported in a subject of Welsh ancestry in the United States.[144] Since then it has been found at polymorphic frequency in Sardinia,[145] Greece,[146] the Canary Islands,[147] and southern Italy.[133,148] We have identified it also in subjects from Algeria, Germany, and Ireland. Thus, although we cannot say where the mutation happened to occur, it must be very ancient, because it appears to predate the radiation of European and North African populations. G6PD Union[149] had been reported in the Chinese[150] and in southern Italy,[133] and it has since turned up in many parts of the world (we had at one point called it G6PD Maewo because it is polymorphic in the Maewo island of the Vanuatu archipelago[151]). Unlike the mutations of G6PD A−, G6PD Mediterranean, and G6PD Seattle, the mutation of G6PD Union consists of a C → T replacement in a CpG doublet, and its presence in disparate parts of the globe might result from independent mutational events in a mutational hot spot rather than from the spread of a single mutation.

With respect to the set of polymorphic alleles that account for the overall prevalence of G6PD deficiency in individual populations, it is interesting that in most areas of high prevalence, multiple polymorphic alleles are found. For instance, this is true in the Mediterranean,[124,133,148,152–154] the Middle East,[141,142,155] India,[156,157] Southeast Asia,[158–161] China,[162–164] Algeria,[139] Papua New Guinea,[165] and Vanuatu.[151] The notable exception is tropical Africa, where G6PD A− accounts for at least 90 percent of G6PD deficiency,[166] and about 90 percent of G6PD A− is accounted for by the allele with the V68M mutation (in *cis* to the N126D G6PD A mutation).

Structure-Function Relationships

G6PD deficiency can arise through either instability or altered catalytic activity, and the former mechanism is by far the more common. The fact that mutations causing loss of enzyme activity are scattered throughout the protein sequence must mean that amino acid replacements in many different positions can reduce intracellular stability (which may or may not be reflected by in vitro stability tests), either by affecting the conformation of the G6PD molecule or by increasing its susceptibility to proteolytic enzymes. It is more difficult to make a general statement about changes in substrate binding. However, the corresponding mutations appear not to be randomly distributed. Indeed, there is a cluster of low-K_mG6P values in variants with mutations in the neighborhood of lysine 205, the catalytic active center. It is intriguing that a variety of amino acid replacements increase rather than decrease substrate affinity; this may mean that the normal K_mG6P is optimal for the purposes of erythrocyte physiology. Increased affinity for NADP is also seen in several variants, such as G6PD Mediterranean; the basis for this is not yet known, because the mutation is distant from the NADP binding site. By contrast, a significant decrease in NADP binding may be important in the pathophysiology of G6PD Orissa, which has a replacement within the NADP binding site.[35]

The model for the 3-D structure of human G6PD has provided insight into the significance of some other mutations as well, such as with respect to the cluster of class I mutations in exons 10 and 11. These two exons encode the protein region that constitutes the

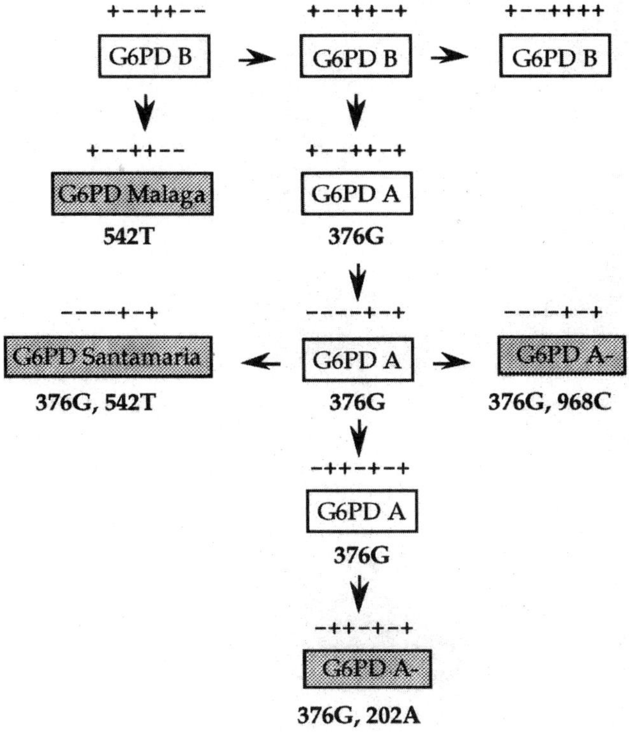

Fig. 179-9 A proposed scheme of evolution for A, A−, and related variants.

interface between the two identical subunits of the enzyme. As a result, any mutation in this region causes the respective amino acid replacements in the two subunits to be quite near each other in the dimer structure, thus potentially increasing their deleterious effects. Even more important, because there is no covalent link between the subunits, it stands to reason that any interference with the shape of the interface surfaces may affect their mutual fit, and thus dramatically destabilize the active form of the enzyme. Indeed, most class I variants are highly unstable. By systematic replacement of a negatively charged residue located at the center of the subunit interface in the dimeric structure (421D), with either neutral or positively charged residues, Bautista's group pinpointed a link between dimer stability and reactivity with NADP.[167] Another cluster of mutations has been noticed in the 3-D model of the G6PD monomer.[168]

Now that a physical structure for human G6PD is available,[26] we should be able to understand much better G6PD deficiency by either solving or modelling individual G6PD mutants. Some examples are already at hand. G6PD Nara has a deletion of residues 319 to 326, some of which are part of a surface loop that was found to be highly mobile in *L. mesenteroides* G6PD. The great flexibility of this loop may allow for the removal of the 8 residues, and for a direct connection between residues 318 and 327 to be accommodated by a local rearrangement of the main chain, without disruption of the overall structure,[31] but at the expense of exposing otherwise buried residues. This would explain how G6PD Nara causes CNSHA, but is compatible with life. Another example is that of G6PD Neapolis, where modelling of the P467R replacement has provided a possible explanation as to why this mutation causes milder disease than others located nearby in the αe helix.[169] A special case is that of G6PD A−. Because, as stated above, this deficient variant of G6PD results from a second mutation in the nondeficient variant G6PD A, one might surmise that the second mutation is responsible for loss of enzyme activity, as well as for subtle changes in enzyme kinetics.[170] However, when either of the two mutations was introduced into the normal gene by site-directed mutagenesis, and the single mutants were expressed in *E. coli*, the enzyme activity recovered was almost normal — only the two mutations together caused severe enzyme deficiency.[171] Thus, the two mutations appear to have a synergistic effect on enzyme stability. We can now see that the two mutations of G6PD A−, V68M and N126D, are spatially very close (on βB and αc respectively), with the side chains of Val68 and Met125 in direct contact.[31] We may surmise that the two substitutions interact specifically with each other causing disruption in the protein structure, possibly in the β-sheet of the coenzyme domain. Recently, it was shown that after denaturation under controlled conditions, G6PD B and G6PD A are able to fold and form active enzyme dimer molecules, but G6PD A− is almost unable to do so, providing a good molecular explanation for its in vivo instability.[172] The mechanism of folding may be relevant to the stability of both normal and mutant G6PD molecules. The role of GroEL has been studied on *L. mesenteroides* G6PD,[173] and there is some evidence that α-crystallin, a chaperone-like protein, may be important in stabilizing G6PD in the mammalian lens.[174,175]

G6PD Haplotypes

Apart from mutations causing changes in the primary structure of the G6PD molecule, two synonymous codon polymorphisms[145,176] and several polymorphic sites in introns[145,177–179] have been identified. Not surprisingly, these exhibit marked linkage disequilibrium among themselves and with coding sequence polymorphisms. For instance, in a study of African populations, only 7 of 128 possible haplotypes have been observed and, as in other systems, they have been used in an attempt to infer the evolutionary history of the G6PD gene.[177] In this case, it appears that the mutation underlying G6PD A− is the most recent in a sequence of mutational events that have spread in the population (Fig. 179-7). Linkage disequilibrium has been revealed over a much larger region (about 3 Mb) surrounding the G6PD gene and extending from the factor VIII gene to the color vision genes. Again, haplotype analysis in a southern Italian population indicates that the mutation underlying the deficient variant G6PD Mediterranean is more recent than other polymorphic sites not associated with enzyme deficiency.[180] Different frequencies of the same haplotypes are found in China, both in the general population and in *cis* with the G6PD Canton mutation.[181,182] It can be presumed in both cases that the more ancient mutations spread by genetic drift and migration, whereas the most recent (A−, Mediterranean, Canton) were selected by malaria.

CLINICAL MANIFESTATIONS

The vast majority of individuals with G6PD deficiency are asymptomatic and go through life without being aware of their genetic abnormality. The only common clinical manifestation is acute hemolysis, which may be rapidly compensated and often remains undetected. Clinical expression results from an interaction of the molecular properties of each individual G6PD variant with exogenous factors and, possibly, with additional genetic factors specific for a certain population. No significant adverse effects of G6PD deficiency were discernible on the health and military performance of young, enlisted U.S. Black males.[183,184] However, G6PD deficiency can cause much human pathology, and the following clinical syndromes are recognized:

- Drug-induced hemolysis
- Infection-induced hemolysis
- Favism
- Neonatal jaundice (NNJ)
- Chronic nonspherocytic hemolytic anemia (CNSHA)

Episodes of hemolysis have also been reported in G6PD-deficient subjects in concomitance with a variety of clinical situations, including diabetic ketoacidosis,[185,186] hypoglycemia,[187] myocardial infarction with pericardial tamponade,[188] and strenuous exercise;[189,190] however, coexistent infection and/or oxidant drug exposure cannot always be excluded.[191] Pregnancy does not, of itself, precipitate hemolysis.[192]

Drug-Induced Hemolytic Anemia

G6PD deficiency was discovered as a direct consequence of investigations into the development of hemolysis in some individuals, usually Blacks, who had received primaquine (30 mg daily), which, in other individuals, causes no red cell destruction.[193,194] Thus, the acute hemolytic anemia associated with G6PD deficiency has become virtually a prototype of hemolytic episodes arising from a unique interaction between genetic and exogenous factors.[6] Clinical hemolysis and jaundice typically begin within 2 to 3 days of starting the drug.[195] The hemolysis is largely intravascular (although to what extent was recently questioned[196]), and it is characteristically associated with hemoglobinuria. The anemia worsens until days 7 to 8. Heinz bodies (Fig. 179-10) are a characteristic finding in the peripheral blood. A reticulocyte response then sets in, and the hemoglobin level begins to recover on the days 8 to 10. A self-limited course is characteristic with some G6PD variants,[193–195] because newly produced red cells, having higher G6PD activity, are less susceptible than the older cells, which have been selectively destroyed. However, a high drug dosage or the presence of a severely deficient G6PD variant will cause more protracted hemolysis.[197] A critical analysis of the data whereby individual drugs have been implicated in the causation of hemolysis in G6PD-deficient subjects was conducted by Beutler,[198,199] who uncovered a discrepancy between the relatively small list of drugs for which there is strong evidence linking them to hemolytic anemia (Table 179-5) and a much larger list of agents for which the evidence is less secure. This discrepancy arises for two reasons. First, clinical hemolysis is not always reproducible after administration of a particular drug, presumably because a number of factors influence both its interaction with the erythrocyte and the clinical consequences of the interaction (Table 179-6). Certain drugs are reported to cause oxidative hemolysis (but not necessarily anemia) in some populations, but not in others (e.g., chloramphenicol[200,201] and vitamin K[202,203]). Probably for the same reason, the same dose of primaquine given to G6PD-deficient subjects of different ethnic origins gives rise to different degrees of hemolysis.[204] Genetic differences in drug metabolism and pharmacokinetics may also affect drug toxicity, while concurrent infection is an important source of additional oxidant stress, particularly in the neonate. Because the oldest red cells have the lowest enzyme activity, the preexisting hemoglobin and reticulocyte count will influence the severity of hemolysis.[166]

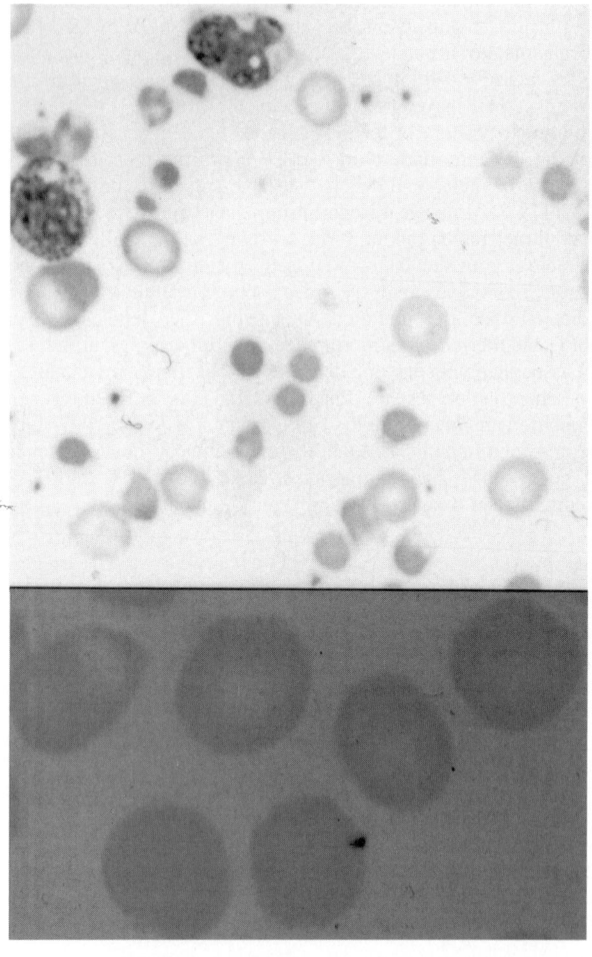

Fig. 179-10 Morphologic changes in the red cells during an acute hemolytic attack induced by fava bean ingestion in a G6PD-deficient boy. *Top*: Romanovsky-stained blood smear showing marked anisocytosis, poikilocytes, "bite" cells, spherocytes, polychromatic cells, and a shift to the left in the granulocytes. *Bottom*: Red cells stained supravitally with methyl violet; one red cell has a purple body, called a Heinz body. This consists of denatured protein, mainly hemoglobin, adhering to the red-cell membrane. Heinz bodies can be also produced in vitro in both G6PD-deficient and normal red cells after incubation with certain oxidant chemicals such as acetylphenylhydrazine.

Second, clinical and hematologic assessment of hemolysis has notoriously low sensitivity, in that even a two- to threefold increase in red cell destruction may not produce a significant anemia or reticulocytosis. In addition, mere clinical association is not an ideal way of assessing the hemolytic potential of drugs in G6PD deficiency, because clinical situations are often complex. For instance, antibiotic, antipyretic, or analgesic drugs[205] are often administered to patients with infection, which may itself precipitate hemolysis. Similarly, it is unclear whether lead poisoning[198] or dimercaprol therapy[206] causes hemolysis in G6PD deficiency. Simultaneous administration of more than one drug makes it particularly difficult to assess the contribution of each. Thus, while the clinical association is very convincing for some agents (e.g., naphthalene,[206] nalidixic acid[207]) it is less so for others (e.g., sodium metasolphan noramidipyrine[208]). The most reliable technique to assess the hemolytic potential of a drug would be to administer it to a normal volunteer who has received a transfusion of ^{51}Cr-labeled G6PD-deficient cells and to follow the cells' survival.[194,209] It was always difficult to do this type of experiment in statistically valid numbers of cases, and it would be regarded today as unethical. Because of these difficulties, in vitro tests (Table 179-7) have been developed that aim to predict whether a drug will cause hemolysis in vivo.[210–213] Although these tests have been generally validated by analysis of drugs already known to cause hemolysis in vivo, they have not been widely used or made compulsory. In our view, they should be carried out before a new drug is introduced to a population in which G6PD deficiency is prevalent.

A practical problem arises when several drugs indicated for a particular condition all carry the risk of hemolysis. Usually an alternative can be found; for example, for an acute inflammatory condition high-dose aspirin and acetaminophen may be risky, but ketoprofen is safe.[214] When there is no known safe alternative, clinical judgment must dictate whether the drug or the disease to be treated is the greater danger. If the disease is the greater danger, then one may have to accept a hemolytic attack and be prepared to manage it. Hemolysis in G6PD-deficient subjects has also been reported upon exposure to volatile nitrites.[215]

Infection-Induced Hemolysis

Outside the areas where favism is prevalent, infection is probably the most common cause of hemolysis in subjects with G6PD deficiency. One estimate attributed up to a third of these episodes of hemolysis to coincidentally administered drugs,[216] but that was probably an overestimate;[217] the true precipitant is usually infection. The severity and clinical consequences of hemolysis

Table 179-5 Drugs and Chemicals Associated with Significant Hemolysis in Subjects with G6PD Deficiency*

Drugs	Definite association	Possible association	Doubtful association
Antimalarials	Primaquine	Chloroquine	Quinacrine
	Pamaquine		Quinine
Sulfonamides	Sulfanilamide	Sulfadimidine	Sulfoxone
	Sulfacetamide	Sulfasalazine	Sulfadiazine
	Sulfapyridine	Glyburide†	Sulfisoxazole
	Sulfamethoxazole		
Sulfones	Dapsone‡		
Nitrofurantoin	Nitrofurantoin		
Antipyretic/analgesic	Acetanilid	Aspirin¶	Acetaminophen§
			Phenacetin
Other drugs	Nalidixic acid	Ciprofloxacin	PAS
	Niridazole	Chloramphenicol	Doxorubicin
	Methylene blue	Vitamin K analogues	Probenecid
	Phenazopyridine	Ascorbic acid	Dimercaprol
	Septrin	p-Aminosalicylic acid	
Other chemicals	Naphthalene	Acalypha** indica	
	Trinitrotoluene		

*From Luzzatto and Mehta[121]
†See Meloni[532]
‡Hemolysis can also occur in patients who are not G6PD deficient
¶High doses[533]
§Overdose causes hemolysis[534]
**An herbal remedy[535]

are, again, influenced by a number of factors, including concurrent administration of oxidant drugs, the preexisting level of hemoglobin, hepatic function, and age. Numerous bacterial, viral, and rickettsial infections have been reported as precipitants, but particularly important are infectious hepatitis,[216,218,219], including hepatitis A,[220] pneumonia,[216,221,222] and typhoid fever.[200,201] Viral infections that affect the upper respiratory or gastrointestinal tract are reported[218] to cause more severe hemolysis than bacterial infections in G6PD-deficient children. Hemolysis is nearly four times more frequent in children with G6PD deficiency who develop viral hepatitis than in normal children,[223] but the degree and duration of jaundice in such children[224] and in adults is frequently out of proportion to the degree of hemolysis,[225] suggesting that the jaundice is in part of hepatocellular origin. Indeed, hepatic dysfunction may contribute to the hyperbilirubinemia seen in G6PD deficiency complicated by viral hepatitis[224–226] and pneumonia.[227] On the other hand, erythrocyte G6PD activity is reported to be transiently depressed in individuals with normal G6PD and typhoid or paratyphoid fever.[227] Renal failure is a well-recognized complication in adults,[216,221,222,228–230] whereas it is rare in children.[231] It may be particularly common after urinary tract infection[222] and in patients with preexisting renal disease,[229] while the concurrent administration of nephrotoxic drugs and pathologic changes in the kidney directly attributable to the underlying infection[232] may contribute to its severity. Acute renal failure is a serious complication in patients with viral hepatitis and G6PD deficiency,[218,228,233–235] but it also occurs in subjects with normal G6PD.[236] The pathogenesis is likely to be multifactorial, but the pathologic lesion is probably acute tubular necrosis caused by renal ischemia. Tubular obstruction by hemoglobin casts may also be important in pathogenesis.[237] Most patients with infection-induced hemolysis make a complete recovery, even when the course has been complicated by renal failure, provided hemodialysis is instituted promptly when indicated. The mechanism of infection-induced hemolysis is not well understood. Incubation of influenza A virus with normal red cells leads to increased hexose monophosphate shunt activity. In contrast, this increase is not seen upon incubation of the virus with

Table 179-6 Factors That Influence Individual Susceptibility to, and Severity of, Drug-Induced Oxidative Hemolysis

Inherited
- Metabolic integrity of the erythrocyte
- Precise nature of enzyme defect
- Genetic differences in pharmacokinetics

Acquired
- Age
- Dose, absorption, metabolism, and excretion of drug
- Presence of additional oxidative stress, e.g., infection
- Effect of drug or metabolite on enzyme activity
- Preexisting hemoglobin level
- Age distribution of red blood cell population

Table 179-7 Techniques Used to Evaluate the Hemolytic Potential of Drugs Administered to G6PD-Deficient Subjects

Clinical association
- The occurrence of otherwise unexplained hemolysis in an individual known to be G6PD-deficient

Clinical challenge
- Administration of drugs in controlled studies to individuals known to be G6PD-deficient[193]
- Administration of drugs to normal volunteers transfused with ^{51}Cr-labeled G6PD-deficient erythrocytes[536]
- Administration of drugs to animals followed by in vitro studies of erythrocytes[537]

In vitro studies
- GSH stability test[39]
- Effect of drug metabolites on mechanical fragility of erythrocytes[538,539]
- Measurement of $^{14}CO_2$ evolution and glucose utlization of normal erythrocytes suspended in homologous serum before and after drug ingestion[381,540]
- Measurement of hydrogen peroxide levels within erythrocytes after incubation with drugs[44]

G6PD-deficient cells, which, instead, show increased autohemolysis with Heinz body formation.[238] Generation of hydrogen peroxide by activated polymorphonuclear neutrophils in close apposition to G6PD-deficient red cells in vitro can lead to a reduction in the reduced form of glutathione (GSH) content and diminished survival of red cells thus treated.[239] The phenomenon of "immune adherence,"[240] whereby opsonized bacteria adhere to red cells in a process mediated by complement, may be important in promoting close apposition of neutrophils to red cells.[241] Hepatic dysfunction may further aggravate the oxidant stress on red cells by permitting accumulation of metabolites capable of oxidizing red-cell SH groups.[233] Activated neutrophils can also mediate lipid peroxidation of red-cell membranes, but G6PD-deficient red cells seem no more susceptible than normal red cells.[242] A variable degree of marrow suppression frequently accompanies infection and may delay recovery of the hemoglobin level. Hemolysis has been reported after vigorous exercise[189] and after pericardial tamponade,[188] even in the absence of infection.

Favism

The occurrence of acute hemolysis after ingestion of broad beans (*Vicia faba*) has been noted since antiquity.[2,4] It has occurred on an epidemic scale, particularly in Mediterranean countries (Italy,[5] Greece,[243] Spain, Portugal, and Turkey[244,245]), but also in the Middle East, the Far East, and North Africa.[245] This geographic distribution correlates best with the geography of customary consumption of fava beans. Most,[246–248] but not all,[249,250] of the patients reported in North America and the United Kingdom have direct Mediterranean ancestry. Once the similarity between favism and primaquine-induced hemolytic anemia was noticed,[251] it became clear that all patients with favism are G6PD deficient.[10,252,253] However, it appears that not all G6PD-deficient subjects are sensitive to fava beans,[254,255] and even those who are show striking variability from one exposure to the next. When ^{51}Cr-labeled G6PD-deficient cells from individuals with a clinical history of favism are infused into normal subjects, challenge with primaquine always leads to hemolysis of the deficient cells, whereas challenge with fava beans leads to hemolysis only in some cases.[256,257] One or more factors in addition to G6PD deficiency may therefore be required for the development of favism,[258] and they may influence the severity of the individual attack. At the same time, it should be noted that the content of offending agents in fava beans is highly variable, and the size of fava bean dishes even more so. The amount and quality of fava beans ingested may play a major role.

Clinical favism presents characteristically with sudden onset of acute hemolytic anemia within 24 to 48 h of ingesting the beans. Pallor and hemoglobinuria are the hallmarks. Jaundice is always present, because not all the hemolysis is intravascular,[259] but the bilirubin level is less than in hemolytic attacks triggered by drugs or infection, presumably because the hemoglobinuria is more massive and hemoglobin catabolism within the body is therefore relatively reduced. The anemia is often severe.[243] Acute renal failure may supervene in adults,[260] but it is very rare in children.[231] However, fatalities in children were not uncommon prior to the availability of transfusion therapy.[4] An increase in the proportion of young erythrocytes leads to a decrease in the level of glycosylated hemoglobin (HbA1).[261] The highest incidence is in children aged 2 to 6 years. Boys are affected two to three times more often than girls[262] because of the greater number, in every population, of hemizygous males than heterozygous females. However, it is well documented that heterozygous girls are affected, although the condition is usually milder in these subjects.[250,263] Favism can occur after ingestion of fresh,[262] dried,[243] or frozen[262] beans, but fresh beans are by far the most common offender, and, therefore, favism is most common during the spring. Hemolysis in breast-fed babies whose mothers have eaten fava beans is well documented.[243,264,265]

The pathophysiology of hemolysis in favism has been authoritatively reviewed.[266] The injury to red cells in favism is likely to consist in oxidant damage due to a chemical agent. On the basis of studies of the effect of fractionated extracts on erythrocyte metabolism, it has been suggested that the toxic components of fava beans are the pyrimidine aglycones divicine and isouramil[267–270] in combination with ascorbic acid. Possible bases for the erratic development of favism might then be variable absorption of toxic compounds from the gut or variability of the concentrations in the beans of the toxic glucosides themselves or of glucosidases required for their release. The levels of this enzyme activity in small intestinal biopsies of subjects with favism do not differ from those in normal and G6PD-deficient control subjects.[271] However, important determinants of intrapersonal variability in clinical expression include the amount and form in which the bean is eaten, the season of consumption,[245] and gastric pH.[266] On the other hand, interpersonal variability may have an additional and possibly genetic component (inherited perhaps as an autosomal recessive gene or as part of the genetic heterogeneity of G6PD deficiency itself[271–273]). The activity of erythrocyte acid phosphatase has been suggested to be lower in G6PD-deficient males sensitive to fava beans than in the general population, owing to a higher frequency of the Pa and Pc alleles of the acid phosphatase gene.[274] Decreased urinary D-glutaric acid and defective hepatic glucuronide formation[275,276] have also been reported in these subjects. A reduction in the number of sheep red-cell rosetting lymphocytes[277] and inversion of the peripheral blood helper T cell (CD4) to suppressor T cell (CD8) ratio owing to a decrease of CD4+ and an increase of CD8+ cells[278] have been described during the hemolytic crisis of favism. These changes may be the consequence of the hemolysis rather than an important pathogenic factor in favism, and similar changes have been reported in hypertransfused subjects with hemoglobinopathies.[279]

Oxidant damage causes cross-linking of erythrocyte membrane proteins, leading to the formation of distorted erythrocytes. It has been suggested that disturbed erythrocyte calcium homeostasis (specifically, reduced activity of the membrane Ca^{2+}-ATPase, leading to increased intraerythrocytic calcium and decreased intraerythrocytic potassium) mediates activation of proteolytic activity in erythrocytes in favic subjects.[280,281] Inhibition of catalase may also play an important role.[282] The distorted erythrocytes are rapidly cleared from the circulation,[283] and there is increasing evidence that extravascular mechanisms are important in this process. They include opsonization by immunoglobulins and complement and phagocytosis within the reticuloendothelial system and bone marrow.

The mainstay of prevention is avoidance of fava beans. Experience in Sardinia has demonstrated the value of neonatal screening and health education in reducing the incidence of favism in that community.[284] The mainstay of treatment remains blood transfusion in severe cases.[231] The original observation suggesting arrest of hemolysis by desferrioxamine[285] has been disputed,[286] but a larger study appears to confirm that a single bolus of desferrioxamine may be useful as an adjuvant to red-cell transfusion.[287] The proposed mechanism is that desferrioxamine reduces iron-dependent formation of damaging oxidant radicals (e.g., hydroxyl ions).

It is widely believed that favism is only associated with the more severely deficient variants of G6PD (particularly G6PD Mediterranean), and, specifically, that G6PD A− is not associated with favism. That is not correct, as typical attacks of favism have been well documented with many other variants, including subjects of African origin with the A− variant.[288] In addition, favism in Spain,[134] Portugal,[244] and Algeria [289] is quite prominent in G6PD-deficient individuals who have been shown to have G6PD A−.

Neonatal Jaundice

G6PD deficiency is the most common red-cell enzymopathy to cause neonatal hemolysis and jaundice.[290] The earliest reports[291,292] gave the impression that this complication occurred particularly in Greece, Sardinia, and the Far East, but the condition subsequently emerged as a major problem in Africa,[293] and it has been reported in North America[294] and elsewhere. Jaundice usually appears by 1 to 4 days of age, at about the same time as or slightly earlier than so-called physiological jaundice,[290,295] and later than in blood group alloimmunization. There may be a slightly higher threshold for its clinical detection in black infants.[296] The relative contributions of red-cell destruction and impaired hepatic function to the pathogenesis of unconjugated neonatal hyperbilirubinemia are disputed.[246] Reports of abnormal red-cell morphology,[297] mild anemia,[298] and reticulocytosis suggest hemolysis, but impaired hepatic function, similar to that seen in normal neonates, may well be the major cause[299,300] in both premature and full-term[301] G6PD-deficient infants. Several distinctive features of neonatal erythrocytes may contribute to the degree of jaundice,[290,297] including elevated levels of ascorbic acid[302] and depressed levels of vitamin E,[303] glutathione reductase,[304] and catalase.[305] Recent measurements of carbon monoxide production in jaundiced newborns confirm that hemolysis accounts only in part for the hyperbilirubinemia of G6PD-deficient newborns.[306–308]

A striking feature of neonatal jaundice (NNJ) in association with G6PD deficiency is the wide variation in its frequency and severity in different populations (Table 179-8). Thus, in West Africa and Southeast Asia, G6PD deficiency accounts for a very high proportion (more than 30 percent) of all NNJ and for more than 50 percent of all cases of otherwise unexplained NNJ. Although kernicterus is a rare complication, the most common cause of it in both Africa[309] and Southeast Asia[310,311] is G6PD deficiency. In communities with a culturally and genetically heterogeneous population (e.g., Singapore[298,312] and Israel[313,314]), these differences in incidence seem to be population-specific.

The cause of this variability is incompletely understood, and both genetic and environmental factors are likely to be important. Severe NNJ can occur probably with any G6PD-deficient variant.[315] However, the type of G6PD variant that is prevalent in a population is likely to be relevant, and is clearly of importance with respect to unusual or sporadic variants in the USA.[316,317] In Sardinia, where at least three polymorphic variants are associated with NNJ, the severity of NNJ does not correlate with red-cell G6PD activity, suggesting that additional variables (e.g., the expression and activity of the G6PD-deficient variant in the liver) may be important. Theoretically, a superimposed red-cell incompatibility between mother and infant might play a role, but this was not the case with respect to ABO blood groups in one series from Israel.[318] Ethnic differences in plasma bilirubin levels of full-term neonates may also reflect genetic differences in the activity of liver and red-cell enzymes. In this respect, a most interesting recent finding is that the genetic variant of uridinediphosphoglucuronate glucuronyltransferase (UDPGT1) that causes Gilbert disease interacts with G6PD deficiency in causing a much-increased risk of NNJ.[319]

Environmental factors are likely to be at least as important as genetic factors. G6PD deficiency is a less frequent cause of NNJ among individuals of African descent in the U.S., and of Greek ancestry in Australia, than in the countries of origin of these populations,[320] although the differences are perhaps less marked than originally thought. Among these environmental factors are maternal exposure to oxidant drugs,[321,322] herbal remedies,[298] and naphthalene (mothballs),[323] all of which may precipitate or exacerbate NNJ, and possibly aflatoxins.[324] Gestational age and maturity is an important consideration, as NNJ is more common, severe, and potentially harmful in premature infants.[297,325] Environmental factors will also affect the incidence of neonatal infection, hypoglycemia, acidosis, and the normal level of neonatal hemoglobin in a population.[166] Cultural factors, including exposure to icterogenic agents, have been identified as important precipitants of NNJ in the G6PD-deficient population of Nigeria.[326] In Bedouin families, the birth of the first baby boy is traditionally celebrated by applying henna dye to his body. Unfortunately, this has been shown to be associated with hemolysis , especially if the baby is G6PD deficient.[327] Severe neonatal jaundice can occur in girls heterozygous for G6PD deficiency. [328]

Management of NNJ generally includes avoiding oxidant drugs and promptly treating hypoxia, sepsis, and acidosis in newborns. Specific measures include eliminating the use of mothballs, prophylactic administration of phenobarbital to at-risk infants to improve hepatic conjugation of bilirubin,[329] and exchange transfusion if the bilirubin level is 20 mg/dl or more.[330,331] With respect to neonatal jaundice in general, there has been recent controversy on treatment policies in relation to the levels of bilirubin.[332] At the moment there is not sufficient evidence for NNJ associated with G6PD deficiency to be regarded as less dangerous than that associated with classical hemolytic disease of the newborn (HDN). Indeed, one can only speculate as to whether the basal nuclei cells from G6PD-deficient babies may be more vulnerable to hyperbilirubinemia than those of G6PD-normal babies. With respect to phototherapy, although it has been suggested that it could worsen hemolysis by leading to riboflavin deficiency and consequent loss of antioxidant activity,[333,334]

Table 179-8 G6PD Deficiency and Neonatal Jaundice (NNJ)*

Population	Incidence of G6PD deficiency	Incidence of NNJ among G6PD-deficient individuals	Incidence of NNJ in control groups	Incidence of G6PD deficiency among NNJ patients
Africa				
W. Africa[541,542]	21	26	10	31
S. Africa[301,543]	1.3	–	–	3.1 (All)
(Bantu)				10 (Full-term)
America				
Jamaica[544]	14.7	–	–	20.5
USA[203,545]	7.2	6	11.6	12.5
	11.2			
Asia				
China/Hong Kong[310,311]	3.6	–	1.2	15–30
Thailand[544,546]	7.5	30	3.0	30–60
Singapore[292,547–549]	1.3	20	25	–
Europe				
Greece[202,550–552]	3	30	9.1	15
Sardinia[329,553]	8.8	20–30	10	8.5

*All figures are percentage values in males only.

several studies have shown conclusively that this treatment is effective in reducing hyperbilirubinemia,[330,335,336] and phototherapy remains a mainstay of the treatment of NNJ whenever the bilirubin level is not so high as to warrant exchange blood transfusion. Recently a single administration of Sn-mesoporphyrin (see reference 337) has been proposed as an effective alternative to phototherapy in both prevention and treatment of NNJ associated with G6PD deficiency.[338]

Chronic Nonspherocytic Hemolytic Anemia

Although a slight degree of chronic hemolysis invariably accompanies G6PD deficiency, the vast majority of individuals with G6PD deficiency experience significant hemolysis and anemia only under conditions of oxidant stress. Some G6PD variants (class I, Table 179-4), however, are characterized by overt chronic hemolytic anemia that is further exacerbated by oxidant stress (see Fig. 179-11). Such variants have been described (almost invariably in males) in many parts of the world, regardless of whether the common types of G6PD deficiency are endemic in the region. For instance, many cases have been reported from Japan.[339] Mostly a single kindred is known for each variant, but sometimes what is apparently the same variant (e.g., G6PD Chicago) has been reported in unrelated individuals in different parts of the world.[340–343] Because the clinical phenotype is similar in affected members of a family and also among unrelated individuals having the same variant, it has been suggested that these variants represent structural and functional changes in the enzyme caused by mutations in the G6PD gene.[166] However, additional factors (genetic or environmental) may also operate to influence the clinical picture, and severe-deficiency variants can cause more severe hemolysis in some family members than in others.[344–346] The causative link of a G6PD variant with chronic nonspherocytic hemolytic anemia (CNSHA) is usually based on clinical evidence. The degree of enzyme deficiency may be very severe, and detailed biochemical characterization of the residual enzyme is often made even more difficult by its instability. In rare cases with associated granulocyte dysfunction,[347] hemolysis can be made worse by increased susceptibility to infection. Sometimes chronic hemolysis may arise from an association of mild G6PD deficiency with an unrelated, genetically transmitted erythrocyte abnormality, such as congenital dyserythropoietic anemia,[348] hereditary spherocytosis,[349] pyruvate kinase deficiency,[350,351] or 6-phosphogluconolactonase deficiency.[352]

Since the original descriptions,[353] a large number of detailed clinical observations have been reported. Many patients present with or give a history of neonatal jaundice, often requiring exchange transfusion.[316,354–358] A history of infection or drug-induced hemolysis is also common.[358,359] Gallstones may be a prominent feature.[360] Splenomegaly is usually (but not always) present.[358,361] While occasionally the hemoglobin concentration is normal and the hemolysis well compensated,[345,354,362] oxidant stress can lead to a dramatic fall in the hemoglobin level.[363] The ^{51}Cr-labeled red-cell half life is shortened to 2 to 17 days, and all patients have a reticulocytosis (4 to 34 percent),[355] which may become extreme after splenectomy. Occasionally, the level of reticulocytosis is inappropriately low (3 percent) in relation to the shortening of the ^{51}Cr-labeled red-cell half-life (12 days[364]); the cause is not clear, but folic acid deficiency[344] could be a factor. The increase in red-cell production at puberty can ameliorate the clinical findings. Red cells usually show no abnormal osmotic fragility, whereas a moderate increase in autohemolysis (with partial correction by added glucose) is reported.[356,358,365] Female heterozygotes have been shown to have two populations of cells,[366] one with normal and one with severely deficient G6PD; because the severely deficient red cells disappear from the circulation rapidly, these individuals usually have normal G6PD levels in peripheral blood cells[444].

Hemolysis in CNSHA is only partly intravascular (in contrast to the acute hemolysis caused by G6PD deficiency), and studies with ^{51}Cr usually indicate increased uptake in both liver and spleen.[358] Splenic sequestration has occasionally been demonstrated,[367] although markedly increased osmotic fragility was also

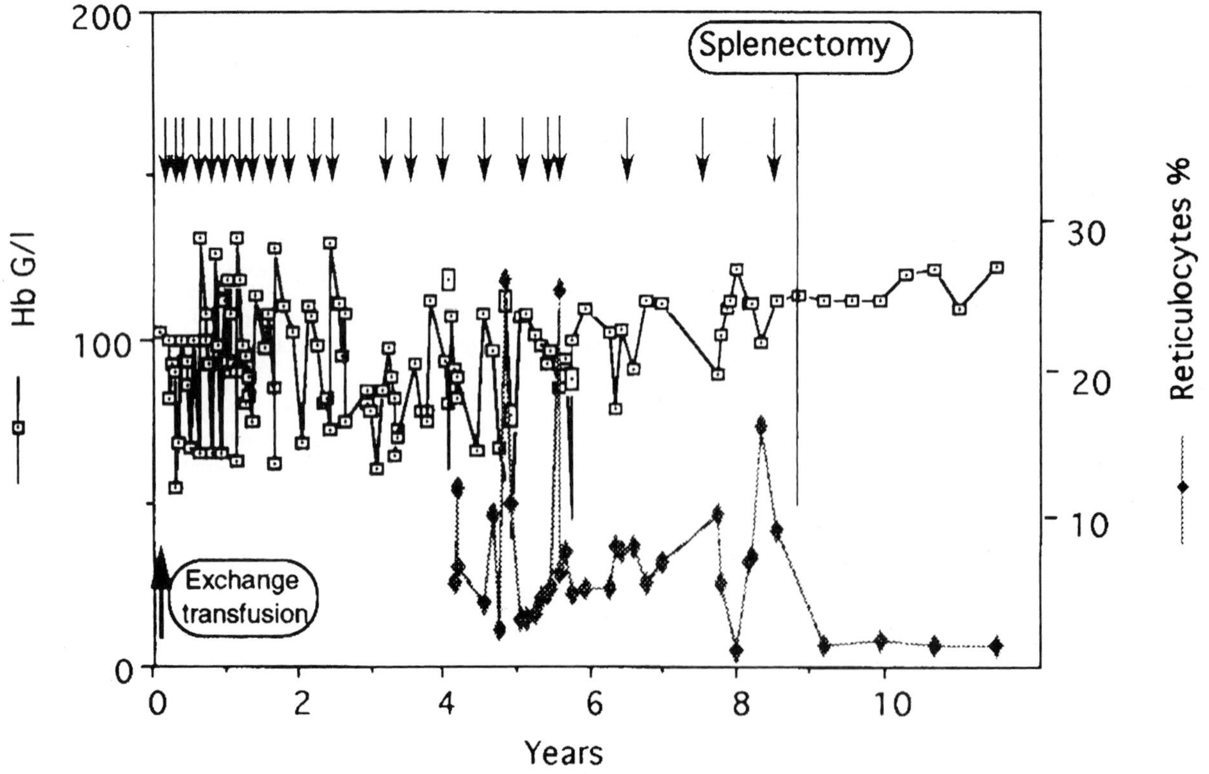

Fig. 179-11 Outline of the clinical course of CNSHA associated with G6PD deficiency (a class I variant called G6PD Harilaou, F216L[508]).

present in that patient, and hereditary spherocytosis cannot be excluded as a coexistent abnormality.[198] Accelerated red-cell aging also implies a role for the spleen in steady-state hemolysis. Increased levels of membrane cholesterol and phospholipids are also reported.[368]

There have been claims that high-dose vitamin E, by acting as an antioxidant, may be useful in the management of chronic hemolysis due to G6PD deficiency,[369,370] and that oral selenium may have an additive beneficial effect.[371] The reported benefit is only modest (e.g., an increase in red-cell half-life from a mean of 15.6 days to 24.3 days, as measured by ^{51}Cr labeling), and such therapy may perhaps be useful in individuals who are deficient in vitamin E. Other studies have failed to show any benefit,[372] and no change in erythrocyte membrane polypeptide aggregates was observed after such treatment.[373] A therapeutic option, especially in severe cases, is splenectomy. On theoretical grounds, one might question its advisability, because selective red-cell destruction in the spleen is seldom documented. In fact, little or no benefit has been reported in some patients,[345,355,362,374–376] but significant improvement has been reported in others.[354–356,365,377] We are personally aware of at least three patients who needed regular blood transfusions before splenectomy but needed few or none over several years after splenectomy (see Fig. 179-11 also Luzzatto[166]).

There is considerable variability in almost every manifestation of CNSHA associated with G6PD deficiency. This variability makes it somewhat problematic to give firm guidelines on management. Unlike the G6PD variants without CNSHA, many of which are polymorphic, those associated with CNSHA are all sporadic, and most, if not all, result from independent mutations (see Table 179-4). It is, therefore, not surprising that the red-cell pathophysiology and, ultimately, the clinical manifestations are subtly different in different cases.

MECHANISM OF HEMOLYSIS

The mammalian red cell is notorious for having a very limited biochemical apparatus and therefore an equally limited range of responses to pathologic changes. Typically, the failure of any metabolic pathway will cause the cell as a whole to fail — in other words, to be destroyed prematurely. In essence, G6PD deficiency entails failure of the glutathione GSH pathway (Fig. 179-3), and the result is hemolysis. Because a large number of G6PD-deficient variants (classes II and III) are not associated with chronic hemolysis, we can infer that a small amount of residual G6PD activity is sufficient for the steady state requirements of the red cells. Below that level (class I variants), it is evident that NADPH production has become inadequate, although we do not yet know precisely how this leads to hemolysis. A reasonable model is that the GSH level becomes so low that critical sulfhydryl groups in some key proteins are not maintained in reduced form, and intramolecular or intermolecular disulfides are formed. The most pertinent observation is probably that of membrane-cytoskeletal protein aggregates in red cells from patients with class I variants.[378,379] Such aggregates decrease red-cell deformability,[380] and they may alter the cell surface-sufficiently to make it recognizable by macrophages as abnormal (much like an aged red cell), thus leading to extravascular hemolysis. With class II and class III variants, hemolysis depends, by definition, on an exogenous trigger. Again, the exact sequence of events is incompletely known, but the following points are well established:

1. Some of the agents that can cause hemolysis stimulate the hexose monophosphate shunt pathway in normal red cells, indicating that in their presence increased NADPH production is required.[381]
2. A fall in GSH is invariably associated with hemolytic events in G6PD-deficient individuals.
3. In some cases, particularly in favism, acute hemolysis is associated with massive formation of Heinz bodies (consisting of denatured hemoglobin) that, by their very presence, certainly mediate red-cell destruction (Fig. 179-10).
4. Oxygen radicals generated by the auto-oxidation of hemoglobin and in other ways also cause Heinz body formation,[382] intracellular proteolysis, and peroxidation of membrane lipids.[383,384]

These facts, taken together, indicate clearly that acute hemolysis in G6PD deficiency results from a failure of the cell, when challenged, to supply enough NADPH for the detoxification of hydrogen peroxide and oxygen radicals, thus justifying the popular phrase "oxidative hemolysis."[385] The question of why some G6PD-deficient variants are associated with CNSHA (class I) while others are not (classes II and III), is not yet fully answered. Residual G6PD activity is certainly a factor, but the values in classes I and II overlap extensively. Analysis of kinetic data has revealed that variants in class II often have abnormally high substrate affinities for G6P, NADP, or both, whereas variants in class I often have low substrate affinities and decreased affinity for the inhibitor NADPH.[386] For reasons explained more fully elsewhere,[73] we think it is likely that residual enzyme activity and the K_m for G6P may be the most important determinants of whether a particular G6PD-deficient variant causes CNSHA or not.

OTHER CLINICAL STUDIES

Given that G6PD is a housekeeping gene, that is, its expression is ubiquitous, G6PD deficiency could affect, in principle, all tissues. In this respect, two issues are important: (a) How severe is the biochemical defect in various somatic cells? and (b) Are there clinical consequences arising from reduced G6PD activity in cells other than blood cells? As mentioned above, there are two reasons why red cells are much more vulnerable than other cells. First, unlike most other somatic cells, they are not competent for protein synthesis, and therefore cannot renew their supply of G6PD; second, they are highly exposed to oxidant stress. However, other cells can suffer as well. Actual data on G6PD levels in different organs of G6PD-deficient subjects are very scanty (see Table 179-1). We know that the shortage of G6PD in leukocytes from G6PD-deficient people is much less than in erythrocytes[386] (Table 179-1), and a decreased leukocyte G6PD level has no clinical consequences in most cases.[387,388] However, it may be important in patients with very rare mutants,[347,389–391] because a residual G6PD activity less than 5 percent of normal may be associated with defective neutrophil function. The functional defect in these cases is similar to that seen in chronic granulomatous disease, and it arises through disturbance of an NADPH-linked pathway required for killing ingested bacteria. Low levels of leukocyte G6PD in chronic granulomatous disease[392,393] are not due to a mutation at the G6PD locus, and they probably do not contribute to the neutrophil dysfunction. Low levels of G6PD activity in platelets are variably associated with in vitro abnormalities,[394,395] but with no demonstrable clinical consequences.

Occasional patients have been described in whom deficiency of G6PD in tissues other than blood cells contributes to the clinical picture (Table 179-9). Most well-designed population studies provide little or no evidence that any disorders other than hemolytic anemia arise more frequently in G6PD-deficient individuals than in nondeficient control subjects.[183] Previous claims that G6PD deficiency may protect from certain malignant tumors, diabetes, or celiac disease have not been confirmed. However, there have been exceptions. For instance, a 10-year follow-up study of a cohort of G6PD-deficient men revealed a death rate lower than in a control group, due to decreased standardized mortality ratios for ischemic heart disease, cerebrovascular disease, and liver cirrhosis.[396] A number of other associations have been reported, both from patient studies and from population studies (Table 179-10).

Reported genetic associations may arise in part because an ethnically heterogeneous population (African-Americans) has

Table 179-9 G6PD Deficiency in Nonerythroid Tissues

Tissue	Clinical effects	References
Hematologic		
Leukocytes	Increased susceptibility	347, 389–391
Granulocytes	to infection	277, 278, 394, 395, 544, 555
Lymphocytes	Probably none	
Platelets	Probably none	
Nonhematologic		
Lens	Cataracts	556–558
Liver	Possible contributory factor in hyperbilirubinemia, e.g., of NNJ	226, 559
Renal, adrenal, myocardial, sperm, saliva	Probably none	559–561
Muscle	Myopathy?	190, 562, 563

*See also reference 386.

been studied; in such cases, an apparent association of a disorder with G6PD deficiency may simply reflect the presence of more than one gene of African origin in the population. The bulk of evidence from Africa[293,397–399] and from the United States[400–402] suggests that there is no true and independent association of G6PD deficiency and sickle cell anemia. In some cases, the association was proposed based on coinheritance of linked X-chromosome loci (e.g., optic atrophy[122,403]), but in these, as with most other single-case reports, there are no detailed family and molecular studies to support a genuine association. At a phenotypic level, the biochemical changes of G6PD deficiency in certain tissues (hematopoietic and nonhematopoietic) may predispose to the development of other conditions. In the presence of another abnormality, G6PD deficiency may act in an additive or synergistic way to influence clinical expression. Thus, the coexistence of G6PD deficiency with another cause of hemolytic anemia may exacerbate the clinical picture. The clinical effects of deficient G6PD levels in nonhematopoietic tissues are largely a topic of speculation, but may be important, for example, in the development of cataracts (Table 179-9).

Table 179-10 Reported Clinical and Genetic Associations of G6PD Deficiency*

	References
Hematologic	
Heterozygosity for sickle cell anemia, beta-thalassemia, and alpha-thalassemia	397–402, 564, 565
Nonhematologic	
Case reports	
Optic atrophy	125, 403
Malignant hyperthermia	566
Xeroderma pigmentosum	567
Cystic fibrosis	568
Population studies	
Schizophrenia	569, 570
Abnormal glucose tolerance	569, 571
Abnormal steroid metabolism	572
Pernicious anemia	573
Regional enteritis	574
Coronary artery disease	575
Hypertension	576
Gilbert disease	577

*We do not consider that a significant effect of G6PD deficiency on any of these conditions has been proven.

G6PD activity in malignant cells from a variety of human tumors (breast,[404,405] prostate,[406] colon, and stomach[407]) is often higher than in benign cells, and this difference forms the basis for cytochemical tests used in the characterization of these tumors.[407,408] The high G6PD activity of tumors, which has been known for 30 years,[113] is presumably related to a high rate of cell division. Perhaps it is this idea that led to studies in which the incidence of G6PD deficiency was reported to be lower in cancer patients than in control individuals,[409,410] as though G6PD deficiency afforded a degree of protection against cancer. However, a controlled study failed to demonstrate a protective effect of G6PD deficiency against the development of hematologic neoplasm.[411]

DIAGNOSIS

The diagnosis of G6PD deficiency is easy. However, careful attention must be paid to methodology and to the interpretation of the results. Prenatal diagnosis has been reported.[412] Important considerations include:

1. There is broad geographical distribution of this defect and a high prevalence in developing countries, which makes it important to adopt tests that are simple and inexpensive.
2. The actual enzyme activity of G6PD must be measured, rather than the amount of G6PD protein.
3. The level of activity in young erythrocytes is higher than in older ones. Thus, a reticulocytosis can lead to a false normal result. One way of circumventing this difficulty is to centrifuge the sample to be tested and to assay separately the enzyme activity in erythrocytes from the bottom (older cells) and from the top (younger cells) of the resulting column of cells, as well as the activity of the whole unfractionated sample.[413,414] Alternatively, or additionally, one can determine the ratio of G6PD activity to the activity of another age-dependent enzyme, e.g., hexokinase.
4. Because of red-cell mosaicism arising from random X-chromosome inactivation, heterozygotes have a mixture of normal and deficient erythrocytes, and the proportions of the two cell types (maternally and paternally derived) can vary enormously, ranging from completely normal activity to complete deficiency. A cell lysate may not reveal heterozygosity if the proportion of enzyme-deficient cells is small. Microscopic examination of individual cells on a blood film slide is preferable. All the existing methods for measuring G6PD activity depend essentially on the production of NADPH. The direct enzyme assay gives an accurate quantitative measurement. A number of other procedures provide convenient screening tests, aiming only to classify subjects as G6PD-normal or G6PD-deficient. Some of them are semi-quantitative (Table 179-11).

G6PD DEFICIENCY, BLOOD TRANSFUSION, AND PUBLIC HEALTH

The vast majority of individuals with G6PD deficiency do not need treatment, as they suffer no ill effects in the steady state. Screening of all newborns, except in areas where low-risk populations predominate (e.g., in northern Europe and among South American Indians), has been proposed,[290,331] and detection of male hemizygotes and most female heterozygotes has been shown to be feasible.[415,416] Such a program would obviously make it possible for susceptible individuals to avoid potentially hemolytic agents (certain drugs and fava beans) or, in the case of necessary drugs, to ensure they are used in subhemolytic doses. Active immunization against hepatitis A has been suggested,[417,418] and active immunization against pneumococcus might be desirable.

Because the viability of G6PD-deficient erythrocytes after storage may not be as high as that of normal erythrocytes,[419] it has been suggested that blood from G6PD-deficient donors should not

Table 179-11 Diagnosis of G6PD Deficiency

Method	Comments	References
Definitive assay	Spectrophotometer required. Measures 6PGD as well as G6PD (activities can be separated).	198, 571, 578–580
Screening assays	Same principle as definitive assay, but special equipment not required.	581–583
Fluorescent spot test	Cheap, simple, reliable. Stored blood usable.	
Ascorbate cyanide test	Semiquantitative results available. Cheap and simple.	584,585
MTT (tetrazolium) staining test	Fresh blood required.	586–589
Methemoglobin reduction methods	Highly reliable cytochemical technique for detecting heterozygotes.	590,591
	Cheap and simple, but prolonged incubation time required.	
	Fresh blood required. False positives reported.	592,593
Dye decolorization	Lends itself to cytochemical modification suitable for heterozygote detection. Cheap, simple, reliable, and extensively used, but prolonged incubation time required. Fresh blood required.	

be used for transfusion purposes.[420,421] There have also been occasional reports of hemolysis of transfused G6PD-deficient erythrocytes,[420–422] although it was not proven that hemolysis was the result of this enzyme defect. Indeed, G6PD-deficient erythrocytes have been shown to be perfectly satisfactory for transfusion purposes,[423] and refusing to use deficient individuals as blood donors would severely deplete the number of available donors in parts of the world where the deficiency is common.[293] Thus, with the exception of exchange transfusion in severe neonatal jaundice and in the management of severe hemolytic anemia due to favism,[231] G6PD-deficient blood should be considered safe for transfusion purposes. Exchange transfusion has been used in a G6PD-deficient child who needed treatment for life-threatening malaria.[424]

SOMATIC CELL SELECTION AND G6PD AS A CLONAL MARKER

Somatic cells in females heterozygous for the G6PD locus will be of two types, each type expressing only one or the other allele[73] (Fig. 179-12). There is a wide variation in the ratio between the two arising cell populations, partly due to drift, but sometimes due to cell section. If a tumor arises by neoplastic transformation of a single cell, all its cells will be expected to express a single G6PD allele. The product of this locus can therefore be used as a clonal marker. Since the original studies of uterine tumors using this approach,[425] a large number of other neoplasms have been studied,[426–430] and most have been shown to be of clonal origin. In the case of hematologic malignancies,[431,432] it has been shown that neoplastic cells that have differentiated along different pathways (e.g., erythrocytes, granulocytes, and platelets in chronic myeloid leukemia[433,434] and polycythemia rubra vera[435]) nevertheless have a common stem-cell origin. Paroxysmal nocturnal hemoglobinuria is a nonmalignant hematologic disorder that has also been shown to be of clonal origin,[436] and clonal proliferation may be important in the pathogenesis of atheromatous plaques.[437] G6PD has been used as a marker in experiments aiming to investigate somatic mutations in intestinal crypts of the mouse.[438] There are several possible sources of error in the interpretation of G6PD phenotypes as clonal markers.[386,439] An admixture of normal cells (e.g., in a solid tumor biopsy), which will have both G6PD phenotypes, may mask the presence of a single G6PD phenotype in the malignant cells. The relative activity of the two phenotypes may vary from one tissue to another and at different sites within the same tissue and, thus, may not be the same in the tissue from which the tumor originated as in other tissues. It is also possible that the tumor arose by clonal proliferation of more than one cell (i.e., is of multicentric origin) but that the original cells were by coincidence of the same G6PD phenotype. A further consideration (Fig. 179-12) is somatic cell selection,[439–441] whereby X-linked genes other than that for G6PD may influence the proliferation of cells after the inactivation process has taken place. Sequence differences between parental G6PD alleles that can be used as clonal markers of high sensitivity by RT-PCR[442] have been used to show that transcripts from paternal genes can be detected in human embryos after in vitro fertilization as early as the four-cell stage.[443] G6PD deficiency itself, if severe, can produce cell selection against G6PD-deficient cells in heterozygous mothers of patients with CNSHA.[444]

G6PD DEFICIENCY AND MALARIA

The now classic notion that G6PD deficiency has become widespread as a result of malaria selection[445] can be visualized easily by comparing the geographic distribution of this red-cell phenotype (Fig. 179-8) with an epidemiologic map of *P. falciparum* malaria (see, for instance, reference 86). Several discrepancies are easy to explain. In southern Europe, G6PD deficiency is common and there is no malaria, but the latter has been eradicated only over the last two generations. In North America there is no malaria, but the prevalence of G6PD deficiency on this continent is entirely accounted for by migrations that have taken place in relatively recent times. Geographic correlation alone is of course no proof of the "malaria hypothesis." The body of more compelling evidence has been reviewed elsewhere,[446,447] and it can be only briefly summarized here.

Micromapping

Analysis of relatively narrow geographic areas has consistently shown a good correlation between the frequency of G6PD deficiency and the intensity of malaria transmission, for instance, in East Africa,[448] Papua New Guinea,[449] the Vanuatu archipelago,[151] Sardinia,[450] and Greece.[451] In some of these areas, the evidence is strengthened by the fact that the population is genetically relatively homogeneous, and the variance of frequencies of other genes was shown to be significantly lower than that of G6PD deficiency.[452]

Genetic Heterogeneity of Polymorphic G6PD Variants

If G6PD deficiency had spread by genetic drift, the same mutant would be found everywhere. Instead, diverse point mutations (see above) must have arisen independently and then spread centrifugally to establish themselves at polymorphic frequencies — a good example of convergent microevolution in the human species. In this respect, the G6PD deficiency polymorphism is more reminiscent of the highly heterogeneous thalassemia system than of the unique mutation of hemoglobin S.

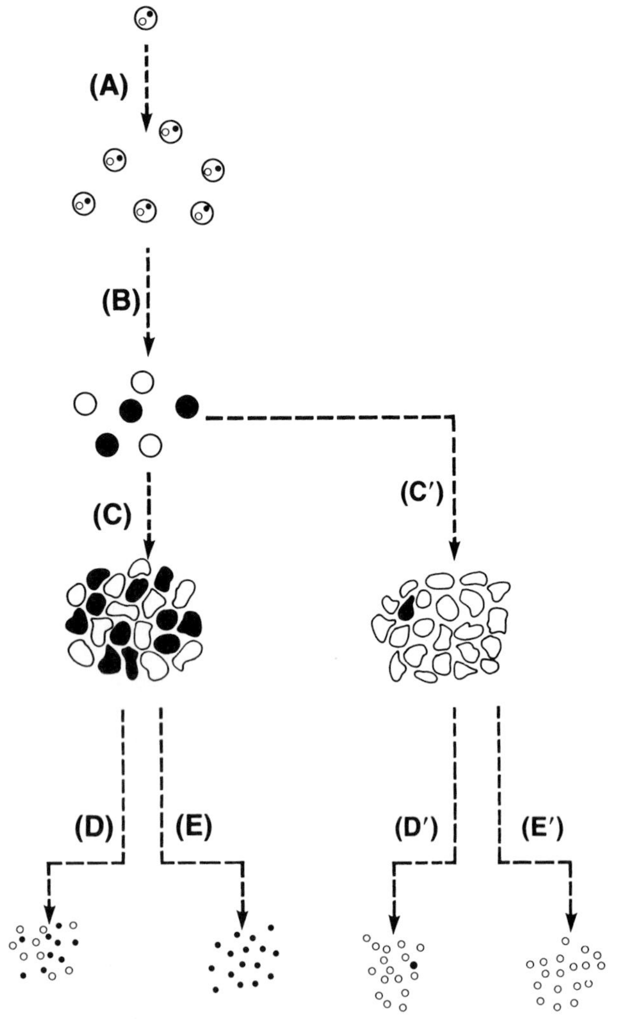

Fig. 179-12 The phenotype in heterozygotes can yield information on clonal proliferation and somatic cell selection. At the top, embryonic cells (*A*) before X-chromosome inactivation; the two dots represent expression of two different alleles of *B*. Inactivation of one X chromosome per cell produces two cell populations (empty and filled circles) distinguishable by their phenotype. *C*, Proliferation of cells at about even rates produces mosaicism in the adult. *C′*, Differential growth rate of the two cell types arising from X inactivation (somatic cell selection) may produce in the adult a (nearly) homogeneous population. This could apply to the whole body, or it may occur in one tissue and not in another, because a particular X-linked gene, for which the subject is heterozygous, may confer a growth advantage only in a tissue where the gene is expressed. *D*, Pathologic tissue (for instance, an inflammatory process or the healing of a wound) will still produce a mosaic. *E*, Pathologic proliferation arising from a single cell ("monoclonal") of an adult tissue (for instance, a tumor) will produce a homogeneous population. *D′* and E′, If pathologic proliferation arises in a tissue that is already homogeneous as a result of *C′*, the resulting cell population will still be homogeneous, regardless of whether the proliferative process is monoclonal or polyclonal.

Clinical Studies

Studies in the field have yielded ambiguous data when prevalence of malaria or malaria parasitemia was compared between normal and G6PD-deficient males or in subjects of both sexes.[453–457] However, in a study in which girls heterozygous for G6PD deficiency (GdB/GdA−) in Nigeria were rigorously classified, a significantly lower *P. falciparum* parasitemia was observed.[458,459] A similar study was repeated more than 20 years later; in Kenya and in the Gambia protection against severe malaria (defined as being associated with either severe anemia or neurologic signs) was seen in both heterozygotes and hemizygotes.[460]

In Vitro Studies

Once a culture system for the intraerythrocytic cycle of *P. falciparum* was developed by Trager and Jensen,[461] it became possible to test, in controlled experiments, whether the G6PD genotype of red cells affected their ability to host the parasite. Several groups have independently reported that the growth of *P. falciparum* was impaired in G6PD-deficient red cells,[462–464] although in some studies, the difference was apparent only when the cultures were subjected to oxidative stress,[465] and in others it could not be detected at all.[466] At least in part the discrepancies could depend on methodology (for instance, the time of storage of G6PD-deficient host red cells is critical). However, the type of G6PD deficiency and variations in the parasite might also play a role (although in some cases, discrepancies arose even when the same strain of *P. falciparum* was used). At any rate, it is clear that intracellular schizogony rather than invasion is affected in G6PD-deficient red cells,[464] probably because they cause or allow oxidative injury to the parasite.[467,468] The preferential development of parasites in G6PD-normal as opposed to G6PD-deficient red cells is in keeping with previous evidence obtained in vivo.[469]

Mechanism of Protection Against Malaria

In view of the above, it seems unlikely that inhibition of parasite growth can be the entire explanation for resistance against malaria of G6PD-deficient people. In some experiments, the parasite was shown to adapt to the G6PD-deficient environment of the host cell, with its growth restored to normal within a few cycles, and it was suggested that this might result from overinduction of a *P. falciparum* G6PD gene.[470] When this gene was eventually cloned,[471] it proved quite interesting, because it has an N-terminal extension of some 300 amino acids, and this may mean that the molecule has another enzyme activity in addition to G6PD.[472] However, there was no obvious difference in the respective levels of the parasite's own G6PD mRNA, when it was grown in vitro, in either normal or G6PD-deficient red cells.[466] Because all strains of *P. falciparum* adapted to in vitro culture have probably accumulated a significant number of mutations, it seems important to validate these data by analysis of parasites from patients with different G6PD genotypes.

An intriguing twist to malaria selection has been noted. Because fava beans are a popular crop in certain areas where malaria and G6PD deficiency are also prevalent, a three-way interaction has been suggested.[473,474] Indeed, both fava beans and primaquine cause hemolysis because they generate oxygen radicals; oxidative stress may play a role in the chemotherapeutic action of primaquine against malaria parasites.[475,476] Ultimately, the way G6PD deficient red cells protect against malaria must depend on the fact that they are sensitive to oxidative stress. However, it is quite clear that fava beans are not required for selection of G6PD-deficient genes (e.g., they have not been grown traditionally in Africa, where both *P. falciparum* and G6PD deficiency are highly endemic).

The findings summarized above leave little doubt that the G6PD deficiency polymorphism is balanced by malaria selection. At the same time, the mechanism that effects this is not fully explained. Recently, it was shown that parasitized G6PD-deficient red cells undergo phagocytosis by macrophages at an earlier stage than parasitized normal red cells,[466] supporting the notion that also in this case, as for AS heterozygotes,[477] suicidal infection is one protective mechanism.

ACKNOWLEDGMENTS

We are immensely indebted to Dr. Ernest Beutler who, having been a pioneer of research in this area, has authoritatively reviewed G6PD deficiency in the first five editions of this textbook over a span of 23 years. We are grateful to many colleagues for sharing in experimental work and many discussions: particularly E. A. Usanga in Ibadan; G. Battistuzzi, M. D'Urso, G. Martini, Graziella Persico, Daniela Toniolo, Viola Calabrò, Stefania Filosa, and E. Poggi in Napoli; P. M. Mason, N. Foulkes, J. S. Kaeda, Margaret Town, E. O'Brien, D. Roper, and B. Kurdi-Haidar in London; Margaret Adams in Oxford; R. Notaro, Ana Rovira, Letizia Longo, P. P. Pandolfi, and Maria De Angioletti in New York; and David Schlessinger in all of these places. Valerie Charles and Rosario Notaro were immensely helpful in the preparation of the manuscript. Work in the authors' laboratory has been supported by grants from the National Institutes of Health (U.S.A.) and the Medical Research Council (G.B.).

REFERENCES

1. Beutler E: Study of glucose-6-phosphate dehydrogenase: History and molecular biology. *Am J Hematol* **42**:53, 1993.
2. Fermi C, Martinetti P: Studio sul favismo. *Annali di Igiene Sperimentale* **15**:76, 1905.
3. Gasbarrini A: Il favismo. *Policlinico Sezione Pratica* **22**:1505, 1915.
4. Luisada L: Favism: A singular disease affecting chiefly red blood cells. *Medicine* **20**:229, 1941.
5. Sansone G, Piga AM, Segni G: *Il Favismo*. Torino, Minerva Medica, 1958.
6. Beutler E: The hemolytic effect of primaquine and related compounds. *Blood* **14**:103, 1959.
7. Beutler E: Glucose 6-phosphate dehydrogenase deficiency, in Stanbury JB, Wyngaarden JB, Fredrickson DS (eds): *The Metabolic Basis of Inherited Disease*. New York, McGraw-Hill, 1960.
8. Carson PE, Flanagan CL, Ickes CE, Alving A: Enzymatic deficiency in primaquine-sensitive erythrocytes. *Science* **124**:484, 1956.
9. Waller HD, Löhr GW, Tabatabai M: Hämolyse und Fehlen von glucose-6-phosphate-dehydrogenase in roten Blutzellen (eine Fermentanomalie der Erythrozyten). *Klinische Wochenschrift* **35**:1022, 1957.
10. Sansone G, Segni G: Nuovi aspetti dell'alterato biochimismo degli eritrociti dei favici: Assenza pressochè completa della glucoso-6-P deidrogenasi. *Bollettino della Societá Italiana di Biologia Sperimentale* **34**:327, 1958.
11. Marks PA: Glucose 6-phosphate dehydrogenase, in Bishop C (ed): *The Red Blood Cell*. New York, Academic Press, 1964.
12. Shows TB, Tashian RE, Brewer GJ: Erythrocyte glucose 6-phosphate dehydrogenase in Caucasians: New inherited variant. *Science* **145**:1056, 1964.
13. Beutler E: G6PD: Population genetics and clinical manifestations. *Blood Rev* **10**:45, 1996.
14. Chang JG, Liu TC: Glucose-6-phosphate dehydrogenase deficiency. *Crit Rev Oncol Hematol* **20**:1, 1995.
15. Bautista JM, Luzzatto L: Glucose 6-phosphate dehydrogenase, in Swallow DM, Edwards YH (eds): *Protein Dysfunction and Human Genetic Disease*. Oxford, BIOS, 1997, p 33.
16. Luzzatto L: Glucose-6-phosphate dehydrogenase deficiency and the pentose phosphate pathway, in Handin RI, Thomas SEL, Stossel P (eds): *Blood: Principles & Practice of Hematology*. Philadelphia, JB Lippincott, 1995, p 1897.
17. Beutler E: *Glucose 6-Phosphate Dehydrogenase Deficiency*, 5th ed. New York, McGraw-Hill, 1995.
18. Glader BE, Lukens JN: *Glucose 6-Phosphate Dehydrogenase Deficiency and Related Disorders of Hexosose Monophosphate Shunt and Glutathione Metabolism*, 10th ed. Philadelphia, Lippincott-Williams & Wilkins, 1998.
19. Cohen P, Rosemeyer MA: Subunit interactions of human glucose 6-phosphate dehydrogenase from human erythrocytes. *Eur J Biochem* **8**:8, 1969.
20. Babalola AOG, Beetlestone JG, Luzzatto L: Genetic variants of human erythrocyte glucose 6-phosphate dehydrogenase. Kinetic and thermodynamic parameters of variants A, B, and A− in relation to quaternary structure. *J Biol Chem* **251**:2993, 1976.
21. Bonsignore A, Cancedda R, Nicolini A, Damiani G, De Flora A: Metabolism of human erythrocyte glucose 6-phosphate dehydrogenase. VI. Interconversion of multiple molecular forms. *Arch Biochem Biophys* **147**:493, 1971.
22. De Flora A, Morelli A, Giuliano F: Human erythrocyte G6PD. Content of bound coenzyme. *Biochem Biophys Res Commun* **59**:406, 1974.
23. Jeffery J, Soderling-Barros J, Murray LA, Wood I, Hansen RJ, Szepesi B, Jornvall H: Glucose 6-phosphate dehydrogenase. Characteristics revealed by the rat liver enzyme. *Eur J Biochem* **186**:551, 1989.
24. Camardella L, Damonte G, Carratore V, Benatti U, Tonetti M, Moneti G: Glucose 6-phosphate dehydrogenase from human erythrocytes: Identification of *N*-acetyl-alanine at the N-terminus of the mature protein. *Biochem Biophys Res Commun* **207**:331, 1995.
25. Luzzatto L, Afolayan A: Enzymic properties of different types of human erythrocyte glucose-6-phosphate dehydrogenase, with chracterization of two new genetic variants. *J Clin Invest* **47**:1833, 1968.
26. Au SWN, Naylor CE, Gover S, Vandeputte-Rutten L, Scopes DA, Mason PJ, Luzzatto L, et al.: Solution of the structure of tetrameric human glucose 6-phosphate dehydrogenase by molecular replacement. *Acta Crystallogr* **D55**:826, 1999.
27. Notaro R, Afolayan A, Luzzatto L: Human mutations in glucose 6-phosphate dehydrogenase reflect evolutionary history. *FASEB J* **14**:485, 2000.
28. De Flora A, Morelli A, Frascio M, Corte G, Curti B, Galliano M, Gozzer C, et al:. Radioimmunoassay and chemical properties of glucose-6-phosphate dehydrogenase and of a specific NADP(H)-binding protein (FX) from human erythrocytes. *Biochim Biophys Acta* **500**:109, 1977.
29. Camardella L, Carratore V, Ciardiello MA, Damonte G, Benatti U, De Flora A: Primary structure of human erythrocyte nicotinamide adenine dinucleotide phosphate (NADP[H])-binding protein FX: Identification with the mouse tum-transplantation antigen P35B. *Blood* **85**:264, 1995.
30. Rowland P, Basak A, Gover S, Levy RH, Adams M: The three-dimensional structure of glucose 6-phosphate dehydrogenase from *Leuconostoc mesenteroides* refined at 2.0 Å resolution. *Structure* **2**:1073, 1994.
31. Naylor CE, Rowland P, Basak AK, Gover S, Mason PJ, Bautista JM, Vulliamy TJ, et al.: Glucose 6-phosphate dehydrogenase mutations causing enzyme deficiency in a model of the tertiary structure of the human enzyme. *Blood* **87**:2974, 1996.
32. Camardella L, Caruso C, Rutigliano B, Romano M, di Prisco G, Descalzi F: Identification of a reactive lysine residue in human erythrocyte glucose-6-phosphate dehydrogenase, in Yoshida A, Beutler E (eds): *Glucose-6-Phosphate Dehydrogenase*. New York, Academic, 1986.
33. Bautista JM, Mason PJ, Luzzatto L: Human glucose-6-phosphate dehydrogenase. Lysine 205 is dispensable for substrate binding but essential for catalysis. *FEBS Lett* **366**:61, 1995.
34. Cosgrove MS, Naylor C, Paludan S, Adams MJ, Levy HR: On the mechanism of the reaction catalyzed by glucose 6-phosphate dehydrogenase. *Biochemistry* **37**:2759, 1998.
35. Kaeda JS, Chootray GP, Ranjit MR, Bautista JM, Reddy PH, Stevens D, Naidu JM, et al.: A new glucose-6-phosphate dehydrogenase variant, G6PD Orissa (44 Ala → Gly), is the major polymorphic variant in tribal populations in India. *Am J Hum Genet* **57**:1335, 1995.
36. Levy HR, Vought VE, Adams MJ: Identification of an arginine residue in the dual coenzyme-specific glucose 6-phosphate dehydrogenase from Leuconostoc mesenteroides that plays a key role in binding NADP+ but not NAD. *Arch Biochem Biophys* **326**:145, 1996.
37. Rosenstraus M, Chasin LA: Isolation of mammalian cell mutants deficient in glucose-6-phosphate dehydrogenase activity: Linkage tohypoxanthine phosphoribosyl tansferase. *Proc Natl Acad Sci U S A* **72**:493, 1975.
38. Town M, Athanasiou Metaxa M, Luzzatto L: Intragenic interspecific complementation of glucose 6-phosphate dehydrogenase in human-hamster cell hybrids. *Somat Cell Mol Genet* **16**:97, 1990.
39. Beutler E: The glutathione instability of drug-sensitive red cells. A new method for the in vitro detection of drug sensitivity. *J Lab Clin Med* **49**:84, 1957.
40. Salvemini F, Franze A, Iervolino A, Filosa S, Salzano S, Ursini MV: Enhanced glutathione levels and oxidoresistance mediated by increased glucose-6-phosphate dehydrogenase expression. *J Biol Chem* **274**:2750, 1999.
41. Kuo WY, Tang TK: Effects of G6PD overexpression in NIH3T3 cells treated with tert-butyl hydroperoxide or paraquat. *Free Rad Biol Med* **24**:1130, 1998.
42. Tian WN, Braunstein LD, Apse K, Pang J, Rose M, Tian X, Stanton RC: Importance of glucose-6-phosphate dehydrogenase activity in cell death. *Am J Physiol* **276**:C1121, 1999.
43. Preville X, Salvemini F, Giraud S, Chaufour S, Paul C, Stepien G, Ursini MV, et al.: Mammalian small stress proteins protect against oxidative stress through their ability to increase glucose-6-phosphate dehydrogenase activity and by maintaining optimal cellular detoxifying machinery. *Exp Cell Res* **247**:61, 1999.
44. Cohen G, Hochstein P: Generation of hydrogen peroxide in erythrocytes by haemolytic agents. *Biochemistry* **3**:895, 1964.

45. Aebi HE, Wyss SR: Acatalasemia, in Stanbury JB, Wyngaarden JB, Fredrickson DS (eds): *The Metabolic Basis of Inherited Disease*, New York, McGraw-Hill, 1978, 1792.
46. Kirkman HN, Gaetani GF: Catalase: A tetrameric enzyme with four tightly bound molecules of NADPH. *Proc Natl Acad Sci U S A* **81**:4343, 1984.
47. Kirkman HN, Gaetani GF, Clemons EH: NADP-binding proteins causing reduced availability and sigmoid release of NADP+ in human erythrocytes. *J Biol Chem* **261**:4039, 1986.
48. Gaetani GF, Galiano S, Canepa L, Ferraris A-M, Kirkman HN: Catalase and glutathione peroxidase are equally active in detoxification of hydrogen peroxide in human erythrocytes. *Blood* **73**:334, 1989.
49. Gaetani GF, Ferraris AM: Recent developments on Mediterranean G6PD. *Br J Haematol* **68**:1, 1988.
50. Tsai KJ, Hung IJ, Chow CK, Stern A, Chao SS, Chiu DT: Impaired production of nitric oxide, superoxide, and hydrogen peroxide in glucose 6-phosphate-dehydrogenase-deficient granulocytes. *FEBS Lett* **436**:411, 1998.
51. Fraenkel DG: Selection of *Escherichia coli* mutants lacking glucose-6-phosphate dehydrogenase or gluconate-6-phosphate dehydrogenase. *J Bacteriol* **95**:1267, 1968.
52. Lobo Z, Maitra PK: Pentose phosphate pathway mutants of yeast. *Mol Gen Genet* **185**:367, 1982.
53. Izawa S, Maeda K, Miki T, Mano J, Inoue Y, Kimura A: Importance of glucose-6-phosphate dehydrogenase in the adaptive response to hydrogen peroxide in saccharomyces cerevisiae. *Biochem J* **330**:811, 1998.
54. Pandolfi PP, Sonati F, Rivi R, Mason P, Grosveld F, Luzzatto L: Targeted disruption of the housekeeping gene encodinbg glucose 6-phosphate dehydrogenase (G6PD): G6PD is dispensable for pentose synthesis but essential for defense against oxidative stress. *EMBO J* **14**:5209, 1995.
55. Longo L, Rosti V, Gaboli M, Tabarini D, Pandolfi PP, Luzzatto L: Mice heterozygous for complete glucose 6-phosphate dehydrogenase (G6PD) deficiency are viable and show somatic cell selection. *Blood* **Suppl I**:408a, 1997.
56. Neifer S, Jung A, Bienzle U: Characterization of erythrocytic glucose-6-phosphate dehydrogenase in a mouse strain with reduced G6PD activity. *Biomed Biochim Acta* **3**:233, 1991.
57. Sanders S, Smith DP, Thomas GA, Williams ED: A glucose-6-phosphate dehydrogenase (G6PD) splice site consensus sequence mutation associated with G6PD enzyme deficiency. *Mutat Res* **374**:79, 1997.
58. Nicol CJ, Zielenski J, Tsui L-C, Wells PG: An embryoprotective role for glucose-6-phosphate dehydrogenase in developmental oxidative stress and chemical teratogenesis. *FASEB J* **14**:111, 2000.
59. Winn LM, Wells PG: Phenytoin-initiated DNA oxidation in murine embryo culture, and embryo protection by the antioxidative enzymes superoxide dismutase and catalase: Evidence for reactive oxygen species mediated DNA oxidation in the molecular mechanism of phenytoin teratogenicity. *Mol Pharmacol* **48**:112, 1995.
60. Wells PG, Kim PM, Laposa RR, Nicol CJ, Parman T, Winn LM: Oxidative damage in chemical teratogenesis. *Mutat Res* **396**:65, 1997.
61. Tian WN, Braunstein LD, Pang J, Stuhlmeier KM, Xi QC, Tian X, Stanton RC: Importance of glucose-6-phosphate dehydrogenase activity for cell growth. *J Biol Chem* **273**:10609, 1998.
62. Kletzien RF, Harris PK, Foellmi LA: Glucose-6-phosphate dehydrogenase: A "housekeeping" enzyme subject to tissue-specific regulation by hormones, nutrients, and oxidant stress. *FASEB J* **8**:174, 1994.
63. Hodge DL, Salati LM: Nutritional regulation of the glucose-6-phosphate dehydrogenase gene is mediated by a nuclear posttranscriptional mechanism. *Arch Biochem Biophys* **348**:303, 1997.
64. Tepperman HM, Tepperman J: On the response of hepatic G6PD activity to changes in diet compostion and food intake pattern, in Weber G (ed): *Advances in Enzyme Regulation*. New York, Pergamon, 1963, p 121.
65. Kletzien RF, Fritz RS, Prostko CR, Jones EA, Dreher KL: Hepatic glucose-6-phosphate dehydrogenase: Nutritional and hormonal regulation of mRNA levels, in Yoshida A, Beutler E (eds): *Glucose-6-Phosphate Dehydrogenase*. Orlando, FL, Academic, 1986.
66. Battistuzzi G, D'Urso M, Toniolo D, Persico GM, Luzzatto L: Tissue specific levels of G6PD correlate with methylation at the 3′ end of the gene. *Proc Natl Acad Sci U S A* **82**:1465, 1985.
67. Persico M, Battistuzzi G, Mareni C, Nobile C, D'Urso M, Toniolo D, Luzzatto L: Genetic variants of human glucose 6-phosphate dehydrogenase (G6PD): Studies of turnover and of G6PD-specific mRNA, in Weatherall DJ, Fiorelli G, Gorini S (eds): *Advances in Red Blood Cell Biology*. New York, Raven, 1982, p 309.
68. Piomelli S, Corash LM, Davenport DD, Miraglia J, Amorosi EL: In vivo lability of glucose-6-phosphate dehydrogenase in Gd A and Gd Mediterranean deficiency. *J Clin Invest* **47**:940, 1968.
69. Cramer CT, Cooke S, Ginsberg LC, Kletzien RF, Stapleton SR, Ulrich RG: Upregulation of glucose-6-phosphate dehydrogenase in response to hepatocellular oxidative stress: Studies with diquat. *J Biochem Toxicol* **10**:293, 1995.
70. Ursini MV, Parrella A, Rosa G, Salzano S, Martini G: Enhanced expression of glucose-6-phosphate dehydrogenase in human cells sustaining oxidative stress. *Biochem J* **323**:801, 1997.
71. Bonsignore A, Lorenzoni I, Cancedda R, Consulich ME, De Flora A: Effect of divalent cations on the structure of human erythrocyte G6PD. *Biochem Biophys Res Commun* **42**:159, 1971.
72. Yoshida A: Haemolytic anaemia and G6PD deficiency. *Science* **179**:532, 1973.
73. Luzzatto L, Testa U: Human erythrocyte glucose 6-phosphate dehydrogenase: Structure and function in normal and mutant subjects. *Curr Top Hematol* **1**:1, 1978.
74. Luzzatto L: Regulation of the activity of glucose-6-phosphate dehydrogenase by NADP+ and NADPH. *Biochim Biophys Acta* **146**:18, 1967.
75. Morelli A, Benatti U, Giuliano F, De Flora A: Human erythrocyte glucose-6-phosphate dehydrogenase. Evidence for competitive binding of NADP and NADPH. *Biochem Biophys Res Commun* **70**:600, 1976.
76. Kirkman HN, Gaetani GD, Clemons EH, Mareni C: Red cell NADP and NADPH in glucose-6-phosphate dehydrogenase deficiency. *J Clin Invest* **55**:875, 1975.
77. Gaetani GF, Parker JC, Kirkman HN: Intracellular restraint: A new basis for the limitation in response to oxidation stress in human erythrocytes containing low activity variants of glucose 6-phosphate dehydrogenase. *Proc Natl Acad Sci U S A* **71**:3584, 1975.
78. Marks PA: Glucose-6-P dehydrogenase stability, activation and inactivation. *Cold Spring Harb Symp Quant Biol* **26**:343, 1961.
79. Oertel GW, Rebelein I: Effects of dehydroepiandrosterone and its conjugates upon the acitivity of glucose-6-phosphate dehydrogenase in human erythrocytes. *Biochim Biophys Acta* **184**:459, 1969.
80. Gordon G, Mackow MC, Levy HR: On the mechanism of interaction of steroids with human glucose 6-phosphate dehydrogenase. *Arch Biochem Biophys* **318**:25, 1995.
81. Schwartz AG, Pashko LL: Cancer prevention with dehydroepiandrosterone and non-androgenic structural analogs [Review]. *J Cell Biochem Suppl* **22**:210, 1995.
82. Di Monaco M, Pizzini A, Gatto V, Leonardi L, Gallo M, Brignardello E, Boccuzzi G: Role of glucose-6-phosphate dehydrogenase inhibition in the antiproliferative effects of dehydroepiandrosterone on human breast cancer cells. *Br J Cancer* **75**:589, 1997.
83. Sartori E: Elementi per la genetica del favismo. *Studi Sassar* **35**:I, 1957.
84. Luzzatto L: Glucose-6-phosphate dehydrogenase deficiency, in Brown MJ (ed): *Advanced Medicine, 21*. London, Churchill Livingstone, 1986, p 398.
85. Nora JJ, Frazer FC: *Medical Genetics*. Philadelphia, Lea & Febiger, 1974.
86. Beutler E, Yeh M, Fairbanks VF: The normal human female as a mosaic of X-chromosome activity: Studies using the gene for G6PD deficiency as a marker. *Proc Natl Acad Sci U S A* **48**:9, 1962.
87. Davidson RG, Nitowsky HM, Childs B: Demonstration of two populations of cells in the human female heterozygous for glucose-6-phosphate dehydrogenase variants. *Proc Natl Acad Sci U S A* **50**:481, 1963.
88. Adam A: Linkage between deficiency of glucose 6-phosphate dehydrogenase and colour-blindness. *Nature* **189**:686, 1961.
89. Keats B: Genetic mapping: X chromosome. *Hum Genet* **64**:28, 1983.
90. Pai GS, Sprenkle JA, Do TT, Mareni CE, Migeon BR: Localization of the loci for hypoxanthine phosphoribosyltransferase and glucose-6-phosphate dehydrogenase and biochemical evidence of non-random X-chromosome expression from studies of human X-autosome translocation. *Proc Natl Acad Sci U S A* **77**:2810, 1980.
91. Szabo P, Purrello M, Rocchi M, Archidiacono N, Alhadeff B, Filippi G, Toniolo D, et al.: Cytological mapping of the human glucose-6-phosphate dehydrogenase gene distal to the fragile-X site suggests a high rate of meiotic recombination across this site. *Proc Natl Acad Sci U S A* **81**:7855, 1984.

92. Trask BJ, Massa H, Kenwrick S, Gitschier J: Mapping of human chromosome Xq28 by two-color fluorescence in situ hybridization of DNA sequences to interphase cell nuclei. *Am J Hum Genet* **48**:1, 1991.
93. Patterson M, Schwartz C, Bell M, Sauer S, Hofker M, Trask B, Van den Engh G, et al.: Physical mapping studies on the human X chromosome in the region Xq27-Xqter. *Genomics* **1**:297, 1987.
94. Freije D, Schlessinger D: A 1.6-Mb contig of yeast artificial chromosomes around the human factor VIII gene reveals three regions homologous to probes for the DXS115 locus and two for the DXYS64 locus. *Am J Hum Genet* **51**:66, 1992.
95. Chen EY, Zollo M, Mazzarella R, Ciccodicola A, Chen C, Zuo L, Heiner C, et al.: Long-range sequence analysis in Xq28: Thirteen known and six candidate genes in 219.4 kb of high GC between RCP/GCP and G6PD loci. *Hum Mol Genet* **5**:659, 1996.
96. Rivella S, Tamanini F, Bione S, Mancini M, Herman G, Chatterjee A, Toniolo D: A comparative transcriptional map of a region of 250 kb on the human and mouse X chromosome between the G6PD and the FLN1 genes. *Genomics* **28**:377, 1995.
97. Martini G, Toniolo D, Vulliamy TJ, Luzzatto L, Dono R, Viglietto G, Paonessa G, et al.: Structural analysis of the X-linked gene encoding human glucose 6-phosphate dehydrogenase. *EMBO J* **5**:1849, 1986.
98. Hodge DL, Charron T, Stabile LP, Klautky SA, Salati LM: Structural characterization and tissue-specific expression of the mouse glucose-6-phosphate dehydrogenase gene. *DNA Cell Biol* **17**:283, 1998.
99. Persico MG, Viglietto G, Martini G, Toniolo D, Paonessa G, Moscatelli C, Dono R, et al.: Isolation of human glucose-6-phosphate dehydrogenase (G6PD) cDNA clones; primary structure of the protein and unusual 5′ non-coding region. *Nucleic Acids Res* **14**:2511, 1986.
100. Chen EY, Cheng A, Lee A, Kuang W-J, Hillier L, Green P, Schlessinger D, et al.: Sequence of human glucose 6-phosphate dehydrogenase cloned in plasmids and a yeast artificial chromosome. *Genomics* **10**:792, 1991.
101. Toniolo D, Filippi M, Dono R, Lettieri R, Martini G: The CpG island in the 5′-region of the G6PD gene of man and mouse. *Gene* **102**:197, 1991.
102. Bird AP: CpE rich islands and the function of DNA methylation. *Nature* **321**:209, 1986.
103. Reynolds GA, Basu SK, Osborne TF, Chin DJ, Gil G, Brown MS, Goldstein JL, et al.: HMG CoA reductase: A negatively regulated gene with unusual promoter and 5′ untranslated regions. *Cell* **38**:275, 1984.
104. Bruce-Chwatt LJ: *Essential Malariology.* London, Heinemann, 1988.
105. Dynan WS, Tjian R: Control of eukaryotic messenger RNA synthesis by sequence-specific DNA-binding proteins. *Nature* **316**:774, 1985.
106. Ursini MV, Scalera L, Martini G: High level of transcription driven by a 400-bp segment of the human G6PD promoter. *Biochem Biophys Res Commun* **170**:1203, 1990.
107. Franze A, Ferrante MI, Fusco F, Santoro A, Sanzari E, Martini G, Ursini MV: Molecular anatomy of the human glucose 6-phosphate dehydrogenase core promoter. *FEBS Lett* **437**:313, 1998.
108. Philippe M, Larondelle Y, Lemaigre F, Mariam, B, Delhez H, Mason P, Luzzatto L, et al.: Promoter function of the human glucose-6-phosphate dehydrogenase gene depends on two GC boxes that are cell specifically controlled. *Eur J Biochem* **226**:377, 1994.
109. Ursini MV, Lettieri T, Braddock M, Martini G: Enhanced activity of human G6PD promoter transfected in HeLa cells producing high levels of HIV-1 Tat. *Virology* **196**:338, 1993.
110. Morikawa N, Nakayawa R, Holtein D: Dietary induction of glucose-6-phosphate dehydrogenase synthesis. *Biochem Biophys Res Commun* **120**:1022, 1984.
111. Manos P, Taylor N, Rudach-Garcia D, Morikawa N, Nakayawa R, Holten D: Signals regulating G6PD levels in rat liver, in: Yoshida A, Beutler E (eds): *Glucose-6-phosphate dehydrogenase*. New York, Academic, 1986.
112. Richards AH, Hilf R: Influence of pregnancy, lactation and involution on glucose 6-phosphate dehydrogenase and lactant dehydrogenase isoenzymes in the rat mammary gland. *Endocrinology* **91**:287, 1972.
113. Weber G, Cantero A: Glucose-6-phosphate utilization in hepatoma, regenerating and newborn rat liver, and in the liver of fed and fasted normal rats. *Cancer Res* **17**:995, 1957.
114. Corcoran CM, Fraser P, Martini G, Luzzatto L, Mason PJ: High-level regulated expression of the human G6PD gene in transgenic mice. *Gene* **173**:241, 1996.
115. Tang TK, Tam KB, Huang SC: High-level and erythroid-specific expression of human glucose-6-phosphate dehydrogenase in transgenic mice. *J Biol Chem* **268**:9522, 1993.
116. Hendriksen PJM, Hoogerbrugge JW, Baarends WM, de Boer P, Vreeburg JTM, Vos EA, van der Lende T, et al.: Testis-specific expression of a functional retroposon encoding glucose-6-phosphate dehydrogenase in the mouse. *Genomics* **41**:350, 1997.
117. McCarrey JR, Thomas K: Human testis-specific PGK gene lacks introns and possesses characteristics of a processed gene. *Nature* **326**:501, 1987.
118. Yoshida A, Lebo RV: Existence of glucose-6-phosphate dehydrogenase-like locus on chromosome 17. *Am J Hum Genet* **39**:203, 1986.
119. Betke K, Beutler E, Brewer GJ, Kirkman HN, Luzzatto L, Motulsky AG, Ramot B, et al.: Standardisation of procedures for the study of glucose-6-phosphate dehydrogenase. Report of a WHO Scientific Group. *WHO Tech Rep Ser* **366**:53, 1967.
120. WHO Working: Glucose-6-phosphate dehydrogenase deficiency. *Bull WHO Working* **67**:601, 1989.
121. Luzzatto L, Mehta A: Glucose 6-phosphate dehydrogenase deficiency, in Scriver CR, Beaudet AL, Sly WS, Valle D (eds): *The Metabolic and Molecular Bases of Inherited Disease*. New York, McGraw-Hill, 1995, p 3367.
122. Vergnes HA, Bonnet LG, Grozdea JD: Genetic variants of human erythrocyte glucose-6-phosphate dehydrogenase: New characterization data obtained by multivariante analysis. *Ann Hum Genet* **49**:1, 1985.
123. Fiorelli G, Manoussakis C, Sampietro M, Pittalis S, Guglielmino CR, Cappellini MD: Different polymorphic variants of glucose-6-phosphate dehydrogenase (G6PD) in Italy. *Ann Hum Genet* **53**:229, 1989.
124. Cappellini MD, Martinez Di Montemuros F, De Bellis G, Debernardi S, Dotti C, Fiorelli G: Multiple G6PD mutations are associated with a clinical and biochemical phenotype similar to that of G6PD Mediterranean. *Blood* **87**:3953, 1996.
125. Escobar MA, Heller P, Trobaugh FE Jr: "Complete" erythrocyte glucose 6-phosphate dehydrogenase deficiency. *Arch Int Med* **113**:428, 1964.
126. Junien C, Kaplan JC, Heienhofer HC, Malgret P, Sender A: G6PD Baudelocque: A new unstable variant characterized in cultured fibroblasts. *Enzyme* **18**:48, 1974.
127. Morelli A, Grasso M, Meloni T, Forteleoni G, Zocchi E, De Flora A: Favism: Impairment of proteolytic systems in red blood cells. *Blood* **69**:1753, 1987.
128. Mason PJ, Sonati MF, MacDonald D, Lanza C, Busutil D, Town M, Corcoran CM, et al.: New glucose 6-phosphate dehydrogenase mutations associated with chronic anemia. *Blood* **85**:1377, 1995.
129. Hirono A, Fujii H, Takano T, Chiba Y, Azuno Y, Miwa S: Molecular analysis of eight biochemically unique glucose-6-phosphate dehydrogenase variants found in Japan. *Blood* **89**:4624, 1997.
130. Vulliamy TJ, Kaeda JS, Ait-Chafa D, Mangerini R, Roper D, Barbot J, Mehta AB, et al.: Clinical and haematological consequences of recurrent G6PD mutations and a single new mutation causing chronic nonsperocytic haemolytic anaemia. *Br J Haematol* **101**:670, 1998.
131. Vlachos A, Westwood B, Lipton JM, Beutler E: G6PD Mount Sinai: A new severe hemolytic variant characterized by dual mutations at nucleotides 376G and 1159T (N126D). *Hum Mut* **Suppl 1**:S154, 1998.
132. Vulliamy TJ, D'Urso M, Battistuzzi G, Estrada M, Foulkes NS, Martini G, Calabro V, et al.: Diverse point mutations in the human glucose-6-phosphate dehydrogenase gene cause enzyme deficiency and mild or severe hemolytic anemia. *Proc Natl Acad Sci U S A* **85**:5171, 1988.
133. Calabrò V, Mason PJ, Civitelli D, Cittadella R, Filosa S, Tagarelli A, Martini G, et al.: Genetic heterogeneity at the glucose 6 phopshate dehydrogenase locus revealed by single-strand conformation and sequence analysis. *Am J Hum Genet* **52**:527, 1993.
134. Beutler E, Kuhl W, Vives-Corrons JL, Prchal JT: Molecular heterogeneity of glucose 6-phosphate dehydrogenase A−. *Blood* **74**:2550, 1989.
135. Pinto FM, Gonzalez AM, Hernandez M, Larruga JM, Cabrera VM: Sub-Saharan influence on the Canary Islands population deduced from G6PD gene sequence analysis. *Hum Biol* **68**:517, 1996.
136. Saad ST, Salles TS, Carvalho MH, Costa FF: Molecular characterization of glucose-6-phosphate dehydrogenase deficiency in Brazil. *Hum Hered* **47**:17, 1997.
137. Marques J, Luzzatto L, Vulliamy T, Barretto OCO, Nonoyama K: Mutation of G6PD gene in Brazilian blood samples. *Blood* **82(Suppl 1)**:465a, 1993.
138. Weimer TA, Salzano FM, Westwood B, Beutler E: G6PD variants in three South American ethnic groups: Population distribution and description of two new mutations. *Hum Hered* **48**:92, 1998.
139. Nafa D, Reghis A, Osmani N, Baghli L, Ait-Abbes H, Benabadji M, Kaplan J-C, et al.: At least five polymorphic mutants account for the prevalence of glucose-6-phosphate dehydrogenase deficiency in Algeria. *Hum Genet* **94**:513, 1994.

140. Oppenheim A, Jury CL, Rund D, Vulliamy TJ, Luzzatto L: G6PD Mediterranean accounts for the high prevalence of G6PD deficiency in Kurdish Jews. *Hum Genet* **91**:293, 1993.
141. Daar S, Vulliamy TJ, Kaeda J, Mason PJ, Luzzatto L: Molecular characterization of G6PD deficiency in Oman. *Hum Hered* **46**:172, 1996.
142. Bayoumi RAL, Nur-E-Kamal MSA, Tadayyon M, Mohammad KKA, Mahboob BHS, Qureshi MM, Lakhani MS, et al.: Molecular characterization of erythrocyte glucose-6-phosphate dehydrogenase deficiency among school boys of Al-Ain district, United Arab Emirates. *Hum Hered* **46**:136, 1996.
143. Kotea R, Kaeda JS, Yan SL, Sem Fa N, Beesoon S, Jankee S, Ramasawmy R, et al.: Three major G6PD-deficient polymorphic variants identified among the Mauritian population. *Br J Haematol* **104**:849, 1999.
144. Kirkman HN, Simon ER, Pickard BM: Seattle variant of glucose 6-phosphate dehydrogenase. *J Lab Clin Med* **66**:834, 1965.
145. DeVita G, Alcalay M, Sampietro M, Cappellini MD, Fiorelli G, Toniolo D: Two point mutations are responsible for G6PD polymorphism in Sardinia. *Am J Hum Genet* **44**:233, 1989.
146. Rattazzi MC, Lenzerini L, Meera Khan P, Luzzatto L: Characterization of glucose 6-phosphate dehydrogenase variants. II. G6PD Kephalonia, G6PD Attica and G6PD "Seattle-like" found in Greece. *Am J Hum Genet* **21**:154, 1969.
147. Cabrera VM, Gonzalez P, Salo WL: Human enzyme polymorphism in the Canary Islands. VII. G6PD Seattle in Canarians and North African Berbers. *Hum Hered* **46**:197, 1996.
148. Calabrò V, Giacobbe A, Vallone D, Montanaro V, Cascone A, Filosa S, Battistuzzi G: Genetic heterogeneity at the glucose 6-phosphate dehydrogenase locus in southern Italy: A study on a population from the Matera district. *Hum Genet* **86**:49, 1990.
149. Rovira A, Vulliamy TJ, Pujades A, Luzzatto L, Vives-Corrons J-L: The glucose 6-phosphate dehydrogenase (G6PD)-deficient variant G6PD Union (454 Arg → Cys) has a worldwide distribution possibly due to recurrent mutation. *Hum Mol Genet* **3**:833, 1994.
150. Perng L, Chiou S-S, Liu TC, Chang JG: A novel C to T substitution at nucleotide 1360 of cDNA which abolishes a natural *Hha*I site accounts for a new G6PD deficiency gene in Chinese. *Hum Mol Genet* **1**:205, 1992.
151. Ganczakowski M, Town M, Kaneko A, Bowden DK, Clegg JB, Luzzatto L: Multiple glucose-6-phosphate dehydrogenase deficient variants correlate with malaria endemicity in the Vanuatu archipelago (south-western Pacific). *Am J Hum Genet* **56**:294, 1995.
152. Corcoran CM, Calabro V, Tamagnini G, Town M, Haidar B, Vulliamy TJ, Mason P, et al.: Molecular heterogeneity underlying the G6PD Mediterranean phenotype. *Hum Genet* **88**:688, 1992.
153. di Montemuros FM, Dotti C, Tavazzi D, Fiorelli G, Cappellini MD: Molecular heterogeneity of glucose-6-phosphate dehydrogenase (G6PD) variants in Italy. *Haematologica* **82**:440, 1997.
154. Cittadella R, Civitelli D, Manna I, Azzia N, Di Cataldo A, Schiliro G, Brancati C: Genetic heterogeneity of glucose-6-phosphate dehydrogenase deficiency in south-east Sicily. *Ann Hum Genet* **61**:229, 1997.
155. Samilchuk E, D'Souza B, Al-Awadi S: Population study of common glucose-6-phosphate dehydrogenase mutations in Kuwait. *Hum Hered* **49**:41, 1999.
156. Ahluwalia A, Corcoran CM, Vulliamy TJ, Ishwad CS, Naidu JM, Argusti A, Stevens DJ, et al.: G6PD Kalyan and G6PD Kerala: Two deficient variants in India caused by the same 317Glu → Lys mutation. *Hum Mol Genet* **1**:209, 1992.
157. Kaeda JS. Molecular genetics of G6PD deficiency in India: A major new variant, G6PD Orissa. University of London, Ph.D. thesis. London, 1997, p 291.
158. Vulliamy TJ, Beutler E, Luzzatto L: Variants of glucose 6-phosphate dehydrogenase are due to missense mutations spread throughout the coding region of the gene. *Hum Mutat* **2**:159, 1993.
159. Ainoon O, Joyce J, Boo NY, Cheong SK, Hamidah NH: Nucleotide 1376 G → T mutation in G6PD-deficient Chinese in Malaysia. *Malays J Pathol* **17**:61, 1995.
160. Soemantri AG, Saha S, Saha N, Tay JS: Molecular variants of red cell glucose-6-phosphate dehydrogenase deficiency in Central Java, Indonesia. *Hum Hered* **45**:346, 1995.
161. Saha N, Hong SH, Low PS, Tay JS: Biochemical characteristics of four common molecular variants in glucose-6-phosphate dehydrogenase-deficient Chinese in Singapore. *Hum Hered* **45**:253, 1995.
162. Chiu DTY, Zuo L, Chao L, Chen E, Louie E, Lubin B, Liu TZ, et al.: Molecular characterization of glucose-6-phosphate dehydrogenase (G6PD) deficiency in patients of Chinese descent and identification of new base substitutions in the human G6PD gene. *Blood* **81**:2150, 1993.
163. Chiu DTY, Zuo L, Chen E, Chao LT, Louie E, Lubin B, Liu TZ, et al.: Two commonly occurring nucleotide base substitutions in Chinese G6PD variants. *Biochem Biophys Res Commun* **180**:988, 1991.
164. Tang TK, Huang WY, Tang CJ, Hsu M, Cheng TA, Chen KH: Molecular basis of glucose-6-phosphate dehydrogenase (G6PD) deficiency in three Taiwan aboriginal tribes. *Hum Genet* **95**:630, 1995.
165. Wagner G, Bhatia K, Board P: Glucose-6-phosphate dehydrogenase deficiency mutations in Papua New Guinea. *Hum Biol* 68:383, 1996.
166. Luzzatto L: Inherited haemolytic states: Glucose-6-phosphate dehydrogenase deficiency. *Clin Haematol* **4**:83, 1975.
167. Scopes DA, Bautista JM, Naylor CE, Adams MJ, Mason PJ: Amino acid substitutions at the dimer interface of human glucose-6-phosphate dehydrogenase that increase thermostability and reduce the stabilising effect of NADP. *Eur J Biochem* **251**:382, 1998.
168. Cheng YS, Tang TK, Hwang M: Amino acid conservation and clinical severity of human glucose-6-phosphate dehydrogenase mutations. *J Biomed Sci* **6**:106, 1999.
169. Alfinito F, Cimmino A, Ferraro F, Cubellis MV, Vitagliano L, Francese M, Zagari A, et al.: Molecular characterization of G6PD deficiency in southern Italy: Heterogeneity, correlation genotype-phenotype and description of a new variant (G6PD Neapolis). *Br J Haematol* **98**:41, 1997.
170. Adediran SA: Kinetic and thermodynamic properties of two electrophoretically similar genetic variants of human erythrocyte glucose-6-phosphate dehydrogenase. *Biochemie* **78**:165, 1996.
171. Town M, Bautista JM, Mason PJ, Luzzatto L: Both mutations in G6PD A− are necessary to produce the G6PD deficient phenotype. *Hum Mol Genet* **1**:171, 1992.
172. Gomez-Gallego F, Garrido-Pertierra A, Mason PJ, Bautista JM: Unproductive folding of the human G6PD-deficient variant A−. *FASEB J* **10**:153, 1996.
173. Pløczi K, Mihalik R, Remnyi P, Milosevits J, Petrnyi GG, Demeter J: GPI-linked molecules on lymphoid cells of allogeneic BMT patients. *Immunol Today* **16**:302, 1995.
174. Ganea E, Harding JJ: Molecular chaperones protect against glycation-induced inactivation of glucose-6-phosphate dehydrogenase. *Eur J Biochem* **231**:181, 1995.
175. Ganea E, Harding JJ: Alpha-crystallin protects glucose-6-phosphate dehydrogenase against inactivation by malondialdehyde. *Biochim Biophys Acta* **1500**:49, 2000.
176. D Urso M, Luzzatto L, Perroni L, Ciccodicola A, Gentile G, Peluso I, Persico MG, et al.: An extensive search for restriction fragment length polymorphisms (RFLP) in the human glucose-6-phosphate dehydrogenase locus has revealed a silent mutation in the coding sequence. *Am J Hum Genet* **42**:735, 1988.
177. Vulliamy TJ, Othman A, Town M, Nathwani A, Falusi AG, Mason PJ, Luzzatto L: Polymorphic sites in the African population detected by sequence analysis of the glucose 6-phosphate dehydrogenase gene outline the evolution of the variants A and A−. *Proc Natl Acad Sci U S A* **88**:8568, 1991.
178. Yoshida A, Takizawa T, Prchal JT: RFLP of the X chromosome linked glucose-6-phosphate dehydrogenase locus in Blacks. *Am J Hum Genet* **42**:872, 1988.
179. Maestrini E, Rivella S, Tribioli C, Rocchi M, Camerino G, Santachiara-Benerecetti S, Paolini O, et al.: Identification of novel RFLPs in the vicinity of CpG islands in Xq28: Application to the analysis of the pattern of X chromosome inactivation. *Am J Hum Genet* **50**:156, 1992.
180. Filosa S, Calabrò V, Lania G, Vulliamy TJ, Brancati C, Tagarelli A, Luzzatto L, et al.: G6PD haplotypes spanning Xq28 from F8C to red/green color vision. *Genomics* **17**:6, 1993.
181. Cai W, Filosa S, Martini G: DNA haplotypes in the G6PD gene cluster studied in the Chinese Li population and their relationship to G6PDCanton. *Hum Hered* **44**:279, 1994.
182. Chen HL, Huang MJ, Huang CS, Tang TK: Two novel glucose-6-phosphate dehydrogenase deficiency mutations and association of such mutations with F8C/G6PD haplotype in Chinese. *J Formos Med Assoc* **96**:948, 1997.
183. Heller P, Best WR, Nelsen RB, Becktel J: Clinical implications of sickle cell trait and glucose-6-phosphate dehydrogenase deficiency in hospitalized Black male patients. *N Engl J Med* **300**:1001, 1979.
184. Hoiberg A, Ernst J, Uddin DE: Sickle cell trait and glucose-6-phosphate dehydrogenase deficiency. Effects on health and military performance in Black naval enlistees. *Arch Int Med* **141**:1485, 1981.

185. Gant FL, Winks GFJ: Primaquine sensitive hemolytic anaemia complicating diabetic acidosis. *Clin Res* **9**:27, 1961.
186. Gellady A, Greenwood RD: G6PD hemolytic anaemia complicating diabetic ketoacidosis. *J Pediatr* **80**:1037, 1972.
187. Shalev O, Eliakim R, Lugassy GZ, Menczel J: Hypoglycemia-induced hemolysis in glucose-6-phosphate dehydrogenase deficiency. *Acta Haematol* **74**:227, 1985.
188. Lee DH, Warkentin TE, Neame PB, Ali MA: Acute hemolytic anemia precipitated by myocardial infarction and pericardial tamponade in G6PD deficiency [Letter]. *Am J Hematol* **51**:174, 1996.
189. Kimmick G, Owen J: Rhabdomyolysis and hemolysis associated with sickle cell trait and glucose-6-phosphate dehydrogenase deficiency. *South Med J* **89**:1097, 1996.
190. Ninfali P, Bresolin N: Muscle glucose 6-phosphate dehydrogenase (G6PD) deficiency and oxidant stress during physical exercise [Letter]. *Cell Biochem Funct* **13**:297, 1995.
191. Shalev O, Wollner A, Menczel J: Diabetic ketoacidosis does not precipitate haemolysis in patients with the Mediterranean variant of glucose-6-phosphate dehydrogenase deficiency. *BMJ* **288**:179, 1984.
192. Perkins RP: The significance of glucose-6-phosphate dehydrogenase deficiency in pregnancy. *Am J Obstet Gynecol* **125**:215, 1976.
193. Dern RJ, Beutler E, Alving AS: The hemolytic effect of primaquine II. The natural course of the hemolytic anemia and the mechanism of its self-limiting character. *J Lab Clin Med* **44**:171, 1954.
194. Beutler E, Dern RJ, Alving AS: The hemolytic effect of primaquine. IV. The relationship of cell age to hemolysis. *J Lab Clin Med* **44**:439, 1954.
195. Tarlov AR, Brewer GJ, Carson PE, Alving AS: Primaquine sensitivity. Glucose-6-phosphate dehydrogenase deficiency: An inborn error of metabolism of medical and biological significance. *Arch Int Med* **109**:209, 1962.
196. Arese P, Mannuzzo L, Turrini F, Faliano S, Gaetani GE: Etiological aspects of favism, in Yoshida A, Beutler E (eds): *Glucose-6-Phosphate Dehydrogenase*. New York, Academic, 1986, p 45.
197. Pannacciulli IM, Tizianello A, Ajmar F, Salvidio E: The causes of experimentally induced haemolytic anaemia in a primaquine sensitive Caucasian. *Blood* **25**:92, 1965.
198. Beutler E: Glucose 6-phosphate dehydrogenase deficiency, in Beutler E (ed): *Hemolytic Anemia in Disorders of Red Cell Metabolism*. New York, Plenum, 1978, p 23.
199. Beutler E: Sensitivity to drug-induced hemolytic anemia in glucose-6-phosphate dehydrogenase deficiency, in Omenn GS, Gelboin HV (eds) *Barnbury Report 16: Genetic Variability in Responses to Chemical Exposure*. New York, Cold Spring Harbor Laboratory, 1984, p 205.
200. McCaffrey RP, Halsted CH, Wahab MFA, Robertson RP: Chloramphenicol-induced hemolysis in Caucasian glucose-6-phosphate dehydrogenase deficiency. *Ann Intern Med* **74**:722, 1971.
201. Chan TK, Chesterman CN, McFadzean AJS, Todd D: The survival of glucose-6-phosphate dehydrogenase-deficient erythrocytes in patients with typhoid fever on chloramphenicol therapy. *J Lab Clin Med* **77**:177, 1971.
202. Doxiadis SA, Valaes F: The clinical picture of glucose-6-phosphate dehydrogenase deficiency in early childhood. *Arch Dis Child* **39**:545, 1964.
203. Zinkham WH: Peripheral blood and bilirubin values in normal full term primaquine-sensitive Negro infants effects of vitamin K. *Pediatrics* **31**:983, 1963.
204. George JN, Sears DA, McCurdy PR, Conrad ME: Primaquine sensitivity in Caucasians: Hemolytic reactions induced by primaquine in G6PD deficient subjects. *J Lab Clin Med* **70**:80, 1967.
205. Herman J, Ben-Meir S: Overt hemolysis in patients with glucose-6-phosphate dehydrogenase deficiency. A survey in general practice. *Isr J Med Sci* **11**:340, 1975.
206. Janakiraman N, Seeler RA, Royal JE, Chen ME: Hemolysis during BAL chelation therapy for high blood lead levels in two G6PD deficient children. *Clin Pediatr* **17**:485, 1978.
207. Mandal BK, Stevenson J: Haemolytic crisis produced by nalidixic acid. *Lancet* **i**:614, 1970.
208. Sansone G, Reali S, Sansone R, Allegranza F: Acute hemolytic anemia induced by a pyrazolonic drug in a child with glucose-6-phosphate dehydrogenase deficiency. *Acta Haematol* **72**:285, 1984.
209. Chan TK, Todd D, Tso SC: Red cell survival studies in glucose-6-phosphate dehydrogenase deficiency. *Bull Hong Kong Med Assoc* **26**:41, 1974.
210. Gaetani GF, Mareni C, Ravazzolo R, Salvidio E: Haemolytic effect of two sulphonamides evaluated by a new method. *Br J Haematol* **32**:183, 1976.
211. Magon AM, Leipzig RM, Zannoni VG, Brewer GJ: Interactions of glucose-6-phosphate dehydrogenase deficiency with drug acetylation and hydroxylation reactions. *J Lab Clin Med* **97**:764, 1981.
212. Luzzatto L: Glucose-6-phosphate dehydrogenase and other genetic factors interacting with drugs, in Kalow W, Goedde HW, Agarwal DP (eds). *Ethnic Differences in Reactions to Drugs and Xenobiotics*. New York: Liss, 1986, p 385.
213. Grossman S, Budinsky R, Jollow D: Dapsone-induced hemolytic anemia: role of glucose-6-phosphate dehydrogenase in the hemolytic response of rat erythrocytes to *N*-hydroxydapsone. *J Pharmacol Exp Ther* **273**:870, 1995.
214. Corda R, Carnelli V: Use of the NSAID ketoprofen lysine salt in glucose-6-phosphate dehydrogenase (G6PD) deficiency in inflammatory disease in children. *Pediatr Med Chir* **18**:391, 1996.
215. Beaupre SR, Schiffman FJ: Rush hemolysis. A "bite-cell" hemolytic anemia associated with volatile liquid nitrite use. *Arch Fam Med* **3**:545, 1994.
216. Burka ER, Weaver Z, Marks PA: Clinical spectrum of hemolytic anemia associated with glucose-6-phosphate dehydrogenase deficiency. *Ann Intern Med* **64**:817, 1966.
217. Shannon K, Buchanan GR: Severe hemolytic anemia in black children with glucose-6-phosphate dehydrogenase deficiency. *Pediatrics* **70**:364, 1982.
218. Agarwal RK, Moudgil A, Kishore K, Srivastava RN, Tandon RK: Acute viral hepatitis, intravascular haemolysis, severe hyperbilirubinaemia and renal failure in glucose-6-phosphate dehydrogenase deficient patients. *Postgrad Med J* **61**:971, 1985.
219. Huo TI, Wu JC, Chiu CF, Lee SD: Severe hyperbilirubinemia due to acute hepatitis A superimposed on a chronic hepatitis B carrier with glucose-6-phosphate dehydrogenase deficiency [Review]. *Am J Gastroenterol* **91**:158, 1996.
220. Siddiqui T, Khan AH: Hepatitis A and cytomegalovirus infection precipitating acute hemolysis in glucose-6-phosphate dehydrogenase deficiency [Citation]. *Mil Med* **163**:434, 1998.
221. Mengel CE, Metz E, Yancey WS: Anemia during acute infections. Role of glucose-6-phosphate dehydrogenase deficiency in Negroes. *Arch Intern Med* **119**:287, 1967.
222. Owusu SK, Addy J, Foli AK, Janosi M, Konotey-Ahulu FID, Larbi EB: Acute reversible renal failure associated with glucose-6-phosphate dehydrogenase deficiency. *Lancet* **i**:1255, 1972.
223. Kattamis CA, Tjortjatou F: The hemolytic process of viral hepatitis in children with normal or deficient glucose 6-phosphate dehydrogenase activity. *J Pediatr* **77**:422, 1970.
224. Choremis C, Kattamis CA, Kyriazakou M, Gavrillidou E: Viral hepatitis in G6PD deficiency. *Lancet* i:269, 1966.
225. Morrow RH, Smetana HE, Sai FT, Edgcomb JH: Unusual features of viral hepatitis in Accra, Ghana. *Ann Intern Med* **68**:1250, 1968.
226. Oluboyede L, Francis TI, Esan GJF, Luzzatto L: Genetically determined deficiency of glucose 6-phosphate dehydrogenase (type A−) is expressed in the liver. *J Lab Clin Med* **93**:783, 1979.
227. Crowell SB, Crowell EB, Mathew M: Depression of erythrocyte glucose-6-phosphate dedhydrogenase (G6PD) activity in enteric fever. *Trans R Soc Trop Med Hyg* **78**:183, 1984.
228. Phillips SM, Silvers NP: Glucose-6-phosphate dehydrogenase deficiency, infectious hepatitis, acute hemolysis and renal failure. *Ann Intern Med* **70**:99, 1969.
229. Selroos O: Reversible renal failure and G6PD deficiency. *Lancet* **ii**:284, 1972.
230. Angle CR: Glucose-6-phosphate dehydrogenase deficiency and acute renal failure. *Lancet* **ii**:134, 1972.
231. Luzzatto L, Meloni T: Hemolytic anemia due to glucose 6-phosphate dehydrogenase deficiency, in Brain MC, Carbone PP (eds): *Current Therapy in Hematology-Oncology: 1985–1986*. Toronto, BC Decker, CV Mosby, 1985, p 21.
232. Walker DH, Hawkins HK, Hudson P: Fulminant Rocky Mountain Spotted fever. Its pathologic characteristics associated with glucose-6-phosphate dehydrogenase deficiency. *Arch Pathol Lab Med* **107**:121, 1984.
233. Salen G, Goldstein F, Haurani F, Wirts CW: Acute hemolytic anemia complicating viral hepatitis in patients with glucose-6-phosphate dehydrogenase deficiency. *Ann Intern Med* **65**:1210, 1966.
234. Chan TK, Todd D: Haemolysis complicating viral hepatitis with glucose-6-phosphate dehydrogenase deficiency. *Br J Haematol* **1**:131, 1975.
235. Al-Rasheed SA, Al-Mugeiren MM, Al-Salloum AA, Al-Fawaz IM, Al-Sohaibani MO: Acute viral hepatitis, glucose-6-phosphate

dehydrogenase deficiency and prolonged acute renal failure: A case report. *Ann Trop Paediatr* **15**:255, 1995.
236. Wilkinson SP, Davis MH, Portman B, Williams R: Renal failure in otherwise uncomplicated viral hepatitis. *Br J Haematol* **2**:338, 1978.
237. Gulati PD, Rizvi SNA: Acute reversible renal failure in G6PD deficient siblings. *Postgrad Med J* **52**:83, 1976.
238. Necheles TF, Gorshein D: Virus-induced hemolysis in erythrocytes deficient in glucose-6-phosphate dehydrogenase. *Science* **160**:535, 1968.
239. Baehner RL, Nathan DG, Castle WB: Oxidant injury of Caucasian glucose-6-phosphate dehydrogenase-deficient red blood cells by phagocytosing leukocytes during infection. *J Clin Invest* **50**:2466, 1971.
240. Nelson RA: The immune adherence phenomenon — An immunologically specific reaction between microorganisms and erythrocytes leading to phagocytosis. *Science* **118**:733, 1953.
241. Kaser ML, Miller WJ, Jacob HS: G6PD deficiency infectious hemolysis: A complement dependent innocent bystander phenomenon. *Br J Haematol* **63**:85, 1986.
242. Claster S, Tsun-Yee Chiu D, Quintanilha A, Lubin B: Neutrophils mediate lipid peroxidation in human red cells. *Blood* **64**:1079, 1984.
243. Kattamis CA, Kyriazakou M, Chaidas S: Favism: clinical and biochemical data. *J Med Genet* **6**:34, 1969.
244. Kahn A, Marie J, Desbois JC, Boivin P: Favism in a Portuguese family due to a deficient glucose-6-phosphate dehydrogenase variant of Canton or Canton like type 1. *Acta Haematol* **56**:58, 1976.
245. Belsey MA: The epidemiology of favism. *Bull WHO* **48**:1, 1973.
246. Dacie JV: Hereditary enzyme deficiency haemolytic anaemias. III: Deficiency of glucose-6-phosphate dehydrogenase, in Dacie JV (ed): *Haemolytic Anaemias. The Hereditary Haemolytic Anaemias*. London, Churchill Livingstone, 1985, 364.
247. Discombe G, Meslitz W: Favism in an English-born child. *Br Med J* **i**:1023, 1956.
248. Holt JM, Sladden RA: Favism in England. Two more cases. *Arch Dis Child* **40**:271, 1965.
249. Davies P: Favism: A family study. *Q J Med* **122**:157, 1962.
250. Stockley R, Dawson A, Slade R: Favism in two British women. *Lancet* **ii**:1013, 1985.
251. Crosby WH: Favism in Sardinia [Newsletter]. *Blood* **11**:91, 1956.
252. Szeinberg A, Sheba C, Hirschorn N, Bodonyi E: Studies on erythrocytes in cases with past history of favism and drug induced acute hemolytic anemia. *Blood* **12**:603, 1957.
253. Gross AT, Hurwitz RA, Marks PA: A hereditary enzymatic defect in erythrocyte metabolism. Glucose-6-phosphate dehydrogenase deficiency. *J Clin Invest* **37**:1176, 1958.
254. Siniscalco M, Bernini L, Latte B, Motulsky AG: Favism and thalassaemia in Sardinia and their relationship to malaria. *Nature* **190**:1179, 1961.
255. Kattamis CA, Chaidas A, Chaidas S: G6PD deficiency and favism in the island of Rhodes. *J Med Genet* **6**:286, 1969.
256. Vullo C, Panizon F: The mechanism of hemolysis in favism. Transfusion experiments with ^{51}Cr tagged erythrocytes. *Acta Haematol* **26**:337, 1961.
257. Panizon F, Vullo C: The mechanism of hemolysis in favism. Researches on the role of non corpuscular factors. *Acta Haematol* **26**:337, 1961.
258. Sartori E: On the pathogenesis of favism. *J Med Genet* **8**:462, 1971.
259. Arese P, Mannuzzu L, Turrini F: Pathophysiology of favism. *Folia Haematol* **116**:745, 1989.
260. Symvoulidis A, Voudiclaris S, Mountokalakis TH, Pougounias H: Acute renal failure in G6PD deficiency. *Lancet* **ii**:819, 1972.
261. Baule GM, Onorato D, Tola G, Forteleoni G, Meloni T: Hemoglobin A1 in subjects with G6PD deficiency during and after hemolytic crisis due to favism. *Acta Haematol* **69**:15, 1983.
262. Meloni T, Forteleoni G, Dore A, Cutillo S: Favism and hemolytic anemia in glucose-6-phosphate dehydrogenase deficiency subjects in North Sardinia. *Acta Haematol* **70**:83, 1983.
263. Ruggo G, Mollica G, Pavone L, Schiliro G: Hemolytic crisis of favism in Sicilian females heterozygous for G6PD deficiency. *Pediatrics* **49**:854, 1972.
264. Schiliro G, Russo A, Curreri R, Marino S, Sciotto A, Russo G: Glucose-6-phosphate dehydrogenase deficiency in Sicily. Incidence biochemical characteristics and clinical implications. *Clin Genet* **15**:183, 1979.
265. Kattamis C: Favism in breast-fed infants. *Arch Dis Child* **46**:741, 1971.
266. Arese P, De Flora A: Pathophysiology of hemolysis in glucose 6-phosphate dehydrogenase deficiency. *Semin Hematol* **27**:1, 1990.
267. Chevion M, Navok T, Glaser G, Mager J: The chemistry of favism-inducing compounds. The properties of isouramil and divicine and their reaction with glutathione. *Eur J Biochem* **127**:405, 1982.
268. Arese P: Favism: a natural model for the study of haemolytic mechanisms. *Rev Pure Appl Pharmacol Sci.* **3**:1234, 1982.
269. Lin JY, Ling KH: Studies on favism. 1. Isolation of an active principle from fava beans (Vicia faba). *J Formosan Med Assoc* **61**:484, 1962.
270. Mager J, Glaser G, Razin A, Izak G, Bien S, Noam M: Metabolic effects of pyrimidines derived from fava bean glycosides on human erythrocytes deficient in glucose-6-phosphate dehydrogenase. *Biochem Biophys Res Commun* **20**:235, 1965.
271. Mareni C, Repetto, Foreteleoni G, Meloni T, Gaetani GF: Favism: Looking for a autosomal gene associated with glucose-6-phosphate dehydrogenase deficiency. *J Med Genet* **21**:278, 1984.
272. Stamatoyannopoulos G, Fraser GR, Motulsky AG, Fessas PH, Akrivakis A, Papayannopoulou T: On the familial predisposition to favism. *Am J Hum Genet* **18**:253, 1966.
273. Battistuzzi G, Morellini M, Meloni T, Gandini E, Luzzatto L: Genetic factors in favism, in Weatherall DJ (ed): *Advances in Red Blood Cell Biology*. New York: Raven Press, 1982, p 339.
274. Bottini E, Lucarelli P, Agostino R, Palmarino R, Businco L, Antognoni G: Favism: Association with erythrocyte acid phosphatase phenotype. *Science* **171**:409, 1971.
275. Cassimos CHR, Malaka-Zafiriu K, Tsiures J: Urinary D-glucaric acid excretion in normal and G6PD deficient children with favism. *J Pediatr* **84**:871, 1974.
276. Cutillo S, Costa S, Vintuledou MC, Meloni T: Salicylamide glucuronide formation in children with favism and their parents. *Acta Haematol* **55**:296, 1976.
277. Schiliro G, Sciotto A, Russo A, Bottard G, Minniti C, Musumeci S, Russo G: Lymphocyte changes in favism: in vitro evidence of a modifying effect of bilirubin and hemoglobin on T-lymphocyte receptors. *Acta Haematol* **69**:230, 1983.
278. Schiliro G, Minniti C, Sciotto A, Bellino A, Russo A: T lymphocyte subpopulation changes during haemolysis in glucose-6-phosphate dehydrogenase (G6PD) deficient children. *Am J Hematol* **21**:73, 1986.
279. Kaplan J, Sarnaik S, Gitlin J, Lusher J: Diminished helper/suppressor rations and natural killer activity in recipients of repeated blood transfusions. *Blood* **64**:308, 1984.
280. De Flora A, Benatti U, Guida L, Forteleoni G, Meloni T: Favism: Disordered erythrocyte calcium hemostatis. *Blood* **66**:294, 1985.
281. Lorani L, Weissman LB, Epel DL, Bruner-Lorand J: Role of intrinsic transglutaminase in the Ca^{++} mediated cross-linking of erythrocyte proteins. *Proc Natl Acad Sci U S A* **73**:4479, 1976.
282. Gaetani GF, Rolfo M, Arena S, Mangerini R, Meloni GF, Ferraris AM: Active involvement of catalase during hemolytic crises of favism. *Blood* **88**:1084, 1996.
283. Fischer TM, Pescarmona GP, Bosia A, Maitana A, Turrini F, Arese P: Membrane cross-banding in red cells in favic crisis — a missing link in the mechanism of extravascular haemolysis. *Br J Haematol* **66**:294, 1985.
284. Meloni T, Forteleoni G, Meloni GF: Marked decline of favism after neonatal glucose-6-phosphate dehydrogenase screening and health education: The northern Sardinian experience. *Acta Haematol* **87**:29, 1992.
285. Ekert U, Rawlinson I: Deferoxamine and favism. *N Engl J Med* **312**:1260, 1985.
286. Meloni T, Forteleoni G, Gaetani GF: Desferrioxamine and favism. *Br J Haematol* **63**:394, 1986.
287. Khalifa AS, El-Alfy MS, Mokhtar G: Effect of desferroxiamine B on hemolysis in glucose 6-phosphate dehydrogenase deficiency. *Acta Haematol (Basel)* **82**:113, 1989.
288. Galiano S, Gaetani GF, Barabino A, Cottafava F, Zeitlin H, Town M, Luzzatto L: Favism in the African type of glucose-6-phosphate dehydrogenase deficiency (A−). *BMJ* **300**:236, 1990.
289. Hirono A, Fujii H, Shima M, Miwa S: G6PD Nara: a new class I glucose 6-phosphate dehydrogenase variant with an eight amino acid deletion. *Blood* **82**:3250, 1993.
290. Matthay KK, Mentzer WC: Erythrocyte enzymopathies in the newborn. *Clin Haematol* **10**:31, 1981.
291. Smith GD, Vella F: Erythrocyte enzyme deficiency in unexplained kernicterus. *Lancet* **1**:1133, 1960.
292. Panizon F: Erythrocyte enzyme deficiency in unexplained kernicterus. *Lancet* **ii**:1093, 1960.
293. Bienzle U: Glucose-6-phosphate dehydrogenase deficiency. Part 1: Tropical Africa. *Clin Haematol* **10**:785, 1981.

294. Karayalcin G, Acs H, Lanzkowsky P: G6PD deficiency and hyperbilirubinaemia in black American full-term infants. *N Y State J Med* **79**:22, 1979.
295. Ling IT, Wilson RJM: G6PD activity of the malarial parasite Plasmodium falciparum. *Mol Biochem Parasitol* **31**:47, 1988.
296. Tarnow-Mordi WO, Pickering D: Missed jaundice in black infants a hazard? *BMJ* **286**:463, 1983.
297. Lopez R, Cooperman JM: Glucose-6-phosphate dehydrogenase deficiency and hyperbilirubinaemia in the newborn. *Am J Dis Child* **122**:66, 1971.
298. Brown WR, Boon WH: Hyperbilirubineamia and kernicterus in glucose-6-phosphate dehydrogenase deficient infants in Singapore. *Pediatrics* **41**:1055, 1968.
299. Meloni T, Costa S, Cutillo S: Haptoglobin, hemopexin, hemoglobin and hematocrit in newborns with erythrocyte glucose-6-phosphate dehydrogenase deficiency. *Acta Haematol* **54**:284, 1975.
300. Malaka-Zafiriu K, Tsiures I, Danielides B, Cassimos C: Salicylamide glucuronide formation in newborns with severe jaundice of unknown aetiology and due to glucose-6-phosphate dehydrogenase deficiency in Greece. *Helv Paediatr Acta* **28**:323, 1973.
301. Levin SE, Charlton RW, Freiman I: Glucose-6-phosphate dehydrogenase deficiency and neonatal jaundice in South African Bantu infants. *J Pediatr* **65**:757, 1964.
302. Hamil BM, Munks B, Moyer EZ, Kaucher M, Williams HH: Vitamin C in the blood and urine of the newborn and in the cord and maternal blood. *Am J Dis Child* **74**:417, 1947.
303. Gross S: Hemolytic anemia in premature infants: Relationship to vitamin E, selenium, glutathione peroxidase and erythrocyte lipids. *Semin Hematol* **3**:187, 1976.
304. Bienzle U, Effiong CE, Aimaku VE, Luzzatto L: Erythrocyte enzymes in neonatal jaundice. *Acta Haemat* **55**:10, 1976.
305. Jones PEH, McCance RA: Enzyme activities in the blood of infants and adults. *Biochem J* **45**:464, 1949.
306. Seidman DS, Shiloh M, Stevenson DK, Vreman HJ, Gale R: Role of hemolysis in neonatal jaundice associated with glucose-6 phosphate dehydrogenase deficiency [Comments]. *J Pediatr* **127**:804, 1995.
307. Slusher TM, Vreman HJ, McLaren DW, Lewison LJ, Brown AK, Stevenson DK: Glucose-6-phosphate dehydrogenase deficiency and carboxyhemoglobin concentrations associated with bilirubin-related morbidity and death in Nigerian infants. *J Pediatr* **126**:102, 1995.
308. Kaplan M, Rubaltelli FF, Hammerman C, Vilei MT, Leiter C, Abramov A, Muraca M: Conjugated bilirubin in neonates with glucose-6-phosphate dehydrogenase deficiency [Comments]. *J Pediatr* **128**:695, 1996.
309. Ifekwunigwe AE, Luzzatto L: Kernicterus in G6PD deficiency. *Lancet* **i**:667, 1966.
310. Lai HC, Lai MPY, Leung KS: Glucose-6-phosphate dehydrogenase deficiency in Chinese. *J Clin Pathol* **21**:44, 1968.
311. Lu T-C, Wei H, Blackwell RQ: Increased incidence of severe hyperbilirubineamia among newborn Chinese infants with G6PD deficiency. *Pediatrics* **37**:994, 1966.
312. Ho CY, Otterud B, Legare RD, Varvil T, Saxena R, DeHart DB, Kohler SE, et al.: Linkage of a familial platelet disorder with a propensity to develop myeloid malignancies to human chromosome 21q22.1-22.2. *Blood* **87**:5218, 1996.
313. Szeinberg A, Oliver M, Schmidt R, Adam A, Sheba C: Glucose-6-phosphate dehydrogenase deficiency and hemolytic disease of the newborn in Israel. *Arch Dis Child* **38**:23, 1963.
314. Milbauer B, Peled N, Svirsky S: Neonatal hyperbilirubineamia and glucose-6-phosphate dehydrogenase deficiency. *Isr J Med Sci* **9**:547, 1973.
315. Niazi GA, Adeyokunnu A, Westwood B, Beutler E: Neonatal jaundice in Saudi newborns with G6PD Aures. *Ann Trop Paediatr* **16**:33, 1996.
316. Beutler E, Grooms AM, Morgan SK, Trinidad F: Chronic severe hemolytic anemia due to G-6-PD Charleston: A new deficient variant. *J Pediatr* **80**:1005, 1972.
317. Feldman R, Gromisch DS, Luhby AL, Beutler E: Congenital nonspherocytic hemolytic anemia due to glucose-6-phosphate dehydrogenase East Harlem: A new deficient variant. *J Pediatr* **90**:89, 1977.
318. Kaplan M, Vreman HJ, Hammerman C, Leiter C, Rudensky B, MacDonald MG, Stevenson DK: Combination of ABO blood group incompatibility and glucose-6-phosphate dehydrogenase deficiency: effect on hemolysis and neonatal hyperbilirubinemia. *Acta Paediatr* **87**:455, 1998.
319. Kaplan M, Renbaum P, Levy-Lahad E, Hammerman C, Lahad A, Beutler E: Gilbert syndrome and glucose-6-phosphate dehydrogenase deficiency: A dose-dependent genetic interaction crucial to neonatal hyperbilirubinemia. *Proc Natl Acad Sci U S A* **94**:12128, 1997.
320. Drew JH, Smith MB, Kitchen WH: Glucose-6-phosphate dehydrogenase deficiency in immigrant greek infants. *J Pediatr* **90**:659, 1977.
321. Brown AK, Cevik N: Hemolysis and jaundice in the newborn following maternal treatment with sulfamethoxypyridazine (Kynex). *Pediatrics* **36**:742, 1965.
322. Perkins RP: Hydrops fetalis and stillbirth in a male glucose-6-phosphate dehydrogenase deficient fetus possibly due to maternal ingestion of sulfisoxazole. *Am J Obstet Gynecol* **11**:379, 1971.
323. Valaes T, Dokiadis S, Fessas PH: Acute hemolysis due to naphthalene inhalation. *J Pediatr* **63**:904, 1963.
324. Sodeinde O, Chan MCK, Maxwell SM, Familusi JB, Hendrickse RG: Neonatal jaundice, aflatoxins and naphthols: Report of a study in Ibadan, Nigeria. *Ann Trop Paediatr* **15**:107, 1995.
325. Eshaghpour E, Oski FA, Williams M: The relationship of erythrocyte glucose-6-phosphate dehydrogenase deficiency to hyperbilirubineamia in Negro premature infants. *J Pediatr* **70**:595, 1967.
326. Owa JA: Relationship between exposure to icterogenic agents, glucose-6-phosphate dehydrogenase deficiency and neonatal jaundice in Nigeria. *Acta Paediatr Scand* **78**:848, 1989.
327. Kandil HH, Al-Ghanem MM, Sarwat MA, Al-Thallab FS: Henna (Lawsonia inermis Linn.) inducing haemolysis among G6PD-deficient newborns. A new clinical observation. *Ann Trop Paediatr* **16**:287, 1996.
328. Corchia C, Balata A, Meloni GF, Meloni T: Favism in a female newborn infant whose mother ingested fava beans before delivery [Comments]. *J Pediatr* **127**:807, 1995.
329. Meloni T, Cagnazzo G, Dore A, Cutillo S: Phenobarbital for prevention of hyperbilirubinemia in glucose 6-phosphate dehydrogenase-deficient newborn infants. *J Pediatr* **82**:1048, 1973.
330. Luzzatto L, Meloni T: Hemolytic anemia due to glucose 6-phosphate dehydrogenase deficiency, in Brain MC, Carbone PP (eds): *Current Therapy in Hematololgy-Oncology, 1985–1986*. Philadelphia, Marcel Dekker, 1985. p. 21.
331. Mallouh AA, Imseeh G, AbuOsba YK, Hamdan JA: Screening for glucose-6-phosphate dehydrogenase deficiency can prevent severe neonatal jaundice. *Ann Trop Paediatr* **12**:391, 1992.
332. Newman TB, Maisels MJ: Evaluation and treatment of jaundice in the term infant: A kinder, gentler approach. *Pediatrics* **89**:809, 1992.
333. Koperman EY, Ey JL, Lee H: Phototherapy in newborn infants with glucose-6-phosphate dehydrogenase deficiency. *J Pediatr* **93**:497, 1978.
334. Lopez R, Gromisch DS, Cole HS, Cooperman JM: Phototherapy in G6PD deficient infants. *J Pediatr* **102**:326, 1983.
335. Meloni T, Costa S, Dore A, Cutillo S: Phototherapy for neonatal hyperbilirubinemia in mature newborn infants with G6PD deficiency. *J Pediatr* **85**:560, 1974.
336. Meloni T, Corti R, Naitana AF, Arese P: Lack of effect of phototherapy on glucose 6-phosphate dehydrogenase activity in normal and G6PD deficient subjects with neonatal jaundice. *J Pediatr* **100**:972, 1982.
337. Rubaltelli FF: Current drug treatment options in neonatal hyperbilirubinaemia and the prevention of kernicterus. *Drugs* **56**:23, 1998.
338. Valaes T, Drummond GS, Kappas A: Control of hyperbilirubinemia in glucose-6-phosphate dehydrogenase-deficient newborns using an inhibitor of bilirubin production, Sn- mesoporphyrin. *Pediatrics* **101**:E1, 1998.
339. Miwa S, Fujii H: Glucose 6-phosphate dehydrogenase variants in Japan, in Yoshida A, Beutler E (eds): *Glucose 6-phosphate dehydrogenase*. New York, Academic Press, 1986, 261.
340. Fairbanks VF, Nepo AG, Beutler E, Dickson ER, Honig G: Glucose-6-phosphate dehydrogenase variants: Reexamination of G6PD Chicago and Cornell and a new variant (G6PD Pea Ridge) resembling G6PD Chicago. *Blood* **55**:216, 1980.
341. Kirkman HN, Rosenthal IM, Simon ER, Carson PE, Brinson AG: "Chicago I" variant of glucose-6-phosphate dehydrogenase in congenital hemolytic disease. *J Lab Clin Med* **63**:715, 1964.
342. McCurdy PR, Kamel K, Selim O: Heterogeneity of red cell glucose 6-phosphate dehydrogenase (G6PD) deficiency in Egypt. *J Lab Clin Med* **84**:673, 1974.
343. McCurdy PR, Maldonado N, Dillon DE, Conrad ME: Variants of glucose-6-phosphate dehydrogenase (G-6-PD) associated with G-6-PD deficiency in Puerto Ricans. *J Lab Clin Med* **82**:432, 1973.
344. Karadsheh NS, Awibi AS, Tarawneh MS: Two new glucose-6-phosphate dehydrogenase (G6PD) variants associated with hemolytic anemia. *Am J Hematol* **22**:185, 1986.

345. Beutler E, Mathai CK, Smith JE: Biochemical variants of glucose-6-phosphate dehydrogenase giving rise to congenital nonspherocytic hemolytic disease. *Blood* **31**:131, 1968.
346. Ben-Ishay D, Izak G: Chronic hemolysis associated with glucose-6-phosphate dehydrogenase deficiency. *J Lab Clin Med* **63**:1002, 1964.
347. Vives-Corrons JL, Feliu E, Pujades MA, Cardellache, Rozman C, Carreras A, Jou JM, et al.: Severe glucose-6-phosphate dehydrogenase (G6PD) deficiency associated with chronic hemolytic anaemia, granulocyte dysfunction and increased susceptibility to infections. Description of a new molecular variant (G6PD Barcelona). *Blood* **59**:428, 1982.
348. Ventura A, Panizon F, Soranzo MR, Veneziano G, Sansone G, Testa U, Luzzatto L: Congenital dyserythropoietic anaemia Type II associated with a new type of G6PD deficiency (G6PD Gabrovizza). *Acta Haematol (Basel)* **71**:227, 1984.
349. Alfinito F, Calabrò V, Cappellini MD, Fiorelli G, Filosa S, Iolascon A, Miraglia del Giudice E, et al.: Glucose 6-phosphate dehydrogenase deficiency and red cell membrane defects: Additive or synergistic interaction in producing chronic haemolytic anaemia. *Br J Haematol* **87**:148, 1994.
350. Mahendra P, Dollery CT, Luzzatto L, Bloom SR: Pyruvate kinase deficiency: Association with G6PD deficiency. *BMJ* **305**:760, 1992.
351. Zanella A, Colombo M, Mintero R, Perroni L, Meloni T, Sirchia G: Erythrocyte pyruvate kinase deficiency — 11 new cases. *Br J Haematol* **69**:399, 1988.
352. Beutler E, Kuhl W, Gilbart T: 6-phosphogluconolactonase deficiency, a hereditary erythrocyte enzyme deficiency: Possible interaction with glucose 6-phosphate dehydrogenase deficiency. *Proc Natl Acad Sci U S A* **82**:3876, 1985.
353. Newton WAJ, Frajola WJ: Drug-sensitive chronic hemolytic anemia: Family studies. *Clin Res* **6**:392, 1958.
354. Miller DR, Wollman MR: A new variant of glucose-6-phosphate dehydrogenase deficiency hereditary hemolytic anemia, G6PD Cornell: Erythrocyte, leukocyte, and platelet studies. *Blood* **44**:323, 1974.
355. Rattazzi MC, Corash LM, Van Zanen GE, Jaffe ER, Piomelli S: G6PD deficiency and chronic hemolysis: Four new mutants — Relationships between clinical syndrome and enzyme kinetics. *Blood* **38**:205, 1971.
356. Balinsky D, Gomperts E, Cayanis E, Jenkins T, Bryer D, Bersohn I, Metz J: Glucose-6-phosphate dehydrogenase Johannesburg: A new variant with reduced activity in a patient with congenital nonspherocytic haemolytic anaemia. *Br J Haematol* **25**:385, 1973.
357. Sonnet J, Lievens M, Verpoorten C, Kriekemans J, Eeckels R: Sporadic G6PD deficiency with haemolytic anemia in two children of West European ancestry. *Br J Haematol* **28**:299, 1974.
358. Mohler DN, Crockett CLJ: Hereditary hemolytic disease secondary to glucose-6-phosphate dehydrogenase deficiency. Report of 3 cases with special emphasis on ATP metabolism. *Blood* **23**:427, 1964.
359. Kirkman HN, Riley HD: Congenital non-spherocytic hemolytic anemia. Studies on a family with a qualitative defect in glucose-6-phosphate dehydrogenase. *Am J Dis Child* **102**:313, 1961.
360. Engstrom PF, Beutler E: G-6-PD Tripler: A unique variant associated with chronic hemolytic disease. *Blood* **36**:10, 1970.
361. Huskisson EC, Murphy B, West G: Glucose-6-phosphate dehydrogenase deficiency and chronic hemolysis in an English family. *J Clin Pathol* **23**:135, 1970.
362. Vuopio P, Harkonen M, Helske T, Naveri H: Red cell glucose-6-phosphate dehydrogense deficiency in Finland. Characterisation of a new variant with severe enzyme deficiency. *Scand J Haemat* **15**:145, 1975.
363. Johnson GJ, Kaplan ME, Beutler E: G6PD Long Prairie: A new mutant exhibiting normal sensitivity to inhibition by NADPH and accompanied by non-spherocytic hemolytic anaemia. *Blood* **49**:247, 1977.
364. Ramot B, Ben-Bassat I, Shchory M: New glucose-6-phosphate dehydrogenase variants observed in Israel and their association with congenital nonspherocytic hemolytic disease. *J Lab Clin Med* **74**:895, 1969.
365. Greenberg LH, Tanaka KR: Hereditary hemolytic anemia due to glucose-6-phosphate dehydrogenase deficiency. *Am J Dis Child* **110**:206, 1965.
366. De Mars R: A temperature sensitive glucose-6-phosphate dehydrogenase in mutant cultured human cells. *Proc Natl Acad Sci U S A* **61**:562, 1968.
367. Ben-Bassat J, Ben-Ishay D: Hereditary hemolytic anemia associated with glucose-6-phosphate dehydrogenase deficiency Mediterranean type. *Isr J Med Sci* **5**:1053, 1969.
368. Bapat JP, Baxi AJ: Mechanism of hemolysis of G6PD deficient red cells: Changes in membrane lipids and polypeptides. *Blut* **44**:355, 1979.
369. Corash L, Spielberg S, Bartsocas C, Boxer L, Steinhertz R, Sheetz M, Egan M, et al.: Reduced chronic haemolysis during high dose vitamin E administration in Mediterranean-type glucose-6-phosphate dehydrogenase deficiency. *N Engl J Med* **303**:416, 1980.
370. Spielberg SP, Boxer LA, Corash LM, Schulman JD: Improved erythrocyte survival with high dose vitamin E in chronic haemolyzing G6PD and glutathione synthetase deficiency. *Ann Intern Med* **90**:53, 1979.
371. Hafez M, Amar ES, Zedan M, Hammad H, Sorour AH, Eldesouky ESA, Gamil N: Improved erythrocyte survival with combined vitamin E and selenium therapy in children with glucose-6-phosphate dehydrogenase deficiency and mild chronic haemolysis. *J Pediatr* **108**:558, 1986.
372. Johnson GJ, Vatassery GR, Finkel B, Allen DW: High-dose vitamin E does not decrease the rate of chronic hemolysis in G6PD deficiency. *N Engl J Med* **303**:432, 1983.
373. Newman GJ, Newman TB, Bowie LJ, Mendlesohn J: An examination of the role of vitamin E in G6PD deficiency. *Clin Biochem* **12**:149, 1979.
374. Tanaka KR, Beutler E: Hereditary hemolytic anemia due to glucose-6-phosphate dehydrogenase Torrance: A new variant. *J Lab Clin Med* **73**:657, 1969.
375. Mentzer WCJ, Warner R, Addiego J, Smith B, Walter T: G6PD San Francisco: A new variant glucose-6-phosphate dehydrogenase associated with congenital nonspherocytic hemolytic anemia. *Blood* **55**:195, 1980.
376. Blackburn EK, Lorber J: Chronic hemolytic anemia due to glucose-6-phosphate dehydrogenase deficiency. *Proc R Soc Med* **56**:505, 1963.
377. Zinkham WH, Lenhard RE: Metabolic abnormalities of erythrocytes from patients with congenital non-spherocytic hemolytic anemia. *J Pediatr* **55**:319, 1959.
378. Allen DW, Johnson GJ, Cadman S, Kaplan ME: Membrane polypeptide aggregates in glucose-6-phosphate dehydrogenase deficient and in vitro aged red blood cells. *J Lab Clin Med* **91**:321, 1978.
379. Johnson GJ, Allen DW, Cadman S, Fairbanks VF, White JG, Lampkin BC, Kaplan ME: Red cell membrane polypeptide aggregates in glucose-6-phosphate dehydrogenase mutants with chronic haemolytic disease: A clue to the mechanism of haemolysis. *N Engl J Med* **301**:522, 1979.
380. Tillman W, Gahr M, Labitke N, Schroter W: Membrane deformability of erythrocytes with glucose-6-phosphate dehydrogenase Hamburg. *Acta Haematol (Basel)* **57**:162, 1977.
381. Welt SI, Jackson EH, Kirkman HN, Parker JC: The effects of certain drugs on the hexose monophosphate shunt of human red cells. *Ann N Y Acad Sci* **179**:625, 1971.
382. Carrell RW, Winterbourn CC, Rachmilewitz EA: Activatated oxygen and haemolysis. *Br J Haematol* **30**:259, 1975.
383. Winterbourn CC: Free radical production and oxidative reactions of hemoglobin. *Environ Health Perspect* **64**:321, 1985.
384. Davies KJ, Goldberg AL: Oxygen radicals stimulate intracellular proteolysis and lipid peroxidation by independent mechanisms in erythrocytes. *J Biol Chem* **262**:8220, 1987.
385. Jandl JH: *Blood: Textbook of Hematology*. Boston, Little, Brown, 1987.
386. Luzzatto L, Battistuzzi G: Glucose-6-phosphate dehydrogenase. *Adv Hum Genet* **14**:217, 1985.
387. Schiliro G, Russo A, Mauro L, Pizzarelli G, Marino S: Leucocyte function and characterisation of leukocyte glucose-6-phosphate dehydrogenase in Sicilian mutants. *Pediatr Res* **10**:739, 1976.
388. Cowan JM, Ammann AJ: Immunodeficiency syndromes associated with inherited metabolic disorders. *Clin Haematol* **10**:139, 1981.
389. Cooper MR, De Chatelet LR, McCall CE, La Via MF, Spurr CL, Baehner RL: Complete deficiency of leukocyte glucose-6-phosphate dehydrogenase with defective bactericidal activity. *J Clin Invest* **51**:769, 1972.
390. Gray FR, Klebanoff SJ, Stamatoyannopoulos G, Austin T, Naiman SC, Yoshida A, Kilman MR, et al.: Neutrophil dysfunction, chronic granulomatous disease and non-spherocytic haemolytic anemia caused by complete deficiency of glucose-6-phosphate dehydrogenase. *Lancet* **ii**:530, 1973.
391. Baehner RL, Johnston RB, Nathan DG: Comparative study of the metabolic and bactericidal characteristics of severely glucose-6-phosphate dehydrogenase deficient polymorphonuclear leucocytes and leucocytes from children with chronic granulomatous disease. *J Reticuloendothel Soc* **12**:150, 1972.

392. Bellanti JA, Cantz BE, Schlegel RJ: Accelerated decay of glucose-6-phosphate dehydrogenase activity in chronic granulomatous disease. *Pediatr Res* **4**:405, 1970.
393. Corberand J, De Larrard B, Vergnesh, Carriere JP: Chronic granulomatous disease with leukocyte glucose-6-phosphate dehydrogenase deficiency in a 28-month-old girl. *Am J Clin Pathol* **70**:296, 1978.
394. Hoffmann J, Bosia A, Arese P, Losche W, Pescarmona GP, Tazartes O, Till U: Glucose-6-phosphate dehydrogenase deficiency in human platelets and its effect on platelet aggregation. *Acta Biol Med Germ* **40**:1707, 1981.
395. Schwartz JP, Cooperberg AA, Rosenberg A: Platelet function studies in patients with glucose-6-phosphate dehydrogenase deficiency. *Br J Haematol* **27**:273, 1974.
396. Cocco P, Todde P, Fornera S, Manca MB, Manca P, Sias AR: Mortality in a cohort of men expressing the glucose-6-phosphate dehydrogenase deficiency. *Blood* **91**:706, 1998.
397. Bienzle U, Sodeinde O, Effiong CE, Luzzatto L: G6PD deficiency and sickle cell anemia: Frequency and features of the association in an African community. *Blood* **46**:591, 1975.
398. Luzzatto L, Allan NC: Relationship between the genes for glucose 6-phosphate dehydrogenase and haemoglobin a Nigerian population. *Nature* **219**:1041, 1968.
399. Nhonoli AM, Kujwalile JM, Kigoni EP, Masawe A: Correlation of glucose-6-phosphate dehydrogenase (G6PD) deficiency and sickle cell trait (Hb-AS). *Trop Geogr Med* **30**:99, 1978.
400. Steinberg MH, Dreiling BJ: Glucose-6-phosphate dehydrogenase deficiency in sickle cell anemia. A study in adults. *Ann Intern Med* **80**:217, 1974.
401. Beutler E, Johnson C, Powars D, West C: Prevalence of glucose-6-phosphate dehydrogenase deficiency in sickle cell disease. *N Engl J Med* **280**:826, 1974.
402. Steinberg MH, West MS, Gallagher D, Mentzer W: Effects of glucose-6-phosphate dehydrogenase deficiency upon sickle cell anemia. *Blood* **71**:748, 1988.
403. Snyder LM, Necheles TF, Reddy WJ: G-6-PD Worcester: A new variant, associated with x-linked optic atrophy. *Am J Med* **49**:125, 1970.
404. Petersen OW, Briand P, van Deurs S: Identification of malignant cells in primary monolayer cultures of human breast tumours. *Acta Pathol Microbiol Immunol Scand* **92**:103, 1984.
405. Bezwoda WR, Derman DP, See N, Mansoor N: Relative value of oestogen receptor assay, Lactoferrin content and glucose-6-phosphate dehydrogenase activity as prognostic indicators in primary breast cancer. *Oncology* **42**:7, 1985.
406. Zampella EJ, Bradley EL, Pretlow TG: Glucose-6-phosphate dehydrogenase: A possible indicator for prostatic carcinoma. *Cancer* **49**:384, 1982.
407. Ibrahim KS, Husain OAN, Bitensky L, Chayen J: A modified tetrazolium reaction for identifying malignant cells from gastric and colonic cancer. *J Clin Pathol* **36**:133, 1983.
408. Petersen OW, Hoyer PE, van Deurs B: Effect of oxygen on the tetrazolium reaction for glucose-6-phosphate dehydrogenase in cryosections of human breast carcinoma, fibrocystic disease and normal breast tissue. *Virchows Arch* **50**:13, 1985.
409. Naik SN, Anderson DE: G6PD deficiency and cancer. *Lancet* **i**:1060, 1970.
410. Sulis E: G6PD deficiency and cancer. *Lancet* **i**:1185, 1972.
411. Ferraris AM, Broccia G, Meloni T, Forteleoni G, Gaetani GF: Glucose 6-phosphate dehydrogenase deficiency and incidence of hematologic malignancy. *Am J Hum Genet* **42**:516, 1988.
412. Beutler E, Kuhl W, Fox M, Tabsh K, Crandall BF: Prenatal diagnosis of glucose 6-phosphate dehydrogenase deficiency. *Acta Haematol* **87**:103, 1992.
413. Herz F, Kaplan E, Scheye ES: Diagnosis of erythrocyte glucose-6-phosphate dehydrogenase deficiency in the Negro male despite hemolytic crisis. *Blood* **35**:90, 1970.
414. Ringelhahn B: A simple laboratory procedure for the recognition of the A− (African type) G6PD deficiency in acute haemolytic crisis. *Clin Chim Acta* 36:272, 1972.
415. Solem E: Glucose-6-phosphate dehydrogenase deficiency: An easy and sensitive quantitative assay for the detection of female heterozygotes in red blood cells. *Clin Chim Acta* **142**:153, 1984.
416. Solem E, Pirzer C, Siege M, Kollman F, Romero-Saravia O, Barktsch-Trefs O, Kornhuber B: Mass screening for glucose-6-phosphate dehydrogenase deficiency. Improved fluorescent spot test. *Clin Chim Acta* **152**:135, 1985.
417. Ackerman Z, Ablin J, Shouval D: Active immunization against hepatitis A is now warranted in glucose-6-phosphate dehydrogenase-deficient subjects [Letter]. *Am J Gatroenterol* **91**:413, 1996.
418. Chau TN, Lai ST, Lai JY, Yuen H: Haemolysis complicating acute viral hepatitis in patients with normal or deficient glucose-6-phosphate dehydrogenase activity. *Scand J Infect Dis* **29**:551, 1997.
419. Orlina AR, Josephson AM, McDonald BJ: The poststorage viability of glucose-6-phosphate dehydrogenase deficient erythrocytes. *J Lab Clin Med* **75**:930, 1970.
420. van der Saar A, Schouter H, Struyker Boudier AM: Glucose-6-phosphate dehydrogenase deficiency in red cells. Incidence in the Curacao population, its clinical and genetic aspects. *Enzyme* **27**:289, 1964.
421. Mimouni F, Shohat S, Reismer SH: G6PD-deficient donor blood as a cause of haemolysis in two pre-term infants. *Isr J Med Sci* 22:120, 1986.
422. Shalev O, Manny N, Sharon R: Posttransfusional hemolysis in recipients of glucose-6-phosphate dehydrogenase deficient erythrocytes. *Vox Sang* **64**:94, 1993.
423. McCurdy PR, Morse EE: Glucose-6-phosphate dehydrogenase deficiency and blood transfusion. *Vox Sang* **28**:230, 1975.
424. Rahimy MC, Dan V, Akpona S, Massougbodji A, Falanga PB: Partial exchange transfusion prior to treating cerebral malaria in an African child with glucose-6-phosphate dehydrogenase deficiency [Letter]. *Transfusion* **37**:984, 1997.
425. Linder D, Gartler SM: Glucose 6-phosphate dehydrogenase mosaicism. Utilization as a cell marker in the study of leiomyomas. *Science* **150**:67, 1965.
426. Liu S-C, Derick LH, Agre P, Palek J: Alteration of the erythrocyte membrane skeletal ultrastructure in hereditary spherocytosis, hereditary elliptocytosis, and pyropoikilocytosis. *Blood* **76**:198, 1990.
427. Vogels IMC, Van Noorden CJF, Worf BHM, Saelman DEM, Tromp A, Schutgens RBH, Weening RS: Cytochemical determination of heterozygous glucose-6-phosphate dehydrogenase deficiency in erythrocytes. *Br J Haematol* **63**:402, 1986.
428. Ramot B, Szeinberg A, Adam A, Sheba C, Gafni D: A study of subjects with glucose-6-phosphate dehydrogenase deficiency. I. Investigation of platelet enzyme. *J Clin Invest* **38**:1659, 1959.
429. Beutler E, Collins Z, Irwin LE: Value of genetic variants of glucose-6-phosphate dehydrogenase in tracing the origin of malignant tumors. *N Engl J Med* **176**:389, 1967.
430. Fialkow PJ: Clonal origin of human tumors. *Ann Rev Med* **30**:135, 1979.
431. Povey S, Hopkinson DA: The use of polymorphic enzyme markers of human blood cells in genetics. *Clin Haematol* 10:161, 1981.
432. Adamson JW: Analysis of hemopoiesis: The use of cell markers and in vitro culture techniques in studies of clonal hemopathies in man. *Clin Haematol* **13**:489, 1984.
433. Fialkow PJ, Gartler SM, Yoshida A: Clonal origin of chronic myelocytic leukemia in man. *Proc Natl Acad Sci U SA* **58**:1468, 1967.
434. Fialkow PJ, Jacobsen RJ, Papyannopoulou T: Chronic myelocytic leukemia: Clonal origin in a stem cell common to the granulocyte, erythrocyte, platelet and monocyte/macrophage. *Am J Med* **63**:125, 1977.
435. Adamson JW, Fialkow PJ, Murphy S, Prchal JF, Steinmann L: Polycythemia vera: Stem-cell and probable clonal origin of the disease. *N Engl J Med* **295**:913, 1976.
436. Oni SB, Osunkoya BO, Luzzatto L: Paroxysmal nocturnal hemoglobinuria: evidence for monoclonal origin of abnormal red cells. *Blood* **36**:145, 1970.
437. Pearson TA, Dillman J, Hepinstall RH: The clonal characteristics of human aortic intima. Comparison with fatty streaks and normal media. *Am J Pathol* **113**:33, 1983.
438. Griffiths DFR, Davies SJ, Williams D, Williams GT, Williams ED: Demonstration of somatic mutation and colonic crypt clonality by X-linked enzyme histochemistry. *Nature* **333**:461, 1988.
439. Fialkow PJ: Clonal origin of human tumors. *Biochim Biophys Acta* **458**:283, 1976.
440. Luzzatto L, Usanga EA, Bienzle U, Esan GJF, Fasuan FA: Imbalance in X-chromosome expression: evidence for a human X-linked gene affecting growth of haemopoietic cells. *Science* **205**:1418, 1979.
441. Williams CKO, Esan GJF, Luzzatto L, Town MM, Ogunmola GB: X-linked somatic-cell selection and polycythemia rubra vera. *N Engl J Med* **310**:1265, 1984.

442. Liu Y, Phelan J, Go RC, Prchal JF, Prchal JT: Rapid determination of clonality by detection of two closely-linked X chromosome exonic polymorphisms using allele-specific PCR. *J Clin Invest* **99**:1984, 1997.
443. Taylor DM, Ray PF, Ao A, Winston RM, Handyside AH: Paternal transcripts for glucose-6-phosphate dehydrogenase and adenosine deaminase are first detectable in the human preimplantation embryo at the three- to four-cell stage. *Mol Reprod Dev* **48**:442, 1997.
444. Filosa S, Giacometti N, Wangwei C, De Mattia D, Pagnini D, Alfinito F, Schettini F, et al.: Somatic-cell selection is a major determinant of the blood-cell phenotype in heterozygotes for glucose-6-phosphate dehydrogenase mutations causing severe enzyme deficiency. *Am J Hum Genet* **59**:887, 1996.
445. Motulsky AG: Metabolic polymorphisms and the role of infectious diseases in human evolution. *Hum Biol* **32**:28, 1960.
446. Luzzatto L: Genetics of red cells and susceptibility to malaria. *Blood* **54**:961, 1979.
447. Ruwende C, Hill A: Glucose-6-phosphate dehydrogenase deficiency and malaria. *J Mol Med* **76**:581, 1998.
448. Allison AC: Glucose 6-phosphate dehydrogenase deficiency in red blood cells of East Africans. *Nature* **186**:531, 1960.
449. Yenchitsomanus P, Summers KM, Board PG, Bhatia KK, Jones GL, Johnston K, Nurse GT: Alpha-thalassemia in Papua New Guinea. *Hum Genet* **74**:432, 1986.
450. Siniscalco M, Bernini L, Filippi G, Latte B, Khan PM, Piomelli S, Rattazzi M: Population genetics of haemoglobin variants, thalassaemia and glucose-6-phosphate dehydrogenase deficiency, with particular reference to the malaria hypothesis. *Bull WHO* **34**:379, 1966.
451. Stamatoyannopoulos G, Panayotopoulos A, Motulsky AG: The distribution of glucose 6-phosphate dehydrogenase deficiency in Greece. *Am J Hum Genet* **18**:296, 1966.
452. Piazza A, Mayr WR, Contu L, Amoroso A, Borelli I, Curtoni ES, Marcello C, et al.: Genetic and population structure of four Sardinian villages. *Ann Hum Genet* **49**:47, 1985.
453. Martin SK, Miller LH, Alling D: Severe malaria and glucose 6-phosphate dehydrogenase deficiency: A reappraisal of the malaria/G6PD hypothesis. *Lancet* **i**:524, 1979.
454. Luzzatto L, Bienzle U: The malaria/G6PD hypothesis. *Lancet* **i**:1183, 1979.
455. Segal HE, Noll WW, Thiemanun W: Glucose 6-phosphate dehydrogenase deficiency and falciparum malaria in two northeast Thai villages. *Proc Helminth Soc Wash* **39**:79, 1972.
456. Gilles HM, Fletcher KA, Hendrickse RG, Lindner R, Reddu S, Allan N: Glucose-6-phosphate dehydrogenase deficiency, sickling, and malaria in African children in South Western Nigeria. *Lancet* **1**:138, 1967.
457. Oo M, Tin-Shwe, Marlar-Than, O'Sullivan WJ: Genetic red cell disorders and severity of falciparum malaria in Myannamar. *Bull WHO* **73**:659, 1995.
458. Bienzle U, Ayeni O, Lucas AO, Luzzatto L: Glucose-6-phosphate dehydrogenase deficiency and malaria. Greater resistance of females heterozygous for enzyme deficiency and of males with non-deficient variant. *Lancet* **i**:107, 1972.
459. Guggenmoos-Holzmann I, Bienzle U, Luzzatto L: Plasmodium falciparum malaria and human red cells. II. Red cell genetic traits and resistance against malaria. *Int J Epidemiol* **10**:16, 1981.
460. Ruwende C, Khoo SC, Snow RW, Yates SN, Kwiatkowski D, Gupta S, Warn P, et al.: Natural selection of hemi- and heterozygotes for G6PD deficiency in Africa by resistance to severe malaria. *Nature* **376**:246, 1995.
461. Trager W, Jensen JB: Human malaria parasites in continuous culture. *Science* **193**:673, 1976.
462. Luzzatto L: Genetics of human red cells and susceptibility to malaria, in: Michal F (ed): *Modern Genetic Concepts and Techniques in the study of parasites*. Basel, Schwabe & Co. AG, 1980, 257.
463. Roth EF Jr., Raventos-Suarez C, Rinaldi A, Nagel RL: Glucose-6-phosphate dehydrogenase deficiency inhibits in vitro growth of *Plasmodium falciparum*. *Proc Natl Acad Sci U S A* **80**:298, 1983.
464. Miller J, Golenser J, Spira DT, Kosower NS: Plasmodium falciparum: Thiol status and growth in normal and glucose-6-phosphate dehydrogenase deficient human erythrocytes. *Exp Parasitol* **57**:239, 1984.
465. Friedman MJ: Oxidant damage mediates variant red cell resistance to malaria. *Nature* **280**:245, 1979.
466. Cappadoro M, Giribaldi G, O'Brien E, Turrini F, Mannu F, Ulliers D, Simula G, et al.: Early phagocytosis of glucose-6phosphate dehydrogenase (G6PD)-deficient erythrocytes parasitized by *Plasmodium falciparum* may explain malaria protection in G6PD deficiency. *Blood* **92**:2527, 1998.
467. Eckman JR, Eaton JW: Dependence of plasmodial glutathione metabolism on the host cells. *Nature* **278**:754, 1979.
468. Clark IA, Hunt NH: Evidence for reactive oxygen intermediates causing hemolysis and parasite death in malaria. *Infect Immun* **39**:1, 1983.
469. Luzzatto L, Usanga EA, Reddy S: Glucose-6-phosphate dehydrogenase deficient red cells: resistance to infection by malarial parasites. *Science* **164**:839, 1969.
470. Usanga EA, Luzzatto L: Adaptation of *Plasmodium falciparum* to glucose 6-phosphate dehydrogenase deficient host red cells by production of parasite-encoded enzyme. *Nature* **313**:793, 1985.
471. O'Brien E, Kurdi-Haidar B, Wanachiwanawin W, Carvajal JL, Villiamy TJ, Cappadoro M, Mason PJ, et al.: Cloning of the glucose 6-phosphate dehydrogenase gene from *Plasmodium falciparum*. *Mol Biochem Parasitol* **64**:313, 1994.
472. Scopes DA, Bautista JM, Vulliamy TJ, Mason PJ: *Plasmodium falciparum* glucose-6-phosphate dehydrogenase (G6PD)—the N-terminal portion is homologous to a predicted protein encoded near to G6PD in *Hemophilus influenzae*. *Mol Microbiol* **23**:847, 1997.
473. Jackson F: Ecological modeling of human-plant-parasite coevolutionary triads: Theoretical perspectives on the interrelationships of human HbβS, G6PD, *Manihot esculenta*, *Vicia faba* and *Plasmodium falciparum*, in Greene LS, Danubio ME (ed): *Adaptation to Malaria. The Interaction of Biology and Culture*, Amsterdam, Gordon and Breach, 1997, p 177.
474. Greene LS, Danubio ME: Adaptation to Malaria, in Greene LS, Danubio ME (ed): *The Interaction of Biology and Culture*. Amsterdam, Gordon and Breach, 1997, p 1.
475. Golenser J, Chevion M: Oxidant stress and malaria: Host-parasite relationships in normal and abnormal erythrocytes. *Semin Hematol* **26**:313, 1989.
476. Golenser J: Malaria and blood genetic disorders with special respect to glucose-6-phosphate dehydrogenase (G6PD deficiency), in Greene LS, Danubio ME (ed): *Adaptation to Malaria. The Interaction of Biology and Culture*, Amsterdam, Gordon and Breach, 1997, p 127.
477. Luzzatto L, Pinching AJ: Commentary to R Nagel—Innate resistance to malaria: The intraerythrocytic cycle. *Blood Cells* **16**:340, 1990.
478. Galanello R, Loi D, Sollaino C, Dessi S, Cao A, Melis MA: A new glucose 6 phosphate dehydrogenase variant G6PD Sinnai (34 G $\rightarrow$ T). Mutations in brief no. 156 [Online]. *Hum Mutat* **12**:72, 1998.
479. Chao L, Du CS, Louie E, Zuo L, Chen E, Lubin B, Chiu TY: A to G substitution identified in exon 2 of the G6PD gene among G6PD deficient Chinese. *Nucleic Acids Res* **19**:6056, 1991.
480. Hirono A, Ishii A, Kere N, Fujii H, Hirono K, Miwa S: Molecular analysis of glucose-6-phosphate dehydrogenase variants in the Solomon Islands [Letter]. *Am J Hum Genet* **56**:1243, 1995.
481. MacDonald D, Town M, Mason PJ, Vulliamy T, Luzzatto L, Goff MC: Deficiency in red blood cells. *Nature* **350**:115, 1991.
482. Vulliamy T, Luzzatto L, Hirono A, Beutler E: Hematologically important mutations: Glucose 6-phosphate dehydrogenase. *Blood Cells Mol Dis* **23**:292, 1997.
483. Nafa K, Reghis A, Osmani N, Baghli N, Benabadji M, Vulliamy T, Luzzatto L: G6PD Aures: A new mutation (48 Ile $\rightarrow$ Thr) causing mild G6PD deficiency is associated with favism. *Hum Mol Genet* **2**:81, 1993.
484. Beutler E, Kuhl W, Ramirez E, Lisker R: Some Mexican glucose 6-phosphate dehydrogenase (G-6-PD) variants revisited. *Hum Genet* **86**:371, 1991.
485. Hirono A, Beutler E: Molecular cloning and nucleotide sequence of cDNA for human glucose-6-phosphate dehydrogenase variant A(−). *Proc Natl Acad Sci U S A* **85**:3951, 1988.
486. Cappellini MD, Sampietro M, Toniolo D, Carandina G, Martinez di Montemuros F, Tavazzi D, Fiorelli G: G6PD Ferrara I has the same two mutations as G6PD A− but a distinct biochemical phenotype. *Hum Genet* **93**:139, 1994.
487. Rovira A, Vulliamy T, Pujades MA, Luzzatto L, Vives-Corrons JL: Molecular genetics of glucose 6-phosphate dehydrogenase (G6PD) deficiency in Spain: Identification of two new point mutations in the G6PD gene. *Br J Haematol* **91**:66, 1995.
488. Hirono A, Fujii H, Miwa S: Molecular abnormality of G6PD Konan and G6PD Ube. *Hum Genet* **91**:507, 1993.
489. Ninfali P, Baronciani L, Ruzzo A, Fortini C, Amadori E, Dallara G, Magnani N, et al.: Molecular analysis of G6PD variants in northern Italy: A study on the population from the Ferrara district. *Hum Genet* **92**:139, 1993.

490. Hirono A, Fujii H, Miwa S: Identification of two novel deletion mutations in glucose-6-phosphate dehydrogenase gene causing hemolytic anemia. *Blood* **85**:1118, 1995.
491. Maeda M, Constantoulakis P, Chen CS, Stamatoyannopoulos G, Yoshida A: Molecular abnormalities of a human glucose 6-phosphate dehydrogenase variant associated with undetectable enzyme activity and immunologically cross-reacting material. *Am J Hum Genet* **51**:386, 1992.
492. Takizawa T, Yoneyama Y, Miwa S, Yoshida A: A single nucleotide base transition is the basis of the common human glucose-6-phosphate dehydrogenase variant A(+). *Genomics* **1**:228, 1987.
493. Zarza R, Pujades A, Rovira A, Saavedra R, Fernandez J, Aymerich M, Vives Corrons JL: Two new mutations of the glucose-6-phosphate dehydrogenase (G6PD) gene associated with haemolytic anaemia: clinical, biochemical and molecular relationships. *Br J Haematol* **98**:578, 1997.
494. Menounos P, Zervas C, Garinis G, Doukas C, Kolokithopoulos D, Tegos C, Patrinos GP: Molecular heterogeneity of the gluscose-6-phosphate dehydrogenase deficiency in the Hellenic population. *Hum Hered* **50**:237, 2000.
495. Vulliamy TJ, Wanachiwanawin W, Mason PJ, Luzzatto L: G6PD Mahidol, a common deficient variant in South East Asia is caused by a (163) Glycine → Serine mutation. *Nucleic Acids Res* **17**:5868, 1989.
496. Tang TK, Yeh C-H, Huang C-S, Huang M-J: Expression and biochemical characterization of human glucose-6-phosphate dehydrogenase in *Escherichia coli*: A system to analyze normal and mutant enzymes. *Blood* **83**:1436, 1994.
497. Khan PM, Ploem JR, Wijnen JT, Breukel C, Korthof G, Weening RS: G6PD Volendam: De novo mutation of unusual mechanism in a severely deficient Dutch female born to apparently normal parents. *Seventh International Congress of Human Genetics* 418a, 1986.
498. Chen HL, Huang MJ, Huang CS, Tang TK: G6PD NanKang (517 T → C; 173 Phe → Leu): A new Chinese G6PD variant associated with neonatal jaundice. *Hum Hered* **46**:201, 1996.
499. Tang TK, Chen H-L, Tzou W-S, Huang M-J: Structural and functional analysis of Chinese G6PD mutations on the basis of a three dimensional structural model of human enzyme. *Blood* **88**:307A, 1996.
500. Hirono A, Miwa S, Fujii H, Ishida F, Yamada K, Kubota K: Molecular study of eight Japanese cases of glucose 6-phosphate dehydrogenase deficiency by non-radioisotopic single-strand conformation polymorphism analysis. *Blood* **83**:3363, 1994.
501. Vulliamy TJ, Rovira A, Yusoff N, Colomer D, Luzzatto L, Vives-Corrons JL: Independent origin of single and double mutations in the huiman glucose 6-phosphate dehydrogenase gene. *Hum Mutat* **8**:311, 1996.
502. Beutler E, Kuhl W, Saenz GF, Rodriguez W: Mutation analysis of G6PD variants in Costa Rica. *Hum Genet* **87**:462, 1991.
503. Beutler E, Kuhl W: The NT 1311 polymorphism of G6PD: G6PD Mediterranean mutation may have arisen more than once. *Am J Hum Genet* **47**:1008, 1990.
504. Beutler E, Westwood B, Prchal JT, Vaca G, Bartsocas CS, Baronciani L: New glucose 6-phosphate dehydrogenase mutations from various ethnic groups. *Blood* **80**:255, 1992.
505. Calabrò V, Mason PJ, Filosa S, Civitelli D, Cittadella R, Tagarelli A, Martini G, et al.: Genetic heterogeneity of glucose 6-phosphate dehydrogenase deficiency revealed by single-strand conformation and sequence analysis. *Am J Hum Genet* **52**:527, 1993.
506. Beutler E, Kuhl W, Gelbart T, Forman M: DNA sequence abnormalities of human glucose 6-phosphate dehydrogenase variants. *J Biol Chem* **266**:4145, 1991.
507. Beutler E, Prchal JT, Westwood B, Kuhl W: Definition of the mutations of G6PD Wayne, G6PD Viangchan, G6PD Jammu and G6PD "LeJeune." *Acta Haematol (Basel)* **86**:179, 1991.
508. Poggi V, Town M, Foulkes NS, Luzzatto L: Identification of a single base change in the G6PD gene by PCR amplification of the entire coding region from genomic DNA. *Biochem J* **271**:157, 1990.
509. Jablonska-Skwiecinska E, Lewandowska I, Plochocka D, Topczewski J, Zimowski JG, Klopocka J, Burzynska B: Several mutations including two novel mutations of the glucose-6-phosphate dehydrogenase gene in Polish G6PD deficient subjects with chronic nonspherocytic hemolytic anemia, acute hemolytic anemia, and favism. *Hum Mutat* **14**:477, 1999.
510. Zimmerman SA, Ware RE, Forman L, Westwood B, Beutler E: Glucose-6-phosphate dehydrogenase Durham: a de novo mutation associated with chronic hemolytic anemia. *J Pediatr* **131**:284, 1997.
511. Xu W, Westwood B, Bartsocas CS, Malcorra-Azpiazu JJ, Indrk K, Beutler E: Glucose 6-phosphate dehydrogenase mutations and haplotypes in various ethnic groups. *Blood* **85**:257, 1995.
512. Costa E, Cabeda JM, Vieira E, Pinto R, Pereira SA, Ferraz L, Santos R, et al.: Glucose-6-phosphate dehydrogenase Aveiro: A de novo mutation associated with chronic nonspherocytic hemolytic anemia. *Blood* **95**:1499, 2000.
513. Beutler E, Westwood B, Kuhl W, Hsia YE: Glucose 6-phosphate dehydrogenase variants in Hawaii. *Hum Hered* **42**:327, 1992.
514. Ninfali P, Bresolin N, Baronciani L, Fortunato F, Comi G, Magnani M, Scarlato G: Glucose 6-phosphate dehydrogenase Lodi 844 C: A study on its expression in blood cells and muscle. *Enzyme* **45**:180, 1991.
515. Cappellini MD, Martinez Di Montemuros F, Dotti C, Tavazzi D, Fiorelli G: Molecular characterisation of the glucose-6-phosphate dehydrogenase (G6PD) Ferrara II variant. *Hum Genet* **95**:440, 1995.
516. Cappellini MD, Sampietro M, Toniolo D, Carandina G, Pittalis S, Martinez di Montemuros F, Tavazzi D, et al.: Biochemical and molecular characterization of a new sporadic glucose-6-phosphate dehydrogenase variant described in Italy: G6PD Modena. *Br J Haematol* **87**:209, 1994.
517. Viglietto G, Montanaro V, Calabro V, Vallone D, D'Urso M, Persico MG, Battistuzzi G: Common glucose 6-phosphate dehydrogenase (G6PD) variants from the Italian Population: Biochemical and molecular characterization. *Ann Hum Genet* **54**:1, 1990.
518. Beutler E, Westwood B, Melemed A, Dal Borgo P, Margolis D: Three new exon 10 glucose-6-phosphate dehydrogenase mutations. *Blood Cells Mol Dis* **21**:64, 1995.
519. Hirono A, Kuhl W, Gelbart T, Forman L, Fairbanks VF, Beutler E: Identification of the binding domain for NADP+ of human glucose-6-phosphate dehydrogenase by sequence analysis of mutants. *Proc Natl Acad Sci U S A* **86**:10015, 1989.
520. Vaca G, Ibarra B, Romero F, Olivares N, Cantu JM, Beutler E: G-6-PD Guadalajara: A new mutant associated with chronic non-spherocytic hemolytic anemia. *Hum Genet* **61**:175, 1982.
521. Ohga S, Higashi E, Nomura A, Matsusaki A, Hirono A, Miwa S, Fujii H, et al.: Haptoglobin therapy for acute favism: A Japanese boy with glucose-6-phosphate dehydrogenase Guadalajara. *Br J Haematol* **89**:421, 1995.
522. Gaetani GF, Galiano S, Melani C, Miglino M, Forni GL, Napoli G, Perrone L, et al.: A new glucose-6-phosphate dehydrogenase variant with congenital nonspherocytic hemolytic anemia (G6PD Genova). Biochemical characterization and mosaicism expression in the heterozygote. *Hum Genet* **84**:337, 1990.
523. Kanno H, Takano T, Fujii H: A new glucose 6-phopshate dehydrogenase variant, G6PD Iwate, associated with CNSHA. *Acta Haematol Japonica* **51**:715, 1988.
524. Filosa S, Calabrò V, Vallone D, Poggi V, Mason P, Pagnini D, Alfinito F, et al.: Molecular basis of chronic non-spherocytic haemolytic anaemia: a new G6PD variant (393Arg → His) with abnormal Km G6P and marked in vivo instability. *Br J Haematol* **80**:111, 1992.
525. Hirono A, Fujii H, Hirono K, Kanno H, Miwa S: Molecular abnormality of a Japanese Glucose 6-phosphate dehydrogenase variant (G6PD Tokyo) associated with hereditary non-spherocytic hemolytic anemia. *Hum Genet* **88**:347, 1992.
526. Saad ST, Salles TS, Arruda VR, Sonati MF, Costa FF: G6PD Sumare: a novel mutation in the G6PD gene (1292 T → G) associated with chronic nonspherocytic anemia. *Hum Mut* **10**:245, 1997.
527. Hsia YE, Miyakawa F, Baltazar J, Ching NSP, Yuen J, Westwood B, Beutler E: Frequency of glucose-6-phosphate dehydrogenase (G6PD) mutations in Chinese, Filipinos, and Laotians from Hawaii. *Hum Genet* **92**:470, 1993.
528. Kugler P, Hofer D, Mayer B, Drenckhahn D: Nitric oxide synthase and NADP-linked glucose-6-phosphate dehydrogenase are co-localized in brush cells of rat stomach and pancreas. *J Histochem Cytochem* **42**:1317, 1994.
529. Vives-Corrons J-L, Kuhl W, Pujades MA, Beutler E: Molecular genetics of the glucose-6-phosphate dehydrogenase (G6PD) Mediterranean variant and description of a new G6PD mutant, G6PD Andalus1361A. *Am J Hum Genet* **47**:575, 1990.
530. Stevens DJ, Wanachiwanawin W, Mason PJ, Vulliamy TJ, Luzzatto L: G6PD Canton: a common deficient variant in South East Asia cause by a 459 Arg→Leu mutation. *Nucleic Acids Res* **18**:7190, 1990.
531. Baronciani L, Tricta F, Beutler E: G6PD "Campinas:" A deficient enzyme with a mutation at the far 3′ end of the gene. *Hum Mutat* **2**:77, 1993.
532. Meloni G, Meloni T: Glyburide-induced acute haemolysis in a G6PD-deficient patient with NIDDM. *Br J Haematol* **92**:159, 1996.

533. Khurana V, Bradley TP: Adult-onset Still's disease associated with G6PD deficiency: A case report and literature review. *J Assoc Acad Minor Phys* **9**:56, 1998.
534. Wright RO, Perry HE, Woolf AD, Shannon MW: Hemolysis after acetaminophen overdose in a patient with glucose-6-phosphate dehydrogenase deficiency. *J Toxicol Clin Toxicol* **34**:731, 1996.
535. Senanayake N, Sanmuganathan PS: Acute intravascular haemolysis in glucose-6-phosphate dehydrogenase deficient patients following ingestion of herbal broth containing Acalypha indica. *Trop Doct* **26**:32, 1996.
536. Zail SS, Charlton RW, Bothwell TH: The haemolytic effect of certain drugs in Bantu subjects with a deficiency of glucose-6-phosphate dehydrogense. *S Afr J Med Sci* **27**:95, 1962.
537. Ham TH, Grauel JA, Dunn RF, Murphy JR, White JG, Kellermeyer RW: Physical properties of red cells as related to effects in vivo. IV. Oxidant drugs producing abnormal intracellular concentration of hemoglobin (eccentrocytes) with a rigid-red-cell hemolytic syndrome. *J Lab Clin Med* **82**:898, 1973.
538. Fraser IM, Vesell ES: Effects of drugs and drug metabolites on erythrocytes from normal and glucose-6-phosphate dehydrogenase deficient individuals. *Ann N Y Acad Sci* **151**:777, 1968.
539. Fraser IM, Tilton BE, Vesell ES: Effects of some metabolites of hemolytic drugs on young and old, normal and G6PD deficient human erythrocytes. *Ann N Y Acad Sci* **179**:644, 1971.
540. Gaetani GD, Mareni C, Ravazzolo R, Salvidio E: Hemolytic effect of two sulphonamides evaluated by a new method. *Br J Haematol* **32**:183, 1976.
541. Capps FPA, Gilles HM, Jolly H, Worlledge SM: Glucose-6-phosphate dehydrogenase deficiency and neonatal jaundice in Nigeria. Their relation to the prophylactic use of vitamin K. *Lancet* **ii**:379, 1963.
542. Bienzle U, Effiong CE, Luzzatto L: Erythrocyte glucose 6-phosphate dehydrogenase deficiency (G6PD type A−) and neonatal jaundice. *Acta Paediatr Scandin* **65**:701, 1976.
543. Bernstein RE: Occurrence and clinical implications of red cell glucose-6-phosphate dehydrogenase deficiency in South African racial groups. *S Afr Med J* **37**:447, 1963.
544. Gibbs WN, Gray R, Lowry M: Glucose 6-phosphate dehydrogenase deficiency and neonatal jaundice in Jamaica. *Br J Haematol* **43**:263, 1979.
545. O'Flynn MED, Hsia DY: Serum bilirubin levels and glucose-6-phosphate dehydrogenase deficiency in newborn American Negros. *J Pediatr* **63**:160, 1963.
546. Phornphutkul C, Whitaker JA, Worathumrong N: Severe hyperbilirubinemia in Thai newborns in association with erythrocyte G6PD deficiency. *Clin Pediatr* **8**:275, 1969.
547. Weatherall DJ: Enzyme deficiency in hemolytic disease of the newborn. *Lancet* **ii**:835, 1960.
548. Vella F: The incidence of erythrocyte glucose-6-phosphate dehydrogenase deficiency in Singapore. *Experientia* **17**:181, 1961.
549. Lie-Injo LE, Virjk HK, Lim PW, Lie AK, Ganesan J: Red cell metabolism and severe neonatal jaundice in West Malaysia. *Acta Haematol (Basel)* **58**:152, 1977.
550. Doxiadis SA, Fessas PH, Valaes T: Erythrocyte enzyme deficiency in unexplained kernicterus. *Lancet* **ii**:44, 1960.
551. Doxiadis SA, Valaes T, Karaklis A, Stavrakakis D: Risk of severe jaundice in glucose 6-phosphate dehydrogenase deficiency of the newborn. Differences in population groups. *Lancet* **ii**:1210, 1964.
552. Fessas PH, Doxiadis SA, Valaes T: Neonatal jaundice in glucose-6-phosphate dehydrogenase deficient infants. *BMJ* **ii**:1359, 1962.
553. Meloni T, Forteleoni G, Dore A, Cutillo S: Neonatal hyperbilirubinaemia in heterozygous glucose-6-phosphate dehydrogenase deficient females. *Br J Haematol* **53**:241, 1983.
554. Wurzel H, McGeary T, Baker L, Gumerman L: Glucose-6-phosphate dehydrogenase deficiency in platelets. *Blood* **17**:314, 1961.
555. Gray GR, Naiman SC, Fobinson GCF: Platelet function and G6PD deficiency. *Lancet* **i**:997, 1974.
556. Zinkham WH: A deficiency of glucose-6-phosphate dehydrogenase activity in lens from individulas with primaquine-sensitive erythrocytes. *Johns Hopkins Med J* **109**:206, 1961.
557. Westring DN, Pisciotta AV: Anemia, cataracts and seizures in a patient with glucose-6-phosphate dehydrogenase deficiency. *Arch Int Med* **118**:385, 1966.
558. Moro F, Gorgone G, Li-Volti S, Cavallaro N, Faro S, Curreri R, Mollica F: Glucose 6-phosphate dehydrogenase deficiency and incidence of cataract in Sicily. *Ophthalmic Paediatr Genet* **5**:197, 1985.
559. Chan TK, Todd D, Wong CC: Tissue enzyme levels in erythrocyte glucose-6-phosphate dehydrogenase deficiency. *J Lab Clin Med* **66**:937, 1965.
560. Sarkar S, Nelson AJ, Jones OW: Glucose-6-phosphate dehydrogenase (G6PD) activity of human sperm. *J Med Genet* **14**:250, 1977.
561. Ramot B, Sheba C, Adam A, Ashkenasi I: Erythrocyte glucose-6-phosphate dehydrogenase deficient subjects: Enzyme-level in saliva. *Nature* **185**:931, 1960.
562. Bresolin N, Bet L, Moggio M, Meola G, Comi G, Gilardi A, Scarlato G: Muscle G6PD deficiency. *Lancet* **ii**:212, 1987.
563. Ninfali P, Baronciani L, Bardoni A, Bresolin N: Muscle expression of glucose-6-phosphate dehydrogenase deficiency in different variants. *Clin Genet* **48**:232, 1995.
564. Masson P, Rigot A, Cecile W: Hydrops fetalis and G-6-PD deficiency. *Arch Pediatr* **2**:541, 1995.
565. Oner C, Oner R, Birben E, Balkan H, Gumruk F, Gurgey A, Altay C: HB H disease with homozygosity for red cell G6PD deficiency in a Turkish female. *Hemoglobin* **22**:157, 1998.
566. Younker D, De Vore M, Hartzage PL: Malignant hyperthermia and glucose-6-phosphate dehydrogenase deficiency. *Anesthesiology* **60**:601, 1984.
567. Harper JI, Coperman PWM: A child with xeroderma pigmentosum and G6PD deficiency. *Clin Exp Dermatol* **7**:213, 1982.
568. Dern RJ, Glynn MF, Brewer GJ: Studies on the correlation of the genetically determined trait, glucose-6-phosphate dehydrogenase deficiency with behavioral manifestations in schizophrenia. *J Lab Clin Med* **62**:319, 1963.
569. Chanmugan D, Frumin AM: Abnormal oral glucose tolerance response in erythrocyte glucose-6-phosphate dehydrogenase deficiency. *N Engl J Med* **271**:1202, 1964.
570. Bowman J, Brewer GJ, Frischer H, Carter JL, Eisentein RB, Bayrakci C: A re-evaluation of the relationship between glucose-6-phosphate dehydrogenase deficiency and behaviorial manifestations. *J Lab Clin Med* **65**:222, 1965.
571. Eppes RB, Brewer GJ, De Gowin RL, Manamara JY, Flanagan CL, Schrier SL, Tarlov AR, et al.: Oral glucose tolerance in Negro men deficient in G6PD. *N Engl J Med* **275**:855, 1966.
572. Borkowski AJ, Marks PA, Katz FH, Lipman MM, Christty NP: An abnormal pathway of steroid metabolism in patient with glucose-6-phosphate dehydrogenase deficiency. *J Clin Invest* **41**:1346, 1962.
573. McCurdy PR: An apparent association between red cell glucose-6-phosphate dehydrogenase deficiency and pernicious anemia in negro males. *Clin Res* **14**:91, 1966.
574. Sheehan RG, Lindeman RJ, Meyer J, Patterson JF, Nechelles TF: The possible association of erythrocyte glucose-6-phosphate dehydrogenase deficiency and regional enteritis. *J Clin Invest* **44**:1098, 1965.
575. Long WK, Wilson SW, Frenkel EP: Associations between red cell glucose-6-phosphate dehydrogenase variants and vascular diseases. *Am J Hum Genet* **19**:35, 1967.
576. Wiesenfeld SL, Petrakis NL, Sams BJ, Collen MF, Cutler JL: Elevated blood pressure, pulse rate and serum creatinine in Negro males deficient in glucose-6-phosphate dehydrogenase. *N Engl J Med* **282**:1001, 1970.
577. Sampietro M, Lupica L, Perrero L, Comino A, Martinez Di Montemuros F, Cappellini MD, Fiorelli G: The expression of uridine diphosphate glucuronosyltransferase gene is a major determinant of bilirubin level in heterozygous beta-thalassaemia and in glucose-6-phosphate dehydrogenase deficiency. *Br J Haematol* **99**:437, 1997.
578. Deutsch J: Maleimide as an inhibitor in measurement of erythrocyte glucose-6-phosphate dehydrogenase activity. *Clin Chem* **24**:885, 1978.
579. Catalano EW, Johnson GF, Solomon HM: Measurement of erythrocyte glucose-6-phosphate dehydrogenase activity with a centrifugal analyzer. *Clin Chem* **21**:134, 1975.
580. Ardern JC, Edwards N, Hyde K, Jardine-Wilkinson C, Cintokai KI, Power DN, MacIver JE: A proposal for further standardization of red blood cell glucose 6-phosphate dehydrogenase determinations. *Clin Lab Haematol* **10**:409, 1988.
581. Beutler E: A series of new screening procedures for pyruvate kinase deficiency, glucose-6-phosphate dehydrogenase deficiency. *Blood* **32**:816, 1968.
582. Beutler E, Blume KG, Kaplan JC, Lohr GW, Ramot B, Valentine WN: International Committee for Standardization in Haematology: Recommended screening test for glucose-6-phosphate dehydrogenase (G6PD) deficiency. *Br J Haematol* **43**:465, 1979.
583. Beni A, Fortini G, Salvati AM, Tentori L, Torlontano G: Quantitation of the ultraviolet light test for erythrocyte glucose-6-phosphated

dehydrogenase, pyruvate kinase and glutathione reductase. *Clin Chim Acta* **49**:41, 1973.
584. Jacob H, Jandl JH: A simple visual screening test for glucose-6-phosphated dehydrogenase deficiency employing ascorbate and cyanide. *N Engl J Med* **274**:1162, 1966.
585. Fairbanks VF, Fernadez MN: The identification of metabolic errors associated with hemolytic anemia. *JAMA* **208**:316, 1969.
586. Fairbanks VF, Lampe LT: A tetrazolium-linked cytochemical method for estimation of glucose 6-phosphate dehydrogenase activity in individual erythrocytes: Applications in the study of heterozygotes for glucose 6-phosphate dehydrogenase deficiency. *Blood* **31**:589, 1968.
587. Van Noorden CJF, Vogels IMC, James J, Tas J: A sensitive cytochemical staining method for glucose 6-phosphate dehydrogenase activity in individual erythrocytes. *Histochemistry* **75**:493, 1982.
588. Gordon PA, Stewart J: Red cell cytochemistry in glucose-6-phosphate dehydrogenase deficiency. *Br J Haematol* **27**:358, 1974.
589. Van Noorden CJF, Vogels IMC: A sensitive cytochemical staining method for glucose-6-phosphate dehydrogenase activity in individual erythrocytes. *Br J Haematol* **60**:57, 1985.
590. Brewer GJ, Tarlov AR, Alving AS: The methemoglobin reduction test for primaquine-type sensitivity of erythrocytes. A simplified procedure for detecting a specific hypersusceptibility to drug hemolysis. *JAMA* **180**:386, 1962.
591. Bapat JP, Baxi AJ, Bhatia HM: Is methemoglobin reduction test a true index of G6PD deficiency? *Indian J Med Res* **64**:1687, 1976.
592. Motulsky AG, Campbell-Kraut JM: Population genetics of glucose 6-phosphate dehydrogenase deficiency of the red cell, in Blumberg BS (ed): *Proceedings of Conference on Genetic Polymorphisms and Geographic Variations in Disease*. New York, Grune & Stratton, 1961, p 159.
593. Bernstein RE: Brilliant cresyl blue screening test for demonstrating glucose-6-phosphate dehydrogenase deficiency in red cells. *Clin Chim Acta* **8**:158, 1963.
594. Usanga EA, Bienzle U, Cancedda R, Fasuan FA, Ajayi O, Luzzatto L: Genetic variants of human erythrocyte glucose 6-phosphate dehydrogenase: New variants in West Africa characterized by column chromatography. *Ann Hum Genet* **40**:279, 1976.

CHAPTER 180

Cytochrome b_5 Reductase Deficiency and Enzymopenic Hereditary Methemoglobinemia

Ernst R. Jaffé ■ Donald E. Hultquist

1. **The major pathway for the reduction of methemoglobin to functional hemoglobin in human erythrocytes involves a NADH-dependent methemoglobin reductase system. In addition to NADH, this system requires the presence in the cytosol of both cytochrome b_5 reductase, a 32,000-dalton protein, and cytochrome b_5, a 12,000-dalton protein. These proteins are presumed to arise from larger parent molecules in the erythroid precursors by proteolytic cleavage of their hydrophobic tails.**
2. **Enzymopenic hereditary methemoglobinemia (MIM 250800) is a rare recessively inherited disorder caused, in most cases, by deficiency of cytochrome b_5 reductase only in erythrocytes (type I). Generalized cytochrome b_5 reductase deficiency, demonstrable in all tissues that have been examined, occurs in 10 to 15 percent of cases and is accompanied by methemoglobinemia and severe, progressive, lethal neurologic disability (type II). Cytochrome b_5 reductase deficiency limited to hematopoietic cells is also manifested by methemoglobinemia, but without neurologic effects (type III). Deficiency of cytochrome b_5 may also lead to methemoglobinemia (type IV).**
3. **The gene regulating the synthesis of cytochrome b_5 reductase has been assigned to chromosome 22. Deficiency of cytochrome b_5 reductase has a worldwide distribution, and electrophoretic variants of the enzyme with normal catalytic properties may have an incidence as high as 1:100. Heterozygotes for cytochrome b_5 reductase deficiency are asymptomatic but have an increased propensity to develop toxic methemoglobinemia induced by drugs or other chemicals.**
4. **The diagnosis of enzymopenic hereditary methemoglobinemia may be made by relatively simple laboratory determinations, but definition of the specific defect requires more sophisticated studies.**
5. **Effective treatment may be provided by the administration of methylene blue, ascorbic acid, or riboflavin but is often not indicated, except for cosmetic reasons. Such therapy, however, has had no demonstrable effect on the neurologic aberrations in the generalized type II disorder.**

HISTORY

Hereditary methemoglobinemia, an interesting albeit rare disorder (MIM 250800), has a worldwide distribution and has been known for a century and a half. In 1845, François[1] described a patient with long-standing congenital cyanosis without obvious cardiac or pulmonary disease. Although altered hemoglobin pigments and drug-induced cyanosis had been reported frequently, it was 1891 before Dittrich[2] established that the methemoglobinemia that developed in dogs given *Blutgifte*, such as nitroglycerine and acetanilide, eventually disappeared without the occurrence of anemia. He also pointed out that the methemoglobinemic cyanosis that developed in patients receiving certain medicines tended to disappear and suggested that the methemoglobin was reduced to hemoglobin within the circulating erythrocytes. Subsequently, other authors described "enterogenous cyanosis" attributed to the absorption of toxic substances from the gastrointestinal tract.[3] Sulfhemoglobin present in some of these patients' erythrocytes was differentiated from methemoglobin in 1905.[4]

Hitzenberger,[5] in 1932, was probably the first to describe a familial incidence of idiopathic cyanosis. He suggested the possibility of congenital, familial methemoglobinemia. Between 1943 and 1945, Gibson[6] and his associates[7] suggested that there was a decreased ability of the erythrocytes to reduce methemoglobin formed continuously at a normal rate in patients with familial, idiopathic methemoglobinemia. The classic investigations of Gibson[8] in 1948 provided substantial experimental evidence for a deficiency of a factor (a methemoglobin reductase) in the erythrocytes of patients with idiopathic methemoglobinemia. In 1959, Scott and Griffith[9] identified an enzyme in normal human erythrocytes that catalyzed the reduction of methemoglobin with NADH and called this enzyme a "diaphorase." The enzyme was subsequently named and assayed as a NADH dehydrogenase, NADH-methemoglobin reductase, NADH-methemoglobin-ferrocyanide reductase, NADH-ferricyanide reductase, and, most recently, NADH-cytochrome b_5 reductase. Scott et al. described a severe deficiency of this enzyme in the erythrocytes of native Alaskans with methemoglobinemia, and intermediate levels of activity in the cells of their acyanotic parents and children.[10,11] To explain the typically recessive pattern of inheritance of idiopathic methemoglobinemia suggested by the family histories of many patients, they proposed that affected individuals inherited one abnormal gene from each parent. These observations have been extended and confirmed by other investigators.[12]

Hultquist and Passon[13] subsequently identified the NADH-dependent enzyme as a cytochrome b_5 reductase and demonstrated that the catalysis of methemoglobin reduction by this reductase involved the participation of a cytochrome b_5 present in normal human erythrocytes. This enzyme system is considered the most important one for the conversion of any methemoglobin formed in normal human erythrocytes to functional, oxygen-carrying hemoglobin. The activity of this system is markedly reduced in the erythrocytes of most patients with enzymopenic hereditary methemoglobinemia.

A list of standard abbreviations is located immediately preceding the index in each volume. Additional abbreviations used in this chapter include: DPG = 2,3-diphosphoglycerate; DCIP = 2,6-dichlorophenolindophenol.

More than 500 cases of hereditary methemoglobinemia have been cited in the literature. Those patients with family histories suggesting dominant inheritance of the methemoglobinemia have usually been proved or presumed to have a hemoglobin M, a hemoglobin that results from a mutation in the hemoglobin gene which makes the hemoglobin more susceptible to oxidation and/or makes the resulting methemoglobin more resistant to reduction (see Chap. 181). More than half of the total reported cases, however, have had family histories or laboratory evidence consistent with inheritance of an autosomal recessive abnormality. With rare exceptions, these latter patients have been presumed or demonstrated to have an abnormality in the methemoglobin reductase activity of their erythrocytes. Their disorder has become known as enzymopenic hereditary methemoglobinemia to differentiate it from the hemoglobin M disorders.

STRUCTURE AND PROPERTIES OF METHEMOGLOBIN

Fully Oxidized Hemoglobin

Methemoglobin is the derivative of hemoglobin obtained by oxidizing the iron of the heme group of deoxyhemoglobin or oxyhemoglobin from the ferrous (Fe^{2+}) state to the ferric (Fe^{3+}) state. For tetrameric hemoglobin, this transformation corresponds to a four-electron loss. Because methemoglobin is incapable of binding molecular oxygen, oxidation of hemoglobin leads to loss of its biologic function and, when carried out to a sufficient extent, leads to pathologic consequences.

Structural and physical studies have established that in methemoglobin, the sixth coordination position of the iron is occupied by a water molecule, whereas this axial position is empty in deoxyhemoglobin and is occupied by O_2 in oxyhemoglobin. The coordinated water molecule of methemoglobin dissociates with a pK of approximately 8 to form a hydroxide ion which remains bound to the iron.[14] Thus, under physiological conditions, methemoglobin is present predominantly as the "aquo" form; the "hydroxy" form becomes more prevalent as the pH is raised.

The differences in valence and axial ligand between ferrous and ferric hemoglobin are the basis for the differences in the chemical, physical, and biologic properties of these forms of the protein. In contrast to ferrous forms of hemoglobin, methemoglobin has a net charge of +1 on the iron atom of each heme moiety, with the consequence that ferrous and ferric forms can be readily separated by electrophoretic techniques. Moreover, the net positive charge on the iron of methemoglobin causes it to bind small anionic ligands such as CN^-, N_3^-, F^-, and Cl^-, but methemoglobin has little affinity for the classic hemoglobin ligands O_2 and CO. The valence and ligand changes that accompany oxidation of hemoglobin also explain the dramatic change in color. In contrast to the bright red color of oxyhemoglobin, aquomethemoglobin is chocolate brown and has absorbance maxima at 500 and 631 nm, and hydroxymethemoglobin is dark red with absorbance maxima at 540 and 575 nm. These spectral differences are responsible for the slate-blue skin color of Caucasian individuals with elevated methemoglobin levels.

X-ray diffraction studies carried out by Perutz and coworkers have established that the protein structure of the tetrameric methemoglobin molecule is very similar to that of the "R-state" conformation of oxyhemoglobin but different from the "T-state" conformation of deoxyhemoglobin.[15] Methemoglobin, like deoxyhemoglobin, binds to polyanionic compounds such as 2,3-diphosphoglycerate (DPG), and the accompanying conformational shift has been termed an "R-to-T-state shift."[16] This binding of polyanions results in changes in physical properties which have been interpreted by some as an increase in the spin state of the hemes.

Valence Hybrids of Hemoglobin

The conversion of tetrameric hemoglobin to tetrameric methemoglobin is a four-step oxidation. Both the oxidation of hemoglobin and the reduction of methemoglobin proceed in sequential one-electron steps, and thus there exist valence hybrids in which one, two, or three hemes are in the ferric form. These valence hybrids, rather than fully oxidized hemoglobin, are central participants in methemoglobin homeostasis. Because the hemoglobin molecule comprises two α chains and two β chains and because each of the two $\alpha\beta$ dimers is relatively stable, eight different valence hybrids should exist (Fig. 180-1). This number of forms can be detected in a partially oxidized sample of hemoglobin under conditions that minimize the interconversion of hybrid forms.[17] However, under physiological conditions that allow for the dissociation of tetramers to $\alpha\beta$ dimers, dimer dissociation, electron exchange, and heme exchange reactions, only two valence hybrids accumulate in appreciable amounts[18,19]; these are the two symmetric forms $(\alpha^+\beta)_2$ and $(\alpha\beta^+)_2$, each of which comprises two identical half-oxidized dimers.

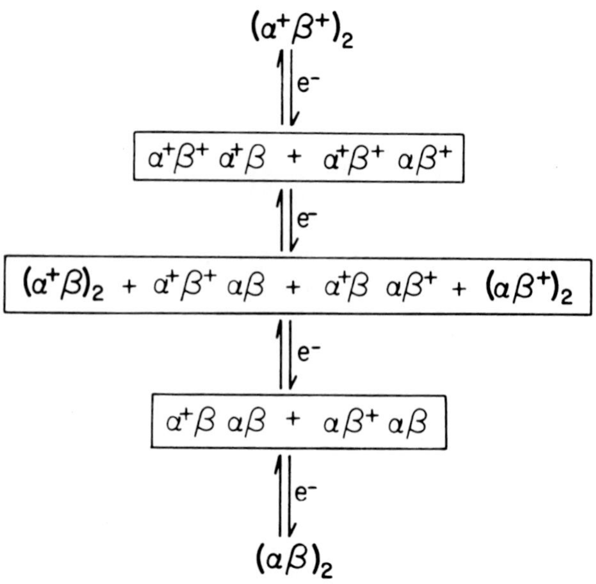

Fig. 180-1 Valence hybrids of hemoglobin A.

The stepwise *oxidation* of hemoglobin subunits, like the stepwise *oxygenation* of hemoglobin, shows cooperativity, has a Bohr (pH) effect, and is influenced by the binding of polyanions (see reviews in references 20 and 21). Both the standard reduction potential (E'_0) and the degree of cooperativity (n, from a Hill plot) depend on pH. The reduction potential is increased by adding polyanions or lowering the pH. Under physiological conditions, tetrameric hemoglobin A shows an $E'_0 = +0.14$ V. In the tetramer, α chains are slightly stronger reductants than the β chains ($E'_0 = +0.12$ and $+0.16$ V, respectively). Valence hybrids of hemoglobin show a greater affinity for oxygen than does hemoglobin.[20,22] This "left shift" of the oxygen saturation curve by ferric subunits has been interpreted as a shifting of the conformational equilibrium of the tetramer to its high-oxygen-affinity R state by the ferric subunits, which themselves are present in an "R-type" conformation.

Throughout this chapter, *methemoglobin* is used in a general sense to include all forms of hemoglobin in which one or more of the subunits are in the ferric form, and *methemoglobinemia* includes those states in which the valence hybrids are elevated in intact, circulating erythrocytes.

METHEMOGLOBIN HOMEOSTASIS

Observations from the nineteenth century demonstrated that methemoglobin can be generated in red blood cells as a consequence either of hereditary disorders or of the ingestion of toxic compounds and that normal red blood cells possess the

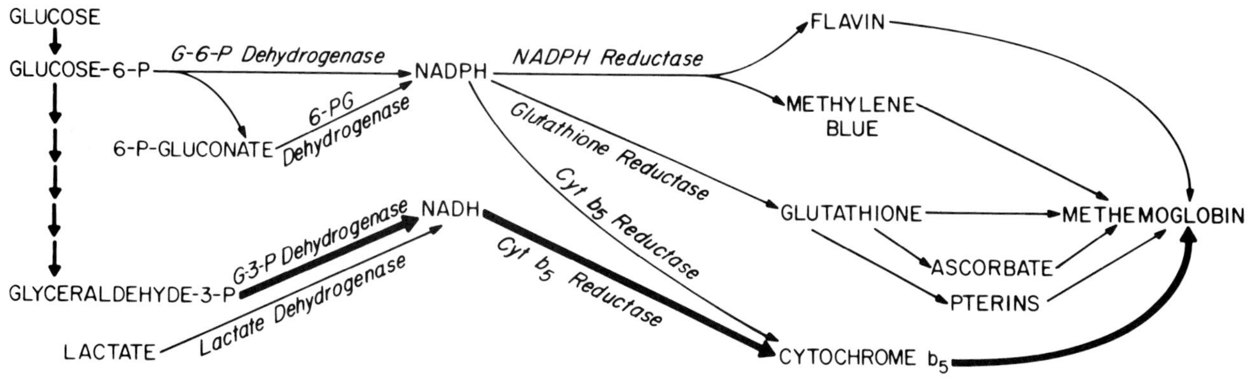

Fig. 180-2 Erythrocyte pathways for the transfer of electrons from metabolites to methemoglobin.

capacity to restore methemoglobin to its functional ferrous form. Subsequent studies have demonstrated that methemoglobin is present at low concentrations in normal human erythrocytes and that both generation and reduction of methemoglobin are normal processes for the erythrocyte.[20,23] Moreover, the evidence that hemoglobin is synthesized in reticulocytes as the ferric form suggests that methemoglobin reduction may be a part of the normal biosynthesis of this hemeprotein.[24]

The steady-state level of methemoglobin in normal erythrocytes is low, with most methods of measurement giving values of less than 1 percent of the total hemoglobin. This finding indicates that the capacity to reduce methemoglobin far exceeds the normal rate of hemoglobin oxidation. In isolated, intact erythrocytes, methemoglobin reduction proceeds at a rate of about 5 percent total hemoglobin per hour (1 μmol hemoglobin subunit per hour per milliliter);[8] the normal rate of hemoglobin oxidation is believed to be 0.02 to 0.12 percent total hemoglobin per hour.

The sustained reduction of methemoglobin in suspensions of intact erythrocytes proceeds only in the presence of a metabolite which can enter the cell and be used in a process that leads to the generation of reduced pyridine nucleotide. Among the substrates that allow for rapid methemoglobin reduction are glucose and a variety of other sugars, lactate, malate, and purine nucleosides such as inosine.[3,23] Studies of the stoichiometry of hemoglobin and pyruvate production in reactions with glucose or lactate as substrate, together with metabolic inhibitor studies, have demonstrated that electrons for methemoglobin reduction are generated primarily by glycolysis and primarily in the form of NADH (Fig. 180-2). However, the rapid methemoglobin reduction that is observed with xylitol and other nonglycolytic substrates[25] suggests that pathways other than glycolysis may be involved with the generation of the NADH used for methemoglobin reduction, at least under conditions where levels of methemoglobin are high.

The steady-state level of methemoglobin is a consequence of all the methemoglobin-reducing reactions (Fig. 180-2) and methemoglobin-generating reactions (Fig. 180-3) in erythrocytes. The major pathway of methemoglobin reduction is catalyzed by erythrocyte cytochrome b_5 reductase and cytochrome b_5; deficiencies of these proteins lead to methemoglobinemia. More difficult to evaluate is the possible role of an erythrocyte NADPH reductase that requires flavin or a redox dye in order to reduce methemoglobin. Likewise, it has been difficult to assess the physiological significance of nonenzymatic reduction reactions, which methemoglobin has been shown to undergo with a number of intracellular compounds. Because methemoglobin reduction proceeds to some extent in red cells severely deficient in cytochrome b_5 reductase activity, the minor pathways, collectively, may be of some importance to the erythrocyte.

A variety of reactions oxidize deoxyhemoglobin and oxyhemoglobin. Among the endogenous compounds that have been identified as reacting with hemoglobin to form methemoglobin are molecular oxygen, hydrogen peroxide (H_2O_2), and a number of free radicals, including superoxide anion ($O_2^{\cdot -}$) and hydroxyl radical ($HO^{\cdot}$). The rate of methemoglobin formation depends on the concentrations of these compounds. The steady state concentrations of these oxidants, in turn, depend on the rates at

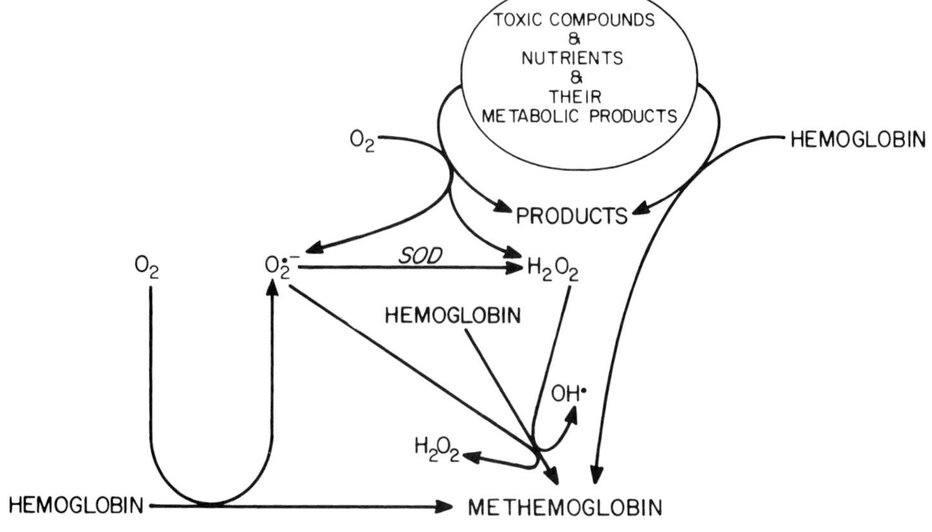

Fig. 180-3 Generation of methemoglobin in erythrocytes.

which they are generated during metabolism, are consumed by reactions with other cellular components, and are destroyed by protective erythrocyte enzymes such as catalase, superoxide dismutase, and glutathione peroxidase.

Elevation of methemoglobin in erythrocytes results either from acceleration of an oxidation reaction or from diminution of a reduction reaction. Such alterations in reaction rates may arise from a hereditary defect or from an environmental stress. The most frequent cause of methemoglobinemia is rapid oxidation arising from ingestion of a toxic compound which either is an oxidant itself or gives rise to oxidants during its metabolism. Methemoglobinemia also arises from rapid autoxidation of a mutant hemoglobin belonging to the hemoglobin M class. Methemoglobinemia due to depressed reduction usually results from deficiency of erythrocyte cytochrome b_5 reductase. A case of methemoglobinemia due to deficiency of cytochrome b_5 has recently been reported.[26] Diminished methemoglobin reduction rates and methemoglobinemia have been observed with hemoglobins $N_{BALTIMORE}$, $I_{TOULOUSE}$, and $M_{MILWAUKEE\text{-}1}$. These mutant hemoglobins presumably fail to interact efficiently with the cytochrome b_5 reductase/cytochrome b_5 system.[27,28] In contrast, methemoglobinemia has not been reported in cases of hereditary hemolytic disorders associated with severe deficiencies of glycolytic enzymes, although an impaired ability to reduce NAD^+ might have been expected to lead to an impaired capacity to reduce methemoglobin, just as inhibition of glycolysis with iodoacetate diminishes methemoglobin reduction.[8]

Methemoglobinemia may also develop if a modest decrease in the ability to reduce methemoglobin is coupled with an environmental stress. The erythrocytes of individuals who are heterozygous for cytochrome b_5 reductase deficiency reduce methemoglobin at approximately 50 percent of the normal rate[29] and are especially susceptible to the methemoglobin-inducing effects of exogenous oxidant agents.[30–32] Similarly, the erythrocytes of newborns have about half the methemoglobin-reducing ability of adults' cells[33,34] and show an increased susceptibility to methemoglobin-producing drugs and chemicals.

OXIDATION OF HEMOGLOBIN

Although the conversion of a ferrous subunit of hemoglobin to the ferric subunit by the removal of an electron can be written as the simplest of chemical reactions, it actually involves a number of complex reactions. In the absence of foreign compounds, much of the oxidation of hemoglobin results from its interaction with O_2 or the partially reduced forms of oxygen, $O_2^{\cdot-}$, H_2O_2, and $HO^{\cdot}$. Following ingestion of foreign compounds, methemoglobin is formed by mechanisms which include direct oxidation by the ingested compound, oxidation by a metabolite derived from the compound, and oxidation by $O_2^{\cdot-}$ and H_2O_2 generated during the metabolism of the compound. The subject of hemoglobin oxidation has been reviewed comprehensively.[21,23,35]

Auto-Oxidation of Hemoglobin

Hemoglobin reacts slowly with molecular oxygen to yield methemoglobin and superoxide anion. The reaction corresponds to the transfer of an electron from the iron of the ferrous heme to molecular oxygen. Because oxyhemoglobin apparently exists as a ferric-superoxide anion complex,[36] auto-oxidation may be visualized as the release of the $O_2^{\cdot-}$ from this complex. Whereas auto-oxidation of free ferrous heme in aqueous solution proceeds very rapidly, the auto-oxidation of hemoglobin is slow. The hydrophobic environment provided by the globin is envisioned as hindering the release of the superoxide anion while allowing rapid release of molecular oxygen. This hypothesis is supported by the observation that mutant hemoglobins in which the heme environment is modified show altered rates of autoxidation. Auto-oxidation is accelerated by chloride and other small anions, which may function by displacing the superoxide anion from the oxyhemoglobin. Polyanions and reduced pH also accelerate the reaction. In tetrameric hemoglobin, the α subunits auto-oxidize more rapidly than the β subunits, with the result that the valence hybrid $(\alpha^+\beta)_2$ is the predominant intermediate in auto-oxidation.[37,38]

The mechanism of auto-oxidation is more complex than the simple release of $O_2^{\cdot-}$ described above. The rate of auto-oxidation increases as the oxygen tension decreases. A maximum rate is achieved when approximately two molecules of oxygen are bound per tetramer.[39] This observation can be interpreted either as evidence that heme is more readily oxidized in deoxyhemoglobin than in oxyhemoglobin or as evidence that $O_2^{\cdot-}$ is more readily released from oxyhemoglobin in the T conformation than in the R conformation. Regardless of the correct mechanism for auto-oxidation, it is clear that the $O_2^{\cdot-}$ generated by auto-oxidation, together with the H_2O_2 and $HO^{\cdot}$ derived from the $O_2^{\cdot-}$, react with hemoglobin to generate additional methemoglobin.

Reactions of Hemoglobin with $O_2^{\cdot-}$ and H_2O_2

$O_2^{\cdot-}$ is generated in erythrocytes not only by the auto-oxidation of hemoglobin but by the auto-oxidation of a number of redox proteins, including cytochrome b_5 and cytochrome b_5 reductase. H_2O_2 is derived from the $O_2^{\cdot-}$ both by a rapid nonenzymatic dismutation reaction and by an even more rapid catalysis of this reaction by superoxide dismutase. H_2O_2 is also an expected end product of oxidase reactions in erythrocytes.

Both $O_2^{\cdot-}$ and H_2O_2 oxidize oxyhemoglobin to methemoglobin. The reaction with $O_2^{\cdot-}$ is a slow one in which the bound molecular oxygen of oxyhemoglobin receives one electron from $O_2^{\cdot-}$ and a second electron from the heme iron:

$$HbFeO_2 + O_2^{\cdot-} + 2H^+ \rightarrow HbFe^+ + H_2O_2 + O_2$$

The overall reaction of H_2O_2 with oxyhemoglobin and deoxyhemoglobin may be written as follows:

$$2HbFeO_2 + H_2O_2 \rightarrow 2HbFe^+ + 2OH^- + 2O_2$$

$$HbFe + H_2O_2 \rightarrow HbFe^+ + OH^- + HO^{\cdot}$$

The highly reactive $HO^{\cdot}$ generated in the latter reaction may react with additional ferrous hemoglobin to form methemoglobin.

The generation of $O_2^{\cdot-}$, H_2O_2, and $HO^{\cdot}$ not only leads to the formation of more methemoglobin but may also promote further oxidation of both the globin and the heme of methemoglobin. One intermediate in this pathway is *hemichrome*, a derivative of methemoglobin in which a functional group of the protein replaces the water molecule bound to the heme. The additional oxidative changes lead to denaturation of the hemoglobin, the formation of intracellular Heinz bodies, and ultimately cell lysis.

The concentrations of $O_2^{\cdot-}$, H_2O_2, and $HO^{\cdot}$ in erythrocytes are normally maintained at low levels by the actions of superoxide dismutase, catalase, and glutathione peroxidase. Superoxide dismutase catalyzes the dismutation of $O_2^{\cdot-}$, catalase the dismutation of H_2O_2, and glutathione peroxidase the reduction of H_2O_2 by reduced glutathione. Because of the relative affinity of catalase and glutathione peroxidase for the substrate H_2O_2, glutathione peroxidase is presumed to be the main agent of the destruction of H_2O_2 under physiological conditions. The ingestion of toxic compounds can lead to rates of $O_2^{\cdot-}$ and H_2O_2 production that overwhelm the protective enzymatic mechanisms.

Oxidation of Hemoglobin by Toxic Compounds

Many drugs, commercial products, other chemical compounds, and metabolic derivatives of such compounds react with hemoglobin to form methemoglobin. If such compounds gain entry into the human circulation, the rate of methemoglobin formation may be several orders of magnitude faster than the rate resulting from the reaction of hemoglobin with oxygen and oxidants generated by normal metabolism. Under such oxidative stress, the erythrocyte methemoglobin reduction systems may be unable to maintain hemoglobin in its functional ferrous form.

The direct reaction of ferrous hemoglobin with various oxidants proceeds with remarkably different reaction rates, reaction mechanisms, preference for α or β chains, and capacity to cause methemoglobinemia. Ferricyanide is an example of an oxidant that accepts one electron from a ferrous heme of hemoglobin. Although this reaction is very rapid, ferricyanide does not lead to methemoglobinemia because it cannot penetrate the red cell membrane. Ferricyanide oxidizes the β subunit somewhat faster than the α subunit, with the result that the $(\alpha\beta^+)_2$ valence hybrid predominates.[40] The reaction of ferricyanide contrasts with that of cupric ion, which exclusively oxidizes the β subunit,[41] and with that of O_2, which favors α-subunit oxidation.

While oxidation of hemoglobin by metal ions results in a valence change of the metal, direct reaction of hemoglobin with organic oxidants yields free radicals. Thus, a variety of oxidant drugs, dyes, and industrial products (including paraquat, menadione, doxorubicin, and methylene blue) react with hemoglobin to form methemoglobin and a free radical; for a quinone, the product is a semiquinone. Many of the free radicals are highly reactive reductants that react with O_2 to form $O_2^{\cdot-}$.

$$R + HbFe \rightarrow HbFe^+ + R^{\cdot-}$$

$$R^{\cdot-} + O_2 \rightarrow R + O_2^{\cdot-}$$

The resulting $O_2^{\cdot-}$ leads to further oxidation of hemoglobin and cell damage. Cell damage may also result from direct reaction with the free radicals.

A number of methemoglobinemia-inducing compounds are reducing rather than oxidizing agents. Nitrites, hydrazines, hydrazides, thiols, phenylenediamines, and aminophenols are among the classes of compounds that oxidize hemoglobin indirectly by reducing O_2 to $O_2^{\cdot-}$, H_2O_2, or $HO^{\cdot}$. With several of these toxic compounds, reduction of O_2 to H_2O_2 proceeds with the bound O_2 of oxyhemoglobin in a reaction analogous to the reaction of oxyhemoglobin with $O_2^{\cdot-}$.

Methemoglobinemia also results from the ingestion of inorganic and organic compounds that are metabolized in vivo to oxidants or reductants that oxidize hemoglobin either directly or indirectly. Nitrate, aniline, and a number of drugs including primaquine, sulfanilamide, dapsone, phenacetin, acetanilide, benzocaine, and phenazopyridine are among the compounds that exert their toxic effects in this manner. Thus, the toxic effect of nitrate in infants arises from its transformation to nitrite in the digestive tract. Likewise, the methemoglobin-forming effect of aniline is dependent on its prior metabolic conversion to phenylhydroxylamine.

REDUCTION OF METHEMOGLOBIN BY MINOR PATHWAYS

Under normal conditions, most of the methemoglobin reduction carried out by the erythrocyte is catalyzed by the cytochrome b_5/cytochrome b_5 reductase system. Only a small fraction of methemoglobin reduction can be attributed to direct reduction of methemoglobin with endogenous reductants in the cell or to catalysis by another methemoglobin reductase system. In individuals with cytochrome b_5 reductase deficiency or in the presence of oxidant stress, these minor pathways may become more important (or even essential) to the cell. These minor pathways also provide the basis for the therapy of methemoglobinemia.

Direct Reaction with Endogenous and Ingested Reductants

Methemoglobin is reduced directly by ascorbic acid, reduced glutathione, reduced flavin, tetrahydropterin, cysteine, cysteamine, and the tryptophan metabolites 3-hydroxyanthranilic acid and 3-hydroxykynurenine.[12,21,23] In order for these endogenous compounds to function in methemoglobin reduction, their reduced forms must be regenerated in the erythrocyte. Indeed, in erythrocytes, reduction of oxidized glutathione is catalyzed by a NADPH-dependent reductase, oxidized ascorbic acid by a glutathione-dependent reductase, and free flavin by a NADPH-dependent reductase, while dihydropterin reacts with reduced glutathione. Under normal conditions, these pathways contribute little to the overall reduction of methemoglobin. The reactions are slow at the concentrations of reductants present in the cell. Methemoglobinemia is not associated with ascorbic acid deficiency (scurvy)[12] or with glutathione deficiency.[42] An increase in the ascorbic acid concentration, however, leads to an increase in the rate of the nonenzymatic reaction between methemoglobin and ascorbic acid both in vitro and in vivo.[6,43] After ingestion of ascorbic acid, the rate of this reaction is sufficiently fast to allow this reductant to be used therapeutically in patients with hereditary methemoglobinemia due to cytochrome b_5 reductase deficiency. Ascorbic acid reduces the β subunit faster than the α subunit, with the result that partial reduction of methemoglobin yields predominantly the $(\alpha^+\beta)_2$ valence hybrid.[44] Polyanions markedly stimulate this reaction.

A number of foreign redox compounds also accelerate the rate of methemoglobin reduction in vitro and in vivo. Methylene blue, Nile blue, and divicine (2,6-diamino-4,5-dihydroxypyrimidine) are among the compounds that are reduced in the erythrocyte and whose reduced forms then reduce methemoglobin directly. Reductions of such foreign redox compounds involve glutathione, cytochrome *b5* reductase, cytochrome b_5, or the NADPH-reductase. The action of many of these reducing agents is complicated by side reactions that alter the amount of H_2O_2 generated.

Role of NADPH-Dependent Reductase of Erythrocytes

A NADPH-dependent reductase present in the cytoplasm of erythrocytes rapidly catalyzes the reduction of methemoglobin, but only in the presence of an electron transfer mediator such as methylene blue or free flavin. By analogy with the erythrocyte NADH-dependent enzyme, this NADPH-dependent enzyme has been variously referred to in the literature as an erythrocyte "dehydrogenase," "reductase," "diaphorase," "methemoglobin reductase," or "ferrihemoglobin reductase." More recently, it has been called "NADPH-flavin reductase." Under normal conditions and in the absence of exogenous redox mediators, the role of this enzyme in methemoglobin reduction is minor, as evidenced by the fact that deficiency of the enzyme does not lead to methemoglobinemia.[45] The extent to which this enzyme catalyzes methemoglobin reduction in cytochrome b_5 reductase deficiency is debatable, but its central role in the treatment of methemoglobinemia is unequivocal.

The studies of Kiese,[23,46] Gibson,[8] and Warburg et al.[47] led to the conclusion that this reductase transferred electrons form NADPH to methylene blue and that the resulting leukomethylene blue then transferred electrons directly to methemoglobin (see Fig. 180-2). Two forms of the NADPH-dependent enzyme with similar properties have been described. Purification procedures have led to increasingly pure enzyme preparations.[23] The enzyme appears to be present in the erythrocyte at nearly 10 μM concentration. The activity does not appear to decline with aging of the cell.

One form of the enzyme has been isolated as a homogeneous protein of 22,000 daltons.[48] The enzyme is unrelated to erythrocyte cytochrome b_5 reductase. Although the isolated protein contains no prosthetic group, it binds FMN or riboflavin and catalyzes either the rapid reduction of these flavins with NADPH as electron donor or a slower reduction with NADH.[49] The resulting reduced form of the flavin rapidly reduces methemoglobin. The β chain is reduced more rapidly than the α chain with the consequence that the $(\alpha^+\beta)_2$ hybrid is an intermediate form.[50] This NADPH-dependent, flavin-mediated pathway (Fig. 180-2) has been presented as a physiological pathway of methemoglobin reduction. The low concentration of flavin in the erythrocyte relative to the K_m values for flavin, however, relegates the pathway to a minor role under normal conditions. When methemoglobin concentration or flavin concentration is high, NADPH-flavin reductase might be expected to play a more significant role.

ERYTHROCYTE CYTOCHROME b_5 REDUCTASE

The early studies of Kiese[46] and Gibson[8] provided the insight that electrons for methemoglobin reduction were transferred from glyceraldehyde-3-phosphate or lactate to NADH by specific dehydrogenases of the glycolytic pathway, and then transferred from NADH to methemoglobin by a reductase (Fig. 180-2). Gibson demonstrated a deficiency of this "methemoglobin reductase" in the red blood cells of two families with idiopathic methemoglobinemia and correctly deduced that this was the basic defect of hereditary methemoglobinemia.

Scott and his colleagues isolated two forms of NADH-dependent reductase from the cytoplasm of normal human erythrocytes and demonstrated that one of these enzymes was absent in an individual with hereditary methemoglobinemia.[51,52] The normal reductase that was deficient in methemoglobinemic individuals rapidly catalyzed the reduction of 2,6-dichlorophenolindophenol (DCIP) and ferricyanide. Further purification of this human erythrocyte reductase has been achieved by Hegesh and Avron,[53] Niethammer and Huennekens,[54] Sugita et al.,[55] Passon and Hultquist,[56] Kuma and Inomata,[57] and Yubisui and Takeshita.[58]

The ability of the enzyme to catalyze the reduction of DCIP and ferricyanide has been used to detect, quantitate, and study the enzyme. These "diaphorase" activities are much faster with NADH than with NADPH as electron donor. In contrast to the very rapid electron transfer to the artificial acceptors, the reductase catalyzes the direct transfer of electrons from NADH to methemoglobin very slowly; the rate of methemoglobin reduction is approximately 0.01 percent of the rate of DCIP reduction. The catalysis of methemoglobin reduction is greatly facilitated by ferricyanide.[59] Ferricyanide is believed to act by transferring electrons between the reductase and methemoglobin.[60] DPG and other polyanionic effectors of hemoglobin stimulate the ferricyanide-facilitated reduction of methemoglobin,[61] suggesting that the T state of methemoglobin is more readily reduced by ferricyanide than is the R state.

The purified reductase is a flavoprotein with a noncovalently bound FAD prosthetic group.[51,56,57] The flavoprotein shows absorbance maxima at 390 and 462 nm and a shoulder at 488 nm. During isolation or storage, the protein may develop electrophoretic heterogeneity owing either to protein alteration or, in the absence of EDTA, to loss of the FAD prosthetic group.

Human erythrocyte cytochrome b_5 reductase is a 32,000-dalton protein comprising a single peptide chain and one FAD residue. Amino acid sequence analysis[62] has recently established that the structure of the enzyme corresponds to the sequence of 275 residues shown in Fig. 180-4. Notable structural features include four cysteine residues and a high content of proline. Although this slightly acidic protein is water soluble, several regions of its peptide chain are highly hydrophobic.

In normal adult human erythrocytes, cytochrome b_5 reductase is present at approximately a 0.1 μM concentration. The mean, standard deviation, and range of reported values vary considerably from laboratory to laboratory and depending on the method of analysis. The more recent studies have shown a standard deviation from the mean of approximately ±15 percent. The reductase activity decreases slowly as erythrocytes age in the circulation, with a half-life of 240 days.[63] Modest changes in the kinetic parameters of the enzyme also occur during aging in vivo.[64] The activity in erythrocytes of cord blood and newborns is normally 50 to 60 percent of the activity in the adult, and activity in the premature infant is even lower. Within a few months of birth, the levels have risen to those of an adult. The reductase activity is very low in individuals homozygous for deficiency of erythrocyte cytochrome b_5 reductase. Individuals heterozygous for the deficiency generally have 50 to 60 percent of normal activity.

In addition to cytoplasmic cytochrome b_5 reductase, erythrocytes contain membrane-bound, NADH-dependent reductase activities.[65,66] One of these activities present in erythrocyte ghosts have been shown to be related to the cytoplasmic cytochrome b_5 reductase.[67–70] This membrane-bound reductase is an integral part of the red cell membrane, and detergent is required to extract it. The detergent-solubilized reductase is a flavoprotein with enzymatic properties indistinguishable from the erythrocyte cytoplasmic cytochrome b_5 reductase. The two forms of the enzyme are immunologically cross-reactive. They appear to be encoded by the same gene, since both enzymes have been reported to be deficient in six patients with enzymopenic hereditary methemoglobinemia.[68] The solubilized membrane reductase differs from the cytoplasmic reductase in that it has a measurably larger molecular weight and undergoes aggregation to form high-molecular-weight forms. Proteolytic digestion of erythrocyte ghosts releases the reductase from the membrane in a lower molecular weight form. This proteolyzed form has full enzymatic activity but does not aggregate.

The fraction of erythrocyte cytochrome b_5 reductase present in the membrane-bound form varies markedly among species. This form represents only 2 percent of the activity of rat erythrocytes, but nearly 100 percent of the activity of bird, reptile, and fish erythrocytes. In the erythrocytes of adult humans, 20 to 35 percent of the activity is bound to the membrane. The erythrocytes of human adults and newborns contain the same level of

```
                5                10                15                20                25
Phe-Gln-Arg-Ser-Thr-Pro-Ala-Ile-Thr-Leu-Glu-Ser-Pro-Asp-Ile-Lys-Tyr-Pro-Leu-Arg-Leu-Ile-Asp-Arg-Glu-
               30                35                40                45                50
Ile-Ile-Ser-His-Asp-Thr-Arg-Arg-Phe-Arg-Phe-Ala-Leu-Pro-Ser-Pro-Gln-His-Ile-Leu-Gly-Leu-Pro-Val-Gly-
               55                60                65                70                75
Gln-His-Ile-Tyr-Leu-Ser-Ala-Arg-Ile-Asp-Gly-Asn-Leu-Val-Val-Arg-Pro-Tyr-Thr-Pro-Ile-Ser-Ser-Asp-Asp-
               80                85                90                95               100
Asp-Lys-Gly-Phe-Val-Asp-Leu-Val-Ile-Lys-Val-Tyr-Phe-Lys-Asp-Thr-His-Pro-Lys-Phe-Pro-Ala-Gly-Gly-Lys-
              105               110               115               120               125
Met-Ser-Gln-Tyr-Leu-Glu-Ser-Met-Gln-Ile-Gly-Asp-Thr-Ile-Glu-Phe-Arg-Gly-Pro-Ser-Gly-Leu-Leu-Val-Tyr-
              130               135               140               145               150
Gln-Gly-Lys-Gly-Lys-Phe-Ala-Ile-Arg-Pro-Asp-Lys-Lys-Ser-Asn-Pro-Ile-Ile-Arg-Thr-Val-Lys-Ser-Val-Gly-
              155               160               165               170               175
Met-Ile-Ala-Gly-Gly-Thr-Gly-Ile-Thr-Pro-Met-Leu-Gln-Val-Ile-Arg-Ala-Ile-Met-Lys-Asp-Pro-Asp-Asp-His-
              180               185               190               195               200
Thr-Val-Cys-His-Leu-Leu-Phe-Ala-Asn-Gln-Thr-Glu-Lys-Asp-Ile-Leu-Leu-Arg-Pro-Glu-Leu-Glu-Glu-Leu-Arg-
              205               210               215               220               225
Asn-Lys-His-Ser-Ala-Arg-Phe-Lys-Leu-Trp-Tyr-Thr-Leu-Asp-Arg-Ala-Pro-Glu-Ala-Trp-Asp-Val-Gly-Gln-Gly-
              230               235               240               245               250
Phe-Val-Asn-Glu-Glu-Met-Ile-Arg-Asp-His-Leu-Pro-Pro-Pro-Glu-Glu-Glu-Pro-Leu-Val-Leu-Met-Cys-Gly-Pro-
              255               260               265               270               275
Pro-Pro-Met-Ile-Gln-Tyr-Ala-Cys-Leu-Pro-Asn-Leu-Asp-His-Val-Gly-His-Pro-Thr-Glu-Arg-Cys-Phe-Val-Phe
```

Fig. 180-4 Primary structure of humane erythrocyte cytochrome b_5 reductase.

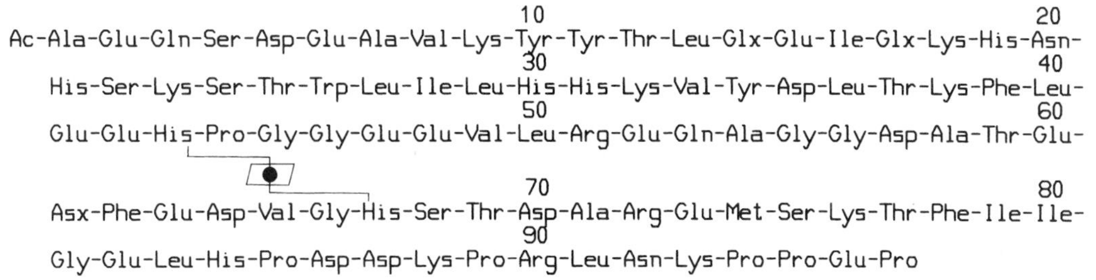

Fig. 180-5 Primary structure of human erythrocyte cytochrome b_5.

membrane-bound cytochrome b_5 reductase, but this form constitutes a larger fraction of the total activity in the newborn because of the lower levels of cytosolic enzyme in such erythrocytes.[69]

ERYTHROCYTE CYTOCHROME b_5

A hemeprotein with spectral properties of cytochrome b_5 and a flavoprotein that catalyzed the reduction of this hemeprotein were detected in the cytoplasm of human erythrocytes in 1969.[71] Erythrocyte cytochrome b_5 at physiological concentrations markedly enhanced the ability of the cytochrome b_5 reductase to catalyze the transfer of electrons from NADH to methemoglobin.[13,72] One major and two minor forms of human erythrocyte cytochrome b_5 have been isolated,[73] and the major form has been purified to homogeneity.[74] Cytochrome b_5 has also been isolated from the cytoplasm of rabbit, mouse, and steer erythrocytes.[73,75–77] Another "*b*-type" cytochrome was isolated from the membrane of human erythrocytes in relatively large amounts, but this "S-protein"[78] did not appear to be structurally or functionally related to erythrocyte cytochrome b_5.

Erythrocyte cytochrome b_5 is a small red protein of approximately 12,000 daltons. It is highly anionic with an isoelectric point of 4.9 and is readily water-soluble. It contains a single protoheme IX prosthetic group, present as a low-spin complex that does not bind carbon monoxide. The hemeprotein, isolated in its ferric state, shows a sharp absorbance maximum at 413 nm. The spectrum of the ferrous form shows sharp maxima at 423, 527, and 556 nm, and a prominent shoulder at 560 nm. The standard reduction potential at pH 7.0 is −2 mV.[79] The ferrous form autoxidizes at a moderate rate.

Erythrocyte cytochrome b_5 comprises 97 amino acid residues in a single peptide chain. No carbohydrate or other nonamino acid groups, other than the heme, are bound to the protein. The protein has a blocked N terminus, which recently has been identified as an *N*-acetylalanine residue.[80] Bovine erythrocyte cytochrome b_5 was the first of these proteins for which it was possible to deduce the amino acid sequence.[81] The sequences have now been deduced for the rabbit,[82] human,[80,83] and pig[80] erythrocyte proteins. The structure of human erythrocyte cytochrome b_5 is shown in Fig. 180-5.

Erythrocyte cytochrome b_5 can be quantitated on the basis of its distinct spectral properties or on the basis of its ability to stimulate the cytochrome b_5 reductase-catalyzed reduction of methemoglobin.[73,79,84–86] Mean values for cytochrome b_5 concentration in erythrocytes range from 0.2 to 0.6 μM. The protein is present in higher concentration in reticulocytes than in erythrocytes. Cytochrome b_5 concentrations decrease both during cell aging in the circulation and during cell storage under blood-bank conditions. The apparent half-life in vivo is 44 days.[63]

RELATIONSHIP BETWEEN THE ERYTHROCYTIC AND MICROSOMAL PROTEINS

The erythrocyte cytochrome is named cytochrome b_5 on the basis of its similarity to microsomal cytochrome b_5. They have identical visible spectra, EPR spectra, prosthetic groups, chemical reactivity at the iron atom, and ability to serve as substrate for cytochrome b_5 reductase.[73] The erythrocyte reductase has been identified as a cytochrome b_5 reductase on the basis of its capacity to catalyze the reduction of cytochrome b_5 and its similarity to microsomal cytochrome b_5 reductase in terms of prosthetic group, substrate specificity, and effects of ionic strength, pH, and EDTA on catalytic activity.[56] The erythrocyte and microsomal proteins differ, however, in that the erythrocyte proteins are smaller, are water soluble, and are located in the cytoplasm rather than the endoplasmic reticulum. These comparisons have led to the suggestion that erythrocyte cytochrome b_5 and cytochrome b_5 reductase correspond to the microsomal proteins without their hydrophobic tails.[56] In liver and other tissues, it is the hydrophobic domains of these proteins that are embedded in the endoplasmic reticulum.

Erythrocyte cytochrome b_5 has been shown to be structurally related to the hydrophilic domain of liver microsomal cytochrome b_5. Trypsin degrades *human* cytochrome b_5 from liver and erythrocytes to electrophoretically identical heme peptides.[74] Likewise, trypsin degrades the 97-residue *bovine* erythrocyte cytochrome b_5 and the 133-residue bovine liver cytochrome b_5 to the same 82-residue heme peptide.[76] The amino acid sequence of the bovine erythrocyte protein corresponds precisely to the sequence of 97 residues starting at the blocked N terminus of the liver protein,[87] with the possible exception that an asparagine residue in the liver is present as an aspartate residue in the erythrocyte. Like the bovine erythrocyte protein, *rabbit* erythrocyte cytochrome b_5 is a 97-residue protein with near identity to residues 1 to 97 of the 133-residue rabbit liver protein. Of the 97 residues, only the one at position 97 differs; it is C-terminal proline in rabbit erythrocyte cytochrome b_5 and threonine in the liver protein.[82] Likewise, *pig* and *human* cytochrome b_5 molecules comprise 97-residue erythrocyte proteins and 133-residue liver microsomal proteins in which there is identity between the first 96 residues but a difference at residue 97.[80] In the pig, residue 97 is serine in erythrocytes and threonine in liver. In humans, residue 97 is proline in erythrocytes (Fig. 180-5) and threonine in liver.

Erythrocyte cytochrome b_5 reductase has been shown to be structurally related to microsomal cytochrome b_5 reductase. The two proteins are immunologically cross-reactive.[67,88,89] They are genetically related, as evidenced by the finding that both erythrocyte cytochrome b_5 reductase and the microsomal enzyme of other tissues are defective in the generalized cytochrome b_5 reductase deficiency of humans.[90] The reductases from bovine erythrocytes and liver are degraded by cathepsin D to electrophoretically identical flavopeptides.[91,92] Nucleotide sequencing of cDNA that codes for human liver cytochrome b_5 reductase has recently established that human erythrocyte cytochrome b_5 reductase is a piece of the liver microsomal cytochrome b_5 reductase.[93] These human liver cDNA sequence data, together with amino acid sequence data for bovine liver cytochrome b_5 reductase, establish that the 275-residue sequence of the human erythrocyte protein corresponds precisely to the 275 residues at the C terminus of the human liver protein. The erythrocyte reductase does not possess the membrane-binding, hydrophobic peptide of approximately 25 residues that is present at the N terminus of the liver reductase.

The structural relationship between the erythrocyte and microsomal proteins led to the proposition that erythrocyte cytochrome b_5 and cytochrome b_5 reductase were derived during erythroid maturation from microsomal precursor proteins.[74,94] This postulate was supported by the finding that an immature erythroid cell line contained only the amphipathic forms of cytochrome b_5 and cytochrome b_5 reductase, whereas mature erythrocytes contained the cytoplasmic forms of these proteins.[77] Moreover, a cathepsin D isolated from a membranous fraction of rabbit reticulocytes was shown to catalyze efficiently the proteolytic removal of the hydrophobic tails of microsomal cytochrome b_5 and cytochrome b_5 reductase without causing cleavage in their hydrophilic domains.[91,95,96] With rabbit liver cytochrome b_5 as substrate, the cathepsin removed peptides sequentially from the C terminus and generated a 98-residue limit heme peptide which was one residue longer than rabbit erythrocyte cytochrome b_5; the extra residue was leucine-98.[82] Similarly, an ATP-dependent protease of rabbit reticulocytes released cytochrome b_5 and cytochrome b_5 reductase as water-soluble proteins from rat liver microsomes.[97] The cytoplasmic form of erythrocyte cytochrome b_5 reductase was postulated by Kaplan and coworkers[70,98] to arise from proteolysis of the reductase that was bound to the erythrocyte membrane. Autoincubation of erythrocyte membranes released a solubilized form of the reductase, a process stimulated by calcium ion.

Thus, acidic, ATP-dependent, and calcium-dependent proteases of reticulocytes are potential candidates for the putative enzyme responsible for converting microsomal proteins of immature erythroid cells to the cytoplasmic forms found in mature erythrocytes. If indeed such a proteolytic event occurs, the processing would be responsible for the conversion of amphiphatic, membrane-bound proteins that function in the desaturation of fatty acids to water-soluble proteins that function to reduce methemoglobin. However, the detection of the structural difference between the two forms of cytochrome b_5 at residue 97 brings into question whether such protein processing actually occurs during erythroid maturation. If it does occur, a form of microsomal cytochrome b_5 distinct from liver microsomal cytochrome b_5 (with a proline residue at position 97) must be present in immature erythroid cells.

THE MECHANISM OF METHEMOGLOBIN REDUCTION BY CYTOCHROME b_5 REDUCTASE AND CYTOCHROME b_5

The marked stimulation of the erythrocyte cytochrome b_5 reductase-catalyzed reduction of methemoglobin by physiological concentrations of erythrocyte cytochrome b_5 led to the postulate that methemoglobin is reduced in vivo by the following sequence of electron transfers:

$$\text{NADH} \xrightarrow{e-} \text{cytochrome } b_5 \text{ reductase} \xrightarrow{3-} \text{cytochrome } b_5 \xrightarrow{e-} \text{methemoglobin}$$

These findings had been anticipated in 1959 by Petragnani and coworkers,[99] who demonstrated that solubilized forms of pig liver cytochrome b_5 reductase and cytochrome b_5 together catalyzed the reduction of methemoglobin. Unaware that cytochrome b_5 or cytochrome b_5 reductase was present in erythrocytes, these workers uncannily suggested that " . . . the erythrocyte methemoglobin reductase may be a similar multienzymatic system. . . . "

The mechanism of this major pathway of methemoglobin reduction has been deduced from studies in many laboratories.[13,51,55–57,79,91,100–105] The rate of methemoglobin reduction in intact cells can be reproduced in crude hemolysates or in systems reconstituted from purified NADH, cytochrome b_5 reductase, cytochrome b_5, and methemoglobin, demonstrating that no additional component plays an essential role in this pathway. Under conditions close to physiological, the rate of methemoglobin reduction is first-order with respect to methemoglobin and cytochrome b_5 reductase and second-order with respect to cytochrome b_5. Thus, methemoglobin reduction proceeds more rapidly when the concentration of methemoglobin is elevated and more slowly when either cytochrome b_5 reductase or cytochrome b_5 is present at less than normal concentration.

The results of the mechanistic studies are compatible with the scheme depicted in Fig. 180-6. After NADH binds to the oxidized flavoprotein (step 1), a pair of electrons is transferred from NADH to FAD (step 2). The reduced flavoprotein sequentially binds and reduces first one and then a second molecule of ferric cytochrome b_5, with the resulting formation of ferrous cytochrome b_5 and oxidized flavoprotein (steps 3 and 4). The generation of a complex between cytochrome b_5 reductase and cytochrome b_5 involves ionic interactions between anionic residues of cytochrome b_5 and cationic residues of cytochrome b_5 reductase. These first four steps are presumably identical with the extensively studied reduction of microsomal cytochrome b_5 catalyzed by microsomal cytochrome b_5 reductase.[106,107]

The reduction of methemoglobin is accomplished by the formation of an ionic complex between ferrous cytochrome b_5 and a ferric subunit of a hemoglobin tetramer (step 5) and the subsequent electron transfer in this complex between the hemes of these proteins (step 6). The cytochrome b_5-methemoglobin complex has been detected by isoelectric focusing[108] and by spectral perturbation of the absorbance spectra.[109,110] The formation of the complex and the transfer of electrons between the proteins of this complex have been separated kinetically.[91,101,103] Computer modeling studies by Poulos and

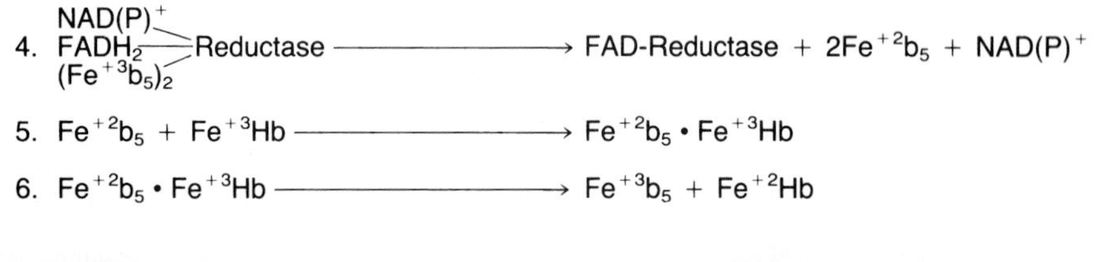
1. NAD(P)H + FAD-Reductase → NAD(P)H / FAD > Reductase
2. NAD(P)H / FAD > Reductase → NAD(P)+ / FADH2 > Reductase
3. NAD(P)+ / FADH2 > Reductase + 2Fe+3 b5 → NAD(P)+ / FADH2 / (Fe+3b5)2 > Reductase
4. NAD(P)+ / FADH2 / (Fe+3b5)2 > Reductase → FAD-Reductase + 2Fe+2b5 + NAD(P)+
5. Fe+2b5 + Fe+3Hb → Fe+2b5 • Fe+3Hb
6. Fe+2b5 • Fe+3Hb → Fe+3b5 + Fe+2Hb

Fig. 180-6 Scheme for the reduction of methemoglobin by cytochrome b_5 reductase and cytochrome b_5.

Mauk[111] suggest that the complex is stabilized by ionic interactions between carboxylate anions on the face of a cytochrome b_5 molecule from which the heme group protrudes and lysyl cations on the face of methemoglobin subunits from which their heme groups protrude. Optimization of four such ionic bonds with the α subunit and five ionic bonds with the β subunit places the interacting hemes in a coplanar orientation, which presumably leads to facile electron transfer. Support for the validity of this model is provided by the observations that mutant hemoglobins in which one of these cationic residues is not present have decreased capacities to be reduced by the cytochrome b_5 reductase/cytochrome b_5 system.[27,28]

The overall rate of methemoglobin reduction in vivo depends on the concentration of the ferrous cytochrome b_5-ferric hemoglobin complex. The interaction between these proteins is weak, and under physiological conditions the concentration of the complex depends on the concentrations of ferrous cytochrome b_5 and methemoglobin. The fraction of cytochrome b_5 present in the ferrous form, in turn, is determined by the concentration of cytochrome b_5 reductase. Complex formation between ferric hemoglobin and cytochrome b_5 appears to be inhibited by ferrous hemoglobin. Complexation proceeds more readily with the R state of methemoglobin than with the T state,[103] and the β subunit of methemoglobin is reduced preferentially in the presence of inositol hexaphosphate.[101] The concentrations of cytochrome b_5 reductase, cytochrome b_5, methemoglobin, and polyanionic effector determine the concentration of the ferrous cytochrome b_5-methemoglobin complex and in this manner determine the rate of methemoglobin reduction in vivo.

The significance of NADPH as an electron donor for this system is debatable. The reduction of cytochrome b_5 reductase (steps 1 and 2) proceeds so much slower in vitro with NADPH than with NADH that the role of NADPH has been assumed to be insignificant. However, the transfer of electrons from reductase to methemoglobin (steps 3 through 6) is rate limiting as a consequence of the very low concentration of cytochrome b_5 in the erythrocyte (far below the K_m of the reductase). In a crude hemolysate or in a system reconstituted from purified cytochrome b_5 reductase and cytochrome b_5, methemoglobin reduction proceeds nearly as rapidly with a saturating level of NADPH as with a saturating level of NADH. Thus, it appears that in vivo steps 1 and 2 are the fast steps in the pathway, even with NADPH as electron donor. This conclusion in not compatible with other studies, which indicate only a minor role for NADPH in methemoglobin reduction.

CLINICAL ASPECTS AND CLASSIFICATION

Subjects with enzymopenic hereditary methemoglobinemia present with persistent slate-gray cyanosis, often dating from birth. A concentration of 1.5 to 2.0 g/dl of methemoglobin (10 to 15 percent of total hemoglobin) produces visible cyanosis, whereas 5 g/dl of deoxygenated hemoglobin is required to produce a comparable degree of cyanosis.[112] In most instances, the patients are really more blue than sick (see, however, type II, below). They lack evidence of cardiac or pulmonary disease. Significant erythrocytosis is observed only occasionally, and the oxygen dissociation curve is normal or shifted only slightly to the left.[3] The absence of manifestations of anoxia may be due to differences in the proportions of valence hybrids in the erythrocytes.[20,22] Hardly any systemic symptoms are reported when the methemoglobin level is 25 percent or less, except for the subjects' odd "cyanotic" appearance. Even with levels up to 40 percent, the only complaints may be headache, easy fatigue, and exertional dyspnea. Life expectancy is normal, and pregnancies are not compromised. The methemoglobinemia is quite well tolerated, and may be readily controlled with appropriate therapy.

Recently, a clinical-biochemical classification of enzymopenic hereditary methemoglobinemia has been proposed on the basis of important differences in the pathophysiology of the disorder.[113]

Type I Enzymopenic Hereditary Methemoglobinemia (Erythrocyte Reductase Deficiency)

Most patients appear to have type I, the classic syndrome with the signs and symptoms described above, that has been extensively studied since the pioneering investigations of Gibson[8] and Scott and Griffith.[9] The subjects have methemoglobinemia alone because the deficiency of cytochrome b_5 reductase is limited to the erythrocytes. Their erythrocytes' metabolic machinery is otherwise intact, so there is no hemolysis.

Type II Enzymopenic Hereditary Methemoglobinemia (Generalized Reductase Deficiency)

A much more severe and lethal disorder occurs in perhaps 10 to 15 percent of patients with enzymopenic hereditary methemoglobinemia; it is referred to as "type II." In addition to methemoglobinemia, signs of a progressive neurologic abnormality become apparent before age 1 year and may be observed even at birth. The association of these two aberrations was described in 1953.[114] The fully expressed syndrome is characterized by severe mental retardation, microcephaly, retarded growth, opisthotonus, attacks of bilateral athetoid movements, strabismus, and generalized hypertonia.[12,29] Death usually supervenes soon. Pathologic examinations of the brains of three sibs with this disorder have revealed only nonspecific alterations, including reduced numbers of nerve elements and retarded myelinization.[29] Not only is the activity of cytochrome b_5 reductase markedly reduced in the patients' erythrocytes, but nearly total deficiency of microsomal cytochrome b_5 reductase is demonstrable in their leukocytes, muscle, liver, fibroblasts, and brain.[90,115,116] Because the microsomal cytochrome b_5/cytochrome b_5 reductase system participates in other tissues in the desaturation of fatty acids, it has been suggested that impairment of fatty acid desaturation, especially in the central nervous system, may account for the generalized systemic manifestations.[90] Lipid analyses of tissues from a child with the type II disorder have revealed decreased cerebroside (48 percent of normal) in the white matter of the brain,[117] decreased linoleic acid and increased palmitic acid in adipose tissue, decreased proportions of unsaturated fatty acids in the ethanolamine phosphoglycerides of the liver, and less than half of normal concentrations of linoleic acid in the ethanolamine phosphoglycerides of the liver, kidney, and spleen.[118] Cholesterol and lipid phosphorus concentrations, however, were normal in the liver, kidney, spleen, muscle, and adrenals. Thus, the effect of the generalized cytochrome b_5 reductase deficiency was unexpectedly slight but the reduction in cerebroside content might have caused a decrease in myelination, leading to mental retardation.[118] The generalized deficiency of cytochrome b_5 reductase activity in patients with type II, as well as in their fetal amniotic cells, has made antenatal diagnosis feasible.[119]

Type III Enzymopenic Hereditary Methemoglobinemia (Hematopoietic Reductase Deficiency)

In addition to a German family reported only in an abstract,[120] a detailed study of a Japanese family has provided evidence for the occurrence of enzymopenic hereditary methemoglobinemia without neurologic involvement but with cytochrome b_5 reductase deficiency demonstrable in erythrocytes, platelets, lymphocytes, and granulocytes.[121] The enzyme stained normally in the two male sibs' hair root and buccal cells. The only clinical manifestations were their cyanotic appearance with methemoglobin concentrations of about 25 percent. These reports have made it necessary to exercise caution in drawing conclusions from assays of cytochrome b_5 reductase activities in detergent-treated leukocytes, the procedure advocated for making the diagnosis of the generalized type II disorder in infants younger than 1 year old or in newborns.

Type IV Enzymopenic Hereditary Methemoglobinemia (Cytochrome b_5 Deficiency) (MIM 250790)

The discovery of a patient with long-standing methemoglobinemic cyanosis (methemoglobin concentrations 12 to 19 percent) associated with an erythrocyte cytochrome b_5 concentration about 23 percent of normal has completed the current roster of pathophysiological mechanisms for this disorder.[26] This observation has provided direct evidence for the physiological role of cytochrome b_5 in the reduction of methemoglobin to hemoglobin in vivo in human erythrocytes. The precise nature of this currently unique abnormality remains to be defined.

THE GENETICS OF CYTOCHROME b_5 REDUCTASE

The gene coding for soluble NADH-cytochrome b_5 reductase has been assigned to chromosome 22. This assignment is based on studies of the electrophoretic mobility and isoelectric focusing patterns of soluble enzyme in the cytosol of rodent-human fibroblast hybrids and concurrent cytogenetic analyses.[122,123] The same gene is assumed to code for the full length of the microsomal enzyme polypeptide chain (i.e., polar plus membrane segments).

The diaphorase activity of cytochrome b_5 reductase has been exploited to permit its visualization after electrophoresis of hemolysates or tissue extracts on starch or polyacrylamide gels.[12,124] A survey of 2783 healthy subjects has revealed five electrophoretic phenotypes with normal staining intensity and suggests an incidence of variants of about 1 in 100.[125] Studies of patients with enzymopenic hereditary methemoglobinemia have disclosed at least 14 different phenotypes, based on electrophoretic mobility and/or kinetic aberrations.[12,126] Thus, the mutations causing reductase deficiency are heterogeneous, with several different mutant alleles occurring at the reductase locus. The molecular basis of these mutations is as yet unknown.

An unusually high incidence of enzymopenic hereditary methemoglobinemia is reported among Alaskan Eskimos and Indians, Navajo Indians, Puerto Ricans, people of Mediterranean origins, and natives of the Yakutsk region of Siberia, 1000 miles west of the Bering Sea.[12]

Type I, uncomplicated, benign enzymopenic hereditary methemoglobinemia is attributable to mutations that affect the catalytic activity or stability of the enzyme in the erythrocytes. Clinically affected subjects are homozygous or genetic compounds for cytochrome b_5 reductase deficiency. Exaggerated lability characterizes at least five enzyme variants.[127,128] The role of altered proteolytic processes in erythrocyte precursors in enzymopenic hereditary methemoglobinemia remains to be defined.[129] The asymptomatic heterozygote may have an increased tendency to develop toxic methemoglobinemia on exposure to methemoglobin-inducing drugs or chemicals, such as malaria chemoprophylaxis,[30] phenazopyridine administration,[32] or the "recreational" sniffing of volatile nitrites.[130]

Type II, severe, lethal enzymopenic hereditary methemoglobinemia is a generalized disorder with defective cytochrome b_5 reductase in all tissues. This disorder is presumed to result from mutation(s) that affect the enzyme's activity, thermal stability, or resistance to proteolysis in all tissues.

The apparently rather benign type III disorder may simply be a variant of type II in that the enzyme is altered by selective activity of proteolytic enzymes only in the hematopoietic tissues.[121,129] On the other hand, it may represent a catalytically less significant mutation affecting cytochrome b_5 reductase, analogous to the variants observed in glucose 6-phosphate dehydrogenase deficiency.

The type IV disorder is a deficiency of cytochrome b_5 alone; the activity of cytochrome b_5 reductase is normal.[26] The concentration of cytochrome b_5 is normal in the erythrocytes of the parents and sibs of the only known patient with this form of hereditary methemoglobinemia. The genetics of cytochrome b_5 deficiency, therefore, remain to be determined.

DIAGNOSIS OF CYTOCHROME b_5 REDUCTASE DEFICIENCY

Blood with more than about 10 percent methemoglobin appears unusually dark red or even brown. It does not become bright red upon vigorous shaking with air, and it leaves a dark reddish brown stain on white filter paper or a white laboratory coat. The presence of methemoglobin may be established by the characteristic absorption spectrum of a clear, stroma-free hemolysate with peaks at 500 and 631 nm at an acid pH.[126] The latter peak should disappear promptly after the addition of a neutralized cyanide solution.

If the spectrum in the 600- to 640-nm region is atypical and the peak near 631 nm is shifted toward a lower wavelength and does not change significantly or quickly on the addition of cyanide, hemoglobin M should be suspected. A hemoglobin M should also be suspected if there is a family history of apparent parent-to-child transmission of longstanding, unexplained cyanosis. Electrophoresis of the methemoglobin form and amino acid analysis of the globin are required for the confirmation of the diagnosis of a hemoglobin M.

Congenital cyanosis in sibs, especially with a history of consanguinity, is suggestive of enzymopenic hereditary methemoglobinemia. Presumptive evidence for cytochrome b_5 reductase deficiency may be obtained by comparing the rate of reduction of methemoglobin in a patient's nitrite-treated, washed erythrocytes incubated with glucose or other substrates before and after the addition of methylene blue with the rate observed with cells from a normal subject.[12] Reductase deficiency may be confirmed by direct assay for NADH-diaphorase,[10] NADH-methemoglobin-ferrocyanide reductase,[131] cytochrome b_5 reductase,[56] or NADH-ferricyanide reductase[132] activity in hemolysates of the patient's erythrocytes. Assay of NADH-ferricyanide reductase activity has been advocated as the simplest because of the ready availability of the substrate potassium ferricyanide. A rapid screening spot test for NADH-diaphorase deficiency has also been described.[133]

TREATMENT OF CYTOCHROME b_5 REDUCTASE DEFICIENCY

Because subjects with type I cytochrome b_5 reductase deficiency have only mild symptoms from the methemoglobinemia, therapy is mainly cosmetic. It may be indicated, however, for psychological reasons. A single dose of methylene blue, 1 mg/kg intravenously, will rapidly reduce the methemoglobin concentration to normal, provided that the subject is not glucose 6-phosphate dehydrogenase-deficient, since the methylene blue-stimulated NADPH-methemoglobin reductase system requires the reduction of $NADP^+$. Methylene blue has been reported to cause urinary tract irritation and, of course, makes the urine blue or bright green. Oral ascorbic acid, 500 to 1000 mg daily, can maintain the methemoglobin concentration at acceptable levels, but its prolonged administration may be responsible for hyperoxaluria and renal stone formation. Oral riboflavin, 20 to 60 mg daily, has been reported to be as effective as ascorbic acid in keeping the methemoglobin level at about 5 percent.[134] These therapeutic agents would also be expected to be effective in patients with the type III and type IV disorders. Although methylene blue will control the methemoglobinemia in the type II disorder, it has had no effect on the progressive neurologic dysfunction.

ADDENDUM

David Valle

Since the appearance of the sixth edition of this text there has been a limited number of publications on the hereditary methemoglobinemias including a concise review.[135] Most of the reports have been on the molecular biology and genetic defects of cytochrome b_5 reductase. What follows is a summary of this recent work.

Clinical

A patient with type I methemoglobinemia who was started on methylene blue, 150 mg/day at age 18, developed carcinoma *in situ* of the bladder at age 47 (Jaffe, personal communication, 1993). Dusky cyanosis recurred with cessation of therapy. The relationship of the methylene blue therapy to the carcinoma, if any, is uncertain.

Yawata and colleagues reported an interesting Japanese male with type II methemoglobinemia whose clinical phenotype included short stature, deformation of both small and large joints, cyanosis, and mild mental retardation.[136] Partial deficiency of cytochrome b_5 reductase was demonstrated in red cells, platelets, lymphocytes, and cultured skin fibroblasts. The molecular defect(s) was not described.

In an important paper, Nagai et al. reevaluated the standard classification of hereditary methemoglobinemia phenotypes into types I to III.[137] They pointed out that earlier assays of NADH-reductase activity used artificial electron acceptors, such as 2,6-dichloroindophenol, which give high background activity, making it difficult to detect mild reductions in b_5 reductase activity in nonerythyroid cells. Recent assays by the authors and others utilizing cytochrome b_5 as the electron acceptor showed a decrease in b_5 reductase activity in platelets and leukocytes as well as in the erythrocytes of patients with type I. This result suggested that the separation of types I and III methemoglobinemia was based on an artifact caused by the way b_5 reductase activity was assayed in the past. Furthermore, Nagai et al. reevaluated the best characterized type III patient using a cytochrome b_5-based assay, and found lymphocyte and platelet b_5 reductase activities in the range of those of patients with type I methemoglobinemia. The authors conclude that it now seems "unnecessary" to have a type III category for the classification of hereditary methemoglobinemia phenotypes.

Cytochrome b_5 reductase activity is reduced ($\sim$65 percent of normal) in the erythrocytes of extremely low-birth-weight infants (birth weight < 1000 g) as compared to adults.[153]

Biochemistry

Mutagenesis studies of bovine and human cytochrome b_5 reductase have investigated the roles of specific residues in the catalytic function of the enzyme. Lysine-110 appears to be involved in the interactions of the enzyme with NADH,[138] as does the nearby serine-127.[139] The latter residue was investigated when it was found to be involved in a naturally occurring mutation (see below). Cysteines-273 and 283 also appear to interact with the NADH binding site but are not essential for catalytic function.[140]

The interaction of b_5 reductase with cytochrome b involves electrostatic interactions between positive residues in the reductase with negatively charged residues in the cytochrome. Mutagenesis studies of the human genes implicate lysine residues at positions 41, 125, 162, and 163 in the reductase and Glu41, Glu42, Asp57, and Glu63 in the cytochrome.[140a] The latter residues are located around the heme of the cytochrome.

Additional studies implicate Glu44 and Glu56 of the cytochrome in electrostatic interactions between cytochrome b_5 and cytochrome c.[140b]

NADPH-dependent methemoglobin reductase has been reviewed and compared to NADH-dependent b_5 reductase.[141] Under normal circumstances the former plays no role in methemoglobin reduction but does contribute when the latter is deficient (see also "A Cytochrome b-Type NADPH Oxidoreductase" below).

Molecular Genetics

Biochemical studies described in the foregoing chapter had shown two forms of NADH-cytochrome b_5 reductase: a 34-kDa myristylated, membrane-associated enzyme found in hepatocytes and other cells, and involved in the desaturation and elongation of fatty acids; and a soluble, 31-kDa erythrocyte enzyme crucial for methemoglobin reduction. The question of how these two forms of the enzyme are generated required molecular studies of the b_5 reductase gene to be answered.

Human, rat, and bovine liver, and human placental NADH-cytochrome b_5 reductase cDNAs have been cloned[141–144] and alignments described.[143] The human liver cDNA has a 903-bp open-reading frame predicting a protein of 301 residues. The N-terminal methionine is followed by a myristylation consensus sequence (G-X-X-X-S/T), which, together with the observation that the bovine enzyme is myristylated, suggests that the human enzyme also undergoes cotranslational myristylation. As in the bovine enzyme, there is an N-terminal hydrophobic domain of 14 amino acids (residues 11 to 24 of the primary translation product). This domain and the myristyl moiety form an anchor that tethers nonerythrocyte b_5 reductase to the outer mitochondrial membrane and the membrane of the endoplasmic reticulum. Borgese et al. showed that myristolation of b_5 reductase has a role in both targeting and membrane-anchoring of the protein.[144a] Similarly, the hydrophobic C-terminal of cytochrome b_5 appears to be involved in localization to the membrane of the endoplasmic reticulum.[144b] The sequence of the C-terminal 275 residues of the protein predicted by the liver cDNA coincides perfectly with the complete sequence of the enzyme purified from erythrocytes,[142] in agreement with the notion that one gene encodes both forms of the enzyme.

The organization of the NADH-cytochrome b_5 reductase gene has been determined in rats[143] and humans.[145] The human gene is about 31 kb in length and initially was thought to contain 9 exons. The translational start site is in exon 1 and exon 2 encodes the junction of the hydrophobic membrane binding domain with the downstream catalytic portion of the protein. The promoter region resembles that of a constitutively expressed gene in that it lacks a TATAA box, has five GC box elements (GGGCGG), and is, overall, very GC rich (86 percent).[145] Primer extension experiments indicate multiple transcription start sites. The promoter of the rat gene has a similar organization.[143] In both species, the mature mRNA produced by the b_5 reductase gene is $\sim$2.0 kb in length.

To investigate the origin of the erythrocyte form of the enzyme, Pietrini and colleagues compared b_5 reductase cDNAs cloned from rat reticulocyte and liver cDNA libraries.[144] They showed that b_5 reductase cDNAs isolated from reticulocytes (R-cDNA) differed from those isolated from liver (L-cDNA) in the 5′ noncoding and early coding region where the 7 codons specifying the myristylation consensus sequence of the liver protein were replaced by an erythrocyte-specific sequence of 13 noncharged amino acids. This observation lead them to reexamine the gene structure looking in particular for sequences corresponding to the 5′ end of the R-cDNA. Ultimately, they found that the rat b_5 reductase gene has two promoters: an upstream constitutive GC-rich promoter responsible for the ubiquitous or liver transcript, and a downstream, erythroid-specific promoter with TATAA and GATA boxes located in what was previously considered to be intron 1 (see Fig. 180-7). The upstream promoter drives expression of a transcript that originates in exon 1, which encodes the N-terminal 25 amino acids, including the myristylation consensus sequence, and splices to exon 3. The downstream promoter directs expression of a transcript originating in the newly recognized exon 2 and encodes two erythrocyte-specific forms of the enzyme that differ at their N-terminal due to alternative translation start sites in the erythrocyte-specific message. The quantitatively minor translation product has 307 amino acids and includes a sequence of 13 noncharged N-terminal residues that is found only in this form of the erythrocyte enzyme. The quantitatively major erythrocyte translation product starts from an internal methionine that corresponds to methionine-24 of the liver transcript and methionine-30 of the longer erythrocyte protein (see Fig. 180-7).

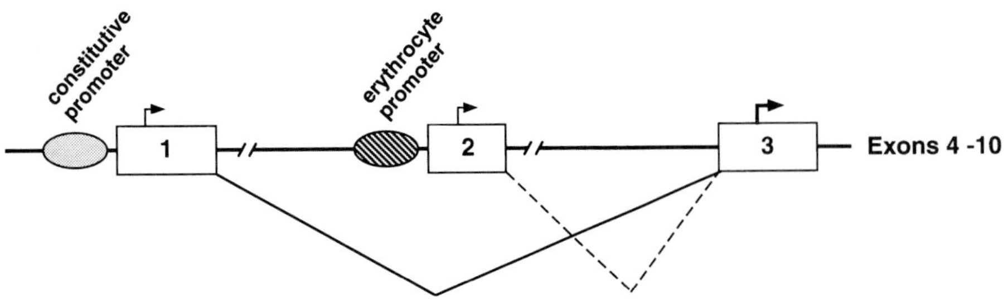

Fig. 180-7 The b_5 reductase gene structure at the 5′ end. The gene has two promoters, one upstream for the ubiquitous (liver) transcript, the other downstream for erythroid cell-specific transcript. The upstream promoter is GC-rich, the downstream promoter has TATAA and GATA boxes. See Addendum text for details.

This methionine is two residues upstream of the phenylalanine which is the N-terminal residue of the mature soluble erythrocyte protein. Thus, in rats, and presumably in humans, a combination of transcriptional and translational mechanisms produce, from one gene, three forms of NADH-cytochrome b_5 reductase differing at their N-terminals. These include a widely expressed membrane-bound protein of 301 residues (processed to 300 residues coincident with myristylation), an erythrocyte-specific, presumptive membrane-associated minor form of 307 residues, and an erythrocyte-specific soluble form of 275 residues. The latter is entirely contained within the C-terminal 275 residues of the former two.

Interestingly, consideration of the structure and function of the b_5 reductase gene predicts that mutations affecting the constitutive promoter and/or exon 1 and leaving the erythrocyte promoter and downstream exons intact will produce an autosomal recessive neurologic phenotype without accompanying methemoglobinemia. No such examples have been recognized to date.

Genetic Variants

Six missense mutations have been described in the NADH-cytochrome b_5 reductase gene in patients with types I to III hereditary methemoglobinemia (see Table 180-1). Thus, allelic heterogeneity is sufficient to account for the phenotypic differences of the various types of the disorder. Mutations that reduce stability and leave catalytic function intact mainly cause a problem in the erythrocyte that depends on enzymes synthesized in the reticulocyte persisting for the ~120-day life span of the enucleate red cell.[146] Conversely, mutations that markedly reduce catalytic function cause problems in all cells expressing cytochrome b_5 reductase and result in the type II phenotype. Presumably, the neurologic involvement derives from loss of the fatty acid desaturation and elongation function, whereas the cyanosis results from an inability to reduce methemoglobin to hemoglobin.

In their studies of methemoglobinemia, Jenkins and Prchal identified an apparently functionally neutral missense mutation, T116S (347C > G), at polymorphic frequency in African-American populations.[149] In subsequent studies they found a T116S allele frequency of 0.23 in African-Americans. The allele was not detected in Caucasian, Asian, Indo-Aryan, and Arabic chromosomes.[150] It would be interesting to determine whether the T116S polymorphism plays any role in the modest, but statistically significant, difference in mean erythrocyte b_5 reductase activity between American Caucasians and African-Americans (3.19 vs. 2.89 IU/gHb, respectively, $p = 0.03$).[151]

A Cytochrome *b*-Type NADPH Oxidoreductase

Using consensus sequences for NADPH and flavin binding sites to screen dbEST, Bunn and colleagues identified a ubiquitiously expressed NADPH-dependent homolog of b_5 reductase.[152] The full-length (~2.4 kb) human transcript (GenBank AF169803) encodes a 487-amino-acid fusion protein (designated "b5+b5R") with an N-terminal domain homologous to cytochrome b_5 and a C-terminal domain homologous to b_5 reductase separated by a "hinge-region" of about 100 amino acids. The hinge-region has no counterpart in b_5 reductase or cytochrome b_5. There is no membrane-anchoring structure; that is, neither a membrane-spanning domain nor a myristylation site. Expression studies

Table 180-1 Missense and Nonsense Mutations Described in Patients with Hereditary Methemoglobinemia

N	Allele*	Phenotype	Pedigrees	Ethnic origin	Nucleotide change†	Comment	Reference
1	S128P	II	1	Japanese	382 T>C	Unstable	139, 147
2	R58Q	I	3	Japanese	173 G>A	Mutant enzyme has 62% of normal activity but is unstable	146
3	L149P	I	1	Japanese	446 T>C	Patient previously classified as type III mutant enzyme has 60% of normal activity but is unstable	137, 148
4	V106M	I	1	Italian	316 G>A	Mutant enzyme has 77% of normal activity but is unstable	146
5	Q213K	I	1	African-American	637 G>A	Unstable, b5R-Shreveport	149
6	Y43X	II	1	Northern European	129 C>A	Truncated, inactive	154
7	P96H	II	1	Northern European	287 C>A	Alters a residue in the FAD binding domain	154
8	Q77X	II	1	Hindoostani Surinese	229 C>T	Severe deficiency	155
9	R160X	II	1	Hindoostani Surinese	478 C>T	Severe deficiency	155

*By convention, codons are numbered based on the amino acid sequence of the mature membrane-bound constitute or liver enzyme with the initiation methionine removed; that is, codon 1 refers to the N-terminal glycine of the mature myristylated enzyme. For reference, the N-terminal amino acid of the soluble erythrocyte enzyme is Phe-26.

†The A of the initiation methionine codon equals +1.

showed that the b5+b5R protein is cytosolic and can be reduced by NADPH. The authors suggest that this enzyme plays a role in the respiratory burst that takes place in mammalian neutrophils and macrophages when they engulf microbes. They also speculate that the protein could function as an oxygen sensor.

REFERENCES

1. François: Cas de cyanose congeniale sans cause apparente. *Bull Acad Roy Med Belg* **4**:698, 1845.
2. Dittrich P: Ueber methamoglobinbildende Gifte. *Naunyn-Schmiedeberg's Arch Exp Pathol Pharmacol* **29**:247, 1891.
3. Jaffe ER: Hereditary methemoglobinemias associated with abnormalities in the metabolism of erythrocytes. *Am J Med* **41**:786, 1966.
4. van den Bergh AAH: Enterogene cyanose. *Dtsch Arch Klin Med* **83**:86, 1905.
5. Hitzenberger K: Autotoxische zyanose (intraglobulare methamoglobinamie). *Wien Arch Inn Med* **23**:85, 1932.
6. Gibson QH: The reduction of methaemoglobin by ascorbic acid. *Biochem J* **37**:615, 1943.
7. Barcroft H, Gibson QH, Harrison DC, McMurray J: Familial idiopathic methaemoglobinaemia and its treatment with ascorbic acid. *Clin Sci* **5**:145, 1945.
8. Gibson QH: The reduction of methaemoglobin in red blood cells and studies on the cause of idiopathic methaemoglobinaemia. *Biochem J* **42**:13, 1948.
9. Scott EM, Griffith IV: The enzymic defect of hereditary methemoglobinemia: Diaphorase. *Biochim Biophys Acta* **34**:584, 1959.
10. Scott EM: The relation of diaphorase of human erythrocytes to inheritance of methemoglobinemia. *J Clin Invest* **39**:1176, 1960.
11. Balsamo P, Hardy WR, Scott EM: Hereditary methemoglobinemia due to diaphorase deficiency in Navajo Indians. *J Pediatr* **65**:928, 1964.
12. Schwartz JM, Reiss AL, Jaffe ER: Hereditary methemoglobinemia with deficiency of NADH cytochrome b_5 reductase, in Stanbury JB, Wyngaarden JB, Fredrickson DS, Goldstein JL, Brown MS (eds): *The Metabolic Basis of Inherited Disease*, 5th ed. New York, McGraw-Hill, 1983, p 1654.
13. Hultquist DE, Passon PG: Catalysis of methaemoglobin reduction by erythrocyte cytochrome b_5 and cytochrome b_5 reductase. *Nature* **229**:252, 1971.
14. Haurowitz F: Zur chemie des blutfarbstoffes; zur kenntnis das methamoglobins und seiner derivative. *Z Physiol Chem* **138**:68, 1924.
15. Ladner RC, Heidner EJ, Perutz MF: The structure of horse methaemoglobin at 2.0 Å resolution. *J Mol Biol* **114**:385, 1977.
16. Perutz MF, Fersht AR, Simon SR, Roberts GCK: Influence of globin structure on the state of the heme. II. Allosteric transitions in methemoglobin. *Biochemistry* **13**:2174, 1974.
17. Perrella M, Cremonesi L, Benazzi L, Rossi-Bernardi L: Isolation of intermediate valence hybrids between ferrous and methemoglobin at subzero temperatures. *J Biol Chem* **256**:11098, 1981.
18. Itano HA, Robinson E: Electrophoretic separation of intermediate compounds in two reactions of ferrihemoglobin. *Biochim Biophys Acta* **29**:545, 1958.
19. Bunn HF, Drysdale JW: The separation of partially oxidized hemoglobins. *Biochim Biophys Acta* **229**:51, 1971.
20. Bodansky O: Methemoglobinemia and methemoglobin-producing compounds. *Pharmacol Rev* **3**:144, 1951.
21. Bunn HF, Forget BG: *Hemoglobin: Molecular, Genetic, and Clinical Aspects*. Philadelphia, WB Saunders, 1986, p 638.
22. Darling RC, Roughton FJW: The effect of methemoglobin on the equilibrium between oxygen and hemoglobin. *Am J Physiol* **137**:56, 1942.
23. Kiese M: *Methemoglobinemia: A Comprehensive Treatise*. Cleveland, CRC Press, 1974.
24. Schulman HM, Martinez-Medellin J, Sidloi R: The oxidation state of newly synthesized hemoglobin. *Biochem Biophys Res Commun* **56**:220, 1974.
25. Asakura T, Adachi K, Minakami S, Yoshikawa H: Non-glycolytic sugar metabolism in human erythrocytes. I. Xylitol metabolism. *J Biochem (Tokyo)* **62**:184, 1967.
26. Hegesh E, Hegesh J, Kaftory A: Congenital methemoglobinemia with a deficiency of cytochrome b_5. *N Engl J Med* **314**:757, 1986.
27. Nagai M, Yubisui T, Yoneyama Y: Enzymatic reduction of hemoglobins M Milwaukee-1 and M Saskatoon by NADH-cytochrome b_5 reductase and NADPH-flavin reductase purified from human erythrocytes. *J Biol Chem* **255**:4599, 1980.
28. Gacon G, Lostanlen D, Labie D, Kaplan J-C: Interaction between cytochrome b_5 and hemoglobin: Involvement of β66 (E10) and β95 (FG2) lysyl residues of hemoglobin. *Proc Natl Acad Sci U S A* **77**:1917, 1980.
29. Jaffe ER, Neumann G, Rothberg H, Wilson FT, Webster RM, Wolff JA: Hereditary methemoglobinemia with and without mental retardation: A study of three families. *Am J Med* **41**:42, 1966.
30. Cohen RJ, Sachs JR, Wicker DJ, Conrad ME: Methemoglobinemia provoked by malarial chemoprophylaxis in Vietnam. *N Engl J Med* **279**:1127, 1968.
31. Horne MK, Waterman MR, Simon LM, Garriott JC, Foerster EH: Methemoglobinemia from sniffing butyl nitrite. *Ann Intern Med* **91**:417, 1979.
32. Daly JS, Hultquist DE, Rucknagel DL: Phenazopyridine induced methaemoglobinaemia associated with decreased activity of erythrocyte cytochrome b_5 reductase. *J Med Genet* **20**:307, 1983.
33. Ross JD: Deficient activity of DPNH-dependent methemoglobin diaphorase in cord blood erythrocytes. *Blood* **21**:51, 1963.
34. Kanazawa Y, Hattori M, Kosaka K, Nakao K: The relationship of NADH-dependent diaphorase activity and methemoglobin reduction in human erythrocytes. *Clin Chim Acta* **19**:524, 1968.
35. Winterbourn CC: Free-radical production and oxidative reactions of hemoglobin. *Environ Health Perspect* **64**:321, 1985.
36. Wittenberg JB, Wittenberg BA, Peisach J, Blumberg WE: On the state of the iron and the nature of the ligand in oxyhemoglobin. *Proc Natl Acad Sci U S A* **67**:1846, 1970.
37. Mansouri A, Winterhalter KH: Nonequivalence of chains in haemoglobin oxidation. *Biochemistry* **12**:4946, 1973.
38. Tomoda A, Yoneyama Y, Tsuji A: Changes in intermediate haemoglobins during autoxidation of haemoglobin. *Biochem J* **195**:485, 1981.
39. Brooks J: The oxidation of haemoglobin to methaemoglobin by oxygen. II. The relation between the rate of oxidation and the partial pressure of oxygen. *Proc R Soc London (B)* **118**:560, 1935.
40. Tomoda A, Yoneyama Y: Analysis of intermediate hemoglobins in solutions of hemoglobin partially oxidized with ferricyanide. *Biochem Biophys Acta* **581**:128, 1979.
41. Winterbourn CC, Carrell RC: Oxidation of human haemoglobin by copper. *Biochem J* **165**:141, 1977.
42. Mohler DN, Majerus PW, Minnich V, Hess CE, Garrick MD: Glutathione synthetase deficiency as a cause of hereditary hemolytic disease. *N Engl J Med* **283**:1253, 1970.
43. Vestling CS: The reduction of methemoglobin by ascorbic acid. *J Biol Chem* **143**:439, 1942.
44. Tomoda A, Tsuji A, Matsukawa S, Takeshita M, Yoneyama Y: Mechanism of methemoglobin reduction by ascorbic acid under anaerobic conditions. *J Biol Chem* **253**:7420, 1978.
45. Sass MD, Caruso CJ, Farhangi M: TPNH-methemoglobin reductase deficiency: A new red-cell enzyme defect. *J Lab Clin Med* **70**:760, 1967.
46. Kiese M: Die Reduktion des hamiglobins. *Biochem Z* **316**:264, 1944.
47. Warburg O, Kubowitz F, Christian W: Über die katalytische Wirkung von Methylenblau in lebenden Zellen. *Biochem Z* **227**:245, 1930.
48. Yubisui T, Matsuki T, Takeshita M, Yoneyama Y: Characterization of the purified NADPH-flavin reductase of human erythrocytes. *J Biochem (Tokyo)* **85**:719, 1979.
49. Yubisui T, Takeshita M, Yoneyama Y: Reduction of methemoglobin through flavin at the physiological concentration by NADPH-flavin reductase of human erythrocytes. *J Biochem (Tokyo)* **87**:1715, 1980.
50. Tomoda A, Yubisui T, Tsuji A, Yoneyama Y: Changes in intermediate haemoglobins during methaemoblobin reduction by NADPH-flavin reductase. *Biochem J* **179**:227, 1979.
51. Scott EM, McGraw JC: Purification and properties of diphosphopyridine nucleotide diaphorase of human erythrocytes. *J Biol Chem* **237**:249, 1962.
52. Scott EM, Duncan IW, Ekstrand V: The reduced pyridine nucleotide dehydrogenases of human erythrocytes. *J Biol Chem* **240**:481, 1965.
53. Hegesh E, Avron M: The enzymatic reduction of ferrihemoglobin. II. Purification of a ferrihemoglobin reductase from human erythrocytes. *Biochim Biophys Acta* **146**:397, 1967.
54. Niethammer D, Huennekens FM: Electrophoretic separation and characterization of the multiple forms of methemoglobin reductase. *Arch Biochem Biophys* **146**:564, 1971.
55. Sugita Y, Nomura S, Yoneyama Y: Purification of reduced pyridine nucleotide dehydrogenase from human erythrocytes and methemoglobin reduction by the enzyme. *J Biol Chem* **246**:6072, 1971.

56. Passon PG, Hultquist DE: Soluble cytochrome b_5 reductase from humane erythrocytes. *Biochim Biophys Acta* **275**:62, 1972.
57. Kuma F, Inomata H: Studies on methemoglobin reductase. II. The purification and molecular properties of reduced nicotinamide adenine dinucleotide-dependent methemoglobin reductase. *J Biol Chem* **247**:556, 1972.
58. Yubisui T, Takeshita M: Characterization of the purified NADH-cytochrome b_5 reductase of humane erythrocytes as a FAD-containing enzyme. *J Biol Chem* **255**:2454, 1980.
59. Hegesh E, Avron M: The enzymatic reduction of ferrihemoglobin. I. The reduction of ferrihemoglobin in red blood cells and hemolysates. *Biochim Biophys Acta* **146**:91, 1967.
60. Reiss A, Schwartz JS, Patel S: Mechanism of the enzyme-dependent reduction of methemoglobin in the presence of NADH and ferrocyanide. *Blood* **50(Suppl 1)**:84, 1977.
61. Taketa F, Chen JY: Activation of the NADH-methemoglobin reductase reaction by inositol hexaphosphate. *Biochem Biophys Res Commun* **75**:389, 1977.
62. Yubisui T, Miyata T, Iwanaga S, Tamura M, Takeshita M: Complete amino acid sequence of NADH-cytochrome b_5 reductase purified from human erythrocytes. *J Biochem (Tokyo)* **99**:407, 1986.
63. Takeshita M, Tamura M, Yubisui T, Yoneyama Y: Exponential decay of cytochrome b_5 and cytochrome b_5 reductase during senescence of erythrocytes: Relation to the increased methemoglobin content. *J Biochem (Tokyo)* **93**:931, 1983.
64. Yubisui T, Tamura M, Takeshita M: Studies on NADH-cytochrome b_5 reductase activities in hemolysates of human and rabbit red cells by isoelectric focusing. *Biochem Biophys Res Commun* **102**:860, 1981.
65. Zamudio I, Canessa M: Nicotinamide-adenine dinucleotide dehydrogenase activity of human erythrocyte membranes. *Biochim Biophys Acta* **120**:165, 1966.
66. Wang C-S, Alaupovic P: Isolation and partial characterization of human erythrocyte membrane NADH: (acceptor) oxidoreductase. *J Supramol Str* **9**:1, 1978.
67. Goto-Tamura R, Takesue Y, Takesue S: Immunological similarity between NADH-cytochrome b_5 reductase of erythrocytes and liver microsomes. *Biochim Biophys Acta* **423**:293, 1976.
68. Choury D, Leroux A, Kaplan J-C: Membrane-bound cytochrome b_5 reductase (methemoglobin reductase) in human erythrocytes. Study in normal and methemoglobinemic subjects. *J Clin Invest* **67**:149, 1981.
69. Kitajima S, Yasukochi Y, Minakami S: Purification and properties of human erythrocyte membrane NADH-cytochrome b_5 reductase. *Arch Biochem Biophys* **210**:330, 1981.
70. Choury D, Reghis A, Pichard A-L, Kaplan J-C: Endogenous proteolysis of membrane-bound red cell cytochrome b_5 reductase in adults and newborns: Its possible relevance to the generation of the soluble "methemoglobin reductase." *Blood* **61**:894, 1983.
71. Hultquist DE, Reed DW, Passon PG: Isolation, characterization, and enzymatic reduction of cytochrome B (556) from human erythrocytes. *Fed Proc* **28**:862, 1969.
72. Passon PG, Hultquist DE: Participation of erythrocyte cytochrome b_5 in methemoglobin reduction and evidence for the occurrence of erythrocyte P-420. *Fed Proc* **29**:732, 1970.
73. Passon PG, Reed DW, Hultquist DE: Soluble cytochrome b_5 from human erythrocytes. *Biochim Biophys Acta* **275**:51, 1972.
74. Hultquist De, Dean RT, Douglas RH: Homogeneous cytochrome b_5 from human erythrocytes. *Biochem Biophys Res Commun* **60**:28, 1974.
75. Capalna S: The erythrocyte cytochrome b_5. *Physiologie* **14**:85, 1977.
76. Douglas RH, Hultquist DE: Evidence that two forms of bovine erythrocyte cytochrome b_5 are identical to segments of microsomal cytochrome b_5. *Proc Natl Acad Sci U S A* **75**:3118, 1978.
77. Slaughter SR, Hultquist DE: Membrane-bound redox proteins of the murine Friend virus-induced erythroleukemia cell. *J Cell Biol* **83**:231, 1979.
78. Hultquist DE, Reed DW, Passon PG, Andrews WE: Purification and properties of S-protein (hemoprotein 559) from human erythrocytes. *Biochim Biophys Acta* **229**:33, 1971.
79. Abe K, Sugita Y: Properties of cytochrome b_5 and methemoglobin reduction in human erythrocytes. *Eur J Biochem* **101**:423, 1979.
80. Abe K, Kimura S, Kizawa R, Anan FK, Sugita Y: Amino acid sequences of cytochrome b_5 from human, porcine, and bovine erythrocytes and comparison with liver microsomal cytochrome b5. *J Biochem (Tokyo)* **97**:1659, 1985.
81. Slaughter SR, Williams CH, Hultquist DE: Demonstration that bovine erythrocyte cytochrome b_5 is the hydrophilic segment of liver microsomal cytochrome b_5. *Biochim Biophys Acta* **705**:228, 1982.
82. Schafer DA, Hultquist DE: Purification and structural studies of rabbit erythrocyte cytochrome b_5. *Biochem Biophys Res Commun* **115**:807, 1983.
83. Imoto M: The purification and primary structure of human erythrocyte cytochrome b5. *Juzen Igakkai Zasshi* **86**:256, 1977.
84. Hultquist DE, Slaughter SR, Douglas RH, Sannes LJ, Sahagian GG: Erythrocyte cytochrome b_5; Structure, role in methemoglobin reduction, and solubilization from endoplasmic reticulum. *Prog Clin Biol Res* **21**:199, 1978.
85. Takeshita M, Yubisui T, Tanishima K, Yoneyama Y: A simple enzymatic microdetermination of cytochrome b_5 in erythrocytes. *Anal Biochem* **107**:305, 1980.
86. Kaftory A, Hegesh E: Improved determination of cytochrome b_5 in human erythrocytes. *Clin Chem* **30**:1344, 1984.
87. Ozols J, Strittmatter P: Correction of the amino acid sequence of calf liver microsomal cytochrome b_5. *J Biol Chem* **244**:6617, 1969.
88. Leroux A, Kaplan J-C: Presence of red cell type NADH-methemoglobin reductase (NADH-diaphorase) in human nonerythroid cells. *Biochem Biophys Res Commun* **49**:945, 1972.
89. Kuma F, Prough RA, Masters BSS: Studies on methemoglobin reductase. Immunochemical similarity of soluble methemoglobin reductase and cytochrome b_5 of human erythrocytes with NADH-cytochrome b_5 reductase and cytochrome b_5 of rat liver microsomes. *Arch Biochem Biophys* **172**:600, 1976.
90. Leroux A, Junien C, Kaplan J-C, Bamberger J: Generalised deficiency of cytochrome b5 reductase in congenital methaemoglobinemia with mental retardation. *Nature* **258**:619, 1975.
91. Hultquist DE, Sannes LJ, Schafer DA: The NADH/NADPH-methemoglobin reduction system of erythrocytes. *Prog Clin Biol Res* **55**:291, 1981.
92. Hultquist DE, Peters CL, Schafer DA: Proteolytic generation of erythrocyte cytochrome b_5 and cytochrome b_5 reductase from endoplasmic reticulum (ER). *Proc XIth Intl Cong Biochem* 490, 1979.
93. Yubisui T, Naitoh Y, Zenno S, Tamura M, Takeshita M, Sakaki Y: Molecular cloning of cDNAs of human liver and placenta NADH-cytochrome b_5 reductase. *Proc Natl Acad Sci U S A* **84**:3609, 1987.
94. Hultquist DE, Douglas RH, Dean RT: The methemoglobin reduction system of erythrocytes. *Prog Clin Biol Res* **1**:297, 1975.
95. Schafer DA, Hultquist DE: Isolation of an acid protease from rabbit reticulocytes and evidence for its role in processing redox proteins during erythroid maturation. *Biochem Biophys Res Commun* **100**:1555, 1981.
96. Schafer DA, Hultquist DE: Isolation and characterization of cathepsin D from reticulocyte membranes. *Prog Clin Biol Res* **165**:549, 1984.
97. Raw I, Difini F: The possible role of ATP-dependent proteolysis on the solubilization of methemoglobin reductase during reticulocyte maturation. *Biochem Biophys Res Commun* **116**:357, 1983.
98. Choury D, Wajcman H, Boissel JP, Kaplan J-C: Evidence for endogenous proteolytic solubilization of human red-cell membrane NADH-cytochrome b_5 reductase. *FEBS Lett* **126**:172, 1981.
99. Petragnani N, Nogueira OC, Raw I: Methaemoglobin reduction through cytochrome b_5. *Nature* **184**:1651, 1959.
100. Sannes LJ, Hultquist DE: Effects of hemolysate concentration, ionic strength and cytochrome b_5 concentration on the rate of methemoglobin reduction in hemolysates of human erythrocytes. *Biochem Biophys Acta* **544**:547, 1978.
101. Tomoda A, Yubisui T, Tsuji A, Yoneyama Y: Kinetic studies of methemoglobin reduction by human red cell NADH cytochrome b_5 reductase. *J Biol Chem* **254**:3119, 1979.
102. Kuma F: Properties of methemoglobin reductase and kinetic study of methemoglobin reduction. *J Biol Chem* **256**:5518, 1981.
103. Juckett DA, Hultquist DE: Magnetic circular dichroism studies of hemoglobin. The reduction of ferrihemoglobin by ferrocytochrome b_5 and characterization of the high-spin hydroxy species of mixed-valence hemoglobin. *Biophys Chem* **19**:321, 1984.
104. Hultquist DE, Sannes LJ, Juckett DA: Catalysis of methemoglobin reduction, in DeLuca M, Lardy H, Cross RL (eds): *Current Topics in Cellular Regulation*, vol 24. New York, Academic, 1984, p 287.
105. Lostanlen D, Gacon G, Kaplan J-C: Direct enzyme titration curve of NADH:cytochrome b_5 reductase by combined isoelectric focusing/electrophoresis. *Eur J Biochem* **112**:179, 1980.
106. Strittmatter P: NADH-cytochrome b_5 reductase, in Slater EC (ed): *Flavins and Flavoproteins*. New York, Elsevier, 1966, p 325.

107. Dailey HA, Strittmatter P: Modification and identification of cytochrome b_5 carboxyl groups involved in protein-protein interaction with cytochrome b_5 reductase. *J Biol Chem* **254**:5388, 1979.
108. Righetti PG, Gacon G, Gianazza E, Lostanlen D, Kaplan J-C: Titration curves of interacting cytochrome b_5 and hemoglobin by isoelectric focusing-electrophoresis. *Biochem Biophys Res Commun* **85**:1575, 1978.
109. Mauk MR, Mauk AG: Interaction between cytochrome b_5 and human methemoglobin. *Biochemistry* **21**:4730, 1982.
110. Mauk MR, Reid LS, Mauk AG: Conversion of oxyhaemoglobin into methaemoglobin by ferricytochrome b_5. *Biochem J* **221**:297, 1984.
111. Poulos TL, Mauk AG: Models for the complexes formed between cytochrome b_5 and the subunits of methemoglobin. *J Biol Chem* **258**:7369, 1983.
112. Finch CA: Methemoglobinemia and sulfhemoglobinemia. *N Engl J Med* **239**:470, 1948.
113. Jaffe ER: Enzymopenic hereditary methemoglobinemia: A clinical/biochemical classification. *Blood Cells* **12**:81, 1986.
114. Worster-Drought C, White JC, Sargent F: Familial idiopathic methaemoglobinaemia associated with mental deficiency and neurological abnormalities. *BMJ* **2**:114, 1953.
115. Kaplan JC, Leroux A, Beauvais P: Formes cliniques et biologiques du deficit en cytochrome b_5 reductase. *CR Seances Soc Biol* **173**:368, 1979.
116. Kaplan JC, Leroux A, Bakouri S, Grangaud JP, Benabadji M: La lesion enzymatique dans la methemoglobinemie congenitale recessive avec encephalopathie. *Nouv Rev Fr Hematol* **14**:755, 1974.
117. Hirono H: Lipids of myelin, white matter and gray matter in a case of generalized deficiency of cytochrome b_5 reductase in congenital methemoglobinemia with mental retardation. *Lipids* **15**:272, 1980.
118. Hirono H: Lipids of liver, kidney, spleen and muscle in a case of generalized deficiency of cytochrome b_5 reductase in congenital methemoglobinemia with mental retardation. *Lipids* **19**:60, 1984.
119. Junien C, Leroux A, Lostanlen D, Reghis A, Boue J, Nicolas H, Boue A, Kaplan JC: Prenatal diagnosis of congenital enzymopenic methaemoglobinaemia with mental retardation due to generalized cytochrome b_5 reductase deficiency: First report of two cases. *Prenat Diagn* **1**:17, 1981.
120. Arnold H, Botcher HW, Hufnagel D, Lohr GW: Hereditary methemoglobinemia due to methemoglobin reductase deficiency in erythrocytes and leukocytes without neurological symptoms [Abstracts]. Paris, XVII Congress of the International Society of Hematology, 1978, p 752.
121. Tanishima K, Tanimoto K, Tomoda A, Mawatari K, Matsukawa S, Yoneyama Y, Ohkuwa H, Takazakura E: Hereditary methemoglobinemia due to cytochrome b_5 reductase deficiency in blood cells without associated neurologic and mental disorders. *Blood* **66**:1288, 1985.
122. Fisher RA, Povey S, Borrow M, Solomon E, Boyd Y, Carritt B: Assignment of the DIA/1 locus to chromosome 22. *Ann Hum Genet* **41**:151, 1977.
123. Junien C, Vibert M, Weil D, Van-Cong N, Kaplan J-C: Assignment of NADH-cytochrome b_5 reductase (DIA1 locus) to human chromosome 22. *Hum Genet* **42**:233, 1978.
124. Kaplan J-C, Beutler E: Electorphoresis of red cell NADH- and NADPH-diaphorases in human subjects and patients with congenital methemoglobinemia. *Biochem Biophys Res Commun* **29**:605, 1967.
125. Hopkinson DA, Corney G, Cook PJL, Robson EB, Harris H: Genetically determined electrophoretic variants of human red cell NADH diaphorase. *Ann Hum Genet* **34**:1, 1970.
126. Jaffe ER: Methemoglobinemia in the differential diagnosis of cyanosis. *Hosp Pract* **20**:92, 1985.
127. Schwartz JM, Paress PS, Ross JM, Dipillo F, Rizek R: Unstable variant of NADH methemoglobin reductase in Puerto Ricans with hereditary methemoglobinemia. *J Clin Invest* **51**:1594, 1972.
128. Feig SA,Nathan DG, Gerald PS, Zarkowski HS: Congenital methemoglobinemia: The result of age-dependent decay of methemoglobin reductase. *Blood* **39**:407, 1972.
129. Beutler E: Selectivity of proteases as a basis for tissue distribution of enzymes in hereditary deficiencies. *Proc Natl Acad Sci U S A* **80**:3767, 1983.
130. Sharp CW, Stillman RC: Blush not with nitrites [Editorial]. *Ann Intern Med* **92**:700, 1980.
131. Hegesh E, Calmanovici N, Avron M: New method for determining ferrihemoglobin reductase (NADH-methemoglobin reductase) in erythrocytes. *J Lab Clin Med* **72**:339, 1968.
132. Board PG: NADH-ferricyanide reductase, a convenient approach to the evaluation of NADH-methaemoglobin reductase in human erythrocytes. *Clin Chim Acta* **109**:233, 1981.
133. Kaplan J-C, Nicolas AM, Hanzlickova-Leroux A, Beutler E: A simple spot screening test for fast detection of red cell NADH-diaphorase deficiency. *Blood* **36**:330, 1970.
134. Kaplan JC, Chirouze M: Therapy of recessive congenital methaemoglobinaemia by oral riboflavine. *Lancet* **2**:1043, 1978.
135. Mansouri A, Lurie AA: Methemoglobinemia. *Am J Hematol* **42**:7, 1993.
136. Yawata Y, Ding L, Tanishima K, Tomoda A: New variant of cytochrome b_5 reductase deficiency ($b_5R_{KURASHIKI}$) in red cells, platelets, lymphocytes and cultured fibroblasts with congenital methemoglobinemia, mental and neurologic retardation and skeletal anomalies. *Am J Hematol* **40**:299, 1992.
137. Nagai T, Shirabe K, Yubisui T, Takeshita M: Analysis of mutant NADH-cytochrome b_5 reductase: Apparent "type III" methemoglobinemia can be explained as type I with an unstable reductase. *Blood* **81**:808, 1993.
138. Strittmatter P, Kittler JM, Coghill JE: Characterization of the role of lysine 110 of NADH-cytochrome b_5 reductase in the binding and oxidation of NADH by site-directed mutagenesis. *J Biol Chem* **267**:20164, 1992.
139. Yubisui T, Shirabe K, Takeshita M, Kobayashi Y, Fukumaki Y, Sakaki Y, Takano T: Structural role of serine 127 in the NADH-binding site of human NADH-cytochrome b_5 reductase. *J Biol Chem* **266**:66, 1991.
140. Shirabe K, Yubisui T, Nishino T, Takeshita M: Role of cysteine residues in human NADH-cytochrome b_5 reductase studied by site-directed mutagenesis. *J Biol Chem* **266**:7531, 1991.
140a. Shirabe K, Nagai T, Yubisui T, Takeshita M: Electrostatic interaction between NADH-cytochrome b_5 reductase and cytochrome b_5 studied by site-directed mutagenesis. *Biochim Biophys Acta* **1384**:16, 1998.
140b. Qian W, Sun Y-L, Wang Y-H, Zhuang J-H, Xie Y, Huang Z-H: The influence of mutation at Glu44 and Glu56 of cytochrome b_5 on the protein's stabilization and interaction between cytochrome *c* and cytochrome b_5. *Biochem* **37**:14137, 1998.
141. Hultquist DE, Xu F, Quandt KS, Shlafer M, Mack CP, Till GO, Seekamp A, Betz AL, Ennis SR: Evidence that NADPH-dependent methemoglobin reductase and administered riboflavin protect tissues from oxidative injury. *Am J Hematol* **42**:13, 1993.
141a. Ozols J, Korza G, Heinemann FS, Hediger MA, Strittmatter P: Complete amino acid sequence of steer liver microsomal NADH-cytochrome b_5 reductase. *J Biol Chem* **260**:11953, 1985.
142. Yubisui T, Naitoh Y, Zenno S, Tamura M, Takeshita M, Sakaki Y: Molecular cloning of cDNAs of human liver and placenta NADH-cytochrome b_5 reductase. *Proc Natl Acad Sci U S A* **84**:3609, 1987.
143. Zenno S, Hattori M, Misumi Y, Yubisui T, Sakaki Y: Molecular cloning of a cDNA encoding rat NADH-cytochrome b_5 reductase and the corresponding gene. *J Biochem* **107**:810, 1990.
144. Pietrini G, Carrera P, Borgese N: Two transcripts encode rat cytochrome b_5 reductase. *Proc Natl Acad Sci U S A* **85**:7246, 1988.
144a. Borgene N, Aggujaro D, Carrera P, Pietrini G, Bassetti M: A role for N-myristoylation in protein targeting: NADH-cytochrome b_5 reductase requires myristic acid for association with outer mitochondrial but not ER membranes. *J Cell Biol* **135**:1501, 1996.
144b. Pedrazzini E, Villa A, Borgene N: A mutant cytochrome b_5 with a lengthened membrane anchor escapes from the endoplasmic reticulum and reaches the plasma membrane. *Proc Natl Acad Sci U S A* **93**:4207, 1996.
145. Tomatsu S, Kobayashi Y, Fukumaki Y, Yubisui T, Orii T, Sakaki Y: The organization and the complete nucleotide sequence of the human NADH-cytochrome b_5 reductase gene. *Gene* **80**:353, 1989.
146. Shirabe K, Yubisui T, Borgese N, Tang C, Hultquist DE, Takeshita M: Enzymatic instability of NADH-cytochrome b_5 reductase as a cause of hereditary methemoglobinemia type I (red cell type). *J Biol Chem* **267**:20416, 1992.
147. Kobayashi Y, Fukumaki Y, Yubisui T, Inoue J, Sakaki Y: Serine-proline replacement at residue 127 of NADH-cytochrome b_5 reductase causes hereditary methemoglobinemia, generalized type. *Blood* **75**:1408, 1990.
148. Katsube T, Sakamoto N, Kobayashi Y, Seki R, Hirano M, Tanishima K, Tomoda A, Takazakura E, Yubisui T, Takesha M, Sakaki Y, Fukumaki Y: Exonic point mutations in NADH-cytochrome b_5 reductase genes of homozygotes for hereditary methemoglobinemia, types I and III: Putative mechanisms of tissue-dependent enzyme deficiency. *Am J Hum Genet* **48**:799, 1991.

149. Jenkins MM, Prchal JT: A novel mutation found in the 3′ domain of NADH-cytochrome b_5 reductase in an African-American family with type I congenital methemoglobinemia. *Blood* **87**:2993, 1996.
150. Jenkins MM, Prchal JT: A high frequency polymorphism of NADH-cytochrome b_5 reductase in African-Americans. *Hum Genet* **99**:248, 1997.
151. Mansouri A, Nandy I: NADH-methemoglobin reductase (cytochrome b_5 reductase) levels in two groups of American blacks and whites. *J Investig Med* **46**:82, 1998.
152. Zhu H, Yoon H-W, Huang S, Bunn HF: Identification of a cytochrome *b*-type NAD(P)H oxidoreductase ubiquitously expressed in human cells. *Proc Natl Acad Sci U S A* **96**:14742, 1999.
153. Miyazono Y, Hirono A, Miyamoto Y, Miwa S: Erythrocyte enzyme activities in cord blood of extremely low-birth-weight infants. *Am J Hematol* **62**:88, 1999.
154. Manabe J, Arya R, Sumimoto H, Yubisui T, Bellingham AJ, Layton DM, Fukumaki Y: Two novel mutations in the reduced nicotinamide adenine dinucleotide (NADH)-cytochrome b_5 reductase gene of a patient with generalized type, hereditary methemoglobinemia. *Blood* **88**:3208, 1996.
155. Aalfs CM, Salieb-Beugelaar GB, Wanders RJA, Mannens MMAM, Wijburg FA: A case of methemoglobinemia type II due to NADH-cytochrome b_5 reductase deficiency: Determination of the molecular basis. *Hum Mut* **16**:18, 2000.

CHAPTER 181

The Hemoglobinopathies

D.J. Weatherall ▪ J.B. Clegg ▪ D.R. Higgs ▪ W.G. Wood

1. **The inherited disorders of hemoglobin fall into three overlapping groups: structural variants; thalassemias characterized by a reduced rate of synthesis of one or more of the globin chains of hemoglobin; and conditions in which fetal hemoglobin synthesis persists beyond the neonatal period, known collectively as hereditary persistence of fetal hemoglobin. Taken together, they are the commonest single-gene disorders in the world population.**
2. **Because the different hemoglobin disorders co-exist at a high frequency in many populations, and because individuals may inherit more than one type, hemoglobin disorders are responsible for an extremely complex series of clinical phenotypes. Their molecular pathology has been elucidated in many subjects and a start has been made in relating primary molecular defects to associated clinical phenotypes.**
3. **Although some 750 structural hemoglobin variants have been identified, only three—hemoglobins S, C, and E—reach very high frequencies in some populations. The various interactions of the hemoglobin S gene may result in chronic hemolytic anemia and vasculo-occlusive episodes. Hemoglobin C is associated with a mild hemolytic anemia, while hemoglobin E is synthesized at a reduced rate and results in the phenotype of a mild form of β thalassemia. There are other groups of much rarer variants that are of clinical significance, including the unstable hemoglobins associated with hemolytic anemia, high oxygen affinity variants that cause congenital polycythemia, and variants associated with methemoglobinemia.**
4. **The β thalassemias are divided into β^+ thalassemia, in which some β globin chains are produced, and β^o thalassemia in which there is no β chain synthesis. The α thalassemias are similarly divided into α^o and α^+ thalassemias. Over 170 different mutations have been identified as the cause for β thalassemia, most of which interfere with the transcription of β globin mRNA or its processing or translation. A few types of β thalassemia result from the production of highly unstable β globin chains. The common forms of α thalassemia result from deletions that involve either one or both of the linked α globin genes. Some less common forms of α thalassemia result from point mutations which interfere with the translation or transcription of the α globin genes.**
5. **The development of rapid methods for studying the globin genes has also made it possible to analyze their population genetics and the mechanisms underlying their high gene frequencies.**
6. **The carrier states for most of the important hemoglobin disorders are easily identified. Their homozygous or compound heterozygous states can be identified in fetal life by fetal blood sampling or analysis of DNA obtained from chorionic villi. Hence, the disease can be avoided in an affected family by reproductive counseling and a choice of options.**
7. **Apart from marrow transplantation, there is no definitive treatment, and management is symptomatic.**

McKusick (OMIM) numbers have been assigned to the various globin genes. The entries also document the allelic series that cause the corresponding hemoglobinopathies; the alleles are given numbers after the decimal point. The OMIM numbers are: alpha () locus-1 (141800); locus-2 (141850); beta (B) locus (141900); gamma locus (142200); delta locus (142000); epsilon locus (142100) zeta locus (142310). Three hemoglobin variants that reach polymorphic frequencies in some populations are: HbC (141900.0038); HbE (141900.0071); HbS (141900.0243). HbM variants are numbered by locus and allele (e.g., HbM_{BOSTON} (141800.0092), $HbM_{HYDE\ PARK}$ (141900.0164). The unstable Hb variants are also an allelic series, e.g., Hb_{ZURICH} 141900.0310. HbF (Hereditary Persistence of Fetal Hb) (HPFH) is a separate entry (141790); as is HbH-related mental retardation, deletion type (141750).

The GenBank accession numbers for the nucleotide sequences of the globin genes are: globin genes, Z84721; globin genes, UO1317.

The most comprehensive website for mutation of globin genes is http://globin.cse.psu.edu.

INTRODUCTION

The inherited disorders of hemoglobin are the commonest single-gene conditions in man. The World Health Organization has suggested that, at a conservative estimate, about 5 percent of the world's population are carriers for different inherited disorders of hemoglobin, and that about 370,000 severely affected homozygotes or compound heterozygotes are born each year.[1] In the developing countries, in which there is still a very high mortality from infection and malnutrition in the first year of life, many of these conditions are unrecognized. However, as economic conditions improve and infant death rates fall, they pose an increasingly heavy burden on health services.

As the result of mass migrations of populations from high prevalence areas, the hemoglobin disorders are being seen with increasing frequency in parts of the world in which they have not been recognized previously. Because some of them, particularly sickle cell anemia and the more severe forms of thalassemia, can produce life-threatening medical emergencies or chronic ill health, it is important for clinicians in all countries to have a working knowledge of their clinical features, genetic transmission, management, and prevention. The other reason why the hemoglobin disorders are of particular interest is that they were the first diseases to be analyzed by the methods of recombinant DNA technology. More is known about their molecular pathology than about the molecular pathology of any other genetic disease, and it is likely that their study has already given us a relatively complete picture of the repertoire of mutations that underlie single gene disorders.

This chapter reviews the main clinical, genetic, and population aspects of these conditions. It is not possible to provide an all-encompassing picture of the enormous amount of work that has been done in this field. Readers who wish to study this subject in greater depth are referred to two extensive monographs on the subject.[2,3]

HISTORICAL BACKGROUND

The fascinating story of the evolution and development of the human hemoglobin field is the subject of several reviews and monographs that contain extensive bibliographies.[2,4–6]

In trying to understand why the human hemoglobin field has paved the way for the application of molecular biology to the study of human disease, it is helpful to trace three historical threads that finally came together in the 1950s. The first is the story of the discovery of hemoglobin and the elucidation of its structure and function. The second encompasses the early description of sickle cell anemia, the realization that it is an inherited disease, and the characterization of its molecular pathology. And, finally, there is the even more complex saga of the gradual amalgamation of observations from many parts of the world that led to the notion that the thalassemias are also genetic disorders of hemoglobin with many features in common with the structural hemoglobin variants. The final chapter of this biological detective story, which is not yet complete, is how, given all this diverse information and the new tools of molecular and cell biology, it has been possible in less than 20 years to describe so much of the molecular pathology of hemoglobin that it is likely that we already have a very good idea about the repertoire of the molecular defects that underlie single-gene disorders.

Following the studies of William Harvey on the circulation of the blood, two English workers, Robert Boyle and Richard Lower, established that the function of the pulmonary circulation is to aerate venous blood. The mechanism of the binding of oxygen to blood was a subject of intense interest during the second half of the 19th century, and in 1862, Hoppe-Seyler first used the term "hemoglobin" to describe the oxygen-carrying pigment. The structure of heme was worked out by Kuster in 1912, but it was not until the mid-1950s, following pioneering work on protein structure by Sanger, that Ingram, Rhinesmith, Schroeder, Pauling, and others established that hemoglobin is a tetramer composed of two pairs of unlike peptide chains, α and β. Using the newly developed techniques of amino acid sequence analysis, the primary structures of these chains were rapidly determined. At the same time, Perutz and his colleagues were arriving at a solution for the three-dimensional structure of hemoglobin by x-ray analysis. Thus by the early 1960s a start could be made in relating the structure of hemoglobin to its functional properties that had been so elegantly described by Bohr and Krogh in Denmark, Barcroft, Haldane, Hill, and Roughton in England, and Henderson in the United States.

This new knowledge, together with the discovery of the abnormal hemoglobins, led to rapid progress toward an understanding of the genetic control of human hemoglobin. But part of the work that laid the basis for this remarkably productive period of hemoglobin research had started half a century before with the discovery of sickle cell anemia.

The first description of sickle cell anemia appeared in 1910 in Herrick's classic paper.[7] The genetic basis of this disease was established by workers in the United States, particularly Neel, and in Africa, notably Lambotte-Legrands and Beet. Following the famous conversation between Castle and Pauling in 1945,[4] the discovery that sickle cell anemia results from a structural change in hemoglobin was announced by Pauling and his colleagues in 1949,[8] and the amino acid substitution in Hb S was determined by Ingram in 1956.[9] After it was realized that there are two globin chains, α and β, and that the amino acid substitution in sickle hemoglobin is in the β chain, the one gene-one enzyme (or peptide chain) concept, which had been proposed earlier by Beadle and Tatum from their work on *Neurospora*, was confirmed for higher organisms. More hemoglobin variants were soon discovered by electrophoresis, and by studying families in which genes for both α and β globin variants segregated, the independent genetic control of the α and β chains was established. The different chains of fetal and the adult minor hemoglobin, A_2, were characterized, and by careful analysis of families with different genetic variants, and appropriate linkage studies, a reasonable working model of the order of the α-like and β-like globin genes on their respective chromosomes was obtained.

The third thread in the story starts in 1927 with the first description of thalassemia by Cooley and Lee.[10] Although milder forms of this condition were probably identified at about the same time in Italy,[6] it was more than 25 years before the genetic transmission of thalassemia was fully appreciated. During this period reports of the disease appeared from all over the world, and soon after hemoglobin analysis became part of the armamentarium of clinicians during the 1950s it was realized that thalassemia is one of the commonest genetic diseases and also extremely heterogeneous. Studies of the hemoglobin patterns of patients with different types of thalassemia and structural hemoglobin variants done in the late 1950s led to the suggestion by Ingram and Stretton[11] that there might be two main types, α and β thalassemia. The development of a method for studying hemoglobin synthesis in the test tube[12,13] led to the experimental validation of this hypothesis and to the further analysis of thalassemia, so that by the early 1970s it was known that there are many different forms, and it was also possible to make a guess at their underlying defects.

Thus, by the mid-1970s a great deal was known about the genetic control of human hemoglobin, its structural variants, and the biosynthetic defects and remarkable heterogeneity of the thalassemias. The field was ready for the techniques of recombinant DNA. Over the last 20 years, these techniques have been used successfully to determine the molecular pathology of the globin disorders, paving the way toward an understanding of the molecular basis for many single-gene disorders.

THE STRUCTURE, GENETIC CONTROL, AND SYNTHESIS OF HEMOGLOBIN

Structure

All normal hemoglobins have a tetrameric structure consisting of two pairs of unlike peptide chains (Fig. 181-1). In normal adults, the major component, comprising about 97 percent of the total is Hb A ($\alpha_2\beta_2$) with the remainder being Hb A_2 ($\alpha_2\delta_2$). The main hemoglobin in fetal life is Hb F ($\alpha_2\gamma_2$) (although traces of it [$\sim$0.5 percent] are found in adults) and this is preceded in the embryo by Hbs Gower 1 ($\zeta_2\varepsilon_2$) and 2 ($\alpha_2\varepsilon_2$) and hemoglobin Portland ($\zeta_2\gamma_2$). There are also various minor components that are the result of postsynthetic modifications that take place *in vivo*. The most common of these are Hb A_{IC}, which is formed by the reaction of glucose with hemoglobin, and Hb F_I, which is an acetylated form of fetal hemoglobin. The amino acid sequences of all the normal globins are known and they are clearly related to each other, retaining many key features in common. Broadly speaking, they can be regarded as "α-like" (ζ and α, each of 141 amino acids) and "β-like" (ε, γ, δ, and β, 146 amino acids), and it appears that they arose from a single ancestral globin by successive duplications and divergence of the duplicated genes (see below).

The three-dimensional structure of human hemoglobin has been determined by Perutz and colleagues to a resolution better than 2.7Å by x-ray crystallography.[14,15] It consists of an ellipsoid approximately $64 \times 55 \times 50$Å in which the subunits are oriented in a unit with a twofold symmetry axis running down a central water-filled cavity. Seventy-five percent of the native hemoglobin molecule is in the form of α-helix. Where the α-helix is interrupted (for example by a proline residue) the polypeptide chains can turn corners, thus enabling them to fold and take up the compact shape seen in the tetrameric molecule. Within the tetramer, individual polypeptide chains have only a limited contact with each other, and there is relatively little interaction between them compared with the forces that maintain their individual secondary and tertiary structures. The individual subunit chains of hemoglobin have similar three-dimensional structures with analogous helical segments. Eight helical regions (A-H) are present in the β chain and seven are present in the α chain, which lacks a region corresponding to the β chain D helix. Amino acids can thus be identified with specific helical positions.

The interiors of the subunits are made up almost entirely of nonpolar (hydrophobic) residues, which contact neighboring

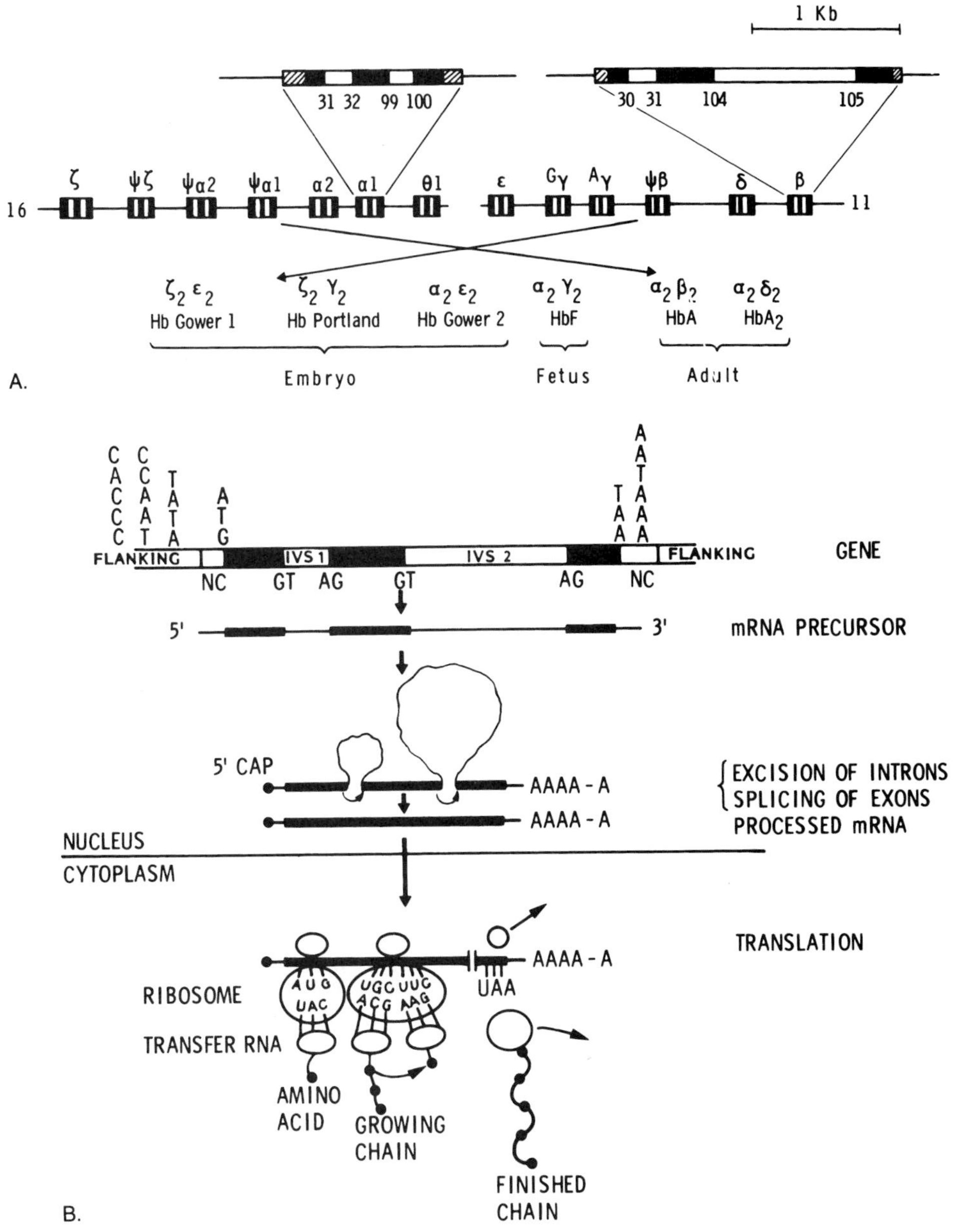

Fig. 181-1 Genetic control of human hemoglobin. *A.* The human hemoglobins and globin gene clusters. *B.* The mechanism of globin synthesis. The exons are shown in dark shading and the introns (IVS1 and IVS2) unshaded. The positions of the 5′ regulatory boxes and the 5′ and 3′ noncoding (NC) regions are also shown. Further details, including location of RFLPs, VNTRs and *Alu* repeats, are given in refs. 3, 51, 52, and 471.

residues by low energy, short-range (van der Waals) forces. All the side chains that are ionizable under normal physiological conditions are on the surface of the subunits, as are most of the polar (hydrophilic) side groups. The exterior surface of hemoglobin is thus covered with polar groups that generally interact with water rather than other hydrophilic groups.

Oxygen Binding

Binding of oxygen to hemoglobin is mediated by the prosthetic group heme, a ferroporphyrin molecule in which the iron atom is located at the center of the porphyrin ring (Fig. 181-2). The heme is situated within clefts in the globin subunits that are lined with nonpolar residues. The heme lies between two histidines, the "proximal histidine," which is bonded directly to the heme iron atom through the nitrogen atom of its imidazole group, and the "distal" histidine, which lies opposite the oxygen binding site but is not directly attached to the heme (Fig. 181-2). The orientation of the heme within the pocket enables its nonpolar vinyl groups to be buried within the hydropic interior while the polar propionic acid groups reside on the hydrophilic surface of the globin subunit. A large number of interatomic contacts (<4Å) between the heme and side chains of amino acid residues of the E and F helices stabilize this structure.

The residues that surround the heme group are invariant throughout the animal kingdom, suggesting a highly conservative structure that is essential if it is to function normally as an oxygen carrier. Indeed, hemoglobin variants with mutations in the heme pocket often show profound alterations in their stability or oxygen-binding properties.

There is a marked difference in the three-dimensional structures of the oxy- and deoxy forms of hemoglobin, implying that the subunit chains change their relative orientation with respect to each other during oxygenation and vice versa. In the tetramer, each α chain is in contact with the two β chains; the two contacts can be defined as $\alpha_1\beta_1$ and $\alpha_1\beta_2$, and the twofold symmetry generates the structurally identical $\alpha_2\beta_1$ and $\alpha_2\beta_2$ contacts (Fig. 181-3). Most of the movement during oxygenation/deoxygenation takes place at the $\alpha_1\beta_2$ ($\alpha_2\beta_1$) interfaces, while the

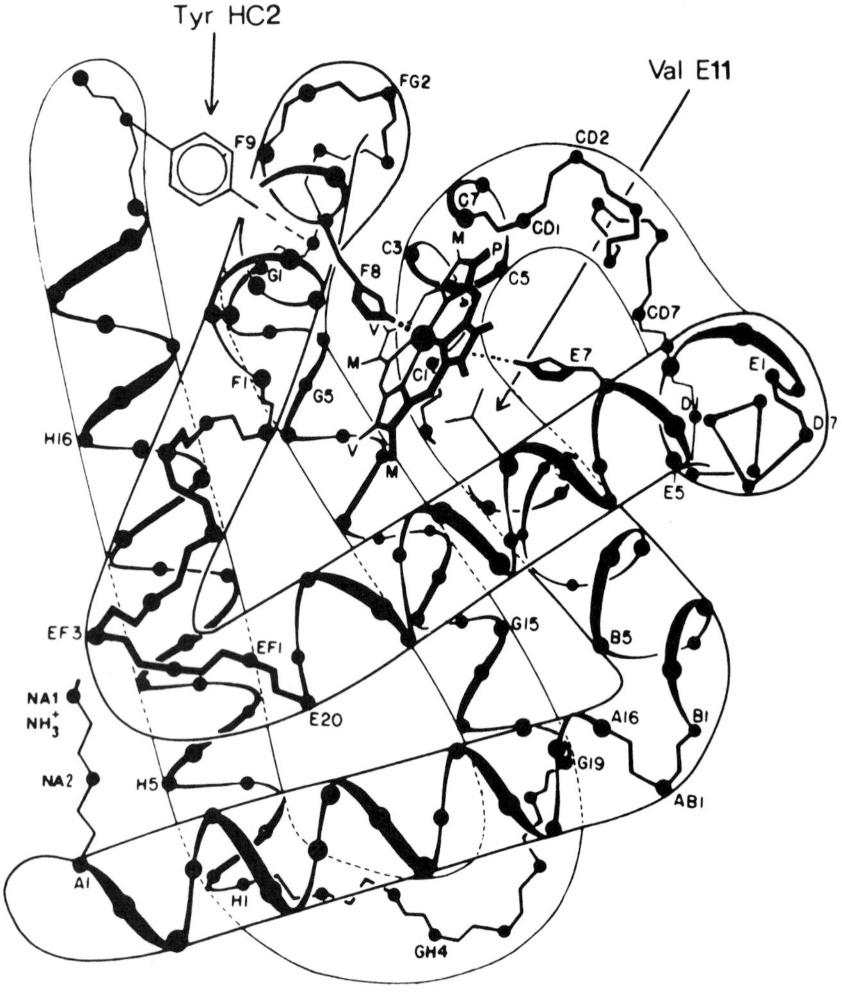

Fig. 181-2 The α-globin subunit showing the structure and relationships of the heme pocket.

$\alpha_1\beta_1$ ($\alpha_2\beta_2$) interfaces remain relatively immobile, in keeping with the 40 contacts at the latter interface as compared to the 17 contacts at the weaker $\alpha_1\beta_2$ interface.[16]

Good contacts between subunits can only be made when key regions of the two $\alpha\beta$ dimers are in the same relative orientation, thus favoring the formation of two specific quaternary states, oxy or "relaxed" (R) and deoxy or "tense" (T), without any stable intermediates.[17,18] Owing to the movement that occurs at the $\alpha_1\beta_2$ interface, the nature and number of contacts change during oxygen/deoxygenation. In the deoxy (T) state there are about 40 contacts (which include 19 hydrogen bonds), which drops by almost half (to 22 and 12, respectively) in the oxy (R) state. Not surprisingly, the $\alpha_1\beta_2$ contact, like the heme pocket, is a highly conserved structure, which has remained unchanged through long periods of evolutionary time. Mutations involving residues in this contact can have drastic functional consequences.

Deoxyhemoglobin has a more stable quaternary structure than oxyhemoglobin because of the increased number of contacts at the $\alpha_1\beta_2$ interface, and because there are additional inter- and intrasubunit salt linkages that are absent or much weaker in oxyhemoglobin. Thus the carboxyl group of the C-terminal arginine of one α chain interacts with the ε-amino group of a lysine residue at position 132 (H10) in the other α chain, and the guanidine group of this same C-terminal arginine interacts with the carboxyl group of the aspartic acid residue at position 131 (H9) of the other α chain. There is also a chloride ion-mediated link between the C-terminal guanidine group and the opposite α chain's α-NH_2 group. None of these α-α salt linkages can be formed in oxyhemoglobin because of steric hindrance effects.[18] In a similar manner, the β-chain C-terminal histidines are involved in two interactions: through the imidazole group, with the aspartate residue at position 94 (FG1) of the same β chain, and through the carboxyl group, with the ε-NH_2 group of lysine α40 (C5) forming a salt bridge that spans the $\alpha_1\beta_2$ interface. In oxyhemoglobin, these residues are displaced too far apart for these interactions to occur, and no salt bridges are formed.

Physiological measurements indicate that there is a free energy change of 10 to 12 cal per mole of tetramer on the transition of oxy to deoxy states, a figure in accordance with the energy estimated to residue in the salt bridges of 1 to 2 cal/bond. The salt bridges thus represent a considerable reservoir of stored energy, maintaining the deoxyhemoglobin molecule in a high-energy or "tense" (T) state.

Structure-Function Relationships

The role of hemoglobin as oxygen carrier depends on its ability to absorb and release oxygen in response to the relatively small changes in partial pressures encountered under physiological conditions. The function of oxygen bound versus partial pressure is sigmoid, a property that depends crucially on a heterotetrameric structure (it does not occur in monomeric myoglobin or in the homotetrameric hemoglobins H [β_4] and Bart's [γ_4]) and which is achieved by cooperative interactions between the heme groups as the oxygenation at one enhances the subsequent O_2 binding at the others. Hemoglobin thus behaves as an allosteric molecule. In addition, O_2 binding is influenced by the interaction of small molecules such as 2,3 diphosphoglycerate (2,3DPG) and is sensitive to changes in pH, a phenomenon known as the Bohr effect.

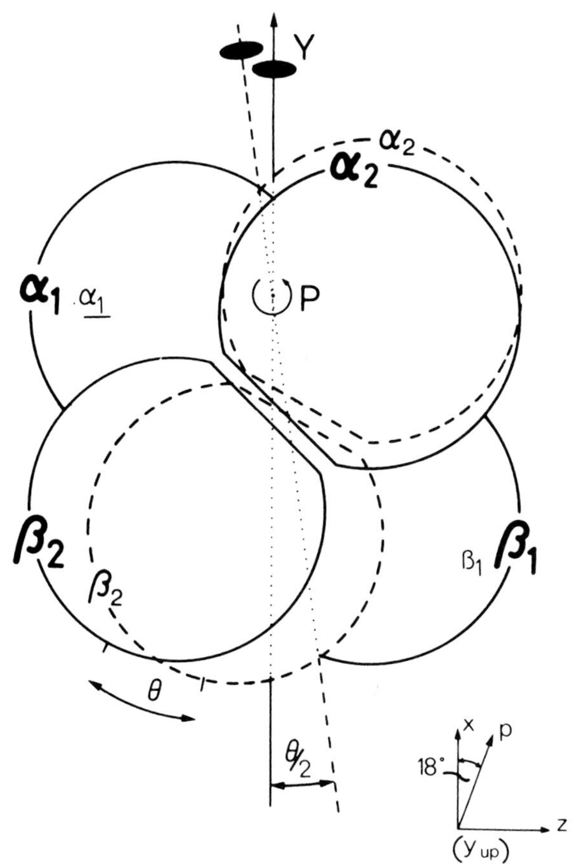

Fig. 181-3 Schematic diagram of quarternary structure of hemoglobin and the relative changes in orientation fo the subunits during oxygenation. ***Bold*****: deoxy;** ***light*****: oxy. (*****From Fermi G, Perutz MF:*** **Haemoglobin and Myoglobin.** ***Oxford University Press. Used by permission.*****)**

Heme-Heme Interaction. The heme-heme interaction that promotes the cooperative binding of oxygen is dependent on small rearrangements that occur when oxygen is taken up. During oxygenation the β-chain hemes move apart by about 7Å in a process that is dependent on interactions between the α and β subunits. It is likely that the $\alpha_1\beta_2$ contact is particularly important in these cooperative interactions. The three-dimensional structure indicates that α_1 and β_2 (or α_2 and β_1) subunits can have much more direct interaction than can α_1 and β_1 (or α_2 and β_2). Furthermore, oxygenation of the β_2 subunit causes it to rotate much more with respect to α_1 than does oxygenation of the β_1 subunit. And, as we have seen earlier, the overall structure of the $\alpha_1\beta_2$ contact has remained invariant throughout mammalian evolution. Most hemoglobin variants with abnormalities in heme-heme interactions have mutations in or close to the $\alpha_1\beta_2$ interface.

The molecular origin for the conformational changes that take place in the subunits during oxygenation lies in the heme molecule. When no O_2 molecule is bound, the atomic diameter of the iron atom is too great to allow it to sit flush in the plane of the porphyrin ring and it is thus displaced 0.6Å towards the proximal histidine residue. When the heme iron binds oxygen, the resulting changes in the distribution of electrons orbiting the iron atom nucleus lead to an effective reduction in its atomic diameter and it can move into the plane of the porphyrin ring. This movement results in a tilt of the heme into its pocket. This tilt is amplified as a change in the tertiary structure of the subunit, which ultimately pushes the penultimate tyrosine from between the F and H helices, resulting in rupture of the C-terminal salt bridges. The transition of the quaternary structure from the deoxy (T) to oxy (R) conformation occurs abruptly as the salt bridges successively break apart, and constraints on the $\alpha_1\beta_2$ interface are relaxed. Because the α subunit hemes are relatively more accessible to oxygen, they are probably oxygenated first. The shift from T to R structure then opens up the clefts of the unliganded β-chain hemes, greatly increasing their affinity for oxygen.

Modification of Oxygen-Binding Properties by 2,3DPG and Chloride. Some organic phosphates increase the stability of deoxyhemoglobin. In human erythrocytes, the major effector of this type is 2,3 diphosphoglycerate (2,3DPG).[19,20] This binds specifically to the β chains of hemoglobin in the T state through electrostatic bonds between the 2,3DPG phosphate groups and the N-terminal amino and imidazole groups of the β_2 and β143 histidine residues and the ε-amino group of β82 lysine.[21] When the structure changes from the T to R state, the bound 2,3DPG molecules are released because the β-chain H helices are now too close and the N-terminal amino groups too far apart for the 2,3DPG to bind. Thus 2,3DPG and oxygen binding are mutually exclusive, and the overall effect is that 2,3DPG reduces the oxygen affinity of hemoglobin by stabilizing the deoxy (T) form. The cellular concentrations of 2,3DPG and chloride thus have an important influence on oxygen affinity.

Chloride has a similar effect on O_2 affinity to 2,3DPG, by neutralizing electrostatic repulsion of excess positive charges in the central cavity of the Hb molecule.[22,23] This stabilizes the quaternary T (deoxy) structure, thereby lowering the O_2 affinity. Unlike 2,3DPG and other allosteric effectors of Hb, however, chloride ions do not bind to any particular sites. Differences in oxygen affinity between fetal and adult red cells are largely due to 2,3DPG having only a weak affinity for deoxyhemoglobin F.[24,25] A weak chloride effect may be responsible for the high O_2 affinity of embryonic Hb relative to adult Hb.[23]

The Bohr Effect. The binding of oxygen to hemoglobin is sensitive to changes in pH, a phenomenon that has physiological importance through its effect on the transport of CO_2 in the blood. Carbon dioxide released on respiration is too insoluble to be transported in any quantity in the blood except as bicarbonate ion, produced by reaction with water;

$$CO_2 + H_2O \rightarrow HCO_3^- + H^+$$

The released protons can combine with hemoglobin, forcing the reaction towards bicarbonate formation. Protons stabilize the deoxy (T) state of the hemoglobin molecule, thus favoring oxygen release in the tissues. On oxygen binding (in the lungs) the converse occurs. Protons are released, driving the bicarbonate/ CO_2 reaction towards CO_2 formation, thus releasing from the blood. The Bohr effect mediates a reciprocal CO_2/O_2 exchange.[17,26]

Hemoglobin is also responsible for the direct transport of about 10 percent of respired CO_2 through the formation of a carbamate linkage with the N-terminal amino groups. Because CO_2 binds more readily to the deoxy form, this, again, facilitates the removal of CO_2 from the circulation.

The Hemoglobin Genes

Organization and Chromosomal Location. Six different types of globin chain (α, β, γ, δ, ε, ζ) are found in normal human hemoglobins at different stages of development, requiring a minimum of six different structural genes.[27] Genetic analysis of families in which abnormal Hb variants were segregating established that the α and β globin genes are on separate chromosomes, and that it was likely that the fetal and adult non-α genes were present in a single cluster. The relationships between the amino acid sequences of the ζ and α chains, and ε, γ, δ and β chains, suggested that they had arisen by successive duplications and divergences of ancestral genes.

The localization of these groups of genes to specific chromosomes was achieved by the use of hybrid rodent/human somatic cell lines containing one or a few human chromosomes. The α gene cluster was found on chromosome 16, and the β-like genes on chromosome 11[28–30] (Fig. 181-1). These assignments have been refined by *in situ* hybridization studies and by gene mapping of cell lines containing different translocations and deletions. Such analyses place the β-like cluster distal to band p14 on the short arm of chromosome 11,[31–35] and the α-like cluster in band 16p13.3 at the tip of chromosome 16.[36,37]

Restriction enzyme mapping of genomic DNA coupled with fine structure mapping of cloned DNA from the globin gene complexes on chromosomes 11 and 16 has enabled a very detailed picture to be built of the precise chromosome organization of the two complexes. The conclusions that had been reached by conventional genetic and structural analyses of hemoglobin variants have been vindicated by the molecular analyses. In addition, the loci for the embryonic ζ and ε genes were found to be linked to the clusters containing the adult genes (Fig. 181-1).[38–40]

Unexpectedly, other genes or gene-like structures, unsuspected prior to these molecular analyses, and with considerable structural homology to the "real" genes, have been identified within the clusters; one ($\psi\beta$[41,42]) between the $^{A}\gamma$ and δ genes, and no fewer than four ($\psi\zeta 1$,[43] $\psi\alpha 1$,[41] $\psi\alpha 2$,[44] and $\theta 1$[45]) in the α cluster (Fig. 181-1). With the exception of $\theta 1$ these (nonfunctional) genes are designated pseudogenes, and are thought to be relics of past evolutionary changes within the globin gene clusters. The conserved structure of $\theta 1$ and the fact that it contains no inactivating mutations suggest that it may be functional. However, no protein product has been identified, and protein structural considerations indicate that the predicted protein could not form a viable globin.[46] The role of $\theta 1$ is thus presently enigmatic.

Several regions of the α (but not β) cluster contain highly polymorphic tandemly repeated segments of DNA (HVRs, VNTRs) varying from a few to hundreds of repeat units. Both α and β clusters contain *Alu*-family elements, some of which are polymorphic at their 3′ ends. References to more detailed descriptions of these structural aspects of the globin gene are given in the caption to Fig. 181-1.

Evolution. By comparing the nucleotide sequences of the genes and using estimates of the average rates of nucleotide substitution derived from species comparisons, it is possible to establish an evolutionary history for the human globin genes. Various estimates put the time of α and β gene divergence from a single ancestral gene at approximately 450 million years (my) ago, during early vertebrate evolution.[5,47] In birds and mammals, the α and β gene clusters subsequently became established on different chromosomes. The ζ-α gene split was probably the most ancient of the subsequent duplications[48] followed by β/γ at 200 my, and γ/ε at 100 my.[47] The δ/β divergence appears at 40 my, although this is probably the time of a gene conversion following on from a much more ancient duplication event.[49] Duplication of the α genes, like the ζ-α split, appears to have been a relatively early event, whereas the γ duplication is more recent, with the subsequent near-identity of the two α genes and two γ genes being maintained by rounds of gene conversion. It is inferable from this history that developmental patterns of hemoglobin synthesis have changed considerably during evolution, presumably a reflection, in part, on the changing physiological and environmental circumstances that hemoglobin has had to respond to.

It can be seen from Fig. 181-1 that the globin genes are arranged in the order in which they are expressed during development and are all in the same transcriptional orientation. The significance of this, which is a feature of many (but not all; chicken and goat are exceptions) animal species, in terms of the changes in gene expression that take place during development is at present unclear.

Individual Variation of Globin Gene Structure. The effort involved in producing very fine structure (down to the nucleotide level) maps of the globin gene clusters has been considerable. Consequently, most of the sequence information available has come from intensive analyses of just one or two chromosomes, and it gives little indication of the variation that might be found if large numbers of individuals were to be studied. The initial indications that sequence variations might be relatively common came from the work of Jeffreys[50] who found two *Hind*III polymorphisms in the γ genes of a number of individuals and estimated that perhaps 1 percent of nucleotide sites might be polymorphic. Subsequent studies have shown many such polymorphisms throughout the globin gene clusters. Some of these are common, and present in all racial groups while others may have a much more restricted distribution.

Of particular interest and importance is that the polymorphisms do not normally occur in association with each other in a random fashion; rather they are present in linked groups called haplotypes[51,52] (Fig. 181-4). Within any given population there are usually a small number of common haplotypes and a larger number of rarer ones, only some of which are clearly related to the more common types, for example, by a difference at a single site. The frequency and types of haplotype present in various populations can provide some interesting insights into racial affinities and evolution.[52–56] At a more practical level, that haplotypes exist at all implies that, in the region defined by the restriction enzyme cleavage sites comprising the haplotype, there

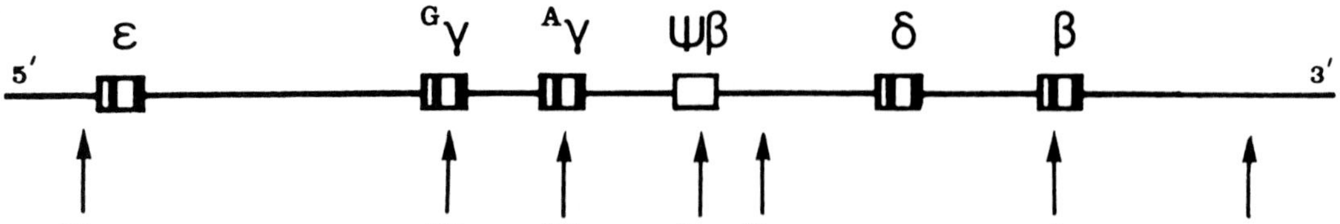

	Hc	Hd	Hd	Hc	Hc	A	B
I	+	−	−	−	−	+	+
II	−	+	+	−	+	+	+
III	−	+	−	+	+	+	−
IV	−	+	−	+	+	−	+
V	+	−	−	−	−	+	−
VI	−	+	+	−	−	−	+
VII	+	−	−	−	−	−	+
VIII	−	+	−	+	−	+	−
IX	−	+	−	+	+	+	+

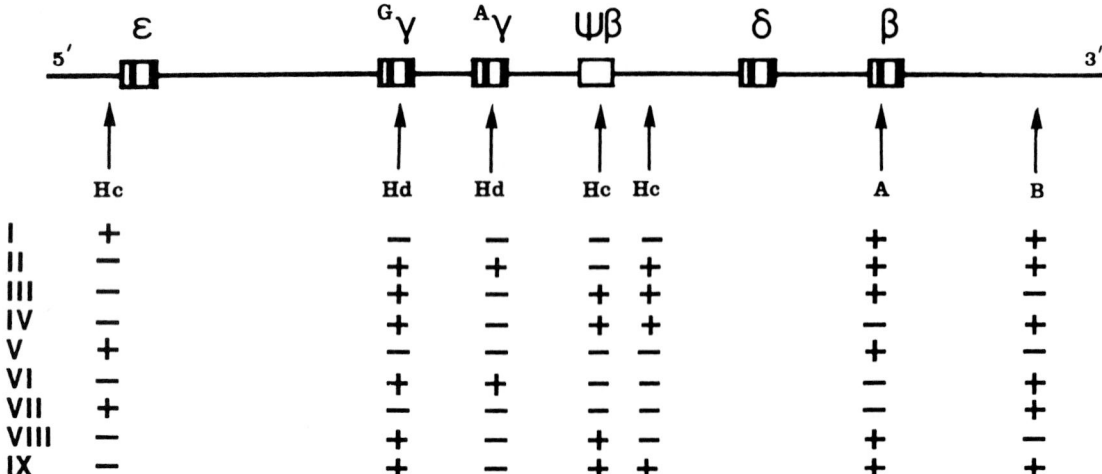

Fig. 181-4 Polymorphic restriction enzyme sites in the human β-globin complex and nine of the common haplotypes derived from them.

has been little, if any, recombination between chromosomes (because if there had been the nonrandom association between polymorphic sites would have been destroyed). The knowledge that these chromosome arrangements are relatively stable has thus enabled the polymorphisms comprising the various haplotypes to be used in linkage analysis of hereditary disorders affecting globin genes. For example, establishing the particular haplotype carrying a β-thalassemia defect enables the affected chromosome to be followed within a pedigree, and it can also be used for prenatal diagnostic purposes by analysis of DNA from fetuses at risk.[57–59]

Although the features of the α- and β-like gene clusters noted in Fig. 181-1 are the norm, many examples are now known of individuals with various rearrangements in the clusters, most of which have little or no phenotypic effects of clinical significance. Most often seen are the variations in copy number of those genes that are usually duplicated (or have an associated, nearly identical, pseudogene such as ζ). Thus many individuals with triplicated ζ,[60] γ,[61] and α[62] genes have been documented and even quadruplicate α and γ arrangements are known. Likewise, there are numerous examples of single ζ,[60] i.e., lacking $\psi\zeta$, α,[63,64] and γ[65] gene chromosomes that have probably arisen through unequal crossing-over events. While most of these rearrangements are found at very low frequency in most populations, the single α gene chromosomes are extremely common in many tropical countries because they appear to be at a selective advantage in malarial environments[66,67] (see below).

Rare cases of homogenization of the $^{G}\gamma$ or $^{A}\gamma$ genes, to form $^{G}\gamma$-$^{G}\gamma$ or $^{A}\gamma$-$^{A}\gamma$ arrangements[68] and of $\psi\zeta$ by ζ to form a ζ-ζ arrangement,[69] are also known, possibly the result of localized gene conversion events.

Structural Features of Globin Genes. It has been apparent since 1977 that the coding regions of most mammalian genes—and globin genes are no exception—are interrupted by stretches of noncoding DNA, usually referred to as "intervening sequence" or "intron" DNA. All globin genes possess two introns in identical positions relative to the coding sequence but of variable length, the shortest being the first intron (IVS1) of the α genes at 117 bp and the largest of 1264 bp in IVS1 of the ζ gene. That introns are found in identical positions in all globin genes suggests that they were in place before the expansion of the globin gene repertoire from an ancestral gene occurred. Molecular sequence analysis of the β-like genes reveals little or no homology among the larger IVS2 introns except in the case of the duplicated $^{G}\gamma$ and $^{A}\gamma$ genes, and variable homology among the small IVS1 introns. Within the α-like genes, the duplicated α_1 and α_2 genes show considerable homology between IVS1 and IVS2 of those genes, but very little with the linked upstream ζ gene or the $\psi\zeta$ gene.

Comparisons of the sequences of introns from many different genes reveal only a few common features, most notably in the sequences immediately adjacent to and around the coding sequences they interrupt[70] and a sequence 20 to 40 bases from the 3′ end that is involved in the formation of the branched splicing intermediate. Intron sequences are removed (spliced out) of the initial precursor mRNA transcript in order to form the final mature mRNA product. The necessary signals for correct splicing reside at the 5′ (consensus sequence $_{C}$AG↓GU$_{G}$AGU) and 3′ (consensus ($_{C}$) X($_{C}$)AG↓G) ends of the introns.[71] The importance of these sequences is illustrated by the fact that mutations in them can interfere with, or even abolish, correct splicing, leading to abnormal processing of globin mRNA precursors, the molecular basis of a number of the thalassemias (see below).

The regions flanking the coding sequences of globin genes contain a number of sequence motifs that are necessary for correct expression[72] (Fig. 181-1*B*). The first of these is the ATA box that serves to accurately locate the site of transcription initiation at the "cap" site, usually about 30 bases downstream, and which also appears to influence the level of transcription. Natural mutations within the ATA region can reduce transcription quite markedly (see below). Seventy or 80 base pairs upstream is a second conserved sequence, the CCAAT box (in δ the sequence is CCAAC, and the γ genes have a duplicated structure). In model systems, mutations introduced into CCAAT sequences also lead to reductions in the level of transcription.[73] Further 5′, approximately 80 to 100 bp from the cap site, is a GC-rich region with general structure GGGG$_{C}$G or C$_{G}$CCCCC, which can be inverted and/or duplicated. These sequences resemble those required for optimal transcription of the SV40 early region, and mutations within this region in β globin genes adversely affect expression.[74,75]

Other nonglobin mammalian genes contain similar conserved sequences upstream of the mRNA cap sites, each of which is necessary for normal gene expression, presumably because they provide binding sites for transcription factors that influence the rate of interaction of transcription by RNA polymerase II. *In vitro* experiments involving modification or deletion of the sequences are consistent with this, and natural mutations within them may result in decreased expression of the associated gene (see below).

Globin Gene Expression. The mechanism of protein synthesis in eukaryotes has been elucidated in considerable detail (for reviews see references 27, 72, 76, and 77). In this section, only those aspects of globin gene expression that are particularly relevant to the molecular basis of the hemoglobinopathies are considered.[27,72]

Transcription of the globin genes initiates at the cap site, which is ~50 bp upstream of the AUG initiation codon, and which becomes the 5′ end of the mature mRNA after processing. Although mature mRNA terminates 10 to 20 bp downstream of the AATAAA, there is evidence from *in vitro* studies that the initial transcript may extend beyond this site and that the specific cleavage distal to the polyadenylation signal takes place subsequently. Supporting this is evidence from a case of β thalassemia with a mutation in the AATAAA sequence,[78] in which elongated β gene transcripts were observed in RNA isolated from erythroid cells of the affected individual, and in *in vitro* experiments in a similar case of α thalassemia.[79]

The large initial precursor mRNA transcript is rapidly processed after synthesis. The first events, capping the 5′ end and polyadenylation of the 3′ end, probably serve to stabilize the transcript and prevent attack by exonucleases. Capping involves a GTP-mediated modification of the 5′ residue, usually an A or G, to form a 5′ppp5′ linkage, while polyadenylation, as the term implies, results in the addition of a long string of A residues (>50) to the 3′ end of the transcript formed by cleavage of the initial precursor 10 to 20 bp downstream of the AATAAA signal.

Subsequent to these steps, the intervening sequences are removed from the pre-mRNA in a two-stage process. In the first stage, pre-mRNA is cut at the 5′ splice site to generate two intermediates, a linear first exon and a branched lariat-type molecule containing the intron and second exon. In the second step, the 3′ splice site is cleaved, the lariat intron released, and the two exons are joined.[71] Introns may be removed in a sequential manner until the mature mRNA is produced. The mature mRNA is then transported from the nucleus to the cytoplasm where ribosomal translation of mRNA to globin occurs. The details of the translational phase of protein synthesis are well known and have been extensively reviewed.[76,77] The synthesis of globin closely follows the pattern of other eukaryotic proteins; indeed, many aspects of the general mechanism were elucidated with cell-free systems synthesizing rabbit globins.

Regulation of Globin Gene Expression

Recent experimental work has begun to dissect the important elements involved in both tissue-specific and developmental-stage-specific regulation of gene expression from the two globin-gene complexes. It is clear that this involves critical regulatory sequences around and within the genes themselves, as well as at the 5′ end of each gene cluster. These sequences interact with a number of transcriptional factors, some of which have a ubiquitous tissue distribution, while others are more-or-less erythroid-cell restricted. An outline of current understanding of globin gene

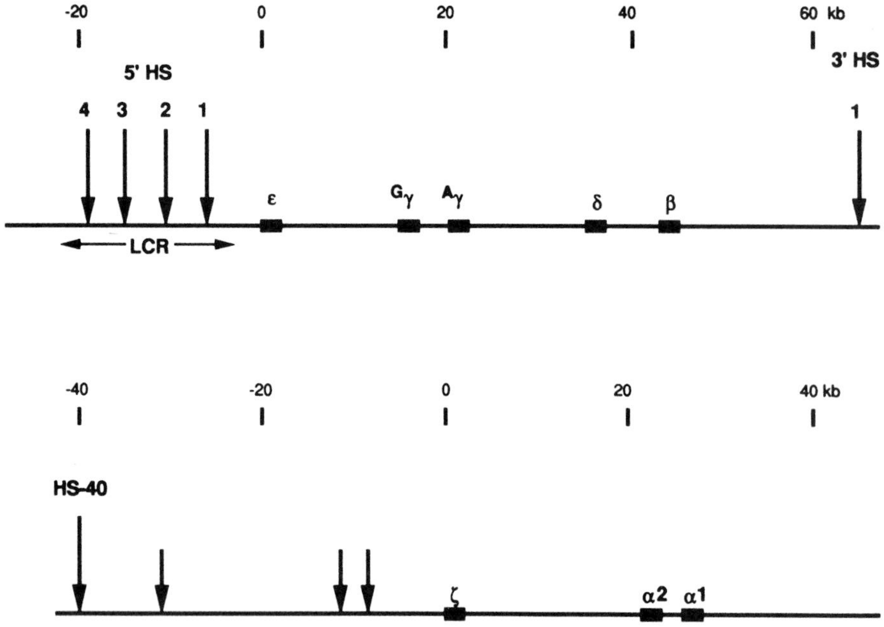

Fig. 181-5 Location of the erythroid-specific DNase I hypersensitive sites in the human α- and β-globin gene complexes. The major regulatory regions, the β locus control region and α hypersensitivity site 40 kb upstream of the ζ globin gene are indicated.

regulation is given below; more detailed reviews can be found in references 27, 80, and 81.

The β Globin LCR and the α Globin HS-40 Sequences. (See Fig. 181-5.) Transfection of human α or β globin genes into mouse erythroleukemia cells and analysis of their expression in stable cell lines has demonstrated variable, but generally low, levels of expression which appear to be dependent on the site of their integration into the mouse chromosomes.[82,83] Similar results were obtained when the human γ or β genes were injected into fertilized mouse eggs and expression analyzed in the resulting transgenic mice; human globin mRNA was either undetectable or present at low levels.[84,85] In most cases, expression was confined to erythroid cells, suggesting that the sequences around the genes contained elements important in tissue specificity. Furthermore both the γ and β genes showed developmental-stage specificity, the fetal γ gene being transcribed during the embryonic stage of erythropoiesis in the mouse (which lacks a true fetal hemoglobin), while the adult β gene was expressed only in postembryonic erythroid cells.[86,87] Again, this suggests that information relating to the appropriate time of gene expression is contained in the sequences in and around the genes themselves.

In these experiments, high-level expression of human genes was only achieved when they were attached to a 20-kb region from immediately upstream of the ε globin gene.[88] This region, now known as the β globin locus control region (LCR), is marked by four sites that are hypersensitive (HS) to digestion with DNase I but only in erythroid cells.[89,90] The importance of this region has been confirmed by analysis of patients in whom the LCR is deleted, but the globin genes have been spared; there is no expression from globin genes on chromosomes carrying LCR deletions[91] (see below).

The LCR confers high-level, tissue-specific expression on attached genes (globin or heterologous). In transgenic mice, the LCR confers position independence and shows copy-number dependent expression. Individually, HSs 2, 3, and 4 are capable of enhancing the expression of the globin genes (to ~20 to 40 percent of the activity of the intact LCR), whereas HS1 is much less active and may be dispensable. Similarly, when individual HSs are deleted from the mouse β LCR, expression is reduced by ~20 to 30 percent.[92,93] It has been suggested that the individual elements of the LCR are combined into a single functional complex (holocomplex) that loops round and interacts with the promoters of the globin genes to activate their transcription.[94] Direct evidence to prove this is still awaited.

Deletions of a region upstream of the α globin genes also result in lack of expression from the genes *cis* to the lesion, indicating that there is an equivalent regulatory element in the α globin gene cluster.[95,96] Experimental analysis in transfected cell lines and transgenic mice have suggested that the region around a DNase I hypersensitive site 40 kb upstream of the ζ globin gene (HS-40) is the major regulator of α globin gene expression.[97,98] Other erythroid-specific hypersensitive sites, as well as several constitutive sites, have been found in this region but as yet have not been shown to affect expression levels, either alone or in combination with HS-40.

Sequence analysis of the hypersensitive sites combined with binding studies using nuclear protein extracts (*in vitro* "footprinting") have demonstrated that each region is rich in sequence motifs that form the recognition sites for the binding of various proteins involved in transcription. The β LCR 5′ HSs 2, 3, and 4, as well as α HS-40 have binding sites for two proteins, GATA-1 and NFE-2, whose tissue distribution is limited largely to erythroid cells, as well as sites for other less well-characterized erythroid-restricted proteins. In addition, these regions, which span a few hundred base pairs, contain multiple binding sites for ubiquitously expressed transcription factors. It appears that cooperative activity between the proteins bound at these sites is necessary for full function of the region.

Chromatin Structure. In nonerythroid cells, the β globin cluster exists in a chromatin structure that is insensitive to digestion with DNase I, whereas in erythroid cells, the whole region is in a more open conformation that is more readily susceptible to DNase I digestion.[99] In addition to the hypersensitive sites that mark the LCR, the promoter regions at the 5′ end of the genes also display hypersensitive sites; in fetal liver, these sites are found in front of the $^{G}\gamma^{A}\gamma\delta$ and β genes, whereas in adult bone marrow the γ gene sites are no longer present.[100] The LCR seems to be an essential element in setting up this chromatin structure, because in somatic erythroid cell hybrids containing a chromosome 11 with most of the LCR deleted, the whole region around the β globin gene cluster is DNase I insensitive and the remaining DNase hypersensitive sites are no longer present.[100] Furthermore, while in hybrids containing a normal chromosome 11 the β globin cluster replicates in an early S phase of the cell cycle, this region becomes late replicating when the LCR is absent, as is the case for the normal chromosome in nonerythroid cells.

There are marked differences in the structure of the α and β complexes. The α gene cluster lies in a GC-rich region, contains several CpG islands, and, unlike the β gene complex, has no potential sites for binding to the nuclear matrix.[101] However, like the β gene complex, the α gene region is more sensitive to DNase I digestion in erythroid cells compared to nonerythroid cells[102] although the presence of constitutive DNase I hypersensitive sites within the cluster suggests that its chromatin structure may be less tightly compacted in nonerythroid cells than that of the β gene complex. In addition to the upstream DNase hypersensitive sites, the α gene cluster also has hypersensitive sites at the 5′ end of the genes when they are expressed. Interestingly, four other genes have been detected in the region at the 5′ end of the α gene cluster, all of which are expressed in a wide variety of different cell types, and the major regulatory region of the α genes, HS-40, actually lies in the intron of one of these genes. The significance of these observations and their relationship to the concept that the α and β gene clusters might lie in distinct regulatory "domains" is discussed elsewhere.[103]

Methylation. The role of DNA methylation, the only known chemical modification of DNA, in the regulation of gene expression, is still unclear. The methylation of cytosine residues in CpG dinucleotides is frequently associated with inactive genes, although whether this relationship is causal or a secondary response to gene repression is unclear. The β globin gene cluster is extensively methylated in nonerythroid cells, while the pattern of methylation in erythroid cells varies with stages of development.[104] In embryonic erythroblasts, the ε gene is unmethylated, while the ${}^{G}\gamma$,${}^{A}\gamma$ and β genes remain methylated. This situation is reversed in fetal liver erythroblasts where both γ and β genes are active, while in adult bone marrow, the γ genes become remethylated and the β gene remains unmethylated.

In the α globin gene cluster the expressed genes themselves show little or no methylation in any tissue. This is in keeping with other CpG-rich areas and is also compatible with the concept that the α globin gene complex has a more open conformation in nonerythroid cells than the β genes.

***Trans*-acting Factors.** Protein-DNA interactions are of major importance in the regulation of tissue-specific gene expression and may well be critical in the differential expression of genes in clusters at different developmental stages. Erythroid cells contain general transcription factors common to all cell types but, in addition, contain DNA-binding proteins with a very restricted tissue distribution. The best characterized of these is GATA-1,[105–107] found in megakaryocytes and mast cells as well as erythroid cells, and a member of a family of at least six proteins recognizing the consensus sequence ${}_{W}GATA_{R}$. Two other members, GATA-2 and GATA-3 are also expressed in erythroid cells, albeit at lower levels than GATA-1, but have a wider tissue distribution.[108] The GATA-1 protein regulates expression of its own gene as well as a wide range of erythroid-specific genes. In mice, it shows higher levels in fetal and adult erythroid cells than in embryonic erythroblasts, and it also increases in amount during erythroid differentiation.[109] Its major role in erythroid cell development has been demonstrated in chimeric mice produced by injecting blastocysts with embryonic stem (ES) cells from which the GATA-1 was deleted. Chimeric mice showed variable anemia (leading to fetal death in some cases), and although the ES cells contributed 15 to 50 percent of the cells in most tissues, no detectable erythroid cells were derived from these cells.[110] When the inactivated GATA-1 allele was transmitted through the germ line, male embryos died at ~10.5 to 11.5 d gestation, with erythropoiesis arrested at the early proerythroblast stage.[111] The GATA-1 factor is required, therefore, for both primitive and definitive erythropoiesis but different sequence elements may be required for its activation in the two cell types.[112,113] GATA-1 interacts with other transcription factors, including FOG,[114] and may be part of a large oligomeric DNA-binding complex involving Lmo2, Tal1, Ldb1, and E2A.[115,116]

Binding sites for the basic leucine zipper transcription factor NFE-2 are found in the βLCR HSs 2 and 4 and in αHS-40, as well as in the regulatory regions of other erythroid genes. Deletion or mutation of the NFE-2 sites generally leads to significant reduction in globin gene expression in experimental systems.[117,118] However, when the *NF-E2p45* gene was knocked out in mice, it resulted in only mild effects on erythropoiesis and globin gene expression, while a major effect was seen in platelet production, leading to death from hemorrhage.[119] It is now clear that NF-E2 sites bind a range of basic leucine zipper proteins such as Nrf1, Nrf2, and Bach1, all of which, like NF-E2, form heterodimers with small proteins of the Maf family. Their binding sites are now known to be Maf recognition elements, or MAREs.[120,121] It seems likely that functional redundancy within this group of proteins accounts for the lack of an erythroid phenotype in NF-E2-deficient mice.

It is clear that *trans*-acting factors play a major role in determining tissue-specific gene expression, but the role of putative stage-specific factors in developmental gene regulation has yet to be clarified. A number of genetic disorders that decrease expression of the β globin gene have been described that do not segregate with the gene cluster, suggesting that a gene-specific *trans*-acting factor is involved.[122–124] Several families also have been described that have a syndrome of mental retardation and α thalassemia due to mutations in the X-linked *ATR-X* gene (see below). Considerable down-regulation of α gene expression is observed from both chromosomes 16, yet they function normally after fusion with mouse erythroleukemia cells.[125] Because the β globin genes remain unaffected it is clear that the *ATR-X* gene has a specific role in α globin gene expression.

Heterokaryons formed between erythroid and nonerythroid cells or between erythroid cells expressing different globin genes can result in the induction of previously silent globin genes. In the K562 cell line, the β globin genes are inactive yet they are fully functional when transferred to other erythroid cell lines by cell fusion. Conversely, normal β genes transferred to K562 are inactive. This suggests that K562 cells either lack an essential *trans*-activating factor or contain a suppressor of β globin gene expression.

In chicks, a protein that binds to the β globin gene promoter is found in extracts from adult erythroid nuclei but not in nuclear extracts from embryonic cells, a stage at which the β gene is not expressed.[126] This heteromeric protein contains CP2, a ubiquitous transcription factor together with an unknown partner. CP2 also forms part of the stage selector protein (SSP), which binds to the stage selector element found in the γ gene promoter and also in the ε promoter and HS2 and HS3 of the β LCR. This protein is believed to play a role in the selective expression of γ and β genes.[127]

An erythroid transcription factor specific for the β globin gene is the erythroid Kruppel-like factor (EKLF).[128] It binds to the CACCC box in the promoter of this gene but not to the similar binding sites in other globin genes. Loss of EKLF activity severely down-regulates expression of the β globin gene.[129,130] However, EKLF is expressed throughout all stages of development[131] and is active in embryonic cells, even though the β gene is not normally expressed there.[132,133] Its precise role, if any, in globin gene switching remains to be determined.

Developmental Changes in Globin Gene Expression

The pattern of Hb synthesis changes during development. In the very early embryo, Hb synthesis is restricted to the yolk sac and the production of Hbs Gower 1 ($\zeta_2\varepsilon_2$) and Gower 2 ($\alpha_2\varepsilon_2$) and Portland ($\zeta_2\gamma_2$). Subsequently, at about 8 weeks of gestation, the fetal liver takes over, synthesizing predominantly Hb F ($\alpha_2\gamma_2$) and a small amount (< 10 percent) of Hb A. Between about 18 weeks

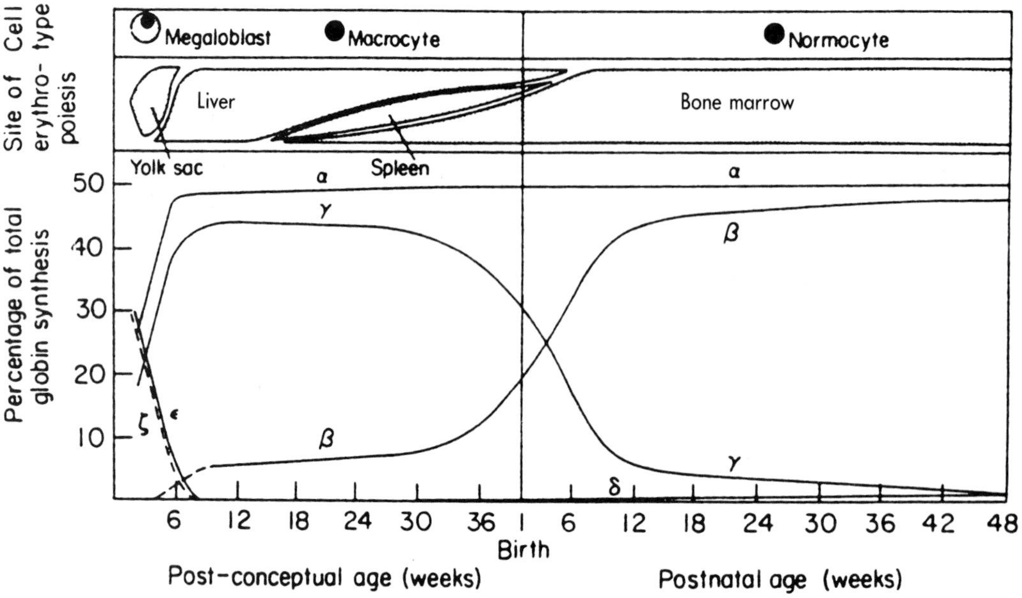

Fig. 181-6 Globin synthesis at various stages of embryonic and fetal development.

and birth, the liver is progressively replaced by bone marrow as the major site of red cell production; this is accompanied in the later stages of gestation with a reciprocal switch in production of Hbs F and A, which continues until by the end of the first year Hb F production has dropped to less than 2 percent (Fig. 181-6).

The mechanism by which fetal erythroid cells switch from the production of Hb F to Hb A remains elusive, and has been (and still is) the subject of a considerable research effort, not only for its own intrinsic interest, but also because of the important therapeutic implications that would arise from the ability to manipulate the switching process.

In humans, the switch from Hb F to Hb A production seems to be closely related to the gestational age of the fetus, and largely independent of environmental factors. Experiments in sheep (which provide a good model system with close developmental parallels to humans) have shown that while various treatments, such as fetal hypophysectomy in the lamb, may alter the *rate* at which the developmental changes occur, they do not affect the *time* of switching.[134] Infants of diabetic mothers show a delayed pattern of hemoglobin switching, possibly due to butyric acid. Injection of butyric acid analogues in fetal sheep *in utero* can delay switching.[135] Thus, environmental factors may play a role in fine-tuning the time of switching.

Transplantation experiments involving the introduction of fetal (liver) cells into lethally irradiated adult animals show that the pattern of hemoglobin synthesis in the treated adults is that expected of a fetus of the same age as the donor cells, with switching to the production of adult hemoglobin only at the appropriate time.[136] The reverse experiments, transplanting adult cells into a fetus *in utero*, showed continued production of adult (Hb) in the fetal environment, until the appropriate time for switching when the fetus began producing its own adult Hb.[137] These observations provide evidence for preprogrammed globin gene expression that is not appreciably affected by environmental changes. However, when adult hematopoietic stem cells are injected in mouse blastocysts, they are reprogrammed and express their embryonic genes appropriately.[138] This suggests that developmental plasticity remains and can be reactivated in the right environment.

The use of transgenic mouse models has enabled a start to be made in dissecting the processes that govern the developmental regulation of the globin genes. The βLCR and αHS-40 regions are essential for high-level expression of all the genes in their respective complexes, but it is not clear whether they play a determinative role in selective gene expression at different stages of development. The embryonic ζ and ε genes appear to be autonomously regulated; the ε gene alone, or attached to the βLCR, is only expressed during the embryonic period of erythropoiesis in transgenic mice.[139] A similar situation appears to apply to γ gene or LCR-γ gene constructs in transgenic mice, at least when they are present in only one to two copies.[140] The adult β gene is developmentally regulated in transgenic mice in the absence of the βLCR, but is expressed at all stages of development in the presence of the LCR and in the absence of the other β-like genes. Developmental regulation of the β gene is restored in mice carrying larger LCR-γ-β constructs, suggesting that there may be competition between the γ and β genes that is necessary for down-regulating β gene transcription during early developmental stages.[141,142] However, there is evidence that the organization of the genes in such constructs, their distance from the LCR and their order, for example, affects their pattern of expression.[143,144] Therefore, caution must be exercised in the interpretation of experiments using artificial gene constructs, often present in multiple tandem arrays in these transgenic mice.

Experiments using artificial constructs in transgenic mice suggest that individual hypersensitive site elements of the βLCR might interact with specific genes during the developmental regulation of the β cluster.[145,146] However, deletions of specific sites from the mouse βLCR *in situ* do not have developmental consequences,[92,93] and so the question of whether there is a change in the structure of the putative LCR holocomplex during development remains unresolved.

In the α gene complex, no expression of the genes has been reported in transgenic mice in the absence of HS-40 except when βLCR elements are substituted for HS-40. Embryonic ζ gene expression is restricted to the embryonic phase of erythropoiesis in βLCR-ζ constructs and also shows a similar pattern of transcription in mice bearing HS-40 ζ α constructs. Both mouse and human α globin genes are expressed at the earliest stages of erythropoiesis in these transgenic mice.

At this stage, therefore, our understanding of the developmental regulation of globin genes is extremely limited. It is clear that the overall organization of the complexes is important, and it is likely that sequences specifying developmental stage-specific expression lie in the vicinity of the genes, but the role of the upstream regulatory regions, the importance of *trans*-acting

Table 181-1 Genetic Disorders of Hemoglobin

Sructural hemoglobin variants
α Chain
β Chain
γ Chain
δ Chain
Fusion chains
δβ
βδ
γβ
Thalassemias
α Thalassemia
β Thalassemia
δβ Thalassemia
γδβ Thalassemia
γ Thalassemia
δ Thalassemia
Hereditary persistence of fetal hemoglobin
Deletion
Nondeletion
Linked to β-globin gene cluster
Unlinked to β-globin gene cluster

factors, and the possible effects of developmentally induced epigenetic modifications of the complexes[147] have yet to be clarified.

CLASSIFICATION OF HEMOGLOBIN DISORDERS

The main groups of hemoglobin disorders are summarized in Table 181-1. They are divided into those in which there is a structural change in a globin chain and those in which there is a reduced rate of production of one or more of the globin chains, the thalassemias. In addition, there is a group of conditions that are characterized by a defect in the normal switching of fetal to adult hemoglobin production, known collectively as hereditary persistence of fetal hemoglobin. Although they are of no clinical significance, they are useful models for studying the regulation of gene switching during development.

Although offering a useful conceptual framework on which to describe the hemoglobin disorders this classification is not entirely satisfactory. In particular, there is an overlap between the structural hemoglobin variants and the thalassemias; some abnormal hemoglobins are produced at a reduced rate or are highly unstable, and are associated with the clinical phenotype of thalassemia.

It should be remembered that in many populations there is a high incidence of structural hemoglobin variants *and* different forms of thalassemia. It is not uncommon, therefore, for an individual to have inherited more than one genetic determinant for a hemoglobin variant and/or different forms of thalassemia. In some countries, these interactions produce a bewildering collection of genetic disorders of hemoglobin production with widely varying clinical phenotypes; in Thailand, for example, over 60 different combinations have been observed.[2]

THE STRUCTURAL HEMOGLOBIN VARIANTS

Extensive population studies using hemoglobin electrophoresis and analyses of the hemoglobin of patients with specific hematologic conditions have led to the discovery of some 750 structural hemoglobin variants. In this section, only those abnormal hemoglobins that are associated with clinical disorders are described in detail. Complete lists of the human hemoglobin variants together with their structural alterations and functional properties are listed in a monograph on the subject.[148]

Nomenclature

When the first hemoglobin variants were described, after the discovery of sickle cell hemoglobin in 1949,[8] they were designated by letters of the alphabet. By the late 1950s, all the letters of the alphabet had been used up and it became customary to name a new hemoglobin by its place of origin. There is no consistent usage. Names range from the exotic (Hb_{AIDA}), through the chauvinistic ($Hb_{BRIGHAM}$) or parochial ($Hb_{RIVERDALE\text{-}BRONX}$), to the patriotic ($Hb_{ABRAHAM\ LINCOLN}$); they could also have added the poetic ($Hb_{CONSTANT\ SPRING}$).

Although for many years there have been no formal recommendations for nomenclature of the abnormal hemoglobins, certain conventions are observed in the hemoglobin literature. Heterozygotes for hemoglobin variants are usually described as having the trait; for example, sickle cell trait, Hb C trait. Homozygotes are described as having the "disease;" for example, sickle cell disease, Hb C disease, Hb D disease. In fact, with the exception of the three β globin variants that occur in polymorphic frequencies in many populations, Hbs S, C, and E, the homozygous states for other β chain variants are extremely rare and have usually been encountered in consanguineous marriages.[3] Individuals who inherit a different β globin chain variant from each parent, that is compound heterozygotes, are described as having SC, SD, or SE disease, and so on. Similarly, a person who has inherited a β globin chain variant, such as Hb S from one parent and a β thalassemia gene from the other, is said to have Hb S β thalassemia. The homozygous state for α chain variants is also extremely uncommon and, because there are two α globin genes per haploid genome, such individuals also have Hb A.

There are a number of γ and δ chain variants that result from single amino acid substitutions.[3] Abnormal fetal hemoglobins that contain γ chain variants are usually described after their place of origin; Hb F_{MALTA}, Hb F_{POOLE}, for example. The first structural δ chain variant was called Hb A_2', or B_2. Subsequently they were named after their place of discovery, Hb $A_{2CANADA}$ for example.

Because α chains are shared by Hbs F, A, and A_2, it follows that heterozygotes for α chain variants will have both normal Hbs F, A, and A_2 and variant forms composed of abnormal α chains combined with normal γ, β, and δ chains, respectively. These abnormal fetal and adult hemoglobins are usually named after the α chain variant. For example, individuals heterozygous for the α chain variant Hb $G_{PHILADELPHIA}$ have an abnormal fetal hemoglobin variant, Hb GF ($\alpha_2{}^G\gamma_2$), and an abnormal Hb A_2 called Hb G_2 ($\alpha^G\delta_2$).

The situation becomes even more complex when an individual is heterozygous for both an α chain variant and a β chain variant. Random association of subunits produces four main hemoglobin species. For instance, an individual who has inherited an α globin variant designated X and a β chain variant Y, would have these hemoglobins: $\alpha_2\beta_2$, $\alpha_2{}^X\beta_2$, $\alpha_2\beta_2{}^Y$, and $\alpha_2{}^X\beta_2{}^Y$. If the β chain variant was Hb S and the α chain variant was Hb G, these hemoglobins would become A, G, S, and SG. Of course things are even more complicated because such individuals also have an abnormal form of Hb A_2 and an abnormal fetal hemoglobin due to the association of abnormal α chains with δ and γ chains. They would have six hemoglobins in adult life, but during the switch from fetal to adult hemoglobin, there would be eight!

Molecular Pathology

The majority of the 750 or more human hemoglobin variants that have been isolated to date result from single amino acid substitutions in one of the globin chains. In addition, there are a few variants with either elongated or shortened globin chains, chains that are fusion products, part β and part δ or part β and part γ, and chains that contain more than one amino acid substitution.

Single-Base Substitutions. The single amino acid replacements that are found in the structural hemoglobin variants nearly all result from a single base substitution in the corresponding triplet

Table 181-2 Examples of Hemoglobin Variants with Elongated or Shortened Subunits

Elongated globin chains	
Chain termination mutations	$\text{Hbs}_{\text{CONSTANT SPRING, ICARIA, KOYA DORA, SEAL ROCK}}$
Frameshift mutations	$\text{Hbs}_{\text{WAYNE, SAVERNE, TAK, CRANSTON}}$
Reduplication	Hb_{GRADY}
Persistent *N*-terminal Met	$\text{Hbs}_{\text{MARSEILLE, S. FLORIDA, LONG ISLAND}}$
Shortened globin chains	
Deletions	$\text{Hbs}_{\text{LEIDEN, LYON, FREIBURG, GUNN HILL, MCKEES ROCKS}}$, and others

NOTE: A full list is given in Reference 148.

codon of the particular globin gene. A few variants have amino acid replacements at two different sites on the same subunit. Three variants involve the Hb S substitution. It is believed that they arose either by a new mutation on the β^S gene or by crossing over between the β^S gene and a β gene containing another structural variant.[3]

There are 2583 single base substitutions possible for the 140 residues of the α chain and the 146 residues of the β chain.[3] Of these, 1690 would result in an amino acid replacement, only one-third of which would cause a change in charge enabling the identification of the variant by electrophoresis. Remarkably, about 45 percent of these charged variants have already been identified. The relatively few known hemoglobin variants with neutral mutations that have been discovered were discovered because the amino acid substitution altered the stability of the hemoglobin molecule causing a hemolytic anemia.

Elongated Globin Chain Variants. Thirteen different elongated globin chain variants have been discovered (Table 181-2). They are caused by either single base substitutions in a chain-termination codon, by frameshift mutations, or by mutations that cause failure of cleavage of the initiator methionine residue.

The chain-termination mutants are all α chain variants in which there is a single base substitution in the chain-termination codon UAA[149] (Fig. 181-6). Thus, instead of coding for "termination," an amino acid is inserted in the growing peptide chain. Messenger RNA that is not normally translated is then read through until another in-phase chain-termination codon is reached. The result is an elongated α chain. For example, $\text{Hb}_{\text{CONSTANT SPRING}}$ has an α chain with 31 additional amino acid residues at its C-terminal end. The residue at position 142, next to what is normally the C-terminal arginine residue, is glutamine. This is because of a single base change in the chain termination codon UAA to CAA; the latter codes for glutamine. In fact, there is a family of α chain-termination variants, all of which differ at position 142, but which have identical residues in their elongated portions (Fig. 181-7). These variants all reflect different base substitutions in the chain-termination codon. Because $\text{Hb}_{\text{CONSTANT SPRING}}$ and its related family of elongated α chain variants are all associated with the clinical phenotype of α thalassemia,[149] they are considered further in a later section.

Several elongated hemoglobin variants have been found that appear to result from frameshift mutations. Hb_{WAYNE} is an α chain variant that has five additional amino acid residues at its C-terminal end.[150] This results from the loss of a single base at codons 138 or 139 that throws the reading frame out of phase, generating a completely new sequence. Because the α chain-termination codon is also out of phase, translation continues until a new in-phase termination codon is reached. The elongated β globin chain variant Hb_{TAK} also appears to arise by a frameshift mutation involving the duplication of two bases: CA at positions 146/147 or AC at position 147.[151] Other elongated β chain

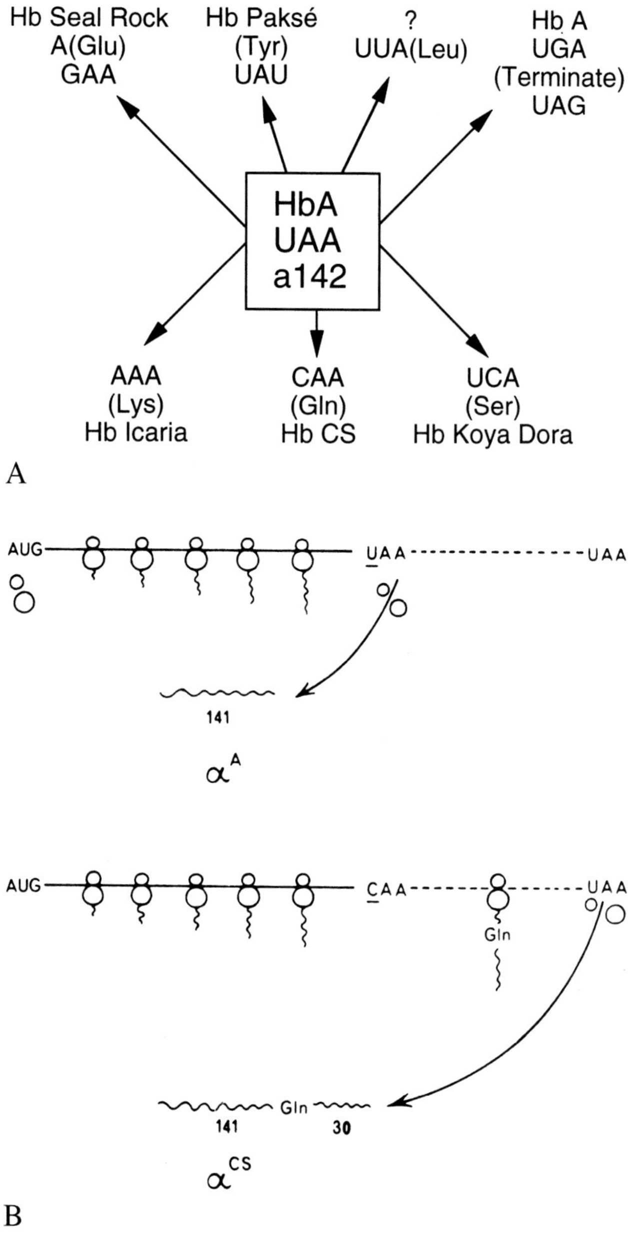

Fig. 181-7 The α-chain termination mutants. *A.* The various replacements in the α-chain termination codon which give rise to the family of termination mutants. *B.* Schematic representation of the synthesis of the elongated α chain of $\text{Hb}_{\text{CONSTANT SPRING}}$ (α^{CS}).

variants — $\text{Hb}_{\text{CRANSTON}}$ and $\text{Hb}_{\text{SAVERNE}}$ — also arise from frameshift mutations.[152,153]

There are five hemoglobin variants with elongated globin chains due to amino acid insertions. For example, Hb_{GRADY} has an α chain which is normal in every way except for the insertion of nine bases that result in repetition of the Glu-Phe-Thr sequence between α118 and α119.[154] Several mechanisms have been suggested for its generation, including unequal crossing-over between allelic α chain genes or, as seems more likely, the production of a break in a DNA strand; mispairing at an adjacent short repeated dinucleotide sequence; and filling in and repairing with the insertion of the additional bases, in this case, the in-phase codons for Glu-Phe-Thr.

Several hemoglobin variants with elongated amino terminal ends have been found; in each case, there is an additional methionine residue. For example, $\text{Hb}_{\text{LONG ISLAND-MARSEILLE}}$[155,156] has two amino acid substitutions in the β chain; an extension of the amino terminus by a methionine residue and a histidine to proline (CAC → CCC) change at the normal second position. Hb$_{SOUTH\ FLORIDA}$[157] has an extra N-terminal methionine, and the normal N-terminal valine is replaced by methionine. Methionine is the first residue to be incorporated during translation of globin chains and many other peptide chains. During translation of the nascent peptide chain, the amino terminal methionine is normally cleaved leaving, in the case of the β globin chain, valine as the amino terminal residue. It has been suggested that the amino acid substitutions in these variants somehow inhibit the activity of a peptidase that normally cleaves the amino terminal methionine.[155] Thus they are all single amino-acid replacements; the additional N-terminal methionine reflects posttranslational modification.

None of these elongated globin chain variants, with the exception of the α chain termination mutants, is associated with any major hematologic abnormality.

Shortened Globin Chains.[3] Several hemoglobin variants with shortened globin chains have been described (Table 181-2). In each case, one-to-five adjacent amino acids are missing from the abnormal chains and the remainder of the chain is completely normal. These variants probably involve deletion of one or more intact codons; if an entire codon is lost, the reading frame will remain in-phase and the remainder of the amino acid sequence will not differ from normal. In some cases, Hb$_{GUN\ HILL}$,[158] for example, the deletion results in molecular instability and the clinical picture of an unstable hemoglobin disorder (see below). Interestingly, the sequence of globin mRNA in the regions where these deletions have occurred may show a reiterated nucleotide sequence from two to eight bases in length. These deletion mutants may have arisen by chromosomal mispairing and nonhomologous crossing over in these regions.

One hemoglobin variant with a shortened β chain, Hb$_{MCKEES\ ROCKS}$, may have arisen from a nonsense mutation, that is a single base change that results in a chain termination codon within the coding region of the β globin gene.[159] Although, as shown later, this is the cause of several forms of β thalassemia, in the case of this variant the premature termination codon is at position 145, thus producing a viable globin chain lacking its two C-terminal residues, tyrosine and histidine.

Fusion Hemoglobins. There are several hemoglobin variants that contain fused or hybrid globin chains. The first to be discovered, Hb$_{LEPORE}$, contains normal α chains and non-α chains that consist of the first 50 to 80 amino acid residues of the δ chains and the last 60 to 90 residues of the normal C-terminal amino acid sequence of the β chains.[160] Thus the Hb$_{LEPORE}$ non-α chain is a $\delta\beta$ fusion chain. Three different varieties of Hb$_{LEPORE}$ have been described in which the transition from δ to β sequences occurs at different points.[160–162] Hb$_{KENYA}$ is analogous to Hb$_{LEPORE}$ except that the abnormal hybrid chain contains γ and β sequences; that is, it is a $\gamma\beta$ fusion chain.[163]

The fusion chains have probably arisen by nonhomologous crossing-over between part of the δ locus on one chromosome and part of the β locus on the complementary chromosome (Fig. 181-8). This event results from misalignment of chromosome pairing during meiosis so that a δ chain gene pairs with a β chain gene instead of its homologous partner. As shown in Fig. 181-8, such a mechanism should give rise to two abnormal chromosomes; the first, the Lepore chromosome, has no normal δ or β loci but simply a $\delta\beta$ fusion gene. At the opposite of the homologous pairs of chromosomes there should be an anti-Lepore ($\beta\delta$) fusion gene together with normal δ and β loci. Similarly, in the case of Hb$_{KENYA}$ there should be an anti-Kenya chromosome with intact

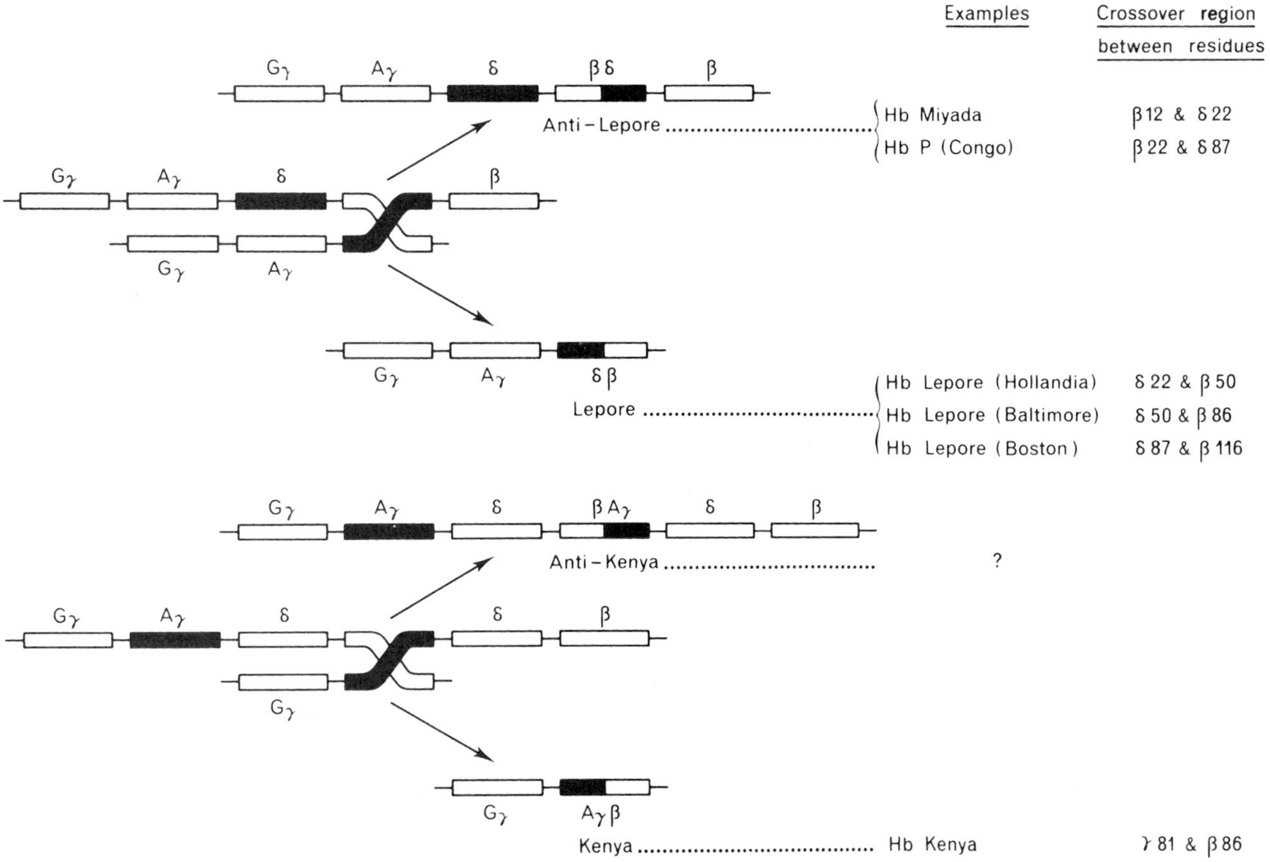

Fig. 181-8 **The generation of Hb$_{LEPORE}$ and Hb$_{KENYA}$.** ***(From Weatherall and Clegg.[2] Used by permission.)***

Table 181-3 Spectrum of Clinical Disorders Due to Structural Hemoglobin Variants

Hemolytic anemia
Sickling disorders
Hb C
Unstable variants
Abnormal oxygen transport
High affinity variants
Low affinity variants
Thalassemia phenotypes
Ineffectively synthesized variants
Hb E
$Hb_{KNOSSOS}$
Chain termination variants
Fusion variants
Highly unstable variants

Table 181-4 Common Sickling Disorders

Disorder	Genotype	Hemoglobins
Homozygous for Hb S		
Sickle cell disease	$\alpha\alpha/\alpha\alpha\beta^S\beta^S$	S, F, A_2
With α thalassemia	$-\alpha/-\alpha\beta^S\beta^S$	S, F, $A_2\uparrow$
	$-\alpha/\alpha\alpha\beta^S\beta^S$	S, F, A_2
Heterozygous for Hb S		
Sickle cell trait	$\alpha\alpha/\alpha\alpha\beta^A\beta^S$	A, S, A_2
With α thalassemia	$-\alpha/-\alpha\beta^A\beta^S$	A, S$\downarrow$, A_2
	$-\alpha/\alpha\alpha\ \beta^A\beta^S$	A, S, A_2
With β thalassemia*	$\alpha\alpha/\alpha\alpha\ \beta^0\beta^S$	S, F, $A_2\uparrow$
	$\alpha\alpha/\alpha\alpha\ \beta^+\beta^S$	S, A, F, A_2, $\uparrow$
With β-chain variants	$\alpha\alpha/\alpha\alpha\ \beta^S\beta^C$	S, C, A_2
	$\alpha\alpha/\alpha\alpha\ \beta^S\beta^D$	S, D, A_2
	$\alpha\alpha/\alpha\alpha\ \beta^S\beta^O{}_{ARAB}$	S, O_{ARAB}, A_2
	Many others	
With α-chain variants	$\alpha^G\alpha/\alpha\alpha\ \beta^A\beta^S$	A, S, G, A_2, G_2, SG
	Several other interactions	
With HPFH†	$\alpha\alpha/\alpha\alpha\ \beta^S -$	S, F, A_2

* β^0 and β^+ indicate β thalassemia with complete and partial deficiency of β-chain genes.
† Represents a chromosome with a deleted β-chain.

$^A\gamma$, δ, and β loci. A variety of anti-Lepore hemoglobins have been discovered, including Hb_{MIYADA}, $Hb_{P\text{-}CONGO}$, $Hb_{LINCOLN\ PARK}$, and $Hb_{P\text{-}NILOTIC}$.[164–167]

Another variant with fusion chains, $Hb_{PARCHMAN}$, is more complex in that the non-α chain has a δ sequence at the N- *and* C-terminal ends and a β sequence in the middle. It seems likely that this arose by a double-crossover or gene conversion.[168]

The Lepore variants result in the clinical phenotype of β or $\delta\beta$ thalassemia and are considered further in a later section. The anti-Lepore variants and Hb_{KENYA} are not associated with any significant hematologic changes.[2]

Structural Hemoglobin Variants of Clinical Importance

The structural hemoglobin variants that cause clinical disorders are summarized in Table 181-3. The three that reach polymorphic frequencies, causing a major public health problem, are Hbs S, C, and E. The other clinically important variants are much less common. They fall into two major groups. The first group is comprised of those variants that alter the oxygen-carrying properties of hemoglobin and result either in hereditary polycythemia or methemoglobinemia. The second group is comprised of unstable variants that produce a hemolytic anemia of varying severity. Finally, there are several hemoglobin variants that are ineffectively synthesized and that are, therefore, associated with the clinical phenotype of α or β thalassemia.

The Sickling Disorders

Hb S was the first hemoglobin variant to be discovered[8] and the first to have its amino acid substitution determined.[9] Sickle cell anemia is the cause of considerable mortality and morbidity in Africa and in every population that has had a migration of individuals of African descent, in parts of the Mediterranean region, in the Middle East, and in the Indian subcontinent. Despite the fact that the molecular lesion has been known for over 30 years, many questions remain about its pathophysiology, clinical heterogeneity, prognosis, and, above all, its clinical management.

Classification. The sickling disorders include the heterozygous state (sickle-cell trait (AS)), the homozygous condition (sickle cell disease (SS)), and the compound heterozygous states for the sickle cell gene in association with other β globin chain variants such as Hbs C and D (SC and SD disease) or β thalassemia (Hb S β thalassemia) (Table 181-4). The sickle cell gene is also found in association with α chain variants and different forms of α thalassemia.

Molecular Pathology. Hb S differs from Hb A by the substitution of valine for glutamic acid at position 6 of the β globin chain.[9] This reflects an A$\rightarrow$T substitution in the triplet codon for the sixth residue of the β globin chain. In concentrated hemoglobin solutions that are partially or fully deoxygenated, this amino acid substitution leads to polymerization and the formation of intracellular fibers that cause the sickle-cell deformity. The latter results in reduced deformability of the red cell and hence in its defective passage through the microcirculation. This is the basis for the vaso-occlusive manifestations of sickle cell disease. In addition, these structural changes of the red cell lead to a shortened survival and a chronic hemolytic anemia.

Despite an enormous amount of work over the last half-century, the final story of how sickle cells sickle remains to be told.[169,170] Early workers in the field observed that sickling is associated with the formation of liquid crystals or tactoids.[171] Electron micrographs of sickled erythrocytes show long thin bundles of Hb S fibers that tend to run parallel to the long axis of the cell and which are probably responsible for its abnormal morphology[172,173] (Fig. 181-9). The precise ultrastructure of these fibers is the subject of considerable controversy. A number of different models have been proposed in which 6, 8, or, more probably, 14 strands are twisted in a helical configuration to form hollow fibers with an external diameter of 170 to 220 Å.[174,175] The stabilization of these structures is dependent on interactions between individual globin chains. The precise localization of the contact points and the identification of the amino acid residues involved has been derived from a variety of techniques, particularly x-ray defraction studies. One of the most important contacts is made by the β6 Val of one molecule and the hydrophobic acceptor pocket of the β subunit of another molecule formed by Leu88 and Phe85 surrounded by hydrophilic Asp73, Thr84, and Thr87 residues.[176] Changing Leu88 to Ala by site-directed mutagenesis increases the solubility of Hb S Ala88 dramatically and reduces its polymerization rate compared to normal Hb S[177] (see below).

Polymer Formation. The way in which Hb S polymerizes to form a large molecular weight gel that is in equilibrium with monomeric hemoglobin solution is not fully understood. Monomers are stable in solution at a particular concentration of Hb S, pH, ionic strength, and temperature. However, small alterations in any of these variables lead to a rapid change to the gel form of Hb S. It is probably this sol-to-gel transition that leads to the viscosity changes, abnormalities of cell morphology, and sludging in the microcirculation and organ infarction, which are the hallmarks of the sickling disorders.

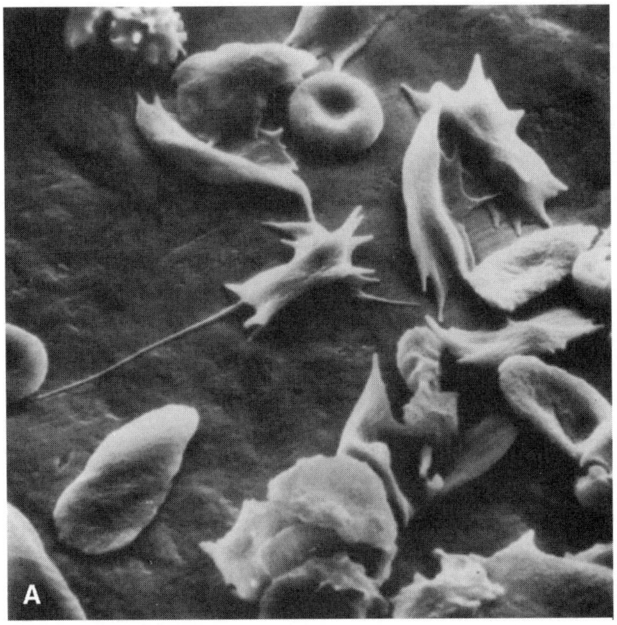

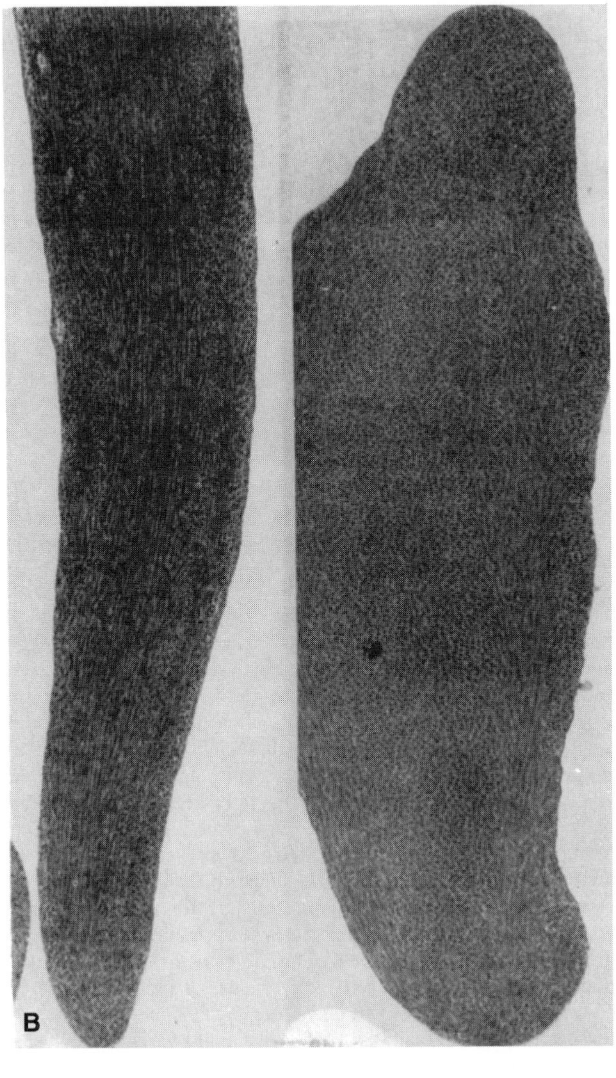

The sol-to-gel transformations have been studied using many different techniques including light scattering and turbidimetry,[178,179] sedimentation,[180] birefringence optics,[181] calorimetry,[182] and nuclear magnetic resonance.[183] Although no unifying model has arisen from these studies, several important factors emerge. There appear to be two distinct steps in the transition. The first is a lag phase that corresponds to the construction of a polymer of a critical size. Once this has occurred the reaction proceeds more rapidly and results in the formation of a high molecular weight polymer with closely aligned fibers. Recent x-ray structural data and microscopic observations suggest that the contacts responsible for the interfiber exponential polymerization are a subset of those responsible for the formation of the basic 14-stranded polymer unit.[184] The delay time varies as much as from the 30th to 50th power of the initial hemoglobin concentration; it has been calculated that by decreasing the intracellular hemoglobin concentration from 35 to 34 g/dl the delay phase is doubled. The sol-to-gel transformation is also extremely sensitive to changes in temperature and pH.

Further studies resulted in a model for the kinetics of Hb S polymerization based on a double-nucleation mechanism. Gelation is initiated by a process called homogenous nucleation in which single deoxy-Hb S molecules aggregate. These aggregates are thermodynamically unstable, and after a critical number of molecules aggregate, termed the critical nucleus, addition of further molecules produces a more stable aggregate or polymer. A second nucleation phase, termed heterogeneous nucleation, then takes place on the surface of a preexisting polymer. As this process proceeds, more surface area becomes available and the reaction becomes autocatalytic (see reference 170 for further discussion).

The kinetics of gel formation by Hb S in red cells is probably similar to that in solution. In some models of the pathophysiology of sickling, the delay time is thought to have important pathophysiological consequences. Oxygenation and deoxygenation of red cells in the circulation takes approximately the same time the sol-to-gel transformation of Hb S in solution.[185] This means that in the pulmonary circulation, at a high-oxygen tension, Hb S gels melt in less than half a second. They remain more or less in this state in the arterial circulation, but in the microcirculation, where oxygen saturation rapidly declines, there is a concomitant reduction in hemoglobin solubility. The red cell spends approximately 1 s in the capillary circulation; if the delay time is less than 1 s, cells could sickle and occlude the microcirculation. On the other hand, if the delay time is prolonged, sickling should not occur in the capillaries and the microcirculation remains patent. In other words, if the transit time is shorter than the delay time, occlusion does not occur. The type of environment that red cells may encounter in the renal medulla or spleen, where there may be a low pH, high hemoglobin concentration, and high ionic strength, all of which shorten the delay time, favors sickling. But although this type of mechanism may be important, other interpretations of the kinetics of sickling, which are considered later, suggest that the situation may be more complex than this. In particular, the physiological significance of the delay time has been questioned.[186]

Interactions Between Sickle and Other Hemoglobins. If known proportions of solutions of purified Hb S and other hemoglobins are mixed under appropriate conditions and are then completely deoxygenated, the degree of interaction of a particular hemoglobin in the sickling process can be assessed by determining the

Fig. 181-9 Sickle cells. *A.* Scanning electron microscopy appearance showing deoxygenated sickle cells with bizarre shapes and long filaments, short spicules, and chiseled surfaces. *B.* Electron microscopy (×20,770). The cells are shown in longitudinal section on the left and in cross section on the right. The figures are of deoxygenerated irreversibly sickled cells (ISC). In contrast to a more random pattern or filaments on deoxygenated non-ISC there is a distinctive regularity of filament arrangements. (*From Bertles and Dobler.*[188] *Used by permission.*)

minimum concentration of the final mixture in grams per deciliter at which gelling occurs (minimum gelling concentration or MGC).[187] Hence, a low MGC indicates an increased tendency to sickle and a high MGC indicates a decreased tendency to sickle. For example, mixtures of Hb S and Hb C have a higher MGC than solutions of Hb S alone, indicating that the substitution of the basic lysine does not cause sickling as efficiently as a hydrophobic valine. Hbs D and O Arab involve substitutions in the $\beta 121$ region, an area that x-ray data suggest is an important contact region. Gelation studies show that these variants interact with sickle cell hemoglobin and support sickling as efficiently as Hb S. On the other hand, experiments of this type show that Hb F has an inhibitory effect on sickling. This is probably a reflection of the fact that the glutamine residue ($\gamma 87$) prevents an important lateral contact in the double strand of the sickle fiber. Interestingly, x-ray studies that have analyzed contacts between double strands provide information that agrees with the location of mutations that affect gelation. The extensive data that have been generated on the various contact points and intermolecular interactions that may be important in the genesis of sickling are all consistent with a 14-strand structure of the sickle cell fiber (reviewed in references 3 and 186).

Cellular Heterogeneity. Films prepared from well-oxygenated blood samples from patients with sickle cell anemia show a number of sickled forms. Such irreversibly sickled cells (ISCs) are derived from a relatively young erythrocyte population with a low content of Hb F.[188] They are thought to be the end result of cycles of sickling and unsickling, leading to polymerization-induced damage to the red cell membrane. The ISC is a particularly rigid cell that is partly responsible for the abnormal viscosity of oxygenated whole blood of patients with sickle cell anemia. The ISC's decreased deformability is related directly to the degree of cellular dehydration.

The formation of the ISC is thought to occur in several stages. Cycles of sickling cause damage to the red cell membrane that becomes abnormally permeable to cations, resulting in a low K^+, high Na^+, high Ca^{++} concentration. In an effort to restore cation homeostasis, ATP-dependent pumps are activated, with a consequent decrease in intracellular ATP. At this stage, the erythrocyte is calcium loaded and ATP depleted, and may undergo the "Gardos effect," that is, gross dehydration with loss of potassium and water (reviewed in references 170 and 186). There has been considerable progress in defining the roles of the different red cell cation channels in determining the MCHC of sickle cells.[189,190] Probably the most important contributors to the dehydration of sickle cells are potassium-chloride cotransport and Ca^{++}-activated K^+ efflux. It is believed that the dehydrated cell, with its high MCHC, has a decreased delay time and tends to remain in the sickled configuration. It seems likely that the low level of Hb F in dehydrated cells is a major factor in their termination in the irreversibly sickled state.

The Role of the Vascular Endothelium.[191] Because of the ill-understood and unpredictable nature of the vaso-occlusive episodes that characterize all the sickling disorders, there is an increasing interest in the interaction between sickle cells and vascular endothelium. Under a variety of conditions, it is quite clear that these cells are "sticky" and adhere more readily than normal red cells to cultured endothelial cells. There appears to be a correlation between the severity of the sickling disorders and the degree of adherence.

At least some progress has been made toward the identification of some of the molecules involved in these interactions. Reticulocytes have on their surface an integrin complex, $\alpha_4\beta_1$, which apparently binds to both fibronectin and vascular cell adhesion molecule 1; the latter is expressed on the surface of all endothelial cells particularly after activation by inflammatory cytokines such as tumor necrosis factor-α. In addition, both vascular endothelial cells and subpopulations of sickle cell reticulocytes express CD36, which binds to thrombospondin secreted by activated platelets. Thrombospondin also interacts with sulfated glycans on sickle cells.

There are several other plasma proteins, including very-high-molecular weight varieties of von Willebrand factor, which also have the potential to make important contributions to adhesion. Particularly during inflammatory stress, a number of these different molecular interactions may result in increased adhesion of sickle cells to vascular endothelium. It also seems likely that leukocytes may be directly and indirectly involved in some of these interactions. Although the full significance of these studies is not yet clear, it seems likely that these interactions may be of considerable clinical importance in the generation or perpetuation of the vaso-occlusive phenomena and its consequences.

Rheology.[186] The transition from the sol to gel state is accompanied by a marked increase in viscosity. Hemoglobin, whether in free solution or in red cells, is a non-Newtonian fluid. This means that its viscosity is critically dependent on shear rate. Above minimum gelling concentration of deoxy Hb S, the viscosity increases dramatically; the rheologic properties of the gel are probably the most immediate cause of the vaso-occlusive manifestations of the sickling disorders.

Oxygen Affinity. Although Hb S in dilute solution has a normal oxygen dissociation curve, blood from patients with sickle cell anemia shows a decreased oxygen affinity.[3] There are probably several factors responsible for the shift in the oxygen dissociation curve. Although individuals with sickle cell anemia have higher levels of red cell 2,3-DPG, the major cause is intracellular polymerization of Hb S.

Pathophysiology. The sickling disorders are all characterized by two major pathologic processes, anemia and vaso-occlusion. Over the years, thinking about the pathophysiology of sickling disorders has changed.[186] Originally, it was thought to be the result of a vicious circle whereby the sickling of cells in the circulation led to stasis, decreased oxygen saturation, further sickling, and further stasis. In the 1970s, this view was modified to develop a more kinetic concept of what happens in the vasculature of patients with the sickling disorders. It was suggested that the delay time of intracellular polymerization is determined by the intracellular Hb S concentration and by other factors, including temperature, pH, and the circulatory dynamics. Obstruction might be viewed as the end result of the interaction of a number of variables; but overall, as the reflection of the relationship between delay and transit times. However, it was pointed out that the extremely rapid polymerization time expected to occur in the body, especially if there is preexisting polymer in many cells, makes it unlikely that this delay time is physiologically critical.

An alternate view[186] suggests that the actual sickling of red cells is relatively unimportant and that the major pathologic mechanisms in the sickling disorders reflect the rheologic effects of continuous variations in intracellular deoxy Hb S polymers. Because of the low mixed-arterial saturation in sickle cell anemia patients due to pulmonary ventilatory abnormalities and shunting, and the right shift in the oxygen dissociation curve caused by sickle hemoglobin, sickle erythrocytes are below 85 to 90 percent oxygen saturation even in the aorta. It is likely, therefore, that many cells will contain polymer while on the arterial side of the microcirculation. This will produce a marked decrease in the flexibility of red cells. Hence resistance to flow increases in the terminal arterioles and there is a tendency for stasis leading to local anoxia and tissue damage. In this model, hemolysis is visualized as the end result of chronic impedence of relatively inflexible cells as they try to negotiate areas of high resistance.[186]

Whatever the precise pathophysiological mechanisms involved, it is necessary to explain both the anemia and vascular occlusion that characterize the sickling disorders. It is likely that similar mechanisms are involved in both processes.

Anemia and Vaso-Occlusion. The anemia of sickle cell disease has an extremely complex pathophysiology. It seems likely that physical trapping of erythrocytes in the microcirculation plays a major role in shortening red cell survival. Even when fully oxygenated, sickle cells exhibit decreased deformability. Both static and dynamic deformability of oxygenated sickle cells decrease with increasing dehydration.[192] Because polymerization of Hb S is highly dependent on hemoglobin concentration, dehydrated sickled red cells show the most marked changes during partial deoxygenation. The decreased deformability is thought to cause trapping of rigid cells in small vessels.

There are other mechanisms that may be of importance in causing premature red cell destruction. As already mentioned, sickle cells have a tendency to adhere to vascular endothelial cells.[191,193] Furthermore, *in vitro* studies show that these cells are recognized more actively by monocytes and macrophages, suggesting that one component of the anemia of the sickling disorders is accelerated erythrophagocytosis.[194] It is also likely that oxidative damage to the red cell membrane plays a role in the destruction of sickle cells (reviewed in references 170 and 194 to 196). Sickle hemoglobin is unstable and dissociates with the production of hemichromes, which have the property of targeting auto-oxidative damage to red cell membrane components. Free-heme and iron may also mediate similar oxidative damage.[195,196] Excessive amounts of the byproducts of lipid peroxidation and the modification of membrane constituents by potential cross-linking agents, such as malondialdehyde, have also been demonstrated. Small aggregates of precipitated sickle hemoglobin may, like excess α chains in β thalassemia, attach with high affinity to the cytoplasmic portion of the membrane component, band 3. The resulting clustering of the band 3 protein may be associated with the deposition of specific antiband-3-protein antibodies on the red cell surface, a process linked to normal red cell senescence and possibly contributing to the shortened life span of sickle cells.[197] Sickle hemoglobin also has a tendency to auto-oxidize to form methemoglobin, therefore generating superoxide and losing heme. Overall, it appears that membrane damage due to oxidation may be a major factor in the shortened survival of sickle cells, linking the pathophysiology of the sickling disorders to the thalassemias (see below).

Irreversibly sickled cells are dehydrated, have a high calcium and low potassium content, and are extremely rigid. It seems likely, therefore, that the anemia of the sickling disorders reflects a shortened red cell survival consequent on decreased deformability, adherence to endothelial cells, erythrophagocytosis, auto-oxidation, and gross membrane abnormalities. Finally, it was observed that there might be a suboptimal proliferative response by the bone marrow in this condition, probably because of the low oxygen affinity of Hb S in red cells.[198] Thus, part of the anemia of patients with sickle cell anemia may be a physiological adaptation to the altered oxygen carrying properties of their blood.

The vaso-occlusive manifestations of the sickling disorders probably result from the altered rheologic properties of red cells containing a high concentration of Hb S. As already described, it is likely that the tendency for sickle cells to adhere to vascular endothelium may also be involved, and that plasma constituents may play a role in their interaction with endothelial cells.[191,199] Adherent cells may retard the flow of other sickle cells thereby increasing the time available for sickling as cells pass through hypoxic tissues. Ultimately, the mass of adherent red cells and rigid cells free in small vessels may lead to microvascular occlusion and subsequent tissue infarction. To this complicated picture must be added the flow properties and regulation of the diameter of the microcirculation itself. This important topic has not been studied extensively although such evidence as there is suggests that there are important differences in microcirculation flow kinetics in patients with sickle cell anemia as compared with normal individuals (reviewed in references 170, 186, and 189).

Although these mechanisms may well contribute to vascular occlusion in sickle cell disease, the triggering mechanisms for the acute occlusive episodes that are the basis for the painful crises of the disease are still not understood. Similarly, we have no information about the factors that cause the curious hypertrophic changes in some of the cerebral vessels that seem to be responsible for the neurologic complications of sickle cell anemia (see below). There is some epidemiologic evidence that cold may be a precipitating factor in the painful crisis[200] and it seems likely that other factors which alter the dynamics of the microcirculation, either generally or regionally, may be important triggering mechanisms.[186] But all this is speculation and virtually nothing is known about what precipitates a painful crisis.

The Sickle Cell Trait. The life expectancy of individuals with the sickle cell trait is probably the same as the life expectancy of nonaffected persons.[200] Although a number of clinical abnormalities have been reported in individuals with the trait, most of the reports are anecdotal and the association may be coincidental. It seems likely that such persons are at risk for splenic infarction when flying at high altitudes under conditions of inadequate cabin pressurization. Except in very unusual circumstances, this problem should not be encountered in commercial aircraft. There is no justification for denial of employment or life insurance to individuals with the sickle cell trait who fly in normally pressurized aircraft.

There is some evidence that otherwise unexplained hematuria may be associated with the sickle cell trait, as may the ability to concentrate urine. Other associations, that are based on less firm data, include a slightly increased risk of pulmonary embolism, renal papillary necrosis, and avascular necrosis of bone. There are a few reports of infarctive episodes following the application of a limb tourniquet for orthopedic procedures, or following a poorly administered anesthetic.

Sickle Cell Anemia. Sickle cell anemia is characterized by a lifelong hemolytic anemia, the occurrence of acute exacerbations called crises, and a variety of complications resulting from an increased propensity to infection and the deleterious effects of repeated vaso-occlusive episodes. Despite so much knowledge about the molecular pathology of the condition, why the course of the illness is so variable, even within individual sibships let alone between different racial groups, is poorly understood. In this section, we describe the typical features of sickle cell anemia and then define what is known about the factors that modify the clinical phenotype.

Clinical and Hematologic Features and Course of the Illness.[170,186,200] Sickle cell anemia usually presents during the first or second year of life, although in milder cases later presentation is common and some patients may only be ascertained as adults during family studies or by chance. The usual presenting features are failure to thrive, repeated infections in infancy, attacks of painful dactylitis (the hand-foot syndrome; see below), or pallor. At this stage, the infant looks pale, there may be slight icterus, the spleen is usually palpable, and the typical hematologic findings of sickle cell anemia are established. The hemoglobin value varies between 7 and 11 g/dl, although higher levels are encountered with unusually mild forms of the illness. There are typical features of hemolysis with a raised reticulocyte count in the 10 to 20 percent range, marked variation in the depth of staining of the red cells, and some sickled erythrocytes on the blood film. The serum bilirubin level is slightly elevated and the urinary urobilinogen level is increased.

The subsequent course is variable. Overall, patients with this disorder show early retardation of growth; weight is affected more than height. Although the mean height is generally reduced in childhood, data from studies in older children and adolescents are less clear. Usually by the age of 20 years, the height curves in males approach those of control groups and in females may actually exceed those of normal individuals.[200] Although there has been much controversy, it appears that patients with sickle cell disease have an abnormal body habitus characterized by long limbs and hence a decrease in the upper to lower segment ratio. Other features of abnormal anthropometry include narrow pectoral and pelvic girdles, increased anteroposterior chest diameters, a reduced arm circumference, and thinner skin folds. The onset of puberty is often delayed.

Splenomegaly is usually present in infancy and early childhood; in a large Jamaican study, 77 percent of patients had palpable spleens by the age of 24 months.[200] In the majority of patients, the organ gradually becomes impalpable during later childhood; persistent splenomegaly occurs in patients with high levels of Hb F and in those who are homozygous for α^+ thalassemia (see below). The gradual splenic fibrosis and atrophy reflects repeated infarction of the organ. These changes in spleen size are mirrored by the presence of pitted red cells that result from reduced splenic function;[201] the pitted red cell count in sickle cell anemia correlates with other assessments of splenic function, such as the clearance of heat-damaged autologous red cells and the uptake of labeled sulfacolloid.[202]

Because of the right-shifted oxygen dissociation curve, patients with sickle cell anemia tend to compensate well for their anemia and exercise tolerance is good. The main clinical problems that are encountered early in life are crises (see below) and an increased propensity to infection.

It is clear that children with this condition have an increased susceptibility to infection, although many of the published studies lack adequate controls. There is no doubt, however, that they are prone to infections due to *Streptococcus pneumoniae, Salmonella, Escherichia coli*, and *Hemophilus influenzae*.[186,200] The *Salmonella* infections may be gastrointestinal, but osteomyelitis is also common and probably results from infection of infarcted bone. The pattern of other infections is also variable but pneumococcal pneumonia and septicemia are particularly important; overwhelming septicemia and shock is a common cause of death, particularly during infancy and childhood.

Undoubtedly a major factor in this proneness to infection is impaired splenic function together with generalized reticuloendothelial blockade; the pattern of infection in childhood is very similar to that of children who have had their spleens removed for other causes. The precise mechanism whereby splenic hypofunction increases susceptibility to infection is not clear; both antibody production and antigen processing may be involved. There may be other factors, particularly in children with sickle cell anemia, including defective neutrophil function and abnormalities of the alternative pathway of complement activation, although such changes are only found in a small proportion of patients.[200] Infection is a major cause of death at all ages, which suggests that hyposplenism is not the only factor involved in increased susceptibility.

Crises. Acute exacerbations of the illness in patients with sickle cell anemia are called *crises*, which can take many clinical forms. Although the subdivision of crises into specific entities is useful for descriptive purposes it should be emphasized that in many sickling crises a number of different pathophysiological mechanisms seem to be involved.

The *painful crisis*[200] is the most common and important manifestation of sickle cell anemia. These episodes are characterized by the rapid onset of pain in the limbs, back, abdomen, or chest. The mechanism is still unknown. There is good epidemiologic evidence that cold may be a factor; in some cases, there may also be an underlying infection. But in many instances, no precipitating factor is found. There are no consistent changes in blood platelets or coagulation factors. It is clear, however, that these are vaso-occlusive episodes; bone marrow biopsy over regions of bone pain invariably shows infarcted marrow. On theoretical grounds, a vaso-occlusive episode of this type could be caused either by enhancement of intravascular sickling or an alteration in the flow kinetics in the microcirculation. Other factors that may be involved include acidosis, hypoxia, and dehydration, all of which are known to potentiate intracellular polymerization.

The clinical course of the painful crisis is characteristic. The pain follows no particular pattern and tends to be severe for 2 or 3 days, after which it settles spontaneously. It is quite common to observe mild pyrexia on the second or third day, even in patients in whom an extensive search has not demonstrated any source of infection. Presumably, the pyrexia is due to bone infarction. In an uncomplicated painful crisis, the hematologic findings remain unchanged.

One particularly important form of painful crisis, which occurs early in infancy, is the so-called *hand-foot* syndrome. This is a dactylitis characterized by the sudden onset of painful swelling of the dorsum of the hands and feet. Two pathophysiological mechanisms are involved. First, at this age bones are growing rapidly and may have a limited blood supply. Second, the occlusion of vessels by sickled cells may not be easily compensated for by a coaxial blood supply to the bone. Autopsy studies have shown complete necrosis of the marrow and the inner third of the cortex, lesions similar to those that can be produced in experimental animals by interruption of both the metaphyseal and nutrient artery supplies to long bones. In later life, almost any bone can be involved in a painful crisis, and local swelling of the bone, which presumably reflects a periosteal reaction over an infarct, is commonly observed. Although painful crises always settle, repeated vaso-occlusive episodes may lead to destruction of bone and soft tissue.

Although painful crises are usually self-limiting and not life-threatening, there are other forms of acute exacerbation of the clinical course of sickle cell anemia that are more serious and, together with infection, are the most common causes of death. There are a variety of *sequestration crises*. The commonest type involves the spleen in the first two years of life.[200,203] The clinical picture is characterized by a rapid enlargement of the spleen that becomes engorged with sickled erythrocytes. This may progress to a stage at which a large proportion of the circulating blood volume is entrapped in the spleen leading to profound anemia and death. These episodes may occur more than once, particularly in children with persistent splenomegaly. A similar type of sequestration may occur in the liver in later life; the organ rapidly enlarges, while at the same time there is a dramatic fall in the hematocrit.[204]

Another important type of sequestration crisis is called the *chest syndrome*.[205] Chest syndrome is increasingly recognized as a cause of morbidity and mortality in patients of all ages. Pleuritic pain, fever, cough, and increasing dyspnea characterize it. These symptoms reflect widespread blockage of the pulmonary arteries with sickled cells leading to pulmonary infarction. Initially there may be no radiologic findings, but as the condition develops, pulmonary infiltrates appear and may progress to an almost complete "white-out" of the lung fields. Blood gas analysis shows increasing hypoxemia. It is often very difficult to distinguish between an acute chest syndrome and a chest infection, and it is possible that infection may precipitate the syndrome in some cases. A previous history of an upper respiratory infection, infected sputum, a marked leukocytosis on presentation, and lower lobe disease is more in keeping with a pneumonia, but these features are by no means always present and the distinction may be extremely difficult. A falling hematocrit and/or platelet count, and rapidly deteriorating pO_2 values are useful indicators of an impending chest syndrome.[205]

Attacks of acute abdominal pain resembling a "surgical abdomen" occur frequently in patients with sickle cell anemia and constitute an *abdominal crisis*.[200] The pain is usually widespread and may be associated with tenderness without guarding, distension, and a reduction or absence of bowel sounds. These features may be difficult to distinguish from peritonitis, although in the abdominal crisis, rebound tenderness is absent and the patient's general condition is usually not so poor as in those with peritonitis. It is very important that this syndrome be recognized if unnecessary surgical exploration is to be avoided.

Another important cause of death in patients of all ages with sickle cell anemia is the *aplastic crisis*. Extensive studies implicate a human parvovirus-like agent as the commonest cause of this condition.[206] Infection with this agent in normal people causes transient erythroid hypoplasia and a slight drop in the hemoglobin level. In patients with sickle cell anemia who have a very short red cell survival, temporary marrow aplasia may lead to profound anemia. A very sudden drop in the hematocrit and the disappearance of reticulocytes from the peripheral blood characterizes profound anemia. The bone marrow shows a marked reduction or absence of erythroid precursors. Recovery occurs in a few days, heralded by a rising reticulocyte count. Aplastic crises occur in epidemics and often involve more than one family member. This reflects the periodic epidemicity of parvovirus infections in the general population.

Acute neurologic episodes or *neurologic crises* are a particularly important and distressing accompaniment of sickle cell anemia.[207] The prevalence has ranged in different series from 5.5 to 17 percent.[208] These episodes usually reflect cerebral infarction in younger patients and hemorrhage in older ones. Angiographic studies suggest that these neurologic episodes may be the result of occlusion or stenosis of large arteries in the carotid distribution. Histologic studies have shown both thrombosis and intimal thickening in the large and small arteries.[209] It has been suggested that these changes result from intimal damage from a combination of high velocity flow, rigidity of the red cells, and their adherence to the vessel wall, all associated with intravascular sludging. The clinical features of these disorders are very similar to those that result from carotid occlusion due to atherosclerotic disease, including premonitory transient ischemic attacks.[210] Regular monitoring of the cerebral vessels using Doppler ultrasonography, possibly with magnetic resonance angiography, is a valuable approach to assessing the likely occurrence of this important complication.[208]

Hemolytic crisis is often used to describe an acute exacerbation of the hemolytic component of sickle cell anemia. In patients with intercurrent infection or painful crises, the reticulocyte count may rise, but it is doubtful if the hemolytic crisis is a separate entity. *Priapism* occurs acutely, and results from occlusion of the outflow vessels from the corpora cavernosa by sickled cells. This is an extremely distressing complication that may last for several days and that may lead to permanent deformity of the penis.[200]

Chronic Organ Damage. Repeated vaso-occlusive episodes may lead to chronic organ damage resulting from repeated infarction with subsequent healing and fibrosis.

Renal involvement occurs in virtually every patient with sickle cell anemia.[200] In early life, there is impairment of renal function that is correctable by blood transfusion. In later life, this defect is irreversible. It probably results from derangement of the normal countercurrent distributor in the medullary circulation; blood flow to the glomeruli is maintained whereas flow to the vasa recta in the medulla is reduced. Injection of kidneys at autopsy has demonstrated decreased filling of these vessels, with dilated capillaries and extravasation of contrast media from ruptured vessels. In addition, there may be a mild form of distal tubular acidosis. Otherwise unexplained hematuria is common, and probably results from lesions of the papillae. It appears that chronic progressive renal failure is a common form of death in adults with the sickling disorders.[200]

In early life, the concentrating defect of the kidney may be reflected in thirst and polyuria, and it is thought that nocturnal enuresis is common. In addition, there have been a number of reports of a true nephrotic syndrome, although recent analyses have cast doubt on the true association between the sickling disorders and nephrosis.[200]

Many other organs may be involved in the chronic damage resulting from vascular blockage. Permanent penile deformity has already been mentioned. *Avascular necrosis* of the femoral or humoral heads occurs (Fig. 181-10) although it is not clear whether this is as common in sickle cell disease as in Hb SC disease (see below). Involvement of the mandible, skull, ribs, and sternum, and vertebral bodies may all give rise to deformity or chronic bone tenderness. Chronic *leg ulceration* is also very common. The lesions occur just above the medial or lateral malleoli; presumably, this reflects the precarious vascularization of the skin of this region. *Proliferative retinopathy* also occurs in sickle cell anemia, although it is commoner in hemoglobin SC disease; it is described in a later section. As mentioned earlier, the *central nervous system* may be involved in a variety of chronic complications following acute vaso-occlusive episodes. Stroke is the most important; two thirds of strokes occur in children, and in many cases, there are recurrent episodes.[210] Although there may be a remarkable degree of restoration of neurologic function, many children are left with permanent defects in cognitive, sensory, and motor function.

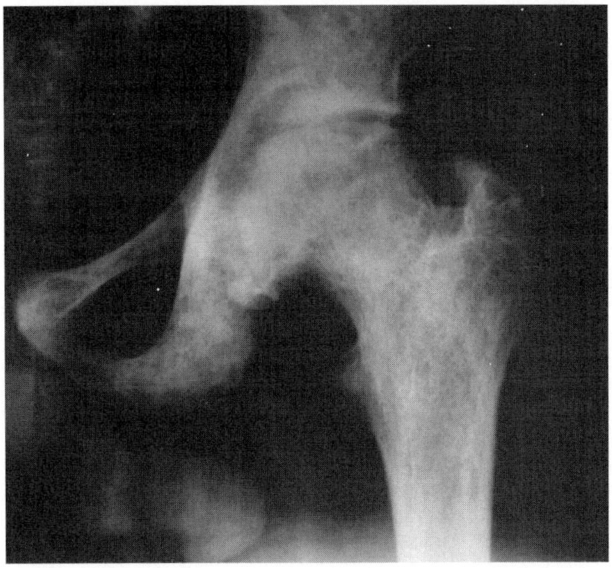

Fig. 181-10 Aseptic necrosis of the head of the left humerus in a patient with HB SC disease. (*From Weatherall and Clegg.*[2] *Used by permission.*)

Hepatic involvement occurs in a variety of forms. There is invariably iron loading of the Kupffer cells and hepatocytes, and true macronodular cirrhosis has been observed although the frequency of this condition seems to vary; for example, it is very rare in Jamaica. *Chronic pulmonary involvement* with progressive obliteration of the pulmonary vascular bed, associated pulmonary hypertension, and right ventricular hypertrophy is being recognized as shunting, with increasing frequency in adults.[211] Similarly, the *heart* seems to escape infarction. There is nearly always some degree of cardiac enlargement and a variety of flow murmurs have been described, together with all the other manifestations of a hyperdynamic circulation. It is surprising that although the myocardium extracts more oxygen than any other tissue, vaso-occlusive episodes involving the myocardium do not seem to occur and coronary occlusion is not a recognized complication. This probably reflects the rapidity of blood flow in the myocardium, especially in a hyperdynamic heart. The question of whether there is a specific sickle *cardiomyopathy* remains open, although autopsy series reveal only minor histologic changes in cardiac muscle.[200]

Other Complications. There is a large literature on the effects of sickle cell anemia on *pregnancy*. The most recent series estimate a very low maternal mortality, although it should be noted that most of these studies were done in developed Western societies.[200] Such data as are available from Nigeria indicate that there is still a high maternal mortality.[212] Fetal wastage from abortion, stillbirth, and neonatal death is increased in all populations.[200] The anemia is exacerbated and there appears to be an increased incidence of crises during pregnancy; the acute chest syndrome is particularly important. The association of preeclamptic toxemia remains controversial.

Because of the chronic hemolysis and high turnover of bilirubin, the formation of pigment stones in the gall bladder is extremely common. It seems likely that this complication has been underrecognized in the past, and many patients with sickle cell anemia have attacks of biliary colic and cholecystitis and require cholecystectomy.[200]

Because of the rapid marrow turnover, *folate deficiency* may occur, particularly in pregnancy, although this seems to be uncommon in patients maintained on adequate diets. Although *Plasmodium falciparum* malaria may be less severe in sickle cell heterozygotes, there is no doubt that it is a major cause of morbidity and mortality in homozygotes living in endemic areas. Audiometry has revealed *sensorineural hearing loss* in about 12 percent of patients with sickle cell anemia.[200] However this is usually subclinical; rarely, sudden deafness may occur during a painful crisis.

Factors that Influence Prognosis. Until recently, with the exception of the pioneering studies of Serjeant and his colleagues in Jamaica,[200] surprisingly little was known about the prognosis of sickle cell anemia. Serjeant's studies suggested that there was a mortality of approximately 10 percent in the first few years of life, the most important causes of death being infection and splenic sequestration, with a smaller number of sudden, unexpected deaths of uncertain etiology. More recent studies,[213] and data from the Cooperative Study of Sickle Cell Disease in the United States,[214] found a peak incidence of death between 1 and 3 years of age, again caused by infection. The overall mortality rate was 2.6 percent and the probability of surviving to the age of 29 years was about 85 percent. These figures are similar to those in Jamaica, which show a 10-year survival of 84 percent with the suggestion of a second peak in the mortality curve in the 20- to 24-year-old group. Data about longevity are extremely sparse. Similarly, little is known about the prognosis for the disease in rural Africa although such data as are available suggest that there is a high mortality in early life. Infection seems to be the commonest cause of death at all ages, but at least in Jamaica, progressive renal failure is being seen with increasing frequency in older age groups.[200]

Unfortunately, knowledge about the factors that modify the course of sickle cell anemia is extremely scanty. In certain populations, such as those of eastern Saudi Arabia and Orissa, India, there is a relatively mild form of the disease,[215,216] which is characterized by higher hemoglobin levels, lower reticulocyte counts, and persistence of splenomegaly into adult life. In both these populations, the majority of patients have unusually high levels of fetal hemoglobin in the 15 to 25 percent range, and there is high prevalence of α thalassemia. While overall it appears that elevated levels of fetal hemoglobin are protective in sickle cell anemia, the relationship is not straightforward.[217] Studies in Saudi Arabia that compared the clinical course in low versus high fetal-hemoglobin-producing populations of patients with sickle cell anemia confirmed that the disease is milder in some respects in those with the higher levels of fetal hemoglobin. These studies also demonstrated that this group might not be protected against certain complications, particularly painful crises and bone disease.[218] The occurrence of severe, destructive aseptic necrosis of the femoral heads was equally common in both groups. Much may depend on the intracellular level and distribution of Hb F. It is only in those who are compound heterozygotes for the sickle cell and hereditary persistence of fetal hemoglobin genes that there is a relatively uniform distribution of Hb F among the red cells; this disorder is particularly mild. Even in the populations of Saudi Arabia and Orissa, India, where there may be fetal hemoglobin levels of similar magnitude, the Hb F is much less uniformly distributed.

While the elevated level of Hb F in patients with sickle cell anemia undoubtedly results from selection of cells containing relatively greater amounts of this hemoglobin in the peripheral circulation, there is no doubt that many different genetic factors are involved in setting the final level of fetal hemoglobin.[189] This question is addressed in more detail below when the genetic factors responsible for the variable elevation of Hb F in different forms of β thalassemia are described.

Another factor that modifies the course of sickle cell anemia is the coinheritance of α thalassemia.[189,219] About 2 percent of African American and Jamaican populations are homozygous for the deletion form of α^+ thalassemia. Comparison of such individuals, who also have sickle cell anemia, with individuals who have sickle cell anemia without α thalassemia, shows that the α thalassemic group has higher hemoglobin levels, typical thalassemic red cell indices, a greater likelihood of splenomegaly after childhood, and fewer episodes of the acute chest syndrome and chronic leg ulceration. The α thalassemic group also has lower levels of Hb F. *In vitro* studies show that the deformability of sickle cells is enhanced if α thalassemia is also present, providing a cellular basis for these observations.[220] Evidence about the effect on survival of the coinheritance of α thalassemia remains conflicting.

But if high levels of Hb F and α thalassemia are excluded, the clinical picture of sickle cell anemia still remains remarkably heterogeneous and the factors that are involved in modifying the course are not understood. As shown later, a second mutation in the β globin gene occasionally accounts for some of this heterogeneity, but undoubtedly many other factors remain to be identified.

The Hemoglobin Constitution. In the sickle cell trait there is usually about 30 percent Hb S with a normal Hb A_2 level (Fig. 181-11). The relative amount of Hb S varies. The main factor that seems to be responsible is the number of active α globin genes. Individuals with the sickle cell trait who are also heterozygous for α^0 thalassemia, or heterozygous or homozygous for α^+ thalassemia have lower levels of Hb S. Those with triplicated α globin genes have higher levels.[221]

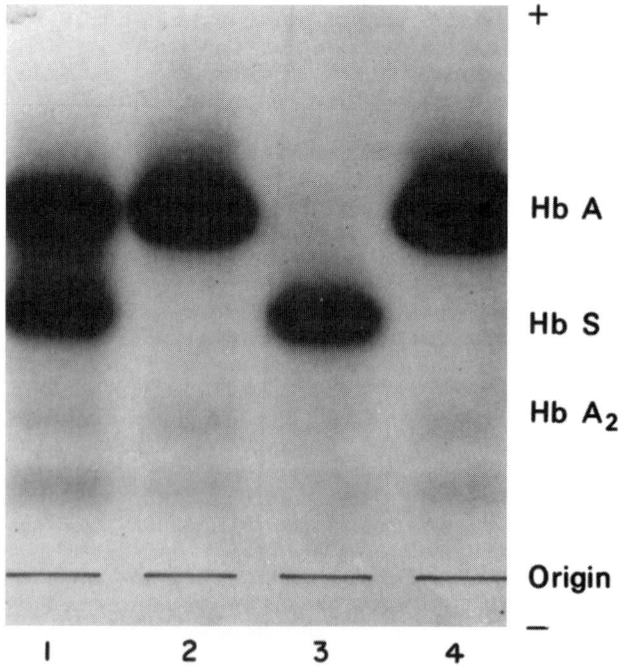

Fig. 181-11 Hemoglobin electrophoresis (starch gel; protein stain, pH 8.6). The following are shown from left to right: 1 = sickle cell trait; 2 = normal; 3 = sickle cell anemia; 4 = normal. (*From Weatherall and Clegg.[2] Used by permission.*)

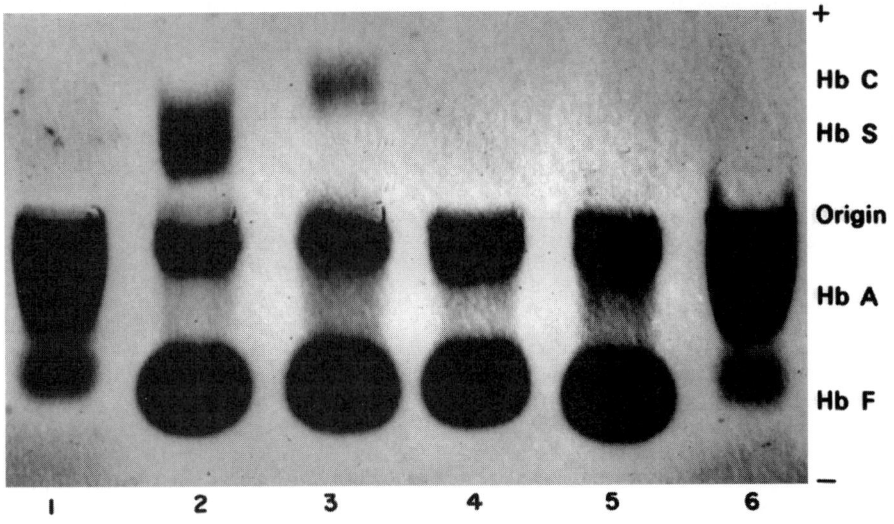

Fig. 181-12 Hemoglobin electrophoresis (agar gel, pH 6.0). The following are shown from left to right: 1 = normal; 2 = sickle cell trait in newborn period; 3 = Hb C trait in newborn period; 4 and 5 = normal newborns; 6 = normal adult. (*From Weatherall and Clegg.*[2] *Used by permission.*)

In sickle cell anemia, the hemoglobin consists mainly of Hb S with a normal Hb A_2 level and a variable amount of Hb F ranging from 1 or 2 percent to 30 percent. Hemoglobin S can be distinguished from other variants with a similar electrophoretic migration on standard electrophoresis at alkaline pH by its different properties on agar gel electrophoresis (Fig. 181-12). However, the presence of Hb S should always be confirmed by a test for sickling. Individuals homozygous for Hb S who also have α thalassemia have slightly raised Hb A_2 levels.

Other Sickling Disorders. The sickle cell gene has been associated with many structural hemoglobin variants.[3,200,222] Only a minority of these conditions, however, are common enough to warrant separate description. Recently, a new sickling syndrome has been described that is symptomatic in the heterozygous state and that results from the coinheritance of a second mutation in a β globin gene containing the sickle cell mutation.

Hemoglobin SC Disease. This condition[3,186,200,222] occurs in individuals of West African origin. It is a milder disorder than sickle cell anemia, although almost all the complications of the latter have been observed. Growth, development, and body habitus are normal, and the only abnormal physical sign is splenomegaly that occurs in about 65 percent of cases. The disease may not present with one of the complications until middle or late in life. The blood picture shows a mild anemia with hemoglobin levels in the 11 to 13 g/dl range, and a reticulocytosis of 3 to 5 percent. The peripheral blood film is particularly striking, showing sickled cells, many target cells, and cells that contain linear crystalline structures that tend to lie across their centers.

The main importance of Hb SC disease is that it often goes unrecognized until a serious complication occurs because it is mild. These complications include otherwise unexplained hematuria, aseptic necrosis of the femoral or humoral heads, and, particularly, ocular manifestations. All these changes reflect the abnormal rheology of red cells that contain both Hbs S and C; the pathophysiology of Hb C is considered below.

The ocular complications are particularly important and are characterized by what is termed a proliferative sickle retinopathy (PSR).[200] The latter seems to develop through successive stages, starting with peripheral arteriolar occlusions, the development of arteriolar-venular anastomoses, neovascularization, and, finally, the development of vitreous hemorrhages and retinal detachment. In a large series studied in Jamaica, about one-third of patients with Hb SC disease had PSR at varying stages of development, and this complication seems to be more prevalent in those with higher steady state hematocrits.[200]

The other serious complication of Hb SC disease is the development of widespread pulmonary vaso-occlusion with the rapid onset of a typical chest syndrome as described in the section on sickle cell anemia. This complication occurs particularly commonly during pregnancy or the puerperium.

Sickle Cell β Thalassemia.[3] The coinheritance of the sickle cell and β thalassemia genes generates a wide spectrum of clinical disorders, the severity of which range from a disorder identical to sickle cell anemia to a completely asymptomatic condition that is only identified by chance. Much of this heterogeneity depends on the type of β thalassemia mutation (see the β thalassemia section). In those who inherit β^o thalassemia the clinical disorder is very similar to sickle cell anemia. In those who have a mild β^+ thalassemia mutation there may be as much as 30 percent Hb A in the red cells and the clinical picture is no more severe than sickle cell or β thalassemia trait.

Other Compound Heterozygous Disorders.[13,200] Hb S/ $D_{LOS\ ANGELES}$ is a relatively severe disorder that resembles sickle cell anemia; this reflects the enhanced copolymerization of Hb $D_{LOS\ ANGELES}$ with Hb S due to the β121 substitution at an important contact point in the sickle cell fiber. Hb S/O_{ARAB} is also a severe disorder that is very similar to sickle cell anemia. The various combinations of *Hb S with hereditary persistence of fetal hemoglobin* are all extremely mild. There are numerous other examples of the interaction of α or β globin chain variants with Hb S. In most cases they result in an asymptomatic disorder identical to the sickle cell trait. The effects of α thalassemia on the course of sickle cell anemia are considered in an earlier section.

Sickle Cell Disease in Heterozygotes; Hb $S_{ANTILLES}$. This sickling hemoglobin with two substitutions in *cis* in the β globin chain, 6 Glu $\rightarrow$ Val and 23 Val $\rightarrow$ Ile,[223] is of particular phenotypic interest. This variant has the same electrophoretic mobility as Hb S and the erythrocytes of heterozygotes tend to sickle at partial pressures of oxygen similar to those that induce sickling in Hb SC disease. Heterozygotes have a mild hemolytic anemia, splenomegaly, and, in some cases, painful crises. Thus, the condition resembles Hb SC disease. Nuclear magnetic spin resonance studies suggest that the β23 substitution induces slight structural perturbations throughout the β subunit.

The discovery of this mutation is of particular interest because it raises the possibility that some of the reported heterogeneity of the sickle cell trait and sickle cell anemia might result from substitutions of this type that do not alter the charge of sickle hemoglobin and hence cannot be identified on routine electrophoresis. However, several other hemoglobins with the sickle mutation and a second mutation, including Hb $S_{PROVIDENCE}$, Hb S_{OMAN}, and Hb S_{TRAVIS}, all of which contain the sickle mutation together with a second substitution,[148] appear to be symptomless in heterozygotes. Presumably, the key to these interesting mutations is the functional properties of the second mutation.

Other Common Hemoglobin Variants

The only other hemoglobin variants that are encountered commonly are Hbs C, D, and E.

Hemoglobin C. This was the second variant to be identified electrophoretically. It results from the substitution of lysine for glutamic acid at position 6 in the β chain.[224] It is restricted in its distribution to areas of West Africa and to countries in which there has been movement of populations from this region. The gene frequency in African Americans, for example, ranges from 0.01 to 0.02.

A number of observations suggest that Hb C is less soluble than Hb A, with the result that it tends to crystallize in red cells.[225] This is probably due to intermolecular interactions arising from the $\beta 6$ substitution. Interestingly, crystal formation is favored by the oxyhemoglobin configuration and the crystals tend to melt when red cells undergo deoxygenation in the capillaries.[226] The red cells of Hb C homozygotes contain less water than normal and have an enhanced rate of potassium efflux. It was suggested that these changes result from the direct interaction of the positively charged Hb C with negatively charged proteins on the cytoplasmic surface of the red cell membrane.[227] Because of the increased MCHC and the tendency to crystal formation, red cells containing Hb C are less deformable than normal. It seems likely that this is the major mechanism whereby their survival is shortened in the circulation. They also have decreased oxygen affinity.

Hemoglobin C heterozygotes have no hematologic changes except for an increased number of target cells on a stained blood film. The homozygous state for Hb C is characterized by a mild hemolytic anemia with splenomegaly. The blood film shows nearly 100 percent target cells and there is a slightly elevated reticulocyte count. The peripheral blood film also shows a number of intracellular crystals.

The important interactions of Hb C are with Hb S (see previous section) and with β thalassemia. The compound heterozygous state with β^o thalassemia produces a clinical picture very similar to Hb C disease.

Hemoglobin D. Hemoglobin D is the term used to describe a number of hemoglobin variants that have an identical rate of migration to Hb S on electrophoresis at an alkaline pH. The only common abnormal hemoglobin with these properties is Hb $D_{LOS\ ANGELES}$ (D_{PUNJAB}). This variant occurs frequently in the Punjab region and a number of homozygotes have been reported.[228] Their hemoglobin pattern shows almost all Hb D with normal levels of Hb A_2 and normal or only slightly elevated levels of Hb F. They have normal or only slightly reduced hemoglobin levels and their red cells are normal except for increased numbers of target forms.

Hemoglobin E. This is probably the most common hemoglobin variant in the world population. It results from the substitution of glutamic acid by lysine at position 26 in the β chain.[229] It occurs mainly in a region stretching east from Bangladesh through Burma and reaches its highest frequency in eastern Thailand and Laos. It is also found in parts of China and its distribution extends south down to the Indonesian islands. Gene frequencies in these populations are considered below.

The pathophysiology of Hb E is still not fully understood. There seems little doubt that it is synthesized inefficiently compared with Hb A and hence is associated with the clinical phenotype of a mild form of β thalassemia.[230] One reason for this is that the base substitution that is responsible for Hb E activates a cryptic splice site within exon 1 leading to abnormal splicing of β globin mRNA.[231]

The heterozygous state for Hb E is associated with no clinical disability and with normal hemoglobin levels, even though the red cells are slightly microcytic and hypochromic. There is usually 30 to 35 percent Hb E. Similarly, Hb E homozygotes are asymptomatic and are only slightly anemic, even though they have red cell indices that are very similar to those of heterozygous β thalassemics.

The importance of Hb E lies in the different phenotypes that result from its interaction with β thalassemia.[232] Compound heterozygotes for Hb E and β thalassemia have a variable clinical picture ranging from a condition indistinguishable from homozygous β thalassemia to a mild form of β thalassemia intermedia (see the thalassemia section). The hemoglobin pattern varies; in Hb E β^o thalassemia compound heterozygotes there is usually 50 to 70 percent Hb F, the remainder being Hb E. Compound heterozygotes for Hb E and β^+ thalassemia tend to have a milder disorder and produce variable amounts of Hb A. The reason for the severity of these interactions is not absolutely clear but may be related to the gross chain imbalance together with the unusual properties of Hb E that make it more sensitive to oxidant stress and that render it less stable than normal.[233]

In Southeast Asia, there is a family of disorders due to the coinheritance of Hb E with different forms of α thalassemia. Heterozygotes for Hb E who inherit either α^+ or α^o thalassemia have unusually low levels of Hb E.[232] The heterozygous state for Hb E in association with the genotype that produces Hb H disease (see the α thalassemia section) is responsible for a well-defined clinical syndrome that is characterized by moderate anemia, splenomegaly, and a hemoglobin pattern consisting of Hbs A, E, and Bart's. The reason why such patients produce Hb Bart's and no Hb H is not clear, although one factor may be the increased affinity of α chains for normal β chains as compared with β^E chains and the inability of the latter to form stable tetramers. Another complex group of anemias result from the various interactions of α thalassemia with the homozygous state for Hb E.[2,232]

The Unstable Hemoglobin Disorders

Over 90 different unstable hemoglobins have been reported.[3] However, the term *unstable hemoglobin disorder* is usually reserved for the clinical phenotype associated with variants, the instability of which is sufficient to cause clinically recognizable hemolysis; about 40 abnormal hemoglobins fall into this category. The clinical picture associated with such abnormal hemoglobins is also called *congenital Heinz body hemolytic anemia* (CHBA).

Molecular Basis of Hemoglobin Instability.[3,234–236] There are several different classes of mutations that can result in instability of the hemoglobin molecule (Fig. 181-13). The first is comprised of amino acid substitutions near the heme pocket. The binding of heme to globin involves specific interactions with particular nonpolar amino acid residues in the CD, E, F, and FG regions of the globin subunits. Most of these residues are invariant and hence it is not surprising that their substitution leads to a decrease in the stability of the binding of heme to globin; some examples are summarized in Fig. 181-13. At least three of these variants have amino acid substitutions at the proximal (heme-linked) histidine; two others have substitutions at the distal histidine. Some abnormal hemoglobins of this type are particularly susceptible to drug-induced precipitation and hemolysis. $Hb_{ZÜRICH}$, for example, has a substitution that leaves the heme pocket wide open, allowing drugs, such as sulfonamides, ready access to the heme iron.

A second group of unstable variants results from amino acid substitutions that disrupt the secondary structure of the globin chains. About 75 percent of globin is in the form of α helix in which proline cannot participate except as part of one of the initial three residues. Many unstable hemoglobin variants result from the substitution of proline. Another group of variants that cause

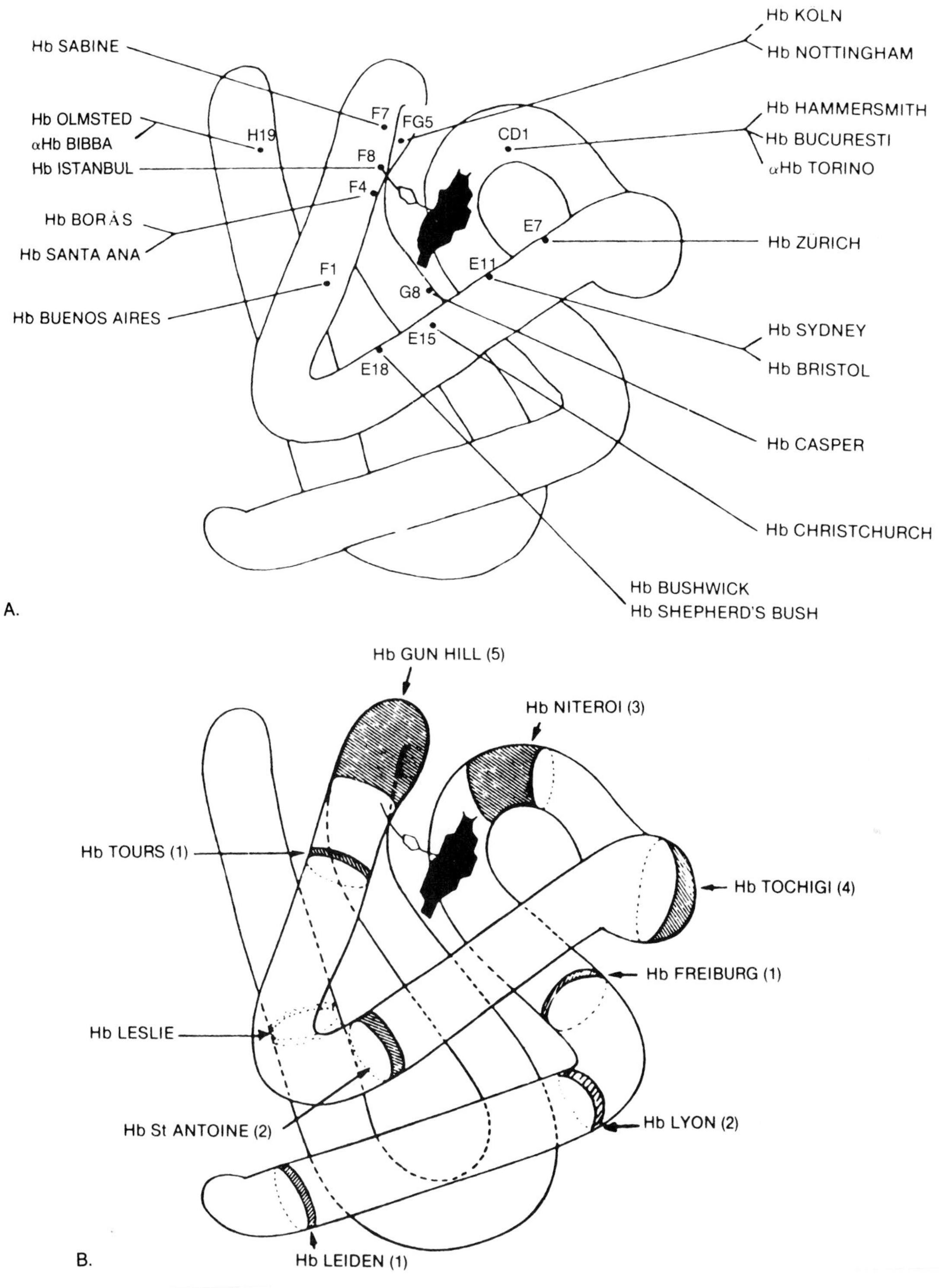

Fig. 181-13 Unstable hemoglobin variants. *A.* Three-dimensional representation of the β chain, showing sites of amino acid deletions that cause unstable hemoglobins. (*From Milner and Wrightstone.*[236] *Used by permission.*)

disruption of the normal configuration of the hemoglobin molecule involves internal substitutions that interfere with the hemoglobin molecule's stabilization by hydrophobic interactions. Some of these variants result in alterations in tertiary structure, allowing water access to the hydrophobic interior of globin subunits.

Finally, there are two groups of unstable hemoglobins that result from gross structural abnormalities of the globin subunits. Some variants have deletions ranging from one to five residues, many of which involve regions at or near interhelical corners. A few unstable variants have elongated globin chains. For example, $Hb_{CRANSTON}$ and $Hb_{SAVERNE}$ are associated with a mild hemolysis that is probably due to the hydrophobic segments attached to the C-terminal ends of their β globin chains.

The Mechanism of Hemoglobin Denaturation.[234–236] The major result of these substitutions is the precipitation of hemoglobin with the formation of rigid Heinz bodies. Although the precise details of the mechanisms of hemoglobin precipitation in these disorders are unknown, some general conclusions can be drawn. Hemoglobin can auto-oxidize to methemoglobin with the dissociation of superoxide anion. The latter, and its reduction product, hydrogen peroxide, are able to generate more methemoglobin. The unstable hemoglobins show a more rapid rate of auto-oxidation than normal hemoglobin. Furthermore, methemoglobin can be converted to hemichrome in which globin undergoes sufficient internal distortion to enable direct bonding of an amino acid side chain to the distal aspect of the heme iron. Initially, this process is reversible, but ultimately irreversible hemichrome formation occurs, which is followed by precipitation of hemoglobin with the production of a Heinz body. In addition, some unstable variants interact with glutathione to form mixed disulfides. Furthermore, as mentioned above, the formation of methemoglobin favors the dissociation of heme from globin.

Mechanism of Hemolysis.[236–238] Red cells that contain Heinz bodies have decreased pliability and negotiate the microcirculation with difficulty. These cells are trapped during their transit between the cords and sinuses of the spleen. In this way, a Heinz body may be "pulled out" of the cell during its passage through the spleen after which the remainder of the cell reseals. This process causes membrane damage that also may be mediated by the adherence of Heinz bodies to the inner surface of the red cell membrane. The red cells of patients with unstable hemoglobin disorders show an increased rate of potassium leak and may show reduced levels of ATP. Furthermore, because unstable hemoglobins may favor release of reactive oxidants such as hydrogen peroxide, superoxide, and free hydroxyl radical, these toxic side products may also damage the red cell membrane by causing lipid peroxidation and crosslinking of membrane proteins. Some of the mechanisms of damage to the red cell membrane may be similar to those observed in β thalassemia (see below).

Clinical and Hematologic Findings. Patients with CHBA have a varying degree of hemolysis that is inherited as an autosomal dominant. In several cases, no affected relatives have been found and the hemoglobin variants are thought to be the result of new mutations.[237]

Anemia, splenomegaly, and the intermittent passage of dark urine characterize the clinical course. The latter is not due to hemoglobinuria but to pigmenturia; the pigments have not been identified with certainty but may be related to dipyrrolmethanes of the mesobilifuscin group. Hematologic studies show the features of a hemolytic anemia with a raised reticulocyte count and variation in the shape and size of the red cells. In patients with an intact spleen, this may be all that is found. However, after splenectomy many of the red cells contain Heinz bodies.

The hemoglobin variants that are associated with this condition often have neutral mutations, that is, they cannot be identified by electrophoresis. However, if dilute hemoglobin solutions are incubated in a neutral phosphate buffer at 50°C for 1 to 2 h, unstable variants precipitate. A similar effect can be induced by incubation of hemolysates in 17 percent isopropanol at 37°C. Hemoglobin electrophoresis may show no abnormality, but sometimes after the red cell lysate has been stored for a few days a variety of bands appear, some of which are heme depleted and seen only with a protein stain. The hemoglobin A_2 level may be slightly increased in patients with unstable β chain variants. The position of the oxygen dissociation curve varies; both high- and low-affinity unstable hemoglobins have been reported.

Course and Prognosis. The majority of patients with CHBA have a mild anemia and are not incapacitated. Because oxidant drugs precipitate some of these variants, exacerbations may occur after drug therapy or with intercurrent illnesses, particularly infection. Rarely, there may be progressive splenomegaly with hypersplenism. Sustained thrombocytosis has been observed after splenectomy.

Table 181-5 Some Hemoglobin Variants with Altered Oxygen Affinity

High-oxygen-affinity variants	
Mutations at $\alpha_1\beta_2$ contacts	
$Hb_{CHESAPEAKE}$	α92 Arg → Leu
$Hb_{J\text{-}CAPE\ TOWN}$	α92 Arg → Gln
$Hb_{TARRANT}$	α126 Asp → Asn
$Hb_{LEGNANO}$	α141 Arg → Leu
Mutations at 2,3-DPG binding sites	
Hb_{RAHERE}	β86 Lys → Thr
$Hb_{HELSINKI}$	β82Lys → Met
$Hb_{PROVIDENCE}$	β82Lys → Asn
Heme binding site	
$Hb_{HEATHROW}$	β103 Phe → Leu
Low-oxygen-affinity variants	
Mutations at $\alpha_1\beta_2$ contact	
Hb_{KANSAS}	β102 Asn → Thr
$Hb_{BETH\ ISRAEL}$	β102 Asn → Ser
Mutations at 2,3-DPG binding site	
$HB_{RALEIGH}$	β1 Val → Acet. Ala

NOTE: A complete list with references is given in reference 148.

Hemoglobin Variants with Abnormal Oxygen Binding

Several clinical syndromes result from abnormalities of oxygen binding by abnormal hemoglobins (Table 181-5). Both low and high oxygen-affinity variants have been encountered. About a third of the unstable variants described in the previous section have increased oxygen affinity, but in those disorders the clinical manifestations are due to accelerated red cell destruction; the hemoglobin level may be modified by the oxygen affinity of the particular variant. There are, however, over 70 abnormal hemoglobins in which increased oxygen affinity occurs without instability.[148] These variants are sometimes associated with the clinical syndrome of genetic polycythemia. On the other hand, variants characterized by a low oxygen affinity may result in a dominantly inherited form of cyanosis.

High Oxygen-Affinity Variants and Hereditary Polycythemia.[3,239–241] As mentioned earlier, hemoglobin exists in equilibrium between two quaternary conformations, R and T. When it is fully deoxygenated it assumes the T (tense) state in which it has a low affinity for oxygen and a relatively high affinity for allosteric molecules such as Bohr protons and 2,3-DPG. On the other hand, oxyhemoglobin exists in the R (relaxed) state in which it has a high affinity for oxygen and a low affinity for allosteric effectors. The transition between these two conformations requires cooperativity between the subunits that is the molecular basis for heme-heme interaction. Most of the high affinity variants result from mutations that cause amino acid substitutions that affect the equilibrium between the R and T states. Many are found at the $\alpha_1\beta_2$ interface, the C-terminal end of the β chain, and at the 2,3-DPG binding sites (Table 181-5).

The clinical findings vary in patients with high oxygen-affinity hemoglobin variants. There is usually erythrocytosis with an elevated hemoglobin level, but no changes in the white cell or platelet counts and no splenomegaly, features that distinguish these conditions from polycythemia vera, a myeloproliferative disorder involving hemopoietic stem cells. The whole blood oxygen dissociation curve is shifted to the left with a reduced p50; many of the high-affinity hemoglobins also show a decreased alkaline Bohr effect. In some cases, there is reduced interaction with 2,3-DPG. The other physiological properties of these variants are the subject of a number of extensive reviews.[3,240,241]

The majority of patients with high oxygen-affinity variants are asymptomatic and are only ascertained because they are found to have a modest erythrocytosis on routine hematologic examination. The diagnosis is made by ruling out other causes of polycythemia and by demonstrating a decreased p50 associated with a hemoglobin variant. Remember that there are other causes of a left-shifted oxygen-dissociation curve, such as methemoglobin or carboxyhemoglobin, that must be excluded by spectroscopic analysis.

Low Oxygen-Affinity Variants. There are fewer hemoglobin variants with low oxygen affinities (Table 181-5). Some unstable variants fall into this group, and some of the M hemoglobins also have decreased oxygen affinity.

Hb_{KANSAS} is a typical variant of this kind.[242] Carriers have normal hemoglobin levels but are cyanosed from birth. The condition is associated with a reduced oxygen saturation of the arterial blood despite a PaO_2 of 100 mm Hg. When these individuals breathe 100 percent oxygen, the oxygen saturation increases by about 30 percent, suggesting that there is a marked decrease in whole-blood oxygen affinity. Hb_{KANSAS} has a threonine substitution for asparagine at position 102 in the β chain. Interestingly, this residue is at the $\alpha_1\beta_2$ interface, which is similar to some of the high-affinity variants described earlier. The low affinity of Hb_{KANSAS} seems to be due in part to a relatively unstable R structure, although the precise mechanism is not understood. The clinical picture associated with other low-affinity variants, $Hb_{BETH\ ISRAEL}$, $Hb_{ST.\ MANDE}$, and Hb_{DENVER} is similar.

Congenital Cyanosis Due to Hemoglobin Variants. Congenital methemoglobinemia may result from either an inherited structural hemoglobin or from a defect in one of the enzyme systems involved in maintaining a normal level of reduced hemoglobin in the red cells; the latter group of conditions is considered in Chap. 180.

The structural hemoglobin variants that are associated with methemoglobinemia are all designated HbM [148]; they are further defined by their place of discovery; for example, Hb M_{BOSTON}, Hb $M_{HYDE\ PARK}$, and so on. Their structure-function relationships are the subject of several reviews.[3,243] As mentioned earlier in this chapter, the iron atom of heme is normally linked to the imidazole group of the proximal histidine residue of the α and β chains. There is another histidine residue on the opposite side, near the sixth coordination position of the heme iron; this, the so-called distal histidine residue, is the normal binding site for oxygen. The imidazole group of the distal histidine does not form a bond with heme iron except in the pathologic conditions, in which hemichrome is formed.

Many of the M hemoglobins result from the substitution of a tyrosine for either the proximal or distal histidine residues in either the α or β chains. It is likely that the phenolic group of the abnormal tyrosine residue forms a covalent link with the heme iron, stabilizing the iron atom in the oxidized (Fe^{3+}) configuration. X-ray crystallographic studies confirm that these amino acid substitutions stabilize the heme group of the mutant hemoglobins in the oxidized forms. Once in this state, the abnormal subunit is resistant to reduction by both enzymes and reducing agents.

Individuals who are heterozygous for the M hemoglobins are cyanosed from early in life but are otherwise asymptomatic. The condition can often be distinguished from congenital methemoglobinemia due to an enzyme defect by the family history; the pattern of inheritance of Hb M is typically dominant. Furthermore, if the cyanosis is present from birth, it is usually due to an α-chain Hb M methemoglobin variant; alternatively, if cyanosis appears only during the first few months of life, the disorder is likely to be due to a β-chain variant. It is interesting that conjunctival cyanosis is present in children with methemoglobin but not in those in whom the cyanosis is due to defective oxygenation of the blood. The conjunctival sac provides such close apposition of the red cells to air that it acts as a "second lung." Even in cases of severe cyanotic heart disease or pulmonary disease, conjunctival cyanosis is usually absent.

Demonstrating increased amounts of methemoglobin in the red cells makes the diagnosis of methemoglobinemia. The M hemoglobins give a characteristic spectral abnormality provided the hemoglobin is completely oxidized to the Fe^{3+} state with ferricyanide. They are not demonstrable by hemoglobin electrophoresis under routine conditions, although some of them separate on agar gel at pH 7.1. The M hemoglobins can be demonstrated more effectively if the red cell lysate is first oxidized with ferricyanide.

No treatment is required for congenital methemoglobinemia due to M hemoglobin. Affected individuals tolerate major surgery without difficulty; the clinician's primary task is to arrive at an accurate diagnosis and to provide adequate reassurance.

THALASSEMIA

The thalassemias are the commonest single gene disorders in the world population. They are the subject of several monographs[2,6,244] and recent reviews.[245–248] After defining and classifying these conditions, this section describes the thalassemia pathophysiology as a group; because they are very heterogeneous, they share much in common with respect to the mechanisms of disordered erythropoiesis and red cell destruction. The molecular pathology and clinical and hematologic features of each of the main varieties is then described.

Definition and Classification

The thalassemias are a heterogenous group of inherited disorders of hemoglobin synthesis, all characterized by the absence or reduced output of one or more of the globin chains of hemoglobin. This leads to imbalanced globin chain synthesis that is the hallmark of all the thalassemia syndromes.[3]

The main types of thalassemia are summarized in Table 181-6. The commonest and clinically most important forms are α,β, and $\delta\beta$ thalassemia. Each is classifiable into disorders in which no chains are produced from the affected chromosomes, α^o, β^o and $(\delta\beta)^o$ thalassemia, and those in which some chains are synthesized, but at a reduced rate, α^+, β^+, and $(\delta\beta)^+$ thalassemia. The related condition, hereditary persistence of fetal hemoglobin, can be

Table 181-6 Thalassemias and Related Disorders

α Thalassemia
α^0
α^+ Deletion, nondeletion
With α-chain Hb variants
With β-chain Hb variants
With β thalassemia
β Thalassemia
β^0
β^+
With β-chain Hb variants
With α-chain Hb variants
With α thalassemia
$\delta\beta$ Thalassemia
$(\delta\beta)^0$ Thalassemia
$(^A\gamma\delta\beta)^0$ Thalassemia
$(\epsilon\gamma\delta\beta)^0$ Thalassemia
δ Thalassemia
γ Thalassemia
Hereditary persistence of fetal hemoglobin
Deletion
$(\delta\beta)^0$ HPFH
Nondeletion
Linked to β-globin gene cluster
Unlinked to β-globin gene cluster

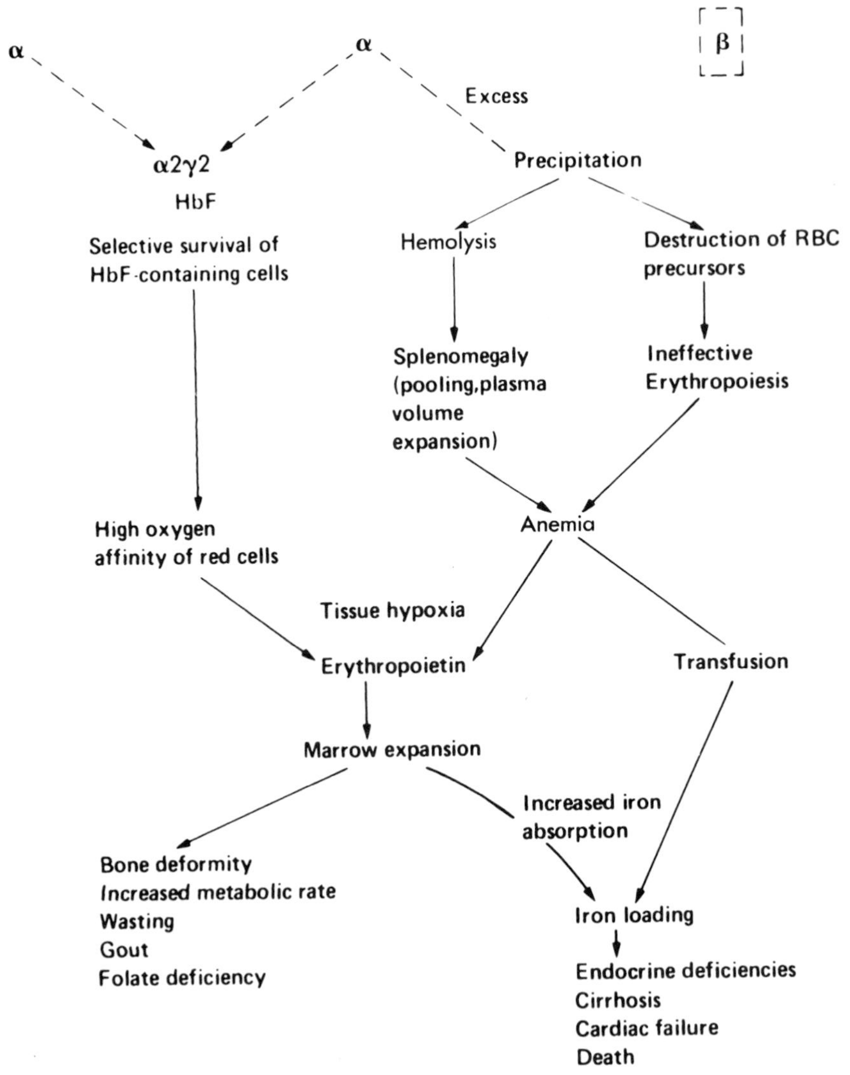

Fig. 181-14 Pathophysiology of β thalassemia.

regarded as a particularly mild form of β or $\delta\beta$ thalassemia in which defective β chain production is fully compensated by persistent γ chain synthesis beyond the neonatal period.

In many populations, the thalassemias coexist with a variety of different structural hemoglobin variants. Thus, it is quite common to inherit both types of condition. Furthermore, it is equally common for individuals to receive genes for more than one type of thalassemia. These complex interactions give rise to an extremely diverse series of clinical disorders that, taken together, constitute the thalassemia syndromes.[2]

Pathophysiology

One of the most remarkable aspects of the thalassemia field is how feasible it has been to relate the diverse clinical manifestations that may affect almost any organ system to primary molecular defects in the α or β globin genes. It is possible to trace almost all of the pathophysiological features of these conditions back to a primary imbalance of globin chain synthesis (Fig. 181-14). It is this phenomenon that makes the thalassemias fundamentally different from all the other genetic and acquired disorders of hemoglobin production and, to a large extent, explains their extreme severity in the homozygous or compound heterozygous states.

Imbalanced Globin Chain Synthesis. Measurements of *in vitro* globin chain synthesis in the peripheral blood or bone marrows of patients with different types of thalassemia,[12] together with genetic studies that enable the action of the thalassemia genes to be examined in patients who have also inherited α or β globin structural variants, provide a clear picture of the action of the thalassemia determinants.[2] In homozygous β thalassemia, β globin synthesis may either be absent or markedly reduced. This results in the production of an excess of α globin chains. Unpaired α globin chains are incapable of forming a viable hemoglobin tetramer and hence precipitate in red cell precursors.[249,250] The resulting inclusion bodies can be demonstrated by both light and electron microscopy (Fig. 181-15). In the bone marrow, precipitation can be seen in the earliest hemoglobinized precursors, and right through the erythroid maturation pathway. These large inclusions are responsible for the intramedullary destruction of red cell precursors and the ineffective erythropoiesis that characterizes all the β thalassemias. It has been calculated that a large proportion of the developing erythroblasts is destroyed within the bone marrow in severe cases.[2] Such red cells as are released are prematurely destroyed by the mechanisms considered below.

β Thalassemia heterozygotes also have imbalanced globin chain synthesis, but in this case, the magnitude of the excess of α chains is much less and presumably can be dealt with successfully by the proteolytic enzymes of the red cell precursors.[251] Notwithstanding, there is a mild degree of ineffective erythropoiesis.

From these considerations it is clear that the anemia of β thalassemia has three major components. First and most important, is ineffective erythropoiesis with intramedullary destruction of a variable proportion of the developing red cell precursors. Second,

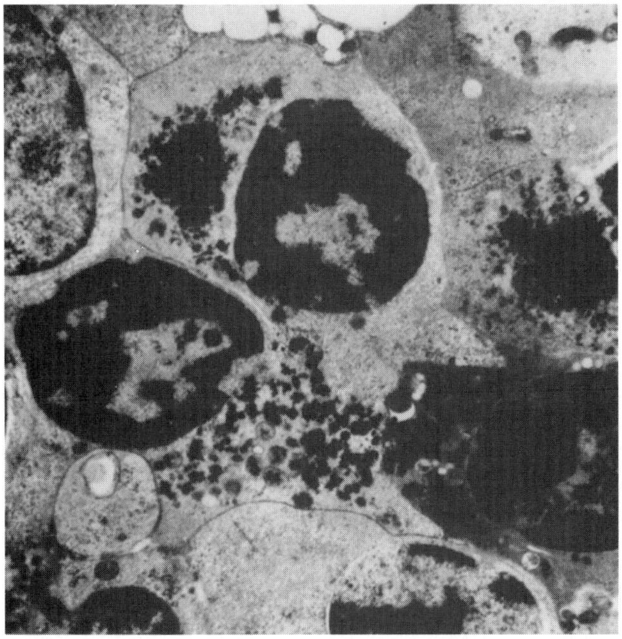

Fig. 181-15 Inclusion bodies in the red-cell precursors in homozygous β thalassemia (electron microscopy ×9000). (*From Weatherall and Clegg.*[2] *Used by permission; original preparations supplied by Dr. A. Polliack.*)

is a hemolytic component due to destruction of mature red cells containing α chain inclusions. Finally, because of the overall reduction in hemoglobin synthesis, the red cells are hypochromic and microcytic.

Because the primary defect in β thalassemia is in β chain production, the synthesis of hemoglobins F and A_2 should be unaffected. Fetal hemoglobin production *in utero* is normal and it is only when the neonatal switch from γ to β chain production occurs that the clinical manifestations of β thalassemia first appear. However, fetal hemoglobin synthesis persists beyond the neonatal period in nearly all forms of β thalassemia; the reasons for this are discussed below. In β thalassemia heterozygotes, there is an elevated level of Hb A_2. This appears to reflect both a relative decrease in Hb A due to defective β chain synthesis and an absolute increase in the output of δ chains both *cis* and *trans* to the mutant β globin gene.[2] The question of Hb A_2 production in homozygous β thalassemia is extremely complex and is discussed below.

The consequences of excess non-α chain production in the α thalassemias are quite different. Alpha chains are shared by both fetal and adult hemoglobin; therefore, defective α chain production is manifest in both fetal and adult life.[245] In the fetus, a reduced output of α chains leads to excess γ chain production; similarly, in the adult, excess β chains are produced. Excess γ chains combine to form γ_4 homotetramers, or Hb Bart's; excess β chains form β_4 homotetramers or Hb H. This ability of γ and β chains to form homotetramers is the basis of the fundamental difference in the pathophysiology of α and β thalassemia.[245] Because γ_4 and β_4 tetramers are soluble, they do not precipitate to any significant degree in the bone marrow and the α thalassemias are not characterized by a severe degree of ineffective erythropoiesis. However, β_4 tetramers precipitate as red cells age, with the formation of inclusion bodies. Thus, the anemia of the more severe forms of α thalassemia in the adult is due mainly to a shortened red cell survival consequent on their damage in the microvasculature of the spleen due to the presence of the inclusions. In addition, because of the defect in hemoglobin synthesis the cells are hypochromic and microcytic. Hb Bart's is more stable than Hb H, and does not appear to form inclusions.

But there is another factor that exacerbates the tissue hypoxia of the anemia of the α thalassemias. Both Hb Bart's and Hb H show no heme-heme interaction and have almost hyperbolic oxygen dissociation curves with very-high oxygen affinities. Thus they are not able to give up oxygen at physiological tissue tensions and are, in effect, useless as oxygen carriers.[2]

It follows that infants with high levels of Hb Bart's have severe intrauterine hypoxia. This is a major component of the clinical picture of homozygous α^0 thalassemia, which results in the stillbirth of hydropic infants late in pregnancy or at term. Severe intrauterine oxygen deprivation is reflected by the grossly hydropic state of the infant, presumably due to an increase in capillary permeability consequent on hypoxia and severe erythroblastosis. Deficient fetal oxygenation is probably responsible for the enormously hypertrophied placentas that occur with the severe forms of intrauterine α thalassemia.[245]

Cellular Mechanisms for Damage Induced by Globin Chain Excess. The mechanisms whereby excess globin chains damage the red cell precursors and their progeny in the peripheral blood in the different forms of thalassemia are extremely complex and multifactorial (Fig. 181-16). As excess α chains accumulate at the membrane and its skeleton they cause alterations in deformability, stability, and cellular hydration.[252,253] Many of these changes seen to follow the early accumulation of α globin and its co-localization with band 4.1 and spectrin at sites of membrane discontinuity in the red cell precursors. It seems likely that these changes reflect the fact that heme, hemichromes, and iron components of α globin serve as foci for generation of reactive oxygen species that result in partial oxidization of band 4.1 and a decrease in spectrin/band 3 ratios. The deficiency of band 3 in the youngest erythroid precursors occurs without any evidence of interaction with α globin and is thought to result from excess α chains interfering at an earlier stage in the complex processes of synthesis, trafficking and membrane insertion of band 3.[254] Damaged red cell precursors may undergo apoptosis[255] or destruction by macrophages.

Damage to the membrane of mature red cells seems to occur similarly and reflects the action of hemichromes and the degradation products of α chains, notably heme, hemin, and free iron.[256–258] The formation of membrane-bound hemichromes creates a copolymer of macromolecular dimensions which promotes clustering of band 3 in the membrane. It seems likely that these clusters are opsonized with autologous IgG and complement and removed by macrophages.[259] As in the case of the red cell precursors, there is partial oxidation of band 4.1 and widespread lipid peroxidation involving the red cell membrane and its organelles as a result of the formation of a variety of reactive oxygen species through the actions of heme and excess iron. The end result of these insults to the membrane is to produce a potassium- and energy-depleted red cell that tends to be dehydrated.

Interestingly, the mechanisms of red cell damage are different in the presence of excess β chain as occurs in α thalassemia. While the membranes in β thalassemia are more mechanically unstable, probably due to oxidation of protein 4.1, in α thalassemia, the membranes are hyperstable and there is no evidence of oxidation or any dysfunction of this protein. Furthermore, the state of cellular hydration is different in the two forms of thalassemia. As mentioned earlier, accumulation of α chains leads to cellular dehydration, whereas the accumulation of β chains leads to increased hydration. It is believed that these findings reflect the results of the action of different kinds of oxidized globin chains on the K:Cl cotransporter, and possibly on other cotransport pathways.

Further details of the mechanisms of red cell destruction and the differences between the two main forms of thalassemia are the subject of a number of recent reviews.[256,260,261] Shinar and Rachmilewitz[258] suggest that the fundamental difference in behavior between α and β subunits in generating damage to the red cell precursors and red cells reflects their different patterns of

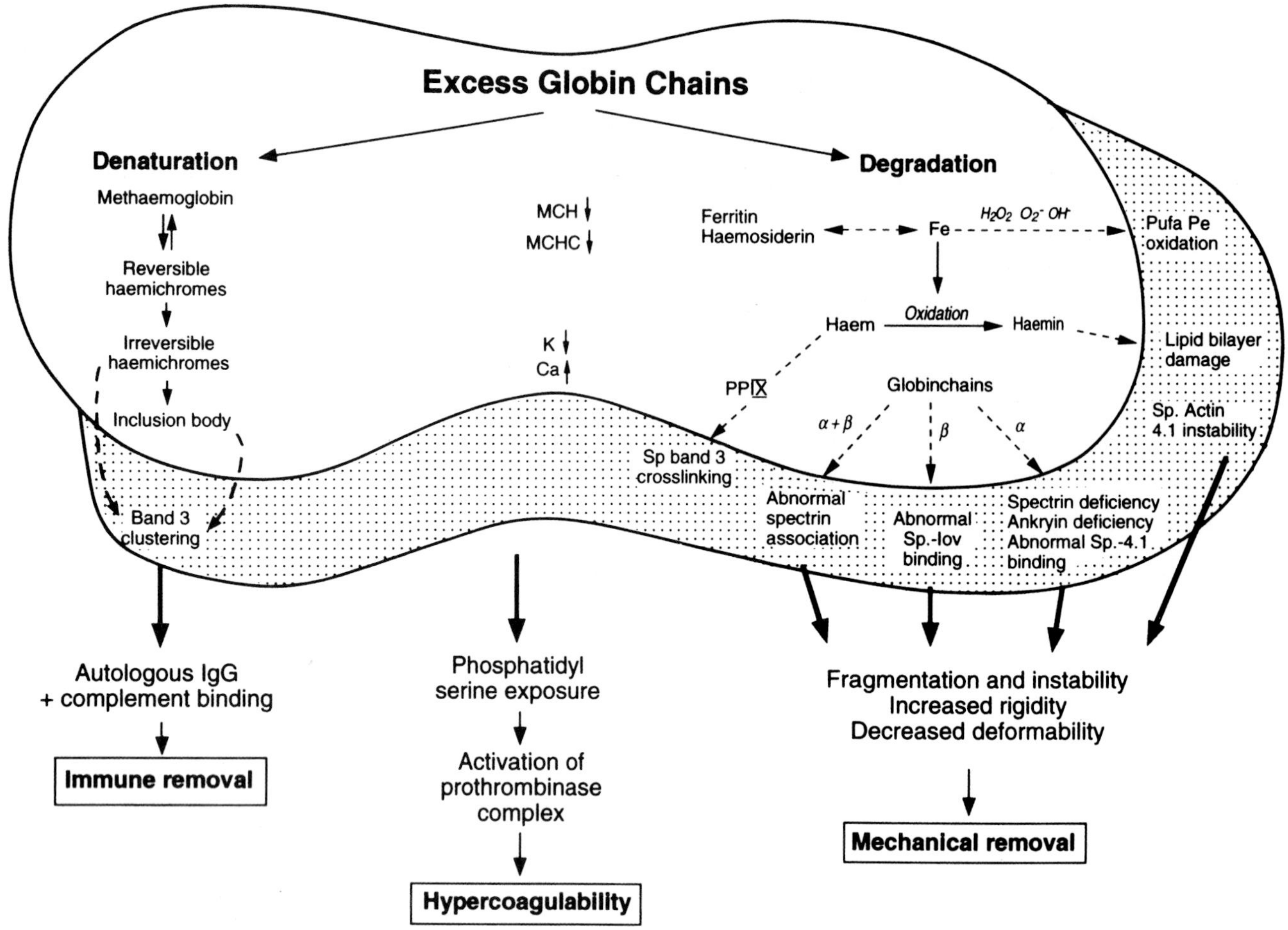

Fig. 181-16 A schematic summary of the various metabolic and biochemical consequences of globin chain precipitation in thalassemia. From Weatherall[509] based on reviews in references 256 to 258. Sp = spectrin. Pufa = polyunsaturated fatty acids. Pe = phosphatidylethanolamine. Iov = inside out vesicles.

precipitation. The larger β subunits, which precipitate in α thalassemia and in the unstable β chain hemoglobinopathies, tend to bind more tightly to protein band 3, the native binding site on the membrane. On the other hand, small α subunits, which precipitate early in the life span of red cells in β thalassemia, are more widely dispersed over the cytoplasm before reacting with specific sites on the membrane. These observations are certainly in keeping with the different electron microscopic appearances of α and β chain binding to thalassemic red cell membranes.[262]

Persistent Fetal Hemoglobin Production and Cellular Heterogeneity. One of the earliest observations regarding the hemoglobin patterns of children with severe thalassemia was that there is a variable amount of Hb F production that persists into childhood and later.[2] Indeed, in the β thalassemias, except for small amounts of Hb A_2, Hb F is the only hemoglobin produced. Examination of the peripheral blood using staining methods that are specific for Hb F show that it is heterogenously distributed among the red cells. Persistent Hb F production is not a feature of the more severe forms of α thalassemia, although in some cases, persistent γ chain synthesis is reflected by the presence of Hb Bart's after the first 6 months of life.

There are still many unanswered questions about the mechanisms of persistent γ chain synthesis in the thalassemias. Normal adults have small quantities of Hb F that are heterogeneously distributed among the red cells; cells with demonstrable Hb F are called F cells. It is clear that one important mechanism for persistent Hb F production in β thalassemia is cell selection.[3,248] The major cause of ineffective erythropoiesis and shortened red cell survival in β thalassemia is the deleterious effects of excess α chains on erythroid maturation, and survival of red cells in the blood. It follows that any red cell precursors that produce significant numbers of γ chains have an advantage in an environment in which there is excess α chains; the latter will combine with γ chains to produce Hb F, making the magnitude of α chain precipitation less. Differential centrifugation experiments and *in vivo* labeling studies show that populations of red cells with relatively large amounts of Hb F are more efficiently produced and survive longer in the peripheral blood than those with low levels or no Hb F (reviewed in reference 2). The peripheral blood of homozygous β thalassemics shows remarkable cellular heterogeneity with respect to red cell survival times. There are populations of cells that contain predominantly Hb A that are very rapidly destroyed in the spleen and elsewhere, cells with a much longer survival that contain relatively more Hb F, and populations of intermediate age and hemoglobin constitution.

Whether cell selection of this type is the only mechanism for persistent γ chain production in β thalassemia is not clear. It is possible that there may be an absolute increase in Hb F production. This is certainly so in some milder forms of homozygous β thalassemia, but in these cases, there may be other genetic factors that are responsible for the relatively high level of γ chain synthesis (see below).

Because there is a reciprocal relationship between γ and δ chain synthesis, it follows that the red cells of β thalassemia homozygotes that contain large amounts of Hb F have relatively low levels of Hb A_2.[2] Thus the measured percent Hb A_2 in these individuals is the average of a very heterogeneous cell population. This probably accounts for the extreme variability in the levels of Hb A_2 reported in patients with this disorder.

A further consequence of the persistence of Hb F in β thalassemia is that the red cells have a high oxygen affinity. Thalassemic red cells adapt poorly to anemia, as reflected by inappropriately low levels of 2,3 DPG and a high oxygen affinity.[2]

Consequences of Compensatory Mechanisms for the Anemia of Thalassemia. The profound anemia of homozygous β thalassemia combined with the high oxygen affinity of such blood as is produced causes severe tissue hypoxia. Because of the properties of Hb Bart's and Hb H, a similar defect in tissue oxygenation occurs in the more severe forms of α thalassemia. The major response is erythropoietin production and expansion of the dyserythropoietic bone marrow. This, in turn, leads to deformities of the skull and face, and porosity of the long bones.[2] In extreme cases, extramedullary hemopoietic tumors may develop. Apart from the production of severe skeletal deformities, bone marrow expansion may cause pathologic fractures, sinus disease, and chronic middle ear infection.

Another effect of the enormous expansion of the marrow mass in severe thalassemia is to divert calories required for normal development to the ineffective red cell precursor population. Thus, severely affected thalassemics show poor development and wasting. The massive turnover of erythroid precursors may result in secondary hyperuricemia and gout, and severe folate deficiency.

The effects of gross intrauterine hypoxia in homozygous α^0 thalassemia were described earlier. In the symptomatic forms of α thalassemia, such as Hb H disease, that are compatible with survival into adult life, bone changes and other consequences of erythroid expansion are seen, although to a much lesser degree than in β thalassemia.

Splenomegaly; Dilutional Anemia. The constant bombardment of the spleen with abnormal red cells gives rise to the phenomenon of "work hypertrophy." Progressive splenomegaly occurs in both α and β thalassemia, and may exacerbate the anemia.[2,244] Large spleens act as a sump for red cells and may sequestrate a considerable proportion of the peripheral red cell mass. Furthermore, splenomegaly may also cause plasma volume expansion, a complication that may be exacerbated by massive expansion of the erythroid bone marrow. The combination of pooling of the red cells in the spleen and plasma volume expansion may cause worsening of the anemia in both α and β thalassemia. The same process may occur in an enlarged liver, particularly after splenectomy.

Abnormal Iron Metabolism. In β thalassemia homozygotes who are anemic, there is an increase in intestinal iron absorption that is related to the degree of expansion of the red cell precursor population; iron absorption is decreased by blood transfusion.[244] Increased absorption causes a steady accumulation of iron, first in the Kupffer cells of the liver and in the RE cells of the spleen, then later in the parenchymal cells of the liver (Fig. 181-17). Most homozygous β thalassemics require regular blood transfusion, thus transfusional siderosis adds to the iron accumulation. In addition to the liver, iron accumulates in the endocrine glands, particularly the parathyroids and adrenals, pancreas, skin, and, most importantly, the myocardium. The latter leads to death, either by involving the conducting tissues or by causing intractable cardiac failure. Other consequences of iron loading include diabetes, hypoparathyroidism, and hypogonadism, mainly due to end-organ failure.[3,244] Disordered iron metabolism is less common in the adult forms of α thalasemia.

It is beyond this chapter's scope to discuss details of the mechanisms of tissue damage by iron loading. Advances in free radical chemistry that have clarified the toxic properties of iron

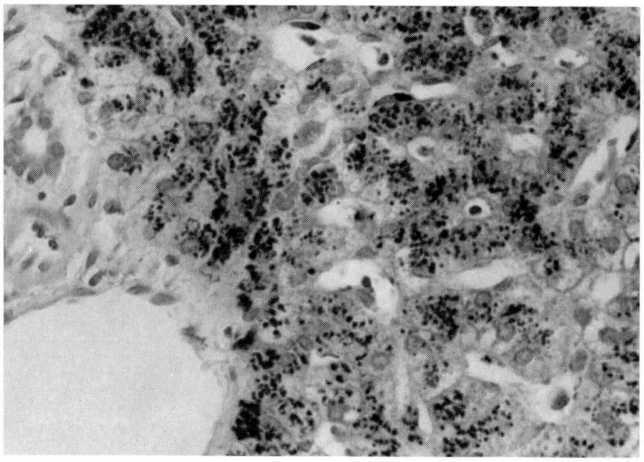

Fig. 181-17 Iron loading of the liver in β thalassemia intermedia (×600, iron stain).

and the effects of free radical damage mediated by iron have been reviewed extensively.[263,264]

Infection. There appears to be an increased susceptibility to bacterial infection in all forms of severe thalassemia.[2,244] The reason is not known. It has been suggested that the relatively high serum iron levels may favor bacterial growth. Another possible mechanism is blockage of the RE system due to the increased rate of destruction of red cells. No consistent defects in white cell or immune function have been demonstrated, but it remains to be shown unequivocally that high serum levels are an important factor.

Clinical Heterogeneity. The pathophysiological mechanisms outlined in the previous sections provide a basis for the remarkable clinical diversity of the thalassemia syndromes. It is clear that all the clinical manifestations of β thalassemia can be related to excess α chain production. It follows that any mechanism that tends to reduce the excess of α chains in β thalassemia should modify the clinical course of the disease. A number of elegant experiments of nature have shown that this is the case. For example, β thalassemia homozygotes who inherit one or more α thalassemia genes tend to run a much milder course than those with β thalassemia alone.[265,266] Similarly, the coinheritance of one or more genetic determinants that favor persistent γ chain synthesis after the neonatal period ameliorates the condition.[267] In other words, if α thalassemia is coinherited, the magnitude of excess α chains is less; if there is a higher than usual output of γ chains, some of the excess α chains combine with γ chains to produce Hb F. In either case, the overall excess of α chains is less, reducing the degree of ineffective erythropoiesis and hemolysis. These clinical observations provide strong support for the various pathophysiological concepts outlined in the previous sections.

It is clear that if patients with β thalassemia are adequately transfused, most of the consequences of excess α chain production can be overcome. The drive to erythroid expansion is diminished and the skeletal and growth abnormalities do not develop. Iron absorption from the gastrointestinal tract is reduced, and because endogenous red cell production is turned off, hepatosplenomegaly does not occur. Thus adequately transfused thalassemic children grow and develop normally, although if iron is not removed by chelation therapy, they succumb to the effects of iron loading of the tissues in the second or third decade.

α Thalassemia

Classification. Until the late 1970s, the various determinants of α thalassemia could only be defined in terms of their effect on the phenotype (MCV, MCH, α/β globin chain synthesis ratio) and the way in which they interact to produce the carrier states for α

Table 181-7 Genotype/Phenotype Relations in the α Thalassemias

Phenotype	Equivalent Number of Functional α Genes	Level of Hb Bart's at Birth, %*	% HbH (Inclusions)	MCV (fl)†	MCH (pg)†	α/β-Globin Chain Synthesis Ratio	Interacting‡ Haplotypes	Most Frequently Encountered Genotypes
Normal	4	0§	0 (none)	90 ± 5	30 ± 2	~1.0	α/α	$\alpha\alpha/\alpha\alpha$
α thalassemia¶ minor (mild)	3	0–2	0 (rare)	81 ± 7	26 ± 2	~0.8	α^+/α	$-\alpha/\alpha\alpha$
α Thalassemia¶ minor (severe)	2	2–8	0 (occasional)	69 ± 4	22 ± 2	~0.6	α^0/α or $\alpha^T\alpha/\alpha\alpha$	$--/\alpha\alpha$ $\alpha^T\alpha/\alpha\alpha$ $-\alpha/-\alpha$
HbH disease	1	10–40	2–40 (many)	65 ± 7	19 ± 2	~0.3	α^0/α^+ or α^+/α^+	$--/-\alpha$ $--/\alpha^T\alpha$ $\alpha^T\alpha/\alpha^T\alpha$
Hb Bart's hydrops fetalis	0	~80	Present (present)	110–120	Reduced	0.0	α^0/α^0 α^0/α^+	$--/--$ $--/\alpha^T\alpha$

*Hb Bart's gradually disappears from peripheral blood in the 3 to 6 months following birth.

†These values vary considerably depending on the age of the patient, and the figures given are a guide to the indices seen in adults with the deletion forms of α thalassemia (from reference 245).

‡α=normal haplotype; $\alpha^+ = \alpha^+$ thalassemia; $\alpha^0 = \alpha^0$ thalassemia.

§Very small amounts of Hb Bart's have been detected in normal infants at birth.

¶The mild and severe forms of α-thalassemia trait are often referred to as α-thalassemia-2 and α-thalassemia-1, respectively.

thalassemia (α thalassemia minor), Hb H disease, or the Hb Bart's hydrops fetalis syndrome (Table 181-7).[2] More recently, many of the underlying molecular defects have been identified, making it possible to establish a more comprehensive system for classifying the mutant alleles.[245,248,268]

α Thalassemias in which no normal α-globin is produced from the α gene complex, are called α^o thalassemias, and those in which the output is reduced are referred to as α^+ thalassemias. This brings the classification of the α thalassemias in line with that for the β-thalassemias. The α^o and α^+ thalassemias can be further subdivided, according to the precise nature of the underlying molecular defect, into deletion and nondeletion types.

The α-globin haplotype may be written $\alpha\alpha$, representing the α_2 and α_1 genes, respectively. A normal individual has the genotype $\alpha\alpha/\alpha\alpha$. A deletion involving one ($-\alpha$) or both ($--$) α genes may be further classified on the basis of its size, written as a superscript; thus $-\alpha^{3.7}$ indicates a deletion of 3.7-kb DNA including one α gene. Where the size of a deletion is not yet established, a superscript describing the geographical or individual origin of the deletion is used; thus $--^{MED}$ describes a deletion of both α genes first identified in individuals of Mediterranean origin.[269] In those thalassemic haplotypes where both genes are intact, the nomenclature $\alpha^T\alpha$ or $\alpha\alpha^T$ is given, depending on whether the α_2 or α_1 gene is affected. When the precise molecular defect is known, as in Hb$_{\text{CONSTANT SPRING}}$,[149] for example, $\alpha^T\alpha$ can be replaced by the more informative $\alpha^{CS}\alpha$ or $\alpha^{TER;T\rightarrow C}\alpha$.

This system provides an accurate shorthand way of describing various interactions. For example the genotype $--^{SEA}/\alpha^{TER;T\rightarrow C}\alpha$ (or $--^{SEA}/\alpha^{CS}\alpha$) denotes an interaction of the Hb$_{\text{CONSTANT SPRING}}$ mutation with the common Southeast Asian α^o defect. The relationship of these genotypes to the commonly observed phenotypes of α thalassemia is outlined in Table 181-7 and discussed in detail below.

Molecular Pathology

α^+ Thalassemia Due to Deletions. The most common molecular defects underlying α thalassemia ($-\alpha^{3.7}$ and $-\alpha^{4.2}$) involve the deletion of one or other of the duplicated α globin genes[63,64] (Fig. 181-18). One or both of these determinants occur in all populations in which thalassemia is common.

The mechanism by which some of the α^+ thalassemia deletions occur has been established and it is clearly related to the underlying molecular structure of the α globin complex.[40,270] Each α gene is located within a region of homology approximately 4 kb long, interrupted by small nonhomologous regions (Fig. 181-18). It is thought that the homologous regions result from an ancient duplication event. Subsequently, during evolution these homologous segments were subdivided, presumably by insertions and deletions, to give three homologous subsegments, which are referred to as X, Y, and Z (Fig. 181-18). The duplicated Z boxes are 3.7 kb apart and the X boxes are 4.2 kb apart. Misalignment and reciprocal crossover between these segments at meiosis can give rise to chromosomes with either single $(-\alpha)^{270}$ or triplicated $(\alpha\alpha\alpha)^{62,271-273}$ α globin genes (Fig. 181-19). Such an occurrence between homologous Z boxes deletes 3.7 kb of DNA (referred to as a rightward deletion, $-\alpha^{3.7}$), whereas a similar crossover

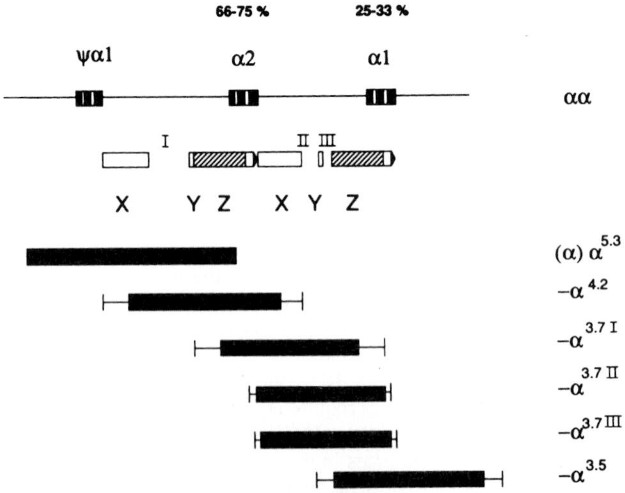

Fig. 181-18 Fine structure around the duplicated α-globin genes (above). The pseudo-α gene ($\psi\alpha1$) and duplicated α genes ($\alpha1$ and α 2) are shown. Above, the relative levels of expression of the $\alpha2$ and $\alpha1$ genes are shown. Black boxes indicate exons; white boxes show the size and positions of introns. Below, the X, Y, and Z boxes are shown, marking the positions and extent of the duplication that gave rise to the two α genes. The deletions that involve one or other of the α genes are shown below. Thick black bars indicate the extent of the deletions and thin bars the regions of uncertainty for the breakpoints.

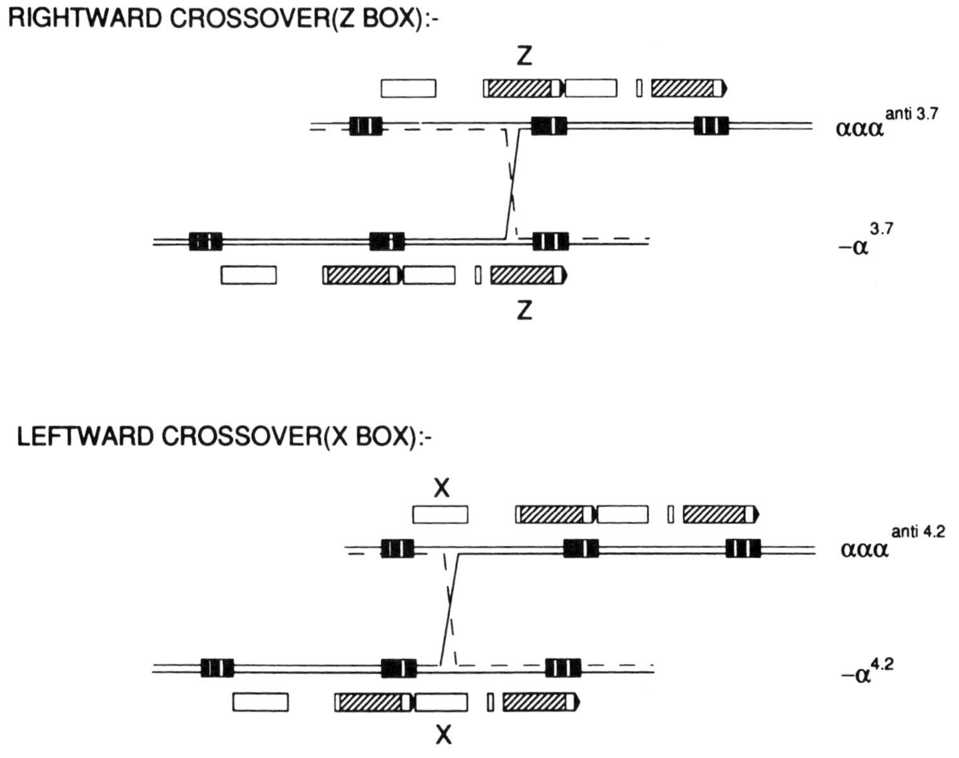

Fig. 181-19 Mechanism of the unequal crossover that gives rise to the $-\alpha^{3.7}$ and $-\alpha^{4.2}$ deletions. The rightward crossover occurs when genetic exchange takes place between the misaligned homologous Z boxes, giving rise to chromosomes with either one ($-\alpha^{3.7}$) or three ($\alpha\alpha\alpha^{anti\ 3.7}$) α-globin genes. The leftward crossover occurs when genetic exchange takes place between the misaligned homologous X boxes, giving rise to chromosomes with either one ($-\alpha^{4.2}$) or three ($\alpha\alpha\alpha^{anti\ 4.2}$) α-globin genes.

between the two X blocks deletes 4.2 kb of DNA (referred to as a leftward deletion, $-\alpha^{4.2}$). The corresponding triplicated α gene arrangements are referred to as $\alpha\alpha\alpha^{anti\text{-}3.7}$ and $\alpha\alpha\alpha^{anti\text{-}4.2}$. Further examples of chromosomes with four α genes ($\alpha\alpha\alpha\alpha^{anti\text{-}3.7}$ and $\alpha\alpha\alpha\alpha^{anti\text{-}4.2}$) presumably result from similar crossovers involving the $\alpha\alpha\alpha^{anti\text{-}3.7}$ and $\alpha\alpha\alpha^{anti\text{-}4.2}$ chromosomes, respectively.[274] Crossovers between single −α and duplicated αα chromosomes have also been described.[275] Indeed, several independent lines of evidence suggest that this type of homologous genetic recombination occurs relatively frequently in globin[276,277] and other loci.[278,279] At present it is not known whether such rearrangements take place between misaligned chromosomes or between chromatids during meiosis.

The mechanism by which two rare deletions that cause α^+ thalassemia (Fig. 181-18) have arisen are not clear. In one of them, $(\alpha)\alpha^{5.3}$ described in an Italian patient,[280] recombination appears to have occurred by an illegitimate process involving partially homologous sequences (see next section). In the other, $-\alpha^{3.5}$ described in an Asian patient,[281] sequence data across the breakpoint are not available.

Based on the geographical distribution and relative frequencies of the common −α chromosomes, it appears that rearrangements involving the Z box are more frequent than those involving the X or Y regions. It is possible to subdivide the common Z box rearrangements into three types ($-\alpha^{3.7I}$, $-\alpha^{3.7II}$, $-\alpha^{3.7III}$) depending on exactly where the crossover occurred with respect to three restriction enzyme sites that differ between the α_2 and α_1 Z boxes[276] (see Fig. 181-18). In general, it appears that the frequency of each of these subtypes ($\alpha^{3.7I}$, $-\alpha^{3.7II}$, $-\alpha^{3.7III}$, and $-\alpha^{4.2}$; Y box crossovers have not been identified) are simply related to the length of homology within each subsegment. It remains to be seen whether more complex physical constraints also play a role in determining the relative frequency of recombination in this region.

The level of expression of the remaining α gene from these chromosomes (−α) can be assessed by the effect of the deletions on phenotype (see Table 181-7) and more directly by measuring the production of α-specific mRNA from such chromosomes. The level of expression of the α_2 gene is two to three times greater than that of the α_1 gene and this appears to be controlled at the level of transcription.[282–285] All six deletions ($-\alpha^{3.7I}$, $-\alpha^{3.7II}$, $-\alpha^{3.7III}$, $-\alpha^{4.2}$, $-\alpha^{3.5}$, $(\alpha)\alpha^{5.3}$) reduce α chain production from the affected chromosome. The similar phenotypes of homozygotes for the $-\alpha^{4.2}$ determinant, in which both α_2 genes are removed, and $-\alpha^{3.7II}$ homozygotes, in which the α_1 genes are effectively deleted, suggests that removal of the α_2 gene results in a partial, compensatory increase in the expression of the remaining α_1 gene on the $-\alpha^{4.2}$ chromosome;[286] increase in expression of the α_1 gene has been clearly demonstrated at the level of mRNA.[287] The mechanism by which this change in gene expression occurs is not understood, although clearly this observation may be of importance in understanding the molecular mechanisms that normally maintain the difference in expression of the α_2 and α_1 genes. At present, there are insufficient phenotypic data to compare the relative levels of expression of the less common −α chromosomes.

α^o Thalassemia Due to Deletions. To date, 19 deletions have been described that involve both α genes and thereby abolish α chain production from the affected chromosome (see Fig. 181-20 and references therein). In addition, several rare deletions extending much further beyond the α cluster have also been described.[288–291] Unlike the $-\alpha^{3.7}$ and $-\alpha^{4.2}$ defects, there seem to be several different ways in which deletions associated with α^o thalassemia can arise.

Some of them have been analyzed in detail to determine whether the underlying mechanisms could be established.[292] Most frequently, the α^o thalassemia defects result from illegitimate recombination. One of the deletions ($--^{MED}$) involves a complex rearrangement that introduces a new piece of DNA bridging the two breakpoints in the α cluster (Fig. 181-20). This new DNA originates upstream from the α cluster and appears to have been replicated into the junction in a manner suggesting that the upstream segment of DNA may lie at the base of a replication loop.

Sequence analysis shows that members of the dispersed family of *Alu* repeats[293] are frequently found at or near the breakpoints of the α^o thalassemia deletions. These repeats may simply provide partially homologous sequences that promote DNA strand

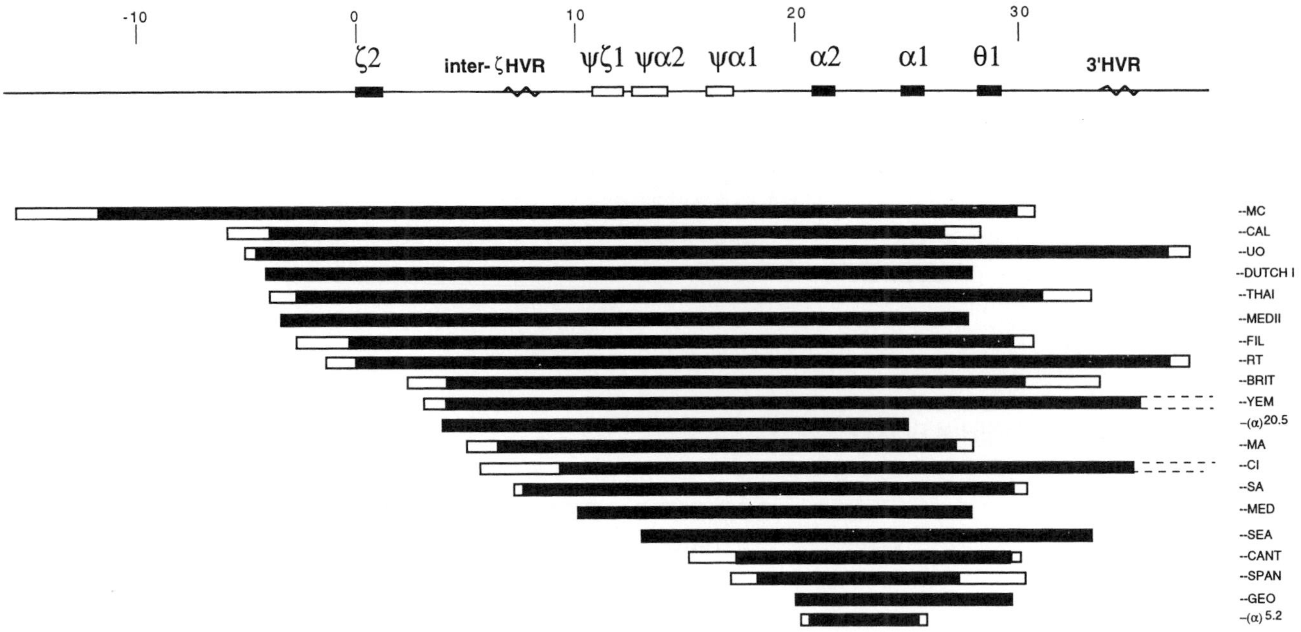

Fig. 181-20 The deletions that are responsible for α° thalassaemia. Full details of the original reports and nomenclature are given in references 2 and 246.

exchanges during replication, or possibly a subset of *Alu* sequences may be more actively involved in the process, particularly if they function as origins of replication.[293] To date, at least eight deletions causing α thalassemia have been shown to have one or both breakpoints lying in *Alu* sequences. It is interesting that similar illegitimate recombination events in the β locus do not seem to involve *Alu* sequences, suggesting that this type of recombination may be to some extent locus specific.[294]

In contrast to the $-\alpha^{3.7}$ and $-\alpha^{4.2}$ defects, the set of deletions that cause α° thalassemia are of limited geographical distribution[245] and each probably represents a single example of an uncommon type of genetic mishap. Perhaps the most extreme example of this is the $--^{BRIT}$ mutation, which is predominantly seen in individuals originating from the north of England.[295,296]

Because both α genes are involved in this group of deletions, α globin synthesis is abolished by these mutants. The similarity of these deletions to those of the β cluster that give rise to HPFH, $\delta\beta$ thalassemia, and $\gamma\delta\beta$ thalassemia raises the question of whether they affect the expression of neighboring genes. In heterozygotes for the two common α° thalassemia determinants ($--^{SEA}/\alpha\alpha$ and $--^{MED}/\alpha\alpha$) it has been shown, using a sensitive radioimmunoassay, that there is a very small increase in ζ globin expression.[297,298] In homozygotes for these mutants ($--^{SEA}/--^{SEA}$ and $--^{MED}/--^{MED}$), large amounts ($\sim$20 to 30 percent) of $Hb_{PORTLAND}$ ($\zeta_2\gamma_2$) are produced. However, it seems more likely that this results from intensive cell selection rather than specific enhancement of ζ globin expression. Hence the change in pattern of gene expression in these deletions may not be comparable to the more dramatic changes in γ expression associated with HPFH. Perhaps it is more relevant to ask why the expression of the embryonic genes ζ and ε is not much changed by these deletions of the α and β globin cluster, whereas γ gene expression is markedly altered.

α Thalassemia Due to Deletions of the α Globin Regulatory Element. It has been shown that expression of the α genes is critically dependent on a segment of DNA that lies 40 kb upstream of the ζ globin gene.[97] This region is associated with an erythroid-specific DNAse I hypersensitive site and is referred to as HS-40. Detailed analysis of HS-40 shows that this segment of DNA contains multiple binding sites for the erythroid restricted *trans*-acting factors GATA-1 and NF-E2.[98,299]

The first indication that such a remote regulatory sequence might exist came from the observation of a patient with α thalassemia.[95] Analysis of the abnormal chromosome, $(\alpha\alpha)^{RA}$, from this patient demonstrated a 62-kb deletion from upstream of the α complex (Fig. 181-21), which includes HS-40. Although both α genes on this chromosome are intact and entirely normal, they appear to be nonfunctional. Since this observation, 11 more patients with α thalassemia due to a deletion of HS-40 and a variable amount of the flanking DNA have been described (Fig. 181-21 and references therein). All of these mutations give rise to the phenotype associated with α° thalassemia.

The mechanisms by which these mutations arose are quite diverse. In the $(\alpha\alpha)^{RA}$ chromosome, the deletion resulted from a recombination event between partially homologous *Alu* repeats that are normally 62 kb apart. Another of these mutations $(\alpha\alpha)^{TI}$ involved truncation of the tip of chromosome 16 so that all material between the deletion breakpoint and the end (telomere) of the chromosome was deleted. This truncated chromosome was healed by the addition of telomere repeat sequence, $(TTAGGG)_n$, to give a stable chromosome.[96]

In the $(\alpha\alpha)^{MB}$ chromosome,[300] the deletion arose via a subtelomeric rearrangement. The chromosomal breakpoint was found in an *Alu* element located $\sim$105 kb from the 16p subtelomeric region. The broken chromosome was stabilized with a new telomere acquired by recombination between this *Alu* element and a subtelomeric *Alu* repeat associated with the newly acquired chromosome end.

In five cases ($(\alpha\alpha)^{CMO}$, $(\alpha\alpha)^{IdF}$, $(\alpha\alpha)^{TAT}$, $(\alpha\alpha)^{IC}$, and $(\alpha\alpha)^{TI}$) the chromosomes appear to have been broken and then stabilized by the direct addition of telomeric repeats to nontelomeric DNA.[301] Sequence analysis suggests that these chromosomes are "healed" via the action of telomerase, an enzyme that is normally involved in maintaining the integrity of telomeres.[301,302]

In the three remaining examples ($(\alpha\alpha)^{IJ}$, $(\alpha\alpha)^{MCK}$, and $(\alpha\alpha)^{SN}$, Fig. 181-21) the mechanism has not yet been established. However, it is interesting that in both $(\alpha\alpha)^{IJ}$ and $(\alpha\alpha)^{MCK}$ the deletions appear to have arisen *de novo*, because neither parent has the abnormal chromosome.

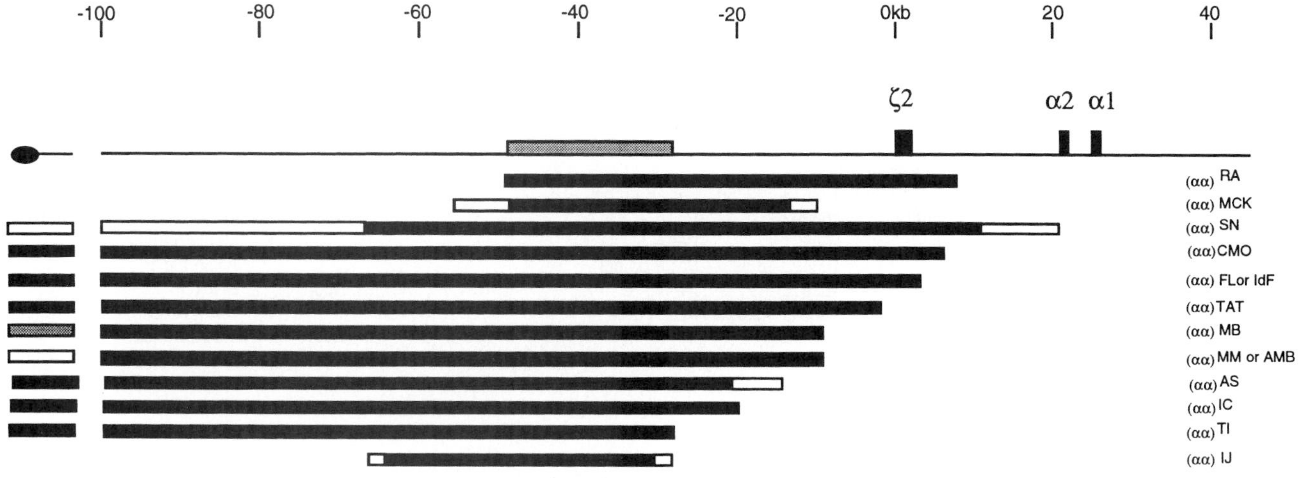

Fig. 181-21 The deletions that remove the HS-40 regulatory region of the α globin gene complex and result in α° thalassemia. As shown, many of these deletions do not involve the complex itself. References and nomenclature are given in reference 2.

α^+ Thalassemia Due to Nondeletion Defects. The nondeletion α thalassemias are classified in this way because analysis of DNA from patients with these disorders reveals no gross abnormality by Southern blotting. In most cases, they result from single or oligonucleotide mutations at regions of the α gene sequence that are critical for normal expression (Table 181-8). Similar mutations in the β globin gene are much more common and are discussed in detail below.

Because expression of the α_2 gene is two to three times greater than that of the α_1 gene[282–285] it is not surprising that most of the nondeletion mutants predominantly affect expression of the α_2 gene. Clearly, such mutations have a greater effect on phenotype, and presumably a greater selective advantage. Unlike the deletion of the α_2 gene in the $-\alpha^{4.2}$ defect, that results in a compensatory increase in expression of the remaining α_1 gene, there appears to be no increase in expression of the α_1 gene when the α_2 gene is inactivated by a point mutation. Therefore the nondeletion α thalassemias have a greater effect on phenotype than the $-\alpha$ mutants.

Mutants that Affect RNA Splicing. Three nondeletion α thalassemia variants affect RNA splicing. One ($\alpha^{IVSI;5bp\ del}\alpha$) results from a pentanucleotide deletion at the 5′ donor site of IVS 1 of the α_2 globin gene.[303,304] This mutation affects the invariant GT sequence and eliminates splicing from the normal donor site while activating a cryptic donor consensus that lies in exon 1. Heterozygotes for this mutation have the phenotype of α thalassemia trait and homozygotes have a correspondingly more severe form of α thalassemia trait.

A mutation of the acceptor site of IVS1 of the α_2 gene ($\alpha^{IVS1;116(A\rightarrow G)}\alpha$) was recently described by Harteveld *et al.* (1996).[305] Abnormal splicing leads to the retention of IVS1, which introduces a premature stop at codon 31. Although all 11 carriers for this mutation have reduced α/β globin chain synthesis ratios their hematologic indices appear remarkably normal.[305] It remains to be seen whether this applies to all carriers of the mutation.

A third splicing defect is caused by mutation of IVS1-117 of the α_1 globin gene ($\alpha^{IVSI\ 117;G\rightarrow A}\alpha$).[306] In this case, the precise nature of the abnormal splicing has not been established.

Mutations Affecting the Poly(A) Addition Signal. The highly conserved sequence motif AATAAA is present 10 to 30 bp upstream of most poly(A) addition sites, and forms part of the signal for mRNA cleavage and polyadenylation of primary transcripts. This sequence is required for transcriptional termination and some evidence suggests that, when mutated, transcription may proceed into neighboring genes and "interfere" with their expression.

At present there are four known mutations of the α_2 gene polyadenylation signal (Table 181-8). The first to be identified (AATAA<u>A</u> → AATAA<u>G</u>) was found in the Saudi Arabian population. Heterozygotes have the hematologic phenotype of severe carriers of α thalassemia trait, but homozygotes have Hb H disease with 5 to 15 percent Hb H in their peripheral blood.[307,308] The mechanisms by which this mutation causes such a severe phenotype are not fully understood.

Homozygotes for other nondeletion mutations that inactivate the α_2 gene do not always have Hb H disease and when present it is often mild with low levels of Hb H (see below). In contrast, homozygotes for the $\alpha^{PA6:A\rightarrow G}\alpha$ haplotype always have Hb H disease with high levels of Hb H. It is interesting that in these individuals α_2 mRNA is reduced but not absent; thus, if the α_1 gene were fully active, one would expect to see a severe form of α thalassemia trait, not Hb H disease. The implication of these findings is that the poly(A) site mutation down-regulates both α_2 and α_1 genes on the same chromosome. In rare individuals, the $\alpha^{PA6:A\rightarrow G}$ mutation is duplicated, producing a chromosome with three α genes $\alpha^{PA6:A\rightarrow G}\alpha^{PA6:A\rightarrow G}\alpha$ which still interacts with the $\alpha^{PA6:A\rightarrow G}\alpha$ chromosome to produce Hb H disease.[309]

Analysis of the $\alpha^{PA6:A\rightarrow G}$ mutation has shown that it has at least two effects. It reduces the amount of α_2 mRNA that accumulates and in a transient assay, readthrough transcripts extending beyond the mutated poly(A) addition site are detected. Recently, extended transcripts were also detected in reticulocytes of patients with this defect using RT-PCR.[310] It seems possible that transcription extending through the normal termination point could run on and interfere with expression of the linked α_1 gene.

Since the original description of the $\alpha^{PA6:A\rightarrow G}$ allele, three other poly(A) signal mutations have been described (Table 181-8). Insufficient data exist to know whether these mutations down-regulate α gene expression in a similar way. In particular, no homozygotes for these mutations have been identified. Compound heterozygotes for these mutations and α^o thalassemia have Hb H disease as expected.[311,312]

Mutations Affecting Initiation of mRNA Translation. Several nondeletion mutations affect mRNA translation and five of the mutations disrupt the initiation consensus sequence CCRCC<u>ATG</u> (Table 181-8). Two mutations occur on chromosomes with a single α gene. In one ($-\alpha^{IN;A\rightarrow G}$) the mutation abolishes translation of mRNA from the gene. It was identified via its interaction with a second α thalassemia chromosome ($-\alpha^{IN;A\rightarrow G}/-\alpha$); affected

Table 181-8 Nondeletion Mutants that Cause α Thalassemia

	Affected Gene	Affected Sequence	Location‡	Mutation	Alternative Notation	Identification	Distribution
mRNA processing	$\alpha 2$	IVS 1 (donor)	163008-163012	IVS 1; 5 bp del	$\alpha^{Hph}\alpha$	R: Hph 1	Mediterranean
	$\alpha 2$	IVS1-116 (Acceptor)	163122	IVS 1; 116 (A → G)		C: Sac 2	Dutch Caucasian
	$\alpha 1$	IVS-1-117 (Acceptor)	166927	IVS 1; 117 (G → A)		R: Fok 1	Asian Indian
	$\alpha 2$	Poly(A) signal	163673-163688	PA; 16 bp del		R: Hae III	Arab
	$\alpha 2$*	Poly(A) signal	163693	PA; 6 A → G	$\alpha^{TSaudi}\alpha$		Middle East, Mediterranean
	$\alpha 2$	Poly(A) signal	163691	PA; 4 A → G			Mediterranean
	$\alpha 2$	Poly(A) signal	163692-163693	PA; 2 bp del			Asian Indian
mRNA Translation§	$-\alpha$	Initiation codon	163912	IN; A → G		R: Nco 1	Black
	$-\alpha^{3.7II}$	Initiation codon	162909-162910	IN; 2 bp del			North African, Mediterranean
	$\alpha 2$	Initiation codon	162913	IN; T → C		R: Nco 1	Mediterranean
	$\alpha 1$	Initiation codon	166716	IN; A → G		R: Nco 1	Mediterranean
	$\alpha 2$	Initiation codon	162913	IN; 1 bp del		R: Nco 1	Vietnam
	$-\alpha$	Exon I	163005-163006	Cd 30/31; 2 bp del			Black
	$\alpha 2$	Exon II	163146-163154	Cd 39/41; del/ins			Yemenite-Jewish
	$\alpha 1$	Exon II	166986-167000	Cd 51-55; 13 bp del		R: Bst NI	Spain
	$\alpha 2$	Exon III	163509-163520	Cd 113-116; 12 bp del			Spanish
	$\alpha 2$	Exon III	163519	Cd 116; G → T		C: Bfa 1	Black
	$\alpha 2$	Termination Codon	163597	TER; T → C (Constant Spring)	$\alpha^{CS}\alpha$	R: Mse 1	Southeast Asian
	$\alpha 2$	Termination Codon	164597	TER; T → A (Icaria)	$\alpha^{Ic}\alpha$	R: Mse 1	Mediterranean
	$\alpha 2$	Termination Codon	163598	TER; A → C (Koya Dora)	$\alpha^{KD}\alpha$	R: Mse 1	Indian
	$\alpha 2$	Termination Codon	163597	TER; T → G (Seal Rock)	$\alpha^{SR}\alpha$	R: Mse 1	Black
	$\alpha 2$	Termination Codon	163599	TER; A → T (Paksé)		R: Mse 1	Laotian
Post translational	$-\alpha$	Exon I	162954	Cd 14; T → G (Evanston) {W > R}			Black
	$\alpha 2$	Exon I	163000	Cd 29; T → C (Argrinio) {L > P}			Mediterranean
	$\alpha 2$	Exon I	163002-163004	Cd 30; 3 bp del {ΔE}			China
	$\alpha 1$	Exon II	163143-163145	Cd 38/39; 3 bp del; (Taybe) {ΔT}			Arabia
	$\alpha 1$	Exon II	167011	Cd 59; G → A (Adana) {G > D}			Turkey
	$\alpha 2$	Exon II	163207	Cd 59; G → A (Adana) {G → D}			China
	$\alpha 1$	Exon II	167013-167018	Cd 60/61; 3 bp del (Clinic) {ΔK}		C: Dde 1	Spain
	$\alpha 2$	Exon II	163215-163217	Cd 62; 3 bp del			Greece
	$\alpha 2$	Exon III	163484	Cd 104; G → A (Sallanches) {C > Y}		C: Bsp M1	French
	$\alpha 2$	Exon III	163499	Cd 109; T → G (Suan Dok) {L > R}	$\alpha^{SD}\alpha$	C: Sma 1	Southeast Asia
	α	Exon III	(163502)	Cd 110; C → A (Petah Tikva) {A > D}	$\alpha^{PT}\alpha$		Middle East
	$\alpha 2$	Exon III	163547	Cd 125; T → C (Quong Sze) {L > P}	$\alpha^{QS}\alpha$	C: Msp 1	Southeast Asia
	$-\alpha^{3.7}$	Exon III	163547	Cd 125; T → A {L > Q}			Israel
	$\alpha 1$	Exon III	167370	Cd 129; T → C (Tunis-Bizerte) {L > P}		C: Nci 1	Tunisia
	$\alpha 2$	Exon III	163559	Cd 129; T → C (Utrecht) {L > P}		C: Hpa II	Netherlands
	$\alpha 2$	Exon III	163561	Cd 130; G → C (Sun Prarie) {A > P}			Asian Indian
	$\alpha 2$	Exon III	163564	Cd 131; T → C (Questembert) {S > P}			Yugoslavia
	$\alpha 2$	Exon III	163580	Cd 136; T → C (Hb Bibba) {L > P}			Caucasian
Uncharacterized	α	Unknown	Unknown	Not determined			Black
	α	Unknown	Unknown	Not determined			Greek**
	α	Unknown	Unknown	Not determined			Pacific

*This mutation has been found in both $\alpha 2$-like genes on an $\alpha\alpha\alpha^{3.7}$ chromosome present in Saudi Arabian individuals.

§The elongated α chains associated with Hb Wayne, which results from a frameshift (deletion of either C at α138 or A at α139 of the α2-globin gene) and Hb Grady which results from a crossover in phase (with insertion of three residues at α118) are not known to be associated with α thalassaemia although the critical interactions that would clearly reveal this have not been described.

**Its interaction with α°-thalassaemia determinants to produce the Hb Bart's Hydrops fetalis syndrome suggests that both α-globin genes may be affected.

R Removes.

C Creates.

‡These numbers refer to the sequence published in Ref. 510; location in brackets assumes α_2 defect.

Original data appear in references 2 and 246.

patients had the typical hematologic features of Hb H disease.[313] In the other case ($-\alpha^{IN;2bp\ del}$), a 2-bp deletion from the consensus sequence reduces the level of mRNA translation by 30 to 50 percent.[314,315] This mutation produces Hb H disease in homozygotes ($-\alpha^{IN;2bp\ del}/-\alpha^{IN;2bp\ del}$) who have a mild hypochromic microcytic anemia (Hb 9.7–9.9, MCV 63, MCH 18–20) with 4.5 to 5.6 percent Hb H.[316]

Two mutations ($\alpha^{IN;T\rightarrow C}\alpha$ and $\alpha^{IN;1bp\ del}\alpha$) abolish translation of mRNA from the α_2 gene. Six of seven homozygotes for the $\alpha^{IN;T\rightarrow C}\alpha$ haplotype have a severe form of α thalassemia trait, but one has a mild form of Hb H disease with 2.6 percent Hb H.[317,318] Compound heterozygotes for this mutation with common α^o thalassemia defects have Hb H disease with substantial amounts of Hb H (~8 to 24 percent) in the peripheral blood.

One mutation $\alpha\alpha^{IN;A\rightarrow G}$ abolishes translation of mRNA from the α_1 globin gene.[319] In the single family reported with this mutation compound, heterozygotes ($--/\alpha\alpha^{IN;A\rightarrow G}$) had relatively low levels of Hb H (1.5 percent and 3 percent) suggesting that mutation of the α_1 gene causes a less severe degree of α chain deficit than a similar mutation of the α_2 gene. This mutation adds weight to the argument that the α_2 gene is expressed at a higher level than the α_1 gene.

In-Frame Deletions, Frameshifts, and Nonsense Mutations. In 1988, Safaya *et al.*[320] described an African American with Hb H disease and Hb $G_{PHILADELPHIA}$ ($-\alpha^{68Asn\rightarrow Lys}$) who synthesized only α^G and no α^A chains. The patient was shown to have the genotype $-\alpha/-\alpha^G$, leading Safaya *et al.* to conclude that the $-\alpha$ chromosome was inactivated by a further mutation. Sequence analysis showed that this single α gene has a dinucleotide deletion from one or other of the Glu (GAG) or Arg (AGG) codons (30 and 31). The loss of two nucleotides leads to a frameshift and a novel protein sequence in exon 2 from codons 31–54 followed by a new, in-phase termination codon (TAA) at position 55. Hence the $-\alpha^{Cd30/31;2bp\ del}$ haplotype is an inactive α^o thalassemia determinant.

Mutations affecting the α globin translational reading frame have also been noted on chromosomes with two α genes (αα). Three affect the α_2 globin gene. In one ($\alpha^{Cd39/41\ del/ins}\alpha$), there is a deletion of 9 bp (codons 39–41) replaced by an 8-nucleotide insertion that duplicates the adjacent downstream sequence. The mutation changes the mRNA reading frame introducing a new termination signal (TGA) 10 codons downstream.

In another patient, a 12-bp deletion of the α_2 gene results in the loss of 4 amino acids (codons 113–116) from the α chain, reducing it from its normal length of 141 amino acids to 137 amino acids. It is thought that this produces an unstable α chain that is rapidly broken down and unable to form a Hb tetramer, like some of the mutants described below. In a heterozygote, this mutation produced the phenotype of α thalassemia trait.

The third mutation in this group has a single base change ($\alpha^{Cd116;G\rightarrow T}\alpha$), which results in a premature termination codon and inactivation of the α_2 gene. Again, carriers for this mutation have α thalassemia trait.

A single Spanish family with a frameshift mutation in the α_1 globin gene was described by Ayala *et al.*[321] Two affected individuals ($\alpha\alpha^{Cd51-55;13bp\ del}/\alpha\alpha$) have the α thalassemia trait. Direct sequence analysis of the α_1 gene reveals a 13-bp deletion between codons 51 and 55. This mutation results in a mRNA reading frameshift, which introduces a new stop signal at codon 62.

Chain Termination Mutants. There are potentially nine single-nucleotide variants of the natural termination codon (TAA) of the α_2 globin gene (Table 181-8). Two (TGA and TAG) encode stop (nonsense) mutations; the others encode amino acids. When mutations change the stop codon to one of these amino acids, the mutations enable mRNA translation to continue to the next in-phase termination codon (UAA) located within the polyadenylation signal (AAUAAA); in each case extending the α chain by 31 amino acids from the natural C-terminal arginine (codon 141). Of the six predicted α_2 variants, five have been described, each with a unique amino acid at α142. These are: $Hb_{CONSTANT\ SPRING}$ (α142 Gln), Hb_{ICARIA} (α142 Lys), $Hb_{KOYA\ DORA}$ (α142 Ser), $Hb_{SEAL\ ROCK}$ (α142 Glu), and $Hb_{PAKSÉ}$ (α142 Tyr) (Fig. 181-6). An extended α globin variant with leucine at position 142 is predicted but has not yet been described.

The mechanism by which chain termination mutants cause α thalassemia has been difficult to elucidate. $Hb_{CONSTANT\ SPRING}$ (CS) is the most extensively studied of this group. Currently, it is suggested that α^{CS} mRNA is unstable, possibly due to disruption of a sequence(s) in the 3′ noncoding region that is translated inappropriately as a result of the chain termination mutant.[322] Recent experimental data support this interpretation; translational readthrough disrupts a putative RNA/protein complex associated with the α_2 globin 3′UTR which is required for mRNA stability in erythroid cells.[323]

Unstable α Chain Variants Associated with α Thalassemia. It is well-established that some globin variants alter the tertiary structure of the hemoglobin molecule making the dimer (αβ) or tetramer ($\alpha_2\beta_2$) unstable. Such molecules may precipitate within the red cell, forming insoluble inclusions (Heinz bodies) that damage the red cell membrane. This situation causes a chronic hemolytic anemia with equal loss of α- and β-like globin chains from the red cell.

Over the past few years, it has become apparent that some α globin variants are so unstable that they undergo very rapid, postsynthetic degradation. In this case, because the α chains probably do not form dimers or tetramers, there is no associated loss of normal β chains which remain, in excess, within the red cell; such patients, by definition, have α thalassemia. Many of these α globin variants are so unstable, that they cannot be detected by conventional protein analysis. Therefore, affected patients often present with nondeletional α thalassemia that can only be explained when the mutation is identified by DNA sequence analysis.

To date, 17 unstable α variants have been shown to produce the phenotype of α thalassemia to a greater or lesser extent (Table 181-8). The mutations most frequently affect the heme pocket, internal hydrophobic regions of the molecule that normally maintain its conformation or hydrophobic residues involved in the formation of $\alpha_1\ \beta_1$ contacts.

Interactions of α Thalassemia Haplotypes

At present, over 100 α haplotypes have been described and thus there are a large number of potential interactions. Phenotypically, these result in one of four broad categories: a normal phenotype; α thalassemia minor, in which there are mild hematologic changes but no major clinical abnormalities; Hb H disease; and the Hb Bart's hydrops fetalis syndrome. These clinical syndromes and the broad classes of interactions that underlie them are summarized in Table 181-7 and are reviewed in detail in the following sections.

Normal Phenotype. Although the majority of normal individuals have four α globin genes (αα/αα), between 1 and 2 percent in most populations have five genes (ααα/αα). Furthermore, in populations where α thalassemia is common, the genotype $-\alpha/\alpha\alpha\alpha$ also occurs.[221] It has been shown that the additional α gene in the ααα haplotype produces a slight excess of α_2 mRNA[283] although this is not always reflected in the α/β globin chain synthesis ratio[61] or at the phenotypic level; individuals with these interactions are often indistinguishable from normal.[61] Rare individuals with αααα/αα or ααα/ααα may produce excess α globin, but again, their phenotype is essentially normal.[274]

Within normal individuals there is a considerable amount of variation in the sequence and structure of the α-globin complex with no apparent effect on the expression of the α globin genes.[52]

α Thalassemia Minor. This most frequently results from the interaction of a normal haplotype (αα) with one of the α^+ or α^o

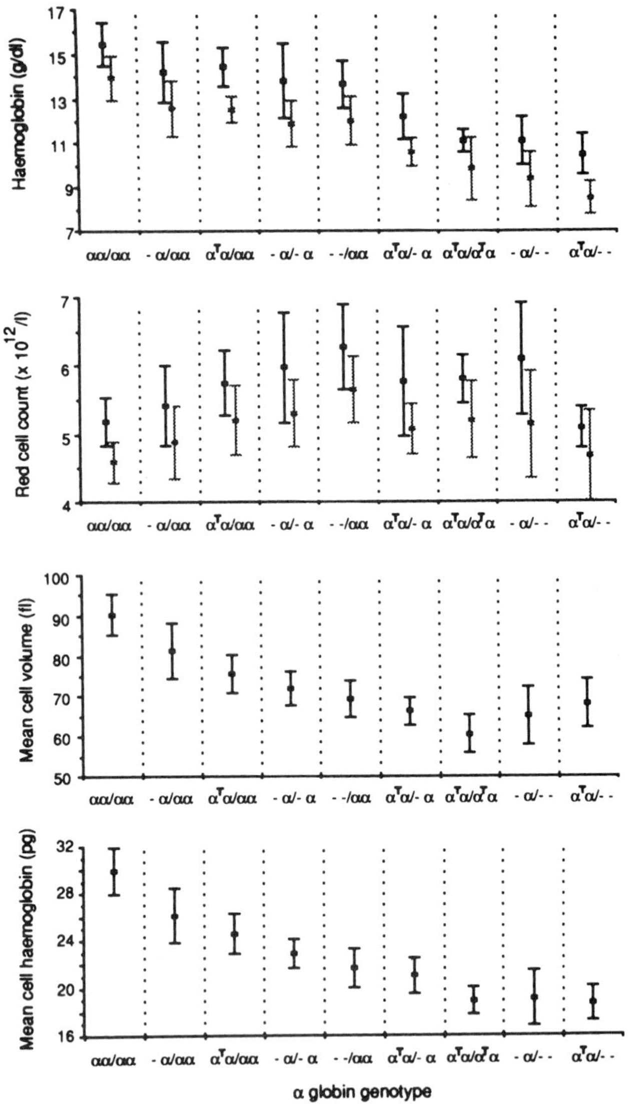

Fig. 181-22 Mean and standard deviation of the Hb, RBC, MCV, and MCH are plotted for each of nine possible genotypes, arranged in order of increasing severity from $\alpha\alpha/\alpha\alpha$ (left) to $\alpha^T\alpha/$ - - (right). Fro Hb and RBC, results are shown separately for males (black bars) and females (gray bars). (*We are grateful to Dr. A.O.M. Wilkie who collated the data presented in this figure.*)

thalassemia determinants (e.g., $-\alpha^{3.7}/\alpha\alpha$, $-\alpha^{4.2}/\alpha\alpha$, $\alpha^T\alpha/\alpha\alpha$, or $--/\alpha\alpha$). In populations where α thalassemia is common, two α^+ thalassemias can also interact to produce α thalassemia minor, $-\alpha^{3.7}/-\alpha^{3.7}$. Because each α thalassemia determinant may be associated with a different degree of suppression of α globin chain synthesis, these interactions produce a range of disorders spanning a clinical and hematologic spectrum from a normal phenotype to Hb H disease (see Table 181-7). The variation in severity of the α^+ and α^o mutations is demonstrated by the degree of anemia, MCV, MCH, α/β globin chain synthesis ratio, and level of Hb Bart's at birth when different determinants interact with each other or a normal chromosome (Fig. 181-22).

In general, chromosomes with a single α gene ($-\alpha$) produce the mildest phenotype, with $-\alpha^{4.2}$ producing a greater reduction in α globin chain synthesis than $-\alpha^{3.7}$.[286] Nondeletion mutants ($\alpha^T\alpha$) that affect the predominant α_2 gene (see Table 181-8) cause a more pronounced reduction in α chain synthesis and deletion mutants involving both α genes (e.g., $--^{MED}$ and $--^{SEA}$) lead to the most severe phenotype. As Fig. 181-22 shows, it is not possible to predict accurately the genotype from any given phenotype and in some cases, such as $-\alpha/\alpha\alpha$, it may be impossible to diagnose a carrier of α thalassemia using any of the conventional phenotypic criteria. Therefore, to perform accurate genetic counseling in families with α thalassemia, genotype determination is essential.

Homozygotes for Nondeletion Types of α Thalassemia. The chain-termination mutant $Hb_{CONSTANT\ SPRING}$ causes a severe reduction in α_2 globin expression from the affected chromosome. Sufficient homozygotes ($\alpha^{TER;T\rightarrow C}\alpha/\alpha^{TER;T\rightarrow C}\alpha$) have been described to establish that the phenotype is more severe than α thalassemia minor, but not as severe as most cases of Hb H disease.[324] The subjects are anemic with thalassemic red cell changes and a reticulocytosis. Basophilic stippling of the red cells is often prominent. They have mild jaundice and a variable degree of hepatosplenomegaly and are therefore quite unlike patients with α thalassemia minor. Patients homozygous for the chain-termination mutant Koya Dora ($\alpha^{TER;A\rightarrow C}\alpha/\alpha^{TER;A\rightarrow C}\alpha$) have been described, but their phenotype was not given.[325]

The only other homozygotes for mutations affecting the predominant α_2 gene are a single Sardinian patient with a very mild form of Hb H disease ($\alpha^{IN;T\rightarrow C}\alpha/\alpha^{IN;T\rightarrow C}\alpha$)[326] and Saudi Arabian patients with typical Hb H disease ($\alpha^{PA;6A\rightarrow G}\alpha/\alpha^{PA;6A\rightarrow G}\alpha$).[79,327] A comparison of the phenotype of homozygotes for $Hb_{CONSTANT\ SPRING}$ ($\alpha^{TER;T\rightarrow C}\alpha/\alpha^{TER;T\rightarrow C}\alpha$) with the Sardinian patient ($\alpha^{IN;T\rightarrow C}\alpha/\alpha^{IN;T\rightarrow C}\alpha$) indicates that these interactions may lie on either side of a critical level of α chain synthesis, below which the syndrome of Hb H disease occurs.

Hb H Disease. Hb H disease most frequently results from the interaction of α^+ and α^o thalassemia; therefore, it is predominantly found in Southeast Asia (commonly $--^{SEA}/-\alpha^{3.7}$) and the Mediterranean basin (commonly $--^{MED}/-\alpha^{3.7}$) where both α^+ and α^o thalassemia are common. Hb H disease may also result from the interaction of nondeletion mutations affecting the predominant α_2 globin gene ($\alpha^{IN;T\rightarrow C}\alpha/\alpha^{IN;T\rightarrow C}\alpha$, $\alpha^{PA;6A\rightarrow G}\alpha/\alpha^{PA;6A\rightarrow G}\alpha$). In Algeria, homozygotes for the $-\alpha^{3.7II}$ defect ($-\alpha^{3.7II\ IN;2bp\ del}/-\alpha^{3.7II\ IN;2bp\ del}$) (see Table 181-8) have typical Hb H disease.[328]

The genetic basis for Hb H disease is diverse and as more molecular defects are characterized, the underlying interactions will inevitably reveal more complexity. It is not yet clear to what extent this molecular diversity is reflected in the variable clinical and hematologic features of Hb H disease. The clinical picture of Hb H disease is usually thalassemia intermedia, although there is considerable variation in the severity of this condition. The predominant features are a hypochromic, microcytic anemia with jaundice and hepatosplenomegaly. Because the main mechanism of the anemia is hemolysis rather than dyserythropoiesis, only one-third of patients have clinical evidence of an expanded erythron. The commonest complication is the development of severe splenomegaly with hypersplenism. Other complications include infection, leg ulcers, gallstones, and folic acid deficiency.

The hematologic features of Hb H disease are also quite variable.[2,232] Hemoglobin levels ranging from 2.6 to 12.4 g/dl have been recorded, in association with reticulocytosis and typical thalassemic changes of the red cell indices. The hemoglobin consists of Hb A with a variable amount of Hb H and sometimes Hb Bart's. The proportion of Hb H varies from 2 to 40 percent. When peripheral blood is incubated with redox dyes, this variablility is reflected in the number of cells that contain typical Hb H inclusions (Fig. 181-23).

As yet, there have been few systematic attempts to correlate the genotype with the phenotype of Hb H disease. However, it appears that, as expected, patients with a nondeletion defect (affecting the predominant α_2 gene) interacting with an α^o thalassemia determinant ($--/\alpha^T\alpha$) have higher levels of Hb H (β_4), a greater degree of anemia and, anecdotally, a more severe clinical course than patients with the $--/-\alpha$ genotype.[329–332] At the extreme of this spectrum, a few patients have been described in whom severe Hb H disease was associated with hydrops fetalis (Hb H hydrops fetalis; see below).

In Thailand, where there is an abundance of well-documented cases of Hb H disease, it is known that despite the relatively

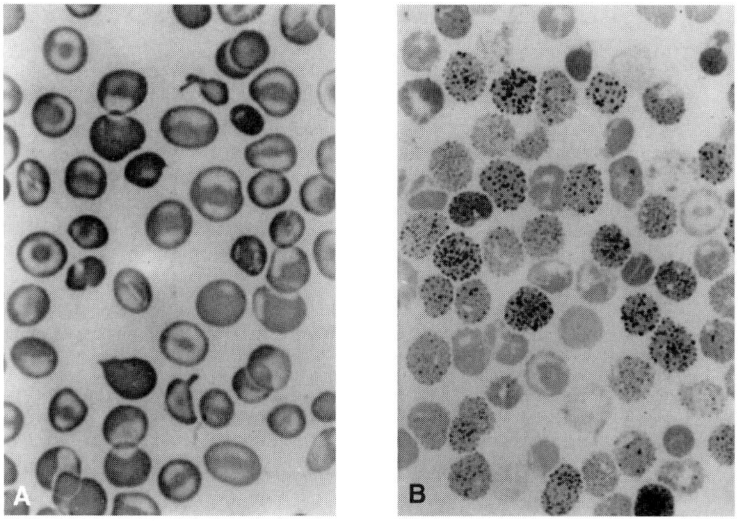

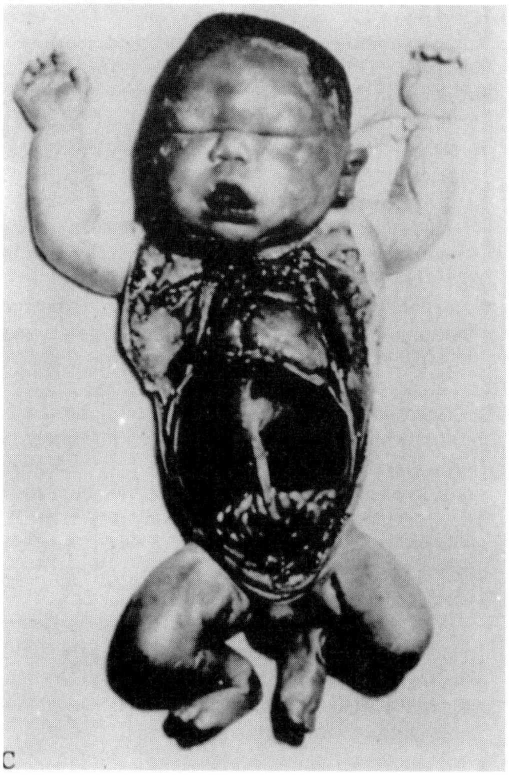

Fig. 181-23 Clinical manifestations of α thalassemia. *A.* A blood smear of a patient with Hb H disease. *B.* The cells were supravitally stained with brilliant cresyl blue to demonstrate Hb H inclusions. *C.* An infant with the hemoglobin Bart's hydrops fetalis syndrome.

homogeneous nature of the molecular basis ($--^{SEA}/-\alpha^{3.7}$ in 80 percent of affected patients)[333] the clinical course is quite variable. This suggests that other genetic and environmental factors play an important role in clinical and hematologic variation seen in this syndrome.

The Hemoglobin Bart's Hydrops Fetalis Syndrome. Nearly all cases of this syndrome are due to the interaction of two α^o thalassemia determinants. As with Hb H disease, this condition is almost exclusively seen in patients of Southeast Asian (commonly $--^{SEA}/--^{SEA}$) or Mediterranean (commonly $--^{MED}/--^{MED}$) origin. Infants with this syndrome either die *in utero* (30 to 40 weeks gestation) or soon after birth (Fig. 181-23). However, long-term survival has been recorded (see below).

Usually, the clinical picture is that of a pale edematous infant with signs of cardiac failure and prolonged intrauterine hypoxia (Fig. 181-23). Hepatosplenomegaly is always present and often there are other congenital abnormalities. The hemoglobin levels range from 3 to 20 g/dl, and the blood film is characterized by anisopoikilocytosis with large hypochromic macrocytes; many nucleated cells are present in the peripheral blood. The hemoglobin consists of ~80 percent Hb Bart's, the remainder being hemoglobins H and Portland. Of these hemoglobins, only $Hb_{PORTLAND}$ transports oxygen efficiently, hence the severe degree of fetal hypoxia. There is a high incidence of maternal complications including toxemia and postpartum hemorrhage.

Hb H Hydrops Fetalis. Nearly all babies with the Hb Bart's hydrops fetalis syndrome inherit no α genes from their parents (genotype $--/--$). However, three reports describe seven rare neonates with severe anemia and various changes associated with hydrops fetalis due to the coinheritance of α^o and α^+ thalassemia.[334–337] In three well-characterized cases, the α^+ thalassemia resulted from mutations in the α_2 gene associated with highly unstable α globin variants ($--/\alpha^{Cd30;3pbdel}\alpha$, $--/\alpha^{Cd59;G\rightarrow A}\alpha$, $--/\alpha^{Cd125;T\rightarrow C}\alpha$).[335,337]

Mothers of these children gave a history of previous neonatal deaths due to anemia. At birth all affected infants were anemic (Hb, 3.4 to 9.7 g/dl) with large amounts of Hb Bart's (31 to 65 percent). Five of the seven infants died at birth and two survived following intrauterine blood transfusion but remain transfusion dependent.

Long-Term Survival of α^o Thalassemia Homozygotes. There is considerable variability in the clinical course of infants with the Hb Bart's hydrops fetalis syndrome. Although most die *in utero*, during delivery, or within 1 to 2 h of birth, others may survive for several days;[338] in some cases, the diagnosis may not be immediately obvious in a newborn infant. It is not surprising, therefore, that during the last 10 years or so, as neonatal care has improved, several homozygotes for α^o thalassemia have survived either as a result of treatment prior to confirmation of the diagnosis or as a result of preplanned intervention.

Six such cases have been reported.[339] Most were delivered prematurely by Caesarean section and transfused soon after birth. Two were transfused *in utero* from ~25 weeks onwards. Most infants have a stormy postnatal period with cardiopulmonary problems and there is a disturbingly high frequency of congenital abnormalities, including patent ductus arteriosus (PDA), limb deformities, and urogenital abnormalities in male infants. Subsequent development has been abnormal in at least half the children, and all require regular blood transfusion and chelation therapy for survival.

α Thalassemia Associated with Mental Retardation. In 1981, three northern European families were described in which a severely mentally retarded son also had Hb H disease.[340] Whereas the common forms of Hb H disease are always inherited in a Mendelian fashion, in these families this appeared not to be so. By 1990, a total of 13 subjects with various forms of α thalassemia and mental retardation (ATR) had been identified and two distinct syndromes delineated.[341,342] One group of patients had large (1 to 2 megabase) deletions of the tip of chromosome 16, including the α globin gene cluster. The clinical features of this so-called ATR-16 syndrome are rather variable, in part because some patients have additional chromosomal aneuploidy. For example, one child with the ATR-16 syndrome inherited an unbalanced submicroscopic 16:1 chromosomal translocation from one of his parents.[343] Thus, this child is monosomic for the tip of chromosome 16p, giving rise to α thalassemia, and trisomic for the tip of

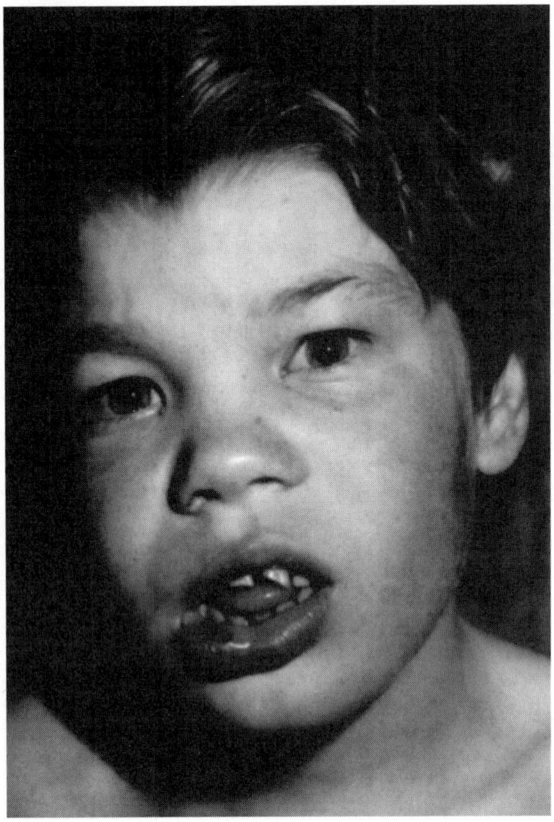

Fig. 181-24 Characteristic facial features of an individual with ATR-X syndrome.

chromosome 1. Some cases of the ATR-16 syndrome have pure monosomy for the tip of 16p,[291] which suggests that there are other genes that are critical for normal development in the vicinity of the α genes at the tip of chromosome 16. Deletion of these genes together with the α globin genes may give rise to the combination of mental retardation and α thalassemia.

In contrast, a second group of patients with α thalassemia and mental retardation has no deletions or any other apparent abnormalities of the α globin gene cluster. These patients have a remarkably uniform phenotype, comprising severe mental retardation, characteristic dysmorphic faces (Fig. 181-24), genital abnormalities, and an unusually mild form of Hb H disease. We currently know of more than 100 cases of this syndrome (for examples, see Gibbons. *et al.*;[125] the major clinical features are summarized in Table 181-9).

Table 181-9 Summary of the Major Clinical Manifestations of the ATR-X Syndrome

Clinical Feature	Total	%
Severe MR*	108/110	98
Normal birth weight	65/72	90
Neonatal hypotonia	59/68	87
Seizures	36/104	35
Characteristic face	86/96	90
Microcephaly	67/88	76
Genital abnormalities	83/94	88
Skeletal abnormalities	83/91	91
Cardiac defects	21/98	21
Renal/urinary abnormalities	16/98	16
Gut dysmotility	66/86	77
Short stature	51/74	69

$n = 112$ patients.
Total represents no. of patients on whom appropriate information is available and patients who do not have thalassemia but in whom ATRX mutations have been identified.
*2 patients too young (<1 year) to assess degree of MR (mental retardation).

It has been shown that this disorder maps to the X chromosome and the disease gene encodes a novel member of the SNF2 family of helicases and DNA-dependent ATPases.[344,345] This family of proteins is thought to exert its effects on DNA transcription, repair, and recombination via an effect on chromatin structure. Circumstantial evidence suggests that the ATRX gene may also influence chromatin structure and when mutated (see references 345 and 346) down-regulates expression of the α globin genes (on chromosome 16) in addition to exerting pleiotropic effects throughout development, giving rise to mental retardation and dysmorphism. Further elucidation of the molecular basis of this disorder promises to be of great value in advancing our understanding of globin gene expression and our knowledge of the molecular basis of some forms of mental handicap.

The Acquired Form of α Thalassemia Associated with Myelodysplasia (ATMDS). Most cases of Hb H disease result from inheritance of the α thalassemia determinants described above. Rarely, patients with myelodysplasia develop an unusual form of Hb H disease that has a striking hypochromic microcytic anemia, classical Hb H inclusions, and detectable levels of Hb H in the peripheral blood. Most cases are of North European origin and in all cases where archival data are available, there is no evidence of preexisting α thalassemia.

The first cases to be reported were diagnosed as having a variety of hematologic malignancies including leukemias, myelofibrosis, myeloproliferative diseases, and acquired sideroblastic anemias. Most of these reports preceded the accurate definition of myelodysplasia (MDS) set out by the French/American/British (FAB) group.[347] A recent review of 14 cases of acquired α thalassemia[348] demonstrated that all these patients have a form of MDS; thus, this condition is now referred to as the α thalassemia/myelodysplasia syndrome (ATMDS).

We currently know of 54 patients with ATMDS. The patients are predominantly males (50/54) with a mean age of 66 years at presentation. The course of this disease is quite variable. The predominant clinical features are those associated with myelodysplasia; ~30 percent have splenomegaly. Most patients eventually develop acute myeloid leukemia or refractory cytopenias, as is expected in a group of patients with MDS.

The structure of the α-globin complex appears to be normal but there is a severe reduction in α-specific mRNA and α globin chain synthesis. The molecular basis for this syndrome appears to involve an acquired defect in transcription of the α genes,[349] although the precise mechanism and its relationship to the hematologic malignancy is not yet known.

The β and δβ Thalassemias and Hereditary Persistence of Fetal Hemoglobin

The β and $\delta\beta$ thalassemias show considerable heterogeneity, not only in clinical severity, but also in the phenotypic characteristics revealed by hematologic measurements and hemoglobin analysis. When the underlying defect is studied at the DNA level, it is clear that the phenotypic diversity hides even further molecular heterogeneity. The equally diverse group of conditions called, collectively, *hereditary persistence of fetal hemoglobin* (HPFH), can be regarded as very mild β or $\delta\beta$ thalassemias in which defective β chain production is compensated for by γ chain production.

Classification. There are two approaches to subdividing this group of disorders. For clinical purposes they can be described as thalassemia major (transfusion dependent), intermedia (of intermediate severity), and minor (asymptomatic). At the biosynthetic level, they are categorized by the affected globin chains and whether there is a partial or complete defect in chain production (see Table 181-6).

The β thalassemias are subdivided into β^o and β^+, representing disorders with complete or partial defects in β chain production.

Table 181-10 Molecular Pathology of the β Thalassemias*

- β° or β^{+} Thalassemia
  - Gene deletions
  - Promoter regions
  - CAP-site
  - 5′ untranslated region
  - Intron/exon boundaries
  - Splice site consensus sequences
  - Cryptic sites in exons
  - Cryptic sites in introns
  - Poly(A) signal
  - Translation of β globin mRNA
    - Initiation
    - Nonsense
    - Frameshift
  - Unstable β globin chains
- Normal Hb A_2 β Thalassemia
  - β thalassemia + δ thalassemia, *cis* or *trans*
  - "Silent" β thalassemia
    - Some promoter mutations
    - CAP + 1
    - CAP + 33
    - 5′ untranslated regions
    - Splice mutation IVS 2 844 C → G
    - Termination codon + 6
- Dominant β Thalassemia
  - Single-base substitutions—highly unstable products
  - Codon deletions
  - Premature termination; Exon 3
  - Frameshifts—elongated, unstable products

* Full list of mutations given in reference 246.

Similarly, the $\delta\beta$ thalassemias are divided into $(\delta\beta)^{+}$ and $(\delta\beta)^{\circ}$ thalassemia depending on whether there is any output of δ or β chains from the affected chromosome. The $(\delta\beta)^{+}$ thalassemias are the result of the production of $\delta\beta$ fusion genes. The $(\delta\beta)^{\circ}$ thalassemias are further divided according to the structure of the Hb F that is produced into the $(\delta\beta)^{\circ}$ thalassemias, in which the Hb F contains both $^{G}\gamma$ and $^{A}\gamma$ chains, and $(^{A}\gamma\delta\beta)^{\circ}$ thalassemia, in which only $^{G}\gamma$ chains are produced.

The different forms of HPFH are classified into three groups according to the underlying defect (Table 181-6): (a) deletions of the δ and β genes (as well as sequences 3′ to these genes) with continued high level expression of the $^{G}\gamma$ and $^{A}\gamma$ genes (5 to 25 percent Hb F) in adult life ($\delta\beta^{\circ}$ HPFH); (b) point mutations in the promoter-regions of a γ gene resulting in increased expression (2 to 20 percent Hb F) of that gene in adults but with persistent β gene expression in *cis* ($^{G}\gamma\beta^{+}$ or $^{A}\gamma\beta^{+}$ HPFH); and (c) a heterogeneous group of disorders with persistent Hb F in adult life (usually low levels) in which the determinant may segregate independently of the β globin gene complex. Previous classifications of these disorders were also based on whether the intercellular distribution of hemoglobin F was pancellular or heterocellular. It now appears that such differences are more likely to be related to the overall Hb F level than to fundamental differences in the underlying molecular pathology.

Molecular Pathology

β Thalassemia. The deficiency or absence of the β chains that characterize β thalassemia could potentially arise from defects affecting any of the stages in the complex process by which the β globin gene is transcribed into RNA, processed into mRNA, and transported to the cytoplasm for translation into polypeptide chains. The molecular basis has been determined in over 170 different β thalassemia alleles, largely by cloning the abnormal gene and then comparing its sequence with that of the normal β^{A} gene. The identification of new defects was originally facilitated by the observation that within any population, each mutation is in strong linkage disequilibrium with specific RFLP haplotypes.[75] Some of the mutations characterized to date are listed in Table 181-10, grouped according to the mechanism by which they inactivate β gene expression, and illustrated in Figs. 181-25 and 181-26.

Gene Deletions. Several different deletions that affect only the β globin gene have been described[350–356] (Fig. 181-26). Of these, only the 619 bp deletion at the 3′ end of the β gene is common, and even that is restricted to the Sind populations of India and Pakistan, where it accounts for ~30 percent of the β thalassemia alleles.[350]

The other deletions are rare and result in the phenotype of β thalassemia with an unusually high Hb A_2.[351–356] In these cases, the 5′ end of the β gene is missing but the δ gene remains intact. It seems that the increased δ chain production results mainly from increased δ gene transcription from the gene in *cis* to the deletion.

Mutations Affecting Transcription. A number of β^{+} thalassemia genes have a single base substitution in two regions immediately in front of the cap site close to or within the CCAAT and ATA boxes that are known to be important in transcriptional efficiency.[74,357–359] These mutant genes show decreased β mRNA production in transient expression systems ranging from 10 to 25 percent of the output from a normal gene, indicating that these substitutions are responsible for the associated thalassemia phenotype.[357] In general, the level of expression *in vitro* correlates well with the clinical severity of the condition, where this is known.

One mutation of this type, C → T at position −101 nt to the β globin gene appears to cause an extremely mild deficit of β globin mRNA.[359] This allele is so mild that it is completely silent in carriers; it can be identified, however, by its interaction with more severe β thalassemia alleles in compound heterozygotes.

Splice Site Mutations Involving the Intron/Exon Boundaries. The boundaries of exons and introns are marked by almost invariant dinucleotides, GT at the donor (5′) site and AG at the acceptor (3′) site (see above). Base substitutions that affect either of those sites totally abolish normal splicing and result in β° thalassemia.[75,247,358] Transcription of these genes appears to be normal but abnormal processing products accumulate at low levels, both in erythroid cells *in vivo* and in *in vitro* expression

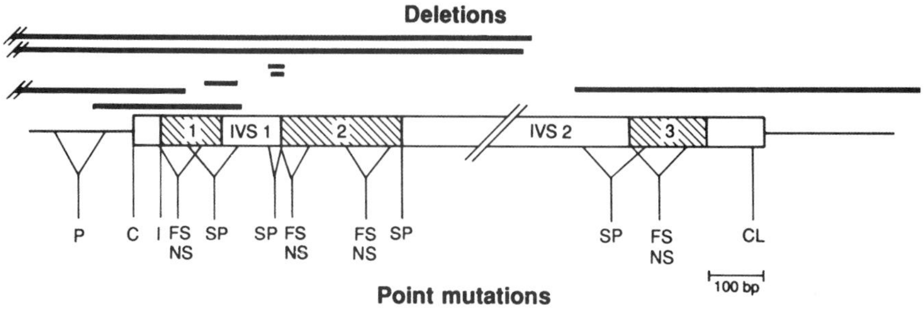

Fig. 181-25 Major classes of mutations of the β-globin gene that cause β thalassemia. P = promoter boxes; C = cap site; I = initiation codon; FS = frameshift; NS = nonsense; SP = splice junction, consensus sequence, or cryptic splice site; CL = RNA cleavage [poly(A)] site.

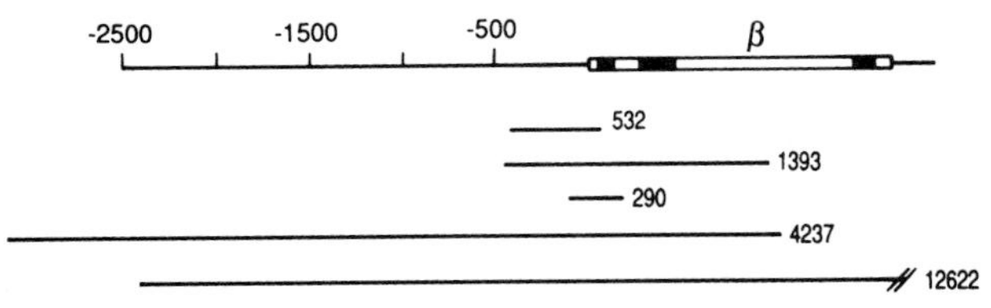

Fig. 181-26 Some of the deletions of the β-globin gene that results in β thalassemia.

systems, as a result of splicing to cryptic splice sites in the surrounding exon or intron.

Splice Site Consensus Sequence Mutations. Although only the GT dinucleotide is invariant at the donor splice site, there is conservation of the surrounding nucleotides and a consensus sequence of these regions can be derived. Mutations within this sequence can reduce the efficiency of splicing to varying degrees, with alternative splicing occurring at the surrounding cryptic splice sites.[75,247,360–365] Mutations of the G at position 5 of IVS1 to C or T result in moderately severe β^+ thalassemia[360] whereas the substitution of C for T at position 6 leads to the very mild β^+ thalassemia (Portuguese type) that is fairly common in the Mediterranean.[266,361]

Mutations in Cryptic Splice Sites in Exons. One of the cryptic splice sites used for alternative splicing in mutations affecting the IVS1 donor site covers codons 24–27 of exon 1 (Fig. 181-27). This site contains a GT dinucleotide. Substitutions that surround this dinucleotide and that alter the cryptic site so that it more closely resembles the consensus donor splice site, result in some use of this site, even though the normal splice site is intact. For example, mutation of codon 24 from GGT to GGA does not alter the amino acid (glycine), but because some splicing occurs at this site instead of at the exon-intron boundary, it results in a moderately severe β^+ thalassemia phenotype.[366]

Mutations of codons 19 (A → G), 26 (G → A), and 27 (G → T) result in both reduced production of mRNA and an amino acid substitution when the mRNA which is spliced normally is translated into protein. The abnormal hemoglobins produced are Hb_{MALAY}, Hb E, and $Hb_{KNOSSOS}$, respectively.[231,367,368] It may be the mild thalassemic nature of the β^E allele that is responsible for its high prevalence in Southeast Asia, rather than an altered property resulting from the amino acid change.

Mutations at Cryptic Sites in Introns. Cryptic splice sites in introns can also undergo mutations that cause them to be used even though the normal site remains intact. The first β thalassemia mutation characterized was of this type, a base substitution at position 110 in IVS 1.[369,370] This region contains a sequence similar to a 3′ acceptor splice site, but lacks the invariant AG dinucleotide. Mutation of the G at 110 to an A supplies the dinucleotide, and ~ 90 percent of the RNA transcripts splice to this site and only ~10 percent splice at the normal site, resulting in a phenotype of severe β^+ thalassemia. The result of the abnormal splicing is a nonfunctional mRNA molecule containing an extra 19 nucleotides from IVS 1 that can be detected in low amounts in reticulocyte or marrow RNA. This lesion is the most common β^+ thalassemia mutation among Mediterranean populations.[75]

Several β thalassemia mutations have been described that generate new donor sites within IVS 2 of the β globin gene.[75,362] In each case, a cryptic acceptor site within IVS 2 following nucleotide 580 is used for processing abnormal transcripts. No normal β globin mRNA appears to be processed from a gene with an A → G substitution at IVS 2 position 654; hence, the clinical phenotype is β^o thalassemia. This is a curious finding because the IVS 2 donor and acceptor sites are entirely normal. It appears that all stable transcripts are spliced from the normal IVS 2 donor to the cryptic acceptor site and from the abnormal new donor site to the normal IVS 2 acceptor. The processed β globin mRNA contains an insertion derived from IVS 2. It is not clear why splicing from the normal donor to acceptor sites does not occur.

CAP Site Mutations. One example of a mutation involving the β globin mRNA CAP site has been described.[371] This involves the substitution of the first A residue by C. It is not clear how this change leads to defective β globin production. It could be mediated by a reduction in the rate of transcription or by slowing down the 5′ capping process which, in turn, might reduce β globin mRNA stability.

Polyadenylation Signal Mutations. The sequence AAUAAA in the 3′ untranslated region of β globin mRNA is the signal for cleavage and polyadenylation of the β gene transcript. Several different mutations of this region have been described.[78,247,372,373] For example, a T → C substitution in the β globin gene in this sequence leads to only one-tenth the normal amount of β globin mRNA transcript and hence to a phenotype of severe β^+ thalassemia. A small amount of an extended β globin mRNA molecule can be found in reticulocytes, presumably polyadenylated at a downstream site.[78]

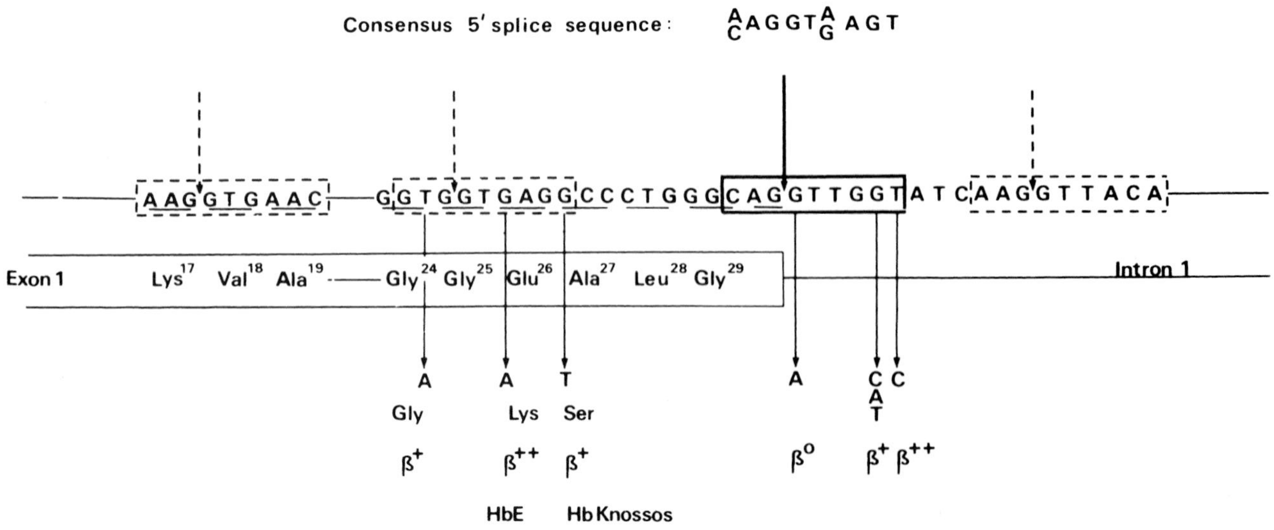

Fig. 181-27 Normal and abnormal splicing at the boundary of exon 1 and intron 1 of the β-globin gene. Solid box and arrow: normal splice site showing consensus sequence and site of cleavage.

Table 181-11 Molecular Forms of Some Dominant β Thalassemias and Structural Variants Associated with a β Thalassemia Phenotype

Mutation	Exon	Phenotype	Designation	Race
		Dominant β Thalassemia		
Codons 128 −4 bp, +5 bp, −11 bp Frameshift terminates codon 154	III	Thalassemia intermedia Inclusion bodies	–	Irish
Codon 121 GAA→TAA*	III	Thalassemia intermedia Inclusion bodies	–	Swiss-French Greek-Polish
Codon 127 CAA→TAA	III	Thalassemia intermedia	–	English
Codon 114 −CT +G Frameshift terminates codon 157	III	Thalassemia intermedia	β Geneva	Swiss-French
Codon 126–T Frameshift terminates codon 157*	III	Thalassemia intermedia Inclusion bodies	β Vercelli	Italian
Codon 94 +TG Frameshift terminates codon 157*	II	Severe thalassemia intermedia Inclusion bodies	β Agnana	Italian
Codon 123–A Frameshift terminates codon 157	III	Thalassemia intermedia Inclusion bodies	β Makabe	Japanese
Codons 123 to 125 −8 bp β-chain 135 residues	III	Severe thalassemia intermedia with Hb E Inclusion bodies	β Khon Kaen	Thai
Codon 127 Gln→Pro	III	Thalassemia intermedia	β Houston	British
Codons 109 to 110–G Frameshift terminates codon 157	III	Thalassemia intermedia	β Manhattan	Ashkenazi Jew
Codons 32/34-GGT*	II	Thalassemia intermedia	β Korea	Korean
Codon 106 Leu→Arg†	III	Thalassemia intermedia	β Terre Haute	European
Codon 28 Leu→Arg	I	Thalassemia intermedia Inclusion bodies	β Chesterfield	English
Codon 60 Val→Glu	II	Thalassemia intermedia	β Cagliari	Italian
		Thalassemia Trait		
Codon 110 Leu→Pro	III	β-thalassemia trait	β Showa-Yakushiji	Japanese
Codon 127 and 128 −3 bp β-chain 145 residues	III	β-thalassemia trait	β Gunma	Japanese
β132 Lys→Gln	III	β-thalassemia trait	$\beta^{K\ Woolwich}$	British
β134 Lys→Gln	III	Mild microcytosis S/β thalassemia interaction with Hb S	Hb North Shore-Caracas	

**De novo* mutations.
† Originally reported as $Hb_{INDIANAPOLIS}$.
SOURCE: Original descriptions given in reference 248.

Mutations to Termination Codons. Base substitutions that change an amino acid codon to a chain termination codon, prevent translation of the mRNA and result in β^o thalassemias. Several mutations of this type have been described, a codon 17 mutation[374] being common in Southeast Asia and the codon 39 mutation[375] occurring at a high frequency in the Mediterranean. The low levels of nuclear and cytoplasmic RNA found in cells with these mutations have yet to be explained.[376]

Frameshift Mutations. The insertion or deletion of one or a few nucleotides in the coding region of the β globin gene disrupts the normal reading frame and results, on translation of the mRNA, in the addition of anomalous amino acids until a termination codon is reached in the new reading frame.[75,247,373] The abnormal mRNA is only found in very low levels in erythroid cells. This type of mutation leads to β^o thalassemia, and one mutation, the deletion of 4 nucleotides in codons 41 and 42, is common in Southeast Asia.

Unstable β Globin Chain Products. Recent studies have shed some light on the complex clinical phenotypes that may result from synthesis of unstable β globin products.[248,377,378] The phenotypic effects of termination codon or frameshift mutations in the β globin gene seem to depend on their particular position. Mutations that produce truncated β chains up to 72 residues in length are usually associated with a mild phenotype in heterozygotes; presumably the short fragments are degraded and the resulting excess of α chains removed in the same way. However, many exon 3 mutations produce longer truncated products and it is likely that the severe heterozygous phenotypes associated with them reflect their heme-binding properties and stability. Truncated products of 120 or more residues should bind heme because only helix H is missing. Furthermore, such heme-containing products should have secondary structure and be less susceptible to proteolytic degradation. These mutations are associated with a dominantly inherited form of thalassemia.[379,380] Presumably the large inclusion bodies which are seen in the erythroid precursors in the marrow of heterozygotes result from both excess α chains and aggregates and precipitated β chain products. Some unstable β globin variants are associated with a milder phenotype similar to heterozygous β thalassemia. A partial list of these mutations is shown in Table 181-11.

Deletions Causing $\delta\beta$ Thalassemia or HPFH. The unequal crossover events that give rise to the Lepore-like hemoglobins and the phenotype of $(\delta\beta)^+$ thalassemia were described earlier. The majority of the $(\delta\beta)^o$ and $(^A\gamma\delta\beta)^o$ thalassemias, as well as different forms of $(\delta\beta)^o$ HPFH (including Hb_{KENYA}), are the result of deletions affecting various parts of the β globin locus. These disorders have attracted considerable interest, because an understanding of how the deletions result in the γ genes remaining active in adult life may provide valuable insights into the normal developmental regulation of the globin genes. Many deletions have now been characterized and the breakpoints have been cloned and sequenced; they are summarized in Fig. 181-28 and reviewed in detail in reference 381. The mechanisms by which they arose

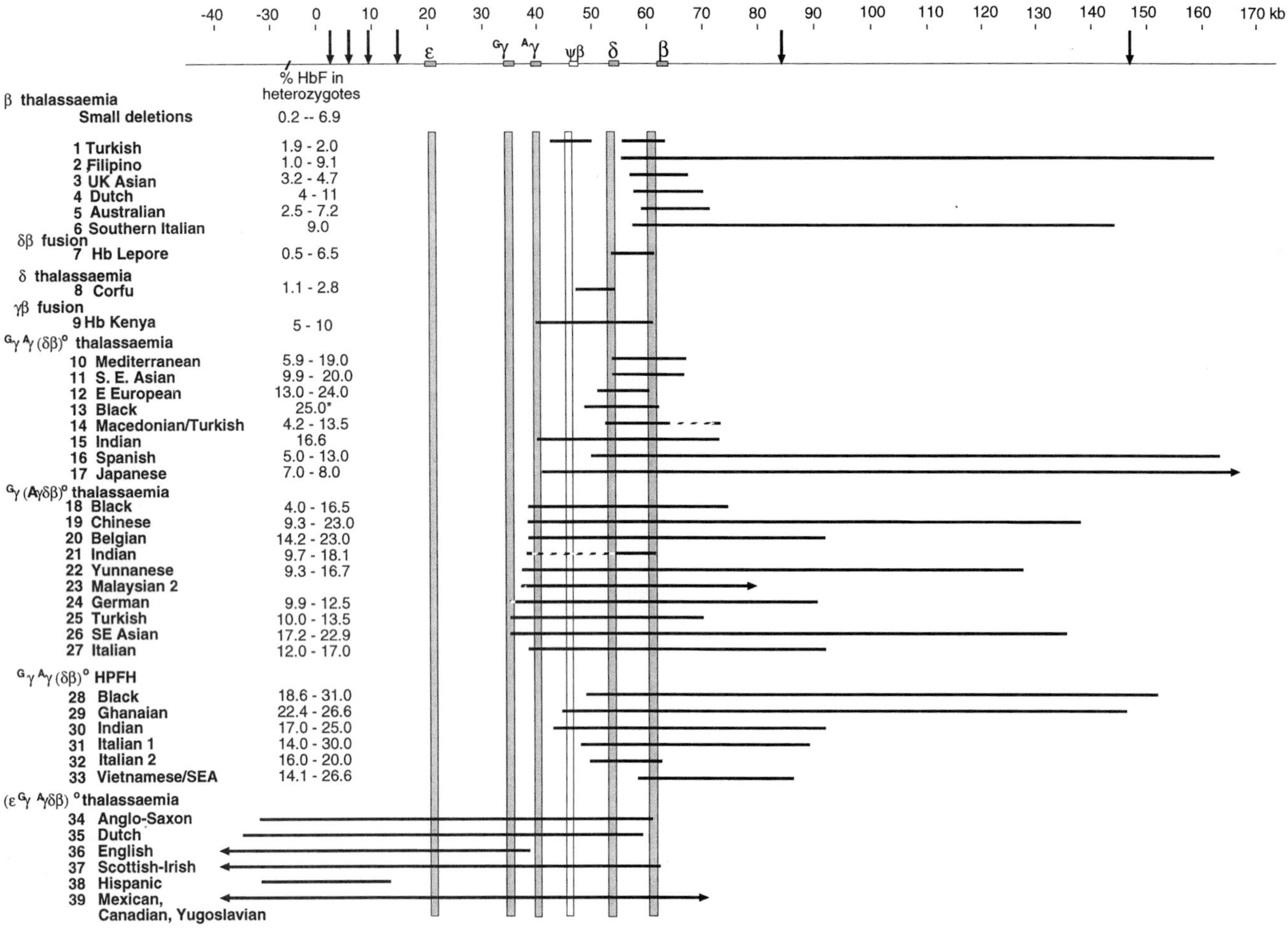

Fig. 181-28 The various deletions of the $\varepsilon\gamma\delta\beta$ globin gene complex that produce different forms of $\delta\beta$ and $\varepsilon\gamma\delta\beta$ thalassemia and hereditary persistence of fetal hemoglobin. Original descriptions are found in references 2 and 246.

are largely unknown. While Hb_{LEPORE}, Hb_{KENYA}, and the γ thalassemias occur as a result of misaligned crossovers between homologous genes, the remaining deletions all involve some type of illegitimate recombination, with little or no sequence homology at the breakpoints.

The $(\delta\beta)^o$ thalassemia deletions remove or inactivate only the δ and β genes, but may extend to a considerable distance on the 3′ side of the cluster. Phenotypically they are all similar, except that Hb_{LEPORE} is associated with only a minimal increase in Hb F production.

The $({}^A\gamma\delta\beta)^o$ thalassemia deletions start in or to the 5′ side of the ${}^A\gamma$ gene, and extend to a variable distance beyond the δ and β genes. The Indian form is not a simple linear deletion but a complex rearrangement with two deletions, one affecting the ${}^A\gamma$ gene and the other the δ and β genes; the intervening region remains but is inverted.[382,383] Again, the phenotypic results of these very different deletions are quite similar. The overall level of Hb F production is similar to that in the $(\delta\beta)^o$ thalassemias, but in this case, only the ${}^G\gamma$ gene is active, not both. $({}^A\gamma\delta\beta)^o$ thalassemia appears to act more like $(\delta\beta)^o$ HPFH in terms of output per gene.

The two African forms of $(\delta\beta)^o$ HPFH are both due to extensive deletions, of similar length ($\sim$105 kb) but with staggered ends, differing phenotypically only in the proportions of ${}^G\gamma$ and ${}^A\gamma$ chains produced.[384] A third type (Indian), although producing a similar amount of Hb F in heterozygotes, has a more severe phenotype than the other two when coinherited with β thalassemia.[385] Two different HPFH deletions have been described in Italy. In addition, there is a Southeast Asian type that spares the δ globin gene.

Deletions of the β Globin LCR; $(\varepsilon\gamma\delta\beta)^o$ Thalassemia. This rare group of thalassemias result from several different long deletions which start approximately 50 to 100 kb upstream from the β globin gene cluster and extend 3′ where they remove all or part of the cluster.[27,248,381,386,387] The approximate extent of these deletions is shown in Fig. 181-28. In cases in which the deletion leaves the β globin gene intact, the Dutch and English forms for example, no β chain production occurs, even though the gene is expressed in heterologous systems.[388–390] The Hispanic form of this condition[91] results from a deletion that includes most of the LCR, including three of four DNase I hypersensitive sites. It is clear, therefore, that any deletion that involves the LCR completely inactivates the downstream globin gene complex. Loss of the LCR also appears to shut down the chromatin domain, which is usually open in erythroid tissues, and also delays the replication of the β genes in erythroid cells.

Deletion Phenotype Analysis. Analysis of the size and position of deletions of the β-like globin gene cluster are of considerable interest because of their potential for demonstrating critical regulatory regions of this gene complex.[391] Although much remains to be learned about the reasons for their phenotypic effect, certain conclusions can be drawn. It is clear that deletions that either completely or partially remove the β globin LCR inactivate the entire complex. On the other hand, deletions starting within the gene cluster and extending 3′ to it, appear to leave the surviving γ genes active in adult life when they would normally be repressed. There is no correlation between the size of the deletion and the amount of Hb F produced.

Comparison of $(\delta\beta)^o$ thalassemia and $(\delta\beta)^o$ HPFH does not identify any region between the $^A\gamma$ and β genes that remains intact in the one but is lost in the other, precluding any simple explanation for the difference in phenotype. Furthermore, there are several deletions that result in β thalassemia, with little or no increase in Hb F, that overlap all of the regions encompassed by the smallest $(\delta\beta)^o$ thalassemia deletions. It appears, therefore, that there is no single element whose loss can account for the persistent γ gene expression in these conditions. The possibility remains that there are a number of regulatory sequences within and downstream of the cluster, with positive or negative effects, and that the balance of these elements that remain determines the probability that the γ promoter will interact with the βLCR in adult cells.

Competition between the γ and β gene promoters for activation by the LCR appears to be important during normal development and in the nondeletion HPFH conditions (see below). The loss of the β or β and δ promoters in these deletions could itself predispose to γ gene activation. If this were the case, additional explanations would be needed to explain the differences in Hb F levels between $(\delta\beta)^o$ thalassemia and $(\delta\beta)^o$ HPFH.

An alternative explanation for the increased Hb F in these conditions is that the newly apposed sequences at the 3′ end contain regulatory elements capable of activating the γ globin genes. This is likely to be the case for the two Black HPFH deletions which terminate close to an erythroid-specific DNase I hypersensitive site that has enhancer activity in a classical transient transcription assay.[392] In transgenic mice, constructs containing the βLCR, the two γ genes, and this 3′ region produced significant levels of Hb F in adult life.[393] Two other regions with similar enhancer activity in transient assays have been found downstream of the β gene, but whether these will behave in the same way remains to be seen. It is also not clear over what distance such enhancers work or whether there are enough such sequences to explain the increased Hb F in all of the $(\delta\beta)^o$ thalassemia and $(\delta\beta)^o$ HPFH deletions.

Overall, analysis of the deletions has yet to explain their phenotypic consequences. It is likely, however, that there is more than one mechanism by which deletions within the complex affect the expression of the surviving genes. An important lesson that can be learned from these conditions is that within this cluster the genes are not regulated solely by the sequences immediately surrounding them; instead, they are subject to control acting over a considerable distance.

Nondeletion HPFH. Analysis of the nondeletion $^G\gamma\beta^+$ and $^A\gamma\beta^+$ forms of HPFH by cloning and sequencing of the overexpressed γ gene has revealed, in each case, a single base substitution in the promoter region upstream from the transcription start site (Table 181-12).[394–398] The clustering of these substitutions and the lack of similar changes in normal γ genes suggests that they are responsible for the persistent Hb F production. That transgenic mice containing constructs with mutated γ gene promotors express the HPFH phenotype strengthens this interpretation.[399] It seems likely that these mutations affect the binding of a *trans*-acting protein involved in the normal developmental repression of γ gene expression, either by decreasing the affinity for an inhibitory factor normally present in adult life, or increasing the affinity for a factor promoting gene expression. The mutations affect binding to the distal CCAAT box (−114 – −117), an Oct1/GATA-1 site (−175) or are close to a GC box (−195 – −202). Thus disruption of several different proteins appear to influence the persistent γ gene expression.

In individuals with nondeletion HPFH, the output of β chains from the chromosome in *trans* is unaffected; these individuals have normal MCHs and balanced globin chain synthesis. It is clear, therefore, that there must be a decrease in β chain production from the gene in *cis* to compensate for the persistent γ chain synthesis. This *cis* active reciprocity between the γ and β genes implies that they are in competition for activation by the βLCR.[399]

Nondeletion HPFH Unlinked to the β Globin Cluster. In some cases of nondeletion HPFH, the genetic determinant is unlinked to the β globin gene cluster. There is genetic heterogeneity in these conditions[400] and there may be incomplete penetrance. The Hb F level is only slightly raised in otherwise normal individuals and its distribution may overlap between normal and affected cases, making phenotypic identification difficult. Nevertheless, multiple regression analysis of a single large pedigree demonstrated the presence of a major gene affecting F-cell levels in this family. It has been localized to band 6q22.3-q24 on chromosome 6.[401] An X-linked gene affecting Hb F levels has also been postulated.[402] Analysis of sib pairs with sickle cell anemia suggested this could be a codominant, bi-allelic gene located at Xp22.2-22.3.[403]

As shown in Table 181-11, and discussed below, it is becoming clear that nondeletion HPFH is very heterogeneous. In some cases, the genetic determinant is unlinked to the β globin gene cluster, but so far the genes have not been isolated. Thus, the molecular basis for these conditions remains to be determined.

$\delta\beta$ Thalassemia-like Disorders Due to Two Mutations in the β Globin Gene Cluster. Several disorders with features similar to $\delta\beta$ thalassemia in which more than one mutation in the β globin gene cluster is found have been described. For example, in the Sardinian form of $\delta\beta$ thalassemia, the β globin gene has the common Mediterranean codon 39 nonsense mutation, which leads to an absence of β globin synthesis.[404] However, there is a relatively high expression of the $^A\gamma$ gene in *cis,* which gives this condition the phenotype of $\delta^+\beta^o$ thalassemia because there is a point mutation at position −196 upstream from the $^A\gamma$ gene. Another condition that was originally designated $\delta\beta$ thalassemia was described in the Corfu population.[405,406] Again, this results from two different mutations. First, there is a 7201-bp deletion that starts in the δ globin gene and extends upstream to a 5′ breakpoint located 1719 to 1722 bp 3′ to the $\psi\beta$ gene termination codon. In addition there is a C → A mutation at position 5 in the donor site consensus region of IVS 1 of the β globin gene. The output from this novel chromosome consists of relatively high levels of γ chains in homozygotes, and extremely low levels of β chains.

Clinical and Hematologic Characteristics of the β Thalassemias[2,244]

β Thalassemia Major. This condition may result from the homozygous state for a β thalassemia mutation or, more commonly, from the compound heterozygous state for two different β thalassemias.

At birth, when Hb F production is still high, β thalassemia homozygotes are asymptomatic, but as Hb F production declines, affected infants present with severe anemia, usually during the first 1 to 2 years of life. Left untreated, they are incapable of maintaining a hemoglobin level above 5 g/dl and show marked growth retardation. The skin shows pallor and icterus, often accompanied by brown pigmentation. Expansion of the bone marrow in response to anemia leads to characteristic skeletal changes including the development of "thalassemic" facies due to frontal bossing of the skull and protrusion of the jaws and cheekbones. On radiography, the skull has a "hair on end" appearance, while the long bones show considerable thinning and trabeculation and are prone to repeated fractures. The magnitude of the increase in erythropoiesis (estimated to be as much as twenty- to thirtyfold) may result in extramedullary masses, arising usually from the sternum and ribs. Progressive hepatosplenomegaly is a constant finding, often leading to secondary dilutional anemia, leukopenia, and thrombocytopenia. Gallstones, leg ulcers, and osteoporosis with pathologic fractures are common. Intercurrent infections are a frequent complication and a major cause of morbidity and mortality in inadequately transfused patients. Transfusion-associated infections, particularly hepatitis B and C, and, in some populations, HIV, are still a major problem.

With frequent transfusions to maintain a hemoglobin level above 9 to 11 g/dl, growth and development are relatively normal

Table 181-12 Non-deletional HPFH: Mutations Characterized in the Promoters of the $^G\gamma$ or $^A\gamma$ Genes and the Hematologic Data (Mean ± SD) in Heterozygotes.

Condition	Mutation	No. of Families/ Individuals*	Hb g/dl	MCV fl	MCH pg	HbA_2 %	HbF %	$^G\gamma$ or $^A\gamma$ %	α/Nonα Synthesis	Xmn I at −158 *in cis*	Distribution
$^G\gamma$ mutations											
Black	−202 C→G	1/5	13.3 ± 1.3	82.0 ± 6.5	27.7 ± 2.0	1.7 ± 0.4	15.6 ± 1.2	99.0 ± 0.5	0.87 ± 0.02	−	Pancellular
Tunisian	−200 +C	1/5	13.1 ± 0.9	95.9 ± 1.8	31.9 ± 0.4	1.5 ± 0.3	25.2 ± 4.1	100 ± 0		+	
Black/Sardinian/British	−175 T→C	2/3	12.7 ± 1.1	85.2 ± 3.1	28.4 ± 1.8	1.3 ± 0.2	20.3 ± 2.8	94.0 ± 5.2	0.97 ± 0.17	−	Pancellular
Japanese	−114 C→T	1/2					12.5 ± 2.1	89.0 ± 4.2		+	
Australian	−114 C→G	1/1	14.2	92		2.3	8.6	90		−	
$^A\gamma$ mutations											
Black	−202 C→T	1/5	12.9 ± 0.9	84.4 ± 5.9	30.0 ± 2.3	2.7 ± 1.0	2.5 ± 0.9	92.8 ± 2.8		−	
British	−198 T→C	3/22	14.2 ± 1.2	83.1 ± 3.3	29.0 ± 1.0	2.5 ± 0.4	6.9 ± 2.2	92.2 ± 1.8	1.05 ± 0.13	−	Heterocellular
Italian/Chinese	−196 C→T	4/8	Normal	Normal	30.0 ± 0.9	1.8 ± 0.6	13.7 ± 2.0	95.0 ± 0.2	1.06 ± 0.05	−	Heterocellular
Brazilian	−195 C→G	1/3	Nnormal	Normal	Normal	2.1	5.4 ± 1.4	89.0 ± 2.5			
Black	−175 T→C	3/7	Normal	Normal	Normal	1.5 ± 0.2	37.4 ± 1.0	78.0 ± 5.5		+	Pancellular
Greek/Black	117 G→A	64/144	14.2 ± 1.1	85.9 ± 4.5	28.4 ± 2.4	2.0 ± 0.3	12.1 ± 2.8	93.4 ± 4.7	0.95 ± 0.10	−	Pancellular
Black†	−114 to −102 del	2/2	11.4 ± 2.9	75.5 ± 2.1	26.8 ± 0.3	2.1 ± 0.0	31.0 ± 1.2	85.7 ± 5.7		−	
Georgia	−114 C→T	1/2	Normal	Normal	Normal	2.5 ± 0.4	3.8 ± 1.3	90.9 ± 0.8			

Source from references 3 and 246.

until early puberty. Splenectomy is often necessary during this period to reduce the transfusion requirements but is associated with an increased incidence of septicemia. By the age of 10 to 11 years, patients begin to show signs of progressive hepatic, cardiac, and endocrine disturbances, associated with a reduced or absent pubertal growth spurt and failure of sexual maturation. These changes are due largely to accumulation of iron from transfusion and its deposition in the tissues. Unless iron overload is controlled by chelation therapy, it results in death in the second or third decade, usually from cardiac failure.

There is increasing evidence that if transfusion-dependent patients are adequately chelated, and compliance is good, they may develop normally, go through normal puberty, and, in some cases, have children of their own. Many of them remain short, and although this is partly explained by the side effects of chelating agents (see below) there is evidence that, because the pituitary is particularly sensitive to iron toxicity, in many cases growth retardation and bone disease reflect hypogonadotrophic hypogonadism (review in reference 503).

The peripheral blood shows grossly abnormal red cell morphology (Fig. 181-24). There is marked anisocytosis and poikilocytosis, target cells, and red cell fragments, all associated with extreme hypochromia. Nucleated red cells are usually present in the blood and often contain inclusion bodies, particularly after splenectomy. White cell and platelet counts are usually normal or elevated, unless there is hypersplenism.

The bone marrow shows intense erythroid hyperplasia (M/E ratio $\sim$0.1) with a shift to the less mature basophilic forms. Hypochromia is evident and inclusion bodies of precipitated α chains can be demonstrated in many of the normoblasts.[249,250] Nuclear and cytoplasmic abnormalities typical of ineffective erythropoiesis and increased phagocytic activity are also prominent. This pattern of highly expanded but ineffective erythropoiesis is reflected by the results of ferrokinetic and erythrokinetic studies.[2] Those cells that do survive to enter the circulation show a markedly reduced red cell life span of 7 to 22 days.

Hemoglobin analysis in untransfused patients usually shows a high proportion of Hb F. In those patients with no β chain production, there is a corresponding lack of Hb A, and except for a small proportion of Hb A_2 (1 to 3 percent) the remainder is Hb F. In those patients with reduced β chain output, a variable amount of Hb A is present, but this rarely exceeds 30 percent. The Hb A_2 level is variable and of no diagnostic help. After transfusion, endogenous erythropoiesis is suppressed and analysis of hemoglobin composition, even immediately prior to transfusion, is an unreliable indicator of the type of β thalassemia.

Detailed clinical descriptions of severe β thalassemia are found in two monographs.[2,244]

Thalassemia Intermedia. Thalassemia intermedia is an ill-defined clinical term used to describe patients with anemia and splenomegaly, but without the full spectrum of clinical severity found in thalassemia major.[2,123,244,407,408] Although far less common than thalassemia major, the condition encompasses a much broader clinical spectrum ranging from a disease similar to the major form to a symptomless condition. The criteria on which the diagnosis is made are a late presentation and the ability to maintain a hemoglobin level above 6 g/dl without transfusion.

At the extreme end of the spectrum, patients present between the ages of 2 and 6 years, and although they are capable of surviving with a hemoglobin level of 5 to 7 g/dl, it is clear that they will not develop normally and will show many of the skeletal and facial changes seen in untreated thalassemia major. Thus, they are treated with transfusion, although their blood requirement may not be as great as the requirement of those patients with thalassemia major. In general, patients with thalassemia intermedia are prone to the same complications as patients with thalassemia major although the complications may occur later in life.

At the other end of the spectrum, patients may not become symptomatic until they reach adult life, and they may remain transfusion free, with hemoglobin levels of 8 to 10 g/dl except at times of infection. There is always some degree of splenomegaly and the development of hypersplenism may render patients transfusion dependent; this complication may be reversed by splenectomy. Sexual development may be normal and many successful pregnancies have been reported although the anemia is exacerbated in the later stages. Folate deficiency is common, and is not confined to pregnancy.

Table 181-13 Causes of β Thalassemia Intermedia

Mild β thalassemia allele interactions
Homozygosity for mild alleles,
E.g., β-88 C $\rightarrow$ T, β-29 A $\rightarrow$ G, β IVS-1-6 T $\rightarrow$ C
Compound heterozygosity for severe and mild alleles,
E.g., as above
Compound heterozygosity for severe and silent alleles,
E.g., β-101 C $\rightarrow$ T, β CAP+1 A $\rightarrow$ C
Dominant β thalassemia
Interactions of severe or mild β thalassemia alleles with α^+ or α° thalassemia
Heterozygous β thalassemia with coinheritance of $\alpha\alpha\alpha$ or $\alpha\alpha\alpha\alpha$
Severe or mild β thalassemia alleles with increased Hb F production
Determinant of Hb F within β globin gene cluster
Determinant of Hb F unlinked to β globin gene cluster
Compound heterozygosity for severe or mild β thalassemia allele and β globin structural variant
Hb E β thalassemia
Hb O Arab β thalassemia
Coinheritance of β thalassemia with unstable β chain variant

Even those who have few transfusions accumulate iron with age, presumably as a result of increased absorption in response to the chronic anemia. Thus, evidence of iron overload may develop in the third and fourth decades, with diabetes mellitus and impairment of other endocrine functions. The chronic hemolysis and ineffective erythropoiesis leads to a high incidence of gallstones. Presumably because of extreme marrow expansion, some patients also develop bone and joint disease later in life.

The hematologic picture of thalassemia intermedia, except for the severity of the anemia, is similar to thalassemia major. The hemoglobin composition is extremely variable. Rare cases are homozygous for β° thalassemia and hence have only Hbs F and A_2, while in others the level of Hb F may be as low as 5 to 10 percent. This variability reflects the wide genetic heterogeneity that can produce this clinical picture and is summarized in Table 181-13.

The main causes of a relatively mild phenotype in β thalassemia homozygotes or compound heterozygotes are "mild" β thalassemia mutations, the coinheritance of α thalassemia, and various genetic determinants that increase Hb F production (Table 181-13). The latter interactions are described below. However, there are many cases in which the mild course remains unexplained.

Heterozygous β Thalassemia. The heterozygous state for β thalassemia is asymptomatic except for a mild anemia of pregnancy and, despite the genetic heterogeneity, is remarkably uniform hematologically. The diagnosis is usually straightforward and is based on a low MCV and MCH, together with an increased proportion of Hb A_2. This is an important consideration for genetic counseling and prenatal diagnosis. The hematologic findings are listed in Table 181-14. The peripheral blood film shows hypochromia and microcytosis with some aniso- and poikilocytosis and basophilic stippling. Red cell survival is normal.

Hemoglobin analysis shows a raised level of Hb A_2, 3.5 to 6.5 percent (mean $\sim$5 percent), that is only found in this condition, and occurs in nearly all patients (see below). It may be accompanied by a slight increase (1 to 3 percent) in Hb F in

Table 181-14 Phenotypic Characteristics of Some Different Types of β Thalassemia

		Heterozygotes			Homozygotes		
Condition	Molecular Defect	MCH (pg)	MCV (fl)	Hb A_2 (%)	Hb A	Hb F	Clinical Status
*β^o	β COD39 C→T	21	63	5.1	0	~98	Thal. major
*β^+ severe	β IVS1-110 G→A	21	64	4.5	10–20	~70–80	Thal. major
*β^+ mild	β IVS1-6 T→C	23	70	3.9	70–80	20–30	Thal. intermedia
*β^+ 'silent'	β-101 C→T	26	80	3.3	–	–	–
†β^+ dominant	β 128/129 – 4bp+5bp β 132-135 – 11bp	25–35	80–100	3.9–4.1	–	–	–
‡β^+ High Hb A_2/F	12,620 bp deletion including 5′ end of β gene	18–24	65–70	6.1–8.6	0	98	Thal. intermedia

* Mean values based on series reviewed in reference 2.
† Most dominant β thalassemias rare. In this family several members had been splenectomized, probably explaining the range of red cell indices. Data from reference 379.
‡ Most dominant β thalassemias are single family reports. These data from references 2 and 388.

about half of patients. Although there is globin chain imbalance, with an α chain excess of about twofold, there is little evidence of ineffective erythropoiesis or of free α chains remaining in the red cell. It appears that the proteolytic mechanisms within the red cell have the capacity to deal with this degree of chain imbalance.

Subtypes of β Thalassemia. The phenotypes of the various forms of β thalassemia that are detectable by hemoglobin analysis are listed in Table 181-13. Numerically, the β^o and β^+ forms are by far the most important; the other types shown in Table 181-13, although widespread, do not usually account for more than 10 percent of the β thalassemia alleles within a population.

β^o Thalassemia genes are found in all affected populations although they are rare in those of African origin. In the homozygous state, they are detected by the lack of Hb A in untransfused patients, whose hemoglobin pattern comprises Hb F plus 1 to 3 percent Hb A_2. The β^o thalassemia gene can also be identified in compound heterozygotes with a β chain variant such as Hb S by the absence of Hb A. In populations with both β^o and β^+ alleles, distinguishing between β^o/β^+ compound heterozygotes and β^+/β^+ homozygotes is not usually possible because of the considerable overlap in the amount of Hb A produced in the two conditions. Heterozygotes for β^o thalassemia cannot be distinguished from individuals heterozygous for the common β^+ forms of thalassemia.

There are numerous β^+ thalassemia alleles with variable levels of residual β chain production and several may be relatively common within the same population. Largely, the extent of the β chain deficit determines the clinical severity but homozygosity or compound heterozygosity for most of the common alleles causes thalassemia major. The extent of the deficiency in β chain production dictated by specific β^+ thalassemia alleles can only be determined by the amount of Hb A in compound heterozygotes with β chain structural variants. Because many alleles have not been observed in such an association, and the molecular defect has not been established in all of those that have, the correlation between the molecular lesion and the extent of β chain deficit remains to be established in many cases.

In some cases, the deficit in β chain production is so mild that a separate category of β^{++} thalassemia may be warranted. Homozygotes may not come to clinical attention and compound heterozygotes with β^o or the more severe β^+ alleles have thalassemia intermedia.

Normal Hb A_2 β Thalassemia. Family studies of β thalassemia patients occasional reveal a parent without the raised Hb A_2 level characteristic of most heterozygotes. Two forms of this condition have been described:[409] type 1 in which the red cell indices are almost normal but in which deficient β chain production is observed when the globin chain synthesis ratio is measured, and type 2 in which only the Hb A_2 level differs from the usual heterozygous β thalassemia picture.

The type 1 form of normal Hb A_2 β thalassemia is heterogeneous at the molecular level. Heterozygotes show no abnormalities and therefore this condition is sometimes called *silent β thalassemia*. Some cases, as mentioned earlier, result from point mutations upstream from the β globin gene.[359] One of the commonest varieties is associated with the abnormal β chain variant, $Hb_{KNOSSOS}$, which is undetectable on standard hemoglobin electrophoresis although it can be demonstrated by isoelectric focussing. The $Hb_{KNOSSOS}$ β chain is produced at a slightly reduced rate resulting in a mild thalassemia phenotype.[368,410] The low Hb A_2 level in this condition occurs because in many cases the $Hb_{KNOSSOS}$ mutation occurs on the same chromosome as a form of δ thalassemia.[411]

There is also heterogeneity within type 2 normal Hb A_2 β thalassemia and several different defects have been observed. Many cases are likely to be due to the coinheritance of a defective δ gene (δ thalassemia), which may occur either in *cis* or *trans* to the β thalassemia gene, which itself may be of the β^o or β^+ type.[411,412] Deletion of the complete complex results in this phenotype[413,414] as do deletions that remove the ε and $^G\gamma$ or ε, $^G\gamma$ $^A\gamma$, and δ genes but spare the β gene.[388,390,415] These conditions, the εγδβ thalassemias, may result in an unusually severe hemolytic anemia at birth that disappears within the first few months.[416] Heterozygotes for the conditions such as the Corfu form of δβ thalassemia, described earlier, also have the clinical phenotype of normal Hb A_2 β thalassemia; the β globin gene is partially inactivated by a mutation and the δ globin gene in *cis* is deleted.

Unusually High Hb F or A_2 Thalassemia. Several β thalassemias have been described in which the proportion of Hb F and/or Hb A_2 in heterozygotes is unusually high. These phenotypes appear to identify certain specific β^o thalassemia mutations in which there is a deletion involving at least the 5′ end of the β gene but sparing the δ gene (see above).

Severe Heterozygous β Thalassemia. Many families have been described in which the inheritance of a mild thalassemia intermedia phenotype follows a dominant pattern.[379,380] The molecular pathology that underlies these dominantly inherited forms of β thalassemia was described earlier (Table 181-11). Many, but not all of the dominantly inherited forms of β thalassemia result from exon 3 mutations of the β globin gene. There is a spectrum of disorders, ranging from severe ineffective erythropoiesis and splenomegaly through a moderately severe hypochromic anemia to heterozygous β thalassemia with more severe anemia than usual. This phenotypic variability seems to reflect the properties of the unstable gene products that underlie these conditions.[248]

The coinheritance of the $\alpha\alpha\alpha$ gene arrangement with heterozygous β thalassemia may also produce this phenotype.[417–419]

Summary of Phenotype/Genotype Relationships in β Thalassemia. While the conditions described in the previous sections at first appear to be distinct and easily definable entities, at least as judged by hematologic or hemoglobin analyses, recent work that relates the genotypes to associated phenotypes shows that the situation is more complex. Some of these problems are summarized in Table 181-14. This question is easier to address in the heterozygous state where the hematology and hemoglobin analyses are not clouded by problems of cell selection. It is apparent that, overall, the Hb A_2 levels in β thalassemia are higher in association with the more severe alleles and significantly lower in the mild alleles. Similarly, in the so-called "silent" alleles the Hb A_2 level, while often normal, may, if enough cases are studied, be seen to be slightly elevated. Thus, in effect, there is a continuum of Hb A_2 levels ranging from normal to the typical level of about 5 percent which is observed in carriers of the more severe β thalassemia alleles. While for diagnostic and screening purposes this does not usually raise problems, it is becoming increasingly clear that there is a distinct "no-man's-land" for Hb A_2 levels in the 3 to 3.5 percent range, and that these levels cannot be ignored and require further investigation. There is also some correlation, although not so good, between the different β thalassemia alleles and associated Hb F levels in heterozygotes.

In homozygous or compound heterozygous β thalassemia, there is a reasonable correlation between the severity of the β thalassemia alleles and the clinical phenotype. Similarly, many of the mild alleles are associated with relatively low levels of Hb F in homozygotes. There are exceptions, however. In the common promoter mutations that are frequently found in African populations, relatively high levels of Hb F, in the 50 to 70 percent range, are found in homozygotes despite the mildness of this particular allele. Thus, although much work remains to be done, it is becoming apparent that ultimately it should be possible to provide reasonably confident predictions of β thalassemia phenotypes from the associated genotype. However, as described below, there are other interactions at different loci that also have to be considered when attempting to relate genotype to phenotype.

Clinical and Hematologic Features of the $\delta\beta$ Thalassemias (Table 181-15)

Hb_{LEPORE}. The structures and molecular mechanisms underlying the Lepore hemoglobins were described earlier.

Homozygotes for Hb_{LEPORE} produce only Hb_{LEPORE} (15 to 20 percent) and Hb F. Clinically, their phenotype is either thalassemia major or thalassemia intermedia; the basis for this variable picture is not understood.[2,420] Although cases have been described from many racial groups, it appears to be relatively common only in the Campagna region of Italy.

$(\delta\beta)^o$ Thalassemias. $(\delta\beta)^o$ Thalassemias are widely distributed but relatively rare, reaching a significant proportion of the β thalassemias only in the Mediterranean region. They are characterized in the homozygous state by a clinical picture of thalassemia intermedia, while hemoglobin analysis shows 100 percent Hb F containing a mixture of both $^G\gamma$ and $^A\gamma$ chains. Hematologic changes are less marked than in β thalassemia homozygotes.

Heterozygotes are distinguished from β thalassemia heterozygotes by normal levels of Hb A_2 together with an increased Hb F level of 5 to 20 percent. The Hb F is heterogeneously distributed, with only a proportion of cells positive after acid elution. The red cell indices of heterozygotes are reduced, but not as severely as in β thalassemia heterozygotes.[421]

In general, the clinical and hematologic findings appear to be very similar in all these disorders, regardless of their underlying defects, although too few cases have been studied in which the underlying lesion is known to be sure that there are no phenotypic differences.

$(^A\gamma\delta\beta)^o$ Thalassemia. These are also rare but widespread disorders. Clinically and hematologically they are very similar to the $(\delta\beta)^o$ thalassemias, with a similar amount and distribution of Hb F. They can be distinguished only by analysis of the γ chain composition of the Hb F, which in the $(^A\delta\beta)^o$ thalassemias consists only of $^G\gamma$ chains. Again, there are few, if any, phenotypic differences between the various types that have been distinguished by the size and position of the underlying gene deletions.[422]

Hematological Features of Hereditary Persistence of Fetal Hemoglobin (HPFH) (Table 181-15)

HPFH is the term used to describe genetically determined increase in Hb F in adult life, a nomenclature that was introduced before the nature of these varied disorders was understood. There are three major types of lesion that come under this definition, each with distinctive phenotype: (a) deletions similar to those observed in $(\delta\beta)^o$ and $(^A\gamma\delta\beta)^o$ thalassemia that remove the δ and β genes and differ from $\delta\beta$ thalassemia only in that the resulting level of Hb F is sufficient to make the condition asymptomatic; (b) nondeletion forms in which fairly high levels of Hb F in heterozygotes (5 to 15 percent) are associated with continued, but reduced, β chain output from the same chromosome; and (c) a group of conditions, probably heterogeneous, in which much lower levels of Hb F (2 to 5 percent) are found in otherwise normal families. There is evidence that in some of these cases the genetic determinant may not be linked to the β globin gene cluster.

$(\delta\beta)^o$ HPFH. This condition is usually found in individuals of African origin, although cases have been described from India and Southeast Asia. Homozygotes have 100 percent Hb F, containing a mixture of both $^G\gamma$ and $^A\gamma$ chains, but are asymptomatic. Their red cells are microcytic and hypochromic, and globin chain imbalance can be demonstrated ($\alpha/\gamma \sim 2.0$) but they maintain Hb levels above 15 g/dl, compensating for the increased oxygen affinity associated with having only Hb F. Heterozygotes have normal hematology and 20 to 35 percent Hb F, which has a pancellular, but uneven, distribution. Three different deletions of the globin gene complex have been found in Africans, affecting the phenotype only in the proportion of $^G\gamma$ chains (30 or 70 percent). A fourth similar

Table 181-15 Characteristics of the Deletion Forms of $\delta\beta$ Thalassemia and HPFH

	Heterozygotes			Homozygotes		
Condition	MCH, pg	% Hb F	% $^G\gamma$	% Hb F	%$^G\gamma$	Clinical Status
Hb_{LEPORE}	22 ± 2	1–3	20–45	70–90	48–62	Intermedia/major
$(\delta\beta)^\circ$ Thalassemia	23 ± 2	5–18	25–56	100	47–64	Intermedia
$(^A\gamma\delta\beta)^\circ$ Thalassemia	24 ± 2	9 ± 18	96–100	100	100	Intermedia
$(\delta\beta)^\circ$ HPFH	27 ± 3	17 ± 35	25–75	100	52–65*	Normal
Hb_{KENYA}	26 ± 3	4–9	100	–	–	–

*African type I 51 ± 4%, type II 32 ± 5% Indian type 69 ± 4%.

SOURCE: From reference 2.

deletion underlies the Indian form, giving ~50 percent $^{G}\gamma$. While the phenotype of the Indian heterozygotes is similar to their African counterparts, the two conditions produce different effects on interaction with β thalassemia. The African compound heterozygotes are similar to β thalassemia heterozygotes while Indians with this combination have thalassemia intermedia, similar to that seen in a $(\delta\beta)^{o}/\beta^{o}$ thalassemia combination. This emphasizes the overlap in the clinical and hematologic effects of $(\delta\beta)^{o}$ thalassemia and $(\delta\beta)^{o}$ HPFH (Table 181-14).

Hb_{KENYA}. Misaligned crossing over between the $^{A}\gamma$ and β genes results in a fusion $^{A}\gamma\beta$ gene, which produces the non-α chain of Hb_{KENYA}.[163] This condition has not been observed in the homozygous state but heterozygotes and compound heterozygotes with Hb S have been found in East Africa.

In the few families studied, the level of Hb_{KENYA} in heterozygotes appears to fall into two groups, comprising 7 to 12 and 20 to 23 percent of the total;[423–425] it is not clear whether this reflects further genetic heterogeneity. This condition is also accompanied by persistent Hb F, with levels of 5 to 10 percent containing only $^{G}\gamma$ chains. Red cell morphology is normal and globin synthesis is balanced.

Nondeletion Types of HPFH. Compound heterozygotes for HPFH and β globin chain variants do not usually produce any Hb A but several conditions have been found in which this is not the case. Family studies have made it clear that these genetic defects are tightly linked to the β globin locus and that there is β chain production from the chromosome responsible for the increased γ chain output. Several types have been described (Table 181-12); sequencing of the overproduced γ gene has demonstrated various single case substitutions within the promoter region in each of these types (see above).

Compound heterozygotes for $^{G}\gamma\beta^{+}$ HPFH[426–428] and Hb S or Hb C produce 45 percent of the abnormal hemoglobin, 30 percent Hb A, and 20 percent Hb F containing only $^{G}\gamma$ chains. Similar Hb F levels are seen in simple heterozygotes. Globin synthesis is balanced, making the combined output of $^{G}\gamma$ and β^{A} chains from the affected chromosome equal to the normal β chain output. This rare condition, which has been found mainly in persons of African origin, is not associated with any hematologic abnormalities.

The most common of the nondeletion types of HPFH, a form of $^{A}\gamma\beta^{+}$HPFH,[429–431] is found most commonly in Greeks. Heterozygotes are hematologically normal but have 10 to 20 percent Hb F, almost all of the $^{A}\gamma$ type. Homozygotes have about 25 percent Hb F and 0.8 percent Hb A_2.[431] Compound heterozygotes with β thalassemia have a hematologic phenotype slightly more severe than β thalassemia trait, and the presence of Hb A in compound heterozygotes with β^{o} thalassemia confirms that the β gene in *cis* to the HPFH defect is active. Conditions with a similar phenotype have also been described in several other racial groups (see reference 387).

It has been possible to study the behavior of the γ genes at birth and during the transition from fetal to adult hemoglobin production in a British family with $^{A}\gamma\beta^{+}$ HPFH.[398,432] Heterozygotes have 3.5 to 10 percent F consisting mostly of $^{A}\gamma$ chains, and homozygotes, who are hematologically normal, show balanced globin chain synthesis, low normal levels of Hb A_2, and Hb F levels of ~20 percent. The offspring of these homozygotes, obligate heterozygotes, have normal levels of Hb F and normal $^{G}\gamma/^{A}\gamma$ ratios at birth, suggesting that the $^{A}\gamma$ gene functions normally during fetal life.[433] After birth, however, there is a markedly delayed decline in Hb F ($^{A}\gamma$) production accompanied by a rapid decline in $^{G}\gamma$ chain production.

Nondeletion HPFH with Low Levels of Hb F. The majority of normal adults have less than 1 percent Hb F. However, it has been recognized for many years that slightly elevated levels of Hb F (1 to 3 percent) can be traced through families and hence have a genetic component.[434] Later studies have confirmed this,[435] although neither the pattern of inheritance nor the amount of genetic heterogeneity which might underlie the condition has been elucidated. It has been suggested, for example, that an X-linked determinant may be involved in setting the level of Hb F at these low levels.[402] The importance of this (or these) condition(s) is that their coinheritance with the more severe forms of β thalassemia can lead to a considerable amelioration in clinical severity through the increased ability to produce Hb F.[401,436]

It is clear from family studies of some cases of β thalassemia or Hb S with unusually high F levels that the high F level is genetically determined and that the determinant is not linked to the β globin locus.[401] Other families, however, have been reported in which the high Hb F determinant does appear to be linked to the cluster (reviewed in reference 387). In most of these cases, only the nuclear family has been studied and the small numbers of individuals give limited opportunities for assortment. Given the possibility of genetic heterogeneity of this condition, combining results from several families for genetic analysis may be misleading and it is not clear to what degree ascertainment bias may have contributed to the published reports.

A further difficulty in genetic studies of such families is whether the determinant shows complete penetrance. In the largest family of this type studied to date,[401] there appeared to be clearcut examples of impenetrance, which may be why the genetics of this disorder have not been clarified in Mendelian terms, even within single families. This may be related to the observation that the high Hb F determinant may be expressed to a much greater degree under conditions of erythroid stress. Thus, families in which β thalassemia heterozygotes coinherit a high Hb F determinant and produce ~5 percent Hb F may contain β thalassemia homozygotes whose level of Hb F production (10 to 12 g/dl) is sufficient to produce a very mild or asymptomatic condition.

Summary of Genetic Factors Associated with Increased Hb F Production in β Chain Globin Disorders

Even though it has been evident for a long time that genetic factors play a major role in determining the level of Hb F production in sickle cell anemia and β thalassemia, knowledge about their nature remains incomplete. However, from such information as is available it appears that they fall into three major groups (reviewed in reference 248). First, there is growing evidence that the mutations that involve the β globin genes in some forms of thalassemia may themselves have some effect on the output of Hb F. Second, it appears that certain polymorphisms involving the $\varepsilon\gamma\delta\beta$ globin gene cluster may be associated with increased Hb F production in response to defective β chain production. And, finally, there are genetic determinants unlinked to the cluster that seem to modify the level of Hb F production in adult life, both in normal individuals and those with β thalassemia or sickle cell anemia. These different mechanisms for modifying Hb F production in the β globin disorders are summarized in Fig. 181-29.

There is some evidence that individuals who are homozygous or compound heterozygotes for promoter mutations of the β globin

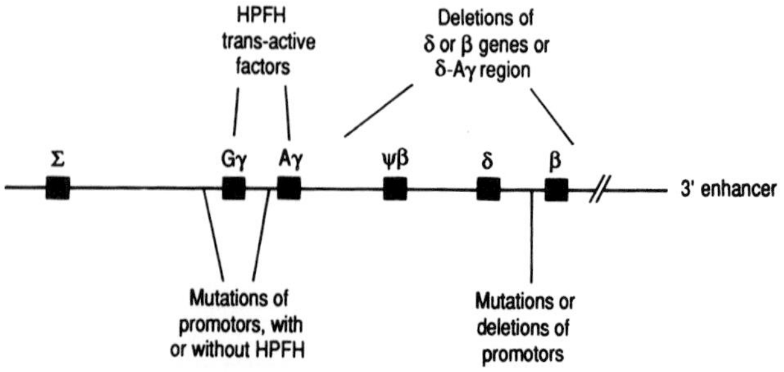

Fig. 181-29 Summary of some of the genetic mechanisms which modify the level of Hb F production in β thalassemia.

gene may have a relatively high output of Hb F.[248] It is possible, therefore, that in conditions of relative hemopoietic stress in which γ chain synthesis is more likely to occur, the level of γ chain production may be modified by competition for transcriptional regulatory sequences between the γ and β chain loci; mutations in or near these transcriptional boxes that cause β thalassemia may favor γ chain production.

Another approach to determining whether *cis*-acting sequences can modify γ chain production is to determine whether there are any particular β globin RFLP haplotypes associated with β thalassemia or sickle cell anemia and unusually high levels of Hb F. There has been particular interest in the relationship between Hb F production and a C $\rightarrow$ T polymorphism at the position 158 in the $^{G}\gamma$ globin gene.[437] This substitution can be identified with a restriction enzyme *Xmn*-I, which makes it possible to analyze large populations for its presence or absence. Studies in Asia, the Mediterranean region, and the Middle East have shown that this polymorphism is associated predominantly with one β globin RFLP haplotype.[438–441] Extensive analyses of β thalassemics and patients with sickle cell anemia of African, Asian, Mediterranean, and Turkish backgrounds have shown a strong, though not absolute, correlation between increased γ chain production and the presence of *Xmn*-I polymorphisms.[442–445] It is not clear whether this change at position −158 is responsible for increased γ chain production in these cases. The whole relationship between this polymorphism and increased γ chain production remains to be clarified.

Recent studies suggest that other polymorphisms, including those that involve the β globin LCR may be involved in increased γ chain production in sickle cell anemia.[446]

Finally, there is clear evidence that the inheritance of some forms of HPFH, the determinants of which are not linked to the β globin gene cluster, may cause an increased output of Hb F in patients with sickle cell anemia or β thalassemia.

In summary, Hb F response to the β globin disorders probably reflects a complex series of genetic variables including the nature of the individual globin gene mutations, polymorphisms of the γ globin gene *cis* to the affected β globin gene, and the interaction of other genes unlinked to the β globin gene cluster, all set against a background of variable intra- or extramedullary selection of red cell precursors or red cells with an increased amount of γ chains.

The Interaction of β Thalassemia with α Gene Mutations

The geographical distribution of α and β thalassemias is largely coincident, and relatively high frequencies of both occur in many populations. The clinical and hematologic consequences of coinheritance have been established among Mediterranean peoples and the findings are likely to be applicable to other groups (Table 181-16).

Homozygous β Thalassemia and α Thalassemia. Early studies established that β thalassemia homozygotes who also inherited an α thalassemia allele sometimes ran a milder clinical course.[2] Because much of the pathology of β thalassemia is due to the pool of excess α chains, this observation can be readily explained, because the effect of α thalassemia is to reduce α chain synthesis and hence the degree of excess α chains. However, until gene mapping enabled the ready detection of α thalassemia, it was not clear to what extent α thalassemia played a part in producing the milder forms of the disease.

Extensive data collected from the populations of the Mediterranean and Southeast Asia indicate that the coexistence of α thalassemia may modify the phenotype of homozygotes or compound heterozygotes for different β thalassemia mutations.[248] The resulting phenotypes are complex and depend on the number of α globin genes that are inactivated, together with whether the β thalassemia is of the β^{o} or β^{+} variety.[265,266,447–449] For example, it is clear that the coexistence of the heterozygous state for α^{+} thalassemia with homozygous β^{o} thalassemia has very little effect on the phenotype of the latter. On the other hand, individuals that are either α^{+} thalassemia homozygotes or α^{o} thalassemia heterozygotes and who also are homozygous for β^{+} thalassemia may have a mild form of β thalassemia intermedia. The same applies to patients who have the genotype of Hb H disease together with homozygous β^{+} thalassemia. These remarkable experiments of nature are the best evidence that the most important factor in determining the phenotype of β thalassemia is the degree of imbalanced globin chain synthesis.

Heterozygous β Thalassemia and α Thalassemia. Studies of β thalassemia heterozygotes who also have α thalassemia (as determined by gene mapping) have a reduced amount of chain imbalance and fewer hematologic abnormalities.[450,451] Hemoglobin levels, MCV, and MCH increase across the series $\alpha\alpha/\alpha\alpha$ and $\alpha-/\alpha-$ but decrease again in those with $\alpha-/--$ (Table 181-16). These results point to a potential problem in screening for β thalassemia on electronic counters by the reduced MCV, because in β thalassemia heterozygotes with an $\alpha-/\alpha-$ genotype there is considerable overlap with normal values. However, screening by Hb A_2 levels should not be affected because the levels remain raised in all these groups. This question is discussed further when population screening is considered.

Homozygous β Thalassemia and ααα. Given the frequency of the $\alpha\alpha\alpha$ genotype in many populations, it undoubtedly occurs in β thalassemia homozygotes and individuals with this interaction and the picture of thalassemia major have been reported. Unexpectedly, four homozygotes with this genotype were described with the milder pattern of thalassemia intermedia. It is probable that in at least some of these cases, there are nondeletion α thalassemia mutations affecting genes within the triplicated α gene arrangement.[452]

Heterozygous β Thalassemia and ααα. The clinical and hematologic picture of double heterozygotes for β thalassemia and the triplicated α gene arrangement (Table 181-16) may be indistinguishable from simple heterozygotes for β thalassemia in

Table 181-16 Hematologic Findings in Heterozygous β Thalassemia with Normal or Abnormal α-Gene Numbers

Condition	n	Hb, g/dl	MCV, fl	MCH, pg	Hb A_2, %	Hb F, %	$\alpha:\beta$ ratio
$\alpha\alpha/\alpha\alpha$	53	12.5 ± 1.2	65 ± 4	21 ± 1	4.9 ± 0.7	1.3 ± 1.1	2.2 ± 0.3
$\alpha\alpha/-\alpha$	36	13.0 ± 1.4	67 ± 4	22 ± 1	5.2 ± 0.7	1.2 ± 0.3	1.4 ± 0.1
$-\alpha/-\alpha$	11	13.9 ± 1.1	77 ± 3	25 ± 1	5.1 ± 0.6	1.1 ± 0.7	0.8 ± 0.1
$-\alpha/--$	6	11.8 ± 0.8	55 ± 3	18 ± 1	4.6 ± 0.2	–	0.5 ± 0.1
$\alpha\alpha/\alpha\alpha\alpha$*	7	11.7 ± 1.9	65 ± 5	21 ± 2	5.0 ± 0.9	2.3 ± 1.5	2.1 ± 0.4
	11	9.1 ± 0.9	70 ± 8	21 ± 2	4.9 ± 0.6	4.3 ± 2.1	2.9 ± 0.6
$\alpha\alpha\alpha/\alpha\alpha\alpha$	3	9.3 ± 0.9	65 ± 3	21 ± 1	4.6 ± 0.3	6.8 ± 2.9	4.0 ± 0.4

*Seven cases presenting with phenotype of thalassemia trait, 11 presenting as thalassemia intermedia.
Data from reference 2.

some cases,[452] while others present with thalassemia intermedia.[417,418] The reason for this difference remains unexplained; it does not seem to be due to the nature of the β thalassemia allele, and in several of the asymptomatic patients all three α genes on the triple α chromosome appeared to be active. Both phenotypes may coexist within the same family.[453]

β thalassemia heterozygotes who are homozygous for the $\alpha\alpha\alpha$ arrangement usually have the clinical phenotype of thalassemia intermedia.[454,455]

The Interaction of β Thalasemia with Structural Variants[2,3]

The association of β thalassemia with Hbs S, C, and E was described earlier.

Although β thalassemia has been reported in association with several other hemoglobin variants, few of such associations result in any clinical disability. Hb $D_{\text{LOS ANGELES (PUNJAB)}}/\beta$ thalassemia is not uncommon in parts of India and elsewhere but, apart from a mild anemia which may be exacerbated in pregnancy, is largely asymptomatic.

Hb $O_{\text{ARAB}}/\beta^{\text{o}}$ thalassemia causes a moderately severe disorder with a hemoglobin level of 6 to 8 g/dl and splenomegaly. Several cases with this combination have been reported from Bulgaria. It is not clear why this interaction is so severe, but homozygotes for Hb O_{ARAB} are also anemic. There have been numerous other interactions with β structural hemoglobin variants described, of which particularly those in which the β variant is unstable, are associated with the clinical picture of β thalassemia intermedia.[2]

WORLD DISTRIBUTION AND POPULATION GENETICS

Although our knowledge of the prevalence and distribution of the hemoglobin disorders is still scanty, enough information is available to suggest that they are the commonest single-gene disorders. Very conservative data compiled by WHO indicate that about 5 percent of the world population are carriers for important hemoglobin disorders.[1] Because these data were compiled before anything was known about the distribution of α thalassemia, as assessed by more recently developed gene mapping techniques, these figures represent a considerable underestimate of the total problem.

The Structural Hemoglobin Variants

The only structural hemoglobin variants to reach polymorphic frequencies are Hbs S, C, and E. The sickle cell gene is most concentrated in West Africa, although its distribution spreads across central Africa, and it is found at lower frequencies in some non-African Mediterranean populations.[3,200,456] It also occurs patchily throughout the Middle East and central India, but apart from some Indian populations in north Malaysia, it has not been observed in Southeast Asia. Hemoglobin C is restricted to parts of West Africa,[3] while Hb E is distributed in a region stretching from the eastern parts of India through Burma to southeast Asia where it reaches its highest frequency in parts of Thailand, Laos, and Cambodia. Hemoglobin E is found sporadically in parts of southern China and it extends in a line stretching south through Thailand, down the Malay peninsula, and into some of the island populations of Indonesia.[3]

Several workers have catalogued the approximate gene frequencies for the structural hemoglobin variants, where known.[3,456] In parts of west central Africa, Nigeria, Ghana, Gabon, and Zaire, for example, the gene frequency for Hb S can exceed 0.15; in other words, heterozygotes comprise over 25 percent of the newborn population. Similar frequencies are found in parts of eastern Saudi Arabia and the condition is almost as common in parts of central India. Hemoglobin C is found exclusively in African populations and reaches its highest frequency in Ghana and Upper Volta with gene frequencies approaching 0.15. The gene frequency for Hb E in Thailand and Myanmar is 0.05 to 0.10, although higher values have been recorded in parts of eastern Thailand near the Vietnamese border, the so-called "Hb E triangle." Minimum estimates are about 30 million heterozygotes for Hb E and about 1 million homozygotes in Southeast Asia. For more extensive population data, broken down into different racial groups, see Livingstone's catalogue.[456]

These remarkably high gene frequencies pose two important questions: How did these variants become distributed among the high incidence populations? What are the factors that have maintained these polymorphisms?

Population Distribution. Before it was possible to analyze human DNA directly, a great deal was written about the distribution of the sickle cell gene and other hemoglobin variants under the assumption that population movements could be derived from the distribution of genetic markers of this type. It was reasonably believed that the distribution of the β^S gene in the New World is based entirely on emigration from West Africa during the transportation of slaves. But it was also thought that the high prevalence of the sickle cell gene in Saudi Arabia and India may have reflected migration out of East Africa; the transport of slaves from East Africa to the Persian Gulf flourished from 200 to 1500 A.D.

Later, however, it was possible to analyze the origins of the sickle cell gene and other structural hemoglobin variants by examining the pattern of restriction fragment length polymorphisms (RFLPs) in and around the β globin gene carrying the sickle mutation. The first study of this type employed a single polymorphism identified by the enzyme *Hpa* I.[457] Nearly all Caucasians and about 97 percent of individuals of African origin with a normal hemoglobin phenotype have a 7.6-kb or, less commonly, a 7.0-kb *Hpa* I fragment that encompasses the entire β globin gene. Only 3 percent have a 13-kb fragment. In contrast, among African Americans who have Hb S, nearly 70 percent have the 13-kb fragment. Similarly, African Americans with Hb C nearly all have the 13-kb fragment. How can this type of linkage disequilibrium be explained? It seems likely that the β^S and β^C mutations both arose on a β gene carrying the 13-kb mutation that may have arisen in a relatively small geographical area corresponding to what is now called Upper Volta and Ghana. Presumably because the β^S and β^C genes offered protection against malaria (see below) their frequency increased, and the linked 13-kb mutation "hitchhiked" along with them. On the other hand, the prevalence of the ancestral 13-kb β^A gene remained low because it lacked a selective advantage. The β^S/13-kb fragment association has also been found in North Africans and Sicilians, although not in individuals from East Africa, Saudi Arabia, or India. These observations suggested an independent origin of the sickle cell gene in West and East Africa.[441]

More recently, extensive RFLP analyses using a variety of single-point polymorphisms in the β globin gene cluster have been done in many populations in an attempt to obtain further information about the origins of both the sickle cell and Hb E mutations.[189,441,458–460] The particular arrangement of RFLPs is referred to as the β globin gene haplotype. Studies in Jamaica and West Africa indicate that the β^S mutation can be found in association with a wide variety of haplotypes, SS_{BENIN}, SS_{BANTU}, SS_{SENEGAL}, $SS_{\text{ARAB-INDIA}}$, for example. At first, these results suggest that the mutation may have had multiple origins. However, these data must be interpreted with caution because the 5′ end of the β gene is known to be affected by an upstream recombination hot spot, so it is possible that a number of gene conversion events could have given rise to at least some of the variability in β^S/haplotype associations.[461,462] However, the occurrence of a common haplotype associated with a β^S gene in parts of eastern Saudi Arabia and Orissa, India, and the finding of completely different haplotypes in some African populations, make it more likely that the β^S mutation had at least two origins, one in East Africa and the other in the Middle East or India[441] (Fig. 181-25).

Similar haplotype data suggest that the β^E mutation may have occurred on more than one occasion.[463] The same reservations apply as in the case of Hb S; gene conversion events might also account for these different haplotypes.

Maintenance of the Polymorphisms for Structural Hemoglobin Variants. In 1949, Haldane suggested that individuals with red cell disorders such as thalassemia might be protected against malaria.[464] Early epidemiologic studies in Africa suggested that Hb S heterozygotes are protected against *P. falciparum* malaria.[465] More recent work in Nigeria and Gambia confirms these studies.[466,467] For example, the prevalence of the sickle cell trait in Nigerian newborns was 24 percent compared with 29 percent over the age of 5 years. Above this age, no differences were noted. These data suggest that the Hb S trait confers a relative fitness of about 0.20 compared with normal individuals in the same population. This figure gives a calculated gene frequency of about 0.15, a value very close to that observed in Nigeria. Furthermore, it can be calculated that it would take about 50 generations (representing 1000 years) to reach the present equilibrium, assuming that the homozygous condition is 100 percent lethal.

If protection against *P. falciparum* malaria is the major mechanism for maintaining the Hb S polymorphism, how is this effect mediated? This problem has been approached by studying the rates of sickling of parasitized and nonparasitized cells under reduced oxygen tension and by examining the patterns of invasion and growth of parasites in red cells containing Hb S using *in vitro* culture systems. At least three possible protective mechanisms have been demonstrated. First, it has been found that under low oxygen tensions AS cells containing *P. falciparum* sickle more readily than nonparasitized cells. It has been suggested, therefore, that *in vivo* sickling may provide a mechanism for the rapid clearance of parasitized cells and their subsequent destruction in the RE system. It would follow that the parasite could not complete its life cycle.[468] *In vitro* culture studies show that under ambient oxygen tensions, parasites invade and grow in sickle cells at the same rate as in normal cells. However, under reduced oxygen conditions both invasion and growth are inhibited.[469] It has been suggested that the relatively low levels of potassium in AS cells that have undergone sickling may mediate this effect.[470]

It is possible that several mechanisms are involved. The major reason the entrapment of sickle cells is favored is that individuals who are homozygous for the sickle cell gene undergo severe malarial infection, which would be hard to explain if parasites could not survive adequately in cells containing a large concentration of Hb S. On the other hand, even a mild malaria infection might have catastrophic consequences for a child with sickle cell anemia.

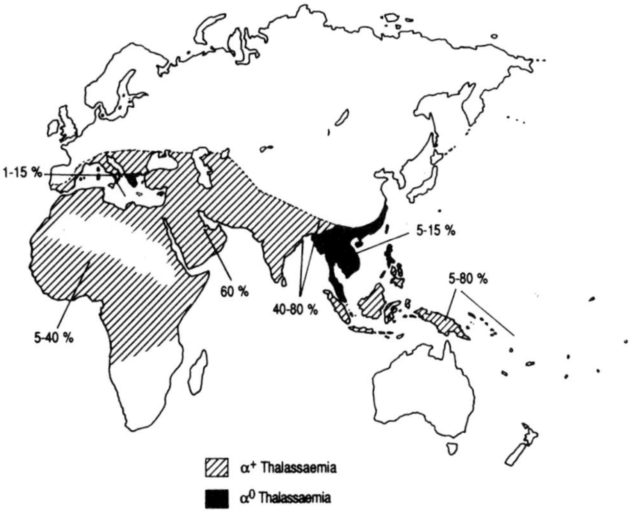

Fig. 181-30 World distribution of α thalassemia.

In vitro studies of invasion and growth of *P. falciparum* in the cells of Hb E heterozygotes or homozygotes have not provided a clear answer as to why Hb E might be protective against malaria. However, because the Hb E mutation produces a thalassemic phenotype, we return to this problem in a later section.

The Thalassemias

The world distribution of the α and β thalassemias is summarized in Figs. 181-30 and 181-31. A detailed breakdown of published data for the gene frequencies of different forms of thalassemia is found in several monographs and review.[2,245–247,456,471]

Adequate gene frequency data for β thalassemia are available for only a small number of populations. It is clear that, with a few

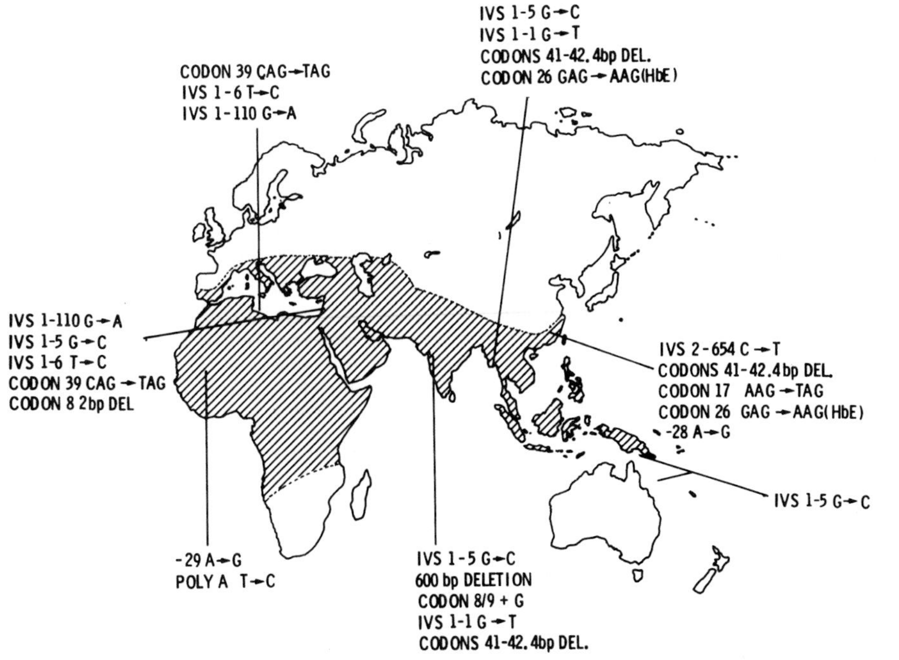

Fig. 181-31 World distribution of β thalassemia.

exceptions such as Liberia, the condition occurs at only a low frequency throughout tropical Africa although higher frequencies have been observed in North Africa. The disease is common throughout the Mediterranean region, parts of the Middle East, India, and Myanmar, although accurate gene frequency data are sparse. It is also common throughout Southeast Asia in a line starting in southern China, stretching through Thailand, Cambodia, and Laos, and down the Malay peninsula into some of the island populations. It is distributed sporadically in Melanesia.

The world distribution of the α thalassemias is summarized in Fig. 181-30. The α^+ thalassemias are extremely common in parts of Africa, the Mediterranean region, the Middle East, and throughout Southeast Asia and the Pacific island populations. Indeed, α^+ thalassemia appears to be reaching fixation in some regions, notably the coastal regions of Papua New Guinea. On the other hand, α^o thalassemia is restricted to the Mediterranean region and Southeast Asia.

Population Distribution. As was the case for the sickle cell gene, much was written about the movement of populations based on the distribution of the β-thalassemia mutations before the advent of DNA technology and the realization of the remarkable heterogeneity of β thalassemia. However, more recent work, in which the precise molecular lesions were defined and β-globin gene RFLP haplotypes determined, has provided a much clearer picture about the population distribution of the β thalassemias.[75,247,471–475]

It is now apparent that in each of the high frequency areas there are a few common mutations together with varying numbers of rare ones (Fig. 181-27). Furthermore, in each of these regions, the pattern of mutations is different. And even where the same mutation occurs in different populations, it is usually found together with a different β-globin gene RFLP haplotype. It seems likely, therefore, that the β-thalassemia mutations arose independently in different populations and then achieved their high frequency by selection. Although there may have been some movement of the β-thalassemia genes between populations, by drift and so on, there is little doubt that the independent mutation and selection provide the overall basis for the world distribution of β thalassemia.

Recent molecular studies of the α thalassemias lead to similar conclusions.[66,67,245,475] The deletions that cause α^o thalassemia in the Mediterranean region and Southeast Asia are different.[269] Furthermore, detailed analysis of the RFLP haplotypes in the α globin gene cluster, together with studies of the crossover events that produce the α^+ thalassemias, show that the common form of α^+ thalassemia due to a 3.7-kb deletion (type I) has occurred on many different occasions in different populations.[67] α^+ Thalassemia type III is, on the other hand, confined to parts of Melanesia. Haplotype analysis suggests that the α^+ thalassemias arose *de novo* in Melanesia and reached their high frequencies by selection;[67] haplotypes of the α^+ thalassemias in Southeast Asia are completely different. These studies suggest that, even allowing for a certain amount of drift and founder effect, the different types of α^+ thalassemia arose independently in different populations.

Maintenance of the Thalassemia Polymorphism. Haldane's suggestion that thalassemia was maintained at a high frequency by the protection of heterozygotes against *P. falciparum* malaria was an extremely attractive hypothesis, but until recently it has been very difficult to provide the experimental data with which to validate it.

Studies in Sardinia, which showed that β thalassemia is less common in the mountainous regions where malaria transmission is relatively low, suggested that β thalassemia might have reached its high frequency because of protection against malarial infection.[476] For many years, these data remained the only convincing evidence for the protective effect of thalassemia against malaria. However, recent studies utilizing malaria endemicity data and globin gene mapping have shown a very clear altitude-related effect on the frequency of α thalassemia in Papua New Guinea.[67] Furthermore, a sharp decline in the frequency of α thalassemia was found in a region stretching north from Papua New Guinea, through the island populations of Melanesia to New Caledonia. A similar gradient in the distribution of malaria has been demonstrated from parasite and spleen-size data collected in this region over many years. This relationship might, of course, have resulted from gene drift and founder effect in these island populations. In other words, a population with a high frequency of α thalassemia might have moved through the islands from the north, with the gene frequency diluted during the migration southward. This explanation is unlikely, however, because there is a random pattern of the distribution of other DNA polymorphisms throughout these island populations.[67] Thus, the frequency of α^+ thalassemia, but not other DNA polymorphisms, shows an altitude- and latitude-dependent correlation with malarial endemicity throughout Melanesia.

These findings suggest that the α^+ thalassemia determinants found throughout this malaria cline originated in Melanesia and were amplified to a high frequency by a locally operated selective mechanism rather than being imported by population migrations from outside the region, from Southeast Asia, for example. In a series of control studies, α thalassemia gene frequencies have been analyzed in areas where malaria has never been recorded,[54,477] including Iceland and Japan and many of the island archipelagoes of Micronesia and Polynesia as Oceanic controls. There is virtually no α thalassemia in either Iceland or Japan but, surprisingly, gene frequencies as high as 12 percent are seen in parts of Polynesia. However, recent population studies suggest that the variant was carried to the eastern Pacific during the migrations of proto-Polynesian colonizers.[54]

The remarkable diversity of the different thalassemia mutations and their widespread distribution, together with population data that indicate that heterozygotes are protected against *P. falciparum* malaria, suggests that there may be properties common to the cells of carriers for different forms of thalassemia that make them less attractive to the malarial parasite.[478] However, an epidemiologic study of α thalassemia in the southwest Pacific[479] suggests, surprisingly, quite the reverse. In children with the homozygous form of α^+ thalassemia ($-\alpha/-\alpha$), both the incidence of uncomplicated malaria and the prevalence of splenomegaly (as an index of malaria infection) were significantly higher than in normal nonthalassemic children. Moreover, the effect was most marked in the youngest children and for the nonlethal parasite *P. vivax*. It seems possible that *P. vivax* may be acting as a natural vaccine by inducing a degree of cross-species protection against the more severe effects of *P. falciparum* malaria. Both *P. vivax* and *P. falciparum* have a preference for invading very young metabolically active red cells. Like other mild forms of thalassemia, α^+ thalassemia homozygotes, and to a lesser extent heterozygotes ($-\alpha/\alpha\alpha$), probably have a degree of ineffective erythropoiesis and reduced red cell survival. Consequently, invasion of thalassemic red cells by *P. vivax* and *P. falciparum* may be more efficient than in normal red cells.

Another intriguing facet to the malaria-thalassemia relationship comes from a case control study aimed at determining the magnitude of the protective effect.[480] α Thalassemia homozygotes ($-\alpha/-\alpha$) enjoyed greater than 60 percent protection against the risk of having severe *P. falciparum* malaria. Unexpectedly, the risk of hospital admissions with infections other than malaria was also reduced to a similar degree. Thus, the survival advantage of thalassemia may extend well beyond direct malaria mortality.

These observations raise completely new avenues of investigation for the protective effect of thalassemia against *P. falciparum* malaria, and suggest that it could be immune-mediated rather than due to the particular properties of the small thalassemic red cell.

DIAGNOSIS, PREVENTION, AND TREATMENT

The practical aspects of the diagnosis, prevention, and management of the hemoglobinopathies are the subject of a number of monographs and reviews,[2,3,169,170,200,244] and are only outlined here.

Diagnosis

The diagnosis of a hemoglobin disorder involves the characterization of the homozygous or compound heterozygous state for a structural hemoglobin variant, or a form of thalassemia in a patient with an appropriate clinical picture, or the identification of a heterozygote as part of a family study or population screening program. In the routine clinical laboratory, a few relatively simple investigations will suffice in the majority of cases, such as the preparation of a well-stained blood film, analysis of the hemoglobin level and hematocrit together with a determination of the red cell indices with an electronic cell counter, hemoglobin electrophoresis, estimation of the Hb F level by alkali denaturation, and a quantitative assessment of the Hb A_2 level. To this list may be added a heat stability or isopropanol test for unstable hemoglobin. Figure 181-32 is a flow chart of the order in which these investigations should be done to obtain maximum information. In addition, it may be necessary to do confirmatory investigations for the sickling disorders, such as the metabisulfite or solubility tests, and, in cases of suspected high or low affinity hemoglobin variants, to determine the p50.

This simple battery of investigations enables identification of the important sickling disorders, hemoglobins C and E, the high-oxygen-affinity variants, and the unstable hemoglobins. For unequivocal structural identification, it is necessary to determine the amino acid or nucleotide base substitution, but this is rarely required in clinical practice.

The diagnosis of the common sickling disorders is usually straightforward. In sickle cell anemia, the Hb A_2 level is normal, and both parents show the sickle cell trait. The other common sickling disorders, such as SC, SD, and S/O_{ARAB} diseases, can be identified provisionally by agar gel electrophoresis or isoelectric focusing. Sickle cell β^o thalassemia is diagnosed by finding the β thalassemia trait in one parent and a raised Hb A_2. It is important to do family studies when a raised Hb A_2 is found in an individual who is apparently homozygous for the sickle cell gene because the coexistence of α thalassemia and homozygous Hb S can also produce a raised Hb A_2 level; in this case, both parents have the sickle cell trait and hematologic evidence of coexistent α thalassemia.

It is usually easy to diagnose the homozygous or compound heterozygous states for the important forms of β and $\delta\beta$ thalassemia by measuring Hb F and A_2 levels and doing a family study. The hemoglobin pattern of heterozygotes for these conditions is quite characteristic; β-thalassemia heterozygotes have typical thalassemic indices and a raised Hb A_2, whereas $\delta\beta$-thalassemia heterozygotes have a normal Hb A_2 but Hb F levels in the 5 to 15 percent range. In homozygous β-thalassemia patients who have been transfused before referral, it may be necessary to repeat the investigations after an interval or to do globin chain synthesis studies on the marrow or blood.

The diagnosis of Hb Bart's hydrops syndrome and Hb H disease usually presents no difficulties. Remember that the level of Hb H varies considerably in Hb H disease and that, because Hb H is unstable, it is necessary to examine fresh red cell lysates. It is also important to do hemoglobin electrophoresis on concentrated red cell lysates so as not to miss the form of Hb H disease associated with $Hb_{CONSTANT\ SPRING}$ or one of the other α chain-termination mutants.

The diagnosis of the α thalassemia carrier states is more difficult. Heterozygous α^o thalassemia is characterized by typical thalassemic red cell indices with a normal Hb A_2; a small proportion of the cells may contain Hb H bodies. Heterozygous α^+ thalassemia is extremely difficult to identify as the red cell indices may be normal. The heterozygous state for α^o thalassemia and the homozygous state for α^+ thalassemia produce identical red cell changes, and the two conditions can be distinguished only in an individual patient by a family study or, better, by α gene mapping.

Screening. Screening for the hemoglobin variants and thalassemias is needed for the prenatal identification of the carrier states for important disorders such as Hb S, β thalassemia, and α^o thalassemia. It may also be required for identification of the sickling disorders or thalassemia in newborn infants or as part of a population screening program.

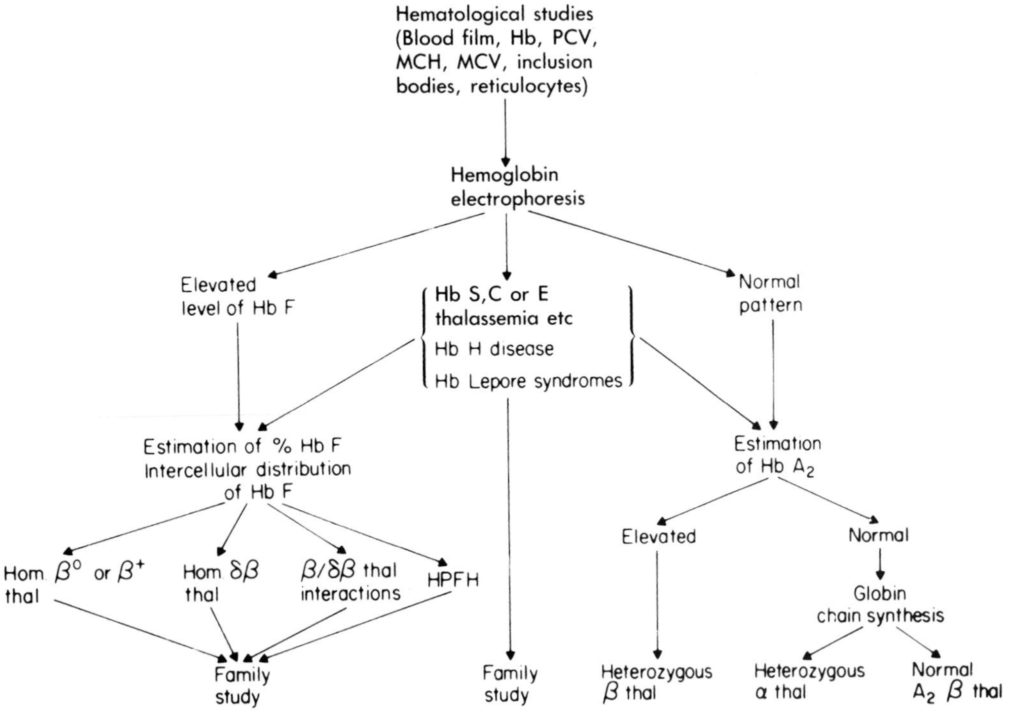

Fig. 181-32 Flow chart showing the approach to the laboratory diagnosis of the hemoglobin disorders. (*From Weatherall and Clegg.*[2] *Used by permission.*)

Screening for the sickle cell trait in adults can be done by hemoglobin electrophoresis or one of the solubility tests for Hb S. Screening for thalassemia is best done by determining the red cell indices and, if the MCV or MCH is less than 80 fl or 27 pg, by doing a serum iron or ferritin estimation to exclude iron deficiency. After thalassemia is suspected, a Hb A_2 estimation should be done. In most cases, this distinguishes β-thalassemia trait from α^o-thalassemia trait. In populations in which β thalassemia with a normal Hb A_2 level is common, it is necessary to do globin chain synthesis or gene mapping analysis to distinguish this condition from heterozygous α^o thalassemia. There is one pitfall that may be encountered in populations in which α and β thalassemia are common. Individuals who are heterozygous for both α and β thalassemia may have relatively normal red cell indices. In these populations, it is wise to use a Hb A_2 estimation as the initial screening procedure because such doubly affected heterozygotes have an elevated Hb A_2.[450,451] Typical red cell indices for the different heterozygous forms of thalassemia are summarized in Table 181-15.

Neonatal screening for the sickle cell gene is best done using agar gel electrophoresis. Screening for α thalassemia can be done by estimating Hb Bart's levels in cord blood, although this will miss many cases of heterozygous α^+ thalassemia. The diagnosis of β thalassemia can be made at birth, but only by globin chain synthesis; where heterozygous or homozygous β thalassemia is suspected it is better to delay hemoglobin analysis until after the first 6 months of life, at which time the typical changes are usually well established.

Avoidance

Programs for the avoidance of the common hemoglobinopathies can be carried out either by population screening of school-leavers or young adults followed by marital advice, or by screening pregnant women and, in cases in which their partners are also carriers, offering prenatal diagnosis followed, where appropriate, by termination of pregnancy. The former approach has been extremely successful in the Montreal program,[481] and in some countries, a major adult education program has led to widespread premarital screening;[482] in others, the antenatal clinic is still the major site for prenatal screening.

Prenatal diagnosis can be done in either the second trimester of pregnancy by fetal blood sampling or examination of the DNA of amniotic fluid cells, or by chorion villus sampling and DNA analysis in the first trimester.[483] Fetal blood sampling followed by globin chain synthesis analysis has been applied widely for the prenatal diagnosis of the hemoglobin disorders.[483] The method is extremely effective for the recognition of the sickling disorders and α and β thalassemias. It carries a 1 to 2 percent risk of fetal loss and there is about a 1 percent error rate. It has been used widely throughout the Mediterranean region, the Middle East, Britain, and North America. The application of this method has reduced considerably the incidence of homozygous β thalassemia in a number of Mediterranean populations.[484–486]

Recently, fetal DNA analysis following chorion villus sampling was developed and is now being widely used for the prenatal diagnosis of all the important hemoglobin disorders.[482,484,487] It is currently estimated that there is a 1 to 2 percent fetal loss following this procedure.[483] It is possible to obtain 20 to 100 μg of fetal DNA from chorion villus material and, if the procedure is carried out correctly, it is usually uncontaminated by maternal cells.

The diagnostic techniques used for fetal DNA analysis have evolved over the last 10 years.[59,482] The first approach involved Southern blotting of fetal DNA using either RFLP linkage analysis[487,488] or, in those cases in which the mutation was known, a restriction enzyme that identifies the base change or an oligonucleotide probe.[489] The use of RFLP analysis for prenatal detection of genetic disease entails three steps. First, an appropriate RFLP marker is chosen that is either within or closely linked to the disease locus and for which an individual at risk of transmitting the disease is heterozygous. Second, it is necessary to determine which of the marker alleles is on the chromosome carrying the disease allele; this involves a study of family members, ideally a previously affected or normal child. Finally, using the markers, fetal DNA is examined to see whether the fetus has inherited the chromosomes carrying the genes for the particular form of hemoglobin disorder, or its normal allele. The disadvantage of this method is that it is necessary to establish, by a family study, that the appropriate markers are available. Although it is largely superseded by more direct approaches for identifying thalassemia mutations in fetal DNA, it is still a valuable fallback in families at risk for having children with rare forms of thalassemia. α^o Thalassemia and a few forms of β^o thalassemia that result from gene deletions can also be identified directly by Southern blotting. Many different β thalassemic mutations alter a particular restriction-enzyme site and can, therefore, be identified directly.[483] Sickle cell anemia and many structural hemoglobin variants can also be diagnosed using this approach.

The development of the polymerase chain reaction (PCR) has greatly facilitated the identification of thalassemia mutations and those for structural hemoglobin variants in fetal DNA. For example, PCR can be used for the rapid detection of mutations that alter restriction-enzyme cutting sites.[490] The appropriate fragment of the β globin gene is amplified for approximately 30 cycles, after which the DNA fragments are digested with the particular enzyme and separated by electrophoresis. Either ethidium bromide or silver staining of DNA bands on gels can detect these fragments; radioactive probes are not required.

Now that the mutations are known for so many different forms of α and β thalassemia, most prenatal diagnosis programs are based on the direct detection of these mutations as the first-line approach.[482] The development of PCR, combined with the use of oligonucleotide probes to detect individual mutations, has offered a variety of new approaches for increasing the speed and accuracy of carrier detection and prenatal diagnosis.[491–493] For example, diagnoses can be made using hybridization of specific ^{32}P-end-labeled oligonucleotides to an amplified region of the β globin gene dotted on a nylon membrane. A number of variations on this theme have been developed. For example, mutations can be rapidly identified using a modification of PCR called the amplification refractory mutation system (ARMS).[494] This is based on the observation that, in many cases, oligonucleotides for the 3′ mismatched residue will, under appropriate conditions, not function as primers in the PCR. Two primers are prepared. The normal one is refractory to PCR on mutant template DNA; the mutant sequence is refractory to PCR on normal DNA. The difference between normal DNA and that carrying a particular mutation is identified by size differences of the amplified fragments (Fig. 181-33). Other modifications of PCR involve the use of nonradioactively labeled probes. For example, it is possible to use horseradish-peroxidase-labeling of the 5′ end of oligonucleotides designed to detect individual mutations.

To develop a comprehensive prenatal diagnosis program for β thalassemia, the first step is to determine the common mutations in the population.[482] After this has been done, a large proportion of cases can be identified by one of these PCR methods. For those in which the mutation is not known, RFLP linkage analysis can be performed. In those rare cases in which DNA analysis is unsuccessful, it is still possible to carry out second trimester diagnosis by fetal blood sampling. Several large series of first-trimester prenatal diagnosis have now been published and it is quite clear that the approach is feasible.[482,485–487] Potential difficulties include plasmid or maternal tissue contamination, crossovers, and nonpaternity. In these series the error rate is about the same or lower than that for fetal blood sampling followed by globin chain synthesis.

Programs of prenatal diagnosis have been extremely successful in some of the Mediterranean island populations[482] where the birth of new patients with β thalassemia has dropped dramatically. Whether this is possible for the large mainland rural populations,

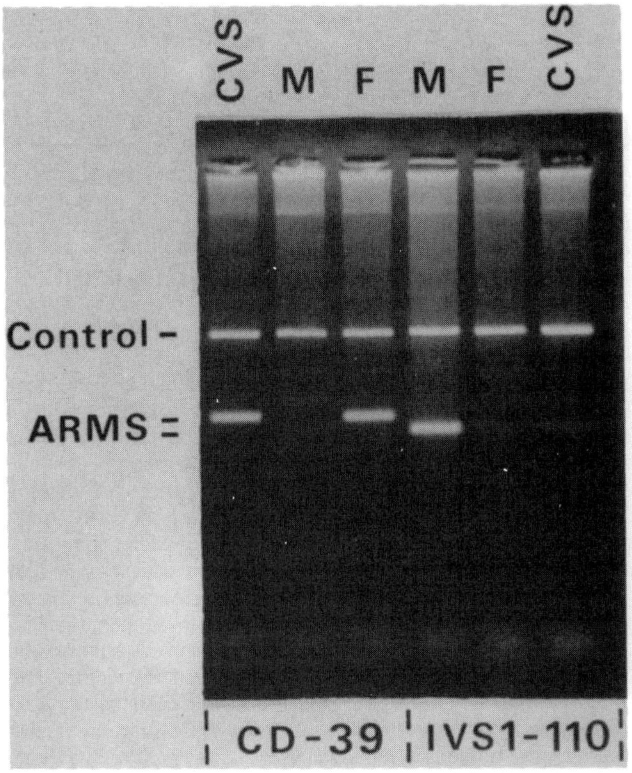

Fig. 181-33 Rapid prenatal diagnosis β thalassemia by ARMS, a development for the rapid identification of mutations based on the PCR. One parent has the common Mediterranean codon 39 (CD) mutation, the other the IVS1 110 G→A mutation. The fetus is heterozygous for the codon 39 mutation. M = mother; F = father; CVS = fetal DNA from chorionic villus sampling. (*Kindly prepared by Dr. John Old.*)

particularly those of the Indian subcontinent and Southeast Asia, remains to be seen.

Treatment

Apart from bone marrow transplantation, there is no definitive treatment for any of the important hemoglobin disorders, but there has been considerable improvement in their symptomatic management.

The Sickling Disorders.[169,170,200,210,495] Individuals with the sickle cell trait require no treatment beyond simple genetic counseling and the avoidance of conditions of extreme oxygen deprivation or dehydration.

Because so many of the serious complications occur in the first 2 years of life, the diagnosis of sickle cell anemia should be made as early as possible. After the diagnosis is established, the parents should be counseled about the dangers of infection during the early years of life. Oral penicillin should be given daily and maintained at least throughout childhood and early adolescence. It is now common practice to also vaccinate against pneumococcus, meningococcus, and *Haemophilus influenzae*. The parents and family physician should be advised to seek hospital advice at the onset of any unusual symptoms. Mothers can be counseled about splenic sequestration and taught to assess spleen size. No other treatment is required for sickle cell anemia in the steady state; folic acid supplements are often given but are probably unnecessary if the infant is receiving a good diet.

The management of all but the mildest sickle cell crises requires hospital admission and an extremely competent level of clinical care. Bed rest, hydration, and adequate analgesia manage the painful crisis. Although it may be possible to manage mild painful crises with first-line analgesics such as paracetamol, more powerful agents are often required, at least for a few days; although there is a risk of addiction patients cannot be left in excruciating pain. Strong analgesics such as diamorphine should be administered by slow, titrated intravenous infusion and should be monitored by close observation of respiration together with regular blood-gas analysis. A source of infection should be sought and the hematocrit and reticulocyte count monitored twice daily. There is no indication for blood transfusion unless the hematocrit is falling. Splenic or hepatic sequestration crises should be managed by prompt transfusion; if the spleen remains large, there is a good case for splenectomy to prevent second episodes. Lung crises should be managed by treatment of any associated infection, adequate oxygenation and hydration, and if the patient is deteriorating despite these measures, exchange transfusion. Neurologic crises should be treated by hypertransfusion or, if the initial hematocrit is relatively high, by exchange transfusion. It is important to maintain these patients on transfusion to avoid recurrence.[496] The management of priapism is difficult. If treated conservatively the condition usually fails to respond and there may be permanent penile deformity. It has been suggested that the best approach is to use adequate hydration and analgesia for 24 h followed by an exchange transfusion or hypertransfusion for a further 24 h. If the condition does not resolve after these measures, consider a cavernosal-spongiosal shunt.[200]

Recently, the whole question of the methods of transfusion of patients with sickle cell anemia has come under review. Hitherto, it has been suggested that blood transfusion should not be given unless the hemoglobin is unusually low, because of the potential danger of raising the blood viscosity unless the number of sickleable red cells can be reduced to less than 30 percent. Thus, exchange transfusion is usually used in situations in which urgent control of sickling is required, such as a lung crisis or neurologic episode. However, recent clinical trials suggest that it may be safe to transfuse children who require regular replacement, those who have had strokes for example, without reverting to exchange transfusion.[497] Clearly, further work is required before a definitive statement about the pattern of transfusion in sickle cell anemia can be made.

Genuine progress toward developing regimens for the prevention of painful crises has been made. Because of its potential for raising fetal hemoglobin levels, a trial of hydroxyurea was established in adult patients with sickle cell anemia. The treated group had significantly fewer crises, higher fetal hemoglobin levels, and a marked increase in the mean cell volume.[498] Encouraging results have also been obtained in trials of children with sickle cell anemia treated in this way.[499] It should be emphasized that the long-term safety of maintaining patients with sickle cell anemia on hydroxyurea is yet to be determined, but the drug is licensed for use in adult patients with sickle cell anemia in the United States.

Hemoglobin SC disease should be managed in the same way as sickle cell anemia. There is increasing evidence that the retinal complications of this disorder may progress to blindness; therefore, all patients with this condition, and probably sickle cell anemia as well, should have regular ophthalmologic surveillance and laser therapy when indicated.

The management of pregnancy in sickle cell anemia is still controversial. Although hypertransfusion regimens have been advocated in the UK, there is no evidence that they are effective. The best compromise is to follow the patient very carefully and transfuse only if there are recurrent crises or a fall in the hematocrit during late pregnancy.

The observation that aplastic crises in sickle cell anemia result from parvovirus infections has important implications. This condition should be suspected in any patient with sickle cell anemia with a falling hematocrit, particularly if the reticulocyte count is also reduced. It requires very careful hospital observation and early transfusion. The possibility of developing a vaccine may make it feasible to prevent this life-threatening complication.

Unstable Hemoglobin Variants. The majority of patients require no treatment. If there is severe hemolysis with a large spleen, splenectomy may be helpful. There are, however, insufficient data to fully evaluate the likely benefit.

Thalassemia. No treatment is required for α or β thalassemia heterozygotes although they should be followed carefully during pregnancy because they may become anemic during the second and third trimesters. They should receive appropriate genetic counseling.

The clinical management of homozygous β thalassemia is unsatisfactory. It is the subject of an enormous amount of work;[3,500–502] only a few principles can be outlined here. When the condition is suspected in early infancy, the patient should be observed carefully to make sure that the patient falls into the transfusion-dependent category. This usually becomes obvious by the end of the first year of life; the infant fails to thrive, feeding is difficult, and the hemoglobin level falls below 6 to 7 g/dl. It is important not to transfuse before this stage because a child with thalassemia intermedia may be wrongly categorized. Transfusion-dependent homozygous β thalassemics require blood, chelating agents, and, in some cases, splenectomy.

It is current practice to maintain children on a "moderate transfusion" program with a baseline level of 9 to 10 g/dl; this is less demanding on blood and reduces the amount of iron load. Because of sensitization, it is essential to carry out a complete blood group genotype before the first transfusion is given. Febrile and urticarial reactions can be minimized by the use of leukocyte-depleted red cells. Donor screening can markedly reduce the risk of acquisition of HIV; hepatitis B and C virus transmission is also preventable in this way.

The chelating agent of choice is still desferrioxamine, the dose of which should not exceed 20 to 30 mg/kg of body weight. The methods of monitoring body iron and the side effects of desferrioxamine and the way they should be avoided have been reviewed extensively.[2,503,504] These reviews also contain details of the use of ascorbate in patients on regular chelation. The present role of oral chelating agents, notably deferiprone (L1), was reviewed recently.[503,504] Its effect on maintaining iron balance does not appear to be sustained in a proportion of patients, it suffers from the disadvantage of causing neutropenia and occasional agranulocytosis, and recent data indicate that it may be associated with the risk of causing hepatic fibrosis.[503] There is increasing evidence that children maintained on adequate transfusion who comply with desferrioxamine regimens grow and develop normally and that secondary sexual development at puberty is often achieved.[505]

Hypersplenism is unusual in children who have been adequately transfused. However, in those who have not been so fortunate, or in nontransfusion-dependent patients with β thalassemia intermedia, hypersplenism is common and the spleen should be removed. Overall, a blood requirement of more than 200 ml/kg/year suggests that splenectomy should be considered. The operation should be avoided in the first few years of life, and in any case, should be followed up by the use of prophylactic penicillin and the same immunization program described earlier for sickle cell anemia. Splenectomy is also occasionally indicated in patients with Hb H disease, although it should be done only if there is severe hypersplenism. There are several reports of migrating thrombophlebitis and more severe thromboembolic disease in splenectomized patients with Hb H disease.[2]

Good general pediatric care is essential for thalassemic children. If they are inadequately transfused, they are prone to infection and to a variety of skeletal complications due to expansion of the bone marrow. Where iron-loading leads to delayed puberty, patients should have a hormone profile done and, if indicated, careful replacement therapy instituted. Unfortunately, this is not always successful because sexual underdevelopment is often due to target-organ unresponsiveness due to iron deposition.

Marrow Transplantation. In recent years, there has been increasing success for bone marrow transplantation, particularly for β thalassemia, but also for selected cases of sickle cell anemia.[501,506,507] Encouraging results have been obtained if the procedure is done early in life, although recent experiences suggest that it is possible to transplant patients up to the age of 20 years or over. Unfortunately, however, successful engraftment requires the availability of a sib or relative with a complete HLA match, making this form of treatment available only to a proportion of children with thalassemia. Lucarelli's group reviews the staging and prognosis for different stages in detail.[507]

Experimental Procedures. Several different therapeutic approaches to the hemoglobin disorders are being explored. Because it is clear that the production of high levels of fetal hemoglobin have the potential to protect patients with β thalassemia and sickle cell anemia, there is much interest in finding ways to stimulate Hb F production. The methods being explored are based on the old observation that there is a transient reversal to fetal hemoglobin synthesis during recovery from marrow suppression after the use of cytotoxic drugs for the treatment of leukemia or after bone marrow transplantation.[508] It is assumed that cytotoxic agents alter the pattern of erythropoiesis in such a way as to favor the expression of the γ globin genes. Several agents have been used, including the demethylating agent 5-azacytidine, hydroxyurea, erythropoietin, and a variety of butyric acid analogues. The current status of these studies is the subject of several recent reviews.[127,508] The success of the hydroxyurea trial in preventing painful crises in sickle cell anemia was described above. The experiences in β thalassemia are less encouraging although in one or two cases there has been a spectacular response to butyrate compounds and hydroxyurea. The reason for these unusual Hb F responses is not clear and it is important to learn whether it is related to particular thalassemia mutations or to other genetic factors that might produce a more favorable response for the pharmacologic manipulation of fetal hemoglobin.

In previous editions of this book, we discussed the potential role of gene therapy in the management of the hemoglobin disorders. Although there has been steady progress on all fronts in gene therapy, the hemoglobinopathies, because of the high level of gene expression that is required and the problems of treating enough hemopoietic stem cells, offer a particular challenge; gene therapy for these conditions still appears to be a long way off.

REFERENCES

1. Angastiniotis M, Modell B: Global epidemiology of hemoglobin disorders. *Proc Natl Acad Sci USA* **850**:251, 1998.
2. Weatherall DJ, Clegg JB: *The Thalassaemia Syndromes*, 4th Ed. Oxford, Blackwell Science, 2000.
3. Forget BG, Higgs DR, Nagel RL, Steinberg MH: *Disorders of Hemoglobin*. New York, Cambridge University Press, 2000.
4. Conley CL: Sickle-cell anemia — the first molecular disease, in Wintrobe MM (ed): *Blood, Pure and Eloquent*. New York, McGraw-Hill, 1980, p 319.
5. Weatherall DJ: Toward an understanding of the molecular biology of some common inherited anemias: The story of thalassemia, in Wintrobe MM (ed): *Blood, Pure and Eloquent*, New York, McGraw-Hill, 1980, p 373.
6. Bannerman RM: *Thalassemia. A Survey of Some Aspects*. New York, Grune and Stratton, 1961.
7. Herrick JB: Peculiar elongated and sickle-shaped red blood corpuscles in a case of severe anemia. *Arch Intern Med* **6**:517, 1910.
8. Pauling L, Itano HA, Singer SJ, Wells IG: Sickle-cell anemia, a molecular disease. *Science* **110**:543, 1949.
9. Ingram VM: Specific chemical difference between the globins of normal human and sickle-cell anaemia haemoglobin. *Nature* **178**:792, 1956.
10. Cooley TB, Lee P: A series of cases of splenomegaly in children with anemia and peculiar bone changes. *Trans Am Pediatr Soc* **37**:29, 1925.
11. Ingram VM, Stretton AOW: Genetic basis of the thalassaemia diseases. *Nature* **184**:1903, 1959.

12. Weatherall DJ, Clegg MA, Naughton MA: Globin synthesis in thalassaemia: An *in vitro* study. *Nature* **208**:1061, 1966.
13. Clegg JB, Naughton MA, Weatherall DJ: Abnormal human haemoglobins. Separation and characterisation of the α- and β-chains by chromatography, and the determination of two new variants, Hb. Chesapeake and Hb. J (Bangkok). *J Mol Biol* **19**:91, 1966.
14. Fermi G, Perutz MF, Shaanan B, Fourme B: The crystal structure of human deoxyhemoglobin at 1.7Å resolution. *J Mol Biol* **175**:159, 1984.
15. Baldwin JM: The structure of human carbon monoxyhaemoglobin at 2.7 Å resolution. *J Mol Biol* **136**:103, 1980.
16. Perutz MF: Stereochemistry of cooperative effects in haemoglobin. *Nature* **228**:726, 1970.
17. Perutz MF: Stereochemical mechanism of oxygen transport by haemoglobin. *Proc R Soc Lond B Biol Sci* **208**:135, 1980.
18. Baldwin J: Structure and cooperativity of haemoglobin. *Trends Biochem Sci* **5**:224, 1980.
19. Chanutin A, Curnish RR: Effect of organic and inorganic phosphates on the oxygen equilibrium of human erythrocytes. *Arch Biochem Biophys* **121**:96, 1967.
20. Benesch R, Benesch RE: The effect of organic phosphates from the human erythrocyte on the allosteric properties of hemoglobin. *Biochem Biophys Res Commun* **26**:162, 1967.
21. Arnone A: X-ray diffraction study of binding of 2,3 diphosphoglycerate to human deoxyhaemoglobin. *Nature* **237**:146, 1972.
22. Perutz MF, Shih DT-b, Williamson D: The chloride effect in human haemoglobin. *J Mol Biol* **239**:555, 1994.
23. Sutherland-Smith AJ, Baker HM, Hofmann OM, Brittain T, Baker EN: Crystal structure of a human embryonic haemoglobin: The carbonmonoxy form of Gower II ($\alpha_2\varepsilon_2$) haemoglobin at 2.9 Å resolution. *J Mol Biol* **280**:475, 1998.
24. Bauer C, Ludwig I, Ludwig M: Different effects of 2,3 diphosphoglycerate and adenosine triphosphate on the oxygen affinity of adult and foetal human haemoglobin. *Life Sci* **7**:1339, 1968.
25. Tyuma I, Shimizu K: Different response to organic phosphates of human fetal and adult hemoglobins. *Arch Biochem Biophys* **129**:404, 1969.
26. Perutz MF: The Bohr effect and combination with organic phosphates. *Nature* **228**:734, 1970.
27. Stamatoyannopoulos G, Nienhuis AW: Hemoglobin switching, in Stamatoyannopoulos G, Nienhuis AW, Majerus PW, Varmus H (eds): *The Molecular Basis of Blood Disease*, 2nd ed. Philadelphia, W.B. Saunders, 1994, p 107.
28. Deisseroth A, Velez R, Nienhuis AW: Hemoglobin synthesis in somatic cell hybrids. Independent segregation of the human alpha- and beta-globin genes. *Science* **191**:1262, 1976.
29. Deisseroth A, Nienhuis A, Turner P et al: Localization of the human α-globin structural gene to chromosome 16 in somatic cell hybrids by molecular hybridization. *Cell* **12**:205, 1977.
30. Deisseroth A, Nienhuis A, Lawrence J, Riles R, Turner P, Ruddle F: Chromosomal localization of human β globin gene on chromosome 11 in somatic cell hybrids. *Proc Natl Acad Sci U S A* **75**:1456, 1978.
31. Gusella JF, Varsanyi-Breiner A, Kao FT, et al: Precise localisation of human β-globin gene complex on chromosome 11. *Proc Natl Acad Sci U S A* **76**:5239, 1979.
32. Jeffreys AJ, Craig IW, Francke U: Localisation of the GγAγ δ and β globin genes on the short arm of chromosome 11. *Nature* **281**:606, 1979.
33. Lebo RV, Carrano AV, Burkhardt-Schultz K, Dozy AM, Yu L-C, Kan YW: Assignment of human β-, γ-, and ζ-globin genes to the short arm of chromosome 11 by chromosome sorting and DNA restriction analysis. *Proc Natl Acad Sci U S A* **76**:5804, 1979.
34. Sanders-Haigh L, Anderson WF, Francke U: The β-globin gene is on the short arm of chromosome 11. *Nature* **283**:683, 1980.
35. Scott AF, Phillips JA, Migeon BR: DNA endonuclease analysis for localisation of human β- and δ-globin genes on chromosome 11. *Proc Natl Acad Sci U S A* **76**:4563, 1979.
36. Koeffler HP, Sparkes RS, Stang H, Mohandas T: Regional assignment of genes for human α globin and phosphoglycerate phosphatase to the short arm of chromosome 16. *Proc Natl Acad Sci U S A* **78**:7015, 1981.
37. Nicholls RD, Jonasson JA, McGee JOD, et al: High resolution mapping of the human α-globin locus. *J Med Genet* **24**:39, 1987.
38. Lawn RM, Fritsch EF, Parker RC, Blake G, Maniatis T: The isolation and characterization of linked δ and β-globin genes from a cloned library of human DNA. *Cell* **15**:1157, 1978.
39. Fritsch EF, Lawn RM, Maniatis T: Molecular cloning and characterization of the human β-like globin gene cluster. *Cell* **19**:959, 1980.
40. Lauer J, Shen C-KJ, Maniatis T: The chromosomal arrangement of human α-like globin genes: Sequence homology and α-globin gene deletions. *Cell* **20**:119, 1980.
41. Jagedeeswaran P, Pan J, Forget BG, Weissman SM: Sequences of human repetitive DNA, non-α-globin genes, and major histocompatibility locus genes. II. Sequences of non-α-globin genes in man. *Cold Spring Harb Symp Quant Biol* **XLVII**:1081, 1983.
42. Chang L-YE, Slightom JL: Isolation and nucleotide sequence analysis of β-type globin pseudogene from human, gorilla and chimpanzee. *J Mol Biol* **180**:767, 1984.
43. Proudfoot NJ, Gil A, Maniatis T: The structure of the human ζ-globin gene and a closely linked, nearly identical pseudogene. *Cell* **31**:553, 1982.
44. Hardison RC, Sawada I, Cheng J-F, Shen C-KJ, Schmid CW: A previously undetected pseudogene in the human alpha globin gene cluster. *Nucleic Acids Res* **14**:1903, 1986.
45. Marks J, Shaw J-P, Shen C-KP: Sequence organization and genomic complexity of primate θ globin gene, a novel α-like gene. *Nature* **321**:785, 1986.
46. Clegg JB: Can the product of θ gene be a real globin. *Nature* **329**:465, 1987.
47. Efstratiadis A, Posakony JW, Maniatis T, et al: The structure and evolution of the human β-globin gene family. *Cell* **21**:653, 1980.
48. Goodman M, Koop BF, Czelusniak J, Weiss ML: The η-globin gene. Its long evolutionary history in the β-globin glue family of mammals. *J Mol Biol* **180**:803, 1984.
49. Hardison RL, Morgot JB: Rabbit-globin pseudogene $\psi\beta_2$ is a hybrid of δ- and β-globin gene sequences. **1**:302, 1984.
50. Jeffreys AJ: DNA sequences in the Gγ-, Aγ-, δ- and β-globin genes of man. *Cell* **18**:1, 1979.
51. Antonarakis SE, Boehm CD, Giardina PVJ, Kazazian HH: Nonrandom association of polymorphic restriction sites in the β-globin gene complex. *Proc Natl Acad Sci U S A* **79**:137, 1982.
52. Higgs DR, Wainscoat JS, Flint J, et al: Analysis of the human α-globin gene cluster reveals a highly informative genetic locus. *Proc Natl Acad Sci U S A* **83**:5165, 1986.
53. Wainscoat JS, Hill AVS, Boyce A, et al: Evolutionary relationships of human populations from an analysis of nuclear DNA polymorphisms. *Nature* **319**:491, 1986.
54. O'Shaughnessy DF, Hill AVS, Bowden DK, Weatherall DJ, Clegg JB: Globin genes in Micronesia: Origins and affinities of Pacific Island peoples. *Am J Hum Genet* **46**:144, 1990.
55. Lang JC, Chakravarti A, Boehm CD, Antonarakis S, Kazazian HH: Phylogeny of human β-globin haplotypes and its implication for recent human evolution. *Am J Phys Anthropol* **81**:113, 1992.
56. Chen LZ, Easteal S, Board PG, Kirk RL: Evolution of β-globin haplotypes in human populations. *Mol Biol Evol* **7**:423, 1990.
57. Boehm CD, Antonarakis SE, Phillips JA, Stetten G, Kazazian HH: Prenatal diagnosis using DNA polymorphisms. *N Engl J Med* **308**:1054, 1983.
58. Old JM, Wainscoat JS: A new DNA polymorphism in the β-globin gene cluster can be used for antenatal diagnosis of β thalassaemia. *Br J Haematol* **53**:336, 1983.
59. Embury SH: Advances in the prenatal and molecular diagnosis of the hemoglobinopathies and thalassemias. *Hemoglobin* **19**:237, 1995.
60. Winichagoon P, Higgs DR, Goodbourn SEY, Lamb J, Clegg JB, Weatherall DJ: Multiple arrangements of the human embryonic ζ-globin genes. *Nucleic Acids Res* **10**:5853, 1982.
61. Trent RJ, Bowden DK, Old JM, Wainscoat JS, Clegg JB, Weatherall DJ: A novel rearrangement of the human β-like globin gene cluster. *Nucleic Acids Res* **9**:6723, 1981.
62. Higgs DR, Old JM, Pressley L, Clegg JB, Weatherall DJ: A novel α-globin gene arrangement in man. *Nature* **284**:632, 1980.
63. Higgs DR, Old JM, Clegg JB, et al: Negro α-thalassaemia is caused by deletion of a single α-globin gene. *Lancet* **ii**:272, 1979.
64. Dozy AM, Kan YW, Embury SH, et al: α-globin gene organisation in blacks precludes the severe form of α-thalassaemia. *Nature* **280**:605, 1979.
65. Sukumaran PK, Nakatsuji T, Gardiner MB, Reese AL, Gilman JG, Huisman THJ: Gamma thalassaemia resulting from the deletion of a γ-globin gene. *Nucleic Acids Res* **11**:46354643, 1983.
66. Hill AVS: The population genetics of α-thalassemia and the malaria hypothesis. *Cold Spring Harb Symp Quant Biol* **LI**:489, 1986.
67. Flint J, Hill AVS, Bowden DK, et al: High frequencies of α thalassaemia are the result of natural selection by malaria. *Nature* **321**:744, 1986.

68. Powers PA, Altay C, Huisman THJ, Smithies O: Two novel arrangements of the human fetal globin genes: $^{G}\gamma$-$^{G}\gamma$ and $^{A}\gamma$-$^{A}\gamma$. *Nucleic Acids Res* **12**:7023, 1984.
69. Hill AVS, Nicholls RD, Thein SL, Higgs DR: Recombination within the human embryonic ζ-globin locus: A common ζ-ζ chromosome produced by gene conversion of the ψζ gene. *Cell* **42**:809, 1985.
70. Mount SM: A catalogue of splice junction sequences. *Nucleic Acids Res* **10**:459, 1982.
71. Green MR: Pre-mRNA splicing. *Annu Rev Genet* **20**:671, 1986.
72. Collins FS, Weissman SM: The molecular genetics of human hemoglobin, in Cohn WE, Moldave K (eds): *Progress in Nucleic Acids Research and Molecular Biology.* New York, Academic Press, 1984, p 315.
73. Grosveld GC, DeBoer E, Shewmaker CK, Flavell RA: DNA sequences necessary for transcription of the rabbit β-globin gene *in vitro*. *Nature* **295**:120, 1982.
74. Orkin SH, Antonarakis SE, Kazazian HHJ: Base substitution at position −88 in a β-thalassemic globin gene. Further evidence for the role of distal promoter element ACACCC. *J Biol Chem* **259**:8679, 1984.
75. Orkin S, Kazazian HH, Antonarakis SE, et al: Linkage of β-thalassaemia mutations and β-globin gene polymorphisms with DNA polymorphisms in human β-globin gene cluster. *Nature* **296**:627, 1982.
76. Lewin B: *Genes. V.* Oxford, Oxford University Press, 1994.
77. Alberts B, Bray D, Lewis J, Raff M, Roberts K, Watson JD: *Molecular Biology of the Cell.* 3rd ed. New York, Garland, 1994.
78. Orkin SH, Cheng T-C, Antonarakis SE, Kazazian HH: Thalassaemia due to a mutation in the cleavage-polyadenylation signal of the human β-globin gene. *EMBO J* **4**:453, 1985.
79. Higgs DR, Goodbourn SEY, Lamb J, Clegg JB, Weatherall DJ, Proudfoot NJ: α-Thalassaemia caused by a polyadenylation signal mutation. *Nature* **306**:398, 1983.
80. Evans T, Felsenfeld G, Reitman M: Control of globin gene transcription. *Ann Rev Cell Dev Biol* **6**:95, 1990.
81. Abel T, Maniatis T, in Stamatoyannopoulos G, Nienhuis AW, Leder P, Majerus PW (eds): *The Molecular Basis of Blood Diseases*, 2nd ed. Philadelphia, W.B. Saunders, 1994, p 33.
82. Wright S, de Boer E, Grosveld FG, Flavell RA: Regulated expression of the human beta-globin gene family in murine erythroleukaemia cells. *Nature* **305**:333, 1983.
83. Charnay P, Treisman R, Mellon P, Chao M, Axel R, Maniatis T: Differences in human alpha- and beta-globin expression in mouse erythroleukemia cells: The role of intragenic sequences. *Cell* **38**:251, 1984.
84. Costantini F, Radice G, Magram J, Stamatoyannopoulos G, Papayannopoulou T: Developmental regulation of human globin genes in transgenic mice. *Cold Spring Harb Symp Quant Biol* **50**:361, 1985.
85. Townes TM, Lingrel JB, Chen HY, Brinster RL, Palmiter RD: Erythroid-specific expression of human β globin genes in transgenic mice. *EMBO J* **4**:1715, 1985.
86. Chada K, Magram J, Costantini F: An embryonic pattern of expression of a human fetal globin gene in transgenic mice. *Nature* **319**:685, 1986.
87. Kollias G, Hurst J, de Boer E, Grosveld F: Regulated expression of human Aγ-, β- and hybrid γβ-globin genes in transgenic mice: Manipulation of the developmental expression patterns. *Cell* **46**:89, 1986.
88. Grosveld F, Blom van Assendelft G, Greaves DR, Kollias G: Position independent, high level expression of the human β globin gene in transgenic mice. *Cell* **51**:975, 1987.
89. Tuan D, Solomon W, Li Q, London I: The β-like globin gene domain in human erythroid cells. *Proc Natl Acad Sci U S A* **82**:6384, 1985.
90. Forrester W, Thompson C, Elder JT, Groudine M: A developmentally stable chromatin structure in the human β-globin gene cluster. *Proc Natl Acad Sci U S A* **83**:1359, 1986.
91. Driscoll C, Dobkin CS, Alter BP: γδβ Thalassemia due to a *de novo* mutation deleting the 5′ β-globin locus activating region hypersensitive sites. *Proc Natl Acad Sci U S A* **86**:7470, 1989.
92. Fiering S, Epner E, Robinson K, et al: Targeted deletion of 5′HS2 of the murine β-globin LCR reveals that it is not essential for proper regulation of the β-globin locus. *Genes Dev* **9**:2203, 1995.
93. Hug BA, Wesselschmidt RL, Fiering S, et al: Analysis of mice containing a targeted deletion of β-globin locus control region 5′ hypersensitive site 3. *Mol Cell Biol* **16**:2906, 1996.
94. Wijgerde M, Grosveld F, Fraser P: Transcription complex stability and chromatin dynamics *in vivo*. *Nature* **377**:209, 1995.
95. Hatton C, Wilkie AOM, Drysdale HC, et al: Alpha thalassemia caused by a large (62-kb) deletion upstream of the human α globin gene cluster. *Blood* **76**:221, 1990.
96. Wilkie AOM, Lamb J, Harris PC, Finney RD, Higgs DR: A truncated human chromosome 16 associated with α thalassaemia is stabilized by addition of telomeric repeat $(TTAGGG)_n$. *Nature* **346**:868, 1990.
97. Higgs DR, Wood WG, Jarman AP, et al: A major positive regulatory region located far upstream of the human α-globin gene locus. *Genes Dev* **4**:1588, 1990.
98. Jarman AP, Wood WG, Sharpe JA, Gourdon G, Ayyub H, Higgs DR: Characterization of the major regulatory element upstream of the human α-globin gene cluster. *Mol Cell Biol* **11**:4679, 1991.
99. Groudine M, Kohwi-Shigematsu T, Gelinas R, Stamatoyannopoulos G, Papayannopoulou T: Human fetal-to-adult globin gene switching: changes in chromatin structure of the β globin locus. *Proc Natl Acad Sci U S A* **80**:7551, 1983.
100. Forrester WC, Epner E, Driscoll MC, et al: A deletion of the human β-globin locus activation region causes a major alteration in chromatin structure and replication across the entire β-globin locus. *Genes Dev* **4**:1637, 1990.
101. Jarman AP, Higgs DR: Nuclear scaffold attachment sites in the human globin gene complexes. *Eur Mol Biol Org J* **7**:3337, 1988.
102. Yagi M, Gelinas R, Elder JT, et al: Chromatin structure and developmental expression of the human α-globin cluster. *Mol Cell Biol* **6**:1108, 1986.
103. Vyas P, Vickers MA, Simmons DL, Ayyub H, Craddock CF, Higgs DR: Cis-acting sequences regulating expression of the human α globin cluster lie within constitutively open chromatin. *Cell* **69**:781, 1992.
104. Mavilio F, Giampaolo A, Care A, et al: Molecular mechanisms of human hemoglobin switching: Selective undermethylation and expression of globin genes in embryonic, fetal and adult erythroblasts. *Proc Natl Acad Sci U S A* **80**:6907, 1983.
105. Wall L, deBoer E, Grosveld F: The human β-globin gene 3′ enhancer contains multiple binding sites for an erythroid-specific protein. *Genes Dev* **2**:1089, 1988.
106. Evans T, Felsenfeld G: The erythroid specific transcription factor Eryf1: A new finger protein. *Cell* **58**:877, 1989.
107. Martin DIK, Tsai S-F, Orkin SH: Increased γ-globin expression in a nondeletion HPFH mediated by an erythroid-specific DNA-binding factor. *Nature* **338**:435, 1989.
108. Yamamoto M, Ko LJ, Leonard MW, Beng H, Orkin S, Engel JD: Activity and tissue specific expression of the transcription factor NF-E1 multigene family. *Genes Dev* **4**:1650, 1990.
109. Whitelaw E, Tsai S-F, Hogben P, Orkin SH: Regulated expression of globin chains and the erythroid transcription factor GATA-1 during erythropoiesis in the developing mouse. *Mol Cell Biol* **10**:6596, 1990.
110. Pevny L, Simon MC, Robertson E et al: Erythroid differentiation in chimaeric mice blocked by a targeted mutation in the gene for transcription factor GATA-1. *Nature* **349**:257, 1991.
111. Fujiwara Y, Browne CP, Cunniff K, Goff SC, Orkin SH: Arrested development of embryonic red cell precursors in mouse embryos lacking transcription factor GATA-1. *Proc Natl Acad Sci U S A* **93**:12355, 1996.
112. Onodera K, Takahashi S, Nishimura S, et al: GATA-1 transcription is controlled by distinct regulatory mechanisms during primitive and definitive erythropoiesis. *Proc Natl Acad Sci U S A* **94**:4487, 1997.
113. McDevitt MA, Fujiwara Y, Shivdasani RA, Orkin SH: An upstream, DNase I hypersensitive region of the hematopoietic-expressed transcription factor GATA-1 gene confers developmental specificity in transgenic mice. *Proc Natl Acad Sci U S A* **94**:7976, 1997.
114. Tsang AP, Visvader JE, Turner CA, et al: FOG, a multitype zinc finger protein, acts as a cofactor for transcription factor GATA-1 in erythroid and megakaryocytic differentiation. *Cell* **90**:109, 1997.
115. Wadman IA, Osada H, Grütz GG, et al: The LIM-only protein Lmo2 is a bridging molecule assembling an erythroid, DNA-binding complex which includes the TAL1, E47, GATA-1 and Ldb1/NLI proteins. *EMBO J* **16**:3145, 1997.
116. Visvader JE, Mao X, Fujiwara Y, Hahm K, Orkin SH: The LIM-domain binding protein Ldb1 and its partner Lmo2 act as negative regulators of erythroid differentiation. *Proc Natl Acad Sci U S A* **94**:13707, 1997.
117. Ney PA, Sorrentino BP, McDonagh KT, Nienhuis AW: Tandem AP-1-binding sites within the human β-globin dominant control region function as an inducible enhancer in erythroid cells. *Genes Dev* **4**:993, 1990.

118. Kotkow KJ, Orkin SH: Dependence of globin gene expression in mouse erythroleukaemia cells on the NF-E2 heterodimer. *Mol Cell Biol* **15**:4640, 1995.
119. Shivdasani RA, Rosenblatt MF, Zucker-Franklin D, et al: Transcription factor NF-E2 is required for platelet formation independent of the actions of thrombopoietin/MGDF in megakaryocyte development. *Cell* **81**:695, 1995.
120. Motohashi H, Shavit JA, Igarashi K, Yamamoto M, Engel JD: The world according to Maf. *Nucleic Acids Res* **25**:2953, 1997.
121. Igarashi K, Hoshino H, Muto A, et al: Multivalent DNA binding complex generated by small Maf and Bach1 as a possible biochemical basis for β-globin locus control region complex. *J Biol Chem* **273**:11783, 1998.
122. Thein SL, Wood WG, Wickramasinghe SN, Galvin MC: β-thalassemia unlinked to the β-globin gene in an English family. *Blood* **82**:961, 1993.
123. Ho PJ, Hall GW, Luo LY, Weatherall DJ, Thein SL: Beta thalassaemia intermedia: Is it possible to predict phenotype from genotype? *Br J Haematol* **100**:70, 1998.
124. Gasperini D, Perseu L, Melis MA, et al: Heterozygous beta-thalassemia with thalassemia intermedia phenotype. *Am J Hematol* **57**:43, 1998.
125. Gibbons RJ, Wilkie AOM, Weatherall DJ, Higgs DR: A newly defined X-linked mental retardation syndrome associated with α thalassaemia. *J Med Genet* **28**:729, 1991.
126. Gallarda JL, Foley KP, Yang Z, Engel JD: The β-globin stage selector element factor is erythroid-specific promoter/enhancer binding protein NF-E4. *Genes Dev* **3**:1845, 1989.
127. Jane SM, Cunningham JM: Understanding fetal globin gene expression: a step towards effective Hb F reactivation in haemoglobinopathies. *Br J Haematol* **102**:415, 1998.
128. Miller IJ, Bieker JJ: A novel, erythroid cell-specific murine transcription factor that binds to the CACCC element and is related to the Krüppel family of nuclear proteins. *Mol Cell Biol* **13**:2776, 1993.
129. Perkins AC, Sharpe AH, Orkin SH: Lethal β-thalassaemia in mice lacking the erythroid CACCC-transcription factor EKLF. *Nature* **375**:318, 1995.
130. Nuez B, Michalovich D, Bygrave A, Ploemacher R, Grosveld F: Defective haematopoiesis in fetal liver resulting from inactivation of the EKLF gene. *Nature* **375**:316, 1995.
131. Southwood CM, Downs KM, Bieker JJ: Erythroid Krüppel-like factor exhibits an early and sequentially localized pattern of expression during mammalian erythroid ontogeny. *Dev Dyn* **206**:248, 1996.
132. Guy L-G, Mei Q, Perkins AC, Orkin SH, Wall L: Erythroid Krüppel-like factor is essential for β-globin gene expression even in absence of gene competition, but is not sufficient to induce the switch from γ-globin to β-globin gene expression. *Blood* **91**:2259, 1998.
133. Teware R, Gillemans N, Wijgerde M, et al: Erythroid Krüppel-like factor (EKLF) is active in primitive and definitive erythroid cells and is required for the function of 5′HS3 of the β-globin locus control region. *EMBO J* **17**:2334, 1998.
134. Wood WG, Pearce K, Clegg JB, et al: The switch from foetal to adult haemoglobin synthesis in normal and hypophysectomised sheep. *Nature* **264**:799, 1976.
135. Perrine SP, Rudolph A, Faller DV, et al: Butyrate infusions in the ovine fetus delay the biologic clock for globin gene switching. *Proc Natl Acad Sci U S A* **85**:8540, 1988.
136. Wood WG, Bunch C, Kelly S, Gunn Y, Breckon G: Control of haemoglobin switching by a developmental clock? *Nature* **313**:320, 1985.
137. Zanjani ED, Lim G, McGlave PB, et al: Adult haemopoietic cells transplanted to sheep foetuses continue to produce adult globins. *Nature* **295**:244, 1982.
138. Geiger H, Sick S, Bonifer C, Müller AM: Globin gene expression is reprogrammed in chimeras generated by injecting adult hematopoietic stem cells into mouse blastocysts. *Cell* **93**:1055, 1998.
139. Raich N, Enver T, Nakamoto B, Josephson B, Papayannopoulou T, Stamatoyannopoulos G: Autonomous developmental control of human embryonic globin gene switching in transgenic mice. *Science* **250**:1147, 1990.
140. Dillon N, Grosveld F: Human γ-globin genes silenced independently of other genes in β-globin locus. *Nature* **350**:252, 1991.
141. Behringer RR, Ryan TM, Palmiter RD, Brinster RL, Townes TM: Human γ- to β-globin gene switching in transgenic mice. *Genes Dev* **4**:376, 1990.
142. Enver T, Raich N, Ebens AJ, Papayannopoulou T, Costantini F, Stamatoyannopoulos G: Developmental regulation of human fetal-to-adult globin gene switching in transgenic mice. *Nature* **344**:309, 1990.
143. Hanscombe O, Whyatt D, Fraser P, et al: Importance of globin gene order for correct developmental expression. *Genes Dev* **5**:1387, 1991.
144. Dillon N, Trimborn T, Strouboulis J, Fraser P, Grosveld F: The effect of distance on long-range chromatin interactions. *Mol Cells* **1**:131, 1997.
145. Fraser P, Pruzina S, Antoniou M, Grosveld F: Each hypersensitive site of the human β-globin locus control region confers a different developmental pattern of expression on the globin genes. *Genes Dev* **7**:106, 1993.
146. Navas PA, Peterson KR, Li Q et al: Developmental specificity of the interaction between the locus control region and embryonic or fetal globin genes in transgenic mice with an HS3 core deletion. *Mol Cell Biol* **18**:4188, 1998.
147. Stanworth SJ, Roberts NA, Sharpe JA, Sloane-Stanley J, Wood WG: Established epigenetic modifications determine the expression of developmentally regulated globin genes in somatic cell hybrids. *Mol Cell Biol* **15**:3969, 1995.
148. Huisman THJ, Carver HFH, Efremov G: *A Syllabus of Hemoglobin Variants*. Augusta, GA, Sickle Cell Anemia Foundation, 1998.
149. Weatherall DJ, Clegg JB: The α chain termination mutants and their relationship to thalassaemia. *Philos Trans R Soc Lond (B)* **271**:411, 1975.
150. Seid-Akhaven M, Winter WP, Abramson RK, Rucknagel DL: Hemoglobin Wayne: A frameshift mutation detected in human hemoglobin alpha chains. *Proc Natl Acad Sci U S A* **73**:882, 1976.
151. Lehmann H, Casey R, Lang A, et al: Haemoglobin Tak: A β-chain elongation. *Br J Haematol* **31**:119, 1975.
152. Bunn HF, Schmidt GJ, Haney DN, Dluhy RG: Hemoglobin Cranston, an unstable variant having an elongated β chain due to nonhomologous crossover between two normal β chain genes. *Proc Natl Acad Sci U S A* **72**:3609, 1975.
153. Delanoe-Garin J, Blouquit Y, Arous N, et al: Hemoglobin Saverne: A new variant with elongated β chains: Structural and functional properties. *Hemoglobin* **12**:337, 1988.
154. Huisman THJ, Wilson JB, Gravely M, Hubbard M: Hemoglobin Grady: The first example of a variant with elongated chains due to an insertion of residues. *Proc Natl Acad Sci U S A* **71**:3270, 1974.
155. Prchal JT, Cashman DP, Kan YW: Hemoglobin Long Island is caused by a single mutation (adenine to cytosine) resulting in a failure to cleave amino-terminal methionine. *Proc Natl Acad Sci U S A* **83**:24, 1986.
156. Blouquit Y, Lena-Russo D, Delanoe J, et al: Hb Marseille ($\alpha_2\beta_2$ 1(A1) NH $\rightarrow$ met, 2(A2) His $\rightarrow$ 3(A3) Pro: First variant having an N-terminal elongated β chain. *Blood* **64**:55, 1984.
157. Broissel J-P, Kasper T, Shah S, Malone T, Bunn HF: NH_2-terminal processing of protein: Hb South Florida. *Proc Natl Acad Sci U S A* **82**:8448, 1987.
158. Rieder RF, Bradley TB: Hemoglobin Gunn Hill: An unstable protein associated with chronic hemolysis. *Blood* **32**:355, 1968.
159. Winslow RM, Swenberg ML, Gross E, Chervenick P, Buchman RR, Anderson WF: Hemoglobin McKees Rocks ($\alpha_2\beta_2$145Tyr-Term), a human "nonsense" mutation leading to a shortened β-chain. *Am J Hum Genet* **27**:95, 1975.
160. Baglioni C: The fusion of two peptide chains in hemoglobin Lepore and its interpretation as a genetic deletion. *Proc Natl Acad Sci U S A* **48**:1880, 1962.
161. Barnabus J, Muller CJ: Haemoglobin Lepore (Hollandia). *Nature* **194**:931, 1962.
162. Ostertag W, Smith EW: Hemoglobin Lepore Baltimore, a third type of $\delta\beta$ crossover (δ50, β86). *Eur J Biochem* **10**:371, 1969.
163. Huisman THJ, Wrightstone RN, Wilson JB, Schroeder WA, Kendall AG: Hemoglobin Kenya, the product of fusion of γ and β polypeptide chains. *Arch Biochem Biophys* **153**:850, 1972.
164. Ohta Y, Yamaoka K, Sumida I, et al: Two structural and synthetical variants, Hb Miyada and homozygous δ-thalassaemia, discovered in *Japanese Proceedings of the XIIth International Congress on Haematology* p. 233. Munich, Verlag, 1970.
165. Lehmann H, Charlesworth D: Observations on hemoglobin P (Congo type). *Biochem J* **119**:43, 1970.
166. Honig GR, Mason RG, Tremaine LM, Vida LN: Unbalanced globin chain synthesis by Hb Lincoln Park (anti-Lepore) reticulocytes. *Am J Hematol* **5**:335, 1978.
167. Badr FM, Lorkin PA, Lehmann H: Haemoglobin P-Nilotic containing β-δ chain. *Nat N Biol* **242**:107, 1973.
168. Adams JG, Morrison WT, Steinberg MH: Double crossover within a single human gene. *Science* **218**:291, 1982.
169. Bunn HF: Pathogenesis and treatment of sickle cell disease. *N Engl J Med* **337**:762, 1997.

170. Dover GJ, Platt OS: Sickle cell disease, in Nathan DG, Orkin SH (eds): *Hematology in Infancy & Childhood,* 5th ed., Philadelphia, W.B. Saunders, 1998, p 762.
171. Harris JW: Studies on the destruction of red blood cells. VII. Molecular orientation in sickle cell hemoglobin solutions. *Proc Soc Exp Biol Med* **75**:197, 1950.
172. Edelstein SJ, Telford JN, Crepeau RH: Structures of fibers of sickle cell hemoglobin. *Proc Natl Acad Sci U S A* **70**:1104, 1973.
173. Finch JT, Perutz MF, Bertles JF, Dobler J: Structure of sickled erythrocytes and of sickle-cell hemoglobin fibers. *Proc Natl Acad Sci U S A* **70**:718, 1973.
174. Garrell RL, Crepeau RH, Edelstein SJ: Cross-sectional views of hemoglobin S fibers by electron microscopy and computer modeling. *Proc Natl Acad Sci U S A* **76**:1140, 1979.
175. Dykes G, Crepeau R, Edelstein SJ: Three-dimensional reconstruction of the fibres of sickle cell haemoglobin. *Nature* **272**:506, 1978.
176. Padlan AE, Love WE: Refined crystal structure of deoxyhemoglobin S. *J Biol Chem* **260**:8280, 1985.
177. Cao Z, Liao D, Mirchev R, et al: Nucleation and polymerisation of sickle hemoglobin with Leu88 substituted by Ala. *J Mol Biol* **265**:580, 1997.
178. Wilson WW, Luzzana MR, Penniston JT, Johnson CS: Pregelation aggregation of sickle cell hemoglobin. *Proc Natl Acad Sci U S A* **71**:1260, 1974.
179. Morrat K, Gibson QH: The rates of polymerization and depolymerization of sickle cell hemoglobin. *Biochem Biophys Res Commun* **61**:237, 1974.
180. Williams RC: Concerted formation of the gel of hemoglobin S. *Proc Natl Acad Sci U S A* **70**:1506, 1973.
181. Hofrichter J, Ross PD, Eaton WA: Supersaturation in sickle cell hemoglobin solution. *Proc Natl Acad Sci U S A* **73**:3035, 1976.
182. Ross PD, Hofrichter J, Eaton WA: Calorimetric and optical characterization of sickle cell hemoglobin gelation. *J Mol Biol* **96**:239, 1975.
183. Zipp A, James TL, Kuntz ID, Shohet ID: Water proton magnetic resonance studies of normal and sickle erythrocytes. Temperature and volume dependence. *Biochim Biophys Acta* **428**:291, 1976.
184. Mirchev R, Ferrone FM: The structural link between polymerisation and sickle cell disease. *J Mol Biol* **265**:475, 1997.
185. Eaton WA, Hofrichter J, Ross PD: Delay time in gelation: A possible determinant of clinical severity in sickle cell disease. *Blood* **47**:621, 1976.
186. Noguchi CT, Schechter AN, Rodgers GP: Sickle cell disease pathophysiology. *Baillieres Clin Haematol* **6**:57, 1993.
187. Singer K, Singer L: Studies on abnormal hemoglobins. VIII. The gelling phenomenon of sickle cell hemoglobin: Its biologic and diagnostic significance. *Blood* **8**:1008, 1953.
188. Bertles JF, Dobler J: Reversible and irreversible sickling; a distinction by electron microscopy. *Blood* **33**:884, 1969.
189. Nagel RL: Severity, pathobiology, epistatic effects, and genetic markers in sickle cell anemia. *Semin Hematol* **28**:180, 1991.
190. Canessa M: Red cell volume-related ion transport systems in hemoglobinopathies. *Hematol Oncol Clin North Am* **5**:495, 1991.
191. Hebbel RP, Vercellotti GM: The endothelial biology of sickle cell disease. *J Lab Clin Med* **129**:288, 1997.
192. Kaul DK, Fabry ME, Windisch P, Baez S, Nagel RL: Erythrocytes in sickle cell anemia are heterogeneous in their rheological and hemodynamic characteristics. *J Clin Invest* **72**:22, 1983.
193. Hebbel RP, Schwartz RS, Mohandas N: The adhesive sickle erythrocyte: Cause and consequence of abnormal interactions with endothelium, monocytes, macrophages and model membranes. *Baillieres Clin Haematol* **14**:141, 1985.
194. Hebbel RP, Miller WJ: Phagocytosis of sickle erythrocytes: Immunologic and oxidative determinants of hemolytic anemia. *Blood* **64**:733, 1984.
195. Kuross SA, Hebbel RP: Nonheme iron in sickle erythrocyte membranes: Association with phospholipids and potential role in lipid peroxidation. *Blood* **72**:1278, 1988.
196. Hebbel RP: Auto-oxidation and a membrane-associated "Fenton Reagent": A possible explanation for development of membrane lesions in sickle erythrocytes. *Baillieres Clin Haematol* **14**:129, 1985.
197. Kay MMB, Goodman SR, Sorensen K, et al: Senescent cell antigen is immunologically related to band 3. *Proc Natl Acad Sci U S A* **80**:1631, 1983.
198. Sherwood JB, Goldwasser E, Chilcote E, Carmichael E, Charmichael LD, Nagel RL: Sickle cell anemia patients have low erythropoietin levels for their degree of anemia. *Blood* **67**:46, 1986.
199. Mohandas N, Evans E: Sickle cell adherence to vascular endothelium: Morphologic correlates and the requirement for divalent cations and collagen-binding plasma proteins. *J Clin Invest* **76**:1605, 1985.
200. Serjeant GR: *Sickle Cell Disease*. 2nd ed. Oxford, Oxford University Press, 1992.
201. Rogers DW, Serjeant BE, Serjeant GR: Early rise in "pitted" red cell count as a guide to susceptibility to infection in childhood sickle cell anaemia. *Arch Dis Child* **57**:338, 1982.
202. Zago M, Bottura C: Splenic function in sickle-cell diseases. *Clin Sci* **65**:297, 1983.
203. Rogers DW, Clarke JM, Cupidore L, Ramlal AM, Sparke BR, Serjeant GR: Early deaths in Jamaican children with sickle cell disease. *BMJ* **i**:1515, 1978.
204. Hatton CSR, Bunch C, Weatherall DJ: Hepatic sequestration in sickle cell anaemia. *BMJ* **290**:744, 1985.
205. Davies SC, Luce PJ, Win AA, Riordan JF, Brozovic M: Acute chest syndrome in sickle-cell disease. *Lancet* **i**:36, 1984.
206. Pattison JR, Jones SE, Hodgson J, et al: Parvovirus infections and hypoplastic crises in sickle-cell anaemia. *Lancet* **i**:664, 1981.
207. Powars D, Wilson B, Imbus C, Pegelow C, Allen J: The natural history of stroke in sickle cell disease. *Am J Med* **65**:461, 1978.
208. Mohr JP: Sickle cell anemia, stroke, and transcranial studies. *N Engl J Med* **326**:637, 1992.
209. Rothman SM, Fulling KH, Nelson JS: Sickle cell anemia and central nervous system infarction: A neuropathological study. *Ann Neurol* **20**:684, 1986.
210. Ohene-Frempong K: Stroke in sickle cell disease: Demographic, clinical, and therapeutic considerations. *Semin Hematol* **28**:213, 1991.
211. Powars D, Weidman JA, Odom-Maryon T, Niland JC, Johnson C: Sickle cell chronic lung disease: Prior morbidity and the risk of pulmonary failure. *Medicine (Baltimore)* **67**:66, 1988.
212. Hendrickse RG, Harrison KA, Watson-Williams EJ, Luzzatto L, Ajabor LN: Pregnancy in homozygous sickle-cell anaemia. *J Obstet Gynaecol Br Commonwealth* **79**:396, 1972.
213. Leikin SL, Gallagher D, Kinney TR, Sloane D, Klug P, Rida W: Mortality in children and adolescents with sickle cell disease. *Pediatrics* **84**:500, 1989.
214. Platt OS, Brambilla DJ, Rosse WF et al: Mortality in sickle cell disease. Life expectancy and risk factors for early death. *N Engl J Med* **330**:1639, 1994.
215. Perrine RP, Brown MJ, Clegg JB, Weatherall DJ, May A: Benign sickle-cell anaemia. *Lancet* **ii**:1163, 1972.
216. Kar BC, Satapathy RK, Kulozik AE, et al: Sickle cell disease in Orissa State, India. *Lancet* **ii**:1198, 1986.
217. Powars DR, Weiss JN, Chan LS, Schroeder WA: Is there a threshold level of fetal hemoglobin that ameliorates morbidity in sickle cell anemia. *Blood* **63**:921, 1984.
218. Padmos MA, Roberts GT, SAckey K, et al: Two different forms of homozygous sickle cell disease occur in Saudi Arabia. *Br J Haematol* **79**:93, 1991.
219. Higgs DR, Aldridge BE, Lamb J, et al: The interaction of alpha-thalassemia and homozygous sickle cell disease. *N Engl J Med* **306**:1441, 1982.
220. Noguchi CT, Dover GJ, Rodgers GP, et al: α thalassemia changes erythrocyte heterogeneity in sickle cell disease. *J Clin Invest* **75**:1632, 1985.
221. Higgs DR, Clegg JB, Weatherall DJ, Serjeant BE, Serjeant GR: Interaction of the $\alpha\alpha\alpha$-globin gene haplotype and sickle haemoglobin. *Br J Haematol* **58**:671, 1984.
222. Nagel RL, Lawrence C: The distinct pathobiology of sickle cell-hemoglobin C disease. *Hematol Oncol Clin North Am* **5**:433, 1991.
223. Monplaisir N, Merault G, Poyart C, et al: Hemoglobin S Antilles: A variant with lower solubility than hemoglobin S and producing sickle cell disease in heterozygotes. *Proc Natl Acad Sci U S A* **83**:9363, 1986.
224. Itano HA, Neel JV: A new inherited abnormality of human hemoglobin. *Proc Natl Acad Sci U S A* **36**:613, 1950.
225. Diggs LW, Kraus AO, Morrison DB, Rudnicki RPT: Intra-erythrocyte crystals in a white patient with hemoglobin C in the absence of other types of hemoglobin. *Blood* **9**:1172, 1954.
226. Hirsch RE, Raventos-Suarez C, Olson JA, Nagel RL: Ligand state of intraerythrocyte circulating Hb C crystals in homozygote CC patients. *Blood* **66**:775, 1985.
227. Reiss G, Ranney HM, Shaklai N: The association of hemoglobin C with red cell ghosts. *J Clin Invest* **70**:946, 1982.
228. Vella F, Lehmann H: Haemoglobin D Punjab (D Los Angeles). *J Med Genet* **11**:341, 1974.

229. Hunt JA, Intram VM: Abnormal human haemoglobins. VI. The chemical difference between haemoglobins A and E. *Biochim Biophys Acta* **49**:520, 1961.
230. Traeger J, Wood WG, Clegg JB, Weatherall DJ, Wasi P: Defective synthesis of Hb E is due to reduced levels of β^E mRNA. *Nature* **288**:497, 1980.
231. Orkin SH, Kazazian HH, Antonarakis SE, Ostrer H, Goff SC, Sexton JP: Abnormal RNA processing due to the exon mutation of β^E-globin gene. *Nature* **300**:768, 1982.
232. Wasi P, Na-Nakorn S, Pootrakul S, Sookanek M, Disthasongchan P, Panich V: Alpha- and beta-thalassemia in Thailand. *Ann N Y Acad Sci* **165**:60, 1980.
233. Weatherall DJ, Clegg JB, Na-Nakorn S, Wasi P: The pattern of disordered haemoglobin synthesis in homozygous and heterozygous β-thalassaemia. *Br J Haematol* **16**:251, 1969.
234. Winterbourn CC, Carrell RW: Studies of hemoglobin denaturation and Heinz body formation in the unstable hemoglobins. *J Clin Invest* **54**:678, 1974.
235. Rachmilewitz EA: Denaturation of the normal and abnormal hemoglobin molecule. *Semin Hematol* **11**:441, 1974.
236. Milner PF, Wrightstone RN: The unstable hemoglobins: a review, in Wallach DFH (eds): *The Function of Red Blood Cells: Erythrocyte Pathobiology*. New York, Alan R. Liss, 1981, p 197.
237. Miller DR, Weed RI, Stamatoyannopoulos G, Yoshida A: Hemoglobin Koln disease occurring as a fresh mutation: Erythrocyte metabolism and survival. *Blood* **38**:715, 1971.
238. Flynn TP, Allen DW, Johnson GJ, White JC: Oxidant damage of the lipids and proteins of the erythrocyte membranes in unstable hemoglobin disease. Evidence for the role of lipid peroxidation. *J Clin Invest* **71**:1215, 1983.
239. Charache S, Weatherall DJ, Clegg JB: Polycythemia associated with a hemoglobinopathy. *J Clin Invest* **45**:813, 1966.
240. Charache S: Haemoglobins with altered oxygen affinity. *Baillieres Clin Haematol* **3**:357, 1974.
241. Adamson JW: Familial polycythemia. *Semin Hematol* **12**:383, 1975.
242. Bonaventura J, Riggs A: Hemoglobin Kansas, a human hemoglobin with a neutral amino acid substitution and an abnormal oxygen equilibrium. *J Biol Chem* **243**:980, 1968.
243. Nagel RL, Bookchin RM: Human haemoglobin mutants with abnormal oxygen binding. *Semin Hematol* **11**:385, 1974.
244. Modell CB, Berdoukas VA: *The Clinical Approach to Thalassemia*. New York, Grune and Stratton, 1981.
245. Higgs DR, Vickers MA, Wilkie AOM, Pretorius I-M, Jarman AP, Weatherall DJ: A review of the molecular genetics of the human α-globin gene cluster. *Blood* **73**:1081, 1989.
246. Huisman THJ, Carver MFH, Erol Baysal E: *A Syllabus of Thalassemia Mutations*. Augusta, GA, The Sickle Cell Anemia Foundation, 1997.
247. Kazazian HH: The thalassemia syndromes: Molecular basis and prenatal diagnosis in 1990. *Semin Hematol* **27**:209, 1990.
248. Weatherall DJ: Thalassemia, in Stamatoyannopoulos G, Nienhuis AW, Majerus PW, Varmus H (eds): *The Molecular Basis of Blood Diseases*, 2nd ed. Philadelphia, WB Saunders Co., 1994, p 157.
249. Fessas P: Inclusions of hemoglobin in erythroblasts and erythrocytes of thalassemia. *Blood* **21**:21, 1963.
250. Wickramasinghe SN, Hughes M: Some features of bone marrow macrophages in patients with homozygous β-thalassaemia. *Br J Haematol* **38**:23, 1978.
251. Chalevalakis G, Clegg JB, Weatherall DJ: Imbalanced globin chain synthesis in heterozygous β-thalassemia bone marrow. *Proc Natl Acad Sci U S A* **72**:3853, 1975.
252. Shinar E, Shalev O, Rachmilewitz RA, Schrier SL: Erythrocyte membrane skeleton abnormalities in severe β-thalassemia. *Blood* **70**:158, 1987.
253. Schrier SL, Rachmilewitz EA, Mohandas N: Cellular and membrane properties of alpha and beta thalassemia erythrocytes are different: Implication for differences in clinical manifestations. *Blood* **74**:2194, 1989.
254. Aljurf M, Ma L, Angelucci E, et al: Abnormal assembly of membrane proteins in erythroid progenitors of patients with beta-thalassemia major. *Blood* **87**:2049, 1996.
255. Yuan J, Angelucci E, Lucarelli G, et al: Accelerated programmed cell death (apoptosis) in erythroid precursors of patients with severe beta-thalassemia (Cooley's anemia). *Blood* **82**:374, 1993.
256. Schrier SL: Thalassemia: Pathophysiology of red cell changes. *Ann Rev Med* **45**:211, 1994.
257. Shinar E, Rachmilewitz EA: Oxidative denaturation of red blood cells in thalassemia. *Semin Hematol* **27**:70, 1990.
258. Shinar E, Rachmilewitz EA: Haemoglobinopathies and red cell membrane function. *Clin Haematol* **6**:357, 1993.
259. Yuan J, Angelucci E, Lucarelli G, Aljurf H, Ma L, Schrier SL: Abnormal assembly of membrane proteins in erythroid progenitors of patients with beta thalassemia. *Blood* **80**:18a, 1992.
260. Advani R, Rubin E, Mohandas N, Schrier SL: Oxidative red blood cell membrane injury in the pathophysiology of severe mouse beta-thalassemia. *Blood* **79**:1064, 1992.
261. Schrier SL: Pathobiology of thalassemic erythrocytes. *Curr Opin Hematol* **4**:75, 1997.
262. Rachmilewitz EA, Shinar E, Shalev O, Galili U, Schrier SL: Erythrocyte membrane alterations in beta-thalassaemia. *Clin Haematol* **14**:163, 1985.
263. Gutteridge JMC, Halliwell B: Iron toxicity and oxygen radicals. *Clin Haematol* **2**:195, 1989.
264. Hershko C, Weatherall DJ: Iron-chelating therapy. *Crit Rev Clin Lab Sci* **26**:303, 1988.
265. Weatherall DJ, Pressley L, Wood WG, Higgs DR, Clegg JB: The molecular basis for mild forms of homozygous β thalassaemia. *Lancet* **i**:527, 1981.
266. Wainscoat JS, Old JM, Weatherall DJ, Orkin SH: The molecular basis for the clinical diversity of β thalassaemia in Cypriots. *Lancet* **i**:1235, 1983.
267. Weatherall DJ: Mechanisms for the heterogeneity of the thalassemias. *Int J Pediatr Hematol Oncol* **4**:3, 1997.
268. Higgs DR: α-thalassaemia, in Higgs DR, Weatherall DJ (eds): *Baillière's Clinical Haematology. International Practice and Research: The Haemoglobinopathies*, vol 6 No. 1. London, Baillière Tindall, 1993, p 117.
269. Pressley L, Higgs DR, Clegg JB, Weatherall DJ: Gene deletions in α thalassaemia prove that the $5'$ ζ locus is functional. *Proc Natl Acad Sci U S A* **77**:3586, 1980.
270. Embury SH, Miller JA, Dozy AM, Kan YW, Chan V, Todd D: Two different molecular organizations account for the single α-globin gene of the α-thalassemia-2 genotype. *J Clin Invest* **66**:1319, 1980.
271. Goossens M, Dozy AM, Embury SH, et al: Triplicated α-globin loci in humans. *Proc Natl Acad Sci U S A* **77**:518, 1980.
272. Trent RJ, Higgs DR, Clegg JB, Weatherall DJ: A new triplicated α-globin gene arrangement in man. *Br J Haematol* **49**:149, 1981
273. Lie-Injo LE, Herrera AR, Kan YW: Two types of triplicated α globin loci in humans. *Nucleic Acids Res* **9**:3707, 1981.
274. Gu YC, Landman H, Huisman THJ: Two different quadruplicated α-globin gene arrangements. *Br J Haematol* **66**:245, 1987.
275. Ramsay M, Jenkins T: The $\alpha\alpha\alpha^{anti\text{-}3.7}$ globin haplotype with an additional *Bgl* III site mutation ($\alpha\alpha\alpha^{anti\text{-}3.7}$ *Bgl* II(−)). *Hemoglobin* **9**:385, 1985.
276. Higgs DR, Hill AVS, Bowden DK, Weatherall DJ, Clegg JB: Independent recombination events between duplicated human α-globin genes: Implications for their concerted evolution. *Nucleic Acids Res* **12**:6965, 1984.
277. Powers PA, Smithies O: Short gene conversions in the human fetal globin gene region: A by-product of chromosome pairing during meiosis? *Genetics* **112**:343, 1986.
278. Nathans J, Piantanida TP, Eddy RL, Shows TB, Hogness DS: Molecular genetics of inherited variation in human color vision. *Science* **232**:203, 1986.
279. Taub RA, Hollis GF, Hieter PA, Korsmeyer S, Waldmann TA, Leder P: Variable amplification of immunoglobulin κ light-chain genes in human populations. *Nature* **304**:172, 1983.
280. Lacerra G, Fioretti G, De Angioletti M, et al: $(\alpha)\alpha^{53}$: A novel α+-thalassemia deletion with the breakpoints in the α_2-globin gene and in close proximity to an Alu family repeat between the $\psi\alpha_2$- and $\psi\alpha_1$-globin genes. *Blood* **78**:2740, 1991.
281. Kulozik A, Kar BC, Serjeant BE, Serjeant GR, Weatherall DJ: α-thalassemia in India: Its interaction with sickle cell disease. *Blood* **71**:467, 1988.
282. Orkin SH, Goff SC: The duplicated human α-globin genes: Their relative expression as measured by RNA analysis. *Cell* **24**:345, 1981.
283. Liebhaber SA, Kan YW: Differentiation of the mRNA transcripts originating from the α_1- and α_2-globin loci in normals and α-thalassemics. *J Clin Invest* **68**:439, 1981.
284. Shakin SH, Liebhaber SA: Translational profiles of α_1-, α_2-, and β-globin messenger ribonucleic acids in human reticulocytes. *J Clin Invest* **78**:1125, 1986.
285. Liebhaber SA, Cash FE, Ballas SK: Human α-globin gene expression. The dominant role of the α_2-locus in mRNA and protein synthesis. *J Biol Chem* **261**:15327, 1986.

286. Bowden DK, Hill AVS, Higgs DR, Oppenheimer SJ, Weatherall DJ, Clegg JB: Different hematologic phenotypes are associated with leftward ($-\alpha^{4.2}$) and rightward ($-\alpha^{3.7}$) α^+-thalassemia deletions. *J Clin Invest* **79**:39, 1987.
287. Liebhaber SA, Cash FE, Main DM: Compensatory increase in α_1-globin gene expression in individuals heterozygous for the α-thalassemia-2 deletion. *J Clin Invest* **76**:1057, 1985.
288. Harteveld KL, Losekoot M, Heister AJ, van der Weilen M, Giordano PC, Bernini LF: α-thalassemia in The Netherlands: A heterogeneous spectrum of both deletions and point mutations. *Hum Genet* **100**:465, 1997.
289. Waye JS, Eng B, Chui DHK: Identification of an extensive ζ-α globin gene deletion in a Chinese individual. *Br J Haematol* **80**:378, 1992.
290. Harris PC, Barton NJ, Higgs DR, Reeders ST, Wilkie AOM: A long range restriction map between the α-globin complex and a marker closely linked to the polycystic kidney disease I (PKDI) locus. *Genomics* **7**:195, 1990.
291. Lamb J, Harris PC, Wilkie AOM, Wood WG, Dauwerse JG, Higgs DR: De novo truncation of chromosome 16p and healing with $(TTAGGG)_n$ in the α-thalassemia/mental retardation syndrome (ATR-16). *Am J Hum Genet* **52**:668, 1993.
292. Nicholls RD, Fischel-Ghodsian N, Higgs DR: Recombination at the human α-globin gene cluster: Sequence features and topological constraints. *Cell* **49**:369, 1987.
293. Jelinek WR, Schmid CW: Repetitive sequences in eukaryotic DNA and their expression. *Annu Rev Biochem* **51**:813, 1982.
294. Henthorn PS, Smithies O, Mager DL: Molecular analysis of deletions in the human β-globin gene cluster: Deletion junctions and locations of breakpoints. *Genomics* **6**:226, 1990.
295. Higgs DR, Ayyub H, Clegg JB, et al: α-thalassaemia in British people. *BMJ* **290**:1303, 1985.
296. Bhavnani M, Wickham M, Ayyub H, Higgs DR: α-thalassaemia in the North West of England. *Clin Lab Haematol* **11**:293, 1989.
297. Chung S-W, Wong SC, Clarke BJ, Patterson M, Walker WHC, Chui DHK: Human embryonic ζ-globin chains in adult patients with α-thalassemias. *Proc Natl Acad Sci U S A* **81**:6188, 1984.
298. Chui DHK, Wong SC, Chung S-W, Patterson M, Bhargava S, Poon M-C: Embryonic ζ-globin chains in adults: A marker for α-thalassemia-1 haplotype due to a $>$17.5-kb deletion. *N Engl J Med* **314**:76, 1986.
299. Strauss EC, Andrews NC, Higgs DR, Orkin SH: *In vivo* footprinting of the human α-globin locus upstream regulatory element by guanine/adenine ligation-mediated PCR. *Mol Cell Biol* **12**:2135, 1992.
300. Flint J, Rochette J, Craddock CF, et al: Chromosomal stabilisation by a subtelomeric rearrangement involving two closely related *Alu* elements. *Hum Mol Genet* **5**:1163, 1996.
301. Flint J, Craddock CF, Villegas A et al: Healing of broken human chromosomes by the addition of telomeric repeats. *Am J Hum Genet* **55**:505, 1994.
302. Blackburn EH: Telomerases. *Annu Rev Biochem* **61**:113, 1992.
303. Felbar BK, Orkin SH, Hamer DH: Abnormal RNA splicing causes one form of α-thalassemia. *Cell* **29**:895, 1982.
304. Orkin SH, Goff SC, Hechtman RL: Mutation in an intervening sequence splice junction in man. *Proc Natl Acad Sci U S A* **78**:5041, 1981.
305. Harteveld CL, Heister JGAM, Giordano PC, et al: An IVS-1-116 (A $\rightarrow$ G) acceptor splice site mutation in the α_2-globin gene causing α^+-thalassemia in two Dutch families. *Br J Haematol* **95**:461, 1996.
306. Çürük MA, Baysal E, Gupta RB, Huisman THJ: An IVS-I-117 (G $\rightarrow$ A) acceptor splice site mutation in the α1-globin gene is a nondeletional α-thalassaemia-2 determinant in an Indian population. *Br J Haematol* **85**:148, 1993.
307. Pressley L, Higgs DR, Clegg JB, Perrine RP, Pembrey ME, Weatherall DJ: A new genetic basis for hemoglobin-H disease. *N Engl J Med* **303**:1383, 1980.
308. Al-Awamy BH: Thalassemic syndromes in Saudi Arabia. *Saudi Med* **21**:8, 2000.
309. Thein SL, Wallace RB, Pressley L, Clegg JB, Weatherall DJ, Higgs DR: The polyadenylation site mutation in the α-globin gene cluster. *Blood* **71**:313, 1988.
310. Molchanova TP, Smetanina NS, Huisman THJ: A second, elongated, α_2-globin mRNA is present in reticulocytes from normal persons and subjects with terminating codon or poly A mutations. *Biochem Biophys Res Commun* **214**:1184, 1995.
311. Fei YJ, Liu JC, Walker ELDI, Huisman THJ: A new gene deletion involving the α_2-, α_1-, and θ_1-globin genes in a Black family with Hb H disease. *Am J Hematol* **39**:299, 1992.
312. Yüregir GT, Aksoy K, Curuk MA, et al: Hb H disease in a Turkish family resulting from the interaction of a deletional α-thalassaemia-1 and a newly discovered poly A mutation. *Br J Haematol* **80**:527, 1992.
313. Olivieri NF, Chang LS, Poon AO, Michelson AM, Orkin SH: An α-globin gene initiation codon mutation in a Black family with Hb H disease. *Blood* **70**:729, 1987.
314. Morlé F, Lopez B, Henni T, Godet J: α-thalassaemia associated with the deletion of two nucleotides at position -2 and -3 preceding the AUG codon. *EMBO J* **4**:1245, 1985.
315. Morlé F, Starck J, Godet J: α-thalassemia due to the deletion of nucleotides -2 and -3 preceding the AUG initiation codon affects translation efficiency both *in vitro* and *in vivo*. *Nucleic Acids Res* **14**:3279, 1986.
316. Tabone P, Henni T, Belhani M, Colonna P, Verdier G, Godet J: Hemoglobin H disease from Algeria: Genetic and molecular characterisation. *Acta Haematol* **65**:26, 1981.
317. Galanello R, Aru B, Dessì C et al: Hb H disease in Sardinia: Molecular, haematological and clinical aspects. *Acta Haematol* **88**:1, 1992.
318. Cao A, Rosatelli C, Pirastu M, Galanello R: Thalassemias in Sardinia: Molecular pathology, phenotype-genotype correlation and prevention. *Am J Pediatr Hematol Oncol* **13**:179, 1991.
319. Moi P, Cash FE, Liebhaber SA, Cao A, Pirastu M: An initiation codon mutation (AUG $\rightarrow$ GUG) of the human α_1-globin gene: Structural characterization and evidence for a mild thalassemia phenotype. *J Clin Invest* **80**:1416, 1987.
320. Safaya S, Rieder RF: Dysfunctional α-globin gene in hemoglobin H disease in blacks. *J Biol Chem* **263**:4328, 1988.
321. Ayala S, Colomer D, Aymerich M, Abella E, Vives Corrons JL: First description of a frameshift mutation in the α_1-globin gene associated with α-thalassaemia. *Br J Haematol* **98**:47, 1997.
322. Hunt DM, Higgs DR, Winichagoon P, Clegg JB, Weatherall DJ: Haemoglobin Constant Spring has an unstable α chain messenger RNA. *Br J Haematol* **51**:405, 1982.
323. Weiss IM, Liebhaber SA: Erythroid cell-specific determinants of α-globin mRNA stability. *Mol Cell Biol* **14**:8123, 1994.
324. Lie-Injo LE, Ganesan J, Clegg JB, Weatherall DJ: Homozygous state for Hb Constant Spring (slow moving Hb X components). *Blood* **43**:251, 1974.
325. de Jong WW, Khan PM, Bernini LF: Hemoglobin Koya Dora: High frequency of a chain termination mutant. *Am J Hum Genet* **27**:81, 1975.
326. Pirastu M, Saglio G, Chang JC, Cao A, Kan YW: Initiation codon mutation as a cause of α-thalassemia. *J Biol Chem* **259**:12315, 1984.
327. Thein SL, Wallace RB, Pressley L, Clegg JB, Weatherall DJ, Higgs DR: Phenotypic expression of the polyadenylation site mutation in the α-globin gene cluster. *Blood* **71**:313, 1988.
328. Henni T, Morlé F, Lopez B, Colonna P, Godet J: α-thalassemia haplotypes in the Algerian population. *Hum Genet* **75**:272, 1987.
329. Kattamis C, Tzotzos S, Kanavakis E, Synodinos J, Metaxotou-Mavrommati A: Correlation of clinical phenotype to genotype in haemoglobin H disease. *Lancet* **i**:442, 1988.
330. Galanello R, Pirastu M, Melis MA, Paglietti E, Moi P, Cao A: Phenotype-genotype correlation in haemoglobin H disease in childhood. *J Med Genet* **20**:425, 1983.
331. Fucharoen S, Winichagoon P, Pootrakul P, Piankijagum A, Wasi P: Differences between two types of Hb H disease, α-thalassemia 1/α-thalassemia 2 and α-thalassemia 1/Hb Constant Spring. *Birth Defects: Orig Article Ser* **23**:309, 1988.
332. George E, Ferguson V, Yakas J, Kronenberg H, Trent RJ: A molecular marker associated with mild hemoglobin H disease. *Pathology* **21**:27, 1989.
333. Winichagoon P, Higgs DR, Goodbourn SEY, Clegg JB, Weatherall DJ, Wasi P: The molecular basis of α-thalassaemia in Thailand. *EMBO J* **3**:1813, 1984.
334. Chan V, Chan TK, Liang ST, Ghosh A, Kan YW, Todd D: Hydrops fetalis due to an unusual form of Hb H disease. *Blood* **66**:224, 1985.
335. Chan V, Chan VWY, Tang M, Lau K, Todd D, Chan TK: Molecular defects in Hb H hydrops fetalis. *Br J Haematol* **96**:224, 1997.
336. Trent RJ, Wilkinson T, Yakas J, Carter J, Lammi A, Kronenberg H: Molecular defects in 2 examples of severe HbH disease. *Scand J Haematol* **36**:272, 1986.
337. Ko T-M, Hsieh F-J, Hsu P-M, Lee T-Y: Molecular characterization of severe α-thalassemias causing hydrops fetalis in Taiwan. *Am J Med Genet* **39**:317, 1990.

338. Isarangkura P, Siripoonya P, Fucharoen S, Hathirat P: Hemoglobin Bart's disease without hydrops manifestation. *Birth Defects: Orig Article Ser* **23**:333, 1987,
339. Chui DHK, Waye JS: Hydrops fetalis caused by α-thalassemia: An emerging health care problem. *Blood* **91**:2213, 1998.
340. Weatherall DJ, Higgs DR, Bunch C, et al: Hemoglobin H disease and mental retardation. A new syndrome or a remarkable coincidence? *N Engl J Med* **305**:607, 1981.
341. Wilkie AOM, Buckle VJ, Harris PC, et al: Clinical features and molecular analysis of the α thalassaemia/mental retardation syndromes. I. Cases due to deletions involving chromosome band 16p13.3. *Am J Hum Genet* **46**:1112, 1990.
342. Wilkie AOM, Zeitlin HC, Lindenbaum RH, et al: Clinical features and molecular analysis of the α thalassaemia/mental retardation syndromes. II. Cases without detectable abnormality of the α globin complex. *Am J Hum Genet* **46**:1127, 1990.
343. Lamb J, Wilkie AOM, Harris PC, et al: Detection of breakpoints in submicroscopic chromosomal translocation, illustrating an important mechanism for genetic disease. *Lancet* **ii**:819, 1989.
344. Gibbons RJ, Picketts DJ, Villard L, Higgs DR: Mutations in a putative global transcriptional regulator cause X-linked mental retardation with α-thalassemia (ATR-X syndrome). *Cell* **80**:837, 1995.
345. Picketts DJ, Higgs DR, Bachoo S, Blake DJ, Quarrell OWJ, Gibbons RJ: *ATRX* encodes a novel member of the SNF2 family of proteins: Mutations point to a common mechanism underlying the ATR-X syndrome. *Hum Mol Genet* **5**:1899, 1996.
346. Gibbons RJ, Bachoo S, Picketts DJ, et al: Mutations in a transcriptional regulator (hATRX) establish the functional significance of a PHD-like domain. *Nat Genet* **17**:146, 1997.
347. Bennett JM, Catovsky D, Daniel MT, et al: Proposals for the classification of the myelodysplastic syndromes. *Br J Haematol* **51**:189, 1982.
348. Craddock CF. *Normal and Abnormal Regulation of Human α Globin Expression*. Oxford, University of Oxford, 1994.
349. Higgs DR, Wood WG, Barton C, Weatherall DJ: Clinical features and molecular analysis of acquired Hb H disease. *Am J Med* **75**:181, 1983.
350. Thein SL, Old JM, Wainscoat JS, Petrou M, Modell B: Population and genetic studies suggest a single origin the for the Indian deletion β^o thalassaemia. *Br J Haematol* **57**:271, 1984.
351. Gilman JG, Huisman THJ, Abels J: Dutch β^o-thalassaemia: A 10-kilobase DNA deletion associated with significant γ-chain production. *Br J Haematol* **56**:339, 1984.
352. Padanilam BJ, Felice AE, Huisman THJ: Partial deletion of the 5′ β globin gene region causes β^o thalassemia in members of an American black family. *Blood* **64**:941, 1984.
353. Popovich BW, Rosenblatt DS, Kendall AG, Nishioka Y: Molecular characterization of an atypical β-thalassemia caused by a large deletion in the 5′ β-globin gene region. *Am J Hum Genet* **39**:797, 1986.
354. Diaz-Chico JC, Yang KG, Kutlar A, Reese AL, Aksoy M, Huisman THJ: A 300-bp deletion involving part of the 5′ β-globin gene region is observed in members of a Turkish family with β-thalassemia. *Blood* **70**:583, 1987.
355. Anand R, Boehm CD, Kazazian HH, Vanin EF: Molecular characterization of a β^o-thalassemia resulting from a 1.4-kb deletion. *Blood* **72**:636, 1988.
356. Aulehla-Scholtz C, Spielberg R, Horst J: A β-thalassemia mutant caused by a 300-bp deletion in the human β-globin gene. *Hum Genet* **81**:298, 1989.
357. Orkin SH, Sexton JP, Cheng TC, et al: TATA box transcription mutation in β-thalassemia. *Nucleic Acids Res* **11**:4727, 1983.
358. Antonarakis SE, Orkin SH, Cheng T-C, et al: β-Thalassemia in American blacks: Novel mutations in the TATA box and IVS-2 acceptor splice site. *Proc Natl Acad Sci U S A* **81**:1154, 1984.
359. Gonzalez-Redondo JH, Stoming TA, Kutlar A et al: A C→T substitution at nt −101 in a conserved DNA sequence of the promoter region of the β-globin gene is associated with "silent" β-thalassemia. *Blood* **73**:1705, 1989.
360. Kazazian HH, Orkin SH, Antonarakis SE et al: Molecular characterization of seven β-thalassemia mutations in Asian Indians. *EMBO J* **3**:593, 1984.
361. Tamagnini GP, Lopes MC, Castanheira ME, Wainscoat JS, Wood WG: β^+ thalassaemia—Portuguese type: clinical, haematological and molecular studies of a newly defined form of β thalassaemia. *Br J Haematol* **54**:189, 1983.
362. Cheng T, Orkin SH, Antonarakis SE, et al: β-Thalassemia in Chinese: Use of *in vivo* RNA analysis and oligonucleotide hybridization in systematic characterization of molecular defects. *Proc Natl Acad Sci U S A* **81**:2821, 1984.
363. Gonzalez-Redondo JH, Stoming TA, Lanclos KD, et al: Clinical and genetic heterogeneity in Black patients with homozygous β-thalassemia from the southeastern United States. *Blood* **72**:1007, 1988.
364. Hill AVS, Bowden DK, O'Shaughnessy DF, Weatherall DJ, Clegg JB: β-Thalassemia in Melanesia: Association with malaria and characterization of a common variant. *Blood* **72**:9, 1988.
365. Lapoumeroulie C, Pagnier J, Bank A, Labie D, Kirshnamoorthy R: β-Thalassemia due to a novel mutation in IVS-1 sequence donor site consensus sequence creating a restriction site. *Biochem Biophys Res Commun* **139**:709, 1986.
366. Goldsmith ME, Humphries RK, Bey T, Cline A, Kantor JA, Nienhuis AW: "Silent" nucleotide substitution in β^+ thalassemia globin gene activated splice site in coding sequence RNA. *Proc Natl Acad Sci U S A* **88**:2318, 1983.
367. Yang KG, Kutlar F, George E, et al: Molecular characterization of β-globin gene mutations in Malay patients with Hb E-β-thalassaemia major. *Br J Haematol* **72**:73, 1989.
368. Orkin SH, Antonarakis SE, Loukopoulos D: Abnormal processing of β Knossos RNA. *Blood* **64**:311, 1984.
369. Spritz RA, Jagadeeswaran P, Choudary PV, et al: Base substitution in an intervening sequence of a β^+ thalassemic human globin gene. *Proc Natl Acad Sci U S A* **78**:2455, 1981.
370. Busslinger M, Moschanas N, Flavell RA: β^+ thalassemia: Aberrant splicing results from a single point mutation in an intron. *Cell* **27**:289, 1981.
371. Wong C, Antonarakis SE, Goff SC, Orkin SH, Gowhm CD, Kazazian HH Jr: On the origin and spread of β-thalassemia: Recurrent observation of four mutations in different ethnic groups. *Proc Natl Acad Sci U S A* **83**:6529, 1986.
372. Jankovic L, Efremov GD, Petkov G, et al: Three novel mutations leading to β-thalassemia. *Blood* **74**:226A, 1989.
373. Rund D, Filon D, Rachmilewitz EA et al: Molecular analysis of β-thalassemia in Kurdish Jews: Novel mutations and expression studies. *Blood* **74**:821A, 1989.
374. Chang JC, Kan YW: β^o thalassemia, a nonsense mutation in man. *Proc Natl Acad Sci U S A* **76**:2886, 1979.
375. Trecartin RF, Liebhaber SA, Chang JC et al: β Thalassemia in Sardinia is caused by a nonsense mutation. *J Clin Invest* **68**:1012, 1981.
376. Takeshita K, Forget BG, Scarpa A, Benz EJ: Intranuclear defect in β globin mRNA accumulation to a premature termination codon. *Blood* **64**:13, 1984.
377. Thein SL, Hesketh C, Taylor P et al: Molecular basis for dominantly inherited inclusion body β thalassemia. *Proc Natl Acad Sci U S A* **87**:3924, 1990.
378. Kazazian HH, Dowling CE, Hurwitz RL, Coleman M, Adams JGI: Thalassemia mutations in exon 3 of the β-globin gene often cause a dominant form of thalassemia and show no predilection for malarial-endemic regions of the world. *Am J Hum Genet* **45**:A242, 1989.
379. Weatherall DJ, Clegg JB, Knox-Macaulay HHM, Bunch C, Hopkins CR, Temperley IJ: A genetically determined disorder with features both of thalassaemia and congenital dyserythropoietic anaemia. *Br J Haematol* **24**:681, 1973.
380. Stamatoyannopoulos G, Woodson R, Papayannopoulou T, Heywood D, Kurachi MS: A form of β thalassemia producing clinical manifestations in simple heterozygotes. *N Engl J Med* **290**:939, 1974.
381. Bollekens JA, Forget BG: δβ thalassemia and hereditary persistence of fetal hemoglobin. *Hematol Oncol Clin North Am* **5**:399, 1991.
382. Jones RW, Old JM, Trent RJ, Clegg JB, Weatherall DJ: Major rearrangement in the human β-globin gene cluster. *Nature* **291**:39, 1981.
383. Jennings MW, Jones RW, Wood WG, Weatherall DJ: Analysis of an inversion within the human beta globin gene cluster. *Nucleic Acids Res* **13**:2897, 1985.
384. Kutlar A, Gardiner MB, Headlee MG et al: Heterogeneity in the molecular basis of three types of hereditary persistence of fetal hemoglobin and the relative synthesis of the $^G\gamma$ and $^A\gamma$ types of γ chain. *Biochem Genet* **22**:21, 1984.
385. Wainscoat JS, Old JM, Wood WG: Characterization of an Indian $(\delta\beta)^o$ thalassemia. *Br J Haematol* **58**:353, 1984.
386. Poncz M, Henthorn P, Stoeckert C, Surrey S: Globin gene expression in hereditary persistence of fetal haemoglobin and $(\delta\beta)^o$ thalassemia, in MacLean N (ed): *Oxford Surveys on Eukaryotic Genes*, vol 5. Oxford, Oxford University Press, 1988, p 163.
387. Orkin SH, Goff SC, Nathan DG: Heterogeneity of the DNA deletion in gamma-delta-beta thalassemia. *J Clin Invest* **67**: 878, 1981.

388. Van Der Ploeg LHT, Konings A, Cort M, Roos D, Bernini L, Flavell RA: $\gamma\delta\beta$-thalassaemia studies showing that deletion of the γ- and δ-genes influence β-globin gene expression in man. *Nature* **283**:637, 1980.
389. Taramelli R, Kioussis D, Vanin E, et al: $\gamma\delta\beta$-thalassaemias 1 and 2 are the result of a 100-kbp deletion in the human β-globin cluster. *Nucleic Acids Res* **14**:7017, 1986.
390. Curtin P, Pirastu M, Kan YW, Gobert-Jones JA, Stephens AD, Lehmann H: A distant gene deletion affects β-globin gene function in an atypical $\gamma\delta\beta$-thalassemia. *J Clin Invest* **76**:1554, 1985.
391. Wood WG: Increased HbF in adult life, in Higgs DR, Weatherall DJ (eds): *Baillière's Clinical Haematology: The Haemoglobinopathies*, vol. 6 No 1. London, Baillière Tindall, 1993, p 177.
392. Feingold EA, Forget BG: The breakpoint of a large deletion causing hereditary persistence of fetal hemoglobin occurs within an erythroid DNA domain remote from the β-globin gene cluster. *Blood* **74**:2178, 1989.
393. Arcasoy MO, Romana M, Fabry ME, Skarpidi E, Nagel RL, Forget BG: High levels of human γ-globin gene expression in adult mice carrying a transgene of deletion-type hereditary persistence of fetal hemoglobin. *Mol Cell Biol* **17**:2076, 1997.
394. Collins FS, Stoeckert CJ, Serjeant GR, Forget BG, Weissman SM: ${}^{G}\gamma\beta^{+}$ Hereditary persistence of fetal hemoglobin: Cosmid cloning and identification of a specific mutation 5′ to the ${}^{G}\gamma$ gene. *Proc Natl Acad Sci U S A* **81**:4894, 1984.
395. Giglioni B, Casini C, Mantovani R, et al: A molecular study of a family with Greek hereditary persistence of fetal hemoglobin and β-thalassemia. *EMBO J* **3**:2641, 1984.
396. Collins FS, Metherall JE, Yamakawa M, Pan J, Weissman SM, Forget BG: A point mutation in the ${}^{A}\gamma$-globin gene promoter in Greek hereditary persistence of fetal haemoglobin. *Nature* **313**:325, 1985.
397. Gelinas R, Endlich B, Pfeiffer C, Yagi M, Stamatoyannopoulos G: G to A substitution in the distal CCAAT box of the ${}^{A}\gamma$ globin gene in Greek hereditary persistence of fetal haemoglobin. *Nature* **313**:323, 1985.
398. Tate VE, Wood WG, Weatherall DJ: The British form of hereditary persistence of fetal haemoglobin results from a single base mutation adjacent to an S1 hypersensitive site 5′ to the ${}^{A}\gamma$ globin gene. *Blood* **68**:1389, 1986.
399. Ronchi A, Berry M, Raguz S, et al: Role of the duplicated CCAAT box region in γ-globin gene regulation and hereditary persistence of fetal haemoglobin. *EMBO J* **15**:143, 1996.
400. Craig JE, Rochette J, Sampietro M, et al: Genetic heterogeneity in heterocellular hereditary persistence of fetal hemoglobin. *Blood* **90**:428, 1997.
401. Craig JE, Rochette J, Fisher CA, et al: Dissecting the loci controlling fetal haemoglobin production on chromosomes 11p and 6q by the regressive approach. *Nat Genet* **12**:58, 1996.
402. Miyoshi K, Kaneto Y, Kawai H, et al: X-linked dominant control of F-cells in normal adult life: Characterization of the Swiss type as hereditary persistence of fetal hemoglobin regulated dominantly by gene(s) on X chromosome. *Blood* **72**:1854, 1988.
403. Dover GJ, Smith KD, Chang YC, et al: Fetal hemoglobin levels in sickle cell disease and normal individuals are partially controlled by an X-linked gene located at Xp22.2. *Blood* **80**:816, 1992.
404. Ottolenghi S, Giglioni B, Pulazzini A, et al: Sardinian $\delta\beta^{o}$-thalassemia: A further example of a C to T substitution at position −196 of the ${}^{A}\gamma$ globin gene cluster. *Blood* **69**:1058, 1987.
405. Wainscoat JS, Thein SL, Wood WG et al: A novel deletion in the β globin gene complex. *Ann N Y Acad Sci* **445**:20, 1985.
406. Kulozik A, Yarwood N, Jones RW: The Corfu $\delta\beta^{o}$ thalassemia: A small deletion acts at a distance to selectively abolish β globin gene expression. *Blood* **71**:457, 1988.
407. Camaschella C, Cappellini MD: Thalassemia intermedia. *Haematologica* **80**:58, 1995.
408. Rund D, Oron-Karni V, Filon D, Goldfarb A, Rachmilewitz E, Oppenheim A: Genetic analysis of β-thalassemia intermedia in Israel: Diversity of mechanisms and unpredictability of phenotype. *Am J Hematol* **54**:16, 1997.
409. Kattamis C, Metaxatou-Mavromati A, Wood WG, Nash JR, Weatherall DJ: The heterogeneity of normal Hb A_2-β thalassaemia in Greece. *Br J Haematol* **42**:109, 1979.
410. Fessas P, Loukopoulos D, Loutradi-Anagnostou A, Komes G: "Silent" β thalassemia caused by a "silent" β chain mutant: The pathogenesis of a syndrome of thalassemia intermedia. *Br J Haematol* **51**:577, 1982.
411. Olds RJ, Sura T, Jackson B, Wonke B, Hoffbrand AV, Thein SL: A novel δ^{o} mutation in *cis* with Hb Knossos: A study of different interactions in three Egyptian families. *Br J Haematol* **78**:430, 1991.
412. Pirastu M, Ristaldi MS, Loudianos G, et al: Molecular analysis of atypical β-thalassemia heterozygotes. *Ann N Y Acad Sci* **612**:90, 1990.
413. Fearon EF, Kazazian HH, Waber PG et al: The entire β-globin gene cluster is deleted in a form of $\gamma\delta\beta$-thalassemia. *Blood* **61**:1269, 1983.
414. Pirastu M, Kan YW, Lin CC, Baine R, Holbrook CT: Hemolytic disease of the newborn caused by a new deletion of the entire β-globin cluster. *J Clin Invest* **72**:602, 1983.
415. Orkin SH, Goff SC, Nathan DG: Heterogeneity of DNA deletion in $\gamma\delta\beta$-thalassemia. *J Clin Invest* **67**:878, 1981.
416. Kan YW, Forget BG, Nathan DG: Gamma-beta thalassemia: A cause of hemolytic disease of the newborn. *N Engl J Med* **286**:129, 1972.
417. Sampietro M, Cazzola M, Cappellini MD, Fiorelli G: The triplicated alpha-gene locus and heterozygous beta thalassaemia: A case of thalassaemia intermedia. *Br J Haematol* **55**:709, 1983.
418. Kulozik AE, Thein SL, Wainscoat JS, et al: Thalassaemia intermedia; interaction of the triple α-globin gene arrangement and heterozygous β-thalassaemia. *Br J Haematol* **66**:109, 1987.
419. Camaschella C, Bertero MT, Serra A, et al: A benign form of thalassaemia intermedia may be determined by the interaction of triplicated α locus and heterozygous β thalassaemia. *Br J Haematol* **66**:103, 1987.
420. Efremov GD: Hemoglobins Lepore and anti-Lepore. *Hemoglobin* **2**:197, 1978.
421. Wood WG, Clegg JB, Weatherall DJ: Hereditary persistence of fetal haemoglobin (HPFH) and $\delta\beta$-thalassaemia. *Br J Haematol* **43**:509, 1979.
422. Trent RJ, Jones RW, Clegg JB, Weatherall DJ: $({}^{A}\gamma\delta\beta)^{o}$ thalassaemia: Similarity of phenotype in four different molecular defects, including one newly described. *Br J Haematol* **57**:279, 1984.
423. Kendall AG, Ojwang PJ, Schroeder WA, Huisman THJ: Hemoglobin Kenya, the product of a γ-β fusion gene: Studies of the family. *Am J Hum Genet* **25**:548, 1973.
424. Smith DH, Clegg JB, Weatherall DJ, Gilles HM: Hereditary persistence of foetal haemoglobin associated with a $\gamma\beta$ fusion variant, Haemoglobin Kenya. *Nat New Biol* **246**:184, 1973.
425. Nute PE, Wood WG, Stamatoyannopoulos G, Olweny C, Fialkow PJ: The Kenya form of hereditary persistence of fetal haemoglobin; Structural studies and evidence for homogeneous distribution of haemoglobin F using fluorescent anti-haemoglobin F antibodies. *Br J Haematol* **32**:55, 1976.
426. Huisman THJ, Miller A, Schroeder WA: A ${}^{G}\gamma$ type of hereditary persistence of fetal hemoglobin with β chain production in *cis*. *Am J Hum Genet* **27**:765, 1975.
427. Friedman S, Schwartz E: Hereditary persistence of foetal haemoglobin with β-chain synthesis in *cis* position (${}^{G}\gamma$-β^{+}-HPFH) in a Negro family. *Nature* **259**:138, 1976.
428. Higgs DR, Clegg JB, Wood WG, Weatherall DJ: ${}^{G}\gamma\beta^{+}$ Type of hereditary persistence of fetal haemoglobin in association with Hb C. *J Med Genet* **16**:288, 1979.
429. Fessas P, Stamatoyannopoulos G: Hereditary persistence of fetal hemoglobin in Greece. A study and a comparison. *Blood* **24**:223, 1964.
430. Clegg JB, Metaxatou-Mavromati A, Kattamis C, Sofroniadou K, Wood WG, Weatherall DJ: Occurrence of ${}^{G}\gamma$ Hb F in Greek HPFH: Analysis of heterozygotes and compound heterozygotes with β thalassaemia. *Br J Haematol* **43**:521, 1979.
431. Camaschella C, Oggiano L, Sampietro M, et al: The homozygous state of G to A −117 ${}^{A}\gamma$ hereditary persistence of fetal hemoglobin. *Blood* **73**:1999, 1989.
432. Weatherall DJ, Cartner R, Clegg JB, Wood WG, Macrae I, Mackenzie A: A form of hereditary persistence of fetal haemoglobin characterised by uneven cellular distribution of haemoglobin F and the production of haemoglobins A and A_2 in homozygotes. *Br J Haematol* **29**:205, 1975.
433. Wood WG, Macrae IA, Darbre PD, Clegg JB, Weatherall DJ: The British type of non-deletion HPFH: Characterisation of developmental changes *in vivo* and erythroid growth *in vitro*. *Br J Haematol* **50**:401, 1982.
434. Marti HR: *Normale und Abnormale Menschliche Haemoglobine*. Berlin, Springer Verlag, 1963.
435. Zago MA, Wood WG, Clegg JB, Weatherall DJ, O'Sullivan M, Gunson HH: Genetic control of F-cells in human adults. *Blood* **53**:977, 1979.
436. Cappellini MD, Fiorelli G, Bernini LF: Interaction between homozygous β^{o} thalassaemia and the Swiss type of hereditary persistence of fetal haemoglobin. *Br J Haematol* **48**:561, 1981.
437. Gilman JG, Huisman THJ: DNA sequence variation associated with elevated fetal ${}^{G}\gamma$ globin production. *Blood* **66**:783, 1985.

438. Thein SL, Sampietro M, Old JM, et al: Association of thalassaemia intermedia with a beta-globin gene haplotype. *Br J Haematol* **65**:370, 1987.
439. Thein SL, Hesketh C, Wallace RB, Weatherall DJ: The molecular basis of thalassaemia major and thalassaemia intermedia in Asian Indians: Application to prenatal diagnosis. *Br J Haematol* **70**:225, 1988.
440. Diaz-Chico JC, Yang KG, Stoming TA, et al: Mild and severe β-thalassaemia among homozygotes from Turkey: Identification of the types by hybridization of amplified DNA with synthetic probes. *Blood* **71**:248, 1988.
441. Kulozik AE, Wainscoat JS, Serjeant GR, et al: Geographical survey of β^S-globin gene haplotypes: Evidence for an independent Asian origin of the sickle-cell mutation. *Am J Hum Genet* **39**:239, 1986.
442. Nagel RL, Fabry ME, Pagnier J, et al: Hematologically and genetically distinct forms of sickle cell anemia in Africa. *N Engl J Med* **312**:880, 1985.
443. Labie D, Dunda-Belkhodja O, Rouabhi F, Pagnier J, Ragusa A, Nagel RL: The −158 site 5′ to the $^G\gamma$ gene and $^G\gamma$ expression. *Blood* **66**:1463, 1987.
444. Kulozik AE, Kar BC, Satapathy RK, Serjeant BE, Serjeant GR, Weatherall DJ: Fetal hemoglobin levels and β^S globin haplotypes in an Indian population with sickle cell disease. *Blood* **69**:1742, 1987.
445. Kulozik AE, Thein SL, Kar BC, Wainscoat JS, Serjeant GR, Weatherall DJ: Raised Hb F levels in sickle cell disease are caused by a determinant linked to the β globin gene cluster, in Stamatoyannopoulos G (ed): *Hemoglobin Switching*, vol 5. New York, Alan R. Liss, 1987, p 427.
446. Oner C, Dimovski AJ, Altay C, et al: Sequence variations in the 5′ hypervariable site-2 of the locus control region of β^S chromosomes are associated with different levels of fetal globin in hemoglobin S homozygotes. *Blood* **79**:813, 1992.
447. Wainscoat JS, Kanavakis E, Wood WG, et al: Thalassaemia intermedia in Cyprus—the interaction of α- and β-thalassaemia. *Br J Haematol* **53**:411, 1983.
448. Wainscoat JS, Bell JI, Old JM, et al: Globin gene mapping studies in Sardinian patients homozygous for β^o thalassaemia. *Mol Biol Med* **1**:1, 1983.
449. Galanello R, Dessi E, Melis MA, et al: Molecular analysis of β^o-thalassemia intermedia in Sardinia. *Blood* **74**:823, 1989.
450. Kanavakis E, Wainscoat JS, Wood WG, et al: The interaction of α thalassaemia with heterozygous β thalassaemia. *Br J Haematol* **52**:465, 1982.
451. Rosatelli C, Falchi AM, Scalas MT, Tuveri T, Furbetta M, Cao A: Hematological phenotype of double heterozygous state for alpha and beta thalassemia. *Hemoglobin* **8**:25, 1984.
452. Kanavakis E, Metaxatous-Mavromati A, Kattamis C, Wainscoat JS, Wood WG: The triplicated α gene locus and β thalassaemia. *Br J Haematol* **54**:201, 1983.
453. Galanello R, Ruggeri R, Paglietti E, Addis M, Melis A, Cao A: A family with segregating triplicated alpha globin loci and beta thalassemia. *Blood* **62**:1035, 1983.
454. Acuto S, Buttice G, Saitta B, et al: $\alpha\alpha\alpha^{anti\text{-}4.2}$ Haplotype and heterozygous β^o thalassemia in a Sicilian family. *Hum Genet* **70**:31, 1985.
455. Thein SL, Al-Hakin I, Hoffbrand AV: Thalassaemia intermedia—A new molecular basis. *Br J Haematol* **56**:333, 1984.
456. Livingstone FB: *Frequencies of Hemoglobin Variants*. New York, Oxford University Press, 1985.
457. Kan YW, Dozy AM: Evolution of the hemoglobin S and C genes in world populations. *Science* **209**:388, 1980.
458. Mears JG, Lachman HM: Sickle gene: Its origin and diffusion from West Africa. *J Clin Invest* **68**:606, 1981.
459. Antonarakis SE, Boehm CD, Serjeant GR, Theisen CE, Dover GJ, Kazazian HH: Origin of the β^S-globin gene in blacks: The contribution of recurrent mutation or gene conversion or both. *Proc Natl Acad Sci U S A* **81**:853, 1984.
460. Wainscoat JS, Bell JI, Thein SL, et al: Multiple origins of the sickle mutation: Evidence from β^S globin gene cluster polymorphisms. *Mol Biol Med* **1**:191, 1983.
461. Fullerton SM, Harding RM, Boyce AJ, Clegg JB: Molecular and population genetic analysis of allelic sequence diversity at the human β globin locus. *Proc Natl Acad Sci U S A* **91**:1805, 1994.
462. Smith RA, Ho PJ, Clegg JB, Kidd JR, Thein SL: Recombination breakpoints in the human β globin gene cluster. *Blood* **92**:4415, 1998.
463. Kazazian HH, Waber PG, Boehm CD, Lee JI, Antonarakis SE, Fairbank VF: Hemoglobin E in Europeans—Further evidence for multiple origins of the beta-E-globin gene. *Am J Hum Genet* **36**:212,1984.
464. Haldane JBS: The rate of mutation of human genes. *Hereditas* **1**(Suppl 35):267, 1948.
465. Allison AC: Protection afforded by sickle cell trait against subtertian malarial infection. *BMJ* **i**:290, 1954.
466. Fleming AF, Storey J, Molineaux L, Iroko EA, Attai EDE: Abnormal haemoglobins in the Sudan savanna of Nigeria. I. Prevalence of haemoglobins and relationships between sickle cell trait, malaria and survival. *Ann Trop Med Parasitol* **73**:161, 1979.
467. Hill AVS, Allsopp CEM, Kwiatkowski D, et al: Common West African HLA antigens are associated with protection from severe malaria. *Nature* **352**:595, 1991.
468. Luzzatto L, Nwachuku-Jarrett ES, Reddy S: Increased sickling of parasitized erythrocytes is mechanism of resistance against malaria in the sickle trait. *Lancet* **i**:319, 1970.
469. Pasvol G, Weatherall DJ: A mechanism for the protective effect of haemoglobin S against *P. falciparum* malaria. *Nature* **274**:701, 1978.
470. Friedman MJ, Roth EF, Nagel RL, Trager W: *Plasmodium falciparum*: Physiological interactions with the human sickle cell. *Exp Parasitol* **47**:73, 1979.
471. Flint J, Harding RM, Boyce AJ, Clegg JB: The population genetics of the haemoglobinopathies. *Baillieres Clin Haematol* **6**:215, 1993.
472. Kazazian HHJ, Boehm CD: Molecular basis and prenatal diagnosis of β-thalassemia. *Blood* **72**:1107, 1988.
473. Orkin SH, Antonarakis SE, Kazazian HH: Polymorphisms and molecular pathology of the human β-globin gene. *Prog Hematol* **13**:49, 1983.
474. Orkin SH, Kazazian HH: The mutation and polymorphism of the human β-globin gene and its surrounding DNA. *Annu Rev Genet* **18**:131, 1984.
475. Flint J, Harding RM, Boyce AJ, Clegg JB: The population genetics of the haemoglobinopathies, in Rogers GP (ed): *Sickle Cell Disease and Thalassaemia. Baillière's Clinical Haematology, 11*, 1, 1998. London, Baillière Tindall.
476. Siniscalo MLB, Filippi G, et al: Population genetics of haemoglobin variants, thalassaemia and glucose-6-phosphate dehydrogenase deficiency, with particular reference to the malaria hypothesis. *Bull World Health Organ* **34**:379, 1966.
477. Flint J, Hill AVS, Weatherall DJ, Clegg JB, Higgs DR: Alpha globin genotypes in two North European populations. *Br J Haematol* **63**:796, 1986.
478. Pasvol G, Wilson RJM: The interaction of malaria parasites with red blood cells. *Br Med Bull* **38**:133, 1982.
479. Williams TN, Maitland K, Bennett S, et al: High incidence of malaria in α-thalassaemic children. *Nature* **383**:522, 1996.
480. Allen SJ, O'Donnell A, Alexander NDE et al: α^+-thalassaemia protects children against disease due to malaria *and* other infections. *Proc Natl Acad Sci U S A* **94**:14736, 1997.
481. Mitchell JJ, Capua A, Clow C, Scriver CR: Twenty-year outcome analysis of genetic screening programs for Tay-Sachs and β-thalassemia disease carriers in high schools. *Am J Hum Genet* **59**:793, 1996.
482. Cao A, Rosatelli MC: Screening and prenatal diagnosis of the haemoglobinopathies. *Clin Haematol* **6**:263, 1993.
483. Weatherall DJ: Prenatal diagnosis of haematological disease, in Hann IM, Gibson BES, Letsky EA (eds): *Fetal and Neonatal Haematology*. London, Baillière Tindall, 1991, p 285.
484. Cao A, Rosatelli MC, Battista G, et al: Antenatal diagnosis of β-thalassemia in Sardinia. *Ann N Y Acad Sci* **612**:215, 1990.
485. Loukopoulos D, Hadji A, Papadakis M, et al: Prenatal diagnosis of thalassemia and of the sickle cell syndromes in Greece. *Ann N Y Acad Sci* **612**:226, 1990.
486. Alter BP: Antenatal diagnosis: Summary of results. *Ann N Y Acad Sci* **612**:237, 1990.
487. Old JM, Fitches A, Heath C, et al: First trimester fetal diagnosis for haemoglobinopathies: Report on 200 cases. *Lancet* **ii**:763, 1986.
488. Kazazian HH, Phillips JAI, Boehm CD, Vik T, Mahoney MJ, Ritchey AK: Prenatal diagnosis of β-thalassemia by amniocentesis: Linkage analysis of multiple polymorphic restriction endonuclease sites. *Blood* **56**:926, 1980.
489. Pirastu M, Kan YW, Cao A, Conner BJ, Teplitz RL, Wallace RB: Prenatal diagnosis of β-thalassemia: Detection of a single nucleotide mutation in DNA. *N Engl J Med* **309**:284, 1983.
490. Chehab F, Doherty M, Cai S, Cooper S, Rubin E: Detection of sickle cell anaemia and thalassaemia. *Nature* **329**:293, 1987.

491. Saiki RK, Chang C-A, Levenson CH, et al: Diagnosis of sickle cell anemia and β-thalassemia with enzymatically amplified DNA and non-radioactive allele-specific oligonucleotide probes. *N Engl J Med* **319**:537, 1988.
492. Cai SP, Chang CA, Zhang JZ, Saiki RK, Erlich HA, Kan YW: Rapid prenatal diagnosis of β-thalassemia using DNA amplification and nonradiactive. *Blood* **73**:372, 1989.
493. Saiki RK, Walsh PS, Levenson Ch, Erlich HA: Genetic analysis of amplified DNA with immobilized sequence-specific oligonucleotide probes. *Proc Natl Acad Sci U S A* **86**:6230, 1989.
494. Old JM, Varawalla NY, Weatherall DJ: The rapid detection and prenatal diagnosis of β-thalassaemia in the Asian Indian and Cypriot populations in the UK. *Lancet* **336**:834, 1990.
495. Bunn HF: Sickle cell hemoglobin and other hemoglobin mutations, in Stamatoyannopoulos G, Nienhuis AW, Majerus PW, Varmus H (eds): *The Molecular Basis of Blood Diseases*, 2nd ed. Philadelphia, WB Saunders, 1994, p 207.
496. Adams RJ, McKie VC, Hsu L, et al: Prevention of a first stroke by transfusions in children with sickle cell anemia and abnormal results on transcranial Doppler ultrasonography. *N Engl J Med* **339**:5, 1998.
497. Vichinsky EP, Haberkern CM, Neumayr L, et al: A comparison of conservative and aggressive transfusion regimens in the perioperative management of sickle cell disease. The Preoperative Transfusion in Sickle Cell Disease Study Group. *N Engl J Med* **333**:206, 1995.
498. Charache S, Terrin ML, Moore RD, et al: Effect of hydroxyurea on the frequency of painful crises in sickle cell anemia. *N Engl J Med* **332**:1317, 1995.
499. Scott JP, Hillery CA, Brown ER, Misiewicz VM, Labotka RJ: Hydroxyurea therapy in children severely affected with sickle cell disease. *J Pediatr* **128**:820, 1996.
500. Piomelli S: Management of Cooley's anaemia. *Clin Haematol* **6**:287, 1993.
501. Giardini C: Treatment of β-thalassemia. *Curr Opin Hematol* **4**:79, 1997.
502. Orkin SH, Nathan DG: The thalassemias, in Nathan DG, Orkin SH (eds): *Hematology of Infancy and Childhood*. Philadelphia, WB Saunders, 1997 p 811.
503. Olivieri NF, Brittenham GM: Iron chelating therapy and the treatment of thalassemia. *Blood* **89**:739, 1997.
504. Hershko C, Konijn AM, Link G: Iron chelators for thalassaemia. *Br J Haematol* **101**:399, 1998.
505. Olivieri NF, Nathan DG, MacMillan JH et al: Survival in medically treated patients with homozygous β-thalassemia. *N Engl J Med* **331**:574, 1994.
506. Kirkpatrick DV, Barrios NJ, Humbert JH: Bone marrow transplantation for sickle cell anemia. *Semin Hematol* **28**:240, 1991.
507. Lucarelli G, Giardini C, Baronciani D: Bone marrow transplantation in β-thalassaemia. *Semin Hematol* **32**:297, 1995.
508. Olivieri NF, Weatherall DJ: The therapeutic reactivation of fetal haemoglobin. *Hum Mol Genet* **7**:1655, 1998.
509. Weatherall DJ: Pathophysiology of thalassaemia. *Clin Haematol* **11**:127, 1998.
510. Flint J, Thomas K, Micklem G, et al: The relationship between chromosome structure and function at a human telomeric region. *Nat Genet* **15**:252, 1997.

CHAPTER 182

Pyruvate Kinase Deficiency and Other Enzymopathies of the Erythrocyte

Akira Hirono ■ Hitoshi Kanno ■ Shiro Miwa ■ Ernest Beutler

1. **Pyruvate kinase (PK) deficiency (MIM 266200) is the most common enzyme deficiency resulting in hereditary hemolytic anemia. The disorder has a worldwide distribution and is characterized clinically by lifelong chronic hemolysis of variable severity. Splenectomy often results in amelioration of the hemolytic process in more severely affected patients, but is less effective in milder cases. Defective PK catalysis in affected erythrocytes generally results in elevated concentrations of 2,3-diphosphoglycerate (2,3-DPG) and decreased ATP levels relative to cells of comparable age.**
2. **PK is encoded by two genes, *PKLR* and *PKM*. *PKLR* is expressed in the liver and in red cells; different splice forms are found in liver and in erythrocytes. *PKM* is expressed in muscle, leukocytes, and many other tissues. Allosteric (M_2) and nonallosteric (M_1) splice forms of PKM exist. The erythrocyte enzyme deficiency is due to mutations of the *PKLR* gene. Many different mutations have been identified, but more than one-half of the PK deficiency mutations among Europeans are 1529G → A (Arg510Gln). PK deficiency is inherited as an autosomal recessive disorder. The red cells of heterozygotes usually have 40 to 60 percent of the PK activity of normal red cells, and heterozygotes are almost always clinically normal.**
3. **Deficiencies of other red cell glycolytic enzymes are less common than is PK deficiency. Severe deficiencies of hexokinase (MIM 235700), glucosephosphate isomerase (GPI) (MIM 172400), phosphofructokinase (PFK) (MIM 171850), aldolase (MIM 103850), triosephosphate isomerase (TPI) (MIM 190450), phosphoglycerate kinase (PGK) (MIM 311800), bisphosphoglycerate mutase/phosphatase (BPGM/BPGP) (MIM 222800), and lactate dehydrogenase (LDH) (MIM 150100) have been documented, and in most cases, mutations have been identified at the DNA level. All of these enzyme deficiencies are autosomal except for PGK, which is X-linked. Deficiencies of BPGM and bisphosphoglycerate phosphatase are associated with mild erythrocytosis secondary to virtual absence of 2,3-DPG. LDH deficiency is also not associated with hemolysis, but in one form there is myopathy. All others are associated with hemolytic anemia of variable severity with partial response to splenectomy, except for PFK deficiency, which usually has a compensated hemolytic process.**
4. **GPI deficiency is second to PK deficiency in frequency; all tissues have decreased GPI activity, but clinical manifestations are usually limited to a chronic hemolytic process, although in some instances, mental retardation and myopathy may occur. In PFK deficiency (glycogen storage disease type VII), clinical hallmarks are male predominance with early onset gout, compensated hemolytic process, and prominent myopathy. Severe deficiency of aldolase activity has been documented in only four patients. TPI deficiency is clinically usually the most severe of the enzymatic defects of the glycolytic pathway; it is characterized by multisystem disease, including progressive neurologic dysfunction, increased susceptibility to infections, cardiomyopathy, and death usually during early childhood. All body tissues investigated are deficient in TPI. Hemolytic anemia and a variety of neurologic abnormalities most frequently accompany PGK deficiency in hemizygous males; the phenotypic picture is variable. Heterozygous females may exhibit only hemolytic anemia of variable degree depending on random X inactivation.**
5. **Glucose-6-phosphate dehydrogenase deficiency (Chap. 179) is the only common enzyme deficiency affecting the hexose monophosphate pathway. In addition, rare instances of deficiencies of enzymes of glutathione synthesis, γ-glutamylcysteine synthetase (MIM 230450) and glutathione synthetase (MIM 226130, 231900, and 601002) have been identified. Deficiency of γ-glutamylcysteine synthetase is manifested by a virtual lack of red-cell glutathione and moderate hemolytic anemia. Deficiency of the second enzyme of glutathione synthesis, glutathione synthetase, presents as two phenotypes. The first exhibits hemolytic anemia alone; the second, presumably due to a generalized deficiency of the enzyme, is characterized by multisystem disease with metabolic acidosis, massive 5-oxoprolinuria, and often neurologic dysfunction accompanying a hemolytic syndrome. Only a single consanguineous kindred with severe glutathione reductase deficiency (MIM 138300) has been documented. There were episodes of hemolysis**

A list of standard abbreviations is located immediately preceding the index in each volume. Additional abbreviations used in this chapter include: AK = adenylate kinase; BPGM = bisphosphoglycerate mutase; DHAP = dihydroxyacetone phosphate; 2,3-DPG = 2,3-diphosphoglycerate; F-6-P = fructose 6-phosphate; F-1,6-P_2 = fructose 1,6-diphosphate; GA-3-P = glyceraldehyde 3-phosphate; G-6-P = glucose 6-phosphate; GPI = glucose phosphate isomerase; HK = hexokinase; HMP = hexose monophosphate shunt; ICSH = International Committee for Standardization in Hematology; M,L,P = muscle, liver, and platelet forms of PFK; PEP = phosphoenolpyruvate; PFK = phosphofructokinase; PGK = phosphoglycerate kinase; PK = pyruvate kinase; *PKLR* = gene symbol for PK locus encoding L and R isozymes; *PKM* = gene symbol for PK locus encoding M isozymes; P5N = pyrimidine 5′-nucleotidase; R, L, M_1, and M_2 = red cell, liver, and muscle isozymes; TPI = triosephosphate isomerase.

associated with fava bean ingestion and possible cataracts in affected members.

6. **Disturbances in erythrocyte nucleotide metabolism that are clearly associated with shortened red-cell life span and hemolytic anemia of variable severity include (a) overproduction of biochemically normal adenosine deaminase (MIM 102730) and (b) severe deficiency of pyrimidine 5′ nucleotidase (MIM 266120). Overproduction of adenosine deaminase is a dominantly inherited disorder characterized by decreases in total erythrocyte adenine nucleotides (less than half-normal values), elevations in pyrimidine nucleotidase activity (three- to fourfold), and approximately one hundred-fold elevations in adenosine deaminase activity. Severe deficiency of pyrimidine nucleotidase is inherited as an autosomal recessive disorder or is acquired secondary to lead toxicity. It is characterized by ineffective clearance of RNA degradation products from maturing reticulocytes with consequent accumulation of diverse pyrimidine conjugates and ribonucleotides, prominent basophilic stippling, and twofold increased concentrations of erythrocyte.**
7. **Adenylate kinase deficiency (MIM 103000), previously thought to induce hemolytic anemia, may not do so without other coexistent abnormalities, since a severe deficiency state has been observed with no adverse hematologic effects.**
8. **Erythrocyte enzymopathies may also have hematologic expression other than hemolysis, may have no obvious deleterious consequences, or may be associated with clinical disorders affecting other than hematopoietic tissue.**

Erythrocytes are highly differentiated cells that have evolved specifically for the purpose of transporting O_2 and CO_2. They contain a saturated solution of hemoglobin, and their deformable biconcave shape is well suited for efficient gas exchange in every narrow capillary. Because erythrocytes lose their nuclei and cytoplasmic organelles during maturation in the marrow, they are unable to generate ATP by oxidative phosphorylation. Nevertheless, the cells can provide sufficient energy for maintenance of membrane plasticity and active cation transport, replenishment of nucleotides and membrane components, and synthesis of glutathione solely by anaerobic glycolysis. Using their economical but effective metabolic pathways, they can perform these tasks and survive as fully functional cells for their intravascular life span of 120 days.

Anaerobic glycolysis of one molecule of glucose through the Embden-Meyerhof pathway can result in the phosphorylation of two molecules of ADP to ATP (Fig. 182-1). The overall velocity of erythrocyte glycolysis is regulated by three rate-limiting kinases,

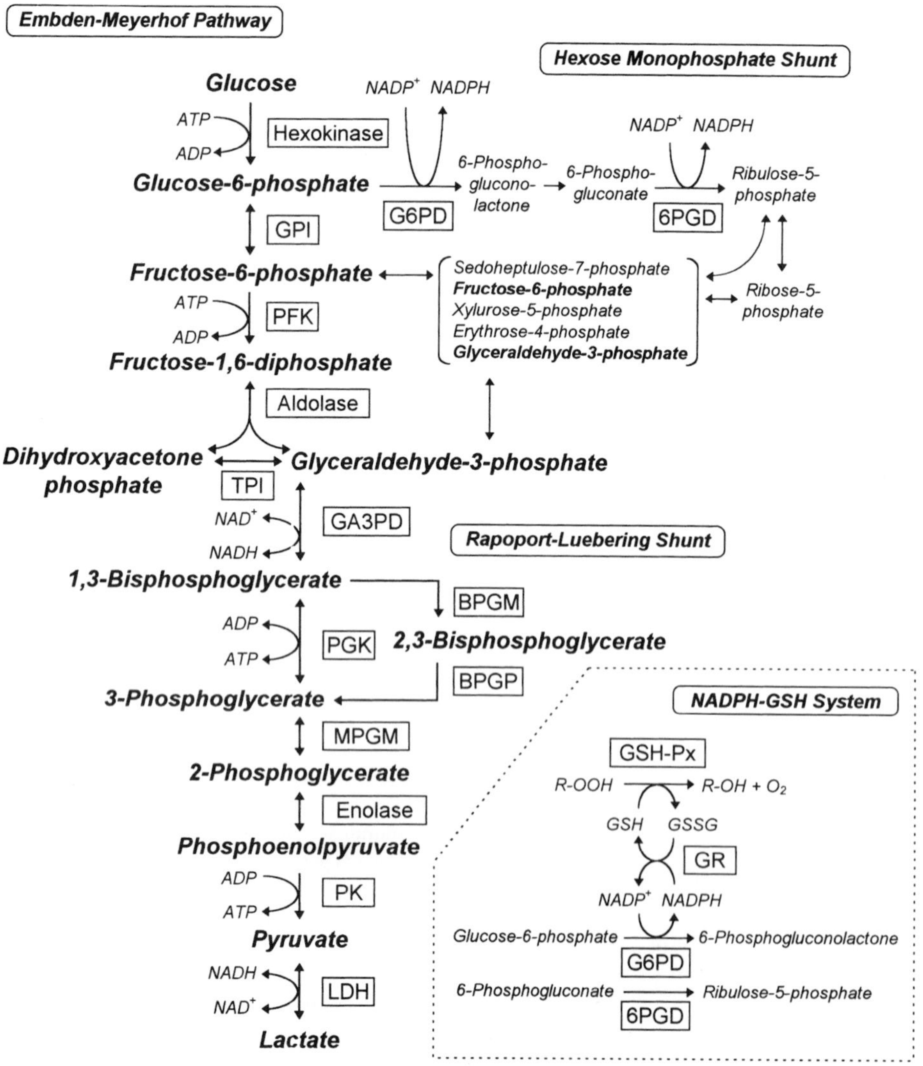

Fig. 182-1 Major pathways in human erythrocytes. The Embden-Meyerhof pathway (glycolytic pathway) converts one molecule of glucose to two molecules of lactate generating two net molecules of ATP. Rapoport-Luebering shunt is a unique pathway to generate 2,3-bisphosphoglycerate. Human erythrocyte hexose monophosphate (HMP) shunt functions mainly for producing NADPH, which is essential for maintaining a high concentration of GSH. BPGM = bisphosphoglycerate mutase; BPGP = bisphosphoglycerate phosphatase; GA-3-PD = glyceraldehyde-3-phosphate dehydrogenase; GPI = glucosephosphate isomerase; GR = glutathione reductase; GSH-Px = glutathione peroxidase; G6PD = glucose-6-phosphate dehydrogenase; LDH = lactate dehydrogenase; MPGM = monophosphoglycerate kinase; PFK = phosphofructokinase; PGK = phosphoglycerate kinase; PK = pyruvate kinase; 6PGD = 6-phosphogluconate dehydrogenase; TPI = triosephosphate isomerase.

hexokinase (HK), phosphofructokinase (PFK), and pyruvate kinase (PK), and by the availability of NAD and of ADP. Erythrocytes have a unique shunt in the glycolytic pathway (Rapoport-Luebering shunt) that bypasses the phosphoglycerate kinase step and that accounts for the synthesis and regulation of 2,3-diphosphoglycerate (2,3-DPG), which is present in very high concentrations (about 4 mM) in these cells and decreases the oxygen affinity of hemoglobin.[1]

Highly toxic superoxide (O_2^-) generated in erythrocytes is converted to H_2O_2 by superoxide dismutase. Because H_2O_2 may also seriously damage essential cell components, a mechanism for its detoxification is needed. Erythrocytes have two enzymes, catalase and glutathione peroxidase, that serve this purpose. Recent studies have suggested that catalase may play the more important role.[2,3] NADPH, which is generated through the hexose monophosphate (HMP) shunt, is a potent electron donor essential for maintaining a high concentration of GSH and preserving catalase activity (see Fig. 182-1). GSH exhibits its antioxidant activity via several redox reactions, including glutathione peroxidase and thioltransferase (glutaredoxin).

When normal peripheral blood is stained vitally by new methylene blue or brilliant cresyl blue, a few erythroid cells may be seen to contain a fine basophilic network. These cells, called reticulocytes, are very young erythrocytes that have lost their nuclei shortly before entering the circulation but are not yet completely mature. Their maturation in the circulation requires 1 to 2 days. Reticulocytes comprise 0.5 to 1.7 percent of the total erythrocytes in normal individuals, which ratio reflects both increased erythropoiesis and the reduced life span of mature erythrocytes. An increase in reticulocytes (reticulocytosis) is an important sign of hemolysis. Reticulocytes still preserve cytoplasmic organelles including ribosomes and mitochondria, and are capable of synthesizing protein and producing ATP by oxidative phosphorylation. On the other hand, reticulocytes may be more severely compromised than mature erythrocytes in the spleen, particularly in patients with glycolytic enzymopathies.[4] Splenectomy in those patients usually results in marked reticulocytosis as well as improvement of anemia, in contrast to patients with hereditary spherocytosis in whom splenectomy leads to normal reticulocyte count. Because reticulocytes are less dense than mature cells, they can easily be concentrated by centrifugation. Several enzymes including HK, PK, G-6-PD, aldolase, and pyrimidine 5′-nucleotidase (P5N) (often called "age-dependent" enzymes) exhibit much higher activities in the reticulocyte-rich fraction.[5]

PYRUVATE KINASE DEFICIENCY

Clinical Aspects

Prevalence. Pyruvate kinase (PK) and glucose-6-phosphate dehydrogenase (G-6-PD) (see Chap. 179) deficiencies are the most prevalent causes of hereditary nonspherocytic hemolytic anemia.[6–10] Both PK and G-6-PD deficiency have been reported in several hundred families, while other rare erythroenzymopathies, such as glucose phosphate isomerase (GPI), P5N, hexokinase (HK) or triosephosphate isomerase, have each been encountered in only 15 to 40 families. Thus, over 80 percent of erythroenzymopathies seem to be accounted for by these two relatively common enzyme deficiencies.[8]

Since it was initially reported in 1961,[11] PK deficiency has been most commonly diagnosed in the United States, northern Europe, and Japan, but it has been reported in several other ethnic populations, showing no remarkable predominance in either races or geographic area. The prevalence rate of PK deficiency is nearly 1/10,000, suggesting allelic frequency of about 1 percent.[12–14] Mass screening studies showed that low erythrocyte PK activity was found in 1/697 (0.143 percent) newborn infants in the United States[15] and in 37/3069 (1.21 percent) of Japanese.[16]

Clinical Features. PK deficiency is inherited as an autosomal recessive disorder (Table 182-1), and patients are usually either compound heterozygotes or homozygotes. In most instances, heterozygotes have no clinical manifestation and are hematologically normal. However, exceptional cases of heterozygotes who were clinically affected have been reported previously.[17–20]

The clinical severity of PK-deficient hemolytic anemia varies from mild and fully compensated hemolysis to severe cases that are transfusion-dependent.[21] In the most severe cases, the affected fetus died in utero with anemia.[22–24] Newborn infants often require exchange transfusion, but subsequently the severity of the PK-deficient hemolytic anemia is moderate.[6] Most patients are diagnosed in infancy or early childhood, but in some cases, mild chronic hemolysis, jaundice, mild to moderate splenomegaly, or cholelithiasis are noticed in adulthood, sometimes at examination incidental to acute viral infection or evaluation in pregnancy.[25–28] Severely affected individuals may require multiple transfusions or splenectomy in early childhood, and generally requirements for transfusion become spontaneously reduced during childhood or after splenectomy has been performed.[8] Even at relatively low

Table 182-1 Clinical Summary of Erythroenzymopathies

Enzyme	GenBank	No. of kindreds	Inheritance*	Hemolysis	Neurologic symptoms	Myopathy
Hexokinase	M75126, X61091	17	AR	chronic	–	–
Glucosephosphate isomerase	K03515	60	AR	chronic	–†	–†
Phosphofructokinase	Liver = X15573 Muscle = Y00698	49	AR	compensated	–	+
Aldolase	M11560	3	AR	chronic	–†	–†
Triosephosphate isomerase	M10036, X69723	38	AR	chronic	+	–†
Phosphoglycerate kinase	M11958	21	XR	chronic	+	+
Bisphosphoglycerate mutase	X04327	1	AR	–	–	–
Pyruvate kinase	D10326, D90465	>400	AR	chronic	–	–
Glucose-6-phosphate dehydrogenase	X03674 X55448	$>10^7$	XR	acute, chronic	–	–
Glutathione reductase	X15772	1	AR	acute	–	–
γ-Glutamylcysteine synthetase	M90656	6	AR	chronic	–†	–
Glutathione synthetase	U34683	~30	AR	chronic	+	–
Adenylate kinase	J04809	7	AR	chronic†	–†	–
Adenosine deaminase	X02994 AF053356	5	AD	chronic	–†	–
Pyrimidine 5′-nucleotidase	–	36	AR	chronic	–†	–

*AD = autosomal dominant; AR = autosomal recessive; XR = X-linked recessive

†Although several patients manifest these sympoms, the causal relationship with enzymopathies has not been established.

hemoglobin levels, the anemia of PK deficiency seems to be well tolerated by most patients, because the metabolic block leads to accumulation of 2,3-DPG, known to lower the affinity of hemoglobin for oxygen.[29–31] The elevated concentration of 2,3-DPG also inhibits pentose phosphate shunt activity, possibly contributing to the acute exacerbation of hemolysis that occurs in infection.[32] Aplastic crises have been described in PK deficiency.[33] Pregnancy may increase the transfusion requirements even in individuals who did not previously require transfusion therapy.[6,25] Iron overload in association with transfusions has been reported in PK deficiency.[34–40] Growth and development of PK-deficient subjects usually is normal, and when delayed may improve after splenectomy.[41]

Other clinical manifestations, such as kernicterus,[42,43] chronic leg ulcers,[44] acute pancreatitis secondary to biliary tract disease,[45] splenic abscess,[46] extramedullary hematopoietic tissues,[47,48] Zieve syndrome (hemolytic anemia, jaundice, hyperlipidemia, and alcohol-induced liver disease),[49] or migratory phlebitis[50] have been reported as rare complications of PK deficiency.

PK deficiency has been diagnosed as combined enzyme deficiency with G-6-PD,[51,52] hereditary spherocytosis,[52a] sickle cell trait,[52b] or α-thalassemia.[53]

Hereditary hemolytic anemia due to erythrocyte PK deficiency has also been identified in dogs[54,55] and mice.[56] Canine PK deficiency was characterized by diverse systemic abnormalities including not only chronic hemolytic anemia, but also osteosclerosis and panmyelofibrosis.[54] Murine PK deficiency has been identified in an inbred colony of the CBA/N strain; life span and fertility were shown to be preserved.[56]

Hematologic Findings. Patients with PK deficiency show normocytic and sometimes macrocytic anemia reflecting the reticulocytosis that is almost invariably present. Hemoglobin concentrations generally range from 6 to 12 g/dl, and packed cell volumes from 17 to 37 percent.[8] Even in well-compensated cases, reticulocytosis is almost always observed with a range of 4 to 15 percent, and splenectomy characteristically induces a paradoxic increase of the reticulocyte counts to levels as high as 40 to 90 percent[57,58] because reticulocytes and young erythrocytes are selectively sequestrated in spleen[4] (see "Pathology," below). Leukocyte and platelet counts are generally normal or modestly increased.[8]

As in most other erythroenzymopathies, specific changes of erythrocyte morphology are not observed in PK deficiency. However, echinocytes and dehydrated and spiculated erythrocytes are often present, particularly in blood films prepared from severely affected individuals. These morphologic changes become more prominent after splenectomy, and siderocytes, target cells, and Pappenheimer and Howell-Jolly bodies are also observed.[8] Shrunken echinocytes on a postsplenectomy blood film have been considered to be suggestive of the presence of PK deficiency.[59] A newborn PK-deficient infant with Pelger-Huet leukocyte anomaly has been reported.[60]

The osmotic fragility of fresh erythrocytes is usually normal, but the incubated osmotic fragility test may be variably abnormal.[8] Direct antiglobulin (Coombs) and acid serum (Ham) tests are negative, and hemoglobin F and A_2 are within normal range. Incubated Heinz body formation is increased.[32] The erythrocyte cytoskeleton has been studied, but no specific skeletal defect has been identified.[61–66]

Erythrocyte life span measured with ^{51}Cr labeling shows moderate to severely shortening of the half-life of affected erythrocytes.[6] A biphasic ^{51}Cr clearance curve, signifying the existence of two populations of erythrocytes has been observed in several studies of humans and in mutant mice.[67–70]

Ferrokinetic studies with ^{59}Fe demonstrate a short plasma clearance time and usually rapid maximal appearance of ^{59}Fe in circulating erythrocytes.[41] Surface scanning shows that both spleen and liver are the organs in which major sequestration of PK-deficient erythrocytes occurs.[4] Experiments derived from ^{51}Cr-labeling seem somewhat conflicting regarding splenic sequestration, but PK-deficient reticulocytes and young erythrocytes may be selectively sequestrated in the spleen. This is because their metabolism depends mainly on mitochondrial oxidative phosphorylation, and it is presumed that under the hypoxic conditions that exist in the spleen, anaerobic glycolysis in these cells is insufficient to provide the membrane flexibility to allow passage through the sinusoids of the spleen.[65]

Other Laboratory Findings. Although L (liver)- and R (red cell)-type PK isozymes are products of a common structural gene,[71,72] and decreased PK activity has been demonstrated both in erythrocytes and liver in several cases,[73,74] PK deficiency has never been shown to be associated with specific organ dysfunction other than hemolytic anemia.[6] Routine laboratory tests of liver function, as well as pathologic findings, showed no abnormalities except for hyperbilirubinemia and hepatic iron deposition, even in one of the most severely affected patients.[75,76] The L-type PK is known to be expressed in pancreatic β cells of Langerhans islet;[77,78] however, diabetes or glucose intolerance has never been described as a complication of PK deficiency. Bone changes accompanied with expansion of bone marrow space due to erythroid hyperplasia have been roentgenologically demonstrated in severe cases.[79]

Pathology. Bone marrow shows normoblastic erythroid hyperplasia. No specific pathologic findings have been described in the spleen or liver by light microscopy; variable degrees of congestion, hemosiderosis, or erythrophagocytosis are present.[6] It is apparently reticulocytes that are phagocytosed by cordal macrophages as visualized by electron microscopy.[80–82] Markedly increased number of erythroid cells have been noted in the spleen of the PK deficient mouse.[56] In rare instances, marked iron deposition not associated with hereditary hemochromatosis was prominent on histologic examination.[8,35,37]

Diagnosis

Diagnosis of PK deficiency depends on erythrocyte enzyme assay,[83–85] measurement of glycolytic intermediates,[86] demonstration of abnormalities in enzymatic characteristics,[87] or identification of gene mutations.[10,88]

A quantitative decrease of enzymatic activity can be documented by spectrophotometric assay of erythrocyte lysates that are prepared by carefully removing leukocytes and platelets.[89] A leukocyte contains as much as 300 times the PK as an erythrocyte,[90] and leukocytes and platelets contain the M_2-type isozyme, the product of a different gene than the R-type expressed in erythrocytes. Therefore, contamination of erythrocytes by platelets and leukocytes can lead to a false negative result in enzymatic diagnosis. The PK activities of clinically affected individuals usually range from less than 10 percent to 25 percent of the normal mean value. However, in some cases, in vitro assay may merely show mildly subnormal activity, or sometimes even higher than normal values.[91] A number of PK variants with abnormally low affinities for phosphoenolpyruvate (PEP) have been identified,[57,92–94] and these variants could be diagnosed by use of assay systems with low concentration of PEP with or without fructose-1,6-diphosphate (F-1,6-DP), the allosteric effector, because in vitro assays contain PEP and F-1,6-DP concentrations far above those existing under in vivo conditions.[91] To avoid false negative results, examination of the enzyme at low substrate concentrations is preferable whenever a high K_m for PEP variant is suspected.[6] Heterozygotes usually show 40 to 60 percent of the PK activities of normal controls. Reticulocytes and young erythrocytes contain higher PK activities than old erythrocytes.[95–98] Thus, when patients are encountered whose erythrocytes show a slight decrease of PK activity but markedly elevated activities of other age-dependent enzymes, such as HK, GPI, or G-6-PD, PK deficiency should be considered. The erythrocytes of fetuses and preterm infants also have higher PK activity than do normal adults.[99]

Thus, the levels of erythrocyte enzyme need to be carefully interpreted in making the diagnosis of PK deficiency. A marginally normal PK activity with a concomitant increase of other age-dependent enzymes in the usual assay system may suggest that a family study be conducted and/or that measurements of glycolytic intermediates be made for confirmation of the existence of PK deficiency.[100] Examination of glycolytic intermediates and adenine nucleotides requires prompt deproteinization of whole blood after blood sampling[86] and preservation of deproteinized sample at −80°C or below before measurements, so that appropriate sampling is somewhat complicated under some circumstances. However, the demonstration of accumulated intermediates upstream of the PK step is important because it constitutes direct evidence of a metabolic block of glycolysis as a consequence of PK deficiency.

Methods of enzymatic characterization of variant PK have been standardized by the International Committee for Standardization in Haematology (ICSH) in 1979.[87] Though there are some difficulties in purification and characterization of unstable mutant enzyme with the limited amount of enzyme usually available in clinical samples, the demonstration of aberrant biochemical characteristics is quite useful not only for definitive diagnosis but in considering the structure-function relationship of PK.[10,101–104]

Biochemistry and Molecular Genetics

Pyruvate kinase (ATP: Pyruvate 2-*O*-phosphotransferase; EC 2.7.1.40) is a key enzyme of the Embden-Meyerhof anaerobic glycolytic pathway. The enzyme catalyzes the irreversible conversion of PEP to pyruvate with the phosphorylation of ADP to ATP (see Fig. 182-1). Because of the essential role of the glycolytic pathway, PK activity can be detected in virtually all tissues and in organisms ranging from bacteria to mammals. Four isozymes of mammalian pyruvate kinase, designated as M_1, M_2, L, and R-type, have been delineated in a rat system,[105,106] and later identified also in humans[74] (Table 182-3). The amino acid sequence of PK is highly conserved among all organisms so far analyzed. All isozymes are active as tetramers consisting of identical subunits of about 60 kDa. M_1-PK is expressed mainly in muscle and brain; M_2-PK is the only isozyme that is active in early fetal tissues[106] and also almost ubiquitously expressed in adult tissues including leukocytes and platelets; L-PK is a major hepatic isozyme and is detected as a minor component in kidney, small intestine, and pancreas; R-PK is exclusively expressed in erythrocytes.

All PK isozymes except the M_1-type are allosterically regulated, and F-1,6-DP is known to act as a heterotropic allosteric effector.[107–109] L-PK[110] and a R-PK[111] are both regulated by phosphorylation of a serine residue near the N-terminus of the subunit. This lowers the affinity for the substrate PEP. Magnesium and potassium are bound to the PK subunits, and the enzyme with bound potassium has an increased affinity for PEP in the presence of magnesium.[112] ATP, a product of the PK reaction, exerts feedback inhibition. Structural analysis by x-ray crystallography was achieved by use of cat muscle M_1-PK,[113] rabbit muscle PK,[114] *E. coli* type-I PK,[115] and yeast PK,[104] the latter two of which are allosterically regulated. Each subunit is composed of four distinct domains: the N-terminal, A, B, and C domains.[113] The active site of PK lies in the pocket between domains A and B,[113] and the allosteric site is entirely located in the C domain.[104] The allosteric properties of the PK isozymes have been considered to be a typical model of the $R \leftrightarrow T$ transformation equilibrium proposed by Monod-Wyman-Chageux.[116] However, recent observations obtained from studies on allosteric PK have suggested a model for cooperativity that incorporates an intermediate R′ state with properties intermediate between those of the T and R states,[117] and in which allosteric activation involves simultaneous and concerted rotations of entire domains of each of the subunits, causing dynamic conformational changes induced by the allosteric regulator.[101] The structure and location of the allosteric site of yeast PK have been elucidated and have successfully explained the differences in structure and regulatory properties between allosteric (M_2) and nonallosteric (M_1) PK.[104]

The similarity in the structure between L- and R-PK was originally suggested the common qualitative abnormality that is detected in the erythrocytes and liver of PK-deficient subjects,[73] and by antigenic identity between the purified isozymes.[118] Later, the primary structure of human M_1-, M_2-, L- and R-type PK[119–122] deduced from the cDNA and genomic sequence have shown that a common structural gene *PKLR*[71,72] encoded the L- and R-PK isozymes and that another gene *PKM* encoded M_1 and M_2-PK. The specific N-terminal amino acid sequences for R- and L-PK are encoded in exons 1 and 2 of the *PKLR* gene respectively; the cDNA for the R enzyme encodes 574 amino acid residues and that for the L enzyme 543 residues (Table 182-3). Both the M_1 and M_2-PK isozymes are comprised of 531 amino acids.[119,123] Chromosomal loci have been assigned in humans: the *PKLR* gene is located at 1q21;[124] the *PKM* gene is located at 15q22.2-q22.3.[125] Fine mapping of this regions shows the *PKLR* gene to be 71 kb distant from the glucocerebrosidase locus,[126] which encodes the enzyme that is deficient in Gaucher disease (see Chap. 146). Both the human *PKLR* and the *PKM* genes have 12 exons. The *PKLR* gene spans about 9.5 kb and *PKM* gene about 32 kb. The primary transcript generated from M gene is alternatively spliced, resulting that mature transcripts of the M_1 and M_2 type specifically include exon 9 or 10 sequence, respectively.[119,123] Native polyacrylamide electrophoresis and staining PK activity can separate human R-PK into two bands; R_1 and R_2. R_1 predominates in reticulocytes and young erythrocytes, whereas the major form of mature erythrocytes is R_2.[74,127] The molecular basis of the difference in the mobility of these two fractions is not known.

The *PKLR* gene has two promoters that direct tissue-specific transcription. The R-type promoter is located upstream of exon 1 and is highly and exclusively active in the erythroid lineage of hematopoietic cells.[72,128,129] The L-type promoter in intron 1 has been found to be transcriptionally active in hepatocytes[130,131] as well as in pancreatic β cells.[77,78,132] Rat and human R-PK promoter activities have been analyzed in erythroleukemia cell lines[72,128,129] and transgenic mice.[133,134] Recent observations indicated that in the rat system a 5′-upstream enhancer was required to drive transgenes at a transcription level similar to that of the endogenous PK gene in erythroid cells of the fetal liver.[135] The human and rat R-PK promoter as well as the rat erythroid-specific enhancer contain multiple GATA motifs. In addition a transactivation experiment demonstrated that GATA-1 transcription factor was involved in activation of the rat R-PK promoter, leading the conclusion that GATA-1,[129] the key regulatory nuclear protein for erythroid-specific genes, is also an essential trans-acting factor for tissue-specific expression of the R-PK. CACCC motifs in close proximity of GATA motifs in erythroid-specific promoter have been recognized, and the CACCC in the rat R-PK promoter has been shown to interact more strongly to Sp-1 than EKLF.[136] Additional experimental evidence using mice lacking EKLF showed that this factor was not involved in R-PK transcription,[137,138] and a recent study showed binding of the BKLF transcription factor to the rat R-PK promoter, suggesting that the nuclear protein which existed abundantly in erythroid progenitors in yolk sac and fetal liver may be one of the factors involved in R-PK transcription.[139] Multiple in vivo footprints have been found in the enhancer, located 3.5 kb upstream of the R-PK promoter. One footprint is similar to NF-E4, a stage-specific erythroid transcription factor.[135] An important difference in regulation between L- and R-PK is the role of hormonal and dietary factors on the expression of L-PK.[140]

The change of the isozyme composition in the process of erythroid differentiation/maturation from M_2- to R-PK (Fig. 182-2) has been demonstrated by several strategies. Immunologically R-PK can be detected at the basophilic erythroblast stage by isozyme-specific antibody.[141] Both M_2- and R-PK are detectable in isolated colony forming units-erythroids (CFU-Es), and the M_2-PK activity disappears in the process of erythroid differentiation

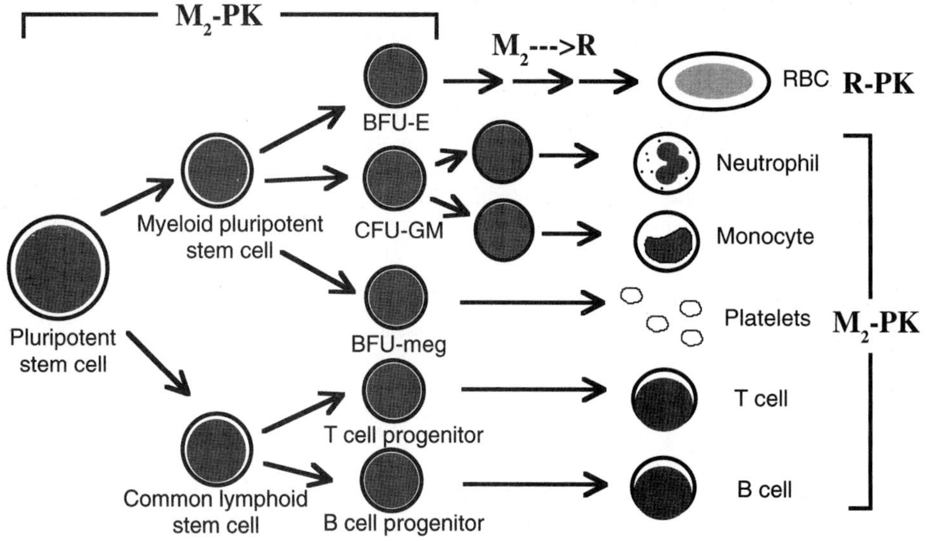

Fig. 182-2 Hematopoietic differentiation and pyruvate kinase isozymes.

induced by erythropoietin.[142] The alteration of the proportion of M_2 to R isozymes in erythrocytes is partly attributable to changes in rates of degradation as well as to changes in synthesis.[143] Persistent expression of the M_2-PK isozyme has been documented in the mature erythrocytes of several PK deficient subjects,[98,144–147] as well as in the animal models.[70,148] One may postulate that the M-gene is reactivated or that it escapes from extinction in order to compensate for the decreased R-PK activity; however, the existence of M_2-PK in erythrocytes does not correlate with severity of hemolysis nor any specific gene mutations, and the mechanisms and significance of the phenomenon remains unknown.

Erythrocyte Metabolism in PK Deficiency

As a result of PK deficiency, the glycolytic rates of PK-deficient erythrocytes are always reduced when erythrocyte age is taken into account, and erythrocyte ATP is usually decreased, but some patients with PK deficiency as well as the PK mutant mice with extremely elevated reticulocyte counts show normal or even increased ATP concentrations.[56,58] The existence of elevated ATP levels despite the impairment of glycolysis is explained by the fact that PK-deficient reticulocytes rely almost entirely on mitochondrial oxidative phosphorylation.[58] Erythrocytes with significant residual PK activity can escape from splenic sequestration under hypoxic circumstances. Consequently, ATP levels in mildly affected cases may be anomalously lower than severe cases.[58]

Glycolytic intermediates proximal to the PK step, such as 2,3-DPG and 3-phosphoglycerate accumulate in enzyme-deficient erythrocytes, whereas the concentration of pyruvate and lactate generally shows only a slight decrease, very likely because they are in near-equilibrium with plasma lactate and pyruvate. The markedly elevated 2,3-DPG level shifts the oxyhemoglobin dissociation curve to the right, and suppresses the pentose phosphate shunt.[8]

Molecular Abnormalities and Structure-Function Relationship of PK Deficiency

To date, over 200 PK alleles of the PK-deficient subjects have been analyzed at the DNA level, and nearly 130 mutations have been identified.[76,103,149–152] Although some specific mutations are found frequently, for example, 1529G → A in Europeans and 1468 → T in Japanese, PK gene mutations responsible for hereditary nonspherocytic hemolytic anemia are quite heterogenous. Screening of gene mutations in PK deficiency has been extensively performed in several countries including the United States, Germany, Italy, France, and Japan.[24,150–155] In five independent comprehensive reports, 184 PK alleles have been screened for mutations altogether, and structural mutations were identified in 164 alleles. Frequencies of specific mutations are shown in Fig. 182-3. In persons of European ancestry 1529G → A (Arg510Gln)[156] is the most common mutation, and over 50 percent of the PK gene abnormalities in those populations can be explained by three common mutations, 1456C → T (Arg486Trp),[156] 994G → A (Gly332Ser)[157] and 1529G → A. In the Japanese population 1468C → T (Arg490Trp),[158,159] 1261C → A (Gln421Lys),[160] 1151C → T (Thr384Met),[122,161] and a three-bases insertion (664insGAC)[158] account for approximately 50 percent of the mutant PK alleles. Although there are

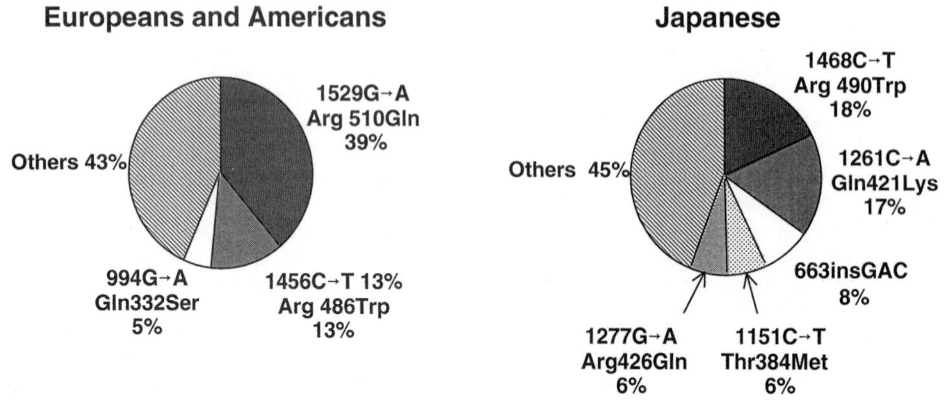

Fig. 182-3 Allelic frequency of the common pyruvate kinase gene mutations. Frequency of the *PKLR* gene mutations in the United States and Europe are calculated from the studies reported by Baronciani,[153] Lenzner,[150] Zanella,[151] Rouger,[24] and Pastore.[152] Frequency of those in the Japanese shown here is based on reports from Miwa and colleagues[76,122,158,160,164,165,168,169] and unpublished results.[192]

some mutations such as 1151C → T, 1436G → A, or 1552C → A that are identified in other populations, among Europeans and the Japanese PK deficiency is caused mostly by population-specific mutations. Several nucleotide polymorphisms have been found in the human L-PK gene,[88,149,160] and haplotype analysis showed that the common mutations are linked with distinct haplotypes, indicating that each may have had a single founder. If heterozygotes for the 1529G → A nor 1468C → T have a selective advantage it has not been identified; therefore, the high gene frequency of these mutations remain unexplained.

As described in the previous section, a subunit of PK consists of four domains; the functional significance of each domain has been discussed. X-ray crystallographic studies of cat muscle and yeast PK,[104,113] have been used to identify putative amino acid residues important in the catalytic site as well as the allosteric site, and the development of mutants was employed to identify the key amino acid residues that determine the allosteric properties of the enzyme.[162,163] The amino acids comprising the active site are located in seven clusters, encoded in exons 5, 7, 8, and 9 of human R-PK.[72,113] The majority of missense mutations are identified in and near these clusters.[10,88,149] Single amino acid substitutions may alter hydrophobicity or secondary structure in vicinity of mutated sites, disturbing contacts of either substrate or cations with the subunit.[164] These structural changes are reflected in an elevated Michaelis constant for PEP, measurable by the ICSH standardized procedure.[87] Homozygotes for 487C → T (Arg163Cys; PK Linz),[161] 941T → C (Ile314Thr; PK Hong Kong),[165] 1151C → T (Thr384Met; PK Tokyo, Nagasaki, Beirut, Mosul)[122,160,161,166] as well as the murine PK gene mutation (1013G → A, Gly338Asp)[167] are categorized in this group. The mutation most frequently identified in the homozygous state in Japanese PK deficiency is 1261C → A, causing Gln421Lys in Aα8 (eighth alpha helix of A domain).[160] This amino acid substitution causes a dramatic increase of hydrophobicity, and may affect not only the active site but also the allosteric site, since the region is close to the Cα1, where the tetramer interface close to the F-1,6-dP$_2$ binding site is located. Consequently, this mutant PK manifests a decrease in the allosteric activation by F-1,6-DP as well as impaired substrate affinities. The 1276C → T (Arg426Tyr; PK Naniwa)[158] and 1277G → A (Arg426Gln; PK Sapporo)[168] mutations also belong to this group. The 3′ half of exon 10 region encodes the amino acids essential for the allosteric regulation of PK. Two human R-PK mutation have been implied to be examples of allosteric mutations: 1403C → T (Ala468Val; PK Hadano)[165] and 1436G → A (Arg479Pro; PK Amish, PK Shinshu).[165,169] Ala468 is located in the turn between Cα2 and Cβ1, the region important for the allosteric site and the tetramer interface, and the Arg479 is on the phosphate-binding loop that binds to F-1,6-dP$_2$. Biochemical characteristics of the homozygous PK variants with the 1436G → A revealed a profoundly decreased response to the allosteric effector,[170,171] despite normal affinities for the substrate, being compatible with the structural studies of the allosteric yeast PK.[104]

Among all PK gene mutations so far elucidated, approximately 70 percent are missense mutations. In addition, nonsense mutations, deletions, insertions, and splice-site mutations, which induce more drastic structural changes, have been reported in the PK deficiency. Because the *PKLR* gene is on the autosome, null mutations are apparently harmless in heterozygotes because normal PK is expressed by the normal PK allele. However, several homozygous PK null mutations have been identified in patients during the past few years (Fig. 182-4). PK Beppu is a variant with one base deletion at 434C,[158] causing a frameshift and premature termination of translation. The mutant subunit encodes the 144 N-terminal amino acids of R-PK plus 33 aberrant amino acids. Interestingly, the canine PK variant found in the Basenji has a one-base deletion of R-PK at the corresponding site.[172] Similarly, a one-base deletion at one of the four G bases from 1231 through 1234 (1231delG) was detected in PK Mondor[173] through prenatal diagnosis of the affected fetus, because the previous pregnancy had terminated with hydrops fetalis. PK Kowloon is one of the most severe PK variants diagnosed in the homozygous state in the Nepalese.[75] Genetic analysis of the variant showed that both twins were homozygous for a transition at the 5′-splice site intron 7. The mutation caused the retention of intron 7 in mature R-PK transcripts, resulting in premature termination at the 321st amino acid residue. The patients were transfusion-dependent, and immunologically the aberrant L-PK could not be detected in liver extracts.[76] Uneven crossing over between the homologous sequence of introns 10 and 11 is thought to be a cause of deletion of exon 11 and flanking regions of PK Gypsy.[153] The 1149-bp deletion of the *PKLR* gene results in prematurely termination after translation of 513 amino acids with an addition of 35 aberrant amino acid residues at the C-terminal. Although the "null" R-PK expression of each variant has not been directly established, the changes that these drastic mutations cause surely prevent the formation of significant quantities of active enzyme. The fact that patients with these variants survive implies that the *PKLR* genes are not necessary for survival. In PK Beppu, M$_2$-PK could be detected in zymogram of mature erythrocytes as the exclusive form of PK activity. These observations allowed us to speculate that the extinction of M gene that normally occurs in the course of erythroid maturation may be inhibited, and that the persistence of the M$_2$ enzyme consequently ameliorated the PK deficiency of the patient. Hematologic examination of the neonatal PK mutant mice revealed that the mutant erythrocytes maintain an erythrocyte life span similar to that of control CBA/N mice until the M$_2$-PK activity comparable to that of R-PK can be demonstrable in the erythrocytes by the age of 2 weeks.[70]

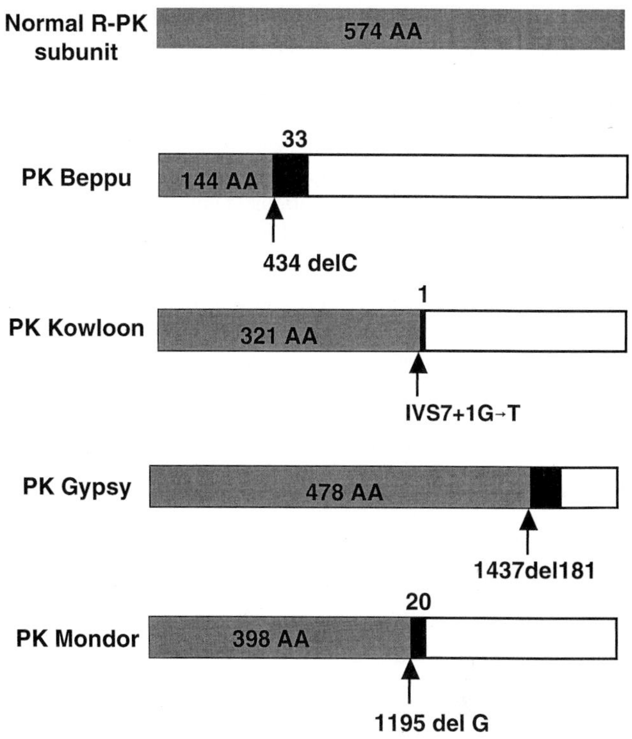

Fig. 182-4 Representation of the aberrant PK subunits responsible for null expression of the PK L-gene. The variants shown here are homozygous for either deletions (PK Beppu, Gypsy, and Mondor) or a single nucleotide substitution at the splice site (PK Kowloon), resulting in frameshifts of translation. Shaded and closed boxes depict authentic and aberrant amino acid residues, respectively, of the human R-type pyruvate kinase.

Pyruvate Kinase and the High ATP Syndrome

Hyperactivity of PK, which ranges from a two- to fourfold increase in the oxygen dissociation curve, has been reported in association with elevated ATP and lowered 2,3-DPG concentrations of the erythrocytes.[174–178] Some affected members show erythrocytosis secondary to a left shift due to elevated 2,3-DPG levels in erythrocytes. The phenomenon is inherited as an autosomal dominant trait, and has been designated the high ATP syndrome. The elevated PK levels are attributable in some cases to the presence of M_2-PK in addition to normal expression of R-PK. Recent molecular analysis of the original family revealed a G to T transition at the 110th nucleotide of R-PK, which interfered with the phosphorylation of Ser104, increasing the affinity for PEP.[179]

Acquired Alterations of Pyruvate Kinase Activity

Acquired PK deficiency is more common than hereditary PK deficiency. A variety of hematologic disorders, such as acute or chronic leukemia, myelodysplastic syndrome, and sideroblastic anemia,[180–183] have been reported as causes of secondary PK deficiency. Among acquired erythrocyte enzymopathies, PK and P5N deficiencies are the most prevalent.[8] Usually PK activity is moderately decreased in acquired or secondary PK deficiency; however erythrocyte life span may not be shortened, sometimes despite some accumulation of glycolytic intermediates.[184] The causal mechanism of acquired PK deficiency remains poorly understood.[185–186]

Elevated PK activity has been reported to be associated with the myelodysplastic syndrome.[187]

Treatment

Because PK deficiency cannot be cured except by marrow transplantation, nonspecific supportive therapies, such as erythrocyte transfusion or splenectomy, have been the mainstay of treatment. Splenectomy does not usually result in normalization of the hemoglobin, but frequently results in clinically significant improvement of anemia as well as better growth and development in very young children.[41] In contrast to hereditary spherocytosis, the response to splenectomy is not predictable, suggesting that recommendations should be based on severity of hemolysis.[188] Severe hemolytic anemia due to PK deficiency in the Basenji dog has been successfully treated by marrow transplantation.[189] The administration of erythropoietin is not beneficial. In one patient being treated for anemia of renal failure an unusually delayed response to erythropoietin led to the unexpected demonstration that the patient had PK deficiency.[190]

Retrovirus-mediated transfer of the cDNA encoding PK into murine hematopoietic cells has been performed experimentally,[191] and when gene transfer into hematopoietic stem cells becomes practical, correction of the defect in patients using this approach may be feasible.

OTHER ERYTHROENZYMOPATHIES OF THE GLYCOLYTIC PATHWAY

Hexokinase Deficiency

Hexokinase (EC 2.7.1.1; HK) is a regulatory enzyme of the Embden-Meyerhof pathway, which catalyzes the phosphorylation of glucose to glucose-6-phosphate (G-6-P) by ATP (see Fig. 182-1). There are four major isozymes of human HK, each encoded by a separate gene (Table 182-2). HK-I is a monomer of 108 kDa that is ubiquitously expressed in many tissues including erythrocytes. It is strongly inhibited by G-6-P, glucose-1,6-diphosphate, and 2,3-DPG, and partially activated by P_i. HK-II and -III are major forms in muscle and fat tissues, and liver, lung and spleen, respectively. The liver isozyme HK-IV, or glucokinase, has higher K_m for glucose and is not inhibited by G-6-P. The HK-I gene is located at 10q22[193] and its 18 exons span more than 75 kb.[194] Human red cells have another isozyme HK_R that appears to be specific for erythrocyte.[195] Both HK-I and HK_R show similar kinetics for glucose and ATP. HK_R, which has a half-life of about 10 days, is the major form in reticulocytes, whereas HK-I is more stable with a half-life of about 66 days, and predominates in mature erythrocytes.[195] The different half-life of each isozyme may explain the biphasic decay[196,197] of total HK activity during erythrocyte maturation.[195] HK_R cDNA[198] is identical to HK-I cDNA[199] except for the 5′ end of the coding sequence and upstream noncoding sequence. Human HK-I and HK_R thus appears to be produced from a single gene using different tissue-specific promoters.[194]

Since the first description by Valentine et al.[200] in 1967, HK deficiency has been reported in 18 cases from 17 families (see Table 182-1).[200–216] The clinical manifestations are characterized by chronic hemolytic anemia of variable severity (median Hb: 9.7 g/dl, range: 6.5 to 13.8; n = 14). Splenectomy is beneficial and may increase hemoglobin concentrations by 2 to 3 g/dl in association with marked reticulocytosis. Three propositi also

Table 182-2 Molecular Genetics of Erythroenzymopathies

Enzyme	Isozymes*	Erythrocyte isozymes	Chromosome locus	Molecular mass (kDa)	No. of mutations† M	N	D/I	S	P	T
Hexokinase	I, II, III, IV, R	I, R	10q22	1 × 108	1	0	2	1	0	4
Glucosephosphate isomerase	single form	–	19cen-q13	2 × 63	23	2	0	2	0	27
Phosphofructokinase	M, L, P	M, L	1cen-q32; 21q22.3	4 × 85	7	1	1	6	0	15
Aldolase	A, B, C	A	16q22-q24	4 × 36	2	0	0	0	0	2
Triosephosphate isomerase	single form	–	12p13	2 × 27	6	2	1	0	0	9
Phosphoglycerate kinase	I, II	I	Xq13.3	1 × 48	9	0	1	2	0	12
Bisphosphoglycerate mutase	single form	–	7q34-7q22	1 × 30	1	0	1	0	0	2
Pyruvate kinase	L, R, M_1, M_2	R	1q21	4 × 58	97	9	16	11	2	135
Glucose-6-phosphate dehydrogenase	single form	–	Xq28	2 × 59	113	1	6	1	0	121
Glutathione reductase	single form	–	8p21	2 × 52	–	–	–	–	–	
γ-Glutamylcysteine synthetase	single form	–	6p12; 1p21	73 + 28	2	0	0	0	0	2
Glutathione synthetase	single form	–	20q11.2	2 × 52	15	1	2	1	0	18
Adenylate kinase	1, 2, 3, 4, 5	1	9q32	1 × 22	2	0	0	0	0	3
Adenosine deaminase‡	L, S	S	20q13.11	1 × 36	–	–	–	–	–	–
Pyrimidine 5′-nucleotidase	single form	–	?	1 × 36	–	–	–	–	–	–

*Some minor tissue specific forms are not included.
†M = missense mutations; N = nonsense mutations; D/I = deletions or insertions; S = splicing site mutations; P = promoter mutations; T = total
‡Overproduction

Table 182-3 Tissue-Specific Expression of Human Pyruvate Kinase Isoenzymes

	M1-type	M-2 type	L-type	R-type
Chromosomal Locus	15q22		1q21	
Structural gene	M gene (32 kb, 12 exons)		LR gene (9.5 kb, 12 exons)	
Promoter	M-type		L-type	R-type
RNA processing	Alternative splicing		Splicing	Splicing
Amino acid residues	531	531	543	574
Subunit molecular weight	58,000	58,000	59,000	62,000
Tissue distribution	Skeletal muscle	Fetal tissue	Liver	Erythrocytes
	Brain	Leukocytes	Kidney	
		Platelets	Pancreas (β cell)	
		Hematopoietic stem cells	Small intestine	
		Other most tissues		

showed multiple malformations[204,208] and/or psychomotor retardation.[208,214] Causal relationship between these symptoms and HK deficiency is unclear. The inheritance of HK deficiency is autosomal recessive.

Because HK is an age-dependent enzyme, it shows much higher activity in reticulocytes than in mature cells. HK activities in affected erythrocytes are 42 to 179 percent of normal controls, but are only 16 to 75 percent when compared with controls with a similar degree of reticulocytosis. This makes diagnosis of HK deficiency difficult in some situations. Calculation of the HK/PK ratio or HK/G-6-PD ratio is useful to avoid the false negative result.[200] Reduced levels of 2,3-DPG and G-6-P in erythrocytes are the common metabolic features. ATP is modestly decreased if patients' reticulocytosis is taken into account.

The molecular study of HK deficiency has just begun. A missense mutation 1667T $\rightarrow$ C (Leu529Ser), and a 96-bp (577 to 672) deletion resulting in deletion of 32 amino acids (166 to 197) have been identified in a compound heterozygous Italian patient with HK "Melzo".[217] The latter is possibly caused by aberrant splicing. An expression study revealed that Leu529Ser completely abolished the HK activity, and the 32-residue deletion drastically reduced the activity.[218] The molecular defect of a HK deficient fetus has been reported.[216] The fetus showed intrauterine growth retardation and severe hemolytic anemia (Hb: 3.7 g/dl; reticulocyte counts: 42.1 percent) with marked reduction of erythrocyte HK activity (17 percent of a normal fetus), and died in utero at 37 weeks of gestation. Analysis of cDNA revealed a 0.5-kb and a 1.8-kb deletion in each transcript, which corresponded to exons 5 to 8, and 3 to 14 in the HK-1 gene, respectively.

Glucosephosphate Isomerase Deficiency

Glucosephosphate isomerase (EC 5.3.1.9; GPI) catalyzes the interconversion of G-6-P and fructose-6-phosphate (F-6-P) (see Fig. 182-1). Tissue-specific isozymes of GPI do not exist. A homodimer composed of two identical 63-kDa subunits is expressed in all human tissues (Table 182-2). The gene encoding human GPI located on the long arm of chromosome 19[219] spans in excess of 40 kb including 18 exons.[220,221] The cDNA sequence coding 558 amino acids has been published (GenBank K03515). It is noteworthy that GPI may also function as a bioactive polypeptide. Neuroleukin,[222] a neurotrophic factor and a lymphokine, is known to be identical with GPI monomer.[223,224] Interestingly, dimeric GPI, which is active as an enzyme, has no neuroleukin activity.[102] Recently, a tumor-secreted cytokine that stimulates cell migration and metastasis (autocrine motility factor) in vivo,[225,226] and a maturation mediator[227] that is capable of differentiating human myeloid leukemic cells to terminal monocytic cells have been reported to be closely related to GPI.

Since the first report by Baughan et al.,[228] hereditary hemolytic anemia associated with GPI deficiency has been described in 74 cases from 60 kindreds.[228–274] It is the third most common erythroenzymopathy after G-6-PD deficiency and PK deficiency. The inheritance of GPI deficiency is autosomal recessive (Table 182-1). The GPI activity of erythrocytes of affected patients is reduced to 7 to 60 percent (median: 22.5 percent; $n = 58$) of normal. The G-6-P/F-6-P ratio is significantly elevated in affected erythrocytes. Benign polymorphic variants of GPI have also been reported.[275]

The main clinical manifestation of GPI deficiency is chronic hemolytic anemia of variable severity (median Hb: 9.8 g/dl, range: 4.5 to 16.8; $n = 49$). Affected individuals often exhibit hemolytic crises triggered by viral or bacterial infections.[273] It has been proposed that these episodes might be due to the metabolic block at the F-6-P $\rightarrow$ G-6-P step, which prevents pentose from cycling more than once through the HMP shunt.[228] Impaired recycling was confirmed by in vitro experiments using [2-^{14}C] glucose in three cases,[228,229,242] but in another study this defect could not be confirmed.[276] Unlike G-6-PD deficiency, which also causes impaired shunt activity, drug-induced hemolysis is quite rare in GPI deficiency and was observed in only two cases.[242,243] Hydrops fetalis seems more common in GPI deficiency than other enzyme deficiencies.[255,263,277] Splenectomy results in significant clinical improvement particularly in childhood. The enzyme deficiency is also found in nonerythroid tissues. A few patients showed manifestations suggestive of dysfunction of such tissues, including mental retardation,[243,257] neuromuscular symptoms,[243,257,261,278] and impaired granulocyte function.[261,264,278]

Molecular analysis has been performed in 22 propositi (10 homozygotes and 12 compound heterozygotes), and 23 different mutations, scattered throughout the coding sequence, have been identified.[266,268–272,279] So far overall heterogeneity of GPI mutations is remarkable compared with PK or triosephosphate isomerase (TPI) mutations. Even the most frequent mutation, 1039C $\rightarrow$ T (Arg347Cys), has been found in no more than five unrelated patients.[268,272] What is more surprising is that there is evidence indicating that the same mutation has arisen independently more than once.[272,280] In 6 of 12 compound heterozygous variants, including Elyria,[238,272] Nordhorn,[102,239,271,281] Bari,[269] Mola,[269] and Zwickau,[102,271] one allele is inactive bearing either a nonsense mutation or a splicing mutation. In GPI Nordhorn, the existence of an inactive allele had been predicted from its biochemical properties.[239,281] A study using recombinant mutants suggests that the impaired kinetics as well as the instability may cause metabolic perturbations in affected cells.[282] An animal model of GPI deficiency has been developed in mice.[283]

Phosphofructokinase Deficiency

Phosphofructokinase (EC 2.7.1.11; PFK) catalyzes the phosphorylation of F-6-P to fructose-1,6-diphosphate (F-1,6-DP$_2$) by ATP. PFK activity is considered to play a major role in the regulation of the rate of glycolysis. PFK is a typical allosteric enzyme that is inhibited by various metabolic intermediates, including ATP, citrate, and 2,3-DPG.[284] Human PFK is a tetramer of 340 kDa with variable combinations of three unique subunits, muscle (M), liver (L), and platelet (P) types (Table 182-2).[285–288] These subunits are encoded by separate loci (M: 1cen-q32;[289] L: 21q22.3;[290] and P: 10p15[291]), and are ubiquitously expressed, but in a tissue-specific manner. Human muscle and liver express homotetramers M_4 and L_4, respectively, while erythrocytes express M and L subunits composing five tetramers, M_4, M_3L, M_2L_2, ML_3, and L_4.[289] M_4 is less sensitive to inhibition by ATP and manifests a greater affinity for F-6-P than does L_4,[288] which might be advantageous in muscle and probably in erythrocytes. The cDNAs for the M[292] and L[293] subunits, both encoding 779 amino acids have been cloned. The 24 exons of the human M subunit gene spans 30 kb,[294] and the L subunit gene spans more than 28 kb with 22 exons.[295] Several alternative splicing products of the human M subunit gene have been found in a tissue-specific manner.[296,297] Mammalian PFK is considered to have evolved by duplication of a gene that originated in prokaryotes.[298]

PFK deficiency (glycogen storage disease type VII, Tarui disease; see Chap. 71) has been reported at least 64 cases from 49 kindreds, since the first description by Tarui et al. in 1965.[299–334] Major clinical manifestations of PFK deficiency are myopathy and fully compensated hemolytic anemia. Many patients experience fatigue and pain with exercise from early childhood. In typical cases, strenuous exercise causes severe muscle cramps and myoglobinuria associated with abdominal pain and nausea. The severe muscle symptoms often make patients avoid vigorous exercise, and myopathy is prone to be overlooked in those cases.[316] Although hemolysis is evident (median reticulocyte counts: 5.2 percent; n = 23), hemoglobin levels are normal or increased in most patients (median: 13.7 g/dl, range: 9.8 to 17.4; n = 18). PFK deficiency is transmitted as an autosomal recessive trait. One-third of reported patients are Jewish origin.

Muscle PFK activities are almost nil in most patients, while the erythrocyte exhibits partial deficiency (median: 51 percent, range: 8 to 75; n = 21), reflecting the complete loss of M subunit. Affected muscle shows a metabolic block at the PFK step and accumulation of glycogen to twice normal levels. Although ischemic forearm exercise causes no appreciable increase of venous lactate in patients, marked increases in plasma ammonia, inosine, and hypoxanthine levels are observed. The accelerated degradation of muscle purine nucleotides may subsequently lead to hyperuricemia particularly in males.[335] Affected erythrocytes, which express only L_4 isozyme, also show a metabolic block at the PFK step with a reduced 2,3-DPG level. Because of its effect on the oxygen dissociation curve the low 2,3-DPG level may account for the fully compensated or often overcompensated hemolysis.

Besides the classical Tarui disease, which manifests both early onset myopathy and hemolysis, several variant types of PFK deficiency have been reported.[316] The isolated hemolytic type has been described in three probands.[303,305,306] Although myopathic symptoms are possibly masked by the patients' aversion to exercise, these cases have unusual features including moderate to severe hemolytic anemia,[305] a normal ischemic exercise test,[303] very-low erythrocyte PFK activity,[303] and/or normal muscle PFK activity.[306] The fatal infantile type is a variant characterized by severe myopathy and early death before the age of 4.[309,314,318,320,321,333] Unfortunately, molecular analysis has not been performed in both of these types at the time of this writing. Although some investigators have proposed that a distinct late onset type exists,[313,319,325,330,332] recent molecular studies have provided evidence that the mutations in the late onset type are indistinguishable from those found in the classical type.[325,330,336] Hereditary deficiency of the L subunit, documented through chromatographic analysis of the erythrocytes, has been found in two asymptomatic individuals.[316,337] Family studies indicate that these individuals are heterozygous for L subunit deficiency.[316,337]

Molecular abnormalities causing PFK deficiency have been studied in more than 30 patients and 15 different mutations have so far been identified.[322–328,331,334,336,338,339] In the Jewish population, a splicing mutation IVS5 + 1G → A causing a deletion of the exon 5 sequence,[322,323,325,331] and a single nucleotide deletion 2003delC leading to a premature stop codon at 684[323,331] are the most frequent. IVS15 + 1G → T causing deletion of 25 residues (423 to 447) has been identified in the first Japanese family described by Tarui et al.,[299,338] and IVS19 + 1G → A which results in skipping of the exon 19 was found in another Japanese family.[324] IVS6 − 2A → C documented in an Italian patient[326] is an interesting mutation because it activates two different cryptic splice sites and leads to the production of 2 different species, one with a deletion of 4 amino acids (codons 143 to 146) and the other with premature termination at 145 amino acid residues. Four subjects in a Swedish family are compound heterozygotes for an intronic mutation IVS16 − 64A → G and an exonic splicing site mutation 1127G → A,[339] each of which generates a truncated peptide with 376 residues and 488 residues, respectively. A nonsense mutation 283C → T predicting a polypeptide of only 94 residues has been described in three homozygous individuals in a Jewish kindred.[336] All of the above mutations may produce completely inactive M subunits.

Missense mutations 116G → T (Arg39Leu), and 116G → C (Arg39Pro) have been identified in a Jewish[323] and two unrelated Italian patients,[326,334] respectively. Arg39 may be one of the essential residues for ATP binding.[298] The complete loss of muscle PFK activity that was found in homozygous individuals with Arg39Pro[326,334] is consistent with the importance of this residue. The mutant with Arg39Leu expressed in yeast showed marked instability.[328] Gly209Asp caused by 626G → A was found in a homozygous French Canadian patient.[328] Gly209 is a highly conserved residue, and it is located adjacent to the Met208 that is essential for F-6-P binding,[298] suggesting that a Gly209Asp might be quite deleterious. Indeed, the mutant enzyme expressed in yeast was completely inactive.[328] Asp543Ala caused by 1628A → C, and Trp686Cys by 2058G → T have been found in an Italian[326] and a Japanese patient,[327] respectively. Both Asp543 and Trp686 are conserved residues, but neither are involved in F-6-P or ATP binding. It is of interest that the patient with Trp686Cys exhibited a small but positive lactate response in forearm exercise test.[327] Although the patient's muscle PFK activity was virtually nil, the mutant enzyme may function to a very minor extent. The other allele of the patient with Asp543Ala was not expressed for some unknown reason.[326] A pair of mutant alleles, 299G → A and 2087G → A, causing Arg100Gln and Arg696His substitutions, were found in a compound heterozygous Swiss patient. Neither of Arg100 and Arg696 is phylogenetically conserved and neither is involved in active site regions. The mutants expressed in yeast were functional but slightly thermolabile.[328] The less deleterious nature of these mutations may account for the detectable PFK activity (8 percent of normal) in the patient's muscle. Hereditary PFK M-subunit deficiency has also been found in dogs.[340]

Aldolase Deficiency

Aldolase (EC 4.1.2.13) catalyzes a reversible reaction, cleaving F-1,6-P_2 into glyceraldehyde-3-phosphate (GA-3-P) and dihydroxyacetone phosphate (DHAP) (see Fig. 182-1). In mammals, there are three distinct isozymes, A, B, and C, each of which is encoded by a separate gene (Table 182-2). Erythrocytes, muscle, brain, and developing embryos express aldolase-A, which is a tetramer composed of four identical subunits of 36 kDa. Deficiency of liver aldolase-B causes hereditary fructose intolerance (see Chap. 70). Aldolase-C is expressed in brain and other nerve tissues. The cDNA for aldolase-A coding 364 amino acids has been cloned.[341] The aldolase-A gene, located at 16q22-q24[342] extends over 7.5 kb and encompasses 12 exons.[343] Several pseudogenes have been identified.[344]

Hereditary deficiency of aldolase-A has been reported in only four patients from three kindreds.[345–347] The common manifestation is moderate chronic hemolytic anemia. The initial Canadian-Jewish boy reported in 1973,[345] showed mild mental retardation and diverse malformations, and a German boy in the third kindred[347] exhibited psychomotor retardation and myopathy in addition to hemolytic anemia. Two Japanese boys in the second kindreds[346] showed no symptoms other than anemia. Erythrocyte aldolase activities in affected individuals were reduced to 4 to 16 percent of normal. Muscle aldolase was assayed in the German patient, and found to be reduced to 11 percent of normal.[347] Accumulation of F-1,6-P_2 in affected erythrocytes was remarkable in the Japanese patients (632- and 878-fold),[346] but only modest in the German patient (1.8-fold).[347] Interestingly, the former patients showed mild but overt hemolytic anemia (Hb: 9.5 g/dl and 11.3 g/dl), while hemolysis was fully compensated in the latter (Hb: 14.6 g/dl). It is not clear whether the modest metabolic block accounts for the mild anemia of the latter.

Molecular analysis has revealed that the Japanese patients are homozygous for the missense mutation 386A → G (Asp129Gly)[348] (note that amino acids are counted from the methionine coded by an initiation codon). The patient's enzyme expressed in *E. coli* showed marked instability, indicating that the phylogenetically conserved Asp129 is important for maintaining enzyme stability.[348] Another mutation 619G → A (Glu207Lys) was identified in the German kindred.[347] Glu207 is located in a helix essential for the subunit interaction, and the Glu207Lys mutation may disturb this interaction leading to the unstable quaternary structure,[347] a conclusion consistent with the marked instability of the patient's enzyme. The inheritance of aldolase deficiency is autosomal recessive mode, and it is of interest that the parents of the first case reported[345] had normal enzyme activity. This finding was interpreted as indicating that the mutant subunit may function normally when incorporated into a tetramer with normal subunits.

Triosephosphate Isomerase Deficiency

Triosephosphate isomerase (EC 5.3.1.1; TPI) catalyzes the interconversion of GA-3-P and DHAP (see Fig. 182-1). The equilibrium favors the formation of DHAP by 20:1. Human TPI is a homodimer of 54 kDa comprised of two identical subunits of 248 amino acids. The cDNA has been cloned from a human liver library.[349] The TPI gene, which extends over 5 kb, is divided into seven exons,[350] and has been localized at 12p13 (Table 182-2).[351] Three processed pseudogenes have been identified.[350]

TPI is expressed in all tissues, and the deficiency is a multisystem disorder that is characterized by chronic hemolytic anemia, progressive neuromuscular dysfunction, and increased susceptibility to infection. The mode of inheritance is autosomal recessive (Table 182-1). Since the first description by Schneider et al.[352] in 1965, it has been reported in nearly 50 cases from 38 kindreds.[352–371]

Hemolytic anemia is the first symptom and is often associated with neonatal hyperbilirubinemia requiring exchange transfusion. Although hemolysis is precipitated by the frequent episodes of infections, anemia in the chronic phase is rather mild (median Hb: 10.4 g/dl; n = 18). Splenectomy was performed in one patient with no improvement of the anemia.[354]

Detailed neurologic information is available in 18 propositi.[352–354,357–362,365–368,370] Retardation of motor development usually appears within a year after birth (median: 7 months, range: 1 to 24). Progressive weakness and hypotonia were the cardinal symptoms in 15 cases, often preceded by spasticity. Other neurologic manifestations included dystonic-dyskinetic syndrome,[358] tremor,[354] opisthotonus,[357] and optic nerve atrophy.[370] The neuromuscular symptoms are progressive in early infantile period, but may stabilize later in surviving patients.[354,366,368] Sensory impairment is absent. Intellectual status has been described in 12 kindreds,[353,354,357–360,362,366,368,370] and 5 propositi were mentally retarded.[353,360,362,366,370] Neuropathologic findings are available only in one patient.[353,372] These were characterized by olivary and cerebellar neuron loss, and axonal spheroids in midbrain and cerebellum. The latter might reflect a nonspecific axonal reaction to various factors including toxins.[372] Cardiac complications have been reported in three propositi.[353,360,362]

Increased susceptibility to infection is observed in most patients. Granulocyte function was impaired in one propositus,[359] but normal in two.[357,358] The patients with TPI deficiency rarely survive beyond childhood (median survival: 20.5 months, range 11 months to 12 years; n = 16). Although the reported causes of death include respiratory failure, cardiac failure, and severe infections, patients often die suddenly without obvious cause. It is noteworthy that several patients have shown an unusually mild clinical course with stable neuromuscular symptoms[354,366,368] and/or absence of increased susceptibility to infection.[366,368] The most striking is a Hungarian family.[368] The 15-year-old propositus had exhibited no neurologic symptoms until the age of 12, and his 23-year-old brother is free of any clinical signs and symptoms except for well-compensated chronic hemolysis.[368] An additional case without neuromuscular symptom has been described briefly in an abstract.[371] Prenatal diagnosis has been performed in several cases.[361,365,367,373]

TPI activities of the erythrocytes of affected individuals are reduced to 2 to 33 percent (median: 12 percent; n = 24) of normal. Markedly reduced enzyme activities are also found in other tissues. The striking increase in DHAP concentration (eighteen- to ninety-sixfold) that has been documented[357–360,365–368] is consistent with a metabolic block at the TPI step. Except in one patient, the residual TPI has been found to be thermolabile,[371] and in most cases the residual enzyme has normal kinetics for GA-3-P. The mechanism of TPI deficiency causing multisystem dysfunction is poorly understood. A hypothesis that the accumulation of DHAP might be toxic for tissues and responsible for the dysfunction is attractive,[374] but there has been no sufficient experimental evidence to support it. In the two Hungarian brothers with markedly discordant neurologic phenotypes, there were roughly 100 percent and 30 percent more 16:0/20:4 and 18:0/20:4 diacylphosphatidylcholine species in the erythrocytes than in normal controls, and the membrane fluidity was increased, more so in the mildly affected brother than in the one with severe neurologic impairment. This led to the speculation that differences in membrane fluidity and enzyme activities between the erythrocytes from the phenotypically differing TPI-deficient might reflect the state of the membranes elsewhere, as in the nervous system and thus be related to the neurologic disorder that was observed.[375]

Molecular analysis of TPI variants has been performed in 19 patients, and 9 different mutations have been identified.[363,364,367,369–371,375–377] The most frequent is a missense mutation 315G → C (Glu105Asp) (note that nucleotide numbers are for cDNA sequence, and that amino acids are counted from the methionine coded by an initiation codon), that was identified in 17 of 19 patients[353,363,364,367,369–371,376,377] and accounted for 74 percent of the total pathogenic TPI mutations. An extensive haplotypic analysis showed that there had been no crossovers over a considerable physical distance, suggesting that all subjects with 315G → C are descendants of a common ancestor in northern Europe who probably lived more than 1000 years ago.[378] This is consistent with the fact that almost all TPI-deficient individuals are of European origin and none of Asian or African origin have ever been reported. A Glu105Asp mutant expressed in cultured Chinese hamster ovary cells as well as the erythrocyte enzyme from the patients was thermolabile.[363] Daar et al.[363] and Mande et al.[379] suggested that the molecular mechanism of the Glu105Asp mutation was perturbation of the local structure of the active site. Glu105 is located near the active site and shields Arg99 from Lys113.[379] Arg99 is very important residue involved in intersubunit binding and is also in contact with the catalytic His96. The shortening of the Glu105 side chain by the substitution to aspartic acid may lead to an unfavorable interaction between Arg99 and Lys113, reducing the stability of the mutant enzyme. All homozygotes for the Glu105Asp variant and compound heterozygotes for Glu105Asp and another allele coding an inactive mutation exhibit progressive neuromuscular symptoms, indicating the deleterious nature of this mutation.

Phe241Leu caused by 721T → C, which has been identified in Hungarian patients with mild phenotype,[368] is another mutation studied molecularly in detail.[369,379] In the crystal structure,

Phe241 is located proximal to the active site.[379] The phenyl ring of Phe241 contacts with residues on a helix, which is important for the phosphate binding. Although the substitution of phenylalanine by leucine is conservative, it may thus alter the direction or the position of the helix and lead to a change in the substrate binding property.

Val232Met caused by 694G → A has been found in a homozygous patient with typical neuromuscular symptoms.[367] Val232 is one of a series of seven highly conserved residues (codons 231 to 237). Cys42Tyr caused by the 125G → A mutation has been found in three unrelated compound heterozygous patients in combination with Glu105Asp.[371,378] Cys42 is not highly conserved, but it is located in the β barrel structure.[379] Ile171Val produced by the 511A → G mutation is of great interest because this mutation was found in a compound heterozygote who did not manifest neurologic symptoms.[371] Moreover, the patient's enzyme is unique in that its thermostability is normal.[371] Considering that the patient has another allele coding a drastic Glu105Asp mutation,[371] the stable enzyme must be the one with the Ile171Val substitution, and one might then expect that this mutation is less deleterious than the common Glu105Asp substitution. However, Ile171 is located in the highly conserved active site loop including the catalytic Glu166,[379] indicating that the residue should be important for the catalytic function. Two nonsense mutations, 568C → T (Arg190Ter) and 436G → T (Glu146Ter), have been found in two compound heterozygotes together with Glu105Asp[353,363,376] or Phe241Leu,[368,369,375] respectively. These nonsense mutations may not only produce inactive premature polypeptides but also reduce the abundance of nuclear mRNA.[376,380] Another type of premature termination caused by a two-nucleotide deletion 86delGT that produces a frameshift results in the deduced production of a truncated chain with only 70 residues has been described.[377] This deletion mutation was found in a compound heterozygote together with Glu105Asp.[377]

Four coding mutations have been identified in asymptomatic heterozygous individuals: 367G → A (Gly123Arg),[381] 218G → C (Gly73Ala),[382] 463G → A (Val155Met),[382] 315G → C (Glu105Asp).[382,378] Gly123Arg is known to cause a thermolabile variant TPI Manchester. In 1982, using a large-scale automated enzyme estimations, Mohrenweiser[383] reported that he found seven putative heterozygotes, infants with reduced enzyme activity, among 146 African-Americans. The absence of clinically affected homozygotes in the African-American population suggested that it was likely that the defect would prove to be a null allele, incompatible with life in the homozygous state. This suggestion is consistent with a subsequent observation in mice of a series of induced mutations with nucleotide substitutions; null alleles were found to be lethal in homozygotes at an early postimplantation stage of embryonic development (see immediately below). Almost 15 years later[382] the DNA from all of these infants was reported to have base substitutions in each of two sites, −5 and −8 base pairs upstream of the transcription start site. The substitutions were A → G at position −5, G → A at position −8 (−40A → G and −43G → A, counting backward from the A of the methionine start codon), mutations that were in the cap site of the TPI gene. Three subjects were found to have an additional T → G substitution −24 base pairs upstream of the start of transcription, in the TATA-box. It was suggested that the −3 and −8 mutations markedly reduced TPI activity and were lethal in the homozygous state. Further studies have shown that this not to be the case. All three of these mutations are polymorphisms in the African-American population. Three haplotypes (−5G), (−5G, −8A), and (−5G, −8A, −24G) with gene frequencies of 0.111, 0.101, and 0.0047, respectively, were found to be associated with a statistically significant, but very modest, reduction in enzyme activity. Indeed, among 424 African-American adults, no cases of one-half normal activity were found as one would have expected if a severe deficiency gene were polymorphic in this population. None of the haplotypes were restricted to subjects with reduction of enzyme activity. Normal homozygotes for the −5G, −8A haplotype were found, ruling out the possibility that these mutations were responsible for lethal TPI deficiency.[384]

An animal model of TPI deficiency has been developed in 1-ethyl-1-nitrosourea-treated mice. All the homozygous mutations are lethal at embryonic stage. Three missense mutations and one terminal codon mutation (Ter → Cys) have been identified.[385]

Phosphoglycerate Kinase Deficiency

Phosphoglycerate kinase (EC 5.3.1.9; PGK) catalyzes the interconversion of 1,3-bisphosphoglycerate (1,3-DPG) and 3-phosphoglycerate. ATP is generated in the forward reaction 1,3-DPG → 3-phosphoglycerate (see Fig. 182-1). In addition to a ubiquitous enzyme PGK-1, that is a 48-kDa monomer, a tissue-specific intronless isoform PGK-2 has been found in spermatozoa (Table 182-2).[386] The human PGK-1 gene is located on the X chromosome (Xq13.3),[387] 11 exons spanning 23 kb.[388] Several pseudogenes have been identified.[388,389] The cDNA sequence for PGK-1, encoding 417 amino acids, has been cloned from a human fetal liver library.[390] Structural investigations have revealed that PGK consists of two domains (the N- and C-terminal domains) connected by a well-conserved hinge region.[391] The binding site for ATP/ADP is located on the C-terminal domain, while the site for the phosphoglycerates is on the opposite domain. These binding sites are distant from each other in the native enzyme or in the presence of only one substrate. However, when both substrates are present, the enzyme undergoes a conformational rearrangement, bending the hinge to bring the substrates close enough for a direct phosphorylation.[392]

Since the first description by Kraus et al.[393] in 1968, symptomatic deficiency of PGK-1 has been reported in 26 patients from 21 kindreds.[393–415] The mode of inheritance is X-linked, and most of the affected individuals are hemizygous males (Table 182-1). Due to random inactivation of the X-chromosome,[416,417] heterozygous females may exhibit various degrees of enzyme deficiency, and sometimes clinical symptoms as well. PGK deficiency is a multisystem disorder characterized by three major clinical manifestations: chronic hemolytic anemia, central nervous system dysfunction, and myopathy.

Chronic hemolytic anemia was found in 12 of 19 hemizygous propositi,[394,397,399–403,407,409–411,413] usually mild (median Hb: 10 g/dl; n = 9), and often fully compensated. Splenectomy was beneficial in three hemizygous patients,[394,399,400] but ineffective in one affected heterozygote.[393]

Slowly progressive central nervous system dysfunction was apparent in 11 of 19 propositi.[394,397,400–403,408,410–412] Speech difficulties in early childhood are often the first sign. Mild to moderate mental retardation has been found in all the reported cases with central nervous system abnormalities. Emotional instability,[394,401,410] convulsion,[394,402,403,408,411] ataxia,[401,402] and tremor[401,402] are also found in some patients, but sensory impairment is absent. Neuropathologic findings are not available.

Myopathy characterized by recurrent episodes of exercise intolerance, cramps, and myoglobinuria has been reported in 9 of 19 propositi.[405,406,408,409,411,412,414,415] Strangely, no PGK-deficient case with myopathy had been described until the first report of such a patient by Rosa et al.[404] in 1979, although it has been reported frequently thereafter. The typical episode with massive myoglobinuria is triggered by a short but vigorous exercise including running and dancing, and in one case, by a generalized tonic-clonic convulsion.[408] The episode is often associated with nausea, vomiting, abdominal pain, and dizziness, and may lead to acute renal failure. Although the first typical episode occurs usually in adolescence, patients often have mild myalgia or muscle weakness since childhood. Muscle biopsy specimens have shown only nonspecific findings.[405,406,408,412,414] Muscle glycogen levels were found to be increased in two patients,[405,408] but normal in two others.[406,414] Most of the patients with myopathy show no increase of lactate after ischemic forearm exercise.

It should be noted that PGK-deficient patients seldom manifest all three cardinal clinical feature of the disease, chronic hemolytic anemia, central nervous system dysfunction, and myopathy.[418] Most patients show only one or two of them in various combinations. The lack of myopathy in several patients may be explained by the fact that patients who are very young or severely limited by mental retardation are unable to perform muscular exercise sufficiently intense to trigger myoglobinuria.[405] It is also possible that symptoms associated with myopathy have been overlooked or misdiagnosed. Symptoms such as "black-colored urine associated with convulsion."[402] "intense fatigue."[397] or "dizziness associated with nausea and vomiting."[410] which were originally interpreted as symptoms associated with hemolytic episodes, may also be consistent with myopathic episodes. Another possibility is that patients' aversion to exercise masks the myopathic symptoms. Such situations are not rare in PFK deficiency.[316]

Erythrocyte PGK activities in hemizygous individuals are decreased to 0 to 23 percent (median: 6.5 percent; $n = 18$) of normal. Heterozygous females may exhibit various degrees of enzyme deficiency. Muscle PGK activities in hemizygotes are 1.5 to 25 percent (median: 5 percent; $n = 9$) of normal. There is no evidence that clinical severity is related to the degree of residual activity. The reduced ATP level and the accumulation of intermediates above PGK step, particularly DHAP (five- to eighteenfold) and F-1,6-dP_2 (four- to twenty-onefold), are observed in affected erythrocytes. The increased levels of DHAP (twenty-onefold) and F-1,6-dP_2 (seventy-fivefold) have also been found in the muscle of a hemizygous individual.[419] The 2,3-DPG content in affected erythrocytes is almost doubled, probably due diversion of 1,3-DPG from the PGK reaction to the bisphosphoglycerate mutase reaction. The right shift in the oxygen dissociation curve that results may improve oxygen delivery to body tissues thereby compensating, to some extent, for the decreased hemoglobin level of the blood.[395] As in the case of other glycolytic enzymopathies, the mechanism of hemolysis in PGK deficiency is unclear. A hypothesis has been proposed that hemolysis is caused by impaired HMP shunt activity resulting from inhibition of 6-phosphogluconate dehydrogenase by the high concentration of 2,3-DPG.[397] However, in one study,[396] no decrease in the HMP shunt activity of affected erythrocytes was found.

Amino acid sequence alterations have been documented in 12 disease-causing variants, 2 by peptide mapping[420,421] and the others by nucleotide sequencing.[409,410,412,413,415,422–425] The mutations are highly heterogeneous, and 11 different mutations have been identified. A 492A → T (Asp164Val) substitution has been found in a Chinese boy with PGK New York[394,424] and a French patient with PGK Amiens[403,423] (note that amino acids are counted from the methionine coded by an initiation codon). Although both probands show moderate hemolytic anemia associated with mental retardation and convulsions, the clinical course is much more progressive with the Asp164Val mutation. Most of the affected males in this family have shown frequent episodes of infection-induced hemolytic crisis and have died before reaching adulthood,[394–396] while the French patient has survived for more than 20 years despite the marked mental retardation and frequent seizures.[403,423] It is of interest that granulocyte function was impaired in one hemizygote of the Chinese family,[426] but appeared intact in the French propositus.[403] Asp164 is located proximal to the binding site for the phosphoglycerates on the N-terminal domain. The replacement of the negatively charged aspartic acid by a hydrophobic valine may cause drastic structural alteration of the active site.[423,424] Gly158Val found in a Japanese male with PGK Shizuoka[409] is another substitution that was identified in the vicinity of Asp164. Although neither Asp164Val nor Gly158Val is a conservative substitution, the latter is located in a random coil apart from the active site.[409] This may explain the much milder clinical consequence of PGK Shizuoka.

The amino acid substitution, Arg206Pro, causing PGK Uppsala[397,420] is of special interest because its possible effect on enzyme function has been studied in detail by using a recombinant yeast mutant.[427] Although the overall three-dimensional structure was not modified, and neither the specific activity nor the kinetic parameters was greatly affected, the Arg206Pro mutant showed a decreased stability. Tertiary structural analysis suggested that the decreased stability may result from the loss of the interaction between Arg206 and Lys229, which might be crucial for stability of the enzyme.[427]

A missense mutation 755A → C, which changes a consensus 5′ splice sequence AGgt to a nonconsensus CGgt, found in a Belgian patient with PGK Antwerp,[415] is interesting because it causes not only an amino acid substitution Glu252Ala but also aberrant splicing leading to the production of an inactive enzyme lacking most of the C-terminal domain. Because Glu252 is not a conserved residue and is located in the region that is involved in neither substrate nor ATP binding of PGK, the aberrant splicing should be responsible for the reduced activity of PGK Antwerp.[415] Indeed, the PGK mRNA content in patient's lymphoblastoid cells was only 10 percent of that of normal,[415] a finding that would be unusual in a variant caused solely by a missense mutation. Ile253 which is replaced by a threonine in PGK Hamamatsu[408,425] is located next to the Glu252. Although both PGK Antwerp and PGK Hamamatsu cause myopathy and lack hemolytic anemia, only the latter is associated with central nervous system dysfunction.

Besides the mutations causing clinical symptoms, two non-disease-causing mutations have been identified: Asp268Asn in PGK München[428] and Thr352Asn in PGK II.[429] Electrophoretic variants of PGK with normal enzyme activity have also been found.[430,431,432]

Bisphosphoglycerate Mutase Deficiency

Bisphosphoglycerate mutase (diphosphoglycerate mutase) (EC 2.7.5.4; BPGM) is a multifunctional enzyme that catalyzes the synthesis and the degradation of 2,3-DPG in the erythrocyte by virtue of its bisphosphoglycerate mutase and bisphosphoglycerate phosphatase activities[433,434] (Rapoport-Luebering shunt). This erythrocyte specific enzyme also has a phosphotransferase activity for the interconversion of 3-phosphoglycerate and 2-phosphoglycerate.[433,434] However, 95 percent of the phosphoglyceromutase activity in erythrocytes may be attributed to another glycolytic enzyme monophosphoglycerate mutase (see Fig. 182-1). Bisphosphoglycerate mutase is a dimer of 60 kDa composed of two identical subunits each of which consists of 258 residues. The cDNA has been cloned from reticulocyte mRNA.[435] The human bisphosphoglycerate mutase gene has been assigned to region 7q34-7q22,[436] where its 3 exons spans more than 22 kb (Table 182-2).[437]

Complete deficiency of bisphosphoglycerate mutase has been found in only a French family reported by Rosa et al.[438] in 1978. The affected individuals, a 42-year-old propositus and his three sisters, had no clinical symptoms except for ruddy cyanosis. They had no hemolytic anemia, but rather erythrocytosis with the hemoglobin levels 17 to 19 g/dl. Bisphosphoglycerate mutase and bisphosphoglycerate phosphatase activities were undetectable in erythrocytes. The patients also showed severe depletion of 2,3-DPG (<3 percent of normal), increased ATP (twofold), and marked accumulation of triosephosphates (fifteenfold) and F-1,6-P_2 (tenfold). These metabolic alterations are consistent with a metabolic block at the bisphosphoglycerate mutase step. The increased ATP level may reflect the increased utilization of 1,3-DPG by PGK in the absence of bisphosphoglycerate mutase. The erythrocytosis is presumably due to the decreased oxygen affinity of hemoglobin caused by the depletion of 2,3-DPG. Immunochemical analysis revealed that the patients' bisphosphoglycerate mutase was very thermolabile if 2,3-DPG is absent.[439] Erythrocytes of heterozygotes showed half-normal enzyme activities (bisphosphoglycerate mutase: 41 to 46 percent ; bisphosphoglycerate phosphatase: 44 to 63 percent) and 2,3-DPG levels (41 to 75 percent).[438,440] Some of them exhibited abnormal oxygen dissociation curves and erythrocytosis.[438,440]

Molecular analysis revealed that the affected patients are compound heterozygous for a missense mutation 268C → T and a deletion of cytidine (60delC)[441] (note that nucleotide numbers are for cDNA sequence, and amino acids are counted from the methionine coded by an initiation codon). The missense mutation generates a variant enzyme with Arg90Cys (bisphosphoglycerate mutase Créteil I), while the deletion causes a frameshift and produces a truncated protein with only 47 residues (bisphosphoglycerate mutase Créteil II). Although Arg90 has not been described as part of the active site, its functional importance may be expected from the strict conservation of the residue.[441] Garel et al.[442] have revealed that the guanidinium group of Arg90 may play an essential role both in the stability and in the catalytic functions of the enzyme, probably by maintaining the correct three-dimensional structure in this region of the molecule. The loss of the guanidinium group associated with the Arg90Cys substitution may thus perturb the local structure and abolish bisphosphoglycerate mutase and bisphosphoglycerate phosphatase activities.

Other Enzyme Abnormalities of the Glycolytic Pathway

Partial deficiency of erythrocyte enolase (EC 4.2.1.11) (see Fig. 182-1) has been documented in association with hemolytic anemia in two unrelated individuals.[443,444] Although the enzyme deficiency was found in three generations in the second family, no one but the propositus showed apparent signs of hemolytic anemia.[444]

Hereditary deficiency of the H (B) subunit of lactate dehydrogenase (EC 1.1.1.27; LDH) (see Fig. 182-1) causes a remarkable reduction of LDH activity (<10 percent of normal) and accumulation of glycolytic intermediates above GA-3-PD step in affected erythrocytes.[445] The latter is considered to be due to the inhibition of GA-3-PD step by a high concentration of NADH associated with LDH deficiency. Despite the remarkable metabolic alteration, affected individuals do not show any symptoms including hemolytic anemia, although in one case minimal reticulocyte count elevations were noted.[446] Patients with LDH M (A) subunit deficiency are known to manifest myopathy and skin lesions, but no hemolysis.[447] It is of interest that, in contrast to human, mice homozygous for LDH M subunit deficiency exhibit chronic hemolytic anemia.[448]

Human monophosphoglycerate mutase (EC 2.7.5.3; MPGM) is composed of two distinct subunits, M and B. Muscle contains the homodimer MM, and many tissues, including erythrocytes, express BB. Hereditary deficiency of the M subunit causes myopathy,[449] but deficiency of B subunit has not been reported.

ENZYMOPATHIES IN THE HEXOSE MONOPHOSPHATE SHUNT AND IN PATHWAYS RELATED TO GLUTATHIONE METABOLISM

6-Phosphogluconate Dehydrogenase Deficiency and Glutathione Peroxidase Deficiency

6-Phosphogluconate dehydrogenase (EC 1.1.1.44; 6-PGD) is the second NADPH-generating enzyme in the HMP shunt (see Fig. 182-1). Hereditary deficiency of 6-phosphogluconate dehydrogenase has been reported as a genetic polymorphism that does not cause hemolytic anemia even in the homozygous state.[450]

An activity of selenoenzyme glutathione peroxidase (EC 1.11.1.9.) (see Fig. 182-1) shows ethnic variation. Individuals of Jewish or Mediterranean origin exhibit lower activities.[451] Selenium-deficient diet may cause reduced glutathione peroxidase activity as low as 15 percent without any signs of hemolysis.[452]

Although a considerable number of individuals with 6-phosphogluconate dehydrogenase deficiency or glutathione peroxidase deficiency have been documented in association with hemolytic syndromes, their enzyme deficiencies are only in a heterozygous level, and some family members also show reduced enzyme activities without symptoms.[453] There is no conclusive evidence that these deficiencies cause hemolytic anemia.[454]

Hereditary deficiency of 6-phosphogluconolactonase (EC 3.1.1.31) has been found to be associated with hemolytic anemia when combined with a nonhemolytic variant of G-6-PD.[455] However, a kinetic considerations make it unlikely that a cause-and-effect relationship exists between this deficiency and hemolytic anemia, even when G-6-PD deficiency is present.[456]

Glutathione Reductase Deficiency

Glutathione reductase (EC 1.6.4.2; GR) catalyzes the reduction of GSSG to GSH (see Fig. 182-1). Mammalian erythrocyte glutathione reductase reaction greatly prefers NADPH as a hydrogen donor, and this is supplied by both G-6-PD and 6-phosphogluconate dehydrogenase in the HMP shunt. Because glutathione reductase contains flavin adenine dinucleotide (FAD), glutathione reductase activity in erythrocytes is markedly influenced by riboflavin intake.[457] Virtually complete erythrocyte glutathione reductase deficiency has been documented in only one consanguineous family.[458] Although the propositus showed an isolated episode of favism, no evidence of chronic hemolysis was obtained. In addition, affected erythrocytes maintained normal GSH level. An in vitro study using a selective glutathione reductase inhibitor has revealed that the reserve capacity of glutathione reductase in human erythrocytes is extremely large, and the relatively mild clinical expression of this patient is consistent with the severe enzyme deficiency.[459]

γ-Glutamylcysteine Synthetase Deficiency and Glutathione Synthetase Deficiency

The initial step of glutathione (GSH) synthesis, glutamic acid + cysteine → γ-glutamylcysteine, is catalyzed by γ-glutamylcysteine synthetase (EC 6.3.2.2; GC-S). This reaction is irreversible and requires ATP. γ-Glutamylcysteine is a rate-limiting enzyme of GSH synthesis and inhibited by GSH. Tissue-specific isozymes of γ-glutamylcysteine probably do not exist. Human γ-glutamylcysteine is a heterodimer composed of a heavy catalytic subunit of 73 kDa and a light regulatory subunit of 28 kDa. The cDNA for both subunits encoding 637 and 274 amino acids have been cloned.[460,461] Genes for heavy and light subunits have been assigned to 6p12[462] and 1p21,[463] respectively.

Hereditary GC-S deficiency has been reported in five patients from four unrelated families.[464–467] The patients showed mild to compensated chronic hemolytic anemia since early childhood. Two siblings in the initial family manifested progressive late onset (after age 29) spinocerebellar degeneration,[464,465] while the other three patients were free from neurologic symptoms.[466,467] Because the latter patients are relatively young (all under age 22), it is difficult to rule out the possibility of the late onset spinocerebellar degeneration secondary to γ-glutamylcysteine synthetase deficiency. Generalized aminoaciduria was found in the first family described,[465] but urinary amino acid levels were not reported in the others. γ-Glutamylcysteine synthetase activities in affected erythrocytes were reduced to 6 to 23 percent of normal and there was marked depletion of GSH (2 to 13 percent of normal). In spite of the expected deterioration of antioxidative potential, affected erythrocytes are not as sensitive to oxidative stress as G-6-PD–deficient cells. In the first and second patients, the Heinz body test was negative.[465] In the fourth and fifth patients, Heinz body test was not performed, but no Heinz body was seen in the blood.[467] There is no description of Heinz body in the third patient.[466] Heinz body formation after incubation with acetylphenylhydrazine is usually negative, and patients have no history of favism or drug-induced hemolytic crisis. The recycling activity of GSSG to GSH rather than the total GSH content is presumably crucial for the protection against the acute oxidative stress. Patients also show erythrocyte glutathione-S-transferase deficiency secondary to the GSH depletion.[466,467] The mode of inheritance is autosomal recessive. Most of the heterozygous individuals exhibit slightly reduced GC-S activities but normal GSH contents in erythrocytes. Recently, the first molecular abnormalities were identified in two additional patients.[467a,b]

The next step of GSH synthesis, γ-glutamylcysteine + glycine $\rightarrow$ GSH, is catalyzed by glutathione synthetase (EC 6.3.2.3; GSH-S). This reaction is also irreversible and requires ATP. Hereditary deficiency of GSH-synthetase causes either isolated hemolytic anemia or a multisystem disorder characterized by severe metabolic acidosis with 5-oxoprolinuria, usually accompanied by hemolytic anemia. Several disease-causing mutations have been identified.[468,469] GSH- synthetase deficiency is discussed in greater detail in Chap. 96.

ENZYMOPATHIES IN THE NUCLEOTIDE METABOLISM

Adenylate Kinase Deficiency

Adenylate kinase (EC 2.7.4.3; AK) is a ubiquitous enzyme that catalyzes the interconversion of three adenine nucleotides: ATP + AMP$\leftrightarrow$2ADP. In the erythrocyte, AK is particularly important because it may be the only enzyme capable of converting AMP to ADP. Vertebrates possess three distinct isozymes — AK1, AK2, and AK3 — which are encoded by separate genes. AK1 is a cytosolic enzyme present in erythrocytes, skeletal muscle and brain, whereas AK2 and AK3 are located in mitochondria (Table 182-2). Human AK1 is a monomer of 22 kDa composed of 194 amino acids.[470] The AK1 gene located at 9q32[471] is comprised of 7 exons extending over a distance of about 12 kb.[472]

Hereditary deficiency of erythrocyte AK has been reported in 14 individuals from six unrelated kindreds since the first description by Szeinberg et al. in 1969.[473–479] The clinical severity of AK deficiency is very variable. Szeinberg et al.[473] and Toren et al.[474] studied six related Arab families in Israel which belong to a large pedigree with complicated consanguineous marriages. All the homozygotes for AK deficiency in this pedigree had moderate to severe hemolytic anemia (Hb: 5.8 to 9.8 g/dl) associated with remarkably reduced erythrocyte AK activities (1 to 9 percent of normal). Two patients in one family have not shown mental retardation,[473] whereas six homozygotes from other families are retarded,[474] although they all presumably carry the same deficient AK variant. In five of the six patients, splenectomy has resulted in complete remission of hemolysis,[474] which is quite unusual in other erythroenzymopathies. Individuals with combined AK and G-6-PD deficiency showed more severe hemolytic anemia than those with AK deficiency alone.[474]

A French boy had severe AK deficiency (3.5 percent of normal) associated with fully compensated hemolytic anemia.[475] He also showed psychomotor retardation which was possibly due to neonatal trauma. A Japanese girl is unique because she had only partial AK deficiency (44 percent of normal) despite her apparent hemolytic anemia.[476] No evidence of hemolytic anemia was found in other heterozygous family members. Two African-American siblings are most unusual.[477] The propositus had undetectable erythrocyte AK activity using spectrophotometric assay and only about 1/2000 of normal activity when studied using sensitive radioisotopic techniques. Moderate hemolytic anemia was present in the patient, but her brother with similar vanishingly low residual enzyme activity showed no evidence of hemolysis. Two other cases have been reported in a Syrian[478] and in an Italian[479] family. Both had undetectable erythrocyte AK activities associated with hemolytic anemia precipitated by infections. The mode of inheritance of AK deficiency is compatible with autosomal recessive mode.

Molecular defects causing AK deficiency have been identified in two cases.[472,476,479] The Japanese girl with partial AK deficiency was found to be heterozygous for a missense mutation 382C $\rightarrow$ T (Arg128Trp), inherited from her mother.[472] The mutant chicken AK with the Arg128Trp mutation expressed in *E. coli* showed reduced catalytic activity. Another missense mutation 491A $\rightarrow$ G (Tyr164Cys) was found in a homozygous Italian patient.[479] The functional role of Tyr164 has not been established. Overall heterogeneity in clinical pictures even within an identical pedigree[473,474,477] raises questions about the causal relationship between AK deficiency and hemolytic anemia.

Adenosine Deaminase Overproduction

Adenosine deaminase (EC 3.5.4.4; ADA) catalyzes the irreversible deamination of adenosine to inosine: Adenosine + H_2O $\rightarrow$ inosine + NH_3. Deoxyadenosine is also can serve as a substrate for ADA. Human tissues display at least two distinct ADA species with molecular mass of 298 kDa and 36 kDa (Table 182-2).[480] The large form is a complex of two small forms and a noncatalytic binding protein of 220 kDa. Human erythrocytes express only the small form composed of 362 amino acids.[480] The human ADA gene has been assigned to 20q13.11[481] its 12 exons spanning 32 kb.[482]

Hereditary deficiency of ADA (see Chap. 109) leads to severe combined immunodeficiency disease without hemolysis, whereas the ADA overproduction in erythrocytes causes hemolytic anemia. Since the first description of a kindred with 12 affected individuals by Valentine et al.[476] in 1977, ADA overproduction has been reported in 4 unrelated families.[483–486] One of us (EB), has encountered a fifth family that has not been published. Except for mental retardation found in an Algerian boy,[485] chronic hemolytic anemia of variable severity is the only clinical manifestation. Stomatocytosis was remarkable in peripheral blood of two Japanese propositi.[484,486] Splenectomy was beneficial in two children with moderate to severe hemolytic anemia.[485,486] ADA activities are strikingly increased in affected erythrocytes (40- to 110-fold), but are normal in other tissues; the overproduction is erythroid-specific. The ATP content of affected erythrocytes is reduced to 50 to 70 percent of reticulocyte-rich controls, with normal or slightly decreased ADP and AMP levels. ADA overproduction is clearly transmitted as an autosomal dominant mode in the American family,[483] but somewhat ambiguous in others. In one Japanese family,[484] the parents had no evidence of hemolysis, and only the mother showed modest increase (fourfold) in ADA activity. The parents in the other Japanese family[486] showed neither hemolytic anemia nor increased ADA activity.

Two reactions compete for adenosine, which is an important substrate for the replenishment of the adenine nucleotide pool. One of these is adenosine kinase, which forms AMP; the other is ADA. The greatly increased ADA activity may interfere with nucleotide salvage via the adenosine kinase reaction by depleting adenosine, leading to the decreased ATP content in affected erythrocytes.[483] The profound depression of ATP synthesis from adenosine has been confirmed in patients' erythrocytes by using radioactive adenosine.[485] Biochemical and immunochemical studies revealed that the increased erythrocyte ADA activity results from the overproduction of the structurally normal enzyme.[487,488] The rate of ADA synthesis in erythroid progenitors was increased elevenfold in a patient.[488] It is of interest that ADA activity in density separated erythrocytes from a patient was twice as high in the top fraction (reticulocyte counts: 4.0 percent) than in the bottom fraction (reticulocyte counts: 1.4 percent), although it was similar in both fractions from normal controls.[488] This may suggest the accelerated decay of overproduced ADA in affected reticulocytes.

In spite of extensive investigations,[486,489–492] the molecular basis of ADA overproduction remains unclear. Southern blot analysis has revealed no evidence for major structural alterations and gene amplification in patients' ADA gene.[486,489] RNAse mapping and northern blot analysis have indicated at least a one hundredfold increase in ADA mRNA in reticulocytes from patients, but cDNA sequencing has shown no abnormality in the coding region and 5′- and 3′-untranslated regions.[489,490] From linkage analysis using a polymorphic TAAA repeat located 1.1 kb upstream of the ADA gene, Chen et al.[491] showed that the mutation causing ADA overproduction is likely to exist within or near the ADA locus. They examined relative reporter gene activity using constructs containing 10.6 kb of 5′ flanking sequence and

12.3 kb of the first intron of the ADA gene from the normal and mutant alleles. However, no difference in expression between normal and mutant alleles was found in transient transfection experiments using erythroid cells.[492] Neither was there a difference in expression in a transgenic mouse model.[492]

Acquired overproduction of erythrocyte ADA has been found in various disorders, including hypoplastic anemia[493] and acquired immunodeficiency syndrome.[494] The degree of overproduction is mild (less than fourfold), except for a patient with primary acquired sideroblastic anemia who showed a seventeenfold increase in erythrocyte ADA activity, but no hemolysis.[495]

Pyrimidine 5′-Nucleotidase Deficiency

Pyrimidine 5′-nucleotidase (P5N, or P5N-I) is a member of cytosolic 5′-nucleotidases (EC 3.1.3.5).[496] It is a monomer of 36 kDa with strict substrate specificity towards pyrimidine 5′-monophosphates. Erythrocytes have another cytosolic pyrimidine nucleotidase (P5N-II) that has a relatively broad specificity utilizing some 2′- and 3′-nucleotides as well as 5′-nucleotides.[497,498] Because of its extremely low content in erythrocytes and marked instability, P5N had not been purified to homogeneity until recently.[499] The primary structure, cDNA sequence, or genomic structure of P5N has not yet been elucidated.

Since its discovery by Valentine and associates[500] in 1974, P5N deficiency has so far been reported in 51 cases from 36 unrelated kindreds.[497,500–522] Mild to moderate chronic hemolytic anemia (median Hb: 10.0 g/dl; n = 31) is the only symptom in most patients. Anemia is usually stable and often fully compensated particularly in adults. Splenectomy has been beneficial in half of the patients.[505,510,511,516,517,519,522] Coarse basophilic stippling of erythrocytes is a hallmark of P5N deficiency, which is usually occur in as many as 5 percent of all erythrocytes. Propositi in five families showed mental retardation,[509,519] although the causal relationship to P5N deficiency is not clear.

During the maturation of erythrocytes, most of the DNA can be released from the cell by denucleation, while the RNA in ribosomes must be degraded through biochemical pathways. AMP and GMP produced by RNA degradation may be utilized metabolically by the maturing erythrocyte, but pyrimidine products such as CMP and UMP play no further known role in the erythrocyte and are normally dephosphorylated to diffusable nucleosides. P5N may be the only enzyme responsible for this process, because another pyrimidine nucleotidase P5N-II does not hydrolyze CMP and UMP.[497,498] Affected erythrocytes show decreased P5N activity to 1 to 56 percent of normal (median: 10 percent; n = 49), and accumulation of pyrimidine mono-, di-, and triphosphates and their derivatives including CDP-choline, CDP-ethanolamine, and UDP-glucose.[500,523,524] Pyrimidine nucleotides account for only 3 percent of the total nucleotides in normal erythrocytes,[500,523] while they are increased to 39 to 86 percent (median: 66 percent; n = 13) in affected erythrocytes. A shift in maximum absorbance from the usual 256–257 to 265–270 nm is observed in patients' deproteinized erythrocyte extract, and forms the basis of a useful rapid diagnostic test for P5N deficiency.[500,525] Most of the patients show increased GSH levels in erythrocytes, probably due to the inhibition of ATP-dependent oxidized glutathione transport by increased levels of pyrimidine nucleotides.[526] Although heterozygotes show modestly reduced P5N activities, they show neither detectable levels of abnormal nucleotides nor hemolytic anemia.

The mechanism by which P5N deficiency causes hemolytic anemia remains to be elucidated. It has often been speculated, without conclusive evidence, that the high concentrations of pyrimidine compounds would interfere with adenine nucleotide dependent reactions such as glycolysis or cation transport.[500] Affected erythrocytes show no significant metabolic block in glycolysis,[507,509] and results of an in vitro study[527] do not fully support the inhibitory effect of pyrimidine compounds on glycolytic kinases in vivo. Tomoda et al.[513] proposed that the high concentrations of pyrimidine nucleotides in affected erythrocytes may depress the HMP shunt activity leading to hemolysis. They found that CTP inhibits G-6-PD competitively with G-6-P in vitro, and noncompetitively with $NADP^+$. It has also been shown that the intraerythrocytic pH is decreased in P5N deficient patients, which may also suppress the HMP shunt activity.[513] There have been some other findings that support this hypothesis.[506,521,522,528] Despite the in vitro evidence,[513] the clinical picture of P5N deficiency is not consistent with the concept that HMP shunt inhibition is the cause of hemolysis. Drug- or infection-induced hemolytic crises, which might be a sign of impaired shunt activity, have been observed only in isolated cases. In addition, erythrocyte GSH was not unstable in four[508,510,512] of five patients examined,[507,508,510,512] and Heinz body formation after incubation with acetylphenylhydrazine was positive in three patients,[506,508,513] but negative in three.[500,501,511]

Because of the marked sensitivity of P5N to inactivation by lead, individuals exposed to lead may develop acquired erythrocyte P5N deficiency. In subjects with chronic lead intoxication, decreased erythrocyte P5N activity is observed in lower blood lead levels,[529] but basophilic stippling and accumulation of pyrimidine nucleotides may become apparent when blood lead levels are as high as 200 μg/dl of erythrocytes.[530,531] Acquired P5N deficiency is also uniformly encountered in patients with transient erythroblastopenia of childhood. This appears to be the case because P5N is unique among erythrocyte enzymes in continuing to decline in activity throughout erythrocyte life span; other age-dependent enzymes lose activity rapidly during the first few days in the circulation and subsequently maintain a relatively constant level of activity. Thus, in very old erythrocyte populations, as are found in erythroblastopenia of childhood and aplastic anemia, it is the P5N activity that decreases the most.[532]

REFERENCES

1. Benesch R, Benesch RE: The effect of organic phosphates from the human erythrocyte on the allosteric properties of hemoglobin. *Biochem Biophys Res Commun* **26**:162, 1967.
2. Gaetani GF, Ferraris AM, Rolfo M, Mangerini R, Arena S, Kirkman HN: Predominant role of catalase in the disposal of hydrogen peroxide within human erythrocytes. *Blood* **87**:1595, 1996.
3. Mueller S, Riedel HD, Stremmel W: Direct evidence for catalase as the predominant H_2O_2-removing enzyme in human erythrocytes. *Blood* **90**:4973, 1997.
4. Mentzer WC Jr, Baehner RL, Schmidt-Schönbein H, Robinson SH, Nathan DG: Selective reticulocyte destruction in erythrocyte pyruvate kinase deficiency. *J Clin Invest* **50**:688, 1971.
5. Beutler E: The relationship of red cell enzymes to red cell life span. *Blood Cells* **14**:69, 1988.
6. Valentine WN, Tanaka KR, Paglia DE: Pyruvate kinase and other enzyme deficiency disorders of the erythrocyte, in Scriver CR, Beaudetal AL, Sly WS, Valle D (eds): *The Metabolic Basis of Inherited Disease*, 6th ed. New York, McGraw-Hill, 1989, p 2341
7. Tanaka KR, Zerez CR: Red cell enzymopathies of the glycolytic pathway. *Semin Hematol* **27**:165, 1990.
8. Tanaka KR, Paglia DE: Pyruvate kinase and other enzymopathies of the erythrocyte, in Scriver CR, Beaudet AL, Sly WS, Valle D (eds): *The Metabolic and Molecular Bases of Inherited Disease*, 7th ed. New York, McGraw-Hill, 1995, p 3485.
9. Lukens JN: Hereditary hemolytic anemias associated with abnormalities of erythrocyte anaerobic glycolysis and nucleotide metabolism, in Lee GR, Bithell TC, Foerster J, Athens JW, Lukens JN (eds): *Wintrobe's Clinical Hematology*, 9th ed. Philadelphia, Lea & Febiger, 1993, p 990.
10. Miwa S, Kanno H, Fujii H: Pyruvate kinase deficiency. Historical perspectives and molecular genetics. *Am J Hematol* **42**:31, 1993.
11. Valentine WN, Tanaka KR, Miwa S: Specific glycolytic enzyme defect (pyruvate kinase) in three subjects with congenital nonspherocytic hemolytic anemia. *Trans Assoc Am Physicians* **74**:100, 1961.
12. Akin H, Baykal-Erkiliç A, Aksu A, Yucel G, Gümüslü S: Prevalence of erythrocyte pyruvate kinase deficiency and normal values of enzyme in a Turkish population. *Hum Hered* **47**:42, 1997.

13. De Medicis E, Ross P, Friedman R, Hume H, Marceau D, Milot M, Lyonnais J, De BM: Hereditary nonspherocytic hemolytic anemia due to pyruvate kinase deficiency: A prevalence study in Quebec (Canada). *Hum Hered* **42**:179, 1992.
14. Feng C-S, Tsang SS, Mak Y-T: Prevalence of pyruvate kinase deficiency among the Chinese: Determination by the quantitative assay. *Am J Hematol* **43**:271, 1993.
15. Mohrenweiser HW: Frequency of enzyme deficiency variants in erythrocytes of newborn infants. *Proc Natl Acad Sci U S A* **78**:5046, 1981.
16. Satoh C, Neel JV, Yamashita A, Goriki K, Fujita M, Hamilton HB: The frequency among Japanese of heterozygotes for deficiency variants of 11 enzymes. *Am J Hum Genet* **35**:656, 1983.
17. Bossu M, Laurenti F, Marzetti G: Neonatal hemolysis in subjects with transitory defects of erythrocyte metabolism. *Riv Clin Pediatr* **81**:493, 1968.
18. Sachs JR, Wicker DJ, Gilcher RO: Familial hemolytic anemia resulting from an abnormal red blood cell pyruvate kinase. *J Lab Clin Med* **72**:359, 1968.
19. Paglia DE, Valentine WN, Williams KO, Konrad PN: An isozyme of erythrocyte pyruvate kinase (PK-Los Angeles) with impaired kinetics corrected by fructose-1,6-diphosphate. *Am J Clin Pathol* **68**:229, 1977.
20. Etiemble J, Picat C, Dhermy D, Buc HA, Morin M, Boivin P: Erythrocytic pyruvate kinase deficiency and hemolytic anemia inherited as a dominant trait. *Am J Hematol* **17**:251, 1984.
21. Bowman HS, McKusick VA, Dronamraju KR: Pyruvate kinase deficient hemolytic anemia in an Amish isolate. *Am J Hum Genet* **17**:1, 1965.
22. Hennekam RCM, Beermer FA, Cats BP, Jansen G, Staal GEJ: Hydrops fetalis associated with red cell pyruvate kinase deficiency. *Genet Couns* **1**:75, 1990.
23. Gilsanz F, Vega MA, Gomez-Castillo E, Ruiz-Balda JA, Omenaca F: Fetal anemia due to pyruvate kinase deficiency. *Arch Dis Child* **69**:523, 1993.
24. Rouger H, Valentin C, Craescu CT, Galactéros F, Cohen-Solal M: Five unknown mutations in the LR pyruvate kinase gene associated with severe hereditary nonspherocytic haemolytic anaemia in France. *Br J Haematol* **92**:825, 1996.
25. Amankwah KS, Dick BW, Dodge S: Hemolytic anemia and pyruvate kinase deficiency in pregnancy. *Obstet Gynecol* **55**:42, 1980.
26. Dente L, D'Urso M, Di Maio S, Brancaccio V, Luzzatto L: Pyruvate kinase deficiency: Characterization of two new genetic variants. *Clin Chim Acta* **126**:143, 1982.
27. Fanning J, Hinkle RS: Pyruvate kinase deficiency hemolytic anemia: Two successful pregnancy outcomes. *Am J Obstet Gynecol* **153**:313, 1985.
28. Levinski U, Fajnholc N, Djaldetti M, De Vries A: Hemolytic anemia in pregnancy associated with erythrocyte pyruvate kinase deficiency. *Clin Sci* **11**:43, 1974.
29. Oski FA, Marshall BE, Cohen PJ, Sugerman HJ, Miller LD: Exercise with anemia. The role of the left-shifted or right-shifted oxygen-hemoglobin equilibrium curve. *Ann Intern Med* **74**:44, 1971.
30. Delivoria-Papadopoulos M, Oski FA, Gottlieb AJ: Oxygen-hemoglobin dissociation curves: Effect of inherited enzyme defects of the red cells. *Science* **165**:601, 1969.
31. Van Eys J, Garms P: Pyruvate kinase deficiency hemolytic anemia: A model for correlation of clinical syndrome and biochemical anomalies. *Adv Pediatr* **18**:203, 1971.
32. Tomoda A, Lachant NA, Noble NA, Tanaka KR: Inhibition of the pentose phosphate shunt by 2,3-diphosphoglycerate in erythrocyte pyruvate kinase deficiency. *Br J Haematol* **54**:475, 1983.
33. Duncan JR, Potter CG, Cappellini MD, Kurtz JB, Anderson MJ, Weatherall DJ: Aplastic crisis due to parvovirus infection in pyruvate kinase deficiency. *Lancet* **2**:14, 1983.
34. Noel D, Duron F, Thomas M: Hemochromatose et deficit en pyruvate kinase. *Ann Med Interne* **130**:679, 1979.
35. Salem HH, Van der Weyden MB, Firkin BG: Iron overload in congenital erythrocyte pyruvate kinase deficiency. *Med J Aust* **1**:531, 1980.
36. Rowbotham B, Roeser HP: Iron overload associated with congenital pyruvate kinase deficiency and high dose ascorbic acid ingestion. *Aust N Z J Med* **14**:667, 1984.
37. Nagai H, Takazakura E, Oda H, Tsuji H, Terada Y, Makino H, Yamauchi H, Saitoh K: An autopsy case of pyruvate kinase deficiency anemia associated with severe hemochromatosis. *Intern Med* **33**:56, 1994.
38. De Braekeleer M, St Pierre C, Vigneault A, Simard H, de ME: Hemochromatosis and pyruvate kinase deficiency. Report of a case and review of the literature. *Ann Hematol* **62**:188, 1991.
39. Vukelja SJ: Erythropoietin in the treatment of iron overload in a patient with hemolytic anemia and pyruvate kinase deficiency. *Acta Haematol* **91**:199, 1994.
40. Zanella A, Berzuini A, Colombo MB, Guffanti A, Lecchi L, Poli F, Cappellini MD, Barosi G: Iron status in red cell pyruvate kinase deficiency: Study of Italian cases. *Br J Haematol* **83**:485, 1993.
41. Tanaka KR, Paglia DE: Pyruvate kinase deficiency. *Semin Hematol* **8**:367, 1971.
42. Bowman HS, Procopio F: Hereditary non-spherocytic hemolytic anemia of the pyruvate-kinase deficient type. *Ann Intern Med* **58**:567, 1963.
43. Gilman PA: Hemolysis in the newborn infant resulting from deficiencies of red blood cell enzymes: Diagnosis and management. *J Pediatr* **84**:625, 1974.
44. Muller-Soyano A, De Roura ET, Duke PR, De Acquatella GC, Arends T, Guinto E, Beutler E: Pyruvate kinase deficiency and leg ulcers. *Blood* **47**:807, 1976.
45. Mahour GH, Lynn HB, Hill RW: Acute pancreatitis with biliary disease in erythrocyte pyruvate-kinase deficiency. *Clin Pediatr* **8**:608, 1969.
46. Linos DA, Nagorney DM, McIlrath DC: Splenic abscess—The importance of early diagnosis. *Mayo Clin Proc* **58**:261, 1983.
47. Rutgers MJ, Van der Lugt PJ, Van Turnhout JM: Spinal cord compression by extramedullary hemopoietic tissue in pyruvate-kinase-deficiency-caused hemolytic anemia. *Neurology* **29**:510, 1979.
48. Schon HR, Emmerich B, Arnold H, Maubach PA, Becker K, Rastetter J: Hemolytic anemia with pyruvate kinase deficiency presenting as paravertebral myelolipoma. *Klin Wochenschr* **62**:133, 1984.
49. Goebel KM, Goebel FD, Muhlfellner G, Kaffarnik H: Red cell metabolism in transient haemolytic anaemia associated with Zieve's syndrome. *Eur J Clin Invest* **5**:83, 1975.
50. Bertrand P, Feremans WW, Barroy JP, Dereume JP, Goldstein M: Vascular complications in a case of hemolytic anemia due to pyruvate kinase deficiency. *Acta Chir Belg* **82**:533, 1982.
51. Vives Corrons JL, García AM, Sosa AM, Pujades A, Colomer D, Linares M: Heterozygous pyruvate kinase deficiency and severe hemolytic anemia in a pregnant woman with concomitant, glucose-6-phosphate dehydrogenase deficiency. *Ann Hematol* **62**:190, 1991.
52. Mahendra P, Dollery CT, Luzzatto L, Bloom SR: Pyruvate kinase deficiency: Association with G6PD deficiency. *Br Med J* **305**:760, 1992.
52a. Zarza R, Moscardo M, Alvarez R, Garcia J, Morey M, Pujades A, Vives-Corrons JL: Co-existence of hereditary spherocytosis and a new red cell pyruvate kinase variant: PK Mallorca. *Haematologica* **85**:227, 2000.
52b. Cohen-Solal M, Prehu C, Wajcman H, Poyart C, Bardakdjian-Michau J, Kister J, Prome D, Valentin C, Bachir D, Galacteros F: A new sickle cell disease phenotype associating Hb S trait, severe pyruvate kinase deficiency (PK Conakry), and an alpha2 globin gene variant (Hb Conakry). *Br J Haematol* **103**:950, 1998.
53. Beutler E, Forman L: Coexistence of α-thalassemia and a new pyruvate kinase variant: PK Fukien. *Acta Haematol* **69**:3, 1983.
54. Searcy GP, Miller DR, Taskeer JB: Congenital hemolytic anemia in the Basenji dog due to erythrocyte pyruvate kinase deficiency. *Can J Comp Med* **35**:67, 1971.
55. Prasse KW, Crouser D, Beutler E, Walker M, Schall WD: Pyruvate kinase deficiency anemia with terminal myelofibrosis and osteosclerosis in a Beagle. *J Am Vet Med Assoc* **166**:1170, 1975.
56. Morimoto M, Kanno H, Asai H, Tsujimura T, Fujii H, Moriyama Y, Kasugai T, Hirono A, Ohba Y, Miwa S, Kitamura Y: Pyruvate kinase deficiency of mice associated with nonspherocytic hemolytic anemia and cure of the anemia by marrow transplantation without host irradiation. *Blood* **86**:4323, 1995.
57. Miwa S, Fujii H, Takegawa S, Nakatsuji T, Yamato K, Ishida Y, Ninomiya N: Seven pyruvate kinase variants characterized by the ICSH recommended methods. *Br J Haematol* **45**:575, 1980.
58. Keitt AS: Pyruvate kinase deficiency and related disorders of red cell glycolysis. *Am J Med* **41**:762, 1966.
59. Leblond PF, Lyonnais J, Delage JM: Erythrocyte populations in pyruvate kinase deficiency anaemia following splenectomy. I. Cell morphology. *Br J Haematol* **39**:55, 1978.
60. O'Connor TA, Monzon CM, Clark FI: Erythrocyte pyruvate kinase deficiency. A case of severe congenital hemolytic anemia. *Mo Med* **86**:92, 1989.

61. Allen DW, Groat JD, Finkel B, Rank BH, Wood PA, Eaton JW: Increased adsorption of cytoplasmic proteins to the erythrocyte membrane in ATP-depleted normal and pyruvate kinase deficient mature cells and reticulocytes. *Am J Hematol* **14**:11, 1983.
62. Zanella A, Brovelli A, Mantovani A, Izzo C, Rebulla P, Balduini C: Membrane abnormalities of pyruvate kinase deficient red cells. *Br J Haematol* **42**:101, 1979.
63. Schröter W, Tillmann W: Membrane-localized pyruvate kinase of red blood cells in hemolytic anemia associated with pyruvate kinase deficiency. *Klin Wochenschr* **53**:1101, 1975.
64. Lakomek M, Tillmann W, Scharnetzky M, Schröter W, Winkler H: Erythrocyte pyruvate kinase deficiency. A kinetic study of the membrane-localised and cytoplasmatic enzyme from six patients. *Enzyme* **29**:189, 1983.
65. Leblond PF, Coulombe L, Lyonnais J: Erythrocyte populations in pyruvate kinase deficiency anaemia following splenectomy. II. Cell deformability. *Br J Haematol* **39**:63, 1978.
66. Marik T, Brabec V, Kodocek M, Jarolim P: Pyruvate kinase-deficiency anemia: Membrane approach. *Biochem Med Metab Biol* **39**:55, 1988.
67. Nathan DG, Oski FA, Miller DR, Gardner FH: Life span and organ sequestration of the red cells in pyruvate kinase deficiency. *N Engl J Med* **278**:73, 1968.
68. Bowman HS, Oski FA: Laboratory studies of erythrocytic pyruvate kinase deficiency. *Am J Clin Pathol* **70**:259, 1978.
69. Wazewska-Czyzewska M, Guminska M: Congenital non-spherocytic haemolytic anaemia variants with primary and secondary pyruvate kinase deficiency. I. Erythrokinetic patterns. *Br J Haematol* **41**:115, 1979.
70. Tsujino K, Kanno H, Hashimoto K, Fujii H, Jippo T, Morii E, Lee YM, Asai H, Miwa S, Kitamura Y: Delayed onset of hemolytic anemia in *CBA-Pk-1^{slc}/Pk-1^{slc}* mice with a point mutation of the gene encoding red blood cell type pyruvate kinase. *Blood* **91**:2169, 1998.
71. Noguchi T, Yamada K, Inoue H, Matsuda T, Tanaka T: The L- and R-type isozymes of rat pyruvate kinase are produced from a single gene by use of different promoters. *J Biol Chem* **262**:14366, 1987.
72. Kanno H, Fujii H, Miwa S: Structural analysis of human pyruvate kinase L-gene and identification of the promoter activity in erythroid cells. *Biochem Biophys Res Commun* **188**:516, 1992.
73. Imamura K, Tanaka T, Nishina T, Nakashima K, Miwa S: Studies on pyruvate kinase (PK) deficiency. II. Electrophoretic, kinetic, and immunological studies on pyruvate kinase of erythrocytes and other tissues. *J Biochem* **74**:1165, 1973.
74. Nakashima K, Miwa S, Oda S, Tanaka T, Imamura K, Nishina T: Electrophoretic and kinetic studies of mutant erythrocyte pyruvate kinase. *Blood* **43**:537, 1974.
75. Wei DC, Chan LC, Li A: Homozygous pyruvate kinase deficiency in Hong Kong ethnic minorities. *J Paediatr Child Health* **28**:334, 1992.
76. Kanno H, Fujii H, Wei DC, Chan LC, Hirono A, Tsukimoto I, Miwa S: Frame shift mutation, exon skipping, and a two-codon deletion caused by splice site mutations account for pyruvate kinase deficiency. *Blood* **89**:4213, 1997.
77. Noguchi T, Yamada K, Yamagata K, Takenaka M, Nakajima H, Imai E, Wang Z, Tanaka T: Expression of liver type pyruvate kinase in insulinoma cells: Involvement of LF-B1 (HNF1). *Biochem Biophys Res Commun* **181**:259, 1991.
78. Marie S, Diaz-Guerra M-J, Miquero L, Kahn A, Iynedjian PB: The pyruvate kinase gene as a model for studies of glucose-dependent regulation of gene expression in the endocrine pancreatic β-cell type. *J Biol Chem* **268**:23881, 1993.
79. Becker MH, Genieser NB, Piomelli S, Dove D, Mendoza RD: Roentgenographic manifestations of pyruvate kinase deficiency hemolytic anemia. *Am J Roentgenol Radium Ther Nucl Med* **113**:491, 1971.
80. Bowman HS, Oski FA: Splenic macrophage interaction with red cells in pyruvate kinase deficiency and hereditary spherocytosis. *Vox Sang* **19**:168, 1970.
81. Matsumoto N, Ishihara T, Nakashima K, Miwa S, Uchino F, Kondo M: Sequestration and destruction of reticulocyte in the spleen pyruvate kinase deficiency hereditary nonspherocytic hemolytic anemia. *Acta Haematol Jpn* **35**:525, 1972.
82. Matsumoto N, Ishihara T, Miwa S, Uchino F: The mechanism of mitochondrial extrusion from reticulocyte in the spleen from patients with erythrocyte pyruvate kinase (PK) deficiency. *Acta Haematol Jpn* **37**:25, 1974.
83. Tanaka KR: Pyruvate kinase, in Yunis JJ (ed): *Biochemical Methods in Red Cell Genetics*. New York, Academic, 1969, p 167.
84. Beutler E: Red Cell Metabolism. *A Manual of Biochemical Methods*, 3rd ed. Orlando, FL, Grune and Stratton, 1984.
85. Fujii H, Miwa S: Pyruvate kinase; Assay in serum and erythrocytes, in Bergmeyer HU (ed): *Methods of Enzymatic Analysis*, 3rd ed. London, , Grune and Stratton, 1983, p 496.
86. Minakami S, Suzuki C, Saito T, Yoshikawa H: Studies on erythrocyte glycolysis. I. Determinations of the glycolytic intermediates in human erythrocytes. *J Biochem* **58**:543, 1965.
87. Miwa S, Boivin P, Blume KG, Arnold H, Black JA, Kahn A, Staal GEJ, Nakashima K, Tanaka KR, Paglia DE, Valentine WN, Yoshida A, Beutler E: Recommended methods for the characterization of red cell pyruvate kinase variants. International Committee for Standardization in Haematolgy. *Br J Haematol* **43**:275, 1979.
88. Beutler E, Baronciani L: Mutations in pyruvate kinase. *Hum Mutat* **7**:1, 1996.
89. Beutler E, West C, Blume KG: The removal of leukocytes and platelets from whole blood. *J Lab Clin Med* **88**:328, 1976.
90. Tanaka KR, Valentine WN, Miwa S: Pyruvate kinase (PK) deficiency hereditary nonspherocytic hemolytic anemia. *Blood* **19**:267, 1962.
91. Beutler E, Forman L, Rios-Larrain E: Elevated pyruvate kinase activity in patients with hemolytic anemia due to red cell pyruvate kinase "deficiency." *Am J Med* **83**:899, 1987.
92. Paglia DE, Valentine WN, Baughan MA, Miller DR, Reed CF, McIntyre OR: An inherited molecular lesion of erythrocyte pyruvate kinase. Identification of a kinetically aberrant isozyme associated with premature hemolysis. *J Clin Invest* **47**:1929, 1968.
93. Brandt NJ, Hanel HK: Atypical pyruvate kinase in a patient with haemolytic anemia. *Scand J Haematol* **8**:126, 1971.
94. Nakashima K: Further evidence of molecular alteration and aberration of erythrocyte pyruvate kinase. *Clin Chim Acta* **55**:245, 1974.
95. Konrad PN, Valentine WN, Paglia DE: Enzymatic activities and glutathione content of erythrocytes in the newborn: Comparison with red cells of older normal subjects and those with comparable reticulocytosis. *Acta Haematol* **48**:193, 1972.
96. Beutler E: How do red cell enzymes age? A new perspective. *Br J Haematol* **61**:377, 1985.
97. Lakomek M, Schröter W, De Maeyer G, Winkler H: On the diagnosis of erythrocyte enzyme defects in the presence of high reticulocyte counts. *Br J Haematol* **72**:445, 1989.
98. Rijksen G, Veerman AJP, Schipper-Kester GPM, Staal GEJ: Diagnosis of pyruvate kinase deficiency in a transfusion-dependent patient with severe hemolytic anemia. *Am J Hematol* **35**:187, 1990.
99. Gahr M, Meves H, Schröter W: Fetal properties in red blood cells of new born infants. *Pediatr Res* **13**:1231, 1979.
100. Lestas AN, Bellingham AJ: A logical approach to the investigation of red cell enzymopathies. *Blood Rev* **4**:148, 1990.
101. Mattevi A, Bolognesi M, Valentini G: The allosteric regulation of pyruvate kinase. *FEBS Lett* **389**:15, 1996.
102. Lakomek M, Winkler H: Erythrocyte pyruvate kinase- and glucose phosphate isomerase deficiency: Perturbation of glycolysis by structural defects and functional alterations of defective enzymes and its relation to the clinical severity of chronic hemolytic anemia. *Biophys Chem* **66**:269, 1997.
103. Van Solinge WW, Kraaijenhagen RJ, Rijksen G, van Wijk R, Stoffer BB, Gajhede M, Nielsen FC: Molecular modelling of human red blood cell pyruvate kinase: Structural implications of a novel G_{1091} to A mutation causing severe nonspherocytic hemolytic anemia. *Blood* **90**:4987, 1997.
104. Jurica MS, Mesecar A, Heath PJ, Shi WX, Nowak T, Stoddard BL: The allosteric regulation of pyruvate kinase by fructose-1,6-bisphosphate. *Structure* **6**:195, 1998.
105. Tanaka T, Harano Y, Sue F, Morimura H: Crystallization, characterization and metabolic regulation of two types of pyruvate kinase isolated from rat tissues. *J Biochem* **62**:71, 1967.
106. Imamura K, Tanaka T: Multimolecular forms of pyruvate kinase from rat and other mammalian tissues. *J Biochem* **71**:1043, 1972.
107. Koler RD, Vanbellinghen P: The mechanism of precursor modulation of human pyruvate kinase I by fructose diphosphate. *Adv Enzyme Regul* **6**:127, 1968.
108. Black JA, Henderson MH: Activation and inhibition of human erythrocyte pyruvate kinase by organic phosphates, amino acids, dipeptides and anions. *Biochim Biophys Acta* **284**:115, 1972.
109. Staal GEJ, Koster JF, Kamp H, van Milligen-Boersma L, Veeger C: Human erythrocyte pyruvate kinase. Its purification and some properties. *Biochim Biophys Acta* **227**:86, 1971.

110. Ljungström O, Ekman P: Glucagon-induced phosphorylation of pyruvate kinase (type L) in rat liver slices. *Biochem Biophys Res Commun* **78**:1147, 1977.
111. Marie J, Buc H, Simon MP, Kahn A: Phosphorylation of human erythrocyte pyruvate kinase by soluble cyclic-AMP-dependent protein kinases. Comparison with human liver L-type enzyme. *Eur J Biochem* **108**:251, 1980.
112. Nowak T, Mildvan AS: Nuclear magnetic resonance studies of the function of potassium in the mechanism of pyruvate kinase. *Biochemistry* **11**:2819, 1972.
113. Muirhead H, Clayden DA, Barford D, Lorimer CG, Fothergill-Gilmore LA, Schlitz E, Schmitt W: The structure of cat muscle pyruvate kinase. *EMBO J* **5**:475, 1986.
114. Larsen TM, Laughlin LT, Holden HM, Rayment I, Reed GH: Structure of rabbit muscle pyruvate kinase complexed with Mn^{2+}, K^+, and pyruvate. *Biochemistry* **33**:6301, 1994.
115. Mattevi A, Valentini G, Rizzi M, Speranza ML, Bolognesi M, Coda A: Crystal structure of *Escherichia coli* pyruvate kinase type I: Molecular basis of the allosteric transition. *Structure* **3**:729, 1995.
116. Monod J, Wyman J, Changeux JP: On the nature of allosteric transitions: A plausible model. *J Mol Biol* **12**:88, 1965.
117. Murcott THL, Gutfreund H, Muirhead H: The cooperative binding of fructose-1,6-bisphosphate to yeast pyruvate kinase. *EMBO J* **11**:3811, 1992.
118. Marie J, Kahn A, Boivin P: Human erythrocyte pyruvate kinase. Total purification and evidence for its antigenic identity with L-type enzyme. *Biochim Biophys Acta* **481**:96, 1977.
119. Takenaka M, Noguchi T, Sadahiro S, Hirai H, Yamada K, Matsuda T, Imai E, Tanaka T: Isolation and characterization of the human pyruvate kinase M gene. *Eur J Biochem* **198**:101, 1991.
120. Tani K, Fujii H, Nagata S, Miwa S: Human liver type pyruvate kinase: Complete amino acid sequences and the expression in mammalian cells. *Proc Natl Acad Sci U S A* **85**:1792, 1988.
121. Tani K, Yoshida MC, Satoh H, Mitamura K, Noguchi T, Tanaka T, Fujii H, Miwa S: Human M_2-type pyruvate kinase: cDNA cloning, chromosomal assignment and expression in hepatoma. *Gene* **73**:509, 1988.
122. Kanno H, Fujii H, Hirono A, Miwa S: cDNA cloning of human R-type pyruvate kinase and identification of a single amino acid substitution ($Thr^{384} \rightarrow Met$) affecting enzymatic stability in a pyruvate kinase variant (PK Tokyo) associated with hereditary hemolytic anemia. *Proc Natl Acad Sci U S A* **88**:8218, 1991.
123. Noguchi T, Inoue H, Tanaka T: The M_1- and M_2-type isozymes of rat pyruvate kinase are produced from the same gene by alternative RNA splicing. *J Biol Chem* **261**:13807, 1986.
124. Tani K, Fujii H, Tsutsumi H, Sukegawa J, Toyoshima K, Yoshida MC, Noguchi T, Tanaka T, Miwa S: Human liver-type pyruvate kinase: cDNA cloning and chromosomal assignment. *Biochem Biophys Res Commun* **143**:431, 1987.
125. Satoh H, Tani K, Yoshida MC, Sasaki M, Miwa S, Fujii H: The human liver-type pyruvate kinase (PKL) gene is on chromosome 1 at band q21. *Cytogenet Cell Genet* **47**:132, 1988.
126. Demina A, Boas E, Beutler E: Structure and linkage relationships of the region containing the human L-type pyruvate kinase (*PKLR*) and glucocerebrosidase (*GBA*) genes. *Hematopathol Mol Hematol* **11**: 63–71, 1998.
127. Oda S, Oda E, Tanaka KR: Relationship of density distribution and pyruvate kinase electrophoretic pattern of erythrocytes in sickle cell diseases and other disorders. *Acta Haematol* **60**:201, 1978.
128. Lacronique V, Boquet D, Lopez S, Kahn A, Raymondjean M: In vitro and in vivo protein-DNA interactions on the rat erythroid-specific L′ pyruvate kinase gene promoter. *Nucleic Acids Res* **20**:5669, 1992.
129. Max-Audit I, Eleouet JF, Romeo PH: Transcriptional regulation of the pyruvate kinase erythroid-specific promoter. *J Biol Chem* **268**:5431, 1993.
130. Yamada K, Noguchi T, Matsuda T, Takenaka M, Monaci P, Nicosia A, Tanaka T: Identification and characterization of hepatocyte-specific regulatory regions of the rat pyruvate kinase L gene. The synergistic effect of multiple elements. *J Biol Chem* **265**:19885, 1990.
131. Cognet M, Bergot MO, Kahn A: *Cis*-acting DNA elements regulating expression of the liver pyruvate kinase gene in hepatocytes and hepatoma cells. Evidence for tissue-specific activators and extinguisher. *J Biol Chem* **266**:7368, 1991.
132. Odagiri H, Wang J, German MS: Function of the human insulin promoter in primary cultured islet cells. *J Biol Chem* **271**:1909, 1996.
133. Tremp GL, Boquet D, Ripoche MA, Cognet M, Lone YC, Jami J, Kahn A, Daegelen D: Expression of the rat L-type pyruvate kinase gene from its dual erythroid- and liver-specific promoter in transgenic mice. *J Biol Chem* **264**:19904, 1989.
134. Yamada K, Noguchi T, Miyazaki J, Matsuda T, Takenaka M, Yamamura K, Tanaka T: Tissue-specific expression of rat pyruvate kinase L/chloramphenicol acetyltransferase fusion gene in transgenic mice and its regulation by diet and insulin. *Biochem Biophys Res Commun* **171**:243, 1990.
135. Lacronique V, Lopez S, Miquerol L, Porteu A, Kahn A, Raymondjean M: Identification and functional characterization of an erythroid-specific enhancer in the L-type pyruvate kinase gene. *J Biol Chem* **270**:14989, 1995.
136. Gregory RC, Taxman DJ, Seshasayee D, Kensinger MH, Bieker JJ, Wojchowski DM: Functional interaction of GATA1 with erythroid Kruppel-like factor and SP1 at defined erythroid promoters. *Blood* **87**:1793, 1996.
137. Nuez B, Michalovich D, Bygrave A, Ploemacher R, Grosveld F: Defective haematopoiesis in fetal liver resulting from inactivation of the EKLF gene. *Nature* **375**:316, 1995.
138. Perkins AC, Sharpe AH, Orkin SH: Lethal β-thalassaemia in mice lacking the erythroid CACCC-transcription factor EKLF. *Nature* **375**:318, 1995.
139. Crossley M, Whitelaw E, Perkins A, Williams G, Fujiwara Y, Orkin SH: Isolation and characterization of the cDNA encoding BKLF/TEF-2, a major CACCC-box-binding protein in erythroid cells and selected other cells. *Mol Cell Biol* **16**:1695, 1996.
140. Kahn A: Transcriptional regulation by glucose in the liver. *Biochimie* **79**:113, 1997.
141. Takegawa S, Miwa S: Change of pyruvate kinase (PK) isozymes in classical type PK deficiency and other PK deficiency cases during red cell maturation. *Am J Hematol* **16**:53, 1984.
142. Nijhof W, Wierenga PK, Staal GEJ, Jansen G: Changes in activity and isozyme patterns of glycolytic enzymes during erythroid differentiation in vitro. *Blood* **64**:607, 1984.
143. Max-Audit I, Kechemir D, Mitjavila MT, Vainchenker W, Rotten D, Rosa R: Pyruvate kinase synthesis and degradation by normal and pathologic cells during erythroid maturation. *Blood* **72**:1039, 1988.
144. Miwa S, Nishina T: Studies on pyruvate kinase (PK) deficiency. I. Clinical, hematological and erythrocyte enzyme studies. *Acta Haematol Jpn* **37**:1, 1974.
145. Miwa S, Nakashima N, Ariyoshi K, Shinohara K, Oda E, Tanaka T: Four new pyruvate kinase (PK) variants and a classical PK deficiency. *Br J Haematol* **29**:157, 1975.
146. Black JA, Rittenberg MB, Bigley RH, Koler RD: Hemolytic anemia due to pyruvate kinase deficiency: Characterization of the enzymatic activity from eight patients. *Am J Hum Genet* **31**:300, 1979.
147. Shinohara K, Tanaka KR: Pyruvate kinase deficiency hemolytic anemia: Enzymatic characterization studies in twelve patients. *Hemoglobin* **4**:611, 1980.
148. Tasker JB, Severin GA, Young SY, Gillette EL: Familial anemia in the Basenji dog. *J Am Vet Med Assoc* **154**:158, 1966.
149. Baronciani L, Bianchi P, Zanella A: Hematologically important mutations: Red cell pyruvate kinase. *Blood Cells Mol Dis* **22**:259, 1996.
150. Lenzner C, Nürnberg P, Jacobasch G, Gerth C, Thiele BJ: Molecular analysis of 29 pyruvate kinase-deficient patients from central Europe with hereditary hemolytic anemia. *Blood* **89**:1793, 1997.
151. Zanella A, Bianchi P, Baronciani L, Zappa M, Bredi E, Vercellati C, Alfinito F, Pelissero G, Sirchia G: Molecular characterization of PK-LR gene in pyruvate kinase-deficient Italian patients. *Blood* **89**:3847, 1997.
152. Pastore L, Della Morte R, Frisso G, Alfinito F, Vitale D, Calise RM, Ferraro F, Zagari A, Rotoli B, Salvatore F: Novel mutations and structural implications in R-type pyruvate kinase-deficient patients from Southern Italy. *Hum Mutat* **11**:127, 1998.
153. Baronciani L, Beutler E: Molecular study of pyruvate kinase deficient patients with hereditary nonspherocytic hemolytic anemia. *J Clin Invest* **95**:1702, 1995.
154. Baronciani L, Magalhães IQ, Mahoney DH Jr, Westwood B, Adekile AD, Lappin TRJ, Beutler E: Study of the molecular defects in pyruvate kinase deficient patients affected by nonspherocytic hemolytic anemia. *Blood Cells Mol Dis* **21**:49, 1995.
155. Miwa S, Fujii H: Molecular basis of erythroenzymopathies associated with hereditary hemolytic anemia: Tabulation of mutant enzymes. *Am J Hematol* **51**:122, 1996.
156. Baronciani L, Beutler E: Analysis of pyruvate kinase-deficiency mutations that produce nonspherocytic hemolytic anemia. *Proc Natl Acad Sci U S A* **90**:4324, 1993.

157. Lenzner C, Nürnberg P, Thiele B-J, Reis A, Brabec V, Sakalova A, Jacobasch G: Mutations in the pyruvate kinase L gene in patients with hemolytic anemia. *Blood* **83**:2817, 1994.
158. Kanno H, Fujii H, Miwa S: Molecular heterogeneity of pyruvate kinase deficiency identified by single strand conformational polymorphism (SSCP) analysis. *Blood* **84**:13a, 1994.
159. Uenaka R, Nakajima H, Noguchi T, Imamura K, Hamaguchi T, Tomita K, Yamada K, Kuwajima M, Kono N, Tanaka T, Matsuzawa Y: Compound heterozygous mutations affecting both hepatic and erythrocyte isozymes of pyruvate kinase. *Biochem Biophys Res Commun* **208**:991, 1995.
160. Kanno H, Fujii H, Hirono A, Omine M, Miwa S: Identical point mutations of the R-type pyruvate kinase (PK) cDNA found in unrelated PK variants associated with hereditary hemolytic anemia. *Blood* **79**:1347, 1992.
161. Neubauer M, Lakomek M, Winkler M, Parke S, Hofferbert S, Schröter W: Point mutations in the L-type pyruvate kinase gene of two children with hemolytic anemia caused by pyruvate kinase deficiency. *Blood* **77**:1871, 1991.
162. Walker D, Chia WN, Muirhead H: Key residues in the allosteric transition of Bacillus stearothermophilus pyruvate kinase identified by site-directed mutagenesis. *J Mol Biol* **228**:265, 1992.
163. Ikeda Y, Tanaka T, Noguchi T: Conversion of non-allosteric pyruvate kinase isozyme into an allosteric enzyme by a single amino acid substitution. *J Biol Chem* **272**:20495, 1997.
164. Kanno H, Fujii H, Tsujino G, Miwa S: Molecular basis of impaired pyruvate kinase isozyme conversion in erythroid cells: A single amino acid substitution near the active site and decreased mRNA content of the R-type PK. *Biochem Biophys Res Commun* **192**:46, 1993.
165. Kanno H, Wei DC, Chan LC, Mizoguchi H, Ando M, Nakahata T, Narisawa K, Fujii H, Miwa S: Hereditary hemolytic anemia caused by diverse point mutations of pyruvate kinase gene found in Japan and Hong Kong. *Blood* **84**:3505, 1994.
166. Lakomek M, Huppke P, Neubauer B, Pekrun A, Winkler H, Schröter W: Mutations in the R-type pyruvate kinase gene and altered enzyme kinetic properties in patients with hemolytic anemia due to pyruvate kinase deficiency. *Ann Hematol* **68**:253, 1994.
167. Kanno H, Morimoto M, Fujii H, Tsujimura T, Asai H, Noguchi T, Kitamura Y, Miwa S: Primary structure of murine red blood cell-type pyruvate kinase (PK) and molecular characterization of PK deficiency identified in the CBA strain. *Blood* **86**:3205, 1995.
168. Kanno H, Fujii H, Miwa S: Low substrate affinity of pyruvate kinase variant (PK Sapporo) caused by a single amino acid substitution (426 Arg → Gln) associated with hereditary hemolytic anemia. *Blood* **81**:2439, 1993.
169. Kanno H, Ballas SK, Miwa S, Fujii H, Bowman HS: Molecular abnormality of erythrocyte pyruvate kinase deficiency in the Amish. *Blood* **83**:2311, 1994.
170. Muir WA, Beutler E, Wasson C: Erythrocyte pyruvate kinase deficiency in the Ohio Amish: Origin and characterization of the mutant enzyme. *Am J Hum Genet* **36**:634, 1984.
171. Tani K, Tsutsumi H, Takahashi K, Ogura H, Kanno H, Hayasaka K, Narisawa K, Nakahata T, Akabane T, Morisaki T, Fujii H, Miwa S: Two homozygous cases of erythrocyte pyruvate kinase (PK) deficiency in Japan: PK Sendai and PK Shinshu. *Am J Hematol* **28**:186, 1988.
172. Whitney KM, Goodman SA, Bailey EM, Lothrop CD: The molecular basis of canine pyruvate kinase deficiency. *Exp Hematol* **22**:866, 1994.
173. Rouger H, Girodon E, Goossens M, Galacteros F, Cohen-Solal M: PK Mondor: Prenatal diagnosis of a frameshift mutation in the LR pyruvate kinase gene associated with severe hereditary nonspherocytic haemolytic anaemia. *Prenat Diagn* **16**:97, 1996.
174. Zurcher C, Loos JA, Prins HK: Hereditary high ATP content of human erythrocytes. *Folia Haematol* **83**:366, 1965.
175. Brewer GJ: A new inherited abnormality of human erythrocytes-elevated erythrocytic adenosine triphosphate. *Biochem Biophys Res Commun* **18**:430, 1965.
176. Max-Audit I, Rosa R, Marie J: Pyruvate kinase hyperactivity genetically determined: Metabolic consequences and molecular characterization. *Blood* **56**:902, 1980.
177. Rosa R, Max-Audit I, Izrael V, Beuzard Y, Thillet J, Rosa J: Hereditary pyruvate kinase abnormalities associated with erythrocytosis. *Am J Hematol* **10**:47, 1981.
178. Staal GEJ, Janse G, Roos D: Pyruvate kinase and the "high ATP syndrome." *J Clin Invest* **74**:231, 1984.
179. Beutler E, Westwood B, van Zweiten R, Roos D: G → T transition at cDNA nt 110 (K37Q) in the PKLR (pyruvate kinase) gene is the molecular basis of a case of hereditary increase of red blood cell ATP. *Hum Mutat* **9**:576, 1997.
180. Boivin P, Galand C, Hakim J, Kahn A: Acquired erythroenzymopathies in blood disorders: Study of 200 cases. *Br J Haematol* **31**:531, 1975.
181. Boivin P, Galand C, Hakim J, Kahn A: Acquired red cell pyruvate kinase deficiency in leukemias and related disorders. *Enzyme* **19**:294, 1975.
182. Goebel KM, Goebel FD, Janzen R, Kaffarnik H: Haemolytic anaemia with hereditary pyruvate kinase instability developing acute leukaemia. *Scand J Haematol* **14**:249, 1975.
183. Gherardi M, Bierme R, Corberand J, Vergnes H: Heterogeneity of erythrocyte pyruvate kinase deficiency and related metabolic disorders in patients with hematological diseases. *Clin Chim Acta* **78**:465, 1977.
184. Abe S: Secondary red cell pyruvate kinase deficiency. I. Study of 30 subjects of malignant hematological disorders. *Acta Haematol Jpn* **39**:247, 1976.
185. Morse EE, Jilani F, Brassel J: Acquired pyruvate kinase deficiency. *Ann Clin Lab Sci* **7**:399, 1977.
186. Kahn A, Cottreau D, Boyer C, Marie J, Galand C, Boivin P: Causal mechanisms of multiple acquired red cell enzyme defects in a patient with acquired dyserythropoiesis. *Blood* **48**:653, 1976.
187. Tani K, Fujii H, Takahashi K, Kodo H, Asano S, Takaku F, Miwa S: Erythrocyte enzyme activities in myelodysplastic syndromes: Elevated pyruvate kinase activity. *Am J Hematol* **30**:97, 1989.
188. Coon WW: Splenectomy in the treatment of hemolytic anemia. *Arch Surg* **120**:625, 1985.
189. Weiden PL, Hackman RC, Deeg J, Graham TC, Thomas ED, Storb R: Long-term survival and reversal of iron overload after marrow transplantation in dogs with congenital hemolytic anemia. *Blood* **57**:66, 1981.
190. Zachee P, Staal GEJ, Rijksen G, Bock RD, Couttenye MM, De Broe ME: Pyruvate kinase deficiency and delayed clinical response to recombinant human erythropoietin treatment. *Lancet* **1**:1327, 1989.
191. Tani K, Yoshikubo T, Ikebuchi K, Takahashi K, Tsuchiya T, Takahashi S, Shimane M, Ogura H, Tojo A, Ozawa K, Takahara Y, Nakauchi H, Markowitz D, Bank A, Asano S: Retrovirus-mediated gene transfer of human pyruvate kinase (PK) cDNA into murine hematopoietic cells: Implications for gene therapy of human PK deficiency. *Blood* **83**:2305, 1994.
192. Kanno H, Miwa S: Unpublished results, 1998.
193. Shows TB, Eddy RL, Byers MG, Haley LL, Henry WM, Nishi S, Bell GI: Localization of the human hexokinase I gene (HK1) to chromosome 10q22. *Cytogenet Cell Genet* **51**:1079a, 1989.
194. Ruzzo A, Andreoni F, Magnani M: Structure of the human hexokinase type I gene and nucleotide sequence of the 5′ flanking region. *Biochem J* **331**:607, 1998.
195. Murakami K, Blei F, Tilton W, Seaman C, Piomelli S: An isozyme of hexokinase specific for the human red blood cell (HK_R). *Blood* **75**:770, 1990.
196. Zimran A, Torem S, Beutler E: The *in vivo* ageing of red cell enzymes: Direct evidence of biphasic decay from polycythaemic rabbits with reticulocytosis. *Br J Haematol* **69**:67, 1988.
197. Piomelli S, Seaman C: Mechanism of red blood cell aging: Relationship of cell density and cell age. *Am J Hematol* **42**:46, 1993.
198. Murakami K, Piomelli S: Identification of the cDNA for human red blood cell-specific hexokinase isozyme. *Blood* **89**:762, 1997.
199. Nishi S, Seino S, Bell GI: Human hexokinase: Sequence of amino- and carboxyl-terminal halves are homologous. *Biochem Biophys Res Commun* **157**:937, 1988.
200. Valentine WN, Oski FA, Paglia DE, Baughan MA, Schneider AS, Naiman JL: Hereditary hemolytic anemia with hexokinase deficiency: Role of hexokinase in erythrocyte aging. *N Engl J Med* **276**:1, 1967.
201. Keitt AS: Hemolytic anemia with impaired hexokinase activity. *J Clin Invest* **48**:1997, 1969.
202. Moser K, Ciresa M, Schwarzmeier J: Hexokinasemangel bei hämolytischer Anämie. *Med Welt* **21**:1977, 1970.
203. Necheles TF, Rai US, Cameron D: Congenital nonspherocytic hemolytic anemia associated with an unusual erythrocyte hexokinase abnormality. *J Lab Clin Med* **76**:593, 1970.
204. Goebel KM, Gassel WD, Goebel FD, Kaffarnik H: Hemolytic anemia and hexokinase deficiency associated with malformations. *Klin Wochenschr* **50**:849, 1972.

205. Semenuk M, Wicks P, Toews CJ, Brain MC: Hexokinase Hamilton: An enzyme variant with abnormal Km for Adenosine triphosphate (ATP) in non-spherocytic hemolytic anemia. *Clin Res* **23**:628a, 1975.
206. Board PG, Trueworthy R, Smith JE, Moore K: Congenital nonspherocytic hemolytic anemia with an unstable hexokinase variant. *Blood* **51**:111, 1978.
207. Beutler E, Dyment PG, Matsumoto F: Hereditary nonspherocytic hemolytic anemia and hexokinase deficiency. *Blood* **51**:935, 1978.
208. Gilsanz F, Meyer E, Paglia DE, Valentine WN: Congenital hemolytic anemia due to hexokinase deficiency. *Am J Dis Child* **132**:636, 1978.
209. Rijksen G, Staal GEJ: Human erythrocyte hexokinase deficiency. Characterization of a mutant enzyme with abnormal regulatory properties. *J Clin Invest* **62**:294, 1978.
210. Siimes MA, Rahiala E-L, Leisti J: Hexokinase deficiency in erythrocytes: A new variant in 5 members of a Finnish family. *Scand J Haematol* **22**:214, 1979.
211. Newman P, Muir A, Parker C: Non-spherocytic haemolytic anaemia in mother and son associated with hexokinase deficiency. *Br J Haematol* **46**:537, 1980.
212. Paglia DE, Shende A, Lanzkowsky P, Valentine WN: Hexokinase "New Hyde Park": A low-activity erythrocyte isozyme in a Chinese kindred. *Am J Hematol* **10**:107, 1981.
213. Rijksen G, Akkerman JWN, Van den Wall Bake AWL, Hofstede DP, Staal GEJ: Generalized hexokinase deficiency in the blood cells of a patient with nonspherocytic hemolytic anemia. *Blood* **61**:12, 1983.
214. Magnani M, Stocchi V, Canestrari F, Dachà M, Balestri P, Farnetani MA, Giorgi D, Fois A, Fornaini G: Human erythrocyte hexokinase deficiency: A new variant with abnormal kinetic properties. *Br J Haematol* **61**:41, 1985.
215. Magnani M, Stocchi V, Cucchiarini L, Novelli G, Lodi S, Isa L, Fornaini G: Hereditary nonspherocytic hemolytic anemia due to a new hexokinase variant with reduced stability. *Blood* **66**:690, 1985.
216. Kanno H, Ishikawa K, Fujii H, Miwa S: Severe hexokinase deficiency as a cause of hemolytic anemia, periventricular leucomalacia and intrauterine death of the fetus. *Blood* **90**:8a, 1997.
217. Bianchi M, Magnani M: Hexokinase mutations that produce nonspherocytic hemolytic anemia. *Blood Cells Mol Dis* **21**:2, 1995.
218. Bianchi M, Crinelli R, Serafini G, Giammarini C, Magnani M: Molecular bases of hexokinase deficiency. *Biochim Biophys Acta* **1360**:211, 1997.
219. McMorris FA, Chen TR, Ricciuti F, Tischfield J, Creagan R, Ruddle F: Chromosome assignments in man of the genes for two hexosephosphate isomerases. *Science* **179**:1129, 1973.
220. Walker JIH, Morgan MJ, Faik P: Structure and organization of the human glucose phosphate isomerase gene (GPI). *Genomics* **29**:261, 1995.
221. Xu W, Lee P, Beutler E: Human glucose phosphate isomerase: Exon mapping and gene structure. *Genomics* **29**:732, 1995.
222. Gurney ME, Heinrich SP, Lee MR, Yin H-S: Molecular cloning and expression of neuroleukin, a neurotrophic factor for spinal and sensory neurons. *Science* **234**:566, 1986.
223. Chaput M, Claes V, Portetelle D, Cludts I, Cravador A, Burny A, Gras H, Tartar A: The neurotrophic factor neuroleukin is 90 percent homologous with phosphohexose isomerase. *Nature* **332**:454, 1988.
224. Faik P, Walker JIH, Redmill AAM, Morgan MJ: Mouse glucose-6-phosphate isomerase and neuroleukin have identical 3′ sequences. *Nature* **332**:455, 1988.
225. Watanabe H, Takehana K, Date M, Shinozaki T, Raz A: Tumor cell autocrine motility factor is the neuroleukin/phosphohexose isomerase polypeptide. *Cancer Res* **56**:2960, 1996.
226. Niinaka Y, Paku S, Haga A, Watanabe H, Raz A: Expression and secretion of neuroleukin/phosphohexose isomerase/maturation factor as autocrine motility factor by tumor cells. *Cancer Res* **58**:2667, 1998.
227. Xu W, Seiter K, Feldman E, Ahmed T, Chiao JW: The differentiation and maturation mediator for human myeloid leukemia cells shares homology with neuroleukin or phosphoglucose isomerase. *Blood* **87**:4502, 1996.
228. Baughan MA, Valentine WN, Paglia DE, Ways PO, Simons ER, DeMarsh QB: Hereditary hemolytic anemia associated with glucosephosphate isomerase (GPI) deficiency — A new enzyme defect of human erythrocytes. *Blood* **32**:236, 1968.
229. Paglia DE, Holland P, Baughan MA, Valentine WN: Occurrence of defective hexosephosphate isomerization in human erythrocytes and leukocytes. *N Engl J Med* **280**:66, 1969.
230. Cartier P, Temkine H, Griscelli C: Etude biochimique d'une anémie hémolytique avec déficit familial en phosphohexo-isomérase. *Enzymol Biol Clin* **10**:439a, 1969.
231. Arnold H, Blume KG, Busch D, Lenkeit U, Löhr GW, Lübs E: Klinische und biochemische Untersuchungen zur Glucosephosphatisomerase normaler menschlicher Erythrocyten und bei Glucosephosphatisomerase-Mangel. *Klin Wochenschr* **48**:1299, 1970.
232. Schröter W, Brittinger G, Zimmerschmitt E, König E, Schrader D: Combined glucosephosphate isomerase and glucose-6-phosphate dehydrogenase deficiency of the erythrocytes: A new haemolytic syndrome. *Br J Haematol* **20**:249, 1971.
233. Oski F, Fuller E: Glucose-phosphate isomerase (GPI) deficiency associated with abnormal osmotic fragility and spherocytes. *Clin Res* **19**:427a, 1971.
234. Blume KG, Hryniuk W, Powars D, Trinidad F, West C, Beutler E: Characterization of two new variants of glucose-phosphate-isomerase deficiency with hereditary nonspherocytic hemolytic anemia. *J Lab Clin Med* **79**:942, 1972.
235. Miwa S, Nakashima K, Oda S, Oda E, Matsumoto N, Ogawa H, Fukumoto Y: Glucosephosphate isomerase (GPI) deficiency hereditary nonspherocytic hemolytic anemia. Report of the first case found in Japanese. *Acta Haematol Jpn* **36**:65, 1973.
236. Miwa S, Nakashima K, Oda S, Matsumoto N, Ogawa H, Kobayashi R, Kotani M, Harata A, Onaya T, Yamada T: Glucosephosphate isomerase (GPI) deficiency hereditary nonspherocytic hemolytic anemia. Report of the second case found in Japanese. *Acta Haematol Jpn* **36**:70, 1973.
237. Arnold H, Engelhardt R, Löhr GW, Jacobi H, Liebold I: Glucosephosphat-Isomerase Typ Recklinghausen: Eine neue Defektvariante mit hämolytischer Anämie. *Klin Wochenschr* **51**:1198, 1973.
238. Beutler E, Sigalove WH, Agnus Muir W, Matsumoto F, West C: Glucosephosphate-isomerase (GPI) deficiency: GPI Elyria. *Ann Intern Med* **80**:730, 1974.
239. Schröter W, Koch HH, Wonneberger KB, Kalinowsky W, Arnold A, Blume KG, Hüther W: Glucose phosphate isomerase deficiency with congenital nonspherocytic hemolytic anemia: A new variant (type Nordhorn). I. Clinical and genetic studies. *Pediatr Res* **8**:18, 1974.
240. Hutton JJ, Chilcote RR: Glucose phosphate isomerase deficiency with hereditary nonspherocytic hemolytic anemia. *J Pediatr* **85**:494, 1974.
241. Müller E, Marti HR, Bach J, Micheli JL, Gasser C: Hereditäre nichtsphärozytäre hämolytische Anämie durch Glukosephosphatisomerase-Mangel: Der erste in der Schweiz beobachtete Fall. *Schweiz Med Wochenschr* **104**:1379, 1974.
242. Paglia DE, Paredes R, Valentine WN, Dorantes S, Konrad PN: Unique phenotypic expression of glucosephosphate isomerase deficiency. *Am J Hum Genet* **27**:62, 1975.
243. Van Biervliet JPGM: Glucosephosphate isomerase deficiency in a Dutch family. *Acta Paediatr Scand* **64**:868, 1975.
244. Miwa S, Nakashima K, Tajiri M, Ono J, Abe S, Oda E, Nonaka H, Matsuoka I, Shimoyama S, Hirata Y, Amaki I, Horiuchi A, Yamaguchi H, Nishina T: Three cases in two families with congenital nonspherocytic hemolytic anemia due to defective glucosephosphate isomerase: GPI Matsumoto. *Acta Haematol Jpn* **38**:238, 1975.
245. Van Biervliet JP, Vlug A, Bartstra H, Rotteveel JJ, de Vaan GAM, Staal GEJ: A new variant of glucosephosphate isomerase deficiency. *Humangenetik* **30**:35, 1975.
246. Kahn A, Vives J-L, Bertrand O, Cottreau D, Marie J, Boivin P: Glucose-phosphate isomerase deficiency due to a new variant (GPI Barcelona) and to a silent gene: Biochemical, immunological and genetic studies. *Clin Chim Acta* **66**:145, 1976.
247. Staal GEJ, Akkerman JWN, Eggermont E, Van Biervliet JP: A new variant of glucosephosphate isomerase deficiency: GPI-Kortrijk. *Clin Chim Acta* **78**:121, 1977.
248. Cayanis E, Penfold GK, Freiman I, MacDougall LG: Haemolytic anaemia associated with glucosephosphate isomerase (GPI) deficiency in a Black South African child. *Br J Haematol* **37**:363, 1977.
249. Arnold H, Dodinval-Versie J, Lambotte C, Löhr GW, van der Hofstadt J: Glucosephosphate isomerase deficiency type Liège: A new variant with congenital nonspherocytic hemolytic anemia. *Blut* **35**:187, 1977.
250. Galand C, Torres M, Boivin P, Bourgeaud JP: A new variant of glucosephosphate isomerase deficiency with mild haemolytic anaemia (GPI-MYTHO). *Scand J Haematol* **20**:77, 1978.
251. Kahn A, Buc H-A, Girot R, Cottreau D, Griscelli C: Molecular and functional anomalies in two new mutant glucose-phosphate-isomerase variants with enzyme deficiency and chronic hemolysis. *Hum Genet* **40**:293, 1978.

252. Steiman I, Kaufman S, Zaidman JL, Leiba H: Combined glucose phosphate isomerase and glucose-6-phosphate dehydrogenase deficiency of erythrocytes. *Isr J Med Sci* **14**:1186, 1978.
253. Zanella A, Rebulla P, Izzo C, Zanuso F, Kahane I, Molinari E, Sirchia G: A new mutant erythrocyte glucosephosphate isomerase (GPI) associated with GSH abnormality. *Am J Hematol* **5**:11, 1978.
254. Isacchi G, Cottreau D, Mandelli F, Papa G, Ciccone F, Kahn A: "GPI Roma," a new glucose phosphate isomerase-deficient variant: In vivo occurrence of postsynthetic modifications of the mutant enzyme. *Hum Genet* **46**:219, 1979.
255. Whitelaw AGL, Rogers PA, Hopkinson DA, Gordon H, Emerson PM, Darley JH, Reid C, Crawfurd Md'A: Congenital haemolytic anaemia resulting from glucose phosphate isomerase deficiency: Genetics, clinical picture, and prenatal diagnosis. *J Med Genet* **16**:189, 1979.
256. Arnold H, Löhr GW, Hasslinger K, Podgajny T: Augsburg-type glucosephosphate isomerase deficiency: A new variant causing congenital nonspherocytic hemolytic anemia in a German family. *Blut* **40**:107, 1980.
257. Zanella A, Izzo C, Rebulla P, Perroni L, Mariani M, Canestri G, Sansone G, Sirchia G: The first stable variant of erythrocyte glucose-phosphate isomerase associated with severe hemolytic anemia. *Am J Hematol* **9**:1, 1980.
258. Takegawa S, Fujii H, Miwa S, Ohba Y, Yamauchi H, Miyata H: A case of congenital nonspherocytic hemolytic anemia associated with glucosephosphate isomerase (GPI) deficiency-GPI "Kinki." *Acta Haematol Jpn* **46**:11, 1983.
259. Arnold H, Hasslinger K, Witt I: Glucosephosphate-isomerase type Kaiserslautern: A new variant causing congenital nonspherocytic hemolytic anemia. *Blut* **46**:271, 1983.
260. Rijksen G, Jansen G, Manaster J, Ezekiel E, Streichman S, Staal GEJ: Glucose-6-phosphate isomerase deficiency-Nahariya: Extreme in vitro and in vivo lability of the mutant enzyme. *Isr J Med Sci* **20**:529, 1984.
261. Bardosi A, Eber SW, Roessmann U: Ultrastructural and histochemical abnormalities of skeletal muscle in a patient with a new variant (type Homburg) of glucosephosphate isomerase (GPI) deficiency. *Clin Neuropathol* **4**:72, 1985.
262. Eber SW, Gahr M, Lakomek M, Prindull G, Schröter W: Clinical symptoms and biochemical properties of three new glucosephosphate isomerase variants. *Blut* **53**:21, 1986.
263. Ravindranath Y, Paglia DE, Warrier I, Valentine W, Nakatani M, Brockway RA: Glucose phosphate isomerase deficiency as a cause of hydrops fetalis. *N Engl J Med* **316**:258, 1987.
264. Neubauer BA, Eber SW, Lakomek M, Gahr M, Schröter W: Combination of congenital nonspherocytic hemolytic anemia and impairment of granulocyte function in severe glucosephosphate isomerase deficiency: A new variant enzyme designated GPI Calden. *Acta Haematol* **83**:206, 1990.
265. Shalev O, Shalev RS, Forman L, Beutler E: GPI Mount Scopus—A variant of glucosephosphate isomerase deficiency. *Ann Hematol* **67**:197, 1993.
266. Walker JIH, Layton DM, Bellingham AJ, Morgan MJ, Faik P: DNA sequence abnormalities in human glucose 6-phosphate isomerase deficiency. *Hum Mol Genet* **2**:327, 1993.
267. Alfinito F, Ferraro F, Rocco S, De Vendittis E, Piccirillo G, Sementa A, Colombo MB, Zanella A, Rotoli B: Glucose phosphate isomerase (GPI) "Morcone": A new variant from Italy. *Eur J Haematol* **52**:263, 1994.
268. Xu W, Beutler E: The characterization of gene mutations for human glucose phosphate isomerase deficiency associated with chronic hemolytic anemia. *J Clin Invest* **94**:2326, 1994.
269. Baronciani L, Zanella A, Bianchi P, Zappa M, Alfinito F, Iolascon A, Tannoia N, Beutler E, Sirchia G: Study of the molecular defects in glucose phosphate isomerase-deficient patients affected by chronic hemolytic anemia. *Blood* **88**:2306, 1996.
270. Kanno H, Fujii H, Hirono A, Ishida Y, Ohga S, Fukumoto Y, Matsuzawa K, Ogawa S, Miwa S: Molecular analysis of glucose phosphate isomerase deficiency associated with hereditary hemolytic anemia. *Blood* **88**:2321, 1996.
271. Huppke P, Wünsch D, Pekrun A, Kind R, Winkler H, Schröter W, Lakomek M: Glucose phosphate isomerase deficiency: Biochemical and molecular genetic studies on the enzyme variants of two patients with severe haemolytic anaemia. *Eur J Pediatr* **156**:605, 1997.
272. Beutler E, West C, Britton HA, Harris J, Forman L: Glucosephosphate isomerase (GPI) deficiency mutations associated with hereditary nonspherocytic hemolytic anemia (HNSHA). *Blood Cells Mol Dis* **23**:402, 1997.
273. Paglia DE, Valentine WN: Hereditary glucosephosphate isomerase deficiency: A review. *Am J Clin Pathol* **62**:740, 1974.
274. Arnold H: Inherited glucosephosphate isomerase deficiency. A review of known variants and some aspects of the pathomechanism of the deficiency. *Blut* **39**:405, 1979.
275. Mohrenweiser HW, Wade PT, Wurzinger KH: Characterization of a series of electrophoretic and enzyme activity variants of human glucose-phosphate isomerase. *Hum Genet* **75**:28, 1987.
276. Chilcote RR, Baehner RL: Red cell (RBC) glucose phosphate isomerase deficiency (GPI): Clinical and laboratory evidence of increased blood viscosity. *Pediatr Res* **8**:398a, 1974.
277. Matthay KK, Mentzer WC: Erythrocyte enzymopathies in the newborn. *Clin Haematol* **10**:31, 1981.
278. Schröter W, Eber SW, Bardosi A, Gahr M, Gabriel M, Sitzmann FC: Generalised glucosephosphate isomerase (GPI) deficiency causing haemolytic anaemia, neuromuscular symptoms and impairment of granulocytic function: A new syndrome due to a new stable GPI variant with diminished specific activity (GPI Homburg). *Eur J Pediatr* **144**:301, 1985.
279. Fujii H, Kanno H, Hirono A, Miwa S: Hematologically important mutations: Molecular abnormalities of glucose phosphate isomerase deficiency. *Blood Cells Mol Dis* **22**:96, 1996.
280. Xu W, Beutler E: An exonic polymorphism in the human glucose phosphate isomerase (GPI) gene. *Blood Cells Mol Dis* **23**:377, 1997.
281. Arnold H, Blume KG, Löhr GW, Schröter W, Koch HH, Wonneberger B: Glucose phosphate isomerase deficiency with congenital nonspherocytic hemolytic anemia: A new variant (type Nordhorn). II. Purification and biochemical properties of the defective enzyme. *Pediatr Res* **8**:26, 1974.
282. Kanno H, Fujii H, Miwa S: Expression and enzymatic characterization of human glucose phosphate isomerase (GPI) variants accounting for GPI deficiency. *Blood Cells Mol Dis* **24**:54, 1998.
283. Merkle S, Pretsch W: Glucose-6-phosphate isomerase deficiency associated with nonspherocytic hemolytic anemia in the mouse: An animal model for the human disease. *Blood* **81**:206, 1993.
284. Layzer RB, Rowland LP, Bank WJ: Physical and kinetic properties of human phosphofructokinase from skeletal muscle and erythrocytes. *J Biol Chem* **244**:3823, 1969.
285. Kahn A, Meienhofer M-C, Cottreau D, Lagrange J-L, Dreyfus J-C: Phosphofructokinase (PFK) isozymes in man: I. Studies of adult human tissues. *Hum Genet* **48**:93, 1979.
286. Vora S, Seaman C, Durham S, Piomelli S: Isozymes of human phosphofructokinase: Identification and subunit structural characterization of a new system. *Proc Natl Acad Sci U S A* **77**:62, 1980.
287. Vora S: Isozymes of human phosphofructokinase in blood cells and cultured cell lines: Molecular and genetic evidence for a trigenic system. *Blood* **57**:724, 1981.
288. Dunaway GA, Kasten TP, Sebo T, Trapp R: Analysis of the phosphofructokinase subunits and isoenzymes in human tissues. *Biochem J* **251**:677, 1988.
289. Vora S, Durham S, de Martinville B, George DL, Francke U: Assignment of the human gene for muscle type phosphofructokinase (PFKM) to chromosome 1 (region cen → q32) using somatic cell hybrids and monoclonal anti-M antibody. *Somat Cell Genet* **8**:95, 1982.
290. Van Keuren M, Drabkin H, Hart I, Harker D, Patterson D, Vora S: Regional assignment of human liver-type 6-phosphofructokinase to chromosome 21q22.3 by using somatic cell hybrids and a monoclonal anti-L antibody. *Hum Genet* **74**:34, 1986.
291. Morrison N, Simpson C, Fothergill-Gilmore L, Boyd E, Connor JM: Regional chromosomal assignment of the human platelet phosphofructokinase gene to 10p15. *Hum Genet* **89**:105, 1992.
292. Nakajima H, Noguchi T, Yamasaki T, Kono N, Tanaka T, Tarui S: Cloning of human muscle phosphofructokinase cDNA. *FEBS Lett* **223**:113, 1987.
293. Levanon D, Danciger E, Dafni N, Bernstein Y, Elson A, Moens W, Brandeis M, Groner Y: The primary structure of human liver type phosphofructokinase and its comparison with other types of PFK. *DNA* **8**:733, 1989.
294. Yamasaki T, Nakajima H, Kono N, Hotta K, Yamada K, Imai E, Kuwajima M, Noguchi T, Tanaka T, Tarui S: Structure of the entire human muscle phosphofructokinase-encoding gene: A two-promoter system *Gene* **104**:277, 1991.
295. Elson A, Levanon D, Brandeis, Dafni N, Bernstein Y, Danciger E, Groner Y: The structure of the human liver-type phosphofructokinase gene. *Genomics* **7**:47, 1990.

296. Nakajima H, Kono N, Yamasaki T, Hamaguchi T, Hotta K, Kuwajima M, Noguchi T, Tanaka T, Tarui S: Tissue specificity in expression and alternative RNA splicing of human phosphofructokinase-M and -L genes. *Biochem Biophys Res Commun* **173**:1317, 1990.
297. Sharma PM, Reddy GR, Babior BM, McLachlan A: Alternative splicing of the transcript encoding the human muscle isoenzyme of phosphofructokinase. *J Biol Chem* **265**:9006, 1990.
298. Poorman RA, Randolph A, Kemp RG, Heinrikson RL: Evolution of phosphofructokinase — Gene duplication and creation of new effector sites. *Nature* **309**:467, 1984.
299. Tarui S, Okuno G, Ikura Y, Tanaka T, Suda M, Nishikawa M: Phosphofructokinase deficiency in skeletal muscle: A new type of glycogenosis. *Biochem Biophys Res Commun* **19**:517, 1965.
300. Layzer RB, Rowland LP, Ranney HM: Muscle phosphofructokinase deficiency. *Arch Neurol* **17**:512, 1967.
301. Serratrice G, Monges A, Roux H, Aquaron R, Gambarelli D: Forme myopathique du déficit en phosphofructokinase. *Rev Neurol* **120**:271, 1969.
302. Waterbury L, Frenkel EP: Hereditary nonspherocytic hemolysis with erythrocyte phosphofructokinase deficiency. *Blood* **39**:415, 1972.
303. Miwa S, Sato T, Murao H, Kozuru M, Ibayashi H: A new type of phosphofructokinase deficiency hereditary nonspherocytic hemolytic anemia. *Acta Haematol Jpn* **35**:113, 1972.
304. Tobin WE, Huijing F, Porro RS, Salzman RT: Muscle phosphofructokinase deficiency. *Arch Neurol* **28**:128, 1973.
305. Lutcher CL, Bigley RL: Hemolytic anemia due to phosphofructokinase (PFK) deficiency. *Clin Res* **22**:66a, 1974.
306. Etiemble J, Kahn A, Boivin P, Bernard JF, Goudemand M: Hereditary hemolytic anemia with erythrocyte phosphofructokinase deficiency: Studies of some properties of erythrocyte and muscle enzyme. *Hum Genet* **31**:83, 1976.
307. Oda S, Oda E, Tanaka KR: Erythrocyte phosphofructokinase (PFK) deficiency: Characterization and metabolic studies. *Clin Res* **25**:344a, 1977.
308. Dupond J-L, Robert M, Carbillet J-P, Leconte des Floris R: Glycogénose musculaire et anémie hémolytique par déficit enzymatique chez deux germains: Forme familiale de maladie de Tarui, par déficit en phosphofructokinase musculaire et érythrocytaire. *Nouv Presse Med* **6**:2665, 1977.
309. Guibaud P, Carrier H, Mathieu M, Dorche C, Parchoux B, Béthenod M, Larbre F: Observation familiale de dystrophie musculaire congenitale par deficit en phosphofructokinase. *Arch Fr Pediatr* **35**:1105, 1978.
310. Tarlow MJ, Ellis DA, Pearce GW, Anderson M: Muscle phosphofructokinase deficiency (Tarui's disease). *Proc Nutr Soc* **38**:110a, 1979.
311. Vora S, Corash L, Engel WK, Durham S, Seaman C, Piomelli S: The molecular mechanism of the inherited phosphofructokinase deficiency associated with hemolysis and myopathy. *Blood* **55**:629, 1980.
312. Agamanolis D, Askari AD, DiMauro S, Hays A, Kumar K, Lipton M, Raynor A: Muscle phosphofructokinase deficiency: Two cases with unusual polysaccharide accumulation and immunologically active enzyme protein. *Muscle Nerve* **3**:456, 1980.
313. Hays AP, Hallett M, Delfs J, Morris J, Sotrel A, Shevchuk MM, DiMauro S: Muscle phosphofructokinase deficiency: Abnormal polysaccharide in a case of late-onset myopathy. *Neurology* **31**:1077, 1981.
314. Danon MJ, Carpenter S, Manaligod JR, Schliselfeld LH: Fatal infantile glycogen storage disease: Deficiency of phosphofructokinase and phosphorylase b kinase. *Neurology* **31**:1303, 1981.
315. Zanella A, Mariani M, Meola G, Fagnani G, Sirchia G: Phosphofructokinase (PFK) deficiency due to a catalytically inactive mutant M-type subunit. *Am J Hematol* **12**:215, 1982.
316. Vora S, Davidson M, Seaman C, Miranda AF, Noble NA, Tanaka KR, Frenkel EP, DiMauro S: Heterogeneity of the molecular lesions in inherited phosphofructokinase deficiency. *J Clin Invest* **72**:1995, 1983.
317. Tani K, Fujii H, Takegawa S, Miwa S, Koyama W, Kanayama M, Imanaka A, Imanaka F, Kuramoto A: Two cases of phosphofructokinase deficiency associated with congenital hemolytic anemia found in Japan. *Am J Hematol* **14**:165, 1983.
318. Servidei S, Bonilla E, Diedrich RG, Kornfeld M, Oates JD, Davidson M, Vora S, DiMauro S: Fatal infantile form of muscle phosphofructokinase deficiency. *Neurology* **36**:1465, 1986.
319. Vora S, DiMauro S, Spear D, Harker D, Danon MJ: Characterization of the enzymatic defect in late-onset muscle phosphofructokinase deficiency: New subtype of glycogen storage disease type VII. *J Clin Invest* **80**:1479, 1987.
320. Amit R, Bashan N, Abarbanel JM, Shapira Y, Sofer S, Moses S: Fatal familial infantile glycogen storage disease: Multisystem phosphofructokinase deficiency. *Muscle Nerve* **15**:455, 1992.
321. Pastoris O, Dossena M, Vercesi L, Scelsi R, Torcetta F, Savasta S, Bianchi E: Muscle phosphofructokinase deficiency in a myopathic child with severe mental retardation and aplasia of cerebellar vermis. *Childs Nerv Syst* **8**:237, 1992.
322. Raben N, Sherman J, Miller F, Mena H, Plotz P: A 5′ splice junction mutation leading to exon deletion in an Ashkenazic Jewish family with phosphofructokinase deficiency (Tarui disease). *J Biol Chem* **268**:4963, 1993.
323. Sherman JB, Raben N, Nicastri C, Argov Z, Nakajima H, Adams EM, Eng CM, Cowan TM, Plotz PH: Common mutations in the phosphofructokinase-M gene in Ashkenazi Jewish patients with glycogenesis VII and their population frequency. *Am J Hum Genet* **55**:305, 1994.
324. Hamaguchi T, Nakajima H, Noguchi T, Ono A, Kono N, Tarui S, Kuwajima M, Matsuzawa Y: A new variant of muscle phosphofructokinase deficiency in a Japanese case with abnormal RNA splicing. *Biochem Biophys Res Commun* **202**:444, 1994.
325. Argov Z, Barash V, Soffer D, Sherman J, Raben N: Late-onset muscular weakness in phosphofructokinase deficiency due to exon 5/intron 5 junction point mutation: A unique disorder or the natural course of this glycolytic disorder? *Neurology* **44**:1097, 1994.
326. Tsujino S, Servidei S, Tonin P, Shanske S, Azan G, DiMauro S: Identification of three novel mutations in non-Ashkenazi Italian patients with muscle phosphofructokinase deficiency. *Am J Hum Genet* **54**:812, 1994.
327. Nakagawa C, Mineo I, Kaido M, Fujimura H, Shimizu T, Hamaguchi T, Nakajima H, Tarui S: A new variant case of muscle phosphofructokinase deficiency, coexisting with gastric ulcer, gouty arthritis, and increased hemolysis. *Muscle Nerve* **3**:S39, 1995.
328. Raben N, Exelbert R, Spiegel R, Sherman JB, Nakajima H, Plotz P, Heinisch J: Functional expression of human mutant phosphofructokinase in yeast: Genetic defects in French Canadian and Swiss patients with phosphofructokinase deficiency. *Am J Hum Genet* **56**:131, 1995.
329. Rudolphi O, Ek B, Ronquist G: Inherited phosphofructokinase deficiency associated with hemolysis and exertional myopathy. *Eur J Haematol* **55**:279, 1995.
330. Sivakumar K, Vasconcelos O, Goldfarb L, Dalakas MC: Late-onset muscle weakness in partial phosphofructokinase deficiency: A unique myopathy with vacuoles, abnormal mitochondria, and absence of the common exon 5/intron 5 junction point mutation. *Neurology* **46**:1337, 1996.
331. Vorgerd M, Karitzky J, Ristow M, Van Schaftingen E, Tegenthoff M, Jerusalem F, Malin J-P: Muscle phosphofructokinase deficiency in two generations. *J Neurol Sci* **141**:95, 1996.
332. Massa R, Lodi R, Barbiroli B, Servidei S, Sancesario G, Manfredi G, Zaniol P, Bernardi G: Partial block of glycolysis in late-onset phosphofructokinase deficiency myopathy. *Acta Neuropathol* **91**:322, 1996.
333. Swoboda KJ, Specht L, Jones HR, Shapiro F, DiMauro S, Korson M: Infantile phosphofructokinase deficiency with arthrogryposis: Clinical benefit of a ketogenic diet. *J Pediatr* **131**:932, 1997.
334. Bruno C, Minetti C, Shanske S, Morreale G, Bado M, Cordone G, DiMauro S: Combined defects of muscle phosphofructokinase and AMP deaminase in a child with myoglobinuria. *Neurology* **50**:296, 1998.
335. Mineo I, Kono N, Hara N, Shimizu T, Yamada Y, Kawachi M, Kiyokawa H, Wang YL, Tarui S: Myogenic hyperuricemia: A common pathophysiologic feature of glycogenosis types III, V, and VII. *N Engl J Med* **317**:75, 1987.
336. Vasconcelos O, Sivakumar K, Dalakas MC, Quezado M, Nagle J, Leon-Monzon M, Dubnik M, Gajdusek DC, Goldfarb LG: Nonsense mutation in the phosphofructokinase muscle subunit gene associated with retention of intron 10 in one of the isolated transcripts in Ashkenazi Jewish patients with Tarui disease. *Proc Natl Acad Sci USA* **92**:10322, 1995.
337. Etiemble J, Simeon J, Buc HA, Picat C, Boulard M, Boivin P: A liver-type mutation in a case of pronounced erythrocyte phosphofructokinase deficiency without clinical expression. *Biochim Biophys Acta* **759**:236, 1983.
338. Nakajima H, Kono N, Yamasaki T, Hotta K, Kawachi M, Kuwajima M, Noguchi T, Tanaka T, Tarui S: Genetic defect in muscle phosphofructokinase deficiency: Abnormal splicing of the muscle phosphofructokinase gene due to a point mutation at the 5′-splicing site. *J Biol Chem* **265**:9392, 1990.

339. Nichols RC, Rudolphi O, Ek B, Exelbert R, Plotz PH, Raben N: Glycogenosis type VII (Tarui disease) in a Swedish family: Two novel mutations in muscle phosphofructokinase gene (PFK-M) resulting in intron retentions. *Am J Hum Genet* **59**:59, 1996.
340. Smith BF, Stedman H, Rajpurohit Y, Henthorn PS, Wolfe JH, Patterson DF, Giger U: Molecular basis of canine muscle-type phosphofructokinase deficiency. *J Biol Chem* **271**:20070, 1996.
341. Sakakibara M, Mukai T, Hori K: Nucleotide sequence of a cDNA clone for human aldolase: A messenger RNA in the liver. *Biochem Biophys Res Commun* **131**:413, 1985.
342. Kukita A, Yoshida MC, Fukushige S, Sakakibara M, Joh K, Mukai T, Hori K: Molecular gene mapping of human aldolase A *(ALDOA)* gene to chromosome 16. *Hum Genet* **76**:20, 1987.
343. Izzo P, Costanzo P, Lupo A, Rippa E, Paolella G, Salvatore F: Human aldolase A gene: Structural organization and tissue-specific expression by multiple promoters and alternate mRNA processing. *Eur J Biochem* **174**:569, 1988.
344. Serero S, Maire P, Van Cong N, Cohen-Haguenauer O, Gross MS, Jégou-Foubert C, de Tand MF, Kahn A, Frézal J: Localization of the active gene of aldolase on chromosome 16, and two aldolase A pseudogenes on chromosomes 3 and 10. *Hum Genet* **78**:167, 1988.
345. Beutler E, Scott S, Bishop A, Margolis N, Matsumoto F, Kuhl W: Red cell aldolase deficiency and hemolytic anemia: A new syndrome. *Trans Assoc Am Phys* **86**:154, 1973.
346. Miwa S, Fujii H, Tani K, Takahashi K, Takegawa S, Fujinami N, Sakurai M, Kubo M, Tanimoto Y, Kato T, Matsumoto N: Two cases of red cell aldolase deficiency associated with hereditary hemolytic anemia in a Japanese family. *Am J Hematol* **11**:425, 1981.
347. Kreuder J, Borkhardt A, Repp R, Pekrun A, Göttsche B, Gottschalk U, Reichmann H, Schachenmayr W, Schlegel K, Lampert F: Inherited metabolic myopathy and hemolysis due to a mutation in aldolase A. *N Engl J Med* **334**:1100, 1996.
348. Kishi H, Mukai T, Hirono A, Fujii H, Miwa S, Hori K: Human aldolase A deficiency associated with a hemolytic anemia: Thermolabile aldolase due to a single base mutation. *Proc Natl Acad Sci U S A* **84**:8623, 1987.
349. Maquat LE, Chilcote R, Ryan PM: Human triosephosphate isomerase cDNA and protein structure: Studies of triosephosphate isomerase deficiency in man. *J Biol Chem* **260**:3748, 1985.
350. Brown JR, Daar IO, Krug JR, Maquat LE: Characterization of the functional gene and several processed pseudogenes in the human triosephosphate isomerase gene family. *Mol Cell Biol* **5**:1694, 1985.
351. Law ML, Kao F-T: Induced segregation of human syntenic genes by 5-bromodeoxyuridine plus near-visible light. *Somat Cell Genet* **4**:465, 1978.
352. Schneider AS, Valentine WN, Hattori M, Heins HL Jr: Hereditary hemolytic anemia with triosephosphate isomerase deficiency. *N Engl J Med* **272**:229, 1965.
353. Valentine WN, Schneider AS, Baughan MA, Paglia DE, Heins HL Jr: Hereditary hemolytic anemia with triosephosphate isomerase deficiency: Studies in kindreds with coexistent sickle cell trait and erythrocyte glucose-6-phosphate dehydrogenase deficiency. *Am J Med* **41**:27, 1966.
354. Harris SR, Paglia DE, Jaffé ER, Valentine WN, Klein RL: Triosephosphate isomerase deficiency in an adult. *Clin Res* **18**:529a, 1970.
355. Freycon F, Lauras B, Bovier-Lapierre F, Dorche C, Goddon R: Anémie hémolytique congénitale par déficit en triose-phosphate-isomérase. *Pediatrie* **30**:55, 1975.
356. Skala H, Dreyfus JC, Vives-Corrons JL, Matsumoto F, Beutler E: Triose phosphate isomerase deficiency. *Biochem Med* **18**:226, 1977.
357. Vives-Corrons J-L, Ribunson-Skala H, Mateo M, Estella J, Feliu E, Dreyfus J-C: Triosephosphate isomerase deficiency with hemolytic anemia and severe neuromuscular disease. Familial and biochemical studies of a case found in Spain. *Hum Genet* **42**:171, 1978.
358. Poll-The BT, Aicardi J, Girot R, Rosa R: Neurological findings in triosephosphate isomerase deficiency. *Ann Neurol* **17**:439, 1985.
359. Zanella A, Mariani M, Colombo MB, Borgna-Pignatti C, De Stefano P, Morgese G, Sirchia G: Triosephosphate isomerase deficiency: 2 new cases. *Scand J Haematol* **34**:417, 1985.
360. Rosa R, Prehu M-O, Calvin M-C, Badoual J, Alix D, Girod R: Hereditary triose phosphate isomerase deficiency: Seven new homozygous cases. *Hum Genet* **71**:235, 1985.
361. Poinsot J, Parent P, Alix D, Toudic L, Castel Y: Un cas d'anémie hémolytique congénitale non sphérocytaire, par déficit en triose phosphate isomérase diagnostic prénatal. *J Genet Hum* **34**:431, 1986.
362. Clark ACL, Szobolotzky MA: Triose phosphate isomerase deficiency: Report of a family. *Aust Paediatr J* **22**:135, 1986.
363. Daar IO, Artymiuk PJ, Phillips DC, Maquat LE: Human triosephosphate isomerase deficiency: A single amino acid substitution results in a thermolabile enzyme. *Proc Natl Acad Sci U S A* **83**:7903, 1986.
364. Elouet JF, Raich N, Rosa J, Roméo PH, Rosa R: New case of codon 104 (Glu → Asp) mutation in homozygous triose phosphate isomerase deficiency and possible prenatal diagnosis of this disease. *Blood* **72**:40a, 1988.
365. Bellingham AJ, Lestas AN, Williams LHP, Nicolaides KH: Prenatal diagnosis of a red-cell enzymopathy: Triose phosphate isomerase deficiency. *Lancet* **2**:419, 1989.
366. Bardosi A, Eber SW, Hendrys M, Pekrun A: Myopathy with altered mitochondria due to a triosephosphate isomerase (TPI) deficiency. *Acta Neuropathol* **79**:387, 1990.
367. Neubauer BA, Pekrun A, Eber SW, Lakomek M, Schröter W: Relation between genetic defect altered protein structure, and enzyme function in triose-phosphate isomerase (TPI) deficiency. *Eur J Pediatr* **151**:232a, 1992.
368. Hollán S, Fujii H, Hirono A, Hirono K, Kanno H, Miwa S, Harsányi V, Gyócs M: Hereditary triosephosphate isomerase (TPI) deficiency: Two severely affected brothers. One with and one without neurological symptoms. *Hum Genet* **92**:486, 1993.
369. Chang M-L, Artymiuk PJ, Wu X, Hollán S, Lammi A, Maquat LE: Human triosephosphate isomerase deficiency resulting from mutation of Phe-240. *Am J Hum Genet* **52**:1260, 1993.
370. Schneider A, Westwood B, Yim C, Prchal J, Berkow R, Labotka R, Warrier R, Beutler E: Triosephosphate isomerase deficiency: Repetitive occurrence of point mutation in amino acid 104 in multiple apparently unrelated families. *Am J Hematol* **50**:263, 1995.
371. Arya R, Lalloz MRA, Bellingham AJ, Layton DM: Molecular pathology of human triosephosphate isomerase. *Blood* **86**:585a, 1995.
372. Clay SA, Shore NA, Landing BH: Triosephosphate isomerase deficiency: A case report with neuropathological findings. *Am J Dis Child* **136**:800, 1982.
373. Pekrun A, Neubauer BA, Eber SW, Lakomek M, Seidel H, Schröter W: Triosephosphate isomerase deficiency: Biochemical and molecular genetic analysis for prenatal diagnosis. *Clin Genet* **47**:175, 1995.
374. Schneider AS, Dunn I, Ibsen KH, Weinstein JM: The pattern of glycolysis in erythrocyte triosephosphate isomerase deficiency. *Clin Res* **13**:282, 1965.
375. Hollán S, Magónyi M, Harsányi V, Farkas T: Search for the pathogenesis of the differing phenotype in two compound heterozygote Hungarian brothers with the same genotypic triosephosphate isomerase deficiency. *Proc Natl Acad Sci U S A* **94**:10362, 1997.
376. Daar IO, Maquat LE: Premature translation termination mediates triosephosphate isomerase mRNA degradation. *Mol Cell Biol* **8**:802, 1988.
377. Schneider A, Cohen-Solal M: Hematologically important mutations: Triosephosphate isomerase. *Blood Cells Mol Dis* **22**:82, 1996.
378. Schneider A, Westwood B, Yim C, Cohen-Solal M, Rosa R, Labotka R, Eber S, Wolf R, Lammi A, Beutler E: The 1591C mutation in triosephosphate isomerase (TPI) deficiency. Tightly linked polymorphisms and a common haplotype in all known families. *Blood Cells Mol Dis* **22**:115, 1996.
379. Mande SC, Mainfroid V, Kalk KH, Goraj K, Martial JA, Hol WGJ: Crystal structure of recombinant human triosephosphate isomerase at 2.8 Å resolution. Triosephosphate isomerase-related human genetic disorders and comparison with the trypanosomal enzyme. *Protein Sci* **3**:810, 1994.
380. Cheng J, Maquat LE: Nonsense codons can reduce the abundance of nuclear mRNA without affecting the abundance of pre-mRNA or the half-life of cytoplasmic mRNA. *Mol Cell Biol* **13**:1892, 1993.
381. Perry BA, Mohrenweiser HW: Human triosephosphate isomerase: Substitution of Arg for Gly at position 122 in a thermolabile electromorph variant, TPI-Manchester. *Hum Genet* **88**:634, 1992.
382. Watanabe M, Zingg BC, Mohrenweiser HW: Molecular analysis of a series of alleles in humans with reduced activity at the triosephosphate isomerase locus. *Am J Hum Genet* **58**:308, 1996.
383. Mohrenweiser HW, Fielek S: Elevated frequency of carriers for triosephosphate isomerase deficiency in newborn infants. *Pediatr Res* **16**:960, 1982.
384. Schneider A, Forman L, Westwood B, Yim C, Lin J, Singh S, Beutler E: The relationship of the −5, −8, and −24 mutations in African-Americans to triosephosphate isomerase (TPI) enzyme activity and to TPI deficiency. *Blood* **92**:2959, 1998.

385. Zingg BC, Pretsch W, Mohrenweiser HW: Molecular analysis of four ENU induced triosephosphate isomerase null mutants in *Mus musculus*. *Mutat Res* **328**:163, 1995.

386. McCarrey JR, Thomas K: Human testis-specific PGK gene lacks introns and possesses characteristics of a processed gene. *Nature* **326**:501, 1987.

387. Willard HF, Goss SJ, Holmes MT, Munroe DL: Regional localization of the phosphoglycerate kinase gene and pseudogene on the human X chromosome and assignment of a related DNA sequence to chromosome 19. *Hum Genet* **71**:138, 1985.

388. Michelson AM, Blake CF, Evans ST, Orkin SH: Structure of the human phosphoglycerate kinase gene and the intron-mediated evolution and dispersal of the nucleotide-binding domain. *Proc Natl Acad Sci U S A* **82**:6965, 1985.

389. Tani K, Singer-Sam J, Munns M, Yoshida A: Molecular cloning and structure of an autosomal processed gene for human phosphoglycerate kinase. *Gene* **35**:11, 1985.

390. Michelson AM, Markham AF, Orkin SH: Isolation and DNA sequence of a full-length cDNA clone for human X chromosome-encoded phosphoglycerate kinase. *Proc Natl Acad Sci U S A* **80**:472, 1983.

391. Banks RD, Blake CCF, Evans PR, Haser R, Rice DW, Hardy GW, Merrett M, Phillips AW: Sequence, structure and activity of phosphoglycerate kinase: A possible hinge-bending enzyme. *Nature* **279**:773, 1979.

392. Bernstein BE, Michels PAM, Hol WGJ: Synergistic effects of substrate-induced conformational changes in phosphoglycerate kinase activation. *Nature* **385**:275, 1997.

393. Kraus AP, Langston MF Jr, Lynch BL: Red cell phosphoglycerate kinase deficiency: A new cause of non-spherocytic hemolytic anemia. *Biochem Biophys Res Commun* **30**:173, 1968.

394. Valentine WN, Hsieh H-S, Paglia DE, Anderson HM, Baughan MA, Jaffé ER, Garson OM: Hereditary hemolytic anemia associated with phosphoglycerate kinase deficiency in erythrocytes and leukocytes: A probable X-chromosome-linked syndrome. *N Engl J Med* **280**:528, 1969.

395. Dodgson SJ, Lee CS, Holland RAB, O'Sullivan WJ, Vowels MR: Erythrocyte phosphoglycerate kinase deficiency: Enzymatic and oxygen binding studies. *Aust N Z J Med* **10**:614, 1980.

396. Svirklys LG, O'Sullivan WJ: Lack of effect of increased 2,3-diphosphoglycerate on flux through the oxidative pathway in phosphoglycerate kinase deficiency. *Clin Chim Acta* **148**:167, 1985.

397. Hjelm M, Wadam B, Yoshida A: A phosphoglycerate kinase variant, PGK Uppsala, associated with hemolytic anemia. *J Lab Clin Med* **96**:1015, 1980.

398. Arese P, Bosia A, Gallo E, Mazza U, Pescarmona GP: Red cell glycolysis in a case of 3-phosphoglycerate kinase deficiency. *Eur J Clin Invest* **3**:86, 1973.

399. Cartier P, Habibi B, Leroux J-P, Marchand J-C: Anémie hémolytique congénitale associée a un déficit en phosphoglycérate-kinase dans les globules rouges, les polynucléaires et les lymphocytes. *Neuv Rev Fr Hematol* **11**: 565, 1971.

400. Miwa S, Nakashima K, Oda S, Ogawa H, Nagafuji H, Arima M, Okuna T, Nakashima T: Phosphoglycerate kinase (PGK) deficiency hereditary nonspherocytic hemolytic anemia: Report of a case found in Japanese family. *Acta Haematol Jpn* **35**:571, 1972.

401. Konrad PN, McCarthy DJ, Mauer AM, Valentine WN, Paglia DE: Erythrocyte and leukocyte phosphoglycerate kinase deficiency with neurologic disease. *J Pediatr* **82**:456, 1973.

402. Akatsuka J, Saito F, Okabe N, Maekawa K, Kitani N, Nishina T, Hashimoto F: Studies on erythrocyte and leukocyte phosphoglycerate kinase deficiency with neurologic disease [in Japanese with English Abstract]. *Jpn J Clin Hematol* **14**:1189, 1973.

403. Boivin P, Hakim J, Mandereau J, Galand C, Degos F, Schaison G: Déficit en 3-phosphoglycérate kinase érythrocytaire et leucocytaire: Étude des propriétés de l'enzyme, de la fonction phagocytaire des polynucléaires et revue de la littérature. *Nouv Rev Fr Hematol* **14**:495, 1974.

404. Rosa R, George C, Rosa J: Severe deficiency of red cell phosphoglycerate kinase (PGK) without concomitant hemolysis. *Blood* **54**:35a, 1979.

405. Rosa R, George C, Fardeau M, Calvin M-C, Rapin M, Rosa J: A new case of phosphoglycerate kinase deficiency: PGK Creteil associated with rhabdomyolysis and lacking hemolytic anemia. *Blood* **60**:84, 1982.

406. DiMauro S, Dalakas M, Miranda AF: Phosphoglycerate kinase deficiency: Another cause of recurrent myoglobinuria. *Ann Neurol* **13**:11, 1983.

407. Guis MS, Karadsheh N, Mentzer WC: Phosphoglycerate kinase San Francisco: A new variant associated with hemolytic anemia but not with neuromuscular manifestations. *Am J Hematol* **25**:175, 1987.

408. Sugie H, Sugie Y, Nishida M, Ito M, Tsurui S, Suzuki M, Miyamoto R, Igarashi Y: Recurrent myoglobinuria in a child with mental retardation: Phosphoglycerate kinase deficiency. *J Child Neurol* **4**:95, 1989.

409. Fujii H, Kanno H, Hirono A, Shiomura T, Miwa S: A single amino acid substitution (157 Gly → Val) in a phosphoglycerate kinase variant (PGK Shizuoka) associated with chronic hemolysis and myoglobinuria. *Blood* **79**:1582, 1992.

410. Maeda M, Bawle EV, Kulkarni R, Beutler E, Yoshida A: Molecular abnormalities of a phosphoglycerate kinase variant generated by spontaneous mutation. *Blood* **79**:2759, 1992.

411. Sugie H, Sugie Y, Tsurui S, Ito M: Phosphoglycerate kinase deficiency. *Neurology* **44**:1364, 1994.

412. Tsujino S, Tonin P, Shanske S, Nohria V, Boustany R-M, Lewis D, Chen Y-T, DiMauro S: A splice junction mutation in a new myopathic variant of phosphoglycerate kinase deficiency (PGK North Carolina). *Ann Neurol* **35**:349, 1994.

413. Yoshida A, Twele TW, Davé V, Beutler E: Molecular abnormality of a phosphoglycerate kinase variant (PGK-Alabama). *Blood Cells Mol Dis* **21**:179, 1995.

414. Tonin P, Shanske S, Miranda AF, Brownell AK, Wyse JP, Tsujino S, DiMauro S: Phosphoglycerate kinase deficiency: Biochemical and molecular genetic studies in a new myopathic variant (PGK Alberta). *Neurology* **43**:387, 1993.

415. Ookawara T, Davé V, Willems P, Martin J-J, de Barsy T, Matthys E, Yoshida A: Retarded and aberrant splicings caused by single exon mutation in a phosphoglycerate kinase variant. *Arch Biochem Biophys* **327**:35, 1996.

416. Lyon MF: Gene action in the X-chromosome of the mouse (*Mus musculus* L.). *Nature* **190**:372, 1961.

417. Beutler E, Yeh M, Fairbanks VF: The normal human female as a mosaic of X-chromosome activity: Studies using the gene for G-6-PD deficiency as a marker. *Proc Natl Acad Sci U S A* **48**:9, 1962.

418. Tsujino S, Shanske S, DiMauro S: Molecular genetic heterogeneity of phosphoglycerate kinase (PGK) deficiency. *Muscle Nerve* **3**:S45, 1995.

419. Miwa S, Nakashima K, Oda S, Takahashi K, Morooka K, Nakashima T: Evidence of the decreased muscle enzyme activity in erythrocyte phosphoglycerate kinase deficiency. *Acta Haematol Jpn* **37**:59, 1974.

420. Fujii H, Yoshida A: Molecular abnormality of phosphoglycerate kinase-Uppsala associated with chronic nonspherocytic hemolytic anemia. *Proc Natl Acad Sci USA* **77**:5461, 1980.

421. Fujii H, Chen S-H, Akatsuka J, Miwa S, Yoshida A: Use of cultured lymphoblastoid cells for the study of abnormal enzymes: Molecular abnormality of a phosphoglycerate kinase variant associated with hemolytic anemia. *Proc Natl Acad Sci U S A* **78**:2587, 1981.

422. Maeda M, Yoshida A: Molecular defect of a phosphoglycerate kinase variant (PGK-Matsue) associated with hemolytic anemia: Leu → Pro substitution caused by T/A → C/G transition in exon 3. *Blood* **77**:1348, 1991.

423. Cohen-Solal M, Valentin C, Plassa F, Guillemin G, Danze F, Jaisson F, Rosa R: Identification of new mutations in two phosphoglycerate kinase (PGK) variants expressing different clinical syndromes: PGK Créteil and PGK Amiens. *Blood* **84**:898, 1994.

424. Turner G, Fletcher J, Elber J, Yanagawa Y, Davé J, Yoshida A: Molecular defect of a phosphoglycerate kinase variant associated with haemolytic anaemia and neurological disorders in a large kindred. *Br J Haematol* **91**:60, 1995.

425. Sugie H, Sugie Y, Ito M, Fukuda T: A novel missense mutation (837T → C) in the phosphoglycerate kinase gene of a patient with a myopathic form of phosphoglycerate kinase deficiency. *J Child Neurol* **13**:95, 1998.

426. Baehner RL, Feig SA, Segel GB, Anderson HM, Jaffé ER: Metabolic phagocytic, and bactericidal properties of phosphoglycerate kinase deficient (PGK) polymorphonuclear leukocytes (PMN). *Blood* **38**:833a, 1971.

427. Tougard P, Le TH, Minard P, Desmadril M, Yon JM, Bizebard T, Lebras G, Dumas C: Structural and functional properties of mutant Arg203Pro from yeast phosphoglycerate kinase, as a model of phosphoglycerate kinase-Uppsala. *Protein Eng* **9**:181, 1996.

428. Fujii H, Krietsch KG, Yoshida A: A single amino acid substitution (Asp → Asn) in a phosphoglycerate kinase variant (PGK München) associated with enzyme deficiency. *J Biol Chem* **255**, 6421, 1980.
429. Yoshida A, Watanabe S, Chen S-H, Giblett ER, Malcom LA: Human phosphoglycerate kinase II. Structure of a variant enzyme. *J Biol Chem* **247**:446, 1972.
430. Chen S-H, Malcom LA, Yoshida A, Giblett ER: Phosphoglycerate kinase: An X-linked polymorphism in man. *Am J Hum Genet* **23**:87, 1971.
431. Le Gall JY, Mubamba C, Godin Y: The red cell 3-phosphoglycerate kinase polymorphism. Report of a new allele. *Hum Genet* **34**:311, 1976.
432. Omoto K, Blake NM: Distribution of genetic variants of erythrocyte phosphoglycerate kinase (PGK) and phosphohexose isomerase (PHI) among some population groups in southeast Asia and Oceania. *Ann Hum Genet* **36**:61, 1972.
433. Rosa R, Audit I, Rosa J: Evidence for three enzymatic activities in one electrophoretic band of 3-phosphoglycerate mutase from red cells. *Biochimie* **57**:1059, 1975.
434. Sasaki R, Ikura K, Sugimoto E, Chiba H: Purification of bisphosphoglyceromutase, 2,3-bisphosphoglycerate phosphatase and phosphoglyceromutase from human erythrocytes: Three enzyme activities in one protein. *Eur J Biochem* **50**:581, 1975.
435. Joulin V, Peduzzi J, Roméo P-H, Rosa R, Valentin C, Dubart A, Lapeyre B, Blouquit Y, Garel M-C, Goossens M, Rosa J, Cohen-Solal M: Molecular cloning and sequencing of the human erythrocyte 2,3-bisphosphoglycerate mutase cDNA: Revised amino acid sequence. *EMBO J* **5**:2275, 1986.
436. Barichard F, Joulin V, Henry I, Garel M-C, Valentin C, Rosa R, Cohen-Solal M, Junien C: Chromosomal assignment of the human 2,3-bisphosphoglycerate mutase gene (BPGM) to region 7q34 → 7q22. *Hum Genet* **77**:283, 1987.
437. Joulin V, Garel M-C, Le Boulch P, Valentin C, Rosa R, Rosa J, Cohen-Solal M: Isolation and characterization of the human 2,3-bisphosphoglycerate mutase gene. *J Biol Chem* **263**:15785, 1988.
438. Rosa R, Prehu M-O, Beuzard Y, Rosa J: The first case of a complete deficiency of diphosphoglycerate mutase in human erythrocytes. *J Clin Invest* **62**:907, 1978.
439. Rosa R, Prehu M-O, Albrecht-Ellmer K, Calvin MC: Partial characterization of the inactive mutant form of human red cell bisphosphoglyceromutase and comparison with an alkylated form. *Biochim Biophys Acta* **742**:243, 1983.
440. Galacteros F, Rosa R, Prehu MO, Najean Y, Calvin MC: Déficit en diphosphoglycérate mutase: Nouveaux cas associés à une polyglobulie. *Nouv Rev Fr Hematol* **26**:69, 1984.
441. Lemarchandel V, Joulin V, Valentin C, Rosa R, Galactéros F, Rosa J, Cohen-Solal M: Compound heterozygosity in a complete erythrocyte bisphosphoglycerate mutase deficiency. *Blood* **80**:2643, 1992.
442. Garel M-C, Lemarchandel V, Calvin M-C, Arous N, Craescu CT, Prehu M-O, Rosa J, Rosa R: Amino acid residues involved in the catalytic site of human erythrocyte bisphosphoglycerate mutase. Functional consequences of substitutions of His10, His187 and Arg89. *Eur J Biochem* **213**:493, 1993.
443. Boulard-Heitzmann P, Boulard M, Tallineau C, Boivin P, Tanzer J, Bois M, Barriere M: Decreased red cell enolase activity in a 40-year-old woman with compensated haemolysis. *Scand J Haematol* **33**:401, 1984.
444. Lachant NA, Jennings MA, Tanaka KR: Partial erythrocyte enolase deficiency: A hereditary disorder with variable clinical expression. *Blood* **65**:55a, 1986.
445. Miwa S, Nishina T, Kakehashi Y, Kitamura M, Hiratsuka A, Shizume K: Studies on erythrocyte metabolism in a case with hereditary deficiency of H-subunit of lactate dehydrogenase. *Acta Haematol Jpn* **34**:228, 1971.
446. Wakabayashi H, Tsuchiya M, Yoshino K, Kaku K, Shigei H: Hereditary deficiency of lactate dehydrogenase H-subunit. *Intern Med* **35**:550, 1996.
447. Miyajima H, Takahashi Y, Kaneko E: Characterization of the glycolysis in lactate dehydrogenase-A deficiency. *Muscle Nerve* **18**:874, 1995.
448. Kremer J-P, Datta T, Pretsch W, Charles DJ, Dörmer P: Mechanisms of compensation of hemolytic anemia in a lactate dehydrogenase mouse mutant. *Exp Hematol* **15**:664, 1987.
449. Tsujino S, Shanske S, Sakoda S, Toscano A, DiMauro S: Molecular genetic studies in muscle phosphoglycerate mutase (PGAM-M) deficiency. *Muscle Nerve* **3**:S50, 1995.
450. Parr CW, Fitch LI: Inherited quantitative variations of human phosphogluconate dehydrogenase. *Ann Hum Genet* **30**:339, 1967.
451. Beutler E, Matsumoto F: Ethnic variation in red cell glutathione peroxidase activity. *Blood* **46**:103, 1975.
452. Cohen HJ, Brown MR, Hamilton D, Lyons-Patterson J, Avissar N, Liegey P: Glutathione peroxidase and selenium deficiency in patients receiving home parenteral nutrition: Time course for development of deficiency and repletion of enzyme activity in plasma and blood cells. *Am J Clin Nutr* **49**:132, 1989.
453. Dacie J: *The Haemolytic Anaemias*, 3rd ed, vol 1.New York, Churchill Livingstone, 1985, p 424.
454. Beutler E: Red cell enzyme defects as nondiseases and as diseases. *Blood* **54**:1, 1979.
455. Beutler E, Kuhl W, Gelbart T: 6-Phosphogluconolactonase deficiency, a hereditary erythrocyte enzyme deficiency: Possible interaction with glucose-6-phosphate dehydrogenase deficiency. *Proc Natl Acad Sci U S A* **82**:3876, 1985.
456. Thorburn DR, Kuchel PW: Computer simulation of the metabolic consequences of the combined deficiency of 6-phosphogluconolactonase and glucose-6-phosphate dehydrogenase in human erythrocytes. *J Lab Clin Med* **110**:70, 1987.
457. Beutler E: Glutathione reductase: Stimulation in normal subjects by riboflavin supplementation. *Science* **165**:613, 1969.
458. Loos H, Roos D, Weening R, Houwerzijl J: Familial deficiency of glutathione reductase in human blood cells. *Blood* **48**:53, 1976.
459. Frischer H, Ahmad T: Consequences of erythrocytic glutathione reductase deficiency. *J Lab Clin Med* **109**:583, 1987.
460. Gipp JJ, Chang C, Mulcahy RT: Cloning and nucleotide sequence of a full-length cDNA for human liver γ-glutamylcysteine synthetase. *Biochem Biophys Res Commun* **185**:29, 1992.
461. Gipp JJ, Bailey HH, Mulcahy RT: Cloning and sequencing of the cDNA for the light subunit of human liver γ-glutamylcysteine synthetase and relative mRNA levels for heavy and light subunits in human normal tissues. *Biochem Biophys Res Commun* **206**:584, 1995.
462. Sierra-Rivera E, Summar ML, Dasouki M, Krishnamani MRS, Phillips JA, Freeman ML: Assignment of the gene (GLCLC) that encodes the heavy subunit of γ-glutamylcysteine synthetase to human chromosome 6. *Cytogenet Cell Genet* **70**:278, 1995.
463. Sierra-Rivera E, Dasouki M, Summar ML, Krishnamani MRS, Meredith M, Rao PN, Phillips JA III, Freeman ML: Assignment of the human gene (GLCLR) that encodes the regulatory subunit of γ-glutamylcysteine synthetase to chromosome 1p21. *Cytogenet Cell Genet* **72**:252, 1996.
464. Konrad PN, Richards F II, Valentine WN, Paglia DE: γ-Glutamylcysteine synthetase deficiency: A cause of hereditary hemolytic anemia. *N Engl J Med* **286**:557, 1972.
465. Richards F II, Cooper MR, Pearce LA, Cowan RJ, Spurr CL: Familial spinocerebellar degeneration, hemolytic anemia, and glutathione deficiency. *Arch Intern Med* **134**:534, 1974.
466. Beutler E, Moroose R, Kramer L, Gelbart T, Forman L: Gamma-glutamylcysteine synthetase deficiency and hemolytic anemia. *Blood* **75**:271, 1990.
467. Hirono A, Iyori H, Sekine I, Ueyama J, Chiba H, Kanno H, Fujii H, Miwa S: Three cases of hereditary nonspherocytic hemolytic anemia associated with red blood cell glutathione deficiency. *Blood* **87**:2071, 1996.
467a. Beutler E, Gelbart T, Kondo T, Matsunaga AT: The molecular basis of a case of γ-glutamylcysteine synthetase deficiency. *Blood* **94**:2890, 1999.
467b. Ristoff E, Augustson C, Geissler J, de Rijk T, Carlsson K, Luo JL, Andersson K, Weening RS, van Zwieten R, Larsson A, Roos D: A missense mutation in the heavy subunit of gamma-glutamylcysteine synthetase gene causes hemolytic anemia. *Blood* **95**:2193, 2000.
468. Shi Z-Z, Habibi GM, Rhead WJ, Gahl WA, He X, Sazer S, Lieberman MW: Mutations in the glutathione synthetase gene cause 5-oxoprolinuria. *Nat Genet* **14**:361, 1996.
469. Dahl N, Pigg M, Ristoff E, Gali R, Carlsson B, Mannervik B, Larsson A, Board P: Missense mutations in the human glutathione synthetase gene result in severe metabolic acidosis, 5-oxoprolinuria, hemolytic anemia and neurological dysfunction. *Hum Mol Genet* **6**: 1147, 1997.
470. Von Zabern I, Wittmann-Liebold B, Untucht-Grau R, Schirmer RH, Pai EF: Primary and tertiary structure of the principal human adenylate kinase. *Eur J Biochem* **68**:281, 1976.
471. Zuffardi O, Caiulo A, Maraschio P, Tupler R, Bianchi E, Amisano P, Beluffi G, Moratti R, Liguri G: Regional assignment of the loci for adenylate kinase to 9q32 and for alpha(1)-acid glycoprotein to 9q31-q32. A locus for Goltz syndrome in region 9q32-qter? *Hum Genet* **82**:17, 1989.

472. Matsuura S, Igarashi M, Tanizawa Y, Yamada M, Kishi F, Kajii T, Fujii H, Miwa S, Sakurai M, Nakazawa A: Human adenylate kinase deficiency associated with hemolytic anemia: A single base substitution affecting solubility and catalytic activity of the cytosolic adenylate kinase. *J Biol Chem* **264**:10148, 1989.
473. Szeinberg A, Kahana D, Gavendo S, Zaidman J, Ben-Ezzer J: Hereditary deficiency of adenylate kinase in red blood cells. *Acta Haemat* **42**:111, 1969.
474. Toren A, Brok-Simoni F, Ben-Bassat I, Holtzman F, Mandel M, Neumann Y, Ramot B, Rechavi G, Kende G: Congenital haemolytic anaemia associated with adenylate kinase deficiency. *Br J Haematol* **87**:376, 1994.
475. Boivin P, Galand C, Hakim J, Simony D, Seligman M: Une nouvelle érythroenzymopathie: Anémie hémolytique congénitale non sphérocytaire et déficit héréditaire en adénylate-kinase érytrocytaire. *Presse Med* **79**:215, 1971.
476. Miwa S, Fujii H, Tani K, Takahashi K, Takizawa T, Igarashi T: Red cell adenylate kinase deficiency associated with hereditary nonspherocytic hemolytic anemia: Clinical and biochemical studies. *Am J Hematol* **14**:325, 1983.
477. Beutler E, Carson D, Dannawi H, Forman L, Kuhl W, West C, Westwood B: Metabolic compensation for profound erythrocyte adenylate kinase deficiency: A hereditary enzyme defect without hemolytic anemia. *J Clin Invest* **72**:648, 1983.
478. Lachant NA, Zerez CR, Barredo J, Lee DW, Savely SM, Tanaka KR: Hereditary erythrocyte adenylate kinase deficiency: A defect of multiple phosphotransferases? *Blood* **77**: 2774, 1991.
479. Qualtieri A, Pedace V, Bisconte MG, Bria M, Gulino B, Andreoli V, Brancati C: Severe erythrocyte adenylate kinase deficiency due to homozygous A → G substitution at codon 164 of human AK1 gene associated with chronic haemolytic anaemia. *Br J Haematol* **99**:770, 1997.
480. Daddona PE, Shewach DS, Kelley WN, Argos P, Markham AF, Orkin SH: Human adenosine deaminase: cDNA and complete primary amino acid sequence. *J Biol Chem* **259**:12101, 1984.
481. Petersen MB, Tranebjaerg L, Tommerup N, Nygaard P, Edwards H: New assignment of the adenosine deaminase gene locus to chromosome 20q13.11 by study of a patient with interstitial deletion 20q. *J Med Genet* **24**:93, 1987.
482. Valerio D, Duyvesteyn MGC, Dekker BMM, Weeda G, Berkvens TM, van der Voorn L, van Ormondt H, van der Eb AJ: Adenosine deaminase: Characterization and expression of a gene with a remarkable promoter. *EMBO J* **4**:437, 1985.
483. Valentine WN, Paglia DE, Tartaglia AP, Gilsanz F: Hereditary hemolytic anemia with increased red cell adenosine deaminase (45- to 70-fold) and decreased adenosine triphosphate. *Science* **195**:783, 1977.
484. Miwa S, Fujii H, Matsumoto N, Nakatsuji T, Oda S, Asano H, Asano S: A case of red-cell adenosine deaminase overproduction associated with hereditary hemolytic anemia found in Japan. *Am J Hematol* **5**:107, 1978.
485. Pérignon J-L, Hamet M, Buc HA, Cartier PH, Derycke M: Biochemical study of a case of hemolytic anemia with increased (85-fold) red cell adenosine deaminase. *Clin Chim Acta* **124**:205, 1982.
486. Kanno H, Tani K, Fujii H, Iguchi-Ariga SMM, Ariga H, Kosaki T, Miwa S: Adenosine deaminase (ADA) overproduction associated with congenital hemolytic anemia: Case report and molecular analysis. *Japan J Exp Med* **58**:1, 1988.
487. Fujii H, Miwa S, Suzuki K: Purification and properties of adenosine deaminase in normal and hereditary hemolytic anemia with increased red cell activity. *Hemoglobin* **4**:693, 1980.
488. Fujii H, Miwa S, Tani K, Fujinami N, Asano S: Overproduction of structurally normal enzyme in man: Hereditary haemolytic anaemia with increased red cell adenosine deaminase activity. *Br J Haematol* **51**:427, 1982.
489. Chottiner EG, Cloft HJ, Tartaglia AP, Mitchell BS: Elevated adenosine deaminase activity and hereditary hemolytic anemia: Evidence for abnormal translational control of protein synthesis. *J Clin Invest* **79**:1001, 1987.
490. Chottiner EG, Ginsburg D, Tartaglia AP, Mitchell BS: Erythrocyte adenosine deaminase overproduction in hereditary hemolytic anemia. *Blood* **74**:448, 1989.
491. Chen EH, Tartaglia AP, Mitchell BS: Hereditary overexpression of adenosine deaminase in erythrocytes: Evidence for a *cis*-acting mutation. *Am J Hum Genet* **53**:889, 1993.
492. Chen EH, Mitchell BS: Hereditary overexpression of adenosine deaminase in erythrocytes: Studies in erythroid cell lines and transgenic mice. *Blood* **84**:2346, 1994.
493. Glader BE, Backer K, Diamond LK: Elevated erythrocyte adenosine deaminase activity in congenital hypoplastic anemia. *N Engl J Med* **309**:1486, 1983.
494. Cowan MJ, Brady RO, Widder KJ: Elevated erythrocyte adenosine deaminase activity in patients with acquired immunodeficiency syndrome. *Proc Natl Acad Sci U S A* **83**:1089, 1986.
495. Kanno H, Fujii F, Tani K, Morisaki T, Takahashi K, Horiuchi N, Kizaki M, Ogawa T, Miwa S: Elevated erythrocyte adenosine deaminase activity in a patient with primary acquired sideroblastic anemia. *Am J Hematol* **27**:216, 1988.
496. Paglia DE, Valentine WN: Characteristics of a pyrimidine-specific 5′-nucleotidase in human erythrocytes. *J Biol Chem* **250**:7973, 1975.
497. Hirono A, Fujii H, Natori H, Kurokawa I, Miwa S: Chromatographic analysis of human erythrocyte pyrimidine 5′-nucleotidase from five patients with pyrimidine 5′-nucleotidase deficiency. *Br J Haematol* **65**:35, 1987.
498. Amici A, Emanuelli M, Ferretti E, Raffaelli N, Ruggieri S, Magni G: Homogeneous pyrimidine nucleotidase from human erythrocytes: Enzymic and molecular properties. *Biochem J* **304**:987, 1994.
499. Amici A, Emanuelli M, Magni G, Raffaelli N, Ruggieri S: Pyrimidine nucleotidases from human erythrocyte possess phosphotransferase activities specific for pyrimidine nucleotides. *FEBS Lett* **419**:263, 1997.
500. Valentine WN, Fink K, Paglia DE, Harris SR, Adams WS: Hereditary hemolytic anemia with human erythrocyte pyrimidine 5′-nucleotidase deficiency. *J Clin Invest* **54**:866, 1974.
501. Vives-Corrons JL, Montserrat-Costa E, Rozman C: Hereditary hemolytic anemia with erythrocyte pyrimidine 5′-nucleotidase deficiency in Spain. *Hum Genet* **34**:285, 1976.
502. Ben-Bassat I, Brok-Simoni F, Kende G, Holtzmann F, Ramot B: A family with red cell pyrimidine 5′-nucleotidase deficiency. *Blood* **47**:919, 1976.
503. Miwa S, Nakashima K, Fujii H, Matsumoto M, Nomura K: Three cases of hereditary hemolytic anemia with pyrimidine 5′-nucleotidase deficiency in a Japanese family. *Hum Genet* **37**:361, 1977.
504. Torrance JD, Karabus CD, Shnier M, Meltzer M, Katz J, Jenkins T: Haemolytic anaemia due to erythrocyte pyrimidine 5′-nucleotidase deficiency. *S Afr Med J* **52**:671, 1977.
505. Rosa R, Rochant H, Dreyfus B, Valentin C, Rosa J: Electrophoretic and kinetic studies of human erythrocytes deficient in pyrimidine 5′-nucleotidase. *Hum Genet* **38**:209, 1977.
506. Shinohara K, Tanaka KR: Kinetic and electrophoretic studies of human erythrocytes deficient in pyrimidine 5′-nucleotidase. *Hum Genet* **51**:107, 1979.
507. Buc H-A, Kaplan J-C, Najman A: Study of a case with severe red-cell pyrimidine 5′-nucleotidase deficiency. *Clin Chim Acta* **95**:83, 1979.
508. Paglia DE, Fink K, Valentine WN: Additional data from two kindreds with genetically induced deficiencies of erythrocyte pyrimidine nucleotidase. *Acta Haematol* **63**:262, 1980.
509. Beutler E, Baranko PV, Feagler J, Matsumoto F, Miro-Quesdada M, Selby G, Singh P: Hemolytic anemia due to pyrimidine-5′-nucleotidase deficiency: Report of eight cases in six families. *Blood* **56**:251, 1980.
510. Ozsoylu S, Gurgey A: A case of hemolytic anemia due to erythrocyte pyrimidine 5′-nucleotidase deficiency. *Acta Haematol* **66**:56, 1981.
511. McMahon JN, Lieberman JE, Gordon-Smith EC, Egan EL: Hereditary haemolytic anaemia due to red cell pyrimidine 5′-nucleotidase deficiency in two Irish families with a note on the benefit of splenectomy. *Clin Lab Haematol* **3**:27, 1981.
512. Miwa S, Ishida Y, Kibe A, Uekihara S, Kishimoto S: Two cases of hereditary hemolytic anemia with pyrimidine 5′-nucleotidase deficiency. *Acta Haematol Jpn* **44**:187, 1981.
513. Tomoda A, Noble NA, Lachant NA, Tanaka KR: Hemolytic anemia in hereditary pyrimidine 5′-nucleotidase deficiency: Nucleotide inhibition of G6PD and the pentose phosphate shunt. *Blood* **60**:1212, 1982.
514. Hirono A, Fujii H, Miyajima H, Kawakatsu T, Hiyoshi Y, Miwa S: Three families with hereditary hemolytic anemia and pyrimidine 5′-nucleotidase deficiency: Electrophoretic and kinetic studies. *Clin Chim Acta* **130**:189, 1983.
515. Hansen TWR, Seip M, de Verdier C-H, Ericson Å: Erythrocyte pyrimidine 5′-nucleotidase deficiency: Report of 2 new cases, with a review of the literature. *Scand J Haematol* **31**:122, 1983.

516. Paglia DE, Valentine WN, Keitt AS, Brockway RA, Nakatani M: Pyrimidine nucleotidase deficiency with active dephosphorylation of dTMP: Evidence for existence of thymidine nucleotidase in activities among normal isozymes of 5′-nucleotidase in human erythrocytes. *Blood* **62**:1147, 1983.
517. Dvilansky A, Hezkelson L, Wolfson M, Nathan I, Bashan N, Meyerstein N: Haemolytic anaemia due to pyrimidine-5′-nucleotidase deficiency. *Int J Tiss Reac* **6**:351, 1984.
518. De Korte D, Sijstermans JM, Seip M, Van Doorn CCH, Van Gennip AH, Roos D: Pyrimidine 5′-nucleotidase deficiency: improved detection of carriers. *Clin Chim Acta* **184**:175, 1989.
519. Li JY, Wan S-D, Ma Z-M, Zhao Y-H, Zhou G-P: A new mutant erythrocyte pyrimidine 5′-nucleotidase characterized by fast electrophoretic mobility in a Chinese boy with chronic hemolytic anemia. *Clin Chim Acta* **200**:43, 1991.
520. Ghosh K, Abdulrahman HI, Torres EC, Wahab AA, Hassanein AA: Report of the first case of pyrimidine 5′ nucleotidase deficiency from Kuwait detected by a screening test. A case report. *Haematologia* **24**:229, 1991.
521. David O, Ramenghi U, Camaschella C, Vota MG, Comino L, Pescarmona GP, Nicola P: Inhibition of hexose monophosphate shunt in young erythrocytes by pyrimidine nucleotides in hereditary pyrimidine 5′ nucleotidase deficiency. *Eur J Haematol* **47**:48, 1991.
522. Rees DC, Duley J, Simmonds HA, Wonke B, Thein SL, Clegg JB, Weatherall DJ: Interaction of hemoglobin E and pyrimidine 5′ nucleotidase deficiency. *Blood* **88**:2761, 1996.
523. Torrance JD, Whittaker D: Distribution of erythrocyte nucleotides in pyrimidine 5′-nucleotidase deficiency. *Br J Haematol* **43**:423, 1979.
524. Ericson Å, de Verdier C-H, Hansen TWR, Seip M: Erythrocyte nucleotide pattern in two children in a Norwegian family with pyrimidine 5′-nucleotidase deficiency. *Clin Chim Acta* **134**:25, 1983.
525. Miwa S, Luzzatto L, Rosa R, Paglia DE, Schröter W, De Flora A, Fujii H, Board PG, Beutler E: Recommended screening test for pyrimidine 5′-nucleotidase deficiency. International Committee for Standardization in Haematology. *Clin Lab Haematol* **11**:55, 1989.
526. Kondo T, Ohtsuka Y, Shimada M, Kawakami Y, Hiyoshi Y, Tsuji Y, Fujii H, Miwa S: Erythrocyte-oxidized glutathione transport in pyrimidine 5′-nucleotidase deficiency. *Am J Hematol* **26**:37, 1987.
527. Oda E, Oda S, Tomoda A, Lachant NA, Tanaka KR: Hemolytic anemia in hereditary pyrimidine 5′-nucleotidase deficiency. II. Effect of pyrimidine nucleotides and their derivatives on glycolytic and pentose phosphate shunt enzyme activity. *Clin Chim Acta* **141**:93, 1984.
528. David O, Vota MG, Piga A, Ramenghi U, Bosia A, Pescarmona GP: Pyrimidine 5′-nucleotidase acquired deficiency in β-thalassemia: Involvement of enzyme-SH group in the inactivation process. *Acta Haematol* **82**:69, 1989.
529. Paglia DE, Valentine WN, Dahlgren JG: Effects of low-level lead exposure on pyrimidine 5′-nucleotidase and other erythrocyte enzymes: Possible role of pyrimidine 5′-nucleotidase in the pathogenesis of lead-induced anemia. *J Clin Invest* **56**:1164, 1975.
530. Valentine WN, Paglia DE, Fink K, Madokoro G: Lead poisoning: Association with hemolytic anemia, basophilic stippling, erythrocyte pyrimidine 5′-nucleotidase deficiency, and intraerythrocytic accumulation of pyrimidines. *J Clin Invest* **58**:926, 1976.
531. Buc H-A, Kaplan J-C: Red-cell pyrimidine 5′-nucleotidase and lead poisoning. *Clin Chim Acta* **87**:49, 1978.
532. Beutler E, Hartman G: Age-related red cell enzymes in children with transient erythroblastopenia of childhood and hemolytic anemia. *Pediatr Res* **19**:44, 1985.

CHAPTER 183

Hereditary Spherocytosis and Hereditary Elliptocytosis

William T. Tse ▪ Samuel E. Lux

1. **The red-blood-cell membrane is composed of a bilayer of lipids and integral membrane proteins laminated to an underlying protein skeleton. The membrane skeleton is a two-dimensional meshwork of spectrin tetramers and oligomers cross-linked by protein 4.1 and short actin filaments. It is attached to the membrane via the binding of spectrin to ankyrin and ankyrin to band 3 protein and via an interaction between protein 4.1 and glycophorin C. The membrane skeleton is a major determinant of membrane shape, strength, and flexibility and helps to control lipid organization and integral protein mobility and topography. Genetic defects in the red cell membrane or its skeleton cause congenital hemolytic disorders or inherited abnormalities in red cell morphology such as hereditary elliptocytosis and hereditary spherocytosis.**
2. **Hereditary elliptocytosis (HE) is a heterogeneous group of congenital red cell disorders characterized by ellipsoidally shaped cells. Hereditary pyropoikilocytosis (HPP) is a related and more severe group of disorders characterized by fragmented red cells and poikilocytes. The clinical phenotypes of HE and HPP are a continuous spectrum with varying degrees of severity. Common HE is usually a mild, dominantly inherited condition with prominent elliptocytosis but little or no hemolysis. Acute hemolytic episodes sometimes occur in patients when splenomegaly develops in response to exogenous stimuli. Some patients with common HE present with poikilocytosis and hemolysis in infancy but later improve and are clinically mild after the first year of life. In the occasional patients with homozygous HE, severe hemolysis is observed. Similar features are observed in HPP, an uncommon, usually sporadic disorder manifest by severe hemolysis, marked poikilocytosis, and increased sensitivity of red cells to heat-induced fragmentation. HPP patients often have family members who have common HE, and their severe phenotype can be explained by the coinheritance of an HE allele and a disease-modifying gene.**
3. **Many defects in membrane skeletal proteins have been identified in patients with HE and HPP. Isolated skeletons from these patients retain the elliptocytic or poikilocytic shape of the original red cells, indicating that the defect causing the abnormal shape is intrinsic to the membrane skeleton. Many HE/HPP patients have spectrins that are heat-sensitive and defective in spectrin tetramer formation, and that cleave abnormally with proteases. Molecular analysis often demonstrate point mutations or small deletions in the α- or β-spectrin genes that interfere with tetramer formation. A low-expression α-spectrin allele, α^{LELY} spectrin, is found at a high frequency in most populations. When α^{LELY} spectrin is coinherited in trans to an HE α-spectrin allele, it markedly aggravates the clinical severity of the disease, explaining the sporadic occurrence of clinically severe HPP patients in common HE families. Other HE/HPP patients have deficient or abnormal protein 4.1 that weakens the skeleton protein meshwork. A small number of patients with very mild HE have glycophorin C deficiency.**
4. **Hereditary spherocytosis (HS) is a congenital hemolytic anemia characterized by spheroidally shaped red cells with a reduced surface area-to-volume ratio, due to a progressive loss of the plasma membrane. These spherocytes are mechanically rigid, osmotically fragile, and selectively retained in the spleen and destroyed. Patients with the common, autosomal dominant form of HS typically have mild to moderate anemia, modest splenomegaly, and intermittent jaundice. Individuals with compensated hemolysis and no anemia are common, and occasionally severe, transfusion-dependent anemia occurs. Other complications associated with HS include neonatal jaundice, gallbladder disease, and aplastic crises. Approximately 25 percent of HS cases occur sporadically, about half of which are cases with *de novo* mutations and the other half, a recessive form of HS. Patients with severe HS respond well to splenectomy clinically, but the underlying red cell abnormalities persist.**
5. **Red blood cells from most HS patients are deficient in spectrin and ankyrin. In these patients clinical severity and response to splenectomy correlate well with the degree of spectrin deficiency. Red cell osmotic fragility is also proportional to spectrin content. In most cases the spectrin deficiency is secondary to ankyrin loss, because primary defects in ankyrin are the major cause of HS in Europeans and Americans (≈50 percent of cases), but mutations in the**

A list of standard abbreviations is located immediately preceding the index in each volume. Additional abbreviations used in this chapter include: 4.1 or 4.1R or *EPB41* for red cell form, 4.1N or *EPB41L1* for nervous system form, 4.1G or *EPB41L2* for general form, 4.1B or *EPB41L3* for brain specific form; AE1, 2 etc. = anion exchanger 1, 2, etc.; Ank, *Ank*, and *ANK* = ankyrin protein, mouse gene symbol, and human gene symbol, respectively; BFU-E = erythroid blast-forming units; CFU-E = erythroid colony forming units; 2,3-DPG = 2,3-diphosphoglycerate; ERM protein family = family of proteins including ezrin, radixin, moesin, merlin, and others; G-3-PD = glyceraldehyde 3-phosphate dehydrogenase; GP = glycophorin, including GPA, GPB, etc.; HE = hereditary elliptocytosis; HPP = hereditary pyropoikilocytosis; HS = hereditary spherocytosis; *ja* = mouse locus for jaundiced anemia; LELY = low expression Lyon, including LELY allele and α^{LELY}; MAGUKs = membrane-associated guanylate kinase homologues; MARCKs = myristoylated alanine-rich C kinase substrate proteins; *nb* = mouse locus for normoblastic anemia; OF = osmotic fragility; PGK = phosphoglycerate kinase; RTA = renal tubular acidosis; SAO = Southeast Asian ovalocytosis; *SLA4A1,2, etc.* = gene symbols for solute carrier family 4 members (anion exchangers); *Sph* = mouse locus for spherocytic anemia; *SPTA, SPTAN1* = gene symbols for αI and αII spectrin, respectively; *SPTB, SPTBN1, SPTBN2* = gene symbols for βI, βII, and βIII spectrin, respectively.

β-spectrin gene are also fairly common (≈25 percent). In both cases most of the mutations are private and differ in each family. They are often null mutations that produce an unstable or truncated peptide. Variable compensation occurs by the normal allele, in trans, which may account for the variable severity of similar null mutations. Mutations in α-spectrin are rare (≈5 percent), but they cause some of the more severe, recessive forms of HS and the most severe degrees of spectrin deficiency. About 30 percent of HS patients have normal red cell spectrin content. Most have combined band 3 and protein 4.2 deficiency due to dominant mutations in the band 3 gene (≈20 percent). The remainder have isolated 4.2 deficiency due to recessive mutations in the protein 4.2 gene. This is an uncommon mutation in western countries (≈5 percent) but is common, as is band 3 deficiency, in Japan.

During its 4-month life span, the average human red blood cell travels around the circulation about 500,000 times, a distance of several hundred miles. To complete this journey, it must be durable enough to withstand strong circulatory shearing forces and flexible enough to negotiate repetitively the narrow portals connecting the splenic cords and sinuses. The flexibility and durability of the red cell are largely determined by the shape, strength, and pliancy of its membrane, and these properties, in turn, are controlled by a submembranous meshwork of proteins termed the "red cell membrane skeleton." All of the major skeletal proteins have been cloned and characterized, and many of their interconnections have been defined. This chapter focuses on the structure of the normal membrane skeleton and on two groups of disorders that are caused by genetic alterations of this structure: hereditary elliptocytosis and hereditary spherocytosis.

Reviews are available covering various aspects of normal and abnormal red cell membrane structure[1–7] and selected specific subjects, including membrane lipids,[8] integral membrane proteins,[9–11] and disorders of red cell permeability.[12] The many brilliant reviews in the 1992–1993 issues of the *Seminars in Hematology*[13] are particularly outstanding and, though several years old now, are often the most authoritative source.

THE RED CELL MEMBRANE AND ITS SKELETON

General Aspects of Membrane Structure

The red cell membrane contains approximately equal parts of proteins and lipids (Table 183-1). Phospholipids and cholesterol predominate and are present in nearly equal proportions (cholesterol/phospholipid = 0.8). These and the other lipids are organized in an asymmetric planar bilayer. The glycolipids and most of the choline phospholipids (phosphatidylcholine and sphingomyelin) are located in the outer half of the bilayer, while phosphatidylinositols and the aminophospholipids (phosphatidylethanolamine and phosphatidylserine) are concentrated in the inner half (see Table 183-1).[8,15,16] The 10 to 12 major membrane proteins are conventionally separated and classified by sodium dodecyl sulfate polyacrylamide gel electrophoresis (SDS-PAGE) (Fig. 183-1) and fall into two general classes: integral and peripheral (Table 183-2).

Integral membrane proteins penetrate or traverse the lipid bilayer and interact with the hydrophobic lipid core. They characteristically have hydrophobic surfaces exposed at such contact points and tend to aggregate or denature in aqueous solution. Red cell band 3 (anion exchanger 1, or AE1), which forms the anion exchange channel, and the sialic acid-bearing glycophorins are the major examples of this class (see Table 183-2). These proteins have an external carbohydrate-bearing region, a membrane-spanning hydrophobic portion, and an internal, hydrophilic domain. Integral membrane proteins form the randomly distributed 8 to 10 nM intramembranous particles seen on freeze-cleave electron microscopy of red cell membranes.

Peripheral proteins are bound to the membrane via interactions with integral proteins or lipids or by posttranslational addition of lipid moieties (myristoylation, palmitoylation, prenylation, or addition of an inositol lipid side-chain). In the red cell, the major peripheral proteins are located on the cytoplasmic membrane

Table 183-1 Composition of Human Erythrocyte Membranes (Ghosts)

Component	Wt %	G/Ghost × 10^{13}	Number of Molecules/ Ghost × 10^6	% in Outer Half of Bilayer*	% in Inner Half of Bilayer*
Proteins and glycoproteins	55	5.7†	5‡		
Lipids					
Phospholipids§	28	3.0	250¶		
Sphingomyelin	6.8	0.73	60	80	20
Phosphatidylcholine	7.0	0.75	63	75	25
Phosphatidylethanolamine	7.4	0.79	65	20	80
Phosphatidylserine	4.3	0.46	40	0	100
Phosphatidylinositols	1.0	0.10	8	0	100
Phosphatidylinositol	0.34	0.036	3		
Phosphatidylinositol-4-P	0.22	0.024	2		
Phosphatidylinositol-4,5-PP	0.39	0.042	3		
Phosphatidic acid	1.0	0.10	8	Unknown	Unknown
Other	0.6	0.06	6	Unknown	Unknown
Cholesterol§	13	1.3	195	~50	~50
Glycolipids**	3	0.3	10	100	0
Free fatty acids††	1	0.1	20	Unknown	Unknown
	100	10.4	480		

* Based on data in references 14 to 16.
†An average of three reported values compiled in reference 17.
‡Calculated from the data in Table 183-2.
§Based on compiled data in reference 18.
¶Number of phospholipids per ghost based on an average molecular weight of 723 calculated from the average red cell phospholipid polar head group and fatty acid side chain composition (see reference 19).
**Based on data in reference 20.
††An average of two reported values compiled in reference 21.

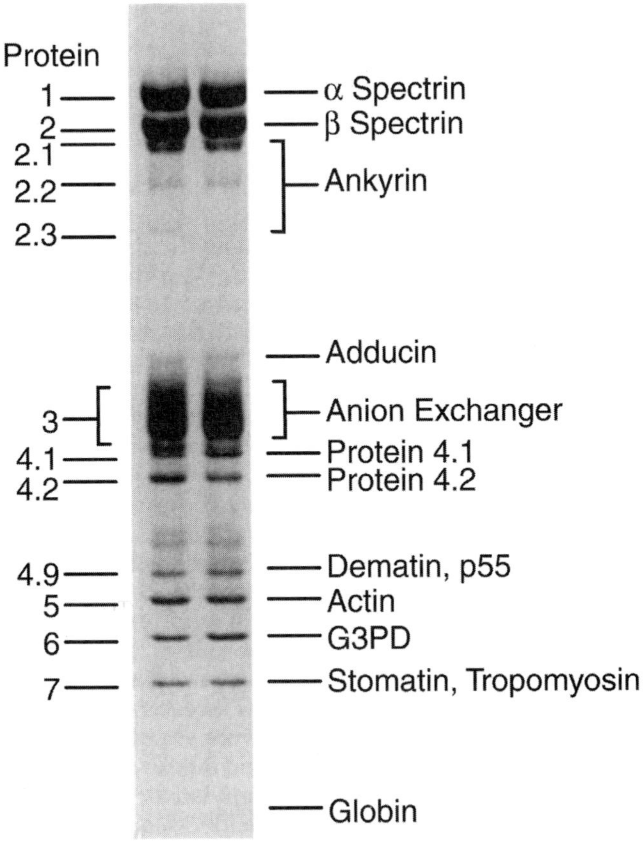

Fig. 183-1 Protein composition of the red blood cell membrane. The major components of the erythrocyte membrane are separated by sodium dodecyl sulfate-polyacrylamide gel electrophoresis (SDS-PAGE) and visualized by Coomassie blue staining. (*From Gallagher PG, Tse WT, Forget BG.*[22] *Used by permission.*)

surface and include enzymes such as glyceraldehyde 3-phosphate dehydrogenase (G-3-PD) and the structural proteins of the membrane skeleton, which will be discussed in detail below.

Glycophorins

The glycophorins are a class of transmembrane red cell glycoproteins that bear large amounts of sialic acid and several types of red cell antigens, as well as certain receptors (Fig. 183-2).[9,10,37] There are four types identified by gel electrophoresis, designated glycophorins A, B, C, and D (abbreviated GPA, GPB, GPC, and GPD), and a fifth type, glycophorin E (GPE), found by molecular cloning. GPB and GPE appear to have arisen by gene duplication from GPA (Fig. 183-2), and these types carry the MN and Ss blood group antigens. GPA was the first membrane protein for which the amino acid sequence was ascertained, yet the precise physiological role of GPA and GPB is unclear, because individuals lacking one or both of these genes exhibit no functional erythrocyte abnormalities.[9] Glycophorins C and D carry the Gerbich (Ge) antigens. GPD is a shortened form of GPC, lacking its N-terminal region (Fig. 183-2), and arises from the same mRNA as GPC by use of an alternative initiation codon.[10] There is a subset of patients with Ge-negative red cells, known as the Leach phenotype, who have elliptocytosis, but without significant hemolysis.[38–40] In patients with homozygous protein 4.1 deficiency and elliptocytosis, there is about 70 percent deficiency of glycophorin C, implying that protein 4.1 in some way regulates the glycophorin C content of the red cell (see sections on "Protein 4.1" and "p55" below).

Band 3 or Anion Exchanger 1 (AE1)

Band 3, the major red cell membrane protein ($\approx 1.2 \times 10^6$ molecules/cell), is the anion exchanger of the red cell membrane and the major anchorage site for the membrane skeleton. It is a 102-kDa transmembrane glycoprotein that exists in the membrane as a noncovalently linked dimer and tetramer. It migrates as a diffuse band on SDS gels due to heterogeneous glycosylation. The 911-amino acid protein is divided into two structural domains that mediate its two distinct biological functions.[11] The first 403 residues form the cytoplasmic domain and the last 508 residues form the 12 to 14 transmembrane segments of the membrane domain (Fig. 183-3).[41]

Membrane Domain. The 52-kDa membrane domain forms the physiologically important anion exchange channel that enables the red cell to exchange Cl^- for HCO_3^-. This allows much of the HCO_3^- produced in red cells by carbonic anhydrase to be carried in the plasma and increases CO_2 transport from the tissues to the lungs by about 60 percent. Exchange is extremely rapid ($T_{1/2} = 50$ msec) for Cl^- and HCO_3^-, the physiologic anions. The specificity of the channel is quite broad and larger anions such as sulfate, phosphate, pyruvate, and superoxide are also transported, though at much slower rates. It appears that anions move by a "ping-pong" mechanism in which an intracellular anion enters the transport channel and is translocated outwards and released, with the channel remaining in the outward conformation until an extracellular anion enters and triggers the reverse cycle.[42] The transmembrane segments of the protein presumably cluster together to form the transport channel. In fact, image analysis of negatively stained, two-dimensional crystals of band 3 dimers shows an apparent channel in the center, where the two monomers abut.[43] It is unclear whether the apparent morphologic channel is actually one or two functional channels. A variety of studies suggest that each monomer contains a functional anion channel.[44] If two channels exist, their location, at the interface of band 3 monomers, raises the possibility that two anions may be translocated simultaneously in opposite directions and/or that allosteric interactions between the subunits may regulate transport.

There is recent evidence that CO_2 may move through the channel, as well as HCO_3^-.[45] Interestingly, carbonic anhydrase II, which interconverts CO_2 and HCO_3^-, is bound to the C-terminus of band 3,[46] in the perfect position to perform this function.

A large number of potent and useful anion transport inhibitors are known, especially various stilbene disulfonates such as DIDS (4,4′-diisothiocyanostilbene-2,2′-disulfonate). These bind to two lysine residues, probably Lys 539 and Lys 851, on externally exposed portions of the protein in or near the entrance of the channel.[47]

A single carbohydrate side chain attached to the outer membrane surface at Asn 642 binds concanavalin A and bears the I/i blood group antigens. The extracellular portion of band 3 also carries the antigens of the Diego blood group system.[48]

Glycophorin A-Band 3 Interactions. There is persuasive evidence that glycophorin A (GPA) and band 3 are associated in the membrane: (1) The expression of the Wright blood group antigen, a receptor for *Plasmodium falciparum* malaria, requires the interaction between GPA and band 3, probably via its extracellular loop.[49] (2) A monoclonal antibody to the Wr^b blood group antigen immunoprecipitates both proteins.[50] (3) The coexpression of GPA in *Xenopus* oocytes enhances expression of band 3, by facilitating transport of band 3 from the endoplasmic reticulum to the cell surface.[51] And (4) GPA is absent from red cell membranes of mice that lack band 3.[52]

Cytoplasmic Domain. The 43-kDa N-terminal, cytoplasmic domain is a water soluble, 403-amino acid segment, with a pliant hinge near the center. The domain extends at high pH and contracts at low pH, presumably flexing about the hinge region.[53]

The cytoplasmic domain contains the binding sites for a large number of red cell proteins. Hemoglobin,[54] hemichromes,[55] and the glycolytic enzymes glyceraldehyde-3-phosphate dehydrogenase (G-3-PD),[56] phosphofructokinase,[57] phosphoglycerate kinase

Table 183-2 Major Erythrocyte Membrane Proteins

SDS Gel Band[a]	Protein	Molec. Mass (kDa) Gel	Cal[b]	Monomer Molecules/ Cell[c] × 10^3	Oligomeric State	Proportion[d] %	Peripheral or Integral	Chromosome Location	Genbank Accession	MIM	Associated Diseases[e]
1	α-Spectrin	240	281	242 ± 20	Heterodimer/tetramer/	14	P	1q21	M61877	182860 266140 270970	HE, HPP, HS
2	β-Spectrin	220	246	242 ± 20	oligomer	13	P	14q22-q23.2	J05500	182870	HS, HE, HPP
2.1[f]	Ankyrin[f]	210	206	124 ± 11[f]	Monomer	5[f]	P	8p11.2	X16609	182900	HS
2.9[g]	α-Adducin	103	81	~30	Heterodimer/tetramer	1	P	4p16.3	X58141	102680	EH
	β-Adducin	97	80	~30		1	P	2p13-p14	X58199	102681	?HS
3[g]	Band 3, AE1	90 to 100[h]	102[i]	~1200	Dimer or tetramer	26	I	17q21-q22	M27819	109270 179800	HS, SAO, RTA, HAc, ?CDAII
4.1	Protein 4.1	80 + 78[j]	66[k]	~200	Monomer	3	P	1p36.1	M14993	130500	HE
4.2	Protein 4.2	72	77	~250	?Dimer or trimer	4	P	15q15	M60298	177070	HS[l]
4.9[g]	Dematin[m]	48 + 52	43 + 45	~140	Trimer	1	P	8p21.1	L19713	125305	—
	p55	55	53	~80	?Dimer	1	P	Xq28	M64925	305360	—
5[f]	β-Actin	43	42	~500	Oligomer (~14)	5	P	7p12-p22	X00351	102630	—
	Tropomodulin	43	41	~30	Monomer		P	9q22.2-q22.3	M77016	190930	—
6	G3PD	35	36	~500	Tetramer	5[n]	P	12p13.1-13.31	X01677	138400	—
7[g]	Stomatin	31	32	—	—	4	I	9q34.1	X60067	133090	None
	Tropomyosin	27 + 29	—[o]	~70	Heterodimer[o]	< 1	P	—[o]	M19713	191010	—
8	Protein 8	23	—	~200	—	1-2	P	—	—		—
PAS-1[p]	Glycophorin A	36[q]	14[i]	~1000	Dimer	3[p]	I	4q28.2-q31.1	M12857	111300	None
PAS-2[p]	Glycophorin C	32[q]	14[i]	~150	—	0.3[p]	I	2q14-q21	M11802	110750	HE
PAS-3[p]	Glycophorin B	20[q]	8[i]	~200	?Dimer	0.4[p]	I	4q28.2-q31.1	J02982	111740	None
	Glycophorin D	23[q]	11[i]	~50	—	0.1[p]	I	2q14-q21	M11802	110750	HE
	Glycophorin E	—[s]	6[i]	—[s]	—[s]	—[s]	I	4q28.2-q31.1	M29610	138590	—

[a]Numbering system of Fairbanks et al. [17]. Bands 1 to 8 refer to gels stained with Coomassie blue. PAS-1 to PAS-3 refer to gels stained with PAS.
[b]Calculated from amino acid sequences.
[c]Based on an estimate of 5.7×10^{-13}g protein/ghost[17] and on the approximate proportion of each protein, estimated from densitometry of SDS gels. The data for spectrin and ankyrin were measured directly by radioimmunoassay,[23] as were the data for glycophorins.[24]
[d]Proteins 1 to 8 were estimated from published[3,17,25]and unpublished (Lux SE and John KM) data.
[e]Abbreviations: CDAII, congenital dyserythropoietic anemia, type II (or HEMPAS); EH, essential hypertension; HAc, hereditary acanthocytosis; HE, hereditary elliptocytosis; HPP, hereditary pyropoikilocytosis; HS, hereditary spherocytosis; RTA, renal tubular acidosis; SAO, Southeast Asian ovalocytosis.
[f]Protein 2.1 is full length ankyrin and is the major isoform. Other isoforms are evident on SDS gels, including band 2.2 = 195 kDa, band 2.3 = 175 kDa, and band 2.6 = 145 kDa. Band 2.2 is produced by alternate splicing. The origin of the other bands is unknown. The data shown are for ankyrin 2.1 except for the number of copies/cell and approximate proportion (wt%), which includes all isoforms.
[g]The α- and β-adducins lie at the high molecular weight end of SDS gel band 3, a region that is sometimes called band 2.9. Band 4.9 contains both dematin and p55; band 5 contains β-actin and tropomodulin; band 7 contains stomatin and tropomyosin.
[h]The protein runs as a broad band on SDS gels because of heterogeneous glycosylation.
[i]The calculated molecular weight does not include the contribution of the carbohydrate chains.
[j]Protein 4.1 is a doublet (4.1a and 4.1b) on SDS gels. Protein 4.1a is derived from 4.1b by slow deamidation.[26] Its proportion is a measure of red cell age.
[k]Protein 4.1 homologues are encoded by at least four genes[27,28] and exist in a very large number of isoforms.[29–32] The major erythroid gene product is listed here.
[l]Deficiency of protein 4.2 is associated with a variety of red cell morphologies, but spherocytes predominate.
[m]The 52-kDa isoform of dematin contains a 22 amino acid, N-terminal, ATP binding domain that 48 kDa dematin lacks.[33,34] The two proteins are derived from the same gene. They form a trimer containing two 48-kDa subunits and one 52-kDa subunit.[33]
[n]The amount of G3PD associated with the membrane varies from person to person (~3 to 6 wt%).
[o]Red cell tropomyosin is a heterodimer of 27- and 29-kDa subunits. There are about 70,000 copies of each chain/red cell. The calculated molecular weight and gene location are not given because, while it is clear that red cells express the hTM5 isoform,[35,36] it is not clear which of the four tropomyosin genes this represents.
[p]The glycophorins are visible only on PAS-stained gels.
[q]Molecular weights, including carbohydrate, estimated from mobilities on SDS gels.[9,10]
[r]Glycophorins C and D are synthesized from the same mRNA using different translational start sites.[10] The number of copies is for the total of glycophorins C and D.
[s]Glycophorin E mRNA has been identified but it is not certain that the mRNA is translated.

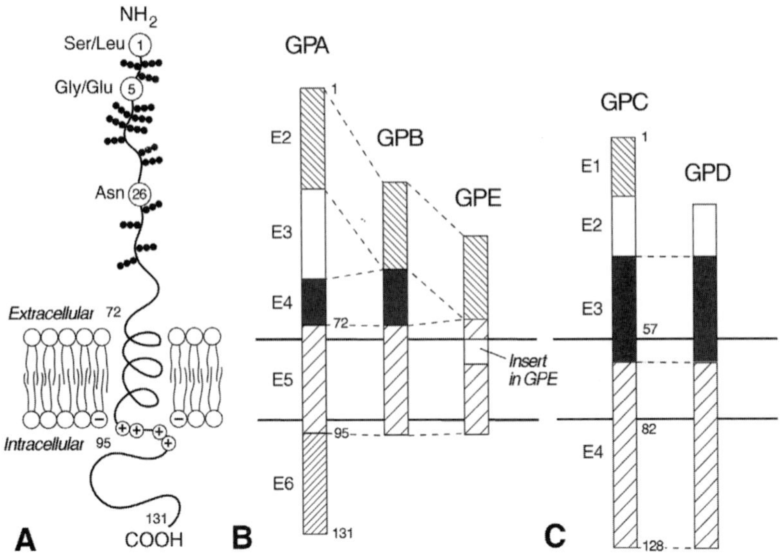

Fig. 183-2 Structure of red cell glycophorins. *A.* Organization of glycophorin (GP) A, the major red cell sialoglycoprotein. The external domain has 15 tetrasaccharides attached to serine or threonine residues and one complex oligosaccharide attached to asparagine 26. Residues 1 and 5 are Ser and Gly in blood group M red cells and Leu and Glu in blood group N cells. *B.* Schematic representation of the exons (E1–E6) that contribute to GPA, GPB, and GPE. Each box represents the portion of each protein encoded by a specific exon or insertion sequence. *C.* Exons that contribute to GPC and GPD. (*Adapted from Lux and Palek.*[4] *Used by permission.*)

(PGK),[58] and aldolase[57] bind to a very acidic segment located at the extreme N-terminus.[54] About 65 percent of G-3-PD, 50 percent of PGK, and 40 percent of aldolase are bound in the intact red cell.[56,57] Membrane attachment inhibits enzyme activity[59,60] and is regulated by substrates, cofactors, and inhibitors of the three enzymes, and by phosphorylation[61] of tyrosine 8. The observations suggest that the protein may be an important regulator of red cell glycolysis. In fact, mild oxidants, which stimulate tyrosine phosphorylation in intact red cells, elevate glycolytic rates.[62] Hemoglobin binds weakly ($K_d < 10^{-4}$ M);[63] nevertheless, because the concentration of hemoglobin is so high, roughly half of the band 3 molecules will have hemoglobin attached under physiological conditions.[63] Hemichromes, a partially denatured form of hemoglobin, bind much better[64] and copolymerize with band 3, forming an aggregate.[64]

Membrane Skeleton Binding. Three peripheral membrane proteins, ankyrin,[65] protein 4.1,[66,67] and protein 4.2,[68] also bind to the cytoplasmic domain of band 3 (Fig. 183-3). Usually one ankyrin molecule binds avidly ($K_d \approx 10^{-8}$ M) to each band 3 tetramer.[69] With this stoichiometry, approximately 30 to 40 percent of the band 3 molecules are attached to ankyrin and the membrane skeleton. The ankyrin binding site on band 3 has been partially characterized[70–73] and includes sequences from the proximal, middle, and distal portions of the cytoplasmic domain. This and other evidence indicates that the domain has a complex folded structure. Ankyrin binds only to band 3 tetramers; band 3 tetramers dissociate to dimers when ankyrin is removed or is genetically missing, and they reassociate when ankyrin is restored.[74,75] In vitro studies show that protein 4.1 binds to two sites—one near the N-terminus of band 3[66] and one near the start of the transmembrane domain[67] (Fig. 183-3)—and competes with ankyrin for attachment.[66] However, extraction of nb/nb RBCs, which lack ankyrin, with Triton X-100 removes virtually all of the band 3, indicating that either ankyrin is the only skeletal protein that binds to band 3 *in situ*, or that 4.1 links are too weak to withstand Triton treatment.[75]

Band 3 Oligomerization. Band 3 forms stable dimers, tetramers and higher oligomers in solutions of the nonionic detergent $C_{12}E_8$ (octaethylene glycol n-dodecyl monoether). These can be separated on sizing columns and quantitated.[76] Normally 70 percent is in the dimer form and 30 percent is tetramers and oligomers. Almost all of the latter is associated with the membrane skeleton,[76] and is immobile,[77] which fits with other evidence that ankyrin binds preferentially to band 3 tetramers.[74] The band 3 dimers are not directly bound to the membrane, but they are corralled by the skeleton meshwork in spaces about 110 nm in diameter. Individual dimers hop from corral to corral every 350 ms, on average.[77]

Related Anion Transporters. Red cell band 3 is a member of a family of homologous anion transport exchangers designated the SLA4A (solute carrier family 4A) gene family, or sometimes the AE (anion exchanger) gene family (reviewed in Alper[78]). SLC4A1 (or AE1) is the erythrocyte form. It is also expressed in the kidney; however, the N-terminal 66 amino acids are not included in the kidney isoform.[79] SLA4A2 (AE2) is widely distributed and is probably the general tissue anion antiporter. SLA4A3 (AE3) is restricted to the heart and the brain.

Defects. Defects in protein 3 are associated with hereditary spherocytosis,[80,81] Southeast Asian ovalocytosis,[82] distal renal tubular acidosis,[83,84] hereditary acanthocytosis,[85] and, possibly, CDAII (congenital dyserythropoietic anemia, type II or HEMPAS [hereditary erythroblast multinuclearity with positive acid serum test]).[86] It is remarkable that mutations in a single protein can produce so many different phenotypes.

The Membrane Skeleton

Operationally, the red cell membrane skeleton is the insoluble proteinaceous residue that remains after extraction of red cells[87] or their ghosts[88] with the nonionic detergent Triton X-100. It comprises 55 to 60 percent of the membrane protein mass and includes all the spectrin, ankyrin, actin, protein 4.1, dematin, adducin, p55, tropomyosin, tropomodulin, and a portion of band 3, protein 4.2, and stomatin (Fig. 183-1). Spectrin, actin, protein 4.1, and dematin form the core of the structure, because the skeleton retains its shape when other components are eluted with hypertonic KCl but disintegrates if spectrin or actin is removed.[87] The chromosomal locations of all the membrane skeletal proteins are now known and are listed in Table 183-2.

Spectrin

Erythrocyte spectrin ($\alpha I\beta I\Sigma 1$ spectrin) is the major red cell skeleton protein and accounts for about 50 to 75 percent of the skeletal mass.[87,88] It contains two large polypeptide chains that are structurally similar but functionally distinct: the α chain (280-kDa) and β chain (246-kDa).[89–91] The two chains are aligned side by side in an antiparallel arrangement with respect to their N-and C-terminal ends.[92] Electron microscopy (EM) shows spectrin to be a slender, twisted worm-like molecule that extends to a total length

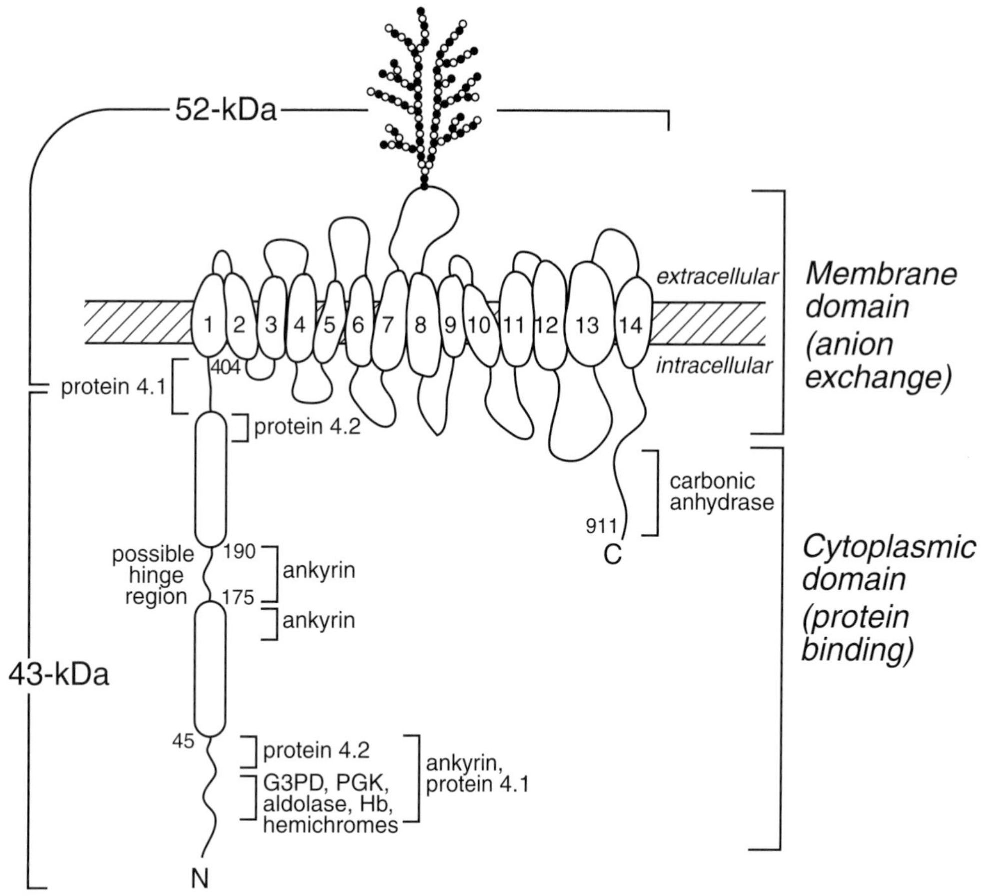

Fig. 183-3 Organizational model of band 3, the erythrocyte anion exchange protein. The protein is divided into two domains: a 43-kDa cytoplasmic domain, which contains binding sites for numerous cytoplasmic and membrane skeleton proteins, and a 52-kDa transmembrane domain that forms the anion exchange channel and provides a binding site for carbonic anhydrase. (*Adapted from Lux and Palek.*[4] *Used by permission.*)

of about 100 nM.[93] The protein is highly flexible and assumes a variety of conformations, an unusual property that may be critical for normal membrane pliancy.

Spectrin Genes. Humans have at least five spectrin genes. Four of these genes form plasma membrane spectrins:[94] αI Spectrin, which is only found in red cells; αII spectrin, which is present in all, or almost all cells except mature red cells; βI spectrin, which is limited to red cells (the S1 isoform), and to muscle and brain (the S2 isoform); and βII spectrin, which is widely distributed, like αII spectrin. Erythrocyte spectrin (spectrin$_R$) contains the αI and βIS1 chains. Muscle spectrin is believed to be αIIβIS2. Most other tissues contain αIIβII spectrin, which is also called fodrin, tissue spectrin, brain spectrin, or spectrin$_G$. Recently, a βIII spectrin was discovered, which is found on Golgi membranes and intracellular vesicles, but not on plasma membranes.[95] It is not yet known whether it forms heterodimers with an alpha spectrin or functions as an isolated chain.

Spectrin Structure. The αI spectrin gene (SPTA) is located on chromosome 1q22-q23, near the Duffy blood group; αII spectrin (SPTAN1) is on chromosome 9q34.1. βI spectrin (SPTB) is on chromosome 14q23-q24.2, βII spectrin (SPTBN1) is on chromosome 2p21,[94] and βIII spectrin (SPTBN2) is on chromosome 11q13.[95]

Each spectrin chain contains a series of 106-amino acid repeats linked end to end (Fig. 183-4). The primary sequence of each repeat shows extensive heptad (7-residue) symmetry, with conserved hydrophobic residues situated in the first and fourth position of each 7-residue motif (Fig. 183-5, panel *A*).[91,97,98] Each segment folds into three helices, designated helix A, B, and C, connected by short nonhelical portions. The helices fold back against each other to form a triple helical bundle (panel *B*),[96] which is stabilized by interaction of hydrophobic side-chains of conserved residues in each helix (panel *C*). Helices in adjacent repeat segments also interact with each other, which probably limits the range of motion between repeats and strengthens the spectrin chain (panel *D*). The start and end of the crystallographic spectrin repeat,[96] which begins with the A helix and ends with the C helix (ABC pattern), is different from the definition of a repeat in earlier publications, where each repeat began with the C helix (CAB pattern).[91,98]

α-Spectrin begins with an isolated, unpaired C helix followed by nine typical spectrin repeats, a tenth "repeat" that is actually a src homology (SH3) domain, and twelve more repeats (nos. 11 to 22) (Fig. 183-4). The SH3 domain presumably serves as an attachment site for a protein, like other SH3 domains, but the specific ligand has not been identified with certainty, although there is a recent candidate that belongs to a family of tyrosine kinase binding proteins.[99] The C-terminus of α-spectrin is a unique region that is related to the actin-binding protein, α-actinin. It contains two "EF hands"—structures that participate in calcium binding and regulate calcium action in other proteins, including α-actinin and probably fodrin (αIIβII spectrin).[100] However, there is no evidence that erythrocyte spectrin (αIβI spectrin) binds calcium or that its interactions with actin and protein 4.1 are regulated by calcium, so the EF hands may be vestigial.

β-Spectrin contains 17 conformational repeats (Fig. 183-4). The fifteenth and the first part of the sixteenth repeats are modified and form the binding site for ankyrin.[101] The N-terminal region (272 residues) contains the actin-binding site[102–104] and the binding site for protein 4.1.[103,105] It is homologous to other actin-binding proteins, including α-actinin, dystrophin, filamin, gelation factor (ABP 120), adducin, and fimbrin. The actin-binding site in gelation factor has been traced to a 27-amino acid sequence within

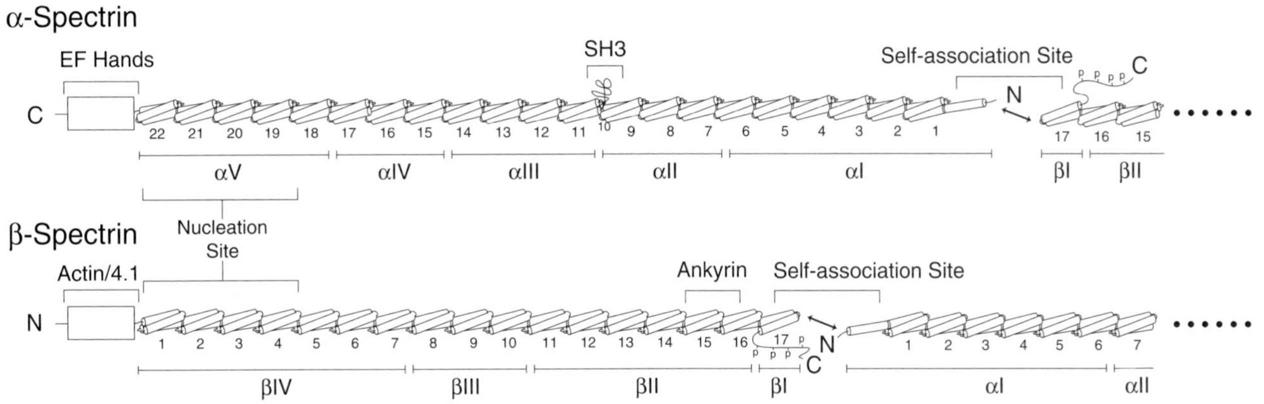

Fig. 183-4 Spectrin structural domains. The α- and β-spectrin chains have sequential, triple helical "spectrin repeats," numbered from the N-terminus of each chain. There are nonrepeat segments, including the actin/protein 4.1 binding sites (Actin/4.1), a potential calcium-binding region (EF Hands), and a Src-homology domain (SH3). Binding to ankyrin occurs at repeat 15 of the β chain (Ankyrin). The α and β chains align antiparallel to each other and form a heterodimer by interacting at a "nucleation site" near one end of each chain. Two heterodimers associate to form a heterotetramer by interaction at "self-association sites" at the C-terminus of the β chain and the N-terminus of the α chain. Each chain can be divided into large structural domains by limited tryptic digestion, denoted as the αI to αV domains in the α chain and the βI to βIV domains in the β chain. For clarity, only a portion of the heterodimer on the right is shown.

the conserved actin binding domain.[106] Presumably the same site is used by spectrin. The C-terminal end of erythrocyte β-spectrin contains a 52-amino acid extension that is phosphorylated (3 P-Ser, 1 P-Thr)[107] by a membrane-associated casein kinase I.[108] Increasing phosphorylation decreases membrane mechanical stability.[109]

Tryptic digestion of the spectrin peptides reveals a series of proteolytically resistant domains joined by protease-sensitive regions.[92,110] There are nine such domains, five on the α chain, designated αI through αV, and four on the β chain, βI through βIV (Fig. 183-4).[110,111] As described later in the chapter, many of the molecular defects in HE have been identified as abnormalities in spectrin domain maps after proteolytic digestion.

Spectrin Oligomerization. The α- and β-spectrin chains assemble into a heterodimer by a side-to-side interaction (see Fig. 183-4). The pairing of the two chains occurs in a zipper-like fashion, beginning with a defined nucleation site composed of four repeats from each chain at the end opposite the self-association site, repeats α19 to α22 and β1 to β4.[112] Two of the four α repeats and one of the four β repeats have an eight-residue insertion in the 106-amino acid repeat unit that are believed to be important. The model suggests that after the initial tight association of the complementary nucleation sites, a conformational change is propagated that promotes pairing of the rest of the two chains.[112] A common α-spectrin allele, α^{LELY}, produces α chains that lack one of the nucleation sites and do not form stable heterodimers. This allele is clinically important and will be discussed in detail later in the "Hereditary Elliptocytosis" section.

Spectrin heterodimers self-associate to form tetramers and higher oligomers by interacting in a head-to-head configuration.[93,113,114] Tetramers predominate in vivo,[115] probably because the association constant for formation of tetramers is substantially higher than for the larger species.[116] At low ionic strength and physiologic temperatures (37°C), spectrin dissociates into dimers,[114,116] while physiologic ionic strength and lower temperatures (25°C) favor tetramers. At 4°C the equilibrium is nearly kinetically frozen because of its high activation energy.[113] It is possible to extract spectrin from the membrane at such temperatures and examine its association state directly. Formation of spectrin tetramers and higher oligomers is essential in maintaining the mechanical strength of the membrane skeleton.[117]

The structure of the spectrin self-association site has been deciphered by analysis of mutant spectrins[118] and synthetic spectrin fragments,[119–121] and by proteolytic studies.[122] The isolated C helix at the N-terminus of α-spectrin combines with the isolated A and B helices at the C-terminus of β-spectrin to form a stable triple helical spectrin repeat and a head-to-head orientation of the spectrin molecules (Fig. 183-4). The isolated helices alone are not sufficient for this interaction. At least one adjacent triple-helical spectrin repeat must be present.[121] Mutations in α- or β-spectrin that disrupt this triple helical coil interaction interfere with the formation of spectrin tetramers and higher oligomers and weaken the membrane skeleton. As will be shown later, such defects are the most common cause of hereditary elliptocytosis (HE) and hereditary pyropoikilocytosis (HPP).

The C-terminal end of β-spectrin is phosphorylated[107] just beyond the site of self-association. Phosphorylation of β-spectrin has no effect on spectrin self-association in vitro,[113,123–125] but in vivo it markedly decreases membrane mechanical stability.[109]

The tail ends of spectrin tetramers and oligomers bind to short, double helical "protofilaments" of F-actin with the aid of protein 4.1, which greatly strengthens the interaction.[126] About six spectrins can be accommodated on each actin protofilament, which leads to the characteristic hexagonal network (Fig. 183-6) that is the basic framework of the membrane skeleton. The actin-protein 4.1 complexes, which reside at the nodal junctions of the network, are associated with multiple other proteins, including adducin, dematin, tropomyosin, tropomodulin, and p55. Each of these is discussed below.

It is thought that spectrin functions as a kind of spring—that in vivo the tetramers are coiled up with an end to end distance of about 76 nM.[128] It appears the spectrin molecules condense by twisting their α and β subunits around a common axis, and that the degree of condensation is regulated by varying the pitch and diameter of the twisted double strand.[129] The coiled spectrin tetramers can extend reversibly when the membrane is stretched but can not exceed their 200 nM contour length without rupturing.

Spectrin Synthesis. Spectrin is synthesized very early in erythroid development. It is plentiful in pronormoblasts[130] and is detectable in undifferentiated erythroleukemia cells, and possibly in immature committed erythroid stem cells, erythroid blast-forming units (BFU-E), and erythroid colony forming units (CFU-E).[131] As shown in chickens, mice, and humans, α-spectrin is normally synthesized in at least threefold excess relative to β-spectrin[132–134] and is degraded by a different, slower pathway.[135] The limited synthesis and more rapid degradation of β-spectrin suggests that its association with the membrane is the rate limiting step in spectrin assembly.[132,135] This difference in the rate of production of α- and β-spectrin is important in explaining

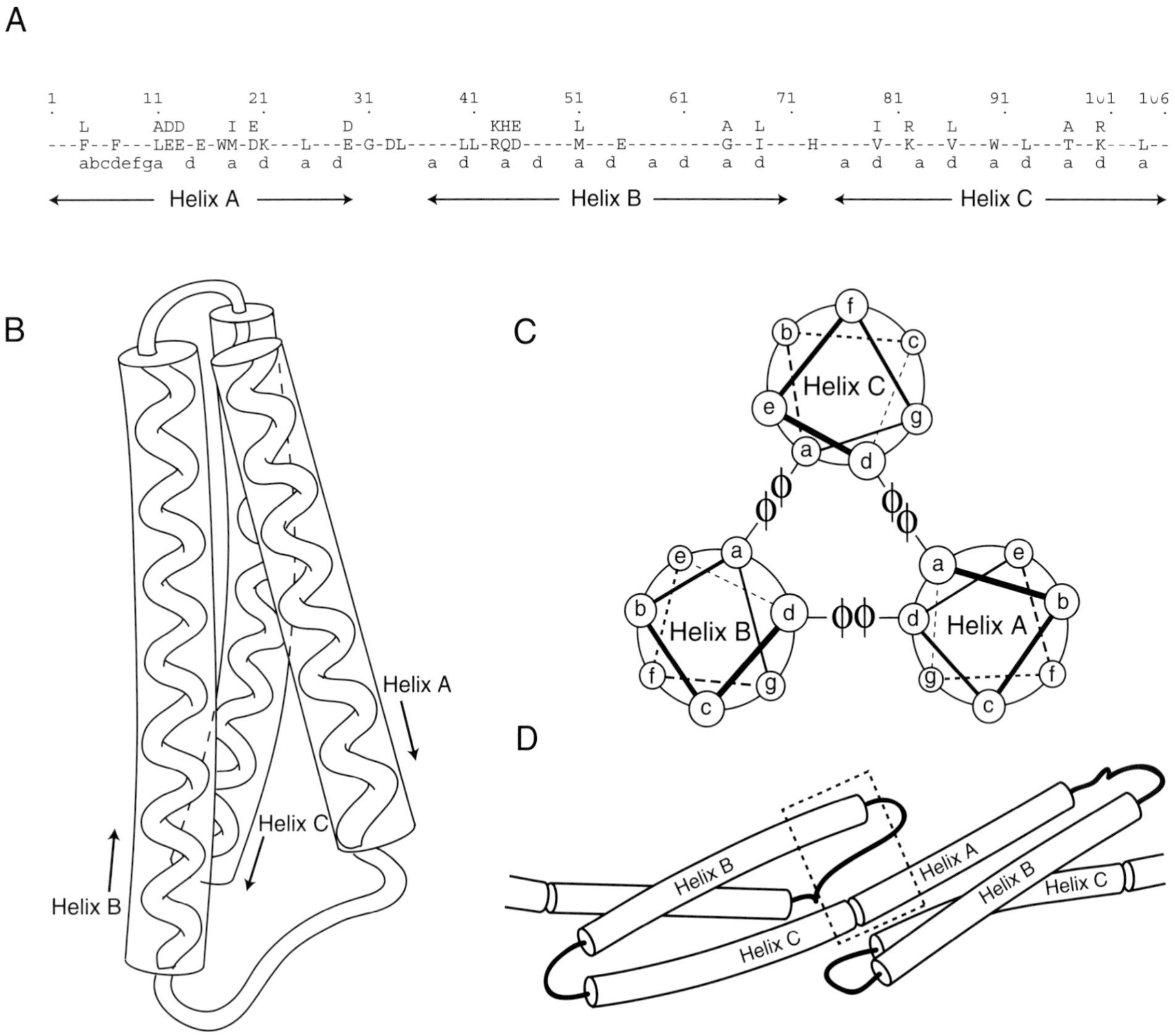

Fig. 183-5 Model of the spectrin repeat. *A.* Consensus sequence of a human erythrocyte spectrin repeat, typically 106 amino acids in length, with the less conserved residues marked by dashes. The primary structure features sequential heptad motifs (a-b-c-d-e-f-g), with hydrophobic residues situated at the first and fourth positions (a and d). The secondary structure consists of three α helices, termed A, B, and C. *B.* The α helices of each repeat fold back twice to form a triple helical, coiled-coil structure. The structure shown here is based on the crystal structure of a single repeat from Drosophila α-fodrin,[96] but other spectrin repeats are believed to have an essentially identical structure. *C.* Hydrophobic residues in positions a and d lie on one face of each helix and interact with each other (f-f) to stabilize the helical bundle. *D.* Helices C and A of two adjacent repeats connect to form one long helix and helix B of the proximal repeat overlaps helix A of the following repeat (dashed box). These interactions stabilize the connection between repeats and probably limit mobility at the repeat junction. (*From Lux and Palek.*[4] *Used by permission.*)

the molecular pathophysiology of red cell membrane disorders involving spectrin (see "Molecular Etiology").

Spectrin Defects. Mutations of spectrin are the major cause of hereditary elliptocytosis and are important in hereditary spherocytosis.

Ankyrin

Ankyrin is a 206-kDa protein that serves as the high affinity ($K_d \approx 10^{-7}$ M) binding site for the attachment of spectrin to the inner membrane surface.[136] Ankyrin binds to spectrin at repeat β15 near the end of the molecule involved in dimer-tetramer interactions (Fig. 183-4).[101] Judging from its relative abundance (see Table 183-2), each spectrin tetramer probably binds on average only one ankyrin molecule, even though two binding sites are available. This is probably because ankyrin binds about 10 times more avidly to spectrin tetramers than to spectrin dimers.[137] Ankyrin, in turn, binds with high affinity ($K_d \approx 10^{-7}$ to 10^{-8} M) to the cytoplasmic portion of band 3,[69,138] at sites near the N-terminus[71,72] and near the postulated hinge[70,73] (Fig. 183-3). Selective disruption of the ankyrin-band 3 interaction in intact red cells, at alkaline pH,[139] markedly decreases membrane stability, emphasizing the importance of the interaction.

Ank1 is detectable at the CFU-E stage of erythroid differentiation, after spectrin synthesis begins, but before band 3 is made.[140]

Ankyrin Structure and Function. Molecular cloning, combined with proteolysis and binding studies, reveals that ankyrin has three domains: an 89-kDa "membrane" domain (amino acids 2 to 827) that binds band 3 and other integral membrane proteins, a 62-kDa spectrin binding domain (amino acids 828 to 1382), and a 55-kDa "regulatory" domain (amino acids 1383 to 1881) (Fig. 183-7).[143,144]

Membrane Domain and Ankyrin Repeats. The 89-kDa membrane domain contains 24 tandem subunits of 33 amino acids, termed "ankyrin repeats." They are thought to be organized into four subdomains of six repeats each,[145] which form two distinct but

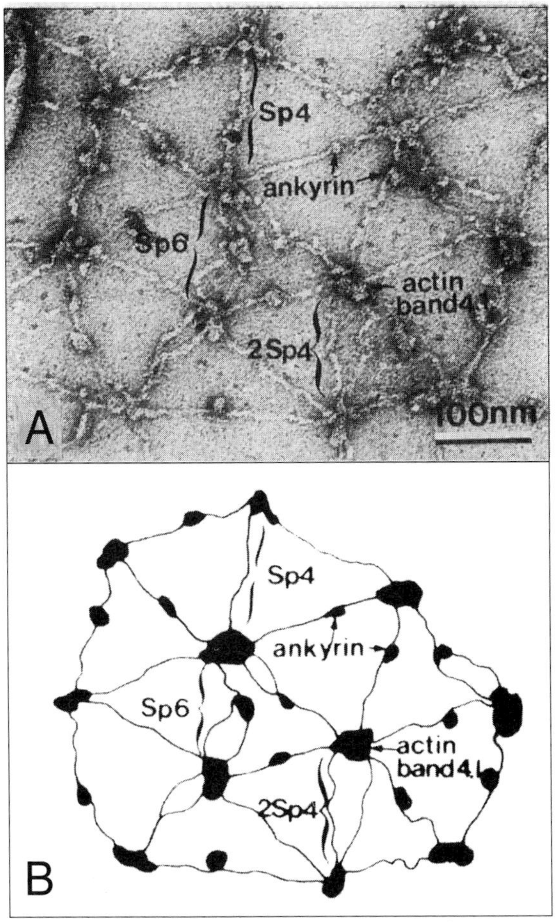

Fig. 183-6 Electron microscopy of the spectrin-based erythrocyte membrane skeleton. The negatively stained skeleton has been artificially expanded to reveal details of its structure. The electron micrograph *A.* and schematic diagram *B.* show the predominantly hexagonal organization of the skeleton. Spectrin tetramers (Sp4) and hexamers (Sp6) interact with each others at nodal junctional complexes, where short actin filaments, protein 4.1 and a variety of other proteins are found. (*From Palek and Sahr.*[127] *Used by permission.*)

cooperative binding sites for band 3.[146] One site utilizes repeats 7 to 12 (subdomain 2); the other uses repeats 13 to 24 (subdomains 3 and 4). Because band 3 is a dimer in the membrane, the presence of two sites on ankyrin allows ankyrin to bind band 3 into a tetramer, its state when associated with ankyrin.[76]

Similar ankyrin repeats are found in hundreds of proteins in all phyla, including bacteria and viruses. These proteins have little in common except the ability to interact with other proteins. The ankyrin repeat must have been an evolutionarily convenient solution to this recurring need. In several crystallized proteins the ankyrin repeats form a novel L-shaped structure consisting of a β hairpin (bottom of the letter L) followed by two α helices that pack side-to-side in an antiparallel fashion (stem of the L)[141,147–152] (Fig. 183-7). In erythrocyte ankyrin, the repeats start at the tip of the β hairpin.[142] The repeats line up side to side, like overlapping Ls, with the hairpins forming a β sheet that is perpendicular to the plane of the α helices. This nonglobular structure explains why the ankyrin repeat is such a versatile protein-binding partner (see below). The concave and convex surfaces of the connected repeats offer many possibilities for interactions. Because the crystallized proteins have only four to six repeats, it is not known how the 24 repeats of the ankyrins pack. As noted above, there is evidence, using fragments containing different combinations of repeats, that the repeats pack in four groups of six.[145,146] If so, there is nothing distinguishing about the boundaries of these groups to suggest that ankyrin folds or changes direction at these points. At the moment our best guess is that all 24 repeats resemble the repeats in the p53-binding protein (53BP) and the other crystallized ankyrin repeat-containing proteins, and that they align in tandem, like a twisted piano keyboard.

Spectrin Domain. The 62-kDa spectrin domain binds to spectrin. The binding site appears to involve regions at both the beginning[153] and middle[154] of the domain. The site in the middle is highly conserved and may be the principal point of attachment, while the nonconserved site at the beginning of the domain may provide specificity and allow ankyrins to discriminate among spectrin molecules.[154] The complementary binding site for ankyrin on spectrin is formed by spectrin repeat 15.[101] As noted earlier, there is considerable evidence that ankyrin and band 3 are the major sites of skeletal attachment in mature erythrocytes. However, nb/nb mice, which lack ankyrin 1,[155] have a normal membrane skeleton,[75] as do mice that lack band 3,[81] suggesting that spectrin can attach to the membrane by some other means during erythropoiesis.

Regulatory Domain. The 55-kDa regulatory domain contains numerous alternative splice sites. At least 15 ankyrin variants result[142] (Fig. 183-7) that differ in size, and, presumably, in function. The only well-studied example is ankyrin 2.2 ("protein 2.2" in Fig. 183-1). It lacks an acidic, 162-amino acid sequence that is present in full-sized ankyrin ("protein 2.1").[143] Ankyrin 2.2 is an activated ankyrin, with enhanced binding to band 3 and spectrin,[156] and the ability to bind to new sites on some other plasma membranes.[157] The 162-amino acid "repressor sequence," expressed as a separate protein, binds to ankyrin 2.2 and inhibits its interaction with band 3.[156] Muscle cells contain small (20 to 26-kDa) "ankyrins" composed of a unique hydrophobic sequence attached to the C-terminal end of the regulatory domain. They appear to be inserted into the sarcoplasmic reticulum membrane. Their function is unknown.[158,159] The regulatory domain of all ankyrins (see below) also contains a region that is homologous to the death domains of proteins involved in apoptosis signaling.[160] It is not known whether ankyrins are involved in this pathway.

Other Ankyrins. There is a family of ankyrins, each encoded by a different gene.[2] They include the erythroid type, designated ankyrin 1 or ankyrin$_R$ (gene symbol, *ANK1*), which is also found in muscle, cerebellum, macrophages, and endothelial cells; a neural protein, called ankyrin 2 or ankyrin$_B$ (*ANK2*) that is localized to neuronal cell bodies, dendrites, and glial cells;[161,162] and a broadly distributed ankyrin, termed ankyrin 3 or ankyrin$_G$ (*ANK3*),[163,164] which is found in most epithelia, axons, postsynaptic membranes at the neuromuscular junction, lymphocytes, megakaryocytes, and muscle cells. Ankyrins 1 and 2 are limited to plasma membranes, but isoforms of ankyrin 3 that lack all or part of the membrane domain localize to intracellular organelles, such as the Golgi apparatus (ankyrin G_{119})[165] and some lysosomes.[166] A 195-kDa Golgi ankyrin has also been described.[167] It is recognized by an antibody to erythrocyte ankyrin, but it is not clear that it derives from the ANK1 gene.

The 220-kDa forms of ankyrin 2 and ankyrin 3 have the same three-domain structure as ankyrin 1. The membrane and spectrin domains are highly conserved, suggesting similar binding functions, but the regulatory domains differ greatly. Ankyrins 2 and 3 also exist as 440-kDa isoforms, due to the insertion of a 220-kDa rod-like sequence between the spectrin and regulatory domains.[164,168] This extra domain targets these giant ankyrins to regions of neurite outgrowth (ankyrin 2) or to axon initial segments and the nodes of Ranvier (ankyrin 3).

Ankyrins bind to a large number of integral membrane proteins, besides band 3 (AE1). Examples include transporters such as anion exchanger 2 (AE2),[169] Na^+/K^+-ATPase,[170–172] the electrogenic and amiloride-sensitive Na^+ channels,[173,174] the Na^+/Ca^{2+} exchanger,[175] H^+/K^+-ATPase,[176] and the hepatic

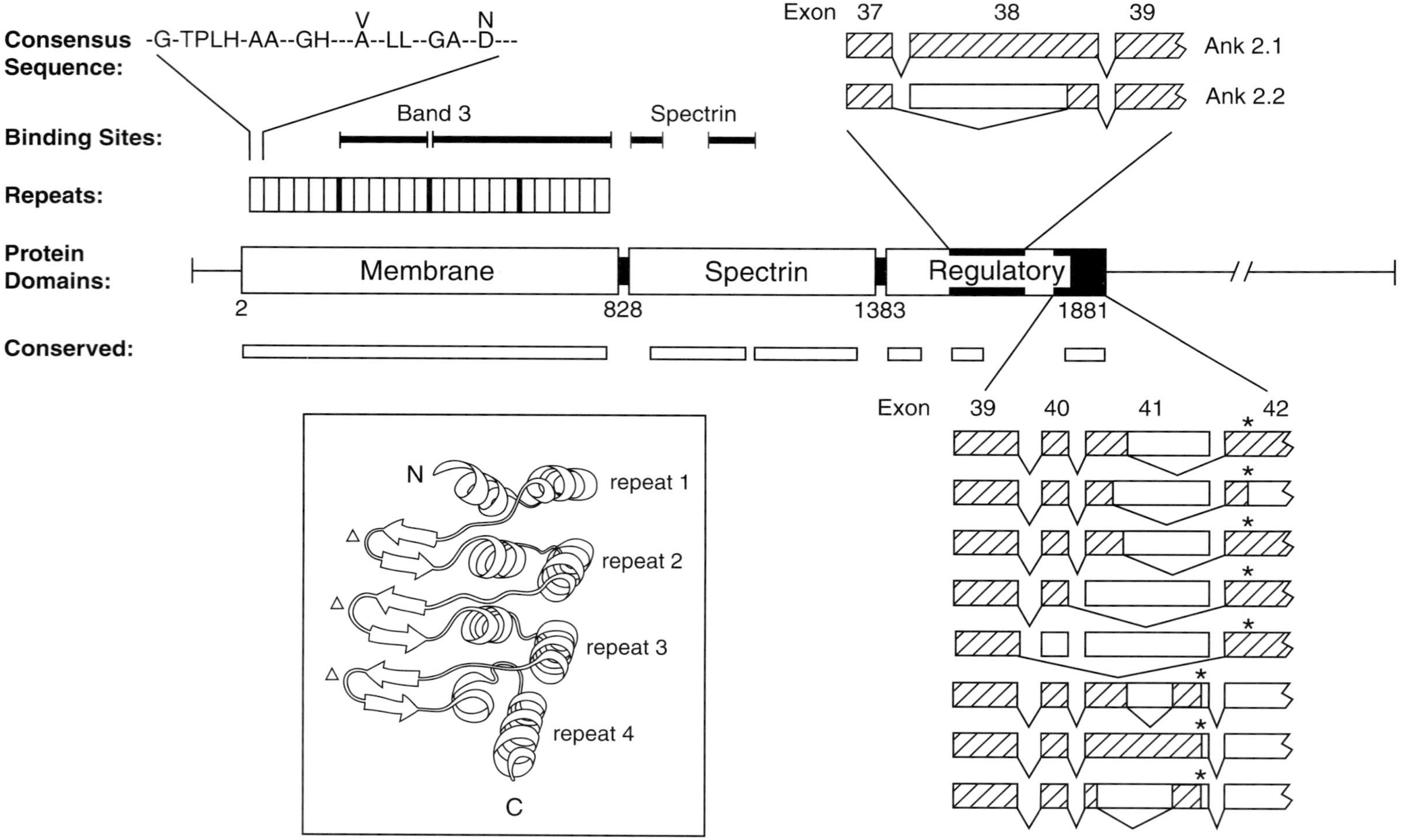

Fig. 183-7 Structure of erythrocyte ankyrin (Ank-1). The 89-kDa membrane domain contains 24 repeats of 33 amino acids, grouped in subdomains of six repeats. Their consensus sequence is shown at the top left in single letter amino acid code. Dashes indicate less conserved residues. The second six ankyrin repeats and the last 12 repeats each bind band 3. The 62-kDa spectrin domain contains the binding sites for spectrin. The 55-kDa regulatory domain is thought to modulate the binding functions of the other two domains. In the middle of this domain a highly acidic inhibitory region is spliced out of full-length ankyrin (ankyrin 2.1) to make ankyrin 2.2. At least eight isoforms of the last three exons exist. The last three isoforms contain a basic sequence that is common in brain Ank-1 but is rare in the red cell protein. In addition isoforms lacking exons 38 and 39, 36 through 39, and 36 through 41 have been detected. The asterisk indicates the location of the translation terminator codon. The inset shows a structural model of four consecutive ankyrin repeats, based on crystallographic data of the p53 binding protein 53BP2.[141] Each repeat forms an L-shaped structure. A β hairpin loop (arrows) makes up the bottom of the L and two antiparallel α helical coils form the vertical stem. The hairpin loops of neighboring repeats interact to create an antiparallel β sheet and the α helices interact to form helical bundles. The small triangles in the inset indicate the junction between adjacent repeats.[142] (*Modified from Lux and Palek.[4] Used by permission.*)

System A amino acid transporter;[177] receptors such as the inositol 1,4,5-triphosphate receptor,[178] and the ryanodine receptor;[179] and adhesive proteins such as CD44[180,181] and the neural cell adhesion molecules neurofascin, L1, NrCAM, NgCAM, and neuroglian.[182–185] For the most part, it is not clear which ankyrins bind which of these membrane proteins in vivo.

Ankyrin Defects. Defects in ankyrin 1 cause hereditary spherocytosis and, as will be discussed, are the most common cause of the disease.

Protein 4.2

Protein 4.2 (reviewed in Cohen[186]) is a 77-kDa erythroid-specific,[187] peripheral membrane protein that helps link the membrane skeleton to band 3 and the lipid bilayer. There are about 200,000 to 250,000 molecules of protein 4.2 per cell.

Protein 4.2 binds to band 3 at sites near the N-terminus of both proteins,[188–190] and may help attach band 3 to the membrane skeleton.[191,192] The interaction is important for the expression of both proteins. Protein 4.2 is absent from the red cells of mutant mice that lack band 3, despite normal 4.2 synthesis,[81] and human red cells that are partially deficient in band 3 are proportionally deficient in protein 4.2. Apparently, protein 4.2 is stabilized by binding to band 3 and is rapidly degraded in its absence. Conversely, band 3 is partially deficient ($\approx$30 percent) in mice that lack protein 4.2,[193,194] suggesting that protein 4.2 may facilitate band 3 synthesis or transport to the membrane.

Protein 4.2 probably also binds to ankyrin.[195] It has been difficult to show that this interaction occurs *in situ*,[195] but in nb/nb mice, which lack red cell ankyrin (Ank1), and in patients with a deletion of one ANK1 gene, the amount of red cell 4.2 is reduced.[196,197]

Protein 4.2 is myristylated[198] and palmitoylated,[199] which suggests it also interacts directly with the lipid bilayer, and it has an ATP binding site,[34] whose function is unknown.

Protein 4.2 is homologous to transglutaminases but lacks transglutaminase activity.[200] The 4.2 gene[201] resembles transglutaminases in its intron-exon organization. Four isoforms exist due to alternative splicing of 90 bp and 234 bp exons in the N-terminal end of the protein. The respective proteins are 80-kDa (both exons present), 78-kDa (small exon absent), 71-kDa (large exon absent), and 69-kDa (both exons absent). The 78-kDa protein is the predominant species (97 percent) in normal red cells; isoforms lacking the 234 bp exon are rare.

In the mouse, protein 4.2 maps to chromosome 2 close to pallid, a pigment disorder with platelet storage pool deficiency.[202] Initial evidence suggested that pallid was caused by a mutation in protein 4.2,[202] and the name pallidin was suggested for 4.2, but recently a genetic cross has shown conclusively that the two loci are distinct.[203]

Absence of protein 4.2 is associated with hereditary spherocytosis or ovalostomatocytosis.

Protein 4.1

Protein 4.1 (reviewed in Conboy[29]) is a core skeletal component that interacts with spectrin and actin, and with proteins in the overlying lipid bilayer. There are about 200,000 copies per red cell (Table 183-2). It is also called protein 4.1R to indicate its red cell origins and to distinguish it from other 4.1 homologues, 4.1N, 4.1G, and 4.1B, described below. The 4.1R (EPB41) gene was originally localized to chromosome 1p33-p34.2[204] but has recently been reassigned to 1p36.1.[205]

Alternate Splicing of Protein 4.1. The large (>200-kb), complex gene contains at least 24 exons, including 13 alternatively spliced exons.[29,30,32,206] This leads to a remarkably diverse collection of 4.1 isoforms (Fig. 183-8) in erythroid and nonerythroid cells, each containing different peptide cassettes or "motifs."[29–32]

An upstream 17-bp sequence located at the 5′ end of exon 2 contains an in-frame ATG codon that is included in 4.1R isoforms produced in most nonerythroid cells[29] (Fig. 183-8). The resulting protein contains extra 209 amino acids at the N-terminus and has an apparent molecular weight of 135-kDa on SDS gels. This sequence is omitted early in erythroid differentiation, and a downstream ATG is used instead, leading to the typical 80-kDa form of protein 4.1 observed in mature red cells[207,208] (Fig. 183-8). Curiously, the cloned protein[209] is only 66-kDa, which suggests it contains a large posttranslational substituent or binds SDS poorly or adopts an unusual conformation in SDS.

Alternate splicing of exon 16 is triggered late in erythroid differentiation and inserts a 21-amino acid sequence into the 10-kb domain that is essential for spectrin-actin binding (see below).[210–212]

Protein 4.1 Structure. Red cell protein 4.1 contains four structural domains, defined by proteolysis.[213] They are aligned: NH_2-(30-kDa)-(16-kDa)-(10-kDa)-(22/24-kDa)-COOH (Fig. 183-8). The 30-kDa domain is conserved in other 4.1-like proteins (see below) and contains binding sites for calmodulin,[214] CD44,[215] glycophorin C,[24,216–219] band 3[66,67] and protein p55.[217–219] The 10-kDa domain binds myosin[220] as well as spectrin and actin. The 22/24-kDa domain contains two posttranslational modifications (Fig. 183-8). One is Asn 502,[26] which is gradually and spontaneously amidated as the red cell ages, converting protein 4.1b (apparent molecular weight of 78-kDa) to 4.1a (80-kDa). This change can occasionally be a useful measure of red cell age. The second modification is an O-linked monosaccharide, *N*-acetylglucosamine, which is found on "cytoplasmic" protein 4.1.[221] The function of this unusual alteration is unknown.

Spectrin-Actin-4.1 Interactions. Protein 4.1 binds to β-spectrin,[103] very near the actin-binding site[102,105] (Fig. 183-4) and greatly amplifies the otherwise weak spectrin-actin interaction.[126,222] This activity can be traced to the 10-kDa domain,[223] which is encoded by a 21-amino acid (aa) alternatively spliced exon (exon 16) and a constitutive exon (exon 17).[210–212] Microdissection of this region shows that the 21-aa sequence and residues 37 to 43 in the constitutive exon form the spectrin-binding site and straddle an actin-binding site located at the beginning of the constitutive sequence.[211,212] Other work confirms that protein 4.1 binds directly to F-actin.[224] The reaction is saturable at one molecule of 4.1 per actin monomer and is highly cooperative,[211,224] which means that the binding of one 4.1 molecule causes conformational changes in the actin filament that promote further 4.1 binding. Overall, the data suggest that protein 4.1 works by bridging spectrin and actin, although other mechanisms have not been excluded.

The interaction of protein 4.1 with spectrin and actin is blocked by protein kinase A phosphorylation, which labels residues in the 16-kDa (Ser 331) and 10-kDa (Ser 467) domains,[225] and by tyrosine kinase phosphorylation, which labels a site (Tyr 418) in the 10-kDa domain[226] (Fig. 183-8). The ternary complex also appears to be regulated by Ca^{2+} and calmodulin.[214,227] Calmodulin binds to protein 4.1 in a Ca^{2+}-independent manner but, once bound, the calmodulin-4.1 complex confers Ca^{2+}-sensitivity on spectrin-actin-4.1 binding.[214]

Protein 4.1 is necessary for normal membrane stability. Patients who lack protein 4.1 have marked hemolysis and very fragile membranes,[228] but normal membrane stability is restored when the ghosts are reconstituted with protein 4.1[229] or even with a fusion protein containing only 64 amino acids (the 21-amino acid spectrin-actin binding site plus the next 43 amino acids).[211]

Glycophorin C/D-4.1-p55 Interaction. Protein 4.1 associates with the cytoplasmic portions of both glycophorin A (GPA)[230] and glycophorins C and D (GPC/D) in vitro.[24,216–219]And both proteins are close enough to 4.1 on the membrane to be modified by a radioactive cleavable crosslinker attached to protein 4.1.[66] But there is considerable evidence that the interaction with GPC/D

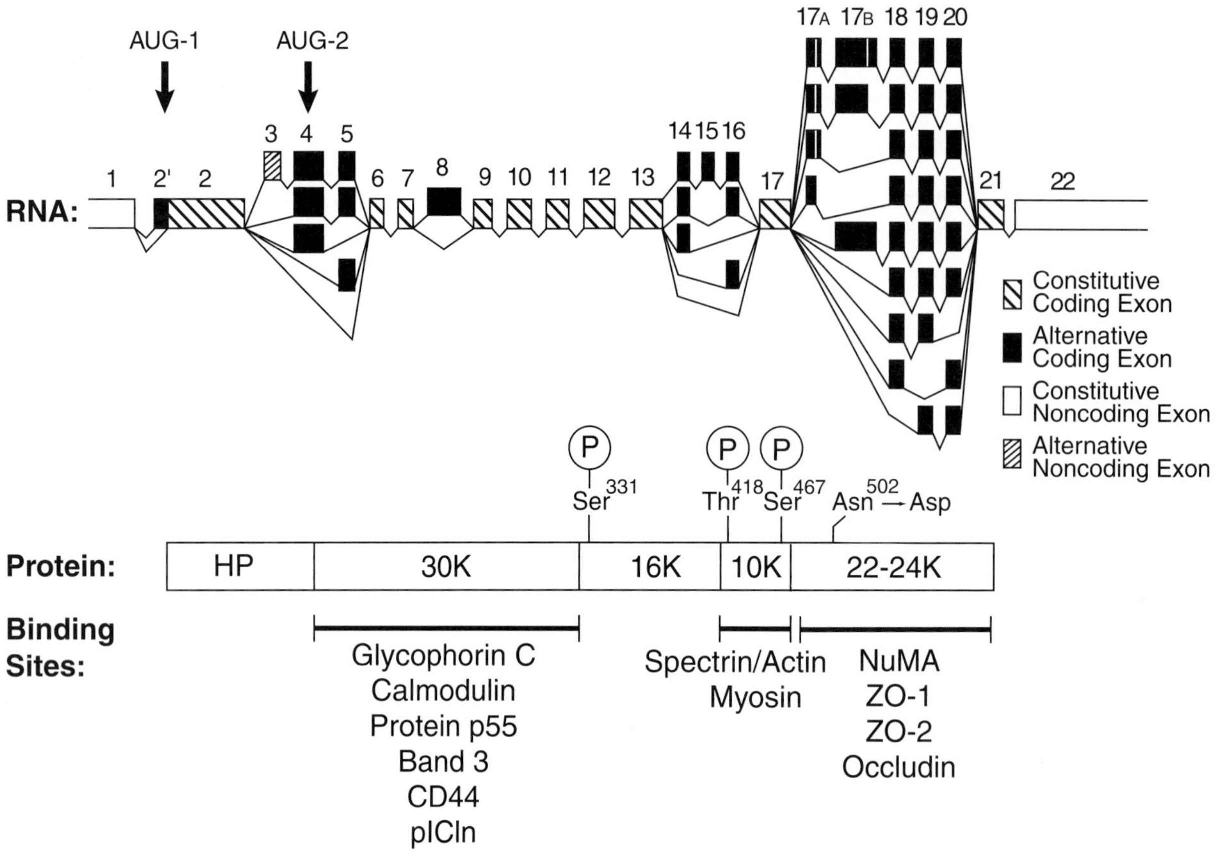

Fig. 183-8 Protein 4.1. ***Top.*** **Alternative splicing map of protein 4.1 mRNA. Erythrocyte 4.1 is translated from the downstream AUG and includes a 63-bp (21-amino acid) erythroid-specific sequence, contributed by exon 16, that is spliced into 4.1 transcripts late in erythropoiesis and is required for protein 4.1 to bind spectrin and actin. Many combinations of exons are expressed, though some are only observed in nonerythroid tissues.** ***Bottom.*** **Domain map of the "80-kDa" (erythroid) form of protein 4.1, indicating binding sites, phosphorylation sites, and the location of a C-terminal asparagine (Asn) that is deamidated in old red cells. HP, headpiece added to 4.1 when the upstream AUG is used. (*Modified from Lux and Palek.*[4] *Used by permission.*)**

is the physiologically important one:[24,37,216,231] (1) 4.1-deficient red cells are also deficient in GPC/D but not GPA;[231] (2) the residual GPC/D in 4.1-deficient cells is only loosely bound to the skeleton, but becomes tightly bound if the cells are reconstituted with protein 4.1;[231] (3) stripped, inside-out membranes vesicles from normal red cells bind more than five times as much protein 4.1 as vesicles from red cells that lack GPC/D;[24] (4) treatment of membrane vesicles with antibodies that block 4.1-binding sites on GPC/D reduces, by 85 percent, the ability of 4.1 to promote binding of [^{125}I]-spectrin and actin to the vesicles;[232] and (5) GPC/D-deficient red cells are elliptocytic and structurally unstable, while GPA-deficient cells are morphologically and mechanically normal.[37]

In addition, both protein 4.1 and GPC bind p55,[217–219,233] which may augment and/or regulate their interaction. Recent studies show that the ternary interactions are complex. GPC/D contains two sites for 4.1 in its cytoplasmic domain. Protein 4.1 binds directly to the proximal site, which is positively charged and located near the lipid bilayer.[218,219] The distal site, near the C-terminus of GPC/D, is where p55 binds.[218] Protein 4.1, in turn, binds to a positively charged region in the middle of p55.[219] It is not clear whether two molecules of 4.1 normally bind to GPC/D at one time, one directly and one through p55, or whether one molecule of 4.1 simultaneously binds to p55 on the distal site and independently to the proximal site.[218]

Band 3-4.1 Interaction. Protein 4.1 also binds to band 3.[218,234,235] The interaction is blocked by phosphorylation of 4.1 by protein kinase C but not by protein kinase A.[236] The binding site(s) is controversial. There is evidence for a site near the N-terminus of band 3[66] and for two sites containing positively charged motifs (LRRRY and IRRRY) near the start of the transmembrane domain.[67] In vitro, glycophorin C/D accounts for most of the 4.1 binding sites on stripped red cell membrane vesicles.[24,216,218] Probably only 20 percent[218] or less of the protein 4.1 is bound to band 3 on the membrane. However, band 4.1 interferes with the attachment of ankyrin to band 3,[66,235] and selective displacement of protein 4.1 from band 3 with charged peptides increases red cell membrane stability and decreases membranes deformability, apparently due to increased ankyrin binding.[235] Whether protein 4.1 modulates ankyrin binding in vivo is not known.

Other Interactions of Protein 4.1R. Protein 4.1R interacts with many other proteins, including myosin,[220] tubulin,[237] the neuronal membrane protein paranodin,[238] the immunophilin FKBP13,[239] the volume-regulated chloride channel pICln,[240] CD44,[215] the nuclear mitotic apparatus protein NuMA,[241] and three tight junction proteins (ZO-1, ZO-2, and occludin).[242]

The interaction with myosin is particularly interesting because the myosin-binding site lies within the 10-kDa domain that regulates spectrin-actin-4.1 complex formation, and because protein 4.1 inhibits the actin-activated Mg^{2+}-ATPase activity of myosin.[220] CD44 is also interesting because it is reasonably abundant in red cells, because it also binds ankyrin, and because in lymphocytes, where it serves as the hyaluronic acid receptor, its interaction with hyaluronic acid on the outside of the cell is regulated by ankyrin binding on the inside. In the red cell, 4.1 binding to CD44 is reduced by Ca^{2+} and calmodulin, and 4.1 interferes with ankyrin binding to CD44.[215]

Isoforms of protein 4.1R, containing an alternatively spliced nuclear localization signal,[215] attach to the nuclear matrix,[243,244] and colocalize with some proteins involved in mRNA splicing.[243] Protein 4.1 also associates with centrosomes, in resting cells, and is found in the mitotic spindle and the midbody during various parts of the cell cycle.[244,245] The functions of 4.1 in all these locations are unknown.

Finally, protein 4.1 binds phosphatidylserine[246] and probably polyphosphoinositides.[216] These negatively charged phospholipids are likely to account for some of the low-affinity binding of protein 4.1 to membranes and may have a regulatory function.

Protein 4.1 Superfamily. In addition to erythrocyte protein 4.1 (gene symbol, *EPB41*), three new protein 4.1 genes have recently been identified:[27] 4.1N (*EPB41L1*), a homologue that is strongly expressed in the nervous system; 4.1G (*EPB41L2*), a general form that is widely expressed;[28] and 4.1B, (*EPB41L3*), another brain-specific analogue. In addition, the 4.1 proteins are part of a superfamily of "ERM" proteins (reviewed in Tsukita and Yonemura[247]) that includes ezrin, radixin, moesin, merlin (or schwannomin), talin, coracle, and several tyrosine phosphatases (e.g., PTPH1, PTPMEG). They share homology to the N-terminal (30-kDa) domain. Merlin, one of the most interesting family members, is the gene responsible for neurofibromatosis, type 2, and is absent in virtually all schwannomas and many meningiomas and ependymomas. It is a tumor suppressor protein that binds to the C-terminal end of βII spectrin (fodrin)[248] and regulates cell growth[249] and the organization of the actin cytoskeleton. As noted earlier, it appears that the N- and C-terminal halves of the ERM proteins interact with, and inhibit each other (reviewed in Tsukita and Yonemura[247]). Perhaps protein 4.1 adopts a similar conformation.

Diseases. Absence of protein 4.1 results in hereditary elliptocytosis in humans and spherocytosis in the mouse.

Protein p55

Protein p55 is a heavily palmitoylated protein with a guanylate kinase-like domain that binds directly to both protein 4.1 and glycophorin C (GPC) to form a tight, ternary complex.[217,250] Patients who lack either protein 4.1 or GPC also lack p55.[251] p55 contains five domains: an N-terminal PDZ domain that binds to the C-terminus of GPC, an SH3 domain, a central 4.1B domain that binds to the 30-kDa domain of protein 4.1, a tyrosine phosphorylation region, and a C-terminal guanylate kinase domain.[252,253] The latter domain places p55 among the family of signaling proteins called MAGUKs (membrane-associated guanylate kinase homologues), which includes the Drosophila tumor suppressor protein Dlg (Drosophila discs large).[233] It is not clear whether p55 has any of the signaling functions that characterize other MAGUKs or whether it simply exists to stabilize the interaction between protein 4.1 and GPC. There are 80,000 copies of p55 per red cell, probably assembled into dimers.[250] This is less than the available binding sites for p55 on protein 4.1 and glycophorin C. It is not known whether 4.1-GPC/D complexes that contain p55 are functionally different from those that do not. The p55 gene is located on the long arm of the X chromosome, at Xq28, just beyond the factor VIII gene. It is expressed throughout erythroid differentiation and is widely expressed in nonerythroid tissues.

Actin

Red cell actin is very similar to other actins, both structurally[254] and functionally.[255] It is the β type,[25] a subtype that is found in a variety of other nonmuscle cells. Unlike the actin in other cells, red cell actin appears to be organized as short, double helical F-actin filaments ("protofilaments") about 12 to 18 monomers long.[256] It appears that these short filaments are stabilized by their interactions with spectrin, protein 4.1, and tropomyosin, by capping of the slow growing or "pointed" end of actin by tropomodulin,[257] and by capping the fast growing, or "barbed" end by adducin.[258] Spectrin dimers bind to the side of actin filaments at a site near the tail end of the spectrin molecule[102] (Fig. 183-4). Spectrin tetramers are therefore bivalent and can crosslink actin filaments; however, binding is weak ($K_d \approx 10^{-3}$ M) and ineffectual in the absence of protein 4.1,[126] which binds both spectrin and actin[224] and crosslinks the two proteins. As discussed in the following paragraph, adducin may also facilitate spectrin-actin interactions.[259]

Adducin

Adducin is a heterodimer or heterotetramer containing α(81-kDa) and β (80-kDa) or α and γ (70-kDa) subunits.[259–261] The $\alpha_2\beta_2$ protein appears to be the major species in the erythrocyte. The subunits are homologous[260,261] and are divided into three domains:[260,262] an N-terminal globular "head" domain and a small linking peptide (the "neck") that both may be involved in oligomerization,[262,263] and a long, protease-sensitive C-terminal "tail" that binds spectrin, actin, and calmodulin.[262,264] The end of the tail is very positively charged and is similar to so-called MARCKS (myristoylated alanine-rich C kinase substrate proteins).

Actin Capping, Spectrin-Actin Interactions. Adducin appears at the proerythroblast stage, but is not stably incorporated into the membrane skeleton until later in erythroid development.[265] It binds to the barbed, or fast-growing, end of actin filaments and blocks filament extension.[258] This activity requires the intact protein and cannot be provided by either end alone. One adducin is probably sufficient because there are 30,000 adducins per cell or one per actin protofilament. Red cells contain capping protein, CapZ, the major barbed end capping protein in most cells, but it is confined to the cytoplasm and only binds to the membrane after adducin is removed.[266]

Adducin increases the binding of spectrin to actin,[259] like protein 4.1. However, unlike protein 4.1, adducin does not interact directly with spectrin in the absence of actin. The tails of both α- and β-adducin bind to the actin-binding domain at the N-terminus of β-spectrin, and to the second spectrin repeat.[267] The adducin-spectrin-actin complex fosters binding of a second spectrin, a reaction that is blocked by calmodulin.[259]

Phosphorylation. Both adducin subunits are phosphorylated by protein kinase C (PKC) and protein kinase A (PKA) on a single serine residue in the C-terminal MARCKS domain.[264] PKA also phosphorylates α-adducin at three sites in the neck domain. Phosphorylation of the C-terminal MARCKS site reduces spectrin-actin interactions,[264,268] and inhibits calmodulin binding. Calmodulin, in turn, slows phosphorylation of β-adducin by PKA and of both subunits by PKC.[264] In addition, Rho-associated kinase, which acts downstream of the GTPase Rho, phosphorylates α-adducin and promotes its interaction with actin.[269] These complex associations suggest that adducin is tightly regulated.

Adducin is widely expressed in nonerythroid tissues[260] and is concentrated at sites of cell-to-cell contact.[270] The protein assembles at these sites in response to extracellular calcium and dissociates after treatment of the cells with phorbol esters,[270] which stimulate phosphorylation of adducin by protein kinase C.[270] The data suggest that adducin allows local regulation of the membrane skeleton by calcium and protein kinase C and attachment of the skeleton to certain parts of the membrane, such as sites of cell contact, that require reinforcement.

Defects

Spherocytosis. β-Adducin has recently been knocked-out by gene targeting.[271] Interestingly, α-adducin levels are low, at least in red cells, suggesting that the α subunit is unstable in the absence of its companion. The mice are born alive and are fertile, but they have a mild hemolytic anemia characterized by loss of membrane surface and a mixture of spherocytes, rounded elliptocytes, and stomatocytes. The phenotype suggests that adducin stabilizes the lipid bilayer by some mechanism that needs to be better defined.

Essential Hypertension. Finally, there is evidence in rats that missense mutations in α-, β-, and γ-adducins are genetically linked to and probably responsible for a form of essential hypertension.[272,273] An amino acid change in α-adducin (G460W) is also linked to hypertension in some populations.[274] Humans who carry the mutant allele are 1.6 times more likely to be hypertensive, their blood pressure is more salt sensitive, and they are more likely to respond to chronic diuretic treatment.[274] The mechanism is unknown but may involve renal salt handling. Expression of rat adducin carrying the α- and β-adducin mutations in rat kidney epithelial cells alters actin polymerization and upregulates Na^+/K^+-ATPase activity.[275]

Other Actin-Associated Proteins

Dematin (Protein 4.9). Dematin is a 48-kDa core skeletal component (dematin[48]) that binds actin and bundles actin filaments into cables.[276] It is related to villin, an actin bundling protein in epithelia. The protein has two domains: an actin binding headpiece at the C-terminus and an N-terminal, rod-shaped tail.[277] A 52-kDa isoform (dematin[52]), derived from the same gene, has an additional 22-amino acid insert in the headpiece[33] that binds ATP.[34] The native protein is a trimer composed of two dematin[48] subunits and one dematin[52] held together by disulfide bonds.[33] It is phosphorylated by protein kinases A and C.[278] The cAMP-dependent phosphorylation abolishes actin bundling.[33] The dematin gene is located at 8p21.1[33] and is widely expressed.

Tropomyosin. Erythrocyte tropomyosin is a heterodimer of 27- and 29-kDa subunits that run on SDS gels in the region of band 7.[279,280] The red cell analogue, hTM5,[35,36] is similar to other nonmuscle tropomyosins by many criteria. There is one copy of erythrocyte tropomyosin for each six to eight actin monomers, which is just enough to cover all of the red cell actin protofilaments. The length of tropomyosin and the length of the protofilaments also correspond. This suggests a model in which each protofilament bears two tropomyosin molecules, one associated with each of the two filaments. The possible functions include stabilization of the short actin filament and conferring specificity to the site of spectrin interactions along the actin protofilaments.

Tropomodulin. Tropomodulin is a 41-kDa protein that binds to the N-terminal end of tropomyosin in a 2:1 molar ratio.[36,281] In erythrocytes, there are 30,000 copies per cell, suggesting that one associates with each actin filament. Evidence indicates that it associates with the pointed end of the filament and blocks growth at that end.[257] Tropomyosin amplifies this effect. Tropomodulin remains attached to the membrane when spectrin, actin, and tropomyosin are removed. Its binding site has not yet been identified.

Myosin. Red cells contain a nonmuscle myosin composed of two light chains (19-kDa and 25-kDa) associated with a 200-kDa heavy chain.[282] The protein forms bipolar filaments and has typical ATPase activities.[282] There are about 4300 myosin in adult red cells and 2.5 times as many in neonatal erythrocytes,[283] or about one myosin per 50 to 100 actin monomers. This may explain the greater motility of neonatal reticulocytes. As noted earlier, myosin, spectrin, and actin all bind near each other on protein 4.1, and protein 4.1 inhibits the actin-activated Mg^{2+}-ATPase activity of myosin.[220] It is hard to believe that this is just coincidental, but it may be that the implied regulatory system is more important in nonerythroid cells.

Caldesmon. Red cells also contain caldesmon,[284] a 71-kDa protein that, together with tropomyosin, has the ability to regulated the actin-activated myosin ATPase activity. There is one caldesmon for each tropomyosin in the red cell. The data suggest that actin-bound caldesmon might be the inhibitory component of a, so far incompletely characterized, contractile system in the erythrocyte.

Organization of the Membrane Skeleton

A model of spectrin and the membrane skeleton is shown in Fig. 183-9. Spectrin heterodimers are depicted as twisted, flexible polymers joined head to head to form heterotetramers and higher-order oligomers. The N-terminal end of the spectrin α chain and the C-terminal end of the spectrin β chain create the self-association site, as described earlier (see "Spectrin" above).

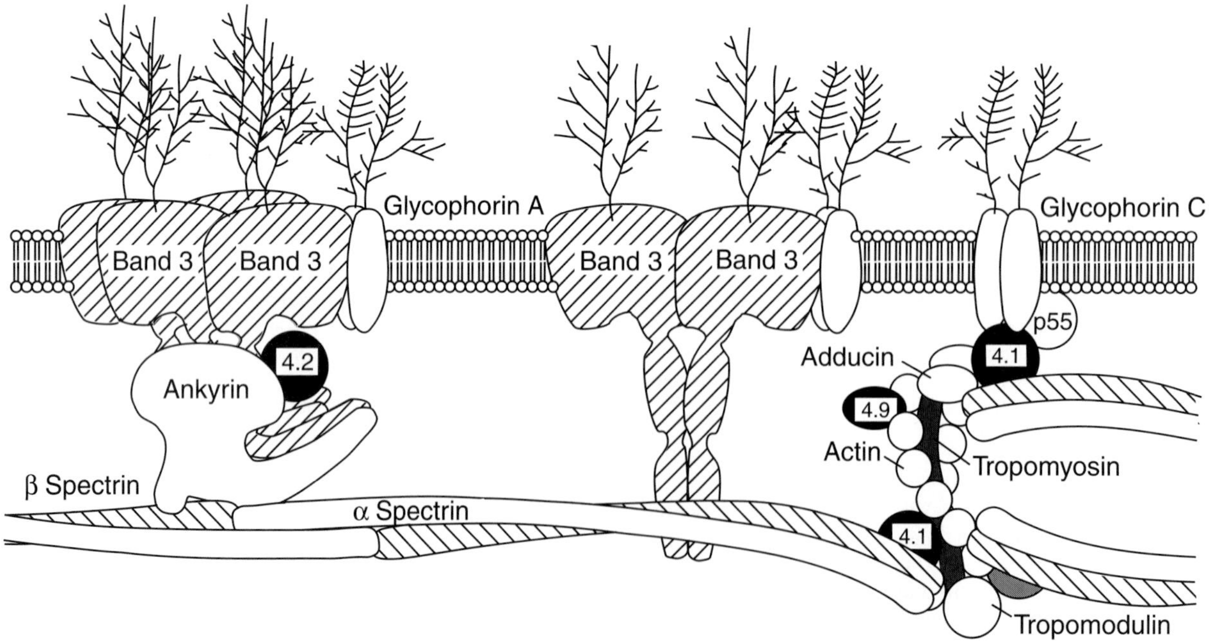

Fig. 183-9 Model of the red cell membrane skeleton. The relative position of the various proteins is correct, but the proteins and lipids are not drawn to scale. (*Modified from Lux and Palek.*[4] *Used by permission.*)

Spectrin molecules are linked into a two-dimensional network by interactions with a complex of actin protofilaments, protein 4.1, dematin, adducin, tropomyosin, and tropomodulin. These associations occur at the tail ends of the bifunctional spectrin tetramer. The predicted complexes are morphologically similar to isolated spectrin-actin-protein 4.1 complexes[285] and to structures observed *in situ* in normal ghosts.[256,286] They appear to serve as a molecular junction or branch point in skeletal construction. Individual spectrin tetramers and oligomers are attached to the overlying lipid bilayer through high affinity interactions with ankyrin and band 3 tetramers. About 30 percent of the band 3 molecules are anchored to the membrane skeleton. Interactions between protein 4.1 and either glycophorin C/D-p55 or band 3 provide secondary sites of attachment.

Complexes of F-actin crosslinked by spectrin molecules are visible by high-resolution, negative-stain electron microscopy (Fig. 183-6).[256,286] Dematin, adducin, and protein 4.1 colocalize with these complexes on immunoelectron microscopy.[1] Most of the complexes are joined by spectrin tetramers and hexamers. The resulting skeleton is a fairly regular hexagonal spectrin network (Fig. 183-6),[286] which implies that the junctional complexes must ordinarily accommodate only six spectrin molecules. The way this stoichiometry is achieved is not understood. Ankyrin and band 3-containing globular complexes are also visible in the electron micrographs (Fig. 183-6).[286] These attach to spectrin close to the site of self-association. If, as it appears, the skeleton is only one or two molecules thick on average, simple calculations show it must cover almost all of the inner membrane surface (140 μ^2 per red cell).

Modulation of Membrane Skeletal Structure

Polyanions. Physiological concentrations of organic polyanions such as 2,3-diphosphoglycerate (2,3-DPG) and ATP weaken and dissociate the membrane skeleton[287,288] and increase the lateral mobility of band 3 in ghosts.[289] At the molecular level 2,3-DPG binds to protein 4.1[290] and inhibits 4.1-actin interactions[224] and 4.1 binding to glycophorin C and band 3.[290] It also binds to band 3 and inhibits ankyrin binding.[290] At physiological concentrations of 2,3-DPG ($\approx$5.9 mM) there is about a 65 percent inhibition of 4.1-glycophorin C interactions and a 15 percent reduction of ankyrin-binding sites.[290] The importance of these effects in adult red cells in vivo is uncertain,[291] but the high levels of free 2,3-DPG in fetal red cells may explain why infants with hereditary elliptocytosis sometimes have augmented hemolysis in the neonatal period (see section on "HE in Infancy").[288]

Phosphorylation. Almost all of the red cell membrane skeletal proteins are phosphorylated by one or more protein kinases. These include casein kinases (spectrin, ankyrin, band 3, protein 4.1, and dematin); protein kinase A (spectrin, ankyrin, adducin, protein 4.1, and dematin); protein kinase C (adducin, protein 4.1, and dematin); tyrosine kinases (band 3 and protein 4.1); and Rho-associated kinase (α-adducin).[269,292]

In all cases except one, phosphorylation inhibits membrane protein interactions: (1) Ankyrin phosphorylation (casein kinase) abolishes the preference of ankyrin for spectrin tetramer[137,293] and decreases binding to band 3.[294] (2) Phosphorylation of protein 4.1 (several kinases) diminishes its binding to spectrin and its ability to promote spectrin-actin binding[225,226,295,296] and decreases its attachment to the membrane.[297] (3) Phosphorylation by protein kinase C also inhibits binding of protein 4.1 to band 3.[236] (4) Phosphorylation of adducin by protein kinases C or A reduces spectrin-actin interactions[264,268] and inhibits calmodulin binding. (5) Phosphorylation of protein 4.9 by PKA prevents actin bundling.[33] (6) Phosphorylation of Tyr 8 at the N-terminus of band 3 blocks the binding of glycolytic enzymes[61] and presumably hemoglobin, and results in increased glycolysis.[62] (7) Spectrin phosphorylation has no detectable effect on spectrin binding assays in vitro,[113,123–125] but it decreases membrane mechanical stability in vivo.[109] The one exception is Rho-associated kinase, which phosphorylates α-adducin, promoting its interaction with actin.[269]

Calcium and Calmodulin. There is good evidence that calmodulin modifies the membrane properties of the red cell.[227] Physiological concentrations of calmodulin, sealed in red cell ghosts, destabilize membranes in the presence, but not absence, of micromolar concentrations of Ca^{2+}. The effect may result from interactions of calmodulin with protein 4.1.[214] Submicromolar concentrations of calmodulin, even lower than those that exist in the red cell ($\approx$3 to 6 μM), block protein 4.1-induced gelation of actin in the presence of spectrin[214] The effect is Ca^{2+}-dependent. It begins at a Ca^{2+} concentration of 10^{-6} to 10^{-7} M, which is relatively low, but still higher than the free Ca^{2+} concentration in the erythrocyte (20 to 40 nM).

Calmodulin also binds to the spectrin β chain in a Ca^{2+}-dependent manner;[298] however the affinity of spectrin for calmodulin is not great and it is unclear whether this effect occurs at the concentrations of calmodulin that exist in erythrocytes.

β-Adducin also binds calmodulin ($K_d = 2.3 \times 10^{-7}$ M).[299] Adducin that is bound to spectrin and actin fosters the attachment of a second, neighboring spectrin. This reaction is blocked by calmodulin in the presence of Ca^{2+} ($> 10^{-7}$ M).[259] Calmodulin also slows phosphorylation of β-adducin by PKA and of both subunits by PKC.[264] The physiological consequences of these effects are unclear.

Functions of the Membrane Skeleton

Membrane Flexibility and Durability. Biochemical analyses of the red cell membrane suggest that its structural properties are determined almost entirely by the membrane skeleton. Historically, the evidence for this hypothesis comes from studies of four mouse mutants with very severe, inherited hemolytic anemias (see section on "Animal Models" under "Hereditary Spherocytosis" below). The red cells of these mice are extraordinarily fragile and spontaneously vesiculate in the circulation. Red cells from mice with a targeted deletion of band 3 have similar sensitivity.[81] Red cells from sph/sph mice, one of the spectrin-deficient mutants lack elasticity, show marked plastic deformation, and mechanically resemble lipid bilayers. Reconstitution of these mutant ghosts with normal spectrin restores membrane stability.[300] Numerous other observations attest to the structural importance of the skeleton. In isolated membranes vesiculation occurs when spectrin is extracted at low ionic strength.[301] Similarly, isolated skeletons become mechanically fragile when spectrin tetramers are converted to dimers by in vitro manipulations of temperature and ionic strength.[117] And, as shown below, hereditary elliptocytosis and pyropoikilocytosis is often due to α- or β-spectrin mutations that weaken spectrin self-association (see below). In such cells, the hexagonal skeletal lattice is disrupted,[302] usually in association with red cell fragmentation and poikilocytosis.

Red Cell Shape. In general, isolated membrane skeletons retain the shape of the ghosts from which they are derived.[303,304] This and other observations[305] confirm the shape-maintaining role of the skeleton. The red cell normally assumes a biconcave shape spontaneously and rapidly regains this shape if it is temporarily deformed. But if the distortion is maintained for some time, the cell will remain misshaped. This phenomenon, known as "plastic deformation," is probably due to realignment of dynamic skeletal interactions in response to the stress of distortion. Diminished skeletal interactions would presumably accelerate this process and foster poikilocytosis.

Integral Protein Distribution and Mobility. Perturbations that cause spectrin molecules to precipitate or aggregate on the inner membrane surface immobilize integral proteins in clusters directly over the spectrin aggregates.[306] Conversely, in congenital absence of spectrin in mice[307] or humans,[308] partial displacement of spectrin from the membrane by a proteolytic fragment of ankyrin,[139] or selective release of ankyrin from band 3 at high pH,[309] enhances the lateral diffusion of integral proteins in the bilayer plane. These experiments clearly show that the membrane skeleton normally restricts the mobility of some integral membrane proteins. This is at least partially due to band 3 binding to the spectrin-ankyrin complex, but only about 30 percent of the band 3 molecules participate in this interaction,[74,77] However, the unattached band 3 dimers are corralled by the spectrin strands and only hop from corral to corral very slowly, about three times per second, on average.[77]

Membrane Endocytosis and Fusion. In addition to its probable importance in cell-cell interactions, skeletal control of integral protein topography appears to help regulate membrane endocytosis and fusion. Studies have shown that endocytic vacuoles in red cells and ghosts are spectrin-depleted and arise from spectrin-free areas of the membrane, produced by rearrangement of the membrane skeleton.[310,311] It appears that a similar process occurs during membrane fusion. Early in the fusion process integral membrane proteins cluster to produce areas of protein-free lipid bilayer.[312] Apparently, fusion results when such bare areas contact each other if the lipids are in the proper configuration.[312] In addition, spectrin-deficient mouse red cells readily fuse with one another in the absence of any inducing agent,[300] a defect that is corrected by reconstituting the cells with normal mouse spectrin.[300] Thus, by immobilizing integral proteins in a diffuse distribution, the membrane skeleton probably protects the red cell from fusing with the many other cells it encounters in the circulation.

HEREDITARY ELLIPTOCYTOSIS

Hereditary elliptocytosis (HE) is a relatively common, clinically heterogeneous disorder characterized by the presence of a large number of elliptically shaped red cells in the peripheral blood. In the more severe forms of the disease, spherocytes or bizarre-shaped poikilocytes are also present, and sometimes these shapes predominate. Hereditary pyropoikilocytosis (HPP), which refers to the fragmented and irregularly shaped erythrocytes also seen in patients with severe cutaneous burns (*pyro-*, fire; *poikilo-*, variegated), is an example of the latter situation. Although HE and HPP were previously considered to be separate entities, emerging evidence clearly indicates that they can properly be considered different manifestations of the same clinical syndrome (HE/HPP). They will be discussed together in this section.

History

According to Lambrecht,[313] elliptocytosis was first observed by Göltz in Königsburg, Germany, in 1860, but no written report of this observation is known. The disease was first reported in 1904 by Dresbach, a physiologist at Ohio State University, in one of his histology students during a laboratory exercise in which the students were examining their own blood.[314] His brief report elicited some controversy as the student died soon thereafter, leading the prominent American physician Austin Flint to suggest that he had actually had incipient pernicious anemia.[315] Dresbach replied that the student died of acute rheumatic carditis and took his slides to Germany, where famous pathologists such as Ewig, Ehrlich, and Arneth supported his view that the red cell disorder was primary.[316] This was substantiated during the next two decades by the reports of Bishop,[317] Sydenstricker,[318] and Huck and Bigelow.[319] Hunter's demonstration of elliptocytosis in three generations of one family firmly established the hereditary nature of the disease.[320]

In the 1930s and early 1940s there was considerable debate about whether HE was a disease or simply a morphologic curiosity. In retrospect, this is surprising because numerous individuals with hemolytic HE were described during this interval[313,321–323] and some authors had clearly differentiated hemolytic and nonhemolytic forms.[313,323] In fact as early as 1928, van den Bergh even reported that anemia and jaundice cleared following splenectomy in one patient.[321] Early on, some confusion also existed in differentiating HE from sickle-cell anemia[324,325] and "hypochromic elliptocytosis" (probably thalassemia)[326] and later in differentiating hemolytic HE from hereditary spherocytosis.[327] These reports illustrate a point that will be emphasized later—namely, that HE, particularly its hemolytic variants, can sometimes be morphologically deceptive.

The recognition of HPP as a clinical entity came more recently. Zarkowsky and coworkers first described children with congenital hemolytic anemia who had fragmented and irregularly shaped erythrocytes that resembled red cells seen in patients with severe cutaneous burns.[328] They showed that these red cells were thermally unstable, and called them pyropoikilocytes. Other reports described patients presenting with a similar clinical picture but the thermal properties of their erythrocytes were not examined.[329] In a follow-up study, Zarkowsky noted that neonates with elliptocytosis and hemolysis also have heat-induced fragmentation of their red cells, prompting the author to suggest that elliptocytosis and pyropoikilocytosis may be caused by a similar defect in the red cell membrane.[330] This predication turned out to be true when the molecular defects of the two disorders were later elucidated.

Prevalence and Genetics

The prevalence of all forms of HE in the United States has been estimated to be between 1 in 2000 to 1 in 5000.[327,331] HE is observed in all racial and ethnic groups but is more prevalent in Africans, with an incidence as high as 1 percent in some groups.[332–334] The high frequency of the gene in these populations suggests the disease may confer some protection against malaria. There is some preliminary evidence supporting this idea,[335] but it has not been adequately tested. Southeast Asian ovalocytosis (SAO) is a distinct and homogeneous subgroup of elliptocytosis that is very prevalent in some parts of Asia and will be discussed separately.[336]

HE is generally inherited as an autosomal dominant trait. It is clinically variable in severity, reflecting a genetic heterogeneity at the molecular level. Patients who are homozygous or compound heterozygous for HE usually have a more severe phenotype with significant hemolysis and splenomegaly. The clinical picture may be indistinguishable from HPP.

Classical genetic studies show that an elliptocytosis locus (*EL1*) is closely linked to the Rh locus on chromosome 1p34-p36.[337,338] The best example of the Rh-linked disease is the large Dutch-American family originally described by Hunter and Geerdink.[320,338] This locus is now known to be the gene for protein 4.1.[209] A second locus (*EL2*) exists on chromosome 1 near the Duffy blood group locus (1q24),[339] and is assigned to the α-spectrin gene (1q22-q25). There may also be an X-linked elliptocytosis locus, which is discussed further below.[340]

Compared with HE, HPP is a much rarer disorder. It usually occurs sporadically, but not infrequently one of the parents or sibs of the proband can be shown to have typical mild elliptocytosis.[328,341,342] The pattern of inheritance of HPP in most cases cannot be explained by the transmission of a single genetic determinant, but can often be explained by the cosegregation of two genetic determinants, one of which may be silent in the carrier state. Recent research suggests that the HPP phenotype is produced by either homozygosity for certain HE genes, compound heterozygosity for two different HE alleles, or coinheritance of an HE mutation and a modifier, such as the α^{LELY} allele (see section "Molecular Etiology" below).[343]

Clinical Features

The HE/HPP syndrome can be divided into different categories on the basis of clinical severity and other characteristic features. These appellations denote clinical phenotypes and not specific molecular or genetic etiologies. Mutations in different membrane

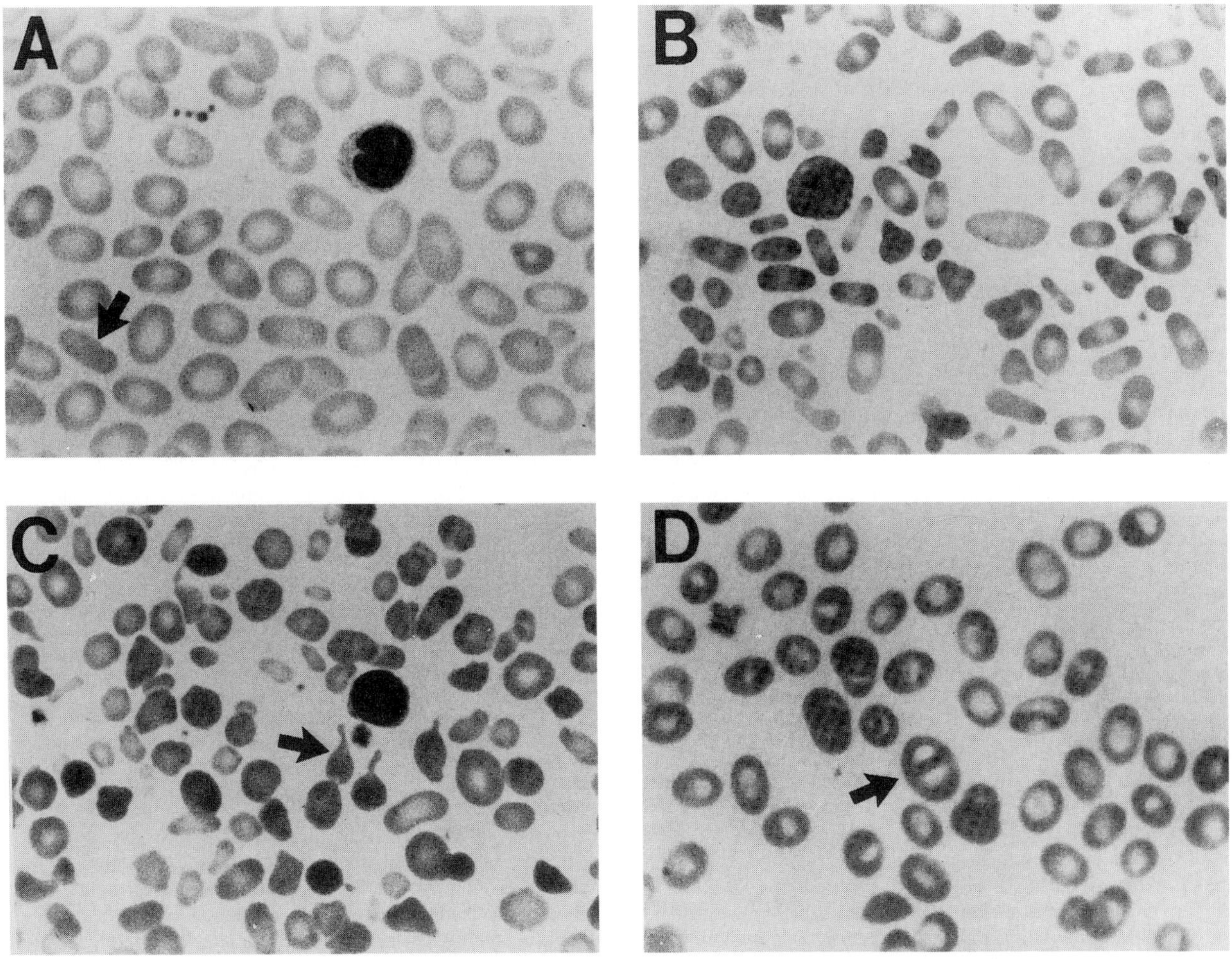

Fig. 183-10 Blood films of subjects with various form of HE/HPP. *A.* Simple heterozygote with mild common HE associated with elliptogenic spectrin mutation. Note predominant elliptocytosis with some rod-shaped cells (arrow) and virtual absence of poikilocytes. *B.* "Homozygous" common HE due to compound heterozygosity for two α-spectrin mutations. Both parents have common HE. There are many elliptocytes as well as numerous fragments and poikilocytes. *C.* HPP. The patient is a compound heterozygote for a mutant α-spectrin and a defect characterized by reduced synthesis of α-spectrin. Note prominent microspherocytosis, micropoikilocytosis, and fragmentation. Only a few elliptocytes are present. Some poikilocytes are in the process of budding (arrow). *D.* Southeast Asian ovalocytosis. The majority of cells are oval, some of them containing either a longitudinal slit or transverse ridge (arrow). (*From Palek and Jarolim.*[3] *Used by permission.*)

proteins may result in a similar clinical phenotype, suggesting that they disrupt red cell membrane integrity by a common mechanism.

Common HE. The common form of HE[327,344–347] is typically dominantly inherited and clinically mild. Affected individuals have no anemia and rarely have splenomegaly. Sometimes red cell survival is normal,[345,348] but more often there is very mild, compensated hemolysis with a slight reticulocytosis and a decreased haptoglobin level.[327,346,347] In these patients HE is little more than a morphologic curiosity. The peripheral blood smear shows prominent elliptocytosis (Fig. 183-10; panel *A*) with little red cell budding, fragmentation, or spherocytosis. Elliptocytes almost always exceed 30 percent of the red cells and sometimes approach 100 percent.[327,344,346] Very elongated elliptocytes (rod forms) are common (>10 percent). According to the older literature, normal individuals have less than 15 percent elliptocytes,[327,344,346] but in our experience this number is too high. We and others[349,350] find that the upper limit of normal is 2 to 5 percent elliptocytes. Somewhat higher proportions are seen in patients with anemia, particularly megaloblastic and hypochromic-microcytic anemias, but even in these individuals elliptocytes and rod forms do not exceed 35 percent and 15 percent, respectively.[344] Hence, the morphologic diagnosis of common HE is rarely difficult. This may not be true in the neonatal period. Early investigators noted that elliptocytes are infrequent in the cord blood of infants with common HE and become more prominent with time.[327,351] For example, Wyandt and coworkers detected only 11 percent elliptocytes at birth in one infant, whereas by 4 months of age, 80 percent of the cells were elliptical.[327] These observations, although few, suggest that the disease may be expressed differently in fetal red cells.

In many large kindreds with typical common HE, a minority (5 to 20 percent) of the patients have a more severe, uncompensated anemia punctuated by episodes of acute hemolysis.[352] Occasionally, acute hemolytic episodes are triggered by various stimuli, such as viral or bacterial infections,[347,352–354] malaria,[355,356] cirrhosis,[357] pregnancy,[347,358] or cobalamin (vitamin B12) deficiency.[359] In other cases, chronic uncompensated hemolysis exists in the absence of any detectable disease process and may be caused by a genetic modifying factor. One frequent factor is the low-expression α^{LELY} allele (see "Molecular Etiology" below).

HE in Infancy. Infants with common HE sometimes begin life with moderately severe hemolytic anemia, characterized by marked red cell budding, fragmentation, and poikilocytosis, and by neonatal jaundice.[288,330,360–362] As discussed above, elliptocytosis may not be prominent in infancy, and the disorder may be mistaken for a microangiopathic or oxidant-induced hemolytic anemia[361,362] or infantile pyknocytosis.[363] The correct diagnosis is easily made if the parents' smears are examined, because one of them is likely to have HE. In most cases, fragmentation and hemolysis decline with time, and the clinical picture of common HE emerges. This transition requires from 4 months to 2 years. The change in morphology often occurs somewhat faster than the decline in hemolysis.[330] Subsequently, the disease is clinically indistinguishable from typical common HE. In other cases, the hemolysis and red cell fragmentation persist and the patients may in fact have a more severe form of HE or HPP, which are discussed in the next section.

It is still not clear why some patients with common HE have a more severe clinical picture in the neonatal period. The dense poikilocytic red cells found in these infants are rich in hemoglobin F,[364] which suggests that the change in the course of the disease is due to the conversion from fetal to adult erythropoiesis. If so, interactions between the defective protein and other skeletal proteins, must differ in fetal and adult red cells. Mentzer has made the interesting suggestion that 2,3-DPG is the critical agent.[288] Free 2,3-DPG is elevated in fetal red cells because it is not bound by hemoglobin F. The free anion is known to weaken actin-4.1,[224] 4.1-GPC,[290] and to a lesser extent ankyrin-band 3 interactions.[290] 2,3-DPG increases the fragility of isolated ghosts at physiological concentrations,[288] although it is controversial whether it does so at physiological concentrations in intact red cells.[291] If so, this would certainly aggravate the underlying defect in spectrin self-association (discussed in "Laboratory Abnormalities" below).

Severe HE and HPP. A few patients with homozygous or compound heterozygous HE have been reported.[118,228,327,365–370] Most have had a very severe or even fatal[368] transfusion-dependent hemolytic anemia (Hemoglobin (Hb) = 2 to 5 g/dl) with marked fragmentation, poikilocytosis, spherocytosis, and elliptocytosis (Fig. 183-10; panel *B*), but in a few patients hemolysis was less rampant (Hb = 7 to 11 g/dl).[327,365] These differences reflect variations in the effect of the molecular defects that produce HE in the different families. Clinically, the disease is very similar to HPP. All treated patients have responded dramatically to splenectomy.

HPP is a rare, usually sporadic disease that presents in infancy or early childhood as a severe hemolytic anemia characterized by extreme poikilocytosis with budding red cells, fragments, spherocytes, elliptocytes, triangulocytes, and other bizarre-shaped cells (Fig. 183-10; panel *C*).[3,328,349,371–374] The morphology is similar to that observed in homozygous HE and HE with poikilocytosis in infancy. Family history may be negative but often there are family members who are affected with common HE. Hemolytic anemia may be severe, requiring acute or chronic transfusion. Long-term complications of severe anemia including growth retardation, frontal bossing, and early gallbladder disease are reported.[329] Laboratory tests, discussed further below, show very abnormal osmotic fragility tests, particularly after incubation,[228,328,329,342,370] and greatly elevated autohemolysis.[328,329,342] In severely affected patients, the MCV is very low (40- to 60 fl) because of the large number of fragmented red cells.

Another characteristic feature of these cells is their remarkable thermal sensitivity. Hereditary pyropoikilocytes fragment at 45 to 46°C (normal = 49°C) after short periods of heating (10 to 15 min).[328] With prolonged heating (> 6 h) they fragment even at body temperatures.[328] In addition, in patients with severe HE or HPP the red cells are spectrin-deficient (≈30 percent less than the normal quantity).[375] This associated spectrin deficiency may explain why these patients often have features seen in patients with HS, such as the presence of microspherocytes and an abnormal osmotic fragility. Also, like patients with HS, these patients often require splenectomy to control their symptoms. Following splenectomy, hemolysis is greatly lessened but not eliminated. Typically, the hemoglobin after splenectomy is 7.5 to 10 g/dl with 3 to 7 percent reticulocytes.

Spherocytic HE. This form of HE is a phenotypic hybrid of HE and HS. It is relatively uncommon, probably accounting for no more than 5 percent of all HE kindreds. Unlike common HE, almost all the affected patients have some hemolysis. This is usually mild to moderate and is often incompletely compensated. The elliptocytes are less prominent and less elongated than in common HE, and some spherocytes, microspherocytes, and microelliptocytes are usually present. Red cell morphology varies, even within the same family. Some family members may have relatively prominent spherocytes and as few as 10 to 25 percent elliptocytes, while in others elliptocytes predominate and spherocytes are rare.[376,377] This may cause diagnostic confusion initially, particularly if the propositus has few elliptocytes.

Spherocytic HE patients share many clinical features with HS patients (discussed further in "Hereditary Spherocytosis" below) The red cells in spherocytic HE are osmotically fragile, particularly after incubation.[376,378,379] Excessive mechanical fragility and increased autohemolysis that responds to glucose are also characteristic.[376,378,379] Gallbladder disease is common,[376,379] and aplastic crises are possible. The splenic pathology also mimics HS.[380,381] Splenic sequestration is evident,[376] red cells are conditioned during splenic passage, and hemolysis abates following splenectomy.[376,379,380]

HE with Dyserythropoiesis. In a small number of families with otherwise typical common HE, the sporadic occurrence of hemolysis and anemia is at least partially due to the development of dysplastic and ineffective erythropoiesis. All the reported patients[382,383] are from central and southern Italy, have somewhat less elongated red cells than is typical for common HE, and show the characteristic findings of ineffective erythropoiesis (high bilirubin, serum iron, and plasma iron turnover; relatively low reticulocyte count; and low incorporation of iron into circulating erythroid cells).[382,383] Their bone marrows are hyperplastic, with excessive intermediate erythroblasts and some dysplastic features, including asynchrony of nuclear-cytoplasmic maturation, binuclearity, and small numbers of ringed sideroblasts. Anemia and presumably erythroid dysplasia usually commence during adolescence or early adult life and advance gradually over a number of years. Because dysplasia persists after splenectomy, response to the operation is incomplete. The available data suggest that dysplasia and elliptocytosis cosegregate, as no individuals with dysplasia have been observed who did not also carry the elliptocytosis gene. If so, these families must represent a unique subtype of common HE. However, the numbers are small, and it is not clear that the nonelliptocytic members of the reported kindreds have been thoroughly examined.

Southeast Asian Ovalocytosis (SAO). This fascinating disease, also known as hereditary ovalocytosis, Melanesian elliptocytosis, or stomatocytic elliptocytosis, is a dominantly inherited condition observed in the aboriginal populations of Melanesia, Indonesia, Papua New Guinea, and the Philippines.[384–386] SAO is very common in Melanesia, particularly in lowland tribes, where 5 to 25 percent of the natives are affected. The affected individuals are often asymptomatic but may have mild compensated hemolysis.[387,388] Homozygosity is probably lethal.[389,390] Microscopy of blood films shows 20 to 50 percent round elliptocytes or "ovalocytes," some of which have one or more transverse bars that divide the central clear space, a morphological feature unique to this condition (Fig. 183-10; panel *D*).[384,391] In contrast to other forms of elliptocytosis, SAO is associated with increased rigidity and decreased deformability of the red cell membrane.[392,393] SAO cells are also heat-resistant, do not undergo drug-induced endocytosis, and strongly resist crenation.[394,395] Many blood group antigens are poorly expressed on the surface of these cells, and the cells are osmotically resistant.[396] The geographical distribution of SAO coincides with endemic malaria,[336] and there is a clear pattern of decreasing SAO prevalence in malaria patients with more severe disease,[390] suggesting that the condition conveys some protection against malaria.[397] This may be explained by the observation that the rigid SAO red cells are resistant to invasion by malaria parasites in vitro.[394,395,398] These properties all suggest that the intrinsic defect involves a component of the red cell membrane.

X-linked Elliptocytosis. One recent report describes a potential new elliptocytosis locus on the X chromosome.[340] Four members of an English family with a submicroscopic deletion of band q22 in the X chromosome have Alport syndrome due to deletion of the COL4A5 gene. The two affected male members also have mental retardation, dysmorphic facies with midface hypoplasia, and prominent elliptocytosis, but no anemia, reticulocytosis, or red cell membrane fragility. These individuals probably have a contiguous gene syndrome that involves a previously unknown elliptocytosis locus.

Laboratory Abnormalities

Isolated ghosts and membrane skeletons of erythrocytes from HE/HPP patients retain the elliptocytic or poikilocytic shape of the parent red cells.[304] The membrane skeletons are unstable when exposed to mechanical shaking[399] or shear stress,[400] suggesting that the primary defects of these disorders lie in the red cell membrane skeleton.

Red Cell Morphology and Indices. Morphological changes of erythrocytes associated with HE/HPP have been described above for each subgroup. In patients with severe disease and ongoing hemolysis, additional laboratory abnormalities can be found, including anemia, reticulocytosis, and hyperbilirubinemia. In these patients, a distinct subpopulation of microcytes with low MCV, or of hyperdense cells with high MCHC, may be evident in histograms of red cell profiles, as a result of red cell fragmentation.[401]

Osmotic Fragility Test. The osmotic fragility test, which measures the surface area-to-volume ratio of red cells, is discussed in more detail under "Hereditary Spherocytosis." Osmotic fragility is usually normal in common HE and abnormal in spherocytic HE or severe HE/HPP, reflecting a loss of erythrocyte membranes in the latter conditions.

Ektacytometry. The ektacytometer is a diffraction viscometer that can be used to assess cell deformability and membrane fragility in patients with hemolytic disorders.[400] It combines a concentric cylinder viscometer with a laser diffractometer (Fig. 183-11). The technique is highly sensitive and is an excellent tool to detect the usually dramatic changes in red cell membrane stability seen in patients with HE (Fig. 183-11, bottom).

Thermal Sensitivity of Red Cells and Spectrin. It has been known for at least 135 years that red cells, when heated to temperatures approaching 50°C for short periods, become unstable and fragment spontaneously.[402] This phenomenon is probably due to the denaturation of spectrin. Normal spectrin denatures after incubation for 10 min at 49°C and normal red cells fragment at the same temperature.[304,403] All patients with HPP and some patients with other forms of HE have thermally sensitive red cells. The thermal instability of the diseased red cells appears to be proportional to the clinical severity of the disorder. Hereditary pyropoikilocytes and red cells from infants with common HE and poikilocytosis fragment after 10 min at 44° to 46°C.[328,330] Red cells from some but not all patients with common HE fragment at 47° to 48°C.[304] Purified spectrin from these red cells is also heat-sensitive.[304,403] This suggests that an increased sensitivity of spectrin to heat denaturation may be related to the underlying cause of HE/HPP.

Abnormal Spectrin Oligomerization. In most cases of HE/HPP, there is a defect in oligomerization of spectrin, which may explain the red cell thermal instability. The ability of spectrin to form oligomers can be assessed in spectrin extracted from the membrane at 0°C. At this low temperature the formation and dissociation of spectrin tetramers and oligomers are greatly slowed, almost kinetically frozen.[113] If the 0°C extracts are carefully protected from warming during separation of spectrin dimers, tetramers, and oligomers (usually on nondenaturing polyacrylamide gels), the proportion of each spectrin species reflects its relative proportion on the membrane.[115] Thirty percent of patients with HE and all patients with HPP thus far tested have a defect in their ability to associate spectrin dimer to tetramers and higher-order oligomers (Fig. 183-12).[404–408] This suggests that the underlying defect of HE/HPP may lie in the spectrin heterodimer self-association site. Analysis of isolated spectrin peptides from these patients confirms that structural abnormalities in either α- or β-spectrin can frequently be found in this region.

Spectrin Peptide Structural Analysis. When spectrin is partially digested by trypsin at 0°C, and the resulting peptides are separated by two-dimensional isoelectric focusing-SDS gel electrophoresis, reproducible peptide maps are obtained.[92,110] As described in the section on "Spectrin," there are five trypsin-resistant domains on the α chain, designated αI through αV, and four on the β chain, designated βI through βIV. Fig. 183-13 shows an example of a normal spectrin domain map. Analysis of spectrin isolated from patients with HE/HPP by this method often shows abnormal peptide fragments that appear at variant positions when compared with the normal, due to the generation of new, abnormal tryptic cleavage sites in the mutant spectrin chains.

The majority of the α-spectrin variants are characterized by a decrease or absence of the normal 80-kDa αI domain and the appearance of smaller proteolytic fragments, including: (1) a new 78-kDa peptide ($\alpha^{I/78}$ variant),[410] (2) a new 74-kDa peptide ($\alpha^{I/74}$ variant),[406,411–414] (3) a new 65-kDa peptide ($\alpha^{I/65}$ variant),[370,414–416] (4) a new 61-kDa peptide ($\alpha^{I/61}$ variant),[417] (5) two new 46- and 17-kDa (or, in other reports, 50 and 21-kDa) peptides ($\alpha^{I/46}$ or $\alpha^{I/50}$ variant),[406,408,414,418] (6)another 50-kDa peptide with a more basic isoelectric point ($\alpha^{I/50}$ variant),[409] (7) a variant with two new peptides ($\alpha^{I/42-43}$ variant),[419] or (8) a new peptide of 36-kDa ($\alpha^{I/36}$ variant).[420]

There are also a few variants associated with other α-spectrin domains. Two αII domain variants have been associated with HE: the $\alpha^{II/31}$ variant (spectrin$_{JENDOUBA}$)[421] and the $\alpha^{II/21}$ variant (spectrin$_{ORAN}$).[422] These both cause asymptomatic HE in the heterozygous state. Another abnormality is a short α-spectrin chain (234 kDa).[423] Although spectrin containing this mutant chain also fails to properly self-associate, studies so far, surprisingly, suggest the primary defect may lie at the opposite end of the molecule, in the αIV domain.[423] Another variant, spectrin $\alpha^{V/41}$, is a very common spectrin polymorphism at the αIV-αV domain junction.[343] Even though this variant itself does not cause HE/HPP, it is closely linked to α^{LELY}, a low-expression α-spectrin allele that significantly affects the clinical manifestation of any HE/HPP allele inherited *in trans*.[343] This variant is discussed in detail under "Low-expression α-spectrin allele" below.

The molecular defects causing most of these variants are now known and are described in the section "Molecular Etiology." In most cases, the abnormal cleavage sites that produce the variant peptides are not the primary defects but are due to conformational changes of the spectrin chains associated with these defects. In general, there is an inverse relationship between the distance of the defect from the spectrin dimer self-association site and its associated clinical severity. The closer to the self-association site, the greater the functional defect, and the more severe the clinical illness. For example, $\alpha^{I/74}$ defects, which are located right at the spectrin dimer self-association site, produce severe disease with a greater proportion of spectrin dimers in heterozygotes, and life-threatening hemolysis in the homozygous state. In contrast, $\alpha^{I/65}$ defects, which are located further from the self-association site, are associated with milder hemolysis and a lesser defect in spectrin self-association. In the $\alpha^{II/21}$ variant, in which the defect

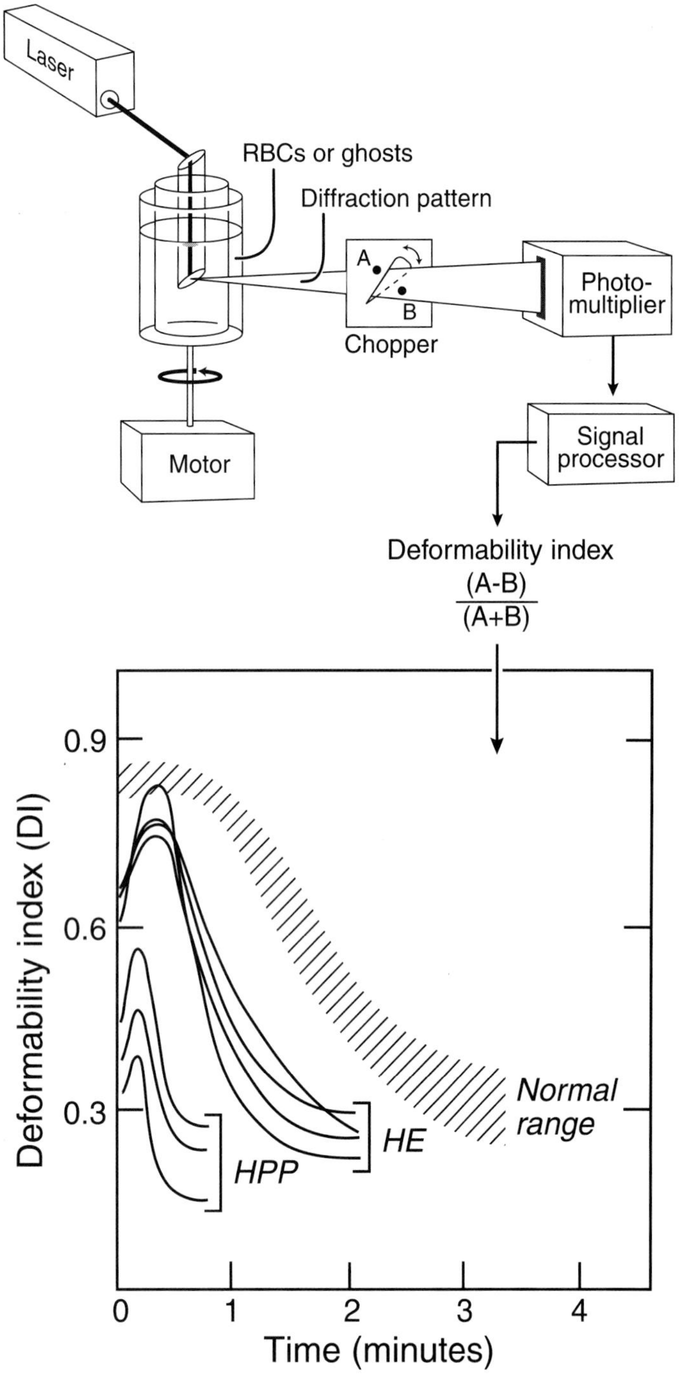

Fig. 183-11 ***Top.*** **Membrane fragility of HE/HPP red cells measured with the ektacytometer. The ektacytometer combines a concentric cylinder viscometer with a laser diffractometer. The outer cylinder of the viscometer is spun to produce a uniform shear stress on a sample of red cells or ghosts placed in between the cylinders. A laser beam diffracted by the sample gives diffraction patterns that depend on the amount of deformation of the sheared cells. The intensity of the beam is alternately sampled, using a chopper, at points A and B, located near the edge of the diffraction patterns. As the shear stress is increased the red cells elongate, the diffraction pattern changes, and the strength of the signal at points A and B varies. A signal processor converts this information into a deformability index (DI), defined by (A−B)/(A+B), which measures the elliptical shape of the sheared cells.** ***Bottom.*** **To measure red cell membrane stability, isolated membranes are subjected to a constant high shear stress (600 dyn/cm^2) and the DI is followed with time. The DI falls as the membranes fragment and become more spheroidal. Fragmentation occurs more rapidly in the fragile red cells found in HE and HPP and is reflected in the sharp drop of the curves in those cases. (*From Mohandas et al.*[400] *Used by permission.*)**

lies at a distance from the self-association site, the disease is very mild even when homozygous.

In a small number of patients with HE/HPP, peptide maps of β-spectrin disclose a truncated β chain. While the normal β-spectrin peptide runs as a 220-kDa band on SDS gels, the variant peptides, named after the city where the proband is located, are shortened to 214-kDa (spectrins$_{\text{LEPUY}}$[424] and $_{\text{GÖTTINGEN}}$[425]), 216-kDa (spectrins$_{\text{NICE}}$,[426] $_{\text{TOKYO}}$,[427] $_{\text{TANDIL}}$,[428] and $_{\text{NAPOLI}}$[429]), or 218-kDa (spectrin$_{\text{ROUEN}}$[430]). In all cases, the spectrin heterodimers containing the shortened β chains do not form tetramers well. Interestingly, in some of these patients, tryptic analysis also shows an αI/74 variant peptide.[426]

Protein 4.1 Deficiency. Protein 4.1 is partially or fully deficient in several reported HE kindreds.[229,407,431–434] This variant is apparently more common in North Africa and Japan.[407,431,435] Protein 4.1 is decreased about 50 percent in heterozygotes and is absent in homozygotes. Clinically, the heterozygotes have common HE with prominent elliptocytosis, no red cell fragmentation, and little or no hemolysis. In contrast, homozygotes have a severe transfusion-dependent hemolytic anemia with marked osmotic fragility, normal thermal stability, bizarre red cell morphology, and a very good response to splenectomy.[228,407,436] The homozygous protein 4.1-deficient membranes are very fragile, but stability can be restored by reconstitution with purified protein 4.1[229] or even by a recombinant peptide containing the region critical for spectrin-actin binding.[210,212]

Interestingly, protein 4.1R, the red cell form, is also expressed in granule cells in the cerebellum and in neurons in the dentate gyrus. Mice that lack 4.1R have subtle defects in movement,

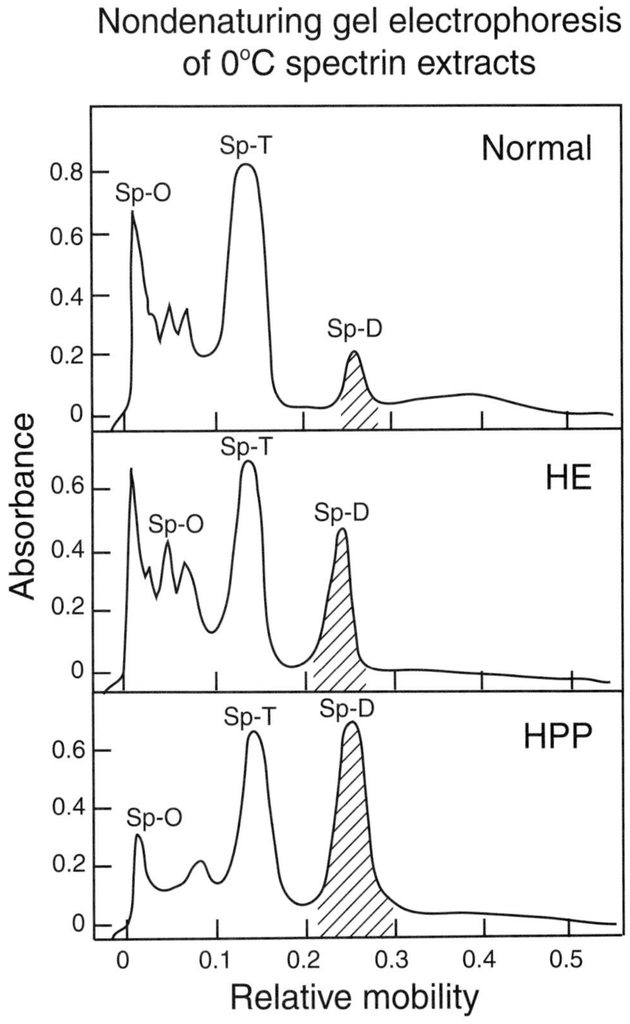

Fig. 183-12 Defective spectrin oligomerization in HE/HPP. Analysis of spectrin dimers (Sp-D), tetramers (Sp-T), and higher-order oligomers (Sp-O) in a normal individual (top panel), an HPP patient (bottom), and his mother, who has HE (middle). The densitometric tracing of the scanned gel is shown. The fraction of spectrin dimers is increased in the HPP patient (≈50 percent) and his mother (HE) (≈30 percent) compared with normal (≈8 percent), indicating a defect in spectrin oligomerization in the patient. (*From Liu, Palek, Prchal, and Castleberry.*[404] *Used by permission.*)

coordination, balance, and learning in addition to the expected hemolytic anemia.[437] It is not known whether humans with homozygous HS due to defects in protein 4.1 have similar abnormalities, as careful neurobehavioral testing has not been done.

Glycophorin C Deficiency. Glycophorin C (GPC) is absent in patients with homozygous protein 4.1 deficiency and in patients with the rare Leach phenotype of Gerbich-negative (Ge−) red cells. The Gerbich antigen system is carried on GPC and GPD. Patients with the Leach subtype of Ge− lack both GPC and GPD.[438,439] These patients, but not other patients with Ge− red cells (who lack the antigen but not GPC and GPD), have mild elliptocytosis[438,439] with increased osmotic fragility (i.e., a form of spherocytic HE). Their red cells contain only 30 percent of the normal amount of protein 4.1,[231] which probably accounts for the elliptocytic phenotype. This and other information, discussed earlier, strongly suggests that GPC is an important binding site for protein 4.1 in normal red cells. In contrast to GPC deficiency, patients lacking GPA, GPB, or both are entirely asymptomatic and have normal red cell morphology.

Molecular Etiology

DNA analysis of the genes of the major membrane skeleton proteins has led to the identification of many molecular defects in HE/HPP and an improved understanding of the molecular pathophysiology. The defects in these disorders appear to lie mainly in the components of the erythrocyte membrane skeleton that are responsible for the horizontal interactions within the skeleton network, specifically, α- and β-spectrin and protein 4.1.

α-Spectrin Defects. Most of the α-spectrin mutations lie in the N-terminal, αI domain that forms part of the spectrin self-association site (Fig. 183-14). The nomenclature used to describe the mutations is defined in Antonarkis et al.[440] In the majority of cases, the mutations alter tryptic maps and lie close to the site of abnormal tryptic cleavage site. Most reside in helix C of the spectrin repeats and presumably disrupt the triple helical structure of the repeats (Fig. 183-15).

The $\alpha^{I/78}$ defect arises due to substitutions in codons 41 or 45 of the α-spectrin peptide.[445–447] The $\alpha^{I/74}$ defect is heterogeneous and is caused by mutations in codons 24, 28, 31, 34, 46, 48, or 49.[441–444,448,449,472] Codon 28, containing a CpG dinucleotide, may be a mutation "hot spot" and is associated with four different mutations. Curiously, the mutations arising in codon 45 or 48 result in severe HPP, whereas those arising in codons 41, 46, or 49 result in a milder HE condition. The $\alpha^{I/65}$ defect is a mild condition arising from the duplication of a leucine residue in codon 154[409,451] or from a missense mutation in codon 151 (spectrin$_{\text{PONTE DE SOR}}$).[450] The mutation responsible for the $\alpha^{I/61}$ defect has not yet been defined. The $\alpha^{I/50}$ defect often results from substitution of a proline, an amino acid known to disrupt α helix formation.[409,453,454] Spectrin$_{\text{DAYTON}}$, which has a 48 residue deletion in codons 178 to 226, also gives rise to an $\alpha^{I/50}$ phenotype.[452] The $\alpha^{I/50}$ defect originates either by proline substitutions[409,454,456] or by a single residue deletion in codon 469.[455] The $\alpha^{I/36}$ mutation (spectrin$_{\text{SFAX}}$) derives from deletion of codons 363 to 371 due to activation of a cryptic splice site.[420] The $\alpha^{II/31}$ mutation (spectrin$_{\text{JENDOUBA}}$) is caused by a point mutation in codon 791,[421] whereas the $\alpha^{II/21}$ defect (spectrin$_{\text{ORAN}}$) is produced by a deletion of amino acids 822 to 862, from a mutation in the acceptor splice site for exon 18, resulting in skipping of exon 18.[457]

Unlike mutations associated with β-spectrin, which often result in premature chain termination (see below), very few truncated α-spectrin peptides have been described in patients with HE/HPP. They would presumably lack the spectrin dimer nucleation site located near the C-terminus and not be incorporated into the membrane skeleton. Because α-spectrin synthesis is normally three- to fourfold more than β-spectrin, enough α-spectrin chains would be still be produced by the single normal α-spectrin allele to bind all of the β-spectrin chains and form a complete membrane skeleton. This point is illustrated by spectrin$_{\text{ST.CLAUDE}}$, in which a splice site mutation causes premature termination of the α-spectrin chains, abolishing the spectrin dimer nucleation site.[458] The proband, homozygous for the mutation, has severe hemolytic anemia with poikilocytosis, microspherocytosis, and elliptocytosis. In contrast, his parents and a brother, all heterozygotes, are completely asymptomatic and have normal red cell morphology.

Low-expression α-spectrin allele (α^{LELY}). In some kindreds with α-spectrin defects and typical common HE, there are individuals with severe hemolytic anemia consistent with a diagnosis of severe HE or HPP. Many, perhaps all of these patients inherit a second, low-expression allele, which is silent in carriers but contributes to the severity of the disease when present *in trans* (on the opposite chromosome) to a structurally mutant allele. This idea emerged from the discovery that a common polymorphism, $\alpha^{V/41}$, is associated with reduced incorporation of α-spectrin chains into the membrane skeleton.[343] The low-expression α-spectrin allele is

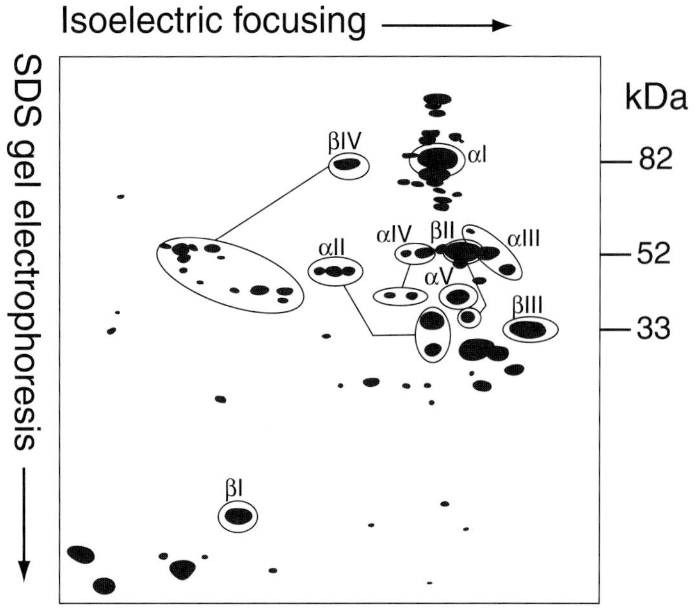

Fig. 183-13 Diagram showing normal tryptic domains of spectrin. The partial tryptic digest is separated by two-dimensional isoelectric focusing (pH 7.2 to 4.5, left to right), followed by SDS gel electrophoresis (*top to bottom*). The major α- and β-chain domain peptides are circled and labeled. These correspond to the domains defined in Fig. 183-4. Connected circles indicate peptides that are related to each other. The smaller peptides in each connected pair result from additional cleavages. (*From Marchesi et al.*[409] *Used by permission.*)

now designated α^{LELY} (Low Expression Lyon), after the peptide that is produced in diminished quantity.

Two linked abnormalities result in the α^{LELY} allele:[459] (1) a Leu 1867 to Val mutation in exon 40 that causes an abnormal tryptic cleavage after amino acid 1920, at the αIV-V junction, resulting in the variant $\alpha^{V/41}$ peptide, and (2) a C-to-T substitution in an acceptor splice site 12 nucleotides before the splice junction that leads to 50 percent in-frame skipping of exon 46. This exon is only 18 bp long, and thus the change in the protein is too small to be observed on SDS gel electrophoresis, but the exon lies within the nucleation site for α to β chain association. Because of the resulting interference with the nucleation site, α-spectrin chains lacking exon 46 (i.e., α^{LELY}) probably fail to bind to β-spectrin chains or be incorporated into the membrane skeleton, and are instead destroyed.[473] The remaining α chains (≈50 percent), which contain the exon, function normally.

Because α-spectrin peptides are normally produced in excess and the α^{LELY} splicing mutation causes only partial skipping of exon 46, the α^{LELY} allele is completely silent by itself, even when homozygous. If the α^{LELY} allele occurs *in trans* to a second allele encoding a structurally abnormal α-spectrin associated with HE, however, the mutant peptide with the structural defect will be preferentially incorporated into the membrane, aggravating the severity of the disease dramatically.[343] Fig. 183-16 details how the α^{LELY} allele can affect the relative expression of the normal and HE alleles, and thus, the clinical severity. If an HE mutation is on a chromosome bearing the α^{LELY} mutation, a mild defect can be converted into a silent one or a severe one into a mild one.[475] In contrast, a defective HE allele inherited in trans to the α^{LELY} allele results in a more severe clinical condition, such as severe HE or HPP.[476]

The α^{LELY} allele is found in a very high frequency in all ethnic groups examined. Its frequency ranges between 16 percent and 31 percent among Caucasians, Africans, Japanese, Chinese, and Amazon Indians, suggesting that it is of a very ancient origin.[477,478] Coinheritance of this allele with an HE allele is therefore frequently encountered and may account for much of the clinical variability seen within HE/HPP families.

β-Spectrin Defects. At least 19 mutations in β-spectrin associated with HE/HPP have been described. They all cluster near the C-terminus of β-spectrin, where the spectrin dimer self-association site is situated. The abnormalities identified include truncations that delete various amounts of the C-terminus as well as missense mutations (Fig. 183-14). Both kinds of mutations presumably alter spectrin self-association by disrupting the coiled-coil triple helical structure that forms the spectrin dimer self-association site (Fig. 183-15). For example, for one of the β-spectrin truncated variants, $\beta^{220/216}$, where about 4-kDa is lost from the C-terminus, low-temperature spectrin extracts contain increased spectrin dimer (≈50 percent of the dimer-tetramer pool as compared with normal [5 to 10 percent]) and nearly all of the abnormal β^{216} spectrin is found in the dimer fraction,[424,425,479] indicating that the inability of the β^{216} peptide to oligomerize is responsible for the functional defect.

Several molecular defects causing truncated β-spectrin chains have been characterized. They include frameshift mutations,[427–429,468,471] exon skipping,[460–463,480] and a nonsense mutation (Fig. 183-14).[470] Defective β-spectrins with missense mutations in the partial repeat that forms the spectrin dimer association site (repeat 17) have also been identified (Fig. 183-14).[118,334,441,464–467,469] Several of these missense mutations result in substitution of a proline residue in the mutant peptide. Because proline is known to disrupt the α helices, this fact underscores the importance of the triple helical conformation of spectrin in maintaining its structural stability. In many of these β-spectrin mutations, an associated α-spectrin abnormality, $\alpha^{I/74}$, can also be seen on tryptic maps.[426] This is now believed to be a secondary effect, a result of the exposure of the N-terminus of the α-spectrin peptide to increased tryptic digestion because of the abnormal spectrin self-association caused by the β-spectrin mutations.[118,481,482]

Clinically, patients with β-spectrin defects have mild to moderate hemolysis with rounded elliptocytes and some fragmented red cells. Where measured, osmotic fragility is often increased, suggesting that these disorders should be classified as examples of spherocytic elliptocytosis. Thermal stability is unusual; the red cells become echinocytic at 47°C (normal, 49°C), but do not fragment. In the occasional patients who are homozygous for these mutations, a clinical picture of HPP with severe neonatal hemolysis, or even lethal hydrops fetalis, has been described.[118,466,467]

Protein 4.1 Defects. Several molecular defects in protein 4.1 associated with HE have been described (Fig. 183-17). In one Algerian kindred, the disease is caused by a 318-bp deletion in the 4.1R gene that eliminates the downstream initiation codon utilized by the 80-kDa erythroid isoform of protein 4.1.[483] Two families

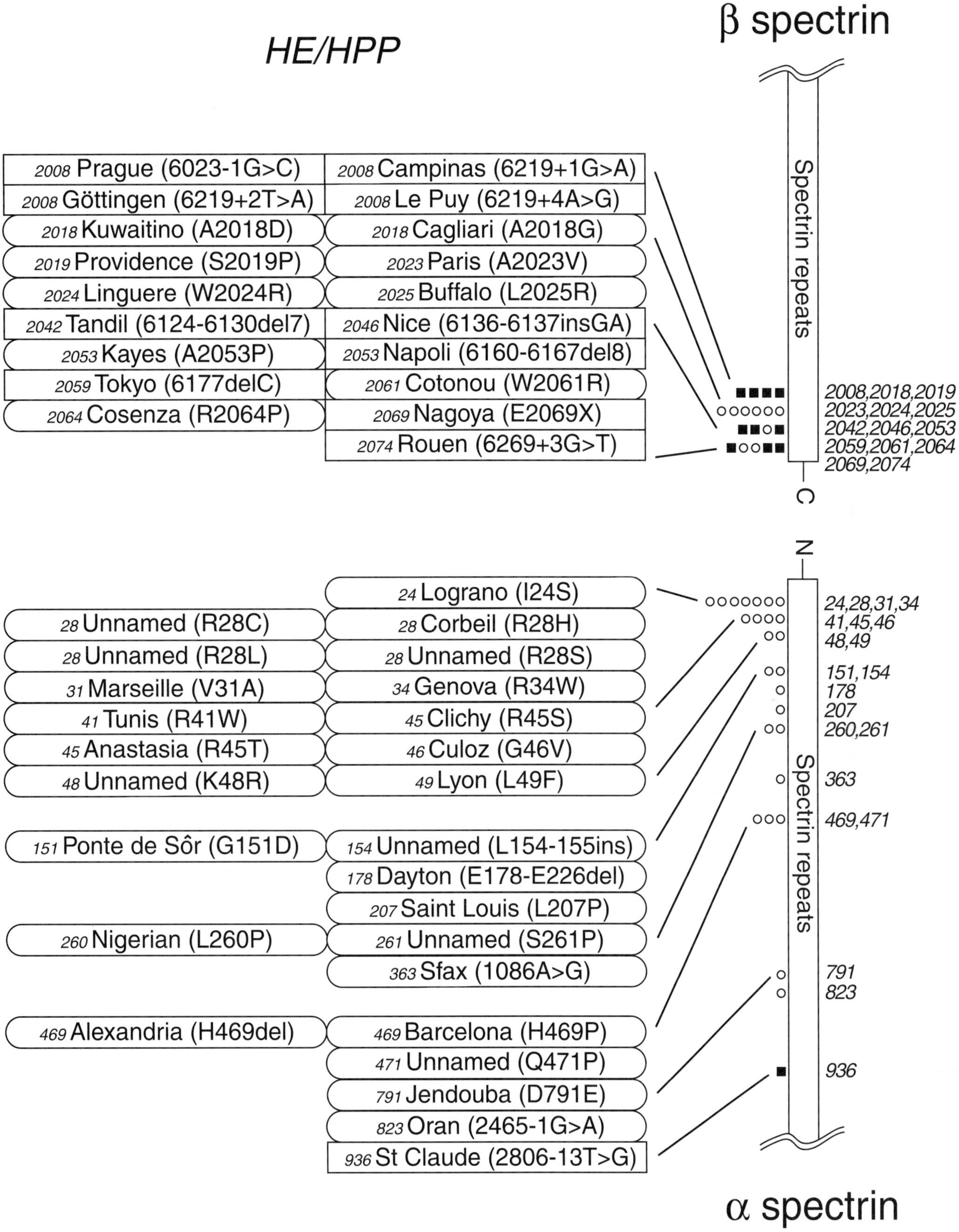

Fig. 183-14 α- and β-spectrin mutations associated with HE/HPP are shown alongside a schematic representation of the N-terminus of α-spectrin and the C-terminus of β-spectrin. On the left, missense mutations are shown in ellipses and mutations causing peptide truncation are shown in rectangles. The common name of each mutation is followed in brackets by its systemic name.[440] The nucleotide numbers of the mutations may be different from those in published reports. The codon number of the spectrin residue affected by each mutation (or the first of several residues affected) is indicated in italics to the left of the common name and on the spectrin model on the right. The data in this figure are compiled from published and unpublished reports of α-spectrin mutations[420,421,441–459] and β-spectrin mutations.[118,334,427–429,441,460–471] A catalogue of the mutations is available at the Web site http://www.kidscancer.net/membrane.

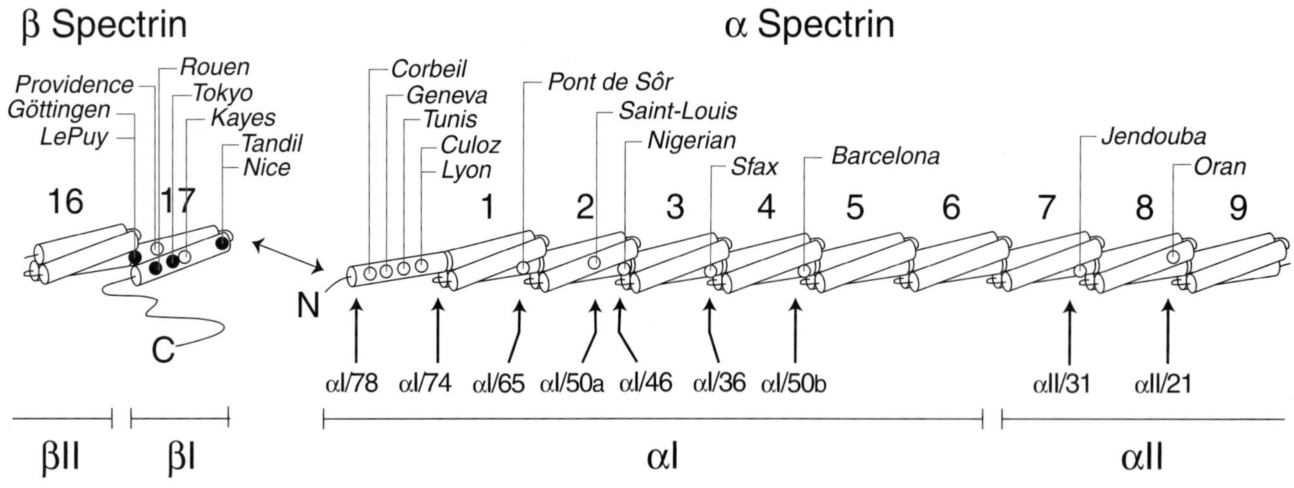

Fig. 183-15 Three-dimensional representation of spectrin defects in HE/HPP. The location of representative mutations causing HE/HPP are shown schematically on a triple helical model of the spectrin chains, clustered around the α- and β-spectrin association site. Open circles denote amino acid substitutions and solid circles denote chain truncations. Spectrin$_{SFAX}$ has a small, in-frame deletion of 9 codons and is also indicated by an open circle. Shown below the model are the tryptic cleavage sites that produce variant peptide fragments associated with the α-spectrin defects. (*Adapted from Gallagher, Tse, and Forget.*[22] *Used by permission.*)

have point mutations in the same initiation codon (protein 4.1_{MADRID} and protein 4.1_{LILLE})[436,485] that also prevent expression of erythroid 4.1. A large 70-kb deletion of the gene causes the deficiency seen in protein 4.1_{ANNERY},[484] and deletion of a single residue in the spectrin-binding domain in protein 4.1_{ARAVIS} abolishes its capacity to bind spectrin.[486]

In addition to deficiency in protein 4.1, some patients are also missing (partially) other proteins, such as protein 4.9[407] or glycophorin C.[432] Patients with complete protein 4.1 deficiency have only 9 percent of the normal amount of glycophorin C. This lends strong support to the theory that protein 4.1 binds to glycophorin C in the membrane.[231]

Several structural defects of protein 4.1 have been described. One occurred in two generations of a French family with common HE and moderate chronic hemolysis.[487] SDS gels showed a 50 percent decrease in protein 4.1 and two faint new bands, 65- and 68-kDa, that are immunologically related to protein 4.1.[487] Functionally, the protein 4.1 from the patient bound to a crude mixture of normal spectrin and actin only 40 percent as well as normal. A similar variant has been observed in dogs (76/78-kDa).[488] Molecular studies demonstrate that protein$4.1^{68/65}$ is caused by a deletion of 80 amino acids, from residue 407 to 486, which includes the entire spectrin-actin binding domain,[489,490] whereas canine protein $4.1^{78/76}$ results from deletion of exon 16 (Fig. 183-8), an alternatively spliced exon that encodes a 21-amino acid peptide required for spectrin-actin binding.[210,491] Another defect has been identified in a single kindred with common HE. The patients are heterozygous for a large (95-kDa) variant of protein 4.1, designated protein 4.1_{95}, that comigrates with band 3 and is detected by immunoblotting.[489,490] This anomaly results from the internal duplication of a 369-bp segment consisting of three exons that encode Lys 407 to Gln 529, thus producing two spectrin-actin binding domains. Fortunately, the insertion does not markedly alter spectrin-actin binding, which probably accounts for its mild phenotype. A third human variant, designated $4.1_{PRESLES}$, is a shortened protein 4.1 that migrates as a doublet with apparent sizes of 73- and 74-kDa.[492] This is caused by skipping one exon that encodes 34 amino acids near the beginning of the C-terminal 22/24-kDa domain.[493] The condition is clinically silent, even in the homozygous state, and so technically is a benign variant of protein 4.1.

Band 3 Defects. Defects in band 3 have not been identified in HE/HPP, except in Southeast Asian ovalocytosis (SAO). Molecular analysis of the band 3 gene in patients with SAO reveals two abnormalities: a known polymorphism, band $3_{MEMPHIS}$,[494] and deletion of amino acid residues 400 to 408 at the junction between the cytoplasmic and membrane domains.[82,495] This deletion removes part of the first transmembrane α helix, which is thought to serve as an internal signal sequence, and probably disrupts the structure of the membrane domain.[496] As a consequence, band 3 SAO lacks anion transport activity.[497] This may explain why homozygous band 3 SAO is not observed and is probably lethal.[389,390]

SAO red cells are extraordinarily rigid, by far the most rigid red cells known.[392,393] This impedes entry of malarial parasites and accounts for the high frequency of the mutations in the indigenous populations of Southeast Asia. How the 400 to 408 deletion causes this rigidity is less clear. Liu and his colleagues found that SAO band 3 binds more ankyrin than normal,[386] and tends to form linear aggregates in the membrane.[498] The aggregates restrict rotational and lateral diffusion of SAO band 3 in the lipid bilayer, and could account for the observed rigidity because band 3 must move, along with spectrin and ankyrin, when the red cell deforms.[498] The enhanced ankyrin binding of SAO band 3, however, has not been detected by others.[496,497]

An alternative hypothesis, advanced by several groups,[495–497] is that the SAO deletion makes the flexible section of the cytoplasmic domain just proximal to the membrane more rigid, which would tend to extend the cytoplasmic domain of band 3 and cause it to become entangled in the spectrin network. In fact, Moriyama and colleagues[496] have observed that band 3 is nonspecifically trapped in isolated skeletons from SAO red cells, which supports this hypothesis. It is reasonable to expect that such entanglement would impede the movement of spectrin chains when the membrane is stretched, leading to membrane rigidity. This concept is supported by recent measurements, using laser tweezers, of the movement of band 3 in normal red cells.[77] One-third of the molecules are immobile and presumably bound to the skeleton. But the remaining two-thirds move discontinuously, as though they are corralled by the spectrin network in spaces 110 nm in diameter. They hop from corral to corral about three times per second. If normal band 3 molecules are already entangled in the skeleton, it is easy to imagine that even a small extension of the cytoplasmic domain, as is postulated in SAO red cells, could aggravate band 3 movement when the cell is deformed and impair membrane flexibility.

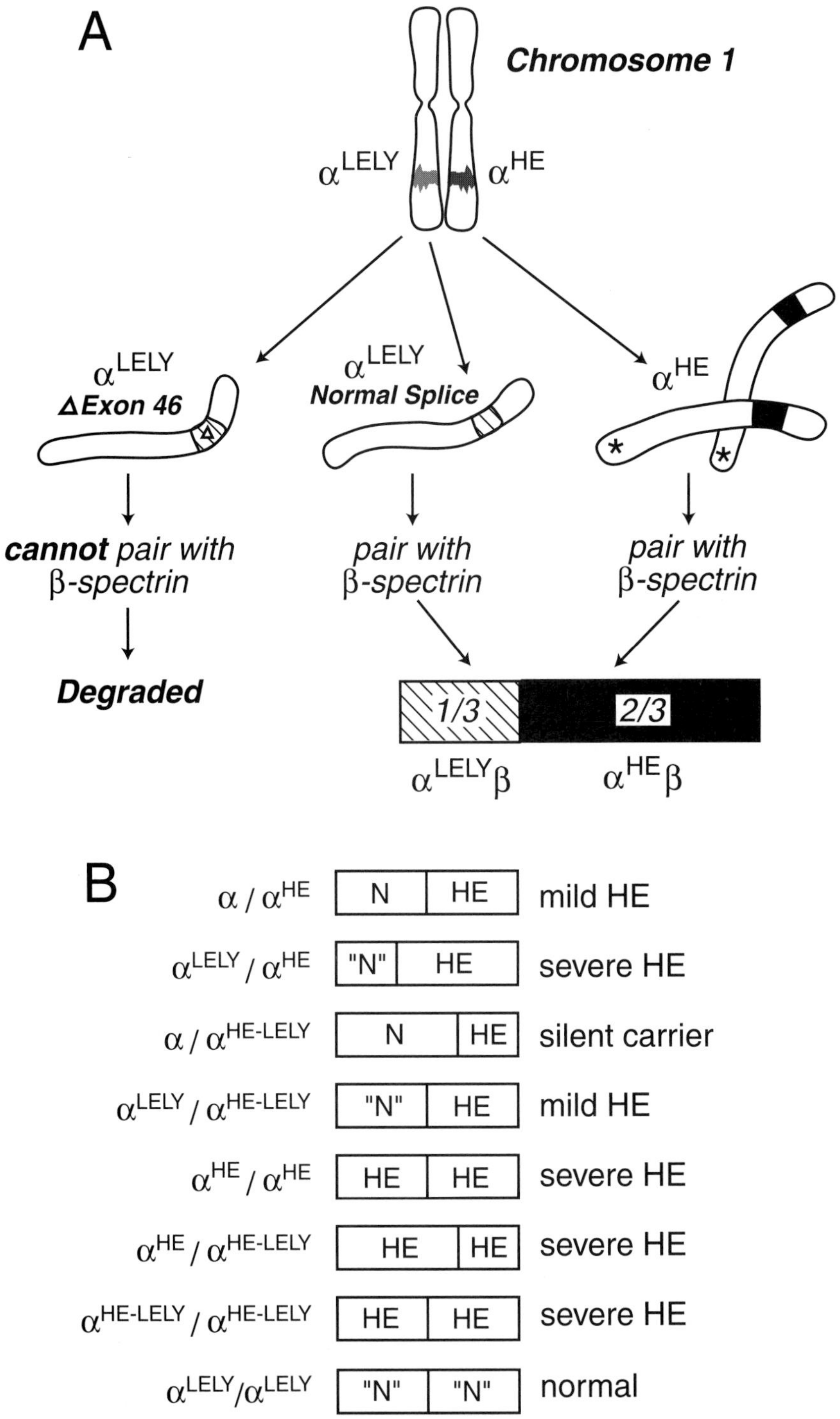

Fig. 183-16 Effect of the α^{LELY} allele on the proportion of spectrins containing normal and HE α chains. *A.* When an α^{LELY} allele pairs with an α allele bearing an HE mutation (asterisk), the abnormal splicing associated with the α^{LELY} allele decreases the amount of normal α chains that can pair with β chains and results in an increased proportion of HE α chain being incorporated into the membrane skeleton. *B.* Interactions of a normal α allele (α), a low-expression allele (α^{LELY}), an HE allele (α^{HE}), and an HE mutation developing on a low-expression allele ($\alpha^{HE\text{-}LELY}$). The resulting proportion of normal (N) and elliptocytic (HE) spectrins and expected clinical phenotype in each case is illustrated. Note that patients who are homozygous for the α^{LELY} mutation are clinically normal This is because α-spectrin synthesis normally exceeds β-spectrin synthesis by so much (three- to fourfold), that α^{LELY} homozygotes still have enough α-spectrin chains to bind all of the β-spectrin. (*Adapted from Delaunay and Dhermy.*[474] *Used by permission.*)

Remarkably, the rigid SAO red cells negotiate the circulation normally and do not impair tissue perfusion or result in hemolysis.

Pathophysiology

Despite our increasing knowledge of the defective structure and function of the specific membrane proteins, we still do not understand how those abnormalities lead to an elliptical shape. Any explanation of the various forms of HE erythrocytes must consider the fact that nucleated elliptocytic precursors are round, and elongate or fragment only gradually as they circulate. This resembles the gradual development of spherocytosis in hereditary spherocytes, and is consistent with the concept that the change in shape is secondary to the intrinsic structural instability of the skeleton. According to this hypothesis, skeletal defects lead to elliptocytosis by increasing membrane plasticity (i.e., plastic deformation). Normal red cells rapidly regain their shape after they are transiently deformed, but they remain misshaped if the distortion is maintained for long periods (minutes to hours).[499,500] Presumably, spectrin-spectrin or spectrin-actin interactions realign in response to prolonged stress. In a cell with defective "horizontal" skeletal interactions, like the hereditary elliptocyte, this realignment process should be accelerated, and may result in an irreversible change in shape of the membrane skeleton. In vivo, red cells are deformed into a stable elliptical or

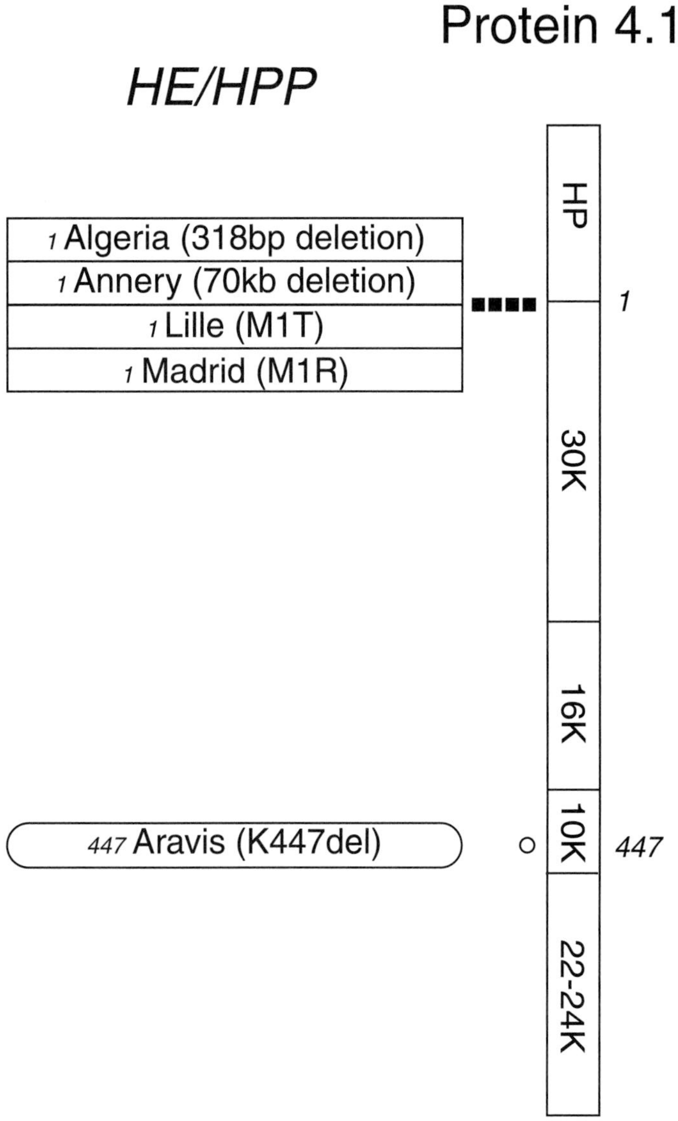

Fig. 183-17 Protein 4.1 mutations associated with HE/HPP are shown alongside a schematic representation of the peptide. On the left, four mutations abolishing the translation start site are shown in shaded rectangles and a missense mutation at codon 447 is shown in an open ellipse. The common name of each mutation is followed in brackets by its systemic name.[440] The data in this figure are compiled from published reports of protein 4.1 mutations.[436,483–486]

torpedo shape when passing through very small capillaries. It is easy to imagine how this distortion, repeated thousands of times per day, could cause red cells gradually to elongate and assume their characteristic elliptical shape. Whether this is, in fact, the pathophysiological mechanism remains to be proved.

Red cells with more severe horizontal skeletal defects would also tend to elongate, but if skeletal instability were sufficiently compromised, they would be unable to withstand the shear stresses experienced in the normal circulation, and fragmentation or combinations of fragmentation and shape change induced by plastic deformation (i.e., bizarre-shaped poikilocytes) would predominate. This process would explain the nearly identical morphology observed in homozygous HE and hereditary pyropoikilocytosis and in neonates with common HE and poikilocytosis.

In spite of the uncertainties about the molecular mechanisms involved in the different subtypes of HE, the available information suggests that red cell death in the various hemolytic forms follows a similar pathway. In all cases hemolysis is markedly ameliorated by splenectomy, and where examined, splenic pathology shows cordal congestion essentially identical to that observed in HS.[380,381,501,502] As in HS, the specific pathophysiologic mechanism(s) responsible for splenic sequestration and red cell destruction remain to be defined.

Clinical Management

Diagnosis. Diagnosis of common HE is usually not difficult if there are obvious morphological changes on the peripheral smear and if there is a positive family history. There are situations when a diagnosis of HE/HPP is more difficult. As discussed above, elliptocytosis may not be prominent in infancy, and morphological or ektacytometric analysis of the parents red cells may be necessary for the diagnosis. Similarly, in sporadic cases of severe hemolytic anemia resembling HPP, careful evaluation of the parents with specialized techniques like ektacytometry and biochemical studies may be needed to make the diagnosis. In HE patients who have a particularly severe phenotype compared to other affected family members, molecular detection of a second genetic determinant, such as the low-expression α^{LELY} allele, may help predict the natural course of the disease. Elliptocytosis may also be secondary to other systemic diseases such as myelodysplasia[503,504] and those causes must be ruled out.

Treatment. Because the clinical severity of the HE/HPP syndrome is variable, the appropriate treatment differs greatly.

Most individuals with common HE are asymptomatic and require no treatment. In the event of hemolytic episodes triggered by infection or other acute events, supportive care alone usually suffices. Splenectomy is almost never indicated. Because red cell survival is near normal, aplastic crises from parvovirus infection (discussed under "Hereditary Spherocytosis") are uncommon, though not unknown.[505] In infants with common HE who present with neonatal hemolysis and poikilocytosis, treatment of hyperbilirubinemia may be necessary and regular red cell transfusions may be needed until the condition improves.

On the other end of the spectrum, patients with severe HE or HPP and uncompensated anemia may be chronically transfusion-dependent and may require splenectomy to control the hemolysis (see "Hereditary Spherocytosis"). In the neonatal period, infants with severe HE/HPP may be critically ill and require intensive care.[467] They may even present as hydrops fetalis and require in utero transfusions to survive.[466] In all patients with chronic hemolysis, oral folate supplements (1 mg daily) are recommended. And in patients requiring chronic transfusion, monitoring of iron overload and transfusion-related infection is warranted and consideration should be given to extended red cell typing and transfusion of cells matched for all Rh antigens (instead of just D) and for Kell, Duffy, and Kidd antigens. Postsplenectomy management is discussed in the relevant section in "Hereditary Spherocytosis."

HEREDITARY SPHEROCYTOSIS

Hereditary spherocytosis (HS), is an important, usually autosomal dominant hemolytic anemia, in which defects in spectrin or the proteins that attach spectrin to the membrane (ankyrin, band 3, protein 4.2) lead to spheroidal, osmotically fragile, often spectrin-deficient cells that are selectively trapped in the spleen and that survive almost normally after splenectomy.

History

HS was first described more than 120 years ago by the Belgian physicians Vanlair and Masius.[506] They reported on a young woman in whom recurrent abdominal pain developed over her enlarged spleen, with associated prostration, vomiting, jaundice, anemia, and muscular weakness. At the time of this attack (presumably a hemolytic crisis), the authors noted that the majority of the red cells were spherical and much smaller than normal. They termed these cells "microcytes" and named the disease "microcythemia." The unstained cells were illustrated in a lithograph drawn and tinted by Vanlair (Fig. 183-18). The drawing clearly shows spherocytosis, although the relatively large number of elliptocytes (19 percent of the evaluable cells) raises the question whether the true diagnosis may not have been spherocytic elliptocytosis. Later, when the patient had improved, her red cells were somewhat larger, but still abnormal, and her spleen remained enlarged.

Vanlair and Masius thought the microcytes were senile normal cells ("globules atrophiques") and that the spleen assisted in their aging. They argued that when red cells are sequestered in the pulp of the spleen, they are removed from the active circulation, lose volume, and become dense, spherical, and microcytic. They believed an enlarged spleen produces even more of such cells than a normal spleen and that the liver completes the work of the spleen by destroying the microcytes it receives via the splenic vein. They suggested that the large number of microcytes in their patient was due in part to splenomegaly and in part to atrophy of the liver. Finally, they noted that the patient's older sister had suffered from an identical illness and had died during an apparent crisis. The mother was also subject to jaundice.

This remarkable paper must rank among the most prescient in hematology. Not only did the authors describe the first example of a hereditary hemolytic anemia well before the microscope was in general use in the analysis of blood diseases, but their deductions concerning the pathophysiology, particularly the role of the spleen, predated Ham and Castle's concept of erythrostasis[507] by more than two-thirds of a century. Their analysis is placed in better perspective when one realizes that 40 to 65 years later HS was ascribed to causes as diverse as hereditary syphilis[508] and splenic hemolysins.[509]

Unfortunately, Vanlair and Masius' report and subsequent descriptions of HS by Wilson and Stanley in the 1890s[510,511] went largely unnoticed. The latter authors clearly recognized the hereditary nature of the disease and were the first to describe the pathology of the spleen, which at autopsy was grossly firm and dark and microscopically engorged with red cells.

A report by Minkowski in 1900[512] received wide attention, and additional papers soon appeared,[513,514] including Chauffard's historic definition of osmotic fragility[515] and reticulocytosis[516] as hallmarks of the disease. At about the same time, Widal et al.[517] differentiated an acquired form of "congenital hemolytic jaundice" (now recognizable as Coombs' test-positive immunohemolytic anemia). Because Hayem had previously reported similar cases,[518] the acquired form of the disease soon became the Hayem-Widal type, while the congenital form was given the eponym Minkowski-Chauffard.

The use of splenectomy was soon advocated, and in 1911 Micheli[519] removed the spleen from a patient with acquired hemolytic jaundice. The fortunately brilliant result, combined with the subsequent success of splenectomy in the congenital disease,[520] soon led to widespread acceptance of the procedure. Actually, the first successful splenectomy for HS was unintentionally performed by Spencer Wells in England in 1887 (3 years before Wilson's description of the disease in that country).[521]

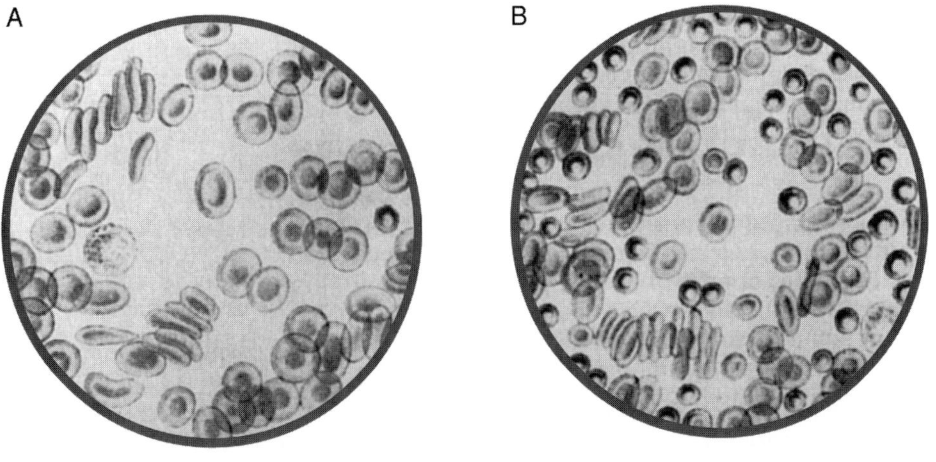

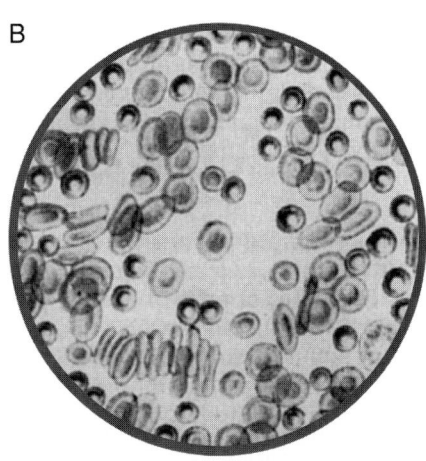

Fig. 183-18 Lithograph of normal blood cells (A) and cells from a patient with "microcythemia" (B) described by Vanlair and Masius in 1871.[506]

Operating on a jaundiced woman for a supposed uterine fibroid, he instead encountered and removed an enormous spleen. The patient recovered and the jaundice disappeared. Forty years later Lord Dawson restudied the woman and her son and found the characteristic osmotic fragility.[521]

Thus, by the time of Tileston's[522] and Gänsslen's[523] reviews in 1922, almost all the major clinical features of HS were documented, the spleen was thought to be involved in the hemolysis, and splenectomy was known to be curative. Nevertheless, with the exception of Vanlair and Masius' farsighted (and still unrecognized) premonitions, nothing substantive was known about the basic mechanism of the disorder or its pathogenesis. These aspects of the disease will be discussed in the sections that follow.

Prevalence and Genetics

HS is the most common hemolytic anemia in people of Northern European extraction. In this population the prevalence is roughly 1 in 5000,[524] and there is evidence, based on data obtained with sensitive diagnostic tests, that very mild forms of the disease may be much more common.[525,526] The disease occurs, but is less frequent, in other races and ethnic groups; this may reflect poor ascertainment or a true difference in incidence.

Approximately 75 percent of HS families have an autosomal dominant inheritance pattern.[524] Homozygotes for dominant HS are rare. In the few reported cases the parents have had a mild phenotype,[527–529] which suggests that homozygosity for typical dominant HS is probably incompatible with life.[530] There is nearly complete penetrance of the dominant disease, but clinical variability is common.

Approximately 25 percent of HS occurs sporadically in patients without a family history of spherocytosis. About half of these cases are *de novo* examples of dominant HS.[531–533] Parental mosaicism occurs and must be considered in genetic counseling.[534] The rest are likely to be examples of a recessive form of the disease, caused by coinheritance of two genetic determinants, one from each of the patient's parents. Patients with recessive HS are often more severely affected,[535,536] but there is also considerable clinical variability.

The first clue that pointed to a genetic locus for congenital spherocytosis was the identification of HS families with balanced translocations involving the short arm of chromosome 8.[537,538] Chilcote and his colleagues also identified two sisters with moderate to severe splenectomy-responsive anemia, spherocytosis, dysmorphic features, micrognathia, nystagmus, psychomotor retardation, and deletion of chromosome bands 8p11.1-p21.2.[539] Together, these observations provide evidence for a genetic locus for congenital spherocytosis in the proximal part of 8p. The nature of this HS locus was clarified when it was shown that the gene for ankyrin resides in this region and that the individuals reported by Chilcote, and another unrelated patient with a similar condition, lacked the ankyrin gene on the abnormal chromosome.[196] This conclusion was supported by genetic analysis of a large kindred with typical autosomal dominant HS and no chromosome deletion. Spherocytosis was linked to an RFLP in the ankyrin gene, while linkage to other candidate genes (α-spectrin, β-spectrin, or protein 4.1 genes) was excluded.[540]

In an analysis of 15 other families with HS, Kimberly et al. observed a weak association of HS with the immunoglobulin Gm type, which is located on 14q34.[537] This observation suggested that the cause of HS is heterogeneous and that there is at least one other genetic locus. This turns out to be true. The second genetic locus is probably the β-spectrin gene, which was later mapped to chromosome 14q23-q24.2.[541] As will be shown, other loci involve the genes for band 3, protein 4.2, α-spectrin, and, possibly, β-adducin.

Clinical Features

The characteristic clinical features of HS are pallor, jaundice, and splenomegaly. The presence of spherocytes in peripheral blood smears is almost the sine qua non of the disease, but HS must be distinguished from other nonhereditary causes of spherocytosis. A positive family history is often present, particularly in dominant HS. The disease typically presents in infancy or childhood, but may present at any age.[542]

Neonatal HS. HS frequently presents as jaundice in the first few days of life.[543,544] The combination of hemolysis and the reduced capacity of the neonatal liver to conjugate bilirubin can cause serum concentrations of unconjugated bilirubin to rise rapidly. Because there is a risk of kernicterus,[543] exchange transfusions are sometimes necessary, though usually phototherapy suffices. Mild anemia is common at this time, but severe anemia occasionally occurs. There is no evidence that patients with HS who are symptomatic as neonates have a more severe form of the disease. Indeed most become asymptomatic within the first few weeks of life. However, some infants become progressively more anemic during the first few months of life and require transfusion. In our experience, this usually occurs because the marrow response to anemia is more sluggish than normal. Fortunately, the problem is usually transient and remits after one or two transfusions, except in the rare patients with severe HS. It is not known if erythropoietin would work, and avert transfusion, but this possibility should be formally tested. The subsequent course of the disease depends on the equilibrium established between the rates of red cell production and destruction. An interesting recent observation points out that the presence or absence of the Gilbert syndrome variation (see Chap. 125),[545] situated in the promoter of the UDP-glucuronyl transferase gene, significantly influences whether an infant with HS has neonatal jaundice.[546]

Mild HS. Once beyond the neonatal period, patients with mild HS typically have a hemoglobin of 11 to 15 g/dl, a reticulocyte count of 3 to 8 percent, and a serum bilirubin of 1 to 2 mg/dl.[531] A surprisingly large numbers ($\approx$20 to 30 percent) have balanced red cell production and destruction and no anemia.[547,548] These individuals are said to have "compensated" hemolysis. They are often asymptomatic, and in some cases diagnosis may be difficult, because hemolysis, spherocytosis, and splenomegaly are usually mild. Many of these patients are diagnosed during family studies or are discovered as adults when splenomegaly or gallstones are detected or when transient episodes of jaundice appear.

Hemolysis may become severe with illnesses that cause the spleen to enlarge, such as infectious mononucleosis.[549] Hemolysis is also exacerbated by pregnancy[550,551] and by intensive physical effort, to the point at which athletic performance in endurance sports may be impaired, even in patients with mild disease.[552] In between these occasional hemolytic episodes, the patients again become asymptomatic.

Although HS is usually consistent within families, mild cases may also occur in families with more severely affected members.[547] Presumably this is due to the inheritance of modifying genetic factors, such as those affecting splenic function or the expression of either the normal or mutant allele of the disease gene. The precise nature of these factors remains to be elucidated.

One of the interesting mysteries is why patients with compensated hemolysis continue to have erythroid hyperproduction when their hemoglobin levels are normal. The phenomenon is difficult to reconcile with the generally accepted theory that erythropoiesis is controlled by tissue hypoxia. One possibility is that the concentration of 2,3-DPG, which is low in hereditary spherocytes prior to splenectomy,[553] increases oxygen affinity and promotes erythropoiesis. An alternative explanation can be found in recent studies which show that serum erythropoietin levels are elevated up to eightfold in HS patients with compensated hemolysis, compared with normal subjects who have similar hemoglobin levels.[554,555] The force driving this overproduction of erythropoietin is unknown. One untested possibility is that the dehydrated HS red cells poorly perfuse the erythropoietin-producing juxtaglomerular cells of the kidney, due to their relative rigidity. If true, then erythropoietin production at any hemoglobin level should correlate inversely with red cell deformability, and compensated hemolysis should mostly occur in disorders with dehydrated erythrocytes (e.g., HS, sickle cell disease, Hb CC disease, and hereditary xerocytosis).

Moderate HS. The majority of HS patients ($\approx$60 to 75 percent) have moderate disease with incompletely compensated hemolysis and mild to moderate anemia. By definition, baseline hemoglobin concentrations are 8- to 12 g/dl, reticulocytes are $\geq$8 percent, and bilirubin levels are usually $\geq$2 mg/dl.[531] Intermittent mild jaundice is common, particularly in children, often associated with viral infections, and is presumably due to reticuloendothelial stimulation and an increase in hemolysis. The spleen is palpable in about 50 percent of these patients during infancy and childhood and in 75 to 95 percent during adult life.[547,556,557] Splenomegaly is usually modest, but it may be massive.[521,522,558,559] There is no published evidence that the size of the spleen correlates with the severity of HS, although such a correlation probably exists, considering the pathophysiology of the disease.

Severe HS. A small proportion of HS patients ($\approx$5 to 10 percent) have severe hemolytic anemia. Their hemoglobin concentrations are $\geq$6 to 8 g/dl, reticulocytes are $\geq$10 percent, and bilirubin concentrations are usually 2 to 3 mg/dl or more.[531] A subset of these patients ($<$5 percent) have life-threatening disease and are transfusion-dependent.[535] In this group particularly, acanthocytes, irregular, shrunken spherocytes, and other bizarre forms may be seen in addition to typical spherocytes.[535] These individuals may present diagnostic difficulties if transfusions are begun before HS is diagnosed, because in the most severe cases the abnormal cells may be destroyed so rapidly that only transfused cells are available for testing. Besides the risks of recurrent transfusions, these patients occasionally suffer from complications of their chronic severe anemia, such as growth retardation, delayed sexual maturation, and frontal bossing or other changes in the facial bones similar to those observed in thalassemia.[558,559] Most of these severely affected patients have the recessive form of HS. Unlike typical dominant HS, anemia may not be completely eliminated by splenectomy in these patients.[535,560]

Laboratory Abnormalities

The first clue to the diagnosis of HS is usually the characteristic morphological change of red cells on peripheral blood smears. Other laboratory findings include those common to all hemolytic processes: an increased number of reticulocytes, a slight to moderate rise in indirect bilirubin in the plasma, an elevated fecal excretion of urobilinogens, and hyperplasia of erythroid precursors in the bone marrow. Plasma hemoglobin is normal and haptoglobin is only variably reduced, because most of the red cells are destroyed extravascularly. Laboratory tests that distinguish HS from other causes of hemolysis usually measure the biophysical properties of the affected red cells, among which the osmotic fragility test is the standard test. Biochemical analysis and DNA analysis of the membrane skeleton proteins in HS, done mainly in a few research laboratories, allow determination of the primary molecular defects underlying HS.

Red Cell Morphology. Spherocytes are the hallmark of HS. They are dense, round and hyperchromic, lack central pallor, and have a decreased mean cell diameter. They are almost always present on smears from patients with moderately severe HS, but are subtle in about 25 to 35 percent of patient with mild HS.[531,547,557] While hereditary spherocytes appear spheroidal in conventional dried smears, most are actually thickened diskocytes or spherostomatocytes when examined in the scanning electron microscope.[561] Although the morphologic defect is mostly acquired in the circulation, and HS erythroblasts are morphologically normal, emerging reticulocytes are more dehydrated and more spherical than normal reticulocytes, implying that, assembly of HS membranes during erythropoiesis is defective.[562]

The various subtypes of HS, discussed below, have subtle differences in red cell morphology. Patients with ankyrin defects and combined spectrin and ankyrin deficiency, the most common subtype,[23,563,564] have typical round spherocytes and microspherocytes (Fig. 183-19; panel *A*). Most patients with band 3 deficiency also have rare (0.2 to 2.3 percent) mushroom-shaped (or "pincered") red cells in their peripheral blood smears (panel *B*).[565,566] Patients with more severe spectrin deficiency have proportionally more misshaped spherocytes, spiculated red cells, and bizarre poikilocytes, which may dominate the blood smear in the most severe cases (panel *C*).[535,567] Combinations of spiculated red cells (acanthocytes) and spherocytes are observed in HS due to defects in β-spectrin (panel *D*).[461,568,569] Red cell morphology is variable in protein 4.2 deficiency and may even be normal.[570] Most patients appear to have mild spherocytosis, but acanthocytes, poikilocytes, and ovalostomatocytes are sometimes observed.[571] Oblong spherocytes, combined with elliptocytes, suggest spherocytic HE, which is most often associated with truncated β-spectrin chains.

Red Cell Indices. There are characteristic changes in the red cell indices associated with HS. The mean corpuscular hemoglobin concentration (MCHC) is increased, owing to mild cellular dehydration, and exceeds the upper limit of normal (36 gm/dl) in about half of patients.[547] Mean corpuscular hemoglobin (MCH) and mean corpuscular volume (MCV) may fall within the normal range,[547] because young red cells, which are increased in HS patients with ongoing hemolysis and which have a high cell volume, skew the distribution. However, the MCV is usually at the lower end of the normal range and sometimes is low. In addition the reticulocyte MCV is also low, which contrasts with the spherocytosis of autoimmune hemolytic anemia, where reticulocyte indices are *normal* and total cellular MCV is *increased*.[562] The profile of the volume and hemoglobin concentration of individual red cells can now be measured with automated blood counters using dual angle laser light scattering (Technicon H-1).[572] In HS blood samples, there is often a right shift of the hemoglobin concentration curve due to red cell dehydration, and a broadening of the volume curve, due to the mixture of small microspherocytes and large young erythrocytes (Fig. 183-20).[573,574] Similar diagnostic information can be obtained from the data generated by aperture impedance (Coulter) analyzers.[575] The combination of a high MCHC, a widened red cell distribution width (RDW), and shifts in distribution curves is often enough to suggest a diagnosis of HS.[575] Studies also show that in nonsplenectomized HS patients, the percentage of microcytes best reflects the severity of the disease, whereas the percentage of hyperdense cells best discriminates HS patients from normal individuals.[574] The presence of hyperdense cells is, however, not specific to HS, as it is also seen in other disorders such as Hb SC and Hb CC disease, hereditary xerocytosis, and autoimmune hemolytic anemia.

Osmotic Fragility Test. The osmotic fragility (OF) test is the most useful test generally available for the diagnosis of HS. The test is performed by suspending the cells in buffered saline solutions of various concentrations.[576] In hypotonic solutions, red cells swell until they become spheres and then burst. Cells with a decreased surface-to-volume ratio, such as hereditary spherocytes, can tolerate less swelling than normal. A curve plotting the percentage of hemolysis at different salt concentrations documents the osmotic fragility profile of the red cells. With HS erythrocytes, there is a shift of the curve away from the direction of hypotonicity, indicating increased osmotic fragility of the cells (Fig. 183-21). For nonsplenectomized HS patients, the osmotic fragility curve shows a major population of cells only slightly more spheroidal than normal and a "tail" of very fragile cells representing a minor population of hyperchromic microspherocytes. The microspherocytes result

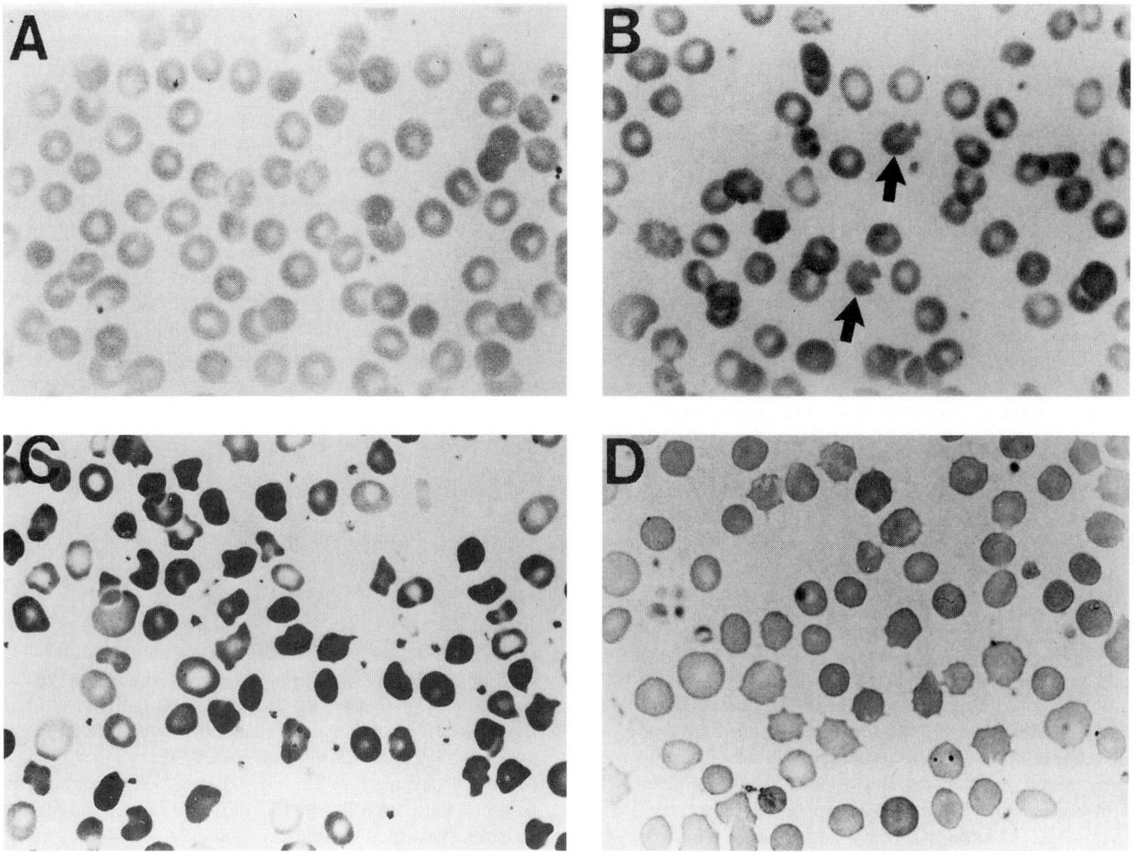

Fig. 183-19 Blood films from patients with different types of HS. *A.* Typical HS with a mild deficiency of red cell spectrin and ankyrin. Although many cells have a spheroidal shape, some of them retain a central concavity. *B.* HS with a small number of mushroom-shaped red cells (arrows), the typical picture in band 3 deficiency. Occasional spiculated cells are also present. *C.* Severe HS with marked spectrin and ankyrin deficiency. In addition to spherocytes, many red cells are misshaped and have irregular contours. *D.* HS associated with a β-spectrin mutation. Echinocytes and acanthocytes (5 to 15 percent) are usually observed in addition to typical spherocytes. (*From Palek and Jarolim.*[3] *Used by permission.*)

from "splenic conditioning," a topic that is discussed in more detail in a later section. Increased osmotic fragility is also observed in autoimmune hemolytic anemia, whereas red cells from patients with thalassemia and sickle cell disease may have decreased osmotic fragility.

In about 25 percent of HS patients, particularly the mildly affected, the OF test lies within the normal range.[556] In most of these cases, the disease is revealed by the "incubated" OF test. Whole blood is preincubated under sterile conditions at 37°C for 24 hours before the OF test is performed. During the incubation, hereditary spherocytes become metabolically depleted and lose membrane surface more rapidly than normal cells, which accentuates their spheroidicity and enhances the sensitivity of the test. HS patients with a normal incubated OF have been described,[577] and such patients may be even more common than reported,[574] but the incubated OF test remains the gold standard in the diagnosis of HS.

Glycerol Lysis Test. Because the OF test is cumbersome to perform and requires 2 ml or more of whole blood, a one-tube glycerol lysis test has been developed.[578] In this test, red blood cells are incubated in a glycerol-sodium phosphate-buffered hypotonic saline solution. The glycerol slows the entry of water into the cells, so that the time for the cells to lyse is prolonged and can be measured accurately. The glycerol lysis time is shortened for hereditary spherocytes because of the reduced surface-to-volume ratio. The sensitivity of the glycerol lysis test is enhanced by using a low pH[577] or by a 24-hour preincubation,[579] and subsequent modifications of the method have improved the sensitivity, reproducibility, and accuracy.[526,580] The simplicity of the glycerol lysis test and its sensitivity make it an excellent test for rapid screening of large numbers of micro blood samples.[526]

Autohemolysis Test. The autohemolysis test was originally described by Ham and Castle.[507] Incubation of red cells in their plasma for 48 hours results in autohemolysis, and the rate of autohemolysis is increased in red cells from HS patients. In general, the autohemolysis test lacks specificity but is relatively sensitive, and is occasionally useful in confirming the diagnosis of mild or sporadic cases of HS.

Hypertonic Cryohemolysis Test. The hypertonic cryohemolysis test is a relatively new method.[581] Spherocytes are particularly sensitive to cooling at 0°C in hypertonic conditions, which causes them to lyse and release their hemoglobin. This is the basis for the test. Hypertonic cryohemolysis is said to be more sensitive than other tests, especially in mild cases of HS,[582] but it can also be positive in some patients with other hemolytic anemias, and with elliptocytosis and some forms of congenital dyserythropoietic anemia.[583] The advantages of the test include its simplicity, high sensitivity, and the ability to use EDTA-preserved blood samples obtained for routine hematological studies. However, the hypertonic cryohemolysis test is still new and its limitations are not yet fully understood. As an example, most of the published studies using the test were done in adult HS patients, so the test still needs be validated in children.

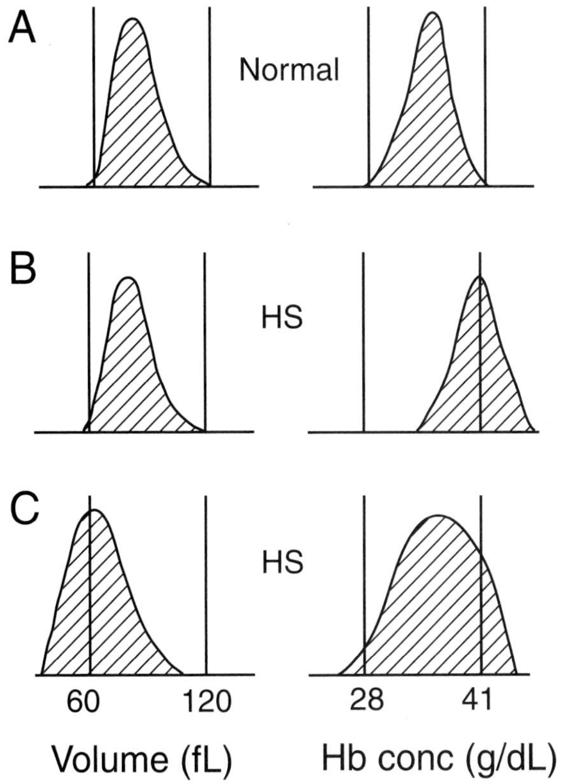

Fig. 183-20 Representative volume and hemoglobin concentration profiles of blood samples from a normal individual (A) and two different HS patients (B and C), obtained using a Technicon H-1 counter. The signposts in the volume distribution separate microcytic (<60 fl) and macrocytic (>120 fl) cells from normocytic red cells (60 to 120 fl), whereas the sign posts in the hemoglobin concentration distribution separate hypochromic (<28 gm/dl) and hyperdense (>41 gm/dl) cells from normochromic red cells (28 to 41 gm/dl). In *B*, the right shift of the hemoglobin concentration indicates cell dehydration. In *C*, the left shift of the volume distribution and the broadening of the hemoglobin distribution indicate the presence of both microcytic and dehydrated red cells. (*From Cynober, Mohandas, and Tchernia.*[574] *Used by permission.*)

Ektacytometry. Ektacytometry, described above in the section on HE/HPP, is the best available method to measure the biophysical properties of intact erythrocytes.[584] "Osmotic gradient ektacytometry," a modification of the original technique, is particularly useful in the diagnosis of HS. In this method, the deformability index of the red cell sample is measured as a function of the osmolarity of the suspending medium, which is continuously varied (Fig. 183-22). The osmolality of the suspending medium at which the red cell deformability index reaches a minimum is the same as the osmolarity at which 50 percent of the red cells hemolyze in an osmotic fragility test.[585,586] This value indirectly measures the surface area-to-volume ratio of the red cells. The maximum deformability index of the curve quantitatively reflects the surface area of the red cells.[574] In patients with HS, there is a shift of the curve to right, demonstrating the reduced surface area-to-volume ratio of the cells, and a decline in the height of the curve, reflecting a decrease of the absolute surface area. Even though this technique is only available in a small number of laboratories at present, it provides useful diagnostic information that cannot be obtained otherwise, and deserves greater availability. Cynober and coworkers, for instance, showed that increased osmotic fragility is only detected in 66 percent of nonsplenectomized HS patients, whereas decreased membrane surface area can be demonstrated in all the patients by osmotic gradient ektacytometry.[574]

Membrane Protein Analysis. Cross-transfusion experiments have clearly shown that defects in HS are intrinsic to the red cells.[576,587] Many of the abnormalities formerly described in HS red cells are now believed to be secondary and do not present primary hereditary defects. These include metabolic derangements, alterations in cation transport, abnormal membrane protein phosphorylation, and altered membrane lipid composition.[588] More recent studies have shown that the primary defects in HS lie in the membrane skeleton proteins, as is the case in HE/HPP. However, the pathophysiology differs. HS involves proteins that attach the skeleton to the membrane (ankyrin, protein 4.2, and band 3), while HE/HPP affects the bonds that hold the skeleton together. Spectrin is the only protein that causes both disorders. But the spectrin defects that cause HS lead to spectrin deficiency, while those that cause HE/HPP affect the function of spectrin, especially self-association, as previously discussed. Similarly, the defects in ankyrin, protein 4.2 and band 3 that cause HS are usually associated with absence of the mutant protein rather than a functionally defective mutant.

Combined Spectrin and Ankyrin Deficiency. Using a sensitive radioimmunoassay (RIA), Agre and coworkers first reported that spectrin is deficient in patients with HS.[560,589] The degree of spectrin deficiency correlates closely with the severity of the disease and with the degree of spherocytosis and osmotic fragility. The degree of spectrin deficiency also predicts the patient's status postsplenectomy, as judged by reticulocyte count, haptoglobin level, and hematocrit.[560] Other studies confirm that spectrin deficiency is a prominent feature in most patients with HS, and accounts for the decreased membrane mechanical stability and the loss of surface area associated with the disease (Fig. 183-23).[531,585] However, more recent evidence shows that the spectrin deficiency is usually secondary to other skeletal protein defects.

Coetzer and her colleagues first described two patients with an atypical, severe form of spherocytosis, who were deficient in both spectrin and ankyrin. The clinical picture of these patients was characterized by transfusion-dependent hemolytic anemia, marked spherocytosis, bizarre poikilocytosis, and only a partial response to splenectomy.[567] The authors showed that red cell membranes from the patients were deficient in both spectrin and ankyrin. Each was reduced to about 50 to 60 percent of normal. They studied the synthesis, assembly and turn-over of spectrin and ankyrin in the reticulocytes in one of the patients and found that a defect in ankyrin synthesis was the primary abnormality.

Other studies showed that combined spectrin and ankyrin deficiency is not limited to these atypical patients but is common in patients with typical HS.[23,563] Savvides and coworkers used RIA to measure the spectrin and ankyrin content in 20 kindreds with dominant HS.[23] Spectrin and ankyrin levels were less than the normal range in 75 percent and 80 percent of the kindreds, respectively, and, with one exception, the degree of deficiency of the two proteins in each kindred correlated strictly with each other (Fig. 183-24). Pekrun and coworkers used an enzyme-linked immunosorbent assay (ELISA) to measure the ankyrin and spectrin contents in erythrocytes of 45 patients with typical HS.[563] They found concomitant deficiency of both proteins in all of the patients, and showed that the degree of deficiency is proportional to the clinical severity.

Several surveys have used SDS gel electrophoresis to estimate the relative frequencies of different membrane protein deficiencies in HS.[566,590–592] They found that about 30 to 45 percent of HS patients have combined ankyrin and spectrin deficiency and about 30 percent have isolated spectrin deficiency. However, SDS-PAGE probably underestimates the degree of ankyrin deficiency in many patients, especially compared with RIA or ELISA measurement. Presumably this occurs because ankyrin runs so close to β-spectrin on SDS gels that it is hard to quantitate. No patients with isolated spectrin deficiency were identified among about 80 tested by RIA

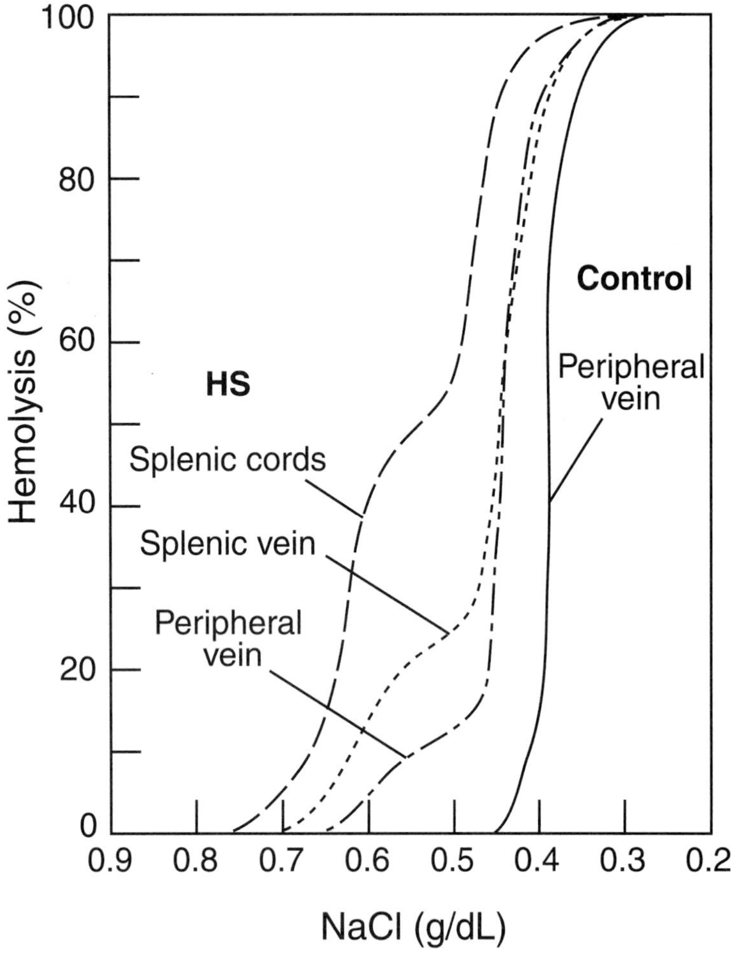

Fig. 183-21 Osmotic fragility in HS. In the osmotic fragility test, red cells are suspended in salt solutions of varying tonicities between isotonic saline (0.9 g/dl NaCl; left) and distilled water (right). Normal red cells swell in hypotonic media and eventually reach a limiting spherical shape, beyond which they hemolyze. Spherocytes, which begin with a lower than normal surface/volume ratio, can swell less before they reach their limiting volume; hence, their osmotic fragility curve is shifted to the left (higher salt concentrations). The spherocytes are said to be osmotically fragile. Before splenectomy, a small proportion of the red cells are extra fragile and produce a tail on the osmotic fragility curve. These cells have been conditioned by the spleen, as shown by their higher concentration in the splenic vein and especially in the splenic cords.[576] (*From Lux and Palek.*[4] *Used by permission.*)

or ELISA.[23,563] A high reticulocyte count may also mask the detection of ankyrin deficiency.[593]

Band 3 Deficiency. Two groups first reported that there are patients with dominant HS who have normal spectrin content in their red cells but have a deficiency in protein band 3 instead.[594,595] These initial observations were confirmed by other reports.[596–598] Estimates suggest that 15 to 25 percent of dominant HS patients have a primary deficiency of band 3.[564,566,591,592] Their red cells contain 20 to 40 percent less band 3 than

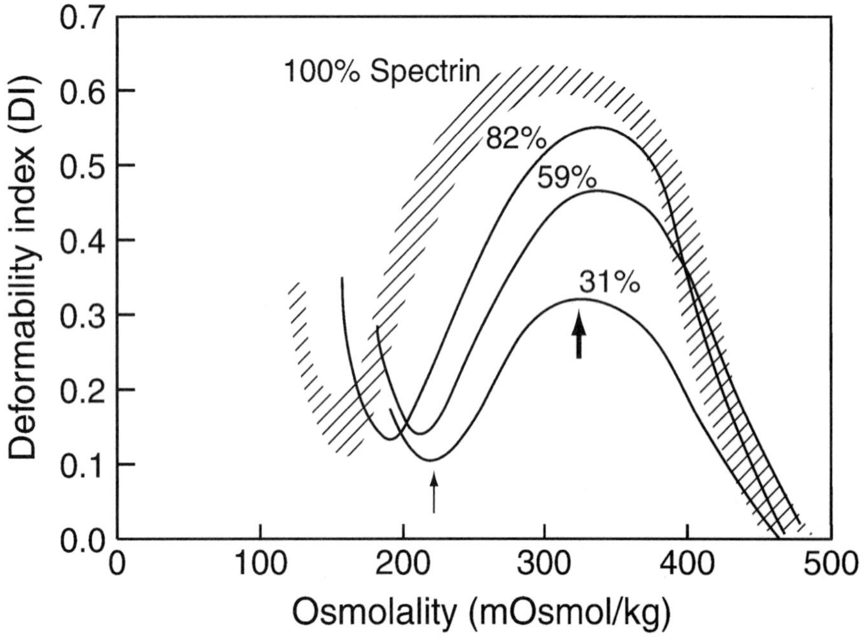

Fig. 183-22 Osmotic gradient ektacytometry of red blood cells with varying degrees of spectrin deficiency. In the spectrin-deficient cells, the minimum deformability index observed in the hypotonic region (thin arrow) is shifted to the right of the control (shaded area), indicating a decrease in the cell surface area-to-volume ratio. The maximum deformability index (DI_{max}) associated with the spectrin-deficient cells (thick arrow) is less than that of control cells, implying reduced surface area. The more pronounced the spectrin deficiency, the greater is the loss of surface area and the lower is the DI_{max}. The osmolality in the hyperosmolar region at which the DI reaches half its maximum value is a measure of the hydration state of the red cells. It is decreased in the patient with the lowest spectrin content, indicating cellular dehydration. (*Adapted from Chasis, Agre, and Mohandas.*[585] *Used by permission.*)

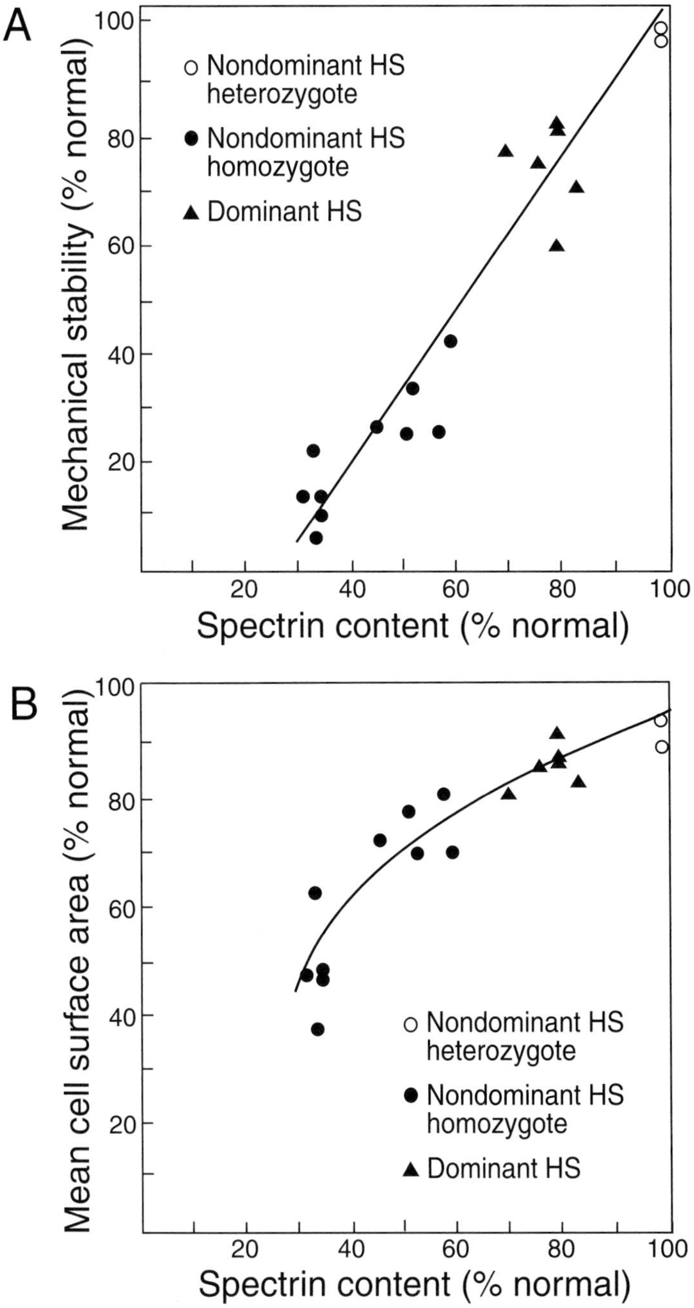

Fig. 183-23 ***A.*** **Membrane spectrin content and mechanical stability. The decrease in membrane mechanical stability is proportional to the decrease in membrane spectrin content as measured by RIA for individuals homozygous (solid circles) or heterozygous (open circles) for nondominant HS. The data for individuals with dominant HS (solid triangles) fall on the same curve in between these two groups.** ***B.*** **Membrane spectrin content and mean cell surface area. The decrease in cell surface area is similarly proportional to the decrease in membrane spectrin content in these groups of patients. (*From Chasis, Agre, and Mohandas.*[585] *Used by permission.*)**

normal.[594–596] These patients appear to form a relatively homogeneous clinical subgroup.[564,566,591,592] They have typical dominant HS with mild to moderate hemolysis, and many nonsplenectomized patients have a small population (0.2 to 2.3 percent) of mushroom-shaped erythrocytes (Fig. 183-19, panel *B*).[565,566]

Protein 4.2 Deficiency. Partial deficiency of protein 4.2 is often seen in patients who have a primary deficiency of ankyrin or band 3, secondary to the underlying defect.[196,592] Protein 4.2 is also absent in a mouse model with targeted deletion of the band 3 gene.[81] Some other HS patients have been described with an isolated deficiency of protein 4.2 in their red cell membranes. They have an apparently recessive disease characterized by moderately severe, splenectomy-responsive hemolytic anemia and complete or nearly complete absence of protein4.2.[570,599–601] The red cell morphology is different from classic HS[599,600] and varies from normal[570] to spherocytes, elliptocytes, or ovalostomatocytes.[571,599,600] Isolated protein 4.2 deficiency is rare in American and European HS patients but is quite common among Japanese.[602]

Molecular Etiology

With the cloning of most of the genes encoding the membrane skeleton proteins in the past several years, many of the molecular defects that cause HS have been identified.

Ankyrin Defects. As discussed above, genetic linkage analyses and cytogenetic evidence first showed that a defect in ankyrin is the primary cause of HS in some families.[196,540] Using a dinucleotide repeat polymorphism in the ankyrin cDNA as a marker to distinguish between the two ankyrin alleles, Jarolim and coworkers showed that one ankyrin allele has reduced expression in a third of HS patients with combined spectrin and ankyrin deficiency.[603] This may be caused by either reduced transcription of one of the ankyrin alleles or instability of its mRNA. By the

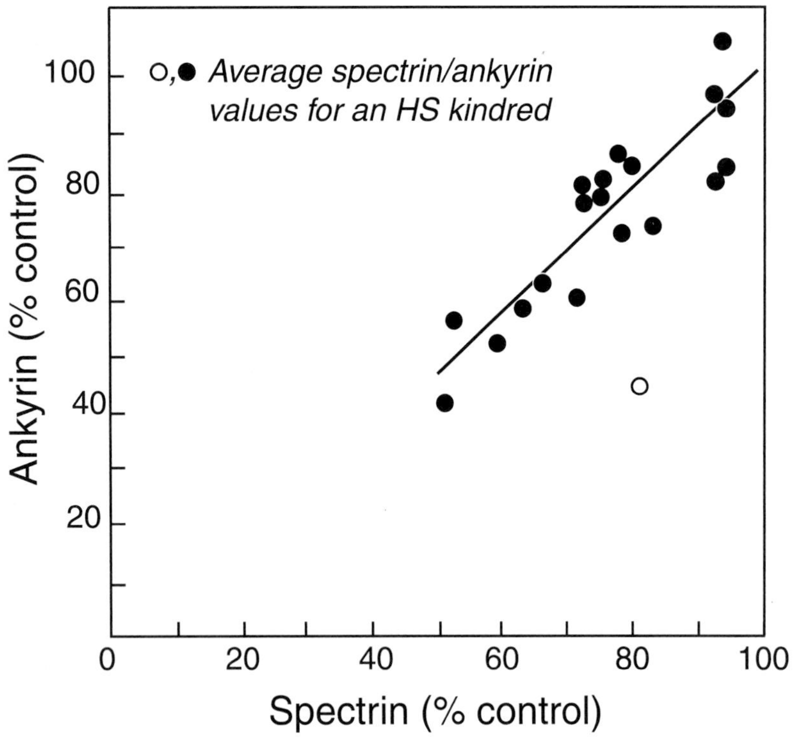

Fig. 183-24 Correlation of spectrin and ankyrin deficiencies in 20 dominant HS kindreds. Each data point represents the mean value for a kindred for both spectrin and ankyrin levels, expressed as a percentage of control. Nineteen kindreds (solid circles) showed very similar degrees of spectrin and ankyrin deficiencies. One otherwise typical HS family (open circle) has marked ankyrin deficiency and a relatively mild spectrin deficit. (*From Savvides, Shalev, John, and Lux.*[23] *Used by permission.*)

same method, it has been shown that *de novo* mutations in one of the ankyrin alleles leading to decreased expression are frequent in HS patients without a positive family history.[532]

Eber et al. examined 46 kindreds with both dominant and recessive spherocytosis and identified 12 different ankyrin mutations in 13 kindreds.[564] Other investigators have reported additional mutations.[604–608] Most of these are family-specific, private mutations. Null mutations (frameshift and nonsense mutations) that result in either unstable ankyrin transcripts or truncated peptides predominate in dominant HS. They are located throughout the ankyrin peptide (Fig. 183-25). One of the more interesting is ankyrin$_{\mathrm{RAKOVNIK}}$, a nonsense mutation within the regulatory domain that leads to selective deficiency of the major ankyrin isoform, band 2.1 (preserving the minor isoform, band 2.2).[613]

All of the ankyrin defects lead to combined and equivalent deficiencies of ankyrin and spectrin. Most of the null mutations are not detectable in reticulocyte mRNA, suggesting instability of the mutant transcript. The clinical manifestations are quite variable and range from mild hemolysis to severe transfusion-dependent anemia.[564] This variability may be explained by different degrees of compensation for the null mutation, either from overproduction of the normal ankyrin allele or diminished ankyrin degradation.

Several ankyrin defects have been identified in patients with recessive HS.[564] These are mostly missense or promoter mutations. A point mutation in the ankyrin promoter, −108T → C, is particularly common and was found in four of seven families with recessive HS. However, so far the mutation has not had a detectable effect on in vitro promoter assays.[614] Two of four families carry a second mutation on the other allele: ankyrins$_{\mathrm{WALSRODE}}$ and $_{\mathrm{BOCHOLT}}$. Ankyrin$_{\mathrm{WALSRODE}}$ contains a missense mutation (V463I) in the band 3 binding domain and has a decreased affinity for band 3.[615] It is present in a patient whose red cells are more deficient in band 3 than in spectrin or ankyrin, which is opposite the trend in other ankyrin defects. Ankyrin$_{\mathrm{BOCHOLT}}$ bears a missense mutation in a rare alternative splice product that may result in aberrant splicing.

HS patients with ankyrin defects have prominent spherocytosis without other morphological defects. Hemolysis and anemia vary from mild to severe.[564,604–607] In general, patients with dominant defects are less affected than those with recessive mutations; however, there is considerable overlap.

Band 3 Defects. Molecular defects have been described in many patients with HS and band 3 deficiency (Fig. 183-26). Conserved arginine residues in band 3 are frequent sites of mutations. Examples include arginines 490, 518, 760 (two mutations found), 808, and 870.[80,564,591] These highly conserved residues are positioned at the internal boundaries of transmembrane segments and substitution probably interferes with co-translational insertion of band 3 into the membranes of the endoplasmic reticulum during synthesis of the protein. In one case, mRNAs for both alleles were present but the mutant band 3 protein was not detected in the membrane, demonstrating either a functional defect in incorporation of the protein into the membrane or instability of the mutant protein.[80] Missense mutations or short in-frame deletions affecting other residues in the transmembrane domain of band 3 have been identified, and presumably also impair insertion of the mutant band 3 into the membrane.[564,566,617,618,624,625,627] A 10 nucleotide duplication near the C-terminal end of band 3$_{\mathrm{PRAGUE}}$ leads to a shift in the reading frame and an altered C-terminus after amino acid 821. This mutation affects the last transmembrane helix and may eliminate the carbonic anhydrase II binding site on band 3.[46] It may also impair insertion of band 3 into the membrane and abolish anion transport function.[626]

Mutations in the cytoplasmic domain of band 3 can interfere with its binding to other membrane skeleton proteins, resulting in a functional defect. A deletion of five amino acids from the ankyrin binding site in band 3$_{\mathrm{NACHOD}}$ presumably disrupts this interaction.[566] An amino acid substitution (Gly → Arg) at residue 130 in the cytoplasmic domain in band 3$_{\mathrm{FUKUOKA}}$ affects protein 4.2 binding.[618] Patients with band 3$_{\mathrm{MONTEFIORE}}$ and $_{\mathrm{TUSCALOOSA}}$ also

Fig. 183-25 Ankyrin mutations associated with HS are shown alongside a schematic representation of the ankyrin peptide. Null mutations, arising from frameshifts or nonsense mutations, are shown in rectangles. Missense and putative promoter mutations are shown in ellipses. The data are compiled from published and unpublished reports.[534,564,604–613]

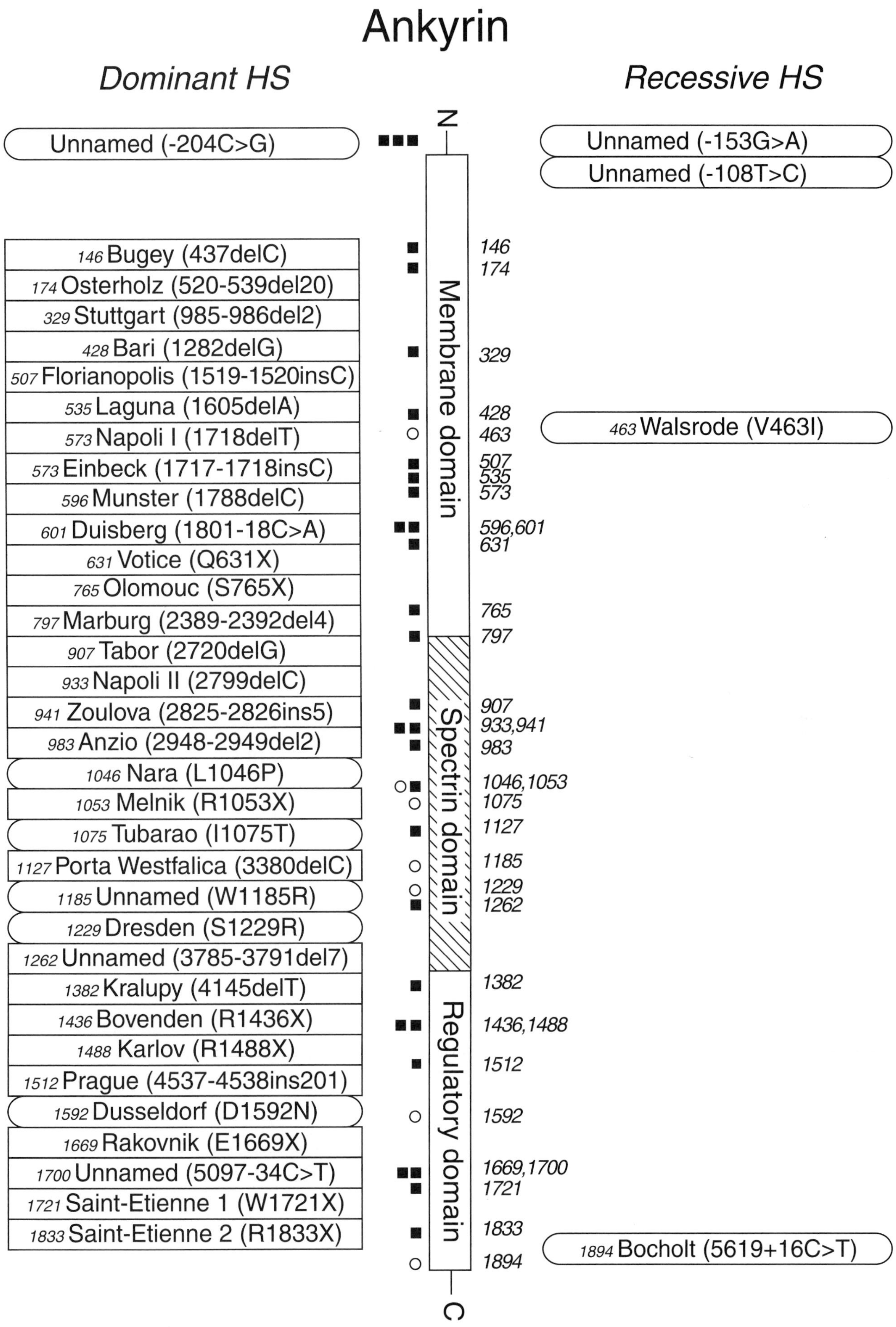
Ankyrin
Dominant HS
Recessive HS
N
C
Membrane domain
Spectrin domain
Regulatory domain
Unnamed (-204C>G)
Unnamed (-153G>A)
Unnamed (-108T>C)
146 Bugey (437delC)
174 Osterholz (520-539del20)
329 Stuttgart (985-986del2)
428 Bari (1282delG)
507 Florianopolis (1519-1520insC)
535 Laguna (1605delA)
573 Napoli I (1718delT)
573 Einbeck (1717-1718insC)
596 Munster (1788delC)
601 Duisberg (1801-18C>A)
631 Votice (Q631X)
765 Olomouc (S765X)
797 Marburg (2389-2392del4)
907 Tabor (2720delG)
933 Napoli II (2799delC)
941 Zoulova (2825-2826ins5)
983 Anzio (2948-2949del2)
1046 Nara (L1046P)
1053 Melnik (R1053X)
1075 Tubarao (I1075T)
1127 Porta Westfalica (3380delC)
1185 Unnamed (W1185R)
1229 Dresden (S1229R)
1262 Unnamed (3785-3791del7)
1382 Kralupy (4145delT)
1436 Bovenden (R1436X)
1488 Karlov (R1488X)
1512 Prague (4537-4538ins201)
1592 Dusseldorf (D1592N)
1669 Rakovnik (E1669X)
1700 Unnamed (5097-34C>T)
1721 Saint-Etienne 1 (W1721X)
1833 Saint-Etienne 2 (R1833X)
463 Walsrode (V463I)
1894 Bocholt (5619+16C>T)
146
174
329
428
463
507
535
573
596,601
631
765
797
907
933,941
983
1046,1053
1075
1127
1185
1229
1262
1382
1436,1488
1512
1592
1669,1700
1721
1833
1894

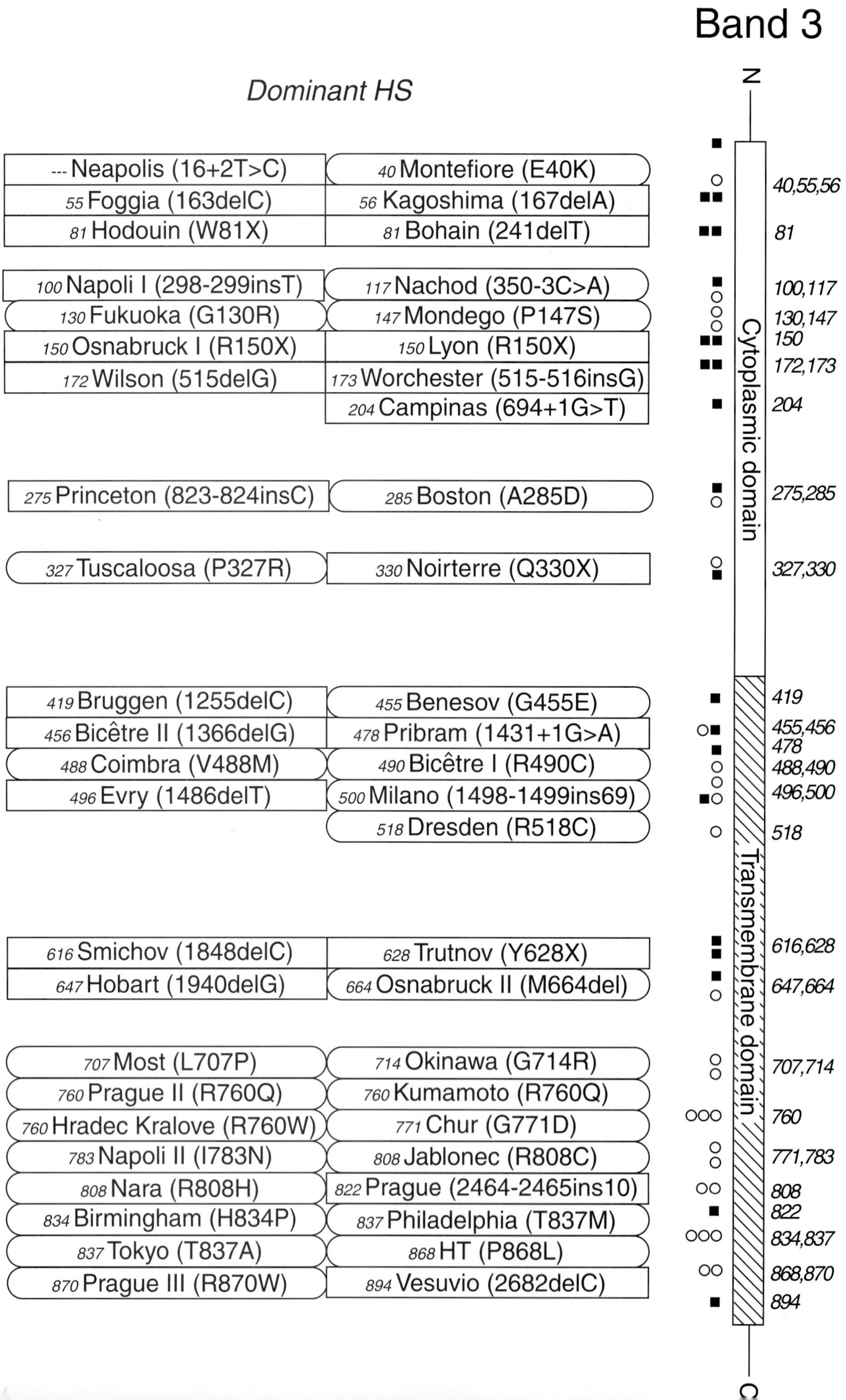

Band 3
Dominant HS
N
C
Cytoplasmic domain
Transmembrane domain
--- Neapolis (16+2T>C)
40 Montefiore (E40K)
55 Foggia (163delC)
56 Kagoshima (167delA)
81 Hodouin (W81X)
81 Bohain (241delT)
100 Napoli I (298-299insT)
117 Nachod (350-3C>A)
130 Fukuoka (G130R)
147 Mondego (P147S)
150 Osnabruck I (R150X)
150 Lyon (R150X)
172 Wilson (515delG)
173 Worchester (515-516insG)
204 Campinas (694+1G>T)
275 Princeton (823-824insC)
285 Boston (A285D)
327 Tuscaloosa (P327R)
330 Noirterre (Q330X)
419 Bruggen (1255delC)
455 Benesov (G455E)
456 Bicêtre II (1366delG)
478 Pribram (1431+1G>A)
488 Coimbra (V488M)
490 Bicêtre I (R490C)
496 Evry (1486delT)
500 Milano (1498-1499ins69)
518 Dresden (R518C)
616 Smichov (1848delC)
628 Trutnov (Y628X)
647 Hobart (1940delG)
664 Osnabruck II (M664del)
707 Most (L707P)
714 Okinawa (G714R)
760 Prague II (R760Q)
760 Kumamoto (R760Q)
760 Hradec Kralove (R760W)
771 Chur (G771D)
783 Napoli II (I783N)
808 Jablonec (R808C)
808 Nara (R808H)
822 Prague (2464-2465ins10)
834 Birmingham (H834P)
837 Philadelphia (T837M)
837 Tokyo (T837A)
868 HT (P868L)
870 Prague III (R870W)
894 Vesuvio (2682delC)
40,55,56
81
100,117
130,147
150
172,173
204
275,285
327,330
419
455,456
478
488,490
496,500
518
616,628
647,664
707,714
760
771,783
808
822
834,837
868,870
894

have spherocytic hemolytic anemia with protein 4.2 deficiency, and missense mutations in the cytoplasmic domain of band 3, at residues 40 and 327, respectively.[188,622]

Null mutations in the band 3 gene also occur. They include nonsense mutations, single nucleotide insertions or deletions, and splicing defects.[529,564,566,591,616,617,621,623] These mutations presumably lead to mRNA instability and protein deficiency.[623]

Distal Renal Tubular Acidosis. Because band 3 functions as an anion exchanger and is expressed in the acid-secreting intercalated cells of the kidney cortical collecting ducts, patients with HS and band 3 deficiency have been tested for a defect in acid-base homeostasis. Two HS patients with Band $3_{PRIBRAM}$ have incomplete distal renal tubular acidosis (RTA)(see Chap. 195),[83] but most other HS patients with band 3 deficiency have no evidence of metabolic acidosis.[83,84] In HS patients with Band $3_{CAMPINAS}$, there is increased basal urinary bicarbonate excretion but efficient urinary acidification.[621] A bovine model of band 3 deficiency exhibits only mild acidosis,[629] and there are no obvious metabolic disturbances in mice that have a targeted deletion of band 3 that eliminates both the red cell and kidney isoform.[81] Band 3 missense mutations have been found in patients with dominant distal renal tubular acidosis, but these patients have no red cell abnormality and the mutations identified are different from those associated with HS.[84,630–632] Mutations affecting Arg 589 are particularly common (8 of 11 families). The mechanism by which these mutations produce RTA is a mystery. The disease does not correlate with the anion transport activity of the band 3 mutants,[84,630] and the one tested mutant (R589H) does not have a dominant negative effect when coexpressed with normal band 3.[84] The best possibility is that the mutant proteins may impair trafficking of band 3.[632]

***β*-Spectrin Defects.** Although spectrin deficiency has long been associated with HS, it is only recently that specific mutations in spectrins have been described as a primary cause of the disorder. Because α-spectrin is normally produced in excess in red cells[132–134] and β-spectrin production is the rate limiting step in the formation of the membrane skeleton, most spectrin mutations found in HS are in the β-spectrin gene.

Monoallelic expression of β-spectrin occurs frequently in HS patients with spectrin deficiency,[533] suggesting that null mutations are common defects. About 13 null mutations have been described in patients with dominant HS. The defects include initiation codon disruption,[633] frameshift and nonsense mutations,[569,634] gene deletions,[635] and splicing defects[461,634] (Fig. 183-27). A 4.6 kb genomic deletion in spectrin_{DURHAM} results in a truncated peptide that is inefficiently incorporated into the red cell.[635] A splice site mutation in $\text{spectrin}_{WINSTON\text{-}SALEM}$ leads to exon skipping and an unstable truncated β-spectrin peptide.[634] A similar defect in $\text{spectrin}_{GUEMENE\text{-}PENFAO}$ causes an intron to be retained and blunts the accumulation of β-spectrin transcripts.[636]

Several missense mutations in the β-spectrin gene have been described in dominant HS.[105,569] In most of these cases, it is not known if the mutations cause a functional defect or destabilize the mRNA or protein. One exception is $\beta\text{-spectrin}_{KISSIMMEE}$, which has been well-characterized on the protein level and is defective in its capacity to bind protein 4.1.[568,639] Heterozygotes have two types of spectrin. The abnormal fraction, approximately 40 percent, cannot bind protein 4.1 and therefore binds weakly to actin.[568,639] Peptide mapping shows the defect resides near the N-terminus of the β-spectrin chain,[639] near the site where protein 4.1 binds.[102,103,640] The mutant spectrin is unstable and susceptible to thiol oxidation.[639] This either causes or exacerbates the defect in binding to protein 4.1, because chemical reduction almost completely restores normal binding activity.[639] Interestingly, very mild oxidation of normal spectrin[641] or storage of normal cells under aerobic conditions in the blood bank[642] produces similar defects in spectrin-4.1 interactions. Patients with the spectrin-4.1 binding defect have only 80 percent of normal red cell spectrin,[639] which may be the real explanation of why they have spherocytosis. Presumably, the defective spectrin detaches from the membrane more easily than normal and falls prey to proteases that specifically degrade unbound or oxidized spectrin chains.[459,643] Loss of the abnormal spectrin explains why the ratio of normal to abnormal spectrin is 60:40 instead of the expected 50:50.

Molecular analysis shows a Trp to Arg substitution at position 202 of the β-spectrin cDNA in the three affected members of one of these kindreds[105] but not in the other two described kindreds with a similar functional defect.[644] The mutation inserts a positively charged amino acid in a highly conserved region of largely hydrophobic amino acid sequence and could thus disrupt a region that is critical for protein 4.1 binding. Two other mutations, $\text{spectrins}_{ATLANTA}$ and $_{OAKLAND}$, have missense mutations at positions 182 and 220 of the β-spectrin cDNA, flanking the position of the $\text{spectrin}_{KISSIMMEE}$ mutation. These mutations may potentially also cause defective protein 4.1 binding, but this hypothesis has not been tested.

A mutation in β-spectrin has only been identified in one case of recessive HS. A point mutation in position 1684 of the β-spectrin chain in $\text{spectrin}_{BIRMINGHAM}$ changes an arginine to cystine.[569] There presumably is another mutation in the second allele to account for the recessive nature of the disease, but it has not been found.

***α*-Spectrin Defects.** As discussed above, α-spectrin is normally synthesized in excess (three- to fourfold).[645] Defective α-spectrin production in one allele is not expected to cause disease. It is therefore not surprising that α-spectrin defects have not been described in patients with dominant HS.

Defects in α-spectrin have been implicated in a subset of patients with a life-threatening form of nondominant HS associated with marked spectrin deficiency (25 to 50 percent of normal).[535] Many, but not all, of these families carry a variant α-spectrin peptide, designated αIIa or $\alpha\text{-spectrin}_{BUGHILL}$.[646] It bears an amino acid substitution, alanine to asparagine, at residue 309 of the α-spectrin chain.[647] Peptide analysis of the α-spectrin peptides from the affected HS patients shows only the αIIa variant, but genomic DNA analysis reveals both an allele with the αIIa/α-$\text{spectrin}_{BUGHILL}$ mutation and one without, indicating that the second α-spectrin allele in these patients may be functionally silent.[647] A candidate gene for this silent mutation was discovered in a family with severe, nondominant HS.[536] One of alleles, designated $\alpha\text{spectrin}_{PRAGUE}$, has a mutation in the penultimate position of intron 36, leading to skipping of exon 37 and premature termination of the α-spectrin peptide (Fig. 183-28). The other α-spectrin allele has a partial splicing abnormality in intron 30, and produces only about one-sixth of the normal amount of α-spectrin. This low-expression allele, named $\alpha\text{-spectrin}_{LEPRA}$ (low-expression allele Prague), is linked to the αIIa/$\alpha\text{-spectrin}_{BUGHILL}$ variant in this patient and several other patients with nondominant HS.[648] The interaction of $\alpha\text{-spectrin}^{LEPRA}$ and an α-spectrin allele encoding a nonfunctional peptide may be a frequent cause of severe nondominant HS.

Protein 4.2 Defects. The molecular etiology of protein 4.2 deficiency has been defined in several cases. The most common mutation is protein 4.2_{NIPPON} (Ala 142 → Thr) (Fig. 183-29).[599,651] It affects the processing of 4.2 mRNA, so that red cells contain only traces of the 72/74-kDa isoforms of protein 4.2 instead of the usual abundant 72-kDa species. This mutation is

Fig. 183-26 Band 3 mutations associated with HS are shown alongside a schematic representation of the band 3 peptide. Null mutations arising from either frameshift or nonsense mutations are shown in rectangles, as is a mutation associated with loss of the translation start site (band $3_{NEAPOLIS}$). Missense mutations or short in-frame deletions or insertions are shown in ellipses. The data are compiled from published and unpublished reports.[80,85,188,529,564,566,591,616–628]

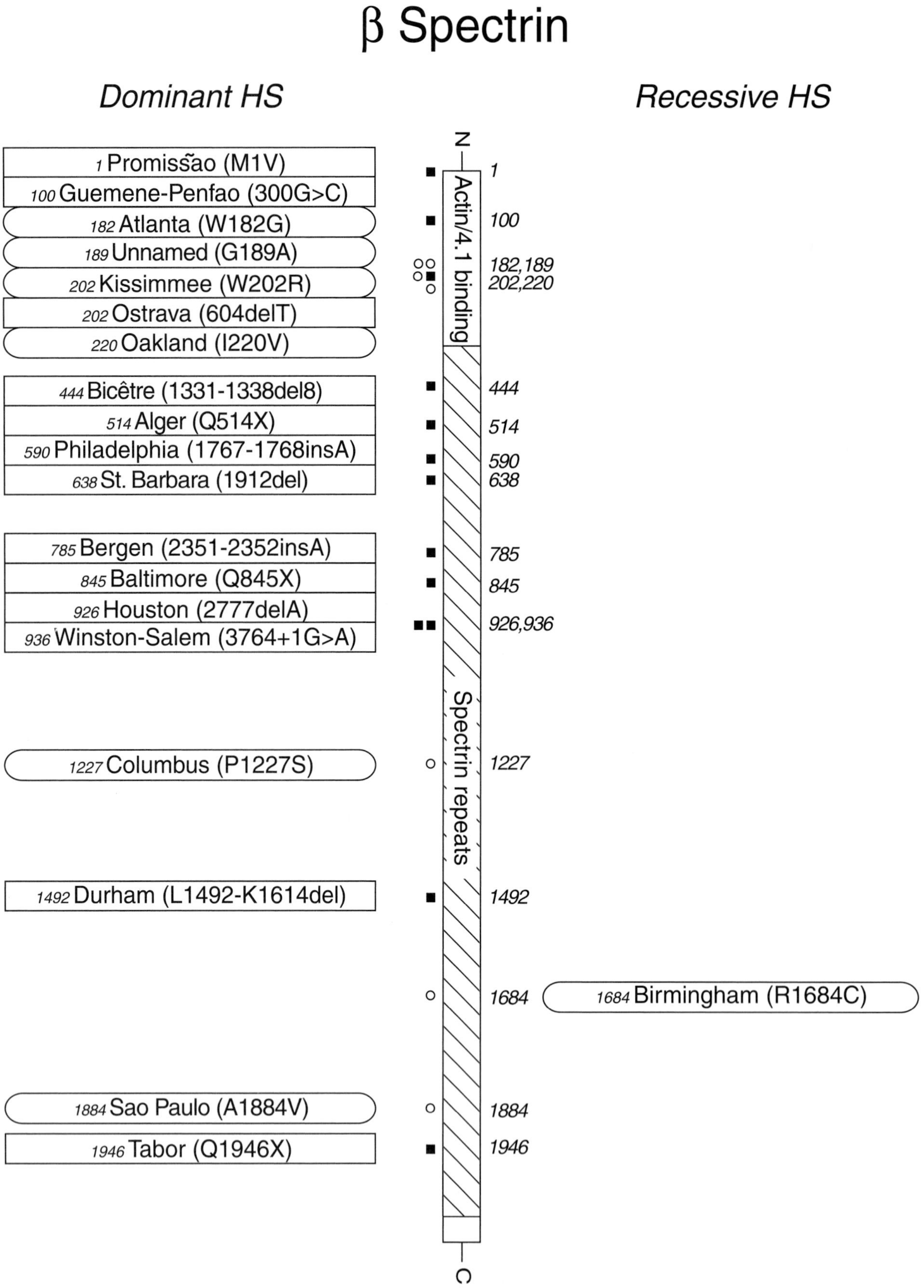

Fig. 183-27 *β*-Spectrin mutations associated with HS are shown alongside a schematic representation of the *β*-spectrin peptide. Null mutations, arising from frameshifts, nonsense mutations, large deletions, or substitution of the initiation codon, are shown in rectangles. Missense mutations are shown in ellipses. The data are compiled from published and unpublished reports.[105,569,633–638]

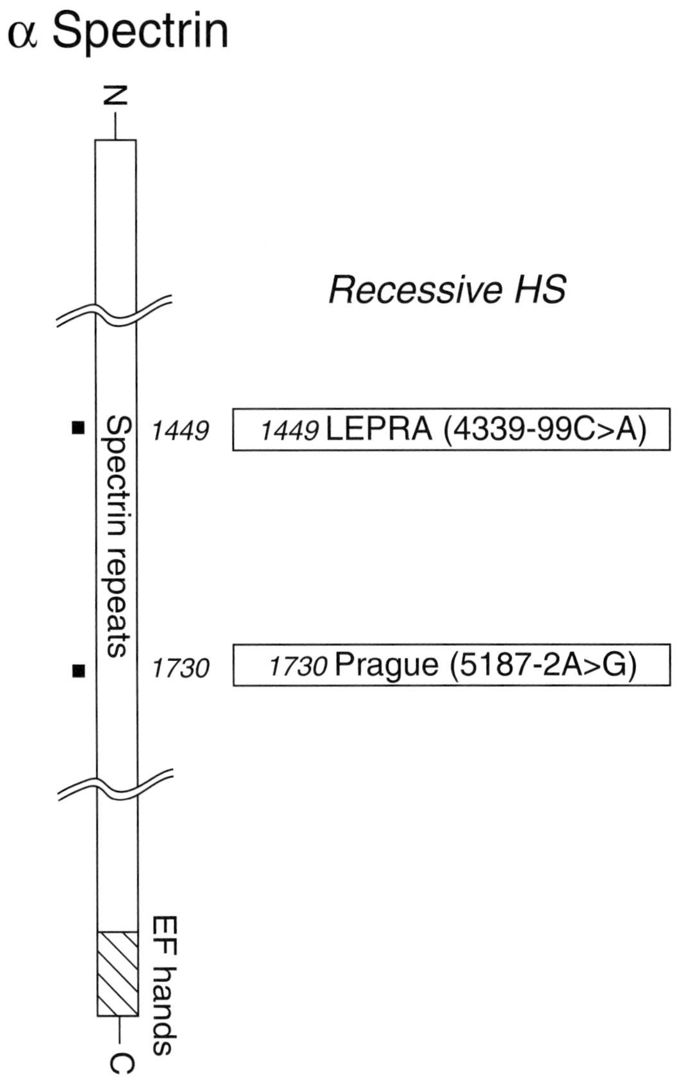

Fig. 183-28 Two α-spectrin mutations associated with recessive HS are shown alongside a schematic representation of the α-spectrin peptide.[536]

very common in Japanese HS patients. It is homozygous in some patients[651,655] or compound heterozygous with a second mutant allele such as protein $4.2_{FUKUOKA,\ NOTAME}$ or $_{SHIGA}$.[650,652,654] Band $4.2_{KOMATSU}$ contains an amino acid substitution in codon 175 that causes a moderate hemolytic anemia with ovalostomatocytosis and increased osmotic fragility in the homozygous state.[571]

The only two protein 4.2 mutations reported outside the Japanese population are protein4.2_{TOZEUR} and protein 4.2_{LISBOA}, found in homozygous form in Tunisian and Portuguese patients, respectively.[649,653] In protein 4.2_{TOZEUR},[570,653] the propositus and her sister had a chronic hemolytic anemia and no protein 4.2 in their red cells. Molecular analysis showed a missense mutation in codon 310, in a region that is conserved in protein 4.2 and other members of the transglutaminase family. A recombinant protein bearing the mutation was abnormally sensitive to proteolysis, which may explain the absence of protein 4.2 in the patients' erythrocytes. In protein 4.2_{LISBOA},[649] a single nucleotide deletion at nucleotide 264 of the cDNA causes a frameshift mutation and premature termination of the peptide. The heterozygous parents are clinically asymptomatic. The proband presented with a hemolytic anemia and splenomegaly at the age of 20. Peripheral blood films showed only a few spherocytes. Her symptoms improved markedly after splenomegaly.

Relative Frequency of Defects. Based on results of both protein and molecular studies, it is estimated that, in Caucasian populations, about 50 percent of HS defects are found in ankyrin, 20 percent are in band 3, 25 percent are in β-spectrin, and 5 percent are in α-spectrin and protein 4.2. Among Japanese, band 3 and protein 4.2 defects are much more prevalent.

Animal Models. The availability of several well-characterized mouse models has contributed to our understanding of the pathophysiology of HS. Six types of hereditary hemolytic anemia have been identified in the common house mouse, *Mus musculus*.[656] These anemias resemble human hereditary spherocytosis and are designated *ja/ja* (jaundice), *sph/sph* (spherocytosis), sph^{ha}/sph^{ha} (hemolytic anemia), sph^{2BC}/sph^{2BC}, sph^{1J}/sph^{1J}, sph^{2J}/sph^{2J}, *sph-Dem/sph-Dem*, and *nb/nb* (normoblastosis). The nomenclature indicates that anemia is observed only in the homozygous state and that the six mutants represent three loci: *ja, sph*, and *nb*. All of the mutants have severe hemolysis, with reticulocyte counts >70 percent, along with marked spherocytosis, jaundice, bilirubin gallstones, and massive hepatosplenomegaly. The defects are autosomal recessive, and the homozygotes have drastically impaired viability.[133,657] There is a similar but much milder condition in the deer mouse, *Peromyscus maniculatus*, designated *sp/sp*.[658] The mice have mild (≈20 percent) spectrin deficiency[659] and a phenotype that resembles typical human HS.

Spectrin Mutants. Studies of the Mus mutants have revealed abnormalities in the erythrocyte membrane skeleton. The *ja/ja*

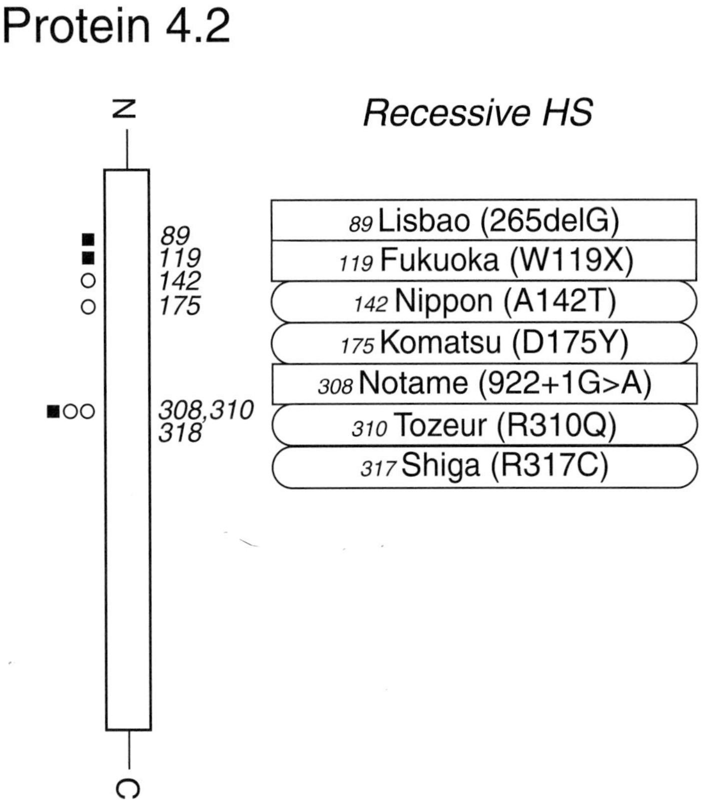

Fig. 183-29 4.2 mutations associated with recessive HS are shown alongside a schematic representation of the peptide. Null mutations, arising from frameshifts or nonsense mutations are shown in rectangles. Missense mutations are shown in ellipses. The data are compiled from published reports.[571,649–654]

mutant has no detectable spectrin. The mice carry a nonsense mutation in the β-spectrin gene[660] and lack the ability to produce stable β chains.[133]

The *sph/sph* variants lack α-spectrin but have small amounts of β-spectrin. They have defects in α-spectrin synthesis, function, and/or stability.[133] The *sph* and *sph*^{2BC} alleles are frameshift mutations and null alleles.[661] In contrast, *sph*^{1J}/*sph*^{1J} mice synthesize normal amounts of spectrin mRNA and protein, however, the protein is not stably incorporated into the membrane skeleton. Surprisingly, the *sph*^{1J} allele contains a nonsense mutation near the C-terminus that deletes the last 13 amino acids from the protein. Apparently these amino acids, in the EF hand region at the spectrin tail (Fig. 183-4), are functionally important in attaching spectrin to actin. The *sph-Dem/sph-Dem* mutation arose spontaneously in CeS3/Dem strain and is missing exon 11 and 46 amino acids from spectrin repeat 5. The mice have both spherocytes and elliptocytes, and some poikilocytes, and are a mixture of HS and HPP.[662]

Cardiac thrombi, fibrotic lesions, and renal hemochromatosis are found in *ja/ja* and *sph/sph* mice in adulthood.[663] Transplantation of hematopoietic cells from *sph/sph* mice are sufficient to induce thrombotic events in the recipients.[664] One possibility is that the membrane vesicles released from the very unstable mouse red cells expose phosphatidyl serine on their outer surface, which would be very thrombogenic.[665]

Ankyrin Mutants. The *nb/nb* mice have 50 to 70 percent of the normal quantity of spectrin and no ankyrin.[657] They have normal spectrin synthesis[133] but are moderately spectrin deficient because their ankyrin is very unstable. The *nb* mutation maps to the Ank-1 locus, indicating a primary ankyrin defect.[155,659] The specific defect has not been identified. Interestingly, fetal *nb/nb* mice have normal reticulocyte counts[666] and no anemia at birth, apparently due to expression of Ank-1-related (165-kDa) and Ank-2-related (155-kDa) proteins in utero.[667]

The *nb/nb* mice develop ataxia when they reached maturity, due to loss of cerebellar Purkinje cells.[668] Ank-1 protein is markedly reduced in the Purkinje cells, which may explain their fragility. The significance of these findings and their relationship to human HS is unknown.

Band 3. New mouse mutants with defects in membrane skeleton proteins have been generated by targeted mutagenesis in embryonic stem (ES) cells. Mice completely deficient in band 3 survive gestation but tend to die in the neonatal period,[81] often from thrombotic complications.[669] Those that survive have a severe spherocytic hemolytic anemia, closely resembling severe HS in humans. The mice have undetectable amounts of protein 4.2 and glycophorin A,[52,81] but have normal amounts of spectrin, actin, and protein 4.1 in their red cell membrane skeletons, and normal membrane skeleton architecture by electron microscopy.[81] Despite their normal skeletons, the band 3 deficient red cells shed astonishing amounts of membrane surface in small vesicles and long tubules. These observations indicates that band 3 is, surprisingly, not required for membrane skeleton assembly, but has a critical function in stabilizing membrane lipids. Loss of this function may be critical to the pathogenesis of HS.

These mice also provide an unexpected clue about the genetic control of reticulocyte response to anemia. The first two generations of the band 3 knockout mice, in a C57BL/6J and 129/Sv (B6/129) hybrid genetic background, had over 70 percent reticulocytes, but later generations of the mice, outcrossed to other genetic backgrounds, show a striking decrease in reticulocytosis and survival.[670] A newly discovered mouse mutant (*wan*) in a C3H/HeJ background that has a null defect in the band 3 gene also has severe anemia without reticulocytosis. But when the *wan/wan* mice are crossed with the band 3 gene knock-out mice in the B6/129 background, there is an elevation of reticulocytes to over 65 percent.[670] These observations suggest that a genetic modifier segregating in the B6/129 background controls a strong reticulocyte response in the absence of band 3. Understanding this modifier will provide important insight into the role of band 3 in the late stages of erythroid differentiation and reticulocyte formation.

In addition to mouse models, there is a recessive form of HS in cattle with moderate hemolytic anemia and complete deficiency of band 3, due to a nonsense mutation at codon 646.[629] The cattle, like band 3 deficient mice, have defective anion transport, lack protein 4.2, and have reduced numbers of intramembrane particles by electron microscopy.

Protein 4.2. The absence of protein 4.2 is not responsible for the severe phenotype observed in band 3 knockout mice, because mice with a targeted deletion of the protein 4.2 gene survive normally and have only a mild spherocytic hemolytic anemia.[193] Surprisingly, however, cation transport pathways are markedly disturbed. In homozygotes, the maximal rate of $Na^+/K^+/Cl^-$ co-transport is increased seven- to eightfold, Na^+/H^+ exchange is increased up to fiftyfold, K^+/Cl^- co-transport is increased by two- to threefold, and K^+ transport via the Gardos channel is enhanced three- to fourfold. In contrast Na^+/K^+-ATPase activity is normal. The data suggest that protein 4.2 directly or indirectly suppresses the activities of these transporters, a function of the protein that was previously unknown.

Protein 4.1. Mice lacking erythrocyte protein 4.1 (protein 4.1R) have also been generated by gene targeting.[671] Homozygotes have mild to moderate hemolysis with increased fragmentation and decreased red cell membrane stability. In addition to the total absence of protein 4.1, there are reduced levels of protein p55 and glycophorin C. There is also partial deficiency in ankyrin and spectrin, suggesting that loss of protein 4.1 compromises membrane skeleton assembly. Erythrocyte morphology shows spherocytosis instead of elliptocytosis, probably related to the spectrin deficiency. Interestingly, these mice also have neurological deficits in movement, coordination, and learning, presumably because neuronal isoforms of erythroid protein 4.1 are also disrupted.[437]

β-Adducin. Mice deficient in β-adducin, due to a targeted gene deletion, have recently been described.[271] The mice have a mild hemolytic anemia characterized by spherocytes, spherostomatocytes, and rounded elliptocytes, and a partial deficiency of α-adducin, indicating that β-adducin is also necessary for the synthesis or stability of its partners, and that adducin is needed for the maintenance of normal red cell surface area. This is an original observation, as no human patient deficient in adducin has yet been described.

Pathophysiology

Irrespective of its molecular cause, the major problem of the hereditary spherocyte is the rheologic consequences of its decreased surface-to-volume ratio. The red cell membrane is very flexible, but it can expand its surface area only about 3 percent before rupturing.[672] The loss of surface area and decreased deformability of the spherocyte causes it to be trapped in the hostile environment of the splenic cords, leading to its early demise.

Loss of Membrane Surface. As discussed above, molecular defects in HS appear to disrupt components of the membrane skeleton that are responsible for attaching the skeleton to the lipid bilayer. How this results in membrane loss is not entirely clear. Two hypotheses have been advanced (Fig. 183-30). In the first, the lipid bilayer and integral membrane proteins are directly stabilized by their interaction with ankyrin or the spectrin skeleton. Deficiency in spectrin or ankyrin would result in the lack of skeletal support in some areas of the membrane, which would then bud off and be lost. In the second hypothesis, membrane surface area is stabilized by interactions of band 3 with neighboring lipids. In band 3 deficiency, more of the lipids lack this interaction and are lost, while in spectrin or ankyrin deficiency, band 3 molecules would more rapidly diffuse and might transiently cluster, with the same consequences.

In spectrin-deficient red cells, the force required to fragment HS membranes is diminished and proportional to the density of spectrin. Cell surface area and membrane stability are proportional to red cell spectrin content and are reduced in HS erythrocytes (Fig. 183-23).[585] This may explain why spectrin-deficient spherocytes fail to withstand circulatory stresses and become trapped in the spleen.

Splenic Trapping. In the spleen most of the arterial blood empties directly into the splenic cords, a narrow, honeycombed

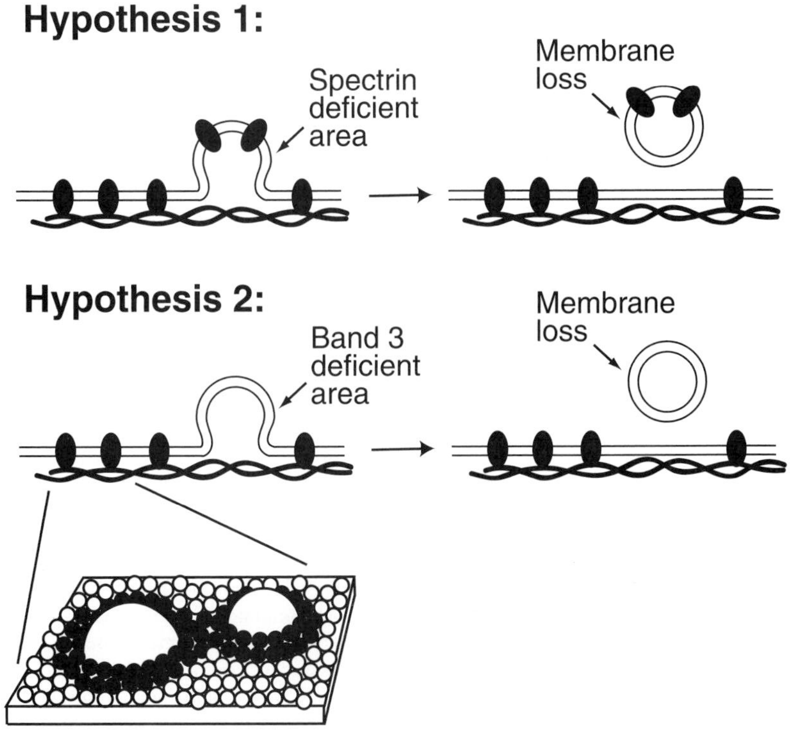

Fig. 183-30 Two hypotheses concerning the mechanism of membrane loss in HS. Hypothesis 1 assumes that the lipid bilayer and integral membrane proteins are directly stabilized by interactions with the spectrin membrane skeleton. Spectrin-deficient areas, lacking support, bud off, leading to spherocytosis. Hypothesis 2 assumes that the membrane is stabilized by interactions of band 3 with neighboring lipids. The influence of band 3 extends into the lipid milieu because the first layer of immobilized lipids slows the lipids in the next layer, and so on. In band 3-deficient cells, the area between lipid molecules increases and unsupported lipids are lost. Spectrin-ankyrin deficiency allows band 3 molecules to diffuse and transiently cluster, with the same consequences. (*From Lux and Palek.*[4] *Used by permission.*)

maze of passages formed by reticular cells and phagocytes.[673–675] If flow through these passages is impeded, red cells are diverted deeper into the labyrinthine portions of the cords, where blood flow is slow and the cells may be detained for minutes to hours. To exit and return to the venous circulation, red cells must squeeze between the endothelial cells that form the walls of the venous sinusoids. Even when maximally distended, these narrow, elliptical fenestrations are much smaller than red cells, which must undergo considerable contortion during their passage.[674,675]

It is clear that spherocytic red cells are significantly hindered at this point in the circulation. Isolated hereditary spherocytes are poorly deformable and pass through 3- to 5-mm filters with difficulty, sometimes bursting in the process.[676] HS red cells are trapped in the cords during in vitro perfusion through spleens removed from patients with idiopathic thrombocytopenic purpura,[677] and ^{51}Cr-labeled spherocytes are selectively sequestered in the spleen in vivo.[678,679] HS spleens characteristically show massively congested cords and relatively empty venous sinuses on light microscopy,[673,680] and electron microscopy shows relatively few spherocytes traversing the sinus wall,[673,680] in contrast to normal spleens, where such cells are easily found.[674]

Although it was known as early as 1913 that red cells obtained from the splenic vein were more osmotically fragile than those in the peripheral circulation,[681] the significance of this observation was not fully appreciated until the classic studies of Emerson[576] and Young[677] and their colleagues. These investigators showed that osmotically fragile microspherocytes are concentrated in the splenic pulp. After splenectomy the tail of hyperfragile cells in the osmotic fragility curve disappears, although the major population of moderately fragile spherocytes persists.[576,677] These results led to the conclusion that the spleen detains and conditions circulating HS red cells in a way that increases their spheroidicity, aggravates loss of their membranes and hastens their demise.[576,677] The kinetics of this process of "splenic conditioning" were beautifully illustrated in vivo by Griggs and his coworkers,[679] who showed that a cohort of ^{59}Fe-labeled HS red cells gradually shifted from the major, less fragile population to the minor, more fragile population during their circulation in vivo.

Splenic Conditioning. The mechanism of splenic conditioning is less clear. It is difficult to obtain precise information about the environment in the splenic cords, but existing data suggest that the climate is inhospitable. Arteries supplying the white pulp skim off plasma and increase congestion in the cords, where the crowded red cells must compete with metabolically voracious phagocytes for limited supplies of glucose. Because of the stagnant circulation, lactic acid accumulates and extracellular pH falls, probably to between 6.5 and 7.0.[576] Intracellular pH must also decline, inhibiting rate limiting enzymes of glycolysis and retarding glucose utilization. Under these conditions stores of 2,3-DPG will be metabolized to provide energy for the cell. The loss of this polyvalent anion, combined with the decreased anionic charge on hemoglobin that occurs in an acid environment, is compensated by the entry of monovalent chloride ions. The resulting increase in osmolarity causes water to enter the HS red cell and worsen its already compromising spheroidicity. Thus, the spherocyte, detained in the splenic cords because of its surface deficiency, is severely stressed by erythrostasis in a metabolically threatening environment.

In summary, it is clear that HS red cells are selectively detained by the spleen during their passages through that organ, leading to a progressive loss of membrane surface, further splenic trapping, and eventual destruction (Fig. 183-31). Indeed, studies have shown that the mean splenic transit time correlates inversely ($r = -0.96$) with red cell survival in HS.[683]

Clinical Management

Diagnosis. The diagnosis of HS is usually easy if there are typical laboratory findings of spherocytosis, Coombs-negative hemolysis, increased osmotic fragility, and a positive family history. There are several situations in which the diagnosis can be more difficult.

In the neonatal period it may be hard to differentiate HS from ABO incompatibility since microspherocytosis is prominent in both conditions and the Coombs' test is frequently negative in ABO disease.[684] Fortunately, in most affected infants with ABO incompatibility, anti-A (or anti-B) antibodies can be eluted from the red cells, and free anti-A or anti-B IgG antibodies can be detected in the infant's serum. Occasionally, older patients with immunohemolytic anemias and spherocytosis also have so few antibody molecules attached to their red cells that the Coombs' test is negative and differentiation of the disease from HS is possible only with the use of radioactive antiglobulin reagents.[685]

Diagnostic difficulties also arise in patients who present during an aplastic crisis (see below). Early in the crisis the acute nature of the symptoms may suggest an acquired process, and the absence of reticulocytes may divert the physician from a diagnosis of hemolytic anemia. Later, as marrow function returns, the physician may be misled by the fact that the emerging young HS red cells are initially less spherocytic and osmotically fragile than usual[686] and acquire their typical microspherocytic form only with age and reticuloendothelial conditioning. If a transfusion has been given, the transfused red cells can also make diagnosis of the underlying HS disease difficult until they are cleared.

HS may also be camouflaged by association with disorders that increase the surface-to-volume ratio of the red cells, such as iron deficiency[687] or obstructive jaundice.[688] Iron deficiency corrects the abnormal shape and fragility of hereditary spherocytes but does not improve their life span,[687] whereas obstructive jaundice improves both shape and survival.[688] The clinical expression of HS may also be modulated by interaction with other hematologic disorders. Coinheritance of HS and β- or α-thalassemia trait, appears to cause a milder disease in some families,[598,689,690] whereas the presence of glucose 6-phosphate dehydrogenase deficiency and HS in the same patient may result in a more severe hemolytic anemia.[691] A patient with Hb SC disease, α-thalassemia trait and HS presented with recurrent acute splenic sequestration crisis, probably because of splenic trapping and intrasplenic sickling of the spherocytic erythrocytes.[692] HS patients with coexisting sickle cell trait may also experience life-threatening acute splenic sequestration crisis.[693] Fortunately, HS is relatively rare in African populations, so these dangerous combinations do not often occur.

Crises. Patients with HS, like patients with other hemolytic processes, are subject to various crises.

Hemolytic Crises. Mild hemolytic crises are probably most frequent and are usually triggered by common viral syndromes,[547] especially in children. They are characterized by a mild, transient increase in jaundice, splenomegaly, anemia, and reticulocyte count. Severe hemolytic crises[558] are less common. Hemolysis can also be aggravated during pregnancy.[550,551] For most patients with a hemolytic crisis, supportive care is all that is needed; red cell transfusions are rarely required. Corticosteroids can be beneficial during episodes of acute hemolysis,[694] but are generally not indicated.

Aplastic Crises. Aplastic crises occur less frequently than hemolytic crises but are more serious, as severe anemia and even death can result.[521,558] They typically present with fever, vomiting, abdominal pain, arthralgias, headache, pallor, and symptoms of anemia.[695] Sometimes multiple family members are affected simultaneously.[696] During the aplastic phase, the hematocrit level and reticulocyte count fall, marrow erythroblasts disappear, and unused iron accumulates in the serum. Mild granulocytopenia and thrombocytopenia are common but are not invariably present. Because production of new HS red cells is halted, the cells that remain age, and microspherocytosis and osmotic fragility increase.[697] The bilirubin level declines because

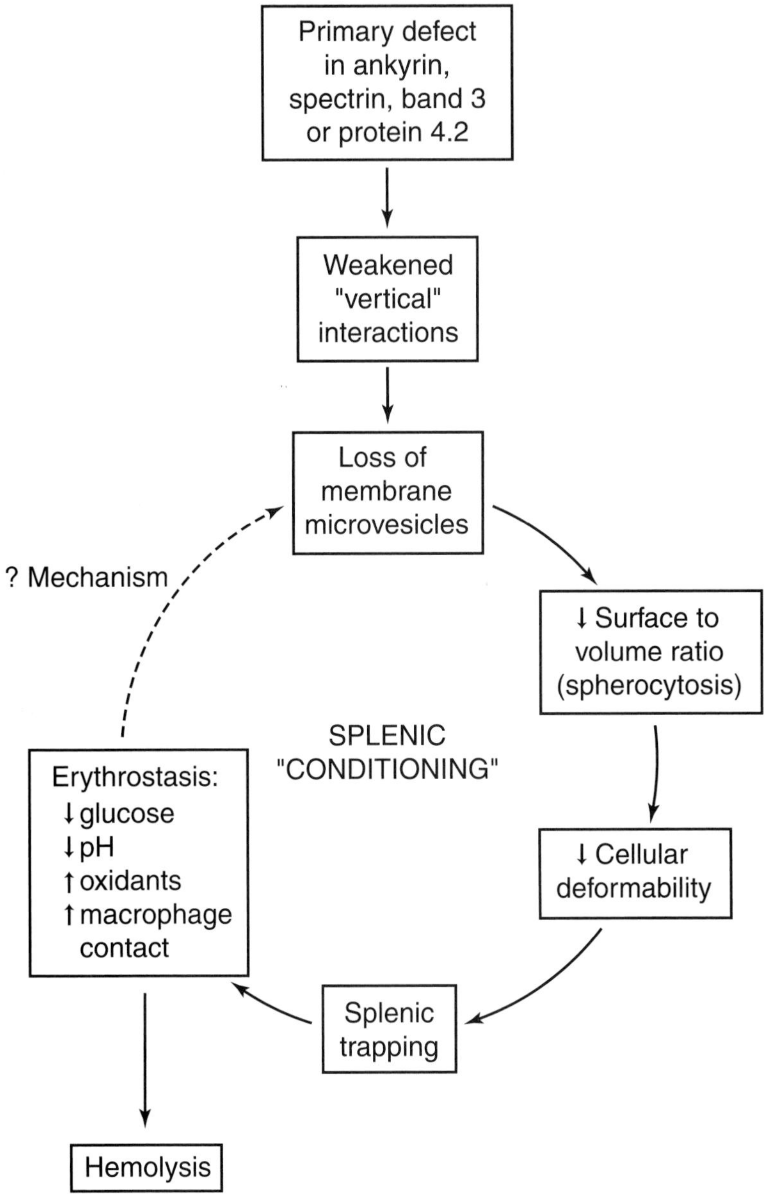

Fig. 183-31 Pathophysiology of the splenic conditioning and destruction of hereditary spherocytes. (*Adapted from Becker and Lux.*[682] *Used by permission.*)

of a decrease in the number of abnormal red cells that have to be destroyed. Because the usual aplastic crisis lasts 10 to 14 days (about half the life span of HS red cells), the hemoglobin concentration typically falls to about half its usual value before recovery ensues. The return of marrow function is heralded by a fall in serum iron concentration, a rise in granulocytes and platelets to normal levels, and reticulocytosis.[695]

It is now known that aplastic crises in HS patients are caused by infection with the human parvovirus B19.[698,699] The B19 parvovirus causes erythema infectiosum or "fifth disease" in small children, and fever, rash, and polyarthropathy in older children and adults. The virus infects and kills early erythroid precursors[700] and drastically impairs red cell production, resulting in aplastic crises in patients who have erythrocytes with a shortened life span, as in HS patients. Occasionally, parvovirus infection can also cause pancytopenia, hemophagocytosis, myelodysplasia, or even autoimmune disorders in HS patients.[701–704] It is not uncommon for an aplastic crisis to be the first sign of HS in previously well-compensated patients.[705,706] Multiple HS members in a family often come down with aplastic crises at the same time because of the infectious nature of the causative agent.[696,707] The infection is diagnosed by immunologic tests or by the polymerase chain reaction. Examination of the bone marrow shows loss of erythroblasts beyond the pronormoblast stage, and, in some cases, characteristic giant pronormoblasts with cytoplasmic vacuoles.

Treatment is supportive until the aplastic episode is over, which usually lasts seven to ten days. Red cell transfusions may be necessary if the anemia is severe. Intravenous immunoglobulin helps clear persistent parvovirus infection in immunocompromised patients but is not necessary for most HS patients. Persons with erythema infectiosum are infectious before the onset of illness and not infectious once the rash appears, but patients in aplastic crisis are contagious from before the onset of symptoms to at least a week afterward.[708] HS patients should avoid exposure to affected family members during this period. Droplets and contact precautions to prevent spread of parvovirus through respiratory secretions are necessary.[708] A parvovirus vaccine is currently undergoing phase I trials and may be available in the future for patients with HS.

Megaloblastic Crises. Megaloblastic crises are rare. They result when the dietary intake of folic acid is insufficient for the increased needs of the erythroid HS bone marrow. The risk is

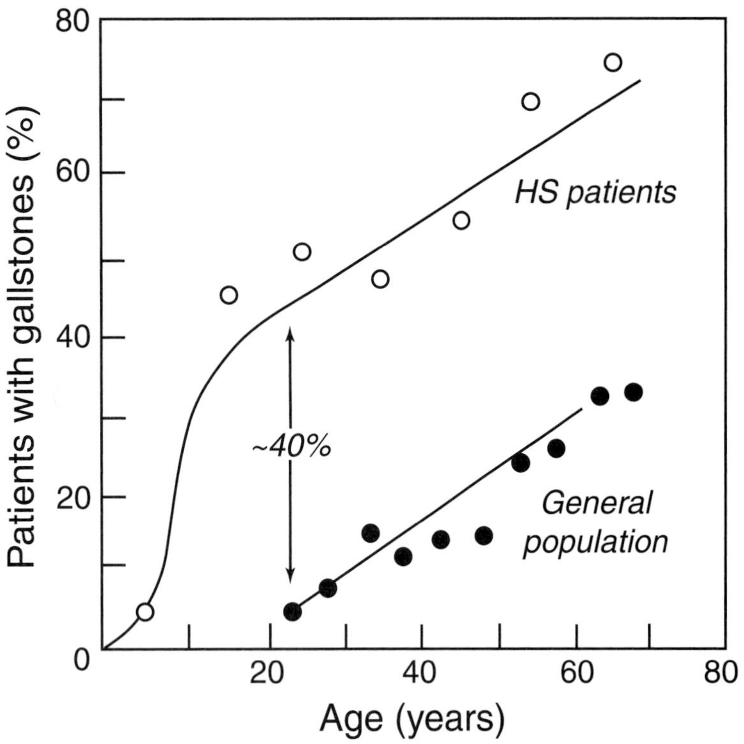

Fig. 183-32 Proportion of normal (solid circles) and HS (open circles) patients with gallstones as a function of age. The prevalence of gallstones rises sharply between the ages of 10 and 30 in HS patients. The subsequent increase then parallels that of the general population after the age of 30, suggesting that cholelithiasis due to HS is primarily manifest in the second and third decades. The HS curve is derived from the data of Bates and Brown;[711] the normal curve is from autopsy data.[712] (*From Lux and Palek.[4] Used by permission.*)

increased during pregnancy, when the need for folic acid is particularly high.[709,710] It is recommended that HS patients with ongoing hemolysis take folic acid supplements of at least 1mg per day.

Gallbladder Disease. Gallbladder disease is the most common complication of HS. Pigment gallstones are reported in patients as young as 3 years[697] but are most prevalent in adolescents and adults.[711] The incidence of gallstones rises rapidly in the second and third decades of life, after which its increase parallels that of the general population[712] (Fig. 183-32). The limited data available indicate that 55 to 85 percent of untreated HS patients will eventually acquire stones[556,711] and that roughly half of these individuals will have symptoms of cholecystitis or, less commonly, biliary obstruction. However, the data were gathered before the common use of ultrasonography to assess gallbladder disease and the risk of complications is based primarily on the experience with cholesterol gallstones. More accurate data on the incidence of these complications in patients with bilirubin gallstones are needed to assess accurately the risk/benefit ratio of cholecystectomy (and splenectomy) in HS.[713]

The incidence of gallstones in HS patients is apparently related to the ability of the liver to metabolize bilirubin. A very common mutation in the promoter of the UDP-glucuronyl transferase gene (*UGT-1A*) has recently been shown to be associated with reduced UDP-glucuronyl transferase activity in heterozygotes and to cause Gilbert syndrome in homozygotes (see Chap. 125).[545] A study of the frequency of gallstones in 103 HS children showed that the rate of gallstone formation in patients homozygous for the mutated *UGT-1A* allele is 2.1 times that of heterozygous patients and 4.5 times that of normals.[714] If this result is confirmed, analysis of this allele should be useful in predicting the risk of gallstones in HS.

The treatment of gallbladder disease in HS is debatable, especially in patients with mild hemolytic disease or asymptomatic gallstones. An initial period of observation is advisable.[715] Surgery may be necessary if there are recurrent symptoms or complications such as cholecystitis or biliary obstruction. Laparoscopic cholecystectomy is the procedure of choice among most surgeons and the general public.[716] If a patient needs splenectomy for ongoing hemolysis or its complications (see below), gallbladder ultrasound should be done first and concomitant cholecystectomy considered if gallstones are present.[717] Splenectomy solely as a prophylaxis for gallstone development is probably not indicated, nor is prophylactic cholecystectomy.

Other Complications. Adult patients with HS occasionally have gout,[522] indolent leg ulcers, or a chronic erythematous dermatitis on the legs.[718] These complications occur mainly in the elderly and usually resolve after splenectomy.

Rarely, patients also have extramedullary masses of hematopoietic tissue, particularly along the posterior thoracic or lumbar spine.[521,719] These gradually enlarge with time and may be mistaken for neoplasms.[719]

Interestingly, Schafer and his colleagues have suggested that untreated HS may predispose patients to a true neoplasm, multiple myeloma.[720] Several patients with HS and myeloma have been reported.[720] It was argued that the association may be due to chronic reticuloendothelial stimulation, because splenic clearance of abnormal red cells induces proliferation of lymphocytes and plasma cells as well as macrophages. HS patients often have a mild, polyclonal hypergammaglobulinemia,[721] and there is evidence favoring the association of myeloma and chronic gallbladder disease.[722] However, it is still unclear if this proposed association of HS and myeloma is a real phenomenon.

There are reports of HS patients who died from liver failure or hepatoma secondary to iron overload.[723,724] While HS may lead to excessive iron uptake in some patients who are clinically heterozygous for hereditary hemochromatosis,[725,726] this is not a problem in most HS patients.

Even though splenomegaly is often seen in patients with HS, traumatic rupture of the enlarged spleen in HS patient is very rare.[727] This contrasts with the higher frequency of splenic rupture in patients with EBV infection, and may reflect the different pathophysiology of splenic enlargement in the two conditions.

Splenectomy. It is one of the rare absolutes in medicine that patients with true, uncomplicated HS always respond dramatically to splenectomy. The degree of response correlates closely with the degree of spectrin deficiency and is incomplete in the most severely affected patients.[531,560] The major issues today are who should have a splenectomy, what kind of operation should be done, and how the patients should be treated postoperatively.

Following splenectomy, spherocytosis persists, but conditioned microspherocytes disappear, and changes typical of the post-splenectomy state—including Howell-Jolly bodies, target cells, acanthocytes, pitted cells, and siderocytes—appear in the peripheral smear.[574,728,729] Reticulocyte counts fall to normal or near-normal levels, although red cell life span, if carefully measured, remains slightly shortened (96 ± 13 days).[730] Abnormal osmotic fragility persists, but the "tail" of the osmotic fragility curve, created by conditioning of a subpopulation of spherocytes by the spleen, disappears. Clinically, patients have better energy and an improved quality of life, and complications such as leg ulcers and extramedullary hematopoiesis resolve. In most cases, anemia and jaundice remit and do not recur, except in the rare case of regrowth of a missed accessory spleen. This is the only proven cause of postsplenectomy failure in HS and is sometimes overlooked, as it may not become evident for years.[731]

Immediate Postsplenectomy Complications. Immediate postoperative complications include bleeding and subphrenic abscess. Hemorrhage usually comes from peritoneal and diaphragmatic surfaces of the splenic bed rather than from identifiable blood vessels. Subphrenic abscess is more likely to occur when adjacent organs are injured during the surgery. Acute pancreatitis can also occur in the postoperative period.[732] A reactive thrombocytosis is commonly seen after splenectomy, with platelet counts as high as 1000 K/dl. The platelets peak 7 to 12 days after the procedure but elevated levels may persist indefinitely. The thrombocytosis is generally benign. It is probably not associated with venous thromboembolic complications,[732,733] and antiplatelet therapy is probably not necessary. Portal vein thrombosis has been reported after splenectomy for hemolytic diseases, but it is probably not related to thrombocytosis.[734–736] The high frequency of thrombotic complications in mice with membrane skeletal defects[663,669] and in patients with membrane disorders such as hereditary stomatocytosis and xerocytosis after splenectomy[737,738] suggest that released membrane fragments may be a major factor. Such fragments are highly thrombogenic if phosphatidyl serine is exposed.[665,669]

Postsplenectomy Sepsis. One of the most serious complications of splenectomy is overwhelming postsplenectomy infection. The absence of a functional spleen puts these patients at an increased risk of infection by bacterial and parasitic pathogens. Among bacterial infections, the risk is particularly high for encapsulated organisms, specifically, *S. pneumoniae*, *N. meningitidis*, and *H. influenzae*. The course of bacterial infection in splenectomized patient can be extremely rapid and potentially fatal, and can occur years or decades after the procedure.[739] It is difficult to estimate the true incidence of overwhelming postsplenectomy infection. The seminal study of King and Shumacker first drew attention to the high risk of fulminant sepsis in infants who had undergone splenectomy for HS,[740] and numerous reports of serious postsplenectomy infection have since been published (results summarized in several reviews[741–744]). The incidence of overwhelming postsplenectomy infection has been estimated to be 0.2 to 0.5 per 100 person-years of follow-up, with a death rate of 0.1 per 100 person-years in adults,[745,746] and a much higher figure in children, particularly younger children.[747–749] The majority of the available studies, however, have serious methodological problems.[744,750] Most are retrospective studies or case reports, which may have a inherent bias towards reporting the more serious cases. The duration of observation is often poorly documented and a large fraction of patients may be lost to follow-up. Most of the patients underwent splenectomy before pneumococcal vaccine was generally available or antibiotic prophylaxis routinely prescribed. The underlying diseases of the patients and the reasons for splenectomy are highly varied.

In our experience, overwhelming postsplenectomy sepsis can be a serious and devastating problem but is relatively uncommon in HS patients, unlike patients with underlying immunological dysfunction, such as Hodgkin disease, or with continuing extravascular hemolysis (e.g., thalassemia).[732,741,748,751] A recent, 30-year follow-up of more than two hundred splenectomized HS adult patients found four patients dead from overwhelming sepsis, making the mortality rate from postsplenectomy sepsis 0.073 per 100 person-years.[752] Three of the four deaths occurred 18 or more years after the operation and none of the patients who died had received pneumococcal vaccine or antibiotic prophylaxis. There is evidence of a dramatic decrease in the incidence of postsplenectomy sepsis in children who are given pneumococcal vaccine and prophylactic antibiotics.[753] This suggests that the incidence of postsplenectomy sepsis may continue to decline, even though failures of the preventive measures may still occur.[754] Continued research is needed to quantitate the true risk of overwhelming postsplenectomy sepsis in HS patients treated according to current practice guidelines.[739]

Babesiosis and Malaria. After splenectomy HS patients are also at risk for serious parasitic infections, such as babesiosis and malaria. Babesiosis is a tick-transmitted zoonotic infection by an intraerythrocytic protozoan that is endemic in Europe and in the northeastern, north central, and western United States.[755] The causative agents include *Babesia microti*, *B. divergens*, and a related organism designated "WA1." In healthy individuals the infection is usually mild and often asymptomatic, but in patients without a functional spleen, it can be rapidly progressive and life-threatening.[756] Patients may have malaise, headache, fever, shaking chills, profuse sweating, jaundice, and dark urine. There may be intravascular hemolysis and, occasionally, pancytopenia[757] and hemophagocytosis.[758] Diagnosis is made by finding the parasites in blood smears, or by serologic tests or amplification of parasitic DNA using the polymerase chain reaction. Current treatment of symptomatic cases is quinine plus clindamycin, but treatment failures have been reported in asplenic patients. Splenectomized HS patients, when traveling in endemic areas, should take measures to avoid tick bites by, for instance, wearing long pants and using tick repellents. The nymphal ticks that cause the disease are only 1 to 2 mm in size and are difficult to detect.

Animal experiments have shown that the spleen is essential for limiting malaria parasitemia in the acute stage of infection,[759,760] but, surprisingly, other than anecdotal reports,[761–763] there are no studies that definitively demonstrate an increased risk of severe malaria in asplenic individuals. It is nevertheless prudent for postsplenectomy HS patients to adhere strictly to malaria chemoprophylaxis protocols when traveling to endemic areas and take measures to reduce exposure to malaria parasites.

Thrombosis and Atherosclerosis. There are occasional reports of thromboembolic events occurring many years after splenectomy,[764] but their causal relationship to splenectomy has not been convincingly demonstrated, except for patients with hereditary stomatocytosis, where the risk of thrombotic complications after splenectomy approaches 100 percent.[737]

On the other hand, there is some evidence that the incidence of atherosclerosis is elevated after splenectomy. A carefully controlled, long-term follow up of splenectomy in 740 WW II servicemen following battlefield injuries, showed excess mortality from pneumonia (see above) and atherosclerotic heart disease (1.9 times relative risk) in the splenectomized patients.[765] The authors suggest that the chronically elevated platelet counts that occur after splenectomy may have contributed to vascular disease. A more recent study found that the cumulative incidence of atherosclerosis after the age of 40 was six times higher in patients who had a splenectomy compared to those who had not had the

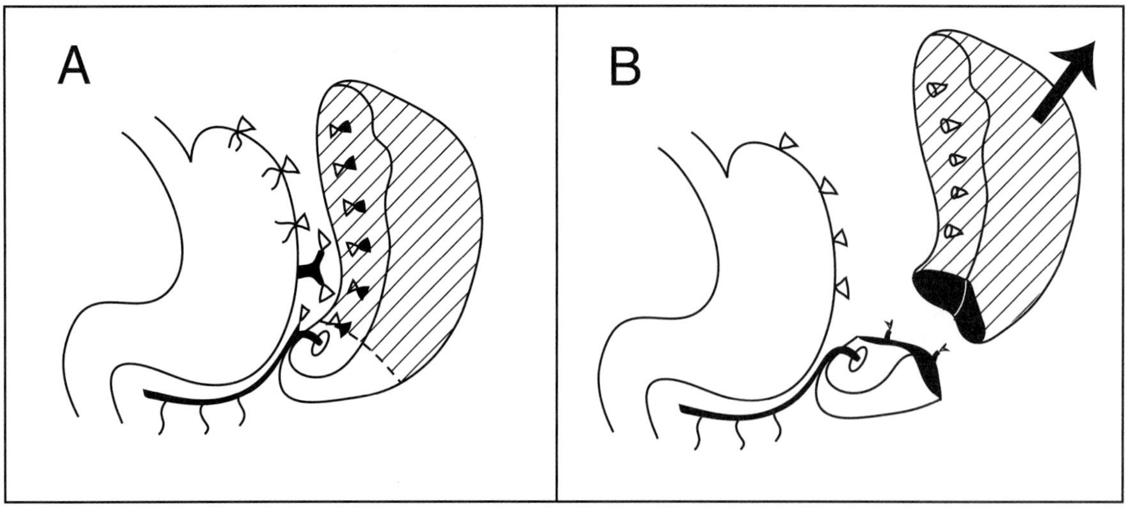

Fig. 183-33 Surgical technique used in partial splenectomy. *A.* All vascular pedicles supplying the spleen are divided except those arising from the left gastroepiploic vessels. *B.* the upper pole of the spleen is removed at the boundary between the well perfused and poorly perfused tissue. (*From Tchernia et al.*[772] *Used by permission.*)

procedure.[766] While these results need to be confirmed by other studies, they support a conservative approach to splenectomy.

Indications for Splenectomy. In view of the many potential complications, splenectomy should be done only if there are clear indications. We believe the procedure is clearly warranted for the rare patients with severe HS who require transfusions or who have serious complications, such as growth failure or thalassemic facies. It may also be indicated for patients with moderate or moderately severe disease who are symptomatic with, for instance, chronic fatigue, decreased physical stamina, or, later in life, compromised perfusion of vital organs, leg ulcers, or extramedullary hematopoietic tumors. Whether patients with moderate HS and asymptomatic anemia should have a splenectomy remains controversial. Subtotal splenectomy (see below) may have a particular role in these patients. Splenectomy can be deferred, probably indefinitely, in patients with mild HS and compensated hemolysis. The presence of gallbladder disease may influence the decision, as discussed above. In young children, the procedure, if indicated, should be delayed until at least 3 years of age, and, if possible, until 5 years or more. There is probably no additional benefit in postponing splenectomy beyond the age of 10 years, because the risk of gallstone development rises sharply after that. In some patients, the procedure may not be needed until old age, when complications like leg ulcers and extramedullary hematopoietic tumors develop.

Surgical Procedures. Laparoscopic splenectomy, sometimes with concomitant laparoscopic cholecystectomy, has now become a viable alternative to open splenectomy.[767,768] The pros for this approach include its minimal invasiveness, a shortened hospital stay, a lower need for narcotic pain control, and a more appealing cosmetic result. The cons include a longer operation time, potential difficulty in control of bleeding, and the chance of missing an accessory spleen. Experience with the procedure has accumulated tremendously in the past few years, although there are few multicenter, controlled trials comparing it with the traditional open surgical approach.[769–771] The current consensus is that if the surgical staff is experienced with the procedure and the spleen is not very large, laparoscopic splenectomy may be the method of choice.

Because of the risk of postsplenectomy sepsis, partial splenectomy (or subtotal splenectomy) has been advocated as an alternative to total splenectomy for HS.[772–774] In this procedure, about 90 percent of the enlarged spleen is removed, leaving behind a remnant with about 25 percent of the volume of a normal spleen (Fig. 183-33). The procedure is safe and decreases the rate of hemolysis while preserving some of the phagocytic function of the spleen.[772–774] Presumably the risk of postsplenectomy sepsis is also decreased, although this may be impossible to prove. After partial splenectomy, the mean hemoglobin in a group of HS patients increased from 9.8 to 12.2 g/dl and the absolute reticulocyte count decreased from 560 to 270 $\times$ 10^9 cells/liter[772,774] There was improved quality of life and gain in physical growth in most of these patients. However, the reduction in hemolytic rate was not as great as that observed after total splenectomy and partial splenectomy did not prevent the development of gallstones completely (3 of 24 patients in one series).[773] The need for secondary total splenectomy was 10 percent at 5 years and 33 percent at 10 years, and the patients have not been followed long enough to determine if there is really a lower risk for subsequent development of overwhelming sepsis. The high rate of subsequent complete splenectomy in these patients may reflect the fact that the procedure was often used in patients with severe disease. In our view it is more suited for patients with mild to moderate HS, in whom splenectomy is often not done. It is likely that the prevalence of gallstones and the need for a second operation will be much lower in these patients. Overall, partial splenectomy shows promise, but it should still be considered investigational at this time.

Partial splenic artery embolization has been done as an alternative to splenectomy in patients with hypersplenism and has been performed in a child with HS.[775] The experience with this procedure in HS is limited and cannot be recommended as a routine procedure.

Vaccination and Antibiotic Prophylaxis. All HS patients undergoing splenectomy should receive vaccines against encapsulated bacteria. Polyvalent (23 strains) pneumococcal vaccine is highly effective[753] after 2 years of age and should be given at least 2 weeks before splenectomy.[776] A conjugated, heptavalent pneumococcal vaccine, effective at all ages, is currently completing clinical trials[777–779] and should be available in the near future. Conjugated *H. influenzae* type b vaccine is now given to all children and should also be given to splenectomized adult HS patients.[780] *N. meningitidis* vaccine currently is effective against only serogroup a and c strains, not the common serogroup b, but probably should still be given to patients undergoing splenectomy.[780] Revaccination with pneumococcal vaccine in 5 years and meningococcal vaccine in 2 years is advised. Yearly influenza vaccination may help reduce the chance of secondary bacterial infection.

Prophylactic antibiotics against *S. pneumoniae* should be given to HS patients after splenectomy. Penicillin V (125 to 250 mg twice per day) is usually used, but some physicians recommend amoxicillin because of its improved absorption.[780] Patients who are allergic to penicillin may be offered erythromycin.[781] Antibiotic prophylaxis should be given to splenectomized patients throughout their childhood, or, for teenagers and adults, in the first 2 to 5 years after splenectomy when the risk of overwhelming infection is highest. Some authorities recommend lifelong antibiotics prophylaxis,[781] but there are concerns of poor patient compliance and emergence of resistant organisms.[782] Patients not on prophylaxis should have a supply of oral antibiotics at hand, which they should take immediately if fever or other symptoms of infection develop. They should then seek medical attention right away.

CONCLUSIONS

HE/HPP and HS are examples of human diseases in which the defects lie in the structural proteins of the red blood cell membrane skeleton. HE and HPP are caused by defective "horizontal" interactions between proteins that hold the membrane skeleton together. HS is caused by defects in the "vertical" interactions that link the membrane skeleton to the overlying lipid bilayer. These molecular defects translate on a cellular level into mechanical instability of the red cell membrane, and, in the cases of HS and severe HE/HPP, to membrane loss. In those disorders, defective red cells are selectively retained and destroyed in the spleen, resulting in hemolysis, anemia, and splenomegaly. Even though much has already been learned, further research is needed to understand how each type of defect causes its associated disease, how abnormal red cells are recognized and removed in the spleen, how modifying factors influence the clinical severity in a patient, and what constitutes the best diagnostic and therapeutic approach for these diseases.

REFERENCES

1. Liu SC, Derick LH: Molecular anatomy of the red blood cell membrane skeleton: Structure-function relationships. *Semin Hematol* **29**:231, 1992.
2. Peters LL, Lux SE: Ankyrins: Structure and function in normal cells and hereditary spherocytes. *Semin Hematol* **30**:85, 1993.
3. Palek J, Jarolim P: Clinical expression and laboratory detection of red blood cell membrane protein mutations. *Semin Hematol* **30**:249, 1993.
4. Lux SE, Palek J: Disorders of the red cell membrane, in Handin RJ, Lux SE, Stossel TP (eds): *Blood: Principles and Practice of Hematology*. Philadelphia, Lippincott-Raven, 1995, p 1701.
5. Delaunay J: Genetic disorders of the red cell membrane. *Crit Rev Oncol Hematol* **19**:79, 1995.
6. Hassoun H, Palek J: Hereditary spherocytosis: A review of the clinical and molecular aspects of the disease. *Blood Rev* **10**:129, 1996.
7. Iolascon A, Miraglia del Giudice E, Perrotta S, Alloisio N, Morlé L, Delaunay J: Hereditary spherocytosis: From clinical to molecular defects. *Haematologica* **83**:240, 1998.
8. Schwartz RS, Chiu DT, Lubin B: Plasma membrane phospholipid organization in human erythrocytes. *Curr Top Hematol* **5**:63, 1985.
9. Fukuda M: Molecular genetics of the glycophorin A gene cluster. *Semin Hematol* **30**:138, 1993.
10. Cartron JP, Le Van Kim C, Colin Y: Glycophorin C and related glycoproteins: Structure, function, and regulation. *Semin Hematol* **30**:152, 1993.
11. Tanner MJ: The structure and function of band 3 (AE1): recent developments. *Mol Membr Biol* **14**:155, 1997.
12. Lande WM, Mentzer WC: Haemolytic anaemia associated with increased cation permeability. *Clin Haematol* **14**:89, 1985.
13. Palek J (ed): Cellular and Molecular Biology of the RBC Membrane Proteins. *Semin Hematol* **29**:229, **30**:1, **30**:85, **30**:169, **30**:249, 1992/1993.
14. Blair L, Bittman R: Cholesteol distribution between the two halves of the lipid bilayer of human erythrocyte ghost membranes. *J Biol Chem* **253**:8366, 1978.
15. Low MG, Finean JB: Modification of erythrocyte membranes by a purified phosphatidylinositol-specific phospholipase. *Biochem J* **162**:235, 1972.
16. Verkleij AJ, Zwaal RFA, Roelofsen B, Comfurius P, Kastelijn D, van Deenen LLM: The asymmetric distribution of phospholipids in the human red cell membrane. A combined study using phospholipases and freeze-etch electron microscopy. *Biochim Biophys Acta* **323**:178, 1973.
17. Fairbanks G, Steck TL, Wallach DFH: Electrophoretic analysis of the major polypeptides of the human erythrocyte membrane. *Biochemistry* **10**:2606, 1971.
18. Ferrel JE Jr, Huestis WH: Phosphoinositide metabolism and the morphology of human erythrocytes. *J Cell Biol* **98**:1992, 1984.
19. Van Deenen LLM, DeGier J: Lipids of the red blood cell membrane, in Surgenor DM (ed): *The Red Blood Cell*, 2d ed. New York, Academic Press, 1974, p 148.
20. Sweeley CC, Dawson G: Lipids of the erythrocyte, in Jamieson GA, Greenwalt TJ (eds): *Red Cell Membrane Structure and Function*. Philadelphia, Lippincott, 1969, p 172.
21. Cooper RA: Lipids of human red cell membrane: normal composition and variability in disease. *Semin Hematol* **7**:296, 1970.
22. Gallagher PG, Tse WT, Forget BG: Clinical and molecular aspects of disorders of the erythrocyte membrane skeleton. *Semin Perinatol* **14**:351, 1990.
23. Savvides P, Shalev O, John KM, Lux SE: Combined spectrin and ankyrin deficiency is common in autosomal dominant hereditary spherocytosis. *Blood* **82**:2953, 1993.
24. Hemming NJ, Anstee DJ, Mawby WJ, Reid ME, Tanner MJ: Localization of the protein 4.1-binding site on human erythrocyte glycophorins C and D. *Biochem J* **299**:191, 1994.
25. Pinder JC, Gratzer WB: Structural and dynamic states of actin in the erythrocyte. *J Cell Biol* **96**:768, 1983.
26. Inaba M, Gupta KC, Kuwabara M, Takahashi T, Benz EJ Jr, Maede Y: Deamidation of human erythrocyte protein 4.1: Possible role in aging. *Blood* **79**:3355, 1992.
27. Peters LL, Weier HUG, Walensky LD, Snyder SH, Parra M, Mohandas N, Conboy JG: Four paralogous protein 4.1 genes map to distinct chromosomes in mouse and human. *Genomics* **54**:348, 1998.
28. Parra M, Gascard P, Walensky LD, Snyder SH, Mohandas N, Conboy JG: Cloning and characterization of 4.1G (EPB41L2), a new member of the skeletal protein 4.1 (EPB41) gene family. *Genomics* **49**:298, 1998.
29. Conboy JG: Structure, function, and molecular genetics of erythroid membrane skeletal protein 4.1 in normal and abnormal red blood cells. *Semin Hematol* **30**:58, 1993.
30. Huang JP, Tang CJ, Kou GH, Marchesi VT, Benz EJ Jr, Tang TK: Genomic structure of the locus encoding protein 4.1. Structural basis for complex combinational patterns of tissue-specific alternative RNA splicing. *J Biol Chem* **268**:3758, 1993.
31. Gascard P, Lee G, Coulombel L, Auffray I, Lum M, Parra M, Conboy JG, Mohandas N, Chasis JA: Characterization of multiple isoforms of protein 4.1R expressed during erythroid terminal differentiation. *Blood* **92**:4404, 1998.
32. Schischmanoff PO, Yaswen P, Parra MK, Lee G, Chasis JA, Mohandas N, Conboy JG: Cell shape-dependent regulation of protein 4.1 alternative pre-mRNA splicing in mammary epithelial cells. *J Biol Chem* **272**:10254, 1997.
33. Azim AC, Knoll JH, Beggs AH, Chishti AH: Isoform cloning, actin binding, and chromosomal localization of human erythroid dematin, a member of the villin superfamily. *J Biol Chem* **270**:17407, 1995.
34. Azim AC, Marfatia SM, Korsgren C, Dotimas E, Cohen CM, Chishti AH: Human erythrocyte dematin and protein 4.2 (pallidin) are ATP binding proteins. *Biochemistry* **35**:3001, 1996.
35. Sung LA, Lin JJ: Erythrocyte tropomodulin binds to the N-terminus of hTM5, a tropomyosin isoform encoded by the g-tropomyosin gene. *Biochem Biophys Res Commun* **201**:627, 1994.
36. Vera C, Lin JJ-C, Sung LA: The residues at 'a' and 'd' positions in the N-terminal heptad repeats of tropomyosin isoform 5 are critical for its binding to erythrocyte tropomodulin. *Blood* **92(Suppl 1)**:6a, 1998.
37. Chasis JA, Mohandas N: Red blood cell glycophorins. *Blood* **80**:1869, 1992.
38. Daniels GL, Shaw MA, Judson PA, Reid ME, Anstee DJ, Colpitts P, Cornwall S, Moore BP, Lee S: A family demonstrating inheritance of the Leach phenotype: a Gerbich-negative phenotype associated with elliptocytosis. *Vox Sang* **50**:117, 1986.
39. Sondag D, Alloisio N, Blanchard D, Ducluzeau MT, Colonna P, Bachir D, Bloy C, Cartron JP, Delaunay J: Gerbich reactivity in 4.1(−)

hereditary elliptocytosis and protein 4.1 level in blood group Gerbich deficiency. *Br J Haematol* **65**:43, 1987.
40. Telen MJ, Le Van Kim C, Chung A, Cartron JP, Colin Y: Molecular basis for elliptocytosis associated with glycophorin C and D deficiency in the Leach phenotype. *Blood* **78**:1603, 1991.
41. Lux SE, John KM, Kopito RR, Lodish HF: Cloning and characterization of band 3, the human erythrocyte anion- exchange protein (AE1). *Proc Natl Acad Sci U S A* **86**:9089, 1989.
42. Tanner MJ: Molecular and cellular biology of the erythrocyte anion exchanger (AE1). *Semin Hematol* **30**:34, 1993.
43. Wang DN, Kuhlbrandt W, Sarabia VE, Reithmeier RA: Two-dimensional structure of the membrane domain of human band 3, the anion transport protein of the erythrocyte membrane. *EMBO J* **12**:2233, 1993.
44. Lindenthal S, Schubert D: Monomeric erythrocyte band 3 protein transports anions. *Proc Natl Acad Sci U S A* **88**:6540, 1991.
45. Forster RE, Gros G, Lin L, Ono Y, Wunder M: The effect of 4,4′-diisothiocyanato-stilbene-2,2′-disulfonate on CO_2 permeability of the red blood cell membrane. *Proc Natl Acad Sci U S A* **95**:15815, 1998.
46. Vince JW, Reithmeier RA: Carbonic anhydrase II binds to the carboxyl terminus of human band 3, the erythrocyte $C1^-/HCO3^-$ exchanger. *J Biol Chem* **273**:28430, 1998.
47. Jennings ML: Structure and function of the red blood cell anion transport protein. *Annu Rev Biophys Biophys Chem* **18**:397, 1989.
48. Jarolim P, Rubin HL, Zakova D, Storry J, Reid ME: Characterization of seven low incidence blood group antigens carried by erythrocyte band 3 protein. *Blood* **92**:4836, 1998.
49. Bruce LJ, Ring SM, Anstee DJ, Reid ME, Wilkinson S, Tanner MJ: Changes in the blood group Wright antigens are associated with a mutation at amino acid 658 in human erythrocyte band 3: A site of interaction between band 3 and glycophorin A under certain conditions. *Blood* **85**:541, 1995.
50. Telen MJ, Chasis JA: Relationship of the human erythrocyte Wr^b antigen to an interaction between glycophorin A and band 3. *Blood* **76**:842, 1990.
51. Groves JD, Tanner MJ: Glycophorin A facilitates the expression of human band 3-mediated anion transport in *Xenopus* oocytes. *J Biol Chem* **267**:22163, 1992.
52. Hassoun H, Hanada T, Lutchman M, Sahr KE, Palek J, Hanspal M, Chishti AH: Complete deficiency of glycophorin A in red blood cells from mice with targeted inactivation of the band 3 (AE1) gene. *Blood* **91**:2146, 1998.
53. Low PS: Structure and function of the cytoplasmic domain of band 3: Center of erythrocyte membrane-peripheral protein interactions. *Biochim Biophys Acta* **864**:145, 1986.
54. Walder JA, Chatterjee R, Steck TL, Low PS, Musso GF, Kaiser ET, Rogers PH, Arnone A: The interaction of hemoglobin with the cytoplasmic domain of band 3 of the human erythrocyte membrane. *J Biol Chem* **259**:10238, 1984.
55. Kannan R, Labotka R, Low PS: Isolation and characterization of the hemichrome-stabilized membrane protein aggregates from sickle erythrocytes. Major site of autologous antibody binding. *J Biol Chem* **263**:13766, 1988.
56. Kliman HJ, Steck TL: Association of glyceraldehyde-3-phosphate dehydrogenase with the human red cell membrane. A kinetic analysis. *J Biol Chem* **255**:6314, 1980.
57. Jenkins JD, Madden DP, Steck TL: Association of phosphofructokinase and aldolase with the membrane of the intact erythrocyte. *J Biol Chem* **259**:9374, 1984.
58. De BK, Kirtley ME: Interaction of phosphoglycerate kinase with human erythrocyte membranes. *J Biol Chem* **252**:6715, 1977.
59. Tsai IH, Murthy SN, Steck TL: Effect of red cell membrane binding on the catalytic activity of glyceraldehyde-3-phosphate dehydrogenase. *J Biol Chem* **257**:1438, 1982.
60. Strapazon E, Steck TL: Interaction of the aldolase and the membrane of human erythrocytes. *Biochemistry* **16**:2966, 1977.
61. Low PS, Allen DP, Zioncheck TF, Chari P, Willardson BM, Geahlen RL, Harrison ML: Tyrosine phosphorylation of band 3 inhibits peripheral protein binding. *J Biol Chem* **262**:4592, 1987.
62. Harrison ML, Rathinavelu P, Arese P, Geahlen RL, Low PS: Role of band 3 tyrosine phosphorylation in the regulation of erythrocyte glycolysis. *J Biol Chem* **266**:4106, 1991.
63. Chétrite G, Cassoly R: Affinity of hemoglobin for the cytoplasmic fragment of human erythrocyte membrane band 3. Equilibrium measurements at physiological pH using matrix-bound proteins: The effects of ionic strength, deoxygenation and of 2,3-diphosphoglycerate. *J Mol Biol* **185**:639, 1985.
64. Waugh SM, Walder JA, Low PS: Partial characterization of the copolymerization reaction of erythrocyte membrane band 3 with hemichromes. *Biochemistry* **26**:1777, 1987.
65. Bennett V, Stenbuck PJ: Association between ankyrin and the cytoplasmic domain of band 3 isolated from the human erythrocyte membrane. *J Biol Chem* **255**:6424, 1980.
66. Lombardo CR, Willardson BM, Low PS: Localization of the protein 4.1-binding site on the cytoplasmic domain of erythrocyte membrane band 3. *J Biol Chem* **267**:9540, 1992.
67. Jöns T, Drenckhahn D: Identification of the binding interface involved in linkage of cytoskeletal protein 4.1 to the erythrocyte anion exchanger. *Embo J* **11**:2863, 1992.
68. Korsgren C, Cohen CM: Purification and properties of human erythrocyte band 4.2. Association with the cytoplasmic domain of band 3. *J Biol Chem* **261**:5536, 1986.
69. Hargreaves WR, Giedd KN, Verkleij A, Branton D: Reassociation of ankyrin with band 3 in erythrocyte membranes and in lipid vesicles. *J Biol Chem* **255**:11965, 1980.
70. Davis L, Lux SE, Bennett V: Mapping the ankyrin-binding site of the human erythrocyte anion exchanger. *J Biol Chem* **264**:9665, 1989.
71. Willardson BM, Thevenin BJ, Harrison ML, Kuster WM, Benson MD, Low PS: Localization of the ankyrin-binding site on erythrocyte membrane protein, band 3. *J Biol Chem* **264**:15893, 1989.
72. Ding Y, Casey JR, Kopito RR: The major kidney AE1 isoform does not bind ankyrin (Ank1) in vitro. An essential role for the 79 NH_2-terminal amino acid residues of band 3. *J Biol Chem* **269**:32201, 1994.
73. Ding Y, Kobayashi S, Kopito R: Mapping of ankyrin binding determinants on the erythroid anion exchanger, AE1. *J Biol Chem* **271**:22494, 1996.
74. Van Dort HM, Moriyama R, Low PS: Effect of band 3 subunit equilibrium on the kinetics and affinity of ankyrin binding to erythrocyte membrane vesicles. *J Biol Chem* **273**:14819, 1998.
75. Yi SJ, Liu SC, Derick LH, Murray J, Barker JE, Cho MR, Palek J, Golan DE: Red cell membranes of ankyrin-deficient *nb/nb* mice lack band 3 tetramers but contain normal membrane skeletons. *Biochemistry* **36**:9596, 1997.
76. Casey JR, Reithmeier RA: Analysis of the oligomeric state of Band 3, the anion transport protein of the human erythrocyte membrane, by size exclusion high performance liquid chromatography. Oligomeric stability and origin of heterogeneity. *J Biol Chem* **266**:15726, 1991.
77. Tomishige M, Sako Y, Kusumi A: Regulation mechanism of the lateral diffusion of band 3 in erythrocyte membranes by the membrane skeleton. *J Cell Biol* **142**:989, 1998.
78. Alper SL: The band 3-related anion exchanger (AE) gene family. *Annu Rev Physiol* **53**:549, 1991.
79. Brosius FCd, Alper SL, Garcia AM, Lodish HF: The major kidney band 3 gene transcript predicts an amino-terminal truncated band 3 polypeptide. *J Biol Chem* **264**:7784, 1989.
80. Jarolim P, Rubin HL, Brabec V, Chrobak L, Zolotarev AS, Alper SL, Brugnara C, Wichterle H, Palek J: Mutations of conserved arginines in the membrane domain of erythroid band 3 lead to a decrease in membrane-associated band 3 and to the phenotype of hereditary spherocytosis. *Blood* **85**:634, 1995.
81. Peters LL, Shivdasani RA, Liu SC, Hanspal M, John KM, Gonzalez JM, Brugnara C, Gwynn B, Mohandas N, Alper SL, Orkin SH, Lux SE: Anion exchanger 1 (band 3) is required to prevent erythrocyte membrane surface loss but not to form the membrane skeleton. *Cell* **86**:917, 1996.
82. Jarolim P, Palek J, Amato D, Hassan K, Sapak P, Nurse GT, Rubin HL, Zhai S, Sahr KE, Liu SC: Deletion in erythrocyte band 3 gene in malaria-resistant Southeast Asian ovalocytosis. *Proc Natl Acad Sci U S A* **88**:11022, 1991.
83. Rysava R, Tesar V, Jirsa M Jr, Brabec V, Jarolim P: Incomplete distal renal tubular acidosis coinherited with a mutation in the band 3 (*AE1*) gene. *Nephrol Dial Transplant* **12**:1869, 1997.
84. Jarolim P, Shayakul C, Prabakaran D, Jiang L, Stuart-Tilley A, Rubin HL, Simova S, Zavadil J, Herrin JT, Brouillette J, Somers MJ, Seemanova E, Brugnara C, Guay-Woodford LM, Alper SL: Autosomal dominant distal renal tubular acidosis is associated in three families with heterozygosity for the R589H mutation in the AE1 (band 3) Cl^-/HCO_3^- exchanger. *J Biol Chem* **273**:6380, 1998.
85. Bruce LJ, Kay MM, Lawrence C, Tanner MJ: Band 3 HT, a human red-cell variant associated with acanthocytosis and increased anion transport, carries the mutation Pro-868 → Leu in the membrane domain of band 3. *Biochem J* **293**:317, 1993.
86. De Franceschi L, Turrini F, del Giudice EM, Perrotta S, Olivieri O, Corrocher R, Mannu F, Iolascon A: Decreased band 3 anion transport

activity and band 3 clusterization in congenital dyserythropoietic anemia type II. *Exp Hematol* **26**:869, 1998.
87. Sheetz MP: Integral membrane protein interaction with Triton cytoskeletons of erythrocytes. *Biochim Biophys Acta* **557**:122, 1979.
88. Yu J, Fischman DA, Steck TL: Selective solubilization of proteins and phospholipids from red blood cell membranes by nonionic detergents. *J Supramol Struct* **1**:233, 1973.
89. Dunn MJ, Kemp RB, Maddy AH: The similarity of the two high-molecular-weight polypeptides of erythrocyte spectrin. *Biochem J* **173**:197, 1978.
90. Anderson JM: Structural studies on human spectrin. Comparison of subunits and fragmentation of native spectrin. *J Biol Chem* **254**:939, 1979.
91. Speicher DW, Marchesi VT: Erythrocyte spectrin is comprised of many homologous triple helical segments. *Nature* **311**:177, 1984.
92. Speicher DW, Morrow JS, Knowles WJ, Marchesi VT: A structural model of human erythrocyte spectrin. Alignment of chemical and functional domains. *J Biol Chem* **257**:9093, 1982.
93. Shotton DM, Burke BE, Branton D: The molecular structure of human erythrocyte spectrin. Biophysical and electron microscopic studies. *J Mol Biol* **131**:303, 1979.
94. Winkelmann JC, Forget BG: Erythroid and nonerythroid spectrins. *Blood* **81**:3173, 1993.
95. Stankewich MC, Tse WT, Peters LL, Ch'ng Y, John KM, Stabach PR, Devarajan P, Morrow JS, Lux SE: A widely expressed βIII-spectrin associated with Golgi and cytoplasmic vesicles. *Proc Natl Acad Sci U S A* **95**:14158, 1998.
96. Yan Y, Winograd E, Viel A, Cronin T, Harrison SC, Branton D: Crystal structure of the repetitive segments of spectrin. *Science* **262**:2027, 1993.
97. Sahr KE, Laurila P, Kotula L, Scarpa AL, Coupal E, Leto TL, Linnenbach AJ, Winkelmann JC, Speicher DW, Marchesi VT, et al: The complete cDNA and polypeptide sequences of human erythroid α-spectrin. *J Biol Chem* **265**:4434, 1990.
98. Winkelmann JC, Chang JG, Tse WT, Scarpa AL, Marchesi VT, Forget BG: Full-length sequence of the cDNA for human erythroid β-spectrin. *J Biol Chem* **265**:11827, 1990.
99. Ziemnicka-Kotula D, Xu J, Gu H, Potempska A, Kim KS, Jenkins EC, Trenkner E, Kotula L: Identification of a candidate human spectrin Src homology 3 domain-binding protein suggests a general mechanism of association of tyrosine kinases with the spectrin-based membrane skeleton. *J Biol Chem* **273**:13681, 1998.
100. Wallis CJ, Wenegieme EF, Babitch JA: Characterization of calcium binding to brain spectrin. *J Biol Chem* **267**:4333, 1992.
101. Kennedy SP, Warren SL, Forget BG, Morrow JS: Ankyrin binds to the 15th repetitive unit of erythroid and nonerythroid β-spectrin. *J Cell Biol* **115**:267, 1991.
102. Cohen CM, Tyler JM, Branton D: Spectrin-actin associations studied by electron microscopy of shadowed preparations. *Cell* **21**:875, 1980.
103. Becker PS, Schwartz MA, Morrow JS, Lux SE: Radiolabel-transfer cross-linking demonstrates that protein 4.1 binds to the N-terminal region of β spectrin and to actin in binary interactions. *Eur J Biochem* **193**:827, 1990.
104. Karinch AM, Zimmer WE, Goodman SR: The identification and sequence of the actin-binding domain of human red blood cell β-spectrin. *J Biol Chem* **265**:11833, 1990.
105. Becker PS, Tse WT, Lux SE, Forget BG: β spectrin Kissimmee: A spectrin variant associated with autosomal dominant hereditary spherocytosis and defective binding to protein 4.1. *J Clin Invest* **92**:612, 1993.
106. Bresnick AR, Janmey PA, Condeelis J: Evidence that a 27-residue sequence is the actin-binding site of ABP-120. *J Biol Chem* **266**:12989, 1991.
107. Harris HW Jr, Lux SE: Structural characterization of the phosphorylation sites of human erythrocyte spectrin. *J Biol Chem* **255**:11512, 1980.
108. Tao M, Conway R, Cheta S: Purification and characterization of a membrane-bound protein kinase from human erythrocytes. *J Biol Chem* **255**:2563, 1980.
109. Manno S, Takakuwa Y, Nagao K, Mohandas N: Modulation of erythrocyte membrane mechanical function by β-spectrin phosphorylation and dephosphorylation. *J Biol Chem* **270**:5659, 1995.
110. Speicher DW, Morrow JS, Knowles WJ, Marchesi VT: Identification of proteolytically resistant domains of human erythrocyte spectrin. *Proc Natl Acad Sci U S A* **77**:5673, 1980.
111. Morrow JS, Speicher DW, Knowles WJ, Hsu CJ, Marchesi VT: Identification of functional domains of human erythrocyte spectrin. *Proc Natl Acad Sci U S A* **77**:6592, 1980.
112. Speicher DW, Weglarz L, DeSilva TM: Properties of human red cell spectrin heterodimer (side-to-side) assembly and identification of an essential nucleation site. *J Biol Chem* **267**:14775, 1992.
113. Ungewickell E, Gratzer W: Self-association of human spectrin. A thermodynamic and kinetic study. *Eur J Biochem* **88**:379, 1978.
114. Morrow JS, Marchesi VT: Self-assembly of spectrin oligomers in vitro: A basis for a dynamic cytoskeleton. *J Cell Biol* **88**:463, 1981.
115. Liu SC, Windisch P, Kim S, Palek J: Oligomeric states of spectrin in normal erythrocyte membranes: Biochemical and electron microscopic studies. *Cell* **37**:587, 1984.
116. Ralston G, Dunbar J, White M: The temperature-dependent dissociation of spectrin. *Biochim Biophys Acta* **491**:345, 1977.
117. Liu SC, Palek J: Spectrin tetramer-dimer equilibrium and the stability of erythrocyte membrane skeletons. *Nature* **285**:586, 1980.
118. Tse WT, Lecomte MC, Costa FF, Garbarz M, Féo C, Boivin P, Dhermy D, Forget BG: Point mutation in the β-spectrin gene associated with $\alpha^{I/74}$ hereditary elliptocytosis. Implications for the mechanism of spectrin dimer self-association. *J Clin Invest* **86**:909, 1990.
119. DeSilva TM, Peng KC, Speicher KD, Speicher DW: Analysis of human red cell spectrin tetramer (head-to-head) assembly using complementary univalent peptides. *Biochemistry* **31**:10872, 1992.
120. Ursitti JA, Kotula L, DeSilva TM, Curtis PJ, Speicher DW: Mapping the human erythrocyte β-spectrin dimer initiation site using recombinant peptides and correlation of its phasing with the α-actinin dimer site. *J Biol Chem* **271**:6636, 1996.
121. Nicolas G, Pedroni S, Fournier C, Gautero H, Craescu C, Dhermy D, Lecomte MC: Spectrin self-association site: Characterization and study of β-spectrin mutations associated with hereditary elliptocytosis. *Biochem J* **332**:81, 1998.
122. Speicher DW, DeSilva TM, Speicher KD, Ursitti JA, Hembach P, Weglarz L: Location of the human red cell spectrin tetramer binding site and detection of a related "closed" hairpin loop dimer using proteolytic footprinting. *J Biol Chem* **268**:4227, 1993.
123. Shahbakhti F, Gratzer WB: Analysis of the self-association of human red cell spectrin. *Biochemistry* **25**:5969, 1986.
124. Harris HW Jr, Levin N, Lux SE: Comparison of the phosphorylation of human erythrocyte spectrin in the intact red cell and in various cell-free systems. *J Biol Chem* **255**:11521, 1980.
125. Anderson JM, Tyler JM: State of spectrin phosphorylation does not affect erythrocyte shape or spectrin binding to erythrocyte membranes. *J Biol Chem* **255**:1259, 1980.
126. Ohanian V, Wolfe LC, John KM, Pinder JC, Lux SE, Gratzer WB: Analysis of the ternary interaction of the red cell membrane skeletal proteins spectrin, actin, and 4.1. *Biochemistry* **23**:4416, 1984.
127. Palek J, Sahr KE: Mutations of the red blood cell membrane proteins: From clinical evaluation to detection of the underlying genetic defect. *Blood* **80**:308, 1992.
128. Vertessy BG, Steck TL: Elasticity of the human red cell membrane skeleton. Effects of temperature and denaturants. *Biophys J* **55**:255, 1989.
129. McGough AM, Josephs R: On the structure of erythrocyte spectrin in partially expanded membrane skeletons. *Proc Natl Acad Sci U S A* **87**:5208, 1990.
130. Geiduschek JB, Singer SJ: Molecular changes in the membranes of mouse erythroid cells accompanying differentiation. *Cell* **16**:149, 1979.
131. Hasthorpe S: Quantification of spectrin-containing erythroid precursor cells in normal and perturbed erythropoiesis. *Exp Hematol* **8**:1001, 1980.
132. Moon RT, Lazarides E: β-Spectrin limits α-spectrin assembly on membranes following synthesis in a chicken erythroid cell lysate. *Nature* **305**:62, 1983.
133. Bodine DMt, Birkenmeier CS, Barker JE: Spectrin deficient inherited hemolytic anemias in the mouse: characterization by spectrin synthesis and mRNA activity in reticulocytes. *Cell* **37**:721, 1984.
134. Hanspal M, Yoon SH, Yu H, Hanspal JS, Lambert S, Palek J, Prchal JT: Molecular basis of spectrin and ankyrin deficiencies in severe hereditary spherocytosis: Evidence implicating a primary defect of ankyrin. *Blood* **77**:165, 1991.
135. Woods CM, Lazarides E: Degradation of unassembled α- and β-spectrin by distinct intracellular pathways: Regulation of spectrin topogenesis by β-spectrin degradation. *Cell* **40**:959, 1985.
136. Bennett V, Stenbuck PJ: Identification and partial purification of ankyrin, the high-affinity membrane-attachment site for human erythrocyte spectrin. *J Biol Chem* **254**:2533, 1979.
137. Cianci CD, Giorgi M, Morrow JS: Phosphorylation of ankyrin down-regulates its cooperative interaction with spectrin and protein 3. *J Cell Biochem* **37**:301, 1988.

138. Bennett V, Stenbuck PJ: The membrane attachment protein for spectrin is associated with band 3 in human erythrocyte membranes. *Nature* **280**:468, 1979.
139. Low PS, Willardson BM, Mohandas N, Rossi M, Shohet S: Contribution of the band 3-ankyrin interaction to erythrocyte membrane mechanical stability. *Blood* **77**:1581, 1991.
140. Wickrema A, Koury ST, Dai CH, Krantz SB: Changes in cytoskeletal proteins and their mRNAs during maturation of human erythroid progenitor cells. *J Cell Physiol* **160**:417, 1994.
141. Gorina S, Pavletich NP: Structure of the p53 tumor suppressor bound to the ankyrin and SH3 domains of 53BP2. *Science* **274**:1001, 1996.
142. Gallagher PG, Tse WT, Scarpa AL, Lux SE, Forget BG: Structure and organization of the human ankyrin-1 gene. Basis for complexity of pre-mRNA processing. *J Biol Chem* **272**:19220, 1997.
143. Lux SE, John KM, Bennett V: Analysis of cDNA for human erythrocyte ankyrin indicates a repeated structure with homology to tissue-differentiation and cell-cycle control proteins. *Nature* **344**:36, 1990.
144. Lambert S, Yu H, Prchal JT, Lawler J, Ruff P, Speicher D, Cheung MC, Kan YW, Palek J: cDNA sequence for human erythrocyte ankyrin. *Proc Natl Acad Sci U S A* **87**:1730, 1990.
145. Michaely P, Bennett V: The membrane-binding domain of ankyrin contains four independently folded subdomains, each comprised of six ankyrin repeats. *J Biol Chem* **268**:22703, 1993.
146. Michaely P, Bennett V: The ANK repeats of erythrocyte ankyrin form two distinct but cooperative binding sites for the erythrocyte anion exchanger. *J Biol Chem* **270**:22050, 1995.
147. Luh FY, Archer SJ, Domaille PJ, Smith BO, Owen D, Brotherton DH, Raine AR, Xu X, Brizuela L, Brenner SL, Laue ED: Structure of the cyclin-dependent kinase inhibitor $p19^{Ink4}$. *Nature* **389**:999, 1997.
148. Jacobs MD, Harrison SC: Structure of an IkBα/NF-kB complex. *Cell* **95**:749, 1998.
149. Batchelor AH, Piper DE, de la Brousse FC, McKnight SL, Wolberger C: The structure of GABPα/β: an ETS domain-ankyrin repeat heterodimer bound to DNA. *Science* **279**:1037, 1998.
150. Venkataramani R, Swaminathan K, Marmorstein R: Crystal structure of the CDK4/6 inhibitory protein $p18^{INK4}$ provides insights into ankyrin-like repeat structure/function and tumor-derived $p16^{INK4}$ mutations. *Nat Struct Biol* **5**:74, 1998.
151. Yang Y, Nanduri S, Sen S, Qin J: The structural basis of ankyrin-like repeat function as revealed by the solution structure of myotrophin. *Structure* **6**:619, 1998.
152. Baumgartner R, Fernandez-Catalan C, Winoto A, Huber R, Engh RA, Holak TA: Structure of human cyclin-dependent kinase inhibitor $p19^{INK4}$: Comparison to known ankyrin-repeat-containing structures and implications for the dysfunction of tumor suppressor $p16^{INK4a}$. *Structure* **6**:1279, 1998.
153. Davis LH, Bennett V: Mapping the binding sites of human erythrocyte ankyrin for the anion exchanger and spectrin. *J Biol Chem* **265**:10589, 1990.
154. Platt OS, Lux SE, Falcone JF: A highly conserved region of human erythrocyte ankyrin contains the capacity to bind spectrin. *J Biol Chem* **268**:24421, 1993.
155. White RA, Birkenmeier CS, Lux SE, Barker JE: Ankyrin and the hemolytic anemia mutation, *nb*, map to mouse chromosome 8: Presence of the *nb* allele is associated with a truncated erythrocyte ankyrin. *Proc Natl Acad Sci U S A* **87**:3117, 1990.
156. Davis LH, Davis JQ, Bennett V: Ankyrin regulation: An alternatively spliced segment of the regulatory domain functions as an intramolecular modulator. *J Biol Chem* **267**:18966, 1992.
157. Davis J, Davis L, Bennett V: Diversity in membrane binding sites of ankyrins. Brain ankyrin, erythrocyte ankyrin, and processed erythrocyte ankyrin associate with distinct sites in kidney microsomes. *J Biol Chem* **264**:6417, 1989.
158. Zhou D, Birkenmeier CS, Williams MW, Sharp JJ, Barker JE, Bloch RJ: Small, membrane-bound, alternatively spliced forms of ankyrin 1 associated with the sarcoplasmic reticulum of mammalian skeletal muscle. *J Cell Biol* **136**:621, 1997.
159. Gallagher PG, Forget BG: An alternate promoter directs expression of a truncated, muscle- specific isoform of the human ankyrin 1 gene. *J Biol Chem* **273**:1339, 1998.
160. Cleveland JL, Ihle JN: Contenders in FasL/TNF death signaling. *Cell* **81**:479, 1995.
161. Otto E, Kunimoto M, McLaughlin T, Bennett V: Isolation and characterization of cDNAs encoding human brain ankyrins reveal a family of alternatively spliced genes. *J Cell Biol* **114**:241, 1991.
162. Kunimoto M, Otto E, Bennett V: A new 440-kD isoform is the major ankyrin in neonatal rat brain. *J Cell Biol* **115**:1319, 1991.
163. Peters LL, John KM, Lu FM, Eicher EM, Higgins A, Yialamas M, Turtzo LC, Otsuka AJ, Lux SE: Ank3 (epithelial ankyrin), a widely distributed new member of the ankyrin gene family and the major ankyrin in kidney, is expressed in alternatively spliced forms, including forms that lack the repeat domain. *J Cell Biol* **130**:313, 1995.
164. Kordeli E, Lambert S, Bennett V: $Ankyrin_G$. A new ankyrin gene with neural-specific isoforms localized at the axonal initial segment and node of Ranvier. *J Biol Chem* **270**:2352, 1995.
165. Kashgarian M, Morrow JS, Foellmer HG, Mann AS, Cianci C, Ardito T: Na,K-ATPase co-distributes with ankyrin and spectrin in renal tubular epithelial cells. *Prog Clin Biol Res* **268B**:245, 1988.
166. Hoock TC, Peters LL, Lux SE: Isoforms of ankyrin-3 that lack the NH_2-terminal repeats associate with mouse macrophage lysosomes. *J Cell Biol* **136**:1059, 1997.
167. Beck KA, Buchanan JA, Nelson WJ: Golgi membrane skeleton: Identification, localization and oligomerization of a 195-kDa ankyrin isoform associated with the Golgi complex. *J Cell Sci* **110**:1239, 1997.
168. Chan W, Kordeli E, Bennett V: 440-kD $ankyrin_B$: structure of the major developmentally regulated domain and selective localization in unmyelinated axons. *J Cell Biol* **123**:1463, 1993.
169. Jöns T, Drenckhahn D: Anion exchanger 2 (AE2) binds to erythrocyte ankyrin and is colocalized with ankyrin along the basolateral plasma membrane of human gastric parietal cells. *Eur J Cell Biol* **75**:232, 1998.
170. Devarajan P, Scaramuzzino DA, Morrow JS: Ankyrin binds to two distinct cytoplasmic domains of Na,K-ATPase α subunit. *Proc Natl Acad Sci U S A* **91**:2965, 1994.
171. Jordan C, Puschel B, Koob R, Drenckhahn D: Identification of a binding motif for ankyrin on the α-subunit of Na^+,K^+-ATPase. *J Biol Chem* **270**:29971, 1995.
172. Zhang Z, Devarajan P, Dorfman AL, Morrow JS: Structure of the ankyrin-binding domain of α-Na,K-ATPase. *J Biol Chem* **273**:18681, 1998.
173. Srinivasan Y, Elmer L, Davis J, Bennett V, Angelides K: Ankyrin and spectrin associate with voltage-dependent sodium channels in brain. *Nature* **333**:177, 1988.
174. Smith PR, Saccomani G, Joe EH, Angelides KJ, Benos DJ: Amiloride-sensitive sodium channel is linked to the cytoskeleton in renal epithelial cells. *Proc Natl Acad Sci U S A* **88**:6971, 1991.
175. Li ZP, Burke EP, Frank JS, Bennett V, Philipson KD: The cardiac Na^+-Ca^{2+} exchanger binds to the cytoskeletal protein ankyrin. *J Biol Chem* **268**:11489, 1993.
176. Smith PR, Bradford AL, Joe EH, Angelides KJ, Benos DJ, Saccomani G: Gastric parietal cell H^+,K^+-ATPase microsomes are associated with isoforms of ankyrin and spectrin. *Am J Physiol* **264**:C63, 1993.
177. Handlogten ME, Dudenhausen EE, Yang W, Kilberg MS: Association of hepatic system A amino acid transporter with the membrane-cytoskeletal proteins ankyrin and fodrin. *Biochim Biophys Acta* **1282**:107, 1996.
178. Bourguignon LY, Jin H: Identification of the ankyrin-binding domain of the mouse T-lymphoma cell inositol 1,4,5-trisphosphate (IP3) receptor and its role in the regulation of IP3-mediated internal Ca^{2+} release. *J Biol Chem* **270**:7257, 1995.
179. Bourguignon LY, Chu A, Jin H, Brandt NR: Ryanodine receptor-ankyrin interaction regulates internal Ca^{2+} release in mouse T-lymphoma cells. *J Biol Chem* **270**:17917, 1995.
180. Lokeshwar VB, Bourguignon LY: Tyrosine phosphatase activity of lymphoma CD45 (GP180) is regulated by a direct interaction with the cytoskeleton. *J Biol Chem* **267**:21551, 1992.
181. Zhu D, Bourguignon LY: The ankyrin-binding domain of CD44s is involved in regulating hyaluronic acid-mediated functions and prostate tumor cell transformation. *Cell Motil Cytoskeleton* **39**:209, 1998.
182. Davis JQ, Bennett V: Ankyrin binding activity shared by the neurofascin/L1/NrCAM family of nervous system cell adhesion molecules. *J Biol Chem* **269**:27163, 1994.
183. Michaely P, Bennett V: Mechanism for binding site diversity on ankyrin. Comparison of binding sites on ankyrin for neurofascin and the Cl^-/HCO_3^- anion exchanger. *J Biol Chem* **270**:31298, 1995.
184. Dubreuil RR, MacVicar G, Dissanayake S, Liu C, Homer D, Hortsch M: Neuroglian-mediated cell adhesion induces assembly of the membrane skeleton at cell contact sites. *J Cell Biol* **133**:647, 1996.
185. Tuvia S, Garver TD, Bennett V: The phosphorylation state of the FIGQY tyrosine of neurofascin determines ankyrin-binding activity

and patterns of cell segregation. *Proc Natl Acad Sci U S A* **94**:12957, 1997.

186. Cohen CM, Dotimas E, Korsgren C: Human erythrocyte membrane protein band 4.2. *Semin Hematol* **30**:119, 1993.
187. Zhu L, Kahwash SB, Chang LS: Developmental expression of mouse erythrocyte protein 4.2 mRNA: Evidence for specific expression in erythroid cells. *Blood* **91**:695, 1998.
188. Rybicki AC, Qiu JJ, Musto S, Rosen NL, Nagel RL, Schwartz RS: Human erythrocyte protein 4.2 deficiency associated with hemolytic anemia and a homozygous 40glutamic acid → lysine substitution in the cytoplasmic domain of band 3 (band 3 Montefiore). *Blood* **81**:2155, 1993.
189. Rybicki AC, Musto S, Schwartz RS: Identification of a band-3 binding site near the N-terminus of erythrocyte membrane protein 4.2. *Biochem J* **309**:677, 1995.
190. Inoue T, Kanzaki A, Kaku M, Yawata A, Takezono M, Okamoto N, Wada H, Sugihara T, Yamada O, Katayama Y, Nagata N, Yawata Y: Homozygous missense mutation (band 3 Fukuoka: G130R): A mild form of hereditary spherocytosis with near-normal band 3 content and minimal changes of membrane ultrastructure despite moderate protein 4.2 deficiency. *Br J Haematol* **102**:932, 1998.
191. Rybicki AC, Schwartz RS, Hustedt EJ, Cobb CE: Increased rotational mobility and extractability of band 3 from protein 4.2-deficient erythrocyte membranes: Evidence of a role for protein 4.2 in strengthening the band 3-cytoskeleton linkage. *Blood* **88**:2745, 1996.
192. Golan DE, Corbett JD, Korsgren C, Thatte HS, Hayette S, Yawata Y, Cohen CM: Control of band 3 lateral and rotational mobility by band 4.2 in intact erythrocytes: Release of band 3 oligomers from low-affinity binding sites. *Biophys J* **70**:1534, 1996.
193. Peters LL, Gwynn B, Ciciotte SL, Korsgren C, Cohen CM, John KM, Lux SE, Brugnara C: Mild spherocytic anemia and altered red blood cell ion transport in mice deficient in protein 4.2. *Blood* **90(Suppl 1)**: 266a, 1997.
194. Peters LL, Jindel HK, Gwynn B, Korsgren C, John KM, Lux SE, Mohandas N, Cohen CM, Brugnara C: Mild spherocytosis and altered red cell ion transport in protein 4. 2-null mice. *J Clin Invest* **103**: 1527, 1999.
195. Korsgren C, Cohen CM: Associations of human erythrocyte band 4.2. Binding to ankyrin and to the cytoplasmic domain of band 3. *J Biol Chem* **263**:10212, 1988.
196. Lux SE, Tse WT, Menninger JC, John KM, Harris P, Shalev O, Chilcote RR, Marchesi SL, Watkins PC, Bennett V, et al: Hereditary spherocytosis associated with deletion of human erythrocyte ankyrin gene on chromosome 8. *Nature* **345**:736, 1990.
197. Rybicki AC, Musto S, Schwartz RS: Decreased content of protein 4.2 in ankyrin-deficient normoblastosis (*nb/nb*) mouse red blood cells: Evidence for ankyrin enhancement of protein 4.2 membrane binding. *Blood* **86**:3583, 1995.
198. Risinger MA, Dotimas EM, Cohen CM: Human erythrocyte protein 4.2, a high copy number membrane protein, is N-myristylated. *J Biol Chem* **267**:5680, 1992.
199. Das AK, Bhattacharya R, Kundu M, Chakrabarti P, Basu J: Human erythrocyte membrane protein 4.2 is palmitoylated. *Eur J Biochem* **224**:575, 1994.
200. Korsgren C, Lawler J, Lambert S, Speicher D, Cohen CM: Complete amino acid sequence and homologies of human erythrocyte membrane protein band 4.2. *Proc Natl Acad Sci U S A* **87**:613, 1990.
201. Korsgren C, Cohen CM: Organization of the gene for human erythrocyte membrane protein 4.2: Structural similarities with the gene for the a subunit of factor XIII. *Proc Natl Acad Sci U S A* **88**:4840, 1991.
202. White RA, Peters LL, Adkison LR, Korsgren C, Cohen CM, Lux SE: The murine pallid mutation is a platelet storage pool disease associated with the protein 4.2 (pallidin) gene. *Nat Genet* **2**:80, 1992.
203. Gwynn B, Korsgren C, Cohen CM, Ciciotte SL, Peters LL: The gene encoding protein 4.2 is distinct from the mouse platelet storage pool deficiency mutation pallid. *Genomics* **42**:532, 1997.
204. Tang CJ, Tang TK: Rapid localization of membrane skeletal protein 4.1 (EL1) to human chromosome 1p33-p34.2 by nonradioactive *in situ* hybridization. *Cytogenet Cell Genet* **57**:119, 1991.
205. Kim AC, Lutchman M, Pack S, Zhuang Z, Chishti AH: Reassignment of protein 4.1 gene (*EPB4.1*) to human chromosome 1p36.1, a region frequently deleted in neuroblastomas and meningiomas. *Blood* **92(Suppl 1)**:6a, 1998.
206. Baklouti F, Huang SC, Vulliamy TJ, Delaunay J, Benz EJ Jr: Organization of the human protein 4.1 genomic locus: New insights into the tissue-specific alternative splicing of the pre-mRNA. *Genomics* **39**:289, 1997.
207. Chasis JA, Coulombel L, Conboy J, McGee S, Andrews K, Kan YW, Mohandas N: Differentiation-associated switches in protein 4.1 expression. Synthesis of multiple structural isoforms during normal human erythropoiesis. *J Clin Invest* **91**:329, 1993.
208. Baklouti F, Huang SC, Tang TK, Delaunay J, Marchesi VT, Benz EJ Jr: Asynchronous regulation of splicing events within protein 4.1 pre-mRNA during erythroid differentiation. *Blood* **87**:3934, 1996.
209. Conboy J, Kan YW, Shohet SB, Mohandas N: Molecular cloning of protein 4.1, a major structural element of the human erythrocyte membrane skeleton. *Proc Natl Acad Sci U S A* **83**:9512, 1986.
210. Discher D, Parra M, Conboy JG, Mohandas N: Mechanochemistry of the alternatively spliced spectrin-actin binding domain in membrane skeletal protein 4.1. *J Biol Chem* **268**:7186, 1993.
211. Discher DE, Winardi R, Schischmanoff PO, Parra M, Conboy JG, Mohandas N: Mechanochemistry of protein 4.1's spectrin-actin-binding domain: Ternary complex interactions, membrane binding, network integration, structural strengthening. *J Cell Biol* **130**:897, 1995.
212. Schischmanoff PO, Winardi R, Discher DE, Parra MK, Bicknese SE, Witkowska HE, Conboy JG, Mohandas N: Defining of the minimal domain of protein 4.1 involved in spectrin-actin binding. *J Biol Chem* **270**:21243, 1995.
213. Leto TL, Marchesi VT: A structural model of human erythrocyte protein 4.1. *J Biol Chem* **259**:4603, 1984.
214. Tanaka T, Kadowaki K, Lazarides E, Sobue K: Ca^{2+}-dependent regulation of the spectrin/actin interaction by calmodulin and protein 4.1. *J Biol Chem* **266**:1134, 1991.
215. Nunomura W, Takakuwa Y, Tokimitsu R, Krauss SW, Kawashima M, Mohandas N: Regulation of CD44-protein 4.1 interaction by Ca^{2+} and calmodulin. Implications for modulation of CD44-ankyrin interaction. *J Biol Chem* **272**:30322, 1997.
216. Gascard P, Cohen CM: Absence of high-affinity band 4.1 binding sites from membranes of glycophorin C- and D-deficient (Leach phenotype) erythrocytes. *Blood* **83**:1102, 1994.
217. Marfatia SM, Lue RA, Branton D, Chishti AH: *In vitro* binding studies suggest a membrane-associated complex between erythroid p55, protein 4.1, and glycophorin C. *J Biol Chem* **269**:8631, 1994.
218. Hemming NJ, Anstee DJ, Staricoff MA, Tanner MJ, Mohandas N: Identification of the membrane attachment sites for protein 4.1 in the human erythrocyte. *J Biol Chem* **270**:5360, 1995.
219. Marfatia SM, Leu RA, Branton D, Chishti AH: Identification of the protein 4.1 binding interface on glycophorin C and p55, a homologue of the *Drosophila* discs-large tumor suppressor protein. *J Biol Chem* **270**:715, 1995.
220. Pasternack GR, Racusen RH: Erythrocyte protein 4.1 binds and regulates myosin. *Proc Natl Acad Sci U S A* **86**:9712, 1989.
221. Holt GD, Haltiwanger RS, Torres CR, Hart GW: Erythrocytes contain cytoplasmic glycoproteins. *O*-linked GlcNAc on Band 4.1. *J Biol Chem* **262**:14847, 1987.
222. Ungewickell E, Bennett PM, Calvert R, Ohanian V, Gratzer WB: In vitro formation of a complex between cytoskeletal proteins of the human erythrocyte. *Nature* **280**:811, 1979.
223. Correas I, Leto TL, Speicher DW, Marchesi VT: Identification of the functional site of erythrocyte protein 4.1 involved in spectrin-actin associations. *J Biol Chem* **261**:3310, 1986.
224. Morris MB, Lux SE: Characterization of the binary interaction between human erythrocyte protein 4.1 and actin. *Eur J Biochem* **231**:644, 1995.
225. Horne WC, Prinz WC, Tang EK: Identification of two cAMP-dependent phosphorylation sites on erythrocyte protein 4.1. *Biochim Biophys Acta* **1055**:87, 1990.
226. Subrahmanyam G, Bertics PJ, Anderson RA: Phosphorylation of protein 4.1 on tyrosine-418 modulates its function in vitro. *Proc Natl Acad Sci U S A* **88**:5222, 1991.
227. Takakuwa Y, Mohandas N: Modulation of erythrocyte membrane material properties by Ca^{2+} and calmodulin. Implications for their role in regulation of skeletal protein interactions. *J Clin Invest* **82**:394, 1988.
228. Tchernia G, Mohandas N, Shohet SB: Deficiency of skeletal membrane protein band 4.1 in homozygous hereditary elliptocytosis. Implications for erythrocyte membrane stability. *J Clin Invest* **68**:454, 1981.
229. Takakuwa Y, Tchernia G, Rossi M, Benabadji M, Mohandas N: Restoration of normal membrane stability to unstable protein

4.1-deficient erythrocyte membranes by incorporation of purified protein 4.1. *J Clin Invest* **78**:80, 1986.
230. Anderson RA, Lovrien RE: Glycophorin is linked by band 4.1 protein to the human erythrocyte membrane skeleton. *Nature* **307**:655, 1984.
231. Reid ME, Takakuwa Y, Conboy J, Tchernia G, Mohandas N: Glycophorin C content of human erythrocyte membrane is regulated by protein 4.1. *Blood* **75**:2229, 1990.
232. Workman RF, Low PS: Biochemical analysis of potential sites for protein 4.1-mediated anchoring of the spectrin-actin skeleton to the erythrocyte membrane. *J Biol Chem* **273**:6171, 1998.
233. Chishti AH: Function of p55 and its nonerythroid homologues. *Curr Opin Hematol* **5**:116, 1998.
234. Pasternack GR, Anderson RA, Leto TL, Marchesi VT: Interactions between protein 4.1 and band 3. An alternative binding site for an element of the membrane skeleton. *J Biol Chem* **260**:3676, 1985.
235. An XL, Takakuwa Y, Nunomura W, Manno S, Mohandas N: Modulation of band 3-ankyrin interaction by protein 4.1. Functional implications in regulation of erythrocyte membrane mechanical properties. *J Biol Chem* **271**:33187, 1996.
236. Danilov YN, Fennell R, Ling E, Cohen CM: Selective modulation of band 4.1 binding to erythrocyte membranes by protein kinase C. *J Biol Chem* **265**:2556, 1990.
237. Correas I, Avila J: Erythrocyte protein 4.1 associates with tubulin. *Biochem J* **255**:217, 1988.
238. Menegoz M, Gaspar P, Le Bert M, Galvez T, Burgaya F, Palfrey C, Ezan P, Arnos F, Girault J-A: Paranodin, a glycoprotein of neuronal paranodal membranes. *Neuron* **19**:319, 1997.
239. Walensky LD, Gascard P, Fields ME, Blackshaw S, Conboy JG, Mohandas N, Snyder SH: The 13-kD FK506 binding protein, FKBP13, interacts with a novel homologue of the erythrocyte membrane cytoskeletal protein 4.1. *J Cell Biol* **141**:143, 1998.
240. Tang CJ, Tang TK: The 30-kD domain of protein 4.1 mediates its binding to the carboxyl terminus of pICln, a protein involved in cellular volume regulation. *Blood* **92**:1442, 1998.
241. Mattagajasingh SN, Huang SC, Hartenstein JS, Benz EJ Jr: Protein 4.1R associates with mitotic spindle pole organizing protein NuMA, dynein and dynactin. *Blood* **92(Suppl 1)**:5a, 1998.
242. Mattagajasingh SN, Huang SC, Hartenstein JS, Benz EJ Jr: Functional interaction of protein 4.1R with tight junction proteins. *Blood* **92(Suppl 1)**:300a, 1998.
243. De Cárcer G, Lallena MJ, Correas I: Protein 4.1 is a component of the nuclear matrix of mammalian cells. *Biochem J* **312**:871, 1995.
244. Krauss SW, Larabell CA, Lockett S, Gascard P, Penman S, Mohandas N, Chasis JA: Structural protein 4.1 in the nucleus of human cells: Dynamic rearrangements during cell division. *J Cell Biol* **137**:275, 1997.
245. Krauss SW, Chasis JA, Rogers C, Mohandas N, Krockmalnic G, Penman S: Structural protein 4.1 is located in mammalian centrosomes. *Proc Natl Acad Sci U S A* **94**:7297, 1997.
246. Rybicki AC, Heath R, Lubin B, Schwartz RS: Human erythrocyte protein 4.1 is a phosphatidylserine binding protein. *J Clin Invest* **81**:255, 1988.
247. Tsukita S, Yonemura S: ERM proteins: Head-to-tail regulation of actin-plasma membrane interaction. *Trends Biochem Sci* **22**:53, 1997.
248. Scoles DR, Huynh DP, Morcos PA, Coulsell ER, Robinson NG, Tamanoi F, Pulst SM: Neurofibromatosis 2 tumour suppressor schwannomin interacts with βII-spectrin. *Nat Genet* **18**:354, 1998.
249. La Jeunesse DR, McCartney BM, Fehon RG: Structural analysis of *Drosophila* merlin reveals functional domains important for growth control and subcellular localization. *J Cell Biol* **141**:1589, 1998.
250. Ruff P, Speicher DW, Husain-Chishti A: Molecular identification of a major palmitoylated erythrocyte membrane protein containing the *src* homology 3 motif. *Proc Natl Acad Sci U S A* **88**:6595, 1991.
251. Alloisio N, Dalla Venezia N, Rana A, Andrabi K, Texier P, Gilsanz F, Cartron JP, Delaunay J, Chishti AH: Evidence that red blood cell protein p55 may participate in the skeleton-membrane linkage that involves protein 4.1 and glycophorin C. *Blood* **82**:1323, 1993.
252. Kim AC, Metzenberg AB, Sahr KE, Marfatia SM, Chishti AH: Complete genomic organization of the human erythroid p55 gene (*MPP1*), a membrane-associated guanylate kinase homologue. *Genomics* **31**:223, 1996.
253. Marfatia SM, Morais-Cabral JH, Kim AC, Byron O, Chishti AH: The PDZ domain of human erythrocyte p55 mediates its binding to the cytoplasmic carboxyl terminus of glycophorin C. Analysis of the binding interface by in vitro mutagenesis. *J Biol Chem* **272**:24191, 1997.
254. Puszkin S, Puszkin E, Maimon J, Rouault C, Schook W, Ores C, Kochwa S, Rosenfield R: α-actinin and tropomyosin interactions with a hybrid complex of erythrocyte-actin and muscle-myosin. *J Biol Chem* **252**:5529, 1977.
255. Tilney LG, Detmers P: Actin in erythrocyte ghosts and its association with spectrin: Evidence for a nonfilamentous form of these two molecules *in situ*. *J Cell Biol* **66**:508, 1975.
256. Byers TJ, Branton D: Visualization of the protein associations in the erythrocyte membrane skeleton. *Proc Natl Acad Sci U S A* **82**:6153, 1985.
257. Fowler VM, Sussmann MA, Miller PG, Flucher BE, Daniels MP: Tropomodulin is associated with the free (pointed) ends of the thin filaments in rat skeletal muscle. *J Cell Biol* **120**:411, 1993.
258. Kuhlman PA, Hughes CA, Bennett V, Fowler VM: A new function for adducin. Calcium/calmodulin-regulated capping of the barbed ends of actin filaments. *J Biol Chem* **271**:7986, 1996.
259. Gardner K, Bennett V: Modulation of spectrin-actin assembly by erythrocyte adducin. *Nature* **328**:359, 1987.
260. Joshi R, Gilligan DM, Otto E, McLaughlin T, Bennett V: Primary structure and domain organization of human α and β adducin. *J Cell Biol* **115**:665, 1991.
261. Katagiri T, Ozaki K, Fujiwara T, Shimizu F, Kawai A, Okuno S, Suzuki M, Nakamura Y, Takahashi E, Hirai Y: Cloning, expression and chromosome mapping of adducin-like 70 (ADDL), a human cDNA highly homologous to human erythrocyte adducin. *Cytogenet Cell Genet* **74**:90, 1996.
262. Hughes CA, Bennett V: Adducin: a physical model with implications for function in assembly of spectrin-actin complexes. *J Biol Chem* **270**:18990, 1995.
263. Li X, Matsuoka Y, Bennett V: Adducin preferentially recruits spectrin to the fast growing ends of actin filaments in a complex requiring the MARCKS-related domain and a newly defined oligomerization domain. *J Biol Chem* **273**:19329, 1998.
264. Matsuoka Y, Hughes CA, Bennett V: Adducin regulation. Definition of the calmodulin-binding domain and sites of phosphorylation by protein kinases A and C. *J Biol Chem* **271**:25157, 1996.
265. Nehls V, Drenckhahn D, Joshi R, Bennett V: Adducin in erythrocyte precursor cells of rats and humans: Expression and compartmentalization. *Blood* **78**:1692, 1991.
266. Kuhlman PA, Fowler VM: Purification and characterization of an $\alpha 1\beta 2$ isoform of CapZ from human erythrocytes: Cytosolic location and inability to bind to Mg^{2+} ghosts suggest that erythrocyte actin filaments are capped by adducin. *Biochemistry* **36**:13461, 1997.
267. Li X, Bennett V: Identification of the spectrin subunit and domains required for formation of spectrin/adducin/actin complexes. *J Biol Chem* **271**:15695, 1996.
268. Matsuoka Y, Li X, Bennett V: Adducin is an in vivo substrate for protein kinase C: Phosphorylation in the MARCKS-related domain inhibits activity in promoting spectrin-actin complexes and occurs in many cells, including dendritic spines of neurons. *J Cell Biol* **142**:485, 1998.
269. Kimura K, Fukata Y, Matsuoka Y, Bennett V, Matsuura Y, Okawa K, Iwamatsu A, Kaibuchi K: Regulation of the association of adducin with actin filaments by Rho-associated kinase (Rho-kinase) and myosin phosphatase. *J Biol Chem* **273**:5542, 1998.
270. Kaiser HW, O'Keefe E, Bennett V: Adducin: Ca^{++}-dependent association with sites of cell-cell contact. *J Cell Biol* **109**:557, 1989.
271. Gilligan DM, Lozovatsky L, Mohandas N, Gwynn B, Peters LL: The β-adducin knockout mouse has spherocytic anemia and loss of α-adducin from RBC ghosts. *Blood* **92(Suppl 1)**:301a, 1998.
272. Bianchi G, Tripodi G, Casari G, Salardi S, Barber BR, Garcia R, Leoni P, Torielli L, Cusi D, Ferrandi M, et al: Two point mutations within the adducin genes are involved in blood pressure variation. *Proc Natl Acad Sci U S A* **91**:3999, 1994.
273. Tripodi G, Szpirer C, Reina C, Szpirer J, Bianchi G: Polymorphism of g-adducin gene in genetic hypertension and mapping of the gene to rat chromosome 1q55. *Biochem Biophys Res Commun* **237**:685, 1997.
274. Cusi D, Barlassina C, Azzani T, Casari G, Citterio L, Devoto M, Glorioso N, Lanzani C, Manunta P, Righetti M, Rivera R, Stella P, Troffa C, Zagato L, Bianchi G: Polymorphisms of α-adducin and salt sensitivity in patients with essential hypertension. *Lancet* **349**:1353, 1997.

275. Tripodi G, Valtorta F, Torielli L, Chieregatti E, Salardi S, Trusolino L, Menegon A, Ferrari P, Marchisio PC, Bianchi G: Hypertension-associated point mutations in the adducin α and β subunits affect actin cytoskeleton and ion transport. *J Clin Invest* **97**:2815, 1996.
276. Siegel DL, Branton D: Partial purification and characterization of an actin-bundling protein, band 4.9, from human erythrocytes. *J Cell Biol* **100**:775, 1985.
277. Rana AP, Ruff P, Maalouf GJ, Speicher DW, Chishti AH: Cloning of human erythroid dematin reveals another member of the villin family. *Proc Natl Acad Sci U S A* **90**:6651, 1993.
278. Horne WC, Leto TL, Marchesi VT: Differential phosphorylation of multiple sites in protein 4.1 and protein 4.9 by phorbol ester-activated and cyclic AMP-dependent protein kinases. *J Biol Chem* **260**:9073, 1985.
279. Fowler VM, Bennett V: Erythrocyte membrane tropomyosin. Purification and properties. *J Biol Chem* **259**:5978, 1984.
280. Fowler VM: Regulation of actin filament length in erythrocytes and striated muscle. *Curr Opin Cell Biol* **8**:86, 1996.
281. Fowler VM: Tropomodulin: A cytoskeletal protein that binds to the end of erythrocyte tropomyosin and inhibits tropomyosin binding to actin. *J Cell Biol* **111**:471, 1990.
282. Fowler VM, Davis JQ, Bennett V: Human erythrocyte myosin: Identification and purification. *J Cell Biol* **100**:47, 1985.
283. Colin FC, Schrier SL: Myosin content and distribution in human neonatal erythrocytes are different from adult erythrocytes. *Blood* **78**:3052, 1991.
284. der Terrossian E, Deprette C, Lebbar I, Cassoly R: Purification and characterization of erythrocyte caldesmon. Hypothesis for an actin-linked regulation of a contractile activity in the red blood cell membrane. *Eur J Biochem* **219**:503, 1994.
285. Beaven GH, Jean-Baptiste L, Ungewickell E, Baines AJ, Shahbakhti F, Pinder JC, Lux SE, Gratzer WB: An examination of the soluble oligomeric complexes extracted from the red cell membrane and their relation to the membrane cytoskeleton. *Eur J Cell Biol* **36**:299, 1985.
286. Liu SC, Derick LH, Palek J: Visualization of the hexagonal lattice in the erythrocyte membrane skeleton. *J Cell Biol* **104**:527, 1987.
287. Sheetz MP, Casaly J: 2,3-Diphosphoglycerate and ATP dissociate erythrocyte membrane skeletons. *J Biol Chem* **255**:9955, 1980.
288. Mentzer WC Jr, Iarocci TA, Mohandas N, Lane PA, Smith B, Lazerson J, Hays T: Modulation of erythrocyte membrane mechanical stability by 2,3-diphosphoglycerate in the neonatal poikilocytosis/elliptocytosis syndrome. *J Clin Invest* **79**:943, 1987.
289. Schindler M, Koppel DE, Sheetz MP: Modulation of membrane protein lateral mobility by polyphosphates and polyamines. *Proc Natl Acad Sci U S A* **77**:1457, 1980.
290. Moriyama R, Lombardo CR, Workman RF, Low PS: Regulation of linkages between the erythrocyte membrane and its skeleton by 2,3-diphosphoglycerate. *J Biol Chem* **268**:10990, 1993.
291. Waugh RE: Effects of 2,3-diphosphoglycerate on the mechanical properties of erythrocyte membrane. *Blood* **68**:231, 1986.
292. Cohen CM, Gascard P: Regulation and posttranslational modification of erythrocyte membrane and membrane-skeleton proteins. *Semin Hematol* **29**:244, 1992.
293. Lu PW, Soong CJ, Tao M: Phosphorylation of ankyrin decreases its affinity for spectrin tetramer. *J Biol Chem* **260**:14958, 1985.
294. Soong CJ, Lu PW, Tao M: Analysis of band 3 cytoplasmic domain phosphorylation and association with ankyrin. *Arch Biochem Biophys* **254**:509, 1987.
295. Ling E, Danilov YN, Cohen CM: Modulation of red cell band 4.1 function by cAMP-dependent kinase and protein kinase C phosphorylation. *J Biol Chem* **263**:2209, 1988.
296. Eder PS, Soong CJ, Tao M: Phosphorylation reduces the affinity of protein 4.1 for spectrin. *Biochemistry* **25**:1764, 1986.
297. Chao TS, Tao M: Modulation of protein 4.1 binding to inside-out membrane vesicles by phosphorylation. *Biochemistry* **30**:10529, 1991.
298. Anderson JP, Morrow JS: The interaction of calmodulin with human erythrocyte spectrin. Inhibition of protein 4.1-stimulated actin binding. *J Biol Chem* **262**:6365, 1987.
299. Gardner K, Bennett V: A new erythrocyte membrane-associated protein with calmodulin binding activity. Identification and purification. *J Biol Chem* **261**:1339, 1986.
300. Shohet SB: Reconstitution of spectrin-deficient spherocytic mouse erythrocyte membranes. *J Clin Invest* **64**:483, 1979.
301. Marchesi VT, Steers E Jr: Selective solubilization of a protein component of the red cell membrane. *Science* **159**:203, 1968.
302. Liu SC, Derick LH, Agre P, Palek J: Alteration of the erythrocyte membrane skeletal ultrastructure in hereditary spherocytosis, hereditary elliptocytosis, and pyropoikilocytosis. *Blood* **76**:198, 1990.
303. Lux SE, John KM, Karnovsky MJ: Irreversible deformation of the spectrin-actin lattice in irreversibly sickled cells. *J Clin Invest* **58**:955, 1976.
304. Tomaselli MB, John KM, Lux SE: Elliptical erythrocyte membrane skeletons and heat-sensitive spectrin in hereditary elliptocytosis. *Proc Natl Acad Sci U S A* **78**:1911, 1981.
305. Johnson RM, Taylor G, Meyer DB: Shape and volume changes in erythrocyte ghosts and spectrin-actin networks. *J Cell Biol* **86**:371, 1980.
306. Elgsaeter A, Shotton DM, Branton D: Intramembrane particle aggregation in erythrocyte ghosts. II. The influence of spectrin aggregation. *Biochim Biophys Acta* **426**:101, 1976.
307. Sheetz MP, Schindler M, Koppel DE: Lateral mobility of integral membrane proteins is increased in spherocytic erythrocytes. *Nature* **285**:510, 1980.
308. Corbett JD, Agre P, Palek J, Golan DE: Differential control of band 3 lateral and rotational mobility in intact red cells. *J Clin Invest* **94**:683, 1994.
309. Che A, Morrison IE, Pan R, Cherry RJ: Restriction by ankyrin of band 3 rotational mobility in human erythrocyte membranes and reconstituted lipid vesicles. *Biochemistry* **36**:9588, 1997.
310. Hardy B, Bensch KG, Schrier SL: Spectrin rearrangement early in erythrocyte ghost endocytosis. *J Cell Biol* **82**:654, 1979.
311. Tokuyasu KT, Schekman R, Singer SJ: Domains of receptor mobility and endocytosis in the membranes of neonatal human erythrocytes and reticulocytes are deficient in spectrin. *J Cell Biol* **80**:481, 1979.
312. Cullis PR, Hope MJ: Effects of fusogenic agent on membrane structure of erythrocyte ghosts and the mechanism of membrane fusion. *Nature* **271**:672, 1978.
313. Lambrecht K: Die Elliptocytose (Ovalocytose) und ihre klinische Bedeutung. *Ergebn Inn Med Kinderheilkd* **55**:295, 1938.
314. Dresbach M: Elliptical human red corpuscles. *Science* **19**:469, 1904.
315. Flint A: Elliptical human erythrocytes. *Science* **19**:796, 1904.
316. Dresbach M: Elliptical human erythrocytes. *Science* **21**:473, 1905.
317. Bishop FW: Elliptical human erythrocytes. *Arch Intern Med* **14**:388, 1914.
318. Sydenstricker VP: Elliptic human erythrocytes. *JAMA* **81**:113, 1923.
319. Huck JG, Bigelow RM: Poikilocytes in otherwise normal blood (elliptical human erythrocytes). *Bull Johns Hopkins Hosp* **34**:390, 1923.
320. Hunter WC, Adams RB: Hematologic study of three generations of a white family showing elliptical erythrocytes. *Ann Intern Med* **2**:1162, 1929.
321. van den Bergh AAH: Elliptische rote Blutkoperchen Blutköperchen. *Dtsch Med Wochenschr* **54**:1244, 1928.
322. Grzegorzewski H: Über familiäres Vorkommen elliptisher Erythrocyten beim Menschen. *Folia Haematol (Leipz)* **50**:260, 1933.
323. Penfold J, Lipscomb JM: Elliptocytosis in man, associated with hereditary haemorrhagic telangiectasis. *Q J Med* **12**:157, 1943.
324. Lawrence JS: Elliptical and sickle-shaped erythrocytes in the circulating blood of white persons. *J Clin Invest* **5**:31, 1927.
325. Pollock LH, Dameshek W: Elongation of red blood cells in a Jewish family. *Am J Med Sci* **188**:822, 1934.
326. Introzzi P: Anemia ipocromica splenomegalica emolitica con ovalocitosi (ellitticitosi), poichilocitosi ed aumento della resistenza osmotica dei globuli rossi, Splenectomia. *Haematologica* **16**:525, 1935.
327. Wyandt H, Bancroft PM, Winship TO: Elliptic erythrocytes in man. *Arch Intern Med* **68**:1043, 1941.
328. Zarkowsky HS, Mohandas N, Speaker CB, Shohet SB: A congenital haemolytic anaemia with thermal sensitivity of the erythrocyte membrane. *Br J Haematol* **29**:537, 1975.
329. Wiley JS, Gill FM: Red cell calcium leak in congenital hemolytic anemia with extreme microcytosis. *Blood* **47**:197, 1976.
330. Zarkowsky HS: Heat-induced erythrocyte fragmentation in neonatal elliptocytosis. *Br J Haematol* **41**:515, 1979.
331. McCarty SH: Elliptical red blood cells in man. A report of eleven cases. *J Lab Clin Med* **19**:612, 1934.
332. Lecomte MC, Dhermy D, Gautero H, Bournier O, Galand C, Boivin P: Hereditary elliptocytosis in West Africa: Frequency and repartition of spectrin variants. *C R Acad Sci III* **306**:43, 1988.
333. Bashir N, Barkawi M, Sharif L: Prevalence of haemoglobinopathies in school children in Jordan Valley. *Ann Trop Paediatr* **11**:373, 1991.
334. Glele-Kakai C, Garbarz M, Lecomte MC, Leborgne S, Galand C, Bournier O, Devaux I, Gautero H, Zohoun I, Gallagher PG, Forget BG,

Dhermy D: Epidemiological studies of spectrin mutations related to hereditary elliptocytosis and spectrin polymorphisms in Benin. *Br J Haematol* **95**:57, 1996.
335. Facer CA: Erythrocytes carrying mutations in spectrin and protein 4.1 show differing sensitivities to invasion by Plasmodium falciparum. *Parasitol Res* **81**:52, 1995.
336. Mgone CS, Koki G, Paniu MM, Kono J, Bhatia KK, Genton B, Alexander ND, Alpers MP: Occurrence of the erythrocyte band 3 (*AE1*) gene deletion in relation to malaria endemicity in Papua New Guinea. *Trans R Soc Trop Med Hyg* **90**:228, 1996.
337. Goodall HB, Hendry DWW, Lawler SD, Stephen SA: Data on linkage in man: Elliptocytosis and blood groups. II. Family 3. *Ann Eugenet* **17**:272, 1953.
338. Geerdink RA, Nijenhuis LE, Huizinga J: Hereditary elliptocytosis: Linkage data in man. *Ann Hum Genet* **30**:363, 1967.
339. Keats BJ: Another elliptocytosis locus on chromosome 1? *Hum Genet* **50**:227, 1979.
340. Jonsson JJ, Renieri A, Gallagher PG, Kashtan CE, Cherniske EM, Bruttini M, Piccini M, Vitelli F, Ballabio A, Pober BR: Alport syndrome, mental retardation, midface hypoplasia, and elliptocytosis: A new X-linked contiguous gene deletion syndrome? *J Med Genet* **35**:273, 1998.
341. Palek J, Lux SE: Red cell membrane skeletal defects in hereditary and acquired hemolytic anemias. *Semin Hematol* **20**:189, 1983.
342. Dacie JV, Mollison PL, Richardson N, Selwyn JG, Shapir I: Atypical congenital haemolytic anaemia. *Q J Med* **22**:79, 1953.
343. Alloisio N, Morlé L, Maréchal J, Roux AF, Ducluzeau MT, Guetarni D, Pothier B, Baklouti F, Ghanem A, Kastally R, et al: Sp $\alpha^{V/41}$: A common spectrin polymorphism at the αIV-αV domain junction. Relevance to the expression level of hereditary elliptocytosis due to α-spectrin variants located *in trans*. *J Clin Invest* **87**:2169, 1991.
344. Florman AL, Wintrobe MM: Human elliptical red corpuscles. *Bull Johns Hopkins Hosp* **63**:209, 1938.
345. Motulsky AG, Singer K, Crosby WH, Smith V: The life span of the elliptocyte. Hereditary elliptocytosis and its relationship to other familial hemolytic diseases. *Blood* **9**:57, 1954.
346. Geerdink RA, Helleman PW, Verloop MC: Hereditary elliptocytosis and hyperhaemolysis. A comparative study of 6 families with 145 patients. *Acta Med Scand* **179**:715, 1966.
347. Jensson O, Jonasson T, Olafsson O: Hereditary elliptocytosis in Iceland. *Br J Haematol* **13**:844, 1967.
348. Trinick RH: Elliptocytosis. *Lancet* **1**:963, 1948.
349. Coetzer T, Lawler J, Prchal JT, Palek J: Molecular determinants of clinical expression of hereditary elliptocytosis and pyropoikilocytosis. *Blood* **70**:766, 1987.
350. Palek J: Hereditary elliptocytosis and related disorders. *Clin Haematol* **14**:45, 1985.
351. Hunter WC: Further study of a white family showing elliptical erythrocytes. *Ann Intern Med* **6**:775, 1932.
352. McCurdy PR: Clinical, genetic and physiological studies in hereditary elliptocytosis, in *Proceedings of the IX Congress International Society of Hematology*. Mexico City, Universidad Nacional Autonoma de Mexico, 1964, vol 1, p 155.
353. Pui CH, Wang W, Wilimas J: Hereditary elliptocytosis: Morphologic abnormalities during acute hepatitis. *Clin Pediatr (Phila)* **21**:188, 1982.
354. Horiguchi-Yamada J, Fujikawa T, Ideguchi H, Iwase S, Yamazaki Y, Yamada H: Hemolysis caused by CMV infection in a pregnant woman with silent elliptocytosis. *Int J Hematol* **68**:311, 1998.
355. Nkrumah FK: Hereditary elliptocytosis associated with severe haemolytic anaemia and malaria. *Afr J Med Sci* **3**:131, 1972.
356. Kruatrachue M, Asawapokee N: Hereditary elliptocytosis and Plasmodium falciparum malaria. *Ann Trop Med Parasitol* **66**:161, 1972.
357. Ozer L, Mills GC: Elliptocytosis with haemolytic anaemia. *Br J Haematol* **10**:468, 1964.
358. Pajor A, Lehoczky D: Hemolytic anemia precipitated by pregnancy in a patient with hereditary elliptocytosis. *Am J Hematol* **52**:240, 1996.
359. Schoomaker EB, Butler WM, Diehl LF: Increased heat sensitivity of red blood cells in hereditary elliptocytosis with acquired cobalamin (vitamin B12) deficiency. *Blood* **59**:1213, 1982.
360. Josephs HW, Avery ME: Hereditary elliptocytosis associated with increased hemolysis. *Pediatrics* **16**:741, 1965.
361. Austin RF, Desforges JF: Hereditary elliptocytosis: An unusual presentation of hemolysis in the newborn associated with transient morphologic abnormalities. *Pediatrics* **44**:196, 1969.
362. Carpentieri U, Gustavson LP, Haggard ME: Pyknocytosis in a neonate: An unusual presentation of hereditary elliptocytosis. *Clin Pediatr (Phila)* **16**:76, 1977.
363. Maxwell DJ, Seshadri R, Rumpf DJ, Miller JM: Infantile pyknocytosis: A cause of intrauterine haemolysis in 2 siblings. *Aust N Z J Obstet Gynaecol* **23**:182, 1983.
364. Lux SE, John KM: Unpublished observations.
365. Grech JL, Cachia EA, Calleja F, Pullicino F: Hereditary elliptocytosis in two Maltese families. *J Clin Pathol* **14**:365, 1961.
366. Lipton EL: Elliptocytosis with hemolytic anemia; the effects of splenectomy. *Pediatrics* **15**:67, 1955.
367. Pryor DS, Pitney WR: Hereditary elliptocytosis: A report of two families from new guinea. *Br J Haematol* **13**:126, 1967.
368. Nielsen JA, Praktitioner S: Homozygous hereditary elliptocytosis as the cause of haemolytic anemia in infancy. *Scand J Haematol* **5**:486, 1968.
369. Evans JP, Baines AJ, Hann IM, Al-Hakim I, Knowles SM, Hoffbrand AV: Defective spectrin dimer-dimer association in a family with transfusion dependent homozygous hereditary elliptocytosis. *Br J Haematol* **54**:163, 1983.
370. Garbarz M, Lecomte MC, Dhermy D, Féo C, Chaveroche I, Gautero H, Bournier O, Picat C, Goepp A, Boivin P: Double inheritance of an $\alpha^{I/65}$ spectrin variant in a child with homozygous elliptocytosis. *Blood* **67**:1661, 1986.
371. Prchal JT, Castleberry RP, Parmley RT, Crist WM, Malluh A: Hereditary pyropoikilocytosis and elliptocytosis: clinical, laboratory, and ultrastructural features in infants and children. *Pediatr Res* **16**:484, 1982.
372. Mentzer WC, Turetsky T, Mohandas N, Schrier S, Wu CS, Koenig H: Identification of the hereditary pyropoikilocytosis carrier state. *Blood* **63**:1439, 1984.
373. Coetzer T, Palek J, Lawler J, Liu SC, Jarolim P, Lahav M, Prchal JT, Wang W, Alter BP, Schewitz G, et al: Structural and functional heterogeneity of α spectrin mutations involving the spectrin heterodimer self-association site: Relationships to hematologic expression of homozygous hereditary elliptocytosis and hereditary pyropoikilocytosis. *Blood* **75**:2235, 1990.
374. Palek J, Lambert S: Genetics of the red cell membrane skeleton. *Semin Hematol* **27**:290, 1990.
375. Coetzer TL, Palek J: Partial spectrin deficiency in hereditary pyropoikilocytosis. *Blood* **67**:919, 1986.
376. Cutting HO, McHugh WJ, Conrad FG, Marlow AA: Autosomal dominant hemolytic anemia characterized by ovalocytosis. A family study of seven involved members. *Am J Med* **39**:21, 1965.
377. Giffin HZ, Watkins CH: Ovalocytosis with features of hemolytic icterus. *Trans Assoc Am Physicians* **54**:355, 1939.
378. Weiss HJ: Hereditary elliptocytosis with hemolytic anemia. *Am J Med* **35**:455, 1963.
379. Greenberg LH, Tanaka KR: Hereditary elliptocytosis with hemolytic anemia — A family study of five affected members. *Calif Med* **110**:389, 1969.
380. Wilson HE, Long MJ: Hereditary ovalocytosis (elliptocytosis) with hypersplenism. *Arch Intern Med* **95**:438, 1955.
381. Matsumoto N, Ishihara T, Takahashi M, Uchino F, Ono J: Fine structures of the spleen in hereditary elliptocytosis. *Acta Pathol Jpn* **26**:533, 1976.
382. Torlontano G, Fioritoni G, Salvati AM: Hereditary haemolytic ovalocytosis with defective erythropoiesis. *Br J Haematol* **43**:435, 1979.
383. Jankovic M, Sansone G, Conter V, Iolascon A, Masera G: Atypical hereditary ovalocytosis associated with defective dyserythropoietic anemia. *Acta Haematol* **89**:35, 1993.
384. Honig GR, Lacson PS, Maurer HS: A new familial disorder with abnormal erythrocyte morphology and increased permeability of the erythrocytes to sodium and potassium. *Pediatr Res* **5**:159, 1971.
385. Cattani JA: *The ovalocytosis polymorphism and malaria resistance in Papua New Guinea: An epidemiological study*. PhD dissertation, University of California-Berkeley, 1984.
386. Liu SC, Zhai S, Palek J, Golan DE, Amato D, Hassan K, Nurse GT, Babona D, Coetzer T, Jarolim P, et al: Molecular defect of the band 3 protein in southeast Asian ovalocytosis. *N Engl J Med* **323**:1530, 1990.
387. Reardon DM, Seymour CA, Cox TM, Pinder JC, Schofield AE, Tanner MJ: Hereditary ovalocytosis with compensated haemolysis. *Br J Haematol* **85**:197, 1993.
388. Coetzer TL, Beeton L, van Zyl D, Field SP, Agherdien A, Smart E, Daniels GL: Southeast Asian ovalocytosis in a South African kindred with hemolytic anemia. *Blood* **87**:1656, 1996.

389. Liu SC, Jarolim P, Rubin HL, Palek J, Amato D, Hassan K, Zaik M, Sapak P: The homozygous state for the band 3 protein mutation in Southeast Asian Ovalocytosis may be lethal. *Blood* **84**:3590, 1994.
390. Genton B, al-Yaman F, Mgone CS, Alexander N, Paniu MM, Alpers MP, Mokela D: Ovalocytosis and cerebral malaria. *Nature* **378**:564, 1995.
391. O'Donnell A, Allen SJ, Mgone CS, Martinson JJ, Clegg JB, Weatherall DJ: Red cell morphology and malaria anaemia in children with Southeast Asian ovalocytosis band 3 in Papua New Guinea. *Br J Haematol* **101**:407, 1998.
392. Mohandas N, Lie-Injo LE, Friedman M, Mak JW: Rigid membranes of Malayan ovalocytes: A likely genetic barrier against malaria. *Blood* **63**:1385, 1984.
393. Saul A, Lamont G, Sawyer WH, Kidson C: Decreased membrane deformability in Melanesian ovalocytes from Papua New Guinea. *J Cell Biol* **98**:1348, 1984.
394. Kidson C, Lamont G, Saul A, Nurse GT: Ovalocytic erythrocytes from Melanesians are resistant to invasion by malaria parasites in culture. *Proc Natl Acad Sci U S A* **78**:5829, 1981.
395. Hadley T, Saul A, Lamont G, Hudson DE, Miller LH, Kidson C: Resistance of Melanesian elliptocytes (ovalocytes) to invasion by *Plasmodium knowlesi* and *Plasmodium falciparum* malaria parasites in vitro. *J Clin Invest* **71**:780, 1983.
396. Booth PB, Serjeantson S, Woodfield DG, Amato D: Selective depression of blood group antigens associated with hereditary ovalocytosis among Melanesians. *Vox Sang* **32**:99, 1977.
397. Foo LC, Rekhraj V, Chiang GL, Mak JW: Ovalocytosis protects against severe malaria parasitemia in the Malayan aborigines. *Am J Trop Med Hyg* **47**:271, 1992.
398. Bunyaratvej A, Butthep P, Kaewkettong P, Yuthavong Y: Malaria protection in hereditary ovalocytosis: Relation to red cell deformability, red cell parameters and degree of ovalocytosis. *Southeast Asian J Trop Med Public Health* **28**:38, 1997.
399. Liu SC, Palek J, Prchal JT: Defective spectrin dimer-dimer association with hereditary elliptocytosis. *Proc Natl Acad Sci U S A* **79**:2072, 1982.
400. Mohandas N, Clark MR, Health BP, Rossi M, Wolfe LC, Lux SE, Shohet SB: A technique to detect reduced mechanical stability of red cell membranes: Relevance to elliptocytic disorders. *Blood* **59**:768, 1982.
401. Silveira P, Cynober T, Dhermy D, Mohandas N, Tchernia G: Red blood cell abnormalities in hereditary elliptocytosis and their relevance to variable clinical expression. *Am J Clin Pathol* **108**:391, 1997.
402. Schültze M: Ein heizbarer objectisch und seine verwendung bei untersuchungen des blutes. *Arch Mikrok Anat* **1**:1, 1865.
403. Chang K, Williamson JR, Zarkowsky HS: Effect of heat on the circular dichroism of spectrin in hereditary pyropoikilocytosis. *J Clin Invest* **64**:326, 1979.
404. Liu SC, Palek J, Prchal J, Castleberry RP: Altered spectrin dimer-dimer association and instability of erythrocyte membrane skeletons in hereditary pyropoikilocytosis. *J Clin Invest* **68**:597, 1981.
405. Liu SC, Palek J, Prchal J: Defective membrane skeleton assembly in hereditary elliptocytosis. *Prog Clin Biol Res* **56**:157, 1981.
406. Lawler J, Liu SC, Palek J, Prchal J: A molecular defect of spectrin in a subset of patients with hereditary elliptocytosis. Alterations in the α-subunit domain involved in spectrin self-association. *J Clin Invest* **73**:1688, 1984.
407. Knowles WJ, Morrow JS, Speicher DW, Zarkowsky HS, Mohandas N, Mentzer WC, Shohet SB, Marchesi VT: Molecular and functional changes in spectrin from patients with hereditary pyropoikilocytosis. *J Clin Invest* **71**:1867, 1983.
408. Marchesi SL, Knowles WJ, Morrow JS, Bologna M, Marchesi VT: Abnormal spectrin in hereditary elliptocytosis. *Blood* **67**:141, 1986.
409. Marchesi SL, Letsinger JT, Speicher DW, Marchesi VT, Agre P, Hyun B, Gulati G: Mutant forms of spectrin α-subunits in hereditary elliptocytosis. *J Clin Invest* **80**:191, 1987.
410. Morlé L, Alloisio N, Ducluzeau MT, Pothier B, Blibech R, Kastally R, Delaunay J: Spectrin Tunis ($\alpha^{I/78}$): a new αI variant that causes asymptomatic hereditary elliptocytosis in the heterozygous state. *Blood* **71**:508, 1988.
411. Lawler J, Liu SC, Palek J, Prchal J: Molecular defect of spectrin in hereditary pyropoikilocytosis. Alterations in the trypsin-resistant domain involved in spectrin self-association. *J Clin Invest* **70**:1019, 1982.
412. Lecomte MC, Dhermy D, Garbarz M, Gautero H, Bournier O, Galand C, Boivin P: Hereditary elliptocytosis with a spectrin molecular defect in a white patient. *Acta Haematol* **71**:235, 1984.
413. Dhermy D, Lecomte MC, Garbarz M, Féo C, Gautero H, Bournier O, Galand C, Herrera A, Gretillat F, Boivin P: Molecular defect of spectrin in the family of a child with congenital hemolytic poikilocytic anemia. *Pediatr Res* **18**:1005, 1984.
414. Dhermy D, Garbarz M, Lecomte MC, Féo C, Bournier O, Chaveroche I, Gautero H, Galand C, Boivin P: Hereditary elliptocytosis: Clinical, morphological and biochemical studies of 38 cases. *Nouv Rev Fr Hematol* **28**:129, 1986.
415. Lecomte MC, Dhermy D, Solis C, Ester A, Féo C, Gautero H, Bournier O, Boivin P: A new abnormal variant of spectrin in black patients with hereditary elliptocytosis. *Blood* **65**:1208, 1985.
416. Alloisio N, Guetarni D, Morlé L, Pothier B, Ducluzeau MT, Soun A, Colonna P, Clerc M, Philippe N, Delaunay J: Sp $\alpha^{I/65}$ hereditary elliptocytosis in North Africa. *Am J Hematol* **23**:113, 1986.
417. Lawler J, Coetzer TL, Mankad VN, Moore RB, Prchal JT, Palek J: Spectrin $\alpha^{I/61}$: A new structural variant of α-spectrin in a double heterozygous form of hereditary pyropoikilocytosis. *Blood* **72**:1412, 1988.
418. Lecomte MC, Dhermy D, Garbarz M, Féo C, Gautero H, Bournier O, Picat C, Chaveroche I, Ester A, Galand C, et al: Pathologic and nonpathologic variants of the spectrin molecule in two black families with hereditary elliptocytosis. *Hum Genet* **71**:351, 1985.
419. Lambert S, Zail S: A new variant of the α subunit of spectrin in hereditary elliptocytosis. *Blood* **69**:473, 1987.
420. Baklouti F, Maréchal J, Wilmotte R, Alloisio N, Morlé L, Ducluzeau MT, Denoroy L, Mrad A, Ben Aribia MH, Kastally R, et al: Elliptocytogenic $\alpha^{I/36}$ spectrin Sfax lacks nine amino acids in helix 3 of repeat 4. Evidence for the activation of a cryptic 5′-splice site in exon 8 of α-spectrin gene. *Blood* **79**:2464, 1992.
421. Alloisio N, Wilmotte R, Morlé L, Baklouti F, Maréchal J, Ducluzeau MT, Denoroy L, Féo C, Forget BG, Kastally R, et al: Spectrin Jendouba: An $\alpha^{II/31}$ spectrin variant that is associated with elliptocytosis and carries a mutation distant from the dimer self-association site. *Blood* **80**:809, 1992.
422. Alloisio N, Morlé L, Pothier B, Roux AF, Maréchal J, Ducluzeau MT, Benhadji-Zouaoui Z, Delaunay J: Spectrin Oran ($\alpha^{II/21}$), a new spectrin variant concerning the αII domain and causing severe elliptocytosis in the homozygous state. *Blood* **71**:1039, 1988.
423. Lane PA, Shew RL, Iarocci TA, Mohandas N, Hays T, Mentzer WC: Unique α-spectrin mutant in a kindred with common hereditary elliptocytosis. *J Clin Invest* **79**:989, 1987.
424. Dhermy D, Lecomte MC, Garbarz M, Bournier O, Galand C, Gautero H, Féo C, Alloisio N, Delaunay J, Boivin P: Spectrin β-chain variant associated with hereditary elliptocytosis. *J Clin Invest* **70**:707, 1982.
425. Eber SW, Morris SA, Schröter W, Gratzer WB: Interactions of spectrin in hereditary elliptocytes containing truncated spectrin β-chains. *J Clin Invest* **81**:523, 1988.
426. Pothier B, Morlé L, Alloisio N, Ducluzeau MT, Caldani C, Féo C, Garbarz M, Chaveroche I, Dhermy D, Lecomte MC, et al: Spectrin Nice ($\beta^{220/216}$): A shortened β-chain variant associated with an increase of the $\alpha^{I/74}$ fragment in a case of elliptocytosis. *Blood* **69**:1759, 1987.
427. Kanzaki A, Rabodonirina M, Yawata Y, Wilmotte R, Wada H, Ata K, Yamada O, Akatsuka J, Iyori H, Horiguchi M, et al: A deletional frameshift mutation of the β-spectrin gene associated with elliptocytosis in spectrin Tokyo ($\beta^{220/216}$). *Blood* **80**:2115, 1992.
428. Garbarz M, Boulanger L, Pedroni S, Lecomte MC, Gautero H, Galand C, Boivin P, Feldman L, Dhermy D: Spectrin β Tandil, a novel shortened β-chain variant associated with hereditary elliptocytosis is due to a deletional frameshift mutation in the β-spectrin gene. *Blood* **80**:1066, 1992.
429. Wilmotte R, Miraglia del Giudice E, Maréchal J, Perrotta S, de Mattia D, Delaunay J, Iolascon A: A deletional frameshift mutation in spectrin β gene associated with hereditary elliptocytosis in spectrin Napoli. *Br J Haematol* **88**:437, 1994.
430. Lecomte MC, Gautero H, Bournier O, Galand C, Lahary A, Vannier JP, Garbarz M, Delaunay J, Tchernia G, Boivin P, et al: Elliptocytosis-associated spectrin Rouen ($\beta^{220/218}$) has a truncated but still phosphorylatable β chain. *Br J Haematol* **80**:242, 1992.
431. Alloisio N, Morlé L, Dorleac E, Gentilhomme O, Bachir D, Guetarni D, Colonna P, Bost M, Zouaoui Z, Roda L, et al: The heterozygous form of 4.1(−) hereditary elliptocytosis [the 4.1(−) trait]. *Blood* **65**:46, 1985.

432. Alloisio N, Morlé L, Bachir D, Guetarni D, Colonna P, Delaunay J: Red cell membrane sialoglycoprotein β in homozygous and heterozygous 4.1(−) hereditary elliptocytosis. *Biochim Biophys Acta* **816**:57, 1985.
433. Conboy J, Mohandas N, Tchernia G, Kan YW: Molecular basis of hereditary elliptocytosis due to protein 4.1 deficiency. *N Engl J Med* **315**:680, 1986.
434. Féo CJ, Fischer S, Piau JP, Grange MJ, Tchernia G: Premiére observation de l'absence d'une protéine de la membrane érythrocytaire (band-4.1) dans un cas d'anemie elliptocytaire familiale. *Nouv Rev Fr Hematol* **22**:315, 1981.
435. Yawata Y, Kanzaki A, Inoue T, Ata K, Wada H, Okamoto N, Higo I, Yawata A, Sugihara T, Yamada O: Red cell membrane disorders in the Japanese population: Clinical, biochemical, electron microscopic, and genetic studies. *Int J Hematol* **60**:23, 1994.
436. Dalla Venezia N, Gilsanz F, Alloisio N, Ducluzeau MT, Benz EJ Jr, Delaunay J: Homozygous 4.1(−) hereditary elliptocytosis associated with a point mutation in the downstream initiation codon of protein 4.1 gene. *J Clin Invest* **90**:1713, 1992.
437. Walensky LD, Shi ZT, Blackshaw S, DeVries AC, Demas GE, Gascard P, Nelson RJ, Conboy JG, Rubin EM, Snyder SH, Mohandas N: Neurobehavioral deficits in mice lacking the erythrocyte membrane cytoskeletal protein 4.1. *Curr Biol* **8**:1269, 1998.
438. Anstee DJ, Ridgwell K, Tanner MJ, Daniels GL, Parsons SF: Individuals lacking the Gerbich blood-group antigen have alterations in the human erythrocyte membrane sialoglycoproteins β and γ. *Biochem J* **221**:97, 1984.
439. Mueller TJ, Morrison M: Glycoconnectin (PAS 2), a membrane attachment site for the human erythrocyte cytoskeleton. *Prog Clin Biol Res* **56**:95, 1981.
440. Antonarakis SE: Recommendations for a nomenclature system for human gene mutations. *Hum Mutat* **11**:1, 1998.
441. Parquet N, Devaux I, Boulanger L, Galand C, Boivin P, Lecomte MC, Dhermy D, Garbarz M: Identification of three novel spectrin $\alpha^{I/74}$ mutations in hereditary elliptocytosis: Further support for a triple-stranded folding unit model of the spectrin heterodimer contact site. *Blood* **84**:303, 1994.
442. Coetzer TL, Sahr K, Prchal J, Blacklock H, Peterson L, Koler R, Doyle J, Manaster J, Palek J: Four different mutations in codon 28 of α spectrin are associated with structurally and functionally abnormal spectrin $\alpha^{I/74}$ in hereditary elliptocytosis. *J Clin Invest* **88**:743, 1991.
443. Garbarz M, Lecomte MC, Féo C, Devaux I, Picat C, Lefebvre C, Galibert F, Gautero H, Bournier O, Galand C, et al: Hereditary pyropoikilocytosis and elliptocytosis in a white French family with the spectrin $\alpha^{I/74}$ variant related to a CGT to CAT codon change (Arg to His) at position 22 of the spectrin αI domain. *Blood* **75**:1691, 1990.
444. Lecomte MC, Garbarz M, Gautero H, Bournier O, Galand C, Boivin P, Dhermy D: Molecular basis of clinical and morphological heterogeneity in hereditary elliptocytosis with spectrin αI variants. *Br J Haematol* **85**:584, 1993.
445. Morlé L, Morlé F, Roux AF, Godet J, Forget BG, Denoroy L, Garbarz M, Dhermy D, Kastally R, Delaunay J: Spectrin Tunis (Sp $\alpha^{I/78}$), an elliptocytogenic variant, is due to the CGG → TGG codon change (Arg → Trp) at position 35 of the αI domain. *Blood* **74**:828, 1989.
446. Lecomte MC, Garbarz M, Grandchamp B, Féo C, Gautero H, Devaux I, Bournier O, Galand C, d'Auriol L, Galibert F, et al: Sp $\alpha^{I/78}$: A mutation of the αI spectrin domain in a white kindred with HE and HPP phenotypes. *Blood* **74**:1126, 1989.
447. Perrotta S, Iolascon A, De Angelis F, Pagano L, Colonna G, Cutillo S, Miraglia del Giudice E: Spectrin Anastasia ($\alpha^{I/78}$): A new spectrin variant (α45 Arg → Thr) with moderate elliptocytogenic potential. *Br J Haematol* **89**:933, 1995.
448. Morlé L, Roux AF, Alloisio N, Pothier B, Starck J, Denoroy L, Morlé F, Rudigoz RC, Forget BG, Delaunay J, et al: Two elliptocytogenic $\alpha^{I/74}$ variants of the spectrin αI domain. Spectrin Culoz (GGT → GTT; αI40 Gly → Val) and spectrin Lyon (CTT → TTT; αI43 Leu → Phe). *J Clin Invest* **86**:548, 1990.
449. Floyd PB, Gallagher PG, Valentino LA, Davis M, Marchesi SL, Forget BG: Heterogeneity of the molecular basis of hereditary pyropoikilocytosis and hereditary elliptocytosis associated with increased levels of the spectrin $\alpha^{I/74}$ tryptic peptide. *Blood* **78**:1364, 1991.
450. Boulanger L, Dhermy D, Garbarz M, Silva C, Randon J, Wilmotte R, Delaunay J: A second allele of spectrin α-gene associated with the $\alpha^{I/65}$ phenotype (allele α Ponte de Sôr). *Blood* **84**:2056, 1994.
451. Roux AF, Morlé F, Guetarni D, Colonna P, Sahr K, Forget BG, Delaunay J, Godet J: Molecular basis of Sp $\alpha^{I/65}$ hereditary elliptocytosis in North Africa: Insertion of a TTG triplet between codons 147 and 149 in the α-spectrin gene from five unrelated families. *Blood* **73**:2196, 1989.
452. Hassoun H, Coetzer TL, Vassiliadis JN, Sahr KE, Maalouf GJ, Saad ST, Catanzariti L, Palek J: A novel mobile element inserted in the α spectrin gene: spectrin Dayton. A truncated α spectrin associated with hereditary elliptocytosis. *J Clin Invest* **94**:643, 1994.
453. Gallagher PG, Tse WT, Coetzer T, Lecomte MC, Garbarz M, Zarkowsky HS, Baruchel A, Ballas SK, Dhermy D, Palek J, et al: A common type of the spectrin αI 46-50a-kD peptide abnormality in hereditary elliptocytosis and pyropoikilocytosis is associated with a mutation distant from the proteolytic cleavage site. Evidence for the functional importance of the triple helical model of spectrin. *J Clin Invest* **89**:892, 1992.
454. Sahr KE, Tobe T, Scarpa A, Laughinghouse K, Marchesi SL, Agre P, Linnenbach AJ, Marchesi VT, Forget BG: Sequence and exon-intron organization of the DNA encoding the αI domain of human spectrin. Application to the study of mutations causing hereditary elliptocytosis. *J Clin Invest* **84**:1243, 1989.
455. Gallagher PG, Roberts WE, Benoit L, Speicher DW, Marchesi SL, Forget BG: Poikilocytic hereditary elliptocytosis associated with spectrin Alexandria: An $\alpha^{I/50}$ variant that is caused by a single amino acid deletion. *Blood* **82**:2210, 1993.
456. Dalla Venezia N, Alloisio N, Forissier A, Denoroy L, Aymerich M, Vives-Corrons JL, Besalduch J, Besson I, Delaunay J: Elliptopoikilocytosis associated with the α 469 His → Pro mutation in spectrin Barcelona ($\alpha^{I/50-46b}$). *Blood* **82**:1661, 1993.
457. Alloisio N, Wilmotte R, Maréchal J, Texier P, Denoroy L, Féo C, Benhadji-Zouaoui Z, Delaunay J: A splice site mutation of α-spectrin gene causing skipping of exon 18 in hereditary elliptocytosis. *Blood* **81**:2791, 1993.
458. Fournier CM, Nicolas G, Gallagher PG, Dhermy D, Grandchamp B, Lecomte MC: Spectrin St Claude, a splicing mutation of the human α-spectrin gene associated with severe poikilocytic anemia. *Blood* **89**:4584, 1997.
459. Wilmotte R, Maréchal J, Morlé L, Baklouti F, Philippe N, Kastally R, Kotula L, Delaunay J, Alloisio N: Low expression allele α^{LELY} of red cell spectrin is associated with mutations in exon 40 ($\alpha^{V/41}$ polymorphism) and intron 45 and with partial skipping of exon 46. *J Clin Invest* **91**:2091, 1993.
460. Jarolim P, Wichterle H, Hanspal M, Murray J, Rubin HL, Palek J: β spectrin Prague: a truncated β spectrin producing spectrin deficiency, defective spectrin heterodimer self-association and a phenotype of spherocytic elliptocytosis. *Br J Haematol* **91**:502, 1995.
461. Basséres DS, Pranke PH, Sales TS, Costa FF, Saad ST: β-spectrin Campinas: a novel shortened β-chain variant associated with skipping of exon 30 and hereditary elliptocytosis. *Br J Haematol* **97**:579, 1997.
462. Yoon SH, Yu H, Eber S, Prchal JT: Molecular defect of truncated β-spectrin associated with hereditary elliptocytosis. β-Spectrin Göttingen. *J Biol Chem* **266**:8490, 1991.
463. Gallagher PG, Tse WT, Costa F, Scarpa A, Boivin P, Delaunay J, Forget BG: A splice site mutation of the β-spectrin gene causing exon skipping in hereditary elliptocytosis associated with a truncated β-spectrin chain. *J Biol Chem* **266**:15154, 1991.
464. Dhermy D, Galand C, Bournier O, King MJ, Cynober T, Roberts I, Kanyike F, Adekile A: Coinheritance of α-and β-spectrin gene mutations in a case of hereditary elliptocytosis. *Blood* **92**:4481, 1998.
465. Sahr KE, Coetzer TL, Moy LS, Derick LH, Chishti AH, Jarolim P, Lorenzo F, Miraglia del Giudice E, Iolascon A, Gallanello R, et al: Spectrin Cagliari: An Ala → Gly substitution in helix 1 of β spectrin repeat 17 that severely disrupts the structure and self-association of the erythrocyte spectrin heterodimer. *J Biol Chem* **268**:22656, 1993.
466. Gallagher PG, Weed SA, Tse WT, Benoit L, Morrow JS, Marchesi SL, Mohandas N, Forget BG: Recurrent fatal *hydrops fetalis* associated with a nucleotide substitution in the erythrocyte β-spectrin gene. *J Clin Invest* **95**:1174, 1995.
467. Gallagher PG, Petruzzi MJ, Weed SA, Zhang Z, Marchesi SL, Mohandas N, Morrow JS, Forget BG: Mutation of a highly conserved residue of βI spectrin associated with fatal and near-fatal neonatal hemolytic anemia. *J Clin Invest* **99**:267, 1997.
468. Tse WT, Gallagher PG, Pothier B, Costa FF, Scarpa A, Delaunay J, Forget BG: An insertional frameshift mutation of the β-spectrin gene associated with elliptocytosis in spectrin nice ($\beta^{220/216}$). *Blood* **78**:517, 1991.
469. Qualtieri A, Pasqua A, Bisconte MG, Le Pera M, Brancati C: Spectrin Cosenza: A novel β chain variant associated with Sp $\alpha^{I/74}$ hereditary elliptocytosis. *Br J Haematol* **97**:273, 1997.

470. Maillet P, Inoue T, Kanzaki A, Yawata A, Kato K, Baklouti F, Delaunay J, Yawata Y: Stop codon in exon 30 (E2069X) of β-spectrin gene associated with hereditary elliptocytosis in spectrin Nagoya. *Hum Mutat* **8**:366, 1996.
471. Garbarz M, Tse WT, Gallagher PG, Picat C, Lecomte MC, Galibert F, Dhermy D, Forget BG: Spectrin Rouen ($\beta^{220/218}$), a novel shortened β-chain variant in a kindred with hereditary elliptocytosis. Characterization of the molecular defect as exon skipping due to a splice site mutation. *J Clin Invest* **88**:76, 1991.
472. Perrotta S, Miraglia del Giudice E, Alloisio N, Sciarratta G, Pinto L, Delaunay J, Cutillo S, Iolascon A: Mild elliptocytosis associated with the α34 Arg → Trp mutation in spectrin Genova ($\alpha^{I/74}$). *Blood* **83**:3346, 1994.
473. Wilmotte R, Harper SL, Ursitti JA, Maréchal J, Delaunay J, Speicher DW: The exon 46-encoded sequence is essential for stability of human erythroid α-spectrin and heterodimer formation. *Blood* **90**:4188, 1997.
474. Delaunay J, Dhermy D: Mutations involving the spectrin heterodimer contact site: Clinical expression and alterations in specific function. *Semin Hematol* **30**:21, 1993.
475. Randon J, Boulanger L, Maréchal J, Garbarz M, Vallier A, Ribeiro L, Tamagnini G, Dhermy D, Delaunay J: A variant of spectrin low-expression allele α^{LELY} carrying a hereditary elliptocytosis mutation in codon 28. *Br J Haematol* **88**:534, 1994.
476. Lorenzo F, Miraglia del Giudice E, Alloisio N, Morlé L, Forissier A, Perrotta S, Sciarratta G, Iolascon A, Delaunay J: Severe poikilocytosis associated with a *de novo* α 28 Arg → Cys mutation in spectrin. *Br J Haematol* **83**:152, 1993.
477. Maréchal J, Wilmotte R, Kanzaki A, Dhermy D, Garbarz M, Galand C, Tang TK, Yawata Y, Delaunay J: Ethnic distribution of allele α^{LELY}, a low-expression allele of red-cell spectrin α-gene. *Br J Haematol* **90**:553, 1995.
478. Basséres DS, Salles TS, Costa FF, Saad ST: Presence of allele α^{LELY} in an Amazonian Indian population. *Am J Hematol* **57**:212, 1998.
479. Ohanian V, Evans JP, Gratzer WB: A case of elliptocytosis associated with a truncated spectrin chain. *Br J Haematol* **61**:31, 1985.
480. Maréchal J, Wada H, Koffa T, Kanzaki A, Wilmotte R, Ikoma K, Yawata A, Inoue T, Takanashi K, Miura A, et al: Hereditary elliptocytosis associated with spectrin Le Puy in a Japanese family: Ultrastructural aspect of the red cell skeleton. *Eur J Haematol* **52**:92, 1994.
481. Lecomte MC, Gautero H, Garbarz M, Boivin P, Dhermy D: Abnormal tryptic peptide from the spectrin α-chain resulting from α- or β-chain mutations: Two genetically distinct forms of the Sp $\alpha^{I/74}$ variant. *Br J Haematol* **76**:406, 1990.
482. Pothier B, Alloisio N, Maréchal J, Morlé L, Ducluzeau MT, Caldani C, Philippe N, Delaunay J: Assignment of Sp $\alpha^{I/74}$ hereditary elliptocytosis to the α- or β-chain of spectrin through in vitro dimer reconstitution. *Blood* **75**:2061, 1990.
483. Conboy JG, Chasis JA, Winardi R, Tchernia G, Kan YW, Mohandas N: An isoform-specific mutation in the protein 4.1 gene results in hereditary elliptocytosis and complete deficiency of protein 4.1 in erythrocytes but not in nonerythroid cells. *J Clin Invest* **91**:77, 1993.
484. Dalla Venezia N, Maillet P, Morlé L, Roda L, Delaunay J, Baklouti F: A large deletion within the protein 4.1 gene associated with a stable truncated mRNA and an unaltered tissue-specific alternative splicing. *Blood* **91**:4361, 1998.
485. Garbarz M, Devaux I, Bournier O, Grandchamp B, Dhermy D: Protein 4.1 Lille, a novel mutation in the downstream initiation codon of protein 4.1 gene associated with heterozygous 4.1(−) hereditary elliptocytosis. *Hum Mutat* **5**:339, 1995.
486. Lorenzo F, Dalla Venezia N, Morlé L, Baklouti F, Alloisio N, Ducluzeau MT, Roda L, Lefrancois P, Delaunay J: Protein 4.1 deficiency associated with an altered binding to the spectrin-actin complex of the red cell membrane skeleton. *J Clin Invest* **94**:1651, 1994.
487. Garbarz M, Dhermy D, Lecomte MC, Féo C, Chaveroche I, Galand C, Bournier O, Bertrand O, Boivin P: A variant of erythrocyte membrane skeletal protein band 4.1 associated with hereditary elliptocytosis. *Blood* **64**:1006, 1984.
488. Conboy JG, Shitamoto R, Parra M, Winardi R, Kabra A, Smith J, Mohandas N: Hereditary elliptocytosis due to both qualitative and quantitative defects in membrane skeletal protein 4.1. *Blood* **78**:2438, 1991.
489. Marchesi SL, Conboy J, Agre P, Letsinger JT, Marchesi VT, Speicher DW, Mohandas N: Molecular analysis of insertion/deletion mutations in protein 4.1 in elliptocytosis. I. Biochemical identification of rearrangements in the spectrin/actin binding domain and functional characterizations. *J Clin Invest* **86**:516, 1990.
490. Conboy J, Marchesi S, Kim R, Agre P, Kan YW, Mohandas N: Molecular analysis of insertion/deletion mutations in protein 4.1 in elliptocytosis. II. Determination of molecular genetic origins of rearrangements. *J Clin Invest* **86**:524, 1990.
491. Horne WC, Huang SC, Becker PS, Tang TK, Benz EJ Jr: Tissue-specific alternative splicing of protein 4.1 inserts an exon necessary for formation of the ternary complex with erythrocyte spectrin and F-actin. *Blood* **82**:2558, 1993.
492. Morlé L, Garbarz M, Alloisio N, Girot R, Chaveroche I, Boivin P, Delaunay J: The characterization of protein 4.1 Presles, a shortened variant of RBC membrane protein 4.1. *Blood* **65**:1511, 1985.
493. Feddal S, Hayette S, Baklouti F, Rimokh R, Wilmotte R, Magaud JP, Maréchal J, Benz EJ Jr, Girot R, Delaunay J, et al: Prevalent skipping of an individual exon accounts for shortened protein 4.1 Presles. *Blood* **80**:2925, 1992.
494. Yannoukakos D, Vasseur C, Driancourt C, Blouquit Y, Delaunay J, Wajcman H, Bursaux E: Human erythrocyte band 3 polymorphism (band 3 Memphis): Characterization of the structural modification (Lys56→Glu) by protein chemistry methods. *Blood* **78**:1117, 1991.
495. Mohandas N, Winardi R, Knowles D, Leung A, Parra M, George E, Conboy J, Chasis J: Molecular basis for membrane rigidity of hereditary ovalocytosis. A novel mechanism involving the cytoplasmic domain of band 3. *J Clin Invest* **89**:686, 1992.
496. Moriyama R, Ideguchi H, Lombardo CR, Van Dort HM, Low PS: Structural and functional characterization of band 3 from Southeast Asian ovalocytes. *J Biol Chem* **267**:25792, 1992.
497. Schofield AE, Tanner MJ, Pinder JC, Clough B, Bayley PM, Nash GB, Dluzewski AR, Reardon DM, Cox TM, Wilson RJ, et al: Basis of unique red cell membrane properties in hereditary ovalocytosis. *J Mol Biol* **223**:949, 1992.
498. Liu SC, Palek J, Yi SJ, Nichols PE, Derick LH, Chiou SS, Amato D, Corbett JD, Cho MR, Golan DE: Molecular basis of altered red blood cell membrane properties in Southeast Asian ovalocytosis: Role of the mutant band 3 protein in band 3 oligomerization and retention by the membrane skeleton. *Blood* **86**:349, 1995.
499. Hochmuth RM, Evans EA, Colvard DF: Viscosity of human red cell membrane in plastic flow. *Microvasc Res* **11**:155, 1976.
500. Chien S, Sung KL, Skalak R, Usami S, Tozeren A: Theoretical and experimental studies on viscoelastic properties of erythrocyte membrane. *Biophys J* **24**:463, 1978.
501. Blackburn EK, Jordan A, Lytle WJ, Swan HT, Tudhope GR: Hereditary elliptocytic haemolytic anaemia. *J Clin Pathol* **11**:316, 1958.
502. Shneidman D, Kiessling P, Onstad J, Wolf P: Red pulp of the spleen in hereditary elliptocytosis. *Virchows Arch A Pathol Anat Histol* **372**:337, 1977.
503. Rummens JL, Verfaillie C, Criel A, Hidajat M, Vanhoof A, Van den Berghe H, Louwagie A: Elliptocytosis and schistocytosis in myelodysplasia: Report of two cases. *Acta Haematol* **75**:174, 1986.
504. Ishida F, Shimodaira S, Kobayashi H, Saito H, Kaku M, Kanzaki A, Yawata Y, Kitano K, Kiyosawa K: Elliptocytosis in myelodysplastic syndrome associated with translocation t(1;5)(p10;q10) and deletion of 20q. *Cancer Genet Cytogenet* **108**:162, 1999.
505. Mallouh AA, Qudah A: An epidemic of aplastic crisis caused by human parvovirus B19. *Pediatr Infect Dis J* **14**:31, 1995.
506. Vanlair CF, Masius JB: De la microcythemie microcythémie. *Bull R Acad Med Belg* **5**:515, 1871.
507. Ham TH, Castle WB: Studies on destruction of red blood cells. Relation of increased hypotonic fragility and erythrostasis to the mechanism of hemolysis in certain anemias. *Proc Am Phil Soc* **82**:411, 1940.
508. Chauffard A: Pathogénie de l'ictére hémolytique congénitale. *Ann Med (Paris)* **1**:3, 1914.
509. Dameshek W, Schwartz SO: Hemolysins as the cause of clinical and experimental hemolytic anemias. With particular reference to the nature of spherocytosis and increased fragility. *Am J Med Sci* **196**:769, 1938.
510. Wilson C: Some cases showing hereditary enlargement of the spleen. *Trans Clin Soc (London)* **23**:162, 1890.
511. Wilson C, Stanley D: A sequel to some cases showing hereditary enlargement of the spleen. *Trans Clin Soc (London)* **26**:163, 1893.
512. Minkowski O: Ueber eine hereditare, unter dem Bilde eines chronischen Ikterus mit Urobilinurie, Splenomegalie und Nierensiderosis verlaufende Affection. *Verh Dtsch Kongr Med* **18**:316, 1900.

513. Gilbert A, Castaigne J, Lereboullet P: De l'ictere l'ictére familial. Contribution a á l'etude l'étude de la diathese diathése biliaire. *Bull Mem Soc Med Hop Paris* **17**:948, 1900.
514. Barlow T, Shaw HB: Inheritance of recurrent attacks of jaundice and of abdominal crises with hepatosplenomegaly. *Trans Clin Soc (London)* **35**:155, 1902.
515. Chauffard MA: Pathogénie de l'ictére congénital de l'adulte. *Semin Med (Paris)* **27**:25, 1907.
516. Chauffard MA: Les ictéres hemolytique. *Semin Med (Paris)* **28**, 1908.
517. Widal F, Abrami P, Brulé M: Differentiation de plusieurs types d'ictéres hémolytiques par le procédédes hématies déplasmatisées. *Presse Med* **15**:641, 1907.
518. Hayem G: Sur une variété particuliére d'ictére chronique. Ictére infectieux chronique splenomégalique. *Presse Med* **6**:121, 1898.
519. Micheli F: Unmittelbare Effekte der Splenektomie bei einem Fall von erworbenem hämolytischen Splenomegalischen Ikterus Typus-Hayem-Widal (Splenohamolytischer Splenohämolytischer Ikterus). *Wien Klin Wochenschr* **24**:1269, 1911.
520. Giffin HZ: Haemolytic jaundice: A review of 17 cases. *Surg Gynecol Obstet* **25**:152, 1917.
521. Dawson of Penn: The Hume Lectures on haemolytic icterus. *Br Med J* **1**:921 and 1963, 1931.
522. Tileston W: Hemolytic jaundice. *Medicine (Baltimore)* **1**:355, 1922.
523. Gänsslen M: Uber hämolytischen Ikterus. *Dtsch Arch Klin Med* **140**:210, 1922.
524. Morton NE, MacKinney AA, Kosower N, Schilling RF, Gray MP: Genetics of spherocytosis. *Am J Hum Genet* **14**:170, 1962.
525. Godal HC, Heisto H: High prevalence of increased osmotic fragility of red blood cells among Norwegian blood donors. *Scand J Haematol* **27**:30, 1981.
526. Eber SW, Pekrun A, Neufeldt A, Schröter W: Prevalence of increased osmotic fragility of erythrocytes in German blood donors: screening using a modified glycerol lysis test. *Ann Hematol* **64**:88, 1992.
527. Olim G, Marques S, Saldanha C, Santos D, Barroca P, Martins-e-Silva J: Red cell abnormalities in a kindred with an uncommon form of hereditary spherocytosis. *Acta Med Port* **6**:137, 1985.
528. Duru F, Gurgey A, Ozturk G, Yorukan S, Altay C: Homozygosity for dominant form of hereditary spherocytosis. *Br J Haematol* **82**:596, 1992.
529. Perrotta S, Nigro V, Iolascon A, Nobili B, d'Urzo G, Conte ML, Poggi V, Cutillo S, Miraglia del Giudice E: Dominant hereditary spherocytosis due to band 3 Neapolis produces a life-threatening anemia at the homozygous state. *Blood* **92(Suppl 1)**:9a, 1998.
530. Whitfield CF, Follweiler JB, Lopresti-Morrow L, Miller BA: Deficiency of α-spectrin synthesis in burst-forming units-erythroid in lethal hereditary spherocytosis. *Blood* **78**:3043, 1991.
531. Eber SW, Armbrust R, Schröter W: Variable clinical severity of hereditary spherocytosis: Relation to erythrocytic spectrin concentration, osmotic fragility, and autohemolysis. *J Pediatr* **117**:409, 1990.
532. Miraglia del Giudice E, Francese M, Nobili B, Morlé L, Cutillo S, Delaunay J, Perrotta S: High frequency of *de novo* mutations in ankyrin gene *(ANK1)* in children with hereditary spherocytosis. *J Pediatr* **132**:117, 1998.
533. Miraglia del Giudice E, Lombardi C, Francese M, Nobili B, Conte ML, Amendola G, Cutillo S, Iolascon A, Perrotta S: Frequent *de novo* monoallelic expression of β-spectrin gene *(SPTB)* in children with hereditary spherocytosis and isolated spectrin deficiency. *Br J Haematol* **101**:251, 1998.
534. Özcan R, Kugler W, Feuring-Buske M, Schröter W, Lux SE, Eber SW: Parental mosaicism for ankyrin-1 mutations in two families with hereditary spherocytosis. *Blood* **90(Suppl 1)**:4a, 1997.
535. Agre P, Orringer EP, Bennett V: Deficient red-cell spectrin in severe, recessively inherited spherocytosis. *N Engl J Med* **306**:1155, 1982.
536. Wichterle H, Hanspal M, Palek J, Jarolim P: Combination of two mutant α spectrin alleles underlies a severe spherocytic hemolytic anemia. *J Clin Invest* **98**:2300, 1996.
537. Kimberling WJ, Taylor RA, Chapman RG, Lubs HA: Linkage and gene localization of hereditary spherocytosis. *Blood* **52**:859, 1978.
538. Bass EB, Smith SW Jr, Stevenson RE, Rosse WF: Further evidence for location of the spherocytosis gene on chromosome 8. *Ann Intern Med* **99**:192, 1983.
539. Chilcote RR, Le Beau MM, Dampier C, Pergament E, Verlinsky Y, Mohandas N, Frischer H, Rowley JD: Association of red cell spherocytosis with deletion of the short arm of chromosome 8. *Blood* **69**:156, 1987.
540. Costa FF, Agre P, Watkins PC, Winkelmann JC, Tang TK, John KM, Lux SE, Forget BG: Linkage of dominant hereditary spherocytosis to the gene for the erythrocyte membrane-skeleton protein ankyrin. *N Engl J Med* **323**:1046, 1990.
541. Fukushima Y, Byers MG, Watkins PC, Winkelmann JC, Forget BG, Shows TB: Assignment of the gene for β-spectrin (*SPTB*) to chromosome 14q23-q24.2 by *in situ* hybridization. *Cytogenet Cell Genet* **53**:232, 1990.
542. Mandelbaum H: Congenital hemolytic jaundice: Report of a case on congenital hemolytic jaundice. Initial hemolytic crisis occurring at the age of 75: Splenectomy followed by recovery. *Ann Intern Med* **13**:872, 1939.
543. Burman D: Congenital spherocytosis in infancy. *Arch Dis Child* **33**:335, 1958.
544. Trucco JI, Brown AK: Neonatal manifestations of hereditary spherocytosis. *Am J Dis Child* **113**:263, 1967.
545. Bosma PJ, Chowdhury JR, Bakker C, Gantla S, de Boer A, Oostra BA, Lindhout D, Tytgat GN, Jansen PL, Oude Elferink RP, et al: The genetic basis of the reduced expression of bilirubin UDP-glucuronosyltransferase 1 in Gilbert's syndrome. *N Engl J Med* **333**:1171, 1995.
546. Iolascon A, Faienza MF, Moretti A, Perrotta S, Miraglia del Giudice E: *UGT1* promoter polymorphism accounts for increased neonatal appearance of hereditary spherocytosis. *Blood* **91**:1093, 1998.
547. MacKinney AA Jr, Morton NE, Kosower NS, Schilling RF: Ascertaining genetic carriers of hereditary spherocytosis by statistical analysis of multiple laboratory tests. *J Clin Invest* **41**:554, 1962.
548. Zanella A, Milani S, Fagnani G, Mariani M, Sirchia G: Diagnostic value of the glycerol lysis test. *J Lab Clin Med* **102**:743, 1983.
549. Gehlbach SH, Cooper BA: Haemolytic anaemia in infectious mononucleosis due to inapparent congenital spherocytosis. *Scand J Haematol* **7**:141, 1970.
550. Ho-Yen DO: Hereditary spherocytosis presenting in pregnancy. *Acta Haematol* **72**:29, 1984.
551. Pajor A, Lehoczky D, Szakacs Z: Pregnancy and hereditary spherocytosis. Report of 8 patients and a review. *Arch Gynecol Obstet* **253**:37, 1993.
552. Godal HC, Refsum HE: Haemolysis in athletes due to hereditary spherocytosis. *Scand J Haematol* **22**:83, 1954.
553. Palek J, Mircevova L, Brabec V: 2,3-Diphosphoglycerate metabolism in hereditary spherocytosis. *Br J Haematol* **17**:59, 1969.
554. Erslev AJ: Compensated hemolytic anemia. *Blood* **86**:3612, 1995.
555. Guarnone R, Centenara E, Zappa M, Zanella A, Barosi G: Erythropoietin production and erythropoiesis in compensated and anaemic states of hereditary spherocytosis. *Br J Haematol* **92**:150, 1996.
556. Young LE, Izzo MJ, Platzer RF: Hereditary spherocytosis. I. Clinical, hematologic and genetic features in 28 cases, with particular reference to the osmotic and mechanical fragility of incubated erythrocytes. *Blood* **6**:1073, 1951.
557. Krueger HC, Burgert EO Jr: Hereditary spherocytosis in 100 children. *Mayo Clin Proc* **41**:821, 1966.
558. Debre R, Lamy M, See G, Schrameck G: Congenital and familial hemolytic disease in children. *Am J Dis Child* **56**:1189, 1938.
559. Diamond LK: Indications for splenectomy in childhood. Results in fifty-two operated cases. *Am J Surg* **39**:400, 1938.
560. Agre P, Asimos A, Casella JF, McMillan C: Inheritance pattern and clinical response to splenectomy as a reflection of erythrocyte spectrin deficiency in hereditary spherocytosis. *N Engl J Med* **315**:1579, 1986.
561. Leblond PF, de Boisfleury A, Bessis M: Erythrocytes shape in hereditary spherocytosis. A scanning electron microscopic study and relationship to deformability. *Nouv Rev Fr Hematol* **13**:873, 1973.
562. Dacosta L, Tchernia G, Sorette M, Mohandas N, Cyanober T: Mechanistic understanding of spherocyte generation in hereditary spherocytosis and in immune hemolytic anemia - implications for differential diagnosis based on red cell and reticulocyte indices. *Blood* **92(Suppl 1)**:9a, 1998.
563. Pekrun A, Eber SW, Kuhlmey A, Schröter W: Combined ankyrin and spectrin deficiency in hereditary spherocytosis. *Ann Hematol* **67**:89, 1993.
564. Eber SW, Gonzalez JM, Lux ML, Scarpa AL, Tse WT, Dornwell M, Herbers J, Kugler W, Ozcan R, Pekrun A, Gallagher PG, Schröter W, Forget BG, Lux SE: Ankyrin-1 mutations are a major cause of dominant and recessive hereditary spherocytosis. *Nat Genet* **13**:214, 1996.

565. Reinhart WH, Wyss EJ, Arnold D, Ott P: Hereditary spherocytosis associated with protein band 3 defect in a Swiss kindred. *Br J Haematol* **86**:147, 1994.
566. Jarolim P, Murray JL, Rubin HL, Taylor WM, Prchal JT, Ballas SK, Snyder LM, Chrobak L, Melrose WD, Brabec V, Palek J: Characterization of 13 novel band 3 gene defects in hereditary spherocytosis with band 3 deficiency. *Blood* **88**:4366, 1996.
567. Coetzer TL, Lawler J, Liu SC, Prchal JT, Gualtieri RJ, Brain MC, Dacie JV, Palek J: Partial ankyrin and spectrin deficiency in severe, atypical hereditary spherocytosis. *N Engl J Med* **318**:230, 1988.
568. Wolfe LC, John KM, Falcone JC, Byrne AM, Lux SE: A genetic defect in the binding of protein 4.1 to spectrin in a kindred with hereditary spherocytosis. *N Engl J Med* **307**:1367, 1982.
569. Hassoun H, Vassiliadis JN, Murray J, Njolstad PR, Rogus JJ, Ballas SK, Schaffer F, Jarolim P, Brabec V, Palek J: Characterization of the underlying molecular defect in hereditary spherocytosis associated with spectrin deficiency. *Blood* **90**:398, 1997.
570. Ghanem A, Pothier B, Maréchal J, Ducluzeau MT, Morlé L, Alloisio N, Féo C, Ben Abdeladhim A, Fattoum S, Delaunay J: A haemolytic syndrome associated with the complete absence of red cell membrane protein 4.2 in two Tunisian siblings. *Br J Haematol* **75**:414, 1990.
571. Kanzaki A, Yawata Y, Yawata A, Inoue T, Okamoto N, Wada H, Harano T, Harano K, Wilmotte R, Hayette S, et al: Band 4.2 Komatsu: 523 GAT → TAT (175 Asp → Tyr) in exon 4 of the band 4.2 gene associated with total deficiency of band 4.2, hemolytic anemia with ovalostomatocytosis and marked disruption of the cytoskeletal network. *Int J Hematol* **61**:165, 1995.
572. Mohandas N, Kim YR, Tycko DH, Orlik J, Wyatt J, Groner W: Accurate and independent measurement of volume and hemoglobin concentration of individual red cells by laser-light scattering. *Blood* **68**:506, 1986.
573. Ialongo P, Vignetti M, Cigliano G, Amadori S, Mandelli F: Flow cytometric measurement (H-1 Technicon) of microcytic and hyperchromic red cell populations in pediatric patients affected by hereditary spherocytosis. *Haematologica* **74**:547, 1989.
574. Cynober T, Mohandas N, Tchernia G: Red cell abnormalities in hereditary spherocytosis: Relevance to diagnosis and understanding of the variable expression of clinical severity. *J Lab Clin Med* **128**:259, 1996.
575. Michaels LA, Cohen AR, Zhao H, Raphael RI, Manno CS: Screening for hereditary spherocytosis by use of automated erythrocyte indexes. *J Pediatr* **130**:957, 1997.
576. Emerson CP Jr, Shen SC, Ham TH, Fleming EM, Castle WB: Studies on the destruction of red blood cells. IX. Quantitative methods for determining the osmotic and mechanical fragility of red cells in the peripheral blood and splenic pulp; the mechanism of increased hemolysis in hereditary spherocytosis (congenital hemolytic jaundice) as related to the function of the spleen. *Arch Intern Med* **97**:1, 1956.
577. Zanella A, Izzo C, Rebulla P, Zanuso F, Perroni L, Sirchia G: Acidified glycerol lysis test: A screening test for spherocytosis. *Br J Haematol* **45**:481, 1980.
578. Gottfried EL, Robertson NA: Glycerol lysis time of incubated erythrocytes in the diagnosis of hereditary spherocytosis. *J Lab Clin Med* **84**:746, 1974.
579. Bucx MJ, Breed WP, Hoffmann JJ: Comparison of acidified glycerol lysis test, Pink test and osmotic fragility test in hereditary spherocytosis: effect of incubation. *Eur J Haematol* **40**:227, 1988.
580. Acharya J, Ferguson IL, Cassidy AG, Grimes AJ: An improved acidified glycerol lysis test used to detect spherocytes in pregnancy. *Br J Haematol* **65**:343, 1987.
581. Streichman S, Gesheidt Y, Tatarsky I: Hypertonic cryohemolysis: A diagnostic test for hereditary spherocytosis. *Am J Hematol* **35**:104, 1990.
582. Streichman S, Gescheidt Y: Cryohemolysis for the detection of hereditary spherocytosis: Correlation studies with osmotic fragility and autohemolysis. *Am J Hematol* **58**:206, 1998.
583. Melrose W: An evaluation of the hypertonic cryohaemolysis test as a diagnostic test for hereditary spherocytosis. *Aust J Med Sci* **13**:22, 1992.
584. Mohandas N, Chasis JA: Red blood cell deformability, membrane material properties and shape: Regulation by transmembrane, skeletal and cytosolic proteins and lipids. *Semin Hematol* **30**:171, 1993.
585. Chasis JA, Agre P, Mohandas N: Decreased membrane mechanical stability and *in vivo* loss of surface area reflect spectrin deficiencies in hereditary spherocytosis. *J Clin Invest* **82**:617, 1988.
586. Clark MR, Mohandas N, Shohet SB: Osmotic gradient ektacytometry: Comprehensive characterization of red cell volume and surface maintenance. *Blood* **61**:899, 1983.
587. Wiley JS: Red cell survival studies in hereditary spherocytosis. *J Clin Invest* **49**:666, 1970.
588. Lux SE, Becker PS: Disorders of the red cell membrane skeleton: Hereditary spherocytosis and hereditary elliptocytosis, in Scriver CR, Beaudet AL, Sly WS, Valle D (eds): *The Metabolic Basis of Inherited Disease*, 6th ed. New York, McGraw-Hill, 1989, p 2367.
589. Agre P, Casella JF, Zinkham WH, McMillan C, Bennett V: Partial deficiency of erythrocyte spectrin in hereditary spherocytosis. *Nature* **314**:380, 1985.
590. Miraglia del Giudice E, Iolascon A, Pinto L, Nobili B, Perrotta S: Erythrocyte membrane protein alterations underlying clinical heterogeneity in hereditary spherocytosis. *Br J Haematol* **88**:52, 1994.
591. Dhermy D, Galand C, Bournier O, Boulanger L, Cynober T, Schismanoff PO, Bursaux E, Tchernia G, Boivin P, Garbarz M: Heterogenous band 3 deficiency in hereditary spherocytosis related to different band 3 gene defects. *Br J Haematol* **98**:32, 1997.
592. Lanciotti M, Perutelli P, Valetto A, Di Martino D, Mori PG: Ankyrin deficiency is the most common defect in dominant and non dominant hereditary spherocytosis. *Haematologica* **82**:460, 1997.
593. Miraglia del Giudice E, Francese M, Polito R, Nobili B, Iolascon A, Perrotta S: Apparently normal ankyrin content in unsplenectomized hereditary spherocytosis patients with the inactivation of one ankyrin *(ANK1)* allele. *Haematologica* **82**:332, 1997.
594. Lux S, Bedrosian C, Shalev O, Morris M, Chasis J, Davies K, Savvides P, Telen M: Deficiency of band 3 in dominant hereditary spherocytosis with normal spectrin content. *Clin Res* **38**:300a, 1990.
595. Jarolim P, Ruff P, Coetzer TL, Prchal JT, Ballas SK, Poon MC, Brabec V, Palek J: A subset of patients with dominantly inherited hereditary spherocytosis has a marked deficiency of the band 3 protein. *Blood* **76(Suppl 1)**:37a, 1990.
596. Miraglia del Giudice E, Perrotta S, Pinto L, Cappellini MD, Fiorelli G, Cutillo S, Iolascon A: Hereditary spherocytosis characterized by increased spectrin/band 3 ratio. *Br J Haematol* **80**:133, 1992.
597. Iolascon A, Miraglia del Giudice E, Perrotta S, Pinto L, Fiorelli G, Cappellini DM, Vasseur C, Bursaux E, Cutillo S: Hereditary spherocytosis due to loss of anion exchange transporter. *Haematologica* **77**:450, 1992.
598. Miraglia del Giudice E, Perrotta S, Nobili B, Pinto L, Cutillo L, Iolascon A: Coexistence of hereditary spherocytosis (HS) due to band 3 deficiency and β-thalassaemia trait: Partial correction of HS phenotype. *Br J Haematol* **85**:553, 1993.
599. Rybicki AC, Heath R, Wolf JL, Lubin B, Schwartz RS: Deficiency of protein 4.2 in erythrocytes from a patient with a Coombs negative hemolytic anemia. Evidence for a role of protein 4.2 in stabilizing ankyrin on the membrane. *J Clin Invest* **81**:893, 1988.
600. Nozawa Y, Noguchi T, Iida H, Fukushima H, Sekiya T: Erythrocyte membrane of hereditary spherocytosis: alteration in surface ultrastructure and membrane proteins, as inferred by scanning electron microscopy and SDS-disc gel electrophoresis. *Clin Chim Acta* **55**:81, 1974.
601. Hayashi S, Koomoto R, Yano A, Ishigami S, Tsujino G: Abnormality in a specific protein of the erythrocyte membrane in hereditary spherocytosis. *Biochem Biophys Res Commun* **57**:1038, 1974.
602. Inoue T, Kanzaki A, Yawata A, Wada H, Okamoto N, Takahashi M, Sugihara T, Yamada O, Yawata Y: Uniquely higher incidence of isolated or combined deficiency of band 3 and/or band 4.2 as the pathogenesis of autosomal dominantly inherited hereditary spherocytosis in the Japanese population. *Int J Hematol* **60**:227, 1994.
603. Jarolim P, Rubin HL, Brabec V, Palek J: Comparison of the ankyrin (AC)n microsatellites in genomic DNA and mRNA reveals absence of one ankyrin mRNA allele in 20% of patients with hereditary spherocytosis. *Blood* **85**:3278, 1995.
604. Miraglia del Giudice E, Hayette S, Bozon M, Perrotta S, Alloisio N, Vallier A, Iolascon A, Delaunay J, Morlé L: Ankyrin Napoli: A *de novo* deletional frameshift mutation in exon 16 of ankyrin gene *(ANK1)* associated with spherocytosis. *Br J Haematol* **93**:828, 1996.
605. Morlé L, Bozon M, Alloisio N, Vallier A, Hayette S, Pascal O, Monier D, Philippe N, Forget BG, Delaunay J: Ankyrin Bugey: A *de novo* deletional frameshift variant in exon 6 of the ankyrin gene associated with spherocytosis. *Am J Hematol* **54**:242, 1997.
606. Randon J, Miraglia del Giudice E, Bozon M, Perrotta S, De Vivo M, Iolascon A, Delaunay J, Morlé L: Frequent *de novo* mutations of the *ANK1* gene mimic a recessive mode of transmission in hereditary

spherocytosis: Three new ANK1 variants: ankyrins Bari, Napoli II and Anzio. *Br J Haematol* **96**:500, 1997.

607. Hayette S, Carre G, Bozon M, Alloisio N, Maillet P, Wilmotte R, Pascal O, Reynaud J, Reman O, Stephan JL, Morlé L, Delaunay J: Two distinct truncated variants of ankyrin associated with hereditary spherocytosis. *Am J Hematol* **58**:36, 1998.
608. Özcan R, Jarolim P, Brabec V, Lux SE, Eber SW: High frequency of frameshift/nonsense mutations of ankyrin-1 in Czech patients with dominant hereditary spherocytosis. *Blood* **88(Suppl 1)**:5a, 1996.
609. Basséres DS, Bordin S, Csota FF, Gallagher PG, Saad STO: A novel ankyrin promoter mutation associated with hereditary spherocytosis. *Blood* **92(Suppl 1)**:8a, 1998.
610. Gallagher PG, Ferreira JDS, Saad STO, Kerbally J, Costa FF, Forget BG: A recurring frameshift mutation of the ankyrin-1 gene associated with severe hereditary spherocytosis in Brazil. *Blood* **88(Suppl 1)**:11a, 1996.
611. Kanzaki A, Takezono M, Kaku M: Molecular and genetic characteristics in Japanese patients with hereditary spherocytosis: Frequent band 3 mutations and rarer ankyrin mutations. *Blood* **90(Suppl 1)**:6b, 1997.
612. Jarolim P, Rubin HL, Brabec V, Palek J: Abnormal alternative splicing of erythroid ankyrin mRNA in two kindreds with hereditary spherocytosis (Ankyrin^{Prague} and Ankyrin^{Rakovnik}). *Blood* **82(Suppl 1)**:5a, 1993.
613. Jarolim P, Rubin HL, Brabec V, Palek J: A nonsense mutation 1669Glu → Ter within the regulatory domain of human erythroid ankyrin leads to a selective deficiency of the major ankyrin isoform (band 2.1) and a phenotype of autosomal dominant hereditary spherocytosis. *J Clin Invest* **95**:941, 1995.
614. Gallagher PG: Personal communication.
615. Eber SW, Pekrun A, Reinhardt D, Schröter W, Lux SE: Hereditary spherocytosis with ankyrin Walsrode, a variant ankyrin with decreased affinity for band 3. *Blood* **84(Suppl 1)**:362a, 1994.
616. Alloisio N, Maillet P, Carre G, Texier P, Vallier A, Baklouti F, Philippe N, Delaunay J: Hereditary spherocytosis with band 3 deficiency. Association with a nonsense mutation of the band 3 gene (allele Lyon), and aggravation by a low-expression allele occurring in trans (allele Genas). *Blood* **88**:1062, 1996.
617. Miraglia del Giudice E, Vallier A, Maillet P, Perrotta S, Cutillo S, Iolascon A, Tanner MJ, Delaunay J, Alloisio N: Novel band 3 variants (bands 3 Foggia, Napoli I and Napoli II) associated with hereditary spherocytosis and band 3 deficiency: Status of the D38A polymorphism within the *EPB3* locus. *Br J Haematol* **96**:70, 1997.
618. Kanzaki A, Hayette S, Morlé L, Inoue F, Matsuyama R, Inoue T, Yawata A, Wada H, Vallier A, Alloisio N, Yawata Y, Delaunay J: Total absence of protein 4.2 and partial deficiency of band 3 in hereditary spherocytosis. *Br J Haematol* **99**:522, 1997.
619. Alloisio N, Texier P, Vallier A, Ribeiro ML, Morlé L, Bozon M, Bursaux E, Maillet P, Goncalves P, Tanner MJ, Tamagnini G, Delaunay J: Modulation of clinical expression and band 3 deficiency in hereditary spherocytosis. *Blood* **90**:414, 1997.
620. Lux SE: Unpublished data, 1990.
621. Lima PR, Gontijo JA, Lopes de Faria JB, Costa FF, Saad ST: Band 3 Campinas: A novel splicing mutation in the band 3 gene (*AE1*) associated with hereditary spherocytosis, hyperactivity of Na^+/Li^+ countertransport and an abnormal renal bicarbonate handling. *Blood* **90**:2810, 1997.
622. Jarolim P, Palek J, Rubin HL, Prchal JT, Korsgren C, Cohen CM: Band 3 Tuscaloosa: Pro327 → Arg327 substitution in the cytoplasmic domain of erythrocyte band 3 protein associated with spherocytic hemolytic anemia and partial deficiency of protein 4.2. *Blood* **80**:523, 1992.
623. Jenkins PB, Abou-Alfa GK, Dhermy D, Bursaux E, Féo C, Scarpa AL, Lux SE, Garbarz M, Forget BG, Gallagher PG: A nonsense mutation in the erythrocyte band 3 gene associated with decreased mRNA accumulation in a kindred with dominant hereditary spherocytosis. *J Clin Invest* **97**:373, 1996.
624. Bianchi P, Zanella A, Alloisio N, Barosi G, Bredi E, Pelissero G, Zappa M, Vercellati C, Baronciani L, Delaunay J, Sirchia G: A variant of the *EPB3* gene of the anti-Lepore type in hereditary spherocytosis. *Br J Haematol* **98**:283, 1997.
625. Maillet P, Vallier A, Reinhart WH, Wyss EJ, Ott P, Texier P, Baklouti F, Tanner MJ, Delaunay J, Alloisio N: Band 3 Chur: A variant associated with band 3-deficient hereditary spherocytosis and substitution in a highly conserved position of transmembrane segment 11. *Br J Haematol* **91**:804, 1995.
626. Jarolim P, Rubin HL, Liu SC, Cho MR, Brabec V, Derick LH, Yi SJ, Saad ST, Alper S, Brugnara C, et al: Duplication of 10 nucleotides in the erythroid band 3 (*AE1*) gene in a kindred with hereditary spherocytosis and band 3 protein deficiency (band 3 Prague). *J Clin Invest* **93**:121, 1994.
627. Iwase S, Ideguchi H, Takao M, Horiguchi-Yamada J, Iwasaki M, Takahara S, Sekikawa T, Mochizuki S, Yamada H: Band 3 Tokyo: Thr837 → Ala837 substitution in erythrocyte band 3 protein associated with spherocytic hemolysis. *Acta Haematol* **100**:200, 1999.
628. Perrotta S, Nigro V, Polito R, Nobili B, Amendola G, De Vivo M, Conte ML, Cutillo S, Miraglia del Giudice E: Hereditary spherocytosis due to an elongated band 3: Band 3 Vesuvio. *Blood* **90(Suppl 1)**:270a, 1997.
629. Inaba M, Yawata A, Koshino I, Sato K, Takeuchi M, Takakuwa Y, Manno S, Yawata Y, Kanzaki A, Sakai J, Ban A, Ono K, Maede Y: Defective anion transport and marked spherocytosis with membrane instability caused by hereditary total deficiency of red cell band 3 in cattle due to a nonsense mutation. *J Clin Invest* **97**:1804, 1996.
630. Bruce LJ, Cope DL, Jones GK, Schofield AE, Burley M, Povey S, Unwin RJ, Wrong O, Tanner MJ: Familial distal renal tubular acidosis is associated with mutations in the red cell anion exchanger (Band 3, AE1) gene. *J Clin Invest* **100**:1693, 1997.
631. Karet FE, Gainza FJ, Gyory AZ, Unwin RJ, Wrong O, Tanner MJ, Nayir A, Alpay H, Santos F, Hulton SA, Bakkaloglu A, Ozen S, Cunningham MJ, di Pietro A, Walker WG, Lifton RP: Mutations in the chloride-bicarbonate exchanger gene AE1 cause autosomal dominant but not autosomal recessive distal renal tubular acidosis. *Proc Natl Acad Sci U S A* **95**:6337, 1998.
632. Tanphaichitr VS, Sumboonnanonda A, Ideguchi H, Shayakul C, Brugnara C, Takao M, Veerakul G, Alper SL: Novel AE1 mutations in recessive distal renal tubular acidosis: Loss-of-function is rescued by Glycophorin A. *J Clin Invest* **102**:2173, 1998.
633. Basséres DS, Vicentim DL, Costa FF, Saad ST, Hassoun H: β-spectrin Promissão: a translation initiation codon mutation of the β-spectrin gene (ATG → GTG) associated with hereditary spherocytosis and spectrin deficiency in a Brazilian family. *Blood* **91**:368, 1998.
634. Hassoun H, Vassiliadis JN, Murray J, Yi SJ, Hanspal M, Johnson CA, Palek J: Hereditary spherocytosis with spectrin deficiency due to an unstable truncated β spectrin. *Blood* **87**:2538, 1996.
635. Hassoun H, Vassiliadis JN, Murray J, Yi SJ, Hanspal M, Ware RE, Winter SS, Chiou SS, Palek J: Molecular basis of spectrin deficiency in β spectrin Durham: A deletion within β spectrin adjacent to the ankyrin-binding site precludes spectrin attachment to the membrane in hereditary spherocytosis. *J Clin Invest* **96**:2623, 1995.
636. Garbarz M, Galand C, Bibas D, Bournier O, Devaux I, Harousseau JL, Grandchamp B, Dhermy D: A 5′ splice region G → C mutation in exon 3 of the human β-spectrin gene leads to decreased levels of β-spectrin mRNA and is responsible for dominant hereditary spherocytosis (spectrin Guemene-Penfao). *Br J Haematol* **100**:90, 1998.
637. Dhermy D, Galand C, Bournier O, Cynober T, F Mc, Tchemia G, Garbarz M: Hereditary spherocytosis with spectrin deficiency related to null mutations of the β-spectrin gene. *Blood Cells Mol Dis* **24**:251, 1998.
638. Basséres DS, Tavares AC, Bordin S: Novel β-spectrin variants associated with hereditary spherocytosis. *Blood* **90(Suppl 1)**:4b, 1997.
639. Becker PS, Morrow JS, Lux SE: Abnormal oxidant sensitivity and β-chain structure of spectrin in hereditary spherocytosis associated with defective spectrin-protein 4.1 binding. *J Clin Invest* **80**:557, 1987.
640. Coleman TR, Harris AS, Mische SM, Mooseker MS, Morrow JS: β-Spectrin bestows protein 4.1 sensitivity on spectrin-actin interactions. *J Cell Biol* **104**:519, 1987.
641. Becker PS, Cohen CM, Lux SE: The effect of mild diamide oxidation on the structure and function of human erythrocyte spectrin. *J Biol Chem* **261**:4620, 1986.
642. Wolfe LC, Byrne AM, Lux SE: Molecular defect in the membrane skeleton of blood bank-stored red cells. Abnormal spectrin-protein 4.1-actin complex formation. *J Clin Invest* **78**:1681, 1986.
643. Fujino T, Ishikawa T, Inoue M, Beppu M, Kikugawa K: Characterization of membrane-bound serine protease related to degradation of oxidatively damaged erythrocyte membrane proteins. *Biochim Biophys Acta* **1374**:47, 1998.
644. Goodman SR, Shiffer KA, Casoria LA, Eyster ME: Identification of the molecular defect in the erythrocyte membrane skeleton of some kindreds with hereditary spherocytosis. *Blood* **60**:772, 1982.
645. Hanspal M, Palek J: Synthesis and assembly of membrane skeletal proteins in mammalian red cell precursors. *J Cell Biol* **105**:1417, 1987.

646. Marchesi SL, Agre PL, Speicher DW, Tse WT, Forget BG: Mutant spectrin αII domain in recessively inherited spherocytosis. *Blood* **74(Suppl 1)**:182a, 1989.
647. Tse WT, Gallagher PG, Jenkins PB, Wang Y, Benoit L, Speicher D, Winkelmann JC, Agre P, Forget BG, Marchesi SL: Amino-acid substitution in α-spectrin commonly coinherited with nondominant hereditary spherocytosis. *Am J Hematol* **54**:233, 1997.
648. Jarolim P, Wichterle H, Palek J, Gallagher PG, Forget BG: The low expression α spectrin LEPRA is frequently associated with autosomal recessive/nondominant hereditary spherocytosis. *Blood* **88(Suppl 1)**:4a, 1996.
649. Hayette S, Dhermy D, dos Santos ME, Bozon M, Drenckhahn D, Alloisio N, Texier P, Delaunay J, Morlé L: A deletional frameshift mutation in protein 4.2 gene (allele 4.2 Lisboa) associated with hereditary hemolytic anemia. *Blood* **85**:250, 1995.
650. Takaoka Y, Ideguchi H, Matsuda M, Sakamoto N, Takeuchi T, Fukumaki Y: A novel mutation in the erythrocyte protein 4.2 gene of Japanese patients with hereditary spherocytosis (protein 4.2 Fukuoka). *Br J Haematol* **88**:527, 1994.
651. Bouhassira EE, Schwartz RS, Yawata Y, Ata K, Kanzaki A, Qiu JJ, Nagel RL, Rybicki AC: An alanine-to-threonine substitution in protein 4.2 cDNA is associated with a Japanese form of hereditary hemolytic anemia (protein 4.2 Nippon). *Blood* **79**:1846, 1992.
652. Matsuda M, Hatano N, Ideguchi H, Takahira H, Fukumaki Y: A novel mutation causing an aberrant splicing in the protein 4.2 gene associated with hereditary spherocytosis (protein 4.2 Notame). *Hum Mol Genet* **4**:1187, 1995.
653. Hayette S, Morlé L, Bozon M, Ghanem A, Risinger M, Korsgren C, Tanner MJ, Fattoum S, Cohen CM, Delaunay J: A point mutation in the protein 4.2 gene (allele 4.2 Tozeur) associated with hereditary haemolytic anaemia. *Br J Haematol* **89**:762, 1995.
654. Kanzaki A, Yasunaga M, Okamoto N, Inoue T, Yawata A, Wada H, Andoh A, Hodohara K, Fujiyama Y, Bamba T, et al: Band 4.2 Shiga: 317 CGC → TGC in compound heterozygotes with 142 GCT → ACT results in band 4.2 deficiency and microspherocytosis. *Br J Haematol* **91**:333, 1995.
655. Iwamoto S, Kajii E, Omi T, Kamesaki T, Akifuji Y, Ikemoto S: Point mutation in the band 4.2 gene associated with autosomal recessively inherited erythrocyte band 4.2 deficiency. *Eur J Haematol* **50**:286, 1993.
656. Bernstein SE: Inherited hemolytic disease in mice: A review and update. *Lab Anim Sci* **30**:197, 1980.
657. Lux SE: Spectrin-actin membrane skeleton of normal and abnormal red blood cells. *Semin Hematol* **16**:21, 1979.
658. Anderson R, Huestis RR, Motulsky AG: Hereditary spherocytosis in the deer mouse: Its similarity to the human disease. *Blood* **15**:491, 1960.
659. Falcone JC, Lux SE: Unpublished observations.
660. Bloom ML, Kaysser TM, Birkenmeier CS, Barker JE: The murine mutation jaundiced is caused by replacement of an arginine with a stop codon in the mRNA encoding the ninth repeat of β-spectrin. *Proc Natl Acad Sci U S A* **91**:10099, 1994.
661. Wandersee NJ, Birkenmeier CS, Gifford EJ, Barker JE: Identification of three mutations in the murine erythroid α spectrin gene causing hereditary spherocytosis in mice. *Blood* **92(Suppl 1)**:8a, 1998.
662. Wandersee NJ, Roesch AN, Hamblen NR, de Moes J, van der Valk MA, Bronson RT, Demant P, Barker JE: A new spontaneous mouse mutant with severe hereditary elliptocytosis is deficient in erythroid α spectrin. *Blood* **92(Suppl 1)**:8a, 1998.
663. Kaysser TM, Wandersee NJ, Bronson RT, Barker JE: Thrombosis and secondary hemochromatosis play major roles in the pathogenesis of jaundiced and spherocytic mice, murine models for hereditary spherocytosis. *Blood* **90**:4610, 1997.
664. Wandersee NJ, Lee JC, Kaysser TM, Bronson RT, Barker JE: Hematopoietic cells from α-spectrin-deficient mice are sufficient to induce thrombotic events in hematopoietically ablated recipients. *Blood* **92**:4856, 1998.
665. Bevers EM, Comfurius P, Dekkers DW, Harmsma M, Zwaal RF: Transmembrane phospholipid distribution in blood cells: Control mechanisms and pathophysiological significance. *Biol Chem* **379**:973, 1998.
666. Peters LL, Birkenmeier CS, Barker JE: Fetal compensation of the hemolytic anemia in mice homozygous for the normoblastosis *(nb)* mutation. *Blood* **80**:2122, 1992.
667. Peters LL, Turtzo LC, Birkenmeier CS, Barker JE: Distinct fetal Ank-1 and Ank-2 related proteins and mRNAs in normal and *nb/nb* mice. *Blood* **81**:2144, 1993.
668. Peters LL, Birkenmeier CS, Bronson RT, White RA, Lux SE, Otto E, Bennett V, Higgins A, Barker JE: Purkinje cell degeneration associated with erythroid ankyrin deficiency in *nb/nb* mice. *J Cell Biol* **114**:1233, 1991.
669. Hassoun H, Wang Y, Vassiliadis J, Lutchman M, Palek J, Aish L, Aish IS, Liu SC, Chishti AH: Targeted inactivation of murine band 3 (*AE1*) gene produces a hypercoagulable state causing widespread thrombosis in vivo. *Blood* **92**:1785, 1998.
670. Peters LL, Swearingen RA, Gwynn B, Lux SE, Eicher EM, Washburn LL, Ciciotte SL, Goff-Anderson S: Failure of effective reticulocytosis in a new spontaneous band 3 deficient mouse stain (C3H/HeJ-*wan*) and in a subset of targeted band 3 null mice (B6,129 AE−/−) suggests the presence of genetic modifiers of band 3 function in red blood cells. *Blood* **92(Suppl 1)**:301a, 1998.
671. Shi ZT, Afzal V, Coller B, Patel D, Chasis JA, Parra M, Lee G, Paszty C, Stevens M, Walensky L, Peters LL, Mohandas N, Rubin E, Conboy JG: Protein 4.1R-deficient mice are viable but have erythroid membrane skeleton abnormalities. *J Clin Invest* **103**:331, 1999.
672. Evans EA, Waugh R, Melnik L: Elastic area compressibility modulus of red cell membrane. *Biophys J* **16**:585, 1976.
673. Barnhart MI, Lusher JM: The human spleen as revealed by scanning electron microscopy. *Am J Hematol* **1**:243, 1976.
674. Chen LT, Weiss L: Electron microscopy of the red pulp of human spleen. *Am J Anat* **134**:425, 1972.
675. Weiss L: A scanning electron microscopic study of the spleen. *Blood* **43**:665, 1974.
676. Johnsson R, Vuopio P: Studies on red cell flexibility in spherocytosis using a polycarbonate membrane filtration method. *Acta Haematol* **60**:329, 1978.
677. Young LE, Platzer RF, Ervin DM, Izzo MJ: Hereditary spherocytosis II. Observations on the role of the spleen. *Blood* **6**:1099, 1951.
678. Jandl JH, Greenberg MS, Yonemoto R, Castle WB: Clinical determination of the sites of red cell sequestration in hemolytic anemias. *J Clin Invest* **35**:842, 1956.
679. Griggs RC, Weisman R Jr, Harris JW: Alterations in osmotic and mechanical fragility related to in vivo erythrocyte aging and splenic sequestration in hereditary spherocytosis. *J Clin Invest* **39**:89, 1960.
680. Molnar Z, Rappaport H: Fine structure of the red pulp of the spleen in hereditary spherocytosis. *Blood* **39**:81, 1972.
681. Banti G: Splenomegalie hemolytique au hemopoietique: Le role de la rate dans l'hemolyse. *Semin Med (Paris)* **33**:313, 1913.
682. Becker PS, Lux SE: Disorders of the red cell membrane, in Nathan DG, Oski FA (eds): *Hematology of Infancy and Childhood*, 4th ed. Philadelphia, WB Saunders, 1993, p 529.
683. Ferrant A, Leners N, Michaux JL, Verwilghen RL, Sokal G: The spleen and haemolysis: Evaluation of the intrasplenic transit time. *Br J Haematol* **65**:31, 1987.
684. Levine DH, Meyer HB: Newborn screening for ABO hemolytic disease. *Clin Pediatr (Phila)* **24**:391, 1985.
685. Gilliland BC, Baxter E, Evans RS: Red cell antibodies in acquired hemolytic anemia with negative antiglobulin serum tests. *N Engl J Med* **285**:252, 1971.
686. Paolino W: Variations of the mean diameter in the ripening of the erythrocyte. *Acta Med Scand* **136**:141, 1949.
687. Crosby WH, Conrad ME: Hereditary spherocytosis: Observations on hemolytic mechanisms and iron metabolism. *Blood* **15**:662, 1960.
688. Cooper RA, Jandl JH: The role of membrane lipids in the survival of red cells in hereditary spherocytosis. *J Clin Invest* **48**:736, 1969.
689. Pautard B, Féo C, Dhermy D, Wajcman H, Baudin-Chich V, Delobel J: Occurrence of hereditary spherocytosis and β thalassaemia in the same family: Globin chain synthesis and visco diffractometric studies. *Br J Haematol* **70**:239, 1988.
690. Li CK, Ng MH, Cheung KL, Lam TK, Shing MM: Interaction of hereditary spherocytosis and α thalassaemia: A family study. *Acta Haematol* **91**:201, 1994.
691. Alfinito F, Calabro V, Cappellini MD, Fiorelli G, Filosa S, Iolascon A, Miraglia del Giudice E, Perrotta S, Migliorati R, Vallone D, et al: Glucose 6-phosphate dehydrogenase deficiency and red cell membrane defects: Additive or synergistic interaction in producing chronic haemolytic anaemia. *Br J Haematol* **87**:148, 1994.
692. Warkentin TE, Barr RD, Ali MA, Mohandas N: Recurrent acute splenic sequestration crisis due to interacting genetic defects: Hemoglobin SC disease and hereditary spherocytosis. *Blood* **75**:266, 1990.
693. Yang YM, Donnell C, Wilborn W, Goodman SR, Files B, Moore RB, Mohandas N, Mankad VN: Splenic sequestration associated with

sickle cell trait and hereditary spherocytosis. *Am J Hematol* **40**:110, 1992.
694. Duru F, Gurgey A: Effect of corticosteroids in hereditary spherocytosis. *Acta Paediatr Jpn* **36**:666, 1994.
695. Owren PA: Congenital hemolytic jaundice. The pathogenesis of the hemolytic crisis. *Blood* **3**:231, 1948.
696. Robins MM: Familial crisis in hereditary spherocytosis. Report of six affected siblings. *Clin Pediatr* **4**:210, 1965.
697. Gairdner D: The association of gallstones with acholuric jaundice in children. *Arch Dis Child* **14**:109, 1939.
698. Kelleher JF, Luban NL, Mortimer PP, Kamimura T: Human serum "parvovirus": a specific cause of aplastic crisis in children with hereditary spherocytosis. *J Pediatr* **102**:720, 1983.
699. Brown KE, Young NS: Parvovirus B19 in human disease. *Annu Rev Med* **48**:59, 1997.
700. Ozawa K, Kurtzman G, Young N: Productive infection by B19 parvovirus of human erythroid bone marrow cells in vitro. *Blood* **70**:384, 1987.
701. Hanada T, Koike K, Takeya T, Nagasawa T, Matsunaga Y, Takita H: Human parvovirus B19-induced transient pancytopenia in a child with hereditary spherocytosis. *Br J Haematol* **70**:113, 1988.
702. Muir K, Todd WT, Watson WH, Fitzsimons E: Viral-associated haemophagocytosis with parvovirus-B19-related pancytopenia. *Lancet* **339**:1139, 1992.
703. Rinn R, Chow WS, Pinkerton PH: Transient acquired myelodysplasia associated with parvovirus B19 infection in a patient with congenital spherocytosis. *Am J Hematol* **50**:71, 1995.
704. Vigeant P, Menard HA, Boire G: Chronic modulation of the autoimmune response following parvovirus B19 infection. *J Rheumatol* **21**:1165, 1994.
705. Summerfield GP, Wyatt GP: Human parvovirus infection revealing hereditary spherocytosis. *Lancet* **2**:1070, 1985.
706. Lefrere JJ, Courouce AM, Girot R, Bertrand Y, Soulier JP: Six cases of hereditary spherocytosis revealed by human parvovirus infection. *Br J Haematol* **62**:653, 1986.
707. Fridell E, Bekassy AN, Larsson B, Eriksson BM: Polymerase chain reaction with double primer pairs for detection of human parvovirus B19 induced aplastic crises in family outbreaks. *Scand J Infect Dis* **24**:275, 1992.
708. Peter G: Parvovirus B19, in *1997 Red Book: Report of the Committee on Infectious Diseases*, 24th ed. Elk Grove Village, IL, American Academy of Pediatrics, 1997, p 383.
709. Kohler HG, Meynell MJ, Cooke WT: Spherocytic anaemia, complicated by megaloblastic anaemia of pregnancy. *Br Med J* **1**:779, 1960.
710. Delamore IW, Richmond J, Davies SH: Megaloblastic anaemia in congenital spherocytosis. *Br Med J* **1**:543, 1961.
711. Bates GC, Brown CH: Incidence of gallbladder disease in chronic hemolytic anemia (spherocytosis). *Gastroenterology* **21**:104, 1952.
712. Mentzer SH: Clinical and pathologic study of cholecystitis and cholelithiasis. *Surg Gynecol Obst* **42**:782, 1926.
713. Holcomb GW Jr, Holcomb GWd: Cholelithiasis in infants, children, and adolescents. *Pediatr Rev* **11**:268, 1990.
714. Miraglia del Giudice E, Perrotta S, Nobili B, d'Urzo G, Conte ML, Cutillo S, Iolascon A: Co-inheritance of Gilbert syndrome increases the risk for developing gallstones in patients with hereditary spherocytosis. *Blood* **92(Suppl 1)**:470a, 1998.
715. Ransohoff DF, Gracie WA: Treatment of gallstones. *Ann Intern Med* **119**:606, 1993.
716. Holcomb GW 3rd: Laparoscopic cholecystectomy. *Semin Laparosc Surg* **5**:2, 1998.
717. Pappis CH, Galanakis S, Moussatos G, Keramidas D, Kattamis C: Experience of splenectomy and cholecystectomy in children with chronic haemolytic anaemia. *J Pediatr Surg* **24**:543, 1989.
718. Beinhauer LG, Gruhn JG: Dermatologic aspects of congenital spherocytic anemia. *Arch Dermatol* **75**:642, 1957.
719. Hanford RB, Schneider GF, MacCarthy JD: Massive thoracic extramedullary hemopoieses. *N Engl J Med* **263**:120, 1960.
720. Schafer AI, Miller JB, Lester EP, Bowers TK, Jacob HS: Monoclonal gammopathy in hereditary spherocytosis: A possible pathogenetic relation. *Ann Intern Med* **88**:45, 1978.
721. Schilling RF: Hereditary spherocytosis: a study of splenectomized persons. *Semin Hematol* **13**:169, 1976.
722. Isobe T, Osserman EF: Pathologic conditions associated with plasma cell dyscrasias: A study of 806 cases. *Ann N Y Acad Sci* **190**:507, 1971.
723. Barry M, Scheuer PJ, Sherlock S, Ross CF, Williams R: Hereditary spherocytosis with secondary haemochromatosis. *Lancet* **2**:481, 1968.
724. Takegoshi T, Nishino T, Tanino M, Nonokura A, Ohta G: An autopsy case of hemochromatosis and hepatoma combined with hereditary spherocytosis. *Jpn J Med* **23**:48, 1984.
725. Mohler DN, Wheby MS: Hemochromatosis heterozygotes may have significant iron overload when they also have hereditary spherocytosis. *Am J Med Sci* **292**:320, 1986.
726. Fargion S, Cappellini MD, Piperno A, Panajotopoulos N, Ronchi G, Fiorelli G: Association of hereditary spherocytosis and idiopathic hemochromatosis. A synergistic effect in determining iron overload. *Am J Clin Pathol* **86**:645, 1986.
727. Berne JD, Asensio JA, Falabella A, Gomez H: Traumatic rupture of the spleen in a patient with hereditary spherocytosis. *J Trauma* **42**:323, 1997.
728. Dacie JV: Familial haemolytic anaemia (acholuric jaundice), with particular reference to changes in fragility produced by splenectomy. *Q J Med* **12**:101, 1943.
729. Langley GR, Felderhof CH: Atypical autohemolysis in hereditary spherocytosis as a reflection of two cell populations: relationship of cell lipids to conditioning by the spleen. *Blood* **32**:569, 1968.
730. Chapman RG, McDonald LL: Red cell life span after splenectomy in hereditary spherocytosis. *J Clin Invest* **47**:2263, 1968.
731. MacKenzie FAF, Elliot DH, Eastcott HHG, Hughes-Jones NC, Barkhan P, Mollison PL: Relapse in hereditary spherocytosis with proven splenunculus. *Lancet* **1**:1102, 1962.
732. Meekes I, van der Staak F, van Oostrom C: Results of splenectomy performed on a group of 91 children. *Eur J Pediatr Surg* **5**:19, 1995.
733. Gordon DH, Schaffner D, Bennett JM, Schwartz SI: Postsplenectomy thrombocytosis: Its association with mesenteric, portal, and/or renal vein thrombosis in patients with myeloproliferative disorders. *Arch Surg* **113**:713, 1978.
734. McGrew W, Avant GR: Hereditary spherocytosis and portal vein thrombosis. *J Clin Gastroenterol* **6**:381, 1984.
735. Skarsgard E, Doski J, Jaksic T, Wesson D, Shandling B, Ein S, Babyn P, Heiss K, Hu X: Thrombosis of the portal venous system after splenectomy for pediatric hematologic disease. *J Pediatr Surg* **28**:1109, 1993.
736. Kemahli S, Canatan D, Cin S, Uysal Z, Akar N, Arcasoy A: Post-splenectomy thrombosis and haemolytic anaemias. *Br J Haematol* **97**:505, 1997.
737. Stewart GW, Amess JA, Eber SW, Kingswood C, Lane PA, Smith BD, Mentzer WC: Thrombo-embolic disease after splenectomy for hereditary stomatocytosis. *Br J Haematol* **93**:303, 1996.
738. Lane PA, Kuypers FA, Clark MR, Andrews DA, Wagner GM, Butikofer P, Shapiro AD, Chiu DT, Lubin BH, Mentzer WC: Excess of red cell membrane proteins in hereditary high-phosphatidylcholine hemolytic anemia. *Am J Hematol* **34**:186, 1990.
739. Waghorn DJ, Mayon-White RT: A study of 42 episodes of overwhelming post-splenectomy infection: Is current guidance for asplenic individuals being followed? *J Infect* **35**:289, 1997.
740. King H, Shumacker HB Jr: Susceptibility to infection after splenectomy performed in infancy. *Ann Surg* **136**:239, 1952.
741. Eraklis AJ, Filler RM: Splenectomy in childhood: A review of 1413 cases. *J Pediatr Surg* **7**:382, 1972.
742. Singer DB: Postsplenectomy sepsis. *Perspect Pediatr Pathol* **1**:285, 1973.
743. Shaw JH, Print CG: Postsplenectomy sepsis. *Br J Surg* **76**:1074, 1989.
744. Holdsworth RJ, Irving AD, Cuschieri A: Postsplenectomy sepsis and its mortality rate: Actual versus perceived risks. *Br J Surg* **78**:1031, 1991.
745. Schwartz PE, Sterioff S, Mucha P, Melton LJD, Offord KP: Postsplenectomy sepsis and mortality in adults. *JAMA* **248**:2279, 1982.
746. Green JB, Shackford SR, Sise MJ, Fridlund P: Late septic complications in adults following splenectomy for trauma: A prospective analysis in 144 patients. *J Trauma* **26**:999, 1986.
747. Pedersen FK: Postsplenectomy infections in Danish children splenectomized 1969-1978. *Acta Paediatr Scand* **72**:589, 1983.
748. Posey DL, Marks C: Overwhelming postsplenectomy sepsis in childhood. *Am J Surg* **145**:318, 1983.
749. Chaikof EL, McCabe CJ: Fatal overwhelming postsplenectomy infection. *Am J Surg* **149**:534, 1985.
750. Platt R: Infection after splenectomy. *JAMA* **248**:2316, 1982.
751. Musser G, Lazar G, Hocking W, Busuttil RW: Splenectomy for hematologic disease. The UCLA experience with 306 patients. *Ann Surg* **200**:40, 1984.
752. Schilling RF: Estimating the risk for sepsis after splenectomy in hereditary spherocytosis. *Ann Intern Med* **122**:187, 1995.

753. Konradsen HB, Henrichsen J: Pneumococcal infections in splenectomized children are preventable. *Acta Paediatr Scand* **80**:423, 1991.
754. Klinge J, Hammersen G, Scharf J, Lutticken R, Reinert RR: Overwhelming postsplenectomy infection with vaccine-type Streptococcus pneumoniae in a 12-year-old girl despite vaccination and antibiotic prophylaxis. *Infection* **25**:368, 1997.
755. Pruthi RK, Marshall WF, Wiltsie JC, Persing DH: Human babesiosis. *Mayo Clin Proc* **70**:853, 1995.
756. Rosner F, Zarrabi MH, Benach JL, Habicht GS: Babesiosis in splenectomized adults. Review of 22 reported cases. *Am J Med* **76**:696, 1984.
757. Gupta P, Hurley RW, Helseth PH, Goodman JL, Hammerschmidt DE: Pancytopenia due to hemophagocytic syndrome as the presenting manifestation of babesiosis. *Am J Hematol* **50**:60, 1995.
758. Miguelez Morales M, Linares Feria M, del Carmen Mesa M: Haemophagocytic syndrome due to babesiosis in a splenectomized patient. *Br J Haematol* **91**:1033, 1995.
759. Wyler DJ, Miller LH, Schmidt LH: Spleen function in quartan malaria (due to *Plasmodium inui*): Evidence for both protective and suppressive roles in host defense. *J Infect Dis* **135**:86, 1977.
760. Oster CN, Koontz LC, Wyler DJ: Malaria in asplenic mice: Effects of splenectomy, congenital asplenia, and splenic reconstitution on the course of infection. *Am J Trop Med Hyg* **29**:1138, 1980.
761. Looareesuwan S, Suntharasamai P, Webster HK, Ho M: Malaria in splenectomized patients: Report of four cases and review. *Clin Infect Dis* **16**:361, 1993.
762. Boone KE, Watters DA: The incidence of malaria after splenectomy in Papua New Guinea. *Br Med J* **311**:1273, 1995.
763. Le TA, Davis TM, Tran QB, Nguyen VP, Trinh KA: Delayed parasite clearance in a splenectomized patient with falciparum malaria who was treated with artemisinin derivatives. *Clin Infect Dis* **25**:923, 1997.
764. Hayag-Barin JE, Smith RE, Tucker FC Jr: Hereditary spherocytosis, thrombocytosis, and chronic pulmonary emboli: A case report and review of the literature. *Am J Hematol* **57**:82, 1998.
765. Robinette CD, Fraumeni JF Jr: Splenectomy and subsequent mortality in veterans of the 1939-45 war. *Lancet* **2**:127, 1977.
766. Schilling RF: Spherocytosis, splenectomy, strokes, and heat attacks. *Lancet* **350**:1677, 1997.
767. Poulin EC, Mamazza J: Laparoscopic splenectomy: Lessons from the learning curve. *Can J Surg* **41**:28, 1998.
768. Katkhouda N, Hurwitz MB, Rivera RT, Chandra M, Waldrep DJ, Gugenheim J, Mouiel J: Laparoscopic splenectomy: outcome and efficacy in 103 consecutive patients. *Ann Surg* **228**:568, 1998.
769. Esposito C, Corcione F, Garipoli V, Ascione G: Pediatric laparoscopic splenectomy: Are there real advantages in comparison with the traditional open approach? *Pediatr Surg Int* **12**:509, 1997.
770. Rescorla FJ, Breitfeld PP, West KW, Williams D, Engum SA, Grosfeld JL: A case controlled comparison of open and laparoscopic splenectomy in children. *Surgery* **124**:670, 1998.
771. Geiger JD, Dinh VV, Teitelbaum DH, Lelli JL, Harmon CM, Hirschl RB, Polley TZ, Drongowski BA, Coran AG: The lateral approach for open splenectomy. *J Pediatr Surg* **33**:1153, 1998.
772. Tchernia G, Gauthier F, Mielot F, Dommergues JP, Yvart J, Chasis JA, Mohandas N: Initial assessment of the beneficial effect of partial splenectomy in hereditary spherocytosis. *Blood* **81**:2014, 1993.
773. Castillo B, Cynober T, Bader-Meunier B, Gauthier F, Miélot F, Tchernia G, Dommergues JP: Sphérocytose héréditaire. Evolution et intérêt de la splénectomie subtotale. *Arch Pediatr* **4**:515, 1997.
774. Tchernia G, Bader-Meunier B, Berterottiere P, Eber S, Dommergues JP, Gauthier F: Effectiveness of partial splenectomy in hereditary spherocytosis. *Curr Opin Hematol* **4**:136, 1997.
775. Jimenez M, Azcona C, Castro L, Bilbao JI, Leon P, Sierrasesumaga L: Partial splenic embolization in a child with hereditary spherocytosis. *Eur J Pediatr* **154**:501, 1995.
776. Konradsen HB, Rasmussen C, Ejstrud P, Hansen JB: Antibody levels against Streptococcus pneumoniae and Haemophilus influenzae type b in a population of splenectomized individuals with varying vaccination status. *Epidemiol Infect* **119**:167, 1997.
777. Dagan R, Melamed R, Muallem M, Piglansky L, Greenberg D, Abramson O, Mendelman PM, Bohidar N, Yagupsky P: Reduction of nasopharyngeal carriage of pneumococci during the second year of life by a heptavalent conjugate pneumococcal vaccine. *J Infect Dis* **174**:1271, 1996.
778. Black S, Shinefield H: Issues and challenges: Pneumococcal vaccination in pediatrics. *Pediatr Ann* **26**:355, 1997.
779. Rennels MB, Edwards KM, Keyserling HL, Reisinger KS, Hogerman DA, Madore DV, Chang I, Paradiso PR, Malinoski FJ, Kimura A: Safety and immunogenicity of heptavalent pneumococcal vaccine conjugated to CRM197 in United States infants. *Pediatrics* **101**:604, 1998.
780. Waghorn DJ: Prevention of postsplenectomy sepsis. *Lancet* **341**:248, 1993.
781. Guidelines for the prevention and treatment of infection in patients with an absent or dysfunctional spleen. Working Party of the British Committee for Standards in Haematology Clinical Haematology Task Force. *Br Med J* **312**:430, 1996.
782. Lambert HP: Managing patients with an absent or dysfunctional spleen: Guidelines do not discuss resistance to antibiotics among pneumococci. *Br Med J* **312**:1361, 1996.

PART 20

IMMUNE AND DEFENSE SYSTEMS

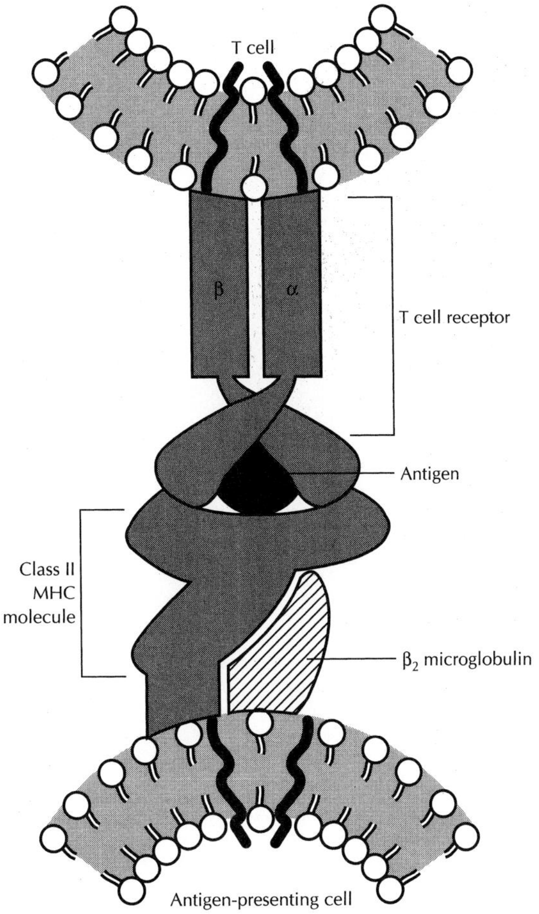

CHAPTER 184

Antibody Deficiencies

Mary Ellen Conley

1. **Antibody deficiencies are a heterogeneous group of disorders characterized by recurrentbacterial infections. Otitis, sinusitis, and pneumonia due to *Streptococcus pneumoniae* or *Haemophilus influenzae* are the most common infections. However, more severe infections such as sepsis, meningitis, cellulitis, and osteomyelitis are not unusual. An antibody deficiency may occur as an isolated finding, or it may be part of a multisystemic disease that affects other limbs of the immune system or other organ systems. Treatment consists of antibody replacement and aggressive use of antibiotics.**
2. **Antibodies are a highly diverse family of serum glycoproteins that bind to and help remove invading microorganisms, extraneous proteins, or foreign cells. Collectively, they account for over a third of the protein found in serum. The typical antibody molecule is made up of two immunoglobulin (Ig) heavy chains and two light chains. There are five major classes of immunoglobulins or antibodies: IgM, IgG, IgA, IgE, and IgD. The IgG class can be further divided into four subclasses (IgG1, IgG2, IgG3, and IgG4), and IgA can be divided into two subclasses (IgA1 and IgA2). The class of the immunoglobulin is defined on the basis of the type of heavy chain. There are two families of light chains, κ and λ, each of which can function with any class of heavy chain.**
3. **The immunoglobulin heavy chain genes are located at the telomere of chromosome 14q32.3. The κ family is at 2p12, and the λ family is encoded at 22q11. At each of these three locations, there are three or four families of gene segments: the variable (V) region, the diversity (D) region, the joining (J) region, and the constant (C) region; these gene segments can be assembled in a myriad of ways to create a highly diverse repertoire of antibodies. Additional variation is introduced by the fact that each heavy chain may be associated with many different light chains.**
4. **Antibodies are produced by plasma cells, the terminally differentiated descendants of the B-cell lineage. The early stages of B-cell development occur in the bone marrow, where pro-B cells, which are derived from hematopoietic stem cells, undergo rearrangement of the immunoglobulin heavy chain genes. This process occurs throughout the life of the individual. At the next stage of B-cell differentiation, in pre-B cells, there is rearrangement of the light chain genes. This allows the expression of the intact immunoglobulin molecule on the cell surface of the B cell. Each B cell and its progeny express only one rearranged immunoglobulin heavy chain and one light chain. When antigen binds to the surface of the B cell, if the appropriate environmental signals are received, the B cell proliferates and differentiates into a memory B cell that can respond more rapidly to future exposures to that antigen, or to a plasma cell that secretes high concentrations of antibodies.**
5. **X-linked, or Bruton, agammaglobulinemia MIM 300300 is associated with the early onset of infections, profound hypogammaglobulinemia, and an absence of B cells in the peripheral circulation. It is caused by mutations in the *BTK* gene encoding the cytoplasmic Bruton tyrosine kinase (Btk). Mutations in Btk are highly variable, but the severity of the disease cannot be predicted by the specific mutation.**
6. **Patients with hyper-IgM syndrome have normal numbers of B cells and normal or elevated serum IgM but markedly decreased IgG and IgA. Approximately 70 percent of patients with this disorder have the X-linked form of the disease MIM 308230, which is due to mutations in the T-cell–derived activation marker, CD40 ligand (also called CD154). The genes responsible for the autosomal dominant, the autosomal recessive, and other forms of the disease are not currently known.**
7. **Common variable immunodeficiency MIM 240500 and IgA deficiency MIM 137100 are multifactorial diseases that are influenced by susceptibility genes. They may occur in the same family and they may be associated with autoimmune disorders.**

Our understanding of host defense has evolved rapidly over the past century. The first Nobel prize for medicine was given to von Behring in 1901 for his studies showing that serum contains factors that can passively transfer immunity to tetanus and diphtheria toxins.[1] In 1908 Paul Ehrlich, who developed methods to quantitate antibodies,[2,3] shared the Nobel prize with Elie Metchnikoff, who first described phagocytes.[4] The award to both men reflected the raging controversy about the relative importance of humoral and cellular immunity and the recognition that both men were correct. The immune system is generally divided into four limbs. The first two are part of the natural, or innate, immune system and include humoral elements in the form of complement and cellular elements in the form of phagocytes. The other two limbs of the immune system represent specific, or acquired, immunity, which is characterized by the more rapid response to the second exposure to antigen. These two limbs also include humoral and cellular components in the forms of antibodies and antigen-specific T cells, respectively. The division of the immune system into these four limbs is also useful for the analysis of immunodeficiencies because defects in each limb of the immune system tend to result in susceptibility to a particular group of

A list of standard abbreviations is located immediately preceding the index in each volume. Additional abbreviations used in this chapter include: *BLNK*/BLNK = B cell linker protein gene symbol/protein, *BTK*/Btk = Bruton tyrosine kinase gene symbol/protein; C, CH1, CH2, CH4, CL = constant region of immunoglobulin including constant heavy (CH) and constant light (CL) regions; CVID = common variable immune deficiency; D, DH = diversity region of immunoglobulin including diversity heavy (DH) regions; Fab = antigen binding fragment of immunoglobulin; Fc = constant fragment of immunoglobulin; J = J region of immunoglobulin; J chain = joining chain of immunoglobulin; **μ** = immunoglobulin heavy chain encoded by *IGHM* gene; PH = pleckstrin homology domain; poly-IgR = polymeric immunoglobulin receptor; pre-B, pro-B = B-lymphocyte precursors, pro-B earlier than pre-B; *RAG1*/*RAG2* = recombination activating genes 1 and 2; SH2, SH3 = Src homology domains 2 and 3; TNF = tumor necrosis factor; V, VH, VL = variable region including variable heavy (VH) and variable light (VL) regions; VDJ = variable, diversity, and joining regions of immunoglobulin; XLA = X-linked agammaglobulinemia.

microorganisms. In this chapter, I focus on antibodies, the genes that are required to produce antibodies, and the disorders of antibody production.

IMMUNOGLOBULINS

Although the terms *antibody* and *immunoglobulin* are often used interchangeably, the term *antibody* is older and was used by Ehrlich to refer to the serum factors that could provide protection against infection. In the late 1930s Tiselius developed the technique of protein electrophoresis[5] and, with Kabat, showed that a fraction of serum proteins that migrated slowly, the γ-globulins, contained antibody activity.[6] Over the next 20 years, studies showed that antibody activity could be found in additional fractions of serum, the macroglobulins and the α-globulins. Thus, these proteins began to be referred to as *immunoglobulins*, and by the 1960s the major classes of serum immunoglobulins, which could be differentiated on the basis of physical, chemical, and antigenic properties, were called IgG, IgM, and IgA.[7] The identification of IgD and IgE, which are present in the serum at much lower concentrations, was aided by studies on myeloma proteins, proteins that are the product of malignancies of antibody-producing cells.[8–11]

The typical immunoglobulin molecule is made up of two identical heavy chains, which are covalently linked to each other, and of two identical light chains, which are covalently linked to the heavy chains (Fig. 184-1). The heavy chains contain the antigenic determinants that define the class of the immunoglobulin (i.e., IgG vs. IgM or IgA). There are two classes of light chains, κ and λ, each of which can combine with any class of immunoglobulin heavy chain. Variable amounts of carbohydrates are linked to the heavy chains and may have a role in maintaining the tertiary structure of the immunoglobulin, its solubility, its resistance to digestion, or its clearance from serum.

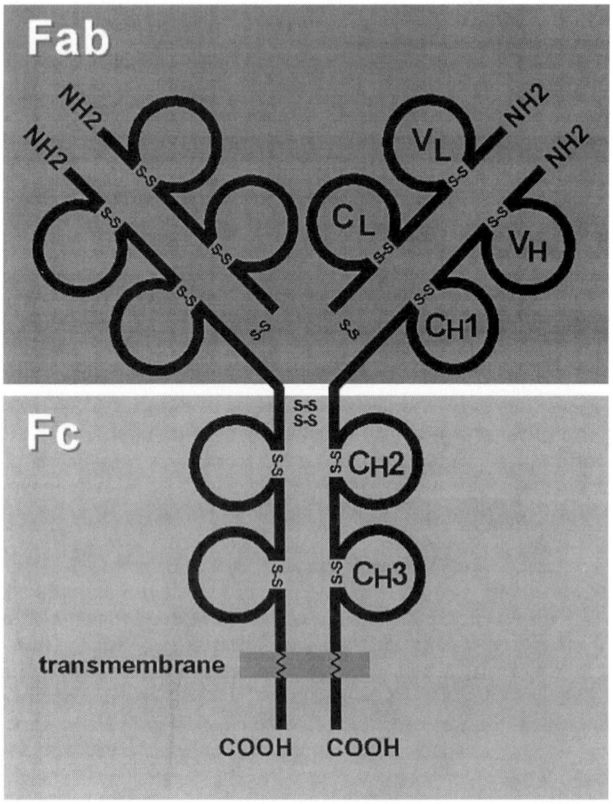

Fig. 184-1 Schematic drawing of an immunoglobulin molecule composed of two immunoglobulin light chains and two immunoglobulin heavy chains. The κ or λ light chains are represented by the variable (VL) and constant (CL) domains, and the heavy chains are shown as the variable (VH) and constant (CH1, CH2, and CH3) domains. The intradomain and intramolecular disulfide bonds are indicated as S–S.

Studies by Porter,[12] Edelman and Poulik,[13] and Nisonoff et al.[14] in the 1950s and 1960s showed that immunoglobulin molecules could be digested with proteases into fragments with distinct functional roles. The highly variable antigen binding portion of the molecule is associated with the N-terminal portions of both the immunoglobulin heavy chain and light chain (Fig. 184-1). This fragment is referred to as the *Fab fragment* (for antigen binding). The C-terminal portion of the heavy chains, the C region, confers the effector functions such as the ability to activate complement and bind to phagoctyes. This fragment is called the *Fc fragment* (the *c* originally referred to the fact that this fragment could be crystallized, but students generally remember it as the constant fragment). The two antigen binding arms of the immunoglobulin molecule pivot around the hinge region, a region that provides both stability and flexibility to the immunoglobulin molecule. Each immunoglobulin class can be produced in a membrane bound form or a secreted form based on alternative splicing at the 3′ portion of the immunoglobulin heavy chain genes.

The basic protein motif of both the immunoglobulin heavy chain and light chain is the immunoglobulin domain,[15–17] a domain of 100 to 110 amino acids that is characterized by an intradomain cysteine–cysteine disulfide bridge that spans approximately 60 amino acids. The immunoglobulin domain evolved from a primordial gene that has duplicated many times and given rise to a variety of cell surface proteins including adhesion molecules such as CD2 and its receptor LFA-3; accessory molecules such as CD19, CD4, and CD8; receptors for immunoglobulins such as poly-IgR; class I and class II major histocompatibility complex (MHC) antigens; the T-cell antigen receptor; and the signal transduction molecules that associate with the antigen receptors, CD3, and the B-cell–specific heterodimer Igα–Igβ. Proteins made up of immunoglobulin domains tend to be involved in cell surface recognition and adhesion, and they often form complexes with other members of the immunoglobulin superfamily.[17] Immunoglobulin heavy chains are composed of four (IgG, IgA, and IgD) or five (IgM and IgE) immunoglobulin domains, and κ and λ each have two immunoglobulin domains. Each domain folds into a compact structure of two antiparallel β pleated sheets, one containing three β strands and the other four β strands.[16] The variable regions of the heavy and light chains are composed of a single immunoglobulin domain in which the amino acids that come together to form the antigen binding site are found in the loops that connect the β strands.

THE IMMUNOGLOBULIN CLASSES

Each of the immunoglobulin classes has evolved to have distinct functional characteristics (Table 184-1). IgM is the first antibody produced in phylogeny and ontogeny. All vertebrates, including fish, have an immune protein that resembles IgM.[18,19] An IgG-like protein is first seen in reptiles and amphibians, but only birds and mammals have an immunoglobulin of the IgA class,[20] and only mammals have IgE. In vertebrates that produce IgG and IgM, the IgM response always precedes the IgG response. Concentrations of serum immunoglobulins are highly dependent on the age of the individual. In a child, serum IgM reaches adult concentrations by the end of the first year of life, IgG reaches adult concentrations by age 8 years, and the concentration of IgA may not reach adult concentrations until adolescence.[21]

IgM

When evaluating patients with suspected antibody deficiency, special attention should be given to the serum concentration of IgM. Although IgM constitutes only 5 to 10 percent of the total serum immunoglobulins, decreased concentrations of IgM are unusual and are almost always associated with significant disease.

Table 184-1 Properties of the Human Immunoglobulin Classes

	IgM	IgG	IgA	IgD	IgE
Serum concentration (mg/100 ml)	65–275	700–1690	70–380	0.5–3	0.01–0.05
Percentage of total serum immunoglobulin	5–10	75–85	5–15	<1	<1
Half-life in days	5	23	6	2.5	2
Molecular mass (kDa)	900	150	160	175	190
Subclasses	—	IgG1, IgG2, IgG3, IgG4	IgA1, IgA2	—	—
Monomer/polymer	Pentamer	Monomer	Monomer (dimer in secretions)	Monomer	Monomer
Percent carbohydrate	10	3	7	9	13
Complement fixation	+++	+	—	—	—
Placental transfer	—	+++	—	—	—
Other biological properties	Primary antibody	Secondary antibody	Mucosal antibody		Allergic antibody

By contrast, low IgG or IgA may reflect transient protein loss or an exaggeration of the normal delay in production of IgG or IgA. Because IgM is produced before IgG or IgA, abnormal serum IgM concentrations can provide an early warning sign in a small child. Further, IgM does not cross the placenta; therefore, IgM found in the serum reflects endogenous production. It should be noted that, as early as the second trimester of gestation, the normal fetus is capable of responding to infection by producing antigen-specific IgM. This is sometimes used as a diagnostic test in a newborn with signs of infection.[22,23]

IgM is expressed as part of the antigen receptor complex on the surface of the majority of B cells. Crosslinking of this IgM by antigen, when coupled with appropriate environmental signals, results in further differentiation of the B cell and ultimately the production of either a memory B cell that can respond more quickly to future challenges from the same antigen or a plasma cell that secretes antigen-specific antibody. The majority of the primary antibody response to any antigen and most of the antibody response to carbohydrate antigens consist of pentameric IgM. Pentameric IgM is made up of five monomers of IgM linked at the C-termini and a single 15-kDa protein called the J chain that facilitates the disulfide linkages that join the monomers. The production of IgM does not require T-cell–mediated signals.

Because of its large size, the majority of IgM, more than 85 percent, remains intravascular. The fact that IgM has 10 antigen binding sites gives it high affinity for microorganisms with repeating antigenic units such as the capsular carbohydrate antigens on the surface of many bacteria. IgM is particularly effective in complement activation, which gives it a prominent role in inflammation. The half-life of IgM is relatively short, 5 days, and the primary IgM response to most antigens is transient; therefore, detection of antigen-specific IgM suggests a recent infection.[24–27]

IgG

IgG constitutes 75 to 85 percent of the immunoglobulin found in serum. It is sometimes referred to as the *secondary antibody*, the antibody that develops after repeated challenges with antigen. In contrast to the IgM response, the IgG response usually persists for years after antigenic stimulation. The half-life of IgG is approximately 23 days, which is considerably longer than that of the other immunoglobulin classes. IgG occurs exclusively as a monomer, and its smaller size allows it to equilibrate between the intravascular and extravascular spaces, so that about 50 percent of the immunoglobulin produced or provided by the intravenous route remains in the blood stream. Because of its longer half-life, a smaller percentage of the total body pool of IgG is produced each day. This lower percentage, when coupled with the smaller size of IgG, results in a disproportionate loss of serum IgG in conditions associated with protein loss, such as nephritis or severe burns.

The interaction of IgG with antigen initiates an inflammatory response. The first component of the complement pathway, C1q, binds to the CH2 region of IgG and activates the complement cascade. In addition, many of the cells involved in host defense, including neutrophils, monocytes, mast cells, and some populations of lymphocytes, express receptors for the Fc portion of IgG. Binding of an antigen–antibody complex to these receptors may result in phagocytosis, activation of antibody-mediated cellular cytotoxicity, release of cytokines, or enhancement or suppression of a lymphocyte response. Placental trophoblasts also express Fc receptors, which are involved in active transport of IgG across the placenta. The majority of the maternal–fetal transfer of IgG occurs during the last trimester of gestation. As a result, premature babies usually have lower concentrations of serum IgG.

The production of IgG requires the close interaction of antigen-specific T cells with B cells specific for antigenic determinants on the same molecule. After repeated antigenic challenge, the IgG response undergoes what is called *affinity maturation*; that is, mutations occur in the variable region of the immunoglobulin molecule, which increase the affinity of the antibody for the antigen that elicited the response. Most antigens elicit a very heterogeneous IgG response in which a single antigenic determinant may induce the production of IgG molecules with many different variable regions.

There are four subclasses of IgG,[28–30] each encoded by a separate gene and numbered according to their relative concentrations in serum. Of total serum IgG, 50 to 70 percent is IgG1, 15 to 25 percent is IgG2, 5 to 15 percent is IgG3, and 1 to 5 percent is IgG4. Although the four subclasses share more than 95 percent of their amino acid sequence, there are some interesting differences. IgG1 and IgG3 fix complement efficiently, IgG2 is less efficient but still active, and IgG4 is unable to activate complement. IgG3 has a short half-life compared with the other IgG subclasses, only about 10 days, in part because it has an unusually long hinge region that makes it vulnerable to proteolysis.[31] Many infectious agents elicit an IgG3 and IgG1 response,[32,33] with IgG3 often preceding IgG1. The response to carbohydrate antigens is predominantly IgG2.[34,35] Prolonged antigen stimulation is sometimes associated with IgG4 production.[36,37]

Caution should be used when trying to determine the significance of an IgG subclass deficiency. Patients with homozygous deletions that include the genes for one or more subclasses may be asymptomatic,[38,39] indicating that other subclasses can compensate. By contrast, patients with Wiskott–Aldrich syndrome (see Chap. 185) fail to make antibody-to-carbohydrate antigens, but they have normal concentrations of IgG2.[40]

IgA

IgA plays a major role in host defense at the mucosal surfaces, where it is the predominant antibody of secretions such as saliva, tears, gastrointestinal secretions, bronchial fluids, and milk.[41] The IgA in secretions is generally locally produced.[42] B cells exposed to antigens at the mucosal surfaces migrate through the lymphatics and the blood steam before they return to the mucosal surfaces.[43] This ensures that the antibody response is not limited to the region where the antigen was initially encountered but instead is more broadly expressed throughout the mucosal surfaces. After this migration, the antigen-specific B cells settle in regions beneath the lamina propria, where they mature into plasma cells that secrete IgA, predominantly in the dimeric form, with the monomeric units of IgA linked end to end with the J chain.[44] Dimeric IgA is transported across the epithelial border by a specialized polymeric immunoglobulin receptor (poly-IgR). At the apical surface of the epithelial cell, the poly-IgR is cleaved into two domains, and the N-terminal domain, which is referred to as the secretory component, remains bound to the dimeric IgA and is released into the secretions as part of the secretory IgA complex.

IgA constitutes about 5 to 15 percent of the immunoglobulin in serum, where it is predominantly in the monomeric form. The majority of this IgA is derived from plasma cells in the bone marrow. IgA does not fix complement well, and it usually does not elicit an inflammatory response. This is an advantage in secretions, where the most important barrier to infection is an intact mucosal surface. Instead, IgA functions by preventing the adherence of foreign antigens and microorganisms and enhancing their removal. In the serum, IgA may help in the removal of food antigens and partially degraded self antigens. Patients with IgA deficiency have an increased incidence of allergies and autoantibodies.[45–52]

There are two subclasses of IgA, IgA1 and IgA2. The IgA in serum is predominantly IgA1, whereas the IgA in secretions is more evenly divided between the two subclasses. The synthesis of IgA is T-cell dependent and is controlled by a variety of cytokines, including TGFβ and interluekin- IL- 10. IgA deficiency, which is the most common immunodeficiency, is a heterogeneous disorder, suggesting that IgA production is very sensitive to perturbations of the immune system. Although serum and secretory IgA are produced at different sites, patients rarely have a significant decrease in one without a similar decrease in the other.

IgE

IgE constitutes less than 0.01 percent of the immunoglobulin in serum, and it has a relatively short half-life of 2 days. Failure to produce IgE does not result in medical problems; however, there are several clinical conditions in which elevated serum IgE is associated with disease. Patients with allergies, in particular eczema, patients with parasitic infections, and patients with an uncommon immunodeficiency referred to as *hyper-IgE syndrome* may have serum concentrations of IgE that are a hundredfold higher than those seen in healthy individuals.

Like IgA, the majority of IgE is produced at the mucosal surfaces.[53,54] It binds to high affinity IgE Fc receptors on mast cells, Langerhans cells, basophils, macrophages, and eosinophils. When this cell bound IgE is crosslinked by antigen, the mast cell releases histamine and inflammatory mediators, resulting in vasodilatation, increased capillary permeability, and smooth-muscle contractions. Depending on the site of the reaction, these responses may be associated with edema, erythema, small airway obstruction and increased intestinal motility. The IgE response may be protective in areas where parasites are endemic; however, in the industrialized world, allergies are troubling and sometimes life threatening. The tendency to make high concentrations of IgE is controlled at least in part by genetic factors.

IgD

IgD has no known unique functional role. It is expressed with IgM on the majority of B cells, and crosslinking of this IgD with antibodies, to simulate the crosslinking that would occur with antigen, induces an activation response that is very similar to that seen after crosslinking of B-cell surface IgM. Mice that are unable to make IgD have only subtle defects in late stages of B-cell maturation.[55] There have been no descriptions of patients or healthy control subjects who lack IgD but who are otherwise normal. About 1 percent of the serum immunoglobulin is IgD. Of interest, this IgD predominantly uses the λ light chain[56] in contrast with the other classes of immunoglobulin, which are more equally divided between the two light chains, κ and λ.

IMMUNOGLOBULIN GENES

The immunoglobulin genes and the genes for the T-cell antigen receptors are encoded in a unique fashion that allows the production of a highly diverse antigen binding repertoire coupled to a highly predictable functional domain. This is achieved by assembling the final gene product from segments of the gene that are arrayed in a highly complex and flexible locus. At each locus there are several gene families that contribute segments to the final gene product.[57]

The immunoglobulin heavy chain locus spans over 1400 kb of DNA at the telomeric end of chromosome 14q32.3[58–66] (Fig. 184-2). Within this locus, there are four separate families of gene segments. Immediately proximal to the telomere, in a 1000-kb span of DNA, there are 50 to 120 VH gene segments, each consisting of a promoter, a leader sequence, and the major portion of an immunoglobulin domain. Approximately half of these VH segments are pseudogenes.[65,66] This 1000-kb stretch of DNA is followed by a 75-kb region that contains five tandem repeats of a cassette containing six DH genes.[61,62] The third family of segments are the six JH genes, which are at the 5′ end of a 20-kb fragment of DNA that also contains a strong enhancer controlling immunoglobulin heavy chain transcription and the CH genes for μ and δ. The remaining C region genes are found in two clusters approximately 60 and 260 kb distal to the genes for μ and δ.[63,64] Each of these CH gene clusters contains two γ C region genes, an ε gene and an α gene. At the 5′ end of each C region gene except δ, there is a repetitive conserved sequence, called the *switch region*, that facilitates a recombination event that allows a VDJ sequence to be transferred from the μ heavy chain gene to one of the other heavy chain genes.[67] Each of the C region genes has exons at the 3′ end of the gene that allow alternative splicing to produce either the membrane bound or secreted form of the immunoglobulin molecule. Downstream of each of the α C region genes, there is an enhancer called the *3′ enhancer* that appears to regulate isotype switching.[68,69,69a]

The genes for the immunoglobulin light chains, κ and λ, are also composed of gene segments that must be assembled; however, they are a bit simpler than the heavy chain genes in that they include V, J, and C regions but no D regions. The κ locus at 2p12 contains about 50 V_κ gene segments, five J_κ gene segments, and a single C_κ region gene.[70,71] Some of the V_κ genes are encoded in the reverse 5′ to 3′ orientation. The λ locus is at 2q11[72] and spans approximately 900 kb.[73] It includes 50 to 60 V region genes and seven to 10 C_λ region genes,[74] each preceded by its own J region. As in the heavy chain locus, all of the V_λ genes are oriented in the same direction.[73]

Immediately 3′ of each V gene, both 5′ and 3′ of the D segments in the heavy chain locus, and 5′ of the J segments, there are conserved sequences, a seven-base sequence and a nine-base sequence, that are recognized by the recombination machinery that assembles the immunoglobulin gene. Parts of the machinery used in the rearrangement of the T-cell antigen receptor genes and the immunoglobulin genes are widely expressed proteins involved in DNA repair. However, at specific points in T- and B-cell differentiation, two enzymes with similarity to transposases, *RAG1* and *RAG2* (recombination activating genes), are transiently produced and play an essential role in the recognition, cleavage, and ligation of the gene segments used to assemble the final

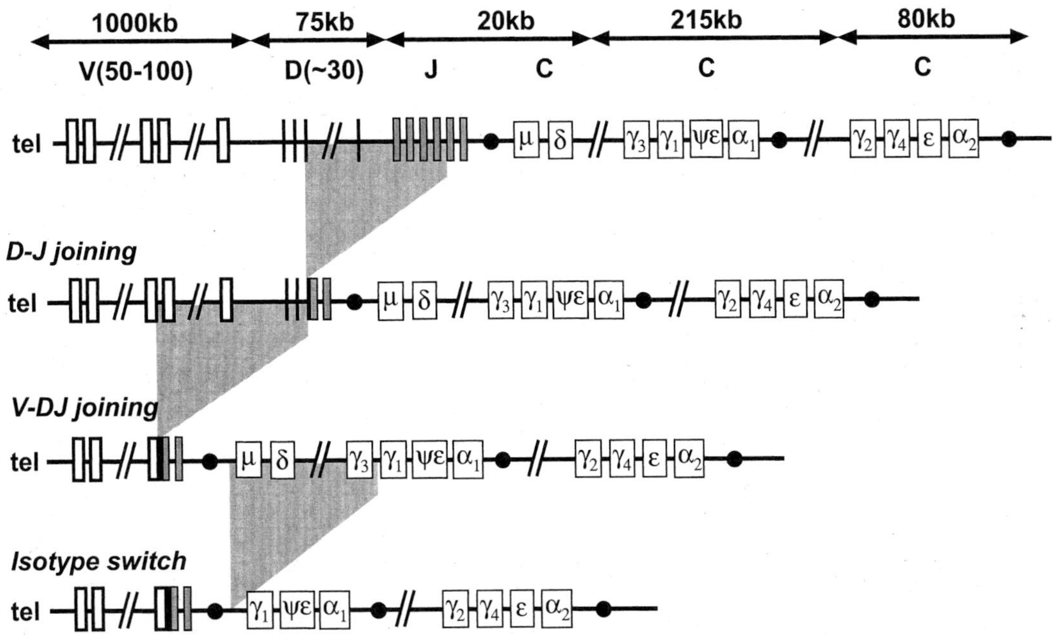

Fig. 184-2 The immunoglobulin heavy-chain locus at 14q32.3 is shown. In the first stage of immunoglobulin gene rearrangement, a D segment is recombined with one of the J segments (DJ joining), and the intervening DNA is deleted. In the next stage, a V region gene is recombined with the DJ segment (VDJ joining). In a mature B cell, the μ C region gene is replaced with a downstream C region (isotype switching).

immunoglobulin gene.[75,76,76a] Immunoglobulin gene rearrangement is a highly inefficient process; approximately two-thirds of rearrangements are out of frame and result in premature stop codons, whereas other rearrangements use nonfunctional variable region pseudogenes.

B-CELL DEVELOPMENT

B cells are produced throughout the life of an individual.[77,78] In the embryo, hematopoietic precursors first appear in the yolk sac at about 4 weeks of gestation. These mesenchymal cells migrate to the fetal liver, and by 8 weeks of gestation, B-cell precursors, cells expressing cytoplasmic μ, can be detected by immunofluorescence.[79] During the second trimester of pregnancy, hematopoiesis and B-cell development move to the bone marrow, and by birth all hematopoiesis and the initial stages of B-cell development occur in the bone marrow. When the genes for both the immunoglobulin heavy and light chains have been successfully rearranged, immature B cells are released from the bone marrow into the bloodstream, where they can migrate into peripheral lymphoid tissues. B cells can travel back into the blood stream by way of the lymphatics and circulate into additional areas of the body. Immature B cells have a very short life span unless they encounter antigen in an appropriate context; however, memory B cells that have been exposed to antigen may persist for many years.

The various stages of B-cell development can be identified based on the status of the immunoglobulin genes and the expression of markers that are specific to the various stages of differentiation[80,81] (Fig. 184-3). The earliest B-cell precursors, which are referred to as *pro-B cells*, still express a marker that is characteristic of hematopoietic stem cells, CD34; but they also express CD19, a cell surface glycoprotein that is specific to the B-cell lineage. RAG expression allows the first step in immunoglobulin gene rearrangement, the juxtaposition of a D gene segment with a J gene segment to occur on both alleles at the immunoglobulin heavy chain locus.[82] At the end of the pro-B–cell stage of differentiation, rearrangement of a V segment with the DJ segment permits the production of an intact μ heavy chain that is immediately expressed on the surface of the cell as part of the pre-B–cell receptor complex, signaling the transition from the pro-B cell to pre-B cell stage of differentiation. Pro-B cells synthesize several proteins that will be used to escort the rearranged μ heavy chain to the cell surface as part of a signal transduction complex. Igα and Igβ are covalently linked transmembrane proteins that have intracytoplasmic domains with motifs that act as docking stations for signaling molecules. They are produced throughout B-cell differentiation, and they assemble with the membrane form of all the immunoglobulin heavy chains. Two proteins designated Vpre B and λ5/14.1 have homology to a light chain variable region and a λ C region, respectively; together they form the surrogate light chain.[83] Before the rearrangement of light chain genes, the surrogate light chain substitutes for a conventional immunoglobulin light chain as part of the pre-B–cell receptor complex. The surrogate light chain may assess the μ chain for its ability to fold correctly and bind a light chain.

Cell surface expression of the pre-B–cell receptor complex plays a critical role in B-cell differentiation. In humans, defects in any of the components of this receptor, or the signaling molecules that respond to this receptor, such as Btk, result in a block in B-cell differentiation and profound hypogammaglobulinemia. Directly or indirectly, the pre-B–cell receptor complex signals the down regulation of RAG expression and cessation of immunoglobulin heavy chain gene rearrangement. This explains, at least in part, "allelic exclusion," that is, the expression of only a single immunoglobulin heavy chain in any B cell and its descendants. Expression of the pre-B–cell receptor complex is also associated with vigorous proliferation. In the normal individual, there are 3 to 10 times more pre-B cells than pro-B cells. At the end of the pre-B–cell stage of differentiation, RAG is again produced and there is rearrangement of the immunoglobulin light chain genes. The rearrangement of the κ-chain genes generally precedes λ light chain gene rearrangement.[84]

Effective rearrangement of a light chain gene permits the cell surface expression of an immunoglobulin molecule in the context of the antigen–receptor complex and release of the immature B cell into the peripheral circulation. At first, the B cell expresses only surface IgM and it is vulnerable to negative selection. This results in the removal of B cells with specificity for self-antigens. Surface IgD is quickly acquired and the B cell has the capacity to respond to antigen stimulation in a variety of ways, depending on

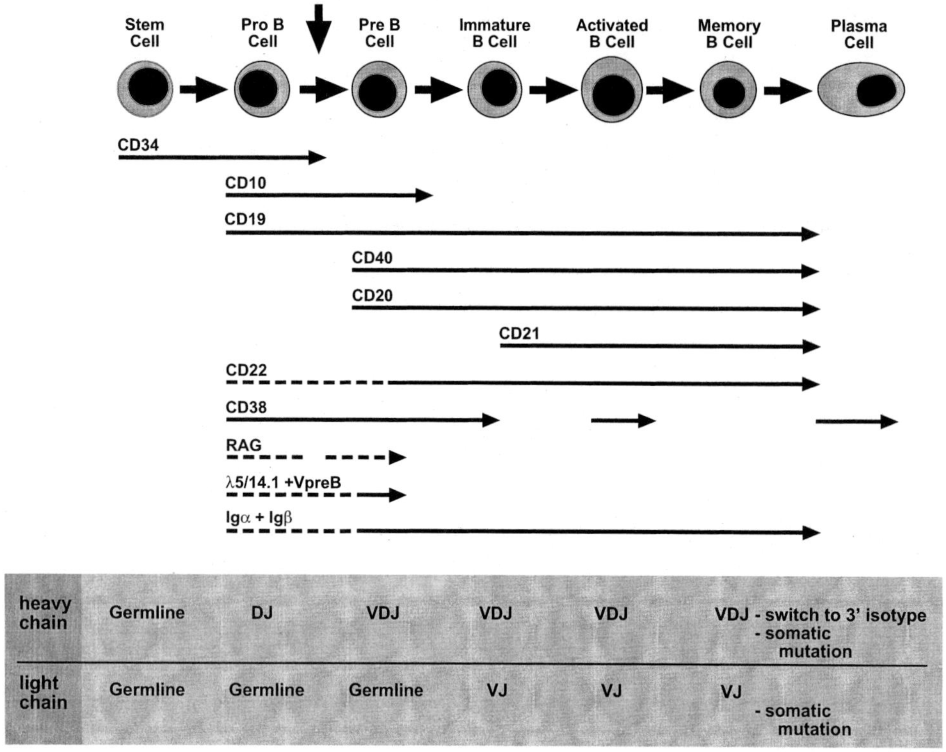

Fig. 184-3 The lymphocyte markers that distinguish the various stages of B-cell differentiation are shown. Markers that are expressed on the cell surface are indicated as solid lines; markers that are predominantly cytoplasmic are shown as dotted lines. Note that some markers may move from the cytoplasm to the cell surface.

the dose of antigen, the presence of preformed antibody to that antigen, the concentration of certain cytokines, and the intensity of activation signals from antigen presenting cells and T cells. After antigen contact, some B cells quickly differentiate into plasma cells that are capable of synthesizing and secreting antigen-specific IgM within 3 to 10 days. Antigen activated B cells in germinal follicles of lymph nodes may be exposed cytokines and CD40 ligand expressing T and undergo "isotype switching." In isotype switching, the rearranged VDJ gene is moved from the μ gene to a downstream IgG, IgA, or IgE C region gene.[85,86,86a] Some switched B cells differentiate into plasma cells; others become memory cells that have the switched isotype on the cell surface instead of IgM and IgD.

Antigen activated mature B cells may undergo a process called *affinity maturation* in which somatic mutations occur within the variable portion of the immunoglobulin heavy and light chain genes but not in the constant portion. Mutations that increase the affinity of the antigen receptor are selected by antigen induced proliferation. Although the mechanisms that focus the somatic mutations on the variable regions are not well understood, it is clear that the DNA proof-reading proteins, referred to as the *mismatch repair system*, play a critical role.[87,88]

ANTIBODY DEFICIENCIES

The term *antibody deficiency* can be used to describe a broad spectrum of disorders that can affect both male and female patients of any age and any ethnic group (Table 184-2). Some antibody deficiencies are part of multisystemic disorders that involve several organ systems, for example, in ataxia telangiectasia, IgA deficiency is associated with neurologic defects and capillary abnormalities.[89] Other antibody deficiencies are due to the failure of T cells to provide essential cytokines or signaling molecules that influence B-cell differentiation. An example of this category would be CD40 ligand deficiency (X-linked hyper-IgM syndrome).[90–94] Still others, such as X-linked agammaglobulinemia, are the result of intrinsic B-cell defects.[95–97] The primary pathogenesis of the most frequent immunodeficiencies, common variable immunodeficiency, IgA deficiency, and IgG subclass deficiency, are not well understood. Several observations suggest that these three disorders may be related.[98] First, IgA deficiency and common variable immunodeficiency may occur in different members of the same family[98–102]; second, IgA deficiency may evolve into common variable immunodeficiency[102,103]; third, about 25 percent of patients with IgA deficiency have IgG subclass deficiencies.[104–106] Finally, certain HLA haplotypes are seen with increased frequency in patients with IgA deficiency and in patients with common variable immunodeficiency.[98,107–113]

In some patients, antibody deficiencies are secondary to other medical conditions or treatments. For example, unusual protein loss, as is seen in extensive skin burns or nephrotic syndrome, is often associated with low concentrations of serum IgG. Chemotherapy and other antimetabolic therapies may result in hypogammaglobulinemia. Irrespective of the cause of antibody deficiency, the most common clinical symptom is recurrent bacterial infections, particularly with the encapsulated bacteria *H. influenzae* and *S. pneumoniae*. Otitis, sinusitis, and pneumonia are the most typical infections. The occurrence of other infections may be influenced by the severity of the antibody deficiency, by defects in other limbs of the immune system, and by scarring in chronically infected tissues.

Not all antibody deficiencies require therapy. Deficiency of serum IgD or IgE is not usually considered clinically significant, and some patients with IgA deficiency or loss of a specific IgG subclass are asymptomatic. The decision about initiation of γ-globulin replacement therapy should be made based on whether the patient is having infections typical of antibody deficiency and whether the patient is able to respond to immunization by making antigen-specific antibodies. The exact concentrations of serum immunoglobulins should not dictate therapy. Although the standard dose of γ-globulin replacements is 400 mg/kg given intravenously once every 4 weeks, some patients do well on lower doses, and other patients, in particular patients with tissue scarring, benefit from higher doses. Many immunologists treat patients with antibody deficiencies with chronic prophylactic antibiotics.

Bone marrow transplantation has been used to treat patients with X-linked hyper-IgM syndrome,[114,114a] and it has been considered in patients with severe complications of common

Table 184-2 Antibody Deficiencies

Disorder*	Alternative Names	Incidence†	Mutant Gene	B-Cell Number	Serum Immunoglobulins	Inheritance‡
X-linked agammaglobulinemia, MIM 300300	Bruton agammaglobulinemia, XLA	1/100,000	Btk	<1%	IgM↓ IgG↓ IgA↓	XL
μ-Chain defect, MIM 147020	Autosomal recessive agammaglobulinemia	1/3,000,000	μ-Heavy chain	Absent	Absent	AR
λ/14.1 Defect MIM 146770	Surrogate light chain defect	1/10,000,000	λ5/14.1	<1%	IgM↓ IgG↓ IgA↓	AR
X-Linked hyper-IgM syndrome, MIM 308230	CD40 ligand defect, XHM	1/300,000	CD40 ligand	Normal	IgM↑ or ↓ or normal IgG↓ IgA↓	XL
Hyper-IgM syndrome	Dysgammaglobulinemia	1/600,000	Unknown	Normal	IgM↑ IgG↓ IgA↓	AR, AD Multifactorial
Common variable immunodeficiency, MIM 240500	Acquired hypogammaglobulinemia CVID	1/50,000	Multifactorial	Normal	IgM↓ or normal IgG↓ IgA↓	Susceptibility genes
IgA deficiency MIM 137100		1/500	Multifactorial	Normal	IgM normal IgG normal; may have ↓ IgG subclasses IgA↓	Susceptibility genes
IgG subclass deficiency (symptomatic)		1/2000	Multifactorial	Normal	Some IgG subclasses low but detectable	Susceptibility genes
IgG subclass deficiency (asymptomatic), MIM 147100	γ-Chain deletion	1/500	γ-Heavy-chain locus	Normal	Some IgG subclasses undectable	AR
κ-Chain deficiency, MIM 147200		?	κ-Light chain	Normal	Normal	AR
Thymoma with hypogammaglobulinemia	Good syndrome	1/500,000	Unknown	<1%	IgM↓ IgG↓ IgA↓	Not inherited

*The Mendelian Inheritance in Man (MIM) identification number is provided if available.
†The incidence figures for X-linked agammaglobulinemia and common variable immunodeficiency are based on population studies. The incidence of the less common disorders are based on a relative comparison with the incidence of XLA or CVID.
‡XL, X-linked; AR, autosomal recessive, AD, autosomal dominant.

variable immunodeficiency. It has not been used to treat patients with X-linked agammaglobulinemia because of the perceived risks associated with transplantation. The identification of the genes responsible for X-linked agammaglobulinemia and X-linked hyper-IgM syndrome has opened the possibility of gene therapy. Although preliminary experiments in animal models of these diseases are in progress,[115,115a,115b] gene therapy is not yet a realistic option.

X-Linked Agammaglobulinemia

X-linked, or Bruton, agammaglobulinemia (gene symbol *BTK*) is frequently thought of as the prototype antibody deficiency because it was the first antibody deficiency described and because the clinical findings are highly specific. Affected patients generally have profound hypogammaglobulinemia and fewer than 1 percent of the normal number of B cells, but other limbs of the immune system are normal. In 1952 Bruton reported the case of an 8-year-old boy with recurrent pneumococcal sepsis and profound hypogammaglobulinemia as detected by protein electrophoresis.[116] The patient was treated with γ-globulin and clinically improved. Over the next few years, it was recognized that the majority of children with agammaglobulinemia were boys and many had a family history of disease compatible with an X-linked pattern of inheritance[117,118]; thus, the disorder came to be known as Bruton, or X-linked, agammaglobulinemia (XLA). In the early 1970s several groups noted that patients with XLA differed from other patients with antibody deficiencies in that XLA patients had almost no B cells in the peripheral circulation.[119–122] However, it was clear by the end of the 1970s that these patients did have B-cell precursors in the bone marrow.[123,124] XLA was mapped to the mid-portion of the X chromosome, at Xq22, in 1986.[125] That same year, carrier detection for XLA became available.[95,126–128] In 1993 two groups reported that mutations in a cytoplasmic tyrosine kinase, which is now called Btk (Bruton tyrosine kinase), were responsible for XLA.[96,97]

Typically, patients with XLA are healthy in the newborn period, but at 6 to 18 months of life, after the loss of transplacentallly acquired maternal immunoglobulin, they begin to develop recurrent bacterial infections, in particular otitis, purulent rhinorrhea, and conjunctivitis due to *H. influenzae* or

S. pneumoniae.[129,130] Diarrhea and poor weight gain are not unusual. Approximately one-third of patients with XLA are first recognized to have an immunodeficiency when they develop a severe, life-threatening infection, such as meningitis, overwhelming pneumonia, or pseudomonas or staphlococcal sepsis. These severe infections are often associated with neutropenia.[131–133] Specific physical findings are limited to signs of past infections and unusually small tonsils and lymph nodes. As would be expected in any X-linked disorder that is lethal without medical intervention, one third to half of all patients with XLA have no family history of immunodeficiency, because they are the first manifestation of a new mutation in their family.[129,134,135] The mean age at diagnosis in a child with no family history of disease is 3 years[129,133]; however, there are patients with mutations in Btk who are not recognized as having immunodeficiency until late adolescence or adulthood.[136,137]

After γ-globulin therapy is started, most patients with XLA have a dramatic improvement in their clinical course. However, some continue to have frequent otitis or sinusitis. Like most patients with antibody deficiencies, patients with XLA have an increased incidence of *Giardia* infections, and they may have pulmonary, joint, or bladder infections due to mycoplasmas and ureoplasmas.[138–142] In the past, as many as 10 percent of patients with XLA developed chronic, progressive infections with enteroviruses,[143] including vaccine associated polio. The use of intravenous γ-globulin, available since 1983, appears to have decreased the frequency of this devastating complication. Patients who had many pneumonias before diagnosis may develop bronchiectasis. In the past, patients with XLA often died of complications of infections in the second or third decade of life[129]; however, earlier diagnosis, better antibiotics, and the capacity to give high doses of γ-globulin have resulted in improved prognosis.

The laboratory findings in XLA usually demonstrate profound hypogammaglobulinemia. The serum IgG is typically below 200 mg/dl, although most patients do have some measurable IgG. The IgM and IgA are usually below 20 mg/dl.[130] The number of B cells in the peripheral circulation is also markedly reduced. In the normal individual, between 5 and 20 percent of the peripheral blood lymphocytes are B cells, whereas in patients with XLA a mean of 0.1 percent of the lymphocytes are B cells. The B cells that can be detected in these patients are blocked at an early stage of differentiation and express an immature phenotype.[127,144] Some patients with mutations in Btk have higher concentrations of serum immunoglobulins, and rare patients have as many as 1 or 2 percent of B cells in the peripheral circulation, but the marked reduction in B-cell number is the most consistent finding in patients with XLA.[144a] Other limbs of the immune system, including T cells and phagocytes, are generally normal; however, occasional abnormalities that may be attributed to chronic infection or secondary changes of the immune system have been reported.[145–147] Bone marrow studies demonstrate that hematopoietic stem cells can differentiate into early B-cell precursors, or pro-B cells, but there is a profound block at the next stage in B-cell maturation, the stage at which an intact μ heavy chain is first expressed on the cell surface as part of the pre-B–cell receptor complex.[124,148]

XLA is caused by mutations in *BTK*, which encodes a 659-amino-acid cytoplasmic tyrosine kinase that is expressed throughout B-cell and myeloid differentiation[96,97,149–151] (Fig. 184-4). Btk is a member of a src-related family of tyrosine kinases that are activated by growth or differentiation factors. Like src, the members of this family have a C-terminal kinase domain preceded by SH2 and SH3 domains. However, Btk and its family members have two additional domains that allow them to interact with other components of signal transduction cascades: an N-terminal pleckstrin homology (PH) domain that binds to phosphoinosides,[152,153] protein kinase C,[154] and the α and β/γ subunits of G proteins[155,156]; and a proline-rich region that binds to SH3 domains.[157] After crosslinking of a variety of cell surface molecules including IgM,[158,159] CD38,[160] IL-5,[161] and IL-6 receptors,[162] and the high affinity IgE receptor on mast cells,[163] Btk moves to the inner side of the plasma membrane, where it is phosphorylated and partially activated by an src family member. Btk then undergoes autophosphorylation[164] and participates in the phosphorylation of phospholipase Cγ.[165] In Btk deficient cell lines, there is reduced calcium mobilization after crosslinking of surface IgM,[166,167] but the exact mechanisms by which mutations in Btk result in abnormal B-cell differentiation are not yet clear.

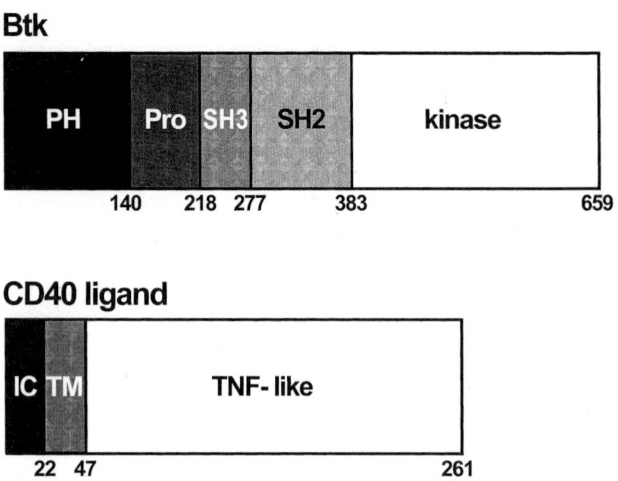

Fig. 184-4 X-linked agammaglobulinemia is caused by mutations in Btk, a cytoplasmic tyrosine kinase with similarities to src family members. The N-terminal portion of Btk contains a pleckstrin homology domain (PH), followed by a proline-rich (Pro) region, an SH3 domain, an SH2 domain, and a kinase domain. X-linked hyper-IgM syndrome is caused by mutations in CD40 ligand, a transmembrane protein expressed on the surface of activated T cells. The N-terminal portion of CD40 ligand is intracellular (IC); the short transmembrane domain (TM) precedes an extracytoplasmic domain with homology to TNF. CD40 ligand is expressed as a trimer. The amino acids that mark the limits of the domains for both molecules are shown below the figures.

The *BTK* gene is encoded in 19 exons spread over 37 kb of DNA at Xq22 (GenBank genomic U78027 and cDNA X58957).[168–171] More than 400 different mutations in Btk have been identified.[135,171a] About one-third of these mutations are amino acid substitutions, one-fourth are premature stop codons, one-fourth are small insertions or deletions resulting in frameshifts, 10 percent are splice defects, and 10 percent are large deletions, inversions or duplications. A high proportion of the amino acid substitutions are found in the kinase domain; the other mutations are more evenly distributed throughout the gene. The premature stop codons, splice defects, and frameshift mutations are usually associated with markedly reduced Btk transcripts in the cytoplasm and thus can be considered functionally equivalent. Amino acid substitutions often result in unstable Btk proteins. The fact that most *BTK* mutations are associated with the absence or marked reduction of Btk protein has been used in diagnostic assays in which monocytes from patients with agammaglobulinemia and absent B cells are assayed by western blot for Btk protein[172] or are indirectly stained with a monoclonal antibody to Btk.[173] There is very little correlation between the specific mutation in *BTK* and the severity of the clinical phenotype.[135,170,174–176] Some patients with premature stop codons early in the gene demonstrate delayed onset of symptoms or higher than expected serum immunoglobulins. This suggests that there are other genetic or environmental factors that influence the severity of XLA.

Several options are now available for families interested in genetic counseling for XLA. In families with a clear X-linked pattern of inheritance, linkage analysis can be used to provide carrier detection and prenatal diagnosis. Useful polymorphic short tandem repeats near Btk are DXS178, DXS101,[177–180] and the flanking markers DXS6797 and DXS6804. If linkage analysis cannot be performed because crucial individuals are not available to assign the specific polymorphic markers to the mutant allele, carrier detection can be provided by using X chromosome inactivation analysis.[95,126,128,181] In the normal female, on average, 50 percent of the cells in any tissue will have the maternally derived X chromosome as the active X and 50 percent will have the paternally derived X as the active X (lyonization). However, if one of the two X chromosomes carries a mutation in a gene required for the proliferation or survival of cells of a particular lineage, then all of the cells of that lineage will be derived from cells having the other X, the nonmutant X, as the active X chromosome. In carriers of XLA, B cells, but not other hematopoietic cells, demonstrate a nonrandom pattern of X chromosome inactivation.[182]

In 90 to 95 percent of males with presumed sporadic XLA, mutations in *BTK* can be identified.[135] The majority of the remaining patients do not have XLA but instead have disorders that are phenotypically similar but genotypically different. As noted below, patients with mutations in μ heavy chain λ5/14.1, Igα, or B cell linker protein (*BLNK*) may be clinically indistinguishable from patients with XLA. When a mutation in *BTK* is found in the DNA of a boy with sporadic XLA, the mother of that patient has an 80 percent risk of carrying that mutation in her genomic DNA.[135] In the remaining patients, it is likely that the new mutation arose in the maternal gamete or the maternal germ line. However, the maternal grandmother of a boy with sporadic XLA has only a 25 percent risk of being a carrier of XLA because, as is true for many genetic disorders,[183–188] the majority of new mutations in *BTK* arise in male gametes.[135]

Autosomal Recessive Agammaglobulinemia

Approximately 10 percent of patients with the early onset of recurrent bacterial infections, profound hypogammaglobulinemia, and absent B cells are girls.[189–193] This suggested that there might be autosomal recessive disorders that are clinically indistinguishable from XLA.[190,194] Recent studies showing that 10 percent of males with presumed sporadic XLA do not have mutations in *BTK*[135] provide additional support for the contention that there are environmental or genetic factors other than Btk that can result in the selective failure of B-cell development.

An approach using linkage analysis to focus on a series of candidate genes was used to study two consanguineous families in which both males and females had hypogammaglobulinemia and absent B cells. Mutations in μ heavy chain were identified in both of these families and in a third family in which the affected male was presumed to have XLA.[148] Four different mutations in μ heavy chain were identified in these families" two large deletions within the immunoglobulin heavy chain locus that removed the entire coding region for the μ heavy chain, and two point mutations that would affect the ability of μ heavy chain to be expressed on the cell surface.[148] The laboratory findings in patients with defects in μ heavy chain are similar to those in patients with XLA, but, in contrast to patients with XLA, the patients with mutations in μ heavy chain had no measurable IgG and they had no detectable B cells. Based on the presumption that defects in other components of the pre-B-cell receptor complex might result in agammaglobulinemia, the genes that encode the surrogate light chain, VpreB and λ5/14.1, and the genes that encode the transmembrane signal transduction module of the antigen receptor, Igα and Igβ, were analyzed. One patient was found to have two different mutations in the gene for λ5/14.1.[195] The clinical and laboratory findings in this boy were almost indistinguishable from those seen in patients with XLA; the patient did have a small amount of IgG and IgM, and he had 0.06% B cells in the peripheral circulation. Another patient, a two-year-old Turkish girl, had a homozygous defect in the gene for Igα.[195a] Like the patients with defects in μ heavy chain, this child had no measurable IgM or IgG and no detectable B cells.

Signaling through the pre-B cell receptor (pre-BCR) results in activation and phosphorylation of a series of signal transduction molecules, including Btk. Several of these signal transduction molecules are assembled on an adaptor or scaffold protein called BLNK (for B cell linker protein). Mutations in *BLNK* can also cause a disorder that is a almost identical to XLA.[195b] Mutations in μ heavy chain, λ5/14.1, Igα, and BLNK do not account for all of the patients with hypogammaglobulinemia and absent B cells, suggesting that there are additional gene defects that result in a failure of B cell development.

Hyper-IgM Syndrome

In the 1960s several groups described patients with "dysgammaglobulinemia," patients who had recurrent infections associated with a marked reduction of serum γ-globulins but an increase in the high molecular weight macroglobulins, the IgM fraction.[196–199] Early studies indicated that this disorder was heterogeneous and that there were autosomal dominant, autosomal recessive, and acquired forms and a more common X-linked form of the disease.[200] Many of the patients with the X-linked form of the disease did not have a family history of disease, and there were no clinical or laboratory signs that clearly differentiated the various forms of hyper-IgM syndrome, which made it difficult to classify individual patients. It was recognized that patients with hyper-IgM syndrome tended to be sicker than patients with X-linked agammaglobulinemia; in addition to bacterial infections, they had a high incidence of opportunistic infections and neutropenia. In 1993 several groups demonstrated that the X-linked form of hyper-IgM syndrome was caused by mutations in CD40 ligand (also called CD154), a member of the TNF family that is expressed on the surface of activated T cells.[90–94] The pathogenesis of hyper-IgM syndrome in the remaining patients is currently unknown.

The majority of patients with X-linked hyper-IgM syndrome show symptoms of their disease in the first year of life.[201] Between 30 and 50 percent of patients develop pneumocystis pneumonia or diarrhea with failure to thrive, symptoms that mimic those seen in patients with severe combined immunodeficiency. However, patients with hyper-IgM syndrome have normal numbers of T cells and B cells and their lymphocytes proliferate normally in response to mitogens. More than 50 percent of patients with defects in CD40 ligand have persistent or recurrent neutropenia. These patients have an increased risk of bacterial sepsis and oral and anal ulcers. Some patients also have mild thrombocytopenia. Only about 50 percent of patients with defects in CD40 ligand actually have elevated concentrations of serum IgM at diagnosis.[201] Young patients, or patients who have had few infections, often have normal or slightly low concentrations of IgM. The serum IgG is consistently very low, but some patients, in particular patients with very active disease, may have detectable or even elevated serum IgA.[201]

In addition to upper and lower respiratory tract infections caused by encapsulated bacteria, patients with X-linked hyper-IgM syndrome have an increased incidence of viral, fungal, and parasitic infections and of infections with nonencapsulated bacteria.[201,201a,201b] Cytomegalovirus, adenovirus, hepatitis C, and hepatitis B may cause significant disease. The chronic diarrhea in patients with X-linked hyper-IgM syndrome may be associated with *Cryptosporidium*, *Giardia lamblia*, *Salmonella*, or *Entamoeba histolytica*. *Cryptosporidium* is a particular problem in patients with X-linked hyper-IgM syndrome because it appears to predispose these patients to sclerosing cholangitis and cancer.[202,202a] A small percentage of patients with X-linked hyper-IgM syndrome are relatively asymptomatic until the second decade of life, when they develop anemia secondary to parvovirus infection.[203]

Degenerative central nervous system disease develops in 10 to 15 percent of patients, sometimes in the absence of a clearly defined etiologic agent. Central nervous system disease, as in the arthritis that is seen in about 10 percent of patients, may be due to infectious organisms that are difficult to identify, or they may be manifestations of autoimmune disease. Patients with defects in CD40 ligand have an increased incidence of autoantibody production and autoimmune disease.[201]

X-linked hyper-IgM syndrome is caused by mutations in CD40 ligand, a 261 amino acid member of the TNF family.[90–94] Like other members of the TNF family, CD40 ligand is a type II transmembrane protein (the extracellular domain is the C-terminus) expressed on the cell surface as a trimer.[204] Activation of T cells results in the transient expression of CD40 ligand on the majority of $CD4^+$ T cells and some $CD8^+$ T cells.[205] CD40 ligand induces the growth, differentiation, and/or activation of cells expressing its cognate receptor, CD40.[206–208] Although CD40 was first detected on B cells, it is now recognized that it can also be found on the surface of epithelial cells, endothelial cells, monocytes, keratinocytes, and dendritic cells.[209–213] The defective interaction of CD40 ligand negative T cells from patients with X-linked hyper-IgM syndrome with endothelial cells, monocytes, and/or dendritic cells may result in a failure to initiate the crosstalk that enhances T-cell activation. This may explain in part the clinical evidence of T-cell deficiency in patients with X-linked hyper-IgM syndrome.

Stimulation of mature B cells with antibody to CD40 or with CD40 ligand results in both short-term and long-term B-cell proliferation[214–216] and increased expression of adhesion molecules and activation markers including CD54, CD23, CD25, and CD80.[217–220] Crosslinking of CD40 protects B cells from apoptosis at some stages of differentiation[221,222] but results in the increased expression of Fas with enhanced susceptibility to apoptosis at other stages of maturation or activation.[223] In the presence of cytokines, CD40 stimulation results in isotype switching.[224,225] B cells from patients with X-linked hyper-IgM syndrome can be stimulated to produce IgG, IgA, and IgE in culture if anti-CD40 and appropriate cytokines are added to the cultures.

The gene for CD40 ligand consists of five exons on a 13-kb fragment of DNA at Xq26 (GenBank L07414).[226–230] More than 100 different mutations in this gene have been identified.[231–233] Approximately 40 percent of the mutations are single amino acid substitutions, the majority of which occur in the TNF-like extracellular domain of CD40 ligand. Some of these mutations would be expected to affect the monomer folding of CD40 ligand, others are likely to inhibit trimerization, and still others interfere with the binding of CD40.[234] Small insertions or deletions that result in frameshifts account for 25 percent of mutations in CD40 ligand. Premature stop codons constitute 20 percent of mutations and 10 percent of splice defects, and gross deletions constitue about 5 percent of mutations. Patients with X-linked hyper-IgM syndrome from the same family, who have the same mutation in CD40 ligand, may have differences in the severity of their disease, suggesting that the precise mutation in CD40 ligand is not the only factor that influences the clinical course of the disease.

Genetic counseling for X-linked hyper-IgM syndrome is similar to that for XLA. In families with multiple affected individuals, linkage analysis can be used for carrier detection or prenatal diagnosis. There is a short tandem repeat within the 3′ untranslated portion of the CD40 ligand mRNA that is polymorphic in 80 percent of women.[93,235] Prenatal diagnosis has been performed using either mutation testing[228] or linkage analysis.[236] Because CD40 ligand does not affect the proliferation or survival of T cells expressing the defective gene, analysis of X chromosome inactivation cannot be used to provide carrier detection of X-linked hyper-IgM syndrome.[237]

Only about 50 percent of patients with the early onset of infections, very low concentrations of serum IgG with normal or elevated IgM, and normal numbers of B cells have defects in CD40 ligand. The remaining patients are a heterogeneous group that includes males and females with autosomal dominant,[99,238] autosomal recessive,[239] or acquired[240,241] disease. Some of these patients have defects in the B-cell response to CD40-mediated signals, although no mutations in CD40 have been identified.[242–244] This group of patients tends not to have the opportunistic infections or neutropenia that are typical of patients with defects in CD40 ligand. They may, however, have severe consequences of their antibody deficiency including bronchiectasis.

Common Variable Immunodeficiency

In the 1950s, when antibody deficiencies were first described, it was recognized that many affected patients had the onset of recurrent infections after early childhood.[245–247] This group of patients included equal numbers of males and females, and, although the onset most often occurred in the third or fourth decade of life, patients of any age might be affected.[248,249] Some of these patients had autoimmune disorders, some had lymphadenopathy, and some had infections that were not typically seen in patients with XLA. Initially, this disorder was called *acquired agammaglobulinemia* to distinguish it from congenital or X-linked agammaglobulinemia; however, as more techniques to study the immune system became available in the 1970s and as the striking heterogeneity in this group of patients became apparent, the disorder was more often called *common variable immunodeficiency* (CVID).[250–254] In general, the term *common variable immunodeficiency* is used to describe patients with detectable numbers of B cells and a marked reduction in at least two of the three major classes of immunoglobulin (IgM, IgG, and IgA).[144a] It is generally believed that the majority of patients with CVID have T-cell and B-cell defects, predisposing them to a wider range of infections and increasing the incidence of autoimmune disease and malignancy. CVID should be considered a diagnosis of exclusion, used only when other known causes of antibody deficiency have been eliminated.

Recurrent pneumonia is the most frequent presenting finding in patients with CVID.[146,191,255–257] In fact, as many as 10 to 20 percent of patients have developed bronchiectasis before they are recognized to have an immunodeficiency. Otitis, sinusitis, and conjunctivitis are also very common. In addition to upper and lower respiratory tract disease, 40 to 50 percent of patients with CVID have significant gastrointestinal disease[255,256,258]; gastritis with achlorhydria, nodular lymphoid hyperplasia, an increased incidence of cholelithiasis, and diarrhea with malabsorption have been reported.[259,260] The gastrointestinal disorders may occur in the absence of obvious infectious agents, and they may persist after the initiation of γ-globulin therapy. *Giardia* infection is also common in patients with CVID. Patients with CVID have an increased incidence of shingles (herpes zoster).[258,259] Autoimmune disorders, including autoimmune hemolytic anemia or thrombocytopenia,[256,261] pernicious anemia,[262,263] arthritis, systemic lupus erythematosus,[264] sarcoidosis,[265] vitiligo, thyroid disease, inflammatory bowel disease, and diabetes, are seen in 20 to 30 percent of patients with CVID but are rarely seen in patients with XLA. Two particular malignancies occur with a high frequency in patients with CVID: non-Hodgkin lymphoma[266] and gastric carcinoma. Gastric carcinoma, which usually occurs more than 10 years after the onset of immunodeficiency, is most likely to occur in patients with chronic gastritis, achylorhydria, and probably *Heliobacter* infection.

The laboratory findings in patients with CVID are highly variable.[267] Some patients have serum immunoglobulin concentrations that are as low as those seen in patients with XLA. The IgG may be below 200 mg/dl, and IgM and IgA are sometimes undetectable. However, in many patients with CVID, the serum immunoglobulins are slightly higher and they may fluctuate during the course of the disease.[102,103,249,264,265,268,269] The concentration of serum IgM is sometimes within normal limits. The B cells in some patients express a normal phenotype,[144] but in others the phenotype indicates abnormal activation[144] or a block in early differentiation.[270,271] When cultured with normal T cells or T-cell factors, B cells from some patients can be stimulated to secrete immunoglobulin.[254,272] B cells from other patients are unresponsive to T-cell–mediated signals.[252,253,273–275] In contrast, T cells from some patients either suppress immunoglobulin production by normal cultured B cells or they fail to provide the required help needed to enhance immunoglobulin secretion.[146,251,271,273,276] Defective antigen presentation has been described in some patients.[146,277]

T cells from a significant proportion of patients with CVID proliferate poorly in response to mitogens.[256,278,279] Some investigators have found that the proliferative response is inversely correlated with the age of the patient, suggesting that CVID may be a progressive disorder in some patients.[256] Antigen challenge with a new antigen, keyhole limpet hemocyanin, fails to elicit antigen specific T cells in some patients.[280] In a subset of patients with CVID, there is a reversed CD4/CD8 ratio due to an increased number of $CD8^+$ T cells.[111,281–285] These $CD8^+$ cells tend to express an activated phenotype. Some patients have been reported to have decreased production of cytokines, such as IL-2, IL-4, IL-5, and γ-interferon,[276,285,286] and others have shown increased production of IL-6.[287] It has been difficult to correlate specific abnormalities in T- or B-cell function with specific clinical findings or serum immunoglobulin concentrations.

Family studies indicate that genetic factors contribute to the etiology of CVID. The relatives of patients with CVID have an increased incidence of autoantibody production and autoimmune disease including hemolytic anemia, rheumatoid arthritis, systemic lupus erythematosus, and thyroid disease.[259,288–290] Abnormalities of immunoglobulin production, with unusually high and unusually low concentrations of serum IgM, IgG, or IgA, have been reported.[259,288] As many as 10 to 20 percent of patients with CVID have first-degree relatives with either CVID or IgA deficiency.[101,256] The affected individual may be sibs, parents, or offspring of the patient. These findings provide support for the hypothesis that CVID is a multifactorial disease influenced by several susceptibility genes.

At least one of the susceptibility genes that contributes to the etiology of CVID resides in the HLA locus at 6p21.3. Several groups have shown an increased frequency of certain unusual HLA haplotypes in patients with CVID or IgA deficiency.[98,107–113] Because the HLA region contains many genes that influence lymphocyte function, the exact nature of the susceptibility gene remains unclear. Haplotypes with deletions of the C4A gene[98,110] and specific alleles of C2 and TNF have been implicated.[111] In the past few years, patients who were previously given the diagnosis of CVID were recognized to have defects in either Btk (X-linked agammaglobulinemia)[291] or CD40 ligand (X-linked hyper-IgM syndrome). There may be additional gene defects that fall under the diagnostic category of CVID.

IgA Deficiency

IgA deficiency is a common disorder, occurring with a frequency of 1 in 500 Caucasian blood donors of Northern European descent.[292–294] It is less common in the Japanese or African American populations, but even in these groups it occurs at a higher frequency than any of the other well-characterized immunodeficiencies.[295] Shortly after IgA deficiency was identified, it was recognized that an absence of serum IgA could be found in otherwise healthy individuals.[296] However, it is clear that people with IgA deficiency have an increased incidence of upper and lower respiratory tract infections, although severe infections resulting in bronchiectasis are rare.[45–50] As with other patients with antibody deficiencies, patients with IgA deficiency have an increased susceptibility to *Giardia* infections. Allergies are also very common in patients with IgA deficiency; large population studies have indicated that 10 percent of the normal population have allergic symptoms, whereas about 50 percent of patients with IgA deficiency have seasonal rhinitis, food or drug allergies, eczema, urticaria, or asthma.[45–50] Autoimmune disorders, for example, rheumatoid arthritis, systemic lupus erythematosus, thyroiditis, hemolytic anemia or thrombocytopenia, celiac disease, and vitiligo, may be seen in 5 to 10 percent of patients with IgA deficiency.[45–50] Decreased serum IgA is almost always associated with absent secretory IgA, and decreased secretory IgA is predictably associated with absent serum IgA.

A developmental delay in the production of IgA is not uncommon.[297,298] Thus, many small children with serum concentrations of IgA that are below the normal range in the first few years of life "grow out" of their disease by 5 to 10 years of age.[297,299] Because of this observation, many immunologists are reluctant to make the diagnosis of IgA deficiency in children younger than 5 years. Children with low but measurable concentrations of serum IgA do have a somewhat higher incidence of upper respiratory tract infections.[300] As the serum IgA concentrations reach normal levels, the number of infections often decreases.

Laboratory studies in patients with IgA deficiency are similar to those in patients with CVID. Most patients have normal numbers of T cells and B cells,[47] but the B cells that express surface IgA are blocked at an early stage of differentiation.[301] Some patients have T cells that suppress IgA synthesis or fail to help IgA production.[302–304] In the presence of CD40 ligand and cytokines, B cells from many IgA-deficient patients can be stimulated to produce IgA in culture.[305,306] Decreased concentrations of serum IgG2, IgG3, or IgG4 are seen in about 25 percent of patients with IgA deficiency[104–106]; this subset of patients has an increased incidence of significant lower respiratory tract infections.[104] In some patients with IgA deficiency, there are increased numbers of IgM or IgD producing plasma cells at the mucosal surfaces,[307–309] and IgM can replace IgA in secretions. IgA-deficient patients who have elevated concentrations of antigen-specific IgM in saliva tend to have a lower frequency of infections.[310] Patients with IgA deficiency, like patients with CVID, are more likely to have inherited a certain unusual HLA haplotypes[98,102,107,108,113,294]; but there is no association with any specific immunoglobulin heavy chain haplotypes, and it is assumed that the immunoglobulin genes are normal in the majority of patients.

A variety of abnormal antibodies can be found in the serum of patients with IgA deficiency. More than 50 percent of patients have milk precipitins, antibodies to bovine albumin, and immunoglobulins.[45–47,311] Antibodies to DNA or RNA have been found in the serum of 20 percent of patients with IgA deficiency.[51,52] About 50 percent of patients with undetectable serum IgA make antibodies to IgA.[311,312] These anti-IgA antibodies can cause anaphylactic reactions in patients who receive transfusions or blood products[313]; however, the high incidence of unrecognized IgA deficiency in the population and the low incidence of anaphylactic reactions to transfusions suggests that the anti-IgA antibodies do not always cause problems. Techniques have been developed to desensitize patients with anti-IgA antibodies who need blood products.[314]

IgA deficiency is seen in 85 percent of patients with ataxia telangiectasia,[89] and it has been seen in association with chromosomal abnormalities, in particular defects in chromosome 18 and partial monosomy 22.[47,315–319] Therapy with certain drugs, such as phenytoins,[320] gold,[321,322] or sulfasalazine,[323] may cause IgA deficiency. IgA deficiency is sometimes seen in patients with congenital rubella infection[324] or after Epstein–Barr virus infection.[325] The occurrence of IgA deficiency in these highly diverse situations suggests that IgA deficiency may be an easily detected sign of perturbations of the immune system. The increased incidence of allergies, autoimmune disease, and respiratory tract infections in patients with IgA deficiency may be due, at least in part, to the absence of IgA in the serum and at the mucosal surfaces, as has been proposed. Alternatively, the infections, allergies, autoimmune diseases, and IgA deficiency may all be signs of less easily detected defects in T cells, B cells, or antigen presenting cells. Studies showing poor production of antigen-specific IgG after immunization[326] and decreased secretion of IgG in culture[327] in patients with IgA deficiency support this hypothesis.

IgG Subclass Deficiency

IgG subclass deficiencies generally can be divided into two groups: those that are identified during evaluations for recurrent infections[328–331] and those that are discovered in population studies that screen large numbers of individuals.[38,332–334] The latter studies indicate that unequal crossovers within the immunoglobulin heavy chain locus can result in large deletions or duplications that involve several heavy chain genes. In Mediterranean populations, large heterozygous deletions that remove one or more IgG subclass genes are seen in as many as 1 in 50 blood donors[334] and homozygous deletions are seen in about 1 in 5000.[332] Duplications occur with an even higher frequency[334]; extra copies of the IgG4 C region gene are seen in 44 percent of normal individuals.[335] Individuals with homozygous deletions that remove genes for several IgG subclasses are usually asymptomatic.[39] This observation suggests that the absence of a particular subclass does not predictably result in immunodeficiency.

Patients with recurrent infections and normal concentrations of serum IgG may have decreased levels of one or more IgG subclasses. Recent studies have indicated that these patients may also have defects within the immunoglobulin heavy chain genes. Two siblings with isolated deficiency of IgG2 were found to have a frameshift mutation within the coding sequence of the $\gamma 2$ gene.[336] Some patients with IgG3 deficiency have unusual sequences in the $\gamma 3$ switch region.[337] However, most patients with IgG subclass deficiencies have normal immunoglobulin genes. As noted above, IgG subclass deficiencies are sometimes seen in patients with IgA deficiency.[104–106] Particular attention has been given to IgG2, the subclass that is largely responsible for the anticarbohydrate antibody response. IgG2 subclass deficiency has been associated with recurrent pneumonias and failure to make antibody to the polysaccharide capsule of *H. influenzae*,[329,338] but IgG2 deficiency has also been identified with otherwise healthy children who are able to make antibody to *H. influenzae* after immunization.[339] As a result, in recent years, there has been an increased emphasis on evaluating antigen-specific antibody responses rather than on concentrations of IgG subclasses in patients being evaluated for immunodeficiency.[330,340] Like IgA deficiency, IgG subclass deficiency may be a reflection of more subtle defects in the immune system.

κ-Chain Deficiency

In 1976 a patient with cystic fibrosis and IgA deficiency was found to have a complete absence of κ light chain in plasma cells in a biopsy from the gut epithelium that was done as a part of an evaluation for malabsorption. Further studies demonstrated that there was no κ in serum immunoglobulins or on the surface of B cells.[341] The patient did not have unusual susceptibility to infections. Later studies showed that this patient had point mutations on both of his alleles for κ C region gene. One mutation replaced an invariant cysteine with glycine and the other alteration replaced an invariant tryptophan with arginine.[342] Because most laboratories do not routinely evaluate the κ/λ ratio, it is difficult to determine how many individuals might have similar mutations. It is unlikely that the κ-chain deficiency in the reported patient was related to cystic fibrosis or IgA deficiency because the gene responsible for cystic fibrosis (*CFTR*) is encoded on chromosome 7 and the κ light chain is encoded on chromosome 2. Alterations in several genes may contribute to the etiology of IgA deficiency, but it is difficult to postulate a mechanism by which mutations in the κ light chain gene would predispose a patient to IgA deficiency. Because there are several copies of the λ C region gene, a point mutation in a single λ light chain gene would not result in the absence of λ light chain; however, one can imagine a deletion of the region encoding all of the λ light chains genes, which would result in λ light chain deficiency.

Transient Hypogammaglobulinemia of Infancy

When evaluating patients with recurrent infections, one occasionally finds a child whose serum immunoglobulin levels fall below the normal range but above the level typically seen in patients with well-characterized immunodeficiencies.[298,343–345] These children usually do not have severe infections; they are able to make antibodies to vaccine and environmental antigens and, with time, their serum immunoglobulins often increase into the normal range. These children are sometimes given the diagnosis of transient hypogammaglobulinemia of infancy because they are thought to have a developmental delay in the normal production of IgG and IgA. Other children may have persistent mild abnormalities and may over time fulfill the diagnostic criteria for IgA deficiency or CVID. Patients should be monitored over time, and their capacity to make antigen specific antibodies should be examined.

Thymoma

Thymomas are uncommon tumors of the thymic epithelium that are often associated with disorders of immune regulation such as myasthenia gravis or pure red cell aplasia.[346,347] Approximately 5 to 10 percent of patients with a thymoma have adult onset hypogammaglobulinemia, an association first recognized by Good.[348] The coincidence of thymoma and hypogammaglobulinemia, which is known as Good syndrome, accounts for about 10 percent of patients with adult onset hypogammaglobulinemia. It may affect individuals of any age,[349] although it is seen most often in patients in the fifth or sixth decade of life.[346] Some patients with Good syndrome have associated anemia or neutropenia and an absence of eosinophils.[346,347,350] The immunodeficiency of Good syndrome is not usually reversed by removal of the thymic tumor and hypogammaglobulinemia may be detected many years after surgical thymectomy.[351]

The majority of patients with Good syndrome have markedly decreased numbers of B cells[123,352] and pre-B cells,[123,353] but exceptions have been noted.[354] The decrease in B-cell numbers is usually associated with reduced numbers of $CD4^+$ T cells and an increase in T-cell suppressor activity. The mechanisms by which thymic tumors influence antibody production are not well understood.

REFERENCES

1. von Behring E, Kitasato S: Über das Zuatendekommen der Diphtherie-Immunität und der Tetanus-Immunität bei Thieren. *Dtsch Med Wochenschr* **16**:1113, 1890.
2. Ehrlich VP: Experimentelle Untersuchungen über Immunität. *Dtsch Med Wochenschr* **17**:1218, 1891.
3. Ehrlich P: Die Wertbemessung des Diphtherieheilserums und deren theoretische Grundlagen. *Klin Jahrb* **6**:299, 1897.
4. Metchnikov E: *Lectures on the Comparative Pathology of Inflammation*. London, Kegan Paul, Trench, Trumber and Company, 1893.
5. Tiselius A: A new apparatus for electrophoretic analysis of colloidal mixtures. *Trans Faraday Soc* **33**:524, 1937.
6. Tiselius A, Kabat EA: Electrophoresis of immune serum. *Science* **87**:1464, 1938.
7. Nomenclature for human immunoglobulins. *Bull WHO* **30**:447, 1964.
8. Rowe DS, Fahey JL: A new class of human immunoglobulins I. A unique myeloma protein. *J Exp Med* **121**:171, 1965.
9. Rowe DS, Fahey JL: A new class of human immunoglobulins II. Normal serum IgD. *J Exp Med* **121**:185, 1965.
10. Ishizaka K, Ishizaka T: Physicochemical properties of reaginic antibody. 1. Association of reaginic activity with an immunoglobulin other than gammaA- or gammaG-globulin. *J Allergy* **37**:169, 1966.
11. Johansson SG, Bennich H: Immunological studies of an atypical (myeloma) immunoglobulin. *Immunology* **13**:381, 1967.
12. Porter RR: The hydrolysis of rabbit γ-globulin and antibodies with crystalline papain. *Biochem J* **73**:119, 1959.
13. Edelman GM, Poulik MD: Studies on structural units of the γ-globulins. *J Exp Med* **113**:861, 1961.
14. Nisonoff A, Wissler FC, Lipman LN: Properties of a major component of peptic digest of rabbit antibody. *Science* **132**:1770, 1960.

15. Edelman GM: The covalent structure of a human γG-immunoglobulin. XI. Functional implications. *Biochemistry* **9**:3197, 1970.
16. Amzel LM, Poljak RJ: Three-dimensional structure of immunoglobulins. *Annu Rev Biochem* **48**:961, 1979.
17. Williams AF, Barclay AN: The immunoglobulin superfamily—domains for cell surface recognition. *Annu Rev Immunol* **6**:381, 1988.
18. Fellah JS, Wiles MV, Charlemagne J, Schwager J: Evolution of vertebrate IgM: Complete amino acid sequence of the constant region of *Ambystoma mexicanum* mu chain deduced from cDNA sequence. *Eur J Immunol* **22**:2595, 1992.
19. Litman GW, Rast JP, Shamblott MJ, Haire RN, Hulst M, Roess W, Litman RT, Hinds-Frey KR, Zilch A, Amemiya CT: Phylogenetic diversification of immunoglobulin genes and the antibody repertoire. *Mol Biol Evol* **10**:60, 1993.
20. Magor KE, Warr GW, Bando Y, Middleton DL, Higgins DA: Secretory immune system of the duck (*Anas platyrhynchos*). Identification and expression of the genes encoding IgA and IgM heavy chains. *Eur J Immunol* **28**:1063, 1998.
21. Stiehm ER, Fudenberg HH: Serum levels of immune globulins in health and disease: A survey. *Pediatrics* **37**:715, 1966.
22. Bromberg K, Rawstron S, Tannis G: Diagnosis of congenital syphilis by combining *Treponema pallidum*–specific IgM detection with immunofluorescent antigen detection for *T. pallidum*. *J Infect Dis* **168**:238, 1993.
23. Guerina NG, Hsu HW, Meissner HC, Maguire JH, Lynfield R, Stechenberg B, Abroms I, Pasternack MS, Hoff R, Eaton RB: Neonatal serologic screening and early treatment for congenital *Toxoplasma gondii* infection. The New England Regional Toxoplasma Working Group [see comments]. *N Engl J Med* **330**:1858, 1994.
24. Harrison HR, Magder LS, Boyce WT, Hauler J, Becker TM, Stewart JA, Humphrey DD: Acute *Chlamydia trachomatis* respiratory infection in childhood. Serologic evidence. *Am J Dis Child* **140**:1068, 1986.
25. Irving WL, Chang J, Raymond DR, Dunstan R, Grattan-Smith P, Cunningham AL: *Roseola infantum* and other syndromes associated with acute HHV6 infection. *Arch Dis Child* **65**:1297, 1990.
26. Clemens JM, Taskar S, Chau K, Vallari D, Shih JW, Alter HJ, Schleicher JB, Mimms LT: IgM antibody response in acute hepatitis C viral infection. *Blood* **79**:169, 1992.
27. Jain VK, Hilton E, Maytal J, Dorante G, Ilowite NT, Sood SK: Immunoglobulin M immunoblot for diagnosis of *Borrelia burgdorferi* infection in patients with acute facial palsy. *J Clin Microbiol* **34**:2033, 1996.
28. Dray S: Three γ-globulins in normal human serum revealed by monkey precipitins. *Science* **132**:1313, 1960.
29. Grey HM, Kunkel HG: H chain subgroups of myeloma proteins and normal 7S γ-globulin. *J Exp Med* **120**:253, 1964.
30. Kunkel HG, Joslin FG, Penn GM, Natvig JB: Genetic variants of G4 globulin. A unique relationship to other classes of G globulin. *J Exp Med* **132**:508, 1970.
31. Michaelsen TE, Frangione B, Franklin EC: Primary structure of the "hinge" region of human IgG3. Probable quadruplication of a 15-amino acid residue basic unit. *J Biol Chem* **252**:883, 1977.
32. Linde GA, Hammarstrom L, Persson MA, Smith CI, Sundqvist VA, Wahren B: Virus-specific antibody activity of different subclasses of immunoglobulins G and A in cytomegalovirus infections. *Infect Immunol* **42**:237, 1983.
33. Hussain R, Dockrell HM, Chiang TJ: IgG subclass antibody to *Mycobacterium leprae* 18,000 MW antigen is restricted to IgG1 and IgG3 in leprosy. *Immunology* **83**:495, 1994.
34. Siber GR, Schur PH, Aisenberg AC, Weitzman SA, Schiffman G: Correlation between serum IgG-2 concentrations and the antibody response to bacterial polysaccharide antigens. *N Engl J Med* **303**:178, 1980.
35. Ambrosino DM, Schiffman G, Gotschlich EC, Schur PH, Rosenberg GA, DeLange GG, Van Loghem E, Siber GR: Correlation between G2m(n) immunoglobulin allotype and human antibody response and susceptibility to polysaccharide encapsulated bacteria. *J Clin Invest* **75**:1935, 1985.
36. Andersen BR, Terry WD: Gamma G4-globulin antibody causing inhibition of clotting factor VIII. *Nature* **217**:174, 1968.
37. Aalberse RC, van der Gaag R, van Leeuwen J: Serologic aspects of IgG4 antibodies. I. Prolonged immunization results in an IgG4-restricted response. *J Immunol* **130**:722, 1983.
38. Lefranc MP, Lefranc G, Rabbitts TH: Inherited deletion of immunoglobulin heavy chain constant region genes in normal human individuals. *Nature* **300**:760, 1982.
39. Smith CIE, Islam KB, Vorechovsky I, Olerup O, Wallin E, Hodjattallah R, Baskin B, Hammarström L: X-linked agammaglobulinemia and other immunoglobulin deficiencies. *Immunol Rev* **138**:160, 1994.
40. Nahm MH, Blaese RM, Crain MJ, Briles DE: Patients with Wiskott-Aldrich syndrome have normal IgG2 levels. *J Immunol* **137**:3484, 1986.
41. Chodirker WB, Tomasi TBJ: Gamma-globulins: Quantitative relationships in human serum and nonvascular fluids. *Science* **142**:1080, 1963.
42. Conley ME, Delacroix DL: Intravascular and mucosal immunoglobulin A: Two separate but related systems of immune defense? *Ann Intern Med* **106**:892, 1987.
43. Czerkinsky C, Prince SJ, Michalek SM, Jackson S, Russell MW, Moldoveanu Z, McGhee JR, Mestecky J: IgA antibody-producing cells in peripheral blood after antigen ingestion: Evidence for a common mucosal immune system in humans. *Proc Natl Acad Sci USA* **84**:2449, 1987.
44. Munn EA, Feinstein A, Munro AJ: Electron microscope examination of free IgA molecules and of their complexes with antigen. *Nature* **231**:527, 1971.
45. Buckley RH, Dees SC: Correlation of milk precipitins with IgA deficiency. *N Engl J Med* **281**:465, 1969.
46. Ammann AJ, Hong R: Selective IgA deficiency: Presentation of 30 cases and a review of the literature. *Medicine (Baltimore)* **50**:223, 1971.
47. Burgio GR, Duse M, Monafo V, Ascione A, Nespoli L: Selective IgA deficiency: Clinical and immunological evaluation of 50 pediatric patients. *Eur J Pediatr* **133**:101, 1980.
48. Burks AWJ, Steele RW: Selective IgA deficiency. *Ann Allergy* **57**:3, 1986.
49. Koskinen S: Long-term follow-up of health in blood donors with primary selective IgA deficiency. *J Clin Immunol* **16**:165, 1996.
50. Burrows PD, Cooper MD: IgA deficiency. *Adv Immunol* **65**:245, 1997.
51. Gershwin ME, Blaese RM, Steinberg AD, Wistar RJ, Strober W: Antibodies to nucleic acids in congenital immune deficiency states. *J Pediatr* **89**:377, 1976.
52. Petty RE, Haddow M, Oen K, Bees W, Cassidy JT, Tubergen DG: Antibodies to nucleic acid antigens in selective IgA deficiency. *Clin Immunol Immunopathol* **13**:182, 1979.
53. Chvatchko Y, Kosco-Vilbois MH, Herren S, Lefort J, Bonnefoy JY: Germinal center formation and local immunoglobulin E (IgE) production in the lung after an airway antigenic challenge. *J Exp Med* **184**:2353, 1996.
54. Cameron LA, Durham SR, Jacobson MR, Masuyama K, Juliusson S, Gould HJ, Lowhagen O, Minshall EM, Hamid QA: Expression of IL-4, Cepsilon RNA, and Iepsilon RNA in the nasal mucosa of patients with seasonal rhinitis: Effect of topical corticosteroids. *J Allergy Clin Immunol* **101**:330, 1998.
55. Roes J, Rajewsky K: Immunoglobulin D (IgD)-deficient mice reveal an auxiliary receptor function for IgD in antigen-mediated recruitment of B cells. *J Exp Med* **177**:45, 1993.
56. Litwin SD, Zehr BD: In vitro studies on human IgD. II. IgD-secreting cells preferentially elaborate IgD, lambda molecules. *Eur J Immunol* **17**:491, 1987.
57. Honjo T: Immunoglobulin genes. *Annu Rev Immunol* **1**:499, 1983.
58. Croce CM, Shander M, Martinis J, Cicurel L, D'Ancona GG, Dolby TW, Koprowski H: Chromosomal location of the genes for human immunoglobulin heavy chains. *Proc Natl Acad Sci USA* **76**:3416, 1979.
59. Cox DW, Markovic VD, Teshima IE: Genes for immunoglobulin heavy chains and for alpha 1-antitrypsin are localized to specific regions of chromosome 14q. *Nature* **297**:428, 1982.
60. Kirsch IR, Morton CC, Nakahara K, Leder P: Human immunoglobulin heavy chain genes map to a region of translocations in malignant B lymphocytes. *Science* **216**:301, 1982.
61. Schroeder HWJ, Walter MA, Hofker MH, Ebens A, Willems van Dijk K, Liao LC, Cox DW, Milner EC, Perlmutter RM: Physical linkage of a human immunoglobulin heavy chain variable region gene segment to diversity and joining region elements. *Proc Natl Acad Sci USA* **85**:8196, 1988.
62. Ichihara Y, Matsuoka H, Kurosawa Y: Organization of human immunoglobulin heavy chain diversity gene loci. *EMBO J* **7**:4141, 1988.

63. Hofker MH, Walter MA, Cox DW: Complete physical map of the human immunoglobulin heavy chain constant region gene complex. *Proc Natl Acad Sci USA* **86**:5567, 1989.
64. Bottaro A, de Marchi M, Migone N, Carbonara AO: Pulsed-field gel analysis of human immunoglobulin heavy-chain constant region gene deletions reveals the extent of unmapped regions within the locus. *Genomics* **4**:505, 1989.
65. Matsuda F, Shin EK, Nagaoka H, Matsumura R, Haino M, Fukita Y, Taka-ishi S, Imai T, Riley JH, Anand R: Structure and physical map of 64 variable segments in the 3′0.8-megabase region of the human immunoglobulin heavy-chain locus. *Nat Genet* **3**:88, 1993.
66. Cook GP, Tomlinson IM, Walter G, Riethman H, Carter NP, Buluwela L, Winter G, Rabbitts TH: A map of the human immunoglobulin VH locus completed by analysis of the telomeric region of chromosome 14q. *Nat Genet* **7**:162, 1994.
67. Davis MM, Kim SK, Hood LE: DNA sequences mediating class switching in alpha-immunoglobulins. *Science* **209**:1360, 1980.
68. Cogne M, Lansford R, Bottaro A, Zhang J, Gorman J, Young F, Cheng HL, Alt FW: A class switch control region at the 3′ end of the immunoglobulin heavy chain locus. *Cell* **77**:737, 1994.
69. Chen C, Birshtein BK: Virtually identical enhancers containing a segment of homology to murine 3′IgH-E(hs1,2) lie downstream of human Ig C alpha 1 and C alpha 2 genes. *J Immunol* **159**:1310, 1997.
69a. Hu Y, Pan Q, Pardali E, Mills FC, Bernstein RM, Max EE, Sideras P, Hammarstrom L: Regulation of germline promoters by the two human Ig heavy chain 3′ alpha enhancers. *J Immunol* **164**:6380, 2000.
70. Hieter PA, Maizel JVJ, Leder P: Evolution of human immunoglobulin kappa J region genes. *J Biol Chem* **257**:1516, 1982.
71. Lorenz W, Straubinger B, Zachau HG: Physical map of the human immunoglobulin K locus and its implications for the mechanisms of VK-JK rearrangement. *Nucleic Acids Res* **15**:9667, 1987.
72. Erikson J, Martinis J, Croce CM: Assignment of the genes for human lambda immunoglobulin chains to chromosome 22. *Nature* **294**:173, 1981.
73. Frippiat JP, Williams SC, Tomlinson IM, Cook GP, Cherif D, Le Paslier D, Collins JE, Dunham I, Winter G, Lefranc MP: Organization of the human immunoglobulin lambda light-chain locus on chromosome 22q11.2. *Hum Mol Genet* **4**:983, 1995.
74. Hieter PA, Hollis GF, Korsmeyer SJ, Waldmann TA, Leder P: Clustered arrangement of immunoglobulin lambda constant region genes in man. *Nature* **294**:536, 1981.
75. Hiom K, Melek M, Gellert M: DNA transposition by the RAG1 and RAG2 proteins: A possible source of oncogenic translocations. *Cell* **94**:463, 1998.
76. Agrawal A, Eastman QM, Schatz DG: Transposition mediated by RAG1 and RAG2 and its implications for the evolution of the immune system. *Nature* **394**:744, 1998.
76a. Fugmann SD, Lee AI, Shockett PE, Villey IJ, Schatz DG: The RAG proteins and V(D)J recombination: Complexes, ends, and transposition. *Annu Rev Immunol* **18**:495, 2000.
77. Kincaide PW, Gimble JM: B lymphocytes, in Paul WE (ed): *Fundamental Immunology* 3d ed. New York, Raven Press Ltd., 1993, p 43.
78. Nunez C, Nishimoto N, Gartland GL, Billips LG, Burrows PD, Kubagawa H, Cooper MD: B cells are generated throughout life in humans. *J Immunol* **156**:866, 1996.
79. Gathings WE, Lawton AR, Cooper MD: Immunofluorescent studies of the development of pre-B cells, B lymphocytes and immunoglobulin isotype diversity in humans. *Eur J Immunol* **7**:804, 1977.
80. Rajewsky K: Clonal selection and learning in the antibody system. *Nature* **381**:751, 1996.
81. Burrows PD, Cooper MD: B cell development and differentiation. *Curr Opin Immunol* **9**:239, 1997.
82. Bertrand FE, Billips LG, Burrows PD, Gartland GL, Kubagawa H, Schroeder HWJ: Ig D(H) gene segment transcription and rearrangement before surface expression of the pan-B-cell marker CD19 in normal human bone marrow. *Blood* **90**:736, 1997.
83. Melchers F, Karasuyama H, Haasner D, Bauer S, Kudo A, Sakaguchi N, Jameson B, Rolink A: The surrogate light chain in B-cell development. *Immunol Today* **14**:60, 1993.
84. Korsmeyer SJ, Hieter PA, Ravetch JV, Poplack DG, Waldmann TA, Leder P: Developmental hierarchy of immunoglobulin gene rearrangements in human leukemic pre-B-cells. *Proc Natl Acad Sci USA* **78**:7096, 1981.
85. Maki R, Traunecker A, Sakano H, Roeder W, Tonegawa S: Exon shuffling generates an immunoglobulin heavy chain gene. *Proc Natl Acad Sci USA* **77**:2138, 1980.
86. Ravetch JV, Kirsch IR, Leder P: Evolutionary approach to the question of immunoglobulin heavy chain switching: Evidence from cloned human and mouse genes. *Proc Natl Acad Sci USA* **77**:6734, 1980.
86a. Kinoshita K, Honjo T: Unique and unprecedented recombination mechanisms in class switching. *Curr Opin Immunol* **12**:195, 2000.
87. Cascalho M, Wong J, Steinberg C, Wabl M: Mismatch repair co-opted by hypermutation. *Science* **279**:1207, 1998.
88. Wiesendanger M, Scharff MD, Edelmann W: Somatic hypermutation, transcription, and DNA mismatch repair. *Cell* **94**:415, 1998.
89. McFarlin DE, Strober W, Wochner RD, Waldmann TA: Immunoglobulin A production in ataxia telangiectasia. *Science* **150**:1175, 1965.
90. Allen RC, Armitage RJ, Conley ME, Rosenblatt H, Jenkins NA, Copeland NG, Bedell MA, Edelhoff S, Disteche CM, Simoneaux DK, Fanslow WC, Belmont JW, Spriggs MK: CD40 Ligand gene defects responsible for X-linked hyper-IgM syndrome. *Science* **259**:990, 1993.
91. Aruffo A, Farrington M, Hollenbaugh D, Li X, Milatovich A, Nonoyama S, Bajorath J, Grosmaire LS, Stenkamp R, Neubauer M, Roberts RL, Noelle RJ, Ledbetter JA, Francke U, Ochs HD: The CD40 ligand, gp39, is defective in activated T cells from patients with X-linked hyper-IgM syndrome. *Cell* **72**:291, 1993.
92. Korthauer U, Graf D, Mages HW, Briere F, Padayachee M, Malcolm S, Ugazio AG, Notarangelo LD, Levinsky RJ, Kroczek RA: Defective expression of T-cell CD40 ligand causes X-linked immunodeficiency with hyper-IgM. *Nature* **361**:539, 1993.
93. DiSanto JP, Bonnefoy JY, Gauchat JF, Fischer A, de Saint Basile G: CD40 ligand mutations in X-linked immunodeficiency with hyper-IgM. *Nature* **361**:541, 1993.
94. Fuleihan R, Ramesh N, Loh R, Jabara H, Rosen FS, Chatila T, Fu SM, Stamenkovic I, Geha RS: Defective expression of the CD40 ligand in X chromosome-linked immunoglobulin deficiency with normal or elevated IgM. *Proc Natl Acad Sci USA* **90**:2170, 1993.
95. Conley ME, Brown P, Pickard AR, Buckley RH, Miller DS, Raskind WH, Singer JW, Fialkow PJ: Expression of the gene defect in X-linked agammaglobulinemia. *N Engl J Med* **315**:564, 1986.
96. Vetrie D, Vorechovsky I, Sideras P, Holland J, Davies A, Flinter F, Hammarstrom L, Kinnon C, Levinsky R, Bobrow M, Smith CIE, Bentley DR: The gene involved in X-linked agammaglobulinemia is a member of the *src* family of protein-tyrosine kinases. *Nature* **361**:226, 1993.
97. Tsukada S, Saffran DC, Rawlings DJ, Parolini O, Allen RC, Klisak I, Sparkes RS, Kubagawa H, Mohandas T, Quan S, Belmont JW, Cooper MD, Conley ME, Witte ON: Deficient expression of a B cell cytoplasmic tyrosine kinase in human X-linked agammaglobulinemia. *Cell* **72**:279, 1993.
98. Schaffer FM, Palermos J, Zhu ZB, Barger BO, Cooper MD, Volanakis JE: Individuals with IgA deficiency and common variable immunodeficiency share polymorphisms of major histocompatibility complex class III genes. *Proc Natl Acad Sci USA* **86**:8015, 1989.
99. Feldman G, Koziner B, Talamo R, Bloch KJ: Familial variable immunodeficiency: Autosomal dominant pattern of inheritance with variable expression of the defect(s). *J Pediatr* **87**:534, 1975.
100. Olerup O, Smith CIE, Bjorkander J, Hammarstrom L: Shared HLA class II–associated genetic susceptibility and resistance, related to the HLA-DQB1 gene, in IgA deficiency and common variable immunodeficiency. *Proc Natl Acad Sci USA* **89**:10653, 1992.
101. Vorechovsky I, Zetterquist H, Paganelli R, Koskinen S, Webster AD, Bjorkander J, Smith CIE, Hammarstrom L: Family and linkage study of selective IgA deficiency and common variable immunodeficiency. *Clin Immunol Immunopathol* **77**:185, 1995.
102. Johnson ML, Keeton LG, Zhu ZB, Volanakis JE, Cooper MD, Schroeder HWJ: Age-related changes in serum immunoglobulins in patients with familial IgA deficiency and common variable immunodeficiency (CVID). *Clin Exp Immunol* **108**:477, 1997.
103. Espanol T, Catala M, Hernandez M, Caragol I, Bertran JM: Development of a common variable immunodeficiency in IgA-deficient patients. *Clin Immunol Immunopathol* **80**:333, 1996.
104. Bjorkander J, Bake B, Oxelius VA, Hanson LA: Impaired lung function in patients with IgA deficiency and low levels of IgG2 or IgG3. *N Engl J Med* **313**:720, 1985.
105. Out TA, van Munster PJ, De Graeff PA, The TH, Vossen JM, Zegers BJ: Immunological investigations in individuals with selective IgA deficiency. *Clin Exp Immunol* **64**:510, 1986.

106. Sandler SG, Trimble J, Mallory DM: Coexistent IgG2 and IgA deficiencies in blood donors. *Transfusion* **36**:256, 1996.
107. Wilton AN, Cobain TJ, Dawkins RL: Family studies of IgA deficiency. *Immunogenetics* **21**:333, 1985.
108. Olerup O, Smith CIE, Hammarström L: Different amino acids at position 57 of the HLA-DQβ chain associated with susceptibility and resistance to IgA deficiency. *Nature* **347**:289, 1990.
109. Volanakis JE, Zhu ZB, Schaffer FM, Macon KJ, Palermos J, Barger BO, Go R, Campbell RD, Schroeder HWJ, Cooper MD: Major histocompatibility complex class III genes and susceptibility to immunoglobulin A deficiency and common variable immunodeficiency. *J Clin Invest* **89**:1914, 1992.
110. Howe HS, So AK, Farrant J, Webster AD: Common variable immunodeficiency is associated with polymorphic markers in the human major histocompatibility complex. *Clin Exp Immunol* **83**:387, 1991.
111. Mullighan CG, Fanning GC, Chapel HM, Welsh KI: TNF and lymphotoxin-alpha polymorphisms associated with common variable immunodeficiency: Role in the pathogenesis of granulomatous disease. *J Immunol* **159**:6236, 1997.
112. Schroeder HWJ, Zhu ZB, March RE, Campbell RD, Berney SM, Nedospasov SA, Turetskaya RL, Atkinson TP, Go RC, Cooper MD, Volanakis JE: Susceptibility locus for IgA deficiency and common variable immunodeficiency in the HLA-DR3, -B8, -A1 haplotypes. *Mol Med* **4**:72, 1998.
113. Cucca F, Zhu ZB, Khanna A, Cossu F, Congia M, Badiali M, Lampis R, Frau F, De Virgiliis S, Cao A, Arnone M, Piras P, Campbell RD, Cooper MD, Volanakis JE, Powis SH: Evaluation of IgA deficiency in Sardinians indicates a susceptibility gene is encoded within the HLA class III region. *Clin Exp Immunol* **111**:76, 1998.
114. Thomas C, de Saint B, Le Deist F, Theophile D, Benkerrou M, Haddad E, Blanche S, Fischer A: Correction of X-linked hyper-IgM syndrome by allogeneic bone marrow transplantation. *N Engl J Med* **333**:426, 1995.
114a. Hadzic N, Pagliuca A, Rela M, Portmann B, Jones A, Veys P, Heaton ND, Mufti GJ, Mieli-Vergani G: Correction of the hyper-IgM syndrome after liver and bone marrow transplantation. *N Engl J Med* **342**:320, 2000.
115. Drabek D, Raguz S, De Wit TP, Dingjan GM, Savelkoul HF, Grosveld F, Hendriks RW: Correction of the X-linked immunodeficiency phenotype by transgenic expression of human Bruton tyrosine kinase under the control of the class II major histocompatibility complex Ea locus control region. *Proc Natl Acad Sci USA* **94**:610, 1997.
115a. Brown MP, Topham DJ, Sangster MY, Zhao J, Flynn KJ, Surman SL, Woodland DL, Doherty PC, Farr AG, Pattengale PK, Brenner MK: Thymic lymphoproliferative disease after successful correction of CD40 ligand deficiency by gene transfer in mice. *Nat Med* **4**:1253, 1998.
115b. Rohrer J, Conley ME: Correction of X-linked immunodeficient mice by competitive reconstitution limiting numbers of normal bone marrow cells. *Blood* **94**:3358, 1999.
116. Bruton OC: Agammaglobulinemia. *Pediatrics* **9**:722, 1952.
117. Janeway CA, Apt L, Gitlin D: Agammaglobulinemia. *Trans Assoc Am Phys* **66**:200, 1953.
118. Good RA: Clinical Investigations in patients with agammaglobulinemia. *J Lab Clin Med* **44**:803, 1954.
119. Siegal FP, Pernis B, Kunkel HG: Lymphocytes in human immunodeficiency states: A study of membrane-associated immunoglobulins. *Eur J Immunol* **1**:482, 1971.
120. Cooper MD, Lawton AR: Circulating B-cells in patients with immunodeficiency. *Am J Pathol* **69**:513, 1972.
121. Geha RS, Rosen FS, Merler E: Identification and characterization of subpopulations of lymphocytes in human peripheral blood after fractionation on discontinuous gradients of albumin. *J Clin Invest* **52**:1726, 1973.
122. Preud'Homme JL, Griscelli C, Seligmann M: Immunoglobulins on the surface of lymphocytes in fifty patients with primary immunodeficiency diseases. *Clin Immunol Immunopathol* **1**:241, 1973.
123. Pearl ER, Vogler LB, Okos AJ, Crist WM, Lawton IAR, Cooper MD: B lymphocyte precursors in human bone marrow: An analysis of normal individuals and patients with antibody-deficiency states. *J Immunol* **120**:1169, 1978.
124. Campana D, Farrant J, Inamdar N, Webster ADB, Janossy G: Phenotypic features and proliferative activity of B cell progenitors in X-linked agammaglobulinemia. *J Immunol* **145**:1675, 1990.
125. Kwan S-P, Kunkel L, Bruns G, Wedgwood RJ, Latt S, Rosen FS: Mapping of the X-linked agammaglobulinemia locus by use of restriction fragment-length polymorphism. *J Clin Invest* **77**:649, 1986.
126. Fearon ER, Winkelstein JA, Civin CI, Pardoll DM, Vogelstein B: Carrier detection in X-linked agammaglobulinemia by analysis of X-chromosome inactivation. *N Engl J Med* **316**:427, 1987.
127. Conley ME: B cells in patients with X-linked agammaglobulinemia. *J Immunol* **134**:3070, 1985.
128. Allen RC, Nachtman RC, Rosenblatt HM, Belmont JW: Application of carrier testing to genetic counseling for X-linked agammaglobulinemia. *Am J Hum Genet* **54**:25, 1994.
129. Lederman HM, Winkelstein JA: X-linked agammaglobulinemia: An analysis of 96 patients. *Medicine* **64**:145, 1985.
130. Ochs HD, Winkelstein J: Disorders of the B-cell system, in Stiehm ER (ed): *Immunologic Disorders in Infants and Children*, 4th ed. Philadelphia, Saunders, 1996, p 296.
131. Good RA, Zak SJ: Disturbances in gamma globulin synthesis as "experiments of nature." *Pediatr Res* **18**:109, 1956.
132. Kozlowski C, Evans DIK: Neutropenia associated with X-linked agammaglobulinemia. *J Clin Pathol* **44**:388, 1991.
133. Farrar JE, Rohrer J, Conley ME: Neutropenia in X-linked agammaglobulinemia. *Clin Immunol Immunopathol* **81**:271, 1996.
134. Haldane JBS: The rate of spontaneous mutation of a human gene. *J Genet* **31**:317, 1935.
135. Conley ME, Mathias D, Treadaway J, Minegishi Y, Rohrer J: Mutations in Btk in patients with presumed X-linked agammaglobulinemia. *Am J Hum Genet* **62**:1034, 1998.
136. Kornfeld SJ, Haire RN, Strong SJ, Tang H, Sung S-SJ, Fu SM, Litman GW: A novel mutation ($Cys^{145\text{-stop}}$) in Bruton's tyrosine kinase is associated with newly diagnosed X-linked agammglobulinemia in a 51-year-old male. *Mol Med* **2**:619, 1996.
137. Ishida F, Kobayashi H, Saito H, Futatani T, Miyawaki T, Kiyosawa K: The oldest case with X-linked agammaglobulinemia in Japan lacking Bruton-type tyrosine kinase protein detected by flow cytometry. *Rinsho Ketsueki* **39**:44, 1998.
138. Roifman CM, Rao CP, Lederman HM, Lavi S, Quinn P, Gelfand EW: Increased susceptibility to *Mycoplasma* infection in patients with hypogammaglobulinemia. *Am J Med* **80**:590, 1986.
139. Meyer RD, Clough W: Extragenital *Mycoplasma hominis* infections in adults: Emphasis on immunosuppression. *Clin Infect Dis* **17(suppl 1)**:S243, 1993.
140. Furr PM, Taylor-Robinson D, Webster AD: Mycoplasmas and ureaplasmas in patients with hypogammaglobulinaemia and their role in arthritis: Microbiological observations over twenty years. *Ann Rheum Dis* **53**:183, 1994.
141. La Scola B, Michel G, Raoult D: Use of amplification and sequencing of the 16S rRNA gene to diagnose *Mycoplasma pneumoniae* osteomyelitis in a patient with hypogammaglobulinemia. *Clin Infect Dis* **24**:1161, 1997.
142. Berglof A, Sandstedt K, Feinstein R, Bolske G, Smith CIE: B cell–deficient muMT mice as an experimental model for *Mycoplasma* infections in X-linked agammaglobulinemia. *Eur J Immunol* **27**:2118, 1997.
143. McKinney RE Jr, Katz SL, Wilfert CM: Chronic enteroviral meningoencephalitis in agammaglobulinemic patients. *Rev Infect Dis* **9**:334, 1987.
144. Tedder TF, Crain MJ, Kubagawa H, Clement LT, Cooper MD: Evaluation of lymphocyte differentiation in primary and secondary immunodeficiency diseases. *J Immunol* **135**:1786, 1985.
144a. Conley ME, Notarangelo LD, Etzioni A: Diagnostic criteria for primary immunodeficiencies. *Clin Immunol* **93**:190, 1999.
145. Krantman HJ, Saxon A, Stevens RH, Stiehm ER: Phenotypic heterogeneity in X-linked infantile agammaglobulinemia with in vitro monocyte supression of immunoglobulin synthesis. *Clin Immunol Immunopathol* **20**:170, 1981.
146. Rozynska KE, Spickett GP, Millrain M, Edwards A, Bryant A, Webster AD, Farrant J: Accessory and T cell defects in acquired and inherited hypogammaglobulinaemia. *Clin Exp Immunol* **78**:1, 1989.
147. Richards SJ, Scott CS, Cole JC, Gooi HC: Abnormal CD45R expression in patients with common variable immunodeficiency and X-linked agammaglobulinaemia. *Br J Haematol* **81**:160, 1992.
148. Yel L, Minegishi Y, Coustan-Smith E, Buckley RH, Trubel H, Pachman LM, Kitchingman GR, Campana D, Rohrer J, Conley MD: Mutations in the mu heavy chain gene in patients with agammaglobulinemia. *N Engl J Med* **335**:1486, 1996.
149. de Weers M, Verschuren MCM, Kraakman MEM, Mensink RGJ, Schuurman RKB, Van Dongen JJM, Hendricks RW: The Bruton's tyrosine kinase gene is expressed throughout B cell differentiation

from early precursor B cell stages preceding immunoglobulin gene rearrangement up to mature B cell stages. *Eur J Immunol* **23**:3109, 1993.

150. Smith CIE, Baskin B, Humire-Greiff P, Zhou J-N, Olsson PG, Maniar HS, Kjellén P, Lambris JD, Christensson B, Hammarström L, Bentley D, Vetrie D, Islam KB, Vorechovsky I, Sideras P: Expression of Bruton's agammaglobulinemia tyrosine kinase gene, *BTK*, is selectively down-regulated in T lymphocytes and plasma cells. *J Immunol* **152**:557, 1994.
151. Genevier HC, Hinshelwood S, Gaspar HB, Rigley KP, Brown D, Saeland S, Rousset F, Levinsky RJ, Callard RE, Kinnon C, Lovering R: Expression of Bruton's tyrosine kinase protein within the B cell lineage. *Eur J Immunol* **24**:3100, 1994.
152. Fukuda M, Kojima T, Kabayama H, Mikoshiba K: Mutation of the pleckstrin homology domain of Bruton's tyrosine kinase in immunodeficiency impaired inositol 1,3,4,5-tetrakisphosphate binding capacity. *J Biol Chem* **271**:30303, 1996.
153. Rameh LE, Arvidsson A, Carraway KL, Couvillon AD, Rathbun G, Crompton A, VanRenterghem B, Czech MP, Ravichandran KS, Burakoff SJ, Wang DS, Chen CS, Cantley LC: A comparative analysis of the phosphoinositide binding specificity of pleckstrin homology domains. *J Biol Chem* **272**:22059, 1997.
154. Yao L, Kawakami Y, Kawakami T: The pleckstrin homology domain of Bruton tyrosine kinase interacts with protein kinase C. *Proc Natl Acad Sci USA* **91**:9175, 1994.
155. Bence K, Ma W, Kozasa T, Huang XY: Direct stimulation of Bruton's tyrosine kinase by G(q)-protein alpha-subunit. *Nature* **389**:296, 1997.
156. Langhans-Rajasekaran SA, Wan Y, Huang XY: Activation of Tsk and Btk tyrosine kinases by G protein beta gamma subunits. *Proc Natl Acad Sci USA* **92**:8601, 1995.
157. Cheng G, Ye Z-S, Baltimore D: Binding of Bruton's tyrosine kinase to Fyn, Lyn or Hck through a Src homology 3 domain-mediated interaction. *Proc Natl Acad Sci USA* **91**:8152, 1994.
158. de Weers M, Brouns GS, Hinshelwood S, Kinnon C, Schuurman RKB, Hendriks RW, Borst J: B-cell antigen receptor stimulation activates the human Bruton's tyrosine kinase, which is deficient in X-linked agammaglobulinemia. *J Biol Chem* **269**:23857, 1994.
159. Aoki Y, Isselbacher KJ, Pillai S: Bruton tyrosine kinase is tyrosine phosphorylated and activated in pre-B lymphocytes and receptor-ligated B cells. *Proc Natl Acad Sci USA* **91**:10606, 1994.
160. Kitanaka A, Mano H, Conley ME, Campana D: Expression and activation of the nonreceptor tyrosine kinase Tec in human B cells. *Blood* **91**:940, 1998.
161. Sato S, Katagiri T, Takaki S, Kikuchi Y, Hitoshi Y, Yonehara S, Tsukada S, Kitamura D, Watanabe T, Witte O, Takatsu K: IL-5 receptor-mediated tyrosine phosphorylation of SH2/SH3- containing proteins and activation of Bruton's tyrosine and Janus 2 kinases. *J Exp Med* **180**:2101, 1994.
162. Matsuda T, Takahashi-Tezuka M, Fukada T, Okuyama Y, Fujitani Y, Tsukada S, Mano H, Hirai H, Witte ON, Hirano T: Association and activation of Btk and Tec tyrosine kinases by gp130, a signal transducer of the interleukin-6 family of cytokines. *Blood* **85**:627, 1995.
163. Kawakami Y, Yao L, Miura T, Tsukada S, Witte ON, Kawakami T: Tyrosine phosphorylation and activation of Bruton tyrosine kinase upon Fc?RI cross-linking. *Mol Cell Biol* **14**:5108, 1994.
164. Rawlings DJ, Scharenberg AM, Park H, Wahl MI, Lin S, Kato RM, Fluckiger A-C, Witte ON, Kinet J-P: Activation of Btk by a phosphorylation mechanism initiated by SRC family kinases. *Science* **271**:822, 1996.
165. Takata M, Kurosaki T: A role for Bruton's tyrosine kinase in B cell antigen receptor- mediated activation of phospholipase C-gamma 2. *J Exp Med* **184**:31, 1996.
166. Genevier HC, Callard RE: Impaired Ca^{2+} mobilization by X-linked agammaglobulinaemia (XLA) B cells in response to ligation of the B cell receptor (BCR). *Clin Exp Immunol* **110**:386, 1997.
167. Fluckiger AC, Li Z, Kato RM, Wahl MI, Ochs HD, Longnecker R, Kinet JP, Witte ON, Scharenberg AM, Rawlings DJ: Btk/Tec kinases regulate sustained increases in intracellular Ca^{2+} following B-cell receptor activation. *EMBO J* **17**:1973, 1998.
168. Rohrer J, Parolini O, Belmont JW, Conley ME: The genomic structure of human *BTK*, the defective gene in X-linked agammaglobulinemia. *Immunogenetics* **40**:319, 1994.
169. Hagemann TL, Chen Y, Rosen FS, Kwan S-P: Genomic organization of the Btk gene and exon scanning for mutations in patients with X-linked agammaglobulinemia. *Hum Mol Genet* **3**:1743, 1994.
170. Ohta Y, Haire RN, Litman RT, Fu SM, Nelson RP, Kratz J, Kornfeld SJ, De La Morena M, Good RA, Litman GW: Genomic organization and structure of Bruton agammaglobulinemia tyrosine kinase: Localization of mutations associated with varied clinical presentations and course in X chromosome-linked agammaglobulinemia. *Proc Natl Acad Sci USA* **91**:9062, 1994.
171. Sideras P, Muller S, Shiels H, Jin H, Khan WN, Nilsson L, Parkinson E, Thomas JD, Branden L, Larsson I, Paul WE, Rosen FS, Alt FW, Vetrie D, Smith CIE, Xanthopoulos KG: Genomic organization of mouse and human Bruton's agammaglobulinemia tyrosine kinase (Btk) loci. *J Immunol* **153**:5607, 1994.

171a. Vihinen M, Kwan SP, Lester T, Ochs HD, Resnick I, Valiaho J, Conley ME, Smith CI: Mutations of the human BTK gene coding for bruton tyrosine kinase in X-linked agammaglobulinemia. *Hum Mutat* **13**:280, 1999.

172. Gaspar HB, Lester T, Levinsky RJ, Kinnon C: Bruton's tyrosine kinase expression and activity in X-linked agammaglobulinaemia (XLA): the use of protein analysis as a diagnostic indicator of XLA. *Clin Exp Immunol* **111**:334, 1998.
173. Futatani T, Miyawaki T, Tsukada S, Hashimoto S, Kunikata T, Arai S, Kurimoto M, Niida Y, Matsuoka H, Sakiyama Y, Iwata T, Tsuchiya S, Tatsuzawa O, Yoshizaki K, Kishimoto T: Deficient expression of Bruton's tyrosine kinase in monocytes from X-linked agammaglobulinemia as evaluated by a flow cytometric analysis and its clinical application to carrier detection. *Blood* **91**:595, 1998.
174. Conley ME, Parolini O, Rohrer J, Campana D: X-linked agammaglobulinemia: New approaches to old questions based on the identification of the defective gene. *Immunol Rev* **138**:5, 1994.
175. de Weers M, Mensink RGJ, Kraakman MEM, Schuurman RKB, Hendriks RW: Mutation analysis of the Bruton's tyrosine kinase gene in X-linked agammaglobulinemia: Identification of a mutation which affects the same codon as is altered in immunodeficient xid mice. *Hum Mol Genet* **3**:161, 1994.
176. Jin H, Webster AD, Vihinen M, Sideras P, Vorechovsky I, Hammarstrom L, Bernatowska-Matuszkiewicz E, Smith CI, Bobrow M, Vetrie D: Identification of Btk mutations in 20 unrelated patients with X-linked agammaglobulinaemia (XLA). *Hum Mol Genet* **4**:693, 1995.
177. Guioli S, Arveiler B, Bardoni B, Notarangelo LD, Panina P, Duse M, Ugazio A, de Saint Basile G, Mandel JL, Camerino G: Close linkage of probe p212 (DXS178) to X-linked agammaglobulinemia. *Hum Genet* **84**:19, 1989.
178. Kwan S-P, Terwilliger J, Parmley R, Raghu G, Sandkuyl LA, Ott J, Ochs H, Wedgwood R, Rosen F: Identification of a closely linked DNA marker, DXS178, to further refine the X-linked agammaglobulinemia locus. *Genomics* **6**:238, 1990.
179. Allen RC, Belmont JW: Dinucleotide repeat polymorphism at the DXS178 locus. *Hum Mol Genet* **1**:216, 1992.
180. Allen RC, Belmont JW: Trinucleotide repeat polymorphism at DXS101. *Hum Mol Genet* **2**:1508, 1993.
181. Conley ME, Puck JM: Carrier detection in typical and atypical X-linked agammaglobulinemia. *J Pediatr* **112**:688, 1988.
182. Conley ME: Molecular approaches to analysis of X-linked immunodeficiencies. *Annu Rev Immunol* **10**:215, 1992.
183. Stephens K, Kayes L, Riccardi VM, Rising M, Sybert VP, Pagon RA: Preferential mutation of the neurofibromatosis type 1 gene in paternally derived chromosomes. *Hum Genet* **88**:279, 1992.
184. Goldberg YP, Kremer B, Andrew SE, Theilmann J, Graham RK, Squitieri F, Telenius H, Adam S, Sajoo A, Starr E: Molecular analysis of new mutations for Huntington's disease: intermediate alleles and sex of origin effects. *Nat Genet* **5**:174, 1993.
185. Palau F, Lofgren A, De Jonghe P., Bort S, Nelis E, Sevilla T, Martin JJ, Vilchez J, Prieto F, van Broeckhoven C: Origin of the de novo duplication in Charcot-Marie-Tooth disease type 1A: Unequal nonsister chromatid exchange during spermatogenesis. *Hum Mol Genet* **2**:2031, 1993.
186. Carlson KM, Bracamontes J, Jackson CE, Clark R, Lacroix A, Wells SAJ, Goodfellow PJ: Parent-of-origin effects in multiple endocrine neoplasia type 2B. *Am J Hum Genet* **55**:1076, 1994.
187. Tuchman M, Matsuda I, Munnich A, Malcolm S, Strautnieks S, Briede T: Proportions of spontaneous mutations in males and females with ornithine transcarbamylase deficiency. *Am J Med Genet* **55**:67, 1995.
188. Becker J, Schwaab R, Moller-Taube A, Schwaab U, Schmidt W, Brackmann HH, Grimm T, Olek K, Oldenburg J: Characterization of the factor VIII defect in 147 patients with sporadic hemophilia A: Family studies indicate a mutation type-dependent sex ratio of mutation frequencies. *Am J Hum Genet* **58**:657, 1996.

189. Aiuti F, Fontana L, Gatti RA: Membrane-bound immunoglobulin (Ig) and in vitro production of Ig by lymphoid cells from patients with primary immunodeficiencies. *Scand J Immunol* **2**:9, 1973.
190. Hoffman T, Winchester R, Schulkind M, Frias JL, Ayoub EM, Good RA: Hypoimmunoglobulinemia with normal T cell function in female siblings. *Clin Immunol Immunopathol* **7**:364, 1977.
191. Sweinberg SK, Wodell RA, Grodofsky MP, Greene JM, Conley ME: Retrospective analysis of the incidence of pulmonary disease in hypogammaglobulinemia. *J Allergy Clin Immunol* **88**:96, 1991.
192. De La Morena M, Haire RN, Ohta Y, Nelson RP, Litman RT, Day NK, Good RA, Litman GW: Predominance of sterile immunoglobulin transcripts in a female phenotypically resembling Bruton's agammaglobulinemia. *Eur J Immunol* **25**:809, 1995.
193. Meffre E, LeDeist F, de Saint-Basile G, Deville A, Fougereau M, Fischer A, Schiff C: A human non-XLA immunodeficiency disease characterized by blockage of B cell development at an early proB cell stage. *J Clin Invest* **98**:1519, 1996.
194. Conley ME, Sweinberg SK: Females with a disorder phenotypically identical to X-linked agammaglobulinemia. *J Clin Immunol* **12**:139, 1992.
195. Minegishi Y, Coustan-Smith E, Wang Y-H, Cooper MD, Campana D, Conley ME: Mutations in the human $\lambda5/14.1$ gene result in B cell deficiency and agammaglobulinemia. *J Exp Med* **187**:71, 1998.
195a. Minegishi Y, Coustan-Smith E, Rapalus L, Ersoy F, Campana D, Conley ME: Mutations in Igalpha (CD79a) result in a complete block in B-cell development. *J Clin Invest* **104**:1115, 1999.
195b. Minegishi Y, Rohrer J, Coustan-Smith E, Lederman HM, Pappu R, Campana D, Chan AC, Conley ME: An essential role for BLNK in human B cell development. *Science* **286**:1954, 1999.
196. Israel-Asselain R, Burtin P, Chebat J: Un trouble biologique nouveau: l'agammaglobulinemie avec $\beta2$ macroglobulinemie (un cas). *Bull Soc Med Hop Paris* **76**:519, 1960.
197. Rosen FS, Kevy SV, Merler E, Janeway CA, Gitlin D: Recurrent bacterial infections and dysgamma-globulinemia: Deficiency of 7S gamma-globulins in the presence of elevated 19S gamma-globulins. *Pediatrics* **28**:182, 1961.
198. Hong R, Schubert WK, Perrin EV, West CD: Antibody deficiency syndrome associated with beta-2 macroglobulinemia. *J Pediatr* **61**:831, 1962.
199. Rosen FS, Craig JM, Vawter G, Janeway CA: The dysgammaglobulinemias and X-linked thymic hypoplasia. *Birth Defects* **4**:67, 1968.
200. Notarangelo LD, Duse M, Ugazio AG: Immunodeficiency with hyper-IgM (HIM). *Immunodef Rev* **3**:101, 1992.
201. Levy J, Espanol-Boren T, Thomas C, Fischer A, Tovo P, Bordigoni P, Resnick I, Fasth A, Baer M, Gomez L, Sanders EA, Tabone MD, Plantaz D, Etzioni A, Monafo V, Abinun M, Hammarstrom L, Abrabamsen T, Jones A, Finn A, Klemola T, DeVries E, Sanal O, Peitsch MC, Notarangelo LD: Clinical spectrum of X-linked hyper-IgM syndrome. *J Pediatr* **131**:47, 1997.
201a. Cunningham CK, Bonville CA, Ochs HD, Seyama K, John PA, Rotbart HA, Weiner LB: Enteroviral meningoencephalitis as a complication of X-linked hyper IgM syndrome. *J Pediatr* **134**:584, 1999.
201b. Tsuge I, Matsuoka H, Nakagawa A, Kamachi Y, Aso K, Negoro T, Ito M, Torii S, Watanabe K: Necrotizing toxoplasmic encephalitis in a child with the X-linked hyper-IgM syndrome. *Eur J Pediatr* **157**:735, 1998.
202. Cosyns M, Tsirkin S, Jones M, Flavell R, Kikutani H, Hayward AR: Requirement of CD40–CD40 ligand interaction for elimination of *Cryptosporidium parvum* from mice. *Infect Immunol* **66**:603, 1998.
202a. Hayward AR, Levy J, Facchetti F, Notarangelo L, Ochs HD, Etzioni A, Bonnefoy JY, Cosyns M, Weinberg A: Cholangiopathy and tumors of the pancreas, liver, and biliary tree in boys with X-linked immunodeficiency with hyper-IgM. *J Immunol* **158**:977, 1997.
203. Seyama K, Kobayashi R, Hasle H, Apter AJ, Rutledge JC, Rosen D, Ochs HD: Parvovirus B19-induced anemia as the presenting manifestation of X-linked hyper-IgM snydrome. *J Infect Dis* **178**:318, 1998.
204. Peitsch MC, Jongeneel CV: A 3-D model for the CD40 ligand predicts that it is a compact trimer similar to the tumor necrosis factors. *Int Immunol* **5**:233, 1993.
205. Lane P, Traunecker A, Hubele S, Inui S, Lanzavecchia A, Gray D: Activated human T cells express a ligand for the human B cell–associated antigen CD40 which participates in T cell–dependent activation of B lymphocytes. *Eur J Immunol* **22**:2573, 1992.
206. Armitage RJ, Fanslow WC, Strockbine L, Sato TA, Clifford KN, Macduff BM, Anderson DM, Gimpel SD, Davis-Smith T, Maliszewski CR, Clark EA, Smith CA, Grabstein KH, Cosman D, Spriggs MK: Molecular and biological characterization of a murine ligand for CD40. *Nature* **357**:80, 1992.
207. Graf D, Korthäuer U, Mages HW, Senger G, Kroczek RA: Cloning of TRAP, a ligand for CD40 on human T cells. *Eur J Immunol* **22**:3191, 1992.
208. Hollenbaugh D, Grosmaire LS, Kullas CD, Chalupny NJ, Braesch-Andersen S, Noelle RJ, Stamenkovic I, Ledbetter JA, Aruffo A: The human T cell antigen gp39, a member of the TNF gene family, is a ligand for the CD40 receptor: Expression of a soluble form of gp39 with B cell co-stimulatory activity. *EMBO J* **11**:4313, 1992.
209. Galy AHM, Spits H: CD40 is functionally expressed on human thymic epithelial cells. *J Immunol* **149**:775, 1992.
210. Yellin MJ, Brett J, Baum D, Matsushima A, Szabolcs M, Stern D, Chess L: Functional interactions of T cells with endothelial cells: the role of CD40L-CD40-mediated signals. *J Exp Med* **182**:1857, 1995.
211. Alderson MR, Armitage RJ, Tough TW, Strockbine L, Fanslow WC, Spriggs MK: CD40 expression by human monocytes: Regulation by cytokines and activation of monocytes by the ligand for CD40. *J Exp Med* **178**:669, 1993.
212. Caux C, Massacrier C, Vanbervliet B, Dubois B, Van Kooten C, Durand I, Banchereau J: Activation of human dendritic cells through CD40 cross-linking. *J Exp Med* **180**:1263, 1994.
213. Peguetnavarro J, Dalbiezgauthier C, Moulon C, Berthier O, Reano A, Gaucherand M, Banchereau J, Rousset F, Schmitt D: CD40 ligation of human keratinocytes inhibits their proliferation and induces their differentiation. *J Immunol* **158**:144, 1997.
214. Clark EA, Ledbetter JA: Activation of human B cells mediated through two distinct cell surface differentiation antigens, Bp35 and Bp50. *Proc Natl Acad Sci USA* **83**:4494, 1986.
215. Gruber MF, Bjorndahl JM, Nakamura S, Fu SM: Anti-CD45 inhibition of human B cell proliferation depends on the nature of activation signals and the state of B cell activation. *J Immunol* **142**:4144, 1989.
216. Banchereau J, De Paoli P, Vallé A, Garcia E, Rousset F: Long-term human B cell lines dependent on interleukin-4 and antibody to CD40. *Science* **251**:70, 1991.
217. Gordon J, Millsum MJ, Guy GR, Ledbetter JA: Resting B lymphocytes can be triggered directly through the CDw40 (Bp50) antigen. A comparison with IL-4-mediated signaling. *J Immunol* **140**:1425, 1988.
218. Barrett TB, Shu G, Clark EA: CD40 signaling activates CD11a/CD18 (LFA-1)–mediated adhesion in B cells. *J Immunol* **146**:1722, 1991.
219. Ranheim EA, Kipps TJ: Activated T cells induce expression of B7/BB1 on normal or leukemic B cells through a CD40-dependent signal. *J Exp Med* **177**:925, 1993.
220. Lederman S, Yellin MJ, Inghirami G, Lee JJ, Knowles DM, Chess L: Molecular interactions mediating T–B lymphocyte collaboration in human lymphoid follicles. Roles of T cell-B-cell–activating molecule (5c8 antigen) and CD40 in contact-dependent help. *J Immunol* **149**:3817, 1992.
221. Liu Y-J, Joshua DE, Williams GT, Smith CA, Gordon J, MacLennan ICM: Mechanism of antigen-driven selection in germinal centres. *Nature* **342**:929, 1989.
222. Valentine MA, Licciardi KA: Rescue from anti-IgM-induced programmed cell death by the B cell surface proteins CD20 and CD40. *Eur J Immunol* **22**:3141, 1992.
223. Schattner EJ, Elkon KB, Yoo DH, Tumang J, Krammer PH, Crow MK, Friedman SM: CD40 ligation induces Apo-1/Fas expression on human B lymphocytes and facilitates apoptosis through the Apo-1/Fas pathway. *J Exp Med* **182**:1557, 1995.
224. Rousset F, Garcia E, Banchereau J: Cytokine-induced proliferation and immunoglobulin production of human B lymphocytes triggered through their CD40 antigen. *J Exp Med* **173**:705, 1991.
225. Spriggs MK, Armitage RJ, Strockbine L, Clifford KN, Macduff BM, Sato TA, Maliszewski CR, Fanslow WC: Recombinant human CD40 ligand stimulates B cell proliferation and immunoglobulin E secretion. *J Exp Med* **176**:1543, 1992.
226. Mensink EJBM, Thompson A, Sandkuyl LA, Kraakman MEM, Schot JDL, Espanol T, Schuurman RKB: X-linked immunodeficiency with hyperimmunoglobulinemia M appears to be linked to the DXS42 restriction fragment length polymorphism locus. *Hum Genet* **76**:96, 1987.
227. Padayachee M, Levinsky RJ, Kinnon C, Finn A, McKeown C, Feighery C, Notarangelo LD, Hendriks RW, Read AP, Malcolm S:

Mapping of the X linked form of hyper IgM syndrome (HIGM1). *J Med Genet* **30**:202, 1993.
228. Villa A, Notarangelo LD, DiSanto JP, Macchi PP, Strina D, Frattini A, Lucchini F, Patrosso CM, Giliani S, Mantuano E, Agosti S, Nocera G, Kroczek RA, Fischer A, Ugazio AG, de Saint-Basile G, Vezzoni P: Organization of the human CD40L gene: Implications for molecular defects in X-linked hyper-IgM syndrome and prenatal diagnosis. *Proc Natl Acad Sci USA* **91**:2110, 1994.
229. Pilia G, Porta G, Padayachee M, Malcolm S, Zucchi I, Villa A, Macchi P, Vezzoni P, Schlessinger D: Human CD40L gene maps between DXS144E and DXS300 in Xq26. *Genomics* **22**:249, 1994.
230. Shimadzu M, Nunoi H, Terasaki H, Ninomiya R, Iwata M, Kanegasaka S, Matsuda I: Structural organization of the gene for CD40 ligand: molecular analysis for diagnosis of X-linked hyper-IgM syndrome. *Biochim Biophys Acta* **1260**:67, 1995.
231. Notarangelo LD, Peitsch MC: CD40lbase: A database of CD40L gene mutations causing X-linked hyper-IgM syndrome. *Immunol Today* **17**:511, 1996.
232. Lin Q, Rohrer J, Allen RC, Larche M, Greene JM, Shigeoka AO, Gatti RA, Derauf DC, Belmont JW, Conley ME: A single strand conformation polymorphism study of CD40 ligand. Efficient mutation analysis and carrier detection for X-linked hyper IgM syndrome. *J Clin Invest* **97**:196, 1996.
233. Macchi P, Villa A, Strina D, Sacco MG, Morali F, Brugnoni D, Giliani S, Mantuano E, Fasth A, Andersson B, Zegers BJM, Cavagni G, Reznick I, Levy J, Zan-Bar I, Porat Y, Airo P, Plebani A, Vezzoni P, Notarangelo LD: Characterization of nine novel mutations in the CD40 ligand gene in patients with X-linked hyper-IgM syndrome of various ancestry. *Am J Hum Genet* **56**:898, 1995.
234. Bajorath J, Chalupny NJ, Marken JS, Siadak AW, Skonier J, Gordon M, Hollenbaugh D, Noelle RJ, Ochs HD, Aruffo A: Identification of residues on CD40 and its ligand which are critical for the receptor-ligand interaction. *Biochemistry* **34**:1833, 1995.
235. Allen RC, Springgs MK, Belmont JW: Dinucleotide repeat polymorphism in the human CD40 ligand gene. *Hum Mol Genet* **2**:828, 1993.
236. DiSanto JP, Markiewicz S, Gauchat J-F, Bonnefoy J-Y, Fischer A, de Saint Basile G: Prenatal diagnosis of X-linked hyper-IgM syndrome. *N Engl J Med* **330**:969, 1994.
237. Hendriks RW, Kraakman MEM, Craig IW, Espanol T, Schuurman RKB: Evidence that in X-linked immunodeficiency with hyperimmunoglobulinemia M the intrinsic immunoglobulin heavy chain class switch mechanism is intact. *Eur J Immunol* **20**:2603, 1990.
238. Brahmi Z, Lazarus KH, Hodes ME, Baehner RL: Immunologic studies of three family members with the immunodeficiency with hyper-IgM syndrome. *J Clin Immunol* **3**:127, 1983.
239. Winfield JB, Cohen PL, Bradley L, Finkelman FD, Eisenberg RA, Wistar R, Whisnant JK: IgM cryoprecipitation and anti-immunoglobulin activity in dysgammaglobulinemia type I. *Clin Immunol Immunopathol* **23**:58, 1982.
240. Gordon DS, Jones BM, Browning SW, Spira TJ, Lawrence DN: Persistent polyclonal lymphocytosis of B lymphocytes. *N Engl J Med* **307**:232, 1982.
241. Slepian IK, Schwartz SA, Weiss JJ, Roth SL, Mathews KP: Immunodeficiency with hyper-IgM after systemic lupus erythematosus. *J Allergy Clin Immunol* **73**:846, 1984.
242. Conley ME, Larché M, Bonagura VR, Lawton III AR, Buckley RH, Fu SM, Coustan-Smith E, Herrod HG, Campana D: Hyper IgM syndrome associated with defective CD40-mediated B cell activation. *J Clin Invest* **94**:1404, 1994.
243. Callard RE, Smith SH, Herbert J, Morgan G, Padayachee M, Lederman S, Chess L, Kroczek RA, Fanslow WC, Armitage RJ: CD40 ligand (CD40L) expression and B cell function in agammaglobulinemia with normal or elevated levels of IgM (HIM). Comparison of X-linked, autosomal recessive, and non-X-linked forms of the disease, and obligate carriers. *J Immunol* **153**:3295, 1994.
244. Durandy A, Hivroz C, Mazerolles F, Schiff C, Bernard F, Jouanguy E, Revy P, DiSanto JP, Gauchat JF, Bonnefoy JY, Casanova JL, Fischer A: Abnormal CD40-mediated activation pathway in B lymphocytes from patients with hyper-IgM syndrome and normal CD40 ligand expression. *J Immunol* **158**:2576, 1997.
245. Sanford JP, Favour CB, Tribeman MS: Absence of serum gamma globulins in an adult. *N Engl J Med* **250**:1027, 1954.
246. Zinneman HH, Hall WH, Heller BI: Acquired agammaglobulinemia; report of three cases. *JAMA* **156**:1390, 1954.
247. Prasad AS, Koza DW: Agammaglobulinemia. *Ann Intern Med* **41**:629, 1954.
248. Hausser C, Virelizier JL, Buriot D, Griscelli C: Common variable hypogammaglobulinemia in children. Clinical and immunologic observations in 30 patients. *Am J Dis Child* **137**:833, 1983.
249. Conley ME, Park CL, Douglas SD: Childhood common variable immunodeficiency with autoimmune disease. *J Pediatr* **108**:915, 1986.
250. Fudenberg H, Good RA, Goodman HC, Hitzig W, Kunkel HG, Roitt IM, Rosen FS, Rowe DS, Seligmann M, Soothill JR: Primary immunodeficiencies: Report of a World Health Organization Committee. *Pediatrics* **47**:927, 1971.
251. Waldmann TA, Durm M, Broder S, Blackman M, Blaese RM, Strober W: Role of suppressor T cells in pathogenesis of common variable hypogammaglobulinaemia. *Lancet* **2**:609, 1974.
252. Geha RS, Schneeberger E, Merler E, Rosen FS: Heterogeneity of "acquired" or common variable agammaglobulinemia. *N Engl J Med* **291**:1, 1974.
253. de la Concha EG, Oldham G, Webster AD, Asherson GL, Platts-Mills TA: Quantitative measurements of T- and B-cell function in "variable" primary hypogammaglobulinaemia: Evidence for a consistent B-cell defect. *Clin Exp Immunol* **27**:208, 1977.
254. Siegal FP, Siegal M, Good RA: Role of helper, suppressor and B-cell defects in the pathogenesis of the hypogammaglobulinemias. *N Engl J Med* **299**:172, 1978.
255. Hermans PE, Diaz-Buxo JA, Stobo JD: Idiopathic late-onset immunoglobulin deficiency. Clinical observations in 50 patients. *Am J Med* **61**:221, 1976.
256. Cunningham-Rundles C: Clinical and immunologic analyses of 103 patients with common variable immunodeficiency. *J Clin Immunol* **9**:22, 1989.
257. Dukes RJ, Rosenow EC, Hermans PE: Pulmonary manifestations of hypogammaglobulinaemia. *Thorax* **33**:603, 1978.
258. Hermaszewski RA, Webster AD: Primary hypogammaglobulinaemia: A survey of clinical manifestations and complications. *Q J Med* **86**:31, 1993.
259. Wolf JK: Primary acquired agammaglobulinemia with a family history of collagen disease and hematologic disorders. *N Engl J Med* **266**:473, 1962.
260. Diaz-Buxo JA, Hermans PE, Elveback LR: Prevalence of cholelithiasis in idiopathic late-onset immunoglobulin deficiency. *Ann Intern Med* **82**:213, 1975.
261. Webster ADB, Plebani A, Jannossy G, Morgan M, Asherson GL: Autoimmune blood dyscrasias in five patients with hypogammaglobulinemia: Response of neutropenia to vincristine. *J Clin Immunol* **1**:113, 1981.
262. Douglas SD, Goldberg LS, Fudenberg HH, Goldberg SB: Agammaglobulinaemia and co-existent pernicious anaemia. *Clin Exp Immunol* **6**:181, 1970.
263. Ehtessabian R, Cassidy JT, Thomas R, Mathews KP, Tubergen DG: Clinical conference: Common variable immunodeficiency with pernicious anemia, asthma, and reactions to gamma globulin; treatment with plasma. *J Allergy Clin Immunol* **58**:336, 1976.
264. Sussman GL, Rivera VJ, Kohler PF: Transition from systemic lupus erythematosus to common variable hypogammaglobulinemia. *Ann Intern Med* **99**:32, 1983.
265. Fasano MB, Sullivan KE, Sarpong SB, Wood RA, Jones SM, Johns CJ, Lederman HM, Bykowsky MJ, Greene JM, Winkelstein JA: Sarcoidosis and common variable immunodeficiency. Report of 8 cases and review of the literature. *Medicine (Baltimore)* **75**:251, 1996.
266. Cunningham-Rundles C, Lieberman P, Hellman G, Chaganti RS: Non-Hodgkin lymphoma in common variable immunodeficiency. *Am J Hematol* **37**:69, 1991.
267. Spickett GP, Farrant J, North ME, Zhang JG, Morgan L, Webster AD: Common variable immunodeficiency: How many diseases? *Immunol Today* **18**:325, 1997.
268. Zielinski CC, Mutschlechner R, Schwarz G, Eibl MM: Transient immunoglobulin and antibody production. Occurrence in two patients with common varied immunodeficiency. *Arch Intern Med* **143**:1937, 1983.
269. Wright JJ, Birx DL, Wagner DK, Waldmann TA, Blaese RM, Fleisher TA: Normalization of antibody responsiveness in a patient with common variable hypogammaglobulinemia and HIV infection. *N Engl J Med* **317**:1516, 1987.
270. Fiorilli M, Crescenzi M, Carbonari M, Tedesco L, Russo G, Gaetano C, Aiuti F: Phenotypically immature IgG-bearing B cells in patients with hypogammaglobulinemia. *J Clin Immunol* **6**:21, 1986.

271. Saxon A, Giorgi JV, Sherr EH, Kagan JM: Failure of B cells in common variable immunodeficiency to transit from proliferation to differentiation is associated with altered B cell surface-molecule display. *J Allergy Clin Immunol* **84**:44, 1989.
272. Mayer L, Fu SM, Cunningham-Rundles C, Kunkel HG: Polyclonal immunoglobulin secretion in patients with common variable immunodeficiency using monoclonal B cell differentiation factors. *J Clin Invest* **74**:2115, 1984.
273. Mitsuya H, Osaki K, Tomino S, Katsuki T, Kishimoto S: Pathophysiologic analysis of peripheral blood lymphocytes from patients with primary immunodeficiency. I. Ig synthesis by peripheral blood lymphocytes stimulated with either pokeweed mitogen or Epstein-Barr virus in vitro. *J Immunol* **127**:311, 1981.
274. Saiki O, Ralph P, Cunningham-Rundles C, Good RA: Three distinct stages of B-cell defects in common varied immunodeficiency. *Proc Natl Acad Sci USA* **79**:6008, 1982.
275. Perri RT, Weisdorf DJ: Impaired responsiveness to B cell growth factor in a patient with common variable hypogammaglobulinemia. *Blood* **66**:345, 1985.
276. Sneller MC, Strober W: Abnormalities of lymphokine gene expression in patients with common variable immunodeficiency. *J Immunol* **144**:3762, 1990.
277. Eibl MM, Mannhalter JW, Zlabinger G, Mayr WR, Tilz GP, Ahmad R, Zielinski CC: Defective macrophage function in a patient with common variable immunodeficiency. *N Engl J Med* **307**:803, 1982.
278. Douglas SD, Kamin RM, Fudenberg HH: Human lymphocyte response to phytomitogens in vitro: Normal, agammaglobulinemic and paraproteinemic individuals. *J Immunol* **103**:1185, 1969.
279. Ichikawa Y, Gonzalez EB, Daniels JC: Suppressor cells of mitogen-induced lymphocyte proliferation in the peripheral blood of patients with common variable hypogammaglobulinemia. *Clin Immunol Immunopathol* **25**:252, 1982.
280. Kondratenko I, Amlot PL, Webster AD, Farrant J: Lack of specific antibody response in common variable immunodeficiency (CVID) associated with failure in production of antigen-specific memory T cells. MRC Immunodeficiency Group. *Clin Exp Immunol* **108**:9, 1997.
281. Pandolfi F, Quinti I, Frielingsdorf A, Goldstein G, Businco L, Aiuti F: Abnormalities of regulatory T-cell subpopulations in patients with primary immunoglobulin deficiencies. *Clin Immunol Immunopathol* **22**:323, 1982.
282. Wright JJ, Wagner DK, Blaese RM, Hagengruber C, Waldmann TA, Fleisher TA: Characterization of common variable immunodeficiency: Identification of a subset of patients with distinctive immunophenotypic and clinical features. *Blood* **76**:2046, 1990.
283. Baumert E, Wolff-Vorbeck G, Schlesier M, Peter HH: Immunophenotypical alterations in a subset of patients with common variable immunodeficiency (CVID). *Clin Exp Immunol* **90**:25, 1992.
284. Jaffe JS, Strober W, Sneller MC: Functional abnormalities of $CD8^+$ T cells define a unique subset of patients with common variable immunodeficiency. *Blood* **82**:192, 1993.
285. North ME, Webster AD, Farrant J: Primary defect in $CD8^+$ lymphocytes in the antibody deficiency disease (common variable immunodeficiency): abnormalities in intracellular production of interferon-gamma (IFN-gamma) in $CD28^+$ ('cytotoxic') and CD28− ('suppressor') $CD8^+$ subsets. *Clin Exp Immunol* **111**:70, 1998.
286. Farrington M, Grosmaire LS, Nonoyama S, Fischer SH, Hollenbaugh D, Ledbetter JA, Noelle RJ, Aruffo A, Ochs HD: CD40 ligand expression is defective in a subset of patients with common variable immunodeficiency. *Proc Natl Acad Sci USA* **91**:1099, 1994.
287. Adelman DC, Matsuda T, Hirano T, Kishimoto T, Saxon A: Elevated serum interleukin-6 associated with a failure in B cell differentiation in common variable immunodeficiency. *J Allergy Clin Immunol* **86**:512, 1990.
288. Fudenberg H, German JLI, Kunkel HG: The occurrence of rheumatoid factor and other abnormalities in families of patients with agammaglobulinemia. *Arthrit Rheum* **5**:565, 1962.
289. Douglas SD, Goldberg LS, Fudenberg HH: Clinical, serologic and leukocyte function studies on patients with idiopathic "acquired" agammaglobulinemia and their families. *Am J Med* **48**:48, 1970.
290. Vorechovsky I, Litzman J, Lokaj J, Sobotkova R: Family studies in common variable immunodeficiency. *J Hyg Epidemiol Microbiol Immunol* **35**:17, 1991.
291. Vorechkovsky I, Zhou J-N, Vetrie D, Bentley D, Björkander J, Hammarström L, Smith CIE: Molecular diagnosis of X-linked agammaglobulinaemia. *Lancet* **341**:1153, 1993.
292. Hobbs JR: Immune imbalance in dysgammaglobulinaemia type IV. *Lancet* **1**:110, 1968.
293. Koistinen J: Selective IgA deficiency in blood donors. *Vox Sang* **29**:192, 1975.
294. Oen K, Petty RE, Schroeder ML: Immunoglobulin A deficiency: genetic studies. *Tissue Antigens* **19**:174, 1982.
295. Kanoh T, Mizumoto T, Yasuda N, Koya M, Ohno Y, Uchino H, Yoshimura K, Ohkubo Y, Yamaguchi H: Selective IgA deficiency in Japanese blood donors: Frequency and statistical analysis. *Vox Sang* **50**:81, 1986.
296. Rockey JH, Hanson LA, Heremans JF, Kunkel HG: Beta-2A aglobulinemia in two healthy men. *J Lab Clin Med* **63**:205, 1964.
297. Plebani A, Ugazio AG, Monafo V, Burgio GR: Clinical heterogeneity and reversibility of selective immunoglobulin A deficiency in 80 children. *Lancet* **1**:829, 1986.
298. Herrod HG: Follow-up of pediatric patients with recurrent infection and mild serologic immune abnormalities. *Ann Allergy Asthma Immunol* **79**:460, 1997.
299. Ostergaard PA: Clinical and immunological features of transient IgA deficiency in children. *Clin Exp Immunol* **40**:561, 1980.
300. Ludviksson BR, Eiriksson TH, Ardal B, Sigfusson A, Valdimarsson H: Correlation between serum immunoglobulin A concentrations and allergic manifestations in infants. *J Pediatr* **121**:23, 1992.
301. Conley ME, Cooper MD: Immature IgA B cells in IgA-deficient patients. *N Engl J Med* **305**:495, 1981.
302. Waldmann TA, Broder S, Krakauer R, Durm M, Meade B, Goldman C: Defect in IgA secretion and in IgA specific suppressor cells in patients with selective IgA deficiency. *Trans Assoc Am Phys* **89**:215, 1976.
303. Atwater JS, Tomasi TBJ: Suppressor cells and IgA deficiency. *Clin Immunol Immunopathol* **9**:379, 1978.
304. Schwartz SA: Heavy chain-specific suppression of immunoglobulin synthesis and secretion by lymphocytes from patients with selective IgA deficiency. *J Immunol* **124**:2034, 1980.
305. Briere F, Bridon JM, Chevet D, Souillet G, Bienvenu F, Guret C, Martinez-Valdez H, Banchereau J: Interleukin 10 induces B lymphocytes from IgA-deficient patients to secrete IgA. *J Clin Invest* **94**:97, 1994.
306. Marconi M, Plebani A, Avanzini MA, Maccario R, Pistorio A, Duse M, Stringa M, Monafo V: IL-10 and IL-4 co-operate to normalize in vitro IgA production in IgA- deficient (IgAD) patients. *Clin Exp Immunol* **112**:528, 1998.
307. Brandtzaeg P, Fjellanger I, Gjeruldsen ST: Immunoglobulin M: local synthesis and selective secretion in patients with immunoglobulin A deficiency. *Science* **160**:789, 1968.
308. Brandtzaeg P, Gjeruldsen ST, Korsrud F, Baklien K, Berdal P, Ek J: The human secretory immune system shows striking heterogeneity with regard to involvement of J chain-positive IgD immunocytes. *J Immunol* **122**:503, 1979.
309. Hahn-Zoric M, Carlsson B, Bjorkander J, Mellander L, Friman V, Padyukov L, Hanson LA: Variable increases of IgG and IgM antibodies in milk of IgA deficient women. *Pediatr Allergy Immunol* **8**:127, 1997.
310. Mellander L, Bjorkander J, Carlsson B, Hanson LA: Secretory antibodies in IgA-deficient and immunosuppressed individuals. *J Clin Immunol* **6**:284, 1986.
311. Koistinen J, Sarna S: Immunological abnormalities in the sera of IgA-deficient blood donors. *Vox Sang* **29**:203, 1975.
312. Petty RE, Palmer NR, Cassidy JT, Tubergen DG, Sullivan DB: The association of autoimmune diseases and anti-IgA antibodies in patients with selective IgA deficiency. *Clin Exp Immunol* **37**:83, 1979.
313. Burks AW, Sampson HA, Buckley RH: Anaphylactic reactions after gamma globulin administration in patients with hypogammaglobulinemia. Detection of IgE antibodies to IgA. *N Engl J Med* **314**:560, 1986.
314. Sundin U, Nava S, Hammarstrom L: Induction of unresponsiveness against IgA in IgA-deficient patients on subcutaneous immunoglobulin infusion therapy. *Clin Exp Immunol* **112**:341, 1998.
315. Richards BW, Hobbs JR: IgA and ring-18 chromosome. *Lancet* **1**:1426, 1968.
316. Feingold M, Schwartz RS, Atkins L, Anderson R, Bartsocas CS, Page DL, Littlefield JW: IgA deficiency associated with partial deletion of chromosome 18. *Am J Dis Child* **117**:129, 1969.
317. Ruvalcaba RH, Thuline HC: IgA absence associated with short arm deletion of chromosome No. 18. *J Pediatr* **74**:964, 1969.
318. Stewart JM, Go S, Ellis E, Robinson A: Absent IgA and deletions of chromosome 18. *J Med Genet* **7**:11, 1970.

319. Smith CA, Driscoll DA, Emanuel BS, McDonald-McGinn DM, Zackai EH, Sullivan KE: Increased prevalence of immunoglobulin A deficiency in patients with the chromosome 22q11.2 deletion syndrome (DiGeorge syndrome/velocardiofacial syndrome). *Clin Diagn Lab Immunol* **5**:415, 1998.
320. Ruff ME, Pincus LG, Sampson HA: Phenytoin-induced IgA depression. *Am J Dis Child* **141**:858, 1987.
321. Stanworth DR, Williamson JP, Shadforth M, Felix-Davies D, Thompson R: Drug-induced IgA deficiency in rheumatoid arthritis. *Lancet* **1**:1001, 1977.
322. Snowden N, Dietch DM, Teh LS, Hilton RC, Haeney MR: Antibody deficiency associated with gold treatment: Natural history and management in 22 patients. *Ann Rheum Dis* **55**:616, 1996.
323. Leickly FE, Buckley RH: Development of IgA and IgG2 subclass deficiency after sulfasalazine therapy. *J Pediatr* **108**:481, 1986.
324. Soothill JF, Hayes K, Dudgeon JA: The immunoglobulins in congenital rubella. *Lancet* **1**:1385, 1966.
325. Saulsbury FT: Selective IgA deficiency temporally associated with Epstein-Barr virus infection. *J Pediatr* **115**:268, 1989.
326. De Graeff PA, The TH, van Munster PJ, Out TA, Vossen JM, Zegers BJ: The primary immune response in patients with selective IgA deficiency. *Clin Exp Immunol* **54**:778, 1983.
327. Cassidy JT, Oldham G, Platts-Mills TA: Functional assessment of a B cell defect in patients with selective IgA deficiency. *Clin Exp Immunol* **35**:296, 1979.
328. Schur PH, Borel H, Gelfand EW, Alper CA, Rosen FS: Selective gamma-g globulin deficiencies in patients with recurrent pyogenic infections. *N Engl J Med* **283**:631, 1970.
329. Umetsu DT, Ambrosino DM, Quinti I, Siber GR, Geha RS: Recurrent sinopulmonary infection and impaired antibody response to bacterial capsular polysaccharide antigen in children with selective IgG-subclass deficiency. *N Engl J Med* **313**:1247, 1985.
330. Hanson LA, Soderstrom R, Avanzini A, Bengtsson U, Bjorkander J, Soderstrom T: Immunoglobulin subclass deficiency. *Pediatr Infect Dis J* **7**:S17, 1988.
331. Shield JP, Strobel S, Levinsky RJ, Morgan G: Immunodeficiency presenting as hypergammaglobulinaemia with IgG2 subclass deficiency. *Lancet* **340**:448, 1992.
332. Migone N, Oliviero S, de Lange G, Delacroix DL, Boschis D, Altruda F, Silengo L, DeMarchi M, Carbonara AO: Multiple gene deletions within the human immunoglobulin heavy-chain cluster. *Proc Natl Acad Sci USA* **81**:5811, 1984.
333. Olsson PG, Rabbani H, Hammarstrom L, Smith CI: Novel human immunoglobulin heavy chain constant region gene deletion haplotypes characterized by pulsed-field electrophoresis. *Clin Exp Immunol* **94**:84, 1993.
334. Brusco A, Cariota U, Bottaro A, Boccazzi C, Plebani A, Ugazio AG, Galanello R, Guerra MG, Carbonara AO: Variability of the immunoglobulin heavy chain constant region locus: A population study. *Hum Genet* **95**:319, 1995.
335. Brusco A, Cinque F, Saviozzi S, Boccazzi C, DeMarchi M, Carbonara AO: The G4 gene is duplicated in 44% of human immunoglobulin heavy chain constant region haplotypes. *Hum Genet* **100**:84, 1997.
336. Tashita H, Fukao T, Kaneko H, Teramoto T, Inoue R, Kasahara K, Kondo N: Molecular basis of selective IgG2 deficiency. The mutated membrane-bound form of gamma2 heavy chain caused complete IGG2 deficiency in two Japanese siblings. *J Clin Invest* **101**:677, 1998.
337. Pan Q, Lindersson Y, Sideras P, Hammarstrom L: Structural analysis of human gamma 3 intervening regions and switch regions: Implication for the low frequency of switching in IgG3-deficient patients. *Eur J Immunol* **27**:2920, 1997.
338. Shackelford PG, Granoff DM, Polmar SH, Scott MG, Goskowicz MC, Madassery JV, Nahm MH: Subnormal serum concentrations of IgG2 in children with frequent infections associated with varied patterns of immunologic dysfunction. *J Pediatr* **116**:529, 1990.
339. Shackelford PG, Granoff DM, Madassery JV, Scott MG, Nahm MH: Clinical and immunologic characteristics of healthy children with subnormal serum concentrations of IgG2. *Pediatr Res* **27**:16, 1990.
340. Gross S, Blaiss MS, Herrod HG: Role of immunoglobulin subclasses and specific antibody determinations in the evaluation of recurrent infection in children. *J Pediatr* **121**:516, 1992.
341. Zegers BJ, Maertzdorf WJ, Van Loghem E, Mul NA, Stoop JW, Van Der Laag J, Vossen JJ, Ballieux RE: Kappa-chain deficiency. An immunoglobulin disorder. *N Engl J Med* **294**:1026, 1976.
342. Stavnezer-Nordgren J, Kekish O, Zegers BJ: Molecular defects in a human immunoglobulin kappa chain deficiency. *Science* **230**:458, 1985.
343. Tiller TLJ, Buckley RH: Transient hypogammaglobulinemia of infancy: Review of the literature, clinical and immunologic features of 11 new cases, and long-term follow-up. *J Pediatr* **92**:347, 1978.
344. McGeady SJ: Transient hypogammaglobulinemia of infancy: need to reconsider name and definition. *J Pediatr* **110**:47, 1987.
345. Dalal I, Reid B, Nisbet-Brown E, Roifman CM: The outcome of patients with hypogammaglobulinemia in infancy and early childhood. *J Pediatr* **133**:144, 1998.
346. Souadjian JV, Enriquez P, Silverstein MN, Pepin JM: The spectrum of diseases associated with thymoma. Coincidence or syndrome? *Arch Intern Med* **134**:374, 1974.
347. Gray GF, Gutowski WT: Thymoma. A clinicopathologic study of 54 cases. *Am J Surg Pathol* **3**:235, 1979.
348. Good RA: Agammaglobulinemia: A provocative experiment of nature. *Bull Univ Minn Hosp* **26**:1, 1954.
349. Watts RG, Kelly DR: Fatal varicella infection in a child associated with thymoma and immunodeficiency (Good's syndrome). *Med Pediatr Oncol* **18**:246, 1990.
350. Degos L, Faille A, Housset M, Boumsell L, Rabian C, Parames T: Syndrome of neutrophil agranulocytosis, hypogammaglobulinemia, and thymoma. *Blood* **60**:968, 1982.
351. Raschal S, Siegel JN, Huml J, Richmond GW: Hypogammaglobulinemia and anemia 18 years after thymoma resection. *J Allergy Clin Immunol* **100**:846, 1997.
352. Platts-Mills TA, De Gast GC, Webster AD, Asherson GL, Wilkins SR: Two immunologically distinct forms of late-onset hypogammaglobulinaemia. *Clin Exp Immunol* **44**:383, 1981.
353. Hayward AR, Paolucci P, Webster AD, Kohler P: Pre-B cell suppression by thymoma patient lymphocytes. *Clin Exp Immunol* **48**:437, 1982.
354. Brenner MK, Reittie JG, Chadda HR, Pollock A, Asherson GL: Thymoma and hypogammaglobulinaemia with and without T suppressor cells. *Clin Exp Immunol* **58**:619, 1984.

CHAPTER 185

T Cell and Combined Immunodeficiency Disorders

John W. Belmont ▪ Jennifer M. Puck

1. Antigen-specific adaptive immune responses require the function of both T and B lymphocytes. These cells express multichain cell-surface receptors, T cell receptor (TCR) and immunoglobulin (Ig), respectively, that specifically recognize antigenic determinants or epitopes. While Ig directly binds antigens, TCR recognition requires presentation of short peptide antigens via interaction with the class I or class II molecules encoded in the major histocompatibility complex (MHC). Growth and activation of T cells require a network of potent extrinsic regulatory factors (cytokines) acting through specific receptors and signal transduction pathways. The major role of B cells is to produce specific immunoglobulins or antibodies. T cells exhibit diverse functions, including direct cellular cytotoxicity and production of helper factors for B cells and other immune cells. Given the central role of T lymphocytes in coordination of the immune response, defects affecting T and B cells or T cells alone cause severe combined immunodeficiency (SCID). The hallmark of SCID is severe or repeated infections, especially with opportunistic microorganisms. Other features may frequently accompany immunodeficiency including autoimmune phenomena, hematologic abnormalities, dermatoses, and neoplasia, depending on the specific genetic etiology. SCID results from failure of lymphocytes to develop and mature, from defects in MHC expression, and from interruption of signals required for growth and activation. Abnormalities restricted to T cell activation and/or apoptosis account for other genetic defects in T cells with less profound immunodeficiency.

2. DNA rearrangement of the immunoglobulin and T cell receptor loci to generate the repertoire of antigen-specific receptors is a critical developmental checkpoint in both B cells and T cells. Rearrangement occurs by a unique site-specific recombination mechanism acting on signal sequences flanking the receptor loci. The process of receptor exon rearrangement is called V(D)J recombination. At least two lymphocyte-specific proteins, recombination-activating genes 1 and 2 (RAG1 and RAG2), as well as several proteins with broader functions in the repair of double-strand breaks (DSB) in DNA mediate V(D)J recombination. Failure of V(D)J recombination leads to developmental blocks in antigen-specific cell surface receptor expression and consequent failure of both T cell and B cell development (T^-B^- SCID). Mutations in both RAG1 and RAG2 have been associated with T^-B^- SCID. Allelic heterogeneity in RAG1 and RAG2 mutations accounts for the milder phenotype of Omenn syndrome (OS). While not directly impairing the process of TCR rearrangement, disorders affecting DSB repair or related cell-cycle checkpoints, ataxia-telangiectasia, Bloom syndrome, and Nijmegen breakage syndrome, lead to T cell immune deficiency and multiple aberrant chromosomal rearrangements of TCR. These disorders are accompanied by high risk of neoplasia, especially lymphoma.

3. Signal transduction after ligand interaction by the TCR involves a complex of proteins, the CD3 complex, that recruits other signal transduction components. CD3 is composed of two ε, two ζ, and one each of δ and γ chains. In addition, T cells express either CD4 or CD8 as coreceptors that influence the interaction of TCR with MHC class II or class I, respectively. Mutations in ZAP70, a protein tyrosine kinase that interacts with the ζ chain of CD3, result in a characteristic deficiency of $CD8^+$ T cells. Lck is a src-family protein tyrosine kinase that interacts with CD4. Rare mutations in lck lead to a specific defect in the maturation of $CD4^+$ T cells.

4. Recognition of antigenic peptides by TCR requires presentation of the peptide by either class I or class II MHC proteins. MHC cell surface expression depends on intracellular association with processed peptide antigens delivered

A list of standard abbreviations is located immediately preceding the index in each volume. Many of the abbreviations used are in standard font for the protein and in italics for the gene locus. Additional abbreviations used in this chapter include: AIRE = autoimmune regulator transcription factor; ALPS = autoimmune lymphoproliferative syndrome; APECED = autoimmune polyendocrinopathy with candidiasis and ectodermal dystrophy; BCG = Bacillus Calmette-Guérin; BLS = bare lymphocyte syndrome; BMT = bone marrow transplantation; BRCT = BRCA2-like protein domain; CHH = cartilage hair hypoplasia; CIITA = class II transactivator; CLIP = class II HLA-associated invariant chain derived peptides; CRD = cysteine rich domain; DNA-PK = DNA-dependent protein kinase; DNMT3B = DNA methyltransferase 3B; DSB = double-strand break; FADD = Fas-associated death domain protein; Fas = tumor necrosis factor receptor superfamily, member 6, gene symbol *TNFRSF6* (formerly apoptosis antigen 1, *APT1*); FasL = CD95L/Fas ligand; GVHD = graft versus host disease; H2 = mouse histocompatibility gene complex; HMG = high mobility group proteins including HMG1, HMG2, etc.; ICF = immune deficiency with centromeric instability and dysmorphic facies; IL1R, IL2Rγ, IL2R, etc. = interleukin 1 receptor, interleukin 2 receptor, etc. (e.g. IL2Rγ, gene symbol *IL2RG*; IL7Rα; gene symbol *IL7RA*); ITAM = immunoreceptor tyrosine-based activation motifs; ITP = immune thrombocytopenia; IVIG = intravenous immunoglobulins; JAK1, JAK3, etc. = Janus kinase 1, Janus kinase 3, etc.; Ku = Ku p70/p80 autoantigen; lck, LCK = lymphocyte specific protein-tyrosine kinase p56(lck); MHC2TA = MHC class II transactivator; OS = Omenn syndrome; PCP = *Pneumocystis carinii* pneumonia; RAG1 or RAG2 = recombination activating gene 1 or 2; RFX1, RFX2, etc. = regulatory factor X1, 2, etc.; RFXANK = RFX, ankyrin repeat containing; RFXAP = RFX-associated protein; RSS = recombination signal sequences; SAP = SLAM-associated protein; SCID = severe combined immunodeficiency; Sir = silent information regulator yeast genes including Sir1, Sir2, etc.; SLAM = signaling lymphocyte activation molecule; STAT = signal transducers and activators transcription; TAP1 or TAP2 = transporter, ATP-binding cassette 1 or 2; T^-B^- SCID and variations = T cell negative, B cell negative SCID and variations; TCR = T cell receptor; TdT = terminal deoxynucleotidyltransferase; Th1, Th2 = T helper type 1,2 lymphocyte; TNFR = tumor necrosis factor receptor; WAS = Wiskott-Aldrich syndrome; WASP = Wiskott-Aldrich syndrome protein; XRCC5, XRCC6, etc.; = X-ray repair, complementing defective, in Chinese hamster cells 5, 6, etc.; XSCID = X linked SCID; XLT = X-linked thrombocytopenia; ZAP70 = zeta-chain-associated protein kinase.

to the lumen of the endoplasmic reticulum by the TAP peptide transporter. The peptide transporter is composed of TAP1 and TAP2 proteins. Failure of proper cell surface expression of either class I or class II proteins or both results in severe humoral and cellular immune deficiency. MHC class I deficiencies are rare disorders with apparent locus heterogeneity. MHC class I deficiency can result from mutations in either TAP1 or TAP2, although the molecular basis for the condition is otherwise unknown. MHC class II deficiency is also heterogeneous with five complementation groups currently identified. MHC class II deficiencies all result from defects in the transcriptional regulation of the class II gene family. Complementation group A results from mutations in the transcription factor MHC class II transactivator (MHC2TA). Complementation groups B, C, and D result from mutations in subunits of the regulatory factor X (RFX) DNA-binding complex (RFXANK, RFX5, and RFXAP, respectively) that regulates MHC class II transcription.

5. **Proper regulation of immune responsiveness requires selection of the T cell repertoire and control of clonal T cell proliferation. Abnormal regulation of T cells underlies rare autoimmune disorders characterized by poorly controlled T cell proliferation and immunodeficiency. Defects in T cell apoptosis caused by mutations in either Fas (tumor necrosis factor receptor superfamily, member 6; (*TNFRSF6*) or caspase 10 lead to autoimmune lymphoproliferative syndrome (ALPS). A rare form of autoimmunity—autoimmune polyendocrinopathy with candidiasis and ectodermal dystrophy (APECED)—is caused by mutations in a novel lymphoid lineage transcription factor, autoimmune regulator (*AIRE*). Finally, autosomal recessive autoimmune syndrome can be caused by mutation in the IL2Rα gene.**
6. **T cell growth and maturation require the activities of multiple cytokines. The hematopoietin family of cytokines is particularly important as evidenced by the severe phenotype associated with defects in receptors and signaling. The most common form of SCID is the X-linked SCID (XSCID) caused by mutations in a subunit, γc, of IL2 receptor (IL2Rγ, *IL2RG*). This subunit is shared with receptors for IL4, IL7, IL9, and IL15. Defects in the function of the IL7-dependent axis may be particularly important in XSCID, because rare patients with mutations in the α chain of the IL7 receptor (IL7Rα, *IL7RA*) component also exhibit SCID. This subfamily of receptors interacts with the protein tyrosine kinases JAK1 and JAK3 that play critical roles in cytokine receptor signal transduction. The γc subunit specifically interacts with JAK3. One form of autosomal recessive SCID results from JAK3 mutations. Interferons constitute another cytokine family. Interferon γ is particularly important in the induction of class II MHC expression. Defects in the interferon γ receptor lead to increased susceptibility to mycobacterial infections.**
7. **Wiskott-Aldrich syndrome (WAS) is an X-linked immune deficiency affecting antigen-specific T cell proliferation. Failure of antibody responses to polysaccharide antigens is a unique characteristic. In addition to the immune deficiency, the classic clinical features include eczema and thrombocytopenia. Patients also commonly exhibit autoimmune phenomena and have increased risk for malignancy. The disorder results from mutations in a novel X-linked gene, *WAS*, that encodes the Wiskott-Aldrich syndrome protein (WASP). WASP contains several peptide motifs that point to a role in coordinating signal transduction and cytoplasmic actin movements. WAS is allelic to the rare X-linked thrombocytopenia (XLT).**
8. **A variety of miscellaneous cellular immune deficiencies remain to be classified based on molecular pathology. These include an autosomal recessive SCID unique to the Athabascan people, reticular dysgenesis, and cartilage hair hypoplasia (CHH). In addition, two inborn errors of purine metabolism, adenosine deaminase deficiency and purine nucleoside phosphorylase deficiency, are responsible for about 15 percent of SCID. Immune deficiency with centromeric instability and dysmorphic facies (ICF) syndrome was recently found to be due to mutations in DNA methyltransferase 3B (DNMT3B), a component necessary for maintenance of chromatin conformation.**

INTRODUCTION AND HISTORY

Adaptive cellular immunity is found only in vertebrates and, unlike more primitive cellular defenses, allows the animal to form antigen-specific receptors and effector molecules. Antigen-specific receptors activate clones of cells with specialized regulatory or effector functions and also provide a basis for immunologic memory via persistence of previously activated cells. Specific cellular immunity primarily involves the activities of T cells in both regulatory and effector functions. Defects in the development and activation of T cells by antigen or cytokines underlie the genetic cellular immunodeficiencies. Because T cells also regulate antibody production by B cells, complete T cell defects generally result in severe combined immunodeficiency (SCID).

Studies of primary immunodeficiencies have traditionally informed the field of immunology by highlighting the consequences of defects in both humoral, or antibody, and cellular defenses. The first clinical recognition of patients with a primary disorder of the immune system can probably be attributed to Wiskott,[1] who, in 1937, described a patient with repeated infections, eczema, and thrombocytopenia. Aldrich reported a similar disorder in a family in 1954,[2] and recognized for the first time the X-linked pattern of inheritance for what became known as Wiskott-Aldrich syndrome. In 1950, Glanzman and Riniker[3] described siblings with candidiasis, severe infections, decreased lymphocytes, and reduced immunoglobulins, that is, SCID. This condition, fatal in infancy and initially called Swiss-type agammaglobulinemia, was more severe than the agammaglobulinemia reported by Bruton (see Chap. 184). Genetic heterogeneity in SCID was demonstrated as some pedigrees suggested autosomal recessive inheritance,[4] while others were typical of X-linked inheritance.[5] The association of congenital absence of the thymus with infection and hypoparathyroidism was first described by DiGeorge in 1965[6] and provided support for a central role of the thymus in the production of thymus-dependent lymphocytes or T cells. Adenosine deaminase deficiency, as reported in 1972 by Giblett,[7] provided the first biochemical etiology for a primary immunodeficiency. The inability to perform tissue-typing using anti-HLA antibodies on a patient's peripheral blood cells led to the descriptive term bare lymphocyte syndrome.[8,9] Further characterization of SCID patient's cellular and functional phenotypes has proceeded in parallel with the development of new cell surface markers and assays for T cell activation. As individual disorders are delineated based on laboratory phenotype, more examples of genetic heterogeneity within phenotypes are documented.[10,11] Clearly, the mutant genes responsible for a number of rare autosomal recessive SCIDs that currently lie outside mechanistic classifications remain to be elucidated. Broadly, we can define groups of SCID and specific T cell defects based on the predominant mechanism: disorders of V(D)J recombination; disorders of major histocompatibility complex (MHC) expression; disorders of T cell receptor signal transduction; disorders of cytokine signal transduction; disorders of apoptosis/autoimmunity; disorders of purine metabolism; abnormalities of thymic organ development (including DiGeorge syndrome); and Wiskott-Aldrich syndrome, a unique abnormality in signal transduction/

cytoskeleton integration. Adenosine deaminase (MIM 102700, 20q13.11) and purine nucleoside phosphorylase (MIM 164050, 14q13.1) deficiencies, which together account for about 15 percent of SCID, are discussed in detail in Chap. 109. The complex cytogenetic basis for DiGeorge syndrome (MIM 188400, 22q11) is described in Chap. 65.

The birth incidence and prevalence of cellular immune deficiencies is not known with certainty, a situation common to most rare genetic disorders. However, efforts to collect data on patients in large registries give a minimum prevalence of all primary immunodeficiencies of ~1 per 100,000 with T cell or combined immunodeficiencies constituting ~20 percent of cases.[12] Data reported by the European Society for Immunodeficiencies Registry (25 countries) indicates that countries with large populations and very active clinical research groups have prevalence estimates two- to fourfold higher. Lower prevalence estimates elsewhere might be explained by early death before immunodeficiency is recognized, incomplete reporting, differences in standards of patient detection, and ethnic differences in carrier frequencies of rare recessive alleles. Given the large contribution of X-linked loci[13] (~60 percent) and the high degree of allelic heterogeneity in primary immune disorders, the latter explanation seems less likely.

CLINICAL AND LABORATORY PRESENTATION

SCID has a mean age at diagnosis of 6 to 7 months,[13,14] indicating that symptomatic infections occur early and frequently (Table 185-1). There is a distinct male predominance (~75 percent) but no particular ethnic risk. Severe, persistent, and opportunistic infections occur due to viruses [cytomegalovirus (CMV), respiratory syncytial virus, adenovirus, parainfluenza], *Pneumocystis carinii*, candida, and bacteria. Persistent diarrhea, rashes, and poor weight gain are the most common presenting features. There is generally peripheral lymphoid hypoplasia with lack of palpable lymph nodes, although B lymphocyte proliferative disorders secondary to Epstein-Barr virus infection are sometimes observed. The thymic shadow may be absent on chest X-ray, and usually there is lymphocytopenia in the peripheral blood. Live-attenuated vaccines, such as polio, should not be given because of the risk of disseminated infection. Graft versus host disease can result either from transplacentally acquired maternal T cell engraftment or following postnatal transfusions. The latter produces, in general, much more severe complications. Therefore, any blood products for patients with suspected immune compromise should be irradiated as well as tested to rule out infection with CMV.

Quantitative immunoglobulins are usually abnormal in patients with SCID, although IgG may be normal in the first 3 months of life as the result of residual maternal antibody. Reduced IgM and IgA are characteristic, while some children may have elevated IgE. Specific antibody responses to vaccines do not occur. Most SCID patients (90 percent) have lymphopenia. Immunophenotyping to determine numbers and types of lymphocytes is helpful in distinguishing various etiologies of SCID; for example, ADA-deficient patients have very low B cells, while those with γc and JAK3 defects have relatively higher levels. Classification of SCID into $T^-B^-NK^-$ and $T^-B^+NK^-$ (typical of γc and JAK3 abnormalities) is helpful.[15] Isolated $CD8^-$ lymphopenia is characteristic of ZAP70 defects.[16] All SCID patients have abnormally low proliferative responses to mitogens and allogeneic cells in vitro.

Table 185-1 **Clinical Presentation of SCID**

Number of patients	116
Age at diagnosis (mean)	142 days
Growth impairment (mean delay)	2.8 months
Persistent diarrhea	61%
Lung infection	58%
Candidiasis	34%
Opportunistic infection	26%
Fever	25%
Upper airway infection	14%
Sepsis	5%
Meningitis	4%

Adapted from Stephan et al: *J Pediatr* **12**:456, 1991.

DISORDERS OF V(D)J RECOMBINATION AND T CELL RECEPTOR SIGNALING

V(D)J Recombination

T cells predominantly recognize short peptide antigens that must be bound by MHC (Chap. 12) on the surface of antigen-presenting cells. MHC proteins are highly polymorphic[17] and most of the amino acid residues contributing to their diversity are adjacent to the peptide-binding/recognition site.[18] This ensures that T cells become activated only when interacting by direct contact with antigen in the context of a MHC molecule on another cell. The T cell receptor (TCR) binding site is similar to the V domains of antibodies (Chap. 184), but binds only a small antigenic determinant in contact with a MHC molecule. On the cell surface, two TCR chains (α and β, or γ and δ) participate in a complex of proteins, the CD3 complex, involved in plasma membrane expression and signal transduction[19] (Fig. 185-1). Physical association of the TCR complex with the MHC is aided by the CD4[20] (MIM 186940, 12pter-p12) and CD8[21] (MIM 186910, MIM 186730, 2p12) accessory molecules that interact with nonpolymorphic domains of the MHC proteins.[22] T cells that express CD4 have TCRs that specifically interact with MHC class II molecules, and T cells that express CD8 have TCRs that interact with class I MHC proteins.[23] The two TCR isoforms, $\alpha\beta$ and $\gamma\delta$, are disulfide-linked heterodimers.[24,25] Each chain is composed of a V and C domain. The V domains interact to form the antigen-binding site and the C domains interact with the cell membrane and with proteins of the CD3 complex to anchor the TCR to the cell surface and to transduce the signal upon TCR binding (see below).

TCR gene assembly is similar to Ig recombination in that distant variable (V) segments are juxtaposed to the constant (C) segments (Fig. 185-2) via a set of joining (J) segments immediately 5′ to C.[26–28] In addition, two of the TCR loci (β and δ) employ short diversity (D) segments 5′ to the J elements that, after V to D rearrangement, sequentially rearrange to J (therefore called V(D)J recombination).[26–31] The recombination process appears to be an adaptation of an ancient transposon that invaded a primordial Ig-domain receptor.[32–38] Rearrangement is accompanied by additional sequence modification at the coding joint. Exonuclease activity may lead to short deletions and terminal deoxynucleotidyl transferase (TdT, MIM 187410, 10q23-24) catalyzes addition of non-germ-line-encoded (N) nucleotides on free 3′OH coding ends.[39] Four TCR loci encode the different peptide chains. The human Cα (MIM 186880, 14q11.2) is composed of 4 exons (Ig domain, 16 amino acid cysteine-rich bridge, transmembrane domain, and 3′ untranslated). It has >50 Jα segments. So far, >100 Vα genes, which can be ordered into 32 subgroups, have been identified.[29] The δ chain genes are embedded within the α locus and are deleted during α rearrangement. The Cδ is also composed of four exons and is associated with two Jδ segments. In addition, there are two Dδ segments, and in adult $\gamma\delta$ T cells, the structure of δ is usually V-D1-D2-J with N regions at each of the three junctions.[30] The β chain locus (MIM 186930, 7q35) is composed of two Cβ genes containing four exons each associated with seven Jβ segments. The entire TCR β locus with V genes has been sequenced and reveals several internal duplications within the V regions.[27,28] Unlike the Ig heavy chain locus, there is no isotype switching in

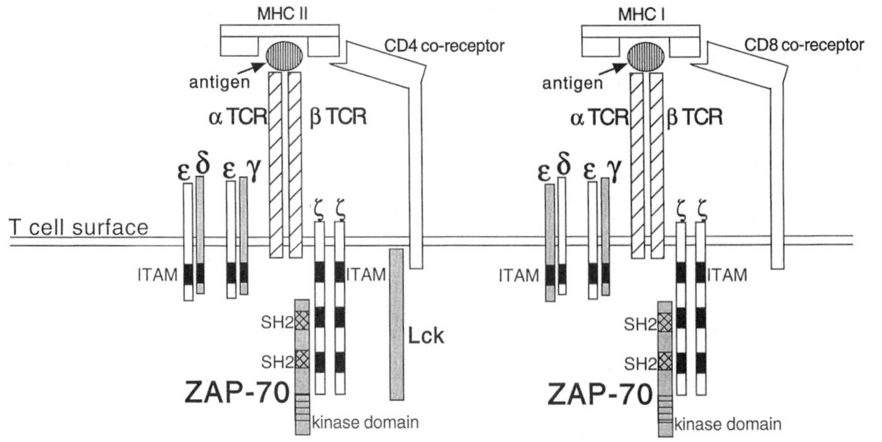

Fig. 185-1 CD3/TCR receptor complex. CD3 receptors contain two variable T cell receptor (TCR) chains ($\alpha\beta$ or $\gamma\delta$, the latter not shown) plus at least six invariant chains δ,γ; two ε chains; and two ζ chains. MHC class I molecules present antigen to CD3 complexes with CD8 coreceptors; MHC class II molecules present antigen to those with CD4 coreceptors. SH2 domains of the intracellular kinase ZAP-70 interact with ITAMs such as those on the ζ chains of the CD3 complex; and the T-cell kinase Lck interacts with the CD4 coreceptor in human cells, and possibly other receptors, including CD8. Shaded molecules indicate those which when defective are known to result in SCID in humans.

TCRβ. All the Vβ segments may rearrange to either Cβ_1 or C$_{\beta 2}$. The human TCR γ locus (MIM 186970, 7p15) is similar to the α locus in that V regions rearrange directly to J without a D. Unlike the other TCR loci, γ gene V-J rearrangements follow a sequential pattern during fetal and adult development,[40–45] and the resulting cells distribute into characteristic intraepithelial locations.[41] Diversity of the TCRs is generated by combinatorial usage of V, D, and J elements within a locus; combinatorial association of the α and β chains or γ and δ chains; and coding joint imprecision at the V(D)J boundaries.[46,47] Because of the imprecision of the coding joint formation only one-third of rearrangements retain a continuous open reading frame for translation. Failure to create a competent coding sequence allows further recombination events on the same or the other allele to proceed. When a T cell successfully rearranges and expresses a functional β chain, a feedback signal is generated that suppresses further β locus recombination.[48–52] These cells proliferate and can then begin α chain locus rearrangement. Expression of an α chain leads to inhibition of further α rearrangement. The resulting allelic exclusion allows one lymphocyte to make a single receptor molecular species. Allelic exclusion involves a recently discovered SLP76-dependent (MIM 601603, 5q33.1-qter) signal transduction pathway.[50]

A unique DNA recombinase system catalyzes the assembly of the Ig and TCR loci.[46,47,53–59] Comparison of DNA sequences at the recombination boundaries identified elements required in *cis* for DNA rearrangement. Recombination signal sequences (RSS) have a stereotypic organization — a heptamer CACTGTG, a 12- or 23-bp spacer, and then a nonamer GGTTTTTGT. RSS with a 12-bp spacer recombine at the site of a 23-bp spacer RSS and vice versa — a process that is called the "12/23 rule." The 12/23 rule confers ordered specificity to the rearrangement process. V(D)J RSS are positioned with the conserved heptamers next to the protein coding segments; that is, downstream of V and upstream of J. Joining of the coding sequences (coding joint) requires a simultaneous joining of heptamers (signal joint). V(D)J recombination generates four DNA ends, two coding and two RSS, held together (synapsis) before strand healing.[60–62] Signal joint formation is extremely precise with all nucleotides preserved at the junction. One difference between the coding ends and the RSS ends is that coding ends are protected by the formation of hairpin structures.[60–64] The existence of these hairpin structures was first inferred by the presence of short palindromic repeat nucleotides (P nucleotides) at the rejoined coding ends.[65] P nucleotides are generated when the hairpin is opened by an endonuclease activity within coding nucleotides.

V(D)J recombination can be considered as a set of ordered steps regulated and catalyzed by multicomponent protein complexes (Fig. 185-3). The steps involve: (a) establishment of locus accessibility to the recombinase; (b) RSS binding and synapsis;

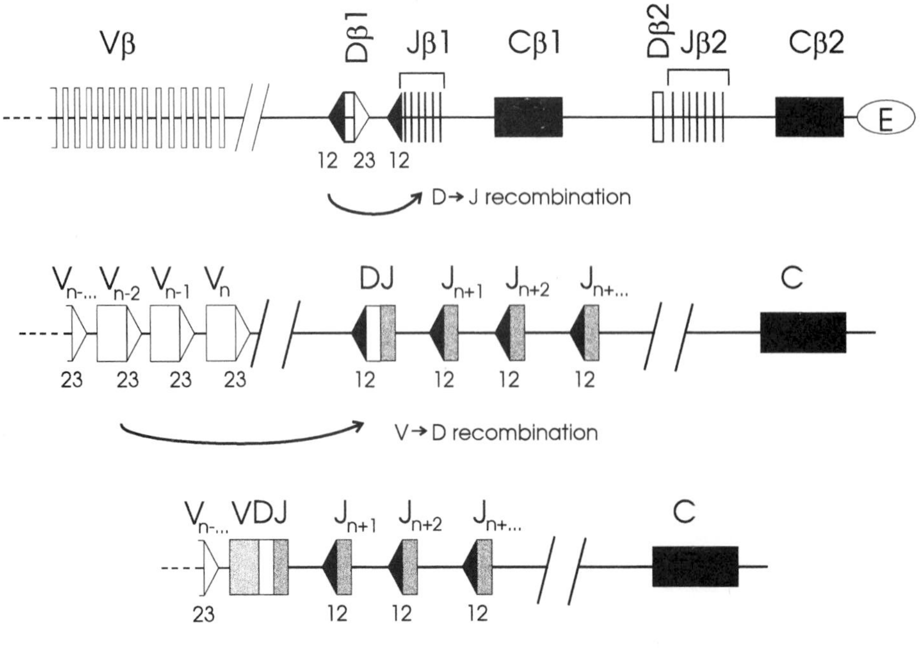

Fig. 185-2 V(D)J recombination generates T cell receptors. TCRβ locus illustrates the DNA rearrangements that assemble the exons encoding the β chain.

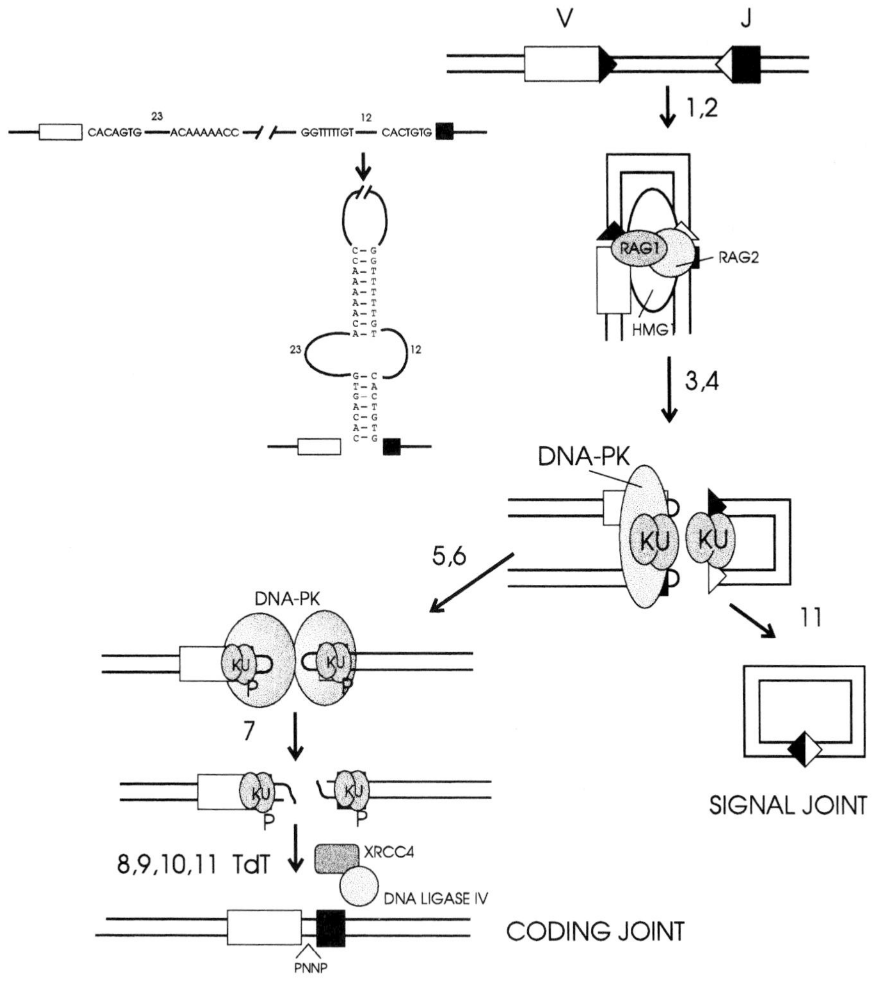

Fig. 185-3 The mechanism of V(D)J recombination. 1. The RAG1:RAG2:HMG1 complex binding to the recombination signal sequences (RSS). 2. Synapsis of the RSS following the 12/23 rule. 3. Strand nicking by RAG the complex. 4. Coding end hairpin formation. 5. KU86:KU70 binding to DNA ends. 6. DNA-PK activation and KU phosphorylation. 7. Hairpin opening. 8. Coding and signal end pairing. 9. TdT addition of N nucleotides with alignment of microhomologies; P nucleotide production as a consequence of filling-in open hairpins. 10. Nucleases and polymerase trimming and filling gaps. 11. Strand ligation by XRCC4:DNA ligase IV complex. (*Adapted in part from Grawunder et al.*[26] *Used with permission.*)

(c) DNA nicking, double-strand cleavage, and coding end hairpin formation; (d) coding end hairpin opening and end modification; (e) ligation of signal and coding joints. Several proteins directly involved in the recombination apparatus have been identified. The recombinase activating genes, RAG-1 and RAG-2 (MIM 179615 and 179616, 11p13) were isolated by transfection of 3T3 cells bearing a selectable rearrangement substrate.[66,67] This suggested that the remaining elements needed for V(D)J recombination were ubiquitous and possibly components of more general recombination or DNA repair pathways. RAG-1 and RAG-2 functionally collaborate[68,69] as a heterotetramer to bring the RSS together and make the initial DNA double-strand break.[70–78] RAG-1 is a zinc-finger protein that appears to have greater affinity for DNA, but it is not known which component actually catalyzes the DNA strand cleavage. RAG1 and RAG2 are responsible for hairpin opening at the coding joint.[79–81] Joining of the coding ends created by V(D)J recombination[82,83] proceeds via an end-joining reaction that requires general cellular double-strand break (DSB) repair functions.[84,85] Joining of the signal ends also requires DSB factors. RAG-mediated DSB formation is initiated by DNA nicking,[86–89] which exposes a 3′ hydroxyl group on each of the coding ends flanking the RSS. RAG1 binds strongly to the conserved nonamer and possibly recruits RAG2 to the complex.[90,91] Both RAG1 and RAG2 then associate with the conserved heptamer of the RSS. The binding of the RAG complex is enhanced by the high mobility group proteins HMG1 and HMG2,[92] and it is the RAG-HMG complex that enforces the 12/23 rule. DNA nicking is stimulated by synapsis formation. The RSS ends are left blunt with a free 3′ hydroxyl. Nucleophilic attack of 3′ hydroxyl allows formation of an intramolecular hairpin on the coding ends. The RAG complex is also intimately involved in the rejoining of both the signal and coding ends.[93–98] These reactions are similar to those accomplished by transposases (the enzymes that mediate hopping of transposable elements and integration of retroviruses). Formation of signal ends and coding joints is substantially impaired by mutations in the DSB machinery. This observation led to the identification of Ku antigen or p70/p80 autoantigen as an important component of the recombination pathway.[99–101] Ku is a heterodimer composed of an 80-kDa component (XRCC5, MIM 194364, 2q35) and a 70-kDa component (XRCC6, MIM 152690, 22q11-13); XRCC signifies X-ray repair, complementary defective, in Chinese hamster cells. Ku binds to DNA ends[102] and is probably involved in a protein complex that permits synapsis of the free coding and signal ends.[101] Ku binds to and probably recruits terminal deoxynucleotidyltransferase (TdT) to the V(D)J coding ends.[103] Mutations in Ku80 lead to severe defects in both coding and signal joint formation.[104–108] The yeast homologue of Ku also binds to Sir4, a component of a transcriptional silencing complex.[109] The Sir complex may have a dual role in transcription and DNA repair.[110] In yeast, the Sir complex plays a role in both nonhomologous end joining[110] and in maintenance of telomeres,[111] but no direct role for Sir in V(D)J recombination has yet been demonstrated. Ku is probably the DNA-targeting component of a larger complex that includes a third and fourth component Xrcc4[112–113] (MIM 194363, 5q13-q14) and DNA-dependent protein kinase (DNA-PK, MIM 600899, 8q11) that are required for V(D)J recombination. Xrcc4 encodes a 25-kDa protein of unknown function and no known similarities. Xrcc4 is required for DSB repair based on analysis of mutant cells. Xrcc4 interacts with DNA ligase IV[114]

(MIM 601837, 13q22-34), the protein component required to complete the strand ligation in V(D)J recombination[115–117] in mice. A cell line derived from a single individual with leukemia and radiation sensitivity, but not immunodeficiency, has been found to have a missense mutation in DNA ligase IV.[118] DNA ligase IV has two unique BRCA2-like motifs (BRCT) in its C-terminal domain.[119,120] The function of the BRCT domains is unknown but may mediate interaction with Xrcc4.[119] Xrcc4 stimulates DNA ligase IV activity in vitro.[114,120] Another Ku interaction partner that plays a critical role in V(D)J recombinations is DNA-PK.[121] DNA-PK is a 350-kDa serine-threonine kinase that is activated upon DNA binding.[121] RAG-1, RAG-2, and Ku are among the physiological targets of DNA-PK phosphorylation.[122,123] DNA-PK is mutated in the classical mouse mutation, severe combined immune deficiency (*scid*),[124–129] as well as the equine autosomal recessive SCID.[130,131] Animals with DNA-PK defects exhibit defective T and B cell development and generalized radiation sensitivity. The primary immunologic defect in *scid* results from failure of coding joint formation in both TCR and Ig. However, signal joint formation, while readily detected, is also reduced tenfold, and its precision diminished.[132] DNA-PK shares some significant protein motifs including the kinase domain with the ataxia telangiectasia mutated (ATM) gene[133,134] (see Chap. 29). Defective immunologic development and incomplete suppression of intermolecular joining in *scid* (DNA-PK), ataxia telangiectasia (*ATM*, MIM 208900, 11q22.3), Bloom syndrome[135] (*BLM*, MIM 210900, 15q26.1), and Nijmegen breakage[136,137] syndrome (*NIBRIN/p95*, MIM 251260, 8q21) mutants suggests similarities in the cellular mechanisms for monitoring free DNA ends. However, the roles of each of the latter proteins in V(D)J recombination and/or lymphocyte developmental checkpoints are unclear. The free DNA ends temporarily formed during the recombination process represent a potential danger to the cell in that they could become involved in aberrant intermolecular joining.[138] This is, in fact, the basis for many characteristic translocations found in human leukemia and lymphoma.[139] Intermolecular joining is suppressed by various mechanisms[140–142] including inaccessibility of the potential target regions and inefficient synapsis formation.

Disorders of V(D)J Recombination

Failure of the recombination machinery leads to arrest of both T cell and B cell development. It can be inferred from animal model studies[68,69,143–147] that successful cell-surface expression of rearranged antigen receptors constitute an important cellular developmental "checkpoint." Cells that fail to express TCR in the thymus are eliminated by apoptosis. Infants with complete defects in recombinase activity would thus be predicted to lack mature B and T cells in peripheral blood and peripheral lymphoid organs. Schwarz et al.[148] observed mutations in RAG1 or RAG2 in a subset of T^-B^- SCID patients (MIM 601457). Clinical problems reflected defects in both humoral and cellular immunity. These included early infection with opportunistic organisms and recurrent respiratory or gastrointestinal infections. These patients were clinically very similar to others with SCID. Partial deficiencies of RAG1 and RAG2 have also been observed in the Omenn syndrome[149–152] (OS, MIM 267700). OS, first described in 1965,[153] is characterized by immunodeficiency, erythroderma, failure to thrive, chronic diarrhea, hepatosplenomegaly, and lymphadenopathy. Patients with OS typically have hypoproteinemia (a consequence of skin and GI losses), anemia, thrombocytopenia, and eosinophilia. More specialized investigation of immune functions demonstrates low serum immunoglobulins, low or absent B lymphocytes, and low specific humoral immune response to vaccination, but paradoxically elevated IgE.[154] The numbers of T cells in the peripheral blood and lymph nodes are variable and the T cells may have an activated phenotype.[155] Tissue culture studies demonstrate low *in vitro* T cell proliferative responses to mitogens or antigens. Lymph node architecture contrasts with that seen in typical SCID in that instead of hypoplasia there is an increased proportion of eosinophils and reticular cells along with the lack of follicles. The disease was originally named "familial reticuloendotheliosis with eosinophilia" because of this pathologic picture. Other peripheral lymphoid tissue is severely involved with hypoplastic Peyer's patches and thymus as well as decreased splenic white pulp. The clinical presentation is in many ways similar to severe graft versus host disease (GVHD). True GVHD may be observed in SCID patients due to maternal cell engraftment or transfusion of nonirradiated blood products. Clinical diagnosis of OS, therefore, requires demonstration of a RAG1 or RAG2 mutation and/or exclusion of GVHD. The activated T cells in OS are skewed to the T-helper type 2 lymphocyte (Th2) phenotype and secrete Th2-type cytokines,[154–156] a fact that may explain elevated levels of serum IL4 and IL5.[154] The abnormal levels of IL4 could account for the elevated serum IgE and the elevated IL5 the eosinophilia. The T cells in OS are oligoclonal, functionally defective, and particularly susceptible to apoptosis, most likely reflecting a general defect in T lymphopoiesis.[157–159] Mutation analysis in seven OS patients revealed mutations in RAG1 in six and RAG2 in one.[152] OS patients were found to have homozygous missense mutations or to be compound heterozygotes for missense and null mutations. It is also possible that mutations causing OS are restricted in their protein domain distribution. Heterodimerization of RAG1 and RAG2 required for RSS binding recognition activity may be affected by the OS mutations. Missense mutations probably allow production of RAG proteins with some residual function in contrast to the severe RAG mutations observed in T^-B^- SCID subjects.[160–163]

Disorders of T Cell Receptor Signaling

The CD3 receptor complex on the surface of T cells consists of multiple components in addition to the polymorphic TCR $\alpha\beta$ or TCR $\gamma\delta$ receptors themselves. The complex collectively referred to as CD3 (Fig. 185-3) includes a single $\alpha\beta$ or $\gamma\delta$ TCR unit plus at least five additional noncovalently associated membrane-spanning protein components, a δ chain, a γ chain, two ε chains—one associated with the δ and one with the γ chain—and two ζ chains.[164,165] Non-TCR chains are important for stabilization, cell-surface expression, and signal transduction through the complex. Extracellularly, these proteins may facilitate docking of antigen on the TCR and/or clustering of receptors to enhance the effectiveness of signal transmission. Their intracellular domains contain immunoreceptor tyrosine-based activation motifs, or ITAMs, which are required to interact with specific intracellular signal transducing molecules. Although the CD3 complex components do not exhibit the sequence diversity of the TCRs, some variations are observed due to alternative splicing of their genomic exons. For example, an alternative splice form of CD3γ may play a special role for the transport and assembly of the pre-TCR/CD3 complex in immature thymocytes.[166] The genes for CD3γ and CD3δ are situated about 1.6 kb apart, organized in a head-to-head orientation. The CD3γ/CD3δ gene pair is within 30 kb of the CD3ε gene; therefore, these genes form a tightly linked cluster on chromosome 11q23.[167] Human immunodeficiency due to autosomal recessive mutations of *CD3G* (MIM 186740) has been described in three individuals from two families,[168] and a single case of immunodeficiency due to *CD3E* mutation (MIM 186830) has been documented.[169] While the original proband with CD3γ deficiency had a severe phenotype and fatal course of uncontrolled infections compatible with SCID, his affected brother had a mild course with only frequent respiratory infections and a suggestion of autoimmune disease later in childhood. In all affected individuals, cell-surface expression of multiple CD3 components was markedly decreased, and *in vitro* proliferation, after exposure to anti-CD3 antibodies and to mitogen phytohemagglutinin, was deficient. Molecular analysis showed homozygous or compound heterozygous mutations in all cases. Studies in mice with targeted deletions of CD3 components have confirmed that all chains are required for normal expression and function of the CD3 T cell receptor system.[170]

A cofactor of the CD3 complex is a lymphocyte-specific protein-tyrosine kinase p56(lck), encoded by the *LCK* locus on human chromosome 1p35-p32.[171] In mice *Lck*, a member of the src oncogene family of kinases, is required for development of both $CD4^+$ and $CD8^+$ lymphocyte lineages in the thymus; and its regulatory role in lymphocyte development is underlined by its involvement in translocations seen in human T-cell lymphoblastic leukemia.[172] An infant with SCID who lacked Lck (MIM 153390) has been reported.[173] Unlike mice with targeted *Lck* deletions that fail to develop any mature $CD4^+$ or $CD8^+$ T cells,[147] this child demonstrated selective $CD4^+$ cell deficiency. He had normal $CD8^+$ cell counts, although these $CD8^+$ cells were unable to proliferate normally in response to mitogens and IL-2.

One of the important intracellular signal transducers in T cells is ZAP70, a 70-kDa protein tyrosine kinase that associates with the ζ chain of the CD3 complex.[174–175] ZAP70 is recruited to the TCR immediately after extracellular engagement of antigen (Fig. 185-4). The two SH2 domains of ZAP70 interact with ITAMs of the ζchain and possibly other chains of CD3. This and additional interactions result in the activation of the kinase domain of ZAP70 and transmission of T cell signals to further protein tyrosine kinases. In humans, autosomal recessive mutations of ZAP70 have been found to cause a type of SCID with distinctive preservation of CD4 cells and absence of CD8 cells (MIM 176947), which, while very rare, has nonetheless yielded important insight into human T cell development in the thymus. The first children recognized to have ZAP70 deficiency were from the genetically isolated Mennonite populations, but the disorder has now been recognized in Caucasian and Hispanic consanguineous matings.[176–179] All patients presented in the first 2 years of life with recurrent and opportunistic infections. Unexpectedly, and with a pattern opposite that seen in human Lck deficiency, above, they had normal to elevated numbers of lymphocytes in peripheral blood, almost all with CD4 coreceptor, as well as normal size and histology of lymph nodes and thymus. The number and function of NK cells were normal, and some patients had intact B cell antibody responses. However, T cell skin test reactivity was absent, and *in vitro* responses to specific antigens and a variety of activation stimuli that require an intact CD3 complex were severely defective. Bone marrow transplantation provided successful immune reconstitution in six cases. Thymic cell analysis revealed a block of lymphocyte maturation from $CD4^+$ $CD8^+$ double-positive immature thymocytes to single-positive $CD8^+$ cells. It remains unclear exactly why human ZAP70 deficient thymocytes can differentiate as far as the double-positive stage, a point at which TCR engagement was already required in the process, which eliminates autoreactive T cells before they can mature. Mice with targeted disruption of ZAP70 do not develop any mature T cells and have severe defects in thymocyte activation.[180] One possible explanation is that redundancy between ZAP70 and other related protein tyrosine kinases, particularly Syk kinase, which is primarily found in developing B cells, can partially make up for the absence of ZAP70 activity.

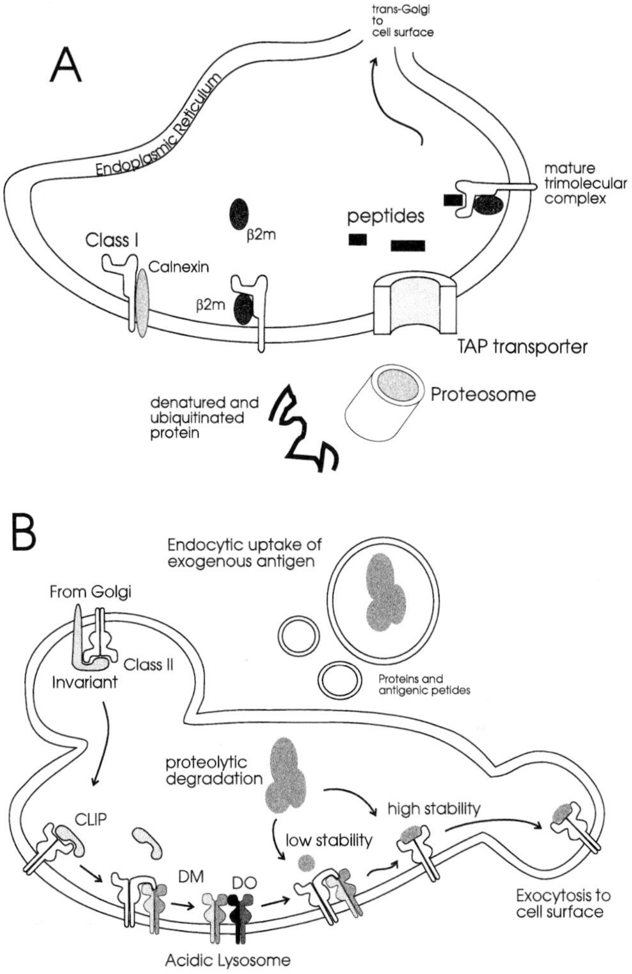

Fig. 185-4 Pathways of antigen processing. *A*: Endogenous antigens. Class I proteins bind peptides originating from endogenous proteins degrade by the ubiquitination-proteasome pathway. These peptides are transported into the ER by the TAP transporter composed of TAP1 and TAP2. Class I proteins bind the chaperone calnexin, which is displaced by β_2-microglobulin (β_{2m}). After peptide binding, the mature complexes are exported to the cell surface. *B*: Exogenous antigens. Class II proteins are bound by the invariant chain (Ii) during synthesis and transport through the Golgi. Ii is processed to CLIP, which is displaced by HLA-DM. HLA-DO binds HLA-DM and is a competitor for HLA-DM binding to other class II proteins. Exogenous proteins and peptides are taken up by the endocytic pathway often aided by antibody binding on B cells and other accessory cells. Exogenous peptides are generated by proteolytic cleavage in the acidic lysosomes. Low affinity interactions with peptides do not displace HLA-DM. High affinity peptide interactions displace HLA-DM and allow export to the cell surface via the exocytic pathway.

DISORDERS OF MAJOR HISTOCOMPATIBILITY COMPLEX PROTEINS

Expression and Function of the MHC

T cells react specifically with antigenic peptides bound to cell-surface MHC molecules. The antigenic peptides are derived from two parallel processing pathways. The endogenous pathway uses ubiquitin-activated proteasome degradation and transport of the resulting peptides into the ER by a specific transporter, TAP. The exogenous pathway involves lysosomal protein degradation and requires specific class II chaperones, invariant chain (Ii), and the MHC-encoded HLA-DM. MHC molecules are divided into three classes (I, II, and III) based on their primary structure and functions in the immune system.[181–191] The class I and class Ib proteins are 44-kDa polymorphic transmembrane glycoprotein α-chains.[192,193] The proteins have three domains—$\alpha1$, $\alpha2$, $\alpha3$—and polymorphic residues occur primarily in the $\alpha1$ and $\alpha2$ domains. These proteins associate at the cell surface with a monomorphic 12-kDa chain, β_2-microglobulin, which is also a member of the Ig superfamily (MIM 109700, 15q21-22). Cell-surface expression of class I α chain is dependent on β_2-microglobulin coexpression. Expression of class I gene products is nearly ubiquitous in various cells and tissues. Class I molecules bind peptides that arise from an intracellular degradation pathway restricted to proteins that are synthesized by the antigen presenting cells (e.g., endogenous or viral antigens). Class I antigen processing involves production of cytosolic peptides, followed by ER peptide transport, and then binding to class I molecules.[194–197] The proteasome is the most important source of antigenic peptides but other cytosolic peptidases may contribute.[198–202] Folding and assembly of class I molecules in the ER involves several accessory proteins. The thiol oxidoreductase, ERp57, is a component of the MHC class I peptide-loading complex and probably controls the folding of class I during peptide loading.[203–205] Peptides are transported from the cytosol into the lumen of the ER by a peptide transporter (Fig. 185-4), TAP,[206–215] that is composed of two chains TAP1 (MIM 170260) and TAP2 (MIM 170261). The assembly of class I α chain and β_2-microglobulin with peptides is facilitated by the chaperone calreticulin (MIM 109091) and tapasin[216,217] (MIM 601962) in a multicomponent "loading complex." Approximately four class I/tapasin complexes bind to each TAP molecule. The trimolecular complex, α chain, β_2-microglobulin, and peptide, is then transported through the secretory pathway to the cell surface. The class I molecules are recognized specifically by T cell receptors that are expressed by CD8$^+$ T cells (CD8a MIM 186910 and CD8b MIM 186730, 2p12). Most CD8$^+$ T cells exhibit cytotoxic killer activity (CTL or cytotoxic T lymphocyte). CD8 is a heterodimeric protein expressed on T cells that interacts through the nonpolymorphic region of the class I molecules.[218] The class Ib genes are homologous in their structure and also require β_2-microglobulin coexpression.[219–221] They are less polymorphic and serve functions in iron metablism,[222] differentiation,[223] immune surveillance,[224,225] and pregnancy[226,227] that are poorly understood compared to the classical class Ia proteins.

The class II molecules also have a heterodimeric structure.[228–232] The α (34 kDa) and β (29 kDa) subunits are each composed of a polymorphic peptide binding region, an Ig superfamily domain, a transmembrane domain, and a short cytoplasmic tail. Class II molecules are expressed only on antigen presenting cells such as dendritic cells, macrophages, B cells, and activated T cells. Their expression can be induced in a variety of other cells by stimulation with γ-interferon. Class II molecules bind and present peptides that are degraded in an endosomal/lysosomal compartment that processes exogenous proteins. During assembly of class II proteins in the endoplasmic reticulum, α and β chains are associated with a 31-kDa protein called the invariant chain[233–243] (Ii or CD74, MIM 142790, 5q32). Ii or its specific proteolytic cleavage products, called class II HLA-associated invariant chain derived peptides (CLIP), stays associated with class II through the Golgi apparatus until it arrives in an endosomal compartment where peptides are encountered. Ii dissociates from class II in this compartment. HLA-DM (a conserved member of the class II family also composed of α and β chains) is required for the normal assembly of peptides with MHC class II molecules.[244–261] HLA-DM catalyzes the release of class II and the opening of the peptide binding site. DM functions as a peptide editor by displacing class II-bound peptides that contain suboptimal side chains and those shorter than 11 amino acids.[259] Mice lacking functional histocompatibility M locus (H2-M) express cell-surface class II associated with CLIP. These mice have elevated CD4$^+$ counts, and they are hyperreactive to wild-type stimulator cells.[253,255,260] In contrast, H2-M-deficient stimulating cells do not elicit proliferative responses from wild-type T cells. Similarly, HLA-DO (yet another MHC-encoded class II family member) inhibits the class II antigen-processing pathway by binding DM and blocking DM-catalyzed peptide loading.[262–268] Analysis of antigen presentation by B cells from mice lacking H2-O (the mouse homolog of HLA-DO), shows that HLA-DO/H2-O decreases the presentation of antigens internalized by fluid-phase endocytosis and concentrates the B cell-mediated antigen presentation on antigens internalized by membrane immunoglobulin.[263,264,267] The T cells that recognize antigen in the context of class II are CD4$^+$ (MIM 186940, 12pter-12). The source of antigen (endogenous vs. exogenous) presented by the class I and class II molecules corresponds to the effector functions of the responding T cells (i.e., class I stimulates CTL and class II stimulates helper T cells).

These proteins (excluding β_2-microglobulin) are encoded in a large multigene locus on chromosome 6 that has been sequenced in full.[269] This is called the HLA complex (human leukocyte antigen). HLA-A, -B, and -C encode class I proteins. HLA-DR, -DQ, and -DP are loci that encode several class II proteins. There are 224 identified gene loci within the MHC of humans, many of which are still of unknown function and about half of which are predicted only from their primary sequence. It is estimated that about 40 percent of the expressed genes have immune system function. Several genes within the MHC have an ancient origin that can be traced to organismal divergence of at least 700 million years. Therefore, some of the MHC functions predate the emergence of the antigen-specific adaptive immune system (vertebrate radiation about 400 million years ago). MHC molecules exhibit extensive polymorphism in the antigen-binding groove; the amino acid sequences of the interacting folds control the spectrum of peptides that may be bound by the MHC molecule. Some of the capacity to generate peptide-binding specificity arises from combinatorial association of the class II α and β chains. In the DR locus, the β chain is nonpolymorphic and associates with either the $\alpha1$ or $\alpha3$ chains. In both DQ and DP, the α and the β chains are polymorphic and can associate in either *cis* (same chromosome) or *trans* (other chromosome) dimers. Individual and population polymorphism plays an important role in immune competence to resist infectious diseases.[270] Some alleles and haplotypes confer a substantial liability to certain autoimmune diseases (Chap. 12).[271,272]

MHC Class I Deficiency

Bare lymphocyte syndromes (BLS, MIM 209920) are rare disorders with variable severity of immunodeficiency.[273–284] Cells from BLS patients cannot be typed with serologic reagents due to low cell-surface expression of class I or II molecules. BLS type I involves only class I expression, while type II and type III refer to deficiency of class II or both class I and class II, respectively.[283] Complete lack of class I expression has never been observed in a patient, consistent with the idea that complete deficiency would be incompatible with embryonic development. Clinically, isolated class I deficiency generally does not present with infantile opportunistic infections, while sinusitis and bronchiectasis due to chronic respiratory tract infection are characteristic.[276] Nasal polyposis is a distinctive finding common to several individuals with the condition. Patients do not tend to suffer with chronic gastrointestinal disease or systemic bacterial infections. Mutations in *TAP2* have been observed in two families.[285,286] Very recently, two cases with *TAP1* mutations were reported.[287,288] TAP1 and TAP2 deficiencies cannot be distinguished clinically, reinforcing the concept that both TAP1 and TAP2 are required for TAP functions. In the remainder of BLS type I cases, the mutant gene is unknown. Failure of peptide loading by TAP leads to retention of the class I and β_2 microglobulin complex within the *cis*-Golgi compartment and a thirty- to one hundredfold decrease in cell surface class I expression. TAP deficiency, interestingly, has different consequences for different HLA class I alleles with some only mildly altered in expression and others more profoundly affected. Expression of class Ib molecules is not affected by TAP deficiency. Although class I is required for maturation of CD8$^+$ T cells, class I-deficient patients do not seem to have an altered CD4 to CD8 ratio. However, increased numbers of CD8$^+$ TCR$^+$ cells were detected in one subject with BLS type I.[286] Antibody responses may be attenuated in class I deficiency, but patients do not have hypogammaglobulinemia and can mount specific antiviral responses. NK cells may be reduced in numbers; although unable to lyse cells expressing HLA class I,[289] NK cells from a class I-deficient patient could perform antibody-dependent cell cytotoxicity (ADCC) and had normal NK cell surface markers.

MHC Class II Deficiency

MHC class II subunit expression is coordinately regulated at the level of mRNA transcription (Fig. 185-5). Several autosomal recessive diseases resulting in global deficits of MHC II (BLS type II, MIM 209920) expression result from defects in the transcrip-

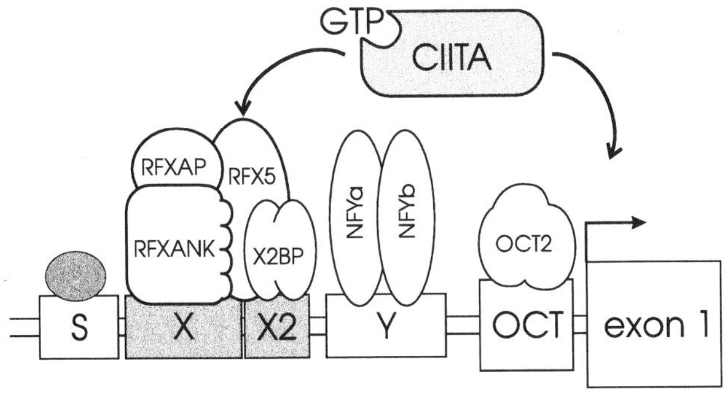

Fig. 185-5 Transcriptional control of class II expression. Schematic of prototypical class II gene promoter. RFX is formed by the heterotrimer of RFX5:RFXAP:RFXANK. GTP binding facilitates CIITA nuclear localization. OCT2, NF-Y, and X2BP are not lymphoid lineage-specific and are not known to be involved in human immunodeficiency. Complementation group A arises from mutations in CIITA; group B from mutations in RFXANK; group C from mutations in RFX5; and group D from mutations in RFXAP. (*Adapted from Kara et al.*[320] *and Masternak et al.*[343] *Used with permission.*)

tional regulation of the gene family. Patients are susceptible to bacterial, viral, fungal, and protozoal infections.[290–293] Common opportunistic agents are the most frequent, but neither the locations nor the spectrum of infections are unique to this condition. Severe respiratory tract infection, gastroenteritis, and central nervous system infections are common. Bacterial respiratory infections, including sinusitis, bronchitis, and pneumonia, are also common complications. Chronic diarrhea and failure to thrive secondary to malabsorption are typically caused by *Crytosporidium* and *Giardia* infections. Chronic viral meningoencephalitis has been seen in approximately half of patients. Autoimmune hematologic disorders and hepatitis complete the clinical picture. Survival is rare beyond the first few years of life.

The absence of MHC class II antigen presentation leads to severe defects in antigen-specific immune responses.[294–306] This includes both humoral and cell-mediated immune responses to most foreign antigens. Not surprisingly, cells from these patients are poor stimulators of mixed lymphocyte reactions in tissue culture. Patients have very reduced serum immunoglobulins, but normal numbers of T and B cells. A disturbed $CD4^+$ to $CD8^+$ T cell ratio is characteristic.[294,299,305] This emphasizes the role of MHC class II in positive selection of the $CD4^+$ lineage of T cells. An unexplained observation is that the residual $CD4^+$ T cells are immunocompetent,[299] but functional abnormalities in the CD40-CD40 ligand axis may help to explain the abnormal T cell-B cell interactions.[306] MHC class II protein expression is generally restricted to antigen-presenting cells, including B lymphocytes, dendritic cells, and monocytes. After stimulation with IFN-γ, almost all cell types can be induced to express cell surface class II. No expression of MHC class II protein is observed in antigen-presenting cells or after IFN-γ stimulation in class II-deficient patients.[295,297,298] Reduced cell-surface expression results almost entirely from failure of class II gene transcription.[300,301] All class II proteins are affected including DP, DQ, and DR, as well as the invariant chain.[297,302,338] The majority of patients also exhibit more mild reductions in class I and β_2-microglobulin cell-surface expression.

Complementation experiments provide evidence that MHC class II deficiency results from mutations in more than one locus. Patients have been found to assort into five complementation groups.[307–315] Approximately half of patients fall into Group B, and there is a predilection for these cases to be of North African origin.[308,311] While groups A to D show a global defect in MHC II expression, a very rare fifth complementation group (represented by a single pair of twins) demonstrates selective expression of some (DRA, DQA, DPB) but not other (DRB, DQB, DPA) class II proteins.[315] There is evidently some tissue specificity to the defect, because the mononuclear cells do express these proteins, while B cell lymphoblasts do not. The defect in class II deficiency results from reduced transcription at the class II loci.[316–327] A short regulatory element of approximately 150 bp contains signals for baseline and induced expression of class II transcripts. The regulatory sequence contains S, X, X2, and Y boxes that are conserved in all the active MHC II genes. Extensive characterization of class II promoter DNA-binding proteins led to the identification of a protein complex RFX that binds the X box.[320,322–324,326] The RFX complex cooperatively forms a stable higher order complex on the class II promoters with NF-Y[325] (a Y box-binding factor) and X2BP (an X2 box-binding factor). RFX is a heteromeric complex composed of 75-kDa[322] (RFX5, MIM 601863, 1q21.1-q21.3), 36-kDa[340] (RFXAP, MIM 601861, 13q14), and 33-kDa[343] (RFXANK, MIM 603200, 19p12) proteins. The discovery of the RFX complex led to biochemical classification of class II deficiency into RFX present[318,320,327] (complementation group A) or absent (complementation groups B to D) categories. The extremely rare complementation group E class II promoters exhibit selective abnormalities in the genes whose expression is reduced. Complementation cloning led to the identification of class II transactivator (CIITA)[328] (MIM 600005, 16p13) that rescues class II expression in group A cells, accounting for 14 percent of bare lymphocyte syndrome II patients.[329–335] CIITA is a transcriptional coactivator, not a part of the RFX complex, and does not independently bind DNA.[329] Recently, CIITA was shown to be a GTP-binding protein, and its nuclear translocation, required for transactivation of class II expression, is dependent on GTP.[336] Interestingly, it has little GTPase activity but rather uses GTP-binding to facilitate its nuclear localization. Complementation group C (7 percent) is caused by mutations in the RFX5 gene,[337–339] while complementation group D (19 percent) is caused by mutation in RFXAP.[340–342] Until recently, the molecular basis of the most common group B (52 percent) patients was unknown.[343–344] Using an efficient copurification scheme, Masternak et al.[343] recently identified the gene responsible for group B defects as RFXANK. RFXANK is required for efficient DNA-binding and transcriptional activation of class II. RFXANK contains three ankyrin repeats that might be responsible for RFX protein interactions or interactions with the other class II locus transcription factors X2BP, NF-Y, and CIITA.

Albinism and immunodeficiency characterize the Chediak-Higashi (CHS) and Griscelli syndromes. CHS is caused by mutations in lysosomal-trafficking regulator, LYST (MIM 214500, Chap. 220). Peptide loading onto major histocompatibility complex class II molecules and antigen presentation are delayed in CHS cells.[345] Late endosomes have reduced levels of class II and HLA-DM, consistent with a defect in transport from the *trans*-Golgi network and/or early endosomes into late multivesicular endosomes. Whether a similar phenomenon is involved in the phenotypically similar Griscelli syndrome (MIM 214450), which is caused by mutations in MYO5A, is not known.

DISORDERS OF CYTOKINE SIGNALING

Enumeration of T and B cells is one method to categorize phenotypic subsets of SCID. Most SCID patients have very few T cells, but normal or increased numbers of functionally impaired B cells (T^-B^+ SCID).[13,346] The preponderance of these patients are males, but the existence of females with T^-B^+ SCID indicates that both autosomal recessive and X-linked gene defects could produce this phenotype. Patients with no T or B cells (T^-B^- SCID) have a much more even ratio of males to females, suggesting autosomal recessive inheritance. It is now known that T^-B^+ SCID can be due to defects in at least three genes. The principal one is *IL2RG*, encoding the common gamma chain γc found in receptors for interleukins IL-2, IL-4, IL-7, IL-9, and IL-15.[347–349] *IL7RA* encodes the partner chain, which, together with γc, makes up the

IL-7 cell-surface receptor.[350] And *JAK3* encodes the cytoplasmic-signaling kinase that interacts intracellularly with the common γ chain.[351,352]

X-linked SCID (XSCID, also known as SCIDX1, MIM 300400) is caused by defects in *IL2RG* (MIM 308380), the gene at Xq13.1 encoding the interleukin-2 receptor γ chain. Roughly half of all SCID cases have *IL2RG* defects.[353,354] Prior to 1970, patients with XSCID almost always died of severe infections within the first year of life. However, immune reconstitution by bone marrow transplantation (BMT) from an HLA identical sibling marked the beginning of successful treatment.[355] Lack of histocompatible donors for the majority of XSCID patients led to isolation in a gnotobiotic environment for David, the "Bubble Boy," the famous Texas patient who came to represent SCID to the general public. Although David succumbed after a haploidentical T cell depleted transplant at age 12,[356] the gnotobiotic environment has now been successfully adapted for BMT of infants with XSCID. Early diagnosis, better antibiotics, and intensive supportive care also contributed to the evolution of XSCID from a fatal to a treatable disease.[346,354]

Males with XSCID are healthy at birth, but as transplacentally transferred maternal antibody levels wane, they develop unremitting diarrhea and infections, generally bringing them to medical attention by 3 to 6 months of age. Presenting complaints are not distinguishable from patients with autosomal forms of SCID except that females can be assumed to have autosomal SCID. Due to a substantial new mutation rate, most patients with XSCID have a negative family history.[353,357] The single most helpful diagnostic clue from a simple laboratory test is a low absolute lymphocyte count, compared to values for age-matched normal infants. While not universally present, a lymphocyte count of $< 2000/\mu l$ should raise the clinician's suspicion of a combined immunodeficiency in an infant with a significant infection. Typically, the small numbers of lymphocytes found in patients with XSCID are predominantly or entirely B cells. In vitro T cell responses to mitogens are absent, and antibody concentrations are extremely low, except that IgG is normal at birth due to transplacental transfer, falling to low levels by 3 months of age. Spontaneous maternal engraftment of lymphocytes in males with XSCID can be found in the majority of XSCID patients if sensitive methods are used. Although there may be no discernible consequences of maternal engraftment, maternal cells may recognize the infant's paternally derived histocompatibility antigens. Florid, and often fatal, graft versus host disease (GVHD) can also arise from transfusions of nonirradiated blood products.

The SCIDX1 locus was linked to polymorphic markers in the proximal long arm of the X chromosome.[358,359] Linkage studies were assisted by the ability to diagnose female carriers by their X inactivation patterns.[360] In contrast to the expected random X chromosome inactivation in female tissues, female carriers of XSCID have only the nonmutated X chromosome as the active X in their lymphocytes. This nonrandom X inactivation (more strictly, nonrandom survival after presumed random inactivation) reflects a selective disadvantage in maturation of lymphocyte progenitors lacking normal γc protein. Nonrandom X inactivation is found in T cells, B cells, and NK cells of XSCID carriers, while normal, random X inactivation patterns are seen in their granulocytes, monocytes, and other tissues.[360–362]

IL2RG, as depicted in Fig. 185-6, spans 4.5 kb of genomic DNA and contains eight exons encoding a typical member of the cytokine-receptor gene family. The extracellular domain contains a 5′ signal sequence, four conserved cysteine residues, and a juxtamembrane conserved hallmark of all cytokine receptors, the WSXWS box. The highly hydrophobic transmembrane domain occupies most of exon 6; and the proximal intracellular domain in exon 7 encodes a box1-box2 domain homologous to SH2 subdomains of Src-related tyrosine kinases. Mutations in 200 unrelated XSCID patients span all eight exons. All except three large deletions are changes of one to a few nucleotides, producing truncations, missense mutations in conserved areas, and splice

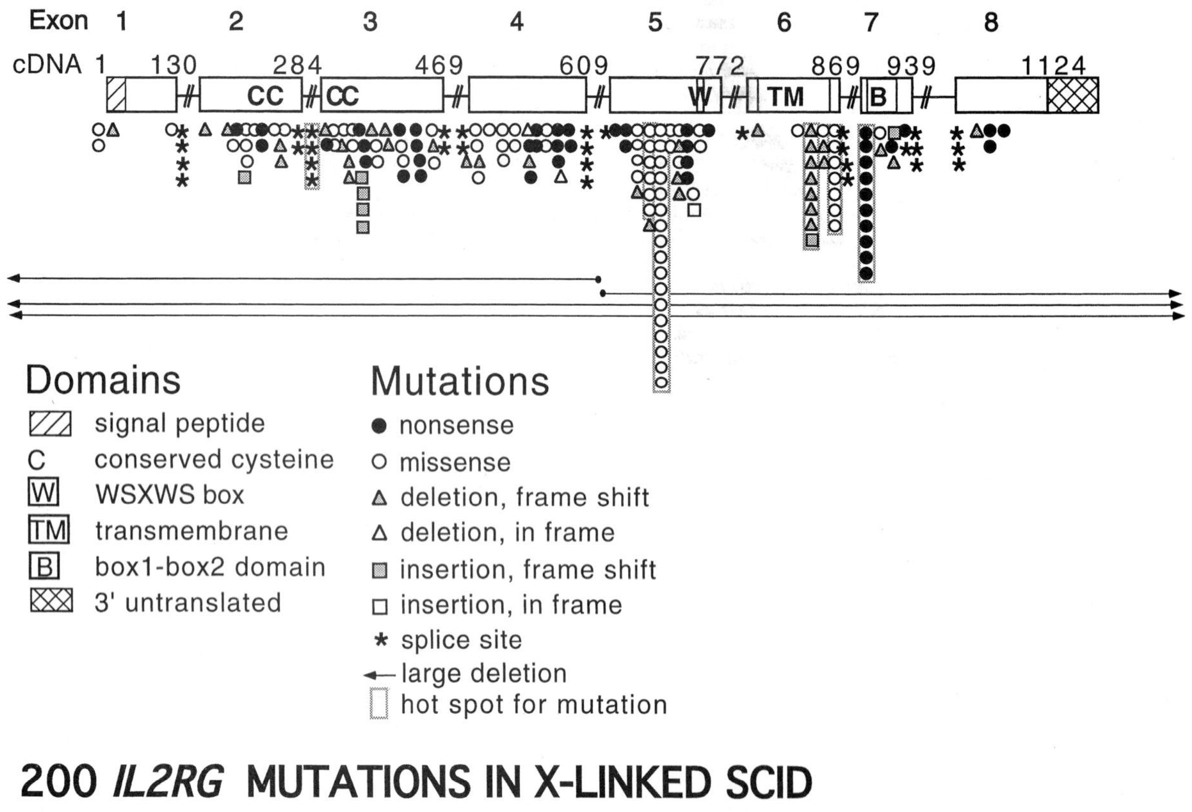

Fig. 185-6 Structure of *IL2RG* and 200 mutations found in patients with X-linked SCID and reported to IL2RGbase (www.nhgri.nih.gov/DIR/LGT/SCID/; Puck et al.[364]); GenBank L19546.

mutations. Five CG dinucleotide hot spots for mutation and one deletion/insertion hot spot are the sites of 25 percent of reported mutations[353,363,364] [also unpublished; see IL2RGbase, a Database of γc-chain Defects Causing Human X-Linked Severe Combined Immunodeficiency (XSCID) at http://www.nhgri.nih.gov/DIR/LGT/SCID/]. Although almost all reported mutations result in severe disease, mild phenotypes are recognized.[365,366] As expected with X-linked disorders that are reproductively lethal, new mutations cause up to one-third of cases (see Chap. 1). Female germ line mosaicism has been documented in XSCID,[367] and women have been identified whose blood lymphocytes had no mutation, but who passed an *IL2RG* mutation on to multiple affected offspring.[367,368]

The first report of γc as a component of IL-2 receptors by Takeshita et al.[369] established its presence in both B and T cell lines. It is expressed in mouse hematopoietic progenitor cells, from the earliest stem-cell-enriched populations throughout development of myeloid and lymphoid lineages,[370] but is not found in liver or epithelial cells. Expression of γc on murine thymocytes increases as they mature from $CD4^-CD8^-$ to double-positive $CD4^+CD8^+$ to single-positive $CD4^+$ helper or $CD8^+$ cytotoxic lymphocytes; further up-regulation occurs after lymphocyte activation, as with mitogen stimulation.[371–373] The recognition that γc is a component of the IL-2 receptor explained why mitogen responses are poor in infants with XSCID. However, mice lacking the cytokine IL-2 have grossly normal T and B cell development, developing autoimmunity later in life.[374,375] This apparent paradox was explained when γc was demonstrated to participate in receptors for additional cytokines. Indeed, as shown in Fig. 185-7, γc is part of the receptor complexes for IL-4,[376,377] IL-7,[378] IL-9,[379] and IL-15.[380]

Data from additional mouse knockout experiments and cellular cytokine activation studies suggested that the interaction between IL-7 and the IL-7 receptor complex, containing γc, is an essential signal for development of lymphocyte lineages from bone marrow hematopoietic stem cells (Fig. 185-7). IL-7 and IL-7 receptor-deficient mice have a SCID phenotype with impaired lymphocyte development,[381] and IL-7 can induce rearrangement of the T cell receptor β locus *in vitro* by promoting expression of the recombinase genes RAG-1 and RAG-2.[382] These findings prompted the prediction that autosomal SCID in humans could be caused by mutation of *IL7RA* on chromosome 5p13 encoding the IL-7 receptor chain (IL-7Rα). Because such patients, unlike γc-deficient XSCID patients, would have intact IL-15 receptors (IL-15 was known to be important for NK cell development), it was further predicted that IL-7Rα-deficient SCID would have a $T^-B^+NK^+$ phenotype. Indeed, a systematic search for mutations in patients with T^-B^+ SCID, who had NK cells and who lacked γc defects, led to identification of compound heterozygous mutations in an IL-7Rα-deficient SCID patient (MIM 600802).[350]

The importance of γc in the IL-4 and IL-9 receptor complexes is less clear. IL-4-deficient mice have T and B cells, although T help for induction of B cell isotype switching to IgE is defective.[383,384] Although IL-4 receptor complexes containing γc mediate optimal signaling from IL-4, there is evidence from γc-defective human XSCID B cell lines that some IL-4 activation can occur even through IL-4 receptors that do not contain γc.[385,386]

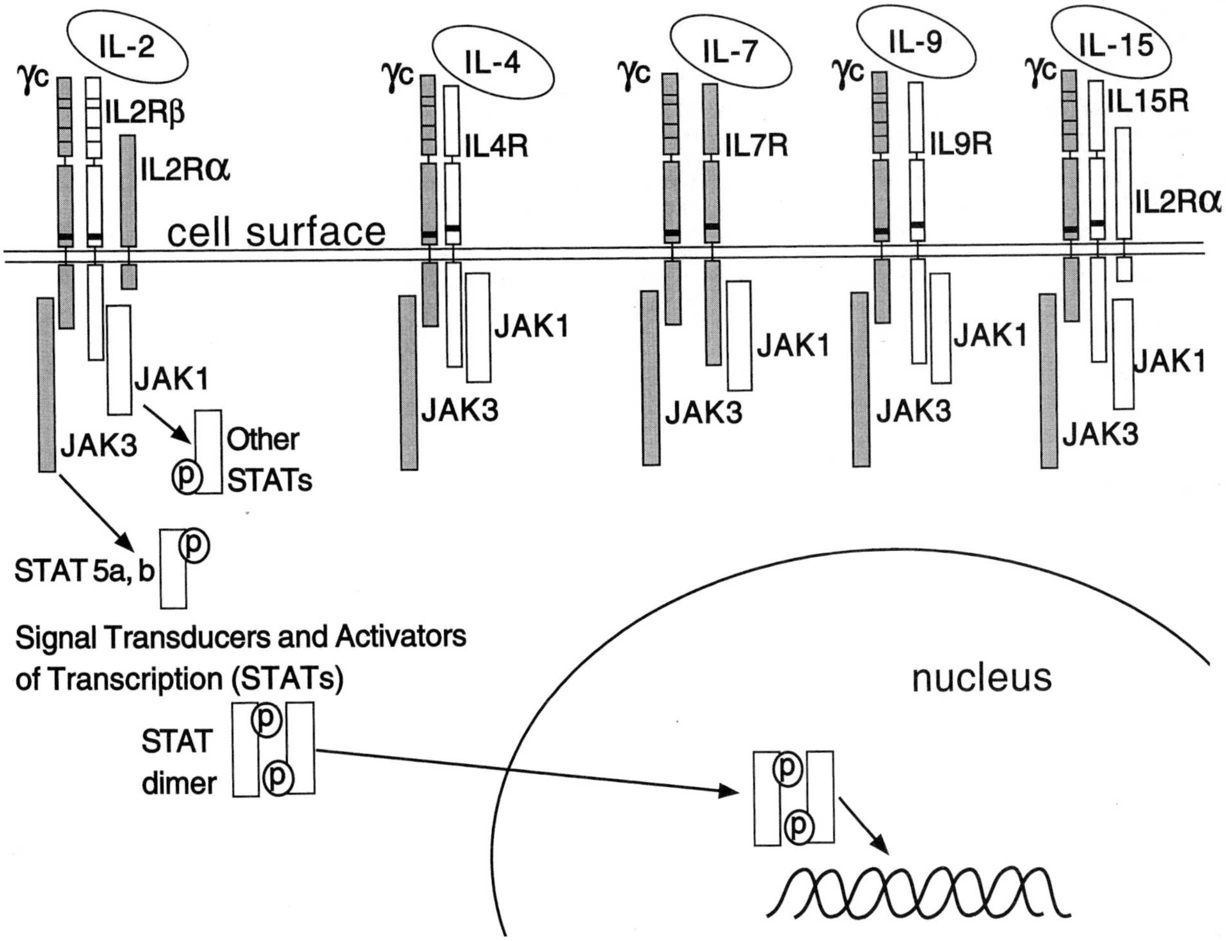

Fig. 185-7 Lymphocyte cytokine receptor complexes and their molecular associations. The common gamma chain, γc, is part of receptor complexes for IL-2, IL-4, IL-7, IL-9, and IL-15. Upon binding of extracellular cytokine, γc interacts intracellularly with JAK3, after which STAT molecules dock with the complex, become phosphorylated, dimerize, and translocate into the nucleus where they bind to DNA promotor sequences. Shaded molecules depict those which when defective result in human SCID.

After interaction with any one of the above cytokines on the surface of a cell, γc passes on an activation signal intracellularly by means of its association with JAK3, a member of the cytoplasmic Janus family of tyrosine kinases (Fig. 185-7).[379,387–389] After cytokine binding, both γc and JAK3 are rapidly phosphorylated at specific tyrosine residues. Immediately following these events signal transducers and activators of transcription (STAT proteins) can be recruited to the phosphorylated tyrosine motifs of γc and undergo phosphorylation themselves. Phosphorylated STATs form dimers and translocate into the cell nucleus, where they alter the cellular transcription program. There is a one-to-one correspondence between cytokine binding to γc and phosphorylation of JAK3; that is, only γc can activate JAK3, and no other JAK-related kinase is activated by γc. These facts predicted that JAK3 gene defects could cause human SCID that, other than its autosomal recessive inheritance pattern, would be indistinguishable from X-linked $T^-B^+NK^-$ SCID.[351,352] SCID patients with homozygous and compound heterozygous mutations in JAK3 in chromosome 19p13 (MIM 600173) have now been found to comprise approximately 7 percent of SCID cases.[354,390]

Hyper-IgM Syndrome

The very rare Hyper-IgM syndrome was classically described as a failure of isotype switching from IgM to IgG or IgA in (predominantly) male patients who had recurrent sinopulmonary infections and diarrhea.[391] High IgM is typical, but not universal; pan-hypogammaglobulinemia may be present. B cells fail to become activated normally and lymph node germinal centers exhibit poor B cell proliferation. It is now clear that there are T cell defects as well as humoral defects, with patients frequently developing pneumocystis pneumonia. Neutropenia is often found as well. Autoimmune phenomena may occur. Laboratory manifestations of T cell defects include impaired IFNγ production and reduced numbers of antigen-primed $CD45RO^+$ T cells.[392] Most cases of hyper-IgM syndrome occur in males and are inherited in an X-linked manner (MIM 308220).[393–397] The gene defect is in *CD40L*, in Xq26.3-q27, encoding the ligand expressed on T cells that interacts with the B cell coreceptor CD40 to induce isotype switching. CD40 ligand, normally expressed upon T cell activation, belongs to the tumor necrosis factor (TNF) family. In T cells from unaffected subjects, expression of CD40 ligand can be demonstrated in vitro after culture with phorbol myristate acetate and ionomycin by staining with soluble CD40, but confirmation of the defect in patients with hyper-IgM syndrome may require mutation detection. There are autosomal recessive and dominant[398] forms of hyper-IgM syndrome, but the causative genetic lesions are not known.

Long-term prognosis is poor, with causes of death including infection, severe biliary and hepatic disease, neurologic degeneration of unclear etiology, and lymphoreticular malignancy. Treatment with regular use of intravenous immunoglobulins (IVIG) and prophylaxis for *Pneumocystis carinii* pneumonia (PCP) is helpful, and BMT can be considered, even from an unrelated matched donor, because of the otherwise serious prognosis. Gene therapy is complicated by the fact that *CD40L* expression is tightly controlled, and overexpression may be harmful.

Hereditary Susceptibility to Mycobacterial Infection

Recent progress has defined several related syndromes characterized by heritable specific susceptibility to infections with mycobacteria and other intracellularly killed organisms such as *Salmonellae* (MIM 209960). Affected patients may appear otherwise in good health, but during infancy or childhood, develop severe mycobacterial infections, often with organisms of limited or absent invasiveness in normal hosts. In countries where Bacillus Calmette-Guérin (BCG) is administered as a live vaccine against tuberculosis, BCG can cause severe, disseminated disease. Genetically isolated and consanguineous families with multiple affected members account for a subset of the cases.

There is a normal, positive feedback cycle, shown by arrows in Fig. 185-8, of activation between lymphocytes and macrophages to accomplish the intracellular killing by macrophages of mycobacteria and certain other classes of microbes. Upon ingestion of live mycobacteria into phagocytic vacuoles, macrophages become activated to secrete IL-12, a dimer of p35 and p40 subunits. IL-12 binds to its divalent receptors on helper and cytotoxic lymphocytes and natural killer cells, inducing activation of these cells. T helper cells of the TH1 subtype secrete interferon γ (IFNγ), a major activator of macrophages. Therefore, when macrophages receive IFNγ signals via their IFNGR1/IFNGR2 receptors, they become more activated, increasing their ability to kill intracellular bacteria as well as their IL-12 secretion.

Recessive susceptibility to mycobacterial disease was first found to be due to mutations in the gene encoding the β1 chain of the interleukin 12 receptor expressed on T cells (*IL12RB1*; MIM 209950, 19p13).[399,400] Subsequently, homozygous recessive mutation[401] was reported in the macrophage receptor 2 chain of the interferon γ receptor gene on chromosome 21q22.1-q22.2 (*IFNGR2*; MIM 147569). A small deletion hotspot in the gene encoding chain 1 of the macrophage interferon γ receptor on chromosome 6q23-q24 (*IFNGR1*; MIM 107470) was recently reported to cause autosomal dominant mutations in 12 unrelated families.[402] The *IFNGR1* mutations all occur at cDNA position 818 in the proximal intracellular domain and cause frameshifts of

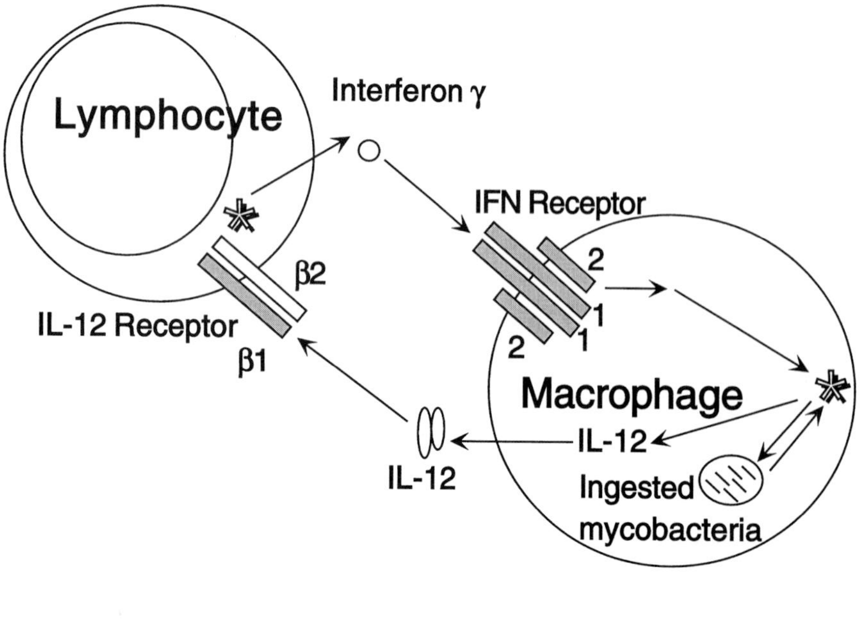

Fig. 185-8 Positive feedback cycle of macrophage and lymphocyte activation. Asterisks indicate intracellular activation pathways. Shaded molecules associated with gene defects causing human susceptibility to mycobacterial disease.

one or four nucleotides; the resulting truncated receptor molecule fails to transduce activation signals, but is expressed at the cell surface at increased concentration because it lacks a normal recycling motif and is not catabolized. Many other cases of susceptibility to mycobacterial disease have none of the above defects. In one family[403] with persistent BCG infection and recurrent salmonellosis, IL-12 production was impaired due to a homozygous intragenic deletion in *IL12B*. Multiple genetic etiologies for these phenotypes can be expected to be discovered in the future.

ADDITIONAL SIGNAL TRANSDUCTION DEFECTS IN T LYMPHOCYTES

X-Linked Lymphoproliferative Disease (XLP)

Lymphoproliferative disease following exposure to the Epstein-Barr virus is a genetic condition affecting 1 to 2 per million individuals and is most often X-linked.[404,405] X-linked lymphoproliferative disease (XLP, MIM 308240) has been associated with deletions or mutations of the gene *SH2D1A* in Xq25-q26.[406,407] This enigmatic disorder is also known as Duncan syndrome for the first family described or Purtillo syndrome for the pathologist who reported it and established a patient registry. Males with XLP are asymptomatic before encountering the Epstein-Barr virus (EBV), but over half die of fulminant mononucleosis and hepatic failure during initial infection. Survivors develop late sequelae, including dysgammaglobulinemia (low IgG, increased IgM), B-cell aplasia, aplastic anemia, or lymphoma of predominantly B cell type. No studies other than linkage analysis in known families or mutation detection can identify presymptomatic males or female carriers with reliability.

The gene SH2D1A (for SH2 domain protein 1A of Duncan disease) was identified as a transcript from the minimal critical linkage region for XLP as part of the Human Genome Project X chromosome sequence.[406] It was independently cloned as the gene encoding SAP, for SLAM-associated protein, SLAM being a signaling lymphocyte activation molecule.[407] SLAM is a self-interacting bidirectional costimulatory molecule expressed by both T and B cells. SAP has been characterized as an inhibitor of T cell/B cell interactions mediated by SLAM. Its absence in patients with XLP may allow normally regulated EBV-induced B cell proliferation to proceed unchecked. It may also prevent T cells from effectively eliminating EBV-infected B cells.

Because of the high risk of fatal complications of EBV infection in XLP, treatment with prophylactic IVIG is generally instituted in males as soon as genotypic diagnosis is made. More drastic prophylactic BMT has also been advocated when an unaffected HLA-matched related donor is available. BMT in males over 15 years of age has led uniformly to fatal complications; benefits of potential cure by BMT in young, healthy males must be balanced against the risk.

Wiskott-Aldrich Syndrome

Wiskott-Aldrich syndrome (WAS; MIM 301000) is one of the classically recognized primary immune deficiencies. The combination of infections, thrombocytopenia, and eczema presents as a very distinctive clinical entity.[1,2,408–411] The excess occurrence of the condition in males led early to the determination that WAS is an X-linked disease. As sophistication in immunologic testing progressed, WAS was found to be a primary disorder of the immune system involving cell-mediated immunity as well as a peculiar failure to produce antibodies to polysaccharide antigens. WAS may present shortly after birth with thrombocytopenia. Often before 6 months of age, the affected child develops persistent respiratory infections, otitis, and diarrhea. Severe viral infections can be observed including varicella or vaccine-associated polio. A smaller percentage of patients may develop pneumocystis infection, a further sign of impaired cell mediated immunity. Fungal infections are relatively uncommon and are usually caused by Candida when present. The eczema may be severe producing chronic superficial skin infections. WAS patients may have autoimmune diseases[412] as well as increased susceptibility to malignancy that is not necessarily restricted to the lymphoid or hematopoietic system.

Thrombocytopenia is one of the diagnostic features of WAS. Platelet counts do not respond to corticosteroids or immunoglobulin infusion, features that help to distinguish WAS from idiopathic or autoimmune thrombocytopenias. The platelets are small and have reduced function.[413–417] The severity of the immune deficit may vary; but in most cases, both the cellular and humoral immune systems are affected. Quantitative immunoglobulins demonstrate dysgammaglobulinemia with reduced IgG and IgM, but elevated IgA and IgE.[418,419] Isohemagglutinins (anti-A and anti-B responses) are persistently low or absent.[420,421] Abnormal response to other polysaccharide antigens is also manifested by poor response to Pneumococcal and to Haemophilus influenza vaccines.[422] The latter is particularly interesting because the vaccine is polysaccharide-protein conjugate unlike other polysaccharide vaccine or antigens. Specific antibody responses are reduced after immunization including diptheria-pertussis-tetanus (DPT) vaccine and bacteriophage ΦX174 antigen. Although the antibody response is impaired, WAS patients with more mild disease may develop true secondary responses and switch from IgM to IgG. Functional abnormalities of T cells are manifested by abnormal response to mitogens, alloantigens, and immobilized anti-CD3 in tissue culture.[423–425] Although initial T cell counts may be within the normal range, as the child becomes older there may be loss of T lymphocytes and peripheral blood lymphopenia.[408,410] Ultrastructural examination of the T lymphocytes indicates a lack of microvillous projections from the T cell surface[423] (Fig. 185-9). In tissue culture, chemotaxis of neutrophils and monocytes is also defective, although the role of these defects in the clinical expression of immune deficiency is unclear.[426,427]

With identification of the gene responsible for WAS, several related but less severe clinical variants have now been proven to result from allelic heterogeneity. A clinical variant of WAS[428] is characterized by eczema, thrombocytopenia, elevated IgA, mild nephropathy, and intact immunity (MIM 314000). Patients with X-linked thrombocytopenia[429,430] (MIM 313900) do not have evidence of immunodeficiency but do have persistently low platelets. Rare females with WAS have been reported.[431,432] This may result from mutation in the WASP gene coincident with constitutional skewing of X chromosome inactivation.[432–434] However, locus heterogeneity has also been suggested by rare pedigrees consistent with both autosomal recessive[431] and dominant inheritance.[435] Such rare patients suggest that mutation in one or more other genes in the WAS pathway may result in a similar clinical phenotype.

Using classical linkage analysis from a large number of independent WAS pedigrees, the *WAS* locus was mapped to Xp11.23.[436–438] The *WAS* gene was identified by positional cloning[439] and found to be composed of 12 exons spanning only 9 kb.[440,441] The mRNA consists of 1821 bp encoding a 502-amino-acid 54-kDa protein called WASP.[442,443] The *WAS* gene is expressed primarily in hematopoietic cells in primitive through mature cell phenotypes.[444,445] A paralogous protein called N-WASP has also been identified and has a broader pattern of expression.[446] Motif similarities of WASP and N-WASP allowed identification of a homologous yeast gene, *Bee1*,[447] as well as homologues in *Dictyostelium*[448] and *Cenorhabditis elegans*. WASP is a cytoplasmic protein but may associate selectively with proteins along the plasma membrane. Extensive studies of WASP have delineated several functional domains that are critical to its physiological functions. The modular nature of the protein strongly suggests that it plays a unique role in coupling signal transduction to actin cytoskeleton functions. The first domain is called the WASP-homology (WH1) domain based on conservation between WASP and N-WASP. *Bee1* and the *Drosophila* protein

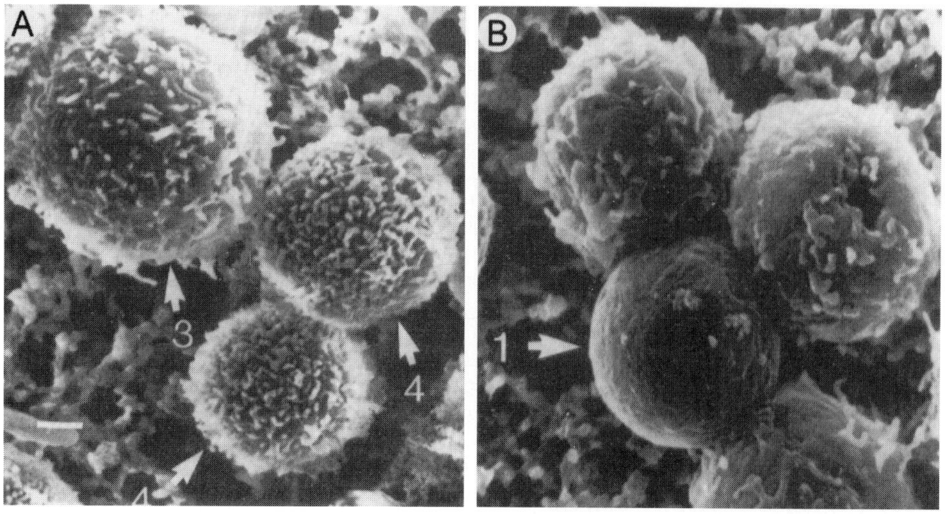

Fig. 185-9 Abnormal T cell morphology in Wiskott-Aldrich syndrome. *A*: Normal lymphocytes. *B*: WAS lymphocytes showing paucity of surface microvillous projections as a consequence of abnormal intracellular actin remodeling. (*From Kenney et al.*[423] *Used with permission.*)

homer are involved in actin cytoskeleton regulation and assembly.[449] The WH1 domain partially overlaps with a pleckstrin homology (PH) domain that binds phosphoinositol 4,5-*bis*-phosphate (PIP_2).[450] N-WASP overexpression alters cellular actin polymerization and is further stimulated by PIP_2.[446] WASP also contains a small GTPase binding domain (Cdc42 or Rac-interactive binding).[451,452] The Cdc42 and related GTPases have pleiotropic roles in cell organization and actin polymerization.[453,454] WASP was found to bind the activated GTP-bound form of Cdc42.[455,456] Like N-WASP, WASP overexpression also stimulates actin polymerization,[457] an effect that can be blocked with dominant a negative mutant Cdc42. This would be consistent with the concept that actin reorganization stimulated by WASP is Cdc42-dependent.[458] Whether Cdc42 is a physiological target of WASP is at present unclear, because the binding activity is low and greater specificity for N-WASP is observed.[459] WASP also contains a proline-rich (PR) motif. The PR domains of WASP are typical for SH3 binding targets. Indeed, interaction of WASP with several SH3 proteins, including Grb2, nck, fyn, fgr, lck, c-src, p47phox, btk, Tec, PLCγ1, and ITK, has been demonstrated.[460–465] Another interesting SH3 protein interaction has been observed with the cytoskeleton-associated protein proline serine threonine phosphatase interacting protein (PSTPIP).[466] These findings suggest that WASP acts to tie intracellular signal transduction pathways to other cellular systems including the cytoskeleton. WASP also associates with shc, yet another signal transduction-coupling protein, in meagakyocytes.[467] WASP also has a verprolin/cofillin homology domain.[468–470] Verprolin and cofilin are yeast proteins that directly bind to actin and are required for cytoskeleton maintenance and organization.[469,471] Another WASP-interacting protein, WIP, was identified by yeast two-hybrid approach.[472–474] Binding studies suggest that WIP acts downstream of WASP in actin polymerization.[475] The C-terminal domain of WASP contains domains that may interact directly with actin.[476] WASP overexpression in cultured cells led to aggregation of F-actin.[454] This was dependent on the C-terminal domain of WASP. The actin-related proteins Arp2 and Arp3 are part of a seven-protein complex that is localized in the lamellipodia of a variety of cell types.[477–479] The Arp2/3 complex enhances actin nucleation and causes branching and crosslinking of actin filaments in vitro.[480–482] N-WASP and Arp2/3 complex has been shown to be an essential linker of Cdc42 signaling to actin assembly.[483] In vivo it is thought to control the formation of lamellipodia and to control actin-driven motility. WASP has been shown to coimmunoprecipitate with activated EGF receptor (EGFR),[465,484] which is enhanced by Grb2. Scar1[485] is a member of a new family of proteins related to WASP; it may also have a role in regulating the actin cytoskeleton. Scarl is the human homologue of *Dictyostelium* Scar, which is thought to connect G-protein-coupled receptors to the actin cytoskeleton.[486] Overexpression of C-terminal fragments of Scarl or WASP in cells causes abnormal localization of the Arp2/3 complex and loss of lamellipodia.[485,487]

Based on these protein interaction domains, it would appear that WASP coordinates signal transduction with cellular actin polymerization.[470,488] WASP seems to act as an adaptor protein in the transmission of signals from tyrosine kinase receptors and small GTPases to the actin cytoskeleton. A specific signaling

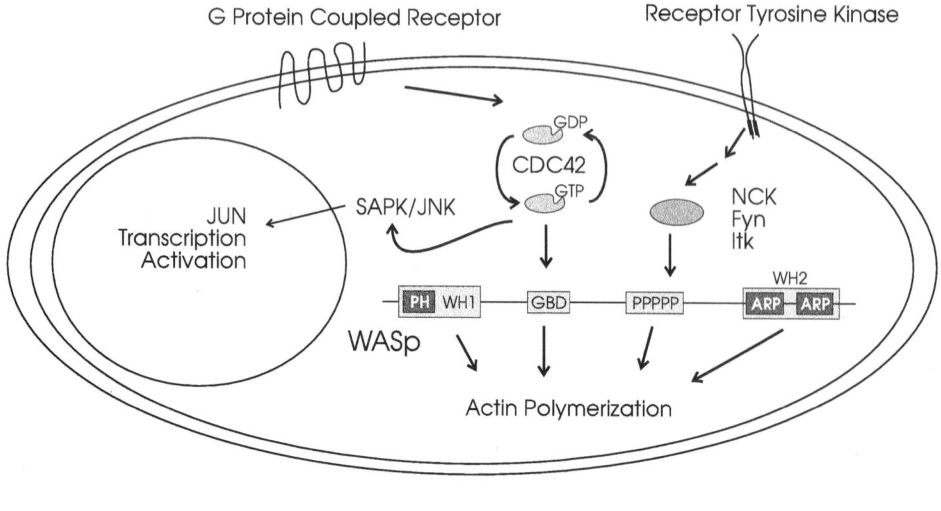

Fig. 185-10 WASP protein domains and interactions. WASP acts as a signal transducer for various cell surface receptors to affect actin polymerization in the cell. PH = pleckstrin homology domain; WH1 = WASP homology domain 1; GBD = GTP binding protein interaction domain; PPPP = proline rich domain; WH2 = WASP homology domain 2 including actin-regulating protein domains (ARP).

defect has not yet been demonstrated in WAS cells, however. How these functions are related to the complex phenotype of WAS remains somewhat of a puzzle. Female carriers of WASP mutations have preferential usage of the X chromosome with the normal allele active in all peripheral blood cells.[434] This demonstrates that WASP plays an essential role in all mature hematopoietic cell types. WASP probably has a required function throughout hematopoietic development[489] as evidenced by the skewed X inactivation pattern observed in primitive bone marrow precursors from carrier females.[433,434] The defect in cellular immunity and T cell proliferation may be the consequence of abnormal signal transduction of required growth pathways.[490–496] The functional significance of abnormal lamellipodia on T cells is unclear, although it is very characteristic of the condition.[497] The dysgammaglobulinemia of WAS has typically been attributed to defects in T cell/B cell interaction, but the inferred B cell growth defect may also explain the poor humoral immune response.[498,499] Some insight can be derived from the unique mutations observed in patients with WAS. The PH/WH1 domains are required for the most important protein functions based on the observation of missense mutations in classic WAS patients within these domains.[500–507] More mild mutations correlate with isolated platelet defect causing the X-linked thrombocytopenia.[508–513] Correlation of mutations with phenotype indicates that patients bearing missense mutations in the WH1 domain may have mild disease. All mutations associated with mild phenotype involve splicing or missense mutations,[501,504] resulting in production of a normal-sized protein or slightly truncated protein. Most other mutations lead to severe WAS.

DISORDERS OF LYMPHOCYTE REGULATION OR APOPTOSIS

Autoimmunity in Inherited Disorders of Lymphocyte Regulation

Immunodeficiency disorders have traditionally been thought of as conditions resulting from the inability to mount effective host responses to infectious agents. However immune dysregulation and autoimmune phenomena are commonly seen both in acquired immunodeficiency syndromes, such as AIDS, and in several primary inherited disorders.[514] Particular alleles of the class I and class II MHC loci are associated with increased susceptibility to a variety of diseases with an autoimmune basis, such as insulin-dependent diabetes mellitus and celiac disease.[515–517] While the exact mechanisms leading to development of immune reactions against one's own tissues are not understood, the selection of lymphocyte repertoire in the thymus, defined in part by the MHC genotype, can confer the potential for cross-reactivity between self-antigens in the tissues and foreign antigens from the environment. Genetic loci other than MHC are now being mapped and identified as important contributors that cooperate with permissive MHC alleles to produce autoimmune diseases with complex inheritance. In addition, immune disorders with Mendelian inheritance are now recognized in which autoimmunity, caused by disruption of lymphocyte regulation, predominates over infectious diathesis due to immunodeficiency. These diseases include autoimmune lymphoproliferative syndrome (ALPS), autoimmune polyendocrinopathy with candidiasis and ectodermal dystrophy (APECED), and IL-2 receptor β-chain deficiency.

After maturation, lymphocytes undergo a life cycle of activation, proliferation, and effector responses followed by apoptosis, or programmed cell death. Apoptosis refers to a characteristic sequence of cellular events including rapid membrane permeabilization; exposure of proteins not normally detectable at the cell surface; DNA cleavage between nucleosome units into fragments of assorted sizes, visible on electrophoresis gels as "ladders"; condensation and segmentation of nuclei; and shedding of nuclear particles encased in membrane, which are rapidly phagocytosed by macrophages.[518,519] Apoptosis, in contrast to necrosis, the other major physiological mechanism for removal of cells in the body, does not incite local inflammation. In the immune system, apoptosis maintains immune homeostasis by limiting lymphocyte accumulation, thus minimizing potential reactions against self-antigens. A major apoptosis pathway for mature lymphocytes involves the cell surface receptor CD95, also known as Fas or APO-1, encoded by the tumor necrosis factor receptor superfamily member 6, gene (*TNFRSF6*; formerly apoptosis antigen 1 or *APT1)* on human chromosome 10q23 (MIM 134673). After lymphocytes have been activated and are proliferating, a second encounter with antigen induces expression of both the transmembrane receptor CD95/Fas and its ligand, CD95 ligand (CD95L) or Fas ligand (FasL). FasL, which occurs in membrane-bound and secreted forms, self-associates into homotrimers with a conical configuration to become functionally active. The FasL trimeric complex engages three Fas molecules that extend and embrace the ligand by means of their extracellular projections. Extracellular engagement of a trimer of FasL with homotrimeric Fas triggers a series of intracellular molecular interactions including recruitment of FADD (Fas-associated death-domain protein) to the Fas trimer complex, activation of a cascade of proteases called caspases, and, ultimately, execution of the apoptosis program.[520]

Fas and FasL are members of two superfamilies of receptors and ligands that play important roles in immune regulation.[518] Fas is a member of the tumor necrosis factor receptor (TNFR) gene family. These membrane-spanning proteins contain variable numbers of conserved extracellular cysteine-rich domains (CRDs). Fas, TNFR-1, and additional recently discovered related proteins also share an intracellular region of homology known as the "death domain," required for communicating intracellular signals for programmed cell death.

The in vivo importance of the Fas apoptosis pathway in maintaining lymphocyte homeostasis was first appreciated in mice with *lpr* and *gld* mutations, which are genetic defects in Fas and FasL expression, respectively.[518,521,522] Mice with these mutations develop lymphoproliferation, autoantibodies, and autoimmune nephritis and arthritis.[523,524] They also have a characteristic expansion of a normally rare subset of T cells that have $\alpha\beta$ TCR, but which do not express either CD4 or CD8 surface antigens (designated double-negative T cells or DNT). In 1992, Sneller et al. described two children with massive, chronic, nonmalignant hyperplasia of spleen and lymph nodes, autoimmune disease, and elevated numbers of double-negative T cells.[525] Subsequently, Rieux-Laucat et al.[526] and Fisher et al.[527] documented that this disorder is associated with inherited mutations in the *TNFRSF6* gene, which encodes CD95/Fas. The syndrome known as autoimmune lymphoproliferative syndrome (ALPS), also called lymphoproliferative syndrome with autoimmunity or Canale-Smith syndrome, has now been reported in over 50 patients from the U.S., Europe, and Japan.[528–534] However, children with idiopathic lymphadenopathy, splenomegaly, and autoimmune phenomena have been described in the literature for at least four decades.[535–539] Several of these individuals are likely to have been suffering from ALPS, and in some cases, ALPS was proved retrospectively by detection of mutations in *TNFRSF6*.[528]

ALPS (Table 185-2) is a disorder with defective lymphocyte apoptosis in which patients manifest chronic, nonmalignant lymphadenopathy, and splenomegaly along with expansion of double-negative T cells in peripheral blood and lymphoid organs. Autoimmune phenomena, including significant titers of autoantibodies and/or overt autoimmune disease are documented in nearly all patients at some point in time. Most patients with ALPS have deleterious mutations in *TNFRSF6*. The great majority of patients have heterozygous mutations resulting in production of a defective Fas protein that can interfere in a dominant manner with apoptosis via normal Fas. Rare, severely affected patients, including one of the original subjects reported,[540] have recessive mutations with complete loss of Fas expression. A few more recently studied patients with ALPS have not had Fas defects, suggesting that

Table 185-2 Genetic Basis of Cellular Immune Deficiencies

Disorder	Gene	Map	Immunophenotype	Other Manifestations
V(D)J Recombination				
SCID or Ommen syndrome	*RAG1*	11p13	T^-B^- or $T\pm\downarrow B\pm\downarrow$	Hypomorphic mutations produce Ommen syndrome
	RAG2	11p13		
CID with complex phenotypes	*ATM*	11q22.3	$T\downarrow B^+$	Neurologic, teleangiectasia
	NIBRIN/p95	8q21	$T\downarrow B^+$	Chromosome instability, malignancy
	BLM	15q26.1	$T\downarrow B^+$	Chromosome instability, malignancy
TCR signal transduction				
Combined immunodeficiency	*CD3G*	11q23	$T\downarrow B^+$, CD3 $\downarrow$	
	CD3E	11q23	$T\downarrow B^+$, CD3 $\downarrow$	
	LCK	1p35	$CD4^-$, $CD8^+$;	
	ZAP70	2q12	$CD4^+$, $CD8^-$	
Antigen presentation				
Bare lymphocyte syndrome type I BLSI	*TAP1*	6p21.3	T^+B^+	Sinopulmonary infections with bronchiectasis
	TAP2	6p21.3	T^+B^+	
BLS II and BLS III A	*CIITA*	16p13	T^+B^+CD4 $\downarrow$	
B	*RFXANK*	19p12	T^+B^+ CD4 $\downarrow$	
C	*RFX5*	1q21.1	T^+B^+CD4 $\downarrow$	
D	*RFXAP*	13q14	T^+B^+, CD4 $\downarrow$	
Cytokine signal transduction				
SCID	*IL2RG*	Xq13	$T^-B^+NK^-$	
	IL7RA	5p13	$T^-B^+NK^+$	
	JAK3	19p13	$T^-B^+NK^-$	
Hyper IgM syndrome	*CD40L*	Xq26	T^+B^+	Elevated IgM, neutropenia
Familial atypical mycobacteriosis	*IFNGR2*	21q22	T^+B^+	Disseminated BCG, salmonellosis
	IFNGR1	6q23	T^+B^+	
	IL12RB1	19p13	T^+B^+	
	IL12B	5q31	T^+B^+	
Additional signal transduction				
X-linked lymphoproliferative syndrome	*SH2D1A*	Xq26	T^+B^+	Fulminant EBV infection, lymphoma
Wiskott-Aldrich syndrome	*WAS*	Xp11	$T\downarrow B^+$	Thrombocytopenia, eczema; isolated thrombocytopenia (XLT)
Apoptosis regulation				
Autoimmune lymphoproliferative syndrome (ALPS)	*APT1*	10q23	$\uparrow\uparrow\uparrow CD4^-CD8^-$	Splenic and lymph node hyperplasia
	Caspase 10	2q33		
Autoimmune polyendocrinopathy with candidiasis and ectodermal dystrophy (APECED)	*AIRE*	21q22		Multiple endocrine abnormalities, skin
	IL2RA	10p15	CD4 $\downarrow$, $CD25^-$	Lymphadenopathy, splenomegaly
Metabolic				
Adenosine deaminase	*ADA*	20q13.11	$T^-B\downarrow$	$\pm$ Skeletal dysplasia
Purine nuceloside phosphorylase	*NP*	14q13.1	T^-B^+	Developmental delay, hypotonia
Biotinidase	*BTD*	3p25	T^+B^+	Rash, acidosis, neurologic impairment
Holocarboxylase synthetase	*HLCS*	21q22.1	T^+B^+	
Methionine synthase (cb1G)	*MTR*	1q43	T^+B^+	Megaloblastic anemia, neurologic impairment
Orotic aciduria	*UMPS*	3q13	T^+B^+	
Thymus development				
DiGeorge syndrome	?	22q11del 10p13del	T^-B^+	Facial dysmorphism, cardiac defects, cleft palate, hypocalcemia
	WHN	17q11-q12	T^-B^-	Congenital alopecia, nail dystrophy, homolog of murine *nude*
Unclassified				
Immunodeficiency-centromeric instability-facial anomalies (ICF)	*DNMT3B*	20q11.2	T^+B^+	Abnormal centromeric chromatin condensation especially chr. 1, 9, 16
Reticular dysgenesis	?	?	T^-B^-	Congenital severe neutropenia
SCID with intestinal atresia	?	?	T^-B^-	
Cartilage hair hypoplasia	*CHH*	9q13	CD4$\pm\downarrow$	Short-limbed dwarfism, with fine hair
Athabascan SCID	*SCID-A*	10p12	T^-B^-	
Chronic mucocutaneous candidiasis	?	?	T^+B^+	

defects in other molecules in the apoptosis pathway may also cause ALPS.[541–543]

Clinical and laboratory features of patients with ALPS are shown in Table 185-3 and Table 185-4. Lymphoproliferation is the most dramatic and consistent feature of ALPS. Presentation with splenomegaly and adenopathy, often of massive proportions, occurs in infancy or early childhood. Splenectomy has been performed in the majority of patients because of hypersplenism. Almost all patients have experienced protracted periods of palpable, nontender lymph node enlargement, but the dimensions of the nodes have fluctuated, and they may regress through adolescence and adulthood. Histopathologic analysis of lymph nodes of patients affected with ALPS shows characteristic pathologic changes, first described by Sneller et al.[525] Although architecture is preserved, there is florid reactive follicular hyperplasia and marked paracortical expansion with immunoblasts and plasma cells. The features resemble those of viral lymphadenitis except for the conspicuous absence of histiocytes. The paracortical expansion is in some cases extensive enough to consider a differential diagnosis of immunoblastic lymphoma, with many cells expressing the Ki-67 antigen indicative of active proliferation.[544] Analysis of splenic tissue demonstrates lymphoid hyperplasia of the white pulp with histologic features similar to those of the lymph nodes. B cells expand the lymphoid follicles while T cells accumulate in the paracortical areas. Although many of the T cells in both spleen and lymph nodes are $CD4^+$ or $CD8^+$, a remarkable and characteristic feature of the lymphoid histology in ALPS is the abnormally large proportion of double-negative T cells in the paracortical areas.

Mild to moderate hepatomegaly is observed in the majority of patients at some point in time, and elevations of transaminases and cholesterol have occurred even in the absence of hepatitis C virus superinfection, which has complicated the course of some who have received blood transfusions. Although less common in humans, but regularly found in Fas-deficient mice, glomerulonephritis does occur, occasionally with renal compromise severe enough to require dialysis. Guillain-Barré polyneuroradiculitis without any recognized predisposing infectious illness has also been reported.[525] In addition, many patients suffer from urticarial rashes and nonspecific cutaneous vasculitis.

Autoimmunity in ALPS is largely directed against blood cells. Coombs-positive hemolytic anemia is most common followed by immune-mediated thrombocytopenia (ITP). Autoimmune neutropenia has been proven less frequently, possibly due to a lack of sensitive standardized tests. Episodes of hemolysis may be severe; many patients have at least one episode of hemoglobin level below 7 mg/dl. Similarly, platelet counts below 10,000/μl are seen in around half of the patients. Autoimmunity can be difficult to document. Not all patients are tested for all types of autoantibodies. Some patients manifest overt autoimmune phenomena

Table 185-3 Defining Features of Autoimmune Lymphoproliferative Syndrome (ALPS)

- I. Required
  - Nonmalignant lymphoproliferation
    - Chronic splenomegaly
    - Chronic noninfectious lymphadenopathy
  - Elevated numbers of $CD4^-/CD8^-$ T cells expressing α/β T cell receptors
    - Peripheral blood, > 1% of T cells
    - Lymphoid tissues
  - Defective lymphocyte apoptosis by *in vitro assay*
- II. Nearly universal
  - Autoimmunity, including one or more of
    - Autoimmune hemolytic anemia
    - Autoimmune thrombocytopenia
    - Autoimmune neutropenia
    - Other autoimmune manifestations
    - Autoantibodies, especially positive direct Coombs test
- III. Supporting
  - Positive family history of
    - Lymphoproliferation, with or without documented autoimmunity
    - B-cell lymphoma
  - Deleterious mutation of Fas
  - Deleterious mutation of caspase 10

Table 185-4 Features of Autoimmune Lymphoproliferative Syndrome*

Clinical Features	
Age of presentation	0–5 years; average 10 months
Sex	males and females
Lymphoproliferation	100%
Splenomegaly	100%
Splenectomy performed	74%
Hepatomegaly	67%
Documented lymph node enlargement	97%
Over Autoimmune Disease	87%
Hemolytic anemia	75%
Thrombocytopenia	54%
Neutropenia	46%
Glomerulonephritis	2 patients
Guillain-Barré syndrome	1 patients
Skin rashes, including urticaria, vasculitis	common
Malignancy	
B cell lymphoma	10%
Other types of malignancy reported; significance currently unclear	
Laboratory Findings	
Immunology	
Lymphocytes	
Impaired apoptosis of lymphocytes cultured in vitro with PHA and IL-2 and then exposed to anti-CD3 or anti-Fas antibodies	
Relative or absolute lymphocytosis involving both B and T cells	
Increased double negative T cells, specifically > 1% $\gamma\delta$ TCR $CD4^-/CD8^-$ cells	
Increased proportions of HLA DR^+ and $CD57^+$ T cells	
Granulocytes	
Neutropenia	
Eosinophilia	
Immunoglobulins	
Elevated levels of IgG, IgA, and/or IgM	
Poor and/or unsustained specific antibody responses to polysaccharide antigens (pneumococcal vaccines)	
Autoantibodies to	
Erythrocytes (direct Coombs)	
Platelets	
Neutrophils	
Phospholipids	
Smooth muscle	
Rheumatoid factor	
Antinuclear antigens	
Cytokines	
Elevated serum IL-10	
Hematology	
Anemia	
Hypersplenism	
Autoimmune hemolysis	
Iron deficiency	
Elevated vitamin B_{12} levels	

*Adapted from Jackson and Puck, 1999.[601]

only after many years of lymph node and spleen enlargement. For example, one patient first developed ITP at age 31, while another had autoimmune hemolysis for the first time at age 54.[544] Finally, in the absence of demonstrable antibodies, one cannot assign with certainty an immune basis for blood cytopenias in the setting of ongoing hypersplenism. Some patients, who were recognized because of their more severely affected sibs, failed to manifest overt autoimmune disease, but do have circulating autoantibodies.[529,540,545]

In some patients with ALPS, an incorrect diagnosis of lymphoreticular malignancy or premalignant state was made, leading in some cases to unwarranted cytotoxic chemotherapy. However, it is now clear that lymphoma can be a late complication of ALPS. B cell lymphomas have been documented in 5 of 192 individuals with Fas mutations who had ALPS or were related to a proband with ALPS, a rate about fifteenfold higher than that of the general population. Occurring between the ages of 16 and 50, these lymphomas included Burkitt's and Hodgkin's lymphomas as well as a histiocyte-rich T cell-rich large B cell lymphoma and an unusual variant of follicular B cell lymphoma. Somatic mutations of Fas have been noted in non-Hodgkin's lymphoma,[546] multiple myeloma,[547] and T cell leukemia,[548] consistent with the hypothesis that resistance to apoptotic elimination may contribute to malignant transformation of lymphocytes.

There is currently insufficient data to assess the risk of other types of malignancy in ALPS. One ALPS patient had hepatocellular carcinoma at age 43, in a setting of hepatitis C and previous cytotoxic chemotherapy for his adenopathy; another had multiple thyroid and breast adenomas and two basal cell carcinomas.[528]

Lymphocyte phenotyping demonstrating double-negative T cells provided the first clues as to the unique nature of ALPS. Unlike immature $CD4^-/CD8^-$ thymocytes, the double-negative T cells of ALPS, when isolated and studied in vitro, are poorly responsive and fail to produce IL-2, although they can produce IL-10.[531,549] They are, therefore, thought to represent a population of aged T cells that have escaped elimination by apoptosis, perhaps serving as a marker for the ALPS disease state rather than constituting a primary cause of autoimmunity. ALPS patients show other abnormalities in their immunologic profile, including a characteristic TH2-oriented cytokine profile, with increased in vitro release of TH2 cytokines IL-4, IL-5, and IL-10 (Table 185-3).[549] However, despite a dramatic, and at times alarming, degree of lymphoid organ enlargement, ALPS is characterized by surprisingly intact immunity.

Although symptoms of ALPS tend to abate in adolescence and adulthood, episodes of autoimmune disease can recur or arise unpredictably at any age.[528,545] Splenectomy has been required in some patients with ALPS because of hypersplenism, severe hemolysis, or refractory thrombocytopenia. However, the risk of splenectomy must be weighed against that of postsplenectomy sepsis, which has been documented in multiple ALPS patients despite prior administration of polysaccharide vaccines and prescription of prophylactic antibiotics.

Many patients with ALPS, even after splenectomy, suffer severe episodes of autoimmune hemolytic anemia, thrombocytopenia, and/or neutropenia requiring immunosuppressive therapy. Most episodes of ITP and some hemolytic crises respond to short courses of high-dose steroids.

In one patient with homozygous *TNFRSF61* mutation and complete Fas deficiency, ALPS manifestations were so severe that HLA haploidentical bone marrow transplantation was performed. There was no recurrence of lymphoproliferation or autoimmunity for over 3 years, although double-negative T cells persisted in the child's blood.[550] Clearly, the role of bone marrow transplantation is not well defined in ALPS, and this treatment should be considered only for severe, life-threatening complications.

By far the most common form of ALPS is that associated with heterozygous Fas defects; 75 percent of the *TNFRSF6* mutations causing ALPS are in the intracellular death domain encoded in *TNFRSF6* exon 9. The dominant interfering effect on apoptosis of Fas proteins with a death domain mutation has been demonstrated by in vitro apoptosis studies after cotransfection of mutant and wild-type cDNAs at varying ratios into a Fas-negative cell line.[527,533] The magnitude of the dominant interference is consistent with the model of Fas as a functional trimer in which a trimer complex containing one or two abnormal components will not transmit a death signal. Transfected *TNFRSF6* cDNAs bearing death domain mutations have a more profound inhibitory effect than those with extracellular mutations.[533,534]

Studies of family members of ALPS probands with defined mutations of *TNFRSF6* have revealed additional individuals who carry the same *TNFRSF6* mutations as ALPS probands.[526–529,531,545] Defective lymphocyte apoptosis is a dominant trait that segregates with *TNFRSF6* mutation in relatives of ALPS probands. Clinical and laboratory abnormalities of ALPS show a wide range of expressivity in mutation bearing relatives. Interestingly, both the penetrance of ALPS features and clinical morbidity are greater in kindreds in which *TNFRSF6* mutations lie in the intracellular death domain rather than the extracellular domains of Fas.[533,534] Nonetheless, variable penetrance and expression within kindreds strongly suggests that other genetic and/or environmental factors are important determinants of the ALPS phenotype. As is the case with humans, the expression of abnormalities in Fas-null mice with *lpr* mutation is strain dependent. For example, C57BL/6 mice with the *lpr* mutation have much less severe disease than MRL/*lpr* mice, and breeding studies have suggested loci that contribute additively to the autoimmune phenotypes.[551,552] These loci may encode members or regulators of apoptosis pathway proteins or may be other genes.

Finally, a minority of patients with ALPS, or very similar clinical syndromes, have no defects in Fas, and are presumed to have mutations in genes encoding other proteins involved in lymphocyte apoptosis.[531,541] A FasL defect, which could account for the autoimmune lymphoproliferation in some of these patients, as was shown in the *gld* mouse, has been reported in an adult with atypical lupus.[553] Another mechanism is the recently identified deficiency of caspase 10.[543] Caspases are cysteine proteases required for apoptosis. Wang et al.[543] described two families with ALPS type II (MIM 603909) each with independent missense mutations in Casp10 (MIM 601762, 2q33-q34). ALPS type II patients had hypergammaglobulinemia with multiple autoantibodies, adenopathy, splenomegaly, fever, and dramatically elevated immature $CD4^-CD8^-$ T cells. In one family, a missense mutation was dominant with much milder phenotypic effects in the mother, but in the second family, the parents were both heterozygous and normal, while the affected child was homozygous for the mutation.

Together, the studies of ALPS suggest that defects in apoptosis pathway proteins other than Fas, particularly downstream proteins and proteins in parallel pathways, might also contribute to a wider variety of syndromes with autoimmunity, lymphoproliferation, and malignancy.

Inherited Autoimmune Polyendocrinopathy and Candidiasis

Autoimmune polyendocrinopathy with candidiasis and ectodermal dystrophy (APECED) (MIM 240300) is a rare, fully penetrant, autosomal recessive condition.[554] In certain isolated populations, including Finns and Iranian Jews, an increased incidence of 1 in 25,000 to 1 in 9000, respectively, has been reported, presumably due to founder effects.[555,556] Starting in childhood, but continuing to progress throughout life, autoimmune diseases of one or more endocrine organs occur in virtually all affected individuals. Typical manifestations are hypoparathyroidism, adrenal cortical destruction, insulin-dependent diabetes from loss of pancreatic β cells, gonadal failure, hypogonadism, hypothyroidism, pernicious anemia due to loss of gastric parietal cells, and autoimmune hepatitis. Chronic mucocutaneous candidiasis is a regular feature of APECED, as is ectodermal dystrophy, manifested by alopecia, vitiligo, dystrophic dental enamel and nails, and keratopathy.[554] Although impaired cellular immunity is suggested by the susceptibility to candidiasis, no specific abnormalities of T cells other than somewhat reduced proliferative responses to mitogens have been found.[557] A wide range of autoantibodies occurs in the sera of patients with APECED.

Linkage studies in kindreds with APECED mapped the disorder to chromosome 21q22.3,[555] and positional cloning was used to identify the gene mutated in APECED, designated *AIRE* for autoimmune regulator.[557,558] *AIRE* encodes a peptide of 545 amino acids that belongs to the family of transcriptional activators that contain zinc finger domains of the PHD type (homologous to the polycomb gene of *Drosophila*), with high cysteine content. In addition to the common Finnish mutation, a premature termination R256X, additional APECED mutations have been reported in patients with German, Italian, Swiss, English, American, Canadian, and Finnish backgrounds.[557–561] *AIRE* mRNA is predominantly expressed in the thymus, and in mouse embryos is localized to a few cells in the thymic medulla,[562] suggesting that the APECED protein may be required for appropriate development of the T cell repertoire. The 58-kDa APECED protein contains a nuclear localizing signal and is expressed in nuclear-speckled domains in transfected cell lines, suggesting that it may be involved in the regulation of gene expression.[563,564] However, more work will be needed to determine what cellular functions the APECED protein is regulating and how its absence invariably leads to autoimmune disease.

Autoimmunity Caused by Lack of Interleukin-2 Receptor α Chain

Another immunodeficiency with more direct evidence of failure of thymic repertoire selection is the recently reported deficiency of IL-2 receptor α chain (IL2Rα) in the son of a marriage of first cousins.[565] Unlike typical SCID patients who generally present in the first months of life, this patient was diagnosed at 3 years of age to have more infections than normal, including chronic diarrhea and *Candida* esophagitis. He had normal IgG and IgM levels and peripheral blood T cell numbers in the low normal range, although his $CD4^+$ T cell count was reduced. He also had lymphadenopathy and hepatosplenomegaly. A thymus biopsy disclosed normal cellularity, but loss of corticomedullary distinction and absence of the CD1 staining normally found on cortical thymocytes. The antiapoptotic protein Bcl-2 was high throughout the thymus, rather than decreasing in the medullary areas thought to be the location where autoreactive cells are normally eliminated through programmed cell death. Dense lymphocytic infiltrates of gut, lung, and liver were found. The patient's lymphocytes lacked cell surface expression of IL2Rα, also known as CD25, due to a homozygous four base-pair deletion of nucleotides 60 to 64, early in the coding sequence of the *IL2RA* gene.

High affinity IL-2 receptor complexes are composed of IL2Rα along with the common γ chain and the IL-2 receptor β chain, both of which are also shared by the IL-15 receptor. While the β and γ chains are constitutively expressed throughout the T cell lineage, IL2Rα is found at only two stages—first, on early thymocytes, and then later on mature, peripheral T cells that have been stimulated. Failure to express IL2Rα, which confers one hundred-fold higher affinity for IL-2 than the $\beta\gamma$ form of the receptor, would be expected to blunt the proliferation of early thymocytes as well as peripheral lymphocytes, as has been shown in mice rendered deficient in IL2Rα by gene targeting.[566,567]

The T cells of the patient with IL2Rα deficiency were indeed unresponsive to exogenously added IL-2, undoubtedly contributing to his susceptibility to infections. However, his thymic histochemical abnormalities strongly suggested an additional defect in the process of thymic T cell repertoire selection, which normally involves intense early thymocyte proliferation followed by programmed destruction of thymocytes that are self-reactive. Lack of IL-2 responsiveness in early thymocytes could result in the survival and maturation of T cells with receptors capable of engaging self-determinants. Although the proliferative potential of these cells would be diminished by nonresponsiveness to IL-2, they might have participated in the extensive autoimmune tissue infiltration experienced by this patient. Another potential mechanism for the production of this patient's lymphocytic infiltrates is failure to remove autoimmune T cells in the periphery because of their IL-2 resistance; direct evidence for impaired peripheral deletion of activated T cells has been shown in the IL2Rα knockout mouse.[565]

Mice lacking the IL-2 receptor β chain (IL2Rβ) have also been constructed,[567] although no human disease has yet been identified to be caused by this genetic defect. Mice lacking IL2Rβ are similar to IL2Rα knockout mice in that they have mature T and B cells and seem to have more autoimmunity than susceptibility to infections. Their T cells are spontaneously activated, and organ infiltration, autoantibody production, and autoimmune anemia accompany defective T cell homeostasis.

UNCLASSIFIED SCID OR CELLULAR IMMUNE DEFICIENCIES

Reticular dysgenesis (MIM 267500) is a rare and extremely severe form of autosomal recessive SCID.[568,569] Newborns have both agranulocytosis and lymphopenia. Limited experience with transplantation could be consistent with primary defects in T lymphopoiesis and granulocytopoiesis, but a normal B cell lineage in these patients. SCID with intestinal atresia (MIM 243150) has been observed in two pedigrees,[571] which suggests autosomal recessive inheritance. Cartilage hair hypoplasia (CHH; MIM 250250) is a form of short-limbed dwarfism accompanied by fine, sparse, and light-colored hair.[571] Many, but not all, CHH patients have immunologic defects characterized by susceptibility to viral infections, lymphopenia, decreased $CD4^+$ cell count, and decreased $CD4^+/CD8^+$ ratio.[572,573] The B lymphocyte and natural killer cell count is usually normal. CHH patients may also have neutropenia and/or anemia, as well as increased risk for malignancy. The CHH gene maps to chromosome 9q13[574,575] and there is no evidence for genetic heterogeneity in either Finnish or Amish populations.[575] Athabascan SCID (SCID-A, MIM 602450) is a unique T^-B^- SCID observed in some Native American groups.[347] The incidence may be as high as 1 in 2000 live births among Navajo Indians. SCID-A maps to 10p with linkage disequilibrium spanning approximately 6.5 cM,[577] which is consistent with a single founder mutation of relatively recent origin. The occurrence of a common haplotype in the Dine, a distinct Athabascan group residing in the Canadian Northwest, suggests that a common mutant allele was present in the original population and has increased in frequency within the Southwest population. Chronic mucocutaneous candidiasis (MIM 114580 and MIM 212050) is a complex and heterogeneous disorder characterized by dermatophytosis, alopecia, loss of teeth, and recurrent viral infections. There may be nongenetic forms along with apparently dominant pedigrees.[578] Some individuals have total skin test anergy, while in others the defect seems restricted to response to *Candida*. A clinically distinctive form has been observed in French-Canadians and is possibly recessive.[579] This condition tends to be generally mild, but fatal *Candida* meningitis occurred in some affected individuals.

An unusual and variable immunodeficiency has been observed in association with centromeric instability of chromosomes 1, 9, and 16.[580] The karyotype may reveal increased mitotic recombination and occurrence of strange multibranched configurations. These children also have facial dysmorphism and developmental delay/mental retardation. IgA deficiency seems to be a consistent feature and alteration in cell-mediated immunity more variable. There are low numbers of T cells and decreased NK cells. Homozygosity mapping in families with a total of only four ICF patients localized the ICF syndrome gene to 20q11-q13.[581] By positional/candidate methods the gene, *DNMT3B*, was recently identified[582] and found to be a novel DNA cytosine-5-methyltransferase. The N-terminal region of DNMT3B contains a cysteine-rich domain closely related to the DNA helicase ATRX

(MIM 300032, associated with X-linked mental retardation with α-thalassemia). The pathophysiology of immune deficiency in ICF syndrome is unknown, but the known importance of local chromatin structure to V(D)J recombination suggests that process as a potential target. Dnmt3b-deficient mouse ES cells show abnormal *de novo* methylation and the null mutation is an embryonic lethal.[583]

Another rare SCID variant has been reported with an association of congenital alopecia, severe T^- cell immunodeficiency, and nail abnormalities. Two siblings had decreased mature $CD4^+$ T cells and mitogen induced proliferative responses.[584] Because the congenital alopecia suggested similarity to the classic mouse and rat *nude* mutations, the WHN gene was screened as a likely candidate. *nu/nu* animals have a severe ectodermal dysplasia with absent thymus. Analysis of the patients revealed a homozygous nonsense mutation in *WHN*, a winged helix transcription factor active in ectodermal derivatives and T cells.[585] One sib was treated successfully with bone marrow transplant consistent with defect intrinsic to the T cell lineage.

In addition to ADA and PNP deficiencies, several other metabolic disorders can be complicated by secondary T cell immune deficiency. These include orotic aciduria type I (MIM 258900, Chap. 113); biotinidase (MIM 253260) and holocarboxylase synthetase deficiencies (MIM 253270, Chap. 156), and possibly methionine synthase deficiency (cblG complementation group of homocystinuria, MIM 250940, Chap. 94 and Chap. 155). These conditions generally are accompanied by macrocytic anemia, neurologic symptoms, and/or dermatologic abnormalities. Because of available treatments, basic metabolic screening in any child with a suspected SCID is warranted.

PREVENTION AND TREATMENT

Prenatal diagnosis of SCID is best performed by specific mutation diagnosis of amniocyte or chorionic villus DNA if the genotype of a proband in the family is known.[586] When the genotype of a deceased proband is unknown, but the phenotype is well documented, fetal blood sampling has been successfully used in at-risk pregnancies. Low numbers of T cells and defective T cell blastogenic responses to mitogens can be definitively demonstrated in affected fetuses by week 17 of gestation.[587]

In one study of utilization of prenatal diagnosis for X-linked SCID, 93 percent of families at risk for having an affected pregnancy desired prenatal testing, whether or not termination of pregnancy was a consideration.[586] In only 2 instances of 13 affected male predictions, did parents choose pregnancy termination. Other families' prepared for optimal treatment of an affected newborn including selection of a BMT center, HLA testing of family members, and initiating a search for a matched unrelated donor for bone marrow. One family chose an experimental *in utero* BMT.[586]

The best current treatment for SCID is HLA-matched BMT.[589–593] Unfortunately, most patients lack a matched, related donor. Haploidentical, T-cell-depleted BMT has been quite successful.[593] Matched unrelated donor transplantation of marrow or cord blood stem cells has also been used. Infants transplanted immediately after birth are less likely to have serious pretransplant infections or failure to thrive. They also have more rapid engraftment, fewer posttransplant infections, and less graft versus host disease than those whose BMT is delayed.[593] Nevertheless, some posttransplant patients have graft versus host disease; many fail to make adequate antibodies and require long-term immunoglobulin replacement; and some develop autoimmune phenomena due to lymphocyte dysregulation. The oldest surviving individuals with SCID received HLA matched related BMT and are now in their twenties and in excellent health. As larger numbers of children are now growing up after BMT for SCID, study of very-long-term outcomes is possible.

The concept of prenatal treatment for XSCID has reemerged after initial low rates of success.[582,588] In two instances, fetuses affected with XSCID were infused intraperitoneally between 17 and 20 weeks of gestation with paternal, T-cell-depleted, or $CD34^+$-enriched paternal bone marrow cells. Infants were born with engrafted, functional T cells from their donors.

XSCID and JAK3 SCID also are promising candidate diseases for gene transfer therapy for several reasons. The success of BMT indicates that stem-cell correction should reverse the phenotype. Ubiquitous hematopoietic cell expression suggests that use of strong promotors in retroviral constructs may not be harmful. A natural in vivo selective advantage exists for lymphocytes expressing functional γc or JAK3, as illustrated by female carrier lymphocytes showing nonrandom X chromosome inactivation in XSCID and a natural reversion of a SCID-causing *IL2RG* mutation in T cells of one patient.[594] Retroviral correction of the defects in human cell lines[596,597] and mouse knockout models[598] has been successful. The major limitation of retroviral gene therapy in humans has been the poor efficiency of gene transduction into self-renewing bone marrow hematopoietic stem cell populations. Nonetheless, a preliminary report from Cavazzana-Calvo et al. indicates development of functional T cells in two infants with XSCID after retroviral transduction of their CD34+ bone marrow cells with a γc retrovirus.[599] Further new approaches offer considerable promise; for example, cytokine administration prior to stem-cell harvest has been shown to amplify the available stem cell pool for transduction by retroviruses.[600]

REFERENCES

1. Wiskott A: Familiarer, angeborener Morbus Werlhofii? *Mschr Kinderheilk* **68**:212, 1937.
2. Aldrich RA, Steinberg AG, Campbell DC: Pedigree demonstrating a sex-linked recessive condition characterized by draining ears, eczematoid dermatitis and bloody diarrhea. *Pediatrics* **13**:133, 1954.
3. Glanzman E, Riniker P: Essentielle Lymphocytophthises. Ein neues Krankheitsbildaus der Sauglings-pathologie. *Ann Pediatr (Basel)* **175**:1, 1950.
4. Tobler R, Cottier H: Familiäre Lymphopenie mit Agammaglobulinamie und schwerer moniliasis: die "essentielle Lymphocytophthises" al besondere Form der frühkindliehen Agammaglobulinämie. *Helv Pediatr Acta* **13**:313, 1958.
5. Gitlin D, Craig JM: The thymus and other lymphoid tissues in congenital agammaglubulinemia. I. Thymic alymphoplasia and lymphocytic hypoplasias and their relation to infection. *Pediatrics* **32**:517, 1963.
6. DiGeorge AM: A new concept of the cellular basis of immunity [Discussion]. *J Pediatr* **67**:907, 1965.
7. Giblett ER, Anderson JE, Cohen F, Pollara B, Meuwissen HJ: Adenosine-deaminase deficiency in two patients with severely impaired cellular immunity. *Lancet* **2(7786)**:1067, 1972.
8. Van Rood JJ, van Leeuwen A, Termitjelen A, Keuning JJ: The genetics of the major histocompatibility complex in man, in the role of the products of the histocompatibility gene complex, in Kåtz DH, Benacceraf B (eds): *Immune Responses*. New York, Academic Press, 1978, p 31.
9. Touraine JL, Betuel H, Souillet G, Jeune M: Combined immunodeficiency disease associated with absence of cell-surface HLA-A and -B antigens. *J Pediatr* **93(1)**:47, 1978.
10. Conley ME: Genetic effects on immunity new genes—How do they fit? *Curr Opin Immunol* **11(4)**:427, 1999.
11. Puck JM: Primary immunodeficiency diseases. *JAMA* **278(22)**:1835, 1997.
12. Lappalainen I, Ollila J, Smith CI, Vihinen M: Registries of immunodeficiency patients and mutations. *Hum Mutat* **10**:261, 1997.
13. Buckley RH, Schiff RI, Schiff SE, Markert ML, Williams LW, Harville TO, Roberts JL, Puck JM: Human severe combined immunodeficiency: Genetic, phenotypic, and functional diversity in one hundred eight infants. *J Pediatr* **130(3)**:378, 1997.
14. Berthet F, Le Deist F, Duliege AM, Griscelli C, Fischer A: Clinical consequences and treatment of primary immunodeficiency syndromes characterized by functional T and B lymphocyte anomalies (combined immune deficiency). *Pediatrics* **93**:265, 1994.
15. Stephan JL, Vlekova V, Le Deist F, Blanche S, Donadieu J, De Saint-Basile G, Durandy A, Griscelli C, Fischer A: Severe combined immunodeficiency: A retrospective single-center study of clinical presentation and outcome in 117 patients. *J Pediatr* **123**:564, 1993.

16. Elder ME: ZAP-70 and defects of T-cell receptor signaling. *Semin Hematol* **35(4)**:310, 1998.
17. Dawkins R, Leelayuwat C, Gaudieri S, Tay G, Hui J, Cattley S, Martinez P, Kulski J: Genomics of the major histocompatibility complex: Haplotypes, duplication, retroviruses and disease. *Immunol Rev* **167**:275, 1999.
18. Mach B: Genetics of histocompatibility. *Curr Opin Hematol* **1**:4, 1994.
19. Malissen B, Ardouin L, Lin SY, Gillet A, Malissen M: Function of the CD3 subunits of the pre-TCR and TCR complexes during T cell development. *Adv Immunol* **72**:103, 1999.
20. Konig R, Fleury S, Germain RN: The structural basis of CD4-MHC class II interactions: Coreceptor contributions to T cell receptor antigen recognition and oligomerization-dependent signal transduction. *Curr Top Microbiol Immunol* **205**:19, 1996.
21. Huang Z, Li S, Korngold R: Immunoglobulin superfamily proteins: Structure, mechanisms, and drug discovery. *Biopolymers* **43**:367, 1997.
22. Jones EY, Tormo J, Reid SW, Stuart DI: Recognition surfaces of MHC class I. *Immunol Rev* **163**:121, 1998.
23. Kaufman J, Salomonsen J, Flajnik M: Evolutionary conservation of MHC class I and class II molecules—Different yet the same. *Semin Immunol* **6**:411, 1994.
24. Garcia KC, Teyton L, Wilson IA: Structural basis of T cell recognition. *Annu Rev Immunol* **17**:369, 1999.
25. Bentley GA, Mariuzza RA: The structure of the T cell antigen receptor. *Annu Rev Immunol* **14**:563, 1996.
26. Grawunder U, West RB, Lieber MR: Antigen receptor gene rearrangement. *Curr Opin Immunol* **10**:172, 1998.
27. Rowen L, Koop BF, Hood L: The complete 685-kilobase DNA sequence of the human beta T cell receptor locus. *Science* **272(5269)**:1755, 1996.
28. Koop BF, Hood L: Striking sequence similarity over almost 100 kilobases of human and mouse T-cell receptor DNA. *Nat Genet* **7**:48, 1994.
29. Jouvin-Marche E, Hue I, Marche PN, Liebe-Gris C, Marolleau JP, Malissen B, Cazenave PA, Malissen M: Genomic organization of the mouse T cell receptor V alpha family. *EMBO J* **9**:2141, 1990.
30. Boysen C, Simon MI, Hood L: Analysis of the 1.1-Mb human alpha/delta T-cell receptor locus with bacterial artificial chromosome clones. *Genome Res* **7**:330, 1997.
31. Ibberson MR, Copier JP, So AK: Genomic organization of the human T-cell receptor variable alpha (TCRAV) gene cluster. *Genomics* **28**:131, 1995.
32. Willerford DM, Swat W, Alt FW: The origins of V(D)J recombination. *Curr Opin Genet Dev* **6(5)**:603, 1996.
33. Lewis SM, Wu GE: The origins of V(D)J recombination. *Cell* **88**:159, 1997.
34. Bernstein RM, Schluter SF, Bernstein H, Marchalonis JJ: Primordial emergence of the recombination activating gene 1 (RAG1): Sequence of the complete shark gene indicates homology to microbial integrases. *Proc Natl Acad Sci U S A* **93**:9454, 1996.
35. Schatz DG: Transposition mediated by RAG1 and RAG2 and the evolution of the adaptive immune system. *Immunol Res* **19**:169, 1999.
36. Rast JP, Litman GW: Towards understanding the evolutionary origins and early diversification of rearranging antigen receptors. *Immunol Rev* **166**:79, 1998.
37. Agrawal A, Eastman QM, Schatz DG: Transposition mediated by RAG1 and RAG2 and its implications for the evolution of the immune system. *Nature* **394**:744, 1998.
38. van Gent DC, Mizuuchi K, Gellert M: Similarities between initiation of V(D)J recombination and retroviral integration. *Science* **271**:1592, 1996.
39. Komori T, Okada A, Stewart V, Alt FW: Lack of N regions in antigen receptor variable region genes of TdT-deficient lymphocytes. *Science* **261(5125)**:1171, 1993.
40. Chen CH, Six A, Kubota T, Tsuji S, Kong FK, Gobel TW, Cooper MD: T cell receptors and T cell development. *Curr Top Microbiol Immunol* **212**:37, 1996.
41. Willerford DM, Swat W, Alt FW: Developmental regulation of V(D)J recombination and lymphocyte differentiation. *Curr Opin Genet Dev* **6**:603, 1996.
42. Itohara S, Mombaerts P, Lafaille J, Iacomini J, Nelson A, Clarke AR, Hooper ML, Farr A, Tonegawa S: T cell receptor delta gene mutant mice: Independent generation of alpha beta T cells and programmed rearrangements of gamma delta TCR genes. *Cell* **72**:337, 1993.
43. Barrett TA, Bluestone JA: Development of TCR gamma delta iIELs. *Semin Immunol* **7**:299, 1995.
44. Hayday AC, Hoffman ES, Douglas N: Signals involved in gamma/delta T cell versus alpha/beta T cell lineage commitment. *Semin Immunol* **11**:239, 1999.
45. Robey E, Fowlkes BJ: The alpha beta versus gamma delta T-cell lineage choice. *Curr Opin Immunol* **10**:181, 1998.
46. Gellert M: Recent advances in understanding V(D)J recombination. *Adv Immunol* **64**:39, 1997.
47. Bogue M, Roth DB: Mechanism of V(D)J recombination. *Curr Opin Immunol* **8**:175, 1996.
48. Aifantis I, Pivniouk VI, Gartner F, Feinberg J, Swat W, Alt FW, von Boehmer H, Geha RS: Allelic exclusion of the T cell receptor beta locus requires the SH2 domain-containing leukocyte protein (SLP)-76 adaptor protein. *J Exp Med* **190**:1093, 1999.
49. Aifantis I, Buer J, von Boehmer H, Azogui O: Essential role of the pre-T cell receptor in allelic exclusion of the T cell receptor beta locus. *Immunity* **7**:601, 1997.
50. O'Shea CC, Thornell AP, Rosewell IR, Hayes B, Owen MJ: Exit of the pre-TCR from the ER/cis-Golgi is necessary for signaling differentiation, proliferation, and allelic exclusion in immature thymocytes. *Immunity* **7**:591, 1997.
51. Xu Y, Davidson L, Alt FW, Baltimore D: Function of the pre-T-cell receptor alpha chain in T-cell development and allelic exclusion at the T-cell receptor beta locus. *Proc Natl Acad Sci U S A* **93**:2169, 1996.
52. Pivniouk V, Tsitsikov E, Swinton P, Rathbun G, Alt FW, Geha RS: Impaired viability and profound block in thymocyte development in mice lacking the adaptor protein SLP-76. *Cell* **94(2)**:229, 1998.
53. Alt FW, Oltz EM, Young F, Gorman J, Taccioli G, Chen J: VDJ recombination. *Immunol Today* **13(8)**:306, 1992.
54. Oettinger MA: Cutting apart V(D)J recombination. *Curr Opin Genet Dev* **6(2)**:141, 1996.
55. Steen SB, Zhu C, Roth DB: Double-strand breaks, DNA hairpins, and the mechanism of V(D)J recombination. *Curr Top Microbiol Immunol* **217**:61, 1996.
56. Ramsden DA, Paull TT, Gellert M: Cell-free V(D)J recombination. *Nature* **388**:488, 1997.
57. Schatz DG: V(D)J recombination moves in vitro. *Semin Immunol* **9**:149, 1997.
58. Ramsden DA, van Gent DC, Gellert M: Specificity in V(D)J recombination: New lessons from biochemistry and genetics. *Curr Opin Immunol* **9**:114, 1997.
59. Roth DB, Craig NL: VDJ recombination: A transposase goes to work. *Cell* **94(4)**:411, 1998.
60. Roth DB, Nakajima PB, Menetski JP, Bosma MJ, Gellert M: V(D)J recombination in mouse thymocytes: Double-strand breaks near T cell receptor delta rearrangement signals. *Cell* **69**:41, 1992.
61. Roth DB, Menetski JP, Nakajima PB, Bosma MJ, Gellert M: V(D)J recombination: Broken DNA molecules with covalently sealed (hairpin) coding ends in SCID mouse thymocytes. *Cell* **70**:983, 1992.
62. Roth DB, Zhu C, Gellert M: Characterization of broken DNA molecules associated with V(D)J recombination. *Proc Natl Acad Sci U S A* **90**:10788, 1993.
63. Zhu C, Roth DB: Characterization of coding ends in thymocytes of SCID mice: Implications for the mechanism of V(D)J recombination. *Immunity* **2**:101, 1995.
64. Steen SB, Gomelsky L, Speidel SL, Roth DB: Initiation of V(D)J recombination in vivo: Role of recombination signal sequences in formation of single and paired double-strand breaks. *EMBO J* **16(10)**:2656, 1997.
65. Lafaille JJ, DeCloux A, Bonneville M, Takagaki Y, Tonegawa S: Junctional sequences of T cell receptor gamma delta genes: Implications for gamma delta T cell lineages and for a novel intermediate of V-(D)-J joining. *Cell* **59**:859, 1989.
66. Schatz DG, Oettinger MA, Baltimore D: The V(D)J recombination activating gene, RAG-1. *Cell* **59**:1035, 1989.
67. Oettinger MA, Schatz DG, Gorka C, Baltimore D: RAG-1 and RAG-2, adjacent genes that synergistically activate V(D)J recombination. *Science* **248**:1517, 1990.
68. Mombaerts P, Iacomini J, Johnson RS, Herrup K, Tonegawa S, Papaioannou VE: RAG-1-deficient mice have no mature B and T lymphocytes. *Cell* **68**:869, 1992.
69. Shinkai Y, Rathbun G, Lam KP, Oltz EM, Stewart V, Mendelsohn M, Charron J, Datta M, Young F, Stall AM: RAG-2-deficient mice lack mature lymphocytes owing to inability to initiate V(D)J rearrangement. *Cell* **68**:855, 1992.
70. van Gent DC, Ramsden DA, Gellert M: The RAG1 and RAG2 proteins establish the 12/23 rule in V(D)J recombination. *Cell* **85**:107, 1996.

71. Eastman QM, Leu TM, Schatz DG: Initiation of V(D)J recombination *in vitro* obeying the 12/23 rule. *Nature* **380**:85, 1996.
72. Sawchuk DJ, Weis-Garcia F, Malik S, Besmer E, Bustin M, Nussenzweig MC, Cortes P: V(D)J recombination: Modulation of RAG1 and RAG2 cleavage activity on 12/23 substrates by whole cell extract and DNA-bending proteins. *J Exp Med* **185(11)**:2025, 1997.
73. West RB, Lieber MR: The RAG-HMG1 complex enforces the 12/23 rule of V(D)J recombination specifically at the double-hairpin formation step. *Mol Cell Biol* **18**:6408, 1998.
74. Hiom K, Gellert M: Assembly of a 12/23 paired signal complex: A critical control point in V(D)J recombination. *Mol Cell* **1**:1011, 1998.
75. Leu TM, Schatz DG: rag-1 and rag-2 are components of a high-molecular-weight complex, and association of rag-2 with this complex is rag-1 dependent. *Mol Cell Biol* **15**:5657, 1995.
76. Agrawal A, Schatz DG: RAG1 and RAG2 form a stable postcleavage synaptic complex with DNA containing signal ends in V(D)J recombination. *Cell* **89**:43, 1997.
77. Eastman QM, Schatz DG: Nicking is asynchronous and stimulated by synapsis in 12/23 rule-regulated V(D)J cleavage. *Nucleic Acids Res* **25**:4370, 1997.
78. Eastman QM, Villey IJ, Schatz DG: Detection of RAG protein-V(D)J recombination signal interactions near the site of DNA cleavage by UV cross-linking. *Mol Cell Biol* **19**:3788, 1999.
79. Kabotyanski EB, Zhu C, Kallick DA, Roth DB: Hairpin opening by single-strand-specific nucleases. *Nucleic Acids Res* **23**:3872, 1995.
80. Shockett PE, Schatz DG: DNA hairpin opening mediated by the RAG1 and RAG2 proteins. *Mol Cell Biol* **19**:4159, 1999.
81. Besmer E, Mansilla-Soto J, Cassard S, Sawchuk DJ, Brown G, Sadofsky M, Lewis SM, Nussenzweig MC, Cortes P: Hairpin coding end opening is mediated by RAG1 and RAG2 proteins. *Mol Cell Biol* **2**:817, 1998.
82. Li W, Swanson P, Desiderio S: RAG-1 and RAG-2-dependent assembly of functional complexes with V(D)J recombination substrates in solution. *Mol Cell Biol* **17(12)**:6932, 1997.
83. Nagawa F, Ishiguro K, Tsuboi A, Yoshida T, Ishikawa A, Takemori T, Otsuka AJ, Sakano H: Footprint analysis of the RAG protein recombination signal sequence complex for V(D)J type recombination. *Mol Cell Biol* **18(1)**:655, 1998.
84. Jeggo PA: DNA breakage and repair. *Adv Genet* **38**:185, 1998.
85. Jeggo PA: Identification of genes involved in repair of DNA double-strand breaks in mammalian cells. *Radiat Res* **150**:S80, 1998.
86. Difilippantonio MJ, McMahan CJ, Eastman QM, Spanopoulou E, Schatz DG: RAG1 mediates signal sequence recognition and recruitment of RAG2 in V(D)J recombination. *Cell* **87**:253, 1996.
87. Bellon SF, Rodgers KK, Schatz DG, Coleman JE, Steitz TA: Crystal structure of the RAG1 dimerization domain reveals multiple zinc-binding motifs including a novel zinc binuclear cluster. *Nat Struct Biol* **4**:586, 1997.
88. Steen SB, Han JO, Mundy C, Oettinger MA, Roth DB: Roles of the "dispensable" portions of RAG-1 and RAG-2 in V(D)J recombination. *Mol Cell Biol* **19**:3010, 1999.
89. McBlane JF, van Gent DC, Ramsden DA, Romeo C, Cuomo CA, Gellert M, Oettinger MA: Cleavage at a V(D)J recombination signal requires only RAG1 and RAG2 proteins and occurs in two steps. *Cell* **83**:387, 1995.
90. Leu TM, Eastman QM, Schatz DG: Coding joint formation in a cell-free V(D)J recombination system. *Immunity* **7**:303, 1997.
91. Akamatsu Y, Oettinger MA: Distinct roles of RAG1 and RAG2 in binding the V(D)J recombination signal sequences. *Mol Cell Biol* **18**:4670, 1998.
92. Aidinis V, Bonaldi T, Beltrame M, Santagata S, Bianchi ME, Spanopoulou E: The RAG1 homeodomain recruits HMG1 and HMG2 to facilitate recombination signal sequence binding and to enhance the intrinsic DNA-bending activity of RAG1-RAG2. *Mol Cell Biol* **19**:6532, 1999.
93. Melek M, Gellert M, van Gent DC: Rejoining of DNA by the RAG1 and RAG2 proteins. *Science* **280**:301, 1998.
94. Weis-Garcia F, Besmer E, Sawchuk DJ, Yu W, Hu Y, Cassard S, Nussenzweig MC, Cortes P: V(D)J recombination: In vitro coding joint formation. *Mol Cell Biol* **17**:6379, 1997.
95. Smider V, Chu G: The end-joining reaction in V(D)J recombination. *Semin Immunol* **9**:189, 1997.
96. Gao Y, Sun Y, Frank KM, Dikkes P, Fujiwara Y, Seidl KJ, Sekiguchi JM, Rathbun GA, Swat W, Wang J, Bronson RT, Malynn BA, Bryans M, Zhu C, Chaudhuri J, Davidson L, Ferrini R, Stamato T, Orkin SH, Greenberg ME, Alt FW: A critical role for DNA end-joining proteins in both lymphogenesis and neurogenesis. *Cell* **95**:891, 1998.
97. Roth DB, Nakajima PB, Menetski JP, Bosma MJ, Gellert M: Double-strand breaks associated with V(D)J recombination at the TCR delta locus in murine thymocytes. *Curr Top Microbiol Immunol* **182**:115, 1992.
98. Kim DR, Oettinger MA: Functional analysis of coordinated cleavage in V(D)J recombination. *Mol Cell Biol* **18**:4679, 1998.
99. Errami A, Smider V, Rathmell WK, He DM, Hendrickson EA, Zdzienicka MZ, Chu G: Ku86 defines the genetic defect and restores X-ray resistance and V(D)J recombination to complementation group 5 hamster cell mutants. *Mol Cell Biol* **16**:1519, 1996.
100. Taccioli GE, Gottlieb TM, Blunt T, Priestley A, Demengeot J, Mizuta R, Lehmann AR, Alt FW, Jackson SP, Jeggo PA: Ku80: Product of the XRCC5 gene and its role in DNA repair and V(D)J recombination. *Science* **265**:1442, 1994.
101. Tuteja N, Tuteja R, Ochem A, Taneja P, Huang NW, Simoncsits A, SusicS, Rahman K, Marusic L, Chen J, Zhang J, Wang S, Pongor S, Falaschi A: Human DNA helicase II: A novel DNA unwinding enzyme identified as the Ku autoantigen. *EMBO J* **13**:4991, 1994.
102. Han JO, Steen SB, Roth DB: Ku86 is not required for protection of signal ends or for formation of nonstandard V(D)J recombination products. *Mol Cell Biol* **17**:2226, 1997.
103. Mahajan KN, Gangi-Peterson L, Sorscher DH, Wang J, Gathy KN, Mahajan NP, Reeves WH, Mitchell BS: Association of terminal deoxynucleotidyl transferase with Ku. *Proc Natl Acad Sci U S A* **96**:13926, 1999.
104. Bogue MA, Wang C, Zhu C, Roth DB: V(D)J recombination in Ku86-deficient mice: Distinct effects on coding, signal, and hybrid joint formation. *Immunity* **7**:37, 1997.
105. Zhu C, Bogue MA, Lim DS, Hasty P, Roth DB: Ku86-deficient mice exhibit severe combined immunodeficiency and defective processing of V(D)J recombination intermediates. *Cell* **86**:379, 1996.
106. Takiguchi Y, Kurimasa A, Chen F, Pardington PE, Kuriyama T, Okinaka RT, Moyzis R, Chen DJ: Genomic structure and chromosomal assignment of the mouse Ku70 gene. *Genomics* **35**:129, 1996.
107. Gu Y, Seidl KJ, Rathbun GA, Zhu C, Manis JP, van der Stoep N, Davidson L, Cheng HL, Sekiguchi JM, Frank K, Stanhope-Baker P, Schlissel MS, Roth DB, Alt FW: Growth retardation and leaky SCID phenotype of Ku70-deficient mice. *Immunity* **7**:653, 1997.
108. Ouyang H, Nussenzweig A, Kurimasa A, Soares VC, Li X, Cordon-Cardo C, Li Wh, Cheong N, Nussenzweig M, Iliakis G, Chen DJ, Li GC: Ku70 is required for DNA repair but not for T cell antigen receptor gene recombination in vivo. *J Exp Med* **186**:921, 1997.
109. Martin SG, Laroche T, Suka N, Grunstein M, Gasser SM: Relocalization of telomeric Ku and SIR proteins in response to DNA strand breaks in yeast. *Cell* **97**:621, 1999.
110. Guarente L: Diverse and dynamic functions of the sir silencing complex. *Nat Genet* **23(3)**:281, 1999.
111. Laroche T, Martin SG, Gotta M, Gorham HC, Pryde FE, Louis EJ, Gasser SM: Mutation of yeast Ku genes disrupts the subnuclear organization of telomeres. *Curr Biol* **8**:653, 1998.
112. Han JO, Erskine LA, Purugganan MM, Stamato TD, Roth DB: V(D)J recombination intermediates and non-standard products in XRCC4-deficient cells. *Nucleic Acids Res* **26**:3769, 1998.
113. Li Z, Otevrel T, Gao Y, Cheng H-L, Seed B, Stamato TD, Taccioli GE, Alt FW: The XRCC4 gene encodes a novel protein involved in DNA double-strand break repair and V(D)J recombination. *Cell* **83**:1079, 1995.
114. Critchlow SE, Bowater RP, Jackson SP: Mammalian DNA double-strand break repair protein XRCC4 interacts with DNA ligase IV. *Curr Biol* **7**:588, 1997.
115. Grawunder U, Zimmer D, Fugmann S, Schwarz K, Lieber MR: DNA ligase IV is essential for V(D)J recombination and DNA double-strand break repair in human precursor lymphocytes. *Mol Cell* **2**:477, 1998.
116. Grawunder U, Zimmer D, Kulesza P, Lieber MR: Requirement for an interaction of XRCC4 with DNA ligase IV for wild-type V(D)J recombination and DNA double-strand break repair in vivo. *J Biol Chem* **273**:24708, 1998.
117. Frank KM, Sekiguchi JM, Seidl KJ, Swat W, Rathbun GA, Cheng HL, Davidson L, Kangaloo L, Alt FW: Late embryonic lethality and impaired V(D)J recombination in mice lacking DNA ligase IV. *Nature* **396**:173, 1998.
118. Riballo E, Critchlow SE, Teo SH, Doherty AJ, Priestley A, Broughton B, Kysela B, Beamish H, Plowman N, Arlett CF, Lehmann AR, Jackson SP, Jeggo PA: Identification of a defect in DNA ligase IV in a radiosensitive leukaemia patient. *Curr Biol* **9**:699, 1999.
119. Zhang X, Morera S, Bates PA, Whitehead PC, Coffer AI, Hainbucher K, Nash RA, Sternberg MJ, Lindahl T, Freemont PS: Structure of an

XRCC1 BRCT domain: A new protein-protein interaction module. *EMBO J* **17**:6404, 1998.
120. Grawunder U, Zimmer D, Leiber MR: DNA ligase IV binds to XRCC4 via a motif located between rather than within its BRCT domains. *Curr Biol* **8**:873, 1998.
121. Fujimori A, Araki R, Fukumura R, Saito T, Mori M, Mita K, Tatsumi K, Abe M: The murine DNA-PKcs gene consists of 86 exons dispersed in more than 250 kb. *Genomics* **45**:194, 1997.
122. Singleton BK, Torres-Arzayus MI, Rottinghaus ST, Taccioli GE, Jeggo PA: The C terminus of Ku80 activates the DNA-dependent protein kinase catalytic subunit. *Mol Cell Biol* **19**:3267, 1999.
123. Chan DW, Ye R, Veillette CJ, Lees-Miller SP: DNA-dependent protein kinase phosphorylation sites in Ku 70/80 heterodimer. *Biochemistry* **38**:1819, 1999.
124. Kirchgessner CU, Patil CK, Evans JW, Cuomo CA, Fried LM, Carter T, Oettinger MA, Brown JM: DNA-dependent kinase (p350) as a candidate gene for the murine SCID defect. *Science* **267**:1178, 1995.
125. Blunt T, Gell D, Fox M, Taccioli GE, Lehmann AR, Jackson SP, Jeggo PA: Identification of a nonsense mutation in the carboxyl-terminal region of DNA-dependent protein kinase catalytic subunit in the SCID mouse. *Proc Natl Acad Sci U S A* **93**:10285, 1996.
126. Araki R, Fujimori A, Hamatani K, Mita K, Saito T, Mori M, Fukumura R, Morimyo M, Muto M, Itoh M, Tatsumi K, Abe M: Nonsense mutation at Tyr-4046 in the DNA-dependent protein kinase catalytic subunit of severe combined immune deficiency mice. *Proc Natl Acad Sci U S A* **94**:2438, 1997.
127. Gao Y, Chaudhuri J, Zhu C, Davidson L, Weaver DT, Alt FW: A targeted DNA-PKcs-null mutation reveals DNA-PK-independent functions for KU in V(D)J recombination. *Immunity* **9**:367, 1998.
128. Jhappan C, Morse HC 3rd, Fleischmann RD, Gottesman MM, Merlino G: DNA-PKcs: A T-cell tumour suppressor encoded at the mouse SCID locus. *Nat Genet* **17**:483, 1997.
129. Taccioli GE, Amatucci AG, Beamish HJ, Gell D, Xiang XH, Torres Arzayus MI, Priestley A, Jackson SP, Marshak Rothstein A, Jeggo PA, Herrera VL: Targeted disruption of the catalytic subunit of the DNA-PK gene in mice confers severe combined immunodeficiency and radiosensitivity. *Immunity* **9**:355, 1998.
130. Wiler R, Leber R, Moore BB, VanDyk LF, Perryman LE, Meek K: Equine severe combined immunodeficiency: A defect in V(D)J recombination and DNA-dependent protein kinase activity. *Proc Natl Acad Sci U S A* **92(25)**:11485, 1995.
131. Shin EK, Perryman LE, Meek K: A kinase-negative mutation of DNA-PK(CS) in equine SCID results in defective coding and signal joint formation. *J Immunol* **158(8)**:3565, 1997.
132. Bogue MA, Jhappan C, Roth DB: Analysis of variable (diversity) joining recombination in DNA-dependent protein kinase (DNA-PK)-deficient mice reveals DNA-PK-independent pathways for both signal and coding joint formation. *Proc Natl Acad Sci U S A* **95**:15559, 1998.
133. Hsieh CL, Arlett CF, Lieber MR: V(D)J recombination in ataxia telangiectasia, Bloom's syndrome, and a DNA ligase I-associated immunodeficiency disorder. *J Biol Chem* **268**:20105, 1993.
134. Xu Y, Ashley T, Brainerd EE, Bronson RT, Meyn MS, Baltimore D: Targeted disruption of ATM leads to growth retardation, chromosomal fragmentation during meiosis, immune defects, and thymic lymphoma. *Genes Dev* **10**:2411, 1996.
135. Ellis NA, Groden J, Ye T-Z, Straughen J, Lennon DJ, Ciocci S, Proytcheva M, German J: The Bloom's syndrome gene product is homologous to RecQ helicases. *Cell* **83**:655, 1995.
136. Varon R, Vissinga C, Platzer M, Cerosaletti KM, Chrzanowska KH, Saar K, Beckmann G, Seemanova E, Cooper PR, Nowak NJ, Stumm M, Weemaes CMR, Gatti RA, Wilson RK, Digweed M, Rosenthal A, Sperling K, Concannon P, Reis A: Nibrin, a novel DNA double-strand break repair protein, is mutated in Nijmegen breakage syndrome. *Cell* **93**:467, 1998.
137. Carney JP, Maser RS, Olivares H, Davis EM, Le Beau M, Yates JR, Hays L, Morgan WF, Petrini JHJ: The hMre11/hRad50 protein complex and Nijmegen breakage syndrome: Linkage of double-strand break repair to the cellular DNA damage response. *Cell* **93**:477, 1998.
138. Han JO, Steen SB, Roth DB: Intermolecular V(D)J recombination is prohibited specifically at the joining step. *Mol Cell* **3**:331, 1999.
139. Hiom K, Melek M, Gellert M: DNA transposition by the RAG1 and RAG2 proteins: A possible source of oncogenic translocations. *Cell* **94**:463, 1998.
140. Danska JS, Guidos CJ: Essential and perilous: V(D)J recombination and DNA damage checkpoints in lymphocyte precursors. *Semin Immunol* **9**:199, 1997.
141. Vanasse GJ, Halbrook J, Thomas S, Burgess A, Hoekstra MF, Disteche CM, Willerford DM: Genetic pathway to recurrent chromosome translocations in murine lymphoma involves V(D)J recombinase. *J Clin Invest* **103**:1669, 1999.
142. Morrison C, Smith GC, Stingl L, Jackson SP, Wagner EF, Wang ZQ: Genetic interaction between PARP and DNA-PK in V(D)J recombination and tumorigenesis. *Nat Genet* **17**:479, 1997.
143. Lam KP, Kuhn R, Rajewsky K: In vivo ablation of surface immunoglobulin on mature B cells by inducible gene targeting results in rapid cell death. *Cell* **90**:1073, 1997.
144. Bories JC, Demengeot J, Davidson L, Alt FW: Gene-targeted deletion and replacement mutations of the T-cell receptor beta-chain enhancer: The role of enhancer elements in controlling V(D)J recombination accessibility. *Proc Natl Acad Sci U S A* **93**:7871, 1996.
145. Turner M, Mee PJ, Costello PS, Williams O, Price AA, Duddy LP, Furlong MT, Geahlen RL, Tybulewicz VL: Perinatal lethality and blocked B-cell development in mice lacking the tyrosine kinase Syk. *Nature* **378**:298, 1995.
146. Kitamura D, Kudo A, Schaal S, Muller W, Melchers F, Rajewsky K: A critical role of lambda 5 protein in B cell development. *Cell* **69**:823, 1992.
147. Molina TJ, Kishihara K, Siderovski DP, van Ewijk W, Narendran A, Timms E, Wakeham A, Paige CJ, Hartmann KU, Veillette A: Profound block in thymocyte development in mice lacking p56lck. *Nature* **357**:161, 1992.
148. Schwarz K, Gauss, G H, Ludwig L, Pannicke U, Li Z, Linder D, Friedrich W, Seger RA, Hansen-Hagge TE, Desiderio S, Lieber MR, Bartram CR: RAG mutations in human B cell-negative SCID. *Science* **274**:97, 1996.
149. Barth RF, Khurana SK, Vergara GG, Lowman JT, Beckwith JB: Rapidly fatal familial histiocytosis associated with eosinophilia and primary immunological deficiency. *Lancet* **II**:503, 1972.
150. de Saint-Basile G, Le Deist F, de Villartay J-P, Cerf-Bensussan N, Journet O, Brousse N, Griscelli C, Fischer A: Restricted heterogeneity of T lymphocytes in combined immunodeficiency with hypereosinophilia (Omenn's syndrome). *J Clin Invest* **87**:1352, 1991.
151. Gomez L, Le Deist F, Blanche S, Cavazzana-Calvo M, Griscelli C, Fischer A: Treatment of Omenn syndrome by bone marrow transplantation. *J Pediat* **127**:76, 1995.
152. Schwarz K, Notarangelo LD, Spanopoulou E, Vezzoni P, Villa A: Recombination defects, in Ochs HD, Smith CIE, Puck JM (eds): *Primary Immunodeficiency Diseases: A Molecular and Genetic Approach*. New York, Oxford University Press, 1999, p 155.
153. Omenn GS: Familial reticuloendotheliosis with eosinophilia. *N Engl J Med* **273**:427, 1965.
154. Melamed I, Cohen A, Roifman CM: Expansion of $CD3^{+}CD4^{-}CD8^{-}$ T cell population expressing high levels of IL-5 in Omenn's syndrome. *Clin Exp Immunol* **95(1)**:14, 1994.
155. Harville TO, Adams DM, Howard TA, Ware RE: J Oligoclonal expansion of $CD45RO^{+}$ T lymphocytes in Omenn syndrome. *Clin Immunol* **17(4)**:322, 1997.
156. Chilosi M, Facchetti F, Notarangelo LD, Romagnani S, Del Prete G, Almerigogna F, De Carli M, Pizzolo G, de Saint-Basile G, Le Deist F, de Villartay J-P, Cerf-Bensussan N, Journet O, Brousse N, Griscelli C, Fischer A: CD30 cell expression and abnormal soluble CD30 serum accumulation in Omenn's syndrome: Evidence for a T helper 2-mediated condition. *Eur J Immunol* **26(2)**:329, 1996.
157. Rieux-Laucat F, Bahadoran P, Brousse N, Selz F, Fischer A, Le Deist F, De Villartay JP: Highly restricted human T cell repertoire in peripheral blood and tissue-infiltrating lymphocytes in Omenn's syndrome. *J Clin Invest* **102(2)**:312, 1998.
158. Brooks EG, Filipovich AH, Padgett JW, Mamlock R, Goldblum RM: T-cell receptor analysis in Omenn's syndrome: Evidence for defects in gene rearrangement and assembly. *Blood* **93(1)**:242, 1999.
159. Brugnoni D, Airo P, Facchetti F, Blanzuoli L, Ugazio AG, Cattaneo R, Notarangelo LD: In vitro cell death of activated lymphocytes in Omenn's syndrome. *Eur J Immunol* **27(11)**:2765, 1997.
160. Notarangelo LD, Villa A, Schwarz K: RAG and RAG defects. *Curr Opin Immunol* **11**:435, 1999.
161. Signorini S, Imberti L, Pirovano S, Villa A, Facchetti F, Ungari M, Bozzi F, Albertini A, Ugazio AG, Vezzoni P, Notarangelo LD: Intrathymic restriction and peripheral expansion of the T-cell repertoire in Omenn syndrome. *Blood* **94**:3468, 1999.
162. Villa A, Santagata S, Bozzi F, Giliani S, Frattini A, Imberti L, Gatta LB, Ochs HD, Schwarz K, Notarangelo LD, Vezzoni P, Spanopoulou E: Partial V(D)J recombination activity leads to Omenn syndrome. *Cell* **93**:885, 1998.

163. Villa A, Santagata S, Bozzi F, Imberti L, Notarangelo LD: Omenn syndrome: A disorder of Rag1 and Rag2 genes. *J Clin Immunol* **19**:87, 1999.
164. Regueiro JR, Pacheco A, Alvarez-Zapata D, Corell A, Sun, J-Y, Millan R, Arnaiz-Villena AA: CD3 deficiencies, in Ochs H, Smith CIE, Puck JM (eds): *Primary Immunodeficiency Diseases, a Molecular and Genetic Approach.* New York, Oxford University Press, 1999, p 189.
165. DeJarnette JB, Sommers CL, Huang K, Woodside KJ, Emmons R, Katz K, Shores EW, Love PE: Specific requirement for CD3-epsilon in T cell development. *Proc Nat Acad Sci U S A* **95**:14909, 1998.
166. Takase K, Okazaki Y, Wakizaka K, Shevchenko A, Mann M, Saito T: Molecular cloning of pTAC12 an alternative splicing product of the CD3 gamma chain as a component of the pre-T cell antigen-receptor complex. *J Biol Chem* **273(46)**:30675, 1998.
167. Lerner A, D'Adamio L, Diener AC, Clayton LK, Reinherz EL: CD3 zeta/eta/theta locus is colinear with and transcribed antisense to the gene encoding the transcription factor Oct-1. *J Immunol* **151(6)**:3152, 1993.
168. Arnaiz-Villena A, Timon M, Corell A, Perez-Aciego P, Martin-Villa JM, Regueiro JR: Brief report: Primary immunodeficiency caused by mutations in the gene encoding the CD3-gamma subunit of the T-lymphocyte receptor. *N Engl J Med* **327**:529, 1992.
169. Soudais C, de Villartay JP, Le Deist F, Fischer A, Lisowska-Grospierre B: Independent mutations of the human CD3-epsilon gene resulting in a T cell receptor/CD3 complex immunodeficiency. *Nat Genet* **3**:77, 1993.
170. Haks MC, Krimpenfort P, Borst J, Kruisbeek AM: The CD3gamma chain is essential for development of both the TCRalphabeta and TCRgammadelta lineages. *EMBO J* **7**:1871, 1998.
171. Anderson SJ, Levin SD, Perlmutter RM: Protein tyrosine kinase p56(lck) controls allelic exclusion of T-cell receptor beta-chain genes. *Nature* **365**:552, 1993.
172. Burnett RC, Thirman MJ, Rowley JD, Diaz MO: Molecular analysis of the T-cell acute lymphoblastic leukemia-associated t(1;7)(p34;q34) that fuses LCK and TCRB. *Blood* **84**:1232, 1994.
173. Goldman FD, Ballas ZK, Schutte BC, Kemp J, Hollenback C, Noraz N, Taylor N: Defective expression of p56lck in an infant with severe combined immunodeficiency. *J Clin Invest* **102**:421, 1998.
174. Chan AC, Iwashima M, Turk CW, Weiss A: ZAP-70: A 70-kd protein tyrosine kinase that associates with the TCR zeta chain. *Cell* **71**:649, 1992.
175. van Oers NS, Weiss A: The Syk/ZAP-70 protein tyrosine kinase connection to antigen receptor signalling processes. *Semin Immunol* **7**:227, 1995.
176. Elder ME: ZAP-70 and defects of T-cell receptor signaling. *Semin Hematol* **35**:310, 1998.
177. Elder ME, Weiss A: SCID resulting from mutations in the gene encoding the protein tyrosine kinase ZAP-70, in Ochs H, Smith CIE, Puck JM (eds): *Primary Immunodeficiency Diseases, a Molecular and Genetic Approach.* New York, Oxford University Press, 1999, p 146.
178. Gelfand EW, Weinberg K, Mazer BD, Kadlecek TA, Weiss A: Absence of ZAP-70 prevents signaling through the antigen receptor on peripheral blood T cells but not on thymocytes. *J Exp Med* **182**:1057, 1995.
179. Roifman CM: A mutation in ZAP-70 protein tyrosine kinase results in a selective immunodeficiency. *J Clin Immunol* **15(Suppl)**:52S, 1995.
180. Negishi I, Motoyama N, Nakayama K, Nakayama K, Senju S, Hatakeyama S, Zhang Q, Chan AC, Loh DY: Essential role for ZAP-70 in both positive and negative selection of thymocytes. *Nature* **376**:435, 1995.
181. Tomlinson IP, Bodmer WF: The HLA system and the analysis of multifactorial genetic disease. *Trends Genet* **11**:493, 1995.
182. Parham P, Ohta T: Population biology of antigen presentation by MHC class I molecules. *Science* **272**:67, 1996.
183. Hughes AL, Yeager M: Natural selection at major histocompatibility complex loci of vertebrates. *Annu Rev Genet* **32**:415, 1998.
184. Hill AV: The immunogenetics of human infectious diseases. *Annu Rev Immunol* **16**:593, 1998.
185. Ohta T: Effect of gene conversion on polymorphic patterns at major histocompatibility complex loci. *Immunol Rev* **167**:319, 1999.
186. Vogel TU, Evans DT, Urvater JA, O'Connor DH, Hughes AL, Watkins DI: Major histocompatibility complex class I genes in primates: Co-evolution with pathogens. *Immunol Rev* **167**:327, 1999.
187. Amadou C, Kumanovics A, Jones EP, Lambracht-Washington D, Yoshino M, Lindahl KF: The mouse major histocompatibility complex: Some assembly required. *Immunol Rev* **167**:211, 1999.
188. Bontrop RE, Otting N, de Groot NG, Doxiadis GG: Major histocompatibility complex class II polymorphisms in primates. *Immunol Rev* **167**:339, 1999.
189. Beck S, Trowsdale J: Sequence organisation of the class II region of the human MHC. *Immunol Rev* **167**:201, 1999.
190. Yeager M, Hughes AL: Evolution of the mammalian MHC: Natural selection, recombination, and convergent evolution. *Immunol Rev* **167**:45, 1999.
191. Jones EY: MHC class I and class II structures. *Curr Opin Immunol* **9**:75, 1997.
192. Collins EJ, Garboczi DN, Wiley DC: Three-dimensional structure of a peptide extending from one end of a class I MHC binding site. *Nature* **371**:626, 1994.
193. Garboczi DN, Ghosh P, Utz U, Fan QR, Biddison WE, Wiley DC: Structure of the complex between human T-cell receptor, viral peptide and HLA-A2. *Nature* **384**:134, 1996.
194. Pamer E, Cresswell P: Mechanisms of MHC class I—Restricted antigen processing. *Annu Rev Immunol* **16**:323, 1998.
195. van Endert PM: Genes regulating MHC class I processing of antigen. *Curr Opin Immunol* **11**:82, 1999.
196. Kovacsovics-Bankowski M, Rock KL: A phagosome-to-cytosol pathway for exogenous antigens presented on MHC class I molecules. *Science* **267**:243, 1995.
197. Lewis JW, Elliott T: Evidence for successive peptide binding and quality control stages during MHC class I assembly. *Curr Biol* **8**:717, 1998.
198. Uebel S, Tampe R: Specificity of the proteasome and the TAP transporter. *Curr Opin Immunol* **11**:203, 1999.
199. Paz P, Brouwenstijn N, Perry R, Shastri N: Discrete proteolytic intermediates in the MHC class I antigen processing pathway and MHC I-dependent peptide trimming in the ER. *Immunity* **11**:241, 1999.
200. Groll M, Ditzel L, Lowe J, et al: Structure of 20S proteasome from yeast at 2.4 Å resolution. *Nature* **386**:463, 1997.
201. Geier E, Pfeifer G, Wilm M, et al: A giant protease with potential to substitute for some functions of the proteasome. *Science* **283**:978, 1999.
202. Fehling HJ, Swa, W, Laplace C, et al: MHC class I expression in mice lacking the proteasome subunit LMP-7. *Science* **265**:1234, 1994.
203. Morrice N, Powis SJ: A role for the thiol-dependent reductase ERp57 in the assembly of MHC class I molecules. *Curr Biol* **8**:713, 1998.
204. Hughes EA, Cresswell P: The thiol oxidoreductase ERp57 is a component of the MHC class I peptide-loading complex. *Curr Biol* **8**:709, 1998.
205. Lindquist JA, Jensen ON, Mann M, Hammerling GJ: ER-60, a chaperone with thiol-dependent reductase activity involved in MHC class I assembly. *EMBO J* **17**:2186, 1998.
206. Powis SJ, Townsend AR, Deverson EV, Bastin J, Butcher GW, Howard JC: Restoration of antigen presentation to the mutant cell line RMA-S by an MHC-linked transporter. *Nature* **354**:528, 1991.
207. Van Kaer L, Ashton-Rickardt PG, Ploegh HL, Tonegawa S: TAP1 mutant mice are deficient in antigen presentation, surface class I molecules, and CD4-8+ T cells. *Cell* **71**:1205, 1992.
208. Kleijmeer MJ, Kelly A, Geuze HJ, Slot JW, Townsend A, Trowsdale J: Location of MHC-encoded transporters in the endoplasmic reticulum and *cis*-Golgi. *Nature* **357**:342, 1992.
209. Shepherd JC, Schumacher TN, Ashton-Rickardt PG, et al: TAP1-dependent peptide translocation in vitro is ATP dependent and peptide selective [published erratum appears in *Cell* **75(4)**:613, 1993]. *Cell* **74**:577, 1993.
210. Neefjes JJ, Momburg F, Hammerling GJ: Selective and ATP-dependent translocation of peptides by the MHC-encoded transporter. *Science* **261**:769, 1993.
211. Aldrich CJ, DeCloux A, Woods AS, Cotter RJ, Soloski MJ, Forman J: Identification of a Tap-dependent leader peptide recognized by alloreactive T cells specific for a class Ib antigen. *Cell* **79**:649, 1994.
212. Suh WK, Cohen-Doyle MF, Fruh K, Wang K, Peterson PA, Williams DB: Interaction of MHC class I molecules with the transporter associated with antigen processing. *Science* **264**:1322, 1994.
213. Ortmann B, Androlewicz MJ, Cresswell P: MHC class I/beta 2-microglobulin complexes associate with TAP transporters before peptide binding. *Nature* **368**:864, 1994.
214. Grandea AG 3rd, Androlewicz, MJ, Athwal RS, Geraghty DE, Spies T: Dependence of peptide binding by MHC class I molecules on their interaction with TAP. *Science* **270**:105, 1995.
215. Knittler MR, Alberts P, Deverson EV, Howard JC: Nucleotide binding by TAP mediates association with peptide and release of assembled MHC class I molecules. *Curr Biol* **9**:999, 1999.

216. Sadasivan B, Lehner PJ, Ortmann B, Spies T, Cresswell P: Roles for calreticulin and a novel glycoprotein, tapasin, in the interaction of MHC class I molecules with TAP. *Immunity* **5**:103, 1996.
217. Ortmann B, Copeman J, Lehner PJ, et al: A critical role for tapasin in the assembly and function of multimeric MHC class I-TAP complexes. *Science* **277**:1306, 1997.
218. Gao GF, Tormo J, Gerth UC, et al: Crystal structure of the complex between human CD8alpha(alpha) and HLA-A2. *Nature* **387**:630, 1997.
219. Stroynowski I, Lindahl KF: Antigen presentation by non-classical class I molecules. *Curr Opin Immunol* **6(1)**:38, 1994.
220. Stroynowski I, Forman J: Novel molecules related to MHC antigens. *Curr Opin Immunol* **7(1)**:97, 1995.
221. Zeng Z, Castano AR, Segelke BW, Stura EA, Peterson PA, Wilson IA: Crystal structure of mouse CD1: An MHC-like fold with a large hydrophobic binding groove. *Science* **277**:339, 1997.
222. Lebron JA, Bennett MJ, Vaughn DE, et al: Crystal structure of the hemochromatosis protein HFE and characterization of its interaction with transferrin receptor. *Cell* **93**:111, 1998.
223. Fiszer D, Ulbrecht M, Fernandez N, Johnson JP, Weiss EH, Kurpisz M: Analysis of HLA class Ib gene expression in male gametogenic cells. *Eur J Immunol* **27(7)**:1691, 1997.
224. Grigoriadou K, Menard C, Perarnau B, Lemonnier FA: MHC class Ia molecules alone control NK-mediated bone marrow graft rejection. *Eur J Immunol* **29(11)**:3683, 1999.
225. Lopez-Botet M, Bellon T: Natural killer cell activation and inhibition by receptors for MHC class I. *Curr Opin Immunol* **11(3)**:301, 1999.
226. Le Bouteiller P, Blaschitz A: The functionality of HLA-G is emerging. *Immunol Rev* **167**:233, 1999.
227. Le Bouteiller P, Rodriguez AM, Mallet V, Girr M, Guillaudeux T, Lenfant F: Placental expression of HLA class I genes. *Am J Reprod Immunol* **35(3)**:216, 1996.
228. Germain RN: Binding domain regulation of MHC class II molecule assembly, trafficking, fate, and function. *Semin Immunol* **7**:361, 1995.
229. Pieters J: MHC class II restricted antigen presentation. *Curr Opin Immunol* **9(1)**:89, 1997.
230. Nandi D, Marusina K, Monaco JJ: How do endogenous proteins become peptides and reach the endoplasmic reticulum. *Curr Top Microbiol Immunol* **232**:15, 1998.
231. Ghosh P, Amaya M, Mellins E, Wiley DC: The structure of an intermediate in class II MHC maturation: CLIP bound to HLA-DR3. *Nature* **378**:457, 1995.
232. Fremont DH, Hendrickson WA, Marrack P, Kappler J: Structures of an MHC class II molecule with covalently bound single peptides. *Science* **272**:1001, 1996.
233. Jasanoff A, Wagner G, Wiley DC: Structure of a trimeric domain of the MHC class II-associated chaperonin and targeting protein Ii. *EMBO J* **17**:6812, 1998.
234. Reinherz EL, Tan K, Tang L, et al: The crystal structure of a T cell receptor in complex with peptide and MHC class II. *Science* **286**:1913, 1999.
235. Cresswell P: Invariant chain structure and MHC class II function. *Cell* **84**:505, 1996.
236. Bertolino P, Rabourdin-Combe C: The MHC class II-associated invariant chain: A molecule with multiple roles in MHC class II biosynthesis and antigen presentation to CD4+ T cells. *Crit Rev Immunol* **16**:359, 1996.
237. Roche PA, Marks MS, Cresswell P: Formation of a nine-subunit complex by HLA class II glycoproteins and the invariant chain. *Nature* **354**:392, 1991.
238. Avva RR, Cresswell P: In vivo and in vitro formation and dissociation of HLA-DR complexes with invariant chain-derived peptides. *Immunity* **1**:763, 1994.
239. Kropshofer H, Vogt AB, Stern LJ, Hammerling GJ: Self-release of CLIP in peptide loading of HLA-DR molecules. *Science* **270**:1357, 1995.
240. Stumptner P, Benaroch P: Interaction of MHC class II molecules with the invariant chain: Role of the invariant chain (81-90) region. *EMBO J* **16**:5807, 1997.
241. Jasanoff A, Wagner G, Wiley DC: Structure of a trimeric domain of the MHC class II-associated chaperonin and targeting protein Ii. *EMBO J* **17(23)**:6812, 1998.
242. Jasanoff A, Song S, Dinner AR, Wagner G, Wiley DC: One of two unstructured domains of Ii becomes ordered in complexes with MHC class II molecules. *Immunity* **10**:761, 1999.
243. Avva RR, Cresswell P: In vivo and in vitro formation and dissociation of HLA-DR complexes with invariant chain-derived peptides. *Immunity* **1(9)**:763, 1994.
244. Fremont DH, Crawford F, Marrack P, Hendrickson WA, Kappler J: Crystal structure of mouse H2-M. *Immunity* **9(3)**:385, 1998.
245. Mosyak L, Zaller DM, Wiley DC: The structure of HLA-DM, the peptide exchange catalyst that loads antigen onto class II MHC molecules during antigen presentation. *Immunity* **9(3)**:377, 1998.
246. Vogt AB, Kropshofer H: HLA-DM — An endosomal and lysosomal chaperone for the immune system. *Trends Biochem Sci* **24(4)**:150, 1999.
247. Sanderson F, Kleijmeer MJ, Kelly A, et al: Accumulation of HLA-DM, a regulator of antigen presentation, in MHC class II compartments. *Science* **266**:1566, 1994.
248. Denzin LK, Cresswell P: HLA-DM induces CLIP dissociation from MHC class II alpha beta dimers and facilitates peptide loading. *Cell* **82**:155, 1995.
249. Sherman MA, Weber DA, Jensen PE: DM enhances peptide binding to class II MHC by release of invariant chain-derived peptide. *Immunity* **3**:197, 1995.
250. Sloan VS, Cameron P, Porter G, et al: Mediation by HLA-DM of dissociation of peptides from HLA-DR. *Nature* **375**:802, 1995.
251. Weber DA, Evavold BD, Jensen PE: Enhanced dissociation of HLA-DR-bound peptides in the presence of HLA-DM. *Science* **274**:618, 1996.
252. Weber DA, Evavold BD, Jensen PE: Enhanced dissociation of HLA-DR-bound peptides in the presence of HLA-DM. *Science* **274**:618, 1996.
253. Fung-Leung WP, Surh CD, Liljedahl M, et al: Antigen presentation and T cell development in H2-M-deficient mice. *Science* **271**:1278, 1996.
254. Riberdy JM, Newcomb JR, Surman MJ, Barbosa JA, Cresswell P: HLA-DR molecules from an antigen-processing mutant cell line are associated with invariant chain peptides. *Nature* **360**:474, 1992.
255. Tourne S, Miyazaki T, Wolf P, Ploegh H, Benoist C, Mathis D: Functionality of major histocompatibility complex class II molecules in mice doubly deficient for invariant chain and H-2M complexes. *Proc Natl Acad Sci U S A* **94**:9255, 1997.
256. Kovats S, Whiteley PE, Concannon P, Rudensky AY, Blum JS: Presentation of abundant endogenous class II DR-restricted antigens by DM-negative B cell lines. *Eur J Immunol* **27**:1014, 1997.
257. Kropshofer H, Hammerling GJ, Vogt AB: How HLA-DM edits the MHC class II peptide repertoire: Survival of the fittest? *Immunol Today* **18(2)**:77, 1997.
258. Morris P, Shaman J, Attaya M, Amaya M, Goodman S, Bergman C, Monaco JJ, Mellins E: An essential role for HLA-DM in antigen presentation by class II major histocompatibility molecules. *Nature* **368(6471)**:551, 1994.
259. Kropshofer H, Vogt AB, Moldenhauer G, Hammer J, Blum JS, Hammerling GJ: Editing of the HLA-DR-peptide repertoire by HLA-DM. *EMBO J* **15**:6144, 1996.
260. Fung-Leung WP, Surh CD, Liljedahl M, Pang J, Leturcq D, Peterson PA, Webb SR, Karlsson L: Antigen presentation and T cell development in H2-M-deficient mice. *Science* **271(5253)**:1278, 1996.
261. Rabinowitz JD, Vrljic M, Kasson PM, et al: Formation of a highly peptide-receptive state of class II MHC. *Immunity* **9**:699, 1998.
262. Denzin LK, Sant'Angelo DB, Hammond C, Surman MJ, Cresswell P: Negative regulation by HLA-DO of MHC class II-restricted antigen processing. *Science* **278**:106, 1997.
263. Tourne S, Miyazaki T, Oxenius A, et al: Selection of a broad repertoire of CD4+ T cells in H-2Ma0/0 mice. *Immunity* **7**:187, 1997.
264. Liljedahl M, Winqvist O, Surh CD, et al: Altered antigen presentation in mice lacking H2-O. *Immunity* **8**:233, 1998.
265. Kropshofer H, Vogt AB, Thery C, Armandola EA, Li BC, Moldenhauer G, Amigorena S, Hammerling GJ: A role for HLA-DO as a co-chaperone of HLA-DM in peptide loading of MHC class II molecules. *EMBO J* **17(11)**:2971, 1998.
266. Jensen PE: Antigen processing: HLA-DO — a hitchhiking inhibitor of HLA-DM. *Curr Biol* **8(4)**:R128, 1998.
267. Liljedahl M, Winqvist O, Surh CD, Wong P, Ngo K, Teyton L, Peterson PA, Brunmark A, Rudensky AY, Fung-Leung WP, Karlsson L: Altered antigen presentation in mice lacking H2-O. *Immunity* **8(2)**:233, 1998.
268. Denzin LK, Sant'Angelo DB, Hammond C, Surman MJ, Cresswell P: Negative regulation by HLA-DO of MHC class II-restricted antigen processing. *Science* **278(5335)**:106, 1997.
269. The MHC Sequencing Consortium: Complete sequence and gene map of a human major histocompatibility complex. *Nature* **401(6756)**:921, 1999.
270. Carrington M, Nelson GW, Martin MP, Kissner T, Vlahov D, Goedert JJ, Kaslow R, Buchbinder S, Hoots K, O'Brien SJ: HLA and HIV-1:

Heterozygote advantage and B*35-Cw*04 disadvantage. *Science* **283(5408)**:1748, 1999.
271. Todd J: From genome to aetiology in a multifactorial disease, type 1 diabetes. *Bioessays* **21(2)**:164, 1999.
272. Nishimura Y, Oiso M, Fujisao S, Kanai T, Kira J, Chen YZ, Matsushita S: Peptide-based molecular analyses of HLA class II-associated susceptibility to autoimmune diseases. *Int Rev Immunol* **17(5-6)**:229, 1998.
273. Touraine JL: The bare-lymphocyte syndrome: Report on the registry. *Lancet* **1**:319, 1981.
274. Deleted in proof.
275. Touraine JL, Betuel H: Immunodeficiency diseases and expression of HLA antigens. *Hum Immunol* **2**:147, 1981.
276. Touraine JL, Betuel H: The bare lymphocyte syndrome: Immunodeficiency resulting from the lack of expression of HLA antigens. *Birth Defects Orig Artic Ser* **19**:83, 1983.
277. Schuurman HJ, van de Wijngaert FP, Huber J, et al: The thymus in "bare lymphocyte" syndrome: Significance of expression of major histocompatibility complex antigens on thymic epithelial cells in intrathymic T-cell maturation. *Hum Immunol* **13**:69, 1985.
278. Chess J, Kaplan S, Rubinstein A, Wang F, Wiznia A: Candida retinitis in bare lymphocyte syndrome. *Ophthalmology* **93**:696, 1986.
279. Taets van Amerongen AH, Golding RP, Veerman AJ: Hypertrophic osteoarthropathy in a young child with cytomegalovirus pneumonia and the bare lymphocyte syndrome. *Pediatr Radiol* **16**:257, 1986.
280. Sugiyama Y, Maeda H, Okumura K, Takaku F: Progressive sinobronchiectasis associated with the "bare lymphocyte syndrome" in an adult. *Chest* **89**:398, 1986.
281. Arens MQ, Knutsen AP, Schwarz KB, Roodman ST, Swierkosz EM: Multiple and persistent viral infections in a patient with bare lymphocyte syndrome. *J Infect Dis* **156**:837, 1987.
282. Will N, Seger RA, Betzler C, et al: Bare lymphocyte syndrome—Combined immunodeficiency and neutrophil dysfunction. *Eur J Pediatr* **149**:700, 1990.
283. Touraine JL, Marseglia GL, Betuel H, Souillet G, Gebuhrer L: The bare lymphocyte syndrome. *Bone Marrow Transplant* **1(Suppl 9)**:54, 1992.
284. de la Salle H, Hanau D, Fricker D, et al: Homozygous human TAP peptide transporter mutation in HLA class I deficiency. *Science* **265**:237, 1994.
285. Donato L, de la Salle H, Hanau D, et al: Association of HLA class I antigen deficiency related to a TAP2 gene mutation with familial bronchiectasis. *J Pediatr* **127**:895, 1995.
286. Raghavan M: Immunodeficiency due to defective antigen processing: The molecular basis for type 1 bare lymphocyte syndrome. *J Clin Invest* **103**:595, 1999.
287. Furukawa H, Yabe T, Watanabe K, et al: Tolerance of NK and LAK activity for HLA class I-deficient targets in a TAP1-deficient patient (bare lymphocyte syndrome type I). *Hum Immunol* **60**:32, 1999.
288. Furukawa H, Murata S, Yabe T, et al: Splice acceptor site mutation of the transporter associated with antigen processing-1 gene in human bare lymphocyte syndrome. *J Clin Invest* **103**:755, 1999.
289. Zimmer J, Donato L, Hanau D, et al: Activity and phenotype of natural killer cells in peptide transporter (TAP)-deficient patients (type I bare lymphocyte syndrome). *J Exp Med* **187**:117, 1998.
290. Klein C, Lisowska-Grospierre B, LeDeist F, Fischer A and Griscelli C: Major histocompatibility complex class II deficiency: Clinical manifestations, immunologic features, and outcome. *J Pediatr* **123**:921, 1993.
291. Ersoy F, Sanal O, Tezcan I, Yel L, Metin A: Bare lymphocyte syndrome with lack of HLA class I and II antigens. Presentation of two cases. *Turk J Pediatr* **37**:141, 1995.
292. Elhasid R and Etzioni A: Major histocompatibility complex class II deficiency: A clinical review. *Blood Rev* **10**:242, 1996.
293. Bejaoui M, Barbouche MR, Mellouli F, Largueche B, Dellagi K: Primary immunologic deficiency by deficiency of HLA class II antigens: Nine new Tunisian cases. *Arch Pediatr* **5**:1089, 1998.
294. Jin Z, Yang SY: Activation of CD8+ T cells by allogeneic class II-deficient B-cell lines derived from patients with bare lymphocyte syndrome. *Tissue Antigens* **35**:136, 1990.
295. Andrien M, Stordeur P, Vamos E, et al: Differential inducibility of HLA class I and II antigens by r-IFN gamma in type III bare lymphocyte syndrome. *Transplant Proc* **23**:441, 1991.
296. Sullivan KE, Stobo JD, Peterlin BM: Molecular analysis of the bare lymphocyte syndrome. *J Clin Invest* **76**:75, 1985.
297. Clement LT, Plaeger-Marshall S, Haas A, Saxon A, Martin AM: Bare lymphocyte syndrome. Consequences of absent class II major histocompatibility antigen expression for B lymphocyte differentiation and function. *J Clin Invest* **81**:669, 1988.
298. Hume CR, Shookster LA, Collins N, O'Reilly R, Lee JS: Bare lymphocyte syndrome: Altered HLA class II expression in B cell lines derived from two patients. *Hum Immunol* **25**:1, 1989.
299. van Eggermond MC, Rijkers GT, Kuis W, Zegers BJ, Van den Elsen PJ: T cell development in a major histocompatibility complex class II-deficient patient. *Eur J Immunol* **23**:2585, 1993.
300. Lambert M, van Eggermond M, Verheij C, Van Ree J, van den Elsen P: Analysis of MHC class II transcription in two type III bare lymphocyte syndrome patients of a single family. *Immunodeficiency* **4**:277, 1993.
301. Nocera A, Barocci S, De Palma R, Gorski J: Analysis of transcripts of genes located within the HLA-D region in B cells from an HLA-severe combined immunodeficiency individual. *Hum Immunol* **38**:231, 1993.
302. Kovats S, Drover S, Marshall WH, et al: Coordinate defects in human histocompatibility leukocyte antigen class II expression and antigen presentation in bare lymphocyte syndrome. *J Exp Med* **179**:2022, 1994.
303. Kovats S, Nepom GT, Coleman M, Nepom B, Kwok WW, Blum JS: Deficient antigen-presenting cell function in multiple genetic complementation groups of type II bare lymphocyte syndrome. *J Clin Invest* **96**:217, 1995.
304. Hauber I, Gulle H, Wolf HM, Maris M, Eggenbauer H, Eibl MM: Molecular characterization of major histocompatibility complex class II gene expression and demonstration of antigen-specific T cell response indicate a new phenotype in class II-deficient patients. *J Exp Med* **181**:1411, 1995.
305. Henwood J, van Eggermond MC, van Boxel-Dezaire AH, et al: Human T cell repertoire generation in the absence of MHC class II expression results in a circulating $CD4^{+}CD8^{-}$population with altered physicochemical properties of complementarity-determining region 3. *J Immunol* **156**:895, 1996.
306. Nonoyama S, Etzioni A, Toru H, Ruggerie DP, Lewis D, Pollack S, Aruffo A, Yata JI, Ochs HD: Diminished expression of CD40 ligand may contribute to the defective humoral immunity in patients with MHC class II deficiency. *Eur J Immunol* **28**:589, 1998.
307. Yang Z, Accolla RS, Pious D, Zegers BJ, Strominger JL: Two distinct genetic loci regulating class II gene expression are defective in human mutant and patient cell lines. *EMBO J* **7**:1965, 1988.
308. Benichou B, Strominger JL: Class II-antigen-negative patient and mutant B-cell lines represent at least three, and probably four, distinct genetic defects defined by complementation analysis. *Proc Natl Acad Sci U S A* **88**:4285, 1991.
309. Seidl C, Saraiya C, Osterweil Z, Fu YP, Lee JS: Genetic complexity of regulatory mutants defective for HLA class II gene expression. *J Immunol* **148**:1576, 1992.
310. Peijnenburg A, Godthelp B, van Boxel-Dezaire A, Van den Elsen PJ: Definition of a novel complementation group in MHC class II deficiency. *Immunogenetics* **41**:287, 1995.
311. Lisowska-Grospierre B, Fondaneche MC, Rols MP, Griscelli C, Fischer A: Two complementation groups account for most cases of inherited MHC class II deficiency. *Hum Mol Genet* **3**:953, 1994.
312. Douhan J 3rd, Hauber I, Eibl MM, Glimcher LH: Genetic evidence for a new type of major histocompatibility complex class II combined immunodeficiency characterized by a dyscoordinate regulation of HLA-D alpha and beta chains. *J Exp Med* **183**:1063, 1996.
313. Lennon A, Ottone C, Peijnenburg A, Hamon-Benais C, Colland F, Gobin S, van den Elsen P, Fellous M, Bono R, Alcaide-Loridan C: The RAG cell line defines a new complementation group of MHC class II deficiency. *Immunogenetics* **43**:352, 1996.
314. Schwartz RS: The case of the bare lymphocyte syndrome—Tracking down faulty transcription factors [Editorial; Comment]. *N Engl J Med* **337**:781, 1997.
315. Villard J, Mach B, Reith W: MHC class II deficiency: Definition of a new complementation group. *Immunobiology* **198**:264, 1997.
316. Glimcher LH, Kara CJ: Sequences and factors: A guide to MHC class-II transcription. *Annu Rev Immunol* **10**:13, 1992.
317. Abdulkadir SA, Ono SJ: How are class II MHC genes turned on and off? *FASEB J* **9**:1429, 1995.
318. Reith W, Steimle V, Mach B: Molecular defects in the bare lymphocyte syndrome and regulation of MHC class II genes. *Immunol Today* **16**:539, 1995.
319. Rohn WM, Lee YJ, Benveniste EN: Regulation of class II MHC expression. *Crit Rev Immunol* **16**:311, 1996.
320. Kara CJ, Glimcher LH: In vivo footprinting of MHC class II genes: Bare promoters in the bare lymphocyte syndrome. *Science* **252**:709, 1991.

321. Durand B, Kobr M, Reith W, Mach B: Functional complementation of major histocompatibility complex class II regulatory mutants by the purified X-box-binding protein RFX. *Mol Cell Biol* **14**:6839, 1994.
322. Moreno CS, Emery P, West JE, et al: Purified X2 binding protein (X2BP) cooperatively binds the class II MHC X box region in the presence of purified RFX, the X box factor deficient in the bare lymphocyte syndrome. *J Immunol* **155**:4313, 1995.
323. Moreno CS, Rogers EM, Brown JA, Boss JM: Regulatory factor X, a bare lymphocyte syndrome transcription factor, is a multimeric phosphoprotein complex. *J Immunol* **158**:5841, 1997.
324. Scholl T, Mahanta SK, Strominger JL: Specific complex formation between the type II bare lymphocyte syndrome-associated transactivators CIITA and RFX5. *Proc Natl Acad Sci U S A* **94**:6330, 1997.
325. Currie RA: Biochemical characterization of the NF-Y transcription factor complex during B lymphocyte development. *J Biol Chem* **273**:18220, 1998.
326. Gobin SJ, Peijnenburg A, van Eggermond M, van Zutphen M, Van den Berg R, Van den Elsen PJ: The RFX complex is crucial for the constitutive and CIITA-mediated transactivation of MHC class I and beta2-microglobulin genes. *Immunity* **9**:531, 1998.
327. DeSandro A, Nagarajan UM, Boss JM: The bare lymphocyte syndrome: Molecular clues to the transcriptional regulation of major histocompatibility complex class II genes. *Am J Hum Genet* **65**:279, 1999.
328. Steimle V, Otten LA, Zufferey M, Mach B: Complementation cloning of an MHC class II transactivator mutated in hereditary MHC class II deficiency (or bare lymphocyte syndrome). *Cell* **75**:135, 1993.
329. Zhou H, Glimcher LH: Human MHC class II gene transcription directed by the carboxyl terminus of CIITA, one of the defective genes in type II MHC combined immune deficiency. *Immunity* **2**:545, 1995.
330. Mahanta SK, Scholl T, Yang FC, Strominger JL: Transactivation by CIITA, the type II bare lymphocyte syndrome-associated factor, requires participation of multiple regions of the TATA box binding protein. *Proc Natl Acad Sci U S A* **94**:6324, 1997.
331. Bontron S, Steimle V, Ucla C, Eibl MM, Mach B: Two novel mutations in the MHC class II transactivator CIITA in a second patient from MHC class II deficiency complementation group A. *Hum Genet* **99**:541, 1997.
332. Peijnenburg A, Gobin SJ, van Eggermond MC, Godthelp BC, van Graafeiland N, Van den Elsen PJ: Introduction of exogenous class II trans-activator in MHC class II-deficient ABI fibroblasts results in incomplete rescue of MHC class II antigen expression. *J Immunol* **159**:2720, 1997.
333. Bradley MB, Fernandez JM, Ungers G, et al: Correction of defective expression in MHC class II deficiency (bare lymphocyte syndrome) cells by retroviral transduction of CIITA. *J Immunol* **159**:1086, 1997.
334. Quan V, Towey M, Sacks S, Kelly AP: Absence of MHC class II gene expression in a patient with a single amino acid substitution in the class II transactivator protein CIITA. *Immunogenetics* **49(11-12)**:957, 1999.
335. Cressman DE, Chin KC, Taxman DJ, Ting JP: A defect in the nuclear translocation of CIITA causes a form of type II bare lymphocyte syndrome. *Immunity* **10**:163, 1999.
336. Harton JA, Cressman DE, Chin KC, Der CJ, Ting JPY: GTP binding by class II trans activator: Role in nuclear import. *Science* **285**:1402, 1999.
337. Steimle V, Durand B, Barras E, et al: A novel DNA-binding regulatory factor is mutated in primary MHC class II deficiency (bare lymphocyte syndrome). *Genes Dev* **9**:1021, 1995.
338. Peijnenburg A, Van Eggermond MJ, Gobin SJ, et al: Discoordinate expression of invariant chain and MHC class II genes in class II transactivator-transfected fibroblasts defective for RFX5. *J Immunol* **163**:794, 1999.
339. Peijnenburg A, Van Eggermond MC, Van den Berg R, Sanal O, Vossen JM, Van den Elsen PJ: Molecular analysis of an MHC class II deficiency patient reveals a novel mutation in the RFX5 gene. *Immunogenetics* **49**:338, 1999.
340. Villard J, Lisowska-Grospierre B, van den Elsen P, Fischer A, Reith W, Mach B: Mutation of RFXAP, a regulator of MHC class II genes, in primary MHC class II deficiency [see comments]. *N Engl J Med* **337**:748, 1997.
341. Durand B, Sperisen P, Emery P, Barras E, Zufferey M, Mach B, Reith W: RFXAP, a novel subunit of the RFX DNA binding complex is mutated in MHC class II deficiency. *EMBO J* **16**:1045, 1997.
342. Fondaneche MC, Villard J, Wiszniewski W, Jouanguy E, Etzioni A, Le Deist F, Peijnenburg A, Casanova JL, Reith W, Mach B, Fischer A, Lisowska-Grospierre B: Genetic and molecular definition of complementation group D in MHC class II deficiency. *Hum Mol Genet* **7**:879, 1998.
343. Masternak K, Barras E, Zufferey M, Conrad B, Corthals G, Aebersold R, Sanchez JC, Hochstrasser DF, Mach B, Reith W: A gene encoding a novel RFX-associated transactivator is mutated in the majority of MHC class II deficiency patients. *Nat Genet* **20**:273, 1998.
344. Nagarajan UM, Louis-Plence P, DeSandro A, Nilsen R, Bushey A, Boss JM: RFX-B is the gene responsible for the most common cause of the bare lymphocyte syndrome, an MHC class II immunodeficiency. *Immunity* **10**:153, 1999.
345. Faigle W, Raposo G, Tenza D, Pinet V, Vogt AB, Kropshofer H, Fischer A, de Saint-Basile G, Amigorena S: Deficient peptide loading and MHC class II endosomal sorting in a human genetic immunodeficiency disease: The Chediak-Higashi syndrome. *J Cell Biol* **141(5)**:1121, 1998.
346. Fischer A: Thirty years of bone marrow transplantation for severe combined immunodeficiency. *N Engl J Med* **340**:559, 1999.
347. Noguchi M, Yi H, Rosenblatt HM, Filipovitch AH, Adelstein S, Modi WS, McBride OW, Leonard WJ: Interleukin-2 receptor γ chain mutation results in X-linked severe combined immunodeficiency in humans. *Cell* **73**:147, 1993a.
348. Puck JM, Deschenes SM, Porter JC, Dutra AS, Brown CJ, Willard HF, Henthorn PS: The interleukin-2 receptor gamma chain maps to Xq13.1 and is mutated in X-linked severe combined immunodeficiency, SCIDX1. *Hum Mol Genet* **2**:1099, 1993.
349. Puck JM: X-linked severe combined immunodeficiency, in Ochs H, Smith CIE, Puck JM, (eds): *Primary Immunodeficiency Diseases, a Molecular and Genetic Approach.* New York, Oxford University Press, 1999, p 99.
350. Puel A, Ziegler SF, Buckley RH, Leonard WJ: Defective IL7R expression in $T(^{-})$ $B(^{+})$ $NK(^{+})$ severe combined immunodeficiency. *Nat Genet* **20**:394, 1998.
351. Macchi P, Villa A, Giliani S, Sacco MG, Frattini A, Porta F, Ugazio AG, Johnston JA, Candotti F, O'Shea JJ, Vezzoni P, Notarangelo LD: Mutations of Jak-3 gene in patients with autosomal severe combined immune deficiency (SCID). *Nature* **377**:65, 1995.
352. Russell SM, Tayebi N, Nakajima H, Riedy MC, Roberts JL, Aman MJ, Migone T-S, Noguchi M, Markert ML, Buckley RH, O'Shea JJ, Leonard WJ: Mutation of Jak3 in a patient with SCID: Essential role of Jak3 in lymphoid development. *Science* **270**:797, 1995.
353. Puck JM, Pepper AE, Henthorn PS, Candotti F, Isakov J, Whitwam T, Conley ME, Fischer RE, Rosenblatt HM, Small TN, Buckley RH: Mutation analysis of IL2RG in human X-linked severe combined immunodeficiency. *Blood* **89**:1968, 1997.
354. Buckley RH, Schiff SE, Schiff RI, Markert L, Williams LW, Roberts JL, Myers LA, Ward FE: Hematopoietic stem-cell transplantation for the treatment of severe combined immunodeficiency. *N Engl J Med* **340**:508, 1999.
355. Gatti RA, Allen HD, Meuwissen HJ, Hong R, Good RA: Immunological reconstitution of sex-linked lymphopenic immunological deficiency. *Lancet* **2**:1366, 1968.
356. Shearer WT, Ritz J, Finegold MJ, Guerra IC, Rosenblatt HM, Lewis DL, Pollack MS, Taber LH, Sumaya CV, Grumet C, Cleary ML, Warnke R, Sklar J: Epstein-Barr virus-associated B-cell proliferations of diverse clonal origins after bone marrow transplantation in a 12-year-old patient with severe combined immunodeficiency. *N Engl J Med* **312**:1151, 1985.
357. Baird AM, Gerstein RM, Berg LJ: The role of cytokine receptor signaling in lymphocyte development. *Curr Opin Immunol* **11**:157, 1999.
358. De Saint Basile G, Arveiler B, Oberlé J, Malcolm S, Levinsky R, Lau Y, Hofker M, Debre M, Fischer A, Griscelli C, Mandel, J-L: Close linkage of the locus for X chromosome-linked SCID to polymorphic markers in Xq11-q13. *Proc Natl Acad Sci U S A* **84**:7576, 1987.
359. Puck JM, Conley ME, Bailey LC: Refinement of localization of human X-linked severe combined immunodeficiency (SCIDX1) in Xq13. *Am J Hum Genet* **53**:176, 1993b.
360. Puck JM, Nussbaum RL, Conley ME: Carrier detection in X-linked severe combined immunodeficiency based on patterns of X chromosome inactivation. *J Clin Invest* **79**:1395, 1987.
361. Conley ME, Lavoie A, Briggs C, Guerra C, Puck JM: Non-random X chromosome inactivation in B cells from carriers of X-linked severe combined immunodeficiency. *Proc Nat Acad Sci U S A* **85**:3090, 1988.
362. Wengler GS, Allen RC, Parolini O, Smith H, Conley ME: Nonrandom X chromosome inactivation in natural killer cells from obligate carriers of X-linked severe combined immunodeficiency. *J Immunol* **150**:700, 1993.

363. Pepper AE, Buckley RH, Small TN, Puck JM: Two CpG mutational hot spots in the interleukin-2 receptor γ chain gene causing human X-linked severe combined immunodeficiency. *Am J Hum Genet* **57**:564, 1995.
364. Puck JM, de Saint Basile G, Schwarz K, Fugmann S, Fischer RE: IL2RGbase: A database of γc-chain defects causing human X-SCID. *Immunol Today* **17**:507, 1996.
365. DiSanto JP, Rieux-Laucat F, Dautry-Varsat A, Fischer A, De Saint Basile G: Defective human interleukin 2 receptor γ chain in an atypical X chromosome-linked severe combined immunodeficiency with peripheral T cells. *Proc Natl Acad Sci U S A* **91**:9466, 1994.
366. Schmalstieg FC, Leonard WJ, Noguchi M, Berg M, Rudloff HE, Denney RM, Dave SK, Brooks EG, Goldman AS: Missense mutation in exon 7 of the common gamma chain gene causes a moderate form of X-linked combined immunodeficiency. *J Clin Invest* **95**:1169, 1995.
367. Puck JM, Pepper AE, Bédard P-M, Laframboise R: Female germ line mosaicism as the origin of a unique IL-2 receptor γ-chain mutation causing X-linked severe combined immunodeficiency. *J Clin Invest* **95**:895, 1995.
368. O'Marcaigh AE, Puck JM, Pepper AE, Cowan MJ: Maternal germline mosaicism for an IL2RG mutation causing X-linked SCID in a Navajo kindred. *J Clin Immunol* **17**:29, 1997.
369. Takeshita T, Asao H, Ohtani K, Ishii N, Kumaki S, Tanaka N, Munakata H, Nakamura M, Sugamura K: Cloning of the gamma chain of the human IL-2 receptor. *Science* **257**:379, 1992.
370. Orlic D, Girard L, Lee D, Anderson S, Puck JM, Bodine DM: Interleukin-7Rα and interleukin-2Rβ mRNA expression increase as stem cells differentiate to T and B lymphocyte progenitors: Implications for X-linked SCID. *Exp Hematol* **25**:217, 1997.
371. DiSanto JP, Certain S, Wilson A, MacDonald HR, Avner P, Fischer A, De Saint Basile G: The murine interleukin-2 receptor γ chain gene: Organization, chromosomal localization and expression in the adult thymus. *Eur J Immunol* **24**:3014, 1994.
372. Nakarai T, Robertson MJ, Streuli M, Wu, Z, Ciardelli TL, Smith KA, Ritz J: Interleukin 2 receptor g chain expression on resting and activated lymphoid cells. *J Exp Med* **180**:241, 1994.
373. Sugamura K, Asao H, Kondo M, Tanaka N, Ishii N, Ohbo K, Nakamura M, Takeshita T: The interleukin-2 receptor γ chain: Its role in the multiple cytokine receptor complexes and T cell development in XSCID. *Annu Rev Immunol* **14**:179, 1996.
374. Schorle H, Holtschke T, Hunig T, Schimpl A, Horak I: Development and function of T cells in mice rendered interleukin-2 deficient by gene targeting. *Nature* **352**:621, 1991.
375. Schimpl A, Hunig T, Elbe A, Berberich I, Kraemer S, Merz H, Feller AC, Sadlack B, Schorle H, Horak I: Development and function of the immune system in mice with targeted disruption of the interleukin 2 gene, in Bluethmann H, Ohashi P (eds): *Transgenesis and Targeted Mutagenesis in Immunology*. New York, Academic Press, 1994, p 191.
376. Russell SM, Keegan AD, Harada N, Nakamura Y, Noguchi M, Leland P, Friedmann MC, Miyajima A, Puri RK, Paul WE, Leonard WJ: Interleukin-2 receptor gamma chain: A functional component of the interleukin-4 receptor. *Science* **262**:1880, 1993.
377. Kondo M, Takeshita T, Ishii N, Nakamura M, Watanabe S, Arai K Sugamura K: Sharing of the interleukin-2 (IL-2) receptor gamma chain between receptors for IL-2 and IL-4. *Science* **262**:1874, 1993.
378. Noguchi M, Nakamura Y, Russell SM, Ziegler SF, Tsang M, Cao X, Leonard WJ: Interleukin-2 receptor γ chain: A functional component of the interleukin-7 receptor. *Science* **262**:1877, 1993.
379. Russell SM, Johnston JA, Noguchi M, Kawamura M, Bacon CM, Friedmann M, Berg M, McVicar DW, Witthuhn BA, Silvennoinen O, Goldman AS, Schmalstieg FC, Ihle JN, O'Shea JJ, Leonard WJ: Interaction of IL-2Rα and γc chains with Jak1 and Jak3: Implications for XSCID and XCID. *Science* **266**:1042, 1994.
380. Giri JG, Ahdieh M, Eisenman J, Shanebeck K, Grabstein K, Kumaki S, Namen A, Park LS, Cosman D, Anderson D: Utilization of the beta and gamma chains of the IL-2 receptor by the novel cytokine IL-15. *EMBO J* **13**:2822, 1994.
381. DiSanto JP, Muller W, Guy-Grand D, Fischer A, Rajewsky K: Lymphoid development in mice with a targeted deletion of the interleukin 2 receptor γ chain. *Proc Natl Acad Sci U S A* **92**:377, 1995.
382. Muegge K, Vila MP, Durum SK: Interleukin-7: A cofactor for V(D)J rearrangement of the T cell receptor β gene. *Science* **261**:93, 1993.
383. Kuhn R, Rajewsky K, Muller W: Generation and analysis of interleukin-4 deficient mice. *Science* **254**:707, 1991.
384. Seder RA, Paul WE: Acquisition of lymphokine-producing phenotype by CD4$^+$ T cells. *Annu Rev Immunol* **12**:635, 1994.
385. Matthews DJ, Clark PA, Herbert J, Morgan G, Armitage RJ, Kinnon C, Minty A, Grabstein KH, Caput D, Ferrara P, et al: Function of the interleukin-2 (IL-2) receptor gamma-chain in biologic responses of X-linked severe combined immunodeficient B cells to IL-2, IL-4, IL-13, and IL-15. *Blood* **85(1)**:38, 1995.
386. Taylor N, Uribe L, Smith S, Jahn T, Kohn DB, Weinberg K: Correction of interleukin-2 receptor function in X-SCID lymphoblastoid cells by retrovirally mediated transfer of the gamma-c gene. *Blood* **87**:3103, 1996.
387. Johnston JA, Kawamura M, Kirken RA, Chen Y-Q, Blake TB, Shibuya K, Ortaldo JR, McVicar DW, O'Shea JJ: Phosphorylation and activation of the Jak-3 Janus kinase in response to interleukin-2. *Nature* **370**:151, 1994.
388. Miyazaki T, Kawahara A, Fujii H, Nakagawa Y, Minami Y, Liu Z-J, Oishi I, Silvennoinen O, Witthuhn BA, Ihle JN, Taniguchi T: Functional activation of JAK1 and JAK3 by selective association with IL-2 receptor subunits. *Science* **266**:1045, 1994.
389. Leonard WJ, O'Shea JJ: JAKs and STATs: Biological implications. *Annu Rev Immunol* **16**:293, 1998.
390. Candotti F, Oakes SA, Johnston JA, Giliani S, Schumacher RF, Mella P, Fiorini M, Ugazio AG, Badolato R, Notarangelo LD, Bozzi F, Macchi P, Strina D, Vezzoni P, Blaese RM, O'Shea JJ, Villa A: Structural and functional basis for JAK3-deficient severe combined immunodeficiency. *Blood* **90**:3996, 1997.
391. Ramesh N, Geha RS, Notarangelo LD: CD40 ligand and the hyper-IgM syndrome, in Ochs H, Smith CIE, Puck JM (eds): *Primary Immunodeficiency Diseases, a Molecular and Genetic Approach*. New York, Oxford University Press, 1999, p 233.
392. Jain A, Atkinson TP, Lipsky PE, Slater JE, Nelson DL, Strober W: Defects of T-cell effector function and post-thymic maturation in X-linked hyper-IgM syndrome. *J Clin Invest* **103**:1151, 1999.
393. Allen RC, Armitage RJ, Conley ME, Rosenblatt H, Jenkins NA, Copeland NG, Bedell MA, Edelhoff S, Disteche CM, Simoneaux DK, et al: CD40 ligand gene defects responsible for X-linked hyper-IgM syndrome. *Science* **259**:990, 1993.
394. Aruffo A, Farrington M, Hollenbaugh D, Li X, Milatovich A, Nonoyama S, Bajorath J, Grosmaire LS, Stenkamp R, Neubauer M, et al: The CD40 ligand, gp39, is defective in activated T cells from patients with X-linked hyper-IgM syndrome. *Cell* **72(2)**:291, 1993.
395. DiSanto JP, Bonnefoy JY, Gauchat JF, Fischer A, de Saint Basile G: CD40 ligand mutations in X-linked immunodeficiency with hyper-IgM. *Nature* **361**:541, 1993.
396. Fuleihan R, Ramesh N, Loh R, Jabara H, Rosen RS, Chatila T, Fu SM, Stamenkovic I, Geha RS: Defective expression of the CD40 ligand in X chromosome-linked immunoglobulin deficiency with normal or elevated IgM. *Proc Natl Acad Sci U S A* **90**:2170, 1993.
397. Korthauer U, Graf D, Mages HW, Briere F, Padayachee M, Malcolm S, Ugazio AG, Notarangelo LD, Levinsky RJ, Kroczek RA: Defective expression of T-cell CD40 ligand causes X-linked immunodeficiency with hyper-IgM. *Nature* **361**:539, 1993.
398. Brahmi Z, Lazarus KH, Hodes M E, Baehner RL: Immunologic studies of three family members with the immunodeficiency with hyper-IgM syndrome. *J Clin Immun* **3**:127, 1983.
399. Altare F, Durandy A, Lammas D, Emile JF, Lamhamedi S, Le Deist F, Drysdale P, Jouanguy E, Doffinger R, Bernaudin F, Jeppsson O, Gollob JA, Meinl E, Segal AW, Fischer A, Kumararatne D, Casanova JL: Impairment of mycobacterial immunity in human interleukin-12 receptor deficiency. *Science* **280**:1432, 1998.
400. de Jong R, Altare F, Haagen IA, Elferink DG, Boer T, van Breda Vriesman PJ, Kabel PJ, Draaisma JM, van Dissel JT, Kroon FP, Casanova JL, Ottenhoff TH: Severe mycobacterial and Salmonella infections in interleukin-12 receptor-deficient patients. *Science* **280**:1435, 1998.
401. Dorman SE, Holland SM: Mutation in the signal-transducing chain of the interferon-gamma receptor and susceptibility to mycobacterial infection. *J Clin Invest* **101**:2364, 1998.
402. Jouanguy E, Lamhamedi-Cherradi S, Lammas D, Dorman SE, Fondaneche MC, Dupuis S, Doffinger R, Altare F, Girdlestone J, Emile JF, Ducoulombier H, Edgar D, Clarke J, Oxelius VA, Brai M, Novelli V, Heyne K, Fischer A, Holland SM, Kumararatne DS, Schreiber RD, Casanova JL: A human IFNGR1 small deletion hotspot associated with dominant susceptibility to mycobacterial infection. *Nat Genet* **21**:370, 1999.
403. Altare F, Lammas D, Revy P, Jouangu E, Doffinger R, Lamhamedi S, Drysdale P, Scheel-Toellner D, Girdlestone, J, Darbyshire P, Wadhwa M, Dockrell H, Salmon M, Fischer A, Durandy A, Casanova J-L, Kumararatne DS: Inherited interleukin 12 deficiency in a child with

bacille Calmette-Guerin and *Salmonella enteritidis* disseminated infection. *J Clin Invest* **102**:2035, 1998.
404. Purtilo DT, Grierson HL, Davis JR, Okano M: The X-linked lymphoproliferative disease: From autopsy toward cloning the gene 1975–1990. *Pediatr Pathol* **11**:685, 1991.
405. Schuster V, Kreth HW: X-linked lymphoproliferative disease, in Ochs H, Smith CIE, Puck JM (eds): *Primary Immunodeficiencies: A Molecular and Genetic Approach.* New York, Oxford University Press, 1999, p 222.
406. Coffey AJ, Brooksbank RA, Brandau O, Oohashi T, Howell GR, Bye JM, Cahn AP, Durham J, Heath P, Wray P, Pavitt R, Wilkinson J, Leversha M, Huckle E, Shaw-Smith CJ, Dunham A, Rhodes S, Schuster V, Porta G, Yin L, Serafini P, Sylla B, Zollo M, Franco B, Bentley DR, et al: Host response to EBV infection in X-linked lymphoproliferative disease results from mutations in an SH2-domain encoding gene. *Nat Genet* **20**:129, 1998.
407. Sayos J, Wu C, Morra M, Wang N, Zhang X, Allen D, van Schaik S, Notarangelo L, Geha R, Roncarolo MG, Oettgen H, De Vries JE, Aversa G, Terhorst C: The X-linked lymphoproliferative-disease gene product SAP regulates signals induced through the co-receptor SLAM. *Nature* **395**:462, 1998.
408. Sullivan KE, Mullen CA, Blaese RM, Winkelstein JA: A multi-institutional survey of the Wiskott-Aldrich syndrome. *J Pediatr* **125**:876.1994.
409. Smith CI, Notarangelo LD: Molecular basis for X-linked immunodeficiencies. *Adv Genet* **35**:57, 1997.
410. Ochs HD: The Wiskott-Aldrich syndrome. *Semin Hematol* **35**:332, 1998.
411. Sullivan KE: Recent advances in our understanding of Wiskott-Aldrich syndrome. *Curr Opin Hematol* **6**:8, 1999.
412. Akman IO, Ostrov BE, Neudorf S: Autoimmune manifestations of the Wiskott-Aldrich syndrome. *Semin Arthritis Rheum* **27**:218, 1998.
413. Ochs HD, Slichter SJ, Harker LA, Von Behrens WE, Clark RA, Wedgwood RJ: The Wiskott-Aldrich syndrome: Studies of lymphocytes, granulocytes, and platelets. *Blood* **55**:243, 1980.
414. Remold-O'Donnell E, Rosen FS, Kenney DM: Defects in Wiskott-Aldrich syndrome blood cells. *Blood* **87**:2621, 1996.
415. Semple JW, Siminovitch KA, Mody M, Milev Y, Lazarus AH, Wright JF, Freedman J: Flow cytometric analysis of platelets from children with the Wiskott-Aldrich syndrome reveals defects in platelet development, activation and structure. *Br J Haematol* **97**:747, 1997.
416. Gross BS, Wilde JI, Quek L, Chapel H, Nelson DL, Watson SP: Regulation and function of WASp in platelets by the collagen receptor, glycoprotein VI. *Blood* **94**:4166, 1999.
417. Shcherbina A, Rosen FS, Remold-O'Donnell E: Pathological events in platelets of Wiskott-Aldrich syndrome patients. *Br J Haematol* **106**:875, 1999.
418. Buckley RH, Fiscus SA: Serum IgD and IgE concentrations in immunodeficiency diseases. *J Clin Invest* **55(1)**:157, 1975.
419. Inoue R, Kondo N, Kuwabara N, Orii T: Aberrant patterns of immunoglobulin levels in Wiskott-Aldrich syndrome. *Scand J Immunol* **41**:188, 1995.
420. Briles DE, Scott G, Gray B, Crain MJ, Blaese M, Nahm M, Scott V, Haber P: Naturally occurring antibodies to phosphocholine as a potential index of antibody responsiveness to polysaccharides. *J Infect Dis* **155**:1307, 1987.
421. Rijkers GT, Sanders LA, Zegers BJ: Anti-capsular polysaccharide antibody deficiency states. *Immunodeficiency* **5**:1, 1993.
422. Barra A, Bremard-Oury C, Bajart A, Griscelli C, Fritzell B, Preud'homme JL: Immunogenicity of *Haemophilus influenzae* type b capsular polysaccharide and its tetanus toxoid conjugate in patients with recurrent infections or humoral immunodeficiency. *Int J Clin Lab Res* **21**:231.1992.
423. Kenney D, Cairns L, Remold-O'Donnell E, Peterson J, Rosen FS, Parkman R: Morphological abnormalities in the lymphocytes of patients with the Wiskott-Aldrich syndrome. *Blood* **68**:1329, 1986.
424. Gallego MD, Santamaria M, Pena J, Molina IJ: Defective actin reorganization and polymerization of Wiskott-Aldrich T cells in response to CD3-mediated stimulation. *Blood* **90**:3089, 1997.
425. Zhang J, Shehabeldin A, da Cruz LA, Butler J, Somani AK, McGavin M, Kozieradzki I, dos Santos AO, Nagy A, Grinstein S, Penninger JM, Siminovitch KA: Antigen receptor-induced activation and cytoskeletal rearrangement are impaired in Wiskott-Aldrich syndrome protein-deficient lymphocytes. *J Exp Med* **190**:1329, 1999.
426. Zicha D, Allen WE, Brickell PM, Kinnon C, Dunn GA, Jones GE, Thrasher AJ: Chemotaxis of macrophages is abolished in the Wiskott-Aldrich syndrome. *Br J Haematol* **101(4)**:659, 1998.
427. Badolato R, Sozzani S, Malacarne F, Bresciani S, Fiorini M, Borsatti A, Albertini A, Mantovani A, Ugazio AG, Notarangelo LD: Monocytes from Wiskott-Aldrich patients display reduced chemotaxis and lack of cell polarization in response to monocyte chemoattractant protein-1 and formyl-methionyl-leucyl-phenylalanine. *J Immunol* **161(2)**:1026, 1998.
428. Bennett CP, Barnicoat AJ, Cotter F, Wang Q, Mathew CG: A variant of Wiskott-Aldrich syndrome with nephropathy is linked to DXS255 [Letter]. *J Med Genet* **32**:757, 1995.
429. Warrier I, Lusher JM: Congenital thrombocytopenias. *Curr Opin Hematol* **2**:395, 1995.
430. Zhu Q, Zhang M, Blaese RM, et al: The Wiskott-Aldrich syndrome and X-linked congenital thrombocytopenia are caused by mutations of the same gene. *Blood* **86**:3797, 1995.
431. Kondoh T, Hayashi K, Matsumoto T, et al: Two sisters with clinical diagnosis of Wiskott-Aldrich syndrome: Is the condition in the family autosomal recessive? *Am J Med Genet* **60**:364, 1995.
432. Parolini O, Ressmann G, Haas OA, et al: X-linked Wiskott-Aldrich syndrome in a girl [see comments]. *N Engl J Med* **338**:291, 1998.
433. Wengler G, Gorlin JB, Williamson JM, Rosen FS, Bing DH: Nonrandom inactivation of the X chromosome in early lineage hematopoietic cells in carriers of Wiskott-Aldrich syndrome. *Blood* **85**:2471, 1995.
434. Puck JM, Willard HF: X inactivation in females with X-linked disease. *N Engl J Med* **338**:325, 1998.
435. Rocca B, Bellacosa A, De Cristofaro R, et al: Wiskott-Aldrich syndrome: Report of an autosomal dominant variant. *Blood* **87**:4538, 1996.
436. Kwan SP, Lehner T, Hagemann T, Lu B, Blaese M, Ochs H, Wedgwood R, Ott J, Craig IW, Rosen FS: Localization of the gene for the Wiskott-Aldrich syndrome between two flanking markers, TIMP and DXS255, on Xp11.22-Xp11.3. *Genomics* **10**:29, 1991.
437. Greer WL, Peacocke M, Siminovitch KA: The Wiskott-Aldrich syndrome: Refinement of the localization on Xp and identification of another closely linked marker locus, OATL1. *Hum Genet* **88**:453, 1992.
438. Cremin SM, Greer WL, Bodok-Nutzati R, Schwartz M, Peacocke M, Siminovitch KA: Linkage of Wiskott-Aldrich syndrome with three marker loci, DXS426, SYP and TFE3, which map to the Xp11.3-p11.22 region. *Hum Genet* **92**:250, 1993.
439. Derry JM, Ochs HD, Francke U: Isolation of a novel gene mutated in Wiskott-Aldrich syndrome. *Cell* **78**:635, 1994.
440. Kwan SP, Hagemann TL, Radtke BE, Blaese RM, Rosen FS: Identification of mutations in the Wiskott-Aldrich syndrome gene and characterization of a polymorphic dinucleotide repeat at DXS6940, adjacent to the disease gene. *Proc Natl Acad Sci U S A* **92**:4706, 1995.
441. Hagemann TL, Kwan SP: The identification and characterization of two promoters and the complete genomic sequence for the Wiskott-Aldrich syndrome gene. *Biochem Biophys Res Commun* **256**:104, 1999.
442. Featherstone C: The many faces of WAS protein. *Science* **275**:27, 1997.
443. Kirchhausen T, Rosen FS: Disease mechanism: Unravelling Wiskott-Aldrich syndrome. *Curr Biol* **6**:676, 1996.
444. Stewart DM, Treiber-Held S, Kurman CC, Facchetti F, Notarangelo LD, Nelson DL: Studies of the expression of the Wiskott-Aldrich syndrome protein. *J Clin Invest* **97**:2627, 1996.
445. Parolini O, Berardelli S, Riedl E, et al: Expression of Wiskott-Aldrich syndrome protein (WASP) gene during hematopoietic differentiation. *Blood* **90**:70, 1997.
446. Miki H, Miura K, Takenawa T: N-WASP, a novel actin-depolymerizing protein, regulates the cortical cytoskeletal rearrangement in a PIP2-dependent manner downstream of tyrosine kinases. *EMBO J* **15**:5326, 1996.
447. Li R: Bee1, a yeast protein with homology to Wiskott-Aldrich syndrome protein, is critical for the assembly of cortical actin cytoskeleton. *J Cell Biol* **136**:649, 1997.
448. Bear JE, Rawls JF, Saxe CL 3rd: SCAR, a WASP-related protein, isolated as a suppressor of receptor defects in late Dictyostelium development. *J Cell Biol* **142**:1325, 1998.
449. Ponting CP, Phillips C: Identification of homer as a homologue of the Wiskott-Aldrich syndrome protein suggests a receptor-binding function for WH1 domains. *J Mol Med* **75**:769, 1997.
450. Insall R, Machesky L: PH domains in WASP — A bug in the system? Wiskott-Aldrich syndrome protein. *Trends Cell Biol* **9**:211, 1999.
451. Rudolph MG, Bayer P, Abo A, Kuhlmann J, Vetter IR, Wittinghofer A: The Cdc42/Rac interactive binding region motif of the

Wiskott-Aldrich syndrome protein (WASP) is necessary but not sufficient for tight binding to Cdc42 and structure formation. *J Biol Chem* **273**:18067, 1998.
452. Abdul-Manan N, Aghazadeh B, Liu GA, et al: Structure of Cdc42 in complex with the GTPase-binding domain of the "Wiskott-Aldrich syndrome" protein. *Nature* **399**:379, 1999.
453. Zhang B, Wang ZX, Zheng Y: Characterization of the interactions between the small GTPase Cdc42 and its GTPase-activating proteins and putative effectors. Comparison of kinetic properties of Cdc42 binding to the Cdc42-interactive domains. *J Biol Chem* **272**:21999, 1997.
454. Castellano F, Montcourrier P, Guillemot JC, et al: Inducible recruitment of Cdc42 or WASP to a cell-surface receptor triggers actin polymerization and filopodium formation. *Curr Biol* **9**:351, 1999.
455. Aspenstrom P, Lindberg U, Hall A: Two GTPases, Cdc42 and Rac, bind directly to a protein implicated in the immunodeficiency disorder Wiskott-Aldrich syndrome. *Curr Biol* **6**:70, 1996.
456. Kolluri R, Tolias KF, Carpenter CL, Rosen FS, Kirchhausen T: Direct interaction of the Wiskott-Aldrich syndrome protein with the GTPase Cdc42. *Proc Natl Acad Sci U S A* **93**:5615, 1996.
457. Symons M, Derry JM, Karlak B, et al: Wiskott-Aldrich syndrome protein, a novel effector for the GTPase CDC42Hs, is implicated in actin polymerization. *Cell* **84**:723, 1996.
458. Miki H, Sasaki T, Takai Y, Takenawa T: Induction of filopodium formation by a WASP-related actin-depolymerizing protein N-WASP. *Nature* **391**:93, 1998.
459. Kato M, Miki H, Imai K, et al: Wiskott-Aldrich syndrome protein induces actin clustering without direct binding to Cdc42. *J Biol Chem* **274**:27225, 1999.
460. Rivero-Lezcano OM, Marcilla A, Sameshima JH, Robbins KC: Wiskott-Aldrich syndrome protein physically associates with Nck through Src homology 3 domains. *Mol Cell Biol* **15**:5725, 1995.
461. Bunnell SC, Henry PA, Kolluri R, Kirchhausen T, Rickles RJ, Berg LJ: Identification of Itk/Tsk Src homology 3 domain ligands. *J Biol Chem* **271**:25646, 1996.
462. Banin S, Truong O, Katz DR, Waterfield MD, Brickell PM, Gout I: Wiskott-Aldrich syndrome protein (WASp) is a binding partner for c-Src family protein-tyrosine kinases. *Curr Biol* **6**:981, 1996.
463. Finan PM, Soames CJ, Wilson L, et al: Identification of regions of the Wiskott-Aldrich syndrome protein responsible for association with selected Src homology 3 domains. *J Biol Chem* **271**:26291, 1996.
464. Guinamard R, Aspenstrom P, Fougereau M, Chavrier P, Guillemot JC: Tyrosine phosphorylation of the Wiskott-Aldrich syndrome protein by Lyn and Btk is regulated by CDC42. *FEBS Lett* **434**:431, 1998.
465. Tang J, Feng GS, Li W: Induced direct binding of the adapter protein Nck to the GTPase-activating protein-associated protein p62 by epidermal growth factor. *Oncogene* **15(15)**:1823, 1997.
466. Wu Y, Spencer SD, Lasky LA: Tyrosine phosphorylation regulates the SH3-mediated binding of the Wiskott-Aldrich syndrome protein to PSTPIP, a cytoskeletal-associated protein. *J Biol Chem* **273**:5765, 1998.
467. Miki H, Nonoyama S, Zhu Q, Aruffo A, Ochs HD, Takenawa T: Cell tyrosine kinase signaling regulates Wiskott-Aldrich syndrome protein function, which is essential for megakaryocyte differentiation. *Growth Differ* **8(2)**:195, 1997.
468. Miki H, Takenawa T: Direct binding of the verprolin-homology domain in N-WASP to actin is essential for cytoskeletal reorganization. *Biochem Biophys Res Commun* **243**:73, 1998.
469. Naqvi SN, Zahn R, Mitchell DA, Stevenson BJ, Munn AL: The WASp homologue Las17p functions with the WIP homologue End5p/verprolin and is essential for endocytosis in yeast. *Curr Biol* **8**:959, 1998.
470. Nonoyama S, Ochs HD: Characterization of the Wiskott-Aldrich syndrome protein and its role in the disease. *Curr Opin Immunol* **10**:407, 1998.
471. Suetsugu S, Miki H, Takenawa T: The essential role of profilin in the assembly of actin for microspike formation. *EMBO J* **17**:6516, 1998.
472. Ramesh N, Anton IM, Martinez-Quiles N, Geha RS: Waltzing with WASP. *Trends Cell Biol* **9**:15, 1999.
473. Ramesh N, Anton IM, Hartwig JH, Geha RS: WIP, a protein associated with Wiskott-Aldrich syndrome protein, induces actin polymerization and redistribution in lymphoid cells. *Proc Natl Acad Sci U S A* **94**:14671, 1997.
474. Anton IM, Lu W, Mayer BJ, Ramesh N, Geha RS: The Wiskott-Aldrich syndrome protein-interacting protein (WIP) binds to the adaptor protein Nck. *J Biol Chem* **273**:20992, 1998.
475. Vaduva G, Martinez-Quiles N, Anton IM, et al: The human WASP-interacting protein, WIP, activates the cell polarity pathway in yeast. *J Biol Chem* **274**:17103, 1999.
476. Miki H, Suetsugu S, Takenawa T: WAVE, a novel WASP-family protein involved in actin reorganization induced by Rac. *EMBO J* **17**:6932, 1998.
477. Carlier MF, Ducruix A, Pantaloni D: Signalling to actin: The Cdc42-N-WASP-Arp2/3 connection. *Chem Biol* **6**:R235, 1999.
478. Higgs HN, Blanchoin L, Pollard TD: Influence of the C terminus of Wiskott-Aldrich syndrome protein (WASp) and the Arp2/3 complex on actin polymerization. *Biochemistry* **38**:15212, 1999.
479. Winter D, Lechler T, Li R: Activation of the yeast Arp2/3 complex by Bee1p, a WASP-family protein. *Curr Biol* **9**:501, 1999.
480. Madania A, Dumoulin P, Grava S, et al: The *Saccharomyces cerevisiae* homologue of human Wiskott-Aldrich syndrome protein Las17p interacts with the Arp2/3 complex. *Mol Biol Cell* **10**:3521, 1999.
481. May RC, Hall ME, Higgs HN, et al: The Arp2/3 complex is essential for the actin-based motility of *Listeria monocytogenes*. *Curr Biol* **9**:759, 1999.
482. Yarar D, To W, Abo A, Welch MD: The Wiskott-Aldrich syndrome protein directs actin-based motility by stimulating actin nucleation with the Arp2/3 complex. *Curr Biol* **9**:555, 1999.
483. Rohatgi R, Ma L, Miki H, Lopez M, Kirchhausen T, Takenawa T, Kirschner MW: The interaction between N-WASP and the Arp2/3 complex links Cdc42-dependent signals to actin assembly. *Cell* **97**:221, 1999.
484. She HY, Rockow S, Tang J, et al: Wiskott-Aldrich syndrome protein is associated with the adapter protein Grb2 and the epidermal growth factor receptor in living cells. *Mol Biol Cell* **8**:1709, 1997.
485. Machesky LM, Insall RH: Scar1 and the related Wiskott-Aldrich syndrome protein, WASP, regulate the actin cytoskeleton through the Arp2/3 complex. *Curr Biol* **8**:1347, 1998.
486. Suetsugu S, Miki H, Takenawa T: Identification of two human WAVE/SCAR homologues as general actin regulatory molecules which associate with the Arp2/3 complex. *Biochem Biophys Res Commun* **260**:296, 1999.
487. Machesky LM, Mullins RD, Higgs HN, Kaiser DA, Blanchoin L, May RC, Hall ME, Pollard TD: Scar, a WASp-related protein, activates nucleation of actin filaments by the Arp2/3 complex. *Proc Natl Acad Sci U S A* **96(7)**:3739, 1999.
488. Bi E, Zigmond SH: Actin polymerization: Where the WASP stings. *Curr Biol* **9**:R160, 1999.
489. Petrella A, Doti I, Agosti V, et al: A 5′ regulatory sequence containing two Ets motifs controls the expression of the Wiskott-Aldrich syndrome protein (WASP) gene in human hematopoietic cells. *Blood* **91**:4554, 1998.
490. Cory GO, MacCarthy-Morrogh L, Banin S, et al: Evidence that the Wiskott-Aldrich syndrome protein may be involved in lymphoid cell signaling pathways. *J Immunol* **157**:3791, 1996.
491. Snapper SB, Rosen FS: The Wiskott-Aldrich syndrome protein (WASP): Roles in signaling and cytoskeletal organization. *Annu Rev Immunol* **17**:905, 1999.
492. Kajiwara M, Nonoyama S, Eguchi M, et al: WASP is involved in proliferation and differentiation of human haemopoietic progenitors in vitro. *Br J Haematol* **107**:254, 1999.
493. Gallego MD, Santamaria M, Pena J, Molina IJ: Defective actin reorganization and polymerization of Wiskott-Aldrich T cells in response to CD3-mediated stimulation. *Blood* **90**:3089, 1997.
494. Miki H, Fukuda M, Nishida E, Takenawa T: Phosphorylation of WAVE downstream of mitogen-activated protein kinase signaling. *J Biol Chem* **274**:27605, 1999.
495. Linder S, Nelson D, Weiss M, Aepfelbacher M: Wiskott-Aldrich syndrome protein regulates podosomes in primary human macrophages. *Proc Natl Acad Sci U S A* **96**:9648, 1999.
496. Baba Y, Nonoyama S, Matsushita M, et al: Involvement of Wiskott-Aldrich syndrome protein in B-cell cytoplasmic tyrosine kinase pathway. *Blood* **93**:2003, 1999.
497. Rawlings SL, Crooks GM, Bockstoce D, Barsky LW, Parkman R, Weinberg KI: Spontaneous apoptosis in lymphocytes from patients with Wiskott-Aldrich syndrome: Correlation of accelerated cell death and attenuated bcl-2 expression. *Blood* **94**:3872, 1999.
498. Snapper SB, Rosen FS, Mizoguchi E, et al: Wiskott-Aldrich syndrome protein-deficient mice reveal a role for WASP in T but not B cell activation. *Immunity* **9**:81, 1998.
499. Thrasher AJ, Jones GE, Kinnon C, Brickell PM, Katz DR: Is Wiskott-Aldrich syndrome a cell trafficking disorder? *Immunol Today* **19**:537, 1998.

500. Kwan SP, Hagemann TL, Blaese RM, Knutsen A, Rosen FS: Scanning of the Wiskott-Aldrich syndrome (WAS) gene: Identification of 18 novel alterations including a possible mutation hotspot at Arg86 resulting in thrombocytopenia, a mild WAS phenotype. *Hum Mol Genet* **4**:1995, 1995.
501. Wengler GS, Notarangelo LD, Berardelli S, et al: High prevalence of nonsense, frameshift, and splice-site mutations in 16 patients with full-blown Wiskott-Aldrich syndrome. *Blood* **86**:3648, 1995.
502. Greer WL, Shehabeldin A, Schulman J, Junker A, Siminovitch KA: Identification of WASP mutations, mutation hotspots and genotype-phenotype disparities in 24 patients with the Wiskott-Aldrich syndrome. *Hum Genet* **98**:685, 1996.
503. Schindelhauer D, Weiss M, Hellebrand H, et al: Wiskott-Aldrich syndrome: No strict genotype-phenotype correlations but clustering of missense mutations in the amino-terminal part of the WASP gene product. *Hum Genet* **98**:68, 1996.
504. Lemahieu V, Gastier JM, Francke U: Novel mutations in the Wiskott-Aldrich syndrome protein gene and their effects on transcriptional, translational, and clinical phenotypes. *Hum Mutat* **14**:54, 1999.
505. Novak K: Mutant WASp stops cells in their tracks [News]. *Nat Med* **5**:1128, 1999.
506. Schwarz K: WASPbase: A database of WAS- and XLT-causing mutations. *Immunol Today* **17**:496, 1996.
507. Stewart DM, Tian L, Nelson DL: Mutations that cause the Wiskott-Aldrich syndrome impair the interaction of Wiskott-Aldrich syndrome protein (WASP) with WASP interacting protein. *J Immunol* **162**:5019, 1999.
508. Derry JM, Kerns JA, Weinberg KI, et al: WASP gene mutations in Wiskott-Aldrich syndrome and X-linked thrombocytopenia. *Hum Mol Genet* **4**:1127, 1995.
509. Kolluri R, Shehabeldin A, Peacocke M, et al: Identification of WASP mutations in patients with Wiskott-Aldrich syndrome and isolated thrombocytopenia reveals allelic heterogeneity at the WAS locus. *Hum Mol Genet* **4**:1119, 1995.
510. Villa A, Notarangelo L, Macchi P, et al: X-linked thrombocytopenia and Wiskott-Aldrich syndrome are allelic diseases with mutations in the WASP gene. *Nat Genet* **9**:414, 1995.
511. de Saint Basile G, Lagelouse RD, Lambert N, et al: Isolated X-linked thrombocytopenia in two unrelated families is associated with point mutations in the Wiskott-Aldrich syndrome protein gene. *J Pediatr* **129**:56, 1996.
512. Zhu Q, Watanabe C, Liu T, et al: Wiskott-Aldrich syndrome/X-linked thrombocytopenia: WASP gene mutations, protein expression, and phenotype. *Blood* **90**:2680, 1997.
513. Thompson LJ, Lalloz MR, Layton DM: Unique and recurrent WAS gene mutations in Wiskott-Aldrich syndrome and X-linked thrombocytopenia. *Blood Cells Mol Dis* **25**:218, 1999.
514. Puck JM, Straus SE, Rieux-Laucat F, Le Deist F, Fischer A: Inherited disorders with autoimmunity and defective lymphocyte regulation, in Ochs H, Smith CIE, Puck JM (eds): *Primary Immunodeficiency Diseases, a Molecular and Genetic Approach.* New York, Oxford University Press, 1999, p 339.
515. Bodmer J: World distribution of HLA alleles and implications for disease. *Ciba Found Symp* **197**:233, 1996.
516. Hammer J, Sturniolo T, Sinigaglia F: HLA class II peptide binding specificity and autoimmunity. *Adv Immunol* **66**:67, 1997.
517. Thorsby E: Invited anniversary review: HLA associated diseases. *Hum Immunol* **53**:1, 1997.
518. Nagata S, Goldstein P: The Fas death factor. *Science* **267**:1449, 1995.
519. Lenardo M: Fas and the art of lymphocyte maintenance. *J Exp Med* **183**:721, 1996.
520. Martin DA, Zheng L, Siegel RM, Huang B, Fisher GH, Wang J, Jackson CE, Puck JM, Dale J, Straus SE, Peter ME, Krammer PH, Fesik S, Lenardo MJ: Defective CD95/APO-1/Fas signal complex formation in the human autoimmune lymphoproliferative syndrome, type Ia. *Proc Natl Acad Sci U S A* **96**:4552, 1999.
521. Watanabe-Fukunaga R, Brannan CI, Copeland NG, Jenkins NA, Nagata S: Lymphoproliferation disorder in mice explained by defects in Fas antigen that mediates apoptosis. *Nature* **356**:314, 1992.
522. Oehm A, Behrmann I, Falk W, Pawlita M, Maier G, Klas C, Li-Weber M, Richards S, Dhein J, Trauth BC, et al: Purification and molecular cloning of the APO-1 cell surface antigen, a member of the tumor necrosis factor/nerve growth factor receptor superfamily. Sequence identity with the Fas antigen. *J Biol Chem* **267**:10709, 1992.
523. Theofilopoulos AN, Balderas RS, Shawler DL, Lee S, Dixon FJ: Influence of thymic genotype on the systemic lupus erythematosus-like disease and T cell proliferation of MRL/Mp-lpr/lpr mice. *J Exp Med* **153**:1405, 1981.
524. Cohen PL, Eisenberg RA: Lpr and gld: Single gene models of systemic autoimmunity and lymphoproliferative disease. *Annu Rev Immunol* **9**:243, 1991.
525. Sneller MC, Straus SE, Jaffe ES, Jaffe JS, Fleisher TA, Stetler SM, Strober W: A novel lymphoproliferative/autoimmune syndrome resembling murine lpr/gld disease. *J Clin Invest* **90**:334, 1992.
526. Rieux-Laucat F, Le Deist F, Hivroz C, Roberts IAG, Debatin KM, Fischer A, de Villartay JP: Mutations in Fas associated with human lymphoproliferative syndrome and autoimmunity. *Science* **268**:1347, 1995.
527. Fisher GH, Rosenberg FJ, Straus SE, Dale JK, Middleton LA, Lin AY, Strober W, Lenardo MJ, Puck JM: Dominant interfering Fas gene mutations impair apoptosis in a human autoimmune lymphoproliferative syndrome. *Cell* **81**:935, 1995.
528. Drappa J, Vaishnaw AK, Sullivan KE, Chu J-L, Elkon KB: Fas gene mutations in the Canale-Smith syndrome, an inherited lymphoproliferative disorder associated with autoimmunity. *N Engl J Med* **335**:1643, 1996.
529. Bettinardi A, Brugnoni D, Quirós-Roldan E, Malagoli A, La Grutta S, Correra A, Notarangelo LD: Missense mutations in the Fas gene resulting in autoimmune lymphoproliferative syndrome: A molecular and immunological analysis. *Blood* **89**:902, 1997.
530. Pensati L, Costanzo A, Ianni A, Accapezzato D, Iorio R, Natoli G, Nisini R: Fas/APO-1 mutations and autoimmune lymphoproliferative syndrome in a patient with type 2 autoimmune hepatitis. *Gastroenterology* **113**:1384, 1997.
531. Sneller MC, Wang J, Dale JK, Strober W, Middelton LA, Choi Y, Fleischer TA, Lim MS, Jaffe ES, Puck JM, Lenardo MJ, Straus SE: Clinical, immunologic and genetic features of an autoimmune lymphoproliferative syndrome associated with abnormal lymphocyte apoptosis. *Blood* **89**:1341, 1997.
532. Kasahara Y, Wada T, Niida Y, Yachie A, Seki H, Ishida Y, Sakai T, Koizumi F, Koizumi S, Miyawaki T, Taniguchi N: Novel Fas (CD95/APO-1) mutations in infants with a lymphoproliferative disorder. *Int Immunol* **10**:195, 1998.
533. Jackson CE, Fischer RE, Hsu AP, Anderson SM, Choi Y, Wang J, Dale JK, Fleisher TA, Middelton LA, Sneller MC, Lenardo MJ, Straus SE, Puck JM: Autoimmune lymphoproliferative syndrome with defective Fas: Genotype influences penetrance. *Am J Hum Genet* **64**:1002, 1999.
534. Vaishnaw AK, Orlinick JR, Chu JL, Krammer PH, Chao MV, Elkon KB: The molecular basis for apoptotic defects in patients with CD95 (Fas/Apo-1) mutations. *J Clin Invest* **10**:355, 1999.
535. Randall DL, Reiquam CW, Githens JH, Robinson A: Familial myeloproliferative disease. *Am J Dis Child* **110**:479, 1965.
536. Holimon JL, Madge GE: A familial disorder characterized by hepatosplenomegaly presenting as preleukemia. *VA Med Monthly* **98**:644, 1971.
537. Canale VC, Smith CH: Chronic lymphadenopathy simulating malignant lymphoma. *J Pediatr* **70**:891, 1967.
538. Cheng DS, Williams HJ, Kitahara M: Hereditary hepatosplenomegaly. *West J Med* **132**:70, 1980.
539. Rao LM, Shahidi NT, Opitz JM: Hereditary splenomegaly with hypersplenism. *Clin Genet* **5**:379, 1974.
540. Le Deist F, Emile J-F, Rieux-Laucat F, Benkerrou M, Roberts I, Brousse N, Fischer A: Clinical, immunological, and pathological consequences of Fas-deficient conditions. *Lancet* **348**:719, 1996.
541. Dianzani U, Bragardo M, DiFranco D, Alliaudi C, Scagni P, Buonfiglio D, Redoglia V, Bonissoni S, Correra A, Dianzani I, Ramenghi U: Deficiency of the Fas apoptosis pathway without Fas gene mutations in pediatric patients with autoimmunity/lymphoproliferation. *Blood* **89**:2871, 1997.
542. Straus SE, Sneller M, Lenardo MJ, Puck JM, Strober W: An inherited disorder of lymphocyte apoptosis: The autoimmune lymphoproliferative syndrome. *Ann Intern Med* **130**:591, 1999.
543. Wang J, Zheng L, Lobito A, Chan FK, Dale J, Sneller M, Yao X, Puck JM, Straus SE, Lenardo MJ: Inherited human caspase 10 mutations underlie defective lymphocyte and dendritic cell apoptosis in autoimmune lymphoproliferative syndrome type II. *Cell* **98(1)**:47, 1999.
544. Gerdes J, Lemke H, Baisch H, Wacker HH, Schwab U, Stein H: Cell cycle analysis of a cell proliferation-associated human nuclear antigen defined by the monoclonal antibody Ki-67. *J Immunol* **133**:1710, 1984.
545. Infante AJ, Britton HA, DiNapoliT, Middelton LA, Lenardo MJ, Jackson CE, Wang J, Fleisher T, Straus SE, Puck JM: The clinical spectrum in a large kindred with autoimmune lymphoproliferative

syndrome (ALPS), due to a Fas mutation that impairs lymphocyte apoptosis. *J Pediatr* **133(5)**:629, 1998.

546. Beltinger C, Kurz E, Bohler T, Schrappe M, Ludwig WD, Debatin KM: CD95 (APO-1/Fas) mutations in childhood T-lineage acute lymphoblastic leukemia. *Blood* **91**:3943, 1998.
547. Landowski TH, Qu N, Buyuksal I, Painter JS, Dalton WS: Mutations in the Fas antigen in patients with multiple myeloma. *Blood* **90**:4266, 1997.
548. Tamiya S, Etoh K, Suzushima H, Takatsuki K, Matsuoka M: Mutation of CD95 (Fas/Apo-1) gene in adult T-cell leukemia cells. *Blood* **91**:3935, 1998.
549. Fuss IJ, Strober W, Dale JK, Fritz S, Pearlstein G, Puck JM, Lenardo M, Straus S: Characteristic T helper 2 T cell cytokine abnormalities in autoimmune lymphoproliferative syndrome, a syndrome marked by defective apoptosis and humoral autoimmunity. *J Immunol* **158**:1912, 1997.
550. Benkerrou M, Le Deist F, de Villartay JP, Caillat-Zucman S, Rieux-Laucat F, Jabado N, Cavazzana-Calvo M, Fischer A: Correction of Fas (CD95) deficiency by haploidentical bone marrow transplantation. *Eur J Immunol* **27**:2043, 1997.
551. Izui S, Kelley VE, Masuda K, Yoshida H, Roths JB, Murphy ED, Kasahara Y, Wada T, Niida Y, Yachie A, Seki H, Ishida Y, Sakai T, et al: Induction of various autoantibodies by mutant gene lpr in several strains of mice. *J Immunol* **133**:227, 1984.
552. Vidal S, Kono DH, Theofilopoulos AN: Loci predisposing to autoimmunity in MRL-Fas^{lpr} and C57BL/6-Fas^{lpr} mice. *J Clin Invest* **101**:696, 1998.
553. Wu J, Wilson J, He J, Xiang L, Schur PH, Mountz JD: Fas ligand mutation in a patient with systemic lupus erythematosus and lymphoproliferative disease. *J Clin Invest* **98**:1107, 1996.
554. Ahonen P, Myllärniemi S, Sipilä I, Perheentupa J: Clinical variation of autoimmune polyendocrinopathy-candidiasis-ectodermal dystrophy (APECED) in a series of 68 patients. *N Engl J Med* **322**:1829, 1990.
555. Aaltonen J, Björses P, Sandkuijl L, Perheentupa J, Peltonen L: An autosomal locus causing autoimmune disease: Autoimmune polyglandular disease type I assigned to chromosome 21. *Nat Genet* **8**:83, 1994.
556. Zlotogora J, Shapiro MS: Polyglandular autoimmune syndrome type I among Iranian Jews. *J Med Genet* **29**:824, 1992.
557. Aaltonen J, Björses P, Perheentupa J, Horelli-Kuitunen N, Palotie A, Peltonen L, Lee YS, Francis F, Hennig S, Thiel C, Lehrach H, Yaspo M-L: An autoimmune disease, APECED, caused by mutations in a novel gene featuring two PHD-type zinc-finger domains. *Nat Genet* **17**:399, 1997.
558. Nagamine K, Peterson P, Scott HS, Kudoh J, Minoshima S, Maarit H, Krohn KJE, Lalioti MD, Mullis PE, Antonarakis SE, Kawasaki K, Asakawa S, Ito F, Shimizu N: Positional cloning of the APECED gene. *Nat Genet* **17**:393, 1997.
559. Pearce SH, Cheetham T, Imrie H, Vaidya B, Barnes ND, Bilous RW, Carr D, Meeran K, Shaw NJ, Smith CS, Toft AD, Williams G, Kendall-Taylor P: A common and recurrent 13-bp deletion in the autoimmune regulator gene in British kindreds with autoimmune polyendocrinopathy type 1. *Am J Hum Genet* **63**:1675, 1998.
560. Scott HS, Heino M, Peterson P, Mittaz L, Lalioti MD, Betterle C, Cohen A, Seri M, Lerone M, Romeo G, Collin P, Salo M, Metcalfe R, Weetman A, Papasavvas MP, Rossier C, Nagamine K, Kudoh J, Shimizu N, Krohn KJ, Antonarakis SE: Common mutations in autoimmune polyendocrinopathy-candidiasis-ectodermal dystrophy patients of different origins. *Mol Endocrinol* **12**:1112, 1998.
561. Ward L, Paquette J, Seidman E, Huot C, Alvarez F, Crock P, Delvin E, Kampe O, Deal C: Severe autoimmune polyendocrinopathy-candidiasis-ectodermal dystrophy in an adolescent girl with a novel AIRE mutation: Response to immunosuppressive therapy. *J Clin Endocrinol Metab* **84**:844, 1999.
562. Blechschmidt K, Schweiger M, Wertz K, Poulson R, Christensen HM, Rosenthal A, Lehrach H, Yaspo ML: The mouse aire gene: Comparative genomic sequencing, gene organization, and expression. *Genome Res* **9**:158, 1999.
563. Bjorses P, Pelto-Huikko M, Kaukonen J, Aaltonen J, Peltonen L, Ulmanen I: Localization of the APECED protein in distinct nuclear structures. *Hum Mol Genet* **8**:259, 1999.
564. Rinderle C, Christensen HM, Schweiger S, Lehrach H, Yaspo ML: AIRE encodes a nuclear protein co-localizing with cytoskeletal filaments: Altered sub-cellular distribution of mutants lacking the PHD zinc fingers. *Hum Mol Genet* **82**:277, 1999.
565. Sharfe N, Dadi HK, Shahar M, Roifman CM: Human immune disorder arising from mutation of the γ chain of the interleukin-2 receptor. *Proc Natl Acad Sci U S A* **94**:3168, 1997.
566. Willerford DM, Chen J, Ferry JA, Davidson L, Ma A, Alt FW: Interleukin-2 receptor γ chain regulates the size and content of the peripheral lymphoid compartment. *Immunity* **3**:521, 1995.
567. Suzuki H, Kündig TM, Furlonger C, Wakeham A, Timms E, Matsuyama T, Schmits R, Simard JJ, Ohashi PS, Griesser H, Taniguchi T, Paig C, Mak TW: Deregulated T cell activation and autoimmunity in mice lacking interleukin-2 receptor beta. *Science* **268**:1472, 1995.
568. Ownby DR, Pizzo SV, Blackmon L, Gall SA, Buckley RH: Severe combined immunodeficiency with leukopenia (reticular dysgenesis) in siblings: Immunologic and histopathologic findings. *J Pediat* **89**:382, 1976.
569. Roper M, Parmley RT, Crist WM, Kelly DR, Cooper MD: Severe congenital leukopenia (reticular dysgenesis): Immunologic and morphologic characterizations of leukocytes. *Am J Dis Child* **139**:832, 1985.
570. Moreno LA, Gottrand F, Turck D, Manouvrier-Hanu S, Mazingue F, Morisot C, Le Deist F, Ricour C, Nihoul-Fekete C, Debeugny P, Griscelli C, Farriaux J-P: Severe combined immunodeficiency syndrome associated with autosomal recessive familial multiple gastrointestinal atresias: Study of a family. *Am J Med Genet* **37**:143, 1990.
571. Makitie O: Cartilage-hair hypoplasia in Finland: Epidemiological and genetic aspects of 107 patients. *J Med Genet* **29**:652, 1992.
572. Makitie O, Kaitila I: Cartilage-hair hypoplasia—Clinical manifestations in 108 Finnish patients. *Eur J Pediatr* **152**:211, 1993.
573. Makitie O, Kaitila I, Savilahti E: Susceptibility to infections and in vitro immune functions in cartilage-hair hypoplasia. *Eur J Pediatr* **157**:816, 1998.
574. Sulisalo T, Sistonen P, Hastbacka J, Wadelius C, Makitie O, de la Chapelle A, Kaitila I: Cartilage-hair hypoplasia gene assigned to chromosome 9 by linkage analysis. *Nat Genet* **3**:338, 1993.
575. Sulisalo T, van der Burgt I, Rimoin DL, Bonaventure J, Sillence D, Campbell JB, Chitayat D, Scott CI, de la Chapelle A, Sistonen P, Kaitila I: Genetic homogeneity of cartilage-hair hypoplasia. *Hum Genet* **95**:157, 1995.
576. Erickson RP: Southwestern Athabaskan (Navajo and Apache) genetic diseases. *Genet Med* **1**:151, 1999.
577. Li L, Drayna D, Hu D, Hayward A, Gahagan S, Pabst H, Cowan MJ: The gene for severe combined immunodeficiency disease in Athabascan-speaking Native Americans is located on chromosome 10p. *Am J Hum Genet* **62**:136, 1998.
578. Sams WM Jr, Jorizzo JL, Snyderman R, Jegasothy BV, Ward FE, Weiner M, Wilson JG, Yount WJ, Dillard SB: Chronic mucocutaneous candidiasis: Immunologic studies of three generations of a single family. *Am J Med* **67**:948, 1979.
579. Germain M, Gourdeau M, Hebert J: Familial chronic mucocutaneous candidiasis complicated by deep *Candida* infection. *Am J Med Sci* **307**:282, 1994.
580. Brown DC, Grace E, Sumner AT, Edmunds AT, Ellis PM: ICF syndrome (immunodeficiency, centromeric instability and facial anomalies): Investigation of heterochromatin abnormalities and review of clinical outcome. *Hum Genet* **96**:411, 1995.
581. Wijmenga C, van den Heuvel LPWJ, Strengman E, Luyten JAFM, van der Burgt IJAM, de Groot R, Smeets DFCM, Draaisma JMT, van Dongen JJ, De Abreu RA, Pearson PL, Sandkuijl LA, Weemaes CMR: Localization of the ICF syndrome to chromosome 20 by homozygosity mapping. *Am J Hum Genet* **63**:803, 1998.
582. Xu G-L, Bestor TH, Bourc'his D, Hsieh C-L, Tommerup N, Bugge M, Hulten M, Qu X, Russo JJ, Viegas-Pequignot E: Chromosome instability and immunodeficiency syndrome caused by mutations in a DNA methyltransferase gene. *Nature* **402**:187, 1999.
583. Okano M, Bell DW, Haber DA, Li E: DNA methyltransferases Dnmt3a and Dnmt3b are essential for *de novo* methylation and mammalian development. *Cell* **99**:247, 1999.
584. Pignata C, Fiore M, Guzzetta V, Castaldo A, Sebastio G, Porta F, Guarino A: Congenital alopecia and nail dystrophy associated with severe functional T-cell immunodeficiency in two sibs. *Am J Med Genet* **65**:167, 1996.
585. Frank J, Pignata C, Panteleyev AA, Prowse DM, Baden H, Weiner L, Gaetaniello L, Ahmad W, Pozzi N, Caerhalmi-Friedman PB, Aita VM, Uyttendaele H, Gordon D, Ott J, Brissette JL, Christiano AM: Exposing the human nude phenotype. *Nature* **398**:473, 1999.
586. Puck JM, Middelton LA, Pepper AE: Carrier and prenatal diagnosis of X-linked severe combined immunodeficiency: Mutation detection methods and utilization. *Hum Genet* **99**:628, 1997.

587. Durandy A, Dumez Y, Griscelli C: Prenatal diagnosis of severe inherited immunodeficiencies: A five year experience, in Vossen J, Griscelli C (eds): *Progress in Immunodeficiency Research and Therapy*, vol 2. Amsterdam, Elsiever, 1986, p 323.
588. Flake AW, Almeida-Porada G, Puck JM, Roncarolo M-G, Evans MI, Johnson MP, Abella EM, Harrison DD, Zanjani ED: Treatment of X-linked SCID by the in utero transplantation of CD34 enriched bone marrow. *N Engl J Med* **355**:1806, 1996.
589. Klein C, Cavazzana-Calvo M, Le Deist F, et al: Bone marrow transplantation in major histocompatibility complex class II deficiency: A single-center study of 19 patients. *Blood* **85**:580, 1995.
590. Godthelp BC, Van Eggermond MC, Peijnenburg A, Tezcan I, van Lierde S, van Tol MJ, Vossen JM, Van den Elsen PJ: Incomplete T-cell immune reconstitution in two major histocompatibility complex class II-deficiency/bare lymphocyte syndrome patients after HLA- identical sibling bone marrow transplantation. *Blood* **94**:348.1999.
591. Ozsahin H, Le Deist F, Benkerrou M, et al: Bone marrow transplantation in 26 patients with Wiskott-Aldrich syndrome from a single center. *J Pediatr* **129**:238, 1996.
592. Fischer A, Haddad E, Jabado N, et al: Stem cell transplantation for immunodeficiency. *Semin Immunopathol* **19**:479, 1998.
593. Buckley RH, Schiff SE, Schiff RI, Markert L, Williams LW, Roberts JL, Myers LA, Ward FE: Hematopoietic stem-cell transplantation for the treatment of severe combined immunodeficiency [see comments]. *N Engl J Med* **340**:508, 1999.
594. Wengler GS, Lanfranchi A, Frusca T, Verardi R, Neva A, Brugnoni D, Giliani S, Fiorini M, Mella P, Guandalini F, Mazzolari E, Pecorelli S, Notarangelo LD, Porta F, Ugazio AG: In-utero transplantation of parental CD34 haematopoietic progenitor cells in a patient with X-linked severe combined immunodeficiency (SCIDXI). *Lancet* **348(9040)**:1484, 1996.
595. Stephan V, Wahn V, Le Deist F, Dirksen U, Broker B, Muller-Fleckenstein I, Horneff G, Schroten H, Fischer A, de Saint Basile G: Atypical X-linked severe combined immunodeficiency due to possible spontaneous reversion of the genetic defect in T cells. *N Engl J Med* **335**:1563, 1996.
596. Candotti F, Johnston JA, Puck JM, Sugamura K, O'Shea JJ, Blaese RM: Retroviral-mediated gene correction for X-linked severe combined immunodeficiency (XSCID). *Blood* **87**:3097, 1996.
597. Hacein-Bey H, Cavazzana-Calvo M, Le Deist F, Dautry-Varsat A, Hivroz C, Riviere I, Danos O, Heard JM, Sugamura K, Fischer A, De Saint Basile G: Gamma-c gene transfer into SCID X1 patients' B-cell lines restores normal high-affinity interleukin-2 receptor expression and function. *Blood* **87**:3108, 1996.
598. Bunting KD, Sangster MY, Ihle JN, Sorrentino BP: Restoration of lymphocyte function in Janus kinase 3-deficient mice by retroviral-mediated gene transfer. *Nat Med* **4**:58, 1998.
599. Cavazzana-Calvo M, Hacein-Bey S, de Saint Basile G, Gross F, Nusbaum P, Yvon E, Casanova JL, Le Deist F, Fischer A: Correction of SCID-X1 disease phenotype following γc gene transfer by a retroviral vector into CD34+ cells in two children. *Blood* **94(Suppl 2)**:367a, 1999.
600. Whitwam T, Haskins ME, Henthorn PS, Kraszewski JN, Kleiman SE, Seidel NE, Bodine DM, Puck JM: Retroviral marking of canine bone marrow: Long term, high level expression of human IL-2 receptor common gamma chain in canine lymphocytes. *Blood* **92**:1565, 1998.
601. Jackson CE, Puck JM: Autoimmune lymphoproliferative syndrome: A disorder of apoptosis. *Curr Opin Pediatr* **11**:521, 1999.

CHAPTER 186

Genetically Determined Disorders of the Complement System

Kathleen E. Sullivan ▪ Jerry A. Winkelstein

1. **The complement system is composed of a series of plasma proteins and cellular receptors that, when functioning in an ordered and integrated fashion, serve as important mediators of host defense and inflammation. In order for the individual components of complement to subserve their biologic functions, however, they must first be activated. Activation of the complement system can occur via the classical pathway, the alternative pathway, or the lectin pathway. Once activated, individual components act as opsonins, possess chemotactic activity, are potent anaphylatoxins, and can assemble into the membrane attack complex and generate cytolytic activity. In addition, the complement system is important in the processing of immune complexes and the generation of a normal antibody response.**
2. **Some of the complement genes have been grouped into supergene families based on similarities in structure, function, and chromosomal location. For example, the genes encoding C2, factor B, and C4 constitute the class III genes of the major histocompatibility complex on chromosome 6; the products of these genes are constituents of the enzymes that activate C3 and C5. The genes for C4-binding protein, factor H, decay-accelerating factor, membrane cofactor protein, and two of the receptors for C3 cleavage products make up another family of complement genes located on the long arm of chromosome 1; the products of these genes share their ability to interact with the activation products of C4 and C3. The synthesis of a number of components of complement is regulated by cytokines such as interleukin 1 (IL-1), tumor necrosis factor (TNF), IL-6, and γ-interferon and by endotoxic lipopolysaccharide.**
3. **Genetically determined deficiencies have been described for most of the individual components of complement. The usual mode of inheritance is autosomal recessive with only two exceptions; C1-inhibitor deficiency is inherited as an autosomal dominant disorder, and properdin deficiency is inherited as an X-linked recessive disorder. The clinical manifestations of individuals with complement deficiencies have varied. Most individuals have had either an increased susceptibility to infection, rheumatic disorders, or angioedema. Patients with a deficiency of C3 or with a deficiency of a component in the pathways necessary for the activation of C3 have an increased susceptibility to infection with encapsulated bacteria, for which C3b-dependent opsonization is an important host defense. Patients with deficiencies of terminal components, C5 through C9, are markedly susceptible to systemic neisserial infections because serum bactericidal activity is an important host defense against these organisms. The prevalence of rheumatic disorders, such as systemic lupus erythematosus, vasculitis, and membranoproliferative glomerulonephritis, is highest in patients who are deficient in components of the classical activating pathway (C1, C4, and C2) and C3. Finally, patients with C1-inhibitor deficiency present with angioedema.**

The complement system was first described around the turn of the century as a cytolytic mechanism responsible for lysing bacteria or erythrocytes sensitized with antibody.[1] The term *complement* was used because the cytolytic principle "complemented" the action of antibody. Nearly 100 years later, it is now appreciated that the complement system is composed of a series of proteins and cellular receptors that, when functioning in an ordered and integrated fashion, serve as important mediators of host defense and inflammation.[2,3] In addition to its cytolytic function, the complement system subserves a variety of other biologically significant functions. Individual components of the complement system act as opsonins, possess chemotactic activity, or are potent anaphylatoxins. In addition, the complement system plays an important role in the processing of immune complexes and the generation of a normal antibody response. When its activation is controlled and directed against invading microorganisms, the complement system is an important mechanism of defense and is beneficial to the host. However, when its activation proceeds in an uncontrolled manner or is directed against the host, the complement system is an important mediator of immunopathologic damage and is detrimental to the host.

The first description of an individual with a genetically determined deficiency of one of the components of complement was in 1960.[4] Since then, genetically determined deficiencies of nearly all the components of the complement system have been described in humans.[5–8] The discovery of individuals with genetically determined abnormalities of the complement system not only has identified a new group of patients with inborn errors

A list of standard abbreviations is located immediately preceding the index in each volume. Nonstandard abbreviations used in this chapter include: C1-INH = C1 inhibitor; C4bp = C4-binding protein; DAF = decay-accelerating factor; MCP = membrane cofactor protein; MBL = mannose-binding lectin; MASP = MBL-associated serine protease; MIRL = membrane inhibitor of reactive lysis; HRF = homologous restriction factor; C8bf = C8-binding factor; IL-8 = interleukin 8; MHC = major histocompatability complex; SCRs = short consensus repeats; C6SD = C6 subtotal deficiency; C7SD = C7 subtotal deficiency; HAE = hereditary angioedema; EACA = ε-aminocaproic acid; RCA = regulation of complement activation; GPI = glycosyl-phosphatidylinositol; MBP = mannose-binding protein.

of metabolism, but elucidation of the pathophysiology in these patients also has led to a better understanding of the physiologic role of complement in normal individuals.

This chapter will review the biochemistry, biology, and molecular genetics of the normal complement system and relate these to the genetically determined disorders of the complement system in humans.

BIOCHEMISTRY OF THE COMPLEMENT SYSTEM

The complement system is composed of a series of proteins and cellular receptors (Table 186-1). The majority of the biologically significant effects of the complement system are mediated by C3 and the terminal components, C5, C6, C7, C8, and C9. In order to subserve their biologic functions, however, C3 and C5–C9 must

Table 186-1 Components of Human Complement

Component	Chromosomal Location	Approximate Molecular Weight	Chains
Classical pathway			
C1q	1p34.1-36.3	460,000	6A, 6B, 6C
C1r	12p13	83,000	Single
C1s	12p13	83,000	Single
C4	6p	200,000	1 alpha, 1 beta, 1 gamma
C2	6p	102,000	Single
Alternative pathway			
Factor D	?	25,000	Single
Factor B	6p	93,000	Single
C3 and terminal components			
C3	19p	185,000	1 alpha, 1 beta
C5	9q32-34	190,000	1 alpha, 1 beta
C6	5q13	128,000	Single
C7	5q13	120,000	Single
C8	1p3.2, 9q	163,000	1 alpha, 1 beta, 1 gamma
C9	5p13	79,000	Single
Control proteins			
C1 inhibitor	11q	105,000	Single
C4 binding protein	1q4	550,000	7-8 identical
Factor H	1q	150,000	Single
Factor I	4q2	100,000	1 alpha, 1 beta
Properdin	Xp11.23-21	223,000	4 identical
Membrane cofactor			
Protein (CD46)	1q	58,000	Single
Membrane inhibitor of reactive lysis (CD59)(HRF 20)	11p13-14	20,000	Single
Membrane/receptor proteins			
Decay accelerating factor (CD55)	1q	70,000	Single
CR1 (CD35)	1q	250,000	Single
CR2 (CD21)	1q	145,000	Single
CR3 (CD11b/18)	16p	250,000	1 alpha, 1 beta
CR4	21q	150,000	1 alpha, 1 beta

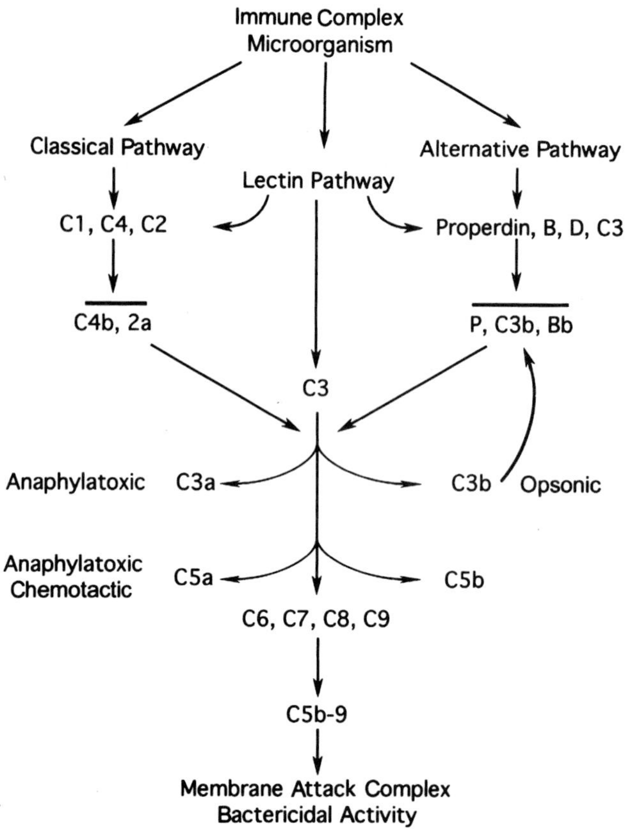

Fig. 186-1 The activation of C3 and the terminal components (C5–C9) of complement by the classical, alternative, and lectin pathways.

first be activated. Activation of C3 and C5–C9 may occur through at least three mechanisms: the classical pathway, the alternative pathway, and the lectin pathway (Fig. 186-1).

The Classical Pathway

Activation of the classical pathway usually is initiated by antigen-antibody complexes (Fig. 186-2). Antibodies of the appropriate class (IgG and IgM) or subclass (IgG_1, IgG_2, IgG_3) combine with an antigen to form an immune complex, which is then capable of binding and activating the first component of complement (C1).[9] Only one molecule of pentameric IgM is needed for activation of C1, but the IgM molecule must combine with the antigen through more than one of its Fab arms. In contrast, two IgG molecules are needed in order for C1 to bind and activation to occur, and they must be in close proximity. The requirements for an IgG doublet greatly reduces the efficiency of immune complexes composed of IgG as compared with IgM to activate C1 and the classical pathway, since hundreds, if not thousands, of IgG molecules must be deposited on a bacterial surface for two of them to be aligned in close proximity.

In its native state, a single molecule of C1 is a macromolecular complex composed of three biochemically distinct subcomponents, designated C1q, C1r, and C1s,[10] which are present in molar ratios of 1:2:2, respectively.[11] It is C1q that binds to the immunoglobulin molecules in the immune complex.[12] Binding of C1q to the immune complex results in a conformational change in C1r, exposing a proteolytic site that initiates the autocatalytic cleavage of C1r and thereby converts the single-chain zymogen to the disulfide-linked heterodimer that is the active enzyme.[13] A serine esterase, C1r then converts C1s to its active form. Native C1s is a single polypeptide chain that on activation by C1r is also cleaved into two disulfide-linked chains, and its serine esterase activity is expressed.[14]

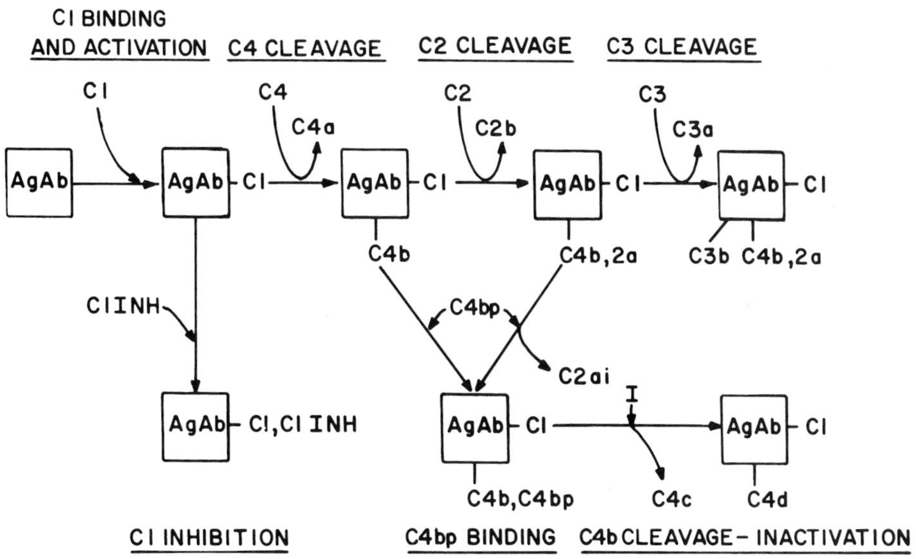

Fig. 186-2 The classical pathway of C3 activation. Activation of the pathway is initiated by immune complexes (AgAb) that activate C1. Activated C1 then cleaves C4 and C2, generating cleavage products that form a bimolecular complex, C4b2a, that is the classical pathway C3-convertase. The generation and expression of the C3-convertase are regulated by the control proteins, C1-INH, C4bp, and factor I (I).

Activated C1s then activates its natural substrate, the fourth component of complement (C4). Native C4 is composed of three disulfide-linked chains (α, β, and γ).[15] Activation of C4 is accomplished by cleaving a peptide (C4a) of 6000 Da from the N-terminal portion of the largest of the three chains, the α chain. This exposes an intrachain reactive thiolester bond in the remaining portion of the α chain of the larger cleavage product (C4b). The nascent C4b is then able to bind covalently to cell surfaces or to immunoglobulins through either esterification of hydroxyl groups on polysaccharides or amidation of amino groups on proteins by the acyl group of the reactive thiolester.[16] The internal thiolester bond of the C4b is highly labile, however, and if transesterification or amidation does not occur quickly, the C4b is inactivated by hydrolysis in the fluid phase and unable to bind to the cell surface or immunoglobulin. It is the lability of the reactive thiolester that confines the binding of the nascent C4b to the immediate vicinity of the immune complex and thereby helps to restrict activation of the complete cascade to the area in which it was initiated.

The reaction continues with the cleavage of the second component (C2) by C1s.[17] In order for most efficient activation of native C2 to occur, however, the C2 must first complex with C4b molecules that are in close proximity to C1s. Cleavage of the C2 results in the liberation of a small peptide (C2b). The larger fragment, C2a, remains complexed with the C4b to form a bimolecular enzyme, C4b2a, which is responsible for activating C3[18] and initiating the assembly of the terminal components (C5–C9) into the membrane attack complex.

If the activation of the classical pathway were to proceed in an uncontrolled fashion, then the generation of the C4b2a enzyme would lead to the continuous activation of C3, C5, and the other terminal components.[19] This, in turn, could result in the generation of excessive amounts of the phlogistic fragments of complement, which could cause widespread immunopathologic damage to the host. Fortunately, a number of mechanisms act to control the assembly and expression of the classical pathway C3-convertase C4b2a. First, the C4b2a enzyme is very labile at physiologic temperatures and undergoes spontaneous decay with release of C2a and loss of enzymatic activity.[18] Second, the enzymatic actions of C1r and C1s can be inhibited by a control protein, C1 inhibitor (C1-INH).[20] C1-INH is a naturally occurring glycoprotein that binds covalently to C1r and C1s, leading to dissociation of the C1 macromolecular complex.[21] Third, another regulatory protein, C4-binding protein (C4bp), inhibits the C4b2a enzyme by limiting the uptake of C2 by C4b, by accelerating the decay/dissociation of the C2a once it has complexed with the C4b, and by enhancing the ability of yet another inhibitor, factor I (C3b/C4b inactivator), to cleave and inactivate C4b.[22,23] Factor I cleaves the α chain of C4b so as to release a large cleavage product (C4c) of C4b into the fluid phase, leaving a smaller fragment of the α chain (C4d) still covalently attached to the cell surface but no longer able to bind native C2.[23] Finally, a fourth inhibitor, decay-accelerating factor (DAF), an integral membrane protein found in erythrocytes and a variety of other cells, also accelerates the release of C2a from the C4b2a enzyme.[24] Thus, in the usual situation, the assembly and expression of the C4b2a enzyme, and thus activation of C3, proceeds in a controlled fashion and is limited to the immediate vicinity of the initiating substance (e.g., a microbial surface or an immune complex).

Activation of the classical pathway usually is initiated by antigen-antibody complexes and therefore is considered to be especially important in acquired immunity. However, some enveloped RNA viruses,[25] some *Mycoplasma* species,[26] and certain strains and species of both gram-negative[27] and gram-positive bacteria[28] can bind C1q directly and activate the classical pathway. Thus, under some circumstances, the classical pathway may be activated in an antibody-independent fashion and function in "natural" immunity.[29]

The Alternative Pathway

Activation of the alternative pathway begins with the C3 molecule[30] (Fig. 186-3). Like C4 (see above), native C3 contains an internal thiolester in its α chain.[31] Under normal physiologic conditions, this internal thiolester undergoes continuous low-grade hydrolysis to create a C3b-like molecule [C3(H_2O)].[32] The "C3b-like" C3 then can bind native factor B and allow its cleavage by a serine protease, factor D.[33] Two cleavage products of factor B are generated, a larger product, Bb, and a smaller product, Ba. The association of the hydrolyzed C3 with Bb then creates a C3-cleaving enzyme, C3Bb (termed the *priming* C3-convertase),[30] that is responsible for a continuous, low-grade cleavage of C3 and hence the generation of nascent C3b. As with the activation of C4, the cleavage of native C3 exposes the reactive thiolester, allowing transesterification with or amidation of suitable acceptor sites on the cell surface. Should a suitable surface not be available, then hydrolysis of the thiolester results in an inactive C3b molecule. On the other hand, if the nascent C3b binds covalently to a suitable surface, it can form a reversible complex with native factor B, which is then cleaved by factor D to create a highly efficient C3-cleaving enzyme, C3bBb, termed the *amplification* C3-convertase.[30]

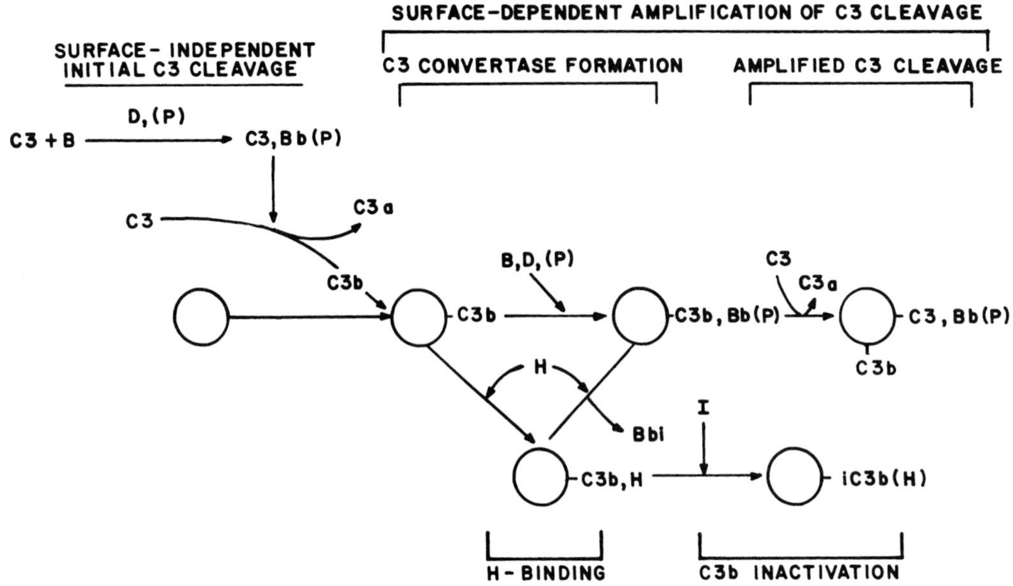

Fig. 186-3 The alternative pathway of C3 activation. There is a continuous, low-grade generation of C3b by a "priming" C3-convertase (C3,Bb,P) in the fluid phase. If the nascent C3b attaches to a cell surface that is an "activator" of the alternative pathway, then the amplification C3-convertase (C3b,Bb,P) is formed, additional C3 is cleaved, and more C3b is deposited on the surface. However, if the nascent C3b attaches to a "nonactivating" surface, then the control proteins, factors H and I, act to prevent the generation and expression of the amplification C3-convertase.

Two points regarding the relationship of the classical and alternative pathways to the activation of C3 and C5–C9 deserve emphasis. First, since C3b is both the product of the alternative pathway C3-convertase and also forms part of the alternative pathway C3-convertase, the activation of C3 via the alternative pathway creates a positive-feedback amplification loop (see Fig. 186-1). Second, activation of the classical pathway, by creating nascent C3b, can lead to activation of the alternative pathway. Thus the alternative pathway can act to amplify the action of the classical pathway.

As with the classical pathway, a number of opposing factors influence the activity of the alternative pathway C3-convertase.[19] The C3bBb enzyme is relatively labile and, under physiologic conditions, rapidly undergoes intrinsic decay through dissociation of the Bb. One of the proteins of the alternative pathway, properdin (P), stabilizes the binding of Bb to C3b and thereby retards its intrinsic decay.[34] Two other control proteins, factor H and factor I, act to inhibit the generation and/or expression of the C3bBb enzyme. Factor H not only competes with B for binding to C3b in the assembly of the alternative pathway C3-convertase[35] but also can displace Bb from the C3bBb complex once the C3-convertase has formed.[36] Factor I inhibits the alternative pathway C3-convertase by inactivating cell-bound C3b through proteolytic cleavage, creating iC3b (Fig. 186-4). The rate of inactivation of C3b by factor I is markedly accelerated by factor H[37] and by an integral membrane protein termed *membrane cofactor protein* (MCP).[38]

Certain particles, such as yeast cells,[39] rabbit erythrocytes,[40] and some bacteria,[29,41] are potent activators of the alternative pathway. They do so, in part, by virtue of their ability to bind nascent C3b and to protect the C3bBb enzyme from the inhibitory actions of factors H and I.[42] At least one molecular mechanism by which a particle protects the alternative pathway C3-convertase from these two control proteins has been elucidated. The binding of factor H to a particle, and thus its inhibitory effects on the alternative pathway C3-cleaving enzyme, is favored by the presence of sialic acid residues on the particle.[35,43]

Antibody is not required for the activation of the alternative pathway, and thus the alternative pathway generally is viewed as

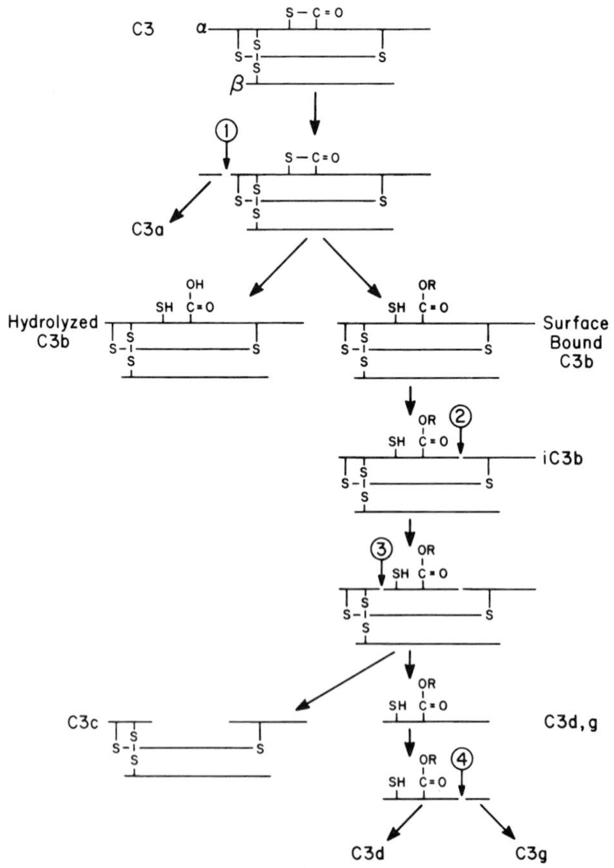

Fig. 186-4 The proteolytic cleavage of C3. Step 1 involves the cleavage of the α chain by either the alternative pathway or classical pathway C3-convertases. Step 2 results from the action of factor I with factor H or the CR1 (C3b) receptor serving as cofactors. Step 3 is also mediated by factor I and CR1. Step 4 involves cleavage by plasmin, trypsin, leukocyte elastase, and cathepsin G. (*Modified with permission from Fearon and Wong.*[70])

an important mechanism of natural immunity.[29] However, antibody can enhance the activation of the alternative pathway by a variety of particles, including bacteria[41,44,45] and virus-infected cells,[46] although the mechanism differs depending on the nature of the initiating particle and class of antibody involved.[45,47,48] Thus the alternative pathway can also participate in "acquired" immunity.

The Lectin Pathway

In recent years, evidence has accumulated that a third mechanism exists by which C3 can be activated.[49,50] Mannose-binding lectin (MBL) is a member of the collectin family of proteins and exists in serum as oligomers composed of identical subunits.[49] The available evidence suggests that each subunit is in turn composed of three identical peptide chains that are linked by disulfide bonds in their N-terminal regions to other subunits, form a typical collagenous triple helix in their middle, and terminate in a C-terminal cluster of three lectin domains capable of recognizing carbohydrate moieties. Although the binding of each carbohydrate-recognition domain is relatively weak, the presence of multiple binding sites probably endows the molecule with significant avidity when it binds to microbial surfaces with repeating sugar groups. MBL is capable of binding to a variety of microorganisms including *Haemophilus influenzae*, *Neisseria meningitidis*, and streptococci, but the binding is significantly impaired by the presence of a capsule.[51]

MBL is capable of activating C3 via the classical pathway without a requirement for C1q.[52,53] Apparently, MBL interacts with a novel serine protease termed MBL-associated serine protease (MASP), a 100-kDa protein that shares 39 percent homology with both human C1r and C1s.[54] Like C1s, MASP can cleave both C4 and C2, thereby generating C4b2a and its C3-cleaving activity. In addition, there is some evidence to support the ability of the MBL-MASP complex to activate C3 via the alternative pathway[55,56] and directly.[57]

Activation of C3

Whether C3 is activated via the classical or alternative pathways, the α chain of the C3 is cleaved, generating two fragments of unequal size, C3a and C3b (Fig. 186-4). In the classical pathway C3-convertase (C4b2a), the C2a contains the active site,[18] whereas in the alternative pathway C3-convertase (C3bBb), the Bb contains the active site.[58] The activation of C3 by either of the two C3-convertases represents an amplification step, since many hundreds of C3 molecules can be cleaved by one C3-convertase. Cleavage of native C3 by either convertase releases a small peptide (C3a) from the α chain into the fluid phase, where it acts as an anaphylatoxin (see below). Most of the nascent C3b is also released into the fluid phase, where it is rapidly inactivated through hydrolysis of the thiolester. Other molecules of C3b, however, bind covalently to the cell surface or immunoglobulins through transesterification with hydroxyl groups of polysaccharides or amidation of amino groups of proteins.[59] The cell-bound C3b may then be degraded by factor I and other proteases, yielding a variety of cleavage products (see Fig. 186-4). If the cell-bound C3b is not degraded, it is able to combine with either of the C3-convertases to create two new enzymes, the alternative pathway and classical pathway C5-convertases.

Activation of the Terminal Components (C5-C9)

The classical pathway C5-cleaving enzyme is composed of C4b2a3b.[60] In this complex, the C3b acts to bind native C5, whereas the C2a carries the active enzymatic site. In the alternative pathway, the C5-cleaving enzyme is composed of $(C3b)_2Bb$.[61] One C3b molecule binds Bb in the proper configuration for expression of its enzymatic activity, whereas the other C3b serves to bind native C5 in the proper location for cleavage by Bb. Activation of C5 by either the alternative or classical pathway C5-convertases results in cleavage of the α chain of the native molecule to create a small-molecular-weight product, C5a, and a larger-molecular-weight product, C5b. The smaller cleavage product, C5a, is released into the fluid phase, where it, like C3a, can act as an anaphylatoxin (see below). In addition, C5a possesses potent chemotactic activity (see below). If the C5b combines with native C6 while it is still attached to the C5-convertase, it is stabilized and can initiate formation of the membrane attack complex, a multimolecular assembly of C5b, C6, C7, C8, and C9 that is capable of cytolytic activity.[62] The initial event is stabilization of the nascent C5b by C6.[63] Addition of C7 to form the C5b,6,7 complex leads to insertion of hydrophobic domains of this trimolecular complex into the cell membrane and results in stable binding to the cell membrane.[64–66] The addition of C8 leads to further insertion of the complex and the generation of small and unstable pores in the membrane through which small molecules can pass.[67] On reaction of C5b,8 with C9 and polymerization of C9, a large and stable transmembrane channel is formed, leading to accelerated lysis of the target cell.[68]

Just as there are regulatory proteins affecting the classical and alternative pathways, there are two membrane proteins that regulate assembly of the membrane attack complex.[19] One is termed *membrane inhibitor of reactive lysis* (MIRL), or *CD59*, and the other is called *homologous restriction factor* (HRF) or *C8-binding protein* (C8bp). Each inhibits cell lysis mediated by C8 and C9 by preventing the polymerization and insertion of C9.[69]

Complement Receptors

Receptors for many of the cleavage products of individual components of complement exist on a variety of cells.[70] In general, two types of receptors exist: receptors that bind small-molecular-weight, diffusible fragments, such as C3a, C4a, and C5a, and receptors that bind large-molecular-weight fragments, primarily C3b and its degradation products, that have become fixed to the activating material.

Receptors for C3a/C4a and C5a are present on mast cells, basophils, eosinophils, neutrophils, monocytes/macrophages, and smooth muscle cells.[71,72] In addition, the receptors for C3a/C4a have been found on platelets and for C5a on endothelial cells. The interactions of C3a, C4a, and C5a with these receptors are capable of initiating the anaphylatoxic and chemotactic responses of these cells.

There are four distinct receptors for C3b and its cleavage products. The CR1 receptor (C3b/C4b receptor, CD35) is found on polymorphonuclear leukocytes, eosinophils, monocytes, macrophages, mast cells, glomerular podocytes, B-lymphocytes, and some T-lymphocytes.[70] In addition, it is found on the erythrocytes of primates, including humans.[73] Although C3b is the primary ligand for the CR1 receptor, it is also capable of binding C4b. One of the more important functions of the CR1 receptor is to enhance the phagocytosis of particles opsonized with C3b.[74] In addition, its presence on erythrocytes allows them to bind circulating immune complexes bearing C3b and transport the immune complexes to cells of the reticuloendothelial system.[75] Finally, CR1 can act to dissociate Bb from the C3bBb enzyme as well as act as a cofactor in the factor I-mediated cleavage of C3b.[76] In an analogous fashion, it can facilitate dissociation of C2a from the C4b2a enzyme of the classical pathway and act as a cofactor in the cleavage of C4b by factor I.[77]

The CR2 receptor (CD21) is found on B-lymphocytes and follicular dendritic cells. It binds C3dg and C3d (see Fig. 186-4) and the Epstein-Barr virus. The CR2 receptor on B cells is important in mediating the role of C3 in enhancing B-cell responses to antigens.[78] The CR3 (CD11b/18) and CR4 (CD11c/18) receptors are members of the integrin family of proteins. CR3 is found on the same cells as the CR1 receptor, but its primary ligand is iC3b. Since iC3b is one of the C3 degradation products formed in the presence of serum, the CR3 receptor also plays an important role in ingestion of opsonized particles. The CR4 receptor is found on monocytes, polymorphonuclear leukocytes, and macrophages, and its primary ligand also appears to be iC3b.

BIOLOGIC CONSEQUENCES OF COMPLEMENT ACTIVATION

Anaphylatoxic Activity

The smaller cleavage products of both C3 and C5 (C3a and C5a) possess anaphylatoxic activity.[79] Each of these small polypeptides (9000 and 11,000 Da, respectively) is cleaved from the N-terminal portion of the α chain of their respective parent molecules. When compared on a molar basis, C5a is approximately 100 to 200 times more potent as an anaphylatoxin than C3a.[80] Both these anaphylatoxins are subject to attack by serum carboxypeptidase-B. This enzyme rapidly cleaves the C-terminal arginine that is common to both C3a and C5a and in each case creates a new molecule (C3a-des Arg and C5a-des Arg, respectively) that is significantly less potent as an anaphylatoxin than the parent molecule. It also should be noted that C4a also possesses some anaphylatoxic activity but with a specific activity much less than either C3a or C5a.[81]

Complement-derived anaphylatoxins possess a variety of activities of biologic importance. They originally were identified through their ability to cause histamine release from basophils and tissue mast cells, to promote smooth muscle contraction, and to increase vascular permeability.[72] More recently, additional functions of these peptides have been identified.[80] Anaphylatoxins can promote the aggregation of platelets and the subsequent release of arachidonic acid metabolites from them. In addition, they can cause neutrophils to aggregate and degranulate, generate arachidonic acid metabolites, produce toxic oxygen radicals, and discharge their granular enzymes.

Chemotactic Activity

The smaller cleavage product of C5, C5a, is also a potent chemotactic factor causing the directed movement of polymorphonuclear leukocytes and monocytes as well as eosinophils and basophils.[82] When the terminal arginine is removed by the action of carboxypeptidase-B, producing C5a-des Arg, the molecule loses approximately 90 percent of its biologic activity due to its decreased affinity for the C5a receptor.[83] In addition to its role in attracting mobile phagocytic cells to foci of complement activation, C5a also promotes adherence of phagocytic cells to vascular endothelium via its capacity to alter surface expression of adhesion molecules,[84] a necessary prerequisite to their exit from the intravascular compartment. A number of in vivo studies have demonstrated that C5a plays an important role in attracting phagocytic cells to local sites of microbial invasion or immune-complex deposition.[85,86] In addition, studies in C5a receptor knockout mice have demonstrated an important role for this G-protein-linked receptor in neutrophil-mediated clearance of bacteria within the pulmonary tree[87] and in the response to immune-complex-mediated pulmonary damage.[88] Finally, engagement of the C5a receptor on human bronchial epithelial cells mediates interleukin 8 (IL-8) release.[89]

Opsonic Activity

The larger cleavage products of C3, C3b and iC3b, act as potent opsonins when fixed to the surface of a microorganism.[90] It appears that they subserve different opsonic functions depending on the nature of the phagocytic cell and its state of activation. In the case of neutrophils and nonactivated macrophages, C3b promotes attachment of the particle, whereas immunoglobulin G acts to promote ingestion.[91] In the case of activated macrophages, C3b serves to aid in both attachment and ingestion.[92]

There are a great deal of data to suggest that C3-dependent opsonic activity is one of the more important activities of the complement system. Studies in experimental animals have shown that C3 is an important opsonin in both nonimmune hosts[93] and hosts who have high levels of antibody.[94]

Bactericidal Activity

The generation of complement-mediated serum bactericidal activity requires the participation of the entire terminal complement sequence.[95] Although bactericidal activity can occur in the absence of C9, killing proceeds at a very much slower rate.[96] Only gram-negative bacteria can be killed by complement. Although protoplasts of gram-positive organisms are susceptible to lysis by complement,[97] intact gram-positive organisms are not, suggesting that their thick cell wall somehow interferes with the bactericidal action of C5–C9. The site of action of C5–C9 appears to be the outer lipid membrane of gram-negative organisms.[98]

Processing of Immune Complexes

The complement system also plays an important role in the processing of immune complexes.[99] There are a number of mechanisms by which the complement system could modify the structure and/or influence the biologic activities of immune complexes. First, opsonically active C3b or iC3b can enhance the uptake of immune complexes by phagocytic cells.[100] Second, the activation of C3 via the classical pathway can retard the formation of large complexes and prevent, to some degree, their precipitation from serum.[101] Third, once complexes are formed, they can be solubilized by the complement system.[102] Apparently, it is much easier to prevent immune precipitation than it is to solubilize the complexes once they have formed. It appears that the covalent binding of C3b to the immune complex is important in both the prevention of precipitation and the solubilization of preformed complexes. In an experimental model of serum sickness, C3 has been shown to facilitate the efficient removal of immune complexes in the kidney, suggesting that C3 may play an important role of solubilization of immune complexes in vivo.[103]

Primates have an additional complement-mediated mechanism available for handling immune complexes. They possess the CR1 receptor for C3b on their erythrocytes,[70,73] and circulating immune complexes bearing C3b will fix to erythrocytes through these receptors.[75] The erythrocyte-bound complexes are then transported to the liver, where the immune complexes are ingested by Kupffer cells and the erythrocytes returned to the circulation.[75] In this manner, erythrocytes serve to capture immune complexes, prevent their deposition in organs such as the kidney, and enhance their clearance by organs of the reticuloendothelial system.

Role of Complement in Antibody Formation

Interest in the role of complement in antibody formation has been stimulated by a number of independent but related observations. Monocytes/macrophages, B-lymphocytes, and a subset of T-lymphocytes all have receptors for C3 and/or C5 cleavage products,[70] making it possible that their participation in the generation of a normal antibody response could be influenced by the complement system. In vivo studies using experimental animals pharmacologically depleted of C3[104]; animals with genetically determined deficiencies of C4,[105] C2,[106] or C3[107]; or animals who have been rendered deficient in C3, C4, or CR2 using recombinant DNA technology[108–110] clearly have shown the complement system to be important in the generation of a normal antibody response. The antibody response to T-dependent antigens is relatively more dependent on an intact complement system than is the response to T-independent antigens. In addition, an intact complement system facilitates the isotype switch from IgM to IgG in the normal immune response.

There are a number of steps in the generation of a normal humoral response in which the complement system could enhance antibody formation. The evidence to this point in time suggests that C3d fixed to antigen and bound to CR2 markedly lowers the activation threshold for the B-cell antigen receptor.[111] In addition, C3 may play a role in increasing the efficiency of antigen uptake and retention by antigen-presenting cells such as follicular dendritic cells and thus provide a reservoir for periodic restimulation of B cells.[112]

MOLECULAR GENETICS OF COMPLEMENT: GENERAL CONSIDERATIONS

Gene Families

The complement genes have been grouped into supergene families on the basis of similarities in structure, function, and chromosomal localization.[113] For instance, the genes encoding C2, factor B, and C4 are class III genes of the major histocompatibility complex (MHC) on human chromosome 6.[114] The 3′ terminus of the C2 gene is just 421 bp upstream of the factor B gene.[115] Factor B and C2 are similar in structural and functional features, suggesting that the genes were derived from a common ancestral gene.[116] The two C4 genes (C4A and C4B) lie approximately 30 kb centromeric from the C2 and factor B genes. The C4 loci are separated by 10 kb, and each has a cytochrome P-450 steroid 21-hydroxylase (21-OH) gene within 1.5 kb of the 3′ terminus.[117–119] The order of the genes in the direction of transcription is C2-BF-C4A-21-OHA-C4B-21-OHB, and they have been mapped within a 0.7-cM region between HLA-B and HLA-DR.[117,118,120] The topology of these MHC class III genes is highly conserved in evolution, as shown in several studies of the syntenic region in mice.[116,121] Other genes in this region include the *DM, TAP*, and *LMP* genes, which are involved in antigen processing, tumor necrosis factor genes A and B, and the heat shock protein 70 gene. This region contains an unusually high density of transcribed genes, and there are many other genes in this region for which a function has yet to be determined.[122]

The genes encoding complement receptors CR1 and CR2, C4bp, factor H, MCP, and DAF are members of another supergene family, the RCA family (regulators of complement activation).[113] They are closely clustered on the long arm of chromosome 1,[123–128] and their products share several structural and functional characteristics. These six genes share the capacity to act as cofactors for factor I, bind C3b, and modulate C3-convertase activity. Direct sequence analyses of genes within this family have demonstrated repeating homology units of approximately 60 amino acids.[123] These repeating units, termed *short consensus repeats* (SCRs), are also seen in the sequence of C2,[129] factor B,[122,130] and C1r/s.[131] One property common to all the complement proteins that have these highly conserved repeating homology units is their capacity to bind fragments of C3 and C4. Therefore, the complement regulatory genes on chromosome 1 and the genes encoded in the class III region of the MHC on chromosome 6 may be considered parts of a larger supergene family related because of their capacity to interact with the activation fragments of C3 and C4 (reviewed in refs. 113 and 131). These repeating homology units also are found in noncomplement proteins such as the IL-2 receptor, β_2-glycoprotein 1, the haptoglobin α chain, and the herpes simplex virus glycoprotein C, none of which interact with C3 or C4. The genes for complement proteins C3, C4, and C5 have been described as a family that shares structural and functional properties at the protein level with α_2-macroglobulin, β_1-inhibitor 3, and the pregnancy zone protein.[113,132] These genes all encode multichain disulfide-linked molecules. Except for C5, a thiolester-reactive site is a distinct characteristic of this family. These genes do not appear to be clustered in a specific chromosomal region, however.

Based on primary sequence homologies, several of the proteins of the membrane attack complex (i.e., C6, C7, C8 α chain, C8 β chain, and C9) also appear to be members of a large gene family[113,133–135] that also includes other proteins with pore-forming functions (i.e., perforin, mellitin, and the pore-forming protein of *Trypanasoma cruzi*).

C1 inhibitor shares structural and functional characteristics with several other serine proteinase inhibitors so that it is often included in the SERPIN (serine proteinase inhibitor) supergene family. The chromosomal localization of several SERPIN genes has been determined, and they are dispersed throughout the genome. For example, C1 inhibitor maps to human chromosome 11,[136] whereas another member of this family, α_1-proteinase inhibitor, is localized on chromosome 14.

Protein Polymorphisms

Many of the individual components of complement demonstrate protein polymorphism (reviewed in refs. 137 and 138). Polymorphic variants of C3 were the first to be identified because the relatively high concentration of C3 in serum permitted direct visualization of C3 variants in prolonged agarose gel electrophoresis. The common C3 variants (C3 fast and C3 slow) are found in all major racial groups. In addition, about 20 rare variants have been detected in one or several populations. Other methods have been used to detect polymorphic variants of other complement proteins, such as factor B, C2, C4, C6, C7, C8, and factor D.[138] In some instances, the structural basis for this genetic variation has been determined by sequence analysis of cDNA clones[139,140] or genomic DNA.[140]

Considerable attention has been given to an analysis of the complement proteins encoded by genes within the MHC. Studies of protein polymorphisms of the C2, factor B, and C4A and C4B loci, together with typing of the class I and class II genes, have generated the concept of "extended" haplotypes.[141,142] This concept derives from data showing a decreased frequency of recombinant events extending over a 7 to 14 $\times$ 10^6 bp region of chromosome 6. Taken together, the extended haplotypes account for nearly 30 percent of haplotypes in normal Caucasian populations studied thus far. Because some of these polymorphic variants have altered function, there has been much interest in understanding whether these polymorphic variants are associated with a predisposition to autoimmune or infectious diseases. For example, there are data to support an association of a dysfunctional C4 allele, *C4F1*, with lepromatous leprosy, and a factor B allele, *BfF1*, has been found to be associated with idiopathic membranous nephropathy.[143] The relationship of polymorphisms of individual components outside the MHC class III region with disease are discussed in the sections dealing with individual component deficiencies.

Regulation of Complement Gene Expression

The delicate balance between activation of the complement system and inhibition of activation is controlled to a certain extent by the production and local concentrations of the individual components and regulatory proteins. Particularly for those components which are present in the serum in small amounts, the capacity to synthesize such components at local sites may be important for host defense and inflammation. Transcription, splicing, translation, and posttranslational modification may all play a role in controlling the local production of complement components. In general, quantitative control of production occurs at the level of transcription, which in turn is regulated by the tissue specificity, developmental pattern, and cytokine responsiveness of the individual genes.

The majority of the complement components found in serum are derived predominantly from liver synthesis. For example, the majority of serum factor B, C4, and C3 is produced by the liver.[144–146] Monocytes, macrophages, fibroblasts, and certain endothelial cells also make small amounts of certain soluble complement components.[147] Additionally, C3 has been detected in epithelial cells of uterus, kidney, small intestine, lung, and vascular endothelium and neutrophils.[148,149]

Liver and bone marrow transplant patients have been used to quantify the amount of extrahepatic complement in serum. Approximately 5 percent of serum C3 is derived from extrahepatic sources, although this increases with inflammation.[150] This is in good agreement with the extrahepatically derived levels of C6 (10 percent) in an experimental rat system.[151] Not only does extrahepatically derived complement contribute to serum levels, but it also is capable of playing a role in local inflammatory responses and in humoral immune responses.[151,152]

COMPLEMENT DEFICIENCIES: GENERAL CONSIDERATIONS

Genetically determined deficiencies have been described for nearly all the individual components of the complement system[5–8] (Table 186-2). The usual mode of inheritance is as an autosomal recessive trait with only two known exceptions. Deficiency of C1 inhibitor has an autosomal dominant mode of inheritance, whereas properdin deficiency is inherited as an X-linked recessive disorder.

Diagnosis

Most of the genetically determined deficiencies of the early components of the classical pathway (C1, C4, and C2), of C3, and of the terminal components (C5, C6, C7, C8, and C9) can be detected using antibody-sensitized sheep erythrocytes in a total serum hemolytic complement (CH_{50}) assay. Since this assay depends on the functional integrity of C1 through C9, severe deficiencies of any of these components lead to a marked reduction or absence of total hemolytic complement activity. There is one exception, however. The lysis of antibody-sensitized erythrocytes can occur in the absence of C9,[67] although at a much slower rate and to a lesser extent than in the presence of C9. Therefore, patients with C9 deficiency do have some serum hemolytic complement activity, but it is reduced to between one-third and one-half of the lower limit of normal.[153]

Deficiencies of factor H, factor I, and properdin of the alternative pathway can be detected by a hemolytic assay that assesses lysis of rabbit erythrocytes mediated by the alternative pathway.[154] Rabbit erythrocytes are potent activators of the alternative pathway,[40] due in part to the fact that they have very low levels of surface sialic acid.[30] Obviously, the sera of patients with deficiencies of C3 or C5–C9 also will be abnormal when tested in the rabbit erythrocyte assay because the lysis of rabbit erythrocytes depends on these components as well as on components of the alternative pathway.

Identification of the specific component that is deficient usually rests on both functional and immunochemical tests. Highly specific functional assays have been developed for each of the individual components.[155] They usually depend on reagents that lack the specific component in question but possess the other components of the hemolytic pathway in excess. Monospecific antibodies are also available for each of the individual components, allowing for their detection by immunochemical techniques. In most cases, either functional or immunochemical assessment of the specific component will identify the deficiency. There are some exceptions, however. For example, one form of C1 inhibitor deficiency[156] and one form of C1q deficiency[157] are characterized by dysfunctional proteins that are present when immunochemical assays are used but are markedly reduced in functional activity. In addition, patients with C8 deficiency lack either one (C8β) or two (C8α-γ) chains of the complete three-chain molecule.[158] This, too, may lead to the detection of C8 antigen in the serum of such patients, while their C8 function is markedly reduced.

Individuals who are heterozygous for a deficiency of a single component usually have normal total serum hemolytic complement (CH_{50}) levels because this assay is not sensitive enough to reliably detect mild to moderate reductions in a single component. As a group, individuals who are heterozygous deficient usually have levels of the specific component that are approximately one-third to one-half the average level of normal. However, assignment of any given individual as a heterozygote based solely on their serum level of a specific component may be difficult because the range of values for normal individuals may be quite wide and the levels in some heterozygotes may overlap the lower limit of normal. In some instances, such as in C2 deficiency[159] and C4 deficiency,[160] the gene for the deficiency is closely linked to the MHC and often is associated with a specific extended haplotype. Thus family members of deficient individuals may be assigned provisionally as heterozygotes based on HLA typing.[161,162] However, recent studies that have identified the molecular genetic basis for most of the complement deficiencies have allowed for more precise detection of heterozygous deficient individuals.[163]

Table 186-2 Genetically Determined Deficiencies of Complement in Humans

Deficiency	Inheritance	Approximate Number of Patients/Kindreds	Major Clinical Manifestations
C1q	Autosomal recessive	24/14	Rheumatic disorders and pyogenic infections
C1r/s	Autosomal recessive	11/7	Rheumatic disorders
C4	Autosomal recessive	21/17	Rheumatic disorders and pyogenic infections
C2	Autosomal recessive	109/79	Rheumatic disorders and pyogenic infections
C3	Autosomal recessive	19/14	Pyogenic infections and rheumatic disorders
C5	Autosomal recessive	27/17	Meningococcal sepsis and meningitis
C6	Autosomal recessive	77/49	Meningococcal sepsis and meningitis
C7	Autosomal recessive	73/50	Meningococcal sepsis and meningitis
C8	Autosomal recessive	73/52	Meningococcal sepsis and meningitis
C9	Autosomal recessive	18/15	Meningococcal sepsis and meningitis
Factor H	Autosomal recessive	13/8	Hemolytic uremic syndrome
Factor I	Autosomal recessive	14/12	Pyogenic infections
Properdin	X-linked recessive	70/23	Meningococcal sepsis and meningitis
Factor D	Unknown	3/2	Meningococcal sepsis and meningitis/sinopulmonary infections
C4-binding protein	Unknown	1/1	Behçet's disease and angioedema
DAF	Unknown	2/2	Inab phenotype
CD59	Unknown	1/1	Paroxysmal nocturnal hemoglobinuria
C1 inhibitor	Autosomal dominant	100s/100s	Angioedema

SOURCES: Some data from Ross and Densen[5] and Figueroa and Densen.[6]

Clinical Presentation

The clinical presentation of individuals with genetically determined deficiencies of complement components has varied. While some individuals are asymptomatic, most have presented with either an increased susceptibility to infection, a variety of rheumatic diseases, or angioedema.[5–8]

Infection. An increased susceptibility to infection has been a prominent clinical finding in patients with complement deficiencies.[5–8] Although a number of studies in experimental animals have shown that the complement system has the potential to contribute to the host's defense against a wide variety of bacteria, fungi, and viruses,[2,3,29] clinical experience would suggest that the greatest susceptibility of complement-deficient patients is to bacterial infections.[5,6] The kinds of bacteria that most commonly cause infection in a specific deficiency reflect the biologic functions of the missing component. For example, C3 is an important opsonin in both the nonimmune and immune host. Therefore, patients with a deficiency of C3 or with a deficiency of a component in the pathways necessary for the activation of C3 have an increased susceptibility to encapsulated bacteria, for which opsonization is the primary host defense (e.g., pneumococcus and *H. influenzae*). Similarly, C5–C9 form the membrane attack complex and therefore are responsible for the bactericidal/bacteriolytic functions of complement. Patients with deficiencies of C5–C9 can opsonize bacteria normally because they possess C3 and the components necessary for its activation. Thus these patients are not unduly susceptible to infection by bacteria for which opsonization is the primary host defense. These patients are, however, markedly susceptible to neisserial species because serum bactericidal activity is an important host defense against these organisms.

Although blood-borne infections such as bacteremia/sepsis and meningitis are the most common infections in patients with complement deficiencies,[5,6] localized infections such as sinusitis and pneumonia also have been reported. Not only do patients with complement deficiencies have an increased frequency of infections, but the infections also may have features that differ from those in the normal population. For example, systemic blood-borne infections with unencapsulated bacteria are extremely rare in normal hosts.[164] However, sepsis and meningitis caused by unencapsulated "avirulent" meningococci have occurred in complement-deficient individuals.[165,166] In addition, although patients with deficiencies of terminal components have a higher risk for recurrence of systemic meningococcal infections than do normal individuals, their mortality rate has been reported to be lower.[5,6,167]

Rheumatic Disorders. Patients with complement deficiencies also have a variety of clinical conditions that can best be characterized as rheumatic disorders.[5,6,168] These include systemic lupus erythematosus and discoid lupus as well as glomerulonephritis, dermatomyositis, anaphylactoid purpura, and vasculitis. The prevalence of these inflammatory disorders is highest in those patients with deficiencies of the classical activating pathway (C1, C4, and C2) and of C3. For example, approximately 80 percent of patients with C4 or C3 deficiency and just over 30 percent of patients with C2 deficiency have had a rheumatic disorder.[5,6] In contrast, fewer than 10 percent of patients with deficiencies of terminal complement components have rheumatic disorders.[5,6]

There are some interesting and important differences between the rheumatic diseases seen in complement-deficient patients and their counterparts in "normal" non-complement-deficient individuals. For example, the systemic lupus erythematosus seen in complement-deficient individuals is usually characterized by an early onset (often in childhood) and prominent annular photosensitive skin lesions resembling discoid lupus (Fig. 186-5). Individuals deficient in C2 have relatively limited renal and pleuropericardial involvement and a relatively infrequent occurrence of immunoglobulin and C3 in the skin.[5,6] In addition, C2-deficient individuals with systemic lupus erythematosus usually have absent or relatively low titers of both antinuclear antibodies and anti-native DNA antibodies, and their lupus preparations are often negative.[161,169,170] In contrast, the incidence of anti-Ro (SSA) antibodies is significantly higher in C2-deficient patients with lupus than it is in non-complement-deficient patients with lupus.[169,170] Thus, both with respect to some of their clinical manifestations and with respect to their serologic findings, C2-deficient patients with lupus bear a striking resemblance to a subgroup of lupus patients who are "antinuclear antibody negative."[171,172] Patients deficient in C1 or C4 also have an early onset with prominent cutaneous manifestations but are more likely

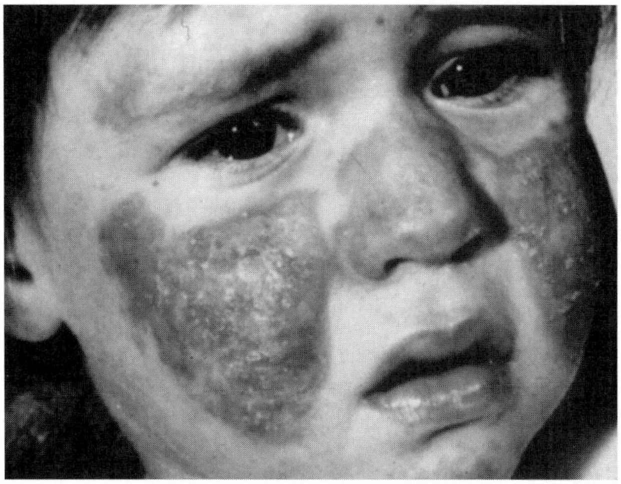

Fig. 186-5 Photosensitive skin lesions on the face of a child with C4 deficiency. (*Courtesy of Dr. Georges Hauptmann.*)

to have the usual array of autoantibodies and the classic end-organ affects of lupus such as cerebritis and nephritis.[173–176]

The pathophysiologic basis for the association between rheumatic disorders and complement deficiencies is unclear, but a number of possibilities exist. First, a number of studies have shown that components of the complement system can neutralize and/or lyse certain viruses in vitro,[177] whereas other studies in experimental animals have shown that C3 and C5 are important mechanisms of antiviral host defense in vivo.[178,179] Thus, in some instances, the rheumatic disorders seen in complement-deficient patients may be the consequence of an altered host response to recurrent or chronic viral infections, although this has never been documented. Second, the genes for three of the individual components of complement (C4, C2, and factor B) are located within the MHC and are in linkage disequilibrium with specific HLA haplotypes.[138,180,181] It is possible, therefore, that in some instances the rheumatic disorders seen in complement-deficient patients are due in part to other genes within the MHC that in some manner influence immune function rather than to the deficiency in complement itself. Third, since the complement system plays an important role in the generation of a normal antibody response,[78] the rheumatic diseases seen in complement-deficient patients could result from disordered humoral immunity. And finally, since C1q may play an important role in the clearance of apoptotic cells,[182] a deficiency of C1q could allow immunologic recognition of intracellular antigens such as Ro and La.

Perhaps the most attractive hypothesis linking rheumatic diseases and complement-deficiency diseases has to do with the role of the complement system in the clearance and processing of immune complexes. A number of studies have shown that the sera of patients with complement deficiencies have altered and/or reduced abilities to process immune complexes and that the inability of the patients' sera to process immune complexes in vitro correlates with their risk for developing a rheumatic disorder. For example, serum from patients with genetically determined deficiencies of C1q, C4, C2, and C3 fails to prevent the precipitation of immune complexes as they are forming,[101,183] has a reduced ability to resolubilize complexes once they have formed,[183–185] and does not support the binding of preformed immune complexes to CR1 receptors on human erythrocytes.[186] In addition, a single C2-deficient individual has been shown to have markedly diminished binding of radiolabeled immune complexes to erythrocytes in vivo and impaired splenic uptake of the complexes from the circulation, both of which normalized after C2 repletion, indicating a direct effect of the complement deficiency.[187] In contrast, in those instances in which they have been tested, the sera of patients with deficiencies of terminal components (C5–C9) are normal with respect to these activities. Thus, for a given complement-deficiency disease, there appears to be an excellent correlation between the inability of the patient to process immune complexes normally and the patient's susceptibility to rheumatic diseases.

Epidemiology

Given the limited clinical manifestations of complement deficiencies, a number of studies have examined series of patients with specific clinical disorders in order to determine the frequency of genetically determined complement deficiencies in these clinical settings and to evaluate the utility of screening for complement deficiencies.

Infection. A number of studies have shown that the prevalence of genetically determined complement deficiencies is significantly higher in children or adults with systemic meningococcal infections than in the general population.[188] Prospective studies have estimated the frequency of complement deficiencies in unselected cases of meningococcal sepsis and/or meningitis to be between 0 and 15 percent,[189–192] the differing estimates probably reflecting the different populations that have been studied. In general, the prevalence is higher among sporadic cases than it is in epidemic cases. The prevalence is also higher in patients who present with unusual serotypes. For example, two different studies have shown that between 20 and 50 percent of patients with uncommon meningococcal serotypes, such as serotypes X, Y, Z, W135, or 29E, have an inherited deficiency of a component of the complement system.[193,194] Similarly, the prevalence is also higher among patients with recurrent meningococcal disease or a positive family history of meningococcal disease.[193] For example, as many as 40 percent of patients with recurrent meningococcal disease and as many as 10 percent of patients with a positive family history of meningitis have genetically determined complement deficiencies.[193] Other genes such as the genes for the Fc receptor may modulate the risk of meningococcal disease in complement-deficient individuals.[195] The severity of meningococcal disease may be less in complement-deficient individuals, although the occurrence of deafness may be higher.[167,188,196]

Although a relatively large number of complement-deficient patients have presented with bacteremia and/or meningitis due to the pneumococcus, streptococcus, and *H. influenzae*,[5,6] inherited disorders of the complement system do not appear to be markedly more common in patients with these infections.[192,197–199]

Rheumatic Disorders. A number of studies have examined the frequency of complement deficiencies in a variety of rheumatic diseases. However, only a few studies have examined a large enough series of patients with a single rheumatic disorder to yield meaningful information.[161,200–202] The prevalence of homozygous C2 deficiency in a the general population has been estimated at 1 in 10,000 (0.01 percent).[161,202,203] In contrast, the prevalence of homozygous C2 deficiency in a large series of patients with systemic lupus erythematosus has varied between 0.4 and 2.0 percent.[161,202] Attempts also have been made to determine whether there is an increased frequency of heterozygous C2 deficiency in lupus. In one such early study, the prevalence of heterozygous C2 deficiency was estimated (indirectly based on C2 levels and HLA typing) to be 5 percent,[161] a figure approximately 5 times the estimate in the general population. However, the identification of a single molecular genetic defect as the basis of C2 deficiency in the overwhelming majority of patients (>95 percent)[163,202] has allowed the precise identification of C2 null alleles, and thus heterozygotes, in a large cohort of lupus patients and controls.[202] Thus, when lupus patients are examined using molecular genetic techniques, the frequency of C2 heterozygotes is not increased.[202]

The most common complement deficiency found in lupus patients is a deficiency of one of the isotypes of C4. The fourth component of complement is encoded by two closely linked genes that give rise to two isotypes, C4A and C4B.[204,205] Although complete C4 deficiency is uncommon, deficiencies of one or the other isotype are not unusual; approximately 1 percent of normal individuals are homozygous C4A deficient, and 3 percent of normal individuals are homozygous C4B deficient.[205,206] A number of studies have demonstrated that both homozygous and heterozygous C4A deficiency is associated with systemic lupus erythematosus.[201,207–209] In one of these studies, the association of C4A deficiency with lupus was found to be independent of other MHC associations and represented a distinct risk factor.[209] Having a C4A null allele also appears to predispose individuals to the development of hydralazine-induced lupus.[210]

COMPLEMENT DEFICIENCIES: SPECIFIC DISORDERS

C1q Deficiency (MIM 120550)

Molecular Biology. As noted earlier, C1 is a macromolecule consisting of three noncovalently bound subcomponents, C1q, C1r, and C1s, that are the products of five genes; three for C1q (A, B, and C chains) and one each for C1r and C1s. The three different polypeptides that constitute the C1q molecule are encoded by three highly homologous, tightly linked 2.6-kDa genes on the long arm of chromosome 1 (1p34.1-36.3) in the order A-C-B ($5' \rightarrow 3'$).[211] The region coding for a collagen-like domain interrupts the sequence exactly at the site at which the triple helix of C1q bends when viewed in the electron microscope.

Pathophysiology and Clinical Expression. Only a limited number of individuals with C1q deficiency have been described.[5,6,212] The deficiency is inherited as an autosomal recessive trait. Individuals with C1q deficiency have markedly reduced levels of both total hemolytic complement (CH_{50}) and C1 functional activity in their serum. There appear to be at least two forms of C1q deficiency.[212] In one form, no C1q can be detected by either functional or immunochemical analysis.[213–215] In the other form, immunochemical C1q is present, but it lacks functional activity (i.e., dysfunctional C1q).[157,216–218] The dysfunctional C1q does not bind to immunoglobulin,[216,217] nor does it interact with C1r and C1s.[217] The dysfunctional C1q found in one family is not always the same as in another because the abnormal molecules may differ in molecular mass from each other as well as from normal C1q[216,217]; i.e., the deficiency is genetically heterogeneous.

The predominant clinical presentation associated with either form of C1q deficiency has been lupus.[5,6,175,212] Approximately 30 patients with C1q deficiency have been described, and all but 2 have developed lupus.[5,6,175,212] In fact, C1q deficiency appears to be the strongest known genetic risk factor for lupus. The clinical manifestations of lupus in patients with C1q deficiency are not markedly different from those seen in complement-sufficient individuals, although the age of onset is somewhat earlier and the disease can be very severe with significant central nervous system manifestations and renal disease. In contrast to C2- or C3-deficient patients, most C1q-deficient patients develop the usual autoantibodies seen in lupus, including ANA, anti-RNP, anti-SM, and anti-Ro; anti-dsDNA is less common. The cutaneous manifestations typically are prominent, and skin biopsies demonstrate IgG, IgM, and C3 deposition, as is characteristic of lupus. The lupus in C1q-deficient patients may be resistant to steroid therapy, and thalidomide has been used successfully in some steroid-resistant patients.[219]

Patients with C1q deficiency also have an increased susceptibility to blood-borne infections with pyogenic organisms, such as sepsis and/or meningitis, presumably due to their inability to generate opsonically active C3b via activation of the classical pathway.

Molecular Genetic Defect. The molecular defects causing C1q deficiency are diverse, although there is a mutation in C1qA that is common among patients from Turkey.[220] Mutations in each of the three chains have been identified.[219–224] In the common Turkish mutation, a premature termination codon results in no detectable A chain being produced. B and C polypeptide chains are also undetectable in these patients, suggesting that C1qA must be present for the formation and secretion of C1q.[222] Other mutations in C1qB and C1qC result in premature stop codons and the absence of C1q protein. Two other mutations have been identified that destabilize the higher-order forms of C1q,[219,222] a theme that is also seen in mannose-binding protein deficiency. These patients exhibit a reduced amount of nonfunctional, low-molecular-weight C1q. Because there are many mutations causing C1q deficiency, carrier detection and prenatal testing will rely on the identification of each individual mutation in a previously affected family member, although allele-specific PCR has been used to identify carriers of the common Mediterranean mutation.[220]

Animal Models. A C1q knockout mouse has defective immune-complex clearance and spontaneously develops membranoproliferative glomerulonephritis with subendothelial deposits of C3 and immunoglobulin,[225] thus mimicking the findings in human C1q deficiency.

C1r/C1s Deficiency (MIM 216950/120580)

Molecular Biology. The genes encoding C1r and C1s map to 12p13.[226,227] They are separated by 9.5 kb and oriented tail to tail. The C1r and C1s genes are highly homologous, and although they share the same pattern of tissue expression, each is separately regulated.[228] C1r and C1s are expressed predominantly in the liver, but extrahepatic tissues also produce low levels of both C1r and C1s.[228]

Pathophysiology and Clinical Expression. Only a few individuals with C1r/C1s deficiency have been described.[5,6,212,229] The disorder is inherited in an autosomal recessive fashion. Patients with C1r/C1s deficiency have markedly reduced total hemolytic complement activity (CH_{50}) and C1 functional activity in their serum. Their C1q levels are normal. C1r levels are markedly reduced (<1 percent of normal), and C1s levels are usually 20 to 50 percent of normal.[229,230] One patient has been described in which C1s is markedly reduced while C1r levels are 50 percent of normal.[231] It is therefore likely that neither monomer is stable in the absence of the other.

Most C1r/C1s-deficient patients have presented with systemic lupus erythematosis, although isolated glomerulonephritis also has been described. In addition, some patients ascertained as part of family studies have been clinically well.

Molecular Genetic Defect. Thus far, the molecular basis for C1r/C1s deficiency has not been determined.

C4 Deficiency

Molecular Biology. The fourth component of complement is a three-chain disulfide-linked glycoprotein. There are two loci within the MHC for C4.[204] Although the products of the two loci (C4A (MIM 120810) and C4B (MIM 120820)) share functional, structural, and antigenic characteristics that identify them as C4, they differ with respect to electrophoretic mobility,[205] molecular weight of the α chain,[232] specific epitopes,[233] and functional hemolytic activity.[232,234] The difference between the two isotypes, with respect to functional activity, relates to their different abilities to transacylate with either hydroxyl or amino groups after activation. Nascent C4A is much more efficient than C4B in transacylating with amino groups of proteins, and nascent C4B is more efficient than C4A in transacylating with hydroxyl groups of carbohydrates.[232,234] There are only four amino acid differences between the *C4A* and *C4B* genes.[139] This variation in sequence is near the thiolester region of the C4 α chain. Substitution of residue 1106 from Asp (*C4A*) to His (*C4B*) by site-directed mutagenesis has established that this site is critical for the functional differences between the *C4A* and *C4B* gene products.[235]

The complete nucleotide sequences of the two human C4 genes, *C4A* and *C4B*, have been determined.[236,237] The *C4A* gene is 22 kDa in size. A variation in size of the *C4B* gene (16 kDa in some individuals and 22 kDa in other individuals) is a result of the presence or absence of a 6.8-kb intron toward the 5′ terminus of the *C4B* gene.[238,239] The variation in sequence between *C4A* and *C4B* does not explain the apparent 2-kDa difference in α-chain size between the two isotypes.[240] A relatively high frequency of duplications, deletions, and rearrangements leads to polymorphic variation in the human C4 genes.[206] Thus far, some 35 allotypic variants of C4 have been described. Many of the variants and null alleles ascribed to these genes are based on electrophoretic mobility of the C4 protein. By direct analysis of gene structure, several additional polymorphic variations have been defined, and estimates of the frequency of homoduplications and deletions have been revised.[241,242]

Hepatic synthesis of the 185-kDa single-chain precursor of C4, prepro-C4[243,244] is directed by a polyadenylated mRNA of approximately 5 kb.[245] C4 message also has been detected in mononuclear phagocytes, as well as in thyroid follicular epithelial cells, salivary gland ductal epithelial cells, renal tubular epithelial cells, brain, and small intestine.[246] Posttranslational modification involves proteolytic excision of two intersubunit-linking peptides,[247,248] sulfation,[249] modification of residues generating the thiolester reactive site,[250] and glycosylation of the α and β subunits.[251,252] There is also a specific proteolytic cleavage of a C-terminal fragment of the C4 α chain that is mediated by a metalloenzyme.[253,254]

Pathophysiology and Clinical Expression. Complete deficiency of C4 is the result of being homozygous deficient at both the *C4A* and *C4B* loci (*C4A**QO, *C4B**QO) and is uncommon.[5,6,206] Patients with C4 deficiency have severely depressed serum levels of both antigenic and functional C4 (<1 percent). Individuals who are heterozygous for C4 deficiency, at either or both of the C4 loci, as a group will have serum C4 levels that generally reflect the number of active genes.[255,256] However, assignment of a given individual as heterozygous for the deficiency is complicated by the fact that the range of C4 levels in normal individuals is quite wide, and a deficiency of C4 at one or the other locus is relatively common.[205,206] Accordingly, assignment of an individual as heterozygous for the deficiency is usually based on kindred analysis using HLA linkage,[160] DNA Southern blot analysis,[241] or electrophoretic analysis of C4 allotypes in serum.[205]

Patients with complete C4 deficiency have a markedly decreased ability to activate the classical pathway. However, those serum activities which can be mediated via the alternative pathway, such as opsonic, chemotactic, and bactericidal activities, are present, although usually reduced because of a lack of an intact classical pathway.[257,258]

The predominant clinical manifestation of complete C4 deficiency has been systemic lupus erythematosis.[5,6,206] The disease onset is early, and cutaneous features, including photosensitive skin rash (see Fig. 186-5), Raynaud's phenomenon, and vasculitic ulcers, are common. Anti-DNA titers are sometimes absent, as is also seen in C2-deficient patients with lupus. Biopsies of inflammatory skin lesions from C4-deficient patients usually demonstrate the presence of immunoglobulin and C1q consistent with immune-complex deposition and complement activation. The deposition of C3 also has been identified in the kidney, suggesting that the alternative pathway also can play a role in the development of these lesions.[259] These patients also have an increased susceptibility to bacterial infections, probably as a consequence of impaired opsonization and possibly because of poor development of humoral immunity. In fact, most deaths in C4-deficient patients are due to infection.[5,6] Because of the high frequency of infection and likelihood of impaired humoral immunity, intravenous immunoglobulin has been used in one patient.[176] As with many of the other complement-deficiency diseases, there also have been a few asymptomatic C4-deficient patients ascertained as the result of family studies.

Although complete C4 deficiency is extremely rare, individuals who are homozygous deficient for either C4A or C4B are quite common.[205,206] There is a relatively high frequency of null alleles at either the *C4A* or *C4B* locus among both African-Americans[260] and Caucasians.[205] For example, the frequency of *C4A*QO* among Caucasians has been estimated as between 13 and 14 percent and that of *C4B*QO* as between 15 and 16 percent. The corresponding frequencies of homozygous null individuals at each locus would be just over 1 percent for *C4A* and just under 3 percent for *C4B*. Because of the differences in functional activity between C4A and C4B, it has been suggested that individuals who are homozygous deficient in one or the other isotype may be predisposed to certain illnesses. For example, individuals with homozygous C4A deficiency lack the isotype that interacts most efficiently with proteins. They therefore may not be able to normally process protein-containing immune complexes and as a consequence may be at an increased risk for developing immune-complex diseases such as lupus. In fact, a number of studies have shown that the prevalence of homozygous C4A deficiency in lupus varies between 10 and 15 percent, a figure 10 to 15 times higher than the prevalence in the general population.[207–209] The lupus patients with C4A deficiency appear to have a lower prevalence of anticardiolipin, anti-Ro, anti-dsDNA, and anti-Sm antibodies, less neurologic and renal disease, and more photosensitivity than other lupus patients.[261,262] *C4A* null alleles also have been associated with a variety of other autoimmune and immune-complex disorders such as Henoch-Schönlein purpura, idiopathic thrombocytopenic purpura, and celiac disease.[263–265]

Individuals with homozygous C4B deficiency lack the isotype that is most efficient in interacting with polysaccharides. They therefore may not be able to assemble the classical pathway C3-cleaving enzyme (C4b2a) and deposit opsonically active C3b on the polysaccharide capsules of pathogenic bacteria, which, in turn, may predispose them to blood-borne bacterial infections. In fact, there is an increased prevalence of homozygous C4B deficiency in children with bacteremia and meningitis.[197,266]

Molecular Genetic Defect. C4A deficiency in Caucasians typically is due to a large gene deletion and arises on the extended haplotype HLA-A1-Cw7-B8-C2C-BfS-C4AQ0-C4B1-DR3.[267] Additionally, a 2-bp insertion in exon 29 has been identified as the most common cause of nonexpression of an intact *C4A* gene in Caucasians and usually is linked to HLA-B60-DR6.[268] Gene conversion can cause either C4A or C4B deficiency, and some *C4B*QO* alleles are the result of gene deletions.[269]

Since many of the molecular genetic causes of C4 null alleles have been identified, they would be amenable to prenatal diagnosis and carrier detection. In addition, C4 allotyping and isotyping have been performed in a number of kindreds to determine carrier status.

Animal Models. There is a naturally occurring strain of guinea pigs completely deficient in C4.[270] These animals provided valuable evidence for the existence of an alternative pathway.[271] They also have been useful in defining the relative roles of the classical and alternative pathways in a variety of complement-mediated biologic activities[94,270] and in the generation of a normal antibody response.[272] Although they have deficient clearance of bacteria,[94] they have not demonstrated any evidence of immune-complex disease.[273] A C4 knockout mouse has confirmed the importance of C4 in humoral immune responses and the clearance of endotoxin.[274–276]

C2 Deficiency (MIM 217000)

Molecular Biology. The C2 gene, consisting of 18 exons within a 14-kb span, is quite similar in overall structure to the closely linked factor B gene, and their products display 35 percent homology in the derived amino acid sequences.[114,116,129] The 3′ terminus of the C2 gene is approximately 500 bp upstream of the factor B gene. As a result, critical transcriptional control elements included in the regulation of factor B expression are embedded within the region encoding the 3′ untranslated region of the C2 mRNA.

C2 mRNA programs the translation of three distinct polypeptides.[277] The three forms of C2 are probably derived from differential transcription or posttranscriptional processing. Translation of the most abundant C2 mRNA (2.8 kb) generates an 84-kDa product that is further modified and secreted within 30 to 60 minutes. Two forms of C2 of lower molecular mass remain cell-associated. These multiple forms of C2 also have been detected in murine L cells transfected with a genomic fragment bearing the human C2 and factor B genes.[278]

Polymorphic variation in C2 and factor B is much less frequent than in C4 or the class I and class II MHC gene products. Nevertheless, several allelic forms of these two proteins have been defined by electrophoretic techniques[138,180] and by restriction endonuclease digestion.[279,280]

Pathophysiology and Clinical Expression. Genetically determined C2 deficiency is the most common of the inherited complement deficiencies, occurring in 1 in 10,000 Caucasians.[5,6,202,281] Individuals homozygous for C2 deficiency generally have less than 1 percent of the normal amount of C2 functional activity and undetectable C2 by standard immunochemical analysis.[282] Heterozygotes for C2 deficiency generally have C2 levels between 30 and 70 percent of the average values for normal individuals.[282] The wide range of C2 levels in both normal individuals and individuals who are heterozygous for C2 deficiency makes assignment of heterozygous status based on C2 levels alone difficult.

Complement-mediated serum activities, such as opsonization and chemotaxis, are present in patients with C2 deficiency, presumably because their alternative pathway is intact.[283–285] However, when assessed carefully and compared with those of normal individuals, these activities are not generated as quickly nor to the same degree as in individuals with an intact classical pathway.[90,285–287]

The clinical manifestations of C2 deficiency have varied from individuals who are asymptomatic to individuals who are clinically affected with either rheumatic diseases and/or an increased susceptibility to infection.[5,6,281] Whether the patient expresses rheumatic diseases or an increased susceptibility to infection does not appear to be determined by linked MHC class I or class II genes.[163,202,288]

Approximately 40 percent of C2-deficient individuals develop systemic lupus erythematosus or discoid lupus. The association of C2 deficiency with systemic lupus is believed to be due to the compromise in immune-complex clearance that results when C2 is deficient.[187] C2-deficient systemic lupus erythematosus patients have immune complexes that contain increased amounts of C4 but which lack C3 and therefore are cleared inefficiently.[187,289] Normalization of serum complement by the administration of fresh-frozen plasma has returned immune-complex clearance to normal in C2-deficient patients.[187] For this reason, some have advocated the use of fresh-frozen plasma for the treatment of systemic lupus erythematosus in complement-deficient patients.[290]

Patients with C2 deficiency express many of the characteristic features of lupus, although severe nephritis, cerebritis, and aggressive arthritis are less common than in complement-sufficient lupus patients.[5,6] Cutaneous lesions are common in C2-deficient patients with lupus, and many have a characteristic annular photosensitive rash. Patients with C2 deficiency and systemic lupus erythematosus have a lower prevalence of anti-DNA and antinuclear antigen antibodies than do other lupus patients,[161,169,170] but their incidence of anti-Ro antibodies is higher.[169,170] A number of other rheumatic disorders also have been described in C2 deficiency, including glomerulonephritis, inflammatory bowel disease, dermatomyositis, anaphylactoid purpura, and vasculitis.[281,285,291–294] A potential explanation for the lower association of lupus with C2 deficiency compared with either C1 or C4 deficiency could be the ability of factor B to substitute for C2 in processing of immune complexes.[295]

Approximately 50 percent of C2-deficient patients have had an increased susceptibility to bacterial infections. The infections are usually blood-borne and systemic (e.g., sepsis, meningitis, arthritis, and osteomyelitis) and caused by encapsulated organisms (e.g. pneumococcus, *H. influenzae*, and meningococcus).[5,6,281,284,296–298]

It is unclear whether patients who are heterozygous for C2 deficiency have any clinical manifestations. An early study demonstrated an increased frequency of heterozygous C2 deficiency in systemic lupus erythematosus and juvenile rheumatoid arthritis.[161] However, assignment of a given individual as heterozygous for C2 deficiency was based on serum levels of C2 and HLA haplotype. More recently, PCR detection of the characteristic 28-bp deletion in ethnically and geographically matched lupus patients and controls found no increased frequency of C2 heterozygotes in lupus.[202] However, a recent study suggested that heterozygous C2 deficiency in combination with C4 null alleles could be associated with an increased predisposition to lupus.[299]

Molecular Genetic Defect. A number of studies have shown that the gene for C2 deficiency (*C2*QO*) is closely linked to genes of the MHC and that it is in linkage disequilibrium with specific alleles of the MHC.[159,161,300–304] Over 95 percent of C2-deficient individuals are homozygous for a 28-bp deletion at the 3′ end of exon 6 that results in premature termination of transcription.[163,202,305] The 28-bp deletion is associated with a conserved MHC haplotype consisting of HLA-B18, C2*QO, Bf*S, C4A*4, C4B*2, and DR*2.[163,202,304–306] The gene frequency of this deletion has been found to be 0.005 to 0.007 in Caucasian populations.[163,202,305] The 28-bp deletion accounts for more than 95 percent of C2-deficient patients.[163,202] In addition, two different missense mutations have been identified that result in impaired secretion of mature C2,[307] and in another kindred a 2-bp deletion results in a premature stop codon.[308]

Detection of the 28-bp deletion using PCR has been used for both carrier detection and prenatal diagnosis.[309]

Animal Models. A C2-deficient guinea pig has been useful in elucidating the role of complement in the generation of a normal humoral immune response.[106]

C3 Deficiency (MIM 120700)

Molecular Biology. The human C3 gene consists of 41 exons spanning 42 kb[310] on chromosome 19.[311] It specifies transcription of a 5.2-kb mature mRNA[312] that encodes the prepro-C3 primary translation product.[313] Serum C3 is synthesized primarily in hepatocytes.[313–315] Monocytes, fibroblasts, endothelium, and epithelial cells of several organs also produce C3.[147–149] In fact, local synthesis of C3 is capable of restoring the defective antibody responses in C3-deficient mice.[152] Co- and postsynthetic processing involves cleavage of the signal peptide and the interchain-linking peptide and glycosylation to generate the heterodimeric disulfide-linked C3 protein. The thiolester bridge is generated by isomerization of a lactam to yield a thiolactone.

Pathophysiology and Clinical Expression. Genetically determined C3 deficiency is inherited as an autosomal recessive trait.[5,6,316] This genetic defect, although relatively rare, has been observed in many different ethnic groups throughout the world. Affected individuals have severely depressed levels of C3 in their sera (<1 percent of normal).[316] In many patients, some C3 antigen and function can be detected using highly sensitive techniques,[317] whereas in others, no C3 protein is detected even when using extremely sensitive assay systems.[318] Those serum functions either directly dependent on C3 or indirectly dependent on C3 because of its role in the activation of C5–C9 are also markedly reduced. That is, serum opsonic, chemotactic, and bactericidal activities are either absent or markedly diminished in patients with C3 deficiency.[317–325]

Infection is the most common finding in C3-deficient individuals.[5,6,316] Patients with C3 deficiency have had a variety of infections, including pneumonia, bacteremia, meningitis, and osteomyelitis, caused by encapsulated pyogenic bacteria, such as the pneumococcus, *H. influenzae*, and the meningococcus.[5,6,316–318,321,323–327] Patients tend to present early in life with recurrent severe infections. Their increased susceptibility to infection emphasizes the important physiologic role of C3 as an opsonin but also may relate to the role of C3 in the generation of a normal humoral immune response.[78]

Approximately 25 percent of C3-deficient patients develop rheumatic diseases.[5,6] A number of patients have presented with arthralgias and vasculitic skin rashes.[322,323] In some patients, a clinical picture consistent with systemic lupus erythematosus is present.[323] Interestingly, although certain clinical features of lupus are present in some patients with C3 deficiency, as with some other complement-deficient patients, they may not have serologic evidence of lupus. Renal disease also has been seen in C3-deficient patients.[320,328,329] Histologically, the lesions most closely resemble membranoproliferative glomerulonephritis with mesangial cell proliferation, an increased mesangial matrix, and electron-dense deposits in both the mesangium and the subendothelium of capillary loops.[328,329] Immunofluorescent studies have revealed all major immunoglobulin classes to be present, but no C3. In one of the cases of renal disease, as well as in some of the cases of vasculitis or lupus in which there was no apparent renal disease, circulating immune complexes have been found in the serum.[323,325,328] The renal disease may reflect the role of C3 in immune-complex clearance. For this reason, administration of fresh-frozen plasma to replete C3 has been advocated as a treatment for the renal disease. However, evidence from C3-deficient dogs with membranoproliferative glomerulonephritis suggests that supplying C3 after the renal disease has occurred may make the glomerulonephritis worse.[330]

The third component of complement is highly polymorphic, with at least 20 allelic variants having been identified.[137,138] The two most common alleles, C3 fast (*C3*F*) and C3 slow (*C3*S*), can be distinguished by their electrophoretic mobility and are found in over 98 percent of the population. A single nucleotide change at position 364 resulting in either a glycine (*C3*F*) or an arginine (*C3S*) underlies this polymorphism.[331] Two particularly rare variants have been described that are indistinguishable from C3 slow and C3 fast by electrophoretic mobility but are associated with decreased staining after electrophoresis and reduced levels of serum C3. Termed *hypomorphic C3 slow* (*C3*s*) and *hypomorphic C3 fast* (*C3*f*), these variants have been identified in patients with a variety of rheumatic disorders. Hypomorphic C3 fast has been described in a patient with glomerulonephritis and arthritis,[332] cutaneous vasculitis,[333] and recurrent hemolytic-uremic syndrome,[334] as well as in normal individuals.[335] Hypomorphic C3 slow has been described in a patient with nephritis as well as in his asymptomatic family members.[336]

Molecular Defect. Approximately 20 patients with C3 deficiency have been described.[5,6,316] In 4 patients the molecular genetic defect has been identified. The first C3-deficient patient was found to have a mutation in the 5′ donor splice site of intron 18 resulting in a premature stop codon.[337] A second C3-deficient patient has a donor splice site mutation in intron 10.[338] In the third patient, a point mutation in exon 13 causes an amino acid change that blocks the maturation of intracellular pro-C3 to mature C3.[316] Finally, an Afrikaans-speaking patient was found to have an 800-bp deletion between two Alu repeats.[318] This 800-bp deletion has been found with a relatively high gene frequency (0.0057) in the Afrikaans-speaking South African population.[318]

Because the mutations causing C3 deficiency are diverse, carrier detection and prenatal diagnosis will rely on the identification of each individual mutation in a previously affected family member. Among the Afrikaans-speaking population of South Africa, RFLP detection of the 800-bp deletion has been used for carrier testing.[318]

Animal Models. Dogs with genetically determined C3 deficiency were discovered in 1981.[339] The mutation responsible for the C3 deficiency is a single-base-pair deletion resulting in a premature stop codon.[340] Affected animals have both an increased susceptibility to infection and membranoproliferative glomerulonephritis, thereby closely resembling their human counterparts.[341] The C3-deficient dog has been useful in demonstrating the role of C3 in a variety of physiologic functions such as the generation of a normal antibody response[107] and in resistance to endotoxic shock and multiple organ failure.[342] A C3 knockout mouse has impaired humoral immune responses and poor germinal center formation.[108] The C3 knockout mouse also demonstrates an increased mortality after endotoxin challenge.[275] Interestingly, administration of C1 inhibitor to endotoxin-challenged C3 knockout mice helps protect them from death.[275]

C5 Deficiency (MIM 120900)

Molecular Biology. C5 is encoded by a relatively large gene (79 kDa) comprising 41 exons on chromosome 9q.[343,344] The 6.0-kb mature C5 mRNA programs synthesis of prepro-C5,[345–347] a precursor with similarities to prepro-C4 and prepro-C3. There appear to be several splice variants of C5, but their function is not clear.[343] Precursor pro-C5 undergoes co- and postsynthetic processing to generate the two-chain disulfide-linked native protein. C5 is synthesized in liver hepatocytes, as well as in alveolar epithelium and mononuclear phagocytes.

Pathophysiology and Clinical Expression. Genetically determined C5 deficiency is inherited as an autosomal recessive trait and has been identified in a number of different families.[5,6,348] Homozygous deficient individuals usually have markedly reduced levels of C5 functional activity (<1 percent), and no C5 antigen is detectable in their serum. In one instance, however, a patient had as much as 1 to 2 percent of the normal amount of C5 functional activity, although her homozygous deficient sister had less than 0.1 percent.[349] The sera of patients with C5 deficiency are unable to generate normal amounts of chemotactic or bactericidal activity.[350,351] As expected, serum opsonic activity is intact, since the activation of C3 can proceed without the participation of C5.[350,351]

Although the initial patient identified as C5-deficient had systemic lupus erythematosus and membranoproliferative glomerulonephritis,[349] subsequent patients have been ascertained because of either meningococcal meningitis, disseminated gonococcal infections, or other autoimmune diseases such as Sjögren syndrome.[350–354] The relationship of C5 deficiency to autoimmune diseases is not clear, although a recent study in mice has demonstrated a linkage of the murine C5 gene with susceptibility to collagen-induced arthritis.[355] A few C5-deficient patients have been asymptomatic, having been ascertained as part of family studies.

Molecular Genetic Defect. Approximately 30 patients with C5 deficiency have been described.[5,6] The specific mutation has been identified in three African-American patients. Two patients from unrelated kindreds had a nonsense mutation in exon 1, and a third patient had a nonsense mutation in exon 36.[356] These patients were all compound heterozygotes for C5 deficiency, and these mutations were not detected in 4 other Caucasian patients, indicating that diverse mutations are associated with C5 deficiency.

Because many mutations are responsible for C5 deficiency, carrier detection and prenatal diagnosis rely on the identification of each individual mutation in a previously affected family member.

Animal Models. A number of inbred strains of mice have a complete deficiency of C5.[357] Mice deficient in C5 have been of value in defining the relative role of C5 in generating a local inflammatory response in response to a variety of stimuli in a variety of organs and in the rejection of skin allografts.[358] In addition, these mice have been useful in delineating the role of C5 in resistance to a variety of infections.[358]

C6 Deficiency (MIM 217050)

Molecular Biology. C6 is a single-chain glycoprotein encoded by a gene on chromosome 5q13.[359] The message for C6 is approximately 6.6 kb and is produced primarily in the liver, with additional expression in neutrophils, endothelial cells, and astroglioma.[360,361] Like many other complement proteins, C6 is an acute-phase reactant and is upregulated at sites of inflammation. Co- and postsynthetic processing results in a protein of 128 kDa. Its molecular architecture has been established by circular dichroism spectroscopy, and its tertiary structure has been revealed by transmission electron microscopy. It has a sickle shape with a small "hook" on one end.[362] C6 contains several thrombospondin repeat motifs that are believed to function in protein-protein and protein-phospholipid interactions during assembly of the membrane attack complex.

Pathophysiology and Clinical Expression. C6 deficiency has been reported in nearly 100 individuals, many of whom are African-Americans.[5,6] Deficiency of C6 is inherited in an autosomal recessive fashion.[5,6,363] The most common form of C6 deficiency is characterized by absent or nearly absent levels of C6 (<1 percent of normal), whether it is assessed immunochemically or functionally.[364] The only abnormality relating to their serum complement system is a marked deficiency of serum bactericidal activity.[365–368] Those complement-mediated serum activities which depend only on the activation of C3 and C5, such as opsonic activity and chemotactic activity, are normal.[365–368]

A C6 subtotal deficiency of C6 (C6SD) also has been described that is characterized by serum levels of C6 that are 1 to 2 percent of normal.[369] This truncated C6 protein has a lower molecular weight, and although it is able to be incorporated into the membrane attack complex, it functions less efficiently. This form of C6 deficiency was first identified in family members of individuals with complete C6 deficiency when the C6SD allele was inherited with a *C6*QO* allele. Patients with C6SD do not appear to have an increased susceptibility to infection.

Two unrelated patients with a genetically determined combined deficiency of both C6 and C7 also have been described.[370,371] The patients had very low levels of both C6 (1–5 percent of normal) and C7 (3–9 percent of normal). In one patient, when concentrated from the serum, the C6 was found to be smaller in size (110,000 Da) than normal C6 (140,000 Da) and antigenically deficient, whereas the C7 appeared normal.[370] The other patient had no detectable C6, even in a concentrated serum sample, although small amounts of normal C7 were present.[371]

The major clinical manifestation of complete C6 deficiency has been disseminated neisserial infections.[5,6] While most patients have had meningococcal sepsis and meningitis, others have had disseminated gonococcal infections. One patient with C6 deficiency has presented with a lupus-like syndrome.[372]

Molecular Genetic Defect. The genetic basis for complete C6 deficiency has been determined in three unrelated patients.[373,374] One African-American patient was homozygous for a single-base-pair deletion in exon 12 that results in premature termination. A second African-American patient was heterozygous for the same exon 12 deletion and a single-base-pair deletion in exon 7. The third patient was Japanese and was a compound heterozygote with a deletion of four nucleotides on one chromosome and an undefined defect on the other.

Complete C6 deficiency occurs most frequently in South Africa, where haplotype determinations of flanking markers have demonstrated that the majority of *C6*QO* alleles in this population arose from the same distant ancestor.[375,376] These haplotype determinations also have been used to identify carriers.

The basis for C6SD is a loss of the splice donor site at intron 15 and premature termination.[369]

Animal Models. Genetically determined C6 deficiency has been described in rats and rabbits.[358,377] The C6-deficient rat has been valuable in demonstrating that the extrahepatic synthesis of complement can contribute significantly to some of the biologic functions of the complement system.[378]

C7 Deficiency (MIM 217070)

Molecular Biology. The gene for C7 is closely linked to the genes for C6 and C9 on chromosome 5.[359,379] Like C6 and C9, it contains domains with homology to thrombospondin, low-density lipoprotein receptor, and the epidermal growth factor receptor.[380]

Pathophysiology and Clinical Expression. Only a few patients with C7 deficiency have been identified.[5,6,381] The defect appears to be inherited as an autosomal recessive trait. Deficient individuals have severely reduced (<1 percent) levels of C7 and have little, if any, total hemolytic complement serum activity. Similarly, serum bactericidal activity is also markedly reduced in those patients in whom it has been tested.[382–384] A second type of C7 deficiency has been described in which the quantity of C7 is diminished but not absent.[385] The C7 that is present exhibits an altered isoelectric point. Interestingly, this form of C7 deficiency, termed *C7 subtotal deficiency* (C7SD), has been seen primarily in association with C6SD (see above).[386]

A number of clinical presentations have been associated with C7 deficiency.[5,6,381] As with the other deficiencies of terminal components, systemic neisserial infections have occurred in most reported cases of C7 deficiency. Individual patients also have presented with lupus,[387] rheumatoid arthritis,[388] scleroderma,[389] and pyoderma gangrenosum.[390] Finally, there have been a few patients with C7 deficiency who have been clinically well.

Molecular Genetic Defect. The molecular genetic defects causing C7 deficiency are heterogeneous. Mutation analysis of two Japanese patients has revealed one patient with a homozygous transversion resulting in a premature stop codon at exon 16.[391] The second patient was homozygous for a 2-bp deletion resulting in a premature stop codon. In another study, an Irish patient had a point mutation in the splice acceptor site of intron 1, and a second Irish person had a deletion of exons 7 and 8.[385] Israeli patients of Sephardic origin have a common missense mutation in exon 9.[385] C7SD has been shown to result from a missense mutation in exon 11 that leads to an arginine-to-serine substitution.[385,386]

C8 Deficiency (MIM 120950, 120960)

Molecular Biology. C8 is composed of three polypeptide chains (α, β, γ).[392] The α and γ chains are covalently joined to form one subunit (C8α,γ), which is joined to the other subunit, the β chain (C8β), by noncovalent bonds.[393] Each of the C8 polypeptides is encoded by separate genes (*C8A*, *C8B*, and *C8G*).[133,134,394,395] *C8A* and *C8B* map to chromosome 1p3.2, and *C8G* maps to 9q.[395] The *C8A* and *C8B* genes each encode 2.4-kb messages. While they have close physical linkage, they are independently regulated. *C8A* and *C8B* contain several thrombospondin repeat motifs that are common to many of the terminal components. *C8G* is most closely related to lipocalin.[396] The precursors of the three C8 polypeptides are translated in liver, co- and postsynthetically processed, assembled and secreted.[397] The rates of α- and γ-chain synthesis are equal, but exceed that for β chain so that in addition to native C8, free C8α,γ is also found in plasma.[398]

Pathophysiology and Clinical Expression. Several variants of C8 deficiency have been recognized. In one form of C8 deficiency (MIM 120950), patients lack the C8α,γ subunit, whereas in the other form (MIM 120960), the C8β subunit is deficient.[399,400]

Two types of C8β-subunit deficiency have been identified thus far. In one form, the C8β chain is present in serum but dysfunctional,[399,401] and in the other form, C8β chain is markedly decreased in serum.[402] In all variants, C8 functional activity is markedly reduced (<1 percent of normal). In the case of C8β-subunit deficiency, C8 antigen can be detected in the serum of affected individuals using standard immunodiffusion techniques, but it lacks antigenic determinants present in the intact C8 molecule.[403] Isolation of the C8 antigen from the serum of patients with C8β-subunit deficiency has shown it to be identical to the normal C8α,γ subunit.[404,405] Addition of C8β subunit, purified from normal C8, to the serum from patients with C8β-subunit deficiency restores C8 functional activity, offering additional evidence that the C8α,γ subunit in these patient's sera is normal.[404,405]

In the case of C8α,γ deficiency, initial analysis of serum from these patients using standard immunodiffusion techniques failed to detect any C8 antigen.[406,407] However, when sera from these patients is immunoprecipitated with antiserum to C8 and the precipitates examined using SDS-page analysis, the C8β subunit can be detected.[400] Addition of purified C8α,γ from normal serum restores C8 functional hemolytic activity to C8α,γ-subunit-deficient sera.[400] As expected, when C8α,γ-subunit-deficient sera is mixed with C8β-subunit-deficient sera, hemolytic activity is also restored.[400]

The only biologically functional defect in C8-deficient sera is a marked reduction in bactericidal activity.[406,408] Other complement-mediated serum activities, such as opsonization, are intact.

The clinical presentation of C8 deficiency has been similar to the other deficiencies in terminal complement components.[5,6,399] Meningococcemia (Fig. 186-6), meningococcal meningitis, and disseminated gonococcal infections have predominated, but systemic lupus erythematosus also has been seen rarely.

Molecular Genetic Defect. Deficiency of C8β is more common in Caucasians, whereas C8α,γ deficiency is more common in African-Americans. Eighty-six percent of C8β null alleles are due to C $\rightarrow$ T transition in exon 9 producing a premature stop codon,[409–411] suggesting a founder effect. Three additional C $\rightarrow$ T transitions and two single-base-pair deletions causing premature stop codons also have been identified in C8β deficiency, implying that there will be many different mutations occurring in the 14 percent of patients who do not carry the common mutation.[410] The molecular basis of C8α,γ deficiency has been identified in three

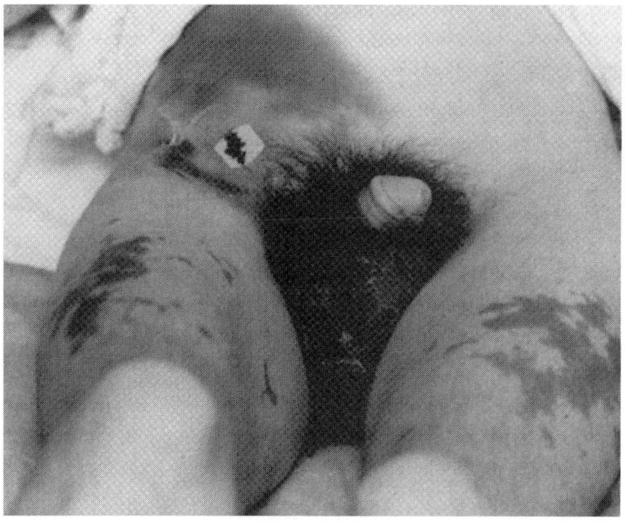

Fig. 186-6 Purpura fulminans in a C8-deficient patient with meningococcal sepsis. (*Courtesy of Dr. Peter Densen.*)

patients. In five of six null alleles, an intronic mutation alters the splicing of exons 6 and 7 of *C8A* and creates a 10-bp insertion that generates a premature stop codon.[412]

C9 Deficiency (MIM 120940)

Molecular Biology. C9 is a 70-kDa glycoprotein that has sequence homology with other members of the membrane attack complex (C8α,γ, C8β, C6, C7, and perforin).[413–415] The C9 gene is approximately 2500 bp from the C6 and C7 genes on chromosome 5p13.[416,417] C9 is produced primarily by the liver and is highly developmentally regulated. Newborn infants produce substantially less than adults.[418] C9 is also cytokine-inducible and behaves as an acute-phase reactant.[419]

Pathophysiology and Clinical Expression. Only a few Occidental patients with C9 deficiency have been identified,[5,6,420] but it appears to be the most common complement deficiency in Japan, with a prevalence of 0.036 to 0.095 percent.[421] In those patients in whom family members have been available for testing, the disease appears to be inherited as an autosomal recessive trait.

Most affected individuals have markedly reduced levels of C9, whether tested immunochemically or by functional analysis. In one case, however, the patient had trace amounts of C9 antigen detectable in her serum and between 10 and 15 percent of the normal amount of C9 functional hemolytic activity.[422] The hemolysis of sensitized erythrocytes can be mediated by a membrane attack complex composed of C5b–C8 and is not therefore strictly dependent on C9.[67] As a result, patients with C9 deficiency have some total hemolytic complement activity, although it is usually between one-third and one-half of the lower limit of normal.[423,424] Similarly, their sera possess some bactericidal activity, although the rate of killing is significantly reduced.[422]

Like patients with deficiencies of other terminal components, patients with C9 deficiency have an increased susceptibility to systemic meningococcal infections.[5,6,420] Although the first few individuals with C9 deficiency were asymptomatic, some subsequent patients with C9 deficiency have presented with systemic meningococcal infections.[5,6,425] In addition, an epidemiologic study of C9 deficiency in Japan has firmly established a relationship between C9 deficiency and meningococcal sepsis and meningitis.[426] A few patients have presented with autoimmune disease, but the relationship of the autoimmune disease to C9 deficiency is unclear.[427,428]

Molecular Genetic Defect. The molecular genetic basis for C9 deficiency has been identified in one Swiss kindred. Two different point mutations in exons 2 and 4 resulted in premature stop codons.[429] The common mutation in Japanese patients is a nonsense mutation in exon 4.[430] RFLP analysis has allowed carrier detection in another kindred.[431]

Factor B Deficiency (MIM 138470)

Molecular Biology. Factor B is a serine protease that is expressed primarily in the liver and macrophages. The gene for factor B is part of the HLA class III region at 6p21.3 and is highly homologous to C2, with which it is closely linked.[114,116,129] Because the two genes are in close proximity and the polyadenylation signal for C2 overlaps the 5′ regulatory region of the factor B gene, it is possible that they share regulatory signals. Interestingly, decreased expression of factor B has been described in association with some kindreds with C2 deficiency,[296,308] and conversely, C2 expression is diminished in a factor B knockout mouse.[432]

Pathophysiology and Clinical Expression. A single patient with factor B deficiency has been described.[433] No functional factor B was detected, and the factor B protein was structurally abnormal. As expected, there was no detectable alternative pathway activity. The patient was ascertained after an episode of meningococcemia. Although it is difficult to be sure in a single patient that the meningococcemia was related to the underlying factor B deficiency, it is likely because most alternative pathway deficiencies have been associated with systemic meningococcal disease.

Molecular Genetic Defect. The molecular genetic defect responsible for this patient's factor B deficiency is unknown.

Animal Models. Two groups have generated factor B knockout mice. In one case, the factor B-deficient mice also had reduced expression of C2 and of D17H6S45.[432] Because both the alternative pathway and the classical pathway are affected, sera from these mice were unable to clear immune complexes efficiently or opsonize sheep red blood cells. Another factor B-deficient knockout mouse demonstrates a normal ability to withstand endotoxin challenge.[434] Unlike animals deficient in C3 or components of the classical pathway, these mice demonstrate normal humoral immunity, suggesting that the alternative pathway is not necessary for the generation of a normal antibody response.

Factor D Deficiency (MIM 134350)

Molecular Biology. Factor D is a serine protease that has a molecular weight of 24 kDa. Also known as adipsin, it is synthesized in adipocytes, muscle cells, lung, and monocytes/macrophages.[435] Unlike other complement components, factor D is not synthesized in the liver. It has a role not only in regulation of the alternative pathway but also in triglyceride metabolism and the regulation of degranulation of neutrophils.[436,437] The genetic locus for factor D has not been identified. Regulation of factor D activity is accomplished by conformational changes induced by its natural substrate, C3bB.[438]

Pathophysiology and Clinical Expression. Two kindreds with factor D deficiency have been described. In one, identical twins were found to have 8 percent of the normal levels of factor D.[439] In the second kindred, neither functional nor antigenic factor D was detectable in the proband and was present in approximately half-normal levels in the mother and sister, suggesting possible X-linked inheritance.[440] As expected the CH_{50} in the patients was mildly depressed, while the AP_{50} was 0 to 5 percent of normal. The presenting manifestations of factor D deficiency have been recurrent neisserial infections and recurrent sinopulmonary infections.[439,440]

Molecular Genetic Defect. The molecular genetic basis for factor D deficiency is unknown.

Animal Models. A factor D-deficient mouse is most remarkable for obesity.[437]

C1-Inhibitor Deficiency (MIM 106100)

Molecular Biology. Genetically determined deficiency of C1-INH is responsible for the clinical disorder termed hereditary angioedema (HAE).[441] C1-INH, a glycoprotein with a molecular mass of 105 kDa and total carbohydrate content of 33 percent,[442] is encoded by a 17-kDa gene on chromosome 11q.[136,443,444] The liver is the major source of plasma C1-INH,[445–448] but mononuclear phagocytes and fibroblasts also synthesize and secrete C1-INH.[449]

The primary sequence of the C1-INH has been determined.[443,444] It shares approximately 20 percent homology with serine protease inhibitors α_1-proteinase inhibitor, α_1-antichymotrypsin, antithrombin III, and angiotensinogen.

Pathophysiology and Clinical Expression. Hereditary angioedema is inherited in an autosomal dominant fashion. There are at least two forms of C1-INH deficiency.[156,450] In the commonest form (type I), accounting for approximately 85 percent of the patients, the sera of affected individuals are deficient in both C1-INH protein (5–30 percent of normal) and C1-INH functional activity.[441,450–452] In the other, less common form (type II), a dysfunctional protein is present in normal or elevated concentrations, but the functional activity of C1-INH is markedly reduced.[441,450–452] In patients with type I HAE, the diagnosis can be established easily by demonstrating a decrease in serum C1-INH protein when assessed by immunochemical techniques. However, in patients with type II HAE, the diagnosis must rest on demonstrating a decrease in C1-INH functional activity. In either case, C4 levels and C2 levels are usually reduced below the lower limit of normal during attacks,[451–454] due to their uncontrolled cleavage by C1s. The level of C4 in serum is also reduced between attacks, making its measurement useful as a diagnostic clue.[451,454]

A number of studies have examined the dysfunctional C1-INH molecules from different families and found that they not only differ from normal C1-INH but from each other with respect to their electrophoretic mobility, ability to bind C1s, and ability to inhibit a synthetic substrate, *N*-acetyl-tyrosine-ethyl-ester.[156,450,455–457] Normal C1-INH also inhibits plasma kallikrein, activated Hageman factor, and plasmin. In one study comparing the dysfunctional C1-INH molecules from eight different kindreds, each dysfunctional C1-INH was unique with respect to its spectrum of inhibitory activities against these enzymes,[457] although none of the dysfunctional proteins inhibited plasmin.

The levels of normal C1-INH function in patients with either type of HAE are lower than one might expect in a hemizygote: 5 to 30 percent of normal in type I C1-INH deficiency and little or none in type II C1-INH deficiency. In addition, the immunochemical levels of the dysfunctional protein in the type II disorder usually are equivalent to normal or higher than normal rather than the expected 50 percent of normal. In an attempt to explain these apparent discrepancies, metabolic studies using both normal and dysfunctional proteins have been performed in both normal and deficient subjects.[458] As expected, the synthesis of the normal C1-INH in the type I disorder was reduced, findings consistent with earlier studies showing reduced content of the normal protein in the livers of patients with C1-INH deficiency.[448] In addition, the fractional catabolic rate of normal C1-INH in both types of patients with HAE was significantly elevated. Finally, the fractional catabolic rates of two different dysfunctional C1-INH proteins were different from each other and from normal; in one the fractional catabolic rate was near normal, and in the other it was strikingly reduced. These studies have been used to create a model to explain the low levels of C1-INH found in the type I disorder and the elevated levels of dysfunctional protein found in the type II disorder.[459] The model proposes that there are two catabolic routes for normal C1-INH, one in which the inhibitor complexes with the enzymes with which it reacts in vivo and another independent of inhibitor-enzyme complexes and representing the normal catabolism of any serum protein. Thus it has been suggested that in the type I disorder the markedly lowered levels of C1-INH are the result of both decreased synthesis and increased catabolism consequent to the complexing of the normal C1-INH with the activated enzymes that it normally inhibits. Similarly, it has been suggested that the low levels of normal C1-INH and elevated levels of dysfunctional C1-INH protein in the type II disorder are the result of decreased synthesis and increased catabolism of the normal C1-INH and, at least in some cases, decreased catabolism of the dysfunctional C1-INH consequent to its inability to complex with C1 and other enzymes.

The pathophysiologic mechanism(s) by which the absence of C1-INH activity leads to the angioedema characteristic of the disorder are still incompletely understood. Neither the mediators responsible for producing the edema nor the mechanisms initiating their production have been clearly identified. There is a great deal of evidence implicating complement in the pathogenesis of the edema. Clearly, C1s activity is present in the sera of patients during an attack.[460] Furthermore, when purified C1s is injected into normal or HAE patients' skin, angioedema is produced.[461] The intradermal response to C1s in C2-deficient individuals is markedly diminished, whereas it is preserved in C3-deficient individuals, suggesting the direct involvement of C2 in the production of the angioedema.[461] Other evidence suggests that the plasma kallikrein system also may be involved in the generation of the edema. C1-INH is capable of inhibiting the ability of activated Hageman factor to initiate kinin generation, fibrinolysis, and coagulation.[462] It also inhibits kallikrein of the kinin system, plasma thromboplastin antecedent (factor XIa) of the clotting system, and plasmin of the fibrinolytic system.[451] It is possible, therefore, that products of the kinin system could be involved in the edema formation. In fact, blister fluids from HAE patients contain active plasma kallikrein,[463] and their sera have decreased amounts of prekallikrein and kininogen,[464] suggesting activation of the kinin system during attacks of edema.

The clinical symptoms of HAE are the result of submucosal or subcutaneous edema. The lesions are characterized by noninflammatory edema associated with capillary and venule dilation.[465] The postcapillary venule also demonstrates gaps between the endothelial cells.[465] The three most prominent areas of involvement are the skin, respiratory tract, and gastrointestinal tract.[451,452,466,467] Although symptoms during attacks may relate to only one of these areas, they are not mutually exclusive and may be seen in combination.

Attacks involving the skin may involve the extremities, the face, or the genitalia (Fig. 186-7). In some instances, there may be changes just preceding the edema, such as mottling, a transient serpinginous erythema, or frank erythema marginatum. The edema usually expands centripetally from a single site and may vary in size from a few centimeters to involvement of a whole extremity. The lesions are pale rather than red, are usually not warm, and are characteristically nonpruritic. There may be, however, a feeling of tightness in the skin due to the accumulation of subcutaneous fluid. Attacks usually progress for 1 to 2 days and resolve over an additional 2 to 3 days.

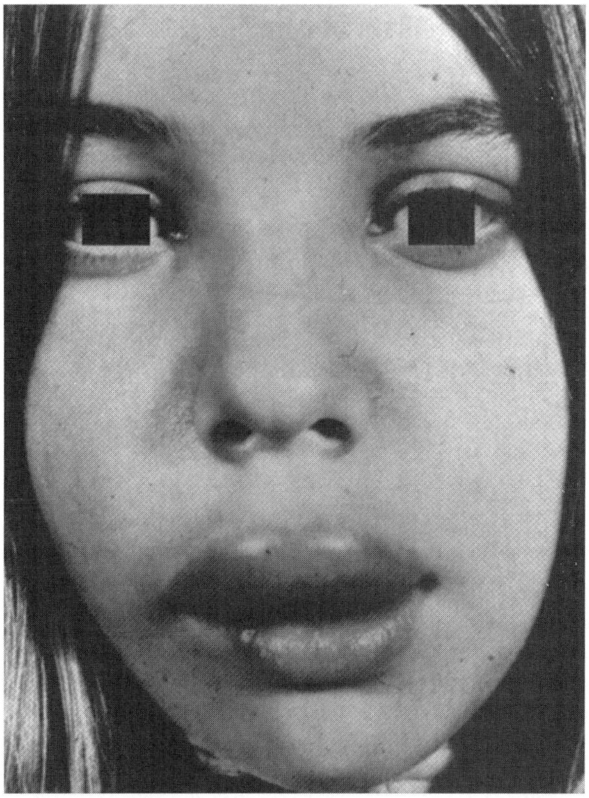

Fig. 186-7 A patient with C1-INH deficiency during an attack of angioedema. (*Courtesy of Dr. Fred S. Rosen.*)

Attacks involving the upper respiratory tract represent a serious threat to the patient with HAE. In one series, pharyngeal edema had occurred at least once in nearly two-thirds of the patients.[451] The patient initially may experience a "tightness" in the throat, and swelling of the tongue, buccal mucosa, and oropharynx follows. In some instances, laryngeal edema, accompanied by hoarseness and stridor, occurs, progresses to respiratory obstruction, and represents a life-threatening emergency. In fact, in a series from 20 years ago, tracheotomies had been performed in one of every six patients with HAE.[451]

The gastrointestinal tract also can be affected by HAE. Symptoms are probably related to edema of the bowel wall and may include anorexia, dull aching of the abdomen, vomiting, and in some cases crampy abdominal pain. Abdominal symptoms can occur in the absence of concurrent cutaneous or pharyngeal involvement. In some instances, abdominal symptoms may be the only symptoms the patient has ever had, leading to difficulty in diagnosis.

The onset of symptoms referable to HAE occurs in over half the patients before adolescence,[451,452,467] but in some patients their first symptoms do not occur until they are well into adult life. Although in just over half of patients no specific events can be clearly identified as initiating attacks, anxiety and/or stress are cited frequently.[451,452,467] Dental extractions and tonsillectomy can initiate edema of the upper airway, and cutaneous edema may follow trauma to an extremity. Some patients report attacks following the use of tight-fitting clothing or shoes, whereas others have related cold exposure to the onset of symptoms.

The therapy of HAE can be conveniently considered to fall into three categories: (1) the long-term prophylaxis of attacks, (2) the short-term prophylaxis of attacks, and (3) the treatment of acute attacks. In those patients who have had laryngeal obstruction or have suffered frequent and debilitating attacks that have interfered with work or other responsibilities, the long-term prevention of attacks may be indicated. Antifibrinolytic agents, such as ε-aminocaproic acid (EACA) or its cyclic analogue, tranexamic acid, have been used with some success in the long-term prevention of attacks, particularly in children, where androgen use may be undesirable (see below).[468,469] Improvement consists of a decreased frequency of attacks in most patients and a decrease in severity in others. The mechanisms by which they exert their protective effect are unclear.

More recently, "impeded" androgens, such as danazol and stanozolol, which have attenuated androgenic potential, have been found to be useful in the long-term prophylaxis of HAE.[470] The basis for their use lies in an earlier observation that methyltestosterone therapy was effective in HAE.[471] During a double-blind, controlled study of danazol, only 1 of 46 courses of danazol therapy was accompanied by attacks of angioedema, whereas 44 of 47 courses of placebo therapy were interrupted by an attack.[470] Danazol therapy appears to be effective for extended periods of time, but because of dose-related adverse reactions (e.g., weight gain, abnormal liver function tests, microscopic hematuria, and altered libido), therapy needs to be closely monitored.[472] Danazol increases serum concentrations of the normal C1-INH in these patients, whether they have the form of the disease characterized by low levels of C1-INH protein (type I) or the form characterized by a dysfunctional protein (type II).[470,473] In some instances, patients may need short-term prophylactic therapy, such as before oral surgery. In these circumstances, danazol therapy may be initiated 1 week before surgery or EACA the day before surgery. There is some controversy concerning the use of fresh-frozen plasma during an acute attack, since the plasma not only supplies the missing C1-INH but also C1 enzyme and substrates such as C4 and C2. Nevertheless, the use of plasma transfusions 12 hours before elective surgery may prevent morbidity from the procedure.[474]

A number of drugs have been used in an attempt to interrupt an attack of HAE once it has begun. Epinephrine, antihistamines, and corticosteroids are of no proven benefit. Trials with partially purified C1-INH have been encouraging. Infusion of C1-INH has been accompanied by resolution of edema and symptoms within a few hours.[475,476]

Molecular Genetic Defect. The division of C1-INH deficiency into two categories based on the presence or absence of a dysfunctional protein has no correlation with clinical phenotype and only limited correlation with genotype because there are some examples of C1-INH mutations in which a dysfunctional protein is produced but is degraded so rapidly that it is not detectable in the serum.[477,478]

Alu-mediated deletions and duplications account for the most common C1-INH null genotypes.[478,479] The C1-INH gene contains a total of 17 *Alu* repetitive DNA elements, and these are responsible for most of the gene rearrangements leading to C1-INH deficiency. A number of single-base changes and smaller deletions and duplications also have been identified.[478] Most patients with type II HAE deficiency have a mutation that replaces the reactive center arginine residue. The other mutations identified in patients with a dysfunctional protein are usually found in the hinge region, thereby inactivating the C1-INH.[478,480] Several mutations just N-terminal to the active site apparently generate changes in the stressed loop confirmation of the C1-INH SERPIN,[481–483] and one located more distantly leads to an abnormal glycosylation signal.[484]

A unique dysfunctional C1-INH has been described that is capable of inhibiting C1s but not C1r. No member of the kindred had angioedema, although the proband was identified due to systemic lupus erythematosus. A codon 443 Ala-Val substitution rendered the molecule dysfunctional in the complement cascade but active as an inhibitor of trypsin.[485]

C4b-Binding Protein Deficiency (MIM 120830, 120831)

Molecular Biology. C4b-binding protein contains seven α chains arrayed radially around a single disulfide-linked β chain. The genes for the α and β chains are tightly linked at 1q32 within the regulation of complement activation (RCA) gene cluster.[486] All the RCA members (MCP, CR1, CR2, DAF, C4b-binding protein α, C4b-binding protein β, and factor H) share sequence homology and contain multiple β-sheet repeat units. The C4bp α chains contain the binding site for C4.[487] C4b-binding protein is synthesized primarily in the liver, and the two genes are differentially induced by interferon-γ and tumor necrosis factor α.[488]

Pathophysiology and Clinical Expression. C4b-binding protein controls classical pathway C3-convertase activity by serving as a cofactor for factor I. A single kindred with a deficiency of C4b-binding protein has been identified.[489] The proband presented with angioedema, cutaneous vasculitis, and arthritis. C4b-binding protein was present at 15 percent of normal levels and appeared to lead to uncontrolled activation of the classical pathway and increased C3 consumption.

Molecular Genetic Defect. The molecular genetic cause of C4b-binding protein deficiency is not known.

Decay Accelerating Factor (MIM 125240)

Molecular Biology. DAF is composed of 4 SCR units and a 70-amino-acid tail. It is encoded by a 35-kDa gene that maps to the RCA region on chromosome 1.[124] Expression of DAF is limited to blood components and vascular endothelial cells.[490] There is also high-level expression on the cornea. DAF is attached to the cell membrane by a glycosyl-phosphatidylinositol (GPI) anchor. The GPI anchor is a posttranslational modification. The GPI anchor associates with SRC family protein tyrosine kinases and may transduce membrane signals.[491]

Pathophysiology and Clinical Expression. Genetically determined deficiency of DAF has been associated with the Inab phenotype.[492,493] Individuals who possess the Inab phenotype lack all blood group antigens of the Cromer complex, antigens that reside on DAF. Acquired DAF deficiency is a manifestation of paroxysmal nocturnal hemoglobinuria in which a series of GPI-anchored proteins are lost from the cell surface, leaving cells abnormally sensitive to lysis by complement. In contrast, genetically determined DAF deficiency and the resulting Inab phenotype are not associated with hemolysis. DAF is completely lacking in Inab patients, and despite increased deposition of C3, hemolysis is not observed.[492] Two patients with the Inab phenotype have had severe protein-losing enteropathies.[493]

Molecular Genetic Defect. Four kindreds with DAF deficiency have been reported. A patient from one kindred with no detectable DAF had a single-nucleotide substitution.[494] Another patient with undetectable DAF was homozygous for a single-nucleotide substitution that resulted in activation of a cryptic splice site in exon 2 followed by a premature stop codon.[495] Members of two other kindreds had some detectable DAF on the surface of their erythrocytes. In one of these two kindreds, a point mutation was identified that altered antigenicity and resulted in use of a cryptic splice site that then altered the reading frame.[494]

Factor I Deficiency (MIM 217030)

Molecular Biology. Factor I is a heterodimer composed of disulfide-linked polypeptides. One polypeptide has homology with complement components C6 and C7 and the low-density lipoprotein receptor. The other chain possesses serine protease activity and cleaves C3b to produce iC3b, a cleavage product that cannot function in the C3-cleaving enzyme of the alternative pathway. The gene for factor I is located on chromosome 4q.[496] Factor I is synthesized in human hepatoma cells as a single-chain precursor, pro-I, and undergoes posttranslational proteolysis to generate the mature protein.[497] It is also synthesized in human mononuclear phagocytes and endothelial cells.[498]

Pathophysiology and Clinical Expression. Genetically determined factor I deficiency has been described in only a few families.[5,6,499] It is inherited as an autosomal recessive trait. Patients with factor I deficiency have an uncontrolled activation of C3 via the alternative pathway.[500–503] As mentioned earlier, there is continuous low-grade generation of the alternative pathway C3-cleaving enzyme, C3bBb, that is inhibited by factors H and I. In the absence of factor I, there is no control imposed on the formation and expression of the alternative pathway C3-convertase, and as a result, there is the continued activation and cleavage of C3.[504] Patients with factor I deficiency therefore have a secondary consumption of native C3 with markedly reduced levels of antigenic C3 in their sera, most of which is not in the form of native C3 but rather in the form of the cleavage product, C3b.[500] Serum levels of other components of the alternative pathway, factor B, factor H, and properdin, are also reduced, reflecting continuing activation of the alternative pathway.[503] As expected, those serum activities which depend on C3, either directly or indirectly, such as bactericidal activity, opsonic activity, and chemotactic activity, are reduced in patients with factor I deficiency.[500] Infusion of purified factor I corrects the defect by reestablishing control of the alternative pathway, stopping the activation and consumption of native C3 and thus restoring serum hemolytic and opsonic activities to normal.[503]

The most common clinical expression of factor I deficiency is an increased susceptibility to infection.[5,6,499,500,505–508] As with primary C3 deficiency, infections have included both localized infections on mucosal surfaces and systemic infections. The organisms most commonly responsible for these infections have been encapsulated pyogenic bacteria, such as the streptococcus, pneumococcus, meningococcus, and *H. influenzae*, organisms for which C3 is an important opsonic ligand. In addition to problems with infection, some patients have had elevated levels of circulating immune complexes.[506,507] There have as yet been no reports of patients with factor I deficiency developing chronic renal disease, as has been the case with C3 deficiency. However, there has been one report of a transient illness resembling serum sickness and characterized by fever, rash, arthralgia, hematuria, and proteinuria.[506]

Molecular Genetic Defect. The molecular genetic basis for factor I deficiency has been identified in four patients and found to be diverse.[509,510] In one patient, mutation of a histidine at position 400 to a leucine suggests that this amino acid may be critical to its function.

Factor H Deficiency (MIM 134370)

Molecular Biology. Factor H is a 150-kDa single-chain glycoprotein that regulates the activity of the alternative pathway. It is composed of 20 homologous repeating units (SCRs) that are also found in C4bp, DAF, MCP, CR1, and CR2.[125] The factor H gene maps to the RCA region of chromosome 1. Additional factor H-related cDNAs and proteins have been characterized. A total of four messages are produced in human liver. The 4.4-kb message encodes the 150-kDa classic factor H protein. A 1.8-kb factor H message is a splice variant that also exhibits factor H activity.[511] Two other highly homologous genes encode factor H-related proteins that do not exhibit cofactor activity. They consist of five SCR units, three of which are highly homologous to those found in factor H. All four messages are constitutively expressed in liver. The two factor H-derived messages are also found in fibroblasts, endothelial cells, and monocytes. The short factor H-related species are found only in liver.[511] Like many other complement components, there are several polymorphic variants.[512]

Pathophysiology and Clinical Expression. Genetically determined factor H deficiency has been described in only a few families.[5,6,513–517] The deficiency appears to be inherited as an autosomal recessive trait. In two families, the parents were first cousins and had approximately half the normal level of factor H as did some of the other family members.[515,516] In two of the cases, factor H has been undetectable,[514,517] whereas in two other families factor H has been detectable but reduced to less than 10 percent of normal.[514,515] The levels of the alternative pathway components factor B and properdin are also reduced, but not to the same degree as factor H. Similarly, serum levels of C3 are also reduced, and the majority of the C3 that is present is in the form of an activation/cleavage product. Presumably, the markedly reduced level of factor H leads to continuous activation of the alternative pathway and the resulting depletion of C3 and other proteins of the alternative pathway.

The clinical manifestations of factor H deficiency have included glomerulonephritis, hemolytic-uremic syndrome, systemic lupus erythematosus, and systemic meningococcal infections.[5,6,513] In addition, some individuals with factor H deficiency have been ascertained because of family studies and have been asymptomatic.[516]

Molecular Genetic Defect. One patient with factor H deficiency was found to be heterozygous for two missense mutations affecting conserved cysteine residues in SCR modules. This resulted in an inability to secrete the full-length protein.[518] In another patient, PCR amplification of factor H cDNA suggested that a truncated mRNA was produced. However, a specific mutation was not identified.[519]

Animal Model. A porcine strain with factor H deficiency spontaneously develops membranoproliferative renal disease.[520] Deposition of complement components occurs along the capillary wall of the renal glomeruli, as is seen in the renal disease associated with factor H deficiency.

Properdin Deficiency (MIM 312060)

Molecular Biology. The gene for properdin has been mapped to Xp11.23-21.1,[521] and the complete structure of properdin has been elucidated.[522,523] The message for properdin is 1.5 kb long and encodes a protein that appears in electron microscopy as a bent rod. The protein is comprised of six thrombospondin repeat motifs, which are also common to many of the terminal complement components. Properdin is synthesized by monocytes, activated macrophages, T cells, and hepatocytes and is a component of secondary granules of neutrophils.[523] Some studies indicate that liver and lung also may synthesize properdin. Properdin circulates as polydispersed aggregates of 56-kDa polypeptide subunits.

Pathophysiology and Clinical Expression. Properdin deficiency is the only complement deficiency that is inherited as an X-linked recessive trait.[5,6] In some families, affected males have markedly reduced levels of properdin (<1 percent of normal),[524,525] whereas in others, properdin is present but in reduced amounts (10 percent of normal).[526,527] Finally, a third form of properdin deficiency has been described in which properdin is present in normal concentrations but is dysfunctional.[528] The sera of patients with properdin deficiency are unable to activate C3 via the alternative pathway, and serum bactericidal activity for some strains of meningococcci is reduced.[524–530]

The most common clinical manifestation of properdin deficiency has been fulminant meningococcemia and meningococcal meningitis, emphasizing the importance of the alternative pathway in host defense against meningococci.[5,6] These patients appear to have a particularly high mortality rate (75 percent) compared with complement-sufficient patients or patients with deficiencies of terminal complement components.[531] Systemic lupus erythematosus and discoid lupus also have been described in isolated patients.[5,6,529]

Molecular Genetic Defect. Mutations have been identified in seven properdin-deficient patients. Mutations resulting in premature stop codons have been identified in three patients with undetectable properdin.[532] In kindreds in whom low levels of properdin can be detected, diverse nonsense mutations have been found that appear to affect the formation of higher order forms.[532] One kindred with normal levels of dysfunctional properdin had a single-base-pair mutation in exon 9 resulting in a substitution of aspartic acid for tyrosine rendering the molecule unable to interact with C3b.[533] Use of direct mutation detection for carrier testing and prenatal diagnosis has been difficult due to the high GC content of the gene. Microsatellite haplotyping has been used in some kindreds for carrier detection.[534]

CD59 Deficiency (MIM 107271)

Molecular Biology. CD59 (HRF 20, MIRL) is a 20-kDa GPI-anchored glycoprotein that maps to chromosome 11p13-14.[535] CD59 is widely expressed on erythrocytes, leukocytes, and endothelial cells, where it functions to prevent intravascular complement mediated lysis.[536] CD59 is a member of the Ly-6 gene family that includes the protooncogenes *Sis* and *Myc*.[535]

Pathophysiology and Clinical Expression. A single patient with CD59 deficiency, the product of a consanguineous marriage, has been described.[537] He presented with hemolytic anemia as a child and had positive HAM and sucrose tests for paroxysmal nocturnal hemoglobinuria. He also suffered recurrent cerebral infarctions. CD59 was consistently undetectable on the surface of his erythrocytes and fibroblasts. Studies of four GPI-anchored proteins that are typically lost in paroxysmal nocturnal hemoglobinuria revealed normal levels of all, except for CD59. His mother and father had half-normal levels of expression, suggesting autosomal recessive inheritance.[537]

Molecular Genetic Defect. The CD59-deficient patient was homozygous for a CD59 allele bearing two mutations in codons 16 and 96.[538]

Mannose-Binding Protein Deficiency (MIM 154545)

Molecular Biology. Mannose-binding protein (MBP) can activate C3 indirectly, via activation of the classical pathway, and directly. The structure of MBP is similar to C1q, with a collagen-like region stabilized by disulfide bonds and a calcium-dependent carbohydrate-recognition domain.[539]

Pathophysiology and Clinical Expression. MBP deficiency is associated with an increased frequency of bacterial infections in both adults and children.[540,541] It also has been found with increased frequency in patients with systemic lupus erythematosus and rheumatoid arthritis.[542–545]

Molecular Genetic Defects. There are five polymorphisms in MBP that affect serum concentrations. Three of these occur in the collagen-like region of the molecule and destabilize the higher-order forms.[546] Two others occur in the promoter region of the gene and result in decreased transcription. The gene frequencies of these polymorphisms are fairly high. The codon 54Asp polymorphism has a gene frequency of 0.19 in England, and the codon 57Glu polymorphism has a gene frequency of 0.29 in Gambians. The two polymorphic promoter variants exist as three haplotypes present in varying proportions in different populations. Due to the high frequency of these polymorphisms in some populations, it is not uncommon to have homozygous deficient individuals.[547] Based on studies that correlated serum levels of MBP with the genotype of the donor, it has been found that the structural variants have a dominant-negative effect, whereas the promoter variants are autosomal codominant.

REFERENCES

1. Mayer MM: Complement: Historical perspectives and current issues. *Complement* **1**:2, 1984.
2. Frank MM: The complement system in host defense and inflammation. *Rev Infect Dis* **1**:483, 1979.
3. Johnston RB Jr: The complement system in host defense and inflammation: The cutting edges of a double edged sword. *Pediatr Infect Dis J* **12**:933, 1993.
4. Silverstein AM: Essential hypocomplementemia: Report of a case. *Blood* **16**:1338, 1960.
5. Ross SC, Densen P: Complement deficiency states and infection: Epidemiology, pathogenesis and consequences of neisserial and other infections in an immune deficiency. *Medicine* **63**:243, 1984.
6. Figueroa JE, Densen P: Infectious diseases associated with complement deficiencies. *Clin Microb Rev* **4**:359, 1991.
7. Lokki ML, Colten HR: Genetic deficiences of complement. *Ann Med* **27**:451, 1995.
8. Colten HR, Rosen FS: Complement deficiencies. *Annu Rev Immunol* **10**:809, 1992.
9. Porter RR, Reid KBM: The biochemistry of complement. *Nature* **275**:699, 1978.
10. Lepow IH, Naff GB, Todd EW, Pensky J, Hinz CF: Chromatographic resolution of the first component of complement into three activities. *J Exp Med* **117**:983, 1963.
11. Gigli I, Porter RR, Sim RB: The unactivated form of the first component of human complement, C1. *Biochem J* **157**:541, 1976.
12. Muller-Eberhard HJ, Kunkel H: Isolation of a thermolabile serum protein which precipitates gammaglobulin aggregates and participates in immune hemolysis. *Proc Soc Exp Biol Med* **106**:291, 1961.
13. Ziccardi RJ, Cooper NR: Activation of C1r by proteolytic cleavage. *J Immunol* **116**:504, 1976.
14. Sakai K, Stroud RM: Purification, molecular properties and activation of C1 proesterase, C1. *J Immunol* **110**:1010, 1973.
15. Schreiber RD, Muller-Eberhard HJ: Fourth component of human complement: Description of a three polypeptide chain structure. *J Exp Med* **140**:1324, 1974.
16. Law SK, Dodds AW: The internal thioester and the covalent binding properties of the complement proteins C3 and C4. *Protein Sci* **6**:263, 1997.
17. Nagasawa S, Stroud RM: Cleavage of C2 by C1s into antigenically distinct fragments, C2a and C2b: Demonstration of binding of C2a to C4b. *Proc Natl Acad Sci USA* **74**:2998, 1977.

18. Shin HS, Mayer MM: The third component of the guinea pig complement system: II. Kinetic study of the reaction of EAC'4,2a with guinea pig C3. *Biochemistry* **7**:2997, 1968.
19. Liszewski MK, Farries TC, Lublin DM, Rooney IA, Atkinson JP: Control of the complement system. *Adv Immunol* **61**:201, 1996.
20. Pensky J, Levy LR, Lepow IH: Partial purification of a serum inhibitor of C'1-esterase. *J Biol Chem* **236**:1674, 1961.
21. Harpel PC, Cooper NR: Studies on human plasma C1 inactivator-enzyme interactions: I. Mechanisms of interactions with C1s, plasmin, and trypsin. *J Clin Invest* **55**:593, 1975.
22. Gigli I, Fujita T, Nussenzweig V: Modulation of the classical pathway C3 convertase by the plasma proteins, C4-binding protein and C3b inactivator. *Proc Natl Acad Sci USA* **76**:6596, 1979.
23. Nagasawa S, Ichibara C, Stroud RM: Cleavage of C4b by C3b inactivator: Production of a nicked form of C4b, C4b', as an intermediate cleavage product of C4b by C3b inactivator. *J Immunol* **125**:578, 1980.
24. Nicholson-Weller A, Burge J, Fearon DT, Weller PF, Austen KF: Isolation of a human erythrocytes membrane glycoprotein with decay-accelerating activity for C3 convertases of the complement system. *J Immunol* **129**:184, 1982.
25. Hirsch RL, Winkelstein, JA, Griffin DE: The role of complement in viral infections: III. Activation of the classical and alternative pathways by Sindbis virus. *J Immunol* **124**:2507, 1980.
26. Bredt W, Wellek B, Brunner H, Loos M: Interactions between *Mycoplasma pneumoniae* and the first component of complement. *Infect Immun* **15**:7, 1977.
27. Loos M, Wellek B, Thesen R, Opferkuch W: Antibody-independent interaction of the first component of complement with gram-negative bacteria. *Infect Immun* **22**:5, 1978.
28. Eads ME, Levy NJ, Kasper DL, Baker CJ, Nicholson-Weller A: Antibody-independent activation of C1 by type 1a group B streptococci. *J Infect Dis* **146**:665, 1982.
29. Winkelstein JA: Complement and natural immunity. *Clin Immunol Allergy* **3**:421, 1983.
30. Fearon DT: Activation of the alternative complement pathway. *CRC Crit Rev Immunol* **1**:1, 1979.
31. Tack BF, Harrison RA, Janotova J, Thomas ML, Prahl JW: Evidence for presence of an internal thiolester bond in third component of human complement. *Proc Natl Acad Sci USA* **77**:5764, 1980.
32. Pangburn MK, Muller-Eberhard HJ: Relation of a putative thioester bond in C3 to activation of the alternative pathway and the binding of C3b to biological targets of complement. *J Exp Med* **152**:1102, 1980.
33. Fearon DT, Austen KF: Initiation of C3 cleavage in the alternative complement pathway. *J Immunol* **115**:1357, 1975.
34. Fearon DT, Austen KF: Properdin: Binding to C3b and stabilization of the C3b-dependent C3 convertase. *J Exp Med* **142**:856, 1975.
35. Kazatchkine MD, Fearon DT, Austen KF: Human alternative complement pathway: Membrane-associated sialic acid regulates the competition between B and B1H for cell-bound C3b. *J Immunol* **122**:75, 1979.
36. Weiler JM, Daha MR, Austen KF, Fearon DT: Control of the amplification convertase of complement by the plasma protein, B1H. *Proc Natl Acad Sci USA* **73**:3268, 1976.
37. Whaley K, Ruddy S: Modulation of the alternative complement pathway by B1H globulin. *J Exp Med* **144**:1147, 1976.
38. Lublin DN, Atkinson JP: Decay-accelerating factor and membrane cofactor protein. *Curr Top Microb Immunol* **153**:124, 1989.
39. Pillemer L, Blum L, Lepow IH, Ross OA, Todd EW, Wardlaw AC: The properdin system and immunity: I. Demonstration and isolation of a new serum protein, properdin, and its role in immune phenomena. *Science* **120**:279, 1954.
40. Platts-Mills TAE, Ishizakah K: Activation of the alternate pathway of human complement by rabbit cells. *J Immunol* **113**:348, 1974.
41. Winkelstein JA, Shin HS, Wood WB Jr: Heat labile opsonins to pneumococcus: III. Participation of immunoglobulin and of the alternative pathway of C3 activation. *J Immunol* **108**:1681, 1972.
42. Fearon DT, Austen KF: Activation of the alternative complement pathway due to resistance of zymosan-bound amplification convertase to endogenous regulatory mechanisms. *Proc Natl Acad Sci USA* **74**:1683, 1977.
43. Fearon DT: Regulation by membrane sialic acid of B1H-dependent decay: Dissociation of amplication C3 convertase of the alternative pathway. *Proc Natl Acad Sci USA* **75**:1971, 1978.
44. Winkelstein JA, Shin HS: The role of immunoglobulin in the interaction of pneumococci and the properdin pathway: Evidence for its specificity and lack of requirement for the Fc portion of the molecule. *J Immunol* **112**:1635, 1974.
45. Edwards MS, Nicholson-Weller A, Baker CJ, Kasper DL: The role of specific antibody in alternative complement pathway mediated opsonophagocytosis of type III, group B streptococcus. *J Exp Med* **151**:1275, 1980.
46. Perrin LH, Joseph BS, Cooper NR, Oldstone MBA: Mechanism of injury of virus-infected cells by antiviral antibody and complement: Participation of IgG, F(ab')2 and the alternative pathway. *J Exp Med* **143**:1027, 1976.
47. Moore FD Jr, Fearon DT, Austen KF: IgG on mouse erythrocytes augments activation of the human alternative complement pathway by enhancing deposition of C3b. *J Immunol* **126**:1805, 1981.
48. Nicholson-Weller A, Daha MR, Austen KF: Different functions for specific guinea pig IgG1 and IgG2 in the lysis of sheep erythrocytes by C4-deficient guinea pig serum. *J Immunol* **126**:1800, 1981.
49. Turner MW: Mannose-binding lectin: The pluripotent molecule of the innate immune system. *Immunol Today* **17**:532, 1996.
50. Ikeda K, Sannoh T, Kawasaki IN, Kawasaki T, Yamashina I: Serum lectin with known structure activates complement through the classical pathway. *J Biol Chem* **262**:7451, 1987.
51. Van Emmerik LC, Kuijper EJ, Fijen CA, Dankert J, Thiel S: Binding of mannan-binding protein to various bacterial pathogens of meningitis. *Clin Exp Immunol* **97**:411, 1994.
52. Lu JH, Thiel S, Wiedemann H, Timpl R, Reid KB: Binding of the pentamer/hexamer forms of mannan-binding protein to zymosan activates the proenzyme C1r2C1s2 complex, of the classical pathway of complement, without involvement of C1q. *J Immunol* **144**:2287, 1990.
53. Ohta M, Okada M, Yamashina I, Kawasaki T: The mechanism of carbohydrate-mediated complement activation by the serum mannan-binding protein. *J Biol Chem* **265**:1980, 1990.
54. Takayama Y, Takada F, Takahashi A, Kawakami M: A 100-kDa protein in the C4-activating component of Ra-reactive factor is a new serine protease having module organization similar to C1r and C1s. *J Immunol* **152**:2308, 1994.
55. Schweinle JE, Ezekowitz RAB, Tenner AJ, Kuklman M, Joiner KA: Human mannose-binding protein activates the alternative pathway and enhances serum bactericidal activity on a mannose-rich isolate of *Salmonella*. *J Clin Invest* **84**:1821, 1989.
56. Suankratay C, Zhang XH, Lint TF, Gewurz H: Requirement for the alternative pathway as well as C4 and C2 in complement-dependent hemolysis via the lectin pathway. *J Immunol* **160**:3006, 1998.
57. Matsushita M, Fujita T: Cleavage of the third component of complement (C3) by mannose-binding protein-associated serine protease (MASP) with subsequent complement activation. *Immunobiology* **194**:443, 1995.
58. Fearon DT, Austen KF, Ruddy S: Formation of a hemolytically active cellular intermediate by the interaction between properdin factors B and D and the activated third component of complement. *J Exp Med* **138**:1305, 1973.
59. Hostetter MK, Gordon DL: Biochemistry of C3 and related thiolester proteins in infection and inflammation. *Rev Infect Dis* **9**:97, 1987.
60. Shin HS, Pickering RJ, Mayer MM: The fifth component of the guinea pig complement system: II. Mechanisms of SAC1,4,2,3,5b formation and C5 consumption by EAC1,4,2,3. *J Immunol* **106**:473, 1971.
61. Daha MR, Fearon DT, Austen KF: C3 requirements for formation of alternative pathway C5 convertase. *J Immunol* **117**:630, 1976.
62. Esser AF: The membrane attack complex of complement: Assembly, structure and cytotoxic activity. *Toxicology* **87**:229, 1994.
63. Thompson RA, Lachman PJ: Reactive lysis: The complement mediated lysis of unsensitized cells: II. The characterization of activated reactor as C5b and the participation of C8 and C9. *J Exp Med* **131**:643, 1970.
64. Shin ML, Paznekas WA, Abromovitz AS, Mayer MM: On the mechanism of membrane damage by complement: Exposure of hydrophobic sites on activated complement proteins. *J Immunol* **119**:1358, 1977.
65. Hammer CH, Nicholson A, Mayer MM: On the mechanism of cytotysis by complement: Evidence on insertion of C5b and C7 subunits of the C5b,6,7 complex into phospholipid bilayers of erythrocyte membranes. *Proc Natl Acad Sci USA* **72**:5076, 1975.
66. Hu VW, Esser SF, Podack ER, Wisnieshis BJ: The membrane attack mechanism of complement: Photolabelling reveals insertion of terminal proteins into target membranes. *J Immunol* **27**:380, 1981.
67. Stolfi RL: Immune lytic transformation: A state of irreversible damage generated as a result of the reaction of the eighth component in the guinea pig complement system. *J Immunol* **100**:46, 1968.

68. Tschopp J, Podack ER, Muller-Eberhard HJ: The membrane attack complex of complement: C5b-8 complex as accelerator of C9 polymerization. *J Immunol* **134**:495, 1985.
69. Lachman PJ: The control of homologous lysis. *Immunol Today* **12**:312, 1991.
70. Fearon DT, Wong WW: Complement ligand-receptor interactions that mediate biological responses. *Annu Rev Immunol* **1**:243, 1983.
71. Wetzel RA: Structure, function and cellular expression of complement anaphylatoxin receptors. *Curr Opin Immunol* **7**:48, 1995.
72. Hugli TE: The structural basis for anaphylatoxin and chemotactic functions of C3a, C4a and C5a. *CRC Crit Rev Immunol* **2**:321, 1981.
73. Fearon DT: Identification of the membrane glycoprotein that is the C3b receptor of the human erythrocyte, polymorphonuclear leukocyte, B lymphocyte and monocyte. *J Exp Med* **152**:20, 1980.
74. Ehlenberger AG, Nussenzweig V: The role of membrane receptors for C3b and C3d in phagocytosis. *J Exp Med* **145**:357, 1977.
75. Cornacoff JB, Hebert LA, Smead WL, van Aman ME, Birmingham DJ, Waxman FJ: Primate erythrocyte-immune complex-clearing mechanism. *J Clin Invest* **71**:236, 1983.
76. Fearon DT: Regulation of the amplification C3 convertase of human complement by an inhibitory protein isolated from human erythrocyte membranes. *Proc Natl Acad Sci USA* **76**:5867, 1979.
77. Iida K, Nussenzweig V: Complement receptor is an inhibitor of the complement cascade. *J Exp Med* **153**:1138, 1981.
78. Carroll MC, Fischer MB: Complement and the immune response. *Curr Opin Immunol* **9**:64, 1997.
79. Cochrane CG, Muller-Eberhard HJ: The derivation of two distinct anaphylatoxins from the third and fifth components of human complement. *J Exp Med* **127**:371, 1968.
80. Vogt W: Anaphylatoxins: Possible roles in diseases. *Complement* **3**:177, 1986.
81. Gorski J, Hugli TE, Muller-Eberhard HJ: C4a: The third anaphylatoxin of the human complement system. *Proc Natl Acad Sci USA* **76**:5299, 1979.
82. Synderman R, Goetzl EJ: Molecular and cellular mechanisms of leukocyte chemotaxins. *Science* **213**:830, 1981.
83. Perez HD, Goldstein IM, Chernoff D, Webster RO, Henson PM: Chemotactic activity of C5a des arg: Evidence of a requirement for an anionic peptide "helper factor" and inhibition by a cationic protein in serum from patients with systemic lupus erythematosis. *Mol Immunol* **17**:163, 1980.
84. Hoover RL, Briggs RT, Karnovsky MJ: The adhesive interaction between polymorphonuclear leukocytes and endothelial cells in vitro. *Cell* **14**:423, 1978.
85. Snyderman R, Phillips JK, Mergenhagen SE: Biological activity of complement in vivo: Role of C5 in the accumulation of polymorphonuclear leukocytes in inflammatory exudates. *J Exp Med* **134**:1131, 1971.
86. Larsen GL, Mitchell BC, Henson PM: The pulmonary response of C5 sufficient and deficient mice to immune complexes. *Am Rev Respir Dis* **123**:434, 1981.
87. Hopken UE, Lu B, Gerard NP, Gerard C: The C5a chemoattractant receptor mediates mucosal defense to infection. *Nature* **383**:86, 1996.
88. Bozic CR, Lu B, Hopken UE, Gerard C, Gerard NP: Neurogenic amplification of immune complex inflammation. *Science* **273**:1722, 1996.
89. Floreani A, Heires AJ, Welniak LA, Miller-Landholm A, Clark-Pierce L, Rennard SI, Morgan EL, Sanderson SD: Expression of receptors for C5a anaphylotoxin (CD88) on human bronchial epithelial cells: Enhancement of C5a-mediated release of IL-8 upon exposure to cigarette smoke. *J Immunol* **160**:5073, 1998.
90. Johnston RB Jr, Klemperer MR, Alper CA, Rosen FS: The enhancement of bacterial phagocytosis by serum: The role of complement components and two co-factors. *J Exp Med* **129**:1275, 1969.
91. Mantovani B, Rabinovitch M, Nussenzweig V: Phagocytosis of immune complexes by macrophages: Different roles of the macrophage receptor sites for complement (C3) and for immunoglobulin (IgG). *J Exp Med* **135**:780, 1972.
92. Bianco C, Griffin FM Jr, Silverstein SC: Studies on the macrophage complement receptor: Alteration of receptor function upon macrophage activation. *J Exp Med* **141**:1278, 1975.
93. Winkelstein JA, Smith MR, Shin HS: The role of C3 as an opsonin in the early stages of infection. *Proc Soc Exp Biol Med* **149**:397, 1975.
94. Hosea SW, Brown EJ, Frank MM: The critical role of complement in experimental pneumococcal sepsis. *J Infect Dis* **142**:903, 1980.
95. Muschel LH, Fong JSC: Serum bactericidal activity and complement, in Day NK, Good RA (eds): *Comprehensive Immunology*. New York, Plenum Press, 1977, p 137.
96. Haniman GR, Esser AF, Podack ER, Wunderlich AC, Braude AI, Lint TF, Curd JG: The role of C9 in complement-mediated killing of *Neisseria*. *J Immunol* **127**:2386, 1981.
97. Saulsbury FT, Winkelstein JA: Activation of the alternative complement pathway by L-phase variants of gram-positive bacteria. *Infect Immun* **23**:711, 1979.
98. Wright SD, Levine RP: How complement kills *E. coli*: I. Location of the lethal lesion. *J Immunol* **127**:1146, 1981.
99. Schifferli JA, Ng YC, Peters DK: The role of complement and its receptor in the elimination of immune complexes. *New Engl J Med* **315**:488, 1986.
100. van Snick JL, Masson PL: The effect of complement on the ingestion of soluble antigen-antibody complexes and IgM aggregates by mouse peritoneal macrophages. *J Exp Med* **148**:903, 1978.
101. Schifferli JA, Bartolotti SR, Peters DK: Inhibition of immune precipitation by complement. *Clin Exp Immunol* **42**:387, 1980.
102. Miller GW, Nussenzweig V: A new complement function: Solubilization of antigen-antibody aggregates. *Proc Natl Acad Sci USA* **72**:418, 1975.
103. Bartolotti SR, Peters DK: Delayed removal of renal-bound antigen in decomplemented rabbits with acute serum sickness. *Clin Exp Immunol* **32**:199, 1978.
104. Pepys MB: The role of complement in induction of antibody production in vivo. *J Exp Med* **140**:126, 1974.
105. Ochs HD, Wedgewood RJ, Frank MM, Heller SR, Hosea SW: The role of complement in the induction of antibody responses. *Clin Exp Immunol* **53**:208, 1983.
106. Bottger EC, Hoffmann T, Hadding V, Bitter-Suermann D: Influence of genetically inherited complement deficiencies on humoral immune response in guinea pigs. *J Immunol* **135**:4100, 1985.
107. O'Neil KM, Ochs HD, Heller SR, Cork LC, Winkelstein JA: Deficient humoral immunity in C3-deficient dogs. *J Immunol* **140**:1939, 1988.
108. Fischer MB, Ma M, Goerg S, Zhou X, Xia J, Finco O, Han S, Kelsoe G, Howard RG, Rothstein TL, Kremmer E, Rosen FS, Carroll MC: Regulation of the B cell response to T-dependent antigens by the classical pathway of complement. *J Immunol* **157**:549, 1996.
109. Ahearn JM, Fischer MB, Croix D, Goerg S, Ma M, Xia J, Zhou X, Rothstein TL, Carroll MC: Disruption of the CR2 locus results in a reduction in B-1a cells and in an impaired B cell response to T-dependent antigen. *Immunity* **4**:251, 1996.
110. Molina H, Holers VM, Li B, Fung Y, Mariathasan S, Goeller J, Strauss-Schoenberger J, Karr R, Chaplin D: Markedly impaired humoral immune response in mice deficient in complement receptor 1 and 2. *Proc Natl Acad Sci USA* **93**:3357, 1996.
111. Dempsey PW, Allison MED, Akkaraju S, Goodnow CC, Fearon DT: C3d of complement as a molecular adjuvant: Bridging innate and acquired immunity. *Science* **271**:348, 1996.
112. Jacquier M, Gabert F, Villiers M, Colomb M: Modulation of antigen processing and presentation by covalently linked complement C3b fragment. *Immunology* **84**:164, 1995.
113. Farries TC, Atkinson JP: Evolution of the complement system. *Immunol Today* **12**:295, 1991.
114. Carroll MC, Campbell RD, Bentley DR, Porter RR: A molecular map of the human major histocompatibility complex class III region linking complement genes C4, C2 and factor B. *Nature* **307**:237, 1984.
115. Wu L-C, Morley BJ, Campbell RD: Cell specific expression of the human complement protein factor B gene: Evidence for the role of two distinct 5′ flanking elements. *Cell* **48**:331, 1987.
116. Ishikawa N, Nonaka M, Wetsel RA, Colten HR: Murine complement C2 and factor B genomic and cDNA cloning reveals different mechanisms for multiple transcripts of C2 and B. *J Biol Chem* **265**:19040, 1990.
117. White PC, Grossberger D, Onufer BJ, Chaplin DD, New MI, Dupont B, Strominger JL: Two genes encoding 21-hydroxylase are located near the genes encoding the fourth component of complement in man. *Proc Natl Acad Sci USA* **82**:5111, 1985.
118. Olaisen B, Teisberg R, Jonassen R, Thorsby E, Gedde-Dahl T: Gene order and gene distance in the HLA regions studied by the haplotype method. *Am Hum Genet* **47**:285, 1983.
119. Whitehead AS, Colten HR, Chang CC, Demars R: Localization of MHC-linked complement genes between HLA-B and HLA-DR by using HLA mutant cell lines. *J Immunol* **134**:641, 1985.

120. Carroll MC, Cambell RD, Porter RR: Mapping of steroid 21-hydroxylase genes adjacent to complement component C4 genes in HLA, the major histocompatibility complex in man. *Proc Natl Acad Sci USA* **82**:521, 1985.
121. Chaplin DD, Woods DE, Whitehead AS, Goldberger G, Colten HR, Seidman JG: Molecular map of the murine S region. *Proc Natl Acad Sci USA* **80**:6947, 1985.
122. Trowsdale J, Ragoussis J, Campbell RD: Map of the human MHC. *Immunol Today* **12**:443, 1991.
123. Klickstein LB, Wong WW, Smith JA, Morton C, Fearon DT, Weis JH: Identification of long homologous repeats in human CR1. *Complement* **2**:44, 1985.
124. Lublin DM, Lemons RS, Lebeau MM, Holers VM, Tykocinski ML, Medof ME, Atkinson JP: The gene encoding decay-accelerating factor is located in the complement regulator locus on the long arm of chromosome 1. *J Exp Med* **165**:1731, 1987.
125. Rodriquez de Cordoba S, Lublin DM, Rubinstein P, Atkinson JP: Human genes for 3 complement components that regulate the activation of C3 are tightly linked. *J Exp Med* **161**:1189, 1985.
126. Kristensen T, Wetsel RA, Tack BF: Structural analysis of human complement protein H: Homology with C4b binding protein, beta-2-glycoprotein 1 and Ba fragment of B. *J Immunol* **136**:3407, 1986.
127. Weis JH, Morton CC, Bruns GAP, Weis JJ, Klickstein LB, Wong WW, Fearon DT: A complement receptor locus: Genes encoding C3b/C4b receptor and C3d/Epstein-Barr virus receptor map to 1q32. *J Immunol* **138**:312, 1987.
128. Campbell RD, Dunham I, Sargent CA: Molecular mapping of the HLA-linked complement genes and the RCA linkage group. *Exp Clin Immunogenet* **5**:81, 1988.
129. Bentley DR: Primary structure of human complement component C2: Homology to two unrelated protein families. *Biochem J* **239**:339, 1986.
130. Morley BJ, Campbell RD: Internal homologies of the Ba fragment from human complement component factor B, a class III MHC antigen. *EMBO J* **3**:153, 1984.
131. Reid KBM, Bentley DR, Campbell RD, Chung LP, Sim RB, Kristensen T, Tack BF: Complement system proteins which interact with C3b or C4b: A super family of structurally related proteins. *Immunol Today* **7**:230, 1986.
132. Suttrup-Jenson L, Stepanik TM, Kristensen T, Conblad PB, Jones CM, Wierzbicki DM, Magnusson S, Domdey H, Wetsel R, Lundwall A, Tack BF, Fey GH: Common evolutionary origen of β_2-macroglobulin and complement components C3 and C4. *Proc Natl Acad Sci USA* **82**:9, 1985.
133. Rao AG, Howard OMZ, Ng S, Whitehead AS, Colten HR, Sodetz JM: cDNA and derived amino acid sequence of the alpha subunit of human complement protein C8: Evidence for the existence of separate alpha subunit mRNA. *Biochemistry* **26**:3556, 1987.
134. Howard OMZ, Rao AG, Sodetz JM: cDNA and derived amino acid sequence of the beta subunit of human complement protein C8: Identification of a close structural and ancestral relationship to the alpha subunit and C9. *Biochemistry* **26**:3565, 1987.
135. Stanley KK, Kocher HP, Luzio JP, Jackson P, Tschopp J: The sequence and topology of human complement component C9. *EMBO J* **4**:375, 1985.
136. Davis AE, Whitehead AS, Harrison RA, Dauphinais A, Bruns GAP, Cicardi M, Rosen FS: Human inhibitor of the first component of complement, C1: Characterization of cDNA clones and localization of the gene to chromosome 11. *Proc Natl Acad Sci USA* **83**:3161, 1986.
137. Morgan BP: *The Genetics of Complement in Complement: Clinical Aspects and Relevance to Disease*. San Diego, Academic Press, 1990.
138. Raum D, Donaldson VH, Rosen FS, Alper CA: Genetics of complement. *Curr Top Hematol* **3**:111, 1980.
139. Yu CY, Belt KT, Giles CM, Campbell RD, Porter RR: Structural basis of the polymorphism of human complement components C4A and C4B: Gene size, reactivity and antigenicity. *EMBO J* **5**:2873, 1986.
140. Daurinche C, Abbal M, Clerc A: Molecular characterization of human complement factor B subtypes. *Immunogenetics* **32**:309, 1990.
141. Awdeh ZL, Raum D, Yunis EJ, Alper CA: Extended HLA/complement allele haplotypes: Evidence for T/t-like complex in man. *Proc Natl Acad Sci USA* **80**:259, 1983.
142. Awdeh ZL, Alper CA, Eynon E, Alosco SM, Stein R, Yunis EJ: Unrelated individuals matched for MHC extended haplotypes and HLA-identical siblings show comparable responses in mixed lymphocyte culture. *Lancet* **2**:853, 1985.
143. Rittner C, Bertrams J: On the significance of C2, C4, and factor B polymorphisms in disease. *Hum Genet* **56**:235, 1981.
144. Alper CA, Raum D, Awdeh ZL, Peterson BH, Taylor PD, Starzl TE: Studies of hepatic synthesis in vivo of plasma proteins, including orosomucoid, transferrin, α-antitrypsin, C8 and factor B. *Clin Immunol Immunopathol* **16**:84, 1980.
145. Wolpl A, Robin-Winn M, Picklmayr R, Goldmann SF: Fourth component of complement (C4) polymorphism in human orthoptic liver transplantation. *Transplantation* **40**:154, 1985.
146. Alper CA, Johnson AM, Birtch AG, Moore FD: Human C3: Evidence for the liver as the primary site of synthesis. *Science* **163**:286, 1969.
147. Colten HR: Tissue specific reglation of inflammation. *J Appl Physiol* **72**:1, 1992.
148. Sundstrom SA, Komm BS, Xu Q, Boundy V, Lyttle CR: The stimulation of uterine complement component C3 gene expression by antiestrogens. *Endocrinology* **126**:1449, 1990.
149. Botto M, Lissandrini D, Sorio C, Walport MD: Biosynthesis and secretion of complement component C3 by activated human polymorphonuclear leukocytes. *J Immunol* **149**:1348, 1992.
150. Naughton MA, Botto M, Carter MJ, Alexander GJM, Goldman JM, Walport MJ: Extrahepatic secreted complement C3 contributes to circulating C3 levels in humans. *J Immunol* **167**:3051, 1996.
151. Brauer RB, Lam TT, Wang D, Horwitz LR, Hess AD, Klein AS, Sanfilippo F, Baldwin WM 3d: Extrahepatic synthesis of C6 in the rat is sufficient for complement-mediated hyperacute rejection of a guinea pig cardiac xenograft. *Transplantation* **59**:1073, 1995.
152. Fischer MB, Ma M, Hsu NC, Carroll MC: Local synthesis of C3 within the splenic lymphoid compartment can reconstitute the impaired immune response in C3 deficient mice. *J Immunol* **160**:2619, 1998.
153. Lint TF, Zeitz HJ, Gewurz H: Inherited deficiency of the ninth component of complement in man. *J Immunol* **125**:2252, 1980.
154. Polhill RB Jr, Pruitt KM, Johnston RB Jr: Kinetic assessment of alternative pathway activity in a hemolytic system: I. Experimental and kinetic analysis. *J Immunol* **121**:363, 1978.
155. Nelson RA Jr, Jensen J, Gigli I, Tamura N: Methods for the separation, purification and measurement of the nine components of the hemolytic complement in guinea pig serum. *Immunochemistry* **3**:111, 1966.
156. Rosen FS, Charache P, Pensky J, Donaldson V: Hereditary angioneurotic edema: Two genetic variants. *Science* **148**:957, 1965.
157. Thompson RA, Haeney R, Reid KBM, Davies JG, White RHR, Cameron AH: A genetic defect of the C1q subcomponent of complement associated with childhood (immune complex) nephritis. *New Engl J Med* **303**:22, 1980.
158. Tedesco F, Densen P, Villa MA, Petersen BH, Sirchia G: Two types of dysfunctional eighth component of complement (C8) molecules in C8 deficiency in man: Reconstitution of normal C8 from the mixture of two abnormal C8 molecules. *J Clin Invest* **71**:183, 1983.
159. Fu SM, Kunkel HG, Brusman HP, Allen FH Jr, Fotino M: Evidence for linkage between HL-A histocompatibility genes and those involved in the synthesis of the second component of complement. *J Exp Med* **140**:1108, 1975.
160. Ochs HD, Rosenfeld SI, Thomas ED, Giblett ER, Alper CA, Dupont B, Schaller JG, Gilliland BC, Hansen JA, Wedgewood RJ: Linkage between the gene (or genes) controlling synthesis of the fourth component of complement and the major histocompatibility complex. *New Engl J Med* **296**:470, 1977.
161. Glass D, Raum D, Gibson D, Stillman JS, Schur P: Inherited deficiency of the second component of complement: Rheumatic disease associations. *J Clin Invest* **58**:853, 1976.
162. Gibson DJ, Glass D, Carpenter CB, Schur PH: Hereditary C2 deficiency: Diagnosis and HLA gene complex associations. *J Immunol* **116**:1065, 1976.
163. Johnson CA, Densen P, Hurford R, Colten HR, Wetsel RA: Type I human complement C2 deficiency: A 28 basepair gene deletion causes skipping of exon 6 during RNA splicing. *J Biol Chem* **267**:9347, 1992.
164. Devoe IW: The meningococcus and mechanisms of pathogenicity. *Microbiol Rev* **162**:46, 1982.
165. Hummel DS, Mocca LF, Frasch CE, Winkelstein JA, Jean-Baptiste HJJ, Canas JA, Leggiardro RJ: Meningitis caused by a non-encapsulated strain of *Neisseria meningitidis* in twin infants with a C6 deficiency. *J Infect Dis* **155**:815, 1987.
166. Kemp AS, Vernon J, Muller-Eberhard HJ, Bau DCK: Complement C8 deficiency with recurrent meningococcemia. *Aust Pediatr J* **21**:169, 1985.
167. Platonov AE, Beloborodov VB, Vershinia IV: Meningococcal disease in patients with late complement component deficiency: Studies in the U.S.S.R. *Medicine* **72**:374, 1993.

168. Kolble K, Reid KB: Genetic deficiencies of the complement system and association with disease: Early components. *Int Rev Immunol* **10**:17, 1993.
169. Provost TT, Arnett FC, Reichlin M: Homozygous C2 deficiency, lupus erythematosis, and anti-Ro (SSA) antibodies. *Arthritis Rheum* **26**:1279, 1983.
170. Meyer O, Hauptmann G, Tappeiner G, Ochs HD, Mascart-Lemone F: Genetic deficiency of C4, C2 or C1q and lupus syndromes: Association with anti-Ro (SS-A) antibodies. *Clin Exp Immunol* **62**:678, 1985.
171. Maddison PJ, Provost TT, Reichlin M: Serologic findings in patients with "ANA-negative" SLE. *Medicine* **60**:87, 1981.
172. Sontheimer RD, Stastny P, Maddison P, Reichlin M, Gilliam JN: Serologic and HLA associations in subacute cutaneous lupus erythematosis (SCLE): A clinical subset of lupus erythematosis. *Ann Intern Med* **97**:664, 1982.
173. Welch TR, Beischel LS, Choi E, Balakrishnan K, Bishof NA: Uniparental isodisomy 6 associated with deficiency of the fourth component of complement. *Complement* **86**:675, 1990.
174. Fredrikson GN, Truedsson L, Sjoholm AG, Kjellman M: DNA analysis in a MHC heterozygous with complete C4 deficiency-homozygosity for C4 gene deletion and C4 pseudogene. *Exp Clin Immunogenet* **8**:29, 1991.
175. Bowness P, Davies KA, Norsworthy PJ, Athanassiou P, Taylor-Wiedeman J, Borysiewicz LK, Meyer PA, Walport MJ: Hereditary C1q deficiency and systemic lupus erythematosus. *Q J Med* **87**:455, 1990.
176. Welch TR, McAdams AJ, Beischel LS: Glomerulonephritis associated with complete deficiency of the fourth component of complement. *Arthritis Rheum* **38**:1333, 1995.
177. Hirsch RL: The complement system: Its importance in the host response to viral infection. *Microbiol Rev* **46**:71, 1982.
178. Hirsch RL, Griffin DE, Winkelstein JA: The effect of complement depletion on the course of sindbis virus infection in mice. *J Immunol* **121**:1276, 1978.
179. Hicks JT, Ennis FA, Kim E, Verbonitz M: The importance of an intact complement pathway in recovery from a primary viral infection: Influenza in decomplemented and in C5-deficient mice. *J Immunol* **121**:1437, 1978.
180. Alper CA: Complement and the MHC, in Dorf ME (ed.): *The Role of the Major Histocompatibility Complex in Immunology.* New York, Garland Press, 1981, p 173.
181. Colten HR: Genetics and synthesis of components of the complement system, in Ross GD (ed.): *Immunobiology of the Complement System.* New York, Academic Press, 1986, p 163.
182. Korb LC, Ahearn JM: C1q binds directly and specifically to surface blebs of apoptotic human keratinocytes: Complement deficiency and systemic lupus erythematosus revisited. *J Immunol* **158**:4525, 1997.
183. Schifferli JA, Steiger G, Hauptmann G, Spaeth PJ, Sjoholm AG: Formation of soluble immune complexes by complement in sera of patients with various hypocomplementemic states. *J Clin Invest* **76**:2127, 1985.
184. Czop J, Nussenzweig V: Studies on the mechanisms of solubilization of immune precipitates by serum. *J Exp Med* **143**:615, 1976.
185. Takahaski M, Takahaski M, Brade V, Nussenzweig V: Requirements for solubilization of immune aggregates by complement. *J Clin Invest* **62**:349, 1978.
186. Paccaud JP, Steiger G, Sjoholm AG, Spaeth PJ, Schifferli JA: Tetanus toxoid-anti-tetanus toxoid complexes: A potential model to study the complement transport system for immune complex in humans. *Clin Exp Immunol* **69**:468, 1987.
187. Davies KA, Erlendsson K, Beynon HL, Peters AM, Steinsson K, Valdimarsson H, Walport MJ: Splenic uptake of immune complexes in man is complement dependent. *J Immunol* **151**:3866, 1993.
188. Figueroa J, Andreoni J, Densen P: Complement deficiency states and meningococcal disease. *Immun Res* **12**:295, 1993.
189. Ellison RT, Kohler PH, Curd JG, Judson FN, Reller LB: Prevalance of congenital and acquired complement deficiency in patients with sporadic meningococcal disease. *New Engl J Med* **308**:913, 1983.
190. Merino J, Rodriquez-Valverde V, Lamelas JA: Prevalence of deficits of complement components in patients with recurrent meningoccoal infections. *J Infect Dis* **148**:331, 1983.
191. Leggiadro RJ, Winkelstein JA: Prevalence of complement deficiencies in children with systemic meningococcal infections. *Pediatr Infect Dis* **6**:75, 1987.
192. Rasmussen JM, Brandslund I, Teisner B, Isager H, Suehag S-E, Maarup L, Willumsen L, Ronne-Rasmussen JO, Permin H, Andesen PL, Skovmann O, Sorensen H: Screening for complement deficiencies in unselected patients with meningitis. *Clin Exp Immunol* **68**:437, 1987.
193. Nielsen HE, Koch C, Magnussen P, Lind I: Complement deficiencies in selected groups of patients with meningococcal disease. *Scand J Infect Dis* **21**:389, 1989.
194. Fijen CA, Juijper EJ, Hannema AJ, Sjoholm AG, van Putten JPM: Complement deficiencies in patients over ten years old with meningococcal disease due to uncommon serogroups. *Lancet* **2**:585, 1989.
195. Platinov AE, Kuijper EJ, Vershinina IV, Shipulin GA, Westerdaal N, Fijen CA, van de Winkel JG: Meningococcal disease and polymorphism of FcgRIIa (CD32) in late complement component-deficient individuals. *Clin Exp Immunol* **111**:97, 1998.
196. Mayatepek E, Grauer M, Hansch GM, Sonntag HG: Deafness, complement deficiencies and immunoglobulin status in patients with meningococcal diseases due to uncommon serogroups. *Pediatr Infect Dis J* **12**:808, 1993.
197. Rowe PC, McLean RH, Wood RA, Leggiardro RJ, Winkelstein JA: Association of homozygous C4B deficiency with bacterial meningitis. *J Infect Dis* **160**:448, 1989.
198. Ernst T, Spath PJ, Aebi C, Schaad UB, Bianchetti MG: Screening for complement deficiency in bacterial meningitis. *Acta Paediatr* **86**:1009, 1997.
199. Ekdahl K, Truedsson L, Sjoholm AG, Braconier JH: Complement analysis in adult patients with a history of bacteremic pneumococcal infections or recurrent pneumonia. *Scand J Infect Dis* **27**:111, 1995.
200. Hartung K, Fontana A, Klar M, Krippner H, Jorgens K, Lang B, Peter HH, Pichler WJ, Schendel D, Robin-Winn M: Association of class I, II, and III MHC gene products with systemic lupus erythematosis. *Rheumatol Int* **9**:13, 1989.
201. Petri M, Watson R, Winkelstein JA, McLean RH: Clinical expression of systemic lupus in patients with C4A deficiency. *Medicine* **72**:236, 1993.
202. Sullivan KE, Petri M, Bias WB, McLean R, Schmeckpepper B, Winkelstein JA: Prevalence of a mutation which causes C2 deficiency in a population of patients with SLE. *J Rheumatol* **21**:1128, 1994.
203. Ruddy S: Component deficiencies: The second component. *Progr Allergy* **39**:250, 1986.
204. O'Neill GJ, Yang SY, Dupont B: Two HLA-linked loci controlling the fourth component of human complement. *Proc Natl Acad Sci USA* **75**:5165, 1978.
205. Awdeh ZL, Alper CA: Inherited structural polymorphism of the fourth component of human complement. *Proc Natl Acad Sci USA* **77**:3576, 1978.
206. Hauptmann G, Tappeiner G, Schifferli JA: Inherited deficiency of the fourth complement. *Immunodef Rev* **1**:3, 1988.
207. Christiansen FT, Dawkins RL, Uko G, McClusky J, Kay PH, Zilko PJ: Complement allotyping in SLE: Association with C4A null. *Aust NZ J Med* **13**:483, 1983.
208. Fiedler AHL, Walport MJ, Batchelor JR, Rynes RI, Black CM, Dodi IA, Hughes GRV: Family study of the major histocompatibility complex in patients with systemic lupus erythematosis: Importance of null alleles of C4A and C4B in determining disease susceptibility. *Br Med J* **286**:425, 1983.
209. Howard PF, Hochberg MC, Bias B, Arnett FC, McLean RH: Relationship between C4 null genes, HLA-D region antigens, and genetic susceptibility to systemic lupus erythematosis in Caucasian and black Americans. *Am J Med* **81**:187, 1986.
210. Speirs C, Fielder AHL, Chapel H, Davey NJ, Batchelor JR: Complement system protein C4 and susceptibility to hydralazine-induced systemic lupus erythematosis. *Lancet* **1**:922, 1989.
211. Sellar GC, Blake DJ, Reid KBM: Characterization and organization of the genes encoding the A-, B- and C-chains of human complement subcomponent C1q. *Biochem J* **272**:481, 1991.
212. Loos M, Heinz HP: Component deficiencies: The first component: C1q, C1r, C1s. *Progr Allergy* **39**:212, 1986.
213. Berkel AI, Loos M, Sanal O, Ersoy F, Yegin O: Selective complete C1q deficiency: Report of two cases. *Immunol Lett* **2**:263, 1981.
214. Leyva-Cobian F, Moneo I, Mampaso R, Sanchez-Boyle M, Ecija JL: Familial C1q deficiency associated with renal and cutaneous disease. *Clin Exp Immunol* **44**:173, 1981.
215. Starsia Z, Buc M, Dluholucky S, Tomicova E, Zitnan D, Niks M, Toth J, Stefanovic J: Inherited deficiency of C1 component of complement in members of gypsy families associated with SLE-like symptoms. *Complement* **3**:28, 1986.
216. Chapuis RM, Hauptmann G, Grosshans E, Isliker H: Structural and functional studies in C1q deficiency. *J Immunol* **129**:1509, 1982.

217. Reid KBM, Thompson RA: Characterization of a non-functional form of C1q found in patients with a genetically linked deficiency of C1q activity. *Mol Immunol* **20**:117, 1983.
218. Hannema AJ, Kluin-Nelemans JC, Hack CE, Erenberg-Belmer AJM, Mallee C, van Helden HPT: SLE-like syndromes and functional deficiency of C1q in members of a large family. *Clin Exp Immunol* **55**:106, 1984.
219. Petry F, Hauptmann G, Goetz J, Grosshans E, Loos M: Molecular basis of a new type of C1q-deficiency associated with a non-functional low molecular weight (LMW) C1q: parallel and differences to other known genetic C1q defects. *Immunopharmacology* **38**:189, 1997.
220. Petry F, Berkel AI, Loos M: Multiple identification of a particular type of hereditary C1q deficiency in the Turkish population: Review of the cases and additional genetic functional analysis. *Hum Genet* **100**:51, 1997.
221. McAdam RA, Goundis D, Reid KBM: A homozygous point mutation results in a stop codon in the C1q B chain of a C1q deficient patient. *Immunogenetics* **27**:259, 1988.
222. Petry F, Le DT, Kirschfink M, Loos M: Non-sense and mis-sense mutations in the structural genes of complement component C1q A and C chains are linked with two different types of complete selective C1q deficiencies. *J Immunol* **155**:4734, 1995.
223. Slingsby JH, Norsworthy P, Peace G, Vaishnaw AK, Issler H, Morley BJ, Walport MJ: Homozygous hereditary C1q deficiency and systemic lupus erythematosus. *Arthritis Rheum* **39**:663, 1996.
224. Berkel AI, Petry F, Sanal O, Tinaztepe K, Ersoy F, Bakkaloglu A, Loos M: Development of systemic lupus erythematosus in a patient with selective complete C1q deficiency. *Eur J Pediatr* **156**:113, 1997.
225. Robson MG, Cook HT, Botto M, Pusey CD, Walport MJ, Davies KA: Accelerated nephrotoxic nephritis: Increased severity in C1q deficient mice. *Mol Immunol* **35**:343, 1998.
226. Tosi M, Duponchel C, Meo T, Julier C: Complement C1s sequence and linkage to C1r. *Biochemistry* **26**:8516, 1987.
227. Kusumoto H, Hirosawa S, Salier JP, Hagen FS, Kurachi K: Human genes for complement components C1r and C1s in a close tail-to-tail arrangement. *Proc Natl Acad Sci USA* **85**:7307, 1988.
228. Bensa JC, Reboul A, Colomb MG: Biosynthesis in vitro of complement subcomponents C1q, C1s and C1 inhibitor by resting and stimulated human monocytes. *Biochem J* **216**:385, 1983.
229. Loos M, Colomb M: C1, the first component of complement: Structure-function-relationship of C1q and collectins (MBP, SP-A, SP-D, conglutinin), C1-esterases (C1r and C1s), and C1-inhibitor in health and disease. *Behring Inst Mitt* **93**:1, 1993.
230. Lee SL, Wallace SL, Barone R, Blum L, Chase PH: Familial deficiency of two subunits of the first component of complement: C1r and C1s associated with a lupus erythematosus-like disease. *Arthritis Rheum* **21**:958, 1978.
231. Suzuki Y, Ogura Y, Otsubo O, Akagi K, Fujita T: Selective deficiency of C1s associated with a systemic lupus-like syndrome. *Arthritis Rheum* **35**:576, 1992.
232. Isenman DE, Young JR: The molecular basis for the difference in immune hemolysis activity of the Chido and Rogers isotypes of human complement components C4. *J Immunol* **132**:3019, 1984.
233. O'Neill GJ, Yang SY, Tegoli J, Berger R, Dupont B: Chido and Rogers blood groups are distinct antigenic components of human complement C4. *Nature* **273**:668, 1978.
234. Law SKA, Dodds AW, Porter RR: A comparison of the properties of two classes, C4A and C4B of the human complement components C4. *EMBO J* **3**:1819, 1984.
235. Carroll MC, Fathallah DM, Bergamaschini L, Alicot EM, Isenman DE: Substitution of a single amino acid (aspartic acid for histidine) converts the functional activity of C4B to C4A. *Proc Natl Acad Sci USA* **87**:6868, 1990.
236. Belt KT, Carroll MC, Porter RR: The structural basis of the multiple forms of human complement component C4. *Cell* **36**:907, 1984.
237. Belt KT, Yu CY, Carroll MC, Porter RR: Polymorphism of the human complement component C4. *Immunogenetics* **21**:173, 1985.
238. Carroll MC, Palsdottir A, Belt KT, Porter RR: Deletion of complement C4 and steroid 21-hydroxylase genes in the HLA class III region. *EMBO J* **4**:2547, 1985.
239. Prentice HL, Schneider PM, Strominger JL: C4B gene polymorphism detected in human cosmid clone. *Immunogenetics* **23**:274, 1986.
240. Roos MH, Mollenhauer E, Demant P, Rittner CH: A molecular basis for the two locus model of human complement component C4. *Nature* **298**:854, 1982.
241. Schneider PM, Carroll MC, Alper CA, Rittner C, Whitehead AS, Yunis EJ, Colten HR: Polymorphism of the human complement C4 and steroid 21-hydroxylase gene: Restriction fragment length polymorphisms revealing structural deletions, homoduplications and size variants. *J Clin Invest* **78**:650, 1986.
242. Whitehead AS, Woods DE, Fleishnick E, Chin JE, Katz AJ, Gerald PS, Alper CA, Colten HR: DNA polymorphism of the C4 gene: A new marker for analysis of the major histocompatibility complex. *New Engl J Med* **310**:88, 1984.
243. Hall RE, Colten HR: Cell-free synthesis of the fourth component of guinea pig complement (C4): Identification of a precursor of serum C4 (pro-C4). *Proc Natl Acad Sci USA* **74**:1707, 1977.
244. Roos MH, Atkinson JP, Shreffler DC: Molecular characterization of SS and Slp (C4) proteins of the mouse H-2 complex subunit composition, chain size, polymorphism and an intracellular (pro-Ss) precursor. *J Immunol* **121**:1106, 1978.
245. Ogata R, Shreffler D, Sepich D, Lilly S: cDNA clone spanning the alpha-gamma subunit junction in the precursor of the murine fourth complement component. *Proc Natl Acad Sci USA* **80**:5061, 1983.
246. Witte DP, Welch TR, Beischel LS: Detection and cellular localization of human C4 gene expression in the renal tubular epithelial cells and other extrahepatic epithelial sources. *Am J Pathol* **139**:717, 1991.
247. Goldberger G, Colten HR: Precursor complement protein (pro-C4) is converted in vitro by plasmin. *Nature* **286**:514, 1980.
248. Goldberger G, Abraham GN, Williams J, Colten HR: Amino terminal sequence analysis of pro-C4, the precursor of the fourth component of guinea pig complement. *J Biol Chem* **250**:7071, 1980.
249. Karp DR: Post-translational modification of the fourth component of complement: Sulfation of the alpha chain. *J Biol Chem* **258**:12745, 1983.
250. Karp DR: Post-translational modification of the fourth component of complement: Effect of tunicamycin and amino acid analogs on the formation of the internal thiolester and disulfide bonds. *J Biol Chem* **258**:14490, 1983.
251. Matthews WJ, Goldberger G, Marino JT, Einstein LP, Gash DJ, Colten HR: Complement proteins C2, C4 and factor B: Effect of glycosylation on their secretion and catabolism. *Biochem J* **204**:839, 1982.
252. Roos MH, Kornfeld S, Shreffler DC: Characterization of the oligosaccharide units of the fourth component of complement (Ss protein) synthesized by murine hepatocytes. *J Immunol* **124**:2860, 1980.
253. Chan AC, Mitchell KR, Munns TW, Karp DR, Atkinson JP: Identification and partial characterization of the secreted form of the fourth component of human complement: Evidence that it is different from the major plasma form. *Proc Natl Acad Sci USA* **80**:268, 1983.
254. Hortin G, Change AS, Fok KF, Strauss AW, Atkinson JP: Sequence analysis of the COOH terminus of the alpha chain of the fourth complement of human complement: Identification of the site of its extracellular cleavage. *J Biol Chem* **261**:9065, 1986.
255. Awdeh ZL, Ochs HD, Alper CA: Genetic analysis of C4 deficiency. *J Clin Invest* **67**:260, 1981.
256. Welch TR, Beischel L, Berry A, Forristal J, West CD: The effect of null C4 alleles on complement function. *Clin Immunol Immunopathol* **34**:316, 1985.
257. Clark RA, Klebanoff SJ: Role of the classical and alternative complement pathways in chemotaxis and opsonization: Studies of human serum deficient in C4. *J Immunol* **120**:1102, 1978.
258. Mascart-Lemone F, Hauptmann G, Goetz J, Duchateau J, Delespesse G, Vray B, Dab I: Genetic deficiency of C4 presenting with recurrent infections and a SLE-like disease. *Am J Med* **75**:295, 1983.
259. Lhotta K, Thoenes W, Glatzl J, Hintner H, Kronenberg F, Joannidis M, Konig P: Hereditary complete deficiency of the fourth component of complement: Effects on the kidney. *Clin Nephrol* **39**:117, 1993.
260. Budowle B, Roseman JM, Go RCP, Louv W, Barger BO, Acton RT: Phenotypes of the fourth component (C4) in black Americans from the southeastern United States. *J Immunogenet* **10**:199, 1983.
261. Petri M, Watson R, Winkelstein JA, McLean RH: Clinical expression of systemic lupus erythematosus in patients with C4A deficiency. *Medicine* **72**:236, 1993.
262. Welch TR, Brickman C, Bishof N, Maringhini S, Rutkowski M, Frenzke M, Kantor N: The phenotype of SLE associated with complete deficiency of complement isotype C4A. *J Clin Immunol* **18**:48, 1998.
263. McLean RH, Wyatt RJ, Julian BA: Complement pheontypes in glomerulonephritis: Increased frequency of homozygous null C4 phenotypes in IgA nephropathy and Henoch-Chonlein purpura. *Kidney Int* **26**:855, 1984.
264. Cahill J, Stevens FM, McCarthy CF: Complement C4 types in coeliacs and controls. *Irish J Med Sci* **160**:168, 1991.

265. Nielsen HE, Truedsson L, Donner M: Partial complement deficiencies in idiopathic thrombocytopenia of childhood. *Acta Paediatr* **83**:749, 1994.
266. Biskof NA, Welch TR, Beischel LS: C4B deficiency: A risk factor for bacteremia with encapsulated organisms. *J Infect Dis* **162**:248, 1990.
267. Kemp ME, Atkinson JP, Skanes VM, Levine RP, Chaplin DD: Deletion of C4A genes in patients with systemic lupus erythematosus. *Arthritis Rheum* **30**:1015, 1987.
268. Barba G, Rittner C, Schneider PM: Genetics basis of human complement C4A deficiency. *J Clin Invest* **91**:1681, 1993.
269. Braun L, Schneider PM, Giles CM, Bertrams J, Rittner C: Null alleles of human complement C4: Evidence for pseudogenes at the C4A locus and gene conversion at the C4B locus. *J Exp Med* **171**:129, 1990.
270. Ellman L, Green I, Frank M: Genetically controlled deficiency of the fourth component of complement in the guinea pig. *Science* **170**:74, 1970.
271. Frank MM, May J, Gaither T, Ellman L: In vitro studies of complement function in C4-deficient guinea pigs. *J Exp Med* **134**:176, 1971.
272. Ochs HD, Wedgwood RJ, Frank MM, Heller SR, Hosea SW: The role of complement in the induction of antibody responses. *Clin Exp Immunol* **53**:208, 1983.
273. Foltz CJ, Cork LC, Winkelstein JA: Absence of glomerulonephritis in guinea pigs deficient in the fourth component of complement. *Vet Pathol* **31**:201, 1994.
274. Reid R, Prodeus AP, Khan W, Hsu T, Rosen FS, Carroll MC: Endotoxin shock in antibody-deficient mice: Unraveling the role of natural antibody and complement in the clearance of immune complexes. *J Immunol* **159**:970, 1997.
275. Fischer MB, Prodeus A, Nicholson-Weller A, Ma M, Murrow J, Reid RR, Warren HB, Lage AL, Moore FD Jr, Rosen FS, Carroll MC: Increased susceptibility to endotoxin shock in complement C3- and C4-deficient mice is corrected by C1 inhibitor replacement. *J Immunol* **159**:976, 1997.
276. Ma M, Fischer MB, et al: Regulation of the B cell response to T-dependent antigens by classical pathway complement. *Mol Immunol* **33**:S78, 1996.
277. Perlmutter DH, Cole FS, Goldberger G, Colten HR: Distinct primary translation products from human liver mRNA give rise to secreted and cell-associated forms of complement C2. *J Biol Chem* **259**:10380, 1984.
278. Perlmutter DH, Colten HR, Grossberger D, Strominger J, Seidman JD, Chaplin DD: Expression of complement proteins C2 and factor B in transfected L cells. *J Clin Invest* **76**:1449, 1985.
279. Cross SJ, Edwards JM, Bentley DR, Cambell RD: DNA polymorphism of the C2 and factor B genes: Detection of a restriction fragment length polymorphism which subdivides haplotypes carrying the C2C and factor B F alleles. *Immunogenetics* **21**:39, 1985.
280. Woods DE, Edge MD, Colten HR: Isolation of a cDNA clone for the human complement protein C2 and its use in identification of a restriction fragment length polymorphism. *J Clin Invest* **74**:634, 1984.
281. Ruddy S: Component deficiencies: The second component. *Prog Allergy* **39**:250, 1986.
282. Ruddy S, Klemperer MR, Rosen FS, Austen KF, Kumate J: Hereditary deficiency of the second component of complement in man: Correlation of C2 hemolytic activity with immunochemical measurements of C2 protein. *Immunology* **18**:943, 1970.
283. Johnson FR, Agnello V, Williams RC Jr: Opsonic activity in human serum deficient in C2. *J Immunol* **109**:141, 1971.
284. Sampson HA, Walchner AM, Baker PJ: Recurrent pyogenic infections in individuals with absence of the second component of complement. *J Clin Immunol* **2**:39, 1982.
285. Friend P, Rapine J, Kim Y, Clawson CC, Michael AF: Deficiency of the second component of complement (C2) with chronic vasculitis. *Ann Intern Med* **83**:813, 1975.
286. Repine JE, Clawson CC, Friend PS: Influence of a deficiency of the second component of complement on the bactericidal activity of neutrophils in vitro. *J Clin Invest* **59**:802, 1977.
287. Geibink GS, Verhoeff J, Peterson PK, Quie PG: Opsonic requirements for phagocytosis of streptococcus pneumoniae types VI, XVIII, XXIII and XXV. *Infect Immun* **18**:291, 1977.
288. Truedsson L, Sturgfelt G, Nived O: Prevalence of the type I complement C2 deficiency gene in Swedish systemic lupus erythematosus patients. *Lupus* **2**:325, 1993.
289. Garred P, Mollnes TE, Thorsteinsson L, Erlendsson K, Steinsson K: Increased amounts of C4-containing immune complexes and inefficient activation of C3 and the terminal complement pathway in a patient with homozygous C2 deficiency and systemic lupus erythematosus. *J Immunol* **31**:59, 1990.
290. Steinsson K, Erlendsson K, Valdimarsson H: Successful plasma infusion treatment of a patient with C2 deficiency and systemic lupus erythematosus: Clinical experience over forty-five months. *Arthritis Rheum* **32**:906, 1989.
291. Kim Y, Friend PS, Dresner IG, Yunis EJ, Michael AF: Inherited deficiency of the second component of complement (C2) with membranoproliferative glomerulonephritis. *Am J Med* **62**:765, 1977.
292. Leddy JP, Griggs RC, Klemperer MR, Frank MM: Hereditary complement (C2) deficiency with dermatomyositis. *Am J Med* **58**:83, 1975.
293. Gelfand EW, Clarkson JO, Minta JO: Selective deficiency of the second component of complement in a patient with anaphylactoid purpura. *Clin Immunol Immunopathol* **4**:269, 1975.
294. Perlemuter G, Chassada S, Soubrane O, Degoy A, Lounal A, Barbet P, Legman P, Kahan A, Weiss L, Couturier D: Multifocal stenosing ulcerations of the small intestine revealing vasculitis associated with C2 deficiency. *Gastroenterology* **110**:1628, 1996.
295. Traustadothi KH, Rafner BO, Steinsson K, Valdimarsson H, Erlandsson K: Participation of factor B in residual immune complex red cell binding activity observed in serum from C2 deficient patient may delay the appearance of clinical symptoms. *Arthritis Rheum* **41**:427, 1998.
296. Newman SL, Vogler LB, Feigen RD, Johnston RB Jr: Recurrent septicemia associated with congenital deficiency of C2 and partial deficiency of factor B of the alternative pathway. *New Eng J Med* **299**:290, 1978.
297. Hyatt AC, Altenburger KM, Johnston RB Jr, Winkelstein JA: Increased susceptibility to severe pyogenic infections in patients with an inherited deficiency of the second component of complement. *J Pediatr* **98**:417, 1981.
298. Fasano MB, Hamosh A, Winkelstein JA: Recurrent systemic bacterial infections in homozygous C2 deficiency. *Pediatr Allergy Immunol* **1**:46, 1990.
299. Hartmann D, Fremeaux-Bacchi V, Weiss L, Meyer A, Blouin J, Haputmann G, Kazatchkine M, Uring-Lambert B: Combined heterozygous deficiency of the classical complement pathway proteins C2 and C4. *J Clin Immunol* **17**:176, 1997.
300. Rhynes RI, Britten AF, Pickering RJ: Deficiency of the second component of complement association with the HLA haplotype A10, B18 in a normal population. *Ann Rheumat Dis* **41**:93, 1982.
301. Fu SM, Stern R, Kunkel HG, Dupont B, Hansen JA, Day NK, Good RA, Jersild C, Fotino M: Mixed lymphocyte culture determinants and C2 deficiency. LD-7a associated with C2 deficiency in four families. *J Exp Med* **142**:495, 1975.
302. Day NK, L'Esperance P, Good RA, Michael AF, Hansen JA, Dupont B, Jersild C: Hereditary C2 deficiency: Genetic studies and association with the HL-A system. *J Exp Med* **141**:1464, 1975.
303. Wolski KP, Schmid FR, Mittal K: Genetic linkage between the HL-A system and a deficiency of the second component (C2) of complement. *Science* **188**:1020, 1975.
304. Awdeh ZL, Raum DD, Glass D, Agnello V, Schur PH, Johnston RB Jr, Gelfand EW, Ballow M, Yunis E, Alper CA: Complement-human histocompatibility antigen haplotypes in C2 deficiency. *J Clin Invest* **67**:581, 1981.
305. Truedsson L, Alper CA, Awdeh ZL, Johansen P, Sjoholm AG, Sturfelt G: Characterization of type I complement C2 deficiency MHC haplotypes: Strong conservation of the complotype/HLA-B region and absence of disease association due to linked class II genes. *J Immunol* **151**:5856, 1993.
306. Hauptmann G, Tongio MM, Goetz J, Mayer S, Fauchet R, Sobel A, Griscel C, Berthoux F, Rivat C, Rother U: Association of the C2-deficiency gene ($C2^*Q0$) with the $C4A^*4$, $C4B^*2$ genes. *J Immunogenet* **9**:127, 1982.
307. Wetsel RA, Kulics J, Lokki ML, Kiepiela P, Akama H, Johnson CA, Densen P, Colten HR: Type II human complement C2 deficiency: Allele-specific amino acid substitutions (Ser189-Phe; Gly444-arg) cause impaired C2 secretion. *J Biol Chem* **271**:5824, 1996.
308. Wang X, Circolo A, Lokki ML, Shackelford PG, Wetsel RA, Colten HR: Molecular heterogeneity in deficiency of complement protein C2 type I. *Immunology* **93**:184, 1998.
309. Sullivan KE, Winkelstein JA: Prenatal diagnosis of heterozygous deficiency of the second component of complement. *Clin Diagn Lab Immunol* **1**:606, 1994.
310. Vik DP, Amiguet P, Moffat GJ, Fey M, Amiguet-Barras F, Wetsel R, Tack BF: Structural features of the human C3 gene: Intron/exon organization, transcriptional start site, and promoter region sequence. *Biochemistry* **30**:1080, 1991.

311. Whitehead AS, Solomon E, Chambers S, Bodmer WF, Povey S, Fey G: Assignment of the structural gene for the third component of human complement to chromosome 19. *Proc Natl Acad Sci USA* **79**:5021, 1982.
312. de Bruijn MHL, Fey G: Human complement component C3: cDNA coding sequence and derived primary structure. *Proc Natl Acad Sci USA* **82**:708, 1985.
313. Morris KM, Goldberger G, Colten HR, Aden DP, Knowles BB: Biosynthesis and processing of a human precursor complement protein, pro-C3, in a hepatoma-derived cell line. *Science* **215**:399, 1982.
314. Alper CA, Johnson AM, Birtch AG, Moore RD: Human C3: Evidence for the liver as the primary site of synthesis. *Science* **163**:286, 1969.
315. Ramadori G, Tedesco F, Bitter-Buermann D, Meyer ZUM, Buschenfelde KH: Biosynthesis of the third (C3), eighth (C8), and ninth (C9) complement components by guinea pig hepatocyte primary cultures. *Immunobiology* **170**:203, 1985.
316. Singer L, Colten HR, Wetsel RA: Complement C3 deficiency: Human, animal, and experimental models. *Pathobiology* **62**:14, 1994.
317. Davis AE III, Davis JS IV, Robson AR, Osofsky SG, Colten HR, Rosen FS, Alper CA: Homozygous C3 deficiency: Detection of C3 by radioimmunoassay. *Clin Immunol Immunopathol* **8**:543, 1977.
318. Botto M, Fong KY, So AK, Rudge A, Walport MJ: Molecular basis of hereditary C3 deficiency. *J Clin Invest* **86**:11581, 1990.
319. Alper CA, Colten HR, Gear JSS, Robson AR, Rosen FS: Homozygous human C3 deficiency: The role of C3 in antibody production, C1s-induced vasopermiability, and cobra venom-induced passive hemolysis. *J Clin Invest* **57**:222, 1976.
320. Pussell BA, Bourke E, Nayef M, Morris S, Peters DK: Complement deficiency and nephritis: A report of a family. *Lancet* **1**:675, 1980.
321. Ballow M, Shira JE, Harden L, Yang SY, Day NK: Complete absence of the third component of complement in man. *J Clin Invest* **56**:703, 1975.
322. Osofsky SG, Thompson BH, Lint TF, Gewurz H: Hereditary deficiency of the third component of complement in a child with fever, skin rash, and arthralgias: Response to transfusion of whole blood. *J Pediatr* **90**:180, 1977.
323. Roord JJ, Daha M, Kuis W, Verbrugh HA, Verhoef J, Zegers BJM, Stoop JW: Inherited deficiency of the third component of complement associated with recurrent pyogenic infections, circulating immune complexes, and vasculitis in a Dutch family. *Pediatrics* **71**:81, 1983.
324. Hsieh K-H, Lin C-Y, Lee T-C: Complete absence of the third component of complement in a patient with repeated infections. *Clin Immunol Immunopathol* **20**:305, 1981.
325. Sano Y, Nishinukai H, Kitamura H, Nagaki K, Inai S, Hamasaki Y, Maruyama I, Igata A: Hereditary deficiency of the third component of complement in two sisters with systemic lupus erythematosis-like symptoms. *Arthritis Rheum* **24**:1255, 1981.
326. Alper CA, Colten HR, Rosen FS, Robson AR, MacNab GM, Gear JSS: Homozygous deficiency of C3 in a patient with repeated infections. *Lancet* **2**:1179, 1972.
327. Grace HJ, Brereton-Stiles GG, Vos GH, Schonland M: A family with partial and total deficiency of complement C3. *S Afr Med J* **50**:139, 1976.
328. Berger M, Balow JE, Wilson CB, Frank MM: Circulating immune complexes and glomerulonephritis in a patient with congenital absence of the third component of complement. *New Engl J Med* **308**:1009, 1983.
329. Borzy MS, Houghton D: Mixed-pattern immune deposit glomerulonephritis in a child with inherited deficiency of the third component of complement. *Am J Kidney Dis* **5**:54, 1985.
330. Cork LC, Morris JM, Olson JL, Krakowka S, Swift AJ, Winkelstein JA: Membranoproliferative glomerulonephritis in dogs with a genetically determined deficiency of the third component of complement. *Clin Immunol Immunopathol* **60**:455, 1991.
331. Botto M, Fong KY: Molecular basis of polymorphisms of human complement component C3. *J Exp Med* **172**:1011, 1990.
332. McLean RH, Weinstein A, Damjanov I, Rothfield N: Hypomorphic variant of C3, arthritis, and chronic glomerulonephritis. *J Pediatr* **93**:937, 1978.
333. McLean RH, Weinstein A, Chapitis J, Lowenstein M, Rothfield N: Familial partial deficiency of the third component of complement (C3) and the hypocomplementemic cutaneous vasculitis syndrome. *Am J Med* **68**:549, 1980.
334. Wyatt RJ, Jones D, Stapleton FB, Roy S, Odom TW, McLean RH: Recurrent hemolytic-uremic syndrome with the hypomorphic fast allele of the third component of complement. *Complement* **107**:564, 1985.
335. Alper CA, Rosen FS: Studies of a hypomorphic variant of human C3. *J Clin Invest* **50**:324, 1971.
336. McLean RH, Bryan RK, Winkelstein JA: Hypomorphic variant of the slow allele of C3 associated with hypocomplementemia and hematuria. *Am J Med* **78**:865, 1985.
337. Botto M, Fong KY, So AK, Barlow R, Routier R, Morley BJ, Walport MJ: Homozygous hereditary C3 deficiency due to a partial gene deletion. *Proc Nat Acad Sci USA* **89**:4957, 1992.
338. Huang JL, Lin CY: A hereditary C3 deficiency due to aberrant splicing of exon 10. *Clin Immunol Immunopathol* **73**:267, 1994.
339. Winkelstein JA, Cork LC, Griffin DE, Griffin JW, Adams RJ, Price DL: Genetically determined deficiency of the third component of complement in the dog. *Science* **212**:1169, 1981.
340. Ameratunga R, Winkelstein JA, Brody L, Binns M, Cork LC, Colombani P, Valle D: Molecular analysis of the third component of canine complement (C3) and identification of the mutation responsible for hereditary canine C3 deficiency. *J Immunol* **160**:2824, 1998.
341. Blum JR, Cork LC, Morris JM, Olson JL, Winkelstein JA: The clinical manifestations of a genetically determined deficiency of the third component of complement in the dog. *Clin Immunol Immunopathol* **34**:304, 1985.
342. Quezado ZMN, Hoffman WD, Winkelstein JA, Ytasiv I, Koev CA, Cork LC, Elin RJ, Eichacker PQ, Natanson C: The third component of complement protects against endotoxin-induced shock and multiple organ failure. *J Exp Med* **179**:569, 1994.
343. Carney DF, Haviland DL, Noack D, Wetsel RA, Vik DP, Tack BF: Structural aspects of the human C5 gene: Intron/exon organization, 5′ flanking features, and characterization of two truncated cDNA clones. *J Biol Chem* **266**:18786, 1991.
344. Wetsel RA, Barnum SR: Molecular biology and biochemistry of the third (C3) and fifth (C5) complement components, in Sim RB (ed.): *Biochemistry and Molecular Biology of Complement*. Lancaster, England, MTP Press, 2000.
345. Ooi YM, Colten HR: Biosynthesis and post-synthetic modification of a precursor (Pro-C5) of the fifth component of mouse complement (C5). *J Immunol* **123**:2494, 1979.
346. Patel F, Minta JO: Biosynthesis of a single chain pro-C5 by normal mouse liver mRNA: Analysis of the molecular basis of C5 deficiency in AKR/J mice. *J Immunol* **123**:2408, 1979.
347. Lundwall AB, Wetsel RA, Kristensen T, Whitehead AS, Woods DE, Ogden RL, Colten HR, Tack BF: Isolation of a cDNA clone encoding the fifth component of human complement. *J Biol Chem* **260**:2108, 1985.
348. McCarty GA, Snyderman R: Component deficiencies: The fifth component. *Progr Allergy* **39**:271, 1986.
349. Rosenfeld SI, Kelly ME, Leddy JP: Hereditary deficiency of the fifth component of complement in man: I. Clinical, immunochemical, and family studies. *J Clin Invest* **57**:1626, 1976.
350. Rosenfeld SI, Baum J, Steigbigel RT, Leddy JP: Hereditary deficiency of the fifth component of complement in man: II. Biological properties of C5-deficient human serum. *J Clin Invest* **57**:1635, 1976.
351. Synderman R, Durack DT, McCarty GA, Ward FE, Meadows L: Deficiency of the fifth component of complement in human subjects: Clinical genetic and immunologic studies in a large kindred. *Am J Med* **67**:638, 1979.
352. McLean R, Peter G, Gold R, Guerra L, Yunis EJ, Kruetzer DL: Familial deficiency of C5 in humans: Intact but deficient alternative complement pathway activity. *Clin Immunol Immunopathol* **21**:62, 1981.
353. Peter G, Weigert MB, Bissel AR, Gold R, Kreutzer D, McLean RH: Meningococcal meningitis in familial deficiency of the fifth component of complement. *Pediatrics* **67**:882, 1981.
354. Schoonbrood TH, Hannema A, Fijen CA, Markusse HM, Swaak AJ: C5 deficiency in a patient with primary Sjögren's syndrome (complement deficiencies). *J Rheumatol* **22**(7):1389, 1995.
355. Mori L, de Libero G: Genetic control of susceptibility to collagen-induced arthritis in T cell receptor β chain transgenic mice. *Arthritis Rheum* **41**:256, 1998.
356. Wang X, Fleischer DT, Whitehead WT, Haviland DL, Rosenfeld SI, Leddy JP, Snyderman R, Wetsel RA: Inherited human complement C5 deficiency: Nonsense mutations in exons 1 (Gln1 to stop) and 36 (Arg1458 to stop) and compound heterozygosity in three African-American families. *J Immunol* **154**:5464, 1995.
357. Rosenberg LT, Tachibana DK: Activity of mouse complement. *J Immunol* **89**:861, 1962.

358. Hammer CH, Gaither T, Frank MM: Complement deficiencies of laboratory animals, in Gershwin ME, Merchant B (eds.): *Immunologic Defects in Laboratory Animals*. New York, Plenum Press, 1981, pp 207–241.
359. Jeremiah SJ, West LF, Abbott CM, Murad Z, Povey S, Thomas HJ, Solomon E, Discipio R, Fey GH: Three genes coding for late acting components of complement assigned to chromosome 5. *Cytogenet Cell Genet* **51**:1019A, 1989.
360. Haefliger JA, Tschopp J, Vial N, Jenne DE: Complete primary structure and functional characterization of the sixth component of the human complement system. *J Biol Chem* **264**:18041, 1989.
361. Gonzalez S, Lopez-Larrea C: Characterization of the human C6 promoter. *J Immunol* **157**:2282, 1996.
362. Di Scipio RG, Hugli TE: The molecular architecture of human complement component C6. *J Biol Chem* **264**:16197, 1989.
363. Rother U: Component deficiencies: The sixth component. *Prog Allergy* **39**:283, 1986.
364. Glass D, Raum D, Balavitch D, Kagan E, Robson A, Schur PH, Alper CA: Inherited deficiency of the sixth component of complement: A silent or null gene. *J Immunol* **120**:538, 1978.
365. Leddy JP, Frank MM, Gaither T, Baum J, Klemperer MR: Hereditary deficiency of the sixth component of complement in man: I. Immunochemical, biologic, and family studies. *J Clin Invest* **53**:544, 1974.
366. Lim D, Gewurz Z, Lint TF, Ghaze M, Sephari B, Gewurz H: Absence of the sixth component of complement in a patient with repeated episodes of meningococcal meningitis. *J Pediatr* **89**:42, 1976.
367. Vogler LB, Newman SL, Stroud RM, Johnston RB Jr: Recurrent meningococcal meningitis with absence of the sixth component of complement: An evaluation of underlying immunologic mechanisms. *Pediatrics* **64**:465, 1979.
368. Lee TJ, Snyderman R, Patterson J, Rauchbach AS, Folds JD, Yount WJ: *Neisseria meningitidis* bacteremia in association with deficiency of the sixth component of complement. *Infect Immun* **24**:656, 1979.
369. Wurzner R, Hobart MJ, Fernie BA, Mewar D, Potter PC, Orren A, Lachmann PJ: Molecular basis of subtotal complement C6 deficiency. *J Clin Invest* **95**:1877, 1995.
370. Lachman PJ, Hobart MJ, Woo P: Combined genetic deficiency of C6 and C7 in man. *Clin Exp Immunol* **33**:193, 1978.
371. Morgan BP, Vara SP, Bennett AJ, Thomas SP, Mathews N: A case of hereditary combined deficiency of complement components C6 and C7 in man. *Clin Exp Immunol* **75**:396, 1989.
372. Tedesco F, Silvani CM, Agelli M, Giovanetti AM, Bombardieri S: A lupus-like syndrome in a patient with deficiency of the sixth component of complement. *Arthritis Rheum* **24**:1438, 1981.
373. Nishizaka H, Horiuchi T, Zhu ZB, Fukumori Y, Nagasawa K, Hayashi K, Krumdieck R, Cobbs CG, Higuchi M, Yasunaga S, et al: Molecular bases for inherited human complement component C6 deficiency in two unrelated individuals. *J Immunol* **156**:2309, 1996.
374. Zhu ZB, Totemchokchyakarn K, Atkinson TP, Volanakis JE: Molecular defects leading to human complement component C6 deficiency. *FASEB J* **10**:A1446, 1996.
375. Fernie BA, Hobart MJ, Delbridge G, Potter PC, Orren A, Lachmann PJ: C6 haplotypes: Associations of a Dde I site polymorphism to complement deficiency genes and the Msp I restriction fragment length polymorphism. *Clin Exp Immunol* **95**(2):351, 1994.
376. Fernie BA, Orren A, Wurzner R, Jones AM, Potter PC, Lachmann PJ, Hobart MJ: Complement component C6 and C7 haplotypes associated with deficiencies of C6. *Ann Hum Genet* **59**:183, 1995.
377. Leenaerts PL, Stad RK, Hall BM, van Damme BJ, Vanrenterghem Y, Daha M: Hereditary C6 deficiency in a strain of PVG/c rats. *Clin Exp Immunol* **97**:478, 1994.
378. Brauer RB, Lam TT, Wang D, Horwitz LR, Hess AD, Klein AS, Sanfilippo F, Baldwin WM 3d: Extrahepatic synthesis of C6 in the rat is sufficient for complement-mediated hyperacute rejection of a guinea pig cardiac xenograft. *Transplantation* **59**:1073, 1995.
379. Setien F, Alvarez V, Coto E, Discipio RG, Lopez-Larrea C: A physical map of the human complement component C6, C7, and C9 genes. *Immunogenetics* **38**:341, 1993.
380. Hobart MJ, Fernie BA, Discipio RG: Structure of the human C7 gene and comparison with the C6, C8B, and C9 genes. *J Immunol* **154**:5188, 1995.
381. Zeitz HJ, Lint TF, Gewurz A, Gewurz H: Component deficiencies: 7. The seventh component. *Prog Allergy* **39**:289, 1986.
382. Wellek B, Opferkuch W: A case of deficiency of the seventh component of complement in man: Biological properties of a C7-deficient serum and description of a C7-inactivating principle. *Clin Exp Immunol* **19**:223, 1975.
383. Lee TJ, Utsinger PD, Synderman R, Yount WJ, Sparling PF: Familial deficiency of the seventh component of complement associated with recurrent bacteremic infections due to *Neisseria*. *J Infect Dis* **138**:359, 1978.
384. Loirat C, Buriot D, Peltier AP, Berche P, Aujard Y, Griscelli C, Mathieu H: Fulminant meningococcemia in a child with hereditary deficiency of the seventh component of complement and proteinuria. *Acta Paediatr Scand* **69**:553, 1980.
385. Fernie BA, Orren A, Sheehan G, Schlesinger M, Hobart MJ: Molecular bases of C7 deficiency: Three different defects. *J Immunol* **159**:1019, 1997.
386. Fernie BA, Wurzner R, Orren A, et al: Molecular basis of combined C6 and C7 deficiency. *Mol Immunol* **S1**:59, 1996.
387. Zeitz HJ, Miller GW, Lint TF, Ali MA, Gewurz H: Deficiency of C7 with systemic lupus erythematosis: Solubilization of immune complexes in complement-deficient sera. *Arthritis Rheum* **24**:87, 1981.
388. Alcalay M, Bontoux D, Peltier A: C7 deficiency, abnormal platelet aggregation and rheumatoid arthritis. *Arthritis Rheum* **24**:102, 1981.
389. Boyer JT, Gall EP, Norman ME, Nilsson UR, Zimmerman TS: Hereditary deficiency of the seventh component of complement. *J Clin Invest* **56**:905, 1975.
390. Friduss SR, Sadoff WI, Hern AE, Fivenson DP: Fatal pyoderma gangrenosum in association with C7 deficiency. *J Am Acad Dermatol* **27**:356, 1992.
391. Nishizaka H, Horiuchi T, Zhu ZB, Fukumori Y, Volanakis JE: Genetic bases of human complement C7 deficiency. *J Immunol* **157**:4239, 1996.
392. Kolb WP, Muller-Eberhard HJ: The membrane attack mechanism of complement: The three polypeptide chain structure of the eighth component (C8). *J Exp Med* **143**:1131, 1976.
393. Steckel EW, York RG, Monahan JB, Sodety JM: The eighth component of human complement: Purification and physicochemical characterization of its unusual subunit structure. *J Biol Chem* **255**:11997, 1980.
394. Rittner C, Schneider PM: Genetics and polymorphism of the complement components, in Rother K, Till GO (eds): *The Complement System*. Heidelberg, Springer-Verlag, 1988, p 80.
395. Kaufman KM, Snider JV, Spurr NK, Schwartz CE, Sodety JM: Chromosomal assignments of genes encoding the α, β, γ subunits of human complement protein C8: Identification of a close physical linkage between the α and γ loci. *Genomics* **5**:475, 1989.
396. Kaufman KM, Sodetz JM: Genomic structure of the human complement protein C8α: Homology to the lipocalin gene family. *Biochemistry* **33**:5162, 1994.
397. Ng SC, Sodetz JM: Biosynthesis of C8 by hepatocytes: Differential expression and intracellular association of the α, β, and γ subunits. *J Immunol* **139**:3021, 1987.
398. Densen P, McRill CM: Differential expression of C8 subunits: Primary role of C8 beta. *Clin Res* **35**:613A, 1987.
399. Tedesco F: Component deficiencies: 8. The eighth component. *Prog Allergy* **39**:295, 1986.
400. Tedesco F, Densen P, Villa MA, Petersen BH, Sirchia G: Two types of dysfunctional eighth component of complement (C8) molecules in C8 deficiency in man: Reconstitution of normal C8 from the mixture of the two abnormal C8 molecules. *J Clin Invest* **71**:183, 1983.
401. Tschopp J, Penea F, Schifferli J, Spath P: Dysfunctional C8 beta chain in patients with C8 deficiency. *Scand J Immunol* **24**:715, 1986.
402. Warnick PR, Densen P: Reduced C8α messenger RNA expression in families with hereditary C8α deficiency. *J Immunol* **146**:1052, 1991.
403. Tedesco F, Bardare M, Giovanetti AM, Sirchia G: A familial dysfunction of the eighth component of complement (C8). *Clin Immunol Immunopathol* **16**:180, 1980.
404. Tschopp J, Esser AF, Spira TJ, Muller-Eberhard HJ: Occurrence of an incomplete molecule in homozygous C8 deficiency in man. *J Exp Med* **154**:1599, 1981.
405. Tedesco F, Villa MA, Densen P, Sirchia G: Beta chain deficiency in three patients with dysfunctional C8 molecules. *Mol Immunol* **20**:47, 1983.
406. Petersen BH, Graham JA, Brooks GF: Human deficiency of the eighth component of complement: The requirement of C8 for serum *Neisseria gonorrhoeae* bactericidal activity. *J Clin Invest* **57**:283, 1976.
407. Jasin HE: Absence of the eighth component of complement in association with system lupus erythematosis-like disease. *J Clin Invest* **60**:709, 1977.
408. Nicholson A, Lepow I: Host defense against *Neisseria meningitidis* requires a complement-dependent bactericidal activity. *Science* **205**:298, 1979.

409. Kaufmann T, Hansch G, Rittner C, Spath P, Tedesco F, Schneider PM: Genetic basis of human complement C8 beta deficiency. *J Immunol* **150**:4943, 1993.
410. Saucedo L, Ackermann L, Platonov AE, Gewurz A, Rakita RM, Densen P: Delineation of additional genetic basis for C8α deficiency. *J Immunol* **155**:5022, 1995.
411. Kotnik V, Luznik-Bufon T, Schneider PM, Kirschfink M: Molecular, genetic and functional analysis of homozygous C8 β-chain deficiency in two siblings. *Immunopharmacology* **38**:215, 1997.
412. Densen P, andAckerman L, et al: The genetic basis of C8α-γ deficiency. *Mol Immunol* **S1**:68, 1996.
413. Discipio RG, Gehring MR, Podack ER, Kan CC, Hugli TE, Fey GH: Nucleotide sequence of human complement component C9. *Proc Natl Acad Sci USA* **81**:7298, 1984.
414. Stanley KK, Luzio JP: Construction of a new family of high efficiency bacterial expression vectors: Identification of cDNA clones for human liver proteins. *EMBO J* **3**:11429, 1984.
415. Stanley KK, Kocher HP, Luzio JP, Jackson P, Tschopp J: The sequence and topology of human complement component C9. *EMBO J* **4**:375, 1985.
416. Marazziti D, Eggersten G, Stanley KK, Fey G: Evolution of the cysteine-rich domains of C9. *Complement* **4**:189, 1987.
417. Abbott C, West L, Povey S, Jeremiah S, Murad Z, Discipio R, Fey G: The gene for human complement component C9 mapped to chromosome 5 by polymerase chain reaction. *Genomics* **4**:606, 1989.
418. Lassiter HA, Wilson JL, Feldhoff RC, Hoffpauir JM, Klueber KM: Supplemental complement component C9 enhances the capacity of neonatal serum to kill multiple isolates of pathogenic *Escherichia coli*. *Pediatr Res* **35**:389, 1994.
419. Adinolfi M, Lehner T: C9 and factor B as acute phase proteins and their diagnostic and prognostic value in disease. *Exp Clin Immunogenet* **5**:123, 1988.
420. Lint TF, Gewurz H: Component deficiencies: The ninth component. *Prog Allergy* **39**:307, 1986.
421. Yoshimura K, Fukumori Y, Ohnoki S, Okubo Y, Yamaguchi H, Tanaka M, Akagaki Y, Inai S: Studies on complement deficiencies in blood donors in Osaka area of Japan. *Jpn J Hum Genet* **28**:120, 1983.
422. Harriman GR, Esser AF, Podack ER, Wunderlich AC, Braude AI, Lint TF, Curd JG: The role of C9 in complement-mediated killing of *Neisseria*. *J Immunol* **127**:2386, 1981.
423. Inai S, Kitamura H, Hiramatsu S, Nagaki K: Deficiency of the ninth component of complement in man. *J Clin Lab Immunol* **2**:85, 1979.
424. Lint TF, Zeitz HJ, Gewurz H: Inherited deficiency of the ninth component of complement in man. *J Immunol* **125**:2252, 1980.
425. Fine DP, Gewurz H, Griffis M, Lint TF: Meningococcal meningitis in a woman with inherited deficiency of the ninth component of complement. *Clin Immunol Immunopathol* **28**:413, 1983.
426. Nagata M, Hara T, Aoki T, Mizuno Y, Akeda H, Inaba S, Tsumoto K, Veda K: Inherited deficiency of the ninth component of complement: An increased risk of meningococcal meningitis. *J Pediatr* **114**:260, 1989.
427. Hironaka K, Makino H, Amano T, Ota Z: Immune complex glomerulonephritis in a pregnant woman with congenital C9 deficiency. *Int Med* **32**:806, 1993.
428. Maruyama K, Arai H, Ogawa T, Hoshino M, Tomizawa S, Morikawa A: C9 deficiency in a patient with poststreptococcal glomerulonephritis. *Pediatr Nephrol* **9**:746, 1995.
429. Witzel-Schlomp K, Spath PJ, Hobart MJ, Fernie BA, Rittner C, Kaufmann T, Schneider PM: The human complement C9 gene: Identification of two mutations causing deficiency and revision of the gene structure. *J Immunol* **158**:5043, 1997.
430. Horiuchi T, Neshizaka H, Jojima T, Sawabe T, Niko Y, Schneider PM, Inaba S, Sakai K, Hayashi K, Hashimura C, Fukumori Y: A nonsense mutation at Arg 95 is predominant in C9 deficiency in Japanese. *J Immunol* **160**:1509, 1998.
431. Alvarez V, Coto E, Setien F, Spath PJ, Lopez-Larrea C: Genetic detection of the silent allele (*Q0) in hereditary deficiencies of the human complement C6, C7, and C9 components. *Am J Med Genet* **55**:408, 1995.
432. Taylor PR, Nash JT, Theodoridis E, Bygrave AE, Walport MJ, Botto M: A targeted disruption of the murine complement factor B gene resulting in loss of expression of three genes in close proximity, factor B, C2, and D17H6S45. *J Bio Chem* **273**:1699, 1998.
433. Densen P, Weiler J, et al: Functional and antigenic analysis of human factor B deficiency. *Mol Immunol* **S1**:68, 1996.
434. Matsumoto M, Fukuda W, et al: Generation and characterization of mice deficient for factor B. *Mol Immunol* **S1**:63, 1996.
435. White RT, Damm D, Hancock N, Rosen BS, Lowell BB, Usher P, Flier JS, Spiegelman BM: Human adipsin is identical to complement factor D and is expressed at high levels in adipose tissue. *J Biol Chem* **267**:9210, 1992.
436. Balke N, Holtkamp U, Horl WH, Tschesche H: Inhibition of degranulation of human polymorphonuclear leukocytes by complement factor D. *FEBS Letts* **371**:300, 1995.
437. Choy LN, Spiegelman BM: Regulation of alternative pathway activation and C3a production by adipose cells. *Obes Res* **4**:521, 1996.
438. Kim S, Narayana SV, Volanakis JE: Mutational analysis of the substrate binding site of human complement factor D. *Biochemistry* **33**:14393, 1994.
439. Kluin-Nelemans HC, van Velzen-Blad H, van Helden HPT, Daha MR: Functional deficiency of complement factor D in a monozygous twin. *Clin Exp Immunol* **58**:724, 1984.
440. Hiemstra PS, Langeler E, Compier B, Keepers T, Leijh PCS, van den Barselaar MT, Overbosch D, Daha MR: Complete and partial deficiencies of complement factor D in a Dutch family. *J Clin Invest* **84**:1957, 1989.
441. Donaldson VH, Evans RR: A biochemical abnormality in hereditary angioneurotic edema: Absence of serum inhibitor of C1-esterase. *Am J Med* **35**:37, 1963.
442. Harrison RA: Human C1 inhibitor: Improved isolation and preliminary structural characterization. *Biochemistry* **22**:5001, 1983.
443. Carter PE, Duponchel C, Tosi M, Fothergill JE: Complete nucleotide sequence of the gene for human C1 inhibitor with an unusually high density of Alu elements. *Eur J Biochem* **197**:301, 1991.
444. Bock SC, Skriver K, Neilson E, Thogersen HC, Wiman B, Donaldson VH, Eddy RL, Muarinan J, Rodziejewska E, Huber R, Shows TB, Magnusson S: Human C1 inhibitor: Primary structure, cDNA cloning and chromosomal localization. *Biochemistry* **25**:4294, 1986.
445. Morris KM, Aden DP, Knowles BB, Colten HR: Complement biosynthesis by the human hepatoma-derived cell line, HepG2. *J Clin Invest* **70**:906, 1982.
446. Colten HR: Ontogeny of the human complement system: In vitro biosynthesis of individual complement components by fetal tissues. *J Clin Invest* **51**:725, 1972.
447. Gitlin D, Biasucci A: Development of gamma G, gamma A, gamma M, beta-1-C/beta-1-A, C1 esterase inhibitor, ceruloplasmin, transferrin, hemopexin, haptoglobin, fibrinogen, plasminogen, alpha1 antitrypsin, orosomucoid, beta-lipoprotein, $alpha_2$ macroglobulin and prealbumin in the human conceptis. *J Clin Invest* **48**:1433, 1969.
448. Johnson AM, Alper CA, Rosen FS, Craig JM: Immunofluorescent hepatic localization of complement proteins: Evidence for a biosynthetic defect in hereditary angioneurotic edema (HANE). *J Clin Invest* **50**:50a, 1971.
449. Bensa JC, Reboul A, Colomb MG: Biosynthesis in vitro of complement subcomponents C1q, C1s, and C1 inhibitor by resting and stimulated human monocytes. *Biochem J* **216**:385, 1983.
450. Rosen FS, Alper CA, Pensky J, Klemperer MR, Donaldson VH: Genetically determined heterogeneity of the C1 esterase inhibitor in patients with hereditary angioneurotic edema. *J Clin Invest* **50**:2143, 1971.
451. Frank MM, Gelfand JA, Atkinson JP: Hereditary angioedema: The clinical syndrome and its management. *Ann Intern Med* **84**:580, 1976.
452. Cicardi M, Bergamaschini L, Marasini B, Boccassini G, Tucci A, Agostini A: Hereditary angioedema: An appraisal of 104 cases. *Am J Med Sci* **284**:2, 1982.
453. Austen KF, Sheffer AL: Detection of hereditary angioneurotic edema by demonstration of a reduction in the second component of human complement. *New Engl J Med* **272**:649, 1965.
454. Pickering RJ, Gewurz H, Kelly JR, Good RA: The complement system in hereditary angioneurotic edema: A new perspective. *Clin Exp Immunol* **3**:423, 1968.
455. Rosen FS, Alper CA, Pensky J, Klemperer MR, Donaldson VH: Genetically determined heterogeneity of C1 esterase inhibitor in patients with hereditary angioneurotic edema. *J Clin Invest* **50**:2143, 1971.
456. Harpel PC, Hugli TE, Cooper NR: Studies on human plasma C1 inactivator-enzyme interactions: II Structural features of an abnormal C1 inactivator from a kindred with hereditary angioneurotic edema. *J Clin Invest* **55**:605, 1975.
457. Donaldson VH, Harrison RA, Rosen FS, Being DH, Kindness G, Canar J, Wagner CJ, Awad S: Variability in purified dysfunctional C1-inhibitor proteins from patients with hereditary angioneurotic edema: Functional and analytical gel studies. *J Clin Invest* **75**:124, 1985.

458. Quastel M, Harrison R, Cicardi M, Alper CA, Rosen FS: Behavior in vivo of normal and dysfunctional C1 inhibitor in normal subjects and patients with hereditary angioneurotic edema. *J Clin Invest* **83**:1041, 1983.
459. Lachman PJ, Rosen FS: The catabolism of C1-inhibitor and the pathogenesis of hereditary angio-edema. *Acta Pathol Microbiol Immunol Scand* **92**:35, 1984.
460. Donaldson VH, Rosen FS: Action of complement in hereditary angioneurotic edema: Role of C1-esterase. *J Clin Invest* **43**:2204, 1964.
461. Klemperer MR, Donaldson VH, Rosen FS: Effect of C1 esterase on vascular permiability in man: Studies in normal and complement-deficient individuals and in patients with hereditary angioneurotic edema. *J Clin Invest* **47**:604, 1968.
462. Schreiber AP, Kaplan AP, Austen KF: Inhibition by C1INH of Hageman factor fragment activation of coagulation, fibrinolysis, and kinin generation. *J Clin Invest* **52**:1402, 1973.
463. Curd JG, Progais LJ Jr, Cochrane CG: Detection of active kallikrein in induced blister fluids of hereditary angioedema patients. *J Exp Med* **152**:742, 1980.
464. Schapira M, Silver LD, Scott CF, Schmaier AH, Prograis LJ, Curd JG, Colman RW: Prekallikrein activation and high-molecular-weight kininogen consumption in hereditary angioedema. *New Engl J Med* **308**:1050, 1983.
465. Sheffer AL, Craig JM, Willms-Kretschmer K, Austen KF, Rosen FS: Histopathological and ultrastructural observations on tissues from patients with hereditary angioneurotic edema. *J Allergy* **47**:292, 1971.
466. Landerman NS: Hereditary angioneurotic edema: I. Case reports and review of the literature. *J Allergy* **33**:316, 1962.
467. Donaldson VH, Rosen FS: Hereditary angioneurotic edema: A clinical survey. *Pediatrics* **37**:1017, 1966.
468. Sheffer AL, Austen KF, Rosen FS: Tranexamic acid therapy in hereditary angioneurotic edema. *New Engl J Med* **287**:452, 1972.
469. Frank MM, Sergent JS, Kane MA, Alling DW: Epsilon aminocaproic acid therapy of hereditary angioneurotic edema: A double blind study. *New Engl J Med* **286**:808, 1972.
470. Gelfand JA, Sherins RJ, Alling DW, Frank MM: Treatment of hereditary angioedema with danazol: Reversal of clinical and biochemical abnormalities. *New Engl J Med* **295**:1444, 1976.
471. Spaulding WB: Methyltestosterone therapy for hereditary episodic edema (hereditary angioneurotic edema). *Ann Intern Med* **53**:739, 1960.
472. Hosea SW, Santaella ML, Brown EJ, Berger M, Katusha K, Frank MM: Long-term therapy of hereditary angioedema with danazol. *Ann Intern Med* **93**:809, 1980.
473. Gadek JE, Hosea SW, Gelfand JA, Frank MM: Response of variant hereditary angioedema phenotypes to danazol therapy. *J Clin Invest* **64**:280, 1979.
474. Jaffe CJ, Atkinson JP, Gelfand JA, Frank MM: Hereditary angioedema: The use of fresh frozen plasma for prophylaxis in patients undergoing oral surgery. *J Allergy Clin Immunol* **55**:386, 1975.
475. Gadek JE, Hosea SW, Gelfand JA, Santaella M, Wickerhauser M, Triantaphyllopoulos DC, Frank MM: Replacement therapy in hereditary angioedema: Successful treatment of acute episodes of angioedema with partly purified C1 inhibitor. *New Engl J Med* **304**:542, 1980.
476. Waytes AT, Rosen FS, Frank MM: Treatment of hereditary angioedema with vapor-heated C1 inhibitor concentrate. *New Engl J Med* **334**:1630, 1996.
477. Agostoni A, Cicardi, M: Hereditary and acquired C1-inhibitor deficiency: Biological and clinical characteristics in 235 patients. *Medicine* **71**:206, 1992.
478. Davis AE 3d, Bissler JJ, Cicardi M: Mutations in the C1 inhibitor gene that result in hereditary angioneurotic edema. *Behring Inst Mitt* **93**:313, 1993.
479. Stoppa-Lyonnet D, Duponchel C, Meo T, Laurent J, Carter PE, Arala-Chaves M, Cohen JH, Dewald G, Goetz J, Hauptmann G, et al: Recombinational biases in the rearranged C1-inhibitor genes of hereditary angioedema patients. *Am J Hum Genet* **49**:1055, 1991.
480. Verpy E, Couture-Tosi E, Eldering E, Lopez-Trascasa M, Spath P, Meo T, Tosi M: Crucial residues in the carboxy-terminal end of C1-inhibitor revealed by pathogenic mutants impaired in secretion or function. *J Clin Invest* **95**:350, 1995.
481. Levy NJ, Ramesh N, Cicardi M, Harrison RA, David AE: Type II hereditary angioneurotic edema that may result from a single nucleotide change in the codon for alanine-436 in the C1 inhibitor gene. *Proc Natl Acad Sci USA* **87**:265, 1990.
482. Skriver K, Wikoff WR, Patston PA, Tausk F, Schapira M, Kaplan AP, Bock SC: Substrate properties of C1 inhibitor Ma (alanine 434-glutamic acid): General and structural evidence suggesting that the P12-region contains critical determinants of serine protease inhibitor/substrate status. *J Biol Chem* **266**:9216, 1991.
483. Davis AE, Aulak KS, Parad RB, Stecklein HP, Eldering E, Hack CG, Kramer J, Strunk RC, Rosen FS: Characterization and expression of C1 inhibitor non-reactive center mutations. *Complement Inflamm* **8**:138A, 1991.
484. Parad RB, Kramer J, Strunk RC, Rosen FS, Davis AE: Dysfunctional C1 inhibitor Ta: Deletion of Lys-251 results in acquisition of an *N*-glycosylation site. *Proc Natl Acad Sci USA* **87**:6786, 1990.
485. Zahedi R, Bissler JJ, Davis AE 3d, Andreadis C, Wisnieski JJ: Unique C1 inhibitor dysfunction in a kindred without angioedema. *J Clin Invest* **95**:1299, 1995.
486. Holers VM, Cole JL, et al: Human C3b- and C4b- regulatory proteins: A new multigene family. *Immunol Today* **6**:188, 1985.
487. Hardig Y, Hillarp A, Dahlback B: The amino terminal module of the C4b-binding protein alpha-chain is crucial for C4b binding and factor I-cofactor function. *Biochem J* **323**:469, 1997.
488. Criado Garcia O, Sanchez-Corral P, Rodriquez de Cordoba S: Isoforms of human C4b-binding protein: II. Differential modulation of the *C4BPA* and *C4BPB* genes by acute phase cytokines. *J Immunol* **155**:4037, 1995.
489. Trapp RG, Fletcher M, Forristal J, West CD: C4 binding protein deficiency in a patient with atypical Behçet's disease. *J Rheumatol* **14**:135, 1987.
490. Ewulonu UK, Ravi L, Medof ME: Characterization of the decay-accelerating factor gene promoter region. *Proc Natl Acad Sci USA* **88**:4675, 1991.
491. Shenoy-Scaria AM, Kwong J, Fujita T, Olszowy MW, Shaw AS, Lublin DM: Signal transduction through decay-accelerating factor. *J Immunol* **149**:3535, 1992.
492. Holguin MH, Martin CB, Bernshaw NJ, Parker CJ: Analysis of the effects of activation of the alternative pathway of complement on erythrocytes with an isolated deficiency of decay accelerating factor. *J Immunol* **148**:498, 1992.
493. Telen MJ, Green AM: The Inab phenotype: Characterization of the membrane protein and complement regulatory defect. *Blood* **74**:437, 1989.
494. Lublin DM, Mallinson G, Poole J, Reid ME, Thompson ES, Ferdman BR, Telen MJ, Anstee DJ, Tanner MJ: Molecular basis of reduced or absent expression of decay-accelerating factor in Cromer blood group phenotypes. *Blood* **84**:1276, 1994.
495. Wang L, Uchikawa M, Tsuneyama H, Tokunaga K, Tadokoro K, Juji T: Molecular cloning and characterization of decay-accelerating factor deficiency in Cromer blood group Inab phenotype. *Blood* **91**:680, 1998.
496. Goldberger G, Bruns GA, Rits M, Edge MD, Kwiatkowski DJ: Human complement factor I: Analysis of cDNA-derived primary structure and assignment of its gene to chromosome 4. *J Biol Chem* **262**:10065, 1987.
497. Goldberger G, Arnaout MA, Aden D, Kay R, Rits M, Colten HR: Biosynthesis and postsynthetic processing of human C3b/C4b inactivator (factor I) in three hepatoma cell lines. *J Biol Chem* **259**:6492, 1984.
498. Whaley K: Biosynthesis of complement components and the regulatory proteins of the alternative complement pathway by human peripheral blood monocytes. *J Exp Med* **151**:501, 1980.
499. Vyse TJ, Spath PJ, Davies KA, Morley BJ, Philippe P, Athanassiou P, Giles CM, Walport MJ: Hereditary complement factor I deficiency. *Q J Med* **87**:385, 1994.
500. Alper CA, Abramson N, Johnston RB Jr, Jandl JH, Rosen FS: Increased susceptibility to infection associated with abnormalities of complement-mediated functions and of the third component of complement (C3). *New Engl J Med* **282**:349, 1970.
501. Alper CA, Abramson N, Johnston RB, Jandl JH, Rosen FS: Studies in vivo and in vitro on an abnormality in the metabolism of C3 in a patient with increased susceptibility to infection. *J Clin Invest* **49**:1975, 1970.
502. Abramson N, Alper CA, Lachmann PJ, Rosen FS, Jandl JH: Deficiency of C3 inactivator in man. *J Immunol* **107**:19, 1971.
503. Zeigler JB, Alper CA, Rosen FS, Lachmann PJ, Sherington L: Restoration by purified C3b inactivator of complement-mediated function in vivo in a patient with C3b inactivator deficiency. *J Clin Invest* **55**:668, 1975.
504. Nicol Pae, Lachmann PJ: The alternative pathway of complement activation: The role of C3 and its inactivator (KAF). *Immunology* **24**:259, 1973.

505. Wahn V, Rother V, Rauterberg EW, Day NK, Laurell AB: C3b inactivator deficiency: Association with an alpha-migrating factor H. *J Clin Immunol* **1**:228, 1981.
506. Solal-Celigny P, Laviolette M, Hebert J, Atkins PC, Sirois M, Brun G, Lehner-Netsch G, Delage JM: C3b inactivator deficiency with immune complex manifestations. *Clin Exp Immunol* **47**:197, 1982.
507. Teisner B, Brandslund I, Folkerson J, Rasmussen JM, Paulsen LO, Svehog SE: Factor I deficiency and C3 nephritic factor: Immunochemical findings and association with *Neisseria meningitidis* infection in two patients. *Scand J Immunol* **20**:291, 1984.
508. Thompson RA, Lachmann PJ: A second case of human C3b inhibitor (KAF) deficiency. *Clin Exp Immunol* **27**:23, 1977.
509. Morley BJ, Vyse TJ, et al: Molecular basis of hereditary factor I deficiency. *Mol Immunol* **S1**:71, 1996.
510. Vyse TJ, Morley BJ, Bartok I, Theodoridis EL, Davies KA, Webster AD, Walport MJ: The molecular basis of hereditary complement factor I deficiency. *J Clin Invest* **97**:925, 1996.
511. Skerka C, Timmann C, Horstmann RD, Zipfel PE: Two additional human serum proteins structurally related to complement factor H. *J Immunol* **148**:3313, 1992.
512. Feifel E, Prodinger WM, Molgg M, Schwaeble W, Schonitzer D, Koistinen V, Misasi R, Dierich MP: Polymorphism and deficiency of human factor H-related proteins p39 and p37. *Immunogenetics* **36**:104, 1992.
513. Sim RB, Kolble K, McAleer MA, Dominguez O, Dee VM: Genetics and deficiencies of the soluble regulatory proteins of the complement system. *Int Rev Immunol* **10**:65, 1993.
514. Nielsen HE, Christensen KC, Koch C, Thomsen BS, Heegaard NHH, Tranum-Jensen J: Hereditary, complete deficiency of complement factor H associated with recurrent meningococcal disease. *Scand J Immunol* **30**:711, 1989.
515. Levy M, Halbwachs-Mecarelli L, Gubler MC, Kohout G, Bensenouci A, Niaudet P, Hauptmann G, Lesavre P: H deficiency in two brothers with atypical dense intramembranous deposit disease. *Kidney Int* **30**:949, 1986.
516. Thompson RA, Winterborn MH: Hypocomplementaemia due to a genetic deficiency of beta-1H globulin. *Clin Exp Immunol* **46**:110, 1981.
517. Brai M, Misiano G, Maringhini S, Cutaja I, Hauptmann G: Combined homozygous factor H and heterozygous C2 deficiency in an Italian family. *J Clin Immunol* **8**:50, 1988.
518. Ault BH, Schmidt BZ, Fowler NL, Kashtan CE, Ahmed AE, Vogt BA, Colten HR: Human factor H deficiency: Mutations in framework cysteine residues and block in H protein secretion and intracellular catabolism. *J Biol Chem* **272**:25168, 1997.
519. Wurzner R, Steinkasserer A, Hunter D, Dominguez O, Lopez-Larrea C, Sim RB: Complement factor H mRNA in Epstein-Barr virus transformed B lymphocytes of a factor H-deficient patient: Detection by polymerase chain reaction. *Exp Clin Immunogenet* **12**:82, 1995.
520. Hogasen K, Jansen JH, Mollnes TE, Hovdenes J, Harboe M: Hereditary porcine membranoproliferative glomerulonephritis type II is caused by factor H deficiency. *J Clin Invest* **95**:1054, 1995.
521. Goundis D, Holt SM, Boyd Y, Reid KBM: Localization of the properdin structural locus to Xp11.23-Xp21.1. *Genomics* **5**:56, 1989.
522. Robson KJH, Halt JRS, Jennings MW, Harris TJR, Marsh K, Newbnold CI, Tate VE, Weatherall DJ: A highly conserved amino-acid sequence in thromobospondin, properdin and in proteins from sporozoites and blood stages of a human malarial parasite. *Nature* **335**:79, 1988.
523. Nolan KF, Schwaeble W, Kaluz S, Dierich MP, Reid KBM: Molecular cloning of the cDNA coding for properdin, a positive regulator of the alternative pathway of human complement. *Eur J Immunol* **21**:771, 1991.
524. Sjoholm AG, Braconier JH, Soderstrom C: Properdin deficiency in a family with fulminant meningococcal infections. *Clin Exp Immunol* **50**:291, 1982.
525. Densen P, Weiler JM, Griffiss JM, Hoffmann LG: Familial properdin deficiency and fatal meningococcemia: Correction of the bactericidal defect by vaccination. *New Eng J med ital* **316**:922, 1987.
526. Nielson HE, Kock C.: Congenital properdin deficiency and meningococcal infection. *Clin Immunol Immunopathol* **44**:134, 1987.
527. Sjoholm AG, Soderstrom C, Nilsson LA: A second variant of properdin deficiency: The detection of properdin at low concentrations in affected males. *Complement Inflamm* **5**:130, 1988.
528. Sjoholm AG, Kuijper EJ, Tijssen CC, Jansz A, Bol P, Spanjaard L, Zanen HC: Dysfunctional properdin in a Dutch family with meningococcal disease. *New Engl J Med* **319**:33, 1988.
529. Holme ER, Veitch J, Johnston A, Hauptmann G, Uring-Lambert B, Seywright M, Docherty V, Morley WN, Whaley K: Familial properdin deficiency associated with chronic discoid lupus erythematosus. *Clin Exp Immunol* **76**:76, 1989.
530. Gelfand EW, Rao CP, Minta JO, Ham T: Inherited deficiency of properdin and C2 in a patient with recurrent bacteremia. *Am J Med* **82**:671, 1987.
531. Densen P, Weiler JM, Griffiss JM, Hoffman LG: Familial properdin deficiency and fatal meningococcemia: correction of the bactericidal defect by vaccination. *New Engl J Med* **316**:922, 1987.
532. Westberg J, Fredrikson GN, Truedsson L, Sjoholm AG, Uhlen M: Sequence-based analysis of properdin deficiency: Identification of point mutations in two phenotypic forms of an X-linked immunodeficiency. *Genomics* **29**:1, 1995.
533. Fredrikson GN, Westburg J, et al: Molecular genetic characterization of properdin deficiency type III: Dysfunction due to a single point mutation in exon 9 of the structural gene causing a tyrosine to aspartic acid interchange. *Mol Immunol* **S1**:1, 1996.
534. Kolble K, Cant AJ, Fay AC, Whaley K, Schlesinger M, Reid KB: Carrier detection in families with properdin deficiency by microsatellite haplotyping. *J Clin Invest* **91**:99, 1993.
535. Forsberg UH, Bazil V, Stefanova I, Schroder J: Gene for human CD59 (likely Ly-6 homologue) is located on the short arm of chromosome 11. *Immunogenetics* **30**:188, 1989.
536. Lehto T, Meri S: Interactions of soluble CD59 with the terminal complement complexes. *J Immunol* **151**:4941, 1993.
537. Yamashina M, Ueda E, Kinoshita T, Takami T, Ojima A, Ono H, Tanaka H, Kondo N, Orii T, Okada N, Okada H, Inoue K, Kitani T: Inherited complete deficiency of 20 kilodalton homologous restriction factor (CD59) as a cause of paroxysmal nocturnal hemoglobinuria. *New Engl J Med* **323**:1184, 1990.
538. Motoyama N, Okada N, Yamashina M, Okada H: Paroxysmal nocturnal hemoglobinuria due to hereditary nucleotide deletion in the HRF20 (CD59) gene. *Eur J Immunol* **22**:2669, 1992.
539. Sastry K, Herman GA, Day L, Deignan E, Bruns G, Morton CC, Ezekowitz RA: The human mannose binding protein gene. *J Exp Med* **170**:1175, 1989.
540. Sumiya M, Super M, Tabona P, Levinsky RJ, Arai T, Turner MW, Summerfield JA: Molecular basis of opsonic defect in immunodeficient children. *Lancet* **337**:1569, 1991.
541. Summerfield JA, Ryder S, Sumiya M, Thursz M, Gorchein A, Monteil MA, Turner MW: Mannose binding protein gene mutations associated with unusual and severe infections in adults. *Lancet* **345**:886, 1995.
542. Davies EJ, Snowden N, Hillarby MC, Carthy D, Grennan DM, Thomson W, Ollier WE: Mannose-binding protein gene polymorphism in systemic lupus erythematosus. *Arthritis Rheum* **38**:110, 1995.
543. Sullivan KE, Wooten C, Goldman D, Petri M: Mannose binding protein genetic polymorphisms in black patients with systemic lupus rythematosus. *Arthritis Rheum* **39**:2046, 1996.
544. Davies EJ, Teh L-S, Ordi-Ros J et al: A dysfunctional allele of the mannose binding protein gene associates with systemic lupus erythematosus in a Spanish population. *J Rheumatol* **24**:485, 1997.
545. Graudal NA, Homann C, Madsen HO, Svejgaard A, Jurik AG, Graudal KH, Garred P: Mannan binding lectin in rheumatoid arthritis. *J Rheumatol* **25**:629, 1998.
546. Madsen HO, Garred P, Thiel S, Kurtzhals JA, Lamm LU, Ryder LP, Svejgaard A: Interplay between promoter and structural gene variants control basal serum level of mannan-binding protein. *J Immunol* **155**:3013, 1995.
547. Kakkanaiah VN, Shen GQ, Ojo-Amaize EA, Peter JB: Association of low concentrations of serum mannose-binding protein with recurrent infections in adults. *Clin Diag Lab Immunol* **5**:319, 1998.

CHAPTER 187

Immotile Cilia Syndrome (Primary Ciliary Dyskinesia), Including Kartagener Syndrome

Björn A. Afzelius ▪ Björn Mossberg ▪ Sten Erik Bergström

1. **The immotile cilia syndrome is a genetically determined disorder characterized by dysmotility or even complete immotility of the cilia in the airways and elsewhere. Usually spermatozoa are also either immotile or poorly motile.**
2. **Kartagener syndrome is a subgroup of the immotile cilia syndrome and is further characterized by situs inversus viscerum. Situs inversus, bronchiectasis, and chronic sinusitis form the classic Kartagener triad.**
3. **The reason for the ciliary immotility or dysmotility usually can be seen with an electron-microscopic investigation of a ciliated mucosal biopsy or of the spermatozoa of an ejaculate. Certain specific defects in the ciliary axoneme are regarded to be pathognomonic of the syndrome, principally a lack of dynein arms. Cilia and sperm tails normally exhibit the same defects in the same patient. Motility can be evaluated by light-microscopic examination of living cilia or spermatozoa and the functional capacity of cilia by measurement of mucociliary transport.**
4. **The clinical consequences of the immotile cilia syndrome include chronic cough and expectoration, bronchiectasis, chronic rhinitis and nasal polyposis, chronic or recurrent sinusitis, and often an agenesis of the frontal sinuses. Otosalpingitis and otitis are common. Obstructive lung disease may develop and is expressed as chronic airflow limitation. Most clinical manifestations date from early childhood. Neonatal asphyxia occurs often.**
5. **Males are usually sterile. Females may be fertile or infertile.**
6. **Treatment is symptomatic and directed against complications in the upper and lower respiratory tract. Physiotherapy often should be started early in life. With modern care and abstinence from smoking, the prognosis in the immotile cilia syndrome is good.**
7. **The immotile cilia syndrome clearly is a genetically heterogeneous disease, although its clinical profile is fairly uniform. Many genes participate in the construction of a cilium, and an error in any one of them will prevent the cilia from working properly. The inheritance in most cases is autosomal recessive. In families in which the immotile cilia syndrome occurs, on average, half the affected siblings have situs inversus. Presumably, chance alone decides between situs inversus and situs solitus in homozygotes of the syndrome.**

In a paper in 1933, Manes Kartagener published the case histories of four persons who all had situs inversus totalis, bronchiectasis, and chronic sinusitis.[1] Siewert previously had described one such patient.[2] This combination of symptoms later came to be known as *Kartagener syndrome* or *Kartagener triad.* It is caused by a structural and generalized abnormality of cilia, making the cilia immotile, feebly motile, or dysmotile[3,4] and, hence, nonfunctional. Ciliary dysmotility is associated with situs inversus in only about half the patients. Because situs inversus per se usually has no serious implications, this chapter will address the immotile cilia syndrome in its entirety and will include Kartagener syndrome as a subgroup of the immotile cilia syndrome.

PREVALENCE

Most authors estimate the prevalence of Kartagener syndrome at 1 in 30,000 to 1 in 60,000 persons.[5,6] The prevalence of the immotile cilia syndrome can be estimated from the following data. Situs inversus has been estimated to have a prevalence in Europe and the United States of 1 in 8000 to 1 in 25,000 persons.[5,7,8] Roughly one-fourth to one-fifth of all persons with situs inversus also have bronchiectasis and chronic sinusitis.[7] A somewhat higher fraction has generalized bronchitis but not bronchiectasis (yet). This gives a figure of the prevalence of Kartagener syndrome on the order of 1 in 40,000 to 1 in 120,000 persons. If it is true, as assumed,[3] that half the patients with the immotile cilia syndrome have situs inversus, then the prevalence of this syndrome will be twice that of Kartagener syndrome, or about 1 in 20,000 to 1 in 60,000 persons.

Geographic and Racial Distribution

Kartagener syndrome has been described in all major races and from all parts of the world. Detailed pedigrees have been published from Austria,[9] Canada,[10] France,[11] Germany,[12,13] Great Britain,[14] Israel,[15] Japan,[16] Sweden,[17] Switzerland,[18] the United States,[19–21] and other countries. In all these publications it was remarked that one or several sibs of the propositus had the same bronchial and sinusoidal symptoms as the propositus but had no situs inversus. Sometimes these sibs have been claimed to have an "incomplete Kartagener syndrome." The seemingly equal number of affected sibs with and without situs inversus supports the idea that the immotile cilia syndrome is inherited as a recessive disorder and that chance alone determines whether the viscera take up the normal or the reversed position during embryogenesis in affected individuals.[3]

CILIA IN THE HUMAN BODY

The symptoms of the immotile cilia syndrome and of its subgroup, Kartagener syndrome, cannot be understood without a knowledge of the distribution in the body of cilia and of the normal ciliary anatomy. Cilia and sperm tails are outgrowths from centrioles

A list of standard abbreviations is located immediately preceding the index in each volume.

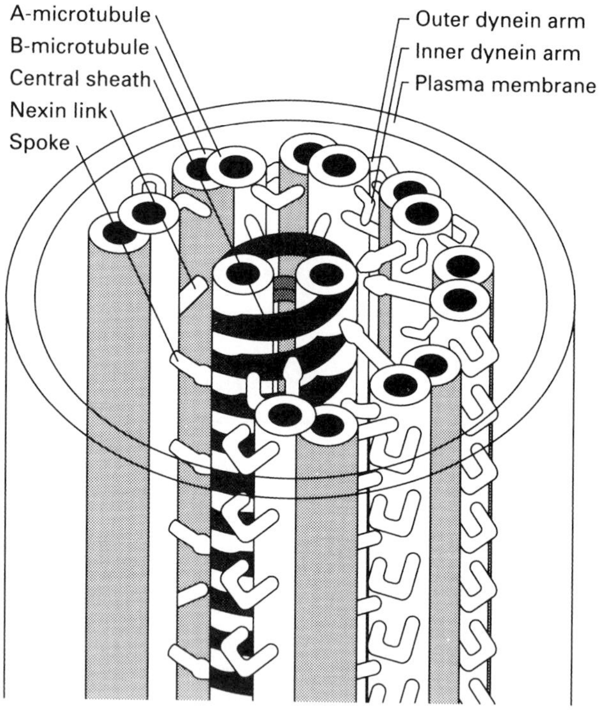

Fig. 187-1 Three-dimensional reconstruction of the cilium. (*From Klaus Hausmann. Reproduced by permission of Biologie in unserer Zeit.*)

(basal bodies) with an architecture as shown in Figs. 187-1 to 187-3. The central axis is called the *axoneme* and consists of nine microtubular doublets in a ring around two single microtubules. These nine plus two units are joined by three types of bonds:

1. Two rows of *dynein arms* along each doublet, which are instrumental in microtubular sliding and ciliary undulation. Cilia or spermatozoa with no outer dynein arms are capable of slow beatings, whereas the inner arms seem to be indispensable for ciliary movements.[22]

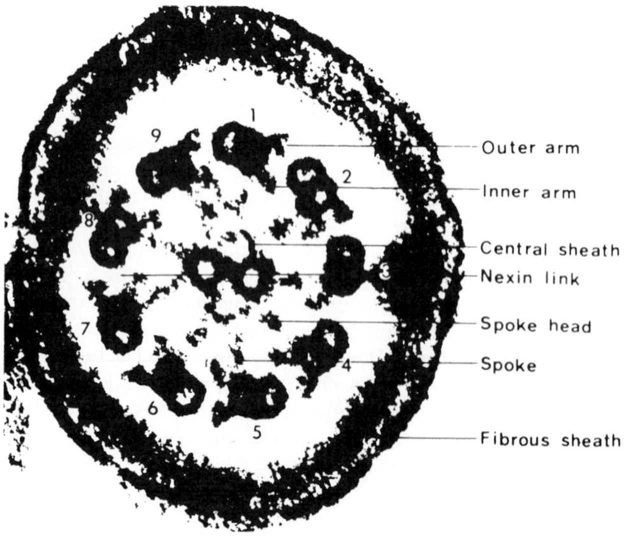

Fig. 187-2 Electron micrograph of a transversely sectioned human sperm tail from a healthy man. The central part of the sperm tail has the same structure as that of a cilium. There are nine outer microtubular doublets in a ring around two central microtubules. The terms used for some of the components are given. (*From Afzelius and Eliasson.[45] Used with permission.*)

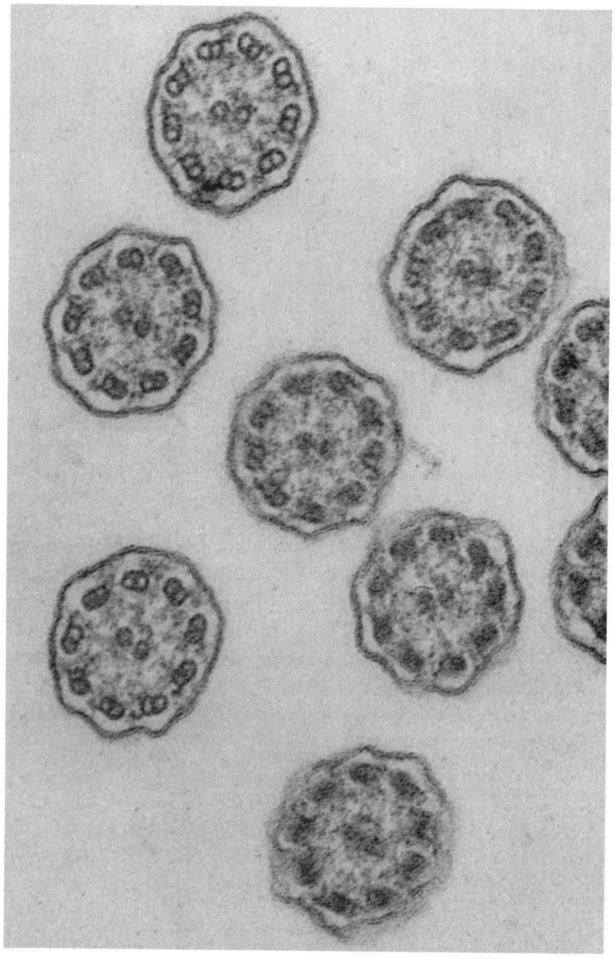

Fig. 187-3 Cilia from the bronchial mucosa of a person who has normal cilia. Note that the cilia have a fairly ordered orientation best seen in the two central microtubules.

2. *Nexin links*, which are responsible for the maintenance of axoneme structure during sliding. They seem to limit the sliding by being stretchable only to a certain degree.
3. *Spokes*, which extend from the outer doublets to a central sheath around the two central microtubules and that participate in the mechanism for converting sliding into bending.

Further details of the ciliary machinery and its mode of action can be found in references 5 and 22 through 27.

Ciliated epithelia are found in the following places in the human body: the upper airways (i.e., nasal passages, paranasal sinuses, Eustachian tubes, middle ear mucosa, and nasopharynx), the trachea and bronchi down to respiratory bronchioles, the lacrimal sac, the ependymal lining of the brain and central canal of the spinal cord, the endometrial lining of the deeper parts of the cervix, the fallopian tubes, and the ductuli efferentes on the border between the testis and the epididymis.

Some epithelia have a single cilium per cell (a monocilium), e.g., the thyroid gland,[28] the inner corneal endothelium, the trabecular meshwork, and the choroid of the eye,[29] as do several of the embryonic epithelia.[5] Such primary cilia have been found to beat, but whether their beatings can perform work is unknown.[30] Certain sensory cells carry a sensory hair that is a modified cilium. The tail of the human spermatozoon has an axoneme, with the typical structure of a cilium, although it is much longer and has a flagellar beat. Cilia are about 6 μm long; sperm tails are about 40 μm long.

The cilia of the airway epithelia beat in a layer of serous fluid that is about 5 μm thick (the sol layer). Overlying this layer and at

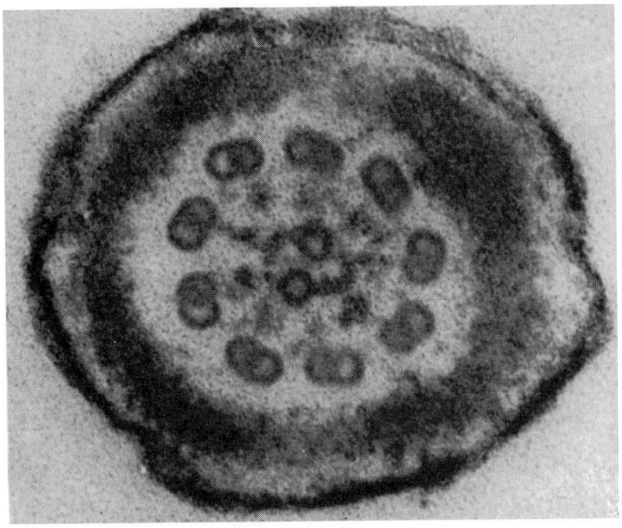

Fig. 187-4 Sperm tail of a man with the immotile cilia syndrome. In this man, the sperm tails and the cilia are characterized by a total or nearly total lack of both the outer and inner dynein arms.

the level of the ciliary tips is a mucous or gel layer that may be either patchy or continuous.[23] Most cilia are oriented in the same general direction, which determines the direction of their effective strokes. The cilia are mechanically coordinated into short metachronal waves and transport the mucous layer with its entrapped inhaled particles and endogenous debris toward the pharynx with a speed of about 2 mm/min in the central bronchi and trachea. The role of cilia in the fallopian tubes, the ductuli efferentes, and the ependyma of the central nervous system is largely speculative.

Ultrastructure of Cilia and Sperm Tails in the Immotile Cilia Syndrome

The essential feature of the immotile cilia syndrome, including Kartagener syndrome, is the abnormal structure and function of cilia. Usually an immotility or a dysmotility can be detected by light microscopic videorecording, and an abnormal ciliary ultrastructure can be seen by electron microscopy. Most—possibly all—clinical data of this syndrome can be explained by defective ciliary work. Cilia and sperm tails from hundreds of persons have been examined as to their motility or immotility and ultrastructure, and the data from different laboratories are in essential agreement. It is evident that the immotile cilia syndrome is a heterogeneous disease and that several subgroups can be found:

1. Dynein arms are practically absent in both rows[3,5,31–39] (Figs. 187-4 and 187-5).
2. Both outer and inner dynein arms are reduced in number, often to about half normal.[17,38–40]
3. The outer dynein arms are short, and the inner dynein arms may be missing.[32,34,41,42]
4. Only the outer dynein arms are missing[33,38,41–43] (Fig. 187-6).
5. Only the inner dynein arms are missing.[38,41,44]
6. The entire spokes or the spoke heads as well as the central sheath are missing; the two inner microtubules often are off-center (the *spoke defect*[5,33,34,45,46]) (Fig. 187-7).
7. The central microtubules are short or absent, and microtubular doublet number 1 is transposed to a central position; the inner dynein arms may be absent (*microtubular transposition defect*[36,47,48]).
8. Nexin links, spokes, and the inner dynein arms are missing, and the circle of microtubular doublets is disrupted (*disorganized axoneme*[33,34]).
9. The two central microtubules and the inner dynein arms are missing.[49]
10. Cilia have a normal ultrastructure as seen in sections[50,51] and may be immotile,[49,50] dysmotile,[39] or *hypermotile* though nonfunctional.[52] In some cases, the cilia have approximately twice the normal length.[53]
11. Cilia and basal bodies may be completely lacking. Ciliated cells in the nasal epithelium only or in the nasal epithelium and tracheobronchial tree may be replaced by cells that have long microvilli[50,54–56]; these cells may be undifferentiated mucous cells or brush cells.[32,57–59] It should be noted here that viral or bacterial infections tend to reduce the number of ciliated cells and that it thus may be difficult to distinguish between inherited and acquired diseases.

Other subgroups may well exist. In many of the patients in subgroups 1 to 7, the cilia are further characterized by the presence of supernumerary or missing microtubules in the axoneme. Cilia also tend to be rather poorly aligned[60–63]; the range of orientation of the basal feet[60] or of the two central microtubules[61–63] thus is wider than in controls. Although it seems that a very accurate alignment of mucus-propelling cilia may be unnecessary, a random orientation of cilia would exclude coordinated activity. About half the patients in most of these subgroups have situs inversus. Cilia from different types of epithelia of the same patient usually have the same ultrastructure, indicating that the defect is a generalized one.[32,45,64,65] It is possible, however, that focal abnormalities may make the diagnosis uncertain; it is thus recommended that cilia from two or more sites be evaluated. One patient has been reported in whom cilia at one site of the bronchi had microtubular transposition to a high percentage and at other sites were close to normal.[66] Viral airway infections may

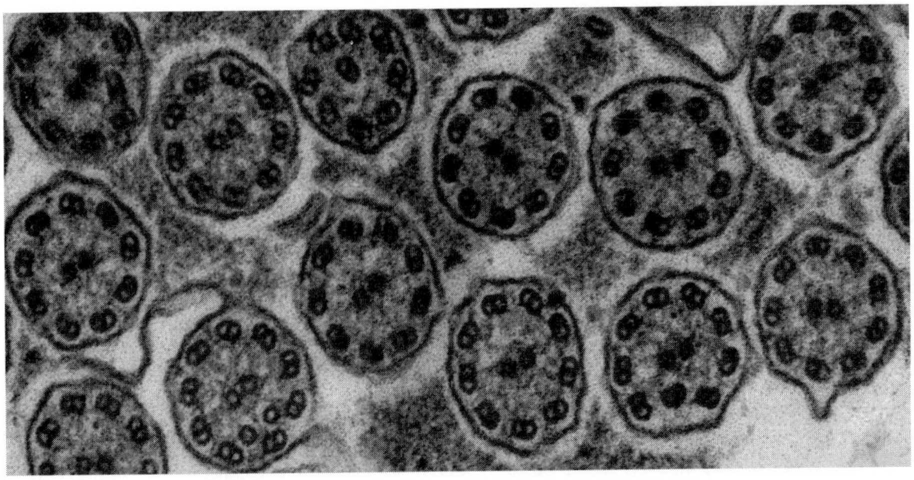

Fig. 187-5 Cilia from the nasal epithelium of a woman with the immotile cilia syndrome. The dynein arms are missing.

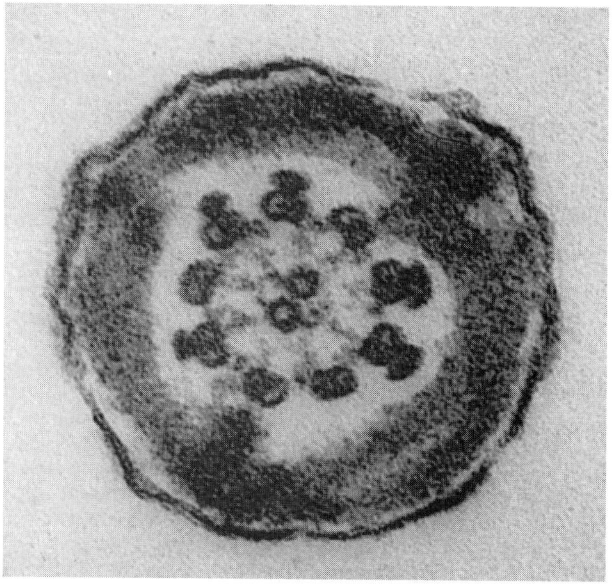

Fig. 187-6 Sperm tail of a man with the immotile cilia syndrome and characterized by the presence of inner dynein arms but no, or very few, outer dynein arms. The spermatozoa had some degree of motility.

reduce the number of ciliated cells,[67–69] as may chronic nasal obstruction.[69] In studies in which repeated biopsies were taken from the same patient, the cilia usually were found to have the same ultrastructure,[70] but in three patients an anomaly (short dynein arms) was found in a first but not a second biopsy.[71]

Cilia and sperm tails tend to display the same type of defect in the same patient, although the spermatozoa may be completely devoid of dynein arms in men who have cilia with a few dynein arms.[3,64,71,72] There are also a few published cases with only the spermatozoa immotile and lacking dynein arms[73] or in which only the cilia display these features.[74] The difference in axonemal ultrastructure between cilia and spermatozoa from the same patient could be due either to a mosaicism, to a separate genetic control of their structural component, or to a variable penetrance.

Some of the ciliary abnormalities listed earlier, and in particular defects other than the listed ones, have been described in patients with infections, allergies, or chemical treatment.[71,75,76] These include the clumping of several axonemes within a common limiting membrane (into "compound cilia") or the presence of supernumerary microtubular doublets or singlets or a deficiency in their number.[75–78] These types of ciliary defects hence are not diagnostic of the immotile cilia syndrome.

Motility of Cilia and Sperm Tails

The immotile cilia syndrome is due to a lack of cilia[55] or to the cilia being completely immotile,[31,32,34,36,45,79] being feebly motile,[80] or displaying erratic movements.[80–82] Because a good correlation usually exists between ciliary motility and spermatozoal motility, an examination of the spermatozoa can be made for diagnostic purposes.[64] Sperm immotility may be due also to other factors: exposure of the ejaculate to cold, immobilization by antibodies, necrospermia (i.e., dead spermatozoa), and certain disorders in which the spermatozoa are grossly abnormal.[64] In order to observe the motility or immotility of cilia, ciliated cells have to be removed and observed *in vitro*. Cilia from persons with the immotile cilia syndrome may be immotile or may have an abnormal and inefficient motility. Several variants of abnormal motility have been described: reduced beat frequency, hyperfrequent low-amplitude vibrations, "windshield wiper movement," multiplanar "egg-beater-like rotations," "corkscrewlike rotation," slow-grabbing movements of the distal portion, and flagella-like undulation.[80–84] Certain dysmotilities can be correlated with specific ultrastructural defects.[85] However, the functional capacity of the cilia measured by mucociliary clearance is absent; this is a hallmark of the syndrome.[86–89]

A relatively simple method has been devised to differentiate between ciliary dysfunctions being the cause of airway disease and such that are a consequence of the disease (thus between primary ciliary dyskinesia and secondary ciliary dyskinesia).[90] Cells taken from a nasal brushing are isolated by pronase treatment and kept in cell culture for some weeks, during which time the old cilia fall off and a new population of cilia emerge. If the ciliated cells rotate, this is a sign of the cilia having coordinated activity and hence the patient having secondary ciliary dyskinesia—if the cells remain stationary, the diagnosis is primary ciliary dyskinesia.

Biopsies or brushings from a ciliated epithelium can be examined with phase-contrast or interference-contrast microscopy.[79,80,84,91] It is difficult, however, to distinguish between normal and erratic types of ciliary beatings with an unaided eye, and analysis has to be performed either with an oscillographic technique[82,92] or by making videorecordings that can be studied in slow motion.[93]

A complete motility study should include three parameters: ciliary beat frequency, ciliary beat coordination, and ciliary beat amplitude.[93] Sometimes, even such a complete study will not be enough. In one patient with immotile spermatozoa and a reduced number of dynein arms in his cilia, ciliary motility *in vitro* was not affected, although mucociliary clearance *in vivo* was, possibly because of the increased load of mucus *in vivo*.[80] It was noticed

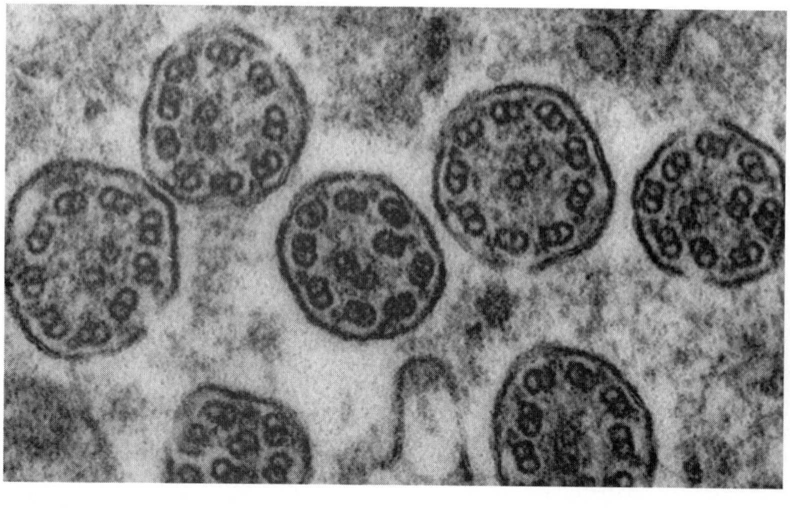

Fig. 187-7 Cilia from the nasal epithelium of a woman with the immotile cilia syndrome. The inner microtubules are off-center, presumably because of defective spokes.

that cilia started beating properly *in vitro* only after the mucus had been washed away.

Some investigators have objected to the term *immotile cilia syndrome* for patients who have some degree of ciliary motility[81,82] or who evidently lack cilia, they have suggested terms such as *primary ciliary dyskinesia*, the *dyskinetic cilia syndrome*, or the *acilia syndrome*. A clinical investigation will not distinguish between immotile and dysmotile cilia or a lack of cilia, however, and hence it is impractical to have different names for different subgroups. Ciliary motility, when present, is ineffective and represents a functionally immotile state. In a clinical context, the disease is an entity.

Situs Inversus and Embryonic Cilia

The following explanation has been suggested for the association between ciliary immotility and situs inversus.[3] Embryonic epithelia often carry a single cilium per cell. In the normal course of events, these cilia are assumed to beat and, by their beatings, cause the heart to be moved to the left side, whereupon the liver goes to the right side of the body. With no ciliary work, chance alone will decide whether the visceral asymmetry will be normal or reversed. In agreement with this hypothesis, Nonaka *et al.* have found that the monocilia in the primitive node of normal mouse embryos rotate in a clockwise fashion (when seen from above) causing a leftward stream of substances in the extraembryonic fluid (and a normal development), whereas in mutated embryos lacking the nodal monocilia, there is a 50 percent chance of situs inversus.[94] In the mouse mutant *iv/iv* with a random determination of situs position,[95] the monocilia have been shown to be rigid and immotile.[96] The *iv* gene of the mouse has a location that would correspond to human chromosome 14q32.

GENETIC CONSIDERATIONS

An examination of published pedigrees[9–21] indicates that the immotile cilia syndrome is inherited as an autosomal recessive trait. Heterozygotes have a normal ciliary ultrastructure, as was shown by an examination of parents of the affected children.[97,98] On average, half the affected persons have situs inversus. As a consequence, the offspring of a mating between two heterozygotes each has a one-eighth chance of having situs inversus. Careful segregation analyses of proband sibships in cases of situs inversus[99] or of the immotile cilia syndrome[46] have been consistent with this mode of inheritance. Approximately 1 in 60 among the population would be a heterozygous carrier if the syndrome were genetically homogeneous.[46] The risk of having a child with the immotile cilia syndrome is apparently not increased with higher age of the mother.[46] One of the pedigrees published by Katsuhara *et al.* is more consistent with a dominant mode of inheritance than with a recessive one,[16] and another seems to be either X-linked or has a dominant pattern of inheritance.[100]

The primary gene products may be the proteins that are seen to be missing in the cilia — dyneins, nexins, spoke proteins, etc. — or the proteins that are responsible for their binding to the microtubules. Nearly 200 different polypeptides have been identified within the ciliary axoneme of lower organisms, and 85 ciliary loci have been identified by over 270 independent mutations.[101] It is likely that various genes responsible for different subgroups of the immotile cilia syndrome are located on most chromosomes in humans. The first gene shown to be responsible for a subgroup of the disease in man is one for an intermediate-chain dynein. Mutations are associated with the absence of outer dynein arms. The gene is located at 9p13-p21.[101a]

Males and females are equally affected. Most males with the syndrome have immotile spermatozoa and are sterile. Male sterility also can be observed in most, but not all, published pedigrees.[21] In rare cases, a Kartagener patient may have normally motile spermatozoa and be capable of fathering a healthy child.[74]

In a Norwegian population, 5 percent of all children with Kartagener syndrome had first-cousin parents, and 16 percent had second-cousin parents.[102] Among the control population, 0.5 percent of parents are first cousins.

CLINICAL FEATURES

Diagnosis

Diagnosis of the immotile cilia syndrome is most reliably performed by the cell culture method mentioned earlier, in which coordinated ciliary activity of regrown cilia is examined.[90] Alternatively, electron microscopy can be used in a search for specific ultrastructural defects of cilia or sperm tails from persons with a clinical picture compatible with the syndrome. The motility of cilia or of spermatozoa also can be examined. With the exception of sperm motility investigations, these tests are too complicated to be used as a first-line screening. Measurements of airway mucociliary clearance are valuable in excluding the diagnosis, since an absence of mucociliary clearance is a hallmark of the syndrome.[86,103] Measurement of the tracheobronchial clearance of inhaled radioactively tagged test particles is also a complicated and expensive method, which moreover has to be interpreted with caution because coughing often obscures the impaired mucociliary clearance in these patients.[89,103] As a first screening method, the saccharin test of nasal mucociliary clearance is much more applicable.[104–106] Saccharin particles are placed on the inferior nasal turbinate about 10 mm from its anterior end, and the time is measured for the sweet taste to appear. A greatly prolonged time — usually to more than 40 to 60 min — is found in patients with nonfunctioning cilia. A reduced mucociliary clearance however, may be an acquired condition and is found also in some other diseases.

Samples of ciliated cells are easily obtained from the inferior nasal turbinate by gentle scraping with a curette or better still with a cytology brush, a procedure that does not require anesthesia.[80,83,91] Alternatively, mucosal biopsies may be obtained by bronchoscopy. Ciliary motility may then be analyzed *in vitro*, by light microscopy and oscillometry or videoscreen recording, by which methods the characteristic immotility or dysmotility may be assessed accurately and ciliary beat frequency measured.[52,84,107,108] The ciliary material also may be prepared for electron microscopy, which is diagnostic in typical patients, such as those with a severe deficiency of dynein arms.[5] In patients with more discrete types of defects, the electron-microscopic evaluation is more problematic and may require quantitative analysis.[109]

A demonstration of specific defects of ciliary ultrastructure and/or motility is unnecessary for purely clinical purposes. The diagnosis may be regarded as established with a sufficient degree of reliability in the following situations: (1) patients with complete Kartagener syndrome, (2) men with the typical clinical signs (chronic bronchitis and rhinitis since early childhood) who have immotile or poorly motile but otherwise normal spermatozoa, and (3) patients with the same clinical signs concerning airway disease who have a sibling who fulfills the criteria of (1) or (2). It should be kept in mind that most persons with situs inversus do not have chronic respiratory tract disease and thus do not have the immotile cilia syndrome, and patients with situs inversus accompanied by other types of respiratory tract disease, such as asthma and atopic rhinitis, should not be confused with immotile cilia syndrome patients.

A very low, nearly absent, amount of exhaled nitric oxide (NO) has been reported from patients with immotile cilia syndrome.[111] Since the same has been reported from some patients with secondary ciliary dyskinesia,[106] the usefulness of this diagnostic tool still remains to be determined.

The immotile cilia syndrome has many features in common with cystic fibrosis, e.g., male infertility. Mucociliary clearance may be retarded in cystic fibrosis but often is present despite the airway disease; this disease, nevertheless, has a more serious prognosis than the immotile cilia syndrome, and the cilia have a normal ultrastructure.[110] Patients with immunoglobulin deficiency also may have a rather similar clinical profile, with mucociliary clearance retarded secondary to the chronic infections; again, ciliary ultrastructure has been found normal.[112] Another differential diagnosis is Young syndrome, defined as obstructive azoospermia and chronic sinopulmonary infections[113]; this condition is the most common cause of the combination of male infertility and chronic airway infections. The respiratory tract disease generally seems to be less severe here than in the immotile cilia syndrome.[113]

Respiratory Tract

Although the immotile cilia syndrome is a heterogeneous condition with regard to ultrastructure, and hence genetics, the clinical profile seems to be fairly or even remarkably uniform—perhaps not surprising when one considers the absence of mucociliary clearance as a common denominator. Characteristically, the respiratory tract disease can be traced back to early childhood or even infancy—often to the very day of birth.[36,38,52,89,114] Neonatal respiratory distress is not uncommon.[114,115] Chronic cough and expectoration of mucoid, mucopurulent, or at times purulent sputum is generally present and often tends to increase during the day rather than being most prominent in the morning as in smoker's chronic bronchitis. Atelectasis and pneumonia are fairly common.

Rhinitis with discharge of a mostly rather thin secretion is also almost universally present, and it is not infrequently complicated by nasal polyposis.[42,114] Chronic or recurrent sinusitis is present, affecting both maxillary and ethmoidal sinuses; the frontal sinuses often fail to develop. The mastoid cells are poorly aerated. Chronic secretory otitis media is constantly present in childhood, with bouts of more acute otitis superimposed.[17,38,65,116–118] In many patients there is a conductive hearing loss of moderate degree—10 to 40 dB.[17,82,116] The ear and nose symptoms usually peak in childhood and adolescence, often with numerous surgical interventions, with a considerable improvement by adult age.[17]

Common colds do not seem to have a much more severe course in patients with the immotile cilia syndrome than in normal subjects. When there is no apparent acute infection, sedimentation rate and serum immunoglobulin levels are usually normal.[89] Sputum cultures may fail to reveal specific pathogens; when such are found, *Haemophilus influenzae* and *Pneumococcus* are common findings, but *Staphylococcus aureus* and *Pseudomonas aeruginosa* also may be found.[50,52,65,119]

Bronchiectasis is probably never present at birth but often develops during childhood and adolescence (Figs. 187-8 and 187-9). In contrast to the situation in cystic fibrosis, it is most commonly found in the middle and lower lobes and lingula. It occurs in dependent parts of the lungs, may be cylindrical or saccular, and on histologic examination shows nonspecific inflammation. The changes are identical to bronchiectasis from other causes.[120,121] When bronchiectasis develops, there may be a marked worsening of the previously often rather discrete endobronchial symptoms, with increased expectoration, infectious episodes with fever, hemoptysis, and development of finger clubbing. The respiratory tract disease of Kartagener syndrome traditionally has been described in terms of bronchiectasis and sinusitis, but now it appears clear that a generalized bronchitis and rhinitis are the more primary features.

Lung function evaluated by spirometry may be normal or show an obstructive impairment of ventilation; in a few cases there may be a restrictive impairment as well, attributable to resectional surgery for bronchiectasis or to generally stiff lungs.[89,122] When obstruction occurs, it is usually of moderate degree and does not seem to progress much over the years,[36,38,89,114,123] especially if the disease is diagnosed at an early stage and is treated properly with intensive physiotherapy and antibiotics. At times, there may be severe airflow obstruction with effort dyspnea by the third decade, and it seems that smokers are at particular risk.[114] Usually there is little reversibility of airflow obstruction, although significant bronchospasm is occasionally present.[65,89,114,122]

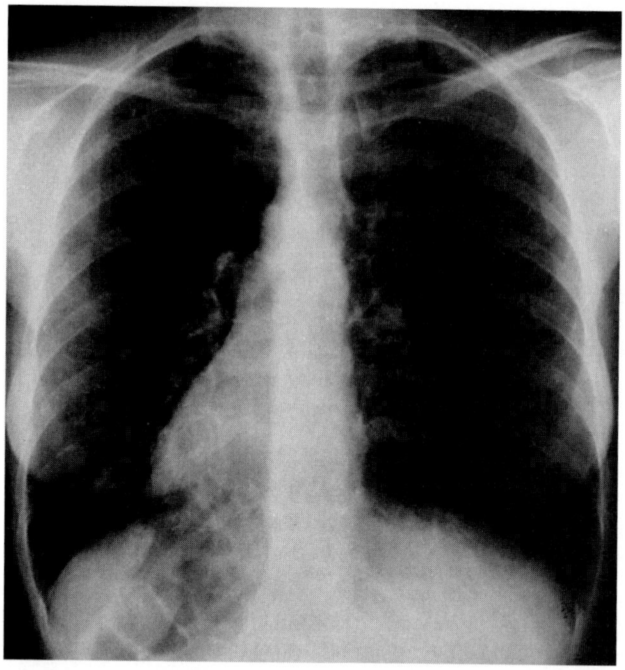

Fig. 187-8 Chest radiograph of a 32-year-old woman with Kartagener syndrome. Changes suggesting bronchiectasis are seen behind the heart. Note the transposition of the heart and also of the abdominal viscera, with part of the colon to the right and the liver to the left.

When significant airways obstruction is present, it is usually expressed as effort dyspnea; asthmatic attacks are not a prominent feature.[114,125] On lung auscultation, crackles are usually heard, wheezing to a lesser extent, mainly in children. Radiography or computed tomography (CT) of the chest often shows a moderate degree of hyperinflation and in more advanced disease peribronchial thickening, atelactasis, and bronchiectasis.[119]

Sensory Organs

For otologic aspects of the immotile cilia syndrome, see the preceding discussion. The sense of balance seems not to be affected in most patients,[5] although about 10 percent of patients claim to have less than a good sense of balance. Most subjects with inborn ciliary immotility are anosmic or have a decreased sense of smell.[5,116]

Examination of the eyes of 10 patients with the syndrome showed corneal abnormalities in 9 but no consistent abnormalities.[125] These abnormalities may be secondary to a developmental disturbance. It may be remembered that the corneal endothelium is a monociliated epithelium. Some patients have been described who suffer from both Kartagener syndrome and retinitis pigmentosa.[50,126–130] This is interesting because it has been claimed that abnormalities in the ultrastructure of human nasal cilia[130] and spermatozoa[131] are found in persons suffering from retinitis pigmentosa.

Central Nervous System

Some patients suffer from fatigue, dull headaches, or endogeneous depression[5]; an association with schizophrenia has been claimed.[132] In the Swedish case reports, two-thirds of the patients complained of chronic headaches, and many had sought medical advice for this complaint. The headaches persisted even during periods free of sinusitis or other infections. Schizophrenia was not seen to be more common than in the general population.

It is likely that patients with the immotile cilia syndrome run a higher than normal risk of neonatal hydrocephalus. Occasionally,

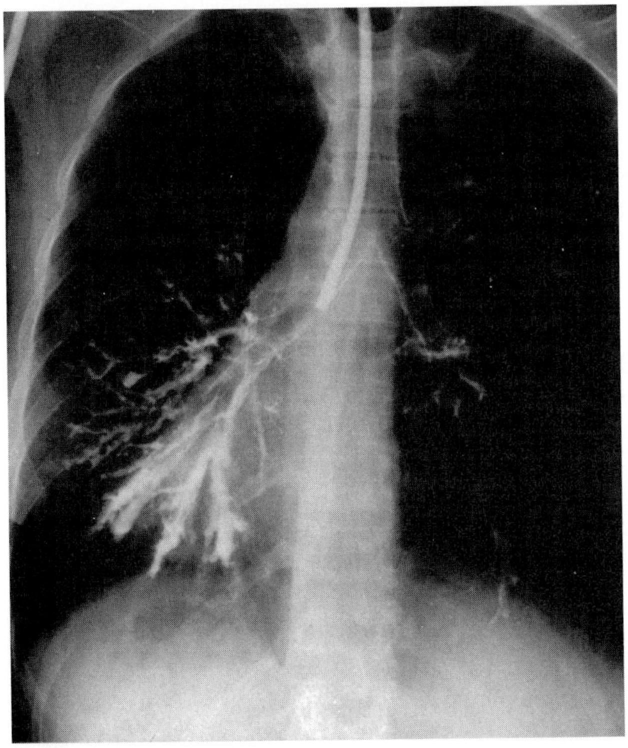

A

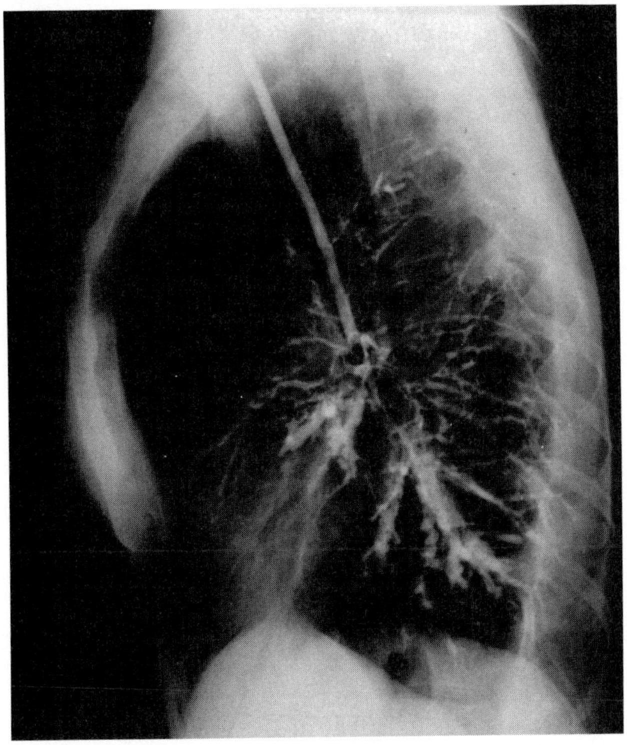

B

Fig. 187-9 ***A, B.*** **Bronchography of the right lung from the same patient as in Fig. 187-7. Large bronchiectasis is seen in the lower lobe and in the right-sided lingula segment of the upper lobe.**

patients with the immotile cilia syndrome have had hydrocephalus.[50,56,133,134] Hydrocephalus developed in one baby at the age of 2 weeks due to exit foramina obstruction but was treated by a ventricular atrial shunt followed by a ventricular peritoneal shunt; the child grew up with normal intelligence.[134] It may be that ependymal cilia normally keep the aqueduct patent and that the risk of stenosis is increased with ciliary immotility.

In one study, the brains of 7 persons with the immotile cilia syndrome were examined by means of CT, and a slight enlargement of the ventricular system and the sulci was found in 2 cases.[5] In another 7 persons, no changes were noted.[135] The brain does not seem to be mirrored in persons with Kartagener syndrome; 3 of 36 patients (8 percent) were left-handed, a conventional frequency.[5]

Reproductive Organs

It has already been remarked that nearly all men with the immotile cilia syndrome are sterile because of immotility or poor motility of their spermatozoa but that some men have motile spermatozoa and are fertile. In typical cases, the volume of the ejaculate and the values for sperm number are within the normal range, and sperm morphology, as evaluated by light microscopy, is likewise normal. Conception with immotile spermatozoa can be achieved by intracytoplasmic sperm injection, which has been performed successfully in some cases.[136]

Some patients have hydrocele,[137] oligospermia, or azoospermia.[138,139] In one patient, the amount of carboxylmethylase in spermatozoa has been measured and found to be decreased.[140] This enzyme plays a role in chemotactic responses in bacteria and also may be involved in animal cell motility.

Women with the immotile cilia syndrome may or may not be fertile.[141–145] In a Swedish series, 9 of 19 women had been unsuccessful in their attempts to become pregnant, 5 had conceived, and 4 had not attempted to become pregnant.[141] In a British study, 4 of 7 women were infertile.[51] The fertility of a woman with immotile cilia in the oviduct has been demonstrated by Bleau *et al.*,[142] whereas in another case a woman who had never conceived had oviductal cilia that were completely immotile.[144] It has been suggested that female fertility varies in the different subgroups of the immotile cilia syndrome,[147] but evidence for this hypothesis has not yet been provided. A priori it would seem likely that women with the immotile cilia syndrome experience a greater than normal risk of ectopic pregnancies, but no evidence of this has been found.[5,6,143,145] In addition, no increased risk of salpingitis has been found so far.

Cardiovascular System

As mentioned earlier, half the persons with the immotile cilia syndrome have situs inversus and may be classified as having Kartagener syndrome. Most of these patients have a complete transposition of the thoracic and abdominal viscera that form a mirror image of the normal condition. Usually no other congenital malformations of the heart or other organs are apparent in Kartagener syndrome, as is common in cases of isolated dextrocardia.[147] Occasional malformations of the heart have been recorded in Kartagener syndrome, as well as in cases of incomplete situs inversus.[6,52]

Leukocytes

The capacity of the leukocytes to orient and to migrate in a chemotactic gradient has been examined in an attempt to find out whether defects in cell motility are restricted to spermatozoa and ciliated cells or have a more general occurrence. It has been reported that the chemotactic migration indeed is significantly reduced in some, but not all, persons investigated and also that the capacity to orient is hampered.[148–152] Whether the decreased chemotactic migration is a primary phenomenon or a consequence of the chronic infections is at present unknown. Most persons with the immotile cilia syndrome do not appear to have an increased incidence of infections at sites outside the airways, although one such case has been reported.[152]

Developmental Anomalies

An extensive list of malformations and diseases that have been observed in patients suffering from Kartagener syndrome is found in Rott.[6] It is likely that the simultaneous occurrence of a certain disease and the syndrome in most cases is purely coincidental. In some instances, a disease or an anomaly may be a direct or indirect consequence of the ciliary malfunction. If so, one might expect to find the anomaly in several patients and a similar defect in the animal models. Some of the congenital cardiac malformations may belong to this category. So may polydactyly, which has been noted in some patients[153,154] and which also is characteristic of *hpy/hpy* mice, a strain in which cilia are abnormal.[95]

TREATMENT AND PROGNOSIS

Treatment is symptomatic and directed against complications in the upper and lower respiratory tract. There is no method available to restore ciliary and spermatozoal motility *in situ*. Antibiotics or chemotherapeutic agents may be given when there are signs of bacterial infection, such as increased purulence of sputum or bouts of sinusitis or otitis. In selected patients, intravenous administration of antibiotics may be necessary as well as extended courses of 1 to 3 months of oral antibiotics.[119,155] The value of mucolytics is uncertain, but they may be tried in selected patients with tenacious secretions. Bronchodilators (β-adrenergics, methylxanthines, or anticholinergics) may be valuable in patients in whom there is airway obstruction with a bronchospastic component.

Physiotherapy is often important and, if started early in life, may prevent or delay the evolution of bronchiectasis and atelectasis. Abandonment of smoking is a most important preventive measure, since smoking probably accelerates deterioration of lung function.

Surgical interventions against maxillary sinusitis, nasal polyposis, and middle ear disease are often performed repeatedly in these patients (e.g., endonasal trepanation, Caldwell-Luc operation, polypectomy, tympanostomy). Such operations doubtless may be necessary in certain patients, but a certain amount of conservatism has been advocated in this context, since there often is a spontaneous remission in adulthood.[17,116]

Thoracic surgical intervention against bronchiectasis is sometimes indicated, although the choice may be difficult in individual patients. Smit *et al.* have reported on 13 adult patients with immotile cilia syndrome, of whom 85 percent considered the resection of bronchiectasis beneficial despite the remaining respiratory symptoms.[155] In another series of 35 adult patients with this disease, bronchiectasis was demonstrated by bronchography in 22 patients, of whom 16 had undergone operation; half of these improved with surgery.[123] The symptoms of chronic bronchitis are not to be expected to be cured by resectional surgery. A heart-lung transplantation has been performed in two patient suffering from the complete Kartagener syndrome.[156,157]

Without access to antibiotics, the average life span may be somewhat reduced owing to severe respiratory tract infections, particularly in childhood and adolescence. The rather frequent occurrence of chronic obstructive pulmonary disease with the risk of development of respiratory insufficiency probably also tends to reduce life span somewhat, although airways obstruction may not be very progressive in most patients. Whether there is an increased risk of lung cancer in the syndrome is not known.

Most persons with the syndrome seem to live an active life.[123] General physical and mental development is usually not retarded by the chronic disease. Situs inversus is usually not combined with congenital malformations. Kartagener syndrome has been described in old age.[158] With modern medical care and abstinence from smoking, the prognosis may be encouraging or even excellent.

REFERENCES

1. Kartagener M: Zur Pathogenese der Bronchiektasien: Bronchiektasien bei Situs viscerum inversus. *Beitr Klin Tuberk* **83**:489, 1933.
2. Siewert AK: Ueber einen Fall von Bronchiektasie bei einem Patienten mit Situs inversus viscerum. *Berl Klin Wochenschr* **41**:139, 1904.
3. Afzelius BA: A human syndrome caused by immotile cilia. *Science* **193**:317, 1976.
4. Eliasson R, Mossberg B, Camner P, Afzelius BA: The immotile-cilia syndrome: A congenital ciliary abnormality as an etiologic factor in chronic airway infections and male sterility. *N Engl J Med* **297**:1, 1977.
5. Afzelius BA: The immotile-cilia syndrome and other ciliary diseases. *Int Rev Exp Pathol* **19**:1, 1979.
6. Rott H-D: Kartagener's syndrome and the syndrome of immotile cilia. *Hum Genet* **46**:249, 1979.
7. Adams R, Churchill ED: Situs inversus, sinusitis and bronchiectasis. *J Thorac Surg* **7**:206, 1937.
8. Svartengren M, Floderus-Myrhed B, Mossberg B, Camner P: Defekta försvars mekanismer i lungorna. *Hjärta Kärl Lungor (Stockh)* **3**:81, 1983.
9. Falser N: Anomalies of kinocilia in Kartagener's syndrome. *Laryngol Rhinol Otol* **62**:128, 1983.
10. Gibney RTN, Herbert FA: Kartagener's syndrome. *Ir Med J* **73**:87, 1980.
11. Monnet P: Situs inversus and bronchopulmonary disease in the neonatal period. *Arch Fr Pediatr* **35**:607, 1978.
12. Weinaug P: Ein Fall von Kartagener-Syndrom bei Geschwistern. *Z Erkr Atmungsorgane* **134**:454, 1971.
13. Rott H-D, Warnatz H, Pasch-Hilgers R, Weikl A: Kartagener's syndrome in sibs: Clinical and immunological investigations. *Hum Genet* **43**:1, 1978.
14. Knox G, Murray S, Strang L: A family with Kartagener's syndrome: Linkage data. *Ann Hum Genet* **24**:137, 1960.
15. Guggenheim F: Kartagener's syndrome in an Arab family. *Isr J Med Sci* **7**:1079, 1971.
16. Katsuhara K, Kawamoto S, Wakabayashi T, Belsky JL: Situs inversus totalis and Kartagener's syndrome in a Japanese population. *Chest* **61**:56, 1972.
17. Ernstson S, Afzelius BA, Mossberg B: Otological manifestations of the immotile cilia syndrome. *Acta Otolaryngol (Stockh)* **97**:83, 1984.
18. Kartagener M, Horlacher A: Zur Pathogenese der Bronchiektasien, Situs viscerum inversus and Polyposis nasi in einem Falle familiarer Bronchiektisien. *Beitr Klin Tuberk* **87**:331, 1935.
19. Perone PM: Situs viscerum inversus, bronchiettasie e sinusiti: Tre casi di sindrome di Kartagener. *Arch Ital Otolaryngol* **67**:653, 1956.
20. Overholt EL, Banman DF: Variants of Kartagener's syndrome in the same family. *Ann Intern Med* **48**:547, 1958.
21. Logan WD, Abbott OA, Hatcher CR: Kartagener's triad. *Dis Chest* **48**:613, 1965.
22. Weaver A, Hard R: Isolation of newt lung ciliated cell models. *Cell Motil* **5**:355, 1985.
23. Sleigh M, Blake JR, Liron N: The propulsion of mucus by cilia. *Am Rev Respir Dis* **137**:726, 1988.
24. Satir P: Dynein as a microtubule translocator in ciliary motility. *Cell Motil Cytoskel* **10**:263, 1988.
25. Sturgess J: Mucous secretion in the respiratory tract. *Pediatr Clin North Am* **26**:481, 1979.
26. Lindemann CB, Kanous KS: A model for flagellar motility. *Int Rev Cytol* **173**:1, 1997.
27. Goodenough UW, Heuser JE: Outer and inner dynein arms of cilia and flagella. *Cell* **41**:341, 1985.
28. Fujita H: Fine structure of the thyroid gland. *Int Rev Cytol* **40**:197, 1975.
29. Svedbergh B, Bill A: Scanning electron microscopic studies of the corneal epithelium in man and monkeys. *Acta Ophthalmol (Copenh)* **50**:321, 1972.
30. Odor DL, Blandau RJ: Observations on the solitary cilium of rabbit oviductal epithelium: Its motility and ultrastructure. *Am J Anat* **174**:437, 1985.
31. Grimfeld JA, Tournier G, Jouannet P, Bisson JP, Salomon JL, Baculard A, Gerbeaux J: Immotile cilia syndrome in infants and children. *Thorax* **34**:709, 1979.
32. Jahrsdoerfer R, Feldman PS, Rubel EW, Guerrant JL, Eggleston PA, Selden RF: Otitis media and the immotile cilia syndrome. *Laryngoscope* **89**:769, 1979.
33. Afzelius BA, Eliasson R: Flagellar mutants in man: On the heterogeneity of the immotile cilia syndrome. *J Ultrastruct Res* **69**:43, 1979.
34. Schneeberger EE, McCormack J, Issenberg H, Schuster SR, Gerald PS: Heterogeneity of ciliary morphology in the immotile-cilia syndrome in man. *J Ultrastruct Res* **73**:34, 1980.
35. Pedersen H, Rebbe H: Absence of arms in the axoneme of immobile human spermatozoa. *Biol Reprod* **12**:541, 1975.
36. Corkey CWB, Levison H, Turner JAP: The immotile cilia syndrome: A longitudinal survey. *Am Rev Respir Dis* **124**:544, 1981.

37. Escalier D, Jouannet P, David G: Abnormalities of the ciliary axonemal complex in children. *Biol Cell* **44**:271, 1982.
38. Levison H, Mindorff CM, Chao J, Turner JAP, Sturgess JM, Stringer DA: Pathophysiology of the ciliary motility syndromes. *Eur J Respir Dis* **64**(suppl 127):102, 1983.
39. Van Der Baan S, Veerman AJP, Bezemer PD, Feenstra L: Primary ciliary dyskinesia. *Ann Otol Rhinol Laryngol*: **96**:264, 1987.
40. Barlocco EG, Valletta EA, Canciano M, Lungarella G, Gardi C, de Santi MM, Mastella G: Ultrastructural ciliary defects in children with recurrent infections of the lower respiratory tract. *Pediatr Pulmonol* **10**:17, 1991.
41. David G, Serres C, Escalier D: Cinematique du spermatozoide humain. *Ann Endocrinol (Paris)* **42**:391, 1982.
42. Woodring JH, Royer JM, McDonagh D: Kartagener's syndrome. *JAMA* **247**:2814, 1982.
43. Nielsen MH, Pedersen M, Christensen B, Mygind N: Blind quantitative electron microscopy of cilia from patients with primary ciliary dyskinesia and from normal subjects. *Eur J Respir Dis* **64**(suppl 127):19, 1983.
44. Chabrolle JP, Euziere P, Bigel P, Blondet P: Syndrome d'immotilite ciliaire chez un enfant de 10 ans. *Arch Fr Pediatr*: **39**:235, 1982.
45. Sturgess JM, Chao J, Turner JAP: Cilia with defective radial spokes: A cause of human respiratory disease. *N Engl J Med* **300**:53, 1979.
46. Sturgess JM, Thompson MW, Czegledy-Nagy E, Turner JAP: Genetic aspects of immotile cilia syndrome. *Am J Med Genet* **25**:149, 1986.
47. Sturgess JM, Chao J, Turner JAP: Transposition of ciliary microtubules. Another cause of impaired ciliary motility. *N Engl J Med* **303**:318, 1980.
48. Neustein HB, Nickerson B, O'Neil M: Kartagener's syndrome with absence of inner dynein arms of respiratory cilia. *Am Rev Respir Dis* **122**:979, 1980.
49. Salomon JL, Grimfeld A, Tournier G, Baculard A, Escalier D, Jouannet P, David G: Ciliary disorders of the bronchi in children. *Rev Fr Malad Respir* **11**:645, 1983.
50. Herzon FS, Murphy S: Normal ciliary ultrastructure in children with Kartagener's syndrome. *Ann Otol Rhinol Laryngol* **89**:81, 1980.
51. Greenstone M, Dewar A, Mackay I, Cole PJ: Primary ciliary dyskinesia—Cytological and clinical features. *Q J Med* **67**:40, 1988.
52. Pedersen M, Stafanger G: Bronchopulmonary symptoms in primary ciliary dyskinesia. *Eur J Respir Dis* **64**(suppl 127):118, 1983.
53. Afzelius BA, Gargani G, Romano C: Abnormal length of cilia as a cause of defective mucociliary clearance. *Eur J Respir Dis*: **66**:173, 1985.
54. Dudley JP, Waelch MJ, Carney JM, Stiehm ER, Soderber M: Scanning and transmission electron microscopic aspects of the nasal acilia syndrome. *Laryngoscope* **92**:297, 1982.
55. de Santi MM, Gardi C, Barlocco G, Canciani M, Mastella G, Lungarella G: Cilia-lacking respiratory cells in ciliary aplasia. *Biol Cell* **64**:67, 1988.
56. de Santi MM, Magni A, Valletta EA, Gardi C, Lungarella G: Hydrocephalus, bronchiectasis, and ciliary aplasia. *Arch Dis Child* **65**:543, 1990.
57. Fonzi L, Lungarella G, Palatresi R: Lack of kinocilia in the nasal mucosa. *Eur J Respir Dis* **63**:558, 1982.
58. Gordon RE, Kattan M: Absence of cilia and basal bodies with predominance of brush cells in the respiratory mucosa from a patient with immotile cilia syndrome. *Ultrastruct Pathol* **6**:45, 1984.
59. Cereso L, Price G: Absence of cilia and basal bodies with predominance of brush cells in the respiratory mucosa from a patient with immotile cilia syndrome. *Ultrastruct Pathol* **8**:381, 1985.
60. Holley MC, Afzelius BA: Alignment of cilia in immotile cilia syndrome. *Tissue Cell* **18**:521, 1986.
61. de Iongh R, Rutland J: Orientation of respiratory tract cilia in patients with primary ciliary dyskinesia, bronchiectasis, and in normal subjects. *J Clin Pathol* **42**:613, 1989.
62. Rautiainen M, Collan Y, Nuutinen J, Afzelius BA: Ciliary orientation in the immotile cilia syndrome. *Eur Arch Otorhinolaryngol* **247**:100, 1990.
63. Rayner CF, Rutman A, Dewar A, Greenstone MA, Cole PJ, Wilson R: Ciliary disorientation alone as a cause of primary ciliary dyskinesia syndrome. *Am J Respir Crit Care Med* **153**:1123, 1996.
64. Camner P, Afzelius BA, Eliasson R, Mossberg B: Relation between abnormalities of human sperm flagella and respiratory tract disease. *Int J Androl* **2**:211, 1979.
65. Turner JAP, Corkey CWB, Lee JYC, Levison H, Sturgess JM: Clinical expression of immotile cilia syndrome. *Pediatrics* **67**:805, 1981.
66. Fox B, Bull TB, Makey AR, Rawbone R: The significance of ultrastructural abnormalities of human cilia. *Chest* **80**(suppl):796, 1981.
67. Hilding AC: The relation of ciliary insufficiency to death from asthma and other respiratory diseases. *Ann Otol Rhinol Laryngol*: **52**:5, 1943.
68. Camner P, Jarstrand C, Philipson K: Tracheobronchial clearance in patients with influenza. *Am Rev Respir Dis* **108**:131, 1973.
69. Pedersen M, Sakakura Y, Winther B, Brofeldt S, Mygind N: Nasal mucociliary transport, number of ciliated cells, and beating pattern in naturally acquired colds. *Eur J Respir Dis* **64**(suppl 128):355, 1983.
70. Pedersen M: Specific types of abnormal ciliary motility in Kartagener's syndrome and analogous respiratory disorders. *Eur J Respir Dis* **64**(suppl 127):78, 1983.
71. Lungarella G, Fonzi L, Burrini AG: Ultrastructural abnormalities in respiratory cilia and sperm tails in a patient with Kartagener's syndrome. *Ultrastruct Pathol* **3**:319, 1982.
72. Escudier E, Escalier D, Pinchon MC, Boucherat M, Bernaudin JF, Fleuryfeith J: Dissimilar expression of axonemal anomalies in respiratory cilia and sperm flagella in infertile men. *Am Rev Respir Dis* **142**:674, 1990.
73. Walt H, Campana A, Balerna M, Domenighetti G, Hedinger C, Jakob M, Pescia G, Sulmoni A: Mosaicism of dynein in spermatozoa and cilia and fibrous sheath aberrations in an infertile man. *Andrologia* **15**:295, 1983.
74. Jonsson MS, McCormick JR, Gillies CG, Gondos B: Kartagener's syndrome with motile spermatozoa. *N Engl J Med* **307**:1131, 1982.
75. Afzelius BA: Immotile cilia syndrome and ciliary abnormalities induced by infection and injury. *Am Rev Respir Dis* **124**:107, 1981.
76. Cornille FJ, Lauweryns JM, Corbeel L: Atypical bronchial cilia in children with recurrent respiratory tract infections. *Pathol Res Pract* **178**:595, 1984.
77. Konradova V, Hlouskova Z, Tomanek A: Atypical kinocilia in human epithelium from large bronchus. *Folia Morphol (Praha)* **23**:293, 1975.
78. Takasaka T, Sato M, Onodera A: Atypical cilia in the human mucosa. *Ann Otol Rhinol Laryngol* **89**:37, 1980.
79. Veerman AJP, van Delden L, Feenstra L, Leene W: The immotile cilia syndrome: Phase contrast light microscopy, scanning and transmission electron microscopy. *Pediatrics* **65**:698, 1980.
80. Rutland J, Cole PJ: Non-invasive sampling of nasal cilia for measurement of beat frequency and study of ultrastructure. *Lancet* **2**:564, 1980.
81. Rossman CM, Forrest JB, Lee RMKW, Newhouse MT: The dyskinetic cilia syndrome: Ciliary motility in immotile cilia syndrome. *Chest* **78**:580, 1980.
82. Pedersen M, Mygind N: Ciliary motility in the immotile cilia syndrome. *Br J Dis Chest* **74**:239, 1980.
83. Sturgess JM, Turner JAP: Ultrastructural pathology of cilia in the immotile cilia syndrome. *Perspect Pediatr Pathol* **8**:133, 1984.
84. Rossman CM, Forrest JB, Lee RMKW, Newhouse AF, Newhouse MT: The dyskinetic cilia syndrome. *Chest* **80**:860, 1981.
85. Rossman CM, Lee RMKW, Forrest JB, Newhouse MT: Nasal ciliary ultrastructure and function in patients with primary ciliary dyskinesia compared with that in normal subjects and in subjects with various respiratory diseases. *Am Rev Respir Dis* **129**:161, 1984.
86. Camner P, Mossberg B, Afzelius BA: Evidence for congenitally non-functioning cilia in the tracheobronchial tract in two subjects. *Am Rev Respir Dis* **112**:807, 1975.
87. Palmblad J, Mossberg B, Afzelius BA: Ultrastructural, cellular, and clinical features of the immotile cilia syndrome. *Annu Rev Med* **35**:481, 1984.
88. Nuutinen J, Karja J, Karjalainen P: Measurements of impaired mucociliary activity in children. *Eur J Respir Dis* **64**:454, 1983.
89. Mossberg B, Afzelius BA, Eliasson R, Camner P: On the pathogenesis of obstructive lung disease: A study in the immotile cilia syndrome. *Scand J Respir Dis* **59**:55, 1978.
90. Jorissen M, Van der Schueren, Van der Berghe H, Cassiman JJ: Ciliogenesis and coordinated ciliary beating in human nasal epithelial cells cultured in vitro. *Acta Otorhinolaryngol Belg* **43**:67, 1990.
91. Boat TF, Wood RE, Tandler B, Stern RC, Orenstein DM, Doershuk CF: A screening test for the immotile cilia syndrome. *Pediatr Res* **13**:531, 1979.
92. Pedersen M, Nielsen MH, Mygind N: Primary ciliary dyskinesia. *Mod Probl Paediatr* **21**:68, 1982.
93. Van Der Baan S, Veerman AJP, Wulffraat N, Bezemer PD, Feenstra L: Primary ciliary dyskinesia. *Acta Otolaryngol (Stockh)* **102**:274, 1986.

94. Nonaka S, Tanaka Y, Okada Y, Takeda S, Harada A, Kanai Y, Kido M, Hirokawa N: Randomization of left-right asymmetry due to loss of nodal cilia generating leftward flow of extraembryonic fluid in mice lacking KIF3B motor protein. *Cell* **95**:829, 1999.
95. Brueckner M, D'Eustachio P, Horwich AL: Linkage mapping of a mouse gene, *iv*, that controls left-right asymmetry of the heart and viscera. *Proc Natl Acad Sci USA* **86**:5035, 1989.
96. Supp DM, Potter S, Brueckner M: Molecular motors: The driving force behind mammalian left-right development. *Trend Cell Biol* **10**:41, 2000.
97. Eavey RD, Nadol JB, Holmes LB, Laird NM, Lapey A, Joseph MP, Strome M: Kartagener's syndrome: A blinded, controlled study of cilia ultrastructure. *Arch Otolaryngol Head Neck Surg* **112**:646, 1986.
98. Antonelli M, Modesti A, Quattrini A, De Angelis M: Supernumerary microtubules in the respiratory cilia of two sibs. *Eur J Respir Dis* **64**:607, 1983.
99. Moreno A, Murphy EA: Inheritance of Kartagener syndrome. *Am JMed Genet* **8**:305, 1981.
100. Narayan D, Krishnan SN, Upender M, Ravikumar TS, Mahoney MJ, Dolan TF, Teebi AS, Haddad GG: Unusual inheritance of primary ciliary dyskinesia (Kartagener's syndrome). *J Med Genet* **31**:493, 1994.
101. Dutcher SK, Lux FG: Genetic interactions of mutations affecting flagella and basal bodies in Chlamydomonas. *Cell Motil Cytoskel* **14**:104, 1989.
101a. Pennarun G, Escudier E, Chapelin C, Bridoux A-M, Cacheux V, Roger G, Clément A, Goossens M, Amselem S, Duriez B: Loss-of-function mutations in a human gene related to *Chlamydomonas reinhandtii* dynein IC78 result in primary ciliary dyskinesia. *Am J Hum Genet* **65**:1508, 1999.
102. Torgersen J: Genic factors in visceral asymmetry and in the development and pathologic changes of lungs, heart and abdominal organs. *Arch Pathol* **47**:566, 1949.
103. Camner P, Mossberg B, Afzelius BA: Measurements of tracheobronchial clearance in patients with immotile-cilia syndrome and its value in differential diagnosis. *Eur J Respir Dis* **64**(suppl 127):57, 1983.
104. Stanley P, McWilliam L, Greenstone M, Mackay I, Cole PJ: Efficacy of a saccharin test for screening to detect abnormal mucociliary clearance. *Br J Dis Chest*: **78**:62, 1984.
105. Canciani M, Barlocco EG, Mastella G, de Santi MM, Gardi C, Lungarella G: The saccharin method for testing mucociliary function in patients suspected of having primary ciliary dyskinesia. *Pediatr Pulmonol* **5**:210, 1988.
106. Lindberg S, Cervin A, Runer T: Low levels of nasal nitric oxide (NO) correlate to impaired mucociliary function in the upper airways. *Acta Otolar (Stockh)* **117**:728, 1997.
107. Burgersdijk FJA, De Groot JCMJ, Graamans K, Rademakers LHPM: Testing ciliary activity in patients with chronic and recurrent infections of the upper airways. *Laryngoscope* **96**:1029, 1986.
108. Chapelin C, Coste A, Reiner P, Boucherat M, Millepied M-C, Poron F, Escudier E: Incidence of primary ciliary dyskinesia in children with recurrent respiratory diseases. *Ann Otol Rhinol Laryngol* **106**:854, 1997.
109. Nielsen MH, Pedersen M, Christensen B, Mygind N: Blind quantitative electron microscopy of cilia from patients with primary ciliary dyskinesia and from normal subjects. *Eur J Respir Dis* **64**(suppl 127):19, 1983.
110. Kollberg H, Mossberg B, Afzelius BA, Philipson K, Camner P: Cystic fibrosis compared with the immotile cilia syndrome: A study of mucociliary clearance, ciliary ultrastructure, clinical picture and ventilatory function. *Scand J Respir Dis*: **59**:297, 1978.
111. Lundberg JON, Weitzberg E, Nordvall SL, Kuylenstierna R, Lundberg JM, Alving K: Primary nasal origin of exhaled nitric oxide and absence in Kartagener's syndrome. *Eur Respir J* **7**:1501, 1994.
112. Mossberg B, Björkander J, Afzelius BA, Camner P: Mucociliary clearance in patients with immunoglobulin deficiency. *Eur J Respir Dis* **63**:570, 1982.
113. Handelsman DJ, Conway AJ, Boylan LM, Turtle JR: Young's syndrome: Obstructive azoospermia and chronic sinopulmonary infections. *N Engl J Med* **310**:3, 1984.
114. Mossberg B, Camner P, Afzelius BA: The immotile cilia syndrome compared to other obstructive lung diseases: A clue to their pathogenesis. *Eur J Respir Dis* **64**(suppl 127):129, 1983.
115. Whitelaw A, Evans A, Corrin B: Immotile cilia syndrome: A new cause of neonatal respiratory distress. *Arch Dis Child*: **56**:432, 1981.
116. Mygind N, Pedersen M: Nose-, sinus-, and ear-symptoms in 27 patients with primary ciliary dyskinesia. *Eur J Respir Dis* **64**(suppl 127):96, 1983.
117. Van Der Baan S: Primary ciliary dyskinesia and the middle ear. *Laryngoscope*: **101**:751, 1991.
118. Pedersen M, Mygind N: Rhinitis, sinusitis and otitis media in Kartagener's syndrome. *Clin Otolaryngol* **7**:373, 1983.
119. Ellerman A, Bisgaaard H: Longitudinal study of lung function in a cohort of primary ciliary dyskinesia. *Eur Respir J* **10**:2376, 1997.
120. Kartagener M, Stucki P: Bronchiectasis with situs inversus. *Arch Pediatr* **79**:193, 1962.
121. Mossberg B, Hanngren Å: Kartagener's syndrome: A ciliary immotility syndrome. *Mt Sinai J Med* **44**:837, 1977.
122. Evander E, Arborelius M, Jonson B, Simonsson BG, Svensson G: Lung function and bronchial reactivity in six patients with immotile cilia syndrome. *Eur J Respir Dis* **64**(suppl 127):137, 1983.
123. Mossberg B, Afzelius BA, Camner P: Mucociliary clearance in obstructive lung diseases: Correlations to the immotile cilia syndrome. *Eur J Respir Dis* **69**(suppl 146):295, 1986.
124. Nadel HR, Stringer DA, Levison H, Turner JAP, Sturgess J: The immotile cilia syndrome: Radiological manifestations. *Radiology* **154**:651, 1985.
125. Svedbergh B, Johnsson V, Afzelius BA: Immotile cilia syndrome and the cilia of the eye. *Graefes Arch Klin Exp Ophthalmol* **215**:265, 1981.
126. Bonneau D, Raymond F, Kremer C, Klossek JM, Kaplan J, Patte F: Usher syndrome type-1 associated with bronchiectasis and immotile nasal cilia in two brothers. *J Med Genet* **30**:253, 1993.
127. Hunter DG, Fishman GA, Kretzer FL: Abnormal axonemes in X-linked retinitis pigmentosa. *Arch Ophthalmol* **106**:362, 1988.
128. Ohga H, Suzuki T, Fujiwara H, Furutani A, Koga H: A case of immotile cilia syndrome accompanied by retinitis pigmentosa. *Acta Soc Ophthalmol Jpn* **89**:795, 1991.
129. Van Dorp DB, Wright AF, Carothers AD, Bleeker-Wagemakers EM: A family with RP3 type of X-linked retinitis pigmentosa: An association with ciliary abnormalities. *Hum Genet* **88**:331, 1992.
130. Fox B, Bull TB, Arden GB: Variations in the ultrastructure of human nasal cilia including abnormalities found in retinitis pigmentosa. *J Clin Pathol* **33**:327, 1980.
131. Gentleman S, Kaiser-Kupfer MI, Sherins RJ, Caruso R, Robison WG, Lloyd-Muhammad RA, Crawford MA, Pikus A, Chader GJ: Ultrastructural and biochemical analysis of sperm flagella from an infertile man with rod-dominant retinal degeneration. *Hum Pathol* **27**:80, 1996.
132. Glick ID, Graubert DN: Kartagener's syndrome and schizophrenia: A report of a case with chromosomal studies. *Am J Psychol* **121**:603, 1964.
133. Zammarchi E, Calzolari C, Pignotti MS, Pezzati P, Lignana E, Cama A: Unusual presentation of the immotile cilia syndrome in two children. *Acta Paediatr* **82**:312, 1993.
134. Greenstone MA, Jones RWA, Dewar A, Neville BGR: Hydrocephalus and primary ciliary dyskinesia. *Arch Dis Child* **59**:481, 1984.
135. Roth Y, Baum GL, Tadmor R: Brain dysfunction in primary ciliary dyskinesia? *Acta Neurol Scand* **78**:353, 1988.
136. Zumbusch von A, Fiedler K, Meyerhofer A, Jessberger B, Ring J, Vogt HJ: Birth of healthy children after intracytoplasmic sperm injection in two couples with male Kartagener's syndrome. *Fertil Steril* **70**:643, 1998.
137. Pellnitz D, Heyland S: Beitrag zur Kartagenerschen Trias (Situs inversus, Bronchiektasis und Nasenpolypen). *HNO* **3**:41, 1952.
138. Bashi S, Khan MA, Guirjis A, Joharjy IA, Abid MA: Immotile cilia syndrome with azoospermia: A case report and review of the literature. *Br J Dis Chest* **82**:194, 1988.
139. Matwijiw I, Thliveris JA, Faiman C: Aplasia of nasal cilia with situs inversus, azoospermia and normal sperm flagella: A unique variant of the immotile cilia syndrome. *J Urol* **137**:522, 1987.
140. Gagnon C, Sherins RJ, Mann T, Bardin W, Amelar RD, Dubin L: Deficiency of protein carboxyl-methylase in spermatozoa of necrospermia patients, in Steinberger A, Steinberger E (eds): *Testicular Development, Structure, and Functions*. New York, Raven Press, 1980, p 491.
141. Afzelius BA, Camner P, Mossberg B: On the function of cilia in the female reproductive tract. *Fertil Steril* **29**:72, 1978.
142. Bleau G, Richer C-L, Bousquet D: Absence of dynein arms in cilia of endocervical cells in a fertile woman. *Fertil Steril* **30**:362, 1978.
143. Lurie M, Tur-Kaspa I, Weill S, Katz I, Rabinovici J, Goldenberg S: Ciliary ultrastructure of respiratory and fallopian tube epithelium in a sterile woman with Kartagener's syndrome. *Chest* **95**:578, 1989.
144. McComb P, Langley L, Villalon M, Verdugo P: The oviductal cilia and Kartagener's syndrome. *Fertil Steril* **46**:412, 1986.

145. Mouriquand P: Dyskinesie ciliaire primitive: Une revue generale. Consequences sur la fertilite. Thesis, University of Lyon, 1985.
146. Jean Y, Langlais J, Roberts KD, Chapdelaine A, Bleau G: Fertility in a woman with non-functional ciliated cells in the fallopian tubes. *Fertil Steril* **31**:349, 1979.
147. Miller RD, Divertie MB: Kartagener's syndrome. *Chest* **62**:130, 1972.
148. Afzelius BA, Ewetz L, Palmblad J, Uden A-M, Venizelos N: Structure and function of neutrophil leukocytes from patients with the immotile cilia syndrome. *Acta Med Scand* **208**:145, 1980.
149. Walter RJ, Malech HL, Oliver JM: Cell motility and microtubules in cultured fibroblasts from patients with Kartagener's syndrome. *Cell Motil* **3**:185, 1983.
150. Valerius NH, Knudsen BB, Pedersen M: Defective neutrophil motility in patients with primary ciliary dyskinesia. *Eur J Clin Invest* **13**:489, 1983.
151. Wolburg H, Dopfer R, Schieferstein G, Thiel E: Immotile cilia syndrome: Reduced chemotaxis and reduced number of intramembranous particles in granulocytes. *Klin Wochenschr* **62**:1044, 1984.
152. Brenner S, Tur E, Fishel B, Alkan M, Topilsky M: Cutaneous manifestations and impaired chemotaxis of polymorphonuclear leukocytes associated with Kartagener's syndrome. *Dermatologica* **183**:251, 1991.
153. Conway DJ: A congenital factor in bronchiectasis. *Arch Dis Child* **26**:253, 1951.
154. Sielicka-Zuber L, Ficer J: Zespol Kartagener. *Przegl Dermatol* **61**:171, 1974.
155. Smit HJM, Scheurs AJM, Van der Bosch MM, Westermann JJ: Is resection of bronchiectasis beneficial in patients with primary ciliary dyskinesis? *Chest* **109**:1541, 1996.
156. Miralles A, Muneretto C, Gandjbakheh I, Lecompte Y, Pavie A, Rabago G, Bracomonte L, Desruennes M, Cabrol A, Cabrol C: Heart-lung transplantation in situs inversus: A case report in a patient with Kartagener's syndrome. *J Thorac Cardiovasc Surg* **103**:307, 1992.
157. Macchiarini P, Chapelier A, Vouve P, Cerrina J, Ladurie FL, Parquin F, Brenot F, Simonneau G. Dartevelle P, Herve P: Double lung transplantation in situs inversus with Kartagener syndrome. *J Thorac Cardiovasc Surg* **108**:86, 1994.
158. Amjad H, Richburg FD, Adler E: Kartagener's syndrome: Case report in an elderly man. *JAMA* **227**:1420, 1974.

CHAPTER 188

Leukocyte Adhesion Deficiencies

Donald C. Anderson ■ C. Wayne Smith

1. A cascade of adhesive events is needed for efficient localization of leukocytes at foci of inflammation. Members of the selectin family of glycoproteins are required for primary adhesion of flowing leukocytes interacting with endothelial cells at venular shear rates. L-selectin (CD62L) is expressed constitutively on neutrophils, monocytes, eosinophils, and subsets of lymphocytes and binds to carbohydrate ligands on endothelial cells and other leukocytes. E-selectin (CD62E) is not constitutively expressed by endothelial cells but is up-regulated following stimulation with inflammatory cytokines such as IL-1. P-selectin (CD62P) is found in α granules of platelets and Wiebel-Palade bodies of venular endothelial cells, and is rapidly up-regulated to the luminal surface following stimulation (e.g., with histamine). The selectins bind to sialylated and fucosylated carbohydrate ligands on cell surface glycoproteins. This interaction at venular shear rates results in rolling of leukocytes along the endothelium. Stationary adhesion and transendothelial migration of leukocytes depends on the interaction of integrins on the leukocyte surface with ligands on the endothelial cells. The integrins of greatest importance to neutrophils are Mac-1 (CD11b/CD18) and LFA-1 (CD11a/CD18), members of the β_2 integrin family. Cell activation is required for effective transition from selectin-dependent rolling to stable integrin-dependent adhesion. Chemotactic substances on the surface of endothelial cells (e.g., IL-8 and platelet-activating factor) stimulate this activation. Intercellular adhesion molecule-1 (CD54) is the principal ligand on endothelial cells for these integrins. It is constitutively expressed on venular endothelium and is markedly up-regulated by stimulation of these cells with inflammatory cytokines. Blockade or absence of individual components can interrupt this cascade of events. Failure of the selectin-dependent step results in failure of leukocytes to effectively bind to endothelial cells, with consequent failure of effective emigration. Failure of the integrin-dependent step allows rolling of leukocytes, but emigration is again prevented.
2. Aberrations in adhesive mechanisms account for several clinical syndromes that involve an increase in susceptibility to bacterial infection. Leukocyte adhesion deficiency I (LAD I) (MIM 116920) was the first to be defined at a molecular level; it results from mutations in CD18, the β subunit of β_2 integrins, leading to partial or complete absence of expression, or dysfunction of these integrins. In addition to their role in neutrophil emigration, these integrins serve additional functions in host defense against infection. LFA-1 is involved in costimulation of lymphocytes during antigen presentation. Mac-1 functions as a receptor for complement opsonized bacteria, enhancing phagocytosis and bactericidal mechanisms (e.g., enhanced reactive oxygen production). Patients with LAD I appear to fall into two phenotypes. The severe phenotype occurs when CD18 expression is absent or extremely low. These patients are subject to overwhelming, life-threatening bacterial infections. The moderate phenotype occurs when either CD18 expression is very low or CD18 integrins are dysfunctional. These patients exhibit increased susceptibility to bacterial infections, but most have survived to adulthood. Numerous CD18 mutations have been defined, and patients are often compound heterozygotes, with differing mutations from the maternal and paternal alleles.
3. A second type of leukocyte adhesion deficiency, called LAD II (MIM 266265), results from dysfunction of the selectin pathway of adhesion. This syndrome results from a general defect in fucose metabolism, causing an absence of key carbohydrate ligands for the selectins [e.g., sialylated Lewis X (sLeX)]. Abnormalities in the inflammatory process are consistent with failure of normal selectin functions. Neutrophils fail to exhibit the typical rolling behavior required for effective localization at sites of inflammation, and skin infections without pus have been observed. While these patients have increased susceptibility to infections, particularly early in life, infections have not been life-threatening as is the case with the LAD I severe phenotype. The exact defect in the *de novo* pathway of fucose production from GDP-mannose to GDP-fucose is not known with certainty, but recent evidence indicates that in cell lysates from a LAD II patient, GDP-D-mannose-4, 6-dehydratase (GMD), the first of the two enzymes of the pathway, has defective activity when compared to control subjects.
4. Two additional patient populations with defective adhesion have been described. One involves neonatal neutrophils, which exhibit defects in adhesion that may enhance susceptibility to infection. Both selectin and integrin adhesive pathways seem to be involved. Specifically,

A list of standard abbreviations is located immediately preceding the index in each volume. Additional abbreviations used in this chapter include: C = complement (e.g., C5a, iC3b, etc.); CD = leukocyte differentiation antigens (e.g., CD11a, CD18, etc.); CLA = cutaneous leukocyte antigen; CR = complement receptor (e.g., CR1, CR3, etc.); Fc = constant immunoglobulin fragment; GM-CSF = granulocyte/monocyte-colony stimulating factor; HEV = high-endothelial venule; HUVEC = human umbilical-vein endothelial cell; ICAM = intercellular adhesion molecule, also ICAM-1, ICAM-2, etc.; IFN = interferon, also IFN; KLH = keyhole limpet hemocyanin; LAD I, LAD II = leukocyte adhesion deficiency types I and II; LFA-1 = lymphocyte function-associated antigen-1; Mac-1 = macrophage-1; MoMuLV = Maloney murine leukemia virus; NCAM = neural cell adhesion molecule; NK cell = natural killer cell; PAF = platelet-activating factor; PSGL-1 = P-selectin glycoprotein ligand-1; SCR = short consensus repeat; sLeX = sialyl Lewis X; TNF = tumor necrosis factor; VCAM = vascular cell adhesion molecule; VLA = very late activation antigen, also VLA-4, etc.

L-selectin levels on neutrophils are significantly reduced compared with adults, and L-selectin contributions to rolling of leukocytes on endothelial cells under flow conditions are significantly reduced. In addition, there are deficits involving Mac-1. The up-regulation of Mac-1 function following chemotactic stimulation is significantly reduced compared with adult neutrophils. There is reduced adhesion to endothelial cells and to ligands recognized by Mac-1. Total cellular levels of Mac-1 appear to be reduced in neonates. Another syndrome associated with defective adhesion is specific granule deficiency (MIM 245480). Several granule populations have been defined in neutrophils, and some, such as specific granules (also called secondary granules), contain preformed adhesion molecules that can be mobilized to the cell surface following stimulation (e.g., chemotactic stimulation). Leukocytes deficient in specific granules also lack secondary granule markers (lactoferrin, B_{12} transport protein, cytochrome b, and lysozyme). There is defective chemotaxis as well as defective accumulation of neutrophils at sites of inflammation, and increased susceptibility to infection. This is a complex abnormality involving much more than simply a deficit in adhesion, and the underlying molecular mechanisms remain obscure.

5. **Animal models with leukocyte adhesion deficiencies have been developed. Targeted deletions of each of the selectins and CD18 integrins in mice reveal inflammatory deficits when animals are specifically challenged. All animals deficient in these specific adhesion molecules are viable and fertile, and only two of the mutations to date have resulted in phenotypes with spontaneous infections of animals maintained in barrier facilities. The CD18-deficient mice mimic most of the features of LAD I, but selective deficiencies of LFA-1 and Mac-1 do not. Mice with combined deficiency of E-selectin and P-selectin develop a syndrome sharing aspects of the inflammatory deficits of patients with LAD II.**

MECHANISMS OF LEUKOCYTE-ENDOTHELIAL INTERACTIONS

The mobility of leukocytes is clearly dependent on two major factors. The first is the flow of blood transporting unstimulated neutrophils throughout the distribution of circulating blood. The second is the adhesion of neutrophils to endothelial cells at sites of leukocyte emigration. This adhesion must be of sufficient strength to initially withstand the shear forces of flowing blood, and then to control the movement of neutrophils through the blood vessel wall. Recent advances reveal a cascade of events where different classes of adhesion molecules play distinct and critical roles that ultimately lead to the emigration of neutrophils at sites of inflammation. The discussion that follows presents some details regarding the molecules involved and their respective roles with special emphasis on neutrophils and other factors relevant to clinical syndromes of leukocyte adhesion deficiencies.

Adhesion Molecules

The CD18 (β_2) Integrins. LFA-1 (CD11a/CD18), Mac-1 (CD11b/CD18) and p150,95 (CD11c/CD18) and αd/CD18 are structurally related $\alpha\beta$ heterodimers which share a common β subunit[1,2] (see Table 188-1). The CD18 integrins are, in turn, related to a larger family of integrin adhesion molecules that include primarily extracellular matrix receptors such as the fibronectin receptor, vitronectin receptor, and platelet glycoprotein IIb-IIIa. The α subunits of the CD18 integrins, like other integrins, contain multiple divalent cation-binding domains which are similar to the Ca^{2+}-binding domains of calmodulin and troponin C.[3–6] Not surprisingly, CD18 adhesion functions are Mg^{2+}- and Ca^{2+}-dependent. The leukocyte integrin α subunits contain a domain, designated "I" or "inserted" domain, which is homologous to similar domains found in von Willebrand factor, complement proteins C2 and B, and cartilage matrix protein. The leukocyte integrin β subunit, like other integrin β subunits, is a cysteine-rich transmembrane protein, with a fourfold repeat of an unusual cysteine motif.[7,8] The crystal structures of the I domains of the α subunits of Mac-1 and LFA-1 show that a conserved cation-binding site is present in each protein. Purified recombinant I domains have intrinsic ligand binding activity. For example, recombinant I domain of CD11b is sufficient to bind to specific peptides in the fibrinogen sequence,[9] and the I domain of integrin LFA-1 interacts with domain 1 of intercellular adhesion molecule-1 (ICAM-1, CD54).[10] In several systems, interactions of the I domain with ligands has been demonstrated to be cation-dependent.[11] The α subunit of Mac-1 contains several distinct regions in its extracellular segment. The N-terminal region has been predicted to fold into a β-propeller domain composed of seven β-sheets, each approximately 60-amino-acid residues long, with the I-domain inserted between β sheets 2 and 3.[12]

CD18 integrin expression is restricted to white blood cells. LFA-1 is expressed by lymphocytes, monocytes, and granulocytes, whereas Mac-1 (also referred to as complement receptor 3 or CR3),[13] and p150,95 (also referred to as CR4)[14] are primarily restricted to myeloid cells, although they are also expressed by some lymphocytes and NK cells. The most recently discovered member of this family, αd/CD18,[2] is restricted to myeloid cells, recently being identified on eosinophils.[15] The CD18 integrins have a broad role in many leukocyte adhesion-related functions. LFA-1 is implicated in cell-mediated cytolysis, antigen presentation, lymphocyte homotypic aggregation, and leukocyte adhesion to a variety of cytokine-activated cells, including endothelial cells as reviewed elsewhere.[1] Mac-1 is implicated in neutrophil homotypic aggregation, adhesion to substrates, binding and phagocytosis of iC3b-coated particles, adhesion-dependent respiratory burst, neutrophil locomotion, and leukocyte adhesion to cytokine-activated cells.

Both LFA-1 and Mac-1 mediate adhesion through multiple ligands. LFA-1 binds to the intercellular adhesion molecules ICAM-1,[16] ICAM-2,[17] and ICAM-3.[18] Mac-1 also binds to ICAM-1,[19] although at a site distinct from that of LFA-1.[20] In addition, Mac-1 recognizes a wide spectrum of unrelated molecules, including the iC3b fragment of complement, fibrinogen, factor X, and several microbial antigens. The molecular basis for the promiscuous nature of ligand recognition is not defined.[1] ICAM-3 serves as a ligand for αd/CD18.[12]

CD18 Regulation. The broad range of functions that the CD18 integrins mediate requires that the functional activity of these receptors be regulated to prevent inappropriate adhesion. Mac-1 (CD11b/CD18) can be regulated both quantitatively and qualitatively. It is stored in intracellular granules of neutrophils and monocytes,[21] and upon stimulation with low levels of chemotactic agents, is rapidly recruited to the cell surface, resulting in a three- to tenfold increase in the quantity of Mac-1 on the cell surface. In addition, the functional activity of Mac-1 is qualitatively regulated by chemoattractant-induced activation of neutrophils.[22,23] On resting neutrophils, Mac-1, LFA-1 (CD11a/CD18), and possibly p150,95 (CD11c/CD18) are in an inactive state, but following stimulation with chemotactic factors, the CD18 integrins undergo a change resulting in high avidity.[24] Signal transduction through phosphoinositide 3-OH kinase (PI 3-kinase) has been implicated in the regulation of lymphocyte adhesion mediated by integrin receptors. Cytohesin-1 appears to be a cytoplasmic regulator of CD18 integrin adhesion to intercellular adhesion molecule 1.[25]

The molecular nature of this change is uncertain. While there is evidence that the I domain of LFA-1 is involved in a conformational change leading to high-affinity binding to ICAM-1,[26] cellular adhesion through the CD18 integrins is a complex event involving activation, ligand binding, and cell-shape changes that

Table 188-1 Cellular Distribution and Functional Activities of β_2 Integrin Heterodimers

	LFA-1 (CD11a/CD18)*	Mac-1 (CD11b/CD18)	p150,95 (CD11c/CD18)	$\alpha_d\beta_2$ (CD11d/CD18)
Leukocyte distribution	T and B lymphocytes, large granular lymphocytes, monocytes, and granulocytes	Granulocytes, monocytes, macrophages, large granular lymphocytes	Macrophages, monocytes, granulocytes	Macrophages, monocytes, granulocytes, lymphocytes
Myeloid cell functions	Antibody-dependent cellular cytotoxicity	Complement receptor 3 functions	Complement receptor 4 functions	Unknown at present but evidence suggests phagocytic functions; adhesion to ICAM-3
	Adhesion to cells expressing ICAM family members (e.g., endothelial cells)	iC3b binding Phagocytosis and intracellular killing	iC3b binding Phagocytosis and intracellular killing	
	Necessary for efficient neutrophil emigration	Binding of microbial determinants (e.g., filamentous hemagglutin)		
		Homotypic aggregation		
		Adhesion to endothelium and various protein substrates		
		Adhesion-dependent oxidative burst and degranulation		
		Cell locomotion in chemotactic gradient		
		Antibody-dependent cellular cytotoxicity		
Lymphoid cell functions	Cytolytic T lymphocyte killing Natural killing Antigen-mitogen- or alloantigen-induced-proliferation T and B cell aggregation T cell helper responses	Cytotoxicity by large granular lymphocytes	Cytolytic T cell-target cell conjugation	

*Genbank accession numbers: CD11a = Y00792; CD18 = M15395; CD11b = J03925; CD11c = M81695; α_d = U37028.

ultimately result in enhanced adhesion. Events after ligand binding are induced by stimulation of leukocytes and require protein tyrosine kinase, phosphatase, and RhoA activities.[27] LFA-1-mediated adhesion, for example, appears to be regulated by cytoskeletal restraint and by the Ca^{2+}-dependent protease calpain.[28] Positive and inhibitory domains exist within the CD18 cytoplasmic tail and apparently regulate α-actinin binding.[29] The high avidity state is transient, allowing adherent leukocytes to detach,[30–32] an event that appears to be necessary for optimal cellular locomotion or repeated target binding in cell-mediated cytolysis. This active state may be recognized and possibly induced by some monoclonal antibodies that bind either to the α or β subunit, and that can hold the CD18 integrins in an active conformation in the absence of cellular activation.[33]

In addition, the β_2 integrins have been implicated in signaling directly or cosignaling through other receptors. For example, signaling through the T-cell receptor is markedly enhanced by coligation of LFA-1,[34–35] and Mac-1 (CD11b/CD18) signals the neutrophil for markedly enhanced hydrogen peroxide production.[36] There is evidence that CD18 integrins can interact in *cis* with other receptors on the cell membrane, allowing integrins and their partner receptors to form distinct membrane complexes that recruit signaling molecules.[37–39]

Intercellular Adhesion Molecules (ICAMs). Three members of the expanding ICAM family[40] were originally defined as ligands for LFA-1. ICAM-1 (CD54), ICAM-2 (CD102), and ICAM-3 (CD50) are known to be structurally related members of the immunoglobulin supergene family. They are most closely related to other Ig-like adhesion molecules such as vascular cell adhesion molecule-1 (VCAM-1, CD106) and neural cell adhesion molecule (NCAM). ICAM-1 has five Ig-like domains, with a short hinge region separating the third and fourth Ig-like domains.[41,42] ICAM-1 is a ligand for Mac-1 as well as LFA-1, but the binding sites for LFA-1 and Mac-1 are distinct. LFA-1 binds to domains 1 and 2,[43] while Mac-1 binds to domain 3.[20] ICAM-1 also serves as a receptor for rhinovirus[44] and malaria-infected red blood cells. ICAM-2, in contrast, has only two Ig-like domains that are most closely related to domains 1 and 2 of ICAM-1.[17] ICAM-3[18] has a five-domain structure similar to that of ICAM-1.

The distribution and regulation of the ICAM molecules are quite distinct. ICAM-1 is expressed basally only at low levels on some vascular endothelial cells and on lymphocytes.[16,45] However, ICAM-1 expression can be induced to high levels on a variety of cells by stimulation with inflammatory cytokines, such as interleukin-1 (IL-1), tumor necrosis factor (TNF), and γ-interferon (INFγ).[45] Induced or greatly increased expression of ICAM-1 has been reported on vascular endothelial cells, keratinocytes, epithelial cells, hepatocytes, and myocytes. In addition, ICAM-1 expression is increased on activated lymphocytes. Induction of ICAM-1 requires *de novo* protein synthesis. As a counterreceptor for LFA-1, ICAM-1 is implicated in guiding leukocyte migration, cell-mediated cytolysis, antigen presentation, and lymphocyte homotypic aggregation. Additionally, ICAM-1 as a receptor for Mac-1 is involved in neutrophil-endothelial cell interactions, and adhesion-dependent respiratory burst.

ICAM-2 expression, in contrast to that of ICAM-1, is constitutive and restricted to endothelial cells and mononuclear leukocytes.[18,46] Functionally, it is not clear what role ICAM-2 plays in the inflammatory response. ICAM-3 is even more restricted in expression. It is expressed on monocytes, lymphocytes, and granulocytes,[47] and functions as a signaling molecule when cross-linked.[48–50]

The Selectins. All three members of the selectin family (see Table 188-2) share common structural features,[51–57] most prominently an N-terminal C-type lectin domain. As discussed below, the lectin domain is central to the carbohydrate-binding properties of all three selectins. The lectin domain motif belongs to the C-type lectin family described by Drickamer et al.[58] This Ca^{2+}-dependent lectin domain accounts for, at least in part, the requirement of Ca^{2+} in adhesion mediated by all three selectins. The lectin domain is followed by a domain homologous to epidermal growth factor, a variable number of short consensus repeats (SCR) (a motif found in many complement regulatory proteins), a conventional transmembrane domain, and a C-terminal cytoplasmic domain. The number of SCRs accounts for much of the size difference between the selectins: L-selectin, the smallest member, has two SCRs; E-selectin has six SCRs; and P-selectin has alternatively spliced forms of eight and nine SCRs. This is a highly conserved gene family, with over 60 percent amino acid identity in the lectin and EGF domains.

L-selectin was first described as a lymphocyte homing molecule involved in tissue-specific migration to peripheral lymph nodes as reviewed elsewhere.[59] More recently, L-selectin has been demonstrated on myeloid cells and is involved in neutrophil-endothelial cell and monocyte-endothelial cell interactions at sites of inflammation. Monoclonal antibodies against L-selectin reduce neutrophil adhesion to cytokine-stimulated endothelial cell cultures. L-selectin mediated adhesion appears to be most readily measured when neutrophils are subjected to shear stress.[60–62] A role for carbohydrate binding by L-selectin was demonstrated by Rosen and colleagues[59] many years before the lectin domain structure was elucidated by gene cloning.

E-selectin was first defined as a cytokine-inducible adhesion molecule on endothelial cells.[63] Monoclonal antibodies against E-selectin specifically block neutrophil and myeloid cell line (HL-60) adhesion to IL-1 and TNF-stimulated endothelial cells.[63,64] E-selectin expression is prominent in acute inflammatory lesions in vivo \ and correlates with the large influx of neutrophils.[65–69] Although E-selectin appears to be primarily associated with acute inflammatory lesions, E-selectin expression occurs in some chronic inflammatory lesions, notably the inflamed skin[68,70] and the synovium from patients with arthritis.[71] Furthermore, a small subset of memory T lymphocytes, defined by the HECA-452, a monoclonal antibody that recognizes a ligand for E-selectin, bind

Table 188-2 Molecular Ligand Receptor Pairs Involved in Leukocyte Adhesion to Vascular Endothelium

Leukocyte Determinants			Endothelial Ligands			
Molecule*	Structure	Cell Distribution	Molecule	Structure	Cell Distribution	Regulatory Factors
Mac-1† (CD11b/CD18)	β_2 integrin	Neutrophils, eosinophils, and monocytes	ICAM-1	Ig family	Unstimulated and activated endothelial and other cell types	Endotoxin, IFNγ, IL-1, and TNFα
LFA-1 (CD11a/CD18)	β_2 integrin	Neutrophils, eosinophils, monocytes, and lymphocytes	ICAM-1 ICAM-2	Ig family Ig family	Unstimulated and activated endothelial and other cell types	Endotoxin, IFNγ, IL-1, and TNFα
VLA-4 ($\alpha_4\beta_1$)	β_1 integrin	Eosinophils, lymphocytes, monocytes, neutrophils	VCAM-1	Ig family	Activated endothelium	Endotoxin, IL-1, TNFα, IL-4
L-selectin (CD62L)	Selectin family	Neutrophils, eosinophils, lymphocytes, monocytes	CD34, MAdCAM CLA-like molecule	Mucin-like Sulfated, HECA-452 binding	High endothelial venules Venular endothelium	 TNFα
ESL-1, PSGL-1, L-selectin, others (?)	Sialylated and fucosylated structures (e.g., SLeX)	Neutrophils, eosinophils, monocytes, lymphocytes (subsets)	E-selectin (CD62E)	Selectin family	Activated endothelial cells	Endotoxin, IL-1, TNFα
PSGL-1, others (?)	Sialylated and fucosylated structures (e.g., SLeX), sulfated tyrosines	Neutrophils, eosinophils, monocytes, lymphocytes (subsets)	P-selectin (CD62P)	Selectin family	Activated endothelial cells and platelets	Histamine, thrombin, IL-4

†Abbreviations: CLA = cutaneous lymphocyte antigen; ESL-1 = E-selectin ligand-1; ICAM-1 = intercellular adhesion molecule-1; LFA-1 = lymphocyte function antigen-1 (CD11a/CD18); Mac-1 = $\alpha_M\beta_2$ integrin; PAF = platelet activating factor; PSGL-1 = P-selectin glycoprotein ligand-1; SLeX = sialyl Lewis X; VCAM-1 = vascular cell adhesion molecule-1 = CD106; VLA-4 = very late antigen-4, also known as $\alpha_4\beta_1$ integrin.

*Genbank accession numbers: α_4 (CD49d), X16988; β_1 (CD29), X07979; VCAM-1 (CD106), M73255; L-selectin (CD62L), M25280; E-selectin (CD62E), M30640; P-selectin (CD62P), M35322; PSGL-1 (CD162), U02297 and U25956.

specifically to E-selectin.[70] These studies indicate that in some circumstances, E-selectin can mediate lymphocyte traffic to chronic inflammatory sites.

P-selectin was first defined as a marker for activated platelets.[72,73] P-selectin was localized to the α-granules of platelets[74,75] and later to the Weibel-Palade bodies of endothelial cells.[76–78] In both cell types, cell activation results in a rapid recruitment of these granules to the cell surface.[74–75,78] P-selectin is involved in mediating neutrophil-platelet interactions[79–81] and in neutrophil-endothelial cell interactions in vitro.[82–84] These results indicate that P-selectin may play a central role in bridging hemostasis and acute inflammation very early in the response to vascular injury or insult.[85–89]

Selectin Ligands. Since L-selectin was first described as a lymphocyte homing receptor, the most intensive search for an L-selectin ligand has been on high endothelial venules of lymph nodes. In a series of elegant studies, Rosen and colleagues demonstrated a clear role for carbohydrates in L-selectin-mediated adhesion.[59] Lymphocyte adhesion to high endothelial venules of peripheral lymph nodes (HEV) is sensitive to neuraminidase treatment of the HEV.[90,91] Charged sugars, such as mannose-6-phosphate, and polymers of charged sugars, such as phosphomanan monoester cove complex (PPME; a polysaccharide rich in mannose 6-phosphate) and fucoidin (fucose-sulfate-rich), bind specifically to L-selectin and block lymphocyte adhesion to HEV.[92,93] A major ligand for selectins is a sialylated and fucosylated tetrasaccharide of the sialylated Lewis X blood group (sLeX, CD15s).[94,95] It is expressed constitutively at high levels on monocyte and neutrophil surface glycoproteins, and up-regulated on some peripheral lymphocytes following stimulation. A closely related molecule found as a major capping group on a well-characterized glycoprotein (GlyCAM-1[96]) recognized by L-selectin is 6′-sulfo-sialyl LeX.[97] In both forms of sLeX, the α 2 → 3-linked sialic acids and α 1 → 3/4 fucosylation are important to selectin recognition. However, the detailed carbohydrate structures for the various physiologic ligands on an array of cell types (e.g., endothelial cells, tumor cells, leukocytes) recognized by the selectin family remain unknown.[98]

Although the affinity of the selectins for small sialylated, fucosylated oligosaccharides is relatively weak, the avidity for carbohydrate structures on some glycoproteins and proteoglycans is much higher. For example, several mucin-like proteins have been identified as possible physiological ligands for L-selectin. GlyCAM-1,[96] CD34,[99] and MadCAM-1[100] have been well characterized. P-selectin glycoprotein ligand-1 (PSGL-1, CD162)[101] is a mucin-like molecule found on the surface of neutrophils, monocytes, and some lymphocytes that serves as a functionally significant ligand for all three selectins, with P-selectin showing the highest affinity.[102] In addition to the carbohydrate residues containing sLeX on PSGL-1,[103] sulfated tyrosines at the N-terminus appear to be critical for high affinity binding of P-selectin to this ligand.[104] An E-selectin ligand has been identified that is prominently expressed on mouse neutrophils.[105] Current evidence indicates that α1 → 3-fucosyltransferases IV and VII are involved in the synthesis of appropriate ligands for the selectins on glycoproteins such as these ligands,[106–109] and the physiologic contribution of the structure of these carbohydrate ligands is evident.[110,111]

Selectin Regulation. L-selectin is constitutively expressed on resting neutrophils in a seemingly functional form. However, within minutes of neutrophil exposure to low levels of chemotactic factors, L-selectin is rapidly down-regulated from the cell surface.[112] Near complete down-regulation of L-selectin can be detected within minutes in vitro. A large fragment of L-selectin is recoverable from the supernatant of activated cells, which suggests that L-selectin is proteolytically clipped close to the transmembrane domain.[112] A broad range of activating agents, including C5a, f-Met-Leu-Phe (fMLP), TNF, granulocyte/monocyte-colony stimulating factor (GM-CSF), and interleukin-8 (IL-8), are effective at inducing this response,[60,112–114,] and the rapid shedding of L-selectin is similar to the kinetics of Mac-1 up-regulation from intracellular stores. Analysis of neutrophils that are recovered from the inflamed peritoneum in vivo[113] and immunohistologic analysis of neutrophils in inflamed skin sites[112] reveals that this inverse regulation of adhesion molecules occurs in vivo as well.

E-selectin is normally absent from endothelial cells. However, upon stimulation with inflammatory cytokines, endothelial cells express E-selectin within several hours. E-selectin is synthesized *de novo* and is blocked by protein synthesis inhibitors.[63] This up-regulation of E-selectin is similar to that seen with other endothelial adhesion molecules, such as ICAM-1 and VCAM-1. However, in contrast to these other adhesion molecules, which remain highly expressed for over 24 h, E-selectin expression peaks at 3 to 4 h and then is diminishes to very low levels by 24 h in vitro.[63,115] The time course of E-selectin expression is similar to the time course of neutrophil infiltration into acute inflammatory sites in vivo. These results suggest that E-selectin is involved primarily in the acute inflammatory response. E-selectin expression is also rapidly inducible in vivo and coincides with the influx of neutrophils.[65–69,116] E-selectin expression is also quite prominent in some chronic inflammatory lesions, notably some inflamed skin and synovial sites.[65,70,71,116]

P-selectin, like E-selectin, is expressed by activated endothelium, but the activation signals and the kinetics of expression differ for these two events. P-selectin is stored in intracellular Weibel-Palade bodies.[76–78,117] Stimulation of endothelial cells with histamine or thrombin induces a rapid recruitment of Weibel-Palade bodies to the cell surface, resulting in surface expression of P-selectin within minutes after stimulation. Similarly, P-selectin is also stored in the α-granules of platelets, which are recruited to the cell surface within seconds of platelet activation.[74,75] This rapid up-regulation of P-selectin suggests a critical role in the earliest events of inflammation and hemostasis. Surface expression of P-selectin on endothelium is also transient. Within 30 min, P-selectin is down-modulated, apparently by receptor endocytosis rather than surface proteolysis.[118]

A Model for Neutrophil-Endothelial Cell Interactions

In 1989, a two-step adhesion model for neutrophil interaction with endothelium was proposed, based primarily on the observation that Mac-1 and L-selectin are inversely regulated by exposure to chemotactic factors.[112,113,119] The rapid down-regulation of L-selectin with a concomitant up-regulation of Mac-1 suggested that these adhesion molecules mediate distinct, but complementary, adhesion events. In this model, L-selectin mediates the initial interaction of the circulating neutrophil with the activated endothelium, thus guiding the unstimulated neutrophil to the appropriate site of inflammation. This initial binding event results in rolling and slows the neutrophil, thereby enhancing exposure to chemotactic factors at the site of inflammation. The chemoattractants trigger the transition from L-selectin-mediated adhesion to CD18-mediated adhesion, an event that must occur rapidly if neutrophils are to localize efficiently in the vessels of inflammatory foci. Enhanced adhesion can be seen within seconds in experimental settings where the time from stimulus to adhesion can be measured with some accuracy.[120,121]

In recent years, this model was expanded as more details of the interactions between leukocytes and endothelial cells have come to light (Table 188-3, Fig. 188-1, and discussion below). A multistep cascade of adhesive and signaling events is evident, the specific components of which provide specificity for localizing each type of leukocyte in different vascular beds. The cascade can be viewed as requiring at least three distinct steps for the leukocyte to make the transition from a flowing cell to one firmly adherent on the apical surface of endothelium.[122,123] Given the large diversity in adhesion molecules and chemotactic factors, a remarkably high

Table 188-3 Proposed Steps in Neutrophil Emigration at Sites of Inflammation

Step	Adhesion Molecules Involved	Regulatory Factors
1. Initial margination, rolling	P-selectin, PSGL-1, and possibly other SLeX-bearing molecules	Stimuli that mobilize Wiebel-Palade bodies containing P-selectin in venular endothelium.
	E-selectin, PSGL-1, ESL-1, possibly L-selectin and other SLeX-bearing molecules	Stimuli that induce expression of new protein (E-selectin) by endothelial cells (e.g., IL-1).
	L-selectin, PSGL-1	Conditions that promote homotypic interactions of neutrophils under flow conditions.
	L-selectin	Stimuli that induce new synthesis (e.g., TNFα) of CLA-like glycoprotein (?) on endothelium.
2. Activation of stable adhesion	LFA-1 (CD11a/CD18), Mac-1 (CD11b/CD18)	Chemotactic factors such as IL-8 and PAF bound to the apical surface of endothelial cells; possible signaling through L-selectin tethers.
	ICAM-1 (CD54), others (?)	Stimuli that induce expression of new protein (ICAM-1) by endothelial cells (e.g., IL-1).
3. Stationary adhesion, emigration into tissues	LFA-1 (CD11a/CD18), Mac-1 (CD11b/CD18)	Chemotactic factors such as IL-8 and PAF bound to the apical surface of endothelial cells; possible signaling triggered by L-selectin tethers.
	ICAM-1 (CD54), others (?)	Stimuli that induce expression of new protein (ICAM-1) by endothelial cells (e.g., IL-1).
	VLA-4 ($\alpha_4\beta_1$), possibly other β_1 integrins	Transmigration in response to chemotactic gradients induces expression of β_1 integrin.

CLA = cutaneous lymphocyte antigen; ESL-1 = E-selectin ligand-1; ICAM-1 = intercellular adhesion molecule-1; LFA-1 = lymphocyte function antigen-1 (CD11a/CD18); Mac-1 = $\alpha_M\beta_2$ integrin; PAF = platelet activating factor; PSGL-1 = P-selectin glycoprotein ligand-1; SLeX = sialyl Lewis X; VLA-4 = very late antigen-4, also known as $\alpha_4\beta_1$ integrin.

number of combinations for these three steps is available for very precise selection of leukocytes to adhere at specific sites in the vascular bed. This model seems robust enough to account for the diverse characteristics of the inflammatory process (e.g., the early arrival of neutrophils in acute inflammation), as well as the physiological trafficking of leukocytes through tissues (e.g., the recirculation of lymphocytes through lymph nodes). It is beyond the scope of this chapter to review the extensive applications of this model. However, some focused explanation is necessary to understand the clinical syndromes of leukocyte adhesion deficiency.

Primary Capture and Rolling of Neutrophils. The first step in this model as it applies to acute inflammation involves the initial capture of flowing neutrophils. If this event occurs in postcapillary venules, all three members of the selectin family can be involved.[86,124–127] If this event occurs in the alveolar capillaries of the lungs,[128] or the sinusoids of the liver,[129,130] an additional factor is particularly important, that is, physical trapping apparently resulting from increased rigidity of the leukocyte.[131] In such vessels, selectins can contribute to the retention of neutrophils.[132] In postcapillary venules, the selectin-dependent capture is characterized by leukocytes rolling on the endothelium, a phenomenon that has been known for over a century in classic intravital microscopy studies.[133,134] Neutrophils can be seen to roll and stop along venules, but not along small arteries or arterioles. Rolling under flow conditions can be observed in vitro on cultured

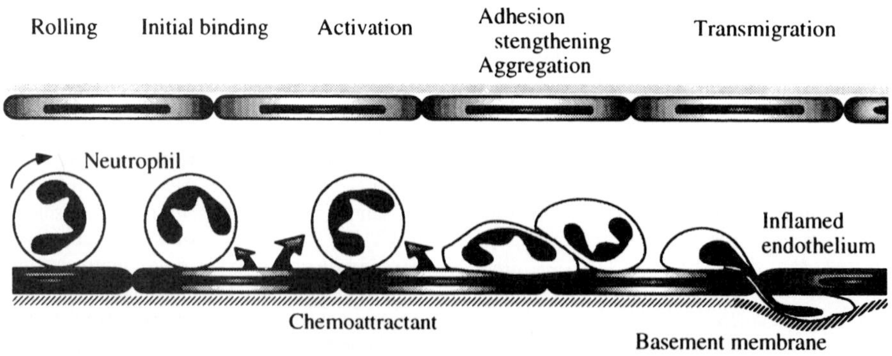

Fig. 188-1 A dynamic model for neutrophil interaction with inflamed endothelium. Neutrophil localization and activation is a multistep process. Endothelial cells adjacent to a site of inflammation are stimulated by cytokines (such as TNF and IL-1) to synthesize E-selectin and ICAM-1. These inducible adhesion molecules provide position-specific information for leukocytes. L-selectin on the neutrophil and E-selectin on the endothelium mediate the initial interaction between the unactivated neutrophil and the stimulated endothelium. This interaction guides the neutrophil to the appropriate site. The transiently bound neutrophil is exposed to low concentrations of chemoattractants. Free-flowing neutrophils are not activated. This activation event induces a rapid transition in neutrophil morphology and adhesiveness. There is a transient increase in L-selectin-mediated adhesion followed by a rapid shedding of the cell-surface L-selectin. Simultaneously, there is activation of Mac-1 adhesiveness accompanied by a rapid increase in cell-surface Mac-1 expression from intracellular stores. Thus, activation rapidly shuts down one adhesion pathway (L-selectin) and turns on another adhesion pathway (Mac-1). Engagement of Mac-1 results in adhesion strengthening, neutrophil aggregation, and transendothelial migration.

endothelial cell monolayers[135] that have been stimulated to express either E-selectin[136] following exposure to cytokines, such as IL-1β, TNFα, or endotoxin, or to mobilize P-selectin from a storage pool in Weibel-Palade bodies[137] by stimulation with histamine.[138] Observations in mice deficient in E-selectin or P-selectin exhibit specific deficiencies in these functions.[86,139–141] The endothelial selectins bind to their carbohydrate ligands at physiologically relevant shear rates.[142] PSGL-1, for example, supports the initial capture of neutrophils under flow conditions[102,143,144] because of its binding affinity for the selectins and its topography. It is concentrated on the tips of membranous folds and microvillus-like projections from the leukocyte surface, a position that appears to mediate enhanced interaction with the endothelium.[102,145]

The topography of L-selectin on unstimulated leukocytes parallels that of PSGL-1,[146,147] being concentrated on the tips of membranous folds and microvillus-like projections. Antibodies to L-selectin reduce the ability of neutrophils to roll on cytokine-stimulated monolayers of endothelial cells,[60] and rolling and localization of neutrophils are impaired in L-selectin-deficient mice.[125] The exact contribution of L-selectin is currently unclear. There are three possible mechanisms by which it could contribute to the primary capture of neutrophils on endothelial cells under conditions of flow. The first possible mechanism involves the recognition of carbohydrate ligands on the endothelial cell. While this is clearly demonstrated for the localization of lymphocytes on high endothelial venules in lymphoid tissue,[148,149] the evidence for such a mechanism with cytokine-stimulated endothelial cells is incomplete. A sulfated, fucosylated ligand on endothelial cells up-regulated by inflammatory cytokines appears to be distinct from L-selectin ligands on high endothelial venules in lymph nodes.[150] This incompletely characterized ligand is recognized by monoclonal antibody HECA-452, which suggests a structural similarity with cutaneous lymphocyte antigen (CLA), a sLeX-like ligand for E-selectin on subsets of lymphocytes.[71] A second possible mechanism involves direct interactions between E-selectin and L-selectin. This interaction is theoretically possible because L-selectin on neutrophils is decorated with sLeX,[146] a ligand for E-selectin. There is evidence for the direct binding of E-selectin and L-selectin.[151] A third possible mechanism involves the potential capture of flowing neutrophils by those neutrophils already bound to the endothelial surface or to some other adhesive substratum.[152] Such an event has been demonstrated in vitro at physiologically relevant shear rates,[153] and shown to promote recruitment of neutrophils onto an adhesive substratum through an L-selectin-dependent mechanism. This homotypic interaction of neutrophils depends on L-selectin binding to carbohydrate ligands of PSGL-1 on the opposing neutrophil.[153]

An additional mechanism for potential primary capture of neutrophils involves the ability of platelets to adhere to neutrophils. Under flow conditions, in vitro monolayers of platelets will catch flowing neutrophils, supporting some rolling and some substantial firm adhesion.[154–156] This interaction appears to depend primarily on P-selectin (mobilized to the platelet surface from a storage pool in α-granules) binding to PSGL-1 on the neutrophils. Thus, platelets adherent to a vessel wall potentially serve as a mechanism for neutrophil localization.

Activation of Rolling Leukocytes. The events described above involve circulating neutrophils that are in a resting state prior to their initial capture at the endothelial surface. Selectin binding alone appears to be unable to promote stationary adhesion under the conditions of flowing blood, and ample evidence confirms the need for a transition to integrin binding for stationary adhesion to occur.[157] This transition requires activation of the leukocytes, and has been demonstrated in vitro in a simplified flow chamber with neutrophils rolling over a planar surface coated with P-selectin and ICAM-1.[158] Significant stationary adhesion in this experimental model was seen only when a chemotactic stimulus was added to the neutrophil suspension immediately before entering the flow chamber and contacting the substratum. The observed stationary adhesion was found to depend on binding of CD18 integrins on the neutrophils to ICAM-1 on the substratum. Flowing neutrophils at physiologically relevant shear rates did not interact with a substratum coated only with ICAM-1, and stationary adhesion did not occur when the substratum was coated with only P-selectin. Such a transition from selectin to integrin adhesion can only be seen under flow conditions, both in vitro[60] and in vivo,[159] and can be induced by an array of stimulants (chemokines and chemotactic factors) showing varying degrees of specificity for different leukocyte subsets (an expansive topic covered in recent reviews[160]).

A key feature of the activation of neutrophils leading to stable adhesion on endothelial cells under conditions of flow is that the activating stimulation occurs in close physical and temporal proximity to the potential site of stable adhesion. Neutrophils that are stimulated minutes prior to contacting cytokine-stimulated endothelial cells exhibit markedly reduced adhesion,[60,159,161] because this stimulation disrupts the mechanisms of selectin adhesion[60,162] (e.g., by inducing shedding of L-selectin[112]). Although stimulation also up-regulates integrin avidity, integrin binding is very inefficient at the shear rates of flowing blood.[158] Thus, stimulation that occurs within seconds of primary selectin-dependent capture is most effective, because its timing promotes transition from selectin to integrin adhesion. Such stimulation is best accomplished by a surface-bound chemotactic factor or chemokine, and current evidence demonstrates that IL-8[163–166] and platelet activating factor (PAF),[165,167] two relevant stimuli known to activate neutrophil integrin adhesion,[168,169] can be presented at the endothelial surface.

Another potentially important aspect of selectin binding comes from recent evidence that L-selectin functions not only as a tether, but also as a signaling molecule.[170–172] Cross-linking L-selectin with monoclonal antibodies results in several functional changes in previously unstimulated neutrophils, and one change of particular interest in the present context is an increase in CD18-dependent adhesion.[173] This cross-linking also increases the sensitivity of neutrophils to chemotactic stimuli, potentiating the rate of CD18-dependent adhesion.[174] Thus, it is possible that signaling through the tethers formed by E-selectin during the initial capture of flowing neutrophils could facilitate the transition to stationary adhesion.

Stationary Adhesion and Emigration into Tissues. Using intravital microscopy, Arfors et al.[175] demonstrated that a monoclonal antibody against CD18 integrins prevented stationary adhesion of leukocytes at inflammatory foci without measurable effect on the rolling behavior of these cells. This was confirmed in vitro for isolated neutrophils flowing over cultured endothelial monolayers.[135] In addition, it has been evident in numerous studies that blocking stationary adhesion prevents transendothelial migration.[176] Humans, cattle, and dogs with severe CD18 deficiency (i.e., with markedly reduced or absent expression of all CD18 integrins, see below) exhibit profound deficiency in neutrophil infiltration at most sites of infection and inflammation. Recent studies in experimental animals reveal that two of the members of the CD18 family can play distinct roles in the acute inflammatory process. Mice with a targeted deletion of CD11a (i.e., lacking expression of functional LFA-1) appear to mobilize neutrophils into sites of acute inflammation much less efficiently than wild-type mice,[177] while mice deficient in CD11b (i.e., lacking expression of functional Mac-1) exhibit no deficit in neutrophil emigration.[178–180] Studies in animal models using anti-CD11a and anti-CD11b monoclonal antibodies confirm the distinctions seen in genetically engineered mice.[178,181,182] In contrast to LFA-1, Mac-1 appears to be more important in effector functions of neutrophils, signaling phagocytosis of complement opsonized particles,[183] and enhanced secretory activity (e.g., generation of reactive oxygen species).[36,184,185] These functions are also shared by p150,95 (CD11c/CD18, CR4), an integrin that is much less abundant on the neutrophil surface.[186]

While members of the CD18 family can bind to several members of the ICAM family,[40] ICAM-1 (CD54)[16] appears to be the most important member of this family for neutrophil adhesion to endothelial cells.[187] Studies with monoclonal antibodies in animal models of inflammation,[188,189] and with mice deficient in ICAM-1,[190,191] reveal the significance of its contribution in vivo. Mac-1 appears to bind to other ligands on endothelial cells,[192] although no molecular definition has been obtained. Other integrins may contribute to stable adhesion of leukocytes on endothelial cells. For example, $\alpha_4\beta_1$ integrin (CD49d/CD29, VLA4) on lymphocytes,[193,194] monocytes,[195] and eosinophils[196] binds to vascular cell adhesion molecule-1 (VCAM-1, CD106). Recent evidence indicates that neutrophils may also use $\alpha_4\beta_1$ for adhesion,[197] but that this integrin is not constitutively expressed on circulating human neutrophils. It is, however, up-regulated following transmigration of neutrophils toward a chemotactic gradient, and would be available for adhesion to extravascular tissues bearing the appropriate ligands (e.g., fibrinectin or VCAM-1).[198]

Chemotactic factors, therefore, not only activate leukocytes for firm adhesion to endothelial surfaces, but activate the mechanisms of locomotion needed for transendothelial migration,[199,200] locomotion through extravascular tissue,[201] and adhesion to tissue components such as parenchymal cells.[198,202,203] Here, again, specificity can be introduced by chemotactic factors selective for distinct subsets of leukocytes. Leukocytes demonstrate essentially no motility in the absence of specific stimuli, but a diverse array of chemotactic factors may modify substantially the speed and direction of locomotion. Stimulated migration with no directional component is termed chemokinesis or random locomotion.[204] When under the influence of concentration gradients of chemotactic factors, however, cells migrate toward the stimulating agent, and individual leukocytes demonstrate a rather uniform orientation toward the origin of the chemotactic gradient.[205,206] Homing of leukocytes migrating in extravascular tissues may be guided by sequential local gradients of different chemotactic factors as suggested by the studies of Foxman et al.[207]

A variety of techniques have been utilized to evaluate the migratory properties of myeloid or lymphoid cells. Evaluations of the kinetics and extent of the mobilization of leukocytes in various tissues of human subjects are limited to histopathologic assessments and applications of "skin window" techniques initially described by Rebuck and Crowley.[208] The skin window technique and several more quantitative modifications[209] are of limited value for several reasons. Difficulties encountered in creating uniform skin lesions, in addition to the pain or possible infectious complications associated with the use of abrasive techniques, limit their overall suitability for clinical application. Findings of large numbers of one or more types of leukocytes in tissue exudates does not exclude the possibility of defective mobility, because these cells may have infiltrated too late to prevent the establishment of infections.[210] The result of these concerns is that evaluations of the migratory functions of leukocytes in clinical samples are most commonly performed in vitro.

Assays of chemotaxis include those evaluating the effect of chemoattractants on a population of cells. Each of these assays, in principle, represents a modification of the micropore filter method[211] originally described by Boyden[212] in which a test cell population migrates into or through a micropore filter toward a test reagent placed in an adjacent stimulant compartment. A modification of the micropore filter method[206] distinguishes chemotaxis from chemokinesis. This is accomplished by the use of protocols in which a range of concentrations of a stimulant reagent is incorporated independently in the cell and stimulant compartments of a culture chamber.[213]

Direct observations reveal that leukocytes, particularly neutrophils, are relatively fast-moving cells compared, for example, with fibroblasts.[205,214,215] Most descriptions of the morphology of leukocytes during locomotion in vitro indicate that they assume a characteristic bipolar shape.[205] This involves the appearance of a veil-like, flattened membrane or lamellipodia at the anterior end of the cell. Migrating cells also generally demonstrate a uropod or tail-like structure with retraction fibers developing as a cell migrates. To study the effects of chemotactic factors on these events, it is necessary to establish experimental conditions that allow exposure of cells to stable and continuous chemical gradients. Under such conditions, the effects on both the rate and the direction of cell orientation or movement can be observed. Most investigators have used microbial point sources such as bacterial clumps or spores of yeast, or specially designed orientation chambers for applications in visual assays.[205,214–216] A conceptually similar technique in which leukocytes migrate toward a chemoattractant source on plastic or glass under agarose[217] has also proved useful.

The bipolar shape seen in migrating cells also occurs if neutrophils[211] and monocytes[218] are exposed to chemotactic stimuli in suspension. Thus, the cells need not be attached to a surface in order to assume a bipolar shape. Using this morphologic change as a sensitive indicator of chemotactic stimulation, abnormal cellular responses have been identified in clinical conditions characterized by increased infections, and the inhibitory action of selected pharmacologic agents has been assessed.[219–221]

CLINICAL DISORDERS OF LEUKOCYTE ADHESION

General Considerations

The rapid localization of phagocytes to sites of microbial invasion or trauma represents a first-line defense mechanism of particular importance in nonimmune hosts. Quantitative or qualitative aberrations of either the cellular or humoral contributions to these adaptive responses may impair inflammatory defenses, and thus, increase infectious susceptibility. Early studies[210] demonstrated a critical 2- to 4-h period after cutaneous invasion by bacterial pathogens during which phagocytic cells must arrive at a site of invasion in order to prevent the establishment of an infectious process. Recurrent bacterial or fungal infections of the skin or mucous membranes are prominent in patients with quantitative deficiencies of peripheral blood leukocytes.[222] Such infections are also evident in patients with qualitative disorders resulting in insufficient accumulation of phagocytes at inflammatory sites, despite normal numbers of leukocytes in the peripheral blood.[223,224] Among both patient groups, common pathogens such as *Staphylococcus aureus*, *Pseudomonas*, other gram-negative enteric species, or *Candida albicans* account for most infectious complications. Infected tissues in these patients are characteristically gangrenous or necrotic, devoid of pus, and contain few granulocytes when examined microscopically. Local inflammatory signs or symptoms in such patients may be minimal, even though chronic infections may eventually lead to the destruction of cutaneous, subcutaneous, periodontal, or other submucosal tissues.

Early reports of clinical disorders typified by susceptibility to recurrent soft tissue infections described patients with abnormalities of leukocyte migration in vitro and/or tissue mobilization in vivo.[225–229] In contrast to observations in patients with chronic granulomatous disease (see Chap. 189), studies of granulocytes or monocytes in these patients demonstrated neither abnormalities of microbicidal functions nor granulomatous inflammation in infected tissues. Initially, at least for purposes of comparison of individual patients, a distinct subclassification of disorders of leukocyte motility or chemotaxis seemed justified. However, an explosion of literature followed in which defects of chemotaxis in vitro were associated with a wide array of clinical disorders or conditions. Such reports clearly implied but rarely documented that diminished chemotaxis in vitro was associated with diminished availability or delayed infiltration of phagocytes into inflamed tissues. Correlations between abnormalities of cellular motility in vitro and altered exudation in tissues of human subjects have been infrequent because of the imprecisions in the techniques used to evaluate cellular infiltration in vivo in humans (e.g., skin window techniques).

A reliable interpretation of leukocyte functions in vitro must consider the clinical status of the individual patient, because it is important to determine whether abnormal functions result in increased susceptibility to infection or simply reflect other factors surrounding the patient's condition. Certain pharmacologic agents as well as the nutritional status of the patient may transiently influence selected functions tested in vitro.[220,230] Blood samples obtained for study during the course of infections may contain an increased percentage of immature myeloid cells that function suboptimally.[231] Also, many investigators have reported enhanced, diminished, or otherwise abnormal motility, phagocytosis, oxidative metabolism, and/or other functions of leukocytes in patients with clinical bacterial infections.[232–235] In most cases, these abnormalities are found to be transient, probably reflecting cellular influences of inflammatory mediators[230,236–238] or products of the infecting organisms. Certain bacterial toxins exert significant inhibitory effects on cellular locomotion as well as on other functions in vitro.[230] Some, such as cholera toxin and certain enterotoxins of *E. coli*, exert primarily intracellular effects (e.g., activate adenyl cyclase and elevate intracellular cyclic AMP levels).[239,240] Others preferentially perturb cell membrane properties and include streptolysin O, the clostridial toxins perfringolysin and phospholipase C, a diverse group of staphylococcal toxins (sphingomyelinase C and leukocidin), and proteases (alkaline protease, elastase) elaborated by pathogenic strains of *Pseudomonas aeruginosa*.[241,242] Suggested pathogenic mechanisms related to microbial toxin exposure include the disruption of receptors for chemotactic factors, ligands for complement proteins or reactions from the Fc portion of IgG, alteration of membrane fluidity, and inhibition of cytoskeletal protein assemblage. Finally, certain microbial proteases or other products act directly on humoral mediators of cellular locomotion. For example, elastases elaborated by *Pseudomonas aeruginosa* cleave C5 (as well as other serum complement proteins) thereby generating complement-derived chemotactic moieties in vitro or in vivo.[241]

The molecular pathogeneses of a limited number of genetic or secondary disorders characterized by defective migration of leukocytes have been defined. Investigation of these clinical syndromes has provided important insights concerning the physiological and pathologic significance of leukocyte trafficking in vivo, as well as the molecular determinants of these events.

Identification of CD18 Deficiency in Human, Canine, and Bovine — Leukocyte Adhesion Deficiency I (LAD I)

Early Studies. An autosomal recessive trait characterized by recurrent bacterial infections, impaired pus formation and wound healing, and a broad spectrum of functional abnormalities of myeloid and lymphoid cells results from heterogenous mutations of the β subunit of CD18 (β_2) integrins. These mutations result in defective biosynthesis of each of heterodimeric glycoproteins of the β_2 subfamily including LFA-1 (CD11a/CD18), Mac-1 (CD11b/CD18), and p150,95 (CD11c/CD18).

Before 1980 several reports documented a group of human patients with recurrent bacterial and fungal infections, defective leukocyte motility and phagocytosis, impaired wound healing, and/or delayed umbilical cord severance.[243–251] Crowley et al.[252] first proposed that defects of neutrophil chemotaxis and associated infectious susceptibility were due to underlying defects of cell adhesion. Moreover, lysates of blood neutrophils in their patient lacked a high-molecular-weight cell-surface glycoprotein termed gp110. Later reports described similar patients lacking leukocyte surface glycoproteins ranging in M_r from 130 to 180 kDa.[253,254] This M_r range for deficient glycoproteins was consistent with that of Mac-1 described by that time in mouse and human as an $\alpha\beta$ complex with subunits of M_r 165,000 (α) and 95,000 (β) present on macrophages, monocytes, neutrophils, and large granular lymphocytes.[255,256] Studies in 1984 by Dana et al.,[257] Anderson et al.,[258] Beaty et al.,[259] and Springer et al.[260] revealed that both the α and β subunits of Mac-1 (also designated Mo-1 or CR3) were deficient on patient leukocytes. Anderson et al.,[258] Springer et al.,[260] and Arnaout et al.[261] also showed that the LFA-1 $\alpha\beta$ complex, which showed a β subunit identical to that of Mac-1,[255] was deficient on patient neutrophils and lymphocytes. A third type of $\alpha\beta$ complex, designated p150,95, was also deficient on patient cells.[262] These findings led to the proposal that the primary defect in this disorder was related to the β subunit, and that biosynthesis of the β subunit was requisite for surface expression of each of the α subunits.[260]

Subsequent to these early reports, numerous patients with similar clinical features were shown to lack the Mac-1, LFA-1, and p150,95 glycoproteins on neutrophils, monocytes, lymphocytes, and/or transformed β lymphoblasts or T-cell lines[21,250,252–254,257,260–283] as reviewed elsewhere.[249] This group of patients, sharing similar clinical features and the same molecular defect, clearly defined a distinct pathologic disorder. Because it was identified in several independent laboratories, it was variably referred to as Mac-1, LFA-1 deficiency disease, Mo-1 deficiency, Leu-cam deficiency, or CR3 deficiency. In the interests of brevity and comprehensiveness, the term leukocyte adhesion deficiency (LAD) was proposed in 1987.[249] The term LAD I was adopted in 1992 following discovery of a similar clinical syndrome due to a distinct molecular defect termed LAD II (see below). Very similar clinical disorders recognized in Irish Setter dogs[284,285] and Holstein cattle[286–290] were subsequently described and shown to be due to defects of the β_2 integrin subunit. Thus, the terms canine LAD and bovine LAD were adopted.

The discovery of bovine LAD occurred as part of studies by the United States Department of Agriculture to develop new methods to prevent mastitis in periparturient dairy cows.[291] As part of these studies, Kehrli et al.[286] identified a Holstein heifer that exhibited marked and progressive blood leukocytosis. Analysis of this animal revealed chronic neutrophilia (exceeding 100,000/FL) associated with the development of fever and chronic diarrhea leading to death at 48 days of age. Prior to death, in vitro studies of blood neutrophils of the calf revealed several functional abnormalities. As the clinical features of this calf were similar to those of human patients with LAD, further postmortem assessments were performed, including immunoblot analyses of neutrophil lysates of the heifer calf, which revealed a total deficiency of Mac-1. Further immunofluorescent analyses indicated diminished amounts of CD18 on blood neutrophils of the calf's dam and sire and diminished amounts of CD18 on neutrophils of 8 of 15 paternal half-sibs, findings that are consistent with an autosomal recessive disorder.[286,292] Antigen-specific immune responses were found to be delayed and impaired.[293] Genealogic studies revealed that the affected proband calf was related to previously reported Holstein cattle with bovine granulocytopathy syndrome, as reviewed elsewhere,[286] and that all shared a common ancestor in their pedigrees. With the availability of cDNA probes to bovine CD18,[294] it was later shown that a single mutant CD18 allele was prevalent among Holstein cattle worldwide (see below). Bovine LAD represents one of several genetic disorders identified in dairy cattle that resulted from highly regulated breeding practices as reviewed elsewhere.[294]

Clinical and Histopathologic Features of LAD I. Clinical and histopathologic features of LAD I are remarkably similar among affected human, canine, and bovine subjects.[249,264,284,287,290] Recurrent necrotic and indolent infections of soft tissues primarily involving skin, mucous membranes, and intestinal tract are the clinical hallmarks of this disease. Superficial infections on body surfaces may invade locally or systemically. Typical small, erythematous, nonpustular skin lesions often progress to large, well-demarcated, ulcerative craters, or "pyoderma gangrenosa," which heal slowly or with dysplastic eschars.[249,264] Staphylococcal or gram-negative enteric bacterial organisms may be cultured from such lesions for up to several weeks despite antimicrobial therapy.

Fulminant progression of gas gangrene of soft tissues of a distal extremity in one patient prompted surgical amputation as a life-saving measure.[254] Septicemia progressing from omphalitis associated with delayed umbilical cord severance has been observed in several families.[244,245,249,264] Perirectal abscess or cellulitis leading to peritonitis and/or septicemia has been reported in multiple patients, and facial or deep neck cellulitis has been observed to progress from ulcerative mucous membrane lesions of the oral cavity.[253,254–264] Recurrent invasive candidal esophagitis, erosive gastritis, acute appendicitis, and necrotizing enterocolitis have been reported in multiple human patients.[249] Recurrent or chronic diarrhea is a common and often lethal complication in affected Holstein cattle.[291] Recurrent otitis media occurs commonly, and progression to mastoiditis and facial nerve paralysis has been reported. Other common respiratory infections include severe bacterial (pseudomonal) laryngotracheitis, recurrent pneumonitis, and sinusitis.[249] Severe gingivitis and/or periodontitis is a major feature among all patients who survive infancy. Acute gingivitis appears in all cases with eruption of the primary dentition. Subsequently, all human and bovine subjects develop characteristic features of a severe, progressive, generalized periodontitis, including gingival proliferation, defective recession, mobility, pathologic migration, and advanced alveolar bone loss associated with periodontal pocket formation and partial or total loss of both the deciduous and permanent dentitions.[264,283,289]

The recurrent infections observed in affected patients appear to reflect a profound impairment of leukocyte mobilization into extravascular inflammatory sites. Skin windows as well as biopsies of infected tissues demonstrate inflammatory infiltrates totally devoid of neutrophils.[254,264,278,288] This histopathologic feature is particularly striking considering that marked peripheral blood leukocytosis (five- to twentyfold normal values) is a constant feature of this disorder.[264,284,291] Transfusions of leukocytes result in the appearance of donor neutrophils and monocytes in skin windows and in skin chambers.[254] Impaired healing of traumatic or surgical wounds observed in several patients represents a clinical feature not generally observed in patients with neutropenia or dysfunctional neutrophils. Unusual paper-thin or dysplastic cutaneous scars have been found in some patients.[264,295] These may reflect the lack of sufficient monocyte infiltration and the lack of inflammatory contributions to healing such as the elaboration of angiogenesis factors.[264] The wide spectrum of gram-positive or gram-negative bacterial and fungal infectious microorganisms[249,296] is also characteristic of patients with primary neutropenia syndromes. These clinical models also demonstrate insufficient tissue leukocyte infiltration. However, deep-seated granulomatous infections typical of chronic granulomatous disease and other examples of oxidative or nonoxidative intracellular killing deficits have not been observed in LAD I.

Some evidence suggests that human patients with LAD I have an increased susceptibility to viral infection. Most patients have demonstrated normal and self-limiting courses of varicella or other viral respiratory infections, and in one report,[264] 5 of 10 patients demonstrated no untoward reactions to live viral vaccine administration. However, one patient died of an overwhelming infection with picornavirus involving oral pharynx, glottis, trachea, and lungs, and three patients of the same series had one or more episodes of aseptic (presumably viral) meningitis.[264]

The severity of clinical infectious complications among human LAD I patients appears to be directly related to the degree of glycoprotein deficiency. Two phenotypes, designated severe and moderate deficiency, are defined.[249,264,281] As measured by immunofluorescence flow cytometry and verified by radioimmunoassay and immunoprecipitation techniques, severely deficient patients had essentially undetectable expression of all three complexes[264] on their neutrophils. Moderately deficient patients expressed 2.5 to 6 percent of all three $\alpha\beta$ complexes. Patients with severe deficiency have either died in infancy or have demonstrated a susceptibility to severe, life-threatening systemic infections (peritonitis, septicemia, pneumonitis, aseptic meningitis). In contrast, among the patients with moderate deficiency, life-threatening infections have been infrequently observed.[264] Patients within a kindred demonstrate similar survival periods. For example, in one study, three with moderate disease died at ages 19, 22, and 32 years.[297] In other studies of patients with severe disease, five died in their first year and one died at 3 years of age.[245,298,299] In some moderately affected patients, skin lesions may disappear after the first few years of life, recurring only with occasional infections. Severe gingivitis is always observed in these patients and may be the presenting symptom.[283] Delayed umbilical cord separation occurs more frequently in patients with the severe phenotype, but it is not universally found. Heterozygous carriers of alleles with CD18 mutations among human kindreds or Holstein cattle do not demonstrate any distinctive clinical features.

Overall, more profound functional abnormalities in vitro have been observed among severely deficient patients.[249,264] Abnormalities of leukocyte adherence to substrates, and adhesion-dependent functions, including chemotaxis and/or aggregation, were observed among almost all patients studied.[223,249,252,264] CD18-deficient neutrophils and monocytes demonstrate profound abnormalities of adhesion to and migration in vitro through endothelial cell monolayers.[19,187,300–302] These reflect deficits of the adhesive interactions of Mac-1 and LFA-1 with ICAM-1 and other ligands expressed on vascular endothelial cells.[19,187] Deficits of neutrophil transendothelial migration as well as egress into experimental inflammatory sites are directly related to the degree of CD18-deficiency observed among severe, moderate, or heterozygote patient groups. Findings of relatively normal neutrophil emigration into experimental skin windows of heterozygotes are consistent with their normal clinical status.[249,264,283]

Chemotaxis of neutrophils appears to be affected because it requires adhesion,[264,303] and abnormalities of chemotaxis by CD18-deficient cells are most evident when employing assay systems which require adhesion for directed migration.[303] Binding and phagocytosis of iC3b-opsonized particles is also deficient, in agreement with the identity of the CR3 with Mac-1.[304] In addition, because particles opsonized with iC3b are phagocytosed poorly, they fail to normally trigger the respiratory burst or degranulation.[244,247,253,258,264,297,305] Abnormalities of neutrophil or monocyte antibody-dependent cellular cytotoxicity have also been observed in several human patients and bovine subjects.[223,264,266,289] In contrast, adherence-independent cellular functions of CD18-deficient cells elicited by chemotactic factors or phorbol esters are generally shown to be normal. These include cell bipolarization,[258] complement receptor type-1 (CR1) upregulation,[258] L-selectin down-regulation,[60] specific granule release,[258,264] superoxide production induced phorbol esters,[264] and actin polymerization.[250] Intracellular microbicidal activity (e.g., the ability to kill *Staphylococcus aureus*) in most reported human patients is relatively normal,[254,258,264,297] although diminished killing of this test organism was reported in studies of one case of bovine LAD.[286] This may reflect the fact that receptors (e.g., FcγR or CR1) other than CR3 (Mac-1) are sufficient to promote a normal level of phagocytosis and intracellular killing in these in vitro assays.[258,260,264,306]

In vitro assessments of bovine CD18-deficient neutrophils have shown diminished phagocytosis-associated oxidative and secretory functions during ingestion of iC3b opsonized zymosan, findings similar to those with CD18-deficient human neutrophils. Endocytosis of IgG-opsonized *Staphylococcus aureus* by bovine CD18-deficient neutrophils is significantly reduced, a phenomenon similar to the reported deficits of IgG-Fc receptor mediated endocytosis by human CD18-deficient neutrophils, and indicative of an apparent cooperative interaction of FcγR and Mac-1.[267,307,308]

The predominance of recurrent bacterial (as opposed to viral or fungal) infections in patients with LAD I implies that the functions of neutrophils or monocytes are more profoundly affected than those of lymphocytes. However, T lymphocyte-mediated killing, proliferative responses, natural killing, and antibody-dependent killing by patients' lymphocytes are deficient compared to adult controls.[223,244,266,269,272,278,293,309–310] In primary mixed lymphocyte culture, lymphocytes in several studies have demonstrated profoundly diminished cytotoxic and proliferative responses and diminished interferon production.[246,259,269,272] After further stimulation, though, these responses increase to nearly normal levels.[269] This may be due to compensatory mechanisms, perhaps alternative accessory adhesion molecules, and may account for the relatively normal functions of B and T lymphocytes observed in most cases. Delayed cutaneous hypersensitivity reactions are normal in most patients tested, and most individuals demonstrate normal specific antibody synthesis.[258,275] However, T lymphocyte-dependent antibody responses in vivo (for example, to repeated vaccination with tetanus, diphtheria toxoids, and polio virus) were impaired in some cases, and antibody production in vivo or in vitro in response to influenza virus was found to be abnormal in one patient.[271] Thus, responses of lymphocytes in vivo may be deficient in only some of the patients whose β subunit mutation is particularly deleterious to the expression of LFA-1.

Collectively, these findings imply that in vivo functions of granulocytes and monocytes including hyperadherence, aggregation, and adhesion-primed cytotoxic functions are facilitated by an increased surface expression, functional activation, and/or alterations of receptor-density distribution of Mac-1, LFA-1, and p150,95 in response to inflammatory mediators. The profound inability of CD18-deficient cells to localize and function normally in inflamed tissues would appear to reflect their inability to upregulate and/or activate β_2 heterodimers normally required for avid ligation with ICAM-1 and other endothelial ligands or substrates. However, CD18-deficient cells appear capable of normal vascular margination-demargination in vivo,[270] findings indicating that CD18-independent adhesive or physical[311] determinants interact with vascular endothelium to mediate this physiologic process.

Definition of the Molecular Basis of LAD I. Prior to the availability of recombinant DNA reagents for phenotypic assessments of LAD I patients and their kindreds, several lines of evidence supported an autosomal recessive pattern of inheritance for this disorder. Both male and female patients were described in initial reports, and applications of monoclonal antibodies to CD18 subunits in family studies showed heterozygous male and female carriers with expression of 50 percent of normal amounts of these proteins on their neutrophils and lymphoid cells.[258,264] In three reported families, all the clinically unaffected mothers and fathers, and some of the sibs, were shown to express intermediate levels of CD18 on their leukocytes.[264] In one family spanning three generations, an affected son was born to heterozygous parents. The affected son married a heterozygote, and the couple bore an affected son and daughter and two heterozygous daughters. These findings, together with the overall equal numbers of male-female patients recognized worldwide[246,249,264,276,297,298,305] and a frequent history of consanguineous matings[244,247,264,272,275,299] strongly suggested that LAD I is inherited as an autosomal trait. In one kindred,[253,261] X-linked inheritance was suggested, but no definitive evidence for an X-linked form of LAD I presently exists.

Clinical studies showed that patients with LAD I were uniformly deficient in the expression of all three leukocyte integrins,[249] suggesting that a primary defect in the common β subunit of Mac-1, LFA-1, and p150,95 accounted for this disease. To date, no patients with LAD I (human, canine, or bovine) have been reported demonstrating a selective deficiency of a single β_2 integrin heterodimer. A defect of the β_2 (CD18) subunit was also evidenced by initial biosynthesis studies using available monoclonal antibodies directed at both subunits of LFA-1. As shown in studies using EBV-transformed B lymphocytes or mitogen-stimulated T-lymphocyte cell lines, normal individuals synthesize LFA-1α (CD11a) and β (CD18) precursors which associate prior to further carbohydrate processing and transport of $\alpha\beta$ complexes to cell surfaces. In contrast, lymphoblasts of patients with LAD I synthesize an apparently normal LFA-1α subunit precursor, but this precursor does not undergo normal carbohydrate processing, does not associate with a β precursor, and is never expressed on the cell surface. Such findings indicated that the α subunit of LFA-1 is apparently degraded in the absence of a normal β subunit.[260]

Somatic cell complementation studies further implicated a pathologic role of the β subunit in LAD I.[265] In hybrids of human and mouse lymphocytes, human LFA-1α and β subunits from healthy individuals associated with mouse LFA-1$\alpha\beta$ subunits to form interspecies hybrid $\alpha\beta$ complexes. In hybrids of patient and mouse lymphocytes, however, the human α subunit (CD11a) but not β subunit (CD18) was rescued by the formation of interspecies complexes that were expressed on the surface of hybrid cells. Thus, the α subunit of LFA-1 in CD18-deficient cells is competent for biosynthesis and surface expression in the presence of the mouse β_2 (CD18) subunit. These same complementation protocols facilitated mapping of the β_2 subunit to chromosome 21.

Heterogeneity among patients with LAD I was first described with respect to the extent of β_2 integrin deficiency on leukocyte surfaces, as shown by flow cytometric or radiolabeled antibody-binding assays.[264] As previously discussed, the severity of clinical features and the magnitude of functional deficits observed in individual patients is directly related to the degree of protein deficiency,[264] but the underlying molecular basis for this heterogeneity often remains undefined. The availability of the CD18 subunit cDNA[7,8] and a rabbit antiserum reactive with the CD18 precursor[312] allowed more precise evaluations of the CD18 subunit of patients' cells. These revealed several distinct phenotypes of CD18 expression and structure among patients previously designated severe or moderate phenotype based on protein expression and clinical features.[264] In one study of six unrelated patients and four related patients and members of their kindred, five distinct variations in CD18 were identified (312): (a) the CD18 subunit mRNA and protein precursor were undetectable; (b) the quantities of CD18 mRNA and protein precursor were diminished; (c) an aberrantly large CD18 subunit precursor possibly due to an extra glycosylation site was observed; (d) an aberrantly small CD18 subunit due to a polypeptide chain defect was found; and (e) no gross abnormality in the CD18 subunit mRNA or protein precursor was detectable. Findings similar to the latter phenotype were evident in studies of four other patients reported by Dana et al.[313] and one patient described by Dimenshe.[248] Despite the presence of apparently normal CD11a and CD18 precursors in this group of patients, neither subunit is normally processed or transported to the cell surface. Among this group of patients, it is unclear why some are of the moderate and some of the severe phenotype.[248,312–315] Tables 188-4A and B list, and Fig. 188-2 illustrates, the known specific mutations with the two phenotypes that are discussed below.

In detailed studies of an extended west Texas kindred, including four patients with moderate phenotype, an aberrantly small CD18 precursor of identical size was identified in each case.[316] Of 10 relatives of this kindred, 9 were typed as heterozygous based on protein expression.[264] Each of these nine relatives showed both normal-sized and abnormally small CD18 precursors. One noncarrier relative with normal neutrophil surface protein values showed only the normal CD18 precursor. Endoglycosidase H digestion of the *N*-linked carbohydrate from the small CD18 precursor showed that the deficit was in the protein backbone rather than glycosylation.

Detailed assessments of this kindred by Kishimoto et al.[316] confirmed that an aberrantly small CD18 precursor is synthesized and degraded in patient cells prior to transport to and processing in the Golgi apparatus. However, studies employing large numbers of ^{125}I-labeled patient lymphoblasts revealed that small amounts of

Table 188-4 CD18 Mutations

A. Identified in Severe Phenotype LAD I Kindreds

Nucleotide	Protein	References
605C → T (CCG → CTG) Transcriptional defect: probable splicing deficiency, no detectable mRNA	P178L	Back et al.,[329] Konno et al.,[330] Ohashi et al.[428]
577G → A (GGG → AGG) Probably homozygous, possible splicing defect (exon 2–3)	G169R	Corbi et al.,[327] Nelson et al.[323]
969 + 1G → A; complex splicing defect on exon 7–8; homozygous	Aberrantly large mRNA due to splicing defect; truncated CD 18	Matsuura et al.,[326] Kobayashi et al.[429]
454G → A (GAC → AAC) Homozygous	D128N	Matsuura et al.,[326] Nunoi et al.[331]
383G → A (GAC → GGC) Homozygous, cattle	D128G	Shuster et al.,[291] Kehrli et al.
922G → A (GGC → AGC) Homozygous	G284S	Wright et al.,[320] Taylor et al.[325]
GGCCCGGCTG191 → 200 deletion and 43 bp insertion at G130-T131; splicing defect of exon 2–3. Homozygous.	41–43 deletion → frameshift → premature stop codon	Lopez Rodriquez et al.,[328] Lisowski-Grospierre et al.[273]
1674C → A (TGC → TGA) No detectable mRNA. Second allele not determined.	C534X	Lopez Rodriquez et al.,[328] Anderson et al.[264]
605C → T (CCG → CTG) 220 bp deletion (G1730-C1950) Genomic mutation not determined	P178L; deletion of exon 13 frameshift → premature stop codon	Back et al.,[329] Bowen et al.[254]
577G → A (GGG → AGG) Homozygous or second undefined allele not expressed	G169R	Wardlaw et al.,[314] Anderson et al.[264]
2142 deletion T (GAT → GA) Second mutant allele not determined	D690 frameshift	Sligh et al.,[318] Anderson et al.[264]
922G → A (CGC → AGC) Homozygous	G284S	Law SK (personal communication), Anderson et al.[264]

B. Identified in Moderate Phenotype LAD I Kindreds

Nucleotide	Protein	References
1155 + 3G → C; deletion of exon 9 (1066–1156) due to defect of 5′ splice acceptor site; homozygous	Deletion of exon 9 (K332-R361) due to aberrant splicing	Kishimoto et al.,[316] Anderson et al.[264]
518T → C (CTA → CCA) Low mRNA expression of an undefined second allele	L149P	Wardlaw et al.,[314] Wright et al.,[320] Anderson et al.[264]
659A → C (AAA → ACA) 1849C → T (CGT → TGT)	K196T R593C	Anderson et al.,[258] Arnaout et al.[315]
74T → A (ATG → AAG) 2142 deletion T (GAT → GA)	M1K D690 frameshift	Sligh et al.,[318] Anderson et al.[264]
1828C → T (CGG → TGG) and 814-14C → A; aberrant 3′ splice acceptor site (exon 6–7)	R586W (benign polymorphism) P247 *ins* (PSSQ)	Nelson et al.,[323] Wright et al.,[320] Ross et al.[295]
1124A → G (AAT → AGT)	N351S	
1327 deletion of GA; homozygous	T418 frameshift	Wright et al.,[320] Lau et al.[322]
922G → A (GGC → AGC) 1849C → T (CGT → TGT)	G284S R593C	Wright et al.,[320] Davies et al.[321]
922G → A (GGC → AGC) Second allele not determined	G284S	Back et al.,[324] Bowen et al.[254]
484T → C (TCC → CCC) 889G → C (GGA → CGA)	S138P G273R	Hogg et al.[336]

normally sized LFA-1$\alpha\beta$ complexes were synthesized and transported to the cell surface, findings consistent with a moderate phenotype.[264] S1 nuclease protection studies revealed a 90-nucleotide deletion in the CD18 subunit mRNA. Sequence analysis of PCR amplified cDNA indicated that the deletion resulted in deletion of 30 amino acids in the extracellular domain. Analysis of genomic DNA showed that this 90-bp region is encoded by a single exon (exon 9) in both patient and normal. Sequence analysis of patient genomic DNA revealed a single G to C substitution in the sequence of the 5N splice site, suggesting aberrant RNA splicing. A small amount of apparently normally spliced message was detected (by PCR amplification) in patient cells, which appears to encode a normal CD18 subunit. This apparently accounts for the low but detectable levels (3 to 6 percent of normal) of CD11/CD18 expression in affected patients.

Of significance, the 30-amino-acid deletion recognized in this kindred is located within a 241-amino-acid region of the extracellular domain of CD18 that is highly conserved in evolution. For example, the β subunit of a *Drosophila* integrin shares 35 percent amino acid identity overall within the entire CD18 subunit, but 50 percent identity in this sequence,[317] which, in turn, shares 63 percent amino acid identity with the corresponding region of the fibronectin receptor.[316] It is noteworthy that a high percentage of CD18 mutations identified among currently reported kindreds with LAD I are located within this highly conserved segment. Domains within this segment (such as the deleted 30-amino-acid domain described above) are presumably required for $\alpha\beta$ precursor association and biosynthesis and may represent critical contact sites between the α and β chain precursors. Notably, the corresponding region of the β_3 integrin has been directly implicated in binding to peptides containing Arg-Gly-Asp (RGD) sequences. Moreover, a mutation in this region of the β_3 integrin causes Glanzmann thrombasthenia (see Chap. 177). Patients with this mutation have normal expression of IIb-IIIa on

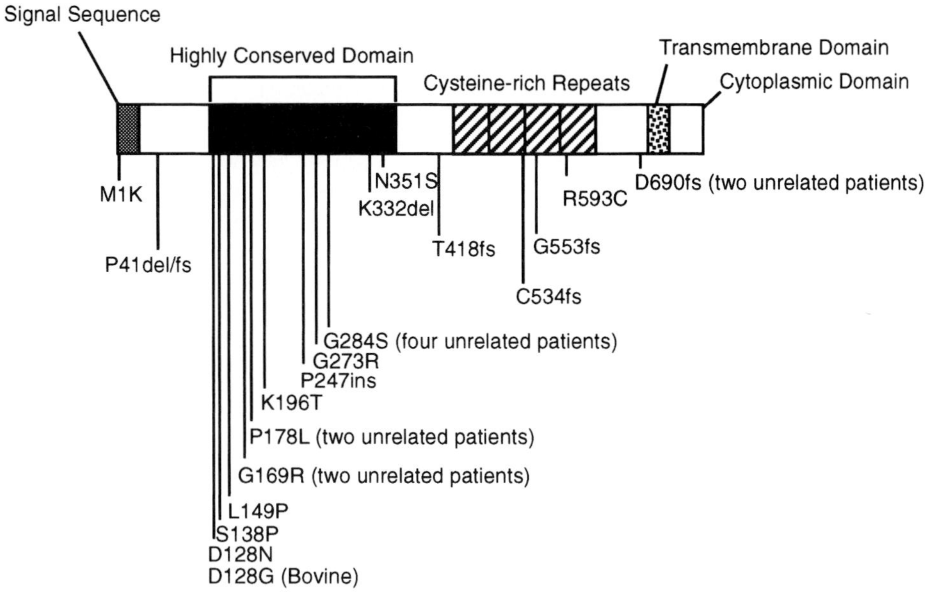

Fig. 188-2 Mutations in the CD18 gene associated with either severe or moderate phenotypes of leukocyte adhesion deficiency.

platelets but defective ligand binding. Thus, this region of the integrin β subunits appears to be critical for both $\alpha\beta$ association and ligand binding.

Detailed studies of another moderate phenotype kindred[318] defined distinct mutant alleles of paternal and maternal origin. The paternal allele includes an ATG-to-AAG substitution in the initiation code of the CD18 mRNA (M1K), and the maternal allele (D690 fs, where fs means frameshift) results from a T deletion in codon 690 (GAT → GA), 31 nucleotides 5′ to the beginning of the transmembrane domain. Studies in expression protocols have not been carried out to define which mutant allele accounts for low levels of apparently normal CD18 protein expressed on the patient's cells. However, it is plausible to suggest that the paternal allele (M1K) allows for low levels of mRNA transcription and biosynthesis of (normal) CD18 protein expressed on the patient's cells, based on the observation that an alternative translation initiation codon consistent with the criteria of Kozak[319] is created by the paternal allele substitution. Translation via this codon could result in low, albeit detectable, amounts of an essentially normal-sized message and CD18 protein subunit as shown by Kishimoto et al.[312] The predicted result of the maternal mutation is a frameshift in the CD18 mRNA predicting a premature termination codon and the biosynthesis of an aberrantly small CD18 subunit lacking a transmembrane domain and cytoplasmic tail. Such an anchorless subunit would possibly be secreted from the cell (unconfirmed), but would not likely target and insert into cell membranes. That this D690 fs mutation (maternal allele) does not allow for any biosynthesis of LFA-1 (and thus can't account for the patient's moderate phenotype) is supported by the observation[318] of an identical mutant allele in another (unrelated) compound heterozygote patient with a severe clinical phenotype. Transfection studies employing each of these mutant cDNAs should facilitate a determination of the extent to which one or both are capable of promoting CD11/CD18 expression.

Distinct and diverse CD18 mutant alleles have been defined in other moderate phenotype kindreds, including homozygous-deficient or compound heterozygote-deficient patients.[314,315,320–323] Studies by Wright[320] of a moderate phenotypic 19-year-male described by Lau et al.,[322] revealed a GA deletion (at nucleotide 1256) *and* an abnormally large (4.3 kb) mRNA. The absence of a normal-sized mRNA and the presence of the 1256-mutant allele in all PCR products from both cDNA and genomic DNA clones, suggest that the patient is homozygous deficient and that both abnormalities are encoded by the same allele. This is in agreement with a history of related parents.[322] The 1256-GA deletion predicts a frameshift in translation and a complete (severe) deficiency of CD18 expression. However, this does not appear to be the case by other criteria.[322] The nature of the 4.3-kb mRNA has not been characterized, and it is not known if it is associated with LAD I.

In another moderate phenotypic patient, Wardlaw et al.[314] defined a 446 T-to-C point mutation (CTA → CCA) resulting in a L149P substitution. Cotransfection of this mutant CD18 cDNA with wild-type LFA-1α (CD11a) cDNA in COS cells showed detectable, although markedly diminished, expression of a functionally defective LFA-1 protein. Additional studies of the same patient by Wright et al.[320] confirmed the L149 P mutation in one predominant species of cDNA associated with the creation of an *MvaI* site. Whereas PCR products from this cDNA showed almost complete cleavage with *MvcI*, only about 50 percent of PCR product from the genomic DNA was cleaved, findings suggesting that this patient has another allele of low mRNA expression yet to be characterized.

Two distinct point mutations including G284S and R593C have been reported by Wright et al.[320] in another moderate patient.[321] PCR fragments covering both locations showed that they were located on different alleles of maternal (G284S) or paternal (R593C) origin. The basis for detectable CD18 protein expression consistent with a moderate phenotype in this case is unclear. A G284S mutation resulting in an aberrantly small (60-kDa) CD18 subunit protein has been reported in another moderate patient;[324] this case presumably represents a compound heterozygote, but the nature of a second mutant allele has not been defined. A G284S mutation has been reported in two additional unrelated severe phenotype patients,[325] but the mutant (G284S) alleles are not identical to those described by Wright et al.,[320] as indicated by distinct polymorphisms. In contrast to the two former (moderate) cases, both severe cases are homozygous for the G284S mutant allele. Nelson et al.[323] defined two distinct mutant CD18 alleles of maternal origin in a male patient with moderate phenotype. These included (a) a 12-bp insertion in the cDNA that added four amino acids (Pro-Ser-Ser-Gln) between Pro247 and Glu248 and arose from a single C-to-A transversion in the 3′ terminus of an intron, which, in turn, generated an aberrant splice receptor site, and (b) an 1828C → T nucleotide transition (CGC → TGG) resulting in an R586W mutation. A third recognized mutation, an 1124A → G nucleotide transition (AAT-AGT) resulting in an N351S substitution, apparently represents a *de novo* mutation not detected in either parent cell line. COS cell transfection protocols using normal CD11a cDNA and these mutant CD18 cDNAs showed that the double-mutant maternal allele allowed essentially no surface expression of CD11b/CD18 complexes. The R586W mutation alone allowed near-normal expression, findings that suggest that it represents a benign polymorphism. Transfections of N351S mutant cDNA allowed only 22 percent of normal CD11b/CD18 expression recognized by a single anti-CD18 Mab; these findings suggest that this mutation may account for the moderate deficiency phenotype.

Investigations of a series of severe phenotype patients have defined several apparently more deleterious point mutations in the coding region of tile CD18 subunit mRNA.[314,320,325–329] As is also true for recognized mutations associated with distinct moderate phenotypes, a disproportionate number of mutant alleles involve the highly conserved domain (exons 5 through 9). These findings provide indirect evidence that this region may be critical to common structural and functional characteristics of β-integrin subunits, including the association of α and β precursors. This cluster includes reported G169R substitutions in two unrelated patients,[314,323] P178L substitutions in two additional and (presumably) unrelated patients,[329,330] and two mutations involving substitutions of the arginine 128-amino-acid residue by asparagine[326,331] or glycine.[291] The latter (D128G) mutation represents the molecular basis of bovine LAD currently prevalent worldwide among Holstein cattle as a result of artificial insemination and inbreeding of this allele in the 1970s.[291] The deleterious nature of the G169R mutation has been demonstrated by an absence of biosynthesis and expression of LFA-1 $\alpha\beta$ complexes following cotransfection of mutant CD18 cDNA of the severe patient described by Wardlaw et al.[314] and wild-type CD11a cDNA into COS cells. Of interest, severe mutations within this cluster involve amino acid residues conserved in all other β subunits, while some of the mutant alleles associated with a moderate phenotype involve nonconserved amino acids (e.g., L149P and K196T). Another cluster of severe mutations is also evident within the CD18 segment encoded by exon 13 within the cysteine-rich repeats proposed to impart structural rigidity to β integrin subunits. These include a G553fs allele[329] and a C534X nonsense mutation.[328]

Various splicing defects contribute to these or other described severe phenotype-associated alleles[326,328,329,332] and involve both the highly conserved domain and cysteine-rich repeats, as well as other domains. They include: (a) a G-to-A substitution in the exon 7 splice site resulting in aberrant splicing and premature chain termination within the highly conserved domain;[326] (b) a probable but undefined splicing defect accounting for a deletion of exon 13[329] or impaired transcription[332] in two unrelated patients each sharing a mutant P178L allele; and (c) a likely defect of splicing involving the 5′ region (intron 2/3–exon 3/4) of the CD18 gene in a patient described by Corbi et al.[327]

While this spectrum of CD18 mutations provides an incomplete explanation for the considerable heterogeneity recognized among LAD I patients, some insights concerning the structural and functional requirements for biosynthetics and expression of CD11/CD18 heterodimers are implicit in these descriptions. The deleterious nature of mutations involving the highly conserved domain and the cysteine-rich repeats (among both severe and moderate phenotype patients) supports the likely requirements for these domains in α-β precursor associations and subsequent processing and cell transport of mature CD11/CD18 complexes. In addition to quantitative defects of expression, the loss of functional activity (reflected by impaired binding of anti-CD18 blocking Mab) as a result of site-directed mutagenesis of selected epitopes within the highly conserved domain of CD18 provides additional support for this concept. Moreover, this domain in the β_3 integrin (gpIIb) subunit contains motifs required for ligand (fibrinogen, RGD, other) binding by gpIIb/IIIa[333] and has been shown to be defective in patients with Glansmann thrombasthenia (see Chap. 177).[334]

The basis for impaired transcription of CD18 among some recognized LAD I alleles is poorly understood. Wright et al.[320] described low levels of mRNA expression associated with undefined[314] or P247 (PSSQ) insertion[323] alleles. Three additional LAD I patients characterized by low mRNA expression[318,326,328] each demonstrate frameshift mutations encoding truncated proteins. Studies of the CD18 promoter elements in a severe phenotypic patient with undetectable CD18 mRNA (by northern blot)[328] revealed no abnormalities, but similar studies in other patients may reveal defects in transcriptional regulatory domains contained within a 1-kb domain 5′ to the first exon. Frameshift mutations may affect the stability of mRNA in some patients, but this explanation is not applicable to others. For example, a 10-bp deletion in the patient described by Lopez Rodriquez et al.[328] has no apparent effect on mRNA levels. An initiation codon mutation (MIK) described by Sligh et al.[318] provides a plausible explanation for a partial deficiency of CD18 expression, but three mutant alleles exclusively associated with partial CD18 expression and a moderate phenotype (L149P, K196T, and R593C) map to regions of the highly conserved or cysteine-rich repeat domains most commonly associated with severe phenotypes.

Kuijpers et al.[335] described a LAD I variant. This patient exhibited a moderate LAD I phenotype. There were bacterial infections without apparent pus formation in the presence of a striking granulocytosis, and for which intravenous treatment with high-dose antibiotics was needed. Delayed-type hypersensitivity reaction upon skin testing was absent, and there was delayed wound healing. Specific antibody generation was abnormal, but normal in vitro T cell proliferation responses after immunization were found. Expression levels of CD11/CD18 proteins were completely normal, but leukocyte activation did not result in CD11/CD18 activation and high-avidity ligand binding. No sequence abnormalities in the CD18 integrin proteins were found. In vitro chemotaxis, endothelial transmigration of the neutrophils, and leukocyte aggregation responses were almost absent. During follow-up, a bleeding tendency, which was related to decreased glycoprotein IIb-IIIa (β_3 integrin) activation on platelets, became clinically apparent; it was different from previously described cellular adhesion molecule variants. This was the first reported case of a clinical combined immunodeficiency syndrome that apparently resulted from nonfunctional CD11/CD18 molecules.

Hogg et al.[336] recently described a patient with clinical features compatible with a moderate phenotype of LAD I, but whose neutrophils expressed LFA-1 and Mac-1 at 40 to 60 percent of normal levels. This level of expression should be adequate for normal integrin function, but both the patient's Mac-1 on neutrophils and LFA-1 on T cells failed to bind ligands such as fibrinogen and ICAM-1, respectively, or to display a β_2 integrin activation epitope after adhesion-inducing stimulation of the cells. Sequencing of the patient's two CD18 alleles revealed the mutations S138P and G273R. Both mutations are within the highly conserved domain of CD18, and S138P is a putative divalent cation-coordinating residue in the metal ion-dependent adhesion site (MIDAS) motif.[1] After cotransfection of a cell line (K562) with normal α subunits, the mutated S138P β_2 subunit was coexpressed but did not support adhesive functions, whereas the G273R mutant was not expressed. This is the second reported example of a LAD I patient exhibiting a failure of β_2 integrin function despite adequate levels of cell-surface expression.

Clinical Management of LAD I. Suggested therapeutic guidelines for LAD I are based on a relatively limited clinical experience. Of major importance is the potential for life-threatening systemic bacterial infections that may extend from commonly infected sites in skin or mucus membranes, especially in severely affected patients. Superficial inflammatory lesions must be managed aggressively with local care and systemic antibiotic regimens. The early use of combination therapy with a staphylocidal agent and an aminoglycoside, or extended-spectrum penicillin agent, is justified in acutely ill or febrile patients in the absence of localizing clinical findings. The use of prophylactic antibiotics for chronic infections (e.g., progressive periodontitis) may be advised, but clinical data documenting the long-term efficacy of this empiric approach is lacking. Trimethoprim B-sulfamethoxazole is widely used in this setting based on its broad antimicrobial spectrum of activity and safety profile.

In patients with progressive and life-threatening infections refractory to antibiotic therapy, granulocyte transfusions are efficacious in attenuating, if not eliminating, infectious episodes. The major limitations of granulocyte transfusions include the short half-life of transfused cells and the need for repeated infusions on a daily basis for the duration of infections, often for several weeks.

Bone marrow transplantation (BMT) with successful engraftment and long-term clinical recovery from disease has been achieved in several patients, although unsuccessful and fatal complications of this approach have been reported.[337,338] Because of the inherent risks of myeloid suppression and graft versus host disease (GVHD), some investigators have advised this approach preferentially for severe phenotype patients. Among patients undergoing transplantation, recipients of HLA B identical, as well as HLA mismatched, bone marrow have shown successful engraftment. In the largest reported experience, Thomas et al.[338] retrospectively analyzed the outcome of BMT in 14 patients with LAD I. Performed between 1981 and 1993 in two European centers, five patients received bone marrow from HLA B identical donors and nine received T-cell-depleted marrow from two HLA B antigen or haplotype mismatched parents. In five cases, failure of engraftment occurred as a result of either insufficient myeloablation or graft rejection (as seen in two cases of moderate phenotype LAD I). These patients were successfully retransplanted using a conditioning regimen that included total body irradiation and chemotherapy, with the use of anti-LFA-1 and anti-CD2 monoclonal antibodies for moderate patients. Eight patients developed acute GVHD, and chronic GVHD occurred in four cases with fatal complications in three of these patients. At the time of this report,[338] 10 patients of the series were alive and well 12 months to 12 years after BMT; chimerism was full in 6 cases, and mixed but stable in 4 cases, with variable proportions of normal and CD18-deficient leukocytes in peripheral blood. Mixed chimerism observed in these cases does not appear to reflect slowly progressive graft failure and is compatible with long-term freedom from infectious complications.

Studies demonstrating the retroviral-mediated gene transfer of the human CD18 subunit into EBV-B cells, mouse bone marrow cells, and human bone marrow cells[339–341] have set the stage for attempts at somatic cell gene therapy for LAD I. Bauer et al.[342] recently reported high levels of transfection of peripheral blood $CD34^+$ cells derived from a patient with severe LAD using a novel retroviral vector. Based on these preliminary observations, it should be possible to engraft autologous cells removed from LAD patients and treated ex vivo with candidate retroviral vectors.

Identification of Leukocyte Adhesion Deficiency II (LAD II, Rambon-Hasharon Syndrome)

Clinical and Histopathologic Features. Frydman et al.[343] described two male Arab patients (ages 5 and 3), both products of unrelated consanguineous matings. Distinctive clinical features of these patients included craniofacial dysmorphism, neurologic deficits (microcephaly, cortical atrophy, central hypotonia, seizures, and developmental delay), and striking peripheral blood neutrophilia. Extreme neutrophilia was noted from the first day of life. Recurrent bacterial infections occurred early in life, and included pneumonia, periodontitis, otitis media, and cellulitis. Mild to moderate skin infections occurred without obvious pus formation. In contrast to most patients with LAD I, these patients' infections were not life threatening.[344] After the age of 3 years, the frequency of infections diminished, with the main infectious events being severe periodontitis, a condition also observed in patients with LAD I (Table 188-5).

That these patients represent examples of a new, presumably autosomal recessive, syndrome was suggested by the finding that both patients lack the red blood cell H antigen and manifest the

Table 188-5 Leukocyte Adhesion Deficiencies

	LAD I		LAD II*
	Severe	Moderate	
Clinical Manifestations			
Severe infections	++++	+	+
Neutrophilia			
Basal	++	+	+++
With infection	++++	+++	+++
Periodontitis	++++	+++	+++
Skin infections	+++	++	+
Developmental abnormalities	–	–	+++
Laboratory Findings			
sLeX expression	normal	normal	absent
CD18 integrins expression	↓↓↓, or absent	↓↓, or dysfunctional	normal
Neutrophil L-selectin	↓↓	↓	normal
Neutrophil motility in vitro	↓↓↓	↓↓	↓↓
Neutrophil rolling	normal	normal	↓↓↓
Neutrophil firm adhesion	↓↓↓	↓↓	↓
Neutrophil emigration	↓↓↓↓	↓↓↓	↓↓
Opsonophagocytosis	↓	↓	normal
Lymphocyte function	↓	↓	normal

*Adapted from Etzioni.[430]

Bombay (hh) phenotype. This phenotype is ordinarily due to homozygosity for a rare recessive (h) allele. Individuals with this phenotype generally lack the H antigen, an intermediate in the production of A and B antigens of red blood cells. The H gene product is an α_2 fucosyltransferase that catalyzes the addition of a GDP fucose to *N*-acetylgalactosamine to produce the H antigen.[345,346] The Hh system is genetically heterogeneous, and both complete (Bombay) and incomplete (Para-Bombay) deficiencies are recognized. In contrast to the patients described here, individuals with these phenotypes do not have any distinctive clinical features.

The findings of markedly elevated blood neutrophil counts (60 to 150,000 FL) in the patients reported by Frydman prompted studies of leukocyte functions. The prolonged intravascular neutrophil survival seen in the LAD I syndrome,[321] which seems to account for the marked leukocytosis, was not seen in LAD II patients.[347] In fact, the intravascular half-disappearance time was much shorter than normal, and the neutrophil turnover rate was markedly elevated. The estimated turnover was eight times normal.[347] In vitro studies revealed significant defects of random or directed neutrophil migration[348] and diminished homotypic aggregation of neutrophils.[349] In contrast, opsonophagocytic and bactericidal activities of patient neutrophils were normal, as were lymphocyte proliferation and natural killer cell activities. However, delayed type hypersensitivity reactions were not observed upon intradermal injections of various antigens.[347] This may be due to the absence of cutaneous lymphocyte antigen (CLA) involved in E-selectin-dependent lymphocyte homing to the skin.[71] Leukocyte surface levels of L-selectin are normal in LAD II, in contrast to observations in LAD I where L-selectin levels on neutrophils are often diminished,[350] most likely due to frequent infections leading to some low-level neutrophil activation and subsequent shedding of this adhesion molecule (see selectin regulation above).[112]

Additional studies were performed to assess the in vivo immune responsiveness and lymphocyte recruitment to the skin in response to keyhole limpet hemocyanin (KLH) in a LAD II patient.[351] There was normal priming of KLH-specific T cells, as well as a strong in vivo anti-KLH antibody response, both indicative of a normal T-B cell function and collaboration. Skin biopsies following KLH injection revealed a large number of T cells recruited to the site of challenge, and up-regulation of the endothelial adhesion molecules ICAM-1 (CD54), VCAM-1 (CD106), and E-selectin (CD62E). The recruited T cell showed a normal subset distribution but lacked cutaneous lymphocyte antigen (CLA), the cutaneous homing receptor. However, the clinical symptoms of delayed-type hypersensitivity in the patient (redness and swelling) were severely depressed compared to that in the controls. It appeared that the LAD II patient showed a normal T cell priming and T cell-dependent antibody response, and a significant T cell recruitment to the site of KLH challenge, indicating that fucosylated sugar determinants, such as SLe(x) and CLA, are not strictly required for immune responsiveness and skin homing of some lymphocytes, although some effector functions appear abnormal, possibly as a result of absence of an important effector subset of lymphocytes.

Several features of this syndrome suggest the possibility of a glycosylation defect that might influence the expression of Sialyl-Lewis X (sLeX) (NeuAcα2,3 Gal β1,4 (Fucα1,3) GlcNac), a carbohydrate ligand of the endothelial adhesion molecules E-selectin and P-selectin. LAD II neutrophils exhibited the ability to be activated for the up-regulation of CD18 integrins in vitro, and exhibited the ability to spread on a protein coated glass surface[352] (in contrast to LAD I neutrophils[264]). In addition to this rare Bombay phenotype, both patients were secretor negative and Lewis negative, blood groups associated with Fucα2, Gal and Fucα1, 3/4 GlcNac linkages, respectively.[353,354] Because each of these carbohydrate structures contain fucose, Etzioni et al.[355] tested the possibility that patient leukocytes were deficient in sLeX, which also contains fucose. Flow cytometric studies using an anti-sLeX monoclonal antibody confirmed a complete absence of this determinant on neutrophils of both patients. Additional studies demonstrated profoundly diminished adherence of patient neutrophils to IL-1 elicited endothelial monolayers bearing high levels of E-selectin. These findings suggest that the clinical features of neutrophilia and recurrent pulmonary infections in this syndrome reflect leukocyte adherence defects due to a lack of sLeX-bearing ligands required for selectin-mediated adhesion to endothelial cells. This concept is supported by intravital microscopic studies of patient neutrophils in rabbit mesenteric venules primed for 4 h with IL-1, a condition in which human neutrophils normally demonstrate rolling margination in vivo.[350] Isolated patient neutrophils exhibited markedly reduced rolling adhesion in this model, a finding consistent with the concept that lectin-carbohydrate interactions are necessary for this phase of localization (see Table 188-3).

Characterizations of this novel syndrome provide strong evidence for important adhesive interactions of sLeX-bearing ligands and E-selectin in neutrophil migration and recruitment at sites of inflammation in vivo. This possibility is also supported by in vitro investigations and in vivo animal model studies demonstrating that selectins mediate adhesion of neutrophils (and other leukocyte cell types) to vascular endothelium under flow conditions of postcapillary venules.[122,158,356–360] Because P-selectin has also been shown to recognize sLeX-containing ligands,[359] it is possible that neutrophils of these patients will be defective in P-selectin-mediated adherence functions. The possibility that sLeX deficiency underlies other neutrophil defects is uncertain, but the observed defects of homotypic aggregation may reflect the requirements for L-selectin interactions with PSGL-1 in this process.[361] Future studies to determine the specific biochemical defects and resulting functional and pathologic consequence in this syndrome should allow additional insights concerning the physiological roles of selectin-dependent adhesion reactions.

Molecular Basis of LAD II. The basic abnormality in LAD II is a general defect in fucose metabolism. Recent observations[362] resulting from prenatal diagnosis of LAD II indicated that at 22 weeks of gestation, the fetus was normal in size and without obvious abnormalities. The finding that the previously identified patients exhibited impaired growth only after birth suggested that fucose transported from the mother may be significant. In this regard, B lymphoblasts and fibroblasts from the LAD II patients failed to show binding of fucose-specific lectins unless fed exogenous fucose in vitro. This indicates that a scavenger pathway is intact in LAD II[363] and that the defect in fucose metabolism is not limited to hematopoietic cells. These observations support the idea that the growth abnormalities and mental retardation are also related to the fucose abnormality. The exact defect in the *de novo* pathway of fucose production from GDP-mannose to GDP-fucose is unknown, but Sturla et al.[364] found that in cell lysates from a LAD II patient, GDP-D-mannose-4,6-dehydratase (GMD), the first of the two enzymes of the pathway, had a defective activity compared to control subjects. GMD in cell lysates from both parents showed intermediate activity levels. Cloning of GMD from patient and control lymphocytes ruled out a mutation affecting the amino acid sequence of this enzyme, and the purified recombinant proteins from both controls and the patient showed identical specific activities. Because the levels of immunoreactive GMD in cell lysates were comparable in the patient and in controls, the biochemical deficiency of intracellular GMD activity in LAD II seems to be due to mutation(s) affecting some still unidentified GMD-regulating protein.

Abnormalities of Adhesion in Neonates

Developmentally related inflammatory deficits observed in human or animal neonates appear to involve defects of neutrophil localization or emigration at sites of inflammation.[365–369] Because specific immunity is limited in the immediate postpartum period, the inflammatory functions of phagocytic cells are an especially important aspect of innate immunity for host defense against microbial invasion.[365] Both quantitative and functional deficits of neutrophils/monocytes appear to contribute to infectious susceptibility.[302,370–372] However, because these functional deficits are observed commonly among healthy neonates, such abnormalities may play a physiological role in limiting inflammatory responses that would be deleterious in immature hosts.[372] For example, injurious pulmonary inflammatory responses to hyperoxia are significantly less in neonatal rats than in adult animals.[373]

The most consistently observed functional abnormalities of neonatal neutrophils are those involving chemotactic migration in vitro. Migration toward gradients of numerous chemotactic factors, including those released by growing *Staphylococcus aureus* and *E. coli* (e.g., f-Met-peptides) and those generated in plasma by antigen-antibody complexes (e.g., C5a),[219,374] is significantly reduced. Visual assays demonstrate that the initial event required for directional migration — the ability to orient toward a gradient of chemotactic factors — is significantly impaired.[219,375] Depressed migration has been found in healthy neonates 1 to 5 days of age,[376,377] although more striking abnormalities have been reported in premature infants. Visual assays using shape change as an index of response to some chemotactic stimuli reveal no deficits[219] in dose-response characteristics of neonatal neutrophils, although receptor numbers for C5a appear to be significantly reduced in neonates.[378] In addition, there is diminished generation of chemotactic activity (chemotaxigenesis) by virulent Type III Group B *Streptococci* in neonatal sera, which is directly related to diminished levels of both type-specific anticapsular antibody and serum complement activity.[379]

The impaired migration of neonatal neutrophils is apparently linked to abnormalities in cell adherence.[219,302,371,372,375,380–384] At least three distinct abnormalities of neutrophil adhesion to endothelial cells or protein substrates in vitro have been recognized. Chemotactic factors fail to stimulate adhesion of neonatal neutrophils to artificial or endothelial substrates[219,302,382,385] apparently as a result of diminished up-regulation and/or functional activation of the Mac-1 heterodimer.[382,384–388] This could be partly due to an increase in the number of immature cells[389] or to a reduction in the total cellular content of Mac-1.[390] The function and levels of LFA-1 on neonatal neutrophils appear to be equivalent to that on adult neutrophils both in vitro[390,391] and in vivo in a neonatal rabbit model of inflammation.[182] Expression of LFA-1 on neonatal cells is normal and contributes to both adhesion and transendothelial migration.[19,302]

Neonatal neutrophils also exhibit diminished adhesion to IL-1 stimulated endothelial cells when studied under conditions of flow (wall shear stress, 2 dynes/cm^2) that select for CD18-independent adhesion mechanisms.[372,392] This abnormality apparently results from markedly diminished surface levels of L-selectin on circulating blood neutrophils or eosinophils of healthy term neonates both human[372,392] and rabbit.[393] Monoclonal antibodies recognizing L-selectin reduced the adhesion of adult neutrophils under these experimental conditions to the level of neonatal neutrophils, and they did not further reduce adhesion of neonatal cells. In a rabbit model of peritoneal inflammation, monoclonal antibodies to L-selectin significantly reduce neutrophil influx in adult animals, but not in neonates.[393] The basis for the reduced L-selectin on neonatal neutrophils is not yet defined, but may relate to high levels of GM-CSF (and/or other plasma factors), as demonstrated in umbilical cord blood and placental tissues in some studies.[394] GM-CSF, similar to chemotactic factors, stimulates the shedding of L-selectin from blood neutrophils in vitro, and significantly diminishes neutrophil emigration into experimental skin windows of adult volunteers.[395] Studies of cord blood or neonatal neutrophils by Koenig et al.[396] have shown that diminished levels of neutrophil L-selectin are inversely related to total blood neutrophil count, and similar relationships have been reported in neonatal rabbits.[393] L-selectin levels are not significantly reduced on neutrophils from healthy premature infants.[397–399] Another deficit of selectin-dependent adhesion of neonatal neutrophils is their significantly reduced ability to interact with P-selectin under conditions of flow.[391] This appears to be due to a reduced level of P-selectin ligands including PSGL-1.[400]

Deficits of Mac-1, L-selectin, and PSGL-1 may contribute to diminished leukocyte sequestration in human neonates, but direct evidence for this is currently insufficient. Rebuck skin window studies[175,401] reveal levels of neutrophil accumulation much like those in adults, as well as two other abnormalities: (a) a slower and less pronounced shift from the early granulocyte to later mononuclear cell predominance, and (b) a marked eosinophilia in some infants 2 to 21 days of age. Diminished leukocyte mobilization in neonatal rats inoculated intraperitoneally with bacteria or chemotactic agents has been reported,[366] and peritoneal influx in a rabbit model was significantly reduced.[393]

Specific Granule Deficiency

Neutrophils contain subpopulations of granules.[402] Azurophil or primary granules appear early in neutrophil development and contain lysosomal enzymes, including lysozyme and myeloperoxidase. Specific or secondary granules develop later, and contain a different set of constituents (e.g., chemotactic receptors, lactoferrin, CD11b/CD18).[403,404] The first example of a deficiency of specific granules was recognized in 1972,[405] and several laboratories subsequently reported other cases.[306,403,406–413] One patient[405] appeared to have had an acquired deficiency (associated with a myeloproliferative syndrome), while all others appeared to have genetically determined disease. Each has demonstrated susceptibility to recurrent and severe infections of the skin, mucous membranes, and lung, most commonly due to *Staphylococcus aureus*, *Pseudomonas aeruginosa*, other enteric pathogens, and *Candida albicans*. Detailed descriptions of the histopathology of infected tissues in all patients are not reported, but skin window studies demonstrated diminished leukocyte sequestration in tissues of some individuals who were not neutropenic.[403,406] A prognosis for this disorder is not well defined, but most individuals have survived the pediatric age group with supportive and antimicrobial therapy.

Neutrophils from each patient studied have shown distinct morphologic abnormalities, including a severe or total deficiency of specific granules and a variety of nuclear abnormalities including bilobed or multilobed nuclei or nuclear blebs, clefts, or pockets. Eosinophils appear to be affected as well.[414] Thus, functional abnormalities in this disorder are not limited to neutrophils, and the secretory proteins absent from patient neutrophils are not limited to specific granules. The membrane-marker alkaline phosphatase is diminished or absent in neutrophils of all but one reported case, and the total cellular content and/or release of the secondary granule markers (lactoferrin, B_{12} transport protein, cytochrome b, and lysozyme) is diminished in most patients. Neutrophils of these patients also lack defensins localized to the azurophil granules.[415] Azurophil granules of patient cells exhibit a decreased density on sucrose gradients when compared with azurophil granules of normal neutrophils.[403]

Somewhat heterogenous abnormalities of in vitro neutrophil functions have been observed. Defects of chemotaxis and intracellular microbicidal activity are most consistently reported. The basis of impaired neutrophil locomotion in vitro or diminished accumulation in skin windows in vivo is uncertain. However, in studies of two patients,[306,403,406] defective neutrophil chemotaxis appeared to be functionally related to abnormalities of adherence. In one patient, there was diminished neutrophil adherence to nylon fibers or endothelial cells, and impaired homotypic aggregation in response to f-Met-Leu-Phe.[406] Neutrophils of another patient failed to enhance CR3 (Mac-1) expression in response to f-Met-Leu-Phe, although up-regulation of the CR1 was normal.[306] Immunoprecipitation studies employing monoclonal antibodies against CD11b and CR1 showed that Mac-1 (but not CR1) cosediments with specific granule fractions of normal neutrophils. CR1 is apparently associated with unique microvesicular bodies in neutrophils unassociated with specific granules.

The molecular basis for the complex cellular abnormalities of these patients is undefined. Indirect evidence implicates abnormalities of the regulation of gene expression during granulopoiesis resulting in a failure to activate a cassette of genes normally expressed at the myelocyte-metamyelocyte stage of maturation.[415,416] Studies of two patients showed no detectable lactoferrin biosynthesis in neutrophils and only trace amounts of lactoferrin transcripts in bone marrow cells.[417] However, lactoferrin biosynthesis in nasal secretory glands and other nonmyeloid tissues was normal in these patients, indicating that the abnormality of lactoferrin gene expression is tissue specific and limited to cells of myeloid lineage. Of interest are mice deficient in PU.1, an ETS family transcription factor that is expressed specifically in hematopoietic lineages, which develop neutrophils expressing neutrophil-specific markers but fail to terminally differentiate, as shown by the absence of messages for neutrophil secondary granule components.[418] While these cells do not mimic exactly those of patients with specific granule deficiency, they provide an interesting model with some parallels.

ANIMAL MODELS OF ADHESION-DEPENDENT INFLAMMATION

Targeted deletions of each of the adhesion molecules in the selectin and CD18 integrin families have been produced in mice. In general, mice with specific deletions of adhesion molecules reveal abnormalities in the inflammatory process when challenged. Absence of individual members of the selectin family leads to defects in leukocyte rolling, and emigration in the early phases of inflammation.[124,141,419,420] Such results were clearly anticipated by earlier studies in vitro using cell culture assays to assess the interactions of leukocytes with endothelial cells under conditions of flow,[60,136,138] and in vivo using blocking monoclonal antibodies.[134] Mice with deletions of either LFA-1 (CD11a/CD18)[177] or Mac-1[178,179] have revealed distinctions in the functions of these two integrins that were not evident from studies using blocking monoclonal antibodies. In contrast to conclusions drawn from early antibody blocking studies,[113,421] Mac-1 does not appear to be necessary for neutrophil emigration,[178,179] although LFA-1 does appear to be necessary for neutrophil emigration.[178] The reduced emigration caused by monoclonal antibodies against Mac-1 was apparently linked to nonspecific effects of intact antibody, because studies with $F(abN)_2$ fragments that are effective in blocking neutrophil adhesion to ligands recognized by Mac-1 revealed no effect of the antibodies on transendothelial migration in vitro or emigration in vivo.[178]

In all cases, mice with targeted deletions of selectins or individual members of the CD18 integrin family are viable and fertile. Except for those with complete CD18 deficiency (i.e., lacking all members of this family as in the case of LAD I)[422] or those with combined deficiency of E-selectin and P-selectin,[423] all animals are healthy when breeding colonies are maintained in a barrier facility. The CD18 null animals[422] have exhibited an increase in perinatal mortality (10 to 40 percent), and survivors have developed progressive perioral soft tissue swelling, facial alopecia, reddening of the skin, and extended facial and submandibular ulcerative dermatitis by approximately 3 months of age. This phenotype was observed in 95 percent of mice.[422] Histopathology of the skin revealed necrotic inflammatory cells and bacterial colonies, with a predominantly mononuclear cell infiltrate and very few neutrophils. Reactive lymphadenopathy involving the nodes that drained the areas of skin erosion was seen. There was splenomegaly with myeloid hyperplasia, bone marrow myeloid hyperplasia, and a 5.5-times increase in blood leukocyte counts when compared with wild-type mice. Blood neutrophil counts were approximately elevenfold those of wild-type mice. Serum IgG levels were ten- to fifteenfold above wild-type levels; serum levels of IL-3 and IL-6 were approximately twentyfold greater than normal. Conjunctival cultures from CD18 null mice were consistently positive for one to three organisms, including *E. coli, Lactobacillus sp., Enterococcus faecalis, Proteus mirabilis, Streptococcus*, and *Staphylococcus epidermidis*. The number of organisms increased with the severity of conjunctivitis. When challenged intraperitoneally with *S. pneumoniae*, CD18 null mice exhibited a marked reduction in survival when compared with wild-type controls. Evaluations of the inflammatory response in the skin of CD18 null mice[422,424] revealed an absence of neutrophil infiltration at sites of inflammatory challenge, and using intravital microscopy, a profound reduction in stable adhesion of leukocytes to the endothelium of venules. Leukocyte rolling, though, was equivalent to wild-type controls. T cell functions were also reduced.

Another feature of the CD18 null mice is the apparent confirmation of a CD18-independent pathway of neutrophil emigration into pulmonary tissues.[425] Studies in these mice reveal substantial pulmonary emigration of neutrophils in response to bacterial challenge,[424] a finding consistent with histopathologic studies of a patient with severe phenotype of LAD I where many foci of bronchopneumonia contained numerous neutrophils, although other infected tissues were devoid of neutrophils.[426] Thus, the LAD I syndrome in CD18 null mice is remarkably consistent with that in humans, cattle, and dogs.

Regarding the selectin-deficient mice, only animals with combined deficiency of E-selectin and P-selectin have exhibited spontaneous illness,[423] although no studies of a triple selectin knockout have been published. Mice with null mutations in both E- and P-selectin did not show increased prenatal or early postnatal mortality, but began to show abnormalities at variable ages after weaning. There was nonulcerative excoriative skin lesions with hair loss in the head and neck, redness and swelling of the oral mucosa, and sevenfold increases in blood neutrophil counts by 6 months of age. Histopathology of the skin and oral mucosa showed loss of the squamous epithelium and superficial colonization with bacteria, and cultures were consistently positive for *Staphylococcus aureus, E. coli, Enterococcus faecium*, and other common floral organisms. The infected regions contained mixed granulocytic and mononuclear cell infiltration. There was periodontitis with chronic leukocytic infiltrate and gingival recession. Some mice developed conjunctivitis with bacterial organisms similar to those recovered from the skin. There was cervical lymphadenopathy, and the node architecture was abnormal, with predominantly plasmacytoid lymphocytes and plasma cells. Serum IgG was approximately tenfold that of wild-type mice. Lung tissue had increased cellularity in the alveolar walls, with a large increase in the number of neutrophils and other leukocytes marginated within the capillary lumina. Neutrophils had not spontaneously migrated into either the interstitium or the alveolar space. Experimental evaluation of inflammatory processes revealed a profound reduction in neutrophil infiltration and edema in *S. pneumoniae* induced peritonitis at 4 h, compared to only moderate reductions in mice deficient in either E-selectin or P-selectin. Although neutrophil influx had returned to normal by 24 h, clearance of the bacteria was significantly reduced at this time in the double-mutant mice. Intravital microscopy studies in the double-mutant mice revealed an absence of rolling leukocytes over an observation time of 2 h. This is in contrast to the high frequency of rolling leukocytes seen in wild-type controls.[141] In P-selectin-deficient mice, rolling is initially reduced, but returns over the 2-h observation time,[427] and rolling is not reduced in E-selectin-deficient mice.[423] Thus, in some respects, the syndrome in mice deficient in both E-selectin and P-selectin exhibits characteristics of the inflammatory deficits of LAD II in humans (i.e., some increased susceptibility to infection, periodontitis, neutrophilia, lack of leukocyte rolling, normal function of CD18 integrins, and reduced leukocyte emigration).

REFERENCES

1. Kishimoto TK, Baldwin ET, Anderson DC: The role of β_2 integrins in inflammation, in Gallin JI, Snyderman, R (eds): *Inflammation. Basic Principles and Clinical Correlates*. Philadelphia, Lippincott-Williams & Wilkins, 1999, p 569.
2. Van der Vieren M, Trong HL, Wood CL, Moore PF, St John T, Staunton DE, Gallatin WM: A novel leukointegrin, $\alpha_d\beta_2$, binds preferentially to ICAM-3. *Immunity* **3**:683, 1995.
3. Corbi AL, Miller LJ, O'Connor K, Larson RS, Springer TA: cDNA cloning and complete primary structure of the alpha subunit of a leukocyte adhesion glycoprotein, p150,95. *EMBO J* **6(13)**:4023, 1987.
4. Corbi AL, Kishimoto TK, Miller LJ, Springer TA: The human leukocyte adhesion glycoprotein Mac-1 (complement receptor type 3, CD11b) alpha subunit: Cloning, primary structure, and relation to the integrins, von Willebrand factor and factor B. *J Biol Chem* **263**:12403, 1988.
5. Arnaout MA, Gupta SK, Pierce MW, Tenen DG: Amino acid sequence of the alpha subunit of human leukocyte adhesion receptor Mol (complement receptor type 3). *J Cell Biol* **106**:2153, 1988.
6. Larson RS, Corbi AL, Berman L, Springer TA: Primary structure of the LFA-1 alpha subunit: An integrin with an embedded domain defining a protein superfamily. *J Cell Biol* **108**:703, 1989.
7. Kishimoto TK, O'Connor K, Lee A, Roberts TM, Springer TA: Cloning of the beta subunit of the leukocyte adhesion proteins: Homology to an extracellular matrix receptor defines a novel supergene family. *Cell* **48**:681, 1987.
8. Law SKA, Gagnon J, Hildreth JEK, Wells CE, Willis AC, Wong AJ: The primary structure of the beta-subunit of the cell surface adhesion glycoproteins LFA-1, CR-3 and p150,95 and its relationship to the fibronectin receptor. *EMBO J* **6**:915, 1987.
9. Ugarova TP, Solovjov DA, Zhang L, Loukinov DI, Yee VC, Medved LV, Plow EF: Identification of a novel recognition sequence for integrin alphaM beta2 within the gamma-chain of fibrinogen. *J Biol Chem* **273**:22519, 1998.
10. Stanley P, Hogg N: The I domain of integrin LFA-1 interacts with ICAM-1 domain 1 at residue Glu-34 but not Gln-73. *J Biol Chem* **273**:3358, 1998.
11. Griggs DW, Schmidt CM, Carron CP: Characteristics of cation binding to the I domains of LFA-1 and MAC-1. The LFA-1 I domain contains a Ca2+-binding site. *J Biol Chem* **273**:22113, 1998.
12. Lu C, Oxvig C, Springer TA: The structure of the beta-propeller domain and C-terminal region of the integrin alphaM subunit. Dependence on beta subunit association and prediction of domains. *J Biol Chem* **273**:15138, 1998.

13. Wright SD, Weitz JI, Huang AJ, Levin SM, Silverstein SC, Loike JD: Complement receptor type three (CD11b/CD18) of human polymorphonuclear leukocytes recognizes fibrinogen. *Proc Natl Acad Sci U S A* **85(2)**:7734, 1988.
14. Myones BL, Dalzell JG, Hogg N, Ross GD: p150,95 has been shown on macrophages to be an iC3b receptor and termed the CR4. *Complement* **4**:199, 1987.
15. Grayson MH, Van der Vieren M, Sterbinsky SA, Gallatin WM, Hoffman PA, Staunton DE, Bochner BS: adβ2 integrin is expressed on human eosinophils and functions as an alternative ligand for vascular cell adhesion molecule 1 (VCAM-1). *J Exp Med* **188**:2187, 1998.
16. Rothlein R, Dustin ML, Marlin SD, Springer TA: A human intercellular adhesion molecule (ICAM-1) distinct from LFA-1. *J Immunol* **137**:1270, 1986.
17. Staunton DE, Dustin ML, Springer TA: Functional cloning of ICAM-2, a cell adhesion ligand for LFA-1 homologous. *Nature* **339**:61, 1989.
18. de Fougerolles AR, Stacker SA, Schwarting R, Springer TA: Characterization of ICAM-2 and evidence for a third counter-receptor for LFA-1. *J Exp Med* **174**:253, 1991.
19. Smith CW, Marlin SD, Rothlein R, Toman C, Anderson DC: Cooperative interactions of LFA-1 and Mac-1 with intercellular adhesion molecule-1 in facilitating adherence and transendothelial migration of human neutrophils in vitro. *J Clin Invest* **83**:2008, 1989.
20. Diamond MS, Staunton DE, Marlin SD, Springer TA: Binding of the integrin Mac-1 (CD11b/CD18) to the third immunoglobulin-like domain of ICAM-1 (CD54) and its regulation by glycosylation. *Cell* **65**:961, 1991.
21. Todd III RF, Arnaout MA, Rosin RE, Crowley CA, Peters WA, Babior BM: Subcellular localization of the large subunit of Mo1 (Mo1$_1$; formerly gp110), a surface glycoprotein associated with neutrophil adhesion. *J Clin Invest* **74**:1280, 1984.
22. Buyon JP, Abramson SB, Philips MR, Slade SG, Ross GD, Weissmann G, Winchester RJ: Dissociation between increased surface expression of Gp165/95 and homotypic neutrophil aggregation. *J Immunol* **140**:3156, 1988.
23. Vedder NB, Harlan JM: Increased surface expression of CD11b/CD18 (Mac-1) is not required for stimulated neutrophil adherence to cultured endothelium. *J Clin Invest* **81**:676, 1988.
24. Newton RA, Thiel M, Hogg N: Signaling mechanisms and the activation of leukocyte integrins. *J Leukoc Biol* **61**:422, 1997.
25. Nagel W, Zeitlmann L, Schilcher P, Geiger C, Kolanus J, Kolanus W: Phosphoinositide 3-OH kinase activates the beta2 integrin adhesion pathway and induces membrane recruitment of cytohesin-1. *J Biol Chem* **273**:14853, 1998.
26. McDowall A, Leitinger B, Stanley P, Bates PA, Randi AM, Hogg N: The I domain of integrin leukocyte function-associated antigen-1 is involved in a conformational change leading to high affinity binding to ligand intercellular adhesion molecule 1 (ICAM-1). *J Biol Chem* **273**:27396, 1998.
27. Petruzzelli L, Maduzia L, Springer TA: Differential requirements for LFA-1 binding to ICAM-1 and LFA-1-mediated cell aggregation. *J Immunol* **160**:4208, 1998.
28. Stewart MP, McDowall A, Hogg N: LFA-1-mediated adhesion is regulated by cytoskeletal restraint and by a Ca2+-dependent protease, calpain. *J Cell Biol* **140**:699, 1998.
29. Sampath R, Gallagher PJ, Pavalko FM: Cytoskeletal interactions with the leukocyte integrin beta2 cytoplasmic tail. Activation-dependent regulation of associations with talin and alpha-actinin. *J Biol Chem* **273**:33588, 1998.
30. Hughes BJ, Hollers JC, Crockett-Torabi E, Smith CW: Recruitment of CD11b/CD18 to the neutrophil surface and adherence-dependent cell locomotion. *J Clin Invest* **90**:1687, 1992.
31. Dustin ML, Springer TA: T-cell receptor cross-linking transiently stimulates adhesiveness through LFA-1. *Nature* **341**:619, 1989.
32. Robinson MK, Andrew D, Rosen H, Brown D, Ortlepp S, Stephens P, Butcher EC: An antibody against the Leu-CAM beta chain (CD18) promotes both LFA-1 and CR3 dependent adhesion events. *J Immunol* **148**:1080, 1992.
33. Keizer GD, Visser W, Vliem M, Figdor CG: A monoclonal antibody (NKL-L16) directed against a unique epitope on the alpha-chain of human leukocyte function-associated antigen 1 induces homotypic cell-cell interactions. *J Immunol* **140**:1393, 1988.
34. Wacholtz MC, Patel SS, Lipsky PE: Leukocyte function-associated antigen 1 is an activation molecule for human T cells. *J Exp Med* **170**:431, 1989.
35. Van Seventer GA, Shimizu Y, Horgan KJ, Shaw S: The LFA-1 ligand ICAM-1 provides an important costimulatory signal for T cell receptor-mediated activation of resting T cells. *J Immunol* **144**:4579, 1990.
36. Shappell SB, Toman C, Anderson DC, Taylor AA, Entman ML, Smith CW: Mac-1 (CD11b/CD18) mediates adherence-dependent hydrogen peroxide production by human and canine neutrophils. *J Immunol* **144**:2702, 1990.
37. Porter JC, Hogg N: Integrins take partners: Cross-talk between integrins and other membrane receptors. *Trends Cell Biol* **8**:390, 1998.
38. Kindzelskii AL, Laska ZO, Todd III RF, Petty HR: Urokinase-type plasminogen activator receptor reversibly dissociates from complement receptor type 3 ($\alpha_M\beta_2$, CD11b/CD18) during neutrophil polarization. *J Immunol* **156**:297, 1996.
39. Petty HR, Kindzelskii AL, Adachi Y, Todd RF: Ectodomain interactions of leukocyte integrins and pro-inflammatory GPI-linked membrane proteins. *J Pharm Biomed Anal* **15**:1405, 1997.
40. Hayflick JS, Kilgannon P, Gallatin WM: The intercellular adhesion molecule (ICAM) family of proteins. New members and novel functions. *Immunol Res* **17**:313, 1998.
41. Staunton DE, Marlin SD, Stratowa C, Dustin ML, Springer TA: Primary structure of intercellular adhesion molecule 1 (ICAM-1) demonstrates interaction between members of the immunoglobulin and integrin supergene families. *Cell* **52**:925, 1988.
42. Simmons D, Makgoba MW, Seed B: ICAM, an adhesion ligand of LFA-1, is homologous to the neural cell adhesion molecule NCAM. *Nature* **331**:624, 1988.
43. Staunton DE, Dustin ML, Erickson HP, Springer TA: The arrangement of the immunoglobulin-like domains of ICAM-1 and the binding sites for LFA-1 and rhinovirus. *Cell* **61**:243, 1990.
44. Staunton DE, Merluzzi VJ, Rothlein R, Barton R, Marlin SD, Springer TA: A cell adhesion molecule, ICAM-1, is the major surface receptor for rhinoviruses. *Cell* **56**:849, 1989.
45. Dustin ML, Rothlein R, Bhan AK, Dinarello CA, Springer TA: Induction by IL-1 and interferon-gamma: Tissue distribution, biochemistry, and function of a natural adherence molecule (ICAM-1). *J Immunol* **137**:245, 1986.
46. Nortamo P, Salcedo R, Timonen T, Patarroyo M, Gahmberg CG: A monoclonal antibody to the human leukocyte adhesion molecule intercellular adhesion molecule-2. Cellular distribution and molecular characterization of the antigen. *J Immunol* **146**:2530, 1991.
47. deFougerolles AR, Springer TA: Intercellular adhesion molecule 3, a third adhesion counter-receptor for lymphocyte function-associated molecule 1 on resting lymphocytes. *J Exp Med* **175**:185, 1992.
48. Campanero MR, del Pozo MA, Arroyo AG, Sanchez-Mateos P, Hernandez-Caselles T, Craig A, Pulido R, Sanchez-Madrid F: ICAM-3 interacts with LFA-1 and regulates the LFA-1/ICAM-1 cell adhesion pathway. *J Cell Biol* **123**:1007, 1993.
49. Campanero MR, Sanchez-Mateos P, del Pozo MA, Sanchez-Madrid F: ICAM-3 regulates lymphocyte morphology and integrin-mediated T cell interaction with endothelial cell and extracellular matrix ligands. *J Cell Biol* **127**:867, 1994.
50. Kessel JM, Hayflick J, Weyrich AS, Hoffman PA, Gallatin M, McIntyre TM, Prescott SM, Zimmerman GA: Coengagement of ICAM-3 and Fc receptors induces chemokine secretion and spreading by myeloid leukocytes. *J Immunol* **160**:5579, 1998.
51. Johnston GI, Cook RG, McEver RP: Cloning of GMP-140, a granule membrane protein of platelets and endothelium: Sequence similarity to proteins involved in cell adhesion and inflammation. *Cell* **56**:1033, 1989.
52. Lasky LA, Singer MS, Yednock TA, Dowbenko D, Fennie C, Rodriguez H, Nguyen T, Stachel S, Rosen SD: Cloning of a lymphocyte homing receptor reveals a lectin domain. *Cell* **56**:1045, 1989.
53. Siegelman MH, Van de Rijn M, Weissman IL: Mouse lymph node homing receptor cDNA clone encodes a glycoprotein revealing tandem interaction domains. *Science* **243**:1165, 1989.
54. Bevilacqua MP, Stengelin S, Gimbrone MA Jr, Seed B: Endothelial leukocyte adhesion molecule 1: An inducible receptor for neutrophils related to complement regulatory proteins and lectins. *Science* **243**:1160, 1989.
55. Siegelman MH, Weissman IL: Human homologue of mouse lymph node homing receptor: Evolutionary conservation at tandem cell interaction domains. *Proc Natl Acad Sci U S A* **86**:5562, 1989.
56. Tedder TF, Isaacs CM, Ernst TJ, Demetri GD, Adler DA, Disteche CM: Isolation and chromosomal localization of cDNAs encoding a novel human lymphocyte cell surface molecule, LAM-1. Homology with the mouse lymphocyte homing receptor and other human adhesion proteins. *J Exp Med* **170**:123, 1989.

57. Bowen BR, Nguyen T, Lasky LA: Characterization of a human homologue of the murine peripheral lymph node homing receptor. *J Cell Biol* **109**:421, 1989.
58. Drickamer K: Two distinct classes of carbohydrate-recognition domains in animal lectins. *J Biol Chem* **263**:9557, 1988.
59. Yednock TA, Rosen SD: Lymphocyte homing. *Adv Immunol* **44**:313, 1989.
60. Smith CW, Kishimoto TK, Abbassi O, Hughes BJ, Rothlein R, McIntire LV, Butcher E, Anderson DC: Chemotactic factors regulate lectin adhesion molecule 1 (LECAM-1)-dependent neutrophil adhesion to cytokine-stimulated endothelial cells in vitro. *J Clin Invest* **87**:609, 1991.
61. Hallmann R, Jutila MA, Smith CW, Anderson DC, Kishimoto TK, Butcher EC: The peripheral lymph node homing receptor, LECAM-1, is involved in CD-18-independent adhesion of human neutrophils to endothelium. *Biochem Biophys Res Commun* **174**:236, 1991.
62. Spertini O, Luscinskas FW, Kansas GS, Munro JM, Griffin JD, Gimbrone MA Jr, Tedder TF: Leukocyte adhesion molecule-1 (LAM-1, L-Selectin) interacts with an inducible endothelial cell ligand to support leukocyte adhesion. *J Immunol* **147**:2565, 1991.
63. Bevilacqua MP, Pober JS, Mendrick DL, Cotran RS, Gimbrone MA Jr: Identification of an inducible endothelial-leukocyte adhesion molecule. *Proc Natl Acad Sci U S A* **84**:9238, 1987.
64. Luscinskas FW, Brock AF, Arnaout MA, Gimbrone MA Jr: Endothelial-leukocyte adhesion molecule-1-dependent and leukocyte (CD11/CD18)-dependent mechanisms contribute to polymorphonuclear leukocyte adhesion to cytokine-activated human vascular endothelium. *J Immunol* **142**:2257, 1989.
65. Cotran RS, Gimbrone MA Jr, Bevilacqua MP, Mendrick DL, Pober JS: Induction and detection of a human endothelial activation antigen in vivo. *J Exp Med* **164**:661, 1986.
66. Munro JM, Pober JS, Cotran RS: Recruitment of neutrophils in the local endotoxin response: Association with *de novo* endothelial expression of endothelial leukocyte adhesion molecule-1. *Lab Invest* **64**:295, 1991.
67. Redl H, Dinges HP, Buurman WA, van der Linden CJ, Pober JS, Cotran RS, Schlag G: Expression of endothelial leukocyte adhesion molecule-1 in septic but not traumatic/hypovolemic shock in the baboon. *Am J Pathol* **139**:461, 1991.
68. Munro JM, Pober JS, Cotran RS: Tumor necrosis factor and interferon-gamma induce distinct patterns of endothelial activation and associated leukocyte accumulation in skin of papio anubis. *Am J Pathol* **135**:121, 1989.
69. Leung DYM, Pober JS, Cotran RS: Expression of endothelial-leukocyte adhesion molecule-1 in elicited late phase allergic reactions. *J Clin Invest* **87**:1805, 1991.
70. Koch AE, Burrows JC, Haines GK, Carlos TM, Harlan JM, Leibovich SJ: Immunolocalization of endothelial and leukocyte adhesion molecules in human rheumatoid and osteoarthritic synovial tissues. *Lab Invest* **64**:313, 1991.
71. Picker LJ, Kishimoto TK, Smith CW, Warnock RA, Butcher EC: ELAM-1 is an adhesion molecule for skin-homing T-cells. *Nature* **349**:796, 1991.
72. McEver RP, Martin MN: A monoclonal antibody to a membrane glycoprotein binds only to activated platelets. *J Biol Chem* **259**:9799, 1984.
73. Hsu-Lin S-C, Berman CL, Furie BC, August D, Furie B: A platelet membrane protein expressed during platelet activation and secretion. Studies using a monoclonal antibody specific for thrombin-activated platelets. *J Biol Chem* **259**:9121, 1984.
74. Stenberg PE, McEver RP, Shuman MA, Jacques YV, Bainton DF: A platelet alpha granule membrane protein (GMP-140) is expressed on the plasma membrane after activation. *J Cell Biol* **101**:880, 1985.
75. Berman CL, Yeo EL, Wencel-Drake JD, Furie BC, Ginsberg MH, Furie B: A platelet alpha granule membrane protein that is associated with the plasma membrane after activation. *J Clin Invest* **78**:130, 1986.
76. McEver RP, Beckstead JH, Moore KL, Marshall-Carlson L, Bainton DF: GMP-140, a platelet alpha-granule membrane protein, is also synthesized by vascular endothelial cells and is localized in Weibel-Palade bodies. *J Clin Invest* **84**:92, 1989.
77. Bonfanti R, Furie BC, Furie B, Wagner DD: PADGEM (GMP140) is a component of Weibel-Palade bodies of human endothelial cells. *Blood* **73**:1109, 1989.
78. Hattori R, Hamilton KK, Fugates RD, McEver RP, Sims PJ: Stimulated secretion of endothelial von Willebrand factor is accompanied by rapid redistribution to the cell surface of the intracellular granule membrane protein GMP-140. *J Biol Chem* **264**:7768, 1989.
79. Hamburger SA, McEver RP: GMP-140 mediates adhesion of stimulated platelets to neutrophils. *Blood* **75**:550, 1990.
80. Larsen E, Celi A, Gilbert GE, Furie BC, Erban JK, Bonfanti R, Wagner DD, Furie B: PADGEM protein: A receptor that mediates the interaction of activated platelets with neutrophils and monocytes. *Cell* **59**:305, 1989.
81. Larsen E, Palabrica T, Sajer S, Gilbert GE, Wagner DD, Furie BC, Furie B: PADGEM-dependent adhesion of platelets to monocytes and neutrophils is mediated by a lineage-specific carbohydrate, LNF III (CD15). *Cell* **63**:467, 1990.
82. Geng JG, Bevilacqua MP, Moore KL, McIntyre TM, Prescott SM, Kim JM, Bliss GA, Zimmerman GA, McEver RP: Rapid neutrophil adhesion to activated endothelium mediated by GMP-140. *Nature* **343**:757, 1990.
83. Patel KD, Zimmerman GA, Prescott SM, McEver RP, McIntyre TM: Oxygen radicals induce human endothelial cells to express GMP-140 and bind neutrophils. *J Cell Biol* **112**:749, 1991.
84. Lorant DE, Patel KD, McIntyre TM, McEver RP, Prescott SM, Zimmerman GA: Coexpression of GMP-140 and PAF by endothelium stimulated by histamine or thrombin: A juxtacrine system for adhesion and activation of neutrophils. *J Cell Biol* **115**:223, 1991.
85. Johnson RC, Mayadas TN, Frenette PS, Mebius RE, Subramaniam M, Lacasce A, Hynes RO, Wagner DD: Blood cell dynamics in P-selectin-deficient mice. *Blood* **86**:1106, 1995.
86. Homeister JW, Zhang M, Frenette PS, Hynes RO, Wagner DD, Lowe JB, Marks RM: Overlapping functions of E- and P-selectin in neutrophil recruitment during acute inflammation. *Blood* **92**:2345, 1998.
87. Yamada S, Mayadas TN, Yuan F, Wagner DD, Hynes RO, Melder RJ, Jain RK: Rolling in P-selectin-deficient mice is reduced but not eliminated in the dorsal skin. *Blood* **86**:3487, 1995.
88. Celi A, Pellegrini G, Lorenzet R, De Blasi A, Ready N, Furie BC, Furie B: P-selectin induces the expression of tissue factor on monocytes. *Proc Natl Acad Sci U S A* **91**:8767, 1994.
89. Palabrica T, Lobb R, Furie BC, Aronovitz M, Benjamin C, Hsu Y-M, Sajer SA, Furie B: Leukocyte accumulation promoting fibrin deposition is mediated in vivo by P-selectin on adherent platelets. *Nature* **359**:848, 1992.
90. Rosen SD, Singer M, Yednock TA, Stoolman LM: Involvement of sialic acid on endothelial cells in organ-specific lymphocyte recirculation. *Science* **228**:1005, 1985.
91. True DD, Singer MS, Lasky LA, Rosen SD: Requirement for sialic acid on the endothelial ligand of a lymphocyte homing receptor. *J Cell Biol* **111**:2757, 1990.
92. Yednock TA, Butcher EC, Stoolman LM, Rosen SD: Receptors involved in lymphocyte homing: Relationship between a carbohydrate-binding receptor and the Mel-14 antigen. *J Cell Biol* **104**:725, 1987.
93. Stoolman LM, Tenforde TS, Rosen SD: Phosphomannosyl receptors may participate in the adhesive interaction between lymphocytes and high endothelial venules. *J Cell Biol* **99**:1535, 1984.
94. Varki A: Selectin ligands. *Proc Natl Acad Sci U S A* **91**:7390, 1994.
95. Foxall C, Watson SR, Dowbenko D, Fennie C, Lasky LA, Kiso M, Hasegawa A, Asa D, Brandley BK: The three members of the selectin receptor family recognize a common carbohydrate epitope, the sialyl $Lewis^X$ oligosaccharide. *J Cell Biol* **117**:895, 1992.
96. Lasky LA, Singer MS, Dowbenko D, Imai Y, Henzel WJ, Grimley C, Fennie C, Gillett N, Watson SR, Rosen SD: An endothelial ligand for L-selectin is a novel mucin-like molecule. *Cell* **69**:927, 1993.
97. Koenig A, Jain R, Vig R, Norgard-Sumnicht KE, Matta KL, Varki A: Selectin inhibition: Synthesis and evaluation of novel sialylated, sulfated and fucosylated oligosaccharides, including the major capping group of GlyCAM-1. *Glycobiology* **7**:79, 1997.
98. Varki A: Selectin ligands: Will the real ones please stand up? *J Clin Invest* **99**:158, 1997.
99. Baumhueter S, Dybdal N, Kyle C, Lasky LA: Global vascular expression of murine CD34, a sialomucin-like endothelial ligand for L-selectin. *Blood* **84**:2554, 1994.
100. Berg EL, McEvoy LM, Berlin C, Bargatze RF, Butcher EC: L-selectin-mediated lymphocyte rolling on MAdCAM-1. *Nature* **366**:695, 1993.
101. Moore KL, Eaton SF, Lyons DE, Lichenstein HS, Cummings RD, McEver RP: The P-selectin glycoprotein ligand from human neutrophils displays sialylated, fucosylated, *O*-Linked poly-*N*-acetyllactosamine. *J Biol Chem* **269**:23318, 1994.
102. Moore KL, Patel KD, Bruehl RE, Fugang L, Johnson DA, Lichenstein HS, Cummings RD, Bainton DF, McEver RP: P-selectin glycoprotein ligand-1 mediates rolling of human neutrophils on P-selectin. *J Cell Biol* **128**:661, 1995.

103. Liu W, Ramachandran V, Kang J, Kishimoto TK, Cummings RD, McEver RP: Identification of N-terminal residues on P-selectin glycoprotein ligand-1 required for binding to P-selectin. *J Biol Chem* **273**:7078, 1998.
104. Wilkins PP, Moore KL, McEver RP, Cummings RD: Tyrosine sulfation of P-selectin glycoprotein ligand-1 is required for high affinity binding to P-selectin. *J Biol Chem* **270**:22677, 1995.
105. Steegmaier M, Borges E, Berger J, Schwarz H, Vestweber D: The E-selectin-ligand ESL-1 is located in the Golgi as well as on microvilli on the cell surface. *J Cell Sci* **110**:687, 1997.
106. Zöllner O, Vestweber D: The E-selectin ligand-1 is selectively activated in Chinese hamster ovary cells by the a(1,3)-fucosyltransferases IV and VII. *J Biol Chem* **271**:33002, 1996.
107. Knibbs RN, Craig RA, Maly P, Smith PL, Wolber FM, Faulkner NE, Lowe JB, Stoolman LM: Alpha(1,3)-fucosyltransferase VII-dependent synthesis of P- and E-selectin ligands on cultured T lymphoblasts. *J Immunol* **161**:6305, 1998.
108. Havenaar EC, Hoff RC, Van den Eijnden DH, van Dijk W: Sialyl Lewis(x) epitopes do not occur on acute phase proteins in mice: Relationship to the absence of alpha3-fucosyltransferase in the liver. *Glycoconj J* **15**:389, 1998.
109. Brandt EJ, Elliott RW, Swank RT: Defective lysosomal enzyme secretion in kidneys of Chediak-Higashi (beige) mice. *J Cell Biol* **67**:774, 1975.
110. Ellies LG, Tsuboi S, Petryniak B, Lowe JB, Fukuda M, Marth JD: Core 2 oligosaccharide biosynthesis distinguishes between selectin ligands essential for leukocyte homing and inflammation. *Immunity* **9**:881, 1998.
111. Swarte VV, Joziasse DH, Van den Eijnden DH, Petryniak B, Lowe JB, Kraal G, Mebius RE: Regulation of fucosyltransferase-VII expression in peripheral lymph node high endothelial venules. *Eur J Immunol* **28**:3040, 1998.
112. Kishimoto TK, Jutila MA, Berg EL, Butcher EC: Neutrophil Mac-1 and MEL-14 adhesion proteins inversely regulated by chemotactic factors. *Science* **245**:1238, 1989.
113. Jutila MA, Rott L, Berg EL, Butcher EC: Function and regulation of the neutrophil MEL-14 antigen in vivo: Comparison with LFA-1 and MAC-1. *J Immunol* **143**:3318, 1989.
114. Griffin JD, Spertini O, Ernst TJ, Belvin MP, Levine HB, Kanakura Y, Tedder TF: Granulocyte-macrophage colony-stimulating factor and other cytokines regulate surface expression of the leukocyte adhesion molecule-1 on human neutrophils, monocytes, and their precursors. *J Immunol* **145**:576, 1990.
115. Pober JS, Gimbrone MA Jr, Lapierre LA, Mendrick DL, Fiers W, Rothlein R, Springer TA: Overlapping patterns of antigenic modulation by interleukin 1, tumor necrosis factor and immune interferon. *J Immunol* **137**:1893, 1986.
116. Norris P, Poston RN, Thomas DS, Thornhill M, Hawk J, Haskard DO: The expression of endothelial leukocyte adhesion molecule-1 (ELAM-1), intercellular adhesion molecule-1 (ICAM-1), and vascular cell adhesion molecule-1 (VCAM-1) in experimental cutaneous inflammation: A comparison of ultraviolet B erythema and delayed hypersensitivity. *J Invest Dermatol* **96**:763, 1991.
117. Disdier M, Morrissey JH, Fugate RD, Bainton DF, McEver RP: Cytoplasmic domain of P-selectin (CD62) contains the signal for sorting into the regulated secretory pathway. *Mol Biol Cell* **3**:309, 1992.
118. Setiadi H, Sedgewick G, Erlandsen SL, McEver RP: Interactions of the cytoplasmic domain of P-selectin with clathrin-coated pits enhance leukocyte adhesion under flow. *J Cell Biol* **142**:859, 1998.
119. Kishimoto TK: A dynamic model for neutrophil localization to inflammatory sites. *J NIH Res* **3**:75, 1991.
120. Taylor AD, Neelamegham S, Hellums JD, Smith CW, Simon SI: Molecular dynamics of the transition from L-selectin- to β2-integrin-dependent neutrophil adhesion under defined hydrodynamic shear. *Biophys J* **71**:3488, 1996.
121. Campbell JJ, Qin S, Bacon KB, Mackay CR, Butcher EC: Biology of chemokine and classical chemoattractant receptors: Differential requirements for adhesion-triggering versus chemotactic responses in lymphoid cells. *J Cell Biol* **134**:255, 1996.
122. Butcher EC: Leukocyte-endothelial cell recognition: Three (or more) steps to specificity and diversity. *Cell* **67**:1033, 1991.
123. Springer TA: Traffic signals for lymphocyte recirculation and leukocyte emigration: The multistep paradigm. *Cell* **76**:301, 1994.
124. Ley K, Tedder TF: Leukocyte interactions with vascular endothelium. New insights into selectin-mediated attachment and rolling. *J Immunol* **155**:525, 1995.
125. Arbones ML, Ord DC, Ley K, Ratech H, Maynard-Curry C, Otten G, Capon DJ, Tedder TF: Lymphocyte homing and leukocyte rolling and migration are impaired in L-selectin-deficient mice. *Immunity* **1**:247, 1994.
126. Mayadas TN, Johnson RC, Rayburn H, Hynes RO, Wagner DD: Leukocyte rolling and extravasation are severely compromised in P-selectin-deficient mice. *Cell* **74**:541, 1993.
127. Dore M, Korthuis RJ, Granger DN, Entman ML, Smith CW: P-selectin mediates spontaneous leukocyte rolling in vivo. *Blood* **82**:1308, 1993.
128. Motosugi H, Graham L, Noblitt TW, Doyle NA, Quinlan WM, Li Y, Doerschuk CM: Changes in neutrophil actin and shape during sequestration induced by complement fragments in rabbits. *Am J Pathol* **149**:963, 1996.
129. Jaeschke H, Farhood A, Fisher MA, Smith CW: Sequestration of neutrophils in the hepatic vasculature during endotoxemia is independent of β2 integrins and intercellular adhesion molecule-1. *Shock* **6**:351, 1996.
130. Wong J, Johnston B, Lee SS, Bullard DC, Smith CW, Beaudet AL, Kubes P: A minimal role for selectins in the recruitment of leukocytes into the inflamed liver microvasculature. *J Clin Invest* **99**:2782, 1997.
131. Worthen GS, Schwab III B, Elson EL, Downey GP: Mechanics of stimulated neutrophils: Cell stiffening induces retention of capillaries. *Science* **245**:183, 1989.
132. Ward PA, Mulligan MS, Vaporciyan AA, Eppinger MJ: Adhesion molecules in experimental lung inflammatory injury, in Ward PA, Fantone JC (eds): *Adhesion Molecules and the Lung*. New York, Marcel Dekker, 1996, p 159.
133. Cohnheim J: *Lectures on General Pathology: A Handbook for Practitioners and Students*. London, The New Sydenham Society, 1989.
134. Granger DN, Kubes P: The microcirculation and inflammation: Modulation of leukocyte-endothelial cell adhesion. *J Leuk Biol* **55**:662, 1994.
135. Lawrence MB, Smith CW, Eskin SG, McIntire LV: Effect of venous shear stress on CD18-mediated neutrophil adhesion to cultured endothelium. *Blood* **75**:227, 1990.
136. Abbassi O, Kishimoto TK, McIntire LV, Anderson DC, Smith CW: E-selectin supports neutrophil rolling in vitro under conditions of flow. *J Clin Invest* **92**:2719, 1993.
137. McEver RP, Moore KL, Cummings RD: Leukocyte trafficking mediated by selectin-carbohydrate interactions. *J Biol Chem* **270**:11025, 1995.
138. Jones DA, Abbassi O, McIntire LV, McEver RP, Smith CW: P-selectin mediates neutrophil rolling on histamine-stimulated endothelial cells. *Biophys J* **65**:1560, 1993.
139. Kunkel EJ, Jung U, Bullard DC, Norman KE, Wolitzky BA, Vestweber D, Beaudet AL, Ley K: Absence of trauma-induced leukocyte rolling in mice deficient in both P-selectin and intercellular adhesion molecule 1. *J Exp Med* **183**:57, 1996.
140. Kunkel EJ, Ley K: Distinct phenotype of E-selectin-deficient mice—E-selectin is required for slow leukocyte rolling in vivo. *Circ Res* **79**:1196, 1996.
141. Ley K: Gene-targeted mice in leukocyte adhesion research. *Microcirc Soc* **2**:141, 1995.
142. Lawrence MB, Kansas GS, Kunkel EJ, Ley K: Threshold levels of fluid shear promote leukocyte adhesion through selectins (CD62L, P, E). *J Cell Biol* **136**:717, 1997.
143. Borges E, Eytner R, Moll T, Steegmaier M, Campbell MA, Ley K, Mossmann H, Vestweber D: The P-selectin glycoprotein ligand-1 is important for recruitment of neutrophils into inflamed mouse peritoneum. *Blood* **90**:1934, 1997.
144. Patel KD, McEver RP: Comparison of tethering and rolling of eosinophils and neutrophils through selectins and P-selectin glycoprotein ligand-1. *J Immunol* **159**:4555, 1997.
145. von Andrian UH, Hasslen SR, Nelson RD, Erlandsen SL, Butcher EC: A central role for microvillous receptor presentation in leukocyte adhesion under flow. *Cell* **82**:989, 1995.
146. Picker LJ, Warnock RA, Burns AR, Doerschuk CM, Berg EL, Butcher EC: The neutrophil selectin LECAM-1 presents carbohydrate ligands to the vascular selectins ELAM-1 and GMP-140. *Cell* **66**:921, 1991.
147. Erlandsen SL, Hasslen SR, Nelson RD: Detection and spatial distribution of the beta-2 integrin (Mac-1) and L-selectin (LECAM-1) adherence receptors on human neutrophils by high-resolution field emission SEM. *J Histochem Cytochem* **41**:327, 1993.
148. Hemmerich S, Butcher EC, Rosen SD: Sulfation-dependent recognition of high endothelial venules (HEV)-ligands by L-selectin and MECA-79, an adhesion-blocking monoclonal antibody. *J Exp Med* **180**:2219, 1994.

149. Lawrence MB, Berg EL, Butcher EC, Springer TA: Rolling of lymphocytes and neutrophils on peripheral node addressin and subsequent arrest on ICAM-1 in shear flow. *Eur J Immunol* **25**:1025, 1995.
150. Tu L, Delahunty MD, Ding H, Luscinskas FW, Tedder TF: The cutaneous lymphocyte antigen is an essential component of the L-selectin ligand induced on human vascular endothelial cells. *J Exp Med* **189**:241, 1999.
151. Zöllner O, Lenter MC, Blanks JE, Borges E, Steegmaier M, Zerwes HG, Vestweber D: L-selectin from human, but not from mouse neutrophils binds directly to E-selectin. *J Cell Biol* **136**:707, 1997.
152. Bargatze RF, Kurk S, Butcher EC, Jutila MA: Neutrophils roll on adherent neutrophils bound to cytokine-induced endothelial cells via L-selectin on the rolling cells. *J Exp Med* **180**:1785, 1994.
153. Walcheck B, Moore KL, McEver RP, Kishimoto TK: Neutrophil-neutrophil interactions under hydrodynamic shear stress involve L-selectin and PSGL-1. A mechanism that amplifies initial leukocyte accumulation on P-selectin in vitro. *J Clin Invest* **98**:1081, 1996.
154. Buttrum SM, Hatton R, Nash GB: Selectin-mediated rolling of neutrophils on immobilized platelets. *Blood* **82**:1165, 1993.
155. Dore M, Simon SI, Hughes BJ, Entman ML, Smith CW: P-selectin- and CD18-mediated recruitment of canine neutrophils under conditions of shear stress. *Vet Pathol* **32**:258, 1995.
156. Diacovo TG, Roth SJ, Buccola JM, Bainton DF, Springer TA: Neutrophil rolling, arrest, and transmigration across activated, surface-adherent platelets via sequential action of P-selectin and the $\beta 2$-integrin CD11b/CD18. *Blood* **88**:146, 1996.
157. Springer TA: Traffic signals on endothelium for lymphocyte recirculation and leukocyte emigration. *Annu Rev Physiol* **57**:827, 1995.
158. Lawrence MB, Springer TA: Leukocytes roll on a selectin at physiologic flow rates: Distinction from and prerequisite for adhesion through integrins. *Cell* **65**:859, 1991.
159. von Andrian UH, Hansell P, Chambers JD, Berger EM, Filho IT, Butcher EC, Arfors K-E: L-selectin function is required for beta-2 integrin-mediated neutrophil adhesion at physiologic shear rates in vivo. *Am J Physiol* **263**:H1034, 1992.
160. Hughes AL, Yeager M: Coevolution of the mammalian chemokines and their receptors. *Immunogenetics* **49**:115, 1999.
161. Gimbrone MA Jr, Obin MS, Brock AF, Luis EA, Hass PE, Hebert CA, Yip YK, Leung DW, Lowe DG, Kohr WJ, Darbonne WC, Bechtol KB, Baker JB: Endothelial interleukin-8: A novel inhibitor of leukocyte-endothelial interactions. *Science* **246**:1601, 1989.
162. Lorant DE, McEver RP, McIntyre TM, Moore KL, Prescott SM, Zimmerman GA: Activation of polymorphonuclear leukocytes reduces their adhesion to P-selectin and causes redistribution of ligands for P-selectin on their surfaces. *J Clin Invest* **96**:171, 1995.
163. Rot A: Endothelial cell binding of NAP-1/IL-8 role in neutrophil emigration. *Immunol Today* **13**:291, 1992.
164. Middleton J, Neil S, Wintle J, Clark-Lewis I, Moore H, Lam C, Auer M, Hub E, Rot A: Transcytosis and surface presentation of IL-8 by venular endothelial cells. *Cell* **91**:385, 1997.
165. Rainger GE, Fisher AC, Nash GB: Endothelial-borne platelet-activating factor and interleukin-8 rapidly immobilize rolling neutrophils. *Am J Physiol* **272**:H114, 1997.
166. Wolff B, Burns AR, Middleton J, Rot A: Endothelial cell "memory" of inflammatory stimulation: Human venular endothelial cells store interleukin 8 in Weibel-Palade bodies. *J Exp Med* **188**:1757, 1998.
167. Zimmerman GA, McIntyre TM, Mehra M, Prescott SM: Endothelial cell-associated platelet-activating factor: A novel mechanism for signaling intercellular adhesion. *J Cell Biol* **110**:529, 1990.
168. Zimmerman GA, Elstad MR, Lorant DE, McIntyre TM, Prescott SM, Topham MK, Weyrich AS, Whatley RE: Platelet-activating factor (PAF): Signalling and adhesion in cell-cell interactions. *Adv Exp Med Biol* **416**:297, 1996.
169. Kukielka GL, Smith CW, LaRosa GJ, Manning AM, Mendoza LH, Hughes BJ, Youker KA, Hawkins HK, Michael LH, Rot A, Entman ML: Interleukin-8 gene induction in the myocardium following ischemia and reperfusion in vivo. *J Clin Invest* **95**:89, 1995.
170. Laudanna C, Constantin G, Baron P, Scarpini E, Scarlato G, Cabrini G, Dechecchi C, Rossi F, Cassatella MA, Berton G: Sulfatides trigger increase of cytosolic free calcium and enhanced expression of tumor necrosis factor-alpha and interleukin-8 mRNA in human neutrophils. Evidence for a role of L-selectin as a signaling molecule. *J Biol Chem* **269**:4021, 1994.
171. Crockett-Torabi E, Fantone JC: L-selectin stimulation of canine neutrophil initiates calcium signal secondary to tyrosine kinase activation. *Am J Physiol Heart Circ Physiol* **272**:H1302, 1997.
172. Kansas GS, Ley K, Munro JM, Tedder TF: Regulation of leukocyte rolling and adhesion to high endothelial venules through the cytoplasmic domain of L-selectin. *J Exp Med* **177**:833, 1993.
173. Gopalan PK, Smith CW, Lu H, Berg EL, McIntire LV, Simon SI: Neutrophil CD18-dependent arrest on ICAM-1 in shear flow can be activated through L-selectin. *J Immunol* **158**:367, 1997.
174. Tsang YTM, Neelamegham S, Hu Y, Berg EL, Burns AR, Smith CW, Simon SI: Synergy between L-selectin signaling and chemotactic activation during neutrophil adhesion and transmigration. *J Immunol* **159**:4566, 1997.
175. Bullock JD, Robertson AF, Bodenbender JG, Kontras SB, Miller CE: Inflammatory response in the neonate re-examined. *Pediatrics* **44**:58, 1969.
176. Smith CW: Endothelial adhesion molecules and their role in inflammation. *Can J Physiol Pharmacol* **71**:76, 1993.
177. Schmits R, Kundig TM, Baker DM, Shumaker G, Simard JJL, Duncan G, Wakeham A, Shahinian A, van der Heiden A, Bachmann MF, Ohashi PS, Mak TW, Hickstein DD: LFA-1-deficient mice show normal CTL responses to virus but fail to reject immunogenic tumor. *J Exp Med* **183**:1415, 1996.
178. Lu H, Smith CW, Perrard J, Bullard D, Tang L, Shappell SB, Entman ML, Beaudet AL, Ballantyne CM: LFA-1 is sufficient in mediating neutrophil emigration in Mac-1 deficient mice. *J Clin Invest* **99**:1340, 1997.
179. Coxon A, Rieu P, Barkalow FJ, Askari S, Sharpe AH, von Andrian UH, Arnaout MA, Mayadas TN: A novel role for the $\beta 2$ integrin CD11b/CD18 in neutrophil apoptosis: A homeostatic mechanism in inflammation. *Immunity* **5**:653, 1996.
180. Tang T, Rosenkranz A, Assmann KJM, Goodman MJ, Gutierrez-Ramos JC, Carroll MC, Cotran RS, Mayadas TN: A role for Mac-1 (CDIIb/CD18) in immune complex-stimulated neutrophil function in vivo: Mac-1 deficiency abrogates sustained Fcgamma receptor-dependent neutrophil adhesion and complement-dependent proteinuria in acute glomerulonephritis. *J Exp Med* **186**:1853, 1997.
181. Rutter J, James TJ, Howat D, Shock A, Andrew D, De Baetselier P, Blackford J, Wilkinson JM, Higgs G, Hughes B, Robinson MK: The in vivo and in vitro effects of antibodies against rabbit $\beta 2$-integrins. *J Immunol* **153**:3724, 1994.
182. Graf JM, Smith CW, Mariscalco MM: Contribution of LFA-1 and Mac-1 to CD18-dependent neutrophil emigration in a neonatal rabbit model. *J Appl Physiol* **80**:1984, 1996.
183. Rothlein R, Springer TA: Complement receptor type 3-dependent degradation of opsonized erythrocytes by mouse macrophage. *J Immunol* **135**:2668, 1985.
184. Ross GD, Cain JA, Lachmann PJ: Membrane complement receptor type 3 has lectin-like properties analogous to bovine conglutinin and functions as a receptor for zymosan and rabbit erythrocytes as well as a receptor for iC3b. *J Immunol* **134**:3307, 1985.
185. Anderson DC, Miller LJ, Schmalstieg FC, Rothlein R, Springer TA: Contributions of the Mac-1 glycoprotein family to adherence-dependent granulocyte functions: Structure-function assessments employing subunit-specific monoclonal antibodies. *J Immunol* **137**:15, 1986.
186. Myones BL, Daizell JG, Hogg N, Ross GD: Neutrophil and monocyte cell surface p150,95 has iC3b-receptor (CR4) activity resembling CR3. *J Clin Invest* **82**:640, 1988.
187. Smith CW, Rothlein R, Hughes BJ, Mariscalco MM, Schmalstieg FC, Anderson DC: Recognition of an endothelial determinant for CD18-dependent human neutrophil adherence and transendothelial migration. *J Clin Invest* **82**:1746, 1988.
188. Kishimoto TK, Rothlein R: Integrins, ICAMs, and selectins: Role and regulation of adhesion molecules in neutrophil recruitment to inflammatory sites. *Adv Pharmacol* **25**:117, 1994.
189. Rothlein R, Barton RW, Winquist R: The role of intercellular adhesion molecule-1 (ICAM-1) in the inflammatory response, in Cochrone CG, Ginabrone MA Jr (eds): *Cellular and Molecular Mechanisms of Inflammation*. New York, Academic Press, 1991, p 171.
190. Sligh JE Jr, Ballantyne CM, Rich SS, Hawkins HK, Smith CW, Bradley A, Beaudet AL: Inflammatory and immune responses are impaired in ICAM-1 deficient mice. *Proc Natl Acad Sci U S A* **90**:8529, 1993.
191. Connolly ES Jr, Winfree CJ, Springer TA, Naka Y, Liao H, Yan SD, Stern DM, Solomon RA, Gutierrez-Ramos JC, Pinsky DJ: Cerebral protection in homozygous null ICAM-1 mice after middle cerebral artery occlusion. Role of neutrophil adhesion in the pathogenesis of stroke. *J Clin Invest* **97**:209, 1996.

192. Lo SK, Van Seventer GA, Levin SM, Wright SD: Two leukocyte receptors (CD11a/CD18) mediate transient adhesion to endothelium by binding to different ligands. *J Immunol* **143**:3325, 1989.
193. Jones DA, McIntire LV, Smith CW, Picker LJ: A two-step adhesion cascade for T cell/endothelial cell interactions under flow conditions. *J Clin Invest* **94**:2443, 1994.
194. Gerszten RE, Luscinskas FW, Ding HT, Dichek DA, Stoolman LM, Gimbrone MA Jr, Rosenzweig A: Adhesion of memory lymphocytes to vascular cell adhesion molecule-1-transduced human vascular endothelial cells under simulated physiological flow conditions in vitro. *Circ Res* **79**:1205, 1996.
195. Luscinskas FW, Kansas GS, Ding H, Pizueta P, Schleiffenbaum BE, Tedder TF, Gimbrone MA Jr: Monocyte rolling, arrest and spreading on IL-4-activated vascular endothelium under flow is mediated via sequential action of L-selectin, β1-integrins, and β2-integrins. *J Cell Biol* **125**:1417, 1994.
196. Patel KD: Eosinophil tethering to interleukin-4-activated endothelial cells requires both P-selectin and vascular cell adhesion molecule-1. *Blood* **92**:3904, 1998.
197. Kubes P, Niu X, Smith CW, Kehrli ME Jr, Reinhardt PH, Woodman RC: A novel β_1-dependent adhesion pathway on neutrophils: A mechanism invoked by dihydrocytochalasin B or endothelial transmigration. *FASEB J* **9**:1103, 1995.
198. Reinhardt PH, Ward CA, Giles WA, Kubes P: Emigrated rat neutrophils adhere to cardiac myocytes via a 4 integrin. *Circ Res* **81**:196, 1997.
199. Huber AR, Kunkel SL, Todd III RF, Weiss SJ: Regulation of transendothelial neutrophil migration by endogenous interleukin-8. *Science* **254**:99, 1991.
200. Furie MB, Tancinco MCA, Smith CW: Monoclonal antibodies to leukocyte integrins CD11a/CD18 and CD11b/CD18 or intercellular adhesion molecule-1 (ICAM-1) inhibit chemoattractant-stimulated neutrophil transendothelial migration in vitro. *Blood* **78**:2089, 1991.
201. Bienvenu K, Harris N, Granger DN: Modulation of leukocyte migration in mesenteric interstitium. *Am J Physiol* **267**:H1573, 1994.
202. Entman ML, Youker KA, Shappell SB, Siegel C, Rothlein R, Dreyer WJ, Schmalstieg FC, Smith CW: Neutrophil adherence to isolated adult canine myocytes: Evidence for a CD18-dependent mechanism. *J Clin Invest* **85**:1497, 1990.
203. Jaeschke H, Smith CW: Mechanisms of neutrophil-induced parenchymal cell injury. *J Leuk Biol* **61**:647, 1997.
204. Keller HU, Wilkinson PC, Abercrombie M, Becker EL, Hirsch JG, Miller ME, Ramsey WS, Zigmond SH: A proposal for the definition of terms related to locomotion of leukocytes and other cells. *Cell Biol Int Rep* **1**:391, 1977.
205. Zigmond SH, Hirsch JG: Leukocyte locomotion and chemotaxis. New methods for evaluation and demonstration of a cell-derived chemotactic factor. *J Exp Med* **137**:387, 1973.
206. Zigmond SH, Levitsky HI, Kreel BJ: Cell polarity: An examination of its behavioral expression and its consequences for polymorphonuclear leukocyte chemotaxis. *J Cell Biol* **89**:585, 1981.
207. Foxman EF, Campbell JJ, Butcher EC: Multistep navigation and the combinatorial control of leukocyte chemotaxis. *J Cell Biol* **139**:1349, 1997.
208. Quie PG, White JG, Holmes B, Good RA: In vitro bactericidal capacity of human polymorphonuclear leukocytes: Diminished activity in chronic granulomatous disease of childhood. *J Clin Invest* **46**:668, 1967.
209. Solberg CO, Halstensen A, Digranes A, Hellum KB: Penetration of antibiotics into human leukocytes and dermal suction blisters. *Rev Infect Dis* **5(3)**:S468, 1983.
210. Miles AA, Miles EM, Burke J: The value and duration of defense reactions of the skin to the primary lodgment of bacteria. *Br J Exp Pathol* **38**:79, 1957.
211. Smith CW, Hollers JC, Patrick RA, Hassett C: Motility and adhesiveness in human neutrophils: Effects of chemotactic factors. *J Clin Invest* **63**:221, 1979.
212. Boyden S: The chemotactic effect of mixtures of antibody and antigen on polymorphonuclear leukocytes. *J Exp Med* **115**:453, 1962.
213. Wilkinson PC, Allan RB: Assay systems for measuring leukocyte locomotion: An overview, in Gallin JI, Quie PG (eds): *Leukocyte Chemotaxis*. New York, Raven Press, 1978, p 1.
214. McCutcheon M: Chemotaxis in leukocytes. *Physiol Rev* **26**:319, 1946.
215. Allan RB, Wilkinson PC: A visual analysis of chemotactic and chemokinetic locomotion of human neutrophil leukocytes. *Exp Cell Res* **111**:191, 1978.
216. Ramsey WS: Analysis of individual leukocyte behavior during chemotaxis. *Exp Cell Res* **70**:129, 1972.
217. Nelson RD, Quie PG, Simmons RL: Chemotaxis under agarose: A new and simple method for measuring chemotaxis and spontaneous migration of human polymorphonuclear leukocytes and monocytes. *J Immunol* **115**:1650, 1975.
218. Verghese MW, Smith CD, Charles LA, Jakoi L, Snyderman RA: A guanine nucleotide regulatory protein controls polyphosphoinositide metabolism, Ca^{2+} mobilization and cellular responses to chemoattractants in human monocytes. *J Immunol* **137**:271, 1986.
219. Anderson DC, Hughes BJ, Smith CW: Abnormal mobility of neonatal polymorphonuclear leukocytes. Relationship to impaired redistribution of surface adhesion sites by chemotactic factor or colchicine. *J Clin Invest* **68**:863, 1981.
220. Anderson DC, Krishna GS, Hughes BJ, Mace ML, Smith CW, Nichols BL: Impaired polymorphonuclear leukocyte motility in malnourished infants: Relationship to functional abnormalities of cell adherence. *J Lab Clin Med* **101**:881, 1983.
221. Anderson DC, Mace ML, Brinkley BR, Martin RR, Smith CW: Recurrent infection in glycogenosis type 1b: Abnormal neutrophil motility related to impaired redistribution of adhesion sites. *J Infect Dis* **143**:447, 1981.
222. Howard MW, Strauss RG, Johnston RB Jr: Infections in patients with neutropenia. *Am J Dis Child* **131**:788, 1977.
223. Kohl S, Loo LS, Schmalstieg FC, Anderson DC: The genetic deficiency of leukocyte surface glycoprotein Mac-1, LFA-1, p150,95 in humans is associated with defective antibody-dependent cellular cytotoxicity in vitro and defective protection against herpes simplex virus in vivo. *J Immunol* **137**:1688, 1986.
224. Gallin JI: Abnormal phagocyte chemotaxis: Pathophysiology, clinical manifestations, and management of patients. *Rev Infect Dis* **3**:1196, 1981.
225. Davis SD, Schaller J, Wedgwood RJ: Job's syndrome: Recurrent "cold" staphylococcal abscesses. *Lancet* **1**:1013, 1966.
226. Miller ME, Oski FA, Harris MB: Lazy-leukocyte syndrome: A new disorder of neutrophil function. *Lancet* **1**:665, 1971.
227. Buckley RH, Wray BB, Belmaker EZ: Extreme hyperimmunoglobulinemia E and undue susceptibility to infection. *Pediatrics* **49**:59, 1972.
228. Snyderman R, Altman LC, Frankel A, Blaese RM: Defective mononuclear leukocyte chemotaxis: A previously unrecognized immune dysfunction. *Ann Intern Med* **78**:509, 1973.
229. Ward PA, Schlegel RJ: Impaired leucotactic responsiveness in a child with recurrent infections. *Lancet* **2**:344, 1969.
230. Wilkinson PC: Leukocyte locomotion and chemotaxis: Effects of bacteria and viruses. *Rev Infect Dis* **2**:293, 1980.
231. Boner A, Zeligs BJ, Bellanti JA: Chemotactic responses of various differentiational stages of neutrophils from human cord and adult blood. *Infect Immun* **35**:921, 1982.
232. Hill HR, Gerrard JM, Hogan NA: Hyperactivity of neutrophil leukotactic responses during active bacterial infections. *J Clin Invest* **53**:996, 1974.
233. Hill HR, Warwick WJ, Dettloff J, Quie PG: Neutrophil granulocyte function in patients with pulmonary infection. *J Pediatr* **84**:55, 1974.
234. McCall CE, Caves J, Cooper R, DeChatelet LR: Functional characteristics of human toxic neutrophils. *J Infect Dis* **124**:68, 1971.
235. Movat AG, Baum J: Polymorphonuclear leukocyte chemotaxis in patients with bacterial infections. *Br Med J* **3**:617, 1971.
236. Gallin JI, Buescher ES: Abnormal regulation of inflammatory skin responses in male patients with chronic granulomatous disease. *Inflammation* **7**:227, 1983.
237. Grinsburg I, Quie PG: Modulation of human polymorphonuclear leukocyte chemotaxis by leukocyte extracts, bacterial products, inflammatory exudates, and polyelectrolytes. *Inflammation* **4**:301, 1980.
238. Hill HR: Clinical disorders of leukocyte functions. *Contemp Top Immunobiol* **14**:345, 1984.
239. Bergman M, Guerrant F, Murad R, et al: Interaction of polymorphonuclear neutrophils with *E. coli:* Effects of enterotoxin on phagocytosis, killing, chemotaxis and cyclic AMP. *J Clin Invest* **61**:227, 1978.
240. Bourne HR, Lehrer RI, Lichtenstein LM, Weissmann G, Zurier R: Effects of cholera enterotoxin on adenosine 3′,5′-monophosphate and neutrophil function: Comparison with other compounds which stimulate leukocyte adenyl cyclase. *J Clin Invest* **52**:698, 1973.
241. Fick RB, Robbins RA, Squier SU, Schoderbek WE, Russ WD: Complement activation in cystic fibrosis respiratory fluids: In vivo and in vitro generation of C5a and chemotactic activity. *Pediatr Res* **20**:1258, 1986.

242. Berger M, Dearborn D, Legris G, Doring G, Sorensen R: Complement receptor expression on neutrophils (PMN) in the lung in cystic fibrosis (CF). *Pediatr Res* **20**:305a, 1986.
243. Boxer LA, Hedley-Whyte T, Stossel TP: Neutrophil actin dysfunction and abnormal neutrophil behavior. *N Engl J Med* **291**:1093, 1974.
244. Fischer A, Descamps-Latscha B, Gerota I, Scheinmetzler C, Virelizier JL: Bone marrow transplantation for inborn error of phagocytic cells associated with defective adherence, chemotaxis, and oxidative response during opsonized particle phagocytosis. *Lancet* **2**:473, 1983.
245. Hayward AR, Leonard J, Wood CBS, Harvey BAM, Greenwood MC, Soothill JF: Delayed separation of the umbilical cord, widespread infections, and defective neutrophil mobility. *Lancet* **1**:1099, 1979.
246. Davies EG, Isaacs D, Levinsky RJ: Defective immune interferon production and natural killer activity associated with poor neutrophil mobility and delayed umbilical cord separation. *Clin Exp Immunol* **50**:454, 1982.
247. Harvath L, Andersen BR: Defective initiation of oxidative metabolism in polymorphonuclear leukocytes. *N Engl J Med* **300**:1130, 1979.
248. Dimanche-Boitrel MT, LeDeist F, Fischer A, Arnaout MA, Giscelli C, Lisowska-Grospierre B: LFA-1 beta-chain synthesis and degradation in patients with leukocyte adhesive protein deficiency. *Eur J Immunol* **17**:417, 1987.
249. Anderson DC, Springer TA: Leukocyte adhesion deficiency: An inherited defect in the Mac-1, LFA-1 and p150,95 glycoproteins. *Ann Rev Med* **38**:175, 1987.
250. Southwick FS, Howard TH, Holbrook T, Anderson DC, Stossel TP, Arnaout MA: The relationship between CR3 deficiency and neutrophil actin assembly. *Blood* **73**:1973, 1989.
251. Abramson JS, Mills EL, Sawyer MK, Regelmann WR, Nelson JD, Quie PG: Recurrent infections and delayed separation of the umbilical cord in an infant with abnormal phagocytic cell locomotion and oxidative response during particle phagocytosis. *J Pediatr* **99**:887, 1981.
252. Crowley CA, Curnutte JT, Rosin RE, Andre-Schwartz J, Gallin JI, Klempner M, Snyderman R, Southwick FS, Stossel TP, Babior BM: An inherited abnormality of neutrophil adhesions: Its genetic transmission and its association with a missing protein. *N Engl J Med* **302**:1163, 1980.
253. Arnaout MA, Pitt J, Cohen HJ, Melamed J, Rosen FS, Colten HR: Deficiency of a granulocyte-membrane glycoprotein (gp150) in a boy with recurrent bacterial infections. *N Engl J Med* **306**:693, 1982.
254. Bowen TJ, Ochs HD, Altman LC, Price TH, Van Epps DE, Brautigan DL, Rosin RE, Perkins WD, Babior BM, Klebanoff SJ, Wedgwood RJ: Severe recurrent bacterial infections associated with defective adherence and chemotaxis in two patients with neutrophils deficient in a cell-associated glycoprotein. *J Pediatr* **101**:932, 1982.
255. Springer TA: The LFA-1, Mac-1 glycoprotein family and its deficiency in an inherited disease. *Fed Proc* **44**:2660, 1985.
256. Springer TA, Galfre G, Secher DS, Milstein C: Mac-1: A macrophage differentiation antigen identified by a monoclonal antibody. *Eur J Immunol* **9**:301, 1979.
257. Dana N, Todd III RF, Pitt J, Springer TA, Arnaout MA: Deficiency of a surface membrane glycoprotein (Mo1) in man. *J Clin Invest* **73**:153, 1983.
258. Anderson DC, Schmalstieg FC, Kohl S, Arnaout MA, Hughes BJ, Tosi MF, Buffone GJ, Brinkley BR, Dickey WD, Abramson JS, Springer TA, Boxer LA, Hollers JM, Smith CW: Abnormalities of polymorphonuclear leukocyte function associated with a heritable deficiency of high molecular weight surface glycoproteins (GP138): Common relationship to diminished cell adherence. *J Clin Invest* **74**:536, 1984.
259. Beatty PG, Ochs HD, Harlan JM: Absence of a monoclonal antibody-defined protein complex in a boy with abnormal leukocyte function. *Lancet* **1**:535, 1984.
260. Springer TA, Thompson WS, Miller LJ, Schmalstieg FC, Anderson DC: Inherited deficiency of the Mac-1, LFA-1, p150,95 glycoprotein family and its molecular basis. *J Exp Med* **160**:1901, 1984.
261. Arnaout MA, Spits H, Terhorst C, Pitt J, Todd III RF: Deficiency of a leukocyte surface glycoprotein (LFA-1) in two patients with Mo1 deficiency. *J Clin Invest* **74**:1291, 1984.
262. Springer TA, Miller LJ, Anderson DC: p150,95, the third member of the Mac-1, LFA-1 human leukocyte adhesion glycoprotein family. *J Immunol* **136**:240, 1986.
263. Miller LJ, Bainton DF, Borregaard N, Springer TA: Stimulated mobilization of monocyte Mac-1 and p150,95 adhesion proteins from an intracellular vesicular compartment to the cell surface. *J Clin Invest* **80**:535, 1987.
264. Anderson DC, Schmalstieg FC, Finegold MJ, Hughes BJ, Rothlein R, Miller LJ, Kohl S, Tosi MF, Jacobs RL, Waldrop TC, Goldman AS, Shearer WT, Springer TA: The severe and moderate phenotypes of heritable Mac-1, LFA-1, p150,95 deficiency: Their quantitative definition and relation to leukocyte dysfunction and clinical features. *J Infect Dis* **152**:668, 1985.
265. Marlin SD, Morton CC, Anderson DC, Springer TA: LFA-1 immunodeficiency disease: Definition of the genetic defect and chromosomal mapping of alpha and beta subunits by complementation in hybrid cells. *J Exp Med* **164**:855, 1986.
266. Kohl S, Springer TA, Schmalstieg FC: Defective natural killer cytotoxicity and polymorphonuclear leukocyte antibody dependent cellular cytotoxicity in patients with LFA-1/OKM-1 deficiency. *J Immunol* **133**:2972, 1984.
267. Arnaout MA, Todd III RF, Dana N, Melamed J, Schlossman SF, Colten HR: Inhibition of phagocytosis of complement C3- or immunoglobulin G-coated particles and of C3bi binding by monoclonal antibodies to a monocyte-granulocyte membrane glycoprotein (Mo1). *J Clin Invest* **72**:171, 1983.
268. Issekutz AC, Lee KY, Bigger WD: Combined abnormality of neutrophil chemotaxis and bactericidal activity in a child with chronic skin infections. *Clin Immunol Immunopathol* **14**:1, 1979.
269. Krensky AM, Mentzer SJ, Clayberger C, Anderson DC, Schmalstieg FC, Burakoff SJ, Springer TA: Heritable lymphocyte function-associated antigen-1 deficiency: Abnormalities of cytotoxicity and proliferation associated with abnormal expression of LFA-1. *J Immunol* **135**:3102, 1985.
270. Buchanan MR, Crowley CA, Rosin RE, Gimbrone MA Jr, Babior BM: Studies on the interaction between GP-180 deficient neutrophils and vascular endothelium. *Blood* **60**:160, 1982.
271. Fischer A, Durandy A, Sterkers G, Griscelli C: Role of the LFA-1 molecule in cellular interactions required for antibody production in humans. *J Immunol* **136**:3198, 1986.
272. Fischer A, Seger R, Durandy A, Grospierre B, Virelizier JL, LeDeist F, Griscelli C, Fischer E, Kazatchkine MD, Bohler MC, Descamps-Latscha B, Trung PH, Springer TA, Oliver D, Mavas C: Deficiency of the adhesive protein complex lymphocyte function antigen 1, complement receptor type 3, glycoprotein p150,95 in a girl with recurrent bacterial infections. *J Clin Invest* **76**:2385, 1985.
273. Lisowska-Grospierre B, Bohler MCh, Fischer A, Mawas C, Springer TA, Griscelli C: Defective membrane expression of the LFA-1 complex may be secondary to the absence of the beta chain in a child with recurrent bacterial infections. *Eur J Immunol* **16**:205, 1986.
274. Ross GD: Characterization of phagocytic and cytotoxic abnormalities in patients who have an inherited deficiency of neutrophil complement receptor type three (CR3) and the related membrane antigens LFA-1 and p150,95, in Aiuti F, Rosen F, Cooper MD (eds): *Recent Advances in Primary and Acquired Immunodeficiencies*. New York, Raven Press, 1986, p 119.
275. Buescher ES, Gaither T, Nath J, Gallin JI: Abnormal adherence-related functions of neutrophils, monocytes, and EB virus-transformed B cells in a patient with C3bi receptor deficiency. *Blood* **65**:1382, 1985.
276. Fujita K, Kobayashi K, Uchida M, Kajii T: Neutrophil adhesion abnormality with deficient surface membrane proteins (gp110 and p98): The effect of their antibodies on the function of normal neutrophils. *Pediatr Res* **20**:361, 1986.
277. Ambruso DR, Johnston RB: Lactoferrin enhances hydroxyl radical production by human neutrophils, neutrophil particulate fractions, and an enzymatic generating system. *J Clin Invest* **67**:352, 1981.
278. Weisman SJ, Berkow RL, Plautz G, Torres M, McGuire WA, Coates TD, Haak RA, Floyd A, Jersild R, Baehner RL: Glycoprotein-180 deficiency: Genetics and abnormal neutrophil activation. *Blood* **65**:696, 1985.
279. Thomas C, Le Dcist F, Cavazzana-Calvo M, Benkerrou M, Haddad E, Blanche S, Hartmann W, Friedrich W, Fischer A: Results of allogeneic bone marrow transplantation in patients with leukocyte adhesion deficiency. *Blood* **86**:1629, 1995.
280. Todd III RF, Freyer DR: The CD11/CD18 leukocyte glycoprotein deficiency. *Hematol Oncol Clin North Am* **2**:13, 1988.
281. Fischer A, Lisowska-Grospierre B, Anderson DC, Springer TA: Leukocyte adhesion deficiency: Molecular basis and functional consequences. *Immunodefic Rev* **1**:39, 1988.
282. Arnaout MA: Leukocyte adhesion molecules deficiency: Its structural basis, pathophysiology and implications for modulating the inflammatory response. *Immunol Rev* **114**:145, 1990.
283. Waldrop TC, Anderson DC, Hallmon WW, Schmalstieg FC, Jacobs RL: Periodontal manifestations of the heritable Mac-1, LFA-1

deficiency syndrome — Clinical, histopathologic and molecular characteristics. *J Periodont* **58(6)**:400, 1987.

284. Giger U, Boxer LA, Simpson PJ, Lucchesi BR, Todd III RF: Deficiency of leukocyte surface glycoproteins Mo1, LFA-1, and Leu M5 in a dog with recurrent bacterial infections: An animal model. *Blood* **69**:1622, 1987.
285. Trowald-Wigh G, Hakansson L, Johannisson A, Norrgren L, Segerstad CH: Leucocyte adhesion protein deficiency in Irish setter dogs. *Vet Immunol Immunopathol* **32**:261, 1992.
286. Kehrli ME Jr, Schmalstieg FC, Anderson DC, Van Der Maaten MJ, Hughes BJ, Ackermann MR, Wilhelmsen CL, Brown GB, Stevens MG, Whetstone CA: Molecular definition of the bovine granulocytopathy syndrome: Identification of a deficiency of the Mac-1 (CD11b/CD18) glycoprotein. *J Am Vet Med Assoc* **51(11)**:1826, 1990.
287. Gilbert RO, Rebhun WC, Kim CA, Kehrli ME Jr, Shuster DE, Ackermann MR: Clinical manifestations of leukocyte adhesion deficiency in cattle: 14 cases (1997–1991). *J Am Vet Med Assoc* **202**:445, 1993.
288. Kehrli ME Jr, Ackermann MR, Shuster DE, Van Der Maaten MJ, Schmalstieg FC, Anderson DC, Hughes BJ: Animal model of human disease. Bovine leukocyte adhesion deficiency. Beta$_2$ integrin deficiency in young Holstein cattle. *Am J Pathol* **140**:1489, 1992.
289. Kehrli ME Jr, Shuster DE, Ackermann M, Smith CW, Anderson DC, Dore M, Hughes BJ: Clinical and immunological features associated with bovine leukocyte adhesion deficiency, in Lipsky PE, Rothlein R, Kishimoto TK, Faanes RB, Smith CW (eds): *Structure and Function of Molecules Involved in Leukocyte Adhesion II*. New York, Springer-Verlag, 1993, p 314.
290. Nagahata H, Masuyama A, Masue M, Yuki M, Higuchi H, Ohtsuka H, Kurosawa T, Sato H, Noda H: Leukocyte emigration in normal calves and calves with leukocyte adhesion deficiency. *J Vet Med Sci* **59**:1143, 1997.
291. Kehrli ME Jr, Shuster DE, Ackermann MR: Genetic abnormalities in leukocyte adhesion deficiency among Holstein cattle. *Cornell Vet* **82**:103, 1992.
292. Cox E, Mast J, MacHugh N, Schwenger B, Goddeeris BM: Expression of beta 2 integrins on blood leukocytes of cows with or without bovine leukocyte adhesion deficiency. *Vet Immunol Immunopathol* **58**:249, 1997.
293. Muller KE, Hoek A, Rutten VP, Bernadina WE, Wentink GH: Antigen-specific immune responses in cattle with inherited beta2-integrin deficiency. *Vet Immunol Immunopathol* **58**:39, 1997.
294. Shuster DE, Kehrli ME Jr, Ackermann MR, Gilbert RO: Identification and prevalence of a genetic defect that causes leukocyte adhesion deficiency in Holstein cattle. *Proc Natl Acad Sci U S A* **89**:9225, 1992.
295. Ross GD, Thompson RA, Walport MJ, Springer TA, Watson JV, Ward RHR, Lida J, Newman SL, Harrison RA, Lachmann PJ: Characterization of patients with an increased susceptibility to bacterial infections and a genetic deficiency of leukocyte membrane complement receptor type 3 and the related membrane antigen LFA-1. *Blood* **66**:882, 1985.
296. Root RK, Metcalf J, Oshino N, Chance B: H_2O_2 release from human granulocytes during phagocytosis. I. Documentation, quantitation, and some regulating factors. *J Clin Invest* **55**:945, 1975.
297. Weening RS, Roos D, Weemaes CMR, Homan-Muller JWT, van Schaik MLJ: Defective initiation of the metabolic stimulation of phagocytizing granulocytes: a new congenital defect. *J Lab Clin Med* **88**:757, 1976.
298. Bissenden JG, Haeney MR, Tarlow MJ, Thompson RA: Delayed separation of the umbilical cord, severe widespread infections, and immunodeficiency. *Arch Dis Child* **56**:397, 1981.
299. Niethammer D, Dieterle U, Kleihauer E, Wildfeuer A, Haferkamp O, Hitzig WH: An inherited defect in granulocyte function: Impaired chemotaxis, phagocytosis and intracellular killing of microorganisms. *Helv Paediatr Acta* **30**:537, 1975.
300. Smith CW, Marlin SD, Rothlein R, Lawrence MB, McIntire LV, Anderson DC: Role of ICAM-1 in the adherence of human neutrophils to human endothelial cells in vitro, in Springer TA, Anderson DC, Rosenthal AS, Rothlein R (eds): *Leukocyte Adhesion Molecules: Structure, Function, and Regulation*. New York, Springer-Verlag, 1990, p 170.
301. Tonnesen MG, Smedly LA, Henson PM: Neutrophil-endothelial cell interactions: Modulation of neutrophil adhesiveness induced by complement fragments C5a and C5a$_{desArg}$ and formyl-methionyl-leucyl-phenylalanine in vitro. *J Clin Invest* **74**:1581, 1984.
302. Anderson DC, Rothlein R, Marlin SD, Krater SS, Smith CW: Impaired transendothelial migration by neonatal neutrophils: Abnormalities of Mac-1 (CD11b/CD18)-dependent adherence reactions. *Blood* **78**:2613, 1990.
303. Schmalstieg FC, Rudloff HE, Hillman GR, Anderson DC: Two-dimensional and three-dimensional movement of human polymorphonuclear leukocytes: Two fundamentally different mechanisms of location. *J Leukoc Biol* **40**:677, 1986.
304. Beller DI, Springer TA, Schreiber RD: Anti-Mac-1 selectively inhibits the mouse and human type three complement receptor. *J Exp Med* **156**:1000, 1982.
305. Thompson RA, Candy DCA, McNeish AS: Familial defect of polymorph neutrophil phagocytosis associated with absence of a surface glycoprotein antigen (OKM1). *Clin Exp Immunol* **58**:229, 1984.
306. O'Shea JJ, Brown EJ, Seligmann BE, Metcalf JA, Frank MM, Gallin JI: Evidence for distinct intracellular pools of receptors for C3b and C3bi in human neutrophils. *J Immunol* **134**:2580, 1985.
307. Gresham HD, Graham IL, Anderson DC, Brown EJ: Leukocyte adhesion deficient (LAD) neutrophils fail to amplify phagocytic function in response to stimulation: Evidence for CD11b/CD18-dependent and -independent mechanisms of phagocytosis. *J Clin Invest* **88**:588, 1991.
308. Worth RG, Mayo-Bond L, van de Winkel JGJ, Todd RF, III, Petty HR: CR3 ($\alpha_m\beta_2$; CD11b/CD18) restores IgG-dependent phagocytosis in transfectants expressing a phagocytosis-defective FcgammaRIIA (CD32) tail-minus mutant. *J Immunol* **157**:5660, 1996.
309. Rich KC, Neumann CG, Stiehm ER: Neutrophil chemotaxis in malnourished Ghanaian children, in Suskind RM (ed): *Malnutrition and Immune Response*. New York, Raven Press, 1977, p 271.
310. Mentzer SJ, Bierer BE, Anderson DC, Springer TA, Burakoff SJ: Abnormal cytolytic activity of lymphocyte function-associated antigen-1-deficient human cytolytic T lymphocyte clones. *J Clin Invest* **78**:1387, 1986.
311. Gebb SA, Graham JA, Hanger CC, Godbey PS, Capen RL, Doerschuk CM, Wagner WW Jr: Sites of leukocyte sequestration in the pulmonary microcirculation. *J Appl Physiol* **79**:493, 1995.
312. Kishimoto TK, Hollander N, Roberts TM, Anderson DC, Springer TA: Heterogenous mutations of the beta subunit common to the LFA-1, Mac-1, and p150,95 glycoproteins cause leukocyte adhesion deficiency. *Cell* **50**:193, 1987.
313. Dana N, Clayton LK, Tennen DG, Pierce MW, Lachmann PJ, Law SA, Arnaout MA: Leukocytes from four patients with complete or partial Leu-CAM deficiency contain the common beta-subunit precursor and beta-subunit messenger RNA. *J Clin Invest* **79**:1010, 1987.
314. Wardlaw AJ, Hibbs ML, Stacker SA, Springer TA: Distinct mutations in two patients with leukocyte adhesion deficiency and their functional correlates. *J Exp Med* **172**:335, 1990.
315. Arnaout MA, Dana N, Gupta SK, Tenen DG, Fathallah DM: Point mutations impairing cell surface expression of the common beta subunit (CD18) in a patient with leukocyte adhesion molecule (Leu-CAM) deficiency. *J Clin Invest* **85**:977, 1990.
316. Kishimoto TK, O'Connor K, Springer TA: Leukocyte adhesion deficiency: Aberrant splicing of a conserved integrin sequence causes a moderate deficiency phenotype. *J Biol Chem* **264**:3588, 1989.
317. MacKrell AJ, Blumberg B, Haynes S, Fessler J: The lethal myospheroid gene of *Drosophila* encodes a membrane protein homologous to vertebrate integrin beta subunits. *Proc Natl Acad Sci U S A* **85**:2633, 1988.
318. Sligh JE Jr, Hurwitz MY, Zhu C, Anderson DC, Beaudet AL: An initiation codon mutation in CD18 in association with the moderate phenotype of leukocyte adhesion deficiency. *J Biol Chem* **267**:714, 1992.
319. Kozak M: Context effects and inefficient initiation at non-AUG codons in eucaryotic cell-free translation systems. *Mol Cell Biol* **9**:5073, 1989.
320. Wright AH, Douglass WA, Taylor GM, Lau YL, Higgins D, Davies KA, Law SK: Molecular characterization of leukocyte adhesion deficiency in six patients. *Eur J Immunol* **25**:717, 1995.
321. Davies KA, Toothill VJ, Savill J, Hotchin N, Peters AM, Pearson JD, Haslett C, Burke M, Law SKA, Mercer NFG, Walport MJ, Webster ADB: A 19-year-old man with leucocyte adhesion deficiency. In vitro and in vivo studies of leucocyte function. *Clin Exp Immunol* **84**:223, 1991.
322. Lau YL, Low LC, Jones BM, Lawton JW: Defective neutrophil and lymphocyte function in leucocyte adhesion deficiency. *Clin Exp Immunol* **85**:202, 1991.
323. Nelson C, Rabb H, Arnaout MA: Genetic cause of leukocyte adhesion molecule deficiency: Abnormal splicing and a missense mutation in a conserved region of CD18 impair cell surface expression of beta-2 integrins. *J Biol Chem* **267**:3351, 1992.

324. Back AL, Kerkering M, Baker D, Bauer TR, Embree LJ, Hickstein DD: A point mutation associated with leukocyte adhesion deficiency type 1 of moderate severity. *Biochem Biophys Res Commun* **193**:912, 1993.
325. Taylor GM, Braddock D, Robson AJ, Fergusson WD, Duckett DP, D'Souza SW, Brenchley P: Expression of LFA-1 by a lymphoblastoid cell line from a patient with monosomy 21: Effects on intercellular adhesion. *Clin Exp Immunol* **81**:501, 1990.
326. Matsuura S, Kishi F, Tsukahara M, Nunoi H, Matsuda I, Kobayashi K, Kajii T: Leukocyte adhesion deficiency: Identification of novel mutation in two Japanese patients with a severe form. *Biochem Biophys Res Commun* **184**:1460, 1992.
327. Corbi AL, Vara A, Ursa A, Garcia-Rodriguez MC, Fontan G, Sanchez-Madrid F: Molecular basis for a severe case of leukocyte adhesion deficiency. Simultaneous occurrence of a point mutation and aberrant splicing. *Eur J Immunol* **22**:1877, 1992.
328. Lopez Rodriguez C, Nueda A, Grospierre B, Sanchez-Madrid F, Fischer A, Springer TA, Corbi AL: Characterization of two new CD18 alleles causing severe leukocyte adhesion deficiency. *Eur J Immunol* **23**:2792, 1993.
329. Back AL, Kwok WW, Hickstein DD: Identification of two molecular defects in a child with leukocyte adherence deficiency. *J Biol Chem* **267**:5482, 1992.
330. Konno T, Tsukamoto J, Terasawa M, Tsuchiya S, Tachibana T: OKM-1(Mol)/LFA-1 deficiency in a Japanese infant with recurrent infection, in Eible MM, Rosen FS (eds): *Primary Immunodeficiency Disease*. Amsterdam, Excerpta Medica, 1986, p 315.
331. Nunoi H, Yanabe Y, Higuchi S, Tsuchiya H, Yamamoto J, Matsuda I, Naito M, Takahashi K, Fujita K, Uchida M, Kobayashi K, Jono M, Malech H: Severe hypoplasia of lymphoid tissues in Mo1 deficiency. *Hum Pathol* **19**:753, 1988.
332. Majima T, Minegishi N, Nagatomi R, Ohashi Y, Tsuchiya S, Kobayashi K, Konno T: Unusual expression of IgG Fc receptors on peripheral granulocytes from patients with leukocyte adhesion deficiency (CD11/CD18 deficiency). *J Immunol* **145**:1694, 1990.
333. Kieffer N, Phillips DR: Platelet membrane glycoproteins: Functions in cellular interactions. *Annu Rev Cell Biol* **6**:329, 1990.
334. Loftus JC, O'Toole TE, Plow EF, Glass A, Frelinger III AL, Ginsberg MH: A $\beta 8$ integrin mutation abolishes ligand binding and alters divalent cation-dependent conformation. *Science* **249**:915, 1990.
335. Kuijpers TW, van Lier RAW, Hamann D, de Boer M, Thung LY, Weening RS, Verhoeven AJ, Roos D: Leukocyte adhesion deficiency type 1 (LAD-1)/variant. A novel immunodeficiency syndrome characterized by dysfunctional $\beta 2$ integrins. *J Clin Invest* **100**:1725, 1997.
336. Hogg N, Stewart MP, Scarth SL, Newton R, Shaw JM, Law SKA, Klein N: A novel leukocyte adhesion deficiency caused by expressed but nonfunctional $\beta 2$ integrins Mac-1 and LFA-1. *J Clin Invest* **103**:97, 1999.
337. Fischer A, Trung PH, Descamps-Latscha B, Lisowska-Grospierre B, Gerota I, Perez N, Scheinmetzler C, Durandy A, Virelizier JL, Griscelli C: Bone-marrow transplantation for inborn error of phagocytic cells associated with defective adherence, chemotaxis, and oxidative response during opsonised particle phagocytosis. *Lancet* **2**:473, 1983.
338. Thomas C, LeDeist F, Cavazzana-Calvo M, Benkerrou M, Haddad E, Blanche S, Hartmann W, Friedrich W, Fischer A: Results of allogeneic bone marrow transplantation in patients with leukocyte adhesion deficiency. *Blood* **84**:1635, 1995.
339. Back AL, Kwok WW, Adam M, Collins SJ, Hickstein DD: Retroviral-mediated gene transfer of the leukocyte integrin CD18 subunit. *Biochem Biophys Res Commun* **171**:787, 1990.
340. Wilson JM, Ping AJ, Krauss JC, Mayo-Bond L, Rogers CE, Anderson DC, Todd III RF: Correction of CD18-deficient lymphocytes by retrovirus-mediated gene transfer. *Science* **248**:1413, 1990.
341. Wilson RW, Yorifuji T, Lorenzo I, Smith CW, Anderson DC, Belmont JW, Beaudet AL: Expression of human CD18 in murine granulocytes and improved efficiency for infection of deficient human lymphoblasts. *Hum Gene Ther* **4**:25, 1993.
342. Bauer TR, Schwartz BR, Conrad LW, Ochs HD, Hickstein DD: Retroviral-mediated gene transfer of the leukocyte integrin CD18 into peripheral blood CD34+ cells derived from a patient with leukocyte adhesion deficiency type 1. *Blood* **91**:1520, 1998.
343. Frydman M, Etzioni A, Eidlitz-Markus T, Avidov I, Varsano I, Shecter Y, Orlin JB, Gershoni-Baruch R: Rambam-Hasharon syndrome of psychomotor retardation, short stature, defective neutrophil motility, and Bombay phenotype. *Am J Med Genet* **44**:297, 1992.
344. Etzioni A, Gershoni-Baruch R, Pollack S, Shehadeh N: Leukocyte adhesion deficiency type II: Long-term follow-up. *J Allergy Clin Immunol* 102:323, 1998.
345. Yunis EJ, Svardal JMK, Bridges RA: Genetics of the Bombay phenotype. *Blood* **33**:124, 1969.
346. Watkins WH: Biochemistry and genetics of the ABO, Lewis, and P blood group systems. *Adv Hum Genet* **10**:1, 1980.
347. Price TH, Ochs HD, Gershoni-Baruch R, Harlan JM, Etzioni A: In vivo neutrophil and lymphocyte function studies in a patient with leukocyte adhesion deficiency type II. *Blood* **84**:1635, 1995.
348. Price TH, Ochs HD, Gershoni-Baruch R, Harlan JM, Etzioni A: In vivo neutrophil and lymphocyte function studies in a patient with leukocyte adhesion deficiency type II. *Blood* **84**:1635, 1994.
349. Etzioni A: Adhesion molecule deficiencies and their clinical significance. *Cell Adhes Commun* **2**:257, 1994.
350. von Andrian UH, Berger EM, Chambers JD, Ramezani L, Ochs H, Harlan JM, Paulson JC, Etzioni A, Arfors K-E: In vivo behavior of neutrophils from two patients with distinct inherited leukocyte adhesion deficiency syndromes. *J Clin Invest* **91**:2893, 1993.
351. Kuijpers TW, Etzioni A, Pollack S, Pals ST: Antigen-specific immune responsiveness and lymphocyte recruitment in leukocyte adhesion deficiency type II. *Int Immunol* **9**:607, 1997.
352. Phillips ML, Schwartz BR, Etzioni A, Bayer R, Ochs HD, Paulson JC: Neutrophil adhesion in leukocyte adhesion deficiency syndrome type 2. *J Clin Invest* **96**:2898, 1995.
353. Lowe JB, Stoolman LM, Nair RP, Larsen RD, Berhend TL, Marks RM: ELAM-1-dependent cell adhesion to vascular endothelium determined by a transfected human fucosyltransferase cDNA. *Cell* **63**:475, 1990.
354. Le Pendu J, Cartron JP, Lemieux RU, Oriol R: The presence of at least two different H-blood-group-related beta-D-Gal-alpha-2-l-fucosyltransferases in human serum and the genetics of blood group H substances. *Am J Hum Genet* **37**:749, 1985.
355. Etzioni A, Frydman M, Pollack S, Avidor I, Phillips ML, Paulson JC, Gershoni-Barugh R: Brief report: Recurrent severe infections caused by a novel leukocyte adhesion deficiency. *N Engl J Med* **327(25)**:1789, 1992.
356. Abbassi O, Kishimoto TK, McIntire LV, Smith CW: Neutrophil adhesion to endothelial cells. *Blood Cells* **19**:245, 1993.
357. von Andrian UH, Chambers JD, McEvoy LM, Bargatze RF, Arfors K-E, Butcher EC: Two step model of leukocyte-endothelial cell interaction in inflammation: Distinct roles for LECAM-1 and the leukocyte beta-2 integrins in vivo. *Proc Natl Acad Sci U S A* **88**:7538, 1991.
358. Ley K, Gaehtgens P, Fennie C, Singer MS, Lasky LA, Rosen SD: LEC-CAM 1 mediates leukocyte rolling in mesenteric venules in vivo. *Blood* **77**:2553, 1991.
359. Polley MJ, Phillips ML, Wayner E, Nudelman E, Singhal AK, Hakomori SI, Paulson JC: CD62 and endothelial cell-leukocyte adhesion molecule 1 (ELAM-1) recognize the same carbohydrate ligand, sialyl-Lewis x. *Proc Natl Acad Sci U S A* **88**:6224, 1991.
360. Phillips ML, Nudelman E, Gaeta FCA, Perez M, Singhal AK, Hakomori S, Paulson JC: ELAM-1 mediates cell adhesion by recognition of a carbohydrate ligand, Sialyl-Le^x. *Science* **250**:1130, 1990.
361. Simon SI, Neelamegham S, Taylor A, Smith CW: The multistep process of homotypic neutrophil aggregation: A review of the molecules and effects of hydrodynamics. *Cell Adhes Commun* **6**:263, 1998.
362. Frydman M, Vardimon D, Shalev E, Orlin JB: Prenatal diagnosis of Rambam-Hasharon syndrome. *Prenat Diagn* **16**:266, 1996.
363. Karsan A, Cornejo CJ, Winn RK, Schwartz BR, Way W, Lannir N, Gershoni-Baruch R, Etzioni A, Ochs HD, Harlan JM: Leukocyte Adhesion Deficiency Type II is a generalized defect of *de novo* GDP-fucose biosynthesis. Endothelial cell fucosylation is not required for neutrophil rolling on human nonlymphoid endothelium. *J Clin Invest* **101**:2438, 1998.
364. Sturla L, Etzioni A, Bisso A, Zanardi D, De Flora G, Silengo L, De Flora A, Tonetti M: Defective intracellular activity of GDP-D-mannose-4,6-dehydratase in leukocyte adhesion deficiency type II syndrome. *FEBS Lett* **429**:274, 1998.
365. Wilson CB: Immunologic basis for enhanced susceptibility of the neonate to infection. *J Pediatr* **108**:1, 1986.
366. Schuit KE, Homisch L: Inefficient in vivo neutrophil migration in neonatal rats. *J Leukoc Biol* **35**:583, 1984.
367. Martin TR, Rubens CE, Wilson CB: Lung antibacterial defense mechanisms in infant and adult rats: Implications for the pathogenesis of Group B streptococcal infections in the neonatal lung. *J Infect Dis* **157**:91, 1988.

368. Cheung AT, Ayin SA, Kessell PR: Functional immaturity in neonatal polymorphonuclear leukocytes of rhesus monkeys. *J Med Primatol* **25**:84, 1996.
369. Wolach B, Sonnenschein D, Gavrieli R, Chomsky O, Pomeranz A, Yuli I: Neonatal neutrophil inflammatory responses: parallel studies of light scattering, cell polarization, chemotaxis, superoxide release, and bactericidal activity. *Am J Hematol* **58**:8, 1998.
370. Christensen RD, Rothstein G: Exhaustion of mature marrow neutrophils in neonates with sepsis. *J Pediatr* **97**:316, 1980.
371. Anderson DC: Neonatal neutrophil dysfunction. *Am J Pediatr Hematol Oncol* **11**:224, 1989.
372. Anderson DC, Abbassi O, Kishimoto TK, Koenig JM, McIntire LV, Smith CW: Diminished lectin-, epidermal growth factor-, complement-binding domain-cell adhesion molecule-1 on neonatal neutrophils underlies their impaired CD18-independent adhesion to endothelial cells in vitro. *J Immunol* **146**:3372, 1991.
373. Keeney SE, Mathews MJ, Haque AK, Schmalstieg FC: Comparison of pulmonary neutrophils in the adult and neonatal rat after hyperoxia. *Pediatr Res* **38**:857, 1995.
374. Miller ME: Chemotactic function in the human neonate: Humoral and cellular aspects. *Pediatr Res* **5**:487, 1971.
375. Anderson DC, Hughes BJ, Wible LJ, Perry GJ, Smith CW, Brinkley BR: Impaired motility of neonatal PMN leukocytes: Relationship to abnormalities of cell orientation and assembly of microtubules in chemotactic gradients. *J Leukoc Biol* **36**:1, 1984.
376. Pahwa SG, Pahwa R, Grimes E, Smithwick E: Cellular and humoral components of monocyte and neutrophil chemotaxis in cord blood. *Pediatr Res* **11**:677, 1977.
377. Klein RB, Fischer TJ, Gard SE, Biberstein M, Rich KC, Stiehm ER: Decreased mononuclear and polymorphonuclear chemotaxis in human newborns, infants, and young children. *Pediatrics* **60**:467, 1977.
378. Nybo M, Sorensen O, Leslie R, Wang P: Reduced expression of C5a receptors on neutrophils from cord blood. *Arch Dis Child Fetal Neonatal Ed* **78**:F129, 1998.
379. Anderson DC, Hughes BJ, Edwards MS, Buffone GJ, Baker CJ: Impaired chemotaxigenesis by type III group B streptococci in neonatal sera: Relationship to diminished concentrations of specific anticapsular antibody and abnormalities of serum complement. *Pediatr Res* **17**:496, 1983.
380. Krause PJ, Maderazo EG, Scroggs M: Abnormalities of neutrophil adherence in newborns. *Pediatrics* **69**:184, 1982.
381. Krause PJ, Herson VC, Boutin-Lebowitz J, Eisenfeld L, Block C, LoBello T, Maderazo EG: Polymorphonuclear leukocyte adherence and chemotaxis in stressed and healthy neonates. *Pediatr Res* **20**:296, 1986.
382. Anderson DC, Freeman KLB, Heerdt B, Hughes BJ, Jack RM, Smith CW: Abnormal stimulated adherence of neonatal granulocytes: Impaired induction of surface Mac-1 by chemotactic factors or secretagogues. *Blood* **70**:740, 1987.
383. Lodge-Patch L: The ageing of cardiac infarcts, and its influence on cardiac rupture. *Br Heart J* **13**:37, 1951.
384. Anderson DC: Neonatal neutrophils. *J Lab Clin Med* **120**:816, 1992.
385. Jones DH, Schmalstieg FC, Dempsey K, Krater SS, Nannen DD, Smith CW, Anderson DC: Subcellular distribution and mobilization of Mac-1 (CD11b/CD18) in neonatal neutrophils. *Blood* **75**:488, 1990.
386. Bruce MC, Bailey JE, Medvik K, Berger M: Impaired surface membrane expression of C3bi, but not C3b receptors in neonatal neutrophils. *Pediatr Res* **21**:306, 1987.
387. Ambruso DR, Bentwood B, Henson PM, Johnston RB Jr: Oxidative metabolism of cord blood neutrophils: Relationship to content and degranulation of cytoplasmic granules. *Pediatr Res* **18**:1148, 1984.
388. Jones DH, Schmalstieg FC, Hawkins HK, Burr BL, Rudloff HE, Krater SS, Smith CW, Anderson DC: Characterization of a new mobilizable Mac-1 (CD11b/CD18) pool that co-localizes with gelatinase in human neutrophils, in Springer TA, Anderson DC, Rosenthal AS, Rothlein R (eds): *Leukocyte Adhesion Molecules: Structure, Function, and Regulation*. New York, Springer-Verlag, 1990, p 106.
389. Reddy RK, Xia Y, Hanikyrova M, Ross GD: A mixed population of immature and mature leucocytes in umbilical cord blood results in a reduced expression and function of CR3 (CD11b/CD18). *Clin Exp Immunol* **114**:462, 1998.
390. McEvoy LT, Zakem-Cloud H, Tosi MF: Total cell content of CR3 (CD11b/CD18) and LFA-1 (CD11a/CD18) in neonatal neutrophils: Relationship to gestational age. *Blood* **87**:3929, 1996.
391. Mariscalco MM, Tcharmtchi MH, Smith CW: P-selectin support of neonatal neutrophil adherence under flow: Contribution of L-selectin, LFA-1, and ligand(s) for P-selectin. *Blood* **91**:4776, 1998.
392. Smith JB, Kunjummen, RD, Kishimoto, TK, Anderson, DC: Neonatal eosinophils and neutrophils have similar abnormalities of expression of leukocyte-endothelial cell adhesion molecule-1 (LECAM-1). *Pediatr Res* **29**:278, 1991.
393. Fortenberry JD, Marolda JR, Anderson DC, Smith CW, Mariscalco MM: CD18-dependent and L-selectin-dependent neutrophil emigration is diminished in neonatal rabbits. *Blood* **84**:889, 1994.
394. Laver J, Duncan E, Abboud M, Gasparetto C, Sahdev I, Warren D, Bussel J, Auld P, O'Reilly RJ, Moore MAS: High levels of granulocyte and granulocyte-macrophage colony-stimulating factors in cord blood of normal full-term neonates. *J Pediatr* **116**:627, 1990.
395. Peters WP, Stuart A, Affronti ML, Kim CS, Coleman RE: Neutrophil migration is defective during recombinant human granulocyte-macrophage colony-stimulating factor infusion after autologous bone marrow transplantation in humans. *Blood* **72**:1310, 1988.
396. Koenig JM, Anderson, DC, Smith, CW: Surface levels of LECAM-1 on neonatal neutrophils are further diminished at 24 hours of life. *Pediatr Res* **29**:276A, 1991.
397. Rebuck N, Gibson A, Finn A: Neutrophil adhesion molecules in term and premature infants: Normal or enhanced leucocyte integrins but defective L-selectin expression and shedding. *Clin Exp Immunol* **101**:183, 1995.
398. Koenig JM, Simon J, Anderson DC, Smith EO, Smith CW: Diminished soluble and total cellular L-selectin in cord blood is associated with its impaired shedding from activated neutrophils. *Pediatr Res* **39**:616, 1996.
399. Koenig JM, Smith CW: Cord blood neutrophils bind less avidly to sulfatide than adult neutrophils. *Pediatr Res* **33**:283A, 1993.
400. Tcharmtchi MH, Mariscalco MM, Smith CW: P-selectin (P-Sel) support of neonatal neutrophil (N-PMN) rolling: Contribution of neutrophil P-selectin-glycoligand-1 (PSGL-1). *Pediatr Res* **41**:228A, 1997.
401. Eitzman DV, Smith RT: The nonspecific inflammatory cycle in neonatal infants. *Am J Dis Child* **97**:326, 1974.
402. Baehner RL, Nathan DG: Quantitative nitroblue tetrazolium test in chronic granulomatous disease. *N Engl J Med* **278**:971, 1968.
403. Gallin JI, Fletcher MP, Seligmann BE, Hoffstein S, Cehrs K, Mounessa N: Human neutrophil-specific granules deficiency: A method to assess the role of neutrophil-specific granules in the evolution of the inflammatory response. *Blood* **59**:1317, 1982.
404. Gallin JI, Wright DG, Schiffmann E: Role of secretory events in modulating human neutrophil chemotaxis. *J Clin Invest* **62**:1364, 1978.
405. Spitznagel JK, Cooper MR, McCall AE, DeChatelet LR, Welsh IRH: Selective deficiency of granules associated with lysozyme and lactoferrin in human polymorphs (PMN). *J Clin Invest* **51**:93A, 1972.
406. Boxer LA, Coates TD, Haak RA, Wolach JB, Hoffstein S, Baehner RL: Lactoferrin deficiency associated granulocyte function. *N Engl J Med* **307**:404, 1982.
407. Gallin JI: Neutrophil specific granule deficiency. *Ann Rev Med* **36**:263, 1985.
408. Parmley RT, Ogawa M, Darby CP Jr, Spicer SS: Congenital neutropenia: Neutrophil proliferation with abnormal maturation. *Blood* **46**:723, 1975.
409. Komiyama A, Morosawa H, Nakahata T, Miyagawa Y, Akabane T: Abnormal neutrophil maturation in a neutrophil defect with morphologic abnormality and impaired function. *J Pediatr* **94**:19, 1979.
410. Breton-Gorius J, Mason DY, Buriot D, Vilde JL, Griscelli C: Lactoferrin deficiency as a consequence of a lack of specific granules in neutrophils from a patient with recurrent infections. *Am J Pathol* **99**:413, 1980.
411. Strauss RG, Bove KE, Jones JF, Mauer AM, Fulginiti VA: An anomaly of neutrophil morphology with impaired function. *N Engl J Med* **290**:478, 1974.
412. Borregaard N, Boxer LA, Smolen JE, Tauber AI: Anomalous neutrophil granule distribution in a patient with lactoferrin deficiency: Pertinence to the respiratory burst. *Am J Hematol* **18**:255, 1985.
413. Tamura A, Agematsu K, Mori T, Kawai H, Kuratsuji T, Shimane M, Tani K, Asano S, Komiyama A: A marked decrease in defensin mRNA in the only case of congenital neutrophil-specific granule deficiency reported in Japan. *Int J Hematol* **59**:137, 1994.
414. Rosenberg HF, Gallin JI: Neutrophil-specific granule deficiency includes eosinophils. *Blood* **82**:268, 1993.
415. Gant T, Metcalf JA, Gallin JI, Boxer LA, Lehrer RI: Microbial/cytoxic proteins of neutrophils are deficient in two disorders: Chediak-Higashi syndrome and "specific" granule deficiency. *J Clin Invest* **82**:552, 1988.

416. Lomax KJ, Malech HL, Gallin JI: The molecular biology of selected phagocyte defects. *Blood Rev* **3**:94, 1989.
417. Lomax KJ, Gallin JI, Rotrosen D, Raphael GD, Kalinir MA, Benz EJ, Boxer LA, Malech HL: Selective defect in myeloid cell lactoferrin gene expression in neutrophil specific granule deficiency. *J Clin Invest* **83**:514, 1989.
418. Anderson KL, Smith KA, Pio F, Torbett BE, Maki RA: Neutrophils deficient in PU.1 do not terminally differentiate or become functionally competent. *Blood* **92**:1576, 1998.
419. Mizgerd JP, Quinlan WM, LeBlanc BW, Kutkoski GJ, Bullard DC, Beaudet AL, Doerschuk CM: Combinatorial requirements for adhesion molecules in mediating neutrophil emigration during bacterial peritonitis in mice. *J Leukoc Biol* **64**:291, 1998.
420. Ley K, Tedder TF, Kansas GS: L-selectin can mediate leukocyte rolling in untreated mesenteric venules in vivo independent of E- or P-selectin. *Blood* **82**:1632, 1993.
421. Rosen H, Gordon S: Monoclonal antibody to the murine type 3 complement receptor inhibits adhesion of myelomonocytic cells in vitro and inflammatory cell recruitment in vivo. *J Exp Med* **166**:1685, 1987.
422. Scharffetter-Kochanek K, Lu H, Norman I, van Nood N, Munoz F, Grabbe S, McArthur M, Lorenzo I, Kaplan S, Ley K, Smith CW, Montgomery CA, Rich S, Beaudet AL: Spontaneous skin ulceration and defective T cell function in CD18 null mice. *J Exp Med* **188**:119, 1998.
423. Bullard DC, Kunkel EJ, Kubo H, Hicks MJ, Lorenzo I, Doyle NA, Doerschuk CM, Ley K, Beaudet AL: Infectious susceptibility and severe deficiency of leukocyte rolling and recruitment in E-selectin and P-selectin double-mutant mice. *J Exp Med* **183**:2329, 1996.
424. Mizgerd JP, Kubo H, Kutkoski GJ, Bhagwan SD, Scharffetter-Kochanek K, Beaudet AL, Doerschuk CM: Neutrophil emigration in the skin, lungs, and peritoneum: Different requirements for CD11/CD18 revealed by CD18-deficient mice. *J Exp Med* **186**:1357, 1997.
425. Doerschuk CM, Winn RK, Coxson HO, Harlan JM: CD18-dependent and independent mechanisms of neutrophil emigration in the pulmonary and systemic microcirculation of rabbits. *J Immunol* **144(6)**:2327, 1990.
426. Hawkins HK, Heffelfinger S, Anderson DC: Leukocyte adhesion deficiency: Clinical and postmortem observations. *Pediatric Pathol* **12**:119, 1992.
427. Ley K, Bullard DC, Arbones ML, Bosse R, Vestweber D, Tedder TF, Beaudet AL: Sequential contribution of L- and P-selectin to leukocyte rolling in vivo. *J Exp Med* **181**:669, 1995.
428. Ohashi Y, Yambe T, Tsuchiya S, Kikuchi H, Konno T: Familial genetic defect in a case of leukocyte adhesion deficiency. *Hum Mutat* **2**:458, 1993.
429. Kobayashi K, Fujita K, Okino F: An abnormality of neutrophil adhesion: Autosomal recessive inheritance associated with missing neutrophil glycoproteins. *Pediatrics* **73**:606, 1984.
430. Etzioni A: Adhesion molecules—their role in health and disease. *Pediatr Res* **39**:191, 1996.

CHAPTER 189

Inherited Disorders of Phagocyte Killing

Mary C. Dinauer ▪ William M. Nauseef ▪ Peter E. Newburger

1. **Phagocytic cells are an essential component of the innate immune system that provides a first line of defense against microbial infection. This protective capacity depends on both oxygen-dependent and oxygen-independent killing mechanisms. The latter includes the release of hydrolytic and cytotoxic proteins from cytoplasmic granules into the phagolysosome. Oxygen-dependent microbial killing by activated phagocytes relies on the generation of toxic oxygen products from molecular oxygen through a series of electron transfers. This process is mediated by a multi-component nicotinamide adenine dinucleotide phosphate (NADPH) oxidase that assembles in the plasma membrane during ingestion of microorganisms. Granules also release myeloperoxidase into the phagolysosome, and the enzyme catalyzes production of the microbicidal agent, hypochlorous acid. These oxygen-dependent events do not occur normally in phagocytes from patients with chronic granulomatous disease, myeloperoxidase deficiency, or deficiency of the enzymes glucose 6-phosphate dehydrogenase (G-6-PD), glutathione synthetase, or glutathione reductase.**
2. **Congenital absence or structural mutation of any one of the four major components of the NADPH oxidase complex in phagocytes results in the clinical syndrome of chronic granulomatous disease, characterized by recurrent pyogenic infections of the skin, soft tissues, liver, spleen, lymph nodes, and respiratory tract. Catalase-positive bacteria and fungi are the common pathogens. Phagocytes from these patients ingest organisms normally but display impaired microbial killing, which is the basis of the clinical syndrome. Chronic granulomatous disease is a heterogeneous disorder with regard to mode of inheritance because the four major oxidase components are encoded at different chromosomal locations (1q25, 7q11.23, 16p23, and Xp21.1); see Table 189-5 for MIM and GenBank data. The disease is also heterogeneous with regard to severity of clinical presentation because the mutations in the gene encoding the most commonly affected component (the major subunit of flavocytochrome b_{558}, encoded on the X chromosome) can lead to different degrees of residual function and, consequently, variability in the capacity to kill ingested microorganisms.**
3. **Severe G-6-PD deficiency in neutrophils, which leads to impaired hexose monophosphate shunt activity, can mimic chronic granulomatous disease. Affected neutrophils are unable to generate the NADPH required to sustain activity of the respiratory burst oxidase and as a result display a defect in intracellular killing.**
4. **Myeloperoxidase, present in the azurophilic granules of mature neutrophils, catalyzes the formation of hypochlorous acid from chloride ion and H_2O_2 generated by the respiratory burst. The partial or complete absence of myeloperoxidase affects about 1 in 2000 apparently healthy individuals. Myeloperoxidase deficiency is usually not associated with clinically significant infections, with the exception of invasive fungal disease in individuals with concomitant diabetes mellitus.**
5. **Glutathione synthetase and glutathione reductase activities are required to maintain adequate intracellular levels of reduced glutathione. This sulfhydryl-containing tripeptide protects the cell from oxidative injury. Deficiency of either of these enzymes permits autooxidative damage, which is associated with abnormal microbicidal activity.**

A list of standard abbreviations is located immediately preceding the index in each volume. Additional abbreviations used in this chapter include: CAP = cationic antimicrobial protein, also CAP37 and CAP57; CGD = chronic granulomatous disease; *CYBA* = symbol for the autosomal cytochrome *b* gene encoding p22-*phox*; *CYBB* = symbol for X-linked gene for cytochrome *b* encoding gp 91-*phox*; GDI = GDP dissociation inhibitor; HAF-1 = hematopoetic-associated factor 1; iNOS = inducible nitric oxide synthase; k, Kp^b, Ku = Kellblood group markers (MIM 314850); MPO = myeloperoxidase; NBT = nitroblue tetrazolium; *phox* = phagocyte oxidase; *NCF1, NCF2* = gene symbols for neutrophil cytosol factors 1 and 2 encoding p47-*phox* and p67-*phox*; NO = nitric oxide; NOS = nitric oxide synthase; PKC = protein kinase C; PU.1 = a transcription factor; Rac1, Rac2 = Rac (related to the A and C kinases) serine/threonine protein kinases 1 and 2; Rap1A = Ras-related protein 1A; Rho = a family of GTPase-activating proteins; SH3 = *src* homology domain 3; TMP-SMX = trimethoprim/sulfamethoxazole; *XK* = gene symbold for McLeod phenotype.

NORMAL MICROBICIDAL MECHANISMS OF PHAGOCYTIC CELLS

The role of phagocytes in host defense against invading microbes has been recognized since Metchnikoff reported his observations in 1883.[1,2] His pioneering studies were made with wandering ameboid mesothelial cells from starfish, for which he coined the term *phagocyte*, after the Greek word, *phagein*, meaning "to eat." In the human, phagocytosis is performed efficiently and rapidly by circulating polymorphonuclear neutrophils, eosinophils, and monocytes, and by fixed tissue macrophages, which are the progeny of monocytes.[3] These professional phagocytes provide the body with a first line of defense against infection. When phagocytes, in response to chemotactic stimuli, migrate to sites of infection and contact invading microorganisms, ingestion ensues.

Ingested microorganisms are sequestered within intracellular vacuoles (phagosomes), into which are released digestive lysosomal enzymes and bactericidal antibiotic proteins from storage granules and highly reactive oxidants generated by the respiratory burst. These complementary methods of microbial destruction can be broadly classified as independent of or dependent on molecular oxygen.

Oxygen-Independent Mechanisms

Phagocytic granules contain a supply of cytotoxic and digestive compounds that participate in killing and digestion of ingested

Table 189-1 Bactericidal Proteins of Human Neutrophils

Bactericidal Protein	Molecular Weight	Chromosomal Location	Granule Location	Susceptible Species
Cathepsin G	~25000	14q11.2[15]	Azurophil	Gram-positive and gram-negative bacteria, certain fungi
Cationic antimicrobial protein. (CAP37. azurocidin)	~37000	19pter[10]	Azurophil	Gram-negative bacteria
Proteinase 3	~29000	19pter[10]	Azurophil	Gram-negative bacteria
Elastase	~28000	19pter[10]	Azurophil	Gram-negative bacteria
Bactericidal/permeability-increasing Protein (BPI.CAP57*)	~55000	20q11–q12[21]	Azurophil	Gram-negative bacteria
Defensins	~3000–4000	8p23[22]	Azurophil	Gram-positive and gram-negative bacteria, many fungi, certain viruses
Lysozyme	~14,500	12[24]	Azurophil and specific	Certain gram-positive bacteria, *Candida albicans*

*Cationic antimicrobial protein.

microbes. Several lines of evidence support a role for microbicidal activity that occurs in the absence of oxygen. First, the efficacy of oxygen-independent mechanisms can be demonstrated by the bactericidal activity of neutrophils in oxygen-depleted systems.[4–6] The inability to achieve complete anoxia in these systems, however, precludes absolute proof for nonoxidative killing. Second, neutrophils from patients with chronic granulomatous disease, which are unable to generate microbicidal oxygen metabolites, can kill at least some of an inoculum of most bacteria.[7,8] Third, constituents of both major neutrophil granules, the primary (azurophilic) and secondary (specific) granules, have intrinsic bactericidal capacity (Table 189-1). Furthermore, mice generated by gene targeting to genetically lack neutrophil elastase have impaired host defense to gram-negative bacteria,[9] clearly demonstrating the importance of nonoxidative mechanisms for microbial killing in vivo.

Neutrophil azurophilic granules contain serpocidins,[10–12] members of the serine protease (possessing chymotryptic activity) superfamily, which include 27-kDa cathepsin G,[13] a 37-kDa cationic antimicrobial protein termed variously CAP37 or azurocidin,[14,15] elastase, and proteinase 3. The genes for azurocidin, elastase, and proteinase 3 are clustered on chromosome 19 pter,[11] whereas cathepsin G is encoded by a gene on 14q11.2.[16] Microbial killing by many of these agents proceeds in vitro in the presence of proteolytic inhibitors, suggesting a nonenzymatic mechanism of action. Experiments with proteinase 3 and azurocidin show antimicrobial activity against a variety of gram-negative bacterial and, to a lesser extent, *Streptococcus faecalis* and *Candida albicans*.[12,13,15] Cathepsin G, one of the first neutrophil-derived proteolytic enzymes noted to exhibit antibacterial properties, is particularly active against fungi and gram-positive bacteria, with less potent activity against gram-negative bacteria.[12,16,17] Also extracted from the azurophilic granule and possessing antimicrobial activity are bactericidal/permeability factor and the family of defensins. Bactericidal/permeability factor is specific for gram-negative bacteria and its functional domain is contained in a 25-kDa fragment of the N-terminus.[18] It avidly binds to lipopolysaccharide, leading to both bacterial killing due to membrane damage and to the neutralization of endotoxin associated with the bacterial cell wall and in serum. Based on sequence analysis, bactericidal/permeability factor and a cationic antimicrobial protein of 57 kDa (CAP57) are likely identical.[19–21] Defensins are small (25 to 29 amino acid residues) basic peptides that constitute more than 5 percent of the total cellular protein of human neutrophils.[13,22] Killing studies indicate a broad spectrum of activity against multiple species of gram-positive and gram-negative bacteria, fungi, and enveloped viruses. Defensins kill by insertion into the cellular membrane and formation of voltage-regulated channels. Defensinlike peptides have also been found in small intestinal Paneth cells and in tracheal epithelium.[10]

The 14.5-kDa cationic protein lysozyme is a bacteriolytic agent found in both the azurophilic and specific granules of neutrophils and is secreted constitutively by monocytes and macrophages.[23,24] The bacteriolytic activity of lysozyme may be enhanced in the presence of complement. It acts by cleaving the $\beta 1 \rightarrow 4$ linkage between *N*-acetylmuramic acid and *N*-acetylglucosamine in the glycan backbone of the bacterial cell wall peptidoglycan. The contribution of lysozyme to the microbicidal activity of the neutrophil is not clear. However, the digestion of bacteria within phagolysosomes correlates with their susceptibility to in vitro lysozyme activity.

Optimal neutrophil antimicrobial activity is also likely to depend on the intraphagolysosomal pH. Microorganisms often do not survive in a low pH environment, and granule-associated antibacterial products that are released into the phagolysosome function within an acid pH range.[23]

Oxygen-Dependent Mechanisms

Respiratory Burst. During phagocytosis, neutrophils undergo a burst of oxidative metabolism,[25–30] which is summarized in Table 189-2. These events include a marked increase in oxygen uptake, increased utilization of glucose via the hexose monophosphate shunt, and release of the bactericidal oxygen metabolites superoxide anion (O_2^-), hydrogen peroxide (H_2O_2), hydroxyl radical ($\cdot OH$), and, perhaps, singlet oxygen. This cyanide-insensitive increase in oxidative metabolic activity is commonly termed the *respiratory burst*. Associated with this burst in oxidative metabolism is the ability of the phagocyte to emit low levels of light (chemiluminescence).[31]

The enhanced oxygen consumption in response to phagocytosis was first described in 1933,[25] but it was almost 30 years before it was appreciated that this process was insensitive to mitochondrial poisons and thus not related to increased energy demands associated with phagocytosis.[32] It was subsequently recognized

Table 189-2 Components of the Respiratory Burst

1. Increased oxygen consumption
2. Enhanced glucose utilization through the nexose monophosphate shunt
3. Generation of O_2^-, H_2O_2 and $\cdot OH$
4. Chemiluminescence
5. Turnover of NADPH and reduced glutathione

that phagocytosing neutrophils produce H_2O_2, previously recognized for its toxicity to *Escherichia coli*.[33] This finding provided a plausible basis for the microbicidal nature of phagocytosis. H_2O_2 was shown to interact with halide ions in the presence of the granule protein myeloperoxidase to generate microbicidal hypohalites, especially hypochlorite anion (OCl^-).[28] In 1973, phagocytosing neutrophils were reported to release O_2^-,[34] and data were later presented to suggest intraphagosomal generation of hydroxyl radical (·OH).[35]

Nicotinamide adenine diculeiotide phosphate (NADPH), or respiratory burst oxidase, is the enzyme complex responsible for catalyzing the formation of O_2^-, now recognized to be the initial conversion product of the consumed oxygen. The NADPH oxidase complex is associated with the plasma and phagolysosomal membrane and reduces oxygen univalently by using NADPH as an electron donor:[29]

$$2O_2 + NADPH \xrightarrow[\text{oxidase}]{\text{NADPH}} 2O_2^- + NADP^+ + H^+$$

Most of this O_2^- is thought to react with itself in a dismutation reaction (either spontaneously or more rapidly in the presence of superoxide dismutase) to form the second product of the respiratory burst, H_2O_2:

$$2O_2^- + 2H^+ \xrightarrow[\text{dismutase}]{\text{superoxide}} H_2O_2 + O_2$$

The list of oxygen metabolites generated in the phagocytosis-dependent respiratory burst now includes OCl^- and hydroxyl radical (·OH).[28] ·OH is a highly potent oxidant formed by the interaction between O_2^- and H_2O_2 in the presence of iron or some other heavy metal (Haber-Weiss reactions), summarized as follows:

$$O_2^- + Fe^{3+} \longrightarrow Fe^{2+} + O_2$$

$$Fe^{2+} + H_2O_2 \longrightarrow Fe^{3+} + HO^- + \cdot OH$$

or by the interaction between H_2O_2 and Fe^{2+} (Fenton reaction above).[36] The Fenton reaction is accelerated by the presence of O_2^-.[37] The physiologic role of the hydroxyl radical and control of its production are still being elucidated.[30,38] It is generally recognized that what is symbolized to exist as ·OH may in fact exist at least in part as one or another potent oxidative radical (i.e., ·OR) formed in the above reactions.

More recently identified as indirect products of the respiratory burst are chloramines, formed by the reaction of hypochlorite with ammonia or amines.[39,40] Other microbicidal products of the reduction of oxygen may be formed by phagocytes, but their roles have not yet been substantiated.

The critical importance of the respiratory burst for killing of microorganisms by phagocytes is demonstrated convincingly by the occurrence of the inherited disorder chronic granulomatous disease (CGD), which results from mutations in different subunits of the NADPH oxidase complex. Neutrophils from patients with CGD lack a respiratory burst and exhibit markedly deficient killing of many bacteria and fungi, which is manifested clinically as frequent and life-threatening infections with these microbes.[41–43]

Structure and Activation of the NADPH Oxidase. The NADPH oxidase is a phagosomal and plasma membrane-associated multicomponent enzyme that is dormant in the resting neutrophil and becomes assembled and catalytically active when neutrophils are activated by a variety of inflammatory stimuli[44–47] (Fig. 189-1). The identification of the components of this enzyme has benefited greatly from the biochemical and molecular genetic analysis of patients with CGD. Four polypeptides that are essential for NADPH oxidase activity have been identified (see below), and mutations in the corresponding genes are responsible for the four different genetic subgroups of CGD.[48–52] The oxidase subunits are referred to by their apparent molecular mass (in kilodaltons) and have been given the designation *phox*, for phagocyte oxidase. Characterization of NADPH oxidase has also been facilitated by the development of a cell-free assay using neutrophil cytosolic and membrane factions, in which the activation of the oxidase can be studied under defined conditions.[53–56]

Membrane Components. An unusual b-type cytochrome, located in the plasma membranes and specific granules of resting neutrophils, is the redox center of the oxidase complex. This cytochrome is a heterodimer comprised of a 91-kDa glycosylated

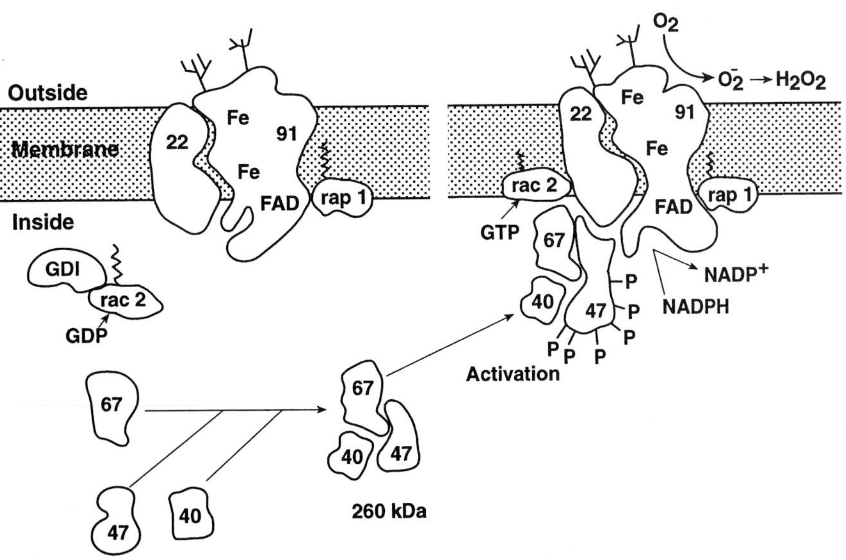

Fig. 189-1 Model of NADPH oxidase activation. In unstimulated neutrophils, NADPH oxidase is in a dormant state, with components distributed in both the membrane and the cytosol (*left side of figure*). The membrane includes the gp91-*phox* and p22-*phox* subunits of cytochrome b_{558} (and possibly Rap1A). The flavin and heme groups (Fe) that mediate the transfer of electrons from NADPH to molecular oxygen are localized in the gp91-*phox* subunit. The cytosolic components p47-*phox* and p67-*phox* may exist as a preformed complex of 260 kDa, which also includes at least one additional protein, p40-*phox*. The small GTPase Rac is also present in the cytosol in its inactive GDP bound state, in a complex with a GDP dissociation inhibitor (GDI). With neutrophil activation (*right side of figure*), the cytosolic complex translocates to the membrane, which may be under the control of the active GTP bound form of Rac, and is further regulated by phosphorylation of p47-*phox*.

protein, gp91-*phox*, and a nonglycosylated 22 kDa subunit, p22-*phox*.[48,51,57–59] The *CYBB* gene for gp91-*phox*, which is the site of mutations in the X-linked form of CGD and located at Xp21.1,[60] was one of the first to be identified by positional cloning.[61] The gene for p22-*phox*, *CYBA*, resides on chromosome 16q24 and is affected in an autosomal recessive form of CGD.[62] The NADPH oxidase cytochrome b_{558} has a very low mid-point potential of −245 mV and, hence, has been referred to as cytochrome b_{-245} and also has a characteristic absorption band at 558 nm when examined spectrophotometrically in its reduced state, accounting for its alternative name of cytochrome b_{558}.[63] Relatively high amounts of cytochrome b_{558} are present in neutrophils, monocytes, eosinophils, and macrophages,[64,65] and low levels are detectable in human glomerular mesangial cells[66] and Epstein–Barr-virus–transformed B lymphocytes.[67]

Based on the redox properties of cytochrome b_{558}, the following pathway has been proposed for the transfer of electrons from NADPH to molecular O_2:

$$\begin{array}{ccccccccc} \text{NADPH} & \longrightarrow & \text{flavin} & \longrightarrow & \text{heme} & \longrightarrow & O_2 & \longrightarrow & O_2^- \\ -330\,\text{mV} & & -256\,\text{mV} & & -245\,\text{mV} & & -160\,\text{mV} & & \end{array}$$

The cytochrome spans the membrane, so that NADPH is oxidized at the cytoplasmic surface and oxygen is reduced to form O_2^- on the outer surface of the plasma membrane (or inner surface of the phagosomal membrane).[48,49,51,68–70]

Current evidence is consistent with a model of cytochrome b_{558} function in which distinct domains within the 570-amino-acid gp91-*phox* subunit provide both the heme components and the flavin-adenine dinucleotide (FAD) binding site. Experimental data indicate that cytochrome b_{558} binds heme and FAD in a molar ratio of 2:1.[71–73] The two heme prosthetic groups have slightly different mid-point potentials[74] and are embedded within the membrane,[75] where they are ligated by histidine residues[76–78] in the gp91-*phox* subunit.[79] The heme groups are likely to reside in the N-terminus of gp91-*phox*, which contains multiple hydrophobic segments that span the membrane multiple times. The flavin and NADPH binding sites also reside in gp91-*phox*. Regions in the hydrophilic C-terminus of gp91-*phox* contain homology with the ferredoxin-$NADH^+$ reductase family of flavoproteins,[72,73,80] and the level of FAD is diminished by half or more in membranes from neutrophils in patients with X-linked CGD.[72,81–84] Several structural models for gp91-*phox* incorporating these features and the sites of N-linked glycosylation have been proposed.[79,85–87] Proteins similar to gp91-*phox*, with homologies in both the putative heme and flavin binding domains, have also been identified in yeast, where they act as a ferric iron reductase involved in transmembrane iron transport,[88] and in plants,[89] where their function is unknown but may be involved in generation of oxidative signals important for signaling pathways and host defense.[90,91]

The role of the p22-*phox* subunit in the superoxide production is less clear. It is also an integral membrane protein and is tightly associated with gp91-*phox*.[71] Heterodimer formation appears to be important for the intracellular stability of each subunit.[92] The p22-*phox* subunit contains 195 residues, and its proline-rich C-terminus includes at least one binding site for an SH3 (*src* homology domain 3) domain in p47-*phox* that is critical for assembly of the oxidase complex.[93–97]

Cytosolic Components. Cytosolic components are also necessary for optimal oxidase activity. Full oxidase activity can be reconstituted in vitro by combining purified cytochrome b_{558} with only three cytosolic proteins: p47-*phox*, p67-*phox*, and a low molecular weight G protein (Rac1 or Rac2).[72,73,98,99] The specific roles of these soluble proteins in enzyme function are currently under investigation.

The p47-*phox* and p67-*phox* subunits appear to normally exist as a complex in the cytoplasm of resting neutrophils[100] with a third protein, p40-*phox*, whose function in the NADPH oxidase is unknown.[101–103] Mutations in the genes encoding either the p47-*phox* or p67-*phox* subunit can result in autosomal recessive forms of CGD. The cDNA for each of these proteins has been cloned, sequenced, and mapped to specific chromosomal locations.[104–108] The gene for p47-*phox*, *NCF1*, is located on chromosome 7q11.23 and encodes a basic, 390-amino-acid polypeptide, whereas the *NCF2* gene encoding p67-*phox*, a basic protein of 526 amino acids, resides on chromosome 1q25.

When neutrophils are stimulated, both p47-*phox* and p67-*phox* translocate from cytosol to the plasma membrane in a fashion that is directly dependent on the concentration of agonist and on the extent of stimulation.[109,110] These proteins apparently dock at the plasma membrane of stimulated cells to form a complex with cytochrome b_{558}.[49,51] It is likely that there are multiple sites of contact between the cytochrome and soluble oxidase subunits.[111–114] These include associations between SH3 domains in p47-*phox* and p67-*phox* and proline-rich target SH3-binding domains in p22-*phox*, p47-*phox*, and p67-*phox*.[94–97] Several other hydrophilic domains in the cytochrome heterodimer may also participate in oxidase assembly based on experiments using peptide inhibitors and phage display library screens.

The factors important in regulating the translocation of p47-*phox* and p67-*phox* for assembly of the active oxidase are incompletely understood. Translocation of p47-*phox* is a prerequisite for the translocation of p67-*phox* because p67-*phox* does not translocate in neutrophils of p47-*phox*–deficient patients, whereas p47-*phox* translocates in neutrophils of p67-*phox*–deficient patients.[115] Oxidase activation is associated with the phosphorylation of both p47-*phox* and p67-*phox*,[47,116–121] which has been postulated to expose SH3 and proline-rich domains that are otherwise inaccessible in resting cells and that control key steps in oxidase assembly.[45,46,97] Pretreatment of neutrophils with staurosporine, which inhibits protein kinase C (PKC), before stimulation with phorbol ester blocks phosphorylation of p47-*phox*, translocation of p47-*phox* to the plasma membrane, and generation of superoxide anion.[110] Phosphorylation of p47-*phox* occurs on multiple serine residues, and those at positions 303 or 304 appear to be particularly important for oxidase activation.[117,122–124] The kinases normally responsible for the phosphorylation of p47-*phox* and p67-*phox* remain to be conclusively identified.

Neither p47-*phox* nor p67-*phox* appears to function in electron transport in the respiratory burst oxidase and more likely serve a regulatory role, perhaps by modulating some aspect of cytochrome b_{558} function at the plasma membrane. Recent studies using cell-free oxidase systems have shown that substantial amounts of superoxide can be generated from neutrophil membranes in the absence of p47-*phox*, provided that high concentrations of p67-*phox* and the small G protein Rac are supplied.[125,126] Hence, it has been postulated that p67-*phox* may participate in the catalytically active complex, whereas p47-*phox* may function as a docking protein to bring p67-*phox* to the membrane.

Several studies have suggested that the active oxidase complex is associated with the cytoskeleton.[110,127] SH3 domains within p47-*phox* and p67-*phox* may also mediate functionally important interactions between these cytosolic NADPH oxidase components and the submembranous cytoskeleton of neutrophils, thereby directing the assembly of the active oxidase at the appropriate site in the plasma membrane.

Investigators at three laboratories have demonstrated that a Ras-related low molecular weight G protein is a third essential cytosolic factor in the oxidase.[98,128,129] GTP is also required for oxidase activity in the cell fraction system,[130,131] which is consistent with findings from previous studies on the augmentation of superoxide production by guanine nucleotides in whole cells that first suggested that a G protein was involved.[132,133] Disagreement exists as to whether Rac1 or Rac2, both of which are 92 percent homologous, is the specific G protein involved in vivo, with sound experimental evidence to support a role for each.[98,128,129] To be active, the G protein must be in the GTP bound form,[129] and posttranslational isoprenoid modification is required for full activity.[134–136] In resting neutrophils, isoprenylated Rac2 is complexed with a GDP dissociation inhibitor (GDI), a novel regulatory protein that interacts with GDP bound forms of Rho proteins[137]; in this way, Rac2 remains cytosolic. With activation, the GTP bound form of Rac2 releases GDI and interacts with the other oxidase components at the plasma membrane. Rac has been shown to bind to the p67-*phox* subunit of the oxidase through an effector domain encompassed within amino acids 30 through 40.[138–140] Translocation of Rac2 is decreased in CGD neutrophils lacking cytochrome b_{558}, suggesting that it also interacts directly with the cytochrome.[141] Full oxidase activity can be reconstituted with recombinant p47-*phox*, recombinant p67-*phox*, and GTP bound recombinant Rac1 or Rac2, a detergent and a source of cytochrome b_{558}.[98,142] Thus, it appears that either Rac1 or Rac2 can support oxidase activity and that processing is important for GDP/GTP nucleotide exchange. Further evidence for the key role of these G proteins in NADPH oxidase function is the finding that the superoxide-generating activity of stimulated Epstein-Barr virus–transformed B lymphocytes is inhibited by introduction of antisense oligonucleotides encoding regions shared by Rac1 and Rac2.[143]

The generation of Rac2-deficient mice by gene targeting has recently shed some light on the relative roles of Rac1 and Rac2 in neutrophil function in vivo.[144] Neutrophils from Rac2−/− mice had multiple defects, with profound abnormalities in chemotaxis and in actin remodeling induced by chemoattractants or ligation of cell surface adhesion receptors. NADPH oxidase activity was also substantially reduced in bone marrow neutrophils isolated from Rac2−/− mice but was near normal in exudate neutrophils and in bone marrow neutrophils stimulated with tumor necrosis factor α. Hence, although Rac2 plays an important role in regulating NADPH oxidase activity in vivo, this function can be partly replaced by Rac1.

Other Putative Factors in the NADPH Oxidase. Although full oxidase activity can be reconstituted by combining recombinant forms of the three cytosolic proteins described above with plasma membranes or lipidated cytochrome b_{558}, other proteins, both cytosolic and membrane associated, may participate in regulating the oxidase in intact cells. The low molecular weight G protein Rap1A is associated with cytochrome b_{558}[145] and shares the same subcellular distribution as the cytochrome.[146,147] The p47-*phox* and p67-*phox* subunits are found in a complex with a 40-kDa protein, p40-*phox*, in the cytoplasm of resting neutrophils, and p40-*phox* translocates to the membrane with neutrophil activation.[101–103] The function of p40-*phox* in NADPH oxidase has not been established.

Activation of the Respiratory Burst. The onset of the respiratory burst requires that appropriate signals be generated to activate the normally dormant NADPH oxidase into an active state capable of catalyzing the conversion of oxygen to O_2^-. A typical time course of the release of O_2^- from neutrophils and monocytes exposed to phorbol myristate acetate or opsonized yeast particles (zymosan) is shown in Fig. 189-2. Superoxide release begins 30 to 60 s after exposure to the stimulus. This delay, or "lag time," is presumably the result of the biochemical steps required to link ligand–receptor interaction with modification of the NADPH oxidase to an active state. A large variety of soluble and particulate stimuli are capable of activating the respiratory burst, including opsonized microorganisms, chemokines, products of arachidonic acid metabolism, and calcium ionophores.[148–150]

The biochemical pathways involved in signal transduction in leukocytes are overlapping and complex.[148–152] A common early downstream event after receptor binding is the activation of membrane phospholipid metabolism to generate two important second messengers, diacylglycerol and inositol 1,4,5-triphosphate,[153,154] which in turn cause release of calcium from intracellular stores and activate PKC. Neutrophil activation is also accompanied by alterations in the phosphorylation status of intracellular proteins, as regulated by PKC,[155] tyrosine kinases,[156,157] and serine and threonine kinases of the mitogen-activated kinase family.[158,159] Guanine nucleotide binding proteins also play important roles in neutrophil signal transduction. These include the heterotrimeric GTP binding proteins that are coupled to the seven transmembrane spanning domain receptors for chemokines and other chemoattractants[160] and the low molecular weight GTPases of the Ras p21 superfamily.[148,150]

The functional oxidase complex is assembled at the plasma membrane and is also incorporated into phagosomes during ingestion. Concomitant with activation, neutrophils degranulate, thereby releasing the granule contents extracellularly (or within the phagosome) and fusing granule membranes with the plasma membrane. Because release of O_2^- occurs largely at the extracellular side of the membrane, oxidants are released at sites of microbial contact or within the phagocytic vacuole,[69,70] where they can interact with granule contents to potentiate their

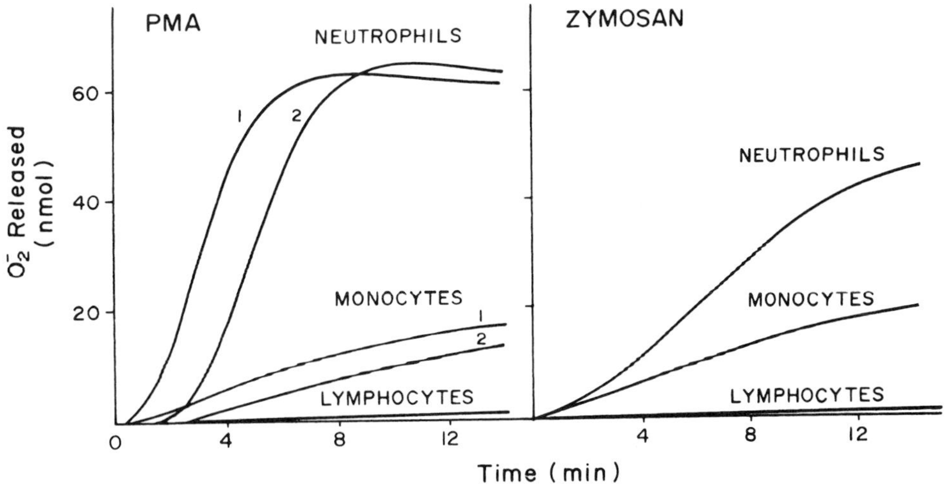

Fig. 189-2 Stimulation of the respiratory burst. Time course of O_2^- generation by 2.5 × 10^6 neutrophils, monocytes, or lymphocytes on contact at 0 min with phorbol myristate acetate (PMA) at concentrations of 67 (*1*) or 33 (*2*) ng/ml (left) or with opsonized zymogen (right). Actual tracings of the recordings by spectrophotometer are represented. Note the typical more vigorous respiratory burst in neutrophils as compared with monocytes. (*Adopted from data of Johnston RB Jr, Lehmeyer JE: The involvement of oxygen metabolites from phagocytic cells in bactericidal activity and inflammation, in Michelson AM, McCord JM, Fridovich I (eds):* Superoxide and Superoxide Dismutases. *New York, Academic, 1977, p 291. Used by permission.*)

microbicidal effects. The membranes of specific granules contain numerous cell surface receptors and cytochrome b_{558}.[161] Thus, degranulation also serves to recruit into the plasma membrane a variety of functionally important molecules, including additional cytochrome b_{558}, presumably to participate in the continued assembly and activation of the oxidase.

Regulation of Expression of NADPH Oxidase. The genes encoding the individual components of the oxidase are separately regulated. Expression of gp91-*phox*, p47-*phox*, and p67-*phox* mRNAs are almost exclusively restricted to differentiated phagocytes, whereas p22-*phox* is more widely expressed.[162,163] For gp91-*phox*, down-regulation of a transcriptional repressor that binds to the promoter CCAAT box appears to be important for increased expression of gp91-*phox* gene during differentiation.[164,165] A region in the gp91-*phox* promotor including nucleotides −53 to −57 upstream of the transcriptional start site influences the binding of the transcription factors hematopoetic-associated factor 1 (HAF-1), PU.1 (a trancription factor), and interferon consensus sequence binding protein.[166–168] Mutations in this region have been associated with an unusual form of CGD[168,169] (see Molecular Basis of CGD below). The myeloid transcription factor PU.1 is also important for up-regulating expression of the p47-*phox* gene.[170]

In cultured human myelomonoblastic cell lines derived from patients with myeloid leukemia, expression of *phox* subunits is low but increases when cells are induced to differentiate into mature neutrophil-like or macrophagelike cells.[104–107,171] The mRNA encoding for gp91-*phox* decreases when primary monocytes become monocyte-derived macrophages in culture.[172] Lipopolysaccharide, an agent known to prime neutrophils for activation,[173,174] up-regulates mRNA for gp91-*phox* but down-modulates that for p47-*phox*.[172] Neutrophils and monocytes cultured in the presence of interferon-γ demonstrate enhanced oxidase activity[175] and concomitantly have up-regulation of mRNA for both gp91-*phox* and p47-*phox*.[172,176,177] Increased expression of neutrophil p47-*phox* has also been observed in vivo in CGD patients receiving interferon-γ prophylaxis.[178] The protein kinase inhibitor staurosporine depresses constitutive and interferon-stimulated levels of mRNA for p47phox and gp91-*phox*, whereas dexamethasone inhibits only mRNA encoding gp91-*phox*,[179] suggesting that the pathways for transcriptional regulation of the various oxidase components are independent.

The issue of cytokine-mediated modulation of gene expression of these factors has special clinical implications because recombinant interferon-γ therapy has been used very effectively for prophylaxis against infection in patients with CGD.[180] Nevertheless, interferon-γ therapy prophylaxis has had no demonstrable effect on the oxidase activity of neutrophils from treated CGD patients.[181]

Antioxidant Mechanisms. Products of the respiratory burst are released into the phagolysosome, where they participate in the destruction of the ingested particle. Figure 189-3 illustrates the biochemical events associated with the respiratory burst and the enzymes required to catalyze the reactions. Because toxic oxygen metabolites can harm other circulating cells and adjacent tissues in addition to the stimulated phagocyte, it is important that the site of action be concentrated in the phagolysosome. Neutrophils possess protective mechanisms to neutralize and rid the cell of oxygen metabolites not consumed in the microbicidal process.

Superoxide dismutase, which is found in the cytoplasm as an enzyme containing copper and zinc and in the mitochondria as a manganoprotein, is the principal scavenger of O_2^-.[182] This enzyme catalyzes the conversion (dismutation) of two O_2^- molecules to H_2O_2 and oxygen. The copper-containing plasma protein ceruloplasmin may also aid in the removal of O_2^- at sites of inflammation.[183]

Several cytoplasmic systems exist to protect phagocytes against the potential oxidative injury of H_2O_2. Glutathione, a tripeptide

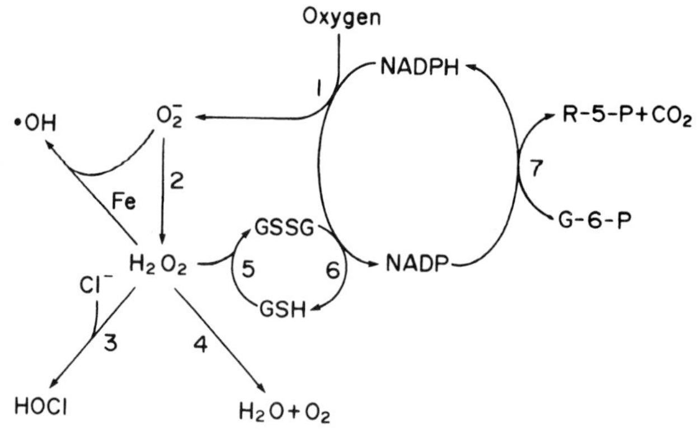

Fig. 189-3 The respiratory burst and associated reactions. Enzymes active in the burst or in protection against its toxic products are indicated by numerals, as follows: 1 = NADPH oxidase; 2 = superoxide dismutase; 3 = myeloperoxidase; 4 = catalase; 5 = glutathione peroxidase; 6 = glutathione reductase; 7 = G-6-PD and 6-phosphogluconate dehydrogenase.

found in all tissues, serves to scavenge H_2O_2 in a reaction catalyzed by glutathione peroxidase.[184] Intracellular glutathione also serves as a source of low molecular weight thiols, which interact with protein sulfhydryl groups in the presence of H_2O_2 to form mixed disulfides.[185] This reversible process, termed *S-thiolation*, may prevent protein denaturation. Catalase enzymatically converts H_2O_2 to H_2O and oxygen.[186,187] Pyruvate, a product of aerobic glycolysis, can increase the survival of cells in tissue culture and has been proposed as an H_2O_2 scavenger.[188]

Other low molecular weight compounds found in cells or plasma can serve as detoxifying agents of harmful oxidants produced by the respiratory burst.[189] Vitamin E (α tocopherol) reacts with toxic oxygen radicals and preserves cell membranes from oxidative damage. Vitamin C (ascorbic acid) combines with oxygen-free radicals to form harmless byproducts and can react with vitamin E radicals to regenerate vitamin E. The nonessential amino acid taurine is a scavenger of hypochlorous acid (HOCl), with the formation of innocuous monochloramine taurine.[184,190]

Myeloperoxidase-Catalyzed System. Since Agner first described myeloperoxidase (MPO) in 1941,[191] numerous investigators have characterized the function and structure of this enzyme,[192–194] located in the azurophilic granules of neutrophils and in the primary lysosomes of monocytes. MPO plays a central role in the phagocyte-dependent innate immune system because stimulated neutrophils generate reactive oxygen species and release granule products, including MPO, into the phagolysosome and extracellular space, thereby creating a milieu cytotoxic to microbes[33,195–197] and tumor cells.[198,199]

MPO shares sequence homology with eosinophil peroxidase, thyroid peroxidase, and lactoperoxidase.[200,201] The sequence homology among these proteins is most striking in the immediate region around the heme.[200–202] Thus, these proteins may be evolutionarily related members of peroxidase superfamily, each with distinctly different physiologic functions as determined by the particular cell type expressing the peroxidase. In addition, homology studies have demonstrated MPO-related proteins in a variety of invertebrates and in specialized functional roles. Peroxinectin, a heme-containing protein in crayfish hemocytes, mediates cell—cell adhesion and exerts peroxidase activity.[203] In squid, an MPO-related peroxidase is expressed only in the symbiotic organ, where it controls the bioactivity of colonizing luminescent bacteria.[204]

Each molecule of mature MPO (140 kDa) is heterotetrameric and is composed of two large α subunits (59 kDa) and two smaller β subunits (13 kDa).[205–210] Native MPO can be cleaved by reductive alkylation into a 78-kDa product with one α and one

β subunit, hemi-MPO, which retains the same specific activity as native MPO.[211] Analytic ultracentrifugation of native and hemi-MPO suggested that the α and β subunits are linked along their long axes,[207] an interpretation confirmed by x-ray crystal structure, which demonstrated this association to be through a disulfide bond between the C319 on each heavy subunit.[202] In addition to the interchain disulfide bonds, there are six intrachain disulfide bonds, five in the heavy subunit and one in the light subunit.

MPO binds calcium ions with high affinity and in an equimolar ratio to iron.[212] Although the functional significance of this property is not understood, it is noteworthy that the calcium-binding loop, a structural feature shared by all four related mammalian peroxidases (MPO, eosinophil peroxidase, thyroid peroxidase, and lactoperoxidase) influences the protein conformation near the heme binding site in MPO.[202] When calcium is chelated from purified MPO, MPO precipitates from solution.[212] There are two iron molecules in each molecule of MPO, with each iron bound to the α subunit. Previous electron spin resonance studies have suggested that the iron in MPO exists linked to a chlorin group and that the chlorin groups are identical.[213–215] However, a number of studies have suggested that the prosthetic group is a formyl substituted porphyrin, akin to that in lactoperxidase, rather than a chlorin.[216–218] The region of heme binding has been difficult to characterize clearly[219] with the techniques of physical chemistry but appears to contain five α helixes and a paucity of β sheets.[202] Analyses of the immediate environment of the heme group indicate that the prosthetic group binds to histidines at codons 261 and 502, the distal and proximal binding sites, respectively. Additional binding through a methionyl sulfonium group at M409 and carboxylates at E260 and E408 completes the interactions between the peptide backbone and the heme group.[220,221]

The presence and significance of different forms of MPO are unsettled issues. Previous studies have suggested there are as many as 10 isozymes,[222–225] but more recent studies have failed to reach a consensus on the presence of isozymic variation.[205,226,227] Using cation exchange chromatography during purification, a number of investigators have identified multiple forms of mature MPO that differ in the size of the α chain,[210,228–231] the susceptibility to inhibition with 3-aminotriazole,[230] or both. Three forms of MPO have been recovered from crystalline MPO[229] and may represent biosynthetic intermediates distributed in different subcellular organelles or artifacts produced during purification.[205,232]

Expression of cDNA for MPO in baby hamster kidney cells[233] and in Sf9 insect cells[234] results in synthesis of immunochemically reactive MPO without enzymatic activity. In contrast, expression of MPO cDNA in Chinese hamster ovary cells produces MPO precursor with spectral and enzymatic properties similar to those of mature, fully processed native MPO.[235,236] A site-directed mutant with His502 mutated to Ala (H502A) loses all enzymatic activity, whereas a mutant at His416 (H416A) is fully active in this system.[237] Crystallographic analysis of mutants derived in this fashion should provide important insights into the structure–function domains in MPO. Application of site-directed mutagenesis to recapitulate specific genotypes has already advanced understanding of the molecular defects in several forms of hereditary MPO deficiency (see Myeloperoxidase Deficiency below).

The most extensively studied functional aspect of the MPO catalyzed system is that involved in antimicrobial activity. Hypochlorous acid and the monochloramines, the long-lived oxidants derived from HOCl, have been best studied in this regard.[38,238–248] The actual mechanisms for the cytocidal activity have not been established, but likely possibilities include destruction of bacterial electron transport,[249] ablation of the bacterial adenine nucleotide pool,[249] oxidation of iron and sulfur centers critical for bacterial viability,[250,251] and modification of sites for bacterial DNA replication.[252] However, recent studies have characterized additional biochemical properties of MPO that may have important biological functions. The MPO-dependent system has been implicated in tyrosyl radical production[253–255] and chlorination,[256] tyrosine nitration,[257] tyrosine peroxide generation,[258] oxidation of lipoproteins,[259–261] or apolipoprotein E,[262] and reactions with peroxynitrite[263] and other nitric oxide (NO)–derived oxidants.[264] Based on this biochemistry, investigators have implicated MPO in a wide range of clinical settings, including atherosclerosis,[265,266] tumorigenesis,[267–271] and degenerative diseases of the nervous system such as multiple sclerosis.[262,272]

Taken together, these data strongly suggest that MPO participates in proinflammatory events that extend beyond those involved in host defense against infection.

Nitric Oxide (NO). The production of NO from the oxidation of L-arginine to L-citrulline is another oxygen-dependent pathway that may be importance for human host defense. This reaction is catalyzed by nitric oxide synthase (NOS), with molecular oxygen supplying the oxygen in NO.[273–275] There are three different NOSs, each encoded by a different gene. Two are constitutively expressed in a variety of tissues, including endothelium, brain, and neutrophils. Expressin of a third form, known as inducible nitric oxide synthase (NOS2, formely iNOS), can be induced by inflammatory stimuli in a variety of cells, including macrophages and neutrophils, where it has a wide spectrum of antimicrobial activity against bacteria, parasites, helminths, and viruses.[273,275,276] Mice with genetic absence of NOS2, generated by targeted disruption of the NOS2 gene in murine embryonic stem cells, have increased susceptibility to infection with *Listeria monocytogenes*.[277] High levels of NOS2 catalyzed NO production are easily elicited in wild-type mouse macrophages by exposure, for example, to endotoxin or interferon-γ. However, it has been difficult to consistently document a similar phenomenon in human macrophages, thus casting doubt on a role for the inducible production of NO in human host defense. However, expression of NOS2 in human macrophages has been elicited with either the crosslinking of CD69, a member of the natural killer cell family of signal transducing receptors,[278] or in activated maacrophages infected by human immunodeficiency virus.[279]

INHERITED DISORDERS OF PHAGOCYTIC KILLING

Chronic Granulomatous Disease

Definition and History. CGD is a heterogeneous group of genetic disorders characterized by recurrent, often severe bacterial and fungal infections most often involving the skin, soft tissues, respiratory tract, lymph nodes, liver, and spleen.[49,51,280] Infectious episodes can be fatal,[281] and therapy generally requires weeks to months of parenteral antibiotics to clear persistent infections.[282] Phagocytes from individuals with CGD can ingest organisms normally but do not undergo a phagocytosis-associated respiratory burst, which is necessary for microbial killing. This defect has been demonstrated in neutrophils,[283,284] monocytes,[285,286] and eosinophils.[287] The inheritance of CGD can be either X linked or autosomal recessive.[48–52]

CGD was probably first noted but not recognized as a distinct syndrome by Janeway in 1954.[288] The first specific identifications of the disease were reported clinically by Good et al.[289,290] and pathologically by Landing and Shirkey[291] in 1957. The clinical papers described four boys with suppurative lymphadenitis, hepatosplenomegaly, pulmonary infiltrates, and eczematoid dermatitis, with findings of granulomas in biopsy and autopsy specimens. The pathology report described the infiltration of viscera by pigmented lipid-laden histiocytes on autopsy of two boys with histories of recurrent, severe infections. The pathogenesis remained in question until the bactericidal and metabolic defects of CGD patients' neutrophils were discovered a decade later.[41,42,283,292] The metabolic defects were accompanied by a failure of affected cells to reduce the redox dye nitroblue

Table 189-3 Infections in Chronic Granulomatous Disease

Infections	Infections (%)†	Infecting Organisms	Isolates (%)
Pneumonia	70–80	*Staphylococcus aureus*	30–50
Lymphadenitis*	60–80	*Aspergillus* species	10–20
Cutaneous infections/impetigo*	60–70	*Escherichia coli*	5–10
Hepatic/perihepatic abscesses*	30–40	*Klebsiella* species	5–10
Osteomyelitis	20–30	*Salmonella* species	5–10
Perirectal abscesses/fistulae*	15–30	*Burkholderia (Pseudomonas) cepacia* and *P.aeruginosa*	5–10
Septicemia	10–20	*Serratia marcescens*	5–10
Otitis media*	≈20	*Staphylococcus epidermidis*	5
Conjunctivitis	≈15	*Streptococcus* species	4
Enteric infections	≈10	*Enterobacter* species	3
Urinary tract infections/pyelonephritis	5–15	*Proteus* species	3
Sinusitis	<10	*Candida albicans*	3
Renal/perinephric abscesses	<10	*Nocardia* species	2
Brain abscesses	<5	*Haemophilus influenzae*	1
Pericarditis	<5	*Pneumocystis carinii*	<1
Meningitis	<5	*Mycobacterium fortuitum*	<1
		Chromobacterium violaceum	<1
		Francisella philomiragia	<1
		Torulopsis glabrata	<1

*Those infections seen most frequently at the time of presentation.
†The relative frequencies of different types of infections in CGD are estimated from data pooled from several large series of patients in the United States, Europe, and Japan. See text for references. These series encompass approximately 550 patients with CGD after accounting for overlap between reports. The list of infecting organisms is also arranged according to the data in these reports and is not paired with the entries in the first column.
SOURCE: From Dinauer.[280] Used by permission.

tetrazolium (NBT), which led to the widespread, and still standard, use of phagocyte NBT reduction tests for the diagnosis of CGD and its X-linked carrier state.[293–296] In 1974–1975, the biochemical basis for abnormal respiratory burst activity and microbial killing in CGD granulocytes was identified as a defect in superoxide generation[284] due to a decrease in phagocyte NADPH oxidase activity.[297–299]

All of the initially reported cases were male,[288,289,291] suggesting an X-linked pattern of inheritance that was confirmed by NBT testing of carrier mothers.[293] However, in 1968, additional papers described CGD in females, noted the lack of abnormalities in parents, and proposed an additional, autosomal recessive mode of inheritance.[293,300] The inheritance of CGD by both X-linked and autosomal recessive patterns derives from the different chromosomal locations of the genes encoding the NADPH oxidase components (see Fig. 189-1 and the Molecular Basis of CGD below). Because the phagocyte cytochrome b_{558} is a heterodimer produced from genes on the X chromosome and chromosome 16, it is absent or inactive in phagocytes from patients with the common, X-linked form and from those with one of the three rarer, autosomal recessive forms of CGD.[49,51,301,302] In the other autosomal recessive forms of CGD, due to defects in cytosolic components of the oxidase,[303–305] phagocytes contain normal amounts of cytochrome b_{558} (see Table 189-5).

Clinical Presentation. CGD should be considered in any individual with recurrent purulent infections caused by catalase-positive bacteria or fungi or with an initial infection by unusual or opportunistic pathogens such as *Burkholderia cepacia* (formerly classified in the *Pseudomonas* genus), *Serratia marcescens*, or *Aspergillus* species.[280,306,307] The hallmark granulomata, sometimes with pigmented histiocytes,[291] may be apparent on biopsy; but nonspecific inflammatory infiltrates are more common early in the course of an infection.

Most, but not all, patients present early in the first decade of life with recurrent acute infections of the types listed in Table 189-3, alone or in combination with one or more of the chronic conditions listed in Table 189-4. There is no "typical presentation," so clinicians need to keep in mind the possibility of CGD underlying any recurrence, persistence, or combination of conditions and infecting organisms listed in these tables. Some patients with autosomal recessive forms of CGD may manifest less severe symptoms,[308] and others with "variant" forms of CGD—due to partial, rather than complete, defects in oxidase activity—may not present until later ages, even well into adulthood.[309–311]

Any organ system can be affected. Cutaneous and mucous membrane surfaces are normally colonized with bacteria and fungi, making these structures and their underlying tissues primary

Table 189-4 Chronic Conditions Associated With Chronic Granulomatous Disease

Condition	Cases (%)
Lymphadenopathy	98
Hypergammaglobulinemia	60–90
Hepatomegaly	50–90
Splenomegaly	60–80
Anemia of chronic disease	Common
Underweight	70
Chronic diarrhea	20–60
Short stature	50
Gingivitis	50
Dermatitis	35
Hydronephrosis	10–25
Ulcerative stomatitis	5–15
Pulmonary fibrosis	<10
Esophagitis	<10
Gastric antral narrowing	<10
Granulomatous ileocolitis	<10
Granulomatous cystitis	<10
Chorioretinitis	<10
Glomerulonephritis	<10
Discoid lupus erythematosus	<10

SOURCE: Dinauer.[280] Used with permission.

targets of microbial invasion. Thus, pneumonia, dermatitis, and perirectal abscess are common forms of infection; and lymphadenitis and hepatic abscesses probably represent extension by regional drainage from the skin, mucous membranes, and gastrointestinal tract. Sepsis is relatively uncommon, except as a terminal event, because the abundant, avidly phagocytic leukocytes rapidly clear circulating microbes to the reticulo-endothelial system.

Staphylococcus aureus and enteric gram negative bacilli cause the majority of infections, but uncommon or opportunistic organisms are also important pathogens for CGD patients (Table 189-3), even at initial presentation or before the use of antibiotics. Gram-negative microbes include not only common pathogens such as *Escherichia coli* and *Klebsiell* species but also *Salmonella* species, *Pseudomonas* species, *S. marcescens*, and *B. cepacia*. The last of these organisms can produce rapidly fatal pneumonia and sepsis; it is highly specific for CGD (or cystic fibrosis) and generally resistant to conventional empirical antibiotics.[306,307] Microbial virulence in CGD correlates in part with the organisms' resistance to nonoxidative killing mechanisms, such as the antibiotic peptides of neutrophil granules.[8] However, CGD patients show no increase in susceptibility to infection by catalase negative organisms such as *Streptococcus pneumoniae* and α-hemolytic *Streptococci*, probably because these bacteria release sufficient amounts of peroxide to provide CGD phagocytes with the weapon for their destruction.[312]

Recurrent or chronic skin and subcutaneous infections occur quite commonly and include eczematoid or pyogenic dermatitis, furunculosis, and abscesses.[313,314] Dermatologic findings can be prominent in adults with otherwise mild disease.[315] Discoid lupus has been recognized in patients with autosomal recessive CGD[316–318] and in carriers of X-linked CGD (see below, this section).[319–321]

Infections of the lower respiratory tract are the most common form of invasive infection in patients with CGD. Organisms responsible for pulmonary infections include *S. aureus*, enteric bacteria, and *Aspergillus* species. The pattern of pneumonia may be lobar, bronchial, or diffuse and generalized (Fig. 189-4) and may be accompanied by consolidation and hilar lymphadenopathy.[322–324] Although most cases of pneumonia are treated empirically with prolonged courses of antibiotics, biopsy and, occasionally, resection of infected tissue may be necessary for infections that are unresponsive or that have a high likelihood of fungal etiology.[325] In particular, pulmonary infections with *Aspergillus* species tend to invade adjacent bone or soft tissues of the chest wall.[322,326–328] Repeated infections may lead to chronic lung disease, with granulomatous infiltration of the lung and pulmonary fibrosis in adult or pediatric patients.[309,322]

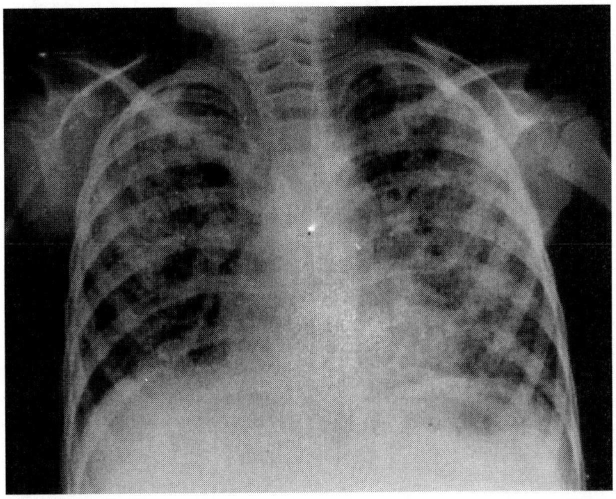

Fig. 189-4 Lower respiratory tract involvement in a boy with CGD. The chest x-ray film shows a diffuse reticulonodular interstital pattern with superimposed alveolar densities in the left midlung field.

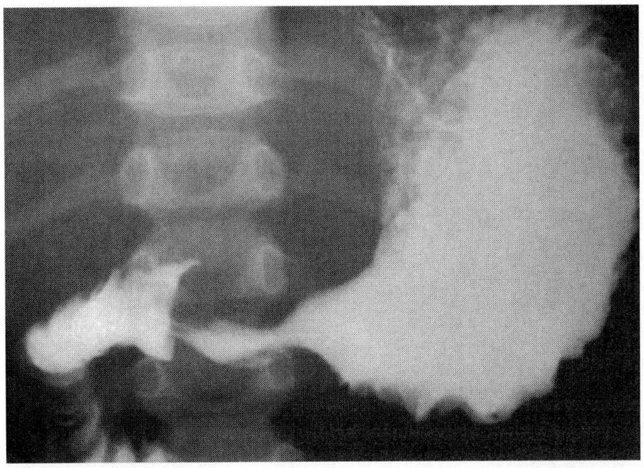

Fig. 189-5 Gastrointestinal involvement in CGD. A 5-year-old boy with X-linked CGD experienced the gradual onset of recurrent vomiting and weight loss. An upper gastrointestinal series showed annular narrowing of the antral lumen, nodular irregularities of the distal greater curvature of the stomach, and delayed gastric emptying.

The oropharynx and gastrointestinal tract[329] are frequent sites of infectious complications. Ulcerative stomatitis and gingivitis can be chronic, and esophagitis may result in strictures and regurgitation.[313,330–333] Involvement of the lower gastrointestinal tract may mimic pyloric stenosis,[334] eosinophilic gastroenteritis,[329] gastrointestinal dysmotility,[335] inflammatory bowel disease,[336] or peritonitis.[337] Granulomatous inflammation of the stomach can lead to a characteristic luminal narrowing of the gastric antrum, as shown in Fig. 189-5, that presents with persistent vomiting.[334,338–340] Similar lesions in the small or large bowel may result in diarrhea, malabsorption, or frank obstruction and may require surgical intervention.[329,341,342] Rectal abscesses, perianal abscesses, and fistulas are common and often extremely persistent.[329] Liver involvement may progress to abscess formation, most commonly with *S. aureus*, and may require surgical drainage.[313] The occurrence of a liver abscess, otherwise rare in children, should suggest the underlying diagnosis of CGD.[322]

Osteomyelitis in CGD patients has been reported to occur, with predilection for the metacarpals, metatarsals, spine, and ribs:[313,328,343–345] *S. aureus*, *S. marcescens*, and *Nocardia* species are the most commonly isolated organisms from primary bone infections. Skeletal involvement may also develop by direct extension of prior infection in lymph nodes, lung, or the gastrointestinal tract, with organisms more likely to include *Aspergillus*, other fungi, or mycobacteria.[328]

Urinary tract involvement has been reported in 7 to 48 percent of patients in three published series.[313,346,347] Cystitis or obstructive uropathy may result from granulomatous involvement of the bladder wall (Fig. 189-6).[338,343,348–350] Urinary tract infections and glomerulonephritis,[347,351,352] renal abscesses,[353] and granulomatous inflammation of the kidney parenchyma have also been reported.[354] Gonadal involvement has been noted with tubo-ovarian abscesses in girls and testicular granulomas reported in a boy.[322]

Disseminated infection, with bacteremia or meningitis (or both), has been reported in 17 percent of 168 early cases, often as a terminal event.[313,355] *Salmonella* species were the most commonly isolated organism,[356] but *B. cepacia* has now been recognized as another important agent of sepsis, usually in the context of severe pneumonia.[306,307] Other rare complications include destructive chorioretinitis,[357] conjunctivitis,[313] thyroiditis,[358] pericarditis,[313] brain abscess,[313] and granulomatous involvement of the brain or spinal cord.[322,359]

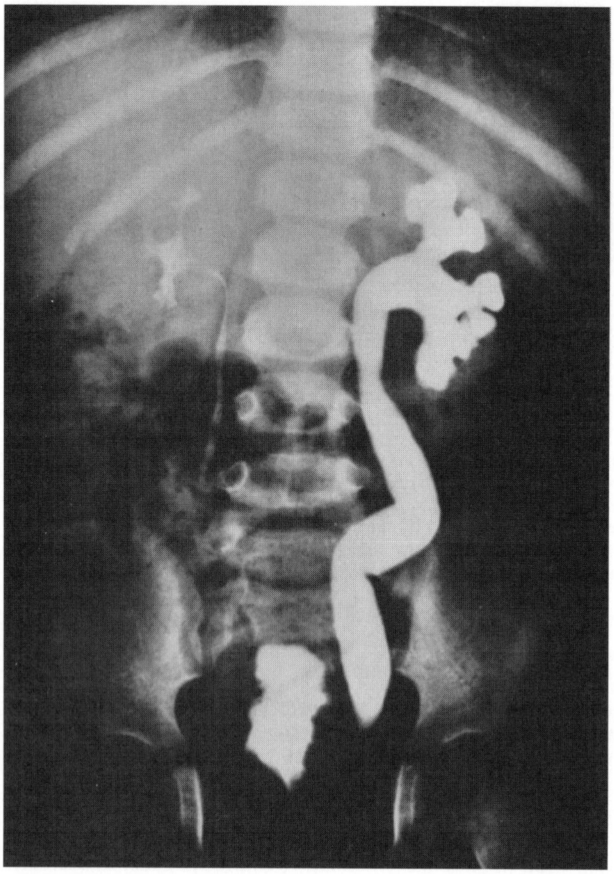

Fig. 189-6 Obstructive uropathy in a patient with CGD. IV pyelogram of a boy with X-linked CGD demonstrating hydronephrosis and hydroureter on the left side. The obstruction was due to compression by a large inflammatory mass in the pelvis between the rectum and the bladder.

Chronic conditions, listed in Table 189-4, are responsible for much of the long-term morbidity of CGD. Most represent nonspecific consequences of chronic infection Others result from the accumulation of granulomas, which can obstruct tubular structures, such as the gastric antrum or ureter, particularly in older patients.

CGD was first described as "fatal granulomatous disease of childhood,"[289] and in the 1970s, surveys of children with CGD reported that one-half to three-fourths of patients had died before 7 years of age.[42,313] Modern treatment modalities (see CGD Treatment below) have greatly reduced, but not eliminated, deaths from infectious complications. More recent reviews of CGD mortality have found that most deaths occurred in the first two decades of life, with actuarial survival of approximately 50 percent at age 20 years.[281,360] Although there were few deaths among survivors reaching their twenties and thirties, the numbers of such patients were small and the duration of follow-up relatively short. The prognosis, with the further refinements in the management of infectious complications coupled with antibiotic and interferon-γ prophylaxis (see CGD Treatment below), is likely to even to be further improved, with survival well into the adult years expected for a majority of patients. Patients with defects in cytosolic oxidase components have often been noted to have a milder disease course than those with cytochrome-negative CGD.[308,361,362]

Most carriers of X-linked CGD are not unduly susceptible to infection because random inactivation of each X chromosome, one containing the normal and the other the CGD allele, produces populations, usually about equal in proportion, of abnormal and normal phagocytes. However, the development of a disease phenotype due to a bias in the X inactivation in CGD carriers has been reported after inactivation with fewer than 10 percent normal granulocytes[363–367] and, indeed, one of the first reported female patients with "autosomal" CGD turned out to have X-linked disease due to complete bias of inactivation of the normal X chromosome in her granulocytes.[368,369] The more usual carrier state can be associated with discoid lupus erythematosus, photosensitivity, or aphthous stomatitis.[316–321] Infiltrative and plaquelike lesions involving the face and distal extremities occur in carriers of X-linked CGD with discoid lupus; but in one series of 14 such patients, none had serologic or clinical evidence of systemic lupus erythematosus.[316–321]

Pathologic Findings. The infectious complications of CGD result in characteristic tissue abnormalities. Specimens from acutely infected sites show a suppurative, sometimes necrotic, inflammatory process. In more prolonged infections, the retention of organisms that are ingested but not killed by CGD phagocytes leads to their accumulation in the lung and reticuloendothelial system, where they are enclosed within characteristic noncaseating granulomata[291,323,370] with multinucleated giant cells, macrophages, lymphocytes, and plasma cells (Fig. 189-7). When organisms are released from a necrotic phagocyte, they are ingested by another. This process recruits additional phagocytes, with the eventual formation of large granulomatous masses. Pigmented lipid-laden macrophages are also commonly seen.[291] The lipid material is yellow or tan in color on specimens stained with hematoxylin and eosin and may result from incomplete degradation of ingested material.[371] The original eliciting organisms may be undetectable on standard or even special stains (e.g., silver stains for fungi) and difficult to culture from biopsy material.

Diagnosis. CGD should be suspected in any individual, whatever the age, with recurrent purulent infections or with any invasive infection involving *B. cepacia*, *S. marcescens*, or opportunistic pathogens such as *Aspergillus* or *Nocardia*. The histochemical NBT test remains the most common and reliable screening test for CGD (Fig. 189-8).[372,373] A positive (i.e., normal) NBT test occurs when yellow, soluble NBT dye is reduced by superoxide to blue, insoluble formazan particles. The assay conditions should be adjusted so that close to 100 percent of the normal control neutrophils reduce the NBT[374,375] to ensure identification of carriers of X-linked CGD and of patients with "variant" CGD (e.g., $X91^-$ subtype; see Molecular Basis of CGD below). Cells from such patients often show homogeneous but faint blue staining; so it is important to read the histochemical test not only by the proportion of "positive" cells but also by the amount of NBT reduction by each cell. Flow cytometric assays of oxidase activity, such as dihydrorhodamine or dichlorofluorescein fluorescence,[376,377] provide both quantitative measurements of peroxide generation and the cell-by-cell distribution of activity.

Other diagnostic tests for CGD include more quantitative measurements of respiratory burst activity, such as measurement of superoxide generation,[284,378] chemiluminescence,[35] oxygen consumption,[379] or hydrogen peroxide production.[380] These methods use pooled cell populations, so they are not appropriate for X-linked CGD carrier detection. Other tests of phagocytic function, such as particle ingestion, are normal or increased.[295,381]

Prenatal diagnosis can be performed with the NBT test by using fetal blood obtained by percutaneous umbilical or placental vessel puncture.[294,382,383] In experienced hands, this procedure can be accomplished safely at 17 to 19 weeks of gestation.[384,385] The prenatal diagnosis of X-linked or autosomal recessive CGD can also be performed in informative kindreds by linkage analysis of DNA samples from chorionic villi or amniocytes.[386–390] These tests offer the advantage of an earlier diagnosis (week 10 of gestation)[391] and no requirement for fetal blood sampling, but many families are not informative at the limited number of polymorphic loci available. Genetic diagnosis from prenatal DNA samples may also be performed by polymerase chain reaction

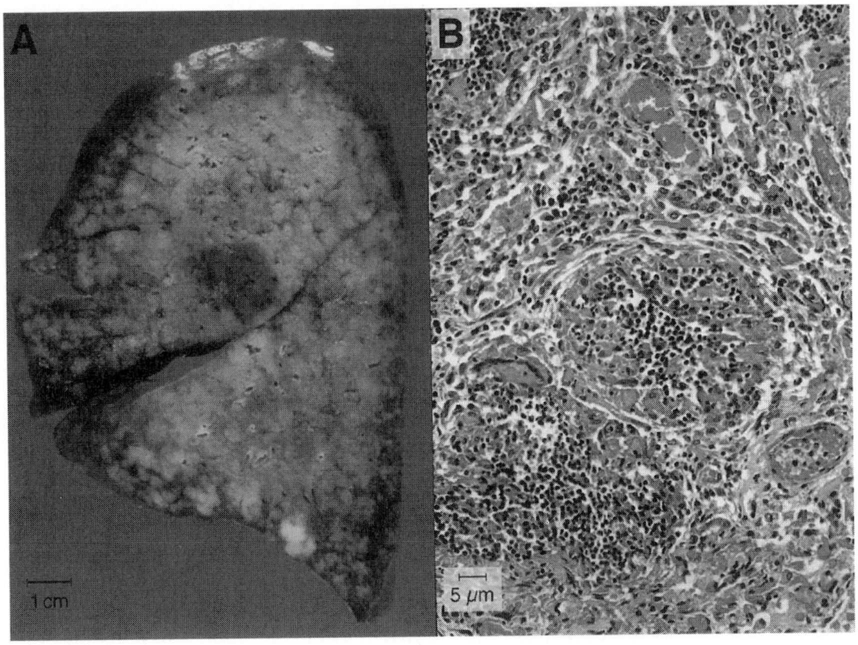

Fig. 189-7 Lung pathology in CGD with *Aspergillus* pneumonia. The patient was a 23-month-old boy with CGD, who died of respiratory failure due to extensive, invasive lung infection with *Aspergillus fumigatus*. *A*. Cut surface of whole lung shows congested, dark purple parenchyma with multiple, bilateral whitish nodules, averaging 0.2 cm in diameter. *B*. Microscopic section of a granuloma, composed of epithelioid histiocytes and giant cells, with a central microabscess. Silver stain (not shown) identified *Aspergillus* hyphae in the central region. The granulomata have obliterated all air spaces. *(Courtesy of Dr. Armando Fraire.)*

detection of the specific CGD mutation in the responsible gene.[387] This method should be applicable to virtually all kindreds because the mutation can generally be identified,[87] even in the absence of material from an affected individual, if sufficient time is available for extensive laboratory analysis.

Other Laboratory Findings. Apart from studies of phagocyte function, laboratory findings reflect the presence of a chronic inflammatory disorder. During infections, a neutrophilic leukocytosis is frequent and may be associated with an elevated erythrocyte sedimentation rate. Anemia appears to be secondary to chronic infections, sometimes with an additional contribution from malabsorption; resolution usually occurs during disease-free intervals, and patients may benefit from iron therapy.[313,338] Polyclonal hypergammaglobulinemia is often present, with elevated serum concentrations of immunoglobulins G, M, and A.[43,288] Other tests of immune function are normal, with the rare exception of abnormal lymphocyte transformation or chemotaxis[392,393] also probably due to chronic infection.

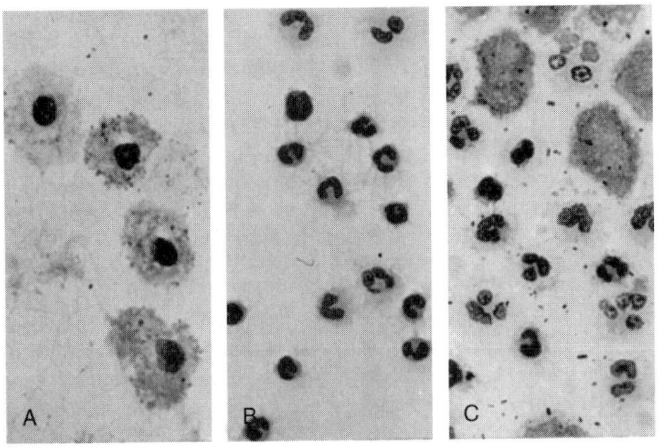

Fig. 189-8 NBT slide test for the diagnosis of CGD. A drop of blood is placed on an endotoxin-coated coverslip and incubated to allow the granulocytes and monocytes to adhere to the glass surface. The coverslip is then incubated with a solution of serum, PMA, and NBT dye and then washed, fixed, counterstained, and mounted. *A*. Normal control; all the granulocytes are NBT-positive and appear as large, degenerated cells with pale-blue cytoplasm. *B*. CGD patient; none of the granulocytes are NBT-positive. The neutrophils retain their typical morphologic appearance and contain no blue (reduced) dye. *C*. Carrier of CGD. Two populations of cells coexist. Some granulocytes are NBT-positive and others are NBT-negative.

Treatment. In the infection-free patient, treatment is aimed at preventing the onset of an infectious process. Successful prophylaxis with trimethoprim/sulfamethoxazole (TMP-SMX), has been reported in several series.[338,360,394] In a retrospective study of 18 patients, treatment with TMP-SMX, 5 mg/kg per day led to increased infection-free periods (3.7 months before therapy, 10.7 months during therapy), primarily by eliminating *S. aureus* infections.[338] The improvement of patients on TMP-SMX may be the result of the cell's ability to concentrate the agents in the phagocytic vacuole.[395–397] Twenty patients with autosomal CGD and 16 with X-linked disease followed at the National Institutes of Health since the 1970s experienced a 2.9-fold ($p < 0.01$) and 2.3-fold ($p = 0.06$) decrease, respectively, in nonfungal infections while being treated with TMP-SMX.[394] There were also less frequent infections with fungal organisms. A retrospective multicenter experience with 34 CGD patients showed similar results, with the average annual incidence of infection per patient improving from 2.06 to 0.43.[360] Patients hypersensitive to TMP-SMX can be treated alternatively with a systemic penicillinase-resistant penicillin.[398] Oral itraconazole may be useful in prophylaxis of *Aspergillus*. One prospective study of 30 patients found an incidence of 3.4 pulmonary *Aspergillus* infections compared with 11.5 in a historical control group not receiving any prophylaxis.[399] Ketoconazole has not been shown to be useful in this setting.[400]

Interferon-γ is a known immunomodulator of respiratory burst activity in normal phagocytic cells.[401,402] In early studies, phagocytes from seven patients with different genetic forms of CGD who had been given interferon-γ by injection exhibited an enhanced respiratory burst and improved killing of *S. aureus*.[176,403,404] Some patients' phagocytes also had a detectable up-regulation of mRNA for the gp91-*phox* subunit of cytochrome b_{558}.[403,404] Based on these observations, a larger multicenter, randomized, double-blind placebo-controlled study of 128 patients was undertaken to test the effectiveness of subcutaneous administration of interferon-γ to control infectious complications common to CGD.[180] Seventy-seven percent of patients receiving interferon-γ, 1.5 μg/kg (body surface area < 0.5 m^2) or 50 μg/m^2 (body surface area $\geq$ 0.5 m^2), by subcutaneous injection three times weekly remained free of serious infection after 12 months of therapy as compared with only 30 percent of those receiving placebo. These beneficial effects were independent of age, mode of inheritance, and concomitant use of prophylactic antibiotics, although patients younger than 10 years had the most pronounced reduction in infectious complications. Side effects were limited to headache, fever and chills, and redness at the injection site. Unlike the preliminary investigations, the reported clinical benefit from interferon-γ was not accompanied by a measurable improvement in phagocytic respiratory burst activity in a majority of patients.[180,181,405] The improvement in the killing of *S. aureus* and *Aspergillus fumigatus* in vitro[406,407] may reflect an alteration in myeloperoxidase-dependent and/or nonoxidative antimicrobial activity.

Granulocyte transfusions have been administered to patients with serious systemic infections, including pneumonia, liver abscesses, and an intramural ileal abscess, all apparently refractory to prolonged administration of parenteral antibiotics.[408–414] Transfusions usually were given as daily infusions of approximately 10^{10} to 10^{11} granulocytes, and recipients tolerated up to 8 weeks of granulocyte therapy without untoward reactions. Careful separation of contaminating red blood cells from donor granulocytes can increase the likelihood of a successful transfusion when compatible blood is not available.[415] The efficacy of granulocyte transfusions is still in question, because the majority of patients were also receiving parenteral antibiotics or were recovering from surgical intervention, and the studies were not controlled.

Patients with CGD and the K_0, or McLeod, phenotypes (see "Mutations in the *CYBB* Gene Encoding gp91-*phox*" below) are susceptible to sensitization by Kell antigens when given blood.[416] One patient with the McLeod phenotype experienced a hemolytic reaction after the sixth leukocyte transfusion.[417]

In most cases, prolonged antibiotic therapy clears the obstruction created by inflammatory granulomatous lesions of the gastrointestinal or genitourinary tract. In patients with protracted severe narrowing of the gastric antrum, esophagus, and urinary tract, corticosteroids in conjunction with antibiotics and nasogastric or intravenous nutritional supplementation can reverse the obstruction.[418–420] The response to corticosteroids can be prompt, but relapse is common. Two patients with progressive respiratory insufficiency responded favorably to corticosteroid therapy.[421]

Allogeneic bone marrow transplantation can be used to treat CGD and has been successfully employed in a number of cases.[422–429] However, because of the risks associated with this procedure and difficulties often encountered in finding a suitable donor, marrow transplantation in the management of CGD is not routine and generally is considered only for those individuals who have frequent and severe infections despite aggressive medical management.

Because CGD results from single gene defects in proteins expressed in myeloid cells, this disorder has been considered a candidate disease for gene therapy targeted at hematopoietic stem cells.[430–432] Female carriers of X-linked CGD can have few or no symptoms even with as little as 5 to 10 percent oxidase-positive neutrophils,[364,365,433,434] which suggests that long-term correction of only a minority of phagocytes could provide substantial clinical benefit. A variety of studies have reported the use of retroviral vectors for transfer of a functional copy of the affected gene in CGD myeloid cell lines and primary hematopoietic cells in vitro.[435–440] At least for the X-linked gene product, gp91-*phox*, it appears that expression of even modest amounts of recombinant protein can lead to considerable reconstitution of superoxide-generating capacity.[437,441] Recently, mouse models for both the X-linked (gp91-*phox*-defecient males) and p47-*phox*-deficient (homozygotes) forms of CGD have been developed by using gene targeting technology.[442,443] Retroviral-mediated gene transfer of the corresponding cDNA into bone marrow cells corrected the neutrophil respiratory burst in vivo and improved the defect in host defense against bacterial and fungal pathogens.[433,437]

A phase 1 clinical trial for gene therapy of p47-*phox*–deficient CGD has been conducted, in which autologous peripheral blood CD34$^+$ cells collected by apheresis were transduced with a p47-*phox*—containing retroviral vector and then reinfused.[444] Peripheral blood neutrophils with respiratory burst oxidase activity were seen for up to 3 to 6 months in all five patients studied, although their frequency was only 0.02 to 0.005 percent of neutrophils. This low percentage most likely reflects the relative inefficiency of current methods for retroviral-mediated gene transfer into human hematopoietic cells capable of engraftment and the fact that patients received no myeloablative conditioning before infusion of transduced cells. However, ongoing research in human hematopoietic stem cell biology, alternative vector systems, and selection strategies for retrovirus-transduced cells is likely to make gene therapy a future option for treatment of CGD and other inherited blood disorders.

Molecular Basis of CGD. The identification of the multiple gene products that form the NADPH oxidase complex has provided the molecular explanation for the genetic heterogeneity of CGD. To date, defects in four of the oxidase components (gp91-*phox*, p22-*phox*, p47-*phox*, and p67-*phox*) have been identified in patients analyzed at the biochemical or molecular level. Deficiencies resulting in a CGD phenotype have not been reported in other components such as p40-*phox*, Rap1A, Rac1, Rac2, or GDI. Based on these findings, the current classification scheme for CGD subdivides the disease according to the specific gene defect (Table 189-5). Additional subtypes within each major group describe the mode of inheritance (abbreviated as A for autosomal or X for X linked), the oxidase component by molecular weight (91, 22, 47, or 67), and the level of that component's protein expression (indicated by a superscripted 0 for absent, + for present, and − for reduced). Thus, the X91^0 CGD subtype refers to the most common form of CGD, derived from defects in the X-linked gene encoding the phagocyte oxidase gp91-*phox* and resulting in undetectable cytochrome b_{558} content and oxidase activity. The less common X91$^-$ subtype is a "variant" form of CGD, usually characterized by a uniform population of neutrophils that exhibit a low level of oxidase activity roughly proportional to the level of cytochrome b_{558} expressed.[50,87,445,446] In X91$^+$ CGD, cytochrome b_{558} is present at normal levels but has either a greatly diminished or absent activity. Most autosomal recessive forms of CGD show no residual expression of the affected component (i.e., subtypes A22^0, A47^0, and A67^0), but occasional autosomal CGD variants have been reported.[447] The molecular basis for these "classic" and "variant" forms of CGD is discussed below.

In two large series of CGD patients, X-linked defects in *CYBB* (the gene encoding gp91-*phox*) account for approximately 65 percent of the cases[52,448] (Table 189-5). Autosomal recessive inheritance is observed in approximately 35 percent of CGD kindreds and most commonly derives from mutations in the gene encoding p47-*phox*. Mutations in the genes for the p22-*phox* and p67-*phox* components each account for approximately 6 percent of the total number of CGD cases.

***Mutations in the* CYBB *Gene Encoding gp91-*phox.** The *CYBB* gene, which encodes the large glycosylated subunit of cytochrome b_{558}, contains 13 exons and spans approximately 30 kb in the Xp21.1 region of the X chromosome.[61,165] Diverse molecular defects producing X-linked CGD have been identified within the coding region, introns, and (rarely) 5′ regulatory region of the *CYBB* gene.[50,75,87,168,169,310,367,369,449–460] A large collection of mutations, identified by an international group of investigators, has recently been compiled by Roos et al. into a computerized database, X-CGDbase,[461] that is accessible through the World

Table 189-5 Classification of Chronic Granulomatous Disease

Component Affected	Gene Symbol	MIM	Chromosome	Inheritance	Subtype Designation*	NBT Score (%Positive)	O_2^- Production (%Normal)	Cytochrome *b* Spectrum (%Normal)	Defect in Cell-Free System	Frequency (% of Cases)†	GenBank
gp91-*phox*	*CYBB*	306400	Xp21.1	XL	$X91^0$	0	0	0	Membrane	56	X04011
					$X91^-$	80–100 (weak)	3–30	3–30	Membrane	5	
					$X91^-$	5–10	5–10	5–10	Membrane	2	
					$X91^-$	0	0	100	Membrane	2	
p22-*phox*	*CYBA*	233690	16p24	AR	$A22^0$	0	0	0	Membrane	6	M21186
					$A22^-$	0	0	100	Membrane	1	
p47-*phox*	*NCFI*	233700	7q11.23	AR	$A47^0$	0	0–1	100	Cytosol	23	M55067
p67-*phox*	*NCF2*	233710	1q25	AR	$A67^0$	0	0–1	100	Cytosol	6	U00776

XL = X-linked inheritance, AR = autosomal recessive inheritance.

*In this nomenclature, the first letter represents the mode of inheritance [X-linked (x) or autosomal recessive (A)] and the number indicates the *phox* component that is genetically affected. The superscript symbols indicate whether the level of protein of the affected component is undetectable (^{0}), diminished($^-$), or normal ($^-$) as measured by immunoblot analysis.

†Represents data from 121 families.[52,448]

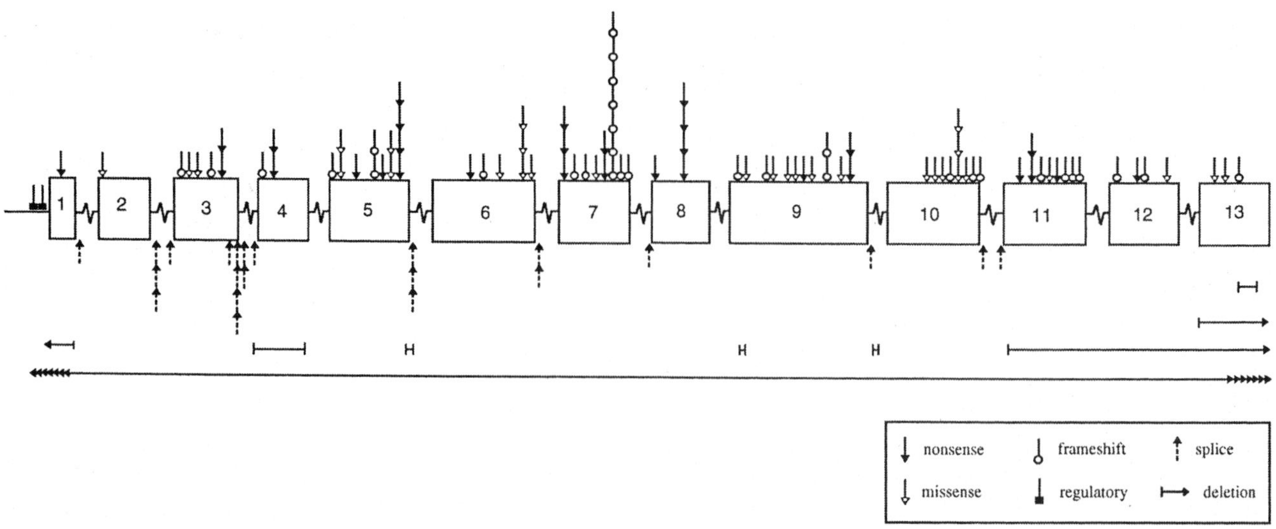

Fig. 189-9 Heterogeneity in positions of CYBB mutations causing X-linked CGD. Each arrow represents a single kindred; the type of arrowhead indicates the type of mutation (as defined in the insert box within the figure). Stacked vertical arrows represent multiple unrelated kindreds with mutations at the same location. Solid horizontal lines indicate deletion mutations; their lengths map the size of the deletion. Arrowheads on the horizontal lines represent unknown deletion length in the direction of the arrow. (*From Rae et al.* American Journal of Human Genetics. *Used with permission.*)

Wide Web site http://www.helsinki.fi/science/signal/databases/x-cgdbase.html. Forms of mutations causing X-linked CGD have included large, multigene deletions, smaller deletions and insertions, missense and nonsense substitutions, and splicing defects. In the two largest series,[50,87] their locations were distributed roughly evenly throughout the gene's exons and intron borders, as illustrated in Fig. 189-9. The combined, nonoverlapping kindreds from these studies provide the basis for calculations of the relative frequencies of different types of mutations in the following paragraphs. The heterogeneity of mutations and the lack of any predominant genotype indicate that the worldwide incidence of CGD represents many different mutational events without any founder effect, as expected for a formerly lethal disorder.

Deletions involving the *CYBB* gene range from single nucleotides to cytogenetically detectable loss of multiple genes. Relatively large deletions in Xp21.1 involving the *CYBB* gene may also affect the adjacent McLeod (*XK*) gene or the Duchenne muscular dystrophy and X-linked retinitis pigmentosa loci.[50,61,87,449,450,462,463] This association is consistent with the known X chromosome map positions of the these genes, in the order: centromere — *CYBB* — *XK* — Duchenne — retinitis pigmentosa — telomere[464] (MIM). The McLeod phenotype includes compensated hemolysis, acanthocytic erythrocyte morphology, and eventual neurologic symptoms including areflexia, dystonia, and choreiform movements.[416] McLeod phenotype is defined hematologically by absent erythrocyte Kx protein and diminished levels of Kell blood group antigens,[416] including k (Cellano), Kp^b (Rautenberg), and Ku (Peltz or anti-total Kell). Importantly, the phenotype is completely distinct from the very common Kell negative and the extremely rare Kell null blood groups. When transfused with red blood cells, McLeod phenotype patients may respond with anti-Kx and anti-Km antibodies that render future transfusion extremely difficult. For this reason, X-linked CGD patients, particularly those with deletion mutations, should be screened for the McLeod phenotype by *quantitative* determination of k, Kp^b, and Ku expression.[465]

Smaller deletions range in size from several kilobases to single base losses. Most result in the $X91^0$ phenotype, i.e., no oxidase function; but small, in-frame interstitial deletions that result in loss of one to six amino acids can preserve partial function as $X91^-$ CGD.[50,87] Deletions and insertions of one or two nucleotides produce a frameshift that inevitably leads to formation of a termination codon in the same or the next downstream exon and, hence, an unstable truncated protein and an $X91^0$ phenotype. Such mutations are relatively common, occurring in 50 of 251 independent kindreds in the two large studies.[50,87]

Nonsense mutations, from a coding to a termination codon, directly cause formation of a truncated protein with an $X91^0$ phenotype. These mutations are also common and were found in 63 of the 251 kindreds.[50,87] Many kindreds shared their mutation with at least one other family. In some, but not all, of the patients' phagocytes, northern blot analysis for *CYBB* transcripts showed reduced or undetectable levels of the mRNA, consistent with the destabilizing effects of nonsense mutations.[466] The locations of these mutations were all 3′ to the positions of the mutations that did not affect mRNA levels, unlike the predominantly upstream positions of destabilizing nonsense codons in transcripts encoding β globin, adenine phosphoribosyltransferase, and triose phosphate isomerase.[466,467]

Missense mutations result from one or two nucleotide changes that alter the DNA sequence to encode a different amino acid. These mutations, which account for CGD in 61 of 251 kindreds,[50,87] are shown in Fig. 189-10, mapped onto a representation of the gp91-*phox* molecule and its functional domains. The putative transmembrane domains and orientation of the N-terminus are based on current and past mutation data, hydropathy plots, and studies with blocking peptides and antipeptide antibodies[468,469] (also Cross, Dinauer, and Curnutte, unpublished data); putative FAD and NADPH binding regions and glycosylation sites are based on gp91-*phox* structural analyses.[85,86] Three regions of the molecule show clusters of mutations: amino acids 209 to 223 (encoded in exon 6), amino acids 309 to 339 (encoded in exon 9), and amino acids 405 to 422 (encoded in exon 10). However, as indicated in Fig. 189-9, these exons do not constitute "hot spots" for other types of mutations. Most "variant" CGD cases come from this category, due to structural derangement without total disruption of the gp91-*phox* molecule. Some such missense mutations partly preserve both cytochrome b_{558} levels and oxidase function. Such $X91^-$ phenotypes indicate positions (shown in Fig. 189-9) in the gp91-*phox* molecule that may be functionally permissive for structural alterations, but at the cost of destabilizing the protein molecule. Others, such as mutations that lead to substitution of histidine for proline at

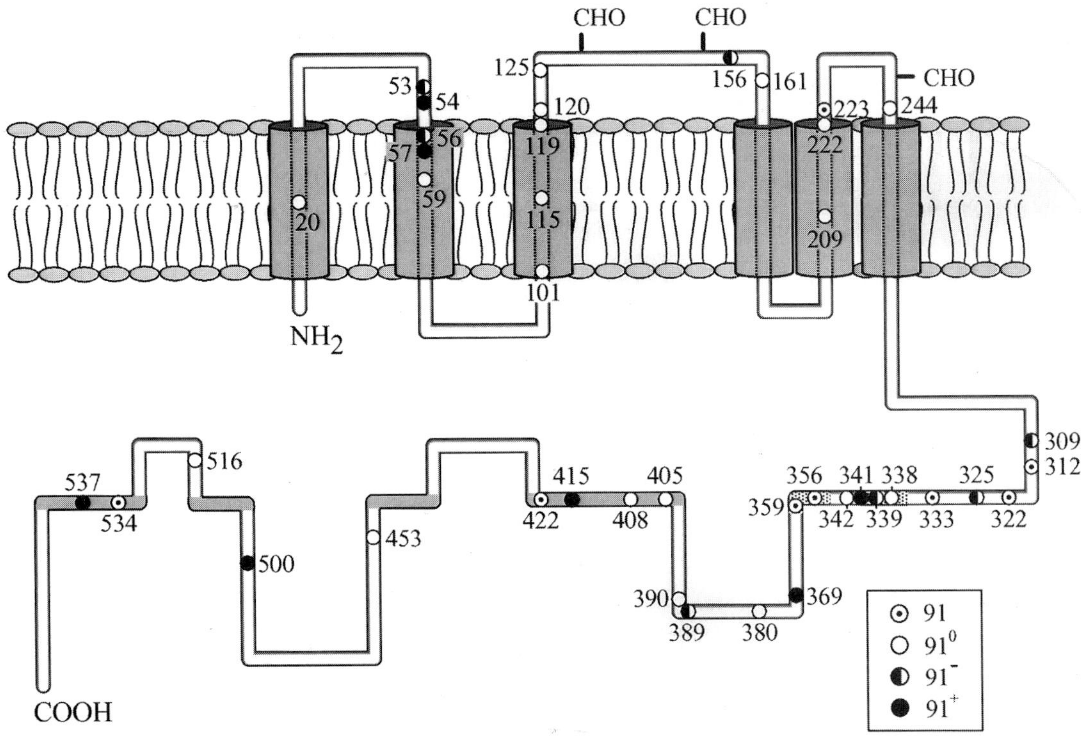

Fig. 189-10 Schematic representation of the gp91-phox protein molecule. Sites of missense mutations are identified by the number of the affected amino acids and types of mutations indicated by symbols (as defined in the insert box within the figure; . = normal). The shaded regions between amino acids 403 and 546 represent the putative NADPH binding site, and the stippled region between amino acids 335 and 360 represents the putative FAD binding site. CHO = indicates glycosylation sites. (*Adapted from Rae et al. American Journal of Human Genetics. Used with permission.*)

position 415 or substitution of arginine for cysteine at residue 537, result in X91$^+$ phenotypes with complete preservation of cytochrome b_{558} but absence of oxidase enzyme activity. Thus, these residues appear essential for function but not for protein stability. Three of the histidines that constitute potential heme binding sites have been altered by missense mutations. Those that have been tested for biochemical function have shown no residual oxidase activity or cytochrome b_{558} protein, as expected from the critical role of heme incorporation in the formation and stability of the cytochrome b_{558} heterodimer.[171] In contrast, several mutations of proline moieties showed partial or complete preservation of cytochrome b_{558} protein (but no function), despite the presumed role of this amino acid in the formation of bends in secondary structure. Benign variants, that is, missense mutations that have no effect on function, are extraordinarily rare.[368,470]

Approximately two-thirds of the "nonsense" and one-third of the missense mutations represented C → T or antisense complementary G → A transitions at CpG dinucleotides.[50,87] The predominance of such mutations has been reported in the factor VIII gene and others[471]; it probably represents spontaneous deamination of methylated cytosines in genomic DNA.[472]

Mutations in or near splice junction sites produce CGD by interfering with mRNA processing and have been found in 39 of 251 (16 percent) kindreds in two large studies. Most occurred at the splice junction and, in those tested, resulted in an X91^0 phenotype due to deletion of one or more exons, as in most previously-reported splicing mutations in X-linked CGD.[452] However, in a small minority of kindreds, such mutations produce X91$^-$ phenotypes due to partial retention of normal splicing.[87] One of these kindreds has proved uniquely responsive to treatment with interferon-γ, with virtually complete restoration of superoxide generating activity in vitro and in vivo, due at least in part to increased levels of normal transcripts.[176,403,473] Other splice site mutations that create novel splice sites within exons can result in X91^0, X91$^+$, or X91$^-$ phenotypes, depending on the severity of the resultant interstitial deletions.[50,87,310] Only three kindreds have been reported with mutations of the regulatory sequence in the 5′ flanking region of the *CYBB* gene.[168,169] Affected patients have a unique form of X91$^-$ CGD, with absent oxidase activity in 90 to 95 percent of their neutrophils and monocytes but normal levels in the remainder[377] and normal activity in all eosinophils.[168] These mutations are located at nucleotide positions −53, −55, and −57 relative to the transcription start site and disrupt the binding of transcription factors HAF-1, PU.1, and interferon consensus sequence binding protein.[166–168] The association of the mutations with CGD thus indicates the probable importance of these transcription factors for expression of the *CYBB* gene.

Carrier detection for X-linked CGD has demonstrated the mutated gene or a functionally abnormal phagocyte population in 85 to 90 percent of mothers.[87,460] The reciprocal apparent spontaneous mutation rate of 10 to 15 percent falls well below Haldane's calculation that, if male and female mutation rates are equal, one-third of cases of X-linked disorders should represent new mutations, if the population is at equilibrium and the viability or fertility of the affected males is very low.[474,475] The difference is consistent with the high frequency of single nucleotide and CpG substitutions that are typical when male gamete mutation rates exceed the female rate and may also reflect some degree of selection bias due to testing of carrier mothers referred for prenatal diagnosis of CGD and to the higher likelihood making the diagnosis of CGD in a patient with a positive family history.

***Mutations in the* CYBA *Gene Encoding p22*-phox.** Mutations in the gene for the p22-*phox* subunit of cytochrome b_{558} account for approximately 6 percent of the cases of CGD (see Table 189-5). The p22-*phox* gene (symbol *CYBA*) resides at chromosome 16q24 and contains six exons that span 8.5 kb.[62] Genetic defects have been investigated in nine different families, with a heterogeneous assortment of 10 different mutations identified.[62,93,390,476,477] The mutations range from large interstitial gene deletions to point mutations associated with missense, frameshift, or RNA splicing defects.[50] In all but two cases, the patients were homozygous for the mutant allele due to consanguinity in the parents.[62,476] The identical mutation was found in only two different patients from different families.[62,476]

Analogous to the cases of $X91^+$ described above, one patient has been reported who is homozygous for a point mutation in the p22-*phox* gene in association with normal levels of cytochrome b_{558} and a nonfunctional oxidase.[93] The mutation predicts the substitution of Gln for Pro156 (P156Q) in the intracytoplasmic C-terminus of p22-*phox*. The patient's neutrophils have undetectable levels of O_2^- production despite the presence of a spectrally normal cytochrome b_{558}. Recent studies have shown that the P156Q mutation disrupts a proline-rich sequence in p22-*phox* that normally interacts with an SH3 domain in p47-*phox* during assembly of the active oxidase complex.[94–96] SH3 motifs, first described in the src tyrosine kinase family, mediate protein–protein interactions by binding to proline-rich sequences in target proteins.[97] The proline substitution in p22-*phox* is at least the second example of a genetic disease caused by disruption of interprotein interactions mediated by means of SH3 domains. A kindred with X-linked agammaglobulinemia due to deletion of the SH3 region of Bruton tyrosine kinase also has been reported.[478]

Mutations in the* NCFI *Gene Encoding p47-phox. The p47-*phox* gene (symbol *NCF1*) is mapped to chromosome 7q11.23 and consists of nine exons spanning 18 kb[479] (Table 189-5). This form of CGD accounts for approximately one-fourth of cases in the United States and Europe but only for approximately 7 percent of the cases in Japan.[480] In contrast to the diversity of mutations seen in patients with cytochrome b_{558} deficiency is the relatively limited number identified in CGD patients with p47-*phox* deficiency.[479–481] Most are homozygous for a mutant allele with a GT deletion at the beginning of exon 2 that predicts a premature stop codon following amino acid residue 50. Four patients have been found to be compound heterozygotes, with each having one allele with the GT deletion.[50] In one of these three individuals, the other allele had an A $\rightarrow$ G substitution at nucleotide 179 that predicts the incorporation of an alanine instead of a threonine at residue 53 (T53A). Another patient had a 502delG mutation predicting a frameshift mutation with premature stop codon. In the other two patients, an A $\rightarrow$ G mutation at nucleotide 425 was identified that predicts a Lys135 to Glu (K135E) substitution.

The high frequency of the p47-*phox* GT deletion mutation in unrelated and racially diverse patients with $A47^0$ CGD now appears to reflect the existence of at least one highly conserved p47-*phox* pseudogene containing the GT deletion mutation.[482] The p47-*phox* gene and pseudogene(s) are closely linked on chromosome 7q11.23. This close physical proximity and the presence within each gene of recombination "hot spots" suggest that the high incidence of the GT deletion mutation in p47-*phox*–deficient CGD results from recombination or gene conversion events between the wild-type gene and the pseudogenes.

***Mutations in the* NCF2 *Gene Encoding p67*-phox.** The 40 kb p67-*phox* gene (symbol *NCF2*) contains 16 exons at its chromosomal location on 1q25.[483] Mutations of this locus account for about 6 percent of cases of CGD (Table 189-5) and have been characterized in a handful of unrelated patients. Most are associated with absence of the p67-*phox* protein and include missense mutations, a dinucleotide insertion producing a frameshift, and a splice junction mutation affecting mRNA processing.[484–487] One interesting patient in whom neutrophils contained about half-normal amounts of p67-*phox* but entirely lacked NADPH oxidase activity was found to be a compound heterozygote for a triplet nucleotide deletion in the p67-*phox* gene, predicting an in-frame deletion of lysine 58 and a larger deletion of approximately 12 kb in the other allele.[488] Translocation of p67-*phox* to the membrane with neutrophil activation failed to occur, and studies with recombinant proteins suggested a defective interaction between the mutant K58Δ p67-*phox* and Rac.

Glucose-6-Phosphate Dehydrogenase (G-6-PD) Deficiency

Leukocyte G-6-PD deficiency can be associated with a phagocytic bactericidal defect as the result of a subnormal respiratory burst, and the clinical presentation can mimic CGD.[489–492] Patients with erythrocyte G-6-PD deficiency suffer bouts of hemolytic anemia as a result of exposure to certain drugs and foods (see Chap. 179). G-6-PD catalyzes the first step in the hexose monophosphate shunt, which is necessary to maintain normal amounts of cellular NADPH. Cells, in particular erythrocytes, that lack adequate levels of NADPH are unable to maintain glutathione in a reduced state (GSH) and, thus are susceptible to oxidative damage on exposure to oxidants in drugs or foods. The disorder is inherited in an X-linked fashion, and affected individuals are usually male, although homozygous affected females are not rare in certain populations, and heterozygous females can express the disorder (see Chap. 179).

G-6-PD activity is present in normal neutrophils and appears to be required to generate the NADPH used as a substrate for the respiratory burst oxidase.[489] Patients whose neutrophils are severely deficient in G-6-PD (with less than 5 percent of normal activity) do not undergo a respiratory burst and suffer recurrent and sometimes fatal bacterial infections with CGD.[489–492] In contrast, individuals with as little as 25 percent of normal G-6-PD activity have not shown an unusual susceptibility to infection.[489] Like neutrophils from individuals with CGD, G-6-PD-deficient neutrophils are unable to reduce NBT and demonstrate an in vitro killing defect against catalase-producing microorganisms. CGD and G-6-PD deficiency can be distinguished by exposing neutrophils to methylene blue, an oxidizing agent that converts NADPH to NADP, thereby activating the hexose monophosphate shunt in CGD but not in G-6-PD deficiency.

Myeloperoxidase Deficiency

Description. Until the late 1970s hereditary deficiency of MPO had been infrequently reported; there were descriptions in the literature of only 15 patients from 12 families.[493–500] However, the diagnosis became common with the widespread application in clinical hematology laboratories of automated flow cytochemistry to quantitate peroxidase activity as a means to enumerate neutrophils in peripheral blood. Application of this technique has demonstrated the true prevalence of MPO deficiency to be approximately 1 in 2000 apparently healthy individuals.[501,502] Histochemical studies of peripheral blood from such individuals showed an absence of peroxidase staining in neutrophils and monocytes, whereas there was normal staining of the peroxidase in eosinophils, consistent with the previous understanding that eosinophil peroxidase is a different protein. Other prominent neutrophil granule proteins, including β glucuronidase, elastase, vitamin B12 binding protein, and lysozyme, are present in normal amounts in MPO-deficient cells.

Clinical Course. Most individuals with MPO deficiency are healthy. In accord with the inability of MPO-deficient neutrophils to kill species of *Candida*, however, four of the six reported patients with MPO deficiency who have had significant infection had disseminated or visceral candidiasis.[494,498,499,502] Of these four patients, three[494,498,502] had concomitant diabetes mellitus. In some cases, MPO deficiency has been part of more complex clinical pictures; some of these have included associated defects in chemotaxis,[503] normal chemotaxis but recurrent and severe skin infection,[504] acne vulgaris,[505] and pustular psoriasis.[506] The contribution of the deficiency of MPO to the clinical syndrome is not clear in these cases. MPO-dependent oxidants appear to be particularly important for the killing of *Candida* species,[39] but there are additional antimicrobial systems that adequately protect the host in most situations. In the absence of MPO, more subtle defects in host defense, such as those present in the antifungal defenses of some diabetics, become clinically significant.

Several studies have suggested that subjects with MPO deficiency have susceptibility to malignant disease and that this susceptibility differs from that in the general population.[507–509] Piedrafita et al.[510] recently identified two forms of the MPO gene promoter that differ in a single base pair 463 nucleotides upstream of the start site. One of the promoter genotypes has been associated with the M3 form of acute leukemia[271] and is twenty-five times more active than the other in in vitro transcription assays. Thus, changes in MPO gene expression may have important etiologic implications in certain forms of hematologic malignancies.[511,512]

In addition to the inherited form of MPO deficiency, there are numerous causes of acquired MPO deficiency. These include pregnancy,[513] lead poisoning,[514] Hodgkin disease,[515] sepsis,[516] megaloblastic anemia,[517–519] ceroid lipofuscinosis,[520,521] and acute nonlymphocytic leukemias, in particular of the M2 to M4 types.[522–527]

Laboratory Diagnosis. Neutrophils and monocytes from individuals with MPO deficiency appear completely normal under the microscope. Thus, the clinician must consider the possibility of MPO deficiency to alert the hematology laboratory to do the appropriate studies. Recurrent, invasive, or disseminated fungal disease in the absence of clearly identifiable risk factors should suggest the possibility of MPO deficiency.

The diagnosis can be easily made by quantitation of the peroxidase activity of isolated cells or by histochemical analysis of peroxidase activity of neutrophils or monocytes in peripheral blood smears. Peroxidase activity can be quantitated using a variety of different substrates,[528–530] but none differentiate eosinophil from neutrophil monocyte peroxidase. If MPO is quantitated in a population of leukocytes, the presence of a disproportionate number of eosinophils could obscure the diagnosis of MPO deficiency[531] because eosinophils contain fourfold more peroxidase than do neutrophils[532] and eosinophil peroxidase is more active than MPO.[533] The diagnosis can be established simply and directly by examining peripheral blood smears stained for peroxidase activity. Currently, substrates such as 3-amino-9-carbazole[534] and 4-chloro-1-naphthol[535] are recommended over the previous standard, benzidine dihydrochloride, which is carcinogenic.[536]

Numerous investigators have characterized the in vitro behavior of MPO-deficient neutrophils and monocytes. These cells have an exuberant respiratory burst, manifested by greater than normal oxygen consumption, increased O_2^- and H_2O_2 release (Fig. 189-11), and greater hexose monophosphate shunt activity.[462,506,537,538] MPO-deficient neutrophils have normal amounts of catalase and glutathione peroxidase,[539] indicating that the detection of supernormal amounts of oxygen products is due to increased production and not to decreased catabolism. In addition, the increase in production is due to a failure in termination of the respiratory burst (Fig. 189-11).

Phagocytosis by MPO-deficient neutrophils of a variety of particles has been reported to be normal.[498,502,538,540] Release of granule products to a variety of stimuli has been reported to be normal or increased.[541] There is increased recovery of granule products from MPO-deficient neutrophils[542–544] because the proteins are not oxidized and inactivated by the MPO—H_2O_2—halide system.

The microbicidal activity of MPO-deficient cells is defective. MPO-deficient cells kill *S. aureus*,[498,501,502,538,540,545,546] *Serratia*,[498] and *E. coli*[547,548] significantly more slowly than do normal cells. However, after 1 h of incubation, MPO-deficient cells have killed the same number of organisms as normal cells. This may reflect the sustained respiratory burst present in MPO-deficient cells and the amplified systems that compensate for the MPO deficiency.[545] Most striking in vitro is the inability of MPO-deficient cells to kill a variety of species of fungi, including the clinically significant *Candida albicans* and *C. tropicalis*[498,499,502,538,540,549] and hyphal forms of *Aspergillus fumigatus*.[550,551] In contrast *T. glabrata*,[503] *C. parapsilosis*,[552] *C. pseudotropicalis*,[553] and the spores of *A. fumigatus* and of *Rhizopus oryzae*[554] are killed normally by MPO-deficient cells.

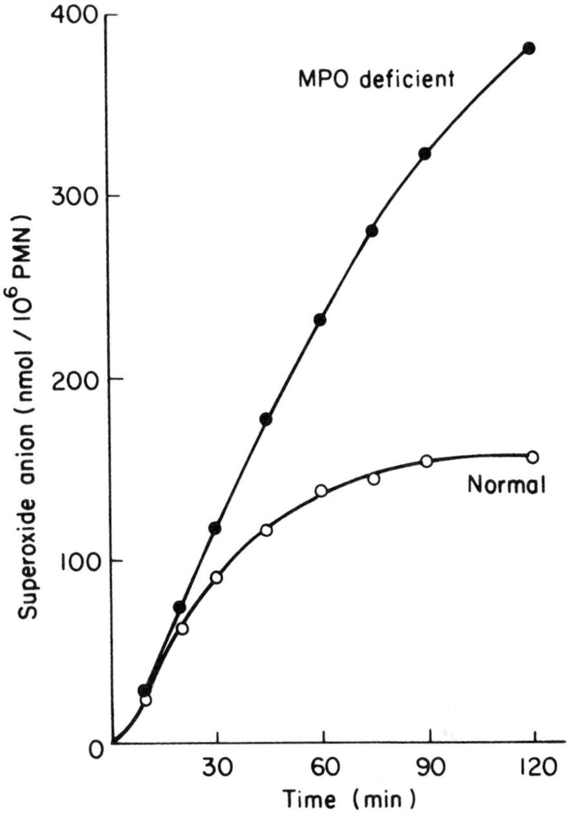

Fig. 189-11 The time course of O_2^- production by neutrophils from a patient with myeloperoxidase deficiency.

Biochemical Defect. The biochemical defect in MPO deficiency is the lack of peroxidase activity in the azurophilic granules of neutrophils and in the primary lysosomes of monocytes. Immunochemical analysis of neutrophils from affected individuals shows that the cells lack the subunits of MPO.[208] However, both normal and MPO-deficient neutrophils contain an immunochemically related protein of a higher molecular weight that has characteristics consistent with its being proMPO. MPO synthesis is under the control of a single gene, although there is evidence of multiple mRNA species in cultured myeloid cells such as the HL-60 cell line,[555] presumably the result of alternative splicing.[556] Expression of mRNA encoding for MPO is restricted to myeloid cells, with other cultured hematopoietic precursors expressing essentially no MPO.[557] Chemical induction of HL-60 cells results in rapid cessation of MPO expression coincident with differentiation into more mature myeloid cells,[558] indicating that transcription of the MPO gene is tightly regulated and temporally linked to myeloid differentiation.[555,558–560] Both demethylation and Dnase I hypersensitivity of the MPO gene are associated with MPO gene expression during myeloid differentiation.[561] The promoter region of the MPO gene has been partly characterized.[562–564] There are regions 5′ to the transcription initiation site in the MPO gene that share sequence homology with 5′ promoter region of the c-myc protooncogene[565] and with 5′ flanking regions of the murine lactoferrin gene,[566] although the significance of these homologies has not been established.

Studies using cultured myeloid cell lines have provided a great deal of information regarding the biosynthesis, processing, and intracellular transport of MPO.[567–574] There is a single primary translation product of approximately 80 kDa that undergoes cotranslational glycosylation to generate apoproMPO, the enzymatically inactive heme-free precursor of MPO. Early in biosynthesis, MPO precursors associate transiently with ER molecular chaperones calreticulin and calnexin[575,576] and apoproMPO is converted to proMPO,[577] also presumably within the endoplasmic reticulum (ER).[574,578] Subsequently, proMPO undergoes proteolytic processing into the mature heterodimer, assembly into dimeric MPO, and subcellular transport to the azurophilic granules. It is clear that inhibition of heme synthesis by addition of succinyl acetone to the culture medium blocks proteolytic maturation into mature MPO,[574,578] suggesting that insertion of the iron-containing prosthetic group and generation of proMPO are necessary for subsequent processing into MPO. Little is known about the factors that mediate this proteolytic processing or the subcellular compartment in which it takes place. Likewise, the mechanism by which MPO is directed to the azurophilic granule is not defined. ProMPO does not bind to a mannose 6-phosphate receptor affinity column,[574] confirming considerable indirect evidence that MPO lysosomal targeting is independent of the mannose 6-phosphate receptor system.

Gene Defect. The gene for MPO is located on chromosome 17 at q22q23,[579,580] near the breakpoint for the 15;17 translocation of promyelocytic leukemia.[581,582] Partial sequence of the MPO gene reveals 12 exons and 11 introns with consensus sequences present for both splice donor and acceptor sites.[565] The genomic sequence spans 14 kb and the full-length cDNA is approximately 3.3 kb, with an open reading frame of 2.2 kb (encoding 745 amino acids). Northern blots of RNA from HL-60 cells or bone marrow cells from humans or mice demonstrate mRNA for MPO at 3.0 to 3.3 kb and 3.5 to 4.0 kb, respectively.

Although one patient has been reported with a likely pretranslational defect underlying MPO deficiency,[583] most patients studied to date have immunochemical evidence of MPO precursor(s) and thus presumably a defect in posttranslational processing as the underlying cause of the deficiency. To date, three genotypes associated with inherited MPO deficiency have been reported.[584–586] The first, and apparently most common, is a missense mutation at codon 569 in which arginine is replaced by tryptophan (R569W).[584] When expressed in a transfected K562 cell line, the R569W mutation results in a maturation arrest in the protein at the level of apoproMPO; apoproMPO is made but fails to incorporate heme and thus remains enzymatically inactive.[587] One family has been recently described with a missense mutation at codon 173 wherein tyrosine is replaced by cysteine.[584] This creates an opportunity for realignment of disulfide bonds within the light subunit and presumably significantly alters folding of the nascent polypeptide precursor. When examined in K562 transfectants, the Y173C mutant generates small amounts of proMPO that remain associated with calnexin much longer than does normal proMPO. The mutant proMPO neither enters the secretory pathway nor undergoes proteolytic maturation and targeting to the azurophilic granule. Instead, mutant proMPO undergoes proteolysis in the cytosolic proteasome. The third genotype described is a compound heterozygote in whom the mutations on each allele were identified.[586] On one allele is a missense mutation in which a methionine at codon 251 is replaced by threonine. The impact of this mutation on the biosynthesis of MPO is unknown at this time, although it is noteworthy that the mutation is close to distal heme binding site. The other allele has a 14-bp deletion from exon 9, although the intracellular impact of this change has not been assessed. It is likely that analyses of such mutations in this sytem will provide important insights into processing and targeting events in the synthesis of myeloid proteins.

Although a number of studies have suggested an autosomal recessive mode of inheritance,[498,531,540,547,588] other studies have suggested variable expression of the gene[501] or defects in structural and regulatory genes.[502] In fact, a recent analysis of the pattern of inheritance of MPO deficiency associated with the R569W mutation suggests that most patients are compound heterozygotes,[589] further complicating studies of the pattern of inheritance based solely on peroxidase activity of neutrophils.

Treatment. There is no specific therapy for MPO deficiency. Given the predilection of diabetics with MPO deficiency for severe fungal infections, it would be prudent to avoid factors that predispose to fungal superinfection (e.g., prolonged use of broad-spectrum antibiotics) and to treat presumed fungal infections earlier in such patients.

Glutathione Synthetase Deficiency

Glutathione (*N*-[*N*-*L*-γ-glutamyl-*L*-cysteinyl]glycine) can be found in high concentrations in most cell types. The ratio of GSH (reduced glutathione) to GSSG (oxidized glutathione) in normal cells is approximately 500:1.[590,591] Its biosynthesis from γ-glutamylcysteine and glycine is catalyzed by the enzyme glutathione synthetase. In the neutrophil, glutathione protects cellular structures from the harmful effects of H_2O_2 and perhaps other oxidizing radicals generated during the phagocytosis-associated respiratory burst. A reduction in the synthesis or regeneration of glutathione in the phagocyte leads to increased oxidative stress and loss of function.[592,593]

Glutathione synthetase deficiency with 5-oxoprolinuria has been described in a 2-year-old boy with two episodes of neutropenia associated with otitis media (see Chap. 96).[593] Hemolytic anemia had been noted at birth. Erythrocytes, leukocytes, and cultured skin fibroblasts had diminished glutathione synthetase activity (5 to 10 percent of normal) and intracellular glutathione content (10 to 20 percent of normal). There was no history of unusual infections. Neutrophil chemotaxis, phagocytosis, and NBT reduction all occurred normally. However, neutrophil bactericidal capacity and iodination were impaired. These defects were thought to be due to deficiency of glutathione, which would be expected to permit accumulation of H_2O_2 intracellularly after stimulation. The resultant increase in oxidative stress was shown to damage the patient's neutrophil membranes and microtubules and to impair phagolysosomal formation.[593]

The oxidant scavenger vitamin E (α tocopherol), 400 IU per day, increased red cell survival, corrected both the bactericidal and

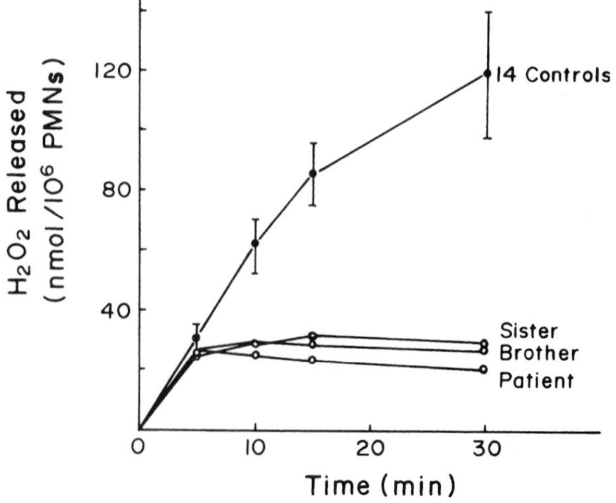

Fig. 189-12 The time course of zymosan-triggered H_2O_2 release by neutrophils from 14 controls and 3 individuals with glutathione reductase deficiency. (*From Roos et al.*[187] *Used by permission.*)

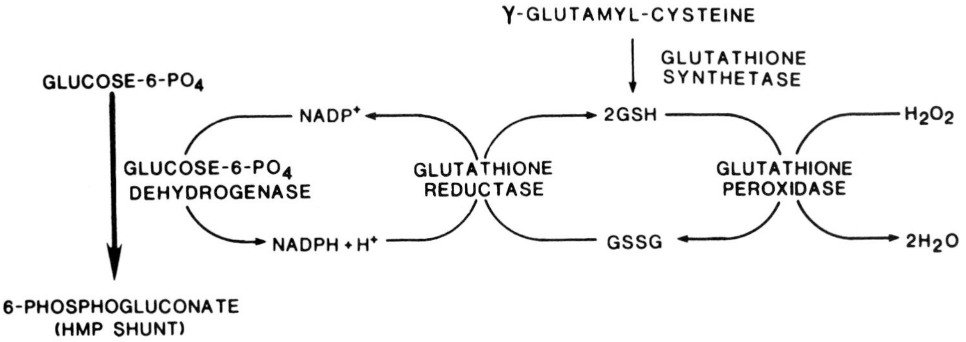

Fig. 189-13 Schematic representation of the glutathione oxidation-reduction cycle. GSH = reduced glutathione; GSSG = oxidized glutathione. (*From Johnston RB Jr: Biochemical defects of polymorphonuclear and mononuclear phagocytes associated with disease, in Sbarra AJ, Strauss R (eds):* The Reticuloendothelial System. *New York, Plenum, 1980, vol 2, p 397. Used by permission.*)

iodination defects, and eliminated the neutropenia that had accompanied certain intercurrent illnesses.[594]

Congenital glutathione synthetase deficiency appears to be inherited in an autosomal recessive fashion.

Glutathione Reductase Deficiency

A 22-year-old woman of parents who were first cousins suffered bouts of hemolysis in association with eating fava beans (see also Chap. 96). Diminished glutathione reductase activity was noted in the erythrocytes and granulocytes. Two sibs with an identical defect of glutathione metabolism were also identified.

There was no history of repeated infections in any of the three kindreds.[595] Chemotaxis, phagocytosis of opsonized *S. aureus*, and degranulation proceeded normally.[592] Intracellular killing appeared normal at low ratios of bacteria to phagocytes, but higher ratios produced defective bacterial killing. The patient's neutrophils phagocytosed opsonized zymosan normally, and oxygen consumption and H_2O_2 production occurred at a normal rate for 5 to 10 min. However, this was followed by complete cessation of respiratory burst activity (Fig. 189-12). Hexose monophosphate shunt activity stopped after 10 min of phagocytosis with a subnormal initial rate.

Glutathione reductase catalyzes the reduction of glutathione disulfide to reduced glutathione by using electrons from NADPH (Fig. 189-13). Absence of glutathione reductase leads to defective generation of reduced glutathione, which permits oxidative damage to the stimulated neutrophil (see Antioxidant Mechanisms above). In contrast to other aspects of the respiratory burst, the release of O_2^-, measured as the reduction of cytochrome c, proceeded normally. Cytochrome c added in vitro scavenges the electrons from O_2^-, which prevents H_2O_2 formation from the dismutation reaction, thereby protecting the cell from oxidative damage.

There is no specific therapy for glutathione reductase deficiency, but avoiding foods and drugs containing potent oxidants will decrease the chance of depleting cellular levels of glutathione. The pattern of inheritance is unknown.

Glutathione Peroxidase Deficiency

In 1968, when CGD was thought to be purely X linked, two females with the disease were described[300] and subsequently reported to have a severe deficiency of leukocyte glutathione peroxidase.[596] The investigators hypothesized that the resultant accumulation of peroxides caused the CGD phenotype in these patients by inhibition of respiratory burst activity. However, a recent study reexamined one of the original females and the sib, also affected by CGD, of the other patient. Application of current molecular and biochemical techniques demonstrated mutations of the phagocyte oxidase genes, as in other cases of cytochrome *b*-negative CGD, along with normal glutathione peroxidase enzyme activity and gene expression.[369] Although acquired glutathione peroxidase deficiency may affect phagocyte function,[597–600] congenital deficiency of the enzyme should no longer be considered a possible cause of the CGD phenotype.

ACKNOWLEDGMENTS

This work was supported in part by USPHS grants DK41625, DK54369, R01HL45635, R01HL52565, P01HL53586, AI34879, and HL53592 and a Merit Review grant from the Veterans Administration. We also thank Dr. John Curnutte and Ms. Julie Rae for their advice, support, and generous sharing of data and figures.

REFERENCES

1. Craddock CG: Defenses of the body: The initiators of defense, the ready reserves, and the scavengers, in Wintrobe M (ed): *Blood, Pure and Eloquent*. New York, McGraw-Hill, 1980, p. 417.
2. Metchnikov I: *Immunity in Infective Diseases*. New York, Dover, 1968.
3. Johnston R: Monocytes and macrophages. *N Engl J Med* **318**:747, 1988.
4. Mandell G: Bactericidal activity of aerobic and anaerobic polymorphonuclear neutrophils. *Infect Immun* **9**:337, 1974.
5. Okamura N, Spitznagel J: Outer membrane mutants of *Salmonella typhimurium* LT2 lipopolysaccharide have resistance to the bactericidal activity of anaerobic human neutrophils. *Infect Immunol* **36**:1086, 1982.
6. Vel W, Namavar F, Verweij A, Pubben A, Maclaren D: Killing capacity of human polymorphonuclear leukocytes in aerobic and anaerobic conditions. *J Med Microbiol* **62**:65, 1984.
7. Weiss J, Victor M, Stendahl O, Elsbach P: Killing of gram-negative bacteria by polymorphonuclear leukocytes. *J Clin Invest* **69**:959, 1982.
8. Odell E, Segal A: Killing of pathogens associated with chronic granulomatous disease by the non-oxidative microbicidal mechanisms of human neutrophils. *J Med Microbiol* **34**:129, 1991.
9. Belaaouaj A, McCarthy R, Baumann M, Gao Z, Ley T, Abraham S, Shapiro S: Mice lacking neutrophil elastase reveal impaired host defense against gram negative bacterial sepsis. *Nat Med* **4**:615, 1998.
10. Weiss J: Leukocyte-derived antimicrobial proteins. *Curr Opin Hematol* **1**:78, 1994.
11. Zimmer M, Medcalf R, Fink T, Mattmann C, Lichter P, Jenne D: Three human elastase-like genes coordinately expressed in the myelomonocyte lineage are organized as a single genetic locus on 19pter. *Proc Natl Acad Sci USA* **89**:8215, 1992.
12. Gabay J, Almeida R: Antibiotic peptides and serine protease homologs in human polymorphonuclear leukocytes: defensins and azurocidin. *Curr Opin Immunol* **5**:97, 1993.
13. Lehrer RI, Ganz T: Antimicrobial polypeptides of human neutrophils. *Blood* **47**:2169, 1990.
14. Morgan J, Sukiennicki T, Pereira H, Spitznagel J, Guerra M, Larrick J: Cloning of the cDNA for the serine protease homolog CAP37/azurocidin, a microbicidal and chemotactic protein from human granulocytes. *J Immunol* **147**:3210, 1991.
15. Spitznagel JK: Antibiotic proteins of human neutrophils. *J Clin Invest* **86**:1381, 1990.
16. Hohn P, Popescu N, Hanson R, Salvesen G, Ley T: Genomic organization and chromosomal localization of the human cathepsin G gene. *J Biol Chem* **264**:13412, 1989.
17. Gabay JE, Scott RW, Campanelli D, Griffith J, Wilde C, Marra MN, Seeger M, et al.: Antibiotic proteins of human polymorphonuclear leukocytes. *Proc Natl Acad Sci. USA* **86**:5610, 1989.
18. Elsbach P, Weiss J: Oxygen-independent antimicrobial systems of phagocytes, in Gallin JI, Goldstein IM, Snyderman R (eds): *Inflammation: Basic Principles and Clinical Correlates*. New York, Raven Press, 1992, p 603.

19. Gray P, Flaggs G, Leong S, Gumina R, Weiss J, Ooi C, Elsbach P: Cloning of the cDNA of a human neutrophil bactericidal protein. Structural and functional correlations. *J Biol Chem* **264**:9505, 1989.
20. Perieira H, Spitznagel J, Winton E, Shafer W, Martin L, Guzman G, Pohl J, et al.: The otogeny of a 57-kd cationic antimicrobial protein of human polymorphonuclear leukocytes: Localization to a novel granule population. *Blood* **76**:825, 1990.
21. Gray P, Corcorran A, Eddy R, Byers M, Shows T: The genes for the lipopolysaccharide binding protein (LBP) and the bacterial permeability increasing protein (BPI) are encoded in the same region of human chromosome 20. *Genomics* **15**:188, 1993.
22. Sparks R, Kronenberg M, Heinzmann C, Daher K, Klisak I, Ganz T, Mohandas T: Assignment of defensin genes to human chromosome 8p23. *Genomics* **5**:240, 1989.
23. Spitznagel J: Nonoxidative antimicrobial reactions of leukocytes. *Contemp Topics Immunobiol* **14**:283, 1984.
24. Peters C, Kruse U, Pollwein R, Grzeschik K, Sippel A: The human lysozyme gene. Sequence organization and chromosomal localization. *Eur J Biochem* **182**:507, 1989.
25. Baldridge CW, Gerard RW: The extra respiration of phagocytosis. *Am J Physiol* **103**:235, 1933.
26. Karnovsky M: Metabolic basis of phagocytic activity. *Physiol Rev* **42**:143, 1962.
27. Badwey J, Karnovsky M: Active oxygen species and the functions of phagocytic leukocytes. *Annu Rev Biochem* **49**:695, 1980.
28. Klebanoff S: Oxygen metabolism and the toxic properties of phagocytes. *Ann Intern Med* **93**:480, 1980.
29. Babior B: The respiratory burst of phagocytes. *J Clin Invest* **73**:599, 1984.
30. Miller R, Britigan B: The formation and biologic significance of phagocyte-derived oxidants. *J Invest Med* **43**:39, 1995.
31. Allen R, Stjernholm R, Steele R: Evidence for the generation of an electronic excitation state(s) in human polymorphonuclear leukocytes and its participation in bactericidal activity. *Biochem Biophys Res Commun* **47**:679, 1972.
32. Sbarra AJ, Karnovsky ML: The biochemical basis of phagocytosis. I. Metabolic changes during the ingestion of particles by polymorphonuclear leukocytes. *J Biol Chem* **234**:1355, 1959.
33. Iyer G, Islam M, Quastfl J: Biochemical aspects of phagocytosis. *Nature* **192**:535, 1961.
34. Babior BM, Kipnes RS, Curnutte JT: Biological defense mechanisms: The production by leukocytes of superoxide, a potential bactericidal agent. *J Clin Invest* **52**:741, 1973.
35. Johnston R, Keele B, Misra H, Lehmeyer J, Webb L, Baehner R, Rajgopalan K: The role of superoxide anion generation in phagocytic bactericidal activity: Studies with normal and chronic granulomatous disease leukocytes. *J Clin Invest* **60**:374, 1975.
36. Weiss S, Rustagi P, Lobuglio A: Human granulocyte generation of hydroxyl radical. *J Exp Med* **147**:316, 1978.
37. Halliwell B: Oxidants and human disease: Some new concepts. *FASEB J* **1**:358, 1987.
38. Ramos C, Pou S, Britigan B, Cohen M, Rosen G: Spin trapping evidence for myeloperoxidase-dependent hydroxyl radical formation by human neutrophils and monocytes. *J Biol Chem* **267**:8307, 1992.
39. Thomas E: Myeloperoxidase-hydrogen peroxide-chloride antimicrobial system: Effect of exogenous amines on antibacterial action against *Escherichia coli*. *Infect Immunol* **25**:110, 1979.
40. Marodi L, Forehand J, Johnston R Jr: Mechanisms of host defense against *Candida* species II. Biochemical basis for the killing of *Candida* by mononuclear phagocytes. *J Immunol* **146**:2790, 1991.
41. Baehner R, Nathan D: Leukocyte oxidase: Defective activity in chronic granulomatous disease. *Science* **155**:835, 1967.
42. Quie P, White J, Holmes B, Good R: *In vitro* bacterial capacity of human polymorhonuclear leukocytes: Diminished activity in chronic granulomatous disease of childhood. *J Clin Invest* **46**:668, 1967.
43. Johnston R, Baehner R: Chronic granulomatous disease: Correlation between pathogenesis and clinical findings. *Pediatrics* **48**:730, 1971.
44. Wientjes F, Segal A: NADPH oxidase and the respiratory burst. *Cell Biol* **6**:357, 1995.
45. DeLeo F, Quinn M: Assembly of the phagocyte NADPH oxidase: molecular of oxidase proteins. *J Leukoc Biol* **60**:677, 1996.
46. Leusen J, Verhoeven A, Roos D: Interactions between the components of the human NADPH oxidase: intrigues in the *phox* family. *J Lab Clin Med* **128**:461, 1996.
47. Chanock S, El Benna J, Smith R, Babior B: The respiratory burst oxidase. *J Biol Chem* **269**:24519, 1994.
48. Smith RM, Curnutte JT: Molecular basis of chronic granulomatous disease. *Blood* **77**:673, 1991.
49. Thrasher A, Keep N, Wientjes F, Segal A: Review: Chronic granulomatous disease. *Biochim Biophys Acta* **1227**:1, 1994.
50. Roos D, de Boer M, Kuribayashi F, Meischl C, Weening R, Segal A, Ahlin A, et al.: Mutations in the X-linked and autosomal recessive forms of chronic granulomatous disease. *Blood* **87**:1663, 1996.
51. Dinauer M: The respiratory burst oxidase and the molecular genetics of chronic granulomatous disease. *Crit Rev Clin Lab Sci* **30**:329, 1993.
52. Curnutte JT: Molecular basis of the autosomal recessive forms of chronic granulomatous disease. *Immunodef Rev* **3**:149, 1992.
53. Bromberg Y, Pick E: Activation of NADPH-dependent superoxide production in a cell-free system of sodium dodecyl sulfate. *J Biol Chem* **260**:13559, 1985.
54. Heyneman R, Vercauteren R: Activation of a NADPH-dependent oxidase from horse polymorphonuclear leukocytes in a cell-free system. *J Leukoc Biol* **36**:751, 1984.
55. Curnutte JT: Activation of human neutrophil nicotinamide adenine dinucleotide phosphate, reduced (triphosphopridine nucleotide, reduced) oxidase by arachidonic acid in a cell-free system. *J Clin Invest* **75**:1740, 1985.
56. McPhail LC, Shirley PS, Clayton CC, Snyderman R: Activation of the respiratory burst enzyme from human neutrophils in a cell-free system: evidence for a soluble cofactor. *J Clin Invest* **75**:1735, 1985.
57. Thrasher A, Chetty M, Casimir C, et al.: Restoration of superoxide generation to a chronic granulomatous disease-derived B-cell like by retrovirus mediated gene transfer. *Blood* **80**:1125, 1992.
58. Huang J, Hitt N, Kleinberg M: Stoichiometry of p22-*phox* and gp91-*phox* in phagocyte cytochrome b_{558}. *Biochemistry* **34**:16753, 1995.
59. Wallach T, Segal A: Stoichiometry of the subunits of flavocytochrome b_{558} of the NADPH oxidase of phagocytes. *Biochem J* **320**:33-38, 1996.
60. Baehner RL, Kunkel LM, Monaco AP, Haines JL, Conneally PM, Palmer C, Heerema N, et al.: DNA linkage analysis of X chromosome-linked chronic granulomatous disease. *Proc Natl Sci Acad USA* **83**:3398, 1986.
61. Royer-Pokora B, Kunkel L, Monaco A, Goff S, Newburger P, Baehner R, Cole F, et al.: Cloning the gene for an inherited human disorder—chronic granulomatous disease—on the basis of its chromosomal location. *Nature* **322**:32, 1986.
62. Dinauer M, Pierce E, Bruns G, Curnutte J, Orkin S: Human neutrophil cytochrome-b light chain (p22-phox): Gene structure, chromosomal location, and mutations in cytochrome-negative autosomal recessive chronic granulomatous disease. *J Clin Invest* **86**:1729, 1990.
63. Cross AR, Jones OTG, Harper AM, Segal AW: Oxidation-reduction properties of the cytochrome *b* found in the plasma-membrane fraction of human neutrophils. *Biochem J* **194**:599, 1981.
64. Segal A, Garcia R, Goldstone A, Cross A, Jones O: Cytochrome b_{-245} of neutrophils is also present in human monocytes, macrophages eosinophils. *Biochem J* **194**:599, 1981.
65. Parkos C, Dinauer M, Walker L, Allen R, Jesaitis A, Orkin S: The primary structure and unique expression of the 22-kDa light chain of human neutrophil cytochrome b. *Proc Natl Acad Sci USA* **85**:3319, 1988.
66. Radeke H, Cross A, Hancock J, Jones O, Nakamura M, Kaever V, Resch K: Functional expression of NADPH oxidase components (a- and b- subunits of cytochrome b_{558} and 45-kDa flavoprotein) by intrinsic human glomerular mesangial cells. *J Biol Chem* **266**:21025, 1991.
67. Volkman D, Buescher E, Gallin J, Fa A: B cell lines as models for inherited phagocytic diseases: abnormal superoxide generation in chronic granulomatous disease and giant granules in Chediak-Higashi syndrome. *J Immunol* **133**:3006, 1984.
68. Cross AR, Jones OTG: Enzymic mechanisms of superoxide production. *Biochim Biophys Acta* **1057**:281, 1991.
69. Dewald B, Baggiolini M, Curnutte J, Babior B: Subcellular localization of the superoxide-forming enzyme in human neutrophils. *J Clin Invest* **63**:21, 1979.
70. Babior G, Rosin R, McMurrich B, Peters W, Baboir B: Arrangement of the respiratory burst oxidase in the plasma membrane of the neutrophil. *J Clin Invest* **67**:1724, 1981.
71. Parkos CA, Allen RA, Cochrane CG, Jesaitis AJ: Purified cytochrome b from human granulocyte plasma membrane is comprised of two polypeptides with relative molecular weights of 91,000 and 22,000. *J Clin Invest* **80**:732, 1987.

72. Segal A, West I, Wientjes F, Nugent J, Chavan A, Haley B, Garcia R, et al.: Cytochrome b_{-235} is a flavocytochrome containing FAD and the NADPH-binding site of the microbicidal oxidase of phagocytes. *Biochem J* **284**:781, 1993.
73. Rotrosen D, Yeung C, Leto T, Malech H, Kwong C: Cytochrome b558: The flavin-binding component of the phagocyte NADPH oxidase. *Science* **256**:1459, 1992.
74. Cross A, Rae J, Curnutte J: Cytochrome b_{-245} of the neutrophil superoxide-generating system contains two non-identical hemes. *J Biol Chem* **270**:17075, 1995.
75. Quinn M, Mullen M, Jesaitis A: Human neutrophil cytochrome *b* contains multiple hemes. *J Biol Chem* **267**:7303, 1992.
76. Miki T, Fujii H, Kakinuma K: EPR signals of cytochrome *b* 558 purified for porcine neutrophils. *J Biol Chem* **267**:19673, 1992.
77. Ueno I, Fujii S, Ohya-Nishiguchi H, Iizuka T, Kanegasaki S: Characterization of neutrophil b-type cytochrome in situ by electron paramagnetic resonance spectroscopy. *FEBS Lett* **281**:130, 1991.
78. Hurst J, Loehr T, Curnutte J, Rosen H: Resonance raman and electron paramagnetic resonance structural investigations of neutrophil cytochrome b558. *J Biol Chem* **266**:1627, 1991.
79. Yu L, Quinn M, Cross A, Dinauer M: $Gp91^{phox}$ is the heme binding subunit of the superoxide-generating NADPH oxidase. *Proc Natl Acad Sci USA* **95**:7993, 1998.
80. Karplus PA, Daniels MJ, Herriott JR: Atomic structure of ferredoxin-NADT+ reductase: Prototype for a structurally novel flavoenzyme family. *Science* **251**:60, 1991.
81. Cross A, Jones O, Garcia R, Segal A: The association of FAD with the cytochrome b_{-245} of human neutrophils. *Biochem J* **208**:759, 1982.
82. Gabig T: The NADPH-dependent O_2-generating oxidase from human neutrophils: identification of a flavoprotein component that is deficient in a patient with chronic granulomatous disease. *J Biol Chem* **258**:6352, 1983.
83. Gabig T, Lefker B: Deficient flavoprotein component of the NADPH-dependent O_2-generating oxidase in the neutrophils from three patients with chronic granulomatous disease. *J Clin Invest* **73**:701, 1984.
84. Bohler M-C, Seger R, Mouy R, Vilmer E, Fischer A, Griscelli C: A study of 25 patients with chronic granulomatous disease: A new classification by correlating respiratory burst, cytochrome b and flavoprotein. *J Clin Immunol* **6**:136, 1986.
85. Wallach T, Segal A: Analysis of glycosylation sites on gp91*phox*, the flavocytochrome of the NADPH oxidase, by site-directed mutagenesis and translation in vitro. *Biochem J* **321**:583, 1997.
86. Taylor W, Jones D, Segal A: A structural model for the nucleotide binding domains of the flavocytochrome b_{-245} b-chain. *Protein Sci* **2**:1675, 1993.
87. Rae J, Newburger P, Dinauer M, Noack D, Hopkins P, Kuruto R, Curnutte J: X-linked chronic granulomatous disease: mutations in the CYBB gene encoding the gp91-phox component of respiratory-burst oxidase. *Am J Hum Genet* **62**:1320, 1998.
88. Shatwell K, Dancis A, Cross A, Klausner R, Segal A: The FRE1 ferric reductase of *Saccharomyces cerevisiae* is a cytochrome *b* similar to that of NADPH oxidase. *J Biol Chem* **271**:14240, 1996.
89. Keller T, Damude H, Werner D, Doerner P, Dixon R, Lamb C: A plant homolog of the neutrophil NADPH oxidase $gp91^{phox}$ subunit gene encodes a plasma membrane protein with Ca^{2+} binding motifs. *Plant Cell* **10**:255, 1998.
90. Lamb C: Plant disease resistance genes in signal perception and transduction. *Cell* **76**:419, 1994.
91. Desikan R, Hancock J, Coffey M, Neill S: Generation of active oxygen in elicited cells of *Arabidopsis thaliana* is mediated by a NADPH oxidase-like enzyme. *FEBS Lett* **382**:213, 1996.
92. Parkos C, Dinauer M, Jesaitis A, Orkin S, Curnutte J: Absence of both the 91 kD and 22 kD subunits of human neutrophil cytochrome b in two genetic forms of chronic granulomatous disease. *Blood* **73**:1416, 1989.
93. Dinauer M, Pierce E, Erickson R, Muhlebach T, Messner H, Orkin S, Seger R, et al.: Point mutation in the cytoplasmic domain of the neutrophil p22-*phox* cytochrome *b* subunit is associated with a nonfunctional NADPH oxidase and chronic granulomatous disease. *Proc Natl Acad Sci USA* **88**:11231, 1991.
94. Leusen J, Bolscher B, Hilarius P, Weening R, Kaulfersch W, Seger R, Roos D, et al.: ^{156}Pro Æ Gln substitution in the light chain of cytochrome b_{558} of the human NADPH oxidase (p22-phox) leads to defective translocation of the cytosolic proteins p47-phox and p67-phox. *J Exp Med* **180**:2329, 1994.
95. Leto T, Adams A, De Mendez I: Assembly of the phagocyte NADPH oxidase: Binding of Src homology 3 domains to proline-rich targets. *Proc Natl Acad USA* **91**:10650, 1994.
96. Sumimoto H, Kage Y, et al: Role of Src homology 3 domains in assembly and activation of the phagocyte NADPH oxidase. *Proc Natl Acad Sci USA* **91**:5345, 1994.
97. McPhail LC: SH3-dependent assembly of the phagocyte NADPH oxidase. *J Exp Med* **180**:2011, 1994.
98. Abo A, Boyhan A, West I, Thrasher A, Segal A: Reconstitution of neutrophil NADPH oxidase activity in the cell-free system by four components: p67-phox, p47-phox, p21rac1, and cytochrome b245. *J Biol Chem* **267**:16767, 1992.
99. Uhlinger D, Inge K, Kreck ML, Tyagi S, Neckelmann N, Lambeth J: Reconstitution and characterization of the human neutrophil respiratory burst oxidase using recombinant p47-*phox*, p67-*phox* and plasma membrane. *Biochem Biophys Res Commun* **186**:509, 1992.
100. Curnutte J, Scott P, Mayo L: Cytosolic components of the respiratory burst oxidase: Resolution of four components, two of which are missing in complementing types of chronic granulomatous disease. *Proc Natl Acad Sci USA* **86**:825, 1989.
101. Wientjes F, Hsuan J, Totty N, Segal A: $p40^{phox}$, a third cytosolic component of the activation complex of the NADPH oxidase to contain src homology 3 domains. *Biochem J* **296**:557, 1993.
102. Tsunawaki S, Mizunari H, Nagata M, Tatsuzawa O, Kuratsuji T: A novel cytosolic component, $p40^{phox}$, of respiratory burst oxidase associates with $p67^{phox}$ and is absent in patients with chronic granulomatous disease who patients with chronic granulomatous disease who lack $p67^{phox}$. *Biochem Biophys Res Commun* **199**:1378, 1994.
103. Tsunawaki S, Kagara S, Yoshikawa K, Yoshida L, Kuratsuji T, Namiki H: Involvement of p40*phox* in activation of phagocyte NADPH oxidase through association of its carboxyl-terminal, but not its amino-terminal, with p67*phox*. *J Exp Med* **184**:893, 1996.
104. Volpp B, Nauseef WM, Donelson JE, Moser DR, Clark RA: Cloning of the cDNA and functional expression of the 47-kilodalton cytosolic component of human neutrophil respiratory burst oxidase. *Proc Natl Acad Sci USA* **86**:7195, 1989.
105. Leto TL, Lomax KJ, Volpp BD, Nunoi H, Sechler JMG, Nauseef WM, Clark RA, et al.: Cloning of a 67-kD neutrophil oxidase factor with similarity to a non-catalytic region of $p60^{c\text{-}src}$. *Science* **248**:727, 1990.
106. Rodaway ARF, Teahan CG, Casimir CM, Segal AW, Bentley DL: Characterization of the 47-kilodalton autosomal chronic granulomatous disease protein: tissue-specific expression and transcriptional control by retinoic acid. *Mol Cell Biol* **10**:5388, 1990.
107. Lomax KJ, Leto TL, Nunoi H, Gallin JI, Malech HL: Recombinant 47-kilodalton cytosol factor restores NADPH oxidase in chronic granulomatous disease. *Science* **245**:409, 1989.
108. Francke U, Hsieh C-L, Foellmer B, Lomax K, Malech H, Leto T: Genes for two autosomal recessive forms of chronic granulomatous disease assigned to Iq25 (*NCF2*) and 7q11.23 (*NCFI*). *Am J Hem Genet* **47**:483, 1990.
109. Clark R, Volpp B, Leidal K, Nauseef W: Two cytosolic components of the human neutrophil respiratory burst oxidase translocate to the plasma membrane during cell activation. *J Clin Invest* **85**:714, 1990.
110. Nauseef W, Volpp B, McCormick S, Leidal K, Clark R: Assembly of the neutrophil respiratory burst oxidase. *J Biol Chem* **266**:5911, 1991.
111. Park M, Imajoh-Ohmi S, Nunoi H, Kanegasaki S: Synthetic peptides corresponding to various hydrophilic regions of the large subunit of cytochrome b_{558} inhibit superoxide generation in a cell-free system from neutrophils. *Biochem Biophys Res Commun* **234**:531, 1997.
112. DeLeo F, Yu L, Burritt J, Loetterle L, Bond C, Jesaitis A, Quinn M: Mapping sites of interaction of p447-phox and flavocytochrome *b* with a random-sequence peptide phage display library. *Proc Natl Acad Sci USA* **92**:7110, 1995.
113. Han C, Freeman J, Lee T, Notalebi S, Lambeth D: Regulation of the neutrophil respiratory burst oxidase: Identification of an activation domain in p67phox. *J Biol Chem* **273**:16663, 1998.
114. De Leo F, Ulman K, Davis A, Jutila K, Quinn M: Assembly of the human neutrophil NADPH oxidase involves binding of $p67^{phox}$ and flavocytochrome *b* to a common functional domain in $p47^{phox}$. *J Biol Chem* **271**:17013, 1996.
115. Heyworth P, Curnutte J, Nauseef W, Volpp B, Pearson D, Rosen H, Clark R: Neutrophil nicotinamide adenine dinucleotide phosphate oxidase assembly. *J Clin Invest* **87**:321, 1991.
116. Bolscher B, van Zwieten R, Kramer I, Weening R, Verhoeven A, Roos D: A phosphoprotein of Mr 47,000, defective in autosomal chronic granulomatous disease, copurifies with one of two soluble components required for NADPH:O_2 oxidoreductase activity in human neutrophils. *J Clin Invest* **83**:757, 1989.

117. Heyworth P, Badwey J: Continuous phosphorylation of both the 47 and the 49 kDa proteins occurs during superoxide production by neutrophils. *Biochem Biophys Acta* **1052**:299, 1990.
118. El Benna J, My-Chan Dang P, Gaudry M, Fay M, Morel F, Hakim J, Gougerot-Pocidalo M: Phosphorylation of the respiratory burst oxidase subunit p67^{phox} during human neutrophil activation. *J Biol Chem* **272**:17204, 1997.
119. Heyworth P, Ding J, Erickson R, Lu D, Curnutte J, Badwey J: Protein phosphorylation in neutrophils from patients with p67-*phox*-deficient chronic granulomatous disease. *Blood* **87**:4404, 1996.
120. Segal AW, Heyworth PG, Cockcroft S, Barrowman MM: Stimulated neutrophils from patients with autosomal recessive chronic granulomatous disease fail to phosphorylate a Mr-44,000 protein. *Nature* **316**:547, 1985.
121. Dusi S, Rossi F: Activation of NADPH oxidase of human neutrophils involves the phosphorylation and the translocation of cytosolic p67phox. *Biochem J* **1**:296, 1993.
122. El Benna J, Faust R, Johnson J, Babior B: Phosphorylation of the respiratory burst oxidase subunit p47phox as determined by two-dimensional phosphopeptide mapping. Phosphorylation by protein kinase C, protein kinase A, and a mitogen-activated protein kinase. *J Biol Chem* **271**:6374, 1996.
123. Inanami O, Johnson J, McAdara J, El Benna J, Faust L, Newburger P, Babior B: Activation of the leukocyte NADPH oxidase by phorbos ester requires the phosphorylation of p47^{PHOX} on serine 303 or 304. *J Biol Chem* **273**:9539, 1998.
124. Faust LRP, El Benna J, Babior BM, Chanock SJ: The phosphorylation targets of p47^{phox}, a subunit of the respiratory burst oxidase. *J Clin Invest* **96**:1499, 1995.
125. Freeman J, Lambeth J: NADPH oxidase activity is independent of p47*phox in vitro*. *J Biol Chem* **271**:22578, 1996.
126. Koshkin V, Lotan O, Pick E: The cytosolic component p47*phox* is not a *sine qua non* participant in the activation of NADPH oxidase but is required for optimal superoxide production. *J Biol Chem* **271**:30326, 1996.
127. Woodman R, Ruedi J, Jesaitis A, Okamura N, Quinn M, Smith R, Curnutte J, et al.: Respiratory burst oxidase and three of four oxidase-related polypeptides are associated with the cytoskeleton of human neutrophils. *J Clin Invest* **87**:1345, 1991.
128. Knaus U, Heyworth P, Evans T, Curnutte J, Bokoch G: Regulation of phagocyte oxygen radical production by the GTP-binding protein rac 2. *Science* **254**:1512, 1991.
129. Mizuno T, Kaibuchi K, Ando S, Musha T, Hiraoka K, Takaishi K, Asada M, et al.: Regulation of the superoxide-generating NADPH oxidase by a small GTP-binding protein and its stimulatory and inhibitory GDP/GTP exchange proteins. *J Biol Chem* **267**:10215, 1992.
130. Peveri P, Heyworth P, Curnutte J: Absolute requirement for GTP in activationof human neutrophil NADPH oxidase in cell-free system: Role of ATP in regenerating GTP. *Proc Natl Acad Sci USA* **89**:2494, 1992.
131. Uhlinger D, Burnham D, Lambell J: Nucleotide triphosphade requirements for superoxide generation and phosphorylation in a cell-free system from human neutrophils: Sodium dodecyl sulfate and diacylglycerol activate independently of protein kinase C. *J Biol Chem* **266**:20990, 1991.
132. Gabig T, English D, Akard L, Schell M: Regulation of neutrophil NADPH oxidase activation in a cell-free system by guanine nucleotides and fluoride. *J Biol Chem* **262**:1685, 1987.
133. Doussiere J, Pilloud M, Vignais P: Activation of bovine neutrophil oxidase in a cell free system. GTP-dependent formation of a complex between a cytosolic factor and a membrane protein. *Biochem Biophys Res Commun* **152**:993, 1988.
134. Bokoch G, Prossnitz V: Isoprenoid metabolism is required for stimulation of the respiratory burst oxidase of HL-60 cells. *J Clin Invest* **89**:402, 1992.
135. Didsbury J, Iyer S, Menard L, Casey P, Tomhave E, Snyderman R, Clark R, et al.: Activation of the NADPH oxidase system in human neutrophils by the rasrelated GTP-binding protein RAC1. *Clin Res* **40**:192A, 1992.
136. Ando S, Kaibuchi K, Sasaki T, Hiraoka K, Nishiyama T, Mizuno T, Asada M, et al.: Post-translational processing of rac p21s is important both for their interaction with the GDP/GTP exchange proteins and for their activation of NADPH oxidase. *J Biol Chem* **267**:25709, 1992.
137. Ueda T, Kikuchi A, Ohga N, Yamamoto J, Takai Y: Purification and characterization from bovine brain cytosol of a novel regulatory protein inhibiting the dissociation of GDP from and the subsequent binding of GTP to rhoB p20, a ras p21-like GTP binding protein. *J Biol Chem* **265**:9373, 1990.
138. Diekmann D, Abo A, Johnston C, Segal A, Hall A: Interaction of Rac with p67phox and regulation of phagocytic NADPH oxidase activity. *Science* **265**:531, 1994.
139. Nisimoto Y, Freeman J, Motalebi S, Hirshberg M, Lambeth D: Rac Binding to p67^{phox}. *J Biol Chem* **272**:18834, 1997.
140. Dorseuil O, Reibel L, Bokoch G, Camonis J, Gacon G: The Rac target NADPH oxidase p67^{phox} interacts preferentially with Rac2 rather than Rac1. *J Biol Chem* **271**:83, 1996.
141. Heyworth P, Bohl B, Bokoch G, Curnutte J: Rac Translocates independently of the neutrophil NADPH oxidase components p47^{phox} and p67^{phox}. *J Biol Chem* **269**:30749, 1994.
142. Heyworth P, Knaus U, Xu X, Uhlinger D, Conroy L, Bokoch G, Curnutte J: Requirement for posttranslational processing of rac gtp-binding proteins for activation of human neutrophil NADPH oxidase. *Mol Biol Cell* **4**:261, 1993.
143. Dorseuil O, Vazquez A, Lang P, Bertoglio J, Gacon G, Leca G: Inhibition of superoxide production in B lymphocytes by rac antisense oligonucleotides. *J Biol Chem* **267**:20540, 1992.
144. Roberts AW, Kim C, Zhen L, Lowe JB, Kapur R, Petryniak B, Spaetti A, Pollock J, Borneo JB, Bradford GB, Atkinson SJ, Dinauer MC Williams DA: Deficiency of the hematopoietic cell-specific Rho-family GTPase, Rac2, is characterized by abnormalities in neutrophil function and host defense. *Immunity* **10**:183, 1999.
145. Quinn M, Parkos C, Walker L, Orkin S, Dinauer M, Jesaitis A: Association of a ras-related protein with cytochrome *b* of human neutrophils. *Nature* **342**:198, 1989.
146. Quinn M, Mullen M, Jesaitis A, Linner J: Subcellular distribution of the Rap1A protein in human neutrophils: Colocalization and cotranslocation with cytochrome b_{559}. *Blood* **79**:1563, 1992.
147. Bokoch G, Quilliam L, Bohl B, Jesaitis A, Quinn M: Inhibition of rap1A binding cytochrome b_{558} of NADPH oxidase by phosphorylation of rap1A. *Science* **254**:1794, 1991.
148. Bokoch GM: Chemoattractant signaling and leukocyte activation. *Blood* **86**:1649, 1995.
149. Mandeville J, Maxfield F: Calcium and signal transduction in granulocytes. *Curr Opin Hematol* **3**:63, 1996.
150. Downey G, Fukushima T, Fialkow L: Signaling mechanisms in human neutrophils. *Curr Opin Hematol* **2**:76, 1995.
151. Cockcroft S: Phospholipid signaling in leukocytes. *Curr Opin in Hematology* **3**:48, 1996.
152. Toker A, Cantley L: Signaling through the lipid products of phosphoinositide-3-OH kinase. *Nature* **387**:673, 1997.
153. Lew PD: Receptors and intracellular signaling in human neutrophils. *Am Rev Respir Dis* **141**:5127, 1990.
154. Thelen M, Wirthmueller U: Phospholipases and protein kinases during phagocyte activation. *Curr Opin Immunol* **6**:106, 1994.
155. Huang C-K: Protein kinases in neutrophils: A review. *Membr Biochem* **8**:61, 1989.
156. Berkow RI, Dodson RW: Tyrosine-specific protein phosphorylation during activation of human neutrophils. *Blood* **75**:2445, 1990.
157. Rollet E, Caon AC, Roberge CJ, Liao NW, Malawista SF, McColl SR, Naccache PH: Tyrosine phosphorylation in activated nehuman neutrophils: Comparison of the effects of different classes of agonists and identification of signalling pathways involved. *J Immunol* **153**:353, 1994.
158. Grinstein S, Furuya W, Butler JR, Tseng J: Receptor-mediated activation of multiple serine/threonine kinases in human leukocytes. *J Biol Chem* **268**:20223, 1993.
159. Ding J, Bawdwey JA: Stimulation of neutrophils with a chemoattractant activates several novel protein kinases that can catalyze the phosphorylation of the 47-kDa protein component of the phagocyte oxidase and the myristoylated alanine-rich C kinase substrate. *J Biol Chem* **268**:17326, 1993.
160. Perez HD: Chemoattractant receptors. *Curr Opin Hematol* **1**:40, 1994.
161. Borregaard N, Cowland J: Granules of the human neutrophilic polymorphonuclear leukocyte. *Blood* **89**:3503, 1997.
162. Tenen D, Hromas R, Licht J, Zhang D-E: Transcription factors, normal myeloid development, and leukemia. *Blood* **90**:489, 1997.
163. Sigurdsson F, Khanna-Gupta A, Lawson N, Berliner N: Control of late neutrophil-specific gene expression: Insights into regulation of myeloid differentiation. *Semin Hematol* **34**:303, 1997.
164. Lievens P, Donady J, Tufarelli C, Neufeld E: Repressor activity of CCAAT displacement protein in HL-60 myeloid leukemia cells. *J Biol Chem* **270**:12745, 1995.

165. Skalnik DG, Strauss EC, Orkin SH: CCAAT displacement protein as a repressor of the myelomonocytic-specific gp91-phox gene promoter*. *J Biol Chem* **266**:16736, 1991.
166. Eklund E, Skalnik D: Characterization of a gp91-phox promoter element that is required for interferon gamma-induced transcription. *J Biol Chem* **270**:8267, 1995.
167. Eklund E, Jalava A, Kakar R: PU.1, interferon regulatory factor 1, and interferon consensus sequence-binding protein cooperate to increase gp91(phox) expression. *J Biol Chem* **273**:13957, 1998.
168. Suzuki S, Kumatori A, Haagen I, Fujii Y, Sadat M, Jun H, Tsuji Y, et al.: PU.1 as an essential activator for the expression of gp91phox gene in human peripheral neutrophils, monocytes, and B lymphocytes. *Proc Natl Acad Sci USA* **95**:6085, 1998.
169. Newburger P, Skalnik D, Hopkins P, Eklund E, Curnutte J: Mutations in the promoter region of the gene gp91-*phox* in X-linked chronic granulomatous disease with decreased expression of cytochrome b_{558}. *J Clin Invest* **94**:1205, 1994.
170. Li S-L, Valente A, Zhao S-J, Clark R: PU.1 is essential for *p47phox* promoter activity in myeloid cells. *J Biol Chem* **272**:17802, 1997.
171. Yu L, Zhen L, Dinauer M: Biosynthesis of the phagocyte NADPH oxidase cytochrome b558. Role of hem incorporation and heterodimer formation in maturation and stability of gp91phox and p22phox subunits. *J Biol Chem* **272**:27288, 1997.
172. Cassatella M, Bazzoni F, Flynn R, Dusi S, Trinchieri G, Rossi F: Molecular basis of interferon-g and lipopolysaccharide enhancement of phagocyte respiratory burst capability. *J Biol Chem* **265**:20241, 1990.
173. Guthrie L, McPhail L, Henson P, Johnston R: Priming of neutrophils for enhanced release of oxygen metabolites by bacterial lipopolysaccharide: evidence for increased activity of the superoxide-producing enzyme. *J Exp Med* **160**:1656, 1984.
174. Forehand J, Pabst M, Phillips W, Johnston R: Lipopolysaccharide priming of human neutrophils for an enhanced respiratory burst: role of intracellular free calcium. *J Clin Invest* **83**:74, 1989.
175. Cassatella M, Della B, Berton G, Rossi F: Activation by gamma interferon of human macrophage capability to produce toxic oxygen molecules is accompanied by decreased Km of the superoxide-generating NADPH oxidase. *Biochem Biophys Res Commun* **132**:908, 1985.
176. Ezekowitz R, Orkin S, Newburger P: Recombinant interferon gamma augments phagocyte superoxide production and X-chronic granulomatous disease gene expression in X-linked variant chronic granulomatous disease. *J Clin Invest* **80**:1009, 1987.
177. Newburger P, Dai Q, Whitney C: In vitro regulation of human phagocyte cytochrome *b* heavy and light chain gene expression by bacterial lipopolysaccharide and recombinant human cytokines. *J Biol Chem* **266**:16171, 1991.
178. Weening R, de Klein A, de Boer M, Roos D: Effect of interferon-g, in vitro and in vivo, on mRNA levels of phagocyte oxidase components. *J Leukoc Biol* **60**:716, 1996.
179. Amezaga M, Bazzoni F, Sorio C, Rossi F, Cassatella M: Evidence for the involvement of distinct signal transduction pathways in the regulation of constitutive and interferon gamma–dependent gene expression of NADPH oxidase components (gp91-phox, p47-phox, and p22-phox) and high-affinity receptor IgG (Fcgammar-I) in human polymorphonuclear leukocytes. *Blood* **79**:735, 1992.
180. The International Chronic Granulomatous Disease Study Group: A controlled trial of interferon gamma to prevent infection in chronic granulomatous disease. *N Engl J Med* **324**:509, 1991.
181. Woodman R, Erickson R, Rae J, Jaffe H, Curnutte J: Prolonged recombinant interferon-g therapy in chronic granulomatous disease: Evidence against enhanced neutrophil oxidase activity. *Blood* **79**:1558, 1992.
182. Michelson A, McCord J, Fridovich I: *Superoxide and Superoxide Dismutases* New York, Academic Press, 1977.
183. Goldstein I, Kaplan H, Edelson H, Weissmann G: Ceruloplasmin: A scavenger of superoxide anion radicals. *J Biol Chem* **254**:4040, 1979.
184. Green T, Fellman J, Eicher A, Pratt K: Antioxidant role and subcellular location of hypotaurine and taurine in human neutrophils. *Biochim Biophys Acta* **1073**:91, 1991.
185. Rokutan K, Thomas J, Johnston R Jr: Phagocytosis and stimulation of the respiratory burst by phorbol diester initiate S-thiolation of specific proteins in macrophages. *J Immunol* **147**:260, 1991.
186. Chance B, Sies H, Boveris A: Hydroperoxide metabolism in mammalian organs. *Physiol Rev* **59**:527, 1979.
187. Roos D, Weening R, Wyss S, Aebi H: Protection of human neutrophils by endogenous catalase: Studies with cells from catalase-deficient individuals. *J Clin Invest* **65**:1515, 1980.
188. O'Donnell-Tormey J, Nathan C, Lanks K, DeBoer C, delaHarpe J: Secretion of pyruvate: An antioxidant defense of mammalian cells. *J Exp Med* **165**:500, 1987.
189. Bast A, Haenen GRMM, Doelman CJA: Oxidants and antioxidants: State of the art. *Am J Med* **91(suppl 3)**:2, 1991.
190. Grisham M, Jefferson M, Melton D, Thomas E: Chlorination of endogenous amines by isolated neutrophils: Ammonia-dependent bactericidal, cytotoxic, and cytolytic activities of the chloramines. *J Biol Chem* **259**:10404, 1984.
191. Agner K: Verdoperoxidase: a ferment isolated from leukocytes. *Acta Physiol Scand* **2(suppl)**:1, 1941.
192. Schultz J: Myeloperoxidase, in Sbarra A, Strauss R (eds): *The Reticuloendothelial System, Biochemistry and Metabolism*. New York, Plenum, 1980, vol 2, p 231.
193. Nauseef W, Olsson I, Stromberg-Arnljots K: Biosynthesis and processing of myeloperoxidase: a marker for myeloid cell differentiation. *Eur J Haematol* **40**:97, 1988.
194. Zgliczynski J: Characteristics of MPO from neutrophils and other peroxidases from different cells, in Sbarra A, Strauss R (eds): *The Reticuloendothelial System, Biochemistry and Metabolism*. New York, Plenum, 1980, vol 2, p 255.
195. Klebanoff S: Myeloperoxidase-halide-hydrogen peroxide antibacterial system. *J Clin Invest* **50**:2226, 1971.
196. Lehrer R: Antifungal effects of peroxidase systems. *J Bacteriol* **95**:2131, 1968.
197. Belding M, Klebanoff S, Ray C: Peroxidase-mediated viricidal systems. *Science* **167**:195, 1970.
198. Clark R, Klebanoff S: Neutrophil-mediated tumor cell cytotoxicity: Role of the peroxidase system. *J Exp Med* **141**:1442, 1975.
199. Clark R, Klebanoff S, Einstein A: Peroxidase–H_2O_2–halide system: Cytotoxic effect on mammalian tumor cells. *Blood* **45**:161, 1975.
200. Kimura S, Kotani T, McBride O, Umeki K, Hirai K, Nakayama T, Ohtaki S: Human thyroid peroxidase: complete cDNA and protein sequence, chromosome mapping, and identification of two alternatively spliced mRNAs. *Proc Natl Acad Sci USA* **84**:5555, 1987.
201. Kimura S, Ikeda-Saito M: Human myeloperoxidase and thyroid peroxidase, two enzymes with separate and distinct physiological functions, are evolutionarily related members of the same gene family. *Proteins* **3**:113, 1988.
202. Zeng J, Fenna R: X-ray crystal structure of canine myeloperoxidase at 3 A resolution. *J Mol Biol* **226**:185, 1992.
203. Johansson M, Lind M, Holmblad T, Thornqvist P-O, Soderhall K: Peroxinectin, a novel cell adhesion protein from crayfish blood. *Biochem Biophys Res Commun* **216**:1079, 1995.
204. Moghaddam A, Rosenzweig M, Lee-Parritz D, Annis B, Johnson R, Wang F: An animal model for acute and persistent Epstein-Barr virus infection. *Science* **276**:2030, 1997.
205. Andersen M, Atkin C, Eyre H: Intact form of myeloperoxidase from normal human neutrophils. *Arch Biochem Biophys* **214**:273, 1982.
206. Andrews P, Krinsky N: The reductive cleavage of myeloperoxidase in half, producing enzymatically active hemi-myeloperoxidase. *J Biol Chem* **256**:4211, 1981.
207. Harrison J, Pabalan S, Schultz J: The subunit structure of crystalline canine myeloperoxidase. *Biochim Biophys Acta* **493**:247, 1977.
208. Nauseef W, Root R, Malech H: Biochemical and immunologic analysis of hereditary myeloperoxidase deficiency. *J Clin Invest* **71**:1297, 1983.
209. Olsson I, Olofsson T, Odeber H: Myeloperoxidase-mediated iodination in granulocytes. *Scand J Haematol* **9**:483, 1972.
210. Yamada M, Mori M, Sugimura T: Purification and characterization of small molecular weight myeloperoxidase forms from human promyelocytic leukemia HL 60 cells. *Biochemistry* **20**:766, 1981.
211. Andrews P, Parnes C, Krinsky N: Comparison of myeloperoxidase and hemi-myeloperoxidase with regard to catalysis, regulation, and bactericidal activity. *Arch Biochem Biophys* **228**:439, 1984.
212. Booth K, Kimura S, Lee H, Ikeda-Saito M, Caughey W: Bovine myeloperoxidase and lactoperoxidase each contain a high affinity binding site for calcium. *Biochem Biophys Res Commun* **160**:897, 1989.
213. Babcock G, Ingle R, Oertling W, Davis J, Averill B, Hulse C, Stufkens D, et al.: Raman characterization of human leukocyte myeloperoxidase and bovine spleen hemoprotein: insight into chromophore structure and evidence that the chromophores of myeloperoxidase are equivalent. *Biochim Biophys Acta* **828**:58, 1985.
214. Ikeda-Saito M, Argade P, Rousseau D: Resonance evidence of chloride binding to the heme iron in myeloperoxidase. *FEBS Lett* **184**:52, 1985.
215. Sibbetts S, Hurst J: Structural analysis of myeloperoxidase by resonance Raman spectroscopy. *Biochemistry* **23**:3007, 1984.

216. Dugad L, LaMar G, Lee H, Ikeda-Saito M, Booth K, Caughey W: A nuclear Overhauser effect study of the active site of myeloperoxidase. Structural similarity of the prosthetic group to that on lactoperoxidase. *J Biol Chem* **265**:7173, 1990.
217. Wever R, Oertling W, Hoogland H, Bolscher B, Kim Y, Babcock G: Denaturation and renaturation of myeloperoxidase. Consequences for the nature of the prosthetic group. *J Biol Chem* **266**:24308, 1991.
218. Sono M, Bracete A, Huff A, Ikeda-Saito M, Dawson J: Evidence that a formyl-substituted iron porphyrin is the prosthetic group of myeloperoxidase: Magnetic circular dichroism similarity of the peroxidase to Spirographies heme reconstituted myoglobin. *Proc Natl Acad Sci USA* **88**:11148, 1991.
219. Lopez-Garriga J, Oertling W, Kean R, Hoogland H, Wever R, Babcock G: Metal-ligand vibrations of cyanoferric myeloperoxidase and cyanoferric horseradish peroxidase: Evidence for a constrained heme pocket in myeloperoxidase. *Biochemistry* **29**:9387, 1990.
220. Fenna R, Zeng J, Davey C: Structure of the green heme in myeloperoxidase. *Arch Biochem Biophys* **316**:653, 1995.
221. Taylor K, Strobel F, Yue K, Ram P, Pohl J, Woods A, Kinkade J Jr: Isolation and identification of a protoheme IX derivative released during autolytic cleavage of human myeloperoxidase. *Arch Biochem Biophys* **316**:635, 1995.
222. Feldberg N, Schultz J: Evidence that myeloperoxidase is composed of isoenzymes. *Arch Biochem Biophys* **148**:407, 1972.
223. Himmelhock S, Evans W, Mage M, Peterson E: Purification of myloperoxidases from the bone marrow of the guinea pig. *Biochemistry* **8**:914, 1969.
224. Schultz J, Feldberg J, John S: Myeloperoxidase, VIII, separation into ten components by free-flow electrophoresis. *Biochem Biophys Res Commun* **28**:543, 1967.
225. Strauven T, Armstrong D, James G, Austin J: Separation of leukocyte peroxidase isoenzymes by agaroseacrylamide disc electrophoresis. *Age* **1**:111, 1978.
226. Nauseef W, Malech H: Immunochemical analysis of myeloperoxidase in normal and MPO-deficient neutrophils and a human promyelocytic cell line. *Clin Res* **30**:560A, 1982.
227. Taylor K, Guzman G, Pohl J, Kinkade J Jr: Distinct chromatographic forms of human hemi-myeloperoxidase obtained by reductive cleavage of the dimeric enzyme. Evidence for subunit heterogeneity. *J Biol Chem* **265**:15938, 1990.
228. Miyasaki K, Wilson M, Cohen E, Jones P, Genco R: Evidence for and partial characterization of three major and three minor chromatographic forms of human neutrophil myeloperoxidase. *Arch Biochem Biophys* **246**:751, 1986.
229. Morita Y, Iwamoto H, Aibara S, Kobayaski T, Hasegawa E: Crystallization and properties of myeloperoxidase from normal human leukocytes. *J Biochem* **99**:761, 1986.
230. Pember S, Fuhrer-Krsi S, Barnes K, Kinkade J: Isolation of three native forms of myeloperoxidase from human polymorphonuclear leukocytes. *FEBS Lett* **140**:103, 1982.
231. Suzuki K, Ota H, Sasagawa S, Sakatani T, Fujikura T: Assay method for myeloperoxidase in human polymorphonuclear leukocytes. *Anal Biochem* **132**:345, 1983.
232. Atkin C, Andersen M, Eyre H: Abnormal neutrophil myeloperoxidase from a patient with chronic myelogenous leukemia. *Arch Biochem Biophys* **214**:284, 1982.
233. Cully J, Harrach B, Hauser H, Harth N, Robenek H, Nagata S, Hasilik A: Synthesis and localization of myeloperoxidase protein in transfected BHK cells. *Exp Cell Res* **180**:440, 1989.
234. Taylor K, Uhlinger D, Kinkade J Jr: Expression of recombinant myeloperoxidase using a baculovirus expression system. *Biochem Biophys Res Commun* **187**:1572, 1992.
235. Moguilevsky N, Garcia-Quintana L, Jacquet A, Tournay C, Fabry L, Pierard L, Bollen A: Structural and biological properties of human recombinant myeloperoxidase produced by Chinese hamster ovary cell lines. *Eur J Biochem* **197**:605, 1991.
236. Jacquet A, Deby C, Mathy M, Moguilevsky N, Deby-Dupont G, Thirion A, Goormaghtigh E, et al.: Spectral and enzymatic properties of human recombinant myeloperoxidase: comparison with the mature enzyme. *Arch Biochem Biophys* **291**:132, 1991.
237. Jacquet A, Deleersnyder V, Garcia-Quintana L, Bollen A, Moguilevsky N: Site-directed mutants of human myeloperoxidase: a topological approach to the heme-binding site. *FEBS Lett* **302**:189, 1992.
238. Grisham M, Jefferson M, Thomas E: Role of monochloramines in the oxidation of erythrocyte hemoglobin by stimulated neutrophils. *J Biol Chem* **259**:6757, 1984.
239. Thomas E, Fishman M: Oxidation of chloride and thiocyanate by isolated leukocytes. *J Biol Chem* **261**:9694, 1986.
240. Thomas E, Jefferson M, Grisham M: Myeloperoxidase-catalyzed incorporation of amino acids into proteins: role of hypochlorous acid and chloramines. *Biochemistry* **21**:6299, 1982.
241. Test S, Lampert M, Ossanna P, Thoene J, Weiss S: Generation of nitrogen-chlorine oxidants by human phagocytes. *J Clin Invest* **74**:1341, 1984.
242. Weiss S, Peppin G, Ortiz X, Ragsdale C, Test S: Oxidative autoactivation of latent collagenase by human neutrophils. *Science* **227**:747, 1985.
243. Weiss S, Regiani S: Neutrophils degrade subendothelial matrices in the presence of alpha-1-protease inhibitor. *J Clin Invest* **73**:1297, 1984.
244. Weiss S, Klein R, Slivka A, Wei M: Chlorination of taurine by human neutrophils. *J Clin Invest* **70**:598, 1982.
245. Weiss S, Slivka A: Monocyte and granulocyte-mediated tumor cell destruction. *J Clin Invest* **69**:225, 1982.
246. Zgliczynski J, Stelmaszynska T: Chlorinating ability of human phagcytosing leukocytes. *Eur J Biochem* **56**:157, 1975.
247. Zgliczynski J, Stelmaszynska T, Domanski J, Ostrowski W: Chloramines as intermediates of oxidation reaction of amino acids by myeloperoxidase. *Biochim Biophys Acta* **235**:419, 1974.
248. Harrison J, Schultz J: Studies on the chlorinating activity of myeloperoxidase. *J Biol Chem* **251**:1371, 1976.
249. Albrich I, McCarthy C, Hurst J: Biological reactivity of hypochlorous acid and implications for microbicidal mechanism of leukocyte myeloperoxidase. *Proc Natl Acad Sci USA* **78**:210, 1981.
250. Rosen H, Klebanorf S: Oxidation of microbial iron-sulfur centers by the MPO–H_2O_2–halide antimicrobial system. *Infect Immun* **47**:613, 1985.
251. Rosen H, Klebanoff S: Oxidation of *Escherichia coli* iron centers by the myeloperoxidase-mediated microbicidal system. *J Biol Chem* **257**:13731, 1982.
252. Rosen H, Michel B, VanDevanter D, Hughes J: Differential effects of myeloperoxidase-derived oxidants on Escherichia coli DNA replication. *Infect Immun* **66**:2655, 1998.
253. Marquez L, Dunford H: Kinetics of oxidation of tyrosine and dityrosine by myeloperoxidase compounds I and II—implications for lipoprotein peroxidation studies. *J Biol Chem* **270**:30434, 1995.
254. Savenkova M, Mueller D, Heinecke J: Tyrosyl radical generated by myeloperoxidase is a physiological catalyst for the initiation of lipid peroxidation in low density lipoprotein. *J Biol Chem* **269**:20394, 1994.
255. Heinecke J, Li W, Francis G, Goldstein J: Tyrosyl radical generated by myeloperoxidase catalyzes the oxidative cross-linking of proteins. *J Clin Invest* **91**:2866, 1993.
256. Domigan N, Charlton T, Duncan M, Winterbourn C, Kettle A: Chlorination of tyrosyl residues in peptides by myeloperoxidase and human neutrophils. *J Biol Chem* **270**:16542, 1995.
257. Sampson J, Rosen H, Beckman J: Peroxynitrite-dependent tyrosine nitration catalyzed by superoxide dismutase, myeloperoxidase, and horseradish peroxidase. *Methods Enzymol* **269**:210, 1996.
258. Winterbourn C, Pichorner H, Kettle A: Myeloperoxidase-dependent generation of a tyrosine peroxide by neutrophils. *Arch Biochem Biophys* **338**:15, 1997.
259. Panasenko O, Evgina S, Aidyraliev R, Sergienko V, Vladimirov Y: Peroxidation of human blood lipoproteins induced by exogenous hypochlorite or hypochlorite generated in the system of "myeloperoxidase+H_2O_2+Cl^-". *Free Radic Biol Med* **16**:143, 1994.
260. Daugherty A, Dunn J, Rateri D, Heinecke J: Myeloperoxidase, a catalyst for lipoprotein oxidation, is expressed in human atherosclerotic lesions. *J Clin Invest* **94**:437, 1994.
261. Hazen S, Hsu F, Duffin K, Heinecke J: Molecular chlorine generated by the myeloperoxidase-hydrogen peroxide-chloride system of phagocytes converts low density lipoprotein cholesterol into a family of chlorinated sterols. *J Biol Chem* **271**:23080, 1996.
262. Jolivalt C, Leininger-Muller B, Drozdz R, Naskalski J, Siest G: Apolipoprotein E is highly susceptible to oxidation by myeloperoxidase, an enzyme present in the brain. *Neurosci Lett* **210**:61, 1996.
263. Floris R, Piersma S, Yang G, Jones P, Wever R: Interaction of myeloperoxidase with peroxynitrite—a comparison with lactoperoxidase, horseradish peroxidase and catalase. *Eur J Biochem* **215**:767, 1993.
264. Eiserich J, Hristova M, Cross C, Jones A, Freeman B, Halliwell B, van der Vliet A: Formation of nitric oxide-derived inflammatory oxidants by myeloperoxidase in neutrophils. *Nature* **391**:393, 1998.

265. Hazell L, Arnold L, Flowers D, Waeg G, Malle E, Stocker R: Presence of hypochlorite-modified proteins in human atherosclerotic lesions. *J Clin Invest* **97**:1535, 1996.
266. Berliner J, Heinecke J: The role of oxidized lipoproteins in atherogenesis. *Free Radic Biol Med* **20**:707, 1996.
267. Petruska J, Mosebrook D, Jakab G, Trush M: Myeloperoxidase-enhanced formation of (±)-*trans*-7, 8-dihydroxy-7, 8-dihydrobenzo [*a*]pyrene-DNA adducts in lung tissue *in vitro*: A role of pulmonary inflammation in the bioactivation of a procarcinogen. *Carcinogenesis* **13**:1075, 1992.
268. Van Rensburg C, Van Staden A, Anderson R, Van Rensburg E: Hypochlorous acid potentiates hydrogen peroxide-mediated DNA-strand breaks in human mononuclear leukocytes. *Mutat Res Fundam Mol Mech Mutagen* **265**:255, 1992.
269. Josephy P: The role of peroxidase-catalyzed activation of aromatic amines in breast cancer. *Mutagen* **11**:3, 1996.
270. Pero R, Sheng Y, Olsson A, Bryngelsson C, Lund-Pero M: Hypochlorous acid/N-chloramines are naturally produced DNA repair inhibitors. *Carcinogenesis* **17**:13, 1996.
271. Reynolds W, Chang E, Douer D, Ball E, Kanda V: An allelic association implicates myeloperoxidase in the etiology of acute promyelocytic leukemia. *Blood* **90**:2730, 1997.
272. Nagra R, Becher B, Tourtellotte W, Antel J, Gold D, Palidino T, Smith R, et al.: Immunohistochemical and genetic evidence of myeloperoxidase involvement in multiple sclerosis. *J Neuroimmunol* **78**:97, 1997.
273. Nathan C: Nitric oxide as a secretory product of mammalian cells. *FASEB J* **6**:3051, 1992.
274. Prince R, Gunson D: Rising interest in nitric oxide synthase. *Trends Biochem Sci* **18**:35, 1993.
275. Marletta MA: Nitric oxide synthase: Aspects concerning structure and catalysis. *Cell* **78**:927, 1994.
276. Nathan C, Xie Q: Nitric oxide synthases: Roles, tolls and controls. *Cell* **78**:915, 1994.
277. MacMicking J, Nathan C, et al.: Altered responses to bacterial infection and endotoxic shock in mice lacking inducible nitric oxide synthase. *Cell* **81**:641, 1995.
278. De Maria R, Cifone MG, Trotta R, Rippo MR, Festucia C, Santoni A, Testi R: Triggering of human monocyte activation through CD69, a member of the NKC family of signal transducing receptors. *J Exp Med* **180**:1999, 1994.
279. Bukrinsky MI, Nottet HSLM, Schmidtmayerova N, Dubrovsky L, Millins ME, Lipton SA, Gendelman HE: Regulation of nitric oxide synthase activity in HIV-1-infected monocytes: Implications for HIV-associated neurological disease. *J Exp Med* **180**, 1994.
280. Dinauer M: The phagocyte system and disorders of granulopoiesis and granulocyte function, in Nathan D, Orkin S (eds): *Hematology of Infancy and Childhood* 5th ed. Philadelphia, WB Saunders, 1998, vol 5, p 889.
281. Finn A, Hadzik N, Morgan G, Strobel S, Levinsky R: Prognosis of chronic granulomatous disease. *Arch Dis Child* **65**:942, 1990.
282. Fischer A, Segal A, Seger R, Weening R: The management of chronic granulomatous disease. *Eur J Pediatr* **152**:896, 1993.
283. Holmes B, Page A, Good R: Studies of the metabolic activity of leukocytes from patients with a genetic abnormality of phagocytic function. *J Clin Invest* **46**:1422, 1967.
284. Curnutte J, Whitten D, Babior B: Defective superoxide production by granulocytes from patients with chronic granulomatous disease. *N Engl J Med* **290**:593, 1974.
285. Davis W, Huber H, Douglas S, Fudenberg H: A defect in circulating mononuclear phagocytes in chronic granulomatous disease of childhood. *J Immunol* **101**:1093, 1968.
286. Rodey G, Park B, Windhorst D, Good R: Defective bactericidal activity of monocytes in fatal granulomatous disease. *Blood* **33**:813, 1969.
287. Lehrer R: Measurement of candidacidal activity of specific leukocyte types in mixed cell populations. II. Normal and chronic granulomatous disease eosinophils. *Infect Immunol* **3**:800, 1971.
288. Janeway C, Craig J, Davidson M, Downey W, Gitlin D, Sullivan J: Hypergammaglobulinemia associated with severe recurrent and chronic non-specific infection. *Am J Dis Child* **88**:388, 1954.
289. Berendes H, Bridges R, Good R: Fatal granulomatosis of childhood: Clinical study of new syndrome. *Minn Med* **40**:309, 1957.
290. Bridges R, Berendes H, Good R: A fatal granulomatous disease of childhood. *Am Med Assoc J Dis Child* **97**:387, 1959.
291. Landing B, Shirkey H: A syndrome of recurrent infection and infiltration of viscera by pigmented lipid histiocytes. *Pediatrics* **20**:431, 1957.
292. Holmes B, Quie P, Windhorst D, Good R: Fatal granulomatous disease of childhood. An inborn abnormality of phagocytic function. *Lancet* **i**:1225, 1966.
293. Beahner R, Nathan D: Quantitative nitroblue tetrazolium test in chronic granulomatous disease. *N Engl J Med* **278**:971, 1968.
294. Newburger P, Cohen H, Rothchild S, Hibbins J, Malawista S, Mahoney M: Prenatal diagnosis of chronic granulomatous disease. *N Engl J Med* **300**:178, 1979.
295. Baehner R, Boxer L, Davis J: The biochemical basis of nitroblue tetrazolium reduction in normal human and chronic granulomatous disease polymorphonuclear leukocytes. *Blood* **48**:309, 1976.
296. Buescher E, Alling D, Gallin J: Use of an X-linked human neutrophil marker to estimate timing of lyonization and size of the dividing stem cell pool. *J Clin Invest* **76**:1581, 1985.
297. Curnutte I, Kipnes R, Barior B: Defect in pyridine nucleotide-dependent superoxide production by a particulate fraction from the granulocytes of patients with chronic granulomatous disease. *N Engl J Med* **293**:628, 1975.
298. Hohn D, Lehrer R: NADPH oxidase deficiency in X-linked chronic granulomatous disease. *J Clin Invest* **55**:707, 1975.
299. McPhail L, Dechatelet L, Shirley P, Wilfert C, Johnston R Jr, McCall C: Deficiency of NADPH oxidase activity in chronic granulomatous disease. *J Pediatr* **90**:213, 1977.
300. Quie P, Kaplan E, Page A, Gruskay F, Malawista S: Defective polymorphonuclear-leukocyte function and chronic granulomatous disease in two female children. *N Engl J Med* **278**:976, 1968.
301. Segal A, Jones O: Novel cytochrome b system in phagocytic vacuoles of human granulocytes. *Nature* **276**:515, 1978.
302. Segal AW, Cross AR, Garcia RC, Borregaard N, Valerius N: Absence of cytochrome b-245 in chronic granulomatous disease: a multicenter European evaluation of its incidence and relevance. *N Engl J Med* **308**:245, 1983.
303. Nunoi H, Rotrosen D, Gallin J, Malech H: Two forms of autosomal chronic granulomatous disease lack distinct neutrophil cytosol factors. *Science* **242**:1298, 1988.
304. Volpp B, Nauseef W, Clark R: Two cytosolic neutrophil oxidase components absent in autosomal chronic granulomatous disease. *Science* **242**:1295, 1988.
305. Clark RA, Malech HL, Gallin JI, Nunoi H, Volpp B, Pearson D, Nauseef W, et al.: Genetic variants of chronic granulomatous disease: prevalence of deficiencies of two cytosolic components of the NADPH oxidase system. *N Engl J Med* **321**:647, 1989.
306. Bottone E, Douglas S, Rausen A, Keusch G: Association of *Pseudomonas cepacia* with chronic granulomatous disease. *J Clin Microbiol* **1**:425, 1975.
307. Speert D, Bond M, Woodman R, Curnutte J: Infection with *Pseudomonas cepacia* in chronic granulomatous disease: Role of nonoxidative killing by neutrophils in host defense. *J Infect Dis* **170**:1524, 1994.
308. Weening R, Adriaansz L, Weemaes C, Lutter R, Roos D: Clinical differences in chronic granulomatous disease inpatients with cytochrome *b*-negative or cytochrome *b* positive neutrophils. *J Pediatr* **107**:102, 1985.
309. Dilworth J, Mandell G: Adults with chronic granulomatous disease of "childhood." *Am J Med* **63**:233, 1977.
310. Schapiro B, Newburger P, Klempner M, Dinauer M: Chronic granulomatous disease in an elderly man: An X-linked cytochrome b positive variant. *N Engl J Med* **325**:1786, 1991.
311. Liese J, Jendrossek V, Jansson A, Petropoulou T, Kloos S, Gahr M, Belohradsky B: Chronic granulomatous disease in adults. *Lancet* **347**:220, 1996.
312. Mandell G, Hook E: Leukocyte bactericidal activity in chronic granulomatous disease: Correlation of bacterial hydrogen peroxide production and susceptibility to intracellular killing. *J Bacteriol* **100**:531, 1969.
313. Johnston R Jr, Newman S: Chronic granulomatous disease. *Pediatr Clin North Am* **24**:365, 1977.
314. Windhorst D, Good R: Dermatologic manifestations of fatal granulomatous disease of childhood. *Arch Dermatol* **103**:351, 1971.
315. Barriere H, Litoux P, Stadler J, Buriot C, Hakim J: Chronic granulomatous disease: Late onset of skin lesions only, in two siblings. *Arch Dermatol* **17**:683, 1981.
316. Stalder J, Dreno B, Bureau B, Hadim J: Discoid lupus erythematosus-like lesions in an autosomal form of chronic granulomatous disease. *Br J Dermatol* **114**:251, 1986.
317. Strate M, Brandrup R, Wand R: Discoid lupus erythematosus-like skin lesions in a patient with autosomal recessive chronic granulomatous disease. *Clin Genet* **30**:184, 1986.

318. Sillevis-Smitt J, Bos J, Weening R, Krieg S: Discoid lupus erythematosus-like skin changes in patients with autosomal recessive chronic granulomatous disease [letter]. *Arch Dermatol* **126**:1656, 1990.
319. Barton L, Johnson C: Discoid lupus erythematosus and X-linked chronic granulomatous disease. *Pediatr Dermatol* **3**:376, 1986.
320. Garioch J, Sampson J, Seywright M, Thomson J: Dermatoses in five related female carriers of X-linked chronic granulomatous disease. *Br J Dermatol* **121**:391, 1989.
321. Yeaman G, Froebel K, Galea G, Ormerod A, Urbaniak S: Discoid lupus erythematosus in an X-linked cytochrome-positive carrier of chronic granulomatous disease. *Br J Dermatol* **126**:60, 1992.
322. Donowitz G, Mandell G: Clinical presentation and unusual infections in chronic granulomatous disease. *Adv Host Defen Mech* **3**:55, 1983.
323. Wolfson J, Quie P, Laxdal S, Good R: Roentgenologic manifestations in children with a genetic defect of polymorphonuclear leukocyte function. *Radiology* **91**:37, 1968.
324. Gold R, Douglas S, Preger L, Steinbach H, Fudenberg H: Roentgenographic features of the neutrophil dysfunction syndrome. *Radiology* **92**:1045, 1969.
325. Pogrebniak H, Gallin J, Malech H, Baker A, Moskaluk C, Travis W, Pas H: Surgical management of pulmonary infections in chronic granulomatous disease of childhood. *Ann Thorac Surg* **55**:844, 1993.
326. Kawashima A, Kuhlman J, Fishman E, Tempany C, Magid D, Lederman H, Winkelstein J, et al.: Pulmonary Aspergillus chest wall involvement in chronic granulomatous disease: CT and MRI findings. *Skel Radiol* **20**:487, 1991.
327. White C, Kwon-Chung K, Gallin J: Chronic granulomatous disease of childhood. An unusual case of infection with *Aspergillus nidulans* var. echinulatus. *Am J Clin Pathol* **90**:312, 1988.
328. Sponseller P, Malech H, McCarthy E Jr, Horowitz S, Jeffe G, Gallin J: Skeletal involvement in children who have chronic granulomatous disease. *J Bone Joint Surg (Am)* **73**:37, 1991.
329. Ament M, Ochs H: Gastrointestinal manifestations of chronic granulomatous disease. *N Engl J Med* **288**:382, 1974.
330. Kelleher D, Bloomfield F, Lenehan T, Griffin M, Geighery C, McCann S: Chronic granulomatous disease presenting as an oculomucocutaneous syndrome mimicking Behcet's syndrome. *Postgrad Med J* **62**:489, 1986.
331. Cohen M, Leong P, Simpson D: Phagocytic cells in periodontal defense. Periodontal status of patients with chronic granulomatous disease of childhood. *J Periodontol* **56**:611, 1985.
332. Dusi S, Poli G, Berton G, Catalano P, Fornasa C, Peserico A: Chronic granulomatous disease in an adult female with granulomatous cheilitis. Evidence for an X-linked pattern of inheritance with extreme lyonization. *Acta Haematol (Basel)* **84**:49, 1990.
333. Renner W, Johnson J, Lichtenstein J, Kirks D: Esophageal inflammation and sticture: complication of chronic granulomatous disease of childhood. *Radiology* **178**:189, 1991.
334. Dickerman J, Colletti R, Tampas J: Gastric outlet obstruction in chronic granulomatous disease of childhood. *Am J Dis Child* **140**:567, 1986.
335. Granot E, Matoth I, Korman S, Ludomirsky A, Lax E: Functional gastrointestinal obstruction in a child with chronic granulomatous disease. *J Pediatr Gastroenterol Nutr* **5**:321, 1986.
336. Fisher J, Khan A, Heitlinger L, Allen J, Afshani E: Chronic granulomatous disease of childhood with acute ulcerative colitis: A unique association. *Pediatr Pathol* **7**:91, 1987.
337. Rossi T, Cumella J, Baswell D, Park B: Ascites as a presenting sign of peritonitis in chronic granulomatous disease of childhood. *Clin Pediatr (Philadelphia)* **26**:544, 1987.
338. Forrest C, Forehand J, Axtell R, Roberts R, Johnston R Jr: Clinical features and current management of chronic granulomatous disease. *Hematol Oncol Clin North Am* **2**:253, 1988.
339. Griscom NT, Kirkpatrick JA Jr, Girdany BR, Berdon WE, Grand RJ, Mackie GG: Gastric antral narrowing in chronic granulomatous disease of childhood. *Pediatrics* **54**:456, 1974.
340. Bowen A, III, Gibson M: Chronic granulomatous disease with gastric antral narrowing. *Pediatr Radiol* **10**:119, 1980.
341. Sty J, Chusid M, Babbitt D, Werlin S: Involvement of the colon in chronic granulomatous disease of childhood. *Radiology* **132**:618, 1979.
342. Mulholland M, Delaney J, Simmons R: Gastrointestinal complications of chronic granulomatous disease: surgical implications. *Surgery* **94**:569, 1983.
343. Tauber A, Borregaard N, Simons E, Wright J: Chronic granulomatous disease: A syndrome of phagocyte oxidase deficiencies. *Medicine (Baltimore)* **62**:286, 1983.
344. Wolfson J, Kane W, Laxdal S, Good R, Quie P: Bone findings in chronic granulomatous disease of childhood. *J Bone Joint Surg (Am)* **51**:1573, 1969.
345. Heinrich S, Finney T, Craver R, Yin L, Zembo M: Aspergillus osteomyelitis in patients who have chronic granulomatous disease. Case report. *J Bone Joint Surg (Am)* **73**:456, 1991.
346. Aliabadi H, Gonzalex R, Quie P: Urinary tract disorders in patients with chronic granulomatous disease. *N Engl J Med* **321**:706, 1989.
347. Walther M, Malech H, Berman A, Choyke P, Venzon D, Linehan W, Gallin J: The urological manifestations of chronic granulomatous disease. *J Urol* **147**:1314, 1991.
348. Cyr W, Johnson H, Balfour J: Granulomatous cystitits as a manifestation of chronic granulomatous disease of childhood. *J Urol* **110**:357, 1973.
349. Young A, Middleton R: Urologic manifestations of chronic granulomatous disease of infancy. *J Urol* **123**:119, 1980.
350. Kontras S, Bodenbender J, McClave C, Smith J: Interstitial cystitis as a manifestation of chronic granulomatous disease. *Clin Exp Immunol* **43**:390, 1981.
351. vanRhenen D, Koolen M, Feltkamp-Vroom T, Weening R: Immune complex glomerulonephritis in chronic granulomatous disease. *Acta Med Complex* **206**:233, 1979.
352. Frifelt J, Schonheyder H, Valerius N, Strate M, Starklint H: Chronic granulomatous disease associated with chronic glomerulonephritis. *Acta Paediatr Scand* **74**:152, 1985.
353. Forbes G, Hartman G, Burke E, Segura J: Genitourinary involvement in chronic granulomatous disease of childhood. *AJR* **127**:683, 1976.
354. Bloomberg S, Neu H, Ehrlich R, Blanc W: Chronic granulomatous disease of childhood with renal involvement. *Urology* **4**:193, 1974.
355. Fleischmann J, Church J, Lehrer R: Case report: primary *Candida* meningitis and chronic granulomatous disease. *Am J Med Sci* **291**:334, 1986.
356. Lazarus G, Heu H: Agents responsible for infection in chronic granulomatous disease of childhood. *J Pediatr* **86**:415, 1975.
357. Martyne L, Lischner H, Pilaggi A, Harley R: Chorioretinal lesions in familial chronic granulomatous disease of childhood. *Am J Ophthalmol* **73**:403, 1972.
358. Halazun J, Lukens J: Thyrotoxicosis associated with aspergillus thyroiditis in chronic granulomatous disease. *J Pediatr* **80**:106, 1972.
359. Walker D, Okiye G: Chronic granulomatous disease involving the central nervous system. *Pediatr Pathol* **1**:159, 1983.
360. Mouy R, Fisher A, Vilmer E, Seger R, Griscelli C: Incidence, severity, and prevention of infections in chronic granulomatous disease. *J Pediatr* **114**:555, 1989.
361. Forrest CB, Forehand JR, Axtell RA, Roberts RL, Johnston J, RB: Clinical features and current management of chronic granulomatous disease. *Hematol Oncol Clin North Am* **2**:253, 1988.
362. Margolis DM, Melnic DA, Alling DW, Gallin JI: Trimethoprim-sulfamethoxazole prophylaxis in the management of chronic granulomatous disease. *J Infect Dis* **162**:723, 1990.
363. Miyazaki S, Shin H, Goya N, Nakagawara A: Identification of a carrier mother of a female patient with chronic granulomatous disease. *J Pediatr* **89**:784, 1976.
364. Mills E, Rholl K, Quie P: X-linked inheritance in females with chronic granulomatous disease. *J Clin Invest* **66**:332, 1980.
365. Johnston RB 3d, Harbeck RJ, Johnston RB Jr: Recurrent severe infections in a girl with apparently variable expression of mosaicism for chronic granulomatous disease. *J Pediatr* **106**:50, 1985.
366. Oez S, Birkmann J, Kalden J: Clonal growth of functionally normal and deficient neutrophils from the bone marrow of a patient with variant chronic granulomatous disease. *Ann Hematol* **66**:21, 1993.
367. Bolscher B, de Boer M, de Klein A, Weening R, Roos D: Point mutations in the b-subunit of cytochrome *b* 558 leading to X-linked chronic granulomatous disease. *Blood* **77**:2482, 1991.
368. Curnutte J, Hopkins P, Kuhl W, Beutler E: Studying X inactivation. *Lancet* **339**:749, 1992.
369. Newburger P, Malawista S, Dinauer M, Gelbart T, Woodman R, Chada S, Shen Q, et al.: Chronic granulomatous disease and glutathione peroxidase deficiency, revisited. *Blood* **84**:3861, 1994.
370. Johnston R Jr: Unusual forms of an uncommon disease (chronic granulomatous disease). *J Pediatr* **88**:172, 1976.
371. Hadfield M, Ghatak N, Laine F, Myer E, Massie F, Kramer W: Brain lesions in chronic granulomatous disease. *Acta Neuropathol (Berl)* **81**:467, 1991.
372. Ochs H, Igo R: The NBT slide test: A simple screening method for detecting chronic granulomatous disease and female carriers. *J Pediatr* **83**:77, 1973.

373. Repine J, Rasmussen B, White J: An improved nitroblue tetrazolium test using phorbol myristate acetate-coated coverslips. *Am J Clin Pathol* **71**:582, 1979.
374. Johnston RI, Harbeck R, Jonhston RI: Recurrent severe infection is a girl with apparently variable expression of mosaicism for chronic granulomatous disease. *J Pediatr* **106**:50, 1985.
375. Meerhof LJ, Roos D: Heterogeneity in chronic granulomatous disease detected with an improved nitroblue tetrazolium slide test. *J Leukoc Biol* **39**:699, 1986.
376. Bass D, Parce J, Dechatelet L, Szejda P, Seeds M, Thomas M: Flow cytometric studies of oxidative product formation by neutrophils: A graded response to membrane stimulation. *J Immunol* **130**:1910, 1983.
377. Woodman R, Newburger P, Anklesaria P, Erickson R, Rae J, Cohen M, Curnutte J: A new X-linked variant of chronic granulomatous disease characterized by the existence of a normal clone of respiratory burst-competent phagocytic cells. *Blood* **85**:231, 1995.
378. Johnston R Jr: Measurement of O_2 secreted by monocytes and macrophages. *Methods Enzymol* **105**:365, 1984.
379. Absolom D: Basic methods for the study of phagocytosis. *Methods Enzymol* **132**:147, 1987.
380. Baggiolini M, Ruch W, Cooper P: Measurement of hydrogen peroxide production by phagocytes using homovanillic acid and horseradish peroxidase. *Methods Enzymol* **132**:395, 1987.
381. Hasui M, Hirabayashi Y, Hattori K, Kobayashi Y: Increased phagocytic activity of polymorphonuclear leukocytes of chronic granulomatous disease as determined with flow cytometric assay. *J Lab Clin Med* **117**:291, 1991.
382. Matthay K, Golbus M, Wara D, Mentzer W: Prenatal diagnosis of chronic granulomatous disease. *Am J Med Genet* **17**:731, 1984.
383. Levinsky R, Harvey B, Nicolaides K, Rodeck C: Antenatal diagnosis of chronic granulomatous disease. *Lancet* **1**:504, 1986.
384. Daffos F, Capella-Pavlovsky M, Forestier F: Fetal blood sampling during pregnancy with use of a needle guided by ultrasound: a study of 606 consecutive cases. *Am J Obstet Gynecol* **153**:655, 1985.
385. Golbus M, McGonigle K, Goldberg J, Filly R, Callen P, Anderson R: Fetal tissue sampling. The San Francisco experience with 190 pregnancies. *West J Med* **150**:423, 1989.
386. Lindlof M, Kere J, Ristola M, Repo H, Leirisalo-Repo M, VonKoskull H, Ammala P, et al.: Prenatal diagnosis of X-linked chronic granulomatous disease using restriction fragment length polymorphism analysis. *Genomics* **1**:87, 1987.
387. DeBoer M, Bolscher B, Sijmons R, Scheffer H, Weening R, Roos D: Prenatal diagnosis in a family with X-linked chronic granulomatous disease with the use of the polymerase chain reaction. *Prenat Diagn* **12**:773, 1992.
388. Pelham A, O'Reilly M-A, Malcolm S, Levinsky R, Kinnon C: RFLP and deletion analysis for X-linked chronic granulomatous disease using the cDNA probe: potential for improved prenatal diagnosis and carrier determination. *Blood* **76**:820, 1990.
389. Kenney R, Malech H, Epstein N, Roberts R, Leto T: Characterization of the p67phox gene: genomic organization and restriction fragment length polymorphism analysis for prenatal diagnosis in chronic granulomatous disease. *Blood* **82**:3739, 1993.
390. Hossle J, de Boer M, Seger R, Roos D: Identification of allele-specific p22-phox mutations in a compound heterozygous patient with chronic granulomatous disease by mismatch PCR and restriction enzyme analysis. *Hum Genet* **93**:437, 1994.
391. D'Alton M, Decharney A: Prenatal diagnosis. *N Engl J Med* **328**:114, 1993.
392. Ward P, Schlegel R: Impaired leukotactic responsiveness in a child with recurrent infections. *Lancet* **2**:344, 1969.
393. Clark R, Klebanoff S: Chronic granulomatous disease: Studies of a family with impaired neutrophil chemotactic, metabolic and bactericidal function. *Am J Med* **65**:941, 1978.
394. Margolis D, Melnick D, Alling D, Gallin J: Trimethoprim-sulfamethoxazole prophylaxis in the management of chronic granulomatous disease. *J Infect Dis* **162**:723, 1990.
395. Johnston R Jr, Wilfert C, Buckley R, Webb L, Dechatelet L, McCall C: Enhanced bactericidal activity of phagocytes from patients with chronic granulomatous disease in the presence of sulfisoxazole. *Lancet* **1**:824, 1975.
396. Gmunder F, Segar R: Chronic granulomatous disease: mode of action of sulfamethoxazole/trimethoprim. *Pediatr Res* **15**:1533, 1981.
397. Ezer G, Soothill J: Intracellular bactericidal effects of rifampicin in both normal and chronic granulomatous disease polymorphs. *Arch Dis Child* **49**:463, 1974.
398. Philippart A, Colodny A, Baehner R: Continuous antibiotic therapy in chronic granulomatous disease: Preliminary communication. *Pediatrics* **50**:923, 1972.
399. Mouy R, Veber F, Blanche S, Donadieu J, Brauner R, Levron JC, Griscelli C, et al.: Long-term itraconazole prophylaxis against *Aspergillus* infections in thirty-two patients with chronic granulomatous disease. *J Pediatr* **125**:998, 1994.
400. Mouy R, Fischer A, Vilmer E, Seger R, Griscelli C: Incidence, severity, and prevention of infections in chronic granulomatous disease. *J Pediatr* **114**:555, 1989.
401. Steinbeck M, Roth J: Neutrophil activation by recombinant cytokines. *Rev Infect Dis* **11**:549, 1989.
402. Gallin J, Malech H: Update on chronic granulomatous diseases of childhood: Immunotherapy and potential for gene therapy. *JAMA* **263**:1533, 1990.
403. Ezekowitz R, Dinauer M, Jaffe H, Orkin S, Newburger P: Partial correction of the phagocyte defect in patients with X-linked chronic granulomatous disease b subcutaneous interferon gamma. *N Engl J Med* **319**:146, 1988.
404. Sechler J, Malech H, White C, Gallin J: Recombinant human interferon-γ reconstitutes defective phagocyte function in patients with chronic granulomatous disease of childhood. *Proc Natl Acad Sci USA* **85**:4874, 1988.
405. Muhlebach T, Gabay J, Nathan C, Erny C, Dopfer G, Schroten H, Wahn V, et al.: Treatment of patients with chronic granulomatous disease with recombinant human interferon-gamma does not improve neutrophil oxidative metabolism, cytochrome b_{558} content or levels of four antimicrobial proteins. *Clin Exp Immunol* **88**:203, 1992.
406. Rex J, Bennett J, Gallin J, Malech H, Melnick D: Normal and deficient neutrophils can cooperate to damage *Aspergillus fumigatus* hyphae. *J Infect Dis* **162**:523, 1990.
407. Bernhisel-Broadbent J, Camargo E, Jaffe H, Lederman H: Recombinant human interferon-gamma as adjunct therapy for Aspergillus infection in a patient with chronic granulomatous disease. *J Infect Dis* **163**:908, 1991.
408. Chusid M, Tomasulo P: Survival of transfused normal granulocytes in a patient with chronic granulomatous disease. *Pediatrics* **61**:556, 1978.
409. Pedersen F, Johansen K, Rosenkvist J, Tygstrup I, Valerius N: Refractory *Pneumocystis carinii* infection in chronic granulomatous disease: Successful treatment with granulocytes. *Pediatrics* **64**:935, 1979.
410. Chusid M, Shea M, Sarff L: Determination of posttransfusion granulocyte kinetics by chemiluminescence in chronic granulomatous disease. *J Lab Clin Med* **95**:168, 1980.
411. Tomtovian R, Abramson J, Quie P, McCullough J: Granulocyte transfusion therapy in chronic granulomatous disease: report of 2 patients and review of the literature. *Transfusion* **21**:739, 1981.
412. Buescher E, Gallin J: Leukocyte transfusions in chronic granulomatous disease. *N Engl J Med* **307**:800, 1982.
413. Elliot G, Clay M, Mills E, Abramson J, McCullough J, Quie P: Granulocyte transfusion kinetics measured by chemiluminescence, nitroblue tetrazolium reduction, and recovery of indium-111-labeled granulocytes. *Transfusion* **27**:23, 1987.
414. Quie P: The white cells: use of granulocyte transfusions. *Rev Infect Dis* **9**:189, 1987.
415. Depalma L, Leitman S, Carter C, Gallin J: Granulocyte transfusion therapy in a child with chronic granulomatous disease and multiple red cell alloantibodies. *Transfusion* **29**:421, 1989.
416. Redman C, Marsh L: The Kell Blood Group System and the McLeod Phenotype. *Semin Hematol* **30**:209, 1993.
417. Brzica S, Rhodes K, Pineda A, Taswell H: Chronic granulomatous disease and the McLeod phenotype: Successful treatment of infection with granulocyte transfusions resulting in subsequent hemolytic transfusion reaction. *Mayo Clin Proc* **52**:153, 1977.
418. Chin T, Steim E, Falloon J, Gallin J: Corticosteroid in treatment of obstructive lesions of chronic granulomatous disease. *J Pediatr* **111**:349, 1987.
419. Collman R, Dickerman J: Corticosteroids in the management of cystitis secondary to chronic granulomatous disease. *Pediatrics* **85**:219, 1990.
420. Danziger R, Goren A, Becker J, Greene J, Douglas S: Outpatient management with oral corticosteroid therapy for obstructive conditions in chronic granulomatous disease. *J Pediatr* **122**:303, 1993.
421. Quie P, Belani K: Corticosteroids for chronic granulomatous disease. *J Pediatr* **111**:393, 1987.
422. Rappeport J, Newburger P, Goldblum P, Goldman A, Nathan D, Parkman R: Allogeneic bone marrow transplantation for chronic granulomatous disease. *J Pediatr* **101**:952, 1982.

423. Kamani N, August C, Douglas S, Burkry E, Etzioni A, Lischner H: Bone marrow transplantation in chronic granulomatous disease. *J Pediatr* **105**:42, 1984.
424. Kamani N, August C, Rausen A, D'Angio G, Douglas S: Marrow transplantation (BMT) form a heterozygous carrier donor in chronic granulomatous disease (CGD). *Pediatr Res* **19**:276A, 1985.
425. DiBartolomeo P, DiGirolamo G, Angrilli F, Schettini F, DeMattia D, Manzionna M, Dragani A, et al.: Reconstitution of normal neutrophil function in chronic granulomatous disease by bone marrow transplantation. *Bone Marrow Transplant* **4**:695, 1989.
426. Hobbs J, Monteil M, McCluskey D, Jurges E, AlTumi M: Chronic granulomatous disease: 100% corrected by displacement bone marrow transplantation from a volunteer unrelated donor. *Eur J Pediatr* **151**:806, 1992.
427. Kamani N, August CS, Campbell DE, Hassan NF, Douglas SD: Marrow transplantation in chronic granulomatous disease: An update, with 6-year follow-up. *J Pediatr* **113**:697, 1988.
428. Calvino M, Maldonado M, Otheo E, Munoz A, Couselo J, Burgaleta C: Bone marrow transplantation in chronic granulomatous disease. *Eur J Pediatr* **155**:877, 1996.
429. Ho C, Vowels M, Lockwood L, Ziegler J: Successful bone marrow transplantation in a child with X-linked chronic granulomatous disease. *Bone Marrow Transplant* **18**:213, 1996.
430. Malech H, Bauer T, Hickstein D: Prospects for gene therapy of neutrophil defects. *Semin Hematol* **34**:355, 1997.
431. Karlsson S: Treatment of genetic defects in hematopoietic cell function by gene transfer. *Blood* **78**:2481, 1991.
432. Weinberg K, Kohn D: Gene therapy for congenital immunodeficiency diseases. *Immunol Allergy Clin North Am* **16**:453, 1996.
433. Mardiney M, Jackson S, Spratt S, Li F, Holland S, Malech H: Enhanced host defense after gene transfer in the murine p47phox-deficient model of chronic granulomatous disease. *Blood* **89**:2268, 1997.
434. Woodman R, Teoh D, Johnston F, Rae J, Sim V, Urton T, Wright B, et al.: X-linked carriers of $gp^{91\text{-}phax}$ chronic granulomatous disease (CGD): Clinical and potential therapeutic implications of extreme unbalanced X chromosome inactivation. *Blood* **86**:27a, 1995.
435. Li F, Linton G, Sekhsaria S, Whiting-Theobald N, Katkin J, Gallin J, Malech H: $CD34^{+}$peripheral blood progenitors as a target for genetic correction of the two flavocytochrome b_{558} defective forms of chronic granulomatous disease. *Blood* **84**:53, 1994.
436. Sekhsaria S, Gallin J, Linton G, Mallory R, Mulligan R, Malech H: Peripheral blood progenitors as a target for genetic correction of $p47^{phox}$-deficient chronic granulomatous disease. *Proc Natl Acad Sci* **90**:7446, 1993.
437. Bjorgvinsdottir H, Ding C, Pech N, Gifford M, Li L, Dinauer M: Retroviral-mediated gene transfer of gp91phox into bone marrow cells rescues in host defense against *Aspergillus fumigatus* in murine X-linked chronic granulomatous disease. *Blood* **89**:41, 1997.
438. Porter C, Parker M, Levinsky R, Collins M, Kinnon C: X-linked chronic granulomatous disease: Correction of NADPH oxidase defect by retrovirus-mediated expression of gp91-*phox*. *Blood* **82**:2196, 1993.
439. Kume A, Dinauer M: Retrovirus-mediated reconstitution of respiratory burst activity in X-linked chronic granulomatous disease cells. *Blood* **84**:3311, 1994.
440. Ding C, Kume A, Bjorgvinsdottir H, Hawley R, Pech N, Dinauer M: High level reconstitution of respiratory burst activity in human X-linked chronic granulomatous disease (X-CGD) cell line and correction of murine X-CGD bone marrow cells by retroviral-mediated gene transfer of human $gp91^{phox}$. *Blood* **88**:1834, 1996.
441. Zhen L, King A, Xiao Y, Chanock S, Orkin S, Dinauer M: Gene targeting of X-linked chronic granulomatous disease locus in a human myeloid leukemia cell line and rescue by expression of recombinant $gp91^{phox}$. *Proc Natl Acad Sci USA* **90**:9832, 1993.
442. Pollock J, Williams D, Gifford M, Li L, Du X, Fisherman J, Orkin S, et al.: Mouse model of X-linked chronic granulomatous disease, an inherited defect in phagocytes superoxide production. *Nat. Genet.* **9**:202, 1995.
443. Jackson SH, Gallin JI, Holland SM: The $p47^{phox}$ mouse knock-out model of chronic granulomatous disease. *J Exp Med* **182**:751, 1995.
444. Malech H, Maples P, Whiting-Theobald N, Linton G, Sekhsaria S, Vowells S, Li F, et al.: Prolonged production of NADPH oxidase-corrected granulocytes after gene therapy of chronic granulomatous disease. *Proc Natl Acad Sci* **94**:12133, 1997.
445. Lew PD, Southwick FS, Stossel TP, Whitin JC, Simons E, Cohen HJ: A variant of chronic granulomatous disease: Deficient oxidative metabolism due to a low-affinity NADPH oxidase. *N Engl J Med* **305**:1329, 1981.
446. Newburger PE, Luscinskas FW, Ryan T, Beard CJ, Wright J, Platt OS, Simons ER, et al.: Variant chronic granulomatous disease: Modulation of the neutrophil by severe infection. *Blood* **68**:914, 1986.
447. Shurin S, Cohen H, Whitin J, Newburger P: Impaired granulocyte superoxide production and prolongation of the respiratory burst due to a low-affinity NADPH-dependent oxidase. *Blood* **62**:564, 1983.
448. Casimir C, Chetty M, Bohler MC, Garcia R, Fischer A, Griscelli C, Johnson B, et al.: Identification of the defective NADPH-oxidase component in chronic granulomatous disease: A study of 57 European families. *Eur J Clin Invest22* **22**:403, 1992.
449. Frey D, Machler M, Seger R, Schmid W, Orkin S: Gene deletion in a patient with chronic granulomatous disease and McLeod syndrome: Fine mapping of the Xk gene locus. *Blood* **71**:252, 1988.
450. DeSaint-Basile G, Bohler M, Fischer A, Cartron J, Dufier J, Griscelli C, Orkin S: Xp21 DNA microdeletion in a patient with chronic granulomatous disease, retinitis pigmentosa, and McLeod phenotype. *Hum Genet* **80**:85, 1988.
451. Dinauer M, Curnutte J, Rosen H, Orkin S: A missense mutation in the neutrophil cytochrome b heavy chain in cytochrome-positive X-linked chronic granulomatous disease. *J Clin Invest* **84**:2012, 1989.
452. DeBoer M, Bolscher B, Dinauer M, Orkin S, Weening R, Roos D: Splice site mutations are a common cause of X-linked chronic granulomatous disease. *Blood* **80**:1553, 1992.
453. Rabbani H, de Boer M, Ahlin A, Sundin U, Elinder G, Hammarstrom L, Palmblad J, et al.: A 40-base-pair duplication in the gp91-*phox* gene leading to X-linked chronic granulomatous disease. *Eur J Haematol* **51**:218, 1993.
454. Ariga T, Sakiyama Y, Matsumoto S: Two novel point mutations in the cytochrome b558 heavy chain gene, detected in two Japanese patients with X-linked chronic granulomatous disease. *Hum Genet* **94**:441, 1994.
455. Ariga T, Sakiyama Y, Furuta H, Matsumoto S: Molecular genetic studies of two families with X-linked chronic granulomatous disease: Mutation analysis and definitive determination of carrier status in patients' sisters. *Eur J Haematol* **52**:99, 1994.
456. Leusen J, de Boer M, Bolscher B, Hilarius P, Weening R, Ochs H, Roos D, et al.: A point mutation in gp91-*phox* of cytochrome b_{558} of the human NADPH oxidase leading to defective translocation of the cytosolic proteins p47-phox and p67-phox. *J Clin Invest* **93**:2120, 1994.
457. Ariga T, Sakiyama Y, Matsumoto S: A 15-base pair (bp) palindromic insertion associated with a 3-bp deletion in exon 10 of the gp91-phox gene, detected in two patients with X-linked chronic granulomatous disease. *Hum Genet* **96**:6, 1995.
458. Azuma H, Oomi H, Sasaki K, Kawabata I, Sakaino T, Koyano S, Suzutani T, et al.: A new mutation on Exon 12 of the gp91-phox gene leading to cytochrome b-positive X-linked chronic granulomatous disease. *Blood* **85**:3274, 1995.
459. Bu-Ghanim H, Segal A, Keep N, Casimir C: Molecular analysis in three cases of X91-variant chronic granulomatous disease. *Blood* **86**:3575, 1995.
460. Ariga T, Furuta H, Cho K, Sakiyama Y: Genetic analysis of 13 families with X-linked chronic granulomatous disease reveals a low proportion of sporadic patients and a high proportion of sporadic carriers. *Pediatr Res* **44**:85, 1998.
461. Roos D: X-CGDbase: A database of X-CGD-causing mutations. *Immunol Today* **17**:517, 1996.
462. Francke U, Ochs H, DeMartinville B, Giacalone J, Lindgren V, Disteche C, Pagon R, et al.: Minor Xp21 chromosome deletion in a male associated with expression of Duchenee muscular dystrophy, chronic granulomatous disease, retinitis pigmentosa, and McLeod syndrome. *Am J Hum Genet* **37**:250, 1985.
463. Kousseff B: Linkage between chronic granulomatous disease and Duchenee's muscular dystrophy? *Am J Dis Child* **135**:1149, 1981.
464. Nagaraja R, MacMillan S, Kere J, Jones C, Griffin S, Schmatz M, Terrell J, et al.: X chromosome map at 75-kb STS resolution, revealing extremes of recombination and GC content. *Genome Res* **7**:210, 1997.
465. Densen P, Wilkinson-Kroovand S, Mandell G, Sullivan G, Oyen R, Marsh W: Kx: Its relationship to chronic granulomatous disease and genetic linkage with Xg. *Blood* **58**:34, 1981.
466. Maquat L: When cells stop making sense: effects of nonsense codons on RNA metabolism in vertebrate cells. *RNA* **1**:453, 1995.
467. Kessler O, Chasin L: Effects of nonsense mutations on nuclear and cytoplasmic adenine phosphoribosyltransferase RNA. *Mol Cell Biol* **16**:4426, 1996.

468. Imajoh-Ohimi S, Tokita K, Ochiai H, Nakamura M, Kanegasaki S: Topology of cytochrome$_{b558}$ in neutrophil membrane analyzed by anti-peptide antibodies and proteolysis. *J Biol Chem* **267**:180, 1992.
469. Burritt J, Quinn M, Jutila M, Bond C, Jesaitias A: Topological mapping of neutrophil cytochrome b epitopes with phage-display libraries. *J Biol Chem* **270**:16974, 1995.
470. Kuribayashi F, De Boer M, Leusen J, Verhoeven A, Roos D: A novel polymorphism in the coding region of CYBB, the human gp91-phox gene. *Hum Genet* **97**:611, 1996.
471. Youssoufian H, Antonarakis S, Bell W, Griffin A, Kazazian H Jr: Nonsense and missense mutations in hemophilia A: Estimate of the relative mutation rate at CG dinucleotides. *Am J Hum Genet* **42**:718, 1988.
472. Cooper D, Krawczak M: The mutational spectrum of single base-pair substitutions causing human genetic disease: Patterns and predictions. *Hum Genet* **85**:55, 1990.
473. Condino-Neto A, Rae J, Padden C, Whitney C, Curnutte J, Newburger P: An intronic mutation in *CYBB* gene leading to RNA instability and variant X-linked chronic granulomatous disease. *Blood* **90**:136a, 1997.
474. Haldane J: The ratio of spontaneous mutation of a human gene. *J Genet* **31**:317, 1935.
475. Lange K, Gladstien K, Zatz M: Effects of reproductive compensation and genetic drift on X-linked lethals. *Am J Hum Genet* **30**:180, 1978.
476. deBoer M, deKlein A, Hossle J-P, Seger R, Corbeel L, Weening R, Roos D: Cytochrome b_{558}-negative, autosomal recessive chronic granulomatous disease: Two new mutations in the cytochrome b_{558} light chain of the NADPH oxidase (p22-*phox*). *Am J Hum Genet* **41**:1127, 1992.
477. Porter C, Parkar M, Kinnon C: Identification of a donor splice site mutation leading to loss of p22-*phox* exon 5 in autosomal chronic granulomatous disease. *Hum Mutat* **7**:374, 1995.
478. Zhu Q, Zhang M, Rawlings DJ, Vihinen M, Hagemann T, Saffran DC, Kwan SP, et al.: Detection within the Src homology domain 3 of Bruton's tyrosine kinase resulting in X-linked agammaglobulinemia (XLA). *J Exp Med* **180**:461, 1994.
479. Chanock S, Barrett D, Curnutte J, Orkin S: Gene structure of the cytosolic component, phox-47 and mutations in autosomal recessive chronic granulomatous disease. *Blood* **78**:165a, 1991.
480. Iwata M, Nunoi H, Yamazaki H, Nakano T, Niwa H, Tsuruta S, Ohga S, et al.: Homologous dinucleotide (GT or TG) deletion in Japanese patients with chronic granulomatous disease with p47-phox deficiency. *Biochem Biophys Res Commun* **199**:1372, 1994.
481. Casimir C, Bu-Ghanim H, Rodaway A, Bentley D, Rowe P, Segal AW: Autosomal recessive chronic granulomatous disease caused by deletion at a dinucleotide repeat. *Proc Natl Acad Sci USA* **88**:2753, 1991.
482. Gorlach A, Lee P, Roesler J, Hopkins P, Christensen B, Green E, Chanock S, et al.: A p47-*phox* pseudogene carries the most common mutation causing p47-*phox*-deficient chronic granulomatous disease. *J Clin Invest* **100**:1907, 1997.
483. Kenney R, Kwon-Chung K, Waytes A, Melnick D, Pass H, Merino M, Gallin J: Successful treatment of systemic *Exophiala dermatitidis* infection in a patient with chronic granulomatous disease. *Clin Infect Dis* **14**:235, 1992.
484. deBoer M, Hilarius-Stokman P, Hossle J-P, Verhoeven A, Graf N, Kenney R, Seger R, et al.: Autosomal recessive chronic granulomatous disease with absence of the 67-kDa cytosolic NADPH oxidase component: identification of mutation and detection of carriers. *Blood* **83**: 531, 1994.
485. Bonizzato A, Russo M, Donini M, Dusi S: Identification of a double mutation (D160V-K161E) in the p67phox gene of a chronic granulomatous disease patient. *Biochem Biophys Res Commun* **231**:861, 1997.
486. Tanugi-Cholley L, Issartel J, Lunardi J, Freycon F, Morel F, Vignais P: A mutation located at the 5′ splice junction sequence of intron 3 in the $p67^{phox}$ gene causes the lack of $p67^{phox}$ mRNA in a patient with chronic granulomatous disease. *Blood* **85**:242, 1995.
487. Nunoi H, Iwata M, Tatsuzawa S, Onoe Y, Shimizu S, Kanegasaki S, Matsuda I: AG dinucleotide insertion in a patient with chronic granulomatous disease lacking cytosolic 67-kD protein. *Blood* **86**:329, 1995.
488. Leusen J, de Klein A, Hilarius P, Ahlin A, Palmblad J, Smith C, Diekmann D, et al.: Disturbed interaction of p21-rac with mutated p67-phox causes chronic granulomatous disease. *J Exp Med* **184**:1243, 1996.
489. Baehner R, Johnston R Jr, Nathan D: Comparative study of the metabolic and bactericidal characteristics of severely glucose-6-phosphate dehydrogenase deficient polymorphonuclear leukocytes from children with chronic granulomatous disease. *J Reticuloendothel Soc* **12**:150, 1972.
490. Cooper M, Dechatelet L, McCall C, Lavia M, Spurr C, Baehner R: Complete deficiency of leukocyte glucose-6-phosphate dehydrogenase with defective bactericidal activity. *J Clin Invest* **51**:769, 1972.
491. Gray G, Klebanoff S, Stamatayannopoulos G, Austin T, Naiman S, Yoshida A, Kliman M, et al.: Neutrophil dysfunction, chronic granulomatous disease and non-spherocytic haemolytica anemia caused by complete deficiency of glucose-6-phosphate dehydrogenase. *Lancet* **2**:530, 1973.
492. Mamlok R, Mamlok V, Mills G, Daeschner C, Schmalstieg F, Anderson D: Glucose-6-phosphate dehydrogenase deficiency, neutrophil dysfunction and *Chromobacterium violaceum* sepsis. *J Pediatr* **111**:852, 1987.
493. Jandl R, Andre-Schwartz J, Borges-DuBois L, Kipnes R, McMurrich B, Babior B: Termination of the respiratory burst in human neutrophils. *J Clin Invest* **61**:1176, 1978.
494. Cech P, Stalder I, Widmann, Rohner A, Meischer P: Leukocyte myeloperoxidase deficiency and diabetes mellitus associated with *Candida albicans* liver abscess. *Am J Med* **66**:149, 1979.
495. Grignaschi V, Sperperato A, Etcheverry M, Macario A: An nuevo cuadio cito guimico: negativad espontanea de las reacciones de peroxidas, oxidas y lipido en la progenia neutrophilia y en los monocitos de dos hermanos. *Rev Assoc Med Argent* **77**:218, 1963.
496. Huhn D, Belohradsky B, Haas R: Familiarer myeloperoxidascdefekt und akute myelloische leukamie. *Acta Haematol (Basel)* **59**:129, 1978.
497. Kitahara M, Stimonian Y, Eyre H: Neutrophil myeloperoxidase: A simple reproducible technique to determine activity. *J Lab Clin Med* **93**:232, 1979.
498. Lehrer R, Cline M: Leukocyte myeloperoxidase deficiency and disseminated candidiasis: The role of myeloperoxidase in resistance to *Candida* infection. *J Clin Invest* **48**:14788, 1969.
499. Moosmann K, Bojanowsky A: Rezidivierende Candidiosis bei myeloperoxidase-mangel. *Monatsschr Kinderheilkd* **123**:408, 1975.
500. Undritz E: Die Alius-Grignaschi-anomalie: der erblich konstitutionelle peroxydasedefekt der neutrophilen und monocyten. *Blut* **14**:129, 1966.
501. Kitahara M, Eyre J, Simonian Y, Atkin C, Hasstedt S: Hereditary myeloperoxidase deficiency. *Blood* **57**:888, 1981.
502. Parry M, Roote R, Metcalf J, Delaney K, Kaplow L, Richar W: Myeloperoxidase deficiency: prevalence and clinical significance. *Ann Intern Med* **95**:293, 1981.
503. Robertson C, Thong Y, Hodge G, Cheney K: Primary myeloperoxidase deficiency associated with impaired neutrophil margination and chemotaxis. *Acta Paedieatr Scand* **68**:915, 1979.
504. Kussenbach G, Rister M: Der Myeloperoxidase-Mangel als Ursache rezidivierende Infektionen. *Klin Padiatr* **197**:443, 1985.
505. Rosen H, Klebanoff S: Chemiluminescence and superoxide production by myeloperoxidase-deficient leukocytes. *J Clin Invest* **58**:50, 1976.
506. Stendahl O, Lindgren S: Function of granulocytes with deficiency of myeloperoxidase-mediated iodination in a patient with generalized pustular psoriasis. *Scand J Haematol* **16**:144, 1976.
507. London S, Lehman T, Taylor J: Myeloperoxidase genetic polymorphism and lung cancer risk. *Cancer Res* **57**:5001, 1997.
508. Lanza F: Pathology of myeloperoxidase deficiency. *J Mol Med* **76**:676, 1998.
509. Lanza F, Fietta A, Spisani S, Castoldi G, Traniello S: Does a relationship exist between neutrophil myeloperoxidase deficiency and the occurrence of neoplasms? *J Clin Lab Immunol* **22**:175, 1987.
510. Piedrafita F, Molander R, Vansant G, Orlova E, Pfahl M, Reynolds W: An Alu element in the myeloperoxidase promoter contains a composite SP1-thyroid hormone-retinoic acid response element. *J Biol Chem* **271**:14412, 1996.
511. Cech P, Schneider P, Bachmann F: Partial myeloperoxidase deficiency. *Acta Haematol (Basel)* **67**:180, 1982.
512. Cech P, Markert M, Perrin L: Partial myeloperoxidase deficiency in preleukemia. *Blut* **47**:21, 1983.
513. El-Maallem H, Fletcher J: Impaired neutrophil function and myeloperoxidase deficiency in pregnancy. *Br J Haematol* **44**:375, 1980.
514. Caldwell K, Taddeini L, Woodburn R, Anderson G, Lobell M: Induction of myeloperoxidase deficiency in granulocytes in lead-intoxicated dogs. *Blood* **53**:588, 1979.
515. Lehrer R, Cline M: Leukocyte candidacidal activity and resistance to system candidiasis in patients with cancer. *Cancer* **27**:1211, 1971.
516. Graham G: The neutrophilic granules of the circulating blood in health and in disease: A preliminary report. *NY State J Med* **20**:46, 1920.

517. Arakawa T, Wada Y, Hayaski T, Kakizaki R, Chiba N, Chida R, Konno T: Uracil-uric refractory anemia with peroxidase negative neutrophils. *Tohoku J Exp Med* **87**:52, 1965.
518. Higashi O, Katsuyama N, Satodate R: A case with hematological abnormalities characterized by the absence of peroxidase activity in blood polymorphonuclear leukocytes. *Tohoku S Exp Med* **87**:77, 1965.
519. Lehrer R, Goldberg L, Apple M, Rosenthal N: Refractory megaloblastic anemia with myeloperoxidase-deficient neutrophils. *Ann Intern Med* **76**:447, 1972.
520. Armstrong D, Dimmit S, van Wormer D: Studies in Batten disease I: Peroxidase deficiency in granulocytes. *Arch Neurol* **30**:144, 1974.
521. Bozdech M, Bainton D, Mustacchi P: Partial peroxidase deficiency in neutrophils and eosinophils associated with neurological disease. *Am J Clin Pathol* **73**:409, 1980.
522. Bendix-Hansen K: Myeloperoxidase-deficient polymorphonuclear leukocytes (VII): Incidence in untreated myeloproliferative disorders. *Scand J Haematol* **36**:8, 1986.
523. Bendix-Hansen K: Myeloperoxidase-deficient polymorphonuclear leukocytes. Longitudinal study during preremission — and the remission phase in acute myeloid leukemia. *Blut* **52**:237, 1986.
524. Bendix-Hansen K, Kerndrup G, Pedersen B: Myeloperoxidase-deficient polymorphonuclear leukocytes (VI): Relation to cytogenetic abnormalities in primary myelodysplastic syndromes. *Scand J Haematol* **36**:3, 1986.
525. Bendix-Hansen K, Kerndrup G: Myeloperoxidase-deficient polymorphonuclear leukocytes (V): Relation to FAB classification and neutrophil alkaline phosphatase activity in primary myelodysplastic syndromes. *Scand J Haematol* **35**:197, 1985.
526. Bendix-Hansen K, Nielsen H: Myeloperoxidase-deficient polymorphonuclear leukocytes I: Incidence in untreated myeloid leukemia, lymphoid leukemia, and normal humans. *Scand J Haematol* **30**:415, 1983.
527. Bendix-Hansen K, Nielson H: Myeloperoxidase-deficient polymorphonuclear leukocytes IV: Relation to FAB classification in acute myeloid leukemia. *Scand J Haematol* **35**:174, 1985.
528. Baggiolini M, Hirsch J, Deduve C: Resolution of granules from rabbit heterophil leukocytes into distinct populations by zonal sedimentation. *J Cell Biol* **40**:529, 1969.
529. Chance B, Mahely A: Assay of catalases and peroxidases. *Methods Enzymol* **2**:764, 1955.
530. *Worthington Enzyme Manual*. Worthington Enzyme, Freehold, NJ, 1972.
531. Dri P, Cramer R, Soranzo M, Comin A, Miotti V, Patriarca P: New approaches to the detection of myeloperoxidase deficiency. *Blood* **60**:323, 1982.
532. Wever R, Hamers M, Weening R, Roos D: Characterization of the peroxidase in human eosinophils. *Eur J Biochem* **108**:491, 1980.
533. Bos A, Wever R, Hamers M, Roos D: Some enzymatic characteristics of eosinophil peroxidase from patients with eosinophilia an from healthy donors. *Infect Immun* **32**:427, 1981.
534. Kaplow L: Substitute for benzidine in myeloperoxidase staining. *Am J Clin Pathol* **63**:451, 1975.
535. Elias J: A rapid, sensitive myeloperoxidase stain using 4-chloro-1-naphthol. *Am J Clin Pathol* **73**:797, 1980.
536. Kaplow L: Simplified myeloperoxidase stain using benzidine dihydrochloride. *Blood* **26**:215, 1965.
537. Klebanoff S, Hamon C: Role of myeloperoxidase-mediated antimicrobial systems in intact leukocytes. *J Reticuloendothel Soc* **12**:170, 1972.
538. Cech P, Papathanassiou A, Boreaux G, Roth P, Miescher P: Hereditary myeloperoxidase deficiency. *Blood* **53**:403, 1979.
539. Nauseef W, Metcalf J, Root R: Role of myeloperoxidase in the respiratory burst of human neutrophils. *Blood* **61**:483, 1983.
540. Larrocha C, Fernandez de Castro M, Fontan G, Viloria A, Fernandez-Chacon J, Jimenez C: Hereditary myeloperoxidase deficiency: study of 12 cases. *Scand J Haematol* **29**:389, 1982.
541. Dri P, Cramer R, Menagazzi R, Patriarca P: Increased degranulation of human myeloperoxidase-deficient polymorphonuclear leukocytes. *Br J Haematol* **59**:115, 1985.
542. Clark R, Borregaard N: Neutrophils autoinactivate secretory products by myeloperoxidase-catalyzed oxidation. *Blood* **65**:375, 1985.
543. Kobayashi M, Tanaka T, Usui T: Inactivation of lysosomal enzymes by the respiratory burst of polymorphonuclear leukocytes: possible involvement of myeloperoxidase–H_2O_2–halide system. *J Lab Clin Med* **100**:896, 1982.
544. Voetman A, Weening R, Hamers M, Meerhof L, Bot A, Roos D: Phagocytosing human neutrophils inactivate their own granular enzymes. *J Clin Invest* **67**:1541, 1981.
545. Klebanoff S: Myeloperoxidase: Contribution to the microbicidal activity of intact leukocytes. *Science* **169**:1095, 1970.
546. Lehrer R, Hanifin J, Cline M: Defective bactricidal activity in myeloperoxidase-deficient human neutrophils. *Nature* **223**:78, 1969.
547. Craner R, Soranzo M, Dri P, Rottini G, Bramezza M, Cirielli S: Incidence of myeloperoxidase deficiency in an area of northern Italy: histochemical, biochemical, and functional studies. *Br J Haematol* **51**:81, 1982.
548. Bos A, Weening, Hamers M, Wever R, Behrendt H, Roos D: Characterization of hereditary partial myeloperoxidase deficiency. *J Lab Clin Med* **99**:589, 1988.
549. Root R, Metcalf J: The role of iodide versus chloride-dependent reactions in myeloperoxidase-mediated microbicidal activity of human neutrophils. *Clin Res* **29**:534A, 1981.
550. Diamond R, Krzesicki R: Mechanisms of attachment of neutrophils to *Candida albicans* pseudohyphae in the absence of serum, and of subsequent damage to pseudohypae by microbicidal processes in neutrophils in vitro. *J Clin Invest* **61**:360, 1978.
551. Diamond R, Clark P, Haudenschild C: Damage to albicans hyphae and pseudohyphae by the myeloperoxidase system and oxidative products of neutrophil metabolism in vitro. *J Clin Invest* **66**:908, 1980.
552. Lehrer R, Ladra K, Hake R: Nonoxidative fungicidal mechanisms of mammalian granulocytes: demonstration of components with candidacidal activity in human, rabbit, and guinea pig leukocytes. *Infect Immunol* **11**:1226, 1975.
553. Lehrer R: Functional aspects of a second mechanism of candidacidal activity by human neutrophils. *J Clin Invest* **51**:2566, 1972.
554. Levitz S, Diamond R: Killing of *Aspergillus fumigatus* spores and *Candida albicans* yeast phase by the iron–H_2O_2–I_2 cytotoxic system: Comparison with MPO–H_2O_2–halide system. *Infect Immunol* **43**:1100, 1984.
555. Johnson K, Nauseef W: Molecular biology of myeloperoxidase, in Everse J, Everse K, Grisham M (eds): *Peroxidases in Chemistry and Biology*. Boca Raton, FL, CRC, 1991, p 63.
556. Hashinaka K, Nishio C, Hur S, Sakiyama F, Tsunasawa S, Yamada M: Multiple species of myeloperoxidase messenger RNAs produced by alternative splicing and differential polyadenylation. *Biochemistry* **27**:5906, 1988.
557. Meier R, Chen T, Friis R, Tobler A: Myeloperoxidase is a primary response gene in HL60 cells, directly regulated during hematopoietic differentiation. *Biochem Biophys Res Commun* **176**:1345, 1991.
558. Tobler A, Miller C, Johnson K, Selsted M, Rovera G, Koeffler H: Regulation of gene expression of myeloperoxidase during myelosis differentiation. *J Cell Physiol* **136**:215, 1988.
559. Sagoh T, Yamada M: Transcriptional regulation of myeloperoxidase gene expression in myeloid leukemia HL-60 cells during differentiation into granulocytes and macrophages. *Arch Biochem Biophys* **262**:599, 1988.
560. Rosmarin A, Weil S, Rosner G, Griffin J, Arnaout M, Tenen D: Differential expression of CD11b/CD18(Mol) and myeloperoxidase genes during myeloid differentiation. *Blood* **73**:131, 1989.
561. Lubbert M, Miller C, Koeffler H: Changes of DNA methylation and chromatin structure in the human myeloperoxidase gene during myeloid differentiation. *Blood* **45**:345, 1991.
562. Austin G, Chan W, Zhao W, Racine M: Myeloperoxidase gene expression in normal granulopoiesis and acute leukemias. *Leuk Lymph* **15**:209, 1994.
563. Austin G, Zhao W, Adjiri A, Lu J: Control of myeloperoxidase gene expression in developing myeloid cells. *Leuk Res* **20**:817, 1996.
564. Zhao W, Lu J, Regmi A, Austin G: Identification and functional analysis of multiple murine myeloperoxidase (MPO) promoters and comparison with the human MPO promoter region. *Leukemia* **11**:97, 1997.
565. Morishita K, Tsuchiya M, Asano S, Kaziro Y, Nagata S: Chromosomal gene structure of human myeloperoxidase and regulation of its expression by granulocyte colony-stimulating factor. *J Biol Chem* **262**:15208, 1987.
566. Shirsat N, Bittenbender S, Kreider B, Rovera G: Structure of the murine lactotransferrin gene is similar to the structure of other transferrin-encoding genes and shares a putative regulatory region with the murin myeloperoxidase gene. *Gene* **110**:229, 1992.
567. Hasilik A, Pohlmann R, Olsen R, VonFigura K: Myeloperoxidase is synthesized as a larger phosphorylated precursor. *EMBO J* **3**:2671, 1984.

568. Koeffler H, Ranyard J, Pertcheck M: Myeloperoxidase: its structure and control of its gene expression during myeloid differentiation. *Blood* **65**:484, 1984.
569. Nauseef W: Myeloperoxidase biosynthesis by a human promyelocytic leukemia cell line: insight into myeloperoxidase deficiency. *Blood* **67**:865, 1986.
570. Stromberg K, Persson A, Olsson I: The processing and intracellular transport of myeloperoxidase. *Eur J Cell Biol* **39**:424, 1986.
571. Yamada M: Myeloperoxidase precursors in human myeloid leukemia HL-60 cells. *J Biol Chem* **257**:5980, 1982.
572. Hur S, Toda H, Tamada M: Isolation and characterization of an unprocessed extracellular myeloperoxidase in HL-60 cell cultures. *J Biol Chem* **264**:8542, 1989.
573. Taylor K, Guzman G, Burgess C, Kinkade J: Assembly of dimeric myeloperoxidase during posttranslational maturation in human leukemic HL-60 cells. *Biochemistry* **29**:1533, 1990.
574. Nauseef W, McCormick S, Yi H: Roles of heme insertion and the mannose-6-phosphate receptor in processing of the human myeloid lysosomal enzyme, myeloperoxidase. *Blood* **80**:2622, 1992.
575. Nauseef W, McCormick S, Clark R: Calreticulin functions as a molecular chaperone in the biosynthesis of myeloperoxidase. *J Biol Chem* **270**:4741, 1995.
576. Nauseef W, McCormick S, Goedken M: Coordinated participation of calreticulin and calnexin in the biosynthesis of myeloperoxidase. *J Biol Chem* **273**:7107, 1998.
577. Stromberg K, Olsson I: Myeloperoxidase precursors incorporate heme. *J Biol Chem* **262**:10430, 1987.
578. Castaneda V, Parmley R, Pinnix I, Raju S, Guzman G, Kinkade J: Ultrastructural, immunochemical, and cytochemical study of myeloperoxidase in myeloid leukemia HL-60 cells following treatment with succinylacetone, an inhibitor of heme biosynthesis. *Exp Hematol* **20**:916, 1992.
579. vanTuinen P, Johnson K, Ledbetter S, Nussbaum R, Merry D, Rovera G, Ledbetter D: Localization of myeloperoxidase to the long arm of human chromosome 17: relationship to the 15, 17 translocation of acute promyelocytic leukemia. *Oncogene* **1**:319, 1987.
580. Inazawa J, Inoue K, Nishigaki H, Tsuda S, Taniwaki M, Misawa S, Abe T: Assignment of the human myeloperoxidase gene (MPO) to bands q21.3aq23 of chromosome 17. *Cytogenet Cell Genet* **50**:135, 1989.
581. Chang K, Schroeder W, Siciliano M, Thompson L, McCredie K, Beran M, Freireich E, et al.: The localization of the human myeloperoxidase gene is in close proximity to the translocation breakpoint in acute promyelocytic leukemia. *Leukemia* **1**:458, 1987.
582. Liang J, Chang K, Schroeder W, Freireich E, Stass S, Trujillo J: The myeloperoxidase gene is translocated from chromosome 17 to 15 in a patient with acute promyelocytic leukemia. *Cancer Genet Cytogenet* **30**:103, 1988.
583. Tobler A, Selsted M, Miller C, Johnson K, Novotny M, Rovera G, Koeffler H: Evidence for a pretranslational defect in hereditary and acquired myeloperoxidase deficiency. *Blood* **73**:1980, 1989.
584. Nauseef W, Brigham S, Cogley M: Hereditary myeloperoxidase deficiency due to a missense mutation of arginine 569 to tryptophan. *J Biol Chem* **269**:1212, 1994.
585. DeLeo F, Goedken M, McCormick S, Nauseef W: A novel form of hereditary myeloperoxidase deficiency linked to endoplasmic reticulum/proteasome degradation. *J Clin Invest* **101**:2900, 1998.
586. Romano M, Dri P, Dadalt L, Patriarca P, Baralle F: Biochemical and molecular characterization of hereditary myeloperoxidase deficiency. *Blood* **90**:4126, 1997.
587. Nauseef W, Cogley M, McCormick S: Effect of the R569W missense mutation on the biosynthesis of myeloperoxidase. *J Biol Chem* **271**:9546, 1996.
588. Salmon S, Cline M, Schultz J, Lehrer R: Myeloperoxidase deficiency: immunologic study of a genetic leukocyte defect. *N Engl J Med* **282**:250, 1970.
589. Nauseef W, Cogley M, Bock S, Petrides P: Pattern of inheritance in hereditary myeloperoxidase deficiency associated with the R569W missense mutation. *J Leukoc Biol* **63**:264, 1998.
590. Meister A: Biochemistry of glutathione, in Greenberg D (ed): *Metabolism of Sulfur Compounds*. New York, Academic Press, 1975, p 101.
591. Meister A, Tate S: Glutathione and related gamma-glutamyl compounds: biosynthesis and utilization. *Annu Rev Biochem* **45**:559, 1976.
592. Roos D, Weening R, Voetman A, vanSchaik M, Bot A, Meerhof L, Loos J: Protection of phagocytic leukocytes by endogenous glutathione: studies in a family with glutathione reductase deficiency. *Blood* **53**:851, 1979.
593. Spielberg S, Boxer L, Oliver J, Allen J, Schulman J: Oxidative damage to neutrophils in glutathione synthetase deficiency. *N Engl J Med* **301**:901, 1979.
594. Boxer L, Oliver J, Spielberg S, Allen J, Schulman J: Protection of granulocytes by vitamin E in glutathione synthetase deficiency. *N Engl J Med* **301**:901, 1979.
595. Loos J, Roos D, Weening R, Houwerzijl J: Familial deficiency of glutathione reductase in human blood cells. *Blood* **48**:53, 1976.
596. Holmes B, Park BH, Malawista SE, Quie PG, Nelson DL, Good RA: Chronic granulomatous disease in females: A deficiency of leukocyte glutathione peroxidase. *N Engl J Med* **283**:217, 1970.
597. Baker S, Cohen H: Altered oxidative metabolism in selenium-deficient rat granulocytes. *J Immunol* **130**:1910, 1983.
598. McCallister J, Harris R, Baehner R, Boxer L: Alteration of microtubule function in glutathione peroxidase-deficient polymorphonuclear leukocytes. *J Reticuloendothel Soc* **27**:59, 1980.
599. Schulman J, Mudd S, Schneider J, Spielberg S, Boxer L, Oliver J, Corash L, et al.: Genetic disorders of glutathione and sulfur amino-acid metabolism. New biochemical insights and therapeutic approaches. *Ann Intern Med* **93**:330, 1980.
600. Speier C, Baker S, Newburger P: Relationships between in vitro selenium supply, glutathione peroxidase activity and phagocytic function in the HL-60 human myeloid cell line. *J Biol Chem* **260**:8951, 1985.

PART 21

MEMBRANE TRANSPORT DISORDERS

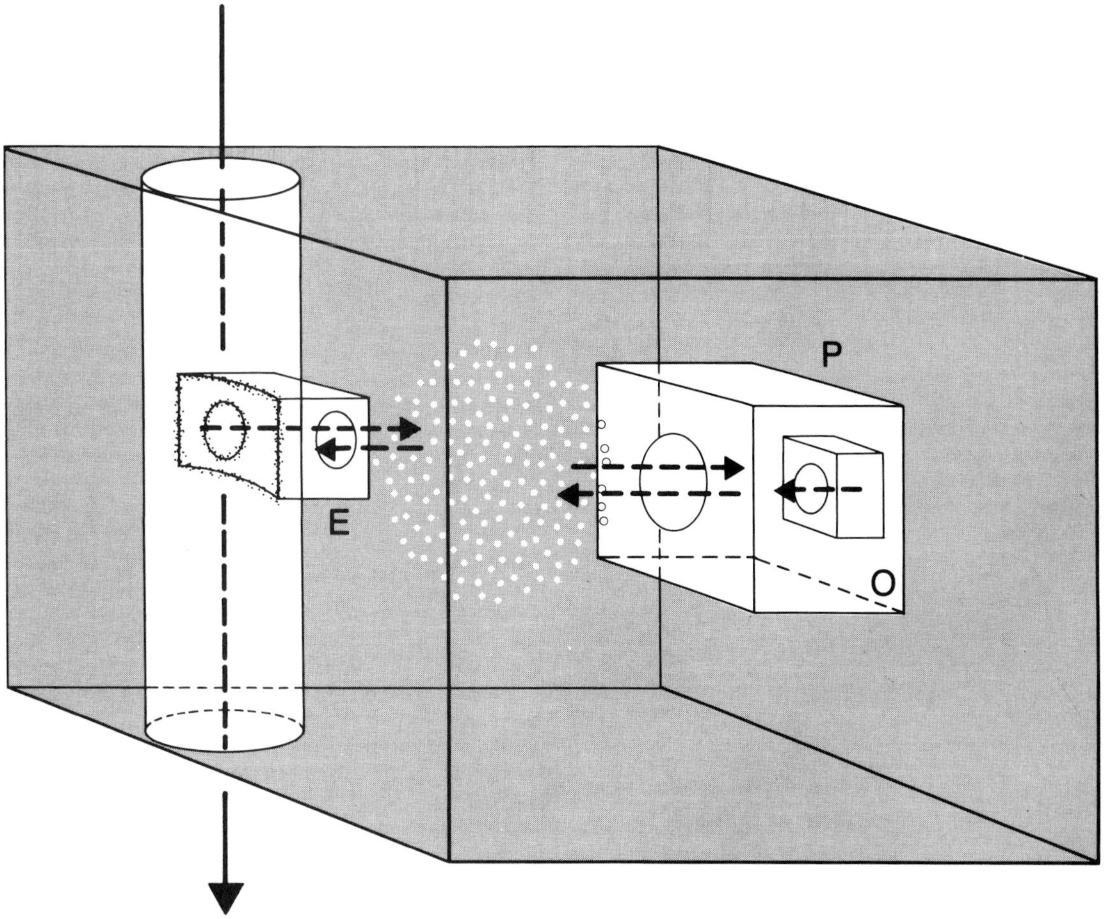

Membrane transport systems affect epithelial cells (E), parenchymal (P) cells, and organelles (O).

CHAPTER 190

Familial Glucose-Galactose Malabsorption and Hereditary Renal Glycosuria

Ernest M. Wright ▪ Martín G. Martín ▪ Eric Turk

1. **Glucose-galactose malabsorption (GGM, OMIM 182380) is a rare autosomal recessive disorder that is due to mutations in the gene coding for the intestinal brush-border sodium-glucose cotransporter (*SGLT1*). It is characterized by the neonatal onset of profuse, watery diarrhea that leads to severe dehydration and death if left untreated. The intestinal absorption of other nutrients such as amino acids and fructose is normal. Frequently, GGM is accompanied by a mild renal glucosuria. The diarrhea is quickly resolved by the elimination of glucose, galactose, and lactose from the diet; the milk sugar lactose is quickly hydrolyzed to glucose and galactose by lactase on the surface of the intestinal mucosa. The malabsorption of glucose and galactose is readily confirmed by the breath hydrogen test. Once the offending sugars are removed from the diet, patients appear to grow and develop normally.**
2. **SGLT1 is present in the brush-border membrane of mature enterocytes lining the upper surface of the intestinal villi. The transporter is responsible for the accumulation of glucose and galactose in the enterocytes, and this occurs by sodium-sugar cotransport. Two sodium ions are transported along with each sugar, and transport is energized by the sodium electrochemical potential gradient across the brush-border membrane. The sodium gradient is maintained by the Na^+/K^+ pump in the basolateral membrane of the enterocyte. This means that sugar in the gut lumen stimulates sodium absorption across the small intestine, and this is followed by anions and water. This process provides the rationalization for oral rehydration therapy used worldwide to treat diarrhea caused by infections. Fructose is not transported by SGLT1, but it uses its own facilitated transporter in the brush-border membrane, GLUT5. Once glucose, galactose, and fructose are within the cell, they exit to the blood across the basolateral membrane of the cell through another facilitated sugar transporter, GLUT2.**
3. **In 46 GGM patients, the *SGLT1* gene has been screened for mutations, and 41 have been identified. These include missense (61 percent), nonsense (10 percent), frameshift (17 percent), and splice-site (12 percent) mutations. About 70 percent have homozygous mutations, whereas the remainder bear compound heterozygous mutations. No mutations have yet been identified in 3 GGM patients. The missense and several of the nonsense mutations have been tested for defects in sugar transport. The mutant proteins were expressed in a heterologous expression system, *Xenopus laevis* oocytes, and all but 3 missense mutations cause a severe reduction in sodium-sugar transport activity. In 2 of the 3 patients with these rather benign mutations, other mutations impaired sugar transport.**
4. **The nonsense, frameshift, and splice-site mutations produce inactive proteins. The missense mutant cRNAs are translated and glycosylated in the oocyte endoplasmic reticulum and remain in the cell at about the same level as the wild-type protein. The majority are retained in the endoplasmic reticulum or Golgi apparatus and are not forwarded to the plasma membrane of the oocyte. This indicates that the mutations cause protein misfolding that impairs proper trafficking to the plasma membrane. Only one missense mutant, *Q457R*, is properly processed in oocytes, but this mutant protein is unable to transport sugar. Immunocytochemical examination of the mucosal biopsies from four GGM patients confirms the conclusions drawn about mutant protein trafficking in the expression system. Thus GGM joins a growing list of disorders in which mutations cause protein folding and trafficking defects.**
5. **Hereditary renal glycosuria (OMIM *8233100) is an autosomal recessive disease that results from the selective inability of the kidney to reabsorb glucose from the glomerular filtrate in the absence of hyperglycemia. The amount of glucose excreted is independent of diet, and oral tolerance tests and plasma insulin levels are normal. These patients only excrete glucose, not galactose, and they store and use carbohydrate normally. Patients with hereditary renal glycosuria do not have a defect in intestinal glucose absorption, and those with GGM do not show a severe renal glycosuria. These characteristics indicate that hereditary renal glycosuria is due to a defect in another sodium-glucose cotransporter in the brush border of the early proximal tubule, i.e., SGLT2. There is some uncertainty about the identity of the human renal SGLT2.**

Glucose-galactose malabsorption (GGM) is a disease resulting from a selective defect in the intestinal absorption of D-glucose and D-galactose, and it is characterized by the neonatal onset of life-threatening diarrhea. The diarrhea is immediately resolved by the elimination of lactose, glucose, and galactose from the diet: "lactose is normally digested to glucose and galactose by lactase on the surface of the small intestine." In the case of lactase deficiency (OMIM 223000; see Chaps. 75 and 76), there is no diarrhea if the patient is fed with a lactose-free formula containing glucose or galactose. The intestinal absorption of the other nutrients, including fructose and amino acids, is normal in GGM patients.

A list of standard abbreviations is located immediately preceding the index in each volume. Nonstandard abbreviations used in this chapter include: GGM = glucose-galactose malabsorption.

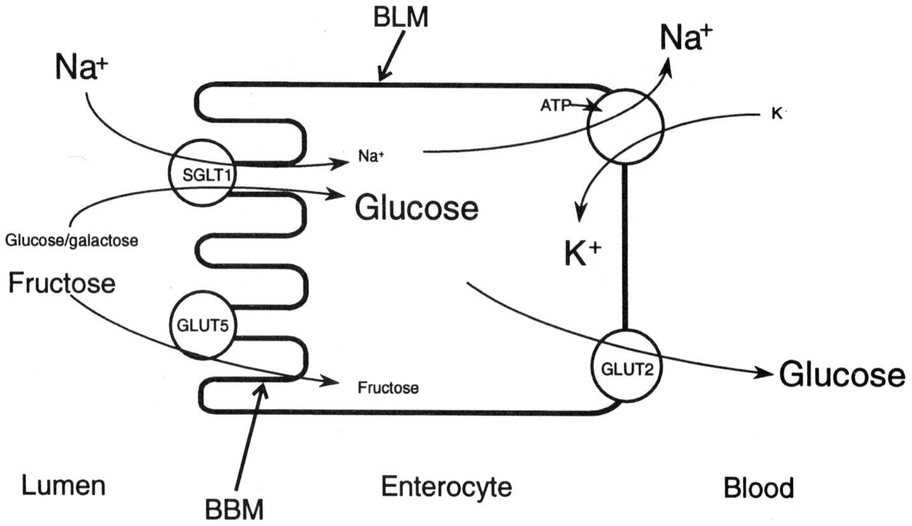

Fig. 190-1 Sugar transport across the mature enterocytes of the small intestine. Glucose and galactose are accumulated within the cell from the intestinal lumen by the sodium-glucose cotransporter (SGLT1) in the brush-border membrane (BBM). SGLT1 is energized by the sodium electrochemical potential gradient across the BBM, and the sodium gradient is maintained by the basolateral membrane (BLM) Na^+/K^+ pump. Addition of glucose or galactose to the gut lumen therefore results in a stimulation of sodium absorption across the intestine. Fructose enters the cell from the lumen down the fructose gradient via the facilitated transporter GLUT5. Glucose, galactose, and fructose then are transported out of the enterocyte into the blood across the BLM by the facilitated sugar transporter GLUT2. (*Courtesy of Dr. B. A. Hirayama.*)

In the 20 years following the first description of this disease in 1962 by Lindguist and Meeuwisse in Sweden[1] and Laplane *et al.* in France,[2] over 40 cases throughout the world have been described in the literature (summarized by Desjeux in an earlier edition of this work).[3] While the disease is considered to be rare, we are aware of around 200 cases. It should be noted that some 10 percent of the normal adult population, first-year medical students, exhibit evidence of glucose malabsorption during breath hydrogen tests.[4] Experimental studies on the first American GGM patient by Kinter and Stirling[5,6] provided compelling evidence that the disease was caused by a defect in the intestinal brush-border sodium-glucose cotransporter. This membrane protein is responsible for the first stage in glucose and galactose transport across the epithelium (Fig. 190-1).

This chapter will focus on studies of GGM done over the past 10 years. The stimulus for our work was our cloning of the rabbit intestinal sodium-glucose cotransporter (SGLT1) in 1987.[7] This was accomplished by a novel strategy that we called *expression cloning,* where the cDNA library was screened for a function in *Xenopus laevis* oocytes. We then isolated the human clone from a human intestinal cDNA library in 1989 using the rabbit cDNA as a probe[8] and shortly thereafter identified the mutation that caused GGM in two patients.[9] We have subsequently screened the *SGLT1* gene for mutations in 46 GGM patients, identified 41 mutations in 43 patients, and studied how these mutations may cause the disease.[10–12] Earlier studies on GGM are summarized in the previous edition.[3]

SUGAR DIGESTION AND ABSORPTION

Milk sugar, lactose, is the sole source of dietary carbohydrate in the newborn, and this is digested to glucose and galactose by lactase on the brush-border surface of the enterocyte. Dietary carbohydrate becomes more varied with age and accounts for about 50 percent of the caloric intake in adults on a Western-type diet. This amounts to about 350 g of carbohydrate consisting of starch, sucrose, and variable amounts of lactose and fructose. The latter is used increasingly as a "low" caloric sweetener in soft drinks. Complex carbohydrates are digested initially by pancreatic amylases in the lumen of the gastrointestinal (GI) tract, and in the final stages, the oligosaccharides and disaccharides are digested to monosaccharides by the hydrolases attached to the brush-border membrane of the mature enterocytes lining the intestinal villi.

The free sugars, glucose, galactose, and fructose, are absorbed across enterocytes in two stages (see Fig. 190-1). Glucose and galactose are first transported across the brush-border membrane by the sodium-glucose cotransporter (SGLT1) and then across the basolateral membrane by the facilitated sugar transporter (GLUT2).[13] Fructose is transported across the brush-border membrane by its own private facilitated carrier (GLUT5) and then exits the cell through the basolateral membrane by GLUT2.

Glucose and galactose are driven across the brush-border membrane by SGLT1 and accumulate within the enterocytes. The accumulation of galactose in humans has been documented by the elegant autoradiographic studies of Kinter and Stirling[5,6] (see Figs. 190-10 and 190-11). The uphill transport of both sugars is blocked by the very specific inhibitor phlorizin (see Fig. 190-11). Phlorizin is a nontransported, competitive inhibitor of SGLT1 with an inhibition constant (K_i) ranging from 10 nM to 1 μM.[14] The energy for uphill glucose and galactose transport is provided by the Na^+ electrochemical potential gradient across the brush-border membrane. Two Na^+ ions are transported along with each sugar molecule,[15] and the sodium that enters the cell is extruded across the basolateral membrane by the Na^+/K^+ pump. The net result is that sugar and sodium are transported across the epithelium, and this is accompanied by an equivalent amount of anions (Cl^- and HCO_3^-) and water. The link between salt, glucose, and water absorption provides the foundation for the oral rehydration therapy used to treat diarrheal diseases such as cholera.[16] Recently, a direct link between sugar and water transport has been established[17,18]; i.e., water is cotransported along with sodium and sugar through SGLT1 and accounts for 4 to 5 liters of water absorption per day.

Crane and colleagues[19] were the first to propose that the active transport of glucose and galactose across the intestinal brush border was due to sodium-sugar cotransport. Over the next decade, this hypothesis was confirmed, refined, and extended to the active transport of other solutes such as amino acids, anions, carboxylic acids, and neurotransmitters.[20] Not until 1984 was the identity of the brush-border sodium-sugar transporter established unequivocally.[21] A major problem was that the transporter accounted only for a minor fraction of the brush-border membrane protein. Shortly thereafter we developed expression cloning to isolate the

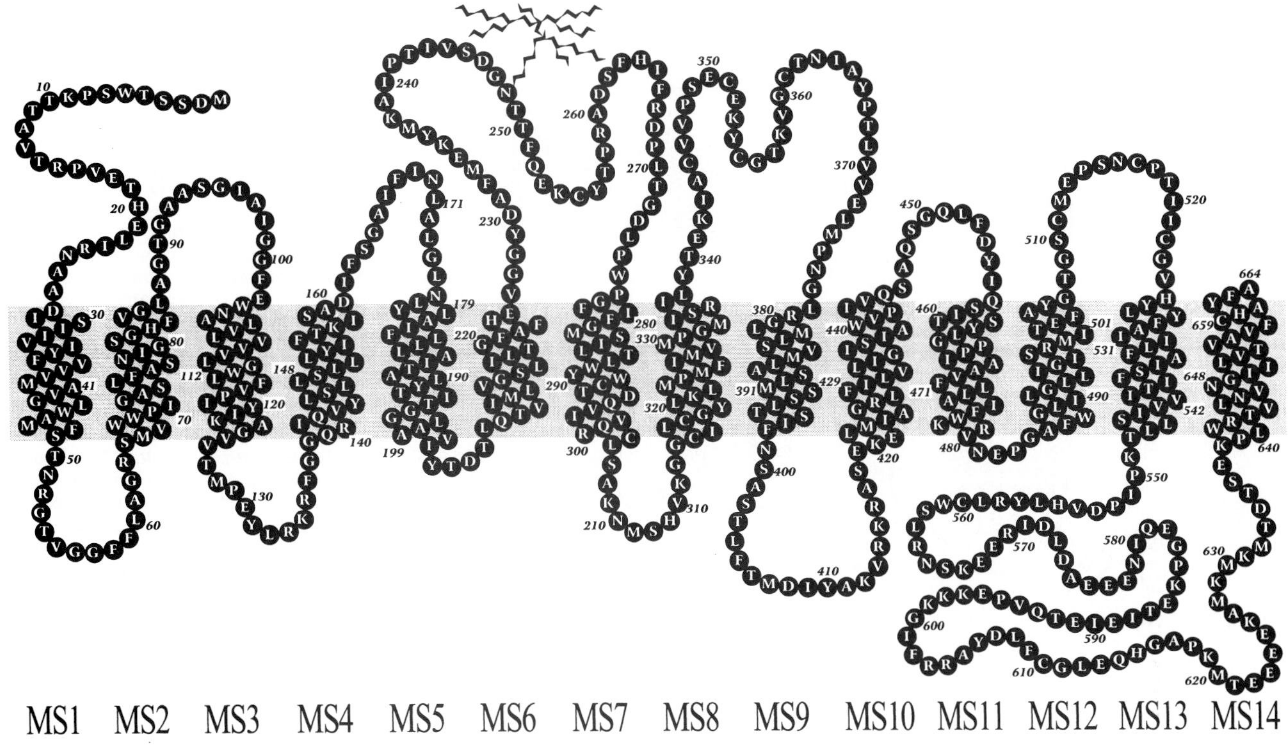

Fig. 190-2 The secondary structure of SGLT1. The 664-amino-acid (73-kDa) protein with 14 transmembrane helices (MS 1–14) is orientated with both the N- and C-termini facing the extracellular side of the membrane. The location of the N-linked glycosylation site (N248) is indicated by the carbohydrate tree. (*From Turk and Wright.*[22] *Used by permission.*)

cotransporter cDNA.[7] Sequencing of the clone revealed that it was the first member of a novel gene family, the *SGLT1* gene family. This family now consists of over 30 sodium cotransporters from animal and bacterial species and includes the thyroid sodium-iodide, the renal sodium-myoinositol, and the *Escherichia coli* sodium-proline cotransporters.[22] These polytopic membrane proteins contain a common core of 13 transmembrane helical spans. SGLT1 protein (Fig. 190-2) contains an additional fourteenth transmembrane helix. This secondary-structure model is consistent with our freeze-fracture electron microscopic examination of SGLT1.[23] Both the N- and C-termini face the extracellular side of the membrane, and the protein is heavily glycosylated at Asn248.[24,25] Glycosylation adds roughly 15,000 Da to the mass of the 73-kDa protein. There are several phosphorylation consensus sites on the cytoplasmic surface of SGLT1, but these do not appear to be used in the short-term regulation of transport.[26,27] Activation of protein kinases indirectly affects sodium-sugar transport by regulating the density of SGLT1 in the plasma membrane by exo- and endocytosis.

The function of SGLT1 has been investigated extensively using heterologous expression systems ranging from *X. laevis* oocytes to insect cells to mammalian cells.[13] These studies have confirmed that both D-glucose and D-galactose are transported by SGLT1 with very similar kinetics (K_m and V_{max} values), voltage dependence, cation dependence (Na^+, H^+, Li^+), and phlorizin sensitivity. Western blot analysis and immunocytochemical studies with antibodies raised against SGLT1 peptides demonstrated that SGLT1 is expressed on the brush-border membrane of mature enterocytes in the small intestine.[28] Such studies provided confidence that indeed SGLT1 is the brush-border sodium-glucose cotransporter. This was bolstered by microsequencing of SGLT1 purified from rabbit intestinal brush borders,[29] where the sequence obtained was identical to the rabbit SGLT1 clone. Additional evidence is provided by our finding that SGLT1 mutations can account for the defect in sugar transport in 43 of the 46 GGM patients we have examined (see below).

Exhaustive biophysical experiments have enabled us to formulate a model for sodium and sugar transport by SGLT1 that accounts for both the observed steady state and pre-steady state kinetics.[30–34] A cartoon form of the model is shown in Fig. 190-3. This is a six-state ordered model where sodium binds first at the external surface, which then causes a conformational change to allow sugar binding. The fully loaded complex then undergoes another conformational change that delivers the sugar- and sodium-binding sites to the internal surface, where first sugar and then sodium dissociate. The final step is the reorientation of the ligand binding sites to the external surface to complete the turnover cycle. The turnover number is 60 per second, and this is largely determined by the reorientation rate of the unloaded ligand-binding sites (reaction $6 \rightarrow 1$ in Fig. 190-3). We have provided direct evidence for three of these conformation changes, and we conclude that the coupling between sodium and sugar transport is determined by ligand- and voltage-induced conformational changes in the protein.[34]

Much effort is directed at resolving the structural basis of sodium-sugar cotransport. There is compelling evidence that the sugar translocation pathway through SGLT1 is formed by four transmembrane helices in the C-terminal domain of the protein. First, it has been observed that the sugar selectivity and affinity of SGLTs is determined by the C-terminal part of the protein (residues 411–662 containing helices 10–14; see Fig. 190-2).[35] Second, the truncated rabbit protein (residues 407–662) behaves as a facilitated sugar uniporter when expressed in oocytes.[36] Third, residues in helices 11 and 12 are important in effecting sugar transport by SGLT1.[34,37] Finally, helix 14 does not appear to be essential for function in this gene family.[22] It follows that sodium binding and transport through SGLT1 must involve the N-terminal half of the protein. Our hypothesis is that sodium-sugar transport involves close interaction between the N-terminal sodium-binding/translocation domain and the C-terminal sugar-binding/translocation domain. Work is in progress to determine how the 14 helices are packed together in the protein. Analysis of the structure

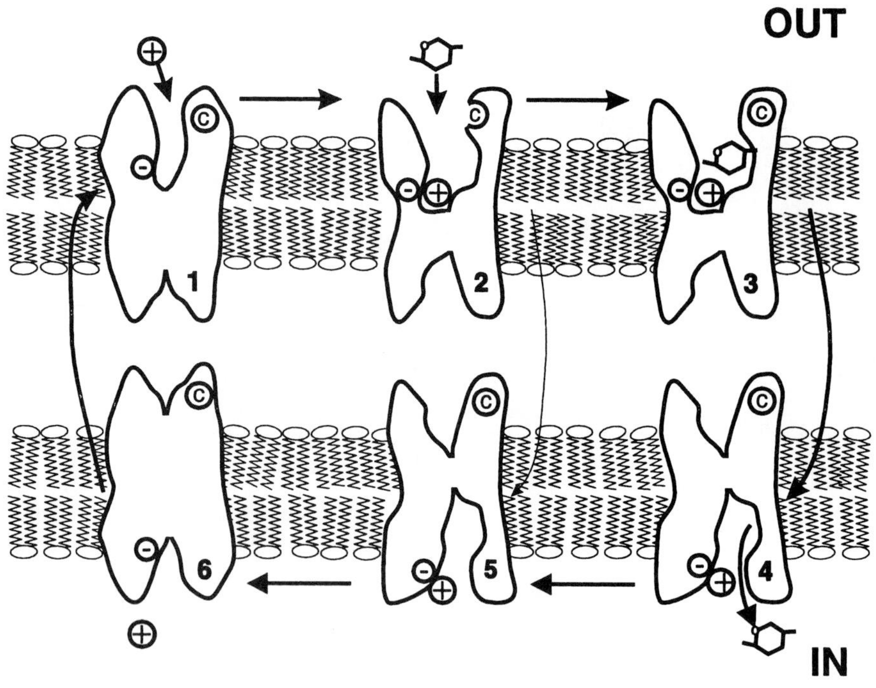

Fig. 190-3 A model for sodium-glucose cotransport by SGLT1. This is an ordered six-state kinetic model where three states (1–3) face the external surface of the membrane and three states (4–6) face the cytoplasm. At the external surface, 2 Na ions bind to form the Na^+-carrier complex (state 2), and this permits the binding of sugar. The fully loaded complex (state 3) undergoes a conformation change resulting in sodium-glucose cotransport across the membrane. The sugar and sodium dissociate from the carrier, and the unloaded form (6) isomerizes to complete the cycle. In the absence of sugar, SGLT1 can transport sodium, the so-called sodium leak, and this is shown as the 2–5 reaction step. Not represented is the cotransport of 230 water molecules during each turnover of the sodium-glucose transport cycle. These conformational changes have been documented in part by measuring the accessibility of a cysteine (C) placed at position 457 in the sugar transport pathway. (*From Loo et al.*[34] *Used by permission.*)

of SGLT1 proteins expressed in the plasma membrane of oocytes by freeze-fracture electron microscopy suggests that SGLT1 functions as a monomer.[23]

Intestinal Sugar Transporter Genes

The human gene *SGLT1* has been mapped to the distal q arm of chromosome 22 using hamster-human hybrid cells.[38] Its localization was later refined[39] to the Giemsa-negative band 22q13.1 by using a cosmid clone for FISH (fluorescence *in situ* hybridization). The exon arrangements have been mapped and reside within a 72-kb genomic region (Fig. 190-4). The 15 exons have been sequenced,[40] and the exon splice sites occur exclusively within protein-encoding sequences. The relatively high density of *Alu* sequences observed while sequencing *SGLT1* exons supports the previous FISH assignment to the Giemsa-negative band 22q13.1, since these nonstaining chromosomal domains are enriched in both active genes and *Alu* sequences.[41] The *SGLT1* transcriptional start site is located 23 bp before the initiator methionine codon and 23 bp 3′ to a putative TATA promoter element.

The human gene *GLUT2* has been assigned to chromosome 3, bands q26.1-26.3, by silver grain distribution after *in situ* hybridization.[42] The exon arrangements have been mapped (see Fig. 190-4), and the 11 exons have been sequenced.[43] Like *SGLT1*, exon splice sites occur exclusively within the protein-encoding sequences. *GLUT2* exons are more compactly arranged within a 29-kb region, with transcription starting 309 bp before the initiator codon and 20 bp after a putative TATA promoter element.

The human gene *GLUT5* initially was assigned to chromosome 1, band p31, by silver grain distribution after *in situ* hybridization.[44] More recent and definitive evidence shows, however, that *GLUT5* resides in fact on the distant band 1p36.2.[45] Using both P1-artificial chromosomes and FISH, *GLUT5* consistently mapped to band 1p36.2, to the exclusion of 1p31. The exon-intron physical distances for only the seven C-terminal exons have been reported (see Fig. 190-4), although all 12 exons have been sequenced.[47] As before, exon splice sites occur exclusively within the protein-encoding sequences. Relative to *GLUT2*, an additional intron appears within the homologous *GLUT2* exon 9. The exons of *GLUT5* reside much closer to one another than those for *GLUT2* (see Fig. 190-4). *GLUT5* transcription starts 96 bp before the initiator codon and 26 bp after a putative TATA promoter element.[46]

Some corresponding features of the *SGLT1, GLUT2,* and *GLUT5* genes are summarized in Table 190-1. There is no homology between SGLT1 and the GLUTs at either the DNA or protein levels. However, human GLUT5 has 41 percent identity at the protein level with GLUT2.[13]

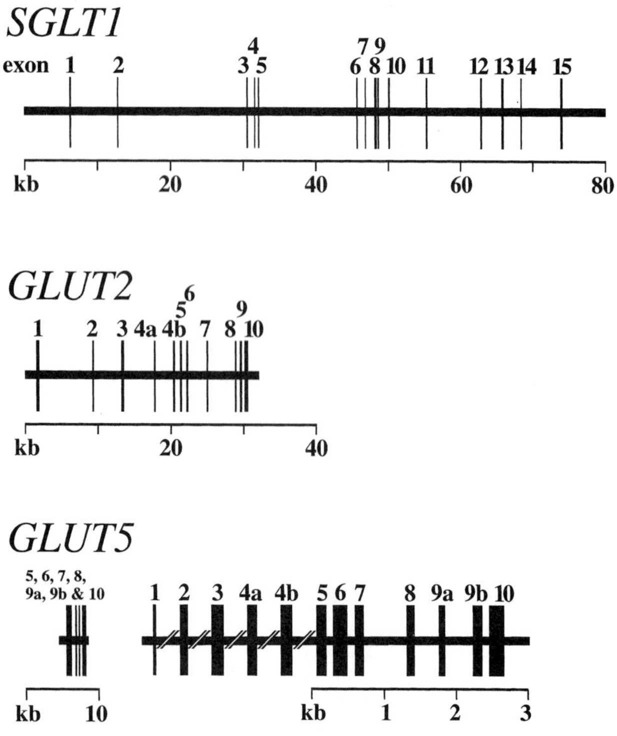

Fig. 190-4 Maps of the human *SGLT1, GLUT2,* and *GLUT5* genes. Positions of the exons are indicated.

Table 190-1 Intestinal Sugar Transporter Genes

	SGLT1	*GLUT2*	*GLUT5*
Chromosome	22q13.1	3q26.1-26.3	1p36.2
Exon number	15	11	12
Exon expanse	72 kb	29 kb	n.a.
5′-UTR	23 bp	309 bp	96 bp
Amino acids	664	524	501
GenBank access	L29328–L29339	L09674–L09684	U05344, U11839–43

GLUCOSE-GALACTOSE MALABSORPTION

Genetics

The family history of GGM is most consistent with an autosomal recessive pattern of inheritance[48] (see Figs. 190-8 and 190-13). Its relative abundance in consanguineous unions and the absence of vertical transmission are most consistent with a recessive pattern of inheritance. Obligate heterozygotes have been reported to have a reduced level of glucose uptake.[49] However, consistent evidence of malabsorption and clinical symptoms have not been well documented.

While the disorder is rare and has not been described to be abundant in any particular ethnic group, it is seen most frequently in populations that have a high incidence of consanguinity. Recent genetic testing was performed on 30 patients in 27 unrelated families from the United States (of North European, African-American, Hispanic-American, and Mediterranean descent), France, Netherlands, Japan, United Kingdom, Belgium, and Sweden.[10] Among the probands, 32 mutations were identified that account for GGM, and all but one patient was determined to have mutations. Identical mutations were identified on both alleles from 18 families, and another 10 were compound heterozygotes. These data were consistent with the family history that showed that 12 of the patients studied were known to be the product of a consanguineous union. Two-thirds of the patients studied in this report were female, consistent with other reports that females are overrepresented among GGM patients.[50]

Clinical Phenotype

The majority of patients with GGM present clinically with severe life-threatening diarrhea during early infancy. On rare occasions, adult patients have been identified with milder symptoms.[51] Mild glycosuria can be identified in most patients. Diarrhea is detected most frequently during the first 2 days of life, while the patient is still hospitalized. Patients usually develop a severe metabolic acidosis and hyperosmolar dehydration. The diarrhea in GGM results from water and electrolyte secretion into the lumen of the intestine in the presence of unabsorbed carbohydrate. If the patients are not diagnosed properly in a timely manner and dietary management implemented, GGM is frequently fatal.

Isolated carbohydrate malabsorption is distinctly unusual during the first several days of life, and its presence should initiate the workup for both GGM and primary lactase deficiency. The osmotic diarrhea seen in GGM patients will persist while they remain on standard formulas, including protein-hydrolysate formula, since such formulas generally contain glucose. Several undiagnosed patients have been managed improperly for long periods of time on home parenteral nutrition.

In a patient with documented carbohydrate malabsorption, the verification of three key features is necessary to establish the diagnosis of GGM. First, the intestinal biopsy of a GGM patient will have normal small bowel histology, including normal villus/crypt ratios, and inflammatory cells in the lamina propria (see Figs. 190-10 and 190-11). Second, a grossly abnormal oral glucose tolerance test and/or glucose breath hydrogen test is found, including glucose-induced diarrhea during the test (Table 190-2 and Fig. 190-5). Finally, eliminating glucose and galactose (and lactose) from the diet results in complete resolution of the diarrheal symptoms. While mucosal glucose uptake and molecular genetic testing are available, they are not necessary to establish the diagnosis in the majority of patients.

Differential Diagnosis

The differential diagnosis of congenital diarrhea is extensive and includes disorders that result in either malabsorption and/or secretory diarrhea.[53] During the first several weeks of life, diarrhea that results from cellular damage is particularly common, and causes include hypersensitivity disorders including cow milk and soybean-protein allergies. Other disorders that result in damage to the intestinal villi are eosinophilic gastroenteritis and a poorly defined autoimmune disorder that results in an intestinal enteropathy. Several clinical features and diagnostic tests should assist

Table 190-2 Oral Tolerance Tests on GGM Patient

Carbohydrate (g/kg)		Blood Concentrations (mg/100 ml)					
		0 h	0.5 h	1 h	2 h	3 h	4 h
Glucose, 1.75	Glucose	74	59	66	70	65	65
	Lactic acid	20	18	18	11	5	11
Galactose, 1.75	Glucose	64	65	68	66	66	nd
	Galactose	0	4	2	0	0	nd
	Lactic acid	9	7	9	7	8	nd
Fructose, 1.75	Glucose	64	120	95	68	47	55
	Fructose	0	0	24	8	8	5
	Lactic acid	16	30	19	14	11	14
Xylose, 0.5	Glucose	55	62	53	63	55	nd
	Xylose	0	21	23	15	13	nd
	Lactic acid	8	7	8	10	10	nd

NOTE: Data on patient from pedigree 28 (Table 190-3) (From Schneider et al., 1966[5]). This is the same GGM patient used in the studies shown in Figs. 190-10 to 190-17. nd, not determined.

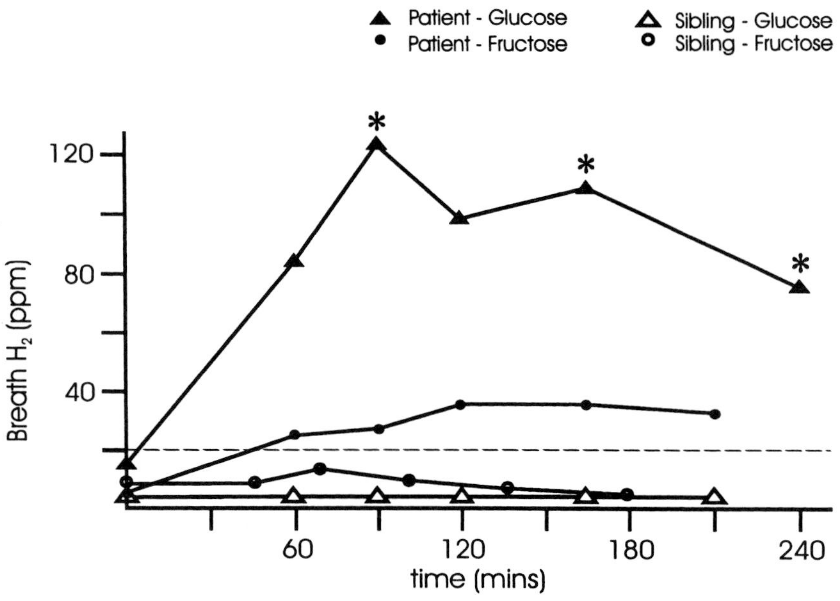

Fig. 190-5 The results of a breath hydrogen test on a GGM patient (pedigree 23 in Table 190-3) and her normal sister. Breath hydrogen was monitored following oral administration of D-glucose (2 g/kg) or D-fructose (1 g/kg). While the GGM patient exhibited a marked rise in breath hydrogen 60 minutes after the ingestion of D-glucose, there was only a modest increase with D-fructose. In the case of the normal sibling, the breath hydrogen remained in the normal range (< 20 ppm) in both tests (Martín Martín, unpublished data).

in distinguishing these disorders from GGM. These disorders result from cellular damage and may present with clinical symptoms of bloody diarrhea with associated colitis as determined by the presence of white blood cells in the stools. Individuals with cow's milk protein allergy generally have a significant family history of atopy, including asthma, eczema, hay fever, and food allergies. The most reliable diagnostic test to distinguish this general group of disorders from GGM is examination of an intestinal mucosal biopsy that has a normal architecture in GGM.

Less common causes of congenital diarrhea to consider are the autosomal recessive disorders congenital chloride diarrhea (OMIM 214700), primary bile acid malabsorption (OMIM 601295), congenital sodium diarrhea (OMIM 270420), and microvillus inclusion disease (OMIM 251850). Congenital chloride diarrhea is caused by a defect in the gene down-regulated in adenomas and results in the excessive excretion of luminal chloride and subsequent secretory diarrhea.[4] Congenital sodium diarrhea has been shown in knock-out mice to be due to defects in the sodium-hydrogen exchanger (NHE3); however, defects in the human isoform have not yet been identified in patients with sodium-secreting diarrhea.[55] Both these congenital secreting diarrheas may be accompanied by excessive intestinal fluid secretion prenatally, as exhibited by polyhydramnios and distended loops of bowel in the fetus.

Primary bile acid malabsorption is another rare diarrheal disorder and is caused by a defect in the bile acid transporter (SLC10A2) located on the apical membrane of the ileum.[56] These patients frequently have steatorrhea, failure to thrive, and low plasma levels of low-density lipoprotein cholesterol. The molecular basis of microvillus inclusion disease has not yet been defined, but presumably it results from a defect in a protein either located in or necessary for the development of the terminal web in the microvillus of the intestine.[57] All these disorders may present with clinical evidence of secretory diarrhea that will distinguish them from GGM. More specifically, patients with congenital chloride and sodium diarrhea will have elevated levels of stool chloride and sodium, respectively. Moreover, the severity of the diarrhea in the congenital ion-secreting diarrheas will not improve when the patient is not fed enterally. Microvillus inclusion disease also presents clinically with severe secretory diarrhea, and microvillus inclusions can be readily diagnosed by electron microscopic evaluation of intestinal biopsy samples.

Other causes of carbohydrate malabsorption that should be considered include primary lactase deficiency (OMIM 223000)[58] and sucrase-isomaltase deficiency (OMIM 222900).[59] Defects in the sucrase-isomaltase gene usually present with clinical symptoms suggestive of diarrhea after the third month of life when sucrose-based diets are usually introduced. The mucosa of individuals with sucrase-isomaltase deficiency has a low sucrase/lactase activity ratio, and sucrose but not glucose malabsorption may be identified by breath hydrogen testing. Primary lactase deficiency may be confused easily with GGM because both will present clinically during the first several days of life with severe osmotic diarrhea while the patient is consuming a lactose-based diet (see Chap. 76). Lactase deficiency is even rarer than GGM and results from defective production of the brush-border enzyme lactase-phlorizin hydrolase (LPH). Primary lactase deficiency should not be confused with hypolactasia, which is very common (20–100 percent of the population) in many parts of the world but usually presents with clinical symptoms generally after the second year of life. Lactase deficiency can be distinguished from GGM by obtaining a low mucosal lactase/sucrase activity ratio and a normal glucose breath hydrogen test. Individuals with GGM cannot tolerate either a glucose or lactose diet, whereas lactase-deficient patients are symptom-free on a glucose-containing diet.

Glucoamylase deficiency (OMIM 154360) is a recently recognized but still poorly defined disorder that may be difficult to distinguish from GGM.[60] Since several formulas contain starch, patients with glucoamylase deficiency may present in early infancy with unexplained osmotic diarrhea. A normal glucose breath hydrogen test should assist in distinguishing this disorder from GGM. Isolated fructose malabsorption has been reported in several kindreds; however, recent attempts to identify mutations in the apically located fructose transporter GLUT5 did not reveal significant disease-causing mutations.[47]

Diagnostic Evaluation

General. When considering the diagnosis of GGM, several general and specific diagnostic tests should be performed. Hospitalized patients should have standard stool analysis including pH, occult blood, and leukocyte analysis, as well as evaluation for the presence of reducing and nonreducing sugars (Clinitest). Carbohydrate malabsorption and subsequent colonic bacterial fermentation result in the synthesis of high concentrations of short-chain fatty acids (e.g., acetate, butyrate, propionate), which leads to the acidification of stool (pH < 4). Stool culture for bacteria and ova/parasites, including analysis for *Clostridium difficile*

Table 190-3 Mutations of *SGLT1* in Glucose-Galactose Malabsorption

Mutation		Exon	Nucleotide	AA	Kindred	Genotype
Missense						
1	*D28N*	1	GAT → AAT @ 92	Asp → Asn	1	Hom
2	*D28G*	1	GAT → GGT @ 93	Asp → Gly	12	Hom
3	*N51S*	2	AAT → AGT @ 162	Asn → Ser	45/9	Hom/Het
4	*R135W*	5	CGG → TGG @ 413	Arg → Trp	16	Het
5	*L147R*	5	CTT → CGT @ 450	Leu → Arg	28	Het
6	*S159P*	5	TCG → CCG @ 485	Ser → Pro	6/24	Het
7	*A166T*	6	GCC → ACC @ 506	Ala → Thr	11	Hom
8	*W276L*	8	TGG → TTG @ 837	Trp → Leu	30	Hom
9	*C292Y*	8	TGC → TAC @ 885	Cys → Tyr	8/48	Hom
10	*Q295R*	8	CAG → CGG @ 893	Gln → Arg	5	Hom
11	*R300S*	9	CGC → AGC @ 908	Arg → Ser	23	Het
12	*A304V*	9	GCC → GTC @ 921	Ala → Val	41	Hom
13	*G318R*	9	GGG → AGG @ 962	Gly → Arg	56	Het
14	*C355S*	10	TGC → AGC @ 1073	Cys → Ser	28	Het
15	*L369S*	10	TTA → TCA @ 1116	Leu → Ser	46	Het
16	*R379Q*	11	CGA → CAA @ 1146	Arg → Gln	24	Het
17	*A388V*	11	GCC → GTC @ 1173	Ala → Val	15	Het
18	*F405S*	11	TTC → TCC @ 1224	Phe → Ser	15	Het
19	*A411T*	11	GCC → ACC @ 1241	Ala → Thr	30	Hom
20	*G426R*	11	GGA → AGA @ 1286	Gly → Arg	6	Het
21	*Q457R*	12	CAG → CGG @ 1380	Gln → Arg	40/49/50	Hom/Het
22	*A468V*	12	GCG → GTG @ 1173	Ala → Val	56	Het
23	*V470N*	12	GTC → GAC @ 1419	Val → Asn	10	Het
24	*R499H*	13	CGT → CAT @ 1506	Arg → His	38	Het
25	*H615Q*	15	CAC → CAG @ 1855	His → Gln	45	Hom
Nonsense						
26	*Y191X*	6	TAC → TAA @ 583	Tyr → Stop	39	Hom
27	*K254X*	8	AAA → TAA @ 770	Lys → Stop	2	Hom
28	*W276X*	8	TGG → TAG @ 837	Trp → Stop	54	Hom
29	*R379X*	11	CGA → TGA @ 1145	Arg → Stop	38	Het
Frameshift						
30	248delG	3	GGA → G_A	FS → Stop	47	Hom
31	273delC	3	GCC → G_C	FS → Stop	55	Het
32	799delC	8	CAC → _AC	FS → Stop	3	Hom
33	1098ins15	10	GGTTGGCTGTACCAA	ins LVGCT	44	Het
34	1265del4	11	T GAG AA → TA	FS → Stop	7/9	Hom
35	1286insT	11	CCG → CCTG	FS → Stop	45	Hom
36	1404insT	12	CCC → TCC C	FS → Stop	35	Hom
Splice site						
37	145+1	I-1	g GTATG → g TTATG		26	Hom
38	382+2de/in	I-4	g GTAAG → g GCTTATATTAAGG		23	Het
39	382+2dupl	I-4	g GTAAG → g		55	Het
40	1458+5	I-12	a GTAGG → a GTAGC		18	Hom
41	1458+2	I-12	a GTAGG → a GCAGC		16	Het

NOTE: Mutations listed are based on the format of internationally accepted nomenclature and are categorized by mutation type. Amino acid and nucleotide residue numbers are based on the methionine initiation codon (ATG). The exon locations of mutations are specified, and the nucleotide mutations are underlined and numbered. The kindered identification number and the patient's number and the patient's genotype are listed.

toxins, should be performed in patients who are at risk for such infections.

Stool electrolytes (sodium, potassium, and chloride) should be determined, and a large osmotic gap of greater than 100 mosm when compared with serum osmolarity would suggest malabsorption. In contrast, a low osmotic gap (< 50 mosm) would be more consistent with a secretory diarrhea. After sufficient stool samples have been obtained and the quantity and characteristics of the diarrheal pattern have been established, a fasting trial should be performed. Diarrhea will continue to persist during the fasting state if it is secretory and will abate if it is osmotic in nature. The stools of a patient with GGM should be acidic, with detectable levels of reducing substance and an electrolyte analysis consistent with osmotic diarrhea while the patient is on a glucose-based diet.

Small Bowel Biopsy. Small bowel biopsies should be performed early in the evaluation of a patient with congenital diarrhea. Analysis of the mucosa should provide several important clues that would assist in establishing the diagnosis. The histologic features from biopsy samples obtained from the duodenum are critically important. Mucosal defects such as flattened villi and a low villus/crypt ratio are inconsistent with the diagnosis of GGM but are characteristic of an individual with food allergies and various forms of enteric infections. GGM patients should have normal-appearing microvilli on electron microscopy, with normal villus architecture on hematoxylin and eosin stains (see Figs. 190-10 and 190-11).

Mucosal biopsies also can be used to assess lactase and sucrase activity, which may be helpful in distinguishing GGM from primary lactase or sucrase deficiency. Glucose and galactose uptake studies of mucosal samples are very useful but are tedious to perform and generally are not readily available. Biopsy samples also may be useful in establishing GGM by immunohistochemical analysis using antisera to SGLT1. As we reported earlier, most SGLT1 mutations result in either targeting defects to the plasma membrane or incomplete synthesis in the form of a nonsense mutation.[10] Immunohistochemical analysis of mucosa has shown an absence of SGLT1 on the apical membrane of individuals with mutations that result in improper targeting to the plasma membrane (see below).

Breath Hydrogen Testing. The glucose breath hydrogen test is another useful test that should be performed in a patient in whom the diagnosis of GGM is being considered. Carbohydrate breath hydrogen testing is an easily performed test that may assist in the diagnosis of several types of carbohydrate malabsorption disorders including lactose, sucrose, and fructose malabsorption. The test relies on the colonic fermentation of unabsorbed carbohydrate by bacteria that produce methane, hydrogen, and carbon dioxide gas. This gas chromatographic analysis quantifies the level of hydrogen gas in exhaled air following the administration of either glucose (or galactose) at 2 g/kg of body weight or a maximum of 50 g for patients who weigh more than 25 kg. While an elevation of more than 20 ppm above the fasting baseline is consistent with the diagnosis of glucose malabsorption, most patients with GGM have levels that are frequently higher than 100 ppm (see Fig. 190-5). Therefore, it is reasonable and probably safer to consider using a much lower glucose load (< 0.5 g/kg) when performing a breath hydrogen test in a patient who is believed to have GGM.

After the administration of antibiotics, the sensitivity of carbohydrate breath hydrogen tests diminishes over the short term. The reliability of breath hydrogen testing in a patient recently treated with antibiotics can be confirmed by administering lactulose, an obligate nonabsorbable carbohydrate. A low-hydrogen breath after a lactulose challenge indicates the absence of significant amounts of colonic bacteria. Moreover, the presence of significant diarrhea either during or shortly after the carbohydrate challenge should raise the suspicion of a false-negative breath hydrogen test. The specificity of an abnormal glucose breath hydrogen test may be confirmed by performing a fructose breath hydrogen test, which should be normal in GGM patients because fructose is absorbed via the unaffected facilitative transporter, GLUT5. However, while slight fructose malabsorption is particularly common in younger children, breath hydrogen levels in a GGM patient will be substantially higher with glucose compared with fructose administration[47] (see Fig. 190-5). Interestingly, 10 percent of healthy individuals have been shown to malabsorb glucose when tested by breath hydrogen methods.[4]

Molecular Genetic Testing

Genetic testing for GGM is currently available. Testing involves the screening of SGLT1's 15 exons for mutations by single-stranded conformational polymorphism (SSCP) and the subsequent sequencing of genomic DNA. All identified missense mutations need to be studied using a heterologous expression system, e.g., *X. laevis* oocytes. This functional test has been essential to distinguish disease-causing mutations from inconsequential polymorphisms.

The abundance of private mutations has made molecular testing costly, cumbersome, and rather slow. Therefore, while genetic testing can be used as a final verification for the diagnosis of GGM, it is clearly not necessary to establish the diagnosis. Genetic testing has been used successfully to perform prenatal diagnosis on a family at risk for GGM[61] (see Fig. 190-8).

Management

GGM patients, like those with other disorders of carbohydrate malabsorption, resolve their symptoms while on a diet free of glucose and galactose. Several formulas are available for managing GGM patients during early infancy. The Ross Carbohydrate-Free Formula (RCF) (Ross Products, Columbus, Ohio) is frequently used in North America and must be supplemented with fructose (4 g fructose per 30 ml of concentrated formula and diluted further with water to a final volume of 60 ml). In Europe, Galactomin 19 (Nutricia, Holland) is generally used and is supplied with fructose. While these formulas are only necessary for the first several years of life, they are frequently used as nutritional supplements well into late childhood.

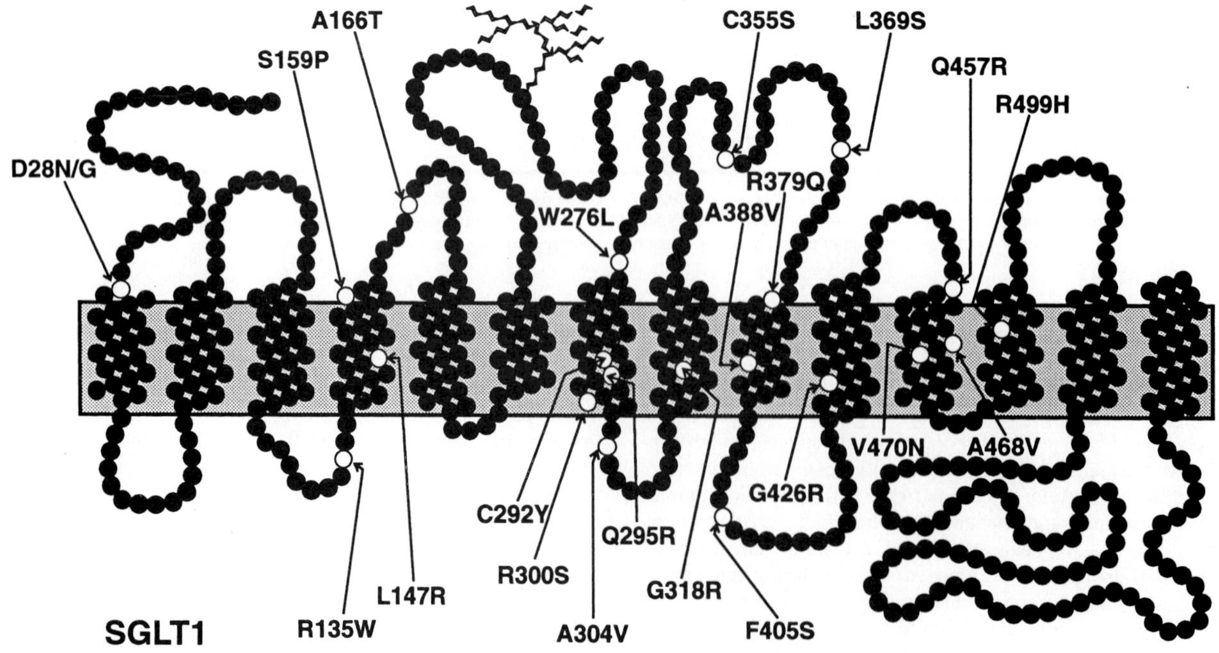

Fig. 190-6 The secondary structure of SGLT1 showing the location of missense mutations causing GGM (see Table 190-3). All these mutant proteins have been assayed for function using the oocyte expression system (see Fig. 190-9).

The dietary management of GGM patients becomes more challenging as they enter into late infancy and begin to exert independence. Guidance from a well-trained dietician is frequently invaluable. Highly motivated parents generally will benefit from dietary manuals[62] that list the sugar content of selected foods. Reviewing with parents such a dietary list will help identify particular foods that have relatively low glucose and galactose contents. Nevertheless, the required diet of a GGM patient is very restricted and inevitably high in fat and protein (see below). The required lifelong glucose- and galactose-free diet may in the long

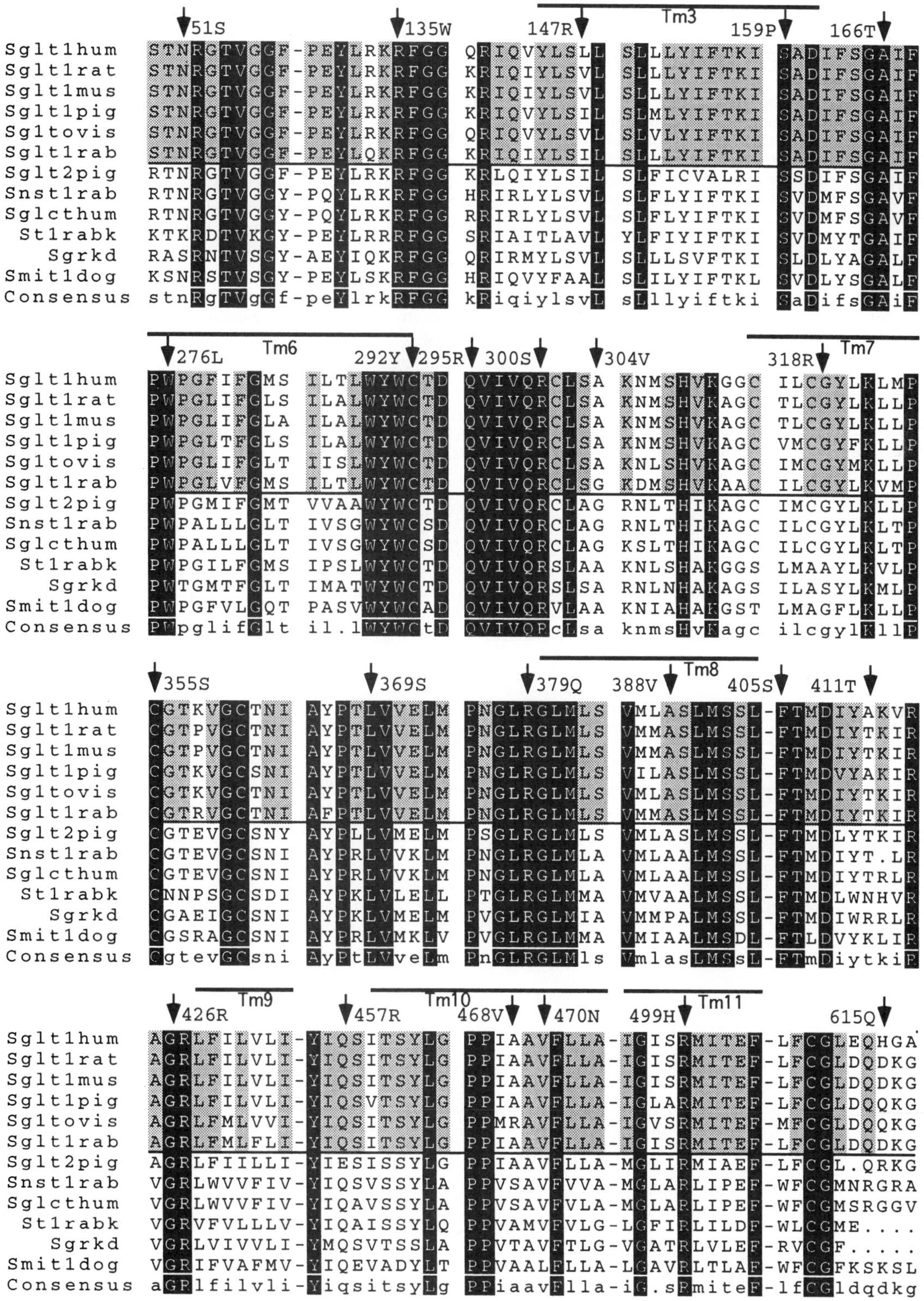

Fig. 190-7 Location of GGM missense mutations in conserved domains of the *SGLT1* gene family. The residues conserved in the gene family are shaded in black, whereas the residues conserved in the sodium-glucose cotransporters are shaded in gray. The family includes the human, rat, mouse, pig, sheep, and rabbit sodium-glucose cotransporters, the pig low-affinity sodium-glucose cotransporter, the rabbit sodium-nucleoside cotransporter, three orphan clones, and the dog sodium-myoinositol cotransporter. (*Modified by permission from Martín et al.*[10])

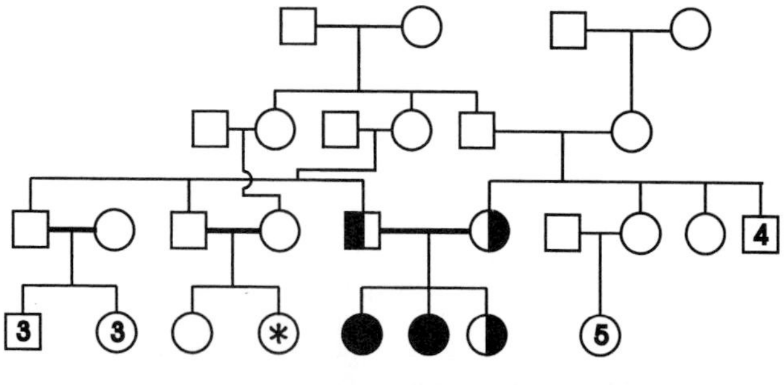

Fig. 190-8 One kindred with two GGM patents. The two sisters (pedigree 1 in Table 190-3) diagnosed with GGM were the first to be screened for mutations in the *SGLT1* gene.[9] Both were homozygous for the *D28N* mutation, and each parent is a carrier for the mutation. A younger sister, screened prenatally for this mutation, also was found to be a carrier.[39] A cousin (*) also was screened prenatally and was normal. The extended family tree was provided by our collaborator Dr. Bernard Zabel of the University of Mainz, Germany.

term have significant renal and cardiovascular consequences; however, thus far no such consequences have been reported in patients with GGM.

Molecular Genetics

The molecular genetics of GGM have been described in several reports and are summarized in Table 190-3.[10–12] A total of 41 significant changes have been detected, including 25 missense, 4 nonsense, 7 frameshift, and 5 splice-site mutations. Transversion mutations accounted for more than a one-quarter of the changes identified, and one in every two mutations occurred at a CpG dinucleotide.

The 25 missense mutations that were identified are dispersed throughout the gene; however, 16 of them were located within exons 8 to 12. Moreover, two particular "hot spots" (residues 276–318 and 355–405) contained a cluster of 11 mutations (Fig. 190-6). Fourteen of the 25 missense mutations were located within the putative transmembrane region of the protein. Five other missense mutations were present within 5 residues of the membrane interface. The majority of the mutations alter residues that are well conserved in the 12 members of the *SGLT1* gene family (Fig. 190-7).

The extended family tree of the first kindred in whom we identified the mutation in *SGLT1* that caused GGM is shown in Fig. 190-8. The parents, who carry the D28N mutation on one allele, are first cousins. The third child of this couple is also heterozygous. Note that the patient in the second kindred has a mutation of the same residue (D28G) (see Table 190-3). Site-directed mutagenesis studies (K. Hager and E. M. Wright, unpublished results) also show that D28Q, D28E, and D28A mutations in *SGLT1* also eliminate sodium-glucose cotransport activity in the oocyte expression system.

Each of the 25 missense mutations was analyzed for its sodium-sugar cotransport activity using the heterologous *Xenopus* oocyte expression system (Fig. 190-9). Transport activity in 16 of the mutant proteins was indistinguishable from that of noninjected oocytes. Moderate sugar uptake, 5 to 12 percent of wild type, was detected in 5 mutations. Of the 4 nonsense mutations identified, the longest and shortest mutants were tested for sugar uptake and were similar to noninjected oocytes. Interestingly, several (A304V, A468V) seemingly minor mutations (i.e., alanine to valine) were shown to completely abolish sugar uptake activity. These mutations must alter residues that are located in the critical regions of the protein, and this underscores the importance of performing functional analysis of mutations identified in patients.

Western blot analysis showed that the expression levels of all missense mutations in oocytes were comparable with those of wild-type SGLT1. These data suggest that in this particular heterologous expression system, the missense and frameshift mutations investigated do not result in a decline in the synthesis of SGLT1 protein. All but one of the missense mutant proteins

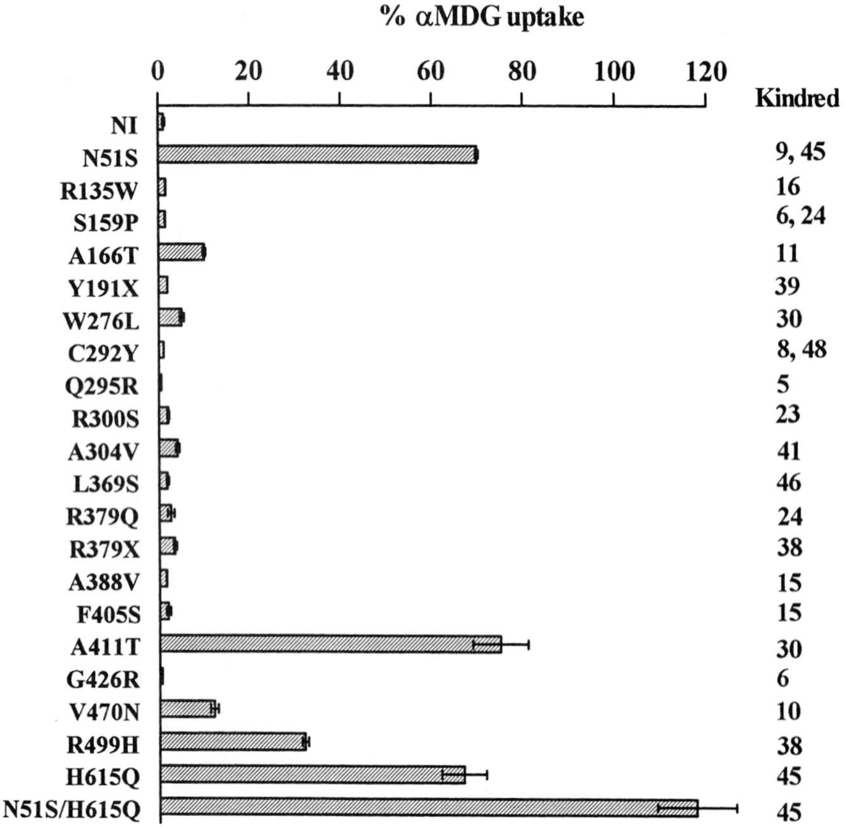

Fig. 190-9 Functional expression of GGM mutants. The mutant proteins were expressed in oocytes and 50 μM [^{14}C]α-methyl-D-glucopyranoside uptakes in sodium were measured after 60 minutes. The uptakes were expressed as a percentage of the uptake obtained with the wild-type SGLT1 expressed in the same batch of oocytes 3 days after cRNA injection. (*From Martín et al.*[10] *Used by permission.*)

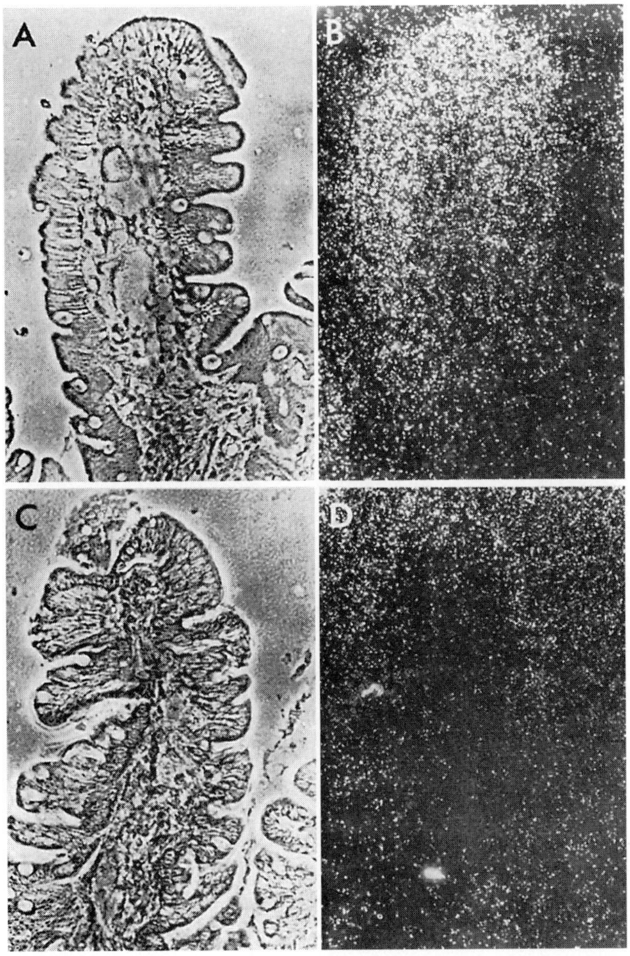

Fig. 190-10 Autoradiographs of intestinal villi from a GGM patient (pedigree 28 in Table 190-3) and a normal individual showing the site of defect in sodium-sugar transport. Intestinal biopsies (10–30 mg) were incubated in physiologic saline containing 1 mM [^{14}C]D-galactose for 3 minutes. The experiments were terminated by freezing the tissue at −160°C, and then frozen sections were cut for autoradiography and histology. In the control (*A, B*) [^{14}C]galactose was accumulated within the enterocytes at the tip of the villi, whereas in the biopsy from the GGM patient (*C, D*) there was no sugar accumulation. Note that the histology of the villus in the GGM patient appeared normal. (Magnification × 110; for higher magnification micrographs, see Figs. 190-11 and 190-12.) (*From Schneider et al.*[5] *Used with permission.*)

failed to be trafficked normally to the plasma membrane, indicating that these proteins were not folded properly for correct targeting.

How Do *SGLT1* Mutations Cause GGM?

We are particularly interested in how the missense mutations identified in the *SGLT1* gene cause GGM. The other mutations—nonsense, frameshift, and splice site—all result in the introduction of premature stop codons, and the truncated protein is not expected to function properly. We have confirmed this for two truncated proteins, Y191X and R379X (see Fig. 190-9), and truncations upstream of residue 407 are anticipated to eliminate the sugar translocation domain of the protein.[39] With the missense mutations it is not immediately obvious why sugar transport is impaired across the brush-border membrane of the intestine. To illustrate one mechanism, we summarize the clinical and experimental studies on one patient and then present functional studies on the *SGLT1* mutations responsible for sugar malabsorption in this patient.

The case we have chosen is the first one reported in North America in 1966.[5] The proband, C.H., was born in 1964 and admitted to hospital at 12 days of age because of diarrhea and dehydration. The diarrhea persisted except when oral feedings were completely withheld. Subsequently, it was discovered that profuse watery diarrhea developed within 8 hours of feeding glucose, and it was reasoned that the patient was unable to absorb glucose. Oral tolerance tests (see Table 190-2) revealed that there was no absorption of glucose or galactose but that absorption of fructose and xylose was normal. The glucose and galactose loads increased stool water and sugar excretion, and diarrhea occurred within 3 hours. Intestinal biopsies showed normal histology of the intestinal mucosa (Figs. 190-10 and 190-11). Sophisticated autoradiographic studies of [^{14}C]D-galactose accumulation in mucosal biopsies from the patient and normal controls (see Figs. 190-10 and 190-11) demonstrated that the patient's mucosa was unable to accumulate galactose across the brush-border membrane from the incubation medium. The enterocytes from the control were able to accumulate galactose to concentrations four to five times higher than the incubation medium within 5 minutes, and this accumulation was blocked by 40 to 71 percent by phlorizin, the specific inhibitor of SGLT1. The patient's intracellular galactose concentration did not rise above this in medium even after 30 minutes of incubation. Autoradiographic experiments to measure [^{3}H]phlorizin binding (see Fig. 190-12) also demonstrated that phlorizin binding to the brush border was reduced dramatically in mucosa from the patient. The density of phlorizin-binding sites on the brush-border membrane was less than 10 percent of the control value. It was concluded that the patient suffered from glucose-galactose malabsorption and that this was due to 90 percent reduction in the density of sugar carriers (phlorizin-binding sites) on the brush-border membrane. The child thrived on a diet free of all carbohydrate except fructose.

This patient, interviewed in 1996, has remained healthy for more than 30 years even though she cannot tolerate glucose and galactose in her diet. She consumes a high-protein, high-fat diet and cannot take a teaspoon (6 g) of table sugar without experiencing symptoms. Blood samples were obtained from the patient, her parents, her brother, and her two children.[11] Genomic DNA was isolated from each sample, and the exons in the *SGLT1* gene were screened for mutations. The patient (kindred 28 in Table 190-3) was a compound heterozygote with a missense mutation on each allele. She inherited the C355S mutation from her mother and the L147R mutation from her father (Fig. 190-13). Her brother carries neither mutation, but each daughter carries one of the two mutations.

Each mutant protein was expressed in *X. laevis* oocytes for functional studies. Radioactive tracer sugar uptake experiments (Fig. 190-14) showed that oocytes injected with *L147R* or *C355S* cRNA did not take up sugar (<1 percent of wild-type uptakes). This was confirmed by electrophysiologic assays (Fig. 190-15) in which no sugar-dependent inward sodium currents were recorded at any membrane voltage between +50 and −150 mV. Furthermore, pre-steady state charge measurements Q in the absence of sugar (see Fig. 190-15*B*) suggested that neither of the mutant proteins was trafficked to the plasma membrane of the oocyte. The Q_{max} measurements for the wild-type protein (25 nC) indicate the presence of the 4.5×10^{10} transporters in the plasma membrane. The absence of detectable charge movements for the mutants indicates that there were less than 5 percent of this number in the membrane. This was confirmed by freeze-fracture electron microscopy (Fig. 190-16). The density of P-face intramembrane particles increased from 200 to 1000/μm^2 in the case of wild-type SGLT1 oocytes, whereas the particle density for the oocytes expressing the mutant proteins was indistinguishable from that of control, noninjected oocytes. Previous studies have determined that the increase in density of P-face particles in SGLT1 cRNA-injected oocytes is due to the trafficking of SGLT1 protein to the plasma membrane.[23,64] Both the charge measurements and freeze-fracture electron microscopic studies led to the conclusion that the lack of transport activity is due to the lack of cotransporter in the plasma membrane.

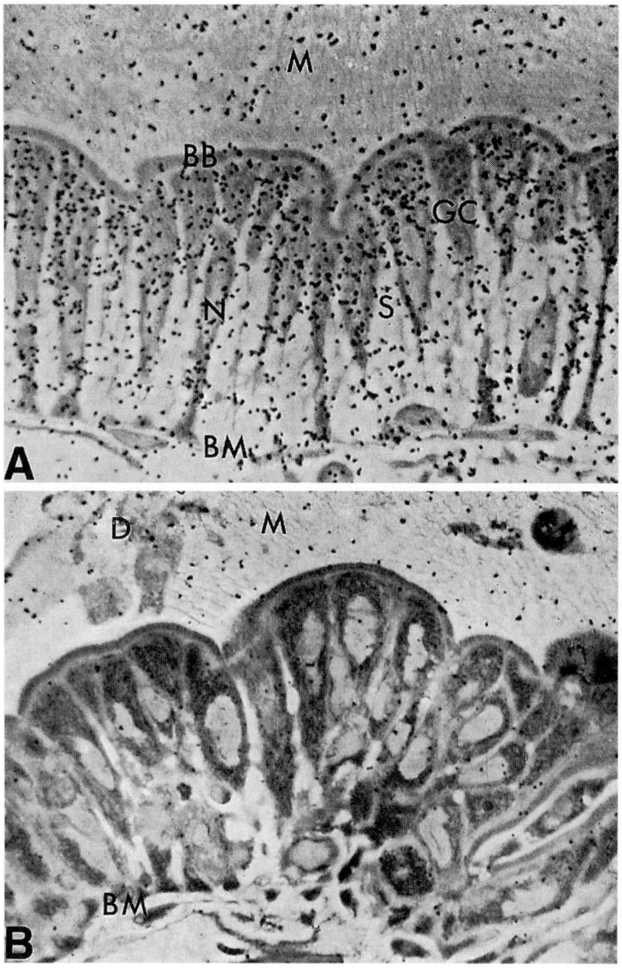

Fig. 190-11 Autoradiographs of [^{14}C]D-galactose accumulation in enterocytes from normal and GGM biopsies. The tissues were incubated in physiologic saline containing 1 mM [^{14}C]D-galactose for 3 to 5 minutes and prepared for autoradiography as described in Fig. 190-10. The grain density (black dots) over the medium (M) respresent the 1 mM labeled sugar. Note the accumulation of galactose (black dots) in the enterocytes of the control biopsy (*A*) but not in the GGM biopsy (*B*). The grain density ratio (cytoplasm/medium) was 4.5 × 0.8^{10} for the control and much less than 1 for the GGM patient. Phlorizin (0.5 mM), a specific blocker of sodium-sugar transport, reduced the galactose accumulation in the control biopsy by 50 percent (magnification 1700–1800). The GGM patient (pedigree 28 in Table 190-3) is the same patient as shown in Figs. 190-10 and 190-12. (*From Stirling et al.*[6] *Used by permission.*)

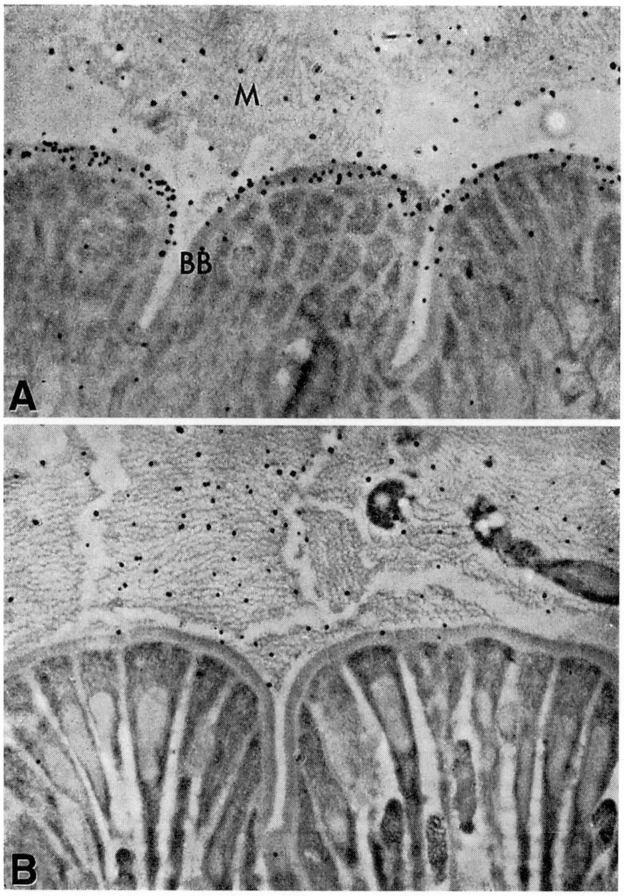

Fig. 190-12 Autoradiographs of [^{3}H]phlorizin binding to the brush-border membrane (BB) of enterocytes from a control subject. Biopsies were incubated in physiologic saline (M) containing [^{3}H]phlorizin and then prepared for autoradiography as described in Fig. 190-10. [^{3}H]Phlorizin (dark grains) was bound to the brush-border membrane when the medium phlorizin concentration was 5 μM (*A*), and this was blocked by increasing the medium phlorizin concentration to 100 μM (*B*) (magnification × 1800). Similar experiments with the GGM biopsy (pedigree 28 in Table 190-3) showed a greater than 10 reduction in [^{3}H]phlorizin binding to the brush-border membrane (the maximum phlorizin binding was reduced from 91 to 8 μmol phlorizin per liter of microvilli). (*From Stirling et al.*[6] *Used by permission.*)

To determine if the low density of mutant SGLT1 protein in the membrane is due to a failure in translation of the cRNA, degradation of the mutant protein, or mistrafficking, we measured the level of SGLT1 protein in the oocytes using Western blotting (Fig. 190-17). This representative blot shows that there are comparable levels of all three SGLT1 proteins in the oocytes, but only the wild-type protein shows both core (60 kDa) and complex (70 kDa) glycosylation. Experiments such as these demonstrate that the mutant SGLT1 proteins are translated and inserted into the endoplasmic reticulum. However, the lack of complex glycosylation suggests that the mutant proteins are retained in the endoplasmic reticulum.

These results with the L147R and C355S SGLT1 mutants are consistent with the earlier autoradiographic studies of the intestinal biopsies from this patient (see Figs. 190-9 through 190-11), where Stirling *et al.*[16] concluded that the cellular defect in glucose and galactose transport across the intestinal brush border is a persistent reduction in the number of functioning sugar carriers at the microvillar membrane.

Improper trafficking of mutant SGLT1 proteins to the plasma membrane appears to be the dominant reason why these mutants cause GGM. Experiments similar to those described above for L147R and C355S have been carried out for all the missense mutations identified.[10–12,64] For all but one of the missense mutations (see Table 190-3), the mutant proteins are present in the oocyte at levels comparable with the wild-type SGLT1 but are not inserted into the plasma membrane. Four nonfunctional mutants, S159P, R300S, A304V, and *A388V,* show complex glycosylation, whereas the remainder are only core glycosylated. This suggests that four are arrested between the trans-Golgi network (Fig. 190-18) and the plasma membrane, whereas the remainder are retained in the endoplasmic reticulum. In the case of one rabbit SGLT1 mutant, A457R,[65] there is evidence that the mutation blocks docking of the transport vesicle bearing the fully glycosylated transporter with the plasma membrane (step 6 in Fig. 190-18).

Are the results obtained in heterologous expression systems such as oocytes of any significance with regard to the intestinal sugar transport in patients? To address this concern, we extended our studies to the intestinal mucosa of GGM patients. The approach was to use immunocytochemical studies on mucosal biopsies of patients with either homozygous missense mutations or compound heterozygous missense mutations with similar defects

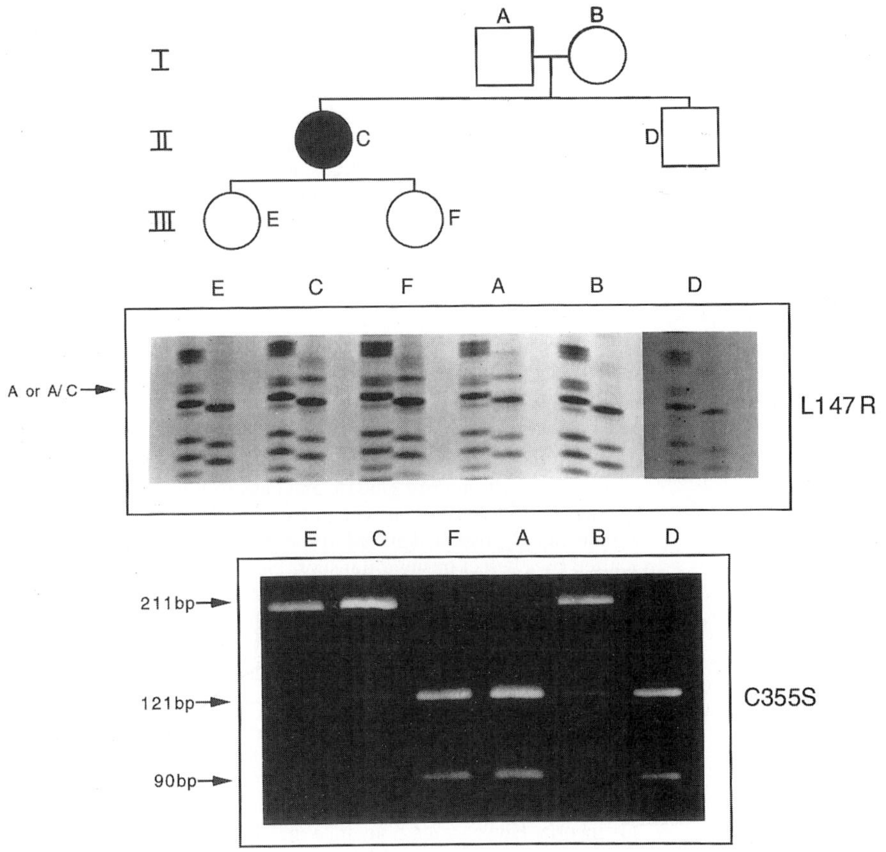

Fig. 190-13 Individual genotypes for the C355S and L147R mutations in one kindred (28 in Table 190-3). (*A*) Each generation is labeled with a roman numeral, with women and men represented by circles and squares, respectively. (*B*) Sequencing of exon 5 is shown with an antisense oligonucleotide primer, which for convenience was limited to the adenine and cytosine nucleotides. Carriers contain both an adenine and cytosine at position 450 (*arrow*), whereas noncarriers contain only adenine (L147C). (*C*) The restriction enzyme (RsaI) digestion of exon 10 (C355S) that was PCR amplified and run on an ethidium bromide-stained agarose gel is shown. The 121- and 90-bp fragments represent digestion of the 211-bp wild-type fragment. Therefore, heterozygotes contain three fragments (211, 121, and 90 bp), whereas noncarriers consist of two fragments (121 and 90 bp). *n,* original proband. (*From Martín et al.*[11] *Used by permission.*)

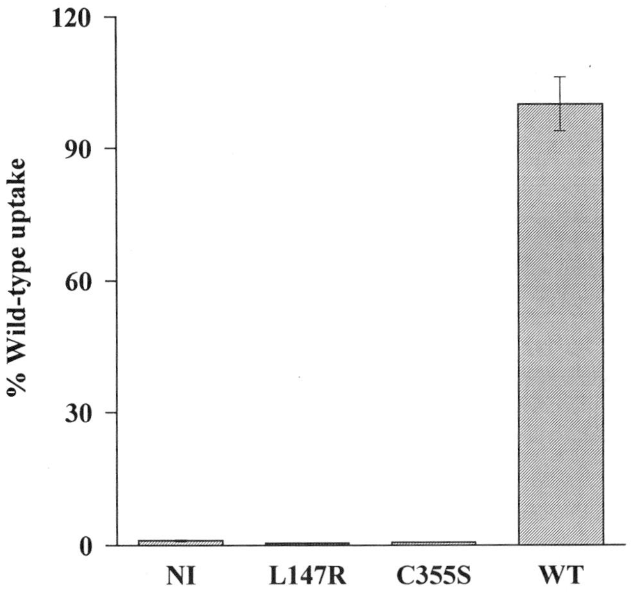

Fig. 190-14 αMDG uptake by human SGLT1, wild type and mutants. Oocytes were injected with 50 ng of complementary RNA coding for wild-type or L47R or C355S mutant SGLT1. Uptakes using 50 mmol/liter of ^{14}C . (MDG was performed and represents the mean of 8 to 10 oocytes expressed as the percentage of the wild-type uptake. Wild-type sugar uptake (*WT*) ranged between 194 ± 14 and 326 ± 18 pmol per oocyte per hour, whereas for both mutants it was less than 1 percent of wild-type sugar uptake. NI, noninjected. (*From Martín et al.*[11] *Used by permission.*)

in the oocyte expression system. So far we have studied four cases (Lostao *et al.*, unpublished data), and the results suggest similar causes for the sugar transport defect in the patients' enterocytes and in oocytes. In patients with homozygous missense mutations D28N and C292Y (see Table 190-3), the SGLT1 immunoreactivity was intracellular between the nucleus and the brush-border membrane, whereas in oocytes these mutants were arrested at a point between the endoplasmic reticulum and the Golgi apparatus. This also was the case with the patient with the compound heterozygous mutations G318R and A468V. It also should be recalled that [^{3}H]phlorizin binding to the brush-border membrane of the patient with the compound heterozygous mutations L147R and C355S was less than 10 percent of controls,[6] and this is consistent with our results in oocytes. In the final case, Q457R, the mutant protein was found at a normal density in both the oocyte plasma membrane and the patient's brush-border membrane, but the mutant protein was unable to transport sugar. Recapitulation of the patient's molecular defect in the oocyte expression system in these five cases validates conclusions drawn from oocyte expression studies about the molecular basis for sugar malabsorption in patients.

How do mutations cause improper trafficking of SGLT1 to the plasma membrane? The majority of the missense mutations involve charged or polar residues, e.g., R300S, L147R, G426R (see Fig. 190-6 and Table 190-3), where it is expected that these will grossly destabilize the protein structure. However, there are three very conservative mutations, A304V, A388V, and A468V, that disrupt normal trafficking of SGLT1 to the plasma membrane. This suggests that changes in bulk at critical residues in the protein are sufficient to alter folding. This is supported by studies where A468 was mutated to a cysteine, which has a molecular volume

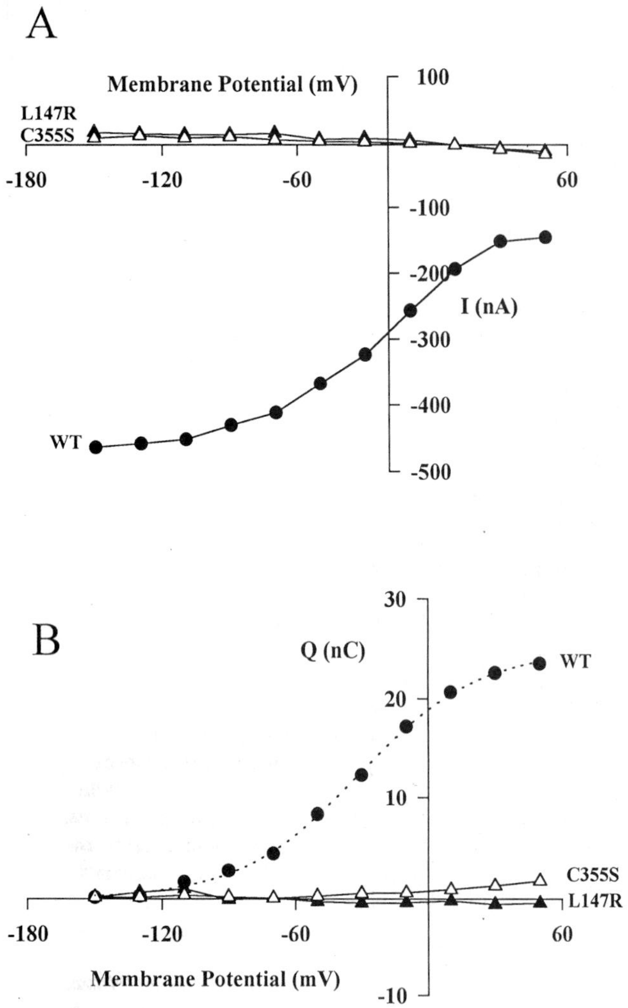

Fig. 190-15 Steady state currents and charge movements produced by wild-type and mutant SGLT1 proteins expressed in oocytes. Wild-type, C355S, and L147R complementary RNA was injected into oocytes, and currents were recorded 4 days after injection. (*A*) Oocytes were incubated in 100 mM NaCl buffer, and the differences in steady state currents were measured in the presence and absence of 25 mmol/liter. (MDG is plotted at each voltage. At V_m = −150 mV, wild type produced −463 nA of inward current, whereas Cys355Ser- and Leu147Arg-injected oocytes did not induce inward current at any membrane potential. (*B*) Charge movement *Q* was obtained by integration of the SGLT1 current transients measured in sugar-free 100 mM NaCl buffer after jumps in the membrane potential. Plotted are the *Q* values obtained at each membrane potential. Q_{max} was 24 and much less than 2.0 nC for wild type, *C355S,* and *L147R,* respectively. The dotted lines in wild type are drawn according to the Boltzman relation. (*From Martín et al.*[11] *Used by permission.*)

intermediate between alanine and valine. The A468C mutant attained a density in the oocyte plasma membrane that was about 25 percent of that for the wild-type protein, and it was fully functional.[37] It follows that the overall conformation is important in the trafficking of SGLT1 from the endoplasmic reticulum to the plasma membrane. Defective protein folding is becoming recognized as the basis of an increasing number of genetic diseases of plasma membrane proteins, e.g., cystic fibrosis and retinitis pigmentosa.[66]

In only one case, the Q457R allele, is the GGM mutant protein in the plasma membrane of oocytes and the brush-border membrane of the patient's enterocytes at normal densities. This conclusion was based on SGLT1 immunocytochemistry of mucosal biopsies in the patient and charge measurements and freeze fracture electron microscopic studies of oocytes expressing the Q457R SGLT1 protein. Nevertheless, this mutant did not transport sugar, as determined from both radioactive sugar uptake tests and current measurements in oocytes (Lostao *et al.*, unpublished data). Sugar binding to the mutant protein was normal, but there was no translocation. Recall that Q457R is located in the sugar-binding/translocation domain of the protein. This phenotype was recapitulated in oocytes expressing the Q457C SGLT1 mutant.[34] Q457C functioned normally in the oocyte plasma membrane, but when treated with alkylating reagents, e.g., MTSEA, sugar transport was fully blocked even though sugar binding was normal.

OTHER POTENTIAL CAUSES OF INTESTINAL SUGAR MALABSORPTION

Fanconi-Bickel Syndrome (OMIM 227810)

This is a rare disorder of glucose and galactose metabolism.[67] It is characterized by glycogen accumulation in the liver and proximal tubule and glycosuria. This led to speculation that the syndrome is caused by a defect in sugar transport. Santer *et al.*[68] screened four patients in three families for mutations in the *GLUT2* gene and found three different homozygous mutations that result in premature stop codons. The truncated gene products are not expected to be functional. It was concluded that *GLUT2* mutations are the probable cause of the Franconi-Bickel syndrome. Given that GLUT2 protein is postulated to play a critical role in glucose, galactose, and fructose transport across the basolateral membrane of the intestinal epithelium (see Fig. 190-1), one would expect that these patients would exhibit sugar malabsorption in addition to glycosuria. However, carbohydrate malabsorption and diarrhea are not seen in all Franconi-Bickel patients. Likewise, in GLUT2-deficient mice[69] the renal reabsorption of glucose is impaired, whereas intestinal glucose absorption appears to be normal. This suggests that there may be another glucose transporter expressed in the intestinal basolateral membrane of both Franconi-Bickel patients and *GLUT2* knock-out mice. It is also of note that a missense mutation in the *GLUT2* gene in a diabetic patient, *V197I,* abolished the transport activity of GLUT2 protein expressed in *Xenopus* oocytes.[70] These investigators suggested that defects in *GLUT2* may be involved in the pathogenesis of non-insulin-dependent diabetes

Fructose Malabsorption

The first step in dietary fructose absorption is transport across the intestinal brush-border membrane by the facilitated transporter GLUT5 (see Fig. 190-1). Patients with isolated fructose malabsorption present with pronounced abdominal pain and diarrhea after ingestion of low amounts of free fructose and give a positive fructose breath hydrogen test.[47] Screening of the *GLUT5* gene in eight patients with this syndrome indicated that mutations in the fructose transporter protein are not responsible for fructose malabsorption. The disorder is most likely due to a reduction in GLUT5 protein expression in the brush-border membrane. Likewise, toddler's diarrhea is probably due to the low expression of GLUT5 protein in early childhood. In healthy adults, about 70 percent fail to completely absorb 50 g of fructose (equivalent to the fructose in two 12-oz cans of soda), as measured by breath hydrogen tests and GI symptoms.[4] This points to a limited expression of GLUT5 protein in the brush-border membrane. Hereditary fructose intolerance is not due to a defect in fructose transport but rather to a defect in fructose-1,6-bisphosphate aldolase B.[71]

HEREDITARY RENAL GLYCOSURIA

Hereditary renal glycosuria (OMIM 233100) is an autosomal recessive disorder in which glucose is excreted in the urine in the absence of hyperglycemia (see ref. 3 for a full discussion). The

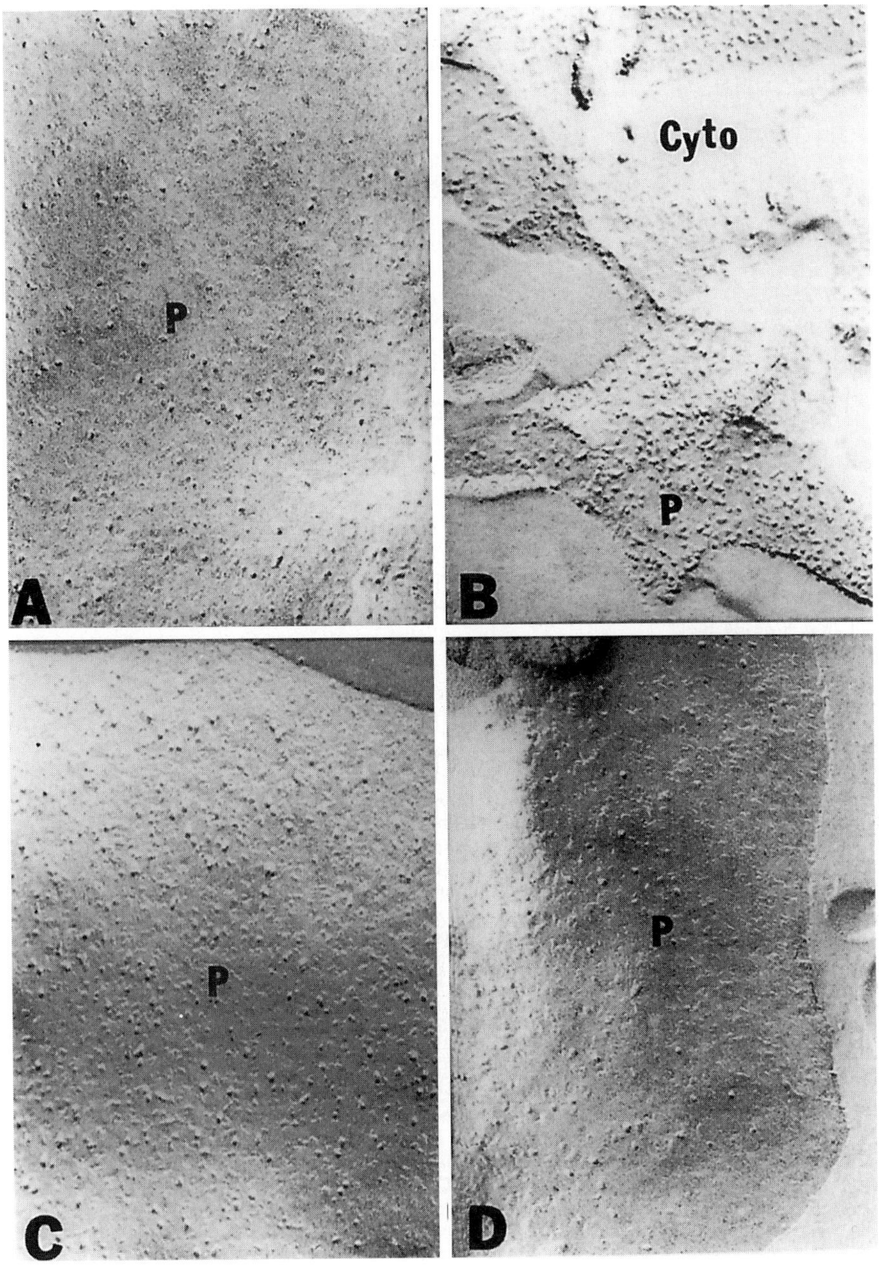

Fig. 190-16 **Freeze-fracture electron microscopy of the L147R and C355S mutants in *Xenopus* oocytes. Freeze-fracture images showing the P-face of the plasma membrane of (*A*) control oocytes and oocytes expressing the human (*B*) wild-type and mutant [(*C*) L147R and (*D*) C355S] SGLT1 proteins. All four oocytes were from the same experiment using oocytes from the same frog, and charge measurements were obtained 10 days after cRNA injection on each oocyte just before fixation. The P-face of the control oocyte shows endogenous intramembrane particles at a density of around 200/mm^2. In the oocyte expressing functional wild-type SGLT1, the density of the intramembrane particles increased to about 1000/mm. In the oocytes expressing the SGLT1 mutant proteins (*C, D*), the density of the P-face intramembrane particles was similar to that of the control oocyte (*A*). The Q_{max} values were 11 nC for oocytes expressing wild-type SGLT1 and much less than 2 nC for both the control oocyte expressing the L147R SGLT1 and C355S SGLT1 (see also Fig. 190-15*B*). P and Cyto refer to the P-face of the plasma membrane and the cytoplasm. The smooth surfaces in *B–D* represent water on the extracellular surface of the oocyte (original magnification × 100,000). (*From Martín et al.*[11] *Used by permission.*)**

amount of glucose excretion is independent of diet, and oral glucose tolerance and plasma insulin levels are normal. This disorder is believed to result from the selective inability of the renal proximal tubule to reabsorb glucose from the glomerular filtrate. These patients, unlike those with the Fanconi-Bickel syndrome (see above), store and use carbohydrate normally. Furthermore, unlike Fanconi-Bickel patients, in these patients only glucose, not galactose, is excreted in the urine.

Several different mutations must be involved in the production of renal glycosuria, since two major phenotypes have been reported: type A, in which there are reductions in both the maximum amount of glucose reabsorption (J_{max}) and the minimum renal glucose threshold (K_m), and type B, in which there is only a reduction in the K_m.[49,72]

To date, the molecular defects responsible for renal glycosuria have not been identified. Glucose is reabsorbed from the glomerular filtrate by the epithelial cells of the proximal tubule, and the mechanisms are very similar to those described for the intestine (see Fig. 190-1), i.e., transport across the brush-border membrane by a sodium-dependent, phlorizin-sensitive transporter and then transport across the basolateral membrane by a facilitated glucose transporter (GLUT2). The major renal sodium-glucose cotransporter is not SGLT1 but another with a low affinity for glucose and a higher selectivity among sugars, i.e., SGLT2.

There is some uncertainty about the identity of SGLT2 in the human kidney. A renal cDNA (HU14) with 59 percent identity to human SGLT1 has been cloned, but this clone functioned poorly when expressed in oocytes.[73] The transport of 500 μM sugar was only two times higher than background, and there also was an increase in 100 μM uridine uptake. HU14 has 91 percent identity to a rabbit sodium-uridine transporter (SNST1), suggesting that they are species variants of the same entity.[22,74] Despite the very low level of functional expression of HU14 in oocytes, Hediger's group has been able to demonstrate that it functions as a low-affinity (2–3 mM) phlorizin-sensitive sugar transporter with a high selectivity for glucose over galactose and that HU14 mRNA is expressed in the early proximal tubules of the rat kidney.[75] Hybrid-depletion studies carried out on oocytes using rat kidney cortex poly(A+) mRNA and the rat homologue of HU14 suggest that the homologue was the major sodium-glucose transporter in

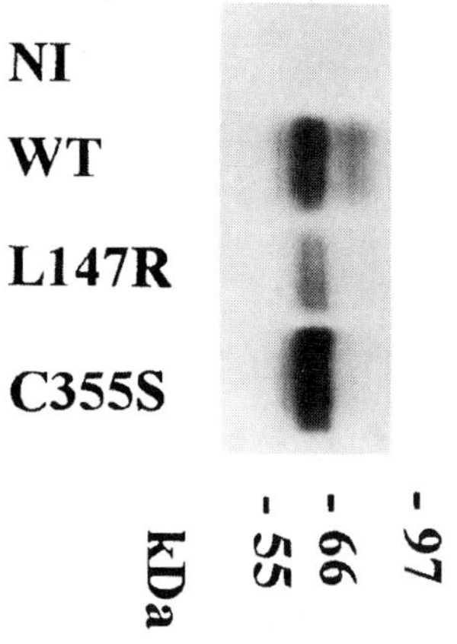

Fig. 190-17 Western blot analysis of wild-type, C355S, and L147R mutant proteins expressed in oocytes. Four days after injection with cRNA coding for wild-type, C355S, and L147R mutants, proteins were extracted from three oocytes. The equivalent to one-third oocyte was run in a 12% SDS-PAGE gel, and after electrotransfer, the nitrocellulose menbrane was probed with antipeptide antibody raised to residues 602–613 at 1:1000 dilution. Lane 1 is a non-injected oocyte. Lane 2 is the wild-type SGLT1 that runs as two bands: one of 70 kDa, the same size as the native complex-glycosylated protein, and a second smaller band (core CHO) of −60 kDa. Lanes 3 and 4 correspond to L147R and C355S mutants, respectively, and only show the core-glycosylated band present in wild type. In this gel, the intensity of the L147R band is lower than in wild type or C355S. (*From Martín et al.*[11] *Used by permission.*)

the rat.[76] Another sodium-glucose cotransporter clone has been isolated from the pig kidney, pSGLT2 or SAAT1, that expresses very well in oocytes — sugar transport rates up to 1000 times higher than HU14 or the rat homologue.[77,78] pSGLT2 has 76 percent identity to SGLT1, and it expresses in oocytes as a low-affinity sodium-glucose transporter that is not able to handle galactose. Apparently pSGLT2 is expressed in humans; a 438-bp cDNA with 86 percent nucleotide identity has been cloned from human brain, and this is also transcribed in kidney carcinomas.[79,80] Evidently, more work is required to determine the identity of the human renal low-affinity sodium-glucose cotransporter and to determine if mutations in this gene cause renal glycosuria.

Relationship Between GGM and Renal Glycosuria

Renal glycosuria is the term used to describe renal excretion of glucose in the urine, particularly when blood glucose levels are normal. Defective renal glucose reabsorption need not be associated with a defect in intestinal sugar absorption, and GGM is generally only accompanied by a mild renal glycosuria. This condition is viewed as benign because it is not associated with significant symptoms or physical consequences. The studies by Elsas *et al.*[49,72] suggest that the familiar form is inherited as an autosomal recessive trait. The most reasonable explanation for the dissociation between the intestinal and renal defects is that there are two separate genes for intestinal and renal sugar transport; the intestinal gene codes for SGLT1, the high-affinity sodium-glucose cotransporter, and the renal gene codes for SGLT2, a low-affinity sodium-glucose cotransporter that does not handle D-galactose. SGLT1 is also expressed at a low level in the late proximal tubule of the kidney, so mutations in this gene would account for the mild glycosuria frequently observed in patients with GGM. However, SGLT2 expressed in the renal proximal tubule is predicted to be responsible for the bulk of renal glucose reabsorption, so mutations in this gene would cause the more severe renal glycosuria.

It is worth noting that mutations in the *GLUT2* gene are also associated with renal glycosuria (the Fanconi-Bickel syndrome)[67,68] and that *GLUT2* knock-out mice[66,69] also exhibit a

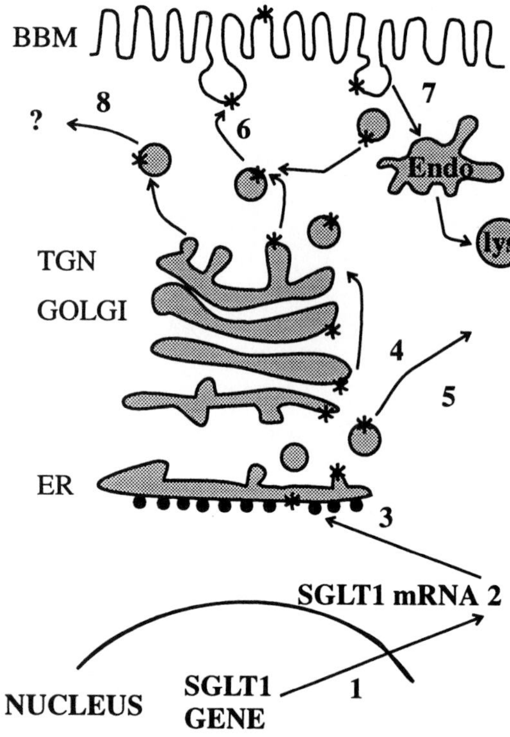

Fig. 190-18 Brush-border membrane sodium-glucose cotransporter (SGLT1) biosynthesis in enterocytes and sites of lesions in GGM patients. The density of brush-border membrane (BBM) SGLT1 proteins (*) is determined by *SGLT1* gene transcription (1), SGLT1 mRNA levels (2), SGLT1 protein translation and insertion into the endoplasmic reticulum (3), SGLT1 protein processing through to the trans-Golgi network (4) and degradation (5), trafficking of SGLT1 protein to the plasma membrane (6), and degradation of BBM SGLT1 protein (7). Mutations in the *SGLT1* gene may cause a reduction in sugar transport across the brush-border membrane by either reducing the density of SGLT1 transporters in the BBM or producing defective BBM SGLT1 transporters. Of the GGM patients studied to date, the SGLT1 mutations include (a) missense (61 percent), (b) nonsense (10 percent), (c) frameshift (17 percent), and (d) splice site (12 percent). The nonsense, frameshift, and splice-site mutations all result in nonfunctional truncated proteins; 22 of the 23 missense mutations cause defects in trafficking of SGLT1 protein between the endoplasmic reticulum and the plasma membrane (steps 4, 6, and 8). One missense mutation results in a defect in sugar translocation across the membrane. The missense mutations to date do not appear to result in any reduction in the level of SGLT1 protein in the cell; i.e., none cause degradation of the protein (step 5 or 7).

severe renal glycosuria. In both cases there are no major abnormalities in intestinal sugar absorption.

CONCLUDING REMARKS

Molecular genetics has made a large impact on our understanding of familial glucose-galactose malabsorption. The disorder has been confirmed to be due to mutations in the gene coding for the sodium-glucose cotransporter and has an autosomal recessive mode of inheritance. As expected, GGM is most frequently observed in populations that have a high incidence of consanguinity. Given that it is a rare disorder, it is perhaps surprising that about 30 percent of the patients have compound heterozygous mutations. This may be correlated with the rather high incidence of glucose malabsorption observed in breath hydrogen tests in the normal population: 10 percent of 460 medical students gave positive glucose breath hydrogen tests.[4] The majority (61 percent) of the *SGLT1* mutations were found to be missense, and these are distributed throughout the protein. Most involve polar residues, but several are conservative changes, e.g., alanine to valine, and the dominant effect of all these mutations is to impair delivery of the transporter to the plasma membrane. GGM thus joins an ever-expanding group of genetic disorders that are caused by protein folding defects. While GGM is fairly simple to treat by removing of the offending sugars from the diet, in practice, this is quite difficult to accomplish. In the future, when more is understood about the trafficking of plasma membrane proteins, it may be possible to devise therapies to restore delivery of the mutant SGLT1 proteins to the patient's brush-border membrane. It is therefore important to determine if the GGM mutant proteins retain their function despite misfolding. The concerted techniques of molecular and cell biology and protein chemistry may be used to address these questions.

ACKNOWLEDGMENTS

We greatly appreciate the editorial assistance of Ms Debra Moorehead. This work was supported by grants from the National Institutes of Health (DK 44582 and DK19567).

REFERENCES

1. Lindquist B, Meeuwisse GW: Chronic diarrhoea caused by monosaccharide malabsorption. *Acta Paediatr* **51**:674, 1962.
2. Laplane R, Polonovski C, Etienne M, Debray P, Lods J-C, Pissarro B: L'intolerance aux sucres a transfert intestinal actif. *Arch Fr Pediatr* **19**:895, 1962.
3. Desjeux J-F, Turk E, Wright EM: Congenital selective Na^+ D-glucose cotransport defects leading to renal glycosuria and congenital selective intestinal malabsorption of glucose and galactose, in Scriver CR, Beaudet AL, Sly WS, Valle D (eds): *Metabolic Basis of Inherited Disease,* 7th ed. New York, McGraw-Hill, 1994, pp 3563–3580.
4. Montes RG, Gottal RF, Bayless TM, Hendrix TR, Perman JA: Breath hydrogen testing as a physiology laboratory exercise for medical students. *Am J Physiol* **262**:S25, 1992.
5. Schneider AJ, Kinter WB, Stirling CE: Glucose-galactose malabsorption: Report of a case with autoradiographic studies of a mucosal biopsy. *N Engl J Med* **274**:305, 1996.
6. Stirling CE, Schneider AJ, Wong M-D, Kinter WB: Quantitative radioautography of sugar transport in intestinal biopsies from normal humans and a patient with glucose-galactose malabsorption. *J Clin Invest* **51**:438, 1972.
7. Hediger MA, Coady MJ, Ikeda TS, Wright EM: Expression cloning and cDNA sequencing of the Na^+/glucose cotransporter. *Nature* **330**:379, 1987.
8. Hediger MA, Turk E, Wright EM: Homology of the human intestinal Na^+/glucose and *E. coli* Na^+/proline cotransporters. *Proc Natl Acad Sci USA* **86**:5748, 1989.
9. Turk E, Zabel B, Mundlos S, Dyer J, Wright EM: Glucose/galactose malabsorption caused by a defect in the Na^+/glucose cotransporter. *Nature* **350**:354, 1991.
10. Martín GM, Turk E, Lostao MP, Kerner C, Wright EM: Defects in Na^+/glucose cotransporter (SGLT1) trafficking and function cause glucose-galactose malabsorption. *Nature Genet* **12**:216, 1996.
11. Martín MG, Lostao MP, Turk E, Lam J, Kreman M, Wright EM: Compound missense mutations in the sodium/D-glucose cotransporter (SGLT1) results in trafficking defects. *Gastroenterology* **112**:1206, 1997.
12. Lam JT, Martín MG, Turk E, Bosshard NU, Steinmann B, Wright EM: Missense mutations in *SGLT1* cause glucose-galactose malabsorption by trafficking defects. *Biochim Biophys Acta* **1453**:297, 1998.
13. Wright EM, Hirayama BA, Loo DDF, Turk E, Hager K: Intestinal sugar transport, in Johnson LR (ed): *Physiology of Gastrointestinal Tract,* vol 2, 3d ed. New York, Raven Press, 1994, 1751–1772.
14. Hirayama BA, Lostao MP, Panayotova-Heiermann M, Loo DDF, Turk E, Wright EM: Kinetic and specificity differences between rat, human and rabbit Na/glucose cotransporters (SGLT1). *Am J Physiol* **270**: G919, 1996.
15. Mackenzie B, Loo DDF, Wright EM: Relations between Na^+/glucose cotransporter (SGLT1) currents and fluxes. *J Membane Biol* **162**:101, 1998.
16. Hirschhorn N, Greenough WB: Progress in oral rehydration therapy. *Sci Am* **264**:50, 1991.
17. Loo DDF, Zeuthen T, Chandy G, Wright EM: Cotransport of water by the Na^+/glucose cotransporter. *Proc Natl Acad Sci USA* **93**:13367, 1996.
18. Meinild A-K, Klaerke D, Loo DDF, Wright EM, Zeuthen T: The human Na^+/glucose cotransporter is a molecular water pump. *J Physiol* **508**:15, 1998.
19. Crane RK, Miller D, Bihler D: The restrictions on possible mechanism of intestinal active transport of sugars, in Kleinzeller A, Kotyk A (eds): *Membrane Transport and Metabolism.* Prague, Academy of Science, 1961, pp 439–449.
20. Schultz SG, Curran PF: Coupled transport of sodium and organic solutes. *Physiol Rev* **50**(4):637, 1970.
21. Peerce BE, Wright EM: Conformational changes in the intestinal brush border Na-glucose cotransporter labeled with fluorescein isothiocyanate. *Proc Natl Acad Sci USA* **81**:2223, 1984.
22. Turk E, Wright EM: Membrane topological motifs in the SGLT cotransporter family. *J Membane Biol* **159**:1, 1997.
23. Eskandari S, Wright EM, Kreman M, Starace DM, Zampighi GA: Structural analysis of cloned membrane proteins by freeze-fracture electron micoscopy. *Proc Natl Acad Sci USA* **95**: 11235, 1998.
24. Hediger MA, Mendlein J, Lee H-S, Wright EM: Biosynthesis of the cloned Na^+/glucose. *Biochim Biophys Acta* **1064**:360, 1991.
25. Hirayama BA, Wright EM: Glycosylation of the rabbit intestinal brush border Na^+/glucose cotransporter. *Biochim Biophys Acta* **1103**:37, 1992.
26. Hirsch JR, Loo DDF, Wright EM: Regulation of Na^+/glucose cotransporter expression by protein kinases in *Xenopus laevis* oocytes. *J Biol Chem* **271**:14740, 1996.
27. Wright EM, Hirsch JR, Loo DDF, Zampighi GA: Regulation of Na^+/glucose cotransporters. *J Exp Biol* **200**:287, 1997.
28. Hwang E-S, Hirayama BA, Wright EM: Distribution of the SLGT1 Na^+/glucose cotransporter and mRNA along the crypt-villus axis of rabbit small intestine. *Biochem Biophys Res Commun* **181**:1208, 1991.
29. Wright EM, Hirayama BA, Hazama A, Loo DDF, Supplisson S, Turk E, Hager KML: The sodium/glucose cotransporter (SGLT1), in *Molecular Biology and Function of Carrier Proteins.* New York, Rockefeller University Press, 1993, chap 18, pp 230–241.
30. Parent L, Supplisson S, Loo DDF, Wright EM: Electrogenic properties of the cloned Na^+/glucose cotransporter: I. Voltage-clamp studies. *J Membane Biol* **125**:49, 1992.
31. Parent L, Supplisson S, Loo DF, Wright EM: Electrogenic properties of the cloned Na^+/glucose cotransporter: II. A transport model under nonrapid equilibrium conditions. *J Membane Biol* **125**:63, 1992.
32. Loo DDF, Hazama A, Supplisson S, Turk E, Wright EM: Relaxation kinetics of the Na^+/glucose cotransporter. *Proc Natl Acad Sci USA* **90**:5767, 1993.
33. Hazama A, Loo DDF, Wright EM: Presteady-state currents of the Na^+/glucose cotransporter (SGLT1). *J Membane Biol* **155**:175, 1997.
34. Loo DDF, Hirayama BA, Gallardo EM, Lam JT, Turk E, Wright EM: Conformational changes couple Na^+ and glucose transport. *Proc Natl Acad Sci USA* **95**:7789, 1998.
35. Panajotova-Heiermann M, Loo DDF, Klong C-T, Lever JE, Wright EM: Sugar binding to Na^+/glucose cotransporters is determined by the C-terminal half of the protein. *J Biol Chem* **271**:10029, 1996.
36. Panayotova-Heiermann M, Eskandari S, Zampighi GA, Wright EM: Five transmembrane helices form the sugar pathway through the Na^+/glucose transporter. *J Biol Chem* **272**:20324, 1997.
37. Loo DDF, Hirayama BA, Gallardo EM, Lam JT, Turk ET, Wright EM: Conformational changes couple Na^+ and glucose transport. *Proc Natl Acad Sci USA* **95**: 7789, 1998
38. Hediger MA, Budarf ML, Emanuel BS, Mohandas TK, Wright EM: Assignment of the human intestinal Na^+/glucose cotransporter gene (*SGLT1*) to the q11.2 → qter region of chromosome 22. *Genomics* **4**:297, 1989.
39. Turk E, Klisak I, Sparkes RS, Wright EM: Assignment of the human Na^+/glucose cotransporter gene *SGLT1* to chromosome 22q13.1. *Genomics* **17**:752, 1993.
40. Turk E, Martín MG, Wright EM: Structure of the human Na^+/glucose cotransporter gene *SGLTI*. *J Biol Chem* **269**:15204, 1994.
41. Korenberg JR, Rykowski MC: Human genome organization: Alu, lines, and the molecular structure of metaphase chromosome bands. *Cell* **53**:391, 1988.
42. Fukumoto H, Seino S, Imura H, Seino Y, Eddy RL, Fukushima Y, Byers MG, Shows TB, Bell GI: Sequence, tissue distribution, and chromosmal localization of mRNA encoding a human glucose transporter-like protein. *Proc Natl Acad Sci USA* **85**:5435, 1988.

43. Takeda J, Kayano T, Fukomoto H, Bell GI: Organization of the human *GLUT2* (pancreatic β-cell and hepatocyte) glucose transporter gene. *Diabetes* **42**:773, 1993.
44. Kayano T, Burant CF, Fukumoto H, Gould GW, Fan YS, Eddy RL, Byers MG, Shows TB, Seino S, Bell GI: Human facilitative glucose transporters: Isolation, functional characterization, and gene localization of cDNAs encoding an isoform (*GLUT5*) expressed in small intestine, kidney, muscle, and adipose tissue and an unusual glucose transporter pseudogene-like sequence (*GLUT6*). *J Biol Chem* **265**: 13276, 1990.
45. White PS, Jensen SJ, Rajalingam V, Stairs D, Sulman EP, Maris JM, Biegel JA, Wooster R, Brodeur GM: Physical mapping of the *CA6, ENO1,* and *SLC2A5* (*GLUT5*) genes and reassignment of *SLC2A5* to 1p36.2. *Cytogenet Cell Genet* **81**(1):60, 1998.
46. Mahraoui L, Takeda J, Mesonero J, Chantret I, Dussaulx E, Bell GI, Brot-Laroche E: Regulation of expression of the human fructose transporter (*GLUT5*) by cyclic AMP. *Biochem J* **301**:169, 1994.
47. Wasserman D, Hoekstra JH, Tolla V, Taylor CJ, Kirschner BS, Takeda J, Bell GI, Taub R, Rand EB: Molecular analysis of the fructose transporter gene (*GLUT5*) in isolated fructose malabsorption. *J Clin Invest* **98**:2398, 1996.
48. Meeuwisse GW, Melin K: Glucose-galactose malabsorption. *Acta Paediatr Scand Suppl* **188**:3, 1969.
49. Elsas LJ, Hillman RE, Patterson JH, Rosenberg LE: Renal and intestinal hexose transport in familial glucose-galactose malabsorption. *J Clin Invest* **49**:576, 1970.
50. Abdullah AMA, El-Mouzan MI, El Shiekh OK, Mazyad AA: Congenital glucose-galactose malabsorption in Arab children. *J Pediatr Gastroenterol Nutr* **23**:561, 1996.
51. Phillips SF, McGill DB: Glucose-galactose malabsorption in an adult: Perfusion studies of sugar, electrolyte, and water transport. *Am J Dig Dis* **18**:1017, 1973.
52. Martín MG: The biology of inherited disorders of the gastrointestinal tract: I. Gastrointestinal disorders. *J Pediatr Gastroenterol Nutr* **6**:321, 1998.
53. Martín MG: The biology of inherited disorders of the gastrointestinal tract: II. Pancreatic and hepatobiliary disorders. *J Pediatr Gastroenterol Nutr* **26**:437, 1998.
54. Höglund P, Haila S, Socha J, Tomaszewski L, Saarialho-Kere U, Karjalainen-Lindsberg ML, Airola K, Holmberg C, de la Chapelle A, Kere, J: Mutations of the down-regulated in adenoma (*DRA*) gene cause congenital chloride diarrhea. *Nature Genet* **14**:316, 1996.
55. Schultheis PJ, Clarke LL, Meneton P, Miller ML, Soleimani M, Gawenis LR, Riddle TM, Duffy JJ, Doetschman T, Wang T, Giebisch G, Aronson PS, Lorenz JN, Shull GE: Renal and intestinal absorptive defects in mice lacking the NHE3 Na^+/H^+ exchanger. *Nature Genet* **19**:282, 1998.
56. Oelkers P, Kirby LC, Heubi JE, Dawson PA: Primary bile acid malabsorption caused by mutations in the ileal sodium-dependent bile acid transporter gene (*SLC10A2*). *J Clin Invest* **99**:1880, 1997.
57. Cutz E, Rhoads JM, Drumm B, Sherman PM, Durie PR, Forstner GG: Microvillus inclusion disease: An inherited defect of brush-border assembly and differentiation. *N Engl J Med* **320**:646, 1989.
58. Savilahti E, Launiala K, Kuitunen P: Congenital lactase deficiency: A clinical study on 16 patients. *Arch Dis Child* **58**(4):246, 1983.
59. Ouwendijk J, Moolenaar CE, Peters WJ, Hollenberg CP, Ginsel LA, Fransen JA, Naim HY: Congenital sucrase-isomaltase deficiency: Identification of a glutamine to proline substitution that leads to a transport block of sucrase-isomaltase in a pre-Golgi compartment. *J Clin Invest* **97**(3):633, 1996.
60. Lebenthal E, Khin-Maung U, Zheng BY, Lu RB, Lerner A: Small intestinal glucoamylase deficiency and starch malabsorption: A newly recognized alpha-glucosidase deficiency in children. *J Pediatr* **124**(4):541, 1994.
61. Martín MG, Turk E, Kerner C, Zabel B, Wirth S, Wright EM: Prenatal identification of a heterozygous status in two fetuses at risk for glucose-galactose malabsorption. *Prenatal Diagn* **16**:452, 1996.
62. Walker WA, Hendricks KM: *Manual of Pediatric Nutrition*. Philadelphia, Saunders, 1985.
63. Zampighi GA, Kreman M, Boorer KJ, Loo DDF, Bezanilla F, Chandy G, Hall JE, Wright EM: A method for determining the unitary functional capacity of cloned channels and transporters expressed in *Xenopus laevis* oocytes. *J Membane Biol* **148**:65, 1995.
64. Lostao MP, Martín MG, Hernell O, Wright EM: Mutation of glutamine 457 to arginine in the Na^+/glucose cotransporter causes glucose-galactose malabsorption in a Swedish family. Presented at the 14th Meeting of the European Intestinal Transport Group. *Physiol Res* **45**:P1, 1996.
65. Lostao MP, Hirayama BA, Panayotova-Heiermann M, Samposna SL, Bok D, Wright EM: Arginine-427 in the Na/glucose cotransporter (SGLT1) is involved in trafficking to the plasma membrane. *FEBS Lett* **377**:181, 1995.
66. Thomas PJ, Qu B-H, Pedersen PL: Defective protein folding as a basis of human disease. *Trends Biochem Sci* **20**:441, 1995.
67. Manz F, Bickel H, Brodehl HJ, Feist D, Gellissen K, GeschollBauer B, Filli G, Harms E, Helwig H, Nutzenadel W: Fanconi-Bickel syndrome. *Pediatr Nephrol* **1**:509, 1987.
68. Santer R, Schneppenheim R, Dombrowski A, Götze H, Steinmann B, Schaub J: Mutations in *GLUT2,* the gene for the liver-type glucose transporter, in patients with Fanconi-Bickel syndrome. *Nature Genet* **17**:324, 1997.
69. Guillam MT, Hummler E, Schaerer Yeh, JI E, Birnbaum MJ, Beermann F, Schmidt A, Deriaz N, Thorens B: Early diabetes and abnormal postnatal pancreatic islet development in mice lacking Glut-2. *Nature Genet* **17**:327, 1997.
70. Mueckler M, Kruse M, Strube M, Riggs AC, Chiu KD, Permutt MA: A mutation in the Glut2 glucose transporter gene of a diabetic patient abolishes transport activity. *J Biol Chem* **269**:17765, 1994.
71. Tolan DR: Molecular basis of hereditary fructose intolerance: Mutations and polymorphisms in the human aldolase B gene. *Hum Mutat* **6**(3):210, 1995.
72. Elsas LJ, Rosenberg LE: Familial renal glycosuria: A genetic reappraisal of hexose transport by kidney and intestine. *J Clin Invest* **48**:1845, 1969.
73. Wells RG, Kanai Y, Pajor AM, Turk E, Wright EM, Hediger MA: The cloning of a human kidney cDNA with similarity to the sodium/glucose cotransporter. *Am J Physiol* **263**:F459, 1992
74. Pajor AM, Wright EM: Sequence, tissue distribution and functional expression of a mammalian Na^+/nucleoside cotransporter. *J Biol Chem* **267**:3557, 1992.
75. Kanai Y, Lee W-S, You G, Brown D, Hediger MA: The human kidney low-affinity Na^+/glucose cotransporter SGLT2. *J Clin Invest* **93**:397, 1994.
76. You G, Lee W-S, Barros E, Kanai Y, Huo T-L, Khawaja S, Wells RG, Nigam SK, Hediger MA: Molecular characterization of Na^+-coupled glucose transporters in adult and embryonic rat kidney. *J Biol Chem* **270**:29365, 1995.
77. Mackenzie B, Panayotova-Heiermann M, Loo DDF, Lever JE, Wright EM: SAAT1 is a low affinity Na^+/glucose cotransporter and not an amino acid transporter. *J Biol Chem* **269**:22488, 1994.
78. Mackenzie BM, Loo DDF, Panayotova-Heiermann M, Wright EM: Biophysical characteristics of the pig kidney Na^+/glucose cotransporter SGLT2 reveal a common mechanism for SGLT1 and SGLT2. *J Biol Chem* **271**:32678, 1996.
79. Poppe R, Karbach U, Gambaryan S, Wiesinger H, Lutzenburg M, Kraemer M, Witte OW, Koepsell H: Expression of the Na^+-D-glucose cotransporter SGLT1 in neurons. *J Neurochem* **69**:84, 1997.
80. Veyhl M, Wagner K, Volk C, Gorboulev V, Baumgarden K, Weber W-M, Schaper M, Bertram B, Wiessler M, Koepsell H: Transport of the new chemotherapeutic agent β-D-glucosylisophosphoramide mustard (D-19575) into tumor cells is mediated by the Na^+-D-glucose cotransporter SAAT1. *Proc Natl Acad Sci USA* **95**:2914, 1998.

CHAPTER 191

Cystinuria

Manuel Palacín ▪ Paul Goodyer
Virginia Nunes ▪ Paolo Gasparini

1. **Cystinuria (OMIM 220200) is a disorder of amino acid transport affecting epithelial cells of the renal tubule and the gastrointestinal tract. The defective transport of cystine, lysine, arginine, and ornithine is transmitted as an autosomal recessive trait. According to the level of urinary excretion of cystine and dibasic amino acids in obligate heterozygotes, two types of cystinuria are envisaged: type I, the fully recessive form, and non-type I (type II, type III), the incomplete recessive form. In the latter type, the affected amino acids are excreted by heterozygotes in urine at levels greater than normal but less than in the homozygous state.**
2. **The only proven clinical manifestation of cystinuria is urolithiasis, due to the low solubility of cystine at low pH. Distinctive hexagonal cystine crystals appear in the urine and radiopaque cystine stones develop repeatedly in affected individuals. Cystinuria is diagnosed by demonstrating selective hyperexcretion of cystine and dibasic amino acids in urine. Stones generally form in acidic urine when urinary cystine concentration exceeds 300 mg cystine per liter (1200 μM). Prevention of urolithiasis is directed at high fluid intake and alkalinizing the urine to maximize cystine solubility. Oral sulfhydryl agents such as D-penicillamine and mercaptopropionylglycine may be used to form soluble mixed disulfides of cystine in the urine. Although effective, these agents are not risk-free and are usually reserved for patients who fail to respond to conservative therapy.**
3. **The corresponding small intestinal transport mechanism for absorption of cystine and dibasic amino acids is also defective in many cystinuria patients; oral loading tests and in vitro studies of jejunal biopsies demonstrate this. However, there are no gastrointestinal symptoms and, under conditions of normal protein intake, plasma amino acid levels are normal. This is presumably due to alternative absorptive mechanisms in the intestine, including direct uptake of dipeptides.**
4. **The renal clearance of cystine varies widely among affected individuals. In both humans and canine mutant phenotypes, fractional excretion of cystine may exceed the glomerular filtration rate, indicating net secretion, or back-leak, of cystine into the tubular fluid. This is particularly true in the first months of life when renal amino acid transport is immature. Thus, some heterozygous infants may initially appear to have homozygous cystinuria and should not be classified until at least 1 year of age.**
5. **In vitro studies of rat renal and intestinal brush-border membrane vesicles, and renal tubular fragments show that cystine and dibasic amino acids share a high-affinity (low K_m) transport mechanism. This transport system, also shared with neutral amino acids, is located at the luminal surface of epithelial cells in the proximal straight tubule (S3 segment). A comparable system ($b^{o,+}$-like) for cystine, dibasic, and neutral amino acids has been demonstrated in the apical membrane of an opossum kidney (OK) cell line. The $b^{o,+}$-like system is an amino acid exchanger that normally mediates influx of cystine and dibasic amino acids and efflux of neutral amino acids or cysteine. A separate low-affinity (high K_m) system for cystine, not shared with dibasic amino acids, is located in the proximal convoluted tubule.**
6. **Direct evidence for a defect in the shared transport mechanism for cystine and the dibasic amino acids derives from in vitro studies of renal cortical slices and jejunal mucosa biopsies from cystinuric patients.**
7. **Expression cloning was used to identify a renal cDNA (rBAT) which induces the $b^{o,+}$ system when expressed in *Xenopus* oocytes. In oocytes, the rBAT ($b^{o,+}$-like) system acts as a tertiary active transport mechanism. rBAT protein has been demonstrated in the brush-border membrane of proximal straight (S3 segment) tubule and small intestinal mucosa; the *rBAT* gene (*SLC3A1*) is responsible for $b^{o,+}$-like activity in OK cells. There is evidence suggesting that rBAT forms a complex with a disulfide-bridged "light" subunit to constitute the luminal high-affinity renal and intestinal cystine holotransporter. Very recently a putative "light" subunit ($b^{o,+}$ AT) has been cloned and characterized.**
8. **To date, 40 unique *SLC3A1* (2p16.3-p21) mutations have been identified in cystinuria patients. In seven missense mutations, loss of function has been demonstrated in oocytes, apparently due to trafficking defects during transfer from endoplasmic reticulum to plasma membrane. Null *SLC3A1* mutations are fully recessive in cystinuria heterozygotes.**
9. **Mutational analysis and linkage studies have demonstrated genetic heterogeneity in cystinuria. The *SLC3A1* gene is only associated with type I (fully recessive) cystinuria. A second cystinuria locus, accounting for type II and type III cystinuria (incomplete recessive forms), has been identified by linkage analysis at chromosome**

A list of standard abbreviations is located immediately preceding the index in each volume. Additional abbreviations used in this chapter include: $b^{o,+}$ = Broad specificity amino acid transporter for neutral (o) and basic (+) amino acid transport system; cRNA = RNA in vitro transcribed from cDNA; D2 = an alias for rBAT and NBAT that refers to the clone name in a ZIP selection screening; 4F2hc = The heavy chain of the surface antigen 4F2 (also named CD98); LAT = L amino acid transporter; NBAT = neutral and basic amino acid transporter; rBAT = *r*elated to $b^{o,+}$ *a*mino acid *t*ransporter; *SLC3A1* = solute carrier family 3 (cystine, dibasic, and neutral amino acid transporter), member 1 (*rBAT*, *NBAT*, and *D2H* are aliases of *SLC3A1*); and y^+ LAT = y^+L amino acid transporter. The GenBank Accession numbers for the relevant nucleotide sequences are: *SLC3A1* (Type 1 cystinuria) = L11696; *SLC7A9* (non-Type 1 cystinuria) = AF141289; *SLC7A7* (Lysinuric protein intolerance) = AF135828, AF135829, AF135830, AF135831.

19q13.1-13.2. The gene for the non-type I cystinuria (*SLC7A9*) most probably represents the light subunit of rBAT, $b^{o,+}$ AT. Patients with the mixed form of cystinuria (type I/III) excrete slightly lower levels of cystine and appear to have lower risk of nephrolithiasis in the first decade. An *SLC3A1* mutation is rarely identified on the fully recessive allele in these patients.

10. **At the cusp of the millennium, it is satisfying that the molecular basis of cystinuria, one of the oldest recognized inborn errors, is finally being unraveled. However, we will still need to determine whether all cases of cystinuria can be explained by mutations of *SLC3A1* and *SLC7A9*, and we will still need a deeper understanding of the structure/function relationship of the transporters, and accurate genotype-phenotype correlations in patients.**

HISTORY

The recognition of cystinuria can be traced back to 1810 when Wollaston recovered two glistening yellowish bladder stones from a patient.[1] Recognizing that the stones represented a "new species of urinary calculus," he noted that the stones were composed of "flat hexagonal plates" and were soluble in strong alkali.[1] His analysis was somewhat errant; believing them to be oxides secreted by the bladder, he named the material "cystic oxide" (from the Greek *kystis*, for bladder). In 1817, Marcet[2] pointed out that similar stones also occurred in the kidneys and were not, therefore, the unique product of bladder secretions. He was also the first to suspect the familial nature of cystinuria, because two of his patients were brothers.[2] In 1830, Berzelius realized that the original chemical analysis was incorrect and that the stones were actually amines, suggesting that the substance be renamed "cystin."[3] By 1838, Thaulow[4] had been able to work out the correct molecular formula, $C_6H_{12}N_2S_2O_4$, and at the turn of the 19th century the proper organic configuration was deduced by Neuberg[5] and Friedman.[6] Thus, both the disease and the amino acid reflect, in their names, an historical link to the bladder stones studied by Wollaston.

The understanding of cystinuria as a disorder of amino acid transport developed slowly. In 1820, Prout[7] and Stromeyer[8] observed that the characteristic hexagonal plates reported by Wollaston were persistently present in the urine of patients with recurrent cystine stones. This prompted Prout to speculate that the disease was caused by a disturbance of kidney function resulting in excessive cystine excretion. In 1851, Toel confirmed this suggestion, reporting up to 1.2 to 1.5 g (5 to 6 mM) of cystine per day in urine from his patients.[9] In 1908, Garrod classified cystinuria among the inborn errors of metabolism, and postulated that a defect in the metabolism of cystine was responsible for the disorder.[10] It was not until 1947, when analytic methods for biologic fluids were more advanced, that cystinuria was found to be associated with excessive urinary arginine, lysine[11] and ornithine.[12] In 1951, Dent and Rose showed that plasma levels of these structurally related amino acids were normal in affected patients, and formulated the seminal hypothesis that cystinuria was caused by a defect in the renal reabsorptive transport mechanism shared by these four amino acids.[13] This idea was important, because it formed the basis for our current understanding of cystinuria and because it heralded the subsequent discovery of many other genetic disorders affecting selective renal transport systems.

Although the observations of Prout and Stromeyer quickly focused attention on the renal manifestations of cystinuria, there were early indications that intestinal absorption of cystine might also be impaired. Brand provided support for this proposition by demonstrating that when two of his cystinuria patients were given an oral load of cystine there was no change in urinary cystine excretion.[14] On the other hand, when they were loaded with methionine, a precursor of other sulfur amino acids, there was a substantial increase in urinary cystine. Other investigators subsequently performed similar loading studies and confirmed the selective failure of cystine (but not cysteine) and dibasic amino acid absorption from the small intestine.[15–20] As early as 1889, von Udransky and Baumann[21] had noted that cystinuria patients also excrete unusually large quantities of cadaverine and putrescine, but this phenomenon remained unexplained until Milne[17] pointed out that the increase in urinary cadaverine and putrescine was additional evidence of an intestinal defect. These compounds are generated from arginine, ornithine, and lysine by decarboxylases that are present in colonic flora but that are not present in human tissues. Thus, failure of dibasic amino acid transport in the small intestine would enhance substrate availability in the colon, generating putrescine and cadaverine which was subsequently absorbed and excreted by cystinuria patients.[17] In the early 1960s, several reports by Thier et al.,[22] Fox et al.,[23] McCarthy et al.,[24] and Rosenberg et al.[25] provided direct *in vitro* evidence of enteric involvement. Biopsies of jejunal mucosa from many cystinuria patients (but not all) failed to concentrate radiolabeled cystine, arginine, and lysine.[25]

The evidence for an intestinal defect in cystinuria is strong, but somewhat puzzling. There are no reports of diarrhea or malabsorption symptoms, suggesting that intestinal transport is not blunted. Similarly, it is unclear how normal plasma amino acid levels are maintained because lysine is an essential amino acid. One possible explanation derives from the 1973 work of Hellier et al.[26] These investigators showed that uptake of low concentrations of lysine perfused through a catheter into the jejunum was substantially lower in cystinuria patients than in controls, but that at high rates of perfusion, the peak plasma level was normal. One interpretation is that alternative low-affinity transporters afford adequate cystine and dibasic amino acid uptake in cystinuria patients taking a normal diet. An alternative interpretation is that sufficient cystine and the dibasic amino acids may be absorbed from the small intestine as dipeptides. Cystinuria patients given oral loads of lysylglycine or casein exhibit a rapid increase in plasma lysine, but not if loaded with equivalent amounts of free lysine or a casein hydrolysate.[27–31] Oligopeptide transporters have been demonstrated in the apical membrane of enterocytes; following apical uptake, dipeptides are cleaved intracellularly and exit the cell as single amino acids via basolateral membrane transporters.[32] These observations also suggest that the defective transporter in cystinuria is normally active at the small intestinal luminal membrane.

CLINICAL ASPECTS

Incidence

The incidence of cystinuria worldwide is estimated to be about 1:7000.[33] In specific populations, the incidence varies considerably: 1:2000 among newborns in England,[60] 1:2500 in Libyan Jews;[34] 1:4000 among newborns in Australia,[35] 1:7200 among newborns in Quebec,[36] 1:17,000 among newborns in the United States,[37] and 1:100,000 in Sweden.[38] However, it is difficult to make these estimates precisely. In some studies, the convenient cyanide-nitroprusside test was used for screening. When sodium cyanide is mixed with alkalinized urine, cystine is reduced to cysteine, which yields a magenta color in the presence of sodium nitroprusside; the test is positive if urine contains more than 75 mg cystine/liter. Thus, Crawhall reported that 1 in 200 medical patients presenting at a hospital in London were positive.[39] Similarly, Lewis found that 1 in 600 college students were positive in the United States.[40] However, the sensitivity of the test detects both stone-forming homozygotes who excrete cystine at concentrations greater than 300 mg/l (the cystine solubility limit in urine at low pH) and incompletely recessive (but not silent) heterozygotes. Consequently, it cannot be used to estimate the disease frequency. Newborn urine-screening programs have provided quantitative information on cystine excretion, but may overestimate the incidence of cystinuria because renal tubular immaturity may confound the issue before 1 year of age.[36]

Excretion of Other Amino Acids in Cystinuria

Although excessive excretion of cystine and the dibasic amino acids are the hallmarks of classical cystinuria, hyperexcretion of several other amino acids has been noted. Frimpter identified the mixed disulfide of cysteine and homocysteine in all cystinuria patients but not in urine from normal controls.[41] It is excreted in amounts of 14 to 225 mg/day but the amount correlates with methionine intake rather than with cystine excretion. The homocysteine-cysteine disulfide is not unique to cystinuria and occurs in most forms of Fanconi syndrome. Homoarginine[42] and citrulline[43] are usually present in urine from cystinuria patients. As well, there has been a case of methioninuria with cystinuria and hyperuricemia[44] and a case of cystinuria with cystathioninuria,[45] but the significance of these isolated reports is unclear. Interestingly, cysteine is not found in the urine of cystinuria patients, but this might be easily overlooked because oxidation of cysteine to cystine could occur during its passage along the urinary tract.[46]

Isolated cystinuria without dibasic aciduria is extremely rare in humans but has been reported in two sibs by Brodehl and coworkers. Cystine clearance was about 30 times normal and tubular reabsorption was only 72 to 80 percent in the sibs; the plasma level of cystine was normal and the parents were unaffected.[47] In contrast to classical cystinuria, oral L-cystine loading was normal in these sibs.[47] Blom and Huijmans identified another case of isolated cystinuria.[48] Stephens and Perrett reported a similar case, but in this patient there was also slight impairment of dibasic amino acid reabsorption,[49] prompting the authors and Brodehl[46] to suggest that this patient might simply fall within the spectrum of type II cystinuria (see description of cystinuria subtypes in "Clinical Aspects" below). Isolated dibasic aminoaciduria without cystinuria (MIM 22690)[50,51] and isolated lysinuria without cystinuria (lysinuric protein intolerance (MIM 222700)) have been reported[52] (see Chap. 192 and reference 53). These observations support the original proposal by Dent and Rose[13] that classical cystinuria is caused by a defect in the specific shared transport mechanism shared by cystine and the dibasic amino acids.

Nephrolithiasis

Although there are numerous reports of cystinuria in combination with a variety of other medical conditions, these combinations appear to be chance associations. At present, the only known manifestation of cystinuria is nephrolithiasis. Cystine, like other amino acids, is freely filtered from glomerular plasma into the tubular fluid. Normally, >98 percent of filtered amino acids are subsequently reabsorbed[54] by transport mechanisms located in the luminal brush border membrane of proximal tubular cells. In cystinuria, however, normal proximal tubule cystine uptake is defective, and patients who inherit two mutant genes excrete cystine in amounts ranging from 50 to 200 percent of the filtered load. Luminal cystine becomes progressively concentrated, as other solutes and water are removed from tubular fluid during its passage along the nephron. In the collecting duct, where hydrogen ion secretory mechanisms can generate a luminal pH as low as 5.0, cystine may exceed its threshold of solubility (about 300 mg/l or 1200 μM).

Nephrolithiasis may be influenced by a variety of factors, including other genes that determine the excretion of stone inhibitors and by environmental factors such as the effective salt balance of the patient. However, characteristic hexagonal cystine crystals indicating cystine precipitation are detectable in nearly every urine specimen from affected patients (Fig. 191-1). These are best identified in early morning urine specimens (which tend to be concentrated and acidic) or by acidification and cooling of the specimen. In reviewing 25 years experience at St. Bartholomew's hospital in London, England, Stephens[55] estimated that 25 to 30 percent of symptomatic patients report their first kidney stone in the first decade of life and another 30 to 35 percent first experience nephrolithiasis in their teens. Interestingly, the remaining patients somehow manage to avoid symptomatic stones until adulthood. Typically, stones range from golden yellow to brown and may be the size of grains of sand or large "staghorn" calculi weighing up to 60 to 70 g and obstructing the renal pelvis. Pure cystine calculi are radiopaque but are less dense than calcium stones; they may be identified by ordinary radiography or by ultrasonography (Fig. 191-1). About 40 to 50 percent of stones recovered from cystinuria patients contain substantial amounts of calcium oxalate or calcium phosphate.[55]

Cystine stones constitute only 1 to 3 percent of all urolithiasis among adults[56] and about 6 to 8 percent of urolithiasis in children.[57] However, cystinuria is a particularly unpleasant form of recurrent stone disease; Martin reported that only 44 percent of his patients remained stone-free 3 months after removal of a cystine stone by surgery or lithotripsy.[58] Among children who inherit two fully recessive cystinuria genes from their parents, at least 50 percent begin to form stones within the first decade of life.[59]

Subtypes

The urinary excretion of cystine, lysine, arginine, and ornithine varies considerably among obligate cystinuria heterozygotes.[60] In 1955, Harris proposed that there were two subtypes of cystinuria families, which could be distinguished by the level of cystine excretion in obligate heterozygotes.[61] In 27 pedigrees, he identified "homozygous" probands who excreted excessive dibasic amino acids and >400 mg cystine/g creatinine. Of these, there were 18 pedigrees whose parents and children all excreted cystine within the normal range; cystine excretion by parents and children of the 9 others was moderately elevated.[61,62] Subsequently, other investigators[25,63,64] provided evidence of a mixed form of cystinuria; that is, probands from families in which one parent excreted cystine in the normal range and one parent excreted moderately elevated levels of cystine. More recently, Scriver et al.,[36] Goodyer et al.,[65] Gasparini et al.,[66] and Calonge et al.[67] used the level of urinary cystine or the sum of urinary cystine plus dibasic amino acids to distinguish fully recessive heterozygotes (type I), incompletely recessive heterozygotes (type III), and dominant heterozygotes excreting cystine in the stone-forming range (type II) (see Table 191-1).

A second approach to the heterogeneity of cystinuria involved an attempt to subclassify patients based on intestinal phenotype. Rosenberg et al.[25] concluded that three cystinuria subtypes could be distinguished by combining urinary excretion patterns in obligate heterozygotes with jejunal biopsy and oral amino-acid-loading studies in the proband. In type I patients, both parents excreted cystine in the normal range, concentrative uptake of cystine and dibasic amino acids by jejunal biopsy tissue was absent, and administration of 0.5 μM cystine per kg of body weight produced no increase in plasma cystine. Among probands with parents who excreted moderately elevated levels of cystine, the jejunal tissue from one group (type II) showed no concentrative uptake of cystine and no plasma response to oral cystine loading, but there was modest uptake of the dibasic amino acids by the jejunal biopsy tissue. In an additional group (type III) there was a substantial plasma response to the oral cystine load and modest jejunal uptake of both cystine and dibasic amino acids was present. Unfortunately, the jejunal biopsies were performed in only a very small number of subjects and some of the distinctions made were not clearcut. Morin et al.[64] later studied another 10 families but found evidence of only the first two subtypes proposed by Rosenberg and colleagues. A few patients with similarities to Rosenberg's type III group were the progeny of one fully recessive and one incompletely recessive parent (based on urinary excretion).

Initially, these various cystinuria subtypes were thought to be allelic; that is, mild, moderate, and severe mutations at a single cystinuria gene locus. However, Goodyer and coworkers noted that children of parents with a mix of fully recessive and incompletely

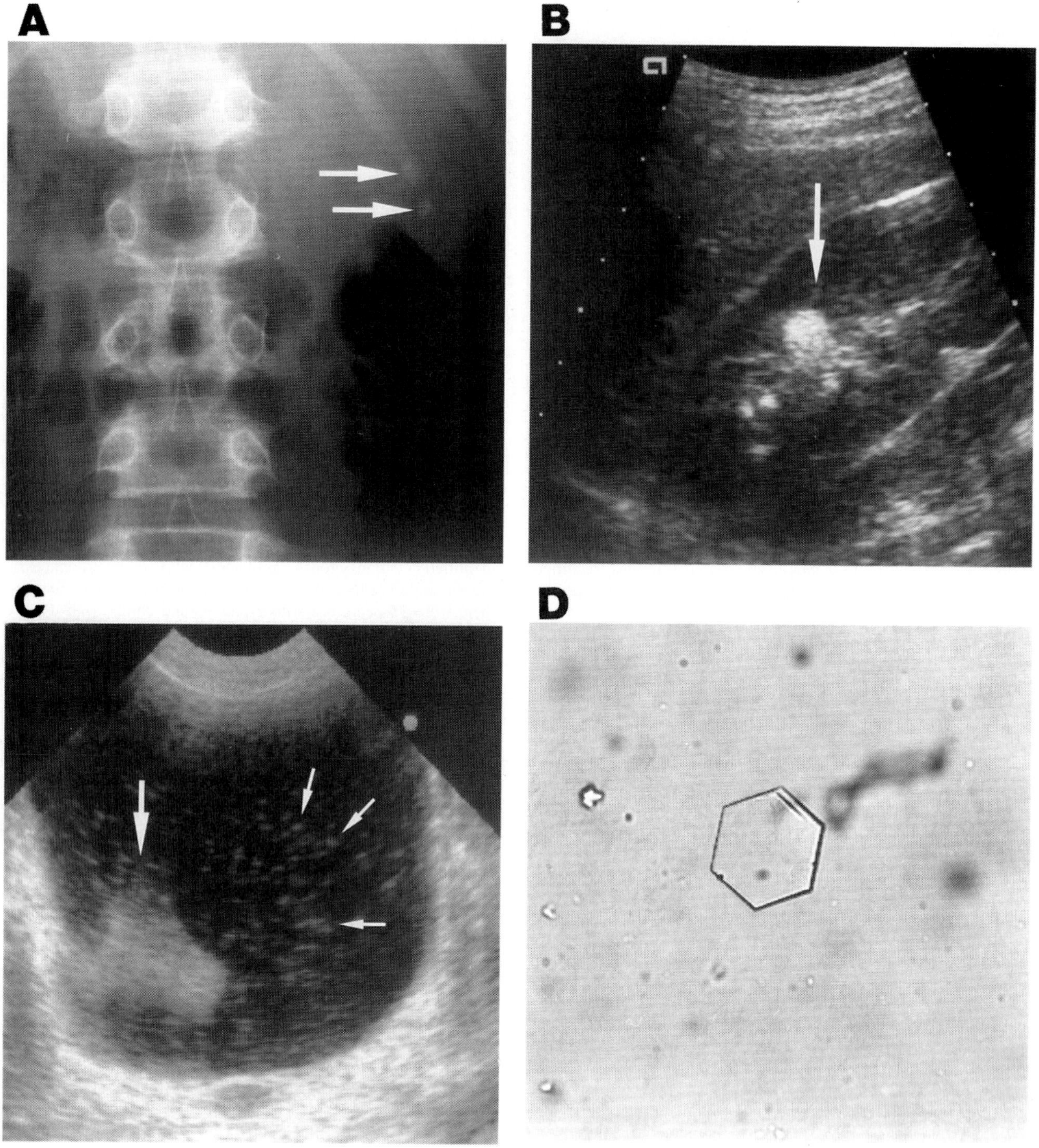

Fig. 191-1 Images of cystine stones and crystals in the urinary tract. *A*, Plain radiograph of the abdomen showing typical cystine stones in the left kidney. *B*, Cystine calculus in the renal collecting system identified by renal ultrasonography. *C*, Multiple small cystine crystal aggregates and a large semisolid consolidation of cystine crystals in the bladder of a cystinuria patient visualized by ultrasonography. *D*, Typical hexagonal cystine crystal seen by standard light microscopy in the urinary sediment.

recessive urinary phenotypes excrete somewhat lower levels of cystine than children of parents who are both fully recessive, and proposed that partial genetic complementation between two or more cystinuria genes might explain this finding.[59,65] In 1992, Tate et al.,[68] Bertran et al.,[69] and Wells et al.[70] used an expression-cloning strategy to isolate a rodent kidney mRNA (GenBank accession numbers L04504, M77345, M80804, and M90096), which induced high-affinity uptake of cystine, the dibasic (and some neutral) amino acids in *Xenopus* oocytes. When the corresponding human cDNA (GenBank accession numbers L11696 and M95548) was isolated,[71,72] it was shown to map to the p16.3-p21 region of chromosome 2.[72–74] At the same time, linkage analysis studies localized the fully recessive cystinuria locus to the same chromosomal region.[67] Finally, two groups reported additional linkage analysis, mapping the incompletely recessive cystinuria genes (type III and probably type II) to a second locus on the long arm of chromosome 19.[75,76] Finally, this gene was found and characterized.[77] This work and its

Table 191-1A Amino Acid Excretion by Cystinuria Children

	C	O	A	L	Total
Normal	< 100	< 100	< 100	< 1000	< 1300
I/N (3)	66 ± 31	36 ± 7	23 ± 3	952 ± 709	1078 ± 731
II/N (8)	1450 ± 273	568 ± 108	310 ± 103	2979 ± 993	8360 ± 1367
III/N (4)	593 ± 68	195 ± 30	140 ± 37	3101 ± 320	4030 ± 632
I/I (7)	3852 ± 435	3135 ± 322	7413 ± 604	11386 ± 901	25787 ± 1570
II/II (0)	N/A	N/A	N/A	N/A	N/A
III/III (5)	2458 ± 247	2624 ± 360	5780 ± 745	6535 ± 613	18398 ± 1132
I/III (15)	1371 ± 119	582 ± 120	330 ± 71	5437 ± 383	7718 ± 626

Mean (± SEM) urinary excretion (μmol/g creatinine) of cystine (C), ornithine (O), arginine (A), lysine (L) and the sum of the four amino acids (Total) by children with various forms of heterozygous and homozygous cystinuria (3 to 15 children per group) vs control values. For each child, 5 to 15 random morning urine specimens were analyzed between 2 and 7 years of age.

Table 191-1B Amino Acid Excretion by Cystinuria Adults

	C	O	A	L	Total
Normals (9)	43 ± 7	22 ± 3	17 ± 5	238 ± 68	323 ± 75
I/N (8)	87 ± 14	40 ± 1	26 ± 3	237 ± 26	390 ± 33
II/N (6)	1035 ± 110	519 ± 82	376 ± 132	3814 ± 655	6369 ± 726
III/N (31)	343 ± 33	126 ± 20	104 ± 20	1488 ± 140	2045 ± 171
I/I (7)	1716 ± 772	2056 ± 534	2610 ± 1171	7380 ± 1390	14000 ± 2922
II/II (4)	1808 ± 566	2290 ± 580	4422 ± 502	9900 ± 1807	18413 ± 3212
III/III (20)	1816 ± 648	1899 ± 402	3833 ± 1401	6963 ± 2039	14511 ± 3286
I/III (6)	1245 ± 517	1382 ± 350	1702 ± 483	5164 ± 800	9489 ± 1964

Mean (± SEM) urinary excretion (μmol/g creatinine) of cystine (C), ornithine (O), arginine (A), lysine (L) and the sum of the four amino acids (Total) by adults (4 to 31 patients/group) vs control values. Data taken from Calonge et al.[67] and Pras et al.[197]

implications for cystinuria are discussed in detail in the sections below.

Ontogeny

Although the process of new nephron formation is completed 1 to 2 months before birth in humans, renal tubular reabsorption of amino acids is reduced in newborns compared to young children or adults.[78] However, in term neonates, the kidney is able to reabsorb at least 95 percent of the filtered load of cystine, the dibasics, and most other amino acids (glycine, histidine, and serine are notably only 85 to 95 percent reabsorbed). In 1985, Scriver et al. reported an important interaction between the ontogeny of tubular transport mechanisms and mutant cystinuria genes.[36] Drawing from the Quebec Newborn Urine Screening Program, Scriver et al. showed that about two-thirds of neonates excreting over 1000 μM cystine per g creatinine at 2 to 4 months of age, were eventually reclassified as partially recessive heterozygotes after the age of 12 months.[36] The same phenomenon is demonstrable for newborns who are eventually classified as completely recessive heterozygotes, but these infants start at values of about 680 ± 420 μM cystine/g creatinine at 2 to 4 months, which values gradually decline to the normal range (< 100).[36] Figure 191-2 depicts the ontogeny of cystine excretion for representative heterozygote and double-heterozygote infants from the Quebec Newborn Urine Screening Program. Note that among infants who inherit two incompletely recessive (non-*rBAT*) alleles, the fractional excretion of cystine (204 percent) often exceeds the calculated filtered load (100 percent), suggesting substantial "back-leak" of cystine into the immature renal tubule.

Treatment

At pH 5 to 7, the theoretic solubility of cystine is about 1250 μM/liter (300 mg/l). The simplest approach to therapy is, therefore, to ensure enough fluid intake to dilute the urinary cystine below this limit. Because many stone-formers excrete 3000 to 4000 μM/day, the goal for a severely cystinuric adult should be to drink about 3 to 3.5 liters in 24 h or about 1.75 to 2.0 liters/m^2/day. This rate of fluid intake (125 to 145 ml/h) is feasible during the daytime, but the problem arises overnight when intake is discontinued and urinary concentration rises. Furthermore, with the normal fall in circulating volume status associated with lack of fluid and salt intake overnight, early morning urine often reaches the lowest pH of the day. To address this issue, Dent and Senior recommend a bolus of fluid before bedtime and at 2 to 3 A.M., believing that this regimen was effective in reducing the frequency of stones in 12 of 18 patients during a 10-year study.[79]

Cystine solubility increases rapidly above pH 7.5. Consequently, another classical approach to the prevention of cystine stones is to alkalinize the urine with oral sodium bicarbonate in three or four divided doses (1.5 to 2.0 mEq/kg/day). Dent and Senior noted that, on occasion, stone dissolution could be achieved by giving 5 to 6 mEq/kg/day for brief periods.[79] Potassium citrate has some theoretic advantages over sodium bicarbonate, because its metabolism consumes hydrogen ions and alkalinizes the urine over a slightly longer period. Because 50 percent of cystine stones contain calcium salts, excess citrate excreted in the urine may also serve to chelate urinary calcium. Citrate therapy would seem to be the logical choice in any patient who happened to have relative hypercalciuria. However, controlled clinical trials have not been performed to compare the two agents directly.

In 1963, Crawhall et al.[80] reported that D-penicillamine could form a mixed disulfide with cystine and prevent its crystallization from urine. When administered orally to adults with cystinuria at a dose of 450 mg every 8 h, free urinary cystine was significantly reduced and about one-third of the penicillamine dose appears as cysteine-penicillamine and penicillamine disulfide. Crawhall et al.[80] and others[55,81,82] have reported stone dissolution. Stephens suggests that penicillamine be introduced gradually at a dose of

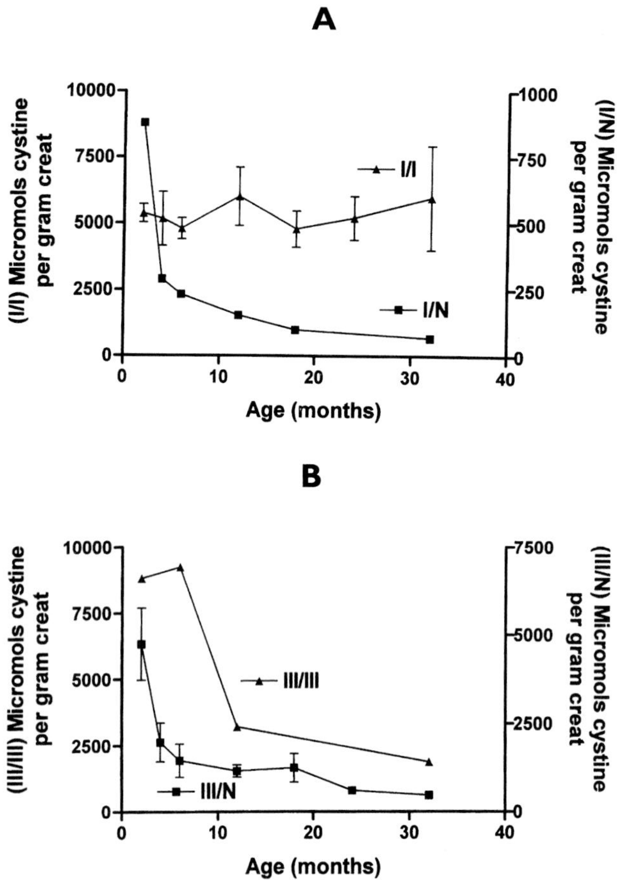

C

Fractional Excretion of Cystine

	< 6 months	>3 years
I/I	74%	103%
III/III	204%	74%
I/III	56%	25%

Fig. 191-2 Ontogeny of cystine excretion in various subtypes of cystinuria. *A*, Mean cystine excretion by children with homozygous Type I/I cystinuria (left Y-axis, N = 5) and heterozygous Type I/N cystinuria (right Y-axis, N = 2). *B*, Mean cystine excretion by children with homozygous Type III/III cystinuria (left axis, N = 1) and heterozygous Type III/N cystinuria (right Y-axis, N = 9). *C*, Fractional urinary cystine excretion by children with various types of cystinuria in infancy (<6 months) versus early childhood (>3 years).

500 to 1000 mg × 3/day, to identify the minimal dose that effectively brings the level of free urinary cystine below the threshold of solubility (<1250 μM cystine/liter).[55] To use this approach, urinary cystine must be measured on an amino acid analyzer under suitable elution conditions to separate free cystine from the cysteine-penicillamine peak. Side effects of penicillamine are not uncommon and may preclude use of the drug in some patients. About 25 percent develop a morbilliform rash and/or fever in the second week of therapy;[55] this complication resolves with discontinuation of therapy with or without oral prednisone and often does not recur if therapy is reintroduced. Occasionally, a more significant rash, which resembles epidermolysis bullosa rash, appears a year or more after onset of therapy. Nearly 25 percent of patients develop proteinuria-associated antibodies to the drug and immune complex-mediated membranous glomerulonephritis. Less frequent side effects include leukopenia, thrombocytopenia, a variety of autoimmune syndromes and loss of taste.[83]

Because of the high incidence of side effects with penicillamine, alternative thiol drugs have been tested. Use of α-mercaptopropionylglycine (MPG) in cystinuria was preliminarily reported by King et al. in 1968,[84] and later by Remien et al. in 1975.[85] In a comparative clinical trial, Pak et al. showed that MPG was as efficacious as penicillamine but only 31 percent of the patients discontinued MPG because of side effects versus 69 percent of patients taking penicillamine.[86] Fortunately, the patients who cannot tolerate penicillamine often have no side effects with MPG,[86] and MPG side effects may be milder or less frequent than with penicillamine.[87,88] Usually patients are started on 15 mg/kg three times a day (250 mg × 3/day in adults); the dose may be increased slightly (20 mg/kg/day to a maximum of 1 g/day) to achieve urinary levels of free cystine below the threshold of solubility. The range of side effects is similar to that reported for penicillamine and includes rash, fever, proteinuria, and hyperlipidemia.[89] Several years ago, Mairino et al. proposed that the familiar agent meso-2,3-dimercaptosuccinic acid (DMSA) might also be a useful chelating agent in cystinuria.[90] Two patients given an oral dose of 10 mg/kg excreted 90 percent of the drug in disulfide linkage with cysteine; this amount would be in the clinically useful range, complexing about 20 to 50 percent of the cystine excreted by a typical patient. No large clinical trials have been attempted with this agent.

A variety of alternative therapeutic approaches have been tried. Sloand and Izzo noted that cystine excretion is significantly reduced when two of their patients were treated with captopril (25 to 50 mg ×3/day).[91] This observation was confirmed by Streem and Hall who noted a decrease in urine cystine excretion of about 50 percent of baseline in eight patients treated with 150 mg/day[92], and by Perazella and Buller who noted a decrease in cystine excretion of 18 percent (100 mg/day) and 89 percent (150 mg/day) in two patients.[93] However, other investigators have been unable to reproduce this finding and Coulthard was unable to find any evidence of captopril-cysteine disulfide in the urine.[94] Because captopril is a powerful inhibitor of angiotensin-converting enzyme, it is possible that variable reduction in urinary cystine excretion seen at high doses may reflect a change in renal perfusion and cystine filtration rate rather than chelation of free urinary cystine.

In 1986, Jaeger studied four cystinuria patients and found that cystine excretion correlated with the sodium concentration urine.[95] In one patient, cystine excretion fell from about 2750 to 2000 μM/g creatinine when the patient was shifted from a high salt to a low salt diet (urine sodium of 300 vs. 50 mM/g creatinine). Others have confirmed this observation and Peces et al. speculated that extracellular volume contraction (produced by sodium depletion) might enhance proximal tubular sodium-coupled amino acid transport and, thus, account for reduced cystine excretion.[96] However, there have been no long-term studies of sodium restriction on the incidence of stone formation. Although Norman and Manette noted no effect on average daily urine pH, low salt diets should increase urine osmolarity and acidity overnight when water intake is low and might actually increase the risk of nephrolithiasis.[97]

The discovery of two cystinuria genes, first, *SLC3A1* and more recently, *SLC7A9* has now opened the door to the possibility of gene therapy for cystinuria. Strategies such as adenovirus expression vectors injected into the renal artery are under investigation to deliver therapeutic cDNAs to the kidney, but thus far, only transient low-level expression has been achieved. However, if an efficient expression system is eventually devised, the *SLC3A1* and *SLC7A9* promoter sequences[98,99] may prove to be useful in targeting expression to the appropriate segment of the proximal tubule.

THE PHYSIOLOGY OF RENAL AND INTESTINAL (RE)ABSORPTION OF CYSTINE AND DIBASIC AMINO ACIDS

Amino acids are ultrafiltered through the renal glomerulus into tubular fluid at plasma concentrations[100] and are subsequently > 98 percent reabsorbed by active transport mechanisms (against an electrochemical gradient), which depend on the lumen-cell sodium gradient and intracellular energy stores.[101] Stop-flow, micropuncture, and microperfusion studies[54,102–104] indicate that reabsorption of amino acids occurs predominantly in the proximal convoluted tubules. In adults, 99 percent of filtered cystine is finally reabsorbed, but the relative contribution of the proximal convoluted (S1 and S2 segments) versus proximal straight tubule (S3 segment) is uncertain.[54] Transport of cystine by rat-kidney brush-border membrane vesicles is relatively sodium-independent compared to other zwitterionic amino acids.[105–108] It is proposed, therefore, that cystine enters the cell down a concentration gradient provided by intracellular systems, which rapidly reduce cystine to cysteine; cysteine then exits the cell by a basolateral transport system.[54] Thus, the main intracellular form of cystine is as the reduced free thiol, cysteine.[109,110] Incubation of kidney cortex slices[110] or isolated renal tubules[111] with (^{35}S) cystine results in the intracellular accumulation of ^{35}S in the form of cysteine and glutathione.[110] Cystine is thought to be reduced by glutathione-cysteine transhydrogenase[112] subsequent to the luminal transport step because cystine taken up by isolated renal brush-border membrane vesicles is not reduced to cysteine.[107,113]

For most amino acids, tubular reabsorption is accomplished by a number of overlapping transport systems (reviewed in references 46 and 54). Although it is clear that proximal tubular amino acid reabsorption is defective in cystinuria, the precise transport mechanism involved was not immediately evident. In 1951, Dent and Rose[13] proposed that cystinuria was due to a defect in the selective renal and intestinal transport system shared by cystine and dibasic amino acids. Robson and Rose produced the first evidence for this postulate by reporting that urinary cystine excretion increased when the filtered load of lysine was increased.[114] Other investigators obtained similar data in humans,[115,116] rats,[117,118] and dogs.[119] In the experiments with dogs, it was noted that lysine infusion resulted in urinary cystine clearance exceeding the glomerular filtration rate (i.e., tubular cystine secretion or back-leak). This was also observed in cystinuric patients[115,116] and in cystinuric dogs.[120] Together these data suggest that dibasic amino acids competitively inhibit cystine reabsorption and also induce or unmask cystine secretion. Bidirectional cystine transport or *trans*-stimulation of this transport by dibasic amino acids might explain these results (see below).

Studies with amino acid infusion *in vivo* have defined multiple renal reabsorptive mechanisms for cystine and dibasic amino acids. Infusion of increasing amounts of lysine in cystinuric patients showed that the reabsorptive defect was no longer evident when the plasma level (and thus the filtered tubular load) was increased to 7 to 10 times normal.[115] This observation suggests at least two transport systems exist for lysine renal reabsorption: (a) a low-capacity (low V_{max}) high-affinity (low K_m) system, which is defective in cystinuria, and (b) a high-capacity (high V_{max}) low-affinity (high K_m) system which is unaffected and becomes the primary determinant of lysine excretion at abnormally high filtered loads. The postnatal maturation of renal dibasic amino acid reabsorption precedes that of cystine, again indicating transporter heterogeneity.[121] It also seems that cystine reabsorption differs from that of cysteine because in rat kidney microperfusion experiments, neutral amino acids inhibit luminal uptake of cystine and cysteine differently.[122]

Studies with rat kidney using microperfusion of tubules, isolated tubule fragments, and brush-border membrane vesicles were used to address the properties of apical membrane cystine transport directly. In those preparations, cystine is transported by a luminal high-affinity system shared with dibasic amino acids and a low-affinity system that is unshared with dibasic amino acids. In microperfusion studies of isolated rat-kidney tubules, arginine was shown to inhibit luminal cystine uptake,[123,124] and Segal's group demonstrated two saturable transport systems for cystine in both brush-border membrane vesicles[113] and tubular fragments.[111] The high-affinity system had an apparent K_m value of about 10 μM and the low-affinity system had an apparent K_m value about 500 μM. This suggests that at typical concentrations of cystine in the ultrafiltrate (50 μM) the contribution of both systems would be similar.[111] The assessment of the low-affinity system *in vitro* is difficult, however, due to the low solubility of cystine (~450 μM in water at 25°C);[125] Volkl and coworkers[122] could not demonstrate saturability of luminal cystine uptake in microperfused rat-kidney tubules up to this limit of solubility. Although dibasic amino acids in isolated tubule fragments and brush-border membrane vesicles inhibit cystine transport via the high-affinity system and cystine inhibits high-affinity lysine uptake by cortical isolated tubules, the low-affinity system shows no interaction with dibasic amino acids.[111,113] Furthermore, the low-affinity cystine transporter is thought to be sodium-dependent,[111,122] whereas the high-affinity system is thought to be sodium-independent.[106] Interestingly, the high-affinity system exhibits heteroexchange of cystine and dibasic amino acids.[107] Thus, the carrier could potentially facilitate cystine movement in either direction across the luminal membrane.

Microperfusion studies and assays with isolated tubule fragments from rat kidney suggest that the high-affinity system is located in the proximal straight tubule (S3 segment), whereas the low-affinity system is located in the proximal convoluted tubule.[122,126] Recently, Riahi-Esfahani et al.[108] reported that luminal membrane vesicles from the outer medulla (i.e., *pars recta* or proximal straight tubules) of rabbit kidney show a conspicuous component of high-affinity cystine transport (apparent K_m 30 μM). Furthermore, cystine transport in proximal tubule brush border membranes from the outer medulla (S3) is less sodium dependent and more sensitive to inhibition by micromolar concentrations of neutral amino acids than in brush border membranes from the outer cortex (*pars convoluta*, S1 and S2) (see Fig. 191-3).

Unlike the kidney, rat-intestinal brush-border membrane vesicles show only a single high-affinity transport system for cystine, shared with dibasic amino acids.[127] Because oral loading studies and jejunal biopsies from cystinuria patients suggest that the small intestine is also affected, it appears to be the sodium-independent, luminal, high-affinity transport mechanism shared by cystine and dibasic amino acids in jejunum and in the S3 segments of the proximal tubule which is defective in cystinuria.

Although there is no evidence of excessive urinary neutral amino acids in cystinuria patients, the renal high-affinity transport system for cystine appears to be shared by neutral amino acids *in vitro*. Transport of cystine at low (μM) concentration by isolated tubule fragments, perfused tubules and brush-border membrane vesicles from rat kidney is inhibited by neutral amino acids.[108,111,122,126,128]

Additional details of this transport mechanism have been derived from studies of the opossum kidney (OK) cell line.[129] Unlike most other immortalized kidney cell lines, OK cells clearly express the apical high-affinity sodium-independent shared cystine and dibasic amino acid transporter.[129] Mora et al.[130] showed that this uptake system in OK cells was similar to the $b^{o,+}$ transport system (broad specificity for neutral (o) and dibasic (+) amino acids) described in mouse blastocysts by Van Winkle and coworkers.[131] Thus, apical transport of cystine in OK cells is mainly sodium independent, and is shared with dibasic amino acids and some neutral amino acids (e.g., L-leucine).[130] Indeed,

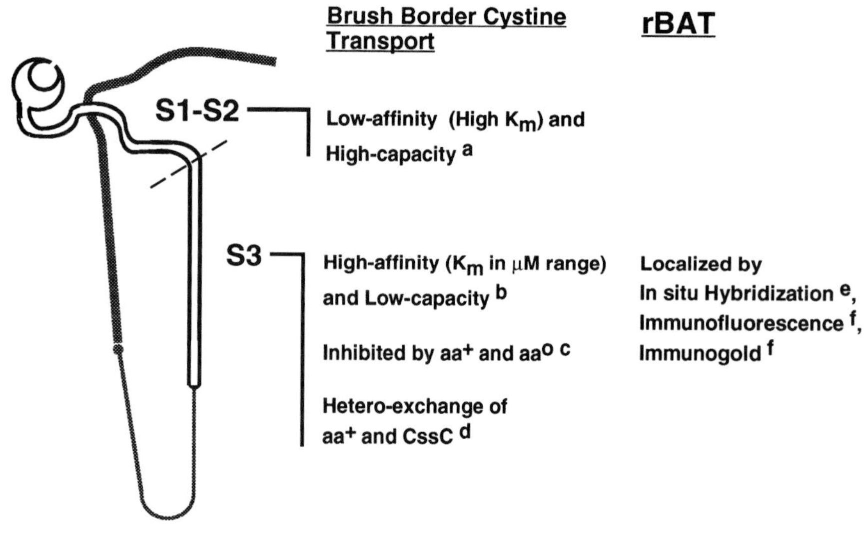

Fig. 191-3 Cystine reabsorption and rBAT/$b^{0,+}$-like system in kidney. The high-affinity and low-capacity reabsorption system for cystine is located predominantly in the brush-border of the epithelial cells of the proximal straight tubule (S3 segment). This transport system is inhibited by dibasic (aa^+) and neutral (aa^o) amino acids, and shows heteroexchange of cystine (CssC) and dibasic (aa^+) amino acids. The rBAT mRNA is expressed in the epithelial cells of the S3 segment, and the rBAT protein in the brush-border of these cells References: a,[113,122]; b,[108,113,126]; c,[111,113,122,126,128]; d,[107], e,[168]; f,[169,170].

100 percent of sodium-independent cystine transport, 80 percent of sodium-independent arginine transport, and 65 percent of the sodium-independent leucine transport occurs via this $b^{o,+}$-like system in OK cells. The transport system also shows[130] the heteroexchange diffusion observed in rat-renal brush-border membrane vesicles studies.[107] Cystine transport by a $b^{o,+}$-like mechanism has also been reported in brush-border membrane vesicles from chicken intestine[132] and in Caco-2 cells.[133]

THE RENAL AND INTESTINAL HIGH-AFFINITY CYSTINE (RE)ABSORPTION MECHANISM (THE rBAT/$b^{o,+}$-LIKE SYSTEM)

Multiple different apical and basolateral amino acid transport systems for cystine and dibasic amino acids have been described in renal or small intestinal epithelial cells.[134,135] Two cystinuria loci have been identified by genetic linkage studies (see "Molecular Genetics of Cystinuria" below): 2p16.3-p21 and 19q13.1-q13.2. There is no evidence for a third cystinuria locus thus far. Of the cloned amino acid transporters potentially participating in renal reabsorption and intestinal absorption of cystine and dibasic amino acids, only the *rBAT* gene (*SLC3A1* in the Human Genome Data base) maps to the 2p16.3-p21 and the *SLC7A9* gene maps to the 19q13.1 cystinuria loci. The other amino acid transporter genes have different locations.[135]

Using an amino acid transport expression cloning strategy in *Xenopus* oocytes, three laboratories independently isolated cDNAs for a putative cystine and dibasic amino acid transporter from rabbit, rat, and human kidney (GenBank accession numbers L04504, M77345, M80804, M90096, L11696, and M95548); homology between the deduced proteins is very high (~85 percent identity).[68–72] A partial rBAT cDNA sequence one from OK (Opossum Kidney) cells has also been reported[130] (GenBank accession number X95475). Each of the three labs assigned different names to these cDNAs: NBAT,[68] rBAT,[69] and D2.[70] For clarity, this chapter uses rBAT (an acronym for "related to $b^{o,+}$ amino acid transporter") for all these cDNAs and proteins.

When a homology search was performed with the deduced rBAT protein amino acid sequence, ~30 percent identity (~50 percent similarity) with the heavy chain of the cell surface antigen 4F2 (4F2hc)[136–140] (GenBank accession numbers J02939, M17430, M18811, M21904, and J03569 for human; U59324 and X89225 for rat; U25708 for mouse) was found. Initially, this was puzzling, because the human 4F2hc cDNA had been isolated as part of an effort to identify lymphoblast cell surface glycoprotein genes.[136–138] However, *rBAT* and *4F2hc* (*SLC3A2* in Human Genome Database) are clearly members of the same family because intron-exon structure is highly conserved; within the open reading frame of human *rBAT* and *4F2hc*, introns 1 and 2 have identical locations, intron 3 in *4F2hc* corresponds to intron 4 in *rBAT*, and intron 8 in *4F2hc* to intron 9 in *rBAT*[98,141,142] (GenBank accession numbers U60810 to U60819 for *rBAT*, and M21898 to M21904 for *4F2hc*). Furthermore, when 4F2hc cRNA was expressed in *Xenopus* oocytes, it induced amino acid uptake with characteristics of the y^+ L-like transport system (versus the $b^{o,+}$-like transport elicited by rBAT); this observation suggests that both molecules are involved in membrane transport.[143,144]

Subunit Structure

Hydrophobicity algorithms suggest that rBAT and 4F2hc contain a single transmembrane domain near the *N*-terminus of each protein.[69,70] Both proteins are *N*-glycosylated integral proteins of the plasma membrane[70,71,145,146] and are considered type II membrane glycoproteins (i.e., intracellular *N*-terminus, a single transmembrane domain, and a bulky extracellular *C*-terminus domain). This is in contrast to the well-known membrane multispanning structure of membrane transporters of polar substrates. However, Moscovitz et al.[147] proposed that rBAT may have three additional amphipathic transmembrane domains (see Fig. 191-4). These results await confirmation; no similar studies have been conducted with 4F2hc. In any event, it seems that rBAT and 4F2hc are not hydrophobic enough to provide a polar pathway for the movement of amino acids across the plasma membrane. This prompted the hypothesis that they are subunits of heteromultimeric transporters.[69,70,143] Thus, induction of amino acid transport by expression of these proteins in oocytes would result from interaction with "silent" complementary subunits already present in the oocytes. A similar expression mechanism has been described for Na^+/K^+ ATPase and multimeric channels.[148–151] Consistent with this, rBAT and 4F2hc form part of a heterodimeric structure. The surface antigen 4F2 is a heterodimer (~125 kDa) with a heavy chain of ~85 kDa (i.e., 4F2hc, the protein which is homologous to rBAT) and a light subunit of ~40 kDa linked by disulfide bridges.[146] Similarly, rBAT in kidney and intestine forms a heterodimeric structure (125 kDa) of a "heavy chain" (~90 kDa) linked by disulfide bridges to a putative "light subunit" of 40 to 50 kDa.[152,153] Several lines of evidence suggest that these heterodimers of rBAT or 4F2hc might be the basic functional units of $b^{o,+}$ and y^+L transporters, respectively.[154] In addition, recent inactivation studies by covalent modification of external cysteine residues showed that 4F2hc is intimately associated, most probably through a disulfide bridge, with a membrane oocyte protein for the expression of system y^+L amino acid transport activity.[155] Finally,

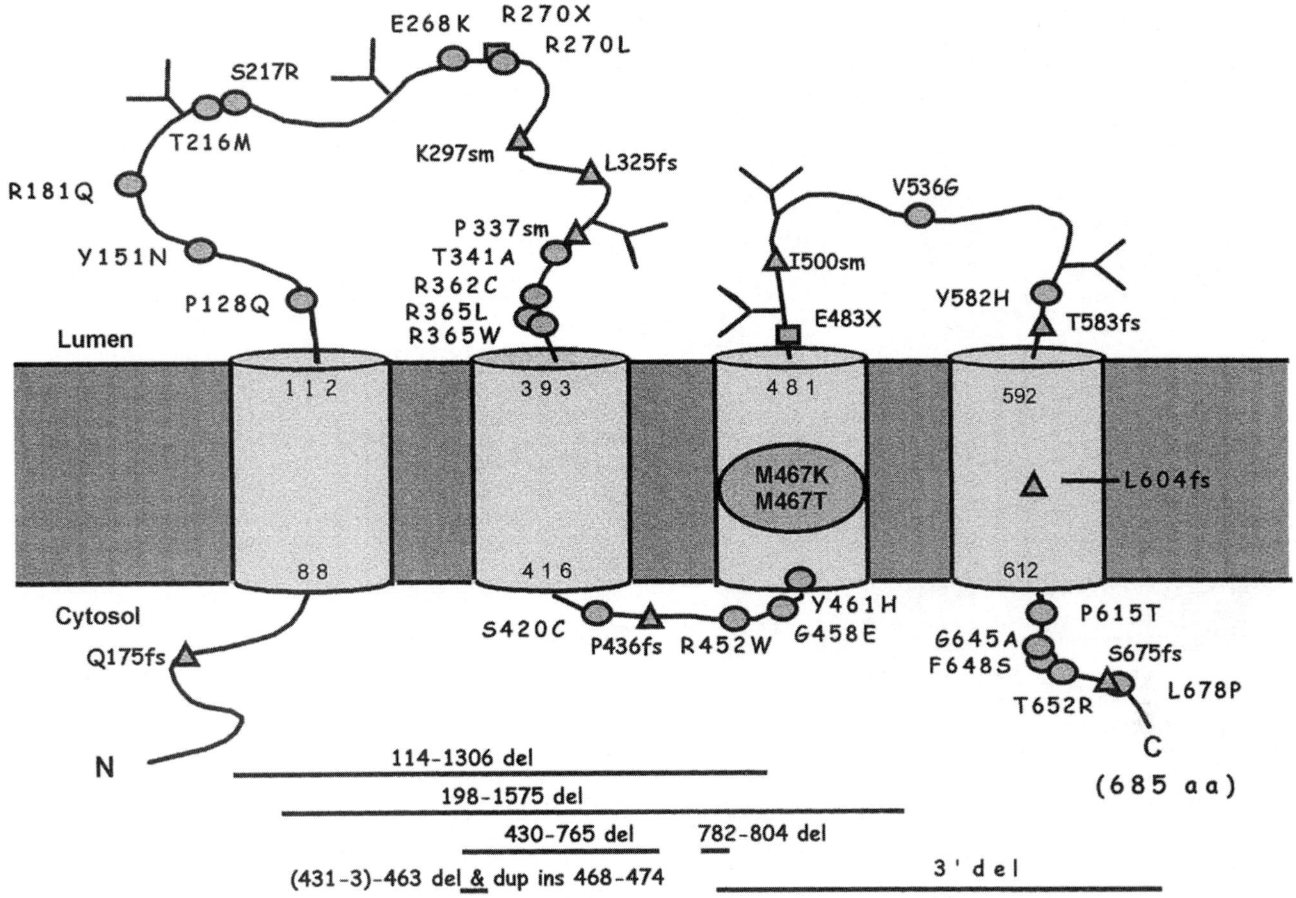

Fig. 191-4 Schematic representation of the human rBAT protein. This four transmembrane topology model of the rBAT protein is based on studies by Tate's group[147] (amino acid residue numbers shown inside the cylinders indicate the limits of the transmembrane segments). Forty cystinuria-specific mutations in the rBAT gene have been reported. This includes 23 missense (circles); 2 nonsense (squares); 3 splice mutations (triangles; K297sm, P337sm, and I500sm correspond to mutations 891 + 4A $\rightarrow$ G, G1011A, and 1500 + 1G $\rightarrow$ T listed in Table 191-2, respectively); 6 frameshift mutations (triangles; Q175fs, L325fs, P436fs, T583fs, L604fs, and S675fs correspond to mutations 163 del C974 del GA, 1306 ins G, 1749 del A, 1810 del TG, and 2922 ins T listed in Table 191-2, respectively); and 6 large deletions (not shown): Δ G38-P436, Δ A66-T525, Δ G144-T255, Δ I145-6204 and dup L159-V161, Δ N261-E268 and Δ E298-C-terminus (amino acid residue numbers indicate the limits of these deletions), which correspond to deletions 114-1306 del, 198-1575 del, 430-765 del, del (431-3)-463, del and dup ins 468-474, 782-804 del and the 3′ deletion listed in Table 191-2, respectively. Closed circles denote the seven missense mutations for which defective amino acid transport activity in oocytes has been reported. Mutations are indicated using the single letter code for amino acids. (Y) indicates six potential *N*-glycosylation sites. (*Adapted from Palacín et al.*[154] *Used by permission.*)

a cDNA from human, rat, and *Xenopus laevis* (LAT-1)[156,157] (GenBank accession numbers AF077866, human; AB015433, rat; and Y12716, *Xenopus laevis*), a rat and human cDNA (LAT-2)[156,158] and two human and mouse cDNAs (y^+LAT-1 and y^+LAT-2)[159] (GenBank accession numbers AF092032 and D87432) and a mouse cDNA (xCT)[160] that associate with 4F2hc to form systems L and y^+L transporters, respectively, have been identified. These proteins represent the first members of LSHAT (**L**ight **S**ubunits of **H**eteromeric **A**mino acid **T**ransporters) family. Human LAT-1, y^+LAT-1, and y^+LAT-2 are homologous proteins (40 to 75 percent amino acid sequence identity among them) with 12 putative transmembrane domains, and represent different light subunits of the cell surface antigen 4F2 and co-express with it amino acid transport activity in oocytes.[157–161] The role of these subunits in amino acid transport was recently highlighted because mutations in y^+LAT-1 cause Lysinuric Protein Intolerance (LPI), an inherited aminoaciduria due to defective renal reabsorption of dibasic amino acids.[162,163]

Due to the functional and structural similarities between 4F2hc and its homologous protein rBAT, it was anticipated that a homolog of the LSHAT family might act as the light subunit required for rBAT to fully express the amino acid transport system $b^{o,+}$ activity. Very recently, a new member ($b^{o,+}$AT) of this family was proposed to be the light subunit of rBAT based on functional expression studies with rBAT (see below: Identification of *SLC7A9* as a cystinuria non-Type I gene). This gene then became an excellent candidate for the non-Type I form of cystinuria.

Tissue Expression

rBAT mRNA is expressed in the kidney and the mucosa of the small intestine.[69–72,164,165] As expected for a tentative rBAT light subunit, $b^{o,+}$AT mRNA has a similar expression pattern.[77] Consistent with this, rBAT antisense oligonucleotides block transport by the $b^{o,+}$-like system induced by injection of renal or intestinal poly(A)$^+$ RNA into oocytes.[70,71,166] Northern blot analysis of human, rat, and rabbit renal and intestinal RNA reveals two rBAT transcripts; ~2.3 kb (which corresponds to the above mentioned cDNAs) and ~4 kb (which represents an alternative polyadenylation of the transcript; GenBank accession number L04504).[145] In situ hybridization and immunohistochemical studies demonstrate that rBAT localizes to the microvilli of the small intestinal mucosa and the epithelial cells of the proximal straght tubules (S3 segment) of the rat nephron[167–169] (Fig. 191-5). Clear rBAT transcripts are also visible in the human pancreas, but the significance of this is unknown.[71] In addition to kidney and intestine, brain tissues show a transcript of ~5 kb that hybridizes

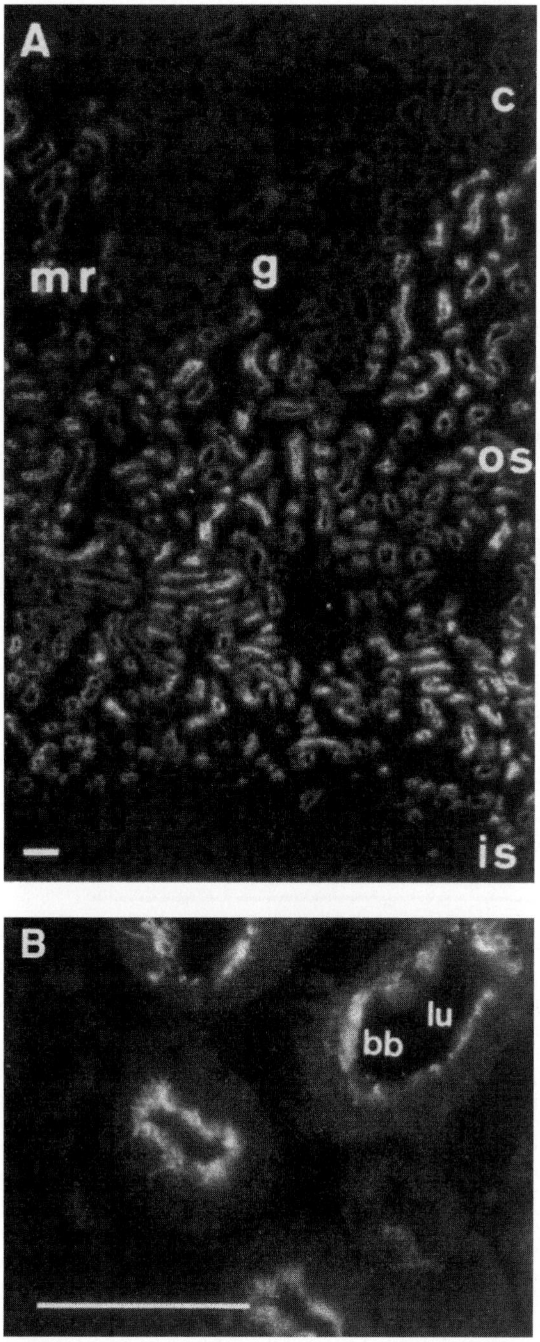

Fig. 191-5 Immunolocalization of rBAT in rat kidney. *A*, General view of part of the cortex (c), outer stripe of the outer medulla (os), and inner stripe of the outer medulla (is). The position of a medullary ray (mr) and a glomerulus (g) is indicated. *B*, Detail of several tubules from the outer stripe of the outer medulla. bb, brush-border; lu, tubular lumen. Cryosections of adult rat kidney were incubated with polyclonal anti-rBAT antibody ManRX and with antibody rhodamine-conjugated swine antirabbit IgG (light signal), as secondary antibody. The rBAT-specific signal is located in the brush-border of the proximal straight tubules in the outer stripe of the outer medulla. Scale bars: 50 μM. (*from Furriols et al.*[168] *Used by permission.*)

with rBAT cDNA probes.[69,71,165] This long transcript is almost ubiquitous, but with a substantially lower abundance in tissues other than brain.[71] RNA protection assays and western immunoblots with some, but not all, anti-rBAT peptide antibodies suggest that this long transcript corresponds to a gene that is homologous to *rBAT*.[165,169] Moreover, rBAT immunoreactivity in hypothalamus is intracellular and it is not located in the plasma membrane as in kidney and intestine.[170]

The expression of *rBAT* is developmentally regulated in kidney. In the rat, rBAT transcripts appear after birth and the onset of the protein expression coincides with postnatal nephron maturation.[168] In humans, the process of nephron formation is completed 4 to 6 weeks prior to birth; rBAT mRNA expression is detectable by 15 to 20 weeks fetal age but renal expression is considerably increased by 3 years of age (Fig. 191-6). This observation may explain why infants who are heterozygous for a mutation at the 19q cystinuria locus (i.e., *SLC7A9* gene) may initially appear to have homozygous cystinuria until the rBAT system matures. A similar phenomenon occurs in infants who inherit one mutant *rBAT* gene (Fig. 191-2). Interestingly, there is minimal evidence of a maturational effect in babies who inherit two mutant *rBAT* alleles from two completely recessive parents (Fig. 191-2). This suggests that the ontogeny effect requires at least one wild-type *rBAT* gene, and developmental regulation of rBAT expression may account in part for the postnatal maturation of renal cystine reabsorption. At present, it is unknown whether the expression of $b^{o,+}$AT is developmentally regulated in kidney, but the ontogeny of rBAT expression appears to be the primary determinant of postnatal maturation of cystine reabsorption in humans.

Transport Properties

The characteristics of the amino acid transport activity associated with rBAT expression have been studied mainly in oocytes. rBAT induces a high-affinity transport with K_m values in the μM range for amino acids such as L-cystine (see Fig. 191-6), L-arginine, L-lysine, L-ornithine, L-leucine, L-histidine, and probably L-cysteine. Kinetic and cross-inhibition studies offer convincing evidence that rBAT induces a single amino acid transport system in *Xenopus* oocytes, at least in sodium-free medium (see below), which is not present in stage VI oocytes.[69,71] This transport activity is sodium independent and is very similar to the amino acid transport system $b^{o,+}$ defined by Van Winkle's group in mouse blastocysts, as a sodium-independent high-affinity system for dibasic and zwitterionic amino acids.[131] Further characterization of the $b^{o,+}$-like (rBAT) transport activity showed that it was independent of external K^+ and Cl^-,[171] changes in the external pH (M. Palacín, unpublished results) and internal ATP.[172] Co-transfection of rBAT and $b^{o,+}$AT in COS cells results in sodium-independent L-arginine transport,[77] but the characteristics of this activity remain to be studied.

Because the $b^{o,+}$-like system appears to be a sodium-, potassium-, proton-, and ATP-independent transporter it was initially unclear how it could participate in an active process such as the reabsorption of cystine and dibasic amino acids. This problem was partially resolved by Busch et al.[171] In oocytes expressing rBAT, the presence of L-arginine in the medium produces an inward positive current, most probably due to an inward flux of this positively charged amino acid. However, with L-leucine in the medium, there was an outward positive current through the oocyte membrane (Fig. 191-7). These results prompted the hypothesis that the $b^{o,+}$-like (rBAT) transporter can exchange amino acids through the plasma membrane—the outward positive current produced by zwitterionic amino acids (e.g., L-leucine) would be due to the concomitant exit of dibasic amino acids from the oocyte. Several laboratories confirmed that the efflux of L-[^{3}H] arginine and L-[^{3}H] leucine is totally dependent on the presence of amino acid substrates in the medium,[173,174] and the electrogenic activity of the transporter is totally dependent on the presence of amino acid substrates with different charges at both sites of the oocyte plasma membrane[172] (Fig. 191-7). Additionally, the $b^{o,+}$-like (rBAT) system is an obligatory exchanger with a stoichiometry of one amino acid (influx) per one amino acid (efflux), and with preference for influx of dibasic amino acids and efflux of neutral amino acids (versus the reverse exchange);[174] a similar exchange activity has been demonstrated in OK cells.[130] Therefore, the $b^{o,+}$-like (rBAT)

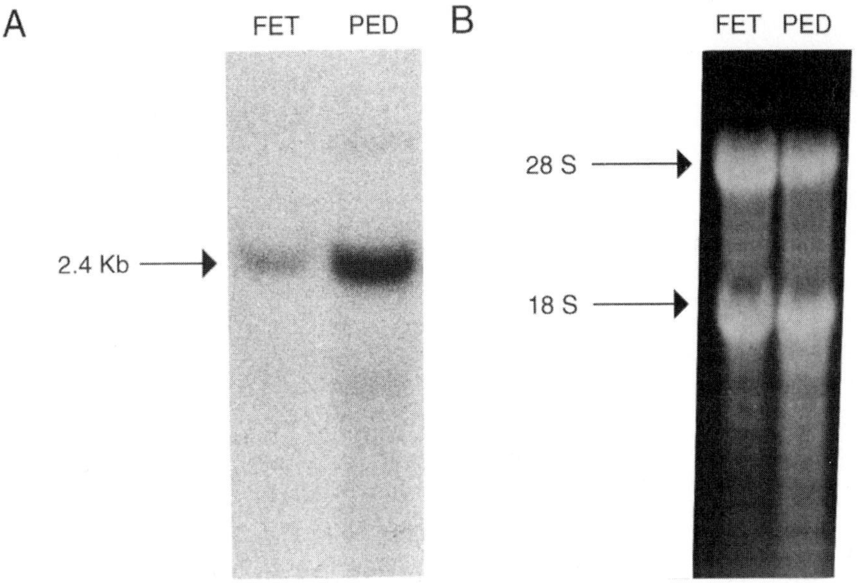

Fig. 191-6 Northern analysis of rBAT mRNA expression. ***A,*** **Total RNA (30 mg/lane) isolated from human fetal (18 weeks fetal age) and pediatric (3 years) kidney was hybridized to a radiolabeled human rBAT cDNA probe.** ***B,*** **Ethidium bromide-stained gel showing approximately equivalent RNA loading in each lane.**

system acts as a tertiary active transporter (see Fig. 191-8).[135] Cystine and dibasic amino acids are probably reabsorbed through the brush-border plasma membrane by exchange with highly concentrated intracellular zwitterionic amino acids. These neutral amino acids are then reclaimed from the tubular fluid by active sodium-dependent mechanisms (Fig. 191-8). In this model, a defective $b^{o,+}$-like (rBAT) system in cystinuria would not affect reabsorption of neutral amino acids because the luminal sodium-dependent neutral amino acid transport system is intact. Similar to rBAT, the y^+ L amino acid transport activity induced by 4F2hc in oocytes behaves as an exchanger, causing efflux of dibasic amino acids and influx of neutral amino acids.[174] 4F2hc is located in the basolateral plasma membrane of proximal tubules[175] and presumably mediates the transfer of dibasic amino acids from cell to blood during transepithelial reabsorption (kidney) or absorption (intestine) (see Fig. 191-8).

RENAL AND INTESTINAL TRANSPORT DEFECTS

All available evidence indicates that the transport defect in cystinuria is restricted to the kidney and the small intestine. Circulating leukocytes, for example, show no abnormalities of amino acid uptake.[176] In kidney, it is the mechanism for reabsorption of cystine and dibasic amino acids from tubular fluid that is affected because aminoaciduria occurs in the presence of normal plasma levels of these amino acids.[15,177] However, the luminal defect has not yet been directly demonstrated with kidney *in vitro* preparations. Brush-border membrane vesicles from kidney possess a high-affinity transport system with properties corresponding precisely to those of the *rBAT* gene when expressed in *Xenopus* oocytes[69–72,171–174] and in OK cells,[135] but brush-border membrane vesicles from cystinuria patients have not yet been studied. Segal and Thier examined steady state accumulation of cystine and dibasic amino acids by slices prepared from cystinuric human kidney. Although accumulation of arginine and lysine was only 50 to 60 percent of normal, there was no apparent defect in concentrative uptake of cystine.[23,178] Initially, this was taken to be evidence against a primary transport defect in cystinuria, but it is now clear that the kidney-slice preparation exposes the basolateral, rather than the apical, surface of tubular cells to substrates in the medium. In retrospect, these studies simply provided good evidence that the defect in cystinuria does not perturb cystine transport at the basolateral cell surface.

In the intestine, the luminal transport defect is better defined. Steady state accumulation of cystine and dibasic amino acids is clearly defective in samples of jejunal mucosa obtained by peroral biopsy.[22,179,180] Coicadan et al. localized the cystinuria transport defect to the apical plasma membrane of intestinal cells by showing that lysine transport is reduced in brush-border membrane vesicles from cystinuric small intestine.[181] Desjeux and coworkers suggested that increased efflux of cystine across the apical plasma membrane of the intestine might be the primary defect in cystinuria.[182] However, because the main intracellular form of cystine is cysteine, and transport of cysteine by mucosal biopsies is unimpaired in cystinuria,[183] this proposal seems unlikely. Furthermore, immunohistochemical studies in mature rodent kidney demonstrate that rBAT protein is localized to the apical membrane of the straight proximal tubule and the small intestine.[168,169]

The fractional excretion of cystine consistently exceeds that of the dibasic amino acids and may be greater than 100 percent of the filtered load in some patients. Furthermore, the fractional excretion of lysine (40 to 70 percent) is usually greater than that of arginine or ornithine.[39,64,116,177,184] One explanation for the apparent secretion of cystine in some patients may derive from the properties of rBAT as an amino acid exchanger. In oocyte expression studies, influx (lumen to cell) of cystine and dibasic amino acids on the rBAT transporter is tightly coupled to efflux (cell to lumen) of cysteine or neutral amino acids.[174] Presumably, the secreted neutral amino acids are then efficiently reabsorbed by sodium-dependent mechanisms in the proximal tubule, but cysteine is rapidly oxidized to cystine and appears in the final urine. In patients with the non-*rBAT* form of cystinuria, the predominance of cystine excretion might be explained by the exchange properties of the intact rBAT exchanger. However, in cystinuria caused by homozygous null mutations of *rBAT,* cystine back-leak must occur via some other pathway. Further studies in animal models or patients with defined cystinuria gene mutations are needed to resolve this issue.

The high fractional excretion of lysine relative to that of other dibasic amino acids in cystinuria cannot readily be explained by the properties of rBAT as an amino acid exchanger. Presumably, alternative transport mechanisms have less capacity to compensate for unreabsorbed lysine than for arginine and ornithine. In normal subjects, arginine infusions induce cystinuria and lysinuria, while lysine infusions induce cystinuria.[117,118] Interestingly, lysine infusion actually increases the intracellular level of cysteine, especially in the outer medulla where rBAT is expressed; this may be due to inhibition of cysteine efflux by intracellular lysine as reported by Schwartzman et al.[185]

Another puzzling aspect of cystinuria is that the renal arteriovenous difference for cystine is minimal both in patients

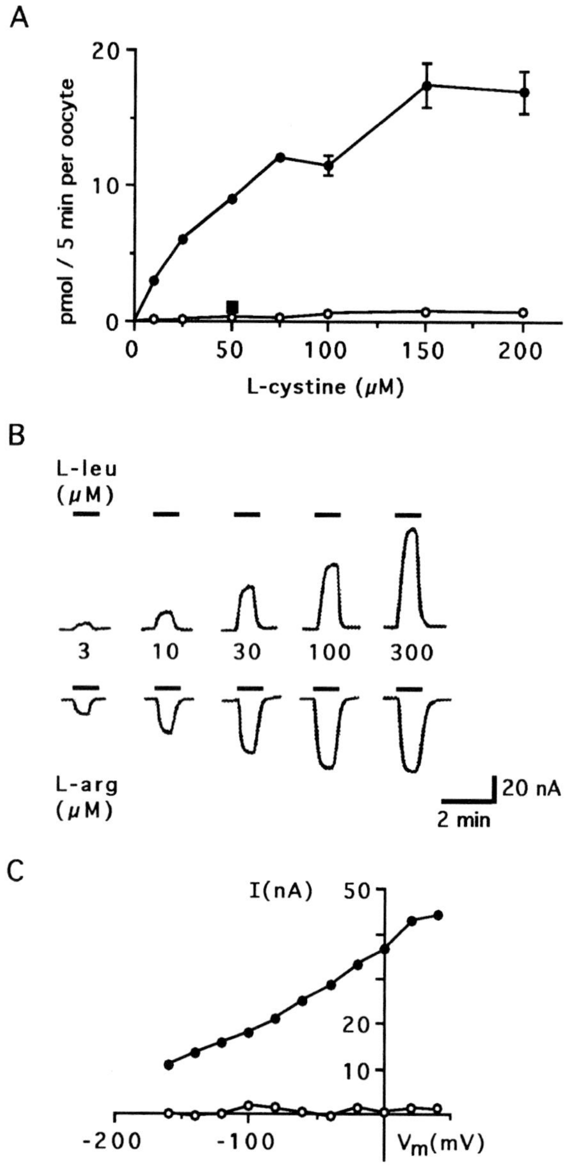

Fig. 191-7 Transport characteristics of the rBAT / $b^{0,+}$-like amino acid transport system. *A*, Kinetics of human rBAT-induced transport of L-[^{35}S] cystine in *Xenopus* oocytes. Oocytes were injected with water (open circles) or 2.5 ng of human rBAT cRNA (closed circles). More than 95 percent of the transport of 50 μM L-cystine induced by rBAT is inhibited by 5 mM L-arginine in the medium (closed square). (*From data in Bertrán et al.*[71] *Used by permission.*) *B*, Concentration-dependent currents induced by the indicated concentrations of L-leucine (outward current; upper panel) and L-arginine (inward current; lower panel) in oocytes expressing rabbit rBAT. Currents were induced at −50 mV by superfusion with the individual amino acids for the period indicated by the horizontal bars. (*From Busch et al.*[153] *Used by permission.*) *C*, Typical alanine-arginine exchange in cut-open oocytes expressing rabbit rBAT. Addition of 500 μM L-alanine to the external medium does not lead to any change in currents (open circles). If 500 μM L-arginine is present in the internal medium, addition of 500 μM L-alanine to the external medium causes a large outward current (closed circles). (*From Coady et al.*[172] *Used by permission.*)

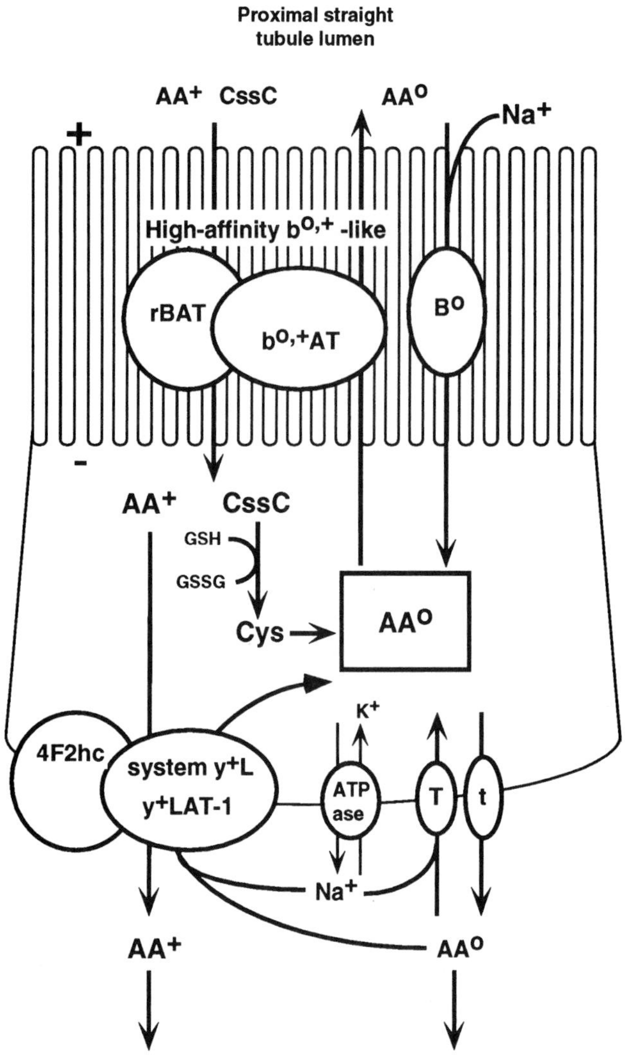

Fig. 191-8 Model for the renal reabsorption of dibasic amino acids via systems $b^{0,+}$-like and Y^+ L-like. The scheme shows an epithelial cell from the proximal straight tubule of the nephron. Obligatory amino acid exchange with neutral amino acids (AA^o) via systems $b^{o,+}$-like (apical) and Y^+ L-like (basolateral) would mediate the active reabsorption of dibasic amino acids (AA^+) and cystine (CssC). Influx of dibasic amino acids and cystine from the lumen would be favored by the negative membrane potential and by the reduction of cystine to cysteine associated with glutathione oxidation (GSH→GssG), respectively. A high intracellular concentration of neutral amino acid would be ensured by concentrative (Na^+ cotransport) neutral amino acid transport activities in the apical pole (system B^o) and the basolateral pole (systems ASC, and others; T transporters shown in the scheme). t, sodium-independent neutral amino acid transporters (e.g., the exchanger system L and facilitated transporters). ATPase, Na^+/K^+ ATPase. The basolateral amino acid transporter Y^+ L (heavy chain: 4Fhc2, light chain Y^+ LAT-1, *SLC7A9* gene) is defective in Lysinuric Protein Intolerance.[162,163] Colocalization of the cell surface antigen 4F2hc and rBAT in the epithelial cells of the proximal straight tubule is hypothetical. (*Adapted from Chillarón et al.*[174] *Used by permission.*)

and controls.[18,41] If nearly all filtered cystine is lost in the urine, one would expect renal venous cystine to be significantly lower than that in the renal artery. This observation suggests that *de novo* renal synthesis of cystine compensates for lack of cystine influx from the tubule. However, studies to confirm or refute this idea have been inconclusive and the paradox remains unresolved.[18,186]

MOLECULAR GENETICS

Identification of *SLC3A1* as a Cystinuria Type I/I Gene

The hypothesis that *SLC3A1* is a cystinuria gene was tested by screening for *SLC3A1* mutations in affected patients. Because the genomic structure of the *SLC3A1* gene was initially unknown, *SLC3A1* mutations were first detected by screening RNAs

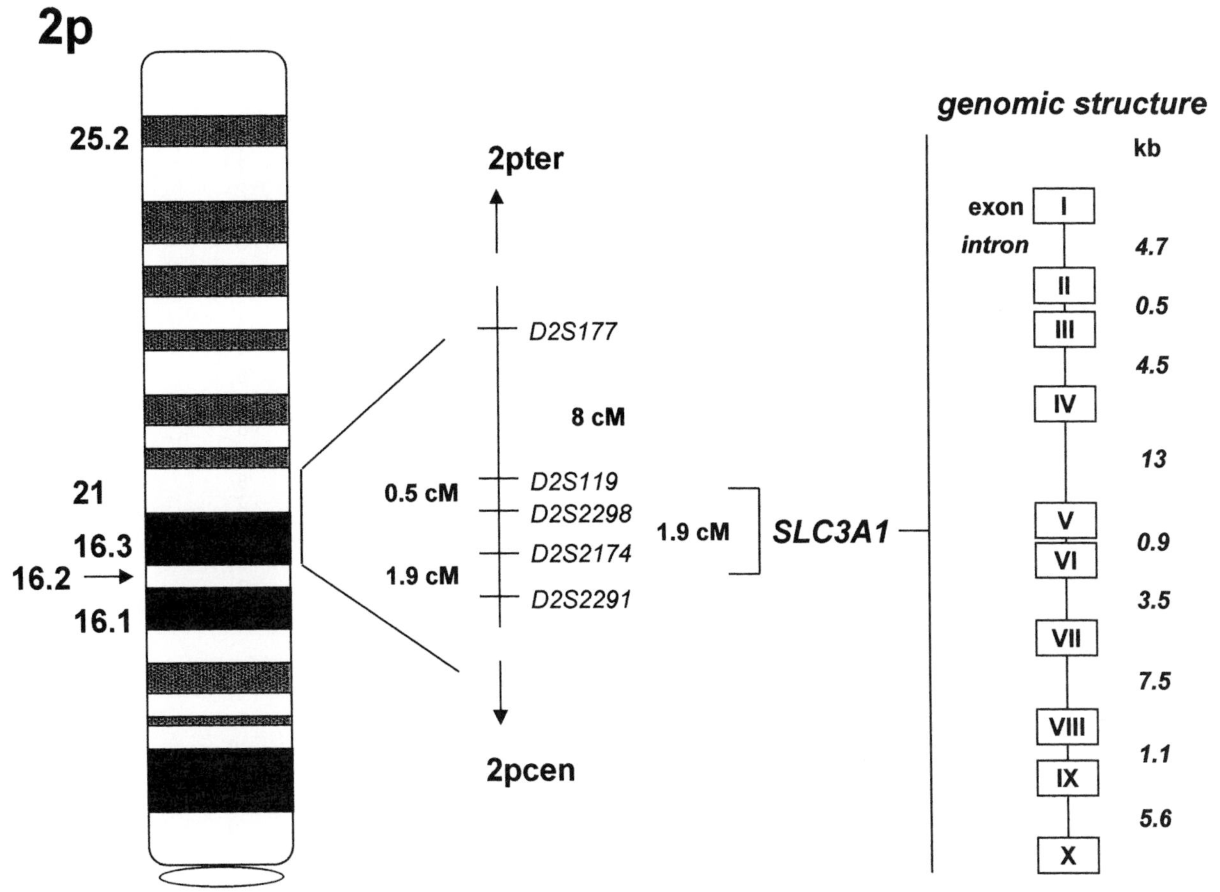

Fig. 191-9 Genetic regional map of the *SLC3A1* cystinuria locus and genomic structure of the *SLC3A1* gene. The short arm of the chromosome 2 with the cytogenetic G bands 2p16.3-p21 in which *SLC3A1* is located.[73,74,190] In the middle of the figure, markers in the vicinity of the *SLC3A1* gene with genetic distance (cM) are indicated. The *SLC3A1* gene is located centromeric to marker *D2S119* and telomeric to *D2S2291*. At the right side of the figure, the genomic structure of the *SLC3A1* gene is shown (not to scale and not oriented), with a length of about 45 kb. The sizes of the introns are taken from Purroy et al.[98]

(illegitimate transcripts) from transformed lymphocytes of cystinuria patients. After RT-PCR with primers designed from the known *SLC3A1* coding region, single-strand conformation polymorphism (SSCP) analysis was performed to identify abnormally migrating fragments. Abnormal bands were then sequenced to define mutations. Using this strategy, six missense mutations in the *SLC3A1* gene that cosegregate with the cystinuria phenotype were identified.[187] The most common mutation (M467T; substitution of methionine residue 467 for threonine) was analyzed functionally in oocytes; reduced $b^{o,+}$-like transport activity was observed. This observation provided the first direct proof that a defect in the *SLC3A1* gene (and thus the $b^{o,+}$-like system) was the cause of cystinuria.[187]

Chromosomal Localization of *SLC3A1* Gene

One case of a *de novo* balanced translocation (14;20) was associated with cystinuria and mental retardation, suggesting that a gene at one of the breakpoints (14q22 and 20q13) might be involved in cystinuria.[188] This suggestion was later discarded when the human *SLC3A1* gene was localized to chromosome 2q32.2-ter.[72] Using a panel of human/rodent somatic cell hybrids, full concordance of the *SLC3A1* gene for chromosome 2 was found. Additional experiments using DNA from hybrids retaining different regions of chromosome 2 assigned *SLC3A1* to 2 pter-p12.[187] Refined chromosomal localization of *SLC3A1* was accomplished by fluorescence in situ hybridization (FISH) that mapped *SLC3A1* to 2p16.3[74] or the adjacent G-band, 2p21[73,189] (Fig. 191-9). These data confirmed that the *SLC3A1* gene maps to the cystinuria locus on chromosome 2p.[67,190]

Genomic Organization of *SLC3A1*

The genomic organization of *SLC3A1* was independently established by two groups in 1996[98,142] and then by Endsley.[99] The gene spans nearly 45 kb on chromosome 2p16.3-p21 and is characterized by 10 exons (Fig. 191-9). The intron sizes range from 500 (intron 2) to 13,000 bp (intron 4). All exon/intron splice junctions conform to the eukaryotic 5′ donor 3′ acceptor consensus splice junctions GT/AG rule. The promotor region has been analyzed and the predicted TATA box, 98 bp upstream of the first coding ATG, was identified. By RNA protection assay the transcription initiation site was determined. One major protected product was observed 48 nucleotides from the ATG initiation codon.[142] Endsley and coworkers subsequently confirmed the details of *SLC3A1*.[99]

Mutations in the *SLC3A1* Gene

After the genomic structure was available, it was possible to investigate the entire *SLC3A1* coding region, all intron/exon boundaries, and some intronic sequences in diverse cystinuria populations. Eleven additional mutations (1 large deletion and 10 point mutations) were described among Italian families.[66,191] In one Italian family, a genomic deletion spans the second half of the *rBAT* gene, while the first part of the corresponding allele was affected by another deletion reported in Eastern Europeans.[192]

Table 191-2 Mutations Described in the *SLC3A1* Gene

Mutation	Nucleotide change	Number of chromosomes	Origin	Exon
Missense				
P128Q	383 C → A	1	Persian Jewish[192]	1
Y151N	451 T → A	1/54	Italian[191]	2
R181Q	542 G → A	1/33	Italian[187]	2
T216M*	647 C → T	1/16	French Canadian[198]	3
		2/54	Italian[191]	3
S217R*	649 A → C	1/16	French Canadian[198]	3
E268K*	802 G → A	1	Japanese[197]	4
R270L*	809 G → T	1/16	French Canadian[198]	4
T341A*	1021 A → G	1	Japanese[197]	6
R362C	1084 C → T	1/54	Italian[191]	6
R365W	1093 C → C	1/142	Italian[66]	6
S240C	1259 C → G	2	American[196]	7
R452W	1354 C → T	1/46	American[99]	8
G458E	1373 G → A	1	American[196]	8
Y461H	1381 T → C	1/46	American[99]	8
M467K*	1400 T → A	1/19	Italian[187,191]	8
M467T*	1400 T → C	6/19	Spanish[187,191]	8
		8/33	Italian[187,191]	
		1/16	French Canadian[193]	
		11/46	American[99]	
		12/56	American[194]	
V536G	1607 T → G	1	American[196]	9
Y582H	1744 T → C	1/142	Italian[66]	10
P615T	1848 C → A	1/19	Spanish[187]	10
G645A	1934 G → C	1	American[196]	10
F648S	1943 T → C	1/33	Italian[66]	10
T652R	1955 C → G	1/33	Italian[187]	10
L678P	2033 T → C	1/33	Italian[187]	10
Stop Mutations				
R270X	808 C → T	1	Jews[192]	4
		1/33	Italian[191]	4
		2/46	American[99]	4
E483X	1447 G → T	2/54	Italian[191]	8
		1/16	French Canadian[193]	8
Frameshift				
163 del C		3	American[196]	1
974 del GA		1/16	French Canadian[193]	5
1306 ins G		1	Jews[192]	7
1749 del A		1/142	Italian[66]	10
1810 del TG		2/16	French Canadian[198]	10
2922 ins T		2	American[196]	10
Splicing				
891+4 A → G		1/16	Israeli Arab[199]	4
1011A → G		1/16	French Canadian[198]	5
1500 +1 G → T		1/16	French Canadian[193]	8
		1/46	American[194]	
Deletions				
114-1306 del		1	Jews[192]	1-7
198-1575 del		1/16	French Canadian[193]	1-9
430-765 del		1	American[189]	1-3
(431-3)-463 del dup ins 468-474		2	American[196]	2
782-804 del		1	American[196]	4
3′ deletion		1/33	Italian[191]	4-10

Mutations in which functional analyses in oocytes had been performed. In the cases where we do not know the number of analyzed chromosomes, we have put the number of positive ones for a given mutation. Mutation nomenclature follows the guidelines by S.E. Antonarakis and the Nomenclature Working Group (*Hum Mut* **11**:1, 1998).

Two more large deletions have been found, one in a French Canadian chromosome and the other in an American chromosome[193–195] A very complex mutation has been found in two American chromosomes consisting of a 36 bp deletion (del C431-3 to T463 and a duplication insertion of 468T to 474A after nucleotide 474 (Table 191-2).[196]

Among the point mutations, one nonsense mutation (E483X) was simultaneously detected in two Italian patients[191] and in a

Table 191-3 Polymorphisms Described in the SLC3A1 Gene

	Frequencies	
Polymorphism/nucleotide change	Cystinurics	Normals
114A/C	20/94	27/100
	9/26*	16/66*
231T/A	12/102	0/160
1136 + 3delT	3/102	5/50
1332 + 7T/C	36/84*	22/88
1398C/T	1/102	0/100
1473C/T	1/102	0/102
1854A/G†	29/94	34/100
	9/26*	22/66*
2189C/T	29/94	34/100

* Data from the French Canadian population.[193] The rest of data obtained from Italian and Spanish populations.[66,191]
† The transport function of this polymorphism has been checked in oocytes, showing no affect on function.[198]

French Canadian patient.[193] The other nonsense mutation (R270X) detected so far has been described in the Druze[192], in Ashkenazi Jews,[192] in two Americans,[99] and in one Italian.[191] In general, the reported missense mutations generate important amino acid changes and affect residues that are highly conserved across species. Additional point mutations, either missense and nonsense, have been described in Persian Jews, Yemenite Jews, Japanese, North Americans, and East Europeans.[99,192,193,196,197] The first splice mutation (1500 + 1G → T) was described in French Canadians;[193] this mutation was later found in another American chromosome.[194] A second splice mutation (1011G → A) was found in a French Canadian chromosome,[198] and a third splice mutation (891 + 4A → G) was recently described in an Israeli Arab family.[199]

At this point, 40 different mutations and 9 polymorphisms have been described within the *SLC3A1* gene (see Tables 191-2 and 191-3). The M467T mutation is the commonest cystinuria allele (found on 38 different chromosomes to date; Table 191-2). Only four other mutated alleles—R270X, E483X, T216M, and 1550 + 1G → T—were distributed worldwide (Table 191-2). Thus, the majority of *SLC3A1* mutations are population specific, suggesting that they have arisen recently or reflect founder effects within genetically isolated groups.

Pathogenicity of *SLC3A1* Mutations

To establish the pathogenicity of missense *SLC3A1* mutations, the aberrant sequences were cloned into plasmid vectors to examine the effect on amino acid transport in the oocyte expression system. Defective transport was shown in seven cystinuria-specific *SLC3A1* missense mutations.[187,197,198,200] Experimental studies were carried out first for the M467T mutation, the most common cystinuric allele, and a less common mutation, M467K, affecting the same amino acid. Initial functional analysis of M467T revealed approximately 20 percent residual transport activity when assayed 2 days after injection of the cRNA.[187] Interestingly, the level of residual function for both mutations depended on the amount of cRNA injected and the timing of the transport assay after injection. Thus, if large amounts of cRNA are injected (>0.5 ng/oocyte) and the transport assay is delayed 6 days, M467T eventually achieves 100 percent of wild-type transport activity.[200] In contrast to wild-type transport activity, M467T and M467K express unique proteins that remain endoglycosidase H sensitive, suggesting a prolonged transit through the endoplasmic reticulum. This results in a very low proportion of the mutant proteins arriving at the oocyte plasma membrane, as demonstrated by biotin surface labeling.[200] However, the mutant protein that does arrive is functional, and expresses system $b^{o,+}$-like activity without change in the apparent affinity of its substrates.[200] Full recovery of M467T-associated transport activity occurs with only 10 percent of the mutated protein at the plasma membrane as compared to the wild-type.[200] This observation is compatible with the view that an endogenous oocyte protein complexes with *SLC3A1* to produce the functional $b^{o,+}$-like transporter; in the oocyte, availability of the *SLC3A1* partner is limited, so that the maximal number of functional units are achieved when only 10 percent of the wild-type protein arrives at the membrane surface. Additional *SLC3A1* mutations have been tested in the oocyte expression system. Miyamoto and coworkers[197] assayed two *SLC3A1* mutations: E268K and T314A. The injection of these cRNAs produced approximately 54 percent and 62 percent of control transport activity, respectively. Coinjection of both mutated cRNAs into oocytes gave only 28 percent of control transport, suggesting interaction between the two mutant proteins. A trafficking defect similar to M467T was suggested by immunofluorescence analysis.

Very recently, Saadi and coworkers expressed three additional missense mutations (T216M, S217R, and R270L) in oocytes.[198] Expression analysis of the T216M mutant showed reduced activity (25 percent of control) at 24 h (this mutation eliminates the first putative *N*-glycosylation site of rBAT). This value was higher after 4 days of expression (75 percent of control). A similar phenomenon was observed for the S217R mutation. This phenomenon suggests another variant of the trafficking defects seen with the M467T, M467K, T216M, and S217R mutants. The R270L mutation retains only 7 percent of control transport activity.[198]

It is intriguing that the majority of dysfunctional *SLC3A1* point mutations (M467T, M467K, E268K, T314A, T216M, and S217R) seem to involve a defect in rBAT trafficking to the oocyte plasma membrane. Because transport activity of the $b^{o,+}$-like system involves a complex between rBAT and $b^{o,+}$AT disulfide-linked "light" (30- to 40-kDa) subunit, the trafficking defect in these six rBAT mutations may be due to improper interactions with the "light subunit" during transport to the oocyte membrane. This suspected defect needs demonstration in affected tissue from cystinuria patients.

Genotype-Phenotype Correlations

To ascertain whether certain *SLC3A1* mutations correlate with mild versus severe forms of type I/I cystinuria, Rizzoni and coworkers[201] and Rousaud (personal communication) examined genotype/phenotype correlations in a cohort of cystinuria families. To some extent, the families having the largest number of stones, stone relapses, and medical interventions per year were those families bearing STOP codon (presumably null) mutations. Some families with a milder clinical picture carried *SLC3A1* point mutations. However, severity among sibs from one family varied considerably, suggesting that other determinants of urolithiasis exert powerful influence over the final clinical impact of *SLC3A1* mutations. Because the number of families analyzed thus far is small, additional work is needed.

Genetic Heterogeneity in Cystinuria

In 1994, the first *SLC3A1* mutations were reported, clearly establishing that it was a cystinuria gene.[187] Clinical and physiological evidence, however, had long suggested that cystinuria might be heterogeneous: Harris had proposed at least two forms of cystinuria (completely recessive and incompletely recessive) based on the level of cystine excretion in obligate heterozygotes.[61] Oral cystine-loading tests suggested that in the completely recessive (type I/I) form of cystinuria, no cystine absorption was present, while in the incompletely recessive form, the intestinal defect was often quite modest.[25] Although the largest fraction of renal reabsorption of cystine seems to occur in the S1-S2 segments of the nephron, rBAT is expressed primarily in the pars recta (S3 segment).[168] Finally, patients who inherit one completely recessive and one incompletely recessive cystinuria gene from their parents were found to excrete lower levels of

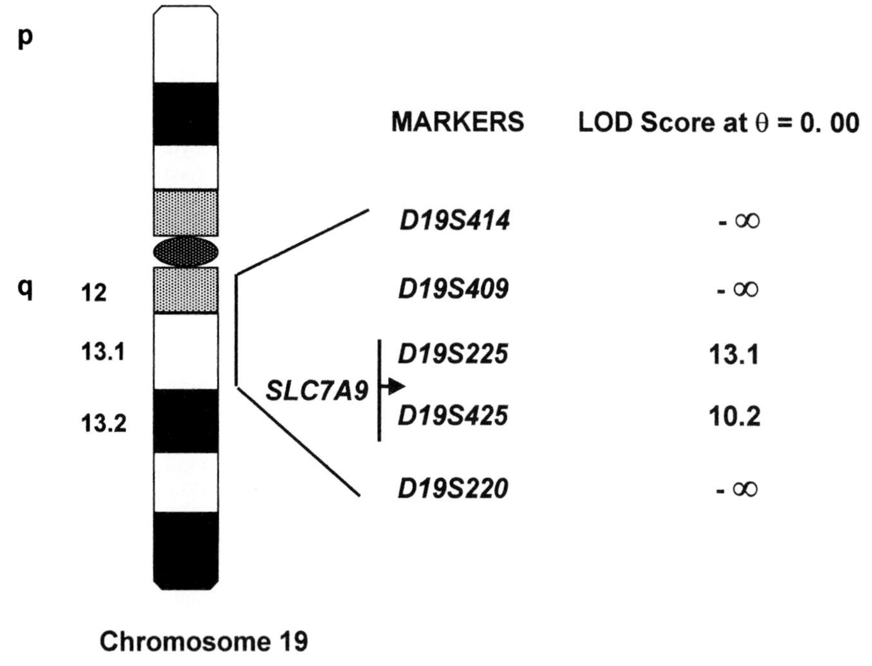

Fig. 191-10 19q cystinuria locus. Pairwise LOD scores. At the left, chromosome 19 with the G bands in which the analyzed markers are located. At the right side of the figure, LOD score data demonstrating that the gene is between markers *D19S409* and *D19S220*. Data taken from Bisceglia et al.[75]

cystine than children with two fully recessive parents, a finding not easily explained by allelic mutations at a single cystinuria locus.[65]

In 1995, two independent studies[66,67] demonstrated clear evidence of genetic heterogeneity in cystinuria. The first data arose from analysis of *SLC3A1* mutations and the corresponding cystinuria phenotypes; the second was a linkage study with markers of chromosome 2p. In the first instance, it became apparent that all known mutant *SLC3A1* alleles were associated only with the fully recessive urinary phenotype. Conversely, an *SLC3A1* mutation was never found in association with the incompletely recessive urinary phenotype[66]. In the second study, linkage data obtained on 22 Italian and Spanish families with the marker *D2S119*, demonstrated that type I/I families showed homogeneous linkage to *SLC3A1*, whereas non-Type I/I families were not linked.[67] Genetic heterogeneity has been also confirmed in the Libyan Jewish population.[76]

The identification of two genetic loci for cystinuria might explain some aspects of proximal tubular transport physiology and data concerning the tissue specificity of rBAT expression. Classical studies with isolated, microperfused segments of the proximal tubule indicate that cystine is transported via a low-affinity system located in the pars convoluta (S1 and S2 segments) and a high-affinity system located in the pars recta (segment S3).[122,126] The early segments of the proximal tubule are believed to be responsible for up to 90 percent of L-cystine resorption, whereas rBAT, located in the S3-segment,[168] is apparently responsible only for the remaining 10 percent of the filtrate. Because many patients bearing two mutant *SLC3A1* alleles excrete more than 100 percent of the filtered load, the S3 segment transporter may also be responsible for a substantial load of cystine delivered to that site via tubular secretion or back-leak. Because it represents the final site of cystine reabsorption, other carriers cannot compensate for dysfunction of the rBAT system. Until the protein product of the 19q cystinuria locus gene is identified, we will not know whether it functions as part of the low-affinity transporter in S1 and S2 segments, as part of the rBAT-associated system in the S3 segment, or in some other unidentified transporter.

Non-Type I/I Cystinuria: The Chromosome 19q locus

To identify non-*SLC3A1* cystinuria loci, a genome-wide search using panels of highly informative microsatellite markers was performed independently by two groups. Each reported, by linkage analysis, a second cystinuria locus on the long arm of chromosome 19 (19q13.1)[75,76] (Fig. 191-10). In the Jewish population, LOD scores were significant, with no recombinant events, using markers *D19S422* and *D19S225* (separated by 8 cM). Marker *D19S225* alone gave significant linkage disequilibrium.[76] The other study was done using the Italian and Spanish families transmitting a type III cystinuria gene, previously excluded from linkage with *SLC3A1*.[67] Pairwise linkage analysis showed a maximum LOD score of 9.65 with the marker *D19S225* at a recombination frequency of 0.0 (Fig. 191-10). A few families transmitting cystinuria genes associated with very high (stone-forming range) cystine excretion in obligate heterozygotes (type II/N) were analyzed separately; significant positive LOD scores with 19q locus markers were obtained.[75] Additional evidence for co-localization of type II and type III alleles at the 19q locus was generated with the HOMOG program to identify genetic homogeneity. However, because the number of patients with type II cystinuria was small, additional studies will be needed for definitive confirmation that it is allelic with type III.

Search for the Gene Responsible for Non-Type I/I Cystinuria

The region of chromosome 19q containing the non-Type I/I cystinuria locus was contained in an available YAC contig.[202] Among the several genes mapped to this region there were initially no good candidate genes for the disease. Polymorphic microsatellite markers used to characterize the haplotype of type III cystinuria alleles among Libyan Jews were useful for confirming the presence of an historical founder effect in this population and identifying recombinants that narrowed the region to a 1.8 Mb on chromosome 19q13.1 between markers *D195430* and *D195874*.[203] The region was further refined by analysis of key recombination events in a heterogeneous group of non-type I cystinuria families. These data placed the gene in an interval flanked by the markers *C13* and *D195587*, which are about 2.8 Mb apart.[204] Together this to studies located the non-type I cystinuria gene between markers *C13* and *D195874*.

Identification of *SLC7A9* as a cystinuria non-Type I/I gene: Once *SLC7A9* was identified, it became an excellent candidate for non-type I/I cystinuria. Co-transfection of *SLC7A9* ($b^{o,+}$AT as an alias for the protein) with rBAT in COS cells brings rBAT to the

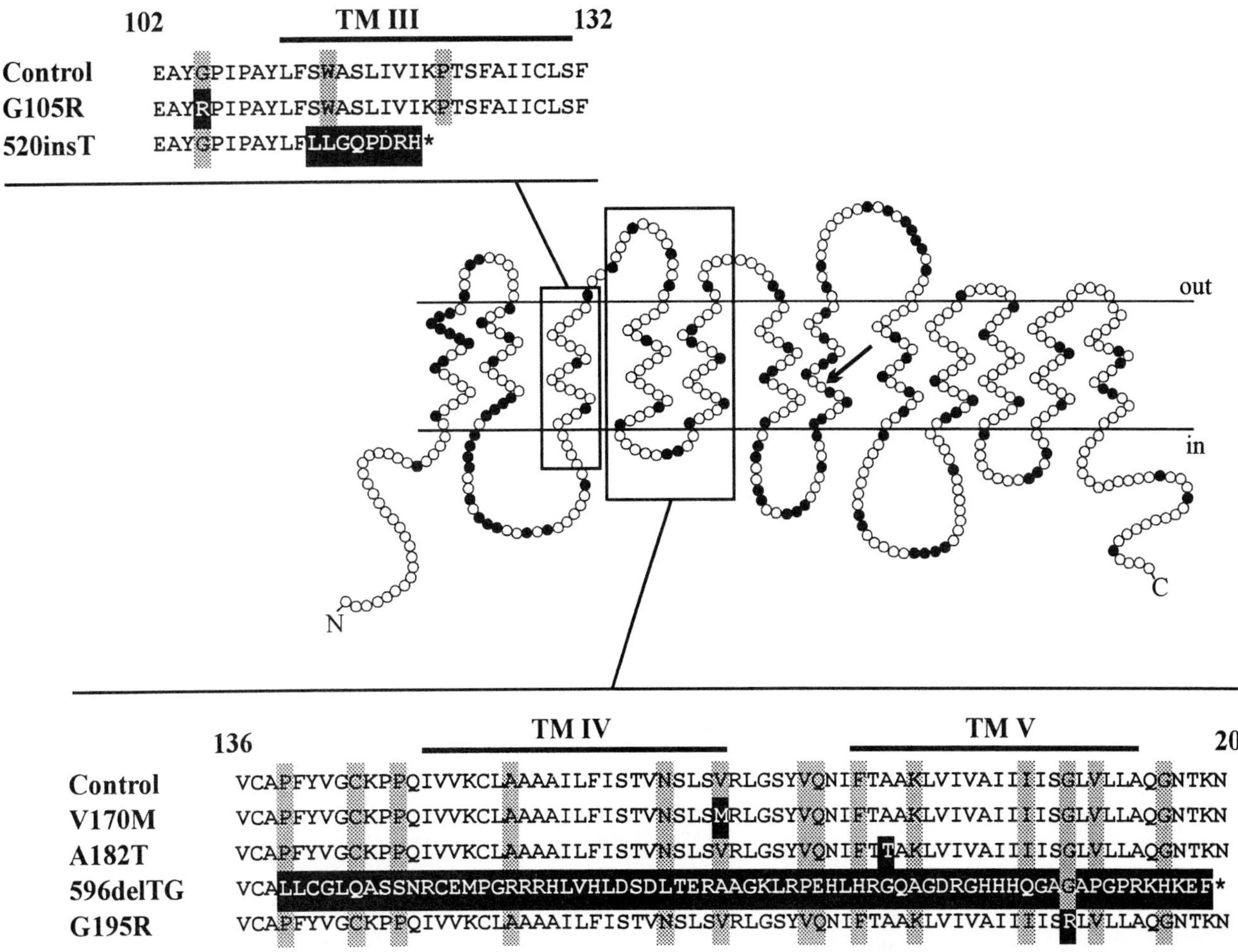

Fig. 191-11 Schematic representation of the *SLC7A9* cystinuria-specific mutations identified in the b$^{o,+}$AT amino acid transporter. Membrane topology prediction algorithms suggest that b$^{o,+}$AT contains 12 transmembrane domains with the N- and C-termini located intracellularly. The mutations found are located in the part of the protein between transmembrane (TM) III and VII. Grey background denotes amino acid residues conserved in the human members of the family. White characters on black background denote sequence alterations versus wild-type sequence. TM, putative transmembrane domain. Amino acid residues are indicated above the alignments. The missense mutations G105R, V170M (The Libyan Jewish mutation) and G159R change residues that are highly conserved in this family of amino acid transporters. The arrow in TMVII indicates the amino acid residue altered in mutation G259R. Control, wild-type sequence, premature STOP codon. (*Adapted from Feliubadaló et al.*[77] *Used by permission*)

plasma membrane and results in the expression of amino acid uptake activity.[77] Similarly to rBAT, *SLC7A9* is expressed in kidney, small intestine, liver and placenta. These data suggested that *SLC7A9* might encode the light subunit of rBAT (b$^{o,+}$AT).[77]

Seven different mutations were found in the *SCL7A9* gene of non-Type I cystinuria families from different populations (Italy, Spain, North America and Israel). These mutations accounted for 48 chromosomes out a total of the 143 independent ones analyzed (Fig. 191-11). Sequencing of the whole coding region of *SLC7A9* in three homozygous Libyan Jews revealed a substitution c693G → A which results in a change of a valine at position 170 to methionine (V170M). This is the mutation carried on the Libyan Jewish ancestral chromosome. Four additional missense mutations (G105R, A182T, G195R and G259R) and two frameshift (520insT and 596delTG) have been identified. Mutations G105R, 520insT and 596delTG were found in American patients. The G105R and the other mutations were found in Spanish and Italian chromosomes (Fig. 191-11). To date, the most frequent mutation in caucasians is G105R.[77]

The two frameshift mutations of *SCL7A9* lead to a truncated b$^{o,+}$AT protein, which lacks the last three-quarters of the molecule. Among the missense mutations, the Libyan Jewish V170M was studied *in vitro* by analyzing sodium-independent uptake of L-arginine after transient cotransfection of rBAT and wild type b$^{o,+}$AT or rBAT and V170M b$^{o,+}$AT in COS cells. V170M abolished the L-arginine uptake associated with the co-transfection of rBAT. These results demonstrated that mutations in *SLC7A9* causes cystinuria non-Type I, and strongly suggest that b$^{o,+}$AT is the light subunit of rBAT.[77]

Clinical Phenotype of non-Type I/I Cystinuria

Among Libyan Jews, the most common form of cystinuria is inherited from parents (Type III/N heterozygotes) who each excrete elevated levels of cystine and dibasic amino acids.[205] The risk of nephrolithiasis is high among adults; clinical features in children have not yet been systematically studied. Because this population is somewhat isolated genetically, it is likely that one mutation accounts for a large portion of the cases.[76] Nevertheless, the level of cystine excretion and the rate of nephrolithiasis vary widely, bespeaking multigenic modifiers of stone formation.

In European and North American populations, a "mixed type" of cystinuria genes has been identified.[67,198] In these families, one parent excretes cystine and dibasic amino acids in the normal range (Type I/N, fully recessive heterozygotes); in the other parent, excretion of cystine and dibasic amino acids is moderately elevated (Type III/N, incompletely recessive heterozygotes). In the first study by Calonge and coworkers,[67] some of these were excluded from linkage to the *SLC3A1* locus and showed no

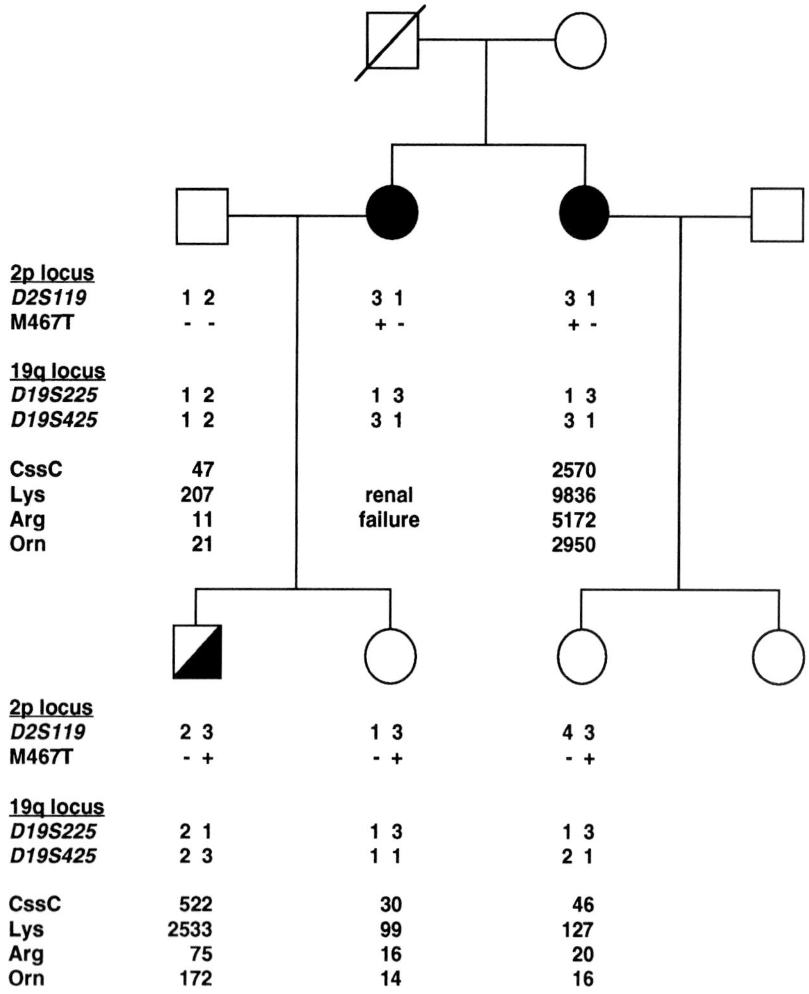

Fig. 191-12 Pedigree of a mixed Type (I/III) cystinuria family. Squares denote males, circles denote females. White symbols denote normal individuals (N/N) with a silent urinary phenotype. Black symbols denote the compound heterozygote individuals (i.e., III/I). Number under individual symbols represent the haplotypes given by these markers: *D2S119* and the *SLC3A1* M467T mutation (+, presence of the mutation; –, absence of the mutation) for the rBAT locus (Type I), and *D19S225* and *D19S425* for the 19q cystinuria locus (Type III). Amino acid excretion values (μmol/g of creatinine) for cystine (CssC), arginine (Arg), lysine (lys), and ornithine (Orn) in the family members are displayed below. Range of values for silent carriers are (μmol/g of creatinine): CssC (20 to 176), Lys (38 to 445); Arg (10 to 55) and Orn (8 to 48) (data taken from Calonge et al.[67]). The two affected sisters in this family carry the M467T mutation; both have passed it on to their progeny. In the third generation, the son (black and white symbol) of one sister shows excretion values higher than normal, suggesting that he has inherited the 19q haplotype corresponding to a mutated allele. Then, there is either an interaction between alleles on chromosome 2 and alleles on chromosome 19, which gives intermediate cystinuria phenotype, or a second unidentified *SLC3A1* mutation has been transmitted along with M467T and the 19q locus mutation. In the latter case, it would not be necessary to postulate an interaction between *SLC3A1* and the *SLC7A9* locus gene products.

cosegregation between the *SLC3A1* locus and either Type I or Type III cystinuria. Saadi et al.[198] screened French Canadian families for *SLC3A1* mutations and were able to identify 15 mutations of 16 Type I alleles. However, among probands with the "mixed type" of cystinuria, only one *SLC3A1* mutation among nine Type I alleles was detected.[198] These observations suggest that non-*SLC3A1* genes could also be responsible for the fully recessive cystinuria Type I. If so, it will be interesting to learn whether these recessive cystinuria genes are simply "mild" genetic variants at the 19q locus. Conceivably, there are two classes of 19q mutants that can interact to cause the mixed type of cystinuria.

It is still an open question as to whether there are examples of digenic cystinuria. A few cases have been identified in which a Type III (incompletely recessive) allele from one parent has combined with a Type I (fully recessive) mutant *SLC3A1* allele from the other parent to produce the mixed type of cystinuria.[66] In some studies,[64,65] patients with the mixed type of cystinuria were found to have somewhat lower amino acid excretion than Type I/I patients. However, this difference in mean cystine excretion between groups is not likely due to digenic complementation, because most of these subjects are now known to lack *SLC3A1* mutations. In one Spanish family with two proven M467T *SLC3A1* heterozygotes, one has a son who excretes cystine in the moderately elevated range phenotype and bears the M467T mutation (Fig. 191-12). Recombination has been excluded for markers at the 19q13.1 locus. Although this is an isolated case, it is possible that the M467T *SLC3A1* mutation may interact with certain mutant Type III mutant 19q alleles to produce mild cystinuria. This hypothesis is currently tested by analyzing the mutations in the *SLC7A9* in those cases.

CURRENT APPROACH TO CLASSIFICATION OF CYSTINURIA STONE FORMERS

Although the relevant gene at 19q (*SLC7A9*) has been isolated, the molecular basis of incompletely recessive cystinuria is not entirely clear, and any system to classify all the subtypes of cystinuria must remain tentative. Nevertheless, studies of the *SLC3A1* gene in combination with clinical phenotype have partially clarified the issues and suggest that patients who consistently excrete cystine (and the dibasic amino acids) in the stone-forming range (>1,000 μmol cystine/g creatinine) can be grouped as follows (Table 191-4):

Type I/I: These patients inherit two fully recessive SLC3A1 mutations from their heterozygous parents; heterozygotes excrete < 100 μmol cystine/g creatinine in the urine. Jejunal uptake of cystine and dibasic amino acids is absent and there is no plasma response to an oral cystine load. Fractional excretion of cystine is very high, often exceeding 100 percent of the filtered load, and the risk of nephrolithiasis in the first decade of life is high.

Type III/III: These patients inherit two incompletely recessive cystinuria genes from their parents. They have two mutations in the SLC7A9 gene.[77] Adults with this form of cystinuria excrete high levels of cystine and produce recurrent stones. The gene is especially common in Libyan Jews. Heterozygotes usually excrete cystine below the stone-forming range. Intestinal absorption of cystine and dibasic amino acids appears to be reduced but is not entirely absent. Cystine uptake by jejunal biopsy tissue varies from very low to the low-normal range. The

Table 191-4 Current Knowledge of the Molecular Basis of Cystinuria and Classification of Cystinuria Stone Formers

Cystine stone formers	Cystine hyperexcretion	Risk of calculi onset	Risk of calculi number	Chromosome	Gene	Defective amino acid transporter
Type I/I	high	early	high	2p16.3-p21	*SLC3A1* (rBAT)	Brush-border system $b^{o,+}$-like
Type I/III	moderate	late	medium	19q13.1	*SLC7A9* ($b^{o,+}$AT)	,,
Type III/III	high	?	high	19q13.1	*SLC7A9* ($b^{o,+}$AT)	,,
Type II/II	high	?	high	19q13.1	*SLC7A9* ($b^{o,+}$AT)	,,
Type II/N	low-moderate	late	low	19q13.1	*SLC7A9* ($b^{o,+}$AT)	,,

The data compiled here suggest that cystinuria is caused by a defect in the brush border system $b^{o,+}$-like amino acid transporter in kidney and intestine, due to mutations in any of the two subunits (heavy chain rBAT; *SLC3A1* gene and light subunit $b^{o,+}$AT; *SLC7A9* gene) of the transporter. The non-Type I cystinuria gene, *SLC7A9*, might be responsible for all cases of this type of cystinuria, but this has not yet been demonstrated. Moreover in some cases of mixed-type cystinuria *SLC7A9* is responsible of the Type I phenotype. Thus, most Type I/III patients inherit the recessive and the incompletely recessive allele at the 19q locus, but some of them inherit a fully recessive mutant rBAT allele from one parent and an incompletely recessive non-rBAT allele (19 q locus) from the other parent.

plasma response to oral cystine loading was near normal in two of Rosenberg's patients, but the plasma response to oral lysine loading was clearly defective in a patient with two SLC7A9 mutations studied by de Sanctis and Ponzone (personal communication).

Mixed Type I/III(A): These patients inherit one fully recessive SLC7A9 gene from one parent and one incompletely recessive SLC7A9 gene from the other parent.[77] The recessive allele does not involve an SLC3A1 mutation. Urinary excretion of cystine is in the stone-forming range, but is slightly lower than in patients bearing two SLC3A1 mutations; the risk of nephrolithiasis in the first decade of life is relatively low. Presumably the intestinal absorption of cystine and dibasic amino acids is affected to some extent but no oral loading studies have yet been performed.

Mixed Type I/III (B): These patients inherit a fully recessive mutant SLC3A1 gene from one parent and an incompletely recessive SLC7A9 gene from the other parent. Urinary cystine excretion is in the stone-forming range, but is slightly less than for SLC3A1 homozygotes; the risk of nephrolithiasis in the first decade of life is low. Only a small number of such patients have been identified thus far and intestinal uptake has not been defined.

Type II/II: A rare type of cystinuria. These patients inherit two incompletely recessive cystinuria genes from their parents, most probably within the 19q locus. Jejunal biopsy tissue from these patients show no accumulation of lysine and markedly reduced accumulation of cystine. The only patient studied by Rosenberg's group showed no plasma cystine elevation in response to oral cystine loading. These patients may simply represent the extreme of the phenotypic range for Type III cystinuria: SLC7A9 mutations have been reported in patients who can be classified as Type II/II on the basis of especially high levels of cystinuria in each heterozygous parent.[77]

Heterozygous Stone-Formers: These patients are heterozygous for a non-SLC3A1 gene but excrete cystine in the stone-forming range at levels comparable to one of their parents. Occasional families have been identified where nephrolithiasis is present in more than one generation, so that the mutant cystinuria gene is clinically autosomal dominant. Linkage analysis suggests a mutant allele at the 19q locus but SLC7A9 mutations in such patients have not yet been demonstrated.

ANIMAL MODELS

Several possible animal models of cystinuria have been identified.[206–209] Canine cystinuria represents a more useful model. Canine cystinuria was described as early as 1823, but no systematic observations were made until the studies from Brand and Cahill in Irish terriers.[210] However, genetic transmission of cystinuria corresponded to a sex-linked inheritance pattern, and the exact amino acid excretion profile was not clear. Isolated cystinuria, cystinuria plus lysinuria, and a full pattern of cystine and dibasic aminoaciduria have been reported.[211–213] Cystinuria has also been found in the maned wolf of Brazil.[214] Eighty percent of the wolves are affected. Amino acid clearance studies in five affected wolves revealed variable cystine reabsorptive defects.

At present, the best animal model of cystinuria is that of the Newfoundland dog. Two families including 11 dogs were studied clinically. Affected dogs persistently excreted an excessive amount of cystine >500 μmol/g of creatinine (normal value 54 ± 38 μmol/g creatinine). Urinary excretion of ornithine, lysine, and arginine was also high. Obligate heterozygotes did not have clinical signs.[215] These data fit perfectly with the Type I/I cystinuria. Researchers have recently isolated and characterized the canine *rBAT* gene and looked for mutations. A STOP codon in exon 2 has been identified. They have also demonstrated a decrease of rBAT mRNA in kidney of affected dogs. (Paula Henthorn, personal communication.)

PERSPECTIVE

Although the two major cystinuria genes have been found several questions remain a) Is *SLC7A9* the only non-rBAT cystinuria gene? b) What is the genetic basis for the mixed Type I/III of cystinuria? c) Is $b^{o,+}$AT indeed the light subunit of rBAT and how do these two molecules interact to achieve cystine reabsorption? Another important point will be to clarify why mutations of *SLC3A1* are recessive whereas mutations in *SLC7A9* are incompletely recessive. One possiblity is that the active $b^{o,+}$ transporter may be constituted by more than one pair of rBAT and $b^{o,+}$AT subunits. In that case certain *SLC7A9* mutations might exert a dominant negative effect even if the multimer contains some wildtype subunits as well.[154] Another possibility is that the light subunit of rBAT ($b^{o,+}$AT) might associate with a protein other than rBAT in different proximal tubular segments. Bulk renal cystine reabsorption occurs in the proximal convoluted tubule via a low-affinity system not yet identified at the molecular level.[123] If *SLC7A9* also participates in this transport system, a partial defect in this major renal reabsorption mechanism would explain the incompletely recessive phenotype of non-Type I cystinuria.

In the future, it will be important to develop animal models which allow study pathophysiology and therapy of cystinuria. This may involve careful characterization of the spontaneous animal models mentioned above as well as "Knockout" mice for *SLC3A1* and *SLC7A9*. No major advances in the therapy of cystinuria have occurred since D-penicillamine and α-mercaptopropionylglycine were introduced. Animal models should help with design and testing of agents to modify excessive cystine excretion or inhibit stone formation.

Although *SLC3A1* expression increases during kidney development, nothing is known about how this gene and *SLC7A9* are regulated; little is known about how the $b^{o,+}$ transporter fits in the overall scheme of amino acid reabsorption in the proximal tubule. Knowledge of these complex mechanisms might help develop therapeutic strategies for cystinuria patients with partial defects in intracellular *SLC3A1* trafficking and might clarify diagnostic issues during infancy.

Since its original description in 1810, cystinuria has served as the prototype of inherited renal transport disorders. The recent discovery of *SLC3A1* and *SLC7A9* may herald the exciting prospect of gene therapy for one of the original "inborn errors of metabolism."

REFERENCES

1. Wollaston WH: On cystic oxide, a new species of urinary calculus. *Philos Trans R Soc Lond B Biol Sci* **100**:233, 1810.
2. Marcet A: *An essay on the Chemical History and Medical Treatment of Calculous Disorders*. London, Longman, Hurst, Rees, Orme and Brown, 1817, pp 79–88.
3. Berzelius D: Calculs urinaires. *Trait Chem* **7**:424, 1833.
4. Thaulow CJ: Sur la composition de la cystine. *J Pharm* **27**:221, 1838.
5. Neuberg C: Uber cysteine. I. *Berichte der Deutschen Chemischen Gesellschaft* **35**:3161, 1902.
6. Friedman E: Der kreislauf des schwefels in der organischen. *Natur Ergebn Physiol* **1**:15, 1902.
7. Prout W: Traite de la gravelle. Paris, , 1823, p 278.
8. Stromeyer L: Oxide cystique. *Ann Chim et Phys* **27**:221, 1824.
9. Toel F: Beobachtungen uber Cystinebildung. *Ann Chem Pharm* **96**:247, 1855.
10. Garrod AE: Inborn errors of metabolism. (Lecture I, p 1; Lecture II, p 73; Lecture III, p 142, Lecture IV, p 214.) *Lancet* 2, 1908.
11. Yeh HL, Frankl W, Dunn MS, Parker P, Hughes B, Gyorgy P: The urinary excretion of amino acids by a cystinuric subject. *Am J Med Sci* **214**:507, 1947.
12. Stein WH: Excretion of amino acids in cystinuria. *Proc Soc Exp Biol Med* **78**:705, 1951.
13. Dent CE, Rose GA: Amino acid metabolism in cystinuria. *QJM* **20**:205, 1951.
14. Brand E, Cahill GF: Further studies on metabolism of sulfur compounds in cystinuria. *Proc Soc Exp Biol Med* **31**:1247, 1934.
15. Dent CE, Senior B, Walshe JM: The pathogenesis of cystinuria. II. Polarographic studies of the metabolism of sulphur-containing amino acids. *J Clin Invest* **33**:1216, 1954.
16. London DR, Foley TH: Cystine metabolism in cystinuria. *Clin Sci* **29**:129, 1965.
17. Milne MD, Asatoor AM, Edwards KDG, Loughridge LW: The intestinal absorption defect in cystinuria. *Gut* **2**:323, 1961.
18. Rosenberg LE, Durant JL, Holland IM: Intestinal absorption and renal excretion of cystine and cysteine in cystinuria. *N Engl J Med* **273**:1239, 1965.
19. Silk DBA, Perrett D, Stephens AD, Clark ML, Scowen EF: Intestinal absorption of cystine and cysteine in normal human subjects and patients with cystinuria. *Clin Sci Mol Med* **47**:393, 1974.
20. Asatoor AM, Lacey BW, London DR, Milne MD: Amino acid metabolism in cystinuria. *Clin Sci* **23**:285, 1962.
21. Von Udransky L, Baumann E: Uber das vorkommen von Diaminen, sogenannten Ptomainen, bei Cystinurie. *Z Physiol Chem* **13**:562, 1899.
22. Thier S, Fox M, Segal S, Rosenberg LE. Cystinuria: In vitro demonstration of an intestinal transport defect. *Science* **143**:482, 1964.
23. Fox M, Thier S, Rosenberg LE, Kiser W, Segal S: Evidence against a single renal transport defect in cystinuria. *N Engl J Med* **270**:556, 1964.
24. McCarthy CF, Borland JL, Lynch HJ, Owen EE, Tyor MPL: Defective uptake of basic amino acids and L-cystine by intestinal mucosa of patients with cystinuria. *J Clin Invest* **43**:15, 1964.
25. Rosenberg LE, Downing S, Durant JL, Segal S: Cystinuria: Biochemical evidence for three genetically distinct diseases. *J Clin Invest* **45**:365, 1966.
26. Hellier MD, Holdsworth CD, Perrett D: Dibasic amino acid absorption in man. *Gastroenterology* **65**:613, 1973.
27. Hellier MD, Perrett D, Holdsworth CD: Dipeptide absorption in cystinuria. *BMJ* 4:782, 1970.
28. Mawer GE, Nixon E: The net absorption of amino acid constituents of a protein meal in normal and cystinuric subjects. *Clin Sci* **36**:463, 1969.
29. Milne MD: Amino acid metabolism in cystinuria. *Proc Biochem Soc* **122**:9P, 1971.
30. Hellier MD, Perrett D, Holdsworth CD, Thirumalai C: Absorption of dipeptides in normal and cystinuric subjects. *Gut* **12**:496, 1971.
31. Asatoor AM, Harrison RDW, Milne MD, Prosser DI: Intestinal absorption of an arginine-containing peptide in cystinuria. *Gut* **13**:95, 1972.
32. Daniel, H: Function and molecular structure of brush-border membrane peptide/H^+ symporters. *J Membr Biol* **154**:197, 1996.
33. Levy HL: Genetic screening, in Harris H, Hirschorn K (eds): *Advances in Human Genetics*, vol. 4. New York, Plenum, 1973, p 1.
34. Weinberger A, Sperling O, Rabinovitch M, Brosh S Adam A, de Vries A: High frequency of cystinuria among Jews of Libyan origin. *Hum Hered* **24**:568, 1974.
35. Turner B, Brown DA: Amino acid excretion in infancy and early childhood: A survey of 200,000 infants. *Med J Aust* **1**:62, 1972.
36. Scriver CR, Clow CL, Reade T, Goodyer P, Auray-Blais C, Giguere R, Lemieux B: Ontogeny modifies expression of cystinuria genes: Implications for counselling. *J Pediatr* **106**:411, 1985.
37. Levy HL, Shih VE, Madigan PM: Massachusetts metabolic disorders screening program. I. Technics, and results of urine screening. *Pediatrics* **49**:825, 1972.
38. Bostrom H, Hambraeus L: Cystinuria in Sweden. VII. Clinical, histopathological and medical-social aspects of the disease. *Acta Med Scand Suppl* **411**:1, 1964.
39. Crawhall JC, Scowen EF, Thompson CJ, Watts RWE: The renal clearance of amino acids in cystinuria. *J Clin Invest* **46**:1162, 1962.
40. Lewis HB: The incidence of cystinuria in healthy young men and women. *Ann Int Med* **6**:183, 1932.
41. Frimpter GW: Cystinuria: Metabolism of the disulfide of cysteine and homocysteine. *J Clin Invest* **42**:1956, 1963.
42. Cox BD, Cameron JC: Homoarginine in cystinuria. *Clin Sci Molec Med* **46**:173, 1974.
43. Milne MD, London DR, Asatoor AM: Citrullinuria in cases of cystinuria. *Lancet* **2**:49, 1962.
44. King JS Jr, Wainer A: Cystinuria with hyperuricemia and methioninuria: Biochemical study of a case. *Am J Med* **43**:125, 1967.
45. Frimpter GW: Cystathioninuria in a patient with cystinuria. *Am J Med* **46**:832, 1969.
46. Brodhehl J: Renal hyperaminoaciduria, in Edelman CM (ed): *Pediatric Kidney Disease*, 2nd ed. Boston, Little, Brown, 1992, p 1811.
47. Brodehl J, Gellissen K, Kowalewski S: Isolated cystinuria (without lysine-ornithine-argininuria) in a family with hypocalcemia tetany. *Klin Wochenschr* **45**:38, 1967.
48. Blom W, Huijmans J: Differential diagnosis of (inherited) amino acid metabolism or transport disorders. *Sci Tools* **332**:10, 1985.
49. Stephens AD, Perrett D: Cystinuria: A new genetic variant. *Clin Sci Mol Med* **5**:27, 1976.
50. Whelan DT, Scriver CR: Hyperdibasic aminoaciduria: An inherited disorder of amino acid transport. *Pediatr Res* **2**:525, 1968.
51. Oyangi K, Miura R, Yamanoughi T: Congenital lysinuria: A new inherited transport disorder of dibasic amino acids. *J Pediatr* **77**:259, 1970.
52. Simell O, Perheentupa J: Renal handling of diamino acids in lysinuria protein intolerance. *J Clin Invest* **54**:9, 1974.
53. Simell O, et al.: Lysinuric protein intolerance, in Scriver CR, Beaudet AL, Sly WS, Valle D (eds): *The Metabolic and Molecular Bases of Inherited Disease. vol. III*, 8th ed. New York, McGraw-Hill, 1995.
54. Silbernagl S: The renal handling of amino acids and oligopeptides. *Physiol Rev* **68**:911, 1988.
55. Stephens AD: Cystinuria and its treatment: 25 years experience at St. Bartholomew's Hospital. *J Inherit Metab Dis* **12**:197, 1989.
56. Singer A: Cystinuria: A review of the pathophysiology and management. *J Urol* **142**:669, 1989.
57. Millner DS: Cystinuria. *Endocr Metab Clin N Am* **19**:889, 1990.
58. Martin X, Salas M, Labeeuw M, Pozet N, Gelet A, Dubernard JM: Cystine stones: The impact of new treatment. *B J Urol* **68**:234, 1991.
59. Goodyer PR, Saadi I, Ong P, Elkas G, Rozen R: Cystinuria subtype and the risk of nephrolithiasis. *Kidney Int* **54**:56, 1998.
60. Crawhall JC, Purkiss P, Watts RWE, Young EP: The excretion of amino acids by cystinuric patients and their relatives. *Ann Hum Genet* **33**:149, 1969.

61. Harris H, Mittwoch U, Robson EB, Warren FL: Phenotypes and genotypes in cystinuria. *Ann Hum Genet* **20**:57, 1955.
62. Harris H, Mittwoch U, Robson EB, Warren FL: Pattern of amino acid excretion in cystinuria. *Ann Hum Genet* **19**:195, 1955.
63. Hershko L, Ben-Ami E, Paciorkovski J, Levin N: Allelomorphism in cystinuria. *Proc Tel-Hashomer Hosp* **4**:21, 1965.
64. Morin CL, Thompson MW, Jackson SH, Sass-Kortsak A: Biochemical and genetic studies in cystinuria: Observations on double heterozygotes of genotype I/II. *J Clin Invest* **50**:1961, 1971.
65. Goodyer PR, Clow C, Reade T, Girardin C: Prospective analysis and classification of patients with cystinuria identified in a newborn screening program. *J Pedriatr* **122**:568, 1993.
66. Gasparini P, Calonge MJ, Bisceglia L, Purroy J, Dianzani I, Notarangelo A, Rousaud F, Gallucci M, Testar X, Ponzone A, Estivill X, Zorzano A, Palacin M, Nunes V, Zelante L: Molecular genetics of cystinuria: Identification of four new mutations and seven polymorphisms, and evidence for genetic heterogeneity. *Am J Hum Genet* **57**:781, 1995.
67. Calonge MJ, Volpini V, Bisceglia L, Rousaud F, DeSantis L, Brescia E, Zelante L, Testar X, Zorzano A, Estivill X, Gasparini P, Nunes V, Palacín M: Genetic heterogeneity in cystinuria: The rBAT gene is linked to type I but not to type III cystinuria. *Proc Natl Acad Sci U S A* **92**:9667, 1995.
68. Tate SS, Yan, N, Udenfriend S: Expression cloning of a Na^+-independent neutral amino acid transporter from rat kidney. *Proc Natl Acad Sci USA* **89**:1, 1992.
69. Bertrán J, Werner A, Moore ML, Stange G, Markovich D, Biber J, Testar X, Zorzano A, Palacín M, Murer, H: Expression cloning of a cDNA from rabbit kidney cortex that induces a single transport system for cystine and dibasic and neutral amino acids. *Proc Natl Acad Sci U S A* **89**:5601, 1992.
70. Wells G, Hediger MA: Cloning of a rat kidney cDNA that stimulates dibasic and neutral amino acid transport and has sequence similarity to glucosidases. *Proc Natl Acad Sci U S A* **89**:5596, 1992.
71. Bertrán J, Werner A, Chillarón J, Nunes V, Biber J, Testar X, Zorzano A, Estivill X., Murer H, Palacín M: Expression cloning of a human renal cDNA that induces high affinity transport of L-cystine shared with dibasic amino acids in *Xenopus* oocytes. *J Biol Chem* **268**:14842, 1993.
72. Lee W-S, Wells. RG, Sabbag RV, Mohandas TK, Hediger MA: Cloning and chromosomal localization of a human kidney cDNA involved in cystine, dibasic, and neutral amino acid transport. *J Clin Invest* **91**:1959, 1993.
73. Zhang X-X, Rozen R, Hediger MA, Goodyer P, Eydoux P: Assignment of the gene for cystinuria (*SLC3A1*) to human chromosome 2p21 by fluorescence in situ hybridization. *Genomics* **24**:413, 1994.
74. Calonge MJ, Nadal M, Calvano S, Testar X, Zelante L, Zorzano A, Estivill X, Gasparini P, Palacin M, Nunes V: Assignment of the gene responsible for cystinuria (rBAT) and of markers D2S119 and D2S177 to 2p16 by fluorescence in situ hybridization. *Hum Genet* **95**:633, 1995.
75. Bisceglia L, Calonge MJ, Totaro A, Feliubadalo L, Melchionda S, Garcia J, Testar X, Gallucci M, Ponzone A, Zelante L, Zorzano A, Estivill X, Gasparini P, Nunes V, Palacin. M: Localization, by linkage analysis, of the cystinuria type III gene to chromosome 19q13.1. *Am J Hum Genet* **60**:611, 1997.
76. Wartenfeld R, Golomb E, Katz G, Bale SJ, Goldman B, Pras M, Kastner DL, Pras E: Molecular analysis of cystinuria in Libyan Jews: Exclusion of the *SLC3A1* gene and mapping of a new locus on 19q. *Am J Hum Genet* **60**:617, 1997.
77. The International Consortium of Cystinuria (Felivbadato L et al.): Non-type I cystinuria caused by mutations in SCL7A9, coding for a subunit ($b^{o,+}$AT) of rBAT. *Nat Genet* **23**:52, 1999.
78. Brodehl J, Gellissen K: Endogenous renal transport of free amino acids in infancy and childhood. *Pediatrics* **42**:395, 1968.
79. Dent C, Senior B: Studies on the treatment of cystinuria. *B J Urol* **27**:317, 1955.
80. Crawhall JC, Scowen EF, Watts RWE: Effect of penicillamine on cystinuria. *BMJ* **1**:588, 1963.
81. McDonald JE, Henneman PH: Stone dissolution in vivo and control of cystinuria with penicillamine. *N Engl J Med* **273**:578, 1965.
82. Combe C, Deforges-Lasseur C, Chehab Z, de Precigout V, Aparicio M: Cystine lithiasis and its treatment with D-penicillamine. The experience in a nephrology service in a 23-year period. Apropos of 26 patients. *Annales d'Urol* **27**:79, 1993.
83. Goodyer P, Khoury M: Cystinuria: Current approaches to medical management. *J Nephrol* **8**:35, 1995.
84. King JS Jr: Treatment of cystinuria with α-mercaptopropionylglycine: A preliminary report with some notes on column chromatography of mercaptans. *Proc Soc Exp Biol Med* **129**:927, 1968.
85. Remien A, Kallistratos G, Burchardt P: Treatment of cystinuria with thiola (alpha-mercaptopropionylglycine) *Eur Urol* **1**:227, 1975.
86. Pak CYC, Fuller C, Sakhaee K, et al.: Management of cystine nephrolithiasis with alpha-mercaptopropionylglycine. *J Urol* **136S**: 1003, 1986.
87. Koide T, Katsuhiro K, Takemoto M, et al.: Conservative treatment of cystine calculi: Effect of oral alpha-mercaptopropionylglycine on cystine stone dissolution and on prevention of stone recurrence. *J Urol* **128**:513, 1982.
88. Harbar JA, Cusworth DC, Lawes LC, Wrong OM: Comparison of 2-mercaptopropionylglycine and D-penicillamine in the treatment of cystinuria. *J Urol* **136**:146, 1986.
89. Siskind MS, Popovtzer MM: Hyperlipidemia associated with alpha-mercaptopropionylglycylglycine therapy for cystinuria. *Am J Kidney Dis* **19**:179, 1992.
90. Mairino RM, Bruce DC, Aposhian HV: Determination and metabolism of dithiol chelating agents. VI. Isolation and identification of the mixed disulfides of meso-2,3-dimercaptosuccinic acid with L-cysteine in human urine. *Toxicol Appl Pharmacol* **97**:338, 1989.
91. Sloand JA, Izzo JL: Captopril reduces urinary cystine excretion in cystinuria. *Arch Int Med* **147**:1409, 1987.
92. Streem SB, Hall P: Effect of captopril on urinary cystine excretion in homozygous cystinuria. *J Urol* **142**:1522, 1989.
93. Perazella MA, Buller GK: Successful treatment of cystinuria with captopril. *Am J Kidney Dis* **21**:504, 1993.
94. Coulthard M, Richardson J, Fleetwood A: Captopril is not clinically useful in reducing cystine load in cystinuria or cystinosis. *Ped Nephrol* **5**:98, 1991.
95. Jaeger P, Portman L, Saunders A, Rosenberg LE, Thier SO: Anticystinuric effects of glutamine and of dietary sodium restriction. *N Engl J Med* **315**:1120, 1986.
96. Peces R, Sanchez L, Gorodstidi M, Alvarez J: Effects of variation in sodium intake on cystinuria. *Nephron* **57**:421, 1991.
97. Norman RW, Manette WA: Dietary restriction of sodium as a means of reducing urinary cystine. *J Urol* **143**:1193, 1990.
98. Purroy J, Bisceglia L, Calonge MJ, Zelante L, Testar X, Zorzano A, Estivill X, Palacín M, Nunes V, Gasparini P: Genomic structure and organization of the human rBAT gene (SLC3A1). *Genomics* **37**:249, 1996.
99. Endsley Jk, Phillipss JA, Hruskaa KA, George AL: Genomic organization of a human cystine transporter gene (SCL3A1) and identification of novel mutations causing cystinuria. *Kidney Int* **51**:1893, 1997.
100. Eisenbach GM, Weise M, Stolte H: Amino acid reabsorption in the rat nephron. Free-flow micropuncture study. *Pflügers Arch* **357**:63, 1975.
101. Ullrich KJ, Rumrich G, Klos S: Sodium dependence on the amino acid transport in the proximal convolution of the rat kidney. *Pfluegers Arch* **351**:49, 1974.
102. Jullia P, Segal S, Thier SO: Renal handling of amino acids, in *Handbook of Physiology. Renal Physiology.* Washington, DC, Am Physiol Soc, Sec. 8, Chap. 20:653, 1973.
103. Silbernagl S: Amino acids and oligopeptides, in Seldin DW, Giebisch G (eds): *Kidney: Physiology and Pathophysiology.* New York, Raven, 1985, p 1677.
104. Silbernagl S, Foulkes EC, Deetjen P: Renal transport of amino acids. *Rev Physiol Biochem Pharmacol* **64**:105, 1975.
105. Jullia P, Foreman JW, Hwang SM, Segal S: Transport interactions of cystine and dibasic amino acids in isolated rat renal tubules. *Metabolism* **29**:53, 1980.
106. McNamara PD, Rea CT, Segal S: Ion dependence of cystine and lysine uptake by rat renal brush border membrane vesicles. *Biochim Biophys Acta* **1103**:101, 1992.
107. McNamara PD, Pepe LM, Segal S: Cystine uptake by rat renal brush-border vesicles. *Biochemistry* **194**:443, 1981.
108. Riahi-Esfahani S, Jessen H, Roigaard, H: Comparative study of the uptake of L-cysteine and L-cystine in the renal proximal tubule. *Amino Acids* **8**:247, 1995.
109. Crawhall JC, Segal S: The intracellular ratio of cysteine and cystine in various tissues. *Biochemistry* **105**:891, 1967.
110. Segal S, Smith I: Delineation of cystine and cysteine transport systems in rat kidney cortex by developmental patterns. *Proc Natl Acad Sci U S A* **63**:926, 1969.

111. Foreman JW, Hwang SM, Segal S: Transport interaction of cystine and dibasic amino acids in isolated rat renal tubules. *Metabolism* **29**:53, 1980.
112. States B, Segal S: Distribution of glutathione-cystine transhydrogenase activity in subcellular fractions of rat intestinal mucosa. *Biochemistry* **113**:443, 1969.
113. Segal S, McNamara PD, Pepe LM: Transport interaction of cystine and dibasic amino acids in renal brush border vesicles. *Science* **197**:169, 1977.
114. Robson EB, Rose GA: The effect of intravenous lysine on the renal clearances of cystine, arginine and ornithine in normal subjects, in patients with cystinuria and their relatives. *Clin Sci* **16**:75, 1957.
115. Lester FT, Cusworth DC: Lysine infusion in cystinuria: Theoretical renal thresholds for lysine. *Clin Sci* **44**:99, 1973.
116. Kato T: Renal handling of dibasic amino acids and cystine in cystinuria. *Clin Sci Mol Med* **53**:9, 1977.
117. Ausiello DA, Segal, S, Thier SO: Cellular accumulation of L-lysine in rat kidney cortex in vivo. *Am J Physiol* **222**:1473, 1972.
118. Greth WE, Thier SO, Segal S: Cellular accumulation of L-cystine in rat kidney cortex in vivo. *J Clin Invest* **52**:454, 1973.
119. Webber WA, Brown JL, Pitts RF: Interactions of amino acids in renal tubular transport. *Am J Physiol* **200**:380, 1961.
120. Bovee KC, Segal S: Renal tubular reabsorption of amino acids after lysine loading of cystinuria dogs. *Metabolism* **33**:602, 1984.
121. Brodehl J: Postnatal development of tubular amino acid reabsorption, in Silbernagl S, Lang F, Greger R (eds): *Amino Acid Transport and Uric Acid Transport*. Stuttgart, Georg Thieme, 1975, p 128.
122. Volkl H, Silbernagl S, Ascher A: Mutual inhibition of L-cystine/L-cysteine and other neutral amino acids during tubular reabsorption. A microperfusion study in rat kidney. *Pflugers Arch* **395**:190, 1982.
123. Silbernagl S, Deetjen P: The tubular reabsorption of L-cystine and L-cysteine: A common transport system with L-arginine or not? *Pfluegers Arch* **337**:277, 1972.
124. Craan AG, Bergeron M: Experimental cystinuria: The cycloleucine model. I. Amino acid interactions in renal and intestinal epithelia. *Can J Physiol* **53**:1027, 1975.
125. Biber J, Stange G, Stieger B, et al.: Transport of L-cystine by renal brush border membrane vesicles. *Pflugers Arch* **396**:335, 1983.
126. Schafer JA, Watkins ML: Transport of L-cystine in isolated perfused proximal straight tubules. *Pfluegers Arch* **401**:143, 1984.
127. Ozegovic B, McNamara PD, Segal S: Cystine uptake by rat jejunal brush border membrane vesicles. *Biosci Rep* **2**:913, 1982.
128. Furlong TJ, Posen S: D-Penicillamine and the transport of cystine by rat renal brush border membrane vesicles. *Am J Physiol* **258**:F321, 1990.
129. States B, Segal S: Cystine and dibasic amino acid uptake by opossum kidney cells. *J Cell Physiol* **143**:555, 1990.
130. Mora C, Chillarón, J, Calonge MJ, Forgo J, Testar X, Nunes V, Murer H, Zorzano A, Palacín M: The rBAT gene is responsible for L-cystine uptake via the $b^{o,+}$-like amino acid transport system in a "renal proximal tubular" cell line (OK cells). *J Biol Chem* **271**:10569, 1996.
131. Van Winkle LJ, Campione AL, Gorman JM: Na^+-independent transport of basic and zwitterionic amino acids in mouse blastocysts by a shared system and by processes which distinguish between these substrates. *J Biol Chem* **263**:3150, 1998.
132. Torras-Llort M, Ferrer R, Soriano-García JF, Moreto M: L-Lysine transport in chicken jejunal brush border membrane vesicles. *J Membr Biol* **152**:183, 1996.
133. Thwaites DT, Markovich D, Murer H, Simmons NL: Na^+-independent lysine transport in human intestinal Caco-2 cells. *J Membr Biol* **151**:21, 1996.
134. Christensen HN: Role of amino acid transport and countertransport in nutrition and metabolism. *Physiol Rev* **70**:43, 1990.
135. Palacín M, Estévez R, Bertrán J, Zorzano A: Molecular biology of mammalian plasma membrane amino acid transporters. *Physiol Rev* **78**:969, 1998.
136. Lumadue JA, Glick AB, Ruddle FH: Cloning, sequence analysis, and expression of the large subunit of the human lymphocyte activation antigen 4F2. *Proc Natl Acad Sci U S A* **84**:9204, 1987.
137. Quackenbush E, Clabby M, Gottesdiener KM, Barbosa J, Jones NH, Strominger JL, Speck S, Leiden JM: Molecular cloning of complementary DNAs encoding the heavy chain of the human 4F2 cell-surface antigen: A type II membrane glycoprotein involved in normal and neoplastic cell growth. *Proc Natl Acad Sci U S A* **84**:6526, 1987.
138. Teixeira S, Di Grandi S, Kühn, LC: Primary structure of the human 4F2 antigen heavy chain predicts a transmembrane protein with a cytoplasmic NH_2 terminus. *J Biol Chem* **262**:9574, 1987.
139. Parmacek MS, Karpinski BA, Gottesdiener KM, Thompson CB, Leiden JM: Structure, expression and regulation of the murine 4F2 heavy chain. *Nucleic Acids Res* **17**:1915, 1989.
140. Bröer S, Bröer A, Hamprecht B: The 4F2hc surface antigen is necessary for expression of system L-like neutral amino acid-transport activity in C6-BU-1 rat glioma cells: Evidence from expression studies in *Xenopus laevis* oocytes. *J Biochem* **312**:863, 1995.
141. Gottesdiener KM, Karpinski BA, Lindstei T, Strominger JL, Jones NH, Thompson CB, Leiden JM: Isolation and structural characterization of the human 4F2 heavy-chain gene, an inducible gene involved in T-lymphocyte activation. *Mol Cell Biol* **8**:3809, 1988.
142. Pras E, Sood R, Raben N, Aksentijevitch I, Chen XY, Kastner DL: Genomic organization of SLC3A1, a transporter gene mutated in cystinuria. *Genomics* **36**:163, 1996.
143. Bertrán J, Magagnin S, Werner A, Markovich D, Biber J, Testar X, Zorzano A, Kühn LC, Palacín M, Murer H: Stimulation of system Y^+-like amino acid transport by the heavy chain of human 4F2 surface antigen in *Xenopus laevis* oocytes. *Proc Natl Acad Sci U S A* **89**:5606, 1992.
144. Wells RG, Lee W, Kanai Y, Leiden M, Hediger MA: The 4F2 antigen heavy chain induces uptake of neutral and dibasic amino acids in *Xenopus* oocytes. *J Biol Chem* **267**:15285, 1992.
145. Markovich DG, Strange G, Bertran J, Palacín M, Werner A, Biber J, Murer H: Two mRNA transcripts (rBAT-1 and rBAT-2) are involved in system $b^{o,+}$-related amino acid transport. *J Biol Chem* **268**:1362, 1993.
146. Haynes BF, Hemler ME, Mann DL, Eisenbarth GS, Shelhamer JH, Mostowski HS, Thomas CA, Strominger JL, Fauci AS: Characterization of a monoclonal antibody (4F2) that binds to human monocytes and to a subset of activated lymphocytes. *J Immunol* **126**:1409, 1981.
147. Mosckovitz R, Udenfriend S, Felix A, Heimer E, Tate SS: Membrane topology of the rat kidney neutral and basic amino acid transporter. *FASEB J* **8**:1069, 1994.
148. Geering K, Theulaz I, Verrey F, Häuptle MT, Rossier BC: A role for the β-subunit in the expression of functional Na^+, K^+-ATPase in *Xenopus* oocytes. *Am J Physiol* **257**:C851, 1989.
149. Hedin KE, Lim NF, Clapham DE: Cloning of a *Xenopus laevis* inwardly rectifying K^+ channel subunit that permits GIRK1 expression of IKACh currents in oocytes. *Neuron* **16**:423, 1996.
150. Barhanin J, Lesag F, Guillemare E, Fink M, Lazdunski M, Romey G: KvLQT1 and ISK (minK) proteins associate to form the IKS cardiac potassium current. *Nature* **384**:78, 1996.
151. Sanguinetti C, Curran ME, Zou A, Shen J, Spector PS Atkinson DL, Keating MT: Coassembly of K(V)LQT1 and minK (ISK) proteins to form cardiac IKS potassium channel. *Nature* **384**:80, 1996.
152. Wang Y, Tate SS: Oligomeric structure of a renal cystine transporter: Implications in cystinuria. *FEBS Lett* **368**:389, 1995.
153. Palacín M, Chillarón J, Mora C: Role of the $b^{o,+}$-like amino acid-transport system in the renal reabsorption of cystine and dibasic amino acids. *Biochem Soc Trans* **24**:856, 1996.
154. Palacín M, Estévez R, Zorzano A: Cystinuria calls for heteromultimeric amino acid transporters. *Curr Opin Cell Biol* **10**:455, 1998.
155. Estévez R, Camps M, Rojas AM, Testar X, Devés R, Hediger MA, Zorzano A, Palacín M: The amino acid transport system Y^+ L/ 4F2hc is a heteromultimeric complex. *FASEB J* **12**:1319, 1998.
156. Kanai Y, Segawa H, Miyamoto K, Uchino H, Takeda E, Endou H: Expression cloning and characterization of a transporter for large neutral amino acids activated by the heavy chain of 4F2 antigen (CD98). *J Biol Chem* **273**:23629, 1998.
157. Mastrobernardino L, Spindler B, Pfeiffer R, Skelly, PJ, Loffing J, Shoemaker CB, Verrey F: Amino acid transport by heterodimers of 4F2hc/CD98 and members of a new permease family. *Nature* **395**:288, 1998.
158. Pineda M, Fernández E, Torrents D, Estévez R, López C, Camps M, Lloberas J, Zorzano A, Palacín M: Identification of a membrane protein (LAT-2) that co-expresses with 4F2hc an L type amino acid transport activity with broad specificity for small and large zwitterionic amino acids. *J Biol Chem* **274**:19738, 1999.
159. Torrents D, Estévez R, Pineda M, Fernández E, Lloberas J, Shi Y-B, Zorzano A, Palacín M: Identification and characterization of a membrane protein Y^+ LAT-1 that associates with 4F2hc to encode the amino acid transport activity Y^+L. A candidate gene for lysinuric protein intolerance. *J Biol Chem* **273**:32437, 1998.
160. Sato H, Tamba M, Ishii T, Bannai S: Cloning and expression of a plsma membrane cystine/glutamate exchange transporter composed of two distint proteins. *J Biol Chem* **274**:11455, 1999.
161. Pfeiffer R, Rossier G, Spindler B, Meier C, Kühn L, Verrey F: Amino acid transport of Y^+ L-type by hetrodimers of 4F2hc/CD98 and

members of the glycoprotein-associated aminoacid transporter family. *EMBO J* **18**:49, 1999.
162. Torrents D, Mykkänen, Pineda M, Feliubadaló L, Estévez R, de Cid R, Sanjurjo P, Zorzano A, Nunes V, Huoponen K, Reinikainen A, Simell O, Savontaus ML, Aula P, Palacín M: Identification of SLC7A7, encoding Y^+ LAT-1, as the lysinuric protein intolerance gene. *Nature Genet* **21**:2983, 1999.
163. Borsani G, Bassi MT, Sperandeo MP, De Grandi A, Buoninconti A, Riboni M, Manzoni M, Incerti B, Pepe A, Andria G, Ballabio A, Sebastio G: SLC7A7, encoding aputative permease-related protein, is mutated in patients with lysinuric protein intolerance. *Nature Genet* **21**:297, 1999.
164. Bertran J, Werner A, Stange G, Markovich D, Biber J, Testar X, Zorzano A, Palacín M, Murer H: Expression of Na^+- independent amino acid transport in xenopus laevis oocytes by injection of rabbit kidney cortex mRNA. *Biochem J* **281**:717, 1992.
165. Yan N, Mosckovitz R, Udenfriend S, Tate S: Distribution of mRNA of a Na^+ independent neutral amino acid transporter cloned from rat kidney and its expression in mammalian tissues and Xenopus laevis oocytes. *Proc Natl Acad Sci USA* **89**:9982, 1992.
166. Magagnin S, Bertran J, Werner A, Markovich D, Biber J, Palacín M, Murer H: Poly (A) + RNA from rabbit intestinal mucosa induces $b^{o,+}$ and Y^+L amino acid transport activities in Xenopus oocytes. *J Bol Chem* **267**:15384, 1992.
167. Kanai Y, Stelzner MG, Lee W-S, Wells RG, Brown D, Hediger MA: Expression of mRNA (D2) encoding a protein involved in amino acid transport in S3 proximal tubule. *Am J Physiol* **263**:F1087, 1992.
168. Furriols M, Chillarón J, Mora C, Castello A, Bertran J, Camps M, Testar X, Vilaró S, Zorzano A, Palacín M: rBAT, related to L-cystine transport, is localized to the microvilli of proximal straight tubules, and its expression is regulated in kidney by development. *J Biol Chem* **268**:27060, 1993.
169. Pickel VM, Niremberg MJ, Chan J, Mosckovitz R, Udenfriend S, Tate S: Ultrastructural localization of a neutral and basic amino acid transporter in rat kidney and intestine. *Proc Natl Acad Sci U S A* **90**:7779, 1993.
170. Hisano S, Haga H, Miyamoto K, Takeda E, Fukui Y: The basic amino acid transporter (rBAT)-like immunoreactivity in paraventricular and supraoptic magnocellular neurons of the rat hypothalamus. *Brain Res* **710**:299, 1996.
171. Busch AG, Herzer T, Waldegger S, Schmidt F, Palacín M, Biber J, Markovich D, Murer H, Lang F: Opposite directed currents induced by the transport of dibasic and neutral amino acids in *Xenopus* oocytes expressing the protein rBAT. *J Biol Chem* **269**:25581, 1994.
172. Coady MJ, Jalal F, Chen X, Lemay G, Berteloot A, Lapointe J-Y: Electrogenic amino acid exchange via the rBAT transporter. *FEBS Lett* **356**:174, 1994.
173. Ahmed A, Peter GJ, Taylor PM, Harper AA, Rennie MJ: Sodium-independent currents of opposite polarity evoked by neutral and cationic amino acids in neutral and basic amino acid transporter cRNA-injected oocytes. *J Biol Chem* **270**:8482, 1995.
174. Chillarón J, Estévez R, Mora C, Wagner CA, Suessbrich H, Lang F, Gelpí JL, Testar X, Buasch AE, Zorzano A, Palacín, M: Amino acid exchange via systems $b^{o,+}$-like and Y^+L-like. A tertiary active transport mechanism for renal reabsorption of cystine and dibasic amino acids. *J Biol Chem* **271**:17761, 1996.
175. Quackenbush EJ, Gougos A, Baumal R, Letarte M: Differential localization within human kidney of five membrane proteins expressed on acute lymphoblastic leukemia cells. *J Immunol* **136**:118, 1986.
176. Rosenberg LE, Downing S: Transport of neutral and dibasic amino acids by human leucocytes: Absence of a defect in cystinuria. *J Clin Invest* **44**:1382, 1965.
177. Arrow VK, Westall RG: Amino acid clearances in cystinuria. *J Physiol* **142**:141, 1958.
178. Rosenberg LE, Albrecht I, Segal S: Lysine transport in human kidney: Evidence for two systems. *Science* **155**:1426, 1967.
179. McCarthy CF, Borland JL, Lynch HJ, Owen EE, Tyor MPL: Defective uptake of basic amino acids and L-cystine by intestinal mucosa of patients with cystinuria. *J Clin Invest* **43**:1518, 1964.
180. Thier S, Segal S, Fox M, Blair A, Rosenberg LE: Cystinuria: Defective intestinal transport of dibasic amino acids and cystine. *J Clin Invest* **44**:442, 1965.
181. Coicadan L, Heyman M, Grasset E, Desjeux JF: Cystinuria: Reduced lysine permeability at the brush-border of intestinal membrane cells. *Pediatr Res* **14**:109, 1980.
182. Desjeux JF, Vonlanthen M, Dumontier AM, Simell O, Legrain M: Cystine fluxes across the isolated jejunal epithelium membrane. *Pediatr Res* **21**:477, 1987.
183. Rosenberg LE, Crawhall JL, Segal S: Intestinal transport of cystine and cysteine in man: Evidence for three separate mechanisms. *J Clin Invest* **46**:30, 1967.
184. Frimpter GW, Horwith M, Furth E, Fellows RE, Thompson DD: Inulin and endogenous amino acid clearances in cystinuria: Evidence for tubular secretion. *J Clin Invest* **41**:281, 1962.
185. Schwartzman L, Blair A, Segal S: A common renal transport system for lysine, ornithine, arginine and cysteine. *Biochem Biophys Res Commun* **23**:220, 1966.
186. Frimpter GW: Cystinuria: Intravenous administration of S^{35} cystine and S^{35} cysteine. *Clin Sci* **31**:207, 1966.
187. Calonge MJ, Gasparini P, Chillarón J, Chillón M, Gallucci M, Rousaud F, Zelante L, Testar X, Dallapiccola B, DiSilverio F, Barceló P, Estivill X, Zorzano A, Nunes V, Palacín M: Cystinuria caused by mutations in rBAT, a gene involved in the transport of cystine. *Nat Genet* **6**:420, 1994.
188. Sharland M, Jones M, Bain M, Chalmers R, Hammond J, Patton MAJ: Balanced translocation (14;20) in a mentally handicapped child with cystinuria. *Med Genet* **29**:507, 1992.
189. Yan N, Mosckovitz R, Gerber LD, Mathew S, Murty VS, Tate SS, Udenfriend S: Characterization of the promoter region of the gene for the rat neutral and basic amino acid transporter and chromosomal location of the human gene. *Proc Natl Acad Sci U S A* **89**:5596, 1994.
190. Pras E, Arber N, Aksentijevitch I, Katz G, Schapiro JM, Prosen L, Gruberg L, Harel D, Liberman U, Weissenbach J, Pras M, Kastner DL: Localization of a gene causing cystinuria to chromosome 2p. *Nat Genet* **6**:415, 1994.
191. Bisceglia L, Calonge MJ, Dello Strologo L, Rizzoni G, de Sanctis L, Gallucci M, Beccia E, Testar X, Zorzano A, Estivill X, Zelante L, Palacín M, Gasparini P, Nunes V: Molecular analysis of cystinuria disease gene: Identification of four new mutations one large deletion and one polymorphism. *Hum Genet* **98**:447, 1996.
192. Pras E, Raben N, Golomb E, Arber N, Aksentijevitch I, Schapiro J, Harel D, Katz G, Liberman U, Pras M, Kastner DL: Mutations of the SLC3A1 transporter gene in cystinuria. *Am J Hum Genet* **56**:1297, 1995.
193. Horsford J, Saadi I, Raelson J, Goodyer PR, Rozen R: Molecular genetics of cystinuria in French Canadians: Identification of four novel mutations in Type I patients. *Kidney Int* **49**:1401, 1996.
194. Gitomer WL, Pak CYC: Recent advances in the biochemical and molecular biological basis of cystinuria. *J Urol* **156**:1907, 1996.
195. Gitomer LW, Reed BY, Ruml LA, Pak YC: 335-Base deletion in the mRNA coding for a dibasic amino acid transporter-like protein (SLC3A1) isolated from a patient with cystinuria. *Hum Mutat* **1(Suppl)**:S69, 1998.
196. Gitomer WI, Redd BY, Ruml LA, Sakhaee K, Pak CYC: Mutation in the genomic deoxyribonucleic acid for SLC3A1 in patients with cystinuria. *J Clin Endocrin Metab* **83**:3688-3694, 1998.
197. Miyamoto K, Katai K, Tatsumi S, Sone K, Segawa H, Yamamoto H, Taketani Y, Takada K, Morita K, Kanayama H, Kagawa S, Takeda E: Mutations of the basic amino acid transporter gene associated with cystinuria. *Biochemistry* **310**:951, 1995.
198. Saadi I, Chen XZ, Hediger M, Ong P, Pereira P, Goodyer P, Rozen R: Molecular genetics of cystinuria: Mutation analysis of SLC3A1 and evidence for another gene in the type I (silent) phenotype. *Kidney Int* **54**:48, 1998.
199. Pras E, Golomb E, Drake C, Aksentijevich I, Katz G, Kastner DL: A splicing mutation (891 + 4A→G) in SLC3A1 leads to exon 4 skipping and causes cystinuria in a Moslem Arab family. *Hum Mutat* **1(Suppl)**:S28, 1998.
200. Chillarón J, Estévez R, Samarzija I, Waldegger S, Testar X, Lang F, Zorzano A, Busch A, Palacín M: An intracellular trafficking defect in type I cystinuria rBAT mutants M467T and M467K. *J Biol Chem* **272**:9543, 1997.
201. Dello Strogolo L, Carbonari D, Gallucci M, Gasparini P, Bisceglia L, Zelante L, Rousaud F, Nunes V, Palacín M, Rizzoni G: Inter- and intrafamilial clinical variability in patients with cystinuria type I and identified mutations [Abstract 1793]. *J Am Soc Nephrol* **8**:388A, 1997.
202. Garcia E, Elliot J, Girvard A, Brandriff B, Gordon L, Soliman K, Ashworth L, et al.: A continuous high resolution physical map spanning 17 megabases of the q12, q13.1 and q13.2 cytogenetic bands of chromosome 19. *Genomics* **27**:52, 1995.
203. Pras E, Pras E, Kreiss Y, Frishberg Y, Prosen L, Aksentijevich I, Kastner DL: Refined mapping of the CSNUIII to a 1.8 Mb region on

chromosome 19q13.1 using historical recombinants in Libyan Jewish cystinuria patients. *Genomics* (in press).
204. Feliubadaló L, Bisceglia L, Font M, Dello Strogolo L, Beccia E, Arslan-KirchnerM, Steinmann B, Zelante L, Estivill X, Zorzano A, palacín M, Gasparini P, Nunes V: Recombinant families locate de gene for Non-type I cystinuria between markers C13 and D19S587 on chromosome 19q13.1. *Genomics* (in press).
205. Pras E, Cochva I, Lubetzky A, Pras M, Sidi Y, Kastner DL: Biochemical and clinical studies in Libyan Jewish cystinuria patients and their relatives. *Am J Med Genet* **80**:173, 1998.
206. Datta SP, Harris H: Urinary amino acid patterns of some mammals. *Ann Eugen* **18**:107, 1953.
207. Crawhall J, Segal S: Sulfocysteine in the urine of the blotched Kenya gene. *Nature* **208**:1320, 1965.
208. Oldfield JE, Allen PH, Adair J: Identification of cystine calculi in mink. *Proc Soc Exp Biol Med* **91**:560, 1956.
209. Di Bartola SP, Chew DJ, Horton ML: Cystinuria in a cat. *J Am Vet Med Assoc* **198**:102, 1991.
210. Brand E, Cahill GF, Kassell B: Canine cystinuria. V: Family history of two cystinuric Irish terriers and cystine determination in dog urine. *J Biol Chem* **133**:431, 1940.
211. Holtzapple PG, Bovee K, Rea CF, Segal S: Amino acid uptake by kidney and jejunal tissue from dogs with cystine stones. *Science* **166**:1525, 1969.
212. Crane CW, Turner AW: Amino acid patterns of urine in blood plasma in a cystinuric Labrador dog. *Nature* **177**:2237, 1956.
213. Goulden BE, Leaver JL: Low-voltage paper electrophoresis as a screening test for the diagnosis of canine cystinuria. *Vet Rec* **80**:244, 1967.
214. Bovee KC, Bush M, Dietz J, Jezyk P, Segal S: Cystinuria in the maned wolf of South America. *Science* **212**:919, 1981.
215. Casal Mlk, Giger U, Bovee KC, Patterson DF: Inheritance of cystinuria and renal defect in Newfoundlands. *Am Vet Assoc* **207**:1585, 1995.

CHAPTER 192

Lysinuric Protein Intolerance and Other Cationic Aminoacidurias

Olli Simell

1. Membrane transport of cationic amino acids lysine, arginine, and ornithine is abnormal in four disease entities: classic cystinuria; lysinuric protein intolerance (hyperdibasic aminoaciduria type 2, or familial protein intolerance); hyperdibasic aminoaciduria type 1; and isolated lysinuria (lysine malabsorption syndrome). Cystinuria, the most common of these, is dealt with in Chap. 191. About 100 patients with lysinuric protein intolerance (LPI) have been reported or are known to me. Almost half of them are from Finland, where the prevalence of this autosomal recessive disease is 1 in 60,000. Autosomal dominant hyperdibasic aminoaciduria type 1 has been described in 13 of 33 members in a French Canadian pedigree, and isolated lysinuria has been described in one Japanese patient.

   Arginine and ornithine are intermediates in the urea cycle; lysine is an essential amino acid. In lysinuric protein intolerance (LPI) (MIM 222700), urinary excretion and clearance of all cationic amino acids, especially of lysine, are increased, and these amino acids are poorly absorbed from the intestine. Their plasma concentrations are low, and their body pools become depleted. The patients have periods of hyperammonemia caused by "functional" deficiency of ornithine, which provides the carbon skeleton of the urea cycle. Consequently, nausea and vomiting occur, and aversion to protein-rich food develops. The patients fail to thrive, and symptoms of protein malnutrition are further aggravated by lysine deficiency.
2. Patients with LPI are usually symptom-free when breast-fed but have vomiting and diarrhea after weaning. The appetite is poor, they fail to thrive, and if force-fed high-protein milk or formulas, they may go into coma. After infancy, they reject high-protein foods, grow poorly, and have enlarged liver and spleen, muscle hypotonia, and sparse hair. Osteoporosis is prominent, and fractures are not uncommon; bone age is delayed. The mental prognosis varies from normal development to moderate retardation; most patients are normal. Four patients have had psychotic periods. The final height in treated patients has been slightly subnormal or low-normal. Pregnancies are risky: Profound anemia develops, platelet count decreases, and severe hemorrhages during labor and a toxemic crisis have occurred, but the offspring are normal if not damaged by delivery-related complications. Acute exacerbations of hyperammonemia have not been a frequent problem in treated patients, but may have been the cause of the sudden death in one adult male after moderate alcohol ingestion. About two thirds of the patients have interstitial changes in chest radiographs. Some patients have developed acute or chronic respiratory insufficiency, which in a few has led to fatal pulmonary alveolar proteinosis and to multiple organ dysfunction syndrome. Patients present with fatigue, cough, dyspnea during exercise, fever, and, rarely, hemoptysis, and may also show signs of nephritis and renal insufficiency. One adult patient with pulmonary symptoms has been treated with high-dose prednisolone and is in remission over 6 years after the occurrence of the symptoms. In another patient, bronchoalveolar lavages have produced immediate relief during several subacute exacerbations.
3. In LPI, the concentrations of the cationic amino acids in plasma are subnormal or low-normal, and the amounts of glutamine, alanine, serine, proline, citrulline, and glycine are increased. Lysine is excreted in urine in massive excess, and arginine and ornithine in moderate excess. Daily urine contains a mean amount of 4.13 mmol lysine (range 1.02 to 7.00), 0.36 mmol arginine (0.08 to 0.69) and 0.11 mmol ornithine (0.09 to 0.13) per 1.73 m^2 body surface area. The mean renal clearances are 25.7, 11.5, and 3.3 ml/min/1.73 m^2, respectively; occasional values suggest net tubular secretion of lysine. Cystine excretion may be slightly increased. Blood ammonia and urinary orotic acid excretion are normal during fasting but are increased after protein meals. The serum urea level is low to normal, and lactate dehydrogenase, ferritin, and thyroid-binding globulin levels are elevated.
4. The transport abnormality is expressed in the kidney tubules, intestine, cultured fibroblasts, and probably in the hepatocytes, but not in mature erythrocytes. In vivo and in vitro studies of the handling of cationic amino acids in the intestine and kidney strongly suggest that the transport defect is localized at the basolateral (antiluminal) membrane of the epithelial cells. In vivo, plasma concentrations increase poorly after oral loading with the cationic amino acids, but also if lysine is given as a lysine-containing dipeptide. Dipeptides and other oligopeptides use a different transport mechanism not shared with that of free amino acids. The dipeptide thus crosses the luminal membrane normally, and is hydrolyzed to free amino acids in the cytoplasm of the enterocyte. An efflux defect at the basolateral membrane explains why the dipeptide-derived lysine is unable to enter the plasma compartment in LPI. Direct measurements and calculations of unidirectional

A list of standard abbreviations is located immediately preceding the index in each volume. Additional abbreviations used in this chapter include: HHH = hyperornithinemia-hyperammonemia-homocitrullinuria; LDH = lactate dehydrogenase; LPI = lysinuric protein intolerance; MCAT-1 and MCAT-2 = mouse cationic amino acid transporter-1 and transporter-2, respectively; TBG = thyroxine-binding globulin.

fluxes of lysine in intestinal biopsy specimens have confirmed that the defect indeed localizes to the basolateral cell surface. Similar cellular localization of the defect in the kidney tubules is suggested by infusions of citrulline, which cause not only citrullinuria but also significant argininuria and ornithinuria. Because citrulline and the cationic amino acids do not share transport mechanisms in the tubules, part of the citrulline is converted to arginine and then to ornithine in the tubule cells during reabsorption. A basolateral transport defect prohibits antiluminal efflux of arginine and ornithine, which accumulate and escape through the luminal membrane into the urine. The genetic mutations in LPI and possibly in all cationic aminoacidurias apparently lead to kinetic abnormalities in the transport protein(s) of the cationic amino acids. This is suggested by the fact that increasing the tubular load of a single cationic amino acid by intravenous infusion increases its tubular reabsorption, but reabsorption remains subnormal even at high loads. he other cationic amino acids are able to compete for the same transport site(s) also in LPI, but an increase in the load of one cationic amino acid frequently leads to net secretion of the others.

The plasma membrane of cultured fibroblasts shows a defect in the trans-stimulated efflux of the cationic amino acids; i.e., their flux out of the cell is not stimulated by cationic amino acids present on the outside of the cell as efficiently as it is in the control fibroblasts. The percent of trans-stimulation of homoarginine efflux in the fibroblasts of the heterozygotes is midway between that of the patients and the control subjects.

5. **The exact cause of hyperammonemia in LPI remains unknown. The enzymes of the urea cycle have normal activities in the liver, and the brisk excretion of orotic acid during hyperammonemia supports the view that N-acetylglutamate and carbamyl phosphate are formed in sufficient quantities. Low plasma concentrations of arginine and ornithine suggest that the malfunctioning of the cycle is caused by a deficiency of intramitochondrial ornithine. This hypothesis is supported by experiments in which hyperammonemia after protein or amino nitrogen loading is prevented by intravenous infusion of arginine or ornithine. Citrulline, a third urea cycle intermediate, also abolishes hyperammonemia if given orally, because, as a neutral amino acid, it is well-absorbed from the intestine. Ornithine deficiency in LPI has recently been questioned because cationic amino acids and their nonmetabolized analogues accumulate in higher-than-normal amounts in intestinal biopsy specimens and cultured fibroblasts from LPI patients in vitro and the concentrations of the cationic amino acids in liver biopsy samples are similar or higher in the patients when compared to these concentrations in the control subjects. If hyperammonemia is not due to simple deficiency of ornithine, it could be caused by inhibition of the urea cycle enzymes by the intracellularly accumulated lysine; by a coexisting defect in the mitochondrial ornithine transport necessary for the function of the urea cycle; or by actual deficiency of ornithine in the cytoplasm caused by abnormal pooling of the cationic amino acids into some cell organelle(s), most likely lysosomes. The latter two explanations imply that the transport defect is expressed also in the organelle(s).**
6. **Lysine is present in practically all proteins, including collagen. Lysine deficiency may cause many of the features of the disease that are not corrected by prevention of hyperammonemia, including enlargement of the liver and spleen, poor growth and delayed bone age, and osteoporosis. Oral lysine supplements are poorly tolerated by the patients because of their poor intestinal absorption. ε-*N*-acetyl-L-lysine, but not homocitrulline, efficiently increases plasma concentration of lysine in the patients, but acetyllysine or other neutral lysine analogues have not been used for supplementation.**
7. **Recently, a 622-amino-acid retroviral receptor (murine leukemia viral receptor REC1) with 12 to 14 potential membrane-spanning domains has been cloned. The physiological role of the receptor was soon found to be that of a cationic amino acid transporter at the cell membrane; the protein was hence renamed MCAT-1, mouse cationic amino acid transporter-1. The functional characteristics of the transporter are similar to those of system y^+, a widely expressed Na^+-independent transport system for cationic amino acids. The human counterpart of the mouse REC1 gene, encoding the retroviral receptor-transport protein, has been assigned to chromosome 13q12-q14 and named ATRC1. MCAT-1 (and y^+) activity is not expressed in rodent liver, but two other related cationic amino acid transport proteins, formed presumably as a result of alternative splicing — Tea (T cell early activation; expressed also in activated T and B lymphocytes) and MCAT-2 — are probably responsible for the low-affinity transport of cationic amino acids that is characteristic of (mouse) liver. Studies addressing the ATRC1 gene as well as the Tea and MCAT-2 genes as candidate genes for LPI are under way.**
8. **Treatment in lysinuric protein intolerance consists of protein restriction and supplementation with oral citrulline, 3 to 8 g daily during meals. Patients are encouraged to increase their protein intake modestly during citrulline supplementation, but aversion to protein in most patients effectively inhibits them from accepting more than the minimal requirement. The treatment clearly improves the growth and well-being of the patients. Pulmonary complications (interstitial pneumonia, pulmonary alveolar proteinosis, cholesterol granulomas, and respiratory insufficiency) have occasionally responded to early treatment with high-dose prednisolone, or to bronchoalveolar lavages. No therapy is known for the associated renal disease and renal failure.**
9. **The clinical and biochemical findings in other cationic aminoacidurias differ slightly from those in lysinuric protein intolerance. The symptoms of the index case with hyperdibasic aminoaciduria type 1 resemble those of LPI, but the other affected members of the pedigree are clinically healthy. The Japanese patient with isolated lysinuria has severe growth failure, seizures, and mental retardation. Her transport defect is apparently limited to lysine, and hyperammonemia is not a feature of the disease.**

Perheentupa and Visakorpi described the first three patients with "familial protein intolerance with deficient transport of basic amino acids" in 1965.[1] The disease is now called lysinuric protein intolerance (LPI) (MIM 222700) or "hyperdibasic aminoaciduria type 2."[2–5] Over 100 patients with this autosomal recessive disease have been described or are known to me; 41 of them are Finns or Finnish Lapps.[6–52] The incidence in Finland is 1 in 60,000 births but varies considerably within the country.[2,53] Patients of black and white American, Japanese, Turkish, Moroccan, Arab, Jewish, Italian, French, Dutch, Irish, Norwegian, Swedish, and Russian origin have also been described. The fascinating combination in the disease of urea cycle failure, expressed as postprandial hyperammonemia, and a defect in the transport of the cationic amino acids lysine, arginine, and ornithine in the intestine and kidney tubules has led to extensive studies of the mechanisms that link these two phenomena. The mechanisms are still partly unresolved, and the sequence of events leading to hyperammonemia is unclear. We can simplify our knowledge by

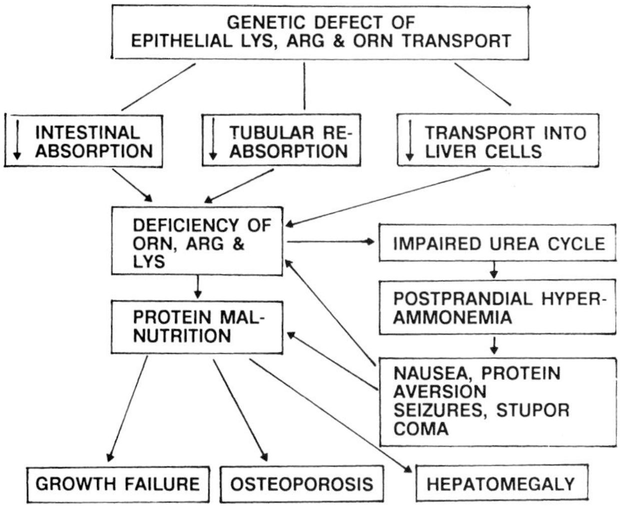

Fig. 192-1 The suggested pathogenesis of lysine, arginine, and ornithine deficiency, hyperammonemia, and aversion to protein in LPI.

saying that hyperammonemia is caused by "functional deficiency" of the urea cycle intermediates arginine and ornithine in the urea cycle[4,11,14,54] (Fig. 192-1). LPI has also been a productive model for studies of cellular transport: It is the first human disease where the transport defect has been localized to the basolateral (antiluminal) membrane of the epithelial cells.[55–57] Further, in LPI the parenchymal cells show a defect in the trans-stimulated efflux of the cationic amino acids, suggesting that the basolateral membrane of the epithelial cells and the plasma membrane of the parenchymal cells have analogous functions.[58,59]

Recently, the first candidate gene for LPI, ATRC1, encoding a human cationic amino acid transporter, has been mapped to the long arm of chromosome 13 (13q12-q14).[60] Without further proof, it is intriguing to hypothesize how a mutation in this or in a functionally similar gene or in genes encoding regulatory proteins of these transporters might lead to the membrane-selective cationic amino acid transport defect of LPI and to the complicated clinical features of the disease.

Several patients with variant forms of cationic aminoaciduria have been described in which the protein tolerance often is better than in LPI and the selectivity and severity of cationic aminoaciduria differs.[23,25,33,61,62] In the report by Whelan and Scriver[61] only the history of the index case suggested hyperammonemia, but other members of the pedigree have been symptom-free. The inheritance of this hyperdibasic aminoaciduria type 1 is autosomal dominant, implying that the patients are heterozygous for LPI or another type of hyperdibasic aminoaciduria.

CLINICAL ASPECTS

Lysinuric Protein Intolerance

Natural Course of the Disease. The gestation and delivery of infants with LPI has been uneventful.[4–6,9–11,35] Breast-fed infants usually thrive because of the low protein concentration in human milk, but symptoms of hyperammonemia may appear during the neonatal period and reflect exceptionally low protein tolerance or a high protein content in the breast milk. Nausea, vomiting, and mild diarrhea appear usually within 1 week of weaning or another increase in the protein content of the meals. Soy-based formulas are perhaps slightly better tolerated than cow's milk. The infants are poor feeders, cease to thrive, and have marked muscular hypotonia. The patient's liver and spleen are enlarged from the neonatal period onward. The association of episodes of vomiting with high protein feeds is not always apparent to the parents and may remain unnoticed even by trained physicians for years. Thus, the diagnosis frequently has been delayed until the school age or even adulthood.[35,47,63]

Around the age of 1 year, most patients begin to reject cow's milk, meat, fish, and eggs. The diet then mainly contains cereals cooked in water, potatoes, rice and vegetables, fruits and juices, bread, butter, and candies. The frequency of vomiting decreases on this diet, but accidental increases in protein intake lead to dizziness, nausea, and vomiting. A few patients have lapsed into coma, to the point where the EEG became isoelectric when the children were tube-fed with high-protein foods.[27,35,40,41,47] Enteral alimentation and total parenteral nutrition may cause symptoms in patients who have remained undiagnosed, because the protein or amino acid loads often exceed patient's tolerance. Prolonged, moderately increased protein intake may lead to dizziness, psychotic periods, chronic abdominal pains, or suspicion of abdominal emergencies.

Bone fractures occur frequently, often after minor trauma.[4,14,30,35,63–66] In a Finnish series, 20 of 29 patients (69 percent) had suffered from fractures of the long bones or of compression fractures of the lumbar spine; 10 (34 percent) had had more than 2 fractures during the 18-year follow-up.[63–65] Most fractures occurred before the age of 5 years. Symptoms of osteoarthrosis often begin at the age of 30 to 40 years. The radiologic signs of osteoporosis are usually severe before puberty but decrease with advancing age. The effect of citrulline therapy on osteoporosis is minimal.

Our accumulating experience with the late complications associated with the disease, together with recent reports of patients from outside Finland, suggest that in a sizable proportion of the patients the classic symptoms of protein intolerance may remain unnoticed. Instead, the patients may present with interstitial lung disease or respiratory insufficiency, or have renal glomerular or glomerulotubular disease with or without renal insufficiency as the first clinical finding (see "Complications and Autopsy Findings" below).

Physical Findings. Muscular hypotonia and hypotrophy are usually noticeable from early infancy but improve with advancing age.[35] Most patients are unable to perform prolonged physical exercises, but acute performance is relatively good. The body proportions of patients after the first couple of years of life are characteristic: the extremities are thin, but the front view of the body is squarelike with abundant centripetal subcutaneous fat. The hair is thin and sparse, the skin may be slightly hyperelastic, and the nails are normal. The liver is variably enlarged, and the spleen is often palpable and is large by ultrasound.

Patients who have remained undiagnosed until the age of several years have had characteristics typical of protein-calorie malnutrition and frequently resemble patients with advanced celiac disease. The subcutaneous fat may be reduced and the skin "loose" and "too large for the body" (Fig. 192-2).

The ocular fundi have been normal by ophthalmoscopy.[35] Of 20 patients studied, 14 had minute opacities in the anterior fetal Y suture of both lenses. In 10 patients, the opacities were surrounded by minute satellites. The opacities were never large enough to cause visual impairment and have remained stable, in some patients now for over 25 years. The mechanism underlying the lens abnormalities is unknown.[67]

The dentition of the patients has been normal, and the patients do not appear to be especially prone to caries, despite the high carbohydrate content of the diet.

Growth. Birth weights and lengths have been normal for gestational age, and postnatal growth is normal before weaning. The growth curves then begin to deviate progressively from the normal mean, and, at the time of diagnosis, 16 of 20 Finnish patients were more than 2 SD below the mean height, 12 patients were more than 3 SD, 6 patients more than 4 SD, 2 patients more than 5 SD, and 1 patient 6 SD below the mean.[35] Skeletal maturation is considerably delayed.[63,64] The bones usually mature

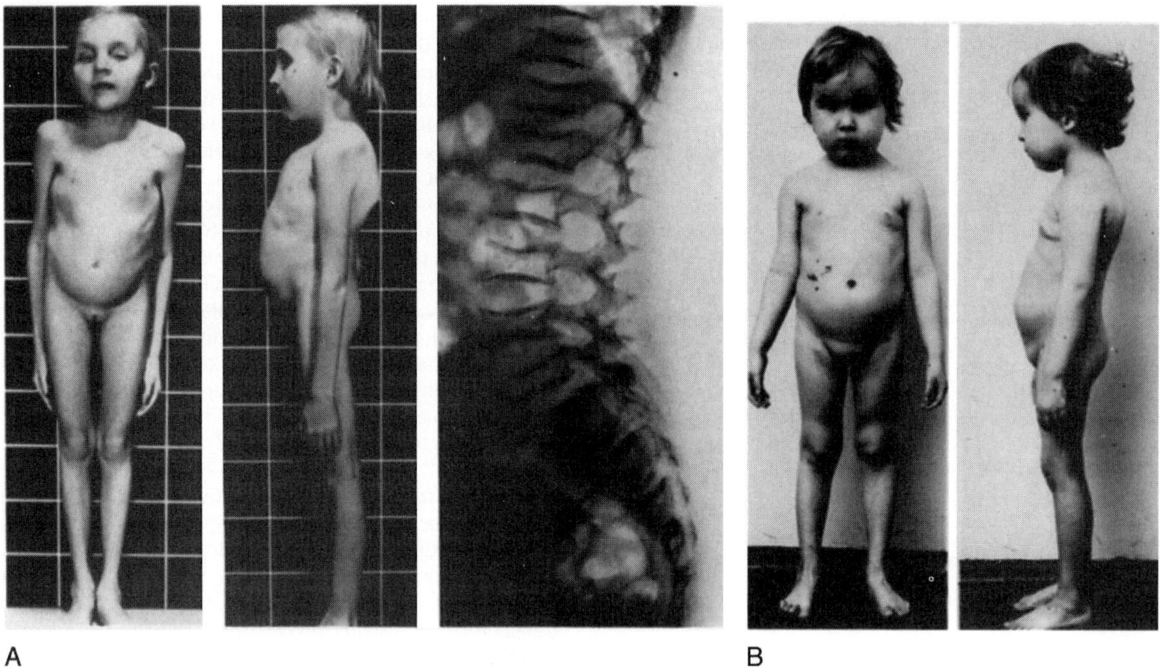

Fig. 192-2 Two children with LPI. The pictures were taken at the time of diagnosis. *A*, Child 12 years old. *B*, Child 6 years old. Note the prominent abdomen, hypotrophic muscles, and "loose" skin. The thorax of the child in A is deformed and her trunk shortened because of osteoporosis and pathologic fractures of the vertebrae.

slowly and linearly without a pubertal catch-up spurt, and most patients have not reached skeletal maturity by the age of 20 years. The final height of the patients has almost invariably been closer to the normal than the height measured at the time of diagnosis, because of therapy and the late cessation of growth. The head circumferences have been normal for age.

The body proportions are normal, but with advancing age the moderate centripetal obesity, which is present from early childhood, becomes more obvious.

Skeletal Manifestations and Bone Metabolism. Osteoporosis is often recognizable in skeletal radiographs and has occasionally been the leading sign of LPI.[30,63–65] Two-thirds of the patients have had fractures, half of which have occurred after insignificant trauma. All fractures have healed properly within a normal time. The skull and sella turcica have been normal in roentgenograms.

Over 70 percent of the patients have some skeletal abnormalities, either osteoporosis, deformations, or early osteoarthrosis.[63–65] In radiographs of 29 Finnish patients, osteoporosis was present in 13; the cortices of the long bones were abnormally thin in 5; the vertebrae had endplate impressions in 8; metaphyses were rickets-like in 2; and cartilage showed early destruction in 3. The cortex of the metacarpal bones was characteristically thickened in 7.[64] Morphometric analyses of bone biopsy samples showed moderate to severe osteoporosis in eight of nine patients studied; trabecular bone and osteoid volume were markedly reduced.[65] After double-labeling of bones with tetracycline *in vivo*, barely identifiable single lines were detected, suggesting poor bone deposition; the findings resembled those in severe malnutrition.[68–74] The number of osteoblasts and osteoclasts was low, and the extent of osteoid along the bone surfaces was low or normal in all specimens studied.

Laboratory tests for evaluation of calcium and phosphate metabolism have given unremarkable results.[35,63–65] Serum calcium and phosphate concentration, urinary excretion of calcium and phosphate, serum magnesium, estradiol, testosterone, thyroid-stimulating hormone, cortisol, vitamin D metabolites [25-$(OH)_2$-D, 1,25-$(OH)_2$-D and 24,25-$(OH)_2$-D], parathyroid hormone, calcitonin, and osteocalcin concentrations have all been within the reference range.

The daily urinary excretion of hydroxyproline is significantly increased during pubertal growth, but half of the adult patients also have supranormal excretion rates (mean of all adults 212 ± 103 μmol/m^2; adult reference range, 60 to 180 μmol/m^2).[65] The serum hydroxyproline concentration is increased in almost all patients irrespective of age. Serum concentrations of the C-terminal propeptide of type I procollagen and of the N-terminal propeptide of type III procollagen have been normal in all pediatric patients, but the concentration of the latter increases during puberty and remains elevated in adult patients.

The incorporation of labeled hydroxyproline into collagen was significantly decreased in cultured LPI fibroblasts as compared with age-matched controls at the ages of 5, 14, and 30 years, but there was no difference at the age of 44 years.[65] Morphometry of the collagen fibrils in electron microscopy showed no differences between patients and controls.

Liver Pathology. In the youngest patients, the histologic findings in liver biopsy specimens have been normal, with only occasional fat droplets in the hepatocytes.[8,35,63,75] In older patients, delimited areas in periportal or central parts of the liver lobules contained hepatocytes with ample pale cytoplasm and small pyknotic nuclei. In these cells, the glycogen content is decreased, and glycogen appears in coarse particles. At the borders of the abnormal areas, many nuclei are ghostlike and have central inclusion bodies staining positively with periodic acid-Schiff. Cytoplasmic fat droplets occur especially in the periportal areas. Children who died of alveolar proteinosis with multiple organ dysfunction syndrome have mostly shown extensive fatty degeneration of the liver but minimal or moderate cirrhosis. Inflammatory cells have always been absent in the liver biopsy samples.

Liver changes in LPI may reflect generalized protein malnutrition, because in kwashiorkor liver fat synthesis is increased, apolipoprotein synthesis is decreased, and lipoprotein lipases are inhibited.[76] Similar liver changes have also been induced in rats by lysine and arginine deprivation.[77]

Performance in Adult Life. Mental development is normal in most subjects. Performance is decreased, particularly in patients with known histories of prolonged hyperammonemia. Altogether, about 20 percent of the patients with LPI reported in the literature or otherwise known to me are mentally retarded. Convulsions are uncommon, but periods of stupor have occasionally been misinterpreted as psychomotor seizures.[18] Four patients have had psychotic periods, which have clearly been precipitated by prolonged moderate hyperammonemia.[35]

Neuropsychologic evaluation of the patients suggests that mathematical and other abstract skills are particularly vulnerable to hyperammonemia. Treatment with a low-protein diet and citrulline supplementation[11,14,63] (see "Treatment" below) has significantly improved the life quality of the patients. Episodes of vomiting and other signs of hyperammonemia have become a rare exception. The patients who underwent prolonged periods of hyperammonemia in early infancy and childhood and who appeared severely retarded at the first presentation have considerably and continuously improved their performance during therapy. All Finnish patients are now able to take care of the activities of daily life, and none of them is institutionalized. The most severely retarded patient, who had an IQ of 40 at the age of 12 years, lives now at the age of 40 in the custody of another family and is capable of taking care of her daily activities; she also works in a protected environment outside the home for a few hours a day and helps routinely in the household. She is talkative, happy, and socially active. At the other end of the spectrum, one patient has graduated from a medical school, works successfully as an internist, is married, and is a mother of one. Several other patients have also graduated from high school or other secondary schools and are permanently employed. The physical fitness of the patients is fair, but their capacity for prolonged heavy work and physical endurance is clearly limited. One patient worked as a construction worker in a building company for a few years, but found the job too heavy; another has been an active jogger for years and is capable of running 15 km without problems. The oldest patient in Finland is now 49 years of age and retired 7 years ago because of back problems. He is mentally and physically active and takes care of the household duties of a small farmhouse. A Finnish-born patient in Sweden is now 58 years old.[16,21,29] One male and seven female patients are married.

Pregnancies of the Patients. The seven married women have had fifteen pregnancies. One of the mothers was treated during the pregnancy only with protein restriction; the other received citrulline supplementation (8 to 14 pills containing 0.414 g L-citrulline daily during meals). Anemia (hemoglobin < 8.5 g/dl) occurred in all, and the platelet count decreased to less than $50 \times 10^3/mm^3$. A severe hemorrhage complicated two deliveries in one patient. Another patient had severe toxemia in her second pregnancy. The blood pressure increased to crisis values and she had prolonged convulsions and unconsciousness, but she recovered totally. In a third patient, an ultrasound-guided amniotic fluid puncture led to a bleed and loss of the fetus at 35 gestational weeks. Despite the mothers' anemia and severely decreased platelet count, other pregnancies and deliveries have been uneventful.

Of the 14 living children born to the patients, 13 are well at the age of 0.5 to 14 years. One child, whose delivery was complicated by a severe maternal hemorrhage, has hemiplegia and slightly delayed mental development, and another one was late in learning to speak but has later developed well.

One male patient has a healthy son.

Complications and Autopsy Findings. Since the first description of LPI in 1965,[1] 4 children and 1 adult of the 39 known Finnish patients have died, and a few pediatric LPI patients have died in other countries. A Moroccan patient died with pulmonary symptoms and autopsy findings similar to those of the four Finnish children (see below),[37] and a Japanese patient has had long-lasting, slowly progressive interstitial changes in the lungs.[36] An American child with LPI presented with interstitial pneumonia at the age of 27 months and later died of pulmonary alveolar proteinosis.[38] More recently, three Italian patients with severe interstitial lung disease have been described.[51] One of them died at the age of 18 months; two others had an accompanying renal glomerular or glomerulotubluar disease. One Arab child had severe respiratory insufficiency as the presenting sign at the age of 11 years, and had had clubbing of the fingers for 5 years.[52] An open lung biopsy showed cholesterol casts surrounded by a granulomatous process and giant cells; there was a small amount of interstitial inflammation and a moderate degree of scarring. Electron microscopy demonstrated cholesterol casts around and within macrophages and within alveolar cells in the alveolar spaces, but no hemorrhage.

Two of the four Finnish children who died had another systemic disease in addition to LPI (SLE; hypothyreosis). In all four, the fatal courses began as acute or subacute respiratory insufficiency, which progressed to multiorgan failure;[63,75,78–80] the symptoms fulfilled the criteria of the multiple organ dysfunction syndrome.[81,82] Progressive fatigue, cough, and mild to high fever were typical, and some children had blood in the sputum.[78–80] Dyspnea with marked air hunger during minimal exercise developed. Hemoglobin and platelet values fell, and the values of serum ferritin and lactate dehydrogenase, which are high in normal circumstances in these patients, increased even further. The sedimentation rate was elevated. Arterial oxygen tension was decreased, and the children had a severe bleeding tendency. The severity of liver, kidney, and pancreas involvement in the multiorgan failure varied. The pulmonary symptoms lasted from 2 weeks to 6 months before death.

The radiologic findings during the acute phase were similar in all patients with a fatal course.[78] Diffuse, reticulonodular densities and, later, signs of rapidly progressing airspace disease appeared in the chest radiographs at the mean age of 5 years (range 1.2 to 10.2 years) (Fig. 192-3). Two children developed acute respiratory insufficiency 2 months after the first radiologic signs of lung involvement, but one patient had densities for over 2 years and another for 12 years before acute exacerbation.

In one patient, a lung biopsy specimen taken at the time of appearance of the reticulonodular densities showed pulmonary alveolar proteinosis (Fig. 192-3*C*). At autopsy, three of the patients showed pulmonary alveolar proteinosis, and one had pulmonary hemorrhage with cholesterol granulomas. The specimens showed accumulations of myelin-like multilamellar structures, simple vesicles, granules, amorphous material, and crystals in transmission electron microscopy (Fig. 192-4).[79] Samples from the patient with pulmonary cholesterol granulomas contained interstitial and intra-alveolar cholesterol crystals and some multilamellar structures. It is interesting that similar pulmonary cholesterol granulomas were described in the lung biopsy sample of the Saudi Arabian child from Israel.[52]

One adult patient developed acute respiratory insufficiency with cough, fever, dyspnea, and hemoptysis at the age of 23 years.[78–80] Chest radiographs showed interstitial densities and airspace disease. Pulmonary function tests showed minimal obstruction of the distal airways but normal diffusing capacity. Extensive microbiologic investigations showed no evidence of infection. An open lung biopsy specimen showed bronchiolitis obliterans with signs of interstitial pneumonia. Granulation tissue polyps obstructed bronchiolar lumina, alveolar septa were thickened, and the sample contained a number of infiltrating lymphocytes and macrophages as well as signs of alveolar hemorrhages; no vasculitis nor full-blown alveolar proteinosis were found. The cytocentrifuge preparation made from the lung biopsy specimen showed 57 percent macrophages, 15 percent neutrophils, and 26 percent lymphocytes of the total cell count. The T-helper to T-suppressor cell ratio was 0.81. Symptoms disappeared rapidly and radiologic findings normalized within two months during high-dose prednisolone treatment. Eight months later, the patient relapsed with hemoptysis, but he responded well again to an increased corticosteroid dose. Now, 5 years later, he is symptom-free; the results of pulmonary function tests,

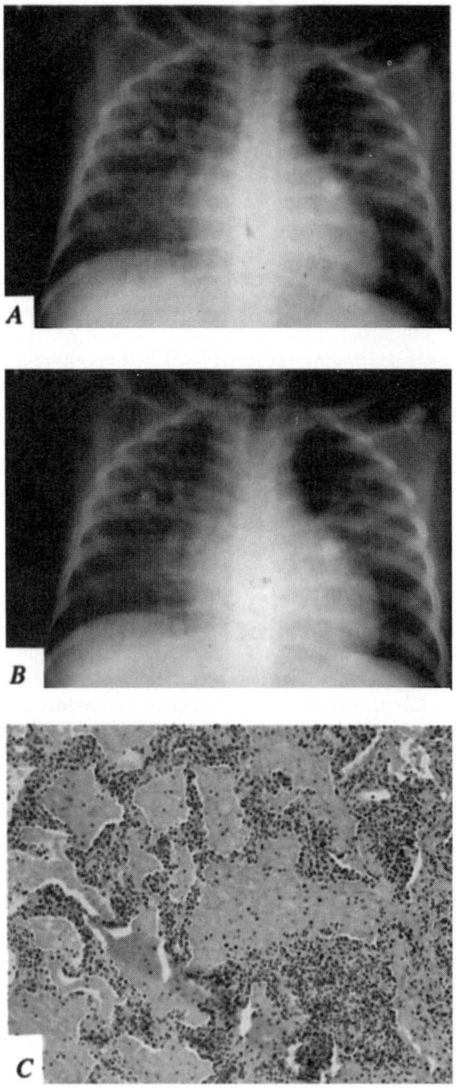

Fig. 192-3 A 13-year-old girl with LPI who developed fatal respiratory insufficiency after a mild respiratory infection. *A*, Chest radiograph at the time of the first respiratory symptoms showed reticulonodular interstitial densities. *B*, Chest radiograph taken two weeks later shows interstitial and alveolar densities. *C*, Pulmonary biopsy specimen shows signs of alveolar proteinosis (hematoxylin-eosin, original magnification ×115). (*From Parto et al.*[78] *Used by permission.*)

high-resolution computed tomography, and radionuclide imaging are normal, but the proportion of erythrocytes in the bronchoalveolar lavage fluid is increased.

Another patient developed chronic, slowly progressive pulmonary insufficiency with dyspnea, cough, chest pain, and hypoxia at the age of 42 years.[78–80] A bronchoalveolar lavage cured clinical symptoms in hours, and the response has been as good in all of the six relapses that have occurred during the 7 years of follow-up. His chest radiographs show increasing interstitial linear and nodular densities. Six years after the initial symptoms, radionuclide perfusion imaging showed a segmental defect and uneven perfusion, and pulmonary function tests suggested slight restriction but normal diffusing capacity. Bronchoscopy showed signs of chronic bronchitis. The relative proportions of cells in the bronchoalveolar lavage fluid were normal.

It is interesting that one-third of the symptom-free patients studied (8 of 25) had findings in chest radiographs that suggested pulmonary fibrosis, and high-resolution computed tomography suggested pulmonary fibrosis in two-thirds of the patients studied

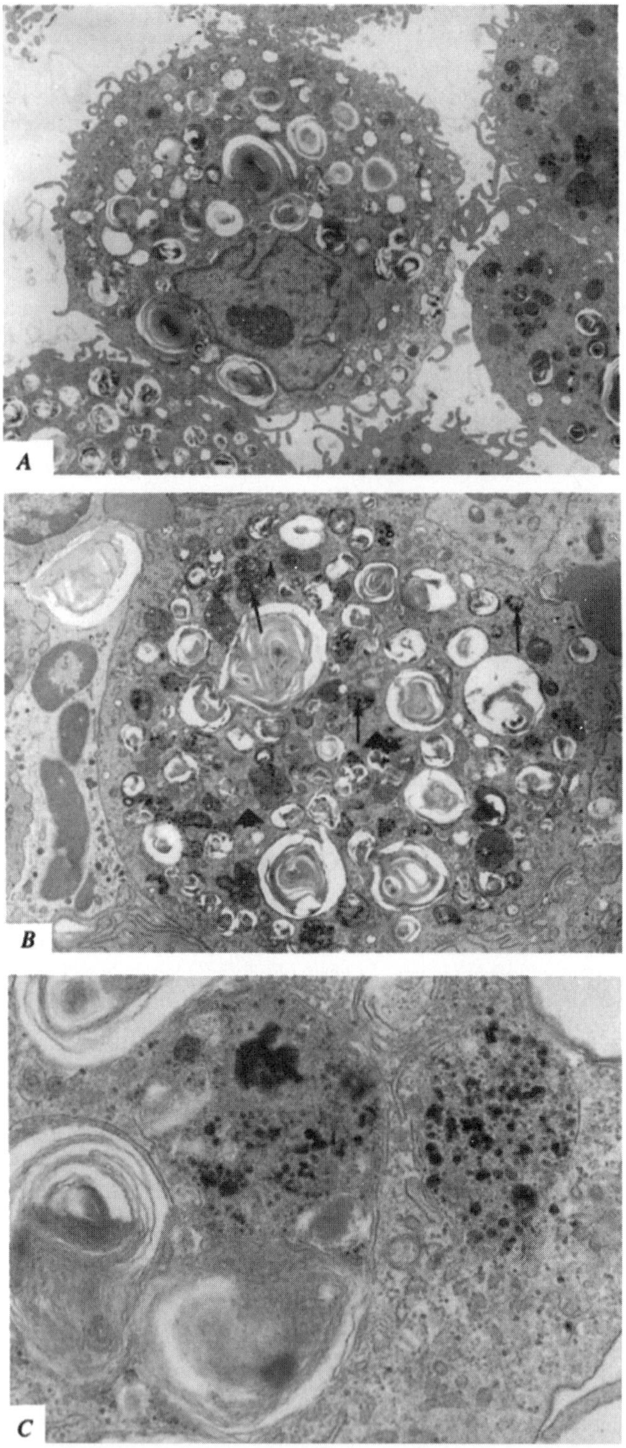

Fig. 192-4 Pulmonary macrophages of patients with LPI. *A*, An electron micrograph shows macrophage containing multilamellar structures and electron-dense bodies that contain iron (magnification ×3100). *B*, The same cell at a greater magnification shows characteristic electron-dense areas which, according to the x-ray spectrum, contained mainly iron (×4600). C. Another pulmonary macrophage containing a number of black-staining, iron-containing precipitations (×27,200). (*From Parto et al.*[79] *Used by permission.*)

(8 of 14).[78] Most of the symptom-free patients (9 of 12) also showed mild abnormalities in perfusion imaging or in pulmonary function tests (8 of 12).

The total cell count in the bronchoalveolar lavage fluid of three adult LPI patients was normal, but two showed markedly increased lymphocyte and decreased macrophage percentages, suggesting alveolar immunoactivation and subclinical alveolitis, as is common in many systemic diseases (Table 192-1).[83] Similar alterations have also been found in lavage fluid of patients with isolated pulmonary alveolar proteinosis.[84] Furthermore, the LPI lavage fluid also contained multilamellar structures of various sizes and shapes, which were absent in control samples. In one patient, the size of macrophages in the lavage fluid was markedly increased, but the size was normal in the others. Macrophages in all patients were filled with multilamellar structures similar to those in type II pneumocytes (Fig. 192-4). The estimated proportional volume of multilamellar structures in pulmonary macrophages was significantly increased, macrophages contained dense inclusions with iron-like material, and the iron content of the cells was elevated (Table 192-1).[63,79] Whether these changes in alveolar macrophages reflect altered iron or phospholipid metabolism in LPI or are a consequence of repeated subclinical pulmonary hemorrhages is unknown. It is possible that increased concentrations of cationic amino acids in the alveolar lining of LPI patients[85,86] may interfere with phospholipid metabolism, change the composition of the surfactant, and lead to the clinical symptoms. Because of their phagocytic nature, normal pulmonary macrophages contain a multitude of inclusions, including round, dense bodies, lamellae, myelin-like figures, and homogeneous lipid-like bodies.[87,88] Multilamellar structures closely resembling those of alveolar macrophages in LPI have been reported in pulmonary alveolar proteinosis associated with other diseases; in abnormalities of phospholipid metabolism; in a silica-induced animal model of alveolar proteinosis; and after experimental use of amphiphilic cationic drugs.[88–91]

Alveolar proteinosis is less common in children than in adults, but the course is usually more aggressive in childhood. Almost 60 pediatric patients with pulmonary alveolar proteinosis have been described, associated in some with alymphoplasia,[92] decreased IgA levels,[93] or various autoimmune diseases.[94,95] It is interesting that there are 10 pairs of siblings with alveolar proteinosis,[93,96–102] suggesting that genetic factors are important or that some of these patients with pulmonary alveolar proteinosis may also have had LPI.

It is apparent that the cascade leading to pulmonary alveolar proteinosis or cholesterol granulomas is part of the symptomatology of LPI. The pathophysiology remains unknown, but the abnormal content of cationic amino acids in the bronchoalveolar lavage fluid of these patients suggests that the transport of cationic amino acids may be abnormal also in the pulmonary alveolar epithelium (Table 192-1).[63,85,86] The transport defect might influence gas exchange or alter the production, composition, or function of surfactant in the alveoli. High-dose prednisolone treatment and bronchoalveolar lavages may slow or prevent disease progression if started early. Thus, all patients and their guardians should be warned of the symptoms.

Two of the patients who died had increased serum creatinine or decreased creatinine clearance values during exacerbation of the symptoms. At autopsy, kidney histology and immunohistochemistry unexpectedly showed immune-mediated glomerulonephritis in all four patients.[63,75] The disease was morphologically classified as diffuse, membranous or mesangial proliferative glomerulonephritis. Histologic findings were similar to those commonly seen in systemic lupus erythematosus. It is interesting that two patients also had onion-skin arteries in spleen tissue, another finding often associated with lupus. The glomeruli were hypercellular, the capillaries were narrowed, and the basement membranes were thickened. The tubules contained granular or homogenous periodic acid-Schiff (PAS)-positive material and, occasionally, calcium crystals. Indirect immunofluorescence studies revealed heavy membranous deposits of IgG, IgM, IgA, complement components C3 and C1q, and immunoglobulin κ and λ light chains in the glomeruli, and electron microscopy revealed large subepithelial and mesangial electron-dense deposits, proliferation of Bowman's epithelium, and tubuloreticular structures in the glomerular endothelial cells. The absence of linear deposition of IgG in glomerular and pulmonary capillaries in all patients and the lack of anti-glomerular basement membrane (anti-GBM) antibodies in the only patient so studied excluded the anti-GBM disease.[103] Other diseases without anti-GBM antibody in which pulmonary hemorrhage and glomerulonephritis have occurred include SLE, Wegener granulomatosis, systemic necrotizing vasculitis, cryoglobulinemia, immune complex-mediated glomerulonephritis, and idiopathic crescentic glomerulonephritis with negative immunofluorescence.[104–107] The recent report by DiRocco and coworkers[51] confirms that renal glomerular involvement in LPI is not uncommon. In their patients, progression of the renal changes (as well as of the pulmonary changes) occurred despite treatment with high-dose prednisone. At this time, there is no known effective treatment of the renal glomerular disease in LPI.

The pediatric patients who died developed symptoms and signs of hepatic insufficiency in the terminal phase of their disease; the liver showed fatty degeneration and mild to severe cirrhosis at autopsy. Excessive amyloid was found in the lymph nodes and spleen. The pancreas showed acinar atrophy and fibrosis, resembling findings in kwashiorkor, and deficiency of cationic amino acids.[77,108] One patient at autopsy had pancreatic necrotizing inflammation, possibly due to shock, terminal pancreatitis,[109] or plugs in pancreatic ducts. However, the possible association of LPI with familial pancreatitis cases is intriguing, as some patients with familial pancreatitis excrete excessive lysine in the urine.[110] Bone marrow was hypercellular at autopsy, but the amount of megakaryocytes was decreased. None of the Finnish patients showed erythroautophagocytosis or erythroblastophagocytosis in the marrow.[20,32,75] Bone specimens showed osteoporosis.

Five adult Finnish patients (age 27 to 49 years) have developed arterial hypertension, and three have hypercholesterolemia (serum cholesterol >9.0 mM), which may represent heterozygous familial cholesterolemia. The one adult Finnish patient who died, died of a cause unrelated to the pulmonary disease.

Other LPI-Associated Features. A few patients with biochemical LPI have had uncommon associated features, which may point to heterogeneity of the syndrome or may be random associations; I have included these patients in the LPI group because of their biochemical identity. A mentally retarded boy with biochemical features typical of LPI showed a peculiar response to phenothiazines, which were prescribed to relieve his hyperactivity.[33] A Japanese 8-year-old girl had a prestage of systemic lupus erythematosus and showed multiple immunologic abnormalities, including impaired function of lymphocyte functioning and the presence of lupus erythematosus cells, antinuclear antibodies, and hypergammaglobulinemia.[31] Interestingly, also, one Finnish patient had systemic lupus erythematosus (see "Complications and Autopsy Findings" above), and another patient had antinuclear antibody-positive rheumatoid arthritis. Two Italian boys with LPI had striking joint hyperextensibility, and three had prominent autophagy of erythroblasts by granulocytes as well as clusters of degenerated erythroblast nuclei in the bone marrow;[20,32,51] autophagy was found also in a patient of Turkish ancestry.[22] The findings in the bone marrow aspirates are interesting and may be a common phenomenon in the disease, but were not found in several Finnish patients studied so far.[35,63,75] The autophagocytosis might be linked with abnormalities in the peripheral red cells of the patients.[35,111] Two Japanese patients with typical LPI findings also had decreased argininosuccinate synthase activity,[45,50] and one patient had glucose 6-phosphate dehydrogenase deficiency.[49]

Other Cationic Aminoacidurias

The proband described by Whelan and Scriver[61] has many clinical features of LPI, including recurrent vomiting during infancy, poor growth, and delayed bone age. The other affected members of the kindred with the dominantly inherited trait were also below the third percentile in height for normals individuals, but they were otherwise healthy. Whelan and Scriver discuss the possibility that

Table 192-1 Cell and Amino Acid Content of Bronchoalveolar Lavage Fluid in Four Adult Patients with Lysinuric Protein Intolerance and in Control Subjects

Case No.	Cell Count × 10^6/liter	Lymphs (%)	Baso (%)	Eos (%)	Polys (%)	Macroph (%)	Eryth (per view)	T_H/T_S	Total Amino Acid Concentration (μ*M*)	Lysine/Total Amino Acids (μmol/μmol)	Arginine/Total Amino Acids (μmol/μmol)	Ornithine/Total Amino Acids (μmol/μmol)	Cross-Sectional Area of Macrophages (mean ± SD)	Volume of Multilamellar Structures/Macrophage Volume	Fe/Cl in Intramacrophage Inclusions
Patients with LPI															
1	77	6	0	3	0	89	>20	1.16	950	55.7	31.8	6.0	128.0 ± 39.9	0.27 ± 0.15	1.63 ± 0.95
2	205	46	1	0	1	52	10	0.96	667	11.7	7.8	3.6			
3	96	59	1	1	0	38	5	0.72	1088	60.8	25.7	9.8	215.4 ± 53.1	0.36 ± 0.10	2.88 ± 5.36
4*	237	3	0	0	0	97	0	1.80	1370	28.5	16.7	5.4	162.8 ± 40.1	0.36 ± 0.11	3.86 ± 2.30
4*	113	18	0	0	0	82	0	1.34	1122	67.6	43.9	4.4			
4*	178	22	0	2	5	71	0	0.65	728	7.8	13.9	5.8			
Mean									905	39.7	14.3	5.8	166.0 ± 57.1	0.32 ± 0.18	2.79 ± 3.48
Control Subjects															
1	821	77	0	0	7	16	0		1370	27.0	17.3	11.8	115.2 ± 32.5	0.09 ± 0.07	0.69 ± 0.98
2	70	5	0	3	3	78	0		761	9.1	0	4.6	112.3 ± 24.7	0.06 ± 0.06	0.27 ± 0.31
3	129	1	0	0	5	93	0		1231	15.4	5.9	5.8	160.3 ± 37.8	0.09 ± 0.05	0.19 ± 0.06
4	165	17	0	3	2	78	0		1232	27.7	15.9	7.2	168.1 ± 35.5	0.02 ± 0.03	0.40 ± 0.15
5	NT	16	0	0	3	81	0		867	10.1	7.2	4.0	138.6 ± 41.9	0.05 ± 0.06	0.48 ± 0.42
Mean									1092	17.9	9.3	6.7	141.1 ± 41.7	0.06 ± 0.06	0.41 ± 0.53

*Bronchoalveolar lavage was performed on one patient with LPI on three separate occasions.

NOTE: NT = not tested; T_H = helper T cells; T_S = suppressor T cells.

SOURCE: From Parto[63] and Parto et al.[79] Used by permission.

the trait was a heterozygous manifestation of the LPI gene or of some other recessive transport disorder. It is interesting that the obligate heterozygotes in the pedigree of Kihara et al.[33] had urinary excretion values similar to those of the subjects with the dominant trait described by Whelan and Scriver,[61] suggesting that the index case might be homozygous for hyperdibasic aminoaciduria type 1. Further pedigrees with the trait of hyperdibasic-aminoaciduria type 1 are needed before firm conclusions concerning this relationship are possible.

In my opinion, the patients described by Kihara et al.,[33] Oyanagi et al.,[24,25] Brown et al.,[23] and others[13,18,20,22,28] have sufficient clinical and biochemical features to be regarded as patients with LPI. The only significant clinical differences are the less marked protein intolerance,[25,28] less significant growth failure,[18,28] and some peculiar features (see below).[20,31–33] We now know that clinical protein tolerance may vary also in LPI, and that vomiting and aversion to high-protein foods are not always prominent in confirmed patients. This variability may depend on the subject's capacity to handle waste nitrogen via other metabolic routes.[112–120] Omura and coworkers[62] described a Japanese 21-month-old girl with severe mental retardation, convulsions, marked growth failure, and clear signs of malnutrition. She excreted excessive lysine in the urine, "but arginine excretion was at the upper limit of normal while ornithine excretion was only slightly increased." Her intestinal absorption of lysine was decreased, but arginine, ornithine, and cystine absorption did not differ from that of control subjects. Fasting blood ammonia and values after loading with cow's milk were normal. LPI cannot with certainty be excluded in this patient, but she likely represents another mutation affecting the transport of the cationic amino acids, and the disease should tentatively be regarded as an entity of its own, best called "isolated lysinuria."

BIOCHEMICAL INVESTIGATIONS

Plasma and Urine Amino Acids

Plasma and urinary amino acid concentrations and the renal clearances of plasma amino acids are given in Table 192-2. Plasma concentrations of lysine, arginine, and ornithine are typically one-third to one-half the normal means values, but occasionally may be well within the normal range.[8,14,19,25,33,35,121] The concentrations of serine, glycine, citrulline, proline, and, especially, alanine and glutamine are increased. The accumulation of amino nitrogen in these pools seems to be a regular feature of LPI. The increase in plasma citrulline is noteworthy.

Urinary excretion and renal clearance of lysine is massively increased, and that of arginine and ornithine is moderately increased. Because of the high plasma concentrations of serine, glycine, citrulline, proline, alanine, and glutamine, they are also found in excess in the urine, but their renal clearances are within the normal range.

In some patients, lysinuria and arginine-ornithinuria have been missed in the thin-layer or paper chromatograms used for screening of inborn errors of metabolism. The reason for the low excretion in these patients has always been that the plasma concentration of the cationic amino acids has been exceptionally low. In such a situation, the molar and relative excretion of the cationic amino acids can be minimal, even though the clearances are high. I have seen this phenomenon a few times in older,

Table 192-2 Plasma Concentration, Urinary Excretion, and Renal Clearance of Free Amino Acids in Patients with Lysinuric Protein Intolerance*

Amino Acid	Plasma Concentration, mM: Range in Normal Children†	Patients with LPI: Mean	Patients with LPI: Range	Urinary excretion (mmol/24 h/1.73 m²): Mean	Urinary excretion: Range	Renal clearance (ml/min/1.73 m²): Mean	Renal clearance: Range
Alanine	0.173–0.305	0.772	0.417–1.017	1.068	0.465–1.586	0.953	0.698–1.324
α-amino-adipic acid	0.002	n.m.		0.609	0.405–0.821		
Arginine	0.023–0.086	0.027	0.012–0.058	0.356	0.076–0.687	11.508	3.175–22.300
Aspartic acid	0.004–0.023	n.m.		n.m.			n.m.
Asparagine and glutamine	0.057–0.467	5.583	3.644–7.161	6.491	4.365–8.542	0.891	0.595–1.628
Citrulline	0.012–0.055‡	0.232	0.141–0.530	0.519	0.155–0.988	1.440	0.762–2.425
Cystine	0.048–0.140‡	0.080	0.057–0.105	0.120	0.059–0.209	0.175	0.050–0.324
Glutamic acid	0.023–0.250	0.049	0.021–0.081	0.047	0.040–0.051	0.853	0.427–0.839
Glycine	0.117–0.223	0.467	0.385–0.530	2.058	1.595–2.808	3.062	2.538–4.067
Histidine	0.024–0.085	0.110	0.084–0.139	0.637	0.155–1.232	4.374	1.184–10.221
Isoleucine	0.028–0.084	0.059	0.029–0.082	0.099	0.071–0.158	1.306	0.598–2.076
Leucine	0.056–0.178	0.090	0.050–0.126	0.101	0.067–0.142	0.830	0.596–1.184
Lysine	0.071–0.151	0.070	0.032–0.179	4.126	1.022–7.000	25.655	11.116–45.877
Methionine	0.011–0.016	0.032	0.021–0.048	0.050	0.038–0.063	1.356	0.976–2.044
Ornithine	0.027–0.086	0.021	0.002–0.083	0.106	0.091–0.134	3.268	2.709–5.357
Phenylalanine	0.026–0.061	0.049	0.033–0.084	0.078	0.056–0.094	1.268	0.574–1.966
Proline	0.068–0.148	0.189	0.158–0.268	n.m.			n.m.
Serine	0.079–0.112	0.251	0.199–0.246	0.607	0.398–0.878	1.900	1.257–2.628
Threonine	0.042–0.095	0.113	0.030–0.172	0.277	0.111–0.554	1.825	1.235–2.578
Tyrosine	0.031–0.071	0.047	0.030–0.072	0.142	0.125–0.158	2.361	1.202–3.688
Valine	0.128–0.283	0.182	0.132–0.244	0.047	0.035–0.059	0.177	0.167–0.186

*The plasma concentrations were measured after an overnight fast, and the respective 24-h urines were collected when the patients were on a self-chosen hospital diet. The clearance values are calculated from the 24-h urinary excretion and from the fasting plasma concentration. Plasma lysine, arginine, and ornithine concentrations were measured on 33 occasions in 20 patients; the other values are from four patients.

†From Dickenson et al.[278]

‡From Scriver and Davies[279]

NOTE: n.m. = not measurable

SOURCE: From Simell et al.[35] Used by permission.

undiagnosed patients who have spontaneously restricted their protein intake to the extreme, and who also have had clear signs of protein malnutrition. When protein intake has been increased, cationic aminoaciduria has become as prominent as in other patients.

The reabsorption defect in kidney tubules is most marked for lysine; arginine is less affected; and ornithine is absorbed best.[121] The measurements of tubular reabsorption of lysine have in some urine collections suggested net secretion. The reabsorption defect for arginine and ornithine and presumably for lysine remains significant also when plasma concentrations of these amino acids are increased, but at extremely high filtered loads, when plasma concentrations are several millimolars, the tubular reabsorption of arginine and ornithine reabsorption resembles normal. At these very high filtered loads, selective transport probably becomes unimportant and physical diffusion phenomena determine the rate of absorption. A significant increase in plasma concentration and, consequently, in the filtered load of one cationic amino acid leads easily to net tubular secretion of the other two cationic amino acids.

Blood Ammonia, Urinary Orotic Acid Excretion, and Serum Urea

Blood ammonium concentration is normal (<70 μM) during fasting, but is elevated (100 to 560 μM) after regular meals.[8,35] The extent of postprandial hyperammonemia depends on the protein content of the meal. The ammonia values usually return to the normal range 2 to 6 h later. Frequent ingestion of high-protein foods, extensive fasting, acute infections (especially gastroenteritis), and severe physical or psychologic stress increase blood ammonia in the patients and easily cause persisting hyperammonemia, which does not disappear during fasting.

Urinary orotic acid is increased more frequently than blood ammonia, suggesting that orotic acid is a better indicator of urea cycle failure in these patients than hyperammonemia.[13,46,122–125] Urine samples collected during fasting frequently contain normal amounts of orotic acid (<0.03 μmol/kg/h, or <11 μmol/mmol creatinine), but values are increased even during a self-chosen low-protein diet (geometric mean, 0.52; range 0.05 to 3.77 μmol/kg/h in 24-h pooled urine samples) and increase massively if the protein intake is increased.[122] Nitrogen loads given in the form of cow's milk protein (0.5 g/kg), ammonium lactate (2.5 mmol/kg) or intravenous alanine (6.6 mmol/kg during 90 min) can be given without clinical risk to the patients. In healthy subjects, blood ammonia is stable after such loads, but blood ammonia and certainly urinary orotic acid excretion increase in the patients (geometric mean and range in the patients: 4.93; 1.61 to 11.19 μmol/kg/h in 4- to 6-h pooled urine; 0.61; 0.10 to 7.22 in 1.5-h urine; and 3.32; 0.30 to 11.73 in 6-h urine after the three loads, respectively). Another advantage in orotic acid measurement is the stability of the compound: Urine samples can be sent via post at room temperature for orotic acid measurement, but blood ammonia has to be measured immediately.[46,122]

Serum urea concentration has been high-normal or even slightly elevated during the first few months of life, but later it has been consistently below the normal mean and often subnormal, the mean of 126 determinations in the patients being 3.7 μM (range, 1.5 to 8.5 μM; normal, 2 to 7 μM).[35] Serum urea increases slowly after nitrogen loading in the patients.[8,35]

Other Laboratory Tests

Slight normochromic or hypochromic anemia with anisocytosis and poikilocytosis is common.[8,35,63,75,111] Most patients have leukopenia, and the platelet count is decreased, in some young patients not uncommonly to less than $30 \times 10^3/m^3$. Reticulocyte count is often slightly elevated, and the osmotic resistance of the erythrocytes, the red cell indexes, and the serum iron level and iron binding capacity are normal. In some patients, autoerythrophagocytosis or erythroblastophagocytosis has been observed in the bone marrow,[20,22,32,51] and the number of megakaryocytes may be increased; in one patient the marrow was hypoplastic with pathologic megaloblastic erythrocyte precursor forms, and in another the marrow was dyserythropoetic, suggesting ineffective erythropoesis.[75] It is interesting that the changes in the peripheral blood cells decrease in intensity during and after puberty, and values in adults are usually within the range of healthy subjects.

The blood pH and the serum concentrations of sodium, potassium, chloride, calcium, and phosphate are normal. Serum low-density lipoprotein (LDL) and high-density lipoprotein (HDL) cholesterol values are often high in older children and adults, probably because the patients replace a large part of their protein calories by fat in the diet. In animals, high orotic acid concentrations influence lipoprotein metabolism,[126] but the possible link between orotic acidemia and hyperlipidemia in LPI is unclear. The triglycerides are usually slightly elevated in the patients. No constant abnormal peaks have been found in analyses of organic acids in the urine.

Interestingly, several of the patients with different ethnic backgrounds and all the Finnish patients have consistently had significantly increased concentrations of lactate dehydrogenase (LDH) and ferritin in serum.[22,35,127] All LDH isoenzymes, but most significantly the liver isoenzyme, are affected; the values are usually two to five times higher than the upper limit of normal. The LDH and ferritin values increase further during complications of the disease, including pulmonary alveolar proteinosis (see "Complications and Autopsy Findings" above). Thyroxine-binding globulin (TBG) is also elevated in the patients, and, consequently, measurements of total T_4 give high values; free T_4 is normal, and the patients are clinically euthyroid.[34,35,128,129] Whether there is a general increase in hormone carrier proteins or only a specific increase in TBG is not known.

In two Japanese patients, growth hormone responsiveness to glucagon, propranolol, arginine, and insulin was studied as a possible cause for the delayed growth and bone age of the patients.[34] The response to insulin was moderately decreased in the one patient studied before arginine supplementation was started, but all responses were normal when the patients had been on arginine supplementation for 8 months.

Kekomäki and coworkers[130] confirmed that the activities of the urea cycle enzymes in liver biopsy samples of the patients were normal. Glutaminase I activity, once suggested to be the basic defect in patients with LPI,[16,21,29] has since been proven to be normal in both leukocytes and liver.[131] Likewise, the activity of ornithine aminotransferase, the enzyme responsible for the main catabolic pathway of ornithine, has been normal or slightly elevated in the liver and cultured fibroblasts of the patients.[57,132,133] The concentration of *N*-acetylglutamine and the rate of its synthesis have not been measured in the patients, but the efficient production of orotic acid by the patients[13,22,122,134] strongly suggests that this cofactor and regulator of the carbamyl phosphate synthase activity[135] is available in sufficient quantities.

PATHOPHYSIOLOGY

Normal Cellular Transport of Cationic Amino Acids

In normal physiology, cationic and other amino acids reach the body only by passing through the intestinal wall in the process of absorption. They do this mainly as free amino acids but also partly as dipeptides and other small peptides, which then are hydrolyzed to free amino acids at the luminal brush border and, predominantly, in the cytoplasm of the epithelial cells.[136–141] During absorption, the amino acids first cross the luminal membrane of the epithelial cell. A fraction of the amino acids is used in cellular metabolism in the cytoplasm ("metabolic runout"),[142,143] and the remainder must cross the basolateral (antiluminal) membrane of the cell to reach the body. In the cytoplasm, the amino acids may also enter the subcellular organelles (mitochondria, lysosomes, other vesicles, etc.), where some amino acids are metabolized. In adult intestine, only free amino acids, not peptides, are able to cross the whole cell in absorption.

Absorption of the cationic amino acids lysine, arginine, and ornithine has been extensively studied in the kidneys,[136,144–157] intestine,[158–160] and some parenchymal tissues[161–163] of animals and human beings. Most studies have included cyst(e)ine, because in cystinuria the transport of all four amino acids is affected.[148,158,164–179] In the kidney, reabsorption occurs along the full length of the nephron. The proximal segment of the tubule receives the highest load of filtered amino acids and, consequently, has to absorb a significant load quickly and efficiently, whereas further down in the tubule a more selective reabsorption system would be more profitable. Such axial heterogeneity[143,180] in absorption has indeed been demonstrated for several amino acids, including the cationic amino acids. The net handling of the cationic amino acids in the kidney and their mutual interactions have been studied by administering amino acid loads and then measuring the urinary excretion and renal clearances of the amino acids.[170,171,174,181–183] Microperfusions of animal nephrons[149,153,177,178] and flux measurements in nephron segments or tubule fragments,[149,150,166,184] in renal cortical slices,[148,151,152,166] in cultured tubule-cells,[185] and in isolated vesicles prepared from the brush border[146,155,172,186,187] or basolateral cell membrane[157] have been performed. The transport of the cationic amino acids across the luminal membrane occurs via a shared, Na^+-dependent system. The system selective for the cationic amino acids in the proximal convoluted tubule has high capacity and low affinity,[150] whereas the system in the proximal straight segment has low capacity and high affinity and is shared with cystine.[149]

At the basolateral membrane in the kidney tubules, the transport of the cationic amino acids is not shared with cystine, and both high- and low-affinity systems are used. The transport from the cell to the pericellular space (efflux) occurs via Na^+-independent exchange diffusion, which may be shared with cystine on the cytoplasmic surface.[143,157,166]

At the brush border of the intestinal epithelium, the cationic amino acids are transported by a single Na^+-dependent system, which has high affinity and is shared by all cationic amino acids and cystine.[188,189]

White and Christensen[162] and others[161,168,185,190] have carefully characterized transport of cationic amino acids in cultured or isolated cells using human fibroblasts,[161,168,191] permanent hepatoma cell lines, rat hepatocytes,[162] and other cells.[185,190] Transport of cationic amino acid into human fibroblasts occurs by a saturable mediation, which they designated "system y^+" (earlier called Ly^+). The system serves the flow of ω-guanidino amino acids and ω, α-diamino acids. The uptake of cationic substrates by system y^+ is Na^+-independent, pH-insensitive, stereoselective, and inhibitable by neutral amino acids in the presence of Na^+ ion. This system is not shared with cystine.[164,168] The uptake and efflux of the substrates are strongly stimulated by cationic amino acids inside and outside the cell, respectively. Arginine and homoarginine accumulate in human fibroblasts and can reach distribution ratios of more than 20 at physiological external amino acid concentrations.[161] The driving force appears to be the transmembrane voltage.

In hepatoma cell lines, the transport of cationic amino acids occurs by the saturable mediation of the system y^+.[162] The influx into hepatoma cells has all the characteristics seen also in the system y^+ of the fibroblasts, including strong stimulation by cationic amino acids inside the cell, that is *trans*-stimulation. In normal hepatocytes, no significant *trans*-stimulation was observed, suggesting that the y^+ system is absent in these cells. The rate at which arginine is transported at the hepatocyte plasma membrane suggests that transport is the rate-limiting step in hydrolysis of arginine by arginase.

Recently, a more detailed analysis of amino acid transport at diverse cellular membranes has led to the discovery of at least three separate transport systems for the cationic amino acids. Furthermore, direct studies of some cationic amino acid transport proteins has become possible after cloning of the respective genes (see "Genetics" below).

Mutations in the Transport of Cationic Amino Acids

In a long series of studies, Segal and coworkers,[176] States and coworkers,[185] and others[160,164,165,169–175,192] have analyzed the interactions of the cationic amino acids and cystine in transport mutations, especially in the cystinuric kidney (see Chap. 191). Scriver and coworkers have provided a detailed review of current knowledge of the transport mutations in cystinuria and other cationic aminoacidurias.[143]

In classic cystinuria, reabsorption of cystine and the cationic amino acids in the kidney tubules is selectively impaired, occasionally to the extent that measurements show net tubular secretion of cystine or lysine.[154,193] In normal tubules, cystine, lysine, arginine, and ornithine mutually compete for transport. Intravenous loading studies in cystinuria suggest that the residual reclamation of cationic amino acids and cystine follows rules of competition similar to those in the normal tubules.[169,174] An absorption defect has also been found in the intestinal epithelium in vivo[175] and in biopsy samples of the jejunum.[158,160] Measurement of unidirectional and net fluxes of cationic amino acids in intestinal biopsy samples of patients with cystinuria clearly shows that the transport defect is localized at the luminal membrane of the epithelial cells.[188] Most likely, the efflux permeability of the luminal membrane is increased, but the influx is normal.[189]

Is the transport defect in patients with LPI similar to that in cystinuria? In their first report on LPI, Perheentupa and Visakorpi[1] had access only to semiquantitative measurement of plasma and urinary amino acids, and they regarded the urinary amino acid excretion as identical to that in cystinuria. It soon became apparent that cystine was excreted in significantly smaller quantities than in cystinuria, and Kekomäki and coworkers[6,8] suggested that the mechanisms of the transport defects differ in the two diseases. Absorption of the cationic amino acids by the kidneys[10,15,25,121,156] and small intestine[9,23,24,33,55,194–196] in LPI has later been carefully characterized. In both organs, absorption of lysine, arginine, and ornithine is defective. The slight increase in renal cystine losses could be explained by the excessive tubular lysine load and normal competition for absorption in the kidney tubules. Oral loading with the dipeptide lysylglycine increased plasma glycine concentrations properly, but plasma lysine remained almost unchanged in the patients[55] (Fig. 192-5). This was in striking contrast to the control subjects, in whom concentrations of both amino acids of the dipeptide increased in plasma. LPI was thus the first human disease in which a defect in peptide absorption was recognized. Because the transport of

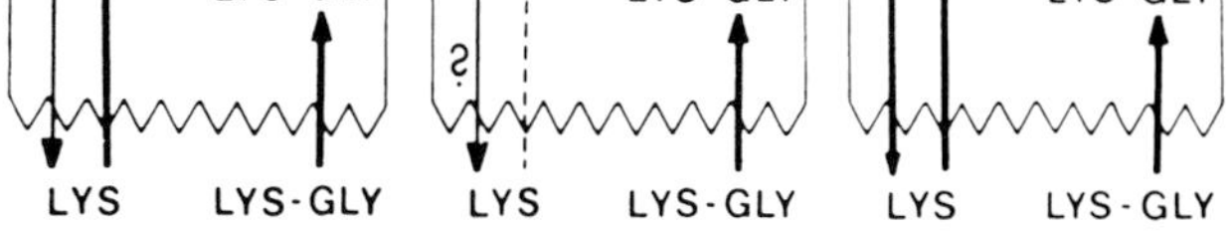

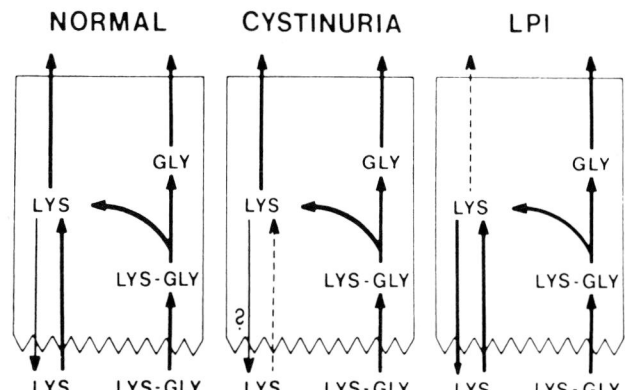

Fig. 192-5 Representation of brush border cells of jejunal mucosa, showing absorption of diamino acids (here lysine, in free and dipeptide form) and suggested sites of defect in cystinuria and LPI. Defective fluxes are indicated by dashed arrows. LYS = lysine. (*From Rajantie et al.*[55] *Used by permission.*)

oligopeptides is not shared with transport of free amino acids at the luminal membrane of the enterocyte, the lysine-containing dipeptide enters the cell normally in LPI. The absorbed peptides are hydrolyzed to free amino acids mainly in the cytoplasm of the enterocyte,[137,138,197] and they are able to cross the basolateral membrane only as free amino acids. The missing increase in plasma lysine after the lysylglycine load but normal increase in plasma glycine shows that the intracellularly released dipeptide-derived lysine is unable to cross the basolateral (antiluminal) membrane of the enterocyte and strongly suggests that the transport defect in LPI is localized at this membrane in the epithelia cells.

In vitro studies of unidirectional and net transport of cationic amino acids in jejunal biopsy samples of the patients soon proved even more directly that the transport defect is situated at the basolateral (antiluminal) membrane of the epithelial cell.[57] These in vitro results differed clearly from identical experiments in cystinuria,[189] where the abnormality in lysine transport was located at the luminal membrane, and the defect in cystine absorption could perhaps best be explained by increased efflux permeability at the luminal membrane of the epithelium. Interestingly, in an earlier study of cationic amino acid accumulation in jejunal biopsy samples and uptake during intestinal perfusion in LPI, no defects could be found.[194] This failure is understandable now, when the defect in LPI has been localized at the antiluminal membrane, and we know that the epithelial cells in LPI accumulate higher-than-normal concentrations of the cationic amino acids (see below).

Rajantie and coworkers[56] gave patients with LPI prolonged intravenous infusions of citrulline and measured plasma and urinary amino acids during the loading. Compared with controls, the plasma citrulline concentration of the patients increased normally, but urinary citrulline excretion increased excessively. Rises in plasma arginine and ornithine during the loading were subnormal, but massive argininuria and moderate ornithinuria appeared (Fig. 192-6). The excretion rates of lysine and other amino acids remained practically unaltered, thus excluding mutual competition as the cause for the increases. This finding is compatible with a transport defect at the basolateral membrane of the renal tubule cells and can be explained as follows: Citrulline as a neutral amino acid does not use the cationic amino acid transport system; citrulline is partly converted to arginine and further to ornithine in the tubule cell as an integral part of the reabsorption process; in LPI, formed arginine and ornithine are unable to exit at the antiluminal membrane, their intracellular concentrations increase, and backflux (argininuria and ornithinuria) into the lumen occurs; high intracellular arginine and ornithine concentrations inhibit citrulline metabolism in the tubule cell; intracellular citrulline concentration increases, and leads to citrullinuria.

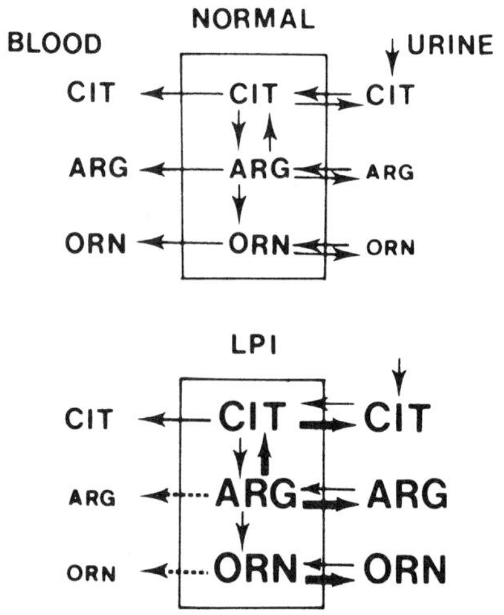

Fig. 192-6 Suggested mechanism of tubular reabsorption of citrulline in human beings and of the pathophysiology of the massive argininuria and moderate citrullinuria and ornithinuria in LPI. Bold type and arrows indicate increased concentrations and fluxes; thin type and dotted arrows indicate decreased concentrations and impaired fluxes. (*From Rajantie et al.*[56] *Used by permission.*)

Table 192-3 Steady State Amino Acid Concentrations in Intact Cultured Fibroblasts of a Control Subject and a Patient with Lysinuric Protein Intolerance

	Concentration Ratio	
Amino Acid	Control	LPI
Lysine/alanine	0.23 ± 0.007	0.35 ± 0.014
Ornithine/alanine	0.11 ± 0.009	0.19 ± 0.008
Arginine/alanine	0.40 ± 0.024	0.54 ± 0.012
Leucine/alanine	0.30 ± 0.016	0.31 ± 0.015

NOTE: Human skin fibroblasts were maintained in culture medium 24 h prior to harvest with a rubber policeman. Cells were resuspended in 1 ml phosphate-buffered saline, sonicated, and deproteinized. The supernatants were assayed for amino acid content with a Durrum D-500 amino acid analyzer. Values are the mean ± SEM, $n = 4$. Amino acid values were normalized to fibroblast alanine concentrations, which were 18 ± 1.3 and 17 ± 1.2 pmol/mg protein in control and LPI cells, respectively.

Reabsorption curves for arginine and ornithine have been produced in patients with LPI by increasing the plasma concentration of arginine or ornithine in a stepwise manner and simultaneously measuring tubular filtration rate and plasma concentration and urinary excretion of the two amino acids.[121] The curves were clearly below those of healthy control subjects at all loads except at values close to the tubular reabsorption maxima of the controls, where the patients' curves approached those of the control subjects. It is possible that at such filtered loads (at plasma concentrations of several millimolars), active transport plays a minor part, and physical factors regulate the amount of reabsorption. The extrarenal metabolic clearances of arginine and ornithine by tissues, calculated from the same infusion experiments, were significantly decreased in the patients.[198] This finding suggests that besides the defect in epithelial transport, transport in LPI is abnormal in other tissues as well.[190]

A direct proof of such an extraepithelial transport defect was obtained in studies of Smith and coworkers,[58] who investigated steady-state amino acid concentrations in intact fibroblasts (Table 192-3), and influx (Figs. 192-7 and 192-8), efflux, and trans-stimulation of the transport of lysine and other cationic amino acids and their nonmetabolized analogues[199] in cultured fibroblasts of the patients (Fig. 192-9). In *trans*-stimulation experiments, the amino acid in question, or another amino acid which uses the same transport system, is present on the other side of the membrane than the labeled amino studied. The influx at the plasma membrane was not different from controls in LPI; *trans*-stimulated efflux was. A defect in *trans*-stimulation was found also in fibroblasts of the heterozygotes with values about 50 percent of that in homozygotes suggesting gene-dosage effect (Fig. 192-10). The results also imply that the basolateral membrane of epithelial cells and the plasma membrane of parenchymal cells are functionally analogous at least in transport of cationic amino acids, but it may well be that this analogy is a general physiological principle. Vesicles prepared from LPI fibroblast plasma membranes failed to show a transport defect for cationic amino acids.[200] This finding possibly is explained by the fact that the preparation of the vesicles favored equally formation of inside-out and right-side-out vesicles. If both forms are present in equal quantities, and the defect is only expressed in efflux, the sum effect in the mixture of the vesicles will be the same as in controls.

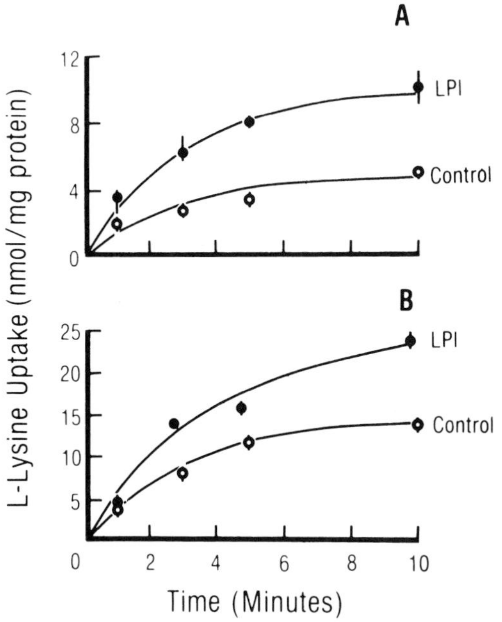

Fig. 192-7 L-Lysine uptake by cultured fibroblasts from a control subject (open circles) and a patient with LPI (solid circles). The cells were incubated for 90 min at 37°C in buffer without arginine (*A*) or in buffer containing 1 mM arginine (*B*), washed twice with PBS (37°C), and then incubated for 1, 3, 5, or 10 min at 37°C in PBS containing 0.1 mM L-[^{3}H]lysine. Data are means and ranges of two or three measurements. (*From Smith et al.*[58] *Used by permission.*)

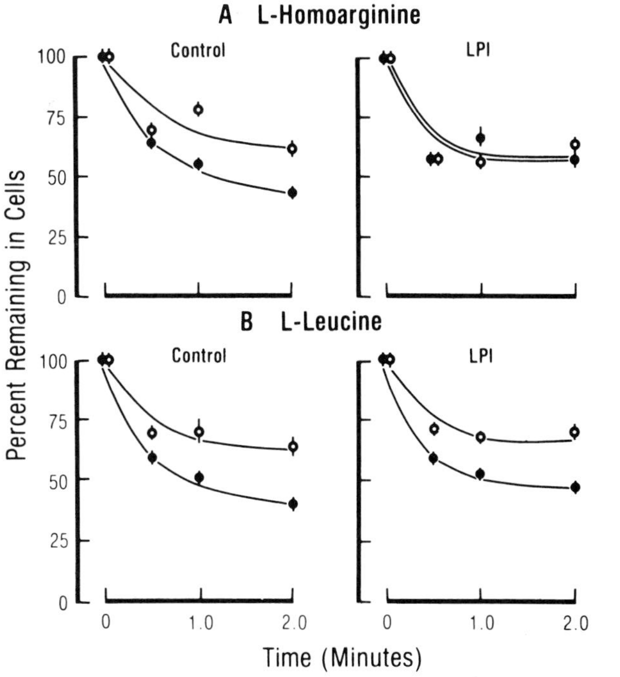

Fig. 192-9 Efflux of L-homoarginine from cultured skin fibroblasts of a control and LPI cell line. The cells were incubated for 40 min at 37°C in buffer containing (*A*) 0.1 mM L-[^{3}H]homoarginine and (*B*) 0.1 mM L-[^{14}C]leucine. The time course of efflux was measured into unlabeled incubation buffer (*trans*-zero condition, open circles) or into buffer containing 1 mM unlabeled amino acid (*trans*-stimulated condition, solid circles). Time course for efflux from the cellular pool is shown. Zero-time homoarginine content (100 percent value) was 2.8 ± 0.16 (control) and 2.9 ± 0.29 (LPI) nmol/mg protein; zero-time leucine content was 8.5 ± 0.37 (control) and 9.8 ± 0.59 (LPI) nmol/mg protein. The difference in the zero-time leucine content for LPI and control cells was not significant. Each point represents the mean and SEM of four determinations. (*From Smith et al.*[58] *Used by permission.*)

Smith and others[201] measured transport of the cationic amino acids and their nonmetabolized analogues in isolated erythrocytes of the patients. The mutant erythrocytes had identical transport characteristics with the controls, and the authors concluded that the mutant transporter is not expressed on the surface of mature human erythrocytes. The findings are in agreement with those of Gardner and Levy,[202] who noticed that the transport of dibasic amino acids in human erythrocytes is temperature-dependent, incapable of uphill transport, and not dependent on extracellular sodium or potassium concentrations or on energy derived from cellular metabolism. They further stated that lysine transport in human erythrocytes comprises two saturable, carrier-mediated processes operating in parallel: One is a high-affinity, low-capacity process that predominates at low lysine concentrations; the other is a low-affinity, high-capacity process that predominates at higher lysine concentrations. Further studies on cationic amino acid

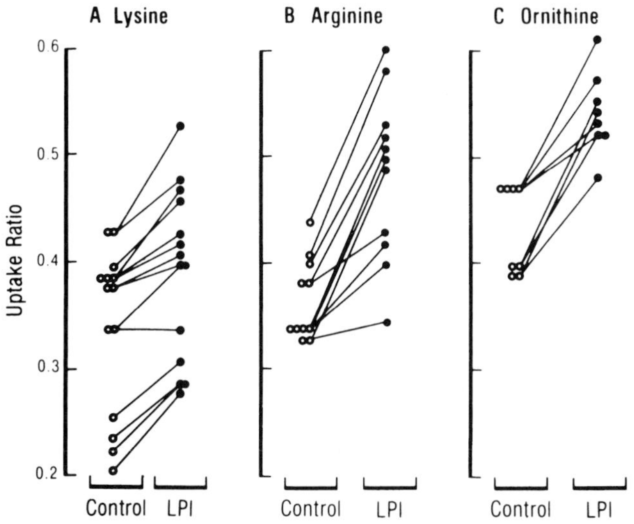

Fig. 192-8 Uptake ratios of the cationic amino acids versus L-leucine at steady state in cultured fibroblasts of control subjects and patients with lysinuric protein intolerance. The cells were incubated for 10 min at 37°C in PBS containing 0.1 mM L-[^{3}H]leucine and (*A*) 0.1 mM L-[^{14}C]lysine, (*B*) L-[^{14}C]arginine, or (*C*) L-[^{14}C]ornithine. Each point represents a single measurement of the net isotopic molar uptake ratio (cationic amino acid/leucine) in paired control and LPI cell strains. The differences between control and LPI cells for uptake of L-lysine (n = 13, p < 0.02), L-arginine (n = 16, p < 0.01), and L-ornithine (n = 8, p < 0.01) are significant by the Wilcoxon signed rank tests. (*From Smith et al.*[58] *Used by permission.*)

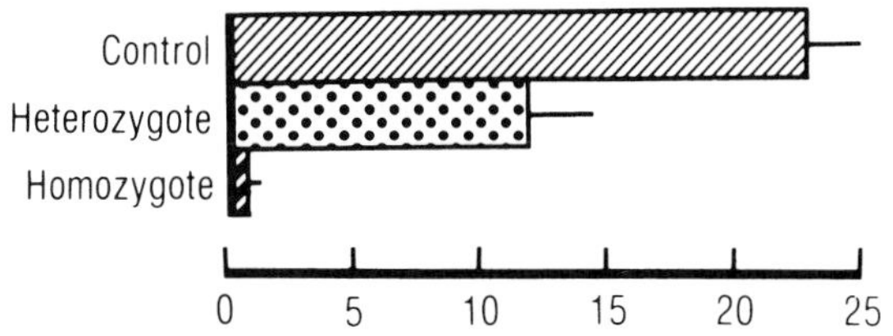

Fig. 192-10 Percent trans-stimulation of homoarginine efflux from cultured skin fibroblasts of control cells and cells from homozygotes and heterozygotes for LPI. The cells were preincubated for 40 min at 37°C in buffer containing 0.1 mM L-[^{3}H]homoarginine and 0.1 mM L-[^{14}C]leucine. The 1-min efflux of label was measured as described in Fig. 192-9. "*Trans*-stimulation" refers to the difference (increase) between *trans*-zero and *trans*-stimulated efflux, normalized to zero-time cellular isotope. Each value represents the mean of three or four determinations on one cell line; error bars indicate the range. (*From Smith et al.*[58] *Used by permission.*)

transport in rabbit reticulocytes[203] and human erythrocytes[204] have clarified details of the transport phenomena in these specialized cells.

Subcellular Transport of Cationic Amino Acids

In the urea cycle, the urea molecule is assembled on an ornithine backbone; cleavage of the urea from arginine regenerates free ornithine. During the cycle, ornithine has to pass from the cytoplasm into the mitochondrial matrix to be carbamylated, and the formed citrulline has to be exported back to the cytoplasm to be further exposed by the enzyme argininosuccinic acid synthase. Whether or not mitochondrial transport processes are involved in the pathophysiology of LPI remains an open question.[205] In rat liver mitochondria and in mitochondria of human cultured fibroblasts, ornithine and citrulline transport has been relatively well characterized. In the classic study of Gamble and Lehninger,[206] the entry of ornithine into the mitochondria of rat liver was mediated by a carrier that was respiratory-dependent and required permeant proton-yielding anions for function.

Ornithine fluxes in mitochondria were earlier measured in the absence of active citrulline synthesis.[207–218] The study of Cohen and coworkers[213] avoided this pitfall: They analyzed the transport phenomena during and without citrulline synthesis in respiring rat liver mitochondria. They were able to characterize both influx of ornithine and efflux of citrulline in the mitochondria. When respiring mitochondria were preloaded with cold ornithine and then incubated in [^{3}H]ornithine, the mitochondria produced citrulline of the same specific activity as that of external ornithine, but ornithine in mitochondrial matrix remained unlabeled. The concentration of ornithine in the matrix was also extremely low when the ornithine concentration in the incubation medium was less than 1 mM. Both findings imply that the ornithine molecule is not transported into the matrix randomly, but is channeled to the intramitochondrial enzymes for further processing to citrulline. The importance of ornithine catabolism by the matrix enzyme ornithine aminotransferase for the net movement of ornithine has remained unclear, but the activity in liver mitochondria is such that all ornithine not immediately used in the urea cycle is transaminated (see Chap. 85).

Studies of citrulline transport in rat liver mitochondria have suggested that the transport mechanisms do not depend on respiratory energy or the presence of permeant cations or anions.[206,212,213] Citrulline transport occurs in liver mitochondria but not in mitochondria of the heart.[206] Some studies have also implied that an ornithine-citrulline antiporter exists in the mitochondrial membrane,[210] but this finding may have been an artifact caused by experimental circumstances in which citrulline was not formed.[211,213]

Recently, increasing evidence has accumulated suggesting that mitochondrial ornithine transport is genetically altered in another human urea cycle disease, the hyperornithinemia-hyperammonemia-homocitrullinuria (HHH) syndrome[112,215,216,218–226] (see Chap. 83). If the plasma membranes of cultured fibroblasts are made permeable to amino acids by digitonin, accumulation of labeled ornithine can be measured in the particulate fraction of the cells, which mainly contains mitochondria.[223,224] Such studies have suggested that ornithine accumulation in mitochondria is decreased in fibroblasts and liver of patients with the HHH syndrome.[220,221,223,224,227] If cultured HHH fibroblasts are incubated with labeled ornithine, a subnormal fraction of label is found in CO_2, implying that ornithine is unable to enter the mitochondria to be further metabolized.[215,216,218–221,225,227]

A mitochondrial transport defect also has been proposed to have a part in the pathophysiology of LPI.[205] This theory has been based on biochemical results that speak against cytoplasmic ornithine deficiency in this disease. First, biopsy samples from the intestinal epithelium accumulate higher-than-normal concentrations of the cationic amino acids in vitro.[57] Second, LPI fibroblasts also accumulate higher-than-normal concentrations of cationic amino acids.[58,59] Third, direct measurements of concentrations

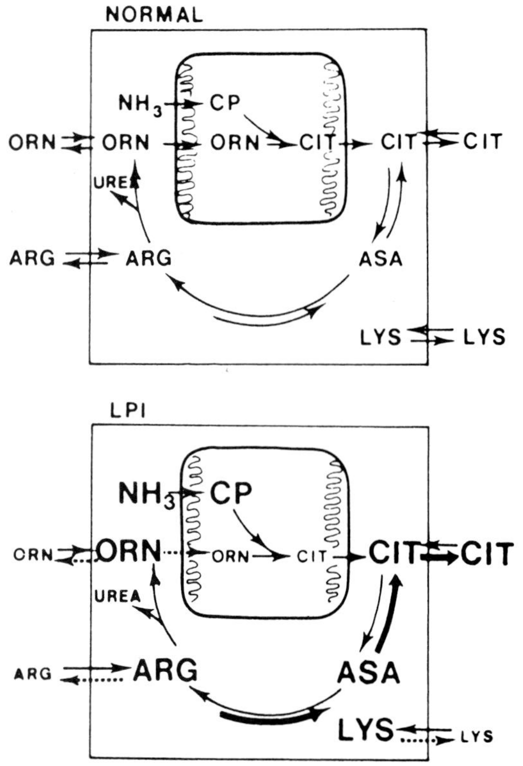

Fig. 192-11 Hypothetical mechanism of the elevated plasma citrulline concentration and the urea cycle failure in LPI. Bold type and arrows indicate supranormal concentrations and fluxes; thin type and dotted arrows, subnormal concentrations and impaired fluxes. For simplicity, only those fluxes are shown that are present at the "basolateral" and mitochondrial membranes of the liver cells. (*From Rajantie et al.*[205] *Used by permission.*)

of the cationic amino acids in liver biopsy samples of the patients contain normal or elevated concentrations of the cationic amino acids, even though their plasma concentrations are decreased.[24,205] Fourth, there is evidence that citrulline formation is not impaired: Plasma concentration of citrulline is constantly high-normal or elevated in the patients;[8,30,31,34,35] citrulline concentration is high-normal or increased in liver biopsy samples of the patients;[24,205] and the extrarenal metabolic clearance of citrulline and conversion of citrulline to arginine and ornithine are retarded[54,205] (Fig. 192-11).

These conflicting findings have been reconciled in a hypothesis which suggests that in LPI a defect in the efflux of the cationic amino acids exists at the plasma membrane of the liver cells or, if the cells retain polarity, at the basolateral membrane, and that the transport defect is expressed also in the mitochondria.[205] Such a mitochondrial defect would further increase cytoplasmic concentrations of arginine and ornithine. Depletion of ornithine in the mitochondria would lead to accumulation of carbamyl phosphate and to hyperammonemia. This theory, though interesting, has recently been questioned because the oxidation of ornithine in cultured LPI fibroblasts proceeds normally.[59]

System y^+ for the cationic amino acids is expressed on the lysosomal membranes and used at least for influx of the cationic amino acids.[228] Normal lysosomes have active and selective efflux mechanisms for cystine, sialic acid, and probably other substances[229–234] (see Chap. 199). Efflux of other amino acids from the lysosomes is strictly limited as is suggested by the disruption of rat liver lysosomes if they are filled by passive diffusion with amino acid methyl esters.[234] These esters are hydrolyzed by lysosomal enzymes, but the liberated amino acids cannot readily escape from the lysosomes, possibly because of their high polarity. They accumulate in the lysosomes and may cause osmotic lysis of the organelles. In LPI, the lysosomes or other vesicular organelles might function as a metabolically excluded pool of lysine and other cationic amino acids, so that the actual cytoplasmic lysine concentration would be relatively normal or even low. No direct proof of such a transport defect has been obtained, but the hypothesis is attractive.

Malfunction of the Urea Cycle

Patients with LPI have decreased nitrogen tolerance and exhibit hyperammonemia after ingestion of even moderate amounts of protein.[8,11,14,35,75,122] The urea cycle failure is clearly less severe than in the "first" enzyme defects of the cycle, that is, in deficiencies of carbamyl phosphate synthase, ornithine transcarbamylase, and *N*-acetylglutamate synthase, or even in a deficiency of argininosuccinate synthase or lyase (see Chap. 85). The clinical impression is that the tendency to hyperammonemia in LPI closely resembles that seen in patients with the HHH syndrome.[112,219,221–223,226]

Already in the first description of the disease, Perheentupa and Visakorpi[1] noticed that intravenous infusion of ornithine during a loading with protein or intravenous L-alanine prevented the hyperammonemia that otherwise followed the loadings. An identical effect has since been shown with arginine and citrulline when given intravenously.[8,11,14,35,123,195]

Oral supplementation with arginine and ornithine has been only minimally effective in these patients, because both amino acids are poorly absorbed from the intestine and easily produce diarrhea.[10,57,196,235] Obviously the absorption defect is not total because a low-protein diet and arginine or ornithine supplementation have improved growth and decreased hyperammonemia in patients with LPI.[6–8,13,17,28,32,63] A few variant patients tolerate arginine or ornithine supplementation well.[13,17,28,32] Awrich et al.[14] showed that the neutral amino acid citrulline, also an intermediate in the urea cycle, when taken as an oral supplement prevents hyperammonemia. It is well tolerated by LPI patients,[11,30] and its effect of preventing hyperammonemia in LPI has now been well documented.[61,122] As a neutral amino acid, it passes the cell membranes normally in LPI and is rapidly converted in the body to arginine and then to ornithine.

Poor intestinal absorption, excessive loss in the urine, and low plasma concentrations of the cationic amino acids arginine and ornithine strongly suggest that the malfunctioning of the urea cycle is caused by deficiencies of these urea cycle intermediates (Fig. 192-1). The finding that hyperammonemia produced by amino nitrogen or protein loads could effectively be prevented by simultaneous intravenous infusion of arginine or ornithine led to the hypothesis that the malfunctioning of the cycle was caused by a deficiency of ornithine in the liver cell.[1,4,236] Even now, when increasing evidence supports the view that the intracellular concentration of the cationic amino acids is increased in these patients in both epithelial and parenchymal cells,[24,205] the malfunction is best explained as a "functional deficiency" of the intermediates. In reality, it is possible that enzymes of the urea cycle are inhibited by an increased intracellular concentration of lysine (see Chap. 85) or that a transport defect at the inner mitochondrial membrane prevents the entry of ornithine into the mitochondria, just as hypothesized in the HHH syndrome (see Chap. 83). Such a defect would decrease the ornithine concentration in the mitochondrial matrix, decrease transcarbamylation, and slow urea production. It is also possible that cytoplasmic concentrations of the cationic amino acids actually are diminished because of accumulation of these substances in lysosomes or some other vesicular organelles. In such a case, cytoplasmic ornithine concentration could be temporarily increased by supplementation with arginine or ornithine. Similar genetic defects are known for transporters in lysosomal membranes (see Chap. 199). These defects all cause reduced efflux from the lysosomes; this is the case at least in cystinosis and Salla disease. An efflux defect could theoretically explain pooling and cytoplasmic depletion of the cationic amino acids in LPI, but our knowledge of amino acid movements into and out of the lysosomes is too sparse, and no direct data to confirm the hypothesis of a lysosomal or vesicular efflux defect exist.

Half of the urea nitrogen originates as free ammonium, which enters the urea cycle by way of carbamyl phosphate synthesis, but this nitrogen does not gain access to the liver cell as free ammonium.[237,238] Animal experiments have suggested that the amide nitrogen of glutamine is an important precursor of urea nitrogen; glutamine functions as a transport and storage form of ammonium ion to keep its tissue levels within tolerable ranges via glutamine synthetase.[16] The ammonium for carbamyl phosphate synthesis is released from glutamine by intramitochondrial glutaminase, which was found to be defective in the leukocytes of one patient.[16,21] The suspected defect in glutaminase led to an interesting hypothesis of the mechanism of the transport disorder in LPI,[16] but later studies did not confirm the deficiency of glutaminase in leukocytes or liver biopsy samples of other patients.[131]

It is possible that during large nitrogen inflow — that is, after protein meals — intrahepatic glutamine synthesis serves to trap free ammonium and amino groups from other amino acids. Plasma glutamine is constantly high in LPI, and its fluctuations seem to be related to the previous nitrogen loading. Exact knowledge of the nitrogen flow in the liver during protein absorption is lacking, and the rate-limiting step in urea formation is not known. It may well be that the rate-limiting step varies and depends on several other factors, including the availability of the substrates.[206,208,213,214,217,239–241]

Patients with LPI efficiently produce orotic acid after nitrogen loading.[22,46,122] This cytoplasmic pathway could theoretically serve as a means to excrete excessive nitrogen from the body via carbamyl phosphate and aspartate, that is, the same substrates as in the urea cycle.[242,243] The level of renal clearance and urinary excretion of orotic acid is high, but the overall capacity of the pathway is limited, and only relatively small amounts of excess nitrogen can be excreted as orotate even during loading conditions.[134] It is interesting that uracil is also excreted in excess in LPI.[22]

Lysine Deficiency

Despite prevention of hyperammonemia by citrulline supplementation and a low-protein diet, several features of the disease have remained unaltered in treated patients. Growth has not totally normalized, bone age is delayed, liver and spleen are enlarged, and liver pathology is unaltered.[11,35] The hematologic abnormalities have also persisted during therapy, osteoporosis persists, and the patients are prone to develop life-threatening pulmonary alveolar proteinosis or pulmonary cholesterol granulomas. These are possibly signs of a continuing deficiency of lysine, whose bioavailability is significantly reduced by the poor intestinal absorption and heavy renal losses.[4,55,121,196] In addition to the transport defects in the epithelial cells, which lead to poor net reclamation of lysine in the body, the transport defect at the plasma membrane of the parenchymal cells and the proposed transport defects in cell organelles also may contribute to the suspected lysine deficiency.[58,205]

Lysine is an integral part of practically all proteins. Relatively speaking, collagen is especially rich in lysine. The pathophysiological mechanisms of the often prominent osteoporosis in patients with LPI have remained un- certain.[63–65] It may well be that the osteoporosis is caused by lysine deficiency, which delays formation of the bone matrix and is an important factor in poor formation of other essential structural proteins and additional proteins.[244–248] Nothing is known of the acute or long-term effects of intravenous lysine infusions or oral supplementation with absorbable lysine derivatives in osteoporosis in LPI. Rajantie and coworkers found that ε-*N*-acetyllysine but not homocitrulline efficiently increases plasma lysine in patients with LPI.[249] Acetyllysine uses a transport system different from that of the cationic amino acids, making it suitable for oral use. Despite the apparently fast metabolism of acetyllysine to lysine in human beings, its suitability for lysine replacement may be limited. In mice fed synthetic amino acid diets, replacement of L-lysine with ε-*N*-methyl-L-lysine, ε-*N*-dimethyl-L-lysine, or ε-*N*-trimethyl-L-lysine resulted in relative replacement values of about $\frac{1}{12}$, $\frac{1}{20}$, and $\frac{1}{25}$, respectively, of the value obtained with the standard lysine diet.[250] α-*N*-acetyl-L-lysine was not used by mice, and the replacement value of the ε-*N*-acetyllysine was about 3 percent that of lysine. Replacement of the charged ε-amino group in lysine with a sulfur-containing group led to weight reduction. *N*-phosphorylated lysine has not been tested in this system.[251]

Arginine is an essential amino acid in inborn errors of the urea cycle and probably in growing children[114,115] and some animals, at least the cat.[252,253] However, arginine deficiency is unlikely to play a role in the symptoms in LPI because ample amounts of arginine should be available during citrulline supplementation.[11,14,63,195]

Serum Ferritin, LDH, and TBG. Serum concentrations of ferritin, LDH, and TBG have been consistently elevated in these patients.[22,35,75] The cause of the high concentration of ferritin is its decreased catabolism in the liver,[111,127] but the reason for this decrease is not known. High ferritin and LDH values have increased further during acute illnesses (see "Complications and Autopsy Findings" above). The increase in TBG and the associated increase in total T4 has in some occasions led to suspicion of hyperthyroidism in these patients.

GENETICS

The inheritance of LPI follows a pattern typical for an autosomal recessive disease.[2,53] The incidence of the disease is 1 in 60,000 in Finland, but the birthplaces of the patients' grandparents are unevenly distributed in the country, and at least three large clusters of families can be recognized.[2,4,35,53] Most patients inother countries have been isolated cases[13–15,18,19,22,23,27,28,30,31,33,44–46,48–52] or multiple affected members of one family.[17,20,25,26,32,34,47,51]

Extensive functional studies have suggested that transport of amino acids into mammalian cells is mediated in different cell lines or tissues by a number of carrier proteins with differing characteristics.[161–163,208,254–259] Competition assays have shown that the cationic amino acids lysine, arginine, and ornithine share the same carrier(s), and that the kinetics of cationic amino acid uptake are similar in many tissues.[161–163,258,260] A widely expressed sodium-independent carrier system designated y^+ has been extensively studied[161–163,258,260] Another carrier, system $b^{o,+}$ is also Na^+-independent and accepts both cationic and neutral amino acids.[256,258] Some mammalian cells express a third, Na^+-dependent transport process, designated $B^{o,+}$.[257,258] The degree to which each of these three systems is expressed varies widely among cell types.[258]

Recently, a cDNA encoding a retroviral receptor (murine leukemia viral receptor REC1) was cloned from NIH 3T3 fibroblasts by expression in human bladder carcinoma cells, which are normally resistant to the virus owing to absence of receptor.[261] The cDNA encoded a 622-amino-acid protein with 12 to 14 potential membrane-spanning domains. The extent of homology between the retroviral receptor and the arginine-histidine transporters of *Saccharomyces cerevisiae* (permeases CAN-1 and HIP-1)[262–264] raised the possibility that the physiological role of the receptor might be mediating cationic amino acid transport at the cell membrane.[265,266] Indeed, this hypothesis was confirmed by expression in *Xenopus* oocytes,[265,266] where the functional characteristics of the transporter were similar to those of the system y^+. Studies using northern blotting showed expression of mouse transporter RNA in a variety of tissues but not in the liver, again supporting the identity with system y^+.[161,258] This transport protein has now been renamed MCAT-1 (mouse cationic amino acid transporter-1) to better represent its physiological function.[267] Using mouse-human somatic cell hybrids, the human version of the mouse REC-1 gene, ATRC1, was soon assigned to chromosome 13, and *in situ* hybridization localized the gene to 13q12-q14.60 The locus shows restriction fragment length polymorphism with *Taq*I. Pairwise and multilocus linkage analyses have shown that the ATRC1 locus is close to the locus ATP1AL1 (ATPase, Na^+K^+, α-polypeptide-like 1) on one side and to the locus D13S6 on the other side.[60]

MCAT-1 is not expressed in freshly isolated rat hepatocytes or in normal rodent liver.[162,258,259] Furthermore, there are data suggesting that murine hepatocytes are resistant to ecotropic retrovirus infection, further suggesting that system y^+ is not expressed in hepatic tissues.[265,268] However, the liver plays a central role in balancing the peripheral amino acid supply after and between meals, and the flux of amino acids between the liver and other tissues is determined, in part, by the activity of specific transport proteins. Recently, a cDNA was isolated from a murine T cell lymphoma cell line that encoded a protein related to MCAT-1, named Tea (T cell early activation).[269] Interestingly, the gene encoding Tea was expressed not only in activated T and B lymphocytes but also in liver. Hypothesizing that the Tea-encoded protein might be the hepatic cationic amino acid transporter, Closs and coworkers[267] found another cationic amino acid carrier (MCAT-2), which was closely related to Tea, was expressed in mouse liver, and had the same substrate specificity as the carrier in extrahepatic tissues. Furthermore, the MCAT-2 protein was encoded by the same gene as Tea, but differed in part of its sequence, presumably as a result of alternative splicing. Functional comparisons of the two transporters (the hepatic MCAT-2 and the more widely expressed MCAT-1 or y^+) in *Xenopus* oocytes showed that, unlike in the extrahepatic transporter, arginine uptake mediated by the MCAT-2 transporter is significant only at substrate concentrations that exceed systemic levels in plasma; its function is also less dependent on the intracellular concentration of the cationic amino acids. Thus, the properties of MCAT-2 suggest that it is the low-affinity transporter of cationic amino acids known to be expressed in the rodent (and human)[190] liver. These properties enable hepatocytes expressing this carrier to remove excess cationic amino acids from the blood without interfering with their uptake by extrahepatic tissues.[267]

Cloning by expression in *Xenopus* oocytes has recently resulted in the isolation of kidney and intestine-specific cDNA clones called rat D2,[270] rat NAA-Tr,[271] and rabbit rBAT.[272] These clones have about 80 percent amino acid sequence identity and induce high-affinity uptake into *Xenopus* oocytes of a broad spectrum of amino acids including cystine, and dibasic and neutral amino acids. These transporters are type II membrane glycoproteins and exhibit similarity to α-glucosidases and to 4F2 cell surface antigen heavy chain. The 4F2 protein also induces amino acid uptake into oocytes, but its substrate specificity is different.[270,273–275] It may well be that D2, rBAT, and the 4F2 heavy chain are not transporters as such but belong to a group of regulatory subunits of heterooligomeric transporters or are independent transport regulators.[270,272–274] Isolation of D2H, the human cDNA counterpart of the rat D2, from a human kidney library, and expression of D2H in Xenopus oocytes, showed that D2H induces uptake of cystine as well as dibasic and neutral amino acids. Furthermore, northern blot analysis demonstrated strong expression of D2H in human kidney and intestine. Mouse-human somatic cell hybrids showed that the human gene for D2H resides on chromosome 2.[273]

The genes for MCAT-1, MCAT-2, and the transporter regulatory units are strong candidate genes for the LPI mutation(s). Our increasing knowledge of the multiplicity and functional diversity of the cationic amino acid transporter proteins and transport regulatory proteins in mammalian tissues allows me to predict that the LPI phenotype will be split into subgroups based on different mutations in one or several transporters; furthermore, mutations in genes encoding transport regulatory proteins may also be involved in some families.

The hyperdibasic aminoaciduria type 1 described by Whelan and Scriver[61] showed autosomal dominant inheritance. Of the 33 subjects in the kindred, 13 had the trait. The suggestion that the affected members of the kindred are heterozygotes of an autosomal recessive disease seems likely, even though no confirmed homozygotes are known. The possibility exists that the patient of Kihara et al.[33] is a homozygote for the trait, as has been suggested by Bergeron and Scriver,[143] but this remains a hypothesis. The original proposal by the authors that the carriers of the trait could be heterozygous for LPI is at least equally attractive.

The expression of the mutant gene in heterozygotes for LPI has been only partially characterized.[2,53,58] The constant finding of decreased epithelial transport of the cationic amino acids in the homozygotes and, especially, the direct measurement of defective cationic amino acid transport in cultured fibroblasts of homozygotes and heterozygotes for LPI,[58] strongly support the view that the mutation affects the transport protein at the basolateral cell membrane of the epithelial cells and at the plasma membrane of the parenchymal cells. Many LPI heterozygotes excrete slightly increased amounts of the cationic amino acids in the urine, but this has not been a constant finding.[2,53] The fact that the heterozygotes have not shown signs and symptoms of protein intolerance suggests that the urea cycle failure is a secondary consequence of the primary defect.[276]

TREATMENT

Hyperammonemia, which occurs in the patients after high-protein meals, during prolonged fasting, or during severe infections, can now be effectively prevented and treated. A diet in which the protein content has been moderately decreased—in children, to 1.0 to 1.5 g/kg/day and, in adults, to 0.5 to 0.7 g/kg/day—forms the basis of successful treatment.[11,14,35] Acute symptoms disappear when the patients are on this diet, but, in many infants, severe protein aversion leads to minimal energy intake as well, and even though nausea and vomiting can be avoided, pediatric patients usually eat very poorly during the first years of life. Supplementation with arginine or ornithine has been moderately helpful in some patients,[6–8,13,17,28,32] but the decreased intestinal absorption of cationic amino acids limits their usefulness, and supplementation often leads to osmotic diarrhea.[55,195,196] Citrulline is a neutral amino acid and uses another transport mechanism at the cell membrane. It is readily absorbed from the intestine and converted to arginine and then to ornithine in the body, especially in the liver. Citrulline supplementation guarantees an adequate supply of urea cycle intermediates at the site of urea synthesis, and, indeed, oral citrulline supplementation has proved clinically to prevent hyperammonemia as efficiently as intravenous arginine or ornithine.[11,14,122] The dose of citrulline supplementation has been 2.5 to 8.5 g (14 to 48 mmol) daily, divided into three to five doses and taken with meals. The individual doses are first calculated according to the protein content of the meals and then adjusted according to the clinical and biochemical responses of the patients. Most patients quickly learn to know how much citrulline they need for a specific portion of each high-protein food. Citrulline can be given as powder dissolved in juice or as pills (ours have 0.414 g L-citrulline) or capsules.

In acute hyperammonemic crisis in LPI, the best treatment has been total removal of protein and nitrogen from the nutrition. Intravenous glucose should be given to supply as much energy as possible. In hyperammonemia, we have also infused ornithine, arginine, or citrulline intravenously, starting with a priming dose of 1 mmol/kg in 5 to 10 min and then infusing at a rate of about 0.5 to 1 mmol/kg/h until the symptoms have subsided. Sodium benzoate and sodium phenylacetate given intravenously or orally[113,116,118,119] appear clinically effective even though they only minimally correct alanine-induced hyperammonemia.[134]

Lysine has been given orally to these patients, but its intestinal absorption is poor and it causes diarrhea and abdominal pains.[11] A few patients have received lysine supplementation for longer periods, but the evidence that lysine can correct signs of protein malnutrition has not been convincing. It is interesting that acute loads of ε-*N*-acetyllysine, a neutral analogue of lysine and a readily absorbed substance, increased plasma lysine concentrations in the patients as well as in the control subjects.[249] Homocitrulline had no effect on plasma lysine. Because of the limited availability and high price of acetyllysine, it has not been used as a long-term supplement in patients.[277] Its usefulness as a replacement for lysine has recently been questioned.[250]

A potentially life-threatening complication of LPI is acute or chronic pulmonary involvement, which may present as interstitial changes on radiographs or as respiratory insufficiency and may progress to pulmonary alveolar proteinosis or cholesterol granulomas[51,52,63,75,78–80] (see "Complications and Autopsy Findings" above). Occasionally, lung involvement may be the presenting sign of the disease.[38,51,52] One adult patient with acute respiratory insufficiency was treated efficiently with high-dose prednisolone immediately after the onset of pulmonary symptoms; the symptoms subsided rapidly after initiation of the therapy. The dose was soon tapered, but a 2.5-mg intermittent-day dose was continued. A relapse 8 months later was again successfully treated by increasing the prednisolone dose. The patient received intermittent-day prednisolone for over 2 years, and has since been symptom-free for over 5 years. However, several pediatric deaths from pulmonary complications suggest either that it is necessary to start the treatment early, or that the response may be variable.[51,52,75,80] Indeed, in two Italian patients aged 5 and 24 years, treatment with prednisolone had no effect on the progression of the pulmonary changes, and the effect was minimal or absent also in an 11-year-old Arab girl.[51,52]

Glomerulonephritis and renal insufficiency, amyloid deposition in the spleen and lymph nodes, and occasionally severe fatty degeneration and cirrhosis of the liver appear to be not uncommon in association with the pulmonary symptoms of LPI; the potentially fatal syndrome fits the criteria of the multiple organ dysfunction syndrome.[81,82] Currently, I have no suggestions for specific treatment of this syndrome in patients with LPI.

ACKNOWLEDGMENTS

This study was supported in part by grants from the Sigrid Juselius Foundation, the Academy of Finland, the Signe and Ane Gyllenberg Foundation, and the University Foundation, Turku, Finland. I am grateful to Dr. Katriina Parto, M.D., Dr. Ilkka Sipilä, M.D., Dr. Jukka Rajantie, M.D., Dr. Martti Kekomäki, M.D., and Prof. Jaakko Perheentupa, M.D., for collaboration, fruitful discussions and help in treating the Finnish patients during a quarter of a century. I want to thank Mrs. Marja Piippo, Mrs. Anneli Enlund, and my wife, Tuula, for help in the processing of the manuscript.

ADDENDUM

David Valle

In the interval since the appearance of this chapter in the seventh edition of this book, the subject of amino acid transport has been the subject of several reviews.[280–282] Additionally, many advances have been made in our understanding of LPI, particularly in the areas of the biochemistry and molecular biology of amino acid transport and in delineation of the molecular basis of LPI. These advances are summarized here.

Clinical Aspects

Additional cases of hemophagocytic lymphohistiocytosis complicating LPI have been described.[283,284] Some have improved in association with immunosuppressive treatment[284] but other regress spontaneously.[285] Thus, the role of immunosuppression for treatment of this complication is uncertain.

Molecular Biology of Amino Acid Transporters

Utilizing the *Xenopus* oocyte expression system to assay amino acid transport, investigators have for some time known that two homologous surface glycoproteins, rBAT and 4F2hc, induce amino acid transport when expressed in oocytes.[280–282] These proteins are only slightly hydrophobic, prompting the hypothesis that they were subunits or modulators of amino acid transporters. This hypothesis was supported by several observations including (a) expression of rBAT or 4Fhc induces transport of several classes of amino acids;[280–282] (b) either rBAT or 4Fhc can be immunoprecipitated as a complex of ≈125 kDa in the absence of reducing agents and as monomers of ≈85 kDa (rBAT or 4F2hc) and ≈40 kDa (unknown subunit) in the presence of reducing agents;[282,286] and (c) in oocytes, the transport activity is less than predicted by the level of either rBAT or 4F2hc expression as if activity is limited by an endogenous factor.[287,288]

A major advance in identification of the partners of rBAT or 4F2hc in the heteromeric complex, came from the isolation by Verrey and colleagues of a *Xenopus* cDNA, designated ASUR4, that encodes a hydrophobic 12-transmembrane-domain protein with homology to yeast and worm amino acid transport proteins and to a partial length human cDNA known as E16.[289] AZUR4 or full-length E16 had no activity when expressed alone in *Xenopus* oocytes. But, when co-expressed with 4F2hc, they induced amino acid transport to a much greater extent than that produced by expression of 4F2hc alone. The substrate specificity and Na^+ dependence of the transport activity induced by co-expression of ASUR4 or E16 with 4F2hc corresponded functionally to the human system.[280] These observations suggested that ASUR4 and E16 encoded members of a family of peptides that formed the small subunit (referred to as the light chain) of the heteromeric complex with 4F2hc. Immunoprecipitation experiments confirmed that the E16 (or AZUR4) peptide was covalently linked to 4F2hc and immunohistochemistry showed this association was required for localization of the light chain in the plasma membrane. Based on these observations, Verrey and colleagues proposed that AZUR4 and E16 were members of a family of light chains that heterodimerize with 4F2hc to form amino acid transporters.[289]

Using a combination of degenerate primer PCR and homology probing of the EST database, Palacin and colleagues identified two newly recognized human cDNAs with homology to AZUR4.[290] Co-expression of either of these with 4F2hc in *Xenopus* oocytes induced amino acid transport with characteristics of the y^+L system (exchanger activity mediating efflux of cationic amino acids and influx of neutral amino acids plus Na^+) and on this basis the cDNAs were designated y^+LAT-1 and y^+LAT-2. The y^+LAT-1 protein has 511 amino acids with 75 percent identity to the 515 amino acid protein encoded by y^+LAT-2 and 51 percent identity to E16, the third membrane of this family in humans. All three are predicted to have 12 transmembrane domains. These investigators showed y^+LAT-1 associates covalently with 4F2hc to form a 135-kDa complex that could be dissociated by reduction to yield a 40-kDa protein specific for y^+LAT-1.[290,291] They suggest that y^+LAT-1, y^+LAT-2 and E16 can each associate with 4F2hc to form heterodimeric amino acid transporters and that the variable light chain confers the specificity of the transporter. The covalent link between the light chain and 4F2hc occurs in segments of the peptides facing the extracellular space. These correspond to a cysteine between the third and fourth transmembrane domains of the light chain (C152 for y^+LAT-1) and C109 of human 4F2hc.[290,291] Interestingly, two additional features of y^+LAT-1 suggested it could be responsible for LPI: the y^+LAT-1 structural gene mapped to 14q11.2, the region implicated for LPI (see below); and northern blot analysis showed high expression in tissues involved in LPI (kidney, peripheral leukocytes, and lung).

Molecular Basis of LPI

The key first step in this success story was localization of the gene responsible for LPI in the Finnish population to 14q11.2 in a linkage study of 20 Finn LPI pedigrees.[292] A second study confirmed the same location for non-Finnish LPI.[293] This mapping result provided a molecular signpost against which all candidates could be tested.

Recognition that the y^+LAT-1 structural gene (designated *SLC7A7* for solute carrier family 7, member 7) maps to the correct location and encodes a subunit of a transporter with the expected functional characteristics, made it an excellent candidate for LPI. Torrents et al. surveyed *SLC7A* in 31 Finnish and 1 Spanish LPI patients.[294] They found a single Finnish mutant allele (1181-2A > T) with an A > T transversion at position −2 of the acceptor splice site in intron 6 of the *SLC7A* gene. This inactivates the normal splice acceptor and activates a cryptic acceptor 10 bp downstream with the result that 10 bp of the ORF are deleted and the reading frame is shifted. All 31 Finnish patients and 10 obligate heterozygotes had this allele. In all but one instance, this was on a common haplotype consistent with the expectation of a founder mutation in the Finnish population. The one exception appeared to result from a recombination between the haplotype markers and the LPI locus. In contrast to the Finnish patients, the Spanish LPI subject was a genetic compound for two *SLC7A* mutations: a missense mutation, L334R (1287T > G); and a 4-bp deletion (1291delCTTT). Expression studies in the oocyte system confirmed that L334R inactivated transporter function.

Simultaneously, Borsani and colleagues used homology probing with the E16 sequence to identify *SLC7A7*[295] independently. They performed mutation analysis in four Finn and five Italian LPI probands. They found 4 of the Italian probands were homozygous for a 4 bp insertion (1625insATAC) that frameshifts the reading frame at codon 462 and predicts translation termination 13 bp downstream. The remaining Italian proband was homozygous for a 543-bp deletion (197del543) that removes the first 168 codons of the reading frame. They also identified the 1181-2A > T mutation in their four Finnish LPI probands.

Together, the reports from these two groups confirmed *SLC7A7* as the gene responsible for LPI. Subsequent studies have delineated the organization of the *SLC7A7* structural gene. The Finnish group finds 11 exons distributed over 18 kb of genomic DNA, with the first two exons encoding 5′ untranslated sequence and the open reading frame beginning in exon 3.[296] The Italian group did not identify the most 5′ exon and therefore reports 10 exons with translation beginning in exon 2.[297] Together, the two groups surveyed 36 non-Finnish LPI probands for *SLC7A7* mutations, including patients of Japanese, Tunisian, Italian, Spanish, Turkish, German, Canadian, Dutch, Norwegian, and Swedish origin. The results are confused by differences in numbering exons and cDNA residues but, in toto, there are at least 5 missense alleles (M1L, G54V, L334R, G338D, S386R), 3 nonsense alleles (W242X, Y384X, R473X), 8 small insertions or deletions, and 4 splice site changes for a total of 20 alleles.[296,297] Five of these alleles were expressed in oocytes to determine their functional consequences. Three of these (1291delCTTT, 1548delC, and the Finnish allele, 1181-2A > T) produced an abnormal protein that did not localize to the plasma membrane. By contrast, two missense alleles (G54V and L334R) produced an abnormal protein that correctly localized to the plasma membrane but was functionally inactive.[296] Interestingly, both groups note that patients with the same genotype at the *SLC7A7* locus may have quite different phenotypic severity. For example, in the Finnish LPI patients, all with the same *SLC7A7* genotype, the severity ranges from nearly normal growth with minimal protein intolerance to severe cases with organomegaly, osteoporosis, alveolar proteinosis, and severe protein intolerance. Thus, there is much work to be done to understand the pathophysiology of the protean manifestations of LPI.

REFERENCES

1. Perheentupa J, Visakorpi JK: Protein intolerance with deficient transport of basic amino acids. *Lancet* **2**:813, 1965.
2. Norio R, Perheentupa J, Kekomaki M, Visakorpi JK: Lysinuric protein intolerance, an autosomal recessive disease. *Clin Genet* **2**:214, 1971.
3. McKusick VA, Francomano CA, Antonarakis SE: *Mendelian Inheritance in Man. Catalogs of Autosomal Dominant, Autosomal Recessive*

and X-linked Phenotypes, 10th ed. Baltimore, Johns Hopkins University Press, 1992, p 1336.
4. Simell O, Rajantie J, Perheentupa J: Lysinuric protein intolerance, in Eriksson AW, Forsius H, Nevanlinna HR, Workman PL, Norio RK (eds): *Population Structure and Genetic Disorders*, London, Academic Press, 1980, p 633.
5. Scriver CR, Simell O: Hyperdibasic-aminoaciduria, in Buyse ML (ed): *Birth Defects Encyclopedia*. Dover, MA, Center for Birth Defects Information Services/Blackwell Scientific, 1990, p 900.
6. Kekomaki M: *Familial protein intolerance. Studies on an inborn error of metabolism and related biochemical problems*. Thesis, Helsinki, 1969.
7. Kekomaki M, Toivakka E, Hakkinen V, Salaspuro M: Familial protein intolerance with deficient transport of basic amino acids. Report on an adult patient with chronic hyperammonemia. *Acta Med Scand* **183**:357, 1968.
8. Kekomaki M, Visakorpi JK, Perheentupa J, Saxen L: Familial protein intolerance with deficient transport of basic amino acids. An analysis of 10 patients. *Acta Paediatr Scand* **56**:617, 1967.
9. Rajantie J: *Lysinuric protein intolerance: Intestinal transport defect and treatment*. Thesis, Helsinki, 1980.
10. Simell O: *Lysinuric protein intolerance*. Thesis. Helsinki, Yliopistokirjapaino, 1975.
11. Rajantie J, Simell O, Rapola J, Perheentupa J: Lysinuric protein intolerance: A two-year trial of dietary supplementation therapy with citrulline and lysine. *J Pediatr* **97**:927, 1980.
12. Perheentupa J, Simell O: Lysinuric protein intolerance. *Birth Defects* **10(4)**:201, 1974.
13. Russell A, Slatter M, Ben-Zvi A: Ornithine administration as a therapeutic tool in dibasic aminoaciduric protein intolerance. *Hum Hered* **27**:206, 1977.
14. Awrich AE, Stackhouse J, Cantrell JE, Patterson JH, Rudman D: Hyperdibasicaminoaciduria, hyperammonemia, and growth retardation: Treatment with arginine, lysine, and citrulline. *J Pediatr* **87**:731, 1975.
15. Kato T, Tanaka E, Horisawa S: Hyperdibasicaminoaciduria and hyperammonemia in familial protein intolerance. *Am J Dis Child* **130**:1340, 1976.
16. Malmquist J, Jagenburg R, Lindstedt G: Familial protein intolerance: Possible nature of enzyme defect. *N Engl J Med* **284**:997, 1971.
17. Yoshimura T, Kato M, Goto I, Kuroiwa Y: Lysinuric protein intolerance—Two patients in a family with loss of consciousness and growth retardation. *Rinsho Shinkeigaku* **23**:140, 1983.
18. Kitajima I, Goto K, Umehara F, Nagamatsu K, Kanehisa Y: A case of lysinuric protein intolerance with intermittent stupor looking like psychomotor seizure in adulthood. *Rinsho Shinkeigaku* **26**:592, 1986.
19. Carson NAJ, Redmond OAB: Lysinuric protein intolerance. *Ann Clin Biochem* **14**:135, 1977.
20. Andria G, Battaglia A, Sebastio G, Strisciuglio P, Auricchio S: Lysinuric protein intolerance. *Rev Ital Pediatr* **2**:386, 1977.
21. Malmquist J, Hetter B: Leucocyte glutaminase in familial protein intolerance. *Lancet* **2**:129, 1970.
22. Behbehani AW, Gahr M, Schroter W: Lysinuric protein intolerance. *Monatsschr Kinderheilkd* **131**:784, 1983.
23. Brown JH, Fabre LF Jr, Farrell GL, Adams ED: Hyperlysinuria with hyperammonemia. *Am J Dis Child* **124**:127, 1972.
24. Oyanagi K, Sogawa H, Minami R, Nakao T, Chiba T: The mechanism of hyperammonemia in congenital lysinuria. *J Pediatr* **94**:255, 1979.
25. Oyanagi K, Miura R, Yamanouchi T: Congenital lysinuria: A new inherited transport disorder of dibasic amino acids. *J Pediatr* **77**:259, 1970.
26. Kato T, Mizutani N, Ban M: Hyperammonemia in lysinuric protein intolerance. *Pediatrics* **73**:489, 1984.
27. Chan H, Billmeier GJ Jr, Molinary SV, Tucker HN, Shin B-C, Schaffer A, Cavallo K: Prolonged coma and isoelectric electroencephalogram in a child with lysinuric protein intolerance. *J Pediatr* **91**:79, 1977.
28. Endres W, Zoulek G, Schaub J: Hyperdibasicaminoaciduria in a Turkish infant without evident protein intolerance. *Eur J Pediatr* **131**:33, 1979.
29. Jagenburg R, Lindstedt G, Malmquist J: Familjar [?] proteinintolerans med hyperammoniemi. *Lakartidningen* **67**:5255, 1970.
30. Carpenter TO, Levy HL, Holtrop ME, Shih VE, Anast CS: Lysinuric protein intolerance presenting as childhood osteoporosis. Clinical and skeletal response to citrulline therapy. *N Engl J Med* **312**:290, 1985.
31. Nagata M, Suzuki M, Kawamura G, Kono S, Koda N, Yamaguchi S, Aoki K: Immunological abnormalities in a patient with lysinuric protein intolerance. *Eur J Pediatr* **146**:427, 1987.
32. Andria G, Sebastio G, Strisciuglio P, Del Giudice E: Lysinuric protein intolerance: Possible genetic heterogeneity? *J Inherit Metab Dis* **4**:151, 1981.
33. Kihara H, Valente M, Porter MT, Fluharty AL: Hyperdibasicaminoaciduria in a mentally retarded homozygote with a peculiar response to phenothiazines. *Pediatrics* **51**:223, 1973.
34. Goto I, Yoshimura T, Kuroiwa Y: Growth hormone studies in lysinuric protein intolerance. *Eur J Pediatr* **141**:240, 1984.
35. Simell O, Perheentupa J, Rapola J, Visakorpi JK, Eskelin L-E: Lysinuric protein intolerance. *Am J Med* **59**:229, 1975.
36. Yamaguchi S: Personal communication, 1987.
37. Saudubray JM: Personal communication, 1987.
38. Fisher M, Roggli V, Merten D, Mulvihill D, Spock A: Coexisting endogenous lipoid pneumonia, cholesterol granulomas, and pulmonary alveolar proteinosis in a pediatric population: A clinical, radiographic, and pathologic correlation. *Pediat Pathol* **12**:365, 1992.
39. Krasnopolskaia KD, Iakovenko LP, Mazaeva IV, Lebedev BV: Lysinuric protein intolerance, a hereditary defect of amino acid transport. *Pediatriia* **6**:78, 1978.
40. Coude FX, Ogier H, Charpentier C, Cathelineau L, Grimber G, Parvy P, Saudubray JM, Frezal J: Lysinuric protein intolerance: A severe hyperammonemia secondary to L-arginine deficiency. *Arch Fr Pediatr* **38(Suppl 1)**:829, 1981.
41. Mori H, Kimura M, Fukuda S: A case of lysinuric protein intolerance with mental-physical retardation, intermittent stupor and hemiparesis. *Rinsho Shinkeigaku* **22**:42, 1982.
42. Mizutani N, Kato T, Maehara M, Watanabe K, Ban M: Oral administration of arginine and citrulline in the treatment of lysinuric protein intolerance. *Tohoku J Exp Med* **142**:15, 1984.
43. Rottem M, Statter M, Amit R, Brand N, Bujanover Y, Yatziv S: Clinical and laboratory study in 22 patients with inherited hyperammonemic syndromes. *Isr J Med Sci* **22**:833, 1986.
44. Takada G, Goto A, Komatsu K, Goto R: Carnitine deficiency in lysinuric protein intolerance: Lysine sparing effect of carnitine. *Tohoku J Exp Med* **153**:331, 1987.
45. Shioya K, Yamamura Y, Kurihara T, Matsukura S: A case of combined lysinuric protein intolerance and hypoactivity of argininosuccinate synthetase (citrullinemia). *Nippon Naika Gakkai Zasshi* **77**:667, 1988.
46. De Parshau L, Vianey-Liaud C, Hermier M, Divry P, Guibaud P: Protein intolerance with lysinuria. Value of orotic aciduria in adjusting treatment with citrulline. *Arch Fr Pediatr* **45**:809, 1988.
47. Shaw PJ, Dale G, Bbates D: Familial lysinuric protein intolerance presenting as coma in two adult sublings. *J Neurol Neurosurg Psychiatry* **52**:648, 1989.
48. Kato T, Sano M, Mizutani N: Homocitrullinuria and homoargininuria in lysinuric protein intolerance. *J Inherit Metab Dis* **12**:157, 1989.
49. Parini R, Vegni M, Pontiggia M, Melotti D, Corbetta C, Rossi A, Piceni-Sereni L: A difficult diagnosis of lysinuric protein intolerance: Association with glucose-6-phosphate dehydrogenase deficiency. *J Inherit Metab Dis* **14**:833, 1991.
50. Ono N, Kishida K, Tokumoto K, Watanabe M, Shimada Y, Yoshinaga J, Fujii M: Lysinuric protein intolerance presenting deficiency of argininosuccinate synthetase. *Intern Med* **31**:55, 1992.
51. DiRocco M, Garibotto G, Rossi GA, Caruso U, Taccone A, Picco P, Borrone C: Role of haematological, pulmonary and renal complications in the long-term prognosis of patients with lysinuric protein intolerance. *Eur J Pediatr* **152**:437, 1993.
52. Kerem E, Elpelg ON, Shalev RS, Rosenman E, Bar Ziv Y, Branski D: Lysinuric protein intolerance with chronic interstitial lung disease and pulmonary cholesterol granulomas at onset. *J Pediatr* **123**:275, 1993.
53. Salonen T: *Lysinuric protein intolerance: Finnish pedigrees and the diagnosis of heterozygotes*. Master's thesis. Turku, University of Turku, 1991.
54. Sogowa H: Studies on the etiology of hyperammonemia associated with inborn errors of amino acid metabolism, part 2: Etiology of hyperammonemia associated with hyperdibasic aminoaciduria. *Sapporo Med J* **47**:215, 1978.
55. Rajantie J, Simell O, Perheentupa J: Basolateral-membrane transport defect for lysine in lysinuric protein intolerance. *Lancet* **1**:1219, 1980.
56. Rajantie J, Simell O, Perheentupa J: Lysinuric protein intolerance. Basolateral transport defect in renal tubuli. *J Clin Invest* **67**:1078, 1981.

57. Desjeux J-F, Rajantie J, Simell O, Dumontier A-M, Perheentupa J: Lysine fluxes across the jejunal epithelium in lysinuric protein intolerance. *J Clin Invest* **65**:1382, 1980.
58. Smith DW, Scriver CR, Tenenhouse HS, Simell O: Lysinuric protein intolerance mutation is expressed in the plasma membrane of cultured skin fibroblasts. *Proc Natl Acad Sci U S A* **84**:7711, 1987.
59. Botschner J, Smith DW, Simell O, Scriver CR: Comparison of ornithine metabolism in hyperornithinemia-hyperammonemia-homocitrullinuria syndrome, lysinuric protein intolerance, and gyrate atrophy fibroblasts. *J Inherit Metab Dis* **12**:33, 1989.
60. Albritton LM, Bowcock AM, Eddy RL, Morton CC, Tseng L, Farrer LA, Cavalli-Sforza LL, Shows TB, Cunninham JM: The human cationic amino acid transporter [ATRC1]: Physical and genetic mapping to 13q12-q14. *Genomics* **12**:430, 1992.
61. Whelan DT, Scriver CR: Hyperdibasicaminoaciduria: An inherited disorder of amino acid transport. *Pediatr Res* **2**:525, 1968.
62. Omura K, Yamanaka N, Higami S, Matsuoka O, Fujimoto A, Issiki G, Tada K: Lysine malabsorption syndrome: A new type of transport defect. *Pediatrics* **57**:102, 1976.
63. Parto K: *Skeletal and visceral findings in lysinuric protein intolerance*. Thesis. Turku, Grafia, 1993.
64. Svedstrom E, Parto K, Marttinen M, Virtama P, Simell O: Skeletal manifestations of lysinuric protein intolerance. *Skeletal Radiol* **22**:11, 1993.
65. Parto K, Penttinen R, Paronen I, Pelliniemi L, Simell O: Osteoporosis in lysinuric protein intolerance. *J Inherit Metab Dis* **16**:441, 1993.
66. Lysinuric protein intolerance: A rare cause of childhood osteoporosis. *Nutr Rev* **44**:110, 1986. (no author)
67. Moschos M, Andreanos D: Lysinuria and changes in the crystalline lens. *Bull Mem Soc Fr Ophtalmol* **96**:322, 1985.
68. Neuberger A, Webster TA: The lysine requirements of adult rat. *J Biochem* **39**:200, 1945.
69. Likens R, Bavetta L, Posner A: Calcification in lysine deficiency. *Arch Biochem Biophys* **70**:401, 1957.
70. Jha G, Deo MG, Ramalingaswami V: Bone growth in protein deficiency, a study in rhesus monkeys. *Am J Pathol* **53**:1111, 1968.
71. Garn SM, Guzman MA, Wagner B: Subperiosteal gain and endosteal loss in protein-calorie malnutrition. *Am J Phys Anthropol* **30**:153, 1969.
72. Shieres R, Avioli LV, Bergfeld MA, Fallon MD, Slatopolsky E, Teitelbaum SL: Effects of semistarvation on skeletal homeostasis. *Endocrinology* **107**:1530, 1980.
73. Orwoll E, Ware M, Sstribrska L, Bikle D, Sanchez T, Andon M, Li H: Effects of dietary protein deficiency on mineral metabolism and bone mineral density. *Am J Clin Nutr* **56**:314, 1992.
74. Branca F, Robin SP, Ferro-Luzzi A, Golden MHN: Bone turnover in malnourished children. *Lancet* **340**:1493, 1992.
75. Parto K, Kallajoki M, Aho H, Simell O: Pulmonary alveolar proteinosis and glomerulonephritis in lysinuric protein intolerance: Case reports and autopsy findings of four pediatric patients. *Hum Pathol* (In press).
76. Dhansay MA, Benade AJ, Donald PR: Plasma lecithin-cholesterol acyltransferase activity and plasma lipoprotein composition and concentrations in kwashiorkor. *Am J Clin Nutr* **53**:512, 1991.
77. Sidransky H, Verney E: Chemical pathology of diamino acid deficiency: Considerations in relation to lysinuric protein intolerance. *J Exp Pathol* **2**:47, 1985.
78. Parto K, Svedstrom E, Majurin ML, Harkonen R, Simell O: Pulmonary manifestations in lysinuric protein intolerance. *Chest* **104**:1176, 1993.
79. Parto K, Maki J, Pelliniemi L, Simell O: Abnormal pulmonary macrophages in lysinuric protein intolerance. Ultrastructural, morphometric and x-ray microanalytical study. *Arch Pathol Lab Med* (In press).
80. Simell OG, Sipila I, Perheentupa J, Rapola J: *Lysinuric protein intolerance: Undefined interstitial pneumonia, a lethal or life-threatening complication* [Abstract]. Sendai, Japan, The Fourth International Congress of Inborn Errors of Metabolism, 1987, p 38.
81. Bone RC, Balk RA, Cerra FB, Dellinger RP, Fein AM, Knaus WA, Schein RMH, Sibbald WJ: Definitions for sepsis and organ failure and guidelines for the use of innovative therapies in sepsis. *Chest* **101**:1644, 1992.
82. Cohen IL: Definitions for sepsis and organ failure—The ACCP/SCCM consensus conference report. *Chest* **103**:656, 1993.
83. Wallaert B: Subclinical alveolitis in immunologic systemic disorders. *Lung* **168(Suppl)**:974, 1990.
84. Milleron BJ, Costabel U, Teschler H, Ziesche R, Cadranel JL, Matthys H, Akoun GM: Bronchoalveolar lavage cell data in alveolar proteinosis. *Am Rev Respir Dis* **144**:1330, 1991.
85. Hallman M, Sipila I: *Lysinuric protein intolerance (LPI): A possible defect in diamino acid transport in pulmonary alveolar epithelium* [Abstract]. Oslo, Norway, European Society for Pediatric Research, Annual Meeting, 1988.
86. Hallman M, Maasilta P, Sipila I, Tahvanainen J: Composition and function of pulmonary surfactant in adult respiratory distress syndrome. *Eur Respir J* **2(Suppl 3)**:104, 1989.
87. Pratt SA, Smith MH, Ladman AJ, Finley TN: The ultrastructure of alveolar macrophages from human cigarette smokers and nonsmokers. *Lab Invest* **24**:331, 1971.
88. Hocking WG, Golde DW: The pulmonary alveolar macrophage. *N Engl J Med* **301**:639, 1979.
89. Heppleston AG: Animal model of human disease. Silica induced pulmonary alveolar lipoproteinosis. *Am J Pathol* **78**:171, 1975.
90. Lullmann H, Lullmann-Rauch R, Wasserman O: Lipidosis induced by amphiphilic cationic drugs. *Biochem Pharmacol* **27**:1103, 1978.
91. Hook GER: Alveolar proteinosis and phospholipidoses of the lung. *Toxicol Pathol* **19**:482, 1991.
92. Colon AR Jr, Lawrence RD, Mills SD, O'Connell EJ: Childhood pulmonary alveolar proteinosis [PAP]. Report of a case and review of the literature. *Am J Dis Child* **121**:481, 1971.
93. Webster JR Jr, Battifora H, Fureay C, Harrison RA, Shapiro B: Pulmonary alveolar proteinosis in two siblings with decreased immunoglobulin A. *Am J Med* **69**:786, 1980.
94. Gray ES: Autoimmunity in childhood pulmonary alveolar proteinosis. *Br Med J* **887**:296, 1973.
95. Samuels MP, Warner JO: Pulmonary alveolar lipoproteinosis complicating juvenile dermatomyositis. *Thorax* **43**:939, 1988.
96. Haworth JC, Hoogstraten J, Taylor H: Thymic alymphoplasia. *Arch Dis Child* **42**:40, 1967.
97. Wilkinson RH, Blanc WA, Hagstrom JWC: Pulmonary alveolar proteinosis in three infants. *Pediatrics* **41**:510, 1968.
98. Danigelis JA, Markarian B: Pulmonary alveolar proteinosis. Including pulmonary electron microscopy. *Am J Dis Child* **118**:871, 1969.
99. Lippman M, Mok MS, Wasserman K: Anesthetic management for children with alveolar proteinosis using extracorporeal circulation. Report of two cases. *Br J Anesthesiol* **49**:173, 1977.
100. Teja K, Cooper PH, Squires JE, Schnatterly PT: Pulmonary alveolar proteinosis in four siblings. *N Engl J Med* **305**:1390, 1981.
101. Schumacher RE, Marrogi AJ, Heidelberger KP: Pulmonary alveolar proteinosis in a newborn. *Pediatr Pulmology* **7**:178, 1989.
102. Moulton SL, Krous HF, Merritt TA, Odell RM, Gangitano E, Cornish JD: Congenital pulmonary alveolar proteinosis: Failure of treatment with extracorporeal life support. *J Pediatr* **120**:297, 1992.
103. Porter KA: The kidneys, in Symmers WS (ed): *Systemic Pathology.* Edinburgh, Churchill Livingstone, 1992, p 217.
104. Marino CT, Pertschuk LP: Pulmonary hemorrhage in systemic lupus erythematosus. *Arch Intern Med* **141**:201, 1981.
105. Hensley MJ, Feldman NT, Lazarus JM, Galvanek EG: Diffuse pulmonary hemorrhage and rapidly progressive renal failure: An uncommon presentation of Wegener's granulomatosis. *Am J Med* **66**:894, 1979.
106. Thomashow BM, Felton CP, Navarro C: Diffuse intrapulmonary hemorrhage, renal failure, and a systemic vasculitis. *Am J Med* **68**:299, 1980.
107. Loughlin GM, Taussig LM, Murphy SA, Strunk RC, Kohnen PW: Immune complex-mediated glomerulonephritis and pulmonary hemorrhage simulating Goodpasture's syndrome. *J Pediatr* **93**:181, 1978.
108. Davies JNP: The essential pathology of kwashiorkor. *Lancet* **1**:317, 1948.
109. Gmaz-Nikulin E, Nikulin A, Plamenac P, Hegenwald G, Gaon D: Pancreatic lesions in shock and their significance. *J Pathol* **135**:223, 1981.
110. Klujber V, Klujber L: Hereditary pancreatitis. *Orv Hetil* **130**:1777, 1989.
111. Rajantie J, Simell O, Perheentupa J, Siimes M: Changes in peripheral blood cells and serum ferritin in lysinuric protein intolerance. *Acta Paediatr Scand* **69**:741, 1980.
112. Simell O, MacKenzie S, Clow CL, Scriver CR: Ornithine loading did not prevent induced hyperammonemia in a patient with HHH syndrome. *Pediatr Res* **19**:1283, 1985.
113. Coude FX, Coude M, Grimber G, Pelet A, Charpentier C: Potentiation by piridoxilate of the synthesis of hippurate from benzoate in isolated rat hepatocytes. An approach to the determination of new pathways of

nitrogen excretion in inborn errors of urea synthesis. *Clin Chim Acta* **136**:211, 1984.
114. Brusilow SW: Arginine, an indispensable amino acid for patients with inborn errors of urea synthesis. *J Clin Invest* **74**:2144, 1984.
115. Visek WJ: Arginine needs, physiological state and usual diets. A reevaluation. *J Nutr* **116**:36, 1986.
116. Brusilow SW, Danney M, Waber LJ, Batshaw M, Burton B, Levitsky L, Roth K, McKeethren C, Ward J: Treatment of episodic hyperammonemia in children with inborn errors of urea synthesis. *N Engl J Med* **310**:1630, 1984.
117. Batshaw ML, Painter MJ, Sproul GT, Schafer IA, Thomas GH, Brusilow S: Therapy of urea cycle enzymopathies: Three case studies. *Johns Hopkins Med* **148**:34, 1981.
118. Brusilow S, Tinker J, Batshaw ML: Amino acid acylation: A mechanism of nitrogen excretion in inborn errors of urea synthesis. *Science* **207**:659, 1980.
119. Smith I: The treatment of inborn errors of the urea cycle. *Nature* **291**:378, 1981.
120. McCormick K, Viscardi RM, Robinson B, Heininger J: Partial pyruvate decarboxylase deficiency with profound lactic acidosis and hyperammonemia: Responses to dichloroacetate and benzoate. *Am J Med Genet* **22**:291, 1985.
121. Simell O, Perheentupa J: Renal handling of diamino acids in lysinuric protein intolerance. *J Clin Invest* **54**:9, 1974.
122. Rajantie J: Orotic aciduria in lysinuric protein intolerance: Dependence on the urea cycle intermediates. *Pediatr Res* **15**:115, 1981.
123. Wendler PA, Blanding JH, Tremblay GC: Interaction between the urea cycle and the orotate pathway: Studies with isolated hepatocytes. *Arch Biochem Biophys* **224**:36, 1983.
124. Milner JA, Prior RL, Visek WJ: Arginine deficiency and orotic aciduria in mammals. *Proc Soc Exp Biol Med* **150**:282, 1975.
125. Milner JA, Visek WJ: Urinary metabolites characteristic of urea-cycle amino acid deficiency. *Metabolism* **24**:643, 1975.
126. Kelley WN, Greene ML, Fox IH, Rosenbloom FM, Levy RI, Seegmiller JE: Effects of orotic acid on purine and lipoprotein metabolism in man. *Metabolism* **19**:1025, 1970.
127. Rajantie J, Rapola J, Siimes MA: Ferritinemia with subnormal iron stores in lysinuric protein intolerance. *Metabolism* **30**:3, 1981.
128. Lamberg B-A, Simell O, Perheentupa J, Saarinen P: Increase in TBG, T4, FT4 and T3 in the lysinuric protein intolerance. *Exerpta Medica Int Congress Series* **378**:232, 1975.
129. Lamberg BA, Perheentupa J, Rajantie J, Simell O, Saarinen P, Ebeling P, Welin M-G: Increase in thyroxine-binding globulin [TBG] in lysinuric protein intolerance. *Acta Endocrinol* **97**:67, 1981.
130. Kekomaki M, Raiha NCR, Perheentupa J: Enzymes of urea synthesis in familial protein intolerance with deficient transport of basic amino acids. *Acta Paediatr Scand* **56**:631, 1967.
131. Simell O, Perheentupa J, Visakorpi JF: Leukocyte and liver glutaminase in lysinuric protein intolerance. *Pediatr Res* **6**:797, 1972.
132. Kekomaki MP, Raiha NCR, Bickel H: Ornithine-ketoacid aminotransferase in human liver with reference to patients with hyperornithinaemia and familial protein intolerance. *Clin Chim Acta* **23**:203, 1969.
133. Valle D: Personal communication, 1988.
134. Simell O, Sipila I, Rajantie J, Valle DL, Brusilow SW: Waste nitrogen excretion via amino acid acylation: Benzoate and phenylacetate in lysinuric protein intolerance. *Pediatr Res* **20**:1117, 1986.
135. Bachmann C, Krahenbuhl S, Colombo JP, Schubiger G, Jaggi KH, Tonz O: N-acetylglutamate synthetase deficiency: A disorder of ammonia detoxication. *N Engl J Med* **304**:543, 1981.
136. Hammerman MR: Na^+-independent L-arginine transport in rabbit renal brush border membrane vesicles. *Biochim Biophys Acta* **685**:71, 1982.
137. Adibi SA: Intestinal transport of dipeptides in man: Relative importance of hydrolysis and intact absorption. *J Clin Invest* **50**:2266, 1971.
138. Matthews DM, Adibi SA: Peptide absorption. *Gastroenterology* **71**:151, 1976.
139. Asatoor AM, Groughman MR, Harrison AR, Light FW, Loughridge LW, Milne MD, Richards AJ: Intestinal absorption of oligopeptides in cystinuria. *Clin Sci* **41**:23, 1971.
140. Ganapathy V, Mendicino JF, Leibach FH: Transport of glycyl-L-proline into intestinal and renal brush border vesicles from rabbit. *J Biol Chem* **256**:118, 1981.
141. Ganapathy V, Mendicino J, Pashley DH, Leibach FH: Carrier-mediated transport of glycyl-L-proline in renal brush-border vesicles. *Biochem Biophys Res Commun* **97**:1133, 1980.
142. Scriver CR, McInnes RR, Mohyuddin F: Role of epithelial architecture and intracellular metabolism in proline uptake and transtubular reclamation in PRO/Re mouse kidney. *Proc Natl Acad Sci U S A* **72**:1431, 1975.
143. Bergeron M, Scriver CR: Pathophysiology of renal hyperaminoacidurias and glucosuria, in Seldin DW, Giebisch G (eds): *The Kidney. Physiology and Pathophysiology*, 2nd ed. New York, Raven, 1992, p 2947.
144. Wilson OH, Scriver CR: Specificity of transport of neutral and basic amino acids in rat kidney. *Am J Physiol* **213**:185, 1967.
145. Webber WA, Brown JL, Pitts RF: Interactions of amino acids in renal tubular transport. *Am J Physiol* **200**:380, 1961.
146. Steiger B, Stange G, Biber J, Murer H: Transport of l-lysine by rat renal brush border membrane vesicles. *Pflugers Arch* **397**:106, 1983.
147. Scriver CR, Clow CL, Reade TM, Goodyer P, Auray-Blais C, Giguere R, Lemieux B: Ontogeny modifies manifestations of cystinuria genes. Implications for counseling. *J Pediatr* **106**:411, 1985.
148. Schwartzman L, Blair A, Segal S: A common renal transport system for lysine, ornithine, arginine and cysteine. *Biochem Biophys Res Commun* **23**:220, 1966.
149. Schafer JA, Watkins ML: Transport of l-cystine in isolated perfused proximal straight tubules. *Pflugers Arch* **401**:143, 1984.
150. Samarzija I, Fromter E: Electrophysiological analysis of rat renal sugar and amino acid transport. IV. Basic amino acids. *Pflugers Arch* **393**:199, 1982.
151. Rosenberg LE, Downing SJ, Segal S: Competitive inhibition of dibasic amino acid transport in rat kidney. *J Biol Chem* **237**:2265, 1962.
152. Rosenberg LE, Albrecht I, Segal S: Lysine transport in human kidney: Evidence for two systems. *Science* **155**:1426, 1967.
153. Bergeron M, Morel F: Amino acid transport in rat renal tubules. *Am J Physiol* **216**:1139, 1969.
154. Crawhall JC, Scowen EF, Thompson CJ, Watts RWE: The renal clearance of amino acids in cystinuria. *J Clin Invest* **46**:1162, 1967.
155. Hilden SA, Sacktor B: L-Arginine uptake into renal brush membrane vesicles. *Arch Biochem Biophys* **210**:289, 1981.
156. Kato T, Mizutani N, Ban M: Renal transport of lysine and arginine in lysinuric protein intolerance. *Eur J Pediatr* **139**:181, 1982.
157. Leopolder A, Burchhardt G, Murer H: Transport of L-ornithine across isolated brush border membrane vesicles from proximal tubule. *Renal Physiol* **2**:157, 1980.
158. McCarthy CF, Borland JL Jr, Lynch HJ Jr, Owen EE, Tyor MP: Defective uptake of basic amino acids and L-cystine by intestinal mucosa of patients with cystinuria. *J Clin Invest* **43**:1518, 1964.
159. Ozegovic B, McNamara D, Segal S: Cystine uptake by rat jejunal brush border membrane vesicles. *Biosci Rep* **2**:913, 1982.
160. Thier SO, Segal S, Fox M, Blair A, Rosenberg LE: Cystinuria: Defective intestinal transport of dibasic amino acids and cystine. *J Clin Invest* **44**:442, 1965.
161. White MF: The transport of cationic amino acids across the plasma membrane of mammalian cells. *Biochim Biophys Acta* **822**:355, 1985.
162. White MF, Christensen HN: Cationic amino acid transport into cultured animal cells. II. Transport system barely perceptible in ordinary hepatocytes, but active in hepatoma cell lines. *J Biol Chem* **257**:4450, 1982.
163. White MF, Gazzola GC, Christensen HN: Cationic amino acid transport into cultured animal cells. I. Influx into cultured human fibroblasts. *J Biol Chem* **257**:4443, 1982.
164. Bannai S: Transport of cystine and cysteine in mammalian cells. *Biochim Biophys Acta* **779**:289, 1984.
165. Dent CE, Rose GA: Aminoacid metabolism in cystinuria. *Q J Med* **79**:205, 1951.
166. Foreman JW, Hwang S-M, Segal S: Transport interactions of cystine and dibasic amino acids in isolated rat renal tubules. *Metabolism* **29**:53, 1980.
167. Foreman JW, Medow MS, Bovee KC, Segal S: Developmental aspects of cystine transport in the dog. *Pediatr Res* **20**:593, 1986.
168. Groth U, Rosenberg LE: Transport of dibasic amino acids, cystine, and tryptophan by cultured human fibroblast: Absence of a defect in cystinuria and Hartnup disease. *J Clin Invest* **51**:2130, 1972.
169. Kato T: Renal handling of dibasic amino acids and cystine in cystinuria. *Clin Sci Mol Med* **53**:9, 1977.
170. Kato T: Renal transport of lysine and arginine in cystinuria. *Tohoku J Exp Med* **139**:9, 1983.
171. Lester FT, Cusworth DC: Lysine infusion in cystinuria: Theoretical renal thresholds for lysine. *Clin Sci* **44**:99, 1973.
172. McNamara D, Pepe M, Segal S: Cystine uptake by rat renal brush border vesicles. *Biochem J* **194**:443, 1981.

173. Morin CL, Thompson MW, Jackson SH, Sass-Kortsak A: Biochemical and genetic studies in cystinuria: Observations on double heterozygotes of genotype I/II. *J Clin Invest* **50**:1961, 1971.
174. Robson EB, Rose GA: The effect of intravenous lysine of the renal clearances of cystine, arginine and ornithine in normal subjects, in patients with cystinuria and Fanconi syndrome and in their relatives. *Clin Sci* **16**:75, 1957.
175. Rosenberg LE: Cystinuria: Genetic heterogeneity and allelism. *Science* **154**:1341, 1966.
176. Segal S, McNamara PD, Pepe CM: Transport interaction of cystine and dibasic amino acids in renal brush border vesicles. *Science* **197**:169, 1977.
177. Volkl H, Silbernagl S: Mutual inhibition of L-cystine/cysteine and other neutral amino acids during tubular reabsorption. A microperfusion study in rat kidney. *Pflugers Arch* **395**:190, 1982.
178. Volkl H, Silbernagl S: Reexamination of the interplay between dibasic amino acids and L-cystine/L-cysteine during tubular reabsorption. *Pflugers Arch* **395**:196, 1982.
179. Thier S, Foc M, Segal S: Cystinuria: In vitro demonstration of an intestinal transport defect. *Science* **143**:482, 1964.
180. Scriver CR, Chesney RW, McInnes RR: Genetic aspects of renal tubular transport. Diversity and topology of carriers. *Kidney Int* **9**:149, 1976.
181. Strauven T, Mardens Y, Clara R, Terheggen H: Intravenous loading with arginine-hydrochloride and ornithine-aspartate in siblings of two families, presenting a familial neurological syndrome associated with cystinuria. *Biomedicine* **24**:191, 1976.
182. Frimpter GW, Horwith M, Furth E, Fellows RE, Thompson DD: Inulin and endogenous amino acid renal clearances in cystinuria: Evidence for tubular secretion. *J Clin Invest* **41**:281, 1962.
183. Bovee KC, Segal S: Renal tubule reabsorption of amino acids after lysine loading of cystinuric dogs. *Metabolism* **33**:602, 1984.
184. Bowring MA, Foreman JW, Lee J, Segal S: Characteristics of lysine transport by isolated rat renal cortical tubule fragments. *Biochim Biophys Acta* **901**:23, 1987.
185. States B, Foreman J, Lee J, Harris D, Segal S: Cystine and lysine transport in cultured human renal epithelial cells. *Metabolism* **36**:356, 1987.
186. Stevens BR, Ross HJ, Wright EM: Multiple transport pathways for neutral amino acids in rabbit jejunal brush border vesicles. *J Membr Biol* **66**:213, 1982.
187. Busse D: Transport of L-arginine in brush border vesicles derived from rabbit kidney cortex. *Arch Biochem Biophys* **191**:551, 1978.
188. Coicadan L, Heyman M, Grasset E, Desjeux J-F: Cystinuria: Reduced lysine permeability at the brush border of intestinal membrane cells. *Pediatr Res* **14**:109, 1980.
189. Desjeux JF, Volanthen M, Dumontier AM, Simell O, Legrain M: Cystine fluxes across the isolated jejunal epithelium in cystinuria: Increased efflux permeability at the luminal membrane. *Pediatr Res* **21**:477, 1987.
190. Simell O: Diamino acid transport into granulocytes and liver slices of patients with lysinuric protein intolerance. *Pediatr Res* **9**:504, 1975.
191. Metoki K, Hommes FA: The uptake of ornithine and lysine by isolated hepatocytes and fibroblasts. *Int J Biochem* **16**:833, 1984.
192. Scriver CR: Cystinuria. *N Engl J Med* **315**:1155, 1986.
193. Frimpter GW: Cystinuria: Metabolism of the disulfide of cysteine and homocysteine. *J Clin Invest* **42**:1956, 1963.
194. Kekomaki M: Intestinal absorption of L-arginine and L-lysine in familial protein intolerance. *Ann Paediatr Fenn* **14**:18, 1968.
195. Rajantie J, Simell O, Perheentupa J: Oral administration of urea cycle intermediates in lysinuric protein intolerance: Effect on plasma and urinary arginine and ornithine. *Metabolism* **32**:49, 1983.
196. Rajantie J, Simell O, Perheentupa J: Intestinal absorption in lysinuric protein intolerance: Impaired for diamino acids, normal for citrulline. *Gut* **21**:519, 1980.
197. Silk DBA: Peptide absorption in man. *Gut* **15**:494, 1974.
198. Simell O, Perheentupa J: Defective metabolic clearance of plasma arginine and ornithine in lysinuric protein intolerance. *Metabolism* **23**:691, 1974.
199. Christensen HN, Cullen AM: Synthesis of metabolism-resistant substrates for the transport system for cationic amino acids; their stimulation of the release of insulin and glucagon, and of the urinary loss of amino acids related to cystinuria. *Biochim Biophys Acta* **298**:932, 1973.
200. Buchanan JA, Rosenblatt DS, Scriver CR: Cultured human fibroblasts and plasma membrane vesicles to investigate transport function and the effects of genetic mutation. *Ann NY Acad Sci* **456**:401, 1985.
201. Smith DW, Scriver CR, Simell O: Lysinuric protein intolerance mutation is not expressed in the plasma membrane of erythrocytes. *Hum Genet* **80**:395, 1988.
202. Gardner JD, Levy AG: Transport of dibasic amino acids by human erythrocytes. *Metabolism* **21**:413, 1972.
203. Christensen HN, Antonioli JA: Cationic amino acid transport in the rabbit reticulocyte. *J Biol Chem* **244**:1497, 1969.
204. Vadgama JV, Christensen HN: Discrimination of Na^+-independent transport systems L, T, and ASC in erythrocytes. Na^+ independence of the latter a consequence of cell maturation? *J Biol Chem* **260**:2912, 1985.
205. Rajantie J, Simell O, Perheentupa J: "Basolateral" and mitochondrial membrane transport defect in the hepatocytes in lysinuric protein intolerance. *Acta Paediatr Scand* **72**:65, 1983.
206. Gamble JG, Lehninger AL: Transport of ornithine and citrulline across the mitochondrial membrane. *J Biol Chem* **248**:610, 1973.
207. Aronson DL, Diwan JJ: Uptake of ornithine by rat liver mitochondria. *Biochemistry* **20**:7064, 1981.
208. Metoki K, Hommes FA: A possible rate limiting factor in urea synthesis by isolated hepatocytes: The transport of ornithine into hepatocytes and mitochondria. *Int J Biochem* **16**:1155, 1984.
209. Hommes FA, Kitchings L, Eller AG: The uptake of ornithine and lysine by rat liver mitochondria. *Biochem Med* **30**:313, 1983.
210. Bradford NM, McGivan JD: Evidence for the existence of an ornithine/citrulline antiporter in rat liver mitochondria. *FEBS Lett* **113**:294, 1980.
211. Raijman L: Citrulline synthesis in rat tissues and liver content of carbamoyl phosphate and ornithine. *Biochem J* **138**:225, 1974.
212. Bryla J, Harris EJ: Accumulation of ornithine and citrulline in rat liver mitochondria in relation to citrulline formation. *FEBS Lett* **72**:331, 1976.
213. Cohen NS, Cheung C-W, Raijman L: Channeling of extramitochondrial ornithine to matrix ornithine transcarbamylase. *J Biol Chem* **262**:203, 1987.
214. Cohen NS, Cheung C-W, Raijman L: The effects of ornithine on mitochondrial carbamyl phosphate synthesis. *J Biol Chem* **255**:10248, 1980.
215. Grays RGF, Hill SE, Pollitt RJ: Studies on the pathway from ornithine to proline in cultured skin fibroblasts with reference to the defect in hyperornithinaemia with hyperammonaemia and homocitrullinuria. *J Inherit Metab Dis* **6**:143, 1983.
216. Grays RGF, Hill SE, Pollitt RJ: Reduced ornithine catabolism in culture fibroblasts and phytohaemagglutinin-stimulated lymphocytes from a patient with hyperornithinaemia, hyperammonaemia and homocitrullinuria. *Clin Chim Acta* **118**:141, 1982.
217. Shih VE: Regulation of ornithine metabolism. *Enzyme* **26**:254, 1981.
218. Shih VE, Mandell R: Defective ornithine metabolism in the syndrome of hyperornithinaemia, hyperammonaemia and homocitrullinuria. *J Inherit Metab Dis* **4**:95, 1981.
219. Vici CD, Bachmann C, Gambarara M, Colombo JP, Sabetta G: Hyperornithinemia-hyperammonemia-homocitrullinuria syndrome: Low creatine excretion and effect of citrulline, arginine, or ornithine supplement. *Pediatr Res* **22**:364, 1987.
220. Inoue I, Saheki T, Kayanuma K, Uono M, Nakajima M, Takeshita K, Koike R, Yuasa T, Miyatake T, Sakoda K: Biochemical analysis of decreased ornithine transport activity in the liver mitochondria from patients with hyperornithinemia, hyperammonemia and homocitrullinuria. *Biochim Biophys Acta* **964**:90, 1988.
221. Inoue I, Koura M, Saheki T, Kayanuma K, Uono M, Nakajima M, Takeshita K, Koike R, Yuasa T, Miyatake T, Sakoda K: Abnormality of citrulline synthesis in liver mitochondria from patients with hyperornithinaemia, hyperammonaemia and homocitrullinuria. *J Inherit Metab Dis* **10**:277, 1987.
222. Gatfield PD, Taller E, Wolfe DM, Haust DM: Hyperornithinemia, hyperammonemia, and homocitrullinuria associated with decreased carbamyl phosphate synthetase I activity. *Pediatr Res* **9**:488, 1975.
223. Hommes FA, Roesel RA, Metoki K, Hartlage PL, Dyken PR: Studies on a case of HHH-syndrome (hyperammonemia, hyperornithinemia, homocitrullinuria). *Neuropediatrics* **17**:48, 1986.
224. Hommes FA, Ho CK, Roesel RA, Coryell ME: Decreased transport of ornithine across the inner mitochondrial membrane as a cause of hyperornithinaemia. *J Inherit Metab Dis* **5**:41, 1982.
225. Oyanagi K, Tsuchiyama A, Itakura Y, Sogawa H, Wagatsuma K, Nakao T: The mechanism of hyperammonaemia and hyperornithinaemia in the syndrome of hyperornithinaemia, hyperammonaemia with homocitrullinuria. *J Inherit Metab Dis* **6**:133, 1983.

226. Shih VE, Efron ML, Moser HW: Hyperornithinemia, hyperammonemia, and homocitrullinuria. A new disorder of amino acid metabolism associated with myoclonic seizures and mental retardation. *Am J Dis Child* **117**:83, 1969.
227. Koike R, Fujimori K, Yuasa T, Miyatake T, Inoue I, Saheki T: Hyperornithinemia, hyperammonemia, and homocitrullinuria: Case report and biochemical study. *Neurology* **37**:1813, 1987.
228. Pisoni RL, Thoene JG, Christensen HN: Detection and characterization of carrier-mediated cationic amino acid transport in lysosomes of normal and cystinotic human fibroblasts. *J Biol Chem* **260**:4791, 1985.
229. Aula P, Autio S, Raivio KO, Rapola J, Thoden C-J, Koskela S-L, Yamashina I: "Salla Disease." A new lysosomal storage disorder. *Arch Neurol* **36**:88, 1979.
230. Gahl WA, Bashan N, Iteze F, Bernardini I, Schulman JD: Cystine transport is defective in isolated leukocyte lysosomes from patients with cystinosis. *Science* **217**:1263, 1982.
231. Renlund M, Aula P, Raivio KO, Autio S, Sainio K, Rapola J, Koskela S-L: Salla disease: A new lysosomal storage disorder with disturbed sialic acid metabolism. *Neurology* **33**:57, 1983.
232. Renlund M, Kovanen PT, Raivio KO, Aula P, Gahmberg CG, Ehnholm C: Studies on the defect underlying the lysosomal storage of sialic acid in Salla disease. Lysosomal accumulation of sialic acid formed from *N*-acetyl-mannosamine or derived from low-density lipoprotein in cultured mutant fibroblasts. *J Clin Invest* **77**:568, 1986.
233. Renlund M, Tietze F, Gahl WA: Defective sialic acid egress from isolated fibroblast lysosomes of patients with Salla disease. *Science* **232**:759, 1986.
234. Reeves JP: Accumulation of amino acids by lysosomes incubated with amino acid methyl esters. *J Biol Chem* **254**:8914, 1979.
235. Desjeux JF, Rajantie J, Simell O, Dumontier AM, Perheentupa J: Flux de lysine a travers l'epithelium du jejunum dans l'intolerance aux proteines avec lysinurie. *Gastroenterol Clin Biol* **4**:31A, 1980.
236. Perheentupa J, Kekomaki M, Visakorpi JK: Studies on amino nitrogen metabolism in familial protein intolerance. *Pediatr Res* **4**:209, 1970.
237. Ratner S: Urea synthesis and metabolism of arginine and citrulline. *Adv Enzymol* **15**:319, 1954.
238. Meister A: Metabolism of glutamine. *Physiol Rev* **36**:103, 1956.
239. Bachmann C, Colombo JP: Computer simulation of the urea cycle: Trials for an appropriate mode. *Enzyme* **26**:259, 1981.
240. Krebs HA, Hems R, Lund P, Halliday D, Read WWC: Sources of ammonia for mammalian urea synthesis. *Biochem J* **176**:733, 1978.
241. Stumph DA, Parks JK: Urea cycle regulation: I. Coupling of ornithine metabolism to mitochondrial oxidative phosphorylation. *Neurology* **30**:178, 1980.
242. Natale PJ, Tremblay GC: On the availability of intramitochondrial carbamylphosphate for the extramitochondrial biosynthesis of pyrimidines. *Biochem Biophys Res Commun* **37**:512, 1969.
243. Pausch J, Rasenack J, Haussinger D, Gerok W: Hepatic carbamoyl phosphate in de novo pyrimidine synthesis. *Eur J Biochem* **150**:189, 1985.
244. Graham GG, MacLean WC Jr, Placko RP: Plasma free amino acids of infants and children consuming wheat-based diets, with and without supplemental casein or lysine. *J Nutr* **111**:1446, 1981.
245. Cree TC, Schalch DS: Protein utilization in growth: Effect of lysine deficiency on serum growth hormone, somatomedins, insulin, total thyroxine [T_4] and triiodothyronine, free T_4 index, and total corticosterone. *Endocrinology* **117**:667, 1985.
246. Borum PR, Broquist HP: Lysine deficiency and carnitine in male and female rats. *J Nutr* **107**:1209, 1977.
247. Jansen GR: Lysine in human nutrition. *J Nutr* **76**:1, 1962.
248. Hwang S-M, Segal S: Developmental and other characteristics of lysine uptake by rat brain synaptosomes. *Biochim Biophys Acta* **557**:436, 1979.
249. Rajantie J, Simell O, Perheentupa J: Oral administration of ε-*N*-acetyllysine and homocitrulline for lysinuric protein intolerance. *J Pediatr* **102**:388, 1983.
250. Friedman M, Gumbmann MR: Bioavailability of some lysine derivatives in mice. *J Nutr* **111**:1362, 1981.
251. Fujitaki JM, Steiner AW, Nichols SE, Helander ER, Lin YC, Smith RA: A simple preparation of *N*-phosphorylated lysine and arginine. *Prep Biochem* **10(2)**:205, 1980.
252. Morris JG, Rogers QR: Ammonia intoxication in the near-adult cat as a result of a dietary deficiency of arginine. *Science* **199**:431, 1978.
253. Morris JG, Rogers QR; Arginine: An essential amino acid for the cat. *J Nutr* **108**:1944, 1978.
254. Christensen HN: A transport system serving mono- and diamino acids. *Proc Natl Acad Sci U S A* **51**:337, 1964.
255. Christensen HN, Handlogten M, Thomas EL: Na^+ facilitated reactions of neutral amino acids with a cationic amino acid transport system. *Proc Natl Acad Sci U S A* **63**:948, 1969.
256. Van Winkle LJ, Christensen HN, Campione AL: Na^+-dependent transport of basic, zwitterionic, and bicyclic amino acids by a broad-scope system in mouse blastocysts. *J Biol Chem* **260**:12118, 1985.
257. Van Winkle LJ, Campione AL, Gorman JM: Na^+-independent transport of basic and zwitterionic amino acids in mouse blastocysts by a shared system and by processes which distinguish between these substrates. *J Biol Chem* **263**:3150, 1988.
258. Kilberg MS, Stevens BR, Novak DA: Recent advances in mammalian amino acid transport. *Ann Rev Nutr* **13**:137, 1993.
259. Metoki K, Hommes FA: The uptake of ornithine and lysine by isolated hepatocytes and fibroblasts. *Int J Biochem* **16**:833, 1984.
260. Christensen HN: Role of amino acid transport and countertransport in nutrition and metabolism. *Physiol Rev* **70**:43, 1990.
261. Albritton LM, Tseng L, Scadden D, Cunningham JM: A putative murine ecotropic retrovirus receptor gene encodes a multiple membrane-spanning protein and confers susceptibility to virus infection. *Cell* **57**:659, 1989.
262. Hoffman W: Molecular characterization of the CAN1 locus in *Saccharomyces cerevisiae*. A transmembrane protein without N-terminal hydrophobic signal sequence. *J Biol Chem* **260**:11831, 1985.
263. Tanaka J, Fink GR: The histidine permease gene (HIP1) of *Saccharomyces cerevisiae*. *Gene* **38**:205, 1985.
264. Weber E, Chevallier M-R, Jund R: Evolutionary relationship and secondary structure predictions in four transport proteins of *Saccharomyces cerevisiae*. *J Mol Evol* **27**:341, 1988.
265. Kim JW, Closs EI, Albritton LM, Cunningham JM: Transport of cationic amino acids by the mouse ecotropic retrovirus receptor. *Nature* **352**:725, 1991.
266. Wang H, Kavanaugh MP, North RA, Kabat D: Cell-surface receptor for ecotropic murine retroviruses is a basic amino-acid transporter. *Nature* **352**:729, 1991.
267. Closs EI, Albritton LM, Kim JW, Cunningham JM: Identification of a low affinity, high capacity transporter of cationic amino acids in mouse liver. *J Biol Chem* **268**:7538, 1993.
268. Jaenisch R, Hoffman E: Transcription of endogenous C-type viruses in resting and proliferating tissues of BALB/Mo mouse. *Virology* **98**:289, 1979.
269. MacLeod CL, Finley K, Kakuda D, Kozak CA, Wilkinson MF: Activated T cells express a novel gene on chromosome 8 that is closely related to the murine ecotropic retroviral receptor. *Mol Cell Biol* **10**:3663, 1990.
270. Wells RG, Hediger MA: Cloning of a rat kidney cDNA that stimulates dibasic and neutral amino acid transport and has sequence similarity to glucosidases. *Proc Natl Acad Sci U S A* **89**:5596, 1992.
271. Tate SS, Yan N, Udenfriend S: Expression cloning of a Na^+-independent neutral amino acid transporter from rat kidney. *Proc Natl Acad Sci U S A* **89**:1, 1992.
272. Bertran J, Werner A, Moore ML, Stange G, Markovich D, Biber J, Testar X, Zorzano A, Palacin M, Murer H: Expression-cloning of a cDNA from rabbit kidney cortex that induces a single transport system for cysteine, dibasic, and neutral amino acids. *Proc Natl Acad Sci U S A* **89**:5601, 1992.
273. Lee W-S, Wells RG, Sabbag RV, Mohandas TK, Hediger MA: Cloning and chromosomal localization of a human kidney cDNA involved in cystine, dibasic, and neutral amino acids transport. *J Clin Invest* **91**:1959, 1993.
274. Bertran J, Magagnin S, Werner A, Markovich D, Biber J, Testar X, Zorzano A, Kuhn LC, Palacin M, Murer H: Stimulation of system y^+-like amino acid transport by the heavy chain of human 4F2 surface antigen in *Xenopus laevis* oocytes. *Proc Natl Acad Sci U S A* **89**:5606, 1992.
275. Wells RG, Lee W-S, Kanai Y, Leiden JM, Hediger MA: The 4F2 antigen heavy chain induces uptake of neutral and dibasic amino acids in *Xenopus* oocytes. *J Biol Chem* **267**:15285, 1992.
276. Kacser H, Burns JA: The molecular basis of dominance. *Genetics* **97**:639, 1981.
277. Li-Chan E, Nakai S: Covalent attachment of N^{ϵ}-acetyl lysine, N^{ϵ}-benzylidene lysine, and threonine to wheat gluten for nutritional improvement. *J Food Sci* **45(3)**:514, 1980.
278. Dickinson JC, Rosenblom H, Hamilton PB: Ion exchange chromatography of the free amino acids in the plasma of the newborn infant. *Pediatrics* **36**:2, 1965.

279. Scriver CR, Davies E: Endogenous renal clearance rates of free amino acids in prepubertal children. *Pediatrics* **36**:592, 1965.
280. Palacín M, Estévez R, Bertran J, Zorzano A: Molecular biology of mammalian plasma membrane amino acid transporters. *Physiol Rev* **78**:969, 1998.
281. Deves R, Boyd CA: Transporters for cationic amino acids in animal cells: Discovery, structure and function. *Physiol Rev* **78**:487, 1998.
282. Verrey F, Jack DL, Paulsen IT, Saier MH Jr, Pfeiffer R: New glycoprotein-associated amino acid transporters. *J Membr Biol* **172**:181, 1999.
283. Duval M, Fenneteau O, Doireau V, Faye A, Yotnda P, Drapier JC, Schlegel N, Sterkers G, de Baulny HO, Vilmer E: Intermittent hemophagocytic lymphohistiocytosis is a regular feature of lysinuric protein intolerance. *J Pediatr* **134**:236, 1999.
284. Bader-Meunier B, Parez N, Muller S: Treatment of hemophagocytic lymphohistiocytosis with cyclosporin A and steroids in a boy with lysinuria protein intolerance. *J Pediatr* **136**:134, 2000.
285. Duval M, de Baulny HO, Vilmer E: Reply. *J Pediatr* **136**:134, 2000.
286. Palacín M, Estévez R, Zorzano A: Cystinuria calls for heteromultimeric amino acid transporters. *Curr Opin Cell Biol* **10**:455, 1998.
287. Chillaron J, Estévez R, Samarzija I, Waldegger S, Testar X, Lang F, Zorzano A, Busch A, Palacín M: An intracellular trafficking defect in type I cystinuria rBAT mutants M467T and M467K. *J Biol Chem* **272**:9543, 1997.
288. Estévez R, Camps M, Rojas AM, Testar X, Deves R, Hediger MA, Zorzano A, PalacÀín M: The amino acid transport system y^+L/4F2hc is a heteromultimeric complex. *FASEB J* **12**:1319, 1998.
289. Mastroberardino L, Spindler B, Pfeiffer R, Skelly PJ, Loffing J, Shoemaker BC, Verrey F: Amino acid transport by heterodimers of 4F2hc/CD98 and members of a permease family. *Nature* **395**:288, 1998.
290. Torrents D, Estévez R, Pineda M, Fernández E, Lloberas J, Shi Y-B, Zorzano A, Palacín M: Identification and characterization of a membrane protein (y^+L amino acid transporter-1) that associates with 4F2hc to encode the amino acid transport activity y^+L. *J Biol Chem* **273**:32437, 1998.
291. Pfeiffer R, Rossier G, Spindler B, Meier C, Kühn L, Verrey F: Amino acid transport of y^+L-type by heterodimers of 4F2hc/CD98 and members of the glycoprotein-associated amino acid transporter family. *EMBO J* **18**:49, 1999.
292. Lauteala T, Sistonen P, Savontaus M-L, Mykkänen J, Simell J, Lukkarinen M, Simell O, Aula P: Lysinuric protein intolerance (LPI) gene maps to the long arm of chromosome 14. *Am J Hum Genet* **60**:1479, 1997.
293. Lauteala T, Mykkanen J, Sperandeo MP, Gasparini P, Savontaus ML, Simell O, Andria G, Sebastio G, Aula P: Genetic homogeneity of lysinuric protein intolerance. *Eur J Hum Genet* **6**:612, 1998.
294. Torrents D, Mykkänen J, Pineda M, Feliubadaló L, Estévez R, de Cid R, Sanjurjo P, Zorzano A, Nunes V, Huoponen K, Reinikainen A, Simell O, Savontaus M-L, Aula P, Palacín M: Identification of SLC7A7, encoding y^+LAT-1, as the lysinuric protein intolerance gene. *Nat Genet* **21**:293, 1999.
295. Borsani G, Bassi MT, Sperandeo MP, De Grandi A, Buoninconti A, Riboni M, Manzoni M, Incerti B, Pepe A, Andria G, Ballabio A, Sebastio G: SLC7A7, encoding a putative permease-related protein, is mutated in patients with lysinuric protein intolerance. *Nat Genet* **21**:297, 1999.
296. Mykkänen J, Torrents D, Pineda M, Camps M, Yoldi ME, Horelli-Kuitunen N, Huoponen K, Heinonen M, Oksanen J, Simell O, Savontaus M-L, Zorzano A, PalacÀín M, Aula P: Functional analysis of novel mutations in y^+LAT-1 amino acid transporter gene causing lysinuric protein intolerance (LPI). *Hum Mol Genet* **9**:431, 2000.
297. Sperandeo MP, Bassi MT, Riboni M, Parenti G, Buoninconti A, Manzoni M, Incerti B, Larocca MR, Di Rocco M, Strisciuglio P, Dianzani I, Parini R, Candito M, Endo F, Ballabio A, Andria G, Sebastio G, Borsani G: Structure of the *SLC7A7* gene and mutational analysis of patients affected by lysinuric protein intolerance. *Am J Hum Genet* **66**:92, 2000.

CHAPTER 193

Hartnup Disorder

Harvey L. Levy

1. **Hartnup disorder is an autosomal recessive impairment of neutral amino acid transport limited to the kidneys and small intestine. It is believed to be caused by a genetic defect in a specific system responsible for neutral amino acid transport across the brush-border membrane of renal and intestinal epithelium. A cell surface receptor for neutral amino acid transport known as ATB^0 has been identified in human kidney and intestine. A cDNA for this transporter has been cloned and the gene mapped to chromosome 19q13.3, but neither the transporter nor the gene has yet been examined in the Hartnup disorder. The diagnostic feature is a striking neutral hyperaminoaciduria. Most affected individuals also have increased excretion of indolic compounds, notably indican (indoxyl sulfate). These indoles originate in the gut from bacterial degradation of unabsorbed tryptophan. Reduced intestinal absorption of tryptophan and increased tryptophan loss in the urine lead to reduced availability of tryptophan for the synthesis of niacin.**
2. **Pellagra-like clinical features have been described in patients with Hartnup disorder. These include a photosensitive skin rash, intermittent ataxia, and psychotic behavior. Some affected individuals have also been mentally retarded or mentally subnormal to a mild degree. Treatment with nicotinamide has been associated with clearing of the rash and, on occasion, disappearance of the ataxia. This has led to the theory that the clinical abnormalities are due to niacin deficiency. Most subjects identified by routine newborn screening, however, as well as most affected sibs of probands, have remained clinically normal without treatment. The most plausible explanation for the disparity in clinical expression is that, while the disorder is monogenic, the "disease" is multifactorial and requires the presence of complicating environmental influences, such as poor diet or diarrhea, and perhaps also a polygenic influence, such as a tendency for low plasma amino acid levels.**
3. **The renal and intestinal defects are not always expressed concordantly. Some individuals with the Hartnup hyperaminoaciduria do not have increased urinary excretion of indolic acids, suggesting that they have the renal defect without the intestinal defect. Conversely, one individual with evidence of an intestinal neutral amino acid transport defect but without the Hartnup hyperaminoaciduria has been reported.**
4. **Maternal Hartnup disorder is probably benign to the fetus and to the pregnancy. At least 14 offspring from women with Hartnup disorder are known, and almost all are normal. One man with Hartnup disorder has fathered two normal children.**

A list of standard abbreviations is located immediately preceding the index in each volume. Additional abbreviations used in this chapter include: 5-HIAA = 5-hydroxyindoleacetic acid; PET = positron emission tomography.

Hartnup disorder is a familial disorder of renal and intestinal amino acid transport. Its constant feature is a specific hyperaminoaciduria that is caused by a diminished capacity for renal reabsorption of a group of monoamino-monocarboxylic ("neutral") acids that share a common, and in this case defective, transport system. In most affected individuals there is also reduced intestinal absorption of at least some of the neutral amino acids, notably tryptophan.

This disorder was once considered to be a rare and usually symptomatic "disease."[1] Information derived from newborn urine screening has widened our view. We now know that Hartnup disorder is one of the most frequent of the hyperaminoacidurias, and that most affected individuals remain asymptomatic,[2] but symptoms can occur when certain factors are present.[3,4]

Jepson, the original author of this chapter, accurately described the place that Hartnup disorder occupies in human biology when he stated, "The disorder has a physiologic interest out of all proportion to its rare clinical occurrence.... Its study has shed light on general problems of renal absorption, amino acid transport, protein digestion, nicotinamide metabolism, and intestinal bacterial reactions."[1]

An interesting historical note is that the name of the disorder is the surname of the family in which the disorder was first found. In the original report[5] the term "H disease" was used; subsequently, the full surname was applied, apparently with the consent of the family.[1]

THE HARTNUP FAMILY

In 1951, a 12-year-old boy, E. Hartnup, was admitted to the Middlesex Hospital, London, England, with mild cerebellar ataxia and a red, scaly rash on the exposed areas of his body. His mother said he had pellagra, because her eldest daughter (P.H.), with identical symptoms, had been treated for that disease. Although the rash in E.H. was quite consistent with pellagra, other findings were not, and a diagnosis of pellagra as a dietary deficiency was untenable.

Apart from variable cerebellar signs and retarded mental development, the only abnormality detected at that time was in the urinary excretion of free amino acids. Paper chromatography of the urine disclosed an excretion pattern of amino acids quite unlike that seen in any other disease.

At the same time, P.H., then 19 years old, had a recurrence of ataxia (without a rash), similar to the episode she had had in childhood when the pellagra-like rash was most severe. The excretion pattern of amino acids in her urine was identical to that of her brother, E.H.

It was then clear that these two sibs were affected by the same disease. An inherited condition seemed probable when it was learned that the parents were first cousins.

Neither parent and none of their other six children gave a clinical history to suggest that they were similarly affected, although one girl (M.H.) was mentally retarded. Two younger sibs, Jh. H. and H.H., also had gross aminoaciduria with the characteristic chromatographic pattern. No abnormality was detected in the urine of the other four sibs or in either parent. In the affected children, the amino acid excretion persisted

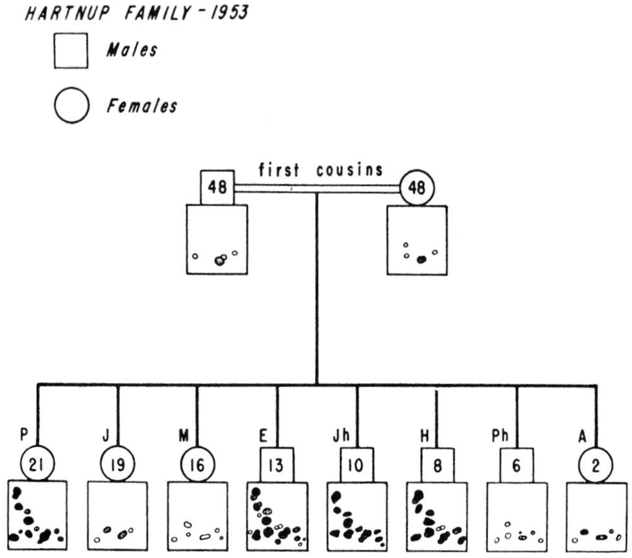

Fig. 193-1 The genealogy of Hartnup disorder as illustrated in the original Hartnup family. The parents were first cousins. The ages of the subjects in 1953 are indicated by the numbers; in the squares are the chromatography patterns of urine samples of two-dimensional chromatograms stained for amino acids.

unchanged in pattern and amount. The skin and neurologic disturbances gradually lessened in P.H. and E.H. but made a fleeting appearance in the younger boys.

The pedigree of the Hartnup family, with a diagrammatic representation of the amino acid chromatographic findings, is given in Fig. 193-1. No other relatives of the Hartnup parents showed the amino acid abnormality.

The publication that first fully reported this family and the existence of this disorder was entitled "Hereditary pellagra-like skin rash with temporary cerebellar ataxia. Constant renal amino-aciduria. And other bizarre biochemical features."[5] As a description of the fully expressed phenotype of the disorder, this title cannot be bettered.

POSSIBLE GENETIC DEFECT

The markedly increased neutral amino acid levels in the urine and feces indicated that the basic defect in Hartnup disorder is in the renal and intestinal transport of these amino acids. Inheritance of the disorder was a further indication of the existence of a specific neutral amino acid transport system in kidney and intestine that was defective in Hartnup disorder (see below). Until recently, however, there was no definitive evidence for such a system. There is now such evidence.

Christensen laid the groundwork for recognition of a renal and intestinal neutral amino acid transport system in the 1960s when he identified a sodium-dependent neutral amino acid transport system in mammalian cells. He termed this system ASC.[5a] In 1993, Arriza et al.,[5b] while screening a human brain cDNA library for sequences related to glutamate transporters, identified a cDNA that was structurally similar to a glutamate transporter gene but, when expressed, transported only neutral amino acids. They named this gene ASCT1 in reference to the ASC plasma-membrane neutral-amino-acid transporter of Christensen.[5a] Three years later, Kekuda et al.,[5c] using the ASCT1 cDNA, isolated from a human placental choriocarcinoma cell library a cDNA that exclusively stimulated the transport of neutral amino acids. They localized this gene to chromosome 19q13.3, which turned out to be the locus of a previously identified gene for a protein with striking sequence similarity to glutamate and neutral amino acid transporters.[5d,5e] Kekuda et al.[5f] have also obtained evidence that this gene expresses a neutral-amino-acid transporter in human kidney and intestine. This transporter and gene are now designated ATB^0. As yet, this gene has not been examined in patients with Hartnup disorder.

Very recently, a gene for a cell surface receptor required for RD114/simian type D retroviral cell entry was identified and found to have sequence and mapping identity to the ATB^0 gene.[5g,5h] These retroviruses produce immunodeficiency and are a major cause of morbidity and mortality in captive primates. A type D virus has also been reported to produce opportunistic infection in a human with AIDS.[5i] The cloned cDNA for the receptor was shown to transport neutral amino acids and it was postulated that the pathogenesis of the immunodeficiency involved viral interference of amino acid transport and resulting intracellular deficiency of neutral amino acids.[5g]

BIOCHEMICAL PHENOTYPE

The diagnosis of Hartnup disorder is based on biochemical rather than clinical abnormalities. The characteristic pattern of neutral hyperaminoaciduria is the one constant feature and is considered the sine qua non for diagnosis. This pattern is a consequence of the defect in renal amino acid transport. The feces contain increased free amino acids, a consequence of the defect in intestinal amino acid transport. The intestinal defect also accounts for the presence of indoles in the urine. Defective absorption of tryptophan allows bacterial enzymes to degrade tryptophan, releasing indole and related metabolites for absorption and further degradation within the body.

Amino Acids

Renal Defect. The pattern of hyperaminoaciduria in Hartnup disorder is distinctive and quite different from other forms of renal hyperaminoaciduria, such as the generalized hyperaminoaciduria of the Fanconi syndrome, cystinuria, or iminoglycinuria. The neutral hyperaminoaciduria of Hartnup disorder consists of striking increases in the monoamino-monocarboxylic amino acids, including alanine, serine, threonine, valine, leucine, isoleucine, phenylalanine, tyrosine, tryptophan, and histidine, as well as glutamine and asparagine, which are neutral monoaminodicarboxylic amides. These free amino acids are excreted in amounts 5 to 20 times normal (Fig. 193-2). The levels of amino acids in the "acidic" (monoaminodicarboxylic) group, such as glutamic acid and aspartic acid, as well as those in the "basic" (diaminomonocarboxylic) group, such as lysine and ornithine, are usually normal or only slightly increased.[6] Methionine, a sulfur-containing neutral amino acid, is also usually normal, although it may be increased. The β-amino acids, taurine and β-aminoisobutyric acid, are not detected in Hartnup urine. It is worth noting that even the most sensitive methods fail to detect increased amounts of proline, hydroxyproline, or arginine. The absence of proline in particular distinguishes the Hartnup pattern from generalized hyperaminoaciduria.[7] The free amino acids are all of the L configuration.[8]

The hyperaminoaciduria is of renal origin, not an "overflow" phenomenon, since plasma amino acid concentrations are not increased. The renal clearances of the excessively excreted amino acids are grossly elevated above normal, both in the fasting state[9] and following an oral load of casein,[10] while the clearances of the amino acids that are not excreted in excess are normal or only slightly elevated. Table 193-1 provides data on renal clearances from several studies.[10–13] The clearance of histidine has been reported to be as high as 140 ml/min,[14] approximating the GFR. One patient excreted 17 percent of an intravenous load of L-histidine unchanged within 4 h, while a control excreted only 0.3 percent.[12] For the other amino acids excreted in excess by Hartnup individuals, the tubular reabsorption of the filtered load at physiological concentrations is about 30 to 60 percent, compared to over 95 percent for normal subjects.

These excretion studies indicate a disturbance in the renal tubular transport of a certain group of amino acids, specifically those of the neutral type, which share a common system for renal

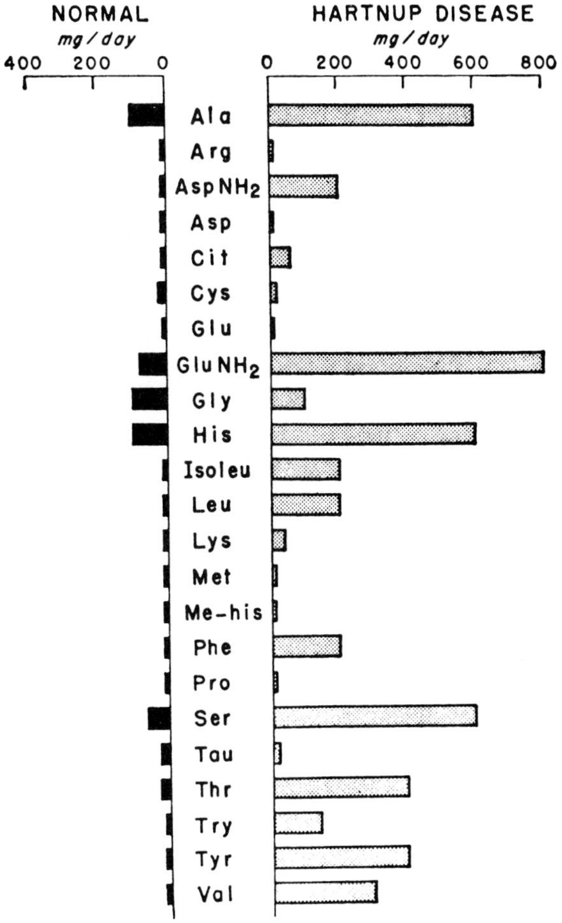

Fig. 193-2 The excretion of free amino acids in the urine of normal subjects and patients with Hartnup disorder.

membrane transport.[15] The quartet of amino acids excreted in cystinuria (cystine, ornithine, lysine, and arginine; see Chap. 191) share another transport system; this system is obviously intact in Hartnup individuals, as is a third distinct transport system, for the glycine-imino acid group, that is defective iminoglycinuria (see Chap. 194). This concept—that Hartnup disorder is one of a trio of genetic disorders each involving only one of the systems for amino acid transport—was first suggested by Milne et al.,[16] who also extended the concept to apply to intestinal transport as well as the renal tubule.

Despite the obvious defect, substantial renal tubular transport of the involved amino acids remains. As noted above, except in rare instances, renal clearances do not approach the GFR. It is possible that the renal tubular defect is far from complete. A more likely explanation is that each amino acid is transported by more than one system.[17] One of these systems transports most of the neutral amino acids. This is most likely a high-capacity system and is defective in Hartnup disorder. Specific low-capacity systems may also exist for each amino acid, as is known to be the case for glycine (see Chap. 194). Thus, in Hartnup disorder, renal tubular reabsorption of neutral amino acids may occur by a combination of specific amino acid transport, passive diffusion, and, perhaps, residual activity of the defective neutral amino acid transport system.

The amino acid excretion pattern is remarkably constant, and is unchanged by nicotinamide or other vitamins, drugs, or antibiotics, despite isolated reports to the contrary.[18,19]

All other tests of renal function have given normal results. One patient was found at autopsy to lack the descending limb of the loop of Henle.[20] This child had unusual features, which included fatty degeneration of the liver with liver failure and terminal myocardial involvement.[21] Microdissection of nephrons was not reported in other patients studied at autopsy.[22,23] The defect is certainly at a subcellular level, but *in vitro* studies of renal amino acid transport in Hartnup individuals have not yet been performed.

Table 193-1 Renal Clearance of Amino Acids in Hartnup Disorder

Amino acid	Excretion in Hartnup disorder	Clearance (ml/min)* Hartnup	Normal
Total amino acid nitrogen			
Fasting	High	6–22	1.5
Maximum on oral protein load	Very high	25–50	3.0
Threonine	High	70	1.0
Tyrosine	High	66	1.5
Histidine	High	122	6.0
Taurine	Low	1.9	5.0
Proline	Low	0.3	0.1
Cystine	Low	0.4	0.5

*Data from references 10–13

Intestinal Defect. Demonstrating a defect in intestinal absorption of free amino acids analogous to the defect in renal transport has been more difficult than identifying the renal defect, but several studies have shown that (a) feces from Hartnup patients contain increased amounts of the affected amino acids; (b) the rise in plasma concentration of several involved amino acids following an oral load is abnormally low or delayed, although normal concentrations are found after intravenous administration; and (c) bacterial degradation products from unabsorbed amino acids are found in excess in urine. The latter feature has been especially investigated for tryptophan.

The first indication of an intestinal defect in Hartnup disorder was the discovery that intestinal transport of tryptophan is affected.[24] This finding will be discussed below in the section on indole compounds. Following this discovery, Scriver and Shaw[25] and then Scriver[26] described a pattern of increased fecal amino acids that almost mirrored the typical Hartnup urinary pattern. Asatoor and coworkers[27] also found that the feces of patients with Hartnup disorder contained greater quantities of tryptophan, phenylalanine, tyrosine, valine, and leucine/isoleucine than did the feces of normal individuals.

In other studies, however, fecal amino acids were not increased when the patients were on regular diets.[28–30] This seemingly conflicting evidence stimulated investigation of transport with orally administered amino acid loads. These studies demonstrated that intestinal transport of leucine, methionine, phenylalanine, and tyrosine is reduced in the Hartnup disorder,[28–33] whereas proline, glycine, and β-alanine, which have normal renal transport in the Hartnup disorder, also have normal intestinal transport.[29–32] On the other hand, studies of intestinal histidine and lysine transport have not produced consistent results, with evidence for reduced transport in Hartnup disorder in some investigations[28,32] and for normal transport in other studies.[12,28,30,34]

Impaired intestinal transport for several free amino acids has been demonstrated in vitro in Hartnup disorder. Tarlow et al.[33,34] found that jejunal biopsy tissue in one patient showed very little accumulation of histidine when incubated with L-histidine. Shih and coworkers[30] studied the uptake of four amino acids by jejunal mucosa obtained through biopsy from two affected brothers. Tryptophan and methionine uptakes were markedly reduced, while lysine and glycine uptakes were only slightly but significantly diminished. Jejunal mucosa has been histologically normal.[20,22,30,32]

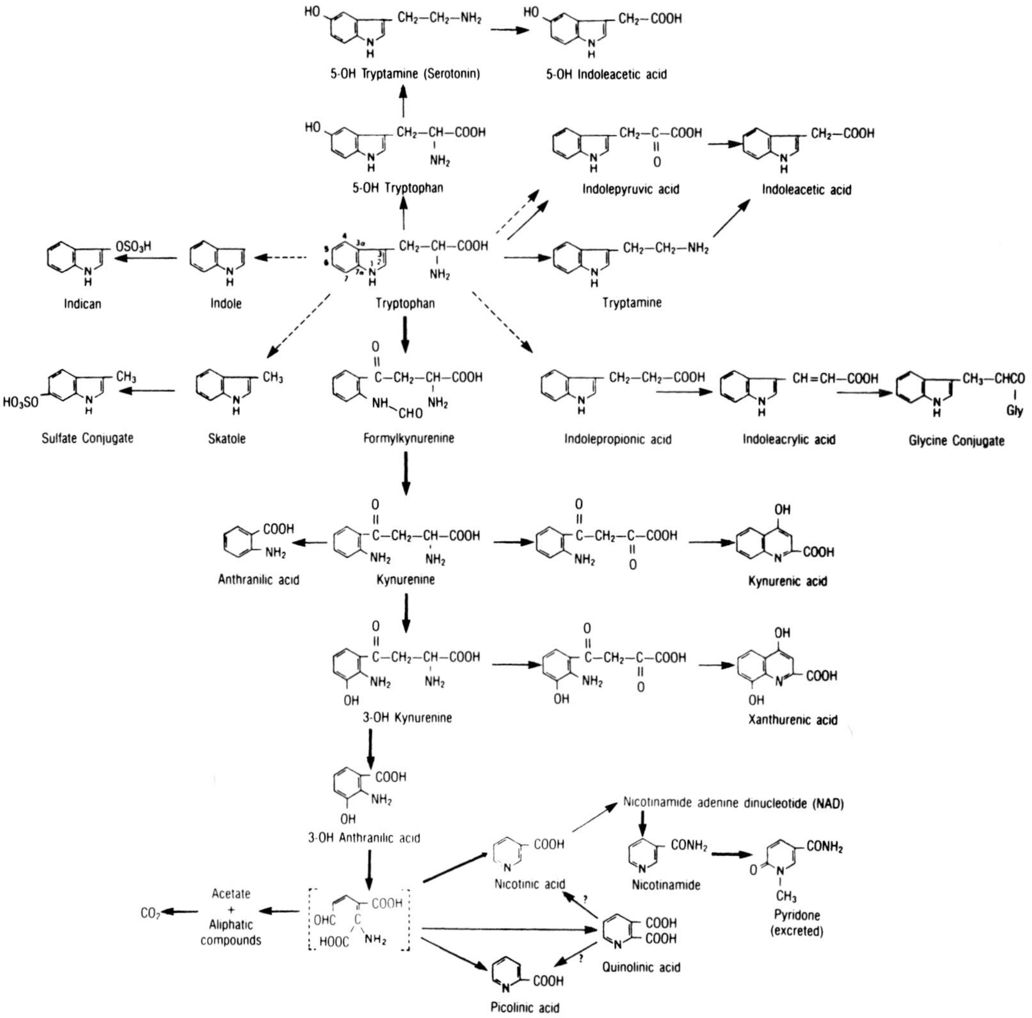

Fig. 193-3 Pathways of tryptophan catabolism. Broken arrows indicate intestinal catabolism by microorganisms.

The defective intestinal absorption of certain neutral amino acids seems not to apply to their ketoacid analogues. Scriver[26] found that transport by the gut of indolepyruvic acid, the ketoacid of tryptophan (Fig. 193-3), was normal in Hartnup disorder, in contrast to the defective transport of tryptophan.

The defect also does not involve intestinal absorption of peptides. When histidine was given to a Hartnup subject in the form of oral carnosine (β-alanyl-L-histidine) rather than as free histidine, the plasma histidine response was normal.[31] This subject also absorbed phenylalanine and tryptophan better when they were in the dipeptide form than as the corresponding mixed free amino acids, while the reverse is true in normal individuals.[32] Analogous results were seen in another affected individual after oral administration of glycyl-tyrosine and free tyrosine.[34] When hydrolyzed casein was given to an individual with Hartnup disorder, there was a rise in plasma amino acids, but when an equivalent mixture of amino acids was given, there was no comparable rise.[35] This suggests that amino acid nutrition in Hartnup disorder (and possibly in analogous situations) is maintained more by absorption of small peptides than by essential amino acids in free form.[36]

An intestinal defect in amino acid transport similar to that noted in the classic Hartnup disorder defect can be present without the renal defect. Drummond et al.[37] reported intestinal malabsorption seemingly limited to tryptophan, with normal urine amino acid excretion in one child and, most probably, also in a deceased sib (see below). Hillman and coworkers[38] described an infant with markedly increased neutral amino acids in the stool and normal or near-normal urine amino acids. These cases, in combination with the diversity in intestinal amino acid transport suggested by the studies in patients with the renal defect, indicate a substantial degree of heterogeneity in the linked renal and intestinal transport of neutral amino acids.

Blood Amino Acids. In all cases in which blood amino acids have been analyzed, the levels have been normal or low, the latter as could be anticipated from diminished absorption and increased excretion.[9,39–41] A study of cases identified by routine screening[3] disclosed slightly lower summed plasma values for the "Hartnup" amino acids in 21 Hartnup subjects as compared to 19 age-matched, unaffected sibs (1552 ± 299 μM and 1657 ± 311 μM, respectively; $p = 0.16$ and 0.06 by Student's t-test and ANOVA, respectively). Summed plasma values for the "non-Hartnup" amino acids were also slightly lower in the Hartnup subjects.

Transport in Other Tissues. Sweat and saliva from Hartnup individuals have a normal amino acid composition.[5] Leukocytes[42] and cultured skin fibroblasts[43] from Hartnup patients transport tryptophan normally. These observations emphasize the conclusion that humans have many genetically independent transport mechanisms and that Hartnup disorder affects only one type and only in specific tissues.

Indole Compounds

Tryptophan Metabolism and Nicotinic Acid (Niacin). Among the clinical abnormalities recognized in the first individuals with Hartnup disorder were psychosis, a photosensitive skin rash, and, occasionally, diarrhea.[5,44,45] Because these are features of pellagra, attention was early directed to the possible role of niacin deficiency in the disorder. However, these patients did not have a dietary history suggesting pellagra nor a deficiency of nicotinic acid derivatives in the urine. Additional tryptophan did not substantially increase the excretion of nicotinic acid derivatives, as would be expected in pellagra.[5] Furthermore, urine amino acids were normal in a patient with diet-induced pellagra.[5] Nevertheless, frequently there seemed to be a clinical response to nicotinamide treatment.[5,44,45] Thus, a defect in the availability of niacin was suspected.

Nicotinic acid and nicotinamide can be synthesized from tryptophan. Figure 193-3 depicts the pathway for this synthesis, the major tryptophan catabolic pathway, as well as some of the many other pathways along which tryptophan catabolism can proceed. Tryptophan is first converted to formylkynurenine by the liver enzyme tryptophan pyrrolase; activity of this enzyme is stimulated by tryptophan administration or by corticoids.[46,47] Formylkynurenine is hydrolyzed to kynurenine by the liver enzyme kynurenine formylase. Kynurenine is hydroxylated to 3-hydroxykynurenine by the mitochondrial enzyme kynurenine-3-hydroxylase. Both kynurenine and 3-hydroxykynurenine are cleared by the pyridoxal-requiring enzyme kynureninase to form anthranilic acid and 3-hydroxyanthranilic acid, respectively. The latter product is oxidized to a labile ring-opened aldehyde intermediate. Ring closure and decarboxylation then occur simultaneously, with the formation of either nicotinic acid or picolinic acid, each by its specific enzyme. Nicotinic acid is further metabolized to nicotinamide adenine dinucleotide (NAD) and nicotinamide.

Under normal conditions, very little tryptophan appears to be converted to nicotinic acid. It is estimated that in the human 60 mg tryptophan is required to replace 1 mg dietary nicotinamide in the form of niacin.[48] Nevertheless, tryptophan may be an important source of niacin, particularly in individuals with relatively poor protein diets.[49]

Evidence that tryptophan is an important source of niacin is seen in patients suspected of having a defect in tryptophan degradation. Common clinical features in several of these patients have included characteristics of niacin deficiency such as a photosensitive rash, ataxia, and mental subnormality.[50–53] In addition, they have often had reduced urinary excretion of *N*-methylnicotinamide,[50,52,53] indicating that the block in tryptophan degradation limited nicotinic acid synthesis.

At least 12 patients with apparent defects in tryptophan catabolism have been reported. Snedden and coworkers[54] described two sibs who had markedly increased plasma and urine tryptophan levels and reduced kynurenine. A block in the conversion of tryptophan to kynurenine was postulated, but enzyme studies to confirm the block were not performed. Tada and colleagues[50] and, later, Wong et al.[51] described children with growth and developmental delay, ataxia, and a photosensitive rash who had very mild increases in plasma tryptophan but that were accentuated by tryptophan loading. Based on reduced urinary kynurenine after tryptophan loading, they also postulated a block in the conversion of tryptophan to kynurenine, but, again, enzyme studies were not done. Komrower et al.[55] reported a child with borderline intelligence, short stature, and headaches who excreted large amounts of both kynurenine and 3-hydroxykynurenine. They suggested that she had a defect in kynureninase, which catalyzes the conversion of kynurenine to anthranilic acid and of 3-hydroxykynurenine to 3-hydroxyanthranilic acid. Clayton and coworkers[56] described a girl with a photosensitive rash, colitis, intellectual deterioration, and severe emotional symptoms who completely recovered with nicotinamide therapy. The increased excretion of kynurenine and kynurenic acid, which was greatly accentuated by tryptophan loading, and the reduced excretion of 3-hydroxykynurenine led these investigators to propose that the defect was at the level of kynurenine-3-hydroxylase. Most recently, Martin et al.[56a] described two sibs with markedly increased fasting plasma and urine tryphophan and massive excretion of indolic acids. The brother had numerous bony abnormalities and severe psychiatric difficulties, including overt hostility, agression, hyperacusis and hyperalgesia. The sister was mentally retarded and had been institutionalized. However, the mother had had rubella during the pregnancy, possibly accounting for the disability. Studies to determine the metabolic block in these sibs were not performed. Other reports include a postulated defect in picolinate carboxylase,[52] a suggested partial defect in kynurenine-3-hydroxylase,[57] the suggestion of an unspecified block proximal to 3-hydroxyanthranilic acid,[53] and an infant with increased tryptophan accompanied by increased blood serotonin who was identified by routine newborn screening.[58]

Other Tryptophan Derivatives. Serotonin (5-hydroxytryptamine), a monoamine neurotransmitter, is an important derivative of tryptophan, although little tryptophan is catabolized in this direction. Serotonin is usually estimated in urine or cerebrospinal fluid as its oxidation product, 5-hydroxyindoleacetic acid (5-HIAA).

Another pathway of tryptophan metabolism is conversion to indolic acids. Normal urine contains a number of indolic acids, the major ones being indoleacetic acid, indolelactic acid, 5-hydroxyindoleacetic acid, and indoleacetylglutamine. [59] The indoleacetic acid is a product of metabolism by intestinal microorganisms and mammalian tissues.[60] This conversion occurs mainly by transamination of tryptophan to indolepyruvic acid, with subsequent decarboxylation to indoleacetic acid. Small amounts of tryptophan are also converted to indoleacetic acid by way of tryptamine. The normal tryptamine excretion by humans is very low, but it can be raised many-fold by the administration of monoamine oxidase inhibitors.[61]

If intestinal absorption of tryptophan is delayed, colonic bacteria can transform tryptophan into indolepropionic acid (Fig. 193-3). This substance is absorbed from the intestine and converted by tissues into indoleacrylic acid, which is excreted as the glycine conjugate.[62,63] Apparently, mammalian tissue cannot produce either indolepropionic acid or indoleacrylic acid directly from tryptophan.

Other important products from the degradation of tryptophan by intestinal microorganisms are indole and skatole (3-methylindole).[64] These microorganisms contain tryptophanase, an enzyme which cleaves tryptophan to indole and pyruvic acid.[65] Indole is absorbed from the intestine, partly oxidized to oxindole and derivatives that are not detectable by standard tests for indoles,[66] and partly hydroxylated in the 3-position to form indoxyl and then its sulfate conjugate (indican). Skatole, the methylated derivative of indole, is converted to 6-hydroxyskatole and likewise conjugated with sulfate for excretion.[67]

Over the years, many correlations have been sought between deranged tryptophan-indole metabolism and mental illness, particularly schizophrenia.[68] Unfortunately, nothing substantial has yet been established.

On the other hand, delayed tryptophan absorption can introduce abnormal urinary excretion of indoles that may mimic metabolic abnormalities.[69] Hartnup disorder is the most extreme of these situations, but many other examples can be found. Africans accustomed to consuming large quantities of matoke (cooked banana) excrete indolylacryloylglycine, presumably because enhanced intestinal motility speeds tryptophan down to colonic bacteria.[70] This effect is also obtained by administering tryptophan orally or per rectum, with a more rapid response by the latter route of administration;[71] sterilization of the gut eliminates this effect.[70,71] Indolylacryloylglycine has also been found in the urine of individuals with unusual intestinal flora.[72,73] Patients with blind-loop syndrome excrete vast amounts of indican.

A familial and specific intestinal malabsorption of tryptophan known as the "blue diaper syndrome" has been described by Drummond et al.[37] (see above). In this disorder, intestinal bacteria convert much of the unabsorbed tryptophan to indican (the

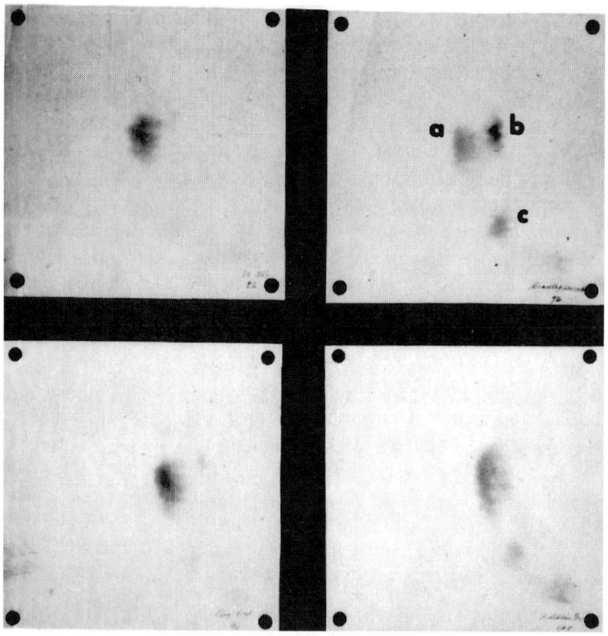

Fig. 193-4 Urine indole patterns (in standardized aliquots) in a normal control (top left), his Hartnup sib (top right), a Hartnup proband with a variant allele (bottom right), and her control sib (bottom left). The typical pattern shows an excess of indoxyl sulfate and tryptophan. The variant pattern shows an excess of tryptophan only. a = urea; b = indoxyl sulfate; c = tryptophan (Scriver, Clow, and Levy, unpublished data.)

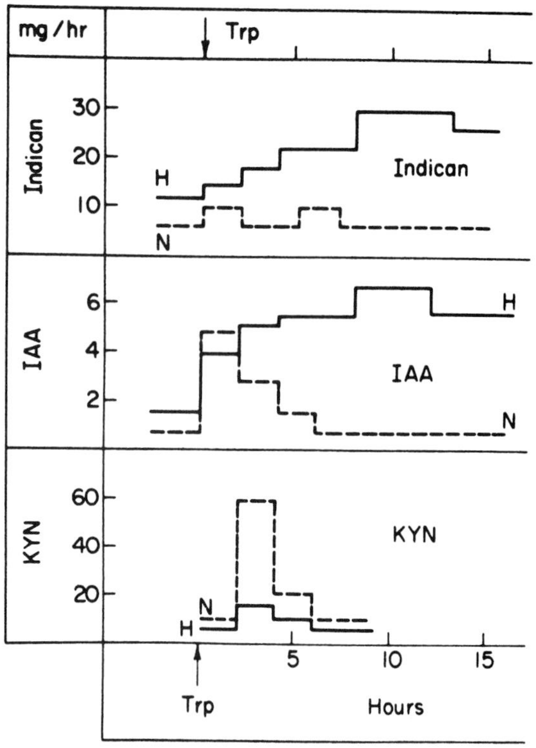

Fig. 193-5 Urinary excretion (mg/h) of tryptophan derivatives following administration of oral L-tryptophan (about 70 mg per kilogram body weight) administered to normal subjects (N-) and to Hartnup patients (H-). These are idealized responses, averaged from the results of several investigators.

designation "blue diaper" comes from indigotin—or indigo blue—the hydrolytic and oxidation product of indican identified in the urine). Other indolic acids are also excreted in abundance. Unlike Hartnup disorder, the defect affects only tryptophan and is expressed only in the intestine, not in the kidney.

Indoles in Hartnup Disorder

Early in the investigations of the Hartnup family, a high but variable excretion of indoxylsulfate (indican) was apparent among affected members. This led to a survey which disclosed increased urinary excretion of other indole compounds as well.[5] Thus, increased excretion of indolic acids derived from tryptophan was revealed in the Hartnup disorder (Fig. 193-4).

Indican has been the most prominent of these urinary indoles; in some instances, Hartnup probands excreted almost 400 mg/day, compared to approximately 100 mg/day excreted by age-matched normal subjects.[74,75] As with normal individuals, urinary indican disappears when the gut is sterilized with antibiotics.[5,19,76–78] Antibiotics do not alter the urinary amino acid excretion, and the indoluria returns to its high level within a few days after cessation of treatment.

Oral administration of L-tryptophan dramatically raises the indicanuria, even in Hartnup patients showing a reasonably normal indican excretion in the basal state,[24] but intravenous L-tryptophan does not have this effect.[19,79] It was the demonstration of this response to oral tryptophan that led Milne and his group[24] to recognize that the transport defect in Hartnup disorder involves the intestine as well as the kidney. Oral tryptophan in normal subjects produces a slight, variable rise in indican, followed by a fall to normal within 12 h, representing a tryptophan-to-indican conversion of no more than 1.6 percent. By contrast, in Hartnup disorder there is a greatly increased indican excretion, which reaches a maximum after 12 h and persists for more than 24 h, with a conversion of 7 to 13 percent[24,79] (Fig. 193-5). A patient investigated by Srikantia et al.[80] is exceptional in showing a fivefold rise in the urinary indican level within 1 h of an oral tryptophan load; the indican level returned to normal within 3 h but peaked again 3 h later. This patient may have a variant of the intestinal defect in Hartnup disorder. In fact, fecal amino acid values and in vitro studies of intestinal transport indicate considerable heterogeneity in the disorder (see "Intestinal Defect" above).

The urinary indoxyl derivatives are final excretion products, formed in the liver from indole absorbed from the colon. Here they must arise from the action of intestinal microorganisms on tryptophan not absorbed from the jejunum because of the transport defect. Studies of the indole-producing bacteria (*Escherichia coli*) from the feces of Hartnup patients failed to show that chronic exposure to tryptophan alters the colonic flora in type or amount from that normally found.[27] On the other hand, there is little or no excretion of 6-hydroxyskatole sulfate, the final product of intestinal skatole formation that may be seen in malabsorption syndromes.[69]

Other urinary indoles that are increased in Hartnup disorder include indoleacetic acid and its conjugate, indoleacetylglutamine.[75,81–83] Indolelactic acid and indoleacetylglucuronide, the other possible conjugate of indoleacetic acid, have also been reported, but only in moderate amounts.[83] The excretion of these indolic acids, especially indoleacetic acid, has been particularly prominent during acute bouts of ataxia and rash in some patients.[5,78]

Nevertheless, the urinary indolic acid pattern has been quite variable in Hartnup individuals and has often been normal under usual conditions as well as during acute clinical episodes.[24,31] Under the stimulus of an oral tryptophan load, however, indolic acid production becomes an obvious feature of Hartnup disorder. The oral administration of L-tryptophan to normal subjects in quantities of about 70 mg per kilogram body weight causes a sharp sixfold rise in free and conjugated urine indoleacetic acid.[24] The peak is reached at 2 h, and the excretion returns to its normal low level in 8 h. The total conversion of such a load to urinary indolic acids is about 0.2 percent. In Hartnup patients, the rise is several times larger, does not reach its peak until 8 or 10 h, and persists at a high level for at least 24 h (Fig. 193-5). The total conversion has been calculated at 1.3 to 1.7 percent in these patients.[24]

Hartnup patients on oral tryptophan loading also excrete large quantities of indolylacryloylglycine with the same 8-h lag period that applies to indoleacetic acid production;[76,84] they may even excrete small amounts of indolylacryloylglycine on a normal diet.[78] In contrast, normal individuals never produce indolylacryloylglycine even with a large oral load of tryptophan, provided the usual intestinal transport mechanisms are operative.

As with indoxyl derivatives, other indolic acids are also derived from bacterial catabolism of tryptophan in the gut. This explanation for their origin is supported by two findings. The first of these findings is the effect of intestinal antibiotics in Hartnup patients. Neomycin (with nystatin) not only lowers the excretion of all indolic acids to somewhat less than the usual level but virtually abolishes any rise after oral tryptophan loading.[19,76,78] It is possible that neomycin slightly inhibits tryptophan or indoleacetic acid absorption from the intestine,[85] but this could not account for more than a small part of the dramatic effect. Second, intravenous tryptophan does not increase indolic acid excretion.[79]

Indolepyruvic acid and its decomposition products have not been detected in the urine of Hartnup patients.[86,87] The urinary excretion of tryptamine is within normal limits in these patients.[1] This may only be tryptamine produced in the kidney and might not reflect tryptamine formation in other tissues or in the intestine.[27] Tryptamine is catabolized to indoleacetic acid by way of the corresponding aldehyde. Experiments to see if oxidation could be diverted through a reductive pathway by the administration of ethanol[88] were unsuccessful; no urinary tryptophol or its conjugates were detectable in Hartnup or control subjects, before or after the consumption of large quantities of alcohol.[1]

Indoluria other than increased tryptophan may not be present in infants during the first 6 months of life.[89,90] This may reflect the more rapid transit of food through the gut during these early months, with less time for bacteria to act upon the tryptophan. After age 6 months, children originally identified by newborn urine amino acid screening have almost always had increased excretion of indolic compounds.[3,89]

Indolic Acids in the Blood. Whole-blood indolic acids have been normal.[75] This finding could be explained by the renal clearance values of indolic acids, which are normally very high.[91] The clearance of indolylacetylglutamine is at least 150 ml/min; the compound may be synthesized, at least in part, from indoleacetic acid in the kidney.[1]

Serotonin Levels. Blood and urine levels for serotonin (5-hydroxytryptamine) have been within normal limits or on the low side of the normal range, in parallel with reduced urinary 5-hydroxyindoleacetic acid excretion.[1,75,77]

Jonas and Butler[41] reported substantially reduced concentrations of 5-hydroxyindoleacetic acid, the oxidation metabolite of serotonin, in the cerebrospinal fluid of a child with Hartnup disorder who had delayed growth and development. Other neurotransmitter metabolite levels were normal. The tryptophan level in cerebrospinal fluid was also reduced, suggesting that this deficiency led to reduced serotonin. Supporting this suggestion was the response to intravenous tryptophan, which increased the level of 5-hydroxyindoleacetic acid in cerebrospinal fluid to a normal value.

Nicotinic Acid Derivatives

The pellagra-like clinical features of some patients with Hartnup disorder led to an early interest in the tryptophan-kynurenine-nicotinic acid pathway.[5] Surprisingly, the urinary excretion of nicotinic acid and derivatives such as nicotinamide and *N*-methylnicotinamide were within normal limits, albeit on the low side. Visakorpi et al.[21] later reported normal niacin concentrations in blood and urine from one patient. Other studies, however, have found that Hartnup subjects may excrete less *N*-methylnicotinamide than normal individuals, both in the basal state[39,42,77,92,93] and after an oral tryptophan load.[39,42,94]

These data might indicate that the amount of nicotinic acid and its derivatives in Hartnup disorder is not necessarily deficient, perhaps because ingested nicotinic acid is absorbed and metabolized normally,[92] but that less comes from ingested tryptophan than in normal individuals. This is not due to a block in the major pathway of tryptophan catabolism through kynurenine (Fig. 193-3), as was once thought might be the case.[5] Notably, tryptophan administered intravenously to Hartnup subjects produces normally enhanced excretion of kynurenine and *N*-methylnicotinamide.[19,79] Rather, it is due to a lower availability of ingested tryptophan, as evidenced by the formation of much less kynurenine[19,24,31,42,79] and xanthurenic acid[76] than in normal controls. Normal individuals converted 3 to 7 percent of oral L-tryptophan to urinary kynurenine, with a peak excretion rate of about 80 mg/h, while Hartnup patients converted only 0.5 to 1.5 percent to kynurenine, with a maximum excretion rate of 10 mg/h.[24] The reduced availability of ingested tryptophan is presumably a result of the defect in intestinal transport (see "Intestinal Defect" above).

CLINICAL PHENOTYPE

The clinical findings in at least two of the four affected children in the original Hartnup family were so much like those seen in pellagra that the investigators performed amino acid analyses on urine specimens from two other English children who had previously been reported as having pellagra.[44,45] In at least one of these children, the diet was much better than that usually ingested by individuals with pellagra.[44] In both children, the amino acid pattern was like that seen in the affected members of the Hartnup family. Thus, it seemed that Hartnup disorder might be phenotypically similar to pellagra.

Subsequent experience has not confirmed such a close association. In fact, children with Hartnup disorder identified by routine newborn urine screening have almost always remained clinically normal.[3,89] This suggests that Hartnup disorder is usually benign. There is little doubt, however, that some individuals with the Hartnup biochemical phenotype develop clinical abnormalities. The unusual combination of a photosensitive rash and neuropsychiatric manifestations has been more often associated with the Hartnup pattern of neutral hyperaminoaciduria than would be expected from coincidence. The most likely explanation for the wide clinical spectrum, proposed by Scriver et al.[3] and Scriver,[4] is that Hartnup disorder represents a monogenic transport defect with which polygenic and environmental factors interact. When these factors are aberrant, as occasionally they are, disease results. Thus, the cause of Hartnup "disease" is multifactorial. Otherwise, the transport disorder is benign.

Skin Lesions

An unusual "pellagra-like" rash has been the most frequent clinical abnormality seen in Hartnup patients. The age of onset has varied from as early as 10 days[95] or 3 months[5,76,96,97] to as late as 13 years.[39] The photosensitive rash has appeared as "severe sunburn," and the patient becomes known as one who should avoid the sun. After unusual exposure to sunlight, blisters have formed much more readily than in normal individuals. The rash has been exclusively or predominantly on the exposed areas of the body, particularly the face, back of neck, back of hands and wrists, external surfaces of the arms and legs, anterior surfaces of the knees, and dorsal surfaces of the feet. In several individuals the rash has been pruritic[39,78,97] and, on occasion, has had the appearance of eczema.[5,21] In three patients the appearance of umbilicated bullae surrounded by erythematous halos suggested the diagnosis of hydroa vacciniforme.[22,98,99] Following the acute erythematous phase, the skin has frequently desquamated, exposing areas of depigmentation. Subsequently, the skin becomes dry and scaly with peripheral depigmentation. The rash has usually been bilateral. Minor skin manifestations were found at slightly higher frequency in Hartnup persons relative to their control sibs in a prospective study.[3]

Neurologic Manifestations

Ataxia. Intermittent ataxia has been the next most frequent abnormality reported among clinically affected patients and the most frequently noted neurologic aberration. The ataxia has usually appeared as unsteadiness while standing and as an unsteady, wide-based gait. In general, no unilaterality has been noted, although in two patients[5,82] the ataxia was more pronounced on the left side and in another patient[80] there was a tendency to fall to one side. The ataxia has usually begun later than the skin abnormalities, but in one case[14] it was the first clinical abnormality noted and in two other cases[80,82] it appeared at the same time as the rash. It has frequently been accompanied by other abnormalities such as nystagmus, diplopia, and tremors, suggesting a cerebellar origin. The most striking characteristic of the ataxia, however, has been its intermittency. In most instances it was present for only a few days or less at a time and then spontaneously disappeared. Precipitating factors in the ataxic episodes have usually not been identifiable, although Shigella dysentery seems to cause an attack in one patient,[5] and exposure to sunlight was implicated in both the rash and ataxia in two other patients.[39]

Mental Development. Although the first two cases identified in the original Hartnup family were mentally retarded, the other two affected members were not retarded.[5] Most of the subsequently reported clinically affected Hartnup patients have not had frank intellectual retardation. School performance has been consistent with intelligence test scores and clinical estimates of intelligence,[5,75,78,87] as have been the types of labor performed.[5,75,82] One of two symptomatic Hartnup patients in a prospective study[3] had delayed cognitive development relative to his non-Hartnup sibs.

Neurologic Signs. Other than the ataxia, there have been few specific neurologic findings. Increased muscle tone and increased deep-tendon reflexes have been reported, usually involving all extremities but, on occasion, only the lower extremities.[39,40,80,93] With the exception of a transient Babinski response in one patient[22] and a persisting response in a child with a progressive encephalopathy,[23] the plantar reflex has been flexor. Pyramidal tract signs have only infrequently been present and when they are present, usually occur during episodes of ataxia. One patient had decreased deep tendon reflexes,[42] and another patient had decreased muscle tone.[100]

Electroencephalographic Findings. Electroencephalographic abnormalities have been described in a number of patients, but there has been no consistent pattern of changes. The abnormalities have ranged from nonspecific slowing[87,101] to variable dysrhythmias, and interpretations of the dysrhythmias have ranged from "electrical immaturity"[100] to "general cerebral dysrhythmia."[78] Increases in theta,[23,31,75] delta,[94] theta-delta,[39,78] and beta[23,39] activities have been mentioned. The abnormalities have usually been generalized, but localized abnormal activities in the parietotemporal,[78] temporal,[23] posterior temporal,[31] and occipital[94] areas have been recorded.

All patients with abnormal EEGs have had clinical abnormalities referable to the central nervous system. In two patients, these findings have been as nonspecific as increased anxiety and irritability.[75] In another case, ataxia and mental retardation were present,[94] while a recently reported child with encephalographic abnormalities died with a progressive encephalopathy.[23] On the other hand, at least two patients with profound central nervous system disease had normal EEGs,[29,87] as did a child with intermittent dystonia and a declining IQ.[93] Electroencephalographic findings have not been recorded in individuals with Hartnup disorder who have not had neurologic disease.

Other Neurologic Findings. One patient had choreiform movements when ataxia was pronounced.[5] Another patient has had intermittent dystonia.[93] Frequent headaches were noted in two patients.[5,78] A patient who had deaf-mutism and was mentally retarded had a history of generalized seizures during early childhood.[29] One patient was prone to vasovagal attacks.[5]

Neuroimaging and Other Studies. Neuroimaging studies have been performed in a few patients with Hartnup disorder. Cranial CT disclosed a small calcification in a frontal subcortical area in an adult with neuropsychiatric illness[101] and minor brain atrophy in a child with progressive encephalopathy,[23] but has also been normal in a child with neurologic disease.[93] MRI of the brain has been described as normal in at least two patients,[23,102] but revealed atrophy, delayed myelination, and dysgenesis of the corpus callosum in a child with intermittent ataxia, developmental delay, and growth failure.[103] Positron emission tomography (PET) revealed "possible bifrontal hypoperfusion" in one adult.[101]

Findings in additional neurologic studies in patients with Hartnup disorder have included normal somatosensory evoked potentials and normal nerve conduction velocities in two patients.[93,101] One child with severe neurologic disease had low-normal nerve conduction velocities.[23]

Psychological Changes

Most of the clinically affected Hartnup patients have had no psychiatric disturbances. Abnormalities of a psychiatric nature suggesting psychosis, however, were among the prominent findings in several of the early cases. The boy described by Hersov[44] was "irritable and morose." The first two members of the Hartnup family had marked emotional instability with depression and outbursts of temper accompanying ataxic episodes. Other patients have been "depressed and depersonalized" with suicidal tendencies,[75] severely anxious,[75] nervous and hallucinatory,[39,78] continuously crying,[78,87] severely confused with hypomania, making meaningless utterances and incontinent,[31] having continuous daytime bruxism,[101] and markedly aggressive.[100] These disturbances have always been episodic and frequently were accompanied by ataxia.

General Somatic Abnormalities

Several different somatic abnormalities have been described in patients with Hartnup disorder. It is doubtful that most are related to the basic defect. Visakorpi et al.[21] described edema and hypoproteinemia with fatty degeneration of the liver and death from liver failure in a child whose affected sister had transient hypoproteinemia and urinary calculi but recovered. Edema and hypoproteinemia were also described in another child who was otherwise well.[104] The patient described by Daute et al.[22] had fever, diarrhea, anemia, and leukopenia and eventually died. Wong and Pillai[79] described recurrent vomiting in one patient. Oyanagi et al.[39] recorded fatty liver in one patient.

Two abnormalities may be related to the Hartnup disorder in some patients. The first of these is atrophic glossitis, present in at least six patients.[22,31,44,45,75,76] The second is small stature, noted in many of the reported cases. Although the general experience from prospective studies of cases identified by newborn screening[3,89] does not support the conclusion of Colliss et al.[105] that Hartnup subjects have a significant reduction in height, occasional children identified prospectively have had growth delay.[3] It is possible that either niacin deficiency or a general deficiency of amino acids[3] complicating certain cases of Hartnup disorder could explain the glossitis and growth retardation.

Characteristics of Individuals Identified by Newborn Screening

Wilcken and her coworkers[89] studied 15 children with Hartnup disorder detected through routine newborn urine screening in New South Wales. Most did not receive nicotinamide treatment. Their intelligence and growth were considered normal and comparable to that of their unaffected sibs. None had abnormal neurologic findings, and only one had a photosensitive rash.

Scriver et al.[3] reported the study of 21 affected children who came to attention through routine urine screening in Massachusetts and Quebec, compared to 19 age-matched unaffected sib controls. None had received continual nicotinamide therapy. Two developed major clinical manifestations, considered to be due to factors acting in concert with the Hartnup defect (see "Is Hartnup Disorder a Disease?" below). Among the remaining 19 affected children, 5 developed skin lesions, which were eczematous in three cases and psoriatic in 2 but not photosensitive in any; 1 unaffected sib had eczema ($p = 0.19$). One Hartnup subject had seizures and an abnormal EEG. The mean $\pm$ SD full-scale IQ scores for 12 Hartnup subjects and 8 sib controls were 103 $\pm$ 10 and 108 $\pm$ 12, respectively. The difference was insignificant. School performances were similar for the two groups. Two Hartnup subjects had learning difficulties, and one of them was subsequently found to also have 47,XXX aneuploidy.[106] Somatic growth was normal in the affected children and comparable to that of their sib controls. Thus, it seems that most Hartnup subjects remain clinically normal.

DIAGNOSIS

The only constant feature of Hartnup disorder is the characteristic excretion of free amino acids, and it is on this that the diagnosis must be based.[1,2] The pattern of urinary amino acids, rather than the total amino acid excretion, is the determining factor. A simple two-dimensional paper or thin-layer chromatographic system with location reagents for amino acids will reveal this pattern,[107] as will quantitative amino acid analysis by column chromatography. Figure 193-2 indicates the urinary amino acids expected in excess in the Hartnup disorder.

Very little else even remotely resembles the Hartnup pattern. In generalized hyperaminoaciduria, with which the Hartnup pattern is most likely confused, proline is always prominent, and cystine and the dibasic amino acids (lysine and ornithine) are excreted in excess. These compounds, particularly proline, are not increased in Hartnup disorder.[5] Fecal contamination of urine, which has often produced factitious results in newborn screening,[108] causes an amino acid pattern much more like generalized hyperaminoaciduria than one resembling Hartnup disorder.[109]

The indolic excretion is not constant enough to be the basis of a diagnostic test. Even increased excretion of indolic acids after an oral tryptophan load might be misleading, since an intestinal defect similar or identical to that in Hartnup disorder may be present without neutral hyperaminoaciduria.[38] Conversely, Hartnup subjects may have only the renal defect.[3] Thus, Hartnup disorder is not excluded by a normal indole excretion, but all patients with a high indican or other indolic acid excretion should be further examined for Hartnup disorder by urine amino acid analysis.

The only alternative diagnoses for the full clinical expression associated with Hartnup disorder would be pellagra or, possibly, a defect in the major pathway of tryptophan catabolism. In pellagra, amino acid excretion is low or normal.[5] Putative defects in tryptophan catabolism include familial disease with pellagra-like skin rash and ataxia, but renal and intestinal amino acid transport is normal.[50–53,110] Hartnup disorder should be suspected in patients with pellagra-like signs but without gross dietary deficiency; photosensitive rash, especially if accompanied by neurologic changes; intermittent ataxia, especially where sibs are similarly affected; or high excretion of indican or other indolic acids.

TREATMENT

The only rational treatment for this disorder is the administration of nicotinic acid or, better, nicotinamide to patients who have signs suggesting a deficiency of this vitamin. This treatment has been used with dosages from 50 to 300 mg/day administered orally. In many instances the rash has cleared with this therapy.[78,111] Several investigators have also reported cessation of ataxia[39,44,82,94] and amelioration of psychotic-type behavior.[31,39,44,75,78,112] Despite reports to the contrary,[18,19] neither the hyperaminoaciduria nor the intestinal transport defect responds to this treatment.[28,92] In addition to nicotinamide, a high-protein diet or protein supplementation might be beneficial in some instances,[1] particularly for patients with low plasma amino acid values[3] in whom symptomatic Hartnup episodes might be prevented. Intravenous nutrition has been beneficial in correcting an eczematoid rash and hypoproteinemic edema associated with low plasma amino acid levels in one patient.[3]

The efficacy of treatment is difficult to evaluate. Because the clinical abnormalities have generally been intermittent, their disappearance in most cases cannot clearly be designated as a therapeutic result. Furthermore, therapy with nicotinamide has not always achieved the desired result. In one patient, the rash disappeared after treatment on one occasion, but did not on another occasion.[5] However, it seems that patients with clinical abnormalities associated with Hartnup disorder should be given at least a trial of nicotinamide therapy.

INHERITANCE

Hartnup disorder has an autosomal recessive inheritance pattern; males and females are about equally represented, sibs are often affected,[1,3,5,89] and parents have normal urine amino acid profiles.[5] Consanguinity between parents, as in the original family,[5] has been reported in a number of families.[1,95,97]

There seems to be widespread distribution of Hartnup disorder with no ethnic predilection. Cases have been found wherever urine amino acid analysis has been conducted, including England, continental Europe, Canada, the United States, Australia, India, Japan, West Africa, and Israel.[113]

Hartnup disorder is not associated with other genetic disorders. Jonxis[14] reported phenylketonuria and Hartnup disorder in one patient. Shih et al.[114] reported the coexistence of Hartnup disorder and methylmalonic aciduria in two families. In one of these families, the proband had both Hartnup disorder and methylmalonic aciduria, and a sib had methylmalonic aciduria alone. The methylmalonic aciduria was B_{12}-unresponsive and was considered to be a benign variant of methylmalonyl CoA mutase deficiency.[115] In the second family, an infant died with severe methylmalonic aciduria; his mother was subsequently found to have Hartnup disorder when she was evaluated for recurrent skin rashes. We are aware of 47,XXX aneuploidy in a girl with Hartnup syndrome,[106] and Tarlow et al.[34] described the coexistence of celiac disease and Hartnup disorder in a boy. One girl identified in newborn screening by Wilcken developed juvenile diabetes mellitus.[116] All of these combinations appear to be purely chance occurrences.

Heterozygotes for the Hartnup mutation, including parents and offspring of Hartnup subjects, have shown no evidence of the renal defect.[1,29,117] The mother of the original Hartnup children had a normal amino acid clearance, even in response to a casein load.[10] Tryptophan loading in heterozygotes, however, might elicit evidence of deficient intestinal transport. The parents of two Hartnup patients had a delayed peak for plasma tryptophan following an oral load.[79] Similarly challenged, the offspring of two Hartnup patients excreted abnormally large amounts of indican, indoleacetic acid, indolylacryloylglycine, indoleacetylglutamine, and indoleacetamide.[29] There may also be a high incidence of photosensitivity among heterozygous individuals.[78,83]

SCREENING AND INCIDENCE

Urine amino acid screening of individuals institutionalized for mental retardation has led to the identification of several Hartnup subjects. Among 729 such individuals screened in India, two

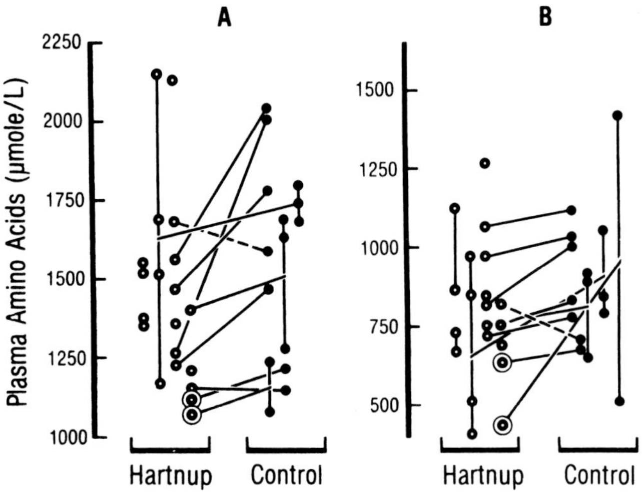

Fig. 193-6 Distributions of plasma amino acid values in Hartnup subjects (circles) and control sibs (black dots). Lines join the corresponding values for sibs (vertical lines, Hartnup vs. Hartnup and control vs. control; solid crossing lines, Hartnup value < control value; interrupted crossing line, Hartnup value > control value). A. Aggregate values (μM) for 10 amino acids (excluding tryptophan) affected by Hartnup mutation. B. Aggregate values for the remaining amino acids. Two symptomatic probands are indicated by the bull's-eye symbol. (*From Scriver et al.*[3] *Used by permission.*)

Hartnup cases were found.[118] Two affected brothers were found among 2100 mentally defective persons screened in a Massachusetts institution.[30] A single case was discovered among an unspecified number of individuals screened in a New Hampshire institution for the mentally retarded.[29]

The fact that the known cases of Hartnup disorder included only these few plus the relatively small number of others identified as a result of amino acid screening for medical indications led to the belief that Hartnup disorder was very rare and, therefore, that the presence of clinical abnormalities in these individuals was highly significant. Routine newborn urine screening has demonstrated, however, that the Hartnup finding is one of the more frequent amino acid disorders.[107] Newborn screening data include incidences of 1:23,000 among 1 million screened in Massachusetts, [119] 1:25,000 among 1 million screened in New South Wales, Australia, [120] 1:32,000 among 193,000 screened in Manitoba,[121] and 1:54,000 among 1.4 million screened in Quebec.[122,123] The combined newborn screening experience is 116 affected infants identified among approximately 3.5 million screened, an incidence of 1:30,000. Additional cases have been identified among sibs of these infants.[3,89] The prevalence of Hartnup disorder seems to be slightly lower than that of cystinuria,[124,125] both of which are about one-half as frequent as phenylketonuria (see Chap. 77).

IS HARTNUP DISORDER A DISEASE?

From prospective and retrospective studies of Hartnup subjects identified by routine newborn screening and followed for many years, most without therapy, it is clear that very few become symptomatic.[3,7,89] On this basis, Hartnup disorder could be considered benign. Furthermore, even the symptomatic few[3] have not had the complete clinical phenotype that was once thought to be characteristic of the Hartnup disorder.[5] These observations and the relatively high frequency of the Hartnup finding in the general population prompt the question of whether the symptoms described in patients with Hartnup disorder might be coincidental and not causally related to the genetic defect.

It is reasonable to propose that this is so. In addition to the preponderance of asymptomatic affected subjects identified by routine screening, the great majority of affected sibs identified by family screening of symptomatic probands have also been clinically normal.[7] Therapeutic correction of niacin deficiency, the factor that is believed to cause clinical abnormalities in the Hartnup disorder, does not always reverse the clinical findings and sometimes produces no benefit whatsoever.[1] Nevertheless, it is difficult to disregard the very striking and unusual pellagra-like phenotype observed in a number of affected individuals.

Attempts to reconcile these quite different observations in Hartnup subjects have produced several hypotheses. The first of these holds that symptomatic cases come from families whose diets are barely adequate for normal individuals or are persons under the stress of temporary malnutrition.[6,124] Thus, a very limited dietary niacin compounds their inherent limited ability to form nicotinamide from its only precursor amino acid, tryptophan.[15] A second hypothesis is that at least the acute attacks of ataxia and, perhaps, psychosis are a result of toxicity to the central nervous system from indolic acids produced in large amounts in some patients by the bacterial degradation of unabsorbed tryptophan in the gut.[24] Supporting this is a report that the ingestion of indoleacetic acid or indolepropionic acid causes irritability and ataxia.[125] In another study, however, indoleacetic acid given in huge quantities did not produce ill effects.[126]

The most recent hypothesis is that of Scriver et al.,[3] which holds that liability to disease in the Hartnup disorder is determined by one or more polygenic factors, notably the associated plasma amino acid value. Accordingly, disease is not likely to occur if the inherent aggregate value for plasma amino acids is normal but will occur, especially in response to environmental stress such as diarrhea, if the aggregate plasma amino acid value is low (Fig. 193-6). In this concept, the cause of disease in the Hartnup disorder is multifactorial.[3] It would seem that this theory is the most reasonable one yet advanced to explain the clinical observations in Hartnup disorder.

MATERNAL HARTNUP DISORDER

Eleven offspring have been reported from four women with the Hartnup disorder.[29,114,117] In addition, Seakins[6] mentions two offspring born to affected women reported before their pregnancies[31,82] and a woman who had two offspring when reported[117] and has subsequently had a third child. Twelve of these 14 offspring are clinically normal, and none has had the Hartnup disorder. Of the two abnormal offspring, one had a meningomyelocele with hydrocephalus and died at age 3 months.[114] The other had methylmalonic acidemia with severe metabolic acidosis and died during early infancy.[114] Pregnancies have been normal in these women, with the exception of one complicated by placenta previa.[117] It seems likely that Hartnup disorder does not adversely affect pregnancy and is harmless to the fetus. The occurrences of methylmalonic acidemia in one offspring and a neural tube defect in another were almost certainly coincidental.[114,117]

In one pregnancy, the ratios between maternal and umbilical vein amino acids at delivery were normal, suggesting that the neutral amino acid transport defect is not expressed in the placenta when the mother has the Hartnup disorder.[117]

One man with Hartnup disorder has fathered two normal non-Hartnup offspring.[29]

REFERENCES

1. Jepson JB: Hartnup disease, in Stanbury JB, Wyngaarden JB, Fredrickson DS (eds): *The Metabolic Basis of Inherited Disease*, 4th ed. New York, McGraw-Hill, 1978, p 1563.
2. Efron M: Comments in Greer M: Hartnup's syndrome. *Trans Am Neurol Assoc* **90**:53, 1965.
3. Scriver CR, Mahon B, Levy HL, Clow CL, Reade TM, Kronick J, Lemieux B, Laberge C: The Hartnup phenotype: Mendelian transport disorder, multifactorial disease. *Am J Hum Genet* **40**:401, 1987.
4. Scriver CR: Nutrient-gene interactions: The gene is not the disease and vice versa. *Am J Clin Nutr* **48**:1505, 1988.

5. Baron DN, Dent CE, Harris H, Hart EW, Jepson JB: Hereditary pellagra-like skin rash with temporary cerebellar ataxia. Constant renal amino-aciduria. And other bizarre biochemical features. *Lancet* **2**:421, 1956.
5a. Christensen HN: Organic ion transport during seven decades. The amino acids. *Biochim Biophys Acta* **779**:255, 1984.
5b. Arriza JL, Kavanaugh MP, Fairmon WA, Wu Y-N, Murdoch GH, North RA, Amara SG: Cloning and expression of a human neutral amino acid transporter with structural similarity to the glutamate transporter gene family. *J Biol Chem* **268**:15329, 1993.
5c. Kekuda R, Prasad PD, Fei Y-J, Torres-Zamorano V, Sinha S, Yang-Feng TL, Leibach FH, Ganapathy V: Cloning of the sodium-dependent, broad-scope, neutral amino acid transporter B° from a human placental choriocarcinoma cell line. *J Biol Chem* **271**:18657, 1996.
5d. Takeda J, Yano H, Eng S, Zeng Y, Bell GI: A molecular inventory of human pancreatic islets: Sequence analysis of 1000 cDNA clones. *Hum Mol Genet* **2**:1793, 1993.
5e. Jones EMC, Menzel S, Espinosa R, LeBeau MM, Bell GI, Takeda J: Localization of a gene encoding a neutral amino acid transporter-like protein to human chromosome band 19q13.3 and characterization of a simple sequence repeat polymorphism. *Genomics* **23**:490, 1994.
5f. Kekuda R, Torres-Zamorano V, Fei Y-J, Prasad PD, Li HW, Mader LD, Leibach FH, Ganapathy V: Molecular and functional characterization of intestinal Na^+-dependent neutral amino acid transporter B°. *Am J Physiol* **272**:G1463, 1997.
5g. Rasko JEJ, Battini J-L, Gottschalk RJ, Mazo I, Miller AD: The RD114/simian type D retrovirus receptor is a neutral amino-acid transporter. *Proc Natl Acad Sci U S A* **96**:2129, 1999.
5h. Tailor CS, Nouri A, Zhao Y, Takeuchi Y, Kabat D: A sodium-dependent neutral amino-acid transporter mediates infections of feline and baboon endogenous retroviruses and simian type D retroviruses. *J Virol* **73**:4470, 1999.
5i. Ford RJ, Donehower LA, Bohannon RC: Studies on a type D retrovirus isolated from an AIDS patient lymphoma. *AIDS Res Hum Retroviruses* **8**:742, 1992.
6. Seakins JWT: Hartnup disease, in Vinken PJ, Bruyn GW (eds): *Metabolic and Deficiency Diseases of the Nervous System*. Amsterdam, North-Holland, 1977, p 149.
7. Levy HL: Hartnup disease, in Goldensohn ES, Appel SH (eds): *Scientific Approaches to Clinical Neurology*. Philadelphia, Lea & Febiger, 1977, p 75.
8. Bonetti E, Dent CE: The determination of optical configuration of naturally occurring amino acids using specific enzymes and paper chromatography. *Biochem J* **57**:77, 1954.
9. Cusworth DC, Dent CE: Renal clearances of amino acids in normal adults and in patients with aminoaciduria. *Biochem J* **74**:550, 1960.
10. Dent CE: The renal aminoacidurias. *Exp Med Surg* **12**:229, 1954.
11. Evered DF: The excretion of amino acids by the human: A quantitative study with ion-exchange chromatography. *Biochem J* **62**:416, 1956.
12. Halvorsen S, Hygstedt O, Jagenburg R, Sjaastad O: Cellular transport of L-histidine in Hartnup disease. *J Clin Invest* **48**:1552, 1969.
13. Tada K, Hirono H, Arakawa T: Endogenous renal clearance rates of free amino acids in prolinuric and Hartnup patients. *Tohoku J Exp Med* **93**:57, 1967.
14. Jonxis JHP: Oligophrenia phenylpyruvica en de hartnupziekte. *Ned Tijdschr Geneeskd* **101**:569, 1957.
15. Scriver CR, Rosenberg LE: *Amino Acid Metabolism and Its Disorders*. Philadelphia, WB Saunders, 1973.
16. Milne MD, Asatoor A, Loughridge L: Hartnup disease and cystinuria. *Lancet* **1**:51, 1961.
17. Scriver CR, Hechtman P: Human genetics of membrane transport with emphasis on amino acids. *Adv Hum Genet* **1**:211, 1970.
18. Fois A, Lecchini L: Acute cerebellar ataxia associated with some features of the Hartnup syndrome. *Helv Paediatr Acta* **19**:42, 1964.
19. De Laey P, Hooft C, Timmermans J, Snoeck J: Biochemical aspects of Hartnup disease. *Ann Paediatr* **202**:145, 1964.
20. Hjelt L, Paatela M, Visakorpi JK: *Autopsy findings in Hartnup disease*. Proceedings of the 13th Northern Pediatrics Congress, Copenhagen, 1961.
21. Visakorpi JK, Hjelt L, Lahikainen T, Ohman S: Hartnup disease in two siblings: Clinical observations and biochemical studies. *Ann Paediatr Fenn* **10**:42, 1964.
22. Daute K-H, Dietel K, Ebert W: Das Hartnupsyndrom. Bericht uber einen todlichen Krankheitsverlauf. *Z Kinderheilkd* **95**:103, 1966.
23. Schmidtke K, Endres W, Roscher A, Ibel H, Herschkowitz N, Bachmann C, Plochl E, Hadorn HB: Hartnup syndrome, progressive encephalopathy and allo-albuminaemia. A clinico-pathological case study. *Eur J Pediatr* **151**:899, 1992.
24. Milne MD, Crawford MA, Girao CB, Loughridge LW: The metabolic disorder in Hartnup disease. *Q J Med* **29**:407, 1960.
25. Scriver CR, Shaw KNF: Hartnup disease: An example of genetically determined defective cellular amino acid transport. *Can Med Assoc J* **86**:232, 1962.
26. Scriver CR: Hartnup disease. A genetic modification of intestinal and renal transport of certain neutral alpha-amino acids. *N Engl J Med* **273**:530, 1965.
27. Asatoor AM, Craske J, London DR, Milne MD: Indole production in Hartnup disease. *Lancet* **1**:126, 1963.
28. Seakins JWT, Ersser RS: Effects of amino acid loads on a healthy infant with the biochemical features of Hartnup disease. *Arch Dis Child* **42**:682, 1967.
29. Pomeroy J, Efron ML, Dayman J, Hoefnagel D: Hartnup disease in a New England family. *N Engl J Med* **278**:1214, 1968.
30. Shih VE, Bixby EM, Alpers DH, Bartsocas CS, Thier SO: Studies of intestinal transport defect in Hartnup disease. *Gastroenterology* **61**:445, 1971.
31. Navab F, Asatoor AM: Studies on intestinal absorption of amino acids and a dipeptide in a case of Hartnup disease. *Gut* **11**:373, 1970.
32. Asatoor AM, Cheng B, Edwards KDG, Lant AF, Matthews DM, Milne MD, Navab F, Richards AJ: Intestinal absorption of two dipeptides in Hartnup disease. *Gut* **11**:380, 1970.
33. Tarlow MJ, Seakins JWT, Lloyd JK, Matthews DM, Cheng B, Thomas AJ: Intestinal absorption and biopsy transport of peptides and amino acids in Hartnup disease. *Clin Sci* **39**:18P, 1970.
34. Tarlow MJ, Seakins JWT, Lloyd JK, Matthews DM, Cheng B, Thomas AJ: Absorption of amino acids and peptides in a child with a variant of Hartnup disease and coexistent coeliac disease. *Arch Dis Child* **47**:798, 1972.
35. Leonard JV, Marrs TC, Addison JM, Burston D, Clegg KM, Lloyd JK, Matthews DM, Seakins JW: Intestinal absorption of amino acids and peptides in Hartnup disorder. *Pediatr Res* **10**:246, 1976.
36. Asatoor AM, Cheng B, Edwards KDG, Lant AF, Matthews DM, Milne MD, Navab F, Richards AJ: Intestinal absorption of dipeptides and corresponding free amino acids in Hartnup disease. *Clin Sci* **39**:1P, 1970.
37. Drummond KN, Michael AF, Ulstrom RA, Good RA: The blue diaper syndrome: Familial hypercalcemia with nephrocalcinosis and indicanuria. *Am J Med* **37**:928, 1964.
38. Hillman RE, Stewart A, Miles JH: Aminoacid transport defect in intestine not affecting kidney. *Pediatr Res* **20**:265A, 1986.
39. Oyanagi K, Takagi M, Kitabatake M, Nakao T: Hartnup disease. *Tohoku J Exp Med* **91**:383, 1967.
40. Nielsen EG, Vedso S, Zimmermann-Nielsen C: Hartnup disease in three siblings. *Dan Med Bull* **13**:155, 1966.
41. Jonas AJ, Butler IJ: Circumvention of defective neutral amino acid transport in Hartnup disease using tryptophan ethyl ester. *J Clin Invest* **84**:200, 1989.
42. Tada K, Morikawa T, Arakawa T: Tryptophan load and uptake of tryptophan by leukocytes in Hartnup disease. *Tohoku J Exp Med* **90**:337, 1966.
43. Groth U, Rosenberg LE: Transport of dibasic amino acids, cystine, and tryptophan by cultured human fibroblasts: Absence of a defect in cystinuria and Hartnup disease. *J Clin Invest* **51**:2130, 1972.
44. Hersov LA: A case of childhood pellagra with psychosis. *J Ment Sci* **101**:878, 1955.
45. Hickish GW: Pellagra in an English child. *Arch Dis Child* **30**:195, 1955.
46. Feigelson P, Feigelson M, Greengard O: Comparison of the mechanisms of hormonal and substrate induction of rat liver tryptophan pyrrolase. *Recent Prog Horm Res* **18**:491, 1962.
47. Schimke RT, Sweeney EW, Berlin CM: The roles of synthesis and degradation in the control of rat liver tryptophan pyrrolase. *J Biol Chem* **240**:322, 1965.
48. Goldsmith GA: Niacin-tryptophan relationships in man and niacin requirements. *Am J Clin Nutr* **6**:479, 1958.
49. Goldsmith GA: The B vitamins: Thiamine, riboflavin, niacin, in Beaton GH, McHenry EW (eds): *Nutrition. A Comprehensive Treatise*. New York, Academic, 1964, vol 2, p 110.
50. Tada K, Ito H, Wada Y, Arakawa T: Congenital tryptophanuria with dwarfism. *Tohoku J Exp Med* **80**:118, 1963.
51. Wong PWK, Forman P, Tabahoff B, Justice P: A defect in tryptophan metabolism. *Pediatr Res* **10**:725, 1976.

52. Salih MAM, Bender DA, McCreanor GM: Lethal familial pellagra-like skin lesion associated with neurologic and developmental impairment and the development of cataracts. *Pediatrics* **76**:787, 1985.
53. Fenton DA, Wilkinson JD, Toseland PA: Family exhibiting cerebellar-like ataxia, photosensitivity, and shortness of stature — A new inborn error of tryptophan metabolism. *J R Soc Med* **76**:736, 1983.
54. Snedden W, Mellor CS, Martin JR: Familial hypertryptophanemia, tryptophanuria and indoleketonuria. *Clin Chim Acta* **131**:247, 1983.
55. Komrower GM, Wilson V, Clamp JR, Westall RG: Hydroxykynureninuria. A case of abnormal tryptophan metabolism probably due to a deficiency of kynureninase. *Arch Dis Child* **39**:250, 1964.
56. Clayton PT, Bridges NA, Atherton DJ, Milla PJ, Malone M, Bender DA: Pellagra with colitis due to a defect in tryptophan metabolism. *Eur J Pediatr* **150**:498, 1991.
56a. Martin IR, Mellor CS, Fraser FC, : Familial hypertryptophanemia in two siblings. *Clin Genet* **47**:180, 1995.
57. Price JM, Yess N, Brown RR, Johnson SAM: Tryptophan metabolism. A hitherto unreported abnormality occurring in a family. *Arch Dermatol* **95**:462, 1967.
58. McCoy EE, Ferreira P: Hypertryptophanemia and hyperserotonemia – Detection in a newborn screening program for PKU. *Clin Res* **35**:212A, 1987.
59. Armstrong MD, Shaw KNF, Gortatowski MJ, Singer H: The indole acids of human urine. *J Biol Chem* **232**:17, 1958.
60. Weissbach H, King W, Sjoerdsma A, Udenfriend S: Formation of indole-3-acetic acid and tryptamine in animals. *J Biol Chem* **234**:81, 1959.
61. Sjoerdsma A, Oates JA, Zaltzman P, Udenfriend S: Identification and assay of urinary tryptamine. *J Pharmacol Exp Ther* **126**:217, 1959.
62. Smith HG, Smith WRD, Jepson JB: Interconversions of indolic acids by bacteria and rat tissue–possible relevance to Hartnup disorder. *Clin Sci* **34**:333, 1968.
63. Smith HG, Smith WRD, Jepson JB, Sorensen K: The metabolism and excretion of indolylacrylic acid in the rat. *Biochem Pharmacol* **19**:1689, 1970.
64. Fordtran JS, Scroggie WB, Polter DE: Colonic absorption of tryptophan metabolites in man. *J Lab Clin Med* **64**:125, 1964.
65. Happold FC: Trytophanase-tryptophan reaction. *Adv Enzymol* **10**:51, 1950.
66. King LJ, Parke DV, Williams RT: Metabolism of indole-2-14C. *Biochem J* **88**:66P, 1963.
67. Nakao A, Ball M: The appearance of a skatole derivative in the urine of schizophrenics. *J Nerv Ment Dis* **130**:417, 1960.
68. Sprince H: Indole metabolism in mental illness. *Clin Chem* **7**:203, 1961.
69. Scriver CR: Abnormalities of tryptophan metabolism in a patient with malabsorption syndrome. *J Lab Clin Med* **58**:908, 1961.
70. Crawford MA: Degradation of aminoacids in the large gut of East Africans and its possible significance. *East Afr Med J* **41**:228, 1964.
71. Crawford MA: Discussion of indole metabolism in Hartnup disease. *Adv Pharmacol* **6B**:176, 1968.
72. Mellman WU, Barness LA, Tedesco TA, Besselman D: Indolylacryloyl-glycine excretion in a family with mental retardation. *Clin Chim Acta* **8**:843, 1963.
73. Szeinberg A, Bar-Or R, Pollack S, Cohen BE, Jepson JB: Observations on urinary excretion of indolylacryloyl-glycine. *Clin Chim Acta* **11**:506, 1965.
74. Rodnight R, McIlwain H: Indicanuria and the psychosis of a pellagrin. *J Ment Sci* **101**:884, 1955.
75. Hersov LA, Rodnight R: Hartnup disease in psychiatric practice: Clinical and biochemical features of three cases. *J Neurol Neurosurg Psychiatry* **23**:40, 1960.
76. Shaw KNF, Redlich D, Wright SW, Jepson JB: Dependence of urinary indole excretion in Hartnup disease upon gut flora. *Fed Proc* **19**:194, 1960.
77. Hooft C, De Laey P, Timmermans J, Snoeck J: La maladie de Hartnup. *Acta Paediatr Belg* **16**:281, 1962.
78. Halvorsen K, Halvorsen S: Hartnup disease. *Pediatrics* **31**:29, 1963.
79. Wong PWK, Pillai PM: Clinical and biochemical observations in two cases of Hartnup disease. *Arch Dis Child* **41**:383, 1966.
80. Srikantia SG, Venkatachalam PS, Reddy V: Clinical and biochemical features of a case of Hartnup disease. *Br Med J* **1**:282, 1964.
81. Jepson JB: Indolylacetyl-glutamine and other indole metabolites in Hartnup disease. *Biochem J* **64**:14p, 1956.
82. Henderson W: A case of Hartnup disease. *Arch Dis Child* **33**:114, 1958.
83. Weyers H, Bickel H: Photodermatose mit Aminoacidurie, Indolaceturie und cerebralen Manifestationen (Hartnup-Syndrom). *Klin Wochenschr* **36**:893, 1958.
84. Jepson JB: Indole metabolism in Hartnup disease. *Adv Pharmacol* **6B**:171, 1968.
85. Hvidt S, Kjeldsen K: Malabsorption induced by small doses of neomycin sulfate. *Acta Med Scand* **173**:699, 1963.
86. Jepson JB: Indolylacetamide, a chromatographic artifact from the natural indoles indolylacetylglucosiduronic acid and indolylpyruvic acid. *Biochem J* **69**:22P, 1958.
87. Lopez F, Velez H, Toro G: Hartnup disease in two Colombian siblings. *Neurology* **19**:71, 1969.
88. Davis VE, Brown H, Huff JA, Cashaw JL: Alteration of serotonin metabolism to 5-hydroxytryptophol by ethanol ingestion in man. *J Lab Clin Med* **69**:132, 1967.
89. Wilcken B, Yu JS, Brown DA: Natural history of Hartnup disease. *Arch Dis Child* **52**:38, 1977.
90. Levy HL, Shih VE, MacCready RA: *Inborn errors of metabolism and transport. Prenatal and neonatal diagnosis. Proceedings of the 13th International Congress of Pediatrics*. Vienna, 1971, vol 5, p 1.
91. Despopoulos A, Weissbach H: Renal metabolism of 5-hydroxyindoleacetic acid. *Am J Physiol* **189**:548, 1957.
92. Wong PWK, Lambert AM, Pillai PM, Jones PM: Observations on nicotinic acid therapy in Hartnup disease. *Arch Dis Child* **42**:642, 1967.
93. Darras BT, Ampola MG, Dietz WH, Gilmore HE: Intermittent dystonia in Hartnup disease. *Pediatr Neurol* **5**:118, 1989.
94. Albers FH, Wadman SK: Een patiente met H-ziekte. *Maandschr Kindergeneeskd* **29**:102, 1961.
95. Somasundaram O, Papakumari M: Hartnup disease. A report on two siblings. *Indian Pediatr* **10**:455, 1973.
96. Haim S, Gilhar A, Cohen A: Cutaneous manifestations associated with aminoaciduria. Report of two cases. *Dermatologica* **156**:244, 1978.
97. Strobel M, Fall M, Kuakuvi N, N'Diaye B, Sanokho A, Marchand J-P: Maladie de Hartnup. *Bull Soc Med Afr Noire Lgue Frse* **23**:118, 1978.
98. Ashurst PJ: Hydroa vacciniforme occurring in association with Hartnup disease. *Br J Dermatol* **81**:486, 1969.
99. Kimmig J: Hartnup-syndrom. *Arch Klin Exp Dermatol* **219**:753, 1964.
100. Guzzetta F, Mazzaglia E: La malattia di Hartnup. *Minerva Pediatr* **22**:480, 1970.
101. Mori E, Yamadori A, Tsutsumi A, Kyotani Y: Adult-onset Hartnup disease presenting with neuropsychiatric symptoms but without skin lesions. *Clin Neurol* **29**:687, 1989.
102. Pomeranz SJ: *Craniospinal Magnetic Resonance Imaging*. Philadelphia, WB Saunders, 1989, p 479.
103. Erly W, Castillo M, Foosaner D, Bonmati C: Hartnup disease: MR findings. *AJNR Am J Neuroradiol* **12**:1026, 1991.
104. Ozalp I, Saatci U, Hassa R: A case of Hartnup disorder with hypoalbuminemia and edema. *Turk J Pediatr* **19**:73, 1977.
105. Colliss JE, Levi AJ, Milne MD: Stature and nutrition in cystinuria and Hartnup disease. *Br Med J* **1**:590, 1963.
106. Levy HL, Kupke KG: Unpublished data.
107. Levy HL: Genetic screening. *Adv Hum Genet* **4**:1, 1973.
108. Levy HL, Coulombe JT, Shih VE: Newborn urine screening, in Bickel H, Guthrie R, Hammersen G (eds): *Neonatal Screening for Inborn Errors of Metabolism*. Heidelberg, Springer-Verlag, 1980, p 89.
109. Levy HL, Madigan PM, Lum A: Fecal contamination in urine amino acid screening. Artifactual cause of hyperaminoaciduria. *Am J Clin Pathol* **51**:765, 1969.
110. Freundlich E, Statter M, Yatziv S: Familial pellagra-like skin rash with neurologic manifestations. *Arch Dis Child* **56**:146, 1981.
111. Milne MD: Hartnup disease. *Biochem J* **111**:3P, 1969.
112. Bartelheimer HK, Gruttner R, Simon HA: Das Hartnup-Syndrom. I. Diagnose, Therapie und klinischer Verlauf. *Monatsschr Kinderheilkd* **119**:52, 1971.
113. Levy HL: Unpublished data.
114. Shih VE, Coulombe JT, Wadman SK, Duran M, Waelkens JJJ: Occurrences of methylmalonic aciduria and Hartnup disorder in the same family. *Clin Genet* **26**:216, 1984.
115. Ledley FD, Levy HL, Shih VE, Benjamin R, Mahoney MT: Benign methylmalonic aciduria. *N Engl J Med* **311**:1015, 1984.
116. Wilcken B: Personal communication.

117. Mahon BE, Levy HL: Maternal Hartnup disorder. *Am J Med Genet* **24**:513, 1986.
118. Rao BS, Narayanan HS, Reddy GN: A clinical and biochemical survey of 729 cases of mental subnormality. *Br J Psychiatry* **118**:505, 1971.
119. Swenson EF, Walraven C, Levy HL: A 25 year experience with newborn urine screening. 9th National Neonatal Screening Symposium [Abstract]. April 7-11, Raleigh, NC, 1992, p 69.
120. Wilcken B, Smith A, Brown DA: Urine screening for aminoacidopathies: Is it beneficial? *J Pediatr* **97**:492, 1980.
121. Stockl E: Personal communication.
122. Lemieux B, Auray-Blais C, Giguere R, Shapcott D, Scriver CR: Newborn urine screening experience with over one million infants in the Quebec Network of Genetic Medicine. *J Inherit Metab Dis* **11**:45, 1988.
123. Lemieux B: Personal communication.
124. Jepson JB: Hartnup disease, in Benson PF (ed): *Cellular Organelles and Membranes in Mental Retardation*. Edinburgh, Churchill Livingstone, 1971, p 55.
125. Greer M: Hartnup's syndrome. *Trans Am Neurol Assoc* **90**:53, 1965.
126. Mirsky JA: Insulinase, insulinase inhibitors and diabetes mellitus. *Recent Prog Horm Res* **13**:429, 1957.

CHAPTER 194

Iminoglycinuria*

Russell W. Chesney

1. Familial iminoglycinuria is a benign inborn error of membrane transport. It involves a membrane carrier in the renal tubule with a preference for L-proline, hydroxy-L-proline, and glycine, resulting in net reabsorption. The iminoglycinuria phenotype is autosomal recessive.

2. Homozygotes retain appreciable tubular reabsorption of the imino acids and glycine. The residual transport function is saturated at endogenous concentrations of substrate, and the normal competitive interactions between the imino acids and glycine during tubular reabsorption are absent. These seemingly paradoxical observations can be explained because multiple carriers participate in the reabsorption of imino acids and glycine. Loss of a carrier shared by the imino acids and glycine, and retention of other carriers with preferences for glycine and imino acids individually, can explain the homozygous iminoglycinuric phenotype.

3. A variant phenotype in which imino acid reabsorption has a normal T_m value and the defect affects glycine reclamation more than proline probably indicates a K_m variant.

4. Impaired intestinal transport of L-proline has been demonstrated in some, but not all, homozygotes. A transport defect has not been shown in the leukocytes or skin fibroblasts.

5. Obligate heterozygotes may be "hyperglycinuric" (incompletely recessive) or "silent" (completely recessive) for expression of the mutant allele. Phenotypic heterogeneity among probands and obligate heterozygotes indicates genetic heterogeneity.

6. The different mutations appear to be allelic. Probands inheriting two "silent" mutant alleles, two "hyperglycinuric" alleles, or two different alleles have the same renal phenotype.

7. Several individual amino acid transport proteins and their corresponding cDNA clones have been isolated and classified into gene families. The Na^+/Cl^--dependent proline transporter (PROT) belongs to a large superfamily of neurotransmitter transporters and is expressed in brain regions containing glutaminergic neurons. The four glycine transporters of the "GLYT family" also are part of the neurotransmitter superfamily and have their most prominent expression in the central nervous system, but can also be found in human kidney.

8. The differential diagnosis of familial iminoglycinuria includes hyperprolinemia, in which iminoglycinuria occurs by a combined saturation-inhibition mechanism; the Fanconi syndrome, in which iminoglycinuria occurs as part of a generalized disturbance of transport; and the newborn, in whom hyperiminoglycinuria occurs in the first 6 months of life. Neonatal iminoglycinuria involves ontogeny of separate transport systems not controlled by the gene locus involved in hereditary iminoglycinuria.

9. Several different forms of renal hyperglycinuria are appreciated that must be distinguished from the hyperglycinuric phenotype of the "incompletely recessive" heterozygote with renal iminoglycinuria.

Familial renal iminoglycinuria is a Mendelian disorder expressed in homozygotes or genetic compounds as a selective hyperaminoaciduria. It is caused by several autosomal alleles, some of which are partially expressed in heterozygotes (incompletely recessive alleles). The disorder is not a disease, although ascertainment of the phenotype in probands with clinical signs suggested to early observers that it might be. Familial iminoglycinuria is significant because it provides evidence for a transport system selective for imino acids† and glycine in the renal tubule and intestine under the control of a single locus. In its medical context, the disorder enters into the differential diagnosis of several hyperaminoacidurias, and because newborn infants have physiological iminoglycinuria, the ontogenetic and Mendelian phenotypes need to be discriminated from each other.

When Dent[4] applied chromatographic methods to the investigation of diseases, he fostered an exponential increase in the discovery of disorders of amino acid metabolism.[5] Renal iminoglycinuria is one of those disorders. Urine was a revealing mirror of metabolic disorders, and chromatography of urine amino acids evinced great interest.[6] It was soon recognized that urine of young infants normally contains a large quantity of the two imino acids proline and hydroxyproline and of the amino acid glycine.[7–10] It then became known that iminoaciduria disappeared as the infant reached about 3 months of age, and therefore the urine normally did not contain detectable amounts of proline or hydroxyproline; the hyperglycinuria had disappeared by about 6 months. Impaired net tubular reabsorption explained neonatal iminoglycinuria (Fig. 194-1).

Persistence of iminoglycinuria beyond 6 months constitutes an abnormality. It occurs under three different clinical situations:

1. As a "combined" aminoaciduria[11] in the presence of hyperprolinemia or hyperhydroxyprolinemia (see Chap. 81).
2. As a component of a generalized disturbance of membrane transport (for example, in the Fanconi syndrome) (see Chap. 196).
3. As a specific inborn error of membrane transport of amino acids now usually known as familial (renal) iminoglycinuria (the subject of this chapter).

Most of the early reports of pathologic iminoglycinuria[12–34] testify that the condition was discovered during retrospective

*Many sections of this chapter remain unaltered from versions in the 6th and 7th editions of this work. Permission has been obtained from the original author, Dr. Charles R. Scriver, for publication.

A list of standard abbreviations is located immediately preceding the index in each volume.

†These compounds are also excreted in bound form as oligopeptides (see Chaps. 81 to 82). Familial iminoglycinuria is a trait affecting only the free forms of proline, hydroxyproline, and glycine. "Imino acid" is a popular term used to distinguish the configuration of the secondary amino group (RC—NHCH—COOH) of the heterocyclic amino acids from the primary amino group (NH_2—CHR—COOH) of other amino acids. The term imino acid is freely used in standard textbooks on the biochemistry and metabolism of amino acids,[1,2] but reservations have been expressed about the accuracy of its use in this way.[3]

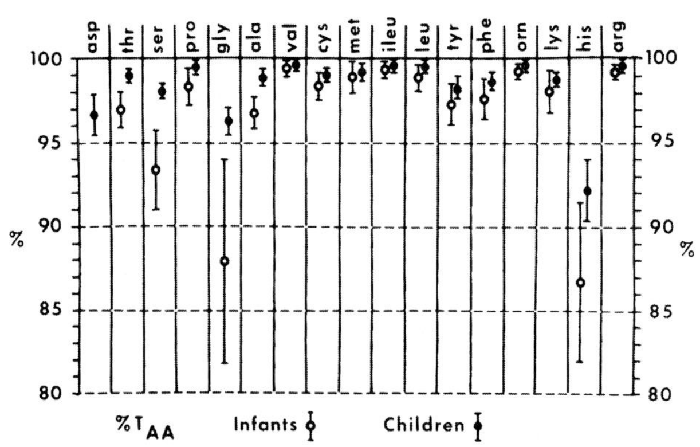

Fig. 194-1 Net tubular reabsorption of amino acids (expressed as percent of filtered load) is less efficient in the newborn human subject than in older subjects. Glycine reabsorption is particularly impaired, and the presence of imino acids in the urine of neonates and young infants is noteworthy. (Redrawn from Brodehl and Gellissen.[10] Reproduced from *Pediatrics* with permission.)

studies carried out for other purposes. Ascertainment bias is still evident in case reports of iminoglycinuria in which the disorder is found in subjects with retardation, propionic acidemia, and 3-methylcrotonylglycinuria.[35,36] The diversity of the clinical abnormalities in probands with familial iminoglycinuria suggests now that there is little or no direct relationship between the inherited disorder of membrane transport and the accompanying illness. It is appropriate to classify familial iminoglycinuria as a benign inborn error of membrane transport,[20–22] a conclusion borne out by the frequent occurrence of healthy iminoglycinuric sibs of probands and by the prospective discovery of probands, through large newborn screening programs,[28,30] in whom follow-up observations have revealed no late-appearing illness.

RENAL TRANSPORT OF IMINO ACIDS AND GLYCINE

Investigation into the cause of iminoglycinuria in another disorder, familial hyperprolinemia[37,38] (see Chap. 81), led to the concept that imino acids and glycine share a specific renal transport system that has preference for these three substrates.[11] Familial renal iminoglycinuria, the phenotype described here, corroborates this hypothesis. Many studies in humans and other mammals indicate that renal transport of amino acids is a complex process apparently involving several carriers, presumably under the control of several genes. Carriers for the imino acids and glycine, of which there are also several, are among them.

Human Studies

There appears to be a maximum rate for net tubular absorption of proline (T_m proline).[38] Hydroxy-L-proline reabsorption also exhibits a T_m value.[39] The capacity of the normal human renal tubule to transport proline and hydroxyproline is shown in Table 194-1. A T_m for glycine has not been demonstrated in human beings, probably because there is extensive paracellular diffusion for glycine in the proximal tubule, but mainly because glycine excretion exceeds 2 percent of filtered load (see Fig. 194-1).[40] This relative hyperexcretion of glycine may also be related to the high K_m for the glycine carrier relative to other amino acid transport systems[35] and to the V_{max} for glycine transport.[41] Infusion of one imino acid increases urinary excretion of the other and of glycine in humans;[38,39] this procedure has little or no influence on the excretion of other amino acids.

Patients with familial hyperprolinemia have hyperiminoglycinuria[37,38] directly proportional to the plasma concentration of proline when it exceeds 1 mM; this is the level at which proline saturates its own transport system and appears in the urine.[38] The data for imino acid and glycine transport by normal human subjects and by patients with disorders of imino acid catabolism are complementary. They indicate the presence of a renal transport process, selective in its preference for proline, hydroxyproline, and glycine, and finite in its capacity.

Reabsorption of substrate is initiated by events at the brush-border membrane (see "Intracellular Events Influencing Proline Reabsorption" below). Transport of imino acids and glycine has been measured in purified brush-border membrane vesicles prepared from human renal cortex samples obtained at operation.[42] Two saturable uptake systems were identified: one has high affinity and is shared both by imino acids and by glycine; the other has low affinity and is not shared by glycine. The high-affinity system can apparently accommodate most of the imino acid load at physiological concentrations in filtrate, and if it were placed distally in proximal nephron, for instance, in the straight segment, it would explain the absence of iminoaciduria in the mature subject (see "Nonhuman Studies" below).

Nonhuman Studies

Amino acid reabsorption in the mammalian nephron is accomplished by a variety of carriers in the brush-border membrane, with selective preferences for particular amino acids and groups of amino acids.[43,44] There exists an axial heterogeneity of carriers located in the more proximal segments of proximal nephron having higher capacity but broader specificity and lower affinity

Table 194-1 Renal Clearance, Net Tubular Absorption, and T_m of Amino Acids and Glycine in Familial Iminoglycinuria

Phenotype	Proline Endogenous Clearance, ml (min·1.73 m²)	Reabsorbed %	T Reabsorbed µmol (min·1.73 m²)	Hydroxyproline Endogenous clearance, ml (min·1.73 m²)	%
Normal	0–0.03	>99.8	180–300	0	100
Homozygous mutant* (classic type):					
Mean	6.7			13	
Range	0.5–19.6	77–99.5	10–18	1–33.6	
65–99					
Heterozygous† ("hyperglycinuric")	0	100	35–117	0	100
Heterozygous‡ ("silent")	0	100	?	0	100
Generic compound (K_m variant)§	~0.3	>99	Normal with "splay"	2–4	<100

*Compiled from Goodman et al.,[18] Scriver,[17] Rosenberg et al.,[21] Hoefnagel and Pomeroy,[19] and Tada et al.[40] Includes genetic compound and homozygous probands.
†Compiled from Goodman et al.,[18] Scriver,[17] Rosenberg et al.,[21] and Hoefnagel and Pomeroy.[19]
‡Compiled from Scriver[17] and Hoefnagel and Pomeroy.[19]
§Compiled from Greene et al.[27]

for substrate and those located more distally having lower capacity but higher affinity and often a narrower specificity.[45] Net reabsorption also uses transport processes that prevent back flux so that the effective concentration of substrate at the luminal pole of the cell is kept lower than the equilibrium concentration; the processes for this situation include intracellular metabolic run out and efflux of substrate at the basolateral pole of the cell by carriers with properties different from those of the carriers in the brush-border membrane.[43,45] While the weight of evidence pertaining to reabsorption of imino acids and glycine is concordant with this general scheme, details have yet to be resolved, and it should be remembered that findings in the nonhuman nephron may not reflect the human case precisely. In fact, it is not possible from current evidence to develop an accurate taxonomy of the tubular transport systems for imino acids and glycine in human beings.

Selective interactions between imino acids and glycine occur *in vivo* during renal reabsorption in rats and dogs.[46,47] Microperfusions *in vivo et situ* in the rat confirm this finding.[48–52] The reabsorption process is saturable, stereospecific (for L-proline), and Na^+-dependent. Electrophysiological studies[53] reveal two mechanisms for reabsorption of imino acids and glycine, both located at the renal brush-border membrane of proximal convolutions: one with low affinity, presumably more proximal, and apparently a general system shared by many neutral amino acids; the other with high affinity, apparently more specific for the triad of substrates, and possibly located more distally in proximal nephron.

In the case of glycine, two Na^+-dependent active transport systems have been demonstrated along the luminal membrane of the isolated perfused proximal tubule: a low-affinity (K_m, 11.8 mM), high-capacity (V_{max}, 28.5 pmol/min/mm tubule length) system in the convoluted segment, and a high-affinity (K_m, 0.7 mM), low-capacity (V_{max}, 2.5 pmol/min/mm) in the straight segment.[54] The latter system, which also operates parallel to a lower apical membrane backflux permeability in the proximal straight tubule,[55] absorbs smaller amounts of glycine against a greater concentration gradient and probably permits the reduction of the luminal glycine concentrations to lower levels than would be achieved in the proximal convoluted tubule.[55] The latter study corroborates earlier findings obtained by the continuous microperfusion technique in rats[50,51] and with the brush-border membrane vesicle preparation from human kidney.[42] The low-capacity, high-affinity system for proline is shared with glycine and hydroxyproline in human kidney.

Glycine transport has been studied in great detail in the isolated perfused rabbit nephron segment.[56,57] Glycine is transported against the chemical gradient, from lumen to cell, by a saturable Na^+-dependent carrier. Two forms of glycine transport were identified: one in the proximal convoluted segments has high capacity and low affinity; the other in the proximal straight segment has low capacity and high affinity. A paracellular, diffusional bidirectional flux was also found. Glycine uptake from peritubular space to cell across the basolateral membrane is both active and Na^+-dependent. The inward-directed basolateral flux is greater in straight segments relative to convoluted segments. The lumen-to-peritubular transcellular flux exceeds the flux in the reverse direction at physiological concentrations of glycine. No observations were made in this work on interactions of imino acids with glycine during transport.

Studies with purified membrane vesicles segregate membrane events from the intracellular events that influence net reabsorption,[43,45] and they are valuable for this reason, provided one recognizes that vesicle and microperfusion experiments measure different properties.[53] The vesicle studies[58–62] are both informative and confusing. Brush-border and basolateral membranes have Na^+-dependent and Na^+-independent systems respectively for L-proline transport (Fig. 194-2). This indicates that brush-border and basolateral membranes have carriers that are different in their function and, presumably, in the genes that control them. Glycine transport by luminal membrane vesicles is Na^+-dependent[61] (see Fig. 194-2); studies of glycine transport by basolateral membrane vesicles have not yet been reported. Imino acids interact with each other[59] but not with glycine[62] during uptake by rabbit renal brush-border membrane vesicles; on the other hand, imino acids and glycine interact on a shared carrier in rat nephron vesicles.[61] It is unclear whether these functional differences reflect differences in species or in methodology, such as the nephron segment from which vesicles were isolated.

Na^+-proline cotransport by rat renal brush-border membrane vesicles appears to be both chloride-dependent and membrane potential-dependent.[63] Hence, both membrane potential and anion-specific properties govern the uptake of L-proline. The imposition of an extravesicular H^+ gradient stimulates L-proline uptake in rabbit kidney[64] but diminishes uptake by rat kidney.[63] Consistent with these findings, agents capable of altering proton accumulation, such as amiloride or carbonyl cyanide p-(trifluoromethoxy) phenyl-hydrazone diminish proline uptake by rabbit kidney but do not influence this process in rat kidney. An inward-directed H^+ gradient stimulates glycine transport across rabbit renal brush-border surface, and this H^+-driven glycine uptake is attenuated by carbonyl cyanide m-chlorophenyl-hydrazone.[65] This H^+ glycine in rabbit is a carrier-mediated electrogenic process whose transport is shared with the imino acids and, to a slight degree, by β-alanine.

The transport characteristics of D-proline were evaluated in rabbit kidney and were found to depend both on an H^+ flux and to be inhibited by L-proline. Hence D-imino acids and their naturally occurring L-isomers probably share a common transport system along the proximal tubule[66] in rabbits, but not in rats, as noted previously.[63]

Renal transport of imino acids and glycine has been studied in rat cortex slices[67] and in isolated tubule fragments from rabbits.[68,69] The slice preparation preferentially exposes the basolateral membrane,[70,71] while the tubule fragment preparation exposes both luminal and antiluminal membranes. There is heterogeneity of carriers for imino acids and glycine in the basolateral membrane with a high-capacity, low-affinity function shared by the three substrates and separate low-capacity, high-affinity functions for imino acids and glycine, respectively.

These descriptions may represent an oversimplification, particularly when one is trying to understand which carrier in which membrane of which nephron segment is affected by the human iminoglycinuria mutation. The apparent distribution of carriers for imino acids and glycine in proximal nephron is summarized in Table 194-2.

Intracellular Events Influencing Proline Reabsorption

A nonhuman mutation (PRO/Re in mouse) affecting renal proline oxidase activity[72] is informative about the overall mechanism for the reabsorption of L-proline. Mammalian renal cortex has a large capacity for proline oxidation.[67,73,74] This provides metabolic run out of proline,[43] which *in vivo et situ* facilitates net reabsorption of the imino acid. Proline oxidation is blocked in the PRO/Re mouse (see Chap. 81), proline content of cortical cells is elevated, and net reabsorption is impaired because backflux from cell to lumen across the brush-border membrane is increased.[72]

A cyclic AMP-dependent protein kinase (protein kinase A) also appears to modulate proline transport across the rat brush-border surface.[75] The exogenous addition of a highly purified catalytic subunit of protein kinase A results in reduced Na^+- and Cl^--linked proline transport across the apical surface. The addition of cAMP reduces proline uptake, which indicates that endogenous protein kinase A activity also influences transport.[76] The activity of both protein kinase C and calmodulin-dependent protein kinase are also found in rat kidney. The activity of both protein kinase C and calmodulin-dependent kinase is reduced in tissue from immature rats;[76] their roles in proline reabsorption are unclear at present.

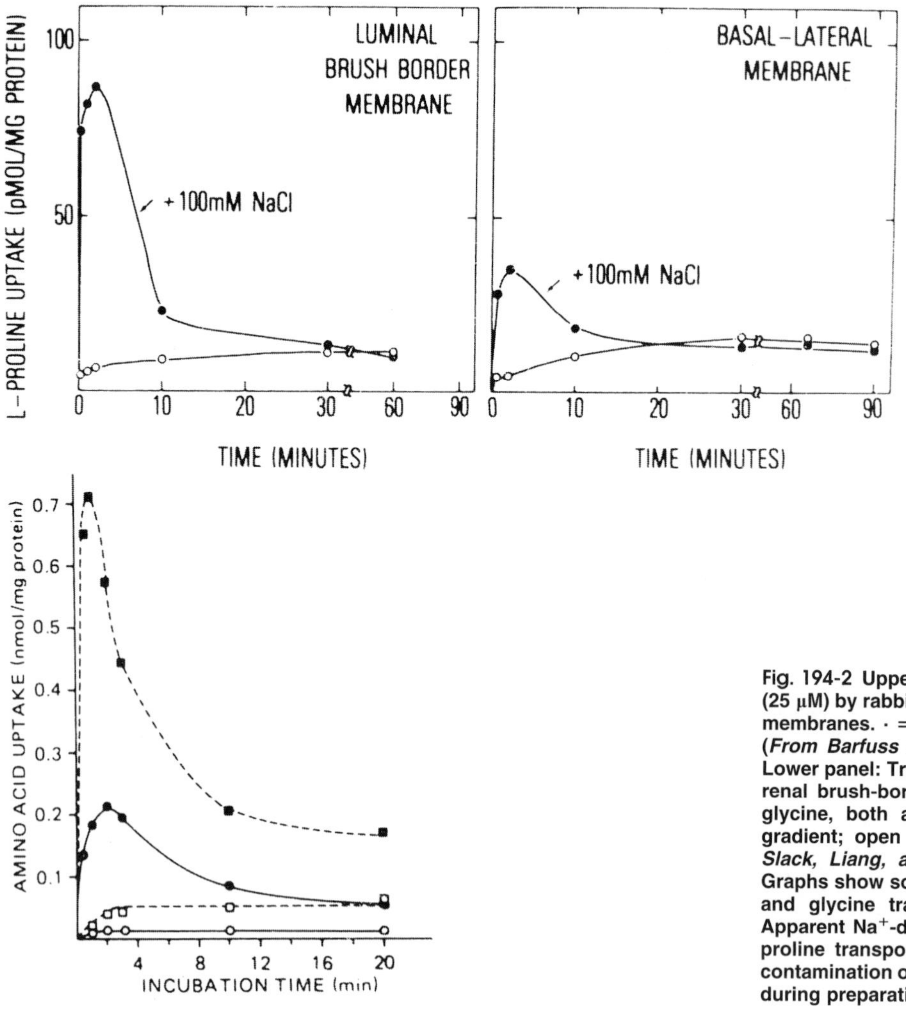

Fig. 194-2 Upper panels: Transport of L-proline (25 μM) by rabbit kidney brush-border and basolateral membranes. · = Na^+ gradient; ° = Na^+-free medium. (*From Barfuss and Schafer.*[56] *Used by permission.*) Lower panel: Transport of L-proline and glycine by rat renal brush-border membranes. né = proline; Im = glycine, both at 0.06 mM; closed symbols = Na^+ gradient; open symbols = no Na^+ gradient. (*From Slack, Liang, and Sacktor.*[58] *Used by permission.*) Graphs show sodium-dependent transport for proline and glycine transport at brush-border membrane. Apparent Na^+-dependence for a small component of proline transport in basolateral membranes reflects contamination of membrane fraction by brush borders during preparation.

Glycine-Specific Transport Proteins

The three roles of glycine in the central nervous system are (a) to serve as an inhibitory neurotransmitter; (b) to interact with the glycine receptor that functions as a ligand-gated Cl-channel activated by glycine; and (c) as an obligatory modulator of glutamate-mediated excitatory neurotransmission.[77] Thus, the movement of glycine into the central nervous system is crucial. Two separate genes, one of which has three isoforms, that encode NA^+/Cl^--dependent glycine transport have been cloned.[78] The high-affinity human glycine transporter GLYT1 possesses 12 putative transmembrane domains, is encoded by an open reading frame of 1914 nucleotides, and consists of a 638-amino acid protein. By alternative splicing, at least three forms—glycine transporter type 1a (GLYT-1a), GLYT1b, and GlYT1c—have been found. The gene for GLYT1c contains an extra exon encoding 54 amino acids in the amino-terminal end of GLYT-1b. All three isoforms are localized on human chromosome 1p31.3. When expressed in COS-7 cells, both human GLYT1b and GLYT-1c show a time- and concentration-dependent uptake of glycine, abolished by the removal of either Na^+ or Cl^-. This glycine uptake is inhibited by glycine (100 percent), sarcosine (65 percent), and proline (30 percent). Northern hybridization analysis demonstrates the strongest labeling in brain and kidney.[78]

Table 194-2 Tentative Classification of Membrane Carriers by Segment, Side of Cell, and Preferences for Imino Acids and Glycine in Mammalian Nephron

Segment	Brush-Border Membrane	Basolateral Membrane
PC	P + HP + (G?)	P + HP + G
	G alone?	p + hp + g
PS	p + hp + (g?)*	
	g	g

*System affected in familial renal iminoglycinuria (hypothesis only).
PC = proximal convoluted; PS = proximal straight; uppercase letters = high-capacity, low-affinity; lowercase letters = low-capacity, high-affinity; G and g = glycine; HP and hp = hydroxyproline; P and p = proline.

A separate high affinity Na^+Cl^--dependent glycine transporter GLYT2 has also been cloned.[79] This transporter is coded by a gene with identical 3′ ends to GLYT1, but 5′ noncoding regions and *N*-termini that differ. This transporter is found in supraspinal regions as well as in the brain. GLYT2 was not found in kidney by *in situ* hybridization.[79] GLYT2 appears to have 48 and 50 percent homology to the previously cloned mouse GLYT-1 and rat proline transporter (PROT).[80] Potential phosphorylation sites for protein kinase C, cAMP-dependent kinase, and calmodulin-dependent kinase were found in the amino-terminal region. The expression of GLYT-1a, b, c, and GLYT-2 are quite different in their ontogeny as well.[81] Neither GLY-T1 or GLYT-2 are found in the kidney of embryonic mouse.[82]

To date, the cloning and characterizations of these glycine transporters derived from kidney tissue in either man or rodent have not been studied. However, the Na^+Cl^--dependent kin of

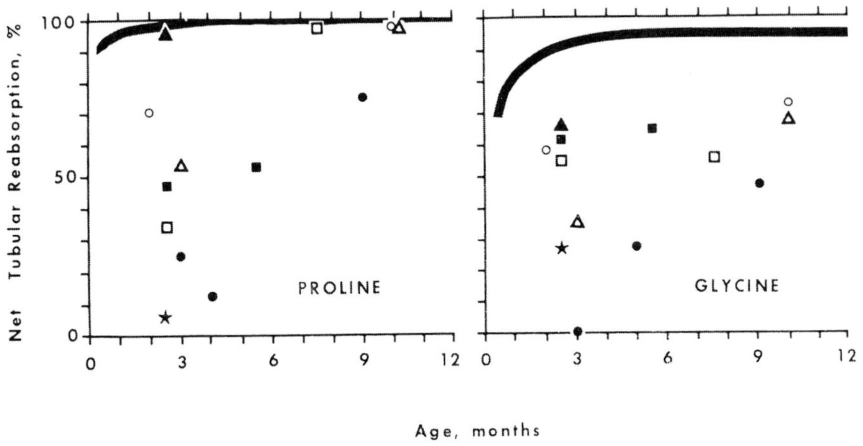

Fig. 194-3 Tubular reabsorption data for proline and glycine in relation to age in seven probands (various symbols, from Lasley and Scriver[90]) with familial renal iminoglycinuria. Shaded region indicates reabsorption values in normal infants. (From Brodehl.[89] Reproduced from *Pediatric Research* with permission.)

uptake in COS-7 cells,[83] inhibitor profile and transport functional similarities to brush border uptake in mammalian kidney membranes suggest that the specific glycine system of brain and kidney are similar if not identical. The ontogenic changes found in mouse brain may explain some of the corresponding differences noted in murine and human kidney that are identified elsewhere in this chapter.

Just as the brain glycine transporters have been cloned, a human brain-specific L-proline transporter has undergone molecular cloning, functional expression,[84] and chromosomal location to human chromosome 5.[85] This brain L-proline transporter is not shared with glycine, nor is it evident in peripheral tissues including kidney. L-Proline uptake is $Na^{+}Cl^{-}$-dependent, and is not inhibited by glycine or other γ amino acids in uptake studies in transfected HeLa cells. Several consensus sequences for protein kinase-mediated phosphorylation are present in this gene, including cAMP-dependent protein kinase phosphorylation, protein-kinase C-dependent protein kinase phosphorylation, and casein kinase II-dependent phosphorylation sites.[86] As yet, the renal isoform of the specific L-proline transporter has not been cloned.

Proline Transporter Protein

Based on work in numerous bacteria and in larval worms,[87,88] there is new evidence for a shared proline, glycine K^{+} symporter. A novel shared symporter was found in the gut of the larval tobacco hornworm *Manduca sexta*.[88] A shared system (demonstrated in midgut brush-border membrane vesicles of this worm) was predicted by Scriver and Wilson.[16]

Ontogeny of Renal Transport of Imino Acids and Glycine

Ontogeny affects renal transport of imino acids and glycine. When ontogeny is combined with Mendelian variation, the findings are informative. Hyperiminoglycinuria in the normal human newborn[6–10] reflects reduced net reabsorption of imino acids and glycine[10,89,90] (see Fig. 194-1). The maturation of tubular transport functions occurs by independent schedules for proline and glycine,[89,90] suggesting that separate carriers are involved. This conclusion is given strong support by findings in probands homozygous for hereditary iminoglycinuria.[90] Such individuals have near-total absence of tubular reabsorption for proline and glycine in the early postnatal period. As tubular function matures, reabsorptive activity for proline appears first, followed by the later appearance of a glycine reabsorptive activity (Fig. 194-3). The profile of maturing proline and glycine transport in the mutant homozygote indicates that there are independent carriers for proline and glycine that are not controlled by the gene locus affected by the mutation.

Transient postnatal iminoglycinuria is characteristic of mammals in general.[89–91] Postnatal maturation of membrane transport activities is believed to involve intensification of specific membrane functions[91] for which an explanation may be improved efficiency in maintaining and coupling the inward-directed Na^{+} gradient, which is the driving force for uptake of amino acids at the brush-border membrane.[92]

Although there is controversy about the process of ontogeny as it involves renal transport of proline and glycine,[93–96] several observations provide an overall insight. First, backflux of amino acids in the immature distal tubule is not a component of postnatal iminoglycinuria.[98] Second, diminished metabolic run out is not a significant cause of diminished net reabsorption.[94–98] Third, postnatal prolinuria in rats is associated with low activity of the high-affinity Na^{+}-dependent proline transport system in nephron[98,99] in the brush-border membrane.[99] Fourth, cortical tubule fragments and slices[91,94,95] from newborn animals have impaired efflux of proline. Together, these findings suggest that ontogeny is associated with deficient activity of high-affinity systems for imino acids and glycine that do not include the system controlled by the familial iminoglycinuria locus.

An alternate explanation is that Na^{+} uptake across the renal brush-border surface is enhanced in younger animals. This rapid entry of Na^{+} tends to reduce the driving force for Na^{+}-proline or Na^{+}-glycine uptake and to reduce Na^{+}-dependent organic solute transport in young animals[100] (Fig. 194-4).

Renal Reabsorption of Imino Acids and Glycine in Familial Iminoglycinuria

Endogenous renal clearance rates are elevated and net reabsorption is decreased in affected probands (see Table 194-1). Of note, however, net tubular absorption of imino acids and glycine is not completely eliminated in homozygotes. Also, the abnormal prolinuria may disappear at low plasma proline concentrations in homozygotes (Fig. 194-5). The venous plasma "threshold" for prolinuria is very low in homozygotes (about 0.1 mM) as compared with normal subjects (about 0.8 mM).

The ability of homozygotes with hereditary iminoglycinuria to retain a considerable fraction of their specific tubular absorptive function is a feature shared by homozygotes with other inborn errors of membrane transport. For example, homozygotes with either classic cystinuria (see Chap. 191), isolated hypercystinuria, or Hartnup disorder (Chap. 193) usually retain some capacity to transport the relevant amino acids. A similar characteristic is also observed for hexose transport in glucose-galactose malabsorption in regard to renal tubular absorption of glucose.[43] One interpretation of this phenomenon in mutant phenotypes is that more than one type of transport protein serves reabsorption of the specific substrate along the nephron, the different systems being controlled by different genes. This theory has not been examined directly in the iminoglycinuria but is upheld in the analogous cystinuria (see Chap. 191).

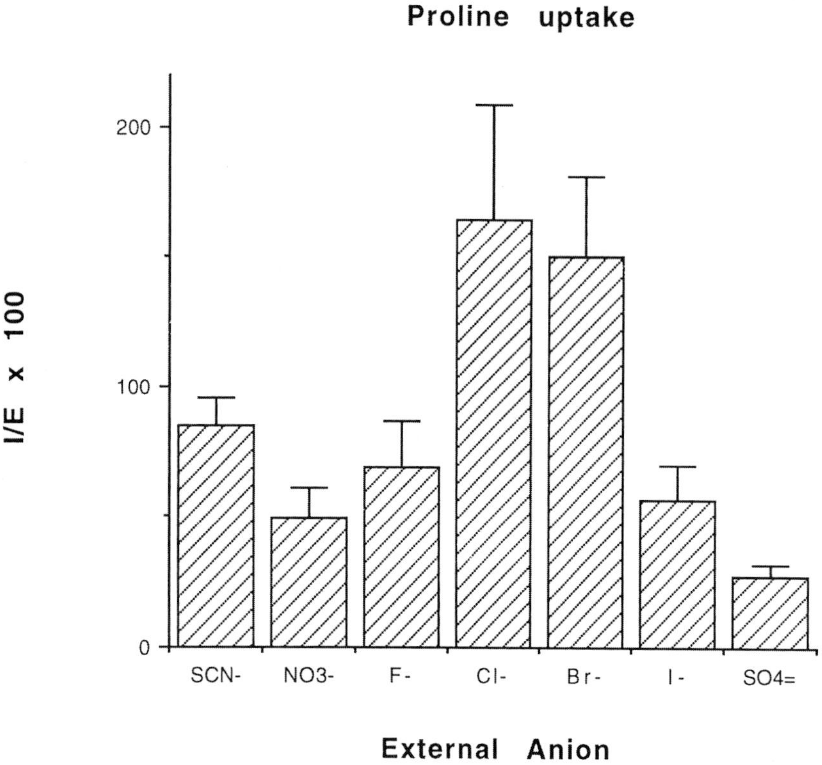

Fig. 194-4 Initial rate/equilibrium (I/E) values for proline uptake in the presence of external anions with varying membrane permeabilities. Incubation media contained 2 mM HEPES/TRIS (pH 7.35), 1 mM $MgSO_4$, 50.53 mM mannitol, and 100 mM NaSCN, $NaNO_3$, NaF, NaCl, NaBr, NaI, or 50 mM Na_2SO_4. Data are the mean ± SE of four determinations performed in triplicate. (From Chesney, Zelikovic, Budreau, and Randle.[64] Used by permission of the *Journal of the American Society of Nephrology*.)

Transport at Saturation in the Mutant Iminoglycinuria Phenotype

T_m values have been measured in mutant homozygotes and obligate heterozygotes infused with L-proline and hydroxy-L-proline.[16,17,21] Imino acid transport is present but saturated at normal plasma concentration of proline and hydroxyproline in the mutant homozygotes (Fig. 194-6). The heterozygote has a T_m value intermediate between normal and homozygous mutant values (see Fig. 194-6); imino acid reabsorption is normal at concentrations below the T_m, suggesting that affinity of the available imino acid transport sites is normal in the heterozygote. Taken together, these findings indicate that the mutation causes functional deletion of a transport system that has a capacity well above the normal concentration of imino acids in filtrate. Another modality of uptake with a small but recognizable capacity and high affinity is retained.

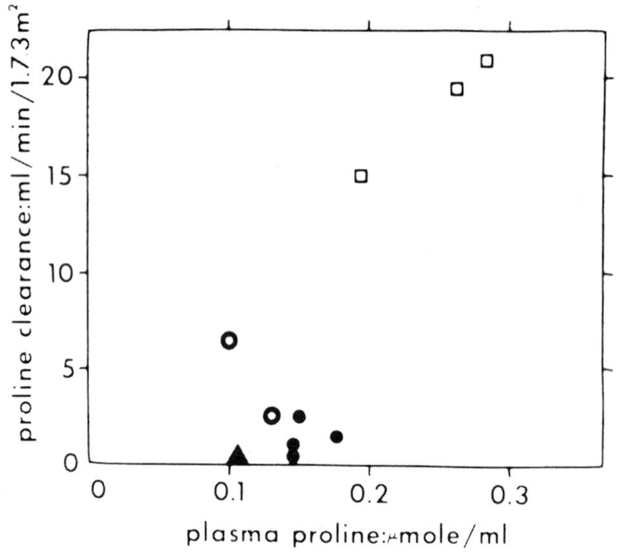

Fig. 194-5 Endogenous renal clearance of L-proline related to its concentration in plasma in homozygotes with familial iminoglycinuria. The "venous plasma threshold concentration" at which prolinuria appears is about 0.1 mM; the normal value is about 0.8 mM.[38] Abnormal prolinuria disappears in mutant homozygotes at low plasma proline concentration, indicating the existence of a small but efficient tubular capacity to transport proline. (Redrawn from Scriver,[17] with permission of the *Journal of Clinical Investigation*, with data (open circles) added from Greene et al.[27] and other data (solid triangle) added from Tada et al.[40])

Greene *et al.*[27] described a proband in whom the mutant allele did not delete the affected transport function but altered its affinity for substrate, so that glycine was very poorly reabsorbed and proline was less avidly transported by the mutant carrier (see Fig. 194-6); a K_m variant was proposed.

Interactions between Imino Acids and Glycine during Tubular Reabsorption in the Mutant Phenotype

Normal adult subjects infused with proline or hydroxyproline show brisk inhibition of glycine reabsorption; mutant homozygotes show no inhibition of the residual activity serving glycine reabsorption[17] (Fig. 194-7). The latter may represent transport of glycine on the high-affinity system in proximal straight tubule or by the diffusional mode in proximal nephron.[56] Loss of a portion of the glycine transport activity in the mutant phenotype is somewhat discordant with the hypothesis[62] that imino acids and glycine do not share a transport system in the brush-border membrane. The latter hypothesis implies that the iminoglycinuria mutation, which is at one locus, affects two transport systems; this could be explained if a polypeptide subunit were common to both carriers. Infusion of one imino acid also impairs reabsorption of the other in normal subjects and in mutant homozygotes.[17] This finding in the mutant phenotype is compatible with inhibition of residual imino acid transport, on the broad-specificity, high-capacity neutral amino acid system in proximal convolutions.[53]

Imino acids and glycine do share transport on a high-capacity, low-affinity system at the basolateral membrane.[67] Some hetero-

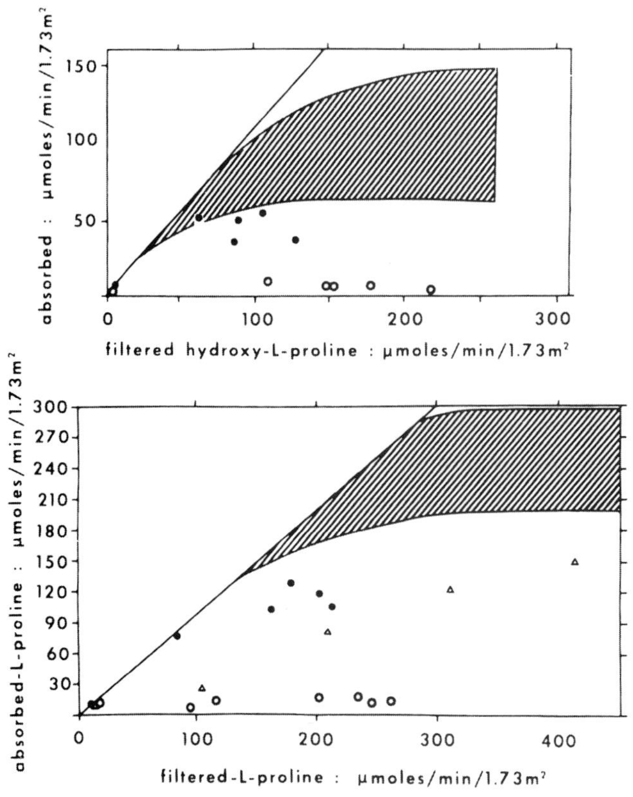

Fig. 194-6 Maximum rates of tubular reabsorption (T_m) of L-proline and hydroxy-L-proline in normal subjects (hatched), heterozygotes (solid circles), and mutant homozygotes (open circles) with classic iminoglycinuria. Data for patient with K_m variant of iminoglycinuria[27] are also shown (Δ). (Redrawn from Scriver[17] and Greene et al.[27] Used by permission.)

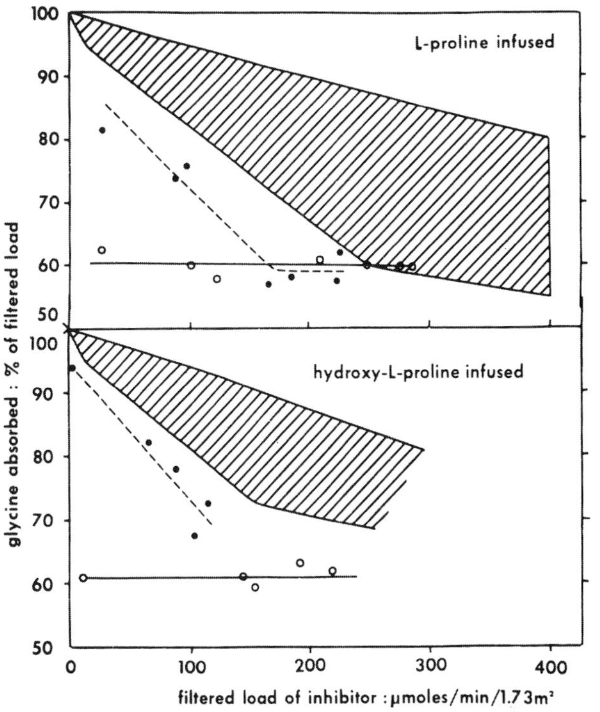

Fig. 194-7 Effect of L-proline and hydroxy-L-proline on net tubular reabsorption of glycine in normal subjects (hatched), heterozygotes (solid circles), and mutant homozygotes with classic iminoglycinuria. (Redrawn from Scriver[17] and Greene et al.[27] Used with permission.)

zygotes, however, have hyperglycinuria at normal plasma glycine concentrations (Figs. 194-6 and 194-7). This finding is compatible with impaired transport activity at the brush-border membrane but less compatible with impairment at the basolateral membrane (see Scriver and Tenenhouse[101] for explanation). Therefore, although we know that familial iminoglycinuria is a disorder involving a carrier selective for imino acids and glycine, it is still uncertain which transport system or site is affected.

Expression of Phenotype in Nonrenal Tissues

Intestine. Intestinal transport of L-proline has been examined *in vivo*[14,15,17,18,21] and in intestinal biopsy material.[21] Fecal excretion of amino acids has also been measured.[17,21] Two phenotypes have been identified. Some homozygotes have normal intestinal transport of L-proline and normal fecal excretion,[14,17,21] while others have impaired absorption and increased fecal excretion of proline.[15,18] The association of different intestinal phenotypes with a single renal phenotype suggests that more than one mutant allele is responsible for the iminoglycinuric trait.

The plasma response to glycine loading by mouth is normal in patients with and without demonstrable impairment of proline absorption.[15,18,21] This may indicate that transport by intestine is qualitatively different from that in kidney or that diffusional uptake of glycine, which would be unaffected by mutation, is significant in the intestine.

Leukocytes and Skin Fibroblasts. Net uptake of isotopically labeled proline at low extracellular concentrations (0.05 mM) by leukocytes and skin fibroblasts was apparently normal in homozygotes.[102] A negative finding has two interpretations: Either the mutant system is not expressed in the plasma membrane of parenchymal cells or the experiment did not test for uptake on the mutant system. The former explanation involves an understanding that plasma membranes of parenchymal cells share homologous transport functions with basolateral membranes of renal and intestinal epithelium but not necessarily with functions in the brush-border membranes,[17,103] and renal iminoglycinuria appears to be a disorder of a brush-border membrane carrier.

Nonmammalian Systems

Studies in yeast[104] and several bacterial species[105–109] indicate that both glycine and proline uptake are important in osmoregulation. When these cells are placed in water, proline or glycine efflux is enhanced. Under salt stress, uptake is rapidly up-regulated. This osmoregulator is a high K_m-system transporter. The low K_m system is used to scavenge low concentrations of these amino acids. Hence, transport systems for these amino acids are found throughout nature.

DIAGNOSIS

Criteria for Abnormal Iminoglycinuria

Any degree of iminoaciduria after 6 months of age may be considered abnormal. Hyperglycinuria may be recognized on partition chromatograms when the glycine spot is disproportionately intense in comparison with other amino acids. The quantitative criteria for hyperglycinuria are urinary excretion exceeding 150 µM per g of total nitrogen,[20] or 150 mg/24 h,[110] or an endogenous clearance rate exceeding 8.6 ml/min/1.73 m²).[111]

Differential Diagnosis

Hyperprolinemia and Hydroxyprolinemia. Iminoglycinuria occurs by a "combined" mechanism when there is hyperprolinemia in excess of about 0.8 mM.[38] Hyperprolinemia, type I or type II (see Chap. 81) is usually accompanied by iminoglycinuria. Patients with hydroxyprolinemia have not exhibited iminoglycinuria because the concentration of hydroxyproline in their

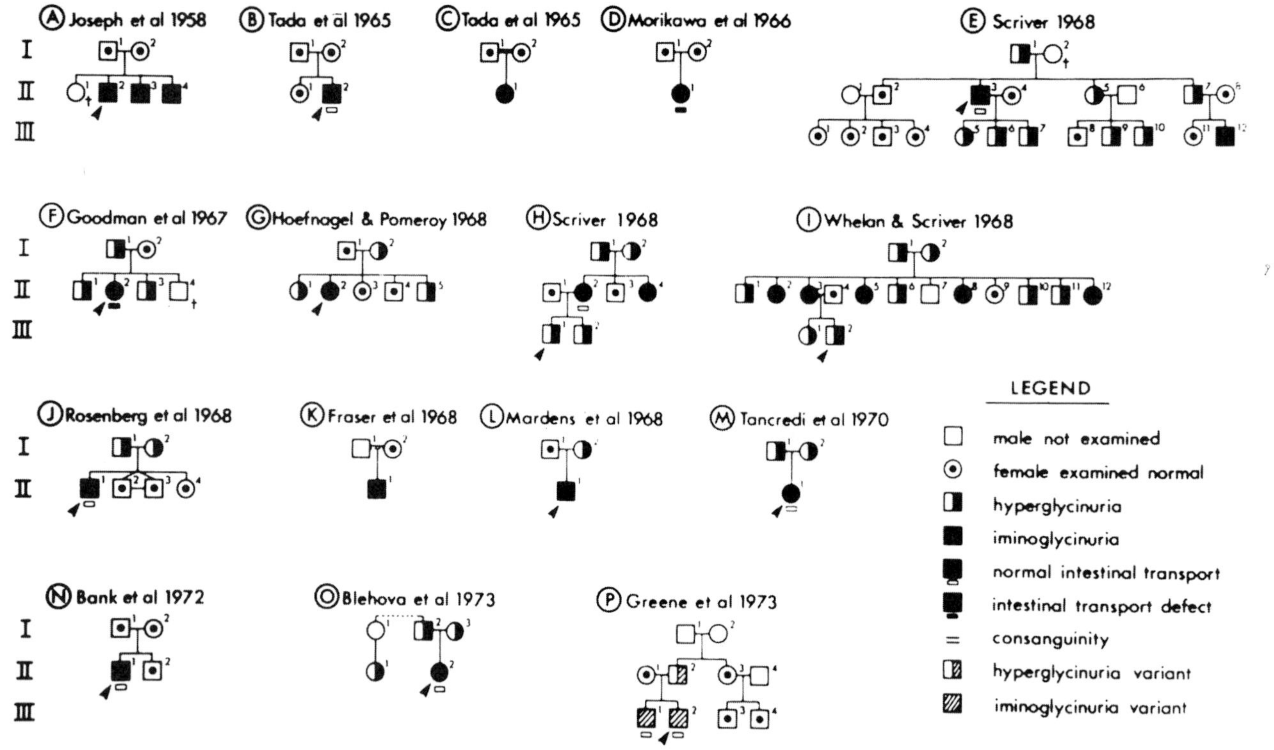

Fig. 194-8 Pedigrees of patients with familial iminoglycinuria. See ref. 12 for pedigree A; ref. 14 for B and C; ref. 15 for D; ref. 17 for E and H; ref. 18 for F; ref. 19 for G; ref. 20 for I; ref. 21 for J; ref. 22 for K; ref. 23 for L; ref. 24 for M; ref. 25 for N; ref. 26 for O; and ref. 27 for P.

plasma has not exceeded 0.4 mM; hydroxyproline must be present in plasma at least at this concentration to competitively inhibit tubular absorption of proline and glycine.[39] Hyperprolinemia and hydroxyprolinemia can be ruled out as a cause of iminoglycinuria if the concentration of both imino acids in plasma is normal in subjects with iminoglycinuria.

Fanconi Syndrome

Iminoglycinuria occurs in Fanconi syndrome as part of a generalized hyperaminoaciduria, in contrast to the selective hyperaminoaciduria in familial iminoglycinuria.

Neonatal Iminoglycinuria

The human infant normally has some degree of hyperiminoaciduria until about the third month of postnatal life; the hyperglycinuria subsides by the sixth month.

Renal Glycinuria

There have been numerous reports of hyperglycinuria without iminoaciduria. This phenotype may represent one form of the heterozygote with the iminoglycinuria mutation or the "K_m variant" form of renal iminoglycinuria.[27] Differential diagnosis includes:

1. Dominantly inherited renal hyperglycinuria and nephrolithiasis.[112,113]
2. Autosomal dominant glucoglycinuria.[114] Glucosuria occurs by the type B mechanism of Reubi; that is, the renal threshold for glucosuria is low (79 mg/dl), but the T_{mG} is normal — 386 mg/min/1.73 m^2. Of the 44 subjects examined,[114] 13 healthy relatives also had glucoglycinuria; no subjects with glucosuria or glycinuria alone were found.
3. X-linked hypophosphatemia with glucoglycinuria.[115,116] Glucosuria is Reubi type A (low T_m). A glycine carrier, shared with imino acids, is present, but it is operating inefficiently. The glucoglycinuria occurs through a mechanism different from that described in the autosomal dominant condition.[114]

These traits should all be distinguished from the "prerenal" form of hyperglycinuria found in hyperglycinemia. Glucoglycinuria in adults with phosphaturia is not significantly elevated when compared to patients with renal disease; it is significantly elevated only when compared to normal controls.[117]

GENETICS

Familial renal iminoglycinuria is the expressed phenotype of alleles at an autosomal locus which controls a membrane carrier shared by imino acids and glycine. Consanguinity in parents of iminoglycinuria probands has been reported[14,22] (Fig. 194-8).

In some pedigrees, obligate heterozygotes have hyperglycinuria (see Fig. 194-8). This represents expression of an "incompletely recessive" allele, and the phenotype must be differentiated from other forms of dominantly inherited hyperglycinuria (see "Renal Glycinuria" above). Most heterozygotes for familial iminoglycinuria do not have hyperglycinuria; their mutant allele is "completely recessive." A third allele[27] is apparent in pedigree P (Fig. 194-8), in which a heterozygote and two affected offspring had hyperglycinuria associated with a mutant transport system expressing lowered affinity for glycine.

There are pedigrees (E, F, G, and L in Fig. 194-8) in which one parent is hyperglycinuric and the other is not; their offspring are indistinguishable from homozygotes with two hyperglycinuric parents or with two "silent" parents. When a proband with the fully expressed phenotype has parents showing phenotypic heterogeneity (for example one is incompletely recessive, the other is completely recessive) the proband is presumed to be a genetic compound for different alleles.

Some mutant homozygotes have impaired intestinal transport of proline (Fig. 194-8), whereas others do not. The intestinal

Table 194-3 Evidence for Allelic Mutations in Familial Renal Iminoglycinuria. Phenotype Heterogeneity Among Homozygotes, "Genetic Compounds," and Obligate Heterozygotes

Presumed Allelic Pair	Renal Phenotype in Homozygote or Compound	Heterozygote	Intestinal Phenotype in Homozygote (or Compound)	Exemplary Pedigrees in Fig. 194-8
I-I	IG	N	Present	D
II-II	IG	N	N	B, N
III-III	IG	G	N	E, H, J, M, O
I-III (or II)	IG	N or G	Present	F
	IG	N or G	Not tested	E, G, L
II-IV	iG (K_m)	N or iG (K_m)	N	P

IG = iminoglycinuria (with loss of "high-K_m" system;) G = glycinuria alone; iG (K_m) = (K_m) variant involving "high-K_m" system affecting glycine more than imino acids; N = normal; "Present" implies defective absorption of proline and/or glycine in test procedure.

phenotype is not consistently associated with any form of the heterozygous phenotypes. From the various combinations of phenotypes, including the K_m variant,[27] one can postulate four mutant alleles (Table 194-3). There has been no opportunity for analysis by molecular genetic methods to confirm this hypothesis.

Prevalence

Newborn screening data[27–29] indicate that the frequency of the presumed homozygote (or genetic compound) among Caucasians is about 1 in 15,000 live births. Of aminoacidurias detected by the screening of 1 million 6-week-old infants, iminoglycinuria was less common than cystinuria, histidinemia, or Hartnup disorder.[118] Accordingly, the frequency of heterozygotes in the population is about 2 percent, about half being incompletely recessive (hyperglycinuric phenotype). The corresponding frequencies of specific alleles (silent, incomplete, and K_m variant) are lower than 1 percent. Because these alleles are presumably all neutral in terms of selection, their high frequency may reflect founder effect or high mutation rate at the locus. However, because of the recent knowledge concerning the brain glycine and proline transporters[77–83] the possibility of some central nervous system lesions in selected subjects with iminoglycinuria exists, as has been suggested in a child with spasticity.[34]

TREATMENT

Familial iminoglycinuria is considered to be a benign condition (with possible rare exceptions[34]) involving nonessential amino acids and no treatment is indicated. The considerable number of healthy subjects in whom iminoglycinuria was discovered quite incidentally (see Fig. 194-8, pedigree E, subjects II.3 and III.12; pedigree H, subjects II.2 and II.4; and all homozygous members of pedigree I) supports this interpretation. The various illnesses that have been associated with the iminoglycinuria trait apparently served only to bring the transport mutation to attention.

REFERENCES

1. Greenstein JP, Winitz M: *Chemistry of the Amino Acid*. New York, John Wiley, 1961.
2. Meister A: *Biochemistry of the Amino Acid*, 2nd ed. New York, Academic Press, 1965.
3. McMillan DE: Letter to the editor. *N Engl J Med* **273**:771, 1965.
4. Dent CE: Detection of amino acids in urine and other fluids. *Lancet* **2**:637, 1946.
5. Scriver CR, Rosenberg LE: *Amino Acid Metabolism and Its Disorders*. Philadelphia, Saunders, 1973.
6. Scriver CR: Hereditary aminoaciduria, in Bearn A, Steinberg AG (eds): *Progress in Medical Genetics,* vol 2. New York, Grune & Stratton, 1962, p 83.
7. Sereni F, McNamara H, Shibuya M, et al: Concentration in plasma and rate of urinary excretion of amino acids in premature infants. *Pediatrics* **15**:575, 1955.
8. Woolf LI, Norman AP: The urinary excretion of amino acids and sugars in early infancy. *J Pediatr* **50**:271, 1957.
9. O'Brien D, Butterfield LJ: Further studies on renal tubular conservation of free amino acids in early infancy. *Arch Dis Child* **38**:437, 1963.
10. Brodehl J, Gellissen K: Endogenous renal transport of free amino acids in infancy and childhood. *Pediatrics* **42**:395, 1968.
11. Scriver CR, Schafer IA, Efron ML: New renal tubular amino acid transport system and a new hereditary disorder of amino acid metabolism. *Nature* **192**:672, 1961.
12. Joseph R, Ribierre M, Job JC, et al: Maladie familiale associante des convulsions a debut tres precoce, une hyperalbuminorachie et uen hyperaminoacidurie. *Arch Fr Pediatr* **15**:374, 1958.
13. Mozziconacci P, Boisse J, Lemonnier A, et al: Les maladies metaboliques des acides amines avec arrieration mentale. Paris, L'Expansion Scientifique Francaise, 1968, p. 249.
14. Tada K, Morikawa T, Ando T, et al: Prolinuria: A new renal tubular defect in transport of proline and glycine. *Tohoku J Exp Med* **87**:133, 1965.
15. Morikawa T, Tada K, Ando T, et al: Prolinuria: Defect in intestinal absorption of imino acids and glycine. *Tohoku J Exp Med* **90**:105, 1966.
16. Scriver CR, Wilson OH: Amino acid transport in human kidney: Evidence for genetic control of two types. *Science* **155**:1428, 1967.
17. Scriver CR: Renal tubular transport of proline, hydroxyproline and glycine. III. Genetic basis for more than one mode of transport in human kidney. *J Clin Invest* **47**:823, 1968.
18. Goodman SI, McIntyre CA, O'Brien D: Impaired intestinal transport of proline in a patient with familial iminoaciduria. *J Pediatr* **71**:246, 1967.
19. Hoefnagel D, Pomeroy J: Personal communication of unpublished data, 1968, p 1969.
20. Whelan DT, Scriver CR: Cystathioninuria and renal iminoglycinuria in a pedigree: A perspective on counseling. *N Engl J Med* **278**:924, 1968.
21. Rosenberg IE, Durant JL, Elsas LJ II: Familial iminoglycinuria: An inborn error of renal tubular transport. *N Engl J Med* **278**:1407, 1968.
22. Fraser GR, Friedmann AI, Patton VM, et al: Iminoglycinuria—A "harmless" inborn error of metabolism? *Humangenetik* **6**:362, 1968.
23. Mardens Y, Andriaenssens K, van Sande M: Glycinurie et iminoacidurie rénales associes a une oligophrenie: Étude clinique et biochimique. *J Neurol Sci* **6**:333, 1968.
24. Tancredi F, Guazzi G, Aurichio S: Renal iminoglycinuria without intestinal malabsorption of glycine and imino acids. *J Pediatr* **7**:386, 1970.
25. Bank H, Crispin M, Ehrlich D, et al: Iminoglycinuria: A defect of renal tubular transport. *Isr J Med Sci* **8**:606, 1972.
26. Blehova B, Pazoutova N, Hyanek J, et al: Iminoglycinuria in a child in Czechoslovakia. *Humangenetik* **19**:207, 1973.
27. Greene ML, Lietman PS, Rosenberg LE, et al: Familial hyperglycinuria: New defect in renal tubular transport of glycine and imino acids. *Am J Med* **54**:265, 1973.

28. Levy HL: Genetic screening, in Harris H, Hirschhorn K (eds): *Advances in Human Genetics,* vol 4. New York, Plenum, 1973, p 1.
29. Turner B, Brown DA: Amino acid excretion in infancy and early childhood: A survey of 200,000 infants. *Med J Aust* **1**:62, 1972.
30. Procopis PG, Turner B: Iminoaciduria: A benign renal tubular defect. *J Pediatr* **79**:419, 1971.
31. Paine RS: Evaluation of familial biochemically determined mental retardation in children, with special reference to aminoaciduria. *N Engl J Med* **262**:658, 1966.
32. Jonxis JHP: Personal communication, 1962.
33. Miller M: Familial cirrhosis with hepatoma. *Am J Dig Dis* **12**:633, 1967.
34. Statter M, Ben-Zvi A, Shina A, et al: Familial iminoglycinuria with normal intestinal absorption of glycine and imino acids in association with profound mental retardation, a possible "cerebral phenotype." *Helv Paediatr Acta* **31**:173, 1976.
35. Purkiss P, Chalmers RA, Borud O: Combined iminoglycinuria and cystine- and dibasic aminoaciduria in patients with propionic acidaemia and 3-methylcrotinylglycinuria. *J Inherit Metab Dis* **3**:85, 1980.
36. Hayasaka S, Mizuno K, Yabata K, et al: Atypical gyrate atrophy of the choroid and retina associated with iminoglycinuria. *Arch Ophthalmol* **100**:423, 1982.
37. Schafer JA, Scriver CR, Efron ML: Familial hyperprolinemia, cerebral dysfunction and renal anomalies occurring in a family with hereditary nephritis and deafness. *N Engl J Med* **267**:51, 1962.
38. Scriver CR, Efron ML, Schafer JA: Renal tubular transport of proline, hydroxyproline and glycine in health and in familial hyperprolinemia. *J Clin Invest* **43**:374, 1964.
39. Scriver CR, Goldman H: Renal tubular transport of proline, hydroxyproline and glycine. II. Hydroxy-L-proline as substrate and as inhibitor in vivo. *J Clin Invest* **45**:1357, 1966.
40. Tada K, Hirono H, Arakawa T: Endogenous renal clearance rates of free amino acids in prolinuric and Hartnup patients. *Tohoku J Exp Med* **93**:57, 1967.
41. Mitch WE, Chesney RW: Amino acid metabolism by the kidney. *Miner Electrolyte Metab* **9**:190, 1983.
42. Foreman JW, McNamara PD, Pepe LM, et al: Uptake of proline by brush border vesicles isolated from human kidney cortex. *Biochem Med* **34**:304, 1985.
43. Scriver CR, Chesney RW, McInnes RR: Genetic aspects of renal tubular transport: Diversity and topology of carriers. *Kidney Int* **9**:149, 1976.
44. Schafer JA, Barfuss DW: Membrane mechanisms for transepithelial amino acid absorption and secretion. *Am J Physiol* **238**:F335, 1980.
45. Scriver CR, Tenenhouse HS: Genetics and mammalian transport system. *Ann N Y Acad Sci* **456**:384, 1985.
46. Wilson OH, Scriver CR: Specificity of transport of neutral and basic amino acids in rat kidney. *Am J Physiol* **213**:185, 1967.
47. Webber WA: Interactions of neutral and acidic amino acids in renal tubular transport. *Am Physiol* **202**:577, 1962.
48. Bergeron M, Morel F: Amino acid transport in rat renal tubules. *Am J Physiol* **216**:1139, 1969.
49. Dubord L, Bergeron M: Multiplicite des systemes transporteurs a la membrane luminale du nephron chez le rat normal. *Rev Can Biol* **33**:99, 1975.
50. Volkl H, Silbernagl S, Deetjen P: Kinetics of L-proline reabsorption in rat kidney studied by continuous microperfusion. *Pflugers Arch* **382**:115, 1979.
51. Volkl H, Silbernagl S: Molecular specificity of tubular reabsorption of L-proline. A microperfusion study in rat kidney. *Pflugers Arch* **387**: 253, 1980.
52. Ulrich KJ, Reimrich G, Kloss S: Sodium dependence of the amino acid transport in the proximal convolution of the rat kidney. *Pflugers Arch* **351**:49, 1974.
53. Somarzija I, Fromter E: Electrophysiological analysis of rat renal sugar and amino acid transport. III. Neutral amino acids. *Pflugers Arch* **393**:199, 1982.
54. Zelikovic I, Chesney RW: Sodium-coupled amino acid transport in renal tubule. *Kidney Int* **36**:351, 1989.
55. Barfuss DW, Schafer JA: Active amino acid absorption by proximal convoluted and proximal straight tubules. *Am J Physiol* **236**:F149, 1979.
56. Barfuss DW, Schafer JA: Active amino acid absorption by proximal convoluted and proximal straight tubules. *Am J Physiol* **236**:F149, 1979.
57. Barfuss DW, Mays JM, Schafer JA: Peritubular uptake and transepithelial transport of glycine in isolated proximal tubules. *Am J Physiol* **238**:F324, 1980.
58. Slack EN, Liang C-CT, Sacktor B: Transport of L-proline and D-glucose in luminal (brush-border) and contraluminal (basal-lateral) membrane vesicles from the renal cortex. *Biochem Biophys Res Commun* **77**:891, 1977.
59. Hammerman MR, Sacktor B: Transport of amino acids in renal brush border membrane vesicles. Uptake of L-proline. *J Biol Chem* **252**:591, 1977.
60. McNamara PD, Ozegovic B, Pepe LM, et al: Proline and glycine uptake by renal brush border membrane vesicles. *Proc Natl Acad Sci U S A* **73**:4521, 1976.
61. McNamara PD, Pepe LM, Segal S: Sodium gradient dependence of proline and glycine uptake in renal brush-border membrane vesicles. *Biochim Biophys Acta* **556**:151, 1979.
62. Hammerman MR, Sacktor B: Na^+-dependent transport of glycine in renal brush border membrane vesicles. *Biochim Biophys Acta* **686**:189, 1982.
63. Schafer JA, Barfuss DW: Membrane mechanisms for transepithelial amino acid absorption and secretion. *Am J Physiol* **238**:F335, 1980.
64. Chesney RW, Zelikovic I, Budreau A, et al: Chloride and membrane potential dependence of sodium ion-proline symport. *J Am Soc Nephrol* **2**:885, 1991.
65. Roigaard-Petersen H, Jessen H, Mollerup S, et al: Proton gradient-dependent renal transport of glycine: Evidence from vesicle studies. *Am J Physiol* **258**:F388, 1990.
66. Radendran VM, Barry JA, Kleinman JG, et al: Proton gradient-dependent transport of glycine in rabbit renal brush-border membrane vesicles. *J Biol Chem* **262**:14974, 1987.
67. Mohyuddin F, Scriver CR: Amino acid transport in mammalian kidney: Identification and analysis of multiple systems for iminoacids and glycine in rat kidney. *Am J Physiol* **219**:1, 1970.
68. Hillman RE, Albrecht I, Rosenberg LE: Identification and analysis of multiple glycine transport systems in isolated mammalian renal tubules. *J Biol Chem* **243**:5566, 1968.
69. Hillman RE, Rosenberg LE: Amino acid transport by isolated mammalian renal tubules. II. Transport systems for L-proline. *J Biol Chem* **244**:4494, 1969.
70. Wedeen RP, Weiner B: The distribution of p-aminohippuric acid in rat kidney slices. I. Tubular localization. *Kidney Int* **3**:205, 1973.
71. Arthus MF, Bergeron M, Scriver CR: Topology of membrane exposure in the renal cortex slice. Studies of glutathione and maltose cleavage. *Biochim Biophys Acta* **692**:371, 1982.
72. Scriver CR, McInnes RR, Mohyuddin F: Role of epithelial architecture and intracellular metabolism in proline uptake and transtubular reclamation in PRO/Re mouse kidney. *Proc Natl Acad Sci U S A* **72**:1431, 1975.
73. Holtzapple P, Genel M, Rea C, et al: Metabolism and uptake of L-proline by human kidney cortex. *Pediatr Res* **7**:818, 1973.
74. Greth WE, Thier SO, Segal S: The transport and metabolism of L-proline-14C in the rat and in vivo. *Metabolism* **27**:975, 1978.
75. Roigaard-Petersen H, Jacobsen C, Jessen H, et al: Electrogenic uptake of D-imino acids by luminal membrane vesicles from rabbit kidney proximal tubule. *Biochim Biophys Acta* **984**:231, 1989.
76. Zelikovic I, Prezkwas J: $Ca(2^+)$-dependent protein kinases modulate proline transport across the renal brush-border membrane. *Am J Physiol* **268(1 pt 2)**:F155, 1995.
77. Malandro MS, Kilberg MS: Molecular biology of mammalian amino acid transporters. *Annu Rev Biochem* **65**:305, 1996.
78. Kim KM, Kingsmore SF, Han H, et al: Cloning of the human glycine transporter type 1: Molecular and pharmacological characterization of novel isoform variants and chromosomal localization of the gene in the human and mouse genomes. *Mol Pharmacol* **45(4)**:608, 1994.
79. Borowsky B, Mezey E, Hoffman B: Two glycine transporter variants with distinct localization in the CNS and peripheral tissues are encoded by a common gene. *Neuron* **10**:851, 1993.
80. Liu QR, Lopez-Corcuera B, Mandiyan S, et al: Cloning and expression of a spinal cord- and brain-specific glycine transporter with novel structural features. *J Biol Chem* **263(30)**:22802, 1993.
81. Adams RH, Sato K, Shimada S, et al: Gene structure and glial expression of the glycine transporter GLYT1 in embryonic adult rodents. *J Neurosci* **15(3 Pt 2)**:2524, 1995.
82. Jursky F, Nelson N: Developmental expression of the glycine transporters GLYT1 and GLYT2 in mouse brain. *J Neurochem* **67(1)**:336, 1996.

83. Bader A, Parthasarathy R, Harvey W: A novel proline, glycine: K^+ symporter in midgut brush-border membrane vesicles from larval *Manduca sexta*. *FEBS Lett* **417(2)**:177, 1997.
84. Fremeau RT, Caron MG, Blakely RD: Molecular cloning and expression of a high affinity L-proline transporter expressed in putative glutamatergic pathways of rat brain. *Neuron* **8(5)**:915, 1992.
85. Shafqat S, Velaz-Faircloth M, Henzi VA, et al: Man brain-specific L-proline transporter: Molecular cloning, functional expression, and chromosomal localization of the gene in human and mouse genomes. *Mol Pharmacol* **48(2)**:219, 1995.
86. Zelikovic I, Prezkwas J: The role of protein phosphorylation in renal amino acid transport. *Pediatr Nephrol* **7(5)**:621, 1993.
87. Yamato I, Kotani M, Oka Y, et al: Site-specific alteration of arginine 376, the unique positively charged amino acid residue in the mid-membrane-spanning regions of the proline carrier of *Escherichia coli*. *J Biol Chem* **269(8)**:5720, 1994.
88. Bader A, Parthasarathy R, Harvey W: A novel proline, glycine: K^+ symporter in midgut brush-border membrane vesicles from larval *Manduca sexta*. *FEBS Lett* **417(2)**:177, 1997.
89. Brodehl J: Postnatal development of tubular amino acid reabsorption, in Silbernagl S, Lang F, Greger R (eds): *Amino Acid Transport and Uric Acid Transport*. Stuttgart, Thieme, 1976, p 128.
90. Lasley L, Scriver CR: Ontogeny of amino acid reabsorption in human kidney. Evidence from the homozygous infant with familial renal iminoglycinuria for multiple proline and glycine systems. *Pediatr Res* **13**:65, 1979.
91. Baerlocher K, Scriver CR, Mohyuddin F: Ontogeny of iminoglycine transport in mammalian kidney. *Proc Natl Acad Sci U S A* **65**:1009, 1970.
92. Christensen HN: On the development of amino acid transport systems. *Fed Proc* **32**:19, 1973.
93. Medow MS, Roth KS, Goldmann DR, et al: Developmental aspects of proline transport in rat renal brush border membranes. *Proc Natl Acad Sci U S A* **83**:7561, 1986.
94. Baerlocher KE, Scriver CR, Mohyuddin F: The ontogeny of amino acid transport in rat kidney II. Kinetics of uptake and effect of anoxia. *Biochim Biophys Acta* **249**:364, 1971.
95. Baerlocher KE, Scriver CR, Mohyuddin F: The ontogeny of amino acid transport in rat kidney I. Effect on distribution ratios and intracellular metabolism of proline and glycine. *Biochim Biophys Acta* **249**:353, 1971.
96. Roth KS, Hwang S-M, London JW, et al: Ontogeny of glycine transport in isolated rat renal tubules. *Am J Physiol* **233**:F241, 1977.
97. Reynolds R, Roth KS, Hwang SM, et al: On the development of glycine transport systems by rat renal cortex. *Biochim Biophys Acta* **511**:274, 1979.
98. Scriver CR, Arthus MF, Bergeron M: Neonatal iminoglycinuria: Evidence that the prolinuria originates in selective deficiency of transport activity in proximal nephron. *Pediatr Res* **16**:684, 1982.
99. Goldmann DR, Roth KS, Langfitt TW Jr, et al: L-Proline transport by newborn rat kidney brush border membrane vesicles. *Biochemistry* **178**:253, 1979.
100. Zelikovic I, Stejskal-Lorenz E, Lohstroh P, et al: Developmental maturation of Na^+/H^+ exchange in rat renal tubular brush border membrane. *Am J Physiol* **261F**:1017, 1991.
101. Scriver CR, Tenenhouse HS: Mendelian phenotypes as "probes" of renal transport system for amino acids and phosphate, in Windhager EE (ed): *Handbook of Physiology, Section 8: Renal Physiology,* vol II. New York, Oxford University Press, 1992, p 1977.
102. Tada K, Morikawa T, Arakawa T: Prolinuria: Transport of proline by leukocytes. *Tohukiu J Exp Med* **90**:189, 1966.
103. Smith DW, Scriver CR, Tenenhouse HS, et al: The lysinuric protein intolerance mutation is expressed in plasma membrane of cultured skin fibroblasts. *Proc Natl Acad Sci U S A* **84**:7711, 1987.
104. Rentsch D, Hirner B, Schmelzer E, et al: Salt stress-induced proline transporters and salt stress-repressed broad specificity amino acid permeases identified by suppression of a yeast amino acid permease-targeting mutant. *Plant Cell* **8(8)**:1437, 1996.
105. Pourkomailian B, Booth IR: Glycine betaine transport by *Staphylococcus aureus:* Evidence for feedback regulation of the activity of the two transport systems. *Microbiology* **140(Pt 11)**:3131, 1994.
106. Glaasker E, Konings WN, Poolman B: Glycine betaine fluxes in *Lactobacillus plantarum* during osmostasis and hyper- and hypo-osmotic shock. *J Biol Chem* **271(17)**:10060, 1996.
107. Townsend DE, Wilkinson BJ: Proline transport in *Staphylococcus aureaus:* A high affinity system and a low-affinity system involved in osmoregulation. *J Bacteriol* **174(8)**:2702, 1992.
108. Molenaar D, Hagting A, Alkema H, et al: Characteristics and osmoregulatory roles of uptake systems for proline and glycine betaine in *Lactococcus lactis*. *Lactococcus lactis* subsp. *J Bacteriol* **175(17)**: 5438, 1993.
109. Glaasker E, Konings WN, Poolman B: Glycine betaine fluxes in *Lactobacillus plantarum* during osmostasis and hyper- and hypo-osmotic shock. *J Biol Chem* **271**:17:10060, 1996.
110. Carver MJ, Paska R: Ion-exchange chromatography of urinary amino acids. I. Normal children. *Clin Chim Acta* **6**:721, 1961.
111. Scriver CR, Davies E: Endogenous renal clearance rates of free amino acids in pre-pubertal children. *Pediatrics* **36**:592, 1965.
112. DeVries A, Kochwa S, Lazebnik J, et al: Glycinuria, a hereditary disorder associated with nephrolithiasis. *Am J Med* **23**:408, 1957.
113. Oberiter V, Pureti CZ, Fabe CI, et al: Hyperglycinuria with nephrolithiasis. *Eur J Pediatr* **127**:279, 1978.
114. Kaser H, Cottier P, Antener I: Glucoglycinuria, a new familial syndrome. *J Pediatr* **61**:386, 1962.
115. Scriver CR, Goldbloom RB, Roy CC: Hypophosphatemic rickets with renal hyperglycinuria, renal glucosuria and glycylprolinuria: A syndrome with evidence for renal tubular secretion of phosphorus. *Pediatrics* **34**:357, 1964.
116. Dent CE, Harris H: Hereditary forms of rickets and osteomalacia. *J Bone Joint Surg [Br]* **38**:204, 1956.
117. Holmgren G, Lindqvist B, Lundberg E: Hyperaminoaciduria in mild phosphate diabetes in adults. *Acta Med Scand* **207(6)**:489, 1980.
118. Wilcken B, Smith A, Brown DA: Urine screening for aminoacidopathies: Is it beneficial? Results of a long-term follow-up of cases detected by screening one million babies. *J Pediatr* **97**:492, 1980.

CHAPTER 195

Renal Tubular Acidosis

Thomas D. DuBose, Jr. ▪ Robert J. Alpern

1. Renal tubular acidosis (RTA) is a clinical syndrome characterized by hyperchloremic metabolic acidosis secondary to an abnormality in renal acidification. The acidification defect may be manifested by an inappropriately high urine pH, bicarbonaturia, and, by definition, reduced net acid excretion. Classical distal renal tubular acidosis and proximal renal tubular acidosis are frequently associated with hypokalemia. Distal renal tubular acidosis can also result from a generalized dysfunction of the distal nephron, in which case it is usually accompanied by hyperkalemia and may be associated with either hypoaldosteronism or aldosterone resistance.

2. Proximal renal tubular acidosis may result from an isolated defect of acidification in the proximal nephron. The isolated defect in acidification could be the result of selective dysfunction of the Na^+/H^+ antiporter, the proximal tubule H^+-ATPase or the $Na^+/HCO_3^-/CO_3^=$ symporter.

3. More commonly, proximal renal tubular acidosis occurs as one manifestation of a generalized defect in proximal tubule function. Patients with this generalized abnormality, the Fanconi syndrome, usually have glycosuria, aminoaciduria, citraturia, and phosphaturia. The acidification defect associated with this generalized tubular dysfunction may be the result of (a) impairment of cellular ATP generation, (b) cellular phosphate depletion, or (c) a selective abnormality of the basolateral Na^+, K^+-ATPase.

4. Vitamin D deficiency is associated with the Fanconi lesion. The transport defect may be due to a combination of factors including reduction in 1,25-dihydroxy vitamin D_3 levels, elevated parathyroid hormone levels, hypocalcemia, and intracellular phosphate depletion.

5. The diagnosis of proximal renal tubular acidosis is based on the demonstration of a chronic hyperchloremic metabolic acidosis and an acid urine pH. Correction of the metabolic acidosis with alkali raises the plasma bicarbonate level above the renal threshold and results in prominent bicarbonaturia and an alkaline urine pH. The fractional excretion of bicarbonate may exceed 15 percent of the filtered load in such conditions, and hypokalemia is common. Bone disease, which commonly accompanies this disorder, is expressed as rickets in children and osteopenia in adults.

6. The goal of therapy in proximal renal tubular acidosis is to maintain a near normal serum bicarbonate concentration while avoiding potassium deficiency. Concomitant administration of thiazide diuretics to reduce intravascular volume, and secondarily to reduce the filtered load of bicarbonate, is often beneficial.

7. The mechanisms underlying hypokalemic classical distal renal tubular acidosis have not been fully elucidated. Nevertheless, important advances in our understanding of the molecular bases of this disorder have been made recently. Distal RTA may be inherited or acquired. The hypokalemia that is particularly prevalent in the acquired forms, suggests a lesion in the medullary collecting duct or a selective lesion in the cortical collecting tubule. Possible mechanisms include an abnormal leak pathway or "gradient" lesion or a "secretory" defect. An example of a leak defect is that induced by amphotericin B in which the urine minus the arterial blood PCO_2 (U−B PCO_2) is normal. Only two patients, both young children, have been reported in which a normal U−B PCO_2 was present in the absence of exposure to amphotericin B, suggesting a nonamphotericin-acquired "gradient" lesion. The observed low U − B PCO_2 gradient in most patients with distal renal tubular acidosis studied thus far argues against a gradient lesion and suggests a rate or secretory defect as the underlying mechanism. The rate of distal H^+ secretion could be impaired as a result of a defect in: (a) the apical H^+-ATPase; (b) the apical H^+,K^+-ATPase; (c) the basolateral HCO_3^-/Cl^- exchanger; or (d) the enzyme carbonic anhydrase present in the cytoplasm of kidney cells (CA II).

8. Most patients with classical hypokalemic distal renal tubular acidosis have the condition in association with a systemic illness (acquired). Most available evidence, derived from studies using renal biopsies in patients with acquired distal RTA, suggests that acquired distal RTA is a result of abnormal function of the H^+-ATPase in the collecting tubule. Classical hypokalemic distal renal tubular acidosis also occurs as an isolated defect inherited as an autosomal dominant trait. Recent studies have demonstrated an association between a missense mutation in the HCO_3^-/Cl^- exchanger or band 3 protein (*AE1* gene) and autosomal dominant distal RTA in several families. It has been proposed that the HCO_3^-/Cl^- exchanger is misdirected to the apical membrane of type A intercalated cells in patients with the inherited form of distal RTA. This hypothesis is not proven. An endemic form of distal RTA, common in northeastern Thailand, appears to be the result of abnormal function of the renal H^+,K^+-ATPase. This association is not proven. Finally, distal RTA is a component of the CA II deficiency syndrome: osteopetrosis, distal RTA, and mental retardation. Patients with this autosomal recessive defect have been demonstrated to have one of several abnormalities in CA

A list of standard abbreviations is located immediately preceding the index in each volume. Additional abbreviations used in this chapter include: CA = carbonic anhydrase; CCT = cortical collecting tubule; IMCD = inner medullary collecting duct; OMCT = outer medullary collecting tubule; RTA = renal tubular acidosis.

II. Most patients, however, appear to have a mixed form of proximal and distal RTA. Therefore, acquired and inherited forms of distal RTA may have diverse etiologies, all of which impair distal acidification and net acid excretion.

9. **Classical hypokalemic distal renal tubular acidosis (type I RTA) is characterized clinically by an inability to acidify the urine appropriately during metabolic acidosis. Most but not all patients have a low U−B PCO_2 gradient. Hypokalemia, hypercalciuria, and hypocitraturia frequently accompany this disorder, but proximal tubular reabsorptive function is preserved. Chronic metabolic acidosis results in calcium, magnesium, and phosphate wasting which may be associated with dissolution of bone and nephrocalcinosis.**
10. **Untreated classical distal renal tubular acidosis produces growth retardation in children and progressive renal and bone disease in adults. Correction of the acidosis by alkali administration leads to correction of the accompanying hypokalemia, sodium depletion, hypercalciuria, and results in an increase in citrate excretion, which decreases the frequency of nephrolithiasis. Restoration of normal growth and prevention of nephrocalcinosis are the major goals of therapy.**
11. **A generalized dysfunction of the distal nephron produces distal renal tubular acidosis in association with hyperkalemia. This type of distal RTA (type 4) is quite common, but may be of diverse etiologies.**
12. **Aldosterone deficiency results in hyperkalemia and metabolic acidosis by decreasing the activity of the apical epithelial sodium channel, the basolateral Na^+,K^+-ATPase, or the force of one of the proton pumps in the collecting tubule. The hyperkalemia has independent effects on net acid excretion by reducing renal ammoniogenesis and ammonium transport in the thick ascending limb of Henle's loop, thereby impairing ammonium excretion.**
13. **Mineralocorticoid resistance also causes hyperkalemic-hyperchloremic metabolic acidosis in children and adults. Pseudohypoaldosteronism type I (PHAI) in children is associated with hyperkalemia, salt wasting, and metabolic acidosis. It was recently reported that PHAI is the result of a loss-of-function mutation of the apical epithelial sodium channel in the cortical collecting tubule (ENaC). Children with PHAI respond to correction of the salt and fluid deficits. Conversely, in adults, pseudohypoaldosteronism type 2 (PHAII), or Gordon syndrome (familial hyperkalemia and hypertension), is associated with volume expansion, hypertension, and hyperkalemic metabolic acidosis. Because these patients respond to dietary salt restriction and thiazide diuretics, it has been suggested that this disorder occurs as a result of a gain-in-function mutation of the electroneutral Na^+-Cl^- cotransporter in the distal convoluted tubule (NCC1). Although linkage analysis has failed to substantiate such an association, recent studies have demonstrated linkage of PHAII to chromosome 1q31-q42 and to chromosome 17p11-q21, a locus that is implicated in blood pressure regulation (QTL).**
14. **In some patients, this defect can be acquired as a result of a "voltage" defect that limits the rate of proton secretion by the cortical collecting tubule at any given luminal pH and impairs potassium secretion. In addition, however, this defect involves compromise in the function of the H^+-ATPase and cannot be ascribed merely to inability to generate a negative transepithelial potential difference.**
15. **Renal insufficiency, especially in association with diabetes and tubulointerstitial disease, may be associated with hyperkalemia and evidence of compromise of distal acidification. The hyperkalemia is out of proportion to the reduction in glomerular filtration rate. Underlying this disorder is either mineralocorticoid deficiency or mineralocorticoid resistance. As in primary mineralocorticoid deficiency, metabolic acidosis is secondary, in part, to the hyperkalemia and to a compromise in the H^+-ATPase or H^+,K^+-ATPase. Correction of the chronic hyperkalemia may result in improvement of the acidosis.**
16. **Patients with hyporeninemic hypoaldosteronism and chronic renal insufficiency may require cation exchange resins, alkali therapy, and a loop diuretic to enhance renal potassium and salt excretion. Mineralocorticoid therapy, which may be necessary in mineralocorticoid deficiency, should be administered in combination with a loop diuretic in edematous or hypertensive patients to avoid volume overexpansion and aggravation of hypertension.**

Renal tubular acidosis (RTA) is a clinical syndrome characterized by a hyperchloremic metabolic acidosis secondary to an abnormality in renal acidification. The abnormality in renal acidification can be manifested as either an inappropriately high urine pH in the face of acidosis or marked bicarbonaturia with near normal serum bicarbonate. Net acid excretion (titratable acid plus ammonium excretion) is, by definition, inappropriately low for the prevailing acidosis in all forms of RTA. The clinical expression of the defect in acidification depends on the specific nephron segment in which the defect arises. The general types of RTA are summarized in Table 195-1. Renal tubular acidosis may occur clinically as a hyperchloremic metabolic acidosis with hypokalemia or hyperkalemia. Classical distal RTA (type I) and proximal RTA (type II) are frequently associated with hypokalemia. In contrast, a generalized dysfunction of the distal nephron, which may be associated with hypoaldosteronism or aldosterone resistance, is usually seen in association with hyperkalemia. Lastly, RTA may occur in patients with renal insufficiency associated with a normal serum potassium. Because all varieties of RTA are associated, when fully expressed, with hyperchloremic metabolic acidosis, the differential diagnosis of hyperchloremia with metabolic acidosis and a normal anion gap is discussed first.

HYPERCHLOREMIC METABOLIC ACIDOSIS

The diverse clinical disorders which may result in a hyperchloremic metabolic acidosis are outlined in Table 195-2. Because a reduced plasma HCO_3^- and elevated Cl^- concentration may also occur in chronic respiratory alkalosis, it is important to confirm an acidemia by measuring arterial pH. In the absence of this information, a slightly elevated anion gap (12 to 15 mEq/liter) and/or signs of pulmonary or hepatic disease suggests the presence of respiratory alkalosis. Hyperchloremic metabolic acidosis occurs most often as a result of loss of HCO_3^- from the gastrointestinal tract or as a result of a renal acidification defect.

Table 195-1 Types of Renal Acidosis

Associated with hypokalemia
Proximal RTA (type II)
Distal RTA (type I)
Associated with hyperkalemia
Aldosterone deficiency or resistance (type IV)
Nonmineralocorticoid voltage defect
Associated with normokalemia
RTA of renal insufficiency

Table 195-2 Differential Diagnosis of Hyperchloremic Metabolic Acidosis

Gastrointestinal bicarbonate loss
Diarrhea
External pancreatic or small bowel drainage
Ureterosigmoidostomy, jejunal loop
Drugs
Calcium chloride
Magnesium sulfate
Cholestyramine
Renal acidosis
Proximal RTA (type II)
Distal ("classical") RTA (type I)
Generalized distal nephron dysfunction (type IV)
Mineralocorticoid deficiency
Mineralocorticoid resistance
Nonmineralocorticoid voltage defects
Renal insufficiency
Other
Acid loads (ammonium chloride, arginine chloride, arginine hydrochloride, hyperalimentation, sulfur)
Loss of potential bicarbonate
Ketosis with ketone excretion
Dilutional acidosis
Posthypocapnic state

Hypokalemia may accompany both gastrointestinal loss of HCO_3^- and proximal and distal RTA.

Diarrhea results in the loss of large quantities of HCO_3^- and HCO_3^- decomposed by reaction with organic acids.[1] Because diarrheal stools contain a higher concentration of HCO_3^- and decomposed HCO_3^- than plasma, volume depletion and metabolic acidosis develop. Hypokalemia exists because large quantities of K^+ are lost from stool and because volume depletion causes elaboration of renin and aldosterone, enhancing renal potassium secretion. Instead of an acid urine pH as anticipated with diarrhea, a pH of 6.0 or more may be found.[2] This occurs because metabolic acidosis and hypokalemia increase renal ammonium synthesis and excretion, thus providing more urinary buffer, which causes an increase in urine pH. Metabolic acidosis due to gastrointestinal losses with a high urine pH can be differentiated from RTA, since urinary NH_4^+ excretion is typically low in RTA while NH_4^+ excretion is high in patients with diarrhea.[3,4]

When renal tubular function is normal, the kidney responds to chronic metabolic acidosis by increasing ammonium production and excretion. In contrast, ammonium production and excretion by the kidney are often impaired by chronic renal failure, hyperkalemia, and routinely in renal tubular acidosis. Therefore, it is important to delineate whether the kidney is responding appropriately to systemic acidosis by increasing ammonium excretion. Urinary NH_4^+ levels can be estimated[4,5] by calculating the urine net charge (UNC):

$$UNC = [Na^+ + K^+]_u - [Cl]_u$$

where "u" denotes urinary electrolyte values on a "spot" urine sample. Because NH_4^+ can be assumed to be present if the sum of the major cations ($Na^+ + K^+$) is less than the sum of major anions in urine, a negative urine net charge is evidence for sufficient ammonium in the urine. In chronic metabolic acidosis of nonrenal origin (such as diarrhea), the expected response by the kidney is to increase ammonium production and excretion. The increase in ammonium $[NH_4^+]$ in the urine in this condition is manifest as an increase in the urine net negative charge (i.e., the urinary Cl^- exceeds the sum of $Na^+ + K^+$). In contrast, in hyperchloremic metabolic acidosis of renal origin (i.e., renal tubular acidosis) the urine net charge is positive, denoting no increase in or minimal NH_4^+ in the urine, signifying an inappropriate renal response to the metabolic acidosis, or a tubular defect in H^+ secretion. The utility of the net negative charge in estimating urinary ammonium has been verified, but caution is urged if NH_4^+ is excreted with an accompanying anion other than Cl^-. For example, ketonuria, the presence of drug anions, or toxins in the urine such as toluene metabolites, invalidate this method. In these circumstances, the urinary ammonium ($U_{NH_4^+}$ may be estimated from the measured urine osmolality (U_{osm}) , urine $[Na^+ + K^+]$, and urine urea and glucose:

$$U_{NH_4^+} = 0.5(U_{osm} - [2(Na^+ = K^+) + \text{urea} + \text{glucose}]$$
$$\text{(all expressed in mmol/L)}$$

In addition, the fractional excretion of sodium would be expected to be low (< 1 to 2 percent) in patients with HCO_3^- loss from the gastrointestinal tract, but usually exceeds 2 to 3 percent in RTA.[2]

External loss of pancreatic and biliary secretions can also cause a hyperchloremic acidosis. Cholestyramine, calcium chloride, and magnesium sulfate ingestion can result in a hyperchloremic metabolic acidosis (Table 195-2), especially in patients with renal insufficiency, but the plasma potassium is typically normal, not depressed.[2,7]

Severe hyperchloremic metabolic acidosis with hypokalemia may occur on occasion in patients with ureteral diversion procedures. Because the ileum and colon are both endowed with Cl^- / HCO_3^- exchanges, when the Cl^- from the urine enters the gut, the HCO_3^- concentration increases as a result of the exchange process.[8] Moreover, K^+ secretion is stimulated which, together with HCO_3^- loss, can result in a hyperchloremic, hypokalemic metabolic acidosis. This defect is particularly common in patients with ureterosigmoidostomies and is more common with this type of diversion because of the prolonged transit time of urine due to stasis in the colonic segment.[9]

Dilutional acidosis, acidosis due to exogenous acid loads and the post hypocapnic state, can usually be excluded by history. When isotonic saline is infused rapidly, particularly in patients with temporary or permanent renal failure, the plasma bicarbonate will decline reciprocally in relation to chloride.[2] Addition of acid or acid equivalents (arginine HCl, lysine HCl, or NH_4Cl) to blood results in metabolic acidosis.[10] A similar situation may arise from endogenous addition of ketoacids during recovery from ketoacidosis when the sodium salts of ketones may be excreted by the kidneys and lost as potential bicarbonate.

Loss of functioning renal parenchyma by progressive renal disease is known to be associated with metabolic acidosis. Typically, the acidosis is hyperchloremic when the GFR is between 20 to 50 ml/min, but may convert to the typical acidosis of uremia with high anion gap with more advanced renal failure, that is, when the GFR is < 15 ml/min.[2,11,12] It is generally assumed that such a progression is observed more commonly in patients with tubulointerstitial forms of renal disease, but hyperchloremic metabolic acidosis can occur with advanced glomerular disease.[13,14] The principal defect in acidification of advanced renal failure is that ammoniogenesis is reduced in proportion to the loss of functional renal mass. In addition, medullary ammonium accumulation and trapping in the outer medullary collecting tubule may be impaired.[4] Because of adaptive increases in potassium secretion by the collecting duct[15] and colon,[16] the acidosis of chronic renal insufficiency is typically normokalemic.[14] Hyperchloremic metabolic acidosis associated with hyperkalemia is almost always associated with a generalized dysfunction of the distal nephron. However, potassium-sparing diuretics, nonsteroidal anti-inflammatory drugs, angiotensin-converting enzyme inhibitors, beta blockers, and heparin may mimic or cause this disorder, resulting in hyperkalemia and a hyperchloremic acidosis. Such drugs should be discontinued before the diagnosis of a nonreversible, generalized defect of the distal nephron is considered.

The diverse clinical disorders associated with hyperchloremic metabolic acidosis should be considered and excluded before embarking upon an extensive evaluation of renal acidification and the diagnosis of RTA (Table 195-2).

PROXIMAL RENAL TUBULAR ACIDOSIS

Mechanism and Regulation of Proximal Acidification

The kidney filters approximately 4000 mEq of HCO_3^- per day. To maintain acid-base balance and to reabsorb the filtered load of HCO_3^-, the renal tubules must secrete 4000 mEq of hydrogen ions. Although the kidney must secrete an additional 50 to 80 mEq of hydrogen ions to titrate urinary buffers, the majority of hydrogen ion secretion is involved in the "reclamation" of filtered HCO_3^-. Approximately 80 to 90 percent of filtered HCO_3^- is reabsorbed in the proximal tubule. Thus, while the distal nephron is responsible for the final acidification of the urine and the generation of large pH gradients, the proximal tubule represents a high-capacity system and secretes the majority of hydrogen ions. Defects in proximal tubular reabsorption of HCO_3^- are typically characterized by large amounts of bicarbonaturia.

Mechanism of H^+ Secretion/HCO_3^- Absorption. Reabsorption of HCO_3^- in the proximal tubule depends on active secretion of hydrogen ions across the apical membrane.[17–19] This process is effected mostly by an apical membrane Na^+/H^+ antiporter, which results in hydrogen ion secretion into the lumen in exchange for sodium ions entering the cell.[20–26] The driving force for hydrogen ion secretion is provided by the low cell-sodium concentration, which is generated by the basolateral membrane Na^+/K^+ ATPase. Thus, ATP indirectly drives this active proton secretion.

Sardet et al. cloned a cDNA for a human Na^+/H^+ exchanger. This cDNA encodes a protein predicted to have a molecular weight of 99 kDa. Its amino-terminal half contains a transmembrane domain, which is predicted to contain 10 to 12 membrane-spanning regions. Using this cDNA as a probe, investigators have now cloned five plasma membrane NHE isoforms, four of which are expressed in the kidney. Of these, NHE2 and NHE3 are apical membrane isoforms. It has now been conclusively demonstrated that the key proximal tubule apical membrane isoform is NHE3. NHE3 mRNA is highly expressed in renal cortex,[27,28] and antibodies against NHE3 label the proximal tubule apical membrane.[29,30] Both NHE3 and the apical membrane Na^+/H^+ exchanger are relatively resistant to agents such as amiloride, amiloride analogs, and HOE694.[31–33] Lastly, in mice in which the NHE3 gene is knocked out, proximal tubule acidification is inhibited by 61 percent and there is a mild metabolic acidosis.[34] By contrast, mice in which NHE2 is knocked out demonstrate no acid/base abnormality.[35]

In parallel with the Na^+/H^+ antiporter is an H^+-ATPase, which mediates a small fraction of apical membrane H^+ secretion.[26,36,37] This H^+-ATPase is believed to be of the vacuolar type, based on staining of the proximal tubule brush border membrane with antibodies against subunits of vacuolar H^+-ATPases.[38] The molecular characteristics of H^+ pumps are discussed further under the distal nephron.

The base generated in the cell by these two transporters then exits the cell across the basolateral membrane via an electrogenic $Na^+/HCO_3^-/CO_3^=$ symporter which transports one sodium, one HCO_3^-, and one CO_3^{-2} ion.[39–44] The driving force for this transporter is the negative cell potential. Romero et al. recently accomplished the expression cloning of an Ambystoma cDNA, which they named aNBC (Ambystoma Na bicarbonate cotransporter).[45] This cDNA encodes a 1035-amino acid protein that shares 25 to 30 percent homology with the AE anion-exchanger family. The hydropathy plot predicts 10 putative membrane-spanning domains. Using aNBC as a probe, a rat homolog, rNBC, was cloned.[46] rNBC mRNA is abundantly expressed in kidney.

Carbonic anhydrase is present in the cytoplasm and on both apical and basolateral membranes of the proximal tubule. The cytoplasmic form is very similar to carbonic anhydrase II of red blood cells.[47,48] The membrane-bound form is a different form, which has been named type IV.[47–49] The molecular characteristics of the carbonic anhydrases are described extensively in Chap. 208. Carbonic anhydrase I, the most prevalent red blood cell carbonic anhydrase, is not present in the kidney.[50] The major function of carbonic anhydrase (CA) in the proximal tubule (and in the kidney in general) is to accelerate the reaction indicated below:

$$CAH^+ + HCO_3^- \leftrightarrow H_2CO_3 \leftrightarrow CO_2 + H_2O$$

Because hydrogen ions are secreted into HCO_3^--containing filtrate in the lumen of the proximal tubule, H_2CO_3 is formed. The H_2CO_3 is rapidly dehydrated by luminal carbonic anhydrase (type IV) to form CO_2 and H_2O.[49] The CO_2 is freely diffusible and is reabsorbed. In the cell, carbonic anhydrase (type II) catalyzes the formation of H_2CO_3 from CO_2 and H_2O. H_2CO_3 then dissociates rapidly to H^+ and HCO_3^-, which are transported across the apical and basolateral membranes, respectively. Thus, carbonic anhydrase allows transmembrane pH gradients to be minimal and facilitates further proton secretion and HCO_3^- reabsorption.[49]

In parallel with the active H^+ secretory mechanism is a leak through the paracellular pathway. Because luminal HCO_3^- concentration is lower than that of blood, HCO_3^- can back diffuse into the lumen. While the proximal tubule is a leaky epithelium with relatively high paracellular permeabilities, the HCO_3^- permeability is comparatively small.[51–55] Diffusion of hydrogen ions is even smaller in magnitude.[56] Thus, leak pathways tend to be unimportant under normal conditions.

Other Proximal Tubular Functions. Proximal renal tubular acidosis is usually associated with defects in other proximal tubule function. The proximal tubule is the major site for reabsorption of glucose, amino acids, organic anions, and phosphate. Each of these solutes is reabsorbed across the apical membrane on transporters coupled to sodium transport. The low intracellular sodium concentration and negative cell voltage which are generated by the basolateral membrane Na^+/K^+-ATPase provide the driving force for these transporters to actively take up these solutes from the lumen. Most of these solutes are then either metabolized within the proximal tubular cell or passively exit across the basolateral membrane. These mechanisms lead to low concentrations of these solutes in the lumen, creating a driving force for back diffusion of these solutes across the paracellular pathway. Once again, under normal conditions, these back-diffusing fluxes are present but small in magnitude.

Of particular relevance to renal tubular acidosis is the proximal tubular transport of citrate. Although citrate is present in plasma in very low concentration, its presence in the urine and tubular fluid is key to the prevention of calcium stones and nephrocalcinosis. Citrate is reabsorbed by the proximal tubule on a Na-coupled transporter, which carries numerous di- and tricarboxylic acids. The cDNA encoding this transporter has now been cloned and is referred to as NaDC-1 (Na dicarboxylate cotransporter-1).[57] After entering the cell, citrate is metabolized by two potential pathways, a cytoplasmic pathway mediated by the enzyme ATP citrate lyase, and a mitochondrial pathway.[58,59] Because citrate is metabolically equivalent to HCO_3^- (its metabolism leads to the generation of HCO_3^-), citrate excretion in the urine is equivalent to HCO_3^- excretion. Thus, in metabolic acidosis, proximal tubular citrate absorption increases leading to hypocitraturia and a predisposition to kidney stones and nephrocalcinosis. This adaption involves an adaptive increase in apical membrane Na/citrate cotransporter activity,[60] the cytoplasmic enzyme ATP citrate lyase,[58] and the mitochondrial enzyme m-aconitase.[61]

Proximal absorption of Na^+ and Cl^- is more complex. High rates of HCO_3^- absorption, preferential to Cl^- in the early proximal tubule, lead to an increased concentration of Cl^- in the late proximal tubule. This provides a chemical gradient for Cl^-

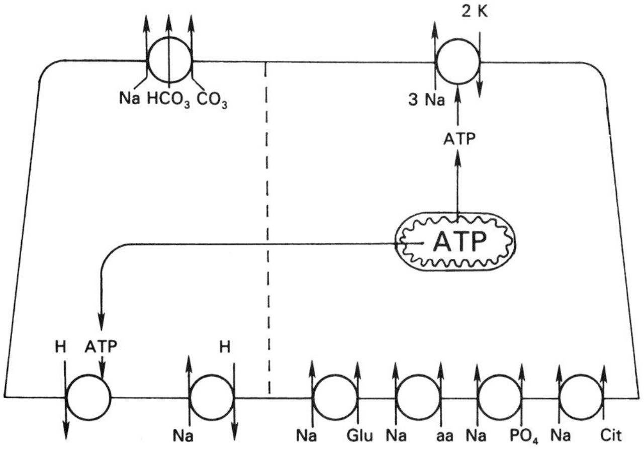

Fig. 195-1 Cell model of proximal tubule. Defects in transporters on the lower membrane of the cell in figure (apical membrane) lead to isolated proximal renal tubular acidosis, while a defect on the basolateral surface leads to generalized dysfunction of the proximal tubule.

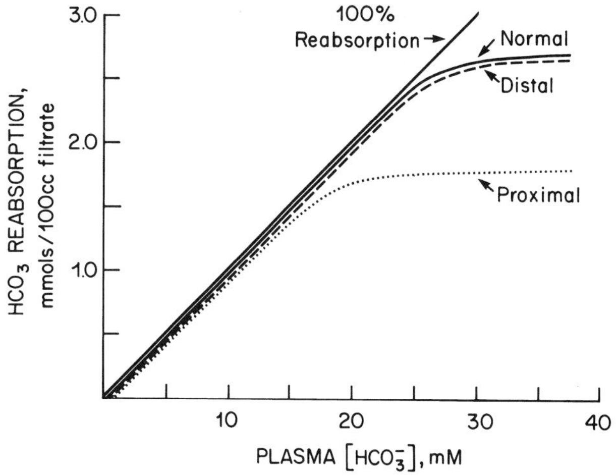

Fig. 195-2 Effect of plasma bicarbonate concentration on renal bicarbonate absorption in normal patients (solid line), patients with hypokalemic distal renal tubular acidosis (broken line), and patients with proximal renal tubular acidosis (dotted line). Bold diagonal line represents 100 percent reabsorption of filtered bicarbonate. In distal renal tubular acidosis, the threshold for bicarbonaturia (i.e., the plasma bicarbonate concentration at which renal bicarbonate absorption is not 100 percent of filtered load) is normal, whereas in patients with proximal renal tubular acidosis the threshold is decreased.

absorption, which drives Cl^- movement and causes a lumen-positive potential difference (P.D.) that secondarily drives Na^+ absorption. While 50 percent of proximal tubular NaCl absorption occurs by such a passive mechanism, there is an additional active transcellular component of NaCl absorption.[62–67] This, however, also appears to be related to acidification in that the apical membrane mechanisms are Na^+/H^+ antiport and Cl^-/base exchange functioning in parallel.[66–69] Figure 195-1 summarizes the transport mechanisms present in the proximal tubule. In Fig. 195-1, defects in transporters on the lower side of the cell lead to isolated proximal RTA, while defects on the upper surface of the cell in the figure lead to generalized dysfunction of the proximal tubule.

Thus, diseases that interfere with HCO_3^- absorption in any manner can interfere secondarily with passive Cl^- absorption by preventing the rise in luminal Cl^- concentrations. In addition, any mechanism that interferes with the Na^+/K^+-ATPase or the Na^+/H^+ antiporter also interfere with transcellular Cl^- absorption. In theory, if the inhibition of HCO_3^- and Cl^- absorption is in proportion to their plasma concentrations (corrected for differences in volume of distribution), the result is a decrease in extracellular fluid volume with no change in the concentrations of HCO_3^- or Cl^-. In reality, the inhibition of HCO_3^- absorption in proximal renal tubular acidosis is proportionately greater than that of Cl^- absorption, resulting in a decrease in plasma HCO_3^- concentration and an increase in plasma Cl^- concentration.

Regulation of Proximal Tubular Bicarbonate Absorption. Pitts and Lotspeich[70] examined the effect of an HCO_3^- infusion on renal HCO_3^- absorption and excretion in normal dogs. As the plasma HCO_3^- concentration rises, renal HCO_3^- absorption also increases. At low plasma bicarbonate concentrations, nearly 100 percent of filtered HCO_3^- is absorbed. However, at higher plasma HCO_3^- concentrations, a threshold is reached where HCO_3^- first appears in the urine (the threshold for bicarbonaturia). As plasma HCO_3^- concentration increases further, HCO_3^- absorption continues to increase until a maximal level is reached, the so-called Tm for HCO_3^- absorption (refer to line labeled "Proximal" in Fig. 195-2).

The initial interpretation of these studies was that HCO_3^- absorption was a saturable process, such that at low-filtered loads of HCO_3^- luminal transporters were able to reabsorb all of the HCO_3^-, but as luminal HCO_3^- concentration increased, the transporters became saturated and fractional HCO_3^- absorption decreased. Tubular microperfusion studies demonstrate that this interpretation is only partly correct.[51,71] While proximal tubular HCO_3^- absorption does saturate as a function of luminal HCO_3^- concentration, a more important regulatory effect is that exerted by the peritubular HCO_3^- concentration. Increases in peritubular HCO_3^- concentration directly inhibit proximal tubular HCO_3^- absorption. Thus, when plasma HCO_3^- is increased, both luminal and peritubular HCO_3^- concentration are increased. While the increase in luminal HCO_3^- concentration leads toward saturation of the system, the increase in peritubular HCO_3^- concentration markedly inhibits proximal tubular HCO_3^- absorption. The net result produces the curve reported by Pitts and Lotspeich.[70]

The studies of Pitts and Lotspeich form the basis for understanding proximal tubular acidification defects. Patients with proximal renal tubular acidosis have apparently normal rates of renal HCO_3^- absorption at low plasma HCO_3^- concentrations. However, even at these low plasma HCO_3^- concentrations, proximal tubular HCO_3^- absorption is probably still subnormal. Distal HCO_3^- delivery is low enough in this setting that the distal nephron can reabsorb the excess HCO_3^-. Because distal nephron acidification is not impaired, the urine can be acidified appropriately. Evidence in support of this is derived from NHE3 knockout mice.[34] In these mice, proximal tubular bicarbonate absorption is inhibited by 61 percent, but serum bicarbonate concentration is only decreased by 3 mEq/liter. Thus, the distal nephron is able to increase the rate of bicarbonate absorption in response to mild metabolic acidosis such that a steady state is achieved. As plasma bicarbonate concentration increases, these patients are found to have a low threshold for bicarbonaturia, as shown in Fig. 195-2. At high plasma HCO_3^- concentrations, distal delivery of HCO_3^- exceeds the capacity of the distal nephron for HCO_3^- absorption and there is significant bicarbonaturia. Patients with distal renal tubular acidification defects, on the other hand, may have small degrees of bicarbonaturia but never have large amounts of bicarbonaturia unless the patients are made alkalotic. Figure 195-2 shows a typical HCO_3^- titration curve for a normal patient, a patient with proximal renal tubular acidosis, and a patient with distal renal tubular acidosis.

Pathogenesis of Proximal Renal Tubular Acidosis

Possible Defects. Proximal renal tubular acidosis can be divided into two general categories, one in which acidification is the only defective function and one in which there is a more generalized proximal tubular dysfunction (Table 195-3). A generalized

Table 195-3 Proposed Pathophysiological Defects in Proximal RTA

Associated with generalized Fanconi syndrome
Abnormality or repression of basolateral Na^+,K^+-ATPase
Intracellular phosphate depletion or sequestration
Intracellular ATP depletion
Associated with selective bicarbonate wasting
Selective lesion of either apical Na^+/H^+ exchanger (NHE 3) or H^+-ATPase
Selective lesion of basolateral $Na^+/HCO_3^-/CO_3^{-2}$ symporter
Carbonic anhydrase deficiency

proximal tubular defect could occur by one of several mechanisms. There could be an increase in the permeability of the paracellular pathway. This would lead to a backleak into the lumen of solutes for which the proximal tubule is the main site of reabsorption and whose concentration is thus low in the lumen. These solutes would include HCO_3^-, phosphate, glucose, amino acids, and organic anions. An alternative mechanism is a generalized disorder of cellular function, which would inhibit absorption of all of these solutes. For example, any disorder that inhibits ATP production in the proximal tubule would lead to a generalized defect in reabsorption. Similarly, because reabsorption of these solutes as well as acidification are coupled to sodium transport, any disorder in which the Na^+/K^+-ATPase is abnormal would lead to a generalized defect in proximal tubular function.

A proximal tubular defect involving only acidification is rare. Such a disorder has to involve a selective defect in the Na^+/H^+ antiporter, the H^+-ATPase, or the $Na^+/HCO_3^-/CO_3^=$ symporter. Abnormalities of cell depolarization or abnormalities in carbonic anhydrase could also present in this manner.

Generalized Proximal Tubular Dysfunction. The majority of cases of proximal renal tubular acidosis fit in the category of generalized proximal tubular dysfunction with glycosuria, generalized aminoaciduria, hypercitraturia, and phosphaturia. The generalized failure of proximal tubular function is referred to as the Fanconi syndrome. As there is a separate chapter in this book dealing with this syndrome (Chap. 196), we only briefly discuss the Fanconi syndrome as it relates to the mechanism of the acidification defect.

In 1950, Berliner, Kennedy, and Hilton,[72] while examining the capacity of organic acids to serve as effective buffers for acidification, accidentally found that maleic acid infused intravenously in dogs caused a syndrome with proximal renal tubular acidosis and glycosuria. This condition, now referred to as maleic acid nephropathy, was subsequently used to study the mechanism of the Fanconi syndrome. Al-Bander et al.,[73] using clearance techniques in dogs undergoing a free-water diuresis, found results suggesting that maleic acid inhibits proximal tubular solute and water absorption. While initial studies raised the possibility of abnormal proximal tubular leaks in the genesis of maleic acid nephropathy,[74] the techniques used were indirect and the conclusions have not been substantiated by subsequently performed more direct studies. Another recent study that found evidence for renal tubular leakage[75] exposed animals to maleic acid 20 hours prior to studying renal function. In this study, tubules were leaky to lissamine green and inulin, suggesting that nephrotoxicity had approached the level of acute tubular necrosis. Hoppe et al.[76] and Gougoux et al.[77] found that the effect of maleate on bicarbonaturia was additive to that of carbonic anhydrase inhibition, suggesting separate mechanisms. Gmaj et al.[78] found no effect of maleate on renal carbonic anhydrase activity.

In studies where the lumen of the proximal tubule was microperfused and rates of acidification measured, Bank et al.[79] found that previous maleic acid treatment inhibited the rates of HCO_3^- absorption and of sodium chloride absorption. These investigators found no inulin leak. In addition, in studies where tubules were perfused in the absence of HCO_3^- and the rate of HCO_3^- entrance was measured (a measure of paracellular HCO_3^- permeability), maleic acid had no effect. Thus, Bank et al. concluded that maleic acid acted by interfering with transcellular active HCO_3^- absorption rather than enhancing HCO_3^- backleak. Reboucas et al.,[80] employing split droplet microperfusion, obtained similar results. Rates of volume absorption were inhibited. In further studies with a pH electrode in the luminal fluid, these investigators measured the rates of luminal acidification and alkalinization. In tubules perfused with alkaline solutions, the rate of acidification was inhibited, a result consistent with either a transcellular defect or enhanced leak. However, in tubules perfused with very acid solutions, the rate of alkalinization was also inhibited, a result consistent only with an inhibited transcellular flux and not consistent with enhanced leakiness. In addition, in these studies, cell voltage was measured and found to be decreased, which is consistent with inhibition of the Na^+/K^+-ATPase.[80] Gunther et al.[81] examined the effect of maleic acid infusion on glycine absorption. Maleic acid infusion inhibited glycine absorption in the microperfused proximal tubule. However, when saturable transcellular glycine absorption was inhibited by excess phenylalanine in the lumen, maleic acid had no effect on glycine absorption.

Salmon and Baum have examined this question utilizing an experimental model of cystinosis.[82] Proximal tubule segments perfused in vitro were incubated with a dimethyl ester of cystine. This compound diffuses in cells where cytoplasmic esterases cleave the ester groups generating intracellular cystine. Proximal tubules incubated with this compound showed decreased rates of volume absorption, HCO_3^- absorption, and glucose absorption, while tubules incubated with methyl esters of leucine or tryptophan demonstrated no abnormalities. Cystine dimethyl ester had no effect on mannitol or HCO_3^- permeability.

These studies demonstrate that the nephropathies associated with maleic acid and cystine involve disruption of active transcellular absorption of HCO_3^-, amino acids, and other solutes. Such a defect could be due to a generalized disorder of apical membrane transporters, a disorder of the basolateral Na^+,K^+-ATPase, or a metabolic disorder that lowers intracellular ATP concentrations. Addition of maleic acid to isolated brush border membrane vesicles did not affect Na^+/glucose cotransport.[83] In addition, the Na^+/glucose cotransporter isolated from either control animals or animals treated in vivo with maleic acid was similar in function. Addition of maleic acid to brush border membranes did not affect transport of α-methylglucoside, alanine, proline, or lysine.[84] Silverman and Huang[85] found that maleic acid addition to vesicles did not affect phlorizin binding to the Na^+/glucose cotransporter. Lastly, LeGrimellec et al.[86] found no effect of maleate on the fluidity of the lipids of brush border membranes. Thus, no abnormality of apical membrane transporters could be demonstrated.

Kramer and Gonick[87] found that maleic acid treatment of rats inhibited Na^+,K^+-ATPase activity in renal cortical homogenates prepared 1 h after treatment. There was no effect on Na^+,K^+-ATPase in medullary homogenates. Thus, inhibition of the Na^+,K^+-ATPase provides one mechanism by which all of the transport defects in maleic acid nephropathy and in Fanconi syndrome could be produced.

In addition to the defect in Na^+,K^+-ATPase, Kramer and Gonick[87] found decreased ATP concentrations in renal cortical homogenates. Coor et al. examined the role of ATP depletion and Na^+,K^+-ATPase inhibition in the above discussed model of cystinosis.[88] Proximal tubules incubated with the dimethyl ester of cystine demonstrated a 60 percent decrease in intracellular ATP, with no change in Na^+,K^+-ATPase activity. Incubation of cystine dimethyl ester-treated tubules with exogenous ATP partially ameliorated the transport defect. These authors thus concluded that the major defect was one of ATP depletion rather than an abnormality in the Na^+,K^+-ATPase. One possible explanation for these decreased ATP levels is inhibition of metabolism by maleic acid. Angielski and Rogulski[89] found that maleic acid interferes with the Krebs cycle. While this effect occurs in many tissues, only kidney cells actively accumulated maleate. Another possible cause of decreased ATP levels is sequestration of intracellular phosphate. Al-Bander et al.,[90] found that previous phosphate loading in dogs could markedly ameliorate the maleic acid-induced bicarbonaturia, natriuresis, and aminoaciduria. There was no effect of previous phosphate loading on the hypercitraturia. In subsequent studies, Al-Bandar et al.[91] found that prior phosphate loading attenuated the increased renal excretion of small molecular weight proteins and lysosomal enzymes seen in maleic acid-treated kidneys.

Production of the Fanconi syndrome by intracellular phosphate depletion has also been proposed in hereditary fructose intolerance where ingestion of fructose leads to accumulation of fructose-1-phosphate in the proximal tubule. Because these patients lack the enzyme fructose-1-phosphate aldolase, the fructose-1-phosphate cannot be further metabolized and intracellular phosphate is sequestered in this form. The renal lesion is confined to the proximal tubule because this is the only segment in the kidney that possesses the enzyme fructokinase.[92] Administration of large parenteral loads of fructose to rats leads to high intracellular concentrations of fructose-1-phosphate and low concentrations of ATP and GTP, as well as of total adenine nucleotides.[92] Prior phosphate loading prevents the reductions in intracellular ATP, total adenine nucleotides, and phosphate.[93]

Vitamin D deficiency, resistance, or dependence, and generalized proximal tubular dysfunction is a clinical association that occurs relatively frequently. Numerous investigators noted an association between vitamin D deficiency and a generalized Fanconi syndrome with proximal renal tubular acidosis, aminoaciduria, and hyperphosphaturia.[94–96] In these studies, correction of the vitamin D deficiency caused correction of the proximal tubular dysfunction.[94,95] Similar results were obtained in patients with vitamin D-dependent and vitamin D-resistant rickets treated with dihydrotachysterol.[97,98] While the existence of this association is undisputed, the mechanisms involved in the proximal tubular dysfunction are not yet clear.

Vitamin D deficiency states are associated with low levels of vitamin D, low levels of serum calcium, and high levels of parathormone (PTH). Parathyroid hormone has been demonstrated to be an important inhibitor of proximal tubular bicarbonate absorption.[99–102] This results from inhibition of active transcellular proton secretion, rather than from an increase in bicarbonate backleak.[101,102] While such an effect may explain proximal RTA, recent studies suggest that chronic parathormone administration does not lead to metabolic acidosis; instead, it leads to metabolic alkalosis.[103,104] This may be due to a stimulation of HCO_3^- absorption in more distal segments, either in Henle's loop[105] or in the collecting tubule. Recent studies suggest that the increased distal phosphate delivery induced by PTH can stimulate distal nephron acidification.[106] In addition, in cell culture, increases in cAMP, as occur with PTH, acutely inhibit but chronically stimulate NHE3.[107,108] Thus, in spite of the marked acute inhibitory effect of parathormone on proximal tubular absorption of HCO_3^-, the effect on whole kidney HCO_3^- absorption appears to be small and, overall, there is a small stimulation of acidification.

Extracellular Ca^{2+} concentration is also a regulator of proximal tubular transport, although less potent than parathormone. In the in vitro perfused proximal convoluted tubule, increases in extracellular Ca^{2+} concentration stimulate HCO_3^- absorption and decreases in extracellular Ca^{2+} concentration inhibit HCO_3^- absorption.[109] However, in these studies, large changes in Ca^{2+} concentrations produced only small effects on HCO_3^- absorption. Although the effects of vitamin D have not yet been studied in the perfused proximal tubule, clearance studies found that administration of 25-hydroxy vitamin D stimulates renal absorption of Ca^{2+}, PO_4^{3-}, sodium, and HCO_3^-.[110,111] The exact nephron segment in which this effect occurs is not established, but is thought to be the proximal tubule.[112]

An additional pathophysiological mechanism for the proximal tubular defect in the Fanconi syndrome could be intracellular phosphate depletion, as discussed above. Intracellular PO_4^{3-} depletion has been proposed as a cause of ATP depletion and the secondary Fanconi syndrome in maleic acid nephropathy and in hereditary fructose intolerance. High levels of PTH will inhibit proximal tubular PO_4^{3-} absorption. In addition, vitamin D may promote proximal tubular phosphate absorption, and its deficiency may reduce PO_4^{3-} absorption, secondarily contributing to intracellular phosphate depletion. Gross and Scriver[113] created an experimental model of vitamin D deficiency in the rat and demonstrated hyperphosphaturia and aminoaciduria. These authors noted that aminoaciduria was not prominent until the animals had been on a vitamin D-deficient diet for 6 weeks. In addition, they noted that the aminoaciduria appeared 2 to 4 weeks after hyperphosphaturia, supporting a role for a more complex scheme than mere hormone presence or absence.

Further support for a role of the Ca^{2+}/PO_4^{3-}/PTH/vitamin D system in proximal RTA can be found from the results of Morris et al.,[114] who found that hypoparathyroidism ameliorated the fructose-induced proximal tubular dysfunction in a patient with hereditary fructose intolerance. Administration of PTH to this hypoparathyroid patient enhanced the fructose-induced renal defect. As discussed above, intracellular PO_4^{3-} depletion has been proposed as the cause of Fanconi syndrome in hereditary fructose intolerance. Decreased levels of PTH could protect these patients by enhancing phosphate uptake by the proximal tubule. An alternative explanation is that the inhibiting effect of PTH on acidification is additive to the effect of fructose-induced intracellular phosphate depletion.

The association between Fanconi syndrome and vitamin D disorders may be partially related to decreased 1 α-hydroxylase activity in disorders of proximal tubule function. 1 α-Hydroxylase, which is present in proximal tubular mitochondria, could be deficient in the Fanconi syndrome. Brewer et al.[115] found that conversion of 25-hydroxy-D_3 to 1,25-hydroxy-D_3 was impaired in maleic acid nephropathy. However, Chesney[116] measured levels of vitamin D metabolites and found them to be normal in three patients with the Fanconi syndrome. In summary, vitamin D deficiency is clearly associated with the Fanconi syndrome. The defect is related to low levels of 1,25-dihydroxy-D_3, high levels of PTH, and low Ca^{2+}. The Fanconi syndrome may be produced in part by intracellular phosphate depletion.

Isolated Proximal Tubular Acidosis. One model for selective inhibition of proximal tubular HCO_3^- absorption is that of lysine infusion. Walker et al.[117] reported that lysine caused marked bicarbonaturia in the dog. Chan and Kurtzman[118] examined the effect of microperfusing rat proximal tubules with lysine. Lysine was found to inhibit HCO_3^- absorption with no effect on volume absorption. This effect was seen only with L-lysine, not with D-lysine, and the dose response for this effect was similar to that of the concentration relationship for lysine absorption from the lumen. Although no specific mechanism for this effect was established, Frömter[119] and Hoshi et al.[120] found that luminal lysine depolarizes the proximal tubular cell. Such an effect could inhibit HCO_3^- efflux across the basolateral membrane, secondarily alkalinizing the cell and inhibiting apical membrane proton secretion.

Isolated proximal renal tubular acidosis could be due to mutations in the apical membrane Na^+/H^+ exchanger or the basolateral membrane $Na^+/HCO_3^-/CO_3^{2-}$ cotransporter. Investigators have now studied animals with mutations in NHE1, NHE2, and NHE3. A strain of mutant mice with slow-wave epilepsy was found to have an inactivating mutation in NHE1.[121] These mice have no acid/base abnormality. Similarly, mice in which NHE2 was knocked out have no acid/base abnormality.[35] As discussed above, NHE3 knockout mice demonstrate a mild metabolic acidosis with proximal RTA.[34] At present, there are no reports of NBC mutations or knockouts.

Another model for isolated proximal tubular acidosis is inherited carbonic anhydrase deficiency. Sly and associates[122,123] have reported an inherited syndrome with osteopetrosis, cerebral calcification, and renal tubular acidosis due to an inherited deficiency of carbonic anhydrase II. These patients may have a combined proximal and distal RTA, but have no other evidence for proximal tubular dysfunction.[124,125] As discussed above, carbonic anhydrase II is present in the cytoplasm of renal cells; thus, an acidification defect occurring in association with its deficiency is not unexpected. This syndrome is discussed extensively in Chap. 208.

An association between renal tubular acidosis and an aberrant carbonic anhydrase I has also been reported.[126,127] These patients appeared to have a combined proximal and distal renal tubular acidosis. While they had normal amounts of carbonic anhydrase I assayed antigenically, carbonic anhydrase I enzyme activity was decreased. Kondo et al.[126] proposed that this defect may be related to abnormal binding of zinc to carbonic anhydrase I. This association may have been a coincidence and not a causal one, because biochemical studies have failed to demonstrate carbonic anhydrase I in the kidney.[50] In addition, in patients with a syndrome of inherited deficiency of carbonic anhydrase I, there is no disorder of renal function.[128]

Brenes and Sanchez noted that patients with isolated proximal tubular acidosis have an abnormally low rate of ammonium excretion (similar to controls) in spite of having metabolic acidosis.[129] Following an acid load, their urine pH was lower than that of control subjects, but urinary ammonium excretion was also lower than in controls. This suggests that lesser amounts of ammonia are available for trapping in the distal nephron. This defect may imply that ammonium synthesis is subnormal in the proximal tubule. It is also possible that a defect in H^+ secretion in the proximal tubule impairs trapping of NH_3 in the lumen of the proximal tubule.

Diagnosis of Proximal Renal Tubular Acidosis. The diagnosis of proximal renal tubular acidosis rests initially on the finding of a hyperchloremic metabolic acidosis. These patients generally present in the steady state with a chronic metabolic acidosis, an acid urine pH, and a small amount of bicarbonate excretion. Upon administration of sodium bicarbonate, as the plasma HCO_3^- rises above the threshold in these patients, bicarbonaturia ensues and the urine becomes alkaline (Fig. 195-2). In its isolated form this metabolic acidosis occurs alone or in association with mild hypokalemia. If bicarbonate intake is high in an attempt to repair the acidosis, patients will have significant bicarbonaturia on presentation and the hypokalemia may be severe.

The diagnosis thus rests on an acid urine (pH < 5.5) in acidotic patients and a high fractional excretion of HCO_3^- (>10 to 15 percent) in patients with a near-normal serum HCO_3^- concentration. An additional clue to the diagnosis is the difficulty with which the plasma HCO_3^- concentration is corrected. In patients with proximal RTA, large amounts of exogenous HCO_3^- are usually required.

In most patients, this acidification defect is part of a generalized proximal tubular dysfunction called the Fanconi syndrome. These patients have hypophosphatemia, hyperphosphaturia, hypouricemia, hyperuricosuria, glycosuria, aminoaciduria, hypercitraturia, hypercalciuria, and proteinuria. In addition, this syndrome is frequently associated with bone disease, which presents as rickets in children or osteopenia in adults.[130] The diagnostic approach to patients with RTA and the use of the fractional excretion of HCO_3^- are discussed later in this chapter in the section on distal RTA.

Clinical Spectrum. Table 195-4 lists the causes of proximal renal acidosis. Isolated proximal renal tubular acidosis occurs either as an idiopathic or as a genetic condition, or is related to carbonic anhydrase insufficiency or inhibition. Syndromes of generalized proximal tubular dysfunction are discussed in depth in Chap. 196, but generally fall into the categories of primary defects, and those associated with inherited disorders of metabolism, dysproteinemic states, nephrotoxins, interstitial nephritis, or vitamin D-deficiency states.

Table 195-4 Disorders Associated with Proximal RTA

Isolated RTA
Primary (sporadic or familial)
Carbonic anhydrase
Inhibition
Acetazolamide
Mafenide (Sulfamylon)
Deficiency
Osteopetrosis with carbonic anhydrase II deficiency
Pyruvate carboxylase deficiency
York-Yendt syndrome
Cyanotic congenital heart disease
Generalized
Primary (sporadic or familial)
Genetically transmitted systemic diseases
Cystinosis
Lowe syndrome
Hereditary fructose intolerance (during fructose ingestion)
Tyrosinemia
Galactosemia
Wilson disease
Mitochondrial phosphoenolpyruvate carboxykinase deficiency
Metachromatic leukodystrophy
Glycogen storage disease
Cytochrome C oxidase deficiency
Acyl-CoA dehydrogenase deficiency
Silver-Russell syndrome
Say syndrome
Dysproteinemic states
Multiple myeloma
Light chain disease
Light chain nephropathy
Amyloidosis
Vitamin D deficiency, dependence, or resistance
Other renal diseases
Sjögren syndrome
Medullary cystic disease
Renal transplantation rejection (early)
Balkan nephropathy
Chronic renal vein thrombosis
Nephrotic syndrome
Paroxysmal nocturnal hemoglobinuria
Toxins/drugs
Outdated tetracycline
Lead
Gentamycin
Cadmium
Maleic acid
Coumarin
Streptozotocin
Ifosfamide
FK506

Associated Findings. Proximal renal tubular acidosis occurs in two forms: (a) as a part of a broader syndrome of proximal tubular dysfunction, namely the Fanconi syndrome, and (b) as an isolated defect. In the Fanconi syndrome, because of the multiple tubular defects, the pathophysiological consequences are complex. In the pure form of proximal renal tubular acidosis, all of the pathophysiological consequences can be explained by inhibition of proximal tubular HCO_3^- absorption.

Rodriguez-Soriano et al.[131] used clearance techniques to examine the distribution of NaCl and volume absorption in patients with proximal RTA. In these studies, the patients were found to have marked inhibition of proximal tubular NaCl and volume absorption with increased distal delivery. Distal NaCl absorption was normal. As discussed above, proximal tubular NaCl absorption is integrally related to proximal tubular acidification mechanisms. First, because proximal tubular bicarbonate absorption establishes the high luminal chloride concentrations that drive passive NaCl absorption, inhibition of acidification will lead to inhibition of passive NaCl absorption. Second, transcellular NaCl absorption is mediated by apical membrane Na^+/H^+ antiport, which may also be defective in proximal RTA.

In patients with proximal RTA who have a significant acidosis but who are not excreting HCO_3^-, potassium handling is normal. Indeed, in two clinical studies of isolated proximal renal tubular acidosis, patients were found to have normal serum potassium, presumably because of a lack of significant bicarbonaturia in the steady state.[132,133] Patients with proximal RTA have renal potassium wasting only during bicarbonaturia. Sebastian et al.[134] found that the magnitude of potassium excretion correlated well with the magnitude of HCO_3^- excretion. The mechanism of the potassium wasting is related to increased distal delivery of sodium with a poorly reabsorbable anion (i.e., bicarbonate). In addition, inhibition of proximal tubular NaCl absorption leads to volume depletion, which leads to increased aldosterone levels and enhanced potassium secretion.

There is presently no evidence to suggest that proximal RTA causes hypercalciuria or hyperphosphaturia.[132,133] Phosphate wasting associated with proximal renal tubular acidosis appears to occur only in association with the Fanconi syndrome. The hypercalciuria frequently seen with chronic metabolic acidosis is not observed in this disorder, probably because increased distal HCO_3^- delivery enhances calcium absorption in the distal nephron.[135] In addition, hypercitraturia helps prevent nephrocalcinosis and nephrolithiasis, which are not seen in proximal RTA. Rickets, which frequently accompanies the Fanconi syndrome, is probably a result of phosphate wasting rather than a result of the proximal renal tubular acidosis per se.

Management and Prognosis. The goal of treatment in proximal renal tubular acidosis is to maintain a normal serum bicarbonate concentration and pH. This can only be achieved by the exogenous administration of large amounts of alkali as HCO_3^- or an equivalent organic anion such as citrate which consumes H^+ during metabolism in the liver (Table 195-5). As described above, such treatment is associated with massive bicarbonaturia in the form of Na^+-HCO_3^- and K^+- HCO_3^-. Thus, the HCO_3^- or citrate administered should be administered as a mixture of the sodium and potassium salts depending on the moieties excreted (K^+-Shohls). One approach to decreasing the magnitude of bicarbonate excretion is to administer thiazide diuretics,[136,137] a maneuver that lowers the filtered load of bicarbonate by decreasing GFR as a result of chronic extracellular fluid volume depletion. Although the prognosis varies according to the specific cause of the proximal tubular dysfunction, proximal renal tubular acidosis per se should not result in major consequences for the patient if the metabolic acidosis is corrected. While growth is stunted in children with isolated proximal RTA, this is corrected by correction of the acidosis and represents one of the major reasons for adequate alkali replacement, especially in children. Some investigators have noted that the tubular defect improves over time in isolated proximal renal tubular acidosis presenting in childhood.

Table 195-5 Forms of Alkali Replacement

Shohl Solution	
Na^+ Citrate 500 mg Citric acid 334 mg/5 mL	Each 1 mL contains 1 mEq sodium and is equivalent to 1 mEq of bicarbonate
$NaHCO_3$ tablets	3.9 mEq/tablet (325 mg) 7.8 mEq/tablet (650 mg)
Baking soda	60 mEq/teaspoon
K-Lyte	25 or 50 mEq/tablet
Polycitra (K-Shohl Solution)	
Na^+ Citrate 500 mg K^+ Citrate 550 mg Citric acid 334 mg/5 mL	Each mL contains 1 mEq potassium and 1 mEq sodium and is equivalent to 2 mEq bicarbonate
Polycitra K Crystals	
K^+ Citrate 3300 mg Citric acid 1002 mg per packet	Each packet contains 30 mEq potassium and is equivalent to 30 mEq bicarbonate
Urocit K tablets Potassium citrate	5 mEq or 10 mEq per tablet

DISTAL RENAL TUBULAR ACIDOSIS

Mechanism and Regulation of Distal Acidification

Because 90 to 95 percent of the filtered HCO_3^- is reabsorbed in the proximal tubule, the distal nephron functions to reabsorb the remaining 5 to 10 percent of filtered HCO_3^-. In addition, the distal nephron must secrete a quantity of protons equal to that generated systemically by metabolism in order to maintain acid-base balance. While this quantity of protons, approximately 50 to 80 mEq/day, is relatively small, it is necessary to buffer this amount to prevent the cumulative development of positive hydrogen ion balance and metabolic acidosis. Ten mEq/liter of hydrogen ions is equivalent to a pH of 2.0 and exposes the urinary tract to extreme acidity if unbuffered. Moreover, to achieve a urine pH of this acidity, proton secretory mechanisms are required to generate large transepithelial H^+ concentration gradients between blood and tubule fluid. To mitigate the development of limiting pH gradients and enable continued acid excretion at a rate commensurate with net acid production, protons secreted in the collecting tubule are buffered by ammonia, phosphate, creatinine, and other miscellaneous buffers. Nonammonium buffers are referred to collectively as titratable buffers because of the manner in which these constituents are measured. The total net acid excretion (NAE) is equal to the sum of titratable acid (TA) and ammonium (NH_4^+) excreted minus any bicarbonate (HCO_3^-) in the urine, or approximately 50 to 80 mEq/day. This amount is equivalent to net acid production daily, illustrating the paramount role of net acid excretion in maintaining acid-base balance.

Anatomic and Physiological Components of the Distal Nephron

The mechanisms of acidification are discussed extensively elsewhere[40] and are reviewed here as pertinent to the distal renal tubular acidoses. For the purpose of this discussion, the distal nephron can be considered to consist of three segments. The first segment is the cortical collecting tubule (CCT), which has three important characteristics. First, it is capable of HCO_3^- absorption and HCO_3^- secretion,[138,139] which are performed by separate cells in this segment.[140] Second, the relative magnitudes of HCO_3^- absorption and secretion can be modulated by the acid-base status of the animal.[140] Third, the CCT actively transports Na^+ and K^+ in addition to H^+-HCO_3^-. The CCT normally has a negative transepithelial voltage due to sodium transport, which can be modulated by variations in the rate of sodium absorption. This segment includes three distinct morphologic segments: the true distal convoluted tubule, the connecting tubule, and the initial cortical collecting tubule. When studied functionally, with respect to acidification, this segment has many characteristics that are similar to the cortical collecting tubule. For example, the superficial distal convoluted tubule actively absorbs sodium and secretes potassium and is capable of absorption or secretion of HCO_3^-, depending on the acid-base status of the animal.[141–143] Thus, the superficial distal tubule and the cortical collecting tubule can be viewed as similar segments of the distal nephron.

The second major segment of the distal nephron, which functions importantly in acidification, is the outer medullary collecting tubule (OMCT). Lombard and colleagues[144] first demonstrated that the outer medullary collecting tubule (inner stripe) was capable of high rates of proton secretion. This segment absorbs HCO_3^- at rates exceeding those observed in the CCT. In addition, this segment does not actively transport sodium or potassium[145] and does not secrete HCO_3^-, but only absorbs HCO_3^-.[135] Moreover, the rate of HCO_3^- absorption is unaffected by the chronic acid-base status of the animal.[135] Finally, as a result of these transport characteristics, specifically, active proton secretion, the luminal electrical potential difference is positive in this segment (see below).[144]

The third distal nephron segment involved in acidification is the inner medullary collecting duct (IMCD). Microcatheter and micropuncture studies have demonstrated a declining pH profile along the length of the IMCD in vivo which occurs in parallel with an increase in net acid secretion. Bicarbonate reabsorption by the terminal IMCD has been substantiated both in vivo and in vitro.[146–148] Apical proton secretion mediates bicarbonate absorption, titrates urinary buffers, and "traps" ammonium. Recent morphologic, immunohistochemical, and immunocytochemical studies helped characterize some features of IMCD cells relevant to acid-base transport, which were reviewed in detail recently.[149] At least two subsegments have been identified: the initial IMCD and the terminal IMCD. The initial subsegment is composed of two cell types, the α intercalated cell and a cell unique to this segment, the IMCD cell. β intercalated cells are not present. The predominant cell type in the distal two-thirds of the IMCD (terminal subsegment) is the "IMCD-cell."[150]

Thus, acidification in the distal nephron can be viewed as occurring predominantly in three segments. The first segment, represented by the CCT, is a low-capacity segment where acidification can be regulated by sodium transport-dependent changes in potential difference, as well as by chronic systemic acid-base balance. H^+ secretion in this segment is regulated importantly by chronic systemic acid-base changes, aldosterone, and systemic K^+ homeostasis.[151] The second segment, represented by the outer medullary collecting tubule, has a higher capacity for proton secretion. Because this segment does not transport sodium actively, H^+ transport is not affected by sodium delivery. Rather, H^+ secretion in this segment is regulated by systemic acid-base changes, the level and effectiveness of aldosterone, and systemic K^+ homeostasis. Finally, while the inner medullary collecting duct has a low capacity for acidification, net proton secretion and ammonium transport are regulated in this segment by systemic acid-base status and potassium balance.[149]

H^+ Secretion/HCO_3^- Absorption

The mechanism of HCO_3^- absorption appears to be similar in all the segments of the distal nephron. Studies measuring disequilibrium pH have demonstrated that HCO_3^- absorption in the superficial distal nephron[17,19] and in the medullary collecting duct is mediated by apical membrane secretion of hydrogen ions.[152] Because of the negative cell potential, secretion of hydrogen ions must be an active process, which requires energy. Numerous studies suggest that an ATP-dependent electrogenic proton pump mediates active proton secretion at the apical membrane. This conclusion is based on studies that demonstrate the electrogenicity and sodium-independence of HCO_3^- absorption.[153–155] An H^+-ATPase was demonstrated in vesicles from renal medulla and was purified.[156–159] This H^+-ATPase is similar to that found in endosomes, clathrin-coated vesicles, Golgi, and endoplasmic reticulum. This type of H^+-ATPase is similar to the F_0-F_1 ATPase of mitochondria in that it is composed of multiple subunits and does not possess a phosphorylated intermediate, but differs in that it is insensitive to oligomycin and is inhibited by *N*-ethylmaleimide[158] and bafilomycin.[151,160] It is referred to as a "vacuolar" pump. The bovine brain clathrin-coated vesicle H^+ pump has been extensively characterized and is a heteroligomer of molecular mass 500 to 700 kDa composed of 9 major polypeptides of 116, 70, 58, 40, 38, 34, 33, 19, and 17 kDa.[161] Similar to the mitochondrial H^+ pump, vacuolar H^+ pumps consist of two components, a transmembranous component and a peripheral component. In the clathrin-coated vesicle H^+ pump, it has been demonstrated that the 70-, 58-, 40-, and 33-kDa polypeptides are required for ATPase activity and most likely contribute to the peripheral component, while the 17-kDa subunit serves as part of a DCCD-sensitive transmembranous H^+ channel.[161] The kidney H^+ pump lacks the 116-kDa component that is a common feature of other vacuolar H^+ pumps, but it contains the polypeptides of 70, 58, 31, and 17 kDa.[162] Antibodies directed against the purified H^+-ATPases of renal medulla stain the apical membrane of the hydrogen-secreting cells in the CCT and OMCT.[163,164]

A second H^+ pump also contributes to apical membrane H^+ secretion in cortical and outer collecting duct cells. This H^+,K^+-ATPase family consists of at least two, and possibly more, isoforms, which are expressed in kidney. One α subunit is similar to that present in gastric parietal cells ("gastric" H^+,K^+-ATPase or $HK\alpha_1$). Another is similar to that present in distal colon ("colonic" H^+,K^+-ATPase or $HK\alpha_2$). Recent studies demonstrate that the colonic H^+,K^+-ATPase is highly regulated by chronic hypokalemia, and by metabolic and respiratory acidosis.[165] Although antibodies against the gastric H^+,K^+-ATPase ($HK\alpha_1$) have been demonstrated to stain intercalated cells of the cortical collecting duct and outer medullary collecting duct of control rat and rabbit kidney slices,[166] more recent studies reveal that neither $HK\alpha_1$ mRNA nor protein abundance is altered by chronic hypokalemia.[167,168] In contrast, both $HK\alpha_2$ mRNA and protein abundance increase significantly in response to chronic hypokalemia, and this increase appears to be localized to the renal medulla.[168] Nevertheless, the overall contribution by both the gastric and colonic isoforms of the H^+,K^+-ATPase α_1 subunit to H^+ transport by the collecting duct and their regulatory roles in chronic hypokalemia and metabolic acidosis have not been established unequivocally. A major problem has been to reconcile differences in pharmacologic sensitivities of the $HK\alpha_2$ isoform in heterologous systems as opposed to cells in culture and in isolated tubules perfused in vitro. Several recent studies demonstrate clearly that colonic (or $HK\alpha_2$) H^+,K^+-ATPase mRNA and protein present in the collecting duct are dramatically up-regulated by chronic hypokalemia.[167,168] Enhanced bicarbonate absorption through augmentation of the H^+,K^+-ATPase in the outer and inner medullary collecting duct has been demonstrated in the rat tIMCD[169] and OMCD.[170] While the H^+,K^+-ATPase remains a candidate gene for distal renal tubular acidosis, and has been implicated in the development of hypokalemic hyperchloremic metabolic acidosis with vanadate intoxication[171] other more recent linkage analysis studies in patients with an inherited form of classical distal RTA have failed to demonstrate linkage with the H^+,K^+-ATPase.[172] The pathophysiological role of the H^+,K^+-ATPases in such acidification defects, if any, has not yet been established.

Active H^+ secretion by the apical membrane generates base in the cell which must exit the basolateral membrane. The mechanism of base exit appears to be Cl^-/HCO_3^- exchange. This conclusion is based on studies that demonstrate that chloride is required for HCO_3^- absorption and proton secretion in the turtle urinary bladder and in the OMCT.[173,174] In addition, Cl^-/HCO_3^- exchange was demonstrated directly on the basolateral membrane of proton secretory cells of the CCT by measuring cell pH.[128] Using antibodies against the red cell anion exchanger (Cl^-/HCO_3^- exchanger, or band 3 protein), an antigenically similar protein was detected in the basolateral membrane.[175] The cDNA encoding this Cl^-/HCO_3^- exchanger has now been cloned.[176,177] This basolateral membrane Cl^-/HCO_3^- exchanger is encoded by

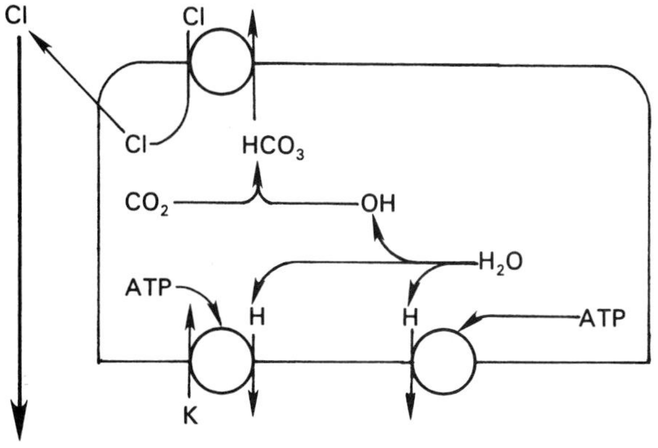

Fig. 195-3 Cell model for hydrogen ion secretion into the lumen of the collecting tubule (and bicarbonate absorption).

the same gene (*AE1*) that encodes band 3 protein in the red cell. However, the two messenger RNAs differ in that exons 1 to 3 of the red cell Cl^-/HCO_3^- exchanger are not present in the renal Cl^-/HCO_3^- exchanger, a difference that is due to alternate initiation sites. Chloride, which enters the cell in exchange for bicarbonate, exits the cell through a basolateral membrane chloride conductance.[178] Chloride then diffuses across the tight junction driven by the positive transepithelial voltage. The mechanism of bicarbonate absorption is summarized in Figs. 195-3 and 195-4.

Bicarbonate Secretion

When animals are pretreated with an alkaline diet, net bicarbonate secretion is observed in the CCT.[179] A similar adaptation occurs in the turtle urinary bladder in which the mechanism of HCO_3^- secretion was investigated extensively. Subsequent studies in the CCT suggest that the turtle urinary bladder and the mammalian CCT share similar transport characteristics. As was true for HCO_3^- absorption, HCO_3^- secretion is dependent on the presence of chloride and independent of sodium.[180–182] Under control conditions, HCO_3^- secretion is electroneutral and active.[183] Based on these findings, it appears that HCO_3^- secretion is mediated by a basolateral membrane H^+-ATPase in series with an apical

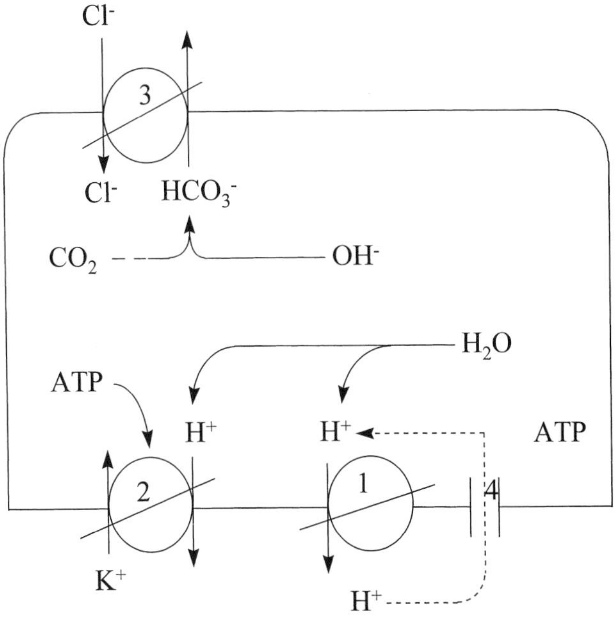

Fig. 195-4 Acid-secreting collecting duct cell displaying four possible pathophysiological defects that might cause classical distal renal tubular acidosis: (1) defective or absent H^+-ATPase; (2) defective or absent H^+,K^+-ATPase; (3) defective HCO_3^-/Cl^- exchanger; and (4) leak pathway for H^+.

membrane Cl^--HCO_3^- exchanger. It is not clear whether the basolateral membrane H^+-ATPase in bicarbonate-secreting cells is identical to the apical membrane H^+-ATPase in bicarbonate-absorbing cells. However, antibodies raised against purified H^+-ATPase label the basolateral membranes of some CCT cells.[163] While apical membrane Cl^--HCO_3^- exchange has been demonstrated in HCO_3^--secreting cells by measuring cell pH, antibodies against the red cell Cl^--HCO_3^- exchanger do not stain the apical membrane in the CCT. The model that best explains the mechanism of electroneutral HCO_3^- secretion is shown in Fig. 195-5A.[22] Here, protons are actively secreted across the basolateral membrane generating base in the cell. Base then exits

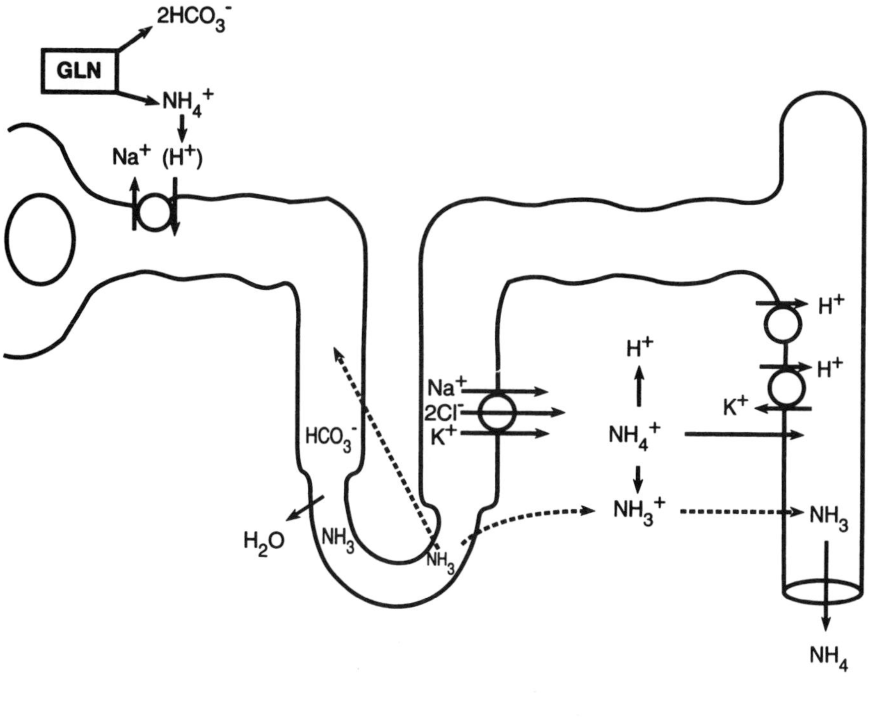

Fig. 195-5 Nephron segments responsible for ammonium excretion. Ammonium excretion is regulated in response to changes in systemic acid-base and potassium balance. Segmental contributions include proximal convoluted tubule; proximal straight tubule; thin descending limb; thick ascending limb; and medullary collecting duct. GLN = glutamine.

across the apical membrane as HCO_3^- in exchange for chloride. The chloride exits across the basolateral membrane chloride conductance. This process is electroneutral because equal proton and chloride currents flow across the basolateral membrane.

It was demonstrated clearly in the turtle urinary bladder that increases in intracellular cAMP levels stimulate HCO_3^- secretion and convert it from electroneutral to electrogenic.[184–186] These data are best explained by activation or appearance of an anion channel in the apical membrane, which is conductive to chloride or HCO_3^-.[158] This has the effect of accelerating HCO_3^- secretion in several ways. First, an additional mechanism for apical membrane HCO_3^- exit is added. Second, an additional mechanism for chloride efflux is added that allows the HCO_3^-/Cl^- exchanger to proceed at a faster rate. Lastly, addition of such a conductance pathway depolarizes the cell, allowing the H^+-ATPase to secrete at a faster rate. Schuster demonstrated that cAMP increased HCO_3^- secretion in the CCT perfused in vitro.[179,187] However, electrogenicity was not demonstrated in these studies. It was shown that the receptor responsible for adenylyl cyclase stimulation was β catecholamine.

Buffers

As discussed above, secreted protons must be buffered to prevent extreme luminal acidity. These buffer systems are conveniently divided into two types: closed and open. A closed buffer system is one in which the concentration of total buffer is fixed. Addition of acid to the solution converts the basic form of the buffer to the acidic form. Such buffers are most efficient at the pK where 50 percent of the total buffer is in the acid form and 50 percent is in the basic form. Because the total concentration of these buffers is fixed, one can calculate the contribution to renal acid secretion by titrating urine from the urinary pH back to blood pH (to simulate the pH of the fluid entering the renal tubules). This is referred to as titratable acidity and represents the contribution of titrated closed buffers to net acid excretion.

An open buffer system is one in which one of the moieties, the acid or the base, can enter or leave the system. The concentration of the other component varies with pH. In biologic systems, the component that enters and leaves the system is lipid-soluble and capable of rapid transepithelial diffusion. Such systems have greatest buffer capacity when the total buffer concentration is greatest. Measuring the concentration in the urine of the impermeable form assesses the contribution of these buffers to acidification. One example of such a buffer system is $CO_2/H_2CO_3/HCO_3^-$. The concentration of carbonic acid is essentially fixed in the presence of the enzyme carbonic anhydrase because of rapid dehydration to CO_2, which is highly permeable. Acid addition merely decreases the concentration of HCO_3^-. However, in the absence of accessibility of tubule fluid at the apical membrane to carbonic anhydrase (type IV carbonic anhydrase), as occurs in the collecting duct, carbonic acid accumulates to concentrations above that predicted if HCO_3^- were in equilibrium with CO_2. Such a condition results in a lower pH *in situ* than at equilibrium (disequilibrium pH).[19]

Ammonium

Another important open buffer system is NH_3/NH_4^+. Because NH_3 permeability is high, proton secretion merely affects the concentration of NH_4^+. This process is referred to as nonionic diffusion. Addition of acid to the lumen causes NH_3 to be converted to NH_4^+, which lowers the concentration of NH_3 and enables NH_3 to diffuse (by nonionic transport) into the lumen.[188] Moreover, a spontaneous acid disequilibrium pH, which prevails in the IMCD, favors NH_3 entry from interstitium to tubule lumen.[152] Recent studies demonstrate that the tubular permeability to NH_3 is not as great as was previously thought, so that in some segments, transport of NH_4^+ can lead to gradients of NH_3.[188]

While several nephron segments have been shown to possess ammoniagenic enzymes, the majority of ammonium excreted in the urine is derived from the metabolism of glutamine in proximal tubule cells.[188,189] Ammonium production in the proximal tubule is regulated homeostatically. The rate-limiting enzyme steps for ammoniagenesis are glutaminase and phosphoenolpyruvate carboxykinase. In states of chronic acidosis, the activities of both of these enzymes increase, as does the abundance of their respective messenger RNAs.[190,191] The increase in glutaminase messenger RNA is secondary to an increase in the stability of the message, while the increase in PEPCK message is secondary to transcriptional activation.[190,191] The precise promoter elements responsible for transcriptional activation of PEPCK have not been defined.[192] At physiological pH, two ammonium ions and the divalent anion α-ketoglutarate are the major products of glutamine metabolism. α-Ketoglutarate serves as a major substrate for the formation of "new bicarbonate" which is transported across the basolateral membrane to the extracellular fluid. This "new bicarbonate" serves to restore the bicarbonate lost in the ECF in the buffering of acid products of metabolism. A major portion of the NH_4^+ produced in the proximal tubule is excreted in the urine. In contrast, any NH_4^+ returned by way of the renal vein to the liver is consumed to produce urea. Thus, the hydrogen ions produced by ureagenesis in the liver neutralize the bicarbonate produced in the kidney from α-ketoglutarate. Therefore, to be effective in maintaining acid-base balance, the ammonium generated by renal ammoniagenesis must be excreted in the urine to avoid hepatic metabolism.

Ammonium is preferentially secreted into the proximal tubule lumen across the apical membrane.[193–196] Quantitatively, the majority of ammonium secretion is accomplished in the earliest portion of the proximal convoluted tubule. Ammonium may then be absorbed to a small extent in the late proximal tubule. The rate of secretion in both the early and late proximal tubules is a highly regulated process, one that is augmented dramatically by systemic metabolic acidosis. In the S_3 segment of the proximal straight tubule, ammonium secretion is enhanced by the presence of an acid disequilibrium pH. The cellular mechanism of ammonium transport involves both NH_3 diffusion and NH_4^+ transport. Direct NH_4^+ secretion may occur via transport of NH_4^+ on the apical membrane Na^+/H^+ exchanger through substitution of NH_4^+ for H^+ (Fig. 195-5).

As tubule fluid leaves the proximal tubule and enters Henle's loop, a number of processes lead to ammonium and ammonia efflux. Accordingly, high medullary interstitial concentrations of ammonium are generated. First, the concentration of bicarbonate in luminal fluid, which issues out of the proximal tubule, increases in the thin descending limb as a result of water abstraction.[197–199] This alkalinization creates a condition favorable for ammonia efflux by nonionic diffusion. In addition, direct NH_4^+ transport by the medullary thick ascending limb of Henle's loop has been demonstrated.[200] This transport process is highly regulated and is responsive to systemic acid-base, potassium, and sodium homeostasis. Specifically, acidosis stimulates and hyperkalemia impairs ammonium absorption on the Na^+, $2Cl^-$, K^+ transporter (through competition for the K^+ site). Ammonia (NH_3) is capable of reentering the proximal straight tubule from the interstitium,[201] thus leading to countercurrent multiplication where the "single effect" involves selective addition of ammonium by the proximal tubule and active ammonium absorption in the ascending limb. The countercurrent system in the loop then multiplies the effect. The net result of this system is a medullary to cortical gradient for ammonium with medullary concentrations exceeding cortical concentrations several fold.[148,188,202] Ammonium concentrations in the inner medullary interstitium reach greatest amplification over cortical levels during chronic metabolic acidosis.[203] Ammonium is secreted from the medullary interstitium into the medullary collecting ducts by a combination of NH_3 diffusion and active H^+ secretion (H^+-ATPase and the H^+-K^+-ATPase) resulting in high concentrations of ammonium in final urine[188,203,204] (Figs. 195-5 and 195-6). Wall recently demonstrated that in addition to this pathway, NH_4^+ can substitute for K^+ on the basolateral (secretory) Na^+, $2Cl^-$, K^+ cotransporter[205] as

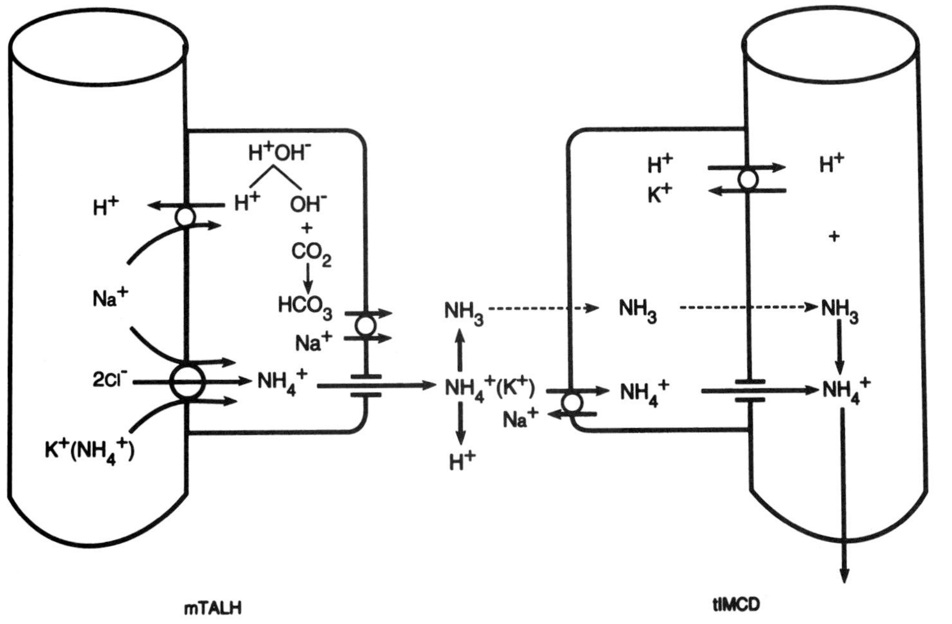

Fig. 195-6 Relationship between ammonium transport in the medullary thick ascending limb of Henle's loop (mTALH) and the terminal inner medullary collecting duct (tIMCD).

well as on the basolateral Na^+,K^+ATPase in the IMCD (Fig. 195-6).[206–208] The net result of both processes is to increase intracellular [NH_4^+], which then diffuses from the terminal IMCD cell across the apical membrane into the tubular lumen as NH_3 in parallel with H^+ secreted by the H^+-ATPase and/or the H^+,K^+-ATPase. The NH_4^+ formed in the lumen is then "trapped" in the final urine because of low NH_4^+ permeability at the IMCD apical membrane. Secretion of NH_4^+ by the Na^+,K^+-ATPase and the $Na^+,2Cl^-,K^+$ co-transporter could serve as an additional means by which NH_4^+ excretion might be regulated by K^+ homeostasis (i.e., increased by hypokalemia and decreased by hyperkalemia).

The decrease in NH_4^+ excretion that accompanies hyperkalemia is a major mechanism through which chronic hyperkalemia is associated with chronic hyperchloremic metabolic acidosis (see section on distal RTA).[209] The relationship between ammonium transport in the medullary thick ascending limb of Henle's loop and the terminal inner medullary collecting duct is summarized in Fig. 195-6.

Maintenance of a high excretion rate of ammonium by the kidney minimizes the amount of ammonium that can exit the kidney via the renal veins into the systemic circulation (where the liver is responsible for conversion of ammonium to glutamine and urea). Such conversion in the liver consumes protons, thus negating the beneficial effects of renal ammoniagenesis, the by-product of which is bicarbonate from α-ketoglutarate.[188] In summary, to generate "new" bicarbonate, the NH_4^+ produced in the proximal tubule must be excreted in the urine through countercurrent multiplication in the renal medulla, and secretion into the medullary collecting duct. Ammonium excretion is uniformly low in renal tubular acidosis when the degree of systemic acidosis is considered. Ammonium excretion in RTA is impaired by medullary interstitial diseases which interrupt the concentration of ammonium in the renal medulla, by impaired H^+ secretion in the distal nephron, and by hyperkalemia which impairs ammonium absorption in Henle's loop and ammonium secretion into the medullary collecting duct.

Regulation of Distal Acidification

As described above, distal acidification involves both HCO_3^- absorption and HCO_3^- secretion, which may be either electroneutral or electrogenic. These mechanisms are subjected to many forms of regulation, which have been reviewed extensively elsewhere.[48] In this section, we discuss some of the aspects of regulation or bicarbonate absorption that are relevant to distal renal tubular acidosis.

The rate of proton secretion is very sensitive to luminal pH. This relationship has been described most extensively in the turtle urinary bladder where the net rate of proton secretion rate is related linearly to luminal pH.[202] Because leak pathways are not significant quantitatively in the distal nephron, this relationship can be assumed to be the result of an effect of luminal pH on active transepithelial proton secretory rate.[202,210]

As discussed above, HCO_3^- absorption or proton secretion is mediated by both an electrogenic mechanism (proton-translocating ATPase) and also by the electroneutral H^+,K^+-ATPase. It would be expected that the rate of the former process would be affected by the transepithelial potential difference. This type of dependency was demonstrated in turtle urinary bladder where transepithelial voltage and transepithelial pH gradients[211] were found to have similar effects on the rate of proton secretion. In the CCT, changes in transepithelial potential difference, which occur secondary to changes in sodium transport, affect the rate of proton secretion.[212] This provides a mechanism by which changes in sodium delivery and changes in the sodium avidity of the CCT, possibly related to mineralocorticoid levels, can affect acidification secondarily. Although the outer medullary collecting tubule also secretes protons by an electrogenic mechanism (H^+-ATPase), this segment does not actively transport sodium; thus, transepithelial voltage is not expected to be affected by sodium delivery. It is not established whether electrogenic HCO_3^- secretion occurs in the CCT. If it does, then the HCO_3^- secretory rate could also be affected by sodium transport and secondary changes in transepithelial voltage. Lastly, it should be noted that anion gradients may affect the transepithelial potential difference in the CCT or OMCT, secondarily affecting the rate of proton secretion. Recent studies demonstrate that the activity of H^+-ATPase in the OMCD is increased by chronic acidosis, while the H^+,K^+-ATPase is up-regulated by chronic hypokalemia.

Mineralocorticoid levels have also been demonstrated to be a potent determinant of proton secretory rate. In the CCT, mineralocorticoids stimulate sodium absorption, increasing the lumen-negative transepithelial potential, secondarily stimulating electrogenic proton secretion.[213,214] In addition, mineralocorticoids stimulate proton secretion directly in the turtle urinary bladder,[215,216] and in the cortical, outer, and inner medullary collecting tubules, even in the absence of sodium.[153,155,217] When examined as a function of luminal pH, mineralocorticoids do not affect the limiting luminal pH gradient; instead, they affect the rate of H^+ secretion at high luminal pH.[215]

Finally, both hypokalemia and hyperkalemia should be regarded as important determinants of the renal response to acid-base balance. While clearance studies suggest that potassium deficiency stimulates distal proton secretion, more direct studies in perfused segments are conflicting.[218,219] Potassium status can affect distal nephron acidification by indirect mechanisms. First, the level of potassium is an important determinant of aldosterone elaboration, which, as discussed above, is an important determinant of distal acidification. Even more important is the effect of potassium on ammonium synthesis in the proximal tubule[220] and on ammonium excretion.[188] Chronic potassium deficiency stimulates ammonium production, whereas hyperkalemia suppresses ammoniagenesis.[188,221] These changes in ammonium production may also affect medullary interstitial ammonium concentration and buffer availability.[148] Recently, the effects of potassium balance on ammonium transport in proximal tubule and the thick ascending limb of Henle's loop were elucidated. Hyperkalemia has no effect on ammonium transport in the superficial proximal tubule, but it does markedly impair ammonium absorption in the thick ascending limb, reducing inner medullary concentrations of total ammonia and decreasing secretion of NH_3 into the inner medullary collecting duct.[221–223]

Chronic hypokalemia, in contrast, is a potent stimulus to the H^+,K^+-ATPase in kidney. This regulatory response appears to be specific for the colonic $\alpha H^+,K^+$-ATPase isoform ($HK\alpha_2$), and not the gastric subunit ($HK\alpha_1$).[167,168,224] Moreover, the site of this regulatory response appears to be the outer and inner medulla rather than the cortex.[225,226]

PATHOGENESIS OF DISTAL RTA

Hypokalemic ("Classical")

The mechanisms involved in the pathogenesis of hypokalemic distal RTA are not yet resolved. Thus far, three lines of evidence have been used to address this question. First, that these patients tend to be hypokalemic (and are not hyperkalemic) demonstrates that generalized CCT dysfunction or aldosterone deficiency is not causative. Some type of lesion in the medullary collecting duct or a selective lesion of the CCT remains a possibility.

The second characteristic, often considered the cardinal feature of this entity, is an inability to acidify the urine maximally (to below pH 5.5). This characteristic has resulted in the designation of hypokalemic distal RTA as a "gradient lesion," which suggests to many investigators the possibility of an abnormal leak pathway (see below).[227,228] Some investigators have also employed the response of urine pH to Na_2SO_4 infusion to classify the defect, arguing that an abnormal leak would result in an inability to maximally acidify the urine that would theoretically respond to Na_2SO_4.[229–231] However, a response to Na_2SO_4 infusion has many interpretations (see below).

The last line of evidence that helps elucidate the pathogenesis of the acidification defect in these patients is the response of the urine PCO_2 to $NaHCO_3$ infusion. In patients given large infusions of $NaHCO_3$ to produce a high HCO_3^- excretion rate, distal nephron hydrogen ion secretion will lead to the generation of a high CO_2 tension in the renal medulla and urine.[232] In fact, the magnitude of the urinary PCO_2 (often referred to as the urine-minus-blood PCO_2 or $U - B$ PCO_2) is quantitatively related to distal nephron hydrogen ion secretion in this setting.[152,233,234] Because of marked bicarbonaturia, the test offers an opportunity to examine distal nephron hydrogen ion secretion in the absence of blood-to-lumen HCO_3^- gradients.

However, it is incorrect to assume that gradients for H^+ ions, H_2CO_3, and non-HCO_3^- buffers are absent in this setting. Because luminal carbonic anhydrase is not present in the collecting tubule, hydrogen ion secretion increases the concentration of these acid moieties in the lumen. Thus, while the luminal HCO_3^- concentrations may exceed that of the interstitium, gradients may exist for backleak of H^+ ions, H_2CO_3, and acid HCO_3^- buffers out of the lumen. Backleak of any of these moieties or decreased rates of hydrogen ion secretion leads to a low $U - B$ PCO_2. While this test has not been routinely performed in all patients with hypokalemic distal RTA, the $U - B$ PCO_2 is usually subnormal except in amphotericin B-induced distal RTA.[232,233,235]

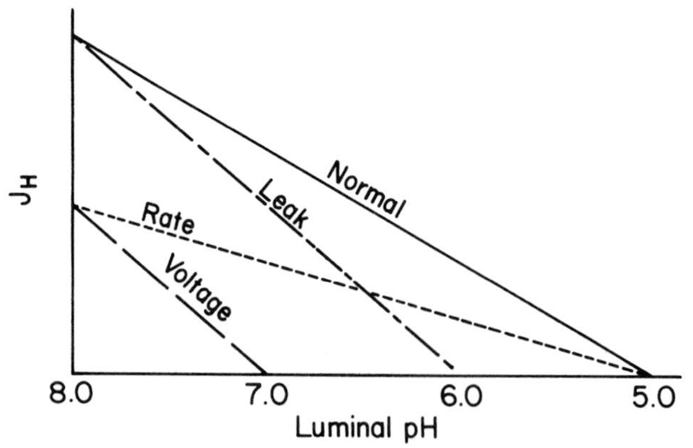

Fig. 195-7 Theoretical mechanisms for defect in hydrogen ion secretion. Rate of hydrogen ion secretion is expressed as a function of luminal pH. See text for explanation.

With this background, we now explore a number of possible mechanisms for defective distal tubular acidification. We orient this discussion along the lines of Fig. 195-7. In this figure, the line labeled "normal" represents the usual relationship between proton secretory rate and luminal pH in the collecting tubule, which is presumed to be similar to the relationship in the turtle bladder, as displayed in Fig. 195-6. When luminal fluid is alkaline, proton secretion is rapid and leads to luminal acidification. The limiting luminal pH represents that pH at which net proton secretion ceases. In the collecting tubule, leak pathways are normally of only minor significance. Thus, the limiting pH represents the pH at which active transepithelial proton secretion ceases.[211]

Pathophysiology of Gradient or "Leak" Defect. In Fig. 195-7, the line labeled *leak* represents an approximation of the expected relationship when an abnormal leak pathway is inserted into the collecting tubule. In the absence of a transepithelial pH gradient, the effect of such a leak is minimal or absent. However, as luminal pH decreases, the leak provides a pathway for base addition and acid efflux from the lumen, which markedly decreases net proton secretion. Thus, a leak appears as a "gradient" defect, in which abnormal acidification is most obvious when the filtered load of HCO_3^- is low and the need to excrete a highly acid urine is great.

The exact acid-base moiety which would leak is not known, but could vary with the type of leak. Possibilities include H^+, OH^- ions, H_2CO_3, HCO_3^-, or nonbicarbonate buffers. Based on Fick's law of diffusion, the rate of diffusion is equal to the permeability times the concentration gradient. The HCO_3^- and non-HCO_3^- buffers, therefore, are likely the moieties to back-diffuse because of the large concentration gradients (millimolar range). Protons, because of high mobility in aqueous solutions, may leak back when the H^+ concentration is sufficiently high (i.e., low luminal pH). Carbonic acid is unlikely to back diffuse through an aqueous pore because of the low concentration in lumen and blood (micromolar). However, if the leak pathway were through lipids, possibly due to an alteration in membrane composition, H_2CO_3 diffusion could be important.

Two additional theoretical mechanisms exist by which a gradient distal renal tubular acidosis could occur. First, in the absence of an abnormal leak pathway, an inability to maximally acidify luminal fluid could represent an energetic problem such as an altered ATP or ADP ratio in the cell or an altered stoichiometry of a transporter (i.e., H^+-ATPase or H^+-K^+-ATPase). Such defects are expected to present as "gradient" lesions and could behave like an abnormal leak (Fig. 195-7). Only one case of an apparent "gradient" lesion not due to amphotericin B has been reported. This case, in an infant with all the features of DRTA but with a normal U – B PCO_2, was described by Bonilla-Felix.[236] Another example was described in a child with Sjögren syndrome.[237] A second possible mechanism of a gradient defect is an enhanced rate of active HCO_3^- secretion. This leads to an inability to maximally acidify the urine along with lower rates of net hydrogen ion secretion.

Pathophysiology of Rate Defect. An alternative to a gradient lesion is denoted in Fig. 195-7 by the line labeled *rate*. In the absence of pH gradients, the rate of proton secretion is markedly depressed. However, the epithelium still retains the capability to achieve normal pH gradients and thus achieve maximal acidification. It is important to note that in the presence of a severe rate defect, achievement of maximal pH gradients may require an extremely long contact time, such that maximal acidification is never achieved. Based on the cell model for HCO_3^- absorption, a rate defect could involve an abnormality in the apical H^+-ATPase or H^+-K^+-ATPase, the basolateral Cl^-/HCO_3^- exchanger, or the chloride conductance, or cell metabolism. All of these possible defects could be present if there were generalized damage to the H^+-secreting cell (see below).

Experimental Models of Gradient and Rate Defects. At present, the best experimental model representative of a "leak" defect is that induced by amphotericin B. Amphotericin B, when inserted in lipid membranes, forms an aqueous channel.[238,239] Animals treated with amphotericin B are unable to maximally acidify their urine under control conditions.[230–233,235,238–240] However, in response to Na_2SO_4 infusion, urinary pH is maximally acidified.[233,240] During HCO_3^- loading in amphotericin-treated rats, the U – B PCO_2 is normal.[233,241] In addition, DuBose[233] found a normal ("acid") disequilibrium pH in the papillary collecting duct (also indicating a normal H^+ secretion rate) in association with a papillary PCO_2 elevated to levels similar to those achieved in control animals. These studies demonstrated that the hydrogen ion secretory rate is normal in this form of distal renal tubular acidosis and that the characteristically inappropriately alkaline urine pH observed spontaneously, after an NH_4Cl challenge, is the result of back diffusion of an acid/base moiety. As amphotericin B is known to form cation selective channels in lipid membranes, the most likely species to backleak is H^+. The occurrence of a normal U – B PCO_2 and normal acid disequilibrium pH during $NaHCO_3$ infusion suggests that, in this setting, $[H^+]$ gradients are not sufficient to generate significant H^+ backleak. However, when the urine pH is lower, significant backleak occurs. Other toxins, such as toluene, have been suggested as producing a similar lesion, but this model has not been studied extensively.[242]

Spectrum of Defects in Patients with Distal RTA. Unlike the situation with the amphotericin B defect, the pathophysiology of the acidification defect in classical hypokalemic distal RTA is unresolved. In part, this is due to the lack of availability of suitable animal models for this disorder. Indeed, the most prevalent accompanying feature of both acquired and inherited forms of distal RTA, nephrocalcinosis, is absent from experimental models. Under a number of different circumstances, including acute acid infusion, patients with classical hypokalemic distal renal tubular acidosis are unable to acidify their urine below pH 5.5.[1,2,14,227,230,235] In most of the reported studies, urine pH remains alkaline after Na_2SO_4 infusion or furosemide administration.[243] In addition, patients with classical hypokalemic distal renal tubular acidosis can enhance net acid excretion in a normal manner in response to buffer infusion. More importantly, the majority of patients with classical hypokalemic distal renal tubular acidosis are reported to display a low U – B PCO_2.[3,230–232,235,243] This finding is not consistent with an enhanced HCO_3^- leak pathway because such a defect would not affect net proton secretion in the absence of a gradient (high tubular fluid HCO_3^- concentration). Moreover, a low U – B PCO_2 rules out enhanced HCO_3^- secretion, as well. Rather, these data are consistent with a rate defect. The inability to acidify the urine below pH 5.5 could be because rates of proton secretion are extremely limited in the most distal segments that can normally secrete protons against large gradients and establish a low urine pH. A normal response of net acid secretion to buffer infusion may be because the diseased segments contribute little quantitatively to whole kidney hydrogen ion secretion in the absence of steep gradients.

An alternative explanation for the defect in classical hypokalemic distal renal tubular acidosis is an enhanced leakiness of the epithelium to H^+ ions (gradient defect). As discussed above, such a leak explains the inability of these patients to create maximal pH gradients and acidify their urine below pH 5.5. In addition, this mechanism explains the normal response in net acid excretion to a buffer infusion.[227] However, as discussed above, such a leak does not explain the low U – B PCO_2 that is reported in most patients with acquired forms of distal RTA. For a significant acid backleak to occur in the presence of significant bicarbonaturia, a large acid disequilibrium pH has to be present leading to large H^+ gradients. However, the normal U – B PCO_2 in the amphotericin model argues against the presence of sufficiently large H^+ gradients in this setting.

Types of "Rate Defects." ***Defective H^+-ATPase.*** Analyses of kidney biopsy specimens in patients with acquired classical distal RTA (Sjögren syndrome)[244] using specific antibodies against one of the subunits of the H^+-ATPase have revealed an absence of this transport protein in the α-intercalated cell apical membrane. The absence of an apical H^+-ATPase in classical distal RTA contrasted with intense staining for the H^+-ATPase in a patient with lupus nephritis, hyperkalemia, and a "voltage" defect (type 4 RTA).[245] Additionally, in one patient with Sjögren syndrome there was no staining for band 3 protein (*AE1*), the HCO_3^-/Cl^- exchanger.[245] Thus, in at least some varieties of acquired classical distal RTA, a defect in the H^+-ATPase is present.

Defective H^+,K^+-ATPase. Based on evidence supporting the existence of K^+-dependent HCO_3^- absorption in the cortical and outer medullary collecting tubule,[246] which was inhibitable by omeprazole or Sch 28080, and the recognition in the same nephron segments by antibodies to the gastric H^+,K^+-ATPase,[166] it is attractive to speculate that a defect in the H^+,K^+-ATPase, which would be predicted to result in both hypokalemia (decrease in K^+ absorption) and metabolic acidosis (decrease in H^+ secretion), could serve as an explanation for classical hypokalemic distal RTA. Initial enthusiasm for this view was prompted by studies suggesting that H^+,K^+-ATPase activity, by indirect enzymatic techniques, was decreased during chronic vanadate administration to rats, which was also associated with metabolic acidosis, hypokalemia, and an inappropriately alkaline urine.[171] Moreover, an unusually high incidence of hypokalemic distal RTA was reported in adults and children in northeastern Thailand (endemic distal RTA).[247] Rather than occurring in an inherited pattern as might be expected if a defect in the H^+,K^+-ATPase gene were present, it is possible that this disorder is the result of vanadate contamination of drinking water.[171,248] Vanadate is a well-known inhibitor of a variety of X^+,K^+-ATPases, including the H^+,K^+-ATPases but not the vacuolar H^+-ATPase. However, this hypothesis seems unlikely because vanadate administered to rats, despite the inhibition of H^+,K^+-ATPase activity in collecting ducts, does not cause distal RTA or renal potassium wasting (reference 249 and author's observation). Alternatively, the association between this disorder and hypokalemia suggests that chronic hypokalemia, which can result in chronic tubulointerstitial disease, could cause the acidification defect. This unique derangement is characterized by generalized muscle weakness, bone pain, nocturia, hypocitraturia, and an increased incidence of urolithiasis, and osteomalacia. Females predominate and the manifestations peak in the summer when potassium deficiency is also most prevalent in this population.[248,250–252] The co-occurrence of hyperchloremic metabolic acidosis and hypokalemia suggests that the H^+,K^+-ATPase could be defective in endemic distal RTA, especially because chronic hypokalemia is one of the most potent stimuli of H^+,K^+-ATPase enzymatic activity, mRNA, and protein expression in the medullary collecting duct.[224] No study thus far has documented genetic linkage between any of the renal H^+,K^+-ATPase genes and inherited forms of classical distal RTA. Acquired abnormalities in the H^+,K^+-ATPase also have not yet been characterized.

Defective* AE1 *or Band 3 Protein. In recent genetic studies using linkage analysis, two groups independently demonstrated a significant association between abnormalities in the *AE1* gene, which encodes band 3 protein or the basolateral HCO_3^-/Cl^- exchanger in the collecting duct, and the occurrence of inherited classical distal RTA in several families in England and in the United States.[172,253] When these abnormal point mutations were expressed in vitro, abnormalities in HCO_3^-/Cl^- transport were not observed. While these studies establish an association between autosomal-dominant DRTA and alterations in the *AE1* gene, the failure to find a parallel functional abnormality represents a dilemma because the disorder cannot be ascribed to abnormal anion transport activity of the mutant protein. Nevertheless, it was proposed that in some inherited forms of distal RTA, misdirection of band 3 protein into the apical, rather than the basolateral, membrane could lead to an acidification defect. If this were the case, a normal or high $U-B\ PCO_2$ would be anticipated. These studies have not been performed in these patients. An enhanced rate of HCO_3^- secretion would be associated with a normal or even elevated $U-B\ PCO_2$. Recently, it was reported that an acidification defect, which is very rarely seen in Southeast Asia ovalocytosis (SAO), was associated with a normal $U-B\ PCO_2$ in a few patients that manifested the features of distal RTA. The normal $U-B\ PCO_2$, in the face of clear evidence for distal renal tubular acidosis, was interpreted by these investigators as indirect proof that the HCO_3^-/Cl^- exchanger, which is abnormal in SAO, was mistargeted to the apical, rather than the basolateral, membrane of the α intercalated cell. That enhanced HCO_3^- secretion, through such a defect, could account for distal RTA in this setting requires additional study (see below).

Impaired NH_4^+ Production and Excretion. Patients with impaired collecting duct hydrogen ion secretion and classical distal RTA also exhibit uniformly low excretory rates of ammonium when the degree of systemic acidosis is considered.[3–5] Low ammonium excretion equates with inappropriately low renal regeneration of bicarbonate, indicating that the kidney is responsible for causing or perpetuating the chronic metabolic acidosis. It would be helpful to understand whether this decrease in excretion of ammonium is the result of, or the cause of, the distal renal tubular acidosis. Low ammonium excretion in classical hypokalemic distal RTA could occur because of the failure to trap ammonium in the medullary collecting duct, as a result of higher than normal tubular fluid pH in this segment and loss of the disequilibrium pH (pH >6.0),[197] as would occur with a defect in the H^+-ATPase, the H^+,K^+-ATPase , or the basolateral HCO_3^-/Cl^- exchanger. However, given the presence of chronic metabolic acidosis and potassium deficiency, it would be expected that rates of ammonium synthesis would be high. In this setting, a urine pH of 5.5 to 6.5 would be sufficient to trap large amounts of ammonium. Because ammonium is normally trapped in the medulla by mechanisms involving the countercurrent system,[188,203] patients with classical distal RTA, who commonly have an associated urinary concentrating defect and/or medullary interstitial disease, could have increased rates of renal ammoniagenesis in the cortex, but an inability to trap ammonium in the medullary countercurrent system.[3,254] This defect reduces the normally favorable ammonia concentration gradient from Henle's loop and medullary interstitium to the outer medullary collecting duct,[203] and is associated with a decrease in NH_4^+ excretion. Whether or not this type of defect contributes to the reduction in ammonium excretion in classical hypokalemic distal RTA requires further investigation. It seems reasonable, however, that an abnormality in medullary ammonium accumulation could occur with nephrocalcinosis and in various forms of tubulointerstitial diseases involving the medulla.

Spectrum of Defects in Classical Hypokalemic DRTA. In summary, hypokalemic distal RTA is characterized by an inability to acidify the urine below pH 5.5. In some patients, this is attributable to an enhanced leakage pathway (amphotericin B lesion or in rare patients without exposure to the antibiotic).[236] However, in most patients the defect cannot be attributed to such a leak. In these patients, a decreased rate of distal H^+ secretion is the likely mechanism. A defect in a cell secreting H^+ by the H^+,K^+-ATPase might be expected to cause hypokalemia, a reduction in NH_4^+ excretion, and metabolic acidosis.[255] To date, such an association has not been documented convincingly. In contrast, if the defect was a result of an abnormal H^+-ATPase, hypokalemia could occur secondarily as a result of volume depletion-induced hyperreninemic hyperaldosteronism. A defect in the H^+-ATPase has been documented in a few patients with acquired distal RTA (see above). Finally, in families with the autosomal dominant form of classical distal RTA, a defect in the basolateral HCO_3^-/Cl^- exchanger which could result in an abnormality in the sorting of this transporter to the apical, rather than the basolateral, membrane was recently reported[172,253] (see above). Therefore, there is no single lesion that explains the acidification defect in classical distal RTA. Autosomal dominant forms appear to be a defect in the *AE1* gene. Acquired forms, especially that seen in Sjögren syndrome appear to be a result of an acquired defect in the H^+-ATPase. Endemic distal RTA appears to be, at least partly, an acquired abnormality of the H^+,K^+-ATPase.

The diverse pathophysiology of distal RTA and what has been learned to date regarding the molecular etiologies are presented in Table 195-6.

Hyperkalemia in Association with an Acidification Defect: Generalized Distal Nephron Dysfunction

Pathophysiology of Voltage Defect. An additional mechanism by which the proton secretory rate can be affected is an altered transepithelial potential difference in the collecting tubule, which has been referred to as "short circuit" or "voltage defect" distal RTA.[256] The expected effect of such a defect on proton secretory rate is denoted by the line in Fig. 195-7 labeled *voltage*. As Fig. 195-7 demonstrates, the effect of transepithelial potential difference and luminal pH are additive. Thus, an altered transepithelial potential shifts the line, thereby affecting both the limiting pH gradient and the rate of proton secretion at any given luminal pH. Any process inhibiting sodium transport in the cortical collecting tubule (CCT) is expected to cause such a defect. Moreover, in this setting, K^+ secretion by the CCT is also decreased.

Three experimental defects have been proposed as models of "voltage" defects in the collecting tubule. The traditional model of such a transport defect is that observed after amiloride administration. It is now appreciated that a similar mechanism results in the generation of hyperkalemia and acidosis in patients receiving trimethoprim and pentamidine.[257] These agents occupy the epithelial sodium channel (ENaC) on the apical membrane of the cortical collecting tubule, thus inhibiting sodium transport, decreasing negative transepithelial voltage, and secondarily inhibiting proton secretion.[258–260] The ability to maximally acidify the urine is clearly impaired and does not respond to sodium sulfate.[230,233,261] Micropuncture studies employing microelectrodes to measure disequilibrium pH as an index of proton

Table 195-6 Molecular Basis of Distal Renal Tubular Acidosis

Classical Distal RTA (type 1)	
Inherited (autosomal dominant)	Defect in *AE1* gene encodes for a single missense mutation (R589H) in the HCO_3^-/Cl^- exchanger (band 3 protein)
	Transporter may be mistargeted to apical membrane
	Other missense mutations reported in some families (R589C and S613F)
(autosomal recessive)	Mutations in ATP6B1, encoding the B-subunit of the collecting duct apical H^+-ATPase or, more commonly, to 7q33–34
Carbonic anhydrase II deficiency syndrome	Defect in enzyme carbonic anhydrase II in RBC, bone, kidney
Endemic (northeastern Thailand)	Possible abnormality in H^+,K^+-ATPase?
Acquired	Reduced expression of H^+-ATPase
Generalized distal nephron dysfunction (type 4)	
Pseudohypoaldosteronism type I (autosomal recessive)	Missense mutation with loss of function of ENaC maps to chromosome 16p12.2-13.11 in six families and to 12p13.1-pter in five additional families
type 1 (autosomal dominant)	Heterozygous mutations of MCR: two frameshift mutations, two premature termination codons, and one splice donor mutation of the mineralocorticoid receptor gene (MLR)
Pseudohypoaldosteronism type II	Linkage to chromosomes 1q31-42 and 17p11-q21; transporter not yet identified

secretion, as well as PCO_2 in the papillary collecting duct in rats receiving amiloride, revealed that the lesion induced by this agent associated with a reduction in proton secretion and, thereby, a reduction in PCO_2.[233] Potassium secretion is also decreased secondary to decreased voltage, and may result in hyperkalemia.[233,262] Studies designed to quantitate enzymatic activity in both the cortical and medullary collecting tubule reveal a decline in H^+-ATPase activity in this same nephron segment after amiloride administration.[255] This finding is compatible with the previous results of DuBose,[233] which suggested that amiloride inhibits acidification by mechanisms other than by simply impairing sodium-dependent transepithelial voltage as evidenced by the observation that amiloride obliterated the acid disequilibrium pH in the inner medullary collecting duct,[233] a segment in which acidification is not dependent on voltage and cannot be dependent, directly or indirectly, on sodium uptake across the apical membrane.[149]

The molecular basis of pseudohypoaldosteronism type I was recently elucidated.[268] This disorder is associated with point mutations in the α and γ subunits of the epithelial sodium channel (ENaC) including, presumably, the apical ENaC in cortical collecting duct principal cells. This defect ENaC impairs Na^+ absorption, reduces transepithelial voltage, and subsequently impairs K^+ and H^+ transport. Therefore, PHAI is the only known example of an inherited "voltage" defect in distal acidification.

The second defect assumed to be an example of a "voltage" lesion is that caused by lithium administration. In contrast to the failure of the amiloride-induced acidification defect to respond to sodium sulfate infusion, the type of distal RTA produced by lithium administration is characterized by an inappropriately alkaline urine pH, which decreases appropriately during sodium sulfate infusion after an acid challenge.[230,233,263] The failure of urinary PCO_2 to increase above blood levels during $NaHCO_3$ infusion in animals with lithium-induced distal RTA demonstrates, however, that proton secretion is impaired.[264] However, studies in the turtle urinary bladder under open-circuit conditions, revealed that lithium impairs proton secretion by virtue of a detrimental effect on the electrical gradient favoring H^+ secretion.[265] As was noted with the amiloride defect, the disequilibrium pH and papillary PCO_2 were also reduced, indicating impaired proton secretion in the lithium defect.[233] In keeping with this observation, recent studies demonstrate a decrease in H^+-ATPase activity in both the cortical and in the medullary collecting ducts after lithium administration.[255,266] This finding is consistent with the observation of obliteration of the disequilibrium pH and reduction in inner medullary collecting duct PCO_2 in lithium intoxication in the rat,[233] and correlates with reports that some patients receiving lithium are unable to increase the $U-B$ PCO_2 during a bicarbonate infusion.[214] Lithium appears then to impair acidification in both CCT[255] and MCT[233] by a mechanism other than simply interfering with sodium-dependent voltage generation. Patients receiving lithium therapy do not, as a rule, develop frank metabolic acidosis, but fulfill the criteria for incomplete distal RTA[267] (see below), and hyperkalemia is not observed.

The third experimental model of distal RTA associated with hyperkalemia assumed to be caused by a "voltage" defect is that induced by unilateral ureteral obstruction. While findings in the postobstructed kidney are similar in many respects to the amiloride defect,[230,233,243] several lines of evidence indicate clearly that this disorder is a result of a nonvoltage-mediated rate defect, not merely a voltage defect. The postobstructed model is associated with an inability to acidify the urine after an acid challenge, a decrease in ammonium excretion, obliteration of the acid disequilibrium pH, and a marked reduction in papillary PCO_2,[233] all features that are compatible with a pump defect. The decrease in ammonium entry into the inner medullary collecting duct appears to be the consequence of the absence of an acid disequilibrium pH. Laski and Kurtzman[212] reported that the decrease in bicarbonate transport (J_tCO_2) observed in rabbit collecting ducts perfused in vitro after obstruction appears first in medullary segments. Only after prolonged obstruction was J_tCO_2 reduced in the CCT. Sabatini and Kurtzman[269] have measured enzymatically the activity of H^+-ATPase in dissected segments of rat collecting ducts 24 hours after unilateral ureteral obstruction (UUO). H^+-ATPase activity was reduced to a greater extent in medullary as opposed to cortical segments. With immunocytochemical techniques, Purcell et al.[270] reported interruption in the cellular distribution of the 31-kDa subunit of H^+-ATPase in rat intercalated cells, suggesting a cytoskeletal defect in UUO resulting in a failure to insert H^+-ATPase into the apical membrane ("gaps" or "discontinuity"). Moreover, with return of acidification, 5 to 10 days after release of UUO, cell convexity and the apical distribution of the proton pump were restored. Sawczuk[271] observed that UUO is associated with induction of growth-related genes (*c-fos*, *c-myc*, *cH-ras*) in the obstructed kidney. It is conceivable that differences in gene expression between the obstructed and contralateral kidney may correlate with expression of pump activity. Thus, biochemical, in vitro microperfusion, and in vivo micropuncture studies support the view that the proton pump is impaired in this defect.

Role of Aldosterone Deficiency in Generation of Hyperkalemic Acidosis: Voltage or Rate Defect? Because the cortical collecting tubule is responsible for sodium reabsorption by an aldosterone-dependent process, which enhances the lumen-negative transepithelial potential difference, thereby favoring the secretion of potassium and hydrogen, it is not surprising that aldosterone deficiency causes hyperkalemia[272] and metabolic acidosis.[273] Moreover, aldosterone stimulates potassium secretion in the distal tubule and whole kidney, and hydrogen ion secretion in both the turtle urinary bladder[215] and medullary collecting tubule, independent of sodium transport.[155,174] Therefore, a decrease in the relative amount of aldosterone or, alternatively, a decrease in responsiveness of the collecting tubule to aldosterone, could result in a reduction in distal sodium reabsorption which would be expected to impair both potassium and hydrogen ion secretion.

Based on the direct and indirect (sodium transport-dependent voltage changes) effects, two mechanisms exist for defective collecting tubule proton secretion in aldosterone deficiency. When examined along the lines displayed in Fig. 195-7, low aldosterone levels cause a "rate" defect.[270] This type of defect is associated with the ability to achieve a normal minimal urine pH, but low rates of proton secretion are observed at higher luminal pH. In contrast, a voltage-dependent lesion is associated with an inability to achieve a normal minimal urine pH (Fig. 195-7). Whole-kidney studies reveal that, during conditions associated with low buffer excretion (i.e., decreased ammonium excretion), a normal minimal urine pH is achievable.[261] Such findings suggest that the "rate" defect is quantitatively more important than the "voltage" defect in hypoaldosteronism and imply that the direct effect of aldosterone on H^+ secretion is quantitatively more important than indirect effects mediated through voltage changes. Additional evidence in this regard is deducible from studies that have examined the effect of spironolactone on acidification. In the turtle urinary bladder, spironolactone blocks aldosterone-stimulated sodium absorption, but serves as an agonist for the direct effect of mineralocorticoid on proton secretion.[274] While it is suggested that spironolactone could cause metabolic acidosis in a single patient with advanced cirrhosis, it is generally assumed that spironolactone administration per se is rarely associated with this acid-base disturbance.[275] Certainly, the decrease in Na^+ delivery to the distal nephron accompanying severe cirrhosis could serve as an additional mechanism for the generation of metabolic acidosis in this patient (voltage defect), the effect of which might be augmented by spironolactone. Nevertheless, the inability of spironolactone to cause a metabolic acidosis in the intact animal supports the view that voltage-mediated changes in mineralocorticoid deficiency-induced distal RTA contribute less to the decrease in net H^+ secretion than aldosterone per se.[276]

Patients with hyperkalemic distal renal tubular acidosis are divided into two groups based on their ability or inability to lower urine pH during acidosis. Using this approach, Batlle's group demonstrated, through the administration of amiloride or bumetanide, that a subset of patients with voltage-dependent RTA has impaired acidification as a result of a derangement other than simply a voltage-dependent defect.[277] All patients in the group unable to maximally acidify the urine during spontaneous metabolic acidosis had low plasma aldosterone levels, suggesting an important role for aldosterone deficiency in the generation of this form of the generalized defect in distal acidification.

The outer medullary collecting duct also serves as a target organ for aldosterone by increasing net proton secretory capacity independent of sodium transport. Selective aldosterone deficiency in the rat has been reported to be associated with impaired H^+ secretion by the IMCD.[217] In this same study, ammonium transfer into the IMCDs was markedly impaired so that ammonium excretion was reduced dramatically. Moreover, as a result of impaired ammonium production, ammonium delivery to Henle's loop was also reduced. Thus, a decrease in inner medullary ammonium accumulation accounted for the reduction in ammonium transfer to the inner medullary collecting duct. Because papillary PCO_2 was reduced during bicarbonate loading, the rate of proton secretion was also clearly compromised.

The importance of mineralocorticoids in the regulation of net acid excretion was also documented in mineralocorticoid-deficient animals and man.[278,279] In adrenalectomized human subjects, net acid excretion and plasma total CO_2 decreased when mineralocorticoid was selectively discontinued, but increased when mineralocorticoid was reinitiated.[279] The change in plasma total CO_2 correlated directly with changes in ammonium excretion, as expected, and inversely with corresponding changes in potassium balance.

Taken together, these findings provide compelling evidence that renal acidification is under the influence of mineralocorticoid and that mineralocorticoid deficiency can cause acidosis and impairment of renal acidification even in the absence of renal disease or glucocorticoid deficiency. The potential for systemic metabolic acidosis in such a setting could be amplified, however, in individuals with renal insufficiency and a decrease in functioning renal mass.

The role of aldosterone deficiency in the pathogenesis of metabolic acidosis in patients with renal insufficiency has been further investigated by the administration of fludrocortisone in the setting of hyperkalemia and hyporeninemic hypoaldosteronism.[279,280] With administration of fludrocortisone in physiological replacement amounts, net acid excretion increased and the hyperkalemia and systemic acidosis improved.[280] Initially, urine pH decreased as a result of mineralocorticoid-mediated enhanced hydrogen ion secretion, but as urinary NH_4^+ excretion increased over several days, urine pH increased as a result of the increase in urinary buffer. Thus, in patients with selective hypoaldosteronism and chronic renal insufficiency, mineralocorticoid administration enhances renal acid excretion directly by increasing renal hydrogen ion secretion, and indirectly by correcting hyperkalemia, which allows ammonium production and excretion to increase.[188]

Role of Hyperkalemia in the Generation of Hyperchloremic Metabolic Acidosis. In addition to impaired hydrogen and potassium secretion as a result of decreased activity of aldosterone, the development of hyperkalemia appears to have independent effects on net acid excretion.[281] Hyperkalemia per se inhibits renal ammoniagenesis and is associated with a decrease in excretion of ammonium, which contributes to the development of metabolic acidosis.[222,272,282] Studies in our laboratory established a critical role for potassium in ammonium excretion and in ammonium synthesis in the proximal tubule.[149,216,282] Hyperkalemia should be regarded, therefore, as an important determinant of the renal response to acid-base balance. Potassium status can affect distal nephron acidification by both direct and indirect mechanisms. First, the level of potassium in systemic blood is an important determinant of aldosterone elaboration which is also an important determinant of distal H^+ secretion. Chronic potassium deficiency stimulates ammonium production while chronic hyperkalemia suppresses ammoniagenesis.[221] These changes in ammonium production may also affect medullary interstitial ammonium concentration and buffer availability.[148,223] Recently, studies from our laboratory demonstrated the effects of potassium balance on ammonium transport in proximal tubule and the thick ascending limb of Henle's loop. Hyperkalemia had no effect on ammonium transport in the superficial proximal tubule but markedly impaired ammonium absorption in the thick ascending limb, reducing inner medullary concentrations of total ammonia and decreasing secretion of NH_3 into the inner medullary collecting duct.[221–223,282] Competition between K^+ and NH_4^+ for the K^+ secretory site on the Na-Cl-2K transporter is the mechanism for impaired absorption of NH_4^+ in the TALH, and perhaps for the apical (and basolateral) K^+ channel, as well. Hyperkalemia may also decrease entry of NH_4^+ into the medullary collecting duct through competition of NH_4^+ and K^+ for the K^+-secretory site on the basolateral membrane sodium pump. The importance of hyperkalemia in the development of metabolic acidosis due to mineralocorticoid deficiency is also demonstrated by correction of hyperkalemia with cation exchange resins. This correction is associated with a significant increase in net acid excretion (ammonium excretion).[280,281] Studies in a rat model of chronic hyperkalemia affirm that whole-kidney ammonium excretion is reduced significantly in vivo in chronic hyperkalemia.[221] This decrease in excretion is associated with a marked reduction in whole-kidney ammonium production, which occurs despite coexistent chronic metabolic acidosis. Nevertheless, chronic hyperkalemia has no effect on net secretion of ammonium by the superficial proximal convoluted tubule. Chronic hyperkalemia, at least in part by inhibition of active NH_4^+ absorption by the medullary TALH,[222] impairs accumulation of ammonium in the inner medulla and significantly compromises the transfer of ammonium into the IMCD.[223]

In summary, hyperkalemia may have a dramatic impact on ammonium production and excretion. Chronic hyperkalemia decreases ammonium production in the proximal tubule and whole kidney, inhibits absorption of NH_4^+ in the mTALH, reduces medullary interstitial concentrations of NH_4^+ and NH_3, and decreases entry of NH_4^+ and NH_3 into the medullary collecting duct. This same series of events leads, in the final analysis, to a marked reduction in $U_{am}V$. The potential for development of a hyperchloremic metabolic acidosis is greatly augmented when renal insufficiency with associated reduction in functional renal mass coexists with the hyperkalemia, or in the presence of aldosterone deficiency or resistance. Such a cascade of events appears to explain the hyperchloremic metabolic acidosis and reduction in net acid excretion characteristic of several experimental models of hyperkalemic-hyperchloremic metabolic acidosis, including obstructive nephropathy, selective aldosterone deficiency, chronic amiloride administration, and chronic dietary hyperkalemia in the rat.

Resistance to Mineralocorticoid Action as a Cause of Metabolic Acidosis. ***Pseudohypoaldosteronism Type I.*** Mineralocorticoid resistance also causes hyperkalemic-hyperchloremic metabolic acidosis in both children and adults.[284] Pseudohypoaldosteronism type I (PHAI) is inherited as either an autosomal recessive or autosomal dominant disorder and is characterized by severe neonatal salt-wasting nephropathy with hyperkalemia, dehydration, and metabolic acidosis. Chronic hyperkalemia and metabolic acidosis may occur in the absence of diffuse renal parenchymal disease or a reduction in glomerular filtration rate.[285] Dehydration and hyponatremia due to renal salt wasting, and hyperkalemia due to renal potassium retention, are typically observed in association with distal renal tubular acidosis.[284,285] Plasma renin activity and plasma aldosterone concentrations are elevated, but deoxycorticosterone and corticosterone concentrations are within the normal rate.[285] The autosomal recessive disorder is caused by mutations in α or β subunits of the amiloride-sensitive epithelial sodium channel (ENaC).[268,286,287] The disease locus has been mapped to chromosome 16p12.2-13.11 in six families and to 12p13.1-pter in five other families[288,289] (Table 195-6). These two chromosomal regions harbor the genes encoding the three subunits of ENaC. The autosomal dominant disorder, in contrast, is a result of a mutation of the mineralocorticoid receptor.[290] Supplemental salt administration can reverse the hyponatremia and hyperkalemia and allow improved growth.[285] After infancy the autosomal dominant disorder typically abates, permitting reduction or discontinuation of sodium chloride supplements. However, it may recur during periods of salt restriction. In contrast, the autosomal recessive disorder persists.

Pseudohypoaldosteronism Type II. Pseudohypoaldosteronism type II (PHAII) (also known as familial hyperkalemia and hypertension or Gordon syndrome) occurs in older children or adults, and is easily distinguished from PHAI by the presence of hypertension, volume expansion, and low to normal plasma aldosterone levels.[290–294] Renal function is usually normal.[250] Recent analysis of linkage in eight PHAII families demonstrated locus heterogeneity of this trait with a multilocus lod score of 8.1 for linkage of PHAII to chromosomes 1q31-q42 and 17p11-q21[296] (Table 195-6). The chromosome 17 locus overlaps a syntenic interval in rat that contains a blood pressure quantitative trait locus.[296] These findings represent what appears to be an important step in the elucidation of the molecular basis of PHAII. In general, it is assumed that the disorder represents a unique abnormality in the distal nephron in which marked avidity for sodium chloride results in volume overexpansion, hypertension, suppressed renin activity, hypoaldosteronism, and reduced potassium secretion.[294]

The primary abnormality in kidney is an increase in the reabsorptive avidity for sodium chloride in the connecting tubule.[295] In contrast to patients with type I pseudohypoaldosteronism, patients with type II pseudohypoaldosteronism respond to thiazide diuretics and salt restriction.[291,297] These patients generally have not exhibited glomerular or tubulointerstitial disease.[298] The acidosis in such patients is mild and can be accounted for by the magnitude of hyperkalemia.[282] Furthermore, renal potassium secretion is resistant to mineralocorticoid administration. Both renin and aldosterone levels increase if volume expansion is corrected by diuretics or salt restriction.[294,299,300] Based on careful studies demonstrating that potassium excretion responds to sodium sulfate infusion but not sodium chloride infusion,[294] it was suggested that this disorder is the result of an early distal tubule "chloride shunt." The "shunt" is viewed as the result of enhanced Cl^- reabsorption in the early distal tubule, which would, by decreasing transepithelial voltage, decrease the driving force for K^+ and H^+ secretion.[294] Therefore, PHAII, like PHAI, but through an entirely separate mechanism, also results in a "voltage" defect. Because thiazide diuretics consistently correct the hyperkalemia and metabolic acidosis, as well as the hypertension, plasma aldosterone and plasma renin levels, it seems likely that this disorder may be the result of increased activity of the Na^+-Cl^- co-transporter in the connecting tubule. To date, such an association has not been proven.

Patients with PHAII respond to either salt restriction,[291] which reduces salt delivery to the connecting tubule, or to thiazide diuretics,[301] which reduce electroneutral sodium chloride cotransport in the connecting tubule.[302] Mineralocorticoid replacement is not required.[291,294,297] PHAII may be distinguished from selective hypoaldosteronism by the presence of normal renal function and hypertension, the absence of diabetes mellitus and salt wasting, and a kaliuretic response to mineralocorticoids.

Hypoaldosteronism. ***Selective (Isolated) Hypoaldosteronism.*** DuBose and associates investigated the pathophysiology of metabolic acidosis in selective hypoaldosteronism in a rat model.[217,257] They demonstrated that acidification was impaired significantly in the inner medullary collecting duct, presumably as a consequence of aldosterone deficiency to decrease the "force" of H^+ secretion (H^+-ATPase or H^+,K^+-ATPase). Moreover, ammonium production and excretion were markedly reduced for the degree of systemic metabolic acidosis. The decrease in net acid excretion was accounted for by the decrease in ammonia production and delivery to Henle's loop, impaired transfer of NH_4^+ from Henle's loop to the collecting duct, and reduced H^+ secretion in the inner medullary collecting duct.[217]

This model is pertinent to the form of isolated hypoaldosteronism seen in critically ill patients on heparin.[303] These patients have elevated levels of ACTH and cortisol, but aldosterone remains suppressed even after angiotensin II infusion.[303] Aldosterone synthesis is impaired because of selective inhibition of aldosterone synthase as a result of hypoxia, TNF-α, IL-1 or increased ANP levels.[304] The clinical features of this disorder have been thoroughly described[305] and are reviewed in the section on disorders of impaired net acid excretion with hyperkalemia (see below).

Hyporeninemic Hypoaldosteronism. Secondary hypoaldosteronism may occur as a result of volume overexpansion,[14,307–311] tubulointerstitial disease, or diabetic nephropathy.[307,308] Aldosterone levels, while reduced, can respond to administration of ACTH and angiotensin II.[309] Both renal salt wasting[310] and volume expansion[311] have been described. Nevertheless, the precise etiology of the decrease in renin elaboration is not firmly established. Primary destruction of cells in the juxtaglomerular

Table 195-7 Diagnostic Studies in RTA

	Type of RTA		
Finding	Proximal (II)	Classical Distal I	Generalized Distal Dysfunction (IV)
Plasma [K^+]	Low	Low	High
Urine pH with acidosis	<5.5	>5.5	<5.5 or >5.5
Urine net charge	Positive	Positive	Positive
Fanconi lesion	Present	Absent	Absent
Fractional bicarbonate excretion	>10–15%	$<5\%$	<5–10%
U – B PCO_2	Normal	Low*	Low
Response to therapy	Least readily	Readily	Less readily
Associated features	Fanconi syndrome	Nephrocalcinosis/hyperglobulinemia	Renal insufficiency

* Except with Amphotericin B

(J-G) apparatus has been reported in diabetic nephropathy.[312,313] Deficient release of renin also occurs in diabetic autonomic insufficiency or in prostaglandin deficiency.[314,315] A defect in conversion of renin precursor to renin was suggested in some patients with diabetes as well.[315]

The pathogenesis of the metabolic acidosis in hyporeninemic-hypoaldosteronism is complex. Proximal HCO_3^- reabsorption was shown to be mildly abnormal and the fractional excretion of HCO_3^- ranges from 3 to 10 percent at a normal plasma HCO_3^- concentration.[272,316] Whether or not this degree of bicarbonate wasting is a result of a defect in proximal bicarbonate reabsorption is not established. The ability to acidify the urine during metabolic acidosis is intact, but there is typically a reduced rate of net acid excretion and ammonium excretion.[272] As mentioned above and outlined in Table 195-7, impaired ammonium excretion is the combined result of hyperkalemia, impaired ammoniagenesis, a reduction in nephron mass, reduced proton secretion, and impaired transport of ammonium by nephron segments in the inner medulla.[307] The clinical features of hyporeninemic hypoaldosteronism are reviewed in the final section of this chapter.

Based on the above discussion, acidification defects in the distal nephron can be grouped into four general categories: (a) an abnormal leak pathway resulting in back diffusion of hydrogen ions (e.g., amphotericin B defect); (b) an abnormality of *AE1* which may result in the mistargeting of the HCO_3^-/Cl^- exchanger to the apical rather than the basolateral membrane of the α-intercalated cell (as in families with inherited distal RTA); (c) a secretory defect in which there are decreased rates of transepithelial proton secretion as a result of an abnormality in the H^+-ATPase (e.g., Sjögren syndrome and most forms of acquired classical distal RTA) or the H^+,K^+-ATPase (e.g., endemic hypokalemic distal RTA); and (d) a voltage-dependent defect associated with intact proton secretion but suppressed net acidification due to an abnormally low negative transepithelial voltage (e.g., PHAI and PHAII). Acquired forms of classical hypokalemic distal RTA (excluding the amphotericin-induced gradient defect and an occasional patient with a nonamphotericin B gradient lesion) appear to be predominantly the result of a defect in the rate of transepithelial proton secretion.[24] The inability to acidify the urine maximally is most likely due to a severe rate defect in the medullary collecting duct, the only segment of the nephron shown to be capable of lowering urine pH below 5.5.

DIAGNOSIS OF TYPE OF DEFECT: TESTS OF URINARY ACIDIFICATION

Urinary Net Charge (Anion Gap) and Ammonium Excretion

All forms of renal tubular acidosis are associated with an inappropriately low excretion of ammonium. Urinary ammonium excretion can be estimated on a spot specimen by consideration of the urinary net charge or urine anion gap.[3–6] This test relies on the assumption that chloride is the most prevalent anion in urine, and that a urine with a low concentration of NH_4^+ has more $Na^+ + K^+$ than Cl^- (net charge is positive).[5] This calculation is based on the constancy of the unmeasured cations, such as magnesium and calcium (excluding NH_4^+), and anions such as phosphate, sulfate, and organic anions present in the urine. In an average American diet, the unmeasured anions exceed the unmeasured cations by approximately 80 mEq/day, so that on a daily basis the sum of urinary

$$Na^+ + K^+ + NH_4^+ = Cl^- + 80.$$

The urinary NH_4^+ concentration is usually estimated from a spot urine by calculating the urine net charge: UNC = $(Na_u^+ + K_u^+ - Cl_u^+)$.[5] Metabolic acidosis due to gastrointestinal losses can be differentiated from renal tubular abnormalities, because urinary NH_4^+ excretion is typically low in renal tubular abnormalities and high in patients with diarrhea. When the urine chloride concentration is greater than the sum of sodium and potassium in the urine (and the urine net charge or gap is negative), the urinary ammonium concentration is usually increased appropriately, suggesting an extrarenal cause for the acidosis. This test is invalid when drug anions or ketones are excreted and appear in the urine. Because the calculation of the urine net charge for a spot urine is derived from consideration of total daily excretion of unmeasured anions and cations, it is most accurate when daily urine volume is 1 liter. The higher the urine output, the more unreliable the urine net charge is in predicting the urinary [NH_4^+]. In polyuric states, the calculation of the urinary osmolal gap may be more precise. The urinary osmolal gap[5,6] can be calculated as follows:

$$\text{Urinary osmolal gap} = U_{osm}(\text{measured}) - U_{osm}(\text{calculated})$$

where:

$$U_{osm}(\text{calculated}) = 2\times[U_{Na^+}] + 2\times[U_{K^+}] + U_{urea}/3 + U_{glucose}/18.$$

This gap is presumed to represent $NH_4^+ + A^-$; therefore, if A^- is monovalent, the estimated urinary ammonium concentration is:

$$[NH_4^+] = \text{urinary osmolal gap}/2$$

This estimate should not be influenced by urinary volume. The net negative charge is also affected by ketonuria or the presence of drug anions in the urine when used to estimate urinary ammonium excretion in metabolic acidosis. Calculation of [NH_4^+] in the urine using the urinary osmolal gap should not be affected by drug anions in the urine (ketoacids, hippurate, or drug anions). Because this method has not been sufficiently validated, it should be remembered that the most reliable method is to measure [NH_4^+] in the urine. Most assays for [NH_4^+] are standardized for the low concentrations anticipated in blood. If the urine sample is diluted 1:100, there should be no problem in measuring urinary [NH_4^+] reliably in a clinical laboratory using routine assays.

When the urine net charge is positive, indicating a low urinary ammonium concentration and a renal origin of the hyperchloremic metabolic acidosis, the minimum urine pH should be measured.

Minimal Urine pH and Maximal Acid Excretion

Historically, the measurement of urine pH is the step applied most commonly to access the ability to acidify the urine in the clinical setting. In the presence of systemic metabolic acidosis, the urine pH should be below 5.5, and is often below 5.0.[3,14,230,243] A urine pH consistently above 5.5 in the presence of systemic metabolic acidosis suggests an acidification defect involving the more distal portions of the nephron. A urine pH below 5.5 is also found in patients with proximal renal tubular acidosis when systemic acidosis is present and the filtered load of bicarbonate is low (i.e., below 15 mEq/liter).[317] The explanation for this finding is that, when the distal nephron is not impaired, reduced filtered loads of HCO_3^- can be reabsorbed in more distal segments so that HCO_3^- does not appear in the urine.[318] A urine pH below 5.5 is also characteristic of patients with selective aldosterone deficiency.[243] In this disorder, low urinary buffer excretion allows the urine pH to reach a limiting pH gradient more rapidly. These findings emphasize that while urine pH is the most commonly used test of renal acidification, it does not measure total hydrogen ion excretion. Patients with chronic metabolic acidosis and normal renal function (as is seen with chronic diarrhea) may have a higher urine pH as a result of the excretion of large quantities of ammonium and other urinary buffers.[3] A low urine pH, therefore, does not insure that the proton secretory mechanism is either intact or appropriate for the level of acidosis, and a high urine pH does not prove an abnormality in acidification. The urine pH should be evaluated in conjunction with an estimate, or precise knowledge of, urine ammonium excretion.[3]

The urine pH should be measured promptly on freshly voided "first morning" urine.[319] If performed in this manner it is not necessary to collect urine under mineral oil. In patients in which systemic acidosis is present, there is no need to perform an ammonium chloride loading test. If systemic acidosis is not present at the time of study, ammonium chloride can be given as a single dose orally (0.1 g/kg body weight) along with food, followed by hourly determinations of urine pH for 2 to 8 h.[320,321] The total CO_2 concentration in plasma should decrease by at least 3 to 5 mEq/liter and the urine pH should fall below 5.5.

Fractional Excretion of HCO_3^-

The fractional excretion of HCO_3^- during $NaHCO_3$ loading, or at a time when the plasma HCO_3^- is normal, is a convenient means of distinguishing proximal renal tubular acidosis from other forms. In patients with distal RTA, HCO_3^- reabsorption, while incomplete at low plasma levels of HCO_3^-, increases with increasing plasma HCO_3^- concentrations. The fractional excretion of HCO_3^- ($FE_{HCO_3^-}$ percent), is calculated as the $(U/P_{[HCO_3^-]} \div U/P_{Cr}) \times 100$. This value is persistently elevated (> 10 to 15 percent) in patients with proximal RTA when the plasma $[HCO_3^-]$ is near the normal range (20 mEq/liter).[14,318] Patients with hyperkalemic distal RTA may have an $FE_{HCO_3^-}$ between 5 to 10 percent. In contrast, in classical hypokalemic distal RTA, the $FE_{HCO_3^-}$ is usually less than 5 percent except in children, where values may exceed 5 to 10 percent.[318,322]

In adults with classical hypokalemic distal RTA, the fractional excretion of bicarbonate is elevated at both normal and reduced plasma bicarbonate concentrations, but is usually less than 5 percent.[318] This contrasts with the typical finding in proximal RTA of frank bicarbonate wasting at a normal plasma bicarbonate concentration (fractional excretion of 10 to 15 percent).[323] The finding of a lower fractional excretion in adults with distal RTA implies that reabsorption of bicarbonate in the proximal tubule is normal. Therefore, adult patients with distal RTA characteristically correct the metabolic acidosis, if the amount of alkali needed to titrate the acid which enters the extracellular fluid from metabolism is replaced. The average alkali replacement requirement in adults usually amounts to 1 to 1.5 mEq/kg.[318] This explains the relative ease with which correction of the acidosis in distal RTA is achieved in contrast to proximal RTA.[2,3,14,318]

In children, however, renal bicarbonate wasting accompanies the otherwise typical features of distal RTA. In infants with distal RTA, frank renal bicarbonate wasting is present initially, but may become apparent only after alkali therapy is initiated.[324] Endogenous acid production in prepubertal children can be as high as 3 mEq/kg/day.[323,325] In older children, renal bicarbonate wasting is often apparent during periods of accelerated growth.[325] McSherry and associates showed that the fractional excretion of bicarbonate in children with classical distal RTA might range as high as 6 to 14 percent.[323,324] Such findings lead initially to the designation of this defect as type III RTA. It is now clear that children with hereditary distal RTA and bicarbonate wasting have affected parents who do not display renal bicarbonate wasting. Because renal bicarbonate wasting in these children usually subsides after puberty, the designation of type III RTA was abandoned. Children with a distal acidification defect and renal bicarbonate wasting are now felt to have classical distal RTA. The important practical point, however, is that renal bicarbonate wasting should be anticipated in children with distal RTA and that adequate alkali replacement must be provided to assure normal growth and maturation.[324]

$NaHCO_3$ Administration and U–B PCO_2

The increment in urinary PCO_2 during $NaHCO_3$ infusion or oral $NaHCO_3$ administration in amounts that result in excretion of highly alkaline urine is a reliable and sensitive index of proton secretion by the terminal nephron.[152,232,233,326,327] After sodium bicarbonate loading, the urine PCO_2 may reach a value approximately 25 mm Hg higher than systemic arterial blood levels. The test is performed by infusing a solution containing 500 mEq of sodium bicarbonate at a rate of 3 ml/min into a peripheral vein.[328] Timed urine collections of approximately 15 to 30 min duration are obtained by having the patient void spontaneously while in the upright position. The test may be terminated after completion of at least three clearance periods when the urine pH is consistently 7.5 or greater. A steady state is usually achieved within 180 to 260 min after initiation of the bicarbonate infusion. Urine should always be collected under mineral oil for measurement of urine PCO_2 and pH. This test may also be performed by administration of acetazolamide, thus avoiding the problems inherent with $NaHCO_3$ loading.[329] Patients with decreased rates of distal hydrogen secretion are expected to display subnormal values during HCO_3^- loading, because the U – B PCO_2 gradient is lower than 10 to 15 mm Hg.[232,327] In contrast, patients with a gradient or "backleak" defect retain the ability to generate high urinary CO_2 tensions during $NaHCO_3$ loading.[233,236,237,241,253,330] The use of the U – B PCO_2 is validated, in both adults and in infants,[331] as well as to distinguish rate-dependent from classical distal renal tubular acidosis in children[332] and adults.[318] Children display an abnormally low U – B PCO_2 alone, whereas adults display an abnormally high urine pH in response to an acid load, and a low U – B PCO_2 in response to bicarbonate loading. In general, patients with inherited distal RTA are predicted to have a normal or elevated U – B PCO_2 (see section on autosomal dominant distal RTA below).

Sodium Sulfate Infusion

If normal subjects are reabsorbing sodium avidly, sodium sulfate administration will result in maximal acidification as assessed by a significant decrease in urine pH.[189] This evaluation requires that the patient be placed on a low-salt diet to enhance distal sodium avidity. The delivery of sodium to the distal nephron is then promoted by administration of sodium accompanied by a poorly reabsorbable anion such as sulfate. This may be accomplished by infusion of 500 ml of 4% Na_2SO_4 over 1 h. One mg of 9-fludrocortisone administered orally 12 h preceding Na_2SO_4 infusion is usually required to insure a sodium-avid state.[243] The typical response to sodium sulfate infusion in control subjects is a decrease in urine pH below 5.5 with or without systemic acidosis.[229,230] Urine collections should be continued for 2 to 3 h after discontinuing the sodium sulfate infusion because of a delayed response in some patients with distal RTA and some with chronic renal insufficiency.[230,243]

Unfortunately, the acidification response to sodium sulfate infusion provides little help in elucidating the mechanisms involved in the acidification defect.[235] A stimulation of proton secretion in response to Na_2SO_4 is expected in (a) the gradient defect, (e.g., amphotericin-B lesion), (b) a sodium-responsive voltage lesion (e.g., lithium-induced RTA), or (c) a rate lesion with decreased pump activity in which the remaining activity is voltage sensitive (e.g., hypoaldosteronism). In addition, if the defect does not involve the cortical collecting tubule (i.e., confined to deeper medullary structures), the normal transport mechanisms in the CCT could still respond to the associated increase in sodium delivery. The only conditions in which one would not anticipate a response to Na_2SO_4 are those in which either Na_2SO_4 cannot alter voltage (e.g., amiloride defect, medullary collecting duct lesion) or those in which acidification mechanisms in the CCT are totally eliminated.

Administration of Loop Diuretics

Because administration of sodium sulfate is cumbersome in the clinical setting and rarely applied except in clinical research centers, Batlle and associates suggest that the response of urine pH and potassium excretion to a single oral dose of 80 mg of furosemide or 2 mg of bumetanide can be employed to characterize the defect in collecting tubule acidification in distal renal tubular acidosis.[235,277] The loop diuretic is administered orally after completing baseline urine collections. Urine is then collected at hourly intervals (or when convenient for the subject) and pH and potassium concentration are determined. In all instances in which the response to furosemide or bumetanide has been evaluated concomitant with administration of sodium sulfate, the two tests have been shown to give the same result.[235] Batlle reported that furosemide, when administered to normal subjects, stimulates voltage-dependent hydrogen and potassium secretion in the collecting tubule.[235] Based on such findings, he suggests that furosemide can be used to disclose the segmental localization of the defect underlying distal RTA. Support for this hypothesis was obtained by observing that the fall in urine pH induced by furosemide was blocked by simultaneous administration of amiloride. In patients with classical hypokalemic distal renal tubular acidosis, furosemide did not produce a decrease in urine pH but potassium excretion increased normally. In hyperkalemic distal renal tubular acidosis, furosemide failed to lower pH below 5.5 and was associated with a blunted increase in potassium excretion.[235] However, the same reservations regarding interpretation of such data as outlined above for Na_2SO_4 infusion pertain to the furosemide effect on acidification.

An Integrated Approach to the Diagnosis of RTA

Whether or not precise localization of the defect in distal renal tubular acidosis can be discerned by the application of such provocative tests of urinary acidification in any given patient, especially those with distal renal tubular acidosis, has not been rigorously tested. Additional evaluation of these maneuvers in experimental models of distal renal tubular acidosis is necessary before wide application can be extended routinely to the clinical setting. As a result of the inherent limitations of these tests and the difficulties encountered when employing these maneuvers in the usual clinical setting, a number of investigators suggest simplified approaches to the evaluation of patients with a suspected defect in acidification.[2,3,328,333] Such an approach is outlined in Table 195-8. Patients with a chronic hyperchloremic metabolic acidosis that cannot be ascribed to bicarbonate loss from the gastrointestinal tract should be suspected of having a defect in urinary acidification. A positive urine net charge or anion gap suggests strongly hyperchloremic metabolic acidosis of renal origin, because the urinary ammonium excretion would be too low for the prevailing acidosis. Patients with either classical distal renal tubular acidosis or proximal RTA usually have hypokalemia, whereas patients with generalized dysfunction of the distal nephron due to aldosterone deficiency or resistance usually have hyperkalemia. Therefore, the serum potassium may provide a clue to the type of defect. If the urine pH with either spontaneous metabolic acidosis, or after an ammonium chloride challenge, is less than 5.0, the defect may reside in either the proximal tubule or may occur as a result of a generalized defect in distal nephron function with hyperkalemia associated with reduced ammoniagenesis, as occurs in hypoaldosteronism.

A urine pH above 5.5 usually denotes a defect in distal nephron hydrogen ion secretion, which can be further examined by evaluating the U − B PCO_2 following bicarbonate loading. The U − B PCO_2 following bicarbonate loading is typically low in hypokalemic distal renal tubular acidosis of the secretory or rate type, but not of the gradient type. Generalized distal nephron dysfunction is associated with a low U − B PCO_2, whereas in proximal RTA the U − B PCO_2 is normal. Hyperkalemia in association with a low U − B PCO_2 and inappropriately low TTKG suggests simultaneous defects in hydrogen ion secretion

Table 195-8 Disorders Associated with Classical Hypokalemic Distal RTA

Primary	
Familial (abnormality of *AE1* gene)	
Sporadic	
Endemic	
Northeastern Thailand	
Secondary to systemic disorders	
Autoimmune diseases	
Hyperglobulinemic purpura	Fibrosing alveolitis
Cryoglobulinemia	Chronic active hepatitis
Sjögren syndrome	Primary biliary cirrhosis
Thyroiditis	Polyarthritis nodosa
HIV nephropathy	
Hypercalciuria and nephrocalcinosis	
Primary hyperparathyroidism	Vitamin D intoxication
Hyperthyroidism	Idiopathic hypercalciuria
Medullary sponge kidney	Wilson disease
Fabry disease	Hereditary fructose intolerance
X-linked hypophosphatemia	Hereditary sensorineural deafness
Drug- and toxin-induced disease	
Amphotericin B	Toluene
Cyclamate	Mercury
Vanadate	Lithium
Hepatic cirrhosis	Classic analgesic nephropathy
Ifosfamide	Foscarnet
Tubulointerstitial diseases	
Balkan nephropathy	Renal transplantation
Chronic pyelonephritis	Leprosy
Obstructive uropathy	Jejunoileal bypass with hyperoxaluria
Vesicoureteral reflux	
Associated with genetically transmitted diseases	
Ehlers-Danlos syndrome	Hereditary elliptocytosis
Sickle cell anemia	Marfan syndrome
Medullary cystic disease	Jejunal bypass with hyperoxaluria
Hereditary sensorineural deficiency	Carnitine palmitoyltransferase I
Osteopetrosis with carbonic anhydrase II deficiency	Hereditary nerve deafness

and potassium secretion. This combination may be due to a failure to generate a normal transepithelial potential gradient in the collecting tubule due to a voltage defect, a generalized defect in CCT function, a defect in permeability to chloride, or low mineralocorticoid levels.

Observing the difficulty with which systemic metabolic acidosis is corrected may also provide more information about the diagnosis of the type of renal tubular acidosis. Proximal RTA is particularly difficult to correct because bicarbonate administration aggravates bicarbonate wasting and also increases urinary potassium excretion. Classical hypokalemic distal renal tubular acidosis typically responds readily to bicarbonate administration. Selective aldosterone deficiency generally responds more readily than proximal RTA but less readily than classical distal RTA. Finally, the accompanying features of the disorder often allow the clinician to categorize the general type of lesion. For example, the Fanconi syndrome is seen in association with proximal RTA; nephrocalcinosis and nephrolithiasis with classical hypokalemic distal RTA; and diabetic nephropathy, obstructive uropathy, or tubulointerstitial disease with a generalized dysfunction of the distal nephron associated with hyperkalemia.

CLINICAL DISORDERS OF IMPAIRED NET ACID EXCRETION WITH HYPOKALEMIA: CLASSICAL DISTAL RTA

Historically, the hallmark of classical hypokalemic distal RTA was an inability to acidify the urine appropriately during spontaneous or chemically induced metabolic acidosis.[334] The defect in acidification by the collecting duct impairs ammonium and titratable acid excretion and results in positive acid balance, hyperchloremic metabolic acidosis, and volume depletion.[320,334] Moreover, medullary interstitial disease, which commonly occurs in conjunction with distal RTA, may impair ammonium excretion by interrupting the medullary countercurrent system for ammonium.[148,188] Proximal tubule reabsorptive function is preserved as evidenced by the conspicuous absence of findings compatible with the Fanconi syndrome.[14,335] The dissolution of bone, which may on occasion accompany distal RTA, appears to be the result of chronic positive acid balance, which causes calcium, magnesium, and phosphate wasting.[2,14] Hypokalemia and hypercalciuria[336] often accompany this disorder. Because chronic metabolic acidosis also decreases renal production of citrate,[336,337] the resulting hypocitraturia in combination with hypercalciuria creates an environment favorable for urinary stone formation and nephrocalcinosis.[336,338] Nephrocalcinosis appears to be a reliable marker of classical distal RTA because this disorder does not occur in proximal RTA or the generalized dysfunction of the nephron associated with hyperkalemia.[339] Nephrocalcinosis aggravates further the reduction in net acid excretion by impairing the transfer of ammonia from Henle's loop to the collecting duct.[148] Pyelonephritis is a common disorder seen in association with distal renal tubular acidosis, especially in the presence of nephrocalcinosis. Eradication of the causative organism may be difficult.[318]

The vast majority of patients with distal renal tubular acidosis have distal RTA in association with a systemic illness, which is referred to as "secondary" distal RTA. Conversely, distal renal tubular acidosis may occur as a part of an inherited defect in which there is no association with systemic disease. The clinical spectrum of classical distal renal tubular acidosis is outlined in Table 195-8.

Primary Complete or Incomplete Distal RTA

Definition and Genetics. Classical distal renal tubular acidosis may occur in the absence of other diseases as an inherited defect (primary distal RTA).[340] This disorder is equally prevalent in males and females and presents at an earlier age than the secondary varieties. Over 30 families with classical hypokalemic distal renal tubular acidosis involving over 300 affected individuals have been reported to date.[172,253,318,324,335,338,341–349] While autosomal dominant and X-linked modes of inheritance have been reported, most patients appear to have an autosomal dominant mode of inheritance.[122,335,345,348–351]

Molecular Biology. It is now recognized that *AE1*, which encodes band 3 or the HCO_3^-/Cl^- exchanger in red blood cells and on the basolateral membrane of type A intercalated cells in the collecting duct, is a candidate gene for this disorder.[172] Two groups of investigators reported that in several families, the affected patients were heterozygous for a single missense mutation in their red cell HCO_3^-/Cl^- exchanger, or *AE1* gene. The most prevalent mutation encodes the mutant *AE1* polypeptide Arg_{589} to His (R589H).[172,253] This mutation changes a positively charged side chain to a titratable group at a position in the cytoplasmic end of transmembrane span 6. This location suggests that R589H might be more susceptible to inhibition by acid pH than wild-type *AE1*.[253] Linkage studies confirmed that the disorder cosegregated, in three of the families, with the microsatellite marker D17S759, which maps to chromosome 17 in proximity to the *AE1* gene.[172,253] *AE1* R589H-associated distal RTA was not associated with any clinically evident abnormality in RBCs.[253]

When distal RTA mutant proteins were expressed in *X. laevis* oocytes, and functionality was monitored by the transport of sulfate or chloride, the most prevalent mutant (R589H) was associated with a reduction in transport of only 20 percent.[172,253] The other variants exhibited transport rates that were indistinguishable from that attained by expression of the wild-type.[172] Coexpression of wild-type and the R589H point mutation failed to substantiate a "dominant-negative" effect.

Based on these findings, it appears that there is an association between autosomal dominant distal RTA and alterations in the *AE1* gene. The failure to find a consistent pattern of abnormal function when the mutants were expressed in *X. laevis* oocytes, as well as the inconsistent pattern of abnormal RBC sulfate transport, represent significant dilemmas when placing these observations in perspective. Both the erythroid and kidney isoforms of the expressed distal RTA variant band 3 proteins showed chloride transport activity similar to that of normal band 3. This finding suggests that the transport activity of band 3 in intercalated cells of distal RTA patients is also expected to be preserved. Assuming that these heterozygotes have equal amounts of normal and abnormal band 3 in type A intercalated cells, only a slight reduction in HCO_3^-/Cl^- exchange across the basolateral membrane is anticipated. It is unlikely that such a small reduction in transport could give rise to a decrease in net acid excretion sufficient to account for the manifestations of distal RTA. Accordingly, these investigators[172,253] were careful to point out that both the disease and its autosomal dominant inheritance could not be ascribed simply to abnormal anion transport activity of the mutant proteins, at least as mimicked in a heterologous expression system.

Loss of polarized targeting of the kidney form of *AE1* could lead to nonpolarized secretion of bicarbonate.[172,253] This arrangement would negate or "titrate" those H^+ ions pumped by the H^+-ATPase or H^+,K^+-ATPase. If this were the case, then it would be anticipated that the U – B PCO_2 would be normal or high in affected family members. Because many of the patients had nephrocalcinosis, it is intriguing to speculate that the inherited defect predisposes the patient, through some undiscovered mechanism, to nephrocalcinosis. Progression of nephrocalcinosis could eventuate in or extend the acidification defect (through damage to either of the three potential membrane transporter proteins or to CA II).[14] The acidosis in the present study population appeared to progress from incomplete to complete dRTA. Indeed, 8 of the 18 patients in this study had evidence of incomplete dRTA and were younger, had lower plasma creatinines, better preservation of urinary concentrating ability, and less nephrocalcinosis.

An enhanced rate of HCO_3^- secretion would be associated with a normal or even elevated U – B PCO_2. Recently, it was reported that the acidification defect, which is only rarely seen in Southeast

Asian ovalocytosis (SAO), was associated with a normal U – B PCO_2 in a family with SAO that manifested the features of distal RTA. The normal U – B PCO_2 in the face of clear evidence for distal renal tubular acidosis was interpreted by these investigators as indirect proof that the HCO_3^-/Cl^- exchanger, which is abnormal in SAO, was mistargeted to the apical, rather than the basolateral membrane of the α intercalated cell. That enhanced HCO_3^- secretion, through such a defect, could account for distal RTA in this setting requires additional study (see below).

Clinical Features. Wrong and Davies were the first to observe that patients with acidification defects evidenced by a failure to lower urine pH during an acid challenge did not always display frank metabolic acidosis (incomplete distal RTA). Patients with "incomplete" distal RTA, who do not have spontaneous acidosis, and in whom the acidification defect is evident only with such provocative tests, are usually diagnosed when testing is extended to members of families with primary classical distal RTA. Most, but not all, patients with inherited distal RTA have hypercalciuria. Those with complete distal RTA usually manifest hypocitraturia in association with the acidosis. Nephrocalcinosis and bone disease are common.[324,341–344,347] Some of the families do not appear to display abnormalities in calcium transport.[335,336,339,348–350] In seven affected members of kindreds studied in San Francisco, nephrocalcinosis was present radiographically as early as age 5, even in patients receiving alkali therapy.[324] However, in a later generation of patients in whom high-dose alkali therapy had been initiated prior to 4 years of age, nephrocalcinosis or nephrolithiasis was not detectable for the period of follow-up which ranged from 10 to 20 years.[347] Moreover, the glomerular filtration rate remained normal during follow-up in these patients.[318] In these children, and in other children treated similarly, with autosomal dominant classical distal renal tubular acidosis, the hypercalciuria and hypocitraturia and stunting of growth are invariably corrected by high-dose alkali therapy.[318,347] Although renal potassium wasting is common in autosomal-dominant distal RTA, hypokalemia is less common and less profound than in acquired distal RTA.

Findings in the families reported by Norman[352] and Coe[336] suggest that hypocitraturia and hypercalciuria may be primary metabolic manifestations of the disorder, but that hypocitraturia in combination with hypercalciuria may be critical in the pathogenesis of nephrocalcinosis and nephrolithiasis with progression to complete distal RTA.

Hamed and associates have reported a large kindred from Oklahoma City in which hypercalciuria was the most frequent finding. The disorder was inherited as an autosomal dominant trait through four generations.[348] The hypercalciuria in this kindred was felt to be a result of augmented intestinal absorption, which appeared to precede both renal tubular acidosis and nephrocalcinosis. Thus, it was proposed that sustained hypercalciuria could damage the renal tubule and ultimately impair acidification, setting the stage for further damage and, ultimately, nephrocalcinosis. In some of the families with hypercalciuria, nephrocalcinosis and renal tubular acidosis (with and without renal failure)[335] inherited as an X-linked disorder, it was postulated that hypercalciuria caused the subsequent development of nephrocalcinosis, renal tubular acidosis, and renal failure. It was recently reported that these patients have a mutation in the voltage-gated chloride channel (CLCN5), which is located on chromosome Xp11. These patients have a missense mutation in the chloride channel (Ser244Leu) and do not have hypophosphatemic rickets or osteomalacia.[353] Thus, this syndrome is not an example of primary renal tubular acidosis, and longitudinal observation reveals that renal acidification abnormalities are not a consistent feature of the phenotype.

Chaabani and associates recently reported finding some of the features of primary distal RTA in 60 of 69 living members of a large family and two unrelated small families.[354] Genetic analysis confirmed the autosomal dominant transmission of this disorder. The acidosis was complete in the majority of cases and was not associated with hypercalciuria, nephrocalcinosis, or growth retardation. These features contrast with acquired varieties of distal RTA, including those associated with hereditary metabolic diseases, in which nephrocalcinosis is common.[355]

In summary, the autosomal dominant form of primary distal RTA is associated with an abnormality in the *AE1* gene which encodes a missense mutation in the HCO_3^-/Cl^- exchanger and impairs net acid excretion by the collecting tubule (α intercalated cell) in an unspecified manner. Presumably, such a defect could occur by mistargeting this "basolateral" transporter to the apical membrane. If this were the case, it would be predicted that the U – B PCO_2 would be normal or high, not low, as is the case with most forms of acquired classical distal RTA. Additional studies are necessary to establish the basis of the cellular defect with certainty and to define the relationship between the defect in distal acidification and its relationship with the development of nephrocalcinosis.

Carbonic Anhydrase II Deficiency

Sly and associates investigated 18 patients in 11 unrelated families with osteopetrosis, renal tubular acidosis, and cerebral calcification.[122,123] Carbonic anhydrase II was shown to be virtually absent from red blood cells in all patients studied.[122] Moreover, reduced levels of carbonic anhydrase II were found in heterozygotes. These findings suggest that carbonic anhydrase II deficiency is the enzymatic basis for this autosomal recessive syndrome. The type of renal tubular acidosis present in this disorder is not clearly delineated. While these patients generally exhibit frank bicarbonate wasting at normal plasma bicarbonate concentrations, suggesting a proximal defect, a number of patients demonstrate an inability to acidify the urine during sustained systemic acidosis.[356] Patients with CA II deficiency exhibit a relatively normal response to acetazolamide, that is, an increase in urinary bicarbonate excretion.[357,358] This observation is important because if the mutation generating CA II deficiency also involves CA IV, acetazolamide would not be expected to elicit bicarbonaturia. Because all patients with CA II deficiency also have osteopetrosis and RTA accompanied by deficiency in CA II in red blood cells, evaluation of the activity of CA II in RBC's is the diagnostic study of choice. It is not clear whether the bicarbonate wasting seen in such patients is a result of a distal defect alone, as is seen in prepubescent children with typical distal renal tubular acidosis (type 3 RTA), or whether a proximal defect is also present. Recently, correction of renal tubular acidosis in CA II-deficient mice by gene therapy was reported.[359] A more detailed analysis of patients with this interesting syndrome is found in Chap. 208.

Endemic Distal RTA (EnRTA)

An extremely high incidence of distal RTA was reported in northeast Thailand. Over 150 patients with strikingly similar symptoms were reported,[248,250,251,360] ranging in age from 18 to 76 years of age, in a female-to-male ratio of 3:1. A recent survey of the prevalence of this condition in the area suggested that 2.8 percent of the general population might be affected based on failure of the urine pH to respond to a standard load.[250] The prevalence of EnRTA and renal stone disease is highest in villagers with poorer socioeconomic status, suggesting that environmental factors may play a major role. Hypokalemia, which is often severe and associated with profound muscle weakness, is a constant feature, as is hyperchloremic metabolic acidosis. Other manifestations include nephrocalcinosis, renal stones, hypocitraturia, osteomalacia, and nocturia. In contrast to normal relatives, these patients exhibit low ammonium excretion rates and an inability to lower urine pH during acidosis, but a significant decrease in pH after furosemide. A spectrum of tubulointerstitial diseases has been described. Because tubulointerstitial damage may be associated with chronic K^+ deficiency, it was postulated that tubulointerstitial disease with interruption of the countercurrent multiplication system for ammonium in the inner medulla might be implicated in the pathogenesis of EnRTA.[360] Is has been suggested that because vanadate inhibits H^+,K^+-ATPase enzyme activity in the rat collecting duct in vitro, and because the soil and well water in this part of Thailand are rich in vanadium, the distal RTA and hypokalemia could be a result of vanadate toxicity causing inhibition of the H^+,K^+-ATPase.[171,248] However, this hypothesis seems unlikely because vanadate administration to rats, despite the inhibition of H^+,K^+-ATPase activity in collecting ducts, does not cause distal RTA or renal potassium wasting (reference 249 and author's observation) (see section on pathophysiology).

Secondary Distal RTA

Table 195-8 outlines the disorders associated with acquired classical distal renal tubular acidosis. The frequency with which hypokalemic distal RTA complicates the hyperglobulinemic states is especially striking. Failure to maximally acidify the urine can be demonstrated in up to 50 percent of patients with Sjögren syndrome and hyperglobulinemic purpura.[361–364] Round cell infiltration of the renal interstitium is frequently found in such disorders and, although not yet proven, the tubular dysfunction may have an immunologic basis. It is not know how dysglobulinemia results in distal RTA, but it is clear that there is no correlation between the class or quantity of the circulating globulin and the renal defect.[361] Recent studies show that hyperglobulinemia, which commonly accompanies HIV disease, is infrequently associated with classical distal RTA.[365] The autoimmune and hyperglobulinemic states reported to be associated with distal RTA include hyperglobulinemic purpura;[361] cryoglobulinemia;[366] fibrosing alveolitis;[367] Sjögren syndrome;[368–370] thyroiditis and Graves disease;[371] primary biliary cirrhosis;[372] chronic active hepatitis;[373–377] systemic lupus erythematosus;[378,379] and, rarely, HIV nephropathy.[365] The association in Sjögren syndrome is particularly striking.[380,381]

The distal acidification defect that complicates the major disorders of calcium metabolism is usually, but not always, associated with nephrocalcinosis. Primary hyperparathyroidism, for example, appears to result in distal RTA only after the development of nephrocalcinosis.[382–385] Similarly, in the absence of nephrocalcinosis, distal RTA does not appear to be a characteristic complication of a number of other disorders, such as vitamin D intoxication;[384,386] hyperthyroidism;[387–389] idiopathic hypercalciuria;[390,391] medullary sponge kidney;[392–394] hereditary fructose intolerance;[395] cryoglobulinemia;[396] Wilson disease; Fabry disease;[403] the syndrome of familial (autosomal recessive) sensorineural deafness;[397–400] X-linked hypophosphatemia;[401] and type 1 glycogen storage disease with nephrocalcinosis.[402] The increased incidence of distal RTA with medullary sponge kidney suggests that cystic dilation of collecting ducts may disrupt acid secretion.[404] Medullary sponge kidney is usually benign unless complicated by nephrocalcinosis, distal RTA, stones, or infection.[393]

Several drugs and toxins can result in a distal tubular acidification defect. These include amphotericin B;[405–408] toluene;[242,409] lithium carbonate;[267] cyclamate;[410] analgesics;[411,412] ifosfamide; foscarnet;[413] and vanadate.[171,248] Amphotericin B, as outlined in the section on pathophysiology, alters the permeability of the distal nephron, allowing backleak of hydrogen ions from blood to lumen and a reduction in net hydrogen secretion ("gradient defect").[233] A concentrating defect due to a direct antagonism by lithium of the effect of antidiuretic hormone on the collecting tubule is commonly observed.[243] Lithium also impairs distal acidification in therapeutic doses and may cause structural tubulointerstitial disease with chronic administration.[267] The renal tubular acidosis associated with renal transplantation may be either of the proximal or distal variety, but the distal variety is more common in association with chronic rejection.[414–417] The RTA of chronic transplant rejection appears to be the result of defective ammonium excretion, generalized distal tubular malfunction, and, in severe cases, reduction in distal nephron H^+-ATPase expression.[417] Other tubulointerstitial diseases associated with distal RTA include leprosy,[337] hyperoxaluria,[419] obstructive uropathy,[420–422] vesicoureteral reflux,[423] and pyelonephritis secondary to urolithiasis.[424]

Finally, distal renal tubular acidosis may occur in association with a variety of genetically transmitted disorders such as Ehlers-Danlos syndrome;[425] hereditary elliptocytosis;[426] hereditary sensorineural deafness (usually with nephrocalcinosis);[397–400,427] sickle cell disease;[428] medullary cystic disease;[329] carnitine palmitoyltransferase I deficiency;[430] type 1 glycogen storage disease;[402] hereditary elliptocytosis;[431] and carbonic anhydrase II deficiency.[122,357,432–434]

Associated Findings in Classical Distal RTA

The pathophysiological basis of the associated clinical features of classical distal RTA are outlined schematically in Fig. 195-8. Abnormal calcium metabolism, as manifest by hypercalciuria, nephrocalcinosis, and nephrolithiasis, is a prominent feature in many patients with classical distal RTA. Low urinary citrate levels are presumed to be the result of chronic metabolic acidosis and facilitate development of nephrolithiasis, and nephrocalcinosis.[435,436] Musculoskeletal complaints are frequent accompanying features of distal RTA and hypocalcemic tetany may occur during alkali therapy.[437] Salt wasting also occurs in distal RTA and is seen more commonly in association with tubulointerstitial disease or advanced nephrocalcinosis.[438,439] Potassium wasting may be particularly severe during acidosis.[440] On occasion, hypokalemia is severe enough to cause paralysis and respiratory depression, and should always be corrected prior to alkali therapy. Chronic alkali therapy usually corrects the potassium wasting, the hypokalemia, and metabolic acidosis.[441]

Renal ammonium excretion in distal RTA is clearly subnormal for the degree of prevailing systemic acidosis and hypokalemia.[320,321] Aldosterone levels are often elevated because of volume contraction and are especially elevated considering the magnitude of hypokalemia.[318,440] In addition to hypercalciuria, the increased renal clearance of phosphate occurs predictably during metabolic acidosis.[442] Calcium phosphate might be expected to be the major constituent of urinary stones in patients with classical distal RTA,[336] but one study reported calcium oxalate stones with equal frequency.[443] Hypocalcemia and hypophosphatemia, when occurring concomitantly, are usually related to the osteomalacia that may occur with chronic metabolic acidosis.[441,444] Chronic metabolic acidosis results in mobilization of skeletal calcium and inhibition of renal conversion of 25 hydroxy-vitamin D_3 to 1,25 dihydroxy-vitamin D_3.[445] In a recent series, radiographic evidence of bone disease was observed in only one of 44 patients with carefully documented classical distal RTA,[339] suggesting that overt bone disease, initially observed commonly in distal RTA, is now less common in this disorder. It also has been emphasized that patients with distal RTA commonly have a urinary concentrating defect, perhaps as a result of tubulointerstitial disease.[446–448] When a concentrating defect of a significant degree accompanies classical distal RTA, it appears to result from the underlying defect, such as tubulointerstitial disease or nephrocalcinosis. Thus, both the concentrating defect and impaired ammonium excretion appear to be the result of interruption of the countercurrent system in the inner medulla.

In infants and young children with untreated distal RTA, abnormal growth is commonly observed.[324] The velocity of growth increases within several weeks of initiating alkali therapy. Within 3 to 6 months, normal stature may be attained.[324] Older children may require several years to achieve normal height.[318,347] Renal HCO_3^- wasting tends to occur and increases in severity during periods of increased growth velocity.[324] As a result, in children with hypokalemic distal RTA, alkali therapy should be provided in an amount that allows sustained correction of the underlying metabolic acidosis. When initiated before 3 years of age, it appears that alkali therapy sufficient to sustain correction of acidosis can prevent nephrocalcinosis.[324]

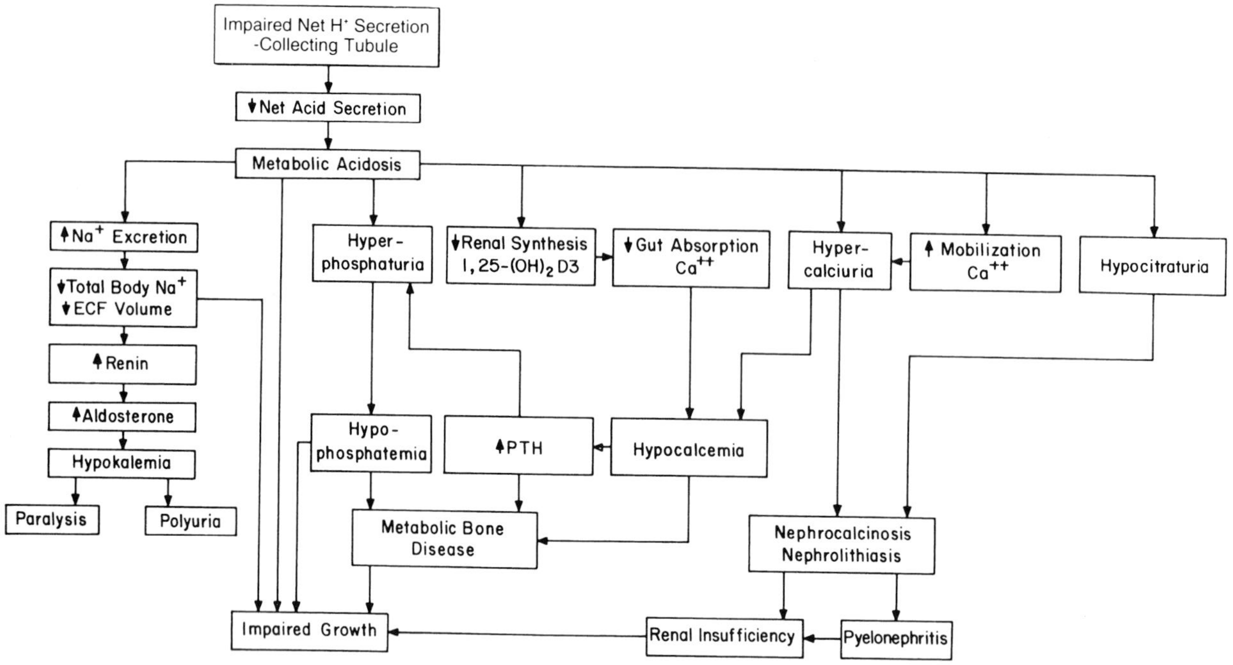

Fig. 195-8 Pathophysiological basis of the numerous clinical features that may accompany classical hypokalemic distal RTA. (*Modified and adapted from Morris and Sebastian.*[318] *Used with permission.*)

Treatment of Classical Hypokalemic Distal RTA

Correction of chronic metabolic acidosis can usually be achieved in patients with classical distal RTA by administration of alkali in an amount sufficient to neutralize the production of metabolic acids derived from the diet. In adult patients with distal RTA, this is usually equal to no more than 1 to 3 mEq/kg/day.[14] In growing children, endogenous acid production is often greater, 2 to 3 mEq/kg/day. However, in children, renal HCO_3^- wasting may occasionally exceed 5 mEq/kg/day. Therefore, larger amounts of bicarbonate must be administered to correct the acidosis and maintain normal growth.[324] Most children with distal RTA are able to take $NaHCO_3$ or bicarbonate precursors orally in amounts necessary to sustain correction of acidosis.[324,347] The various forms of alkali replacement are outlined in Table 195-5. Most patients, especially children, tolerate Shohl's solution more readily than $NaHCO_3$ tablets. Compliance in adults is often limited by taste fatigue with Shohl's solution and by gastrointestinal discomfort with $NaHCO_3$ tablets. Alternating therapy among the numerous forms of alkali may be helpful. In patients with distal RTA, correction of acidosis with alkali therapy reduces urinary potassium excretion, and hypokalemia and sodium depletion may resolve with sustained correction of metabolic acidosis.[317,440,447] Therefore, in most patients with distal RTA, potassium supplement is not necessary. Frank wasting of potassium may occur in a minority of patients in association with secondary hyperaldosteronism despite correction of the acidosis by the alkali therapy.[440] In some children, but not most adults, potassium supplementation may be required even after the acidosis is corrected and may be given as potassium bicarbonate (K-Lyte), potassium citrate (Urocit K), or Polycitra crystals (Table 195-5).

Occasionally, strikingly severe hypokalemia, metabolic acidosis, and hypocalcemia may require immediate therapy. Because hypokalemia may be sufficiently severe to result in paralysis and respiratory depression, immediate therapy with intravenous potassium replacement is necessary and should always be carried out prior to administering alkali.

Prognosis

The goal of therapy in distal RTA is to prevent the relentless progression of renal disease. The prognosis of well-managed patients appears to be excellent, but is determined primarily by the severity of the underlying disease. The glomerular filtration rate should be expected to stabilize and remain constant during replacement with alkali therapy, even if initially reduced.[449]

Hypercalciuria usually disappears on sustained correction of metabolic acidosis; citrate excretion may increase and intestinal reabsorption of calcium increases.[14,435,444,450,451] Moreover, the renal clearance of phosphate decreases and the serum concentration of both phosphate and calcium may reach the normal level.[444] While nephrocalcinosis may persist, nephrolithiasis usually occurs much less frequently with adequate alkali therapy, and may correlate with correction of the hypocitraturia.[336]

DISORDERS OF IMPAIRED NET ACID EXCRETION WITH HYPERKALEMIA: GENERALIZED DISTAL NEPHRON DYSFUNCTION

The coexistence of hyperkalemia and hyperchloremic acidosis suggests that a generalized dysfunction exits in the cortical and/or medullary collecting tubule. In the differential diagnosis of such a patient, it is important to evaluate the functional status of the renin-aldosterone system and the ECF. Table 195-9 outlines the specific disorders causing hyperkalemic-hyperchloremic metabolic acidosis.

Defining the Origin of the Hyperkalemia

Because potassium excretion is primarily the result of regulation of potassium secretion by hyperkalemia, aldosterone, sodium delivery, and nonreabsorbable anions in the cortical collecting duct, it follows that a clinical estimate of K^+ transfer into that segment could be helpful in the recognition of hyperkalemia of renal origin. The transtubular potassium gradient (TTKG)[452] has emerged as a clinically useful tool for estimating the potassium concentration "gradient" between the peritubular capillary and tubule lumen at the level of the the cortical collecting duct. The transtubular potassium gradient is defined as:

$$\mathrm{TTKG} = \frac{[\mathrm{K}]_u/[\mathrm{K}]_p}{\mathrm{U/P_{osm}}}$$

where u and p represent ion concentration in the urine and plasma,

Table 195-9 Generalized Abnormality of Distal Nephron with Hyperkalemia

Mineralocorticoid deficiency
Primary mineralocorticoid deficiency
Combined deficiency of aldosterone, desoxycorticosterone, and cortisol
Addison disease
Bilateral adrenalectomy
Bilateral adrenal destruction
Hemorrhage or carcinoma
Congenital enzymatic defects
21-Hydroxylase deficiency
3β-Hydroxydehydrogenase deficiency
Desmolase deficiency
Isolated (selective) aldosterone deficiency
Chronic idiopathic hypoaldosteronism
Heparin in critically ill patient
Familial hypoaldosteronism
Corticosterone methyloxidase deficiency, types 1 and 2
Primary zona glomerulosa defect
Transient hypoaldosteronism of infancy
Persistent hypotension and/or hypoxemia in critically ill patient
Angiotensin II-converting enzyme inhibition
Endogenous
ACE inhibitors and angiotensin II receptor antagonists
Secondary mineralocorticoid deficiency
Hyporeninemic hypoaldosteronism
Diabetic nephropathy
Tubulointerstitial nephropathies
Nephrosclerosis
Nonsteroidal anti-inflammatory agents
Acquired immunodeficiency syndrome
IgM monoclonal gammopathy
Mineralocorticoid Resistance
Pseudohypoaldosteronism type I (PHAI), autosomal recessive and dominant
Pseudohypoaldosteronism type 2 (PHAII)
Renal Tubular Dysfunction
Hyperkalemic distal RTA
Autosomal recessive PHAI
Drugs which interfere with Na^+ channel function in CCT
Amiloride
Triamterene
Trimethoprim
Pentamidine
Drugs which interfere with Na^+,K^+-ATPase in CCT
Cyclosporin A
Drugs which inhibit aldosterone effect on CCT
Spironolactone
Disorders associated with tubulointerstitial nephritis and renal insufficiency
Lupus nephritis
Methicillin nephrotoxicity
Obstructive nephropathy
Kidney transplant rejection
Sickle-cell disease
William syndrome with uric acid nephrolithiasis

respectively, and osm is osmolality. In this expression, the urine to plasma K^+ concentration ratio is corrected by water abstraction in the more distal segments of the collecting duct because there is usually no additional alteration in K^+ content in the medulla. When the TTKG is low in a hyperkalemic patient (<8) it implies that the collecting tubule is not responding appropriately to the prevailing hyperkalemia and that potassium secretion is impaired. In contrast, in hyperkalemia of nonrenal origin, the kidney should respond "appropriately" by increasing K^+ secretion, as evidenced by a sharp increase in the TTKG. There are numerous assumptions in the derivation of the TTKG, which should be considered. The TTKG assumes no significant net addition or absorption of K^+ between the CCD and final urine; that CCD tubular fluid osmolality is approximately the same as plasma osmolality; that "osmoles" are not extracted between CCD and final urine; and that plasma $[K^+]$ approximates peritubular fluid $[K^+]$. Under certain clinical conditions, some or none of these assumptions may be entirely correct. Particularly problematic is the effect on the TTKG of a dilute urine or of high urine flow rates (polyuria). In these situations, the TTKG underestimates K^+ secretory capacity in the hyperkalemic patient. With consideration for these potential pitfalls, the TTKG appears to be a useful clinical tool to estimate potassium secretory ability, but may be no more useful than the fractional excretion of potassium. Because the hyperkalemia of mineralocorticoid deficiency should respond to mineralocorticoid replacement, the patient with hypoaldosteronism is expected to exhibit an increase in the TTKG after fludrocortisone administration for several days, while the patient with resistance to mineralocorticoid would not be expected to alter the TTKG under this condition. Thus, an increase in the TTKG to >8 after mineralocorticoid suggests aldosterone deficiency, whereas failure of the TTKG to increase suggests tubular insensitivity to mineralocorticoid.

Clinical Disorders

The coexistence of hyperkalemia and hyperchloremic acidosis suggests that a generalized distal tubule dysfunction exists. Generalized distal nephron dysfunction is manifest as a hyperchloremic, hyperkalemic metabolic acidosis in which urinary ammonium excretion is invariably depressed and renal function is often compromised. Although hyperchloremic metabolic acidosis and hyperkalemia occur with regularity in advanced renal insufficiency, patients selected because of severe hyperkalemia (>5.5 mEq/liter) with, for example, diabetic nephropathy and tubulointerstitial disease, have hyperkalemia that is disproportionate to the reduction in glomerular filtration rate. The TTKG emphasized earlier is usually low in patients with this disorder (<8), indicating that the collecting tubule is not responding appropriately to the prevailing hyperkalemia. In such patients, a unique dysfunction of potassium and acid secretion by the collecting tubule coexists and can be attributed to either hypoaldosteronism[306,308] or to a decrease in effectiveness of aldosterone.[306] In patients presenting with this constellation of findings, an evaluation of renin-aldosterone elaboration is indicated. A suggested classification of the clinical disorders associated with hyperkalemia and defects in acidification is summarized in Table 195-9.

Primary Mineralocorticoid Deficiency

Although a growing list of factors can modulate aldosterone secretion (including angiotensin II; ACTH; endothelin; dopamine; acetylcholine; epinephrine; plasma K^+; and Mg^{+2}), angiotensin II and plasma K^+ remain the principal modulators of aldosterone production and secretion. Destruction of the adrenal cortex by hemorrhage, infection, invasion by tumors, or autoimmune processes results in Addison disease. This destruction causes combined glucocorticoid and mineralocorticoid deficiency and is recognized clinically by hypoglycemia, anorexia, weakness, hyperpigmentation, and a failure to respond to stress. These defects can occur in association with renal salt wasting and hyponatremia, hyperkalemia, and metabolic acidosis.[306,308,453] The most common congenital adrenal defect in steroid biosynthesis is 21-hydroxylase deficiency, which is associated with salt wasting, hyperkalemia, and metabolic acidosis in a fraction of the patients. Causes of Addison disease include tuberculosis, autoimmune adrenal failure, fungal infections, adrenal hemorrhage, metastasis, lymphoma, AIDS, amyloidosis, and drug toxicity (ketoconazole, fluconazole, Dilantin, rifampin, and barbiturates).[453] These disorders are associated with low plasma aldosterone levels and high levels of plasma renin activity. The metabolic acidosis of mineralocorticoid deficiency results from a decrease in hydrogen ion secretion in the collecting duct secondary to decreased H^+-ATPase number and function. The hyperkalemia of mineralocorticoid deficiency decreases ammonium production and excretion.

Hyporeninemic-Hypoaldosteronism

In contrast to patients with the primary adrenal disorder, which occurs far less frequently, patients in this group exhibit low plasma renin activity. Patients with this disorder are usually older (mean age 65 years) and almost always exhibit mild to moderate renal insufficiency (70 percent) and acidosis (50 percent) in association with chronic hyperkalemia in the range of 5.5 to 6.5 mEq/liter.[308,454] While the hyperkalemia may be asymptomatic, it is important to recognize that both the metabolic acidosis and the hyperkalemia are out of proportion to the level of reduction in glomerular filtration rate. Cardiac arrhythmias are evident in 25 percent of patients. The most frequently associated renal diseases are diabetic nephropathy and tubulointerstitial disease.[307,308] Additional disorders associated with hyporeninemic-hypoaldosteronism include tubulointerstitial nephritis, systemic lupus erythematosus, and AIDS. For 80 to 85 percent of such patients, there is a reduction in plasma renin activity that cannot be stimulated by the usual physiological maneuvers. The low aldosterone levels, nevertheless, can be increased by administration of angiotensin II or ACTH. The degree of salt wasting associated with hyporeninemic-hypoaldosteronism is generally not severe, and is no worse than that seen in patients with chronic renal insufficiency at comparable levels of GFR. Because approximately 30 percent of patients with hyporeninemic-hypoaldosteronism are hypertensive, the finding of a low plasma renin in such patients suggests a volume dependent form of hypertension with physiological suppression of renin elaboration. In general, patients with more advanced renal insufficiency as a result of glomerular disease, rather than tubulointerstitial disease (e.g., diabetic nephropathy), are more commonly volume expanded.[311]

As mentioned above, impaired ammonium excretion is the combined result of hyperkalemia, impaired ammoniagenesis, a reduction in nephron mass, reduced proton secretion, and impaired transport of ammonium by nephron segments in the inner medulla.[212,217] Hyperchloremic metabolic acidosis occurs in approximately 50 percent of patients with hyporeninemic-hypoaldosteronism. Drugs, which may result in similar manifestations, are reviewed below.

Isolated Hypoaldosteronism in Critically Ill Patients

The pathophysiology of isolated hypoaldosteronism, which may occur in critically ill patients, particularly in the setting of severe sepsis or cardiogenic shock, was described in the section on pathophysiology. This disorder is associated with markedly elevated ACTH and cortisol levels in concert with a decrease in aldosterone elaboration in response to angiotensin II.[302] Selective inhibition of aldosterone synthase is the result of hypoxia or the result of cytokines such as TNF-α, or IL-1. Alternatively, high circulating levels of atrial natriuretic peptide (ANP) may suppress aldosterone synthase.[303] ANP, a powerful suppressor of aldosterone secretion, may be elevated in CHF, with atrial arrhythmias, in subclinical cardiac disease, and in volume expansion. These patients manifest the features of hypoaldosteronism, including hyperkalemia and metabolic acidosis. The development of hyperkalemia may be potentiated by the administration of potassium-sparing diuretics, potassium loads in parenteral nutrition solutions, or as a result of heparin administration. The latter suppresses aldosterone synthesis in the critically ill patient.[305]

Resistance to Mineralocorticoid

Pseudohypoaldosteronism type I (PHAI) is a rare, but often life threatening, autosomal recessive disease characterized by severe neonatal salt wasting, hyperkalemia, metabolic acidosis, and unresponsiveness to mineralocorticoid hormones. The hyperkalemia can be attributed to impaired potassium secretion, despite normal or elevated aldosterone levels. The collecting tubule is unresponsive to aldosterone.[294] Autosomal dominant PHAI is the result of a mutation in the mineralocorticoid receptor.[290] Autosomal recessive PHAI is the result of a loss-of-function mutation in the epithelial sodium channel (ENaC) in the cortical collecting tubule.[268,286–289] This defect compromises channel gating and impairs absorption of sodium across the apical membrane of the principal cell in the cortical collecting duct. PHAI (MIM 264350) was mapped to chromosome 16p12.2-13.11 in six families and to 12p13.1-pter in five additional families.[289] This defect in ENaC secondarily impairs potassium and hydrogen ion secretion, leading to hyperkalemia and metabolic acidosis. Thus, as explained above, both autosomal recessive and autosomal dominant PHAI are examples of "voltage-defect" types of distal RTA.

The clinical features of pseudohypoaldosteronism type II (PHAII) contrast sharply with findings in PHAI. PHAII is a disorder of adults characterized by hyperkalemia, hyperchloremic metabolic acidosis, hypertension, normal renal function, undetectable plasma renin activity, and low aldosterone levels.[249,297,298,456] The molecular basis of this disorder is discussed in the section on pathophysiology. These patients generally have not exhibited glomerular or tubulointerstitial disease.[374] The acidosis is mild and can be accounted for by the magnitude of hyperkalemia. Furthermore, renal potassium secretion is resistant to mineralocorticoid administration. Renin and aldosterone levels both increase if volume expansion is corrected by diuretics or salt restriction.[280,294,300] It has been suggested that this disorder is the result of an early distal tubule "chloride shunt."[294] The "shunt" is viewed as the result of enhanced Cl^- reabsorption in the early distal tubule, which would, by decreasing transepithelial voltage, decrease the driving force for K^+ secretion. Thiazide diuretics consistently correct the hyperkalemia and metabolic acidosis, as well as the hypertension, plasma aldosterone, and plasma renin levels.

Secondary Renal Diseases Associated with Renal Tubular Secretory Defects

Table 195-10 outlines those acquired renal disorders that are commonly associated with hyperkalemia and that often display striking tubulointerstitial involvement.[457–459] In these disorders, the frequency with which hyperkalemia is associated with metabolic acidosis and decreased net acid excretion as a result of impaired ammonium production or excretion cannot be presumed to be a result of the severity of impairment in renal function. While hyperkalemia is more likely to be associated with metabolic acidosis and reduced ammonium excretion when the GFR is below 20 to 50 ml/min, significant hyperkalemia can occur with significantly less renal functional impairment. Hyperkalemia that is out of proportion to the degree of renal insufficiency is typically observed with the nephropathies associated with sickle cell disease, systemic lupus erythematosus, and obstruction of the collecting system; in William syndrome with uric acid nephrolithiasis;[460] in methylmalonic acidemia[461] with acute and chronic renal allograft rejection; in hypoaldosteronism; and, occasionally,

Table 195-10 Acquired Renal Tubular Secretory Defects

Sickle-cell disease
SLE
Renal transplant rejection
Obstructive uropathy
Medullary cystic disease
Drug-induced interstitial nephritis
Analgesic abuse nephropathy
HIV nephropathy
IgM monoclonal gammopathy

Table 195-11 Hyperkalemic Distal RTA

Etiology	
	Voltage defect in the cortical collecting duct (impaired function of ENaC)
Findings	
	Coexistence of alkaline urine pH and hyperkalemia
	Potassium excretion low, urine anion gap positive
	Aldosterone levels low, normal, or elevated
	Acquired in variety of renal diseases and with drugs/toxins
	Autosomal recessive PHAI is best example

in patients with multiple myeloma and amyloidosis (Table 195-9).[459] Some authors describe a third type of PHA, which is associated in adults with overt salt wasting and tubulointerstitial disease but without hypertension. Tubulointerstitial disease with hyperkalemia and hyperchloremic metabolic acidosis with or without salt wasting may be associated with analgesic abuse, sickle cell disease, obstructive uropathy, nephrolithiasis, nephrocalcinosis, and hyperuricemia. Selective hypoaldosteronism has been described in AIDS and in IgM monoclonal gammopathy (Tables 195-9 and 195-10).[459]

Hyperkalemic Distal Renal Tubular Acidosis

A generalized defect in cortical collecting duct secretory function which results in hyperkalemic-hyperchloremic metabolic acidosis has been delineated as hyperkalemic distal RTA because of the coexistence of an inability to acidify the urine ($U_{pH} > 5.5$) during spontaneous acidosis or following an acid load, and hyperkalemia (Table 195-11). The hyperkalemia is the result of impaired renal K^+ secretion and the TTKG and/or the fractional excretion of potassium is invariably lower than expected for the degree of hyperkalemia.[277] Urine ammonium excretion is reduced but aldosterone levels may be low, normal, or even increased. Hyperkalemic distal RTA appears to be the result of a combined voltage and secretory defect in the collecting tubule. This abnormality may be acquired in a wide variety of renal diseases including systemic lupus erythematosus, sickle cell disease, kidney transplant rejection, and amyloidosis, all of which may be associated with an immunologic assault on the collecting tubule. This disorder may also occur in obstructive uropathy in which cortical collecting tubule integrity is compromised. Drugs may be associated with a number of tubular defects which can be manifest as hyperkalemic distal RTA (see below). Hyperkalemic distal RTA can be distinguished from selective hypoaldosteronism because plasma renin and aldosterone levels are usually high or normal. Typically in selective hypoaldosteronism, the U_{pH} is low and the defect in urinary acidification can be attributed to the decrease in ammonium excretion. In contrast to classical hypokalemic distal RTA, patients with hyperkalemic distal RTA do not increase H^+ or K^+ excretion in response to nonreabsorbable anions (Na_2SO_4) or furosemide.[235]

Drug-Induced Renal Tubular Secretory Defects

Impaired Renin-Aldosterone Elaboration. Drugs may impair renin or aldosterone elaboration or produce mineralocorticoid resistance which mimics the clinical manifestations of the acidification defect seen in the generalized form of distal RTA with hyperkalemia (Table 195-9). Cyclooxygenase inhibitors (NSAIDs) can generate hyperkalemia and metabolic acidosis as a result of inhibition of renin release.[462,463] β-Adrenergic antagonists cause hyperkalemia, both as a result of altered potassium distribution and by interference with the renin/aldosterone system. Heparin impairs aldosterone synthesis as a result of direct toxicity to the zona glomerulosa. Angiotensin converting enzyme inhibitors (ACE inhibitors) and angiotensin II receptor (AT_1) antagonists interrupt the RAS and result in hypoaldosteronism with hyperkalemia and acidosis, particularly in the patient with advanced renal insufficiency, or in patients with a tendency to develop hyporeninemic-hypoaldosteronism, such as diabetic nephropathy.[314,315] The combination of potassium-sparing diuretics and ACE inhibitors should be avoided judiciously.

Inhibitors of Potassium Secretion in the Collecting Duct. Spironolactone acts as a competitive inhibitor of aldosterone, inhibits aldosterone biosynthesis, and may be a frequent cause of hyperkalemia and metabolic acidosis when administered to patients with significant renal insufficiency.[259,260,276,464] Similarly, amiloride and triamterene may be associated with this disorder.[465] Both of these potassium-sparing diuretics block the apical Na^+-selective channel in the collecting duct principal cell, which alters the driving force for K^+ secretion (Fig. 195-9). Amiloride is the prototype for a growing number of agents, including trimethoprim and pentamidine, that act similarly to cause hyperkalemia, particularly in patients with AIDS. Trimethoprim and pentamidine are related structurally to amiloride and triamterene because all of these agents are heterocyclic weak bases that exist primarily in the protonated forms in acid urine.[466] The protonated forms of both trimethoprim and pentamidine were demonstrated by Kleyman and Ling[466,467] to inhibit the highly selective Na^+ channel in A6 distal nephron cells. This effect in A6 cells was verified in rat late distal tubules perfused in vivo.[468] Hyperkalemia has been observed in 20 to 50 percent of HIV-infected patients receiving high-dose TMP-SMX or TMP-dapsone for the treatment of opportunistic infections, and in as much as 100 percent of patients with AIDS-associated infections (*Pneumocystis carinii*) receiving pentamidine for more than 6 days.[468] Because both TMP and pentamidine

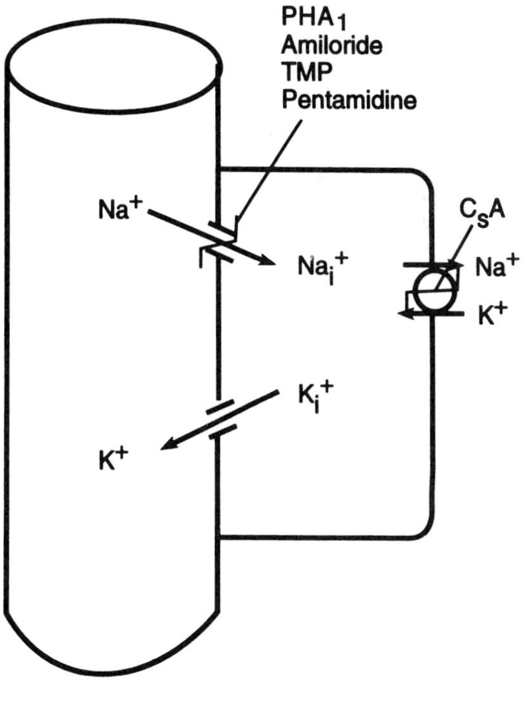

Fig. 195-9 Two examples of "voltage" defects in Na^+ transport across the apical membrane of a principal cell in the cortical collecting tubule: (1) the Na^+ channel (ENaC) is blocked or occupied by amiloride, trimethoprim, or pentamidine and (2) limitation of basolateral Na^+,K^+-ATPase activity by cyclosporin A (CsA). As a consequence of impaired Na^+ uptake, transepithelial K^+ secretion is impaired, leading to hyperkalemia. The pathogenesis of metabolic acidosis, when present, is the result of the unfavorable voltage (which impairs H^+ secretion by the type A intercalated cell, not shown) or through the inhibition of ammonium production and transport as a consequence of hyperkalemia.

decrease the electrochemical driving force for both K^+ and H^+ secretion in the CCT, metabolic acidosis frequently accompanies the hyperkalemia, even in the absence of severe renal failure, adrenal insufficiency, severe tubulointerstitial disease, or hypoaldosteronism. While it has been assumed that such a "voltage" defect could explain the decrease in H^+ secretion, it is likely that hyperkalemia plays a significant role in the development of the metabolic acidosis through a decrease in ammonium production and excretion. Ammonium excretion has not been systematically investigated in patients with hyperkalemia receiving either agent, however.

Cyclosporine A (CsA) and FK506 may be associated with hyperkalemia in the transplant recipient as a result of inhibition of the basolateral Na^+,K^+-ATPase, thereby decreasing intracellular $[K^+]$ and the transepithelial potential, which together decrease the driving force for K^+ secretion (Fig. 195-9).[469,470] It has been suggested that the specific mechanism of CsA inhibition of the Na^+ pump is through inhibition by this agent of calcineurin activity.[471] CsA could also decrease the filtered load of K^+ through hemodynamic mechanisms such as vasoconstriction, which decrease GFR and alter the filtration fraction.

Treatment

In hyperkalemic-hyperchloremic metabolic acidosis, documentation of the underlying disorder is necessary and therapy should be based on a precise diagnosis if possible. Of particular importance is a careful drug and dietary history. Contributing or precipitating factors should be considered and include low urine flow or decreased distal Na^+ delivery; a rapid decline in GFR (especially in acute superimposed on chronic renal failure); hyperglycemia or hyperosmolality; and unsuspected sources of exogenous K^+ intake. The workup should include evaluation of the TTKG; an estimate of renal ammonium excretion (urine net charge, osmolar gap, and urine pH); the U − B PCO_2; and evaluation of PRA and aldosterone secretion. The latter may be obtained under stimulated conditions with dietary salt restriction and furosemide-induced volume depletion, and the response of the TTKG to furosemide and fludrocortisone. The risk for renal stone disease is generally considered to be low in type 4 RTA.[472]

The decision to treat is often based on the severity of the hyperkalemia. Reduction in serum potassium will often improve the metabolic acidosis by increasing ammonium excretion as potassium levels return to the normal range.

Patients with combined glucocorticoid and mineralocorticoid deficiency should receive both adrenal steroids in replacement dosages. Patients with hyporeninemic-hypoaldosteronism may respond to a cation exchange resin (sodium polystyrene sulfonate), alkali therapy, or treatment with a loop diuretic to induce renal potassium and salt excretion (Table 195-12). Volume depletion should be avoided unless the patient is volume overexpanded or hypertensive. Supraphysiological doses of mineralocorticoids may be necessary, but should be administered cautiously in combination with a loop diuretic to avoid volume overexpansion or aggravation of hypertension and to increase potassium excretion.[458]

Infants with pseudohypoaldosteronism type I should receive salt supplement in amounts sufficient to correct the syndrome and allow normal growth,[473] while patients with pseudohypoaldosteronism type II should receive thiazide diuretics along with dietary salt restriction.[295,342]

While it may be prudent to discontinue drugs that are identified as the most likely cause of the hyperkalemia, this may not always be feasible in the patient with a life-threatening disorder; for example, during TMP-SMX or pentamidine therapy in the AIDS patient with PCP. Based on the analysis above of the mechanism by which TMP and pentamidine cause hyperkalemia (voltage defect), it might also be reasoned that the delivery to the CCD of a poorly reabsorbed anion might improve the electrochemical driving force favoring K^+ and H^+ secretion. The combined use of acetazolamide along with sufficient sodium bicarbonate to deliver HCO_3^- to the CCT and thereby increase the negative transepithelial voltage, could theoretically increase K^+ and H^+ secretion.[469] With such an approach, aggravation of metabolic acidosis by excessive acetazolamide or insufficient $NaHCO_3$ administration must be avoided. This approach, while feasible, has not been corroborated by clinical trials.

In summary, hyperkalemia plays a pivotal role in the response of the kidney to metabolic acidosis. Treatment should be directed toward correction of the hyperkalemia, restoration of euvolemia, adequate alkali therapy, loop diuretics, and dietary potassium restriction (Table 195-12). In severe hypoaldosteronism, the effect of loop diuretics can be augmented significantly by administration of small doses of mineralocorticoid. Fludrocortisone should be used cautiously, however, and avoided in the face of hypertension or congestive heart failure.

Table 195-12 Treatment of Generalized Dysfunction of the Nephron with Hyperkalemia

Alkali therapy
Loop diuretic (furosemide, bumetanide)
Sodium polysterene sulfonate (Kayexalate)
Fludrocortisone (0.1–0.3 mg/day)
Avoid in hypertension, volume expansion, heart failure
Combine with loop diuretic
Avoid drugs associated with hyperkalemia in PHAI-NaCl

REFERENCES

1. Teree TM, Mirabal-Font E, Ortiz A, Wallace WM: Stool losses and acidosis in diarrheal disease of infancy. *Pediatrics* **36**:704, 1965.
2. Emmett M, Seldin DW: Clinical syndromes of metabolic acidosis and metabolic alkalosis, in Seldin DW, Giebisch G (eds): *The Kidney: Physiology and Pathophysiology*, 2nd ed. New York, Raven Press, 1992, p 2759.
3. Halperin ML, Goldstein MB, Richardson RMA, Stinebaugh BJ: Distal renal tubular acidosis syndromes: A pathophysiological approach. *Am J Nephrology* **5**:1, 1985.
4. Halperin M, Goldstein MB, Jungas RL, Stinebaugh BJ: Biochemistry and physiology of ammonium excretion, in Seldin DW, Giebisch G (eds): *The Kidney: Physiology and Pathophysiology*, 2nd ed., New York, Raven Press, 1992, p 2645.
5. Goldstein MB, Bear R, Richardson RMA, Marsden PA, Halperin ML: The urine anion gap: A clinically useful index of ammonium excretion. *Am J Med Sci* **292**:198, 1986.
6. Carlisle EJF, Donnelly SM, Halperin ML: Renal tubular acidosis (RTA): Recognize the ammonium defect and pHorget the urine pH. *Pediatr Nephrol* **5**:242, 1991.
7. Kleinman PK: Cholestyramine and metabolic acidosis. *N Engl J Med* **290**:861, 1974.
8. D'Agostino A, Leadbetter WF, Schwartz WB: Alterations in the ionic composition of isotonic saline solution instilled into the colon. *J Clin Invest* **32**:444, 1953.
9. Stamey TA: The pathogenesis and implications of the electrolyte imbalance in ureterosigmoidostomy. *Surg Gynecol Obstet* **103**:736, 1956.
10. Heird WC, Dell RB, Driscoll JM, Grebin B, Winters RW: Metabolic acidosis resulting from intravenous alimentation mixtures containing synthetic amino acids. *N Engl J Med* **287**:943, 1972.
11. DuBose TD Jr: Acid-base balance, in Eknoyan G, Knochel JP (eds): *The Systemic Consequences of Renal Failure*. Orlando, Grune and Stratton, 1984, p 421.
12. Widmer B, Gerhardt RE, Harrington JT, Cohen JJ: The influence of graded degrees of chronic renal failure. *Arch Int Med* **139**:1099, 1979.
13. Gonick HC, Kleeman CR, Rubini ME, Maxwell MH: Functional impairment in chronic renal failure. *Nephron* **6**:28, 1969.
14. Cogan MG, Rector FC Jr: Acid-base disorders, in Brenner BM, Rector FC Jr (eds): *The Kidney*, 4th ed. Philadelphia, WB Saunders, 1991, p 737.
15. Fine LG, Yanagaawa N, Schultz RG, Bricker N: Functional profile of the isolated uremic nephron. Potassium adaptation in the rabbit cortical collecting tubule. *J Clin Invest* **64**:1033, 1979.

16. Van Ypersele de Strihou C: Potassium homeostasis in renal failure. *Kidney Int* **11**:491, 1977.
17. Rector FC Jr, Carter NW, Seldin DW: The mechanism of bicarbonate reabsorption in the proximal and distal tubules of the kidney. *J Clin Invest* **44**:278, 1968.
18. Viera FL, Malnic G: Hydrogen ion secretion by rat renal cortical tubules as studied by an antimony microelectrode. *Am J Physiol* **214**:710, 1968.
19. DuBose TD Jr, Pucacco LR, Carter NW: Determination of disequilibrium pH in the rat kidney in vivo: Evidence for hydrogen secretion. *Am J Physiol* **240**:F138, 1981.
20. Alpern RH, Chambers M: Cell pH in the rat proximal convoluted tubule. Regulation by luminal and peritubular pH and sodium concentration. *J Clin Invest* **78**:502, 1986.
21. Murer H, Hopfer U, Kinne R: Sodium/proton antiport in brush-border membrane vesicles isolated from rat small intestine and kidney. *Biochem J* **154**:597, 1976.
22. Warnock DG, Reenstra WW, Yee VJ: Na^+/H^+ antiporter of brush border vesicles: studies with acridine orange uptake. *Am J Physiol* **238**:F733, 1982.
23. Kinsella JL, Aronson PS: Properties of the Na^+-H^+ exchanger in renal microvillus membrane vesicles. *Am J Physiol* **238**:F461, 1980.
24. Schwartz GJ: Na^+-dependent H^+ efflux from proximal tubule: Evidence for reversible Na^+-H^+ exchange. *Am J Physiol* **241**:F380, 1981.
25. Sasaki S, Shiigai T, Takeuchi J: Intracellular pH in the isolated perfused rabbit proximal straight tubule. *Am J Physiol* **249**:F417, 1985.
26. Preisig PA, Ives HE, Cragoe EJ Jr, Alpern RJ, Rector FC Jr: The role of the Na^+/H^+ antiporter in rat proximal tubule bicarbonate absorption. *J Clin Invest* **80**:970, 1987.
27. Orlowski J, Kandasamy RA, Shull GE: Molecular cloning of putative members of the Na/H exchanger gene family. *J Biol Chem* **267**:9331, 1992.
28. Tse CM, Brant SR, Walker MS, Pouyssegur J, Donowitz M: Cloning and sequencing of a rabbit cDNA encoding an intestinal and kidney-specific Na/H exchanger isoform (NHE-3). *J Biol Chem* **267**:9340, 1992.
29. Biemesderfer D, Pizzonia J, Exner M, Reilly R, Igarashi P, Aronson PS. NHE3: A Na/H exchanger isoform of the renal brush border. *Am J Physiol* **265**:F736, 1992.
30. Amemiya M, Loffing J, Lotscher M, Kaissling B, Alpern RJ, Moe OW: Expression of NHE-3 in the apical membrane of rat renal proximal tubule and thick ascending limb. *Kidney Int* **48**:1206, 1995.
31. Tse CM, Levine SA, Yun CHC, Brant SR, Pouyssegur J, Montrose MH, Donowitz M: Functional characteristics of a cloned epithelial Na/H exchanger (NHE3): Resistance to amiloride and inhibition by protein kinase C. *Proc Natl Acad Sci U S A* **90**:9110, 1993.
32. Orlowski J: Heterologous expression and functional properties of amiloride high affinity (NHE-1) and low affinity (NHE-3) isoforms of the at Na/H exchanger. *J Biol Chem* **268**:16369, 1993.
33. Wu MS, Biemesderfer D, Giebisch G, Aronson P: Role of NHE3 in mediating renal brush border Na^+-H^+ exchange. Adaptation to metabolic acidosis. *J Biol Chem* **271**:32749, 1996.
34. Schultheis PJ, Clarke LL, Meneton P, Miller ML, Soleimani M, Gawenis LR, Riddle TM, et al.: Renal and intestinal absorptive defects in mice lacking the NHE3 Na^+/H^+ exchanger. *Nat Genet* **19**:282, 1998.
35. Schultheis PJ, Clarke LL, Meneton P, Harline M, Boivin GP, Stemmermann G, Duffy JJ, et al.: Targeted disruption of the murine Na^+/H^+ exchanger isoform 2 gene causes reduced viability of gastric parietal cells and loss of net acid secretion. *J Clin Invest* **101**:1243, 1998.
36. Kinne-Saffran E, Beauwens R, Kinne R: An ATP-driven proton pump in brush-border membranes from rat renal cortex. *J Membr Biol* **64**:67, 1982.
37. Chan YL, Giebisch G: Relationship between sodium and bicarbonate transport in the rat proximal convoluted tubule. *Am J Physiol* **240**:F222, 1981.
38. Brown D, Hirsch S, Gluck S: Localization of a proton-pumping ATPase in rat kidney. *J Clin Invest* **82**:2114, 1988.
39. Alpern RJ: Mechanism of basolateral membrane $H^+/OH/HCO_3^-$ transport in the rat proximal convoluted tubule. A sodium-coupled electrogenic process. *J Gen Physiol* **86**:613, 1985.
40. Yoshitomi K, Burckhardt B-CH, Frömter E: Rheogenic sodium-bicarbonate cotransport in the peritubular cell membrane of rat renal proximal tubule. *Pflügers Arch* **405**:360, 1985.
41. Boron WF, Boulpaep EL: Intracellular pH regulation in the renal proximal tubule of the salamander: Basolateral HCO_3^- transport. *J Gen Physiol* **81**:53, 1983.
42. Akiba T, Alpern RJ, Eveloff J, Calamina J, Warnock DG: Electrogenic sodium/bicarbonate cotransport in rabbit renal cortical basolateral membrane vesicles. *J Clin Invest* **78**:1472, 1986.
43. Solemani M, Aronson PS: Ionic mechanism of $Na^+/H^+/CO_3^=$ cotransport in rabbit renal basolateral membranes. *J Biol Chem* **264**:18302, 1989.
44. Sasaki S, Shiigai T, Yoshiyama N, Takeuchi J: Mechanism of bicarbonate exit across basolateral membrane of rabbit proximal straight tubule. *Am J Physiol* **21**:F11, 1987.
45. Romero MF, Hediger MA, Boulpaep EL, Boron WF: Expression cloning and characterization of a renal electrogenic Na^+/HCO_3^- cotransporter. *Nature* **387**:409, 1997.
46. Romero MF, Fong P, Berger UT, Hediger MA, Boron WF: Cloning and functional expression of rNBC, an electrogenic Na^+-HCO_3^- cotransporter from rat kidney. *Am J Physiol* **274**:F425, 1998.
47. Dobyan DC, Bulger RE: Renal carbonic anhydrase. *Am J Physiol* **243**:F311, 1982.
48. Alpern RJ, Stone DK, Rector FC Jr: Renal acidification mechanisms, in Brenner BM, Rector FC Jr (eds): *The Kidney*, 4th ed. Philadelphia, WB Saunders, 1991, p 318.
49. Lucci MS, Tinker J, Weiner I, DuBose TD: Function of proximal tubule carbonic anhydrase defined by selective inhibition. *Am J Physiol* **245**:F535, 1983.
50. Wahlstrand T, Wistrand PJ: Carbonic anhydrase C in the human renal medulla. *Uppsala J Med Sci* **85**:7, 1980.
51. Alpern RJ, Cogan MG, Rector FC Jr: Effect of luminal bicarbonate concentration on proximal acidification in the rat. *Am J Physiol* **243**:F53, 1982.
52. Chan YL, Malnic G, Giebisch G: Passive driving forces of proximal tubular fluid and bicarbonate transport: Gradient -dependence of H^+ section. *Am J Physiol* **245**:F622, 1983.
53. Holmberg C, Kokko JP, Jacobson HR: Determination of chloride and bicarbonate permeabilities in proximal convoluted tubules. *Am J Physiol* **241**:F386, 1981.
54. Sasaki S, Berry CA, Rector FC Jr: Effect of luminal and peritubular HCO_3^- concentrations and PCO_2 on HCO_3^- reabsorption in rabbit proximal convoluted tubules perfused in vitro. *J Clin Invest* **70**:639, 1982.
55. Warnock DG, Yee VJ: Anion permeabilities of the isolated perfused rabbit proximal tubule. *Am J Physiol* **242**:F395, 1982.
56. Hamm LL, Pucacco LR, Kokko JP, Jacobson HR: Hydrogen ion permeability of the rabbit proximal convoluted tubule. *Am J Physiol* **246**:F3, 1984.
57. Pajor AM: Sequence and functional characterization of a renal sodium/dicarboxylate cotransporter. *J Biol Chem* **270**:5779, 1995.
58. Melnick JZ, Srere PA, Elshourbagy NA, Moe OW, Preisig PA, Alpern RJ: Adenosine triphosphate citrate lyase mediates hypocitraturia in rats. *J Clin Invest* **98**:2381, 1996.
59. Simpson DP. Citrate excretion: A window on renal metabolism. *Am J Physiol* **244**:F223, 1983.
60. Jenkins AD, Dousa TP, Smith LH: Transport of citrate across renal brush border membrane: Effects of dietary acid and alkali loading. *Am J Physiol* **249**:F590, 1985.
61. Melnick JZ, Preisig PA, Moe OW, Srere PA, Alpern RJ: Renal cortical mitochondrial aconitase is regulated in hypo- and hypercitraturia. *Kidney Int* **54**:160, 1996.
62. Green R, Bishop JHV, Giebisch G: Ionic requirements of proximal tubular sodium transport. III. Selective luminal anion substitution. *Am J Physiol* **236**:F268, 1979.
63. Jacobson HR: Characteristics of volume reabsorption in rabbit superficial and juxtamedullary proximal convoluted tubules. *J Clin Invest* **63**:410, 1979.
64. Baum M, Berry CA: Evidence for neutral transcellular NaCl transport and neutral basolateral chloride exit in the rabbit proximal convoluted tubule. *J Clin Invest* **74**:205, 1984.
65. Alpern RJ, Howlin KJ, Preisig PA: Active and passive components of chloride transport in the rat proximal convoluted tubule. *J Clin Invest* **76**:1360, 1985.
66. Lucci MS, Warnock DG: Effects of anion-transport inhibitors on NaCl reabsorption in the rat superficial proximal convoluted tubule. *J Clin Invest* **64**:570, 1979.
67. Baum M: Evidence that parallel Na^+-H^+ and Cl^--$HCO_3^-(OH^-)$ antiporters transport NaCl in the proximal tubule. *Am J Physiol* **252**:F338, 1987.

68. Karniski LP, Aronson PS: Chloride/formate exchange with formic acid recycling: A mechanism of active chloride transport across epithelial membranes. *Proc Natl Acad Sci U S A* **82**:6362, 1985.
69. Alpern RJ: Apical membrane chloride/base exchange in the rat proximal convoluted tubule. *J Clin Invest* **79**:1026, 1987.
70. Pitts RF, Lotspeich WD: Bicarbonate and the renal regulation of acid-base balance. *Am J Physiol* **147**:138, 1946.
71. Alpern RJ, Cogan MG, Rector FC Jr: Effects of extracellular fluid volume and plasma bicarbonate concentration on proximal acidification in the rat. *J Clin Invest* **71**:736, 1983.
72. Berliner RW, Kennedy TJ, Hilton JG: Effect of maleic acid on renal function. *Proc Soc Exp Biol Med* **75**:791, 1951.
73. Al-Bander HA, Weiss RA, Humphreys MH, Morris RC Jr: Dysfunction of the proximal tubule underlies maleic acid-induced type II renal tubular acidosis. *Am J Physiol* **243**:F604, 1982.
74. Bergeron M, DuBord L, Hausser C: Membrane permeability as a cause of transport defects in experimental Fanconi syndrome. A new hypothesis. *J Clin Invest* **57**:1181, 1976.
75. Maesaka JK, McCaffery M: Evidence for renal tubular leakage in maleic acid-induced Fanconi syndrome. *Am J Physiol* **239**:F507, 1980.
76. Hoppe A, Gmaj P, Metler M, Angielski S: Additive inhibition of renal bicarbonate reabsorption by maleate plus acetazolamide. *Am J Physiol* **231**:1258, 1976.
77. Gougoux A, Lemieux G, Lavoie N: Maleate-induced bicarbonaturia in the dog: A carbonic anhydrase-independent effect. *Am J Physiol* **231**:1010, 1976.
78. Gmaj P, Hoppe A, Angielski S, Rogulski J: Acid-base behavior of the kidney in maleate-treated rats. *Am J Physiol* **222**:1182, 1972.
79. Bank N, Aynedjian HS, Mutz BF: Microperfusion study of proximal tubule bicarbonate transport in maleic acid-induced renal tubular acidosis. *Am J Physiol* **250**:F476, 1986.
80. Reboucas NA, Fernandes DT, Elias MM, De Mello-Aires M, Malnic G: Proximal tubular HCO_3^-, H^+ and fluid transport during maleate-induced acidification defect. *Pflügrs Arch* **401**:266, 1984.
81. Günther R, Silbernagl S, Deetjen P: Maleic acid induced aminoaciduria, studied by free flow micropuncture and continuous microperfusion. *Pflügers Arch* **382**:109, 1979.
82. Salmon RF, Baum M: Intracellular cystine loading inhibits transport in the rabbit proximal convoluted tubule. *J Clin Invest* **85**:340, 1990.
83. Silverman M: The mechanism of maleic acid nephropathy: investigations using brush border membrane vesicles. *Membr Biochem* **4**:63, 1981.
84. Reynolds R, McNamara PD, Segal S: On the maleic acid induced Fanconi syndrome: Effects on transport by isolated rat kidney brush border membrane vesicles. *Life Sci* **22**:39, 1978.
85. Silverman M, Huang L: Mechanism of maleic acid-induced glucosuria in dog kidney. *Am J Physiol* **231**:1024, 1976.
86. Le Grimellec C, Carriere S, Cardinal J, Giocondi MC: Effect of maleate on membrane physical state of brush border and basolateral membranes of the dog kidney. *Life Sci* **30**:1107, 1982.
87. Kramer HJ, Gonick HC: Experimental Fanconi syndrome. I. Effect of maleic acid on renal cortical Na^+-K^+-ATPase activity and ATP levels. *J Lab Clin Med* **76**:799, 1970.
88. Coor C, Salmon RF, Quigley R, Marver D, Baum M: Role of adenosine triphosphate (ATP) and Na^+-K^+ ATPase in inhibition of proximal tubule transport with intracellular cystine loading. *J Clin Invest* **87**:955, 1991.
89. Angielski S, Rogulski J: Effect of maleic acid on the kidney. I. Oxidation of Krebs cycle intermediates by various tissues of maleate intoxicated rats. *Acta Biochim Pol* **9**:357, 1962.
90. Al-Bander H, Etheredge SB, Paukert T, Humphreys MH, Morris RC Jr: Phosphate loading attenuates renal tubular dysfunction induced by maleic acid in the dog. *Am J Physiol* **248**:F513, 1985.
91. Al-Bander HA, Mock DM, Etheredge SB, Paukert TT, Humphreys MH, Morris RC Jr: Coordinately increased lysozymuria and lysosomal enzymuria induced by maleic acid. *Kidney Int* **30**:804, 1987.
92. Burch HB, Choi S, Dence CN, Alvey TR, Cole BR, Lowry OH: Metabolic effects of large fructose loads in different parts of the rat nephron. *J Biol Chem* **255**:8239, 1980.
93. Morris RC Jr, Nigon K, Reed EB: Evidence that the severity of depletion of inorganic phosphate determines the severity of the disturbance of adenine nucleotide metabolism in the liver and renal cortex of the fructose-loaded rat. *J Clin Invest* **61**:209, 1978.
94. Fraser D, Kooh SW, Scriver CR: Hyperparathyroidism as the cause of hyperaminoaciduria and phosphaturia in human vitamin deficiency. *Pediatr Res* **9**:593, 1975.
95. Guignard JP, Torrado A: Proximal renal tubular acidosis in vitamin D deficiency rickets. *Acta Pediatr Scand* **62**:543, 1973.
96. Vainsel M, Manderlier T, Vis HL: Proximal renal tubular acidosis in vitamin D deficiency rickets. *Biomedicine* **22**:35, 1975.
97. Reade TM, Scriver CR, Glorieux FH, Nogrady B, Delvin E, Poirier R, Holick MF, Deluca HF: Response to crystalline 1 α-hydroxyvitamin D_3 in vitamin D dependency. *Pediatr Res* **9**:593, 1975.
98. Huguenin M, Schacht R, David R: Infantile rickets with severe proximal renal tubular acidosis, responsive to vitamin D. *Arch Dis Child* **49**:955, 1974.
99. Bank N, Aynedjian HS: A micropuncture study of the effect of parathyroid hormone on renal bicarbonate reabsorption. *J Clin Invest* **58**:336, 1976.
100. Iino Y, Burg MB: Effect of parathyroid hormone on bicarbonate absorption by proximal tubules in vitro. *Am J Physiol* **236**:F387, 1979.
101. McKinney TD, Myers P: PTH inhibition of bicarbonate transport by proximal convoluted tubules. *Am J Physiol* **239**:F127, 1980.
102. McKinney TD, Myers P: Bicarbonate transport by proximal tubules: Effect of parathyroid hormone and dibutyryl cyclic AMP. *Am J Physiol* **238**:F166, 1980.
103. Hulter HN, Toto RD, Ilnicki LP, Halloran B, Sebastian A: Metabolic alkalosis in models of primary and secondary hyperparathyroid states. *Am J Physiol* **245**:F450, 1983.
104. Mitnick P, Greenberg A, Coffman T, Kelepouris E, Wolf CJ, Goldfarb S: Effects of two models of hypercalcemia on renal acid base metabolism. *Kidney Int* **21**:613, 1982.
105. Bichara M, Mercier O, Paillard M, Prigent A: Effects of parathyroid hormone on urinary acidification. *Am J Physiol* **251**:F444, 1986.
106. Mercier O, Bichara M, Paillard M, Prigent A: Effects of parathyroid hormone and urinary phosphate on collecting duct hydrogen section. *Am J Physiol* **251**:F802, 1986.
107. Cano A, Preisig P, Alpern RJ: Cyclic adenosine monophosphate acutely inhibits and chronically stimulates Na/H antiporter in OKP cells. *J Clin Invest* **92**:1632, 1993.
108. Cano, Preisig P, Miller RT, Alpern RJ: PTH acutely inhibits and chronically stimulates the Na/H antiporter in OKP cells [Abstract]. *J Am Soc Nephrol* **4**:834, 1993.
109. McKinney TD, Myers P: Effect of calcium and phosphate on bicarbonate and fluid transport by proximal tubules in vitro. *Kidney Int* **21**:433, 1982.
110. Peraino RA, Ghafary E, Rouse D, Stinebaugh BJ, Suki WN: Effect of 25-hydroxycholecalciferol on renal handling of sodium, calcium, and phosphate during bicarbonate infusion. *Miner Electrolyte Metab* **1**:321, 1978.
111. Puschett JB, Moranz J, Kurnick WS: Evidence for a direct action of cholecalciferol and 25-hydroxycholecalciferol on the renal transport of phosphate, sodium, and calcium. *J Clin Invest* **51**:373, 1972.
112. Gekle D, Ströder, Rostock D: The effect of vitamin D on renal inorganic phosphate reabsorption of normal rats, parathyroidectomized rats, and rats with rickets. *Pediatr Res* **5**:40, 1971.
113. Grose JH, Scriver CR: Parathyroid-dependent phosphaturia and aminoaciduria in the vitamin D-deficient rat. *Am J Physiol* **214**:370, 1968.
114. Morris RC Jr, McSherry E, Sebastian A: Modulation of experimental renal dysfunction of hereditary fructose intolerance by circulating parathyroid hormone. *Proc Natl Acad Sci U S A* **68**:132, 1971.
115. Brewer ED, Tsai HC, Szeto KS, Morris RC Jr: Maleic acid-induced impaired conversion of $25(OH)D_3$: Implications for Fanconi's syndrome. *Kidney Int* **12**:244, 1977.
116. Chesney RW, Kaplan BS, Phelps M, Deluca HF: Renal tubular acidosis does not alter circulating values of calcitriol. *J Pediatr* **104**:51, 1984.
117. Walker WG, Dickerman H, Jost LJ: Mechanism of lysine-induced kaliuresis. *Am J Physiol* **206**:409, 1964.
118. Chan YL, Kurtzman NA: Effects of lysine on bicarbonate and fluid absorption in the rat proximal tubule. *Am J Physiol* **242**:F604, 1982.
119. Frömter E: Solute transport across epithelia: What can we learn from micropuncture studies on kidney tubules? *J Physiol* **288**:1, 1979.
120. Hoshi T, Sudo K, Suzuki Y: Characteristics of changes in the intracellular potential associated with transport of neutral, dibasic and acidic amino acids in Trituris proximal tubule. *Biochem Biophys Acta* **44**:492, 1976.
121. Cox GA, Lutz CM, Yang C-L, Biemesderfer D, Bronson RT, Fu A, Aronson PS, et al.: Sodium/hydrogen exchanger gene defect in slow-wave epilepsy mutant mice. *Cell* **91**:139, 1997.
122. Sly WS, Whyte MP, Sundaram V, Tashian RE, Hewett-Emmett D, Guibaud P, Vainsel M, et al.: Carbonic anhydrase II deficiency in 12 families with the autosomal recessive syndrome of osteopetrosis with

renal tubular acidosis and cerebral calcification. *N Engl J Med* **313**:139, 1985.

123. Sly WS, Hewett-Emmett D, Whyte MP, Yu YSL, Tashian RE: Carbonic anhydrase II deficiency identified as the primary defect in the autosomal recessive syndrome of osteopetrosis with renal tubular acidosis and cerebral calcification. *Proc Natl Acad Sci U S A* **80**:2752, 1983.
124. Bregman H, Brown J, Rogers A, Bourke E: Osteopetrosis with combined proximal and distal renal tubular acidosis. *Am J Kidney Dis* II:357, 1982.
125. Bourke E, Delaney VB, Mosawi M, Reavey P, Weston M: Renal tubular acidosis and osteopetrosis in siblings. *Nephron* **28**:268, 1981.
126. Kondo T, Taniguchi N, Taniguchi K, Matsuda I, Murao M: Inactive form of erythrocyte carbonic anhydrase B in patients with primary renal tubular acidosis. *J Clin Invest* **62**:610, 1978.
127. Shapira E, Ben-Yoseph Y, Eyal FG, Russell A: Enzymatically inactive red cell carbonic anhydrase B in a family with renal tubular acidosis. *J Clin Invest* **53**:59, 1974.
128. Kendall AG, Tashian RE: Erythrocyte carbonic anhydrase I: Inherited deficiency in humans. *Science* **197**:471, 1977.
129. Brenes LG, Sanchez MI: Impaired urinary ammonium excretion in patients with isolated proximal renal tubular acidosis. *J Am Soc Neph* **4**:1073, 1993.
130. Brenner RJ, Spring DB, Sebastian A, McSherry EM, Genant HK, Palubinskas AJ, Morris RC Jr: Incidence of radiographically evident bone disease, nephrocalcinosis, and nephrolithiasis in various types of renal tubular acidosis. *N Engl J Med* **307**:217, 1982.
131. Rodriguez-Soriano J, Vallo A, Castillo G, Oliveros R: Renal handling of water and sodium in children with proximal and distal renal tubular acidosis. *Nephron* **25**:193, 1980.
132. Brenes LG, Brenes JN, Hernandez MM: Familial proximal renal tubular acidosis. A distinct clinical entity. *Am J Med* **63**:244, 1977.
133. Nash MA, Torrado AD, Greifer I, Spitzer A, Edelmann CM Jr: Renal tubular acidosis in infants and children. *J Pediatr* **80**:738, 1972.
134. Sebastian A, McSherry E, Morris RC Jr: On the mechanism of renal potassium wasting in renal tubular acidosis associated with the Fanconi syndrome (Type 2 RTA). *J Clin Invest* **50**:231, 1971.
135. Peraino RA, Suki WN: Urine HCO_3- augments renal Ca^2 absorption independent of systemic acid-base changes. *Am J Physiol* **238**:F394, 1980.
136. Callis L, Castello F, Fortuny G, Vallo A, Ballabriga A: Effect of hydrochlorothiazide on rickets and on renal tubular acidosis in two patients with cystinosis. *Helv Paediatr Acta* **6**:602, 1970.
137. Rampini S, Fanconi A, Illig R, Prader A: Effect of hydrochlorothiazide on proximal renal tubular acidosis in a patient with idiopathic "de Toni-Debre-Fanconi syndrome." *Helv Paediatr Acta* **1**:13, 1968.
138. McKinney TD, Burg MG: Bicarbonate transport by rabbit cortical collection tubules; effect of acid and alkali loads in vivo on transport in vitro. *J Clin Invest* **60**:766, 1977.
139. Atkins JL, Burg MB: Bicarbonate transport by isolated perfused rat collecting ducts. *Am J Physiol* **249**:F485, 1985.
140. Schwartz GJ, Barasch J, Al-Awqati Q: Plasticity of functional epithelial polarity. *Nature* **318**:368, 1985.
141. Lucci MS, Pucacco LR, Carter NW, DuBose TD Jr: Evaluation of bicarbonate transport in the rat distal tubule: Effects of acid-base status. *Am J Physiol* **243**:F335, 1982.
142. Levine DZ: An in vivo microperfusion study of distal tubule reabsorption in normal and ammonium chloride rats. *J Clin Invest* **75**:588, 1985.
143. Iacovitti M, Nash L, Peterson LN, Rochon J, Levine DZ: Distal tubule bicarbonate accumulation in vivo. Effect of flow and transtubule bicarbonate gradients. *J Clin Invest* **78**:1658, 1986
144. Lombard WE, Kokko JP, Jacobson HR: Bicarbonate transport in cortical and outer medullary collecting tubules. *Am J Physiol* **244**:F289, 1983.
145. Stokes JB: Na and K transport across the cortical and outer medullary collecting tubule of the rabbit: Evidence for diffusion across the outer medullary portion. *Am J Physiol* **242**:F514, 1982.
146. Ullrich KJ, Papavassiliou F: Bicarbonate reabsorption in the papillary collecting duct of rats. *Pflügers Arch* **289**:271, 1981.
147. Graber ML, Bengele HH, Schwartz JH, Alexander EA: pH and PCO_2 profiles of the rat inner medullary collecting duct. *Am J Physiol* **241**:F659, 1981.
148. DuBose TD Jr, Good DW: Role of the thick ascending limb and inner medullary collecting duct in the regulation of urinary acidification. *Semin Nephrol* **11**:120, 1991.
149. Wall SM, Knepper MA: Acid-base transport in the inner medullary collecting duct. *Semin Nephrol* **10**:148, 1990.
150. Madsen KM, Clapp WL, Verlander JW: Structure and function of the inner medullary collecting duct. *Kidney Int* **34**:441, 1988.
151. Alpern RJ: Renal acidification mechanisms in Brenner BM (ed): *The Kidney*, 6th ed. Philadelphia, WB Saunders, 2000, pp 455–519.
152. DuBose TD Jr: Hydrogen ion secretion by the collecting duct as a determinant of the urine to blood PCO_2 gradient in alkaline urine. *J Clin Invest* **69**:145, 1982.
153. Koeppen BM, Helman SI: Acidification of luminal fluid by the rabbit cortical collecting tubule perfused in vitro. *Am J Physiol* **242**:F521, 1982.
154. McKinney TD, Burg MB: Bicarbonate absorption by rabbit cortical collecting tubules in vitro. *Am J Physiol* **234**:F141, 1978.
155. Stone DS, Seldin DW, Kokko JP, Jacobson HR: Mineralocorticoid modulation of rabbit medullary collecting duct acidification. A sodium-independent acidification. *J Clin Invest* **72**:77, 1983.
156. Gluck S, Al-Awqati Q: An electrogenic proton-translocating adenosine triphosphatase from bovine kidney medulla. *J Clin Invest* **73**:1704, 1984.
157. Stone DK, Xie XS, Racker E: Comparison of the proton ATPase and chloride transporter from bovine clathrin-coated vesicles and renal medullary vesicles [Abstract]. *Kidney Int* **25**:283, 1984.
158. Diaz-Diaz FD, LaBelle EF, Eaton DC, DuBose TD Jr: ATP-dependent proton transport in human renal medulla. *Am J Physiol* **20**:F297, 1986.
159. Kaunitz JD, Gunther RD, Sachs G: Characterization of an electrogenic ATP and chloride-dependent proton translocating pump from rat renal medulla. *J Biol Chem* **260**:11567, 1985.
160. Bowman BJ, Maizer SE, Allen KE, Slayman SW: Effect of inhibitors on the plasma membrane and mitochondrial adenosine triphosphase of *Neurospora crassa*. *Biochim Biophys Acta* **512**:13, 1987.
161. Stone DK, Xie X-S: Proton translocating ATPases: Issues in structure and function. *Kidney Int* **33**:767, 1988.
162. Gluck S, Bastani B: The biochemistry of distal urinary acidification in health and disease, in De Santo NG, Capasso G (eds): *Acid-Base Balance*. Cosenza, Italy, Editoriale Bios, 1991, p 21.
163. Gluck S, Hirsch S, Brown D: Immunocytochemical localization of H^+-ATPase in rat kidney [Abstract]. *Kidney Int* **31**:167, 1987.
164. Silva F, Schulz W, Davis L, Xie X-S, Stone DK: Immunocytochemical localization of the clathrin-coated vesicle proton pump (CCV-PP). [Abstract]. *Kidney Int* **31**:416, 1987.
165. Gifford JD, Ware MW, Crowson S, Shull GE: Expression of a putative rat distal colonic H^+-K^+-ATPase mRNA in rat kidney: Effect of respiratory acidosis. *J Am Soc Nephrol* **2**:700, 1991.
166. Wingo CS, Madsen KM, Smolka A, Tisher CC: H^+-K^+-ATPase immunoreactivity in cortical and outer medullary collecting duct. *Kidney Int* **38**:985, 1990.
167. DuBose TD Jr, Codina J, Burges A, Pressley TA: Regulation of H^+,K^+ATPase expression in kidney. *Am J Physiol* **269**:F500, 1995.
168. Codina J, Delmas-Mata JT, DuBose TD Jr: Colonic H^+,K^+ATPase ($HK\alpha_2$) protein is upregulated selectively in rat renal medulla by chronic hypokalemia. *J Am Soc Nephrol* **8**:31A, 1997.
169. Wall SM, Truong AV, DuBose TD Jr: H^+,K^+-ATPase mediates net acid secretion in rat terminal inner medullary collecting duct. *Am J Physiol* **271**:F1037, 1996.
170. Guntupalli J, Onuigbo M, Wall SM, Alpern RJ, Dubose TD Jr: Adaptation to low K^+ media increases H^+,K^+-ATPase but not H^+,K^+-ATPase-mediated pH_i recovery in $OMCD_1$ cells. *Am J Physiol* **273**:C558, 1997.
171. Dafnis E, Spohn M, Lonis B, Kurtzman NA, Sabatini S: Vanadate causes hypokalemic distal renal tubular acidosis. *Am J Physiol* **262**:F449, 1992.
172. Bruce LJ, Cope DL, Jones GK, Schofield AE, Murley M, Povey S, Unwin RJ, et al.: Familial distal renal tubular acidosis is associated with mutations in red cell anion exchanger (Band 3, *AE1*) gene. *J Clin Invest* **100**:1693, 1997.
173. Fisher JL, Husted RF, Steinmetz PR: Chloride dependence of the HCO_3^- exit step in urinary acidification by the turtle bladder. *Am J Physiol* **245**:F564, 1983.
174. Stone DK, Seldin DW, Kokko JP, Jacobson HR: Anion dependence of rabbit medullary collecting duct acidification. *J Clin Invest* **71**:1505, 1983.
175. Schuster VL, Bonsib SM, Jennings ML: Two types of collecting duct mitochondria-rich (intercalated) cells: Lectin and band 3 cytochemistry. *Am J Physiol* **20**:C347, 1986.

176. Kudrycki KE, Shull GE: Primary structure of the rat kidney band 3 anion exchange protein deduced from a cDNA. *J Biol Chem* **264**:8185, 1989.
177. Brosius FC III, Alper SL, Garcia AM, Lodish HF: The major kidney band 3 gene transcript predicts an amino-terminal truncated band 3 polypeptide. *J Biol Chem* **264**:7784, 1989.
178. Koeppen BM: Conductive properties of the rabbit outer medullary collecting duct: Inner stripe. *Am J Physiol* **17**:F500, 1985.
179. Schuster VL: Bicarbonate reabsorption and secretion in the cortical and outer medullary collecting duct. *Semin Nephrol* **10**:139, 1990.
180. Leslie BR, Schwartz JH, Steinmetz PR: Coupling between Cl^- absorption and HCO_3^- secretion in turtle urinary bladder. *Am J Physiol* **225**:610, 1973.
181. Husted RF, Eyman E: Chloride-bicarbonate exchange in the urinary bladder of the turtle: Independence from sodium ion. *Biochim Biophys Acta* **595**:305, 1980.
182. Star RA, Burg MB, Knepper MA: Bicarbonate secretion and chloride absorption by rabbit cortical collecting ducts: Role of chloride/bicarbonate exchange. *J Clin Invest* **76**:1123, 1985.
183. Oliver JA, Himmelstein AS, Steinmetz PR: Energy dependence of urinary bicarbonate secretion in turtle bladder. *J Clin Invest* **55**:1003, 1975.
184. Satake N, Durham JH, Ehrenspeck G, Brodsky WA: Active electrogenic mechanisms for alkali and acid transport in turtle bladders. *Am J Physiol* **13**:C259, 1985.
185. Ehrenspeck G: Effect of 3-isobutyl-1-methylxanthine on HCO_3^- transport in turtle bladder: Evidence of electrogenic HCO_3^- secretion. *Biochim Biophys Acta* **684**:219, 1982.
186. Stetson DL, Beauwens R, Palmisano J, Mitchell PP, Steinmetz PR: A double-membrane model for urinary bicarbonate secretion. *Am J Physiol* **18**:F546, 1985.
187. Schuster VL: Cyclic adenosine monophosphate-stimulate bicarbonate secretion in rabbit cortical collecting tubules. *J Clin Invest* **75**:2056, 1985.
188. DuBose TD Jr, Good DW, Hamm LL, Wall SM: Ammonium transport in the kidney: New physiologic concepts and their clinical implications. *J Am Soc Nephrol* **1**:1193, 1991.
189. Good DW, Burg MB: Ammonia production by individual segments of the rat nephron. *J Clin Invest* **73**:602, 1984.
190. Hwang J-J, Curthoys NP: Effect of acute alterations in acid-base balance on rat renal glutaminase and phosphoenolpyruvate carboxykinase gene expression. *J Biol Chem* **266**:9392, 1991.
191. Kaiser S, Curthoys NP: Effect of pH and bicarbonate on phosphoenolpyruvate carboxykinase and glutaminase on mRNA levels in cultured renal epithelial cells. *J Biol Chem* **266**:9397, 1991.
192. Pollock AS, Long JA: The 5′ region of the rat phosphoenolpyruvate carboxykinase gene confers pH sensitivity to chimeric genes expressed in renal and liver cell lines capable of expressing PEPCK. *Biochem Biophysi Res Comm* **164**:81, 1989.
193. Kinsella JL, Aronson PS: Interaction of NH_4^+ and L^{i+} with the renal microvillus membrane Na^+-H^+ exchanger. *Am J Physiol* **241**:C220, 1981.
194. Nagami GT, Sonu CM, Kurokawa K: Ammonia production by isolated mouse proximal tubule perfused in vitro. Effect of metabolic acidosis. *J Clin Invest* **78**:124, 1986.
195. Hamm LL, Trigg D, Martin D, Gillespie C, Buerkert J: Transport of ammonia in the rabbit cortical collecting tubule. *J Clin Invest* **75**:478, 1985.
196. Garvin JL, Burg MB, Knepper MA: NH_3 and NH_4^+ transport by rabbit renal proximal straight tubules. *Am J Physiol* **21**:F232, 1987.
197. DuBose TD Jr, Lucci MS, Hogg RJ, Pucacco LR, Kokko JP, Carter NW: Comparison of acidification parameters in superficial and deep nephrons of the rat. *Am J Physiol* **13**:F497, 1983.
198. Buerkert J, Martin D, Trigg D: Segmental analysis of the renal tubule in buffer production and net acid formation. *Am J Physiol* **244**:F442, 1983.
199. Gottschalk CW, Lassiter WE, Mylle M: Localization of urine acidification in the mammalian kidney. *Am J Physiol* **198**:581, 1960.
200. Good DW, Knepper MA, Burge MB: Ammonia and bicarbonate transport by thick ascending limb of rat kidney. *Am J Physiol* **247**:F35, 1984.
201. Kurtz I, Star R, Balaban RS, Garvin JL, Knepper MA: Spontaneous luminal disequilibrium pH in S_3 proximal tubules. Role in ammonia and bicarbonate transport. *J Clin Invest* **78**:989, 1986.
202. Steinmetz PR, Lawson LR: Effect of luminal pH on ion permeability and flows of Na^+ and H^+ in turtle bladder. *Am J Physiol* **220**:1573, 1971.
203. Good DW, Caflisch CR, DuBose TD Jr: Transepithelial ammonia concentration gradients in inner medulla of the rat. *Am J Physiol* **252**:F491, 1987.
204. Knepper MA, Good DW, Burg MB: Mechanism of ammonia secretion by cortical collecting ducts of rabbits. *Am J Physiol* **247**:F729, 1984.
205. Wall SM, Trinh HN, Woodward KE: Heterogeneity of NH_4^+ transport in mouse inner medullary collecting duct cells. *Am J Physiol* **269**:F356, 1995.
206. Wall SM, Koger LM: NH_4^+ transport mediated by Na^+-K^+-ATPase in rat inner medullary collecting duct. *Am J Physiol* **267**:F660, 1994.
207. Wall SM: Ouabain reduces net acid secretion and increases pH_i by inhibiting NH_4^+ uptake on rat tIMCD Na^+-K^+-ATPase. *Am J Physiol* **273**:F857, 1997.
208. Wall SM: NH_4^+ augments net acid secretion by a ouabain-sensitive mechanism in isolated perfused inner medullary collecting ducts. *Am J Physiol* **270**:F432, 1996.
209. DuBose TD Jr: Hyperkalemic hyperchloremic metabolic acidosis: Pathophysiologic insights. *Kidney Int* **51**:591, 1997.
210. Beauwens R, Al-Awqati Q: Active H^+ transport in the turtle urinary bladder: Coupling of transport to glucose oxidation. *J Gen Physiol* **68**:421, 1976.
211. Al-Awqati Q, Muller A, Steinmetz PR: Transport of H^+ against electrochemical gradients in turtle urinary bladder. *Am J Physiol* **233**:F502, 1977.
212. Laski ME, Kurtzman NA: Characterization of acidification in the cortical and medullary collecting tubule of the rabbit. *J Clin Invest* **72**:2050, 1983.
213. O'Neil RG, Helman SI: Transport characteristics of renal collecting tubules: Influences of DOCA and diet. *Am J Physiol* **233**:F544, 1977.
214. Schwartz GJ, Burg MB: Mineralocorticoid effects on cation transport by cortical collecting tubule in vitro. *Am J Physiol* **235**:F576, 1978.
215. Al-Awqati Q, Norby LH, Mueller A, Steinmetz PR: Characteristics of stimulation of H^+ transport by aldosterone in turtle urinary bladder. *J Clin Invest* **58**:351, 1976.
216. Al-Awqati Q: Effect of aldosterone on the coupling between H^+ transport and glucose oxidation. *J Clin Invest* **60**:1240, 1977.
217. DuBose TD Jr, Caflisch CR: Effect of selective aldosterone deficiency on acidification in nephron segments of the rat inner medulla. *J Clin Invest* **82**:1624, 1988.
218. McKinney TD, Davidson KK: Effect of potassium depletion and protein intake in vivo on renal tubular bicarbonate transport in vitro. *Am J Physiol* **21**:F509, 1987.
219. Hays SR, Seldin DW, Kokko JP, Jacobson HR: Effect of K depletion on HCO_3^- transport across rabbit collecting duct segments [Abstract]. *Kidney Int* **29**:268A, 1986.
220. Tannen RL, McGill J: Influences of potassium on renal ammonia production. *Am J Physiol* **231**:1178, 1976.
221. DuBose TD Jr, Good, DW: Effects of chronic hyperkalemia on renal production and proximal tubule transport of ammonium in the rat. *Am J Physiol* **260**:F680, 1991.
222. Good DW: Active absorption of NH_4^+ by rat medullary thick ascending limb. *Am J Physiol* **255**:F78, 1988.
223. DuBose TD Jr, Good DW: Chronic hyperkalemia impairs ammonium transport and accumulation in the inner medulla of the rat. *J Clin Invest* **90**:1443, 1992.
224. DuBose TD Jr, Codina J: H^+,K^+-ATPase. *Curr Opin Nephrol Hypertens* **5**:411, 1996.
225. Ahn KY, Park KK, Kim KK, Kone BC: Chronic hypokalemia enhances expression of the H^+-K^+-ATPase $\alpha 2$ subunit gene in renal medulla. *Am J Physiol* **271**:F314, 1996.
226. Codina J, Delmas-Mata JT, DuBose TD: Expression of $HK\alpha_2$ protein is increased selectively in renal medulla by chronic hypokalemia. *Am J Physiol* **275**:F433, 1998.
227. Seldin DW, Wilson JD: Renal tubular acidosis, in Stanbury JB, Wyngaarden JB, Fredrickson DS (eds): *The Metabolic Basis of Inherited Disease*, 3rd ed. New York, McGraw-Hill, 1972, p 1548.
228. Rector FC Jr: Acidification of the urine, in Orloff J, Berliner RW (eds): *Renal Physiology, Handbook of Physiology*. Baltimore, Williams and Wilkins, 1973, p 431.
229. Schwartz WB, Jenson RL, Relman AS: Acidification of the urine and increased ammonia excretion without change in acid-base equilibrium: Sodium reabsorption as a stimulus to the acidifying process. *J Clin Invest* **34**:673, 1955.
230. Batlle DC, Sehy JT, Roseman MK, Arruda JAL, Kurtzman NA: Clinical and pathophysiologic spectrum of acquired distal renal tubular acidosis. *Kidney Int* **20**:389, 1981.

231. Arruda JAL, Kurtzman NA: Mechanism and classification of deranged distal urinary acidification. *Am J Physiol* **8**:F515, 1980.
232. Halperin ML, Goldstein MB, Haig A, Johnson MD, Steinbaugh BJ: Studies on the pathogenesis of type 1 (distal) renal tubular acidosis as revealed by the urinary PCO_2 tension. *J Clin Invest* **53**:669, 1974.
233. DuBose TD Jr, Caflisch CR: Validation of the difference in urine and blood CO_2 tension during bicarbonate loading as an index of distal nephron acidification in experimental models of distal renal tubular acidosis. *J Clin Invest* **75**:1116, 1985.
234. Berliner RW, DuBose TD Jr: Carbon dioxide tension of alkaline urine. In Seldin DW, Giebisch G (eds): *The Kidney*. New York, Raven Press, 1992, p 2681.
235. Batlle DC: Segmental characterization of defects in collecting tubule acidification. *Kidney Int* **30**:546, 1986.
236. Bonilla-Felix M: Primary distal renal tubular acidosis as a result of a gradient defect. *Am J Kidney Dis* **27**:428, 1996.
237. Zawadzki J: Permeability defect with bicarbonate leak as a mechanism of immune-related distal renal tubular acidosis. *Am J Kidney Dis* **31**:527, 1998.
238. Capasso G, Schultz H, Vickermann B, Kinne R: Amphotericin B and amphotericin B methylester: Effect on brush border membrane permeability. *Kidney Int* **30**:311, 1986.
239. Steinmetz PR, Lawson LR: Defect in acidification induced in vitro by amphotericin B. *J Clin Invest* **49**:596, 1970.
240. Julka N, Arruda JAL, Kurtzman NA: The mechanism of amphotericin-induced distal acidification defect in rats. *Clin Sci* **56**:555, 1979.
241. Garg LC: Lack of effect of amphotericin-B on urine-blood PCO_2 gradient in spite of urinary acidification defect. *Pflügers Arch* **381**:137, 1979.
242. Taher SM, Anderson RJ, McCartney R, Popovtzer MM, Schrier RW: Renal tubular acidosis associated with toluene "sniffing." *N Engl J Med* **290**:765, 1974.
243. Kurtzman NA: Acquired distal renal tubular acidosis. *Kidney Int* **24**:807, 1983.
244. Bastani B, Haragsim L, Gluck SI, Siamopoulos KC: Lack of H^+-ATPase in distal nephron causing hypokalemic distal RTA in a patient with Sjögren's syndrome. *Nephrol Dial Transplant* **10**:908, 1995.
245. Bastani B, Chu N, Yang L, Gluck SI: Presence of intercalated cell H^+-ATPase in two lupus nephritis patients with distal RTA and autoantibody to a kidney peptide. *J Am Soc Nephrol* **4**:283A, 1993.
246. Wingo CS: Active proton secretion and potassium absorption in the rabbit outer medullary collecting duct. *J Clin Invest* **84**:361, 1989.
247. Nimmannit S, Malasit P, Chaovakul V, Susaengrat W, Vasuvattakul S, Nilwarangkur S: Pathogenesis of sudden unexplained nocturnal death (lai tai) and endemic distal renal tubular acidosis. *Lancet* **338**:930, 1991.
248. Sitprija V, Tungsanga K, Eiam-Ong S, Leelhaphunt N, Sriboonlue P: Renal tubular acidosis, vanadium, and buffaloes. *Nephron* **54**:97, 1990.
249. Mujais SK: Transport enzymes and renal tubular acidosis. *Semin Nephrol* **18**:74, 1998.
250. Nimmannit S, Malasit P, Susaengrat W, Ong-Aj-Yooth S, Vasuvattakul S, Pidetcha P, Shayakul C, et al.: Prevalence of endemic distal renal tubular acidosis and renal stone in the northeast of Thailand. *Nephron* **72**:604, 1996.
251. Nilwarangkur S, Malasit P, Nimmannit S, Susaengrat W, Ong-Aj-Yoth S, Vasuvattakul S, Pidetcha P: Urinary constituents in an endemic area of stones and renal tubular acidosis in northeastern Thailand. *Southeast Asian J Trop Med Public Health* **21**:437, 1990.
252. Nilwarangkur S, Nimmannit S, Chaovakul V, Susaengrat W, Ong-Aj-Yooth S, Vasuvattakul S, Pidetcha P, et al.: Endemic primary distal renal tubular acidosis in Thailand. *QJM* **74**:289, 1990.
253. Jarolim P, Shayakul C, Prabakaran D, Jiang L, Stuart-Tilley A, Rubin HL, Simova S, et al.: Autosomal dominant distal renal tubular acidosis is associated in three families with heterozygosity for the R589H mutation in the AE1 (band 3) Cl^-/HCO_3^- exchanger. *J Biol Chem* **273**:6380, 1998.
254. DuBose TD Jr: Experimental models of distal renal tubular acidosis. *Semin Nephrol* **10**:174, 1990.
255. Kurtzman NA: Disorders of distal acidification. *Kidney Int* **38**:720, 1990.
256. Kurtzman NA: "Short-circuit" renal tubular acidosis. *J Lab Clin Med* **95**:633, 1980.
257. DuBose TD Jr: Hyperkalemic hyperchloremic metabolic acidosis: Pathophysiologic insights. *Kidney Int* **51**:591, 1997.
258. Husted RF, Steinmetz PR: The effects of amiloride and ouabain on urinary acidification by turtle bladder. *J Pharmacol Exp Ther* **210**:264, 1979.
259. Lin SH, Kuo AA, Yu FC, Lin YF: Reversible voltage-dependent distal renal tubular acidosis in a patient receiving standard doses of trimethoprim-sulphamethoxazole. *Nephrol Dial Transplant* **12**:1031, 1997.
260. Domingo P, Ferrer S, Cruz J, Morla R, Ris J: Trimethoprim-sulfamethoxazole-induced renal tubular acidosis in a patient with AIDS. *Clin Infect Dis* **20**:1435, 1995.
261. Arruda JAL, Subbarayudu K, Dytko G, Mola R, Kurtzman NA: Voltage dependent distal acidification defect induced by amiloride. *J Lab Clin Med* **95**:407, 1980.
262. Hulter HN, Ilnicki LP, Licht JH, Sebastian A: On the mechanism of diminished urinary carbon dioxide tension caused by amiloride. *Kidney Int* **21**:8, 1982.
263. Nascimento L, Rademacker D, Hamburger R, Arruda JAL, Kurtzman NA: On the mechanism of lithium-induced renal tubular acidosis. *J Lab Clin Med* **89**:445, 1977.
264. Roscoe M, Goldstein MB, Halperin MC, Wilson DR, Stinebaugh BJ: Lithium-induced impairment of urine acidification. *Kidney Int* **9**:344, 1976.
265. Arruda JAL, Dytko G, Mola R, Kurtzman NA: On the mechanism of lithium-induced distal renal tubular acidosis: Studies in the turtle bladder. *Kidney Int* **17**:196, 1980.
266. Daphnis E, Kurtzman NA, Sabatini S: On the mechanism of lithium-induced renal tubular acidosis. *Kidney Int* **37**:534A, 1990.
267. Batlle DC, Gaviria M, Grupp M, Arruda JAL, Wynn J, Kurtzman NA: Distal nephron function in patients receiving chronic lithium therapy. *Kidney Int* **21**:477, 1982.
268. Grunder S, Firsov D, Chang SS, Jaeger NF, Gautschi I, Schild L, Lifton RP, et al.: A mutation causing pseudohypoaldosteronism type 1 identifies a conserved glycine that is involved in the gating of the epithelial sodium channel. *EMBO J* **16**:899, 1997.
269. Sabatini S, Kurtzman NA: Enzyme activity in obstructive uropathy: The biochemical basis for salt wastage and the acidification defect. *Kidney Int* **37**:79, 1990.
270. Purcell H, Bastani B, Harris KPG, Hemken P, Klahr S, Gluck S: Cellular distribution of H^+ATPase following acute unilateral ureteral obstruction in rats. *Am J Physiol* **261**:F365, 1991.
271. Sawczuk I, Hoke G, Olsson C, Connor J, Buttyan R: Gene expression in response to acute unilateral ureteral obstruction. *Kidney Int* **35**:1315, 1989.
272. Schambelan M, Sebastian A, Hulter HN: Mineralocorticoid excess and deficiency syndromes, in Brenner BM, Stein JH (eds): *Contemporary Issues in Nephrology. Acid-Base and Potassium Homeostasis*, Vol 2. New York, Churchill Livingston, 1978, p 232.
273. Hulter HN, Ilnicki LP, Harbottle JA, Sebastian A: Impaired renal H^+ secretion and NH_3 production in mineralocorticoid-deficient glucocorticoid-replete dogs. *Am J Physiol* **326**:F136, 1979.
274. Steinmetz PR: Cellular mechanisms of urinary acidification. *Physiol Rev* **54**:890, 1974.
275. Bruno CM, Neri S, D'Angelo G, D'Amico R, Raciti C, Urso G: Type 4 renal tubular acidosis caused by spironolactone. A case report. *Minerva Medica* **88**:93, 1997.
276. Hulter HN, Bonner EL Jr, Glynn RD, Sebastian A: Renal and systemic acid-base effects of chronic spironolactone administration. *Am J Physiol* **240**:F381, 1981.
277. Schlueter W, Keilani T, Hizon M, Kaplan B, Batlle DC: On the mechanism of impaired distal acidification in hyperkalemic renal tubular acidosis: Evaluation with amiloride and bumetanide. *J Am Soc Nephrol* **3**:953, 1992.
278. Wilcox CS, Cemeriki DA, Giebisch G: Differential effects of acute mineralo- and glucocorticosteroid administration on renal acid elimination. *Kidney Int* **21**:546, 1982.
279. Sebastian A, Sutton JM, Hulter HN, Schambelan M, Poler SM: Effect of mineralocorticoid replacement therapy on renal acid-base homeostasis in adrenalectomized patients. *Kidney Int* **18**:762, 1980.
280. Sebastian A, Schambelan M, Lindenfeld S, Morris RC Jr: Amelioration of metabolic acidosis with fludrocortisone therapy in hyporeninemic hypoaldosteronism. *N Engl J Med* **297**:576, 1977.
281. Szylman P, Better OS, Chaimowitz C, Rosler A: Role of hyperkalemia in the metabolic acidosis of isolated hypoaldosteronism. *N Engl J Med* **294**:361, 1975.
282. Tannen RC: Relationship of renal ammonia production and potassium homeostasis. *Kidney Int* **11**:453, 1977.
283. DuBose TD Jr, Good DW: Effects of chronic chloride depletion metabolic alkalosis on proximal tubule transport and renal production of ammonium. *Am J Physiol* **269**:F508, 1995.
284. Cheek DB, Perry JW: A salt-wasting syndrome in infancy. *Arch Dis Child* **33**:252, 1948.

285. Donnell GN, Litman N, Roldan M: Pseudohypoadrenalocorticism; renal sodium loss; hyponatremia, and hyperkalemia due to renal tubular insensitivity to mineralocorticoids. *Am J Dis Child* **97**:813, 1959.
286. Schild L: The ENaC channel as the primary determinant of two human diseaes: Liddle syndrome and pseudohypoaldosteronism. *Nephrologie* **17**:395, 1996.
287. Chang SS, Grunder S, Hanukoglu A, Rosler A, Mathew PM, Hanukoglu I, Schild L, et al.: Mutations in subunits of the epithelial sodium channel cause salt wasting with hyperkalaemic acidosis, pseudohypoaldosteronism type 1. *Nat Genet* **12**:248, 1996.
288. Strautnieks SS, Thompson RJ, Hanukoglu A, Dillon MJ, Hanukoglu I, Kuhnle U, Seckl J, et al.: Localisation of pseudohypoaldosteronism genes to chromosome 16p12.2-13.11 and 12p13.1-pter by homozygosity mapping. *Hum Mol Genet* **5**:293, 1996.
289. Strautnieks SS, Thompson RJ, Gardiner RM, Chung E: A novel splice-site mutation in the gamma subunit of the epithelial sodium channel gene in three pseudohypoaldosteronism type 1 families. *Nat Genet* **13**:248, 1996.
290. Geller DS, Rodriguez-Soriano J, Vallo Boado A, Schifter S, Bayer M, Chang SS, Lifton RP: Mutations in the mineralocorticoid receptor gene cause autosomal dominant pseudohypoaldosteronism type 1. *Nat Genet* **3**:279, 1998.
291. Arnold JE, Healy JK: Hyperkalemia, hypertension and systemic acidosis without renal failure associated with a tubular defect in potassium excretion. *Am J Med* **47**:461, 1969.
292. Spitzer A, Edelmann CM Jr, Goldberg LD, Henneman PH: Short stature hyperkalemia and acidosis: A defect in renal transport of potassium. *Kidney Int* **3**:251, 1973.
293. Weinstein SF, Allan DME, Mendoza SA: Hyperkalemia, acidosis, and short stature associated with a defect in renal potassium excretion. *J Pediatr* **85**:255, 1974.
294. Schambelan M, Sebastian A, Rector FC Jr: Mineralocorticoid-resistant renal hyperkalemia without salt wasting (type II pseudohypoaldosteronism): Role of increased renal chloride reabsorption. *Kidney Int* **19**:716, 1981.
295. Take C, Ikeda K, Kurasawa T, Kurokawa K: Increased chloride reabsorption as an inherited renal tubular defect in familial type II pseudohypoaldosteronism. *New Engl J Med* **324**:472, 1991.
296. Mansfield TA, Simon DB, Farfel Z, Bia M, Tucci JR, Lebel M, Gutkin M, et al.: Multilocus linkage of familial hyperkalaemia and hypertension, pseudohypoaldosteronism type II, to chromosomes 1q31-42 and 17p11-q21. *Nat Genet* **16**:202, 1997.
297. Lee MR, Ball SG, Thomas TH, Morgan DB: Hypertension and hyperkalemia responding to bendrogluazide. *QJM* **48**:245, 1979.
298. Brautbar N, Levi J, Rosler A, Leitesdorf E, Djaldeti M, Eptstein M, Kleeman CR: Familial hyperkalemia, hypertension and hyporeninemia with normal aldosterone levels. A tubular defect in potassium handling. *Arch Intern Med* **138**:607, 1978.
299. Sebastian A, Schambelan M, Sutton JM: Amelioration of hyperchloremic acidosis with furosemide therapy in patients with chronic renal insufficiency and type 4 renal tubular acidosis. *Am J Nephrol* **4**:287, 1984.
300. Gordon RD, Geddes RA, Pawsey CGK, O'Halloran MW: Hypertension and severe hyperkalemia associated with suppression of renin and aldosterone and completely reversed by dietary sodium restriction. *Aust Ann Med* **4**:287, 1970.
301. Gordon RD, Hodsman GP: The syndrome of hypertension and hyperkalemia without renal failure: long term correction by thiazide diuretic. *Scott Med J* **31**:43, 1986.
302. Shimizu T, Yoshitomi K, Nakamura M, Imai M: Site and mechanism of action of trichlormethiazide in rabbit distal nephron segments perfused in vitro. *J Clin Invest* **82**:721, 1988.
303. Davenport MW, Zipser RD: Association of hypotension with hyperreninemic hypoaldosteronism in the critically ill patient. *Arch Intern Med* **143**:735, 1983.
304. Antonipillai I, Wang Y, Horton R: Tumor necrosis factor and interleukin-1 may regulate renin secretion. *Endocrinology* **126**:273, 1990.
305. O'Kelly R, Magee F, McKenna TJ: Routine heparin therapy inhibits adrenal aldosterone production. *J Clin Endocrinol Metab* **56**:108, 1983.
306. Schambelan M, Sebastian A, Biglieri EG: Prevalence, pathogenesis, and functional significance of aldosterone deficiency in hyperkalemic patients with chronic renal insufficiency. *Kidney Int* **17**:89, 1980.
307. Sebastian A, Schambelan M, Hulter HN, Maher T, Kurtz I, Biglieri EG, Rector FC Jr, Morris RC Jr: Hyperkalemic renal tubular acidosis, in Gonick HC, Buckalew VM Jr (eds): *Renal Tubular Disorders. Pathophysiology, Diagnosis and Management*. New York, Marcel Dekker, 1985, p 307.
308. DeFronzo RA: Hyperkalemia and hyporeninemic hypoaldosteronism. *Kidney Int* **17**:118, 1980.
309. Schambelan M, Stockigt JR, Biglieri M: Isolated hypoaldosteronism in adults. A renin-deficiency syndrome. *N Engl J Med* **287**:573, 1972.
310. Coleman AJ, Arias M, Carter NW, Rector FC Jr, Seldin DW: The mechanism of salt wastage in chronic renal disease. *J Clin Invest* **45**:1116, 1966.
311. Oh MS, Carrol HJ, Clemmons, JE, Vagnucci AH, Levison SP, Whang ESM: A mechanism for hyporeninemic hypoaldosteronism in chronic renal disease. *Metabolism* **23**:1157, 1974.
312. Sparagna M: Hyporeninemic hypoaldosteronism associated with diabetic glomerulosclerosis. *J Steroid Biochem* **5**:369, 1974.
313. Schinder AM, Sommers SC: Diabetic sclerosis of the renal juxtaglomerular apparatus. *Lab Invest* **15**:877, 1966.
314. Tan SY, Shapiro R, Franco R, Stockard H, Mulrow AJ: Indomethacin-induced prostaglandin inhibition with hyperkalemia. A reversible cause of hyperreninemic hypoaldosteronism. *Ann Intern Med* **90**:783, 1979.
315. Norby LH, Ramwell P, Weidig J, Slotkoff L, Flamenbaum W: Possible role for impaired renal prostaglandin production in pathogenesis of hyporeninemic hypoaldosteronism. *Lancet* **2**:1118, 1978.
316. Perez GO, Oster JR, Vaamonde CA: Renal acidosis and renal potassium handling in selective hypoaldosteronism. *Am J Med* **57**:809, 1974.
317. Morris RC Jr: Renal tubular acidosis. Mechanisms, classification and implications. *N Engl J Med* **281**:1405, 1969.
318. Morris RC Jr, Sebastian A: Renal tubular acidosis and Fanconi syndrome, in Stanbury JB, Wyngaarden JB, Fredrickson DS, Goldstein JL, Brown MS (eds): *The Metabolic Basis of Inherited Disease*, 5th ed. New York, McGraw-Hill, 1983, p 1808.
319. Chafe L, Gault MH: First morning urine pH in the diagnosis of renal tubular acidosis with nephrolithiasis. *Clin Nephrol* **41**:159, 1994.
320. Elkington JR, Huth EJ, Webster GD Jr, McCance RA: The renal excretion of hydrogen ion in renal tubular acidosis. *Am J Med* **29**:554, 1960.
321. Wrong O: Urinary hydrogen ion excretion. *J Clin Pathol* **18**:520, 1965.
322. Sebastian A, McSherry E, Morris RC Jr: Metabolic acidosis with special reference to renal acidosis, in BM Brenner, FC Rector Jr (eds): *The Kidney, 2nd ed.* Philadelphia, WB Saunders, 1976, p 615.
323. McSherry E, Sebastian A, Morris RC Jr: Renal tubular acidosis in infants: The several kinds, including bicarbonate wasting classic renal tubular acidosis. *J Clin Invest* **51**:499, 1972.
324. McSherry EM, Morris RC Jr: Attainment and maintenance of normal stature with alkali therapy in infants and children with classic renal tubular acidosis. *J Clin Invest* **61**:509, 1978.
325. Rodriquez-Soriano J, Boichis H, Edelman CM Jr: Bicarbonate reabsorption and hydrogen ion excretion in children with renal tubular acidosis. *J Pediatr* **71**:802, 1967.
326. Kurtzman NA, Arruda JAL: Physiologic significance of urinary carbon dioxide tension. *Miner Electrolyte Metab* **1**:241, 1978.
327. Stinebaugh BJ, Esquenazi R, Schloeder FX, Suki WN, Goldstein MB, Halperin ML: Control of the urine-blood PCO_2 gradient in alkaline urine. *Kidney Int* **17**:31,1980.
328. Batlle DC, Kurtzman NA: The defect in distal (type 1) renal tubular acidosis in HC Gonick, VM Buckalew Jr (eds): *Renal Tubular Disorders. Pathophysiology, Diagnosis and Management*. New York, Marcel Dekker, 1985, p 281.
329. Tesar V, Mokrejsova M, Marecek Z, Petrtyl J: Distal renal tubular acidosis in patients with Wilson's disease. *Sbornik Lekarsky* **93**:315, 1991.
330. Lewis DW: What was wrong with Tiny Tim? *Am J Dis Child* **146**:1403, 1992.
331. Lin JY, Lin JS, Tsai CH: Use of the urine-to-blood carbon dioxide tension gradient as a measurement of impaired distal tubular hydrogen ion secretion among neonates. *J Pediatr* **126**:114, 1995.
332. Strife CF, Clardy CW, Varade WS, Prada AL, Waldo FB: Urine-to-blood carbon dioxide tension gradient and maximal depression of urinary pH to distinguish rate-dependent from classic distal renal tubular acidosis in children. *J Pediatr* **122**:60, 1993.
333. Batlle DC, Kurtzman NA: Renal regulation of acid-base homeostasis; Integrated response, in Seldin DW, Giebisch G (eds): *The Kidney: Physiology and Pathophysiology*. New York, Raven Press, 1985, p 1539.

334. Wrong O, Davies HE: The excretion of acid in renal disease. *QJM* **28**:259, 1959.
335. Buckalew VM Jr, Purvis ML, Shulman MG, Herndon CN, Rudman D: Hereditary renal tubular acidosis. Report of a 64-member kindred with variable clinical expression including idiopathic hypercalcemia. *Medicine* **53**:229, 1974.
336. Coe FL, Parks JH: Stone disease in heredity distal renal tubular acidosis. *Ann Intern Med* **93**:60, 1980.
337. Simpson DP: Influence of plasma bicarbonate concentration and pH on citrate excretion. *Am J Physiol* **206**:875, 1964.
338. Buckalew VM Jr, McCurdy DK, Ludwig GD, Chaykin LB, Elkinton JR: The syndrome of imcomplete renal tubular acidosis. *Am J Med* **45**:32, 1968.
339. Brenner RJ, Spring DB, Sebastian A, McSherry EM, Genant HK, Palubinskas AJ, Morris RC Jr: Incidence of radiographically evident bone disease, nephrocalcinosis, and nephrolithiasis in various types of renal tubular acidosis. *N Engl J Med* **307**:217, 1982.
340. Morris RC Jr, Ives HE: Inherited disorders of the renal tubule, in Brenner BM, Rector FC Jr (eds): *The Kidney, 4th ed.* Philadelphia, WB Saunders, 1991, p 1596.
341. Pitts HH, Schulte JW, Smith DR: Nephrocalcinosis in a father and three children. *J Urol* **73**:208, 1955.
342. Randall RE Jr, Targgart WH: Familial renal tubular acidosis. *Ann Intern Med* **54**:1108, 1961.
343. Randall RE Jr: Familial renal tubular acidosis revisited. *Ann Intern Med* **66**:1024, 1967.
344. Seedat YK: Some observations of renal tubular acidosis: A family study. *S Afr Med J* **38**:606, 1964.
345. Gyory AZ, Edwards KDG: Renal tubular acidosis: A family with an autosomal dominant genetic defect in renal hydrogen ion transport, with proximal tubular and collecting duct dysfunction and increased metabolism of citrate and ammonia. *Am J Med* **45**:43, 1968.
346. Richards P, Wrong OM: Dominant inheritance in a family with familial renal tubular acidosis. *Lancet* **2**:998, 1978.
347. McSherry EM, Pokroy MV: The absence of nephrocalcinosis in children with type 1 RTA on high dose alkali therapy since infancy. *Clin Res* **26**:470A, 1978.
348. Hamed IA, Czerwinski AW, Coats B, Kaufman C, Altmiller DH: Familial absorptive hypercalciuria and renal tubular acidosis. *Am J Med* **67**:385, 1979.
349. Buckalew VM Jr: Familial renal tubular acidosis. *Ann Intern Med* **69**:1329, 1968.
350. Donckerwolcke RA, Van Stehelenburg GJ, Tiddens HA: A case of bicarbonate-losing renal tubular acidosis with defective carbonic anhydrase activity. *Arch Dis Child* **45**:769, 1970.
351. Shapira E, Ben-Yoseph Y, Eyal FC, Russel A: Enzymatically inactive red cell carbonic anhydrase B in a family with renal tubular acidosis. *J Clin Invest* **53**:59, 1974.
352. Norman ME, Cohn RM, McCurdy DK: Urinary citrate excretion in the diagnosis of distal renal tubular acidosis. *J Pediatr* **92**:394, 1978.
353. Kelleher DL, Buckalew VM, Frederickson ED, Rhodes DJ, Conner DA, Seidman JG, Seidman CE: CLCN5 mutation Ser244Leu is associated with X-linked renal failure without X-linked recessive hypophosphatemic rickets. *Kidney Int* **53**:31, 1998.
354. Chaabani H, Hadj-Khlil, Ben-Dhia V Braham H: The primary hereditary form of distal renal tubular acidosis: Clinical and genetic studies in 60-member kindred. *Clin Genet* 45:194, 1994.
355. Report of a Meeting of Physicians and Scientists. Unraveling of the molecular mechanisms of kidney stones. *Lancet* **348**:1561, 1996.
356. Bourke E, Delaney VB, Mosawi M, Reavy P, Weston M: Renal tubular acidosis and osteopetrosis in siblings. *Nephron* **28**:268, 1981.
357. Strisciuglio P, Hu PY, Lim EJ, Ciccolella J, Sly WS: Clinical and molecular heterogeneity in carbonic anhydrase II deficiency and prenatal diagnosis in an Italian family. *J Pediatr* **132**:717, 1998.
358. Sly WS, Whyte MP, Krupin T, Sundaram V: Positive renal response to intravenous acetazolamide in patients with carbonic anhydrase II deficiency. *Pediatr Res* **19**:1033, 1985.
359. Lai LW, Chan DM, Erickson RP, Hsu SJ, Lien YH: Correction of renal tubular acidosis in carbonic anhydrase II-deficient mice with gene therapy. *J Clin Invest* **101**:1320, 1998.
360. Vasuvattakul S, Nimmannit S, Chaovakul V, Susaengrat W, Shayakul C, Malasit P, et al.: The spectrum of endemic renal tubular acidosis in the northeast of Thailand. *Nephron* **74**:541, 1996.
361. Morris RC Jr, Fudenberg HH: Impaired renal acidification in patients with hypergammaglobulinemia. *Medicine* **46**:57, 1967.
362. Cohen A, Way BJ: The association of renal tubular acidosis with hyperglobulinemic purpura. *Australas Ann Med* **11**:189, 1962.
363. Mason AMS, Golding PL: Hyperglobulinaemic renal tubular acidosis: A report of nine cases. *Br Med J* **3**:143, 1970.
364. Marquez-Julio A, Rapoport A, Wilansky DL, Rabinovich S, Chamberlain D: Purpura associated with hypergammaglobulinemia, renal tubular acidosis and osteomalacia. *Can Med Assoc J* **116**:53, 1977.
365. Seux-Levieil ML, Joly V, Veni P, Carbon C, Blanchet F: Evaluation of renal acidification in HIV-infected patients with hypergammaglobulinemia. *Nephron* **75**:196, 1997.
366. Lospalluto J, Dorward B, Biller W, Ziff M: Cryoglobulinemia based on interaction between a gamma macroglobulin and 7S gamma globulin. *Am J Med* **32**:142, 1962.
367. Mason AMS, Mcillmurray MB, Golding PL, Hughes DTD: Fibrosing alveolitis associated with renal tubular acidosis. *Br Med J* **4**:596, 1970.
368. Talal N, Zisman E, Schur PH: Renal tubular acidosis, glomerulonephritis and immunologic factors in Sjögren's syndrome. *Arthritis Rheum* **2**:774, 1968.
369. Talal N: Sjögren's syndrome, lymphoproliferation, and renal tubular acidosis. *Ann Intern Med* **74**:633, 1971.
370. Shioji R, Furuyama T, Onodera S, Saito H, Ito H, Sasaki Y: Sjögren's syndrome and renal tubular acidosis. *Am J Med* **48**:456, 1970.
371. Mason AM, Golding PL: Renal tubular acidosis and autoimmune thyroid disease. *Lancet* **2**:1104, 1970.
372. Golding PL: Renal tubular acidosis in chronic liver disease. *Postgrad Med J* **51**:550, 1975.
373. Bridi, GS, Falcon PW, Brackett NC Jr, Still WJS, Sporn IN: Glomerulonephritis and renal tubular acidosis in a case of chronic active hepatitis with hyperimmunoglobulinemia. *Am J Med* **52**:267, 1972.
374. Reade AE, Sherlock S, Harrison CV: Active "juvenile" cirrhosis considered as part of a systemic disease. *Gut* **4**:378, 1963.
375. Seedat YK, Raine ER: Active chronic hepatitis associated with renal tubular acidosis and successful pregnancy. *S Afr Med J* **39**:595, 1965.
376. Golding PL, Smith M, Williams R: Multisystem involvement in chronic liver disease. Studies on the incidence and pathogenesis. *Ann J Med* **55**:772, 1973.
377. Cochrane AM, Tsantoulos DC, Moussouros A, McFarland IG, Eddleston ALWF, Williams R: Lymphocyte cytotoxicity for kidney cells in renal tubular acidosis of autoimmune liver disease. *Br Med J* **2**:276, 1976.
378. Tu WH, Shearn MA: Systemic lupus erythematosus and latent renal tubular dysfunction. *Ann Intern Med* **67**:100, 1967.
379. Jessop S, Rabkin R, Mumford G, Eales L: Renal tubular function in systemic lupus erythematosus. *S Afr Med J* **47**:132, 1973.
380. Zimhony O, Sthoeger Z, Ben David D, Bar Khayim Y, Geltner D: Sjögren's syndrome presenting as hypokalemic paralysis due to distal renal tubular acidosis. *J Rheumatol* **22**:2366, 1995.
381. Cohen EP, Bastani B, Cohen MR, Kolner S, Hemken P, Gluck SL: Absence of H^+-ATPase in cortical collecting tubules of a patient with Sjögren's syndrome and distal renal tubular acidosis. *J Am Soc Neph* **3**:264, 1992.
382. Reynolds TB, Bethune JE: Renal tubular acidosis secondary to hyperparathyroidism. *Clin Res* **17**:169, 1969.
383. Cohen SI, Fitzgerald MG, Fourman P, Griffiths WJ, Dewardener HE: Polyuria in hyperparathyroidism. *Q J Med* **26**:423, 1957.
384. Ferris T, Kashgarian M, Livitin H, Brandt I, Epstein FH: Renal tubular acidosis and renal potassium wasting acquired as a result of hypercalcemic nephropathy. *N Engl J Med* **265**:924, 1961.
385. Savani RC, Mimouni F, Tsang RC: Maternal and neonatal hyperparathyroidism as a consequence of maternal renal tubular acidosis. *Pediatrics* **91**:661, 1993.
386. Rochman J, Better OS, Winaver J, Chaimovitz C, Carzilai A, Jacobs R: Renal tubular acidosis due to the milk-alkali syndrome. *Isr J Med Sci* **13**:609, 1977.
387. Huth EJ, Mayock RL, Kerr RM: Hyperthyroidism associated with renal tubular acidosis. *Am J Med* **26**:818, 1959.
388. Zisman E, Buccino RA, Gorden P, Bartter FC: Hyperthyroidism and renal tubular acidosis. *Arch Intern Med* **121**:118, 1968.
389. Szeto CC, Chow CC, Li KY, Ko TC, Yeung VT, Cockram CS: Thyrotoxicosis and renal tubular acidosis presenting as hypokalaemic paralysis. *Br J Rheumatol* **35**:289, 1996.
390. Parfitt AM, Higgins BA, Nassim JR, Collins JA, Hilb A: Metabolic studies in patients with hypercalciuria. *Clin Sci* **27**:463, 1964.
391. Dent CE, Harper CM, Parfit AM: The effect of cellulose phosphate on calcium metabolism in patients with hypercalciuria. *Clin Sci* **27**:417, 1964.
392. Deck MDF: Medullary sponge kidney with renal tubular acidosis: a report of 3 cases. *J Urol* **94**:330, 1965.

393. Morris RC Jr, Yamauchi H, Palubinskas AJ, Howenstine J: Medullary sponge kidney. *Am J Med* **38**:883, 1965.
394. Osther PJ, Mathiasen H, Hansen AB, Nissen HM: Urinary acidification and urinary excretion of calcium and citrate in women with bilateral medullary sponge kidney. *Urol Int* **52**:126, 1994.
395. Mass RE, Smith WR, Walsh JR: The association of hereditary fructose intolerance and renal tubular acidosis. *Am J Med Sci* **251**:516, 1966.
396. Koura T, Nishinarita S, Matsukawa Y, Kobayashi T, Shimada H, Takei M, Tomita Y, Baba M, et al.: A case of Sjögren's syndrome complicated with cryoglobulinemia, nephrogenic diabetes insipidus, and renal tubular acidosis. *Nihon Rinsho Meneki Gakkai Kaishi* **18**:221, 1995.
397. Batlle D, Flores G: Underlying defects in distal renal tubular acidosis: New understandings. *Am J Kid Dis* **27**:896, 1996.
398. Stoll C, Gentine A, Geisert J: Siblings with congenital renal tubular acidosis and nerve deafness. *Clin Gen* **50**:235, 1996.
399. Brown MT, Cunningham MJ, Ingelfinger JR, Becker AN: Progressive sensorineural hearing loss in association with distal renal tubular acidosis. *Arch Oto Head Neck Surg* **119**:458, 1993.
400. Bajaj G, Quan A: Renal tubular acidosis and deafness: Report of a large family. *Am J Kid Dis* **27**:880, 1996.
401. Seikaly M, Browne R, Baum M: Nephrocalcinosis is associated with renal tubular acidosis in children with X-linked hypophosphatemia. *Pediatrics* **97**:91, 1996.
402. Restaino K, Kaplan BS, Stanley C, Baker L: Nephrolithiasis, hypocitraturia, and a distal renal tubular acidification defect in type 1 glycogen storage disease. *J Pediatr* **122**:392, 1993.
403. Yeoh SA: Fabry's disease with renal tubular acidosis. *Singapore Med J* **8**:275, 1967.
404. Higashirhara E, Nutahara K, Tago K, Ueno A, Niijima T: Medullary sponge kidney and renal acidification defect. *Kidney Int* **25**:453, 1984.
405. Patterson RM, Ackerman GL: Renal tubular acidosis due to amphotericin B nephrotoxicity. *Arch Intern Med* **127**:241, 1971.
406. Douglas JB, Healy JK: Nephrotoxic effects of amphotericin B, including renal tubular acidosis. *Am J Med* **46**:154, 1969.
407. McCurdy DK, Frederic M, Elkinton JR: Renal tubular acidosis due to amphotericin B. *N Engl J Med* **278**:124, 1968.
408. Sawaya BP, Briggs JP, Schnermann J: Amphotericin B nephrotoxicity: The adverse consequences of altered membrane propertieis. *J Am Soc Nephrol* **6**:154, 1995.
409. Erramouspe J, Galvez R, Fischel DR: Newborn renal tubular acidosis associated with prenatal maternal toluene sniffing. *J Psychoactive Drugs* **28**:201, 1996.
410. Yong JM, Sanderson KV: Photosensitive dermatitis and renal tubular acidosis after ingestion of calcium cyclamate. *Lancet* **2**:1273, 1969.
411. Steele TW, Gyory AZ, Edwards KDG: Renal function in analgesic nephropathy. *Br Med J* **2**:213, 1969.
412. Steele TW, Edwards KDG: Analgesic nephropathy. *Med J Aust* **1**:181, 1971.
413. Navarro JF, Quereda C, Quereda C, Gallego N, Antela A, Mora C, Ortuno J: Nephrogenic diabetes insipidus and renal tubular acidosis secondary to foscarnet therapy. *Am J Kid Dis* **27**:431, 1996.
414. Gyory AZ, Stewart JH, George CRP, Tiller DJ, Edwards KDG: Renal tubular acidosis, acidosis due to hyperkalemia, hypercalcaemia, disordered citrate metabolism and other tubular dysfunctions following human renal transplantation. *Q J Med* **38**:231, 1969.
415. Wilson DR, Siddiqui AA: Renal tubular acidosis after kidney transplantation. *Ann Intern Med* **79**:352, 1973.
416. Better OS, Chaimowitz C, Naveh Y, Stein A, Nahir AM, Barzilai A, Erlik D: Syndrome of incomplete renal tubular acidosis after cadaver kidney transplantation. *Ann Intern Med* **71**:39, 1969.
417. Jordan M, Cohen EP, Roza A, Adams MB, Johnson C, Gluck SL, Bastani B: An immunocytochemical study of H^+ATPase in kidney transplant rejection. *J Lab Clin Med* **127**:310, 1996.
418. Drutz DJ, Gutman RA: Renal tubular acidosis in leprosy. *Ann Intern Med* **75**:475, 1971.
419. Vainder M, Kelly J: Renal tubular dysfunction secondary to jejuno-ileal bypass. *JAMA* **235**:1257, 1976.
420. Better OS, Arieff AI, Massry SG, Kleeman CR, Maxwell MH: Studies on renal function after relief of complete unilateral ureteral obstruction of three months duration in man. *Am J Med* **54**:234, 1973.
421. Earley LE: Extreme polyuria in obstructive uropathy. *N Engl J Med* **255**:600, 1956.
422. Berlyne GM: Distal tubular function in chronic hydronephrosis. *Q J Med* **30**:339, 1961.
423. Guizar JM, Kornhauser C, Malacara JM, Sanchez G, Zamora J: Renal tubular acidosis in children with vesicoureteral reflux. *J Urol* **146**:193, 1996.
424. Cochran M, Peacock M, Smith DA, Nrodin BEC: Renal tubular acidosis of pyelonephritis with renal stone disease. *Br Med J* **2**:721, 1968.
425. Levine AS, Michael AF Jr: Ehlers-Danlos syndrome with renal tubular acidosis and medullary sponge kidneys. *J Pediatr* **71**:107, 1967.
426. Bechner RL, Gilchrist GS, Anderson EJ: Hereditary elliptocytosis and primary renal tubular acidosis in a single family. *Am J Dis Child* **115**:414, 1968.
427. Dunger DB, Brenton DP, Cain AR: Renal tubular acidosis and nerve deafness. *Arch Dis Child* **55**:221, 1980.
428. Oster JR, Lespier LE, Lee SM, Pellegrini EL, Vaamonde CA: Renal acidification in sickle-cell disease. *J Lab Clin Med* **88**:389, 1976.
429. Giselson N, Heinegard D, Holmberg CG, Lindberg LG, Lindstedt G, Schersten B: Renal medullary cystic disease or familial juvenile nephronophthisis: A renal tubular disease. Biochemical findings in two siblings. *Am J Med* **48**:174, 1970.
430. Bergman AJ, Donckerwolcke RA, Duran M, Smeitink JA, Mousson B, Vianey-Saban C: Rate-dependent distal renal tubular acidosis and carnitine palmitoyltransferase I deficiency. *Pediatr Res* **36**:582, 1994.
431. Thong MK, Tan AA, Lin HP: Distal renal tubular acidosis and hereditary elliptocytosis in a single family. *Singapore Med J* **38**:38, 1997.
432. Fathallah DM, Bejaoui M, Sly WS, Lakhoua R, Dellagi K: A unique mutation underlying carbonic anhydrase II deficiency syndrome in patients of Arab descent. *Hum Gen* **94**:581, 1994.
433. Sato S, Zhu XL, Sly WS: Carbonic anhydrase isozymes IV and II in urinary membranes from carbonic anhydrase II-deficient patients. *Proc Natl Acad Sci U S A* **87**:6073, 1990.
434. Fathallah DM, Bejaoui M, Lepaslier D, Chater K, Sly WS, Dellagi K: Carbonic anhydrase II (CA II) deficiency in Maghrebian patients: Evidence for founder effect and genomic recombination at the CA II locus. *Hum Genet* **99**:634-7, 1997.
435. Dedmon RE, Wrong O: The excretion of organic anion in renal tubular acidosis with particular reference to citrate. *Clin Sci* **22**:19, 1962.
436. Morrissey JF, Ochoa M, Lotspeich WD, Waterhouse C: Citrate excretion in renal tubular acidosis. *Ann Intern Med* **58**:159, 1963.
437. Harrington TM, Bunch TW, Van Den Berg C: Renal tubular acidosis. A new look at treatment of musculoskeletal and renal disease. *Mayo Clin Proc* **58**:354, 1983.
438. Sebastian A, McSherry E, Morris RC Jr: Impaired renal conservation of sodium and chloride during sustained correction of systemic acidosis in patients with Type I, classic renal tubular acidosis. *J Clin Invest* **58**:454, 1976.
439. Rodriquez-Soriano J, Vallo A, Castillo G, Oliveros R: Renal handling of water and sodium in children with proximal and distal renal tubular acidosis. *Nephron* **25**:193, 1980.
440. Sebastian A, McSherry E, Morris RC Jr: Renal potassium wasting in renal tubular acidosis (RTA). Its occurence in types 1 and 2 RTA despite sustained correction of systemic acidosis. *J Clin Invest* **50**:667, 1971.
441. Lightwood R, Payne WW, Black JA: Infantile renal acidosis. *Pediatrics* **12**:628, 1953.
442. Lemann J Jr, Litzow JR, Lemmon EJ: The effects of chronic acid loads in normal man: Further evidence for participation of bone mineral in the defense against chronic metabolic acidosis. *J Clin Invest* **45**:1608, 1975.
443. Backman U, Danielson BG, Johansson G, Ljunghall S, Wikstrom B: Incidence and clinical importance of renal tubular defects in recurrent stone formers. *Nephron* **25**:96, 1980.
444. Albright F, Burnett CH, Parson W, Reifenstein ED Jr, Roos A: Osteomalacia and late rickets: The various etiologies met in the United States with emphasis on that resulting in a specific form of renal acidosis, the therapeutic indications for each etiological sub-group, and the relationship between osteomalacia and Milkman's syndrome. *Medicine* **25**:399, 1946.
445. Lee SW, Russel JE, Avioli LV: 25-OHD_3 to 1,25-$(OH)_2D_3$ conversion impaired by systemic acidosis. *Science* **195**:944, 1977.
446. Arruda JAL, Nascimento L, Mehta PK, Rademacher DR, Sehy JT, Westenfelder C, Kurtzman NA: The critical importance of urinary concentration ability in the generation of urinary carbon dioxide tension. *J Clin Invest* **60**:922-**935**, 1977.
447. Sebastian A, McSherry E, Morris RC Jr: Impaired renal conservation of sodium and chloride during sustained correction of systemic

acidosis in patients with type 1, classic renal tubular acidosis. *J Clin Invest* **58**:454, 1976.

448. Rodriguez-Soriano J, Vallo A, Castillo G, Oliveras R: Renal handling of water and sodium in children with proximal and distal renal tubular acidosis. *Nephron* **25**:193, 1980.
449. Morris RC Jr, Sebastian A, McSherry E: Therapeutic experience in patients with classic renal tubular acidosis. *Proceedings VII International Congress of Nephrology*[FES21]. Basel, S Karger, 1978, p 345.
450. Harrington TM, Bunch TW, Van Den Berg C: Renal tubular acidosis. A new look at treatment of musculoskeletal and renal disease. *Mayo Clin Proc* **58**:354, 1983.
451. Harrison HE, Chisolm JJ Jr, Harrison HC: Congenital renal tubular acidosis. *Am J Dis Child* **96**:588, 1958.
452. West ML, Marsden PA, Richardson MA, et al.: New clinical approach to evaluate disorders of potassium excretion. *Miner Electrolyte Metab* **12**:234, 1986.
453. Oetliker OH, Zurbrugg PRP: Renal tubular acidosis in salt-losing syndrome of congenital adrenal hyperplasia (CAH). *J Clin Endocrinol Metab* **31**:447, 1970.
454. Weidmann P, Reinhart R, Maxwell MH, Rowe P, Coburn JW, Massry SG: Syndrome of hyporeninemic hypoaldosteronism and hyperkalemia in renal disease. *J Clin Endocrinol Metab* **36**:965, 1973.
455. Kuhnle U, Hinkel GK, Hubl W, Reichelt T: Pseudohypoaldosteronism: Family studies to identify asymptomatic carriers by stimulation of the renin-aldosterone system. *Horm Res* **46**:124, 1996.
456. Paver WKA, Pauline GJ: Hypertension and hyperpotassemia without renal disease in a young male. *Med J Aust* **2**:305, 1964.
457. Rodriguez-Soriano J, Vallo A, Quintela MJ, Oliveros R, Ubetagoyena N: Normokalemic pseudohypoaldosteronism is present in children with acute pyelonephritis. *Acta Paediatr* **81**:402, 1992.
458. DuBose TD Jr, Alpern R: Renal tubular acidosis. In Scriver CR, Beaudet AL, Sy WS, Valle D (eds): *The Metabolic Basis of Inherited Diseases, 7th ed.* New York, McGraw-Hill, 1995, p 3655.
459. Mehta BR, Cavallo T, Remmers AR Jr, DuBose TD Jr: Hyporeninemic hypoaldosteronism in a patient with multiple myeloma. *Am J Kidney Dis* **4**:175, 1984.
460. DeFerrari ME, Colussi G, Brunati C, Rombola G, Civati G: Type IV renal tubular acidosis and uric acid nephrolithiasis in William's syndrome—an unusual mode of renal involvement. *Nephrol Dial Transplant* **12**:1484, 1997.
461. D'Angio CT, Dillon MJ, Leonar JV: Renal tubular dysfunction in methylmalonic acidaemia. *Eur J Pediatr* **150**:259, 1991.
462. Henrich WL: Nephrotoxicity of nonsteroidal anti-inflammatory agents. *Am J Kidney Dis* **2**:478, 1983.
463. Dunn MJ: Nonsteroidal anti-inflammatory drugs and renal function. *Ann Rev Med* **35**:411, 1984.
464. Gabow PA, Moore S, Schrier RW: Spironolactone-induced hyperchloremic metabolic acidosis in cirrhosis. *Ann Intern Med* **90**:338, 1979.
465. Ponce SP, Jennings AE, Madias NE, Harrington JT: Drug-induced hyperkalemia. *Medicine* **64**:357, 1985.
466. Schlanger LE, Kleyman TR, Ling BN: K^+-sparing diuretic actions of trimethoprim: Inhibition of Na^+ channels in A6 distal nephron cells. *Kidney Int* **45**:1070, 1994.
467. Kleyman TR, Roberts C, Ling BN: A mechanism for pentamidine-induced hyperkalemia: Inhibition of distal nephron sodium transport. *Ann Intern Med* **122**:103, 1995.
468. Velazquez H, Perazella MN, Wright FS, Ellison DH: Renal mechanisms of trimethoprim-induced hyerkalemia. *Ann Intern Med* **119**:296, 1993.
469. Kamel KS, Ethier JH, Quaggin S, Levin A, Albert S, Carlisle EJ, Halperin ML: Studies to determine the basis of hyperkalemia in recipients of a renal transplant who are treated with cyclosporine. *J Am Soc Nephrol* **2**:1279, 1992.
470. Aguilera S, Deray G, Desjobert H, Benhmida M, Le Hoang P, Jacobs C: Effects of cyclosporine on tubular acidification function in patients with idiopathic uveitis. *Am J Neph* **12**:425, 1992.
471. Sands JM, McMahon SJ, Tumlin JA: Evidence that the inhibition of Na^+/K^+-ATPase activity by FK506 involves calcineurin. *Kidney Int* **46**:647, 1994.
472. Uribarri J, Oh MS, Pak CY: Renal stone risk factors in patients with type IV renal acidosis. *Am J Kidney Dis* **23**:784, 1994.
473. New MI, Dupont B, Grumbach K, Levine LS: Congenital adrenal hyperplasia and related conditions, in Wyngaarden JB, Fredrickson DS, Goldstein JL, Brown MS (eds): *Metabolic Basis of Inherited Disease*. New York, McGraw-Hill, 1983, p 973.

CHAPTER 196

The Renal Fanconi Syndrome

Michel Bergeron ▪ André Gougoux
Josette Noël ▪ Lucie Parent

1. **The renal Fanconi syndrome consists of two components: (a) a generalized dysfunction of the proximal renal tubule leading to impaired proximal reabsorption of amino acids, glucose, phosphate, urate, and bicarbonate and therefore increased urinary excretion of all these solutes, and (b) a vitamin D–resistant metabolic bone disease—either rickets in growing children or osteomalacia in adults.**
2. **The renal Fanconi syndrome is either associated with various inborn errors of metabolism or acquired through exposure to various toxic agents. The inherited form may be idiopathic (in the absence of any recognizable metabolic disease) or secondary to various primary Mendelian diseases. Cystinosis is the most common cause of a secondary hereditary Fanconi syndrome in children. The degree of cystine accumulation determines three clinical forms of cystinosis: infantile, adolescent, and adult. The secondary Fanconi syndrome disappears in patients with hereditary fructose intolerance, galactosemia, tyrosinemia, and Wilson disease when these disorders are treated by restriction of fructose, galactose, tyrosine, or copper, respectively. Other metabolic diseases also can be associated with the Fanconi syndrome: vitamin D dependency, glycogen storage disease, and oculocerebrorenal (Lowe) syndrome.**
3. **A wide variety of toxic and immunologic tubular injuries may produce the generalized renal dysfunction characteristic of the Fanconi syndrome. Heavy metals (cadmium, uranium, mercury, lead, and platinum), various drugs (especially antibiotics), the glomerular filtration of abnormal proteins observed in dysproteinemias, and immunologic disorders are all known to induce a Fanconi syndrome. Maleate and cadmium were used to produce experimental models in animals. Finally, the Basenji dog can have a spontaneous Fanconi syndrome.**
4. **The renal Fanconi syndrome theoretically may result either from multiple transport dysfunctions restricted to the proximal tubule or from concomitant proximal and distal tubular dysfunctions. Recent data obtained from the experimental Fanconi syndrome indicate that the initial deleterious effect of maleate (and other toxins) in the proximal cells could be via megalin, a membrane glycoprotein that is a receptor for many ligands. Blockade at any point along the recycling pathway will modify luminal membrane function of the proximal tubular cells by trapping transport proteins and other constituents in endosomes. Some experimental data suggest that in addition to the proximal disturbance, a distal nephron involvement may play a role in the final production of the aminoaciduria, glycosuria, and phosphaturia observed in the Fanconi syndrome; all these transport defects could result from a decreased entry of molecules into the cell, an increased backflux at its luminal pole, or a combination of both. An impaired mitochondrial production of ATP and a reduced activity of the basolateral membrane Na^+, K^+-ATPase also have been suggested as pathogenetic mechanisms. The presence of physiologic intracellular gradients of Na^+, ATP, and ADP may amplify a minor decrease in mitochondrial phosphorylation and translate a modest defect in energy production into a major transport dysfunction.**
5. **In children, the clinical features of the renal Fanconi syndrome are not specific and result from the renal loss of fluid and electrolytes and the characteristic vitamin D–resistant metabolic bone disease. The most frequent manifestations are polyuria, polydipsia, dehydration, hypokalemia, acidosis, impaired growth, and rickets. In the absence of a specific treatment, fluids and electrolytes lost have to be replaced. The metabolic bone disease resulting from Fanconi syndrome must be treated, and renal transplantation can be performed for severely uremic children with nephropathic cystinosis.**

A list of standard abbreviations is located immediately preceding the index in each volume. Nonstandard abbreviations used in this chapter include: GFR = glomerular filtration rate.

DEFINITION

The renal Fanconi syndrome (Lignac-de Toni-Debré-Fanconi syndrome) is characterized by two components:

1. A generalized renal tubular dysfunction leading to increased urinary excretion of amino acids, glucose, phosphate, urate, and bicarbonate. Water[1] and solutes, normally reabsorbed by the kidney, also could be lost in the urine: sodium, potassium, calcium, magnesium,[2–5] carnitine,[6] glyceraldehyde,[7] lysozyme,[8,9] enzymes, peptide hormones, and other low-molecular-weight proteins[10] such as immunoglobulin light chains.
2. A vitamin D–resistant metabolic bone disease, occurring as either rickets in growing children or osteomalacia in adults.

The clinical features are polyuria, dehydration, hypokalemia, acidosis, impaired growth, and rickets.

HISTORICAL SUMMARY

The disease was first recognized in 1903 by Abderhalden,[11] who found cystine crystals in the liver and spleen of a 21-month-old infant and called the disorder a "familial cystine diathesis"—considered to be an inherited susceptibility conferring chemical individuality. In 1924, Lignac[12] described three similar cases in children with severe rickets, dwarfism, renal disease, and progressive wasting. In 1931, Fanconi described rickets and stunted growth in a child with glucosuria and albuminuria.[13] After de Toni[14] in 1933 and Debré et al.[15] in 1934 had reported similar cases, Fanconi in 1936 recognized the similarity between these few reported cases and suggested for this syndrome the name of *nephrotic-glycosuric dwarfism with hypophosphatemic rickets*.[16] This name, which is sometimes referred to in the literature as the *Lignac-de Toni-Debré-Fanconi syndrome*, was reduced to *Fanconi syndrome* by McCune et al.[17] in 1943.

ETIOLOGIC CLASSIFICATION

The Fanconi syndrome can be genetic in origin (Table 196-1) or acquired (Table 196-2).

Genetic Causes

Idiopathic. This form of the syndrome occurs in the absence of any recognized inherited metabolic disease, and its diagnosis can be made only when all the possible acquired causes and various inborn errors of metabolism producing Fanconi syndrome can be excluded. Most cases are sporadic in occurrence, but some familial forms also have been described, most often transmitted in an autosomal dominant fashion.[18–22] Various abnormalities of carbohydrate metabolism have been described in some patients with idiopathic Fanconi syndrome.[23,24]

Known Primary Mendelian Diseases Causing the Fanconi Syndrome. Several inborn errors of metabolism have been reported to induce a Fanconi syndrome, including abnormalities in the metabolism of amino acids (cystinosis, tyrosinemia) and carbohydrates (hereditary fructose intolerance, galactosemia, glycogen storage disease).

Cystinosis. This autosomal recessive disorder associated with the intralysosomal accumulation of cystine in different tissues of the body[25,26] is the inherited metabolic disease most commonly associated with Fanconi syndrome in children.[27] The renal manifestations shown by the patient described by Fanconi in 1936[16] were most likely secondary to cystinosis, as revealed by the presence of cystine crystals in the tissue. According to the degree of cystine accumulation, three clinical forms of the disease have been recognized:

1. The infantile or nephropathic cystinosis, characterized by onset of signs and symptoms within the first year of life and progressive renal failure leading to terminal uremia toward the end of the first decade[28,29]
2. The adolescent or intermediate cystinosis appearing during the second decade of life[30]
3. The adult or benign form of cystinosis without Fanconi syndrome or impaired renal function[31]

Only the infantile and adolescent forms are accompanied by Fanconi syndrome (see also Chap. 199).

Table 196-1 Inherited Fanconi Syndrome

Idiopathic (22770, 22780)	
Known primary Mendelian diseases in the Fanconi Syndrome:	
Cystinosis (219800, 219900, 219750)	Chap. 199
Hepatorenal tyrosinemia (tyrosinemia type I) (276700)	Chap. 79
Hereditary fructose intolerance (229600)	Chap. 70
Galactosemia (230400)	Chap. 72
Glycogen storage disease type I (232200)	Chap. 71
Wilson disease (277900)	Chap. 126
Vitamin D-dependent rickets (277420, 600785)	Chap. 165
Oculocerebrorenal (Lowe) syndrome (309000)	Chap. 252
Dent's disease*	
Cytochrome C oxidase deficiency*	Chap. 99
The Basenji dog	

NOTE: Numbers in parentheses are from the current McKusick catalog and OMIM. Inheritance of all disorders is autosomal recessive except Lowe syndrome, which is X-linked recessive. The chapter numbers indicate where these diseases are described in greater detail in this edition.
*Numerous McKusick entries.

Table 196-2 Acquired Fanconi Syndrome

- Agents
  - Heavy metals
    - Lead
    - Cadmium
    - Uranium
    - Mercury
  - Drugs
    - Outdated tetracyclines
    - Gentamicin
    - Cephalothin
    - Valproate
    - 6-Mercaptopurine
    - Methyl-3-chromone
    - Ifosfamide
    - Toluene
    - Paraquat
    - Lysol
    - Nitrobenzene
    - Salicylates
    - Tributylin oxide
  - Abnormal proteins and unknown factors
    - Multiple myeloma (Bence-Jones protein)
    - Other dysproteinemias
    - Nephrotic syndrome
    - Renal transplantation
    - Malignancies
- Experimental models
  - Maleate
  - Cadmium
  - Cystine dimethylester
  - 4-Pentenoate

Hepatorenal Tyrosinemia (Tyrosinemia Type I). With the ingestion of tyrosine or phenylalanine, the Fanconi syndrome is induced in patients with this autosomal recessive disease but will disappear with appropriate treatment (see Chap. 79). In this disease, an increased urinary excretion of succinylacetone is observed, a substance found to decrease the uptake of glucose and amino acids by rat renal brush-border membrane vesicles.[32]

Hereditary Fructose Intolerance. In this autosomal recessive disorder associated with deficient activity of fructose-1-phosphate aldolase (see Chap. 70), intravenous infusion of fructose rapidly induces an accumulation of fructose-1-phosphate, an intracellular depletion of inorganic phosphate, and a reversible and complete Fanconi syndrome, with the markedly increased urinary excretion of the characteristic substances.[33,34] The renal toxicity is probably related to the depletion of inorganic phosphate and the reduction of ATP[35] in the renal cortex. Because the infusion of fructose induces within minutes a reversible Fanconi syndrome, this is a very useful experimental model used to study the human Fanconi syndrome.

Galactosemia. The autosomal recessively inherited deficiency of galactose-1-phosphate uridyltransferase (catalyzing the transformation of galactose-1-phosphate into glucose-1-phosphate) leads to accumulation of galactose-1-phosphate (see Chap. 72). It is associated with an incomplete Fanconi syndrome that is reversible on removal of lactose or galactose from the diet.[36] The toxic product is presumably the accumulated galactose-1-phosphate, formation of which depletes the intracellular inorganic phosphate in a fashion similar to that observed in hereditary fructose intolerance.

Glycogen Storage Disease (Type I). Type I with autosomal recessive inheritance (see Chap. 71) and galactose intolerance is associated with Fanconi syndrome.[37]

Wilson Disease. This autosomal recessive disorder of copper metabolism (see Chap. 126), primarily affecting the liver and the brain (hepatolenticular degeneration), is accompanied by copper accumulation in the renal cortex and the various tubular defects typical of Fanconi syndrome,[38] both of which can be reversed with chelation therapy.[39] The following clinical triad is characteristic of this disease: (1) hepatic cirrhosis, (2) a wide variety of neurologic symptoms, and (3) the Kayser-Fleischer rings in the cornea.

Vitamin D–Dependency Rickets (Type I). In this autosomal recessive disorder (see Chap. 165), the 1α-hydroxylation of 25-hydroxycholecalciferol in the kidney mitochondria is apparently defective, a phenomenon that induces decreased intestinal absorption of calcium, hypocalcemia, and parathyroid hormone excess.

Oculocerebrorenal (Lowe) Syndrome. Originally described by Lowe et al.[40] in 1952 and characterized by a Fanconi syndrome, rickets (or osteomalacia in a few patients), growth retardation, bilateral congenital cataracts, glaucoma, generalized muscular hypotonia, hyporeflexia, and severe mental retardation, this syndrome often becomes apparent during the first year of life (see Chap. 252). In this X-linked recessive disorder,[41] the great majority of cases have been observed in boys, although a few have been reported in girls.[42] Cortical opacities also can be found in the lenses of heterozygotes.[43,44] There are three distinct phases in the natural history of this inborn error of metabolism: (1) during infancy, neurologic and ophthalmologic manifestations predominate, but the various tubular dysfunctions of the Fanconi syndrome may all appear within the first year of life, (2) during childhood, severe rickets, growth failure, and the Fanconi syndrome are obvious, and (3) later, the patient dies from inanition, pneumonia, and chronic renal failure.

Although the specific defect responsible for Lowe syndrome remains unknown, the increased urinary excretion of mucopolysaccharides, chondroitin sulfate, and hydroxyproline[45,46] either suggests an abnormal metabolism in connective tissue or simply reflects the metabolic bone disease. Early in the course of the disease, renal dysfunction is tubular but is followed by a progressive reduction in glomerular filtration rate (GFR). The finding that the mitochondrial changes and the functional defects are both proximal suggests a relationship between anatomic and physiologic abnormalities.[42] The tubular changes observed with renal biopsy are not specific,[47] whereas variable pathologic changes have been described in the central nervous system, the eyes, the skeletal muscles, and other tissues. Since the possible biochemical abnormality underlying this disorder remains unknown, there is no specific diagnostic test and treatment. However, vitamin D therapy is useful to treat the metabolic bone disease, as is the case for the Fanconi syndrome associated with other inborn errors of metabolism.

Dent's Disease. In recent years, a novel X-linked form of Fanconi syndrome has been described in association with nephrocalcinosis and progressive renal insufficiency by Frymoyer et al.[48] in northern New York. In England, the condition in five families displayed aminoaciduria, hypercalciuria, phosphaturia, and progressive renal failure and was termed *Dent's disease*.[49] Reports of similar families from Italy, the United States, and France focused on elements of the Fanconi syndrome, especially the occurrence of hypophosphatemic rickets.[50] In Japan, a urinary screening program identified a cohort of children with X-linked mild proximal tubular function and hypercalciuria, but rickets and renal insufficiency were not evident.[51] Although initially thought to be distinct entities, the renal syndrome in each set of patients with Dent's disease has now been attributed to mutations of the *CLCN5* gene, which maps to chromosome Xp11.2.[50,52] This gene encodes a putative chloride channel (746 amino acids) expressed, in humans, primarily in kidney.[53] In the rat, the *CLCN5* product is expressed throughout the renal tubule,[54] and hydropathy analysis predicts a macromolecule with 12 transmembrane domains, similar to other members of the voltage-gated chloride channel family.[53] It has been speculated, despite the absence of direct evidence, that *CLCN5* encodes the chloride channel of endocytotic vesicles in tubular cells, accounting for low-molecular-weight proteinuria in X-linked recessive nephrolithiasis (XLRN). At this time, it is not known how mutations in the renal chloride channel result in hypercalciuria and Fanconi-like proximal tubulopathy.[55] There is no proven therapy for the disease at this time, but because nephrocalcinosis is such a striking feature, Schienman has proposed that calcium-sparing diuretics such as hydrochlorothiazide may be of benefit.[50]

Cytochrome C Oxidase Deficiency. The prominence of mitochondria in proximal tubular cells is sufficient to convince one that defects in the electron-transport chain and ATP production may have an impact on active transport in the proximal nephron (see also Chap. 99). Indeed, there are numerous reports of severe renal Fanconi syndrome in association with mitochondrial myopathy[56] or encephalomyopathy among children with autosomal recessive defects in complex III (cytochrome C oxidase) of the respiratory chain.[57] Usually the syndrome appears in the neonatal period with severe lactic acidosis unresponsive to efforts to circumvent the electron-transport block with vitamin C and vitamin K or with ubiquinone.[57] A somewhat milder renal Fanconi syndrome also may be seen in association with deletions of mitochondrial genes contributing to the electron-transport chain, as in the Pearson and MELAS syndromes.[58,59]

Spontaneous Animal Model: The Basenji Dog. A spontaneous animal model resembling the human idiopathic Fanconi syndrome has been found in Basenji dogs.[60–64] They show clinical signs analogous to those found in humans: polydipsia, polyuria, dehydration, weight loss, and weakness; renal failure occurs after months or years. Plasma electrolytes in these dogs were normal, with the exception of a moderate metabolic acidosis. Glucosuria, phosphaturia, and a generalized aminoaciduria, along with elevated sodium, potassium, and urea excretion, were documented in all affected animals. Renal biopsies were normal, but when renal failure was present, various degrees of tubular and glomerular damage were found.

Acquired Causes

Table 196-2 lists a wide variety of toxic and immunologic renal tubular injuries that may produce generalized impairment of net proximal tubular reabsorption characteristic of the Fanconi syndrome. In contrast with the Fanconi syndrome observed with various inherited metabolic diseases, these acquired Fanconi syndromes are seen primarily in adults, although some can occur at any age.

Heavy Metals. Among the heavy metals that can bind to proximal tubular cells and induce the reabsorptive dysfunctions characteristic of the Fanconi syndrome, lead has long been the most frequent cause but is now replaced by cadmium as the agent most often responsible. These induced tubular dysfunctions are completely reversible when exposure to the toxic environment ceases.

Cadmium. After a prolonged occupational or environmental exposure to cadmium for many years, its excessive accumulation in the kidney is responsible for chronic nephrotoxicity.[65] The increased urinary excretion of the low-molecular-weight β_2-microglobulin, an indicator of renal tubular damage, can signal early cadmium nephrotoxicity.[66] Fanconi syndrome appears frequently among workers exposed to cadmium,[67] a finding that has stimulated many investigators to study the experimental cadmium-induced nephropathy in many animal models, including the rabbit[68,69] and the rat.[70–72] Many cases were described after World War II in Japan in middle-aged, postmenopausal, multiparous women; their disease, characterized by severe osteomalacia, is known as the *itai-itai* ("ouch-ouch") *disease*.[73–75] Intoxication came from soil and rice fields contaminated with cadmium in the Jinzu River Basin.

Uranium. Exposure to gaseous uranium compounds also has been associated with Fanconi syndrome. Uranium and cadmium are more toxic than are lead and mercury.[67]

Mercury. The accumulation of mercury in the proximal tubular cells after exposure to inorganic mercury salts or organic mercury compounds (mercurial diuretics) can produce a reversible Fanconi syndrome.[5]

Lead. In lead poisoning, intranuclear inclusion bodies containing lead bound to a protein appear in proximal tubular cells,[76] and a reversible Fanconi syndrome has been observed, especially in acutely intoxicated children.[77]

Platinum. Cisplatin (*cis*-diaminedichloroplatinum II) is a new and potent chemotherapeutic agent used very effectively in the treatment of many carcinomas, particularly testicular and ovarian. Dose-dependent nephrotoxicity with reduced GFR results from the use of this drug.[78] Among the various tubular dysfunctions observed, the most important is the severe urinary loss of magnesium, inducing severe magnesium depletion and hypomagnesemia.[79]

Drugs. The tubular dysfunctions characteristic of the renal Fanconi syndrome also have been described with clinical use of several drugs; all are reversible on drug withdrawal. The ingestion of *outdated tetracycline* produces a reversible Fanconi syndrome.[80,81] Among the degradation products of tetracycline, outdated or stored in a moist warm environment, anhydro-4-epitetracycline has been shown to be the intoxicating substance responsible for the tubulopathy.[82] In rats this metabolite induces mitochondrial injury in the proximal nephron and decreases oxidative enzymatic activity and energy production.[83] Most cases of Fanconi syndrome resulting from *aminoglycoside antibiotics* have been associated with the use of *gentamicin*.[84] Renal magnesium and potassium wasting with severe hypomagnesemia and hypokalemia also have been observed with aminoglycoside antibiotics,[85,86] substances well known to accumulate selectively in proximal tubular cells.[87] A reversible Fanconi syndrome has been reported with the anticonvulsant *valproate*.[88] Some patients with nephrotic syndrome and receiving *6-mercaptopurine* also have had Fanconi syndrome.[89] It is not easy in these patients to dissociate the respective contribution of the nephrotic syndrome and of the 6-mercaptopurine administration. The accidental ingestion of large amounts of *methyl-3-chromone*, a substance structurally related to tetracycline, also has been reported to induce a reversible Fanconi syndrome.[90] Finally, a Fanconi syndrome has been seen following an extensive *Lysol* burn,[91] the ingestion of the herbicide *paraquat*,[92] *toluene* inhalation,[93] and with *ifosfamide* chemotherapy.[94,95]

Urinary Excretion of Abnormal Proteins. *Multiple myeloma* and other *dysproteinemias* are a frequent cause of acquired Fanconi syndrome in adults,[96] which in some patients may even precede by many years the appearance of dysproteinemia.[97] Indeed, this diagnosis of dysproteinemia must be excluded in all adult patients with a Fanconi syndrome of obscure cause. Bence Jones proteinuria is always present[97]; all patients have light chains of the κ variety, except a few with λ light chains.[98] Crystalline inclusion bodies and nonamyloid microfibrils probably representing light-chain accumulation can be observed in the cytoplasm of proximal tubular cells.[96,97,99] These light chains therefore may be directly toxic to the proximal tubular cells,[100] which seem to be the site of their catabolism,[101] or could interfere with megalin (see below), which was shown recently to be a carrier for proteins such as albumin, aprotinin, and others.[102–104] Renal tubular transport abnormalities can disappear after the successful therapy of multiple myeloma and the disappearance of urinary Bence Jones protein.[105] Amyloidosis,[106,107] light-chain nephropathy,[108–110] and benign monoclonal gammopathy[111] are among the dysproteinemias other than multiple myeloma reported to induce Fanconi syndrome and urinary excretion of monoclonal light chains.

Immunologic Disorders. Fanconi syndrome has been reported in nephrotic syndrome,[112] most often with focal and segmental glomerular sclerosis,[113] but the pathogenesis remains uncertain. *Interstitial nephritis with antitubular basement membrane antibodies* (linear deposits along the basement membrane of the proximal tubules) may be accompanied by a Fanconi syndrome. A reversible Fanconi syndrome also has been observed in several patients following *renal transplantation*,[114–116] and the defects of proximal reabsorption, most probably resulting from immunologic tubular injury during acute rejection episodes, seem to disappear during the first year following transplantation. The immunosuppressive drug cyclosporine does not seem to be responsible for the various defects of proximal reabsorption.[117] Some tumors, such as nonossifying fibroma of bone, also can produce Fanconi syndrome, possibly through the release of a humoral factor.[118] Lymphoid *malignancies* with peritubular infiltrates have been associated with a Fanconi syndrome and could result either from immunologic tubular injury or from tubular destruction by tumor infiltration.[119] The simultaneous occurrence of a Fanconi syndrome and other malignancies such as carcinoma of the lung,[120] liver,[121] pancreas,[122] and ovary[123] may be fortuitous. Further investigations need to be performed before clear conclusions can be drawn.

Experimental Models

Maleate, which is an isomer of fumarate, was first used by Berliner et al.[124] in the dog and was found by Harrison and Harrison[125] to induce a Fanconi syndrome in rats. Maleate still remains a model widely used to study the mechanisms and pathogenesis of this complex renal tubular dysfunction.[126] *Cadmium* has been used extensively in rats; the signs, typical of Fanconi syndrome, appear abruptly after 3 weeks of injection and the total administration of about 2.25 mg of cadmium. *Cystine dimethylester* has produced the Fanconi syndrome in rats.[127–130] *4-Pentenoate*, a short-chain fatty acid, also has been shown to produce an experimental Fanconi syndrome in dogs.[131]

MECHANISMS AND PATHOGENESIS

General Characteristics

The pathogenic mechanisms underlying the Fanconi syndrome remain to be elucidated, as do, more specifically, the respective contributions of the proximal and distal nephron, the organelles involved, the membrane-transport defects, and the possibly abnormal enzymatic activities. The role of the endocytotic apparatus and megalin, a membrane glycoprotein that is a receptor for many ligands, may be major, and their disruption by toxins or drugs could be central to explain the resulting Fanconi syndrome. However, many conclusions can be drawn from study of hereditary and acquired diseases, as well as from recent data obtained with the experimental models.

1. The Fanconi syndrome clearly has *two components*: a disorder of multiple renal transport functions and a metabolic bone

disease, i.e., rickets in children or osteomalacia in adults. Since the bone disease is not always present, the primary disturbance in this syndrome is thought to be renal. In fact, some of the etiologic agents may have direct effects on both bone and kidney, whereas others may have an effect only on kidney.

2. Since amino acids, glucose, phosphate, and other molecules are transported into the cells by multiple carriers, it is hard to visualize how defects in a single protein could disturb simultaneously so many substrates. It is more likely that the various mutations associated with the Mendelian forms of the Fanconi syndrome affect components of the transport mechanism other than the carrier(s) per se. The modified critical step has to be *global* enough to affect many transport functions. Such a step could be a disruption of the energy source, a generalized nonspecific membrane permeability defect, or a specific organelle pathology.

3. In many cases, the Fanconi syndrome is expressed only when well-defined factors are present, such as the unrestricted intake of tyrosine and phenylalanine in tyrosinemia[132–134] or the ingestion of fructose in hereditary fructose intolerance.[33,34,135] Reciprocally, when galactose is removed in galactosemia,[36,136] fructose in hereditary fructose intolerance,[33,135] or tyrosine and phenylalanine in tyrosinemia,[137–140] the Fanconi syndrome is no longer expressed. These observations demonstrate the *reversibility* of the abnormality leading to the Fanconi syndrome.

4. The *duration of exposure* to the specific agent also appears to be an important element but varies with the disease underlying the Fanconi syndrome. Intravenous injection of small amounts of fructose to patients with hereditary fructose intolerance increases the excretion of amino acids, phosphate, glucose, and other electrolytes in a dose-dependent fashion.[33,34] On the other hand, patients with galactosemia have to ingest galactose for days[36] before the renal dysfunction occurs, whereas, by contrast, hepatic dysfunction can be noted within minutes.[141] Renal tubular dysfunction caused by cadmium occurs after many years of exposure to a polluted environment or to industrial cadmium (pigment, plastic, alloy, accumulator battery, nuclear, and electronics industries).[65–68] Lead can induce a Fanconi syndrome in acutely intoxicated children almost exclusively,[77,142] in experimental animals,[143] and rarely, in chronic states.

5. A *specific biochemical sequence* of events can take place, as illustrated in patients with hereditary fructose intolerance: Following a fructose infusion, an accumulation of fructose-1-phosphate in proximal tubular cells is postulated to result from the deficiency of aldolase B activity; a severe depletion of inorganic phosphate, ATP, and total adenine nucleotides ensues and may contribute to the multiple transport disorders of the Fanconi syndrome.[144] Any interruption of this sequence of events could prevent the pathologic manifestations. Since in normal humans, rats, and dogs the administration of large amounts of fructose does not induce a Fanconi syndrome, despite the hepatic and renal cortical accumulation of large amounts of fructose-1-phosphate,[145–147] Morris et al.[144] have suggested that the genetic defect is primary and that abnormalities other than the kinetic deficiency of the enzyme are secondarily involved.

Nephron Segment(s) Involved

In normal mammalian kidneys, the reabsorptive capacity of proximal tubular cells is immense for amino acids because most of the filtered load is reabsorbed within the first few millimeters of the proximal nephron[148]; in fact, less than 2 percent of the filtered load of amino acids will appear in the urine, with the exception of aspartic acid, glycine, and histidine, where up to 6 percent may be excreted.[149] In the Fanconi syndrome, the aminoaciduria is generalized.[150] *The absence of selective aminoaciduria* suggests in itself a generalized disease not specific for any carrier or for any nephron segment.

Morphologic Changes. A "swan-neck lesion," resulting from cell atrophy in the earliest portion of the proximal tubule, was found during autopsy in a few patients with cystinosis and was thought for many years to be primarily responsible for the transport dysfunction.[151] This is not likely, since micropuncture studies have demonstrated that the entire length, not only the early part of the proximal nephron, has the capacity to reabsorb amino acids.[148] The one-time popularity of this explanation can be attributed to the beauty of the image given as evidence rather than to a critical assessment of the data, and this hypothesis should now be forgotten. The cell atrophy observed is most probably secondary, since the emergence of the swan-neck lesion in cystinosis is progressive with age and not related to transport dysfunction. Nonspecific tubular and glomerular lesions also were documented in renal biopsies of patients with Lowe syndrome.[41,152] Major morphologic lesions are not found in many other forms of the human Fanconi syndrome such as hereditary tyrosinemia,[134] galactosemia,[36] fructosemia,[144] heavy metal poisoning, and various other forms.[18,153] Renal biopsies from Basenji dogs with the Fanconi syndrome also showed normal histology, and various degrees of tubular and glomerular damage were found only when renal failure was present.[61,62] It should be pointed out, however, that many functional disturbances can be observed in the absence of morphologic lesions; indeed, histologic lesions are seldom observed in most specific transport defects.

In the experimental models of Fanconi syndrome, ultrastructural modifications (Fig. 196-1) always were found in the proximal tubule,[9,154–158] and they seem to follow a time course in parallel with the transport irregularities. The lesions are similar, regardless of the causal toxic agents: extensive cytoplasmic vacuolization, darkening or swelling of the mitochondrial matrix, enlargement of the lysosomes, disruption of cytoplasmic organization, distension of the endoplasmic reticulum cisternae, loss of basolateral membrane infoldings, and even cell necrosis. Many of these lesions are related to cytotoxicity, but as will be described below, some lesions are specific and could explain the transport derangement. Maleate and heavy metals are readily filtered, and the early part of the proximal nephron is therefore first exposed to their deleterious effects; for instance, Gonick and Kramer[72] showed that cadmium specifically accumulates in proximal tubular cells of the renal cortex. Toxic compounds containing heavy metals also yielded similar lesions. All these ultrastructural changes are reversible within a few days after cessation of maleate or cadmium administration. Several investigators have found maleate-induced morphologic injury in proximal tubular cells,[9,154,157–159] but the distal nephron also was found to be damaged when larger doses of maleate were given.[155,156,159]

Functional Changes. Many functional changes observed in the presence of maleate are obviously related to a proximal nephron pathology: decreased uptake of phosphate in rat brush-border membrane vesicles,[160] impairment of the hydroxylation of 25-hydroxyvitamin D_3 in the mitochondria of proximal cells,[161–163] and modification of the γ-glutamyl transpeptidase, a membrane-bound enzyme of the proximal nephron.[164] However, as shown by micropuncture studies in rats[165] and dogs,[166] maleate has additional sites of action located more distally than the proximal convoluted tubule, namely, in thick ascending limb[167] or other parts of the distal nephron.[165] The micropuncture and free-water clearance studies show that maleate,[168,169] like acetazolamide,[170,171] has an effect on the thick ascending limb, whereas sodium chloride and sodium bicarbonate reabsorption are both inhibited in the proximal nephron. Another toxin, 4-pentenoate, has an effect on the proximal tubule but not on the thick ascending limb.[172]

Cell Membranes Involved. The renal Fanconi syndrome impairs net proximal reabsorption of amino acids and other solutes leading to enhanced urinary elimination. Are binding and uptake altered at the luminal membrane? Clinical and laboratory studies indeed suggest that they are not compromised. For example, the studies of Robson and Rose[173] showed that arginine reabsorption is further

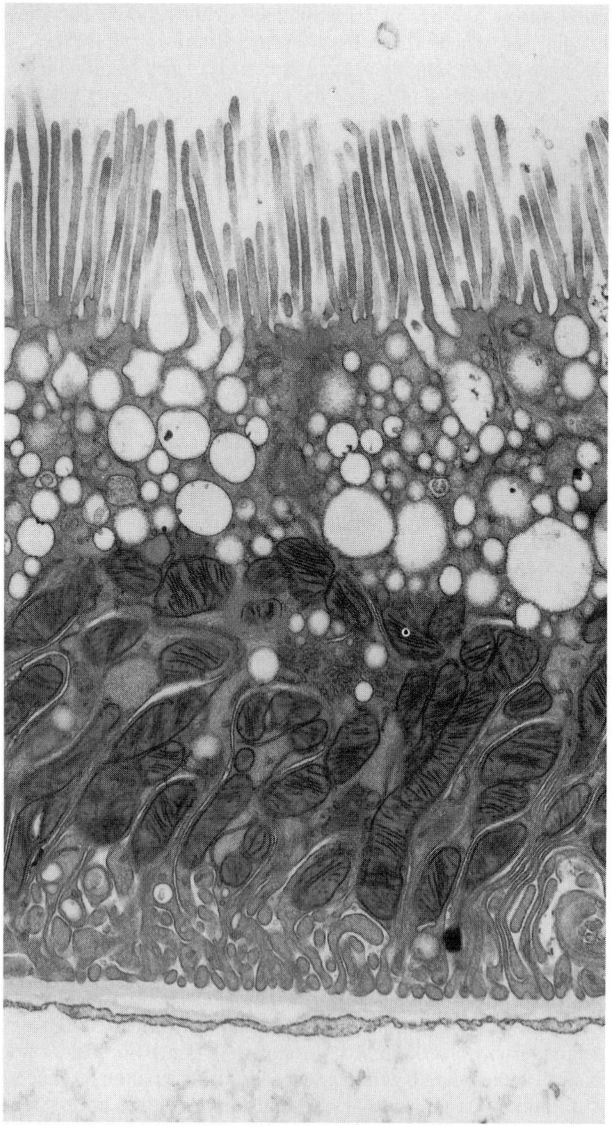

Fig. 196-1 Osmium impregnation of a proximal tubule cell from a rat having received sodium maleate 1 hour before. Note the numerous and large vacuoles at the cell apex, as compared with the normal conditions (see Fig. 196-3). These vesicles are known to contain megalin (see Figs. 196-4 and 196-5) and a variety of associated peptides[161,194,205]; dense apical tubules are conspicuously absent after maleate.[52,161] Fixation by perfusion with 2.5% glutaraldehyde in barbital buffer, citrate-calcium. (Magnification: × 15,000.)

impaired in patients with a Fanconi syndrome when the concentration of lysine, a competitive inhibitor of arginine transport or a shared carrier, is increased in glomerular filtrate. Scriver et al.[174,175] also showed that glycine reabsorption is still normally inhibited by proline in patients with the Fanconi syndrome. Such observations imply that the sites at which amino acids interact with selective carriers are intact and that transport is not attenuated at the interface between tubular fluid and luminal membrane. However, the Basenji dog model is an exception and actually suggests a defect at the substrate-entry step.[61] Since this study was carried out with renal biopsies of affected dogs, it is not clear which renal epithelial cell membrane, luminal or basolateral, is affected. That integrity of carriers is not affected is further supported by studies *in vitro*[176] and *in vivo*[165,177] with the maleic acid model. By microperfusing amino acids of related structure, Bergeron et al.[165] showed that carriers appeared to be intact in maleate-treated kidneys because competition still existed at the luminal membrane. This finding was confirmed by Silverman and Huang[178] who could find no change in the specificity of carrier systems or of their coupling to either the sodium concentration gradient or the membrane potential gradient.

Decreased Uptake or Increased Backflux of Solutes? Since net reabsorption of substrates is still functioning, albeit at a reduced rate,[165] in the syndrome produced experimentally or observed in humans, could the hyperexcretion be better explained by a cellular loss and a backleak into the tubular lumen? In fact, both a decreased reabsorption and an increased backflux appear to contribute to urinary loss of solutes in the maleate model.[165,166,176,178–180] The *in vitro* studies of Rosenberg and Segal,[176] later confirmed by *in vivo* studies of Bergeron et al.,[165,179] showed the preponderant role of cellular exit, as opposed to decreased entry, in explaining the low intracellular concentration of amino acids and sugars in maleate-treated kidneys.[181,182] This increased backflux of amino acids,[176,177,179,180] sugars,[157,166,177,178] potassium,[72,183] and bicarbonate[72,168] seems to occur at both distal and proximal sites (Fig. 196-2, steps 1 and 2). While backflux in the proximal nephron can be corrected downstream, such is not the case in the distal nephron, where there is no reabsorption of amino acids[148] and little absorption of phosphate and glucose.[166] Molecules that exit at this distal site are irrevocably lost in the urine. Thus, in addition to the proximal disturbance, a distal nephron involvement may be a major determinant in the final production of the aminoaciduria, glycosuria, and phosphaturia seen in the Fanconi syndrome. This is further suggested by an increased urinary-minus-blood P_{CO_2} gradient[184–187] and increased kaliuresis in maleate-treated animals[184]; both could reflect accelerated cellular exit of hydrogen and potassium ions into the lumen of the last segments of the nephron. A change in the lipid bilayer of cellular membranes[64,188] would be consistent with a permeability hypothesis for the renal Fanconi syndrome.[165] The membrane could be leaky but still could retain selective permeability, as shown by Obaid et al.[189] in red cell membranes, where maleic anhydride increases sodium and potassium permeabilities while decreasing anion permeability. Other investigators have noted increased potassium efflux from renal cells[165,166,178–180,190] and blood cells,[7] leading to the suggestion that maleate alters membrane permeability, most likely through an effect on membrane phospholipids or through chelation of divalent ions.[177,191]

Pathogenesis: Hypotheses Based on Organelle Dysfunction

Alterations in functions of cellular organelles could be responsible for the backleak of molecules from the cytoplasm to the tubular lumen and hence their excretion in the final urine. The different cellular sites that could be affected in the Fanconi syndrome are illustrated in Fig. 196-2.

Inhibition of Endocytosis and Recycling of Megalin. Inhibition of the endocytotic process mediated by the megalin membrane glycoprotein is presented here as an hypothesis to account for the renal Fanconi syndrome. Increased attention has been given to the role of the endocytotic apparatus, located at the apex of proximal tubular cells (Fig. 196-3), and of megalin, a membrane glycoprotein (gp330) that is a receptor for many ligands.[192–195] Megalin and its associated ligands are normally internalized at the luminal surface in the coated pits and targeted along the endocytotic pathway into early and late endosomes (Figs. 196-4 and 196-5). In these organelles, in the presence of the H^+-ATPase, the ligand is separated from its receptor megalin and transferred to the lysosomes, whereas megalin itself is recycled for reuse at the cell surface (see Fig. 196-5). Bergeron et al.[196] have shown that disruption of this process may account for the generalized permeability defect in tubular function in the maleate model and possibly also in other forms of the Fanconi syndrome. Since maleate and heavy metals are filtered by the glomerulus, the luminal surface of the early segments of the proximal nephron are

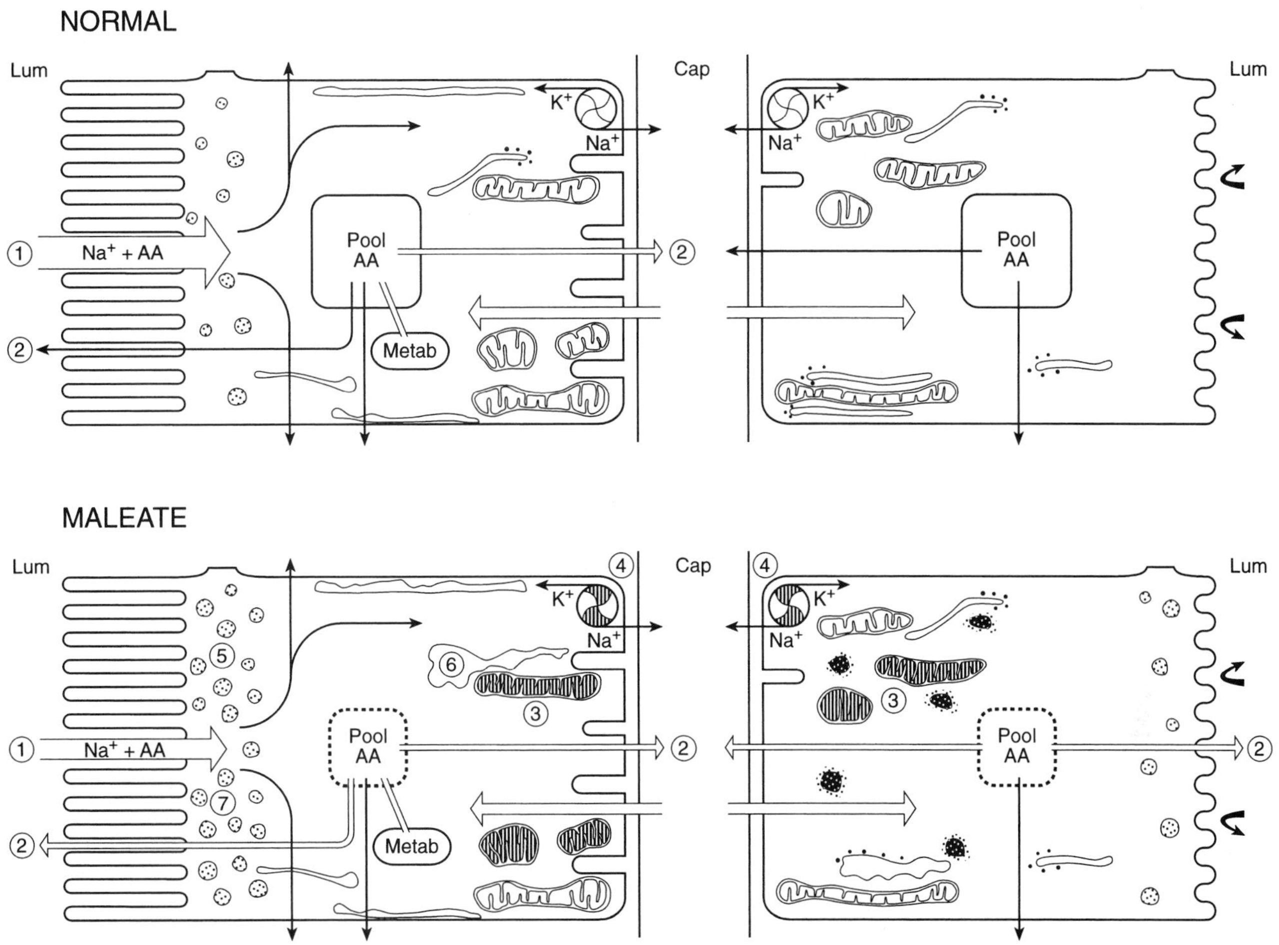

Fig. 196-2 In normal individuals, amino acids gain access to the proximal nephron cells (*left-hand arrows*) through the apical microvilli or through the infoldings of the antiluminal membrane. Intracellular accumulation of amino acids can occur against a concentration gradient. At the brush border, uptake is a carrier-mediated process and, when coupled to a sodium gradient (Na^+ out > Na^+ in), is "secondary active" transport. Exit can occur at all membranes. Amino acids also can be metabolized (metab) in the renal tubular cells. In the distal tubule (*right-hand arrows*), similar amino acid movements occur, except that there is no luminal entry of amino acids and little, if any, luminal entry of glucose and phosphate. In the maleate model of Fanconi syndrome, there is a marked backleak of amino acids and sugar into the tubular lumen. As a consequence, intracellular amino acid levels fall significantly (Pool). In proximal tubular cells, luminal amino acid uptake mechanisms are also disturbed, but residual luminal uptake still exceeds backleak, allowing at least some net amino acid reabsorption. However, in the distal tubule where luminal uptake systems are absent, maleate-induced exit of amino acids into the lumen is completely uncompensated, allowing net amino acid "secretion" into the urine. Other forms of renal Fanconi syndrome have been ascribed to numerous complex mechanisms that might disturb luminal membrane function. These include (1) a defect in some aspect of transport critical to all luminal carrier mechanisms (of note, most solutes lost in urine are coupled to luminal reabsorption of sodium), (2) a disturbance of luminal membrane organization affecting both uptake and backleak of solutes as in the maleate model above, (3) impaired production of metabolic energy or ATP as in the example of human cytochrome C oxidase deficiency, (4) defective Na^+, K^+-ATPase activity at basolateral membranes, affecting the sodium gradient at the luminal membrane, (5) reduced H^+-ATPase activity affecting the endocytotic recycling apparatus, (6) structural disorganization and dysfunction of organelles such as the endoplasmic reticulum or mitochondria, (7) defective megalin-dependent recycling of transport proteins and transporters from endocytotic compartments to the luminal membrane (see Fig. 196-6). *An integrative hypothesis that may link many forms of Fanconi syndrome is that they have in common a toxic effect or a primary cellular dysfunction that disrupts some critical element of endocytotic membrane recycling. Blockade at any point along the recycling pathway will modify luminal membrane function by trapping membrane transport proteins and other constituents in endosomes; depletion of these elements from the luminal membrane may limit reabsorptive transport and allow increased backleak of organic solutes.* Lum lumen; Cap, capillary; AA, amino acids.

the first to be exposed to the toxic effect. At an early stage of toxicity, abundant vacuoles appear beneath the apical surface (see Fig. 196-1). The vesicles are known to contain megalin (see Fig. 196-5) and a variety of associated peptides.[159,197,198] Christensen and Maunsbach[9] demonstrated that transport of lysozyme from endocytotic vesicles to lysosomes is inhibited by maleate. Thus maleate appears to disrupt the endocytotic pathway at the stage of late endosome formation (Fig. 196-6). Megalin is the receptor of many proteins, including albumin.[102,103] A toxic effect on megalin recycling would result in defective uptake of low-molecular-weight proteins from tubular fluid; proteinuria would ensue. Moreover megalin itself is shed into final urine, thus contributing to the proteinuria.[196] Recycling of endocytosed membrane proteins, such as megalin, occurs through dense apical tubules (see Fig. 196-1); the latter are conspicuously absent in the maleate model.[9,159] This observation predicts that toxins such as maleate, which interrupt membrane recycling, could produce widespread dysfunction of reabsorptive mechanisms by trapping membrane receptors (including the glucose and amino acid transporters) in endosomes, thus depleting the pool of transporters at the luminal surface.

Maleate also may involve its chelation effect. Ligand binding to megalin is calcium-dependent.[102,195] By chelating calcium, maleate may disrupt the normal association between megalin and

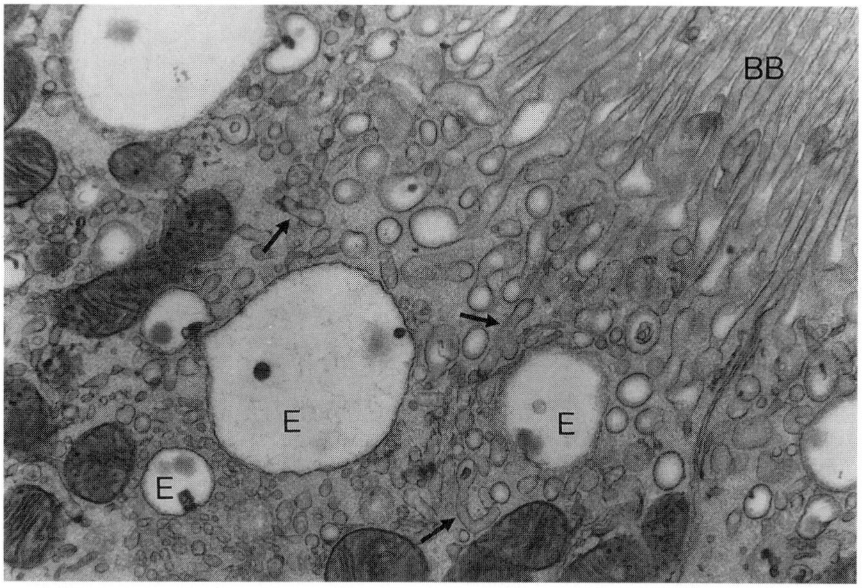

Fig. 196-3 Slightly oblique section through the apex of a proximal tubule cell (S2 segment) below the brush border (BB), showing the normal appearance of the endocytotic apparatus made of vesicles of different sizes (E, endosomes) and dense apical tubules (*arrows*). Fixation by perfusion with 2.5% glutaraldehyde in barbital buffer citrate calcium and post-fixed with imidazole/osmium and lead/copper citrate stain. (Magnification: × 27,000.)

its ligands during endocytosis. Furthermore, by depleting local calcium pools, maleate may block formation of dense apical tubules required for recycling transporters to the apical surface. Calcium depletion has been shown to inhibit exocytosis in other cell types.[199,200]

Intestinal uptake of glucose and amino acids is unaffected by maleate. Megalin is absent from intestinal epithelial cells.[201] Structural and functional aspects of absorption mechanisms thus differ in the renal proximal tubule and in the intestine. Thus the mechanism by which maleate disrupts membrane recycling in the proximal convoluted cell may involve a critical interference with megalin function. Maleate may, in particular, affect the uncoating ATPase or other ATP-dependent processes that are involved in the formation of secondary endosomes[202] or lysosomal transfer. The ATP content, alluded to earlier, is essential for the proper function of these organelles. Another reported manifestation of renal maleate toxicity is the ATP/ADP ratio, which also could be more critical than the actual ATP content because ATP and ADP

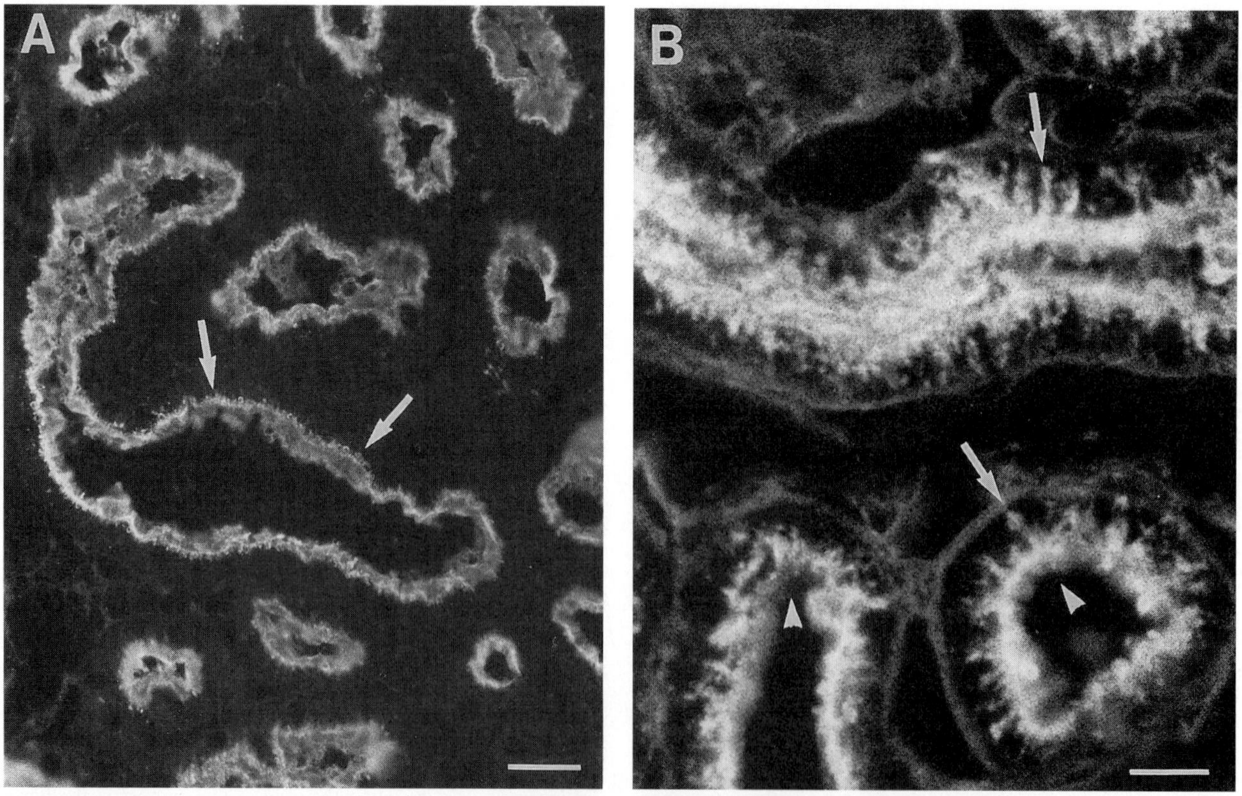

Fig. 196-4 Cryostat sections (3 μm) of rat kidneys incubated with anti-gp330 polyclonal antibody, followed by fluorescein isothiocyanate (FITC)–conjugated goat antirabbit immunoglobulin G (IgG). These two figures show the localization of gp330 in control (*A*) and maleate-treated kidneys (*B*). Note the appearance of the endocytotic vesicles (*arrows*) in the normal proximal convoluted tubule. In the section of maleate-treated rat kidney (3 h), note the many cytoplasmic streaks (*arrows*) below the brush border of proximal cells. The labeling of the brush border is clearly absent (*arrowhead*) in many areas. (Magnifications: A: ×350, bar = 29 μm; B: × 1200, bar = 8 μm.)

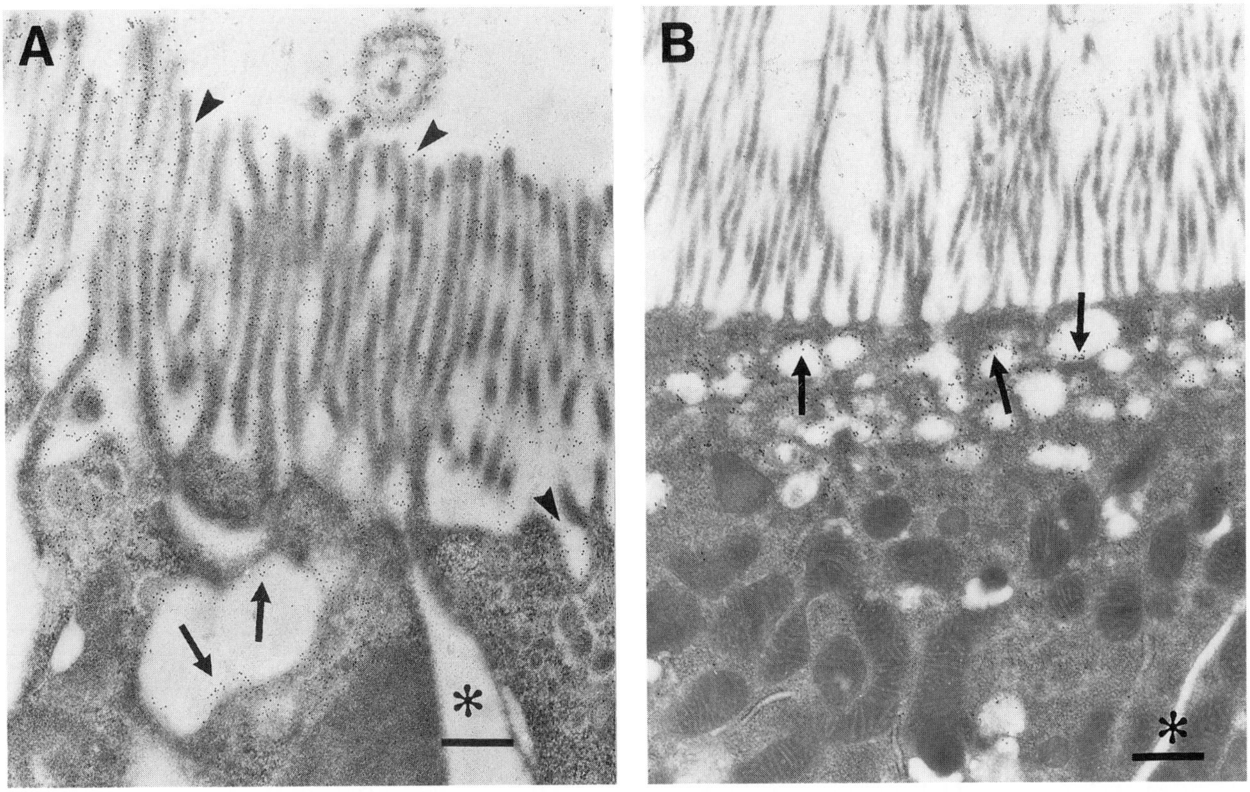

Fig. 196-5 Ultrathin sections of proximal convoluted tubule cells incubated with anti-gp330 antibody followed by protein A–gold, after embedding in Lowicryl K4M, from a control rat (*A*) and after maleate treatment for 45 min (*B*). Panel *A* shows that, in normal rats, gold particles, revealing antigenic sites, are localized on the brush border (*arrowheads*), as well as in apical invaginations and vesicles (*arrows*). Note the uniform distribution of labeling in brush border. All microvilli are labeled. Note presence of gold particles in apical vesicles and their absence from intercellular space (*asterisk*). Panel *B* shows a proximal tubule cell of a maleate-treated kidney (45 min). Gold particles are still present in most apical vacuoles (*arrows*) of this cell and implies that maleate does not inhibit the transfer of megalin and its ligands into the endosomes. (Magnifications: *A*: × 25,000; *B*: × 15,000.)

concentrations, built up by the membrane ATPases and the mitochondrial synthetase, can be established in the cytoplasmic "compartments," and as suggested by Amman et al.,[203] the coexistence of sodium and ATP gradient may amplify the functional consequences of small changes in ATP/ADP ratio on sodium and proton pumps.[203]

These observations on the role of megalin support an hypothesis about a cellular mechanism for the renal Fanconi syndrome. The hypothesis is summarized in Fig. 196-6. Blockade at any point along the recycling pathway will modify luminal membrane function by trapping membrane transport proteins and other constituents in endosomes. Depletion of these elements from the luminal membrane site may limit reabsorptive transport and hence increase excretion of urinary solutes.

Mitochondrial Dysfunction. Maleate, heavy metals, and tetracyclines all have specific, albeit reversible, effects on organelles and their interrelationships.[156,157,204] A major disturbance of the subcellular structures linking mitochondria and the network of perimitochondrial membranes was noted both by Bergeron and Laporte[156] in the maleate model and by Gonick and Kramer[72] in the cadmium model. Mitochondria seem to concentrate cadmium, mercury, and maleate[9,70,72,143]; thus toxins like maleate could impair mitochondrial functions in renal epithelial cells (including the 1-hydroxylation of 25-OH vitamin D_3[161]).

An experimental model of the Fanconi syndrome has been produced in rats by repeated injections of cadmium chloride and was studied extensively by various investigators.[72,204,205] Mitochondrial enlargement and loss of basolateral membrane infoldings were the most conspicuous morphologic changes. Kagi and Vallee[206] described the formation of a low-molecular-weight metalloprotein (metallothionein) that has a high sulfhydryl content (cysteine) and metal content (cadmium and zinc). The cadmium-metallothionein complex is synthesized by the liver, filtered by the glomeruli, and reabsorbed proximally.[207] The proximal tubule appears to be more susceptible to the cadmium-metallothionein[208] or cadmium-cysteine complex[209] than to the inorganic cadmium. Protein degradation in the kidney liberates the metal, which is then incorporated into nascent chains of thionine within the kidney. The delayed onset of renal tubular dysfunction seen in cadmium exposure is most likely related to its interaction with the thionine. Raghavan and Gonick[71] offered the hypothesis that the Fanconi syndrome resulted from a saturation of the cadmium-binding capacity of the renal cortical metallothionein; the excess cadmium was then free to "spill over" from the soluble cytoplasmic fraction to other subcellular fractions, in particular the microsomal and mitochondrial fractions containing cadmium-sensitive enzymes. The mitochondrial oxidation of Krebs cycle intermediates in the kidney,[210] especially the CoA-dependent substrates pyruvate and alphaketoglutarate,[211–213] was decreased by those toxic molecules.

Toxic agents to which renal cells are exposed can impair production of ATP and inhibit the Na^+, K^+-ATPase activity at the basolateral membranes, a phenomenon that would affect the electrochemical sodium gradient across the luminal membrane and decrease net solute reabsorption. Many of the transport functions impaired in the Fanconi syndrome are coupled to the Na^+ gradient, e.g., Na^+-H^+ exchange (bicarbonate reabsorption), Na^+-glucose cotransport, Na^+–amino acid cotransport, and Na^+-PO_4^{2-} cotransport. Although reductions in renal cortical ATP concentration[72,155,204,211] and renal cortical Na^+, K^+-ATPase activity[183,214–218] have been reported following maleate administration, infusion of 4-pentenoate,[131] and intracellular loading of cystine,[219,220] a causal relationship between decreased ATP levels

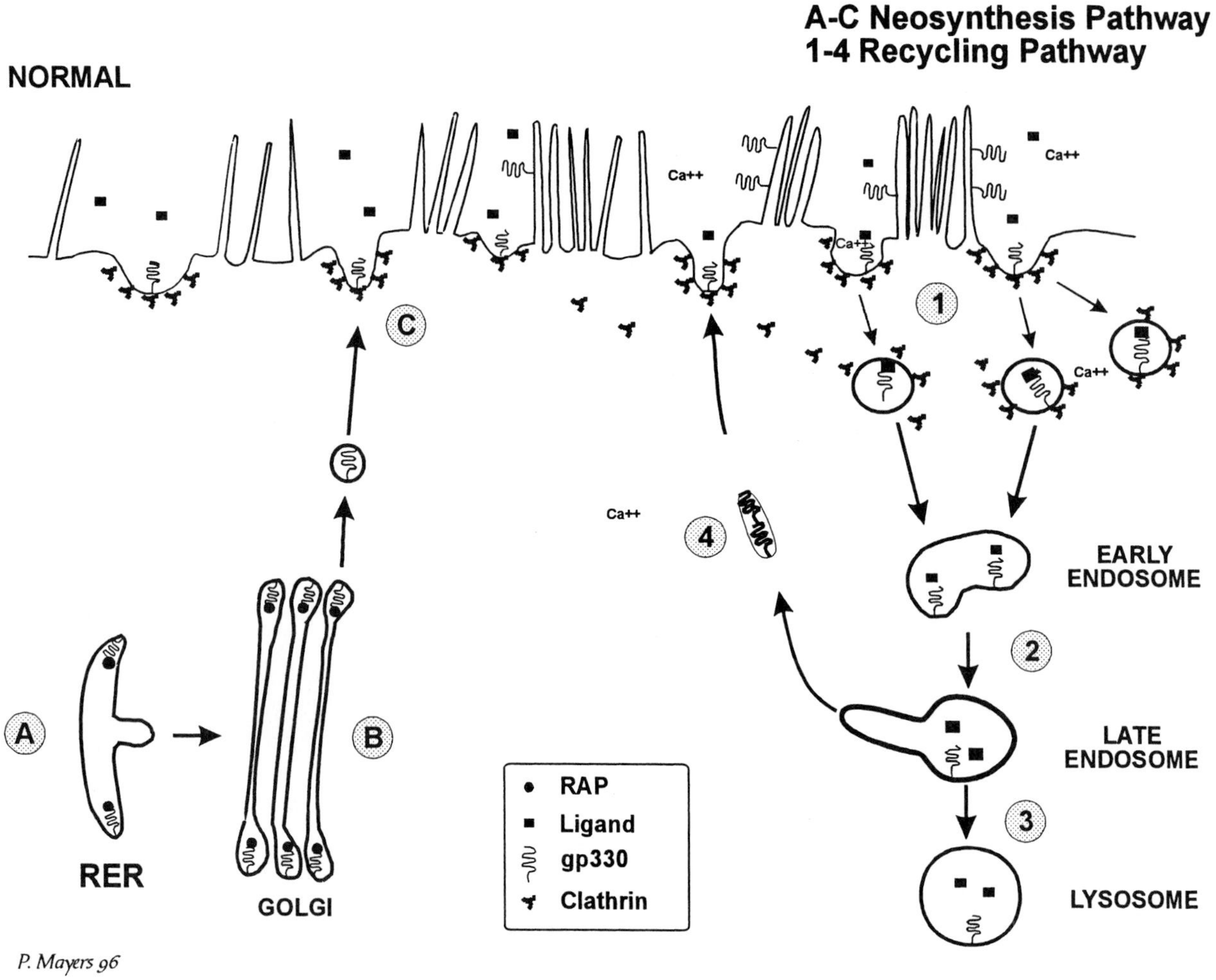

Fig. 196-6 Schematic representation of the *de novo* synthesis pathway (*A–C*) and the recycling pathway (1–4) of megalin in maleate-treated cells. Megalin and RAP, its associated protein, which acts as a chaperon, are synthesized and assembled in the rough endoplasmic reticulum (*A*) and are transported together across Golgi stacks (*B*); megalin then reaches the apical cell surface and is inserted into microvilli and clathrin-coated pits (*C*). Megalin, a receptor for many ligands, is internalized with its ligand (1) into early and late endosomes (2), where it dissociates from its ligand, which is taken up by the lysosome (3). The receptor is recycled back (4), via dense apical tubules, to the cell surface, where it becomes competent again to bind ligands. Maleate could act at the late endosome level (2) and also by blocking the formation of new dense apical tubules (4), which are remarkably absent in maleate-treated rats. Megalin and its ligands are trapped inside fused endosomes. Since there is no recycling of endosomes, there is a widespread dysfunction of reabsorptive mechanism; membrane receptors and transporters (glucose, amino acids, phosphate, etc.) also will be trapped inside these endosomes (see text).

and the inhibited tubular transport of solutes has not been established unequivocally; there are alternative explanations. For instance, in maleate-treated rats, the decrease in Na^+, K^+-ATPase activity appears to be restricted to the proximal convoluted tubule without any corresponding changes in more distal segments of the nephron.[215,217] Moreover, the intestinal transport of glucose and amino acids is unaffected by maleate, even though sodium absorption and Na^+, K^+-ATPase is impaired in this tissue.[221]

Protective Effects of Various Substances

The protective action of certain substances has provided some insights into the mechanism of nephrotoxicity in the renal Fanconi syndrome. For example, the protective effect of acetoacetate on maleate-induced bicarbonaturia and phosphaturia results from competition between acetoacetate (which is the physiologic substrate for succinyl-CoA transferase) and maleate for the transport of CoA.[222] Phosphate loading also can prevent the maleate-induced renal Fanconi syndrome[8,223] and decrease the urinary loss of bicarbonate, amino acids, lysozyme, and lysosomal enzymes. The protective effect of phosphate suggests that a phosphate-dependent membrane abnormality in proximal tubular cells or the loss of intracellular phosphate (and hence of ATP) may play a role in the pathogenesis of the maleate-induced Fanconi syndrome. More recently, a membrane cytoprotective effect of glycine has been documented in different models of experimental Fanconi syndrome, the *in vitro* model of intracellular cystine loading[220,224] and the *in vivo* model in rats treated with intraperitoneal maleate or ifosfamide.[225] As correctly pointed out by Nissim and Weinberg,[225] glycine attenuates, but does not suppress, the abnormalities of tubular function induced by maleate and ifosfamide in rat. This suggests that glycine may act simply by decreasing the uptake of the toxins[226,227]: Less maleate could gain access to the cell membrane, and more important, glycine suppresses the plasma membrane permeability defect,[225,226,228,229] thus reinforcing the permeability hypothesis discussed earlier. Although glycine prevents the fall in renal cortical concentrations of ATP and P_i in maleate-treated rats, it does not do this in ifosfamide-treated rats,[225] illustrating that all models of Fanconi syndrome cannot be explained simply by a single mechanism.

CLINICAL SIGNS AND SYMPTOMS

The clinical manifestations of the Fanconi syndrome result from nonspecific renal losses of fluid and electrolytes and from the vitamin D–resistant metabolic bone disease. The renal loss of other substances such as glucose, amino acids, and uric acid will not induce any clinical signs or symptoms but may contribute in some patients to the diagnosis of Fanconi syndrome.

The age at which a child first becomes symptomatic can provide a clue for the specific inborn error of metabolism. For example, infants with galactosemia or hereditary fructose intolerance can present with acute symptoms within the first few days of life if they ingest galactose or fructose, respectively. Children with nephropathic cystinosis usually present with symptoms only after the age of 6 months. In Wilson disease, symptoms of the renal Fanconi syndrome usually will not appear before the end of the first decade of life. Symptoms induced by acquired forms of the Fanconi syndrome may appear at any age.

Consequences of Renal Losses of Fluid and Electrolytes

The excessive urinary loss of water resulting from the renal concentration defect will produce polyuria and polydipsia and, in infants and young children, dehydration, constipation, and unexplained recurrent fever. The chronic hyperchloremic metabolic acidosis resulting from the associated renal proximal tubular acidosis (see also Chap. 195) can induce anorexia and episodic vomiting. Muscle weakness and even episodic paralysis can result from severe hypokalemia and potassium depletion.

Vitamin D-Resistant Metabolic Bone Disease

Hypophosphatemic rickets (in growing children) or osteomalacia (in adults) is produced at least in part by the exaggerated renal loss of phosphate and may dominate the clinical picture (see also Chap. 197). An impaired renal tubular 1α-hydroxylation of 25-hydroxyvitamin D_3 into 1,25-dihydroxyvitamin D_3 also may play a role in the pathogenesis of this metabolic bone disease; indeed, this biologically active vitamin D metabolite was not found in the blood of five nonazotemic children with Fanconi syndrome.[161] The child with Fanconi syndrome will fail to grow and may present the characteristic clinical findings of rickets: frontal bossing, rachitic rosary, bowing deformities of the legs, metaphyseal widening at the wrists, knees, or ankles, and waddling gait. By contrast, patients with adult-onset Fanconi syndrome often complain of severe bone pain and spontaneous fractures.

THERAPY

Specific Treatment

Although the clinical management of Fanconi syndrome consists mostly of replacing the renal losses of substances not reabsorbed adequately by the kidney, one must always consider the possibility of a dramatic improvement when the responsible metabolite (in some inborn errors of metabolism) or the toxic agent (in acquired Fanconi syndrome) is removed.

In the absence of a specific treatment, such as oral dithiothreitol[230] or cysteamine therapy to reduce intracellular cystine levels in nephropathic cystinosis[231] or NTBC treatment of hereditary tyrosinemia (see Chap. 79), fluids and electrolytes have to be replaced, and the metabolic bone disease resulting from Fanconi syndrome must be treated. Renal transplantation is called for when children with nephropathic cystinosis are severely uremic. By contrast, no therapy is required for the asymptomatic renal loss of substances such as glucose, amino acids, and uric acid.

Correction of Fluid and Electrolyte Disturbances

First, dehydration resulting from polyuria must be prevented by restoring free-water balance. Second, the correction of the hyperchloremic metabolic acidosis usually requires large amounts of alkali (3–20 meq/kg/day depending on the patient), a therapeutic maneuver that will aggravate renal potassium wasting. Extracellular fluid volume contraction also may be induced by the restriction of sodium chloride and water[232] and the long-term administration of hydrochlorothiazide[233] in an attempt to reduce a very large alkali requirement to a level tolerable for the patient. Third, potassium supplements are always necessary in the presence of a severe hypokalemia or during the treatment of metabolic acidosis with alkali therapy. Potassium bicarbonate, citrate, or acetate will simultaneously improve the potassium depletion and the metabolic acidosis.

Treatment of Metabolic Bone Disease

Oral phosphate therapy to replace the renal phosphate loss helps to correct the rickets in children or osteomalacia in adults. Vitamin D therapy, in the form of its more biologically active metabolites, 1,25-dihydroxyvitamin D_3 and 1α-hydroxyvitamin D_3, is preferred because renal production of hormone could be impaired in patients with Fanconi syndrome.[161]

Renal Transplantation

Long-term dialysis and renal transplantation are considered when patients with Fanconi syndrome become terminally uremic. Renal transplantation from either a cadaveric or a living related donor has been especially useful to treat young children with nephropathic cystinosis because the transplanted kidney does not have the genetic defect and consequently there is no recurrence of renal cystinosis and Fanconi syndrome.[234,235] However, these transplanted cystinotic patients remain of short stature, often with photophobia, despite a successful renal transplantation. The severe mental retardation of patients like those with Lowe syndrome may prevent the use of long-term dialysis and/or renal transplantation in the treatment of their end-stage renal disease.

ACKNOWLEDGMENTS

This investigation was supported by the Medical Research Council of Canada. We acknowledge the roles our colleagues Alfred Berteloot, Paul Goodyer, Raynald Laprade, Jennifer McLeese, Philippe Mayers, Stanton Segal, Charles Scriver, Georges Thiéry, and Patrick Vinay have played in the development of the ideas expressed in this chapter; any errors are our sole responsibility, not theirs. We acknowledge the skillful assistance of Christiane Laurier, Daniel Cyr, and Claude Gauthier.

REFERENCES

1. Rodriguez-Soriano J, Vallo A, Castillo G, Oliveros R: Renal handling of water and sodium in children with proximal and distal renal tubular acidosis. *Nephron* **25**:193, 1980.
2. Houston IB, Boichis H, Edelmann CM: Fanconi syndrome with renal sodium wasting and metabolic alkalosis. *Am J Med* **44**:638, 1968.
3. Sebastian A, McSherry E, Morris RC Jr: On the mechanism of renal potassium wasting in renal tubular acidosis associated with the Fanconi syndrome (type 2 RTA). *J Clin Invest* **50**:231, 1971.
4. Rodriguez Soriano J, Houston IB, Boichis H, Edelmann CM Jr: Calcium and phosphorus metabolism in the Fanconi syndrome. *J Clin Endocrinol Metab* **28**:1555, 1968.
5. Lee DBN, Drinkard JP, Rosen VJ, Gonick HC: The adult Fanconi syndrome: Observations on etiology, morphology, renal function and mineral metabolism in three patients. *Medicine* **51**:107, 1972.
6. Bernardini I, Rizzo WB, Dalakas M, Bernar J, Gahl WA: Plasma and muscle free carnitine deficiency due to renal Fanconi syndrome. *J Clin Invest* **75**:1124, 1985.
7. Jonas AJ, Lin SN, Conley SB, Schneider JA, Williams JC, Caprioli RC: Urine glyceraldehyde excretion is elevated in the renal Fanconi syndrome. *Kidney Int* **35**:99, 1989.
8. Al-Bander HAJ, Mock MD, Etheredge SB, Paukert TT, Humphreys MH, Morris RC Jr: Coordinately increased lysozymuria and lysosomal enzymuria induced by maleic acid. *Kidney Int* **30**:804, 1986.
9. Christensen EI, Maunsbach AB: Proteinuria induced by sodium maleate in rats: Effects on ultrastructure and protein handling in renal proximal tubule. *Kidney Int* **17**:771, 1980.
10. Dillard MG, Pesce AF, Pollak VE, Boreisha I: Proteinuria and renal protein clearances in patients with renal tubular disorders. *J Lab Clin Med* **78**:203, 1971.

11. Abderhalden F: Familiare cystindiathese. *Z Physiol Chem* **38**:557, 1903.
12. Lignac GOE: Stooris der Cystine-stofwisseling byj Kinderen. *Ned Tijdschr Geneeskd* **68**:2987, 1924.
13. Fanconi G: Die nicht diabetischen Glykosurien und Hyperglykamien des altern Kindes. *Jahrb Kinderheilk* **133**:257, 1931.
14. De Toni G: Remarks on the relations between renal rickets (renal dwarfism) and renal diabetes. *Acta Paediatr* **16**:479, 1933.
15. Debré R, Marie J, Cleret F, Messimy R: Rachitisme tardif coexistant avec une néphrite chronique et une glycosurie. *Arch Med Enf* **37**:597, 1934.
16. Fanconi G: Der nephrotisch-glykosurische Zwergwuchs mit Hypophosphatamischer Rachitis. *Dtsch Med Wochenschr* **62**:1169, 1936.
17. McCune DJ, Mason HH, Clarke HT: Intractable hypophosphatemic rickets with renal glycosuria and acidosis (the Fanconi syndrome): Report of a case in which increased urinary organic acids were detected and identified, with a review of the literature. *Am J Dis Child* **65**:81, 1943.
18. Hunt DD, Stearns G, McKinley JB, Froning E, Hicks P, Bonfiglio M: Long-term study of family with Fanconi syndrome without cystinosis (DeToni-Debré-Fanconi syndrome). *Am J Med* **40**:492, 1966.
19. Friedman AL, Trygstad CW, Chesney RW: Autosomal dominant Fanconi syndrome with early renal failure. *Am J Med Genet* **2**:225, 1978.
20. Brenton DP, Isenberg DA, Cusworth DC, Garrod P, Krywawych S, Stamp TCB: The adult presenting idiopathic Fanconi syndrome. *J Inherit Metab Dis* **4**:211, 1981.
21. Tolaymat A, Sakarcan A, Neiberger R: Idiopathic Fanconi syndrome in a family: 1. Clinical aspects. *J Am Soc Nephrol* **2**:1310, 1992.
22. Wen SF, Friedman AL, Oberley TD: Two case studies from a family with primary Fanconi syndrome. *Am J Kidney Dis* **13**:240, 1989.
23. Chesney RW, Kaplan BS, Colle E, Scriver CR, McInnes RR, Dupont CH, Drummond KN: Abnormalities of carbohydrate metabolism in idiopathic Fanconi syndrome. *Pediatr Res* **14**:209, 1980.
24. Chesney RW, Kaplan BS, Teitel D, Colle E, McInnes RR, Goldman H, Scriver CR: Metabolic abnormalities in the idiopathic Fanconi syndrome: Studies of carbohydrate metabolism in two patients. *Pediatrics* **67**:113, 1981.
25. Schneider JA, Bradley K, Seegmiller JE: Increased cystine in leukocytes from individuals homozygous and heterozygous for cystinosis. *Science* **157**:1321, 1967.
26. Schneider JA, Rosenbloom FM, Bradley KH, Seegmiller JE: Increased free-cystine content of fibroblasts cultured from patients with cystinosis. *Biochem Biophys Res Commun* **29**:527, 1967.
27. Foreman JW, Roth KS: Human renal Fanconi syndrome—Then and now. *Nephron* **51**:301, 1989.
28. Crawhall JC, Lietman PS, Schneider JA, Seegmiller JE: Cystinosis: Plasma cystine and cysteine concentrations and the effect of D-penicillamine and dietary treatment. *Am J Med* **44**:330, 1968.
29. Schneider JA, Wong V, Seegmiller JE: The early diagnosis of cystinosis. *J Pediatr* **74**:114, 1969.
30. Goldman H, Scriver CR, Aaron K, Delvin E, Canlas Z: Adolescent cystinosis: Comparisons with infantile and adult forms. *Pediatrics* **47**:979, 1971.
31. Lietman PS, Frazier PD, Wong VG, Shotton D, Seegmiller JE: Adult cystinosis: A benign disorder. *Am J Med* **40**:511, 1966.
32. Spencer PD, Medow MS, Moses LC, Roth KS: Effects of succinylacetone on the uptake of sugars and amino acids by brush border vesicles. *Kidney Int* **34**:671, 1988.
33. Morris RC Jr: An experimental renal acidification defect in patients with hereditary fructose intolerance: I. Its resemblance to renal tubular acidosis. *J Clin Invest* **47**:1389, 1968.
34. Morris RC Jr: An experimental renal acidification defect in patients with hereditary fructose intolerance: II. Its distinction from classical renal tubular acidosis; its resemblance to the renal acidification defect associated with the Fanconi syndrome of children with cystinosis. *J Clin Invest* **47**:1648, 1968.
35. Morris RC Jr, Nigon K, Reed EB: Evidence that the severity of depletion of inorganic phosphate determines the severity of the disturbance of adenine nucleotide metabolism in the liver and renal cortex of the fructose-loaded rat. *J Clin Invest* **61**:209, 1978.
36. Holzel A, Komrower GM, Schwarz V: Galactosemia. *Am J Med* **22**:703, 1957.
37. Garty R, Cooper M, Tabachnik E: The Fanconi syndrome associated with hepatic glycogenosis and abnormal metabolism of galactose. *J Pediatr* **85**:821, 1974.
38. Morgan HG, Stewart WK, Lowe KG, Stowers JM, Johnstone JH: Wilson's disease and the Fanconi syndrome. *Q J Med* **31**:361, 1962.
39. Elssas LJ, Hayslett JP, Spargo BH, Durant JL, Rosenberg LE: Wilson's disease with reversible renal tubular dysfunction: Correlation with proximal tubular ultrastructure. *Ann Intern Med* **75**:427, 1971.
40. Lowe CU, Terrey M, MacLachlan EA: Organic-aciduria, decreased renal ammonia production, hydrophthalmos, and mental retardation: A clinical entity. *Am J Dis Child* **83**:164, 1952.
41. Abbassi V, Lowe CU, Calcagno PL: Oculo-cerebro-renal syndrome: A review. *Am J Dis Child* **115**:145, 1968.
42. Sagel I, Ores RO, Yuceoglu AM: Renal function and morphology in a girl with oculocerebrorenal syndrome. *J Pediatr* **77**:124, 1970.
43. Gardner RJM, Brown N: Lowe's syndrome: Identification of carriers by lens examination. *J Med Genet* **13**:449, 1976.
44. Hittner HM, Carroll AJ, Prchal JT: Linkage studies in carriers of Lowe oculo-cerebro-renal syndrome. *Am J Hum Genet* **34**:966, 1982.
45. Akasaki M, Fukui S, Sakano T, Tanaka T, Usui T, Yamashina I: Urinary excretion of a large amount of bound sialic acid and of undersulfated chondroitin sulfate A by patients with the Lowe syndrome. *Clin Chim Acta* **89**:119, 1978.
46. Hayashi S, Nagata T, Kimura A, Tsurumi K: Urinary excretion of acid glycosaminoglycans and hydroxyproline in a patient with oculo-cerebro-renal syndrome. *Tohoku J Exp Med* **126**:215, 1978.
47. Habib R, Bargeton E, Brissaud HE, Raynaud J, Le Ball JC: Constatations anatomiques chez un enfant atteint d'un syndrome de Lowe. *Arch Fr Pediatr* **19**:945, 1962.
48. Frymoyer PA, Scheinman SJ, Dunham PB, Jones DB, Hueber P, Schroeder ET: X-linked recessive nephrolithiasis with renal failure. *New Engl J Med* **325**:681, 1991.
49. Wrong O, Norden AGW, Feest TG: Dent's disease: A familial proximal renal tubular syndrome with low-molecular-weight proteinuria, hypercalciuria, nephrocalcinosis, metabolic bone disease, progressive renal failure and a marked male predominance. *Q J Med* **87**:473, 1994.
50. Scheinman SJ: X-linked hypercalciuric nephrolithiasis: clinical syndromes and chloride channel mutations. *Kidney Int* **53**:3, 1998.
51. Lloyd SE, Pearce SHS, Günther W, Kawaguchi H, Igarashi T, Jentsch TJ, Thakker RV: Idiopathic low molecular weight proteinuria associated with hypercalciuric nephrocalcinosis in Japanese children is due to mutations of the renal chloride channel (*CLCN5*). *J Clin Invest* **99**:967, 1997.
52. Lloyd SE, Pearce SHS, Fisher SE, Steinmeyer K, Schwappach B, Scheinman SJ, Harding B, Bolino A, Devoto M, Goodyer P, Rigden SPA, Wrong O, Jentsch TJ, Craig IW, Thakker RV: A common molecular basis for three inherited kidney stone diseases. *Nature* **379**:445, 1996.
53. Fisher SE, Van Bakel I, Lloyd SE, Pearce SHS, Thakker RV, Craig IW: Cloning and characterization of *CLCN5*, the human kidney chloride channel gene implicated in Dent disease (an X-linked hereditary nephrolithiasis). *Genomics* **29**:598, 1995.
54. Steinmeyer K, Schwappach B, Bens M, Vandewalle A, Jentsch TJ: Cloning and functional expression of rat *CLC-5*, a chloride channel related to kidney disease. *J Biol Chem* **270**:31172, 1995.
55. Morimoto T, Uchida S, Sakamoto H, Kondo Y, Hanamizu H, Fukui M, Tomino Y, Nagano N, Sasaki S, Marumo F: Mutations in *CLCN5* chloride channel in Japanese patients with low molecular weight proteinuria. *J Am Soc Nephrol* **9**:811, 1998.
56. Ning C, Kuhara T, Matsumoto I: Simultaneous metabolic profile studies of three patients with fatal infantile mitochondrial myopathy-de Toni-Fanconi-Debré syndrome by GC/MS. *Clin Chim Acta* **247**:197, 1996.
57. Morris AA, Taylor RW, Birch-Machin MA, Jackson MJ, Coulthard MG, Bindoff LA, Welch RJ, Howell N, Turnbull DM: Neonatal Fanconi syndrome due to deficiency of complex III of the respiratory chain. *Pediatr Nephrol* **4**:407, 1995.
58. Campos Y, Garcia-Silva T, Barrioneuvo CR, Cabello A, Muley R, Arenas J: Mitochondrial DNA deletion in a patient with mitochondrial myopathy, lactic acidosis and stroke-like episodes (MELAS) and Fanconi's syndrome. *Pediatr Nephrol* **13**:69, 1995.
59. Superti-Furga A, Schoenle E, Tuchschmid P, Caduff R, Sakato V, DeMattia D, Getzelmann R, Steinmann B: Pearson bone marrow-pancreas syndrome with insulin-dependent diabetes, progressive renal tubulopathy, organic aciduria and elevated fetal haemoglobin caused by deletion and duplication of mitochondrial DNA. *Eur J Pediatr* **152**:44, 1993.
60. Easley JR, Breitschwerdt EB: Glycosuria associated with renal tubular dysfunction in three Basenji dogs. *J Am Vet Med Assoc* **168**:938, 1976.

61. Bovee KC, Joyce T, Reynolds R, Segal S: The Fanconi syndrome in Basenji dogs: A new model for renal transport defects. *Science* **201**:1129, 1978.
62. Bovee KC, Joyce T, Reynolds R, Segal S: Spontaneous Fanconi syndrome in the dog. *Metabolism* **27**:45, 1978.
63. McNamara PD, Rea CT, Bovee KC, Reynolds RA, Segal S: Cystinuria in dogs: Comparison of the cystinuric component of the Fanconi syndrome in Basenji dogs to isolated cystinuria. *Metabolism* **38**:8, 1989.
64. Hsu BYL, McNamara PD, Mahoney SG, Fenstermacher EA, Rea CT, Bovee KC, Segal S: Membrane fluidity and sodium transport by renal membrane from dogs with spontaneous idiopathic Fanconi syndrome. *Metabolism* **41**:253, 1992.
65. Adams RG, Harrison JF, Scott P: The development of cadmium-induced proteinuria, impaired renal function, and osteomalacia in alkaline battery workers. *Q J Med* **38**:425, 1969.
66. Bernard A, Buchet JP, Roels H, Masson P, Lauwerys R: Renal excretion of protein and enzymes in workers exposed to cadmium. *Eur J Clin Invest* **9**:11, 1979.
67. Clarkson TW, Kench JE: Urinary excretion of amino acids by men absorbing heavy metals. *Biochem J* **62**:361, 1956.
68. Axelsson B, Dahlgren SE, Piscator M: Renal lesions in the rabbit after long-term exposure to cadmium. *Arch Environ Health* **17**:24, 1968.
69. Stowe HD, Wilson M, Goyer RA: Clinical and morphologic effects of oral cadmium toxicity in rabbits. *Arch Pathol* **94**:389, 1972.
70. Nishizumi M: Electron microscopic study of cadmium nephrotoxicity in the rat. *Arch Environ Health* **24**:215, 1972.
71. Raghavan SRV, Gonick HC: Experimental Fanconi syndrome: IV. Effect of repetitive injections of cadmium on tissue distribution and protein-binding of cadmium. *Miner Electrolyte Metab* **3**:36, 1980.
72. Gonick HC, Kramer HJ: Pathogenesis of the Fanconi syndrome, in Gonick HC, Buckalew VM Jr (eds): *Renal Tubular Disorders: Pathophysiology, Diagnosis and Management*. New York, Marcel Dekker, 1985, p 545.
73. Nomiyama K, Sugata Y, Murata I, Nakagawa S: Urinary low-molecular-weight proteins in itai-itai disease. *Environ Res* **6**:373, 1973.
74. Saito H, Shioji R, Hurukawa Y, Nagai K, Arikawa T, Saito T, Sasaki Y, Furuyama T, Yoshinaga K: Cadmium-induced proximal tubular dysfunction in a cadmium-polluted area. *Contrib Nephrol* **6**:1, 1977.
75. Brewer ED: The Fanconi syndrome: Clinical disorders, in Gonick HC, Buckalew VM Jr (eds): *Renal Tubular Disorders: Pathophysiology, Diagnosis and Management*. New York, Marcel Dekker, 1985, p 475.
76. Goyer RA, May P, Cates MM, Krigman MR: Lead and protein content of isolated intranuclear inclusion bodies from kidneys of lead-poisoned rats. *Lab Invest* **22**:245, 1970.
77. Chisolm JJ Jr, Harrison HC, Eberlein WR, Harrison HE: Amino-aciduria, hypophosphatemia, and rickets in lead poisoning. *Am J Dis Child* **89**:159, 1955.
78. Blachley JD, Hill JB: Renal and electrolyte disturbances associated with cisplatin. *Ann Intern Med* **95**:628, 1981.
79. Schilsky RL, Anderson T: Hypomagnesemia and renal magnesium wasting in patients receiving cisplatin. *Ann Intern Med* **90**:929, 1979.
80. Frimpter GW, Timpanelli AE, Eisenmenger WJ, Stein HS, Ehrlich LI: Reversible "Fanconi syndrome" caused by degraded tetracycline. *JAMA* **84**:111, 1963.
81. Gross JM: Fanconi syndrome (adult type) developing secondary to the ingestion of outdated tetracycline. *Ann Intern Med* **58**:523, 1963.
82. Benitz KF, Diermeier HF: Renal toxicity of tetracycline degradation products. *Proc Soc Exp Biol Med* **115**:930, 1964.
83. Lindquist RR, Fellers FX: Degraded tetracycline nephropathy: Functional, morphologic, and histochemical observations. *Lab Invest* **15**:864, 1966.
84. Melnick JZ, Baum M, Thompson JR: Aminoglycoside-induced Fanconi's syndrome. *Am J Kidney Dis* **23**:118, 1994.
85. Bar RS, Wilson HE, Mazzaferri EL: Hypomagnesemic hypocalcemia secondary to renal magnesium wasting: A possible consequence of high-dose gentamicin therapy. *Ann Intern Med* **82**:646, 1975.
86. Kelnar CJH, Taor WS, Reynolds DJ, Smith DR, Slavin BM, Brook CGD: Hypomagnesaemic hypocalcemia with hypokalaemia caused by treatment with high dose gentamicin. *Arch Dis Child* **53**:817, 1978.
87. Kuhar MJ, Mak LL, Lietman PS: Autoradiographic localization of [^{3}H]gentamicin in the proximal renal tubules of mice. *Antimicrob Agents Chemother* **15**:131, 1979.
88. Lenoir GR, Perignon JL, Gubler MC, Broyer M: Valproic acid: A possible cause of proximal tubular renal syndrome. *J Pediatr* **98**:503, 1981.
89. Butler HE Jr, Morgan JM, Smythe CM: Mercaptopurine and acquired tubular dysfunction in adult nephrosis. *Arch Intern Med* **116**:853, 1965.
90. Otten J, Vis HL: Acute reversible renal tubular dysfunction following intoxication with methyl-3-chromone. *J Pediatr* **73**:422, 1968.
91. Spencer AG, Franglen GT: Gross amino-aciduria following a Lysol burn. *Lancet* **1**:190, 1952.
92. Vaziri ND, Ness RL, Fairshter RD, Smith WR, Rosen SM: Nephrotoxicity of paraquat in man. *Arch Intern Med* **139**:172, 1979.
93. Moss AH, Gabow PA, Kaehny WD, Goodman SI, Haut LL, Haussler MR: Fanconi's syndrome and distal renal tubular acidosis after glue sniffing. *Ann Intern Med* **92**:69, 1980.
94. Burk CD, Restaino I, Kaplan BS, Meadows AT: Ifosfamide-induced renal tubular dysfunction and rickets in children with Wilms tumor. *J Pediatr* **117**:331, 1990.
95. Pratt CB, Meyer WH, Jenkins TJ, Avery L, McKay CP, Wyatt RJ, Hancock ML: Ifosfamide, Fanconi syndrome, rickets. *J Clin Oncol* **9**:1495, 1991.
96. Costanza DJ, Smoller M: Multiple myeloma with the Fanconi syndrome: Study of a case, with electron microscopy of the kidney. *Am J Med* **34**:125, 1963.
97. Maldondo JE, Velosa JA, Kyle RA, Wagoner RD, Holley KE, Salassa RM: Fanconi syndrome in adults: A manifestation of a latent form of myeloma. *Am J Med* **58**:354, 1975.
98. Walker BR, Alexander F, Tannenbaum PJ: Fanconi syndrome with renal tubular acidosis and light chain proteinuria. *Nephron* **8**:103, 1971.
99. Orfila C, Lepert JC, Modesto A, Bernadet P, Suc JM: Fanconi's syndrome, kappa light-chain myeloma, non-amyloid fibrils and cytoplasmic crystals in renal tubular epithelium. *Am J Nephrol* **11**:345, 1991.
100. Sanders PW, Herrera GA, Galla JH: Human Bence Jones protein toxicity in rat proximal tubule epithelium *in vivo*. *Kidney Int* **32**:851, 1987.
101. Wochner RD, Strober W, Waldmann TA: The role of the kidney in the catabolism of Bence-Jones proteins and immunoglobin fragments. *J Exp Med* **126**:207, 1967.
102. Christensen EI, Gliemann J, Moestrup SK: Renal tubule gp330 is a calcium binding receptor for endocytic uptake of protein. *J Histochem Cytochem* **40**:1481, 1992.
103. Moestrup SK, Cui S, Vorum H, Bregengard C, Bjorn SE, Norris K, Gliemann J, Christensen EI: Evidence that epithelial glycoprotein 330/megalin mediates uptake of polybasic drugs. *J Clin Invest* **96**:1404, 1995.
104. Tenstad O, Williamson HE, Glausen G, Oien AH, Aukland K: Glomerular filtration and tubular absorption of the basic polypeptide aprotinin. *Arch Physiol Scand* **38**:87, 1994.
105. Uchida S, Matsuda O, Yokota T, Takemura T, Ando R, Kanemitsu H, Hamaguchi H, Miyake S, Marumo F: Adult Fanconi syndrome secondary to κ-light chain myeloma: Improvement of tubular functions after treatment for myeloma. *Nephron* **55**:332, 1990.
106. Finkel PN, Kronenberg K, Pesce AJ, Pollak VE, Pirani CL: Adult Fanconi syndrome, amyloidosis and marked κ-light chain proteinuria. *Nephron* **10**:1, 1973.
107. Rochman J, Lichtig C, Osterweill D, Tatarsky I, Eidelman S: Adult Fanconi's syndrome with renal tubular acidosis in association with renal amyloidosis: Occurrence in a patient with chronic lymphocytic leukemia. *Arch Intern Med* **140**:1361, 1980.
108. Harrison JF, Blainey JD: Adult Fanconi syndrome with monoclonal abnormality of immunoglobulin light chain. *J Clin Pathol* **20**:42, 1967.
109. Smithline N, Kassirer JP, Cohen JJ: Light-chain nephropathy: Renal tubular dysfunction associated with light-chain proteinuria. *New Engl J Med* **294**:71, 1976.
110. Rao DS, Parfitt AM, Villanueva AR, Dorman PJ, Kleerekoper M: Hypophosphatemic osteomalacia and adult Fanconi syndrome due to light-chain nephropathy. *Am J Med* **82**:333, 1987.
111. Dahlstrom U, Marftensson J, Lindstrom FD: Occurrence of adult Fanconi syndrome in benign monoclonal gammopathy. *Acta Med Scand* **208**:425, 1980.
112. van Hooft C, Vermassen A: DeToni-Debré-Fanconi syndrome in nephrotic children: A review. *Ann Pediatr (Paris)* **194**:193, 1960.
113. McVicar M, Exeni R, Susin M: Nephrotic syndrome and multiple tubular defects in children: An early sign of focal segmental glomerulosclerosis. *J Pediatr* **97**:918, 1980.
114. Friedman A, Chesney R: Fanconi's syndrome in renal transplantation. *Am J Nephrol* **1**:45, 1981.
115. Vertuno LL, Preuss HG, Argy WP Jr, Schreiner GE: Fanconi syndrome following homotransplantation. *Arch Intern Med* **133**:302, 1974.

116. Vaziri ND, Nellans RE, Brueggemann RM, Barton CH, Martin DC: Renal tubular dysfunction in transplanted kidneys. *South Med J* **72**:530, 1979.
117. Palestine AG, Austin HA, Nussenblatt RB: Renal tubular function in cyclosporine-treated patients. *Am J Med* **81**:419, 1986.
118. Leehey DJ, Ing TS, Daugirdas JT: Fanconi syndrome associated with a non-ossifying fibroma of bone. *Am J Med* **78**:708, 1985.
119. Goldsweig HG, Brisson De Champlain ML, Davidman M: Proximal tubular dysfunction associated with Burkitt's lymphoma. *Cancer* **41**:568, 1978.
120. Weinstein B, Irreverre F, Watkin DM: Lung carcinoma, hypouricemia and aminoaciduria. *Am J Med* **39**:520, 1965.
121. Stowers JM, Dent CE: Studies on the mechanism of the Fanconi syndrome. *Q J Med* **16**:275, 1947.
122. Myerson RM, Pastor BH: The Fanconi syndrome and its clinical variants. *Am J Med Sci* **228**:378, 1954.
123. Clay RD, Darmady EM, Hawkins M: The nature of the renal lesion in the Fanconi syndrome. *J Pathol Bacteriol* **65**:551, 1953.
124. Berliner RW, Kennedy TJ, Hilton JG: Effect of maleic acid on renal function. *Proc Soc Exp Biol Med* **75**:791, 1950.
125. Harrison HE, Harrison HC: Experimental production of renal glycosuria, phosphaturia, and aminoaciduria by injection of maleic acid. *Science* **120**:606, 1954.
126. Shvil Y, Wald H, Popovtzer MM: Effect of bicarbonate and phosphate on renal phosphate leak in experimental Fanconi syndrome. *Am J Physiol* **252**:F310, 1987.
127. Foreman JW, Bowring MA, Lee J, States B, Segal S: Effect of cystine dimethylester on renal solute handling and isolated renal tubule transport in the rat: A new model of the Fanconi syndrome. *Metabolism* **36**:1185, 1987.
128. Ben-Nun A, Bashan N, Potashnik R, Cohen-Luria R, Moran A: Cystine loading induces Fanconi's syndrome in rats: *In vivo* and vesicle studies. *Am J Physiol* **265**:F839, 1993.
129. Foreman JW, Benson LL, Wellons M, Avner ED, Sweeney W, Nissim I, Nissim I: Metabolic studies of rat renal tubule cells loaded with cystine: The cystine dimethylester model of cystinosis. *J Am Soc Nephrol* **6**:269, 1995.
130. Bajaj B, Baum M: Proximal tubule dysfunction in cystine-loaded tubules: Effect of phosphate and metabolic substrates. *Am J Physiol* **271**:F717, 1996.
131. Gougoux A, Zan N, Dansereau D, Vinay P: Experimental Fanconi's syndrome resulting from 4-pentenoate infusion in the dog. *Am J Physiol* **257**:F959, 1989.
132. Fritzell S, Jagenburg OR, Schnurer LB: Familial cirrhosis of the liver, renal tubular defects with rickets and impaired tyrosine metabolism. *Acta Paediatr* **53**:18, 1964.
133. Halvorsen S, Gjessing LR: Studies on tyrosinosis: 1. Effect of low-tyrosine and low-phenylalanine diet. *Br Med J* **2**:1171, 1964.
134. Harries JT, Seakins JWT, Ersser RS, Lloyd JK: Recovery after dietary treatment of an infant with features of tyrosinosis. *Arch Dis Child* **44**:258, 1969.
135. Levin B, Snodgrass GJAI, Oberholzer VG, Burgess EA, Dobbs RH: Fructosaemia: Observations on seven cases. *Am J Med* **45**:826, 1968.
136. Cusworth DC, Dent CE, Flynn FV: The amino-aciduria in galactosemia. *Arch Dis Child* **30**:150, 1955.
137. Jagenburg R, Lindblad B, De Mare JM, Rodjer S: Hereditary tyrosinemia: Metabolic studies in a patient with partial *p*-hydroxyphenylpyruvate hydroxylase activity. *J Pediatr* **80**:994, 1972.
138. Aronsson S, Engleson G, Jagenburg R, Palmgren B: Long-term dietary treatment of tyrosinosis. *J Pediatr* **72**:620, 1968.
139. Scriver CR, Partington M, Sass-Kortsak A: Hereditary tyrosinemia and tyrosyluria: Clinical report of four patients. *Can Med Assoc J* **97**:1047, 1967.
140. Kang ES, Gerald PS: Hereditary tyrosinemia and abnormal pyrrole metabolism. *J Pediatr* **77**:397, 1970.
141. Isselbacher KJ: Galactosemia, in Stanbury JB, Wyngaarden JB, Fredrickson DS (eds): *The Metabolic Basis of Inherited Disease*, 2d ed. New York, McGraw-Hill, 1966, p 178.
142. Chisolm JJ Jr: Aminoaciduria as a manifestation of renal tubular injury in lead intoxication and a comparison with patterns of aminoaciduria seen in other diseases. *J Pediatr* **60**:1, 1962.
143. Goyer RA: The renal tubule in lead poisoning: I. Mitochondrial swelling and aminoaciduria. *Lab Invest* **19**:71, 1968.
144. Morris RC Jr, McInnes RR, Epstein CJ, Sebastian A, Scriver CR: Genetic and metabolic injury of the kidney, in Brenner BM, Rector FC Jr (eds): *The Kidney*. Philadelphia, Saunders, 1976, p 1193.
145. Burch HB, Lowry OH, Meinhardt L, Max P Jr, Chyu KJ: Effect of fructose, dihydroxyacetone, glycerol, and glucose on metabolites and related compounds in liver and kidney. *J Biol Chem* **245**:2092, 1970.
146. Woods HF, Eggleston LV, Krebs HA: The cause of hepatic accumulation of fructose-1-phosphate on fructose loading. *Biochem J* **119**:501, 1970.
147. Woods HF: Hepatic accumulation of metabolites after fructose loading. *Acta Med Scand Suppl* **542**:87, 1972.
148. Bergeron M, Morel F: Amino acid transport in rat renal tubules. *Am J Physiol* **216**:1139, 1969.
149. Brodehl J, Bickel H: Aminoaciduria and hyperaminoaciduria in childhood. *Clin Nephrol* **1**:149, 1973.
150. Roth KS, Foreman JW, Segal S: The Fanconi syndrome and mechanisms of tubular transport dysfunction. *Kidney Int* **20**:705, 1981.
151. Darmady EM, Stranack F: Microdissection of the nephron in disease. *Br Med Bull* **13**:21, 1957.
152. Witzleben CL, Schoen EJ, Tu WH, McDonald LW: Progressive morphologic renal changes in the oculo-cerebro-renal syndrome of Lowe. *Am J Med* **44**:319, 1968.
153. Schneider JA, Seegmiller JE: Cystinosis and the Fanconi syndrome, in Stanbury JB, Wyngaarden JB, Fredrickson DS (eds): *The Metabolic Basis of Inherited Disease*, 3d ed. New York, McGraw-Hill, 1972.
154. Worthen HG: Renal toxicity of maleic acid in the rat: Enzymatic and morphologic observations. *Lab Invest* **12**:791, 1963.
155. Scharer K, Yoshida T, Voyer L, Berlow S, Pietra G, Metcoff J: Impaired renal gluconeogenesis and energy metabolism in maleic acid-induced nephropathy in rats. *Res Exp Med (Berl)* **157**:136, 1972.
156. Bergeron M, Laporte P: Effet membranaire du maléate au niveau du néphron proximal et distal. *Rev Can Biol* **32**:275, 1973.
157. Rosen VJ, Kramer HJ, Gonick HC: Experimental Fanconi syndrome: II. Effect of maleic acid on renal tubular ultrastructure. *Lab Invest* **28**:446, 1973.
158. Verani RR, Brewer ED, Ince A, Gibson J, Bulger RE: Proximal tubular necrosis associated with maleic acid administration to the rat. *Lab Invest* **46**:79, 1982.
159. McLeese J, Thiéry G, Bergeron M: Maleate modifies apical endocytosis and permeability of endoplasmic reticulum membrane in kidney tubular cells. *Cell Tissue* **282**:29, 1996.
160. Guntupalli J, Delaney V, Weinman EJ, Lyle D, Allon M, Bourke E: Effects of maleic acid on renal phosphorus transport: Role of dietary phosphorus. *Am J Physiol* **261**:F227, 1991.
161. Brewer ED, Tsai HC, Szeto KS, Morris RC Jr: Maleic acid-induced impaired conversion of 25 $(OH)D_3$ to $1,25(OH)_2D_3$: Implications for Fanconi's syndrome. *Kidney Int* **12**:244, 1977.
162. Gray RW, Omdahl JL, Ghazarian JG, Deluca HF: 25-Hydroxycholecalciferol-1-hydroxylase: Subcellular location and properties. *J Biol Chem* **247**:7528, 1972.
163. Akiba T, Endou H, Koseki C, Sakai F: Localization of 25-hydroxyvitamin D_3–1α-hydroxylase activity in the mammalian kidney. *Biochem Biophys Res Commun* **94**:313, 1980.
164. Tate SS, Meister A: Stimulation of the hydrolytic activity and decrease of the transpeptidase activity of γ-glutamyl transpeptidase by maleate; identity of a rat kidney maleate-stimulated glutaminase and γ-glutamyl transpeptidase. *Proc Natl Acad Sci USA* **71**:3329, 1974.
165. Bergeron M, Dubord L, Hausser C: Membrane permeability as a cause of transport defects in experimental Fanconi syndrome: A new hypothesis. *J Clin Invest* **57**:1181, 1976.
166. Wen SF: Micropuncture studies of glucose transport in the dog: Mechanism of renal glycosuria. *Am J Physiol* **231**:468, 1976.
167. Brewer ED, Senekjian HO, Ince A, Weinman EJ: Maleic acid-induced reabsorptive dysfunction in the proximal and distal nephron. *Am J Physiol* **245**:F339, 1983.
168. Bank N, Aynedjian HS, Mutz BJ: Microperfusion study of proximal tubule bicarbonate transport in maleic acid-induced renal tubular acidosis. *Am J Physiol* **250**:F476, 1986.
169. Al-Bander HA, Weiss RA, Humphreys MH, Morris RC Jr: Dysfunction of the proximal tubule underlies maleic acid-induced type II renal tubular acidosis. *Am J Physiol* **243**:F604, 1982.
170. Rosin JM, Katz MA, Rector FC Jr, Seldin DW: Acetazolamide in studying sodium reabsorption in diluting segment. *Am J Physiol* **219**:1731, 1970.
171. Kunau RT Jr: The influence of the carbonic anhydrase inhibitor, benzolamide (C1-11,366), on the reabsorption of chloride, sodium, and bicarbonate in the proximal tubule of the rat. *J Clin Invest* **51**:294, 1972.

172. Gougoux A, Zan N, Dansereau D, Vinay P: Metabolic effects of 4-pentenoate on isolated dog kidney tubules. *Kidney Int* **42**:586, 1992.
173. Robson EB, Rose GA: The effect of intravenous lysine on the renal clearances of cystine, arginine and ornithine in normal subjects, in patients with cystinuria and Fanconi syndrome and in their relatives. *Clin Sci* **16**:75, 1957.
174. Scriver CR, Chesney RW, McInnes RR: Genetic aspects of renal tubular transport: Diversity and topology of carriers. *Kidney Int* **9**:149, 1976.
175. Scriver CR, Goldbloom RB, Roy CC: Hypophosphatemic rickets with renal hyperglycinuria, renal glucosuria and glycyl-prolinuria: a syndrome with evidence for renal tubular secretion of phosphorus. *Pediatrics* **34**:357, 1964.
176. Rosenberg LE, Segal S: Maleic acid-induced inhibition of amino acid transport in rat kidney. *Biochem J* **92**:345, 1964.
177. Bergeron M, Dubord L, Laporte P, Hausser C, Alle-Ando L: On the physiopathology of the Fanconi syndrome, in Silbernagl S, Lang F, Greger R (eds): *Amino Acid Transport and Uric Acid Transport.* Stuttgart, Thieme, 1976, p 46.
178. Silverman M, Huang L: Mechanism of maleic acid-induced glucosuria in dog kidney. *Am J Physiol* **231**:1024, 1976.
179. Bergeron M, Vadeboncoeur M: Microinjections of L-leucine into tubules and peritubular capillaries of the rat: II. The maleic acid model. *Nephron* **8**:367, 1971.
180. Günther R, Silbernagl S, Deetjen P: Maleic acid induced aminoaciduria, studied by free flow micropuncture and continuous microperfusion. *Pflugers Arch* **382**:109, 1979.
181. Bergeron M: Renal amino acid accumulation in maleate treated rats. *Rev Can Biol* **30**:267, 1971.
182. Ausiello DA, Segal S, Thier SO: Cellular accumulation of L-lysine in rat kidney cortex *in vivo*. *Am J Physiol* **222**:1473, 1972.
183. Kramer HJ, Gonick HC: Experimental Fanconi syndrome: I. Effect of maleic acid on renal cortical Na-K-ATPase activity and ATP levels. *J Lab Clin Med* **76**:799, 1970.
184. Gougoux A, Lemieux G, Lavoie N: Maleate-induced bicarbonaturia in the dog: A carbonic anhydrase-independent effect. *Am J Physiol* **231**:1010, 1976.
185. Gmaj P, Hoppe A, Angielski S, Rogulski J: Acid-base behavior of the kidney in maleate-treated rats. *Am J Physiol* **222**:1182, 1972.
186. Gmaj P, Hoppe A, Angielski S, Rogulski J: Effects of maleate and arsenite on renal reabsorption of sodium and bicarbonate. *Am J Physiol* **225**:90, 1973.
187. Hoppe A, Gmaj P, Metler M, Angielski S: Additive inhibition of renal bicarbonate reabsorption by maleate plus acetazolamide. *Am J Physiol* **231**:1258, 1976.
188. Reboucas NA, Fernandes DT, Elias MM, De Mello-Aires M, Malnic G: Proximal tubular $HCO3^-$, H^+ and fluid transport during maleate-induced acidification defect. *Pflugers Arch* **401**:266, 1984.
189. Obaid AL, Rega AF, Garrahan PJ: The effects of maleic anhydride on the ionic permeability of red cells. *J Membrane Biol* **9**:385, 1972.
190. Maesaka JK, McCaffery M: Evidence for renal tubular leakage in maleic acid-induced Fanconi syndrome. *Am J Physiol* **239**:F507, 1980.
191. Laprade R, Beauchesne G, Bergeron M: Effet membranaire du maléate: Etude à l'aide de membranes artificielles lipidiques, in *Proceedings of the VIIth International Congress of Nephrology.* Basel, S. Karger, 1978, p M-6.
192. Christensen EI, Nielson S, Moestrup SK, Borre C, Maunsbach AB, de Heer E, Ronco P, Hammond TG, Verroust P: Segmental distribution of the endocytosis receptor gp330 in renal proximal tubules. *Eur J Cell Biol* **66**:349, 1995.
193. Kerjaschki D, Farquhar MG: The pathogenic antigen of Heymann nephritis is a membrane glycoprotein of the renal proximal tubule brush border. *Proc Natl Acad Sci USA* **79**:5557, 1982.
194. Kerjaschki D, Noronha-Blod L, Sacktor B, Farquhar MG: Microdomains of distinctive glycoprotein composition in the kidney proximal tubule brush border. *J Cell Biol* **98**:1505, 1985.
195. Kounnas MZ, Chappell DA, Strickland DK, Argraves WS: Glycoprotein 330, a member of the low density lipoprotein receptor family, binds lipoprotein lipase *in vitro*. *J Biol Chem* **268**:14176, 1993.
196. Bergeron M, Mayers P, Brown D: Specific effect of maleate on an apical membrane glycoprotein (gp330) in proximal tubule of rat kidneys. *Am J Physiol* **271**:F908, 1996.
197. Pfaller W, Joannidis M, Gstraunthaler G, Kotanko P: Quantitative morphological changes of nephron structures and urinary enzyme activity pattern in sodium maleate-induced renal injury. *Renal Physiol Biochem* **12**:56, 1989.
198. Rodman JS, Seidman L, Farquhar MG: The membrane composition of coated pits, microvilli, endosomes, and lysosomes is distinctive in the rat kidney proximal tubule cell. *J Cell Biol* **102**:77, 1986.
199. Lledo PM, Johannes L, Vernier P, Henry JP, Vincent JD, Darchen F: Calcium-dependent regulated secretion is controlled by GTPase Rab3 in neuroendocrine cells. *CR Seances Soc Biol Fil* **187**:726, 1993.
200. Lledo PM, Vernier P, Vincent JD, Mason WT, Zorec R: Inhibition of Rab3B expression attenuates Ca^{2+}-dependent exocytosis in rat anterior pituitary cells. *Nature* **364**:540, 1993.
201. Chatelet F, Brianti E, Ronco P, Roland J, Verroust P: Ultrastructural localization by monoclonal antibodies of brush border antigens expressed by glomeruli: II. Extrarenal distribution. *Am J Pathol* **122**:512, 1986.
202. Van Weert AWM, Dunn KW, Geuze HJ, Maxfield FR, Stoorvogel W: Transport from late endosomes to lysosomes, but not sorting of integral membrane proteins in endosomes, depends on the vacuolar proton pump. *J Cell Biol* **130**:821, 1995.
203. Ammann H, Noël J, Tejedor A, Boulanger Y, Gougoux A, Vinay P: Could cytoplasmic concentration gradients for sodium and ATP exist in intact renal cells? *Can J Physiol Pharmacol* **73**:421, 1995.
204. Gonick HC, Indraprasit S, Rosen VJ, Neustein H, Van De Velde R, Raghavan SRV: Experimental Fanconi syndrome: III. Effect of cadmium on renal tubular function, the ATP-NA^+, K^+-ATPase transport system and renal tubular ultrastructure. *Miner Electrolyte Metab* **3**:21, 1980.
205. Lee HY, Kim KR, Woo JS, Kim YK, Park YS: Transport of organic compounds in renal plasma membrane vesicles of cadmium intoxicated rats. *Kidney Int* **37**:727, 1990.
206. Kägi JHR, Vallee BL: Metallothionein: A cadmium- and zinc-containing protein from equine renal cortex. *J Biol Chem* **235**:3460, 1960.
207. Foulkes EC: Renal tubular transport of cadmium-metallothionein. *Toxicol Appl Pharmacol* **45**:505, 1978.
208. Nordberg GF, Goyer RA, Nordberg M: Comparative toxicity of cadmium-metallothionein and cadmium chloride on mouse kidney. *Arch Pathol* **99**:192, 1975.
209. Gunn SA, Gould TC, Anderson WAD: Selectivity of organs response to cadmium injury and various protective measures. *J Pathol Bacteriol* **96**:89, 1968.
210. Angielski S, Rogulski J: Effect of maleic acid on the kidney: I. Oxidation of Krebs cycle intermediates by various tissues of maleate intoxicated rats. *Acta Biochim Pol* **9**:357, 1962.
211. Gougoux A, Vinay P, Duplain M: Maleate-induced stimulation of glutamine metabolism in the intact dog kidney. *Am J Physiol* **248**:F585, 1985.
212. Pacanis A, Rogulski J, Ledochowski H, Angielski S: On the mechanism of maleate action on rat kidney mitochondria: Effect on substrate-level phosphorylation. *Acta Biochim Pol* **22**:1, 1975.
213. Rogulski J, Pacanis A, Adamowicz W, Angielski S: On the mechanism of maleate action on rat kidney mitochondria: Effect on oxidative metabolism. *Acta Biochim Pol* **21**:403, 1974.
214. Anner BM, Moosmayer M, Imesch E: Mercury blocks Na-K-ATPase by a ligand-dependent and reversible mechanism. *Am J Physiol* **262**:F830, 1992.
215. Eiam-Ong S, Spohn M, Kurtzman NA, Sabatini S: Insights into the biochemical mechanism of maleic acid-induced Fanconi syndrome. *Kidney Int* **48**:1542, 1995.
216. Imesch E, Moosmayer M, Anner BM: Mercury weakens membrane anchoring of Na^+, K^+-ATPase. *Am J Physiol* **262**:F837, 1992.
217. Mujais SK: Maleic acid-induced proximal tubulopathy: Na:K pump inhibition. *J Am Soc Nephrol* **4**:142, 1993.
218. Nechay BR, Saunders JP: Inhibition of renal adenosine triphosphatase by cadmium. *J Pharmacol Exp Ther* **200**:623, 1977.
219. Coor C, Salmon RF, Quigley R, Marver D, Baum M: Role of adenosine triphosphate (ATP) and Na^+, K^+-ATPase in the inhibition of proximal tubule transport with intracellular cystine loading. *J Clin Invest* **87**:955, 1991.
220. Salmon RF, Baum M: Intracellular cystine loading inhibits transport in the rabbit proximal convoluted tubule. *J Clin Invest* **85**:340, 1990.
221. Wapnir RA, Exeni RA, McVicar M, De Rosas FJ, Lifshitz F: Inhibition of sodium intestinal transport and mucosal Na^+, K^+-ATPase in experimental Fanconi syndrome. *Proc Soc Exp Biol Med* **150**:517, 1975.
222. Szczepanska M, Angielski S: Prevention of maleate-induced tubular dysfunction by acetoacetate. *Am J Physiol* **239**:F50, 1980.

223. Al-Bander H, Etheredge SB, Paukert T, Humphreys MH, Morris RC Jr: Phosphate loading attenuates renal tubular dysfunction induced by maleic acid in the dog. *Am J Physiol* **248**:F513, 1985.
224. Sakarcan A, Aricheta R, Baum M: Intracellular cystine loading causes proximal tubule respiratory dysfunction: effect of glycine. *Pediatr Res* **32**:710, 1992.
225. Nissim I, Weinberg JM: Glycine attenuates Fanconi syndrome induced by maleate or ifosfamide in rats. *Kidney Int* **49**:684, 1996.
226. Baines AD, Shaikh H, Ho P: Mechanisms of perfused kidney cytoprotection by alanine and glycine. *Am J Physiol* **259**:F80, 1990.
227. Heyman SN, Spokes K, Egorin MJ, Epstein FH: Glycine reduces early renal parenchymal uptake of cisplatin. *Kidney Int* **43**:1226, 1993.
228. Venkatachalma MA, Weinberg JM, Patel Y, Davis J, Saikumar P: Functional characterization of a glycine sensitive porous membrane defect in ATP depleted MDCK cells (abstract). *J Am Soc Nephrol* **5**:912, 1994.
229. Weinberg JM, Venkatachalam MA, Roeser NF, Davis JA, Varani J, Johnson KJ: Amino acid protection of cultured kidney tubule cells against calcium ionophore-induced lethal cell injury. *Lab Invest* **65**:671, 1991.
230. Goldman H, Aaron K, Scriver CR, Pinsky L: Use of dithiothreitol to correct cystine storage in cultured cystinotic fibroblasts. *Lancet* **1**:811, 1970.
231. Gahl WA, Reed GF, Thoene JG, Schulman JD, Rizzo WB, Jonas AJ, Denman DW, Schlesselman JJ, Corden BJ, Schneider JA: Cysteamine therapy for children with nephropathic cystinosis. *New Engl J Med* **316**:971, 1987.
232. Arant BS, Greifer I, Edelmann CM, Spitzer A: Effect of chronic salt and water loading on the tubular defects of a child with Fanconi syndrome (cystinosis). *Pediatrics* **58**:370, 1976.
233. Rampini S, Fanconi A, Illig R, Prader A: Effect of hydrochlorothiazide on proximal renal tubular acidosis in a patient with idiopathic "deToni-Debré-Fanconi syndrome." *Helv Paediatr Acta* **23**:13, 1968.
234. Malekzadeh MH, Neustein HB, Schneider JA, Pennisi AJ, Ettenger RB, Uittenbogaart CH, Kogut MD, Fine RN: Cadaver renal transplantation in children with cystinosis. *Am J Med* **63**:525, 1977.
235. West JC, Goodman SI, Schroter GP, Bloustein PA, Hambidge KM, Well R: Pediatric kidney transplantation for cystinosis. *J Pediatr Surg* **12**:651, 1977.

CHAPTER 197

Mendelian Hypophosphatemias

Harriet S. Tenenhouse ▪ Michael J. Econs

1. **Several Mendelian hypophosphatemias have been described. Each has a decrease in net renal tubular phosphate reabsorption as a major underlying abnormality and is associated with rickets and osteomalacia. The disorders differ from one another in their mode of inheritance, clinical features, metabolism of vitamin D, and response to therapy. This chapter describes three Mendelian hypophosphatemias as well as an acquired disorder, oncogenic hypophosphatemic osteomalacia, because of its phenotypic similarities to X-linked hypophosphatemia.**
2. **The most prevalent of the familial hypophosphatemias is inherited as an X-linked dominant trait and referred to as *X-linked hypophosphatemia* (XLH) (OMIM 307800, 307810). It is characterized by reduced TmP/GFR, hypophosphatemia, normocalcemia, normal to low plasma 1,25-dihydroxyvitamin D levels, normal parathyroid gland function, and elevated plasma alkaline phosphatase activity. These changes are associated with growth retardation, lower extremity deformity, radiologic and histomorphometric evidence of rickets and osteomalacia, but no muscle weakness or tetany. This disease appears to result from combined renal defects in tubular phosphate reabsorption and vitamin D metabolism, as well as a functional disorder in bone and teeth. XLH results from inactivating mutations in the *PHEX* gene, a member of the zinc metallopeptidase family of type II integral membrane glycoproteins. PHEX is expressed in bone and teeth and to a lesser extent in lung, ovary, and testis but not in kidney. Nonetheless, the function of PHEX is not understood. The most effective treatment for XLH consists of a combination of oral phosphate (1.0–2.0 g/day in four divided doses) and 1,25-dihydroxyvitamin D_3 (1.0–3.0 μg/day). A specific therapy for XLH has yet to be discovered, and the current modalities are not ideal.**
3. **X-linked *Hyp* and *Gy* mice serve as useful models to study the pathophysiology of XLH. *Hyp* and *Gy* mice harbor large deletions in 3′ and 5′ region of the *Phex* gene, respectively. Both mutants exhibit a defect in renal brush-border membrane Na^+-dependent phosphate transport that is secondary to decreased expression of the type II renal-specific, high-affinity, low-capacity Na^+-phosphate cotransporter Npt2. *Hyp* and *Gy* mice also are characterized by defects in renal vitamin D metabolism and bone mineralization. Studies in *Hyp* mice provide evidence in support of the view that the mutant renal phenotype is humorally mediated, presumably by a factor that is not appropriately processed or degraded by Phex protein. The *Gy* mutation also involves a deletion in the spermine synthase gene that lies upstream of *Phex* and thus is a contiguous gene syndrome. The latter likely accounts for the circling behavior and inner ear abnormalities in *Gy* mice that are not apparent in *Hyp* mice.**
4. **Oncogenic hypophosphatemic osteomalacia (OHO) is an acquired form of isolated phosphate wasting. Clinical and biochemical features of the disease are similar to XLH, except that OHO patients typically exhibit weakness, fatigue, and fractures. Evidence suggests that the phenotypic features in OHO result from the secretion of a humoral factor, since removal of the tumor results in complete correction of the clinical and biochemical manifestations and transplantation of the tumors in mice elicits renal phosphate wasting. The tumors are frequently small and difficult to locate. Therapy consists of oral phosphate and 1,25-dihydroxyvitamin D_3.**
5. **There are two autosomal dominant forms of phosphate wasting, autosomal dominant hypophosphatemic rickets (ADHR; OMIM 193100) and hypophosphatemic bone disease (HBD; OMIM 146350), that may be a forme fruste of ADHR. While most of the clinical and laboratory features of ADHR are similar to those of XLH, ADHR displays incomplete penetrance and variable age of onset. ADHR may present during childhood, with clinical and biochemical features similar to XLH patients, or after puberty, with the additional features of weakness, fatigue, and fracture. Although the pathogenesis of ADHR is unknown and there is no animal model of the disorder, linkage studies in a large kindred have localized the disease gene locus to chromosome 12p13. Therapy for ADHR is the same as therapy for XLH and consists of a combination of oral phosphate and 1,25-dihydroxyvitamin D_3.**
6. **Hereditary hypophosphatemic rickets with hypercalciuria (HHRH; OMIM 241530) is inherited as an autosomal codominant trait. It is characterized by a reduced TmP/GFR, hypophosphatemia, an elevated plasma 1,25-dihydroxyvitamin D concentration, hypercalciuria, a low plasma parathyroid hormone concentration, and elevated plasma alkaline phosphatase activity. These abnormalities are associated with growth retardation, bone pain, muscle weakness, lower extremity deformity, and radiologic and histomorphometric evidence of rickets and osteomalacia. A primary defect in renal phosphate transport, linked to a**

A list of standard abbreviations is located immediately preceding the index in each volume. Nonstandard abbreviations used in this chapter include: PTH = parathyroid hormone; XLH = X-linked hypophosphatemia; ADHR = autosomal dominant hypophosphatemic rickets; HHRH = hereditary hypophosphatemic rickets with hypercalciuria; OHO = oncogenic hypophosphatemic osteomalacia; TmP/GFR = maximum tubular capacity for phosphate reabsorption per glomerular filtration rate; ECF = extracellular fluid; $1,25(OH)_2D$ = 1,25-dihydroxyvitamin D_3; 25(OH)D = 25-hydroxyvitamin D_3; GH = growth hormone; $24,25(OH)_2D$ = 24,25-dihydroxyvitamin D_3; GFR = glomerular filtration rate; HBD = hypophosphatemic bone disease; IH = idiopathic hypercalciuria.

secondary stimulation of the renal 25-hydroxyvitamin D_3-1α-hydroxylase, appears to account for all the biochemical manifestations of the condition. Indeed, disruption of the type II renal Na^+-P_i cotransporter gene *Npt2* by targeted mutagenesis elicits a similar phenotype in mice. Treatment with oral phosphate alone (1.0–2.5 g/day in divided doses) reduces bone pain, heals rickets, and stimulates skeletal growth. Family members with milder degrees of hypophosphatemia have been found to have hypercalciuria and elevated plasma 1,25-dihydroxyvitamin D, without bone disease.

Inorganic phosphate is an essential nutrient in terms of both cell function and skeletal mineralization. It is required for glycolysis, gluconeogenesis, and energy metabolism and for the synthesis of DNA, RNA, membrane phospholipids, and a variety of phosphorylated intermediates. In addition, the phosphorylation of cellular proteins is a major mechanism by which cell function is controlled. Intracellular regulatory roles for the inorganic phosphate anion involve such diverse functions as the control of aerobic metabolism, the control of the O_2 dissociation curve of hemoglobin in the intact red cell, and the regulation of cellular calcium metabolism.

Phosphate is sufficiently abundant in the usual human diet. Thus phosphate deficiency is unlikely to develop except under unusual circumstances, such as extreme starvation or as a consequence of administration of a class of therapeutic agents known as *phosphate binders* that bind phosphate in the intestinal lumen and prevent its absorption. The major portion of ingested phosphate (65–75 percent) is absorbed in the small intestine, and hormonal regulation of this process plays only a minor role in normal phosphate homeostasis. Absorbed phosphate is either eliminated by the kidney, incorporated into organic forms in proliferating cells, or deposited as a component of bone mineral (hydroxyapatite). Bone deposition accounts for a much larger percentage of retained phosphate during the growth period. However, even in the growing organism, only a small percentage of absorbed phosphate is retained, with most of it being excreted in the urine.

Phosphate homeostasis and plasma phosphate concentration depend primarily on renal mechanisms that regulate tubular phosphate transport. In view of the central role of the kidney in phosphate homeostasis, it is not surprising that the mechanisms that determine tubular phosphate reabsorption are complex and are regulated by a multiplicity of factors (for reviews, see refs. 1–13). The two most important determinants of renal phosphate handling are dietary phosphate intake and circulating parathyroid hormone (PTH).

Four well-characterized renal phosphate wasting disorders will be discussed herein. Three, X-linked hypophosphatemia (XLH), autosomal dominant hypophosphatemic rickets (ADHR), and hereditary hypophosphatemic rickets with hypercalciuria (HHRH), are inherited, and the fourth, oncogenic hypophosphatemic osteomalacia (OHO), is acquired. The latter is included in the present discussion because of its possible relevance to our understanding of the pathogenesis of XLH and the regulation of renal phosphate handling.

Despite the fact that all four conditions are characterized by a renal phosphate leak [i.e., a reduced maximum tubular capacity for phosphate reabsorption per glomerular filtration rate (TmP/GFR)] and hypophosphatemia, and are associated with rickets and/or osteomalacia, patients with XLH, OHO, ADHR, and HHRH exhibit different responses to dietary phosphate intake and parathyroid infusion, and they require different therapeutic measures. In the ensuing discussion, a consideration of phosphate homeostasis and renal phosphate handling will be followed by a discussion of the pathogenic mechanisms involved in these conditions. The clinical features of each syndrome and its treatment will be presented. Emphasis is placed on recent positional cloning efforts that have led to identification of the gene responsible for XLH and the demonstration that ADHR is linked to chromosome 12p13. Studies in the *Hyp* and *Gy* murine homologues of XLH are also described because they have contributed significantly to our understanding of the pathogenesis of the human disease. Finally, studies of mice deficient in the renal type II Na^+-phosphate cotransporter gene (*Npt2*) are presented because of their phenotypic similarity to patients with HHRH.

Table 197-1 Mendelian Hypophosphatemias

	McKusick No.
X-linked hypophosphatemia (XLH)	307800, 307810
Autosomal dominant hypophosphatemic rickets (ADHR)	193100
Hypophosphatemic bone disease (HBD)	146350
Hereditary hypophosphatemic rickets with hypercalciuria (HHRH)	241530
Autosomal recessive hypophosphatemic rickets	241520

SOURCE: From McKusick VA: *Mendelian Inheritance in Man*, 10th ed. Baltimore: Johns Hopkins University Press, 1992.

It should be noted that other Mendelian hypophosphatemias have been documented[14] (Table 197-1). Since considerably less information is available about autosomal recessive hypophosphatemic rickets, this condition will not be considered here. Hypophosphatemic bone disease will be discussed in the context of ADHR. For a discussion of earlier work relating to phosphate homeostasis, XLH, OHO, and HHRH, the reader is referred to previous editions in this series.[15–17]

PHOSPHATE HOMEOSTASIS

Under ordinary circumstances, the major determinants of phosphate homeostasis are dietary phosphate intake, the absorption of phosphate from the intestine, and its filtration and reabsorption by the renal tubule. The cellular mechanisms underlying phosphate transport across the intestinal mucosal cell and the renal tubular cell are quite similar. However, their hormonal and dietary controls are different.

Dietary phosphate (approximately 800–1600 mg/d) is absorbed in the small intestine, with the absorptive rate highest in the jejunum and ileum and lowest in the duodenum. Essentially no absorption occurs in the colon.[18] This pattern contrasts with that of calcium, which is absorbed at highest rates in duodenum and ileum and lower rates in jejunum and colon. Intestinal phosphate absorption increases in proportion to the phosphate content of the diet, and vitamin D metabolites play a role in phosphate homeostasis when phosphate intake is significantly reduced.[19,20] The renal excretion of phosphate increases and decreases in direct relation to phosphate intake over a wide range of intakes.[21,22]

The plasma phosphate concentration varies as a function of age in humans: in the range of 3.8 to 5.5 mg/dl (1.23–1.77 mM) in children[23] and 2.7 to 4.5 mg/dl (0.97–1.45 mM) in adults.[24] Of interest is the fact that mice and rats have higher normal plasma phosphate values than humans. This difference in plasma phosphate correlates with differences in basal metabolic rate. In both rodent species, the basal metabolic rate is higher than that in humans.[25]

Although long-term changes in plasma phosphate concentration clearly depend on the balance between intestinal absorption and renal excretion, short-term changes in phosphate concentration can occur as a consequence of the redistribution of phosphate between the extracellular fluid (ECF) and either bone or cell constituents. Since the ECF phosphate represents less than 1 percent of total-body phosphate, either the mobilization of phosphate following tissue destruction or the mobilization of phosphate from bone mineral can lead to temporary increases in plasma phosphate concentration.

In measuring plasma phosphate concentration and relating this value to a clinical situation, it is necessary to bear in mind that there is a diurnal variation in plasma phosphate concentration with a nadir at 9:30 to 10:00 A.M. and a peak at 4 A.M.[26] The change in concentration from nadir to peak may be as much as 1 mg/dl, i.e., a 25 to 35 percent change in concentration.[26] The factors determining this diurnal variation are not known but probably involve extrarenal mechanisms.

Phosphate Homeostasis in States of Altered Mineral Intake

In considering the mechanisms involved in the pathogenesis of XLH, OHO, ADHR, and HHRH, it is useful to discuss our present view of how the organism adapts to severe dietary restrictions of either phosphate or calcium. A discussion of calcium homeostasis within a discussion of disorders of renal phosphate transport is necessary because of (1) the intimate link between the transport of these ions across the intestine and renal tubule, (2) their coexistence as components of bone mineral, (3) their interrelated effects on the regulation of vitamin D metabolism, and (4) the interrelated changes in their metabolism in response to PTH and 1,25-dihydroxyvitamin D_3 [$1,25(OH)_2D$]. The key tissues involved in phosphate and calcium homeostasis are the gut, kidney, and bone, and the key hormonal regulators are PTH and $1,25(OH)_2D$. The reader is referred to Chaps. 164 and 165 in this work for a more complete discussion of PTH and vitamin D, respectively.

Phosphate Deprivation. The kidney adapts to a decrease in phosphate intake with a prompt fall in phosphate excretion. Plasma phosphate may fall only minimally, but with continued phosphate restriction, the plasma phosphate concentration and the filtered load decrease. Either a change in the tubular phosphate transport or a change in the plasma phosphate concentration leads to an increase in 25-hydroxyvitamin D_3 [25(OH)D]-1α-hydroxylase activity in the proximal renal tubule,[27,28] and as a consequence, the plasma concentration of $1,25(OH)_2D$ rises. The fall in plasma phosphate leads to an inhibition of bone mineral deposition, and if bone resorption continues, there is a net shift of phosphate from the skeleton to the ECF. The rise in the plasma $1,25(OH)_2D$ concentration provides an additional stimulus to bone resorption.[29] Moreover, the increase in plasma $1,25(OH)_2D$ also stimulates intestinal phosphate transport by a direct action on the mucosal phosphate transport system[30] and indirectly by the action of $1,25(OH)_2D$ on intestinal calcium absorption.

The rise in plasma $1,25(OH)_2D$ concentration and the resulting increases in both intestinal calcium absorption and bone resorption lead to an increase in the plasma calcium concentration. The latter then acts to inhibit PTH secretion. As a consequence, plasma PTH levels fall, and the distal tubular reabsorption of calcium is decreased. In this way, the increased influx of calcium into the ECF from bone and gut is balanced by an increased renal loss. The decrease in plasma PTH levels also should contribute to renal phosphate retention. However, this is likely not the case because tubular phosphate transport becomes insensitive to the action of PTH under conditions of severe phosphate depletion.[31]

The homeostatic changes in response to phosphate deprivation lead to nearly complete renal phosphate conservation, the mobilization of phosphate and calcium from the skeleton, an increase in intestinal phosphate and calcium absorption, and hypercalciuria. Accordingly, one would predict that a simple renal phosphate leak should lead to a similar sequence of events and in particular to increases in plasma $1,25(OH)_2D$ concentration and intestinal calcium absorption resulting in hypercalciuria. However, in the case of XLH, OHO, and ADHR, the renal phosphate leak coexists with a disordered regulation of renal $1,25(OH)_2D$ synthesis. On the other hand, in HHRH, the phosphate leak is associated with the same tetrad seen during dietary phosphate restriction in animals or humans, namely, high plasma $1,25(OH)_2D$, low plasma PTH, increased intestinal calcium absorption, and hypercalciuria.

Calcium Deprivation. A decrease in calcium intake leads to a slight fall in plasma calcium concentration and a stimulation of PTH secretion. The resulting rise in plasma PTH concentration leads to (1) an increase in bone reabsorption and a net loss of calcium and phosphate from bone, (2) an increase in distal tubular calcium reabsorption, (3) a decrease in proximal tubular phosphate transport, and (4) an increase in the rate of $1,25(OH)_2D$ synthesis by the proximal tubule. The resulting rise in plasma $1,25(OH)_2D$ leads to an increased efficiency of intestinal calcium and phosphate absorption and acts synergistically with PTH to enhance resorption of bone.

Phosphate Excess. A marked increase in dietary phosphate intake can occur without a marked change in plasma phosphate concentration because of the compensatory increase in renal phosphate clearance. However, with very high phosphate intakes, particularly if associated with a reduced calcium intake, plasma phosphate may rise sufficiently to reduce plasma ionized calcium, leading to an increase in PTH secretion, a rise in plasma PTH, and a further reduction in renal tubular phosphate reabsorption. Thus excessive phosphate intake can lead to a state of secondary hyperparathyroidism, an important consideration in the therapeutic use of phosphate in XLH, OHO, ADHR, and HHRH.

RENAL PHOSPHATE TRANSPORT

The renal excretion of phosphate is determined by the balance between the rates of glomerular filtration and tubular reabsorption.[1–13] There is no convincing evidence for net tubular secretion of phosphate by the mammalian nephron under normal conditions. Approximately 90 percent of the phosphate in plasma is ultrafilterable, but as the plasma calcium concentration rises, the percentage of plasma phosphate that is filtered is decreased.[32]

As in the case of many transport processes, the transcellular transport of phosphate is a carrier-mediated, saturable process and a transfer maximum (Tm) for renal phosphate reabsorption can be determined. However, because of the marked effect of phosphate intake on the renal handling of phosphate, the Tm varies considerably with dietary phosphate. The best way to estimate the overall capacity of the renal phosphate transport system is to measure the TmP/GFR during acute phosphate infusion. In practice, an estimate of TmP/GFR can be made by measuring phosphate and creatinine excretion and plasma phosphate concentration and using this information and the nomogram developed by Bijvoet[33] (showing the relationship between plasma phosphate concentration and the fractional excretion of phosphate) to derive this value (Fig. 197-1). Use of this nomogram is limited to situations in which there are significant rates of urinary phosphate excretion.

Tubular Sites of Phosphate Reabsorption, PTH Action, and $1,25(OH)_2D$ Synthesis

Table 197-2 summarizes the tubular sites at which phosphate reabsorption, PTH action, and $1,25(OH)_2D$ synthesis occur.[28,34–40] The bulk of filtered phosphate is reabsorbed in the proximal tubule, with approximately 60 percent of the filtered load reclaimed in the proximal convoluted tubule and 15 to 20 percent in the proximal straight tubule. In addition, a small but variable portion ($<$ 10 percent) of filtered phosphate is reabsorbed in more distal segments of the nephron. The importance of phosphate reabsorption at this latter site is difficult to define because of considerable heterogeneity between the ability of deep and superficial nephrons to conserve phosphate. Nonetheless, it does appear that small amounts of phosphate are reabsorbed distally, and these may be important in disorders involving defects in the

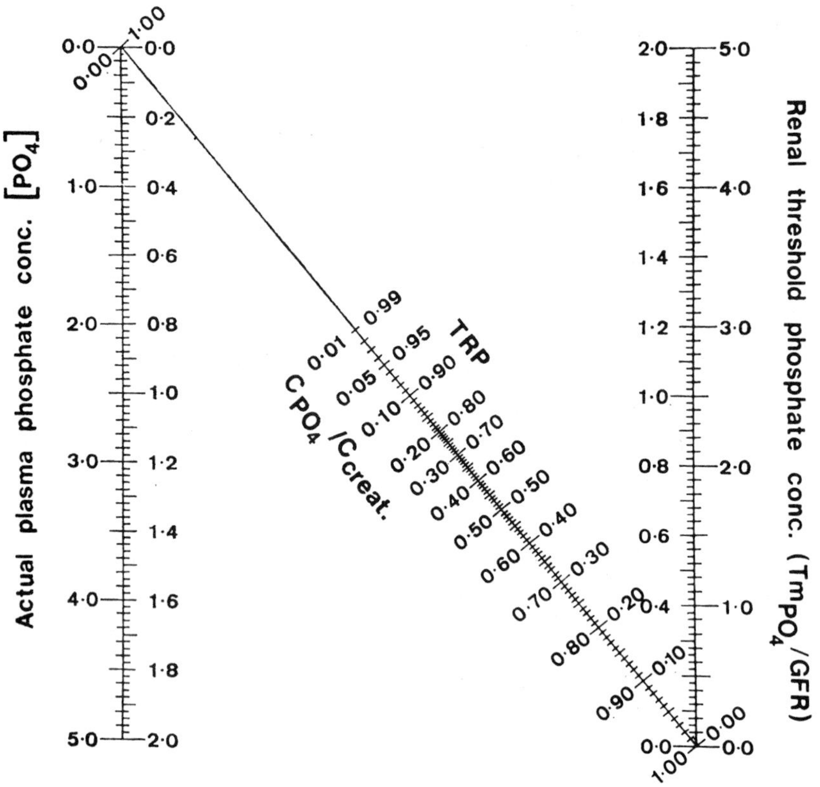

Fig. 197-1 Nomogram for derivation of renal threshold phosphate concentration ($TmPO_4$/GFR). A straight line through the appropriate plasma phosphate and TRP (fractional reabsorption of filtered phosphate load, i.e., phosphate/creatinine clearance) values passes through the corresponding values of $TmPO_4$/GFR. The scales and units of the figures are arbitrary, provided consistent dimensions are used. (*Used with permission from Walton and Bijvoet.*[33])

mechanisms controlling phosphate reabsorption in the proximal nephron.

PTH-sensitive adenylate cyclase is found at all three sites of phosphate transport: proximal convoluted tubule, proximal straight tubule, and distal tubule.[39,40] There is also clear evidence that PTH (or cAMP) will decrease phosphate reabsorption in both the proximal convoluted tubule and the proximal straight tubule but probably not in the distal tubule.[41] From these observations, it has been concluded that PTH inhibits phosphate transport in the proximal tubular segments via a cAMP-dependent process. Further, PTH stimulates 1α-hydroxylase by a cAMP-dependent mechanism in the proximal convoluted tubule[28] and inhibits Na^+-H^+ exchange in this nephron segment.[42,43] Finally, PTH stimulates distal tubular calcium reabsorption by mechanisms that involve both protein kinase A and protein kinase C.[44]

During dietary phosphate deprivation, there is an increase in phosphate transport in all nephron segments and probably an increase in 1α-hydroxylase activity in the proximal convoluted tubule.

Table 197-2 Renal Tubular Site of Phosphate Transport, 1α-Hydroxylase, and Hormone-Sensitive Adenylate Cyclase

	Phosphate Transport	PTH-Sensitive Adenylate Cyclase	PTH-Sensitive 1α-Hydroxylase
PCT*	+++	++	++++
PST	++	+	−−
MTAL	−−	−−	−−
CTAL	−−	++++	−−
DT	+	+++	−−
CT	−−	−−	−−

*PCT, proximal convoluted tubule; PST, proximal straight tubule; MTAL, medullary thick ascending limb; CTAL, cortical thick ascending limb; DT, distal tubule; CT, collecting tubule.

Cellular Mechanisms of Renal Phosphate Transport

A number of experimental systems have been used to characterize proximal tubular phosphate transport systems and to elucidate mechanisms involved in their regulation.[1–13] The process is essentially unidirectional and involves phosphate uptake across the brush-border membrane, translocation across the cell, and efflux at the basolateral membrane (Fig. 197-2). Phosphate uptake at the apical cell surface is the rate-limiting step in the overall phosphate reabsorptive process and the major site of its regulation. It involves secondary active transport of phosphate, driven by a Na^+ gradient (outside > inside) that is maintained by the Na^+,K^+-ATPase or sodium pump on the basolateral membrane. Na^+ increases both the affinity of the cotransporter for phosphate and the V_{max} for Na^+-phosphate cotransport.[45]

Na^+-phosphate stoichiometries of both 2:1 and 3:1 have been documented. Given that divalent phosphate (HPO_4^{2-}) is the predominant anion at physiologic pH ($HPO_4^{2-}/H_2PO_4^{1-} = 4/1$ at pH 7.4), the data suggest that Na^+-phosphate cotransport is both electroneutral and electrogenic. Direct evidence for electrogenic Na^+-phosphate cotransport has been obtained recently by expression studies in *Xenopus laevis* oocytes[45,46] (see "Structural Identification of Renal Na^+-Phosphate Cotransport Systems," below). Na^+-phosphate cotransport across the brush-border membrane is sensitive to changes in pH and is increased 10- to 20-fold when the pH is raised from 6 to 8.5. These findings reflect not only the preferential transport of divalent phosphate but also the action of protons on the cotransporter per se. Indeed, it has been demonstrated that pH has a significant effect on the affinity of the cotransporter for Na^+ ions.[46,47]

The effects of pH on Na^+-phosphate cotransport in isolated brush-border membrane vesicles reflect the effects of systemic acid-base balance on renal phosphate handling.[11] Phosphate reabsorption is decreased by respiratory acidosis and increased by respiratory alkalosis. Because the inhibition of brush-border membrane Na^+-phosphate cotransport during metabolic acidosis depends on intact adrenal glands, it was postulated that adrenal

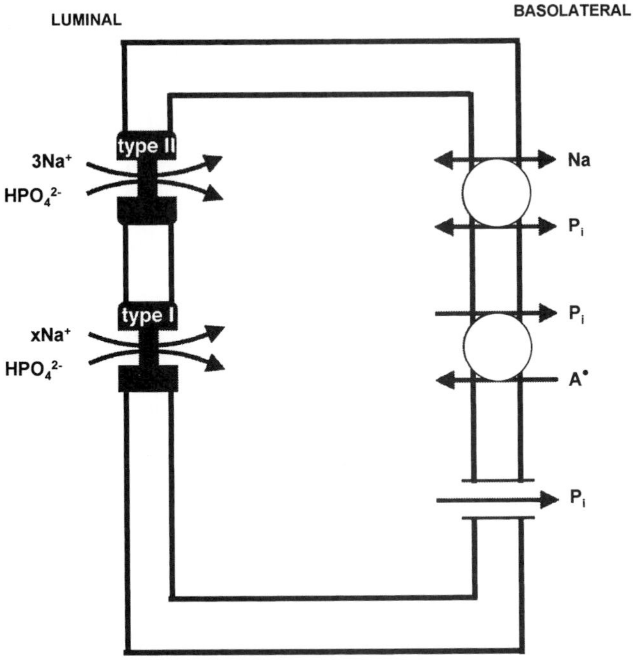

Fig. 197-2 A model of the process of transcellular transport of inorganic phosphate (HPO_4^{2-}) across the proximal convoluted tubule of mammalian kidney. The luminal or brush-border membrane is depicted on the left and the basolateral membrane on the right. Both the type I (NPT1) and type II (NPT2) Na^+-phosphate cotransporters operate in the luminal membrane. A Na^+/phosphate stoichiometry of 3:1 for the type II transporter has been documented. The HPO_4^{2-} that enters the cell across the luminal surface mixes with the metabolic pool of phosphate in the cell and eventually is transported out of the cell across the basolateral membrane via passive diffusion down an electrochemical gradient or via an anion-exchange mechanism. There is also evidence for a Na^+-phosphate cotransporter on the basolateral membrane that is distinct from NPT1 and NPT2. Not shown is the basolateral membrane Na^+, K^+-ATPase that transports Na^+ (which enters the cell on its luminal side) out of the cell, thereby maintaining the Na^+ gradient driving force for luminal phosphate entry.

hormones are necessary for the response.[48] Indeed, metabolic acidosis is associated with increased glucocorticoid levels, and inhibition of Na^+-phosphate cotransport can be achieved by the administration of the glucocorticoid dexamethasone to adrenalectomized rats.[11,48] These results are supported by the demonstration that dexamethasone inhibits Na^+-phosphate cotransport in OK cell cultures[49,50] (Table 197-3) and interferes with the effects of metabolic acidosis in this renal proximal tubular cell line.[50]

There is evidence for two kinetically distinct Na^+-phosphate cotransport systems in the brush-border membrane of several mammalian species.[51] In the early proximal convoluted tubule, a high-capacity, low-affinity system appears to be responsible for reabsorption of the bulk of the filtered load, and a low-capacity, high-affinity system is responsible for the remainder. In the proximal straight tubule, however, a single low-capacity, high-affinity system is found. This topologic arrangement of Na^+-phosphate cotransport systems in series permits highly efficient reabsorption of phosphate in the proximal tubule.

The phosphate that enters the cell is in rapid exchange with intracellular phosphate. There does not appear to be a separate transport pool. The efflux of phosphate out of the cell across the basolateral membrane occurs by a passive process, driven by the electrical gradient existing across this membrane and via an anion-exchange mechanism (see Fig. 197-2). In addition, there appears to be a small component of Na^+-linked secondary active influx of phosphate across the basolateral membrane (see Fig. 197-2) that has a V_{max} only 10 percent of the luminal process.[52] This process can be distinguished from that in the brush-border membrane

Table 197-3 Hormonal Regulation of Phosphate Transport: Evidence from Studies in Cultured Renal Epithelial Cells

Hormone*	Target Cells	Direction of Change	Reference
PTH	OK cells	↓	84
	Mouse primary cultures	↓	338
Glucocorticoids	Chick primary cultures	↓	339
PTHrP	OK cells	↓	340
ANF	OK cells	↓	341
TGF-α	OK cells	↓	342
TGF-β	OK cells	↓	343
$1,25(OH)_2D_3$	Chick primary cultures	↑	344
T3	Chick primary cultures	↑	345
EGF	LLC-PK1 cells	↑	346
IGF-1	OK cells	↑	347
Insulin	OK cells	↑	348

*PTHrP, parathyroid hormone related peptide; ANF, atrial natriuretic factor; TGF-α, transforming growth factor α; TGF-β, transforming growth factor β; EGF, epidermal growth factor; IGF-1, insulin-like growth factor-1; LLC-PK_1, porcine kidney epithelial cells; OK, oppossum kidney epithelial cell line.

because it has a lower K_m for phosphate (0.014 mM), is insensitive to pH, and is more electrogenic. However, this Na^+-dependent entry of phosphate across the basolateral membrane appears to be insufficient to maintain normal intracellular phosphate concentrations in the absence of luminal phosphate entry.

Structural Identification of Renal Na^+-Phosphate Cotransport Systems

Efforts to purify Na^+-P_i cotransport proteins from isolated renal brush-border membrane preparations met with little success because of their low abundance and technical difficulties associated with their solubilization, reconstitution, and purification. More recently, however, cDNAs encoding renal-specific Na^+-phosphate cotransporters have been identified in several species, first by expression cloning in *X. laevis* oocytes and then by homology screening.[47,53–62] The cDNAs, designated type I (NPT1, SLC17A1) and type II (NPT2, SLC34A1), encode two classes of Na^+-phosphate cotransporters that share only 20 percent identity (for reviews, see refs. 12, 13, and 63–66). The NPT1 transporters are approximately 465 amino acids in length with seven to nine member-spanning segments, whereas the NPT2 transporters are comprised of approximately 635 amino acids and are predicted to span the membrane eight times (Fig. 197-3).

The *NPT1* and *NPT2* genes have been mapped to chromosomes 6p22[67] and 5q35,[68,69] respectively, by fluorescence in situ hybridization. The human and murine *NPT2/Npt2* genes have been cloned and characterized (GenBank database accession numbers U5664-U56673, U57491, and U57839 for mouse gene and U56674-U56695 and U57548 for human gene).[70]

The renal localization of *NPT1* and *NPT2* gene expression was determined by immunohistochemistry, in situ hybridization, and reverse transcriptase-polymerase chain reaction (RT-PCR) of RNA prepared from single microdissected nephron segments.[71–74] These studies identified *NPT1* and *NPT2* transcripts in the proximal tubule and immunoreactive protein in the brush-border membrane of proximal tubular cells (see Fig. 197-2). However, while NPT1 protein is uniformly expressed in all segments of the proximal nephron, NPT2 expression is highest in the S_1 segment of the proximal tubule.

Functional studies of NPT1 and NPT2 proteins have been conducted in cRNA-injected oocytes[45,46,53,57,75,76] and in cDNA-transfected renal cell lines.[77–79] Both NPT1 and NPT2 mediate

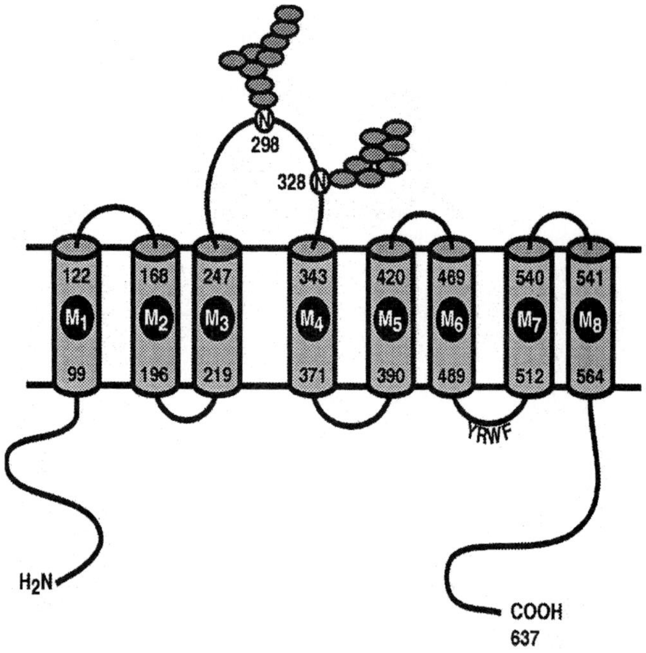

Fig. 197-3 Structural model for the type II Na⁺-phosphate cotransporter (NPT2; rat) based on hydropathy predictions. M1 to M8 refer to the eight transmembrane domains, and the numbers refer to the amino acid residues. Both the N- and C-terminal ends of the NPT2 protein are inside the renal proximal tubular cell. The two glycosylation sites most likely used are indicated. (*Kindly provided by Drs. J. Biber and H. Murer.*)

high-affinity Na^+-phosphate cotransport. However, their pH profiles are significantly different, with that of NPT2 bearing closer resemblance to the pH dependence of Na^+-phosphate cotransport in renal brush-border membrane vesicles. Moreover, NPT1 appears to exhibit a broader substrate specificity than NPT2.[76] NPT1 can induce a Cl^- conductance that is inhibited by Cl^- channel blockers and organic anions, and on this basis it was suggested that NPT1 not only mediates brush-border membrane Na^+-dependent phosphate transport but also serves as an apical channel for Cl^- transport and the excretion of anionic xenobiotics.[76] The precise physiologic role of NPT1 thus will require further study.

Site-directed mutagenesis of *NPT2* cDNA suggested that two major glycosylation sites are used[75] (see Fig. 197-3). While glycosylation of NPT2 does not appear to be crucial for transport activity, it may be required for NPT2 protein biosynthesis and membrane delivery.

Radiation inactivation experiments and electrophoretic separation under reducing and nonreducing conditions suggest that the functionally active conformation of the type II Na^+-phosphate cotransporter may be a homotetramer.[80] In addition, it was suggested that disulfide bonds are involved in the formation of the multimeric structure.[80]

Recent evidence has been obtained for the expression of two novel phosphate transporters in the kidney (designated type III). Both are cell surface viral receptors [gibbon ape leukemia virus (Glvr-1, PiT-1) and murine amphotropic virus (Ram-1, PiT-2)] that mediate high-affinity, electrogenic Na^+-dependent phosphate transport when expressed in oocytes and in mammalian cells.[81] Although neither Glvr-1 nor Ram-1 show any sequence similarity to NPT1 or NPT2, they share 60 percent sequence identity with a putative phosphate permease of *Neurospora crassa*.[81] Since Glvr-1 and Ram-1 are widely expressed in mammalian tissues,[81] it has been suggested that they serve as "housekeeping" Na^+-phosphate cotransporters. Recently, it was shown, by in situ hybridization, that Glvr-1 is expressed throughout the kidney, consistent with its role as a housekeeping cotransporter.[74] However, the relative abundance of Glvr-1 and Ram-1 mRNAs in mouse kidney is approximately 80-fold lower than that of Npt2.[74] Additional studies are necessary to define the renal membrane localization of Glvr-1 and Ram-1 and to determine whether these retroviral receptors contribute significantly to renal phosphate reabsorption.

The *GLVR-1* gene has been mapped to human chromosome 2q11-q14[82] and the *RAM-1* gene to the pericentromeric region of human chromosome 8.[83]

Hormonal Regulation

Phosphate reabsorption by the kidney can be modulated by a variety of peptide and steroid hormones.[3–9,11,12] Growth hormone (GH), insulin-like growth factor I, insulin, epidermal growth factor, thyroid hormone, and 1,25-$(OH)_2D$ all stimulate renal phosphate reabsorption, whereas PTH, PTH-related peptide, calcitonin, atrial natriuretic factor, transforming growth factors α and β, and glucocorticoids inhibit renal phosphate reclamation. From in vitro studies using cultured renal epithelial cells, there is evidence for a direct action of these hormones on the kidney (Table 197-3). With respect to GH, the increase in phosphate transport occurs by virtue of its ability to stimulate insulin-like growth factor I production. Although the mechanisms for hormonal regulation of renal phosphate transport are only beginning to be elucidated, the target for regulation is the high-affinity, type II Na^+-phosphate cotransporter (NPT2) at the apical surface of renal proximal convoluted tubular cells (see Fig. 197-2). Because of the physiologic importance of PTH in the regulation of renal phosphate transport and the vast literature devoted to this subject, the following discussion will focus on the cellular and molecular mechanisms involved in this action of PTH.

The original model for PTH action on proximal tubular phosphate transport was one in which the interaction of PTH with its receptor on the basolateral membrane leads to the activation of adenylate cyclase. This results in an increase in intracellular cAMP that diffuses across the cell and inhibits Na^+-phosphate cotransport by catalyzing protein kinase A-dependent phosphorylation of one or more proteins in the brush-border membrane. More recently, however, there is evidence for PTH receptors in the brush-border membrane as well as in the basolateral membrane[84–86] and for the involvement of the protein kinase C-phosphoinositide signaling pathway in mediating the inhibitory action of PTH on renal Na^+-phosphate cotransport.[87–92] The involvement of the protein kinase C signaling pathway does not preclude the participation of the adenylate cyclase signaling pathway. Indeed, the findings to date suggest that both signal transduction pathways are involved in PTH regulation of renal phosphate transport, with the phosphoinositide pathway operating at low PTH concentrations (10^{-10} – 10^{-12}) and the cAMP cascade at high PTH concentrations (10^{-8} – 10^{-10} M).

Recent studies have provided some insight into events following PTH activation of the regulatory cascades discussed earlier. PTH elicits a decrease in the V_{max} of brush-border membrane Na^+-phosphate cotransport by a mechanism that involves endocytosis and degradation of NPT2 protein. Immunofluorescence studies demonstrated that PTH mediates the retrieval of NPT2 protein from the brush-border membrane[93] and, furthermore, that agents that interfere with the endocytic pathway disrupt the action of PTH on Na^+-phosphate cotransport (see also Chap. 196 for mention of this pathway in renal epithelium). Additionally, evidence was presented for PTH-mediated degradation of NPT2 protein in the lysosomal/endosomal fraction of proximal tubular cells.[94] These findings are consistent with earlier studies showing that recovery of renal Na^+-phosphate cotransport activity following PTH inhibition requires protein synthesis.[95]

A novel hormonal system has been implicated in the regulation of renal phosphate handling. Stanniocalcin, a peptide hormone that counteracts hypercalcemia and stimulates phosphate reabsorption in bony fish,[96] is also produced by humans.[97] The infusion of human stanniocalcin in rats also elicits a stimulation in phosphate reabsorption that is associated with an increase in brush-border membrane Na^+-phosphate cotransport.[98] These findings suggest that stanniocalcin may contribute to the overall maintenance of phosphate homeostasis in mammals as well as fish.

Regulation by Dietary Phosphate

Dietary phosphate intake is an important determinant of renal phosphate reabsorption. Phosphate deprivation elicits an increase in TmP/GFR that is attributable to an adaptive increase in Na^+-phosphate cotransport at the brush-border membrane. The increase in transport is independent of extrarenal factors and has been demonstrated in renal proximal tubular cell cultures grown in low-phosphate medium. While the signal for the adaptive response to phosphate deprivation is not known, it has been suggested that a fall in the concentration of renal cell phosphate plays a role in initiating the phosphate transport response.[99] Both acute and chronic exposure to low phosphate intake elicit an increase in Na^+-phosphate cotransport V_{max}. However, the molecular mechanisms for the adaptive responses to acute and chronic phosphate deprivation are different.

The acute phase (2 h) of the adaptive response is not blocked by inhibitors of protein synthesis, is prevented by colchicine, and is associated with an increase in immunoreactive NPT2 protein in the brush-border membrane.[100] These data suggest that the acute response to low phosphate is mediated by microtubule-dependent recruitment of existing NPT2 protein to the apical membrane.[101] In addition, the acute increase in Na^+-phosphate cotransport and NPT2 protein is rapidly reversed by a high-phosphate diet.[100] The exposure to high phosphate leads to the rapid internalization of cell surface NPT2 protein into the endosomal compartment by a microtubule-independent mechanism.[101] Internalized NPT2 protein is then subject to lysosomal degradation.[102]

The adaptive response to chronic phosphate deprivation depends on protein synthesis and is associated with an increase in renal abundance of both NPT2 mRNA and NPT2 protein.[100] Studies in chronically phosphate-starved opossum kidney cells demonstrated that the increase in NPT2 mRNA can be attributed to an increase in NPT2 mRNA stability rather than to an increase in *NPT2* gene transcription.[103] However, not all studies have been able to document an increase in renal NPT2 mRNA with chronic phosphate deprivation,[74,102,104,105] suggesting that regulation at the mRNA level may not be the only mechanism contributing to the chronic adaptive response. Two recent reports shed some light on the mechanism whereby *NPT2* gene expression is regulated by phosphate. In the first, functional analysis of the *NPT2* promoter showed that reporter gene activity, in cells transfected with *NPT2* promoter-reporter gene constructs, was not responsive to changes in the extracellular phosphate concentration, suggesting that posttranscriptional mechanisms are involved in the chronic adaptive response.[104] In the second, mice heterozygous for the disrupted *Npt2* allele exhibited normal brush-border membrane Na^+-phosphate cotransport and normal Npt2 protein abundance in the face of a 50 percent reduction in Npt2 mRNA. These data are consistent with the notion that the adaptive response to the loss of one copy of the *Npt2* gene occurs at the Npt2 protein and not mRNA level.[106]

In contrast to *NPT2, NPT1* gene expression does not appear to be increased by phosphate restriction.[60] On the other hand, *Glvr-1* and *Ram-1* expressions are regulated by extracellular phosphate at both the mRNA and functional level.[81]

Efforts have been made to identify proteins that play a role in mediating the adaptive response to low phosphate. A new gene product, diphor-1, which is upregulated by dietary phosphate restriction, was identified recently in kidney by differential display-polymerase chain reaction.[107] It is a 52-kDa protein that exhibits a high degree of identity with the Na^+/H^+ exchanger regulatory protein and a tyrosine kinase-activating protein. It is highly expressed in the proximal tubule and intestine and specifically increases Na^+-phosphate cotransport in oocytes coinjected with NPT2 cRNA. Further work is necessary to determine the precise role and mechanism of action of diphor-1 in the renal adaptive response to low phosphate.

X-LINKED HYPOPHOSPHATEMIA

XLH is the most common of the inherited renal phosphate wasting disorders (see Table 197-1). It is an X-linked dominant disease with full penetrance. Other names that have been used for the disorder include *X-linked hypophosphatemic rickets, vitamin D-resistant rickets, familial hypophosphatemic rickets, phosphate diabetes,* and *hypophosphatemic vitamin D-resistant rickets*. The preferred name for the disorder is *X-linked hypophosphatemia* because it best distinguishes this disorder from other Mendelian and acquired hypophosphatemias (see Table 197-1). Vitamin D-resistant rickets, which is still in occasional use, is not an acceptable name because the disorder is not a Vitamin D-resistance syndrome (see also Chap. 165).

Clinical Features

XLH patients frequently present with short stature, lower extremity deformities (valgus or varus), dental abscesses, and bone pain (Fig. 197-4). Joint pain from enthesopathy (calcification of tendons, ligaments, and joint capsules) becomes prominent during middle age.[108–110] Severely affected individuals also may have cranial abnormalities (frontal bossing with increased anteroposterior skull length and decreased transverse diameter) and spinal cord compression.[111] Despite hypophosphatemia, weakness is not a prominent feature of the disease, although patients complain of weakness more than normal controls.[112] However, unlike OHO and some ADHR patients (see "Oncogenic

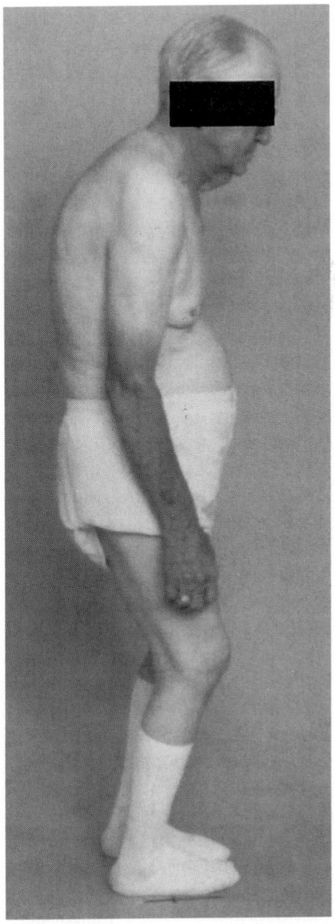

Fig. 197-4 Photograph of an XLH patient demonstrating moderate lower extremity deformity. The most disabling feature of the disease for this individual has been enthesopathic calcifications, which have led to fusion of the sacroiliac joints and lumbar and thoracic vertebrae. The enthesopathy has markedly impaired his mobility and led to a forward leaning of the trunk such that he has to bend his knees to maintain an upright posture.

Hypophosphatemic Osteomalacia" and "Autosomal Dominant Hypophosphatemic Rickets," below), XLH patients do not display objective evidence of weakness.

Disease severity is very variable even among members of the same family. In its mildest form, the disease can present with hypophosphatemia without clinical evidence of bone disease.[113–115] Of note, the variability between members of the same kindred, who presumably all have the same mutation, is similar to the variability observed between members of different kindreds. Although investigators frequently assume that males are more severely affected than females, and although there is some evidence that the radiographic manifestations of the disease are more pronounced in adult males than in adult females,[108,109,116] serum phosphorus values and height Z scores are the same in affected boys and girls.[117] Additionally, disease severity is not influenced by the parental origin of the mutant allele.[117]

The diagnosis of XLH may be difficult to establish during infancy, even in children with an affected parent. Serum phosphorus concentrations may be normal at birth and may remain so for 6 to 9 months. Additionally, it is important to recognize that the normal range for serum phosphorus values (see "Phosphate Homeostasis," above) and TmP/GFR is substantially higher in children than in adults.[23,118] Unfortunately, failure to recognize this fact has led to frequent errors in diagnosis.[112,119]

Although earlier views of the natural history of XLH were that the disease stopped progressing after the cessation of growth, this is clearly not the case. Systematic study of adults of various ages has shown persistent and often progressive evidence of disease, as well as mechanical complications arising from the skeletal deformities acquired during childhood and adolescence.[116] The persistence of disease is evident by the facts that (1) the phosphate-wasting defect persists throughout life, and many, but not all, adults have some elevation in plasma alkaline phosphatase, (2) every adult in whom transiliac crest biopsy has been appraised by histomorphometric analysis has unequivocal evidence of osteomalacia,[108] (3) many adults have radiologic evidence of pseudofractures,[109] (4) most adults have bone pain,[112] and (5) a majority have radiologic signs of bone and/or joint abnormalities (see below). As patients age, joint complaints become a predominant feature of the disease. Patients frequently complain of joint pain and have clinical and radiologic evidence of osteoarthritis, particularly of the ankle and knee.[109] In general, the more evidence there is of bowing of their lower limbs, the greater is the degree of osteoarthritis and joint pain. This is not surprising because mechanical irregularities from lower extremity deformity probably play a major role in the development of osteoarthritis. Additionally, enthesopathy is very common in adult XLH patients.[108–110] Fusion of the sacroiliac joints coupled with spinal hyperostoses, which mimic those seen in diffuse idiopathic skeletal hyperostosis (DISH), can lead to a clinical appearance that is reminiscent of ankylosing spondylitis (see Fig. 197-4). Indeed, stiffness and loss of mobility from enthesopathy may lead to significant disability as patients age.

In addition to bone and joint problems, patients frequently have recurrent dental abcesses.[112,120–124] Hypomineralization of the enamel, associated with a defect in dentin maturation with enlarged pulp chambers, is commonly seen in XLH.[125,126] Under normal circumstances, the dentin matrix calcifies by the formation of calcospheres containing calcium phosphate crystals. These coalesce to form a uniformly calcified dentin. In patients with XLH, the calcospheres fail to coalesce normally so that a distinct pattern of interglobular dentin forms and persists throughout life. It was reported that dental pulp space is highest in treated XLH males, intermediate in treated XLH females, and lowest in age-matched controls, despite near-normal serum phosphate levels in both groups of treated XLH patients, suggesting a possible gene dosage effect in teeth.[127] However, this conclusion is based on the assumption that extracellular phosphate was maintained at normal levels during the long period of tooth development in the treated XLH patients.

Laboratory Findings

The hallmark of XLH is a reduced serum phosphorus concentration and reduced TmP/GFR. As mentioned earlier, the normal range for serum phosphorus and TmP/GFR is substantially higher in children than in adults.[23,118] Proximal tubular reabsorption of other solutes is normal. Specifically, there is no glycosuria, bicarbonaturia, or aminoaciduria (although an occasional patient may have hyperglycinuria). Serum alkaline phosphatase activity is frequently elevated. The serum calcitriol concentration is inappropriately normal, suggesting that the regulation of renal vitamin D metabolism is impaired. Nevertheless, serum calcium, 25(OH)D, and PTH are within the normal range (Table 197-4).

Radiologic Findings

During childhood, the predominant findings are radiographic evidence of rickets with fraying, widening, and cupping of the metaphyseal ends of the tibia, distal femur, radius, and ulna. In general, the knees are a more reliable indicator of disease than the wrists.[128] It is important to note that radiographic evidence of rickets is not an invariant finding in children with XLH. In one study, analysis of pretreatment radiographs from children with XLH demonstrated rachitic abnormalities in only 5 of 11 wrist radiographs and 13 of 15 knee radiographs.[129] Two children did not display evidence of rickets at either the wrist or knee.[129]

Adults display many radiographic abnormalities. A coarse trabecular pattern, consistent with osteomalacia, is often seen on plain films. Pseudofractures, which are seen in many forms of osteomalacia, are rare in children but quite common in adults.[109] Most are located in the femur, and nearly half are located in the midfemoral diaphysis.[109] Calcification of the entheses (tendons, ligaments, and joint capsules) is observed in almost all patients (including those who have not received treatment) after age 40.[109,110,130] In one of these patients, histologic evaluation of an enthesopathic lesion revealed lamellar bone with no inflammatory cells.[110] While the sites of involvement include the hand, ankle, lesser trochanter, pelvis, foot, and greater trochanter,[109,110] the underlying basis for the development of enthesopathy is not clear. Other radiographic findings that may be observed include spinal stenosis[108,111] and Chiari type 1 malformation. Chiari 1 malformation was observed in 7 of 16 cranial magnetic resonance imaging (MRI) scans from "familial hypophosphatemic rickets" patients.[131] However, the significance of this finding is unclear.

Results for bone mineral density studies have been somewhat variable depending on the site measured and the technique used. In general, adults tend to have normal or increased (sometimes markedly increased) bone mineral density of the axial skeleton but normal measurements at peripheral sites.[108,132] Children tend to have a normal bone mineral density of the axial skeleton and low to normal values of the appendicular skeleton.[133,134]

Bone Histomorphometry

Transiliac biopsy demonstrates osteomalacia in both the cortical and trabecular bone, with an increase in osteoid volume, osteoid surface, and mean osteoid seam width.[135–137] Double tetracycline labeling reveals a decrease in calcification rate and a prolongation of mineralization lag time (the time between bone matrix deposition and its eventual calcification). In association with these changes, there are areas of hypomineralization (halos) around osteocytes in the lamellar cortical bone, which are characteristic of XLH.[138] Despite persistent osteomalacia, trabecular calcified bone volume tends to be normal or elevated in affected adults.[108,137,139]

Genetics

As noted earlier, XLH is an X-linked dominant disorder with essentially complete penetrance after 1 year of age (assuming that detailed studies are done to assess renal phosphate handling). Linkage studies mapped the disease locus to Xp22.1.[140,141] Subsequent efforts by the HYP Consortium localized the gene to a few hundred kilobases,[142,143] which allowed the consortium to

Table 197-4 Comparison of the Inherited Hypophosphatemic Rickets with Oncogenic Hypophosphatemic Osteomalacia

	XLH	HHRH	OHO	ADHR
Inheritance	X-linked dominant	Autosomal codominant(?)	−−	Autosomal dominant
Age of onset	Early childhood	Early childhood	Any age	Varies
Clinical features				
Short stature	++	++	++*	++*
Bone pain	++	+++	+++	++
Femoral bowing	++	++	++*	++*
Muscle weakness	−−−	++	++	++†
Radiologic signs				
Rickets	++	++	++*	++*
Pseudofracture	+	++	++	++
Coarse trabeculi	++	++	++	++
Dental abnormalities	++	?	−−	+
Calcium metabolism				
Serum Ca^{2+}	N	N	N	N
iPTH	N-H	LN	N	N
Ca_u	L-N	H	L-N	L-N
Phosphate metabolism				
Serum phosphate	L	L	L	L
TmP/GFR	L	L	L	L
Alkaline phosphatase	H	H	H	N-H
Vitamin D metabolism				
Serum $25(OH)D_3$	N	N	N	N
Serum $1,25(OH)_2D_3$	N	H	L-N	N
$25(OH)D_3$ 1α-hydroxylase				
Response to hypophosphatemia	Abnormal	Normal	Abnormal	Abnormal

*If disorder presents in childhood.
†If disorder presents in adulthood.

identify the gene.[144] The gene codes for a 749-amino-acid protein that has homology to members of the M13 family of membrane-bound metalloendopepidases, which includes neprilysin, endothelin converting enzyme-1, endothelin converting enzyme-2, and the Kell antigen (see GenBank accession nos. Y08111-Y08132 and Y10196 for the human gene sequence and U75645 and U75646 for the human and mouse *PHEX/Phex* cDNA sequences, respectively). The gene originally was referred to as *PEX* (phosphate regulating gene with homologies to endopeptidases on the X chromosome). The name has been changed subsequently to *PHEX* to avoid confusion with genes that are responsible for peroxisomal disorders (see Chaps. 129 to 133).

The predicted amino acid sequence of *PHEX* suggests that its protein structure closely resembles that of other members of the endopeptidase family. These are type II integral membrane glycoproteins with a short N-terminal cytoplasmic domain, a short transmembrane domain, and a large extracellular domain (Fig. 197-5). The membrane localization of PHEX was confirmed recently in COS cells following transfection with *PHEX* cDNA.[145] The extracellular domain of the predicted PHEX protein contains

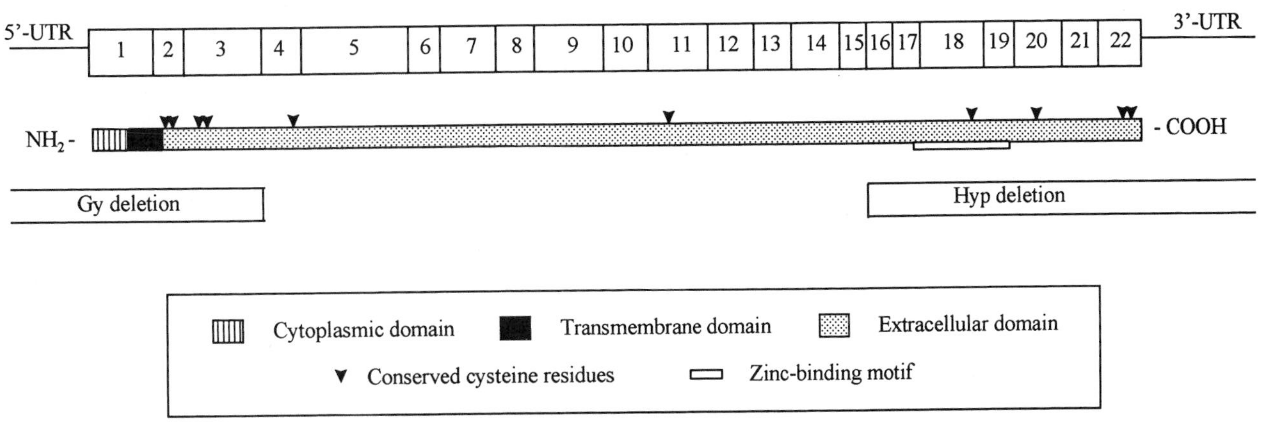

Fig. 197-5 Organization of the coding region of the *PHEX/Phex* gene. *PHEX/Phex* exons, numbered 1 to 22, are represented by boxes. Also shown are the deletion breakpoints in *Hyp* and *Gy* and the three domains of the PHEX/Phex protein: the short cytoplasmic domain at the N-terminal end, the transmembrane domain, and the large extracellular domain with 10 conserved cysteine residues and the zinc-binding motif. (Used with permission from Tenenhouse.[337a])

several highly conserved sequence motifs (see Fig. 197-5). These include a zinc-binding domain with two invariant histidine residues (HEXXH in exon 17) that chelate the metal ion and conserved glutamic acid and aspartic acid residues in exon 19, which are essential for substrate catalysis in the case of NEP. In addition, there are 10 cysteine residues throughout the extracellular domain, which are highly conserved in NEP, ECE-1, ECE-2, and Kell, and appear to be essential for the integrity of the native conformation.

The mouse *Phex* cDNA also was cloned and shown to have high homology with the human *PHEX* cDNA.[147–150] Of interest, neither the human nor murine *PHEX/Phex* genes have "classic" Kozak sequences.[151] The *PHEX/Phex* gene is one of only 3 percent of known genes that does not have a purine at the 3 position before the ATG initiation sequence.[145,147,149,152] This finding may be significant because, in general, genes that do not have good Kozak sequences tend to be posttranscriptionally regulated.[153]

Although little is known about the function of the Kell blood group protein, ECE-1 and NEP function as ectoenzymes. NEP proteolytically inactivates several small peptides including substance P, bradykinin, and enkephalin. ECE-1, on the other hand, plays a role in the proteolytic activation of big endothelin 1 to endothelin 1.[154] It has been suggested that ECE-2 acts as an intracellular enzyme responsible for the conversion of endogenously synthesized big endothelin at the trans-Golgi network.[155] Thus it is likely that PHEX functions to either activate or degrade a peptide hormone. A recent report by Lipman et al.[145] provides evidence that PHEX can degrade PTH and therefore function as an endopeptidase. In this regard, a recent study provided evidence for PHEX expression in the human parathyroid gland and suggested that loss of PHEX function contributes to PTH dysregulation in XLH.[155a]

PHEX/Phex mRNA expression and tissue distribution have been examined by a variety of techniques, including RT-PCR,[145,148,150,156] ribonuclease protection assay,[148] Northern blot analysis[145,148,156–158] and in situ hybridization[158] in human[148,157] and mouse[148,150,156,158] tissues. Evidence for expression was found in mouse bones[148,150,156,158] and teeth[158] and in human fetal bone[145,148] and lung,[148,157] as well as in adult ovary.[157] Northern blots demonstrate a transcript of approximately 6.6 to 7.0 kb in human and mouse bone and human ovary.[145,148,150,156,158] Of note, PHEX/Phex mRNA was not detected in the kidney.[148,156–158] Where relative abundance of PHEX/Phex mRNA expression was estimated, the highest level of expression was apparent in bones[148] and teeth.[158] This is consistent with the abnormalities in bones and teeth in patients with XLH (see above), and the demonstration of an osteoblast defect and dental abnormalities in *Hyp* mice (see "The Murine *Hyp* and *Gy* Models for X-linked Hypophosphatemia," above). PHEX/Phex is a low-abundance transcript and mRNA levels in bone are two orders of magnitude less than β-actin and glyceraldehyde-3-phosphate dehydrogenase mRNAs.[148] It is of interest that PHEX transcripts also were detected in tumors from patients with oncogenic hypophosphatemic osteomalacia[145] (see "Oncogenic Hypophosphatemic Osteomalacia," below). The fact that PHEX is observed in several different tissues suggests that it may play a role in processes other than phosphate homeostasis.

Since the original identification of the *PHEX* gene,[144] many different *PHEX* mutations have been identified in XLH patients.[152,159–162a] There are numerous mutations that lead to premature termination, splice-site mutations, deletions, and insertions. In addition, several missense mutations involve potentially important domains of the molecule. For example, changing the glycine at codon 579, which immediately precedes the zinc-binding motif and which is conserved in NEP and ECE-1 and ECE-2, to either arginine[159,161,162] or valine[160] likely results in the loss of catalytic activity. The reported proline to leucine (codon 534), leucine to proline (codons 138 and 555), and cysteine to serine (codons 77 and 733) missense mutations likely affect protein conformation.[159–162a] Because only a small number of affected individuals with each mutation are available for study, and because there is tremendous variability in the severity of the disease phenotype in members of the same kindred, it is not yet possible to draw conclusions regarding genotype-phenotype correlations.

A *PHEX* mutation database, dedicated to the collection and distribution of information on all *PHEX* gene mutations in one location, has been established (*http://data.mch.mcgill.ca/phexdb*).[162b] PHEXdb provides a submission form for the addition of new mutations, includes links to information pages and publications relevant to *PHEX*, XLH and murine *Hyp* and *Gy* homologues, and is updated continually.

As noted earlier, XLH is an X-linked dominant disorder with little, if any, gene dosage effect. Studies in affected females indicate that they have a normal X-chromosome inactivation pattern.[162c] Thus it is unlikely that preferential inactivation of the normal *PHEX* gene accounts for presence of the XLH phenotype in affected females. The presence of the disease in affected females could be accounted for by either a dominant-negative effect or haploinsufficiency. In either case, one mutant *PHEX* gene would be sufficient to result in the disease phenotype. Several reported mutations appear to shed light on the mechanism by which *PHEX* mutations result in disease. For example, a large ($>$ 50 kb) deletion in the *PHEX* gene that involves exons 1 to 5, which likely results in the absence of PHEX mRNA production, has been identified in one patient.[144,159] Another patient has a potential missense mutation in the 5′ UTR that also could affect PHEX mRNA production.[161] Moreover, a 160- to 190-kb deletion in the *Gy* mouse results in a contiguous gene syndrome that involves the first three *Phex* exons, the entire spermine synthase gene (which lies upstream from *Phex*), and the 39 kb between the two genes[149,164,165] (see "The Murine *Hyp* and *Gy* Models for X-linked Hypophosphatemia," below). This deletion also presumably results in an inability to transcribe Phex mRNA. Thus the available evidence suggests that XLH is not a dominant-negative disorder but rather a haploinsufficiency disorder.

Pathogenesis

Although it is clear that *PHEX* mutations are responsible for XLH, the mechanism whereby loss of PHEX function leads to the disease phenotype is not immediately obvious. However, a few points are noteworthy. First, the absence of detectable PHEX/Phex mRNA expression in the kidney suggests the renal defects in phosphate reabsorption and vitamin D metabolism are humorally mediated. Second, the demonstration of PHEX/Phex expression in bone is consistent with the notion of a primary bone abnormality in XLH. Third, studies in the murine *Hyp* and *Gy* homologues have substantiated these conclusions and have contributed significantly to our understanding of the pathogenesis of XLH. Accordingly, a discussion of the pathogenesis of the human disease will be considered below in the context of a discussion of the *Hyp* and *Gy* mouse models.

The Murine *Hyp* and *Gy* Models for XLH

Like patients with XLH, *Hyp*[166] and *Gy*[167] mice are characterized by hypophosphatemia, decreased growth rate, rickets and osteomalacia, and reduced net tubular reabsorption of phosphate. The traits in *Hyp* and *Gy* mice are inherited as X-linked dominant and map to a locus on the mouse X chromosome that is syntenic to the human XLH locus. Based on these findings, it was postulated that the X-linked mutations causing hypophosphatemia in mice and humans involve homologous genes. Indeed, following the positional cloning of the *PHEX* gene and demonstration that *PHEX* mutations are responsible for XLH (see "X-linked Hypophosphatemia," above), 5′ and 3′ deletions in the homologous gene were identified in *Gy*[149] and *Hyp*[148,149] mice, respectively. The 160- to 190-kb deletion in *Gy* mice also includes the upstream spermine synthase gene.[164,165] *Gy* is thus a contiguous gene syndrome and is not as useful a model for XLH as *Hyp*. While phenotypic evidence was presented for a *Gy* counterpart in a subset of XLH patients,[168] molecular genetic analysis is necessary to confirm these findings. It should be noted that the 3′ boundary of the *Hyp* deletion has not yet been identified.

The ensuing discussion comprises a description of the *Hyp* and *Gy* phenotypes and attempts to demonstrate how the loss of *Phex* gene function contributes to the pathophysiology of this disorder.

General Phenotype. Heterozygous *Hyp* females and hemizygous *Hyp* males can be distinguished from their normal littermates by their shortened hind limbs and tail and reduced body weight. These features persist throughout life and become more obvious with age. Kyphosis of the thoracic vertebrae, rachitic rosary, and prominent bowing of the femur develop with age in mutant mice, and bone ash is significantly reduced.[166,169]

The plasma concentration of inorganic phosphate is significantly reduced in both *Hyp* males and *Hyp* females when compared with that of normal littermates.[166] These differences are apparent by 20 to 49 days of age and persist up to and beyond 400 days of age. Urinary phosphate excretion, in relation to plasma phosphate, is significantly elevated in *Hyp* mice. Mutant mice appear to live a normal life span. *Hyp* females are fertile and raise their young, but not all *Hyp* males can sire offspring.

Gy mice exhibit all the above features as well as abnormalities of the inner ear, deafness, hyperactivity, and circling behavior.[167] These characteristics are likely attributable to the contiguous deletion in the spermine synthase gene upstream from *Phex*.[164,165] The latter results in an abnormality in the metabolism of polyamines, compounds that can affect neuronal receptors, ion channels, and neurotransmitter release and reuptake.[164,165] *Gy* males are sterile and are smaller than *Hyp* males.[170] *Gy* males also have a reduced viability, relative to heterozygous *Gy* females, on the B6C3H genetic background on which they are bred and, in contrast to heterozygous *Gy* females, do not survive on the C57BL/6J background on which *Hyp* mice are bred.[170] The more severe phenotype in *Gy* males has been related to the finding that spermine deficiency occurs as a recessive trait.[164,165] This is in contrast to the dominant expression of the *Phex* mutation.

Renal Phosphate Transport. The defect in phosphate reabsorption in *Hyp* mice was localized to the proximal tubule by micropuncture studies.[171,172] The defect persists after parathyroidectomy of *Hyp* mice[172,173] and involves the brush-border membrane in both *Hyp* and *Gy* mice.[167,174,175] The specificity of the transport defect for phosphate was established by the demonstration that the Na^+-dependent transport of glucose,[174,175] alanine,[167] proline,[176] and sulfate[177] is normal in renal brush-border membrane vesicles derived from mutant mice. Moreover, the phosphate transport defect in *Hyp* mice cannot be attributed to alterations in renal Na^+ transport,[178] brush-border membrane fluidity,[179] or lipid composition.[179]

Kinetic studies in isolated brush-border membrane vesicles demonstrate that while both low-affinity, high-capacity and high-affinity, low-capacity Na^+-phosphate cotransport systems are expressed in *Hyp* mice, only the high-affinity system is impaired by the *Hyp* and *Gy* mutations, with a 50 percent decrease in apparent V_{max} and no change in apparent K_m for phosphate.[180,181] These findings underscore the relative importance of the high-affinity phosphate transport system in the overall maintenance of phosphate homeostasis and suggest that a perturbation of this transport system is sufficient cause for the significant hypophosphatemia that characterizes *Hyp* and *Gy* mice.

Several approaches were undertaken to elucidate the mechanism for the decrease in high-affinity Na^+-phosphate cotransporter V_{max} in the mutant strains.[182–187] First, it was demonstrated that the affinity of the cotransporter for Na^+, the number of Na^+ ions interacting with the cotransport system, and the response of the cotransporter to membrane potential and pH are not different from normal in *Hyp* mice.[182] Second, it was demonstrated by radiation-inactivation analysis that the molecular size of protein(s) mediating Na^+-dependent phosphate transport is similar in brush-border membranes from normal and *Hyp* mice.[183] Third, studies performed with the *Npt2* cDNA probe and an antibody raised against a C-terminal Npt2 peptide demonstrated that the decrease in V_{max} in *Hyp* and *Gy* mice is associated with a corresponding decrease in renal abundance of Npt2 protein and mRNA,[184–186] which in *Hyp* mice is evident as early as 2 weeks of age[188] and is associated with a decrease in *Npt2* gene transcription.[187] Moreover, Na^+-phosphate cotransport, but not Na^+-sulfate cotransport, is significantly decreased in *Xenopus* oocytes injected with renal mRNA isolated from *Hyp* mice when compared with an equivalent amount of renal mRNA from normal mice.[184] In addition, hybrid depletion experiments documented that renal mRNA-dependent expression of Na^+-dependent phosphate transport in *Xenopus* oocytes is indeed related to Npt2.[184] Taken together, the findings clearly indicate that the number of high-affinity Na^+-phosphate cotransporters is significantly reduced in the renal brush-border membrane of *Hyp* and *Gy* mice and that the mechanism for the reduction involves either decreased *Npt2* gene transcription or increased Npt2 mRNA turnover.

Recent studies also have provided evidence for downregulation of renal Npt1 mRNA expression in *Hyp* mice.[74] However, in contrast to Npt2 mRNA, where a 50 percent loss is observed in *Hyp* mice, only a 20 percent loss of Npt1 mRNA abundance is evident.[74] GH, which stimulates renal phosphate conservation (see "Hormonal Regulation," above), does not increase the renal expression of Npt1 or Npt2 mRNA in *Hyp* mice, suggesting that the renal phosphate leak may not be corrected by GH.[74,105] These data are consistent with the findings that GH, in combination with standard therapy, does not improve TmP/GFR over the long term in XLH patients.[189,190]

Despite the reduction in renal *Npt2* gene expression in *Hyp* and *Gy* mice, both mutant strains are able to respond to a low-phosphate challenge with a striking suppression in renal fractional excretion of phosphate and a significant rise in Na^+-phosphate cotransport in renal brush-border membrane vesicles.[181,191,192] However, the difference in renal phosphate transport between the normal and mutant mouse strains persists under these conditions.[180,181,191,192] The adaptive increase in phosphate transport in *Hyp* and *Gy* mice is associated with an increase in V_{max} of high-affinity Na^+-phosphate cotransport and is accompanied by an increase in the abundance of Npt2 protein and mRNA.[185,193] The magnitude of the adaptive increase in Npt2 protein abundance exceeds that for Npt2 mRNA in both normals and mutants, consistent with the notion that regulation at the mRNA level may not be the only mechanism for the adaptive response (see "Regulation by Dietary Phosphate," above).

It is of interest that in vivo assessment of tubular adaptation to phosphate deprivation, by estimation of TmP/GFR, indicates that *Hyp* and *Gy* mice exhibit a blunted response to low-phosphate diet when compared with normal littermates.[194,195] These findings suggest that targets other than Npt2, e.g., the renal 1α-hydroxylase (see "Renal Vitamin D Metabolism," below), may contribute to the abnormal in vivo adaptive response in the mutant mouse strains.

As noted earlier, 5′ and 3′ deletions in the *Phex* gene have been identified in *Gy*[149] and *Hyp*[148,149] mice, respectively. Accordingly, downregulation of renal *Npt2* gene expression must be attributable to the loss of Phex function in the mutant strains. However, the mechanism whereby this occurs is not immediately apparent. Because Phex/PHEX has homology with endopeptidases that are involved in the processing or degradation of biologically active peptides,[196] it has been proposed that Phex/PHEX is involved in the inactivation of a phosphaturic hormone or the activation of a phosphate-conserving hormone.[144,148,197] Thus loss of Phex/PHEX function would be associated with either excess phosphaturic hormone or a deficiency in phosphate-conserving hormone. In either case, renal phosphate wasting would ensue. Since Phex/PHEX is not expressed in the kidney,[148] the Phex/PHEX substrate or product would reach its renal target via the circulation. Indeed, there is considerable evidence to suggest that the defect in renal phosphate transport in *Hyp* mice is mediated by a circulating factor, and the relevant studies are summarized below.

When normal mice are surgically joined to *Hyp* mice, and vascular channels form to permit cross-circulation between the two animals (parabiosis), the normal animals develop significant hypophosphatemia and decreased renal phosphate reabsorption.[198] Furthermore, when brush-border membranes are prepared from the kidneys of these "normal" parabiosed animals, a defect in Na^+-dependent phosphate transport, but not in Na^+-dependent glucose transport, is evident in these vesicles.[199] No such changes in renal phosphate handling are seen in parabiosed normal-normal animals.[199] The changes in renal phosphate handling in normal mice after parabiosis to *Hyp* mice are not dependent on PTH because similar findings are evident in parathyroidectomized normal-*Hyp* pairs.[199] Also, the changes in tubular phosphate handling are reversed on reestablishment of separate circulations in normal mice of normal-*Hyp* pairs.[198]

The simplest interpretation of the parabiosis experiment is that a transacting humoral factor derived from the *Hyp* mouse is perfusing the kidney of the normal animal in the normal-*Hyp* pairs. This factor induces changes in renal phosphate handling both in vivo and in brush-border vesicles studies in vitro, and these changes are the same as those seen in *Hyp* mice. With the current knowledge that the *Hyp* mutation results in loss of function of a putative endopeptidase, Phex, it is not immediately clear why the renal phosphate leak in *Hyp* mice of normal-*Hyp* pairs is not corrected by parabiosis. One possibility is that the wild-type Phex protein in the normal mouse did not have access to the humoral factor before it had a chance to inhibit phosphate transport in the kidney. This is consistent with the findings that Phex mRNA is expressed primarily in bone.[148,150,156,158]

Strong supporting evidence for a transacting humoral factor has come from cross-transplantation experiments between normal and *Hyp* mice. When a kidney from a *Hyp* mouse donor is transplanted into a normal mouse recipient, this kidney functions normally in terms of phosphate handling, and the recipient mouse does not develop hypophosphatemia.[200] In contrast, when a normal mouse is the donor animal and the *Hyp* mouse the recipient, the previously normal kidney does not transport phosphate normally, and the animal displays persistent hypophosphatemia.[200] These findings demonstrate that the defect in *Hyp* mice is neither corrected nor transferred by renal cross-transplantation and also implicate a humoral factor as the cause of the renal phosphate leak.

The data obtained from these renal transplant studies in mice are of particular interest in view of the report that transplantation of a kidney from a normal donor (an unaffected sister) into a 47-year-old man with XLH did not correct the abnormalities in phosphate homeostasis.[201] Hypophosphatemia and disordered renal phosphate handling persisted in the normal kidney after transplantation in the XLH recipient.

Direct evidence for humorally mediated inhibition of renal phosphate transport in *Hyp* mice was provided by the recent demonstration that serum from *Hyp* mice inhibited Na^+-phosphate cotransport in primary mouse renal cell cultures to a significantly greater extent than an equivalent amount of serum from normal littermates.[202] That inhibition by *Hyp* serum was dose-dependent was evident after 24 hours of incubation with target renal cells, and was specific to Na^+-phosphate cotransport.[202] Inhibition of Na^+-phosphate cotransport also was elicited by incubation of target renal cell cultures with conditioned medium from cultured *Hyp* osteoblasts, whereas no inhibition was apparent with conditioned medium from normal osteoblast cultures.[202] These data suggest that the *Hyp* osteoblast is responsible for the release and/or modification of a humoral factor that inhibits Na^+-phosphate cotransport in renal epithelial cells. The demonstration that Phex is expressed predominantly in bone[148,150,156,158] is consistent with these findings (see "Bone Phenotype," below).

The failure to demonstrate the expected gene dose effect in *Hyp* mice is also compatible with a humoral basis for this disorder. Serum phosphate values and renal brush-border membrane Na^+-dependent phosphate transport are similar and half of normal in both heterozygous (*Hyp*/+) and homozygous (*Hyp*/*Hyp*) mutant female mice.[203] Moreover, serum phosphate values and brush-border membrane phosphate transport are similar in mutant hemizygous males and mutant heterozygous females. Male and female patients with XLH also exhibit similar biochemical parameters.[113,117] If the gene dose effect were conventional, heterozygotes should have values intermediate to age-specific values for affected males and unaffected individuals.

Renal Vitamin D Metabolism. The regulation of renal vitamin D metabolism is abnormal in the X-linked *Hyp* and *Gy* mouse, as it is in XLH patients. The plasma concentration of $1,25(OH)_2D$ in both mutant strains is similar to that in normal littermates and thus is inappropriate for the degree of hypophosphatemia.[181,204,205] Moreover, *Hyp* and *Gy* mice respond to dietary phosphate depletion with a paradoxical fall in serum $1,25(OH)_2D$ levels, and *Hyp* mice respond to phosphate supplementation with a paradoxical increase in serum $1,25(OH)_2D$ levels.[181,205] In contrast, in normal mice, serum $1,25(OH)_2D$ levels are increased with phosphate deprivation and unchanged with phosphate supplementation.[205]

The fall in serum $1,25(OH)_2D$ levels in phosphate-deprived *Hyp* mice and the increase in serum $1,25(OH)_2D$ levels in phosphate-supplemented *Hyp* mice can be attributed to corresponding changes in the activity of 1α-hydroxylase, the renal enzyme involved in $1,25(OH)_2D$ synthesis.[206] Moreover, the phosphate-induced changes in serum $1,25(OH)_2D$ levels in both *Hyp* and *Gy* mice are inversely correlated with the rate of renal $1,25(OH)_2D$ catabolism, mediated by the C-24 oxidation pathway.[181,205] The latter is catalyzed by the 24-hydroxylase that converts $1,25(OH)_2D$ through a series of reactions, to its final inactivation product, calcitroic acid.[207,208] A comparison of the relationship between serum phosphate concentration, renal $1,25(OH)_2D$ catabolism, and serum $1,25(OH)_2D$ levels in normal and *Hyp* mice is shown in Fig. 197-6. The increase in renal $1,25(OH)_2D$ catabolism in phosphate-deprived *Hyp* mice is associated with an increase in 24-hydroxylase V_{max} and a corresponding increase in the renal abundance of 24-hydroxylase immunoreactive protein and mRNA.[209] Moreover, the latter occurs as a result of increased 24-hydroxylase gene transcription.[210] It is of interest that GH administration normalizes the 24-hydroxylase mRNA levels but not the serum $1,25(OH)_2D$ concentration in phosphate-deprived *Hyp* mice.[105] It would appear, therefore, that correction of renal 24-hydroxylase gene expression is not sufficient to normalize the serum concentration of $1,25(OH)_2D$ in phosphate-depleted mutants.[105] These findings reaffirm the role of 1α-hydroxylase in the maintenance of the serum $1,25(OH)_2D$ levels and suggest that, in *Hyp* mice, 1α-hydroxylase is likely resistant to regulation by GH. Indeed, defective regulation of renal 1α-hydroxylase in *Hyp* mice is well documented (see below), and GH is essential for the adaptive 1α-hydroxylase response to a low-phosphate diet.[211]

In addition to aberrant regulation by phosphate, the renal 1α-hydroxylase response to vitamin D deficiency[212,213] and calcium restriction[214] is significantly blunted in *Hyp* mice. Reduced synthesis of $1,25(OH)_2D$ in vitamin D-deficient *Hyp* mice is independent of serum calcium[212] and PTH levels[213] and is associated with a decrease in the apparent V_{max} for 1α-hydroxylase, with no change in apparent K_m.[213,215] *Hyp* mice also exhibit a significantly reduced renal 1α-hydroxylase response to infusion of PTH,[216] cAMP,[217] and PTH-related peptide.[218]

Unfortunately, studies of 1α-hydroxylase activity in *Gy* mice are controversial. Davidai et al. demonstrated that serum levels of $1,25(OH)_2D$ and renal production of $1,25(OH)_2D$ in *Gy* mice are appropriately increased by a low-phosphate diet.[219] These data are in sharp contrast to the demonstration that a low-phosphate diet elicits a fall in serum levels of $1,25(OH)_2D$ levels and an increase in renal $1,25(OH)_2D$ catabolism in *Gy* mice[181] (see above). The basis for these conflicting data is not clear, and it has been

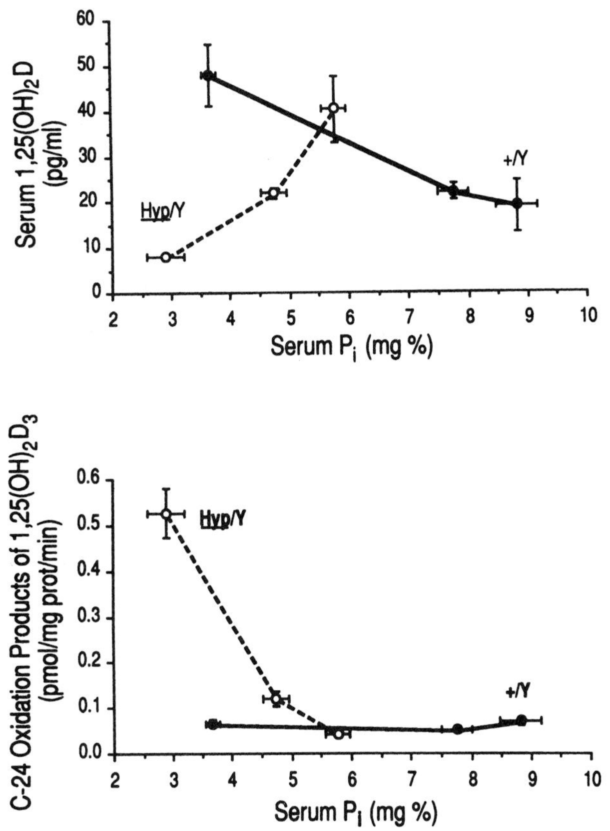

Fig. 197-6 Relationship between serum phosphate concentration and (*A*) the steady-state serum concentration of $1,25(OH)_2D$ and (*B*) the rate of formation of C-24 oxidation products from $1,25(OH)_2D$ by isolated renal mitochondria (●, normal +/Y male mice; ○, mutant *Hyp*/Y male mice). (*Used with permission from Tenenhouse and Jones.*[205])

suggested that differences in background strain and diets may account for the discrepancy.

In summary, the regulation of both renal $1,25(OH)_2D$ synthesis and degradation is impaired in *Hyp* and *Gy* mice. Moreover, both the vitamin D synthetic and catabolic pathways contribute to the inappropriate serum levels of $1,25(OH)_2D$ in the mutant strains. In light of the fact that *Phex* mutations are evident in *Hyp* and *Gy* mice, as well as in XLH patients, Phex/PHEX may play either a direct or indirect role in the regulation of renal vitamin D metabolism. One possibility is that compromised Phex function results in the deficiency (decreased activation) or excess (decreased degradation) of a circulating factor that can directly modulate renal vitamin D metabolism. Alternatively, Phex-mediated downregulation of renal *Npt2* gene expression in *Hyp* and *Gy* mice may be responsible for changes in the renal cell phosphate concentration, which in turn affects the metabolism of vitamin D in the mutant kidneys. Although reduced renal cortical ribonucleoside triphosphate pools in *Hyp* mice have been reported,[220] both chemical and ^{31}P NMR methods have failed to demonstrate genotype differences in the intracellular concentration of inorganic phosphate and phosphorylated compounds.[166,191,221] Moreover, the demonstration of normal phosphate uptake in isolated renal mitochondria derived from *Hyp* mice, under conditions where renal 25(OH)D metabolism is disturbed, suggests that mitochondrial phosphate transport does not contribute to the problems in the regulation of $1,25(OH)_2D$ synthesis and catabolism.[215]

PTH Status and Response to PTH. The persistence of the renal phosphate leak after parathyroidectomy of X-linked *Hyp* mice firmly established that the brush-border membrane phosphate transport defect is not secondary to hyperparathyroidism.[172,173] Indeed, the concurrence of idiopathic hypoparathyroidism in a patient with XLH supports this notion.[222] The PTH status of *Hyp* mice is, nevertheless, a controversial issue, and both normal[166,213] and elevated levels of PTH[223–226] have been reported. Moreover, elevated PTH levels in *Hyp* and *Gy* mice were demonstrated under a variety of dietary conditions.[225,226] While the underlying mechanism for hyperparathyroidism in the mutant strains is not known, it may be directly related to the loss of Phex function.[155a]

Although the relative contribution of hyperparathyroidism to the mutant renal phenotype is difficult to ascertain, there is no evidence for hypersensitivity to PTH.[227] Moreover, differences in brush-border membrane Na^+-phosphate cotransport in normal and *Hyp* mice persist after comparable diet-induced hyperparathyroidism.[228] Renal cAMP-dependent protein kinases[229] and the pattern of cAMP-dependent brush-border membrane protein phosphorylation and dephosphorylation are similar in normal and *Hyp* mice.[230] Finally, parathyroid glands from *Hyp* mice show a normal decrease in PTH mRNA in response to low-phosphate diet and thus adapt appropriately to phosphate restriction.[231]

Intestinal Phenotype. Intestinal phosphate absorption in adult *Hyp* mice is similar to that in normal littermates.[232,233] The absence of an intestinal phosphate transport defect in *Hyp/Gy* mice suggests that Phex is not involved in the regulation of phosphate transport across the intestinal brush-border membrane and is consistent with finding that Npt2 in not expressed in the intestine[57] and that hormonal regulation of intestinal phosphate transport is distinct from that in kidney.

In juvenile *Hyp* mice, however, there is a marked impairment in jejunal phosphate absorption[233] that is secondary to reduced plasma levels of $1,25(OH)_2D$ when compared with age-matched normals.[234] Juvenile *Hyp* mice also exhibit intestinal calcium malabsorption[235,236] that is accompanied by decreased levels of intestinal vitamin D-dependent 9-kDa calcium-binding protein (calbindin-D9k).[237] Since the intestinal phenotype can be corrected by $1,25(OH)_2D$ infusion,[238] it is likely that intestinal abnormalities in juvenile *Hyp* mice are secondary to abnormal renal metabolism of $1,25(OH)_2D$.[204,205,239–241]

Studies of intestinal phosphate uptake by jejunal biopsies derived from patients with XLH have demonstrated both deficient uptake[242] and normal uptake.[243] Genetic heterogeneity between patients and the ages of patients studied are possible explanations for the disparate findings.

Bone Phenotype. Skeletal abnormalities in *Hyp* mice appear to be more uniformly severe in the hemizygous males compared with the heterozygous females.[166,169] Although the basis for the sex difference was thought to be the result of random X-chromosome inactivation in females, recent studies suggest that gonadal hormones contribute to the sexual dimorphism.[244] Gonadectomy of hemizygous mutant males and heterozygous mutant females abolished the sex difference in bone mineral content.[244] Moreover, despite two mutant alleles, bone parameters in homozygous mutant females (*Hyp/Hyp*) are more similar to those in heterozygous mutant females than to those in hemizygous mutant males.[245,246] The absence of gene dosage in *Hyp* mice is also evident for serum phosphate concentration, renal brush-border membrane Na^+-phosphate cotransport, and 24-hydroxylase activity.[247,248]

Hyp mice exhibit craniosynostosis due to premature fusion of the coronal suture[249] and abnormal skull morphology arising mainly from deficient linear growth of the nasal bone.[250] Analytical and histomorphometric methods reveal a shorter than normal vertebral length associated with a wider epiphyseal growth plate in *Hyp* mice.[251] Moreover, impaired endosteal bone mineralization is present in the mutants, as demonstrated by excessive osteoid surface and thickness and decreased extent of the mineralization front.[251]

Several studies have suggested that abnormal bone formation in *Hyp* mice is determined not only by the hypophosphatemic environment, arising from the renal phosphate leak, but also by an intrinsic osteoblast defect in the mutant strain.[252–256] In these studies, bone cells derived from either normal mice or *Hyp* mice were compared histomorphometrically after transplantation into the gluteal muscle of normal or *Hyp* mouse recipients. Bone cells isolated from normal and *Hyp* mice produce abnormal bone when transplanted intramuscularly into mutant mice[253] or into phosphate-deprived normal mice,[255] suggesting that the low-phosphate environment contributes significantly to abnormal bone formation. When bone cells from *Hyp* mice are transplanted into normal mice,[253] into phosphate-supplemented *Hyp* mice,[255] or into 1,25$(OH)_2$D-treated *Hyp* mice,[256] parameters of bone formation are improved significantly, but not normalized. In contrast, bone formation is normal when bone cells from normal mice, with comparable diet-induced hypophosphatemia, are transplanted into normal mice.[254] These findings support the hypothesis that bone cells from *Hyp* mice express an intrinsic mineralization defect and that osteoblast dysfunction cannot be corrected completely by a normal extracellular environment.

Studies in osteoblast cultures derived from normal and *Hyp* mice demonstrate the persistence of biochemical and functional abnormalities in *Hyp* osteoblasts in vitro and thereby support the existence of an intrinsic osteoblast defect in the mutant strain. For example, primary osteoblast cultures derived from *Hyp* mice exhibit a substantial increase in glucose production from several substrates and a significant reduction in intracellular pH when compared with osteoblast cultures from normal mice.[257] Osteoblast cultures derived from mutant mice also exhibit a reduction in casein kinase II activity and a decrease in osteopontin phosphorylation.[258] In addition, the alkaline phosphatase and proliferative responses to 1,25$(OH)_2$D are inappropriately regulated by phosphate in osteoblast cultures derived from *Hyp* mice.[259] More recently, studies in immortalized osteoblasts derived from simian virus 40 transgenic normal mice and *Hyp* mice demonstrate that mineralization of extracellular matrix by *Hyp* osteoblast cultures is significantly impaired when compared with that by normal osteoblast cultures.[260]

Several other parameters measured in osteoblast cultures from *Hyp* mice are, however, not different from normal. These include Na^+-phosphate cotransport,[261,262] 1,25$(OH)_2$D receptor number and affinity,[263] phosphate-stimulated alkaline phosphatase activity and collagen synthesis,[263] synthesis of osteocalcin,[264] and regulation of osteocalcin gene expression by 1,25$(OH)_2$D.[264] The osteocalcin data are discordant with reports of aberrant in vivo regulation of osteocalcin in the *Hyp* mouse[265–267] and suggest that in vivo abnormalities of osteocalcin secretion and regulation may involve systemic factors that would not come into play in osteoblast cultures.

The effect of the *Hyp* mutation on other bone parameters also has been reported. The content of complex acidic phospholipids is significantly reduced in bones of *Hyp* mice relative to normal mice,[268] and marked differences in the mechanical performance of *Hyp* bone are evident.[269] *Hyp* bone undergoes significantly more angular deformation and has significantly lower structural stiffness and failure torque.[269] These differences in mechanical behavior are attributed to the material properties of the bone.[269] *Hyp* bone also has a lower bone ash content, a higher calcium-to-phosphorus ratio, and a reduction in carbonate content.[269]

Hyp mice exhibit dental abnormalities similar to those reported in patients with XLH.[270–273] The molars of *Hyp* males tend to have rather large pulp chambers and a wider predentine band than normal males, with mutant dentine showing prominent interglobular areas of deficient mineralization. Normalization of serum phosphate in *Hyp* mice by feeding a high-calcium, high-phosphate diet for 30 days did not affect the appearance of interglobular dentine in the mutant strain.[274] In addition to these dental abnormalities, exposure of the dental pulp occurs frequently in *Hyp* mice as a result of developmental deficiency of the dentine.

The precise mechanism for abnormal bones and teeth in *Hyp* and *Gy* mice is not immediately apparent, although both phosphate deficiency, secondary to renal phosphate wasting, and an intrinsic bone and tooth defect are postulated to play an important role. Phex mRNA expression was detected in human[148] and mouse[148,150,156,158] bone and in mouse teeth[158] and was localized to osteoblasts and odontoblasts by in situ hybridization of sagittal sections of embryos and newborn mice.[158] Moreover, using this approach, bones and teeth were the only tissues in which Phex mRNA was detected.[158] Phex expression was evident at day 15 of embryonic development, which coincides with the beginning of intercellular matrix deposition in bone, and declined after birth.[158] On the basis of these findings, it is possible that Phex is involved in the processing/degradation of growth factors or cytokines that regulate osteoblast and odontoblast function in a stage-specific manner. The recent demonstration that coculture of immortalized osteoblasts from normal and *Hyp* mice led to decreased extracellular matrix mineralization by the normal osteoblasts suggests that the *Hyp* osteoblasts produce a diffusible inhibitor of bone mineralization.[260] In light of these findings, the authors suggested that *Hyp* osteoblasts fail to degrade an endogenously synthesized, but as yet undefined, inhibitor of bone mineralization that is a substrate for Phex.[260] However, it is also possible that an activator of bone mineralization, which is processed in normal but not *Hyp* osteoblasts, can correct the defect in *Hyp* osteoblasts. Whether the factor that affects bone mineralization is the same factor that is responsible for renal phosphate wasting or an entirely different factor is not known. Clearly, further work is required to elucidate the mechanisms for the mineralization and phosphate-wasting defects in the *Hyp* mouse and to identify the Phex substrate(s)/products(s) involved. In addition, Phex is also a determinant of phosphate availability for bone mineralization by virtue of its role in processing factors that influence renal phosphate handling.

Other Phenotypic Characteristics. Although the phosphate concentration of breast milk was reported to be low in two mothers with XLH,[275,276] the phosphate content of milk from lactating normal and *Hyp/+* females is not significantly different.[277] The data in mice suggest that mutant females can accumulate a normal amount of phosphate in milk, despite significant hypophosphatemia, and provide evidence for the absence of a phosphate-transport defect in mammary glands.[277] Although the phosphate concentration is lower than normal in saliva from *Hyp* mice, salivary phosphate levels in *Hyp* mice are similar to those of normal mice with a comparable degree of diet-induced hypophosphatemia, suggesting that the phosphate-transport defect, which is expressed in the renal brush-border membrane, is not expressed in the salivary gland.[278] In addition, Na^+-phosphate cotransport is not depressed in cultured skin fibroblasts derived from patients with XLH when compared with age-matched controls.[279]

Working Model of How Loss of PHEX/Phex Function Leads to Disease. Although the *PHEX/Phex* mutations responsible for XLH, *Hyp*, and *Gy* have been identified, it is not immediately obvious how loss of PHEX/Phex function elicits the clinical phenotype. We propose that the *PHEX/Phex* gene product in bone is involved either in the activation or degradation of a factor(s) that is (are) essential for osteoblast differentiation and/or mineralization and that loss of PHEX/Phex activity results in abnormal osteoblast function. This hypothesis is consistent with the demonstration, by several groups, of an intrinsic osteoblast defect in *Hyp* mice (see "Bone Phenotype," above). In addition, we hypothesize that the *PHEX/Phex* gene product in bone, or at other sites, is capable of activating or inactivating a humoral factor that has an effect on renal phosphate reabsorption, by modulating *Npt2*, and perhaps *Npt1*, gene expression in the kidney. In this case, loss of PHEX/Phex function would result in impaired activation of a phosphate-conserving hormone or the accumulation of a phosphaturic hormone. This hypothesis is consistent with several reports demonstrating that the renal defect in brush-border membrane Na^+-phosphate cotransport in *Hyp* mice is not intrinsic to the kidney but rather is humorally mediated (see "Renal Phosphate

Transport," above). In this regard, the abnormality in the regulation of the renal $1,25(OH)_2D$ biosynthetic and degradative pathways also may occur as a direct consequence of the same humoral factor that modulates phosphate transport (see "Renal Vitamin D Metabolism," above). The precise relationship between the humoral factor in XLH, *Hyp*, and *Gy* and "phosphatonin," the phosphaturic humoral factor implicated in the pathogenesis of OHO (see "Oncogenic Hypophosphatemic Osteomalacia," below), requires further study.

Use of the *Hyp* Mouse Model to Assess Approaches to Therapy. The *Hyp* mouse has proved to be an invaluable model to assess various therapeutic protocols for the treatment of bone abnormalities in patients with XLH. It was demonstrated that dietary phosphate supplementation of *Hyp* mice from weaning prevented the appearance of severe skeletal abnormalities.[166] Indeed, histomorphometric analysis of bone from phosphate-supplemented *Hyp* mice showed complete correction of endochondral calcification but not of endosteal bone mineralization.[251] Secondary hyperparathyroidism arising from phosphate therapy appeared to stimulate osteoblastic and osteoclastic recruitment and activity and thereby increase endosteal bone turnover.[251] A similar development of secondary hyperparathyroidism occurs in children treated with phosphate alone. However, in contrast to the *Hyp* mouse, phosphate treatment of children with XLH improves endochondral mineralization but does not lead to its normalization.[280] Whether the differences between mouse and human are due to a more uniform and sustained increase in plasma phosphate concentration in the mouse remains to be determined.[251]

Because phosphate supplementation raises plasma $1,25(OH)_2D$ levels in *Hyp* mice, by stimulating renal hormone synthesis[206,281] and inhibiting renal hormone catabolism,[205] it was suggested that the effects of phosphate supplementation on endochondral calcification are attributable in part to the phosphate-induced rise in the plasma $1,25(OH)_2D$ concentration. In this regard, weanling mutant males were infused subcutaneously with the vitamin D hormone for 28 days.[282] This regimen led to the normalization of plasma calcium and phosphorus levels and complete healing of bone mineralization.[282] Subsequent studies examining the effects of phosphate supplementation in combination with either 25(OH)D, 24,25-dihydroxyvitamin D_3 [$24,25(OH)_2D$], or $1,25(OH)_2D$ revealed that neither 25(OH)D nor $24,25(OH)_2D$ could substitute for $1,25(OH)_2D$ in normalizing endosteal bone mineralization in the *Hyp* mouse.[283]

Two recent studies compared the effects of $1,25(OH)_2D$ with high doses of $24,25(OH)_2D$ on bone parameters in *Hyp* mice.[284,285] Both vitamin D metabolites elicited a comparable improvement, but not a normalization, of indices of bone formation. However, there were significant differences in their effects on bone resorption. While both vitamin D metabolites increased indices of bone resorption, $1,25(OH)_2D$, but not $24,25(OH)_2D$, promoted excessive bone resorption; i.e., the values achieved were above those seen in normal mice.[285] These findings suggest that $24,25(OH)_2D$ may be more effective than $1,25(OH)_2D$ in correcting the bone defect in *Hyp* mice and that it may have a unique action on bone. Clearly, additional studies are necessary to establish whether this is indeed the case.[286]

Improved phosphate homeostasis in *Hyp* mice, achieved by the administration of $1,25(OH)_2D$, can be attributed to increased intestinal absorption.[287] Everted gut sacs prepared from all segments of the small intestine of $1,25(OH)_2D$-treated *Hyp* mice exhibited significantly higher phosphate transport activity than sacs from untreated mutants. $1,25(OH)_2D$, however, did not correct the defect in renal brush-border membrane phosphate transport.[287] In contrast, data from studies in XLH patients suggested that $1,25(OH)_2D$ may increase renal phosphate retention.[288,289] Thus it is possible that there is not always a one-to-one correspondence between phosphate handling by the intact kidney and phosphate uptake in isolated renal brush-border membrane vesicles. Furthermore, there is an important difference between phosphate homeostasis in mice and humans: The plasma phosphate concentration is normally maintained at a higher value in mice than in humans. The basis for this difference is not known. Nor is it clear how this difference may affect the expression of a similar genetic defect in the two species.

Treatment of XLH

In light of the fact that the function of the *PHEX* gene is not understood, it is not surprising that a specific therapy directed at the underlying pathophysiology of the disorder has not yet been developed. Thus the current "standard" therapy continues to be a combination of phosphate and $1,25(OH)_2D$ (calcitriol) or 1α-hydroxyvitamin D_3.[280,290,291] Therapy is initiated during childhood and is labor-intensive for the physician, the patient, and the patient's caregiver. In general, therapy is continued at least until growth is completed. The decision as to whether to continue therapy in adulthood must be individualized (see below). To minimize the number of patients who initiate therapy and then discontinue it after a few months, it is necessary to spend a substantial time counseling patients and caregivers about the need for frequent monitoring, the difficulty in taking medications four times per day for many years, and the potential side effects of therapy.

The objectives of therapy in children are to correct or prevent deformity from rickets, enhance growth rate, and lessen bone pain. In some cases, marked improvement in lower extremity deformity is noted with medical therapy. Thus it is advisable to give a course of medical treatment before performing osteotomies to correct deformities. Most affected children probably should be treated if a system exists to administer and monitor therapy. However, in some instances, it may be acceptable not to treat but rather to follow mildly affected children carefully.

In adults, indications for treatment are somewhat more controversial. There are no data to suggest that current treatment regimens slow the rate of calcification of tendons and ligaments (enthesopathy). Indeed, treatment with high-dose $1,25(OH)_2D$ and phosphate conceivably could worsen enthesopathy by improving the environment for mineralization. Pseudofractures are common in moderately to severely affected adult XLH patients. Since pseudofractures are often painful, may lead to fracture, and generally respond well to treatment, we frequently recommend medical therapy for patients with pseudofractures. XLH patients frequently complain of bone pain,[112] presumably due to osteomalacia. Treatment lessens osteomalacia and bone pain, and it is therefore reasonable to treat patients with this complaint. Additionally, it is advisable to treat patients who have nonunion after fractures or osteotomies because treatment may improve fracture healing. In light of the complexity of therapy, possible side effects (see below), and lack of increased risk of fracture in patients without pseudofractures, therapy is not recommended in asymptomatic patients who do not have pseudofractures.

As noted earlier, "standard" therapy continues to be a combination of phosphate and $1,25(OH)_2D$ or 1α-hydroxyvitamin D_3. It is best to start at a low dose of calcitriol and phosphate (to avoid diarrhea from phosphate) and gradually increase therapy over several months. We maintain a "high dose" phase for up to 1 year. During this phase of therapy, the calcitriol dose may be as high as 50 ng/kg per day in two divided doses, but not more than 3.0 μg/day. Also, 1 to 2 g of phosphate is administered in four divided doses. Of note, many patients do not require such a high dose of calcitriol, and we routinely monitor serum calcium, phosphorus, and creatinine levels, as well as urine calcium and creatinine concentrations, on a monthly basis during the high-dose phase. The doses of calcitriol and phosphate are adjusted based on the laboratory results. Hypercalciuria may be the first sign of healing of osteomalacia (theoretically, osteomalacic bone is capable of taking up more calcium and phosphate than bone that is histologically normal). Although some clinicians recommend administering phosphate over five doses per day initially, we do not ask patients to wake up to take medication at night for the following reasons: (1) serum phosphate concentrations tend to rise at night in XLH patients,[292] (2) there is an exaggerated nocturnal rise in PTH concentrations in XLH patients, and (3) it is unrealistic to ask patients to wake up to take medication every night for a chronic condition.

The above treatment plan is more aggressive than recommended by other experienced clinicians[293] who do not use a "high dose" phase. However, using a high-dose phase may lead to normalization of bone histology.[289] After approximately 1 year on high-dose therapy, patients are switched to a long-term "maintenance" phase with approximately 10 to 20 ng/kg per day of calcitriol and no change in the dose of phosphate. While patients are on maintenance therapy, we continue to see them and monitor serum and urine biochemistries at least every 3 to 4 months.

Careful follow-up is required when employing combined therapy because the two agents balance each other's effects. Administration of phosphate alone will lead to secondary hyperparathyroidism, and administration of $1,25(OH)_2D$ alone commonly leads to hypercalciuria and hypercalcemia. Hence a patient on combined therapy can develop hypercalciuria as a consequence of either too much $1,25(OH)_2D$ or too little phosphate. Because of this balance, anytime it becomes necessary to interrupt phosphate administration, it is necessary to discontinue $1,25(OH)_2D$ therapy as well.

Diarrhea and gastrointestinal upset frequently develop from phosphate administration. To minimize diarrhea, the phosphate dose must be increased gradually. If diarrhea develops, decrease (or stop) the dose of phosphate (and calcitriol; see above) and slowly increase therapy as tolerated. Since hypercalcemia may develop from calcitriol therapy, patients should be given instructions on the symptoms of hypercalcemia, such as depression, confusion, anorexia, nausea, vomiting, polyuria, and dehydration. Serum biochemistries should be measured if a patient experiences any symptoms of hypercalcemia. It should not be assumed that patients on high-dose calcitriol who develop nausea, vomiting, and lethargy have food poisoning or another benign etiology of their symptoms. Depending on the type of coverage system available to the physician, patients may need to be instructed to insist on having these measurements made when speaking with health care providers/gatekeepers who have no experience with this disease.

The most common and potentially serious complication of therapy is the development of nephrocalcinosis.[116,294–298] With the widespread use of renal ultrasound, nephrocalcinosis has been noted with increasing frequency. In most cases, the nephrocalcinosis is observed without evident changes in glomerular filtration rate (GFR). Its occurrence may be related to phosphate dosage, and some authors assert that phosphate administration leads to hyperabsorption of oxalate, which results in nephrocalcinosis.[299] However, this assertion remains unproven, and patients who received vitamin D_2, but no phosphate, can develop nephrocalcinosis.[300] Thus hypercalciuria and hypercalcemia may contribute to (or at least aggravate) this problem. Kidney biopsy specimens from three treated patients with nephrocalcinosis showed that renal calcifications are located mainly intratubularly and are composed exclusively of calcium phosphate.[301] Of note, a recent report of two patients with nephrocalcinosis for two decades indicates that it was not associated with impaired renal function.[300] Although these data are somewhat reassuring, the available data are not strong enough to completely allay concerns about renal complications of even carefully monitored therapy.

A second, much rarer complication is the development of tertiary hyperparathyroidism.[15,16,155a,302] Presumably, tertiary hyperparathyroidism results from chronic stimulation of the parathyroid glands by phosphate therapy. Although this complication is more likely in patients who are getting too much phosphate, it also can occur in optimally treated individuals. In tertiary hyperparathyroidism, GFR may decline, necessitating a reduction in the dose of phosphate and calcitriol or cessation of therapy. This will lead to the redevelopment or worsening of the bone disease. A small number of such patients have undergone total parathyroidectomy with autotransplant to the forearm. In a number of these patients, the transplanted tissue has shown a propensity to proliferate and lead to the redevelopment of tertiary hyperparathyroidism. Removal of this hyperplastic tissue from the forearm site leads to a reduction in serum PTH levels. Theoretically, total parathyroidectomy followed by treatment with $1,25(OH)_2D$ and phosphate is a potential option. However, there is insufficient experience with this approach, and it is not recommended because it results in lifelong hypoparathyroidism.

Although treatment complications cannot be prevented entirely, careful monitoring may minimize treatment-related problems. Serum calcium, phosphorus, and creatinine levels and urine calcium and creatinine concentrations should be monitored monthly while patients are on high-dose therapy and every 3 to 4 months while on maintenance therapy. A 24-hour urine phosphorus measurement is often useful to gauge compliance with therapy. Serum PTH concentration should be measured at yearly intervals, as appropriate. We periodically monitor urine oxalate but have not seen patients with elevated urinary oxalate on therapy. A renal ultrasound should be obtained as a baseline at the start of therapy and periodically thereafter.

In light of the difficulty with combined therapy and the complications attributable at least in part to therapy, additional therapeutic options are being explored. These include the use of human GH,[303] $24,25(OH)_2D$,[304] and diuretics.[305] None of these are alternatives to combined therapy, but each has been employed as adjuvant therapy.

The rationale for using GH is based on its ability to increase renal phosphate retention and the fact that short stature is a frequent consequence of XLH. Not all children treated with conventional therapy improve their growth rate. Unfortunately, the available data suggest that children who present with heights over the 15th percentile tend to increase their growth rate in response to therapy, whereas children who present under the 5th percentile (those who need to grow the most) do not increase their growth rate.[306] GH therapy significantly increases growth velocity[189,190,307] and appears to have a positive influence on final height. GH therapy is well tolerated and should be considered in XLH patients with short stature who do not have an adequate growth response on conventional therapy. However, the addition of GH adds substantial expense to an already expensive regimen.

Recent studies by Carpenter et al.[304] examined the effect of adding 5 μg of $24,25(OH)_2D$, two times per day, to standard therapy in 15 patients (4–59 years old). Treatment with $24,25(OH)_2D$ significantly decreased PTH concentrations in these patients and normalized PTH levels in 9 patients. Of note, this treatment abolished the nocturnal surge in PTH.[304] Data from this study indicate that normalization of PTH concentrations was associated with skeletal improvement. Overall, the therapy was well tolerated without significant side effects. Since only one dose of $24,25(OH)_2D$ was studied, the optimal dose remains to be determined. However, $24,25(OH)_2D$ appears to be a useful adjunct to standard therapy,[304] and further studies of this agent are warranted.

Thiazide diuretics and amiloride have been proposed as useful adjuvants to therapy. The rationale for using these agents is that by reducing ECF volume, tubular reabsorption of phosphate is increased, and by giving the thiazide, one enhances tubular calcium reabsorption.[305] Preliminary data indicate that growth rate increases and the radiologic appearance of the epiphyses improves. However, long-term consequences of this very complicated therapeutic program are not yet known, and one must be cautious when administering a therapy that can result in dehydration to a patient who is at risk for hypercalcemia.

A continued search for better therapeutic agents is needed because it is increasingly clear that the present-day combined therapy is not curative and is accompanied by a high complication rate. However, if therapy with combined phosphate and $1,25(OH)_2D$ is monitored carefully, growth rates increase, rickets is corrected, and bowing of the low extremities is significantly reduced.[135,136,280,289,291,298,308]

ONCOGENIC HYPOPHOSPHATEMIC OSTEOMALACIA

OHO is a rare, acquired form of hypophosphatemia that is of importance both because it may be confused with XLH and ADHR and because the changes in proximal tubular function seen in XLH, ADHR and OHO are similar.[16,309–315]

Clinical Features

The disease is characterized by an insidious onset of fatigue and bone pain. Children manifest lower extremity deformities (secondary to rickets) and growth retardation. Adults present with bone pain, pseudofractures, and fractures. In contrast to XLH, proximal muscle weakness is a prominent feature in both children and adults. Unfortunately, delayed diagnosis of OHO is fairly common, and the patient may become bedridden with severe weakness, bone pain, and numerous fractures.[316] Age of onset is usually in adult life but has been reported in patients ranging in age from 5 to 70 years.

OHO patients have the same laboratory findings that are seen in XLH and ADHR: a reduced TmP/GFR, hypophosphatemia, and an inappropriately normal or low plasma $1,25(OH)_2D$ level. The reductions in serum phosphate and $1,25(OH)_2D$ concentrations are usually more severe than those seen in the typical XLH patient. The presence of muscle weakness in OHO may be secondary to the more profound hypophosphatemia or may be related to the fact that these patients have an acquired disease. The serum calcium and 25(OH)D concentrations are normal or low normal with a normal or mildly elevated PTH. Aminoaciduria and glycosuria are occasionally present.[316] Radiologic examination reveals decreased mineral density, occasional rib fractures or pseudofractures at other sites, and in children, rickets. Osteomalacia is present on bone biopsy.

Distinguishing between XLH and OHO is relatively easy because in most cases OHO first appears later in life and leads to progressive disease. Usually the opposite is the case in XLH. It is rare for a patient with XLH who has minimal disease during childhood and adolescence to then display signs of severe disease in adult life. Even when OHO appears in children, its differentiation from sporadic XLH is usually possible based on the facts that (1) XLH is more common than OHO, (2) the signs of XLH usually appear within the first 2 to 3 years of life, and (3) weakness is not a predominant feature in XLH. Unfortunately, it may not always be possible to differentiate OHO from ADHR because in some cases of ADHR there is no family history of phosphate wasting (sporadic cases) and ADHR may present in adulthood.

Pathogenesis

The most intriguing feature of OHO is its association with small mesenchymal tumors. These have been described as hemangiopericytoma, odontogenic tumor of the maxilla, fibroma, angiosarcoma, oat cell carcinoma, myoma, angiofibroma, sclerosing hemangioma, ossifying mesenchymal tumor, or osteoblastoma. Despite this variety of designations, the majority of tumors have been reported to have prominent vascularity and often appear as osteoclast-like multinucleated giant cells. Additionally, patients with the linear sebaceous nevus syndrome have been found to have as a component of their disease a variant of this syndrome. The tumors have been found in the skin, subcutaneous tissue, the nasopharynx, the bone, the paranasal sinuses, and the palm of the hand and sole of the foot.

The tumor is usually small and may be extremely difficult to locate despite the use of numerous imaging procedures. Nevertheless, if the tumor is found and removed, the manifestations of the disease disappear completely. There is a restoration of normal renal function, the TmP/GFR becomes normal, plasma $1,25(OH)_2D$ rises to supranormal values within a few days of surgical removal of the tumor and then falls slowly to normal values, and with time, the osteomalacia heals completely. The working hypothesis is that the tumor produces a humoral factor(s) that acts specifically on the proximal renal tubule to bring about the same, or nearly the same, abnormalities in tubular phosphate transport and $1,25(OH)_2D$ synthesis as seen in XLH and ADHR. The hypothesis is supported by the observation that transplantation of such a human tumor into a nude mouse leads to the development of hypophosphatemia in the mouse.[163,317] The humoral factor also could have a direct effect on bone. However, there is currently insufficient data to address this issue.

We have tentatively referred to the OHO tumor-derived phosphaturic factor(s) as *phosphatonin*.[318] Several investigators have attempted to characterize the factor(s) from tumors excised from OHO patients.[319–321] Although it inhibits Na^+-P_i cotransport in cultured renal cells, it has not been possible to obtain sufficient amounts of the factor from OHO tumors because the tumors lose their phenotype in culture.[321] The available evidence suggests that it is a protein because it is heat-labile[319,321] and trypsin-sensitive.[321] However, estimates of the factor's molecular weight vary considerably, and no one has yet identified the protein(s). Additionally, although phosphatonin leads to renal phosphate wasting, there are no data confirming that it has a role in normal phosphate homeostasis. Indeed, phosphatonin could be analogous to parathyroid hormone-related peptide (PTHrP) in humoral hypercalcemia of malignancy.

Treatment

The obvious therapy for patients with OHO is the surgical removal of the tumor that is the source of the presumed humoral factor. The difficulty is often that of finding the tumor. A recent report of two patients[322] suggests that octreotide scanning may be of use in finding these tumors. However, additional data are needed to assess the sensitivity and general applicability of this technique. If no tumor can be found, then the alternative is treatment with combined phosphate and $1,25(OH)_2D$, as outlined in the section on XLH. These agents may ameliorate some of the signs and symptoms of the disease and may heal the osteomalacia, but they do not cure the disease and must be continued until the tumor is removed.

AUTOSOMAL DOMINANT FORMS OF RENAL PHOSPHATE WASTING

In addition to XLH, two autosomal dominant forms of isolated renal phosphate wasting have been described: ADHR and hypophosphatemic bone disease (HBD). Although both these disorders are less common than XLH and have not been investigated to the same extent, ongoing genetic studies will lead to the identification of the primary defect and improve our understanding of the pathogenesis of these disorders.

Autosomal Dominant Hypophosphatemic Rickets

Clinical Features. Several investigators[146,315,323–326] have described kindreds with isolated renal phosphate wasting and male-to-male transmission, consistent with an autosomal dominant mode of inheritance. A small family with autosomal dominant renal phosphate wasting was described by Bianchine et al.[315,325] The father, who was markedly affected, had isolated renal phosphate wasting, short stature, and an impressive windswept deformity (valgus on one side and varus on the other). He had two affected daughters and one affected son. These investigators reported that the father had a marked tendency toward fracture with or without trauma. Otherwise, the clinical course in these individuals appeared to be similar to that in XLH patients (including hypophosphatemia, bone pain, rickets, and lower extremity deformity).

Econs and McEnery[146] recently described a large ADHR kindred with over 20 affected individuals. This kindred provided an opportunity to explore the phenotypic variability of this disease

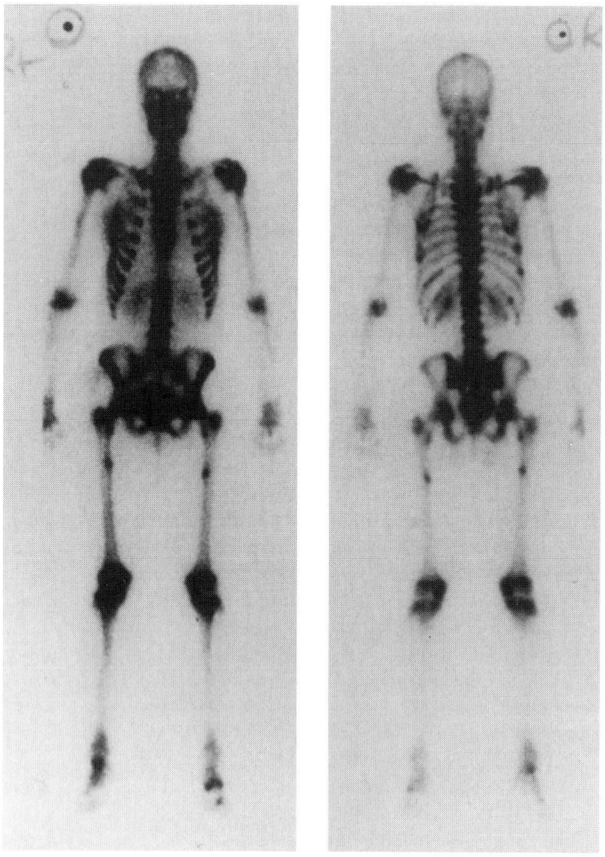

Fig. 197-7 Bone scan from a woman who presented with delayed onset of ADHR that demonstrates increased tracer uptake in several areas, including the ribs, medial aspects of both proximal femurs, and metatarsals. Plain films documented pseudofractures in the medial aspects of the femurs and insufficiency fractures in the metatarsals. Note the absence of lower extremity deformity, consistent with postpubertal onset of disease. (*Used with permission from Econs and McEnery.*[146])

in a large number of individuals who, presumably, all have the same mutation. Affected members of the kindred have isolated renal phosphate wasting, hypophosphatemia, and inappropriately normal serum 1,25$(OH)_2$D concentrations. In contrast to patients with XLH and HHRH, patients with ADHR display variable penetrance. The family contains two subgroups of affected individuals. One subgroup consists of patients who presented with phosphate wasting as adults or adolescents. These individuals complained of bone pain, weakness, and insufficiency fractures but did not have lower extremity deformities (Fig. 197-7). The second group consists of individuals who presented during childhood with phosphate wasting, rickets, and lower extremity deformity in a pattern similar to the classic presentation of XLH. Surprisingly, two of the children in this group lost the phosphate-wasting defect after puberty.[146] In addition to these two groups, there appear to be at least two unaffected individuals who are carriers for the ADHR mutation.[146] Thus the clinical manifestations of ADHR are even more variable than those observed in XLH.

Laboratory Features

Biochemical studies demonstrate that ADHR patients have hypophosphatemia and reduced TmP/GFR, with normal serum concentrations of calcium, bicarbonate, creatinine, and PTH.[146,315,324] Affected individuals do not have glycosuria or aminoaciduria. Of note, affected individuals have inappropriately normal serum calcitriol concentrations and do not have hypercalciuria.[146,324] Thus the data indicate that ADHR is similar to XLH and different from HHRH because the 1,25$(OH)_2$D concentration does not increase in response to hypophosphatemia (see "Hereditary Hypophosphatemic Rickets with Hypercalciuria," below). Whether the defective adaptive response is due to decreased renal production or increased degradation of 1,25$(OH)_2$D is currently unknown. Unfortunately, unlike XLH, there is no animal model of ADHR to gain insight into the mechanism for aberrant vitamin D metabolism in this disorder.

Prevalence and Diagnosis

Although the exact prevalence of ADHR is unknown, it is less common than XLH. However, ADHR is probably not as rare as previously thought. Incomplete penetrance and variable age of onset may hinder a clinician's ability to establish the familial nature of the disease, particularly in patients with a parent who is a silent carrier. Additionally, adult onset of phosphate wasting or sporadic cases of phosphate wasting in children arising from new mutations may be inappropriately labeled as OHO. In this regard, *PHEX* mutations are found in the majority of affected individuals with a family history of XLH but in many fewer sporadic cases.[159–162] While some of these patients may have *PHEX* mutations that are difficult to detect (e.g., upstream elements, the polyadenylation site, etc.), it is likely that many of these patients may not have XLH but have ADHR. Erroneous assumptions about X-linked dominant inheritance may lead to incorrect genetic counseling. Additionally, paternity is often questioned when a male ADHR patient has a daughter that is not affected and the family has been told that family members have XLH.

Positional Cloning Studies

Linkage studies in the large ADHR kindred described earlier indicate that the ADHR locus in this family is on chromosome 12p13.[327] Multilocus analysis places the ADHR gene in the 18-cM interval between the D12S100 and D12S397. Studies in ADHR and HBD (see below) kindreds are in progress to determine if there is genetic heterogeneity for the ADHR phenotype and if ADHR and HBD result from mutations in the same gene. More important, these studies will further localize the gene(s) that are responsible for ADHR and HBD and eventually lead to their identification.

Hypophosphatemic Bone Disease

HBD was described originally by Scriver et al.,[328] who studied five small families in which affected members had isolated renal phosphate wasting, hypophosphatemia, short stature, and lower extremity deformity. In one of the five families there was evidence of male-to-male transmission, indicating an autosomal dominant pattern of inheritance in this family. Children with HBD generally did not display radiographic evidence of rickets. However, in other respects, patients with HBD appeared to be similar to those with other renal phosphate-wasting disorders. Since radiographic evidence of rickets is not always present in XLH,[129] it is possible that radiographic evidence of rickets may not be universal in children with ADHR. Thus HBD may not be distinct from ADHR. However, definitive evidence as to whether ADHR and HBD are distinct clinical entities or forme fruste of one another awaits identification of the gene(s) that cause these disorders. Nevertheless, even if these diseases result from mutations in the same gene, it will be important to characterize the mutations that cause ADHR and HBD because different mutations in the same gene can give rise to different phenotypes. One example of this phenomenon is the dsytrophin gene, in which missense mutations give rise to Beckers muscular dsytrophy and nonsense mutations result in Duchenne muscular dsytrophy[329] (see Chap. 217).

HEREDITARY HYPOPHOSPHATEMIC RICKETS WITH HYPERCALCIURIA

HHRH was first reported in members of a Bedouin tribe in which intermarriage has been widely practiced for many generations[330,331] (Fig. 197-8). HHRH is far less prevalent than XLH, and only a few other sporadic cases have been described in the

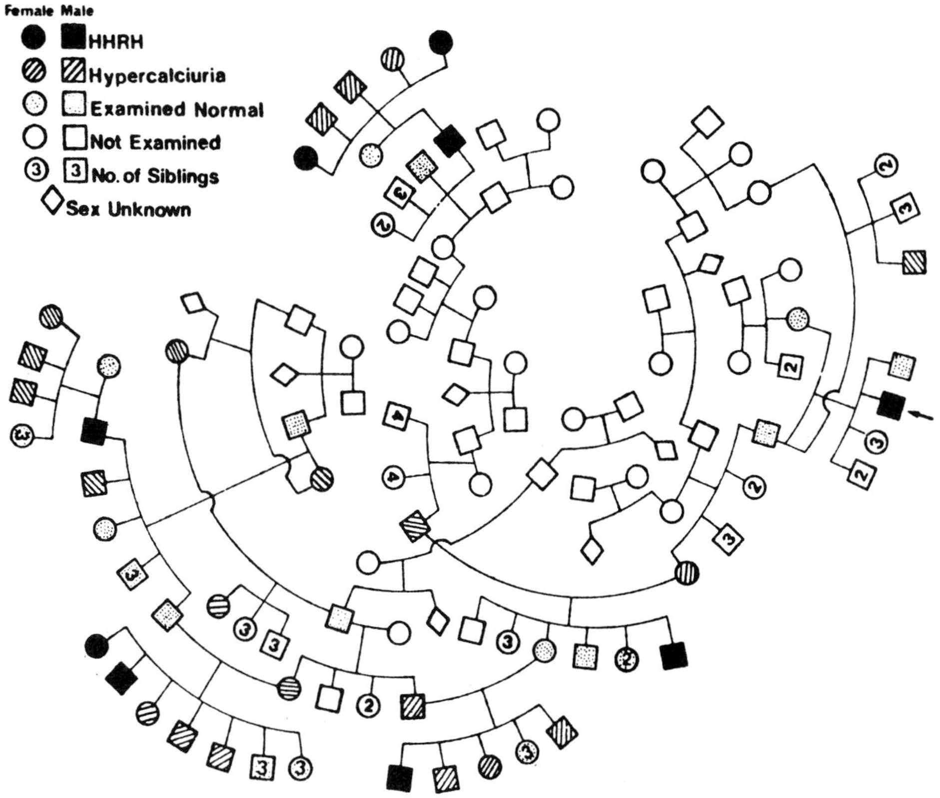

Fig. 197-8 Genetic relationship of 9 patients with hereditary hypophosphatemic rickets and hypercalciuria and 21 subjects with IH alone. Arrow indicates index case. (*Used with permission from Tieder et al.*[331])

literature.[332–335] It has been suggested that the low prevalence of HHRH may be due, in part, to its underdiagnosis, since it shares many of the clinical and biochemical features of other renal phosphate-wasting disorders and of idiopathic hypercalciuria with bone lesions and stunted growth.[335] The cardinal features that distinguish HHRH from other Mendelian hypophosphatemias are increased plasma levels of $1,25(OH)_2D$ with attendant hypercalciuria, and measurement of both parameters is essential for a correct diagnosis and appropriate treatment.

Clinical Features

Presumed Homozygotes. The major clinical features of HHRH are bone pain, skeletal deformities, short stature, and muscle weakness, with X-ray signs of rickets and osteomalacia occurring during infancy and childhood[330] (see Fig. 197-8). The biochemical findings include reduced serum phosphate concentration, reduced TmP/GFR, normal serum calcium concentration, elevated serum alkaline phosphatase activity, low or low-normal serum PTH and urinary cAMP concentrations, normal serum concentrations of 25(OH)D and $24,25(OH)_2D$, and an elevated serum concentration of $1,25(OH)_2D$ that is associated with a marked increase in urinary calcium excretion.

Oral calcium or phosphate loading of HHRH patients demonstrates that there is hyperabsorption of both calcium and phosphate from the intestine. These findings indicate that the intestinal mucosa in HHRH patients is responding normally to the elevated serum levels of $1,25(OH)_2D$. The intravenous injection of parathyroid extract is found to reduce TmP/GFR even further and to increase urinary cAMP excretion.[330]

Presumed Heterozygotes. In an extensive study of 59 closely related members of the Bedouin tribe, 9 individuals were identified with the characteristics described earlier[331] (see Fig. 197-8). However, an additional 21 members were found to be clinically healthy but to display idiopathic hypercalciuria (IH) with slightly reduced plasma phosphate concentrations, elevated plasma $1,25(OH)_2D$ concentrations, and elevated urinary calcium excretion (see Fig. 197-8). The values seen in the subjects with IH are intermediate between normal members of the same tribe and members with HHRH: Urinary calcium concentration was 0.43 ± 0.14 mg/mg Cr in HHRH, 0.34 ± 0.07 in IH, and 0.14 $\pm$ 0.5 in normal individuals; plasma $1,25(OH)_2D$ was 303 pg/ml in HHRH, 145 pg/ml in IH, and 95 pg/ml in normal individuals; TmP/GFR was 3.05 SD units below the mean in HHRH and 1.15 below the mean in IH. Thus the IH individuals appear to have a milder metabolic defect characterized by elevated plasma $1,25(OH)_2D$ concentrations and hypercalciuria without evidence of bone disease or growth retardation.

Based on the phenotypic findings in HHRH and IH subjects in the Bedouin kindred, it has been suggested that HHRH and IH individuals are homozygous and heterozygous, respectively, for the same mutant allele (see "Genetics," below).

Bone Morphology

An examination of transilial biopsies from children with HHRH provides unequivocal evidence for osteomalacia in this disorder.[336] All patients display irregular mineralization fronts, markedly elevated osteoid surface and seam width, increased number of osteoid lamellae, and prolonged mineralization lag time. A significant inverse relationship is evident between plasma phosphate concentration and osteoid parameters, suggesting that the mineralization defect in HHRH is determined primarily by the degree of hypophosphatemia resulting from the renal phosphate leak.[336] In addition, osteoclast surface and osteoclast number are significantly reduced in HHRH.

In contrast to patients with HHRH, bone parameters are within the normal range in hypercalciuric but otherwise asymptomatic family members.[336]

Pathogenesis

HHRH patients exhibit the clinical and biochemical features of isolated renal phosphate wasting. As a consequence, persistent hypophosphatemia develops, and it is of a sufficient degree to lead to a reduction in the rate of bone mineralization and bone growth.

In contrast to patients with XLH, OHO, and ADHR, HHRH patients respond appropriately to the resulting hypophosphatemia with an increase in the serum concentration of $1,25(OH)_2D$, arising from a stimulation in renal 1α-hydroxylase activity. The elevated circulating levels of $1,25(OH)_2D$ lead to hyperabsorption of phosphate and calcium from the gastrointestinal tract and a suppression of PTH secretion. The fact that HHRH patients respond to oral phosphate supplementation with a fall in plasma $1,25(OH)_2D$ concentration, an increase in plasma PTH, and a fall in bone turnover, with improvements in bone growth and a healing of the rickets, fits with this pathogenic mechanism. Unresolved is the location of the renal tubular segment that expresses the disorder in phosphate reabsorption. It is presumed to be the proximal tubule because the bulk of filtered phosphate is reabsorbed in this segment of the nephron [see "Tubular Sites of Phosphate Reabsorption, PTH Action, and $1,25(OH)_2D$ Synthesis," above].

Treatment

The administration of 1 to 2.5 g of neutral phosphate daily, given in five divided doses, leads to an increase in growth rate and the disappearance of bone pain, muscle weakness, and the radiologic signs of rickets. The plasma phosphate concentration rises, and the plasma $1,25(OH)_2D$ concentration falls, as do the plasma calcium concentration and alkaline phosphatase activity. Likewise, urinary calcium excretion falls, the urinary cAMP rises, but TmP/GFR does not change. It is not advisable to treat HHRH patients with $1,25(OH)_2D$ in light of the pathophysiology of the disorder. Bone biopsy of treated subjects reveals complete healing of osteomalacia.

Genetics

A family tree of the original Bedouin tribe in which 9 individuals have HHRH and 21 subjects have IH without clinical evidence of bone disease is shown in Fig. 197-8. The interrelationships emphasize the considerable intermarriage seen within the extended kindred. On the basis of this family tree, it is logical to assume that individuals with HHRH and IH share the same inherited defect which, in IH individuals, leads to a milder degree of phosphate leak and the attendant changes in vitamin D and calcium metabolism. Because of the finding that hypophosphatemia is always accompanied by hypercalciuria, it is likely that only one gene is involved. Nonetheless, the mode of inheritance of HHRH is not clearly apparent. For the majority of HHRH patients, however, the findings are compatible with an autosomal codominant mode of inheritance.

The gene responsible for HHRH has not yet been identified. Based on the assumption that HHRH arises from a primary defect in renal phosphate transport (see "Pathogenesis," above), *NPT1* and *NPT2* are likely candidate genes because both Na^+-phosphate cotransporter genes map to autosomes and are expressed predominantly in the kidney (see "Structural Identification of

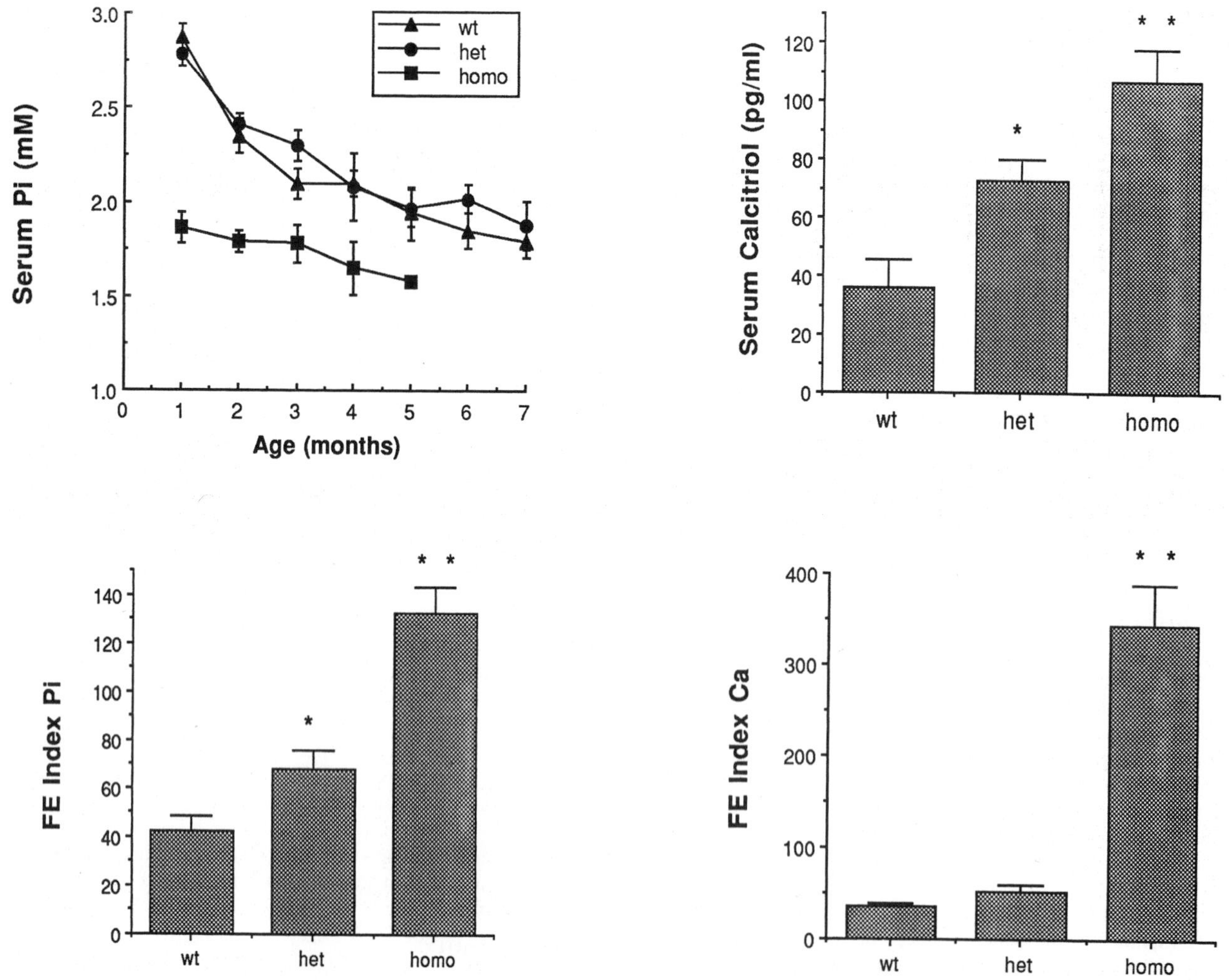

Fig. 197-9 Serum phosphate, serum calcitriol [$1,25(OH)_2D$], fractional excretion (FE) index for phosphate and calcium in wild-type (wt) mice and in mice heterozygous (het) and homozygous (homo) for the disrupted *Npt2* gene. FE index P_i and FE index Ca represent the ratio between urine phosphate or calcium divided by urine creatinine times serum phosphate or calcium. *$p < 0.05$. **$p < 0.01$. (*Data taken from Beck et al.*[106])

Renal Na^+-Phosphate Cotransport Systems," above). Studies have been initiated to genotype DNA from 59 members of the HHRH kindred using polymorphic markers that flank the *NPT1* and *NPT2* genes. Analysis of genotype data for excess homozygosity and allele sharing among affected pedigree members excluded *NPT1* as a candidate gene (CH Kos, PhD thesis, McGill University, 1998). This conclusion is based on the assumption that HHRH is an autosomal codominant disorder and that all the affected individuals possess two copies of the same mutant allele. To date, the data for *NPT2* are not conclusive (see addendum).

Similarities between HHRH and *Npt2* Knockout Mice

To determine whether the loss of Npt2 function in mice elicits the clinical features of HHRH and to define the role of Npt2 in the overall maintenance of phosphate homeostasis, the murine *Npt2* gene was cloned,[70] an *Npt2* targeting vector was constructed, and mice deficient in the *Npt2* gene were generated by homologous recombination.[106] Mice homozygous for the targeted disruption ($Npt2^{-/-}$) exhibit increased urinary phosphate excretion and hypophosphatemia (Fig. 197-9). The latter are associated with an adaptive increase in the serum concentration of $1,25(OH)_2D$ (see Fig. 197-9), hypercalcemia, hypercalciuria (see Fig. 197-9), decreased serum PTH levels, and increased serum alkaline phosphatase activity. In heterozygous mice, urinary phosphate excretion and serum calcitriol levels are intermediate between normal mice and mutant homozygotes (see Fig. 197-9). Thus the biochemical features of $Npt2^{-/-}$ mice are typical of HHRH.

In contrast to the biochemical similarities, the bone manifestations of *Npt2* gene disruption are not similar to those of HHRH. At weaning, $Npt2^{-/-}$ mice are characterized by poorly developed trabecular bone, retarded secondary ossification, and a decrease in osteoclast number. With increasing age, the abnormalities in trabecular bone are no longer apparent in $Npt2^{-/-}$ mice, but the reduction in osteoclast number persists. The data in young and adult $Npt2^{-/-}$ mice are consistent with an osteoclast defect, and in this respect, the bone findings are compatible with those in HHRH patients.

There are several explanations for the differences between the human and murine bone phenotypes. First, the bone response to hypophosphatemia and the phosphate requirement for skeletal mineralization may differ substantially in humans and mice. Indeed, the basal serum phosphate level in mice is strikingly higher than that in humans. Second, bone responses to elevated plasma $1,25(OH)_2D$ levels may differ in both species. The latter is suggested by a recent report demonstrating differences in the regulation of human and murine osteocalcin gene expression by $1,25(OH)_2D$.[337] Third, a mutation in the *NPT2* gene may not be the cause of HHRH. This was indeed the case for XLH, where decreased renal *Npt2* gene expression in the murine *Hyp*[184] and *Gy*[185] homologues of the human disease was attributable to mutations in the *Phex* gene[144,148,149] (see "The Murine *Hyp* and *Gy* Homologues of X-Linked Hypophosphatemia," above). Although the underlying mechanism whereby loss of Phex function causes decreased renal *Npt2* gene expression is not understood, it is clear that the *Phex/PHEX* gene is involved in the regulation of renal Na^+-phosphate cotransport. Nevertheless, the findings in the $Npt2^{-/-}$ mouse model demonstrate unequivocally that Npt2 plays a major role in the maintenance of phosphate homeostasis and is necessary for normal skeletal development.

ADDENDUM

The *NPT2* gene in two affected individuals from the Bedouin kindred (Fig. 197-8) and in HHRH patients from four small families was screened for mutations. No putative disease-causing mutations were found.[349] Two single nucleotide polymorphisms (SNPs), a silent substitution in exon 7 and a nucleotide substitution in intron 4, were identified and neither consistently segregated with HHRH in the Bedouin kindred.[349] Furthermore, linkage analysis demonstrated that these SNPs as well as five microsatellite markers in the chromosome 5q35 *NPT2* gene region, were not linked to HHRH in the Bedouin kindred.[349] These studies thus provide evidence to exclude *NPT2* as a candidate gene for HHRH.

ACKNOWLEDGMENTS

We are indebted to Dr. Howard Rasmussen for his contribution to previous editions of this chapter. Some of this material has been retained in the present chapter. Work done in the authors' laboratories was supported by grants from the Medical Research Council of Canada (GR-13297 and MT-14107) and Fonds pour la Formation de Chercheurs et l'Aide a la Recherche, Quebec, Canada to Harriet S. Tenenhouse, and grants from the National Institutes of Health (AR42228 and AR02095) to Michael J. Econs.

REFERENCES

1. Dennis VW, Brazy PC: Divalent anion transport in isolated renal tubules. *Kidney Int* **22**:498, 1982.
2. Murer H, Burckhardt G: Membrane transport of anions across epithelia of mammalian small intestine and kidney proximal tubule. *Rev Physiol Biochem Pharmacol* **96**:1, 1983.
3. Bonjour J-P, Caverzasio J: Phosphate transport in the kidney. *Rev Physiol Biochem Pharmacol* **100**:161, 1984.
4. Mizgala CL, Quamme GA: Renal handling of phosphate. *Physiol Rev* **65**:431, 1985.
5. Gmaj P, Murer H: Cellular mechanisms of inorganic phosphate transport in kidney. *Physiol Rev* **66**:36, 1986.
6. Hammerman MR: Phosphate transport across renal proximal tubular cell membranes. *Am J Physiol* **251**:F385, 1986.
7. Biber J: Cellular aspects of proximal tubular phosphate reabsorption. *Kidney Int* **36**:360, 1989.
8. Murer H, Werner A, Reshkin S, Wuarin R, Biber J: Cellular mechanisms in proximal tubular reabsorption of inorganic phosphate. *Am J Physiol* **260**:C885, 1991.
9. Berndt TJ, Knox FG: Renal regulation of phosphate excretion, in Seldin DW, Giebisch G (eds): *The kidney: Physiology and Pathophysiology*. New York, Raven Press, 1992, p 2511.
10. Dennis VW: Phosphate homeostasis, in Windhager EE (ed): *Renal Physiology: Handbook of Physiology Series* (sec 8). Bethesda, MD, American Physiological Society, 1992, 2, p 1785.
11. Yanagawa N, Lee DBN: Renal handling of calcium and phosphorus, in Coe FL, Favus MJ (eds): *Disorders of Bone and Mineral Metabolism*. New York, Raven Press, 1992, p 3.
12. Tenenhouse HS: Cellular and molecular mechanisms of renal phosphate transport. *J Bone Miner Res* **12**:159, 1997.
13. Murer H, Forster I, Hilfiker H, Pfister M, Kaissling B, Lotscher M, Biber J: Cellular/molecular control of renal Na/Pi-cotransport. *Kidney Int Suppl* **65**:S2, 1998.
14. McKusick VA, McKusick VA (eds): *Mendelian Inheritance in Man*, 10th ed. Baltimore, Johns Hopkins University Press, 1992.
15. Rasmussen H, Anast C: Familial hypophosphatemic rickets and vitamin D-dependent rickets, in Stanbury JB, Wyngaarden JB, Fredrickson DS, Goldstein JL, Brown MS (eds): *The Metabolic Basis of Inherited Disease*, 5th ed. New York, McGraw-Hill, 1983, p 1743.
16. Rasmussen H, Tenenhouse HS: Hypophosphatemias, in Scriver CR, Beaudet AL, Sly WS, Valle D (eds): *The Metabolic Basis of Inherited Disease*, 6th ed. New York, McGraw-Hill, 1989, p 2581.
17. Rasmussen H, Tenenhouse HS: Mendelian hypophosphatemias, in Scriver CR, Beaudet AL, Sly WS, Valle D (eds): *The Metabolic and Molecular Basis of Inherited Disease*, 7th ed. New York, McGraw-Hill, 1995, p 3717.
18. Walling MW: Intestinal Ca and phosphate transport: Differential responses to vitamin D_3 metabolites. *Am J Physiol* **233**:E488, 1977.
19. Lee DBN, Walling MW, Brautbar N: Intestinal phosphate absorption: Influence of vitamin D and non-vitamin D factors. *Am J Physiol* **250**:G369, 1986.
20. Rizzoli R, Fleisch H, Bonjour J-P: Role of 1,25-dihydroxyvitamin D_3 on intestinal phosphate absorption in rats with a normal vitamin D supply. *J Clin Invest* **60**:639, 1977.
21. Brazy P, McKeown JW, Harris RH, Dennis VW: Comparative effects of dietary phosphate, unilateral nephrectomy, and parathyroid

hormone on phosphate transport by the rabbit proximal tubule. *Kidney Int* **17**:788, 1980.
22. Steele TH, DeLuca HF: Influence of dietary phosphorus on renal phosphate reabsorption in the parathyroidectomized rat. *J Clin Invest* **57**:867, 1976.
23. Greenberg BR, Winters RW, Graham JB: The normal ranges of serum inorganic phosphorus and its utility as a discriminant in the diagnosis of congenital hypophosphatemia. *J Clin Endocrinol Metab* **20**:364, 1960.
24. Scriver CR, Tenenhouse HS: Mendelian phenotypes as "probes" of renal transport systems for amino acids and phosphate, in Windhager EE (ed): *Handbook of Physiology.* New York, Oxford University Press, 1992, p 1977.
25. Sestoft L: Is the relationship between the plasma concentration of inorganic phosphate and the rate of oxygen consumption of significance in regulating energy metabolism in mammals? *Scand J Clin Lab Invest* **39**:191, 1979.
26. Markowitz M, Rotkin L, Rosen JF: Circadian rhythms of blood minerals in humans. *Science* **213**:672, 1981.
27. Gray RW, Napoli JL: Dietary phosphate deprivation increases 1,25-dihydroxyvitamin D_3 synthesis in rat kidney in vitro. *J Biol Chem* **258**:1152, 1983.
28. Kawashima H, Kurokawa K: Metabolism and sites of action of vitamin D in the kidney. *Kidney Int* **29**:98, 1986.
29. Baylink D, Wergedal J, Staeffer M: Formation, mineralization and resorption of bone in hypophosphatemic rats. *J Clin Invest* **50**:2519, 1971.
30. Danisi G, Murer H: Inorganic phosphate absorption in small intestine, in Field M, Frizzel RA (eds): *Handbook of Physiology: The Gastrointestinal System*, vol 4. New York, Oxford University Press, 1991, p 323.
31. Caverzasio J, Bonjour J-P: Resistance to parathyroid hormone-induced inhibition of inorganic phosphate transport in opossum kidney cells cultured in low inorganic phosphate medium. *J Endocrinol* **134**:361, 1992.
32. Harris CA, Sutton RA, Dirks JH: Effects of hypercalcemia and tubular calcium and phosphate ultrafilterability on tubular reabsorption in the rat. *Am J Physiol* **233**:F201, 1977.
33. Walton RJ, Bijvoet OL: Nomogram for the derivation of renal threshold phosphate concentration. *Lancet* **2**:309, 1975.
34. Strickler JC, Thompson DD, Klose RM, Giebisch G: Micropuncture study of inorganic phosphate excretion in the rat. *J Clin Invest* **43**:1596, 1964.
35. Kuntziger H, Amiel C, Gaudebout C: Phosphate handling by the rat nephron during saline diuresis. *Kidney Int* **2**:318, 1972.
36. Legrimellec C: Micropuncture study along the proximal convoluted tubule: Electrolyte reabsorption in the first convolutions. *Pflugers Arch* **354**:133, 1975.
37. Wen S-F: Micropuncture studies of phosphate transport in the proximal tubule of the dog: The relationship to sodium reabsorption. *J Clin Invest* **53**:143, 1974.
38. Greger RF, Lang FC, Marchand G, Knox FG: Site of renal phosphate reabsorption: micropuncture and microinfusion study. *Pfleugers Arch* **369**:111, 1977.
39. Morel F: Sites of hormone action in the mammalian nephron. *Am J Physiol* **240**:F159, 1981.
40. Knox FG, Haramati A: Renal regulation of phosphate excretion, in Seldin DW, Giebisch G (eds): *The Kidney: Physiology and Pathophysiology.* New York, Raven Press, 1985, p 1381.
41. Tenenhouse HS, Gauthier C, Martel J, Gesek FA, Coutermarsh BA, Friedman PA: Na^+-phosphate cotransport in mouse distal convoluted tubule cells: Evidence for *Glvr*-1 and *Ram*-1 gene expression. *J Bone Miner Res* **13**:590, 1998.
42. McKinney TD, Myers P: Bicarbonate transport by proximal tubules: Effect of parathyroid hormone and dibutyryl cyclic AMP. *Am J Physiol* **238**:F166, 1980.
43. Hammerman MR, Klahr S, Cohn DE: Renal failure, metabolic acidosis, and parathyroidectomy in the dog increase Na^+H^+ exchange in isolated renal brush border membrane vesicles, in Forte J, Rector F (eds): *Hydrogen Ion Transport in Epithelia.* New York, Wiley, 1983, p 139.
44. Friedman PA, Coutermarsh BA, Kennedy SM, Gesek FA: Parathyroid hormone stimulation of calcium transport is mediated by dual signaling mechanisms involving protein kinase A and protein kinase C. *Endocrinology* **137**:13, 1996.
45. Forster I, Hernando N, Biber J, Murer H: The voltage dependence of a cloned mammalian renal type II Na^+/P_i cotransporter (NaP_i-2). *J Gen Physiol* **112**:1, 1998.
46. Busch A, Waldegger S, Herzer T, Biber J, Markovich D, Hayes G, Murer H, Lang F: Electrophysiological analysis of Na^+/P_i cotransport mediated by a transporter cloned from rat kidney and expressed in *Xenopus* oocytes. *Proc Natl Acad Sci USA* **91**:8205, 1994.
47. Hartmann CM, Wagner CA, Busch AE, Markovich D, Biber J, Lang F, Murer H: Transport characteristics of a murine renal Na/P_i-cotransporter. *Pflugers Arch* **430**:830, 1995.
48. Boross M, Kinsella J, Cheng L, Sacktor B: Glucocorticoids and metabolic acidosis-induced renal transports of inorganic phosphate, calcium, and NH_4. *Am J Physiol* **250**:F827, 1986.
49. Vrtovsnik F, Jourdain M, Cherqui G, Lefebvre J, Friedlander G: Glucocorticoid inhibition of Na-P_i cotransport in renal epithelial cells is mediated by protein kinase C. *J Biol Chem* **269**:8872, 1994.
50. Jehle AW, Forgo J, Biber J, Lederer E, Krapf R, Murer H: Acid-induced stimulation of Na-P_i cotransport in OK cells: Molecular characterization and effect of dexamethasone. *Am J Physiol* **273**:F396, 1997.
51. Walker JJ, Yan TS, Quamme GA: Presence of multiple sodium-dependent phosphate transport processes in proximal brush-border membranes. *Am J Physiol* **252**:F226, 1987.
52. Schwab SJ, Klahr S, Hammerman MR: Na^+ gradient-dependent P_i uptake in basolateral membrane vesicles from dog kidney. *Am J Physiol* **246**:F633, 1984.
53. Werner A, Moore ML, Mantei N, Biber J, Semenza G, Murer H: Cloning and expression of cDNA for a Na/P_i cotransport system of kidney cortex. *Proc Natl Acad Sci USA* **88**:9608, 1991.
54. Chong SS, Kristjansson K, Zoghbi HY, Hughes MR: Molecular cloning of the cDNA encoding a human renal sodium phosphate transport protein and its assignment to chromosome 6p21.3-p23. *Genomics* **18**:355, 1993.
55. Chong SS, Kozak CA, Liu L, Kristjansson K, Dunn ST, Bourdeau JE, Hughes MR: Cloning, genetic mapping, and expression analysis of a mouse renal sodium-dependent phosphate cotransporter. *Am J Physiol* **268**:F1038, 1995.
56. Miyamoto K, Tatsumi S, Sonoda T, Yamamoto H, Minami H, Taketani Y, Takeda E: Cloning and functional expression of a Na^+-dependent phosphate co-transporter from human kidney: cDNA cloning and functional expression. *Biochem J* **305**:81, 1995.
57. Magagnin S, Werner A, Markovich D, Sorribas V, Stange G, Biber J, Murer H: Expression cloning of human and rat renal cortex Na/P_i cotransport. *Proc Natl Acad Sci USA* **90**:5979, 1993.
58. Sorribas V, Markovich D, Hayes G, Stange G, Forgo J, Biber J, Murer H: Cloning of a Na/P_i cotransporter from opossum kidney cells. *J Biol Chem* **269**:6615, 1994.
59. Werner A, Murer H, Kinne RKH: Cloning and expression of a renal Na-P_i cotransport system from flounder. *Am J Physiol* **267**:F311, 1995.
60. Verri T, Markovich D, Perego C, Norbis F, Stange G, Sorribas V, Biber J, Murer H: Cloning of a rabbit renal Na-P_i cotransporter, which is regulated by dietary phosphate. *Am J Physiol* **268**:F626, 1995.
61. Collins JF, Ghishan FK: Molecular cloning, functional expression, tissue distribution, and in situ hybridization of the renal sodium phosphate (Na^+/P_i) transporter in the control and hypophosphatemic mouse. *FASEB J* **8**:862, 1994.
62. Helps C, Murer H, McGivan J: Cloning, sequence analysis and expression of the cDNA encoding a sodium-dependent phosphate transporter from the bovine renal epithelial cell line NBL-1. *Eur J Biochem* **228**:927, 1995.
63. Murer H, Biber J: Renal sodium-phosphate cotransport. *Curr Opin Nephrol Hypertens* **3**:504, 1994.
64. Murer H, Biber J: Molecular mechanisms of renal apical Na phosphate cotransport. *Annu Rev Physiol* **58**:607, 1996.
65. Levi M, Kempson SA, Lotscher M, Biber J, Murer H: Molecular regulation of renal phosphate transport. *J Memb Biol* **154**:1, 1996.
66. Murer H, Biber J: A molecular view of proximal tubular inorganic phosphate (P_i) reabsorption and of its regulation. *Pflugers Arch* **433**:379, 1997.
67. Kos CH, Tihy F, Murer H, Lemieux N, Tenenhouse HS: Comparative mapping of Na^+-phosphate cotransporter genes, *NPT1* and *NPT2*, in human and rabbit. *Cytogenet Cell Genet* **75**:22, 1996.
68. Kos CH, Tihy F, Econs MJ, Murer H, Lemieux N, Tenenhouse HS: Localization of a renal sodium phosphate cotransporter gene to human chromosome 5q35. *Genomics* **19**:176, 1994.
69. McPherson JD, Krane MC, Wagner-McPherson CB, Kos CH, Tenenhouse HS: High resolution mapping of the renal sodium-phosphate cotransporter gene (*SLC17A2*) confirms its localization to human chromosome 5q35. *Pediatr Res* **41**:632, 1997.

70. Hartmann CM, Hewson AS, Kos CH, Hilfiker H, Soumoumou Y, Murer H, Tenenhouse HS: Structure of murine and human renal type II Na^+-phosphate cotransporter genes (*Npt2* and *NPT2*). *Proc Natl Acad Sci USA* **93**:7409, 1996.
71. Biber J, Custer M, Werner A, Kaissling B, Murer H: Localization of NaP_i-1, a Na/P_i cotransporter, in rabbit kidney proximal tubules: II. Localization by immunohistochemistry. *Pflugers Arch* **424**:210, 1993.
72. Custer M, Lötscher M, Biber J, Murer H, Kaissling B: Expression of Na-P_i cotransport in rat kidney: Localization by RT-PCR and immunohistochemistry. *Am J Physiol* **266**:F767, 1994.
73. Custer M, Meier F, Schlatter E, Greger R, Garcia-Perez A, Biber J, Murer H: Localization of NaP_i-1, a Na-P_i-cotransporter, in rabbit kidney proximal tubules: I. mRNA-localization by RT-PCR. *Pflugers Arch* **424**:203, 1993.
74. Tenenhouse HS, Roy S, Martel J, Gauthier C: Differential expression, abundance and regulation of Na^+-phosphate cotransporter genes in murine kidney. *Am J Physiol* **44**:F527, 1998.
75. Hayes G, Busch A, Lotscher M, Waldegger S, Lang F, Verrey F, Biber J, Murer H: Role of N-linked glycosylation in rat renal Na/P_i-cotransport. *J Biol Chem* **269**:24143, 1994.
76. Busch AE, Schuster A, Waldegger S, Wagner CA, Zempel G, Broer S, Biber J, Murer H, Lang F: Expression of a renal type I sodium/phosphate transporter (NaP_i-1) induces a conductance in *Xenopus* oocytes permeable for organic and inorganic anions. *Proc Natl Acad Sci USA* **93**:5347, 1996.
77. Quabius ES, Murer H, Biber J: Expression of proximal tubular Na-P_i and Na-SO_4 cotransporters in MDCK and LLC-PK1 cells by transfection. *Am J Physiol* **270**:F220, 1996.
78. Quabius ES, Murer H, Biber J: Expression of a renal Na/P_i cotransporter (NaP_i-1) in MDCK and LLC-PK1 cells. *Pflugers Arch* **430**:132, 1995.
79. Timmer RT, Gunn RB: Phosphate transport by the human renal cotransporter NaP_i-3 expressed in HEK-293 cells. *Am J Physiol* **274**:C757, 1998.
80. Xiao Y, Boyer CJ, Vincent E, Dugré A, Vachon V, Potier M, Beliveau R: Involvement of disulphide bonds in the renal sodium/phosphate cotransporter NaP_i-2. *Biochem J* **323**:401, 1997.
81. Kavanaugh MP, Miller DG, Zhang W, Law W, Kozak SL, Kabat D, Miller AD: Cell-surface receptors for gibbon ape leukemia virus and amphotropic murine retrovirus are inducible sodium-phosphate symporters. *Proc Natl Acad Sci USA* **91**:7071, 1994.
82. Kaelbling M, Eddy R, Shows TB, Copeland NG, Gilbert DJ, Jenkins NA, Klinger HP, O'Hara B: Localization of the human gene allowing infection by gibbon ape leukemia virus to human chromosome region 2q11-q14 and to the homologous region on mouse chromosome 2. *J Virol* **65**:1743, 1991.
83. Garcia JV, Jones C, Miller AD: Localization of the amphotropic murine leukemia virus receptor gene to the pericentromeric region of human chromosome 8. *J Virol* **65**:6316, 1991.
84. Caverzasio J, Rizzoli R, Bonjour J: Sodium-dependent phosphate transport inhibited by parathyroid hormone and cyclic AMP stimulation in an opossum kidney cell line. *J Biol Chem* **261**:3233, 1986.
85. Reshkin SJ, Forgo J, Murer H: Functional asymmetry in phosphate transport and its regulation in opossum kidney cells: Parathyroid hormone inhibition. *Pflugers Arch* **416**:624, 1990.
86. Rouleau MF, Warshawsky H, Goltzman D: Parathyroid hormone binding in vivo to renal, hepatic, and skeletal tissues of the rat using a radioautographic approach. *Endocrinology* **118**:919, 1986.
87. Cole JA, Eber AL, Poelling RE, Thorne PK, Forte LR: A dual mechanism for regulation of kidney phosphate transport by parathyroid hormone. *Am J Physiol* **253**:E221, 1987.
88. Quamme G, Pfeilschifter J, Murer H: Parathyroid hormone inhibition of Na^+-phosphate cotransport in OK cells: Generation of second messengers in the regulatory cascade. *Biochem Biophys Res Commun* **158**:951, 1989.
89. Dunlay R, Hruska K: PTH receptor coupling to phospholipase C is an alternate pathway of signal transduction in bone and kidney. *Am J Physiol* **258**:F223, 1990.
90. Quamme G, Pfeilschifter J, Murer H: Parathyroid hormone inhibition of Na^+/phosphate cotransport in OK cells: requirement of protein kinase C-dependent pathway. *Biochim Biophys Acta* **1013**:159, 1989.
91. Miyauchi A, Dobre V, Rickmeyer J, Cole J, Forte LR, Hruska KA: Stimulation of transient elevations of Ca^{2+} is related to inhibition of P_i transport in OK cells. *Am J Physiol* **259**:F485, 1990.
92. Boneh A, Mandla S, Tenenhouse HS: Phorbol myristate acetate activates protein kinase C stimulates the phosphorylation of endogenous proteins and inhibits phosphate transport in mouse renal tubules. *Biochim Biophys Acta* **1012**:308, 1989.
93. Kempson SA, Lotscher M, Kaissling B, Biber J, Murer H, Levi M: Parathyroid hormone action on phosphate transporter mRNA and protein in rat renal proximal tubules. *Am J Physiol* **268**:F784, 1995.
94. Pfister MK, Ruf I, Stange G, Ziegler U, Lederer E, Biber J: Parathyroid hormone leads to the lysosomal degradation of the renal type II Na/P_i cotransporter. *Proc Natl Acad Sci USA* **95**:1909, 1998.
95. Malstrom K, Murer H: Parathyroid hormone regulates phosphate transport in OK cells via an irreversible inactivation of a membrane protein. *FEBS Letts* **216**:257, 1987.
96. Lu M, Wagner GF, Renfro JL: Stanniocalcin stimulates phosphate reabsorption by flounder proximal tubule in primary culture. *Am J Physiol* **267**:R1356, 1994.
97. Olsen HS, Cepeda MA, Zhang Q, Rosen CA, Vozzolo BL, Wagner GF: Human stanniocalcin: A possible hormonal regulator of mineral metabolism. *Proc Natl Acad Sci USA* **93**:1792, 1996.
98. Wagner GF, Vozzolo BL, Jaworski E, Haddad M, Kline RL, Olsen HS, Rosen CA, Davison MB, Renfro JL: Human stanniocalcin inhibits renal phosphate excretion in the rat. *J Bone Miner Res* **12**:165, 1997.
99. Barac-Nieto M, Dowd TL, Gupta RK, Spitzer A: Changes in NMR-visible kidney cell phosphate with age and diet: Relationship to phosphate transport. *Am J Physiol* **261**:F153, 1991.
100. Levi M, Lotscher M, Sorribas V, Custer M, Arar M, Kaissling B, Murer H, Biber J: Cellular mechanisms of acute and chronic adaptation of rat renal phosphate transporter to alterations in dietary phosphate. *Am J Physiol* **267**:F900, 1994.
101. Lotscher M, Kaissling B, Biber J, Murer H, Levi M: Role of microtubules in the rapid regulation of renal phosphate transport in response to acute alterations in dietary phosphate content. *J Clin Invest* **99**:1302, 1997.
102. Pfister MF, Hilfiker H, Forgo J, Lederer E, Biber J, Murer H: Cellular mechanisms involved in the acute adaptation of OK cell Na/P_i-cotransport to high- or low-P_i medium. *Pflugers Arch* **435**:713, 1998.
103. Markovich D, Verri T, Sorribas V, Forgo J, Biber J, Murer H: Regulation of opossum kidney (OK) cell Na/P_i cotransporter by P_i deprivation involves mRNA stability. *Pflugers Arch* **430**:459, 1995.
104. Hilfiker H, Hartmann CM, Stange G, Murer H: Characterization of the 5′-flanking region of OK cell type II Na-P_i cotransporter gene. *Am J Physiol* **274**:F197, 1998.
105. Roy S, Martel J, Tenenhouse HS: Growth hormone normalizes renal 1,25-dihydroxyvitamin D_3-24-hydroxylase gene expression but not Na^+-phosphate cotransporter (Npt2) mRNA in phosphate-deprived *Hyp* mice. *J Bone Miner Res* **12**:1672, 1997.
106. Beck L, Karaplis AC, Amizuka N, Hewson AS, Ozawa H, Tenenhouse HS: Targeted inactivation of *Npt2* in mice leads to severe renal phosphate wasting, hypercalciuria and skeletal abnormalities. *Proc Natl Acad Sci USA* **95**:5372, 1998.
107. Custer M, Spindler B, Verrey F, Murer H, Biber J: Identification of a new gene product (diphor-1) regulated by dietary phosphate. *Am J Physiol* **273**:F806, 1997.
108. Reid IR, Murphy WA, Hardy DC, Teitelbaum SL, Bergfeld MA, Whyte MP: X-linked hypophosphatemia: Skeletal mass in adults assessed by histomorphometry, computed tomography, and absorptiometry. *Am J Med* **90**:63, 1991.
109. Hardy DC, Murphy WA, Siegel BA, Reid IR, Whyte MP: X-linked hypophosphatemia in adults: Prevalence of skeletal radiographic and scintigraphic features. *Radiology* **171**:403, 1989.
110. Polisson RP, Martinez S, Khoury M, Harrell RM, Lyles KW, Friedman N, Harrelson JM, Reisner E, Drezner MK: Calcification of entheses associated with X-linked hypophosphatemic osteomalacia. *New Engl J Med* **313**:1, 1985.
111. Vera CI, Curo JK, Naso WB, Gelven PI, Worsham F, Roof BF, Resnick D, Salinas CF, Gross JA, Pacult A: Paraplegia due to ossification of ligamenta flava in X-linked hypophosphatemia. *Spine* **22**:710, 1997.
112. Econs MJ, Samsa GP, Monger M, Drezner MK, Feussner JR: X-linked hypophosphatemic rickets: A disease often unknown to affected patients. *Bone Miner* **24**:17, 1994.
113. Winters RW, Graham JB, Williams TF, McFalls VW, Burnett CH: A genetic study of familial hypophosphatemia and vitamin D-resistant rickets with a review of the literature. *Medicine* **37**:97, 1958.
114. Burnett CH, Dent CE, Harper C, Warland BJ: Vitamin D-resistant rickets. *Am J Med* **36**:222, 1964.
115. Graham JB, McFalls VW, Winters RW: Familial hypophosphatemia with vitamin D-resistant rickets: II. *Am J Hum Genet* **11**:311, 1959.

116. Reid IR, Hrady DC, Murphy WA, Teitelbaum SL, Bergfeld MA, Whyte MP: X-linked hypophosphatemia: A clinical, biochemical, and histopathologic assessment of morbidity in adults. *Medicine* **68**:336, 1989.
117. Whyte MP, Schrank FW, Armamento-Villareal R: X-linked hypophosphatemia: A search for gender, race, anticipation, or parent of origin effects on disease expression in children. *J Clin Endocrinol Metab* **81**:4075, 1996.
118. Stark H, Eisenstein B, Tieder M, Rachmel A, Albert G: Direct measurement of TP/GFR: A simple and reliable parameter of renal phosphate handling. *Nephron* **44**:125, 1986.
119. Greene WB, Kahler SG: Hypophosphatemic rickets: Still misdiagnosed and inadequately treated. *South Med J* **78**:1179, 1985.
120. Larmas M, Hietala EL, Similia S, Pajari U: Oral manifestations of familial hypophosphatemic rickets after phosphate therapy: A review of the literature and report of a case. *J Dent Child* **58**:328, 1991.
121. Abe K, Ooshima T, Tong SML, Yasufuku Y, Sobue S: Structural deformities of deciduous teeth in patients with hypophosphatemic vitamin D-resistant rickets. *Oral Surg* **65**:191, 1988.
122. McWhorter AG, Seale NS: Prevalence of dental abcess in a population of children with vitamin D-resistant rickets. *Pediatr Dent* **13**:91, 1991.
123. Seow WK: The effect of medical therapy on dentin formation in vitamin D-resistant rickets. *Pediatr Dent* **13**:97, 1991.
124. Tulloch EN, Andrews FFH: The association of dental abscesses with vitamin D-resistant rickets. *Br Dent J* **154**:136, 1983.
125. Rakocz M, Keating JI, Johnson R: Management of the primary dentition in vitamin D-resistant rickets. *Oral Surg* **54**:166, 1982.
126. Herbert FL: Hereditary hypophoshatemic rickets: An important awareness for dentists. *ASCS J Dent Child* **53**:223, 1986.
127. Shields ED, Scriver CR, Reade T, Fujiwara TM, Morgan K, Chiampi A, Schwartz S: X-linked hypophosphatemia: The mutant gene is expressed in teeth as well as in kidney. *Am J Hum Genet* **46**:434, 1990.
128. Swischuk LE, Hayden J, Rickets CK: A roentgenographic scheme for diagnosis. *Pediatr Radiol* **8**:203, 1979.
129. Econs MJ, Feussner JR, Samsa GP, Effman EL, Vogler JB, Martinez S, Friedman NE, Quarles LD, Drezner MK: X-linked hypophosphatemic rickets without "rickets." *Skeletal Radiol* **20**:109, 1991.
130. Burnstein MI, Lawson JP, Kottamasu SR, Ellis BI, Micho J: The enthesopathic changes of hypophosphatemic osteomalacia in adults: Radiologic findings. *AJR* **153**:785, 1989.
131. Caldemeyer KS, Boaz JC, Wappner RS, Moran CC, Smith RR, Quets JP: Chiari I malformation: Association with hypophosphatemic rickets and MR imaging appearance. *Radiology* **195**:733, 1995.
132. Rosenthall L: DEXA bone densitometry measurements in adults with X-linked hypophosphatemia. *Clin Nucl Med* **18**:564, 1993.
133. Block JE, Piel CF, Selvidge R, Genant HK: Familial hypophosphatemic rickets: Bone mass measurements in children following therapy with calcitriol and supplemental phosphate. *Calcif Tissue Int* **44**:86, 1989.
134. Schuster W: Radiological follow-up examination of the mineral salt content in the various vitamin D-resistant forms of rachitis of renal origin. *Pediatr Radiol* **2**:191, 1974.
135. Drezner MK, Lyles KW, Haussler MR, Harrelson JM: Evaluation of a role for 1,25-dihdyroxyvitamin D_3 in the pathogenesis and treatment of X-linked hypophosphatemic rickets and osteomalacia. *J Clin Invest* **66**:1020, 1980.
136. Rausmussen H, Pechet M, Anast C, Mazur H, Gertner J, Broadus AE: Long-term treatment of familial hypophosphatemic rickets with oral phosphate and 1α-hydroxyvitamin D_3. *J Pediatr* **99**:16, 1981.
137. Marie PJ, Glorieux FH: Histomorphometric study of bone remodelling in hypophosphatemic vitamin D-resistant rickets. *Metab Bone Dis Rel Res* **3**:31, 1981.
138. Choufoer JH, Stindjik R: Distribution of the perilacuna hypominrealized areas in cortical bone of patients with familial hypophosphatemic (vitamin D-resistant) rickets. *Calcif Tissue Int* **27**:101, 1979.
139. Harrison JE, Cumming WA, Fornasier D, Fraser D, Kooh SW, McNeill KG: Increased bone mineral content in young adults with familial hypophosphatemic vitamin D refractory rickets. *Metabolism* **25**:33, 1976.
140. Mächler M, Frey D, Gal A, Orth U, Wienker TF, Fanconi A, Schmid W: X-linked dominant hypophosphatemia is closely linked to DNA markers DXS41 and DXS43 at Xp22. *Hum Genet* **73**:271, 1986.
141. Thakker RV, Read AP, Davies KE, Whyte MP, Weksberg R, Glorieux F, Davies M, Mountford RC, Harris R, King A, Kim GS, Fraser D, Kooh SW, O'Riordan JLH: Bridging markers defining the map position of X-linked hypophosphatemic rickets. *J Med Genet* **24**:756, 1987.
142. Econs MJ, Rowe PSN, Francis F, Barker DF, Speer MC, Norman M, Fain PR, Weissenbach J, Read A, Davis KE, Becker PA, Lehrach H, O'Riordan J, Drezner MK: Fine structure mapping of the human X-linked hypophosphatemic rickets gene locus. *J Clin Endocrinol Metab* **79**:1351, 1994.
143. Rowe PSN, Goulding JN, Francis F, Oudet C, Econs MJ, Hanauer A, Lehrach H, Read AP, Mountford RC, Summerfield T, Weissenbach J, Fraser W, Drezner MK, Davies KE, O'Riordan JLH: The gene for X-linked hypophosphatemic rickets maps to a 200–300 kb region in Xp22.1 and is located on a single YAC containing a putative vitamin D response element (VDRE). *Hum Genet* **97**:345, 1996.
144. HYP Consortium: A gene (*PEX*) with homologies to endopeptidases is mutated in patients with X-linked hypophosphatemic rickets. *Nature Genet* **11**:130, 1995.
145. Lipman ML, Panda D, Bennett HPJ, Henderson JE, Shane E, Shen Y, Goltzman D, Karaplis AC: Cloning of human Pex cDNA: Expression, subcellular localization, and endopeptidase activity. *J Biol Chem* **273**:13729, 1998.
146. Econs MJ, McEnery PT: Autosomal dominant hypophosphatemic rickets/osteomalacia: Clinical characterization of a novel renal phosphate wasting disorder. *J Clin Endocrinol Metab* **82**:674, 1997.
147. Du L, Desbarats M, Cornibert S, Malo D, Ecarot B: Fine genetic mapping of the *Hyp* mutation on mouse chromosome X. *Genomics* **32**:177, 1996.
148. Beck L, Soumounou Y, Martel J, Krishnamurthy G, Gauthier C, Goodyer C, Tenenhouse HS: Pex/PEX tissue distribution and evidence for a deletion in the 3′ region of the *Pex* gene in X-linked hypophosphatemic mice. *J Clin Invest* **99**:1200, 1997.
149. Strom TM, Francis F, Lorenz B, Boeddrich A, Econs M, Lehrach H, Meitinger T: Pex gene deletions in *Gy* and *Hyp* mice provide mouse models for X-linked hypophosphatemia. *Hum Mol Genet* **6**:165, 1997.
150. Guo R, Quarles D: Cloning and sequencing of human *PEX* from a bone cDNA library: Evidence for its developmental stage-specific regulation in osteoblasts. *J Bone Miner Res* **12**:1009, 1997.
151. Kozak M: An analysis of 5′ noncoding sequences from 699 vertebrate messenger RNAs. *Nucl Acids Res* **15**:8125, 1987.
152. Francis F, Strom TM, Hennig S, Boddrich A, Lorenz B, Brandau O, Mohnike KL, Cagnoli M, Steffens C, Klages S: Genomic organization of the human *PEX* gene mutated in X-linked hypophosphatemia. *Genome Res* **7**:573, 1997.
153. Kozak M: An analysis of vertebrate mRNA sequences: Intimations of translational control. *J Cell Biol* **115**:887, 1991.
154. Xu D, Emoto N, Giaid A, Slaughter C, Kaw S, deWit D, Yanagisawa M: ECE-1: A membrane-bound metalloprotease that catalyzes the proteolytic activation of big endothelin-1. *Cell* **78**:473, 1994.
155. Emoto N, Yanagisawa M: Endothelin-converting enzyme-2 is a membrane bound, phosphoramidon-sensitiv metalloprotease with acidic pH optimum. *J Biol Chem* **270**:15262, 1995.
155a. Blydt-Hansen TD, Tenenhouse HS, Goodyer P: PHEX expression in parathyroid gland and PTH dysregulation in X-linked hypophosphatemia. *Pediatr Nephrol* **13**:607, 1999.
156. Du L, Desbarats M, Viel J, Glorieux FH, Cawthorn C, Ecarot B: cDNA cloning of the murine *Pex* gene implicated in X-linked hypophosphatemia and evidence for expression in bone. *Genomics* **36**:22, 1996.
157. Grieff M, Mumm S, Waeltz P, Mazzarella R, Whyte MP, Thakker RV, Sclessinger D: Expression and cloning of the human X-linked hypophosphatemia gene cDNA. *Biochem Biophys Res Commun* **231**:635, 1997.
158. Ruchon AF, Marcinkiewicz M, Siegfried G, Tenenhouse HS, DesGroseillers L, Crine P, Boileau G: *Pex* mRNA is localized in developing mouse osteoblasts and odontoblasts. *J Histochem Cytochem* **46**:459, 1998.
159. Rowe PSN, Oudet CL, Francis F, Sindig C, Pannetier S, Econs MJ, Strom T, Meitinger T, Garabedian M, David A, Macher M: *PEX* mutations in families with X-linked hypophosphatemic rickets. *Hum Mol Genet* **6**:539, 1997.
160. Holm IA, Huang X, Kunkel LM: Mutational analysis of the *PEX* gene in patients with X-linked hypophosphatemic rickets. *Am J Hum Genet* **60**:790, 1997.
161. Dixon PH, Christie PT, Wooding C, Trump D, Grieff M, Holm I, Gertner JM, Schmidke J, Shah B, Shaw N, Smith C, Tau C, Schlessinger D, Whyte MP, Thakker RV: Mutational analysis of the

PHEX gene in X-linked hypophosphataemia. *J Clin Endocrinol Metab* **83**:3615, 1998.

161a. Econs MJ, Friedman NE, Rowe PSN, Speer MC, Francis F, Strom TM, Oudet C, Smith JA, Ninomiya JT, Lee BE, Bergen H: A *PHEX* gene mutation is responsible for adult onset vitamin D-resistant hypophosphatemic osteomalacia: Evidence that the disorder is not a distinct entity from X-linked hypophosphatemic rickets. *J Clin Endocrinol Metab* **83**:3459, 1998.

162. Francis F, Strom TM, Hennig S, Boddrich A, Lorenz B, Brandau O, Mohnike KL, Cagnoli M, Steffens C, Klages S, Borzym K, Pohl T, Oudet C, Econs MJ, Rowe PSN, Reinhardt R, Meitinger T, Lehrach H: Genomic organization of the human *PEX* gene mutated in X-linked dominant hypophosphatemic rickets. *Genome Res* **7**:573, 1997.

162a. Filisetti D, Ostermann G, von Bredow M, Strom T, Filler G, Ehrich J, Pannetier S, Garnier JM, Rowe P, Francis F, Julienne A, Hanauer A, Econs MJ, Oudet C: Nonrandom distribution of mutations in the *PHEX* gene, and under-detected missense mutations at non-conserved residues. *Eur J Hum Genet* **7**:615, 1999.

162b. Sabbagh Y, Jones A, Tenenhouse HS: *PHEXdb*, a locus specific database for mutations causing X-linked hypophosphatemia. *Hum Mutat* **16**:1, 2000.

162c. Orstavik KH, Orstavik RE, Halse J, Knudtzon J: X chromosome inactivation pattern in female carriers of X linked hypophosphataemic rickets. *Med Genet* **33**:700, 1996.

163. Chalew SA, Lovchik JC, Brown CM, Sun CC: Hypophosphatemia induced in mice by transplantation of a tumor-derived cell line from a patient with oncogenic rickets. *J Pediatr Endocrinol Metab* **9**:593, 1996.

164. Lorenz B, Francis F, Gempel K, Boddrich A, Josten M, Schmahl W, Schmidt J, Lehrach H, Meitinger T, Strom TM: Spermine deficiency in *Gy* mice caused by deletion of the spermine synthase gene. *Hum Mol Genet* **7**:541, 1998.

165. Meyer RA Jr, Henley CM, Meyer MH, Morgan PL, McDonald AG, Mills C, Price DK: Partial deletion of both the spermine synthase gene and the *Pex* gene in the X-linked hypophosphatemic, Gyro (*Gy*) mouse. *Genomics* **48**:289, 1998.

166. Eicher EM, Southard JL, Scriver CR, Glorieux FH: Hypophosphatemia: Mouse model for human familial hypophosphatemic (vitamin D-resistant) rickets. *Proc Natl Acad Sci USA* **73**:4667, 1976.

167. Lyon MF, Scriver CR, Baker LRI, Tenenhouse HS, Kronick J, Mandla S: The *Gy* mutation: Another cause of X-linked hypophosphatemia in mouse. *Proc Natl Acad Sci USA* **83**:4899, 1986.

168. Boneh A, Reade TM, Scriver CR, Rishikof E: Audiometric evidence for two forms of X-linked hypophosphatemia in humans, apparent counterparts of *Hyp* and *Gy* mutations in mouse. *Am J Med Genet* **27**:997, 1987.

169. Meyer RA Jr., Jowsey J, Meyer MH: Osteomalacia and altered magnesium metabolism in the X-linked hypophosphatemic mouse. *Calcif Tissue Int* **27**:19, 1979.

170. Meyer RA Jr., Meyer MH, Gray RW, Bruns ME: Femoral abnormalities and vitamin D metabolism in X-linked hypophosphatemic (*Hyp* and *Gy*) mice. *J Orthop Res* **13**:30, 1995.

171. Giasson SD, Brunette MG, Danan G, Vigneault N, Carriere S: Micropuncture study of renal phosphorus transport in hypophosphatemic vitamin D-resistant rickets mice. *Pflugers Arch* **371**:33, 1977.

172. Cowgill LD, Goldfarb S, Lau K, Slatopolsky E, Agus ZS: Evidence for an intrinsic renal tubular defect in mice with genetic hypophosphatemic rickets. *J Clin Invest* **63**:1203, 1979.

173. Kiebzak GM, Meyer RA, Mish PM: X-linked hypophosphatemic mice respond to thyroparathyroidectomy. *Miner Electrol Metab* **6**:153, 1981.

174. Tenenhouse HS, Scriver CR, McInnes RR, Glorieux FH: Renal handling of phosphate in vivo and in vitro by the X-linked hypophosphatemic male mouse: Evidence for a defect in the brush border membrane. *Kidney Int* **14**:236, 1978.

175. Tenenhouse HS, Scriver CR: The defect in transcellular transport of phosphate in the nephron is located in brush-border membranes in X-linked hypophosphatemia (*Hyp* mouse model). *Can J Biochem* **56**:640, 1978.

176. Kiebzak GM, Dousa TP: Thyroid hormones increase renal brush border membrane transport of phosphate in X-linked hypophosphatemic (*Hyp*) mice. *Endocrinology* **117**:613, 1985.

177. Tenenhouse HS, Lee J, Harvey N: Renal brush-border membrane Na^+-sulfate cotransport: Stimulation by thyroid hormone. *Am J Physiol* **261**:F420, 1991.

178. Brunette MG, Mernissi GE, Doucet A: Renal sodium transport in vitamin D-resistant hypophosphatemic rickets. *Can J Physiol Pharmacol* **63**:1339, 1985.

179. Ford DM, Molitoris BA: Abnormal proximal tubule apical membrane protein composition in X-linked hypophosphatemic mice. *Am J Physiol* **260**:F317, 1991.

180. Tenenhouse HS, Klugerman AH, Neal JL: Effect of phosphonoformic acid, dietary phosphate and the *Hyp* mutation on kinetically distinct phosphate transport processes in mouse kidney. *Biochim Biophys Acta* **984**:207, 1989.

181. Tenenhouse HS, Meyer RA Jr., Mandla S, Meyer MH, Gray RW: Renal phosphate transport and vitamin D metabolism in X-linked hypophosphatemic *Gy* mice: Responses to phosphate deprivation. *Endocrinology* **131**:51, 1992.

182. Harvey N, Tenenhouse HS: Renal Na^+-phosphate cotransport in X-linked *Hyp* mice responds appropriately to Na^+-gradient, membrane potential and pH. *J Bone Miner Res* **7**:563, 1992.

183. Tenenhouse HS, Lee J, Harvey N, Potier M, Jette M, Beliveau R: Normal molecular size of the Na^+-phosphate cotransporter and normal Na^+-dependent binding of phosphonoformic acid in renal brush border membranes of X-linked *Hyp* mice. *Biochem Biophys Res Commun* **170**:1288, 1990.

184. Tenenhouse HS, Werner A, Biber J, Ma S, Martel J, Roy S, Murer H: Renal Na^+-phosphate cotransport in murine X-linked hypophosphatemic rickets: Molecular characterization. *J Clin Invest* **93**:671, 1994.

185. Beck L, Meyer RA Jr, Meyer MH, Biber J, Murer H, Tenenhouse HS: Renal expression of Na^+-phosphate cotransporter mRNA and protein: Effect of the *Gy* mutation and low phosphate diet. *Pflugers Arch* **431**:936, 1996.

186. Tenenhouse HS, Beck L: Renal Na^+-phosphate cotransporter gene expression in X-linked *Hyp* and *Gy* mice. *Kidney Int* **49**:1027, 1996.

187. Collins JF, Scheving LA, Ghishan FK: Decreased transcription of the sodium-phosphate transporter gene in the hypophosphatemic mouse. *Am J Physiol* **269**:F439, 1995.

188. Muller YL, Collins JF, Ghishan FK: Genetic screening for X-linked hypophosphatemic mice and ontogenic characterization of the defect in the renal sodium-phosphate transporter. *Pediatr Res* **44**:633, 1998.

189. Seikaly MG, Brown R, Baum M: The effect of recombinant human growth hormone in children with X-linked hypophosphatemia. *Pediatrics* **100**:879, 1997.

190. Reusz GS, Miltenyi G, Stubnya G, Szabo A, Horvath C, Byrd DJ, Peter F, Tulassay T: X-linked hypophosphatemia: Effects of treatment with recombinant human growth hormone. *Pediatr Nephrol* **11**:573, 1997.

191. Tenenhouse HS, Scriver CR: Renal adaptation to phosphate deprivation in the *Hyp* mouse with X-linked hypophosphatemia. *Can J Biochem* **57**:938, 1979.

192. Tenenhouse HS, Scriver CR: Renal brush border membrane adaptation to phosphorus deprivation in the *Hyp/Y* mouse. *Nature* **281**:225, 1979.

193. Tenenhouse HS, Martel J, Biber J, Murer H: Effect of P_i restriction on renal Na^+-P_i cotransporter mRNA and immunoreactive protein in X-linked *Hyp* mice. *Am J Physiol* **268**:F1062, 1995.

194. Muhlbauer RC, Bonjour J, Fleisch H: Abnormal tubular adaptation to dietary P_i restriction in X-linked hypophosphatemic mice. *Am J Physiol* **242**:F353, 1982.

195. Thornton SW, Tenenhouse HS, Martel J, Bockian RW, Meyer MH, Meyer RA Jr: X-linked hypophosphatemic *Gy* mice: Renal tubular maximum for phosphate vs brush-border transport after low-P diet. *Am J Physiol* **266**:F309, 1994.

196. Turner AJ, Tanzawa K: Mammalian membrane metallopeptidases: NEP, ECE, KELL and PEX. *FASEB J* **11**:355, 1997.

197. Econs MJ, Francis F: Positional cloning of the *PEX* gene: New insights into the pathophysiology of X-linked hypophosphatemic rickets. *Am J Physiol* **273**:F489, 1997.

198. Meyer RA Jr, Meyer MH, Gray RW: Parabiosis suggests a humoral factor is involved in X-linked hypophosphatemia in mice. *J Bone Miner Res* **4**:493, 1989.

199. Meyer RA Jr, Tenenhouse HS, Meyer MH, Klugerman AH: The renal phosphate transport defect in normal mice parabiosed to X-linked hypophosphatemic mice persists after parathyroidectomy. *J Bone Miner Res* **4**:523, 1989.

200. Nesbitt T, Coffman TM, Griffiths R, Drezner MK: Cross-transplantation of kidneys in normal and *Hyp* mice: Evidence that the Hyp phenotype is unrelated to an intrinsic renal defect. *J Clin Invest* **89**:1453, 1992.

201. Morgan JM, Hawley WL, Chenoweth AI, Retan WJ, Diethelm AG: Renal transplanation in hypophposphatemia with vitamin D-resistant rickets. *Arch Intern Med* **134**:549, 1974.
202. Lajeunesse D, Meyer RA Jr., Hamal L: Direct evidence of a humorally-mediated inhibition of renal phosphate transport in the *Hyp* mouse: Involvement of an osteoblast-derived factor. *Kidney Int* **50**:1531, 1996.
203. Scriver CR, Tenenhouse HS: Conserved loci on the X chromosome confer phosphate homeostasis in mice and humans. *Genet Res Camb* **56**:141, 1990.
204. Meyer RA Jr., Gray RW, Meyer MH: Abnormal vitamin D metabolism in the X-linked hypophosphatemic mouse. *Endocrinology* **107**:1577, 1980.
205. Tenenhouse HS, Jones G: Abnormal regulation of renal vitamin D catabolism by dietary phosphate in murine X-linked hypophosphatemic rickets. *J Clin Invest* **85**:1450, 1990.
206. Yamaoka K, Seino Y, Satomura K, Tanaka Y, Yabuuchi H, Haussler MR: Abnormal relationship between serum phosphate concentration and renal 25-hydroxycholecalciferol-1-alpha-hydroxylase activity in X-linked hypophosphatemic mice. *Miner Electrol Metab* **12**:194, 1986.
207. Akiyoshi-Shibata M, Sakaki T, Ohyama Y, Noshiro M, Okuda K, Yabusaki Y: Further oxidation of hydroxycalcidiol by calcidiol 24-hydroxylase. *Eur J Biochem* **224**:335, 1994.
208. Beckman MJ, Tadikonda P, Werner E, Prahl J, Yamada S, DeLuca HF: Human 25-hydroxyvitamin D_3-24-hydroxylase, a multicatalytic enzyme. *Biochemistry* **35**:8465, 1996.
209. Roy S, Martel J, Ma S, Tenenhouse HS: Increased renal 25-hydroxyvitamin D_3-24-hydroxylase messenger ribonucleic acid and immunoreactive protein in phosphate-deprived *Hyp* mice: A mechanism for accelerated 1,25-dihydroxyvitamin D_3 catabolism in X-linked hypophosphatemic rickets. *Endocrinology* **134**:1761, 1994.
210. Roy S, Tenenhouse HS: Transcriptional regulation and renal localization of 1,25-dihydroxyvitamin D_3-24-hydroxylase gene expression: Effects of the *Hyp* mutation and 1,25-dihydroxyvitamin D_3. *Endocrinology* **137**:2938, 1996.
211. Gray RW, Garthwaite TL: Activation of renal 1,25-dihydroxyvitamin D_3 synthesis by phosphate deprivation: Evidence for a role for growth hormone. *Endocrinology* **116**:189, 1985.
212. Tenenhouse HS: Abnormal renal mitochondrial 25-hydroxyvitamin D_3-1-hydroxylase activity in the vitamin D and calcium deficient X-linked *Hyp* mouse. *Endocrinology* **113**:816, 1983.
213. Tenenhouse HS: Investigation of the mechanism for abnormal renal 25-hydroxyvitamin D_3-1-hydroxylase activity in the X-linked *Hyp* mouse. *Endocrinology* **115**:634, 1984.
214. Tenenhouse HS: Metabolism of 25-hydroxyvitamin D_3 in renal slices from the X-linked hypophosphatemic (*Hyp*) mouse: Abnormal response to fall in serum calcium. *Cell Calcium* **5**:43, 1984.
215. Carpenter TO, Shiratori T: Renal 25-hydroxyvitamin D-1 alpha-hydroxylase activity and mitochondrial phosphate transport in *Hyp* mice. *Am J Physiol* **259**:E814, 1990.
216. Nesbitt T, Drezner MK, Lobaugh B: Abnormal parathyroid hormone stimulation of 25-hydroxyvitamin D-1α-hydroxylase activity in the hypophosphatemic mouse: Evidence for a generalized defect of vitamin D metabolism. *J Clin Invest* **77**:181, 1986.
217. Nesbitt T, Davidai GA, Drezner MK: Abnormal adenosine 3′,5′-monophosphate stimulation of renal 1,25-dihydroxyvitamin D production in *Hyp* mice: Evidence that 25-hydroxyvitamin D-1α-hydroxylase dysfunction results from aberrant intracellular function. *Endocrinology* **124**:1184, 1989.
218. Nesbitt T, Drezner MK: Abnormal parathyroid hormone-related peptide stimulation of renal 25-hydroxyvitamin D-1-hydroxylase in *Hyp* mice: Evidence for a generalized defect of enzyme activity in the proximal convoluted tubule. *Endocrinology* **127**:843, 1990.
219. Davidai GA, Nesbitt T, Drezner MK: Normal regulation of calcitriol metabolism in *Gy* mice: Evidence for biochemical heterogeneity in the X-linked hypophosphatemic diseases. *J Clin Invest* **85**:334, 1990.
220. Sabina RL, Drezner MK, Holmes EW: Reduced renal cortical ribonucleoside triphosphate pools in three different hypophosphatemic animal models. *Biochem Biophys Res Commun* **109**:649, 1982.
221. Brown CE, Wilkie CA, Meyer MH, Meyer RA Jr.: Response of tissue phosphate content to acute dietary phosphate deprivation in the X-linked hypophosphatemic mouse. *Calcif Tissue Int* **37**:423, 1985.
222. Lyles KW, Burkes EJ, McNamara CR, Harrelson JM, Pickett JP, Drezner MK: The concurrence of hypoparathyroidism provides new insights to the pathophysiology of X-linked hypophosphatemia. *J Clin Endocrinol Metab* **60**:711, 1985.
223. Kiebzak GM, Roos BA, Meyer RA Jr.: Secondary hyperparathyroidism in X-linked hypophosphatemic mice. *Endocrinology* **111**:650, 1982.
224. Posillico JT, Lobaugh B, Muhlbaier LH, Drezner MK: Abnormal parathyroid function in the X-linked hypophosphatemic mouse. *Calcif Tissue Int* **37**:418, 1985.
225. Meyer RA Jr, Morgan PL, Meyer MH: Measurement of parathyroid hormone in the mouse: Secondary hyperparathyroidism in the X-linked hypophosphatemic (*Gyro,Gy*) mouse. *Endocrinology* **2**:1127, 1994.
226. Meyer RA Jr, Meyer MH, Morgan PL: Effects of altered diet on serum levels of 1,25-dihydroxyvitamin D and parathyroid hormone in X-linked hypophosphatemic (*Hyp* and *Gy*) mice. *Bone* **18**:23, 1996.
227. Kiebzak GM, Meyer RA Jr.: X-linked hypophosphatemic mice are not hypersensitive to parathyroid hormone. *Endocrinology* **110**:1030, 1982.
228. Tenenhouse HS, Veksler A: Effect of the *Hyp* mutation and diet-induced hyperparathyroidism on renal parathyroid hormone- and forskolin-stimulated adenosine 3′5′-monophosphate production and brush border membrane phosphate transport. *Endocrinology* **118**:1047, 1986.
229. Tenenhouse HS, Henry HL: Protein kinase activity and protein kinase inhibitor in mouse kidney: Effect of the X-linked *Hyp* mutation and vitamin D status. *Endocrinology* **117**:1719, 1985.
230. Hammerman MR, Chase LR: P_i transport, phosphorylation, and dephosphorylation in renal membranes from *Hyp/Y* mice. *Am J Physiol* **245**:F701, 1983.
231. Marks KH, Kilav R, Berman E, Naveh-Many T, Silver J: Parathyroid hormone gene expression in *Hyp* mice fed a low-phosphate diet. *Nephrol Dial Transplant* **12**:1581, 1997.
232. Tenenhouse HS, Fast DK, Scriver CR, Koltay M: Intestinal transport of phosphate anion is not impaired in the *Hyp* (hypophosphatemic) mouse. *Biochem Biophys Res Commun* **100**:537, 1981.
233. Brault BA, Meyer MH, Meyer RA Jr: Malabsorption of phosphate by the intestines of young X-linked hypophosphatemic mice. *Calcif Tissue Int* **43**:289, 1988.
234. Meyer RA Jr., Meyer MH, Gray RW, Bruns ME: Evidence that low plasma 1,25-dihydroxyvitamin D causes intestinal malabsorption of calcium and phosphate in juvenile X-linked hypophosphatemic mice. *J Bone Miner Res* **2**:67, 1987.
235. Meyer MH, Meyer RA Jr, Iorio RJ: A role for the intestine in the bone disease of juvenile X-linked hypophosphatemic mice: Malabsorption of calcium and reduced skeletal mineralization. *Endocrinology* **115**:1464, 1984.
236. Meyer RA Jr., Meyer MH, Erickson PR, Korkor AB: Reduced absorption of calcium-45 from isolated duodenal segments "in vivo" in juvenile but not adult X-linked hypophosphatemic mice. *Calcif Tissue Int* **38**:95, 1986.
237. Bruns ME, Meyer RA Jr, Meyer MH: Low levels of intestinal vitamin D-dependent calcium binding protein in juvenile X-linked hypophosphatemic mice. *Endocrinology* **115**:1459, 1984.
238. Bruns ME, Christakos S, Huang YC, Meyer MH, Meyer RA Jr: Vitamin D-dependent calcium binding proteins in the kidney and intestine of the X-linked hypophosphatemic mouse: Changes with age and responses to 1,25-dihydroxycholecalciferol. *Endocrinology* **121**:1, 1987.
239. Lobaugh B, Drezner MK: Abnormal regulation of renal 25-hydroxyvitamin D-1α-hydroxylase activity in the X-linked hypophosphatemic mouse. *J Clin Invest* **71**:400, 1983.
240. Tenenhouse HS: Effect of age and the X-linked *Hyp* mutation on renal adaptation to vitamin D and calcium deficiency. *Comp Biochem Phys* **81A**:367, 1985.
241. Tenenhouse HS, Yip A, Jones G: Increased renal catabolism of 1,25-dihydroxyvitamin D_3 in murine X-linked hypophosphatemic rickets. *J Clin Invest* **81**:461, 1988.
242. Short EM, Binder HJ, Rosenberg LE: Familial hypophosphatemic rickets: Defective transport of inorganic phosphate by intestinal mucosa. *Science* **179**:700, 1973.
243. Glorieux FH, Morin CL, Travers R, Delvin EE, Poirier R: Intestinal phosphate transport in familial hypophosphatemic rickets. *Pediatr Res* **10**:691, 1976.
244. Soener RA, Meyer MH, Meyer RA Jr.: Ovariectomy abolishes the normalization of femoral mineral content in 40-week-old female X-linked hypophosphatemic mice. *Miner Electrol Metab* **14**:321, 1988.

245. Brault BA, Meyer MH, Meyer RA Jr, Iorio RJ: Mineral uptake by the femora of older female *Hyp* mice but not older male *Hyp* mice. *Clin Orthop* **222**:289, 1987.
246. Shetty NS, Meyer RA Jr: Craniofacial abnormalities in mice with X-linked hypophosphatemic genes (*Hyp* or *Gy*). *Teratology* **44**:463, 1991.
247. Qiu ZQ, Tenenhouse HS, Scriver CR: Parental origin of mutant allele does not explain absence of gene dose in X-linked *Hyp* mice. *Genet Res Camb* **62**:39, 1993.
248. Scriver CR, Tenenhouse HS: X-linked hypophosphatemia: A homologous phenotype in humans and mice with unusual organ-specific gene dosage. *J Inher Metab Dis* **15**:610, 1992.
249. Roy WA, Iorio RJ, Meyer RA: Craniosynostosis in vitamin D-resistant rickets: A mouse model. *J Neurosurg* **55**:265, 1981.
250. Mostafa YA, El-Mangoury NH, Meyer RA Jr, Iorio RJ: Deficient nasal bone growth in the X-linked hypophosphatemic (*Hyp*) mouse and its implication in craniofacial growth. *Arch Oral Biol* **27**:311, 1982.
251. Marie PJ, Travers R, Glorieux FH: Healing of rickets with phosphate supplementation in the hypophosphatemic male mouse. *J Clin Invest* **67**:911, 1981.
252. Yoshikawa H, Masuhara K, Takaoka K, Ono K, Tanaka H, Seino Y: Abnormal bone formation induced by implantation of osteosarcoma-derived bone-inducing substance in the X-linked hypophosphatemic mouse. *Bone* **6**:235, 1985.
253. Ecarot-Charrier B, Glorieux FH, Travers R, Desbarats M, Bouchard F, Hinek A: Defective bone formation by transplanted *Hyp* mouse bone cells into normal mice. *Endocrinology* **123**:768, 1988.
254. Ecarot B, Glorieux FH, Desbarats M, Travers R, Labelle L: Defective bone formation by *Hyp* mouse bone cells transplanted into normal mice: Evidence in favor of an intrinsic osteoblast defect. *J Bone Miner Res* **7**:215, 1992.
255. Ecarot B, Glorieux FH, Desbarats M, Travers R, Labelle L: Effect of dietary phosphate deprivation and supplementation of recipient mice on bone formation by transplanted cells from normal and X-linked hypophosphatemic mice. *J Bone Miner Res* **7**:523, 1992.
256. Ecarot B, Glorieux FH, Desbarats M, Travers R, Labelle L: Effect of 1,25-dihydroxyvitamin D_3 treatment on bone formation by transplanted cells from normal and X-linked hypophosphatemic mice. *J Bone Miner Res* **10**:424, 1995.
257. Rifas L, Gupta A, Hruska KA, Avioli LV: Altered osteoblast gluconeogenesis in X-linked hypophosphatemic mice is associated with a depressed intracellular pH. *Calcif Tissue Int* **57**:60, 1995.
258. Rifas L, Cheng S, Halstead LR, Gupta A, Hruska KA, Avioli LV: Skeletal casein kinase activity defect in the *Hyp* mouse. *Calcif Tissue Int* **61**:256, 1997.
259. Yamamoto T, Ecarot B, Glorieux FH: Abnormal response of osteoblasts from *Hyp* mice to 1,25-dihydroxyvitamin D_3. *Bone* **13**:209, 1992.
260. Xiao ZS, Crenshaw M, Guo R, Nesbitt T, Drezner MK, Quarles LD: Intrinsic mineralization defect in *Hyp* mouse osteoblasts. *Am J Physiol* **38**:E708, 1998.
261. Ecarot B, Caverzasio J, Desbarats M, Bonjour JP, Glorieux FH: Phosphate transport by osteoblasts from X-linked hypophosphatemic mice. *Am J Physiol* **266**:E33, 1994.
262. Rifas L, Halstead LL, Cheng S-L, Scott MJ, Fausto A, Roberts M, Avioli LV: Na^+-dependent phosphate transport in normophosphatemic and hypophosphatemic osteoblasts in an X-linked hypophosphatemic mouse model. *J Bone Miner Res* **6**:437, 1991.
263. Delvin EE, Richard P, Desbarats M, Ecarot-Charrier B, Glorieux FH: Cultured osteoblasts from normal and hypophosphatemic mice: Calcitriol receptors and biological response to the hormone. *Bone* **11**:87, 1990.
264. Carpenter TO, Moltz KC, Ellis B, Andreoli M, McCarthy TL, Centrella M, Bryan D, Gundberg CM: Osteocalcin production in primary osteoblast cultures derived from normal and *Hyp* mice. *Endocrinology* **139**:35, 1998.
265. Gundberg CM, Clough ME, Carpenter TO: Development and validation of a radioimmunoassay for mouse osteocalcin: Paradoxical response in the *Hyp* mouse. *Endocrinology* **130**:1909, 1992.
266. Carpenter TO, Gundberg CM: Osteocalcin abnormalities in *Hyp* mice reflect altered genetic expression and are not due to altered clearance, affinity for mineral, or ambient phosphorus levels. *Endocrinology* **137**:5213, 1996.
267. Tsuji H, Cawthorn C, Ecarot B: Abnormal modulation of serum osteocalcin by dietary phosphate and 1,25-dihydroxyvitamin D_3 in the hypophosphatemic mouse. *J Bone Miner Res* **11**:1234, 1996.
268. Boskey AL, Gilder H, Neufeld E, Ecarot B, Glorieux FH: Phospholipid changes in the bones of the hypophosphatemic mouse. *Bone* **12**:345, 1991.
269. Camacho NP, Rimnac CM, Meyer RA Jr, Doty S, Boskey AL: Effect of abnormal mineralization on the mechanical behavior of X-linked hypophosphatemic mice femora. *Bone* **17**:271, 1995.
270. Iorio RJ, Bell WA, Meyer MH, Meyer RA Jr: Radiographic evidence of craniofacial and dental abnormalities in the X-linked hypophosphatemic mouse. *Ann Dent* **38**:31, 1979.
271. Iorio RJ, Bell WA, Meyer MH, Meyer RA Jr: Histologic evidence of calcification in teeth and alveolae bone of mice with X-linked dominant hypophosphatemia (VDRR). *Ann Dent* **38**:38, 1979.
272. Sofaer JA, Southam JC: Naturally-occurring exposure of the dental-pulp in mice with inherited hypophosphatemia. *Arch Oral Biol* **27**:701, 1982.
273. Abe K, Ooshima T, Masatomi Y, Sobue S, Moriwaki Y: Microscopic and crystallographic examinations of the teeth of the X-linked hypophosphatemic mouse. *J Dent Res* **68**:1519, 1989.
274. Abe K, Masatomi Y, Nakajima Y, Shintani S, Moriwaki Y, Sobue S, Ooshima T: The occurrence of interglobular dentin in incisors of hypophosphatemic mice fed a high-calcium and high-phosphate diet. *J Dent Res* **71**:478, 1992.
275. Reade TM, Scriver CR: Hypophosphatemic rickets and breast milk. *New Engl J Med* **300**:1397, 1979.
276. Jonas AJ, Dominguez B: Low breast milk phosphorus concentration in familial hypophosphatemia. *J Pediatr Gastroenterol Nutr* **8**:541, 1989.
277. Delzer PR, Meyer RA Jr: Normal milk composition in lactating X-linked hypophosphatemic mice despite continued hypophosphatemia. *Calcif Tissue Int* **35**:750, 1983.
278. Delzer PR, Meyer RA Jr: Normal handling of phosphate in the salivary glands of X-linked hypophosphatemic mice. *Arch Oral Biol* **29**:1009, 1984.
279. Escoubet B, Silve C, Balsan S, Amiel C: Phosphate transport by fibroblasts from patients with hypophosphatemic vitamin D-resistant rickets. *J Endocrinol* **133**:301, 1992.
280. Glorieux FH, Marie PJ, Pettifor JM, Delvin EE: Bone response to phosphate salts, ergocalciferol, and calcitriol in hypophosphatemic vitamin D-resistant rickets. *New Engl J Med* **303**:1023, 1980.
281. Davidai GA, Nesbitt T, Drezner MK: Variable phosphate-mediated regulation of vitamin D metabolism in the murine hypophosphatemic rachitic/osteomalacic disorders. *Endocrinology* **128**:1270, 1991.
282. Marie PJ, Travers R, Glorieux PH: Healing of bone lesions with 1,25-dihydroxyvitamin D_3 in the young X-linked hypophosphatemic male mouse. *Endocrinology* **111**:904, 1982.
283. Marie PJ, Travers R, Glorieux FH: Bone response to phosphate and vitamin D metabolites in the hypophosphatemic male mouse. *Calcif Tissue Int* **34**:158, 1982.
284. Yamate T, Tanaka H, Nagai Y, Yamato H, Taniguchi N, Nakamura T, Seini Y: Bone-forming ability of 24*R*,25-dihydroxyvitamin D_3 in the hypophosphatemic mouse. *J Bone Miner Res* **9**:1967, 1994.
285. Ono T, Tanaka H, Yamata T, Nagai Y, Nakamura T, Seino Y: 24*R*,25-Dihydroxyvitamin D_3 promotes bone formation without causing excessive resorption in hypophosphatemic mice. *Endocrinology* **137**:2633, 1996.
286. St-Arnaud R, Glorieux FH: 24,25-Dihydroxyvitamin D: Active metabolite or inactive catabolite? *Endocrinology* **139**:3371, 1998.
287. Tenenhouse HS, Scriver CR: Effect of 1,25-dihydroxyvitamin D_3 on phosphate homeostasis in the X-linked hypophosphatemic (*Hyp*) mouse. *Endocrinology* **109**:658, 1981.
288. Alon U, Chan JCM: Effects of PTH and $1,25(OH)_2D_3$ on tubular handling of phosphate in hypophosphatemic rickets. *J Clin Endocrinol Metab* **58**:671, 1984.
289. Harrell RM, Lyles KW, Harrelson JM, Friedman NE, Drezner MK: Healing of bone disease in X-linked hypophosphatemic rickets/osteomalacia. *J Clin Invest* **75**:1858, 1985.
290. Glorieux FH, Scriver CR, Reade TM, Goldman H, Roseborough A: Use of phosphate and vitamin D to prevent dwarfism and rickets in X-linked hypophosphatemia. *New Engl J Med* **287**:481, 1972.
291. Costa T, Marie PJ, Scriver CR, Cole DEC, Reade TM, Nogrady B, Glorieux FH, Delvin EE: X-linked hypophosphatemia: Effect of calcitriol on renal handling of phosphate, serum phosphate, and bone mineralization. *J Clin Endocrinol Metab* **52**:463, 1981.
292. Carpenter TO, Mitnick MA, Ellison A, Smith C, Insogna KL: Nocturnal hyperparathyroidism: A frequent feature of X-linked hypophosphatemia. *J Clin Endocrinol Metab* **78**:1378, 1994.
293. Carpenter TO: New perspectives on the biology and treatment of X-linked hypophosphatemic rickets. *Pediatr Endcrinol* **44**:443, 1997.

294. Goodyer PR, Kronick JB, Jequier S, Reade TM, Scriver CR: Nephrocalcinosis and its relationship to treatment of hereditary rickets. *J Pediatr* **111**:700, 1987.
295. Stickler GB, Morgenstern BZ: Hypophosphataemic rickets: Final height and clinical symptoms in adults. *Lancet* **2**(8668):902, 1989.
296. Balsan S, Tieder M: Linear growth in patients with hypophosphatemic rickets: Influence of treatment regimen and parental height. *J Pediatr* **116**:365, 1990.
297. Bettinelli A, Bianchi ML, Mazzucchi E, Gandolini G, Appiani AC: Acute effects of calcitriol and phosphate salts on mineral metabolism in children with hypophosphatemic rickets. *J Pediatr* **118**:372, 1991.
298. Verge CF, Lam A, Simpson JM, Cowell CT, Howard NJ, Silink M: Effects of therapy in X-linked hypophosphatemic rickets. *New Engl J Med* **325**:1843, 1991.
299. Reusz GS, Latta K, Hoyer PF, Byrd DJ, Ehrich JHH, Brodehl J: Evidence suggesting hyperoxaluria as a cuase of nephrocalcinosis in phosphate-treated hypophosphatemic rickets. *Lancet* **335**:1240, 1990.
300. Eddy MC, McAlister WH, Whyte MP: X-linked hypophosphatemia: Normal renal function despite medullary nephrocalcinosis 25 years after transient vitamin D_2-induced renal azotemia. *Bone* **21**:515, 1997.
301. Alon U, Donaldson DL, Hellerstein S, Warady BA, Harris DJ: Metabolic and histologic investigation of the nature of nephrocalcinosis in children with hypophosphatemic rickets and in the *Hyp* mouse. *J Pediatr* **120**:899, 1992.
302. Futh RG, Giant CS, Riggs BL: Development of hypercalcemic hyperparathyroidism after long-term phosphate supplementation in hypophosphtemic osteomalacia. *Am J Med* **78**:669, 1985.
303. Wilson DM, Lee PD, Morris AH, Reiter EO, Gertner JM, Marcus R, Quarmby VE, Rosenfeld RG: Growth hormone therapy in hypophosphatemic rickets. *Am J Dis Child* **145**:1165, 1991.
304. Carpenter TO, Keller M, Schwartz D, Mitnick M, Smith C, Ellison A, Carey D, Comite F, Horst R, Travers R, Glorieux FH, Gundberg CM, Poole AR, Insogna K: 24,25-Dihydroxyvitamin D supplementation corrects hyperparathyroidism and improves skeletal abnormalities in X-linked hypophosphatemic rickets: A clinical research study. *J Clin Endocrinol Metab* **81**:2381, 1996.
305. Hanna JD, Niimi K, Chan JCM: X-linked hypophosphatemia: Genetic and clinical correlates. *Am J Dis Child* **145**:865, 1991.
306. Friedman NE, Lobaugh B, Drezner MK: Effects of calcitriol and phosphorus therapy on the growth of patients with X-linked hypophosphatemia. *J Clin Endocrin Metab* **76**:839, 1993.
307. Saggese G, Baroncelli GI, Bertelloni S, Perri G: Long-term growth hormone treatment in children with renal hypophosphatemic rickets: Effects on growth, mineral metabolism, and bone density. *J Pediatr* **127**:395, 1995.
308. Chesney RW, Mazess RB, Rose P, Hamstra AJ, DeLuca HF, Breed AL: Long-term influence of calcitriol (1,25-dihydroxyvitamin D) and supplemental phosphate in X-linked hypophosphatemic rickets. *Pediatrics* **71**:559, 1983.
309. Weidner N: Review and update: Oncogenic osteomalacia-rickets. *Ultrastruct Pathol* **15**:317, 1991.
310. Uchida H, Yokoyama S, Kashima K, Nakayama I, Shimizu K, Masumi S: Oncogenic vitamin D-resistant hypophosphatemic osteomalacia (benign ossifying mesenchymal tumor of bone): Case report. *Jpn J Clin Oncol* **21**:218, 1991.
311. McGuire MH, Merenda JT, Etzkorn JR, Sundaram M: Oncogenic osteomalacia: A case report. *Clin Orthop* **244**:305, 1989.
312. Schultze G, Delling G, Faensen M, Haubold R, Loy V, Molzahn M, Pommer W, Semler J, Trempenau B: Oncogenic hypophosphatemic osteomalacia. *Dtsch Med Wochenschr* **114**:1073, 1989.
313. Nuovo MA, Dorfman HD, Sun CC, Chalew SA: Tumor-induced osteomalacia and rickets. *Am J Surg Pathol* **13**:588, 1989.
314. Leicht E, Biro G, Langer HJ: Tumor-induced osteomalacia: Pre- and postoperative biochemical findings. *Horm Metab Res* **22**:640, 1990.
315. Bianchine JW, Stambler AA, Harrison HE: Familial hypophosphatemic rickets showing autosomal dominant inheritance. *Birth Defects* **7**:287, 1971.
316. Ryan EA, Reiss E: Oncogenous osteomalacia: Review of the world literature of 42 cases and report of two new cases. *Am J Med* **77**:501, 1984.
317. Miyauchi A, Fukase M, Tsutsumi M, Fujita T: Hemangiopericytoma-induced osteomalacia: Tumor transplantation in nude mice causes hypophosphatemia and tumor extracts inhibit renal 25-hydroxyvitamin D-1-hydroxylase activity. *J Clin Endocrinol Metab* **67**:46, 1988.
318. Econs MJ, Drezner MK: Tumor-induced osteomalacia: Unveiling a new hormone. *New Engl J Med* **330**:1679, 1994.
319. Cai Q, Hodgson SF, Kao PC, Lennon VA, Klee GG, Zinsmiester AR, Kumar R: Brief report: Inhibition of renal phosphate transport by a tumor product in a patient with oncogenic osteomalacia. *New Engl J Med* **330**:1645, 1994.
320. Rowe PSN, Ong ACM, Cockerill FJ, Goulding JN, Hewison M: Candidate 56 and 58 kDa protein(s) responsible for mediating the renal defects in oncogenic hypophosphatemic osteomalacia. *Bone* **18**:159, 1996.
321. Nelson AE, Namkung HJ, Patava J, Wilkinson MR, Chang AC, Reddel RR, Robinson BG, Mason RS: Characteristics of tumor cell bioactivity in oncogenic osteomalacia. *Mol Cell Endocrinol* **124**:17, 1996.
322. Jan de Beur SM, Streeten EA, Civelek AC, et al: Identification of tumors producing oncogenic osteomalacia using somatostatin receptor imaging.. *Endocrine Soc* **P3**:161, 1998.
323. Wilson DR, York SE, Jaworski ZF, Yendt ER: Studies in hypophosphatemic vitamin D-refractory osteomalacia in adults. *Medicine* **44**:99, 1965.
324. David L, Pesso JI, Cochat P, Plauchu H, Francois R: Rachitisme hypophosphatemique autosomique type Scriver: Une observation familiale. *Pediatrie* **42**:563, 1987.
325. Harrison HE, Harrison HC: *Rickets and Osteomalacia: Anonymous Disorders of Calcium and Phosphate Metabolism in Childhood and Adolescence*. Philadelphia, Saunders, 1979, p 141.
326. Cabral JM, Rebello V, Econs MJ, et al: Autosomal domiannt hypophosphatemic rickets with major cranio-facial abnormalities.. *Endocrine Soc* **P3**:548, 1998.
327. Econs MJ, McEnery PT, Lennon F, Speer MC: Autosomal dominant hypophosphatemic rickets is linked to chromosome 12p13. *J Clin Invest* **100**:2653, 1997.
328. Scriver CR, MacDonald W, Reade T, Glorieux FH, Nogrady B: Hypophosphatemic non-rachitic bone disease: An entity distinct from X-linked hypophosphatemia in the renal defect, bone involvement and inheritance. *Am J Med Genet* **1**:101, 1977.
329. Koenig M, Beggs AH, Moyer M, Scherpf S, Heindrich K, Bettecken T, Meng G, Muller CR, Lindlof M, Kaariainen H: The molecular basis for Duchenne versus Becker muscular dystrophy: Correlation of severity with type of deletion. *Am J Hum Genet* **45**:498, 1989.
330. Tieder M, Modai D, Samuel R, Arie R, Halabe A, Bab I, Gabizon D, Lieberman UA: Hereditary hypophosphatemic rickets with hypercalciuria. *New Engl J Med* **312**:611, 1985.
331. Tieder M, Modai D, Shaked U, Samuel R, Arie R, Halabe A, Maor J, Weissgarten J, Averbukh Z, Cohen N, Edelstein S, Lieberman UA: "Idiopathic" hypercalciuria and hereditary hypophosphatemic rickets. *New Engl J Med* **316**:125, 1987.
332. Nishiyama S, Inoue F, Matsuda I: A single case of hypophosphatemic rickets with hypercalciuria. *J Pediatr Gastroenterol Nutr* **5**:826, 1986.
333. Proesmans WC, Fabrey G, Marchal GJ, Gillis PL, Bouillon R: Autosomal dominant hypophosphatemia with elevated serum 1,25-dihydroxyvitamin D and hypercalciuria. *Pediatr Nephrol* **1**:479, 1987.
334. Chen C, Carpenter T, Steg N, Baron R, Anast C: Hypercalciuric hypophosphatemic rickets, mineral balance, bone histomorphometry, and therapeutic implications of hypercalciuria. *Pediatrics* **84**:276, 1989.
335. Tieder M, Arie R, Bab I, Maor J, Liberman UA: A new kindred with hereditary hypophosphatemic rickets with hypercalciuria: Implications for correct diagnosis and treatment. *Nephron* **62**:176, 1992.
336. Gazit D, Tieder M, Liberman UA, Passi-Even L, Bab IA: Osteomalacia in hereditary hypophosphatemic rickets with hypercalciuria: A correlative clinical-histomorphometric study. *J Clin Endocrinol Metab* **72**:229, 1991.
337. Clemens TL, Tang H, Maeda S, Kesterson RA, Demayo F, Pike JW, Gundberg CM: Analysis of osteocalcin expression in transgenic mice reveals a species difference in vitamin D regulation of mouse and human osteocalcin genes. *J Bone Miner Res* **12**:1570, 1997.
337a. Tenenhouse HS: X-linked hypophosphatemia: A homologous disorder in humans and mice. *Nephrol Dial Transplant* **14**:333, 1999.
338. Kinoshita Y, Fukase M, Miyauchi A, Takenaka M, Nakada M, Fujita T: Establishment of a parathyroid hormone-responsive phosphate transport system in vitro using cultured renal cells. *Endocrinology* **119**:1954, 1986.
339. Noronha-Blob L, Sacktor B: Inhibition by glucocorticoids of phosphate transport in primary cultured renal cells. *J Biol Chem* **261**:2164, 1986.

340. Pizurki L, Rizzoli R, Moseley J, Martin TJ, Caverzasio J, Bonjour J-P: Effect of synthetic tumoral PTH-related peptide on cAMP production and Na-dependent P_i transport. *Am J Physiol* **255**:F957, 1988.
341. Nakai M, Fukase M, Kinoshita Y, Fujita T: Atrial natriuretic factor inhibits phosphate uptake in opossum kidney cells: As a model of renal proximal tubules. *Biochem Biophys Res Commun* **152**:1416, 1988.
342. Pizurki L, Rizzoli R, Caverzasio J, Bonjour J-P: Effect of transforming growth factor-α and parathyroid hormone-related protein on phosphate transport in renal cells. *Am J Physiol* **259**:F929, 1990.
343. Law F, Rizzoli R, Bonjour JP: Transforming growth factor-β inhibits phosphate transport in renal epithelial cells. *Am J Physiol* **264**:F623, 1993.
344. Liang CT, Barnes J, Balakir R, Cheng L, Sacktor B: In vitro stimulation of phosphate uptake in isolated chick renal cells by 1,25-dihydroxycholecalciferol. *Proc Natl Acad Sci USA* **79**:3532, 1982.
345. Noronha-Blob L, Lowe V, Sacktor B: Stimulation by thyroid hormone of phosphate transport in primary cultured renal cells. *J Cell Physiol* **137**:95, 1988.
346. Goodyer PR, Kachra Z, Bell C, Rozen R: Renal tubular cells are potential targets for epidermal growth factor. *Am J Physiol* **255**:F1191, 1988.
347. Caverzasio J, Bonjour J-P: Insulin-like growth factor I stimulates Na-dependent P_i transport in cultured kidney cells. *Am J Physiol* **257**:F712, 1989.
348. Abraham MI, McAteer JA, Kempson SA: Insulin stimulates phosphate transport in opossum kidney epithelial cells. *Am J Physiol* **258**:F1592, 1990.
349. Jones A, Tzenova J, Fujiwara TM, Frappier D, Crumley MJ, Roslin N, Kos CH, Tieder M, Langman C, Proesmans W, Carpenter TO, Rice D, Anderson D, Morgan K, Tenehhouse HS: Hereditary hypophosphatemic rickets with hypercalciuria is not caused by mutations in the Na/Pi cotransporter *NPT2 (SLC34A1)* gene. *J Am Soc Nephrol*, in press.

CHAPTER 198

Hereditary Renal Hypouricemia

Oded Sperling

1. **Hereditary renal hypouricemia (MIM 242050 and 307830) is an inborn error of membrane transport, presumably in urate reabsorption in the proximal tubule. It is inherited in an autosomal recessive manner. In homozygotes, it manifests as hypouricemia and increased renal urate clearance. Heterozygosity may be detected by moderately decreased serum urate levels and moderately but significantly increased renal urate clearance.**
2. **Homozygosity is associated with moderate or excessive uricosuria, reflecting the diversion of intestinal urate elimination to urinary urate excretion consequent to the hypouricemia. There is no evidence for purine overproduction. Hypercalciuria, probably of the hyperabsorptive type, is associated with renal hypouricemia in about 20 percent of the propositi. The mechanism for this abnormality is not yet clarified. The hyperuricosuria and/or hypercalciuria are etiologic factors in uric acid or calcium oxalate urolithiasis, occurring in about 25 percent of the propositi.**
3. **Transport of urate through the intestinal wall and through the erythrocyte membrane appears to be normal.**
4. **The differential diagnosis of hereditary renal hypouricemia includes familial conditions, in which the defective renal urate transport is one component in a generalized transport abnormality, such as Hartnup syndrome or the group of diseases with Fanconi renal tubulopathy (Wilson disease, cystinosis, galactosemia, and hereditary fructose intolerance).**
5. **The model of the renal handling of urate in humans includes four components: free glomerular filtration, net early proximal tubular reabsorption (segment S1), net tubular secretion (segment S2), and net postsecretory tubular reabsorption (segment S3). It is assumed that reabsorption and secretion of urate in the proximal tubule occur simultaneously and that the manifestation of net reabsorption or secretion at the various segments reflects different intensities of the two processes. The residual urinary urate in the S1 region derives originally from filtration, whereas that in the S3 segment arises from secretion in the S2 segment.**
6. **Several types of renal hypouricemia may be distinguished, according to the nature and site of the transport defect. The classification is based on present knowledge concerning the renal handling of urate in humans and on the mechanism of action of pyrazinamide (assumed to inhibit specifically urate secretion) and probenecid (assumed to inhibit specifically urate reabsorption at the postsecretory site). In hereditary renal hypouricemia, the most common type appears to be that of a presecretory reabsorption defect. Some of patients may have a total transport defect (no reabsorption, no secretion) or total reabsorption defect. A postsecretory reabsorption defect has not been documented in hereditary renal hypouricemia but was found to characterize acquired renal hypouricemia and familial conditions in which renal hypouricemia is a part of a generalized tubular reabsorption defect (Fanconi syndrome). A hypersecretion defect was suggested in one family with hereditary renal hypouricemia and in three patients with isolated renal hypouricemia without evidence for an hereditary basis.**

A list of standard abbreviations is located immediately preceding the index in each volume. Nonstandard abbreviations used in this chapter include: PAH = *para*-aminohippuric acid; SITS = 4-acetamido-4′-isothiocyanostilbene-2,2′-disulfonic acid; GFR = glomerular filtration rate.

It is common knowledge that a certain proportion of the inborn errors of metabolism in humans represent extremely rare and benign diseases. Yet the discovery and study of such defects are very often of utmost importance in that the work contributes to an understanding of the metabolic pathways or processes occurring in the normal human cell or organ. In humans, the renal handling of urate, the final waste product of purine metabolism, is complex; its exact nature has not been clarified conclusively. Hereditary renal hypouricemia is a rare, almost harmless (except for urolithiasis in some patients), inborn error in membrane urate transport in the kidney. It represents "experiments of nature" in the renal handling of urate in humans, furnishing valuable information on urate handling in the normal kidney. Indeed, the first patient reported to be affected with this syndrome (in 1950), although lacking conclusive evidence for familiality,[1] furnished the first indication of renal tubular secretion of urate in humans. The study of the first group of 28 patients with true hereditary renal hypouricemia, documented between 1972 and 1990 (Table 198-1), provided data supporting the four-component model of the renal handling of urate in humans that is accepted at present. Furthermore, the results of these studies suggested that the two reabsorption components in the model — namely, the presecretory and the postsecretory — are controlled by different genes.

DEFINITION AND DIFFERENTIAL DIAGNOSIS

Hereditary renal hypouricemia refers to the hereditary condition of increased renal urate clearance (see Table 198-2 for normal values) caused by a specific (isolated) inborn error of membrane transport for urate in the renal proximal tubule. Patients with this condition present with hypouricemia, as defined by a serum urate level that is less than 149 μM (2.5 mg/dl) for adult men and less than 125 μM (2.1 mg/dl) for adult women using a colorimetric determination.[2–5] Hereditary renal hypouricemia should be differentiated from other hereditary conditions of renal hypouricemia, in which the urate transport defect is only one component of a generalized disturbance of membrane transport, e.g., Fanconi syndrome[6–8] (see Chap. 196) and Hartnup syndrome[9] (see Chap. 193). It also should be distinguished from genetically determined

Table 198-1 Data on Renal Handling of Urate in Hereditary Renal Hypouricemia

		Propositus					
First author	Year	Age at Diagnosis	Sex	Plasma Urate, μM	Urinary Urate, mmol/24 h	C_{ur}, ml/min	FC_{ur} (C_{ur}/GFR), %
1. Greene[48]	1972	23	M	53	3.80	46	38
2. Khachadurian[49]	1973	57	M	12	4.74	173	148
3. Sperling[50]	1974	53	M	35	4.11	55	70.6
4. Akaoka[51]	1975	28	M	24	4.11	88.5	107.3
5. Akaoka[52]	1977	40	M	32	3.55	99	75
6. Akaoka[52]	1977	41	M	28	3.73	114	95
7. Benjamin[53]	1977	37	F	65	3.94	39.5	37.6
8. Benjamin[54]	1978	48	M	71	4.46	553	38.5
9. Frank[55]	1979	39	M	59	5.95	80	47.9
10. Frank[55]	1979	37	M	59	5.95	60	45
11. Weitz[56]	1980	8	M	41	2.11	35.2	43.7
12. Hedley[57]	1980	63	M	77	6.20	—	169
13. Fujiwara[58]	1980	24	M	53	5.72	74.1	56.8
14. Delevelle[59]	1980	74	M	25	3.13	85	80
15. Garty[60]	1981	10	M	89	1.70	45.8	36
16. Matsuda[61]	1982	43	F	29	3.97	83	91.7
17. Tachibana[62]	1982	35	M	24	—	—	—
18. Vinay[63]	1983	43	F	18	6.19	144	77
19. Takeda[64]	1985	3	F	47	3.94	75	90
20. Takeda[64]	1985	10	M	59	7.79	117	88
21. Takeda[64]	1985	12	F	41	9.10	93	102
22. Takeda[64]	1985	4	M	47	6.79	102	146
23. Nakajima[65]	1987	36	M	119	—	31.2	31.9
24. Shichiri[66]	1987	25	F	12	—	54.9	45.2
25. Shichiri[66]	1987	40	F	55	—	74.6	60.6
26. Hisatome[67]	1989	22	M	65	3.55	31.9	46
27. Gafter[68]	1989	60	F	59	4.79	60.5	65.5
28. Tofuku[69]	1990	16	M	41	4.58	76.4	—

NOTE: Values given for serum urate are lowest or average values reported for each subject. Values given for urinary urate excretion, for urate clearance (C_{ur}), and for FC_{ur} are the highest or average values reported for each subject.

metabolic hypouricemia, such as in xanthinuria[10,11] (see Chap. 111) and in purine nucleoside phosphorylase deficiency[12] (see Chap. 109). In the latter conditions, the decreased production of uric acid due to specific enzyme abnormalities is manifest in very low uric acid levels in both serum and urine.

According to the preceding definition, subjects with persistent hypouricemia with normal or somewhat excessive (see below) urinary excretion of uric acid, i.e., increased renal urate clearance, should be investigated for hereditary renal hypouricemia. Hypouricemia is a relatively rare condition; study of hospital

Table 198-2 Effect of Pyrazinamide and Probenecid on FC_{ur} in Control Subjects and Differentiation by These Effects between the Various Types of Renal Hypouricemia*

		Effect on FC_{ur}, %	
No. of Control Subjects	FC_{ur}%	Pyrazinamide	Probenecid
10[a]	9.8±3.4	Decrease to 2.15±1.7	
14[b]	10.3±4	Decrease to 1.2±1.1	
14[c]	8.2±0.6	Decrease to 1.8	Increase to 40.4±8
10[d]	9.3±2.6	Decrease to 1.13±0.35	
5[e]	8.4±2.7		Increase to 46.7±8.3
Type of Renal Hypouricemia			
A. Total transport defect (reabsorption and secretion)	100	No effect	No effect
B. Total reabsorption defect	>100	Attenuated effect Decreasing FC_{ur} to 100%	No effect
C. Presecretory reabsorption defect	?	Attenuated effect	Attenuated effect
D. Postsecretory reabsorption defect	<100	Normal effect	No effect
E. Increased secretion	<100	Normal effect	Normal effect

* Values represent mean±SD.

SOURCES OF DATA: a = Steele and Rieselbach[162]; b = Tofuku et al.[73]; c = Meisel and Diamond[8] (values represent C_{ur} in ml/min instead of FC_{ur} with 1 g probenecid administered intravenously); d = Akaoka et al.,[52] Kawabe et al.,[71] Fujiwara et al. [58] and Shichiri et al.[74]; e = Fujiwara et al.[58]; Shichiri et al.[74]

populations ranging from 2990 to 27,987 patients revealed a rate of from 0.57 to 1 percent.[13–18] In an apparently normal Japanese population (11,499 subjects), only 0.18 percent could be classified as hypouricemic.[19] The frequency of idiopathic renal hypouricemia is even lower—0.12 percent of 3258 Japanese outpatients.[20] In all reported cases of hereditary renal hypouricemia, the classification of hereditary isolated renal hypouricemia was established by demonstration of heredity and by refuting the presence of other renal tubular reabsorption defects. In order to establish the heredity of the defect, siblings and other family members should be screened for hypouricemia (see "Genetics" below). Finding of an additional affected hypouricemic (homozygous) sibling is proof of heredity. Finding of parents or offspring with intermediate blood levels of uric acid (148–208 μM) associated with significantly increased renal urate clearance may be taken to indicate heterozygosity. When familial renal hypouricemia is established, the isolated type can be verified by ruling out the presence of other tubular abnormalities. The presence of the following hereditary diseases should be excluded: Wilson disease,[21–24] cystinosis,[25] galactosemia,[26] and hereditary fructose intolerance[27] (see Chaps. 70, 72, 126, and 200). All these diseases are associated with the Fanconi syndrome, in which uric acid reabsorption in the proximal tubule is decreased along with reabsorption of other crystalloid solutes. Renal hypouricemia is also part of the Hartnup syndrome, which also should be excluded[9] (see Chap. 193).

Subjects with persistent renal hypouricemia who have no siblings or other relatives may be classified as having suspected hereditary renal hypouricemia if they are proved to have the isolated defect in uric acid transport and when the presence of acquired renal hypouricemia is excluded beyond doubt. Acquired renal hypouricemia may accompany conditions of extracellular fluid volume expansion, such as inappropriate antidiuretic hormone secretion,[28–30] and may be seen in various malignancies, such as multiple myeloma,[31] lymphomas,[32,33] cholangiocarcinoma,[34] metastatic breast cancer,[35] undifferentiated retroperitoneal sarcoma of childhood,[35] and pulmonary neoplasms.[36–39] In some of the neoplasms, the renal hypouricemia is part of a broader, Fanconi-like tubulopathy, whereas in others, like Hodgkin disease, it appears as an isolated defect. In the latter disease, the degree of renal urate clearance was found to correlate with the activity of the neoplastic process.[32,33] Renal hypouricemia also may occur in heavy metal intoxication[40,41] and following use of outdated tetracyclines.[45] In both conditions, the renal hypouricemia is part of a general tubulopathy of the Fanconi syndrome type. It also can occur in liver disease, such as jaundice,[43,44] in which the degree of renal urate clearance was shown to improve (decrease) with recovery, and cirrhosis,[45] in which an inverse correlation was found between serum bilirubin and urate levels. Renal hypouricemia also may be found in juvenile diabetes mellitus.[46,47]

Further support (but by no means proof) for the presence of hereditary renal hypouricemia in subjects with persistent renal hypouricemia who have no evidence for acquired conditions but who lack conclusive evidence for heredity may be obtained by demonstration of the presecretory reabsorption type of defect in renal urate handling. This is so because of the apparently characteristic presence of this type of defect in subjects with hereditary renal hypouricemia (see below).

HISTORY

True hereditary renal hypouricemia, due to an isolated tubular defect for urate transport, was first described in humans by Greene et al.[48] in 1972. This condition was described by Praetorius and Kirk[1] in 1950, but in their patient there was no evidence of genetic transmission. The second true case of hereditary renal hypouricemia was documented in 1973 by Khachadurian and Arslanian.[49] In 1974, Sperling et al.[50] reported a new hereditary syndrome that included hypouricemia, hypercalciuria, and decreased bone density. Since then, until 1990, an additional 25 families have been documented with true hereditary renal hypouricemia.[51–69] Many more cases that could fit in this category were reported,[52,70–77] but the genetic transmission was not established.

RENAL HANDLING OF URATE IN NORMAL HUMANS

Since hereditary renal hypouricemia is believed to be caused by a primary defect in the renal handling of urate, the present knowledge of the normal handling of urate in the human kidney is reviewed first. The exact nature of the renal handling of urate in humans has not been clarified conclusively. This is due in part to the lack of an animal model in which the renal handling of urate is identical to that in humans. Experiments in humans were limited to the study of the effects of urate loading[78,79] and of various drugs[79–82] on uric acid excretion. In addition, important information was furnished by the "experiments of nature"—that is, the inborn defects in renal urate reabsorption, the subject of this chapter. In constructing a plausible model for the renal handling of urate in humans, animal information was selected according to its compatibility with the information obtained for humans. Data were obtained from a wide range of laboratory animals, such as reptiles, rats, dogs, *Cebus* monkeys, and chimpanzees. In these animals, stop-flow, micropuncture, and microperfusion experiments in vivo, as well as vesicle studies in vitro, furnished the basic information on the renal handling of urate and the mechanism of renal urate transport.[83] The species that were found to resemble humans most closely were the chimpanzee and the *Cebus* monkey.[84] The first study on urate transport in the proximal tubule of human kidney was published in 1991[85] (and see below).

Components of Renal Handling of Urate

Glomerular Filtration of Uric Acid. Urate is probably bound to plasma proteins, the amount of binding being approximately 5 to 10 percent.[86,87] However, the data regarding binding are conflicting. Practically, urate is freely filtered at the glomerulus, since the binding of urate to plasma proteins is offset by the plasma negative Gibbs-Donnan potential generated across the glomerular membrane.[88] Indeed, determinations of the concentration of urate in glomerular ultrafiltrate and plasma water indicate that they are almost equal.[89–91]

Reabsorption of Uric Acid. In a number of species, the fraction of filtered urate excreted in the urine is less than 100 percent, indicating net reabsorption. This is true for cats, rats, mongrel dogs, the *Cebus* monkey, certain other monkeys, chimpanzees, and humans.[84] In humans, the fractional clearance of urate, in relation to that of inulin or creatinine, is about 7 to 10 percent, indicating very efficient reabsorption. In all animals in which urate reabsorption has been localized, including the *Cebus* monkey,[92] it was found to occur largely in the proximal tubules, although it is possible that some degree of urate reabsorption may occur in some animals in more distal segments. Urate reabsorption may proceed by two mechanisms: a saturable mediated pathway through the cell and a nonsaturable, noninhibitable pathway across the tight junction.[93] That urate reabsorption is an active transport process is evident from several findings. In free-flow micropuncture studies, the ratio between urate concentration in the proximal tubule fluid and that in plasma was shown to be less than 1.[94] Similar results were obtained also in microperfusion studies.[95] In addition, in nonhuman primates and in humans, diuresis and inhibition of urate secretion by pyrazinoate caused the concentration of urate in urine to approach 10 percent of the plasma concentration.[96] In chimpanzees and monkeys, urate concentration in the tubular fluid was found to be from 20 to 60 percent of plasma urate concentration.[97] The relationship between the active absorption of urate and the intraluminal concentration of urate was found to follow first-order kinetics.[93] The urate reabsorption process was found to be affected by alterations in the reabsorption of sodium[98] but could be dissociated from that of the sodium by pharmacologic agents[99,100] and by expansion of the extracellular fluid volume.[101] That the reabsorption of urate and sodium is not linked intimately also was confirmed in vesicle studies.[102,103] Studies in rats in vivo and in vesicles in vitro demonstrated that urate reabsorption is inhibited by a number of substances, such as probenecid, furosemide, *para*-aminohippuric acid (PAH) and the anion exchange inhibitors 4-acetamido-4′-isothiocyanostilbene-2,2′-disulfonic acid (SITS), and 4,4′-diisothiocyanostilbene-2,2′-disulfonic acid and thus that urate reabsorption is mediated by an anion-exchange mechanism.

Secretion of Uric Acid. The first evidence for tubular urate secretion in humans was found in 1950,[1] in the first subject with renal hypouricemia, in whom the fractional urate clearance (FC_{ur}, urate:inulin clearance ratio) was 1.46. This early evidence for the bidirectional tubular transport of urate was augmented subsequently by studies in humans, in which the FC_{ur} was increased artificially to as high as 1.23 by use of urate loading, mannitol diuresis, and probenecid.[79] In humans, the exact localization of urate secretion has not been established conclusively. In one study,[104] the proximal nephron was found to transport urate to the tubular fluid, whereas the distal nephron was unable to do so. Net secretion of urate occurs in many species, such as birds, reptiles, guinea pigs, Dalmatian coach hounds, some individual rabbits, and certain species of monkeys. In virtually all these animals, there is evidence for bidirectional urate transport. In rats, urate secretion occurs by both saturable transcellular and nonsaturable paracellular pathways.[105] The relationship between the mediated secretory flux of urate and the urate concentration in the peritubular capillaries demonstrates first-order kinetics.[105] In vivo microperfusion and microinjection studies indicated that, similar to the reabsorption of urate, the secretory process is a result of an anion-exchange mechanism. The secretory flux of urate was inhibited by probenecid, *p*-chloromercuribenzoate, SITS, PAH, and pyrazinoate.[105–107] Accordingly, it was concluded that the secretory urate exchanger has affinity for PAH and pyrazinoate. Several experiments indicated the presence of an uphill transport step for urate in the rat proximal tubule, probably at the basolateral membrane. When rat kidney slices were incubated in a medium containing urate, the slice-to-medium urate ratio was 0.71.[108] Intravenous loading of rats with urate accompanied by administration of the uricase inhibitor oxonate resulted in a mean fractional delivery of urate to the early proximal tubule of 130 percent.[94] Also in the rabbit, an uphill transport site for urate secretion was firmly implicated in the proximal tubule[109,110] at the basolateral membrane.[108,111] An interesting finding in rabbits is that urate secretion is modulated by a serum protein that affects the basolateral transporter by allosteric modification.[110] This finding may be taken to suggest that abnormalities in renal urate handling also may reflect primary defects in such modulators of secretion or reabsorption (see below). In rabbits, urate secretion was demonstrated to increase markedly with plasma urate concentration.[112,113]

Urate Transport in the Proximal Tubule of the Human Kidney. New data were obtained recently concerning the transport mechanisms of urate in the human proximal tubule.[85,114–117] Studies employing human brush-border membrane vesicles demonstrated that urate is not cotransported with sodium but by a voltage-sensitive pathway and by two urate/anion exchangers. One of the exchangers is less specific, accepting monovalent anions such as lactate, ketone bodies, nicotinate, pyrazinoate, and chloride, whereas the other is more specific, accepting only aromatic compounds, nicotinate, pyrazinoate, and orotate. Hydroxyl ions and PAH were not accepted by the two exchangers. Uricosuric drugs and orotate cis-inhibited urate exchange for lactate or chloride and pyrazinoate cis-inhibited urate exchange for chloride but enhanced its exchange for lactate. Orotate and pyrazinoate, when loaded into brush-border membrane vesicles, stimulated urate uptake. The data obtained for the basolateral membranes are limited, but they indicate that urate is transported through a voltage-sensitive pathway for which PAH has no affinity.[115] The results of these studies were interpreted to suggest that an increase in proximal cell content of substrates for the exchange mechanism should result in enhanced reabsorption.[114,115] Indeed, this may be the mechanism causing the decreased uricosuria in hyperlacticacidemia and in diabetic ketoacidosis, due to the increase in the proximal cell content of acetoacetate and β-hydroxybutyrate. The data concerning the effect of pyrazinoate on urate reabsorption may have significant implications concerning our understanding of the renal handling of urate in humans (see below in the section on the effect of pyrazinamide and probenecide on FC_{ur}).

A Model for Urate Transport. The studies with renal brush-border and basolateral membrane vesicles from rats and brush-border vesicles from dogs[113,118–124] led Kahn and Weinman[88] to construct a model for the bidirectional transport of urate in the proximal tubules of rats. According to this model (Fig. 198-1), urate reabsorption from the lumen to the cell is mediated by the brush-border anion exchanger, exchanging urate for intracellular anions. Anions such as hydroxyl or bicarbonate are above electrochemical equilibrium within the cell; thus their exchange with urate allows uphill reabsorption of urate. Other anions—such as lactate, pyruvate, and succinate—also may exchange with urate. These anions either may be produced in the cell or may be transported from the lumen via a sodium cotransport system. The transport of urate from the cell into the interstitium could occur by simple diffusion or through an anion-exchange mechanism (e.g., for chloride). According to this model of urate reabsorption, compounds such as probenecid, PAH, and furosemide inhibit urate reabsorption from the lumen to the proximal tubule cell by blocking the brush-border anion exchanger. In the secretion process, urate transport from plasma to cell through the basolateral membrane is mediated via anion exchange with cellular chloride or other anions not yet identified. These cellular anions should be above electrochemical equilibrium with respect to the interstitium to allow uphill urate secretion. Another transport mechanism that could mediate uphill urate transport from interstitium to the cell is a sodium-urate transport system. However, this system has not as

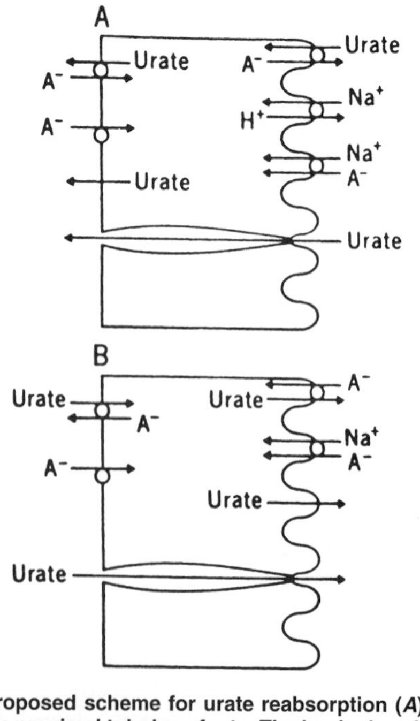

Fig. 198-1 Proposed scheme for urate reabsorption (*A*) and secretion (*B*) in the proximal tubules of rats. The luminal surface is to the right. (*From Kahn and Weinman.[88] Used by permission.*)

yet been demonstrated. The flux of urate from the tubule cell to the lumen could occur by simple diffusion or could be mediated by an anion exchanger, most likely with chloride.

Models for Urate Handling in Humans

Studies on renal handling of urate in humans generated models of a two-, a three-, and finally a four-component system. The first model, suggested in 1950 by Berliner et al.,[78] included glomerular filtration followed by extensive, though incomplete, tubular reabsorption. Eleven years later, following the demonstration of uric acid secretion in humans, this third component was added by Gutman and Yu.[125] More recently, a fourth component, that of postsecretory reabsorption, was added in order to explain the effects of pyrazinamide in some patients or conditions that otherwise, according to the three-component model, could only be interpreted as enhanced tubular secretion of urate. These effects of pyrazinamide included the suppression of the increased uric acid clearance in patients with Wilson disease[24] and Hodgkin disease[32,33] and the suppression in normal subjects, by pretreatment with pyrazinamide, of the probenecid-induced uricosuria, of the uricosuric response to intravenous chlorothiazide,[125] and of the increased urate clearance in volume expansion associated with hypertonic sodium chloride administration.[126] The four-component model (Fig. 198-2) was suggested in 1973 by Steele and Boner,[127] Steele,[128] and Diamond and Paolino[129] and in 1974 by Rieselbach and Steele.[130] It includes glomerular filtration, early proximal reabsorption, later proximal secretion, and extensive postsecretory reabsorption, which could occur at the same location as the secretion, separate and distal to it, or both. Evidence for the existence of the postsecretory reabsorption site with a different mechanism than that of the presecretory reabsorption site was obtained in several patients with renal hypouricemia (see below), in whom the increased urate clearance was attributed to a defect in postsecretory reabsorption.[8,24,32,131,132]

Another model has been proposed[133] (Fig. 198-3). It is similar to the former model, including the same four components, but according to which, reabsorption and secretion of urate occur simultaneously along all the proximal tubule, each at different

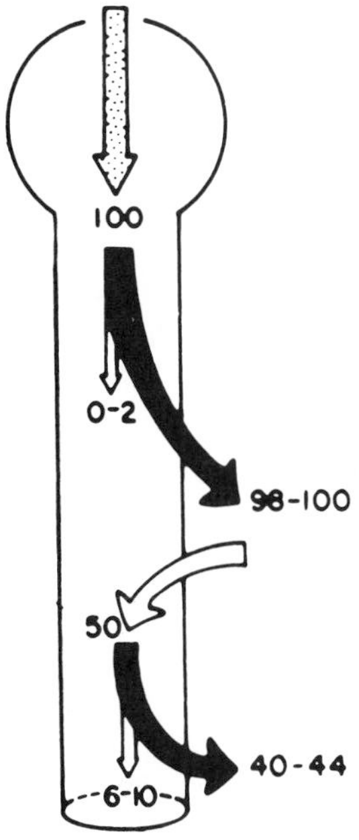

Fig. 198-2 Model for the renal handling of urate in humans. The size and direction of arrows indicate intensity and direction of urate transport. The stippled arrow represents filtered urate; the solid arrow, urate reabsorption; and the open arrow, urate secretion or urate remaining in tubular fluid after reabsorption. Numerical values indicate hypothetical orders of magnitude of the transport processes. (*From Rieselbach and Steele.*[130] *Used by permission.*)

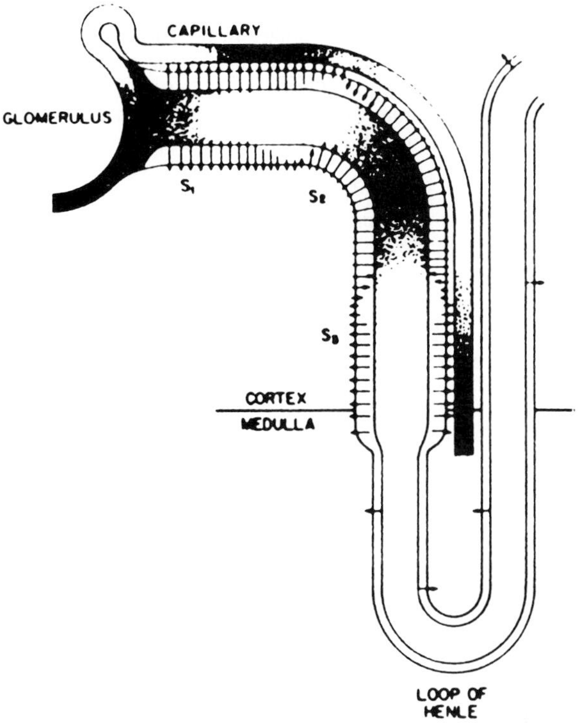

Fig. 198-3 Model of renal handling of urate in humans. The size and direction of arrows indicate intensity and direction of urate transport. The density of shading in the tubule and the capillary indicates the relative amounts of urate (not concentration) in the lumina; see text for details. (*From Grantham and Chonko.*[133] *Used by permission.*)

intensities at the different segments of the tubule. The model suggests a higher density of reabsorption transporters at the S1 segment, as compared with S2 and S3, and a higher intensity of secretion at the S2 region of the tubule. These differences in the intensities of reabsorption and secretion along the tubule result in initial net reabsorption of urate in the S1 segment, followed by net secretion in the S2 segment and by net reabsorption in the S3 segment. According to both models, the residual urinary urate in the S1 region is derived originally from filtration, whereas that in the S3 segment arises from secretion in the S2 segment.

Factors That Affect Renal Handling of Urate in Humans

Age and Sex. Urate excretion becomes less efficient with age.[134–136] Accordingly, plasma urate levels increase with age. This change with maturation was attributed to increased urate reabsorption rather than to a decrease in urate secretion.[136] The mean clearance of urate is 1.2 to 2.3 ml/min higher in females than in males.[137,138] Exogenous estrogen was found to produce a significant increase in urate clearance in transsexual males.[139]

Extracellular Fluid Volume and Urine Flow Rate. The extracellular fluid volume or, more precisely, the volume of the effective arterial circulation is one of the most dominant factors in renal urate handling.[98,140–146] Volume expansion (like that associated with administration of isotonic or hypertonic saline) increases urate clearance, whereas volume contraction (like that associated with restricted sodium chloride intake) decreases urate clearance. Presumably, these effects of changes in extracellular volume are mediated through alterations in urate reabsorption in the proximal tubule.[98,143,144] The rate of urinary flow affects urinary urate concentration and therefore may affect the back-diffusion of urate in the relatively impermeable terminal renal tubules.[145,146] Nevertheless, these effects are probably minor in relation to those of the extracellular fluid volume, as can be judged from the values of renal urate clearance in patients with inappropriate secretion of antidiuretic hormone and in patients with nephrogenic diabetes insipidus. In the former patients with expanded extracellular fluid volume, renal urate clearance is high despite slow urinary flow rate.[28,29,147] In the latter patients with contracted extracellular fluid volume, urinary urate clearance is decreased despite rapid urinary flow rate.[148]

Insulin. Recent data[149,150] indicate that hyperinsulinemia in healthy subjects (physiologic hyperinsulinemia) decreases renal urate clearance, probably by affecting a site beyond the proximal tubule.

Drugs. Many drugs affect renal urate excretion.[133,151] A biphasic effect (different effect at low and high concentrations of the drug) was documented for some of the drugs and suggested for all others.[151] Pyrazinamide, probenecid, phenylbutazone, and salicylate inhibit urate secretion at low doses but inhibit urate reabsorption at high doses.[90,125,152,153] Diuretic drugs are initially uricosuric by direct inhibition of urate reabsorption, but their long-term administration is associated with contraction of the extracellular fluid volume, resulting in antiuricosuria.[125,154–158] An additional property of some of the diuretic drugs is their tendency to compete with tubular urate secretion, decreasing urate excretion further.[156]

RENAL HANDLING OF URATE IN HEREDITARY RENAL HYPOURICEMIA

Renal Clearance of Urate

The data on the renal handling of urate in the propositi of the first 28 families documented to be affected with the true hereditary renal hypouricemia (1972–1990) are summarized in Table 198-1. As can be seen from the table, all the propositi have significantly decreased plasma urate levels, ranging from 12 to 119 μM. In almost all cases, these markedly low serum urate values were found during investigation for unrelated medical problems (to exclude urolithiasis; see below). Urinary urate excretion in the propositi is normal or excessive, renal urate clearance is markedly elevated (ranging from 39.5–173 ml/min), and the fractional clearance of urate (FC_{ur}) ranges from 36 to 169 percent. However, the FC_{ur} was found to exceed 100 percent in only 4 of the 28 propositi. Twenty of the propositi were males, and eight were females; their ages at diagnosis ranged from 3 to 74 years.

The group of subjects with renal hypouricemia in whom no conclusive evidence for heredity could be obtained[1,52,70–77] had similar levels of uric acid in serum and urine as in the propositi with the familial disorder.

Two normouricemic subjects were reported[72,82] to have a renal defect for uric acid handling, which was manifested as increased renal urate clearance only under conditions of purine load. The heredity of this type of defect in the renal handling of urate was not clarified.

Nature of the Renal Transport Defect

Increased renal urate clearance could be caused by defective reabsorption or by increased secretion. Based on the models of urate transport in the proximal tubule (see Fig. 198-1) and of renal handling of urate in humans (see Figs. 198-2 and 198-3), as presented earlier, five main possibilities of specific abnormalities in the active urate transport processes should be considered as causing renal hypouricemia (Fig. 198-4):

A. Total transport defect (no reabsorption and no secretion)
B. Total reabsorption defect
C. Presecretory reabsorption defect
D. Postsecretory reabsorption defect
E. Increased secretion

Being an inborn error, this classification depends, of course, on the genetic control of each of the active transport processes. Accordingly, possibility A is based on the assumption of a common genetic control for all transport processes (i.e., reabsorption and secretion of urate in the renal proximal tubules reflect only inverse positioning of the same mechanism), possibility B on the assumption of a common genetic control for all reabsorption processes, and possibilities C and D on the assumption of separate genetic control for the two reabsorption processes.

Effect of Pyrazinamide and of Probenecid on FC_{ur}. According to the simple model of the renal handling of urate in humans, as depicted in Fig. 198-2, one may distinguish between the preceding types of transport defects by use of drugs inhibiting urate

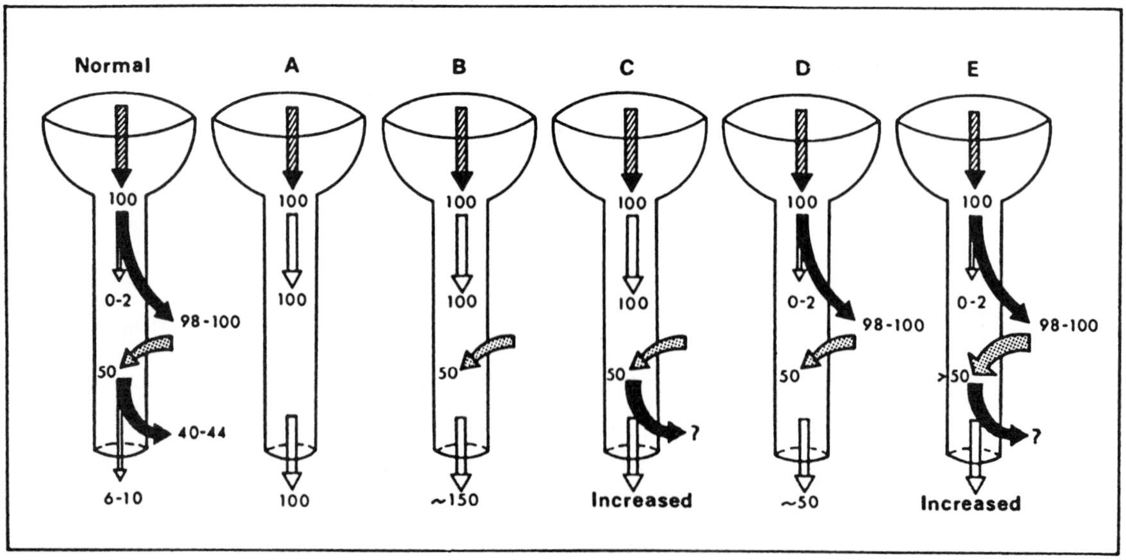

Fig. 198-4 Model for the renal handling of urate in normal humans and the five possible defects (A to E) that may cause renal hypouricemia. See text for detailed explanation. The size and direction of arrows indicate intensity and direction of urate transport. The hatched arrows represent filtered urate; the solid arrows, urate reabsorption; the dotted arrows, urate secretion; and the open arrows, urate remaining in the tubular fluid after reabsorption. Numerical values indicate hypothetical order of magnitude of the transport process. The normal model is based on the model suggested by Rieselbach and Steele.[130] *(From Sperling, Contributions to Nephrology, 100:1, 1992. Used by permission from Karger, Basel)*

reabsorption or secretion. Two drugs, probenecid and pyrazinamide, are employed in the localization of the tubular defect in renal hypouricemia. Probenecid is the generic name for 4-[(dipropylamino)sulfonyl] benzoic acid, which has a dual action on urinary urate excretion. When administered by the oral or intravenous route, at the usual "high" doses, it increases renal urate clearance markedly[48,132,159] (see Table 198-2). On the other hand, at "low" doses, the drug causes a so-called paradoxical urate retention.[159] While the increase of renal urate clearance with high doses of probenecid appears to be due solely to inhibition of tubular reabsorption, the paradoxical urate retention with low doses has been explained by inhibition of tubular secretion. In any event, the net effect of a high probenecid dose (2–3 g orally) is a substantial rise in urate excretion. There are several reasons for the assumption that probenecid inhibits tubular urate reabsorption chiefly at the postsecretory site. First, in the plasma, probenecid is largely bound to albumin[160]; thus the amount filtered is relatively small. Second, probenecid appears in the urine chiefly by tubular secretion, possibly by the same mechanism as uric acid.[161] The tubular secretion of probenecid would explain both its paradoxical urate-retaining action (at low doses) by competition with urate at the secretory site and its reabsorption inhibitory action (at high dose) at a postsecretory tubular site.

Whether and to what extent probenecid also inhibits presecretory tubular reabsorption are still an open question. Evidently, the manyfold increase in urate clearance in response to probenecid in normal subjects is compatible with the dominance of postsecretory absorption in the normal regulation of renal urate excretion. On the other hand, in subjects with renal hypouricemia, the probenecid response should be attenuated, its magnitude depending on the tubular site of the defect, whether postsecretory or presecretory or both. In the case in which the defect is exclusively postsecretory and complete (type D), probenecid will have no effect on urinary urate excretion. However, in cases in which the defect is presecretory (type C), the probenecid response will be maintained but may be of lesser magnitude than normal. When the defect in tubular urate reabsorption is combined presecretory and postsecretory (type B), the probenecid response will be nil.

The separation between the reabsorption sites, as well as the very existence of the postsecretory site, was postulated according to data obtained by the use of pyrazinamide, although the exact effect of this drug on renal urate handling is still under dispute. Following administration of pyrazinamide, urinary uric acid is transiently reduced to very low levels without a change in the glomerular filtration rate (GFR)[162,163] (see Table 198-2). This effect may be attributed to inhibition of urate secretion, a property demonstrated for this drug in dogs[164] and rats.[165] Indeed, this property has been used extensively as a pharmacologic aid in quantitating urate reabsorption and secretion. The pyrazinamide suppression test in humans[128] is based on the assumption that pyrazinamide blocks completely and specifically only urate secretion. It is performed by determining uric acid excretion before and immediately after administration of pyrazinamide, in a dose sufficient to give maximal suppression of uric acid excretion (usually 3 g, administered orally). The difference between the amount of urate filtered and that excreted under maximal effect of the drug is taken to represent urate reabsorption, which was found to be 98 to 99 percent complete in normal humans. On the other hand, the decrement in uric acid excretion, observed under maximal effect of pyrazinamide, is taken to represent tubular urate secretion. The latter was found to account for 80 to 85 percent of excreted urate in normal subjects.[162,166] Data obtained in vivo and in vitro indicate, however, that attribution of the suppression of uric acid excretion by pyrazinamide to a specific effect of blocking tubular urate secretion is an oversimplification. Evidence was first obtained that the effect of pyrazinamide depends on its concentration and that at high concentrations it also inhibits urate reabsorption, increasing urate excretion.[167] Support for the dual effect of the drug was indicated by the findings that pyrazinamide inhibited the precession of [^{14}C]urate relative to [^{3}H]inulin into the urine when both compounds were injected simultaneously into a peritubular capillary[106] and that pyrazinoate inhibited the reabsorption of [^{14}C]urate injected into the rat proximal tubule.[168] In addition to its inhibitory effect on urate reabsorption and secretion, pyrazinamide also was found to enhance urate reabsorption.[169] Thus the suppression effect of pyrazinamide on urate excretion may reflect both inhibition of urate secretion and enhancement of urate reabsorption. Studies in isolated membranes have indicated that pyrazinoate has affinity for the urate anion exchanger in the brush-border membrane.[103,122,170] Accordingly, when in the lumen this drug will inhibit urate reabsorption, but when in the cell it will enhance urate reabsorption. These effects have been demonstrated in studies with dog brush-border vesicles.[88] In view of the new data concerning the effect of pyrazinamide on urate transport in the human proximal tubule,[114–117] the administration of pyrazinamide also should result in enhancement of urate reabsorption. This is so because pyrazinoate can enter the proximal cell, due to the activity of the sodium-pyrazinoate cotransport mechanism, and because pyrazinoate is a favorable substrate for the urate exchanger. Accordingly, the pyrazinamide-induced strong decrease in urate excretion should be considered to reflect enhanced reabsorption rather than inhibition of urate secretion. This new interpretation of the pyrazinamide effect, if correct, will necessitate complete reevaluation of the four-component model of the renal handling of urate in the human, since this model was based mainly on the interpretation of the pyrazinamide effect as a reflection of the inhibition of urate secretion.[128] For the same reason, the presently used algorithm for the classification of the hypouricemic patients to subgroups A to E (see Table 198-2) also will need to be reevaluated.

In view of the foregoing data, the interpretation of the pyrazinamide effect in normal subjects, as well as in subjects with increased renal urate clearance, should be done with reservation and should be regarded as tentative. Nevertheless, for the purpose of classification of patients with renal hypouricemia into the various types (A–E), the pyrazinamide response is still interpreted to reflect mainly the inhibitory effect of the drug on tubular urate secretion, even though the magnitude of the response need not be an exact measure of it. In normal subjects in whom tubular secretion is the main source of urinary urate, pyrazinamide response is expected to be of great magnitude (see Table 198-2). On the other hand, in subjects with increased urate clearance due to a defect in tubular urate reabsorption, the pyrazinamide response could vary according to the site of the defect, whether presecretory or postsecretory. In case of a postsecretory defect in urate reabsorption (type D), pyrazinamide will markedly reduce urinary urate excretion, bringing it to a level similar to that reached in pyrazinamide-treated normal subjects. In the case of a presecretory defect (type C), however, the pyrazinamide response will be attenuated. In the case of combined presecretory and postsecretory defective tubular urate reabsorption (type B), in which the clearance of urate exceeds the GFR, pyrazinamide will reduce the elevated urate clearance to a value close or equal to GFR. In patients with a total transport defect (type A), pyrazinamide will have no effect, but in case of increased secretion (type E), the effect of the drug will be normal.

According to the preceding considerations on renal urate handling and the action of pyrazinamide and probenecid, the five types of renal hypouricemia would be expected to conform to the following responses (see Table 198-2): In a total transport defect (type A), FC_{ur} should be about 100 percent, and this value should not be altered by administration of pyrazinamide or probenecid. In a total reabsorption defect (type B)—i.e., absence of reabsorption at both the presecretory and postsecretory sites but presence of normal secretion—FC_{ur} should be greater than 100 percent. In such a defect, blocking secretion by pyrazinamide will result in an attenuated decrease in FC_{ur}, which should approach 100 percent. Administration of probenecid will not alter FC_{ur}. In a presecretory reabsorption defect (type C), FC_{ur} cannot be estimated, since the maximal rate for net tubular absorption (T_m) for urate at the postsecretory site is unknown. If indeed the excreted urate represents the amount of secreted urate escaping reabsorption at the postsecretory reabsorption site, one can expect a substantial proportion, probably the majority of the filtered load (not reabsorbed at the presecretory site), to escape the postsecretory reabsorption too. If this is the case, then FC_{ur} in a presecretory reabsorption defect will be greater than 100 percent. In a presecretory reabsorption defect, administration of pyrazinamide will decrease FC_{ur} and administration of probenecid will increase this parameter, but both effects will be attenuated. In defective reabsorption at the postsecretory site (type D), FC_{ur} will be less than 100 percent if the amount secreted is less than that filtered. In the presence of such a defect, administration of pyrazinamide will decrease FC_{ur} to normal levels, but administration of probenecid will have no effect. In the case of a defect manifested in increased secretion (type E), FC_{ur} probably will be less than 100 percent (unless the secretion is increased to such a level that its fraction escaping reabsorption will exceed the amounts of filtered urate). In such a defect, the administration of pyrazinamide and probenecid will result in a normal response.

Type of Defect in Hereditary Renal Hypouricemia

Of the 28 propositi reviewed in Table 198-1, the greatest proportion — 15 subjects — had FC_{ur} values between 36 and 85 percent and exhibited an attenuated response to the administration of pyrazinamide and probenecid. These propositi[48,50,52–56,58,59,61,67–69] may be classified as type C — affected with presecretory reabsorption defect. In some of these subjects,[55–57] the effect of pyrazinamide was somewhat greater than in the others, but the lowest FC_{ur} values, obtained under the maximal effect of the drug, did not reach the normal level,[61] and 3 studied by Takeda et al.[64] had FC_{ur} values close to 100 percent, which were not affected significantly by administration of pyrazinamide and probenecid. These 6 subjects may fit with either type C or type A. In only 3 of the propositi, FC_{ur} values were clearly greater than 100 percent. In 2 of them, the pyrazinamide and probenecid tests were not done. In the third patient, a 4-year-old Japanese boy,[64] the tests were done, but under different conditions than those adopted by all other investigators. In this boy, pyrazinamide had almost no effect, whereas benzbromarone (employed instead of probenecid) had an inverse effect, decreasing FC_{ur}. This case could fit with a total reabsorption defect (type B). Two brothers reported by Nakajima et al.[65] exhibited a normal response to pyrazinamide and probenecid and, therefore, were classified with type E (increased secretion). Two subjects reported by Shichiri et al.[66] exhibited resistance to both pyrazinamide and probenecid administration and, therefore, were suggested to represent a subtotal defect in urate transport (subtotal type A). None of the propositi could be classified conclusively with type D. Thus, of the 22 propositi studied for the effects of the drugs, 14 definitely could be classified with type C (presecretory reabsorption defect), 6 with type C or type A (total transport defect), 1 with type B (total reabsorption defect), 1 with type A, and 1 with type E. None of the propositi could be classified with type D (postsecretory reabsorption defect). In the subject reported by Hisatome et al.,[171] renal urate clearance exhibited resistance to both pyrazinamide and probenecid, similar to the 2 subjects reported by Shichiri et al.,[66] justifying classification as type A (subtotal). However, since urate clearance in this patient also did not respond to furosemide or to prednisolone, the patient was suggested to have a drug-resistant rather than defective secretion mechanism.

Nature of the Defect in Other Conditions of Renal Hypouricemia

The pyrazinamide and probenecid tests were done in patients with the Fanconi syndrome,[8] Wilson disease,[24] Hodgkin disease,[32,33] and hyperparathyroidism.[132] In some of these patients the renal hypouricemia was part of a generalized tubular reabsorption defect, such as in the Fanconi syndrome, whereas in the others it represented an isolated defect. Interestingly, most, if not all, of these subjects could be classified as type D (postsecretory reabsorption defect), which was not found in the subjects with hereditary isolated renal hypouricemia. One subject with Hodgkin disease was classified as type D,[33] but two other subjects with Hodgkin disease exhibited a normal response to pyrazinamide and were classified as having increased secretion.[32] Nevertheless, the probenecid effect was not studied in these patients; therefore, the normal pyrazinamide effect also could be interpreted to reflect a postsecretory reabsorption defect. A study of a series of 14 patients with renal hypouricemia associated with type I diabetes mellitus suggested that the increased urate clearance in these patients reflects defective urate reabsorption at both the pre- and postsecretory urate reabsorption sites.[46] The subjects reported with isolated renal hypouricemia but without proof for heredity represent a heterogeneous group. One of these subjects[73] could be classified as type D. Three subjects[74,75] could be classified as type E. They had moderately increased FC_{ur} values, which were normally affected by both pyrazinamide and probenecid or sulfinpyrazone.[75] Three such subjects, studied by Gaspar et al.,[77] exhibited a normal response to pyrazinamide and were classified as affected with impaired postsecretory reabsorption. An additional subject in this group, who demonstrated a normal response to pyrazinamide but also the usual response to probenecid, was classified as affected with enhanced tubular secretion. In two other subjects, studied by Shichiri et al.,[172] administration of probenecid and pyrazinamide did not affect FC_{ur}. These subjects were classified, therefore, as type A — i.e., with total transport defect, including both reabsorption and secretion. Only three of the subjects[73,76] could be classified as type C, the most common type in the group with hereditary renal hypouricemia. In the rest of the subjects of this group, the results of the pyrazinamide and probenecid tests did not allow classification.

In the two normouricemic subjects in whom increased FC_{ur} was found only following purine load,[72,82] the effect of pyrazinamide was normal. In one of these subjects,[72] the defect was suggested to be at the postsecretory reabsorption site, in view of an attenuated response of FC_{ur} to administration of benzbromarone (given instead of probenecid). In the other subject,[82] a high rate of secretion was demonstrated following RNA administration, but the probenecid test was not performed.

The preceding data may be taken to suggest that type C, the presecretory reabsorption defect, is the most common (if not the only type) among subjects with hereditary (isolated) renal hypouricemia, whereas type D (postsecretory reabsorption defect) is the most common in patients with acquired renal hypouricemia and in patients with hereditary renal hypouricemia associated with a generalized renal tubular reabsorption defect. According to the foregoing discussion, in subjects who from all possible aspects appear to be affected with the true hereditary renal hypouricemia but who lack proof for heredity, demonstration of a presecretory reabsorption defect may be taken to support this classification, whereas demonstration of the postsecretory reabsorption defect may be taken to refute it.

Urate Transport in Nonrenal Tissues

Assuming that deletion of a specific carrier is the primary abnormality leading to the defective reabsorption of urate in the renal tubule of subjects with hereditary renal hypouricemia, the tissue specificity of this defect was investigated.[63,173]

Erythrocytes. Uric acid transport into normal human erythrocytes has been shown to be partially inhibited by hypoxanthine,[174] and this is presumed to represent active uric acid transport mediated by an enzymatic system. This active system was suggested to be lacking in the Dalmatian coach hound[175] but was found later to be normal in these dogs.[63] Uric acid transport into erythrocytes was studied in five hypouricemic subjects.[63,173]

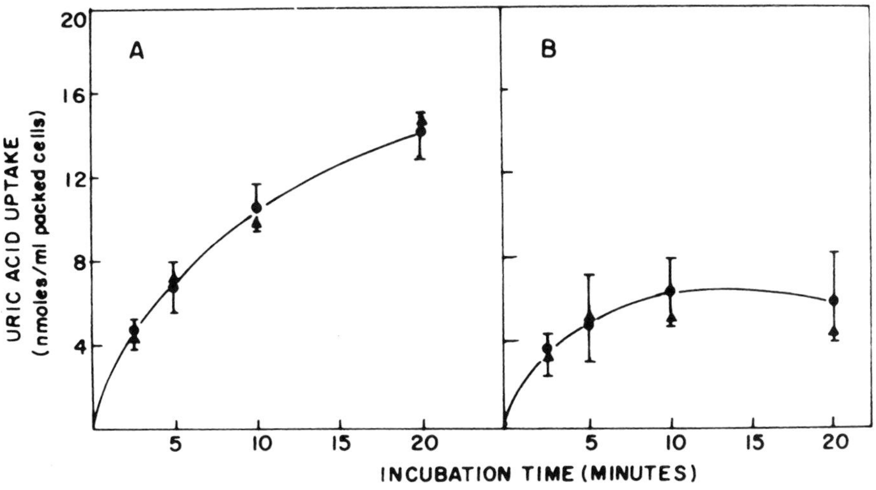

Fig. 198-5 Uptake of uric acid by erythrocytes. The range and mean for five normal subjects (•) and the mean of two experiments for a patient with renal hypouricemia (▲) are presented. A. Total uptake. B. Hypoxanthine-inhibited uptake. (*From Sperling et al.*[173] *Used by permission from Masson.*)

In all these subjects, urate uptake by the erythrocytes — total uptake as well as that inhibited by hypoxanthine — was normal (Figs. 198-5 and 198-6). The lack of expression of the transport defect in the erythrocytes is expected, since to my knowledge the respective transport defect cannot be demonstrated in erythrocytes in any of the known renal tubular transport disorders.

Intestine. Active urate transport through the normal intestinal wall has not been demonstrated.[176,177] Nevertheless, the intestinal uptake of urate was studied in one hypouricemic subject,[173] since genetically determined renal transport defects are often expressed also in the intestinal mucosa, as in cystinuria,[178] iminoglycinuria,[179] and the Hartnup syndrome.[180] The intestinal absorption of uric acid was gauged by the 7 days' cumulative urinary excretion of ^{14}C, following oral administration of [^{14}C]urate (in the presence of bacteriostasis). The value in the hypouricemic subject was similar to that obtained in two control subjects (Fig. 198-7). The apparently accelerated urinary excretion of labeled uric acid in the patient may be taken to reflect his or her increased uric acid clearance.

Presence of an Endogenous Uricosuric Agent

In all the preceding considerations, the existence of an inborn primary renal tubular urate transport defect was presumed. However, in making this assumption and the preceding interpretations as to the location of the tubular defect, caution should be exercised in view of the possibility that the renal tubular abnormalities may be secondary to an abnormal metabolite produced elsewhere in the body or to qualitative or quantitative alterations in modulators affecting urate transport processes. The presence of a humoral uricosuric factor may be possible in some conditions with acquired renal hypouricemia, in which the transitory nature of the defect was demonstrated. In Hodgkin disease, serum uric acid and renal uric acid clearance became normal following chemotherapy, but the hypouricemia and increased renal clearance of urate reappeared with recrudescence of disease.[33] Similarly, in severe burns, the increased renal urate clearance was found to decrease to normal with recovery.[181] Nevertheless, there is no experimental evidence to date for the presence of a uricosuric agent in the plasma of patients with acquired or hereditary renal hypouricemia. Infusing the plasma of a hypouricemic patient with Hodgkin disease into a *Cebus albifrons* monkey did not affect urate clearance.[182] Furthermore, unpublished studies in our laboratory in rabbit kidney slices failed to detect any abnormal uricosuric agent in the plasma of several subjects with renal hypouricemia.

The Dalmatian Coach Hound. This breed of dogs differs from others in that it is relatively hyperuricemic and hyperuricosuric and exhibits increased renal urate clearance.[183–190] The relative hyperuricemia-hyperuricosuria in this breed of dogs was demonstrated to reflect a defective uric acid transport into hepatocytes, the uricase-containing tissue.[191] On the other hand, the reason for the increased renal urate clearance has not yet been clarified. It could reflect a urate transport defect in the kidney or in all tissues.[183,192] Moreover, data are available suggesting that the increased renal urate clearance in this breed of dog reflects the presence of a uricosuric substance produced in the Dalmatian liver. The results of liver transplantation experiments performed by Kuster et al.[192,193] support this hypothesis. These investigators

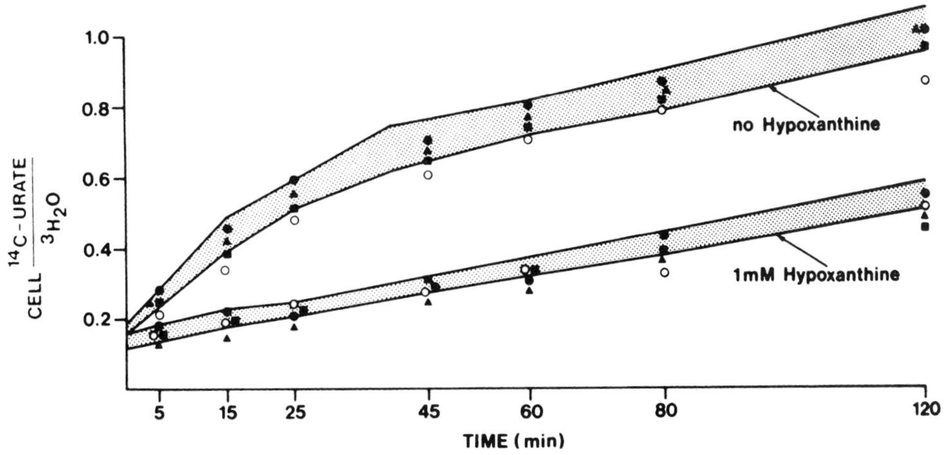

Fig. 198-6 Transport of urate into erythrocytes. The transport is the ratio of ^{14}C-labeled urate space to tritiated water space, with and without hypoxanthine in the buffer. Hatched areas represent ranges for normal controls; symbols represent values for four hypouricemic patients. (*From Vinay et al.*[63] *Used by permission.*)

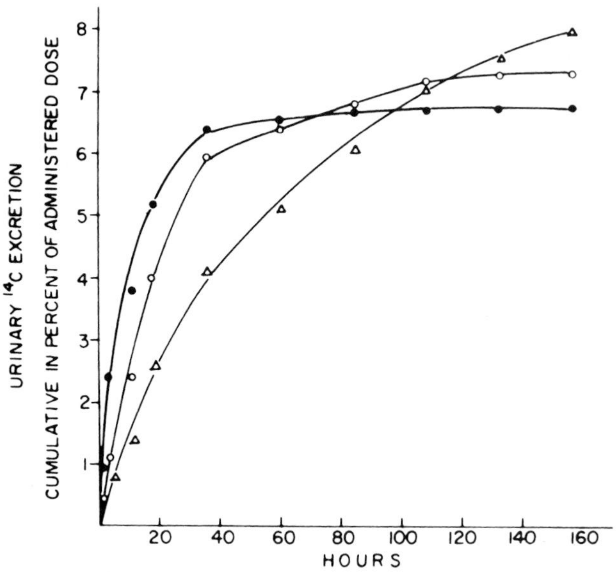

Fig. 198-7 Urine excretion of orally administered ^{14}C-labeled uric acid. Symbols are (•) for a patient with hereditary renal hypouricemia and (○) and (Δ) for normal subjects. ***(From Sperling et al.[173] Used by permission from Masson.)***

found that when non-Dalmatian dogs received Dalmatian livers, the renal clearance and excretion of uric acid increased to values typical of Dalmatians and that when Dalmatians received non-Dalmatian livers, the preceding parameters diminished to those typical for non-Dalmatians. These results were taken to indicate that the Dalmatian liver is responsible for both the increased amount of excreted urate and the increased renal urate clearance. According to the results of this study, the increased renal urate clearance in the Dalmatian is caused by an abnormal metabolite produced in the liver.

An additional support for the possibility that a humoral substance may affect renal urate transport and therefore that abnormality in such a substance may be the primary defect in hereditary renal hypouricemia may be drawn from the finding that in the rabbit a serum protein was found to modulate, by allosteric modification, the basolateral transporter associated with urate secretion (see above).[110]

CLINICAL SIGNIFICANCE

The hypouricemia in the syndrome is generally discovered during screening procedures, mainly for investigation of various diseases such as osteoporosis, familial hypercholesterolemia, urolithiasis, polyarthralgia, stomatitis, neurologic disorders, glomerulonephritis, idiopathic edema, noncongenital colloid goiter, etc. All these diseases, except for urolithiasis, are unrelated to the renal hypouricemia.

Hypouricemia. The hypouricemia as such has, as far as is known, no clinical significance. Indeed, speculatively, the hypouricemia may be advantageous in avoiding the risks associated with hyperuricemia, mainly the various clinical manifestations of urate crystal deposition disease.

Hyperuricosuria. In three of the patients with hereditary renal hypouricemia, reviewed in Table 198-1, the hypouricemia was associated with a marked hyperuricosuria, the urinary uric acid excretion exceeding 5.95 μmol/day. Furthermore, hyperuricosuria, although moderate, was present in many of the other hypouricemic propositi. Thus hyperuricosuria appears to be a constant feature of isolated renal hypouricemia. Principally, the hyperuricosuria may reflect purine overproduction or diversion of intestinal urate elimination to urinary urate excretion consequent to the hypouricemia. There is no evidence in the hypouricemic hyperuricosuric subjects for purine overproduction. Incorporation of [^{15}N]glycine into urinary uric acid was measured in one such patient and was found to be moderately excessive,[52] probably reflecting the decreased intestinal urate disposal. Normal [^{15}N]glycine incorporation was found in another hypouricemic uric acid stone-forming patient as well as in two hypouricemic patients in whom heredity was not proven.[71]

Hypercalciuria. Hypercalciuria was associated with the renal hypouricemia in six of the propositi presented in Table 198-1.[48,50,55,56] In all these subjects, in whom there was no detectable etiology for the hypercalciuria, it may be classified as "idiopathic hypercalciuria." In three of these,[48,55] the hypercalciuria was proven to be of the hyperabsorptive type—i.e., secondary to increased intestinal calcium absorption. Thus far evidence has not been obtained for a primary abnormality in renal calcium handling in any of these hypouricemic, idiopathic hypercalciuric patients. Thus, at this stage of knowledge, the renal tubular defect leading to hypouricemia may be considered as an isolated tubular abnormality in these subjects until proven otherwise. The apparently frequent association between the renal defect for urate handling and the intestinal calcium hyperabsorption is as yet unexplained.

Hematuria. Hematuria was found in 7 females in a series of 16 Japanese patients with isolated renal hypouricemia.[194] Serum urate and urinary urate concentrations were higher in the group with hematuria.

Urolithiasis. Seven of the 28 propositi with inborn isolated renal hypouricemia presented in Table 198-1 had urinary calculi.[48,53,55,57,62] Three had uric acid stones, 3 had calcium oxalate stones, and 1 had a stone of unidentified composition. In 4 other propositi,[64] urolithiasis was present in other family members. In a recently reported family with the true syndrome,[195] the propositus, a 15-month-old boy, presented with acute renal failure, anuria, and sepsis due to bilateral obstructing ureteral uric acid stones. In a series of 36 Japanese patients (33 males and 3 females) with uric acid stones, 2 females showed hypouricemia.[196] The high prevalence of urolithiasis among the subjects with hereditary renal hypouricemia may be explained by the occurrence of hyperuricosuria and hypercalciuria among these subjects. Indeed, the patients who had uric acid stones had the most significant hyperuricosuria (more than 5.95 mmol/day). It is not surprising that only some of the hypouricemic patients had evidence of urolithiasis, since hyperuricosuria and hypercalciuria are important but are not the only determinants in the causation of stone formation.

Of interest is the series of 4 subjects with idiopathic renal hypouricemia (no evidence for heredity or associated abnormalities) reported by Gaspar et al.[77] In this group, 4 had hyperuricosuria, 3 had hypercalciuria, and 3 had calcium oxalate nephrolithiasis.

Uric Acid Nephropathy. Acute uric acid nephropathy may occur in the presence of massive uricosuria, such as in the tumor lysis syndrome. More rarely, it also may occur in some gouty subjects with excessive purine overproduction, especially in association with inborn errors of metabolism, such as the Lesch-Nyhan syndrome (see Chap. 107) and phosphoribosylpyrophosphate synthetase superactivity (see Chap. 106).

In view of the prevalence of hyperuricosuria in renal hypouricemia, the possibility of acute uric acid nephropathy in this syndrome should be taken into consideration, especially under conditions of temporary increased urate excretion (increased purine intake, increased ATP breakdown, etc.). Such cases were first reported in nonhereditary renal hypouricemia. One patient[197] required hemodialysis due to oliguric renal failure. Renal biopsy

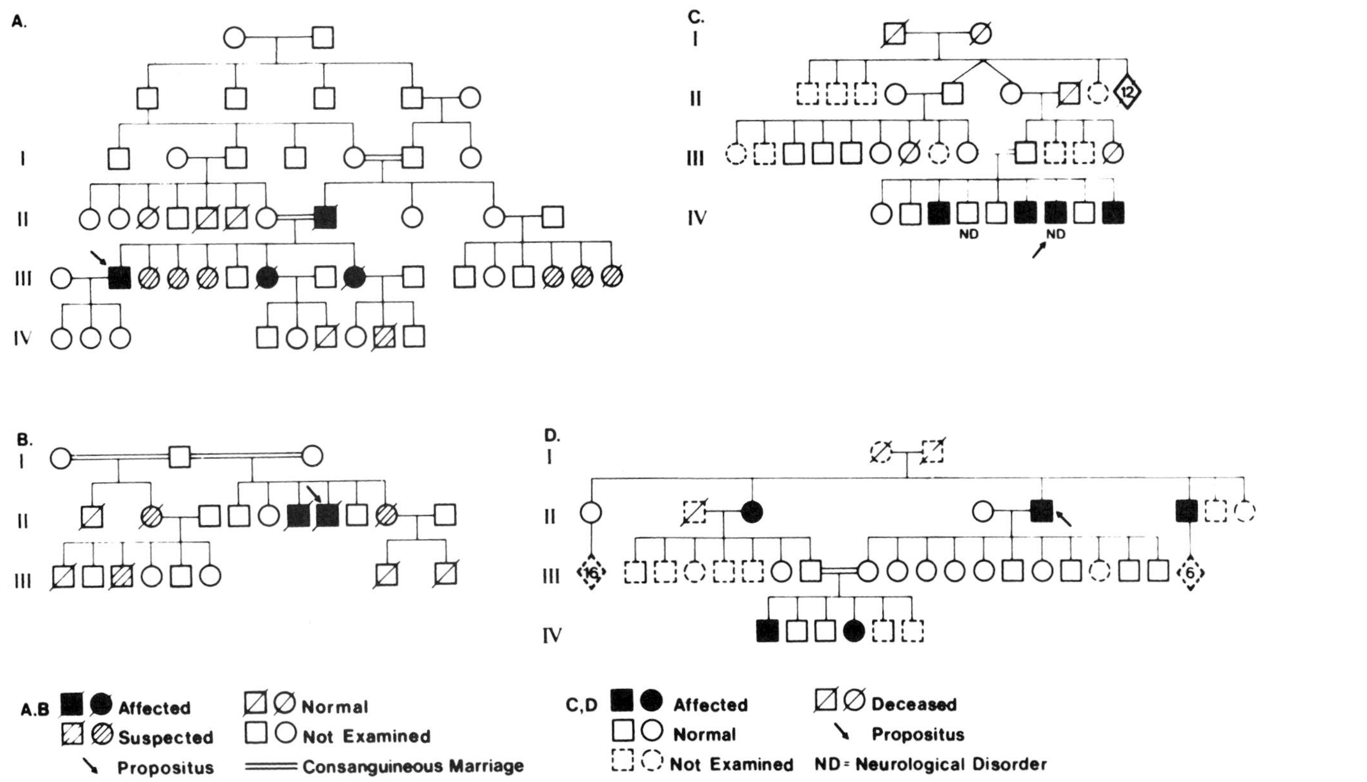

Fig. 198-8 Pedigrees of consanguineous families with hereditary renal hypouricemia. (*A: From Akaoka et al.,*[51] *by permission of the Finnish Medical Society Duodecim. B: From Akaoka et al.*[52] *C: From Weitz and Sperling.*[56] *D: From Sperling et al.*[50] *All used by permission.*)

showed amorphous uric acid crystals in some of the tubular lumina and mild to moderate interstitial inflammation. In this case the hyperuricosuria was attributed to the increased tubular uric acid secretion. Mild acute renal failure induced by exercise in 3 subjects with renal hypouricemia, 1 of whom had familial renal hypouricemia, was reported from Japan.[198] The clinical manifestations in these patients resembled very much the acute renal failure syndrome described by this group in 1982.[199] This syndrome, characterized by patchy renal vasoconstriction, is usually mild and nonoliguric, appears in young healthy subjects, and has a good prognosis. There is only a mild to moderate rise in creatine phosphokinase (CPK), suggesting that massive rhabdomyolysis does not occur. It has been suggested[198,199] that in the 3 reported subjects the renal failure was caused by the precipitation of uric acid. Nevertheless, this could not be demonstrated in the affected patients. An additional case of familial renal hypouricemia associated with acute renal failure was reported by Tofuku et al.[69] The authors speculated that the urinary urate excretion could have been accelerated in the patient due to the increased production of uric acid during physical exercise. In recent years, 12 additional patients were reported with renal hypouricemia who developed exercise-induced acute renal failure.[200–206] Eleven of the new patients were Japanese,[200,202–205] 1 was Pakistani,[201] and 1 was from Korea.[206] In most of the reported patients, data were not available concerning the nature of the renal hypouricemia. Nevertheless, in view of the relatively large number of reports of exercise-induced acute renal failure in renal hypouricemia, this serious complication should be considered in the hereditary syndrome. Most probably, the acute renal failure is caused by precipitation of uric acid. Urinary uric acid content in renal hypouricemia is high. The exercise-induced acceleration of ATP degradation raises uric acid concentration in such patients to levels that exceed supersaturation.[201] Indeed, in 1 patient, an experimental event of exercise-induced hyperuricosuria and acute renal failure could be prevented by allopurinol.[201] Another hypothesis to explain the pathogenesis of the exercise-induced acute renal failure in renal hypouricemia was put forward by Murakami et al.[200] According to them, exercise and subsequent rest are associated with a possible ischemia-reperfusion damage to the kidneys. They suggest that whereas this injury normally is protected against by the high uric acid content in the proximal tubule cell (uric acid being an antioxidant), in renal hypouricemia, because of the markedly lower tissue uric acid level, this protective mechanism is assumed to be less effective.

Decreased Bone Density. Decreased bone density was found to be associated with the hypercalciuria in two renal hypouricemic siblings,[50] and osteoporosis was found in a 4-year-old boy with hereditary renal hypouricemia.[64] Similar abnormalities have not been observed in the other reported hypouricemic families. The association between renal hypouricemia and decreased bone density remains unexplained.

Genetics

Hereditary renal hypouricemia occurs when two mutant autosomal alleles occur at the locus that controls the urate transport site. Known consanguinity in parents of hypouricemic children in 5 of the 28 families[49–52,56] demonstrates the recessive mode of inheritance of the trait (Fig. 198-8). A dominant mode was suggested in one family,[52] in view of the finding that the propositus had three hypouricemic daughters, without consanguinity, and in another family,[65] due to the finding of borderline hypouricemia and increased urate clearance in the mother of two hypouricemic sons. Nevertheless, in the first family,[57] serum uric acid levels reported for these daughters (119, 130, and 142 μM) could very well represent heterozygosity rather than homozygosity. The same is true for the mother of the second family.[65] There is no evidence for X-linkage in the reported pedigrees. In one family,[68] a pseudodominant transmission of a recessive disease was postulated. In at least six of the pedigrees,[49–51,54,55,67] both sexes were affected.

It is of interest that in addition to exhibiting the same mode of inheritance, the vast majority of patients with hereditary renal hypouricemia were classified as being affected with the same type of reabsorption defect — at the presecretory site. Moreover, in none of the families with hereditary renal hypouricemia could an isolated defect for the postsecretory reabsorption site be demonstrated, although such a defect was suggested in other conditions of renal hypouricemia (see above). These findings may be taken to suggest that the presecretory and postsecretory reabsorption sites for urate in the proximal tubule are controlled by different genes.

Another point of interest is that all patients with hereditary renal hypouricemia reported from Israel[50,53–56,60,68] were Jews of non-Ashkenazi (i.e., Sephardic) origin: six were Iraqi, one was Libyan, and one was Turkish. It appears likely, therefore, that hereditary renal hypouricemia is relatively common among non-Ashkenazi Jews.

Treatment

As indicated earlier, urolithiasis is the only clinical manifestation that may be associated with hereditary renal hypouricemia. The urolithiasis is probably the result of the hyperuricosuria and the hypercalciuria found to be common in these patients. Thus it is advisable to study the affected subjects carefully for these parameters and to treat them accordingly. High fluid intake and control of urinary pH may suffice to prevent uric acid stones.[207] In some patients, in whom uric acid excretion is markedly excessive, allopurinol may be needed to reduce uric acid excretion. For prevention of calcium stones, patients exhibiting marked hypercalciuria should be treated by conventional means.

REFERENCES

1. Praetorius E, Kirk JE: Hypouricemia with evidence for tubular elimination of uric acid. *J Lab Clin Med* **35**:856, 1950.
2. Mikkelsen WM, Dodge HJ, Valkenburg H: The distribution of serum uric acid values in a population unselected as to gout or hypouricemia. *Am J Med* **39**:242, 1965.
3. Ramsdell CM, Kelley WN: The clinical significance of hypouricemia. *Ann Intern Med* **73**:239, 1973.
4. Dwosh IL, Roncari DAK, Marliss E, Fox IH: Hypouricemia in disease: A study of different mechanisms. *J Lab Clin Med* **90**:153, 1977.
5. Wyngaarden JB, Kelley WN: Miscellaneous forms of hypouricemia, in Wyngaarden JB, Kelley WN (eds): *Gout and Hyperuricemia*. New York, Grune & Stratton, 1976, p 411.
6. Wallis IA, Eagle RI: The adult Fanconi syndrome: II. Review of eighteen cases. *Am J Med* **22**:13, 1957.
7. Lee DBN, Drinkard JP, Rosen VJ, Gnick HC: The adult Fanconi syndrome: Observation on etiology, morphology, renal functions and mineral metabolism in three patients. *Medicine* **51**:107, 1972.
8. Meisel AD, Diamond HS: Hyperuricosuria in the Fanconi syndrome. *Am J Med Sci* **274**:109, 1977.
9. Baron DN, Dent CE, Harris H, Hard EW, Jebson JB: Hereditary pellagra-like skin rash with temporary cerebellar ataxia, constant renal aminoaciduria and other bizarre biochemical features. *Lancet* **2**:421, 1956.
10. Dent CE, Philpot GR: Xanthinuria, an inborn error (or deviation) of metabolism. *Lancet* **1**:182, 1954.
11. Holmes EW, Wyngaarden JB: Hereditary xanthinuria, in Stanbury JB, Wyngaarden JB, Fredrickson DS, Goldstein JL, Brown MS (eds): *The Metabolic Basis of Inherited Diseases, 5th ed.* New York, McGraw-Hill, 1983, p 1192.
12. Giblett ER, Amman AJ, Sandman R, Wara DW, Diamond LK: Nucleoside phosphorylase deficiency in a child with severely defective T-cell immunity and normal B-cell immunity. *Lancet* **1**:1010, 1975.
13. Cass E, Serrano C, Daimiel E, Michan A, Mateos F, Garcia Puig J: Prevalence, physiopathology and conditions associated with hypouricemia in a hospital population: Analysis of 27,987 analytical determinations. *Rev Clin Esp* **186**:211, 1990.
14. Diaz Curiel M, Zea Mendoza A, Rapado A, Gonzalez Villasante J: Significacion clinica de la hipouicemia en 14,865 determinaciones del autoanalizador. *Rev Clin Esp* **139**:365, 1975.
15. Mikkelsen WM, Dodge HJ, Valkenburg H: The distribution of serum uric acid values in a population unselected as to gout or hyperuricemia, Tecumseh, Michigan 1959–1960. *Am J Med* 39:242, 1965.
16. Ramsdell CM, Kelley WN: The clinical significance of hypouricemia. *Ann Intern Med* **24**:239, 1975.
17. Sperling O, Weinberger A, Pinkhas J, de Vries A: Frequency and causes of hypouricemia in hospital patients. *Isr J Med Sci* **13**:529, 1977.
18. van Pennen HJ: Causes of hypouricemia. *Ann Intern Med* **78**:977, 1973.
19. Yanasze M, Nakahama H, Mikami H, Fukuhara Y, Orita Y, Yoshikawa H: Prevalence of hypouricemia in apparently normal population. *Nephron* **48**:80, 1988.
20. Hisatome I, Ogino K, Kotake H, Ishiko R, Saito M, Hasegawa J, Mashiba H, Nakamoto S: Cause of persistent hypouricemia in outpatients. *Nephron* **51**:13, 1989.
21. Morgan HG, Steewart WK, Lowe KG, Stowers JM, Johnstone JH: Wilson's disease and the Fanconi syndrome. *Q J Med* **31**:361, 1962.
22. Leu ML, Strickland GT, Gutman RA: Renal function in Wilson's disease: Response to penicillamine therapy. *Am J Med Sci* **250**:381, 1970.
23. Elsas LJ, Hayslett JP, Spargo BH, Durant JL, Rosenberg LE: Wilson's disease with reversible renal tubular dysfunction. *Ann Intern Med* **75**:127, 1971.
24. Wilson DB, Goldstein NP: Renal urate excretion in patients with Wilson's disease. *Kidney Int* **4**:331, 1973.
25. Schneider JA, Schulman JD, Seegmiller JE: Cystinosis and the Fanconi syndrome, in Stanbury JB, Wyngaarden JB, Fredrickson DS (eds): *The Metabolic Basis of Inherited Disease, 4th ed.* New York, McGraw-Hill, 1978, p 1660.
26. Cusworth DC, Dent CE, Flynn FV: The amino-aciduria in galactosaemia. *Arch Dis Child* **30**:150, 1955.
27. Lamiere N, Mussche M, Bacle G, Kint J, Ringoir S: Hereditary fructose intolerance: A difficult diagnosis in the adult. *Am J Med* **65**:416, 1978.
28. Beck IH: Hypouricemia in the syndrome of inappropriate secretion of antidiuretic hormone. *New Engl J Med* **301**:528, 1979.
29. Osterlind K, Hansen M, Dombernowsky P: Hypouricemia and inappropriate secretion of antidiuretic hormone in small cell bronchogenic carcinoma. *Acta Med Scand* **209**:289, 1981.
30. Weinberger A, Santo M, Solomon F, Shalit M, Pinkhas J, Sperling O: Abnormality in renal urate handling in the syndrome of inappropriate secretion of antidiuretic hormone. *Isr J Med Sci* **18**:711, 1982.
31. Smithline N, Kassirer JP, Cohen JJ: Light-chain nephropathy. *New Engl J Med* **294**:71, 1976.
32. Bennett JS, Bond J, Singer I, Gottlieb AJ: Hypouricemia in Hodgkin's disease. *Ann Intern Med* **76**:751, 1972.
33. Tykarski A: Mechanism of hypouricemia in Hodgkin's disease: Isolated defect in postsecretory reabsorption of uric acid. *Nephron* **50**:217, 1988.
34. Magoula I, Tsapas G, Kountouras I, Paletas K: Cholangiocarcinoma and severe renal hypouricemia: A study of the renal mechanisms. *Am J Kidney Dis* **18**:514, 1991.
35. Morales M, Garcia-Nieto V: Hypouricemia and cancer: A study of the mechanism of renal urate wasting in two cases. *Oncology* **53**:345, 1996.
36. Weinstein B, Irreverre F, Watkin DM: Lung carcinoma, hypouricemia and aminoaciduria. *Am J Med* **39**:520, 1965.
37. Cooper DS: Oat-cell carcinoma and severe hypouricemia. *New Engl J Med* **288**:321, 1973.
38. Gorshein D, Asbell S: Ectopic production of hormones in tumors. *JAMA* **235**:2716, 1976.
39. Weinberger A, Pinkhas J, Sperling O, de Vries A: Frequency and causes of hypouricemia in hospital patients. *Isr J Med Sci* **13**:529, 1977.
40. Chisholm JJ Jr, Harrison HC, Everlein WR, Harrison HE: Amino-aciduria, hypophosphatemia and rickets in lead poisoning. *Am J Dis Child* **89**:159, 1955.
41. Clarkson TW, Kench JE: Urinary excretion of amino acids by men absorbing heavy metals. *Biochem J* **62**:361, 1965.
42. Gross JM: Fanconi syndrome (adult type) developing secondary to the ingestion of outdated tetracycline. *Ann Intern Med* **48**:523, 1963.
43. Schlosstein L, Kippen I, Bluestone R, Whitehouse MW, Klinenberg JR: Association between hypouricemia and jaundice. *Ann Rheum Dis* **33**:308, 1974.
44. Arranz Caso JA, Fernandez de Paz FJ, Barrio V, Cuadrado Gomez LM, Albarran Hernandez F, Alvarez de Mon M: Severe renal hypouricemia secondary to hyperbilirubinemia. *Nephron* **71**:354, 1995.

45. Michelis MF, Warms PC, Fusco RD, Davis BB: Hypouricemia and hyperuricosuria in Laennec cirrhosis. *Arch Intern Med* **134**:681, 1974.
46. Magoula I, Tsapas G, Paletas K, Mavromatidis K: Insulin-dependent diabetes and renal hypouricemia. *Nephron* **59**:21, 1991.
47. Dura Trave T, Moya Benavent M, Casero Ariza J: Renal hypouricemia in juvenile diabets mellitius. *Ann Esp Pediatr* **44**:425, 1996.
48. Greene ML, Marcus R, Aurbach GD, Kazam ES, Seegmiller JH: Hypouricemia due to isolated renal tubular defect. *Am J Med* **53**:361, 1972.
49. Khachadurian AK, Arslanian MJ: Hypouricemia due to renal uricosuria. *Ann Intern Med* **78**:547, 1973.
50. Sperling O, Weinberger A, Oliver I, Liberman UA, de Vries A: Hypouricemia, hypercalciuria and decreased bone density: A hereditary syndrome. *Ann Intern Med* **80**:482, 1974.
51. Akaoka I, Nishizawa T, Yano E, Takeuchi A, Nishida Y, Yoshimura T, Horiuchi Y: Familial hypouricemia due to renal tubular defect of urate transport. *Ann Clin Res* **7**:318, 1975.
52. Akaoka I, Nishizawa T, Yano E, Kamatani N, Nishida T, Sasaki S: Renal urate excretion in five cases of hypouricemia with an isolated renal defect of urate transport. *J Rheumtol* **4**:86, 1977.
53. Benjamin D, Sperling O, Weinberger A, Pinkhas J, de Vries A: Familial hypouricemia due to isolated renal tubular defect. *Nephron* **18**:220, 1977.
54. Benjamin D, Sperling O, Weinberger A, Pinkhas J: Familial hypouricemia due to isolated renal tubular defect. *Biomedicine* **29**:54, 1978.
55. Frank M, Many M, Sperling O: Familial renal hypouricemia: Two additional cases with uric acid lithiasis. *Br J Urol* **51**:88, 1979.
56. Weitz R, Sperling O: Hereditary renal hypouricemia: Isolated tubular defect of urate reabsorption. *J Pediatr* **96**:850, 1980.
57. Hedley JM, Phillips PJ: Familial hypouricemia and uric acid calculi: Case report. *J Clin Pathol* **33**:971, 1980.
58. Fujiwara J, Takamitsue J, Ueda N, Orita Y, Abe H: Hypouricemia due to an isolated defect in renal tubular urate reabsorption. *Clin Nephrol* **13**:44, 1980.
59. Delevelle F, Trombert JC, Bouvier MF, Canarelli G: Hypouricemie renale idiopathique: 1 observation. *Nouv Presse Med* **35**:2578, 1980.
60. Garty BZ, Nitzan M, Sperling O: Inborn hypouricemia due to isolated defect in renal tubular uric acid transport. *Isr J Med Sci* **17**:295, 1981.
61. Matsuda O, Shiigai T, Ito Y, Aonuma K, Takenchi J: A case of familial renal hypouricemia associated with increased secretion of PAH and idiopathic edema. *Nephron* **30**:178, 1982.
62. Tachibana S, Wakatsuki A, Kamei O, Ochi K, Takeuchi M: A case of idiopathic hypouricemia with recurrent renal stones. *Nish J Urol* **44**:795, 1982.
63. Vinay P, Gatterean A, Moulin B, Gougoux A, Lemieux G: Normal urate transport into erythrocytes in familial renal hypouricemia and in Dalmatian dog. *Can Med Assoc J* **128**:545, 1983.
64. Takeda E, Kuroda T, Ito M, Toshima K, Watanabe T, Ito M, Naiko E, Yokota I, Huwang TJ, Miyao M: Hereditary renal hypouricemia in children. *J Pediatr* **107**:71, 1985.
65. Nakajima H, Gomi M, Iida S, Kono N, Moriwaki K, Tarui S: Familial renal hypouricemia with intact reabsorption of uric acid. *Nephron* **45**:40, 1987.
66. Shichiri M, Iwamoto H, Maeda M, Kanayama M, Shiigai J: Hypouricemia due to subtotal defect in the urate transport. *Clin Nephrol* **28**:300, 1987.
67. Hisatome I, Ogino K, Saito M, Miyamoto J, Hasegawa J, Kotake H, Mashiba H, Nakamoto S: Renal hypouricemia due to an isolated renal defect of urate transport. *Nephron* **49**:81, 1988.
68. Gafter U, Zuta A, Frydman M, Lewinski UH, Levi J: Hypouricemia due to familial isolated renal tubular uricosuria: Evaluation with the combined pyrazinamide-probenecid test. *Minerva Electrol Metab* **15**:309, 1989.
69. Tofuku Y, Ito M, Takasaki H, Koni I, Takeda R: A case of familial renal hypouricemia associated with acute renal failure. *Pur Pyrimid Metabol (Jpn)* **14**:8, 1990.
70. Simkin PA, Skeith DA, Healy LA: Suppression of uric acid secretion in a patient with renal hypouricemia. *Adv Exp Med Biol* **41B**:723, 1974.
71. Kawabe K, Murayama T, Akaoka I: A case of uric acid renal stone with hypouricemia caused by tubular reabsorption defect of uric acid. *J Urol* **116**:690, 1976.
72. Soerensen LB, Levinson DJ: Isolated defect in postsecretory reabsorption of uric acid. *Ann Rheum Dis* **39**:180, 1980.
73. Tofuku Y, Kuroda M, Tekada R: Hypouricemia due to renal urate wasting. *Nephron* **30**:39, 1982.
74. Shichiri M, Matsuda O, Shugai T, Takeuchi J, Kanayama M: Hypouricemia due to an increment in renal tubular urate secretion. *Arch Intern Med* **142**:1855, 1982.
75. Dumont I, Decaux G: Hypouricemia related to a hypersecretional tubulopathy. *Nephron* **34**:256, 1983.
76. Smetana SS, Bar-Khayim J: Hypouricemia due to renal tubular defect: A study with the probenecid-pyrazinamide test. *Arch Intern Med* **145**:1200, 1985.
77. Gaspar GA, Puig TG, Mateos FA, Oria CR, Gomez MEM, Gil AA: Hypouricemia due to renal urate wasting: Different types of tubular transport defects. *Adv Exp Med Biol* **195A**:357, 1986.
78. Berliner RW, Hilton JG, Yu TF, Kennedy TJ Jr: The renal mechanism for urate excretion in man. *J Clin Invest* **29**:396, 1950.
79. Gutman AB, Yu TF, Berger L: Tubular secretion of urate in man. *J Clin Invest* **38**:1778, 1959.
80. Yu TF, Berger L, Stone DJ, Wolf J, Gutman AB: Effect of pyrazinamide and pyrazinoic acid on urate clearance and other discrete renal functions. *Proc Soc Exp Biol Med* **96**:264, 1957.
81. Yu TF, Berger L, Gutman AB: Suppression of tubular secretion of urate by pyrazinamide in the dog. *Proc Soc Exp Biol Med* **107**:905, 1961.
82. Steele TH, Rieselbach RE: The renal mechanism for urate homeostasis in normal man. *Am J Med* **43**:868, 1967.
83. Roch-Ramel F, Werner D: Urate transport in mammalian nephron, in Hatano M (ed): *Nephrology, Proceedings of the 11th International Congress of Nephrology.* Berlin, Springer-Verlag, 1991, p 1399.
84. Weiner IM: Urate transport in the nephron. *Am J Physiol* **237**:F85, 1979.
85. Werner D, Guisan B, Roch-Ramel F: Urate transport in the proximal tubule of human kidney. *Adv Exp Med Biol* **309A**:177, 1991.
86. Abramson RG, Levitt MF: Micropuncture study of uric acid in rat kidney. *Am J Physiol* **228**:1597, 1975.
87. Wyngaarden JB, Kelley WN: Gout, in Stanbury JB, Wyngaarden JB, Fredrickson DS, Goldstein JL, Brown MS (eds): *The Metabolic Basis of Inherited Disease, 5th ed.* New York, McGraw-Hill, 1983, p 1043.
88. Kahn AM, Weinman EJ: Urate transport in the proximal tubule: in-vivo and vesicle studies. *Am J Physiol* **249**:F789, 1985.
89. Roch-Ramel F, Chomety-Diez F, De Rougemont D, Tellier M, Widmer J, Peters G: Renal excretion of uric acid in the rat: A micropuncture and microperfusion study. *Am J Physiol* **230**:768, 1976.
90. Roch-Ramel F, Diez-Chomety F, Roth L, Weiner IM: A micropuncture study of urate excretion by *Cebus* monkeys employing high performance liquid chromatography with amperometric detection of urate. *Pflugers Arch* **383**:203, 1980.
91. Weinman EJ, Steplock D, Sansom SC, Knight TF, Senekjian HO: Use of high-performance liquid chromatography for determination of urate concentrations in nanoliter quantities of fluid. *Kidney Int* **19**:83, 1981.
92. Roch-Ramel F, Weiner IM: Excretion of urate by the kidney of *Cebus* monkeys: A micropuncture study. *Am J Physiol* **224**:1369, 1973.
93. Sansom SC, Senekjian HO, Knight TF, Babino H, Steplock D, Weinman EJ: Determination of the apparent transport constants for urate absorption in the rat proximal tubule. *Am J Physiol* **240**:F406, 1981.
94. de Rougement D, Henchoz M, Roch-Ramel F: Renal urate excretion at various plasma concentrations in the rat: A free-flow micropuncture study. *Am J Physiol* **231**:387, 1976.
95. Weinman EJ, Senekjian HO, Sansom SC, Steplock D, Sheth A, Knight TF: Evidence for active and passive urate transport in the rat proximal tubule. *Am J Physiol* **240**:F90, 1981.
96. Fanelli GM Jr, Weiner IM: Pyrazinoate excretion in the chimpanzee: Relation to urate disposition and the actions of uricosuric drugs. *J Clin Invest* **52**:1946, 1973.
97. Weiner IM, Fanelli GM Jr: Renal urate excretion in animal models. *Nephron* **14**:33, 1975.
98. Weinman EJ, Eknoyan G, Suki WN: The influence of the extracellular fluid volume on the tubular reabsorption of uric acid. *J Clin Invest* **55**:283, 1975.
99. Weinman EJ, Knight TF, McKenzie R, Eknoyan G: Dissociation of urate from sodium transport in the rat proximal tubule. *Kidney Int* **10**:295, 1976.
100. Weinman EJ, Steplock D, Suki WN, Eknoyan G: Urate reabsorption in proximal convoluted tubule of the rat kidney. *Am J Physiol* **231**:509, 1976.
101. Senekjian HO, Knight TF, Sansom SC, Weinman EJ: Effect of flow rate and the extracellular fluid volume on proximal urate and water absorption. *Kidney Int* **17**:155, 1980.
102. Kahn AM, Aronson PS: Urate transport via anion exchange in dog renal microvillus membrane vesicles. *Am J Physiol* **244**:F56, 1983.

103. Kahn AM, Branham S, Weinman EJ: Mechanism of urate and *p*-aminohippurate transport in rat renal microvillus membrane vesicles. *Am J Physiol* **245**:F151, 1983.
104. Podevin R, Ardaillou R, Paillard F, Fontannele J, Richet G: Etude chez l'homme de la cinetique d'apparition dans purine de l'acide urique 2 ^{14}C. *Nephron* **5**:134, 1968.
105. Weinman EJ, Sansom SC, Steplock DA, Sheth AU, Knight TF, Senekjian HO: Secretion of urate in the proximal convoluted tubule of the rat. *Am J Physiol* **239**:F383, 1980.
106. Kramp RA, Lenoir RH: Characteristics of urate influx in the rat nephron. *Am J Physiol* **229**:1654, 1975.
107. Weinman EJ, Sansom SC, Bennett S, Kahn AM: Effect of anion exchange inhibitors and *para*-aminohippurate on the transport of urate in the rat proximal tubule. *Kidney Int* **23**:832, 1983.
108. Platts MM, Mudge GH: Accumulation of uric acid by slices of kidney cortex. *Am J Physiol* **200**:387, 1961.
109. Senekjian HO, Knight TF, Weinman EJ: Urate transport by the isolated perfused S2 segment of the rabbit. *Am J Physiol* **240**:F530, 1981.
110. Shimomura A, Chonko A, Tanner RM, Edwards R, Grantham JJ: Nature of urate transport in isolated rabbit proximal tubules. *Am J Physiol* **241**:F565, 1981.
111. Tanner EJ, Chonko AM, Edwards RM, Grantham JJ: Evidence for an inhibitor of renal urate and PAH secretion in rabbit blood. *Am J Physiol* **244**:F590, 1983.
112. Moller JV: The relation between secretion of urate and *p*-aminohippurate in the rabbit kidney. *J Physiol (Lond)* **192**:505, 1967.
113. Poulsen H, Praetorius E: Tubular excretion of uric acid in rabbits. *Acta Pharmacol Toxicol* **10**:371, 1954.
114. Roch-Ramel F, Werner D, Guisan B: Urate transport in brush-border membrane of human kidney. *Am J Physiol* **266**:F797, 1994.
115. Roch-Ramel F: Renal transport of organic ions and uric acid, in Schreier RW, Gottschalk CW (eds): *Diseases of the Kidney, 6th ed*, Boston, Little, Brown, 1997, p 231.
116. Roch-Ramel F, Guisan B, Schild L: Indirect coupling of urate and *p*-aminohippurate to sodium in human brush-border membrane vesicles. *Am J Physiol* **270**:F61, 1996.
117. Roch-Ramel F, Guisan B, Diezi J: Effects of uricosuric and antiuricosuric agents on urate transport in human brush-border membrane vesicles. *J Pharmacol Exp Ther* **280**:839, 1997.
118. Abramson RG, King VF, Reif MC, Leal-Pinto E, Baruch SB: Urate uptake in membrane vesicles of rat renal cortex: Effect of copper. *Am J Physiol* **242**:F158, 1982.
119. Abramson RG, Lipkowitz MS: Carrier-mediated concentrative urate transport in rat renal membrane vesicles. *Am J Physiol* **248**:F574, 1985.
120. Blomstedt JW, Aronson PS: pH Gradient-stimulated transport of urate and *p*-aminohippurate in dog renal microvillus membrane vesicles. *J Clin Invest* **65**:931, 1980.
121. Boumendil-Podevin EF, Podevin RA, Priol C: Uric acid transport in brush border membrane vesicles isolated from rabbit kidney. *Am J Physiol* **236**:F519, 1979.
122. Guggino SE, Aronson PS: Paradoxical effects of pyrazinoate (PZA) on urate transport in dog renal brush border membrane vesicles (BBMV). *Kidney Int* **23**:256, 1983.
123. Kippen I, Hirayama B, Klinenberg JR, Wright EM: Transport of *p*-aminohippuric acid and glucose in highly purified rabbit renal brush border membranes. *Biochim Biophys Acta* **556**:161, 1979.
124. Nord E, Wright SH, Kippen IM, Wright EM: Pathways for carboxylic acid transport by rabbit renal brush border membrane vesicles. *Am J Physiol* **243**:F456, 1982.
125. Gutman AB, Yu TF: A three-component system for regulation of renal excretion of uric acid in man. *Trans Assoc Am Phys* **74**:353, 1961.
126. Manuel MA, Steele TH: Pyrazinamide suppression of the uricosuric response to sodium chloride infusion. *J Lab Clin Med* **83**:417, 1974.
127. Steele TH, Boner G: Origins of the uricosuric response. *J Clin Invest* **52**:1368, 1973.
128. Steele TH: Urate secretion in man: The pyrazinamide suppression test. *Ann Intern Med* **79**:734, 1973.
129. Diamond HS, Paolino JS: Evidence for a post-secretory reabsorptive site for uric acid in man. *J Clin Invest* **52**:1491, 1973.
130. Rieselbach RE, Steele TH: Influence of the kidney upon urate homeostasis in health and disease. *Am J Med* **56**:665, 1974.
131. Sorensen LB, Levinson DJ: Isolated defect in postsecretory reabsorption of uric acid. *Ann Rheum Dis* **39**:180, 1980.
132. Gibson T, Sims HP, Jimenez SA: Hypouricemia and increased renal urate clearance associated with hyperparathyroidism. *Ann Rheum Dis* **35**:372, 1976.
133. Grantham JJ, Chonko AM: Renal handling of organic anions and cations; metabolism and excretion of uric acid, in Brenner BM (ed): *The Kidney,* 3d ed. Philadelphia, Saunders, 1986, p 663.
134. Harknes RA, Nicol AD: Plasma uric acid levels in children. *Arch Dis Child* **44**:773, 1969.
135. Stapelton FB, Linshawm MA, Hassancin K, Gruskin AB: Uric acid excretion in normal children. *J Pediatr* **92**:911, 1978.
136. Stapelton FB: Renal uric acid clearance in human neonates. *J Pediatr* **103**:290, 1983.
137. Wolfson WO, Hunt HJ, Levine E, Gutterman HS, Cohn C, Rosenberg EF, Huddlestun B, Kadota IC: The transport and excretion of uric acid in man: V. A sex differential in urate metabolism; with a note on clinical and laboratory findings in gouty women. *J Clin Exp* **9**:749, 1949.
138. Scott JT, Pollard AC: Uric acid excretion in relatives of patients with gout. *Ann Rheum Dis* **29**:397, 1970.
139. Nicholls S, Snaith MZ, Scott JT: Effect of estrogen therapy on plasma and urinary levels of uric acid. *Br Med J* **1**:449, 1973.
140. Steele TH: Evidence for altered renal urate reabsorption during changes in volume of the extracellular fluid. *J Lab Clin Med* **74**:288, 1969.
141. Cannon PJ, Svahn DS, Demartini FF: The influence of hypertonic saline infusions upon the fractional reabsorption of urate and other ions in normal and hypertensive man. *Circulation* **41**:97, 1970.
142. Diamond H, Meisel A: Influence of volume expansion, serum sodium and fractional excretion of sodium on urate excretion. *Pflugers Arch* **356**:47, 1975.
143. Steele TH, Oppenheimer S: Factors affecting urate excretion following diuretic administration in man. *Am J Med* **47**:564, 1969.
144. Steele TH, Manuel MA, Boner G: Diuretics, urate excretion and sodium reabsorption: A test of acetazolamide and urinary alkalinization. *Nephron* **11**:48, 1975.
145. Engle JE, Steele TH: Variation of urate excretion with urine flow in normal man. *Nephron* **16**:50, 1976.
146. Meisel A, Diamond H: Effect of vasopressin on uric acid excretion: Evidence for distal nephron reabsorption of urate in man. *Clin Sci Mol Med* **51**:33, 1976.
147. Mees EJD, van Assendelft PB, Nieuvenhuis MG: Elevation of uric acid clearance caused by inappropriate antidiuretic hormone secretion. *Acta Med Scand* **189**:69, 1971.
148. Gordon P, Robertson GL, Seegmiller JE: Hyperuricemia, a concomitant congenital vasopressin-resistant diabetes insipidus in the adult. *New Engl J Med* **284**:1057, 1971.
149. Quinones Galvan A, Natali A, Baldi S, Feascerra S, Sanna G, Ciociaro D, Ferrannini E: Effect of insulin on uric acid excretion in humans. *Am J Physiol* **268**:E1, 1995.
150. Ter Maaten JC, Voorburg A, Heine RJ, Ter Wee PM, Donker AJ, Gans RO: Renal handling of urate and sodium during acute physiological hyperinsulinaemia in healthy subjects. *Clin Sci (Colch)* **92**:51, 1997.
151. Emmerson BT: Abnormal urate excretion associated with renal and systemic disorders, drugs and toxins, in Kelley WN, Weiner IM (eds): *Handbook of Experimental Pharmacology,* vol 51: *Uric Acid.* Berlin, Springer-Verlag, 1978, p 287.
152. Yu TF, Gutman AB: Paradoxical retention of uric acid by uricosuric drugs in low dosage. *Proc Soc Exp Biol Med* **90**:542, 1955.
153. Yu TF, Gutman AB: Study of the paradoxical effects of salicylate in low, intermediate and high dosage on the renal mechanisms for excretion of urate in man. *J Clin Invest* **38**:1298, 1959.
154. Manuel MA, Steele TH: Changes in renal urate handling after prolonged thiazide treatment. *Am J Med* **57**:741, 1974.
155. Demartini FE: Hypouricemia induced by drugs. *Arthritis Rheum* **8**:823, 1965.
156. Stewart RJ, Chonko AM: Pharmacologic inhibition of urate transport across perfused and non-perfused rabbit proximal straight tubules. *Kidney Int* **19**:258, 1981.
157. Reese OG Jr, Steele TH: Renal transport of urate during diuretic-induced hypouricemia. *Am J Med* **60**:973, 1978.
158. Nemati M, Kyle MC, Freis ED: Clinical study of ticrynafen. *JAMA* **237**:652, 1977.
159. Grobner TO, Zollner N: Uricosuria, in Zollner N, Grobner W (eds): *Gicht, Handbuch der Inn Med,* vol 7: *Stoff wechsel krankheiten,* part 3, 5th ed. Berlin, Springer, 1976, p 491.
160. Dayton PG, Yu TF, Chen W, Berger L, Westm LA, Gutman AB: The physiological disposition of probenecid, including renal clearance in man, studied by an improved method for its estimation in biological material. *J Pharmacol Exp Ther* **140**:278, 1963.
161. de Vries A, Sperling O: Implications of disorders of purine metabolism for the kidney and the urinary tract *Ciba Found Symp* **48**:179, 1977.

162. Steele TH, Rieselbach RE: The renal mechanism for urate homeostasis in normal man. *Am J Med* **43**:868, 1967.
163. Yu TF, Berger L, Stone DJ, Wolf J, Gutman AB: Effects of pyrazinamide and pyrazinoic acid on urate clearance and other discrete renal functions. *Proc Soc Exp Biol Med* **96**:264, 1957.
164. Yu TF, Berger L, Gutman AB: Suppression of the tubular secretion of urate by pyrazinamide in the dog. *Proc Soc Exp Biol Med* **107**:905, 1961.
165. Davis BB, Field JB, Rodnan GP, Kedes LH: Localization and pyrazinamide inhibition of distal transtubular movement of uric acid-2-^{14}C with a modified stop-flow technique. *J Clin Invest* **44**:716, 1965.
166. Gutman A, Yu TF, Berger L: Renal function in gout: III. Estimation of tubular secretion and reabsorption of uric acid by use of pyrazinamide (pyrazinoic acid). *Am J Med* **47**:575, 1969.
167. Weiner IM, Tinker JP: Pharmacology of pyrazinamide: Metabolic and renal function studies related to the mechanism of drug-induced urate retention. *J Pharmacol Exp Ther* **180**:411, 1972.
168. Kramp RA, Lassiter WE, Gottschalk CW: Urate-2-^{14}C transport in the rat nephron. *J Clin Invest* **50**:35, 1971.
169. Frankfurt SJ, Weinman EJ: Pyrazinoic acid and urate transport in the rat. *Proc Soc Exp Biol Med* **159**:16, 1978.
170. Guggino SE, Aronson PS: Paradoxical effects of pyrazinoate and nicotinate on urate transport in dog renal microvillus membranes. *J Clin Invest* **76**:543, 1985.
171. Hisatome I, Kato T, Miyakoda H, Takami T, Abe T, Tanaka Y, Kosaka H, Ogino K, Mitani Y, Yoshida A, Kotake H, Shigemasa C, Mashiba H, Sato R, Takeda A: Renal hypouricemia with both drug-insensitive secretion and defective reabsorption of urate: A novel type of renal hypouricemia. *Nephron* **64**:447, 1993.
172. Shichiri M, Itoh H, Iwamoto H, Hirata Y, Marumo F: Renal tubular hypouricemia: Evidence for defect of both secretion and reabsorption. *Nephron* **56**:421, 1990.
173. Sperling O, Boer P, Weinberger A, de Vries A: Transport into erythrocytes and intestinal absorption of uric acid in hereditary renal hypouricemia. *Biomedicine* **23**:157, 1975.
174. Hansen KO, Lassen UV: Active transport of uric acid through the human erythrocyte membrane. *Nature* **4685**:553, 1959.
175. Harvey AM, Christensen HN: Uric acid transport system: Apparent absence in erythrocytes of Dalmatian coach hounds. *Science* **145**:826, 1964.
176. Oh JH, Dossetor JB, Beck IT: Kinetics of uric acid transport and its production in rat small intestine. *Can J Physiol Pharmacol* **45**:121, 1967.
177. Wilson DW, Wilson HC: Studies "in vitro" of the digestion and absorption of purine ribonucleotides by the intestine. *J Biol Chem* **237**:1643, 1962.
178. Thier SO, Segal S: Cystinuria, in Stanbury JB, Wyngaarden, JB, Fredrickson DS (eds): *The Metabolic Basis of Inherited Disease,* 3d ed. New York, McGraw-Hill, 1972, p 1504.
179. Scriver CR: Familial iminoglycinuria, in Stanbury JB, Wyngaarden JB, Fredrickson DS (eds): *The Metabolic Basis of Inherited Disease,* 3d ed. New York, McGraw-Hill, 1972, p 1520.
180. Jepson JB: Hartnup disease, in Stanbury JB, Wyngaarden JB, Fredrickson DS (eds): *The Metabolic Basis of Inherited Disease,* 3d ed. New York, McGraw-Hill, 1972, p 1486.
181. Weinberger A, Weinberger A, Sperling O, Ben-Bassat M, Kaplan I, Pinkhas J: Increased uric acid clearance in patients with burns. *Biomedicine* **27**:277, 1977.
182. Kay NE, Gotlieb AJ: Hypouricemia in Hodgkin's disease: Report of an additional case. *Cancer* **32**:1508, 1973.
183. Briggs OM, Sperling O: Uric acid metabolism in the Dalmatian coach hound. *J S Afr Vet Assoc* **53**:201, 1982.
184. Friedman M, Byers SD: Observations concerning the causes of the excess excretion of uric acid in the Dalmatian dog. *J Biol Chem* **175**:727, 1948.
185. Kessler RH, Hierholzer K, Gurd RS: Localization of urate transport in the nephron of mongrel and Dalmatian dog kidney. *Am J Physiol Ther* **197**:601, 1959.
186. Mudge GH, Gucchi J, Platts M, O'Connell JMB, Berndt WO: Renal excretion of uric acid in the dog. *Am J Physiol* **215**:404, 1968.
187. Mudge GH, Berndt WO, Valtin H: Tubular transport of urea, glucose, phosphate, uric acid, sulphate and thiosulphate, in Orloff J, Berliner BW (eds): *Handbook of Physiology,* sec 8: *Renal Physiology.* Washington, American Physiological Society, 1973, chap 19, p 587.
188. Myers VC, Hanzal RF: The metabolism of methylanthine and their related methyluric acids. *J Biol Chem* **162**:309, 1946.
189. Young EG, Conway CF, Crandall WA: On the purine metabolism of the Dalmatian coach hound. *Biochem J* **32**:1138, 1938.
190. Zins GR, Weiner IM: Bidirectional urate transport limited to the proximal tubule in dogs. *Am J Physiol* **215**:411, 1968.
191. Klemperer FW, Trimble HC, Hastings AB: The uricase of dogs, including the Dalmatian. *J Biol Chem* **125**:445, 1938.
192. Kuster G, Shorter RG, Dawson B, Hallenbeck GA: Uric acid metabolism in Dalmatian and other dogs. *Arch Intern Med* **129**:492, 1972.
193. Kuster G, Shorter RG, Dawson B, Hallenbeck GA: Effect of allogenic hepatic transplantation between Dalmatian and mongrel dogs on urinary excretion of uric acid. *Surg Forum* **18**:360, 1967.
194. Hisatome I, Tanaka Y, Ogino K, Shimoyama M, Hiroe K, Tsuboi M, Yamamoto Y, Hamada N, Kato T, Manabe I, Kinugawa T, Ohtahara A, Yoshida A, Shigemasa C, Takeda A, Sato R: Hematuria in patients with hypouricemia. *Intern Med* **37**:40, 1998.
195. Gofrit O, Verstandig AG, Pode D: Bilateral obstructing ureteral uric acid stones in an infant with hereditary renal hypouricemia. *J Urol* **149**:1506, 1993.
196. Ito H, Kotake T, Nomura K, Masai M: Clinical and biochemical features of uric acid nephrolithiasis. *Eur Urol* **27**:324, 1995.
197. Erley CMM, Hirschberg RR, Hoefer W, Schaefer K: Acute renal failure due to uric acid nephropathy in a patient with renal hypouricemia. *Klin Wochenschr* **67**:308, 1989.
198. Ishikawa I, Sakurai Y, Masuzaki S, Sugishita N, Shinoda A, Shikura N: Exercise-induced acute renal failure in 3 patients with renal hypouricemia. *Jpn J Nephrol* **32**:923, 1990.
199. Ishikawa I, Onoudi Z, Yuri T, Saito Y, Shinoda A, Yamamoto I: Acute renal failure with severe loin pain and patchy renal vasoconstrictions, in Eliahou HE (ed): *Acute Renal Failure*. London, Libbey, 1982, p 224.
200. Murakami T, Kawakami H, Fukuda M, Furukawa S: Patients with renal hypouricemia are prone to develop acute renal failure—why? *Clin Nephrol* **43**:207, 1995.
201. Yeun JY, Hasbargen JA: Renal hypouricemia: prevention of exercise-induced acute renal failure and a review of the literature. *Am J Kidney Dis* **25**:937, 1995.
202. Hisanaga S, Kawamura M, Uchida T, Kondho H, Yoshida T: Exercise-induced renal failure in a patient with hyperuricosuric hypouricemia. *Nephron* **66**:475, 1994.
203. Fujieda M, Yokoyama W, Oishi N, Okada T, Kurashige T, Hamada G: Acute renal failure after exercise in a child with renal hypouricemia. *Acta Paediatr Jpn* **37**:642, 1995.
204. Ninomiya M, Ito Y, Nishi A, Matsumoto T, Koga A, Hori Y, Nishida H, Nomura G, Kato H: Recurrent exercise-induced acute renal failure in renal hypouricemia. *Acta Paediatr* **85**:1009, 1996.
205. Tazawa M, Morooka M, Takeichi S, Minowa S, Yasaki T: Exercise-induced acute renal failure observed in a boy with idiopathic renal hypouricemia caused by postsecretory reabsorption defect of uric acid. *Nippon Jinzo Gakkai Shi* **38**:407, 1996.
206. Yim JJ, Oh KH, Chin H, Ahn C, Kim SH, Han JC, Kim S, Lee JS: Exercise-induced acute renal failure in a patient with congenital renal hypouricemia. *Nephrol Dialysis Transplant* **13**:994, 1998.
207. Sperling O: Uric acid nephrolithiasis, in Wickham JEA, Buck AC (eds): *Renal Tract Stones: Metabolic Basis and Clinical Practice.* London, Churchill-Livingstone, 1990, p 349.

CHAPTER 199

Cystinosis: A Disorder of Lysosomal Membrane Transport

William A. Gahl ▪ Jess G. Thoene ▪ Jerry A. Schneider

1. **Cystinosis is a rare, autosomal recessively inherited lysosomal storage disorder due to defective carrier-mediated transport of the amino acid cystine across the lysosomal membrane. The major clinical manifestation of cystinosis is renal failure at approximately 9 to 10 years of age. The cystinosis gene has been isolated, and several different mutations identified.**
2. **In cystinosis, free, nonprotein cystine accumulates to 10 to 1000 times normal levels and forms crystals within the lysosomes of most tissues, which are damaged at different rates. The diagnosis is made by demonstrating an elevated cystine content in polymorphonuclear leukocytes or cultured fibroblasts or by slit-lamp examination showing corneal crystals which are generally present in patients over 1 year of age. Cystinosis can be diagnosed *in utero* by cystine measurements in amniocytes or chorionic villi, or at birth by cystine measurements of the placenta.**
3. **Children with cystinosis are normal at birth but develop signs of the renal tubular Fanconi syndrome, usually between 6 and 12 months of age. These include dehydration, acidosis, vomiting, electrolyte imbalances, hypophosphatemic rickets, and failure to grow. Weight is proportional to height. Head circumference and intelligence are spared. Other manifestations of cystinosis include photophobia, hypothyroidism, and decreased ability to sweat. Renal glomerular damage progresses inexorably, requiring dialysis or transplantation at 6 to 12 years of age.**
4. **Cystine storage does not occur in the donor kidney, but continued accumulation in the host tissue can result in retinal blindness, corneal erosions, diabetes mellitus, a distal myopathy, swallowing difficulties, decreased pulmonary function, pancreatic insufficiency, primary hypogonadism in males, and neurologic deterioration in a significant number of post-renal transplant patients 13 to 40 years old.**
5. **The cystinosis gene, *CTNS*, is located on chromosome 17p13, has 12 exons spanning 23 kb of genomic DNA, and codes for a 367-amino-acid protein called cystinosin, with 7 transmembrane domains and 8 potential glycosylation sites. Approximately 40 percent of cystinosis patients from northern Europe are homozygous for a 57-kb deletion that disrupts *CTNS*. Twelve percent of the 216 alleles of an American-based cystinosis population contain a 753G → A (W138X) mutation. Twenty-nine other mutations have been identified to date.**
6. **Therapy for cystinosis includes replacement of renal losses due to the Fanconi syndrome; provision of thyroxine, insulin, pancreatic enzymes, and testosterone for deficient patients; and symptomatic care of ophthalmic complaints. Chronic cystine-depleting therapy with the aminothiol cysteamine significantly lowers leukocyte and parenchymal cystine levels, improves growth, and obviates the need for thyroid hormone replacement. More importantly, oral cysteamine therapy preserves renal function and, if initiated in the first 2 years of life, can allow for a net increase in the glomerular filtration rate. Side effects include nausea and vomiting. Cysteamine eyedrops can dissolve corneal crystals in young children and remove the haziness from the corneas of older patients.**
7. **The clinical course and severity of cystine accumulation in cystinosis vary in different kindreds, from ocular cystinosis in adults with corneal crystals but no renal disease to intermediate cystinosis in adolescents with late-onset renal deterioration, and finally to classic nephropathic cystinosis in infants. Heterozygotes for all types of cystinosis are clinically normal.**

A list of standard abbreviations is located immediately preceding the index in each volume. Additional abbreviations used in this chapter include: NICHD = National Institute of Child Health and Human Development; rhGH = recombinant human growth hormone.

Cystinosis is a lysosomal storage disorder resulting from defective transport of cystine (Fig. 199-1) across the lysosomal membrane. The term *cystinosis* can refer to one of several variants of the disease but, unless specified, here denotes nephropathic cystinosis, which results in renal failure at approximately 9 to 10 years of age. Cystinosis is now recognized as a systemic disorder, with variable onset of symptoms for the different tissues affected. Cystinosis represents a prototype for metabolic disorders due to defective integral lysosomal membrane transport proteins. Its gene, *CTNS*, resides on chromosome 17p and has been recently cloned and sequenced.

HISTORICAL ASPECTS

The current understanding of cystinosis as an inherited, multisystemic disease resulting from failure of lysosomal cystine transport follows from more than eight decades of both clinical and laboratory research. Over this time, a number of basic issues were addressed: (a) What is the clinical phenotype of the disease? (b) Is cystinosis different from renal Fanconi syndrome and cystinuria? (c) Where in the cell is the cystine stored? (d) Do the crystals form *in situ* or are they phagocytosed from preformed crystals in the extracellular fluid? (e) What is the source of the stored cystine? (f) Why does the cystine accumulate? (g) What causes the renal failure in cystinosis? (h) How can the disease be

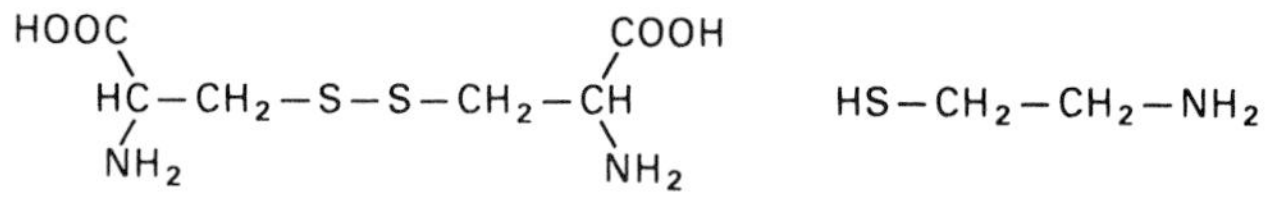

Cystine Cysteamine

Fig. 199-1 Structures of the disulfide amino acid cystine, which is stored in cystinosis, and the aminothiol cysteamine, which depletes cells of cystine.

treated? (i) What is the nature of the molecular pathology accounting for this fatal disease? The answers to all these questions are now known with varying degrees of certitude except what causes the renal failure. The toxic nature of stored lysosomal cystine is still not understood, although plausible hypotheses involving inactivation of critical thiol moieties in intracellular enzymes have been proposed.

Cystinosis was first recognized as a clinical entity by Abderhalden in a 1903 manuscript entitled "Familiare Cystindiathese."[1] He described several children in whom abnormal accumulations of cystine were found. One child demonstrated failure to thrive at 21.5 months of age. In this child's internal organs, white punctate lesions were demonstrated to consist of the amino acid cystine upon classical chemical analysis via formation of the naphthol derivatives. Unfortunately, Abderhalden also reported several children with cystine stones and with excess cystine in the urine, leading to a persistent confusion between cystinosis and cystinuria.[1]

Following Abderhalden's seminal work, the description of this syndrome was enlarged by a number of European authors. Lignac's 1924 report of cystine deposits in each of three infants with rickets, dwarfism, renal disease, and wasting provided some delineation of the clinical aspects of cystinosis.[2] In 1931, Fanconi described nondiabetic glycosuria,[3] and in 1935, de Toni described vitamin D-resistant rickets with spontaneous fractures in a dwarfed child who also had hypophosphatemia, acidosis, albuminuria, and glucosuria.[4] Report of a similar child by Debré et al. in 1934 led to the condition being termed de Toni-Debré-Fanconi syndrome.[5] Nephrotic glucosuria with hypophosphatemic rickets was reported as a distinct clinical entity in 1936, emphasizing the early onset, severe rickets, thermolability, and abnormal tubular vacuolization of the disorder; parental consanguinity suggested autosomal recessive inheritance.[6] In 1937, Beumer and Wepler reemphasized the presence of massive amounts of crystals in the internal organs in children with "renal diabetes," clearly connecting cystine to this clinical entity.[7] Bickel and colleagues provided further evidence of the association of cystinosis with the Fanconi syndrome and with progressive glomerular damage.[8,9]

Experimental work in both rabbits and dogs had previously demonstrated severe renal toxicity when cystine was administered orally or intravenously. The animals developed renal lesions characterized by massive proteinuria, swollen renal tubular cells, and renal casts. All other amino acids spared the kidneys except tyrosine, another relatively insoluble amino acid.[10] The aminoaciduria in cystinosis was extensively studied by Dent who, in 1947, also quantified the extent of polyuria, glucosuria, phosphaturia, and proteinuria.[11] Dent also noted that the generalized aminoaciduria in cystinosis was not due to "overflow" of plasma amino acids and that no obvious error of sulfur amino acid metabolism was present in these patients. The clear distinction between cystinosis and cystinuria was first provided in 1949,[12] when the familial nature of both diseases was recognized, and the rarity of cystine stones in patients with cystinosis was appreciated. Further details on the early investigations of this disorder are available elsewhere.[13–15]

The precise location of the cystine crystals was difficult to ascertain, but Barr[16] and Bickel concluded correctly that they were primarily intracellular and within reticuloendothelial cells. Clay and colleagues demonstrated in histologic studies of cystinotic kidney that many nephrons were hypotrophic, particularly in the proximal convoluted tubules, with narrowing in the first part of the tubule forming a "swan-neck" lesion.[17] Darmady and others showed that these lesions are not specific for cystinosis, but are seen in other renal conditions as well.[9,18] In 1962, electron microscopy of renal biopsy specimens demonstrated hexagonal crystals between tubules in the kidney, and the pathognomonic "swan-neck" deformity of the proximal tubule was confirmed on light microscopy.[19] Vacuolation and swelling of the endoplasmic reticulum were noted, and cytoplasmic bodies were found in the apical and central portions of the cell, frequently with coarse granules in the proximal convoluted tubule. It was concluded that crystallization of cystine between cells, secondary to some unknown primary metabolic or enzymatic defect, led to the renal pathology.

The modern era of clinical investigation into cystinosis began in 1967, when the intracellular location of the stored cystine was identified as the lysosome. This was demonstrated by differential centrifugation of leukocyte[20] and fibroblast[21] subcellular fractions; by electron microscopy in lymph node cells,[22] histiocytes,[23] and rectal mucosal cells;[24] by ferritin labeling;[25] by sucrose density gradients;[26] and by exposure of cystinotic fibroblasts to L-cysteine-D-penicillamine disulfide to selectively induce vacuolation.[27] Next, the metabolism and plasma membrane transport of cysteine and cystine were investigated in cystinotic fibroblasts and leukocytes, with no consistent demonstration of a defect compared with normal.[28] In particular, enzymes involved in cyst(e)ine and glutathione redox reactions were not impaired in cystinotic tissues and cells.[28,29]

These findings, detailed previously,[28] set the stage for pursuit of the hypothesis that transport of small molecules across the lysosomal membrane was carrier-mediated.[30] To directly investigate this possibility for cystine, normal polymorphonuclear leukocytes were loaded to very high cystine concentrations by exposure to cystine dimethylester, which, like other amino acid methylesters,[31,32] was specifically hydrolyzed within lysosomes to methanol and free cystine. This ingenious technique, suggested by Dr. Frank Tietze and exploited in Dr. Joseph Schulman's laboratory in the early 1980s, allowed normal and cystinotic leukocytes to be equivalently loaded with cystine. Subsequent whole cell egress studies, using either ^{35}S-cystine or nonradioactive cystine, revealed rapid losses of cystine from normal cells ($t_{\frac{1}{2}}$ approximately 45 min) and slow losses from cystinotic cells ($t_{\frac{1}{2}}$ approaching infinity).[33] At the same time, investigators in Dr. Jerry Schneider's laboratory were loading cultured fibroblasts with cystine by exposing them to 30 mM cysteine-glutathione mixed disulfide for 24 h. With low, but roughly equal, initial loadings, the normal cells lost half their cystine in 20 min, while the cystinotic cells lost none in 90 min.[34]

Experiments using isolated leukocyte lysosomes verified the whole cell results, with 13 normal granular fractions having a mean $t_{\frac{1}{2}}$ for ^{35}S-cystine of 26.1 ± 1.4 SEM min and 12 cystinotic granular fractions having a mean $t_{\frac{1}{2}}$ of 80.8 ± 0.7 min.[35] Nonradioactive experiments gave similar results, regardless of the initial level of cystine loading.[35] EBV-transformed lymphoblasts, loaded using cystine dimethylester, showed a rate of cystine efflux that was two to three times greater in normal compared with cystinotic granular fractions.[36] Comparable experiments in fibroblasts using either [^{35}S] cystine[37,38] or nonradioactive cystine[38] also revealed short half-times for cystine egress from normal lysosomes and very long half-times using cystinotic lysosomes.

A major advance was the expression of egress rates as initial velocities,[39] which increased linearly with loading of normal lysosomes and then leveled off (Fig. 199-2), indicating saturation kinetics, a hallmark of carrier-mediated transport. Cystinotic granular fractions displayed negligible velocities of cystine egress, regardless of the level of cystine loading. Cystinosis heterozygotes exhibited a V_{max} half that of normals.[39]

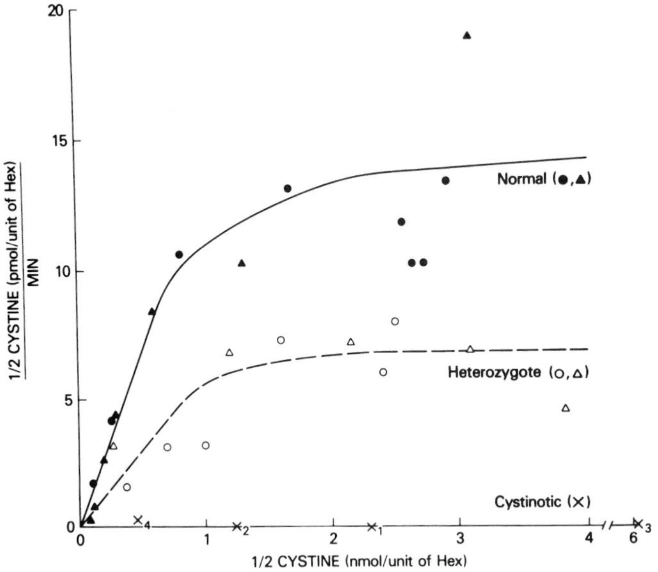

Fig. 199-2 Initial velocity of cystine transport as a function of lysosomal cystine loading using human leukocytes. Normal egress velocity increased with loading and then plateaued, indicating saturation kinetics. Heterozygotes for cystinosis followed a similar pattern but reached only half the normal maximal velocity. Cystinosis patients displayed negligible egress velocity regardless of the level of loading. Values were normalized to the activity of hexosaminidase, a lysosomal enzyme. (*From Gahl et al.*[39] *Used with permission.*)

Finally, the carrier-mediated nature of lysosomal cystine transport was proven definitively by the demonstration of cystine countertransport or *trans*-stimulation. In countertransport, tracer amounts of a radiolabeled substance will cross a membrane at an increased rate if there is a substantial concentration of the nonradioactive substance on the opposite side of the membrane.[40] Thus, normal leukocyte lysosomes loaded with nonradioactive cystine took up [^{3}H]cystine (present in tracer concentrations) more rapidly than lysosomes not loaded with cystine,[41] proving that a carrier for cystine was present in the lysosomal membrane. Cystinotic granular fractions took up virtually no [^{3}H]cystine, regardless of the level of loading.[41] Obligate heterozygotes for cystinosis exhibited half the normal [^{3}H]cystine countertransport.[42]

Following this demonstration, other lysosomal transport systems were rapidly described. At the present writing, more than 20 are known, including systems that recognize all categories of amino acids, inorganic anions and cations, carbohydrates, nucleosides, and cobalamin.[43] Thus, the solution to the cell biology question "Why does lysosomal cystine accumulate?" led to a greatly enhanced understanding of a previously unknown area of cell biology, that of mediated lysosomal transport. The signal role cystinosis has played in allowing delineation of this previously unknown area of cell biology deserves emphasis in the current debate over "translational" research.

In 1995, the cystinosis gene was mapped to chromosome 17p by a consortium of investigators[44] using polymorphic microsatellite repeat markers. In 1998, the cystinosis gene was isolated and a variety of causal mutations identified[45] (see "Genetics" below).

CYSTINE

Chemical Properties

Cystine, the disulfide of the amino acid cysteine, has a molecular weight of 240.3. Cystine and cysteine participate in a reversible oxidation-reduction reaction whose redox potential is -0.22 eV[46] or even more negative. In the presence of oxygen, cysteine is rapidly oxidized to cystine. Cystine's two carboxyl groups and two amine residues have pK_as of <1, 1.7, 7.48, and 9.02, respectively;[47] its net charge at physiological pH is zero, and its pI is 4.60.[47] The disulfide's solubility in water at 25°C approximates 0.5 mM at pH 7.0,[48] but heating or the use of small volumes of dilute (0.01 *N*) acid or alkali facilitates crystal dissolution. The poor solubility of cystine in aqueous solution explains the formation of urinary crystals and renal calculi in cystinuria, a defect of tubular reabsorption of cystine and dibasic amino acids (see Chap. 191). Human plasma at 37°C and pH 7.3 can dissolve approximately 1.67 mM cystine.[13] Cystine's insolubility in alcohol provides the basis for the preservation of cystine crystals in cystinotic tissue by alcohol fixation; the use of aqueous solutions can dissolve the intracellular crystals. The dibasic, diacidic nature of cystine distinguishes it from glutamate and explains the difference between plasma and lysosomal transport of cystine.[43] At neutral pH, both glutamate and cystine are tripolar acidic, and both are recognized by a single transport system in the plasma membrane of fibroblasts.[49] However, at the intralysosomal pH of 5, cystine's second amine is protonated and the compound is now tetrapolar neutral, whereas glutamate, lacking the second amino group, remains tripolar acidic. Hence, the lysosomal membrane transport system distinguishes between the two amino acids, recognizing only cystine.[43]

Metabolism

Cystine forms largely by the direct oxidation of two cysteine molecules. Cysteine is both a precursor in protein synthesis and a product of protein hydrolysis. It is also synthesized *de novo*, deriving its sulfur atom from the essential amino acid, methionine. The transsulfuration of methionine yields homocysteine, which combines with serine to form cystathionine, the proximate precursor of cysteine through the enzymatic activity of cystathionase (see Chap. 88). In conditions in which cystathionine β-synthase or cystathionase is deficient,[50] for example, in homocystinuria or cystathioninuria, or in normal human fetuses and neonates,[51] cysteine becomes an essential amino acid. Cysteine (or cystine) is also required for the growth of normal human fibroblasts,[52] but not normal human lymphoid cells,[53] in culture. In vivo, cysteine is oxidized to inorganic sulfate by one of several pathways[15] for excretion in the urine. It can also be incorporated into free thiols such as glutathione (GSH, γ-glutamylcysteinylglycine), through the γ-glutamyl cycle.

Because of the many cystine-reducing systems present in the cytosol, most cellular cyst(e)ine exists in the free thiol form. It is maintained as cysteine by GSH-disulfide transhydrogenases[54] acting in concert with high cellular concentrations of reduced glutathione (up to 10 mM[55]). Cystine and GSH participate in a disulfide interchange reaction[56] to form cysteine and cysteine-GSH mixed disulfide; a second reaction between reduced GSH and the mixed disulfide produces cysteine and oxidized glutathione. The same type of disulfide interchange reaction provides the basis for the reduction of cystine by cysteamine (see "Mechanism of Cystine Depletion by Cysteamine" below). These disulfide interchange reactions and their products occur within the cytosol, and isolated reports of lysosomal cystine-reducing systems[57] have not been supported in subsequent investigations.[29] Disulfide bonds have been exploited in intermediary metabolism to assist in the maintenance of the tertiary structure of a variety of proteins. Fahey noted that extracellular proteins have a high cystine content (4.1 percent) whereas intracellular proteins have a low concentration (1.6 percent). He suggested that disulfide proteins evolved after the accumulation of oxygen in the atmosphere.[58,59]

Methods of Assay

Cystine can be reduced to cysteine and measured qualitatively by the cyanide-nitroprusside reaction.[60] Semiquantitative assays employ paper[61] or thin-layer[62] chromatography. The routine quantitation of cystine in plasma or urine involves separation from other amino acids by ion-exchange chromatography and identification by ninhydrin staining.[63] The procedure measures total cystine plus cysteine; it cannot differentiate the two. This explains the conventional use of "half-cystine" to express amounts of the disulfide. Most current research employs the *Escherichia coli* cystine-binding protein assay[64] to specifically measure picomole quantities of cystine in protein-free extracts. This assay also allows physicians to diagnose cystinosis and follow cystine depletion by cysteamine. The assay involves competition by unknown quantities of nonradioactive cystine for $[^{14}C]$cystine bound to the protein, with trapping of protein-bound radioactivity on nitrocellulose filters. The less radioactivity that is trapped, the greater the competing nonradioactive cystine.

Cystine Storage in Cystinosis

Plasma cystine concentrations are normal in cystinosis.[13] Intestinal absorption of cystine is normal, and urinary cystine levels are no more elevated than those of other amino acids, differentiating cystinosis from cystinuria (see Chap. 191). Rather, cystine storage in cystinosis is intracellular (Fig. 199-3), with crystal formation in the kidney;[65] liver;[66] lung;[67] pancreas;[68] intestine;[69,70] appendix;[71] spleen;[72] conjunctiva and cornea;[73] retina;[74] lymph node;[22] polymorphonuclear leukocyte and monocyte;[75] bone marrow;[76] thyroid;[77] thymus;[78] muscle;[79] placenta;[80] choroid plexus;[81,82] meninges;[79] and gingival tissue.[83] Pure cystine crystals can be rectangular, in which case they are birefringent[13] or hexagonal. Cystine hydrochloride crystallizes as prismatic needles;[84] this describes the corneal crystals in cystinosis. Various peripheral leukocyte populations[85] and all cells in culture remain devoid of crystals but accumulate 5 to 500 times normal amounts of cystine (Table 199-1). Cystine accumulation and crystal formation occur according to a tissue-specific chronology, with considerable variation among individual patients. Corneal crystals may not be present until 1 year of age, yet crystals have been identified in the Kupffer cells of a 22-week fetus.[86] The brain white and gray matter may be entirely spared of cystine accumulation in a young cystinosis patient,[87] yet show several-fold increased cystine levels in a 25-year-old woman with cystinosis.[88] Both muscle and liver cystine levels increase with age in cystinosis patients who have not received cystine-depleting therapy.[89,90] The reasons for variable rates of cystine accumulation among different tissues are unknown, but may be related to different rates of protein degradation and cell turnover.

Circulating leukocytes from cystinosis patients exhibit normal morphology and normal cysteine concentrations.[20] Cystinotic polymorphonuclear leukocytes, as well as cultured fibroblasts, myoblasts, corneal cells, and renal epithelial and tubular cells, contain fiftyfold to one hundredfold normal amounts of cystine (Table 199-1). Leukocyte cystine values do not change significantly with age in cystinosis patients.[91]

Lysosomal Cystine Transport

Early studies using polymorphonuclear leukocytes delineated several characteristics of lysosomal cystine transport. For example, because *N*-ethylmaleimide did not affect the egress of cystine from normal lysosomes,[39] it was clear that cystine was not being reduced to cysteine and reoxidized to cystine during the transport process; cystine itself was the transported ligand. Moreover, the fact that cystinotic granular fractions cleared tryptophan and methionine in a normal fashion[35] meant that the lysosomal cystine carrier exhibited some specificity.

That specificity was investigated using the powerful technique of countertransport. In particular, normal, cystine-loaded granular fractions did not countertransport other amino acids such as ^{35}S-homocystine except, to a certain extent, ^{35}S-cystathionine.[41] Extralysosomal nonradioactive L-cystine, but not D-cystine, competed with $[^{3}H]$cystine for uptake into cystine-loaded normal granular fractions,[41] establishing the stereo-specificity of the carrier for the L isomer. The carrier presumably also recognized certain sulfur compounds that resembled cystine, such as cystathionine and cystamine, because they competed with cystine for countertransport.[41] Because the dibasic amino acid, arginine, did not compete with cystine, the carrier was presumed to be different from the plasma membrane carrier for dibasic amino

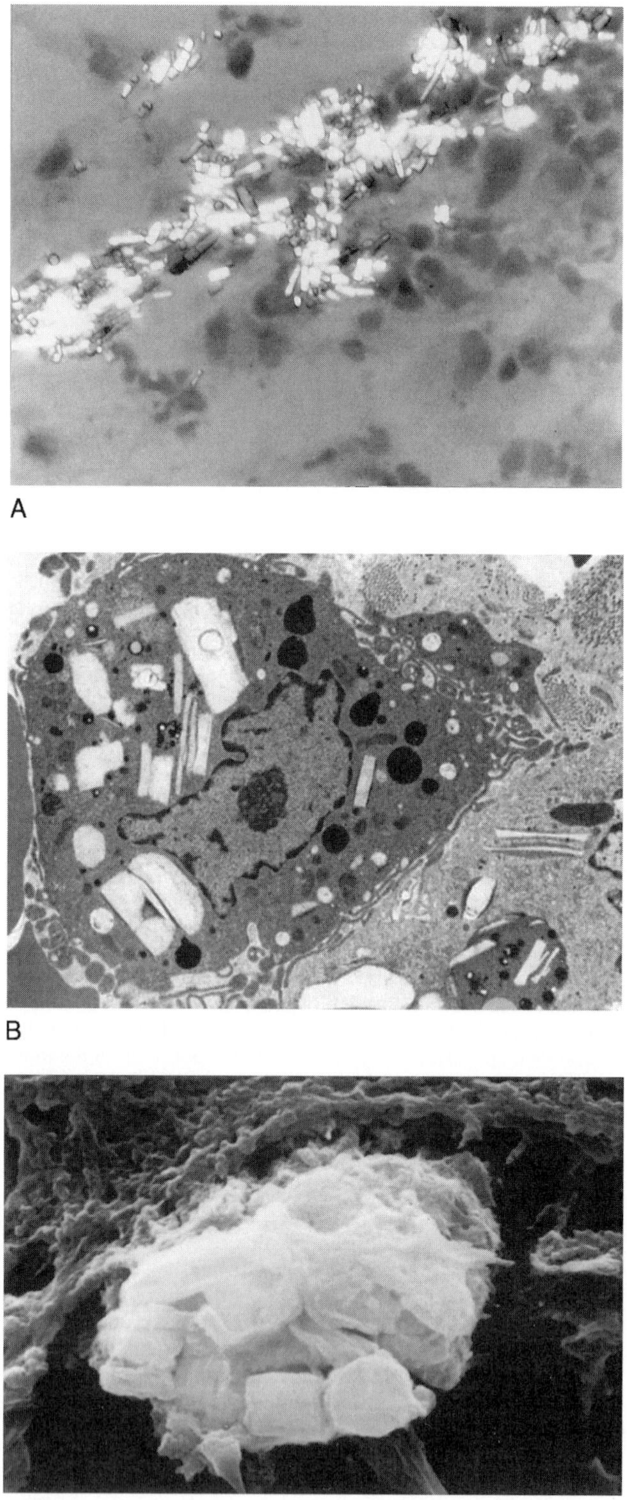

Fig. 199-3 Cystine crystals. *A*, Light microscopy showing conjunctival crystals under cross-polarizing light. *B*, Electron micrograph of hexagonal cystine crystals within lysosomes of a Kupffer cell. ×14,500. *C*, Scanning electron micrograph showing crystals protruding from the surface of a Kupffer cell. ×1800. (*B and C courtesy of K.G. Ishak, M.D., Ph.D., Armed Forces Institute of Pathology, Washington, DC.*)

Table 199-1 Cystine Content of Cystinotic Tissue and Cells

	Cystinotic			Normal			
	N	x̄ ± SD	Range	N	x̄ ± SD	Range	Reference
Tissues		**mol half-cystine/mg wet weight**			**nmol half-cystine/mg wet weight**		
Kidney	1	25.6	—				156
	4	94.8 ± 79.7	24.6–29.5	1	0.25	—	87
	5	51.4 ± 32.6	16.7–101.7	?	—	<0.29	257
	3	64.7 ± 22.2	39.2–80.0	—			338
	1	—	19.8, 21.0	—			339
	1	0.28*	—	—			340
Conjunctiva	7	117.9 ± 115.3	5.2–314.0	13	—	<0.38	203
Muscle	10	0.77 ± 0.53	0.05–1.94	10	0.023 ± 0.003	—	89
	3	0.31 ± 0.23	0.06–0.95	1	0.003	—	211
	12	2.27 ± 3.35	0.23–12.30	1	0.004		79, 90
Brain	2	—	0.02–0.08	1	0.17	—	87
	1	—	0.05–0.20	—			339
	1	—	0.80–4.0	—			79
Lung	1	44.5		—			156
Pancreas	1	35.8					156
	1	40.2					79
Liver	3	73.0 ± 35.0	45.8–112.5	2	—	0.58, 0.92	338
	1	69.1		—			156
	1	—	34.5, 42.4	—			339
	4		2.0–360.0	4	0.04 ± 0.04	0.02–0.10	90
Gallbladder	1	2.1	—	—			156
Spleen	1	132.7					79
	1	119.0					90
Cells		**nmol half-cystine/mg protein**			**nmol half-cystine/mg protein**		
Polymorphonuclear leukocytes	9	6.4 ± 2.8	4.0–13.2	9	0.08 ± 0.06	<0.2	20, 21, 326
	3	—	6.9–10.0	2	—	<0.1	311
	29	8.9 ± 4.7	2.6–23.1	29	0.14 ± 0.06	0.04–0.28	42, 156
Cultured fibroblasts	6	8.4 ± 1.3	6.6–10.6	9	0.07 ± 0.05	<0.2	21, 326
	6	—	6.7–14.3	3	—	<0.1	311
Cultured leukocytes	3	—	0.31–3.10	3	—	<0.03	341
Epstein-Barr virus-transformed lymphoblasts	3	0.46 ± 0.10	—	3	0.10 ± 0.02	—	36
Cultured myoblasts/myotubes	1†	29.8 ± 10.8	16.7–41.2	1	0.31	—	211
Cultured cornea	1	23.2 ± 14.1	11.0–38.7	1	0.27	—	295
Cultured renal cells	1	8.0 ± 0.6	—	1‡	0.06 ± 0.02	—	342
Cultured renal tubular cells	1	3.5	—	1	0.06	—	343

*The patient was receiving long-term cysteamine therapy at the time the biopsy was taken.
†When a single individual's cells were studied, the mean ± SD for at least three separate cultures is given.
‡Madin-Darby canine kidney epithelial cells; human renal cells in culture were not available.

acids in renal tubular and intestinal epithelial cells (see Chap. 191). The lysosomal cystine carrier did not recognize glutamate,[41] indicating that it was genetically distinct from the plasma membrane cystine carrier of fibroblasts that transports both cystine and glutamate.[49] Several other amino acids — that is, methionine, alanine, tryptophan, tyrosine, and homocystine, as well as β-carboxyethyl-L-thiocysteine and other cystine analogues — also did not compete with cystine for transport.[41] The cystine carrier appeared specific for compounds of chain length 6 (not 8) sulfur or methylene units having an amine (but not necessarily a carboxyl) group at each end. Similar ligand preferences have been demonstrated for lysosome cystine transport in mouse L-929 cells, where it was also shown that selenium could substitute for sulfur, and the carrier's recognition site for cystine was dominated by hydrophobic interactions.[92] There were no net charge requirements for ligand binding, but the binding site had both polar and apolar domains. The apolar domain could accommodate branching on the carbon-3 of cystine.

The kinetic properties of lysosomal cystine transport have been loosely defined in at least two different systems. In leukocyte lysosomes, the K_m approximated 0.5 mM with respect to L-cystine,[41] and the V_{max} for egress was approximately 23 pmol half-cystine per unit of hexosaminidase per minute.[39] (Hexosaminidase is a lysosomal enzyme whose activity provides a denominator for expressing transport rates per lysosome.) The Q_{10} approximated 2.0 with an energy of activation of 11.4 kcal/mol.[41] In mouse L-929 cells, the K_m was 0.27 mM, and there appeared to be a component of cystine uptake that could not be saturated.[92]

Normal cystine countertransport, studied in leukocyte lysosomes, was relatively independent of the extralysosomal sodium or potassium ion concentration.[41] However, cystine efflux was greatly enhanced when lysosomal membranes were made permeable to potassium ions either by an ionophore such as valinomycin, or by the presence of a permeant anion.[93] The potassium-valinomycin effects were present in cystinotic lysosomes as well, suggesting that they were not mediated through the carrier system deficient in cystinosis. Moreover, the valinomycin effect was not observed in fibroblast lysosomes,[94] and valinomycin/potassium pretreatment did not enhance cystine egress from rat liver lysosomes.[95] Magnesium chloride did stimulate leukocyte lysosomal cystine transport in a concentration-dependent fashion up to 5 mM at pH 5.5.[96]

The interpretation of ATP effects on lysosomal cystine transport is complicated by the fact that ATP not only provides energy but that it also effects lysosomal acidification through a divalent cation-dependent proton pump.[97] Furthermore, different results and conclusions have emanated from investigations in different cell systems, leaving final analysis for future studies employing artificially expressed CTNS protein. For a detailed discussion of ATP-related work to date, see the previous edition of this chapter.[98]

I-cell fibroblasts, which lack the Golgi enzyme necessary for placement of the mannose-6-phosphate recognition marker on lysosomal enzymes (see Chap. 138), store cystine in their lysosomes.[99,100] I-cell granular fractions have prolonged half-times for cystine clearance,[38] perhaps because optimal cystine carrier function requires lysosomal processing by enzymes deficient in I-cell disease.

Several miscellaneous properties of lysosomal cystine transport have been reported. Polyamines have been shown to stimulate cystine egress from rat liver lysosomes.[101] Stearylamine enhances cystine efflux from cystinotic lysosomes, probably through its detergent properties.[102] Cystinotic fibroblasts lose cystine at above-normal temperatures,[103,104] perhaps because of increased membrane fluidity or because another carrier recognizes cystine at elevated temperatures. Lysosomal cystine transport does not appear to be mediated by γ-glutamyltranspeptidase, because a patient deficient in this enzyme had normal lysosomal cystine transport.[105]

Finally, lysosomal cystine transport has been described in functional rat thyroid (FRTL-5) cells in culture[106] and in *S. cerevisiae* yeast acidic vacuoles.[107]

Mechanism of Cystine Depletion by Cysteamine

Cysteamine, or β-mercaptoethylamine (Fig. 199-1), is an aminothiol that, in 1976, was shown to rapidly and extensively lower the cystine content of cystinotic fibroblasts.[108] It was suggested that cysteamine reacted with cystine to form cysteine and cysteine-cysteamine mixed disulfide (Fig. 199-4). The cysteine would leave cystinotic lysosomes freely,[35] perhaps via a specific lysosomal membrane carrier.[109] The mixed disulfide would also exit the lysosome because its molecular mass was less than 220 daltons, the accepted upper limit for free movement of amino acids and di- and tripeptides across the lysosomal membrane.[110] Subsequent work demonstrated that because cysteine-cysteamine mixed disulfide resembles lysine structurally and because cystinotic fibroblasts have an intact lysosomal transport system for lysine, the mixed disulfide was transported across cystinotic lysosomal membranes in a carrier-mediated fashion, by the intact lysine porter.[37] In fact, experiments in leukocytes demonstrated that cysteine-cysteamine mixed disulfide was cleared at a significant rate from cystinotic granular fractions, in contrast to cystine, which remained trapped inside the lysosomes.[111] These two studies essentially verified the hypothesis put forth several years earlier concerning the mechanism of cystine depletion by cysteamine.[108]

Investigations in isolated human fibroblast lysosomes have now demonstrated that cysteamine is taken up by a specific transport system.[112] It has a biphasic Arrhenius plot with a Q_{10} of 1.2 between 27 and 35°C and 2.2 between 17 and 26°C. The rate of uptake is maximal at pH 8.2 and at pH 5.0 is one-fiftieth of the maximum. The system is specific for aminothiols or aminosulfides containing an amino group and a sulfur atom separated by two carbon atoms. Thus, cystine depletion of cystinotic lysosomes

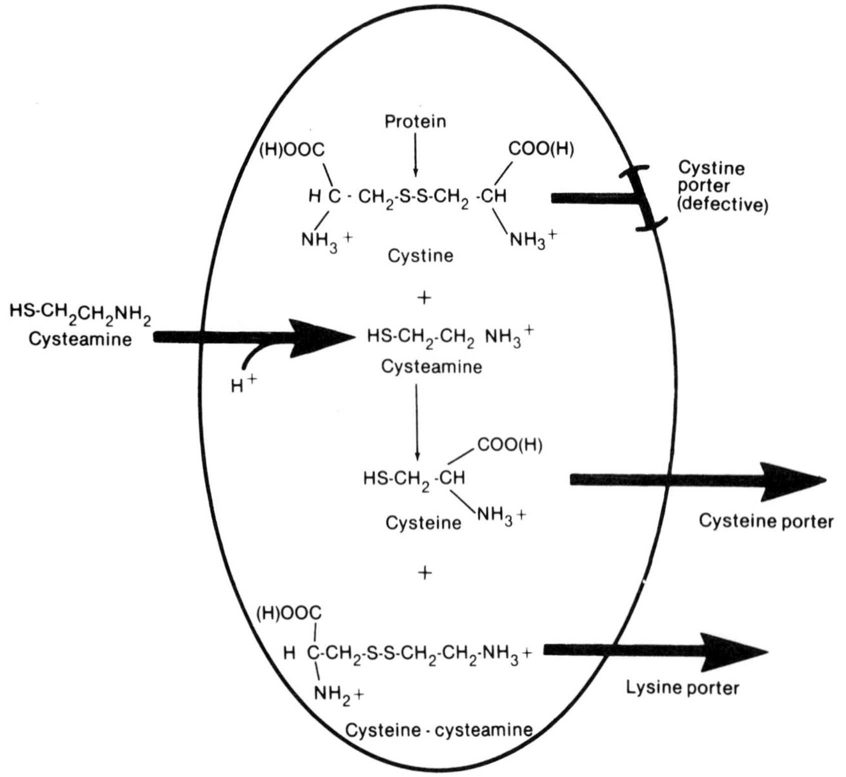

Fig. 199-4 Mechanism of cystine depletion by cysteamine. Cystine is stored inside the cystinotic lysosome because the cystine carrier in the lysosomal membrane is defective. Cysteamine traverses the lysosomal membrane by virtue of its neutral amine group or via a cysteamine carrier. The amine group acquires a positive charge and is "trapped" within the acidic lysosome. Cysteamine then reacts with cystine, producing cysteine and the mixed disulfide cysteine-cysteamine, by disulfide interchange. Cysteine leaves the cystinotic lysosome, perhaps via a cysteine carrier system. The mixed disulfide cysteine-cysteamine is structurally analogous to lysine, and exits the cystinotic lysosome via a lysosomal lysine carrier, which remains functional in cystinosis cells.

utilizes specific carriers for the entry of cysteamine,[112] exodus of the cysteine-cysteamine mixed disulfide via the lysine transport system,[37] and exodus of cysteine, the other product of the intralysosomal reaction, probably by a carrier system of its own.[109]

Several other reagents have been investigated for their cystine-depleting ability, including many which were enclosed in liposomes for presentation to cells.[113] Dithiothreitol lowered the cystine content of intact cystinotic fibroblasts[114] and of leukocyte granular fractions,[111] presumably by penetrating the lysosome and reducing cystine to cysteine. Ascorbic acid caused a 50 percent decrease in the cystine content of cultured fibroblasts, perhaps by its effects on properties of the lysosomal membrane.[115] Other compounds apparently act by producing cysteamine itself. Pantethine, which depletes intact cystinotic fibroblasts[116] but not leukocyte granular fractions of cystine,[111] is degraded to cysteamine by pantetheinase,[117] an enzyme present in human fibroblasts.[118] The aminothiol WR 1065, or *N*-(2′-mercaptoethyl)-1,3-propanediamine, and WR 638, or phosphocysteamine, were also proposed to produce cysteamine as the active cystine-depleting agent.[119,120] Recently, mercaptoethylgluconamide was shown to lower the cystine content of cystinotic cells,[121] again by its breakdown to the active compound, cysteamine.

Cysteamine has other cellular consequences based upon the redox effects of its free thiol. An intact intracellular redox potential is essential for normal cell functioning, and is crucial for the formation of certain viral coat proteins. Cysteamine interferes with HIV replication and may also directly alter the conformation of the gp120 coat protein, thus inhibiting viral transmission. Direct physicochemical effects of cysteamine on critical membrane disulfides may also explain the activity of the free thiol as a topical contraceptive.[122]

Source of Lysosomal Cystine in Cystinosis

The intralysosomal cystine crystals in cystinotic cells are thought to form because of saturating concentrations of cystine within lysosomes[25] rather than the phagocytosis of preformed crystals.[16] In cultured cells, the source of intralysosomal cystine appears to be cystine itself in the presence of exogenous cystine and to be protein catabolism in the absence of exogenous cystine.[123–125] When exogenous cystine serves as the source of lysosomal cystine in cystinotic fibroblasts,[124,126] it may enter via two routes.[127] One is rapid, low-capacity, chloroquine inhibitable, and involves movement through the plasma membrane, cytosol, and lysosomal membrane. The other is slow, high-capacity, stimulated by chloroquine and low medium pH, and might involve pinocytosis, with fusion of pinosomes and lysosomes. There is also evidence that cystine that enters fibroblasts is reduced in the cytoplasm to cysteine,[128] which could enter the lysosome by a known cysteine carrier in the lysosomal membrane.[109] Protein catabolism also gives rise to lysosomal cystine; the lysosomal cystine content has been shown to vary directly with the concentration in the medium of the cystine-rich protein, bovine serum albumin.[129] The process consists of pinocytosis of proteins followed by proteolysis, the rate of which is normal in cystinotic fibroblasts.[129,130] Lloyd pointed out that cysteine could be the physiologic reductant in lysosomal proteolysis facilitating reduction of intrachain disulfides. In this scheme, there would be no net increase or decrease in the amount of disulfide within lysosomes, but the net result would be conversion of an intrachain disulfide to a free cystine molecule.[131] Glutathione may[132] or may not[125] be a source of lysosomal cystine in cystinosis. However, *de novo* cysteine synthesis through the cystathionine β-synthase pathway has been shown not to be the source of stored cystine in cystinosis.[125,133]

We currently do not know why cystine is lost from cystinotic fibroblasts when the fibroblasts are placed at acid pH,[134] in chloroquine-containing medium,[135] at an elevated temperature,[103] or when they are labeled with [^{35}S]cystine and placed in cystine-free medium. This latter occurrence may be due to exocytosis, because the kinetics of [^{35}S]cystine egress resemble those of tritiated sucrose and tritiated mannitol, fluid-phase markers of endocytosis and exocytosis.[28]

GENETICS

All forms of cystinosis, including the unusual variants (see "Cystinosis Variants" below), display autosomal recessive patterns of inheritance, with a male/female ratio near 1.0. In North America, the incidence of infantile nephropathic cystinosis is approximately 1 per 100,000 to 1 per 200,000 live births, with a carrier frequency of roughly 1 in 200 in the general population. An estimated 400 to 500 children in the United States have the disease, but ascertainment is suspected to be incomplete, with undiagnosed infants dying of dehydration. The incidence is higher in certain subpopulations. The French province of Brittany, for example, has an estimated incidence of 1 in 26,000, while in the rest of France, the incidence is 1 per 326,440.[136] The incidence rate of infantile and adolescent cystinosis in the Federal Republic of Germany was approximately 1 per 179,000 live births; of 101 registered patients, 95 had infantile-type cystinosis, 5 had the adolescent type, and 1 had the adult type.[137] A recent study reported the frequency of cystinosis in the West Midlands, United Kingdom, to be 1 in 46,564 among northwest Europeans, and 1 in 3,613 among Pakistanis.[138]

Cystinosis is often considered a disease of fair-skinned individuals of European descent, but it is known to occur in Blacks, Hispanics, and people of Middle Eastern descent, and has also been described in at least one Chinese and several Japanese patients. It is likely that most cases of nonnephropathic (i.e., ocular) cystinosis are never diagnosed, and thus one can only speculate on the incidence of this type of cystinosis.

Only recently has the search for the cystinosis gene reached fruition. In 1995, the Cystinosis Collaborative Research Group used polymorphic microsatellite repeat markers to map the gene for cystinosis to a 4-cM region of chromosome 17p13 by linkage analysis.[44] The lod score for marker *D17S1584*, at a recombination fraction of 0.01, was 10.30. The critical region was progressively narrowed,[139–141] and in 1997, a study of French Canadian cystinosis patients revealed strong linkage disequilibrium for *D17S829*, a specific microsatellite marker in the region.[142] A physical map of the area surrounding this marker was created using a cosmid/P1 artificial chromosome contig. STS analysis indicated that the gene segment deleted in many cystinosis patients was 65 kb in size, and exon trapping followed by cDNA library screening revealed the cDNA of the cystinosis gene *CTNS*.[45] Mutation analysis defining 11 small mutations in cystinosis patients confirmed that this cDNA represented the cystinosis gene.[45] *CTNS* has 12 exons spanning 23 kb of genomic DNA. Its 2.6-kb mRNA codes for the 367-amino-acid protein cystinosin, with homology to a 55.5-kDa *C. elegans* protein and to the yeast transmembrane protein ERS1.[45] Cystinosin has seven transmembrane domains, a GY dipeptide near the C-terminus, and eight potential glycosylation sites.

The most common *CTNS* mutation, involving *D17S829*, consists of a deletion extending from intron 10 upstream 57,257 bases.[142a] This was found in the homozygous state in 23 of 70 patients in the British-French report,[45] and in 48 of 108 American-based patients.[91] Of 82 alleles bearing the 57-kb deletion, 38 derived from Germany, 28 from the British Isles, and 4 from Iceland, suggesting that the deletion arose in Germany prior to 700 AD.[91] The next most common mutation, present in 12 percent of the 216 American alleles studied, was 753G $\rightarrow$ A (W138X). In all, over 30 other mutations have been identified,[45,91,142b,142c,142d,243b] and in one study only 19 percent of patients failed to have one of their mutations determined. The base changes include deletions, insertions, splice site, nonsense, and missense mutations scattered throughout the gene's various exons and domains (Table 199-2). Several polymorphisms were also identified.[91] On northern blot analysis, all patients examined, whether homozygotes or compound heterozygotes, displayed

Table 199-2 *CTNS* Mutations and Frequencies

CTNS Domain	Mutation	# of Alleles*
Exons 1–10	57-kb del	143†
Leader sequence	357delGACT	12
	371delT	1
	397delTG	2
Transmembrane regions	753G → A	27
	845G → A	2
	857delAC	1
	883T → C	1
	985insA	2
	1080delC	1
	1253A → G	1
	1261G → A	2
	1261insG	1
	1354G → A	1
	1367TCGTCTTC → A	1
Nontransmembrane regions	479 + 1G	1
	537del21bp	6
	622G → T	2
	651delTCAC	2
	721C → T	3
	900delG	3
	901-1G → C	1
	908del9bp	1
	950delACG	2
	952G → A	1
	1033insCG	1
	1035insC	2
	1209C → G	2
	1232G → A	1

*Of 356 alleles in 178 individual patients not known to be related.[45,91] Cell repository mutations[91] were not considered.

†This includes one heterozygous patient whose deleted allele was ascertained by inheritance of polymorphic markers. The remaining 71 patients were homozygous for the deletion.

CTNS RNA expression in their cultured fibroblasts, except for homozygotes for the 57-kb deletion.[91]

A previous study in which somatic cell hybrids were prepared between cells from patients with different types of cystinosis suggests that the various forms of cystinosis are allelic.[143] Moreover, inclusion of cystinosis variant families in linkage studies contributed to the lod scores, rather than detracting from them.[44] Finally, preliminary results indicate that intermediate and ocular cystinosis patients have mutations in *CTNS*, but that these mutations differ from those of classical nephropathic cystinosis patients.[144,144a]

CLINICAL FEATURES AND PATHOLOGY

Presentation and General Course (Fig. 199-5)

A recent article reviews the clinical course of cystinosis,[145] and a composite history for a typical child with cystinosis was previously published.[146] As for most lysosomal storage disorders, patients with nephropathic cystinosis are entirely normal at birth, except perhaps for lighter skin and hair pigmentation than their sibs. Development proceeds normally until the second half of the first year of life, when an affected infant generally fails to grow and gain weight, eats poorly, appears fussy, urinates and drinks excessively, and suffers isolated or recurrent episodes of acidosis and dehydration. These findings all result from renal tubular Fanconi syndrome; glucosuria may also eventually lead to a diagnosis of cystinosis. For 55 patients seen at the NIH between 1960 and 1980, the median age at diagnosis was 20 months; for 44 patients seen between 1980 and 1992, the median age at diagnosis was 14 months.[147] The age at diagnosis is constantly decreasing because of increased physician awareness, but some children still probably escape diagnosis when they succumb to severe dehydration during an acute diarrheal illness.

The natural history of cystinosis after infancy dictates that an affected child will manifest normal intelligence but continue to grow poorly. Photophobia usually, but not universally, develops. Renal glomerular function is lost gradually, requiring renal transplantation at approximately 9 to 10 years of age. The child will not have a predisposition to infections, although altered motility and adherence[148] and increased leukotriene C_4 levels[149] have been reported in the phagocytic cells of children with cystinosis. After kidney transplantation, renal function is normalized, but the inexorable accumulation of cystine in other organs creates newly recognized threats to their proper functioning.[146]

Renal Tubular Involvement

The kidney appears particularly susceptible to the adverse effects of cystine accumulation in cystinosis. As early as 1965, three stages of renal damage were recognized in cystinosis: tubular injury with failure to reabsorb; tubular insufficiency with decreased para-aminohippuric acid clearance; and glomerular failure.[150] Impaired tubular reabsorption, known as the renal Fanconi syndrome, apparently correlates with the "swan-neck" deformity of the proximal convoluted tubule.[17] The tubules of a cystinosis patient's kidneys have appeared disorganized and poorly developed even prior to the onset of frank Fanconi syndrome.[151] Cystinosis represents the most common identifiable cause of renal tubular Fanconi syndrome in children, although tyrosinemia, Wilson disease, Lowe syndrome, galactosemia, and glycogen storage disease are part of the differential diagnosis.

The Fanconi syndrome results in excessive urinary losses of glucose, amino acids, phosphate, calcium, magnesium, sodium, potassium, bicarbonate, carnitine, water, and, undoubtedly, other small molecules yet to be identified. Children with cystinosis may initially receive a diagnosis of Bartter syndrome, nephrogenic diabetes insipidus, or pseudohypoaldosteronism.[152–154] A "tubular" proteinuria, in which proteins of molecular weight 10 to 50,000 are excreted in fiftyfold normal amounts, can also develop.[155] Total protein excretion can be up to 5 g per day.[156] Microscopic hematuria is occasionally present. Renal calculi of urate and calcium oxalate have been reported,[157,158] and nephrocalcinosis has been found in association with increased calcium excretion in cystinosis patients.[159] This medullary nephrocalcinosis was documented in 26 of 41 patients age 2 months to 15 years.[160] The mean age of the affected children was 9.4 ± 3.5 years, compared with 5.1 ± 3.8 years for the 15 children without nephrocalcinosis ($p < 0.005$). The nephrocalcinosis, which does not appear to impair glomerular function, was associated with vastly elevated levels of urinary calcium and phosphate, the consequence of renal Fanconi syndrome combined with mineral supplementation.

Although blood glucose levels are normal in cystinosis, glucosuria and polyuria can lead to the mistaken diagnosis of juvenile-onset diabetes mellitus. The polyuria consists of daily excretion of 2 to 6 liters of dilute urine (less than 300 mOsmol/liter), and may contribute to persistent enuresis or may be life-threatening in an infant suffering acute gastroenteritis. Dehydration in such a patient is rapid and can be associated with a mild chronic fever. Acidosis can be profound due to renal losses of bicarbonate. Hyponatremia and hypokalemia, with its risk of arrhythmias, also occur. Muscle weakness due to hypokalemia has led, in some instances, to inappropriate muscle biopsy. Hypocalcemia, and occasionally hypomagnesemia, can result in tetany, especially when acidosis is acutely reversed by alkali therapy or when phosphate supplements bind ionized calcium. Phosphaturia leads to hypophosphatemic rickets with typical metaphyseal widening, rachitic rosary, frontal bossing, genu valgum, and failure to walk. Elevated heat-labile serum alkaline phosphatase

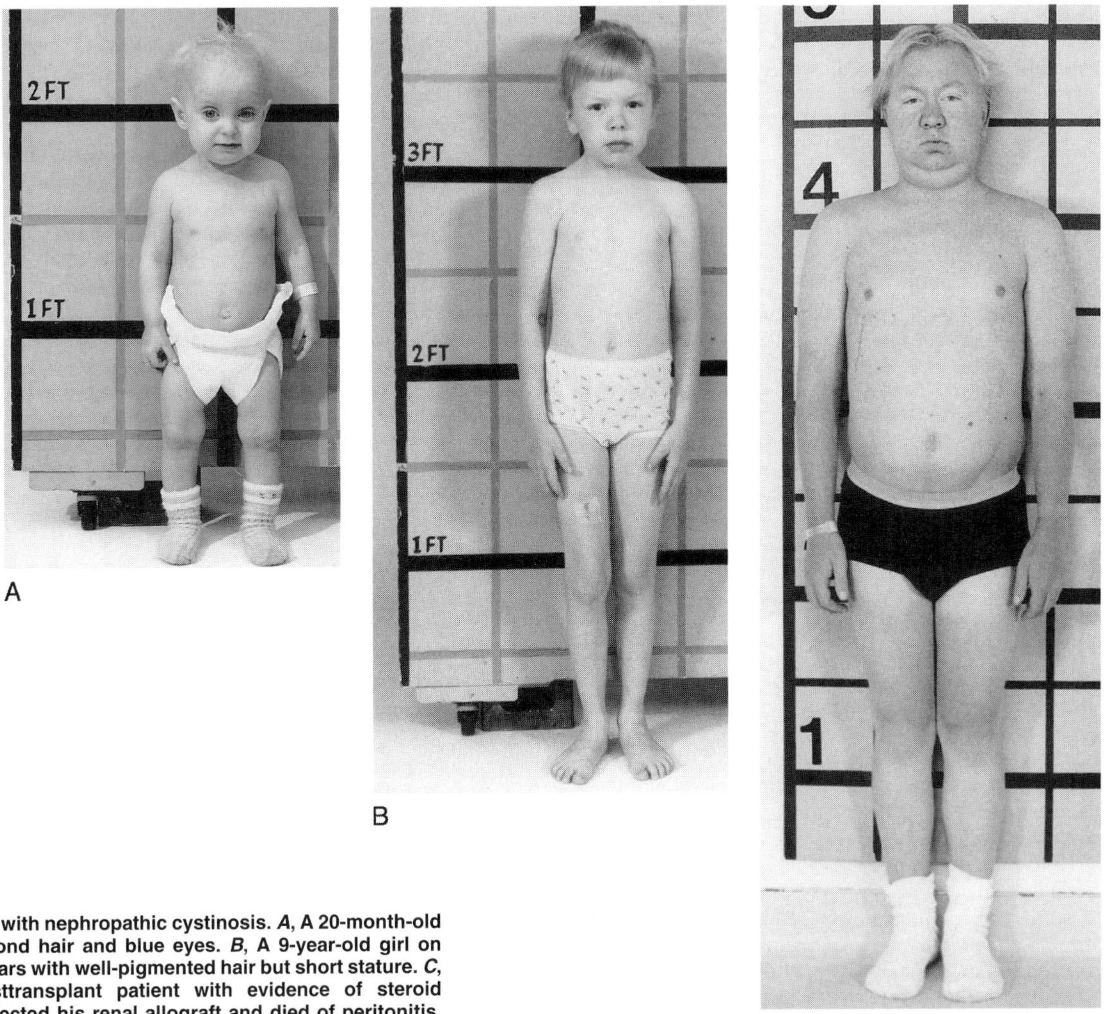

A

B

C

Fig. 199-5 Patients with nephropathic cystinosis. *A*, A 20-month-old girl with sparse blond hair and blue eyes. *B*, A 9-year-old girl on cysteamine for 7 years with well-pigmented hair but short stature. *C*, A 25-year-old posttransplant patient with evidence of steroid effects. He later rejected his renal allograft and died of peritonitis. (*Courtesy of National Institutes of Health Clinical Center.*)

levels reflect active rickets. Vitamin D metabolites are normal in cystinosis.[161] A generalized aminoaciduria[162] results in excretion of, on average, over 1 mmol/kg/day of 21 measurable amino acids; this is over tenfold the normal amino acid excretion.[163] The mean fractional excretions of individual amino acids vary widely,[164] ranging from 0.10 for arginine to 0.71 for histidine;[165] normally, 94 to 99 percent of each amino acid is reabsorbed. Carnitine, a small molecule required for transport of free fatty acids into mitochondria for subsequent energy production, is normally 97 percent reabsorbed. However, because of their Fanconi syndrome, cystinosis patients reabsorb only 70 percent of their carnitine, resulting in plasma and muscle carnitine deficiency.[163] Consequently, lipid droplets accumulate in the muscle, which may appear weak and poorly developed. The full ramifications of the Fanconi syndrome in cystinosis have not yet been determined, but they include the failure to thrive characteristic of this disorder.

Glomerular Damage

The glomerular deterioration that provides the clinical hallmark of cystinosis proceeds inexorably in untreated patients. Pathologically, the cystinotic kidney manifests different stages of destruction[166] with giant-cell transformation of the glomerular epithelium,[167] hyperplasia and hypertrophy of the juxtaglomerular apparatus,[15,89] and occasional "dark" cells and cytoplasmic inclusions.[65] The ultimate result, however, remains a classic end-stage kidney with scarring and fibrosis, chronic interstitial nephritis, and tubular degeneration.[81,168] Crystals, identified as L-cystine,[19] are abundant, but renal stones do not form, as in cystinuria. Clinically, most patients have proteinuria and many have granular casts and microscopic hematuria. Measured creatinine clearances fall monotonically from infancy in untreated patients.[169] Occasionally, renal failure occurs as early as 1 to 3 years of age,[170,171] but renal reserve generally prevents the serum creatinine from rising above 1.0 mg/dl before approximately 5 years of age. As for other renal disease,[172] the reciprocal of serum creatinine decreases linearly with age, predicting renal failure in cystinosis at 9.1[169] or 10.7[173] years of age. For 205 European patients, serum creatinine versus age curves provide standards for the natural history of renal demise;[174] the mean age of renal death was 9.2 years.[175] Many patients approaching renal failure continue to waste large volumes of fluids and electrolytes despite low filtration rates. In others, the Fanconi syndrome appears to improve with the reduced filtration. Some patients have unexplained plateaus in their renal function lasting months to years; others suffer a rapid deterioration of renal function with the onset of an acute infection, acute poststreptococcal glomerulonephritis or, in infants, hypoperfusion secondary to dehydration. Cystinosis patients with uremia can die in congestive heart failure.

Growth

Growth retardation represents a significant part of the clinical picture of nephropathic cystinosis, yet it does not commence *in utero*. Length and weight are normal at birth. During the first year of life, linear growth begins to decrease. Height falls to the third percentile by 1 year of age. In patients who do not receive cystine depletion, growth proceeds at only 50 to 75 percent of the normal rate, so that an 8-year-old patient has the height of a normal 4-year-old.[176] Typically, height velocity is two to three standard deviations below the mean for age when the glomerular filtration rate is above 20 ml/min/1.73 m^2.[177] Bone age follows height age, which soon lags years behind chronologic age.[146,178,179] Because height and weight are equally delayed, the children appear proportional except for a relative macrocephaly caused by sparing of head circumference.

Growth and final height of cystinosis patients after renal transplantation is extremely variable.[89] Mean heights for post-transplant patients age 10 to 18 years are 20 to 30 cm below the fiftieth percentile for age.[163] Of 36 patients age 18 to 34 years seen at the National Institute of Child Health and Human Development (NICHD),[181] the tallest male was 170 cm and the shortest was 129 cm (mean $\pm$ SD, 148 $\pm$ 10 cm); the mean was approximately 30 cm below the average normal adult height. Among females, the range was 117 to 149 cm, with a mean $\pm$ SD of 137 $\pm$ 10 cm, or 26 cm below the mean adult height. Mean values for 33 French patients age 18 to 34 years were 143 cm for males and 128 cm for females.[182] While children transplanted before adolescence have some chance of realizing a growth spurt and achieving near-normal height, this prospect appears remote for patients grafted after 16 years of age, despite a bone age several years delayed.[179] One study found catch-up growth after renal transplant in cystinosis patients receiving cyclosporine A and low-dose prednisone, but not among those receiving azathioprine and high-dose prednisone.[177]

The pathogenesis of the growth retardation in cystinosis remains unresolved. Children with renal failure due to other causes generally do not show the profound impairment of growth exhibited by patients with cystinosis. Renal failure, chronic acidosis, and renal rickets result in growth delays, but even cystinosis patients without these complications grow poorly. The common feeding problems in children with cystinosis[183] may contribute to failure to thrive. In addition, cystine storage in various organs, including growth plates of long bones and developing myofibrils, may inhibit growth, which improves with chronic cystine depletion.[176] Single growth hormone measurements[184] and somatomedin-C levels[178] are normal in patients with cystinosis.

Ocular Damage

Cystinosis eventually affects most of the structures[185] and many of the functions of the eye, but with variable rates of progression. Several reviews have detailed the early[186,187] and late[74,89,179] ocular findings in cystinosis.

Retina. A characteristic peripheral retinopathy, consisting of a patchy depigmentation of the retina with pigment clumps of various sizes, typifies nephropathic cystinosis.[188] This finding is not present at birth, although vacuolization of retinal pigment epithelial cells has been reported in a 21-week cystinotic fetus.[189] A pigment retinopathy has been reported in a 5-week-old girl who was subsequently diagnosed as having cystinosis.[76] Despite the "blond fundus" resulting from degeneration of the retinal pigment epithelium, visual acuity, visual fields, night vision, and electroretinography have been normal in young children with cystinosis.[187] But posttransplant patients, whose retinas have accumulated cystine for one to three decades, exhibit a disconcerting frequency of visual impairment. Although visual acuity was subjectively normal in a series of 10 patients age 11 to 19 years, electroretinography was abnormal in 1 individual.[190] Of 16 patients in a French study, 3 exhibited marked visual impairment and 8 had abnormal electroretinography.[89] In a survey of 80 patients over the age of 10 years in North America, one-third had decreased visual acuity.[191] It is clear that the frequency and severity of visual impairment increase with age. Of six patients over 30 years of age examined at the National Eye Institute, five had visual acuities of 20/200 or worse, with color vision and dark adaptation deficits as well.[179] Electroretinography confirmed the clinical findings in affected patients,[74,179] and retinal crystals were documented by photography in one individual.[74] Color and night vision deficits appear to precede problems with acuity.

Cornea. Corneal crystals, first described in cystinosis in 1941,[192] are pathognomonic of the disorder when seen on slit-lamp examination by a trained ophthalmologist. Descriptions of the pathology of the corneal tissue in cystinosis are numerous.[186,187,193–195] Fusiform crystals involve the anterior portion of the central cornea but occupy the full thickness of the peripheral cornea.[73,187] They are absent at birth and at 3 months of age,[73] but are generally present by 1 year of age.[187] A patchy pattern is occasionally observed between 1 and 2 years of age, and the presence of crystals not apparent on slit-lamp examination in a moving infant can sometimes be documented by photography. By 3 or 4 years, cystinotic corneas are packed with crystals, and by 10 to 20 years of age, corneas often develop a characteristic haziness.[74] At this time, exquisitely painful corneal erosions, documented by fluorescein testing, can recur several times a month and seriously interfere with normal activities.[74,179,196] Decreased tearing, documented by Schirmer testing,[197] can exacerbate this condition. In one patient whose cornea was examined immunohistologically, an inflammatory component appeared to be involved.[198] Of 50 patients over 16 years of age examined at the National Eye Institute, 8 had some degree of band keratopathy, with one 15-year-old girl exhibiting such plaque formation that she was blind to all light perception.[197] Corneal thickness has been reported increased in cystinosis.[199] A keratopathy has been described in rabbits fed L-cystine.[200]

Photophobia of variable onset produces various degrees of discomfort in children with cystinosis,[74,201] who often avoid sunlight. The photophobia probably results from reflections of light off corneal and conjunctival crystals, because it decreases with cysteamine eyedrop therapy[197] and progresses in severity if untreated.[74]

Conjunctiva. The conjunctiva and uvea contain birefringent hexagonal and rectangular crystals[73] shown by x-ray diffraction studies to be made of L-cystine.[195] These can produce a ground-glass appearance on slit-lamp examination, but do not cause inflammation.[187] Electron microscopy of conjunctival tissue has been used to demonstrate the lysosomal location of the crystals.[202] Cystine measurements in conjunctival biopsies have been suggested for the early diagnosis of cystinosis,[203] but leukocyte assays are less invasive.

Other Ocular Tissues. Cystine crystals are present in the uvea and sclera of cystinosis patients.[187] The irides also contain crystals, especially in older individuals,[74] and crystals have been documented overlying the lenses of posttransplant patients.[74,196] The presence of crystals in these locations may give rise to tissue reactions which result in posterior synechiae, observed in nine National Eye Institute patients 16 to 34 years old.[74,179,197] This complication may in turn lead to glaucoma, which has been observed in two patients 19 and 27 years old.[74,179,202] Refractory blepharospasm, apparently a result of constant guarding against painful photophobia, has been found in a few older individuals.[74,179]

Endocrine Involvement

Children with cystinosis frequently develop primary hypothyroidism, with atrophy and crystal formation in follicular cells.[77] This apparently reduces the thyroid's functional reserve and causes compensated hypothyroidism, that is, an increase in thyrotropin (TSH) prior to the onset of frank hypothyroidism.[184,204] In particular, the α subunit of TSH is often elevated.[205] Hypothyroidism clearly represents an age-related phenomenon. In one study, 3 of 15 patients examined before age 13 years were clinically hypothyroid.[77] Fifteen of 27 French children of all ages with cystinosis were hypothyroid.[89] More than 70 percent of 80 North American patients over 10 years of age required thyroid replacement, with an average age of 10 years at the initiation of therapy.[191] Hypothyroidism in cystinosis may be associated with pituitary resistance to thyroid hormone,[206] and histologic studies of cystinotic pituitary glands have revealed occasional hyperplasia of thyrotrophs and refractile crystals.[77] However, growth hormone,[184] somatomedin-C,[178] and cortisol response to ACTH[184] appear normal in children with cystinosis.

The pancreas may also be affected by long-standing cystine accumulation. Although nonsuppressible insulinlike activity is normal in young children with cystinosis,[184] several patients have developed insulin-dependent diabetes mellitus after the age of 10.[68,89,207] Poor glucose tolerance results from impaired insulin production,[68] and is exacerbated by antirejection steroid therapy. Diabetes mellitus has been reported in a 13-month-old infant with cystinosis,[208] and β-cell hyperplasia has been found in cystinotic pancreases examined postmortem.[209]

Females with cystinosis undergo pubertal events in a normal sequence,[179] but at ages which range from normal to late, that is, 16 to 17 years of age. To date, most affected females have undergone a renal transplant before puberty, meaning that uremia, or immunosuppressive therapy, or both, has interfered with normal development. Nevertheless, virtually all the affected females eventually progress,[180] and one 20-year-old woman with cystinosis and a renal transplant gave birth to a normal boy in late 1986.[80]

Male patients with cystinosis have delayed puberty (with a normal sequence of progression), again with some influence exerted by renal failure and transplantation.[210] None of 10 male patients age 15 to 28 years studied at the NICHD reached Tanner stage 5 of pubertal development, but several adult males in a German study did complete sexual development.[177] Three males in the NICHD study had decreased testosterone and seven had elevated FSH and LH levels.[210] In a French study, adult male patients exhibited hypogonadism, with high FSH and LH levels in 9 of 11 individuals tested.[182] These findings suggest primary hypogonadism, and the occurrence of crystals and fibrosis in the testes of a 22-year-old patient is consistent with this diagnosis. Older male patients can experience erections, but three patients who produced a semen sample all proved to be azoospermic.[156,210] To our knowledge, no cystinosis patient has fathered a child, but this may change as treated patients reach adulthood with normal testicular function.

Myopathy

Although the muscle was long considered spared in cystinosis, it recently became apparent that the continued accumulation of cystine in this tissue leads to structural changes and functional impairment. Not only do cystinotic myotubes in culture store cystine,[211] but the cystine content of biopsied muscle increases with age to values 1000 times normal.[79,89,90] The clinical characteristics of the muscle involvement in cystinosis were first recognized in a 22-year-old man with generalized muscle wasting.[79] This posttransplant patient developed hypophonia and dysphagia at age 20, progressed in weakness and wasting, and died of aspiration 2 years later. He had normal nerve conduction studies, but electromyography showed low-amplitude brief-duration polyphasic motor-unit potentials consistent with a myopathy. Muscle biopsy sealed the diagnosis with the appearance of type I fiber atrophy, variation in fiber size, and numerous ring fibers. Cystine crystals were apparent in fibroblastoid cells in the perimysial and endomysial spaces adjacent to muscle fibers.[79] To date, at least five other patients seen at the NIH have had clinically documented myopathies, supported by electrophysiologic evidence.[212] One 21-year-old woman with severe wasting of her hand muscles (Fig. 199-6*A*) underwent a biopsy of one of her abductor digiti minimi muscles, which showed striking vacuolization and a cystine concentration more than one

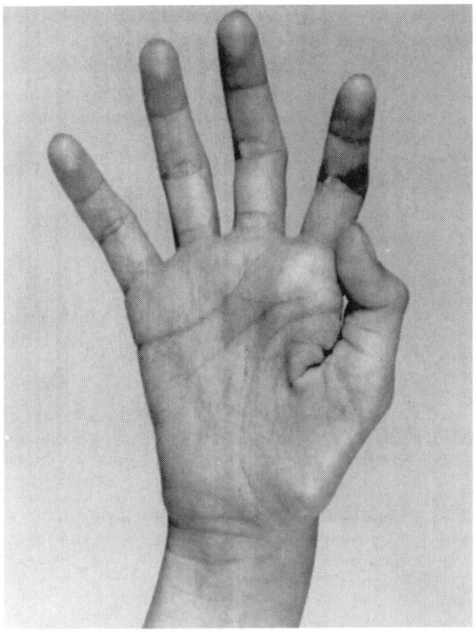

A

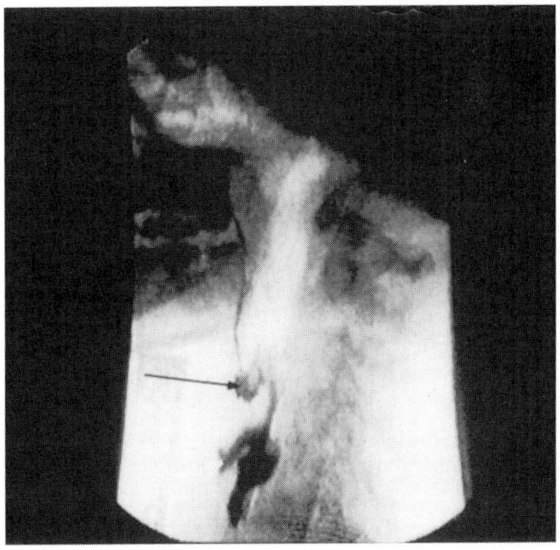

B

Fig. 199-6 Late complications of nephropathic cystinosis. *A*, Right hand of 21-year-old posttransplant patient with a distal myopathy. Note wasting of thenar and hypothenar eminences and interosseous muscles. Fingers are held in partial flexion due to weakness. *B*, Barium study of swallowing in a 22-year-old posttransplant patient. Residual barium coats the pharyngeal wall and remains in the valleculae (arrow). Some barium has penetrated the laryngeal vestibule, and the remainder has pooled in the piriform sinus and cricopharyngeal sphincter. (*From Sonies et al.*[214] *Used with permission.*)

hundredfold elevated.[212] A case of myopathy and corneal crystals reported in the ophthalmic literature appears to represent cystinosis with muscle involvement.[213]

The severe swallowing difficulties observed in older cystinosis patients probably result from impaired muscle function.[214] Affected individuals have decreased tongue and lip strength, hypophonic speech, and abnormal oral structure and anatomy. Swallowing studies (Fig. 199-6*B*) show pooling of barium in the valleculae and piriform sinuses, and some penetration of the laryngeal vestibule, with a significantly increased duration of swallowing. The severity of oral motor dysfunction increased with age. One patient died of his swallowing difficulty,[79] and at least two others are seriously affected.

In a recent study of pulmonary function in cystinosis,[215] 11 of 12 adult patients (mean age 28 $\pm$ 4 years) had restrictive ventilatory defects, with a mean forced vital capacity of 58 $\pm$ 13 percent of predicted. These patients had not received significant chronic cysteamine therapy (see "Therapy" below), and the pulmonary findings were attributed to weak accessory chest and diaphragmatic muscles. Patients under age 20, as a rule, had no pulmonary deficits. It has been suggested that pulmonary cystine crystals can be detected radiographically,[216] but no evidence for this is available. Cardiac muscle has not been extensively examined for abnormal structure, function, or cystine storage in cystinosis. A single report describes elevated myocardial cystine levels and cardiac failure in a 31-year-old posttransplant cystinosis patient.[217]

Nervous System Involvement

Although the central nervous system has also been considered spared in cystinosis, this may be true only early in the disease. Cystine storage is limited in young patients,[87] but one 25-year-old woman accumulated large quantities of cystine in all portions of her central nervous system,[88] and a 28-year-old man had cystine crystals within white matter parenchymal cells.[218] The clinical correlates of central nervous system storage include cerebral atrophy on CT scan, seen in 3 cystinosis patients in chronic renal failure;[219] in 7 of 9[220] and 11 of 17 posttransplant patients;[180] in a group of 10 cystinosis patients with neurologic symptoms such as seizures, tremor, mental retardation, or pyramidal syndrome;[221] in 13 of 14 unselected cystinosis patients age 13 to 25;[222] and in 10 of 11 cystinosis children and adolescents.[223] Cerebral cortical atrophy can be observed in pediatric patients with end-stage renal disease,[224] but the frequency in cystinosis seems excessive, and one study controlled for this.[221] Other cerebral involvement in cystinosis includes nonabsorptive hydrocephalus,[225] demyelination of the internal capsule and brachium pontis,[82] and cystic necrosis with calcification, spongy change, and vacuolization.[218] The patient with the latter problem, a man in his mid-twenties with a renal transplant for 14 years, had difficulty swallowing, slow speech, loss of recent memory, extremity weakness, and a gait disturbance confining him to a wheelchair.[218,222] Despite the cerebral atrophy seen on CT scan, most cystinosis patients have normal neurologic examinations.[222] Neurophysiologic testing of the peripheral nervous system is normal in cystinosis.[226]

Hepatic and Gastrointestinal Complications

Hepatomegaly has been reported in 7 of 16 dialysis and transplant patients with cystinosis[89] and in 42 percent of 80 cystinosis patients over the age of 10.[191] Many children under age 5 also have hepatomegaly, whose etiology is unknown. In general, it is not associated with elevated serum liver enzymes or clinical abnormalities. Esophageal varices in two patients,[89] and bleeding gastric varices in another,[227] did result from portal hypertension. Hypersplenism syndrome has been seen in occasional patients,[89,179] and the incidence of splenomegaly among patients over age 10 is 27 percent.[191]

Liver pathology has demonstrated crystals,[66] hepatic veno-occlusive disease,[226,227] and portal hypertension with fibrosis,[228] but not cirrhosis.[89] The liver has a normal acinar architecture with hypertrophy of Kupffer cells and, to a lesser extent, portal macrophages as a result of cystine crystal formation.[229] The affected Kupffer cells are haphazardly distributed, but may be clustered around terminal hepatic venules in zone 3. There is usually no inflammatory response and little or no fibrosis. Hepatocytes, perisinusoidal lipocytes (Ito cells), bile ducts, and blood vessels usually show no pathologic changes.[229]

Cystine crystals also occur in the appendix,[71] rectal mucosa,[69] and intestinal mucosa.[70] Their presence may contribute to the morning nausea and vomiting observed among some children with cystinosis, many of whom are also poor eaters with penchants for hot, spicy foods.[146] One 7-year-old boy with severe cystinosis has been diagnosed with ulcerative colitis,[230] and a 17-year-old woman,[231] as well as a 21-year-old man,[156] had objective evidence of pancreatic exocrine insufficiency.

Other Clinical and Laboratory Abnormalities

Caucasian (not Hispanic or Black) patients with cystinosis have skin and hair pigmentation that is noticeably lighter than the pigmentation of their unaffected sibs. We speculate that pigment formation may be impaired in the melanosomes, which are the melanocyte counterparts of lysosomes. Deficits of short-term visual memory,[232] tactile recognition,[233] spelling,[234] and arithmetic[235] have been reported in children with cystinosis, although IQ values are in the normal range.[235] Young patients with cystinosis have average intelligence and school performance.[236] Psychosocial problems occur because of their chronic illness, and adjusting to a life of short stature often proves difficult.[146] Some children avoid school and others fail to extricate themselves from dependence on their parents.

Most children with nephropathic cystinosis display an inability to produce a normal volume of sweat, although sweat electrolyte concentrations are normal.[237] This deficiency results in heat intolerance and avoidance, flushing, hyperthermia, and vomiting in small children. The cause is unknown. Stimulated salivary flow rates were also decreased below the normal range in 10 of 18 cystinosis patients tested.[238]

Intraoperative hyperthermia occurred in a child with cystinosis,[239] and feeding problems are common in patients with cystinosis.[183] Polyneuropathy and pulmonary fibrosis have been reported in individual posttransplant patients.[67,240]

For reasons that remain mysterious, several laboratory values are often chronically elevated in cystinosis, including the sedimentation rate, total serum cholesterol (including VLDL and HDL subfractions), and platelet count.[146,179] The platelet count normalizes after renal transplantation.[179] A mild anemia becomes severe with the onset of uremia, with a hematocrit of 15 to 20 percent accompanying a serum creatinine of 3 to 8 mg/dl. The anemia, not due to iron deficiency, may result from decreased erythropoietin production by a damaged kidney and, later, from uremia. Posttransplant patients have normal hematocrits.[179]

Cystinosis as an Adult Disease

Renal allograft procedures have changed the face of cystinosis from a fatal childhood disease followed by pediatric nephrologists to an adult disorder challenging internists and other specialists. The imprint of cystinosis appears immediately on the prematurely aged, jowled faces of young adults, who often have slow, raspy speech,[156] and almost always have short stature.[179] The associated problem of poor self-image is exacerbated in males by the prospect of infertility. Medical catastrophes are also threatening. One enigma of cystinosis is why certain patients suffer severe involvement of a single organ, with sparing of other systems, and other patients suffer complications of a different organ system. Of 36 adult patients seen at the NIH prior to 1993,[181] 7 were deceased, 5 were legally blind, 3 others had poor vision in one eye, 12 had a distal myopathy, 21 had swallowing abnormalities, 8 had cerebral calcifications, and 31 required thyroid hormone replacement. Only 11 were receiving adequate cysteamine therapy (see "Therapy" below). In a similar French study of 33 adult patients,[182] 6 were deceased, 5 were blind, 2 had a distal myopathy, 7 manifested encephalopathy, 5 were insulin-dependent diabetics, and 27 required thyroid replacement. Only 5 were receiving oral cysteamine therapy. Remarkably, despite their medical complications, many of the adults engaged in valuable activities and gainful employment.

Heterozygotes

There are no published reports of any heterozygote for cystinosis having cystine crystals in any tissue or cell, or exhibiting any clinical manifestations of the renal Fanconi syndrome.

Nevertheless, their polymorphonuclear leukocytes contain an increased amount of nonprotein cystine,[241] and peripheral leukocytes of obligate heterozygotes exhibit approximately half-normal rates of lysosomal cystine egress[39] and countertransport.[42] Surprisingly, the free-cystine content of cultured skin fibroblasts from obligate heterozygotes is not significantly different from that found in normal control fibroblasts.[143]

DIAGNOSIS

Postnatal

The first individual diagnosed as having nephropathic cystinosis in a family generally acquires the diagnosis because of suspicion aroused by the presenting renal abnormalities. The diagnosis is confirmed by measuring the white blood cell cystine content. Leukocytes are prepared from as little as 3 ml of heparinized blood by acid citrate-dextran sedimentation, followed by hypotonic lysis of erythrocytes.[242] Cystine is then measured either with an automated amino acid analyzer using column chromatography or by using a specific cystine-binding protein in an isotope dilution assay.[64,243] In normal control individuals, the cystine content of mixed leukocyte preparations is less than 0.2 nmol half-cystine per mg protein. In infantile nephropathic cystinosis, the value averages approximately 8 nmol half-cystine per mg protein (see reference 98 for references). In other forms of cystinosis the value may be lower, but is generally greater than 1 nmol half-cystine per mg protein.

Cystinosis can be diagnosed immediately by ophthalmologic examination, revealing the typical crystalline keratopathy in children over 1 year of age by use of a slit-lamp. The diagnosis can also be made by examination of a bone marrow aspirate with phase microscopy, where the hexagonal and monoclinic cystine crystals are obvious under crossed polarizing prisms (see reference 98 for references). In general, however, patients should be spared invasive biopsies and aspirations, if possible.

The first case of ocular cystinosis in a family (see "Cystinosis Variants" below) is always detected by an ophthalmologist who is doing a slit-lamp examination for some other reason. Again, the diagnosis can be verified by white blood cell cystine assay.

There is no newborn screening program for cystinosis because of the labor-intensive nature of current diagnostic tests.

Prenatal

Prenatal diagnosis can be performed on either cultured amniocytes following amniocentesis or cultured chorionic villi by direct measurement of the intracellular free-cystine. A previous edition of this chapter gives specific values and references.[98] Like cultured skin fibroblasts, cystinotic amniocytes and villus cells store 50 to 100 times the normal concentration of cystine (see Table 199-1). DNA diagnostic techniques may soon be available as well, especially for families in whom the proband is homozygous for the 57-kb deletion in *CTNS*.[243a,243b] The amniotic fluid cystine concentration is normal in affected pregnancies.[98,189]

Because of the success with cysteamine therapy (see "Therapy" below), many families now refuse prenatal diagnosis but ask that the diagnosis be made immediately at birth so that treatment with cysteamine bitartrate can be started as soon as possible. This is done by measuring the cystine content of the placenta and/or white blood cells made from cord blood (see reference 98 for references). DNA diagnostic techniques may soon be available for early diagnosis.

Heterozygotes

Leukocytes from obligate heterozygotes for cystinosis contain, on average, four to five times more free-cystine per milligram of protein than leukocytes from normal control individuals.[20,241] However, when mixed populations of leukocytes are measured, about 10 percent of heterozygotes have values that fall into the normal range. Heterozygote detection is more accurate when cystine is measured in polymorphonuclear cells because most of the cystine is found in these cells and monocytes, and relatively little in the lymphocytes.[85,241] In the future, it may be easier to determine heterozygosity by molecular techniques.

THERAPY

Symptomatic

Patients with cystinosis develop the renal Fanconi syndrome early in life with attendant renal tubular losses of glucose, water, sodium, potassium, bicarbonate, phosphorus, and carnitine. Severe electrolyte imbalances due to renal losses of water and electrolytes can cause fatal dehydration, particularly during summer months and during episodes of gastroenteritis. Children with cystinosis may have extreme polyuria secondary to their renal tubular damage, so that free access to large amounts of water is essential during both day and night. Urinary losses of bicarbonate and electrolytes are replaced orally. Progressive urinary losses of phosphate lead to rickets and generally require oral phosphate replacement, with vitamin D supplementation to enhance gastrointestinal absorption of phosphate. The usual form of vitamin D given these patients in the United States is 1,25-dihydroxycholecalciferol. A typical dose might be 0.25 μg per day, but the dose must be individualized for each patient. Details of management have been published previously.[98,146]

Many European medical centers find indomethacin extremely helpful in managing children with cystinosis.[244–247] Properly used, it markedly reduces abnormal urinary losses.[248] The decreased need for water ingestion may lead to an increased appetite and improved growth.[249] The dose of indomethacin (2 to 3 mg/kg/d) is individualized for each patient so as not to decrease the glomerular filtration rate. Any decrease in GFR appears to be reversible when the drug dosage is reduced.[250] The mechanism of action of indomethacin appears to be related to inhibition of prostaglandin synthesis.[247,248] A recent double-blind trial comparing 2 mg/kg/d of indomethacin to placebo found a small but significant reduction in urine volume in the patients receiving indomethacin.[251] The most impressive finding, however, was that most families believed their child was receiving the active drug because of a placebo effect. Children in both groups ate better and had impressive gains in growth. A weakness of the study was that 2 mg/kg/d was probably too low a dose for optimal effect in many patients.

Carnitine deficiency due to Fanconi syndrome can be treated with oral L-carnitine replacement.[163] Plasma carnitine levels return promptly to normal, but because of enormous ongoing urinary losses, the muscle compartment takes years to replete.[252,253] A mean dose of 92 mg L-carnitine/kg/d, given to six infants for an average duration of 5 years, maintained their muscle free-carnitine in the normal range, but strength was not assessed.[253]

As renal failure supervenes, the basic aspects of medical care are similar to those for any uremic patient. Care must be taken to properly manage serum concentrations of calcium, phosphate, and potassium. However, cystinosis patients have some unique problems. They often develop hypothyroidism by the end of the first decade of life,[184,191] but respond well to standard doses of L-thyroxine. Similarly, insulin-deficient patients are benefited by insulin therapy.[68] As described below, cystine-depletion therapy with cysteamine not only promotes growth and stabilizes renal function, but also prevents hypothyroidism.[254]

Renal Allografts

The natural history of infantile nephropathic cystinosis treated symptomatically is one of unremitting progression of glomerular damage, eventually leading to death in uremia before puberty. In a large European study, the mean age of "renal death" was 9 years.[175] Once uremia ensues in cystinosis, dialysis or renal transplantation becomes essential. Hemodialysis of a boy with cystinosis was reported in 1966[255] and rapidly became part of the standard of care for uremic patients. It has recently been supplanted in some areas by peritoneal dialysis, which can be continuous or intermittent, inpatient or ambulatory. Dialysis represents a temporizing measure for patients awaiting renal transplantation.

Because the primary abnormality leading to renal failure in cystinosis is a genetically determined defect of the intracellular environment, cells without this genetic defect that are transplanted into a cystinosis patient do not accumulate intralysosomal cystine. This knowledge, and the success of the procedure, led to the widespread use of transplantation in cystinosis patients.[89,175,179,180,256–263] Indeed, renal transplantation in cystinosis patients has been more successful than renal transplantation in children with other chronic renal diseases.[89,148,264] One life-table analysis of kidney allografts in cystinosis patients revealed a 50 percent cadaveric graft survival rate 9 years after transplantation.[181] Transplanted kidneys do not develop the series of functional changes of cystinosis,[256,257] but they may reaccumulate cystine, which electron microscopic studies suggest is largely, and perhaps entirely, confined to interstitial and mesangial cells, presumably of host origin.[265] This phenomenon occurs in both heterozygous and cadaver donor kidneys. Despite theoretic concerns that heterozygote donor kidneys might be more prone than cadaver kidneys to cystine reaccumulation,[258] there is no evidence for this, and heterozygotes are routinely accepted as kidney donors. Unfortunately, despite successful renal transplantation, severe late-onset symptoms have occurred in nonrenal tissues in most of these patients.[181,266]

Specific Treatment to Reduce Cystine Storage

Attempts to deplete cystinotic cells of cystine by dietary restriction of cystine and methionine, or use of drugs such as penicillamine, dithiothreitol, or ascorbic acid, have been described in earlier editions of this text.[98] None of these approaches was successful.

Oral Cysteamine Therapy. In contrast to the above experiences, the drug cysteamine (β-mercaptoethylamine), whose mechanism of action has been described (see "Mechanism of Cystine Depletion by Cysteamine" above), has been very effective in removing cystine from cystinotic cells and protecting cystinosis patients' organs from progressive damage. Earlier studies with cysteamine[108,176,267] are reviewed elsewhere.[98,268] The United States Food and Drug Administration approved cysteamine bitartrate capsules (Cystagon) for use in cystinosis in August 1994.[269]

Because cystinosis patients now range in age from infancy to over 40 years, it is best to express the dose of cysteamine in terms of body surface area. Cysteamine, a free thiol, has the odor and taste of rotten eggs, but most patients can tolerate a *daily* dose of 1.3 g/m^2. This is given in divided doses, every 6 h. For patients just starting cysteamine, it is important to begin at a very low dose and slowly increase the dose to the expected final amount over a 4- to 6-week period. In early use of cysteamine, three patients whose cysteamine dose was abruptly started at up to 70 mg/kg per day experienced a Stevens-Johnson-like rash, central nervous system disorientation and lethargy, or neutropenia, all of which resolved on discontinuing the drug.[270] With gradual incremental dosing, the only significant side effects have been nausea and vomiting, which has been observed in approximately 14 percent of patients.[176] A recent study found that cystinosis patients who receive cysteamine experience significant increases in both serum gastrin concentration and gastric acid production.[271] This may play a role in the gastric distress that some patients experience when taking cysteamine.

In 1992, 30 years' experience involving 76 cystinosis patients at the National Institutes of Health was reviewed.[169] Over 2000 24-h urines were collected, and creatinine clearances were measured. Patients who never received cysteamine lost renal function monotonically, reaching renal failure at 9 to 10 years of age. Seventeen patients were considered well treated with oral cysteamine, because they began treatment prior to age 2 years and achieved good leukocyte cystine depletion. These children, selected without knowledge of their ultimate renal function results, exhibited the same, very slow decline in reciprocal serum creatinine that normal individuals display. The well-treated patients were predicted to maintain adequate renal function past 25 years of age. Moreover, they exhibited an *increase* in creatinine clearance in the first 3 years of life, which is consistent with the natural growth of renal function during this period (Fig. 199-7). This increase in glomerular filtration rate translated into vastly prolonged maintenance of renal function later in life, emphasizing the value of early therapy and bolstering hope that some patients may never require a renal allograft procedure. Patients treated less well, or later, with cysteamine therapy, displayed renal function results that were intermediate between those of well-treated patients and those of patients not treated with cysteamine. Well-treated patients grew at approximately a normal rate, approaching the fifth percentile curve for normal children and growing parallel to it. These studies were done with earlier forms of cysteamine (cysteamine hydrochloride, and phosphocysteamine). The form of cysteamine approved by the FDA (cysteamine bitartrate, Cystagon) has led to lower mean levels of leukocyte free-cystine,[272] presumably because of improved patient compliance. Most cystinosis patients who are compliant with Cystagon maintain their leukocyte free-cystine level below 1 nmol half-cystine per mg protein. One patient with intestinal dysmotility received intravenous cysteamine, with leukocyte cystine depletion similar to that achieved by equivalent oral doses of cysteamine.[273]

Other promising results have come from measurements of parenchymal cell cystine concentrations in patients treated for several years with oral cysteamine.[90] In particular, the mean muscle cystine content for 15 patients treated for 4 to 11 years with cysteamine therapy was one-eighth the mean value for 11 patients the same age but not treated with cysteamine. Moreover, a single 9-year-old boy treated from age 1 with oral cysteamine had cystine values in his kidney, liver, lung, and pancreas that were fifty- to one hundredfold less than those of an age-matched cystinosis patient who never received cysteamine. The treated patient also had no crystals in his liver. Cysteamine has been reported to protect against the cystinosis encephalopathy,[274] and one study demonstrated that proper oral cysteamine therapy obviates the requirement for thyroid replacement in cystinosis patients.[254] The combined findings of parenchymal organ cystine depletion, functional improvement in growth and glomerular filtration rate, and prevention of hypothyroidism provide powerful evidence for the efficacy of systemic cysteamine therapy as the treatment of choice for nephropathic cystinosis. The value of early diagnosis cannot be overemphasized, because intervention with cysteamine in the first 2 years of life can allow for critical growth in absolute renal function. In addition, the functional benefit to nonrenal organs indicates that oral cysteamine should be offered to posttransplant as well as pretransplant patients.

The importance of frequent monitoring of the leukocyte free-cystine level was demonstrated when van't Hoff and Gretz studied patients in the U.K. and Ireland at a time when such monitoring was not the standard.[275] Their patients were receiving significantly less cysteamine, and apparently deriving less benefit from this therapy compared with patients in the United States and Canada. Their leukocyte free-cystine values were also higher. This study led to a more aggressive management of cystinosis in the U.K. and Ireland, with more frequent leukocyte cystine measurements. The optimal frequency of cystine dosage remains controversial. Following oral administration of cysteamine, plasma levels peak in approximately 2 h, with a rapid fall to very low levels by 6 h.[272] Consequently, the authors of this chapter urge their patients to take the drug as close to every 6 h as possible. The 20 years of clinical experience that demonstrated cysteamine's effectiveness were based on patients receiving medication every 6 h. Before changing to a different schedule, there should be convincing evidence that the new schedule results in leukocyte cystine depletion to levels

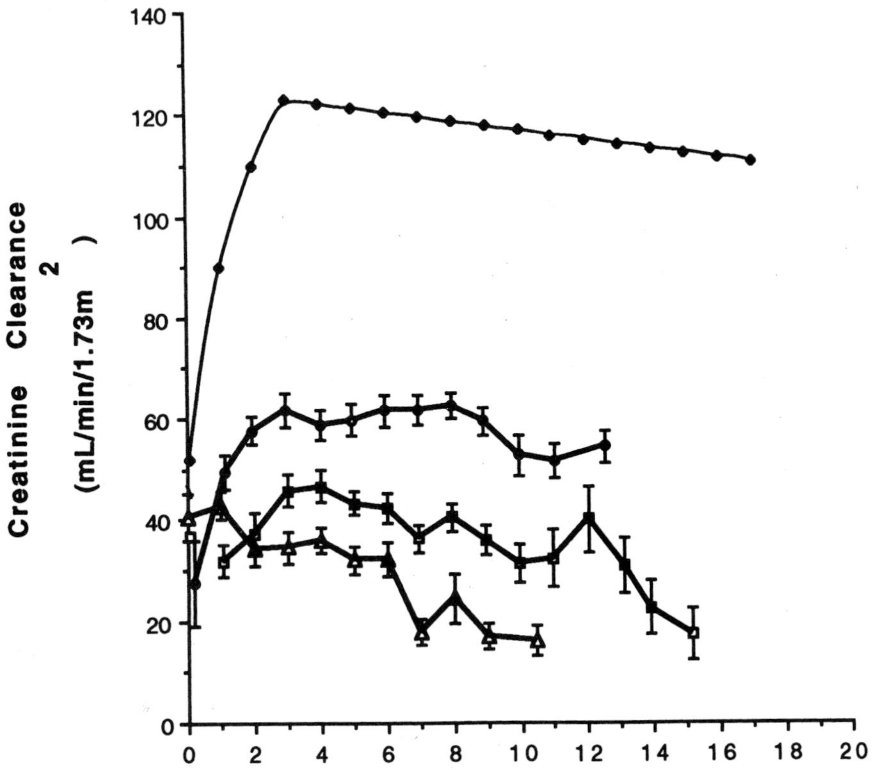

Fig. 199-7 Relationship between creatinine clearance and age in nephropathic cystinosis. The thin line represents the normal increase in renal function for the first three years of life as the kidney grows, followed by a very slow decline in clearance. The triangles represent the natural history of renal deterioration in cystinosis, with end-stage renal disease predicted at 10 years of age. The squares give values for partially treated patients, and the circles represent creatinine clearances for 17 cystinosis patients optimally treated with cysteamine and followed at the National Institute of Child Health and Human Development. This group of patients is predicted to maintain significant renal function through adulthood. (*From Markello et al.*[169] *Used with permission.*)

below 1 nmol half-cystine/mg protein at the end of the longest period between doses.

Cysteamine has served as a duodenal ulcerogenic in rats,[276] and it depletes somatostatin[277,278] and pituitary prolactin[279,280] in rats given doses much larger than those used in humans. (Blood levels of cysteamine in treated cystinosis children reach only 30 to 80 μM 1 h after a dose.[281,282]) Chronic cysteamine administered intraperitoneally to mice has not altered hepatic microsomal aryl hydrocarbon hydroxylase activity compared with controls.[283] Standard treatment of patients with cysteamine has revealed inhibition of glycine turnover,[284] blunting of a prolactin response in thyrotropin-releasing hormone,[285] and conversion of apolipoprotein E_3 to an apolipoprotein E_4 phenotype on isoelectric focusing,[286] but no clinical ramifications have accompanied these laboratory findings. The hepatic veno-occlusive disease that is reportedly due to cysteamine therapy[287] appears more likely to be a complication of cystinosis itself.[288] Hepatomegaly is no more frequent among patients treated with cysteamine than among those who never received cysteamine.[191]

Because of family history, some patients are diagnosed shortly after birth and started on cysteamine at a very early age. Such patients have done extremely well, but in most cases, still developed the renal Fanconi syndrome.[289,290] In addition, older patients treated chronically with oral cysteamine have exhibited no improvement in their renal tubular Fanconi syndrome.[176] The reason why cysteamine is so successful in protecting glomerular, but not tubular, function is not understood.

We have noted that both males and females treated with cysteamine from early childhood progress through puberty in a normal fashion. Moreover, several women with cystinosis and a renal allograft have had successful pregnancies, including one in which placental crystals were documented.[80] To our knowledge, none of these women was receiving significant doses of cysteamine. Recent studies of developmental toxicity of phosphocysteamine in the rat are of concern.[291,292] Pregnant rats were given 1 dose per day of phosphocysteamine from days 6.5 to 18.5 postconception, and fetuses were examined at day 20.5. No apparent developmental toxicity was observed in fetuses receiving doses up to 75 mg cysteamine/kg/day, but at doses of 100 mg, and especially 150 mg, cysteamine/kg/day, fetuses demonstrated cleft palate and kyphosis, as well as intrauterine growth retardation and fetal death.[292] It is difficult to know whether a woman receiving cysteamine would be subject to a similar risk for her fetus. A hypothetical adult woman with cystinosis (60 in, 110 lbs, 1.46 m^2 body surface area) taking 1.3 g/m^2/day of cysteamine would be receiving approximately 38 mg/kg/day of cysteamine.

Recently, cysteamine was demonstrated to inhibit proliferation of neural neoplastic cell lines[293] and replication of human immunodeficiency virus type I,[294] and to have potential as a contraceptive anti-HIV agent.[122]

Cysteamine Eyedrops. Despite years of oral cysteamine therapy, children with cystinosis continued to accumulate corneal crystals, causing painful erosions and ulcerations in older patients. One 12-year-old boy had such debilitating corneal pain that he underwent a penetrating keratoplasty,[196] with marked improvement in his quality of life. The epithelial cells of his cornea were cultured, and exhibited both cystine storage and susceptibility to depletion by cysteamine.[295] This meant that cystinotic corneal cells were intrinsically capable of responding to cysteamine therapy, and that low cysteamine concentrations in the avascular cornea were most likely responsible for the failure of oral cysteamine to lower the corneal crystal content. Delivery might be readily achieved using topically administered cysteamine.

After demonstrating the safety of cysteamine eyedrops in rabbit eyes,[295] two cystinosis patients under age 2 years were enrolled in a randomized, double-blind clinical trial involving a placebo (normal saline) for one eye and 10 mM (0.1 percent) cysteamine plus normal saline for the other eye.[295] Eyedrops were administered every hour while awake, with a marked diminution in corneal crystals in the treated eyes after 4 to 5 months of therapy. By 1990, 29 patients up to 31 years of age had entered the double-masked, randomized, placebo-controlled protocol, which then employed 50 mM (0.5%) cysteamine in normal saline. Eight of 18 patients under 42 months of age, and 2 of 11 patients 4 to 31 years of age, showed marked clearing in one eye, which was subsequently shown to be the cysteamine-treated eye.[296] After breaking the randomization code, both eyes were treated with cysteamine eyedrops. Currently, over 100 patients are under protocol, and there have been no side effects attributable to this therapy. The formulation now contains preservative and is stored frozen before use. A formulation that is stable at room temperature is being investigated. At present, the U.S. Food and Drug Administration has not approved any formulation of cysteamine eyedrops. Other centers have also been successful in clearing corneal cystine crystals with cysteamine eye drops.[297,298]

Some generalizations can be drawn concerning the use of cysteamine eyedrops. First, compliance determines the outcome. When drops are given 10 to 14 times per day, a marked decrease in crystal density is apparent within 4 to 8 months. If given less frequently,[299] such as 3 to 4 times per day,[300] no benefit is evident. Second, young patients with fewer crystals (Fig. 199-8*A* and *B*) respond better and faster than older ones with packed corneas. Several children are now approximately 6 years old with no crystals visible in their corneas. Older patients can lose the haziness to their corneas (Fig. 199-8*C* and *D*) and can experience improved visual acuity. Third, crystal formation appears to be a reversible process. Crystals can be removed at any age, and stopping therapy or reducing the frequency of administration (e.g., to every 4 h) results in recurrence of corneal crystals. Fourth, because the concentration of cysteamine has not been pushed to toxicity, the optimal concentration has not yet been determined. Finally, virtually all compliant patients experience relief of their photophobia.

Use of Growth Hormone

The use of cysteamine/phosphocysteamine has markedly improved the growth of cystinosis patients.[176,254] After starting therapy, patients tend to have a normal growth rate, but do not exhibit "catch-up" growth. Thus, most patients remain below the third percentile for height. There is some evidence that indomethacin also has a positive influence on growth (see reference 249 and "Symptomatic Therapy" above). The long-term efficacy of recombinant human growth hormone (rhGH) for short stature in patients with chronic renal disease is established.[301] Several patients with cystinosis have received rhGH because of its salutary effect on short stature, even in the absence of growth hormone deficiency.[302–306] In 1993, a controversy developed as to whether the increase in muscle mass in cystinosis patients who are treated with rhGH might lead to the earlier need for renal transplantation.[305,307,308] All investigators involved in this debate agreed that further studies were required to answer this

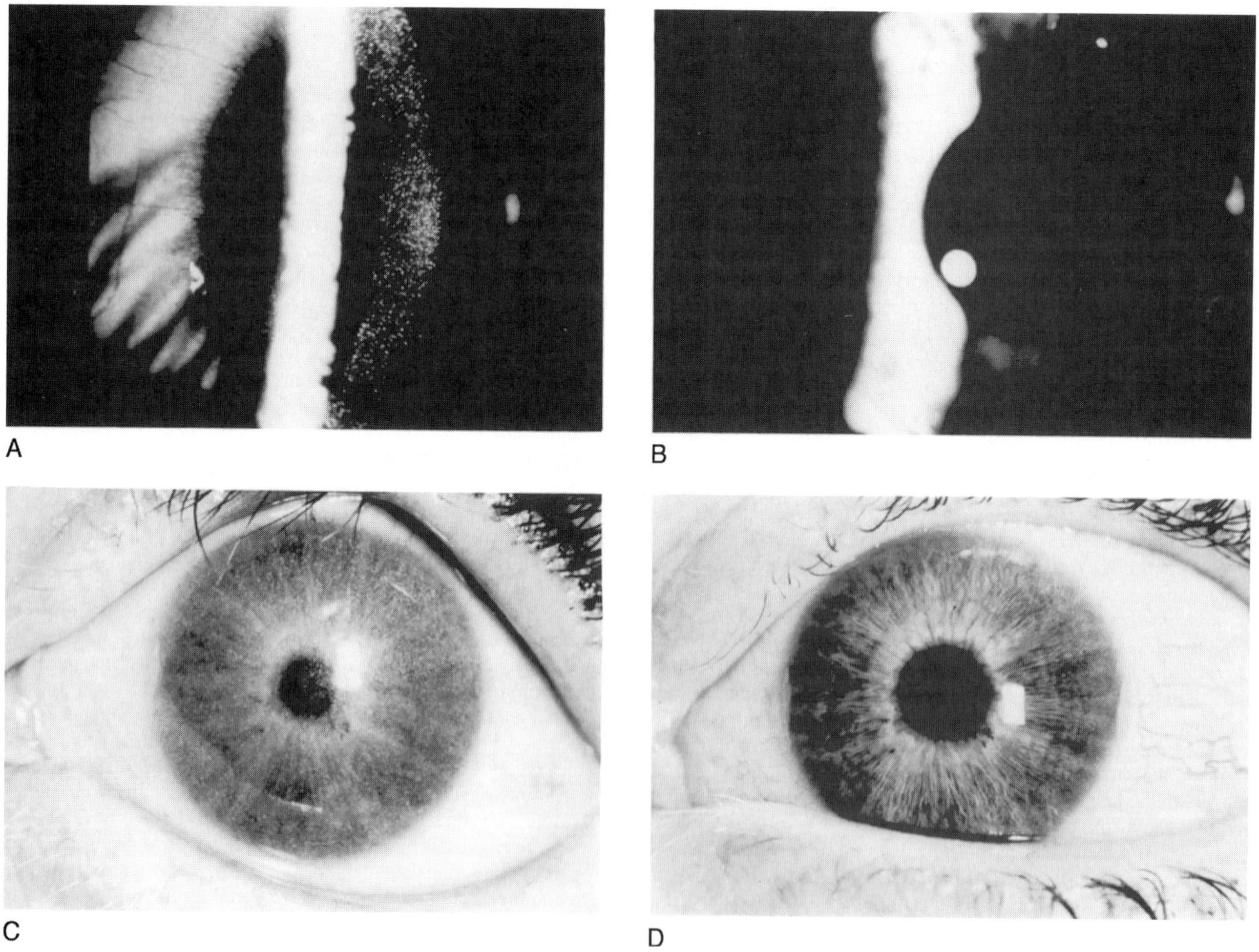

Fig. 199-8 Photographs of corneal cystine crystals before and after cysteamine eyedrop therapy in cystinosis patients. *A*, Right eye of a 28-month-old boy before topical cysteamine therapy, showing abundant crystals. *B*, Same eye as in *A* after 7 months of 0.5% cysteamine eyedrops administered 8 to 12 times per day, with clearing of corneal crystals. *C*, Left eye of 21-year-old woman prior to cysteamine eyedrop therapy. Uniform haziness typifies appearance of cornea at this age. *D*, Same eye as in *C* after several months of diligent therapy with 0.5% cysteamine eyedrops. Cornea is clear to inspection, although crystals remain visible on slit-lamp examination. (*Courtesy of Dr. M.I. Kaiser-Kupfer, National Eye Institute, National Institutes of Health, Bethesda, Maryland.*)

Table 199-3 Different Forms of Cystinosis

Nephrophatic	Nonnephropathic
Infantile (6–18 months)	Ocular (formerly *adult* or *benign*)
Late-onset	
Child (4–5 years)	
Adolescent (12–15 years)	
Adult-onset (26 years)	

question. The European Study Group on Growth Hormone Treatment for Short Children with Nephropathic Cystinosis has completed a study on 36 cystinosis patients. It found an excellent increase in growth velocity (greater than twofold), and no acceleration of the decline in renal function.[309] Their study also provided further evidence that cysteamine therapy reduces the progression of renal failure in cystinosis.

Family Support Group

The Cystinosis Foundation[310] has been active since 1983 in supporting families, physicians, and investigators involved in cystinosis.

CYSTINOSIS VARIANTS

There are two basic cystinosis phenotypes: nephropathic and nonnephropathic. The nephropathic form can be further subdivided, based on age of presentation, as shown in Table 199-3. Each type appears to represent a different, but allelic, mutation, and there likely exists a continuum of disease severity.

The infantile nephropathic form, described above, is the most common and devastating variant of cystinosis, with presentation in the first year or two of life. In the *late-onset forms of nephropathic cystinosis*, the age of presentation ranges from 2 to 26 years.[311–321] Age of onset and symptoms are usually similar in affected siblings or in members of a family. The most usual age of presentation has been 12 to 15 years.[318] These patients have crystalline deposits in the cornea and conjunctiva, and have cystine crystals within bone marrow aspirates. Patients with late-onset cystinosis often do not develop the complete Fanconi syndrome, but their renal disease may progress to end-stage renal failure within a few years of diagnosis. In one family, two sisters were found to have proteinuria during a routine medical examination at 25 years of age.[322] The older sister had rapid deterioration of glomerular function and required a renal transplant at 30 years of age. No specific diagnosis was made at that time. The younger sister had a similar course, also requiring a transplant at 30 years of age. However, the younger sister had a renal biopsy at age 26 that demonstrated cystine crystals. Both patients have late-onset cystinosis, and they exhibit compound heterozygosity for apparently mild mutations in *CTNS*.[144]

Other patients have a *benign, ocular, or nonnephropathic form of cystinosis* that is usually discovered by serendipity when an ophthalmologic examination reveals crystalline opacities within the cornea and conjunctiva. This was first reported in 1957,[323] and since then, many more cases have been reported.[324–333] These patients may suffer from photophobia similar to that of patients with the nephropathic forms of cystinosis, but their photophobia may not begin until middle age, and is usually not debilitating. Because the only patients found to have this condition are those who have had a slit-lamp examination, it is possible that many individuals with this form of cystinosis have no eye symptomatology and are never diagnosed. Patients with ocular cystinosis have crystalline deposits in their bone marrow and elevated leukocyte cystine levels, but never have renal disease. They appear to have a normal life expectancy, but because some patients with late-onset cystinosis do not develop renal dysfunction until their mid-twenties, patients with presumably ocular cystinosis must be followed diligently.

Patients with ocular cystinosis do not appear to accumulate cystine crystals in their kidneys,[325,329] which may explain their lack of kidney pathology. They also do not develop retinopathy. Patients with ocular cystinosis tend to have lower levels of leukocyte cystine than do patients with late-onset cystinosis, who, in turn, have lower levels of leukocyte cystine than do patients with infantile nephropathic cystinosis.[311,326] However, there is much overlap among these values and the measurements were performed using mixed leukocyte preparations, without regard for the fact that the cystine is stored primarily in polymorphonuclear leukocytes.[85,241]

Lysosomes from a patient with late-onset cystinosis exhibited deficient cystine transporting ability. One patient with benign/ocular cystinosis had 9 percent and 29 percent residual lysosomal cystine transporting capacity in two different experiments.[332] This patient has well-defined mutations in *CTNS*.[144a] The transport experiments were also performed with lysosomes from different patients with late-onset and benign cystinosis by a different laboratory with similar results.[334] Thus, it appears that the transport defect is most severe in infantile nephropathic cystinosis and least severe in ocular cystinosis.

Future Research

The major goals of further investigations into cystinosis are to improve treatment, to understand the pathophysiology of the disease, and to expand our knowledge of the cellular mechanisms involved in lysosomal cystine transport.

To improve the clinical care of cystinosis, we must diagnose the disorder earlier by fostering a greater level of suspicion. To prevent extrarenal complications, we should consider treating all cystinosis patients with oral cysteamine. To prevent progressive nephrocalcinosis, we should reduce to a minimum the amount of phosphate supplements we provide our adult, pretransplant patients. To determine how well oral cysteamine depletes cystine from the central nervous system, we should use animal models arising from *CTNS* gene manipulation.

We do not yet understand how cystine accumulation causes clinical disease. Does it destroy cells, such as those in the renal tubules, or merely impair their function? Is it soluble or crystalline cystine that does the damage? How can ocular cystinosis patients store crystalline amounts of cystine in their corneas, and never have renal disease? These questions can be addressed with several available tools. First, renal tubular cells have been cultured from cystinosis patients so that the progression of tubular damage can be studied *in vitro*.[335] Second, whole animals, isolated tubules,[336] and cultured tubular cells can be loaded with cystine dimethylester to simulate the cystinosis condition. In addition, the cloning of *CTNS* means that transgenic mice can be created to investigate the cause of organ and tissue damage. Mice with ocular or intermediate cystinosis will be of particular interest to determine why some tissues are more or less severely affected than others. Expression studies in mammalian or insect cells can also reveal the molecular basis for milder disease in some patients. Looking further into the future, *CTNS* gene therapy for corneal cystine accumulation may serve as an adjunct to oral cysteamine therapy, if vectors can be targeted to stromal keratinocytes.

Regarding lysosomal cystine transport, expression and proteoliposome reconstitution studies can vastly improve our knowledge of the kinetics and structure-function characteristics of the CTNS protein. Antibodies can be used to follow the CTNS protein from synthesis through processing to incorporation into the lysosomal membrane. These findings pertain directly to the hitherto unknown mechanism of intracellular protein sorting and trafficking. Finally, the lysosomal leader sequence of *CTNS* can be exploited to identify other lysosomal membrane transport genes, including that responsible for transport of cobalamin (see reference 337 and Chap. 155).

REFERENCES

1. Abderhalden E: Familiäre cystindiathese. *Z Physiol Chem* **38**:557, 1903.
2. Lignac GOE: Über storung des cystinstoffwechsels bei kindern. *Deutsch Arch Klin Med* **145**:139, 1924.
3. Fanconi G: Die nicht diabetischen glykosurien und hyperglykämien des ältern kindes. *Jahrb Kinderh* **133**:257, 1931.
4. deToni G: Remarks on the relations between renal rickets (renal dwarfism) and renal diabetes. *Acta Paediatr* **16**:479, 1933.
5. Debré R, Marie J, Clétet F, Messimy R: Rachitisme tardif coexistent avec une néphrite chronique et une glycosurie. *Arch Méd Enf* **37**:597, 1934.
6. Fanconi G: Der nephrotisch-glykosurische zwergwuchs mit hypophosphatämischer rachitis. *Dtsch Med Wochenschr* **62**:1169, 1936.
7. Beumer H, Wepler W: Über die cystinkrankheit der ersten lebenzeit. *Klin Wochenschr* **16**:8, 1937.
8. Fanconi G, Bickel H: Die chronische aminoacidurie (aminosäurediabetes oder nephrotisch-glukosurischer zwergwuchs) bei der glykogenose und der cystinkrankheit. *Helv Paediatr Acta* **4**:359, 1949.
9. Bickel H, Baar HS, Astley R, Douglas AA, Finch E, Harris H, Harvey CC, et al.: Cystine storage disease with aminoaciduria and dwarfism (Lignac-Fanconi Disease). *Acta Paed Uppsala* **42(Suppl 90)**:1, 1952.
10. Newburgh LH, Marsh PL: Renal injuries by amino acids. *Arch Intern Med* **36**:682, 1925.
11. Dent CE: The aminoaciduria in Fanconi syndrome. A study making extensive use of techniques based on paper partition chromatography. *Biochem J* **41**:240, 1947.
12. Freudenberg E: Cystinosis: Cystine disease (Lignac's disease) in children. *Adv Pediatr* **4**:265, 1949.
13. Seegmiller JE, Friedmann T, Harrison HE, Wong V, Schneider JA: Cystinosis. Combined clinical staff conference at the National Institutes of Health. *Ann Intern Med* **68**:883, 1968.
14. Schulman JD: Historical perspective, in Schulman JD (ed): *Cystinosis*. Washington, DC, U.S. Dept. of Health, Education, and Welfare, No. (NIH) 72-249, 1973, p 1.
15. Schneider JA, Schulman JD: Cystinosis, in Stanbury JB, Wyngaarden JB, Fredrickson DS, Goldstein JL, Brown MS (eds): *The Metabolic Basis of Inherited Disease*. 5th ed. New York, McGraw-Hill, 1983, p 1844.
16. Baar HS: Pathologie des aminosäuren-diabetes. *Mschr Kinderheilk* **99**:35, 1951.
17. Clay RD, Darmady EM, Hawkins M: The nature of the renal lesion in the Fanconi syndrome. *J Pathol Bacteriol* **65**:551, 1953.
18. Darmady EM: The renal changes in some metabolic diseases, in Mostofi FK, Smith DE (eds): *The Kidney*. Baltimore: Williams & Wilkins, 1966, p 253.
19. Jackson JD, Smith FG, Litman NN, Yuile CL, Latta H: The Fanconi syndrome with cystinosis. Electron microscopy of renal biopsy specimens from five patients. *Am J Med* **33**:653, 1962.
20. Schneider JA, Bradley K, Seegmiller JE: Increased cystine in leukocytes from individuals homozygous and heterozygous for cystinosis. *Science* **157**:1321, 1967.
21. Schneider JA, Rosenbloom FM, Bradley K, Seegmiller JE: Increased free-cystine content of fibroblasts cultured from patients with cystinosis. *Biochem Biophys Res Commun* **29**:527, 1967.
22. Patrick AD, Lake BD: Cystinosis: Electron microscopic evidence of lysosomal storage of cystine in lymph node. *J Clin Pathol* **21**:571, 1968.
23. Wong VG, Kuwabara T, Brubaker R, Olson W, Schulman J, Seegmiller JE: Intralysosomal cystine crystals in cystinosis. *Invest Ophthalmol* **9**:83, 1970.
24. Hummeler K, Zajac BA, Genel M, Holtzapple PG, Segal S: Human cystinosis: Intracellular deposition of cystine. *Science* **168**:859, 1970.
25. Schulman JD, Wong V, Olson WH, Seegmiller JE: Lysosomal site of crystalline deposits in cystinosis as shown by ferritin uptake. *Arch Pathol* **90**:259, 1970.
26. Schulman JD, Bradley KH, Seegmiller JE: Cystine: Compartmentalization within lysosomes in cystinotic leukocytes. *Science* **166**:1152, 1969.
27. Schulman JD, Bradley KH: Cystinosis: Selective induction of vacuolation in fibroblasts by L-cysteine-D-penicillamine disulfide. *Science* **169**:595, 1970.
28. Gahl WA, Renlund M, Thoene JG: Lysosomal transport disorders: Cystinosis and sialic acid storage disorders, in Scriver CR, Beaudet AL, Sly WS, Valle D (eds): *The Metabolic Basis of Inherited Disease*, 6th ed. New York, McGraw-Hill, 1989, p 2619.
29. Tietze F, Bradley KH, Schulman JD: Enzymic reduction of cystine by subcellular fractions of cultured and peripheral leukocytes from normal and cystinotic individuals. *Pediatr Res* **6**:649, 1972.
30. Lucy JA: Lysosomal Membranes, in Dingle JT, Fell HB (eds): *Lysosomes in Biology and Pathology*, vol. 2. New York, American Elsevier, 1969, p 313.
31. Goldman R, Kaplan A: Rupture of rat liver lysosomes mediated by L-amino acid esters. *Biochim Biophys Acta* **318**:205, 1973.
32. Reeves JP: Accumulation of amino acids by lysosomes incubated with amino acid esters. *J Biol Chem* **254**:8914, 1979.
33. Steinherz R, Tietze F, Gahl WA, Triche TJ, Chiang H, Modesti A, Schulman JD: Cystine accumulation and clearance by normal and cystinotic leukocytes exposed to cystine dimethyl ester. *Proc Natl Acad Sci U S A* **79**:4446, 1982.
34. Jonas AJ, Greene AA, Smith ML, Schneider JA: Cystine accumulation and loss in normal, heterozygous, and cystinotic fibroblasts. *Proc Natl Acad Sci U S A* **79**:4442, 1982.
35. Gahl WA, Tietze F, Bashan N, Steinherz R, Schulman JD: Defective cystine exodus from isolated lysosome-rich fractions of cystinotic leucocytes. *J Biol Chem* **257**:9570, 1982.
36. Jonas AJ, Smith ML, Schneider JA: ATP-dependent lysosomal cystine efflux is defective in cystinosis. *J Biol Chem* **257**:13185, 1982.
37. Pisoni RL, Thoene JG, Christensen HN: Detection and characterization of carrier-mediated cationic amino acid transport in lysosomes of normal and cystinotic human fibroblasts. *J Biol Chem* **260**:4791, 1985.
38. Tietze F, Rome LH, Butler JD, Harper GS, Gahl WA: Impaired clearance of free cystine from lysosome-enriched granular fractions of I-cell-disease fibroblasts. *Biochem J* **237**:9, 1986.
39. Gahl WA, Bashan N, Tietze F, Bernardini I, Schulman JD: Cystine transport is defective in isolated leukocyte lysosomes from patients with cystinosis. *Science* **217**:1263, 1982.
40. Christensen HN: *Biological Transport*, 2nd ed. Reading, MA: WA Benjamin, 1975.
41. Gahl WA, Tietze F, Bashan N, Bernardini I, Raiford D, Schulman JD: Characteristics of cystine counter-transport in normal and cystinotic lysosome-rich leucocyte granular fractions. *Biochem J* **216**:393, 1983.
42. Gahl WA, Bashan N, Tietze F, Schulman JD: Lysosomal cystine counter-transport in heterozygotes for cystinosis. *Am J Hum Genet* **36**:277, 1984.
43. Thoene JG: Lysosomal Cystine Transport, in Thoene JG (ed): *Pathophysiology of Lysosomal Transport*. Boca Raton, FL, CRC Press, 1992, p 1.
44. The Cystinosis Collaborative Research Group: Linkage of the gene for cystinosis to markers on the short arm of chromosome 17. *Nat Genet* **10**:246, 1995.
45. Town M, Jean G, Cherqui S, Attard M, Forestier L, Whitmore SA, Callen DF, et al.: A novel gene encoding an integral membrane protein is mutated in nephropathic cystinosis. *Nat Genet* **18**:319, 1998.
46. Jocelyn PC: The standard redox potential of cysteine-cystine from the thiol-disulphide exchange reaction with glutathione and lipoic acid. *Eur J Biochem* **2**:327, 1967.
47. Gorin G, Doughty G: Equilibrium constants for the reaction of glutathione with cystine and their relative oxidation-reduction potentials. *Arch Biochem Biophys* **126**:547, 1968.
48. Meister A: *Biochemistry of the Amino Acids*. New York, Academic Press, 1965.
49. Bannai S, Kitamura E: Transport interaction of L-cystine and L-glutamine in human diploid fibroblasts in culture. *J Biol Chem* **255**:2372, 1980.
50. Brenton DP, Cusworth DC, Dent DE, Jones EE: Homocystinuria: Clinical and dietary studies. *Q J Med* **35**:325, 1966.
51. Sturman JA, Gaull G, Raiha NCR: Absence of cystathionase in human fetal liver: Is cystine essential? *Science* **169**:74, 1970.
52. Eagle H, Piez KA, Oyama VI: The biosynthesis of cystine in human cell cultures. *J Biol Chem* **236**:1425, 1961.
53. Iglehart JD, York RM, Modest AP, Lazarus H, Livingston DM: Cystine requirement of continuous human lymphoid cell lines of normal and leukemic origin. *J Biol Chem* **252**:32767, 1977.
54. Tietze F: Enzymic reduction of cystine and other disulfides, in Schulman JD (ed): *Cystinosis*. Washington, DC, DHEW Publication No. (NIH) 72-249, 1973, p 147.
55. Jocelyn PC: Glutathione metabolism in animals, in Crook EM (ed): *Glutathione*. Cambridge, England, Cambridge University Press, 1959, p 43.
56. Eldjarn L, Pihl A: Equilibrium constants and oxidation-reduction potentials of some thiol-disulfide systems. *J Biol Chem* **79**:4589, 1957.

57. States B, Segal S: Distribution of glutathione-cystine transhydrogenase activity in subcellular fractions of rat intestinal mucosa. *Biochem J* **113**:443, 1969.
58. Fahey RC, Hunt JS, Windham GC: On the cysteine and cystine content of proteins: Differences between intracellular and extracellular proteins. *J Mol Evol* **10**:155, 1977.
59. Fahey RC: Biologically important thiol-disulfide reactions and the role of Cyst(e)ine in proteins: An evolutionary perspective, in Friedman M (ed.): *Protein Crosslinking, Part A*. New York, Plenum, 1977, p 1.
60. Brand E, Harris MM, Biloon S: Cystinuria. The excretion of a cystine complex which decomposes in the urine with the liberation of free cystine. *J Biol Chem* **86**:315, 1930.
61. Schneider JA, Bradley KH, Seegmiller JE: Transport and intracellular fate of cysteine-^{35}S in leukocytes from normal subjects and patients with cystinosis. *Pediatr Res* **2**:441, 1968.
62. States B, Segal S: Thin-layer chromatographic separation of cystine and the *N*-ethylmaleimide adducts of cysteine and glutathione. *Anal Biochem* **27**:323, 1969.
63. Lee PLY: Single-column systems for accelerated amino acid analysis of physiological fluids using five lithium buffers. *Biochem Med* **10**:107, 1974.
64. Oshima RG, Willis RC, Furlong CE, Schneider JA: Binding assays for amino acids. The utilization of a cystine binding protein from *Escherichia coli* for the determination of acid-soluble cystine in small physiological samples. *J Biol Chem* **249**:6033, 1974.
65. Spears GS, Slusser RJ, Tousimis AJ, Taylor CG, Schulman JD: Cystinosis: An ultrastructural and electron-probe study of the kidney with unusual findings. *Arch Pathol* **9**:206, 1971.
66. Scotto JM, Stralin HG: Ultrastructure of the liver in a case of childhood cystinosis. *Virchows Arch [Pathol Anat]* **377**:43, 1977.
67. Almond PS, Matas AJ, Nakhleh RE, Morel P, Troppmann C, Najarian JS, Chavers B: Renal transplantation for infantile cystinosis: Long-term follow-up. *J Pediatr Surg* **28**:232, 1993.
68. Fivush B, Green OC, Porter CC, Balfe JW, O'Regan S, Gahl WA: Pancreatic endocrine insufficiency in posttransplant cystinosis. *Am J Dis Child* **141**:1087, 1987.
69. Holtzapple PG, Genel M, Yakovac WC, Hummeler K, Segal S: Diagnosis of cystinosis by rectal biopsy. *N Engl J Med* **281**:143, 1969.
70. Morecki R, Paunier L, Hamilton JR: Intestinal mucosa in cystinosis. A fine structure study. *Arch Pathol* **86**:297, 1968.
71. Schneider JA, Nolan SP, Seegmiller JE: Appendicitis in a child with cystinosis. *Arch Surg* **97**:565, 1968.
72. Gross U, Masshoff W, Korz R: Die milz in allgemein pathologischer sicht. *Internist (Berlin)* **9**:1, 1968.
73. Cogan DG, Kuwabara T: Ocular pathology of cystinosis, with particular reference to the elusiveness of the corneal crystals. *Arch Ophthalmol* **63**:51, 1960.
74. Kaiser-Kupfer MI, Caruso RC, Minkler DS, Gahl WA: Long-term ocular manifestations in nephropathic cystinosis. *Arch Ophthalmol* **104**:706, 1986.
75. Korn D: Demonstration of cystine crystals in peripheral white blood cells in a patient with cystinosis. *N Engl J Med* **262**:545, 1960.
76. Schneider JA, Wong V, Seegmiller JE: The early diagnosis of cystinosis. *J Pediatr* **74**:114, 1969.
77. Chan AM, Lynch MJ, Bailey JD, Ezrin C, Fraser D: Hypothyroidism in cystinosis. A clinical, endocrinologic and histologic study involving sixteen patients with cystinosis. *Am J Med* **48**:678, 1970.
78. Casey TP: Cystine storage disease. A case report with a note on the extraction of cystine from formalin-fixed tissues. *Aust Ann Med* **15**:61, 1966.
79. Gahl WA, Dalakas MC, Charnas L, Chen KT, Pezeshkpour GH, Kuwabara T, Davis SL, Chesney RW, Fink J, Hutchison HT: Myopathy and cystine storage in muscles in a patient with nephropathic cystinosis. *N Engl J Med* **319**:1461, 1988.
80. Reiss RE, Kuwabara T, Smith ML, Gahl WA: Successful pregnancy despite placental cystine crystals in a woman with nephropathic cystinosis. *N Engl J Med* **319**:223, 1988.
81. Baar HS, Bickel H: Morbid anatomy, histology, and pathogenesis of Lignac-Franconi disease. *Acta Paediatr* **42(Suppl 90)**:171, 1952.
82. Levine S, Paparo G: Brain lesions in a case of cystinosis. *Acta Neuropathol (Berl)* **57**:217, 1982.
83. Heller AN, Heller DS, Schwimmer A, Gordon RE, Cambria RJ: Cystinosis and gingival hyperplasia—Demonstration of cystine crystals in gingival tissue and unusual aspects of management. *J Periodont* **65**:1139, 1994.
84. *Merck Index*, 10th ed. Rahway, NJ, Merck & Co., 1983.
85. Schulman JD, Wong VG, Kuwabara T, Bradley KH, Seegmiller JE: Intracellular cystine content of leukocyte populations in cystinosis. *Arch Intern Med* **125**:660, 1970.
86. Harnes MD, Carter RF, Pollard AC, Carey WF: Light and electron microscopy of infantile and fetal tissues in cystinosis. *Micron* **11**:443, 1980.
87. Schulman JD: Cystine storage disease: Investigations at the cellular and subcellular levels, in Carson NAJ, Raine DN (eds): *Inherited Disorders of Sulphur Metabolism*. Edinburgh, Churchill Livingstone, 1971, p 123.
88. Jonas AJ, Conley SB, Marshall R, Johnson RA, Marks M, Rosenberg H: Nephropathic cystinosis with central nervous system involvement. *Am J Med* **83**:966, 1987.
89. Broyer M, Guillot M, Gubler MC, Habib R: Infantile cystinosis: A reappraisal of early and late symptoms. *Adv Nephrol* **10**:137, 1981.
90. Gahl WA, Charnas LR, Markello TC, Bernardini IM, Ishak KG, Dalakas MC: Parenchymal organ cystine depletion with long-term cysteamine therapy. *Biochem Med Metab Biol* **48**:275, 1992.
91. Shotelersuk V, Larson D, Anikster Y, McDowell G, Lemons R, Bernardini I, Guo J, et al.: *CTNS* mutations in an American-based population of cystinosis patients. *Am J Hum Genet* **63**:1352, 1998.
92. Greene AA, Marcusson EG, Pintos Morell G, Schneider JA: Characterization of the lysosomal cystine transport system in mouse L-929 fibroblasts. *J Biol Chem* **265**:9888, 1990.
93. Bashan N, Gahl WA, Tietze F, Bernardini I, Schulman JD: The effect of ions and ionophores on cystine egress from human leucocyte lysosome-rich granular fraction. *Biochim Biophys Acta* **777**:267, 1984.
94. Smith ML, Greene AA, Potashnik R, Mendoza SA, Schneider JA: Lysosomal cystine transport. Effect of intralysosomal pH and membrane potential. *J Biol Chem* **262**:1244, 1987.
95. Jonas AJ: Cystine transport in purified rat liver lysosomes. *Biochem J* **236**:671, 1986.
96. Gahl WA, Tietze F: pH effects on cystine transport in lysosome-rich leucocyte granular fractions. *Biochem J* **228**:263, 1985.
97. Okhuma S, Moriyama Y, Takano T: Identification and characterization of a proton pump on lysosomes by fluorescein isothiocyanate-dextran fluorescence. *Proc Natl Acad Sci U S A* **79**:2758, 1982.
98. Gahl WA, Schneider JA, Aula PP: Lysosomal transport disorders: Cystinosis and sialic acid storage disorders, in Scriver CR, Beaudet AL, Sly WS, Valle D (eds): *The Metabolic and Molecular Bases of Inherited Disease*, 7th ed. New York, McGraw-Hill, 1995, p 3763.
99. Tietze F, Butler JD: Elevated cystine levels in cultured skin fibroblasts from patients with I-cell disease. *Pediatr Res* **13**:1350, 1979.
100. Greene AA, Jonas AJ, Harms E, Smith ML, Pellett OL, Bump EA, Miller AL, et al.: Lysosomal cystine storage in cystinosis and mucolipidosis type II. *Pediatr Res* **19**:1170, 1985.
101. Jonas AJ, Symons LJ, Speller RJ: Polyamines stimulate lysosomal cystine transport. *J Biol Chem* **262**:16391, 1987.
102. Jonas AJ, Speller RJ: Stearylamine permeabilizes the lysosomal membrane to cystine and sialic acid. *Biochim Biophys Acta* **984**:257, 1989.
103. Lemons RM, Pisoni RL, Christensen HN, Thoene JG: Elevated temperature produces cystine depletion in cystinotic fibroblasts. *Biochim Biophys Acta* **884**:429, 1986.
104. Forster S, Scarlett L, Lloyd JB: The effects of decreased growth temperature on the cystine content of cystinotic fibroblasts. *Biochim Biophys Acta* **1013**:7, 1989.
105. Schulman JD, Patrick AD, Goodman SI, Tietze F, Butler J: Gamma-glutamyl transpeptidase (GGTPase): Investigations in normals and patients with inborn errors of sulfur metabolism. *Pediatr Res* **9**:355, 1975.
106. Harper GS, Kohn LD, Bernardini I, Bernar J, Tietze F, Andersson HC, Gahl WA: Thyrotropin stimulation of lysosomal tyrosine transport in rat FRTL-5 thyroid cells. *J Biol Chem* **263**:9320, 1988.
107. Idriss JM, Jonas AJ: Cystine transport by yeast acidic vacuoles. *Am J Hum Genet* **47**:A159, 1990.
108. Thoene JG, Oshima RG, Crawhall JC, Olson DL, Schneider JA: Cystinosis. Intracellular cystine depletion by aminothiols *in vitro* and *in vivo*. *J Clin Invest* **58**:180, 1976.
109. Pisoni RL, Acker TL, Lisowski KM, Lemons RM, Thoene JG: A cysteine-specific lysosomal transport system provides a major route for the delivery of thiol to human fibroblast lysosomes: Possible role in supporting lysosomal proteolysis. *J Cell Biol* **110**:327, 1990.
110. Ehrenreich BA, Cohn ZA: The fate of peptides pinocytosed by macrophages *in vitro*. *J Exp Med* **129**:227, 1969.

111. Gahl WA, Tietze F, Butler JD, Schulman JD: Cysteamine depletes cystinotic leucocyte granular fractions of cystine by the mechanism of disulphide interchange. *Biochem J* **228**:545, 1985.
112. Pisoni RL, Park GY, Velilla VQ, Thoene JG: Detection and characterization of a transport system mediating cysteamine entry into human fibroblast lysosomes. *J Biol Chem* **270**:1179, 1995.
113. Butler JD: Depletion of cystine in cystinotic fibroblasts by homocysteine. Synergism of cysteamine with various reducing agents in depletion of cystine from cystinotic fibroblasts. *Biochem Pharmacol* **40**:879, 1990.
114. Goldman H, Scriver CR, Aaron K, Pinsky L: Use of dithiothreitol to correct cystine storage in cultured cystinotic fibroblasts. *Lancet* **1**:811, 1970.
115. Kroll WA, Schneider JA: Decrease in free cystine content of cultured cystinotic fibroblasts by ascorbic acid. *Science* **186**:1040, 1974.
116. Butler JD, Zatz M: Pantethine depletes cystinotic fibroblasts of cystine. *J Pediatr* **102**:796, 1983.
117. Butler JD, Zatz M: Pantethine and cystamine deplete cystine from cystinotic fibroblasts via efflux of cysteamine-cysteine mixed disulfide. *J Clin Invest* **74**:411, 1984.
118. Orloff S, Butler JD, Towne D, Mukherjee AB, Schulman JD: Pantetheinase activity and cysteamine content in cystinotic and normal fibroblasts and leukocytes. *Pediatr Res* **15**:1063, 1981.
119. Butler JD, Gahl WA, Tietze F: Cystine depletion by WR-1065 in cystinotic cells. Mechanism of action. *Biochem Pharmacol* **34**:2179, 1985.
120. Thoene JG, Lemons R: Cystine depletion of cystinotic tissues by phosphocysteamine (WR638). *J Pediatr* **96**:1043, 1980.
121. Pisoni RL, Lisowski KM, Lemons RM, Thoene JG: Utilization of mercaptoethylgluconamide for depleting human cystinotic fibroblasts of their accumulated lysosomal cystine. *Pediatr Res* **26**:73, 1989.
122. Anderson RA, Feathergill K, Kirkpatrick R, Zaneveld LJD, Coleman KT, Spear PG, Cooper MD, Waller D, Thoene J: Characterization of cysteamine as a potential contraceptive anti-HIV agent. *J Andrology* **19**:37, 1998.
123. Danpure CJ: The effect of chloroquine on the metabolism of [^{35}S]cystine in normal and cystinotic human skin fibroblasts. *Biochem J* **200**:555, 1981.
124. Thoene JG, Lemons RM: Cystine accumulation in cystinotic fibroblasts from free and protein-linked cystine but not cysteine. *Biochem J* **208**:823, 1982.
125. Thoene JG, Oshima RG, Ritchie DG, Schneider JA: Cystinotic fibroblasts accumulate cystine from intracellular protein degradation. *Proc Natl Acad Sci U S A* **74**:4505, 1977.
126. Schulman JD, Bradley KH: Cystinosis: Therapeutic implications of *in vitro* studies of cultured fibroblasts. *J Pediatr* **78**:833, 1971.
127. Danpure CJ, Jennings PR, Fyfe DA: Further studies on the effect of chloroquine on the uptake, metabolism and intracellular translocation of [^{35}S]cystine in cystinotic fibroblasts. *Biochim Biophys Acta* **885**:256, 1986.
128. Forster S, Scarlett L, Lloyd JB: Mechanism of cystine reaccumulation by cystinotic fibroblasts *in vitro*. *Biosci Rep* **10**:225, 1990.
129. Thoene JG, Lemons R: Modulation of the intracellular cystine content of cystinotic fibroblasts by extracellular albumin. *Pediatr Res* **14**:785, 1980.
130. Kooistra T, Lloyd JB: Pinocytosis and degradation of exogenous proteins by cystinotic fibroblasts. *Biochim Biophys Acta* **887**:182, 1986.
131. Lloyd JB: Disulphide reduction in lysosomes — The role of cysteine. *Biochem J* **237**:271, 1986.
132. Butler JD, Spielberg SP: Accumulation of cystine from glutathione-cysteine mixed disulfide in cystinotic fibroblasts; blockade by an inhibitor of gamma-glutamyl transpeptidase. *Life Sci* **31**:2563, 1982.
133. Crawhall JC, Oshima RG, Schneider JA: Factors controlling the nonprotein cystine content of cystinotic fibroblasts. *Pediatr Res* **11**:41, 1977.
134. Ritchie DG, Jonas AJ, Oshima RG, Neal P, Schneider JA: Cystinotic fibroblasts are depleted of free-cystine by acid pH medium. *Pediatr Res* **15**:1492, 1981.
135. States B, Lee J, Segal S: Effect of chloroquine on handling of cystine by cystinotic fibroblasts. *Metabolism* **32**:272, 1983.
136. Bois E, Feingold J, Frenay P, Briard ML: Infantile cystinosis in France: Genetics, incidence, geographic distribution. *J Med Genet* **13**:434, 1976.
137. Manz F, Gretz N: Cystinosis in the Federal Republic of Germany. Coordination and analysis of the data. *J Inherit Metab Dis* **8**:2, 1985.
138. Hutchesson ACJ, Bundey S, Preece MA, Hall SK, Green A: A comparison of disease and gene frequencies of inborn errors of metabolism among different ethnic groups in the West Midlands, UK. *J Med Genet* **35**:366, 1998.
139. Jean G, Fuchshuber A, Town MM, Gribouval O, Schneider JA, Broyer M, van't Hoff W, et al.: High-resolution mapping of the gene for cystinosis, using combined biochemical and linkage analysis. *Am J Hum Genet* **58**:535, 1996.
140. McDowell G, Isogai T, Tanigami A, Hazelwood S, Ledbetter D, Polymeropoulos MH, Lichter-Konecki U, et al.: Fine mapping of the cystinosis gene using an integrated genetic and physical map of a region within human chromosome band 17p13. *Biochem Mol Med* **58**:135, 1996.
141. Peters U, Senger G, Rahlmann M, DuChesne I, Stec I, Kohler MR, Weissenbach J, et al.: Nephropathic cystinosis (CTNS-LSB): Construction of a YAC contig comprising the refined critical region on chromosome 17p13. *Eur J Hum Genet* **5**:9, 1997.
142. Heick H, McGowan-Jordan J, Podolsky L, Besner-Johnston A, Orrbine E, Goodyer P, MacLaine P, et al.: Fine mapping of cystinosis: Evidence for linkage disequilibrium in French-Canadian families. *Am J Hum Genet* **61**:A279/1624, 1997.
142a. Touchman JW, Anikster Y, Dietrich NL, Maduro VV, McDowell G, Shotelersuk V, Bouffard GG, et al.: The genomic region encompassing the nephropathic cystinosis gene (*CTNS*): Complete sequencing of a 200-kb segment and discovery of a novel gene within the common cystinosis-causing deletion. *Genome Res* **10**:165, 2000.
142b. McGowan-Jordan J, Stoddard K, Podolsky L, Orrbine E, McLaine P, Town M, Goodyer P, et al.: Molecular analysis of cystinosis: Probable Irish origin of the most common French Canadian mutation. *Eur J Hum Genet* **7**:671, 1999.
142c. Anikster Y, Shotelersuk V, Gahl WA: *CTNS* mutations in patients with cystinosis. *Hum Mutat* **14**:454, 1999.
142d. Attard M, Jean G, Forestier L, Cherqui S, van't Hoff W, Broyer M, Antignac C, et al.: Severity of phenotype in cystinosis varies with mutations in the *CTNS* gene: Predicted effect on the model of cystinosin. *Hum Mol Genet* **8**:2507, 1999.
143. Pellett OL, Smith ML, Greene AA, Schneider JA: Lack of complementation in somatic cell hybrids between fibroblasts from patients with different forms of cystinosis. *Proc Natl Acad Sci U S A* **85**:3531, 1988.
144. Thoene J, Lemons R, Anikster Y, Mullet J, Paelicke K, Lucero C, Gahl W, et al.: Mutations of *CTNS* causing intermediate cystinosis. *Mol Genet Metab* **67**:283, 1999.
144a. Anikster Y, Lucero C, Guo JR, Huizing M, Shotelersuk V, Bernardini I, McDowell G, et al.: Ocular nonnephropathic cystinosis: Clinical, biochemical, and molecular correlations. *Pediatr Res* **47**:17, 2000.
145. McDowell GA, Town MM, van't Hoff W, Gahl WA: Clinical and molecular aspect of nephropathic cystinosis. *J Mol Med* **76**:295, 1998.
146. Gahl WA: Cystinosis coming of age. *Adv Pediatr* **33**:95, 1986.
147. Markello TC: Unpublished data.
148. Morell GP, Niaudet P, Jean G, Descamps-Latscha B: Altered oxidative metabolism, motility, and adherence in phagocytic cells from cystinotic children. *Pediatr Res* **19**:1318, 1985.
149. Pintos-Morell G, Salem P, Jean G, Niaudet P, Mencia-Huerta JM: Altered leukotriene generation in leukocytes from cystinotic children. *Pediatr Res* **36**:628, 1994.
150. Brodehl J, Hagge W, Gellissen K: Die veranderungen der nierenfunktion bei der cystinose. Teil I: Die inulin-, PAH-und elektrolyt-clearance in verschiedenen stadien der erkrankung. *Ann Paediatr* **205**:131, 1965.
151. Teree TM, Friedman AB, Kest LM, Fetterman GH: Cystinosis and proximal tubular nephropathy in siblings. Progressive development of the physiological and anatomical lesion. *Am J Dis Child* **119**:481, 1970.
152. Lemire J, Kaplan BS, Scriver CR: Presentation of cystinosis as Bartter's syndrome and conversion to Fanconi syndrome on indomethacin treatment. *Pediatr Res* **12**:544, 1978.
153. O'Regan S, Mongeau JG, Robitaille P: A patient with cystinosis presenting with the features of Bartter syndrome. *Acta Paediatr Belg* **33**:51, 1980.
154. Lemire J, Kaplan BS: The various renal manifestations of the nephropathic form of cystinosis. *Am J Nephrol* **4**:81, 1984.
155. Waldmann TA, Mogielnicki RP, Strober W: The proteinuria of cystinosis: Its pattern and pathogenesis, in Schulman JD (ed): *Cystinosis*. Washington, DC, DHEW Publication No. (NIH) 72-249, 1972, p 55.
156. Gahl WA: unpublished data.

157. Black J, Stapleton FB, Roy S 3d, Ward J, Noe HN: Varied types of urinary calculi in a patient with cystinosis without renal tubular acidosis. *Pediatrics* **78**:295, 1986.
158. Fischsbach M, Terzic J, Cavalier A, Mambrini P, Geisert J: Renal stones in nephropathic cystinosis treated with phosphocysteamine. *Pediatr Nephrol* **11**:787, 1997.
159. Saleem MA, Milford DV, Alton H, Chapman S, Winterborn MH: Hypercalciuria and ultrasound abnormalities in children with cystinosis. *Pediatr Nephrol* **9**:45, 1995.
160. Theodoropoulos DS, Shawker TH, Heinrichs C, Gahl WA: Medullary nephrocalcinosis in nephropathic cystinosis. *Pediatr Nephrol* **9**:412, 1995.
161. Steinherz R, Chesney RW, Schulman JD, DeLuca HF, Phelps M: Circulating vitamin D metabolites in nephropathic cystinosis. *J Pediatr* **102**:592, 1983.
162. Hagge W, Brodehl J: Die veranderungen der nierenfunktion bei der cystinose. Teil II: Die aminosauren-clearances. *Ann Paediatr* **205**:442, 1965.
163. Bernardini I, Rizzo WB, Dalakas M, Bernar J, Gahl WA: Plasma and muscle free carnitine deficiency due to renal Fanconi syndrome. *J Clin Invest* **75**:1124, 1985.
164. Brodehl J, Bickel H: Aminoaciduria and hyperaminoaciduria in childhood. *Clin Nephrol* **1**:149, 1973.
165. Charnas LR, Bernardini I, Rader D, Hoeg JM, Gahl WA: Clinical and laboratory findings in the oculocerebrorenal syndrome of Lowe, with special reference to growth and renal function. *N Engl J Med* **324**:1318, 1991.
166. Spear GS: The pathology of the kidney, in Schulman JD (ed): *Cystinosis*. Washington, DC, DHEW Publication No (NIH) 72-249, 1973, p 37.
167. Spear GS, Slusser RJ, Schulman JD, Alexander F: Polykaryocytosis in the visceral glomerular epithelium in cystinosis with description of an unusual clinical variant. *Johns Hopkins Med J* **129**:83, 1971.
168. Spear GS: Pathology of the kidney in cystinosis. *Pathol Annu* **9**:81, 1974.
169. Markello TC, Bernardini IM, Gahl WA: Improved renal function in children with cystinosis treated with cysteamine. *N Engl J Med* **328**:1157, 1993.
170. Schnaper HW, Cottel J, Merrill S, Marcusson E, Kissane JM, Shackelford GD, So SKS, et al.: Early occurrence of end-stage renal disease in a patient with infantile nephropathic cystinosis. *J Pediatr* **120**:575, 1992.
171. van't Hoff WG, Ledermann SE, Waldron M, Trompeter RS: Early-onset chronic-renal-failure as a presentation of infantile nephropathic cystinosis. *Pediatr Nephrol* **9**:483, 1995.
172. Leumann EP: Progression of renal insufficiency in pediatric patients: Estimation from serum creatinine. *Helv Paediatr Acta* **33**:25, 1978.
173. Gahl WA, Schneider JA, Schulman JD, Thoene JG, Reed GF: Predicted reciprocal serum creatinine at age 10 years as a measure of renal function in children with nephropathic cystinosis treated with oral cysteamine. *Pediatr Nephrol* **4**:129, 1990.
174. Manz F, Gretz N, Broyer M, Geisert J, Grote K, Weber HP, Hennemann H, et al.: Progression of chronic-renal-failure in a historical group of patients with nephropathic cystinosis. *Pediatr Nephrol* **8**:466, 1994.
175. Gretz N, Manz F, Augustin R, Barrat TM, Bender-Götze C, Brandis M, Bremer HJ, et al.: Survival time in cystinosis. A collaborative study. *Proc Eur Dial Transplant Assoc* **19**:582, 1983.
176. Gahl WA, Reed GF, Thoene JG, Schulman JD, Rizzo WB, Jonas AJ, Denman DW, et al.: Cysteamine therapy for children with nephropathic cystinosis. *N Engl J Med* **316**:971, 1987.
177. Winkler L, Offner G, Krull F, Brodehl J: Growth and pubertal development in nephropathic cystinosis. *Eur J Pediatr* **152**:244, 1993.
178. Bercu BB, Rizzo WB, Corden BJ, Reed GF, Schulman JD: Circulating somatomedin-C levels in nephropathic cystinosis. *Isr J Med Sci* **20**:236, 1984.
179. Gahl WA, Kaiser-Kupfer MI: Complications of nephropathic cystinosis after renal failure. *Pediatr Nephrol* **1**:260, 1987.
180. Ehrich JHH, Brodehl J, Byrd DI, Hossfeld S, Hoyer PF, Leipert K-P, Offner G, Wolff G: Renal transplantation in 22 children with nephropathic cystinosis. *Pediatr Nephrol* **5**:707, 1991.
181. Theodoropoulos DS, Krasnewich D, Kaiser-Kupfer MI, Gahl WA: Classic nephropathic cystinosis as an adult disease. *JAMA* **270**:2200, 1993.
182. Broyer M, Tete MJ: Delayed complications of cystinosis, a review of 33 patients older than 18 years. *Anal Pediatrie* **42**:635, 1995.
183. Elenberg E, Norling LL, Kleinman RE, Ingelfinger JR: Feeding problems in cystinosis. *Pediatr Nephrol* **12**:365, 1998.
184. Lucky AW, Howley PM, Megyesi K, Spielberg SP, Schulman JD: Endocrine studies in cystinosis: Compensated primary hypothyroidism. *J Pediatr* **91**:204, 1977.
185. Sanderson PO, Kuwabara T, Stark WJ, Wong VG, Collins EMK: Cystinosis: A clinical, histopathologic, and ultrastructural study. *Arch Ophthalmol* **91**:270, 1974.
186. Francois J, Hanssens M, Coppleters R, Evens L: Cystinosis. A clinical and histopathologic study. *Am J Ophthalmol* **73**:643, 1972.
187. Wong VG: The eye and cystinosis, in Schulman JD (ed): *Cystinosis*. Washington, DC, DHEW Publication No. (NIH) 72-249, 1973, p 23.
188. Wong VG, Lietman PS, Seegmiller JE: Alterations of pigment epithelium in cystinosis. *Arch Ophthalmol* **77**:361, 1967.
189. Schneider JA, Verroust FM, Kroll WA, Garvin AJ, Horger EO 3rd, Wong VG, Spear GS, et al.: Prenatal diagnosis of cystinosis. *N Engl J Med* **290**:878, 1974.
190. Yamamoto GK, Schulman JD, Schneider JA, Wong VG: Long-term ocular changes in cystinosis: Observations in renal transplant recipients. *J Pediatr Ophthalmol Strabismus* **16**:21, 1979.
191. Gahl WA, Schneider JA, Thoene JG, Chesney R: Course of nephropathic cystinosis after age 10 years. *J Pediatr* **109**:605, 1986.
192. Bürki VE: Ueber die cystinkrankheit im klienkindesalter unter besonderer Berücksichtigung des Augenbefundes. *Ophthalmologica* **101**:257, 1941.
193. Cogan DG, Kuwabara T, Kinoshita J, Sudarsky D, Ring H: Ocular manifestations of systemic cystinosis. *Arch Ophthalmol* **55**:36, 1956.
194. Kenyon ER, Sensenbrenner JA: Electron microscopy of cornea and conjunctiva in childhood cystinosis. *Am J Ophthalmol* **78**:68, 1974.
195. Frazier PD, Wong VG: Cystinosis. Histologic and crystallographic examination of crystals in eye tissues. *Arch Ophthalmol* **80**:87, 1968.
196. Kaiser-Kupfer MI, Datiles MB, Gahl WA: Corneal transplant in a twelve-year-old boy with nephropathic cystinosis. *Lancet* **1**:331, 1987.
197. Kaiser-Kupfer MI, Gahl WA: Unpublished data.
198. Kaiser-Kupfer MI, Chan CC, Rodrigues M, Datiles MB, Gahl WA: Nephropathic cystinosis: Immunohistochemical and histopathologic studies of cornea, conjunctiva and iris. *Curr Eye Res* **6**:617, 1987.
199. Katz B, Melles RB, Schneider JA, Rao NA: Corneal thickness in nephropathic cystinosis. *Br J Ophthalmol* **73**:665, 1989.
200. Weber U, Sons HU, Bernsmeier H, Lenz W: Experimentally induced cystine keratopathy in rabbits. *Graefes Arch Clin Exp Ophthalmol* **224**:443, 1986.
201. Richler M, Milot J, Quigley M, O'Regan S: Ocular manifestations of nephropathic cystinosis. The French-Canadian experience in a genetically homogeneous population. *Arch Ophthalmol* **109**:359, 1991.
202. Wan WL, Minckler DS, Rao NA: Pupillary-block glaucoma associated with childhood cystinosis. *Am J Ophthalmol* **101**:700, 1986.
203. Schulman JD, Wong VG, Bradley KH, Seegmiller JE: A simple technique for the biochemical diagnosis of cystinosis. *J Pediatr* **76**:289, 1970.
204. Burke JR, El-Bishti MM, Maisey MN, Chantler C: Hypothyroidism in children with cystinosis. *Arch Dis Child* **53**:947, 1978.
205. Bercu BB, Schulman JD: Pituitary secretion of alpha and beta subunits of thyroid-stimulating hormone (TSH) in nephropathic cystinosis. *Isr J Med Sci* **20**:179, 1984.
206. Bercu BB, Orloff S, Schulman JD: Pituitary resistance to thyroid hormone in cystinosis. *J Clin Endocrinol Metab* **51**:1262, 1980.
207. Chantler C, Carter JE, Bewick M, Counahan R, Cameron JS, Ogg CS, Williams DG, Winder E: 10 years' experience with regular haemodialysis and renal transplantation. *Arch Dis Child* **55**:435, 1980.
208. Ammenti A, Grossi A, Bernasconi S: Infantile cystinosis and insulin-dependent diabetes mellitus. *Eur J Pediatr* **145**:548, 1986.
209. Milner RD, Wirdnam PK: The pancreatic beta cell fraction in children with errors of amino acid metabolism. *Pediatr Res* **16**:213, 1982.
210. Chik CL, Friedman A, Merriam GR, Gahl WA: Pituitary-testicular function in nephropathic cystinosis. *Ann Intern Med* **119**:568, 1993.
211. Harper GS, Bernardini I, Hurko O, Zuurveld J, Gahl WA: Cystine storage in cultured myotubes from patients with nephropathic cystinosis. *Biochem J* **243**:841, 1987.
212. Charnas LR, Dalakas M: Unpublished data.
213. Arnold RW, Stickler GB, Bourne WM, Mellinger JF: Corneal crystals, myopathy, and nephropathy: A new syndrome? *J Pediatr Ophthalmol Strabismus* **24**:151, 1987.

214. Sonies BC, Ekman EF, Andersson HC, Adamson MD, Kaler SG, Markello TC, Gahl WA: Swallowing dysfunction in nephropathic cystinosis. *N Engl J Med* **323**:565, 1990.
215. Anikster Y, Lacbawan F, Bernardini I, Brantly M, Gahl WA: The lungs in cystinosis: Disease in the respiratory muscle [Abstract]. *Am J Hum Genet* **63**:A261/1506, 1998.
216. Chung CJ, O'Connell T, Fordham LA, Specter B, Barker P: Utility of bone imaging in differentiation of pulmonary metastatic calcification from cystine crystal deposition in cystinosis. *Clin Nucl Med* **23**:54, 1998.
217. Edelman M, Silverstein D, Strom J, Factor SM: Cardiomyopathy in a male with cystinosis. *Cardiovasc Path* **6**:43, 1997.
218. Vogel DG, Malekzadeh MH, Cornford ME, Schneider JA, Shields WD, Vinters HV: Central nervous system involvement in nephropathic cystinosis. *J Neuropathol Exp Neurol* **49**:591, 1990.
219. Ehrich JHH, Stoeppler L, Offner G, Brodehl J: Evidence for cerebral involvement in nephropathic cystinosis. *Neuropediatrie* **10**:128, 1979.
220. Brodehl J, Ehrich JHH, Krohn JP, Offner G, Byrd D: Kidney transplantation in nephropathic cystinosis, in Brodehl J, Ehrich JHH (eds): *Pediatric Nephrology*. Berlin, Springer-Verlag, 1984, p 172.
221. Cochat P, Drachman R, Gagnadoux MF, Pariente D, Broyer M: Cerebral atrophy and nephropathic cystinosis. *Arch Dis Child* **61**:401, 1986.
222. Fink JK, Brouwers P, Barton N, Malekzadeh MH, Sato S, Hill S, Cohen WE, Fivush B, Gahl WA: Neurologic complications in long-standing nephropathic cystinosis. *Arch Neurol* **46**:543, 1989.
223. Nichols SL, Press GA, Schneider JA, Trauner DA: Cortical atrophy and cognitive performance in infantile nephropathic cystinosis. *Pediatr Neurol* **6**:379, 1990.
224. Schnaper HW, Cole BR, Hodges FJ, Robson AM: Cerebral cortical atrophy in pediatric patients with end-stage renal disease. *Am J Kidney Dis* **2**:645, 1983.
225. Ross DL, Strife CF, Towbin R, Bove KE: Nonabsorptive hydrocephalus associated with nephropathic cystinosis. *Neurology* **32**:1330, 1982.
226. Swenson MR, Rimmer S, Schneider JA, Melles RB, Trauner DA, Katz B: Neurophysiologic studies of the peripheral nervous system in nephropathic cystinosis. *Arch Neurol* **48**:528, 1991.
227. Avner ED, Ellis D, Jaffe R: Veno-occlusive disease of the liver associated with cysteamine treatment of nephropathic cystinosis. *J Pediatr* **102**:793, 1983.
228. Klenn PJ, Rubin R: Hepatic fibrosis associated with hereditary cystinosis: A novel form of noncirrhotic portal hypertension. *Mod Pathol* **7**:879, 1994.
229. Ishak K: Personal communication, March 9, 1992.
230. Treem WR, Rusnack EJ, Ragsdale BD, Seikaly MG, DiPalma JS: Inflammatory bowel disease in a patient with nephropathic cystinosis. *Pediatrics* **81**:584, 1988.
231. Fivush B, Flick JA, Gahl WA: Pancreatic exocrine insufficiency in a patient with nephropathic cystinosis. *J Pediatr* **112**:49, 1988.
232. Trauner DA, Chase CH, Scheller JM, Fontanesi J, Katz B, Schneider JA: Neurologic and cognitive deficits in cystinosis. *Pediatr Res* **21**:498A, 1987.
233. Colah S, Trauner DA: Tactile recognition in infantile nephropathic cystinosis. *Dev Med Child Neurol* **39**:409, 1997.
234. Williams BLH, Schneider JA, Trauner DA: Global intellectual deficits in cystinosis. *Am J Med Genet* **49**:83, 1994.
235. Ballantyne AO, Scarvie KM, Trauner DA: Academic achievement in individuals with infantile nephropathic cystinosis. *Am J Med Genet* **74**:157, 1997.
236. Wolf G, Ehrich JHH, Offner G, Brodehl J: Psychosocial and intellectual development in 12 patients with infantile nephropathic cystinosis. *Acta Paediatr Scand* **71**:1007, 1982.
237. Gahl WA, Hubbard VS, Orloff S: Decreased sweat production in cystinosis. *J Pediatr* **104**:904, 1984.
238. Fox PC, Baum BJ, Gahl WA: Unpublished data.
239. Purday JP, Montgomery CJ, Blackstock D: Intraoperative hyperthermia in a pediatric patient with cystinosis. *Paediatr Anaesth* **5**:389, 1995.
240. Almond PS, Morel P, Troppmann C, Matas A, Najarian JS, Chavers B: Progression of infantile cystinosis after renal transplantation. *Transplant Proc* **23**:1386, 1991.
241. Smolin LA, Clark KF, Schneider JA: An improved method for heterozygote detection of cystinosis using polymorphonuclear leukocytes. *Am J Hum Genet* **41**:266, 1987.
242. For details on leukocyte preparation, see http://medicine.ucsd.edu/cystinosis.
243. Smith ML, Furlong CE, Greene AA, Schneider JA: Cystine: Binding protein assay. *Methods Enzymol* **143**:144, 1987.
243a. Anikster Y, Lucero C, Touchman JW, Huizing M, McDowell G, Shotelersuk V, Green ED, et al.: Identification and detection of the common 65-kb deletion breakpoint in the nephropathic cystinosis gene (*CTNS*). *Mol Genet Metab* **66**:111, 1999.
243b. Forestier L, Jean G, Attard M, Cherqui S, Lewis C, van't Hoff W, Broyer M, et al.: Molecular characterization of CTNS deletions in nephropathic cystinosis: Development of a PCR-based detection assay. *Am J Hum Genet* **65**:353, 1999.
244. Bëtend B, David L, Vincent M, Hermier M, François R: Successful indomethacin treatment of two paediatric patients with severe tubulopathies. A boy with an unusual hypercalciuria and a girl with cystinosis. *Helv Paediatr Acta* **34**:339, 1979.
245. Haycock GB, Al-Dahhan J, Mak RH, Chantler C: Effect of indomethacin on clinical progress and renal function in cystinosis. *Arch Dis Child* **57**:934, 1982.
246. Betend B, Pugeaut R, David L, Hermier M, François R: Pediatric cystinosis: An experience with indomethacin therapy for nearly 4 years. *Pediatrie* **37**:31, 1982.
247. Parchoux B, Guibaud P, Louis JJ, Benzoni D, Larbre F: Urinary prostaglandins and effect of indomethacin therapy in cystinosis. *Pediatrie* **37**:19, 1982.
248. Usberti M, Pecoraro C, Federico S, Cianciaruso B, Guida B, Romano A, Grumetto L, et al.: Mechanism of action of indomethacin in tubular defects. *Pediatrics* **75**:501, 1985.
249. Broyer M, Tete MJ: [Treatment of cystinosis using cysteamine]. *Ann Pediatr (Paris)* **37**:91, 1990.
250. Lemire J, Kaplan BS: Prolonged use of indomethacin in cystinosis [Abstract]. *Pediatr Res* **15**:696, 1981.
251. Clark KF, Slymen DJ, Schneider JA, Thoene J, Stetz S, Gahl WA, Bernardini I, et al.: A comparative study of indomethacin for treatment of the Fanconi syndrome in cystinosis. *J Rare Dis* **2**:5, 1996.
252. Gahl WA, Bernardini I, Dalakas M, Rizzo WB, Harper GS, Hoeg JM, Hurko O, et al.: Oral carnitine therapy in children with cystinosis and renal Fanconi syndrome. *J Clin Invest* **81**:549, 1988.
253. Gahl WA, Bernardini IM, Dalakas MC, Markello TC, Krasnewich DM, Charnas LR: Muscle carnitine repletion by long-term carnitine supplementation in nephropathic cystinosis. *Pediatr Res* **34**:115, 1993.
254. Kimonis VE, Troendle J, Rose SR, Yang ML, Markello TC, Gahl WA: Effects of early cysteamine therapy on thyroid function and growth in nephropathic cystinosis. *J Clin Endocrinol Metab* **80**:3257, 1995.
255. Mahoney CP, Manning GB, Hickman RO: Hemodialysis in a patient with cystinosis. Effects on amino acid and bone metabolism. *Am J Dis Child* **112**:65, 1966.
256. Mahoney CP, Striker GE, Hickman RO, Manning GB, Marchioro TL: Renal transplantation for childhood cystinosis. *N Engl J Med* **283**:397, 1970.
257. Goodman SI, Hambidge KM, Mahoney CP, Striker GE: Renal homotransplantation in the treatment of cystinosis, in Schulman JD (eds): *Cystinosis*. Washington, DC, DHEW No. (NIH) 72-249, 1973, p 225.
258. West JC, Goodman SI, Schröter GP, Bloustein PA, Hambidge KM, Weil R 3d: Pediatric kidney transplantation for cystinosis. *J Pediatr Surg* **12**:651, 1977.
259. Malekzadeh MH, Neustein HB, Schneider JA, Pennisi AJ, Ettenger RB, Uittenbogaart CH, Kogut MD, et al.: Cadaver renal transplantation in children with cystinosis. *Am J Med* **63**:525, 1977.
260. Chantler C, Carter JE, Bewick M, Counahan R, Cameron JS, Ogg CS, Williams DG, et al.: 10 years' experience with regular haemodialysis and renal transplantation. *Arch Dis Child* **55**:435, 1980.
261. Langlois RP, O'Regan S, Pelletier M, Robitaille P: Kidney transplantation in uremic children with cystinosis. *Nephron* **28**:273, 1981.
262. Ehrich JH, Rizzoni G, Brunner FP, Brynger H, Geerlings W, Fassbinder W, Raine AE, et al.: Combined report on regular dialysis and transplantation of children in Europe, 1989. *Nephrol Dial Transplant* **1(Suppl 6)**:37, 1991.
263. Gagnadoux MF, Charbit M, Guest G, Arsan A, Broyer M: [Clinical evaluation of 70 pediatric renal transplants after 10 to 17 years]. *Ann Pediatr (Paris)* **38**:413, 1991.
264. Kashtan CE, McEnery PT, Tejani A, Stablein DM: Renal allograft survival according to primary diagnosis: A report of the North

American Pediatric Renal Transplant Cooperative Study. *Pediatr Nephrol* **9**:679, 1995.

265. Spear GS, Gubler MC, Habib R, Broyer M: Renal allografts in cystinosis and mesangial demography. *Clin Nephrol* **32**:256, 1989.
266. Broyer M, Tete MJ, Gubler MC: Late symptoms in infantile cystinosis. *Pediatr Nephrol* **1**:519, 1987.
267. Clark KF, Franklin PS, Reisch JS, Hoffman HJ, Gahl WA, Thoene JG, Schneider JA: Effect of cysteamine-HCl and phosphocysteamine dosage on renal function and growth in children with nephropathic cystinosis. *Clin Res* **40**:113A, 1992.
268. Schneider JA: Cysteamine for treatment of cystinosis, in Andreucci VE, Fine LG (eds): *International Yearbook of Nephrology Dialysis Transplantation*, 9th ed. Oxford, Oxford Press, 1994, p 97.
269. Schneider JA: Approval of cysteamine for patients with cystinosis [Letter]. *Pediatr Nephrol* **9**:254, 1995.
270. Corden BJ, Schulman JD, Schneider JA, Thoene JG: Adverse reactions to oral cysteamine use in nephropathic cystinosis. *Dev Pharmacol Ther* **3**:25, 1981.
271. Wenner WJ, Murphy JL: The effects of cysteamine on the upper gastrointestinal tract of children with cystinosis. *Pediatr Nephrol* **11**:600, 1997.
272. Schneider JA, Clark KF, Greene AA, Reisch JS, Markello TC, Gahl WA, Thoene JG, et al.: Recent advances in the treatment of cystinosis. *J Inherit Metab Dis* **18**:387, 1995.
273. Gahl WA, Ingelfinger J, Mohan P, Bernardini I, Hyman PE, Tangerman A: Intravenous cysteamine therapy for nephropathic cystinosis. *Pediatr Res* **38**:579, 1995.
274. Broyer M, Tete MJ, Guest G, Bertheleme JP, Labrousse F, Poisson M: Clinical polymorphism of cystinosis encephalopathy. Results of treatment with cysteamine. *J Inherit Metab Dis* **19**:65, 1996.
275. van't Hoff WG, Gretz N: The treatment of cystinosis with cysteamine and phosphocysteamine in the United Kingdom and Eire. *Pediatr Nephrol* **9**:685, 1995.
276. Selye H, Szabo S: Experimental model for production of perforating duodenal ulcers by cysteamine in the rat. *Nature* **244**:458, 1973.
277. Szabo S, Reichlin S: Somatostatin in rat tissues is depleted by cysteamine administration. *Endocrinology* **109**:2255, 1981.
278. Szabo S, Reichlin S: Somatostatin depletion by cysteamine: Mechanism and implication for duodenal ulceration. *Fed Proc* **44**:2540, 1985.
279. Scammell JG, Dannies PS: Depletion of pituitary prolactin by cysteamine is due to loss of immunological activity. *Endocrinology* **114**:712, 1984.
280. Scammell JG, Burrage TG, Eisenfeld AJ, Dannies PS: Cysteamine causes reduction of prolactin monomers followed by aggregation in the rat pituitary gland. *Endocrinology* **116**:2347, 1985.
281. Jonas AJ, Schneider JA: Plasma cysteamine concentrations in children treated for cystinosis. *J Pediatr* **100**:321, 1982.
282. Smolin LA, Clark KF, Thoene JG, Gahl WA, Schneider JA: A comparison of the effectiveness of cysteamine and phosphocysteamine in elevating plasma cysteamine concentration and decreasing leukocyte free cystine in nephropathic cystinosis. *Pediatr Res* **23**:616, 1988.
283. Peterson TC: Effect of chronic cysteamine treatment on mouse liver aryl hydrocarbon hydroxylase activity. *Can J Physiol Pharmacol* **66**:1433, 1988.
284. Yudkoff M, Nissim I, Schneider A, Segal S: Cysteamine inhibition of [^{15}N]-glycine turnover in cystinosis and of glycine cleavage system in vitro. *Metabolism* **30**:1096, 1981.
285. Gahl WA, Bercu BB: Blunted prolactin response to thyrotropin-releasing hormone stimulation in cystinotic children receiving cysteamine. *J Clin Endocrinol Metab* **60**:793, 1985.
286. Gahl WA, Gregg RE, Hoeg JM, Fisher E: *In vivo* alteration of a mutant human protein using the free thiol cysteamine. *Am J Med Genet* **20**:409, 1985.
287. Avner ED, Ellis D, Jaffe R: Veno-occlusive disease of the liver associated with cysteamine treatment of nephropathic cystinosis. *J Pediatr* **102**:793, 1983.
288. Gahl WA, Schulman JD, Thoene JG, Schneider J: Hepatotoxicity of cysteamine [Letter]? *J Pediatr* **103**:1008, 1983.
289. da Silva VA, Zurbrugg RP, Lavanchy P, Blumberg A, Suter H, Wyss SR, Luthy CM, et al.: Long-term treatment of infantile nephropathic cystinosis with cysteamine. *N Engl J Med* **313**:1460, 1985.
290. Reznik VM, Adamson M, Adelman RD, Murphy JL, Gahl WA, Clark KF, Schneider JA: Treatment of cystinosis with cysteamine from early infancy. *J Pediatr* **119**:491, 1991.
291. Assadi FK, Mullin JJ, Beckman DA: Evaluation of the reproductive and developmental safety of cysteamine in the rat: Effects on female reproduction and early embryonic development. *Teratology* **58**:88, 1998.
292. Beckman DA, Mullin JJ, Assadi FK: Developmental toxicity of cysteamine in the rat: Effects on embryo-fetal development. *Teratology* **58**:96, 1998.
293. Jeitner TM, Renton FJ: Inhibition of the proliferation of human neural neoplastic cell lines by cysteamine. *Cancer Lett* **103**:85, 1996.
294. Bergamini A, Ventura L, Mancino G, Capozzi M, Placido R, Salanitro A, Cappannoli L, et al.: In vitro inhibition of the replication of human immunodeficiency virus type 1 by β-mercaptoethylamine (cysteamine). *J Infect Dis* **174**:214, 1996.
295. Kaiser-Kupfer MI, Fujikawa L, Kuwabara T, Jain S, Gahl WA: Removal of corneal crystals by topical cysteamine in nephropathic cystinosis. *N Engl J Med* **316**:775, 1987.
296. Kaiser-Kupfer MI, Gazzo MA, Datiles MB, Caruso RC, Kuehl EM, Gahl WA: A randomized placebo-controlled trial of cysteamine eye drops in nephropathic cystinosis. *Arch Ophthalmol* **108**:689, 1990.
297. Jones NP, Postlethwaite RJ, Noble JL: Clearance of corneal crystals in nephropathic cystinosis by topical cysteamine 0.5%. *Br J Ophthalmol* **75**:311, 1991.
298. Graf M, Kalinowski HO: [1H-NMR spectroscopic study of cysteamine eyedrops] 1H-NMR-spektroskopische Untersuchung von Cysteamin-Augentropfen. *Klin Monatsbl Augenheilkd* **206**:262, 1995.
299. Lambert SR, Taylor D: Results of a six-month trial of topical cysteamine in two older children with nephropathic cystinosis [Abstract]. *Ophthalmology* **96(Suppl 9)**:131, 1989.
300. MacDonald IM, Noel LP, Mintsioulis G, Clarke WN: The effect of topical cysteamine drops on reducing crystal formation within the cornea of patients affected by nephropathic cystinosis. *J Pediatr Ophthalmol Strabismus* **27**:272, 1990.
301. Fine RN, Kohaut E, Brown D, Kuntze J, Attie KM: Long-term treatment of growth retarded children with chronic renal insufficiency, with recombinant human growth hormone. *Kidney Int* **49**:781, 1996.
302. Wilson DP, Jelley D, Stratton R, Coldwell JG: Nephropathic cystinosis: Improved linear growth after treatment with recombinant human growth hormone. *J Pediatr* **115**:758, 1989.
303. Tönshoff B, Mehls O, Heinrich U, Blum WF, Ranke MB, Schauer A: Growth-stimulating effects of recombinant human growth hormone in children with end-stage renal disease. *J Pediatr* **116**:561, 1990.
304. Rees L, Rigden SP, Ward G, Preece MA: Treatment of short stature in renal disease with recombinant human growth hormone. *Arch Dis Child* **65**:856, 1990.
305. Andersson HC, Markello T, Schneider JA, Gahl WA: Effect of growth hormone treatment on serum creatinine concentration in patients with cystinosis and chronic renal disease. *J Pediatr* **120**:716, 1992.
306. Haffner D, Wuhl E, Nissel R, Schaefer F, Mehls O: Effect of growth hormone treatment on pubertal growth in a boy with cystinosis and growth failure after renal transplantation. *Br J Clin Pract Symp Suppl* **85**:7, 1996.
307. Gretz N, Mehls O: Growth hormone therapy in nephropathic cystinosis [Letter]. *J Pediatr* **122**:328, 1993.
308. Andersson HC, Markello TC, Schneider JA, Gahl WA: Growth hormone therapy in nephropathic cystinosis. Reply [Letter]. *J Pediatr* **122**:329, 1993.
309. Wuhl E, Haffner D, Gretz N, Offner G, van't Hoff WG, Broyer M, Mehls O, et al.: Treatment with recombinant human growth hormone in short children with nephropathic cystinosis: No evidence for increased deterioration rate of renal function. *Pediatr Res* **43**:484, 1998.
310. 2516 Stockbridge Drive, Oakland, CA 94611. http://cystinosisfoundation.ucsd.edu.
311. Goldman H, Scriver CR, Aaron K, Delvin E, Canlas Z: Adolescent cystinosis: Comparisons with infantile and adult forms. *Pediatrics* **47**:979, 1971.
312. Aaron K, Goldman H, Scriver CR: Cystinosis; new observations: 1. Adolescent (type III) form. 2. Correction of phenotypes in vitro with dithiothreitol, in Carson NAJ, Raine DN (eds): *Inherited Disorders of Sulphur Metabolism*. Edinburgh, Churchill Livingstone, 1971, p 150.
313. Hooft C, Carton D, DeSchrijver F, Delbeke MJ, Samijn W, Kint J: Juvenile cystinosis in two siblings, in Carson NAJ, Raine DN (eds): *Inherited Disorders of Sulphur Metabolism*, Edinburgh, Churchill Livingstone, 1971, p 141.

314. Hauglustaine D, Corbeel L, van Damme B, Serrus M, Michielsen P: Glomerulonephritis in late-onset cystinosis. Report of two cases and review of the literature. *Clin Nephrol* **6**:529, 1976.
315. Pabico RC, Panner BJ, McKenna BA, Bryson MF: Glomerular lesions in patients with late-onset cystinosis with massive proteinuria. *Renal Physiol* **3**:347, 1980.
316. Dale RT, Rao GN, Aquavella JV, Metz HS: Adolescent cystinosis: A clinical and specular microscopic study of an unusual sibship. *Br J Ophthalmol* **65**:828, 1981.
317. Manz F, Harms E, Lutz P, Waldherr R, Scharer K: Adolescent cystinosis: Renal function and morphology. *Eur J Pediatr* **138**:354, 1982.
318. Langman CB, Moore ES, Thoene JG, Schneider JA: Renal failure in a sibship with late-onset cystinosis. *J Pediatr* **107**:755, 1985.
319. Hamdoun S, Lebon P, Nivet H, Beaufils H, Babinet F, Kernaonet E: Late onset cystinosis. Apropos of a case. *Nephrologie* **8**:193, 1987.
320. Nakano H, Yamakura Y, Aoyagi K: [A presumed case of "adolescent" cystinosis.] *Nippon Ganka Gakkai Zasshi* **97**:538, 1993.
321. Hory B, Billerey C, Royer J, Saint Hillier Y: Glomerular lesions in juvenile cystinosis: Report of 2 cases. *Clin Nephrol* **42**:327, 1994.
322. Schneider JA, Katz B, Melles RB: Cystinosis. *AKF Neph Letter* **7**:22, 1990.
323. Cogan DG, Kuwabara T, Kinoshita J, Sheehan L, Merola L: Cystinosis in an adult. *JAMA* **164**:394, 1957.
324. Cogan DG, Kuwabara T, Hurlbut CS Jr, McMurray V: Further observations on cystinosis in the adult. *JAMA* **166**:1725, 1958.
325. Lietman PS, Frazier PD, Wong VG, Shotton D, Seegmiller JE: Adult cystinosis — A benign disorder. *Am J Med* **40**:511, 1966.
326. Schneider JA, Wong V, Bradley K, Seegmiller JE: Biochemical comparisons of the adult and childhood forms of cystinosis. *N Engl J Med* **279**:1253, 1968.
327. Brubaker RF, Wong VG, Schulman JD, Seegmiller JE, Kuwabara T: Benign cystinosis. The clinical, biochemical and morphologic findings in a family with two affected siblings. *Am J Med* **49**:546, 1970.
328. Kraus E, Lutz P: Ocular cystine deposits in an adult. *Arch Ophthalmol* **85**:690, 1971.
329. Dodd MJ, Pusin SM, Green WR: Adult cystinosis. A case report. *Arch Ophthalmol* **96**:1054, 1978.
330. Thiel HJ, Voigt GJ, Dorner K, Hake H, von Denffer H: Nephropathic and benign cystinosis [Author's translation]. *Klin Monatsbl Augenheilkd* **177**:324, 1980.
331. Stefani FH, Vogel S: Adult cystinosis: Electron microscopy of the conjunctiva. *Graefes Arch Clin Exp Ophthalmol* **219**:143, 1982.
332. Gahl WA, Tietze F: Lysosomal cystine transport in cystinosis variants and their parents. *Pediatr Res* **21**:193, 1987.
333. Gahl WA, McDowell G, Kaiser-Kupfer MI: Benign cystinosis patients [Letter]. *Cornea* **15**:101, 1996.
334. Greene AA, Schneider JA: Unpublished data.
335. Racusen LC, Wilson PD, Hartz PA, Fivush BA, Burrow CR, Philip ET: Renal proximal tubular epithelium from patients with nephropathic cystinosis — Immortalized cell lines as *in vitro* model systems. *Kid Int* **48**:536, 1995.
336. Bajaj G, Baum N: Proximal tubule dysfunction in cystine-loaded tubules: Effect of phosphate and metabolic substrates. *Am J Physiol* **40**:F717, 1996.
337. Rosenblatt DS, Hosack A, Matiaszuk NV, Cooper BA, Laframboise R: Defect in vitamin B_{12} release from lysosomes: Newly described inborn error of vitamin B_{12} metabolism. *Science* **228**:1319, 1985.
338. Patrick AD: Deficiencies of −SH-dependent enzymes in cystinosis. *Clin Sci* **28**:427, 1965.
339. Depape-Brigger D, Goldman H, Scriver CR, Delvin E, Mamer O: The *in vivo* use of dithiothreitol in cystinosis. *Pediatr Res* **11**:124, 1977.
340. Thoene JG, unpublished data.
341. Schulman JD, Bradley KH, Berezesky IK, Grimley PM, Dodson WE, Al-Aish MS: Biochemical, morphologic, and cytogenetic studies of leukocytes growing in continuous culture from normal individuals and from patients with cystinosis. *Pediatr Res* **5**:501, 1971.
342. Pellet OL, Smith ML, Thoene JG, Schneider JA, Jonas AJ: Renal cell culture using autopsy material from children with cystinosis. *In Vitro* **20**:53, 1984.
343. Racusen LC, Fivush BA, Andersson H, Gahl WA: Culture of renal tubular cells from the urine of patients with nephropathic cystinosis. *J Am Soc Nephrol* **1**:1028, 1991.

CHAPTER 200

Disorders of Free Sialic Acid Storage

Pertti Aula ▪ William A. Gahl

1. **Disorders of free sialic acid storage are characterized by either lysosomal or cytoplasmic accumulation of the negatively charged monosaccharide, sialic acid (*N*-acetylneuraminic acid). The lysosomal free sialic acid storage diseases, Salla disease and infantile free sialic acid storage disease (ISSD), are autosomal recessively inherited disorders with various degrees of psychomotor retardation. Both Salla disease and ISSD result from accumulation of free sialic acid in lysosomes due to an impaired carrier-mediated transport system in the lysosomal membrane. They are allelic disorders of a gene assigned to the proximal portion of the long arm of chromosome 6. The gene was recently cloned and mutations in both phenotypes were identified. The transport system also recognizes other acidic monosaccharides, but structural characteristics of the transport protein are still unknown. The single cytoplasmic free sialic acid storage disease is sialuria, due to impaired feedback inhibition of uridine diphosphate-*N*-acetylglucosamine (UDP-GlcNAc) 2-epimerase by cytidine monophosphate-*N*-acetylneuraminic acid (CMP-Neu5Ac). Its gene was recently cloned.**
2. **The free sialic acid storage disorders include Salla disease and the more severe infantile free sialic acid storage disease, ISSD. Patients with Salla disease, a disorder largely of the Finnish population, are normal at birth, but develop psychomotor delay and ataxia in infancy. Intelligence is moderately to severely impaired, and life span is slightly reduced. In contrast, patients with ISSD can present at birth and often succumb in the first year of life. They have failure to thrive, hepatosplenomegaly, severe mental and motor retardation, and they often have coarse facial features and dysostosis multiplex. Intermediate phenotypes have been reported. Dysmyelination of the brain is a constant and crucial finding in all types of lysosomal free sialic acid storage disorders, as documented by magnetic resonance imaging. There are over 120 Salla disease patients known, mostly with Finnish background, and more than 27 ISSD cases reported.**
3. **Patients with Salla disease and ISSD store, respectively, approximately 10 times and 100 times the normal amounts of free (unbound) *N*-acetylneuraminic acid in their tissues, and excrete 10 and 100 times normal amounts in the urine. Glucuronic acid also accumulates in cultured fibroblasts of patients with Salla disease and ISSD, because the lysosomal monosaccharide carrier defective in these disorders recognizes, in addition to sialic acid, glucuronic acid and other acidic monosaccharides.**
4. **The lysosomal free sialic acid storage disorders can be diagnosed based on increased urinary free sialic acid and histologic and electron microscope evidence of lysosomal storage on skin or conjunctival biopsy. Mutation assay can be applied in the Finnish population because of the high prevalence of the founder mutation. Prenatal diagnosis is based on sialic acid assay of a chorionic villus biopsy or, alternatively, using molecular studies, either genetic linkage analysis or mutation assay. Carriers can be identified in those families or populations in which the disease-causing mutation is known.**
5. **Sialuria, reported in only four patients, is characterized by hepatosplenomegaly, coarse facial features, and various degrees of developmental delay. The symptoms do not appear to progress. The disorder is diagnosed by the finding of gram quantities of free sialic acid in a 24-h urine, and vastly increased concentrations of free sialic acid in the cytoplasm of cultured fibroblasts. The basic defect consists of failure to regulate sialic acid synthesis, due to impaired feedback inhibition of UDP-GlcNAc 2-epimerase by CMP-Neu5Ac. The human epimerase gene has been sequenced, and three sialuria mutations identified; these indicate the region of the enzyme that binds CMP-Neu5Ac. Sialuria appears to be an autosomal dominant disorder. Only symptomatic therapy is available.**

Sialic acid storage disorders can be divided into those in which bound sialic acid accumulates and those in which free sialic acid is stored.[1] Diseases in the former category result from deficient activity of the lysosomal enzyme sialidase, or neuraminidase, and exhibit lysosomal storage of sialic acid-containing glycoconjugates (see Chap. 140). Disorders in the latter category are discussed in the present chapter. They include Salla disease and infantile free sialic acid storage disease (ISSD), in which free sialic acid accumulates in lysosomes, and sialuria, a disorder characterized by extremely high concentrations of free sialic acid in the cytoplasm of cells. All three diseases present with increased urinary excretion of free sialic acid.

SIALIC ACID METABOLISM

The sialic acids are a family of over 30 compounds derived from neuraminic acid, with many biologic roles.[2,3] In humans, the predominant sialic acid is *N*-acetylneuraminic acid (Fig. 200-1), a negatively charged compound of molecular weight 309 and pK 2.6, which we refer to as sialic acid. While a small portion of total sialic acid is free in tissues and body fluids, most is bound by an α-glycosidic linkage to glycoconjugates. Sialic acid provides these macromolecules with a negatively charged terminal sugar that serves many functions,[4] but no direct biologic role is attributed to unbound sialic acid. Human plasma has a low concentration of free

A list of standard abbreviations is located immediately preceding the index in each volume. Additional abbreviations used in this chapter include: CMP-Neu5Ac = cytidine monophosphate-*N*-acetylneuraminic acid; GluAc = glucuronic acid; ISSD = infantile free sialic acid storage disease; ManNAc = *N*-acetylmannosamine; NeuAc = *N*-acetylneuraminic acid, or sialic acid; NeuGc = *N*-glycolylneuraminic acid; and UDP-GlcNAc = uridine diphosphate-*N*-acetylglucosamine.

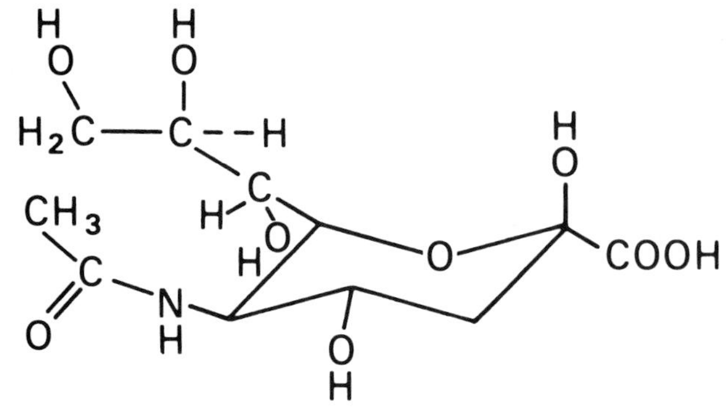

Fig. 200-1 Structure of *N*-acetylneuraminic acid, or sialic acid.

sialic acid, 0.80 nm/ml (±0.28) according to one study.[5] The same study also demonstrated that free sialic acid is filtered by renal glomeruli, but not reabsorbed or secreted by tubules. Free sialic acid clearance paralleled creatinine clearance in individuals with normal, as well as in those with impaired, renal function.

The synthesis of sialic acid begins with glucose, which undergoes several modifications to become activated UDP-*N*-acetyl-D-glucosamine (Fig. 200-2). This central metabolite is converted to *N*-acetylmannosamine (ManNAc) in a reaction that is subject to feedback inhibition by cytidine monophosphate (CMP)-sialic acid.[6,7] ManNAc is modified in stepwise fashion to produce *N*-acetylmannosamine-6-phosphate, *N*-acetylneuraminic acid-9-phosphate, and *N*-acetylneuraminic acid (sialic acid) in reactions apparently not subject to feedback inhibition.[6,8] Sialic acid is then incorporated into glycoconjugates by a *trans*-Golgi process utilizing CMP as a carrier.

The degradation of sialoglycoconjugates occurs within lysosomes by sequential hydrolysis of terminal glycosidic linkages, usually initiated by the removal of one or more sialic acid residues by an acid sialidase. A genetic deficiency of this enzyme leads to accumulation of undegraded sialoglycoconjugates and to an increase of bound sialic acid in sialidosis and galactosialidosis (see Chap. 140). The free sialic acid produced by the action of sialidase can be reutilized or degraded by *N*-acetylneuraminate lyase,[9] a cytoplasmic enzyme apparently not present within lysosomes.[10,11] This suggests that sialic acid must be removed from lysosomes for further metabolism. Prior to the discovery of free sialic acid storage disorders such as Salla disease and ISSD, the requirement for such a transport process was unrecognized.

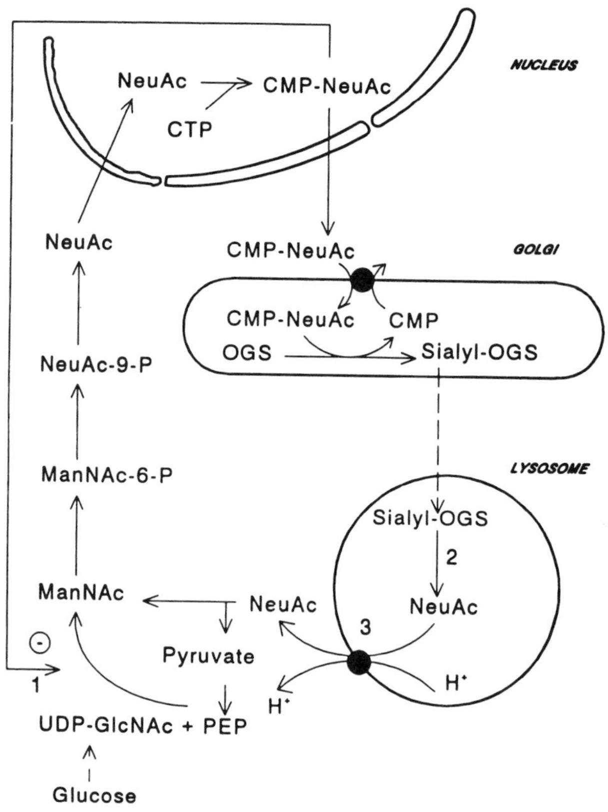

Fig. 200-2 Metabolism of sialic acid. CMP = cytidine-monophosphate; CTP = cytidine-triphosphate; UDP-GlcNAc = Uridine-diphosphate-*N*-acetylglucosamine; ManNac = *N*-acetylmannosamine; PEP = phosphoenolpyruvate; OGS = oligosaccharide. 1, 2, and 3 point to sites of genetic errors of sialic acid metabolism: 1. UDP-GlcNac-2-epimerase; 2. lysosomal sialidase; 3. lysosomal sialic acid carrier. (*Reprinted from Mancini GMS.*[16] *Used with permission of Erasmus University, Rotterdam, The Netherlands.*)

SALLA DISEASE AND ISSD

Historical Aspects

Lysosomal free sialic acid storage disorders have a relatively short history. In 1979, three mentally retarded brothers and their female cousin from northeastern Finland were found to suffer from a hitherto unknown lysosomal storage disorder, which was named Salla disease after the birthplace of the patients.[12] The clinical presentation included early onset of developmental delay, ataxia, and minor dysmorphic features without signs of visceral or ocular involvement. Laboratory studies revealed slightly increased urinary sialic acid excretion, enlarged lysosomal vacuoles in lymphocytes, and skin biopsy fibroblasts, but normal activities of several lysosomal enzymes. Subsequent studies on the urine of the original four patients and nine other patients with similar clinical presentations revealed a ten- to fifteenfold increase in free sialic acid, but no other abnormal oligosaccharides.[13] Studies on cultured fibroblasts indicated that the material stored in the lysosomes was also free sialic acid. A large number of patients, mainly from northeastern Finland, were subsequently detected. Detailed clinical studies enabled the course of the disease to be delineated, from hypotonia in newborns to severe disability in adults with nearly normal life spans.

In 1982, another phenotype was described in severely ill infants with similar, although more pronounced, abnormalities in sialic acid metabolism.[14,15] These infants were characterized by failure to thrive, visceral enlargement, edema, and early death. The disease, which was called infantile free sialic acid storage disease, or ISSD, is less frequent than Salla disease and has no ethnic predilection. More than 15 patients with ISSD have been reported in the literature,[16,17] in contrast to 95 Salla disease patients in Finland, 27 in Sweden, and a few cases elsewhere. A series of studies since 1986 demonstrate that both diseases are caused by a genetic defect of lysosomal membrane transport of free sialic acid.

Sialic Acid Metabolism in Salla Disease and ISSD

The early recognition that free sialic acid is the storage compound in Salla disease patients prompted metabolic studies of the turnover of this molecule. Using cultured fibroblasts and liver from normal and affected individuals, the major enzymes involved in sialic acid metabolism were shown to be normal. These studies included assays of *N*-acetylneuraminate lyase, sialidase, CMP-*N*-acylneuraminate phosphodiesterase, and acylneuraminate cytidylyltransferase.[10,18] In fibroblasts, the activity of sialidase was reported to be normal by most investigators, although two authors reported three- to fivefold increases.[19,20] Sialidase was also reported as increased in the lymphocytes of one patient with Salla disease.[21] All other lysosomal enzymes studied have been normal in ISSD and Salla disease.

The Basic Defect: Impaired Lysosomal Transport of Free Sialic Acid

Several studies in which cultured fibroblasts were loaded with sialic acid demonstrated retention of sialic acid in mutant cells, providing indirect evidence that defective function of the transport system is the primary cause of sialic acid storage disorders. In these experiments, sialic acid precursors,[18] low density lipoprotein,[22] the methylester of sialic acid,[23] fetuin,[24] or *N*-acetylneuraminic acid itself[25,26] were used to load the lysosomes with sialic acid. In each case, retention of free sialic acid in the lysosomal fraction could be shown in the cell strains from sialic acid storage disease patients, suggesting a block in the efflux of free sialic acid through the lysosomal membrane. The rate of sialic acid egress was characterized in more detailed studies with isolated lysosomal fractions from fibroblasts preloaded with ManNAc to yield equal sialic acid concentrations in the lysosomes of normal and mutant cell strains.[27,28] The initial velocity of egress from normal lysosomes increased linearly with loading. The Q_{10} for sialic acid transport was 2.4, suggesting a carrier-mediated mode of transport. Patient cell strains displayed a negligible egress velocity regardless of the initial sialic acid loading. These findings, obtained both with Salla disease[27] and ISSD cell strains,[28] reflect a defective lysosomal membrane transport function in the mutant cells.

Experiments using radiolabeled sialic acid uptake studies in resealed lysosomal membrane vesicles provide direct evidence that a specific carrier facilitates free sialic acid efflux from lysosomes.[29] These studies unequivocally prove that a genetic defect of the sialic acid transport system, presumably a protein, is the primary cause of sialic acid storage disorders. Resealed vesicles from purified rat liver lysosomes and impermeable buffers were employed to produce a pH difference across the lysosomal membrane, thereby mimicking in vivo lysosomal conditions. Cotransport of sialic acid with protons produced by an ATP-dependent proton pump provided the physiological mechanism for sialic acid transport. The K_m for sialic acid transport under the experimental conditions was approximately 0.2 mM. The sialic acid transport system exhibited the properties of both *trans*-stimulation and *cis*-inhibition, demonstrating that it was carrier-mediated. Interestingly, glucuronic acid (GluAc) and some other acidic monosaccharides acted as competitive substrates for the carrier (Table 200-1). Recent studies by the same group further elucidate the characteristics of the transport system and of the putative transport protein itself.[30] Using reconstituted proteoliposomes and the radiolabeled glucuronic acid transport assay,[31] a small amount of a 57-kDa protein was isolated from rat liver homogenates by a combination of chromatographic techniques. Although the final preparation was 432-fold enriched in transport activity, it represented only a 0.1 percent yield and did not allow amino acid sequencing.

Competitive transport assays using the less-purified preparation revealed that not only acidic monosaccharides, that is, sialic acid, glucuronic acid, and iduronic acid, but also several monocarboxylates, that is, lactate, pyruvate, and valproate, employ the same transport system. The lysosomal monosaccharide transporter appears to share many functional properties with the known monocarboxylate transporters of the plasma membrane, that is, MCT1, MCT2, MCT3, and MEV.[32] The carrier for acidic monosaccharides has also been demonstrated in resealed lysosomal vesicles from cultured human fibroblasts and lymphoblasts.[33] The transport could be inhibited to the same extent by the addition of either nonradioactive GluAc or sialic acid. Lysosomal vesicle preparations from cell strains of patients with sialic acid storage disorders were almost completely devoid of the transport activity, both with sialic acid and with glucuronic acid. No differences were observed between the transport activities of Salla disease and ISSD cell strains. Further evidence that deficient carrier-mediated transport of sialic acid is the primary genetic defect in these diseases came from studies of obligate heterozygotes. Transport activity in lysosomal preparations from lymphoblast cell strains of Salla disease parents demonstrated intermediate transport rates for glucuronic acid (Fig. 200-3).

Table 200-1 Substrate Specificity of the Sialic Acid Carrier.

Inhibitor	% of Uninhibited Rate
Sialic acid analogs	
No addition	100
NeuAc	10
NeuGc	12
NeuAc1Me	49
4MU-NeuAc	58
NeuAc2en	50
Other monosaccharides, acidic amino acids	
Glucuronate	10
Gluconate	14
Galacturonate	34
Galactonate	36
Pyruvate	50
Glucose	80
N-Acetylglucosamine	100
N-Acetylmannosamine	100
Gulonolactone	88
Mannuronolactone	86
Aspartate	89
Glutamate	86

Cis-inhibition of NeuAc uptake into lysosomal membrane vesicles by sialic acid analogs, other monosaccharides, and acidic amino acids. Uptake 0.15 mM [^{14}C]NeuAc into lysosome membrane vesicles was studied in the presence of the inhibitors (7 mM) under conditions given in reference 29. Uptake in the presence of inhibitor is expressed as a percentage of the uninhibited rate for duplicate determinations.

SOURCE: From Mancini et al.[29] Used with permission of the American Society for Biochemistry and Molecular Biology.

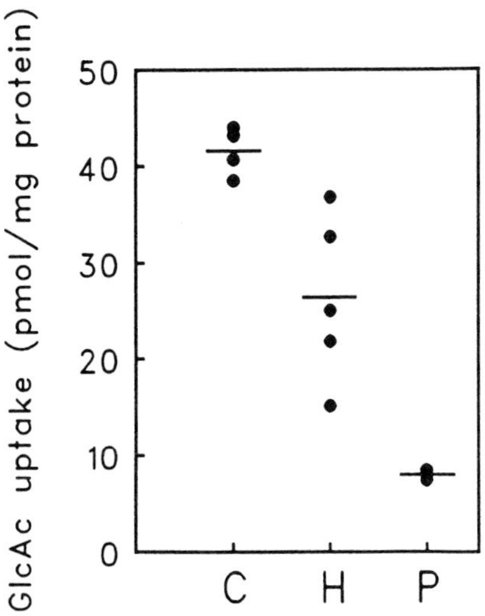

Fig. 200-3 Intermediate glucuronic acid transport of obligate carriers of Salla disease. Lysosomal membrane vesicles from controls (C), from patients with Salla disease (P), and from unrelated parents of Salla disease patients (H) were assayed for transport capacity of 0.055 mM [^{3}H] GlcAc (3 μCi) under conditions given in reference 33. (*From the* Journal of Clinical Investigation, *1991, vol. 87, pp. 1329–35. Used with permission of the American Society for Clinical Investigation.*)

Table 200-2 Urinary Free Sialic Acid in Salla Disease, ISSD, and Sialuria Patients

	Free sialic acid (nM/mg creatinine)			
Disease	N	Mean ± SD	Range	Reference
Salla	22		700–2100	77
	39	713 ± 406	280–1993	49
ISSD	10	6002	1071–14230	15, 20, 25, 56, 60, 78
Sialuria	4		19000–117000	66, 69, 69a
Controls				
Adults	24		7–28	13
	12	58 ± 19	25–88	49
Children	24		100–650	50
	12	131 ± 49	71–220	49

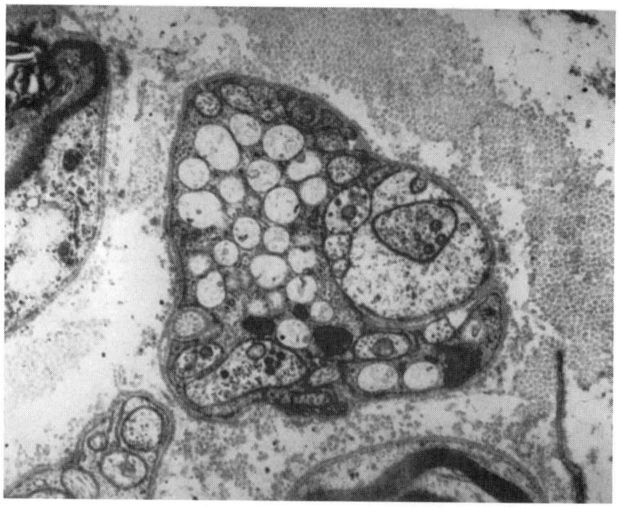

Fig. 200-4 **Electron photomicrograph of unmyelinated dermal nerve Schwann cell from a skin biopsy of a patient with Salla disease. Enlarged single membrane-bound vesicles are filled with amorphous fibrillogranular material. × 11,220 (*From* Archives of Neurology, *1979, vol. 36, pp. 88–94. Used with permission of the American Medical Association.*)**

The significance of defective lysosomal transport of glucuronic acid to the pathogenesis of sialic acid storage diseases remains unknown. Lysosomal accumulation of GluAC, as well as reduced egress from isolated lysosomal fractions of both Salla disease and ISSD cells, has been reported.[34] The amount of glucuronic acid accumulated in the mutant cells averaged only 5 percent of the corresponding amount of free sialic acid. Whether glucuronic acid also accumulates in tissues of patients and is excreted in excess in urine has not been investigated.

Storage of Sialic Acid

A constant finding in both Salla disease and ISSD is the increased urinary excretion (Table 200-2) and cellular concentration of free sialic acid (Table 200-3). Exhaustive characterization of both the urinary excretion product and the storage material in cells almost exclusively identifies *N*-acetylneuraminic acid.[10,13,14,18,19,35] Studies in liver, brain, kidney, placental biopsy, leukocytes, and cultured fibroblasts all give identical results.

In Salla disease, the urinary excretion of free sialic acid is 5 to 20 times normal, and the cellular concentration is 10 to 30 times normal when compared with age-matched controls; in ISSD, there is a twenty- to two-hundredfold increase both in urine and cells (Tables 200-2 and 200-3). In contrast, bound sialic acid levels in the urine and cells of patients have been in the range of controls, or only marginally elevated.

Lysosomal accumulation of free sialic acid has been documented both morphologically and biochemically. Intralysosomal localization of sialic acid was first indicated by immunohistochemical methods using the sialic acid-specific lectin *Limulus polyphemus* agglutinin in cultured fibroblasts from Salla disease patients.[36] Several studies employing cell fractionation of fibroblasts from Salla disease and ISSD patients have demonstrated that the free sialic acid stored in the cells cosediments with the lysosome-enriched fraction.[37]

In EM studies, typical single membrane-bound vacuoles containing amorphous fibrillogranular material were detected in several organs and in various cell types,[12,15,20,21,38,39] including fibrocytes, histiocytes, perithelial cells of capillaries, exocrine and myoepithelial cells of sweat glands, and Schwann cells of peripheral nerves (Fig. 200-4). Lymphocytes and bone marrow cells, as well as hepatocytes and Kupffer cells in hepatic biopsies, have displayed similar storage lysosomes. In two cases of fetuses affected by ISSD, EM studies of chorionic villus biopsies have shown enlarged lysosomal vacuoles supporting the biochemical diagnosis.[40,41] Enlarged lysosomes were not present in an 11-week chorionic villus sample obtained for prenatal diagnosis in a family with Salla disease.[41]

Table 200-3 Free Sialic Acid in Cultured Fibroblasts of Patients with Salla Disease, ISSD, and Sialuria

	Free sialic acid (nM/mg protein)			
Disease	N	Mean ± SD	Range	Reference
Salla	11		6–33	37, 77
	22	15.8 ± 10.9	4–46	49
ISSD	12	75	10–269	20, 37, 56, 60, 78, 79
Sialuria	3	143	75–273	68
Control	10	1.1 ± 1.0		28
	10	2.8 ± 1.8	0.3–6.3	49

Although intralysosomal accumulation of free sialic acid in several organs of patients has been clearly documented, its role in the pathogenesis of the diseases is still largely unknown. Future studies must explain the connection between the severe dysfunction of the brain and free sialic acid storage in the lysosomes.

Genetics and Epidemiology

The mode of inheritance in Salla disease and ISSD is autosomal recessive. Genealogical studies of Salla disease in Finnish families,[42] the high rate of consanguineous families with ISSD, the demonstration of half-normal sialic acid transport activity in the lysosomal membrane preparations of obligate heterozygotes for Salla disease,[33] and finally the recent molecular studies support this.

The gene coding for the transport protein has recently been cloned and the disease-causing mutations have been identified.[43] Earlier, the disease locus was assigned by genetic linkage in Finnish families to chromosome 6q14-15.[44] Allelic association and haplotype analysis with closely linked markers further localized the disease gene to a region of approximately 200 kb and gave strong evidence for presence of a founder mutation in the Finnish population.[45] This is consistent with the existence of founder mutations in several other autosomal recessive diseases enriched in the Finnish population.[46] The common Finnish haplotype found in 94% disease chromosomes was also present in homozygous state in 77% of the Swedish patients with Salla disease, as expected from the known admixture of the two populations. Linkage studies involving ISSD and intermediate phenotype patients having other ethnic backgrounds gave evidence for the same locus on chromosome 6q, suggesting that different phenotypic manifestations of free sialic acid storage are allelic disorders.[47]

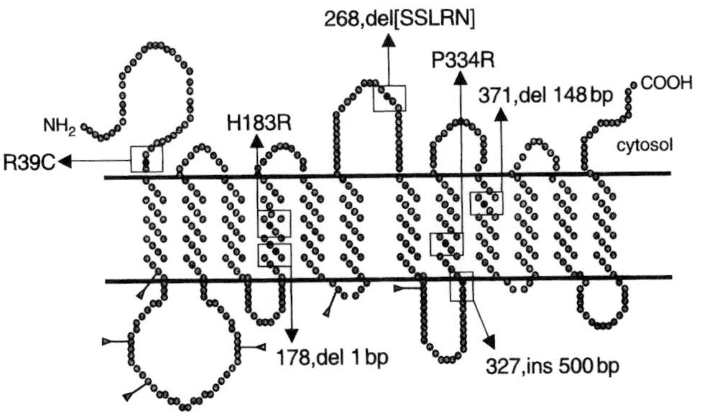

Fig. 200-5 Putative two-dimensional model of the gene product (sialin) encoded by the AST gene depicting mutations found in Salla disease and ISSD patients. Triangles indicate the six potential *N*-glycosylation sites. R39C is the prevalent founder mutation of Finnish Salla disease patients. The other mutations are from ISSD patients. (*From* Nature Genetics, *1999, vol 23, pp 462–465.*)

Sialic acid transporter gene. The chromosomal area harboring the Salla disease gene was further characterized by constructing a physical contig map surrounding the region, thus facilitating the gene identification.[48] Using positional cloning strategy and structural homology comparison with known transporter genes, Verheijen and coworkers were recently able to identify a cDNA clone of 2.5 kb which contained an open reading frame of 1485 base pairs.[43] The gene was designated the AST gene (for Anion and Sugar Transporter).

The gene is expressed most abundantly in heart, kidney, skeletal muscle, liver, placenta, and brain. The gene product, designated as sialin, is predicted to be 495 amino acids long with twelve transmembrane domains in analogy to many other transporter proteins (Fig. 200-5). Both phenotypes of sialic acid storage were found to harbor mutations in the AST gene. Ninety-five percent of the Finnish Salla disease patients had an R39C missense mutation in both alleles, the rest of them being compound heterozygotes. Parents of Salla disease patients were heterozygotes for the R39C mutation. The ISSD patients so far studied carried a variety of mutations including deletions, insertions, and missense mutations. Altogether 15 mutations of the AST gene have so far been identified.

Salla disease displays a strong clustering in the Finnish population, whereas no ethnic predilection exists in the rarer ISSD phenotype. At present, 95 Salla disease patients from 58 Finnish families are known. Most of the families originate from an area in northeastern Finland, but occasionally families come from other areas of the country. An analysis of the birthplace of the grandparents in 45 families with one or more Salla disease patients revealed that 78 of 172 grandparents (45 percent) originated from a region approximately 100 km in diameter in the northeastern part of the country with a present population of approximately 37,000. Several of these families can be traced back to common ancestors.

Twenty-seven patients with the Finnish type of disease are known in Sweden.[49] Most of these families are not recent emigrants from Finland; instead, they reflect the admixture of the populations during earlier centuries. It was recently noted that paucity of characteristic clinical abnormalities and lack of appropriate laboratory confirmation may have led to under-reporting of Salla disease.[50] More than 11 isolated cases in 8 families with the Salla disease phenotype have been described from other countries with a variety of ethnic backgrounds.[16] Some of these patients had intermediate phenotypes with clinical findings typical of both Salla disease and ISSD. Since the first description of ISSD in 1982, more than 15 patients have been reported,[16] largely from Caucasian families with a wide geographic distribution.

Clinical Findings

Salla Disease. Detailed clinical observations of Salla disease patients have been described for 34 adult[42] and 6 pediatric cases.[51] Recent clinical and neuroradiologic evaluations from Finland include 41 patients, 19 under age 20 and 22 over age 20 years.[49] Additional data, less systematically collected, are available from the rest of the 95 Finnish Salla disease patients. These observations allowed a delineation of the clinical course of the disease (Table 200-4) from the normal-appearing newborn to the severely mentally and physically disabled adult.

The pregnancy and newborn period are uneventful for Salla disease patients. The first clinical signs of the disease are muscular hypotonia and ataxia, which usually appear at 6 to 9 months of age. Ocular horizontal nystagmus is frequently seen even earlier, and is replaced later by a divergent squint in about half of the cases. One patient exhibited horizontal nystagmus as early as 3 weeks of age.[42] The ataxia can be truncal as well as in the extremities. The general health of the infants with Salla disease has been unremarkable, without any increased susceptibility to infections or gastrointestinal disturbances. After the age of 1 year, several patients had brisk tendon reflexes and spasticity in the lower limbs. Motor development is always delayed and approximately one-third of the patients never learn to walk. The mean age at walking among the 41 patients was 4 years (range: 1.2 to 9 years). The ataxia is commonly accompanied by athetosis. Speech development is regularly delayed and impaired, with the age at first words varying from 0.8 to 6.0 years.[49] The level of speech development reaches a maximum of that for a 4-year-old child. The majority of patients learned single words or short sentences during the first years of life, but gradual deterioration takes place, and no patient over age 44 could speak even single words. In addition, dysarthria and dyspraxia characterize the speech of all patients; the ability to produce words is affected more than comprehension.

The mental development of Salla disease patients is severely delayed from a young age. By adulthood, patients are severely mentally retarded, with IQs in the range of 20 to 40. The inexorable progression of symptoms that characterizes many

Table 200-4 Clinical Findings and Course of the Disease in Patients with Salla Disease

Neonatal period	
Normal	6/6
Infancy	
Hypotonia	5/6
Ocular nystagmus	4/6
Ataxia	6/6
Sitting at 8 months	1/6
Walking at 2 years	1/6
Words at 15 months	2/6
Childhood	
Developmental delay	34/34
Impaired speech	34/34
Unable to walk	8/34
Growth retardation ($<$ -2SD)	18/34
Adult	
Severe mental retardation	
IQ 20–40	7/34
$<$20	27/34
Ataxia	34/34
Athetosis	22/34
Abnormal tendon reflexes	29/34
Exotrophia	17/34
Convulsions	9/34
Age of death	
(12 cases)	36 years (range 4–70 years)

SOURCE: Adapted from references 42 and 51.

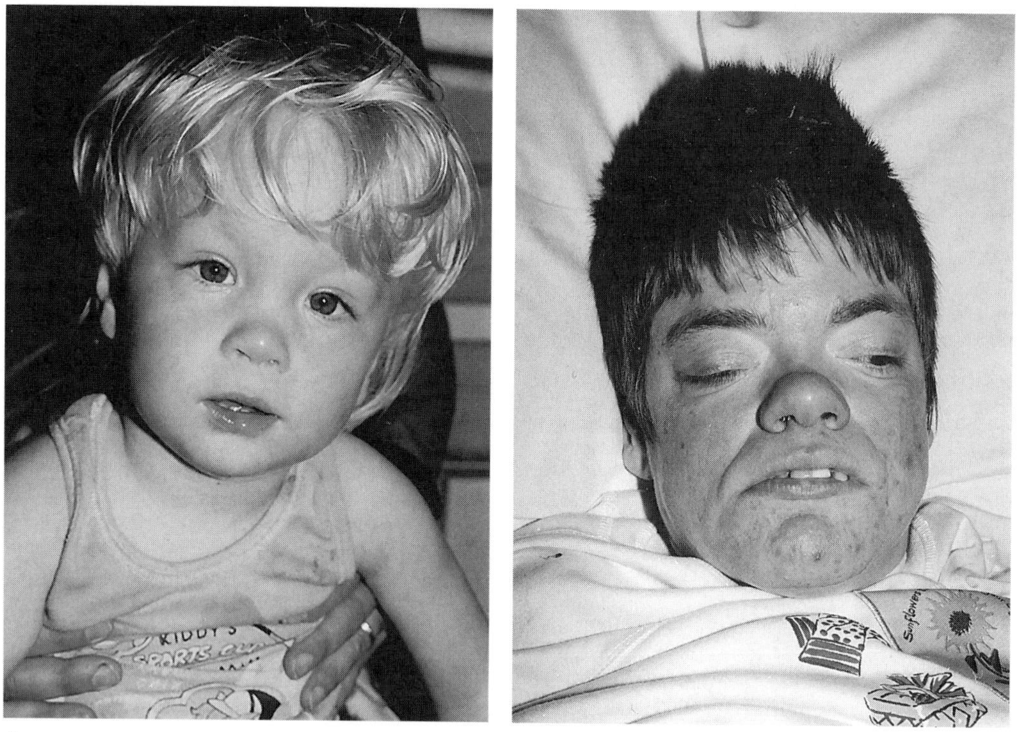

A B

Fig. 200-6 Patients with Salla disease. ***A,*** **An 18-month-old boy with muscular hypotonia, ataxia, and retarded development, but normal facial features.** ***B,*** **A 28-year-old severely affected female patient.**

lysosomal disorders is not a very prominent feature of Salla disease, except in the late stages of the disease. In fact, the plateau in developmental handicap may obscure the true nature of this progressive disease and delay diagnostic evaluation.

Somatic growth is often retarded in Salla disease patients. Eighteen of 34 cases had a height more than 2 standard deviations below the expected height based on parental height and population averages.[42] Two sibs, 21 and 17 years of age, exhibited extreme growth retardation, with heights 8.4 and 5.2 standard deviations below expected. These patients also showed virtually undeveloped secondary sexual features, although most patients have normal pubertal development.

Besides growth retardation and neurologic abnormalities, somatic findings are limited. Facial features (Fig. 200-6) may be coarse in late stages of the disease but to a much lesser extent than in aspartylglucosaminuria and other lysosomal storage disorders. Skeletal dysplasias and other radiologic abnormalities have not been encountered, with the exception of a thickened calvarium present in many patients. Liver and spleen enlargement do not occur despite an abundance of storage lysosomes and excess amounts of free sialic acid in these organs. Corneal clouding and fundal changes, frequent manifestations of lysosomal storage disorders, are absent in Salla disease.

Neurologic examination can reveal ataxia in the extremities and trunk, often accompanied by athetosis and spasticity. Ataxia is more prominent at younger ages, whereas athetosis and spasticity are more frequent in older patients. Hypotonia is often the leading sign during the first year of life. A constant finding in Salla disease patients over 10 years of age has been a low-voltage-type electroencephalographic recording, which is sometimes seen in younger patients. The severity of clinical symptoms and the age of the patient correlate with the decrease in amplitude. Spike waves have been recorded in patients who have seizures. Generalized convulsions are uncommon in Salla disease, but absence-type episodes of short duration do occur. Sixteen of 41 patients were on antiepileptic treatment. Studies of nerve conduction velocity and somatosensory evoked potentials have given evidence suggesting that the peripheral nervous system is also affected by defective myelination. Half of the patients studied had decreased nerve conduction velocities and three severely affected patients had decreased amplitudes as well.

The life span of patients with Salla disease is relatively long. The oldest patient known to us was 72 years old at the time of his death. The mean age at death for 12 patients has been 34.6 years, but in several cases, the cause of death (e.g., accidents or infections) has been only indirectly related to the disease.

Several neuroradiologic studies have been performed. Early CT scans of the head in Salla disease patients revealed cortical and basal atrophy, more pronounced in old than in young patients. Magnetic resonance imaging (MRI) scans have shed new light on the changes in the central nervous system of Salla disease patients.[49,52,53] One girl had a normal brain MRI at 2 months of age, but all other cases have shown abnormalities in myelination. On T2-weighted imaging, a high signal intensity has been observed in white matter areas (Fig. 200-7*A*), with myelin present only in the internal capsule, and in patients with a mild clinical presentation, in the posterior periventricular regions as well. Surprisingly, myelination of the cerebellum has been normal. All patients exhibited an abnormally thin, hypoplastic corpus callosum (Fig. 200-7*B*). There appears to be a good correlation of severity in phenotype with age of the patient and with MRI abnormalities; severely affected and older patients show cortical and cerebellar atrophy and increased periventricular intensity as a sign of a destructive white matter process.

Magnetic resonance spectroscopy (MRS) can yield information about biochemical changes in vivo. MRS was recently performed on 8 Salla disease patients ages 6 to 44 years.[49] The *N*-acetylaspartate signal was consistently increased (34 percent) in the parietal white matter, whereas choline signals were reduced (35 percent) compared with values in healthy individuals. High *N*-acetylaspartate signals are probably related to the increased sialic acid content of the cells, while low choline signals may indicate defective myelination.

The energy metabolism of the brain was recently investigated using positron emission tomography (PET) scanning with a labeled glucose analog (FDG, 2-fluoro-2-deoxy-D-glucose) as a tracer in nine Salla disease patients presenting with different severities of disease.[54] Markedly increased glucose utilization was

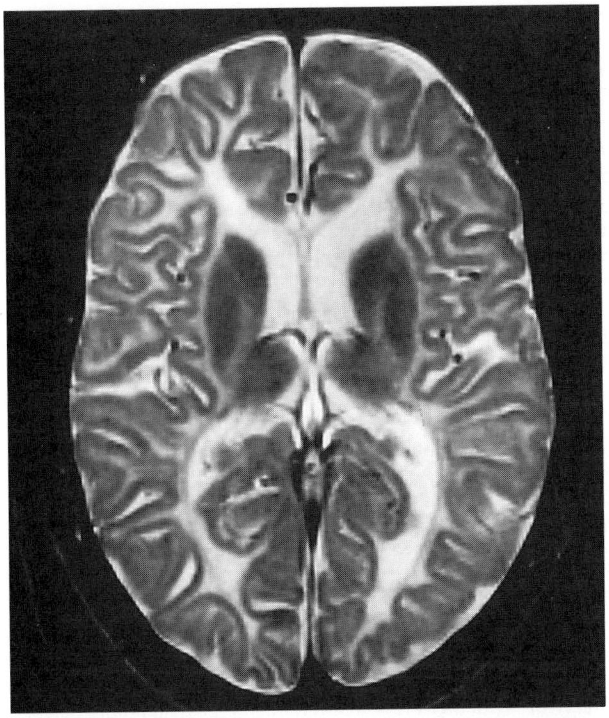

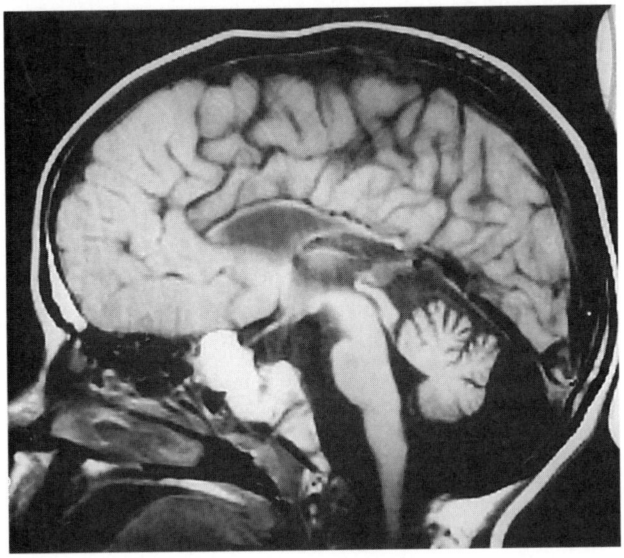

Fig. 200-7 Myelination defects in Salla disease. *A*, Axial T2-weighted MR image of a 9-year-old boy with severe Salla disease showing homogeneous, abnormally high signal intensity in the white matter indicating defective myelination. The basal ganglia are normal (1.5T, 2500/90/20). *B*, Sagittal midline T1-weighted MR image of the same patient illustrating a hypoplastic corpus callosum and atrophic changes, especially in the cerebellum (1.5T, 600/15).

detected in the frontal and sensorimotor cortices and particularly in the basal ganglia of all patients. On the other hand, cerebellar hypometabolism was seen only in patients with severe ataxia and other clinical presentations of the disease. Reduced energy metabolism thus appears to correlate with severity of the disease, but the increased glucose uptake in the frontal cortex and basal ganglia still requires explanation.

The neuropathology of two patients who died of pneumonia at age 41 was reported.[55] The cerebral white matter was severely reduced in both cases, with marked loss of axons and myelin sheaths. Abnormally large amounts of a lipofuscin-like material were seen in the perikaryons of the neurons, particularly in the deep cortical layers. The cerebellum also showed degenerative features and loss of Purkinje cells.

Table 200-5 Clinical Findings and Course of the Disease in Patients with ISSD

In Utero	
Hydrops fetalis	2/15
Neonatal period	
Ascites and edema	4/15
Enlarged liver	8/15
Facial dysmorphism	8/15
Infancy	
Failure to thrive	15/15
Hypotonia	8/15
Enlarged liver/spleen	15/15
Hypopigmentation skin/hair	10/15
Skeletal changes	4/15
Growth retardation	9/9
Age at death (10 cases)	
10 months	(range 1–42 months)

SOURCE: Adapted from references 16 and 17.

ISSD. The clinical presentation of ISSD is more fulminant than that of Salla disease and leads to death during the first years of life. The main features and the course of the disease are outlined in Table 200-5 as compiled from the data of the 15 reported cases of ISSD.[16,17] Four patients manifested the clinical disease at birth, presenting with ascites, hepatosplenomegaly, and coarse facial features. By the age of 3 months, ISSD patients showed failure to thrive, generalized hypotonia, enlarged liver and spleen, mild bone dysplasias, and coarse facial features with hypopigmented skin and fair hair. Psychomotor development was markedly delayed. The age at death in 10 cases reported in the literature has ranged from 1 month to 5 years (mean: 18.1 months). Autopsy reports of two cases describe severe involvement of the central nervous system.[17,56] Widespread neuronal storage was detected with myelin loss, axonal spheroids, and gliosis. Staining with a sialic acid-specific lectin, wheat germ agglutinin, gave direct evidence for sialic acid accumulation in neuronal cells.[17] Cardiac muscle cells, renal tubular cells, fat cells, and macrophages from several organs also contained clear vacuoles with electron-lucent material.

A unique presentation of ISSD was seen in two Austrian siblings, whose sialic acid storage disease was associated with a steroid-resistant congenital nephrosis.[57] On EM of a kidney biopsy, the podocytes, mesangial cells, and endothelial cells displayed numerous membrane-bound vacuoles in addition to typical nephrotic changes. It remains to be seen whether lysosomal sialic acid accumulation can lead to basement membrane dysfunction or whether there exists a specific subtype of ISSD with congenital nephrosis.

Intermediate Phenotypes. A few cases of sialic acid storage disease have been reported with a phenotype intermediate between the classic Salla disease and ISSD.[21,35,58] Considerable variation in the severity of the clinical manifestations has also been observed among the Finnish Salla disease patients. The most severely affected patients are characterized by early-onset muscular hypotonia, leading to spasticity in the lower extremities in more advanced stages, severe growth retardation, absent pubertal development, and profound mental retardation. In fact, a phenotypic continuum can be visualized from the classic fetal-onset ISSD, through an early-onset severely disabled and growth-retarded intermediate phenotype, to the classic Salla disease with ataxia and mental retardation but a long life span. Only biochemical and molecular studies of the transport protein or the corresponding gene will reveal whether phenotypically different types represent specific entities (e.g., allelic mutations) or whether other genes and environmental factors contribute to the phenotypic diversity in free sialic acid storage. Haplotype analysis in the Finnish families supports the hypothesis of allelic heterogeneity, because the severe and intermediate phenotypes had haplotypes different from those of the majority of patients with the classic phenotype.[52]

Diagnosis

The diagnosis of both Salla disease and ISSD is based on clinical findings, increased urinary excretion of free sialic acid, and the presence of storage lysosomes in various types of cells and tissues. Recent identification of the transporter gene (AST) and the disease-causing mutations provide possibilities for accurate molecular diagnosis, particularly for Salla disease in the Finnish population with the prevalent founder mutation R39C. The distinct and early clinical findings and the rapid progression in ISSD easily focus the diagnostic studies toward lysosomal disorders. In Salla disease, however, the paucity of clinical findings and the very slow, or even absent, rate of progression of the disease often hampers the specific diagnosis. Several patients, particularly those with no affected sibs, have reached adulthood before diagnostic studies were undertaken. The association of mental retardation, spasticity, and ataxia was often attributed to brain damage caused by an episode of perinatal asphyxia.

Urinary free sialic acid is most commonly demonstrated with thin-layer chromatography.[59] Patients constantly excrete excess free sialic acid, which was found in the urine of one patient with Salla disease as early as 3 days of age. The enhanced free sialic acid spot on thin-layer chromatography of a patient's sample is usually distinctive enough for diagnosis (see Chap. 141, Fig. 141-12). Normal newborn infants may also show a pronounced sialic acid spot, warranting further studies. More sophisticated techniques, such as HPLC, need to be applied for quantitative assays of urinary free sialic acid, but for diagnostic purposes, such methods are rarely used.[60]

ISSD patients excrete approximately 10 times the free sialic acid that Salla disease patients excrete, and the intermediate types fall between the two. There appears to be a correlation between the severity of the clinical manifestations and the level of sialic acid excretion. A similar correlation has been seen between the severity of clinical disease and the amount of sialic acid stored in tissues.

Lysosomal accumulation of free sialic acid can also be demonstrated by finding vacuolated lymphocytes or enlarged lysosomes on EM of a skin or conjunctival biopsy. Vacuolated lymphocytes may not always be present in Salla disease; young patients, in particular, may not have them.[51] In ISSD, vacuolated lymphocytes are almost always present.

A skin or conjunctival biopsy serves diagnostic purposes very well because of the variety of cell types present in the specimen. Electron-lucent single membrane-bound lysosomes containing fibrillogranular material with some membrane fragments and occasional dark globules have been seen in fibrocytes, Schwann cells, sweat gland cells, myoepithelial cells, and in capillary epithelial cells (Fig. 200-4). The morphology of the enlarged lysosomes in sialic acid storage disorders is similar to that in other glycoproteinoses, such as mannosidosis and aspartylglucosaminuria, and in various types of mucopolysaccharidoses.

Prenatal Diagnosis. Increased intracellular free sialic acid concentrations in fetal specimens allow prenatal detection of both Salla disease and ISSD using quantitative assays. In addition, the presence of vacuoles on EM study of a first-trimester chorionic villus specimen can support the biochemical diagnosis of ISSD, but probably not of Salla disease. Molecular studies have recently become possible in prenatal studies of sialic acid storage disorders. In all families in which the mutation of the index case (or parental mutations) is known, mutation assay on a chorionic villus specimen provides a reliable means of fetal diagnosis. This is particularly important in Salla disease, in which the increase of free sialic acid in chorionic villus specimens is less pronounced than in ISSD. The high prevalence of the R39C founder mutation in the Finnish population undoubtedly will make the mutation assay the method of choice in prenatal diagnosis of Salla disease. Alternatively, in families in which the disease-causing mutation is unknown, genetic linkage analysis using closely linked markers around the disease locus at 6q14-15 can be applied.

The first prenatal diagnosis of sialic acid storage diseases was reported in 1986 in a family with two previous children affected by ISSD.[40] The free sialic acid concentration in cultured amniotic fluid cells, that is, 25.0 nm/mg protein, was approximately 70 times that in control cultures. The cell-free amniotic fluid had a sixfold increase of free sialic acid. The pregnancy was terminated and the diagnosis was confirmed by a nine- to two-hundredfold elevation of free sialic acid in cultured fibroblasts, liver, brain, and kidney of the aborted fetus. Several cell types, including placental trophoblasts, had typical storage lysosomes on EM. At least two other prenatal diagnoses of ISSD have been reported,[41,61] and in one of them, the increase of free sialic acid was also shown in an uncultured first-trimester chorionic villus sample.[41] The chorionic villus cells had numerous vacuoles on EM.

Salla disease is also amenable to intrauterine diagnosis by assay of free sialic acid in a chorionic villus biopsy or by molecular studies. Cultured amniotic fluid cells are less appropriate for prenatal studies because the elevation of free sialic acid content in those cells can be only moderate, leading to false interpretation. A fivefold increase of free sialic acid was seen in cultured amniotic fluid cells in a pregnancy that led to delivery of a child who was later found to be affected by Salla disease.[62] The amniotic fluid supernatant had sialic acid within the range of controls. As in ISSD, sialic acid assay in uncultured first-trimester chorionic villus biopsies has provided reliable prenatal detection of Salla disease.[63] Free sialic acid has been 30 to 100 times normal in pregnancies with affected fetuses as compared to pregnancies that had a normal outcome (Table 200-6). Total sialic acid was only slightly elevated, giving a high ratio of free/total sialic acid.

Carrier Identification. Heterozygotes for Salla disease and ISSD have no clinical manifestations, and their urinary excretion of free sialic acid is within normal limits. The assay of transport activity with resealed lysosomal vesicles from cultured cells can differentiate between the carriers and normals, but the method is not feasible for clinical purposes.[33] The observation of an intermediate free sialic acid level in the granulocyte subpopulation of peripheral blood leukocytes in obligate heterozygotes of Salla disease and ISSD[58] requires further confirmation in a larger series

Table 200-6 Prenatal Diagnosis of Salla Disease by Sialic Acid Assay in First Trimester Chorionic Villus Samples (references 49 and 63)

	(nM/mg protein)					
	Free Sialic Acid		Total Sialic Acid		Ratio	
Outcome	Mean	Range	Mean	Range	Mean	Range
Normal (n = 6)	1.4	1.18–2.08	15.9	14.4–30.0	0.07	0.05–0.14
Salla (n = 3)	63.0	29.7–115.2	84.1	54.4–124.8	0.69	0.55–0.92

of individuals. Mutation assay, if available, provides a reliable carrier test for genetic counseling purposes. A relatively high carrier frequency of the R39C mutation in the Finnish population may justify population-based carrier screening in the future.

Differential Diagnosis. Four clinical entities present with intracellular accumulation and urinary excretion of sialic acid.[1] Sialidosis is due to deficiency of lysosomal neuraminidase leading to storage of undegraded sialyloligosaccharides (see Chap. 140). Sialidosis patients show evidence of lysosomal accumulation, but the storage material, as well as the urinary excretion product, is bound, not free, sialic acid. Definitive diagnosis of sialidosis can be made by assay of neuraminidase activity in leukocytes or cultured fibroblasts. Galactosialidosis is due to a deficiency of a 32-kDa protective protein, and affected patients also excrete sialyloligosaccharides in urine (see Chap. 140). ISSD and Salla disease are allelic mutations of a gene coding for a lysosomal membrane transport protein, and sialuria is a genetic error of impaired feedback inhibition in the synthesis of sialic acid.

The clinical presentations of infantile sialidosis, galactosialidosis, and ISSD may be very similar during the neonatal period, with hepatosplenomegaly, ascites, edema, and dysmorphic features. Cherry-red spots, which are typical ocular findings in sialidosis and galactosialidosis, are not detectable at this early age. Assay of urinary oligosaccharides and enzyme activities in leukocytes or cultured cells usually leads to the correct diagnosis.

The distinction between ISSD and Salla disease is straightforward in typical cases. The severity of the clinical course of the disease and the difference in the amount of sialic acid excreted in the urine and stored in the tissues usually identify the type of disease. Atypical patients, however, may pose diagnostic difficulties. Visceromegaly, dysmorphic features, and hypopigmentation of the skin point to ISSD because these findings have not been described in Salla disease patients.

The final diagnostic consideration is sialuria, characterized by variable degrees of developmental delay, hepatosplenomegaly, coarse facial features, massive urinary excretion, and cytoplasmic storage of free sialic acid (see "Sialuria," below).

Therapy

At present, no specific treatment is available for patients with Salla disease or ISSD. No therapeutic trials with bone marrow transplantation are known. Detailed molecular characterization of the transport mechanism at the lysosomal membrane may pave the way for specific therapeutic modalities.

SIALURIA

Historical Aspects

Sialuria was originally described in 1968 in a mentally retarded French boy with hepatosplenomegaly and coarse facial features.[64,65] He excreted gram quantities of free sialic acid in his urine and his cultured fibroblasts had increased concentrations of free sialic acid in their cytosolic fractions. Three other patients with the same biochemical and clinical presentation were subsequently identified.[66–69] In 1989, the basic defect was demonstrated to be failure of CMP-Neu5Ac to feedback inhibit the initial, rate-limiting enzyme in the sialic acid synthetic pathway.[70] The gene for that enzyme, UDP-GlcNAc 2-epimerase, was cloned in 1998, and three mutations were identified.[71]

Basic Defect

The basic defect in sialuria consists of failure of UDP-GlcNAc 2-epimerase to be feedback inhibited by CMP-Neu5Ac. The epimerase catalyzes the rate-limiting step in sialic acid synthesis (step 1 in Fig. 200-2), that is, the formation of ManNAc from UDP-GlcNAc.[68,70] Lack of feedback inhibition results in unregulated sialic acid synthesis and increased intracellular pools of sialic acid and CMP-Neu5Ac. This latter compound is a central intermediate in sialic acid metabolism and is transported into the Golgi from the cytoplasm to provide sialic acid to glycoconjugates via a sialyltransferase.

The elucidation of the basic defect in sialuria began when Thomas et al.[72] showed that free sialic acid was elevated eighty-sevenfold in fibroblasts cultured from the original sialuria patient. Moreover, when glucosamine was fed to the sialuria fibroblasts, the sialic acid concentrations increased further, in contrast to normal fibroblasts, which did not increase their sialic acid concentrations on glucosamine feeding. This suggested increased activity of the rate-limiting enzyme in sialic acid synthesis, that is, UDP-GlcNAc 2-epimerase. Thomas et al. also showed that sialuria fibroblasts had significantly elevated *cytoplasmic* levels of sialic acid,[73] in contrast to the *lysosomal* storage of sialic acid in ISSD fibroblasts. Finally, Weiss et al.[70] showed that fibroblasts from two patients with sialuria had UDP-GlcNAc 2-epimerase activity that was negligibly inhibited by CMP-Neu5Ac at concentrations that inhibited 85 percent of the epimerase activity of normal fibroblasts. Thus, sialuria represents a rare example of a human disease due to defective allosteric inhibition of an enzyme whose active site is preserved.

In 1991, Seppala et al.[68] verified several key findings in fibroblasts cultured from the three sialuria patients known at the time. First, the excess cellular sialic acid was unbound and cytoplasmic. Second, exposure of the sialuria fibroblasts to D-glucosamine, located proximal to the defective epimerase, increased sialic acid storage in sialuria cells compared with controls. This occurred because feedback inhibition by CMP-Neu5Ac was lacking. Third, exposure to ManNAc had the same effect on sialic acid for sialuria and control cells, because ManNAc is located distal to the epimerase step in the sialic acid synthetic pathway. Fourth, exposure of fibroblast homogenates to 50 μM CMP-Neu5Ac inhibited the sialuria epimerase only 19 to 31 percent compared with 84 to 100 percent for normal epimerase. Finally, cytidine feeding (5 mM, 72 h) reduced the sialic acid content of sialuria cells, probably by increasing the cellular CMP-Neu5Ac concentration and maximizing negative feedback of the mutant epimerase. There was some correlation between the susceptibility of the epimerase to inhibition by CMP-Neu5Ac and the severity of clinical manifestations in patients.[68]

Genetics

All four patients reported with sialuria lack any family history of the disorder,[64–69] which, based solely on molecular studies, is now considered to be inherited in an autosomal dominant fashion.[71] In 1998, the human UDP-GlcNAc 2-epimerase gene was cloned using the known sequence of the homologous rat gene, which codes for a bifunctional enzyme with both the epimerase activity and ManNAc kinase activity.[74,75] The human gene has 722 amino acids, and homology with other epimerase and kinase genes indicates that the amino-terminal 416 amino acids comprise the epimerase portion, while the C-terminal segment encodes the kinase activity. The gene produces a 5.5-kb transcript expressed predominantly in liver and placenta.

Mutation analysis of three sialuria patients revealed heterozygous mutations in the same small region: R263L, R266W, and R266E.[71] This finding essentially defines the allosteric site of the epimerase as the region of codons 263 to 266. Because each patient's other allele had an entirely normal epimerase gene sequence the disorder is considered dominant, as might be expected in a disease involving a mutant enzyme that resists regulation. Moreover, because none of the patients' parents has any symptoms of sialuria, all the abnormal alleles apparently represent new mutations.

Clinical Cases

Clinical characteristics of the four known cases of sialuria are described in detail elsewhere.[1,64–69] Briefly, the original French patient presented at 16 months of age with anemia, rickets, and developmental delay.[64,65] At 21 months he had hypocalcemia and

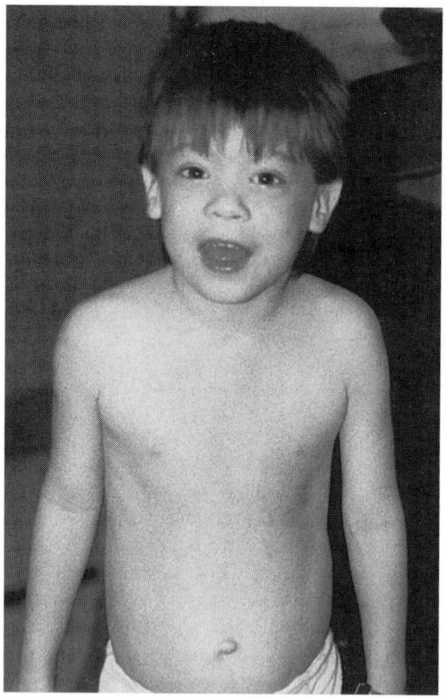

Fig. 200-8 A four-year-old patient with sialuria and mildly dysmorphic facies.

generalized seizures. Over the next few years, he exhibited several episodes of metabolic acidosis, with hepatomegaly, dysmorphic features including mildly coarse facies, a broad nasal bridge, and bilateral epicanthal folds, delayed bone age, and impaired language, fine motor, and cognitive skills. His developmental age was 17 months at 54 months of age. His urinary sialic acid excretion was 13,000 to 15,000 μM/mM creatinine.

An Australian girl with sialuria had hepatosplenomegaly at birth, jaundice until 10 weeks of age, and prominent cortical sulci with normal ventricular size.[66] By 2 years of age, she had moderate developmental delay, slightly coarse facial features, a large tongue, macrocephaly, persistent hepatosplenomegaly, and mild hypotonia. At age 7, the patient attended normal school, although fine motor skills and concentration were impaired.[67] At 69 months of age, she functioned at the level of a 55-month-old, and she continues to have hepatosplenomegaly with mildly elevated liver function tests.

The third sialuria patient had hepatosplenomegaly and dysmorphic facies at 2 months of age and coarse features and a hoarse voice by 10 months of age. Development and growth were normal through 5.5 years of age. Leukocyte free sialic acid was elevated.[1,68]

The fourth patient, born at 30 weeks of gestation, had mild hepatomegaly and rib flaring at 6 months of age. At 4 to 5 years, growth was normal, but dysmorphic facies (Fig. 200-8), generalized hirsutism, and moderate hepatomegaly were noted. Neurologic examination was normal. Developmental assessment at 6 years of age revealed a full scale IQ of 68, with impairment of short-term memory and quantitative reasoning.[69]

To summarize, sialuria patients identified to date have had hepatosplenomegaly, coarse facial features, and various degrees of developmental delay and neurologic impairment. Symptoms of sialuria are nonprogressive in all patients.

Diagnosis

Sialuria can be definitively diagnosed by demonstrating impaired feedback inhibition of UDP-GlcNAc 2-epimerase by CMP-Neu5Ac in cultured fibroblasts. The assay employs UDP-[^{3}H] GlcNAc as substrate, and [^{3}H] ManNAc as the product measured.[68,70] This assay, however, is not commercially performed.

Consequently, sialuria can be practically diagnosed only by analysis of urine and fibroblast sialic acid concentrations. In sialuria, the urine free sialic acid levels are approximately one-hundredfold elevated, that is, 8500 to 18,000 μM/mM creatinine.[67,69] Normal values are <74 μM/mM creatinine;[51] Salla disease levels are 85 to 238 μM/mM creatinine;[51] and ISSD values are up to 1394 μM/mM creatinine.[15,20] Fibroblast studies reveal approximately one-hundredfold elevations in free sialic acid, with approximately 90 percent in the cytosolic fraction (normal is 50 percent).[68,73] This finding makes the diagnosis.

Lysosomal enzymes are normal in sialuria patients, and there is no microscopic evidence of storage in fibroblasts.[64,66,73,76] Urine and plasma amino acids and urine organic acids are normal.[64] There are areas of cytoplasmic clearing on liver biopsy, and EM shows nucleolar degeneration with swollen endoplasmic reticulum. Some mitochondria are enlarged to 20 μM in diameter (normal, 1 μM). These findings[64,66] have not been described in the lysosomal free sialic acid storage disorders.

Therapy

Although the lowering of sialic acid levels in sialuria fibroblasts by cytidine feeding[68] raises the possibility of treatment with this nucleotide, this has not been pursued. Cytidine administration may cause the production of more sialic acid-containing glycoconjugates. Moreover, the symptoms of sialuria are probably largely irreversible. Currently, only symptomatic therapy is available for sialuria patients.

REFERENCES

1. Gahl WA, Krasnewich DM, Williams JC: Sialidoses, in Moser HW (ed): *Handbook of Clinical Neurology*, vol. 22. Amsterdam, Elsevier, 1996, p 353.
2. Schauer R: *Sialic Acids: Chemistry, Metabolism and Function*. New York, Springer-Verlag, 1982.
3. Schauer R: Sialic acids: Chemistry, metabolism and functions of sialic acids. *Adv Carbohydr Chem Biochem* **40**: 131, 1982.
4. Schauer R: Sialic acids and their role as biological masks. *Trends Biochem Sci* **10**:357, 1985.
5. Seppala R, Renlund M, Bernardini I, Tietze F, Gahl WA: Renal handling of free sialic acid in normal humans and patients with Salla disease or renal disease. *Lab Invest* **63**: 197, 1990.
6. Kornfeld S, Kornfeld R, Neufeld EF, O'Brien PJ: The feedback control of sugar nucleotide biosynthesis in liver. *Proc Natl Acad Sci U S A* **52**:371, 1964.
7. Sommar KM, Ellis DB: Uridine diphosphate *N*-acetyl-D-glucosamine 2-epimerase from rat liver. Catalytic and regulatory properties. *Biochim Biophys Acta* **268**:581, 1972.
8. Thomas GH, Scocca J, Miller CS, Reynolds LW: Accumulation of *N*-acetylneuraminic acid (sialic acid) in human fibroblasts cultured in the presence of *N*-acetylmannosamine. *Biochim Biophys Acta* **846**:37, 1985.
9. Kolisis FN, Hervagault JF: Theoretical and experimental studies on the competition of NAN-aldolase and cytidine-5′-monophosphate synthetase for their common substrate *N*-acetylneuraminic acid. *Biochem Int* **13**:493, 1986.
10. Renlund M, Chester AM, Lundblad A, Parkkinen J, Krusius T: Free *N*-acetylneuraminic acid in tissues in Salla disease and the enzymes involved in its metabolism. *Eur J Biochem* **130**:39, 1983.
11. Brunetti P, Jourdian GW, Roseman S: The sialic acids. III. Distribution and properties of animal *N*-acetylneuraminic acid aldolase. *J Biol Chem* **237**:2447, 1962.
12. Aula P, Autio S, Raivio KO, Rapola J, Thoden CJ, Koskela SL, Yamashina I: "Salla disease." A new lysosomal storage disorder. *Arch Neurol* **36**:88, 1979.
13. Renlund M, Chester AM, Lundblad A, Aula P, Raivio KO, Autio S, Koskela SL: Increased urinary excretion of free *N*-acetylneuraminic acid in thirteen patients with Salla disease. *Eur J Biochem* **101**:245, 1979.
14. Hancock LW, Thaler MM, Horwitz AL, Dawson G: Generalized *N*-acetylneuraminic acid storage disease: Quantitation and identification of the monosaccharide accumulating in brain and other tissues. *J Neurochem* **38**:803, 1982.

15. Tondeur M, Libert J, Vamos E, Van Hoff F, Thomas GH, Strecker G: Infantile form of sialic acid storage disorder: Clinical, ultrastructural and biochemical studies in two siblings. *Eur J Pediatr* **139**:142, 1982.
16. Mancini GM: Lysosomal membrane transport. Physiological and pathological events [Abstract]. Thesis Erasmus Universiteit, Rotterdam, The Netherlands, 1991.
17. Pueschel SM, O'Shea PA, Alroy J, Ambler MW, Dangond F, Daniel PF, Kolodny EH: Infantile sialic acid storage disease associated with renal disease. *Pediatr Neurol* **4**:207, 1988.
18. Hancock LW, Horwitz AL, Dawson G: *N*-acetylneuraminic acid sialoglycoconjugate metabolism in fibroblasts from a patient with generalized *N*-acetylneuraminic acid storage disease. *Biochim Biophys Acta* **760**:42, 1983.
19. Thomas GH, Scocca J, Libert J, Vamos E, Miller CS, Reynolds LW: Alterations in cultured fibroblasts of sibs with an infantile form of a free (unbound) sialic acid storage disease. *Pediatr Res* **17**:307, 1983.
20. Stevensson RE, Lubinsky M, Taylor HA, Wenger DA, Schroer RJ, Olmstead PM: Sialic acid storage disease with sialuria: Clinical and biochemical features in the severe infantile type. *Pediatrics* **72**:441, 1983.
21. Ylitalo V, Hagberg B, Rapola J, Mansson JE, Svennerholm L, Sanner G, Tonnby B: Salla disease variants. Sialoylaciduric encephalopathy with increased sialidase activity in two non-Finnish children. *Neuropediatrics* **17**:44, 1986.
22. Renlund M, Kovanen PT, Raivio KO, Aula P, Gahmberg CG, Ehnholm C: Studies on the defect underlying the lysosomal storage of sialic acid in Salla disease. *J Clin Invest* **77**:568, 1988.
23. Mancini GMS, Verheijen FW, Galjaard H: Free *N*-acetylneuraminic acid (NANA) storage disorders: Evidence for defective NANA transport across the lysosomal membrane. *Hum Genet* **73**:214, 1986.
24. Mendla K, Baumkotter J, Rosenau C, Ulrich-Bott B, Cantz M: Defective lysosomal release of glycoprotein-derived sialic acid in fibroblasts from patients with sialic acid storage disease. *Biochem J* **250**:261, 1988.
25. Paschke E, Hofler G, Roscher A: Infantile sialic acid storage disease: The fate of biosynthetically labeled *N*-acetyl(^{3}H) neuraminic acid in cultured human fibroblasts. *Pediatr Res* **20**:773, 1986.
26. Jonas AJ: Studies of lysosomal sialic acid metabolism: Retention of sialic acid by Salla disease lysosomes. *Biochem Biophys Res Commun* **137**:175, 1986.
27. Renlund M, Tietze F, Gahl WA: Defective sialic acid egress from isolated fibroblast lysosomes of patients with Salla disease. *Science* **232**:759, 1986.
28. Tietze F, Seppala R, Renlund M, Hopwood JJ, Harper GS, Thomas GH, Gahl WA: Defective lysosomal egress of free sialic acid (*N*-acetylneuraminic acid) in fibroblasts of patients with infantile free sialic acid storage disease. *J Biol Chem* **264(26)**:15316, 1989.
29. Mancini GMS, De Jong HR, Galjaard H, Verheijen FW: Characterization of a proton-driven carrier for sialic acid in the lysosomal membrane. Evidence for a group-specific transport system for acidic monosaccharides. *J Biol Chem* **264**:15247, 1989.
30. Havelaar AC, Mancini GMS, Beerens CEMT, Souren RMA, Verheijen FW: Purification of the lysosomal sialic acid transporter. Functional characteristics of a monocarboxylate transporter. *J Biol Chem*, **273**:34568, 1998.
31. Mancini GMC, Beerens CEMT, Galjaard H, Verheijen FW: Functional reconstitution of the lysosomal sialic acid carrier into proteoliposomes. *Proc Natl Acad Sci U S A* **89**:6609, 1992.
32. Price NT, Jackson VN, Halestrap AP: Cloning and sequencing of four new mammalian monocarboxylate transporter (MCT) homologues confirms the existence of a transporter family with an ancient past. *Biochem J* **329**:321, 1998.
33. Mancini GMS, Beerens CEMT, Aula PP, Verheijen FW: Sialic acid storage diseases. A multiple lysosomal transport defect for acidic monosaccharides. *J Clin Invest* **87**:1329, 1991.
34. Blom HJ, Andersson HC, Seppala R, Tietze F, Gahl WA: Defective glucuronic acid transport from lysosomes of infantile free sialic acid storage disease fibroblasts. *Biochem J* **268**:621, 1990.
35. Baumkötter J, Cantz M, Mendla K, Baumann W, Frieboli H, Gehler J, Spranger J: *N*-acetylneuraminic acid storage disease. *Hum Genet* **71**:155, 1985.
36. Virtanen I, Ekblom P, Laurila P, Nordling S, Raivio KO, Aula P: Characterization of storage material in cultured fibroblasts by specific lectin binding in lysosomal storage disease. *Pediatr Res* **14**:1199, 1980.
37. Gahl WA, Renlund M, Thoene JG: Lysosomal transport disorders: Cystinosis and sialic acid storage disorders, in Scriver CR, Beaudet AL, Sly WS, Valle D (eds): *The Metabolic Basis of Inherited Disease*, 6th ed. New York, McGraw-Hill, 1989, p 2619.
38. Echenne B, Vidal M, Maire I, Michalski JC, Baldet P, Astruc J: Salla disease in one non-Finnish patient. *Eur J Pediatr* **145**:320, 1986.
39. Wolburg-Bucholz K, Scholte W, Baumkötter J, Cantz M, Holder H, Harzer K: Familial lysosomal storage disease with generalized vacuolization and sialic aciduria. Sporadic Salla disease. *Neuropediatrics* **16**:67, 1985.
40. Vamos E, Libert J, Elkhazen N, Jauniaux E, Hustin J, Wilkin P: Prenatal diagnosis and confirmation of infantile sialic acid storage disease. *Prenat Diagn* **6**:437, 1986.
41. Lake BD, Young EP, Nicolaides K: Prenatal diagnosis of infantile sialic acid storage disease in a twin pregnancy. *J Inherit Metab Dis* **12**:152, 1989.
42. Renlund M, Aula PP, Raivio KD, Autio S, Sainio K, Rapola J, Koskela SL: Salla Disease: A new lysosomal storage disorder with disturbed sialic acid metabolism. *Neurology* **33**:57, 1983.
43. Verheijen FW, Verbeek E, Aula N, Beerens CEMT, Havelaar AC, Joosse M, Peltonen L, et al.: A new gene, encoding an anion transporter, is mutated in sialic acid storage diseases. *Nat Genet* **23**:462, 1999.
44. Haataja L, Schleutker J, Laine A-P, Renlund M, Savontaus M-L, Dib C, Weissenbach J, et al.: The genetic locus for free sialic acid storage disease maps to the long arm of chromosome 6. *Am J Hum Genet* **54**:1042, 1994.
45. Schleutker J, Leine A-P, Haataja L, Renlund M, Weissenbach J, Aula P, Peltonen L: Linkage disequilibrium utilized to establish a refined genetic position of the Salla disease locus on 6q14-15. *Genomics* **27**:286, 1995.
46. De la Chapelle A: Disease gene mapping in isolated human populations: The example of Finland. *J Med Genet* **30**:857, 1993.
47. Schleutker J, Leppanen P, Mensson J-E, Erikson A, Weissenbach J, Peltonen L, Aula P: Lysosomal free sialic acid storage disorders with different phenotypic presentations, ISSD and Salla disease, represent allelic disorders on 6q14-15. *Am J Hum Genet* **57**:893, 1995.
48. Leppanen P, Isosomppi J, Schleutker J, Aula P, Peltonen L: A physical map of the 6q14-15 region harboring the locus for the lysosomal membrane sialic acid transport defect. *Genomics* **37**:62, 1996.
49. Aula P: Unpublished data.
50. Robinson RO, Fensom AH, Lake BD: Salla disease — Rare or underdiagnosed? *Dev Med Child Neurol* **39**:153, 1997.
51. Renlund M: Clinical and laboratory diagnosis of Salla disease in infancy and childhood. *J Pediatr* **104**:232, 1984.
52. Haataja L, Parkkola R, Sonninen P, Vanhanen S-L, Schleutker J, Aarimaa T, Turpeinen U, et al.: Phenotypic variation and magnetic resonance imaging (MRI) in Salla disease, a free sialic acid storage disorder. *Neuropediatrics* **25**:1, 1994.
53. Autti T, Raininko R, Vanhanen S-L, Santavuori P: Magnetic resonance techniques in neuronal ceroid lipofuscinoses and some other lysosomal diseases affecting the brain. *Curr Opin Neurol* **10**:519, 1997.
54. Suhonen-Polvi H, Varho T, Metsahonkala L, Haataja L, Ruotsalainen U, Haaparanta M, Bergman J, et al.: Free sialic acid accumulation causes increased cerebral glucose utilization in Salla disease: An FDG-positron emission tomography study. *J Nucl Med* **40**:12, 1999.
55. Autio-Harmainen H, Oldfors A, Sourander P, Renlund M, Dammert K, Similä S: Neuropathology of Salla disease. *Acta Neuropathol (Berl)* **75**:481, 1988.
56. Stevenson RE, Lubinsky M, Taylor HA, Wenger DA, Schroer RJ, Olmstead PM: Sialic acid storage disease with sialuria: Clinical and biochemical features in the severe infantile type. *Pediatrics* **72(4)**:441, 1983.
57. Sperl W, Gruber W, Quatacker J, Monnens L, Thoenes W, Fink FM, Paschke E: Nephrosis in two siblings with infantile sialic acid storage disease. *Eur J Pediatr* **149**:477, 1990.
58. Mancini GMS, Hu P, Verheijen FW, Van Diggelen OP, Janse HC, Kleijer WJ, Beemer FA, et al.: Salla disease variant in a Dutch patient. Potential value of polymorphonuclear leukocytes for heterozygote detection. *Eur J Pediatr* **151**:590, 1992.
59. Humbel R, Collart M: Oligosaccharides in the urine of patients with glycoprotein storage diseases. Rapid detection by thin-layer chromatography. *Clin Chem Acta* **60**:143, 1975.
60. Romppanen J, Mononen I: Age-related reference values for urinary excretion of sialic acid and deoxysialic acid: Application to diagnosis of storage disorders of free sialic acid. *Clin Chem* **41**:544, 1995.
61. Clements PR, Taylor JA, Hopwood JJ: Biochemical characterization of patients and prenatal diagnosis of sialic acid storage disease for three families. *J Inherit Metab Dis* **11**:30, 1988.

62. Renlund M, Aula P: Prenatal detection of Salla disease based upon increased free sialic acid in amniocytes. *Am J Med Genet* **28**:377, 1987.
63. Renlund M: Unpublished data.
64. Fontaine G, Biserte G, Montreuil J, Dupont A, Ferriaux JP, Strecker G, Spik G, et al.: La sialurie: Un trouble metabolique original. *Helv Paediatr Acta* **23(Suppl XVII)**:3, 1968.
65. Montreuil J, Bisert G, Strecker G, Spik G, Fontaine G, Farriaux J: Description d'un nouveau type de mediturie: La sialurie. *Clin Chem Acta* **21**:61, 1968.
66. Wilcken B, Don N, Greenaway R, Hammond J, Sosula L: Sialuria: A second case. *J Inherit Metab Dis* **10**:97, 1987.
67. Don NA, Wilcken B: Sialuria: A follow-up report. *J Inherit Metab Dis* **14**:942, 1991.
68. Seppala R, Tietze F, Krasnewich D, Weiss P, Ashwell G, Barsh G, Thomas GH, et al.: Sialic acid metabolism in sialuria fibroblasts. *J Biol Chem* **266**:7456, 1991.
69. Krasnewich DM, Tietze F, Krause W, Pretzlaff R, Wenger DA, Diwadkar V, Gahl WA: Clinical and biochemical studies in an American child with sialuria. *Biochem Med Metab Biol* **49**:90, 1993.
69a. Ferreira H, Seppala R, Pinto R, Huizing M, Martins E, Braga AC, Gomes L, Krasnewich DM, Miranda MC, Gahl WA: Sialuria in a Portuguese girl: Clinical, biochemical and molecular characteristics. *Mol Genet Metab* **67**:131, 1999.
70. Weiss P, Tietze F, Gahl WA, Seppala R, Ashwell G: Identification of the metabolic defect in sialuria. *J Biol Chem* **264**:17635, 1989.
71. Seppala R, Lehto V-P, Gahl WA: Mutations in the human UDP-*N*-acetylglucosamine 2-epimerase gene define the disease sialuria and the allosteric site of the enzyme. *Am J Hum Genet* **64**:1563, 1999.
72. Thomas GH, Scocca J, Miller CS, Reynolds LW: Accumulation of *N*-acetylneuraminic acid (sialic acid) in human fibroblasts cultured in the presence of *N*-acetylmannosamine. *Biochim Biophys Acta* **846**:37, 1985.
73. Thomas GH, Scocca J, Miller CS, Reynolds L: Evidence for non-lysosomal storage of *N*-acetylneuraminic acid (sialic acid) in sialuria fibroblasts. *Clin Genet* **36**:242, 1989.
74. Hinderlich S, Stasche R, Zeitler R, Reutter W: A bifunctional enzyme catalyzes the first two steps in *N*-acetylneuraminic acid biosynthesis of rat liver. Purification and characterization of UDP-*N*-acetylglucosamine 2-epimerase/*N*-acetylmannosamine kinase. *J Biol Chem* **272**:24313, 1997.
75. Stasche R, Hinderlich S, Weise C, Effertz K, Lucka L, Moormann P, Reutter W: A bifunctional enzyme catalyzes the first two steps in *N*-acetylneuraminic acid biosynthesis of rat liver. Molecular cloning and functional expression of UDP-*N*-acetylglucosamine 2-epimerase/*N*-acetylmannnosamine kinase. *J Biol Chem* **272**:24319, 1997.
76. Philippart M, Kamensky E, Cancilla P, Callahan J, Zeilstra K, Nakatani S, Farriaux JP: Generalized *N*-acetylneuraminic acid storage with sialuria. *Pediatr Res* **8**:393/119A, 1974.
77. Tietze F: Lysosomal transport of sugars: Normal and pathological, in Thoene JG (ed): *Pathophysiology of Lysosomal Transport*. Boca Raton, FL, CRC Press, 1992 pp 165–200.
78. Cameron PD, Dubowitz V, Besley GTM, Fensom H: Sialic acid storage disease. *Arch Dis Child* **65**:314, 1990.
79. Cooper A, Sardhavalla JB, Thornley M, Ward KP: Infantile sialic acid storage disease in two siblings. *J Inherit Metab Dis* **2**:259, 1988.

CHAPTER 201

Cystic Fibrosis

Michael J. Welsh ▪ Bonnie W. Ramsey
Frank Accurso ▪ Garry R. Cutting

1. **Cystic fibrosis (CF) is a lethal autosomal recessive disease affecting primarily Caucasian populations. The incidence is one in 2000 to 3000 births in various groups.**
2. **CF affects epithelia in several organs. Most of the current morbidity and mortality results from impairment of the pulmonary defense system leading to chronic infection and neutrophil-dominated inflammation of the small and large airways. Persistent infections, especially with *Pseudomonas aeruginosa* and *Staphylococcus aureus* cause chronic sputum production, airway obstruction, and eventually bronchiectasis and lung destruction. Exocrine pancreatic insufficiency occurs in approximately 85 percent of patients. The resulting deficiency of pancreatic enzyme secretion causes malabsorption of fat, steatorrhea, and poor weight gain. Meconium ileus, present in approximately 10 to 20 percent of patients at birth, is often diagnostic of the illness. Almost all males with CF are infertile due to congenital malformation of the reproductive tract. Other manifestations include focal biliary cirrhosis and excessive salt loss from the sweat glands.**
3. **CF is caused by mutations in the gene [FES1]encoding the cystic fibrosis transmembrane conductance regulator (CFTR). The gene contains 27 exons encompassing approximately 250 kb of DNA on chromosome 7q31.2. More than 800 disease-associated mutations have been discovered in the gene. The most common mutation, deletion of phenylalanine at position 508 (ΔF508), accounts for nearly 70 percent of mutations in European-derived Caucasian populations. Only four other mutations individually account for more than 1 percent of CF alleles worldwide. The vast majority of mutations are uncommon worldwide, although they may occur in higher frequency in selected populations.**
4. **The diagnosis of CF is based on two criteria; presence of at least one characteristic clinical feature and evidence of CFTR dysfunction. Clinical features include: (i) chronic sinopulmonary disease including persistent colonization/infection of the airways; (ii) gastrointestinal and nutritional abnormalities including meconium ileus, pancreatic insufficiency, focal biliary cirrhosis, and failure to thrive; (iii) salt loss syndromes; (iv) obstructive azoospermia; (v) a history of CF in a sibling or a positive newborn screening test result. CFTR dysfunction can be documented by: (i) elevated sweat Cl^- concentration; (ii) identification of disease-causing mutations in each CFTR gene; or (iii) demonstration of abnormal ion transport across the nasal epithelium.**
5. **CFTR is a member of the ATP-binding cassette (ABC) transporter family of membrane proteins. CFTR forms a regulated cell membrane Cl^- channel with five domains. Two membrane spanning domains, each comprising six transmembrane sequences, form a Cl^- channel pore. cAMP-dependent phosphorylation of the regulatory (R) domain governs channel activity, and ATP-binding and hydrolysis by two nucleotide binding domains control channel gating. CFTR may also influence the function of other membrane proteins including outwardly-rectifying Cl^- channels, the epithelial Na^+ channel (ENaC), K^+ channels, and the $Cl^-/HCO^-{}_3$ exchanger. Linkage of CFTR to the cytoskeleton may influence its localization and function.**
6. **Mutations in the gene encoding CFTR disrupt CFTR function by four general mechanisms. Class I mutations, including premature termination signals and splicing abnormalities, severely reduce protein production. Class II mutations cause defective folding and disruption of protein biosynthesis. The common ΔF508 mutation does not escape from the endoplasmic reticulum and travel to the apical membrane because of a Class II defect. Class III mutations generate protein that reaches the plasma membrane but the channels show defective regulation. Class IV mutations generate correctly localized CFTR with defective pore properties. Individual mutations may have more than one effect.**
7. **CF epithelia show defective electrolyte transport across the apical membrane, which contributes to the pathogenesis of the disease in the sweat gland, pancreas, intestine, male genital tract, and hepatobiliary system. In the airways, defective electrolyte transport alters the airway surface liquid. The pathogenesis of CF airway disease is complex, but may include defective antimicrobial activity in airway surface liquid, altered mucociliary clearance, abnormal submucosal gland function, an enhanced inflammatory response, and other abnormalities.**
8. **The nature of mutations in CFTR are correlated with the severity of pancreatic disease and degree of sweat Cl^- abnormality. The relationship between genotype and pulmonary phenotype is less robust, likely due to the influence of genetic modifiers and the environmental factors.**
9. **Treatment of CF requires a comprehensive approach to prevention and treatment of pulmonary disease, nutritional status, gastrointestinal disease, and multiple other manifestations in children and adults. Antibiotics, airway clearance techniques, and anti-inflammatories remain the cornerstone for treating lung disease. Pancreatic enzyme replacement is the foundation for treating the pancreatic insufficiency. Recent advances in understanding the cellular and molecular basis of the disease and the pathophysiology are leading to the development of gene therapy and novel pharmacologic approaches to treatment.**

INTRODUCTION AND HISTORICAL PERSPECTIVE

Cystic fibrosis (CF) is an autosomal recessive disorder caused by mutations in the gene encoding the CFTR Cl^- channel. Cystic fibrosis is the most common life-threatening recessive genetic disease in Caucasians, with a carrier frequency of about 1 in 22 to 28 Caucasians, an incidence of 1 in 2000 to 3000, and approximately 30,000 affected persons in the United States. The disease is characterized by chronic infections of the respiratory tract, pancreatic insufficiency, and elevated concentrations of sweat electrolytes.

The clinical and basic study of CF has yielded impressive advances in the lifespan of people who suffer from the disease and in the understanding of the cell and molecular biology of the disease. However, as one of the earliest diseases in which the gene was identified by positional cloning, a review of the history, the advances, the problems, and the opportunities that physicians and scientists have encountered since discovery of the CFTR gene may presage events that will be repeated and varied as an increasing number of disease-associated genes are discovered. Additional historical perspectives can be obtained in other references.[482,651]

Brief History

One of the early references to CF is an adage from northern European folklore: "Woe to that child which when kissed on the forehead tastes salty. They are bewitched and soon will die." That saying describes the salty sweat that is the basis of an important diagnostic test. It also emphasizes the early mortality. Dr. Dorothea Anderson provided one of the first comprehensive descriptions of the disease in 1938 and coined the term "cystic fibrosis of the pancreas" to emphasize the pancreatic lesions.[19] Soon after, she and others began to appreciate the frequency and severity of lung dysfunction. The genetic nature of CF and its autosomal recessive pattern of inheritance were described in 1946.[20] In 1948, a heat wave in New York City allowed Dr. Paul di Sant' Agnese and his colleagues to discover that patients with CF lose excess salt in their sweat, a critical clinical finding.[177] That discovery led to the development of a test that has remained a cornerstone of the diagnosis: measurement of the Cl^- content of sweat.

An understanding of the pathogenesis and molecular bases of CF showed little advancement during the next 30 years (1950s, 60s, and 70s). However, the clinical manifestations ranging from pancreatic insufficiency to chronic bacterial endobronchial infections became better defined resulting in earlier diagnosis and improved therapies. Through these treatment advances the lifespan of patients increased from less than a decade in 1950 to almost 20 years in the 1970s.

The 1980s witnessed impressive advances in understanding the physiology of the disease. Building on the observation that CF sweat contains increased concentrations of Cl^- and Na^+, Dr. Paul Quinton studied the sweat gland duct. He made a landmark discovery: CF sweat gland ducts are relatively impermeable to Cl^-.[483,485] The reduced Cl^- permeability could account for the inability to absorb Cl^- and hence Na^+, producing the salty sweat that is a diagnostic key. Dr. Richard Boucher and colleagues also provided evidence for defective Cl^- transport in CF airway epithelia.[345] In addition, they showed that CF airway epithelia had an enhanced Na^+ permeability. Dr. Jonathan Widdicombe[661]) and colleagues demonstrated that the defect in CF epithelia was predominantly at the apical membrane. In normal airway epithelia, an increase in cAMP opened apical Cl^- channels that provide a pathway for Cl^- to flow across the epithelium. In CF airway epithelia, an increase in cAMP fails to open apical Cl^- channels. Further insight came when Dr. Kenzo Sato showed a defect in cAMP-stimulated, but not Ca^{2+}-stimulated Cl^- secretion in the sweat gland secretory coil.[532] In addition, Dr. Hinda Kopelman[354]) and colleagues suggested defective salt transport by pancreatic duct epithelia. For the first time, these observations began to provide a unifying hypothesis about the disease: CF causes abnormal epithelial Cl^- transport.

The 1980s also saw a major effort to clone the CF gene. In 1985, the gene was localized to chromosome 7. The positional cloning strategy bore fruit in 1989, when Drs. Lap-Chee Tsui, John Riordan, Francis Collins, and their collaborators reported the discovery of the gene that is mutated in CF.[330,509,513] They named the gene product the Cystic Fibrosis Transmembrane Conductance Regulator (CFTR). Convincingly, they learned that the gene was expressed in epithelia affected by the disease and they found mutations that were present on CF chromosomes, but not normal chromosomes. Since then, more than 800 disease-associated mutations have been identified throughout the gene. The ability to detect mutations has allowed individuals to be screened for mutations and has provided the capability of prenatal diagnosis. By 1990, Drs. Alan Smith and Michael Welsh and colleagues,[505] and Drs. James Wilson and Francis Collins and their collaborators[191] expressed the CFTR cDNA in CF epithelial cells and corrected the CF defect in Cl^- transport.

During the 1990s major insights into the function of CFTR, how mutations disrupt its function, and clues to the pathogenesis and pathophysiology emerged. Based on studies from many different laboratories, we now know that CFTR is a regulated Cl^- channel located in the apical membrane of the epithelia affected by CF. Knowledge that CFTR is an epithelial Cl^- channel regulated by phosphorylation began to tie together the clinical observation that epithelia are the site of disease, the physiologic abnormality in epithelial Cl^- transport, and the molecular genetic defect (see "Structure of the CFTR Protein" and "Cl^- Channel Function of CFTR" below). CFTR appears to have additional functions in the regulation of other membrane proteins (see "CFTR as a Regulator of Other Membrane Proteins"). Studies of mutant CFTR showed that there are at least four general mechanisms by which CF-associated mutations disrupt function which are delineated in "Molecular Mechanisms of CFTR Dysfunction."

Understanding the pathogenesis of disease has proven difficult. Knowledge that CF epithelia have defective electrolyte transport may readily explain abnormalities in the sweat gland, pancreas, vas deferens, and intestine. However, it is more difficult to understand the pathogenesis of lung disease. Nevertheless, there has been important recent progress and several intriguing hypotheses (see "Pathogenesis of Airway Infections").

Despite remarkable progress in the genetic, molecular, cellular, and physiologic aspects of CF, lung disease remains a life-threatening and incurable problem. Improved understanding of basic and clinical aspects of the disease will likely lead to advances in the development of gene therapy and several novel pharmacologic approaches in the near future.

Potential Lessons from CF

The history and study of CF research may provide some lessons of value to students of other diseases. First, the identification of people with a distinct clinical syndrome followed by positional cloning brought us the discovery of the CF gene. That knowledge provided those interested in CF with an invaluable resource in the research lab and in the clinic. Without question, identification of genes associated with other diseases will also reap many benefits. Therefore it is critical that we continue to improve our ability to accurately determine clinical phenotypes and our ability to locate and identify genes. Both are essential.

Second, considerable effort has been expended to understand the function of CFTR and its structure. This work has helped relate the molecular biology of CFTR to the physiology of epithelia. Knowledge of CFTR function has provided insight into pathogenesis. These studies have elucidated mechanisms by which disease-associated mutations disrupt function. Discoveries in all these areas have suggested novel therapies. Finally, this work has shed new light on the structure and function of the ABC transporter family; many of these proteins are associated with disease.

Third, a mutation database and examination of the relationship between genotype and phenotype can have several benefits. Knowledge of genotype-phenotype relationships allows prognostication in some cases. It is also critical for identification of genes and environmental factors that modify the CF phenotype. This information may suggest specific preventions and treatments, including therapies targeted to specific mutations.

Fourth, the intense study of a single gene and disease can have an unexpected impact in other areas of medicine. For example, few would have predicted that mutations in the CFTR gene would be related to male infertility and idiopathic pancreatitis. In addition, the basic and clinical research on CF have indirectly impacted work on other diseases.

Fifth, CF stands as a humbling reminder that much work lies between identification of a gene and use of that knowledge to develop effective treatments. Notwithstanding the tremendous progress that has been made, our knowledge of CFTR structure and function remains somewhat superficial, and our understanding of why patients develop lung diseases is not settled. Certainly some genetic diseases will yield their secrets more quickly than CF. But undoubtedly, some will prove more recalcitrant, especially in discovering the function of the gene product and elucidation of the pathogenesis. This predicament is due in part to the necessity of understanding biology at the organ and organism level. Attempts to obtain such knowledge provide a real challenge, because they demand that investigators return to the patient or to model systems that faithfully reproduce *in vivo* biology. In some cases genetically engineered mice will prove instrumental in achieving this goal. However as witnessed by mice with a disrupted CFTR gene, this will not always be the case.

CLINICAL FEATURES

Cystic fibrosis is a complex disease affecting a number of organ systems including the lung and upper respiratory tract, the gastrointestinal tract, pancreas, liver, sweat glands, and the genitourinary tract. Nutritional abnormalities, secondary to the pancreatic insufficiency seen in most patients with CF, have severe consequences for growth and the skeletal system. Pancreatic injury also results in diabetes mellitus in an increasing number of patients. Rheumatic complications are not uncommon and are likely related to chronic airway infection. Organ dysfunction can appear at widely different ages in individuals with CF. Progression of disease is also remarkably variable. Not all patients manifest each of the clinical features, however most patients have evidence of many CF-related abnormalities.

Lung and Upper Respiratory Tract

Although CF is a multisystem disease, lung involvement is the major cause of morbidity and mortality.[9] In CF, a failure of lung defense leads to the establishment of bacterial endobronchitis, particularly with *Pseudomonas aeruginosa*, accompanied by intense inflammation and airway destruction.[161] Cough and sputum production are the common clinical findings. Many patients also have nasal polyps and sinusitis. Evaluation of respiratory status in CF is useful in determining treatment and prognosis and includes imaging techniques, lung function measurements, and monitoring of airway microbial cultures. CF lung disease can result in a host of complications including atelectasis, severe hemoptysis, and pneumothorax and allergic bronchopulmonary aspergillosis. The clinical course of patients with CF is characterized by a progressive decline in lung function leading ultimately to intractable respiratory failure and death or lung transplant. Median cumulative survival in the United States was 32.3 years in 1997 (Fig. 201-1).[9]

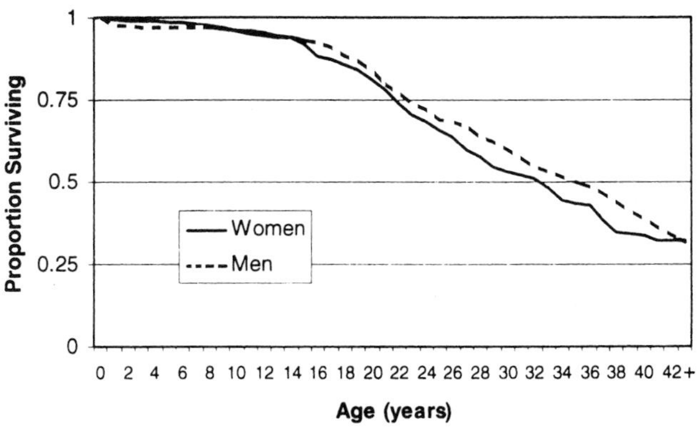

Fig. 201-1 Median survival by sex for CF patients in 1998. Median survival for females is 31.4 years and for males is 34.0 years. Overall median survival is 32.3 years.[9]

Pathology. CF predominantly affects the airways. The hallmarks of airway pathology are mucus plugging, infection, and neutrophil-dominated inflammation.[610] Infection and inflammation are not present in other affected organs such as the pancreas and sweat gland. As the lung disease progresses there is increasing structural injury to airways resulting in bronchiectasis and bronchiolectasis. In end-stage lung disease, there is extensive destruction of airway architecture accompanied by fibrosis of lung parenchyma surrounding the airways. Bronchiectatic cysts and abscesses are prominent. The bronchial circulation becomes hypertrophied and there may be vascular changes associated with pulmonary hypertension. The interstitium and alveoli for the most part are better preserved than the airway.

There is still great interest in the early pathology of the CF lung. In part, this is because it is not clear how mutations in the CFTR lead to infectious endobronchitis and because determining initiating mechanisms of lung disease may provide clues to pathogenesis.[44] There are few pathologic studies of the fetal lung in CF. One study of fetuses, presumed to have CF on the basis of intestinal enzyme elevation and family history, found that tracheal mucus glands were dilated in the CF fetuses and contained less periodic acid Schiff (PAS)-positive material than control fetuses.[451] This suggests that abnormalities in mucus glands occur in utero before infection and inflammation, but this finding has not been confirmed.

Most studies of lung pathology in infants with CF were performed several decades ago when infant patients frequently succumbed to meconium ileus or respiratory disease. An early study of 28 infants with respiratory disease found bacterial infection in 25 but no infection or cellular infiltrate in three infants.[704] Those three infants exhibited extensive mucus plugging. On the basis of the findings in the three infants, the hypothesis was offered that mucus plugging was the initial pathologic event in CF. Viral infection or previous bacterial infection may have contributed to the mucus plugging in these cases; however, viral studies were not performed nor were previous bacterial cultures reported. A series of studies examining the morphology of tracheal glands in infants with CF then followed. Most found no abnormalities in tracheal gland morphology.[120] With improved morphometric techniques, however, a subtle increase in the acinar diameter of tracheal mucus glands was detected, though a number of CF patients had values indistinguishable from controls.[586] Each of the studies of infants reported a few patients with histologically normal lungs in every respect. The weight of the pathologic evidence then is that the lungs are histologically normal at birth in CF except for a small increase in the mean acinar diameter of mucus glands.

By far the majority of infants at postmortem examination, however, had characteristic features of CF including inflammatory infiltrates, epithelial metaplasia, mucopurulent plugging, bronchiectasis, and evidence of some pneumonia. These changes are evident in lungs from older patients with CF. Macroscopically the lungs of older patients with CF exhibit multiple cysts that are for the most part bronchiectatic airways filled with mucopurulent material. Bronchiectatic dilation of the airway in CF encroaches on lung parenchyma significantly. Bronchi make up approximately 13 to 17 percent of the cut surface of the lung in CF compared to less than 5 percent in controls.[568] The upper lobes are more cystic than the lower lobes. Also, the nodularity of the lung apparent macroscopically, on closer inspection corresponds to mucus filled smaller airways. Patchy areas of congestion are often also seen.

Microscopically, there is mucus plugging in the airways with intense neutrophil infiltrates (Fig. 201-2 and Fig. 201-3). Neutrophils are in various stages of degradation. Airway walls show loss of epithelium in spots along with mural inflammatory cell infiltrates. Intramural inflammation often consists of plasma cells and lymphocytes, as opposed to the luminal cell population of neutrophils. Peribronchial and peribronchiolar fibrosis is common. Goblet cell hyperplasia and extension of goblet cells to more peripheral airways occurs. Small airways can be dilated or narrowed. Bronchial vessels are seen next to areas of fibrosis, suggesting an obliterative bronchiolitis. Lung involvement in CF can often be patchy with normal lung adjacent to markedly bronchiectatic areas. Only very rarely is there evidence of emphysema, though hyperinflation of air spaces is commonly encountered. Parenchymal damage occurs, leading to pneumatoceles and interstitial fibrosis in areas close to airways. Peripleural cysts and adhesions are also frequent. Ultrastructural examination of the CF epithelium reveals some disorganization of cilia but no primary ciliary morphologic abnormalities.[102]

Given the importance of infection in CF, the location of bacteria within the airway has received careful scrutiny. It is unusual to find bacteria adherent to the airway epithelium. Bacteria are found immediately next to the airway wall only when the epithelium is denuded or injured.[45] Both *P. aeruginosa* and *Staphylococcus aureus* are located most prominently within the intraluminal mucus.[623] *P. aeruginosa* is commonly seen in microcolonies similar to those encountered in biofilms.[141]

Less typical pathologic findings are associated with some of the infectious complications of CF. Allergic bronchopulmonary aspergillosis is accompanied by bronchocentric granulomatosis and palisading histiocytes. Nontuberculous mycobacteria infection can lead to granuloma formation.

Inflammatory cell products are believed to mediate the extensive fibrosis and tissue injury in the CF airway. In particular, proteolytic activity has been implicated through pathologic studies demonstrating fragmented elastin and elastolysis. A further biochemical description of airway matrix degradation in CF has recently been reported.[195] Monocytes and macrophages appear to be involved in the chondrolysis of bronchi resulting in bronchiectasis, though the pathways of tissue injury are still incompletely understood.[447]

As disease progresses, components of the lung other than the airway become involved. The bronchial circulation is hypertrophied and more tortuous than normal. If chronic hypoxia is untreated, the pulmonary circulation exhibits changes consistent with pulmonary hypertension, including medial hypertrophy and

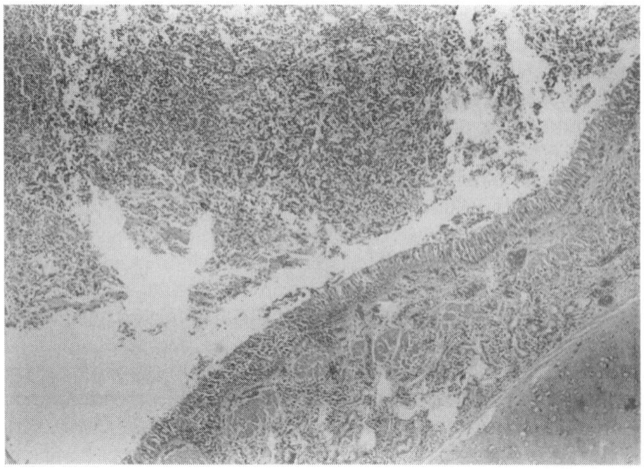

Fig. 201-2 Cartilaginous airway from an eight year old with CF who succumbed to pulmonary involvement. The surface epithelium is relatively well preserved whereas the submucosa is markedly thickened. The lumen contains a striking accumulation of mucus, neutrophils, and bacteria.

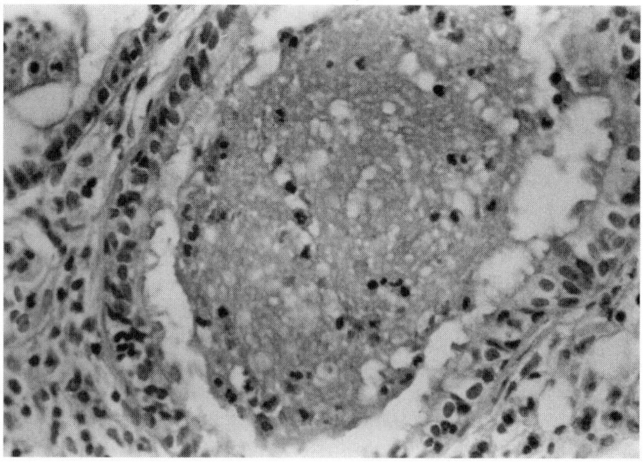

Fig. 201-3 Small airway from the right upper lobe of a four year old child with CF. The lumen is almost totally obstructed by a mucus plug. Inflammatory cells are evident in the plug.

extension of smooth muscle into more peripheral vessels. Interstitial pneumonitis occurs in approximately 10 percent of cases. At postmortem examination regions of pneumonia and pulmonary hemorrhage are frequently seen, but the extensive airways disease is dominant.

The upper respiratory tract in CF is associated with a number of changes that show some similarities with the lungs.[610] Thick, purulent secretions are present in the sinuses. Histologic changes include increased cellular infiltrates in the mucosa particularly with CD4 cells. Bony erosion can also occur. Nasal polyps occur in approximately 15 percent of patients. Polyps are characterized by disordered epithelium with glandular hyperplasia, matrix elements, and inflammatory infiltrates.[282]

Clinical Manifestations. The onset of respiratory symptoms in CF can be variable. Most patients have respiratory symptoms and signs in infancy, but some individuals may not present with respiratory tract involvement until adulthood. Cough is a frequent presenting symptom at any age. Some infants have chronic wheezing that can be resistant to therapy.[324] Chronic wheezing in infancy may predict a more difficult respiratory course in later childhood.[335] In childhood, cough is often first apparent in the morning, presumably because of pooling of secretions over night.

Almost all patients with CF produce sputum at some point. Sputum may be white, yellow, or green in the same patient at different times. In general the more "color," the more respiratory symptoms the patient experiences. Sputum may also be brown in association with allergic bronchopulmonary aspergillosis. Blood tinged sputum, is frequently seen as disease progresses.

In infants and children, increased respiratory rate and inspiratory subcostal retractions are other early signs. Auscultation of the chest frequently reveals wheezes or crackles. However, diminished breath sounds may be the only finding. As the disease progresses, breath sounds become even more faint. Because of hyperinflation secondary to airway obstruction, the chest becomes barrel-shaped with increased anterior-posterior diameter. Patients with advanced disease may have prominent kyphosis.

Several other clinical manifestations of respiratory disease in CF are frequently encountered. A subset of patients with CF experience acute pulmonary exacerbations characterized by increases in cough and sputum production, fall in pulmonary function, and loss of weight. Acute pulmonary exacerbations can occur with viral infection or without identifiable cause. Airways hyperreactivity is also manifest, occurring in up to 90 percent of patients at various times during the course of disease.[602] As disease advances, dyspnea on exertion is prominent, exacerbations are more frequent and quality of life is greatly impaired.

Upper respiratory tract symptoms are common in patients with CF at all ages.[440] Nasal polyps produce airway obstruction leading to mouth breathing. Polyps often recur even after surgery. Chronic sinus obstruction can lead to changes in facial features including broadening of the nasal bridge. Headache is a common presenting sign of sinusitis, although sinus tenderness is unusual. On occasion, sinusitis can be a severely debilitating problem in CF. Chronic sinusitis in children, especially under 5 years of age, is highly suggestive of CF.

Laboratory Evaluation. Laboratory evaluation of lung disease in CF is important in determining the degree of lung impairment, assessing progression of disease, and evaluating response to treatments. Traditionally, the laboratory evaluation has consisted of anatomic assessment of pulmonary involvement through chest radiographs, physiologic assessment through lung function testing, and microbiologic assessment through sputum cultures. These approaches continue to be refined. The application of high resolution computed tomography (HRCT) has increased sensitivity of detection of anatomic abnormalities.[87] Lung function testing has been extended to younger patients.[601] The use of bronchoalveolar lavage to sample airway secretions directly has the potential to aid in microbiologic assessment.[53] Several large data bases that include lung function and microbiology determinations in thousands of individuals with CF have been generated and provide information that is useful in characterizing abnormalities and disease progression.[227,348] Caregivers can use this information to gauge how patients compare to other patients nationwide.

Imaging. Chest x-ray changes are apparent in most patients with CF. In infancy, peribronchial cuffing, increased linear markings, and hyperinflation occur early. Hyperinflation is manifest as flattening of the diaphragm and retro-sternal and retro-cardiac lucency. Atelectasis, particularly of the right upper lobe, also may occur early (Fig. 201-4). With progression of disease there are increased nodular opacities (corresponding to mucus plugs) and increased cystic areas corresponding to bronchiectatic airways (Fig. 201-5 and 201-6). Further progression is accompanied by increases in ill-defined opacities, and subsegmental, segmental, and lobar infiltrates. Interestingly, chest x-rays frequently do not demonstrate change with acute pulmonary exacerbations. Several radiographic scoring systems have been proposed for research, including one to improve sensitivity in detection of early changes.[645]

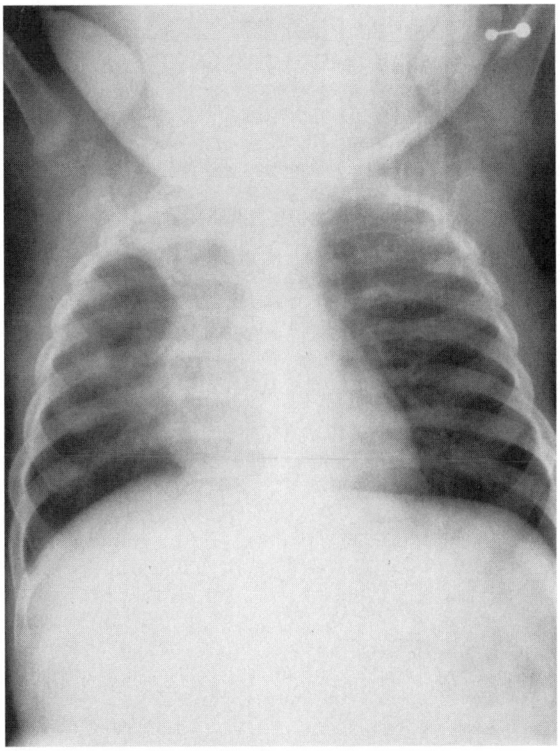

Fig. 201-4 Chest radiograph of an infant with CF and right upper lobe atelectasis.

HRCT allows detection of abnormalities that cannot be determined by x-ray. Bronchiectasis and regional hyperinflation can be seen in patients with "normal" chest x-rays.[87] It is not clear yet whether there is a role for HRCT in routine management of lung disease, however HRCT is often helpful in illustrating the nature of bronchiectasis for families (Fig. 201-7). Ventilation-perfusion scanning can reveal regional impairment in ventilation and perfusion but is not useful in clinical practice.

Lung Function Testing. Lung function testing in CF consistently provides evidence of an obstructive process leading to airflow limitation and elevation of lung volume.[161] Mucus plugging, airway edema, bronchial reactivity, and loss of integrity of airways all contribute to obstruction. Most patients five years and older can cooperate sufficiently to perform spirometry, the most useful approach to measuring lung function in CF. In the growing child it is necessary to normalize data through use of percent predicted values. Early in the disease process forced vital capacity (FVC) and forced expiratory volume in 1 second (FEV1) are preserved. Decreased flows at low lung volumes, for example mid-maximal expiratory flow (MMEF) or forced expiratory flow between 25 percent and 75 percent of vital capacity (FEF25-75), often show the first sign of abnormal lung function (Fig. 201-8). If plethysmography is performed, elevation of residual volume and the ratio of residual volume to total lung capacity are early indicators of obstructive lung disease.

FEV1 has emerged as the most useful measure of lung function in CF because it is reproducible, relatively easily performed, and well studied in a variety of clinical settings. The distribution of FEV1 as a function of age is monitored yearly in the United States by the CF Foundation in approximately 20,000 patients.[227] FEV1 improves following treatment for acute pulmonary exacerbations. In addition, FEV1 is the best predictor of survival. When FEV1 reaches 30 percent predicted, two year survival is less than fifty percent and hence listing for transplant should take place.[336] Improvement in FEV1 has been used as an outcome measure in several large clinical trials of new treatments providing yet more

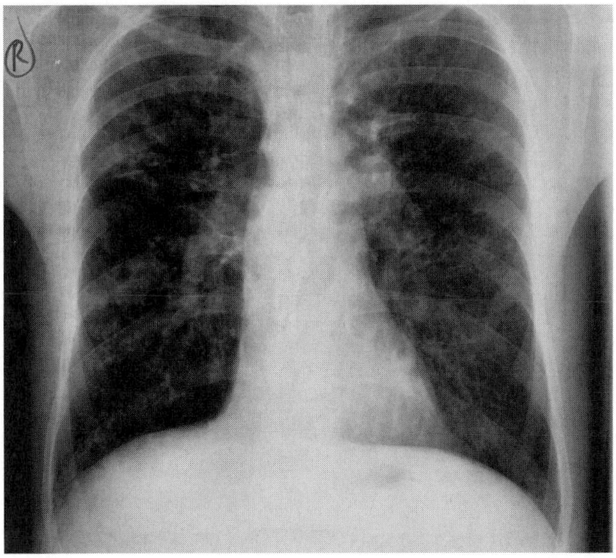

Fig. 201-5 Chest radiograph (PA view) of a 24-year-old male with CF demonstrating hyperinflation, bronchiectasis, and increases in linear markings and round opacifications.

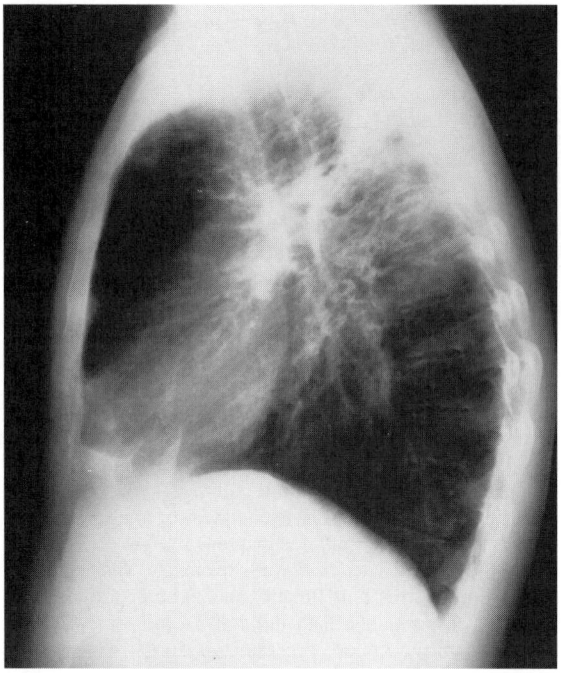

Fig. 201-6 Chest radiograph (lateral view) of a 24-year-old male with CF demonstrating marked retrosternal and retrocardiac lucency consistent with hyperinflation. Bronchiectasis and increased linear markings are also apparent.

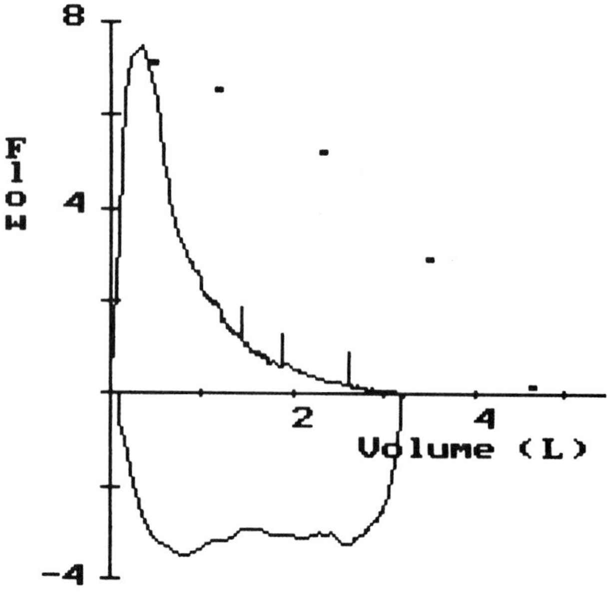

Fig. 201-8 Flow-volume loop from a 28-year-old male with CF. Predicted values indicated by dots. Peak flow is close to normal. There are marked decreases in flows at low lung volumes compared to the predicted values indicating severe airflow limitation. The "scooped" appearance of the expiratory limb of the curve is very characteristic of CF.

data on this pulmonary function measure.[233,491] It is also known that, on average, FEV1 declines steadily with age in CF.[140]

Physiologic evaluation of lung function in infants with CF has recently improved. Early studies employing plethysmography were consistent with airway obstruction and initiation of disease in the small airways. Partial flow-volume loops generated from rapid chest compression during tidal breathing have recently confirmed that infants with CF hospitalized for respiratory symptoms improve in pulmonary function similar to older patients.[127] Partial flow-volume loops have also demonstrated that intravenous corticosteroid treatment improves lung function during respiratory exacerbation in infants.[603] The measurement of expiratory flow rates after chest compression at raised lung volumes appears to be a more sensitive test in detecting airflow limitation than partial flow-volume loops.[621] The improvements in infant lung function testing will likely contribute to evaluation of early interventions. Three and four year olds have been problematic to study because infant techniques cannot be applied to this group and cooperation for standard spirometry has been difficult.

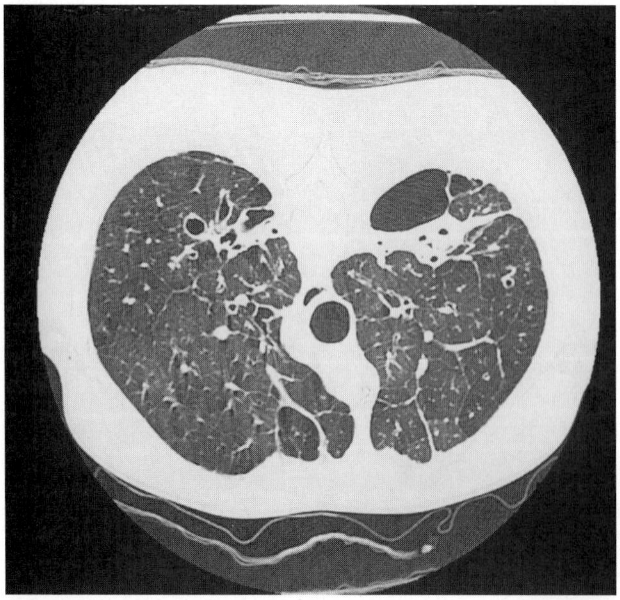

Fig. 201-7 High resolution CT scan of the same 24-year-old male with CF demonstrating inhomogeneity of aeration, mucus plugging of airways, a large cyst in the right posterior lung field, and bronchiectasis in the left posterior lung field.

Several other tests add to the description of functional abnormalities in CF lung disease. Exercise testing can predict survival but is not in widespread use.[441] Respiratory monitoring during sleep is useful in the evaluation of end-stage patients particularly to determine whether noninvasive ventilation is helpful.[101] Blood gases are usually well preserved until the end-stages of disease.

Microbiology. The failure of lung defense in CF leads to chronic endobronchial infection. Organisms commonly encountered in infants and toddlers include *S. aureus* and *Haemophilus influenzae*. As disease progresses, *P. aeruginosa* becomes the most common isolate. In several studies, *Pseudomonas* predominates after two years of age.[33] Early in infection, it exists as a rough or smooth variant, but within a year of so the bacteria take on a mucoid appearance characterized by production of a polysaccharide coat. Once present in this mucoid form, *P. aeruginosa* is only rarely cleared.[612] Other gram negative organisms including *Burkholderia cepacia, Stenotrophomonas maltophilia*, and *Alcaligenes xylosoxidans* have been increasingly isolated from the CF airway.[94] Cultures of CF sputum are also frequently positive for fungus, particularly *Aspergillus fumigatus* and for nontuberculous mycobacteria. Appropriate microbiologic techniques are necessary for adequate identification of organisms. Reference laboratories have been set up to aid with identification and performance of antibiotic sensitivities.[525]

B. cepacia infection is seen in approximately 3 percent of patients. A few patients with *B. cepacia* develop, over several months, a rapid decline in lung function associated with a high mortality. In contrast to *P. aeruginosa*, person-to-person transmission of *B. cepacia* is well documented. The significance of colonization with *S. maltophilia* and *A. xylosoxidans* is still not clear.

Nontuberculous mycobacteria (NTM) infection has been reported to have a prevalence as high as 13 percent in some European and US CF centers.[443] The NTM organisms include *Mycobacterium avium* complex, *M. abscessus*, *M. fortuitum*, *M. gordonae*, and *M. kansasii*. It is not as yet clear whether mycobacterial infection without granulomatosis disease hastens pulmonary decline. Several patients with unsuspected granulomatous disease have been identified at postmortem examination or lung transplantation.

Attempts to better define the colonization status of the airway have led to the use of bronchoalveolar lavage (BAL). This procedure has demonstrated clinical utility in evaluation of patients who cannot expectorate sputum or who are not responding to treatment.[53] BAL studies have also demonstrated that even stable patients with good lung function beyond 12 years of age have airway infection with CF pathogens.[352] It is becoming clear that in young patients throat cultures are poorly predictive of lower airway microbiology identified by BAL.[488,515]

Immunity and Inflammation in CF. The characterization of immunity and inflammation in CF has received considerable attention in view of the importance of these two processes in mediating airway injury. Currently, the only clinically useful assessment of immunity or inflammation in CF is the determination of IgE levels in allergic bronchopulmonary aspergillosis (see "Allergic Bronchopulmonary Aspergillus" below). Other biomarkers of infection and immunity have been noted in CF, including anti-*Pseudomonal* antibodies, reduced levels of opsonizing antibodies circulating markers of inflammation, products of neutrophil degradation, and oxidative stress.[299,350,610] However, the clinical utility of such findings is not clear.

Complications. Mucus plugging, infection, inflammation, and fibrosis in the CF lung can lead to a range of complications including respiratory failure, atelectasis, pneumothorax, hemoptysis and allergic bronchopulmonary aspergillosis.[535]

Respiratory Failure. Respiratory failure is the primary cause of death in over 90 percent of patients with CF. Respiratory failure is characterized by increasing dyspnea, hypoxemia, and elevation of arterial PCO_2. Hypoxemia is often responsive to supplemental oxygen therapy, and thus oxygenation can often be well maintained in patients who are in overt respiratory failure. In infants, respiratory failure is frequently associated with viral infection, and the clinical outcome of mechanical ventilation is very favorable.[238] In the past, mechanical ventilation has been regarded as not beneficial in patients with more advanced disease. With newer techniques of ventilation and intensive care many adults with CF can be successfully ventilated and recover well.

Atelectasis. Atelectasis can occur at any age in CF and often is recalcitrant to treatment. At bronchoscopy, mucus plugs can be seen in the bronchi in some cases, but in other cases plugs are not evident, suggesting that the mucus obstruction is in smaller airways. Hyperinflation of adjacent lobes may also contribute to atelectasis. Some patients with CF will develop severe localized bronchiectasis in atelectatic lobes.[388]

Pneumothorax. Pneumothorax (air in the pleural space) results from rupture of subpleural blebs through the visceral pleura[611] and occurs annually in approximately one percent of patients with CF in the United States.[9] Patients with pneumothorax will frequently complain of sudden onset of dyspnea and chest pain and present in obvious respiratory distress, although occasionally their symptoms are minimal. The diagnosis is based upon frontal and lateral chest radiographs.

Hemoptysis. Minor hemoptysis or blood streaking in expectorated sputum is a common symptom of older patients. It may represent the onset of a pulmonary exacerbation, but requires no specific intervention (see "Hemoptysis" below). Massive hemoptysis, defined as acute bleeding of greater than 240 ml in a 24 hour period or greater than 100 ml per day for 3 to 7 consecutive days[535]) occurs annually in approximately 1 percent of US patients.[9] Like pneumothoraces, the incidence increases with age and illness severity. Hemoptysis is thought to occur because an actively inflamed airway erodes into a hypertrophied bronchial artery. This complication is more common in patients with liver disease who may have disturbances in clotting factors.

Allergic Bronchopulmonary Aspergillosis. Invasive fungal disease is rare in immunocompetent patients with CF, though it has been described in patients receiving long-term corticosteroids or patients who are post-transplantation. By contrast, allergic bronchopulmonary aspergillus (ABPA) occurs in 2 to 5 percent of patients.[60] ABPA will frequently present as refractory wheezing and/or a new infiltrate on chest radiograph. Supportive laboratory criteria include peripheral blood eosinophilia, precipitating antibodies and/or a positive immediate skin test against *Aspergillus fumigatus*, and elevated IgE (150 to >1000 international units/ml).[60] Because of the overlap between the criteria for ABPA and common symptoms of CF, the diagnosis should not be based solely upon laboratory findings, but must be considered in the context of the clinical presentation. There is increasing evidence that the same syndrome may be seen with other fungal organisms.

Pancreas

Exocrine pancreatic insufficiency (PI) is present in the majority (>80 percent) of patients by the time of diagnosis and is highly correlated with genotype (see "CFTR Genotype and Pancreatic Disease").[333,605] Nearly all patients homozygous for ΔF508 have PI, whereas many patients with at least one copy of partial function mutations (e.g., R177H, R334W, A455E) have retained pancreatic exocrine function and are classified as pancreatic sufficient (PS).[362]

The classification of patients as pancreatic insufficient (PI) or sufficient (PS) is based upon the presence (PI) or absence (PS) of steatorrhea secondary to fat maldigestion and malabsorption. All PI patients lack normal exocrine pancreatic function. By contrast, PS patients are a more variable group, consisting of approximately 50 percent with normal and the remaining 50 percent with subnormal zymogen secretion following pancreatic stimulation. Despite their variable pancreatic function, the PS patients are classified as one group, because their clinical course, prognosis, and genotypes are distinct from PI patients.[333]

Pathology. Pathologic changes in the pancreas are evident even by 32 to 38 weeks gestation[587] and progress to virtual destruction of the organ by adulthood in the majority of patients. The distinctive pathologic appearance of this organ led Dorothea Anderson to name the disease "cystic fibrosis of the pancreas" in 1938. Early findings consist of inspissated eosinophilic secretions in pancreatic acini and ducts, which lead to flattening and atrophy of epithelia and dilatation of acini[449] and ducts (Fig. 201-9).

Fibrosis becomes more apparent as the dilatation progresses. In the most advanced stages, the pancreas is replaced with adipose tissues and isolated groups of islets. The islets may be preserved for many years, although it is not known if their total number is normal. Eventually, pancreatic fibrosis leads to disruption of architecture and essential vasculature. In contrast to pulmonary disease, the pancreas has little inflammatory response, with the exception of occasional eosinophilia associated with ruptured acini.

Clinical Manifestations. The exocrine pancreas is responsible for secretion of alkaline pancreatic fluid and for synthesis and release of digestive enzymes. The pancreatic ductal epithelium is the

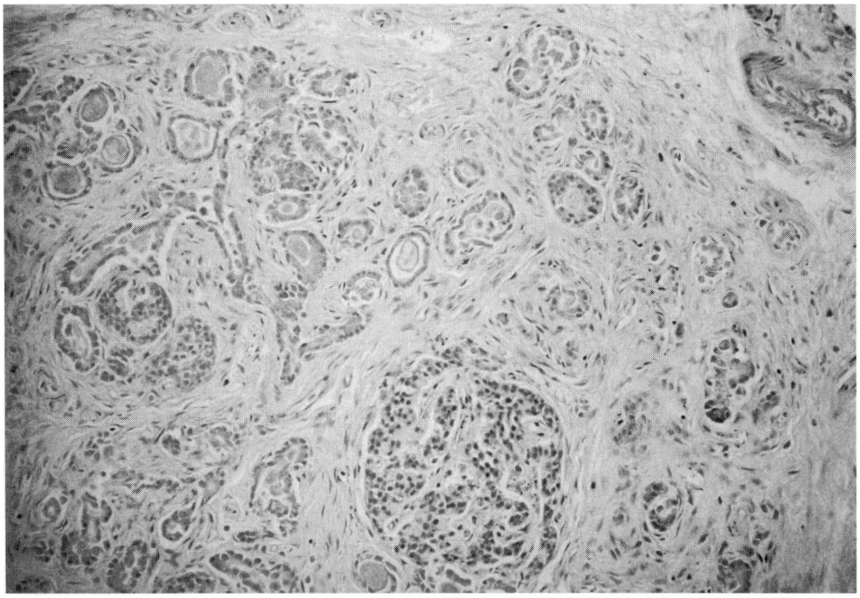

Fig. 201-9 Pancreas, low power: Dense fibrous tissue surrounds degenerating ducts containing inspissating concretions. Residual islet is surrounded by fibrous tissue. Patient one year of age. (*Courtesy of Dr. Joe Rutledge, Children's Hospital & Regional Medical Center, Seattle.*)

likely site of bicarbonate and water secretion. The acinar cells synthesize, store, and secrete enzymes.[145] In CF, loss of function of acini and ducts leads to reduced water, bicarbonate, and enzyme content in the duodenal fluid leaving the pancreas.

Pancreatic enzyme deficiency leads to fat and protein maldigestion, producing a distended abdomen and frequent, bulky, greasy stools. Maldigestion will lead to poor weight gain and stunted linear growth in the young infant who does not receive appropriate enzyme replacement therapy.[214] Failure to thrive secondary to maldigestion is the second most common presenting symptom for infants with CF (after persistent respiratory symptoms). In the United States, 43 percent of patients present with malabsorption at diagnosis.[9] Fat losses in stool may be as high as 50 to 70 percent of total intake and nitrogen malabsorption is quite significant, as well. Carbohydrate digestion and absorption is not severely impaired in this disorder.[290] Although enzyme deficiency and maldigestion are major contributors to malnutrition, growth failure in CF is often the result of multiple contributing factors. Consideration must also be given to inadequate caloric intake[490] and pulmonary infection and inflammation, leading to increased energy requirements. Some infants present with a symptom complex of edema, hypoproteinemia, and anemia.[664] These infants may be severely ill, requiring aggressive nutritional and pulmonary interventions.[12]

Deficient absorption of fat-soluble vitamins A, E, D, and K is a common manifestation of pancreatic insufficiency in CF.[673] Vitamin A deficiency was identified in 21 percent of infants less than 2 months of age (diagnosed by newborn screening). The deficiency was easily corrected with enzyme and vitamin replacement therapy.[571] Symptomatic deficiency, consisting of increased intracranial pressure, xerophthalmia, and night blindness, is rare and seen today only in patients with delayed diagnosis, poorly controlled pancreatic insufficiency, or significant hepatobiliary disease. Although vitamin D deficiency was noted in 35 percent of screened newborns,[571] vitamin D deficiency rickets is now rare in patients on enzyme replacement. Serum levels of vitamin D metabolites may be reduced, although the clinical significance of these reduced values is not known. A much greater problem in the older CF patient, particularly females and individuals receiving chronic steroid therapy, is reduced bone mineral density,[31] leading to osteoporosis and subsequent pathologic fractures (see "Osteoporosis"). Vitamin E deficiency is quite common in untreated patients,[212] potentially leading to neuroaxonal degeneration and decreased red blood cell survival and hemolysis,[212] but is corrected with replacement therapy. Vitamin K deficiency and resultant reduction in vitamin K-dependent coagulation factors (prothrombin) may lead to reduced coagulant activity and prolonged prothrombin time. The severe hemorrhagic disease of infancy is rarely seen with routine administration of vitamin K replacement in the newborn period. In addition to fat malabsorption, important contributing factors to abnormal coagulation function are chronic antibiotic usage, which alters bowel flora required for intestinal metabolism, and hepatic dysfunction, which compromises conversion of vitamin K to prothrombin. Prolongation of prothrombin time should always direct the clinician to evaluation of hepatobiliary function, in addition to correction of pancreatic insufficiency and vitamin K deficiency.

Maldigestion and malabsorption of fats and protein accompanied by a more rapid transit time may lead to losses of a variety of other essential nutrients and source of energy supply. There have been reports of abnormal fatty acid composition of lipid pools, essential fatty acid deficiencies, and deficiency of minerals, such as zinc and selenium. Most of these deficiencies can be corrected by assiduous monitoring of enzyme replacement and nutritional supplementation.[673]

Laboratory Evaluation. The exocrine pancreas has enormous functional reserve, so that steatorrhea may not be observed until lipase output has declined to less than 2 percent of normal values. Steatorrhea is defined as a fecal fat output greater than 7 percent of ingested fat or greater than 5 grams per 24 hours. In most cases, patients with PI present with a history of frequent foul-smelling, bulky stools and inadequate weight gain. Microscopic examination of the stool demonstrates neutral fat droplets.

Pancreatic function may be evaluated by a variety of direct and indirect tests,[147] none of which is ideal. The most widely used indirect test is the 72-hour fecal fat analysis accompanied by a simultaneous 72-hour fat intake record. This test will provide information on daily fat losses but provides no information on pancreatic reserve. This test should be considered for all newly diagnosed patients. In addition, each newly diagnosed patient should also be evaluated to assess the impact of untreated fat and protein malabsorption on nutritional status. This assessment should include review of linear growth, weight gain, fat and muscle stores, serum value for albumin (and prealbumin), hematocrit, and fat soluble vitamins.[490] For patients receiving pancreatic enzyme replacement therapy, periodic fecal fat balance studies may be useful to determine appropriate dose adjustments. Although the nature of this test is odious to families and laboratory staff, no other indirect test is more reliable for longitudinal assessments.

Patients without evidence of steatorrhea by history or microscopic stool examination likely are PS. Assessment of functional pancreatic enzyme reserve and secretory capacity in these patients requires duodenal collection of pancreatic secretions under stimulated conditions utilizing a known secretagogue (e.g., secretin or cholecystokinin).[194] The invasive nature of this test precludes its routine use for serial monitoring of the PS patient. Thus, most clinicians follow growth, nutritional status, and patient history for evidence of the onset of steatorrhea.

Clinical Course. Patients classified as PI generally demonstrate steatorrhea within the first year of life. The nutritional sequelae of fat and protein maldigestion and malabsorption are rapidly apparent but can be corrected with appropriate medical management. Because steatorrhea represents loss of over 98 percent of pancreatic exocrine function, once established there is little change in symptomatology for the remainder of the patient's life. However, enzyme requirements may vary, depending on nutritional intake, growth patterns, physical activity, and other factors. Adults frequently decrease enzyme intake after growth ceases.

Pancreatic sufficient patients often present at an older age with minimal, if any, gastrointestinal or nutritional manifestations. They may develop steatorrhea later in life, but most never require enzyme replacement therapy. PS patients are more likely than insufficient patients to develop pancreatitis during their life-time (see below).

Complications

Recurrent Pancreatitis. Pancreatitis, an uncommon condition among patients with pancreatic insufficiency, occurs most often in adolescent and older patients with CF who have retained exocrine pancreatic function.[517] Pancreatitis presents with severe epigastric or left upper quadrant pain, anorexia, and vomiting associated with elevated serum amylase and lipase levels. It may be chronic or recurring and, at times, can be associated with pancreatic duct stricture or retained gallstone. An association between mutations of the CFTR gene and chronic idiopathic pancreatitis has been identified.[130,549] Both studies identified an increased frequency of CFTR mutations on either one or both alleles in patients with chronic pancreatitis, as well as an increased frequency of the 5T mutation in intron 8 of the CFTR gene, which is associated with reduced proportion of functional CFTR. Although none of these individuals demonstrated pulmonary manifestations of CF or abnormal sweat tests, some did demonstrate abnormalities of ion transport in the nasal epithelium. These cases emphasize that CFTR gene dysfunction likely has a much broader range of phenotypic manifestations than the classic presentation of CF.

Diabetes Mellitus. As patients with CF have longer life spans, both glucose intolerance and CF-related diabetes mellitus (CFRDM) are becoming increasingly common complications. In the 1998 US CFF registry,[9] the prevalence of insulin-requiring CFRDM displayed a strong age association, specifically, 2.2 percent in children less than 18 years and >15 percent in adults 18 years and older. Throughout life, patients with CF have a high probability of insulin deficiency,[703] which may lead to clinical DM by the second or third decade in some patients, with an average onset at 18 to 21 years.[367]

The pathophysiologic basis of CFRDM is not clearly defined. It is widely believed that insulin deficiency is primarily a result of a loss of beta cells from fibrosis and fatty infiltration of the exocrine pancreas, leading to loss of normal islet cell architecture and vascular supply. The total number of islets diminishes and the cellular composition is altered with decreased percentage of beta, alpha and polypeptide cells and increased delta cells.[385] In general, patients with CFRDM have a higher number of beta cells than observed with type 1 DM. Thus, it is likely that other factors, such as insulin insensitivity, contribute to the clinical manifestation of CFRDM. Patients with poor lung function and chronic infection with associated inflammation have greater insulin resistance.[277]

The negative impact of insulin-dependent DM on morbidity and mortality of patients is cause for concern. In one report from a large CF center, 25 percent of patients with CFRDM survived to age 30 years compared with 60 percent of patients without diabetes.[221] CFRDM may also be associated with poorer growth, weight gain, and pulmonary function,[367] although appropriate therapy may lessen these negative effects. CF patients are also at risk for microvascular complications, including retinopathy (5 to 16 percent), nephropathy (3 to 16 percent), and neuropathy (5 to 21 percent).[367,589] Macrovascular complications are not common in CFRDM, which may reflect the younger age of the population.

CFRDM has a distinct clinical presentation that is easily distinguished from types 1 and 2 diabetes. The 1998 American Diabetes Association classification scheme places CFRDM in the category of "Other Specific Types—Diseases of the Exocrine Pancreas".[4] Although some patients may present with the classic constellation of polydipsia, polyuria, polyphagia, and weight loss, the presentation in most patients is much more insidious. Frequent symptoms that may indicate CFRDM are poor weight gain, delayed puberty with poor linear growth, and an unexplained decline in pulmonary function. Abnormal glucose homeostasis may be intermittent in some patients with CF and exacerbated by stresses such as pulmonary infections or oral glucocorticosteroids.

Due to the insidious and often asymptomatic onset of CFRDM and significant increased morbidity in patients with CF having diabetes, a consensus panel recently convened by the Cystic Fibrosis Foundation[428] has recommended annual screening of all patients with a casual (formerly called random) glucose level. If this level is greater than 126 mg/dl, a fasting blood sugar (FBS) must be obtained. An FBS greater than 126 mg/dl is diagnostic for CFRDM, but should be confirmed by a second FBS at a separate occasion. An oral glucose tolerance test (OGTT) should be considered in individuals with a normal FBS who have concurring symptoms, such as poor weight gain or growth velocity. Hemoglobin A_1C is an unreliable measure for the diagnosis of CFRDM.[166,221]

Gastrointestinal Tract

Pathology. Changes in the intestinal tract are not prominent. There are little, if any, primary histologic findings of the esophagus, stomach, or small intestinal tract mucosa. The most prominent finding is dilatation and hyperplasia of submucosal glands throughout the large and small intestinal tracts associated with accumulation of eosinophilic secretions filling the lumen.[179] These findings are prominent in Brunner's glands of the duodenum. The appendix also displays goblet cell hyperplasia of the epithelium and accumulation of secretions within the crypts and in the lumen.[610] Mucoceles have been noted in both the appendix and esophagus. Anatomic anomalies, including ileal and jejunal stenosis and atresia, reduplication, omphalocele, and mesotonic defects are seen in almost half of infants with meconium ileus (see below).[449]

Clinical Manifestations and Complications

Meconium Ileus. Meconium ileus (MI) is present in approximately 10 to 20 percent of CF patients at birth[332] and is often diagnostic of the illness. In 1998, 18.6 percent of CF diagnoses in the United States were based upon MI at birth.[9] These infants in the first days of life fail to pass meconium, in association with abdominal distension and bilious vomiting. Bowel perforation may occur either ante- or post-natally. *In utero* perforation may be associated with intra-abdominal calcifications and anatomic anomalies, such as ileal and jejunal stenosis or atresia. Abdominal radiographs reveal air fluid levels in the small intestine, a "ground glass" appearance in the right lower quadrant, and lack of gas in the colon. Contrast enema with Hypaque or Gastrografin is diagnostic and frequently therapeutic. It demonstrates a small, unused "microcolon," and, if contrast is refluxed into the ileum, the point of ileal obstruction may be identified.[517] Meconium ileus is highly associated with pancreatic insufficiency and the ΔF508 mutation (see "CFTR Genotype and Other Features of the CF Phenotype").[272,332] Meconium ileus should be distinguished from the "meconium plug syndrome" which involves obstruction of the colon[448] in the newborn period. In this syndrome, the colon is normal in size and function. Meconium plug syndrome is less specific for CF and other diagnostic etiologies should be considered.

Distal Intestinal Obstruction Syndrome. Distal intestinal obstruction syndrome (DIOS) is a small bowel obstruction that may occur repeatedly in patients with CF throughout their lives.[524] Approximately 10 to 20 percent of patients experience episodes of crampy right lower quadrant pain associated with decreased defecation. The episodes may have an acute presentation with complete obstruction and bilious vomiting or a more chronic, intermittent presentation over weeks to months. Like meconium ileus of the newborn, obstruction occurs in the terminal ileum and is associated with inspissated, voluminous, partially digested intestinal contents. A fecal mass is usually palpable in the right lower quadrant. Similar to meconium ileus of infancy, contrast enema with Gastrografin is frequently diagnostic and therapeutic.[517]

Abdominal Pain. Chronic abdominal pain is a common symptom of individuals with CF and the differential diagnosis is often quite broad (Table 201-1).[517] It is important to review closely with the patient the location, nature, and duration of the pain, as well as associated symptoms. Epigastric pain is commonly associated with gastroesophageal reflux disease and esophagitis.[450] It may also represent pancreatitis (see "Complications" above). In spite of increased basal gastric acid production in this population, overt peptic ulcer disease and *Helicobacter pylori* infection are not increased, unless patients are receiving therapies such as systemic corticosteroids.[517] Right upper quadrant pain may be associated with gallstones and biliary tract disease.[583] Right lower quadrant pain is most commonly associated with DIOS, but may represent intussusception, intestinal adhesions from previous surgery, appendicitis, ovarian cyst, or irritable bowel syndrome. Diffuse or periumbilical pain is most frequently due to inadequate or incorrect pancreatic enzyme replacement therapy or abdominal wall pain from coughing, but may be referred pain from all the etiologies listed above. Thus, it is very important to methodically evaluate any CF patient with this presenting symptom.

Table 201-1 Abdominal Pain in Patients with CF

Epigastric pain		
	Common diagnosis	Gastritis, duodenitis, ulcer disease, nonulcer dyspepsia, gastroesophageal reflux disease
	Less common diagnoses	Pancreatitis, gallbladder or biliary tract disease, distal intestinal obstruction syndrome (DIOS)
	Usual approach	Trial of H2-receptor antagonist to treat acid peptic disease, upper GI series small bowel follow through or upper GI endoscopy if empirical therapy is unsuccessful
Right upper quadrant pain		
	Common diagnosis	Gallstones or biliary tract disease
	Usual approach	Hepatobiliary ultrasound
Right lower quadrant pain		
	Common diagnosis	DIOS
	Less common diagnoses	Right colon fibrosis or stricture, appendiceal disease, intussusception, partial small bowel obstruction from adhesions from previous abdominal surgery, irritable bowel syndrome, ovarian cyst, renal colic
	Usual approach	Evaluate and treat for DIOS; if no response to DIOS treatment, contrast fluoroscopy may be needed
Periumbilical or diffuse abdominal pain		
	Common diagnosis	Incorrect use of supplemental pancreatic enzymes
	Less common diagnoses	Recurrent abdominal pain of childhood, partial small bowel obstruction, distal intestinal obstruction syndrome, irritable bowel syndrome, lactose intolerance, aerophagia, abdominal wall muscle pain (perhaps related to cough)
	Usual approach	Investigate enzyme use; other evaluation as indicated if this does not reveal the problem

Fibrosing Colonopathy. In the 1990s, there were several reports of some CF patients experiencing chronic abdominal pain who were subsequently found on pathologic examination to have colonic strictures and fibrosis.[565] Contrast enemas revealed a distinct narrowing and lack of distensibility of the right colon. Some individuals underwent partial bowel resections and subsequent pathologic examination of the resected bowel revealed denuded surface epithelium, intermittent disruption of the *muscularis mucosae,* and inflammation with fibrosis of the submucosa.[565] A case-control study consisting of 31 severe cases requiring colectomy identified at 114 US CF care centers between 1991 and 1994 and four, age- and disease-matched controls per case was conducted to investigate the relationship of fibrosing colonopathy with dose and type of enzyme product. This study[228] suggested that fibrosing colonopathy is associated with higher mean daily doses of pancreatic enzymes ($>$24,000 lipase units/kg/day) in younger patients. Based upon these findings, an expert consensus panel[73] recommended that "daily dose of pancreatic enzymes for most patients should remain below 2500 units of lipase per kilogram per meal (10,000 units/kg/day)".

Rectal Prolapse. Rectal prolapse occurs in approximately 20 percent of young patients with a peak incidence between 12 and 30 months of age.[582] Prolapse frequently begins near the time of toilet training and usually resolves by school age. The underlying etiology of prolapse is not entirely understood, but contributing factors include voluminous stools secondary to pancreatic insufficiency, withholding at the time of toilet training, poor nutritional status, and increased intra-abdominal pressure secondary to coughing and/or defecation. In most cases, manual reduction with gentle pressure is sufficient. Adjustment of enzymes to reduce stool bulk will usually prevent recurrences. Surgical intervention is very rare.

Other Complications. Several other gastrointestinal complications have been reported in patients with CF. The appendix is frequently filled with thick, inspissated secretions, which may lead on occasion to a large distended, noninflamed, right lower quadrant mass[146] and appendiceal diverticulosis. Interestingly, the incidence of acute appendicitis is not increased in CF. In fact, patients may frequently present later with either chronic symptoms and/or periappendiceal abscesses, perhaps because of their tolerance of recurrent abdominal pain or misdiagnosis as DIOS. Intussusception occurs in about one percent of patients with a lead point in the terminal ileum. Adenocarcinoma of the colon and pancreas may become more common in CF patients as survival increases (see "Cancer" below).[437]

Hepatobiliary Disease

Hepatic disease is often clinically silent until the emergence of secondary complications related to portal hypertension. For this reason, the importance of liver and biliary tract involvement in the overall morbidity of CF has received less emphasis than pulmonary and pancreatic manifestations. Greater life expectancy has increased the frequency and duration of hepatic complications. In addition, elucidation of the function of CFTR in biliary epithelia has provided a better scientific understanding of the pathogenesis of liver disease, which may lead to more specific therapeutic interventions in the future.

Pathophysiology. Hepatobiliary disease in cystic fibrosis, unlike most inherited disorders of the liver, primarily affects biliary duct epithelial cells rather than hepatocytes. The CFTR gene is expressed in epithelia throughout the intra- and extra-hepatic biliary tract with localization of the protein to the apical surface.[132] Expression in hepatocytes is not evident.[132] CFTR gene mutations lead to reduced or absent cAMP-mediated Cl^- channel function in biliary epithelial cells.[226] Similar to other affected organs, loss of Cl^- efflux likely leads to altered water and Na^+ movement, resulting in abnormal bile hydration and composition. The abnormal biliary secretions lead to sludging and inspissated eosinophilic material in portal biliary ductules with secondary proliferation and chronic inflammation.[449]

Several secondary factors likely effect the rate at which this disease develops. A greater ratio of hydrophobic to hydrophilic bile acids will increase sludging in the biliary tract. With stasis, hydrophilic bile acids are cytotoxic to surrounding epithelial cells, resulting in cell injury, cytokine release, and inflammation.[380] The ongoing cell injury and death leads to collagen deposition and periportal fibrosis. The most specific lesion associated with this process is focal biliary cirrhosis, which may be found even in early childhood and the majority of adults at autopsy.[449] The focal lesion slowly progresses to multilobular cirrhosis over many years and all stages of pathogenesis may be seen as a continuum within the same liver (Fig. 201-10).

Clinical Manifestations. The manifestations of hepatobiliary disease in CF are quite broad, ranging from asymptomatic elevation of liver enzymes to hepatic cirrhosis (Table 201-2).[241] The prevalence of disease is difficult to ascertain due to insensitive diagnostic markers such as serum enzymes and lack of a consistent definition of clinically significant liver disease. As a result, published reports provide a wide variation in prevalence figures depending upon the age group studied and the source of data (i.e., autopsy versus laboratory or physical findings).[136] The 1997 CFF patient registry reported an overall prevalence of hepatic cirrhosis with portal hypertension of 1 percent, ranging from 0.1 percent in patients less than 5 years old to 1.7 percent in those over 18 years old.[9] A retrospective English study[540]) of 1100 patients reported a higher prevalence ranging from 0.3 percent in patients less than 5 year old to 8.7 percent in patients 16 to 20 years old. Elevation in serum liver enzymes is much more common. In several prospective studies,[358] elevated aspartate transferase (AST) and alkaline phosphatase (AP) levels have ranged from 15 to 50 percent, starting in the newborn period and continuing to adulthood.[358] Enzyme elevations are almost always asymptomatic, not associated with elevated bilirubin or jaundice, and frequently transient. The long-term clinical significance of these laboratory findings is not well defined.

Table 201-2 Reported Frequency of Hepatobiliary Diseases in CF

Disease	Frequency (%)
Neonatal liver disease	6–40
Neonatal cholestasis	?
Fatty liver	15–30
Isolated massive statosis	5
Multilobular biliary cirrhosis	2–5
Gallbladder abnormalities (nonfunctional or small)	24–45
Gallstones	4–12
Common bile duct stenosis	?

Several studies have looked at genetic and clinical predictors of liver disease in CF. No studies of genetic mutations have revealed a significant association between specific genotypes and occurrence of liver disease.[196] However, the prevalence of elevated liver enzymes, AST, and AP, was higher (46 percent) in pancreatic insufficient patients homozygous for ΔF508 compared with pancreatic sufficient patients with mild missense mutations (22 percent).[358] There is also an association of meconium ileus and/or distal intestinal obstruction syndrome (DIOS) with subsequent liver disease.[409]

The earliest manifestation of liver disease is neonatal cholestasis, which occurs in approximately 5 percent of newborns with CF.[409] Cystic fibrosis must always be considered in the differential diagnosis of any child with elevated direct

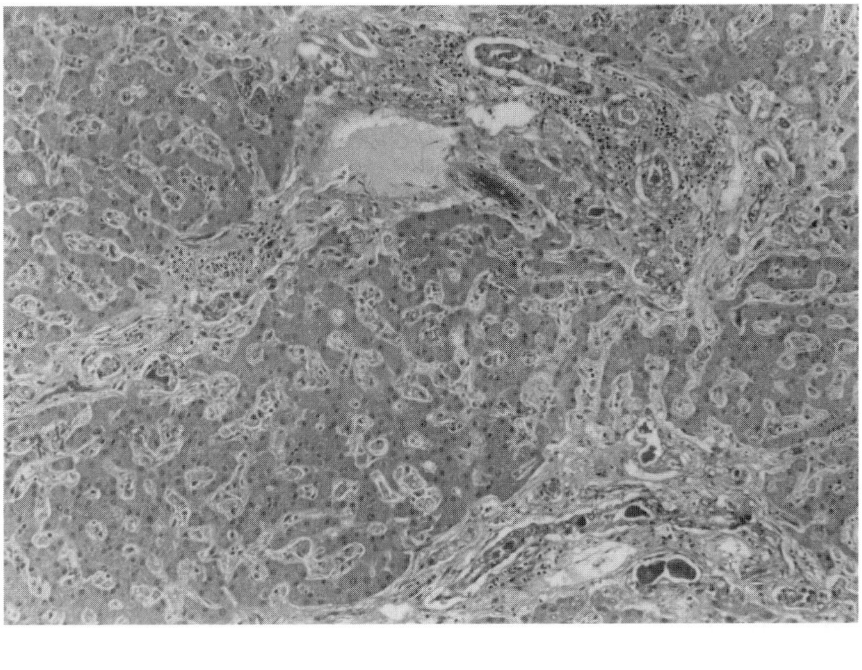

Fig. 201-10 The portal area is distorted by fibrosis and bile duct proliferation. Bile is inspissated in some ducts. (*Courtesy of Dr. Joe Rutledge, Children's Hospital & Regional Medical Center, Seattle.*)

hyperbilirubinemia. Infants present with jaundice, elevated direct bilirubin, hepatomegaly, and acholic stools. Many of the infants (25 to 50 percent) have meconium ileus, as well.[409] The diagnosis of biliary atresia must be considered. However, cholestatic jaundice in CF is self-limited, usually resolving by 2 months of age.

Prior to early aggressive nutritional management, hepatic steatosis or "fatty liver" was a common manifestation and autopsy finding. It is frequently associated with malnutrition and presents as an asymptomatic smooth enlarged liver without splenomegaly. Treatment of nutritional status will resolve hepatomegaly and there is no direct evidence that steatosis progresses to cirrhosis. Earlier diagnosis and initiation of early, nutritional intervention should reduce the prevalence of this clinical manifestation of CF liver disease.

The most common liver disease, biliary cirrhosis, presents as asymptomatic hepatomegaly with or without splenomegaly.[580] Unlike steatosis, the liver is nodular. Elevated liver enzymes, AST, alanine aminotransferase (ALT), AP, or GGT, are usually identified on routine annual screening, but bilirubin is rarely elevated. Another common associated finding is a prolonged prothrombin time secondary to liver disease and/or vitamin K deficiency. In more severe disease, portal hypertension with esophageal or gastric varices will present with sudden onset of hematemesis or melena. Hypersplenism frequently leads to thrombocytopenia and neutropenia, although splenectomy is rarely required. Hepatic synthetic failure and encephalopathy are very late and rare findings.

Although cholelithiasis occurs in 15 to 30 percent of patients, symptomatic disease is reported in less than 5 percent.[583] Gallstones are composed of calcium bilirubinate and protein. Symptoms and presentation are similar to other forms of gallbladder disease. Microgallbladder is a common autopsy and ultrasonic finding, but is asymptomatic in most patients.[583] The diagnosis of cholangiocarcinoma should be considered in biliary obstruction, jaundice, abdominal pain, and weight loss.

Laboratory Evaluation. The key components for identification of clinically significant CF liver disease are careful physical examination of the abdomen for liver and spleen size and texture at each clinic visit and annual screening of liver function tests.[570] These tests should include serum aspartate aminotransferase (AST), alanine aminotransferase (ALT), alkaline phosphatase (AP), gamma glutamyl transpeptidase (GGT), and bilirubin. Any values greater than 1.5 times the upper limit of normal should be repeated in 3 to 6 months. Tests remaining elevated for greater than 6 months, particularly in association with physical findings of hepatomegaly, should lead to further diagnostic work-up. This evaluation should include hepatic synthetic function (serum albumin and prothrombin time) and screening for other etiologies of elevated enzymes, including infections, drugs, and toxins. Ultrasonography of the liver, biliary tract, gallbladder, spleen, and hepatic vasculature is the most useful, noninvasive imaging study[570] and may determine presence of gallstones, ascites, or hepatic vein dilatation. Doppler ultrasonography can detect hepatic flow patterns, which is useful in assessment of portal hypertension. Other imaging techniques, such as computerized tomography and magnetic resonance imaging, which are useful in certain settings, have not been widely validated in controlled studies as screening methods in CF. Hepatobiliary scintigraphy is the best technique to assess bile flow, as well as hepatocyte function.[445]

There is a need to develop better clinical, biochemical, and imaging markers of liver injury, so that early biliary epithelial cell injury can be detected. Such early detection may allow clinicians to predict which patients will develop significant disease and to initiate earlier interventions.

Sweat Glands

Pathology. The most consistent functional alteration in CF has been elevated concentrations of Cl^-, Na^+, and K^+ in eccrine sweat. This abnormality is present at birth and throughout the life of the patient. Interestingly, there is no morphologic correlation for the physiologic abnormality in CF. The sweat glands in CF appear to have normal macroscopic and microscopic morphology,[50] as well as number. Subtle differences in subcellular morphology of unknown physiologic significance have been observed by electron microscopy.[575] Glandular obstruction evident in other affected organs is not observed due to a lack of mucus secretion in this eccrine gland. In contrast, apocrine sweat glands are more dilated and filled with retained secretions when compared with non-CF glands.[204]

Clinical Manifestations. The clinical consequences of sweat gland dysfunction result from excessive water and electrolyte losses. With profuse sweating, all patients may "taste salty" and develop salt crystals on their skin. These periods of salt loss provoke both the release of aldosterone and salt retention by the kidneys. Individuals with CF are also prone to acute heat prostration with excessive heat or exercise. Because infants have an increased surface area to volume ratio, they may be most susceptible. Heat prostration should be considered a medical emergency, as it may lead to rapid cardiovascular collapse. It is preventable by proper education of patients and families on appropriate hydration and salt intake during times of exercise or heat stress. Another chronic manifestation of salt loss presents as hypochloremic alkalosis in infants with CF.[444] The infants often have a history of vomiting, lethargy, weight loss, and diarrhea. These symptoms may be the initial presentation for CF in an undiagnosed infant. In 1998, 5.3 percent of newly diagnosed patients with CF manifested an electrolyte abnormality secondary to salt loss.[9] Oral salt replacement is effective in correcting the metabolic abnormality and intravenous replacement is rarely indicated.

Genitourinary Tract

Males

Pathology. Approximately 97 percent of males with cystic fibrosis are infertile due to azoospermia[90] attributed to congenital bilateral absence of the vas deferens. The pathologic changes occur exclusively in Wolffian duct or mesonephros structures; while metanephric structures, such as the kidney and ureteric bud, are normal, suggesting that injury to the developing duct system occurs after the eighth to twelfth week of gestation.[90,670]

The primary anatomic abnormality is absence, atrophy, or obstruction of the vas deferens (Fig. 201-11), tail and body of the epididymis (globus minor), and seminal vesicles.[610] The head of the epididymis (globus major), consisting of the rete testis and efferent ductules, is spared in most cases. These anatomical changes explain the lack of sperm in the ejaculated semen, in spite of normal spermatogenesis.[449] The prostate is usually normal. The seminal vesicles are either absent or atrophic and fibrotic, often associated with mucus filled cysts. Macroscopically, the testes may be either normal or slightly decreased in size. Other genitourinary manifestations which may occur more commonly in males with CF are inguinal hernias, hydrocele, and undescended testes.[578]

Clinical Manifestations. The physical examination of the testes is normal. However, growth of the testes and other pubertal development is frequently delayed with an associated 2 to 4 year lag in luteinizing and follicle stimulating hormone.[578] This delay may reflect poor pulmonary and nutritional status rather than the primary defect. In postpubertal males, sexual function is normal unless impaired by overall health status. All postpubertal males should be given the option of undergoing a semen analysis to assess fertility. In most cases, the volume of the ejaculate is reduced with complete absence of spermatozoa and altered chemical composition, including decreased fructose, and increased citric acid and acid phosphatase. Infertility may be the initial presentation for male patients with mild disease. Thus, CF must be considered in the differential diagnosis of any male presenting to a

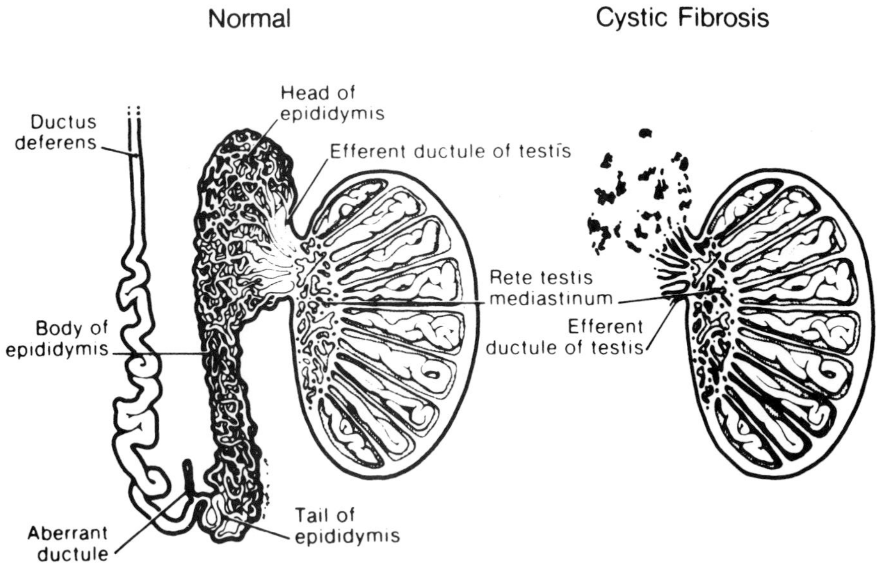

Fig. 201-11 Schematic representation of the testicle, epididymis, and vas deferens in the normal male (left) and CF male (right). Note preservation of the efferent ductule of the epididymis, but the atrophy and absence of the rest of the structures in CF.

fertility clinic with obstructive azoospermia (see "CFTR Genotype and Male Infertility" below).

Females

Pathophysiology. Females with cystic fibrosis may also have reduced fertility, although this has not been thoroughly studied. The ovaries, fallopian tubes, and uterus appear to be normal by gross anatomic and microscopic examination.[449] It is hypothesized that reduced fertility is attributed to thick dehydrated mucus in the cervix, which fails to undergo normal "ferning" during ovulation. Other factors contributing to reduced fertility are both primary and secondary amenorrhea and anovulatory cycles, which may be related to overall pulmonary and nutritional status.[577]

Clinical Manifestations. As more females with CF reach reproductive age, conception and successful pregnancies are increasing in frequency. The CF National Data Registry recorded approximately 30 to 40 annual live births by mothers with CF from 1966 to 1988, with an increase to approximately 100 per annum by the 1990s.[288] Pregnancy imposes physiologic stresses on the respiratory and cardiovascular systems, as well as increasing the nutritional burden by 300 kcal each day.[288] In all women, an increase in minute ventilation, blood volume, and cardiac output, and a decrease in functional residual capacity occurs.[356] Women with CF and mild prepregnancy pulmonary involvement adapt well to these cardiorespiratory stresses, resulting in successful term pregnancies.[99] Appropriate weight gain of 10 kg or greater is easily achieved by women with pancreatic sufficiency,[99] whereas women with pancreatic insufficiency frequently have suboptimal weight gain (mean of 5.2 kg).[230] Poor maternal health, reflected by severe obstructive pulmonary disease, inadequate nutritional status, and/or cor pulmonale prior to pregnancy, is associated with the frequent occurrence of fetal prematurity and low birth weight infants.[356] Pregnancy may also negatively impact the health and survival of women with severe pulmonary disease, although most published reports lack an appropriate nongravid control population to determine whether pregnancy per se or the natural history of the illness is the primary contributing factor.[356] A small case-controlled, retrospective study found no difference in decline in pulmonary function between gravid and matched nongravid females with CF 2 years postpregnancy.[230] Predictive factors for poor maternal and fetal outcomes have included progravid FEV_1 less than 60 percent predicted, and weight less than 15 percent ideal weight for height.[288] There is a critical need for a large prospective study with appropriate controls to better define the impact of pregnancy in women with CF and predictive factors for poor outcome.

Other Manifestations

Osteoporosis. As patients with CF live longer, osteoporosis and its clinical sequelae, fractures, and kyphosis, have become an important cause of pain and disability in adulthood.[31] Osteoporosis, defined as low bone density and fragility fractures, is well documented in CF adults. Children may demonstrate low bone mineral density measured by dual-energy x-ray absorptiometry (DEXA) in the first decade of life and it worsens with increasing age.[283] Several studies,[31,67,283,454,548] which measured lumbar spine bone density by DEXA in patients from ages 2 years to adulthood, demonstrated serious decreases in bone density averaging 1 to 2.5 standard deviations below the normal range, even after correcting for the smaller bone size of these patients compared with age matched controls.

There are multiple risk factors that contribute to bone mineral loss and osteoporosis in CF.[31] These factors include pancreatic insufficiency and maldigestion, poor nutritional status, reduced GI absorption of calcium and vitamin D, reduced physical exercise, delayed and reduced production of sex steroids (e.g., estrogen and androgens), frequent use of corticosteroids, and chronic airway inflammation leading to circulating cytokines that activate osteoclast activity (e.g., tumor necrosis factor and interleukin-1b). Thus, the osteoporosis of CF is likely a combination of both decreased bone formation and increased resorption, which may explain its onset at such a young age.

The clinical sequelae of osteoporosis, increased risk of fractures and kyphosis, has been documented in adults[31] and children.[284] These symptoms are quite frequent in patients with severe pulmonary involvement who are awaiting lung transplantation.[548] These findings are of particular concern in the context of organ transplantation, where chronic use of corticosteroids and other immunosuppressive agents post-transplantation is associated with accelerated bone loss in all patients.[67]

All patients with CF should be considered at risk for bone mineral loss and must be closely monitored for overall nutritional status and adequate calcium and vitamin D intake. Children should be monitored for linear growth and adolescents for pubertal growth and secondary sex changes. High risk patients would include those individuals with short stature, poor nutritional status, delayed puberty, severe pulmonary disease, and frequent or continuous use of corticosteroids. In these individuals, diagnostic tests should include vitamin D levels (25 OH-D), parathyroid hormone levels, sex steroid levels in older children and adults, DEXA scan, and in severe cases, skeletal survey for fracture. Other serum biochemical markers of bone resorption (e.g., N-telopeptide) and formation (e.g., carboxy-terminal propeptide of type 1 procollagen) are currently used as research tools, but not as routine diagnostic tools.

Cancer. The risk of most cancer increases with age in the general population. Thus, a predisposition towards specific types of cancer in the CF population could not be ascertained until the life span extended well into adulthood. In the 1980s, case reports of digestive tract cancers and leukemia began suggesting a possible increased risk of cancer in this population. A large retrospective cohort study examined the occurrence of cancer in over 38,000 patients with CF between 1985 and 1992 in the United States, Europe, and Canada.[437] Thirty seven cancers were observed during 164,764 person-years of follow-up. The relative risk for all cancers was 0.8 compared with the general population, that is, slightly decreased. However, the risk of digestive tract tumors, including cancers of the esophagus, stomach, small and large intestine, colon, liver, biliary tract, pancreas, and rectum was increased with an odds ratio of 6.5 (95 percent C.I. 3.5 to 11.1). There was no increased risk for all other forms of cancer. No specific genetic or phenotypic factors could be identified which predicted which patients with CF would be more likely to acquire a digestive tract tumor. Because the incidence of these neoplasms is rare, there are currently no routine diagnostic screening tests recommended for GI cancer in these patients. However, cancer should be considered in the differential diagnosis of any patient with unexplained abdominal pain, bleeding or jaundice.[417,437]

Rheumatic Disease in CF. Recurrent joint swelling and/or pain are not uncommon symptoms for adolescents and adults with CF.[442] The occurrence of some form of arthropathy is difficult to ascertain because of the variable presentation and reporting by patients. The 1998 CFF Data Registry reported an annual incidence of arthritis as 0.4 percent of patients less than 18 years and 2.3 percent of patients 18 years or older,[9] however clinical reviews of arthropathy have estimated an occurrence of 10 to 15 percent in a patient's lifetime.[78,442] The arthropathies associated with CF can be divided into two major categories, hypertrophic pulmonary osteoarthropathy (HPOA)[128] and episodic arthritis.[222] HPOA is a chronic symmetric periostitis of long bones associated with digital clubbing. It is most commonly observed in young adults with significant pulmonary diseases. The onset of symptoms is often insidious, but may increase during a pulmonary exacerbation. There is often painful swelling of wrists, ankles, or knees. Definitive diagnosis is based upon roentgenographic findings of periosteal new bone formation of the distal ulna, tibia, fibula, or radius.[128]

Episodic arthropathy, is an intermittent symptom complex distinct from HPOA and lacking radiographic changes. Joint swelling and tenderness is usually asymmetric, transient, and may include a single or multiple, small and large joints. Arthropathy may be accompanied by dermatological manifestations, such as a purpuric cutaneous vasculitis or erythema nodosum. Vasculitis may also occur in the absence of joint symptoms. The etiology of this type of arthropathy and vasculitis is thought to be an immunologic mechanism.[84] Chronic bacterial antigenic stimulation in the airway leads to the formation of circulating immune complexes that contain the bacterial antigen. Immunoglobulin deposition has been identified in synovial blood vessels during episodes of arthropathy.[222]

The diagnosis of episodic arthropathy is based upon clinical presentation. There are no specific radiological or serological findings, although some patients have low complement and positive antineutrophilic cytoplasmic antibody (ANCA). Synovial biopsy reveals some congestion of vessels and mild synovial hypertrophy. There is no specific treatment for episodic arthropathy and it is rarely improved by treatment of the underlying pulmonary disease. Short-term anti-inflammatory therapy may relieve symptoms, but do not change the duration of the arthropathy, which eventually resolves spontaneously.

THE CFTR GENE AND GENETICS OF CF

Shortly after CF was recognized as a distinct syndrome, clinicians noted that the disease occurred among siblings, suggesting a genetic etiology.[18] Cloning of the CFTR gene and identification of disease-producing alleles confirmed that CF is an autosomal recessive disorder.[330,509,513] The question has been raised as to whether CF is truly "monogenic" since variation in a number of genes likely contribute to the development of the phenotype.[205] The discovery of genetic "modifier" loci that influence severity of intestinal disease in CF mice and in CF patients support this contention.[520,698] Furthermore, genetic heterogeneity has been suggested by reports of CF-like disease in patients in whom deleterious CFTR mutations could not be found.[421] It appears prudent to regard CF as a single gene disorder, however, until defects in a gene other than CFTR have been shown to produce the CF phenotype.

The CFTR Gene

Gene Mapping and Cloning. The identification of the gene responsible for CF was one of the early triumphs of positional cloning. The availability of a large number of families with two or more affected individuals enabled the use of linkage analysis to localize the gene. Shortly after the first DNA marker (D7515) pinned the CF locus to the long arm of chromosome 7, additional markers MET and D758 were found to be closely linked to the responsible gene.[619,637,656] Identification of these two markers enabled the first genetic diagnosis of CF.[211] These and additional markers were used to demonstrate significant linkage disequilibrium with the CF locus and to indicate that a single mutation in the gene predominated in the Caucasian population.[154,207]

In 1989, the cloning of the gene responsible for CF was reported in a landmark trio of papers.[330,509,513] The investigators used a combination of physical mapping and cross-species hybridization of select DNA fragments derived from the CF locus to detect expressed sequences.[513] After discounting several candidates, a genomic fragment containing the first exon of the gene responsible for CF was isolated. A consensus cDNA sequence was then obtained from overlapping clones isolated from sweat gland, lung, intestine, and pancreas libraries.[509] The concomitant finding of a common mutation ΔF508, and its complete association with the XV2c/KM19 haplotype in linkage disequilibrium with CF provided conclusive proof that the correct gene had been identified.[330]

CFTR Gene Structure. The CFTR gene is composed of at least 27 exons and encompasses about 250 kb of DNA.[702] The gene is transcribed into a mature message RNA of 6.5 kb.[509] The encoded protein contains 1480 amino acids and has a calculated molecular mass of 168 kDa.[509] A number of predictions concerning the possible structure of CFTR were made from the primary amino acid sequence. Hydropathy analysis suggested the presence of twelve transmembrane segments in two groups of six. Homology with Walker motifs A and B suggested two regions that might interact with ATP. Finally, consensus sequences for phosphorylation by cAMP-dependent protein kinase (PKA) were clustered in a region called the R domain (Fig. 201-12). Experimental evidence indicates that most of those predictions are correct (see "Structure of the CFTR Protein").

CFTR Transcription. The expression of CFTR appears to be highly regulated. CFTR is confined to certain tissues where it displays cell-type specificity.[201,616] Analysis of the level of CFTR transcripts during development reveals a distinct temporal pattern of expression.[609] Finally, CFTR expression levels can be

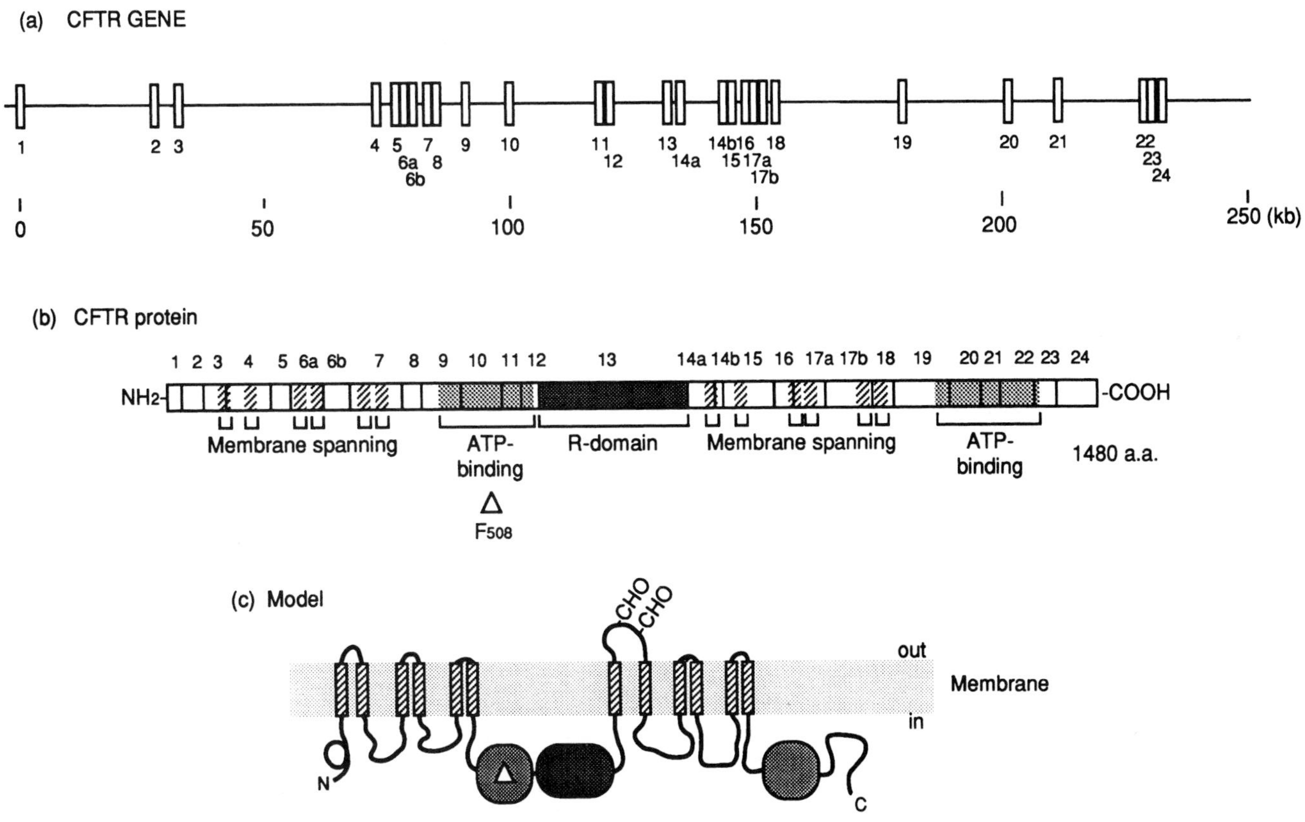

Fig. 201-12 The CFTR gene and its encoded polypeptide. (*From Tsui and Buchwald.*[620] *Used by permission.*)

modulated by cAMP, PKA, PKC, and phorbol esters.[47,414] These observations indicate that the CFTR gene has a sophisticated promoter. However, characterization of the *cis*- and *trans*-acting factors that regulate CFTR transcription has been a complicated affair. For example, the putative promoter region of CFTR reveals sequence characteristics of a housekeeping gene rather than a tissue-specific gene.[119,688] The tissue-specific pattern of CFTR expression is similar among different mammalian species suggesting that transcription regulatory elements may be evolutionarily conserved. Comparison of sequence at the 5′ end of different mammalian CFTR genes has revealed numerous regions of sequence identity. Prominent among these is a 34 bp region that encompasses the first nucleotide (1+ position) of the CFTR cDNA.[171,635] This region contains two consensus sequences from transcriptional control elements, an inverted CCAAT box, and a variant of the cAMP response element (CRE).[414,635]

Multiple transcription initiation sites have been reported for the CFTR gene. Use of these sites appears to be species- and tissue-specific.[349,655] The majority of transcription initiation sites are found within two hundred base pairs surrounding the first nucleotide (+1 position) of CFTR.[349,509,655] Studies of epithelial cell lines and primary epithelial tissues concur on the location of two transcription initiation sites in human CFTR. Transcription starting at the first nucleotide represents a minor start site observed in cell lines expressing high levels of CFTR mRNA (T84, CaCO2, HT-29 cells) and RNA from fetal lung tissue.[349,655,688] The major start site occurs about 60 nucleotides downstream of the putative first nucleotide of CFTR.[119,349,655,688] A small fraction of transcripts in cell lines initiate farther upstream and lead to the incorporation of alternative 5′ exons.[349] These transcripts do not include exon 1 of CFTR. Thus, translation of these alternative transcripts has to begin at the next available methionine codon in exon 4. Functional CFTR appears to be translated from constructs truncated at the 5′ end suggesting that the transcripts containing alternative 5′ exons might encode functional isoforms of CFTR *in vivo*.[426] Inclusion of an untranslated 5′ exon has been observed in CFTR RNA from murine testis, although the biological significance of the use of the alternative transcriptional initiation site is unknown.[655]

Several studies indicate that sequences immediately 5′ of the CFTR gene facilitate basal levels of transcription. Prominent regulatory elements for the basal promoter appear to include the evolutionary conserved inverted CCAAT box and the CRE sequence.[408,414,471] Varying the intracellular levels of cAMP and PKA alters transcription efficiency from each regulatory element, thus providing a rationale for the observed influence of these compounds on cellular levels of CFTR mRNA.[85,414] *Trans*-acting factors such as the CRE-binding protein and the human homeodomain CCAAT displacement protein/*cut* homolog have been shown to bind to their respective consensus sequences derived from the CFTR gene.[377,408] However, the search for *cis*-acting sequences that regulate tissue-specific CFTR transcription has been difficult. The use of different transcriptional-start sites in nonepithelial cells suggests that tissue-specific mechanisms exist.[687] Differences among cell lines in DNase-I hypersensitive sites in the CFTR promoter that correlate with CFTR expression levels indicate that chromatin structure *in vivo* may play a role in tissue-specific regulation.[349,560] Indeed, a putative DNase-I hypersensitive site in intron 1, located 10 kilobases 3′ at the end of exon 1 of CFTR has been shown to facilitate reporter gene expression dependent upon whether CFTR was expressed endogenously.[560] Considerable work remains to characterize the elements governing regulation of CFTR transcription.

CFTR Splicing. The full-length CFTR mRNA transcript is derived from splicing of 27 exons.[702] Alternative splicing of CFTR involving one or two exons has been detected by the RT-PCR method in a variety of epithelial and nonepithelial tissues.[153] Since RT-PCR examines select regions rather than entire transcripts and is highly sensitive, it is not clear whether by-products of the splicing process or biologically relevant alternative transcripts have been identified. Demonstration that an alternatively spliced transcript encodes a functional isoform or conservation across species of an alternative splicing pattern suggest a biologic role. Three types of alternative splicing have been observed for CFTR that meet one, or both, of these criteria.

All detectable CFTR transcripts in cardiac ventricular tissue from rabbit and guinea-pig are missing exon 5 (exon 5−).[279] These exon 5− transcripts appear to encode functional CFTR Cl^- channels because cardiac myocytes have currents like those generated by CFTR, antisense strategies reduce the current, and expression of exon 5− rabbit CFTR in *Xenopus* oocytes generates Cl^- currents.[279,434] Alternative splicing of exon 5 in human CFTR has not been observed, and expression of exon 5− human CFTR produced a misfolded protein that was retained in intracellular membranes.[169,682] Thus, alternative splicing of exon 5 may have evolved to meet specific species and tissue requirements.

Two other forms of alternative splicing may have functional relevance. First, an unusual form of splicing in kidney that is conserved between human and rat leads to the loss of portions of exon 13 and 14a, and introduction of a premature termination codon.[426] The encoded protein retains function as a Cl^- channel, at least in heterologous systems, and as a regulator of other channels.[426] Second, intron 10 of the human CFTR gene contains an exon (10b) that is incorporated into a minor fraction of CFTR transcripts.[422,665] It appears unlikely that a functional isoform would be translated since the exon contains an in-frame stop codon. However, an unused exon with 74 percent nucleotide identity to exon 10b in humans is found in intron 10 of the mouse CFTR gene. Conservation between human and mice suggests that exon 10b may have had some functional role, perhaps in primitive versions of CFTR. Further studies are necessary to confirm whether either form of alternative splicing has functional consequences *in vivo*.

The most common form of alternative splicing of human CFTR generates an in-frame transcript missing exon 9 (exon 9−); this transcript does not produce a functional channel and does not appear to be conserved among species.[123,169] Exon 9− transcripts can range between 0 and 92 percent in airway epithelial cells derived from different individuals.[122] Variation in the length of the polypyrimidine tract of the splice acceptor site preceding exon 9 underlies variability in the efficiency of exon 9 splicing.[121] CFTR genes that posses 5 thymidines (5T) have the lowest efficiency, with 5T/5T homozygotes having 89 to 92 percent of CFTR transcripts missing exon 9. Approximately 5 percent of CFTR genes in Caucasians and African-Americans have the 5T variant.[338] Two other variants, a 7 thymidine (85 percent) (7T) and a 9 thymidine variant (10 percent) (9T) are associated with more efficient exon 9 splicing.121 The efficiency of exon 9 splicing also appears to vary by tissue type. The proportion of CFTR transcripts missing exon 9 is higher in cells from the vas deferens than the nasal epithelium, independent of the 5T/7T/9T status.[398,600] Intriguingly, the 5T variant causes abnormalities in male reproductive status in some men when found in *trans* with a CF mutation (see "CFTR Genotype and Male Infertility"). Furthermore, the 5T variant can affect the severity of the phenotype when found in *cis* with the R117H CF mutation.[338]

Mutations in the CFTR Gene

Over one thousand sequence variations in the CFTR gene had been reported to the CF Genetic Analysis Consortium (CFGAC) database as of September 1999.[11] Nomenclature for CFTR mutations follows standard convention.[59] Table 201-3 shows 22 of the most common mutations. About 83 percent of the sequence changes are associated with disease, while the remainder are classified as polymorphisms. The vast majority of the disease-associated mutations involve one or a few nucleotides. Only 1 percent are genomic rearrangements, such as deletions or insertions that affect hundreds, or thousands of base pairs. Amino acid substitutions (missense) account for 44 percent of disease-associated mutations, while frameshift (22 percent), splice site (16 percent), nonsense (14 percent), and in-frame deletions (2 percent) comprise most of the remaining mutations. About 1 percent of mutations are proposed to be promoter mutations since they occur 5′ of the CFTR gene. However, the effect of these variants upon gene transcription is untested. Indeed, there is a lack of functional correlation for a large fraction of the putative disease-associated mutations; most have been described at the DNA level only. Furthermore, not all of the reported mutations have been discovered in patients with CF. Some were found in phenotypes associated with CFTR dysfunction, such as congenital bilateral absence of the vas deferens. Finally, most reports do not indicate whether an entire gene was sequenced, and whether the reported mutation was the only sequence variation identified. Despite these shortcomings, the list of mutations in the CFGAC database provides a wealth of information for structure/function investigation, genotype/phenotype correlation, and genetic epidemiology.

Mutations that introduce a premature termination codon (e.g., nonsense or frameshift) or alter highly conserved nucleotides of splice sites can be predicted to affect transcript integrity or protein synthesis with reasonable confidence.[274,360] Estimating the consequence of missense mutations is more difficult; five considerations are of value. First, evidence that a substitution alters CFTR function in native tissues or in a heterologous expression system remains the "gold standard". Only a few dozen missense mutations have been evaluated in this fashion (see "Molecular Mechanisms of CFTR Dysfunction"). Second, residues that are highly conserved between species, or between different members of the ABC transporter superfamily are likely to be critical for CFTR function. Third, multiple different mutations of the same amino acid suggest that a particular residue is essential. The 382 amino acid substitutions reported to the Consortium as of September 1999 involve only 305 codons. Two or more substitutions were reported at 64 different codons, suggesting that they cause disease. Fourth, in general, absence of a specific mutation in at least 100 genes from healthy individuals of the same racial and ethnic group as the proband is accepted as evidence that a change is not a polymorphism. This criterion has been met by a substantial fraction of the CFTR missense mutations that have been published. Fifth, analysis of the entire coding region of the CFTR gene using a sensitive technique (e.g., DNA sequencing) can demonstrate that a particular amino acid substitution is the only change in a gene. Reports of complex CF alleles (i.e., genes with more than one mutation) illustrate the importance of studying entire genes.[189,512] Unfortunately, a majority of the missense mutations reported to the CFGAC do not indicate whether the entire gene was screened or not.

Almost 190 polymorphisms have been reported in CFTR (CFGAC). About 55 percent occur in coding regions, half of which result in amino acid substitutions. Most of the substitutions are defined as polymorphisms because they were identified on the non-CF chromosome of a healthy CF heterozygote. However, it cannot be assumed that all polymorphisms are benign in nature. The discovery that certain polymorphisms (e.g., F508C, intron 8 5T) did not cause CF, but were associated with male infertility suggested that context should be considered in the interpretation of polymorphisms.[186] For example, the occurrence of either mutation in the non-CF gene from a healthy female would not uncover the consequence of the mutation upon CFTR function in the male reproductive tract. Furthermore, M470V, the most common amino acid polymorphism has been shown to alter CFTR function.[151] Although M470V does not cause CF, one could speculate that it might act in concert to magnify the functional consequences of a disease-causing mutation.

Population Genetics of CF

CF has traditionally been viewed as one of the most common life threatening inherited disorders in Caucasians. Retrospective epidemiologic studies indicated that the frequency of CF in most European and European-derived populations ranged between 1 in 2000 and 1 in 4000 live births (Table 201-4). Estimates from newborn screening programs and carrier detection in population

Table 201-3 **CF-Causing Mutations That Occur at a Frequency of 0.001 (0.1%) or Higher in Three Samples of Caucasian CF Patients**

		% of CF Alleles		
Mutation	**Consequence**	**Worldwide* (n = 43,849)**	**United States† (n = 25,030)**	**Europe‡ (n = 27,177)**
G85E	Gly → Glu at 85	0.15	0.17	0.21
R117H*	Arg → His at 117	0.30	0.67	0.29
621 + 1G → T	mRNA splicing defect	0.72	0.90	0.54
711 + 1G → T	mRNA splicing defect	0.11	< 0.1	0.11
1078delT	frameshift with premature termination	0.13	< 0.1	0.13
R334W	Arg → Trp at 334	0.12	0.22	0.16
R347P	Arg → Pro at 347	0.24	0.24	0.20
A455E*	Ala → Glu at 455	0.14	0.12	0.20
ΔI507	deletion of Ile at 507	0.21	0.31	0.23
ΔF508	deletion of Phe at 508	66.0	68.8	66.8
1717-1G → T	mRNA splicing defect	0.65	0.28	0.83
G542X	nonsense-mediated mRNA decay	2.42	2.43	2.64
G551D	Gly → Asp at 551	1.64	2.12	1.50
R553X	nonsense-mediated mRNA decay	0.73	0.90	0.75
R560T	Arg → Thr at 560	0.15	0.19	0.18
1898 + 1G → A	mRNA splicing defect	0.12	< 0.1	0.22
2789 + 5G → A*	mRNA splicing defect	0.12	0.31	0.11
R1162X	premature termination	0.29	0.22	0.51
3569delC	frameshift with premature termination	0.12	0.17	0.14
3849 + 10 kbC → T*	mRNA splicing defect	0.24	0.67	0.15
W1282X	nonsense-mediated mRNA decay	1.22	1.41	1.0
N1303K	Asn → Lys at 1303	1.34	1.25	1.64
Total		77.16	81.48	78.54

*CF Genetic Analysis Consortium[204] for worldwide.
†CFF Patient Registry 1997[17] for U.S.
‡Estivill X et al.[661] for European populations.
The number (n) of genes analyzed is shown although some patients were included in more than one sample. Asterisk indicates a mutation that may be associated with normal or borderline sweat Cl^- values. The missense (amino acid substitution), nonsense, and deletion mutations have been shown to disrupt CFTR function by one of the mechanisms discussed in "Molecular Mechanisms of CFTR Dysfunction" and/or not to occur in normal genes from at least 100 carriers of CF mutations of the same ethnic group. These 22 mutations can be used for diagnosis of CF. Two additional mutations (S549N and 2184delA) that account for less than 0.1% of CF alleles may also be used for diagnosis.[240]

samples support these incidence figures. A higher incidence of CF has been reported in certain groups, such as Celts living in Brittany, France (1 in 377), Afrikaners living in southwest Africa (1 in 622), and French-Canadians from the Sauguenay-Lac St. Jean region in Canada (1 in 895).[70,519,591] Presumably, genetic drift and/or founder effect account for the high incidence in these groups.

CF is less frequent in native Asian, African, and American populations, although reliable incidence figures are not available. Our understanding of the disease is primarily through reports of one or a few patients.[79,262,375,394,545] CF has also been reported in individuals of Lebanese, Indian, Arabian, Korean, and Chinese descent.[137]

Deleterious mutations in CFTR have been discovered in all human populations.[3] Disease-causing alterations in CFTR fall into three "frequency" categories; the common mutation (ΔF508); less common mutations, and rare mutations. The ΔF508 mutation was the first CF mutation identified and accounts for about 70 percent of CF alleles in European-derived Caucasian populations.[1,3] The mutation is virtually absent in native African and Asian populations, although it reaches an appreciable frequency in groups with considerable Caucasian admixture, such as African-Americans.[155] The frequency of the ΔF508 mutation varies among European populations with an apparent gradient of increasing frequency from southeast to northwest Europe (30 percent in Turkey and Israel, 40 to 50 percent in southern Italy, 70 percent in middle Europe to 85 to 88 percent in Denmark and parts of the British Isles).[210] This mutation appears to have occurred only once during human evolution.[188,330,431] Estimates of the age of the ΔF508 mutation have been debated, but it probably occurred after divergence of the races, thereby accounting in part for its unequal distribution among human populations.[429,547] The high frequency of the ΔF508 mutation indicates that about half of all Caucasian patients with CF will be homozygous for this mutation. Indeed, in the absence of the ΔF508 mutation, CF would be a relatively rare genetic disorder in Caucasians, and would occur at approximately the same frequency in all races (< 1 in 10,000).

It has been suggested that the high frequency of CF in Caucasians may be due to an advantage of the CF heterozygote. In support of selective advantage, it has been shown that mice carrying a single CF mutation are more resistant to the secretory diarrhea caused by cholera infection.[235] But this observation has been challenged.[152] Cholera and secretory diarrhea occur in all human populations and therefore, it is not clear how this

Table 201-4 The Incidence of CF in Various Populations

Country	Incidence	References
Epidemiologic Studies		
Caucasian		
Australia	1 in 2450; 1 in 2550	662, 663
Czechoslovakia	1 in 2600; 1 in 3300	664, 665
Brittany, France	1 in 1800	195
England: Caucasian	1 in 2400 to 1 in 3000	666–668
Germany	1 in 3300	669
Israel	1 in 5000	670
Italy	1 in 2000	671
Mexico	1 in 8000 to 1 in 9000	672
Northern Ireland	1 in 1700; 1 in 1900	673, 674
South Africa	1 in 6500	675
Sweden	1 in 7700	676
United States	1 in 1900 to 1 in 3700	98
Admixed		
Asian-English	1 in 10,000	677
African-American	1 in 15,000; 1 in 12,000	98, 678
Non-Caucasian		
Asian (Hawaii)	1 in 90,000	679
Asian (Japan)	1 in 323,000	680
Newborn Screening		
Australia: New South Wales	1 in 3060	681
New Zealand	1 in 4140	682
United States: Colorado	1 in 3827	683
United States: Wisconsin	1 in 3431	684
Italy: Veneto	1 in 3944	685, 686
England: Peterboro	1 in 3190	685
England: East Anglia	1 in 2234	687

mechanism would increase the frequency of CF alleles in only one race but not others. Furthermore, one would speculate that any mutation that reduces CFTR function would confer resistance. Why ΔF508 was preferred to other mutations is not explained by the cholera hypotheses. There is also the observation that a different mutation, W1282X, is the most common mutation in the Ashkenazi population.[15,554] Other proposed advantages of heterozygotes include higher fertility, reduced rates of asthma, and resistance to a variety of infectious agents.[501,536] However, each proposal lacks confirmatory evidence.

A mechanism completely different from heterozygote selection has been suggested by the observation that not only ΔF508, but a number of the less common mutations in Caucasians have arisen on the same chromosomal background.[188,330] Thus, CF alleles may have been selected on the basis of a variation elsewhere in the gene or in a nearby gene.[546] The latter phenomenon has been termed the hitch-hiking effect and has been previously suggested as a mechanism for the high frequency of CF.[608,636] Analysis of haplotypes created by DNA markers flanking the CFTR gene in young and elderly individuals from a stable European population revealed that females with the same haplotype found in common with ΔF508 and other CF alleles had the highest survival rate.[396] Studies of another stable Caucasian population is required to confirm that a sequence near the CFTR gene confers a survival advantage to females. Other theories for the high frequency of CF include sex ratio distortion and segregation distortion in favor of mutant alleles.[339,478] Experimental evidence has not supported either theory. Thus, the high frequency of CF and in particular, the ΔF508 mutation, in the Caucasian population remains a mystery.

There are a group of about 20 "less common" mutations that occur with a worldwide frequency of 0.1 percent or higher (Table 201-3). The relative frequencies of each mutation depends upon the population, with certain mutations accounting for 5 percent or more of CF alleles in some groups.[3] DNA haplotype analysis has shown that most of the less common mutations, like ΔF508, have occurred once during human evolution.[504] Therefore, the high frequency of a "less common" CF mutation in a particular group may be due to founder effect (e.g., W1282X in Askenazi populations) or genetic drift (e.g., G551D in Celts, 3120 +1G → A in African/Mediterranean populations).[187,273,334] However, some mutations appear to have occurred more than once.[338,430] In a number of cases (e.g., R117H, R1162X), the codon involved contained a CG dinucleotide, a known hotspot for DNA mutation. The rate of new mutations seems to be quite low, as expected for a recessive disorder. Only one *de novo* mutation (R851X) has been reported so far.[654]

A select set of CF alleles reach an appreciable frequency in non-Caucasian populations. In African-Americans, seven mutations account for 3 to 13 percent of CF alleles. Most of these mutations have not been observed in Caucasians, suggesting African origin.[397] The ΔF508 mutation is found in 37 percent of African-Americans and is the likely result of admixture with Caucasians. Similarly, one mutation (1898+5G → T) has been found in 3 of 10 CFTR genes from Chinese patients.[700] Finally, three mutations have been shown to account for all CF alleles in a tribe of native Americans.[255,424]

The remainder of the mutations (94 percent) are termed rare. Most have been found in only one or a few individuals. However, about 30 mutations reach an appreciable frequency (>0.1 percent) in a specific population probably as a result of founder effect.[3] An excellent example is the Y112X mutation which accounts for 48 percent of CF alleles in the Reunion Island, but is rare elsewhere.[115]

At least two cases of CF have been reported due to inheritance of both copies of chromosome 7 from one parent (uniparental isodisomy).[574,634] The parent in each case was a heterozygous carrier of a CF mutation, thereby giving rise to a homozygous affected child.[57] Although an interesting genetic phenomenon, this form of inheritance is extremely rare and should not be used to alter the risk estimates for healthy carriers of CF alleles.[641]

DIAGNOSIS

Clinical Diagnosis

Until recently, the diagnosis of cystic fibrosis has been based on carefully defined clinical criteria and accurate analysis of sweat Cl^- levels.[161] The availability in the past decade of mutational analyses within the CF gene locus[3] and assessment of the bioelectric properties of respiratory epithelia by measurement of nasal transepithelial electrical potential difference[343] have expanded the clinical spectrum of CF to include individuals with atypical, less severe phenotypic presentations.

To address the evolving diagnosis of this genetic disorder, a panel of clinical and genetic experts was convened in 1997 by the Cystic Fibrosis Foundation (CFF). It was the consensus of this panel that the criteria for the diagnosis of CF should include "the presence of one or more characteristic phenotypic features (Table 201-5), a history of CF in a sibling or a positive newborn screening test result, plus laboratory evidence of a CFTR abnormality as documented by elevated sweat Cl^- concentration, or identification of mutations in each CFTR gene known to cause CF or *in vivo* demonstration of characteristic abnormalities in ion transport across the nasal epithelium."[516]

The majority of patients are still diagnosed because of the presence of clinical features (Table 201-5). The classic symptom constellation includes chronic suppurative sinopulmonary disease and pancreatic insufficiency. The most common clinical presentations in the United States at diagnosis[9] included persistent respiratory symptoms (51.2 percent), failure to thrive (43.0 percent), steatorrhea (35.1 percent), and meconium ileus (18.6 percent). Positive family history, with or without clinical

Table 201-5 Phenotypic Features Consistent with a Diagnosis of CF

1. Chronic sinopulmonary disease manifested by
   a. Persistent colonization/infection with typical CF pathogens including *Staphylococcus aureus*, nontypeable *Haemophilus influenzae*, mucoid and nonmucoid *Pseudomonas aeruginosa*, and *Burkholderia cepacia*
   b. Chronic cough and sputum production
   c. Persistent chest radiograph abnormalities (e.g., bronchiectasis, atelectasis, infiltrates, hyperinflation)
   d. Airway obstruction manifested by wheezing and air trapping
   e. Nasal polyps; radiographic or computed tomographic abnormalities of the paranasal sinuses
   f. Digital clubbing
2. Gastrointestinal and nutritional abnormalities including
   a. Intestinal: meconium ileus, distal intestinal obstruction syndrome, rectal prolapse
   b. Pancreatic: pancreatic insufficiency, recurrent pancreatitis
   c. Hepatic: chronic hepatic disease manifested by clinical or histologic evidence of focal biliary cirrhosis or multilobular cirrhosis
   d. Nutritional: failure to thrive (protein-calorie malnutrition), hypoproteinemia and edema, complications secondary to fat-soluble vitamin deficiency
3. Salt loss syndromes: acute salt depletion, chronic metabolic alkalosis
4. Male urogenital abnormalities resulting in obstructive azoospermia (CBAVD)

symptomatology, was reported in 17 percent of cases. Other presenting symptoms include sinus disease (2.4 percent), liver disease (1 percent), obstructive azoospermia in post-pubertal males (prevalence not provided), and electrolyte imbalance (5.3 percent).

There are several settings where the diagnosis of CF may now be ascertained in the absence of clinical features. A sibling of an affected individual has a 25 percent chance of having the disorder and half siblings are also at increased risk (Caucasians 1:112, African-Americans 1:244, and Asian Americans 1:352).[272] Screening of such individuals with mutational analysis (if both mutations are identified in the affected individual) or sweat test is appropriate in the absence of clinical symptoms. Several newborn screening programs in the United States, as well as worldwide are now including tests for CF (see "Newborn Screening for CF" below). In utero diagnosis, based upon evidence for two CF mutations, has become increasingly common and attributed to 1 percent of new diagnoses in the United States in 1997. Prenatal testing may become even more common as carrier testing of the general population increases.

The sweat test[579] remains the most widely used confirmatory laboratory test in CF, and Cl^- concentration in sweat will accurately diagnose over 90 percent of cases. Guidelines for appropriate performance of the quantitative pilocarpine iontophoresis sweat test procedure have been published by the National Committee for Clinical Laboratory Standards.[371,644] Alternative sweat test procedures are no longer acceptable for the diagnosis of CF. CFF accredited care centers are required to adhere to these guidelines. The test involves collection of sweat by pilocarpine iontophoresis with chemical determination of Cl^- concentration. A minimum acceptable volume (15 μl for the Wescor Maroduct Coil System) or weight (75 mg) of sweat must be collected during a 30 minute period to assure a sweat rate of at least 1 $gm/M^2/min$. A sweat Cl^- level of greater than 60 mM on two separate occasions is considered diagnostic. Levels greater than 160 mM are not physiologically possible and should be considered a technical error. Sweat Na^+ concentrations do not provide additional diagnostic information.

Molecular Diagnosis

Genetic testing for CF generally takes place for one of two reasons; to assist a clinical evaluation or to evaluate an individual who has an increased risk of carrying a CF allele. In the first situation, identification of CF mutations can have diagnostic and prognostic value. New criteria allow genetic information to be used to establish a CF diagnosis in patients with a compatible phenotype (see "Clinical Diagnosis" above).[516] A list of mutations that can be used to confirm a CF diagnosis (Table 201-3) is primarily composed of alterations that have been shown to affect gene function.[516] However, it is anticipated that the list will be expanded considerably in the near future utilizing guidelines outlined in "Mutations in the CFTR Gene" above. Mutation identification can also be useful in patients with atypical CF who have clinical features consistent with CF, but a normal sweat chloride concentration. For example, the splice-site mutation 3849+10 kb C→T has been associated with the atypical phenotype.[285] Other clinical presentations where mutation identification may be useful include male infertility due to congenital bilateral absence of the vas deferens (CBAVD) and idiopathic pancreatitis.[116,130] Knowing that a patient with these phenotypes carries a CF mutation has implications for diagnosis, for family members, and when planning a pregnancy. However, it should be kept in mind that patients with CBAVD and pancreatitis usually carry only one CF mutation. If these patients carry a mutation in their other CFTR gene, it frequently is unusual and therefore not included in the standard CF mutation panel. Therefore, analysis of all coding regions of CFTR may be warranted in patients with CBAVD and idiopathic pancreatitis.

Two conditions in the perinatal period can trigger a genetic evaluation for CF; fetal echogenic bowel and elevated neonatal immunoreactive trypsinogen (IRT) level. Fetal echogenic bowel is a consequence of intestinal blockage which can be due to meconium ileus.[433] Meconium ileus affects 15 to 20 percent of CF infants, however the frequency of echogenic bowel in CF fetuses is unknown. On the other hand, estimates of the frequency of CF in fetuses with echogenic bowel vary between 1 percent and 33 percent.[209,289] Even if the frequency of CF is only 1 percent in patients with echogenic bowel, it is considerably higher than the frequency of CF in a fetus without echogenic bowel (0.03 percent). Genetic testing for CF mutations can be performed upon the parents or upon fetal cells, if available. Neonatal CF screening programs identify infants with elevated IRT levels. Genetic testing is used by many programs as a second step to optimize specificity and sensitivity of the screen for CF (see "Newborn Screening for CF").

For patients with echogenic bowel or elevated IRT, identification of two CF mutations indicates a CF diagnosis, while absence of CF mutations substantially reduces the chance of CF. However, the discovery of a single CF mutation presents a dilemma. For the fetus with echogenic bowel, one must weigh the chance that a second CF mutation is present in the fetus but not detected by the mutation panel, against the possibility that the fetus is a CF carrier and has echogenic bowel due to reasons other than CF. A numerical risk for CF can be derived from a Bayesian calculation. In the case of the neonate with a high IRT level and one CF mutation, a sweat test can be performed to confirm a CF diagnosis. Interestingly, there appears to be a higher than expected rate of CF carriers with high IRT levels.[106,368]

Carrier identification is generally performed to assess the risk of transmitting CF mutations to offspring. Individuals with a family history of CF have a higher risk of being a CF carrier, than the general population; they may therefore desire mutation testing to refine their risk. For example, a Caucasian individual who has a first cousin with CF has a 1 in 16 chance of being a CF carrier versus 1 in 28 in the general Caucasian population. Screening of the family member for the panel of common CF mutations is likely to reveal whether the individual is a carrier. However, to fully evaluate risk when the mutation test is negative, it is important to know the CF genotype of the affected member. Carrier status can be confidently excluded if the administered test included both mutations carried by the affected member. On the other hand, if one or both mutations carried by the affected member are not included in the test, then a negative result may not exclude carrier status. Bayesian analysis can be used to provide a risk estimate that takes into account the relationship of the family member to the affected member and ethnic background.[170] When mutation-based tests are inconclusive, linkage analysis can be performed using DNA markers that flank, or are within, the CFTR gene.[58] Linkage testing requires the involvement of multiple family members to establish inheritance pattern of the DNA markers relative to the mutated CFTR genes. The status of the DNA markers reveals whether an individual has inherited one of the mutated CFTR genes segregating in their family. Linkage analysis can predict carrier status with high accuracy in almost all families but incurs greater effort and expense than mutation analysis. Therefore, linkage studies are used only when mutation analysis is not informative.

Prenatal genetic testing is usually performed for couples where both members are carriers and therefore have a 1 in 4 risk of having a child with CF. Mutation analysis of both parents and the fetus can establish whether the fetus has inherited an at-risk genotype. The counseling situation becomes more complicated for genotypes associated with atypical forms of CF. For example, the parents of a fetus with the genotype ΔF508/R117H-7T will have to be informed that their child might develop mild CF or may be asymptomatic if the fetus is female. On the other hand, this genotype is likely to cause infertility if the fetus is male.[338] Couples in which one member is a known carrier and the other member tests negative also present a challenge. Although a negative test substantially reduces the chance that an individual is a carrier, the lack of a test with 100 percent specificity leaves the couple with residual risk (about 1 in 1000), that is higher than the risk for couples in the general population (1 in 3200 for Caucasians). Infertile men with absent or malformed vas deferens who are considering sperm aspiration for insemination of their partner should be tested for CF mutations. Identification of a mutation in the infertile man should prompt CF mutation screening of the other partner to assess their risk of having a child with CF.

Population-based carrier screening for CF has been debated since the cloning of the CFTR gene.[56,666] A consensus conference was convened by the NIH to review the results of the pilot programs and to assess the issue of population-wide CF screening.[10] The panel of physicians, health care professionals, public policy experts, and lay individuals concurred with the practice of offering screening to family members of a CF patient and to partners of individuals with CF, but extended the recommendation to include couples seeking prenatal testing and those planning a pregnancy.[10]

Genetic testing can be performed upon DNA from a variety of sources; buccal mucosal cells, peripheral blood cells, dried blood cells on Guthrie cards, amniocytes, chorionic villus cells, and surgical specimens preserved in paraffin. Most commercial and academic DNA diagnostic laboratories in Europe and North America test for the ΔF508 mutation and a core of mutations that are found in virtually all Caucasian groups worldwide (e.g., G542X, G551D, R553X, W1282X, N1303K).[175,261] Testing of European Caucasians can be tailored to the mutations know to exist at high frequency in a particular region. For example, 17 mutations account for 94 percent of CF alleles in Belgians, testing for 19 mutations detects 98 percent in Celts living in Brittany while nearly complete detection is attained in Wales by testing for 29 mutations.[112,218,423] Caucasian populations in North America are derived from various parts of Europe and therefore, have a wider range of CF alleles. Some DNA diagnostic laboratories offer a large panel of CF mutations with claims of detection rates approaching 90 percent in the heterogenous US Caucasian population. However, mutation frequency data from several sources indicate that testing for more than 20 to 30 of the common mutations achieves only marginal increases in sensitivity in heterogeneous Caucasian populations (Table 201-3). DNA testing of individuals of Asian or African background for Caucasian CF alleles has a predictably low sensitivity. However, detection rates of 75 percent can be achieved in African-Americans by testing for "Caucasian" CF alleles and mutations that appear to originate from Native Africans.[397] To guide clinicians and testing laboratories in the choice of CF mutation tests, the American College of Medical Genetics has appointed a Laboratory Standards Committee for CF Genetic Testing. The charge of the committee is to provide recommendations for a standard panel of CF mutations that optimizes detection rates for the Caucasian and non-Caucasian populations in North America.

Nasal Potential Difference Measurements

Respiratory epithelia, like epithelial tissues in other organs, regulate the ion and water content of surface fluid by active ion transport mechanisms. These ionic movements create a transepithelial electric potential difference. Absence of functional CFTR at the apical surface and the resultant decreased Cl^- efflux and Na^+ hyperabsorption result in an abnormal electrical potential difference measurement across the epithelia of individuals with CF. Due to the accessibility of nasal epithelial tissue, the distinct pattern of nasal potential differences (PD) recorded from patients with CF is well defined (Fig. 201-13).[343] Nasal PD has been widely utilized as a biologic marker demonstrating correction of CFTR Cl^- channel function in clinical trials of new therapies.[100] It has also been accepted as an alternative diagnostic test, which may complement the use of the sweat test and mutational analysis. Nasal PD is most helpful in patients with an atypical presentation who have a normal or borderline sweat test (Cl^- value 40 to 60 mM) and do not have two identified genetic mutations associated with CF.[672]

There are three features which distinguish CF nasal PD measurements from unaffected individuals:[343,516] (1) raised (more negative) baseline PD reflecting enhanced Na^+ transport across a membrane relatively impermeable to Cl^-, (2) greater change in PD following perfusion of nasal mucosa with amiloride, an inhibitor of Na^+ channel activity, and (3) lack of change in PD in response to perfusion of the epithelial surface with a Cl^--free solution followed by a beta agonist, which results in cAMP-mediated Cl^- transport (via CFTR) in normal epithelia.

The protocol for nasal PD measurement is well described and standardized[343] and safely performed in many accredited CF care centers worldwide. Yet, it is technically difficult and requires extensive experience for proper conduct and interpretation. Development of reference values at each center is also necessary. Several potential pitfalls may lead to misinterpretation of results. Because the nasal mucosal surface is composed of a heterogeneous population of cell types, varying from squamous to ciliated columnar epithelial cells, proper placement of the probe under the anterior turbinate must be strictly adhered. Inflammation will alter bioelectrical properties of nasal mucosa and may result in false negative results. Any test result suggestive of CF must be duplicated at a second time for confirmation.

Ancillary Tests to Support the Diagnosis of CF

With the availability of the three laboratory modalities (sweat test, mutation analysis, and NPD) described above, the diagnosis of cystic fibrosis is readily achieved in almost all cases. Several ancillary tests, such as stool trypsin, used in the past to support the diagnosis are no longer necessary. However, further diagnostic

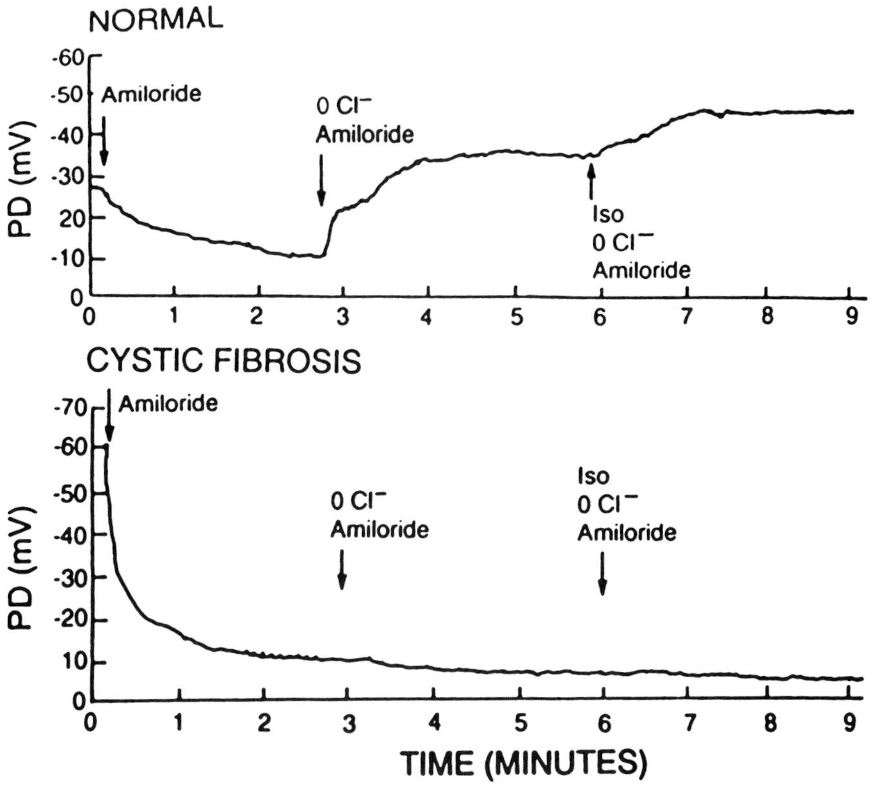

Fig. 201-13 Nasal PD tracing in a normal subject (top panel) and a patient with CF (bottom panel). Tracings illustrate response of nasal PD to perfusion with amiloride (10^{-4} mol/L), addition of a Cl^--free solution (gluconate buffer) to amiloride, and addition of isoproterenol (10^{-5} mol/L) to the Cl^--free solution containing amiloride.

evaluation to define clearly the phenotypic expression and degree of organ dysfunction in each newly diagnosed patient is essential for development of an optimal treatment regimen. Further testing should include assessment of pancreatic and respiratory tract status and in postpubertal males an evaluation of the male genital tract.

An assessment of pulmonary status should include a characterization of respiratory microbial flora, measurement of pulmonary function and imaging studies to define the presence and extent of bronchiectasis. As described above, patients with CF have a predilection for chronic colonization with *P. aeruginosa*, especially mucoid phenotypes, and commonly are colonized with *S. aureus* and *H. influenza*.[161]

Obstructive azoospermia is present in over 97 percent of postpubertal males with CF as a result of absence of the vas deferens. It is essential that all males diagnosed after puberty receive appropriate counseling regarding fertility and a careful urologic examination, including semen analysis. Individuals with the diagnosis of CBAVD usually have no other findings of CF, but may have an elevated or intermediate sweat test.[116] These individuals may require a complete diagnostic evaluation, including sweat test, mutational analysis, and nasal PD measurement. They should only be given the diagnosis of CF if they fulfill the criteria outlined by the CFF consensus group above.

Newborn Screening for CF

Rationale for Newborn Screening. Most individuals with CF are diagnosed conventionally, that is only after symptoms appear. These symptoms frequently are accompanied by conditions that may not be reversible, including poor growth and chronic respiratory infection. In addition, conventional diagnosis is often delayed. Examination of the US Cystic Fibrosis Foundation registry shows that if patients with meconium ileus and family history are removed from consideration, the median age of conventional diagnosis is greater than a year.[9] One quarter of all patients are identified after three years of age. Several problems are associated with this delay in diagnosis. Patients may have had potentially treatable symptoms for months or years before they are diagnosed. Parents are often burdened with not understanding what is wrong with their child leading to frequent physician contacts and sometimes hospitalizations. The rationale for newborn screening for CF, then, stems from the potential benefits of early diagnosis. Anticipated benefits of early diagnosis include improved short and long-term outcomes, avoidance of complications of conventional diagnosis, reduction in parental anxiety before diagnosis is made, and greater choice in reproductive decision making. Before newborn screening and early diagnosis of CF is accepted as public health policy, however, important laboratory, medical and ethical questions need to be addressed. The most important question is whether early diagnosis through newborn screening results in direct benefit to individuals with CF. Studies over the past two decades have addressed many of the issues concerning newborn screening for CF and are briefly reviewed here.

Current Approaches to Newborn Screening for CF. Almost all newborn screening programs for CF begin with determination of immunoreactive trypsinogen (IRT), a presumed marker of pancreatic dysfunction, from a dried blood spot taken within a few days after birth.[663] In general, infants with CF have elevations of IRT (hypertrypsinogenemia) compared to normal infants. Although, the pathophysiology of hypertrypsinogenemia is not completely understood, it is thought that pancreatic acini in infants with CF are capable of producing IRT but ductules are blocked leading to "spillage" into the circulation. As individuals with CF age, IRT decreases and often is below the normal range indicating that pancreatic acini are not functioning well enough to produce enzyme. Thus, IRT is useful in screening for CF only in infancy.

A single elevation of IRT soon after birth is not specific for CF since many normal infants will demonstrate transient elevations. It was soon appreciated that infants with CF have persistent elevations of IRT and hence most early screening programs recalled infants for a second IRT at a few weeks of age greatly increasing the specificity. Sweat testing was then performed to establish the diagnosis of CF. A number of screening programs around the world demonstrated that by measuring two IRT levels (IRT/IRT approach) coupled with sweat testing, a sensitivity in the range of 95 percent in the target population could be achieved.[663] The IRT/IRT approach identifies both pancreatic sufficient and insufficient infants. Interestingly, infants with meconium ileus frequently have values below the threshold for elevated IRT. This is not clinically significant since these patients are almost all identified soon after birth and hence are not targets of screening. It has also become clear from screening programs that sweat testing is easily accomplished in the great majority of term infants after a week of age, laying to rest the concern that sweat tests cannot be performed until several months of age.[213]

There are two major difficulties with the IRT/IRT approach. The very high false positive rate on the first sample leads to anxiety in the large number of parents of infants who turn out not to have CF. In addition, the delay following notification of the need for a second IRT until the test results are back is a period of anxiety for all parents.

Incorporation of mutation analysis into newborn screening for CF deals with the two major problems of the IRT/IRT approach and hence is used by most screening programs.[258] With this approach, patients are identified through elevated IRT and have mutation analysis performed on the same blood spot (IRT/DNA approach). If the infant is found to carry two CF mutations then the diagnosis is made and supported by a sweat test. If the infant carries only one CF mutation then sweat testing is needed for diagnosis. If no mutations are detected then the infant is presumed not to have CF. The sensitivity of this approach depends on the frequency of mutations in a given population and the number of mutations tested. In populations where the incidence of the ΔF508 is greater than 70 percent of alleles, sensitivities of above 90 percent can be achieved by testing for this mutation alone. Several programs have improved sensitivity by adding a panel of mutations.[107] There are two problems with the IRT/DNA approach. One is the obligate false negative rate that arises from the limit on the number of mutations tested. The second problem is that carriers of CF mutations often demonstrate hypertrypsinogenemia. IRT/DNA testing detects carriers at approximately three times the rate it detects infants with CF, greatly increasing the genetic counseling needed as part of the screening program. Most programs view carrier detection as an unwanted side effect of IRT/DNA screening. There has been concern that newborn screening carries the risk of psychological harm to families of infants who are false positive or have presymptomatic CF, but the weight of evidence now is that the psychological effects of screening do not cause undue harm.[49]

Clinical Course of Infants with CF Identified through Newborn Screening. Follow-up of infants identified through newborn screening has provided important information about the natural history of CF as well as insight into early pathophysiology. Most infants have gastrointestinal symptoms at diagnosis.[245] Reduced growth can be appreciated by two months of age. Sixty percent of infants have significant fat malabsorption by that age and the degree of malabsorption is related to reduced growth.[88] This suggests that the mechanism of poor growth is related to early malabsorption. A variety of biochemical markers of undernutrition are abnormally low by two months of age in approximately a third of infants; these include fat soluble vitamins, total body K^+, linoleic acid, albumin, prealbumin, and trace elements.[361] Given this picture, it is not surprising that infants with CF diagnosed conventionally may have severe vitamin deficiency or protein calorie malnutrition leading to edema and hypoproteinemia.[664] In addition to nutritional abnormalities, infants with CF identified through newborn screening often have evidence of marked airway infection and inflammation suggesting that lung disease in infants is similar to that in adults and older children.[34] Taken together these early abnormalities strongly suggest the need for early treatment.

Long-Term Outcome of Infants Identified through Newborn Screening. Several observational studies have suggested improved growth and pulmonary function and decreased morbidity in infants identified through newborn screening. However, the most compelling evidence of benefit from early diagnosis comes from the Wisconsin study.[214] In this study, essentially all infants born in Wisconsin over a period of ten years were screened for CF, but only half of families were informed of the diagnosis soon after birth. The other half of families were informed at four years if their child was not clinically identified before that age. This study showed unequivocally that growth is improved at least through ten years of age through early diagnosis. Given the extent of early malabsorption, it is not surprising that early treatment with pancreatic enzymes and close follow-up of growth, as performed in the Wisconsin study, would lead to an improved outcome.

Current Controversies in Newborn Screening for CF. A recent Center for Disease Control workshop reviewed the current status of newborn screening for CF with respect to laboratory and medical issues.[5] This workshop came to the conclusion that the demonstration of improved growth was not sufficient to recommend newborn screening as a general public health policy. More evidence was needed with respect to pulmonary function or neurodevelopmental outcome before endorsement of screening. The neurodevelopmental outcome is important because at least two studies have shown decreased head circumference in some children with CF that may be related to early impaired growth.[214,244] The workshop did recommend, however, that there is sufficient basis for statewide pilot projects to investigate methods of testing and approaches to clinical care of infants identified through screening. The World Health Organization council on CF has also called for international pilot projects of newborn screening for CF to determine incidence of the disease as well as to identify affected infants.[7] It is generally recognized that improved pulmonary treatments may drive newborn screening and early diagnosis. If it turns out that colonization with *P. aeruginosa* can be delayed by early intervention or if other pulmonary treatments can delay the development of lung disease, then it is likely that screening will be more widely adopted.

CFTR

Structure of the CFTR Protein

The primary amino acid sequence of CFTR509 places it in a family of transport proteins called ATP-binding cassette (ABC) transporters.[183,303] Members of the ABC transporter family are found in all three kingdoms, including archaea, eubacteria, and eukaryotes. In some organisms, such as *Escherichia coli*, they form the largest family of paralogous proteins. Mutations in ABC transporters are increasingly recognized as the cause of human genetic diseases; examples include, hyperinsulinemic hypoglycemia due to mutations in the sulfonylurea receptor (SUR1) (MIM 600509), Stargardt macular dystrophy due to mutations in the retina-specific ABC transporter (ABCR) (Chap. 243), Zellweger syndrome due to mutations in the 70 K peroxisomal membrane protein (Chap. 129),[240] X-linked adrenoleukodystrophy due to mutations in the adrenoleukodystrophy protein (ALDP) (Chap. 131), familial intrahepatic cholestasis due to mutations in the bile salt export pump (BSEP) (MIM 601847, 603201), Dubin Johnson syndrome due to mutations in the canalicular multispecific organic anion transporter (cMOAT) (Chap. 125), and Tangier disease due to mutations in ABC1 (Chap. 122). This list will surely continue to lengthen.

ABC transporters contain two nucleotide-binding domains (NBDs) and two membrane-spanning domain (MSDs). The NBDs, which share sequence similarity among diverse members of the family, are the defining characteristic of ABC transporters. In ABC transporters, the NBDs bind and hydrolyze ATP, using the energy for active transmembrane substrate transport and/or to produce conformational changes in the MSDs. The MSDs share little if any sequence between unrelated family members. However, MSD topology is similar in that most but not all are composed of six transmembrane segments. The MSDs confer specific transport functions on individual ABC transporters. Thus, in ABC transporters the NBDs serve as conserved engines that power a wide variety of different machines, including pumps, regulators, and, in the case of CFTR, a channel.[652]

Similarity to other ABC transporters allowed Riordan et al.[509] to propose a structure for CFTR that turned out to be remarkably prescient. Figure 201-14 shows a model. In the linear amino acid structure of CFTR, the sequence of domains is MSD1, NBD1, R domain, MSD2, and NBD2. The R (regulatory) domain is a unique sequence that contains multiple phosphorylation sites and many charged amino acids. The NBDs, the R domain, and the N- and C-termini are intracellular, and the membrane topology of the six membrane-spanning sequences in each MSD has been elucidated.[110,174] Although the tertiary structure of CFTR domains is not known, insight and clues have come from functional studies of CFTR bearing site-directed mutations. In addition, solution of the NBD structure of the *Salmonella typhimurium* histidine permease[302] provides a starting point for further exploration of CFTR structure.

Cl^- Channel Function of CFTR

Compelling evidence demonstrates that CFTR is a Cl^- channel. When investigators express recombinant CFTR in cells that do not normally express CFTR they generate unique Cl^- currents. These currents have biophysical and regulator properties similar to those observed in epithelial cells expressing endogenous CFTR.[23,323] Moreover, mutation of specific residues in CFTR alters anion permeability and regulation in specific ways.[22,162] In addition, when isolated purified recombinant CFTR is reconstituted into planar lipid bilayers it forms Cl^- channels with properties similar to those in native epithelia.[55]

The CFTR Cl^- channel displays several distinguishing characteristics (Fig. 201-15): (1) It has a small single-channel conductance of 6 to 10 pS. (2) The current-voltage (I-V) relationship is linear. (3) The channel is selective for anions over cations. (4) The anion permeability sequence is $Br^- \geq Cl^- > I^-$. (5) Gating is time- and voltage-independent. (6) Activity is regulated by cAMP-dependent phosphorylation and by intracellular nucleoside triphosphates.

Contribution of the MSDs to Channel Function. The properties of CFTR Cl^- channels have been discovered in studies using the patch-clamp technique. The channels show selectivity for anions over cations, with a Na^+ to Cl^- permeability ratio of 0.1 to 0.03.[162] CFTR is a multi-ion pore that contains at least two anions simultaneously. The anion permeability sequence is $Br^- \geq Cl^- > I^- > F^-$;[22] the apparent I^- to Cl^- permeability is influenced by the ability of I^- to block the pore.[594] This sequence distinguishes CFTR Cl^- channels from several other epithelial Cl^- channels that have a higher permeability to I^- than Cl^-.[24,162] Water and urea may also permeate the channel,[280] and there are conflicting reports about the ability of ATP to permeate through CFTR.[457,498,539,596] Although there are no highly specific agents that block CFTR; DPC, glibenclamide, large anions, and MOPS can block the channel and have been used to probe its structure.[307,537]

A model of the CFTR pore is beginning to emerge.[162,551] Functional studies suggest that the pore has a narrow portion, ≈5.3 Å,[381] that may be flanked by large intracellular and extracellular vestibules. Because mutation of specific residues in M1, M5, M6, and M12 alter conductance, permeation, and open-channel block, these transmembrane segments appear to contribute to the pore.[14,162,550,551] Recent studies have shown that mutations of arginine 347, a site of four CF-associated mutations, alter conduction properties, but not because this residue contributes directly to the pore. Instead, mutations at this site alter pore architecture, possibly by disrupting a salt bridge.[144] Thus, mutations in the MSDs can change the properties of the pore in many different ways. In contrast, mutation of specific residues within the NBDs and R domain have had little discernible effect on conduction and permeation, despite their profound effects on gating. These findings suggest that the NBDs and R domain do not contribute directly to the pore.

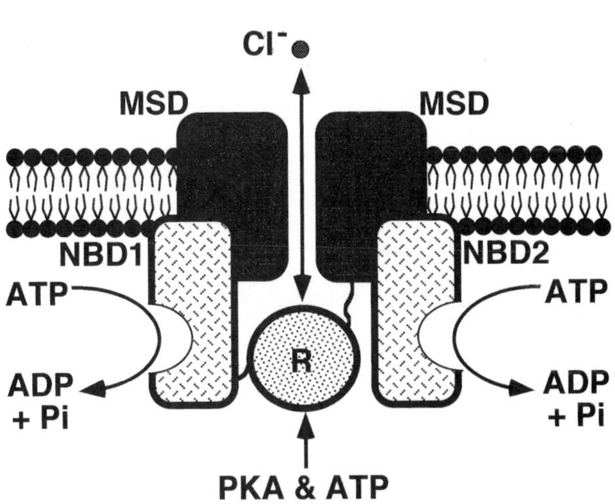

Fig. 201-14 Model showing the proposed domain structure of CFTR. MSD refers to a membrane-spanning domain, NBD refers to a nucleotide-binding domain, and R refers to regulatory domain. PKA refers to cAMP-dependent protein kinase.

Contribution of the NBDs to ATP-dependent Gating. The NBDs contain two highly conserved sequences that bind and hydrolyze intracellular ATP and convert the energy into channel gating; these include the Walker A (G-X-X-G-X-G-K) and Walker B (h-h-h-h-D, where *h* indicates a hydrophobic residue) motifs. CFTR and other ABC transporters also contain a conserved L-S-G-G-Q motif. Intracellular ATP is required for gating of phosphorylated CFTR Cl^- channels; nonhydrolyzable nucleoside analogs are not able to open the channel.[21,236] Figure 201-16 shows the effect of ATP concentration on the channel. As the cytosolic concentration increases, the open state probability increases because the mean closed-time between bursts of activity decreases. Biochemical studies of purified, reconstituted CFTR and NBD1 and NBD2 proteins also indicate that CFTR binds and hydrolyses ATP.[346,376,492] Although ATP interacts with both NBDs to control channel gating, the two NBDs are not functionally equivalent, and there is cooperative behavior between the two NBDs.[236,551]

The nonhydrolyzable ATP analog AMP-PNP, as well as pyrophosphate (PP_i), VO_4, and BeF_3 bind to phosphorylated channels in the presence of ATP, increasing Cl^- current by delaying the termination of bursts of activity.[54,103,264] These agents have asymmetric effects at the two NBDs. Most models of CFTR gating propose that ATP binding and/or hydrolysis at one NBD (probably NBD1) is a prerequisite for channel opening, and that ATP binding and/or hydrolysis at the other NBD (probably NBD2) is a prerequisite for channel closure. However, there is clearly crosstalk or cooperativity between the two NBDs, which makes distinction of their precise roles in gating difficult. There are at least two discrete open states, revealed by MOPS block, and at least two discrete closed states, revealed by kinetic analysis.[265,307] The data link the activity of the NBDs to alterations in the CFTR pore and indicate that input of external energy from ATP binding and/or hydrolysis causes a conformational change in the pore. Current models represent oversimplifications of how NBDs control the complex gating cycle. Additional functional and structural studies are required to better understand this process. Hopefully, the emerging data will also help us understand the function of other ABC transporters.

Contribution of the R Domain to Regulation by Phosphorylation. Regulation of channel activity is precisely controlled by

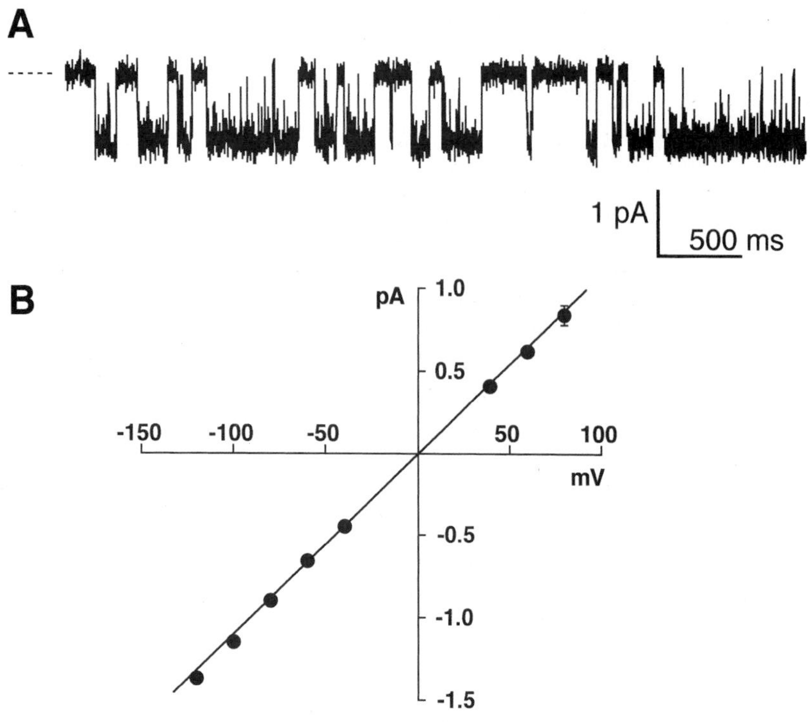

Fig. 201-15 Single-channel tracing and current-voltage relationship of wild-type CFTR. *A.* A 5 sec tracing from an excised, inside-out membrane patch containing a single CFTR Cl^- channel. Channel was activated by 1 mM ATP and 75 nM PKA. Membrane voltage was −80 mV. Dashed line indicates closed state, and downward deflections indicate channel openings. *B.* Current-voltage relationship of channel at 35°C with symmetrical 140 mM *N*-methyl-D-glucamine chloride. (A *was adapted from Cotten and Welsh.*[143] B *was adapted from Ishihara.*[307] *Used by permission.*)

the balance of kinase and phosphatase activity within cells.[236,551] The cAMP-dependent protein kinase (PKA) is the most important kinase responsible for regulating CFTR Cl^- channel activity.[114,464] However, several isoforms of protein kinase C (PKC) can phosphorylate and activate CFTR Cl^- channels, and may facilitate phosphorylation by PKA.[63,313] The type II cGMP-dependent protein kinase (cGKII) and the tyrosine kinase p60$^{c\text{-}src}$ can also phosphorylate and activate CFTR.[224,625] On removal or inactivation of a kinase, channel activity decreases due to dephosphorylation. In airway and intestinal epithelia, protein phosphatase 2A and 2C (PP2A, PP2C) probably play the most important role.[223,391,614] Protein phosphatase 1 (PP1) may play a more important role in dephosphorylating CFTR in the sweat gland duct.[497]

Although the R domain was originally defined as exon 13 (residues 590 to 830), sequence comparisons, deletion studies, and evaluation of site-directed mutations indicate that there are two parts to exon 13, the first shares some sequence with NBDs of ABC transporters, and the second (approximately amino acids 679 to 798) is unique to CFTR and may encompass the majority of the

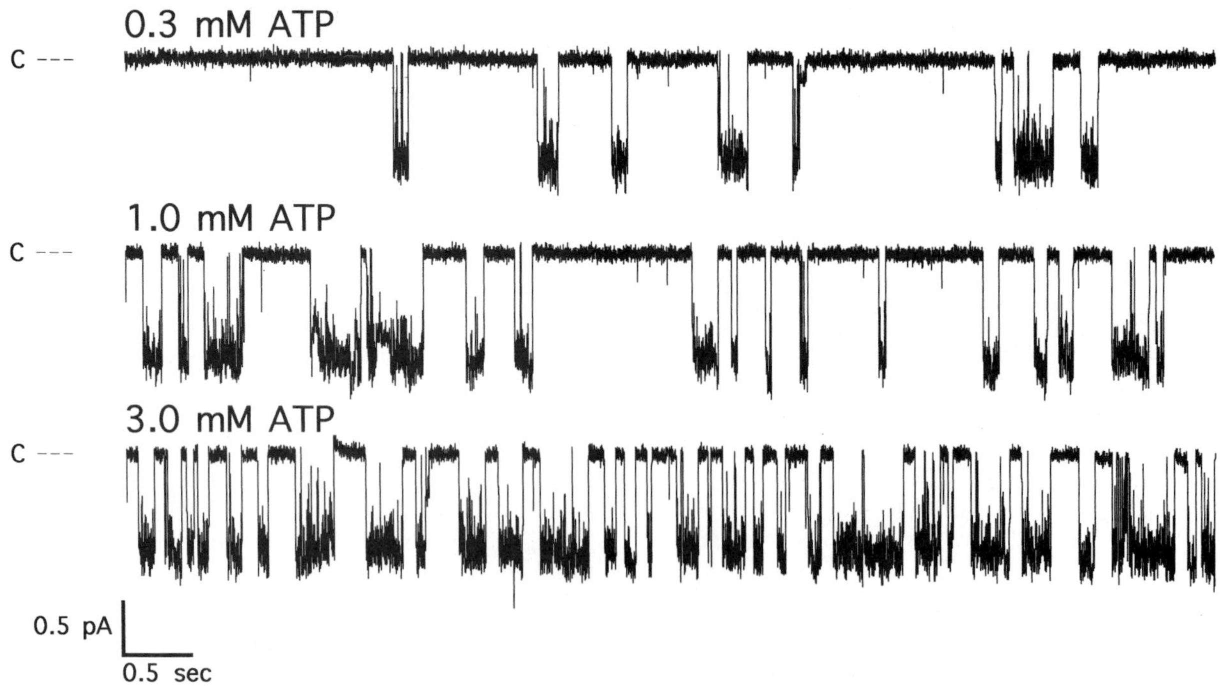

Fig. 201-16 Effect of cytosolic ATP concentration on CFTR Cl^- channel function. Single-channel currents recorded from an excised, inside-out patch. The bath (cytosolic) solution contained the indicated concentration of ATP. Dashed lines indicate the closed state; downward deflections represent channel opening. Voltage was −120 mV. (*Adapted from Winter, et al.*[676] *Used by permission.*)

phosphorylation-dependent "regulatory" function.[193,508] Five serines are phosphorylated by PKA *in vivo*: Ser660, Ser700, Ser737, Ser795, and Ser813.[114,464] When these residues are mutated to alanine, additional residues are phosphorylated.[542,613] PKC phosphorylates at least two serine residues *in vivo*, Ser686 and Ser700.[313,464]

A model of R domain function is now emerging. It appears that the R domain can have both inhibitory and stimulatory effects. Evidence for an inhibitory function came from the finding that deletion of residues 708 to 835 (CFTRΔR) produced Cl^- channels with biophysical properties similar to those of wild-type CFTR, with exceptions that were constitutively active in the presence of ATP, even without phosphorylation.[62,507] However, the activity of CFTRΔR is reduced compared with that of wild-type CFTR; this suggests that the R domain also possesses stimulatory activity. Consistent with this conclusion, adding a phosphorylated recombinant R domain protein (residues 645 to 834) to the intracellular solution stimulates CFTRΔR by increasing the rate of entry into bursts of activity (Fig. 201-17).[393,677] Only the phosphorylated R domain stimulates activity; the unphosphorylated R domain protein fails to stimulate and in some studies inhibits. Mutation of phosphorylation sites in wild-type CFTR had the opposite effect on the same kinetic step; the rate of channel opening into bursts was slowed and the relationship between ATP concentration and activity was altered.[677] Consistent with these data, phosphorylation enhances the ATPase activity of CFTR.[376] Interestingly, the channel is also stimulated when multiple negatively charged aspartates are substituted for serines in the R domain[506] and by covalent modification of the R domain by a neutral hydrophobic adduct, N-ethylmaleimide at residue C832.[143] Thus, multiple different structural alterations of the R domain are able to activate the channel.

These studies show that, the R domain does not function solely as an inhibitor that keeps the channel closed; it is not simply an "on-off" switch. When phosphorylation modifies the R domain, it might have two effects: the first might be permissive, releasing steric inhibition; the second effect might be stimulatory, facilitating interactions of ATP with the NBDs. Moreover, as individual phosphorylation sites do not contribute equally to activity, phosphorylation may have graded effects in stimulating the channel.

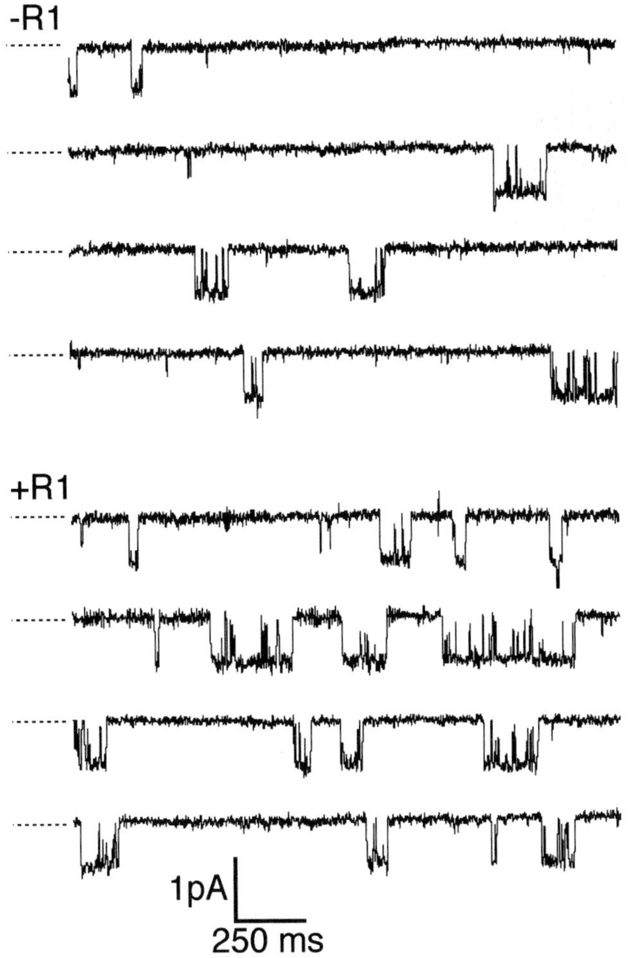

Fig. 201-17 Effect of a recombinant R domain (R1, residues 645 to 834) on CFTR-ΔR/S660A channel in the presence of PKA. Data are example of continuous single-channel tracings before and at 10 min after the addition of R1. (*From Winter and Welsh.[677] Used by permission.*)

CFTR as a Regulator of Other Membrane Proteins

In addition to its function as a Cl^- channel, CFTR appears to regulate the function of several other membrane proteins. Figure 201-18 shows some of the potential mechanisms by which CFTR may regulate other membrane proteins.

CFTR Regulation of Outwardly-Rectifying Cl^- Channel Function. Before the CFTR gene was identified, it was known that cAMP agonists and PKA failed to activate an outwardly-rectifying Cl^- channel (ORCC) in cultured CF epithelial cells.[538] The ORCC channel is a different molecule from the CFTR Cl^- channel; it has a higher single-channel conductance, an outwardly-rectifying current-voltage relationship, a different anion-selectivity sequence, different pharmacologic inhibitor profile, and it is present in CF cells that lack CFTR.[24,538] The principal abnormality of ORCC function in CF cells is that cAMP agonists and PKA fail to activate ORCC channels. Expression of wild-type CFTR corrects this deficiency. Yet how CFTR regulates ORCC is not clear. The Cl^- channel function of CFTR is not required for ORCC activation, and conversely, a CFTR variant containing large deletions is reported to retain Cl^- channel activity but fail to confer normal ORCC regulation. Such studies suggest that NBD1 and the R domain are required for ORCC regulation. A difficulty in understanding how CFTR and ORCC interact is that the molecular identity of the ORCC is unknown.

CFTR Regulation of Cellular ATP Release. In addition to an interaction with CFTR, regulation of ORCC may require extracellular ATP.[538] This requirement was first evidenced by the ability of extracellular ATP scavengers to uncouple ORCC from CFTR. Ensuing work showed that expression of CFTR in some way promoted ATP release from the cell (Fig. 201-18). The mechanism by which CFTR influences ATP release is not understood (see above), it varies from one cell type to another, and it has not been observed in some experimental systems.[315,498,538] A current hypothesis suggests that CFTR facilitates release of ATP, which stimulates a purinergic receptor. The purinergic receptor then acts via a second messenger pathway to regulate ORCC.[538]

CFTR Regulation of Na^+ Channel Function. Cystic fibrosis airway epithelia show amiloride-sensitive Na^+ absorption under voltage-clamped short-circuit conditions that is approximately twice that in non-CF airway epithelia, although there is substantial variability.[77] This increase in short-circuit current is due to increased activity of apical membrane amiloride-sensitive Na^+ channels,[668] likely the epithelial Na^+ channel (ENaC).[97,98] Consistent with this conclusion, *in situ* hybridization has shown ENaC transcripts in airway epithelia,[92,407] and disruption of ENaC genes in mice reduces amiloride-sensitive current in airway epithelia.[48,301,413] However, an unexplained observation is that the conductive and gating properties of ENaC show significant differences from those of Na^+ channels reported in airway epithelia.[118,320] In non-CF airway epithelia, cAMP agonists are reported to reduce or not change amiloride-sensitive short-circuit

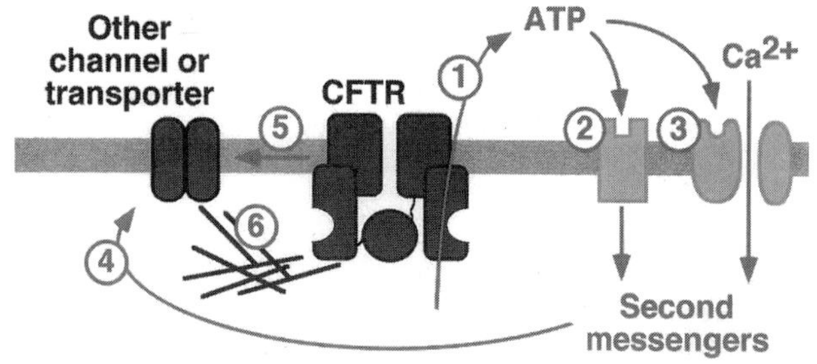

Fig. 201-18 Potential mechanisms by which CFTR may regulate other membrane channels and transporters. Numbers refer to various mechanisms. *1.* CFTR may influence the release of cellular ATP. *2.* ATP can activate membrane receptors, such as P2Y receptors to increase cell Ca^{2+} concentration. *3.* ATP can activate P2X receptors that allow influx of extracellular Ca^{2+}, which will serve as a second messenger. *4.* The effect of second messengers may alter the function of membrane channels and transporters either directly or indirectly, for example via phosphorylation or influencing protein-protein interactions. *5.* There may be direct associations between CFTR and other membrane channels and transporters that influences function. *6.* Regulatory interactions may be mediated by linker and adaptor proteins with connections to the cytoskeleton; examples include proteins containing PDZ domains. See text for details.

current, whereas cAMP agonists are reported to increase this current in CF.[77] These observations suggest an inhibitory or negative effect of CFTR on ENaC function.[539]

The relationship between CFTR and ENaC function is the opposite in the sweat gland duct.[495] In the sweat gland, activity of ENaC required CFTR Cl^- channel function. CFTR and ENaC channels opened together, thereby facilitating salt absorption and maintaining electroneutrality. These findings establish apparently different interactions between CFTR and ENaC in different tissues and place constraints on hypotheses to explain the relationship.

Studies using recombinant ENaC and CFTR suggest that in some heterologous systems cAMP agonists stimulate ENaC Na^+ channel activity in the absence of CFTR; however in the presence of CFTR cAMP agonists reduce Na^+current.[364,588] Studies in which the α, β, and γ subunits of ENaC form Na^+ channels in planar lipid bilayers have also shown a reduced open state probability when incorporated with CFTR Cl^- channels.[309] The molecular mechanisms responsible for functional effects of CFTR on Na^+ channel function remain a mystery. There are many different hypotheses (Fig. 201-18). (a) There may be direct interactions between CFTR and ENaC; this mechanism would be consistent with studies in planar lipid bilayers[309] and results obtained with the yeast two-hybrid system showing an interaction between the C-terminus of α rat ENaC and the NBD1 and R domain of human CFTR.[364] (b) CFTR-dependent ATP release into the extracellular solution might alter ENaC function after activation of purinergic receptors or adenosine receptors (see "CFTR Regulation of Cellular ATP Release"). (c) CFTR might influence ENaC function via attachments to a membrane-associated cytoskeletal web (see "CFTR Interaction with Cytoskeletal and Adaptor Proteins"). A subapical scaffold of proteins that associate with CFTR and ENaC might somehow couple the activity of the two channels. (d) Recent observations suggest that nitric oxide (NO) production is reduced in CF airways and that constitutive NO production inhibits Na^+ transport (see "CFTR Effects on Nitric Oxide Production"). Thus, reduced NO production in CF might increase Na^+ channel activity in airways.

CFTR Regulation of K^+ Channel Function. The apical membrane of the renal collecting duct contains both CFTR and an ATP-sensitive K^+ channel, ROMK2. Although the native collecting duct K^+ channel is inhibited by glibenclamide, when ROMK2 is expressed alone in heterologous systems, it is not inhibited. Coexpression studies show that CFTR confers glibenclamide sensitivity on the ROMK2 channel.[418,419] Glibenclamide inhibition is prevented by cAMP-dependent phosphorylation and requires NBD1 of CFTR.

CFTR Regulation of the Cl/HCO3 Exchanger. In several tissues CFTR plays a key role in HCO_3^- secretion; often CFTR Cl^- channels function in parallel with a Cl^-/HCO_3^- exchanger to effect net HCO_3^- secretion. In heterologous cells expressing CFTR, activation of CFTR by cAMP agonists stimulated Cl^-/HCO_3^- exchanger activity.[370] Pharmacological and mutagenesis studies indicated that expression of CFTR in the plasma membrane was required for activation of the Cl^-/HCO_3^- exchanger. Furthermore, mutations in NBD2 influenced Cl^-/HCO_3^- exchanger activity independent of their effect on Cl^- channel activity.

CFTR Regulation of Gap Junctional Coupling. Gap junctional communication via connexin 45 is increased by cAMP agonists in cells expressing CFTR.[111] The enhancement of junctional conductance did not depend on Cl^- flow through CFTR. The responsible mechanisms are not known.

CFTR Interaction with Cytoskeletal and Adaptor Proteins. The N-terminal cytoplasmic tail of CFTR binds syntaxin 1A, a membrane protein that is a component of the neuronal vesicle fusion machinery.[435,436] Heterologous expression studies showed that when syntaxin 1A binds CFTR, it inhibits its channel activity. The physical and functional interactions between syntaxin 1A and CFTR are blocked by the syntaxin-binding protein, Munc18. Additional studies suggest that syntaxin may participate in regulation of CFTR insertion and retrieval from the cell membrane.[462,477] Thus, syntaxin may fine-tune the regulation of CFTR activity by influencing both the channel activity and the number of channels in the apical membrane.

The last four residues in the C-terminal cytoplasmic tail of CFTR bind the Na^+/H^+ exchanger regulatory factor (NHERF).[268,553,640] NHERF is a multifunctional adaptor protein that contains two PDZ domains, one of which binds the C-terminal tail of CFTR. This interaction may be important in localizing CFTR to the apical membrane[432] placing it in proximity to cellular regulatory factors. PDZ domain proteins are reported to cluster a number of other ion channels and proteins into membrane microdomains. Therefore, it is interesting to speculate that NHERF or related PDZ domain proteins might be responsible for regulatory interactions between CFTR and other membrane proteins such as ORCC, ENaC, and so on (Fig. 201-18).

CFTR Endocytosis and Exocytosis. In addition to its apical location, CFTR lies in an endosomal compartment just beneath the apical membrane. The amount of transepithelial Cl^- current may be controlled by insertion and retrieval of endosomal CFTR from the apical surface. CFTR is efficiently removed from the plasma membrane and the responsible endosomes are predominantly clathrin-coated.[81,390,477] cAMP agonists decrease the rate of CFTR internalization. Moreover, cAMP agonists may increase the membrane insertion rate of endosomes that contain CFTR.[595] The combination of these two effects would generate more CFTR Cl^- channels in the membrane, an effect that would act synergistically with cAMP-dependent CFTR phosphorylation to increase Cl^- current. CFTR may not be just a passenger in endosomes; there are suggestions that CFTR itself may decrease endocytosis, increase exocytosis, and stimulate endosome fusion.[80] An effect of CFTR on endosome insertion and retrieval could have wide-ranging cellular effects. However, not all studies show such an effect and additional studies performed in differentiated epithelia should provide additional insight.[68,174,384]

CFTR Effects on Nitric Oxide Production. Reports of reduced exhaled NO levels in CF led to evaluation of this system in airway epithelia. Examination of the inducible isoform of nitric oxide synthase (iNOS) revealed constitutive expression in non-CF airways, but greatly reduced levels in CF.[326] Additional studies showed that inhibition of iNOS activity or disruption of the iNOS gene in mice reduced Na^+transport.[200] The mechanism by which the loss of CFTR reduces iNOS expression is unknown.

MOLECULAR MECHANISMS OF CFTR DYSFUNCTION

Mutations in the gene encoding CFTR disrupt CFTR function in a number of different ways. Although insights into the mechanism of dysfunction has been obtained for only a small proportion of the more than 800 reported CF-associated mutations, four general mechanisms have been described. Some mutations involve more than one mechanism of dysfunction. Figure 201-19 shows a schematic diagram of the mechanisms and Table 201-6 gives a few examples.

Class I Mutations: Defective or Reduced Protein Production

Many mutations produce premature termination signals due to splicing abnormalities, frame-shifts due to insertions or deletions, and nonsense mutations. CFTR genes bearing these mutations fail to synthesize full-length protein. In many cases (such as R553X), the mutation generates an unstable mRNA and no detectable protein.[274] In other cases, a truncated protein or an aberrant protein missing sequence or containing novel amino acid sequences may be produced. However, such proteins are often unstable and would usually either be degraded rapidly or have little or no function. To date, naturally occurring truncated or aberrant versions of protein have not been detected in CF cells. It is also possible that mutations in the gene promoter could reduce or eliminate protein production.

Class I mutations may also reduce the amount of functional protein, rather than eliminating it completely, by causing abnormal or alternative splicing. A common example occurs with variable in-frame skipping of exon 9 (see "CFTR Splicing" above). Exon 9-transcripts fail to produce functional Cl^- channels because the protein is not processed correctly (see "Class II Mutations" below).[169] Because of variable exon 9 splicing, some apparently normal individuals have only a small percent ($\approx$8 percent) of normal transcripts,[122] suggesting that even very small amounts of functional CFTR are sufficient for normal airway epithelial function. This has significant implications for therapeutic maneuvers designed to restore CFTR function. The 3849+10 kb C to T mutation is another variant that reduces but does not preclude correct mRNA splicing.[285,585] This mutation creates a partially active splice site in intron 19 that inserts a new "exon" containing an in-frame stop codon. Normally spliced transcripts are reduced to approximately 8 percent. The 3849 + 10 kb C to T mutation is associated with less severe disease in the pancreas and vas deferens.

In principle, a mutation in the CFTR promoter could reduce CFTR production and cause CF. However, mutations in the conserved regions of the CFTR promoter have not been identified.[630] This result suggests that the promoter region is not frequently mutated and suggests that CF-causing mutations in the promoter are likely rare.

Class II Mutations: Defective Protein Processing

Several CF-associated mutations, including the most common, ΔF508, cause the protein to misfold during biosynthesis; as a result it fails to traffic to the cell membrane.[113,653] Missense mutations associated with misfolding are scattered throughout the protein, in the NBDs, the MSDs, and the intracellular loops (Table 201-6). CFTR biosynthesis is outlined in Fig 201-20.[355,650] Newly synthesized CFTR is initially glycosylated in the ER (band B).[113] From there it traffics to the Golgi complex, where complex glycosylation occurs (band C), and then on to the cell surface. Studies with brefeldin A (BFA), which disrupts the Golgi complex and inhibits protein export from the ER, indicate that wild-type CFTR forms an intermediate (labeled stable B in Fig. 201-20) before it leaves the ER.[389,642] Surprisingly, only 20 to 30 percent of wild-type CFTR matures; the remaining 70 to 80 percent of the protein is ubiquitinated and degraded by the proteasome.[312,643] The reason for this inefficiency is not known. To protect the newly synthesized protein and to facilitate folding, Hsp70, Hsp90, calnexin, Hdj-2, and likely other chaperones, interact with the immature band B.[387,420] Coincident with its maturation, the protein half-life increases from about 30 minutes for immature band B to 7 to 24 hours for both stable B and mature band C.[389,642] Most studies showing ΔF508 misfolding have been performed *in vitro*; with *in vivo* studies most[135,201,232,692] but not all[321] studies also suggest misfolding.

What is different about ΔF508 that causes its misfolding? Wild-type and ΔF508 CFTR appear to have a similar conformation early during biosynthesis, but whereas wild-type can achieve a more mature conformation, ΔF508 can not. This suggests that ΔF508 does not assume a markedly different conformation that earmarks it for degradation, rather it just cannot complete the folding process. This conclusion is consistent with findings that

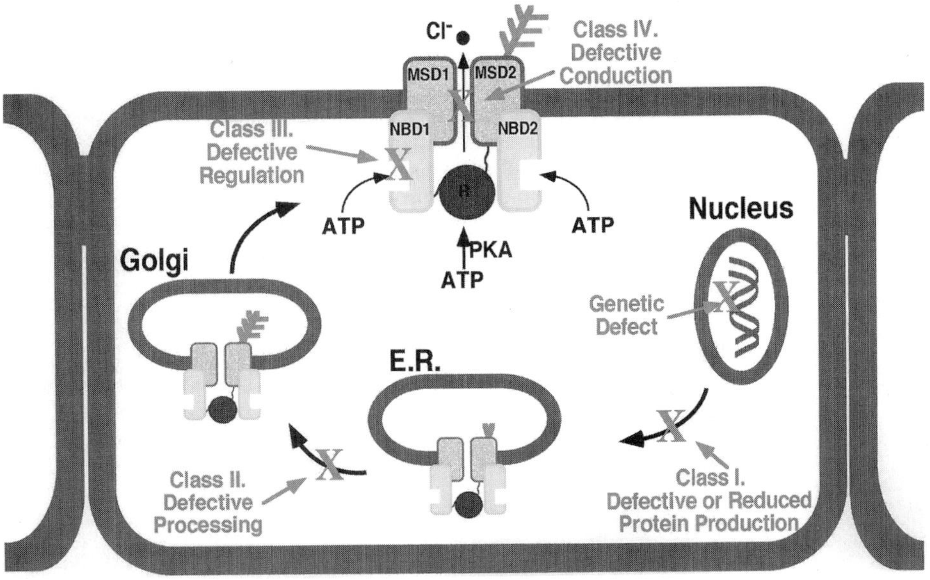

Fig. 201-19 Mechanisms by which CF-associated mutations disrupt CFTR function. See text for details. (*Adapted from Welsh and Smith.[653] Used by permission.*)

Table 201-6 Examples of Class I-IV Mutations

Class	Defect		Example	Domain	Ref
I	Defective or Reduced Protein Production				
	Absent protein	Nonsense	R553X	NBD1	189
		Frameshift	3898insC	NBD2	688
		Splice	621+1G→T	MSD1	689
	Reduced amount		5T tract with exon 9−	NBD1	183
	of protein		3849+10 kb C to T	NBD2	244
II	Defective Processing				
			ΔF508	NBD1	369
			N1303K	NBD2	690
			G85E	MSD1	691
			L1065P	MSD2	692
III	Defective Regulation				
			G551D	NBD1	393
			S1255P	NBD2	394
IV	Defective Conduction				
			R347P	MSD1	298
			R334W	MSD1	298

NOTE: See text for details.

introduction of the ΔF508 mutation into an NBD1 protein reduces the efficiency of folding, but has little effect on protein stability once the protein is folded.[480,481] The fact that ΔF508 remains in an immature conformation accounts for its prolonged association with chaperones. Recent studies suggest that recognition of the

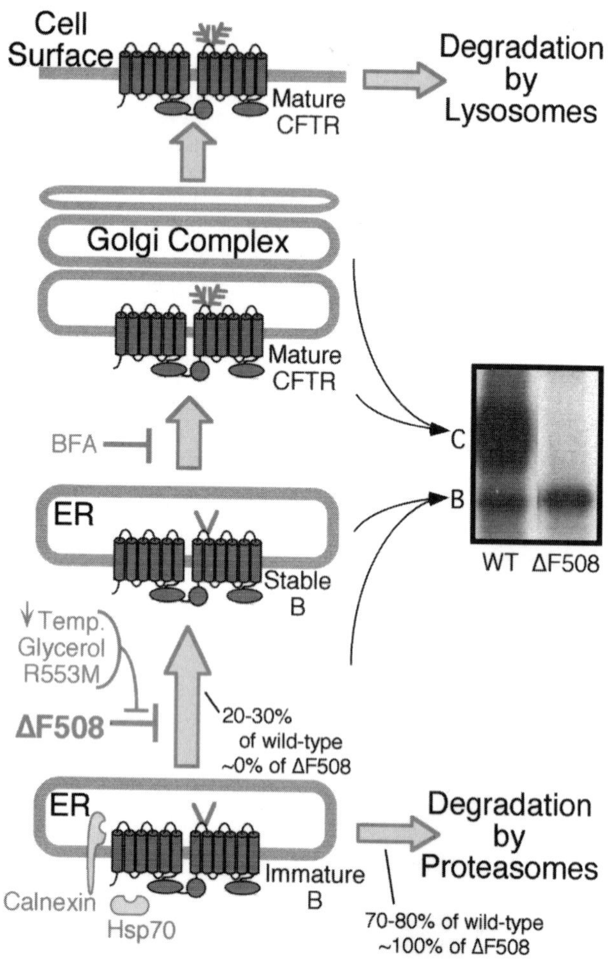

Fig. 201-20 Biosynthesis of wild-type and ΔF508 CFTR. See text for details. (*From Welsh and Ostedgaard.*[650] *Used by permission.*)

ΔF508 mutant as incompetent for export from the ER may depend, at least in part, on arginine-framed tripeptide sequences.[109] Mutation of four such sequences in CFTR allowed the ΔF508 protein to escape ER quality control.

Even though ΔF508 does not fold well enough to escape the ER, folding is sufficient to generate Cl^- channels with relatively normal regulation; ΔF508 channels have one-half to one-third the activity of wild-type.[156,173] The retention of significant activity is important because ΔF508 can be coaxed to the membrane under certain conditions. For example, reducing the incubation temperature to 27°C, which likely affects folding, allows ΔF508 to escape from the ER, traffic to the cell surface, and generate Cl^- currents.[173] Chemical chaperones such as glycerol, trimethylamine N-oxide, and deuterated water can also help ΔF508 escape the ER.[89] Moreover, intragenic suppressor mutations in NBD1 (e.g., R553M and R555K) have been discovered that allow ΔF508 to escape from the ER and generate Cl^- channel activity at the cell surface.[598,599] Interestingly, mutation of both Arg553 and Arg555 disrupt an arginine-framed tripeptide sequence.[109] These data and *in vitro* studies of NBD1[480]) indicate that interventions which enhance folding allow exit from the ER. Thus pharmacologic interventions that coax ΔF508 past its block in folding should theoretically have a beneficial effect. It seems likely that under normal conditions, a few molecules of CFTRΔF508 might escape from the ER and reach the cell surface. The quality control system that degrades misfolded proteins is not likely to be 100 percent effective. For example, some CF-associated mutants, such as P574H have a defect in folding that is less severe than ΔF508, and as a result the protein reaches the plasma membrane, and functions.[328,453] Mutations that produce a misfolded protein that fails to progress to the cell surface occur throughout most of the protein. Although insufficient ΔF508 protein reaches the cell surface to generate Cl^- transport, it remains possible that an increase in the Cl^- channel activity of a small number of molecules might be of some therapeutic benefit.

Class III Mutations: Defective Regulation

Analysis of mutant proteins that are able to reach the plasma membrane indicates that several have mutations in the NBDs. Because intracellular ATP controls the opening of CFTR Cl^- channels, it is perhaps not surprising that mutations in these domains could alter channel function. Several abnormalities have been observed: in some NBD mutants (such as G551D) there is very little function, in some (such as S1255P) ATP is less potent at stimulating activity, and in others (such as G551S, G1244E, and

G1349D) the absolute activity is reduced.[26,192] The defective gating of such mutants and the resulting decrease in net Cl^- channel activity is likely to be responsible for the defective epithelial Cl^- permeability in patients bearing these mutations. Perhaps not surprisingly some mutations that severely disrupt function, such as G551D, are associated with a severe clinical phenotype, and some that cause a moderate impairment of function, such as A455E and P574H, are associated with a less severe clinical phenotype.

CFTR is also regulated by phosphorylation of the R domain. Although missense mutations have been reported to occur in exon 13, there are few missense mutations in the C-terminal portion of the R domain. Mutations in the N-terminal portion cause defective folding and/or defective gating.[458] Although it is less well understood how mutations in the C-terminal portion of the R domain cause CFTR Cl^- channel dysfunction, it appears that they may cause defective regulation.[646]

Class IV Mutations: Defective Conduction

Numerous CF-associated missense mutations have been identified in the MSDs; many of these are correctly processed and delivered to the apical membrane, but they generate reduced Cl^- current.[550] For example, three mutations in MSD1 (R117H, R334W, and R347P) affect arginine residues. Regulation by PKA-dependent phosphorylation and intracellular ATP appear similar to that of wild-type CFTR, however the amount of current is reduced. Studies of single channels in excised, inside-out membrane patches indicate that these proteins generate less Cl^- current because the rate of ion flow through a single open channel is reduced. In addition, the amount of time that the channel is open is reduced for some mutants.

Other Mechanisms of Dysfunction

In principle, CF could be caused by mutations that destabilize the mature protein, markedly reducing its lifetime in the plasma membrane. For example, deletion of 70 to 98 residues from the C-terminus accelerated degradation five- to sixfold.[266] It is possible that sequence alterations may also disrupt CFTR-dependent regulation of other channels and transporters (see "CFTR as a Regulator of Other Membrane Proteins" above), although no variants are reported that do this exclusively. If a mutation completely retargeted CFTR from the apical to the basolateral membrane, it might also cause CF. Interestingly, mutations in the C-terminus disrupt the exclusive apical targeting of CFTR.[432] Moreover, truncation of the last 26 amino acids does not disrupt the Cl^- channel activity of CFTR and does not cause CF but does increase sweat Cl^- levels.[425,508] It seems likely that to cause CF, such a mutation would need to reduce the amount of functional apical protein by 95 percent or more.

Understanding Mechanisms of CFTR Dysfunction

Grouping mutations into different classes is useful for understanding the mechanism of dysfunction. However, it is probably inappropriate to apply it rigidly because a single mutation can cause more than one type of abnormality, and hence fall into multiple classes. For example, defective processing (a Class II abnormality) is the major abnormality found with the ΔF508 mutant, but a reduced open state probability (a Class III abnormality) is also observed. Importantly, many investigators expect that understanding how mutations disrupt function will lead to specific new therapies that restore CFTR activity.

FUNCTION OF CFTR IN EPITHELIA AND PATHOGENESIS OF DISEASE

The organs and tissues clinically involved by CF are all composed of epithelia. In those epithelia, defective electrolyte transport, particularly defective Cl^- transport, is the distinctive characteristic that distinguishes CF from non-CF epithelia. This section discusses the physiology of the affected organs and current ideas about the pathogenesis and pathophysiology.

Sweat Gland

Abnormalities in electrolyte transport by the sweat gland provide us with a most useful clinical test for CF. Studies of ion transport by the sweat gland were also the first to implicate abnormal Cl^- transport by CF epithelia; in doing so, they provided the basis for the first unifying hypothesis about the basic CF defect. The sweat gland is composed of two different regions, the secretory coil and the reabsorptive duct; Fig. 201-21 shows a schematic representation. The secretory coil produces isotonic NaCl. Then, as the sweat passes up through the water-impermeable duct, NaCl is absorbed, leaving a liquid with a low NaCl concentration to emerge at the skin surface.

Sweat Gland Duct. The clinical observation that Cl^- and Na^+ concentrations are increased in CF sweat led Quinton and colleagues to examine the ion transport properties of the sweat duct.[482,484] They found that CF ducts, both *in vivo* and *in vitro*, have a higher transepithelial voltage than normal ducts. Normal isolated, perfused ducts generate a voltage of about −7 mV, whereas CF ducts have a voltage of about −75 mV (lumen voltage with respect to interstitial surface). When luminal Cl^- (or NaCl) concentration is reduced in normal ducts, luminal voltage becomes more negative; indicating that Cl^- transport is electrically conductive. In contrast, when luminal Cl^- is decreased in CF ducts, transepithelial voltage becomes more positive. These results indicate that the CF sweat duct is Cl^--impermeable and suggest that the increased transepithelial voltage results from the presence of Na^+-absorptive mechanisms in the absence of Cl^- permeability.

Subsequent studies confirmed and extended this work. Na^+ absorption in the sweat duct occurs by Na^+ entry into the cell across the apical membrane, driven by a favorable electrochemical gradient (Fig. 201-21). Na^+ then exits across the basolateral membrane in exchange for K^+ on the Na^+-K^+-adenosine-triphosphatase (ATPase). K^+ which enters the cell is predominantly recycled via basolateral membrane K^+ channels. These processes are the same in normal and CF. Na^+ transport establishes the ion concentration and voltage gradients that drive passive Cl^- absorption. In normal ducts, Cl^- flows through the cells, passing through CFTR Cl^- channels located in both the apical and basolateral membranes.[131,322,496] Under basal conditions, CFTR Cl^- channels at both cell membranes are active; this appears to be due either to relatively high basal levels of cAMP or to little specific phosphatase activity that leaves CFTR in a phosphorylated and activated state.[486,496] The loss of CFTR in CF ducts explains the pathophysiology; Cl^- cannot follow Na^+ absorption; hence, NaCl absorption is prevented, the Na^+ and Cl^- concentrations in the sweat increase, and the loss of the Cl^- conductance increases the transepithelial voltage.

Sweat Gland Secretory Coil. In the secretory coil, cholinergic (muscarinic) agonists increase the intracellular Ca^{2+} concentration and stimulate sweat production by opening Ca^{2+}-activated apical membrane Cl^- channels.[531] This process is not affected in CF, and consequently sweat volume in response to agonists such as pilocarpine is normal in CF. β-Adrenergic agonists also stimulate sweating although the volume of sweat produced is a fraction of that generated by cholinergic agonists. β-Adrenergic agonists increase cellular levels of cAMP and open apical membrane CFTR Cl^- channels in the coil cells.[61,533] In patients with CF, cAMP-stimulated sweat secretion is lost. Defective β-agonist-induced sweat production provides the most clear-cut instance in which an abnormality can be demonstrated in carriers; heterozygotes for CF mutations produce approximately half as much sweat as normal subjects in response to β-adrenergic agonists.

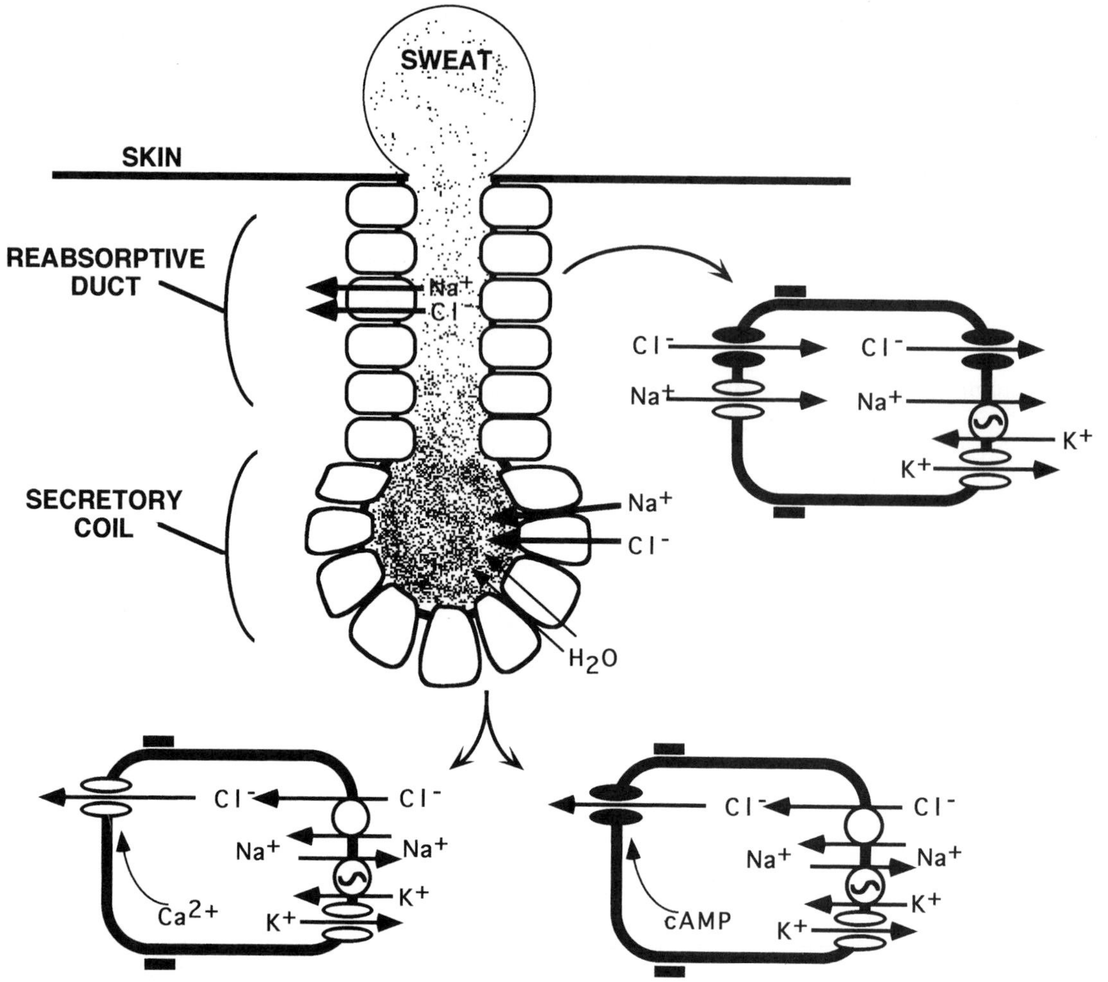

Fig. 201-21 Schematic representation of sweat production and electrolyte transport by the sweat gland. Reabsorptive duct and secretory coil are indicated. Insets show cellular mechanisms of electrolyte transport by duct and coil epithelial cells. Note that cAMP-dependent and Ca^{2+}-dependent Cl^- secretion appear to occur in two different types of cells in the secretory coil. The CFTR Cl^- channel is indicated by shading; all other channels, transporters, and pumps are indicated by open symbols.

Airway Epithelia

CF Causes a Local Pulmonary Defense Defect. As described above, recurrent airway infections are the hallmark of CF pulmonary disease. Several observations indicate that a defect in the local pulmonary defense system causes the repeated infections. (a) Infections are restricted to the lung; other organs are not infected. (b) When non-CF lungs are transplanted into a CF patient, they do not become infected. (c) Antibiotic treatment, including aerosolized antibiotics, is currently the most effective therapy. (d) The defect is subtle with a prolonged period of low-grade bacterial colonization.

The recurrent infections and exuberant inflammation in CF involve both the upper and lower airways. The proximal airway epithelium is a pseudostratified, columnar epithelium composed of ciliated cells, goblet cells, and basal cells.[83] The distal airway epithelia is predominantly composed of ciliated and nonciliated bronchiolar (Clara) cells.[472] In addition, the proximal epithelium contains submucosal glands containing serous and mucous cells and a duct composed of cuboidal ciliated and nonciliated cells.[52,503]

Electrolyte Transport by Airway Epithelia

Cellular and Molecular Mechanisms of Transport. Upper airway epithelia generate a transepithelial electrical potential difference (Vt). When measured with a mucosal solution containing a NaCl concentration similar to that of serum, Vt is approximately −10 to −30 mV *in vitro* and *in vivo* (lumen electrically negative compared to the interstitial surface).[341,343] When the epithelium is studied *in vitro* in Ussing chambers, with symmetrical solutions on both surfaces and Vt clamped to 0 mV, the resulting current (the short-circuit current, Isc) is accounted for by Na+ absorption from the mucosal to the submucosal surface and Cl− secretion from the submucosal to the mucosal surface. Under basal Isc conditions, electrogenic Na+ absorption accounts for the majority of the Isc; observation of electrogenic Cl− secretion requires inhibition of Na+ absorption.

Figure 201-22 shows a model that describes current understanding of electrolyte transport by airway epithelia. All of the various transport processes are shown in a single cell, although the relative contribution of specific cell types to various aspects of electrolyte transport is not certain. It appears that both ciliated and nonciliated epithelial cells contribute to transepithelial Na^+ and Cl^- transport, and there may be coupling between cells through gap junctions. The main features of the model are as follows.

- Na^+ enters the cell across the apical membrane, moving through amiloride-sensitive ENaC Na^+ channels.[97,98,412] Entry is passive, with Na^+ moving down a favorable electrochemical gradient; the intracellular Na^+ concentration (≈ 10 to 25 mM) is lower than that in the apical solution and the intracellular voltage is negative with respect to the apical solution. Regulation of channel activity is not well understood, but may be predomi-

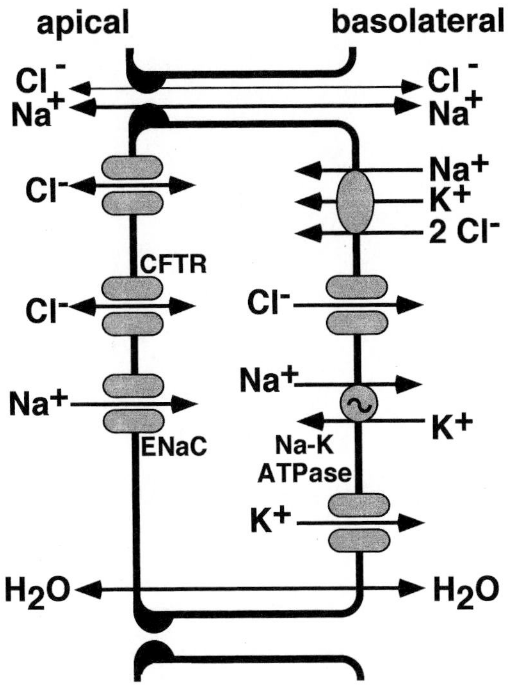

Fig. 201-22 Model of electrolyte transport by airway epithelia. See text for details.

nately controlled by endosomal insertion and retrieval that determine the number of channels in the apical membrane.

- Na^+ is pumped out across the basolateral membrane via the Na^+-K^+-ATPase. This enzyme provides the energy for ion transport by maintaining a low intracellular Na^+ concentration. The Na^+-K^+-ATPase also accumulates K^+ inside the cell.
- K^+ exits passively through a basolateral membrane K^+ channel. The basolateral K^+ conductance and K^+ concentration gradient hyperpolarize the cell, providing the electrical driving force for Na^+ and Cl^- transport. There are likely at least two different basolateral K^+ channels, one type regulated by intracellular Ca^{2+} concentration, $[Ca^{2+}]_c$, and another stimulated when intracellular cAMP levels increase.
- Cl^- enters the cell across the apical membrane through CFTR. CFTR is localized in the apical membrane. The electrochemical gradient for Cl^- entry is small and not far from equilibrium, although the driving force has not been measured under conditions that mimic the *in vivo* situation. As described above, regulation is predominately via phosphorylation. Figure 201-23 shows the immunocytochemical localization of CFTR in the apical membrane of proximal and distal airway epithelia, as well as in the apical membrane of submucosal gland serous cells.[201,202]
- The apical membrane also contains other Cl^- channels that appear to be regulated by $[Ca^{2+}]_c$, although their regulation and molecular identity remain to be established with certainty. Activation of apical Cl^- channels other than CFTR provides a potential mechanism for bypassing the loss of CFTR Cl^- channels.
- Cl^- exits the cell through basolateral membrane Cl^- channels. These channels are just beginning to be evaluated at the molecular level.[624]
- The basolateral membrane contains an electrically neutral cotransporter that can couple entry of 2 Cl^- to 1 Na^+ and 1 K^+. The Na^+ concentration gradient provides the driving force for entry of Cl^- and K^+. The Na/K/2Cl^- cotransporter is regulated by phosphorylation.[378] When apical Na^+ channels are inhibited by amiloride (which hyperpolarizes the apical membrane) and cellular levels of cAMP increase, the epithelium can secrete Cl^-. Under these conditions, Cl^- enters the cell across the basolateral membrane via the Na/K/2Cl^- cotransporter and exits through CFTR.
- The paracellular pathway provides an important route for transepithelial ion movement. As is the case in most epithelia, this pathway appears to be slightly more permeable to cations than to anions.

A variety of neurohumoral and pharmacologic agents regulate transepithelial electrolyte transport through two main second messengers: cAMP and $[Ca^{2+}]_c$. An increase in levels of cAMP activates cAMP-dependent protein kinase (PKA) which phosphorylates and thereby regulates specific membrane transport processes. Agents that increase intracellular levels of cAMP include β-adrenergic agonists, vasoactive intestinal peptide, and specific prostaglandins.[648] An increase in $[Ca^{2+}]_c$ may have direct effects on transport proteins; it may also activate Ca^{2+} and calmodulin-dependent kinases. Several agonists stimulate the hydrolysis of phosphatidylinositol bisphosphate to generate inositol triphosphate, Ins(1,4,5)P_3, which increases $[Ca^{2+}]_c$, and diacylglycerol, thereby activating protein kinase C. Examples include bradykinin, substance P, leukotrienes, and nucleotides, including ATP.[75,648] As in other Na^+-absorbing epithelia, aldosterone and glucocorticoids may regulate Na^+ absorption, although the effects appear to be variable.

Defective Electrolyte Transport in CF. CF airway epithelia manifest defects in two of the membrane transport process shown in Fig. 201-23. One defect is qualitative, the other quantitative. First, the absence of CFTR Cl^- channels markedly reduces the apical membrane Cl^- permeability and abolishes the response to cAMP agonists. Second, the activity of apical Na^+ channels is approximately twice that in non-CF epithelia. As a result, the *in vivo* basal Vt across upper airway epithelia is more negative in CF patients (≈ -50 mV).[341,343] Reductions in the apical Cl^- concentration reveal Cl^- impermeability, and there is a greater response to apical amiloride.[17,345,661] In contrast, Ca2+ activated apical Cl^- transport remains intact.[402,658]

Liquid Transport by Airway Epithelia. Liquid transport by cultured human airway epithelial cells has been measured in several studies.[314,404,563,691] By necessity, in these studies liquid is placed on the apical surface so that changes can be measured. However, this intervention introduces a set of artificial conditions different from those under equilibrium conditions at the air-liquid interface: the composition of ASL is changed, the transepithelial voltage is changed, and the function of the epithelium may be altered. Nevertheless, these studies provide insight into epithelial function.

Under basal conditions, the epithelium absorbs liquid due to active Na^+ absorption. ENaC plays a central role in Na^+ and liquid absorption; addition of amiloride or removal of apical Na^+ inhibits absorption.[314,404,563,691] Moreover, mice lacking α-ENaC as a result of gene targeted disruption die of respiratory distress because they fail to clear liquid at birth.[301] Mice lacking β- or γ-ENaC subunits have delayed lung liquid clearance at birth, but do not die of ventilatory failure.[48,413] As discussed below, it is interesting that humans with mutations in ENaC subunits are not reported to have difficulties at birth, suggesting that they have alternative mechanisms of Na^+ and liquid absorption.

Stimulating the epithelium with cAMP agonists either does not change or increases the rate of liquid absorption[314,404,563,624,691] by activating the Cl^- conductive pathway through the cells. However, when the epithelium is treated with amiloride, cAMP agonists stimulate secretion. Inhibitors of the basolateral Na^+-K^+-2Cl^- cotransporter, such as furosemide, prevent secretion.

Measurements of liquid absorption by CF airway epithelia have suggested that the rate of liquid absorption is less than, the same as, or greater than that in non-CF epithelia.[314,404,561,691] Studies in

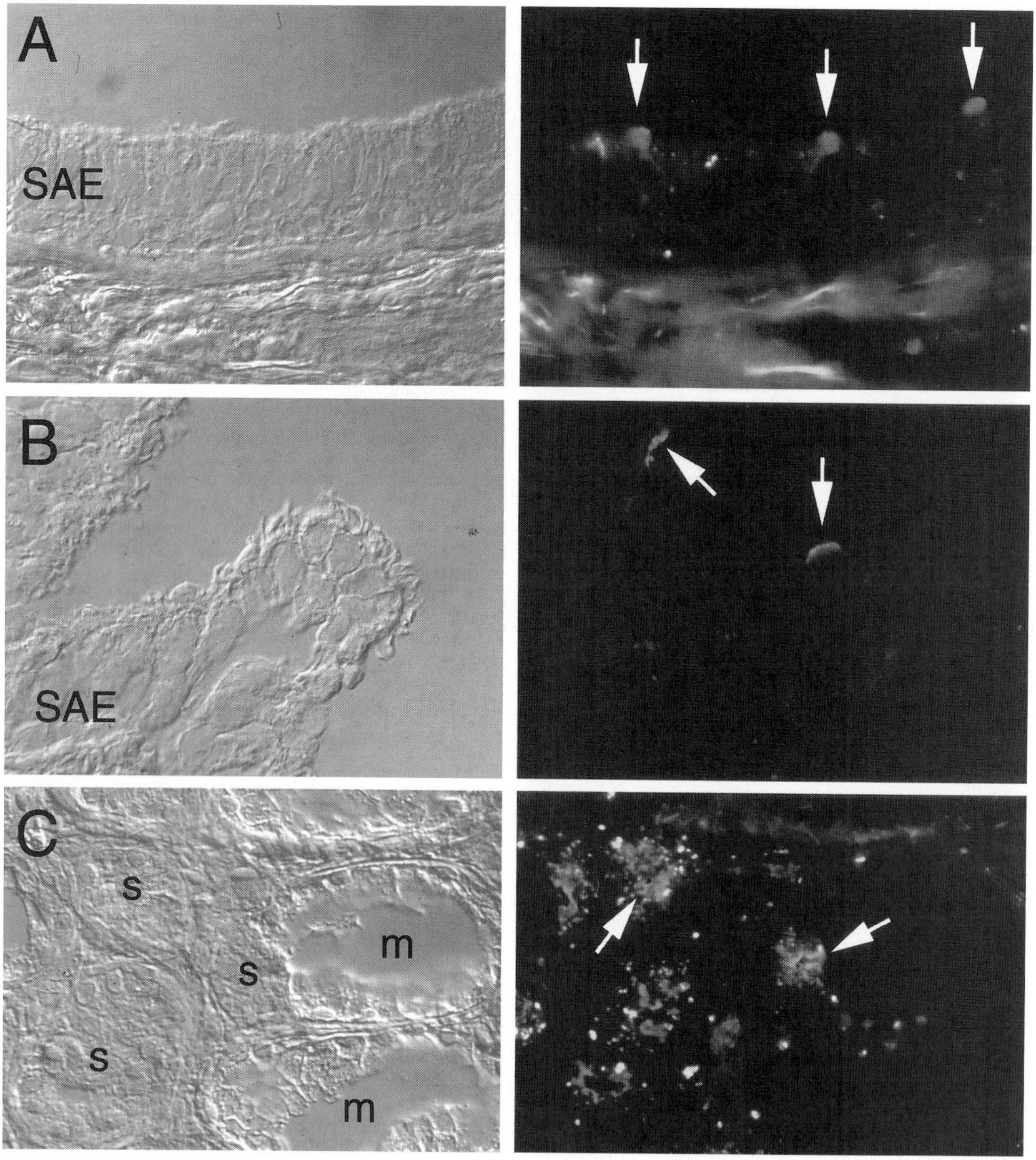

Fig. 201-23 Immunocytochemical localization of CFTR in the apical membrane of human airway epithelia and in serous cells of submucosal glands. Shown are the surface epithelium of the proximal, *A*, and distal, *B*, airways and submucosal glands, *C*. Panels are Nomarski (left) and fluorescent (right) photomicrographs. SAE indicates surface airway epithelium, *s* indicates serous cell, and *m* indicates mucous cell. Bar indicates 35 μm. Arrows point to some areas of CFTR expression. See Color Plate 10. (*From Engelhardt.*[201,202] *Used by permission.*)

xenografts suggest greater absorption rates in CF.[694] Some of the differences may be due to differences in culture methods and models. However more likely are differences in the amount of Na^+ absorption measured as amiloride-sensitive short-circuit current (Isc_{Amil}).[691] When CF epithelia have a greater Isc_{Amil} than non-CF, and the absolute values of Isc_{Amil} are relatively low, CF epithelia show a greater rate of liquid absorption than non-CF. However at high values of Isc_{Amil}, non-CF epithelia have greater rates of liquid absorption than CF. The physiologic significance of these relationships remains uncertain. Less ambiguous and more consistent from one study to another is the failure of CF epithelia to secrete liquid in epithelia treated with amiloride and cAMP agonists.

How does CFTR contribute to liquid absorption in airway epithelia? Transepithelial Na^+ absorption provides the active driving force. Cl^- can follow passively via a transcellular or a paracellular route.[659] It appears that a significant fraction of the Cl^- that follows Na^+ passes through the cells via CFTR Cl^- channels at the apical membrane and novel cAMP-activated Cl^- channels at the basolateral membrane.[624]

There is good agreement that when the apical surface is covered with large volumes of liquid, absorption and secretion are isotonic.[404,691] This result is expected based on the significant water permeability of the epithelium.[229]

ASL volume has been estimated from transmission electron photomicrographs showing the liquid depth.[556,686] In some cases, a distinct watery sol layer can be observed surrounding the cilia, and a gel layer containing mucus can be seen lying above the sol layer. However, the distinction between sol and gel is not always apparent. With an *in vivo* periciliary, sol layer ranging in depth from 2 to 7 μm, the predicted volume is 200 to 700 nl of liquid over each cm^2 of epithelium. The mucus gel may add an additional 2 to 8 μm of depth and 200 to 800 nl liquid/cm^2.

Composition of Airway Surface Liquid. Although many studies have examined transepithelial electrolyte transport by airway epithelia, current knowledge of the composition of the airway surface liquid (ASL) and of how electrolyte transport generates and regulates ASL is inadequate. This is a particular problem because such knowledge will likely influence approaches to therapy. The paucity of knowledge results, in large part, from the inaccessibility and very small volumes of ASL. Thus technical limitations pose a significant obstacle; because the volume is tiny, the process of removing and measuring ASL may change its composition. Moreover, most studies have focused on epithelium of large intrapulmonary airways and upper airways. Sputum has been collected and analyzed, but sputum also contains mucus and may be modified by cellular debris, bacteria, and saliva, especially in subjects with increased respiratory secretions. Moreover sputum is not present in normal individuals. Therefore investigators have attempted to sample ASL from humans, to measure ASL composition in models of human airway epithelia, and to sample ASL in animals.

Table 201-7 shows results from several studies that have attempted to determine ASL Na^+ and Cl^- concentrations. The top part of the table shows *in vivo* measurements. Earlier studies showed that the use of filter paper to collect ASL draws liquid from the serum, thus the more liquid collected, the more the contamination with serum.[203] One study reported ASL Na^+ and Cl^- concentrations less than those in serum and higher values in CF.[318] Two other studies with filter paper reported that ASL Na^+ and Cl^- concentrations were the same in non-CF and CF.[298,344] A potential explanation for the difference is that the first study briefly touched the filter to the airway surface and collected 1 to 10 nl, whereas the second two studies laid the filter paper on the surface for 10 to 20 sec, collecting much larger volumes. Another study collected ASL by aspiration and reported higher values in CF than non-CF. A confounding complication in all these studies is that the collection process and the use of bronchoscopy may stimulate submucosal glands and collect that liquid; estimates are that the NaCl concentration is ≈75 to 90 mM in submucosal gland secretions. Because the volume of submucosal gland secretions may be relatively large compared to the thin ASL layer, gland secretions can have a major impact on estimates of ASL NaCl concentrations. This complication has led some to conclude that ASL has Na^+ and Cl^- concentrations that are the same as those in serum.[344]

A few studies have measured ASL Na^+ and Cl^- concentrations in primary cultures of human airway epithelia grown at the air-liquid interface. Table 201-7 shows that there is good agreement between values obtained with different techniques, and that ASL Na^+ and Cl^- concentrations are much lower than those on the basolateral surface. CF epithelia had higher concentrations than non-CF. Studies have also measured Na^+ and Cl^- concentrations using xenografts implanted subcutaneously in immunocompromised mice. Human airway cells grown in rat xenografts and human fetal tracheal xenografts showed Na^+ and Cl^- concentrations less than values in serum, and CF tended to be higher than non-CF. These *in vitro* and xenograft studies offer the advantage of avoiding some of the many potential artifacts associated with *in vivo* studies in humans, but they also have limitations. Most important is the assumption that the models accurately reflect the *in vivo* condition. In addition, xenografts have significantly more liquid covering their surface than does the airway *in vivo*.

Mice bearing disruptions of the CFTR gene also provide a model in which to evaluate ASL. *In vitro* and *in vivo* studies show Na^+ and Cl^- concentrations significantly lower than serum, and one study suggests that non-CF and CF both have low ASL Na^+ and Cl^- concentrations (Table 201-7). A limitation of *in vivo* studies in mice is that the very small airways pose a significant

Table 201-7 Na^+ and Cl^- Concentration in ASL from CF and non-CF Airway Epithelia

	Non-CF		CF		
Method	Cl^-	Na^+	Cl^-	Na^+	Reference
In vivo studies in humans					
Filter paper, < 1 μl from trachea/bronchus	84	82	129	121	433
Filter paper, ~20 μl from bronchus	82	92	77	82	434
Filter paper	108	85	77	78	435
Aspiration, ~200 μl from bronchus	85	–	170	–	693
Human airway epithelia cultured at the air-liquid interface at steady state					
Isotope equilibration	40	50	85	95	694
Micropipet collection—submucosal glands	27	44	66	79	695
X-ray microanalysis	40	40	–	–	696
Xenografts implanted in mice					
Human cells in rat trachea, expulsion with air	83	83	172	178	443
Human cells in rat trachea, expulsion with air	114	–	125	–	427
Human fetal trachea	65	64	83	80	697
Studies in mice					
In vitro, primary cultures, isotope equilibration	18	–	13	–	698
In vivo, aspiration, ~ 100 nl	57	89			699
In vivo, X-ray microanalysis	2	6			700

Data are concentrations in mM from indicated references. Not included are data from airway epithelia not cultured at air-liquid interface, data from studies in which large volumes of liquid were added to apical surface, studies of expectorated sputum obtained from subjects with disease, or studies in animals other than mice.

technical limitation. Perhaps more importantly, the CF mice do not show a clinical phenotype like that of humans and Cl^- channels other than CFTR may also control ASL composition.[125,126,692] Additional studies of a variety of mouse strains are needed.

The majority of data summarized in Table 201-7 show ASL $Na^+$and Cl^- concentrations much lower than those in serum. A low NaCl concentration in ASL and a high NaCl concentration in basolateral liquid will generate a significant transepithelial osmotic gradient. Because airway epithelia are water permeable,[229] there must be some force to counterbalance the osmotic gradient. If this were not the case, the epithelium could not maintain a salt concentration gradient. Moreover, without counterbalancing forces, the apical surface would be completely dry; all of the liquid would be removed by active transport. At present, the counterbalancing force(s) is not understood. Several potential factors bear consideration. There may be unrecognized nonionic osmolytes in ASL. Because ASL volume is very small, the absolute amount might be very low, yet the concentration could be high. Surface tension also needs to be considered; it will generate pressures at the interfaces between the ciliated surface of the cell and the periciliary sol possibly between the sol and gel, and between the liquid layer and the air. Mucus that covers the epithelium can generate a counterbalancing force, but colloid oncotic pressure is equivalent to only a few mOsm. However, the tangled network of mucus could potentially generate significant pressure if liquid absorption dehydrates it. Additional work and novel approaches are needed in this area. New studies should also address the dynamic nature of the ASL; for example, intermittent secretion from the submucosal glands may transiently alter ASL composition, and the stirring action of the cilia may influence ASL consistency.

Pathogenesis of Airway Infections. It has been difficult to link the loss of CFTR function to the propensity to airway infection. Several hypotheses about the pathogenesis have been proposed. Many of the hypotheses are not mutually exclusive. In fact, CF airway disease may result from the concerted effect of several functional defects that yield the unique clinical picture.

Before considering specific hypotheses, it is necessary to make a distinction between early and late disease. The early defects in the CF airway that predispose to and initiate disease may be significantly different from the factors that perpetuate and fuel the later course. That is, the pathogenesis may have significant differences from the pathophysiology. An analogy would be a viral airway infection that sets in motion a train of events leading to chronic bacterial bronchiectasis. That disease would appear very different early and late in its course. This distinction has important implications. It suggests that the study of patients and airways with well established disease may not give insight into the pathogenesis. Moreover, prevention of lung disease may require very early intervention. It may also be that preventive maneuvers may be different from the interventions used to treat established lung disease. In the end, to develop new preventions and treatments, we need to understand the disease at all stages.

Here we describe several hypotheses to explain the pathogenesis of the lung disease. They are shown schematically in Fig. 201-24.

Defective Antimicrobial Activity in Airway Surface Liquid. The submucosal glands and surface epithelium secrete numerous antimicrobial peptides and proteins into the ASL (Fig. 201-24). These peptides are part of the innate immune system, an evolutionarily ancient system that predates development of the acquired immune system.[373] There is great diversity in the structure of the antimicrobials, and they are widespread throughout the plant and animal kingdom.

In airways, the antimicrobials include lysozyme, lactoferrin, secretory leukoproteinase inhibitor (SLPI), human beta defensins 1 and 2 (HBD-1 and HBD-2), the cathelicidin LL37, secretory phospholipase A2, and NO.[66,372,615] Lysozyme and lactoferrin are the most abundant, with estimated concentrations of 0.01 to 1 mg/ml. Most of the proteins and peptides are cationic. Their mechanism of action is only partially understood; several appear to permeabilize bacteria. The relative antimicrobial spectrum varies for different peptides, although they all show broad specificity, killing gram-positive and gram-negative bacteria, as well as some yeast. Several of the peptides show striking synergy, suggesting that a soup of peptides in the ASL may provide a potent defense against inhaled and aspirated bacteria. Some of the peptides, such as HBD-1, are secreted constitutively from the epithelium, whereas others, such as HBD-2, are secreted in response to inflammatory stimuli.[42,180,248,410]

The relative importance of any one factor to the overall antimicrobial defense system is not certain. Because the potencies of individual factors are not dramatically different, the amount of a specific antimicrobial may be a key variable in the contribution to the airway defense. Thus lysozyme and lactoferrin may be particularly important. However, other peptides play important roles as suggested by several studies. A xenograft model with human airway epithelia produced HBD-1 which showed salt-sensitive bacterial killing.[248] Antisense oligonucleotides to HBD-1 ablated antimicrobial activity in ASL from non-CF grafts, suggesting that HBD-1 plays an important role in innate immunity. In another study, overexpression of LL-37 in CF xenografts increased levels of this peptide in ASL.[43] This treatment restored bacterial killing to normal levels, providing evidence that antimicrobial peptides protect against bacterial infection. Additional insight into the importance of various factors has come from

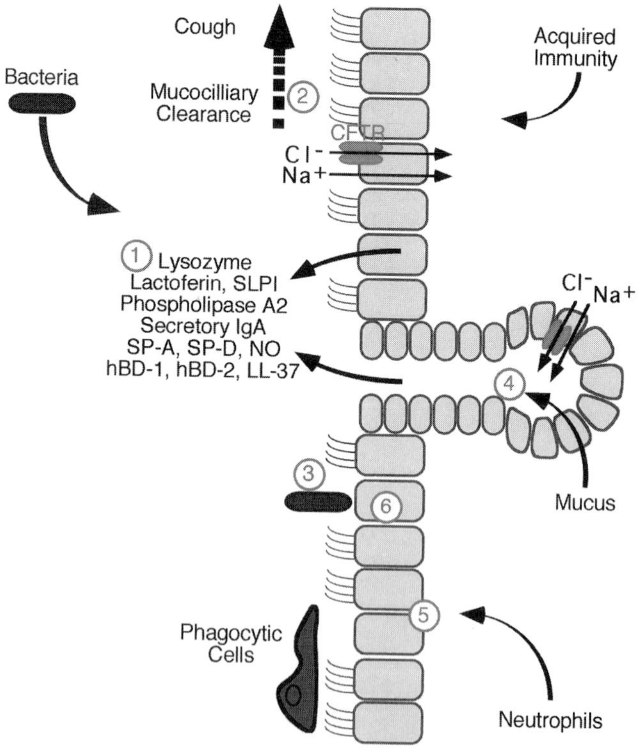

Fig. 201-24 Airway host defense mechanisms and potential sites of pathogenic and pathophysiologic defects in CF. Numbers refer to hypotheses about how the loss of CFTR disrupts airway host defense. *1.* Reduced activity of endogenous antimicrobials because of an elevated NaCl concentration in ASL. *2.* Defective mucociliary clearance because of abnormal electrolyte transport. *3.* Increased binding of bacteria to epithelial surface because of abnormal modification of membrane proteins. *4.* Abnormal function of submucosal glands and abnormal mucus production because of the loss of CFTR Cl^- channel activity. *5.* Enhanced inflammatory response. *6.* Impaired phagocytosis of *P. aeruginosa*. See text for details.

studies of nasal secretions. The antimicrobial activity of these secretions varies between donors, and secretions from a few donors who carry *S. aureus* failed to kill indigenous bacteria.[133] Interestingly, microbicidal activity was corrected by a 1:1 addition of nasal liquid from noncarriers, but not by lysozyme or lactoferrin. This result suggests that factors other than lysozyme and lactoferrin are important in airway defense.

Activity of nearly all ASL antimicrobial peptides is inhibited by high salt concentrations.[42,180,248,410,615,695] The salt concentration, not the osmolarity is important for inhibition, suggesting that high salt concentrations may inhibit binding of peptides to bacteria. Moreover cations seem to have a greater effect than anions. There is no unique NaCl concentration at which activity is inhibited, rather the lower the salt concentration, the greater the activity.[557,615] Conversely increasing the concentration of antimicrobial peptides can at least partially overcome salt-dependent inhibition.

This innate host defense system may be defective in CF airways, because of an increased ASL NaCl concentration. When a small number of the common CF pathogens *P. aeruginosa* and *S. aureus* were applied to the apical surface of normal airway epithelia grown on permeable supports at the air-liquid interface, the bacteria were killed.[562] In contrast, bacteria multiplied when added to CF epithelia. However, when it was removed from the epithelium, ASL from both normal and CF epithelia killed bacteria, suggesting that in CF alterations of the fluid may inhibit a bactericidal factor. The defective killing in CF epithelia was corrected either by artificially lowering ASL NaCl concentration or by adenoviral-mediated expression of CFTR. Virtually identical results have been obtained with a xenograft model of human airway epithelia.[248] Moreover nasal and bronchial liquid from non-CF and CF subjects showed similar antimicrobial activity.[615] Thus in CF, partial impairment of ASL bactericidal activity could predispose to repeated airway infections. As a result, macrophages and neutrophils may be required to clear bacteria, thereby initiating the inflammatory cascade observed in CF airways.

Because endogenous antimicrobials kill many different organisms in a salt-sensitive way, partial disruption of this pulmonary defense system would predispose to bacterial infection. For example, killing of *E. coli* is salt-sensitive. Yet *E. coli* pulmonary infections are rare in both normal and CF individuals. Why is it that CF airways are predisposed to infections with *P. aeruginosa*, *S. aureus*, and *B. cepacia*. Is it possible that other factors contribute to the prominence of specific bacterial species as the disease progresses? For example as described below, differential adherence, specific virulence factors, resistance to pharmaceutical antibiotics, and defects in phagocytosis may favor emergence of common CF pathogens as the disease progresses.

Defective Mucociliary Clearance. Because mucociliary clearance is an important component of the pulmonary defense system, it has attracted significant attention in CF (Fig. 201-24). Several studies using a variety of techniques have measured mucociliary clearance by the CF lung. The data have led to varying conclusions suggesting either normal or reduced mucociliary clearance. Important technical issues can account for some differences between studies, but perhaps most important is the stage of the disease. There is a significant relationship between mucociliary clearance and disease severity; mucociliary clearance decreases with increasing severity, measured as a percentage predicted FEV_1 or clinical score.[502] However, it is not clear whether defects in mucociliary clearance play an important role in the pathogenesis of the lung disease, or whether they are a result of the infection and inflammation. Irrespective of whether the abnormalities are primary or secondary, once lung disease has developed, defective mucociliary clearance plays an important role in the pathophysiology. Impaired clearance contributes to obstruction and delayed removal of the mix of mucin, cell debris, and microorganisms.

A number of factors contribute to normal mucociliary clearance. Cilia are one important component, because they propel mucus up the airways. Studies of ciliary structure and function have shown no primary abnormality in CF, although the products of *P. aeruginosa* and damage to the epithelium can impair ciliary function as the disease progresses. Another important component of mucociliary clearance is the viscoelasticity and physical/chemical properties of mucus derived from submucosal glands; CF abnormalities are discussed below.

It has often been said that CF mucus is dehydrated due to abnormal airway epithelial electrolyte transport, and that defective hydration is responsible for impaired mucociliary clearance. However, it is important to remember that this conclusion relies on the observation that the percent solids in CF sputum is increased compared to "normals." However, "normals" do not raise sputum, and any changes may be more important in the pathophysiology than the pathogenesis. Moreover, it is possibly that dehydration of the mucus alone could under some circumstances increase mucociliary clearance. When ciliary transport of mucus was measured on bovine trachea, inspissation by evaporation or increasing the osmolality of sputum with NaCl or nonelectrolytes raised the transport rate.[667]

Defective ion transport by CF airway epithelia has also been proposed to impair mucociliary clearance by altering the volume of ASL. This hypothesis proposes that in CF, the rate of liquid absorption is abnormally increased which concentrates and thickens the mucus leading to defective mucociliary clearance.[404] The defective mucociliary clearance is proposed to initiate the infection in CF. In support of this hypothesis are data obtained with an *in vitro* model of airway epithelia showing a reduction in mucus velocity and a reduced height of the periciliary sol layer. It is proposed that because of reduced ASL volume, the effectiveness of ciliary beating is impaired in CF.

Ciliary motility, and consequently mucociliary clearance is enhanced by elevated intracellular Ca^{2+} concentrations, $[Ca^{2+}]_c$. One of the most potent agonists that increase $[Ca^{2+}]_c$ is extracellular ATP. Recent data suggest that the ASL Na^+ concentration specifically and competitively inhibits an ATP-gated, $[Ca^{2+}]_c$-permeable channel in airway epithelia, thereby attenuating ATP-induced ciliary motility.[647] These data suggest that an elevated ASL Na^+ concentration could inhibit mucociliary clearance by reducing ciliary motility in the *in vivo* CF airway.

Increased Binding of* P. aeruginosa *to Airway Epithelia Because of Defective Acidification of Intracellular Organelles. Initiation and perpetuation of infection at organ and tissue surfaces is often tied to enhanced bacterial adherence, an example is in urinary tract infections. Thus a number of studies have investigated this issue in CF airways. Most work has focused on *P. aeruginosa*, because of its characteristic prevalence as the disease progresses; *S. aureus* and *H. influenza* have been studied to a lesser extent.

CF epithelial cells in primary culture bind about twice as many *P. aeruginosa* as non-CF cells, and expression of wild-type CFTR in CF epithelia reduced binding (Fig. 201-24).[163,306,526] The basis for increased binding appears to be that the apical surfaces of CF cells contain more asialoganglioside 1 (aGM1), which serves as a receptor for *P. aeruginosa*. Binding was reduced via incubation of *P. aeruginosa* with aGM1 or treatment of epithelia with an anti-aGM1 antibody.

The link between defective CFTR function and increased aGM1 on the cell surface may come from the loss of CFTR Cl^- channel function in intracellular vesicles.[46,306] Cl^- channels located in parallel with an electrogenic H^+-ATPase acidify intracellular organelles. It has been proposed that CFTR aids in acidifying vesicles targeted to the apical surface. Consequently in CF, there is not an optimal pH for trans-Golgi enzymes involved in sialylation of apical membrane glycoproteins and glycolipids. Hence the less fully sialylated cell surface serves as a better receptor for *P. aeruginosa*. Defective CF acidification of the trans-Golgi complex and endosomes has been shown in some airway epithelial cells.[46] Not surprisingly, this is not a universal phenomenon; in 3T3-fibroblasts CFTR expression did not influence acidification of these compartments.[543] Additional studies of the impact of CFTR on this process are needed.

The relative importance of enhanced bacterial binding to CF pathogenesis remains uncertain. In studies of CF lungs the vast majority of *P. aeruginosa* and *S. aureus* are found bound to mucus, rather than to the epithelial surface. However, bacteria do show increased binding to airway surfaces at sites where the epithelium is denuded or regenerating. Consistent with these *in vivo* observations, an *in vitro* model showed much greater *P. aeruginosa* adherence to regenerating epithelial cells.[164] Moreover, binding to regenerating CF epithelia was greater than to non-CF epithelia because of the presence of aGM1. Thus, irrespective of whether enhanced bacterial binding is important as the initial defect in the pathogenesis, it may contribute to the unusual propensity of CF airways to become colonized with *P. aeruginosa* as the disease progresses.

Abnormal Submucosal Gland Function. Submucosal glands play a key role in airway physiology and host defense (Fig. 201-24).[51,469] They produce much of the mucin and glycoconjugates that are critical for mucociliary clearance, and they secrete many antimicrobial substances that protect the lung. Submucosal glands are scattered throughout the cartilaginous airways with ≈100 glands/cm^2 of tracheal surface. Mucus cells, similar to those in the surface epithelium, account for ≈60 percent of cells and produce mucins and high molecular mass glycoproteins. Serous cells account for 40 percent of the cell population; they contain smaller secretory granules and produce lysozyme, lactoferrin, antimicrobial peptides, and perhaps the liquid that expels the secretions from the glands. Collecting ducts and submucosal gland ducts carry the secretory products to the airway lumen, possibly modifying the composition along the way.

The importance of submucosal glands for normal lung function, their hypertrophy and abundant secretion as the disease progresses, and the impaired mucociliary clearance in the disease, has implicated them in the pathogenesis and pathophysiology of CF. Moreover, serous cells in the submucosal glands show quantitatively more CFTR expression than do epithelial cells lining the airways (Fig. 201-23).[201] There tend to be two general ideas of how submucosal glands may be defective in CF. One hypothesis focuses on the role of CFTR in fluid and electrolyte transport. Serous cells tend to lie in the distal portions of the glands where CFTR-mediated liquid secretion may propel gland contents out to the airway lumen. In addition, loss of CFTR function in the gland ducts could modify the composition of the gland output; for example, CFTR may play a key role in HCO_3^- secretion to alkalinize the gland products.[304,369] A CF-associated abnormality could contribute to airway disease in several ways. It could lead to obstruction of the submucosal gland ducts. It could reduce the volume of liquid secretion that is important to the ASL and mucociliary clearance. Or it could alter the electrolyte composition of submucosal gland secretion, thereby altering the viscoelastic properties of the emerging mucus and the composition of ASL.

A second hypothesis suggests that the macromolecular composition of gland secretions is abnormal in CF, impairing mucociliary clearance. CFTR Cl^- channels present in the glands and in the secretory vesicles may contribute to hydration of the secretory products. The degree of surface gel hydration is an important determinant of mucus elasticity and thus effective mucociliary clearance. Sulfation of glycoproteins is also increased in CF;[693] a resulting increase in viscosity may inhibit mucociliary clearance. In addition, abnormal sialylation of glycoproteins as described above may alter the physical properties of the mucus gel that traps and removes inhaled particulates and bacteria.[534] The relative importance of submucosal gland dysfunction to the pathogenesis and pathophysiology remains a central but unresolved issue. In part this is because it is difficult to study the critical determinants in a model that will allow investigators to relate molecular abnormalities to organ physiology and to defects in disease.

Enhanced Inflammatory Response in CF Airways. The inflammatory response in CF airways plays a central role in disease progression and eventual lung destruction. It has usually been considered that inflammation is a response to the infection. However, several studies have begun to suggest that CF airways may exhibit an abnormally profuse inflammatory response (Fig. 201-24). In CF infants, bronchoalveolar lavage has shown evidence of inflammation, even before overt infection can be detected.[337] Interestingly, bronchial epithelial cells obtained from healthy controls produced the anti-inflammatory cytokine IL-10 but little of the pro-inflammatory cytokines IL-8 and IL-6.[71] Another study showed that stimulation of airway epithelia with *P. aeruginosa* generated greater amounts of NF-κB in CF than non-CF cells, suggesting an exaggerated inflammatory response in CF.[181] When *P. aeruginosa*-laden agarose beads were administered to CF mice, mortality and the production of inflammatory mediators was greater than in non-CF mice.[626] However, not all studies suggest increased airway epithelial production of inflammatory cytokines.[403] Additional work is needed to confirm an excessive inflammatory response in CF airways and to tie this phenomenon to CFTR. One intriguing explanation for the enhanced inflammatory response and increased Na^+ transport comes from data suggesting that nitric oxide production may be defective in CF airways.[200,326] These studies showed reduced nitric oxide synthase activity in CF airway epithelia. Yet the connection between these findings and CFTR dysfunction awaits elucidation.

***Impaired Phagocytosis of* P. aeruginosa.** It has been proposed that CFTR serves as a receptor for *P. aeruginosa* binding to airway epithelia and subsequent phagocytosis, and that this process is impaired in CF (Fig. 201-24).[467,468] The frequency with which airway epithelia endocytose bacteria and the importance of this process in the pathogenesis and pathophysiology of CF airway disease are uncertain. When differentiated epithelia have been studied, no intracellular bacteria were detected.[473] Moreover, if defective phagocytosis were responsible for *P. aeruginosa* infection, then it might be predicted that patients bearing mutations that allow CFTR expression on the apical surface would not be predisposed to *P. aeruginosa* infection.

Heterogeneity in Mannose-Binding Lectin. The course of lung disease can vary significantly even in patients with the same mutations. Modifier genes may be responsible (see "Modifiers of the CF Phenotype Independent of CFTR Genotype" below). A recent report suggests that alleles of the mannose-binding lectin (MBL) which reduce MBL serum levels are associated with a more severe pulmonary phenotype.[239] MBL is a serum protein that participates in the innate immune defense and may be particularly important in protecting against bacterial and viral infections. MBL deficiency has been associated with an increased risk of infection in non-CF children and adults. Thus variations in the innate immune system due to variations in MBL levels could be an important factor that modifies the course of CF lung infections.

Relationship to Other Diseases. CF has been compared to several other diseases in an attempt to gain insight into the pathogenesis. Although CF remains unique in terms of its characteristic clinical and physiologic manifestations, such comparisons may help identify factors relevant to the pathogenesis and pathophysiology.

Immotile Cilia Syndrome. Patients with primary defects in cilia structure and function share with CF the propensity to airway infections and the progressive development of bronchiectasis (Chap. 187). However, despite a more severe impairment of mucociliary clearance, these patients often have organisms that are different from those that characterize CF. In addition the disease is not as severe as CF. Thus, it seems unlikely that defective mucociliary clearance alone accounts for CF airway disease.

Liddles Syndrome. Liddles syndrome is caused by gain-of-function mutations that increase the number of Na^+ channels in the apical membrane.[552,567] As a result, renal Na^+ absorption is increased and patients develop salt-sensitive hypertension. Studies are limited, but preliminary data suggest that Na^+ absorption is also increased in the upper airways.[40] If this is the case in the lower airways, it would suggest that an increase in Na^+ channel activity by itself does not account for CF airway disease.

Pseudohypoaldosteronism Type 1 (PHA). PHA is caused by loss-of-function mutations that abolish Na^+ channel activity (Chap. 211). Na^+ channel activity also appears to be disrupted in the PHA airway.[331,476] Although airway infections, including *P. aeruginosa* infections, are reported in some children with PHA, airway disease in adults does not consistently mimic CF.[275,401] These observations suggest that the human airway has mechanisms for salt and liquid absorption other than ENaC. This conclusion is consistent with the finding that mice with a disrupted α-ENaC gene die as neonates because they are unable to clear lung liquid, whereas humans do not have this problem.[301] These observations suggest that humans might develop compensatory mechanisms for Na^+ transport in PHA. The defect in PHA would suggest that patients have an inability to lower the salt concentration in ASL and therefore the activity of ASL antimicrobial factors would be reduced. However the potentially increased volume of ASL and compensatory mechanisms confound this interpretation.

Diffuse Panbronchitis. Diffuse panbronchitis is a chronic inflammatory disease affecting the respiratory bronchioles.[359] The small conducting airways show infiltration with plasma cells and lymphocytes, and bronchoalveolar lavage shows neutrophilia. Patients are typically men who develop chronic mucopurulent cough and exertional dyspnea. Like CF, early in the course of the disease sputum is often positive for *H. influenza* and in many cases this is replaced by *P. aeruginosa*. Chronic sinusitis is also very frequent. The cause of the disease is uncertain; it is not known to have a genetic basis, but it is rarely found outside of Japan. Erythromycin and related macrolides provide effective treatments, although the mechanisms of action are not known. The response to erythromycin suggests that macrolides might possibly be of value in CF even though *P. aeruginosa* is usually resistant to these agents.

Bronchiectasis. Bronchiectasis from a variety of other causes can produce a clinical picture with characteristics similar to CF, including infection with *P. aeruginosa*. This observation serves to highlight the distinction between the pathogenesis and the pathophysiology of CF. It also makes early intervention in CF airway disease a critical goal.

Summary of Pathogenesis and Pathophysiology of Airway Disease. The pathogenesis of CF lung disease is clearly a complex problem. It is difficult to explain all aspects of the disease with a single hypothesis. Part of this difficulty is due to our inability to separate the initiating events from the secondary consequences that are so important to the pathophysiology. This inability is compounded by the fact that the pathogenic mechanism is likely to involve a partial impairment of lung defense, rather than an absolutely complete disruption of function. Moreover, secondary compensatory mechanisms might partially alleviate CF-associated defects. In the end, it seems likely that several of the hypotheses described above will, in combination, cause CF lung disease. If the pathogenesis and pathophysiology are a function of several factors, each subject to modifier genes and environmental influences, it could explain some of the complexity and variability observed in the clinic.

Pancreas

The pancreatic secretory system is composed of two functionally distinct components: the acinar system and the pancreatic ducts. The acinar system secretes pancreatic enzymes when stimulated by cholecystokinin and acetylcholine; this process is not directly affected in CF. Instead, organ dysfunction starts in the small pancreatic ducts which secrete a HCO_3^--rich liquid to increase the volume and pH of the luminal fluid.[253,569] Before total organ failure develops, pancreatic secretions from CF subjects have a higher concentration of protein than controls, primarily because CF pancreatic ducts secrete less liquid.[354] Electrolyte transport by CF pancreatic ducts is disrupted because of the loss of apical CFTR Cl^- channels and perhaps defective Cl/HCO_3 exchanger activity.[400,696] In duct epithelia, apical membrane CFTR Cl^- channels function in parallel with Cl^-/HCO_3^- exchangers. Cl^- enters the duct lumen through CFTR[251,252] and then recycles back into the cell through a Cl^- /HCO_3^- exchanger.[252,569] As a result HCO_3^- is secreted into the lumen, generating an alkaline secretion. Disruption of this process in CF, decreases the alkaline liquid secretion that hydrates, solubilizes, and inactivates acinar secretions. Consequently, the thick secretions obstruct the ducts, leading to destruction of the organ.

Intestine

The most consistent abnormality observed in CF intestine has been the loss of CFTR-mediated cAMP-stimulated Cl^- secretion.[250,597,604] The cellular mechanism of epithelial Cl^- secretion involves electrically neutral Cl^- entry at the basolateral membrane via a Na^+-K^+-$2Cl^-$ cotransport process and Cl^- exit across the apical membrane via CFTR Cl^- channels. The coupled entry of Cl^- with Na^+ provides the driving force for accumulation of Cl^- against its electrochemical gradient. Na^+, which enters the cell at the basolateral membrane coupled to Cl^-, exits across the basolateral membrane via the Na^+-K^+-ATPase, which provides the energy for transepithelial Cl^- secretion by maintaining a low intracellular Na^+ concentration. The Na^+-K^+-ATPase also accumulates K^+ inside the cell. K^+ then exits passively through a basolateral membrane K^+ channel. The basolateral K^+ conductance and the K^+ concentration gradient hyperpolarize the cell, providing the electrical driving force for Cl^- exit at the apical membrane. In contrast to airway epithelium, intestinal epithelia lack apical membrane Ca^{2+}-activated Cl^- channels and thus do not manifest Ca^{2+}-stimulated Cl^- secretion.[25] Because amiloride-sensitive Na^+ current is increased in airway epithelia, Na^+ absorptive processes have been studied in the intestine. In contrast to airway, glucose-coupled Na^+ transport is normal in CF,[629] and the amiloride-inhibitable component of electrogenic Na^+ transport appears to be normal in CF.[249,629]

The abnormal electrolyte transport by CF intestinal epithelia likely alters the composition of the luminal contents. The lack of Cl^- secretion to counterbalance intestinal absorptive processes could reduce the liquid content in the intestinal lumen causing dehydration, and hence impaction. Thus it may contribute to meconium ileus and distal intestinal obstruction syndrome. However, the relative contribution of defective intestinal electrolyte transport and the loss of pancreatic function to gastrointestinal disease are not certain.

Male Genital Tract

The observation that most males with CF are sterile and observations of histologic changes in the epididymis and vas deferens have suggested that ion transport abnormalities in these ducts may occur in CF. Studies of the rat epididymis have shown that the epithelium secretes Cl^- and HCO_3^-.[108,680] The mechanism of secretion is most likely similar to that observed in airway epithelia and in pancreatic ducts, with anion accumulation processes at the basolateral membrane and anion channels at the apical membrane.

Studies of epididymal cells using the patch-clamp technique have demonstrated the presence of a low conductance Cl^- channel (3 to 5 pS) that is activated when cAMP agonists are added to the cells.[474] The channel showed little time-dependent voltage effects and was more permeable to Cl^- than to HCO_3^-; this channel most likely represents the CFTR Cl^- channel. It has been suggested that dysfunction of the CFTR Cl^- channel in CF may result in thickened secretions that plug the small ducts of the male genital tract, thereby producing the pathology and sterility in males with CF.[679]

Hepatobiliary System

Fluid and electrolyte secretion by the small intrahepatic bile ducts is thought to be important for normal hepatic physiology. CFTR is localized in the apical membrane of the intrahepatic bile duct epithelial cells.[132] In these cells it generates Cl^- currents in response to cAMP agonists.[225] Abnormal ductular secretion and subsequent obstruction is likely to be responsible for the cholestatic liver disease in CF.[386]

Mouse Models of CF

Gene targeting has been used to disrupt the CFTR gene in mice and to introduce mutations associated with human disease.[263] Six knockout strains have been developed in which the CFTR gene is disrupted by insertion, duplication, or an in-frame stop codon,[184,281,446,493,520,566] three mouse models have been developed in which the phenylalanine at position 508 has been deleted (ΔF508),[135,627,692] and in one model the glycine at position 551 has been changed to an aspartate (G551D).[168] The study of these mice as well as an examination of differences between strains has improved our understanding of epithelial biology and has provided a model for testing and novel therapeutic strategies including gene transfer.

The most striking phenotype in these mice has been in the intestine. The intestinal pathology is severe, with mucus accumulation in the crypts of Lieberkuhn, goblet cell hypertrophy, hyperplasia, and eosinophilic concretions in the crypts. The mice develop intestinal blockage and perforation. As a result, a large fraction of mice die either within a week of birth or shortly after weaning. Two of the knockout strains have a less severe intestinal phenotype[184,627]); they appear to either make some normal CFTR mRNA or a small amount of the ΔF508 protein is targeted to the membrane. Use of a liquid diet or addition of polyethylene glycol and electrolytes to the drinking water has been able to extend the life of the mice, providing additional time to study the phenotype. The intestinal pathology and abnormal physiology have also been corrected by expression of the human CFTR cDNA under control of an intestinal specific promoter.[697] It is interesting that just as humans with the G551D mutation are reported to have reduced rate of meconium ileus, mice with the G551D tend to have less severe intestinal disease.

The CF mice show intestinal electrolyte transport abnormalities similar to those observed in humans. There is a lack of cAMP-mediated Cl^- secretion due to the loss of CFTR.[263] As previously shown for human intestinal epithelia, mouse intestine does not express a Ca^{2+}-stimulated apical Cl^- channel. It has been speculated that the lack of either a CFTR Cl^- channel or a Ca^{2+}-activated Cl^- conductance accounts for the severe disease.[263]

When CF mice were developed it was hoped that they might recapitulate the airway disease observed in humans. Unfortunately, in all the CF mouse models the lung histology is nearly normal. However, with repeated exposure to *S. aureus* administered over one to two months, it has been reported that there is a significantly increased incidence of goblet cell hyperplasia and bronchiolitis and reduced clearance of bacteria.[159] In addition, when agarose beads containing *P. aeruginosa* have been instilled into the mouse lung, the concentration of inflammatory mediators is reported to be higher and the mortality is greater in the CF mice than in non-CF mice.[626] Thus, future work may be able to establish a pulmonary phenotype of value to investigators.

The CF mice have changes in ion transport similar to those observed in humans. In the upper airways, the animals show a reduced cAMP-stimulated Cl^- current, consistent with the lack of CFTR.[263] There is also increased Na^+ channel activity and normal or increased activity of Ca^{2+}-activated Cl^- channels. In the lower airways there appear to be differences between animals. Some animals have defective cAMP-stimulated Cl^- transport in the trachea, whereas others do not. These observations are complicated by the ability of cAMP to increase Ca^{2+} in the airway cells of some animals. At present, the reason for the marked difference between the pulmonary pathology in mice and in humans remains uncertain.

Histopathology in the pancreas has been observed although it appears to be much less common and less severe than that in humans with CF. Moreover, the reported abnormalities vary in different mouse strains.[263] The reasons for the differences between the mice and humans is not apparent. Liver pathology is not prominent in the CF mouse although the G551D CF mouse is reported to have hyperplasia of biliary duct epithelia.[168] In contrast to the human, there appears to be no pathology of the male reproductive tract, and the males are fertile.

The CF mouse models will continue to provide research opportunities. The CF mice may provide a good model in which to investigate and discover modifier loci that alter the phenotype. For example, a subset of CF mice have prolonged survival and may have an increase in Ca^{2+}-activated Cl^- conductance.[520] In addition, a congenic mouse strain develops a pulmonary phenotype with fibrosis.[327] The CF mice will also be of value in testing novel treatment strategies. Finally, further insight into why disruption of CFTR function produces different pathology in the human and the mouse may yield new insight into the disease.

GENOTYPE-PHENOTYPE CORRELATIONS

Variability in an inherited disorder can be attributed to three factors: the nature of the defect in the responsible gene, the context in which that gene operates, and the influence of environment. Understanding the first factor, the relationship between CFTR genotype and the degree to which it determines phenotype, has been an area of intense study since the cloning of the gene. Two general themes have emerged. The first is that the correlation between genotype and disease severity varies by affected organ system. A close association is observed between CFTR genotype and pancreatic status. A clear but less robust correlation exists between mutations and the degree of sweat chloride abnormality, the severity of sinus disease, and the occurrence of meconium ileus. CFTR genotype has some influence upon the severity of the pulmonary phenotype. Finally, developmental abnormalities in the male reproductive tract appear to correlate with the nature of the mutation in CFTR. The second theme is that different epithelial tissues require different levels of CFTR for normal function. An illustration of the latter correlation can be derived by comparing the level of CFTR RNA found in patients with different splice site mutations and different phenotypes (Table 201-8). It appears that the pancreas has the lowest requirement followed by the sweat gland and lungs, with the vas deferens having the highest requirement.[117]

It is tempting to combine these themes and conclude that tissues with the lowest requirement for functional CFTR will show the greatest correlation with genotype. In other words, partial function mutants are more likely to alleviate disease in the pancreas than the vas deferens. Improved pancreatic status would therefore correlate with specific mutations while the relationship to lung disease should be less robust. One could predict that correlation between CFTR genotype and lung disease may be evident only for mutants that retain substantial function. Indeed, there appears to be evidence to support this concept. However, the multifunctional nature of CFTR and presence of genetic and environmental variables indicate that a simplistic interpretation of genotype/phenotype relationships in CF may be useful for testing hypotheses, but of little value for an individual patient.

CFTR Genotype and Lung Disease

Pulmonary disease is the primary cause of morbidity and mortality in CF. Familial studies involving small numbers of patients

Table 201-8 Correlation of Phenotype with the Level of CFTR mRNA in Respiratory Epithelial Cells

Phenotype*	Mutations	% Normal CFTR mRNA	Pancreas	Sweat [Cl⁻]	Lungs	Vas Deferens	Reference
PI-CF	1811+1.6 kbA→G	1–3%	+	+	+	+	512
	1898+5G→T	<2–5%					231, 701
PS-CF	2789+5G→A	4%	−	+	+	+	702
Atypical CF	3849+10kbC→T	8%	−	−	+	+	244
CBAVD	Intron 8 5T	6-37%	−	−	−	+	185, 703

*PI-CF = pancreatic insufficient CF; PS-CF = pancreatic sufficient CF; CBAVD = congenital bilateral absence of the vas deferens. The (+) and (−) indicate the presence or absence of disease in the indicated organ.

suggested concordance among adult siblings for one measure of lung function (percent FEV_1), hinting that genetic factors, namely CFTR genotype, influence the severity of pulmonary disease.[529,530] Concordance was most evident for sibs with mild pancreatic disease, indicating that better nutritional status rather than CFTR genotype lead to improved lung function. Indeed, several studies have indicated that mild pancreatic disease correlates with less severe lung disease.[242]

The wide variability in pulmonary disease observed in individuals with identical genotypes illustrates the difficulty in correlating this aspect of the CF phenotype with CFTR mutations. Studies involving ΔF508 homozygotes revealed that almost all were pancreatic insufficient, and most had high sweat Cl^- concentrations.[333,605] Yet lung disease, as measured by pulmonary function testing, was highly variable.[605] Furthermore, individuals heterozygous for the ΔF508 mutation and individuals carrying two non-ΔF508 CF mutations showed as much variability in the severity of lung disease as ΔF508 homozygotes.[333,605]

Part of the problem inherent in multicenter genotype/phenotype studies is that grouping patients from different ethnic backgrounds and from different treatment centers may obscure subtle correlations. Indeed, the A455E mutation is relatively common in the Dutch and in French Canadian CF patients.[167,237] Comparison of ΔF508/A455E heterozygotes with ΔF508 homozygotes drawn from the same population reveals that carriers of the A455E mutation have improved pulmonary function compared to the homozygous patients.[167,237] Interestingly, the study of Dutch patients revealed lower rates of colonization with *P. aeruginosa*. The concept that bacterial colonization of the lungs may correlate with the nature and location of CFTR mutations was first suggested by a study of 267 European CF patients.[363] Since the A455E mutation is associated with pancreatic sufficiency, and bacterial colonization was closely correlated with pancreatic status, the possibility remains that less severe lung disease in A455E heterozygotes was a consequence of better nutritional status. However, one mutation, R117H, is associated with pancreatic sufficient phenotypes with and without lung disease. Life-limiting CF lung disease in patients carrying one or two R117H mutations appears to depend upon the presence of a variation in intron 8 of the CFTR gene. Patients with the R117H mutation and the 5 thymidine (5T) in the polypyrimidine tract of the splice acceptor preceding exon 9 generally develop CF lung disease. However, pairing of the R117H mutation with the 7 thymidine variant (7T) permits normal lung function, although male patients manifest abnormalities in the vas deferens characteristic of CF.[338] The R117H-5T and R117H-7T alleles are both associated with pancreatic sufficiency, indicating that pulmonary function is influenced by the nature of the defect in CFTR. These studies suggest that relationships between CFTR genotype and CF lung disease exist, but they exist only in certain contexts such as mutations that permit considerable residual CFTR function.

CFTR Genotype and Pancreatic Disease

Although exocrine pancreatic disease is universal among CF patients, about 5 to 15 percent of patients retain sufficient function to escape the need for replacement of digestive enzymes.[178,220] This feature, termed pancreatic sufficiency (PS), shows concordance of 95 percent or greater in CF siblings with identical CFTR genotypes.[139] The high concordance rates indicate that the nature of the CF mutations have considerable influence upon the degree of pancreatic function.[329] Indeed, the ΔF508 mutation and a series of other mutations that have similarly profound deleterious effects upon CFTR are consistently associated with severe pancreatic disease requiring enzyme replacement (pancreatic insufficiency, PI).[333,605] Conversely, a subset of mutations that permit some CFTR function are associated with PS.[362] The relationship is not mutually exclusive however. For example, a small fraction of ΔF508 homozygotes remain PS into adulthood while the fraction of PS patients carrying partial function mutations R334W, A455E, or R117H ranges from 40 to 78 to 87 percent, respectively (Table 201-9). Therefore, environment and/or genetic background appears to play a role in the severity of pancreatic disease.

CFTR Genotype and Male Infertility

Infertility due to malformation of structures derived from the Wolffian duct affects approximately 97 percent of men with CF.[90] Abnormalities of the testes and of spermatogenesis have also been reported.[172,670] A relationship between CF mutations and infertility has not been evident because virtually all male patients with CF have abnormal development of the reproductive tract. One RNA splicing mutation, 3849 + 10 kbC→T, appears to be associated with preserved fertility in some males with CF.[285] However, other male CF patients with the same mutation are infertile, suggesting that the degree of abnormal CFTR splicing caused by the 3849 mutation may vary, leaving some males with sufficient levels of normal CFTR to escape the infertility phenotype.

The relationship between CFTR genotype and male infertility was elucidated by the identification of CF mutations in men with a distinct genetic disorder called congenital bilateral absence of the vas deferens (CBAVD). This condition affects about 2 percent of men with obstructive azoospermia.[340] Some men with CBAVD have sinopulmonary disease and elevated sweat chloride concentrations suggesting overlap between this condition and CF.[27,134] Other men with CBAVD are apparently healthy without clinical evidence of pulmonary or pancreatic disease.[134] Furthermore, nasal potential difference measurements of males with CBAVD revealed a pattern distinct from normal, and also from CF.[452,672] Thus, men with CBAVD represent a spectrum of conditions ranging from mild CF presenting as male infertility to isolated abnormalities of the male reproductive tract.

Screening of CFTR genes in men with CBAVD confirmed that this condition overlaps with CF, but also represents a distinct entity. The initial report that a significant fraction of males with CBAVD carry CF mutations was followed by several confirmatory studies.[27] Comprehensive studies of 106 German men and 102 men from Europe and the United States with absent vas deferens indicates that 70 to 75 percent carry mutations in each CFTR gene.[116,186] Two observations illustrate that the nature of the

Table 201-9 Association between Mutations and Specific Features of the CF Phenotype

Mutation	% Pancreatic Sufficient	Sweat Chloride Concentration (mM)	Age at Diagnosis in Years	Reference
ΔF508	2.5 (396)	106 ± 22 (328)	1.7 ± 3.0 (392)	68
P67L‡	77 (12)	57 ± 9 (12)	22.5 ± 11.3 (12)	704
R117H	87 (23)§	82 ± 19 (22)§	10.2 ± 10.5 (23)†	68
R334W	40 (15)§	108 ± 16 (15)	7.6 ± 6.6 (15)†	705
A455E	79 (33)§	not reported	15.0 ± 10.6 (33)‡	516
A455E	78 (9)*	80 ± 19 (9)†	5.7 ± 1.6 (9)†	517
3849 + 10 kb C → T‡	67 (15)	62 ± 17 (14)	12.5 ± 8.8 (15)	706
3849 + 10 kb C → T‡	77 (13)	39 (13)	not reported	244

*p < 0.05.
†p < 0.01.
‡Statistical comparison with ΔF508 homozygotes was not performed.
§p < 0.001 compared to a group of age- and sex-matched ΔF508 homozygote controls.

alterations in the CFTR gene correlate with the CBAVD phenotype. First, a distinct group of CFTR mutations are found in men with CBAVD that are not found in CF patients.[27,116,186] For example, the R117H mutation has been reported in both groups, however CF patients with R117H almost invariably have the 5T splicing variant in intron 8 that causes inefficient splicing while CBAVD patients have the more efficient 7T variant.[121,338] Second, the 5T variant by itself occurs at much higher frequency in CBAVD men than in the general population although males carrying a CF mutation and the 5T variant have fathered children.[116,701] The difference in fertility status appears to be explained by a separate genetic variant in intron 8 of CFTR.[151]

CFTR Genotype and Other Features of the CF Phenotype

Attempts have been made to correlate genotype with sweat gland dysfunction. Sweat Cl^- concentrations appear to be lower in PS patients than their PI counterparts.[605,671] However, sweat Cl^- values in PS patients may vary from values in the normal range to values observed in patients homozygous for the ΔF508 mutation. Table 201-9 shows the relationship between different mutations and the sweat Cl^- concentration.

The G551D mutation appears to confer a lower risk of meconium ileus than the ΔF508 mutation.[272,273,332] Moreover, mice with a G551D mutation had a lower rate of fatal intestinal obstruction than mice with a null mutation.[168] A genetic modifier that influences the occurrence of meconium ileus has been identified on chromosome 19 (see below), indicating an interplay between the CFTR genotype and genetic background in determining the risk of meconium ileus.

Upper airways disease may also be related to some mutations. A significant fraction of men with CBAVD due to CFTR mutations also have sinus disease.[105] Several studies have suggested that certain CF mutations may be related to nasal polyp formation and sinus disease.[93,319,628]

Modifiers of the CF Phenotype Independent of CFTR Genotype

Phenotype variability among CF patients with identical CFTR genotypes emphasizes the importance of other factors in the development of disease. These factors can be divided into two broad groups: allelic variants of genes that influence outcome in some fashion and environmental effects. Although each group may be composed of many different factors, progress has been made in the identification of genetic modifiers of CF. Murine CF models provide a tractable system to identify genetic modifiers because selective breeding of mice can isolate a variant of the disease phenotype. For example, intestinal obstruction leading to death in the neonatal period is commonly observed in CF mice.[125,184,566] However, prolonged survival of a fraction of animals was observed in some strains of mice bearing an identical CF genotype. Breeding experiments within and among mouse strains demonstrated that prolonged survival was genetically determined. A genome-wide scan identified the responsible locus on murine chromosome 7.[520] The corresponding locus in humans is on chromosome 19. Haplotypes created from a subset of polymorphic markers from the chromosome 19 locus show a nonrandom distribution among CF sibs with or without meconium ileus.[698] Sibs concordant for meconium ileus have significantly greater allele sharing, while sibs that are discordant have significantly less allele sharing. These data support the existence of a genetic modifier of intestinal disease in mice and humans.

The identified locus encompasses a large amount of DNA, suggesting that the search for specific modifier genes may be difficult. Electrophysiologic studies of mice indicated that prolonged survival was associated with a robust Ca^{2+}-mediated Cl^- conductance.[520] A similar explanation has been proposed for the absence of lung disease in CF mice.[126] Correlation of these findings in CF sibs concordant or discordant for meconium ileus may help refine the search for genes encoding CF modifiers.

The lack of a close correlation between CFTR genotype and the severity of pulmonary disease suggest that genetic and nongenetic determinants independent of CFTR play a significant role in the development of CF lung disease. Although CF mice do not normally exhibit lung disease, inbreeding of mice created a congenic strain that spontaneously developed lung disease, albeit with a phenotype showing fibrosis that was somewhat different from human CF.[327] Unlike CF mice on outbred strains, the nasal potential difference of congenic CF mice did not respond to UTP.[327] This result may be due to abnormal Ca^{2+}-mediated Cl^- conductance, or amiloride-sensitive Na^+ conductance. Homologs of the genetic modifiers of lung disease in mice may have a similar effect in humans.

Small-scale studies of twins and siblings with CF support the existence of modifiers for lung disease in human.[528,530] Since specific loci have not yet been identified by linkage studies, investigators have tested reasonable candidates. Alleles of genes involved in inflammatory and immune response in the lung showed intriguing associations with different degrees of lung disease severity.[35,300] A striking correlation has been reported between variants that reduce the amount of mannose-binding lectin (MBL) and lung function in CF patients chronically infected with *P. aeruginosa*.[239] Furthermore, survival rates and predicted median life expectancy differed significantly among CF patients grouped according to MBL serum levels.[239] The latter observations are expected of a significant modifier of lung disease since lung function is the major determinant of mortality in CF. These results confirm that genetic modifiers of CF lung disease exist, and can be identified using current technology.

Identifying environmental modifiers poses a more difficult task because of the potentially large number of factors. Exposure to cigarette smoke and virulent bacterial pathogens has been shown to affect patient outcome.[523] Smoking in the home causes significant reduction in pulmonary function in children with CF.[357,523,564] Acquisition rates of *Pseudomonas* vary by clinic setting, but the consequence of earlier colonization has been debated.[215,294] However, colonization with *B. cepacia* is associated with shortened median survival and patient-to-patient transmission has been implicated as an environmental risk.[316,607]

TREATMENT

Introduction

The treatment of cystic fibrosis (CF) is primarily directed towards prevention and/or correction of organ dysfunction and alleviation of symptoms. Although several novel therapies targeted to correct or modify CFTR dysfunction are being developed, none are currently available for patient care. Close patient monitoring and optimal management directed towards the secondary effects of CFTR mutations will afford patients the best opportunity to benefit from these novel therapies when they become available in the future.

To realize this goal, the US Cystic Fibrosis Foundation (CFF) has established a network of specialized accredited care centers, which provide multidisciplinary care to patients with CF of all ages. Similar care models have been established by specialists caring for patients with CF in Canada, throughout Europe, Australia, and New Zealand. Over the past decade, the US CFF has convened a series of consensus conferences involving experts in the CF field to establish guidelines for preventative and maintenance care of these patients, as well as treatment of the most common complications.[2,73,489,490,516,535,570,685] This process culminated in published care guidelines,[6] which represent an "explicit description of a national standard of care for patients with CF." The recommendations were based upon previously published scientific studies documenting the efficacy of specific interventions. If scientific evidence was insufficient, recommendations were based upon expert consensus.

The cornerstones of preventative care have been close monitoring of nutritional, gastrointestinal, and pulmonary status to promote normal growth and development in childhood and ongoing health in adulthood. The needs of adults with CF have led to the development of programs with specialized expertise in this area. A major advantage of close monitoring at a multidisciplinary center is the ability to collect longitudinal historical, physical, and laboratory data, allowing detection of subtle changes in health status. These changes will often identify progression of disease before the patients and families perceive it, so that interventions may be initiated early before irreversible organ damage occurs. The standard of care in most US CF care centers is to monitor patients quarterly when stable as assessed by nutritional and pulmonary status, and more frequently when a decline in clinical status is observed. The most common parameters used to monitor health status are height (in growing children), weight, and pulmonary function (e.g., forced expiratory volume in 1 sec, FEV_1, and forced vital capacity, FVC).

Another important aspect of preventative care is ongoing patient education. To assure optimal health and overall well-being, individuals with CF must closely self-monitor health status, as well as adhere to a complex daily medical regimen, which includes both multiple medications and physiotherapy. The patients and families must understand the pathophysiology of the disease and warning signs for disease progression, as well as potential adverse effects and interactions for all medications. The education process should continue throughout the life of the patient, requiring ongoing teaching and communication by all members of a multidisciplinary team.

Lung and Upper Respiratory Tract Therapy

Overview. The primary cause of morbidity and mortality in CF is progressive lung disease due to chronic bacterial endobronchial infections. Until prevention of bronchial colonization is an achievable goal, efforts should be directed towards minimizing other environmental factors that may be injurious to the CF lung and accelerate the pulmonary deterioration process.

Environmental irritants, in particular, cigarette smoking, both active and passive, should be avoided. Children exposed to passive smoking have an increased frequency of hospitalization and other respiratory symptoms similar to asthmatics[96] and a reduction in lung function.[357,523,564]

Respiratory viral infections are commonly associated with pulmonary exacerbations and are particularly injurious to the infant with CF,[13] resulting in prolonged hospitalization, oxygen requirements, wheezing, and potentially contributing to initial bacterial colonization. Respiratory syncytial virus (RSV) is of greatest concern in infants and young children. Efforts to develop RSV vaccines or immunotherapy are actively being pursued. RespiGam, an immunoglobulin preparation enriched with anti-RSV antibodies, has shown efficacy in reducing hospitalization for infants with chronic lung disease.[8] An RSV monoclonal antibody, Palivizumab has demonstrated similar efficacy.[606] Although neither product is specifically approved for infants with CF, it is commonly used in CF patients with established lung disease. A purified fusion protein vaccine (PFP-2) is being developed for annual administration to RSV-seropositive children to prevent subsequent lower respiratory tract illnesses during RSV season. Initial studies in children ages 2 to 9 years have been encouraging, with a reduction in lower respiratory tract infections (LRTI) and hospitalization rate with no evidence of vaccine enhanced disease.[466] Further Phase III studies are in progress. Whether RSV vaccines will eventually be administered to seronegative patients is controversial, because of the significant adverse effects of older vaccine products developed in the 1960s.

Other measures to reduce exposure and morbidity from respiratory viral infections include avoidance of contact with infected individuals and appropriate immunization strategies. In general, infants and preschool patients should not be placed in high density daycare settings and if placed, should be removed during times when respiratory viruses are prevalent. All CF children must receive immunizations using an age appropriate schedule that follows American Academy of Pediatrics guidelines (141 Northwest Point Blvd, Elk Grove Village, IL 60009-0927, www.aap.org). In addition, all patients over 6 months of age should be adequately immunized for influenza virus infection on a yearly basis. Because CF patients are rarely colonized with *S. pneumoniae*, the value of an annual pneumococcal vaccine is not known.

Treatment of the Upper Respiratory Tract. The nose and sinuses are frequently involved in CF. Sinus disease can be particularly severe and greatly impact on quality of life.

Treatment of Nasal Polyps. Several medical approaches have been offered for the treatment of nasal polyps in CF, though none have been proven in controlled trials.[617] Antihistamines and decongestants may provide symptomatic relief. Oral and inhaled corticosteroid treatments have also been tried. Surgical removal is often necessary when polyps cause significant obstruction of the nasal passages.

Treatment of Sinusitis. Treatment of sinusitis in CF is directed at the thick secretions, infection, and inflammation present in sinuses.[269] In addition, sinus polyposis may contribute to obstruction. Nasal irrigations performed on a daily basis as part of outpatient care are often helpful in controlling symptoms.

Antibiotics and anti-inflammatories have also been used systemically and intranasally. If these measures fail, surgery is necessary. The decision to perform surgery is based on clinical assessment, since abnormalities on imaging studies do not correlate with symptoms. Endoscopic irrigation of the sinuses often relieves symptoms for a while. Unfortunately, sinusitis is a recurring problem in CF and patients frequently require a series of procedures. Catheters left in place for irrigation with antibiotics may provide more prolonged relief of symptoms. Stents at the maxillary ostia have also been used but can become infected themselves. Brain abscess can occur in patients with particularly severe chronic sinusitis. Because of the chronic pain and headache accompanying chronic sinusitis, patients often require a great deal of support from CF caregivers.

Airway Clearance Techniques. Clearance of the abnormally viscous airway secretions has long been the mainstay of management for CF pulmonary disease. The major nonpharmacologic approaches to promote clearance has been standard chest physiotherapy (CPT), consisting of postural drainage with vibrations and percussion in 8 to 11 anatomic positions which favor gravitational movement of secretions.[416] This approach is based on the idea that coughing clears mucus from large airways while vibrations remove small airway secretions. Controlled studies have demonstrated that CPT is beneficial in patients with daily secretions and in treatment of pulmonary exacerbations.[82] Long-term effects in mild, asymptomatic patients are less well defined. In recent years a wide array of airway clearance techniques (ACT) have become available which allow patients greater autonomy and the ability to develop an individualized program, which often combines exercise and ACT's adapted to their needs.[278,416] These newer techniques can be divided between methods and/or devices requiring active patient participation and more passive techniques. The active techniques include the forced expiratory technique (e.g., "huff"),[278] autogenic drainage,[415] positive expiratory pressure (PEP),[415] and airway oscillators (e.g., Flutter).[353] Passive techniques include high frequency chest compressions[28] and an intrapulmonary percussive ventilator.[293] Short-term controlled studies have shown that most of these techniques are more efficacious than cough alone in sputum production and improving pulmonary function (FVC or FEV_1),[82] but that no significant difference between techniques may be discerned. A recent comparative trial suggested that an active technique such as positive expiratory pressure may improve lung function more than a passive technique such as conventional CPT during a comparable time period.[415] However, it is difficult to compare efficacy among methods because of small sample sizes and methodological problems in most study designs. Thus, patient satisfaction and compliance are often the most important criteria for selection of techniques.

Bronchodilators. Many patients with CF demonstrate bronchial lability which is variable over time and increases with illness severity. Short-term studies of both inhaled beta-adrenergic[295] agents and ipratropium bromide[527] have demonstrated improved pulmonary function. Long-term usage remains controversial, however.[622] It is also important to remember that one of the major contributing factors to CF airway lability is the underlying inflammation and infection. Thus, close monitoring and treatment of infection must be an integral part of any evaluation of bronchodilator therapy.

Some clinicians recommend limiting bronchodilator usage to those patients who demonstrate an increase of 10 percent or more in FEV_1 in response to a bronchodilator challenge. Sequential bronchodilator studies and repeated clinical evaluation of the patient have been advocated to follow responsiveness to therapy over time.[459] Both inhaled beta-adrenergic and parasympatholytic agents may improve expiratory flow rates, and when given together effects may be potentiated.[527] Oral anticholinergic agents (e.g., atropine) are not recommended because of adverse effects such as blurred vision, dry mouth, and drying of bronchial secretions. These adverse effects have not been a significant problem with the inhaled ipratropium bromide. The dose of inhaled bronchodilators in patients with CF is the same as recommended for patients with asthma (*Guidelines for the Diagnosis and Management of Asthma*, NIH Publication No. 97-4051, July 1997).

Methylxanthines, such as theophylline, may also have a bronchodilatory effect, although their use has decreased in recent years because of potentially lethal adverse effects (arrhythmias and convulsions).[622] Use of these oral agents in the CF population may be problematic because of increased hepatic clearance[308] necessitating larger and more frequent doses and concomitant administration of other medications, such as erythromycin and ciprofloxacin, which decrease theophylline clearance. Theophylline usage should be limited to those patients poorly responsive to inhaled beta-adrenergic or anticholinergic therapy. If initiated, serum concentrations must be closely monitored.

Mucolytic Agents. Abnormal viscoelastic properties of CF mucus contribute to airway obstruction and possibly to eventual structural damage. Several approaches to decrease viscosity have been advocated, including modulation of Cl^- or Na^+ epithelial transport (see "Airway Epithelia" above), hydration of airway secretions, and degradation of mucus or extracellular DNA fibrils.

The most well studied and currently most widely used therapy to reduce sputum viscoelasticity is rhDNase (Pulmozyme). Extracellular DNA derived from lysed polymorphonuclear neutrophils, aggregates to form large insoluble fibrils that increase sputum viscosity. A purified recombinant human deoxyribonuclease I (Pulmozyme) that can digest extracellular DNA reduces the viscosity of sputum specimens from patients with CF. A series of randomized, controlled clinical trials demonstrated rapid improvement in FEV_1 of approximately 14 percent in short-term administration[515] and a sustained improvement of 5 to 6 percent predicted over a six month period.[233] Enzyme administration was also associated with a significant reduction in the risk of respiratory exacerbations requiring intravenous antibiotic therapy.[233]

Pulmozyme at a dose of 2.5 mg administered daily by inhalation has been FDA approved in all patients with CF. This human recombinant protein has not been associated with hypersensitivity reactions and the only consistent adverse reactions have been transient laryngitis and hoarseness.

Use of Pulmozyme has been directed towards patients with evidence of chronic endobronchial bacterial infections associated with purulent secretions and an obstructive pattern on pulmonary function testing. No baseline characteristics have been useful predictors of clinical response, although spirometric improvement at 3 months correlates well with sustained response at 12 months.[160] There are individuals, however, with no spirometric response who may demonstrate a decrease in frequency of respiratory exacerbations and should be considered treatment responsive.[233]

Pulmozyme should be administered as a chronic daily therapy. It was not shown to be beneficial as a short-term intermittent therapy for pulmonary exacerbations[669] and the effect on pulmonary function is not sustained after cessation of the drug.[199]

Antibiotic Therapy. Chronic endobronchial infections are the major cause of morbidity and mortality in CF. Thus, appropriate antimicrobial therapy directed against bacterial pathogens isolated from respiratory tract secretions is the mainstay of treatment of the lung disease and has contributed to the improved life span. Clinicians may administer antibiotics in three distinct clinical settings during the lifetime of a CF patient: (1) intensive antibiotic therapy (frequently in hospital) for treatment of increased respiratory symptomatology, termed a pulmonary exacerbation; (2) chronic maintenance therapy in hopes of reducing the frequency and morbidity of pulmonary exacerbations and decline in pulmonary function; and (3) preventative therapy to delay initial lower airway colonization with the most common pathogen, *P. aeruginosa*.

Treatment of Pulmonary Exacerbation. Although patients are persistently infected with lower airway pathogens, such as *S. aureus* and *P. aeruginosa*, their respiratory symptomatology varies over time. They will experience periodic exacerbations characterized by increased cough and sputum production, decreased exercise tolerance, anorexia, and weight loss.[487]

The standard therapy for an exacerbation is parenteral antibiotic therapy with two antibiotics for 14 to 21 days.[487,500] The choice of antibiotics should be based upon susceptibility testing of bacteria isolated from sputum. The most common antibiotic combinations and appropriate dosage regimens utilized for treatment are displayed in Table 201-10. A combination of an aminoglycoside and beta-lactam provides drug synergy and slows emergence of resistance. Doses of these antibiotics need to be higher than in non-CF populations due to an increased volume of distribution and creatinine clearance in most patients with CF.[559] Intravenous aminoglycoside therapy must be closely monitored with serum drug levels to minimize the risk of renal and ototoxicity. A single administration of the total daily dose of intravenous aminoglycosides has been advocated in non-CF populations as preferable to three divided doses, because bacterial killing is dependent upon peak serum concentrations, whereas toxicity is related to trough antibiotic concentration. Preliminary studies in patients with CF suggest that once daily dosing achieves good aminoglycoside sputum levels without serum accumulation or observed toxicity.[631] Larger, prospective studies are needed to demonstrate equivalency of once and thrice daily administration regimens.

In addition to antibiotics, treatment of an exacerbation requires intensified airway clearance techniques and nutritional support. Some patients require increased bronchodilator therapy and inhaled, oral, or parenteral corticosteroids. Response to therapy is reflected by improved pulmonary function, and overall well-being.[500] Therapy is commonly initiated in the hospital to assure stabilization of respiratory status, although home administration of intravenous therapy is increasingly commonplace. Home care with adequate supervision may be as effective as inpatient therapy, though further studies are needed.[678]

Maintenance Antibiotic Therapy. Patients colonized with bacterial pathogens commonly receive long-term antibiotics in hopes of slowing the progression of obstructive pulmonary disease and reducing the frequency of pulmonary exacerbations. For mild, preschool patients colonized with *S. aureus*, use of chronic oral antistaphylococcal antibiotics was a common practice in the past. Two prospective studies, however, demonstrated no difference in clinical symptom score, lung function, nutritional status or frequency of exacerbation with continuous antibiotics.[487] More concerning, one study observed an increased emergence of *P. aeruginosa* associated with a reduction in *S. aureus* colonization.

Several approaches have been used for maintenance therapy in patients colonized with *P. aeruginosa*. Quarterly administration of intravenous anti-*Pseudomonal* antibiotics has been advocated by Danish physicians based upon a report of slower decline in lung function compared with historical controls.[593] However, an increasing incidence of *P. aeruginosa* resistant to common intravenous antibiotics is cause for concern.[311] Many European and North American care centers have utilized inhaled aminoglycosides as maintenance therapy, based upon reports of improved pulmonary function and decreased hospitalization following chronic administration of aminoglycosides at a dose of 60 to 80 mg thrice daily.[383] Inhaled administration of aminoglycosides is attractive, because of the greater therapeutic index afforded by direct delivery of very high concentrations into airway secretions, with low systemic absorption minimizing toxicity. A large, Phase III multicenter, placebo-controlled efficacy trial in the United States[491]) recently reported a 10 percent increase in forced expiratory volume in one second (FEV_1) and a 36 percent reduction in use of intravenous antibiotics following 6 months intermittent administration of 300 mg inhaled tobramycin (TOBI) twice daily (cycling four weeks on, four weeks off). The study closely monitored *P. aeruginosa* isolates for emergence of tobramycin resistance and found a trend towards higher minimal inhibitory concentration in the treated patients, but this trend had no adverse effect on the improvement in pulmonary function among patients receiving therapy. Aerosolized colistin sulfate, colistimethate, and polymixin B have been chronically administered to stabilize pulmonary status, but published data on long-term efficacy and safety are limited.[383] Inhaled colistin may cause chest tightness and decline in pulmonary function.[182]

Oral antibiotics are frequently used for maintenance therapy or treatment of milder, subacute pulmonary exacerbations in older patients colonized with either *S. aureus* or *P. aeruginosa*. Commonly utilized antibiotics and appropriate doses are shown in Table 201-11. Macrolides, such as erythromycin, clarithromycin, and azithromycin, have been highly effective antibiotics in treatment of diffuse panbronchiolitis,[347] an airway disease also associated with chronic mucoid *P. aeruginosa*. The pathophysiology of this chronic infection is similar to CF, with colonies of *P. aeruginosa* forming a protective antibiotic resistant biofilm of mucoid-alginate that induces immune complex formation and secondary inflammation. In this setting, macrolides appear to have several modes of action, including inhibition of alginate production and host antialginate antibody production, as well as an antimicrobial effect. There is increasing interest in the use of chronic macrolides in CF and several prospective studies are currently in progress.

The most effective oral anti-*Pseudomonal* antibiotics are the quinolones, such as ciprofloxacin, which have excellent bioavailability in airway secretions and may be as effective as intravenous antibiotics in treatment of mild exacerbations.[74] Unfortunately, drug resistance is common after 3 to 4 weeks of monotherapy, so long-term chronic therapy should be discouraged.[541] Quinolones have not been FDA-approved for use in patients less than 18 years of age, because they may cause arthropathy in weight-bearing diarthrodial joints of young animals. However, extensive experience in children with CF on a compassionate basis has shown no evidence of arthropathy.[124]

Preventative Therapy. Initiation of early antibiotic therapy to prevent persistent colonization with *P. aeruginosa* in young patients remains controversial. European studies have reported decreased acquisition of persistent *P. aeruginosa* colonization as measured by either oropharyngeal or sputum cultures and/or development of a serologic response directed against *P. aeruginosa* exotoxins utilizing either aerosolized colistin with oral ciprofloxacin[231] or inhaled tobramycin[662] at the time of initial positive *P. aeruginosa* culture (prior to seropositivity). These reports are provocative, but difficult to interpret, because of the poor sensitivity of oropharyngeal cultures and serology in predicting lower airway microbiologic status.[33,515]

Immunotherapy. An alternative to antibiotic therapy for chronic *P. aeruginosa* endobronchial infections has been the use of either active or passive immunotherapy. Early clinical trials with vaccines directed against *P. aeruginosa* lipopolysaccharide (LPS) were unsuccessful and slowed research efforts for more than a decade. An octavalent *P. aeruginosa* O-polysaccharide-toxin A conjugate is being developed in Europe and appears to be well tolerated and capable of inducing high-affinity anti-LPS antibodies.[366] A *P. aeruginosa* flagella vaccine has also been shown to elicit long-lasting anti-flagella antibody titers and a European Phase III multicenter vaccine trial is currently in progress.[185] Passive immunotherapy utilizing standard intravenous immunoglobulin (IVIG), 100 mg/Kg, has been studied as adjunctive therapy for pulmonary exacerbation in patients colonized with

Table 201-10 Bacteria Associated with Exacerbations of Pulmonary Infection in Patients with CF and Appropriate Intravenous Treatments

	First Choice[1]			Alternative[1]		
		Dose			Dose	
Prevalent Bacteria	Antibiotic	Child	Adult	Antibiotic	Child	Adult
S. aureus	Cefazolin	50 mg/kg every 8 hr	1 g every 8 hr	Vancomycin[2]	15 mg/kg every 6 hr	500 mg every 6 hr Or 1 g every 1 hr
	Nafcillin[3]	25–50 mg/kg every 6 hr	1 g every 6 hr			
H. influenzae and *S. aureus*	Ticarcillin-clavulanate[4]	100 mg/kg of ticarcillin and 3.3 mg/kg of clavulanate every 6 hr	3 g of ticarcillin and 0.1 g of clavulanate every 6 hr	Nafcillin[3] PLUS gentamicin[5]	25–50 mg/kg every 6 hr 3 mg/kg every 8 hr	1 g every 6 hr 3 mg/kg every 8 hr
	PLUS gentamicin[5]	3 mg/kg every 8 hr	3 mg/kg every 8 hr			
S. aureus and *P. aeruginosa*	Ticarcillin-clavulanate	100 mg/kg of ticarcillin and 3.3 mg/kg of clavulanate every 6 hr	3 g of ticarcillin and 0.1 g of clavulanate every 6 hr	Piperacillin-tazobactam PLUS tobramycin[5]	100 mg/kg every 6 hr 3 mg/kg every 8 hr	3 g every 6 hr 3 mg/kg every 8 hr
	PLUS tobramycin[5]	3 mg/kg every 8 hr	3 mg/kg every 8 hr			
P. aeruginosa only	Ticarcillin[4] PLUS	100 mg/kg every 6 hr	3 g every 6 hr	Tobramycin[5] PLUS	3 mg/kg every 8 hr	3 mg/kg every 8 hr
	tobramycin[5]	3 mg/kg every 8 hr	3 mg/kg every 8 hr	ceftazidime	50 mg/kg every 8 hr	2 g every 8 hr
				piperacillin	100 mg/kg every 6 hr	3 g every 6 hr
				imipenem[6] OR	15–25 mg/kg every 6 hr	500 mg-1g every 6 hr
				meropenem[6]	40 mg/kg every 8 hr	2 g every 8 h
				Aztreonam PLUS	50 mg/kg every 6 hr	2 g every 8 hr
				amikacin[8]	5–7.5 mg/kg every 8 hr	5–7.5 mg/kg every 8 hr
P. aeruginosa and *B. cepacia*[7]	Ceftazidime PLUS	50–75 mg/kg every 8 hr	2 g every 8 hr	Meropenem[6] PLUS	40 mg/kg every 8 hr	2 g every 8 hr
	ciprofloxacin	15 mg/kg every 12 hr	400 mg every 12 hr	tobramycin	3 mg/kg every 8 hr	3 mg/kg every 8 hr
				Ceftazidime PLUS	50–75 mg/kg every 8 hr	2 g every 8 hr
				Chloramphenicol[9] OR	15–20 mg/kg every 6 hr	15–20 mg/kg every 6 hr —max 4g/d
				trimethoprim-sulfamethoxazole	5 mg/kg trimethoprim and 25 mg/kg sulfamethoxazole every 6 hr	5 mg/kg trimethoprim and 25 mg/kg sulfamethoxazole every 6 hr
B. cepacia[7] only	Chloramphenicol[9]	15–20 mg/kg every 6 hr	15–20 mg/kg every 6 hr—max 4g/d	Meropenem[6]PLUS	40 mg/kg every 8 hr	2 g every 8 hr
	OR trimethoprim-sulfamethoxazole OR Both	5 mg/kg trimethoprim and 25 mg/kg sulfamethoxazole every 6 hr	5 mg/kg trimethoprim and 25 mg/kg sulfamethoxazole every 6 hr	Chloramphenicol[9]	15–20 mg/kg every 6 hr	15–20 mg/kg every 6 hr —max 4 g/d
				OR trimethoprim-sulfamethoxazole	5 mg/kg trimethoprim and 25 mg/kg sulfamethoxazole every 6 hr	5 mg/kg trimethoprim and 25 mg/kg sulfamethoxazole every 6 hr

[1]Most doses are expressed as milligrams per kilogram of body weight. The dose given to children should not exceed that for adults.
[2]Vancomycin should be infused slowly to avoid histamine release. Serum concentrations should be monitored; target peak concentration ranges from 20–30 μg per milliliter, trough from 5–10 μg per milliliter.
[3]To minimize phlebitis, nafcillin should be diluted to a concentration of less than 20 mg per milliliter.
[4]Ticarcillin may be associated with occasional platelet dysfunction. Its use is limited by the possibility of resistant organisms.
[5]Serum concentrations should be monitored; target peak concentration ranges from 8–12 μg per milliliter, trough concentration less than 2 μg per milliliter.
[6]These drugs should be limited to patients with sensitivity to cephalosporins or multidrug-resistant organisms.
[7]Frequent antibiotic susceptibility testing is recommended to ensure treatment with the optimal combination of antibiotics; synergy testing may be helpful.
[8]Serum concentrations should be monitored; the peak concentration ranges from 15–25 μg per milliliter, and the trough concentration is less than 10 μg per milliliter.
[9]Serum concentrations should be monitored; the peak concentration ranges from 15–25 μg per milliliter, and the trough from 5–10 μg per milliliter.

Table 201-11 Oral antibiotics Commonly Used to Suppress Respiratory Pathogens in Patients with CF*

Pathogen	Antibiotic	Dose: Child	Dose: Adult
S. aureus	Dicloxacillin	6.25 mg/kg every 6 hr	250–500 mg every 6 hr
	Cephalexin	12.5 mg/kg every 6 hr	500 mg every 6 hr
	Amoxicillin-clavulanate†	12.5–22.5 mg/kg of amoxicillin every 12 hr	400–875 mg of amoxicillin every 12 hr
	Erythromycin	15 mg/kg every 8 hr	250 mg every 8 hr
	Clarithromycin	7.5 mg/kg every 12 hr	500 mg every 12 hr
H. influenzae	Cefaclor	10–15 mg/kg every 8 hr	250–500 mg every 8 hr
	Amoxicillin	20–40 mg/kg every 8 hr	500 mg every 8 hr
S. aureus and *H. influenzae*	Cefixime	8 mg/kg/day	400 mg/day
	Amoxicillin-clavulanate	12.5–22.5 mg/kg of amoxicillin every 12 hr	400–875 mg of amoxicillin every 12 hr
	Trimethoprim-sulfamethoxazole	4 mg/kg of trimethoprim and 20 mg/kg sulfamethoxazole every 12 hr	160 mg of trimethoprim and 800 mg of sulfamethoxazole every 12 hr
	Cefpodoxime	5 mg/kg every 12 hr	200 mg every 12 hr
	Cefuroxime	20 mg/kg every 12 hr	250–500 mg every 12 hr
P. aeruginosa	Ciprofloxacin‡	Not approved	500–750 mg every 12 hr
	Ofloxacin‡	Not approved	400 mg every 12 hr
B. cepacia	Trimethoprim-sulfamethoxazole	4 mg/kg of trimethoprim and 20 mg/kg of sulfamethoxazole every 12 hr	160 mg of trimethoprim and 800 mg of sulfamethoxazole every 12 hr
	Doxycycline	5 mg/kg initial dose followed by 2.5 mg/kg every 12 hr§	200 mg initial dose followed by 100 mg every 12 hr
	Minocycline	4 mg/kg initial dose followed by 2 mg/kg every 12 hr§	200 mg initial dose followed by 100 mg every 12 hr

*The list is not intended to be exhaustive. The dose given to children should not exceed that for adults.
†Higher doses of clavulanate are frequently associated with diarrhea.
‡Ciprofloxacin and ofloxacin have not been approved for use in patients under 18 years of age.
§Tetracycline antibiotics are not recommended for children under 8 years of age.

P. aeruginosa and may augment clinical efficacy of antibiotics.[675] Attempts to develop more specific anti-*Pseudomonas* monoclonal antibodies targeted to the CF population for passive immunotherapy have not yet been successful.

Other Pathogens. The risk of all long-term antibiotic therapy in patients with CF, whether directed towards prevention of initial colonization or stabilization of the previously-colonized patient, is the emergence of *P. aeruginosa* pathogens resistant to common antibiotics, or superinfection with new airway pathogens inherently resistant to most antibiotics. A 1996 cross-sectional study of sputum microbiology on almost 4000 isolates from 595 patients colonized with *P. aeruginosa* at 69 US CF care centers reported a prevalence of tobramycin resistance at 21 percent and multiply resistant *P. aeruginosa* (defined as pathogens resistant to at least 2 classes of anti-*Pseudomonal* antibiotics) at 11.6 percent.[94] The emergence of other multiply resistant gram negative pathogens, such as *Stenotrophomonas maltophilia* and *B. cepacia*, is also concerning. The clinician must, therefore, weigh the benefit of stabilization in pulmonary status against the risk of selecting for antibiotic resistant bacteria.

Treatment of infections with multiresistant *P. aeruginosa* is challenging, but use of *in vitro* synergy testing[525] may be useful in defining the optimal drug combinations. In addition, use of high-dose inhaled tobramycin[491] may achieve adequate levels in the airway to overcome even resistant strains.

Several gram-negative pathogens, inherently resistant to multiple antibiotics, have become more common. *B. cepacia* is the most widely reported, but *S. maltophilia* and *Alcaligenes xylosoxidans* have also been identified at multiple CF care centers. The pathogenicity of *S. maltophilia* and *A. xylosoxidans* is not yet well defined. By contrast, *B. cepacia* may cause rapid deterioration and premature death in some patients.[316,607] Infection control is critical to prevent patient to patient transmission of multiresistant pathogens. All CF care centers are now taking precautionary measures to isolate all patients from other patients in both the inpatient and outpatient settings. Antibiotic therapy for treatment of these pathogens must be based upon careful review of *in vitro* susceptibility testing and synergy studies (if available). These pathogens are frequently susceptible to trimethoprim-sulfa or chloramphenicol; some *S. maltophilia* is susceptible to doxycycline.

The clinical significance and treatment guidelines for nontuberculous mycobacteria (NTM) in CF are evolving.[443] There are currently no definitive guidelines to "identify" which patients have active disease, which will benefit from antimicrobial therapy (the optimal treatment regimen), or the duration of therapy. The best available guidelines are now evolving from an ongoing multicenter NTM study. Active infection is best assessed by multiple positive sputum samples collected over several weeks and HRCT evidence of peripheral nodules.[443] In some patients, bronchoscopic collection of specimens for staining and culture or a mucosal biopsy for evidence of granulomatosis disease may be helpful. Multidrug therapy for at least one year's duration is usually necessary to achieve clinical or microbiologic response. A summary of appropriate antibiotic agents and dose regimens for each of the common NTM organisms has been recently published (Table 201-12).[443]

Anti-Inflammatory Treatment. A common characteristic of airway disease in CF is massive influx of neutrophils perpetuating the inflammatory cycle by releasing chemoattractants. This process contributes to airway obstruction and injury (see "Lung and Upper Respiratory Tract" above). A variety of therapeutic approaches has been proposed to limit the adverse consequences of this airway inflammatory response while permitting the immune

Table 201-12 Guidelines for Treatment of Nontuberculosis Mycobacterium in Patients with CF with Well-Defined Pathogenic Infection

General

Start with a single drug, adding sequentially every 3–4 days, observing for side effects with each new drug
Dose at bedtime to improve absorption and to mask gastrointestinal side effects
Because of altered metabolism and absorption in patients with CF,
  Monitor serum levels two weeks after all medications started
  Draw peak serum levels 2 hours post-dosing
Follow-up cultures monthly
Consider adding or changing drugs at 6 mos if adequate levels obtained,
  and yet there is either no clinical response or no microbiologic response
  (no reduction in colony counts, positive smear)
In vitro drug susceptibility testing may be useful in selecting alternate drugs

Specific

Organism	Agent	Dose*	Comments
MAC	Clarithromycin	30 mg/kg/day (max 1,000 mg) po	Levels decreased by rifampicin, rifabutin, increased by azoles
	Rifabutin	5 mg/kg/day (max 300 mg) po	Discontinue if leukocytes < 2000 or granulocytes < 1000
	Ethambutol	25 mg/kg/day po	Baseline eye examination/monitor acuity and color monthly
Duration: Not established, probably 1 yr after negative culture			
Drugs to consider adding include: clofazamine, streptomycin, amikacin three times weekly (serum peaks 40 µg/mL), ciprofloxacin			
M. abscessus (formerly *M. chelonei*, subspecies abscessus)	Cefoxitin	200 mg/kg/day IV	Max 12 g/day
	Amikacin	15 mg/kg/day IV every 12 h audiogram, monitor renal function	Peak 18–24 µg/ml, baseline
M. fortuitum	Clarithromycin	30 mg/kg/day (max 1000 mg)	As above
Duration: 6–12 mos			
If resistance to clarithromycin noted on susceptibility testing, use ciprofloxacin			
M. kansasii	Isoniazid	10–20 mg/kg/day po qd, max 300 mg	LFT's at baseline, then monthly D/C if > 3 x normal
	Rifampin	10–20 mg/kg/day po qd, max 600 mg	LFT's at baseline, then monthly D/C if > 3 x normal
	Ethambutol	25 mg/kg/day po qd x 2 months, then decrease to 15 mg/kg/day po qd	Baseline eye examination/monitor acuity and color monthly
Duration: 18 mos, monthly cultures until negative, then at completion of therapy			

*Doses and maximums are for initial dosing only; subsequent doses guided by peak serum levels.
D/C = discontinue; IV = intravenous; LFT = liver function test; MAC = *Mycobacterium avium* complex; po = by mouth; qd = every day

system to appropriately control infection. These approaches fall into two major categories: agents which inhibit chemotaxis and/or activation of leukocytes, such as corticosteroids and nonsteroidal anti-inflammatory drugs (NSAID's), and agents which inhibit the adverse effects of toxic leukocyte byproducts, such as antiproteases and antioxidants.

Corticosteroids have been extensively studied and utilized for their multiple, potent anti-inflammatory effects.[350] They are routinely prescribed in CF patients with asthma and are the mainstay of therapy for allergic bronchopulmonary aspergillosis.[438]

Long-term administration of steroids to modulate or prevent airway inflammation to all patients remains controversial. A multicenter, 4-year controlled trial of alternate day oral steroids (dose 1 to 2 mg/kg) in children with mild to moderate disease demonstrated beneficial anti-inflammatory effects[198] specifically, better pulmonary function and fewer hospitalizations, but unacceptable side effects included growth retardation, cataracts, and abnormal glucose metabolism.[198] A small subsequent study utilizing a shorter 12 week course of oral prednisolone therapy demonstrated similar benefit with fewer side effects.[254] Smaller studies of inhaled steroids, such as fluticasone, have demonstrated little benefit,[41] but may warrant further study. Thus, physicians continue to utilize oral corticosteroids with close monitoring for growth retardation and other potential adverse effects.

Ibuprofen is the most well established NSAID for use in CF, because of its ability to inhibit neutrophil migration.[350] A 4-year, placebo-controlled study in 85 patients showed less annual decline in FEV_1 among patients receiving ibuprofen (−2.2 percent), than in those in the placebo group (−3.6 percent).[351] The most pronounced effect was observed in children ages 5 to 13 years. Effective use of therapy requires close monitoring of serum values to maintain peak concentrations of 50 to 100 µg/ml. Widespread use of ibuprofen in the CF community has been limited by a lack of long term safety data and the difficulty of on-going monitoring of serum levels.[350] Another NSAID, piroxicam, may also have a beneficial effect on pulmonary function, but data is limited.[572]

The burden of neutrophil-derived free-elastase and other proteolytic enzymes overwhelms the host antiprotease response in the CF airways. To prevent further destruction of lung tissue by proteolytic enzymes, administration of exogenous antiproteases has been proposed to augment the host defense system. The most well studied antiprotease, alpha 1-antitrypsin (α1AT), reduced but did not eliminate the active elastase content in bronchoalveolar lavage fluid after four weeks of aerosol administration in a preliminary study.[64] Commonly available plasma-derived α1AT is limited in supply and carries a small risk of blood borne pathogens. A transgenic human α1AT protein is currently under investigation and may prove more efficacious and safe.[350] Other potential aerosolized and oral antiprotease agents, such as recombinant human secretory leukocyte protease inhibitor (rhSLPI) have been evaluated in early human trials, but no published results are available.[350] A recombinant human monocyte/neutrophil elastase inhibitor which mitigates protease-induced lung injury from CF airway secretions in the rat model, may be a potential therapeutic agent in the future.[499] To prevent the proinflammatory effects of proteases such as elastase, it is likely that all free enzyme in the airways must be neutralized. None of the current therapies has yet achieved this goal.

Oxidant lung injury, another by-product of the intense neutrophilic inflammatory response, has received increased attention as an important factor in the progression of CF lung disease. Endogenous antioxidants, beta-carotene (a precursor of vitamin A), alpha tocopherol (vitamin E), and ascorbic acid (vitamin C) have long been prescribed to patients as nutritional supplements (see "Nutritional management" below). Their antioxidant effects and the appropriate dose regimen to achieve optimal antioxidant therapy must be further studied. Supplementation with glutathione has also been proposed.[518]

In summary, the potential role of anti-inflammatory therapies has gained wide acceptance in the CF community. To date, only corticosteroids and ibuprofen have been closely scrutinized in well controlled, long-term clinical trials.

Treatment of Common Complications of CF Lung Disease. The unrelenting endobronchial bacterial infections and associated inflammation lead to structural airway damage (bronchiectasis), alveolar hypoventilation, and progressive respiratory impairment. The incidence of pulmonary complications, including hypoxemia with hypercapnic respiratory failure, pneumothorax, and hemoptysis increases with age and illness severity. The morbidity and mortality associated with these complications is significant, frequently requiring immediate, aggressive medical interventions, which have been well described in recent reviews.[535,581]

Respiratory Failure. Respiratory failure is the primary cause of death in over 90 percent of patients with CF.[161] In recent years, better management of the associated sequelae of respiratory failure, hypoxemia, and hypercapnia, have significantly improved the quality and duration of life for patients with end-stage disease. Hypoxemia, resulting primarily from the ventilation-perfusion mismatch of chronic airway obstruction, is most effectively treated with supplemental oxygen.[535] Patients should be considered for supplemental oxygen therapy when their ambient oxygen saturation is less than 88 percent while resting, less than 90 percent with exercise, or less than 88 percent for more than 10 percent of sleep time, or they have documented right ventricular hypertrophy.[684] As sleep may worsen hypoxemia in patients with significant airway obstruction, nocturnal oximetry studies are recommended to document the degree of sleep hypoxemia and response to therapy. Oxygen therapy should be titrated to maintain arterial blood above a partial oxygen pressure of 60 mm Hg (oxygen saturations $>$ 88 to 90 percent). Other therapies, such as diuretics, cardiac glycosides, or pulmonary vasodilators are rarely used with early oxygen intervention and have limited additional efficacy.

Hypercapnia resulting from alveolar hypoventilation may occur acutely from a significant intercurrent respiratory infection (viral or bacterial) or secondary complications, such as pneumothorax or hemoptysis. In the setting of acute respiratory failure, the patient's prognosis is dependent upon the severity of the underlying, irreversible lung disease. Patients with milder disease (especially young infants and children)[238] will respond favorably to short-term mechanical ventilation. Patients with severe, end-stage disease will likely not sustain a long-term benefit from endotracheal intubation and mechanical ventilation unless the individual is a previously listed transplantation candidate with a wait list priority that assures availability of a donor organ (or living-related donor) within weeks.

The need for ventilatory support for respiratory failure may be delayed or prevented by assiduous management of the underlying disease, including initiation of oxygen supplementation, rehabilitative exercise programs to improve respiratory muscle strength, enteral nutritional support, aggressive management of lung infection, and clearance of airway secretions. The use of positive pressure ventilation at home via nasal or facial mask has been advocated in some patients with hypercapnic respiratory failure.[470]

Pneumothorax. Small asymptomatic pneumothoraces filling less than 20 percent of the hemithorax are treated conservatively with observation and management of underlying infection.[535] Pneumothoraces of greater size which are symptomatic require chest tube thoracostomy to evacuate air and appose the visceral and parietal pleura. Recurrent or persistent ($>$ 5 days) pneumothoraces require pleurodesis, either surgical or chemical in most cases, to obliterate the pleural space. Surgical approaches with bullectomy and pleurodesis have the greatest success rate[573] and are the preferred management alternative for potential lung transplantation candidates.[176] Chemical pleurodesis should only be considered for patients in whom surgery poses a significant risk.

Hemoptysis. Hemoptysis in the past carried a high mortality. With current approaches, however, acute bleeding is rarely fatal if the patient rapidly reaches a medical facility and is appropriately treated with aggressive therapy to slow the hemorrhaging and assure an adequate airway.[581] Therapy for recurrent episodes of hemoptysis should include appropriate treatment of underlying airway infections, assessment of coagulation status (e.g., prothrombin and partial prothrombin times, platelet count), and cessation of all drugs that interfere with coagulation. Other etiologies of bleeding, such as a gastrointestinal bleeding source, must be considered. The definitive therapy for recurrent hemoptysis is bronchial artery embolization,[86] which has a high success rate with few complications if performed by an experienced angiographer.

Allergic Bronchopulmonary Aspergillosis. Patients with ABPA are treated daily or every other day with oral corticosteroids (0.5 to 1.0 mg/kg) for months, with gradual reduction based upon clinical response and serum IgE levels. The antifungal agent, itraconazole, has recently been used chronically to decrease steroid use.[438]

Lung Transplantation. Since the mid-1980's, bilateral lung or heart-lung transplantation has been a therapeutic option available to some patients with end-stage lung disease. The United Network for Organ Sharing has recorded 1339 lung transplants worldwide in patients with CF through 1998, representing approximately 15 percent of all lung transplant recipients. The mean age among CF recipients is 26 years (range 5 to 59 years) with equal male and female distribution.[685] Survival among patients with CF undergoing transplantation is comparable to other non-CF patients with a one year survival of 70 percent and five year survival of 48 percent.[138] No statistical differences are attributable to age, gender, blood group (A, O, AB/B combined), or cytomegaloviral infection status. Survival rates may be higher, however, at larger centers with a greater frequency of transplantation.[685]

Patients should be considered for transplantation when their progressive lung disease and associated respiratory insufficiency will likely lead to death in a time frame somewhat longer than the expected waiting period for available donor organs.[336,685] Unfortunately, the growing disparity between the availability of donor lungs and the increasing number of potential recipients has lengthened the waiting time at some centers to over 2 years. Selected centers have initiated a living-donor approach[129] to address the increasing obstacle of limited available cadaveric donor organs. The complexity and morbidity of the living-related donor approach may preclude its widespread use. Criteria for patient referral to a transplant center includes an FEV_1 less than 30 percent predicted[336,685] associated with hypoxemia and hypercarbia, increased frequency of and poor response to hospital therapy for pulmonary exacerbation, and increasing resistance to antibiotics for treatment of lung infections.

Contraindications to transplantation may vary based upon the individual experience of each center. Absolute contraindications at all centers are limited to infections with human immunodeficiency virus (HIV), hepatitis B positive surface antigen, and active *Mycobacterium tuberculosis* infection.[685] Relative contraindications at most centers include significant nonpulmonary organ dysfunction (e.g., liver, kidney), infections with pathogens such as *B. cepacia* or some *P. aeruginosa* strains that are resistant to all available antibiotic agents,[29] and psychosocial dysfunction that compromises compliance with medical therapy.

The most widely utilized thoracic transplantation procedure in US centers is bilateral lung transplantation through a transverse "clamshell" incision.[456] This procedure has reduced perioperative mortality and morbidity, in particular massive hemorrhage, in the CF population. The European experience with heart-lung transplant has been equally successful.[165]

The postoperative course and medical management of patients with CF receiving lung transplantation are similar to those of non-CF patients.[685] The reader is referred to a recent review chapter for a more complete summary of common immunosuppression regimens.[455] The most common complications among all transplant recipients are graft rejection, either acute or chronic, and infections. With all transplant recipients, vigilant monitoring for evidence of infection or rejection and early, aggressive intervention are mandatory to optimize survival. After patients have survived greater than six months post-transplantation, the most common cause of morbidity and mortality is bronchiolitis obliterans with an incidence of 20 to 50 percent in both CF and non-CF populations.[618] Bronchiolitis obliterans may be associated with recurrence of *P. aeruginosa* infections and bronchiectasis.

Lung transplantation, with its associated immunosuppressive regimen, leads to unique challenges in the CF population. Common complications include gastrointestinal motility disorders, inadequate nutrition and linear growth in children, exacerbation of glucose intolerance or pre-existing diabetes mellitus, and osteoporosis.[31,65,67] These symptoms are further complicated by the common toxicities of the immunosuppression agents, which include nephro- and neuro-toxicity (e.g., cyclosporin and tacrolimus), and bone marrow suppression (azathioprine and CellCept). Pharmacokinetics of many therapeutic drugs are affected by the altered enteric absorption, volume of distribution, and renal and hepatic clearance in CF.[559] Thus, higher doses of drugs such as cyclosporin may be required, mandating close monitoring of serum levels. In addition, patients are frequently prescribed other drugs that may affect the cytochrome P450 system (e.g., macrolides, phenytoin), altering cyclosporin levels. Finally, patients with CF are a younger population than most transplant recipients and may have a lower prevalence of either cytomegaloviral or Epstein-Barr viral seropositivity prior to transplantation. Patients who acquire these infections post-transplantation may be at increased risk for complications, such as bronchiolitis obliterans and post-transplantation lymphoproliferative disorders (EBV).[30,455]

Although lung transplantation has become an important treatment option for some patients with end-stage disease, successful transplantation is still available only to a minority of patients. The process places an enormous financial and emotional burden on the family, a problem the entire CF and medical community must address.

Pancreas

Pancreatic involvement in CF is associated with three important conditions requiring treatment: exocrine pancreatic insufficiency in 85 percent of patients, diabetes mellitus in 5 to 15 percent, and recurrent pancreatitis in 1 to 3 percent. Treatment of exocrine pancreatic insufficiency is intimately related to achieving the best nutritional status possible—a lifelong struggle for most patients with CF.

Treatment of Exocrine Pancreatic Insufficiency. The goals of treatment of exocrine pancreatic insufficiency in CF are to establish normal growth in children, achieve normal weights in adults, establish normal micronutrient status, and control symptoms (steatorrhea, abdominal pain, and flatulence) at all ages.[73] Treatment for most patients consists primarily of supplementation with pancreatic enzymes and dietary counseling. Enzyme dosage is now carefully monitored because of the risk of fibrosing colonopathy in patients who receive high doses.[228] Most patients can be managed with between 500 and 2500 U of lipase per kg per meal. If growth is impaired or symptoms are present, then further evaluation and additional treatments are necessary. Dietary practices and techniques of enzyme administration should be carefully reviewed. Three-day stool fat collections provide quantitative determination of enzyme efficacy. The use of H2 blockers or proton pump inhibitors often reduces symptoms and improves weight gain. Since commercially available enzyme replacements vary in composition, trying different preparations sometimes makes a difference in individual patients. Abdominal pain can be a symptom of enzyme replacement failure in CF, but it should be kept in mind that there are multiple causes of abdominal pain in CF. Hence not all episodes of pain can be attributed to failure of enzyme supplementation.

Nutritional Management. Nutritional status is frequently impaired in CF for a number of reasons including exocrine pancreatic insufficiency, poor intake, and increased caloric requirements secondary to lung disease. In addition, there are several studies linking improved nutritional status with better pulmonary outcome.[72] Nutritional management is therefore an important part of CF care from the time of diagnosis. Outpatient nutritional follow-up includes careful tracking of growth and caloric intake as well as nutritional counseling aimed at increasing calories and replacing micronutrients. Nutritional regimens often place great stress on families and should be approached with sensitivity.

Nutritional management in infancy presents special problems because of rapid growth rates and the impact of early respiratory symptomatology. Forty-seven percent of infants with CF have height or weight or both below the fifth percentile for normal children.[365] Very close monitoring of growth is therefore necessary in infants. Raising the caloric density of formulas or switching to elemental formulas is often tried. Feeding by gastrostomy can improve weight gain and often diminishes stress around feedings.[514] Breast feeding of infants is encouraged and can achieve good growth with early diagnosis and careful follow-up.[291] Older children with CF are still below normal in height and weight but less so than infants, suggesting that some catch-up growth is possible. This catch-up growth still falls far short of what is required to achieve normal weight and height. Growth falls off again during adolescence, in part because of the increased caloric requirements of this time of life. This frequently necessitates nutritional intervention.

If, despite appropriate enzyme use, patients at any age fall below 15 percent of ideal body weight, then supplemental caloric intervention is warranted.[6] This usually takes the form of oral supplementation, nasogastric tube feeding, or gastrostomy feeding. Impaired growth, manifest by stunting (height less than the fifth percentile and weight greater than the fifth percentile) or wasting (weight less than the fifth percentile and height greater than the fifth percentile) or both, remains a major unsolved problem in CF care.

Before diagnosis, infants are at risk for severe nutritional deficiencies including protein calorie malnutrition, zinc deficiency, and linoleic acid deficiency.[243] Patients with CF at any age are at very real risk for severe complications from micronutrient deficiencies particularly with respect to the fat soluble vitamins.[673] Fat soluble vitamin (A, D, E, K) supplementation is therefore an important part of CF care. It is known that patients with CF have very low circulating levels of other nutrients, including carotene and linoleic acid.[399] It is not yet known whether addition of these nutrients would be beneficial.[292,399] Carotene may improve antioxidant status, for example, and therefore potentially add protection against oxidant-mediated lung injury.

Treatment of Diabetes Mellitus. CF patients manifest a wide range of disturbances of glucose metabolism.[427] The degree of disturbance presumably corresponds to varying stages of pancreatic fibrosis and concomitant loss of endocrine pancreatic function. In the approximately 5 percent of all patients who have overt diabetes mellitus, management consists of several times a day glucose monitoring, insulin administration, and nutritional counseling. Since the incidence of diabetes increases with age in CF, approaching 20 percent in some series of adults, careful monitoring for symptoms is necessary in adolescent and adult patients. The development of diabetes may be insidious, however, and therefore it is likely that more formal testing through serial oral glucose tolerance tests will be recommended in the near future. Diabetic vascular complications have been reported in CF underscoring the need for tight glucose control. Some patients manifest diabetes only when treated with corticosteroids and may require insulin during periods of corticosteroid treatment. The use of oral antihyperglycemic agents has not been studied well in CF. There are potential risks with the oral antihyperglycemic agents, including liver toxicity. Some of these agents are related to compounds that inhibit CFTR and therefore their use might be theoretically deleterious in patients with some mutations.

Many patients with CF who do not have fasting hyperglycemia, the hallmark of diabetes mellitus, will have abnormal glucose tolerance tests. These patients often have increased rates of proteolysis that correlate with impairment of pulmonary function.[276] This suggests that treatment with insulin may be beneficial in these cases although this has not yet been proven in a controlled trial.

Treatment of Recurrent Pancreatitis. Recurrent pancreatitis, which occurs in a subset of pancreatic sufficient patients, can be a painful, debilitating feature of CF.[194] Treatment often includes resting the pancreas by using elemental formulas for alimentation. Use of oral pancreatic enzymes may also decrease symptomatology. Pain management, at times with narcotics, may also be necessary. Since pancreatitis in CF has been associated with some oral antibiotics, discontinuation of their use or substitution with inhaled or intravenous antibiotics may be of benefit. The recognition of CF-related pancreatitis can prevent unnecessary diagnostic procedures and in some cases surgery.

Gastrointestinal Tract

Individuals with CF are prone to gastrointestinal obstructions at any time of life. Management increasingly emphasizes nonsurgical approaches to relief of obstructions and prevention of obstruction by appropriate dietary and bowel regimens.

Management of Fetal Intestinal Abnormalities in CF. Hyperechoic intestine, indicating abnormal fetal intestinal contents, can be detected in a significant number of fetuses with CF in the first trimester.[558] This finding, in cases without a family history, prompts genetic testing in parents and frequently amniocentesis for genetic diagnosis in the fetus. The prenatal diagnosis of CF then allows counseling of families and preparation for postnatal care. Hyperechoic bowel often resolves spontaneously and does not necessarily predict meconium ileus. Some fetuses will go on to have *in utero* intestinal obstruction that may necessitate premature delivery and neonatal intensive care.

Treatment of Meconium Ileus. Advances in neonatal intensive care and pediatric surgery have resulted in greatly increased survival from meconium ileus over the past few decades.[234] Approximately half of patients can now be managed with diluted Gastrografin enemas under fluoroscopy and will not require surgery. If Gastrografin enema fails to relieve the obstruction, surgery is required. Inspection of the gut at surgery will determine whether the intestine can be flushed of its thick meconium contents or whether a section of gut should be removed, most often because of ischemia. If intestine is removed, then a double-barreled ostomy is performed and reanastomosed at a later date. All patients require intravenous hyperalimentation following surgery and therefore a central line is placed. Management following surgery requires vigilance for infection and intestinal obstruction. Feeding is slowly advanced. If feeding is not tolerated, contrast studies of the proximal ostomy site are necessary to look for strictures.

Treatment of Other Neonatal Intestinal Obstruction Syndromes. Neonates with CF may present with intestinal obstructions including jejunal and ileal atresia or stenosis, or volvulus with or without meconium ileus.[510] These conditions most often present in the immediate neonatal period with abdominal distension and feeding intolerance. Intestinal stenosis may present later in life. In cases of intestinal atresia, stenosis, or volvulus, surgery is almost always required. Newborns with CF may, in addition, present with meconium plug syndrome, which is associated with a small colon and usually responds to osmotic enema treatment. The differential diagnosis of meconium plug syndrome is broad and CF infants represent only 5 percent of those presenting with this syndrome.

Treatment of Distal Intestinal Obstruction Syndrome (DIOS) and Chronic Constipation. The classic description of DIOS includes abdominal pain, marked decreased frequency of bowel movements, abdominal distension, and a tubular mass in the right lower quadrant tender to palpation.[382] With this presentation patients have inspissated fecal material at the ileocecal junction that is causing a blockage. However, DIOS represents an extreme form of the chronic constipation that many patients with CF suffer. Patients with chronic constipation may have only vague, periumbilical pain and not report a decreased frequency of stooling. Abdominal films showing increased stool in the colon are helpful in determining that the cause of the pain is related to chronic constipation. Whether the full-blown syndrome of DIOS or the less dramatic chronic constipation is present, the management involves both acute and chronic approaches. If no distension is present, oral or nasogastric administration of polyethylene glycol-electrolyte solutions may be successful. If distention is present it is necessary to perform a contrast enema to determine the type and level of obstruction. Hyperosmolar contrast enemas are not only diagnostic but are often therapeutic relieving the obstruction. If complete obstruction is present and does not yield to enema treatment, then surgery is required. Surgery is also required if patients appear toxic. Since DIOS and chronic constipation are prone to recur, long term management is necessary. Chronic use of fiber supplements is often all that is required. Occasionally, patients will take mineral oil or solutions containing polyethylene glycol on a daily, weekly, or monthly basis. Enterostomy for flushing the intestine with solutions containing polyethylene glycol on a daily basis has occasionally been required.

Treatment of Fibrosing Colonopathy. The use of high dose pancreatic enzyme supplementation has been associated with a noninfectious, noninflammatory fibrosis of the colon referred to as fibrosing colonopathy.[73] This condition very often requires surgical removal of some or all of the colon. If fibrosing colonopathy is suspected, then imaging studies must be performed as soon as possible and enzyme intake decreased to the minimum tolerable level.

Treatment of Rectal Prolapse. Management of rectal prolapse in CF often requires a variety of approaches. Since large bulky stools are thought to contribute to rectal prolapse, attention to appropriate pancreatic enzyme dosing is often helpful. Most children with rectal prolapse have evidence of chronic stool retention and hence the use of fiber and laxatives along with counseling about bowel habits are important. If prolapse does not resolve with medical treatment, sclerosing of the rectum may help. More complex surgery to reconstruct the walls of the rectum is occasionally required.

Treatment of Gastroesophageal Reflux. Gastroesophageal reflux and esophagitis are common causes of epigastric pain in CF. Esophagoscopy and pH monitoring are useful in evaluation. Initial treatment usually consists of counseling to avoid foods and medications that can exacerbate reflux, as well as the use of H2 blockers or proton pump inhibitors. The use of cisapride to decrease gastric stasis may also be of benefit. If symptoms persist, then surgical antireflux procedures are required. There is controversy over whether tipping of infants during chest physical therapy contributes to gastroesophageal reflux, further illustrating how treatments for one aspect of CF can potentially impact other aspects of treatment.[95]

Treatment of Feeding Disorders. Feeding disorders with frank food aversion are not uncommon in infants with CF and can present important psychosocial strains on the family.[576] The causes of food aversion are not completely understood but often follow intestinal complications in early infancy. Gastrostomy feeding is almost always required, often for years. Psychological support and occupational therapy are important aspects of management.

Treatment of Miscellaneous Disorders of the Intestine in CF. Patients with CF are prone to an array of intestinal disorders other than those described above. These disorders include, intussusception, chronic appendicitis, and *Clostridia difficile* related pseudomembranous colitis.[197,382] In addition, adults with CF carry a severalfold risk of developing intestinal neoplasms compared to the general population. Treatment of intussusception, which often involves the appendix, is usually by hyperosmolar enema. Surgery may also be required. Chronic appendicitis has been reported in CF. Medical management includes antibiotics and intestinal lavage but surgery may be needed. *C. difficile* can be cultured from about one half of patients with CF, but only occasionally causes disease and should not be treated without symptoms. Pseudomembranous colitis should be considered immediately for patients presenting with high fever and severe abdominal pain and bloating. The diarrhea that is characteristic of pseudomembranous colitis in non-CF patients may not be seen in CF which makes the diagnosis more difficult.

Management of Hepatobiliary Disease

Patients with CF can develop biliary cirrhosis that is thought to be related to abnormal CFTR function in cholangiocytes. In addition, they may develop hepatic steatosis (fatty liver) secondary to malnutrition and hepatic congestion secondary to cor pulmonale. Management of liver disease in CF requires a team approach bridging several disciplines.[570] CF center physicians and dietitians work closely with hepatologists and hepatobiliary surgeons to provide follow-up and ongoing management.

Management of Biliary Cirrhosis. A key part of CF center care is screening for biliary disease through serial physical examinations and the panel of liver blood tests obtained yearly. A firm or enlarged liver prompts a further evaluation, as does a palpable spleen. Elevations of hepatic enzymes, especially GGT, can alert caregivers to the possibility of biliary disease. If the physical examination or hepatic enzymes are abnormal, ultrasound imaging of the liver and spleen is undertaken. Patchy, echodense regions suggest cirrhosis. Endoscopic retrograde cholangiography is then often performed to determine whether extrahepatic bile duct obstruction is present. This entity has been reported in CF and can be relieved by balloon dilation or surgery. However it is not as common as first reported. If extrahepatic bile duct obstruction is not present, liver biopsy is then performed to determine whether fibrosis and or cirrhosis are present. Once cholestasis, fibrosis, or frank cirrhosis has been demonstrated, therapy is aimed at slowing liver damage, maintaining nutritional status, and treating complications. No treatments have as yet been proven to slow the progression to cirrhosis, however oral administration of ursodeoxycholic acid (URSO) has been targeted as a potential treatment. The mechanisms of action of URSO are complex and could involve improving bile flow, displacing dysfunctional bile acids, increasing bicarbonate secretion into bile, and exerting a direct cytoprotective effect. URSO has decreased GGT and other liver enzymes over 3 to 12 month periods in some studies, but has not shown any effect in others.[379] Decreased symptomatology has been reported with URSO use in some patients with CF. To minimize further hepatic injury with viral infection, hepatitis A and B immunizations have recently been recommended.[570]

Nutritional therapy is a major part of management of liver disease in CF. With impairment of bile acid flow, lipid absorption is often decreased. Treatment with formulas containing medium chain triglycerides, which are absorbed more easily in the presence of decreased bile flow than long chain fats, may be important. Protein intake is not usually restricted but may be if hepatic encephalopathy is seen following high protein intake. Patients with hepatic disease often have a difficulty maintaining normal fat soluble vitamin status with routine replacement. Dosages of vitamins A, D, E, and K often have to be increased over the usual dose. Vitamin K deficiency with elevation of prothrombin time can contribute to hemoptysis in patients with bronchiectasis. A key part of nutritional management is frequent monitoring of vitamin and protein levels along with adjustment of nutritional supplements.

Other complications of biliary disease in CF include the development of portal hypertension, hypersplenism, and hepatic encephalopathy. Portal hypertension is almost always accompanied by esophageal varices and therefore a greatly increased risk of gastrointestinal bleeding. Varices are best treated expectantly through periodic endoscopic evaluation with ligation or sclerosis. Management of acute gastrointestinal bleeding requires close monitoring and acute measures. The gastropathy that often occurs with portal hypertension is usually treated with gastric acid inhibitors. Occasionally, medical management and endoscopic ligation of varices is not sufficient and splenorenal or portacaval shunts are required. The use of β-blockers has not been well studied in CF liver disease and may result in bronchoconstriction. Hypersplenism can also result from portal hypertension. If sequestration of platelets becomes severe, then splenic embolization is performed. Portal hypertension may also be accompanied by ascites. The treatment of ascites includes salt restriction and diuretics. Hepatic encephalopathy occurs when patients have had large protein loads and/or are constipated. Treatment consists of lactulose to speed gut transit time and neomycin to decrease bacterial flora in the gut. Protein restriction may also be necessary.

Biliary disease in CF can progress to liver failure resistant to medical therapy. This state is characterized by uncontrolled ascites, elevated blood ammonia, encephalopathy, hyperbilirubinemia, and prolonged prothrombin time. Referral for liver transplant is then considered. Data on liver transplant in CF is encouraging with survival comparable to other indications for liver transplant. Liver transplant may be performed with lung transplant when indicated.

Treatment of Hepatic Steatosis. Hepatic steatosis (fatty liver) may occur with or without fibrosis or cirrhosis. It often reflects malnutrition and frequently occurs in infants presenting with hypoalbuminemia. Treatment is aimed at correcting nutritional deficits. Institution of proper pancreatic enzyme replacement, vitamins, and caloric intake are the main components of treatment. If steatosis persists after nutritional rehabilitation other potential causes should be sought, possibly diabetes mellitus, drug reaction, or toxin exposure.

Treatment of Hepatic Congestion. Hepatic congestion may occur in patients with cor pulmonale. Treatment is aimed at relief of cor pulmonale through improved pulmonary management, oxygen therapy, and noninvasive ventilation.

Management of Cholelithiasis. Although many patients with CF have evidence of cholelithiasis by imaging studies, only a few have sufficient symptomatology to require treatment. There are conflicting reports as to whether URSO treatment helps with gall bladder disease, but the balance of the evidence suggests it does not. Cholecystectomy is indicated when stones are present and there is chronic abdominal pain consistent with gall bladder disease. Surgery is increasingly performed laparoscopically.

Management of the Sweat Gland Abnormality

Hyponatremia and hypochloremia are common presenting signs of CF likely secondary to salt loss in the sweat. Most patients respond to oral supplements, though occasionally intravenous repletion is necessary. Infants can be supplemented with one-eighth teaspoon of salt daily which corresponds to 11 equivalents of NaCl. Older children and adults are taught to increase salt intake in hot weather or with vigorous physical activity.

Reproductive Issues

Management of Infertility. Most males with CF are infertile because of azoospermia secondary to absence or blockage of the vas deferens.[463] Advances in reproductive medicine, however, have now made treatment of male infertility in CF possible. Sperm can be obtained through microsurgical epididymal aspiration for *in vitro* fertilization. It appears that direct intracytoplasmic injection of sperm into ova may have better results than the standard *in vitro* fertilization technique.[555] Artificial insemination is another potential approach. The mild impairment of fertility in females with CF does not usually require treatment.

Management of Pregnancy. There have been an increasing number of successful pregnancies in women with CF. Pregnancies are classified High Risk because of maternal lung disease and undernutrition, and therefore close monitoring is required. Pregnant women with CF are at risk for decline in lung function and nutritional status as well as for gestational diabetes. Use of intravenous or inhaled antibiotics does not seem to be teratogenic as long as levels are monitored. Nutritional follow-up is required to insure adequate weight gain.

Other Conditions

Management of Osteoporosis. Prevention is the preferred treatment for osteoporosis in this illness. Adequate caloric, vitamin D, and calcium intake in association with optimal pancreatic enzyme replacement is the mainstay of prevention. Documented hypogonadism should be treated with appropriate gonadal hormones. Excessive use of corticosteroids should be avoided. There are no published data on the safety or efficacy of antiresorptive medications, such as bisphosphonates and calcitonin in this patient population. Although bisphosphonates improve bone density in postmenopausal women, there are theoretical concerns for their use in CF. In children, bisphosphonates may impair primary modeling of bones near growth plates. These agents bind tightly to bone and have a half-life greater than 10 years, an additional concern in young patients. Thus, regular usage in this population is discouraged until further data are available. Regular exercise is likely of benefit.[454]

Management of Rheumatic Conditions in CF. Vasculitis in CF, manifest by transitory skin lesions and arthralgias, often responds to anti-inflammatory agents. In general, ibuprofen is tried first. If this fails, then other nonsteroidal anti-inflammatories can be tried. If treatment with nonsteroidal anti-inflammatory agents is not successful, then a trial of oral corticosteroids may be of benefit. Since patients will sometimes have increased symptoms of vasculitis and arthralgias at times of pulmonary exacerbation, increasing pulmonary treatment with antibiotics and secretion clearance may help. Symptoms of hypertrophic pulmonary osteoarthropathy also often improve with analgesic and anti-inflammatory medications in conjunction with treatment of the underlying pulmonary infection.[454]

Management of Chronic Pain in CF. Management of chronic pain in CF demands first that appropriate diagnostic studies be performed based on the site of pain. For headache, the possibilities of hypercarbia, hypoxia, and sinusitis should be considered. Causes of chest wall pain in CF include pneumothorax, empyema, rib fracture, and muscle strains from coughing. CF-related causes of abdominal pain are legion and include malabsorption from inadequate pancreatic enzyme replacement, chronic constipation, distal intestinal obstruction syndrome, intestinal stenosis, *Clostridia* infection, and pseudomembranous colitis, intussusception, and chronic appendicitis. Joint pain suggests evaluation for CF-associated vasculitis. Osteoporosis and kyphosis often are accompanied by back pain. Nonsteroidal anti-inflammatories often will treat musculoskeletal pain. Opiates are occasionally necessary for musculoskeletal pain but low doses are frequently sufficient to control pain. Management is often best performed in conjunction with pain teams.[442]

Therapeutic Strategies Under Investigation

Gene Transfer to CF Airway Epithelia. Conceptually, the simplest approach to treating CF is to express wild-type CFTR in the affected cells. Because lung disease is the current major problem, most work has focused on gene transfer to airway epithelia. There has been substantial progress toward this goal, including an improved understanding of the pathogenesis and pathophysiology of CF, greater knowledge of the biology of the airways, and identification of barriers to gene transfer and strategies to circumvent them.

The potential targets for gene transfer include the sites where CFTR is expressed: large and small airways and submucosal glands (see "Cellular and Molecular Mechanisms of Transport"). Current knowledge does not allow a definitive conclusion about whether correction will be required in airway epithelia, in submucosal glands, or in both. However, the early onset of disease in small airways (see "Lung and Upper Respiratory Tract—Pathology"), where there are no submucosal glands, suggests that superficial airway epithelia should be the initial target. Probably epithelia in both proximal and distal airways will need to be targeted. The cells involved in electrolyte transport include both ciliated and nonciliated cells, suggesting that they are appropriate targets. Access to these cells via the airway lumen also makes them an attractive target for direct vector delivery.

Several studies have shed light on the amount of CFTR that may be needed to prevent lung disease. Knowledge that individual airway cells contain only 1 or 2 CFTR transcripts (see "CFTR Transcription"), that some apparently normal individuals have only ≈8 percent wild-type CFTR transcripts (see "CFTR Splicing"), and that ion channels have very high rates of electrolyte transport (see "Cl^- Channel Function of CFTR") suggest that minimal levels of CFTR will be required. However, there is an important distinction between the amount of CFTR needed and the percentage of cells that must be targeted. Mixing experiments indicate that targeting 5 to 10 percent of cells may be enough to correct the defect in transepithelial Cl^- transport.[317] Correction of enhanced Na^+ transport would require a greater percentage. Although the lack of an *in vivo* model of airway disease prevents a precise determination of the percentage of cells, further insight into the pathogenesis of lung disease (see "Pathogenesis of Airway Infections") should refine these estimates.

The feasibility of expressing CFTR in CF airway epithelia *in vitro* and *in vivo* to correct the CF phenotype is now well established.[16,150,674] Approximately 20 experiments have administered CFTR cDNA to humans using adenovirus, adeno-associated virus (AAV), and cationic lipid vectors. These human experiments and studies in model systems have shown us that CFTR can be expressed in appropriate target tissues, that expression can complement the CF loss of Cl^- transport *in vivo* in humans, and that gene transfer can be relatively safe, at least in initial experiments. However, those experiments have also shown us some significant barriers and limitations. Two challenges that must be met are the limited efficiency of gene transfer and the limited persistence of expression. These two issues are related; if the duration of expression could be increased, a lower transduction rate might be acceptable, and to a lesser extent the converse.

Gene transfer to differentiated airway epithelia is very inefficient.[76,649] As a result, large amounts of vector are required to obtain minimal levels of gene transfer. Hence the therapeutic index is unfavorable. The apical membrane of human airway epithelia provides a significant barrier because it does not express receptors that bind the commonly used adenovirus,[465,638,638] adeno-associated virus (AAV),[590] retrovirus vectors,[639] or nonviral vectors.[217,406] In several cases these receptors are hidden beneath the tight junctions on the basolateral surface where they are not accessible from the airway lumen. Without the advantage of specific high affinity binding and entry into the cell, infection is inefficient. Additional barriers may include limited rates of endocytosis across the apical membrane, the mucus that covers airway epithelia, the glycocalyx covering the apical surface, mucociliary clearance, proteins in airway surface liquid that bind and inactivate vectors, and phagocytosis of vectors by non-epithelial cells such as macrophages.[16]

Identification of these barriers has suggested ways to circumvent the limited apical membrane binding; five general strategies are being investigated (Fig. 201-25).

1. The vector can be delivered from the basolateral surface so that it accesses basolateral receptors. This works well *in vitro*, but *in vivo* it would require blood stream delivery with very specific targeting.[219]
2. The tight junctions can be transiently disrupted by Ca^{2+} chelation or hypotonic solutions, allowing vector to penetrate to basolateral receptors.[639]
3. The apical membrane can be modified so that it binds vector.
4. New formulation and delivery methods can also enhance binding and gene transfer; novel formulation strategies for plasmid DNA as well as viral vectors show promise.[69,216,461,681]
5. The vectors can be engineered or chemically coupled to display new ligands that bind to the apical surface.[190,511,632,657]

Alternatively new viral vectors or serotypes of existing vectors with improved binding and entry could be identified. The five strategies in Fig. 201-25 apply to most vectors. For nonviral vectors, the additional steps of escape of DNA from endosomes and delivery to the nucleus remain significant hurdles.[689]

For a genetic disease like CF, the goal is either a single vector administration with prolonged expression or repeated vector delivery with moderate duration expression. Several important factors may limit persistence of CFTR expression (Fig. 201-26); identification of these problems suggests strategies to circumvent them.[16,76,150,649,674]

1. Promoter "shut-off," first recognized with retroviral constructs, may be overcome using tissue-specific promoters and enhanced viral promoters to achieve sustained expression.
2. Loss of transgene from the cells is a particular problem for nonviral vectors and for some viral vectors. Integrating viruses and vectors that persist in stable episomal forms may provide solutions.
3. Another factor that limits transgene persistence arises because CpG motifs in bacterial DNA contained in plasmid vectors can generate an inflammatory response.
4. Numerous studies have highlighted an immune response that can destroy transduced cells, a problem that is particularly acute when a viral vector retains some viral genes that have leaky transcription or when the transgene expressed is immunogenic.
5. Finally, the life span of differentiated airway cells is limited, and is probably in the range of 3 months. Integrating vectors that target progenitor cells could potentially solve this problem.

The progress outlined above is encouraging for developing gene transfer for CF airway disease. The principle has been proven and barriers and limitations have been identified. The challenge for future work is to discover novel strategies to circumvent remaining barriers.

Pharmacologic Approaches to Correcting the CF Phenotype. An increased understanding of the molecular mechanisms of CFTR dysfunction and the pathogenesis of disease have stimulated attempts to develop new therapeutic interventions. The goal has

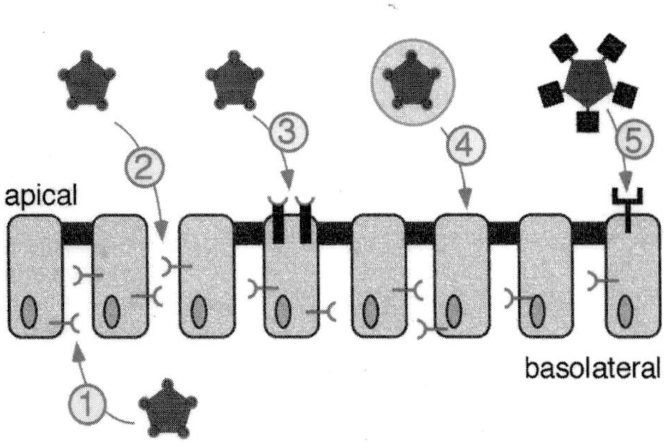

Fig. 201-25 Strategies to enhance gene transfer to airway epithelia. The receptors for currently used viral vectors are shown in red, novel engineered receptors are in dark gray, and potentially useful endogenous apical receptors are in black. The numbered arrows correspond to the strategies listed in the text. Note that these approaches could be applied to many different classes of vectors, hence pentagonal shape of vector. (*From Welsh.*[649] *Used by permission.*)

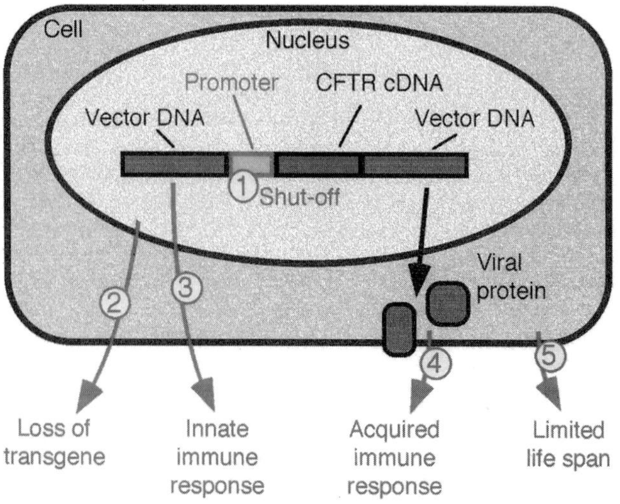

Fig. 201-26 Factors limiting the duration of transgene expression in airway epithelia. The numbered arrows refer to the challenges to persistent expression that are discussed in the text. (*From Welsh.*[649] *Used by permission.*)

been to at least partially correct abnormal function of the mutated protein or to bypass the loss of CFTR function. Much of the effort has been targeted at the four general mechanisms by which mutations disrupt CFTR function (see "Molecular Mechanisms of CFTR Dysfunction"). Targeting pharmacologic approaches toward these mechanisms emphasizes the importance of genotyping each patient at the time of diagnosis. Many potential new drugs are under development, and a few have reached early (Phase I/II) human trials. None of these potential therapies have been shown to be safe and clinically efficacious in large trials. As is frequently the case with new drug development, most of the products in early phase trials will not successfully achieve FDA approval. They will, however, provide valuable data regarding proof of concept, biologic effects, and safety profiles, paving the way for effective therapies in the future. This section contains a short review of some classes of therapeutic agents currently being evaluated. None of these agents are available for patient care at this time.

Class I Mutations: Defective or Reduced Protein Production. Approximately 10 percent of patients carry CFTR mutations that produce premature termination signals resulting in the production of little or no full length functional protein (see "Molecular Mechanisms of CFTR Dysfunction" above). Certain antibiotics in the aminoglycoside family, such as gentamicin, are capable of suppressing these premature stop-mutations with translational read-through, allowing production of a functional protein. *In vitro* exposure of bronchial epithelial cells from patients with Class I mutations to gentamicin has shown evidence of CFTR production.[297] Human trials of both intravenous and topical nasal application of gentamicin are now underway with measurement of nasal PD (see "Nasal Potential Difference Measurements") as an initial endpoint.

Class II Mutations: Defective Protein Processing. Since the ΔF508 mutation is present on at least one chromosome in 88 percent of patients (see "Mutations in the CFTR Gene"), a treatment directed at a Class II defect could be of broad utility. The ΔF508 mutant is misfolded and fails to travel appropriately to the cell surface (see "Class II Mutations: Defective Protein Processing" above). Because the ΔF508 protein retains at least partial function, there is significant interest in developing compounds that may act as chemical chaperones, facilitating delivery to the cell surface where the ΔF508 protein could function. Many compounds have been tested *in vitro* (e.g., glycerol, trimethylamine N-oxide),[89] but human trials have been limited to phenylbutyrate and cyclopentylxanthine (CPX).[32,521] Both compounds are reported to improve biosynthesis of the mutant protein *in vitro*. In a small human trial, oral phenylbutyrate partially corrected Cl^- transport as measured by nasal PD.[522]

Class III/IV Mutations: Defective Regulation or Conduction. There have been several attempts to enhance the activity of mutant CFTR that is present in the apical membrane (see "Class III Mutations: Defective Regulation" and "Class IV Mutations: Defective Conduction" above). In addition to Class III/IV mutations, this approach might also be of value for Class II mutants that reach the cell surface either in small number or in response to a treatment that improves biosynthesis. One strategy designed to do this augments cyclic AMP levels by administering a phosphodiesterase inhibitor, such as IBMX or other methyl xanthines.[325] As yet there are no human studies testing this approach.

Attempts to activate alternative Cl^- channels. The apical membrane of airway epithelia contains Cl^- channels distinct from CFTR (see "Cellular and Molecular Mechanisms of Transport"). The function of some of these channels remains intact in CF airway epithelia. Therefore, drugs that stimulate such channels may be candidates to increase apical membrane Cl^- permeability. The group of compounds most studied to date is nucleotide triphosphates, including uridine triphosphate (UTP). UTP increases Cl^- conductance by activating P2 purinergic receptors. It has been speculated that these agents may be more efficacious if administered in combination with a Na^+ channel antagonist, such as amiloride. Initial human trials with direct nasal application of 10^{-4} molar UTP plus amiloride to nasal epithelial cells partially and transiently corrected the Cl^- transport abnormality as measured by nasal PD.[342] Studies of amiloride alone, while initially encouraging, did not demonstrate any clinical efficacy in a large, multicenter trial.[487]

REFERENCES

1. Cystic Fibrosis Genetic Analysis Consortium: Worldwide survey of the deltaF508 mutation. Report from the Cystic Fibrosis Genetic Analysis Consortium (CFGAC). *Am J Hum Genet* **47**:354, 1990.
2. Consensus Conference: Practical applications of pulmozyme. *Pediatr Pulmonol* **17**:404, 94.
3. Cystic Fibrosis Genetic Analysis Consortium: Population variation of common cystic fibrosis mutations. *Hum Mutat* **4**:167, 1994.
4. American Diabetes Association: Clinical practice recommendations 1997. *Diabetes Care* **20(Suppl 1)**:S1, 1997.
5. Centers for Disease Control and Prevention: Newborn screening for cystic fibrosis: A paradigm for public health genetics policy development-proceedings of a 1997 workshop. *MMWR* **46(RR-16)**:18, 1997.
6. *Clinical Practice Guidelines for Cystic Fibrosis*. Bethesda, MD, Cystic Fibrosis Foundation, 1997.
7. Implementation of cystic fibrosis services in developing countries: Memorandum from a joint WHO/ICF(M)A meeting. *Bull World Health Organ* **75**:1, 1997.
8. The PREVENT Study Group: Reduction of respiratory syncytial virus hospitalization among premature infants and infants with bronchopulmonary dysplasia using respiratory syncytial virus immune globulin prophylaxis. *Pediatrics* **99**:93, 1997.
9. Cystic Fibrosis Foundation: *Patient Registry 1998 Annual Data Report*. Bethesda, MD, 1999.
10. National Institutes of Health Consensus Development Conference statement on genetic testing for cystic fibrosis. *Arch Intern Med* **159**:1529, 1999.
11. www.genet.sickkids.on.ca/cftr/. 1999.
12. Abman SH, Accurso FJ, Bowman CM: Persistent morbidity and mortality of protein calorie malnutrition in young infants with CF. *J Pediatr Gastroenterol Nutr* **5**:393, 1986.
13. Abman SH, Ogle JW, Harbeck RJ, Butler-Simon N, Hammond KB, Accurso FJ: Early bacteriologic, immunologic, and clinical courses of young infants with cystic fibrosis identified by neonatal screening. *J Pediatr* **119**:211, 1991.
14. Akabas MH, Kaufmann C, Cook TA, Archdeacon P: Amino acid residues lining the chloride channel of the cystic fibrosis transmembrane conductance regulator. *J Biol Chem* **269**:14865, 1994.
15. Albeliovich D, Lavon IP, Lerer I, Cohen T, Springer C, Avital A, Cutting GR: Screening for five mutations detects 97% of cystic fibrosis (CF) chromosomes and predicts a carrier frequency of 1:29 in the Jewish Ashkenazi population. *Am J Hum Genet* **51**:951, 1992.
16. Alton EW: Towards gene therapy for cystic fibrosis. *J Pharm Pharmacol* **47**:351, 1995.
17. Alton EW, Currie FWD, Logan-Sinclair R, Warner JO, Hodson ME, Geddes DM: Nasal potential difference: A clinical diagnostic test for cystic fibrosis. *Eur Respir J* **3**:922, 1990.
18. Andersen DH, Hodges RG: Celiac syndrome. *Am J Dis Child* **72**:62, 1946.
19. Anderson D: Cystic fibrosis of the pancreas and its relationship to celiac disease: Clinical and pathologic study. *Am J Dis Child* **56**:344, 1938.
20. Anderson DH, Hodges RG: Celiac Syndrome. V. Genetics of cystic fibrosis of the pancreas with a consideration of etiology. *Am J Dis Child* **72**:62, 1946.
21. Anderson MP, Berger HA, Rich DP, Gregory RJ, Smith AE, Welsh MJ: Nucleoside triphosphates are required to open the CFTR chloride channel. *Cell* **67**:775, 1991.
22. Anderson MP, Gregory RJ, Thompson S, Souza DW, Paul S, Mulligan RC, Smith AE, Welsh MJ: Demonstration that CFTR is a chloride channel by alteration of its anion selectivity. *Science* **253**:202, 1991.
23. Anderson MP, Rich DP, Gregory RJ, Smith AE, Welsh MJ: Generation of cAMP-activated chloride currents by expression of CFTR. *Science* **251**:679, 1991.

24. Anderson MP, Sheppard DN, Berger HA, Welsh MJ: Chloride channels in the apical membrane of normal and cystic fibrosis airway and intestinal epithelia. *Am J Physiol* **263**:L1, 1992.
25. Anderson MP, Welsh MJ: Calcium and cAMP activate different chloride channels in the apical membrane of normal and cystic fibrosis epithelia. *Proc Natl Acad Sci U S A* **88**:6003, 1991.
26. Anderson MP, Welsh MJ: Regulation by ATP and ADP of CFTR chloride channels that contain mutant nucleotide-binding domains. *Science* **257**:1701, 1992.
27. Anguiano A, Oates RD, Amos JA, Dean M, Gerrard B, Stewart C, Maher TA, White MB, Milunsky A: Congenital bilateral absence of the vas deferens a primary genital form of cystic fibrosis. *JAMA* **267**:1794, 1992.
28. Arens R, Gozal D, Omlin KJ, Vega J, Boyd KP, Keens TG, Woo MS: Comparison of high frequency chest compression and conventional chest physiotherapy in hospitalized patients with cystic fibrosis. *Am J Respir Crit Care Med* **150**:1154, 1994.
29. Aris RM, Gilligan PH, Neuringer IP, Gott KK, Rea J, Yankaskas JR: The effects of panresistant bacteria in cystic fibrosis patients on lung transplant outcome. *Am J Respir Crit Care Med* **155**:1699, 1997.
30. Aris RM, Maia DM, Neuringer IP, Gott K, Kiley S, Gertis K, Handy J: Post-transplantation lymphoproliferative disorder in the Epstein-Barr virus-naive lung transplant recipient. *Am J Respir Crit Care Med* **154**:1712, 1996.
31. Aris RM, Renner JB, Winders AD, Buell HE, Riggs DB, Lester GE, Ontjes DA: Increased rate of fractures and severe kyphosis: Sequelae of living into adulthood with cystic fibrosis. *Ann Intern Med* **128**:186, 1998.
32. Arispe N, Mar J, Jacobson KA, Pollard HB: Direct activation of cystic fibrosis transmembrane conductance regulator channels by 8-cyclopentyl-1,3-dipropylxanthine (CPX) and 1,3-diallyl-8-cyclohexylxanthine (DAX). *J Biol Chem* **273**:5727, 1998.
33. Armstrong DS, Grimwood K, Carlin JB, Carzino R, Olinsky A, Phelan PD: Bronchoalveolar lavage or oropharyngeal cultures to identify lower respiratory pathogens in infants with cystic fibrosis. *Pediatr Pulmonol* **21**:267, 1996.
34. Armstrong DS, Grimwood K, Carzino R, Carlin JB, Olinsky A, Phelan PD: Lower respiratory infection and inflammation in infants with newly diagnosed cystic fibrosis. *BMJ* **310**:1571, 1995.
35. Aron Y, Polla BS, Bienvenu T, Dall'ava J, Dusser D, Hubert D: HLA class II polymorphism in cystic fibrosis. *Am J Resp Crit Care Med* **159**:1464, 1999.
36. Audrezet MP, Mercier B, Guillermit H, Quere I, Verlingue C, Rault G, Ferec C: Identification of 12 novel mutations in the CFTR gene. *Hum Mol Genet* **2**:51, 1993.
37. Augarten A, Kerem BS, Yahav Y, Noiman S, Rivlin Y, Tal A, Blau H, Ben-Tur L, Szeinberg A, Kerem E, et al: Mild cystic fibrosis and normal or borderline sweat test in patients with the 3849 + 10 kb C → T mutation. *Lancet* **342**:25, 1993.
38. Baconnais S, Tirouvanziam R, Zahm JM, de Bentzmann S, Peault B, Balossier G, Puchelle E: Ion composition and rheology of airway liquid from cystic fibrosis fetal tracheal xenografts. *Am J Respir Cell Mol Biol* **20**:605, 1999.
39. Baconnais S, Zahm J, Kilian L, Bonhomme P, Gobillard D, Perchet A, Puchelle E, Balossier G: X-ray microanalysis of native airway surface liquid collected by cryotechnique. *J Microsc* **191**:311, 1998.
40. Baker E, Jeunemaitre X, Portal AJ, Grimbert P, Markandu N, Persu A, Corvol P, MacGregor G: Abnormalities of nasal potential difference measurment in Liddle's syndrome. *J Clin Invest* **102**:10, 1998.
41. Balfour-Lynn IM, Klein NJ, Dinwiddie R: Randomised controlled trial of inhaled corticosteroids (fluticasone propionate) in cystic fibrosis. *Arch Dis Child* **77**:124, 1997.
42. Bals R, Wang X, Wu Z, Freeman T, Bafna V, Zasloff M, Wilson JM: Human β-defensin 2 is a salt-sensitive peptide antibiotic expressed in human lung. *J Clin Invest* **102**:874, 1998.
43. Bals R, Weiner DJ, Meegalla RL, Wilson JM: Transfer of a cathelicidin peptide antibiotic gene restores bacterial killing in a cystic fibrosis xenograft model. *JCI* **103**:1113, 1999.
44. Bals R, Weiner DJ, Wilson JM: The innate immune system in cystic fibrosis lung disease. *J Clin Invest* **103**:303, 1999.
45. Baltimore RS, Christie CDC, Walker Smith GJ: Immunohistopathologic localization of *Pseudomonas aeruginosa* in lungs from patients with cystic fibrosis. *Am Rev Respir Dis* **140**:1650, 1989.
46. Barasch J, Kiss B, Prince A, Saiman L, Gruenert D, Al-Awqati Q: Defective acidification of intracellular organelles in cystic fibrosis. *Nature* **352**:70, 1991.
47. Bargon J, Trapnell BC, Chu C-S, Rosenthal ER, Yoshimura K, Guggino WB, Dalemans W, Pavirani A, Lecocq J-P, Crystal RG: Down-regulation of cystic fibrosis transmembrane conductance regulator gene expression by agents that modulate intracellular divalent cations. *Mol Cell Biol* **12**:1872, 1992.
48. Barker PM, Nguyen MS, Gatzy T, Grubb B, Norman H, Hummier E, Rossier B, Boucher RC, Koller B: Role of γENaC subunit in lung liquid clearance and electrolyte balance in newborn mice. *J Clin Invest* **102**:1634, 1998.
49. Baroni MA, Anderson YE, Mischler E: Cystic fibrosis newborn screening: impact of early screening results on parenting stress. *Pediatr Nurs* **23**:143, 1997.
50. Bartman J, Landing BH: Morphology of the sweat apparatus in cystic fibrosis. *Am J Clin Pathol* **45**:455, 1966.
51. Basbaum C, Welsh MJ: Defense mechanisms and immunology: Mucous secretion and ion transport in airways. Philadelphia, PA, W.B. Saunders, 1999, p 323.
52. Basbaum CB, Jany B, Finkbeiner WE: The serous cell. *Annu Rev Physiol* **52**:97, 1990.
53. Baughman RP, Keeton DA, Perez C, Wilmott RW: Use of bronchoalveolar lavage semiquantitative cultures in cystic fibrosis. *Am J Respir Crit Care Med* **156**:286, 1997.
54. Baukrowitz T, Hwang TC, Nairn AC, Gadsby DC: Coupling of CFTR Cl^- channel gating to an ATP hydrolysis cycle. *Neuron* **12**:473, 1994.
55. Bear CE, Li C, Kartner N, Bridges RJ, Jensen TJ, Ramjeesingh M, Riordan JR: Purification and functional reconstitution of the cystic fibrosis transmembrane conductance regulator (CFTR). *Cell* **68**:809, 1992.
56. Beaudet AL: Carrier screening for cystic fibrosis. *Am J Hum Genet* **47**:603, 1990.
57. Beaudet AL, Perciaccante RG, Cutting GR: Homozygous nonsense mutation causing cystic fibrosis with uniparental isodisomy. *Am J Hum Genet* **48**:1213, 1991.
58. Beaudet AL, Spence JE, Montes M, O'Brien WE, Estivill X, Farrall M, Williamson R: Experience with new DNA markers for the diagnosis of cystic fibrosis. *N Engl J Med* **318**:50, 1988.
59. Beaudet AL, Tsui L: A suggested nomenclature for designating mutations. *Hum Mutat* **2**:245, 1993.
60. Becker JW, Burke W, McDonald G, Greenberger PA, Henderson WR, Aitken ML: Prevalence of allergic bronchopulmonary aspergillosis and atopy in adult patients with cystic fibrosis. *Chest* **109**:1536, 1996.
61. Behm JK, Hagiwara G, Lewiston NJ, Quinton PM, Wine JJ: Hyposecretion of beta-adrenergically induced sweating in cystic fibrosis heterozygotes. *Pediatr Res* **22**:271, 1987.
62. Berger HA, Rich DP, Cheng SH, Travis SM, Saxena M, Smith AE, Welsh MJ: Regulation of the cystic fibrosis transmembrane conductance regulator Cl^- channel by negative charge in the R domain. *Jap J Physiol* **44(Suppl 2)**:S167, 1994.
63. Berger HA, Travis SM, Welsh MJ: Regulation of the cystic fibrosis transmembrane conductance regulator Cl^- channel by specific protein kinases and protein phosphatases. *J Biol Chem* **268**:2037, 1993.
64. Berger M, Konstan M, Hilliard J, et al: Aerosolized prolastin (α1-protease inhibitor) in cystic fibrosis. *Pediatr Pulmonol* **20**:421, 1995.
65. Berkowitz N, Schulman LL, McGregor C, Markowitz D: Gastroparesis after lung transplantation. Potential role in postoperative respiratory complications. *Chest* **108**:1602, 1995.
66. Bevins CL: Scratching the surface inroads to a better understanding of airway host defense. *Am J Respir Cell Mol Biol* **20**:861, 1999.
67. Bhudhikanok GS, Lim J, Marcus R, Harkins A, Moss RB, Bachrach LK: Correlates of osteopenia in patients with cystic fibrosis. *Pediatrics* **97**:103, 1996.
68. Biwersi J, Emans N, Verkman AS: Cystic fibrosis transmembrane conductance regulator activation stimulates endosome fusion *in vivo*. *Proc Natl Acad Sci U S A* **93**:12484, 1996.
69. Blessing T, Remy J-S, Behr J-P: Monomolecular collapse of plasmid DNA into stable virus-like particles. *Proc Natl Acad Sci U S A* **95**:1427, 1998.
70. Bois E, Feingold J, Demenais F, Runavot Y, Jehanne M, Toudic L: Cluster of cystic fibrosis cases in a limited area of Brittany (France). *Clin Genet* **14**:73, 1978.
71. Bonfield TL, Panuska JR, Konstan MW, Hilliard KA, Hilliard JB, Ghnaim H, Berger M: Inflammatory cytokines in cystic fibrosis lungs. *Am J Respir Crit Care Med* **152**:2111, 1995.
72. Borowitz D: The interrelationship of nutrition and pulmonary function in patients with cystic fibrosis. *Curr Opin Pulm Med* **2**:457, 1996.

73. Borowitz DS, Grand RJ, Durie PR: Use of pancreatic enzyme supplements for patients with cystic fibrosis in the context of fibrosing colonopathy. Consensus Committee. *J Pediatr* **127**:681, 1995.
74. Bosso JA, Black PG, Matsen JM: Ciprofloxacin versus tobramycin plus azlocillin in pulmonary exacerbations in adult patients with cystic fibrosis. *Am J Med* **82**:180, 1987.
75. Boucher RC: Human airway ion transport. Part one. *Am J Respir Crit Care Med* **150**:271, 1994.
76. Boucher RC: Status of gene therapy for cystic fibrosis lung disease. *J Clin Invest* **103**:441, 1999.
77. Boucher RC, Stutts MJ, Knowles MR, Cantley L, Gatzy JT: Na^+ transport in cystic fibrosis respiratory epithelia. Abnormal basal rate and response to adenylate cyclase activation. *J Clin Invest* **78**:1245, 1986.
78. Bourke S, Rooney M, Fitzgerald M, Bresnihan B: Episodic arthropathy in adult cystic fibrosis. *QJM* **64**:651, 1987.
79. Bowler IM, Estlin EJ, Littlewood JM: Cystic fibrosis in Asians. *Arch Dis Child* **68**:120, 1995.
80. Bradbury NA: Intracellular CFTR: Localization and function. *Physiol Rev* **79**:5179, 1999.
81. Bradbury NA, Clark JA, Watkins SC, Widnell CC, Smith HS IV, Bridges RJ: Characterization of the internatlization pathways for the cystic fibrosis transmembrane conductance regulator. *Am J Physiol* **276**:L659, 1999.
82. Braggion C, Cappelletti LM, Cornacchia M, Zanolla L, Mastella G: Short-term effects of three chest physiotherapy regimens in patients hospitalized for pulmonary exacerbations of cystic fibrosis: A cross-over randomized study. *Pediatr Pulmonol* **19**:16, 1995.
83. Breeze RG, Wheeldon RB: The cells of the pulmonary airways. *Am Rev Respir Dis* **116**:705, 1977.
84. Bresnihan B: Cystic fibrosis, chronic bacterial infection and rheumatic disease. *Br J Rheumatol* **27**:339, 1988.
85. Breuer W, Kartner N, Riordan JR, Cabantchik ZI: Induction of expression of the cystic fibrosis transmembrane conductance regulator. *J Biol Chem* **267**:10465, 1992.
86. Brinson GM, Noone PG, Mauro MA, Knowles MR, Yankaskas JR, Sandhu JS, Jaques PF: Bronchial artery embolization for the treatment of hemoptysis in patients with cystic fibrosis. *Am J Respir Crit Care Med* **157**:1951, 1998.
87. Brody AS: Cystic fibrosis: when should high-resolution computed tomography of the chest be obtained? *Pediatrics* **101**:1071, 1998.
88. Bronstein MN, Sokol RJ, Abman SH, Chatfield BA, Hammond KB, Hambidge KM, Stall CD, Accurso FJ: Pancreatic insufficiency, growth, and nutrition in infants identified by newborn screening as having cystic fibrosis. *J Pediatr* **120**:533, 1992.
89. Brown CR, Hong-Brown LQ, Biwersi J, Verkman AS, Welch WJ: Chemical chaperones correct the mutant phenotype of the ΔF508 cystic fibrosis transmembrane conductance regulator protein. *Cell Stress Chaperon* **1**:117, 1996.
90. Brugman SM, Taussig LM: The reproductive system, in Taussig LM (ed): *Cystic Fibrosis*. New York, Thieme-Stratton, 1984, p 323.
91. Brunecky Z: The incidence and genetics of cystic fibrosis. *J Med Genet* **9**:33, 1972.
92. Burch LH, Talbot CR, Knowles MR, Canessa CM, Rossier BC, Boucher RC: Relative expression of the human epithelial Na^+ channel subunits in normal and cystic fibrosis airways. *Am J Physiol* **269**:C511, 1995.
93. Burger J, Macek M Jr, Stuhrmann M, Reis A, Krawczak M, Schmidtke J: Genetic influences in the formation of nasal polyps. *Lancet* **337**:974, 1991.
94. Burns JL, Emerson J, Stapp JR, Yim DL, Krzewinski J, Louden L, Ramsey BW, Clausen CR: Microbiology of sputum from patients at cystic fibrosis centers in the United States. *Clin Infect Dis* **27**:158, 1998.
95. Button BM, Heine RG, Catto-Smith AG, Phelan PD: Postural drainage in cystic fibrosis: Is there a link with gastro-oesophageal reflux? *J Paediatr Child Health* **34**:330, 1998.
96. Campbell PWI, Parker RA, Roberts BT, Krishnamani MR, Phillips JAI: Association of poor clinical status and heavy exposure to tobacco smoke in patients with cystic fibrosis who are homozygous for the F508 deletion. *J Pediatr* **120**:261, 1992.
97. Canessa CM, Horisberger J-D, Rossier BC: Epithelial sodium channel related to proteins involved in neurodegeneration. *Nature* **361**:467, 1993.
98. Canessa CM, Schild L, Buell G, Thorens B, Gautschi I, Horisberger JD, Rossier BC: Amiloride-sensitive epithelial Na^+ channel is made of three homologous subunits. *Nature* **367**:463, 1994.
99. Canny GJ, Corey M, Livingstone RA, Carpenter S, Green L, Levison H: Pregnancy and cystic fibrosis. *Obstet Gynecol* **77**:850, 1991.
100. Caplen NJ, Alton EW, Middleton PG, Dorin JR, Stevenson BJ, Gao X, Durham SR, Jeffery PK, Hodson ME, Coutelle C: Liposome-mediated CFTR gene transfer to the nasal epithelium of patients with cystic fibrosis [erratum published in *Nat Med* 1(3):272, 1995]. *Nat Med* **1**:39, 1995.
101. Caronia CG, Silver P, Nimkoff L, Gorvoy J, Quinn C, Sagy M: Use of bilevel positive airway pressure (BIPAP) in end-stage patients with cystic fibrosis awaiting lung transplantation. *Clin Pediatr (Phila)* **37**:555, 1998.
102. Carson JL, Collier AM, Gambling TM, Knowles MR, Boucher RC: Ultrastructure of airway epithelial cell membranes among patients with cystic fibrosis. *Hum Pathol* **21**:640, 1990.
103. Carson MR, Winter MC, Travis SM, Welsh MJ: Pyrophosphate stimulates wild-type and mutant CFTR Cl^- channels. *J Biol Chem* **270**:20466, 1995.
104. Carter CO: Genetic aspects of cystic fibrosis of the pancreas. *Mod Probl Pediatr* **10**:372, 1967.
105. Casals T, Bassas L, Ruiz-Romero J, Chillón M, Giménez J, Ramos MD, Tapia G, Narvaez H, Nunes V, Estivill X: Extensive analysis of 40 infertile patients with congenital absence of the vas deferens: In 50% of cases only one CFTR allele could be detected. *Hum Genet* **95**:205, 1995.
106. Castellani C, Benetazzo M, Bonizzato A, Pignatti PF, Mastella G: Cystic fibrosis mutations in heterozygous newborns with hypertrypsinemia and low sweat chloride. *Am J Hum Genet* **64**:303, 1999.
107. Castellani C, Bonizzato A, Cabrini G, Mastella G: Newborn screening strategy for cystic fibrosis: A field study in an area with high allelic heterogeneity. *Acta Paediatr* **86**:497, 1997.
108. Chan HC, Ko WH, Zhao W, Fu WO, Wong PY: Evidence for independent Cl^- and $HCO3^-$ secretion and involvement of an apical $Na(+)$-$HCO3^-$ cotransporter in cultured rat epididymal epithelia. *Exp Physiol* **81**:515, 1996.
109. Chang X, Cui L, Hou Y, Jensen TJ, Aleksandrov AA, Mengos A, Riordan JR: Removal of multiple arginine-framed trafficking signals overcomes misprocessing of delta F508 CFTR present in most patients with cystic fibrosis. *Mol Cell* **4**:137, 1999.
110. Chang X-B, Hou Y-X, Jensen TJ, Riordan JR: Mapping of cystic fibrosis transmembrane conductance regulator membrane topology by glycosylation site insertion. *J Biol Chem* **269**:18572, 1994.
111. Chanson M, Scerri I, Suter S: Defective regulation of gap junctional coupling in cystic fibrosis pancreatic duct cells. *J Clin Invest* **103**:1677, 1999.
112. Cheadle JP, Goodchild MC, Meridith AL: Direct sequencing of the comlete CFTR gene: The molecular characterisation of 99.5% of CF chromosomes in Wales. *Hum Mol Genet* **2**:1551, 1993.
113. Cheng SH, Gregory RJ, Marshall J, Paul S, Souza DW, White GA, O'Riordan CR, Smith AE: Defective intracellular transport and processing of CFTR is the molecular basis of most cystic fibrosis. *Cell* **63**:827, 1990.
114. Cheng SH, Rich DP, Marshall J, Gregory RJ, Welsh MJ, Smith AE: Phosphorylation of the R domain by cAMP-dependent protein kinase regulates the CFTR chloride channel. *Cell* **66**:1027, 1991.
115. Chevalier-Porst F, Chomel JC, Hillaire D, Kitzis A, Kaplan JC, Goutaland R, Mathieu M: A nonsense mutation in exon 4 of the cystic fibrosis gene frequent among the population of the Reunion Island. *Hum Mol Genet* **1**:647, 1992.
116. Chillón M, Casals T, Mercier B, Bassas L, Lissens W, Silber S, Romey M-C, Ruiz-Romero J, Verlingue C, Claustres M, Nunes V, Férec C, Estivill X: Mutations in the cystic fibrosis gene in patients with congenital absence of the vas deferens. *New Engl J Med* **332**:1475, 1995.
117. Chillón M, Dörk T, Casals J, Giménez J, Fonknechten N, Will K, Ramos D, Nunes V, Estivill X: A novel donor splice site in intron 11 of the CFTR gene, created by mutation $1811+1.5kbA \rightarrow G$, produces a new exon: High frequency in Spanish cystic fibrosis chromosomes and association with severe phenotype. *Am J Hum Genet* **56**:623, 1995.
118. Chinet TC, Fullton JM, Yankaskas JR, Boucher RC, Stutts MJ: Sodium-permeable channels in the apical membrane of human nasal epithelial cells. *Am J Physiol* **265**:C1050, 1993.
119. Chou JL, Rozmahel R, Tsui LC: Characterization of the promoter region of the cystic fibrosis transmembrane conductance regulator gene. *J Biol Chem* **266**:24471, 1991.
120. Chow CW, Landau LI, Taussig LM: Bronchial mucous glands in the newborn with cystic fibrosis. *Eur J Pediatr* **139**:240, 1982.

121. Chu C-S, Trapnell BC, Curristin S, Cutting GR, Crystal RG: Genetic basis of variable exon 9 skipping in cystic fibrosis transmembrane conductance regulator mRNA. *Nat Genet* **3**:151, 1993.
122. Chu C-S, Trapnell BC, Curristin SM, Cutting GR, Crystal RG: Extensive posttranscriptional deletion of the coding sequences for part of nucleotide-binding fold 1 in respiratory epithelial mRNA transcripts of the cystic fibrosis transmembrane conductance regulator gene is not associated with the clinical manifestations of cystic fibrosis. *J Clin Invest* **90**:785, 1992.
123. Chu CS, Trapnell BC, Murtagh JJJ, Moss J, Dalemans W, Jallat S, Mercenier A, Pavirani A, Lecocq JP, Cutting GR, et al: Variable deletion of exon 9 coding sequences in cystic fibrosis transmembrane conductance regulator gene mRNA transcripts in normal bronchial epithelium. *EMBO J* **10**:1355, 1991.
124. Chysky V, Kapila K, Hullmann R, Arcieri G, Schacht P, Echols R: Safety of ciprofloxacin in children: worldwide clinical experience based on compassionate use. Emphasis on joint evaluation. *Infection* **19**:289, 1991.
125. Clarke LL, Grubb BR, Gabriel SE, Smithies O, Koller BH, Boucher RC: Defective epithelial chloride transport in a gene-targeted mouse model of cystic fibrosis. *Science* **257**:1125, 1992.
126. Clarke LL, Grubb BR, Yankaskas JR, Cotton CU, McKenzie A, Boucher RC: Relationship of a non-cystic fibrosis transmembrane conductance regulator-mediated chloride conductance to organ-level disease in *Cftr*(−/−) mice. *Proc Natl Acad Sci USA* **91**:479, 1994.
127. Clayton RG Sr, Diaz CE, Bashir NS, Panitch HB, Schidlow DV, Allen JL: Pulmonary function in hospitalized infants and toddlers with cystic fibrosis. *J Pediatr* **132**:405, 1998.
128. Cohen AM, Yulish BS, Wasser KB, Vignos PJ, Jones PK, Sorin SB: Evaluation of pulmonary hypertrophic osteoarthropathy in cystic fibrosis. A comprehensive study. *Am J Dis Child* **140**:74, 1986.
129. Cohen RG, Barr ML, Schenkel FA, DeMeester TR, Wells WJ, Starnes VA: Living-related donor lobectomy for bilateral lobar transplantation in patients with cystic fibrosis. *Ann Thorac Surg* **57**:1423, 1994.
130. Cohn JA, Friedman KJ, Noone PG, Knowles MR, Silverman LM, Jowell PS: Relation between mutations of the cystic fibrosis gene and idiopathic pancreatitis. *N Engl J Med* **339**:653, 1998.
131. Cohn JA, Melhus O, Page LJ, Dittrich KL, Vigna SR: CFTR: Development of high-affinity antibodies and localization in sweat gland. *Biochem Biophys Res Commun* **181**:36, 1991.
132. Cohn JA, Strong TV, Picciotto MR, Nairn AC, Collins FS, Fitz JG: Localization of the cystic fibrosis transmembrane conductance regulator in human bile duct epithelial cells. *Gastroenterology* **105**:1857, 1993.
133. Cole AM, Dewan P, Ganz T: Innate antimicrobial activity of nasal secretions. *Infect Immun* **67**:3267, 1999.
134. Colin AA, Sawyer SM, Mickle J, Oates RD, Milunsky A, Amos J: Pulmonary function and clinical observations in men with congenital bilateral absence of the vas deferens. *Chest* **110**:440, 1996.
135. Colledge WH, Abella BS, Southern KW, Ratcliff R, Jiang C, Cheng SH, MacVinish LJ, Anderson JR, Cuthbert AW, Evans MJ: Generation and characterization of a ΔF508 cystic fibrosis mouse model. *Nat Genet* **10**:445, 1995.
136. Colombo C, Apostolo MG, Ferrari M, Seia M, Genoni S, Giunta A, Sereni LP: Analysis of risk factors for the development of liver disease associated with cystic fibrosis. *J Pediatr* **124**:393, 1994.
137. Conneally PM, Merritt AD, Yu P: Cystic fibrosis: population genetics. *Tex Rep Biol Med* **31**:639, 1973.
138. Cooper JD, Pohl MS, Patterson GA: An update on the current status of lung transplantation: Report of the St. Louis International Lung Transplant Registry. *Clin Transpl* 95, 1993.
139. Corey M, Durie P, Moore D, Forstner G, Levison H: Familial concordance of pancreatic function in cystic fibrosis. *J Pediatr* **115**:274, 1989.
140. Corey M, Edwards L, Levison H, Knowles M: Longitudinal analysis of pulmonary function decline in patients with cystic fibrosis. *J Pediatr* **131**:809, 1997.
141. Costerton JW, Stewart PS, Greenberg EP: Bacterial biofilms: A common cause of persistent infections. *Science* **284**:1318, 1999.
142. Cotten JF, Ostedgaard LS, Carson MR, Welsh MJ: Effect of cystic fibrosis-associated mutations in the fourth intracellular loop of cystic fibrosis transmembrane conductance regulator. *J Biol Chem* **271**:21279, 1996.
143. Cotten JF, Welsh MJ: Covalent modification of the regulatory domain irreversibly stimulates cystic fibrosis transmembrane conductance regulator. *J Biol Chem* **272**:25617, 1997.
144. Cotten JF, Welsh MJ: Cystic fibrosis-associated mutations at arginine 347 alter the pore architecture of CFTR. Evidence for disruption of a salt bridge. *J Biol Chem* **274**:5429, 1999.
145. Cotton CU, Davis PB: The pancreas in cystic fibrosis, in Davis PB (ed.): *Cystic Fibrosis*. New York, Marcel Dekker, 1993, p 162.
146. Coughlin JP, Gauderer MW, Stern RC, Doershuk CF, Izant RJ Jr, Zollinger R M Jr: The spectrum of appendiceal disease in cystic fibrosis. *J Pediatr Surg* **25**:835, 1990.
147. Couper R: Pancreatic function tests, in Walker WA, Durie PR, Hamilton JR, Walker-Smith JA, Watkins JB (eds): *Pediatric Gastrointestinal Disease: Pathophysiology, Diagnosis, Management*. St. Louis, CV Mosby, 1995, p 1621.
148. Cowley EA, Govindaraju K, Lloyd DK, Eidelman DH: Is mouse airway surface fluid hypotonic. *Pediatric Pulmonol* **14(Suppl)**:233, 1997.
149. Crawford J, Labrinidis A, Carey WF, Nelson PV, Harvey JS, Morris CP: A splicing mutation (1898+1G → T) in the CFTR gene causing cystic fibrosis. *Hum Mutat* **5**:101, 1995.
150. Crystal RG: Transfer of genes to humans: Early lessons and obstacles to success. *Science* **270**:404, 1995.
151. Cuppens H, Lin W, Jaspers M, Costes B, Teng H, Vankeerberghen A, Jorissen M, Droogmans G, Reynaert I, Goossens M, Nilius B, Cassiman JJ: Polyvariant mutant cystic fibrosis transmembrane conductance regulator genes. The polymorphic (TG)n locus explains the partial penetrance of the T5 polymorphism as a disease mutation. *J Clin Invest* **101**:487, 1998.
152. Cuthbert AW, Halstead J, Ratcliff R, Colledge WH, Evans MJ: The genetic advantage hypothesis in cystic fibrosis heterozygotes: A murine study. *J Physiol* **482**:449, 1995.
153. Cutting GR: Splicing of the CFTR gene, in Dodge JA, Brock DJH, Widdicombe JH (eds): *Current Topics in Cystic Fibrosis*. Chichester, John Wiley & Sons, 1994, p 55.
154. Cutting GR, Antonarakis SE, Buetow KH, Kasch LM, Rosenstein BJ, Kazazian HH Jr: Analysis of DNA polymorphism haplotypes linked to the cytic fibrosis locus in North American Black and Caucasian families supports the existence of multiple mutations of the cystic fibrosis gene. *Am J Med Genet* **44**:307, 1989.
155. Cutting GR, Curristin SM, Nash E, Rosenstein BJ, Lerer I, Abeliovich D, Hill A, Graham C: Analysis of four diverse population groups indicates that a subset of cystic fibrosis mutations occur in common among Caucasians. *Am J Hum Genet* **50**:1185, 1992.
156. Dalemans W, Barbry P, Champigny G, Jallat S, Dott K, Dreyer D, Crystal RG, Pavirani A, Lecocq JP, Lazdunski M: Altered chloride ion channel kinetics associated with the ΔF508 cystic fibrosis mutation. *Nature* **354**:526, 1991.
157. Danks DM, Allan JR, Anderson CM: A genetic study of fibrocystic disease of the pancreas. *Ann Hum Genet* **28**:323, 1965.
158. Danks DM, Allan JR, Phelan PD, Chapman C: Mutations at more than one locus may be involved in cystic fibrosis-evidence based on first-cousin data and direct counting of cases. *Am J Med Genet* **35**:838, 1983.
159. Davidson DJ, Dorin JR, McLachlan G, Ranaldi V, Lamb D, Doherty C, Govan J, Porteous DJ: Lung disease in the cystic fibrosis mouse exposed to bacterial pathogens. *Nat Genet* **9**:351, 1995.
160. Davies J, Trindade MT, Wallis C, Rosenthal M, Crawford O, Bush A: Retrospective review of the effects of rhDNase in children with cystic fibrosis. *Pediatr Pulmonol* **23**:243, 1997.
161. Davis PB, Drumm M, Konstan MW: Cystic fibrosis. *Am J Respir Crit Care Med* 154:1229, 1996.
162. Dawson DC, Smith SS, Mansoura MK: CFTR: Mechanism of anion conduction. *Physiological Reviews* **79**:S47, 1999.
163. de Bentzmann S, Plotkowski C, Puchelle E: Receptors in the Pseudomonas aerurinosa adherence to injured and repairing airway epithelium. *Am J Respir Crit Care Med* **154**:S155, 1996.
164. de Bentzmann S, Roger P, Dupuit F, Bajolet-Laudinat O, Fuchey C, Plotkowske MC, Puchelle E: Asialo GM1 is a receptor for pseudomonas aeruginosa adherence to regenerating respiratory epithelial cells. *Infect Immun* **64**:1582, 1996.
165. de Leval MR, Smyth R, Whitehead B, Scott JP, Elliott MJ, Sharples L, Caine N, Helms P, Martin I R, Higenbottam T: Heart and lung transplantation for terminal cystic fibrosis. A $4\frac{1}{2}$-year experience. *J Thorac Cardiovasc Surg* **101**:633, 1991.
166. De Schepper J, Dab I, Derde MP, Loeb H: Oral glucose tolerance testing in cystic fibrosis: Correlations with clinical parameters and glycosylated haemoglobin determinations. *Eur J Pediatr* **150**:403, 1991.

167. DeBraekeleer M, Allard C, Leblanc J, Simard F, Aubin G: Genotype-phenotype correlation in cystic fibrosis patients compound heterozygous for the A455E mutation. *Hum Genet* **101**:208, 1997.
168. Delaney SJ, Alton EWFW, Smith SN, Lunn DP, Farley R, Lovelock PK, Thomson SA, Hume DA, Lamb D, Porteous DJ, Dorin JR, Wainwright BJ: Cystic fibrosis mice carrying the missense mutation G551D replicate human genotype-phenotype correlations. *EMBO J* **15**:955, 1996.
169. Delaney SJ, Rich DP, Thomson SA, Hargrave MR, Lovelock PK, Welsh MJ, Wainwright BJ: Cystic fibrosis transmembrane conductance regulator splice variants are not conserved and fail to produce chloride channels. *Nat Genet* **4**:426, 1993.
170. DeMarchi J, Beaudet AL, Caskey CT, Richards CT: Experience of an academic refernce laboratory using automation for analysis of cystic fibrosis mutations. *Arch Pathol Lab Med* **118**:26, 1994.
171. Denamur E, Chehab FF: Analysis of the mouse and rat CFTR promoter regions. *Hum Mol Genet* **3**:1089, 1994.
172. Denning CR, Sommers SC, Quigley HJ: Infertility in male patients with cystic fibrosis. *Pediatrics* **41**:7, 1968.
173. Denning GM, Anderson MP, Amara JF, Marshall J, Smith AE, Welsh MJ: Processing of mutant cystic fibrosis transmembrane conductance regulator is temperature-sensitive. *Nature* **358**:761, 1992.
174. Denning GM, Ostedgaard LS, Cheng SH, Smith AE, Welsh MJ: Localization of cystic fibrosis transmembrane conductance regulator in chloride secretory epithelia. *J Clin Invest* **89**:339, 1992.
175. Dequeker E, Cassiman JJ: Evaluation of CFTR gene mutation testing methods in 136 diagnostic laboratories: Report of a large European external quality assessment. *Eur J Hum Genet* **6**:165, 1998.
176. Detterbeck FC, Egan TM, Mill MR: Lung transplantation after previous thoracic surgical procedures. *Ann Thorac Surg* **60**:139, 1995.
177. Di Sant' Agnese PA, Darling RC, Perera GA, Shea E: Abnormal Electrolyte Composition of Sweat in Cystic Fibrosis of the Pancreas. *Pediatrics* **12**:549, 1953.
178. di Sant 'Agnese PA, Hubbard V: The pancreas, in Taussig LM (ed): *Cystic Fibrosis*. New York, Thieme-Stratton, 1984, p 230.
179. di Sant' Agnese PA, Hubbard VS: The gastrointestinal tract, in Taussig LM (ed): *Cystic Fibrosis*. New York, Thieme-Stratton, 1984, p 213.
180. Diamond G, Bevins CL: Beta-defensins: Endogenous antibiotics of the innate host defense response. *Clin Immunol Immunopath* **88**:221, 1998.
181. DiMango E, Ratner AJ, Bryan R, Tabibi S, Prince A: Activation of NF-κB by adherent *Pseudomonas aeruginosa* in normal and cystic fibrosis respiratory epithelial cells. *J Clin Invest* **101**:2598, 1998.
182. Dodd ME, Abbott J, Maddison J, Moorcroft AJ, Webb AK: Effect of tonicity of nebulised colistin on chest tightness and pulmonary function in adults with cystic fibrosis. *Thorax* **52**:656, 1997.
183. Doige CA, Ames GF: ATP-dependent transport systems in bacteria and humans: Relevance to cystic fibrosis and multidrug resistance. *Annu Rev Microbiol* **47**:291, 1993.
184. Dorin JR, Dickinson P, Alton EW, Smith SN, Geddes DM, Stevenson BJ, Kimber WL, Fleming S, Clarke AR, Hooper ML, et al: Cystic fibrosis in the mouse by targeted insertional mutagenesis. *Nature* **359**:211, 1992.
185. Doring G, Dorner F: A multicenter vaccine trial using the Pseudomonas aeruginosa flagella vaccine IMMUNO in patients with cystic fibrosis. *Behring Inst Mitt* 338, 1997.
186. Dörk T, Dworniczak B, Aulehla-Scholz C, Wieczorek D, Böhm I, Mayerova A, Seydewitz HH, Nieschlag E, Meschede D, Horst J, Pander HJ, Sperling H, Ratjen F, Passarge E, Schmidtke J, Stuhrmann M: Distinct spectrum of CFTR gene mutations in congenital absence of vas deferens. *Hum Genet* **100**:356, 1997.
187. Dörk T, El-Harith EH, Stuhrmann M, Macek M Jr, Egan M, Cutting GR, Tzetis M, Kanavakis E, Carles S, Claustres M, Padoa C, Ramsay M, Schmidtke J: Evidence for a common ethnic origin of cystic fibrosis mutation 3120+1G→A in diverse populations. *Am J Hum Genet* **63**:656, 1998.
188. Dörk T, Neümann T, Wulbrand U, Wulf B, Kalin N, Maass G, Krawczak M, Guillermit H, Ferec C, Horn G, Klinger K, Kerem BS, Zielenski J, Tsui LC, B Tümmler: Intra- and extragenic marker haplotypes of CFTR mutations in cystic fibrosis families. *Hum Genet* **88**:417, 1992.
189. Dörk T, Wulbrand U, Richter T, Neumann T, Wolfes H, Wulf B, Maab G, Tümmler B: Cystic fibrosis with three mutations in the cystic fibrosis transmembrane conductance regulator gene. *Hum Genet* **87**:441, 1991.
190. Drapkin PT, O'Riordan CR, Yi SM, Chiorini JA, Cardella J, Zabner J, Welsh MJ: Targeting the urokinase plasminogen activator receptor enhances gene transfer to human airway epithelia by increasing binding and stimulating endocytosis. *J Clin Invest* **105**:589, 2000.
191. Drumm ML, Pope HA, Cliff WH, Rommens JM, Marvin SA, Tsui L-C, Collins FS, Frizzell RA, Wilson JM: Correction of the cystic fibrosis defect *in vitro* by retrovirus-mediated gene transfer. *Cell* **62**:1227, 1990.
192. Drumm ML, Wilkinson DJ, Smit LS, Worrell RT, Strong TV, Frizzell RA, Dawson DC, Collins FS: Chloride conductance expressed by ΔF508 and other mutant CFTRs in *Xenopus* oocytes. *Science* **254**:1797, 1991.
193. Dulhanty AM, Riordan JR: A two-domain model for the R domain of the cystic fibrosis transmembrane conductance regulator based on sequence similarities. *FEBS Lett* **343**:109, 1994.
194. Durie PR: Inherited and congenital disorders of the exocrine pancreas. *Gastroenterologist* **4**:169, 1996.
195. Durieu I, Peyrol S, Gindre D, Bellon G, Durand DV, Pacheco Y: Subepithelial fibrosis and degradation of the bronchial extracellular matrix in cystic fibrosis. *Am J Respir Crit Care Med* **158**:580, 1998.
196. Duthie A, Doherty DG, Williams C, Scott-Jupp R, Warner JO, Tanner MS, Williamson R, Mowat AP: Genotype analysis for delta F508, G551D and R553X mutations in children and young adults with cystic fibrosis with and without chronic liver disease. *Hepatology* **15**:660, 1992.
197. Eggermont E: Gastrointestinal manifestations in cystic fibrosis. *Eur J Gastroenterol Hepatol* **8**:731, 1996.
198. Eigen H, Rosenstein BJ, FitzSimmons S, Schidlow DV: A multicenter study of alternate-day prednisone therapy in patients with cystic fibrosis. Cystic Fibrosis Foundation Prednisone Trial Group. *J Pediatr* **126**:515, 1995.
199. Eisenberg JD, Aitken ML, Dorkin HL, Harwood IR, Ramsey BW, Schidlow DV, Wilmott RW, Wohl ME, Fuchs HJ, Christiansen DH, Smith AL: Safety of repeated intermittent courses of aerosolized recombinant human deoxyribonuclease in patients with cystic fibrosis. *J Pediatr* **131**:118, 1997.
200. Elmer HL, Brady KG, Drumm ML, Kelley TJ: Nitric oxide-mediated regulation of transepithelial sodium and chloride transport in murine nasal epithelium. *Am J Physiol* **276**:L466, 1999.
201. Engelhardt JF, Yankaskas JR, Ernst SA, Yang Y, Marino CR, Boucher RC, Cohn JA, Wilson JM: Submucosal glands are the predominant site of CFTR expression in the human bronchus. *Nat Genet* **2**:240, 1992.
202. Engelhardt JF, Zepeda M, Cohn JA, Yankaskas JR, Wilson JM: Expression of the cystic fibrosis gene in adult human lung. *J Clin Invest* **93**:737, 1994.
203. Erjefält I, Persson CGA: On the use of absorbing discs to sample mucosal surface liquids. *Clin Exp All* **20**:193, 1990.
204. Esterly NB, Oppenheimer EH, Esterly JR: Observations on cystic fibrosis of the pancreas. The apocrine gland. *Am J Dis Child* **123**:200, 1972.
205. Estivill X: Complexity in a monogenic disease. *Nat Genet* **12**:348, 1996.
206. Estivill X, Bancells C, Ramos C: Geographic distribution and regional origin of 272 cystic fibrosis mutations in European populations. The Biomed CF Mutation Analysis Consortium. *Hum Mutat* **10**:135, 1997.
207. Estivill X, Farrall M, Williamson R, Ferrari M, Seia M, Giunta AM, Novelli G, Potenza L, Dallapicolla B, Borgo G, et al: Linkage disequilibrium between cystic fibrosis and linked DNA polymorphisms in Italian families: A collaborative study. *Am J Hum Genet* **43**:23, 1988.
208. Estivill X, Ortigosa L, Peréz-Frias J, Dapena J, Ferrer J, Pena J, Pena L, Llevadot R, Gimenez J, Nunes V, Cobos N, Vázquez C, Casals T: Clinical characteristics of 16 cystic fibrosis patients with the missense mutation R334W, a pancreatic insufficiency mutation with variable age of onset and interfamilial clinical differences. *Hum Genet* **95**:331, 1995.
209. Estroff JA, Parad RB, Benacerraf BR: Prevalence of cystic fibrosis in fetuses with dilated bowel. *Radiology* **183**:677, 1992.
210. European Working Group on CF Genetics. Gradient of distribution in Europe of the major CF mutation and of its associated haplotype. *Hum Genet* **85**:436, 1990.
211. Farrall M, Law HY, Rodeck CH, Warren R, Stanier P, Super M, Lissens W, Scambler P, Watson E, Wainwright B, Williamson R: First-trimester prenatal diagnosis of cystic fibrosis with linked DNA probes. *Lancet* **1**:1402, 1986.
212. Farrell PM, Bieri JG, Fratantoni JF, Wood RE, di Sant'Agnese PA: The occurrence and effects of human vitamin E deficiency. A study in patients with cystic fibrosis. *J Clin Invest* **60**:233, 1977.

213. Farrell PM, Koscik RE: Sweat chloride concentrations in infants homozygous or heterozygous for F508 cystic fibrosis. *Pediatrics* **97**:524, 1996.
214. Farrell PM, Kosorok MR, Laxova A, Shen G, Koscik RE, Bruns WT, Splaingard M, Mischler EH: Nutritional benefits of neonatal screening for cystic fibrosis. Wisconsin Cystic Fibrosis Neonatal Screening Study Group. *N Engl J Med* **337**:963, 1997.
215. Farrell PM, Shen G, Splaingard M, Colby CE, Laxova A, Kosorok MR, Rock MJ, Mischler EH: Acquisition of Pseudomonas aeruginosa in children with cystic fibrosis. *Pediatrics* **100**:E2, 1997.
216. Fasbender A, Lee JH, Walters RW, Moninger TO, Zabner J, Welsh MJ: Incorporation of adenovirus in calcium phosphate precipitates enhances gene transfer to airway epithelia *in vitro* and *in vivo*. *J Clin Invest* **102**:184, 1998.
217. Fasbender A, Zabner J, Zeiher BG, Welsh MJ: A low rate of cell proliferation and reduced DNA uptake limit cationic lipid-mediated gene transfer to primary cultures of ciliated airway epithelia. *Gene Ther* **4**:1173, 1997.
218. Férec C, Audrézet MP, Mercier B, Guillermit H, Moullier P, Quéré I, Verlingue C: Detection of over 98% cystic fibrosis mutations in a celtic population. *Nat Genet* **1**:188, 1992.
219. Ferkol T, Perales JC, Eckman E, Kaetzel CS, Hanson RW, Davis PB: Gene transfer into the airway epithelium of animals by targeting the polymeric immunoglobulin receptor. *J Clin Invest* **95**:493, 1995.
220. Figarella C, Carrére J: The evolution of pancreatic disease in cystic fibrosis, in Dodge JA, Brock DJH, Widdicombe JH, (eds): *Cystic Fibrosis—Current Topics*. New York, John Wiley, 1994, p 255.
221. Finkelstein SM, Wielinski CL, Elliott GR, Warwick WJ, Barbosa J, Wu SC, Klein DJ: Diabetes mellitus associated with cystic fibrosis. *J Pediatr* **112**:373, 1988.
222. Finnegan MJ, Hinchcliffe J, Russell-Jones D, Neill S, Sheffield E, Jayne D, Wise A, Hodson ME: Vasculitis complicating cystic fibrosis. *QJM* **72**:609, 1989.
223. Fischer H, Illek B, Machen TE: Regulation of CFTR by protein phosphatase 2B and protein kinase C. *Pflugers Arch* **436**:175, 1998.
224. Fischer H, Machen TE: The tyrosine kinase $p60^{c\text{-}src}$ regulates the fast gate of the cystic fibrosis transmembrane conductance regulator chloride channel. *Biophys J* **71**:3073, 1996.
225. Fitz JG, Basavappa S, Mcgill J, Melhus O, Cohn JA: Regulation of membrane chloride currents in rat bile duct epithelial cells. *J Clin Invest* **91**:319, 1993.
226. Fitz JG, Basavappa S, McGill J, Melhus O, Cohn JA: Regulation of membrane chloride currents in rat bile duct epithelial cells. *J Clin Invest* **91**:319, 1993.
227. FitzSimmons SC: The changing epidemiology of cystic fibrosis. *Curr Probl Pediatr* **24**:171, 1994.
228. FitzSimmons SC, Burkhart GA, Borowitz D, Grand RJ, Hammerstrom T, Durie PR, Lloyd-Still JD, Lowenfels AB: High-dose pancreatic-enzyme supplements and fibrosing colonopathy in children with cystic fibrosis. *N Engl J Med* **336**:1283, 1997.
229. Folkesson HG, Matthay MA, Frigeri A, Verkman AS: Transepithelial water permeability in microperfused distal airways. *J Clin Invest* **97**:664, 1996.
230. Frangolias DD, Nakielna EM, Wilcox PG: Pregnancy and cystic fibrosis: A case-controlled study. *Chest* **111**:963, 1997.
231. Frederiksen B, Koch C, Hoiby N: Antibiotic treatment of initial colonization with Pseudomonas aeruginosa postpones chronic infection and prevents deterioration of pulmonary function in cystic fibrosis. *Pediatr Pulmonol* **23**:330, 1997.
232. French PJ, van Doorninck JH, Peters RHPC, Verbeek E, Ameen NA, Marino CR, De Jonge HR, Bijman J, Scholte BJ: A ΔF508 mutation in mouse cystic fibrosis transmembrane conductance regulator results in a temperance-sensitive processing defect *in vivo*. *J Clin Invest* **98**:1304, 1996.
233. Fuchs HJ, Borowitz DS, Christiansen DH, Morris EM, Nash ML, Ramsey BW, Rosenstein BJ, Smith AL, Wohl ME: Effect of aerosolized recombinant human DNase on exacerbations of respiratory symptoms and on pulmonary function in patients with cystic fibrosis. The Pulmozyme Study Group. *N Engl J Med* **331**:637, 1994.
234. Fuchs JR, Langer JC: Long-term outcome after neonatal meconium obstruction. *Pediatrics* **101**:E7, 1998.
235. Gabriel SE, Brigman KN, Koller BH, Boucher RC, Stutts MJ: Cystic fibrosis heterozygote resistance to cholera toxin in the cystic fibrosis mouse model. *Science* **266**:107, 1994.
236. Gadsby DC, Narin AC: Control of CFTR channel gating by phosphorylation and nucleotide hydrolysis. *Physiol Rev* **79**:s77, 1999.
237. Gan KH, Veeze HJ, van den Ouweland AM, Halley DJ, Scheffer H, van der Hout A, Overbeek SE, de Jongste JC, Bakker W, Heijerman HG: A cystic fibrosis mutation associated with mild lung disease. *N Engl J Med* **333**:95, 1995.
238. Garland JS, Chan YM, Kelly KJ, Rice TB: Outcome of infants with cystic fibrosis requiring mechanical ventilation for respiratory failure. *Chest* **96**:136, 1989.
239. Garred P, Pressler T, Madsen HO, Frederiksen B, Svejgaard A, Hoiby N, Schwartz M, Koch C: Association of mannose-binding lectin gene heterogeneity with severity of lung disease and survival in cystic fibrosis. *J Clin Invest* **104**:431, 1999.
240. Gärtner J, Moser H, Valle D: Mutations in the 70K peroxisomal membrane protein gene in Zellweger syndrome. *Nat Genet* **1**:16, 1992.
241. Gaskin K: Liver and biliary tract disease in cystic fibrosis, in Suchy FJ (ed): *Liver Disease in Children*. Philadelphia, Mosby Yearbook, 1994, p 705.
242. Gaskin K, Gurwitz D, Durie P, Corey M, Levison H, Forstner G: Improved respiratory prognosis in patients with cystic fibrosis with normal fat absorption. *J Pediatr* **100**:857, 1982.
243. Gaskin KJ, Waters DL: Nutritional management of infants with cystic fibrosis. *J Paediatr Child Health* **30**:11994.
244. Ghosal S, Taylor CJ, Pickering M, McGaw J: Head growth in cystic fibrosis following early diagnosis by neonatal screening. *Arch Dis Child* **75**:191, 1996.
245. Giglio L, Candusso M, D'Orazio C, Mastella G, Faraguna D: Failure to thrive: The earliest feature of cystic fibrosis in infants diagnosed by neonatal screening. *Acta Paediatr* **86**:1162, 1997.
246. Gilfillan A, Warner JP, Kirk JM, Marshall T, Greening A, Ho L, Hargreave T, Stack B, McIntyre D, Davidson R, Dean JC, Middleton W, Brock DJ: P67L: A cystic fibrosis allele with mild effects found at high frequency in the Scottish population. *J Med Genet* **35**:122, 1998.
247. Gilljam H, Ellin A, Strandvik B: Increased bronchial chloride concentration in cystic fibrosis. *Scand J Clin Lab Invest* **49**:121, 1989.
248. Goldman MJ, Anderson GM, Stolzenberg ED, Kari UP, Zasloff M, Wilson JM: Human β-defensin-1 is a salt-sensitive antibiotic in lung that is inactivated in cystic fibrosis. *Cell* **88**:553, 1997.
249. Goldstein JL, Nash NT, Al-Bazzaz F, Layden TJ, Rao MC: Rectum has abnormal ion transport but normal cAMP-binding proteins in cystic fibrosis. *Am J Physiol* **254**:C719, 1988.
250. Goldstein JL, Shapiro AB, Rao MC, Layden TJ: *In vivo* evidence of altered chloride but not potassium secretion in cystic fibrosis rectal mucosa. *Gastroenterology* **101**:1012, 1991.
251. Gray MA, Greenwell JR, Argent BE: Secretin-regulated chloride channel on the apical plasma membrane of pancreatic duct cells. *J Membr Biol* **105**:131, 1988.
252. Gray MA, Plant S, Argent BE: cAMP-regulated whole cell chloride currents in pancreatic duct cells. *Am J Physiol* **264**:C591, 1993.
253. Gray MA, Winpenny JA, Verdon B, McAlroy H, Argent BE: Chloride channels and cystic fibrosis of the pancreas. *Biosci Rep* **15**:531, 1995.
254. Greally P, Hussain MJ, Vergani D, Price JF: Interleukin-1 alpha, soluble interleukin-2 receptor, and IgG concentrations in cystic fibrosis treated with prednisolone. *Arch Dis Child* **71**:35, 1994.
255. Grebe TA, Doane WW, Richter SF, Clericuzio C, Norman RA, Seltzer WK, Rhodes SN, Goldberg BE, Hernried LS, McClure M, Kaplan G: Mutation analysis of the cystic fibrosis transmembrane regulator gene in Native American populations of the southwest. *Am J Hum Genet* **51**:736, 1992.
256. Grebe TA, Seltzer WK, DeMarchi J, Silva DK, Doane WW: Genetic analysis of hispanic individuals with cystic fibrosis. *Am J Med Genet* **54**:443, 1994.
257. Green MR, Weaver LT, Heeley AF, Nicholson K, Kuzemko JA: Cystic fibrosis identified by neonatal screening: Incidence, genotype and early natural history. *Arch Dis Child* **58**:464, 1993.
258. Gregg RG, Simantel A, Farrell PM, Koscik R, Kosorok MR, Laxova A, Laessig R, Hoffman G, Hassemer D, Mischler EH, Splaingard M: Newborn screening for cystic fibrosis in Wisconsin: Comparison of biochemical and molecular methods. *Pediatrics* **99**:819, 1997.
259. Gregg RG, Wilfond BS, Farrell PM, Laxova A, Hassemer D: Application of DNA analysis in a population-screening program for neonatal diagnosis of cystic fibrosis (CF); Comparison of screening protocols. *Am J Hum Genet* **52**:616, 1993.
260. Gregory RJ, Rich DP, Cheng SH, Souza DW, Paul S, Manavalan P, Anderson MP, Welsh MJ, Smith AE: Maturation and function of cystic fibrosis transmembrane conductance regulator variants bearing mutations in putative nucleotide-binding domains 1 and 2. *Mol Cell Biol* **11**:3886, 1991.

261. Grody WW, Desnick RJ, Carpenter NJ, Noll WW: Diversity of cystic fibrosis mutation-screening practices. *Am J Hum Genet* **62**:1252, 1998.
262. Grove SS: Fibrocystic disease of the pancreas in the Bantu. *S Afr Med J* **5**:113, 1959.
263. Grubb BR, Boucher RC: Pathophysiology of gene-targeted mouse models for cystic fibrosis. *Physiol Rev* **79**:S193, 1999.
264. Gunderson KL, Kopito RR: Effects of pyrophosphate and nucleotide analogs suggest a role for ATP hydrolysis in cystic fibrosis transmembrane regulator channel gating. *J Biol Chem* **269**:19349, 1994.
265. Gunderson KL, Kopito RR: Conformational states of CFTR associated with channel gating: The role ATP binding and hydrolysis. *Cell* **82**:231, 1995.
266. Haardt M, Benharouga M, Lechardeur D, Kartner N, Lukacs GL: C-terminal truncations destabilize the cystic fibrosis transmembrane conductance regulator without impairing its biogenesis. A novel class of mutation. *J Biol Chem* **30**:21873, 1999.
267. Hall BD, Simpkiss MJ: Inheritance of fibrocystic disease in Wessex. *J Med Genet* **5**:262, 1968.
268. Hall RA, Ostedgaard LS, Premont RT, Blitzer JT, Rahman N, Welsh MJ, Lefkowitz RJ: A C-Terminal Motif Found in the beta2-adrenergic receptor, p2y1 receptor and cystic fibrosis transmembrane conductance regulator determines binding to the Na^+/H^+ exchanger regulatory factor family of PDZ proteins. *Proc Natl Acad Sci U S A* **95**:8496, 1998.
269. Halvorson DJ, Dupree JR, Porubsky ES: Management of chronic sinusitis in the adult cystic fibrosis patient. *Ann Otol Rhinol Laryngol* **107**:946, 1998.
270. Hammond K, Naylor E, Wilcken B: Screening for cystic fibrosis, in Therrell BL Jr (ed): *Advances in Neonatal Screening*. New York, Excerpta Medica, 1987, p 377.
271. Hammond KB, Abman SH, Sokol RJ, Accurso FJ: Efficacy of statewide neonatal screening for cystic fibrosis by assay of trypsinogen concentrations. *N Engl J Med* **325**:769, 1991.
272. Hamosh A, Fitz-Simmons SC, Macek M Jr, Knowles MR, Rosenstein BJ, Cutting GR: Comparison of the clinical manifestations of cystic fibrosis in black and white patients . *J Pediatr* **132**:255, 1998.
273. Hamosh A, King TM, Rosenstein BJ, Corey M, Levison H, Durie P, Tsui L-C, McIntosh I, Keston M, Brock DJH, Macek M Jr, Zemková D, Krásnicanová H, Vávrová V, Macek M Sr, Golder N, Schwarz MJ, Super M, Watson EK, Williams C, Bush A, O'Mahoney SM, Humphries P, DeArce MA, Reis A, Bürger J, Stuhrmann M, Schmidtke J, Wulbrand U, Dörk T, Tümmler B, Cutting GR: Cystic fibrosis patients bearing both the common missense mutation GlyØ asp at codon 551 and the ΔF508 mutation are clinically indistinguishable from ΔF508 homozygotes, except for decreased risk of meconium ileus. *Am J Hum Genet* **51**:245, 1992.
274. Hamosh A, Trapnell BC, Zeitlin PL, Montrose-Rafizadeh C, Rosenstein BJ, Crystal RG, Cutting GR: Severe deficiency of cystic fibrosis transmembrane conductance regulator messenger RNA carrying nonsense mutations R553X and W1316X in respiratory epithelial cells of patients with cystic fibrosis. *J Clin Invest* **88**:1880, 1991.
275. Hanukoglu A, Bistritzer T, Rakover V, Mandelber A: Pseudohypoaldosteronism with increased sweat and saliva electrolyte values and frequent lower respiratory tract infections mimicking cystic fibrosis. *J Pediatr* **125**:752, 1994.
276. Hardin DS, LeBlanc A, Lukenbaugh S, Para L, Seilheimer DK: Proteolysis associated with insulin resistance in cystic fibrosis. *Pediatrics* **101**:433, 1998.
277. Hardin DS, LeBlanc A, Lukenbough S, Seilheimer DK: Insulin resistance is associated with decreased clinical status in cystic fibrosis. *J Pediatr* **130**:948, 1997.
278. Hardy KA: A review of airway clearance: New techniques, indications, and recommendations. *Respir Care* **39**:440, 1994.
279. Hart P, Warth JD, Levesque PC, Collier ML, Geary Y, Horowitz B, Hume JR: Cystic fibrosis gene encodes a cAMP-dependent chloride channel in heart. *Proc Natl Acad Sci U S A* **93**:6343, 1996.
280. Hasegawa H, Skach W, Baker O, Calayag MC, Lingappa V, Verkman AS: A multifunctional aqueous channel formed by CFTR. *Science* **258**:1477, 1992.
281. Hasty P, O'Neal WK, Liu KQ, Morris AP, Bebok Z, Shumyatsky GB, Jilling T, Sorscher EJ, Bradley A, Beaudet AL: Severe phenotype in mice with termination mutation in exon 2 of cystic fibrosis gene. *Somat Cell Mol Genet* **21**:177, 1995.
282. Hellquist HB: Nasal polyps update. Histopathology. *Allergy Asthma Proc* **17**:237, 1996.
283. Henderson RC, Madsen CD: Bone density in children and adolescents with cystic fibrosis. *J Pediatr* **128**:28, 1996.
284. Henderson RC, Specter BB: Kyphosis and fractures in children and young adults with cystic fibrosis. *J Pediatr* **125**:208, 1994.
285. Highsmith WE, Burch LH, Zhou Z, Olsen JC, Boat TE, Spock A, Gorvoy JD, Quittel L, Friedman KJ, Silverman LM, Boucher R, Knowles MR: A novel mutation in the cystic fibrosis gene in patients with pulmonary disease but normal sweat chloride concentrations. *N Engl J Med* **331**:974, 1994.
286. Highsmith WE Jr, Burch LH, Zhou Z, Olsen JC, Strong TV, Smith T, Friedman KJ, Silverman LM, Boucher RC, Collins FS, Knowles MR: Identification of a splice site mutation ($2789 + 5$ G $>$ a) associated with small amounts of normal CFTR mRNA and mild cystic fibrosis. *Hum Mutat* **9**:332, 1997.
287. Hill ID, Macdonald WBG, Bowie MD, Ireland JD: Cystic fibrosis in Cape Town. *S Afr Med J* **73**:147, 1988.
288. Hilman BC, Aitken ML, Constantinescu M: Pregnancy in patients with cystic fibrosis. *Clin Obstet Gynecol* **39**:70, 1996.
289. Hodge SE, Lebo RV, Yesley AR, Cheney SM, Angle H, Milunsky J: Calculating posterior cystic fibrosis risk with echogenic bowel and one characterized cystic fibrosis mutation: Avoiding pitfalls in the risk calculations. *Am J Med Genet* **82**:329, 1999.
290. Hoffman RD, Isenberg JN, Powell GK: Carbohydrate malabsorption is minimal in school-age cystic fibrosis children. *Dig Dis Sci* **32**:1071, 1987.
291. Holliday KE, Allen JR, Waters DL, Gruca MA, Thompson SM, Gaskin KJ: Growth of human milk-fed and formula-fed infants with cystic fibrosis. *J Pediatr* **118**:77, 1991.
292. Homnick DN, Cox JH, DeLoof MJ, Ringer TV: Carotenoid levels in normal children and in children with cystic fibrosis. *J Pediatr* **122**:703, 1993.
293. Homnick DN, White F, de Castro C: Comparison of effects of an intrapulmonary percussive ventilator to standard aerosol and chest physiotherapy in treatment of cystic fibrosis. *Pediatr Pulmonol* **20**:50, 1995.
294. Hoogkamp-Korstanje JA, Meis JF, Kissing J, van der Laag J, Melchers WJ: Risk of cross-colonization and infection by Pseudomonas aeruginosa in a holiday camp for cystic fibrosis patients. *J Clin Microbiol* **33**:572, 1995.
295. Hordvik NL, PH Sammut, CG Judy, SJ Strizek, JL Colombo: The effects of albuterol on the lung function of hospitalized patients with cystic fibrosis. *Am J Respir Crit Care Med* **154**:156, 1996.
296. Houstek J, Vavrova V: Notre experience a pros de la mucoviscidose. *Rev Med Llege* **22**:421, 1967.
297. Howard M, Frizzell RA, Bedwell DM: Aminoglycoside antibiotics restore CFTR function by overcoming premature stop mutations. *Nat Med* **2**:467, 1996.
298. Hull J, Skinner W, Robertson C, Phelan P: Elemental content of airway surface liquid from infants with cystic fibrosis. *Am J Respir Crit Care Med* **157**:10, 1998.
299. Hull J, South M, Phelan P, Grimwood K: Surfactant composition in infants and young children with cystic fibrosis. *Am J Respir Crit Care Med* **156**:161, 1997.
300. Hull J, Thomson AH: Contribution of genetic factors other than CFTR to disease severity in cystic fibrosis. *Thorax* **53**:1018, 1998.
301. Hummler E, Barker P, Gatzy J, Beermann F, Verdumo C, Schmidt A, Boucher R, Rossier BC: Early death due to defective neonatal lung liquid clearance in *αENaC*-deficient mice. *Nat Genet* **12**:325, 1996.
302. Hung LW, Wang IX, Nikaido K, Liu PQ, Ames GF-L, Kim SH: Crystal structure of the ATP-binding subunit of an ABC transporter. *Nature* **396**:703, 1998.
303. Hyde SC, Emsley P, Hartshorn MJ, Mimmack MM, Gileadi U, Pearce SR, Gallagher MP, Gill DR, Hubbard RE, Higgins CF: Structural model of ATP-binding proteins associated with cystic fibrosis, multidrug resistance and bacterial transport. *Nature* **346**:362, 1990.
304. Illek B, Fischer H, Machen TE: Genetic disorders of membrane transport. II. Regulation of CFTR by small molecules including HCO3−. *Am J Physiol* **275**:G1221, 1998.
305. Imalzumi Y: Incidence and mortality rates of cystic fibrosis in Japan. *Am J Med Genet* **58**:161, 1995.
306. Imundo L, Barasch J, Prince A, Al-Awqati Q: Cystic fibrosis epithelial cells have a receptor for pathogenic bacteria on their apical surface. *Proc Natl Acad Sci U S A* **92**:3019, 1995.
307. Ishihara H, Welsh MJ: Block by MOPS reveals a conformation change in the CFTR pore produced by ATP hydrolysis. *Am J Physiol* **273**:C1278, 1997.

308. Isles A, Spino M, Tabachnik E, Levison H, Thiessen J, MacLeod S: Theophylline disposition in cystic fibrosis. *Am Rev Respir Dis* **127**:417, 1983.
309. Ismailov II, Awayda MS, Jovov B, Berdiev BK, Fuller CM, Dedman JR, Kaetzel MA, Benos DJ: Regulation of epithelial sodium channels by the cystic fibrosis transmembrane conductance regulator. *J Biol Chem* **271**:4725, 1996.
310. Jacquot J, Tabary O, Baconnais S, Balossier G, Hubert D, Couetil J, Puchelle E: Highly increased levels of constitutive sodium chloride and C-X-C chemokines production by CF human bronchial submucosal gland cells. *Pediatr Pulmonol* **17(Suppl)**:387, 1998.
311. Jensen T, Pedersen SS, Hoiby N, Koch C, Flensborg EW: Use of antibiotics in cystic fibrosis. The Danish approach. *Antibiot Chemother* **42**:237, 1989.
312. Jensen TJ, Loo MA, Pind S, Williams DB, Goldberg AL, Riordan JR: Multiple proteolytic systems, including the proteasome, contribute to CFTR processing. *Cell* **83**:129, 1995.
313. Jia Y, Mathews CJ, Hanrahan JW: Phosphorylation by protein kinase C is required for acute activation of cystic fibrosis transmembrane conductance regulator by protein kinase A. *J Biol Chem* **272**:4978, 1997.
314. Jiang, C, Finkbeiner WE, Widdicombe JH, McCray PB Jr, Miller SS: Altered fluid transport across airway epithelium in cystic fibrosis. *Science* **262**:424, 1993.
315. Jiang Q, Mak D, Devidas S, Schwiebert EM, Bragin A, Zhang Y, Skach WR, Guggino WB, Foskett JK, Engelhardt JF: Cystic fibrosis transmembrane conductance regulator-associated ATP release is controlled by a chloride sensor. *J Cell Biol* **143**:645, 1998.
316. John M, Ecclestone E, Hunter E, Couroux P, Hussain Z: Epidemiology of *Pseudomonas cepacia* colonization among patients with cystic fibrosis. *Pediatr Pulmonol* **18**:108, 1994.
317. Johnson LG, Olsen JC, Sarkadi B, Moore KL, Swanstrom R, Boucher RC: Efficiency of gene transfer for restoration of normal airway epithelial function in cystic fibrosis. *Nat Genet* **2**:21, 1992.
318. Joris L, Dab I, Quinton PM: Elemental composition of human airway surface fluid in healthy and diseased airways. *Am Rev Respir Dis* **148**:1633, 1993.
319. Jorissen M, DeBoeck K, Cuppens H: Genotype-phenotype correlations for the paranasal sinuses in cystic fibrosis. *Am J Resp Crit Care Med* **159**:1412, 1999.
320. Jorissen M, Vereecke J, Carmeliet E, Van Der Berghe H, Cassiman J-J: Identification of a voltage- and calcium-dependent non-selective cation channel in cultured adult and fetal human nasal epithelial cells. *Pflugers Arch* **415**:617, 1990.
321. Kalin N, Claass A, Sommer M, Puchelle E, Tummler B: DeltaF508 CFTR protein expression in tissues from patients with cystic fibrosis. *J Clin Invest* **103**:1379, 1999.
322. Kartner N, Augustinas O, Jensen TJ, Naismith AL, Riordan JR: Mislocalization of delta F508 CFTR in cystic fibrosis sweat gland. *Nat Genet* **1**:321–327, 1992.
323. Kartner, N, JW Hanrahan, Jensen TJ, Naismith AL, Sun S, Ackerley CA, Reyes EF, Tsui L-C, Rommens JM, Bear CE, Riordan JR: Expression of the cystic fibrosis gene in non-epithelial invertebrate cells produces a regulated anion conductance. *Cell* **64**:681, 1991.
324. Katznelson D, Szeinberg A, Augarten A, Yahav Y: The critical first six months in cystic fibrosis: A syndrome of severe bronchiolitis. *Pediatr Pulmonol* **24**:134, 1997.
325. Kelley TJ, al-Nakkash L, Cotton CU, Drumm ML: Activation of endogenous ΔF508 cystic fibrosis transmembrane conductance regulator by phosphodiesterase inhibition. *J Clin Invest* **98**:513, 1996.
326. Kelley TJ, Drumm ML: Inducible nitric oxide synthase expression is reduced in cystic fibrosis murine and human airway epithelial cells. *J Clin Invest* **102**:1200, 1998.
327. Kent G, Iles R, Bear CE, LJ Huan, Griesenbach U, McKerlie C, Frndova H, Ackerley C, Gosselin D, Radzioch D, O'Brodovich H, Tsui LC, Buchwald M, Tanswell AK: Lung disease in mice with cystic fibrosis. *J Clin Invest* **100**:3060, 1997.
328. Kenyon GL, Bruice TW: Novel sulfhydryl reagents. *Methods Enzymol* **47**:407, 1977.
329. Kerem BS, Buchanan JA, Durie P, Corey ML, Levison H, Rommens JM, Buchwald M, Tsui L-C: DNA marker haplotype association with pancreatic sufficiency in cystic fibrosis. *Am J Hum Genet* **44**:827, 1989.
330. Kerem B-S, Rommens JM, Buchanan JA, Markiewicz D, Cox TK, Chakravarti A, Buchwald M, Tsui L-C: Identification of the cystic fibrosis gene: Genetic analysis. *Science* **245**:1073, 1989.
331. Kerem E, Bistritzer T, Hanukoglu A, Hofmann T, Zhou Z, Bennett W, MacLaughlin E, Barker P, Nash M, Quittell L, Boucher R, Knowles MR: Pulmonary epithelial sodium-channel dysfunction and excess airway liquid in pseudohypoaldosteronism. *N Engl J Med* **341**:156, 1999.
332. Kerem E, Corey M, Kerem B, Durie P, Tsui L-C, Levison H: Clinical and genetic comparisons of patients with cystic fibrosis, with or without meconium ileus. *J Pediatr* **114**:767, 1989.
333. Kerem E, Corey M, Kerem BS, Rommens J, Markiewicz D, Levison H, Tsui L-C, Durie P: The relation between genotype and phenotype in cystic fibrosis—Analysis of the most common mutation (delta F508). *N Engl J Med* **323**:1517, 1990.
334. Kerem E, Kalman YM, Yahav Y, Shoshani T, Abeliovich D, Szeinberg A, Rivlin J, Blau H, Tal A, Ben-Tur L, Springer C, Augarten A, Godfrey S, Lerer I, Branski D, Friedman M, Kerem BS: Highly variable incidence of cystic fibrosis and different mutation distribution among different Jewish ethnic groups in Israel. *Hum Genet* **96**:193, 1995.
335. Kerem E, Reisman J, Corey M, Bentur L, Canny G, Levison H: Wheezing in infants with cystic fibrosis: Clinical course, pulmonary function, survival analysis. *Pediatrics* **90**:703, 1992.
336. Kerem E, Reisman J, Corey M, Canny GJ, Levison H: Prediction of mortality in patients with cystic fibrosis. *N Engl J Med* **326**:1187, 1992.
337. Khan TZ, Wagener JS, Bost T, Martinez J, Accurso FJ, Riches DW: Early pulmonary inflammation in infants with cystic fibrosis. *Am J Respir Crit Care Med* **151**:1075, 1995.
338. Kiesewetter S, Macek M Jr, Davis C, Curristin SM, Chu CS, Graham C, Shrimpton AE, Cashman SM, Tsui L-C, Mickle J, et al: A mutation in CFTR produces different phenotypes depending on chromosomal background. *Nat Genet* **5**:274, 1993.
339. Kitzis A, Chomel JC, Kaplan JC: Unusual segregation of cystic fibrosis allele to males. *Nature* **333**:215, 1988.
340. Kleczkowska A, Fryns JP, Steeno O, Van den Berghe H: On the familial occurrence of congenital bilateral absence of vas deferens. *Clin Genet* **35**:268, 1989.
341. Knowles M, Gatzy J, Boucher R: Increased bioelectric potential difference across respiratory epithelia in cystic fibrosis. *N Engl J Med* **305**:1489, 1981.
342. Knowles MR, Clarke LL, Boucher RC: Activation of extracellular nucleotides of chloride secretion in the airway epithelia of patients with CF. *N Engl J Med* **325**:533, 1999.
343. Knowles MR, Paradiso AM, Boucher RC. *In vivo* nasal potential difference: Techniques and protocols for assessing efficacy of gene transfer in cystic fibrosis. *Hum Gene Ther* **6**:445, 1995.
344. Knowles MR, Robinson JM, Wood RE, Pue CA, Mentz WM, Wager GC, Gatzy JT, Boucher RC: Ion composition of airway surface liquid of patients with cystic fibrosis as compared with normal and disease-control subjects. *J Clin Invest* **100**:2588, 1997.
345. Knowles MR, Stutts MJ, Spock A, Fischer N, Gatzy JT, Boucher RC: Abnormal ion permeation through cystic fibrosis respiratory epithelium. *Science* **221**:1067, 1983.
346. Ko YH, Pedersen PL: The first nucleotide binding fold of the cystic fibrosis transmembrane conductance regulator can function as an active ATPase. *J Biol Chem* **270**:22093, 1995.
347. Kobayashi H: Biofilm disease: Its clinical manifestation and therapeutic possibilities of macrolides. *Am J Med* **99**:26S, 1995.
348. Koch C, McKenzie SG, Kaplowitz H, Hodson ME, Harms HK, Navarro J, Mastella G: International practice patterns by age and severity of lung disease in cystic fibrosis: Data from the Epidemiologic Registry of Cystic Fibrosis (ERCF). *Pediatr Pulmonol* **24**:147, 1997.
349. Koh J, Sferra TJ, Collins FS: Characterization of the cystic fibrosis transmembrane conductance regulator promoter region. Chromatin context and tissue-specificity. *J Biol Chem* **268**:15912, 1993.
350. Konstan MW: Therapies aimed at airway inflammation in cystic fibrosis. *Clin Chest Med* **19(6)**:505, 1998.
351. Konstan MW, Byard PJ, Hoppel CL, Davis PB: Effect of high-dose ibuprofen in patients with cystic fibrosis. *N Engl J Med* **332**:848, 1995.
352. Konstan MW, Hilliard KA, Norvell TM, Berger M: Bronchoalveolar lavage findings in cystic fibrosis patients with stable, clinically mild lung disease suggest ongoing infection and inflammation. *Am J Respir Crit Care Med* **150**:448, 1994.
353. Konstan MW, Stern RC, Doershuk CF: Efficacy of the Flutter device for airway mucus clearance in patients with cystic fibrosis. *J Pediatr* **124**:689, 1994.
354. Kopelman H, Durie P, Gaskin K, Weizman Z, Forstner G: Pancreatic fluid secretion and protein hyperconcentration in cystic fibrosis. *N Engl J Med* **312**:329, 1985.
355. Kopito RR: Biosynthesis and degradation of CFTR. *Physiol Rev* **79**:S167, 1999.

356. Kotloff RM, FitzSimmons SC, Fiel SB: Fertility and pregnancy in patients with cystic fibrosis. *Clin Chest Med* **13**:623, 1992.
357. Kovesi T, Corey M, Levison H: Passive smoking and lung function in cystic fibrosis. *Am Rev Respir Dis* 148:1266-1271, 1993.
358. Kovesi T, Corey M, Tsui L-C, Levison H, Durie P: The association between liver disease and mutations of the cystic fibrosis gene. *Pediatr Pulmonol* **8**:244.
359. Koyama H, Geddes DM: Erythromycin and diffuse panbronchiolitis. *Thorax* **52**:915, 1997.
360. Krawczak M, Reiss J, Cooper DN: The mutational spectrum of single base-pair substitutions in mRNA splice junctions of human genes: causes and consequences. *Hum Genet* **90**:41, 1992.
361. Krebs NF, Sontag M, Accurso FJ, Hambidge KM: Low plasma zinc concentrations in young infants with cystic fibrosis. *J Pediatr* **133**:761, 1998.
362. Kristidis P, Bozon D, Corey M, Markiewicz D, Rommens J, Tsui L-C, Durie P: Genetic determination of exocrine pancreatic function in cystic fibrosis. *Am J Hum Genet* **50**:1178, 1992.
363. Kubesch P, Dörk T, Wulbrand U, Kälin N, Neumann T, Wulf B, Geerlings H, Weissbrodt H, von der Hardt H, Tummler B: Genetic determinants of airways' colonisation with *Pseudomonas aeruginosa* in cystic fibrosis. *Lancet* **341**:189, 1993.
364. Kunzelmann K, Kiser GL, Schreiber R, Riordan JR: Inhibition of epithelial Na+ currents by intracellular domains of the cystic fibrosis transmembrane conductance regulator. *FEBS Lett* **400**:341, 1997.
365. Lai HC, Kosorok MR, Sondel SA, Chen ST, FitzSimmons SC, Green CG, Shen G, Walker S, Farrell PM: Growth status in children with cystic fibrosis based on the National Cystic Fibrosis Patient Registry data: Evaluation of various criteria used to identify malnutrition. *J Pediatr* **132**:478, 1998.
366. Lang AB, Schaad UB, Rudeberg A, Wedgwood J, Que JU, Furer E, Cryz SJ Jr: Effect of high-affinity anti-*Pseudomonas aeruginosa* lipopolysaccharide antibodies induced by immunization on the rate of *Pseudomonas aeruginosa* infection in patients with cystic fibrosis. *J Pediatr* **127**:711, 1995.
367. Lanng S: Diabetes mellitus in cystic fibrosis. *Eur J Gastroenterol Hepatol* **8**:744, 1996.
368. Lecoq I, Brouard J, Laroche D, Ferec C, Travert G: Blood immunoreactive trypsinogen concentrations are genetically determined in healthy and cystic fibrosis newborns. *Acta Paediatr* **88**:338, 1999.
369. Lee MC, Penland CM, Widdicombe JH, Wine JJ: Evidence that calu-3 human airway cells secrete bicarbonate. *Am J Physiol* **274**:450, 1998.
370. Lee MG, Wigley WC, Zeng W, Noel LE, Marino CR, Thomas PJ, Muallem S: Regulation of $Cl^-/HCO3^-$ exchange by cystic fibrosis transmembrane conductance regulator expressed in NIH 3T3 and HEK 293 cells. *J Biol Chem* **274**:3414, 1999.
371. LeGrys VA: Sweat testing for the diagnosis of cystic fibrosis: Practical considerations. *J Pediatr* **129**:892, 1996.
372. Lehrer RI, Ganz T: Antimicrobial peptides in mammalian and insect host defence. *Curr Opin Immunol* **11**:23, 1999.
373. Lehrer RI, Ganz T, Selsted ME: Defensins: Endogenous antibiotic peptides of animal cells. *Cell* **64**:229, 1991.
374. Levin S: Fibrocystic disease of the pancreas, in Goldschmidt E (ed): *Genetics of Migrant and Isolate Populations*. Baltimore, Williams & Wilkins, 1963, p 294.
375. Levin SE, Blumberg H, Zamit R, Schmaman A, Wagstaff L: Mucoviscidosis (cystic fibrosis of the pancreas) in Bantu twin neonates. *S Afr Med J* **41**:482, 1967.
376. Li C, Ramjeesingh M, Wang W, Garami E, Hewryk M, Lee D, Rommens JM, Galley K, Bear CE: ATPase activity of the cystic fibrosis transmembrane conductance regulator. *J Biol Chem* **271**:28463, 1996.
377. Li S, Moy L, Pittman N, Shue G, Aufiero B, Neufeld EJ, LeLeiko NS, Walsh MJ: Transcriptional repression of the cystic fibrosis transmembrane conductance regulator gene, mediated by CCAAT displacement protein/cut homolog, is associated with histone deacetylation. *J Biol Chem* **274**:7803, 1999.
378. Liedtke CM, Thomas L: Phorbol ester and okadaic acid regulation of Na-2Cl-K cotransport in rabbit tracheal epithelial cells. *Am J Physiol* **271**:C338, 1996.
379. Lindblad A, Glaumann H, Strandvik B: A two-year prospective study of the effect of ursodeoxycholic acid on urinary bile acid excretion and liver morphology in cystic fibrosis-associated liver disease. *Hepatology* **27**:166, 1998.
380. Lindblad A, Hultcrantz R, Strandvik B: Bile-duct destruction and collagen deposition: A prominent ultrastructural feature of the liver in cystic fibrosis. *Hepatology* **16**:372, 1992.
381. Linsdell P, Tabcharani JA, Rommens JM, Hou Y-X, Chang X-B, Tsui L-C, Riordan JR, Hanrahan JW: Permeability of wild-type and mutant cystic fibrosis transmembrane conductance regulator chloride channels to polyatomic anions. *J Gen Physiol* **110**:355, 1997.
382. Littlewood JM: Cystic fibrosis: Gastrointestinal complications. *Br Med Bull* **48**:847, 1992.
383. Littlewood JM, Smye SW, Cunliffe H: Aerosol antibiotic treatment in cystic fibrosis. *Arch Dis Child* **68**:788, 1993.
384. Loffing JMB, McCoy DD, Stanton BA: Exocytosis is not involved in activation of Cl- secretion via CFTR in Calu-3 airway epithelial cells. *Am J Physiol* **275**:C913, 1998.
385. Lohr M, Goertchen P, Nizze H, Gould NS, Gould VE, Oberholzer M, Heitz PU, Kloppel G: Cystic fibrosis associated islet changes may provide a basis for diabetes. An immunocytochemical and morphometrical study. *Virchows Arch A Pathol Anat Histopathol* **414**:179, 1989.
386. Lomri N, Fitz JG, Scharschmidt BF: Hepatocellular transport: Role of ATP-binding cassette proteins. *Semin Liver Dis* **16**:201, 1996.
387. Loo MA, Jensen TJ, Cui L, Hou Y, Chang XB, Riordan JR: Perturbation of Hsp90 interaction with nascent CFTR prevents its maturation and accelerates its degradation by the proteasome. *EMBO J* **17**:6879, 1998.
388. Lucas J, Connett GJ, Lea R, Rolles CJ, Warner JO: Lung resection in cystic fibrosis patients with localised pulmonary disease. *Arch Dis Child* **74**:449, 1996.
389. Lukacs GL, Mohamed A, Kartner N, Chang XB, Riordan JR, Grinstein S: Conformational maturation of CFTR but not its mutant counterpart (ΔF508) occurs in the endoplasmic reticulum and requires ATP. *EMBO J* **13**:6076, 1994.
390. Lukacs GL, Segal G, Kartner N, Grinstein S, Zhang F: Constitutive internalization of cystic fibrosis transmembrane conductance regulator occurs via clathrin-dependent endocytosis and is regulated by protein phosphorylation. *Biochem J* **328**:358, 1997.
391. Luo J, Pato MD, Riordan JR, Hanrahan JW: Differential regulation of single CFTR channels be PP2C, PP2A, and other phosphatases. *Am J Physiol* **274**:C1397, 1998.
392. Lyon ICT, Webster DR: Newborn screening for cystic fibrosis. *Pediatrics* **87**:954, 1991.
393. Ma J, Zhao J, Drumm ML, Xie J, Davis PB: Function of the R domain in the cystic fibrosis transmembrane conductance regulator chloride channel. *J Biol Chem* **272**:28133, 1997.
394. MacDougall LG: Fibrocystic disease of the pancreas in African children. *Lancet* **1**:409, 1962.
395. MacDougall SL, Grinstein S, Gelfand EW: Activation of $Ca2^+$-dependent K^+ channels in human B lymphocytes by anti-immunoglobulin. *J Clin Invest* **81**:449, 1988.
396. Macek M Jr, Macek M Sr, Krebsova A, Nash E, Hamosh A, Reis A, Varon-Mateeva R, Schmidtke J, Maestri NE, Sperling K, Krawczak M, Cutting GR: Possible association of the allele status of the CS.7/HhaI polymorphism 5′ of the CFTR gene with postnatal female survival. *Hum Genet* **99**:565, 1997.
397. Macek M Jr, Macková A, Hamosh A, Hilman BC, Seldon RF, Lucotte G, Friedman KJ, Knowles MR, Rosenstein BJ, Cutting GR: Identification of common cystic fibrosis mutations in African-Americans with cystic fibrosis increases the detection rate to 75%. *Am J Hum Genet* **60**:1122, 1997.
398. Mak V, Jarvi K, Zielenski J, Durie P, Tsui L-C: Higher proportion of intact exon 9 CFTR mRNA in nasal epithelium compared with vas deferens. *Hum Mol Genet* **6**:2099, 1997.
399. Marcus MS, Sondel SA, Farrell PM, Laxova A, Carey PM, Langhough R, Mischler EH: Nutritional status of infants with cystic fibrosis associated with early diagnosis and intervention. *Am J Clin Nutr* **54**:578, 1991.
400. Marino CR, Matovcik LM, Gorelick FS, Cohn JA: Localization of the cystic fibrosis transmembrane conductance regulator in pancreas. *J Clin Invest* **88**:712, 1991.
401. Marthinsen L, Kornfalt R, Aili M, Andersson D, Westgren U, Schaedel C: Recurrent Pseudomonas bronchopneumonia and other symptoms as in cystic fibrosis in a child with type I pseudohypoaldosteronism. *Acta Pediatr* **87**:472, 1998.
402. Mason SJ, Paradiso AM, Boucher RC: Regulation of transepithelial ion transport and intracellular calcium by extracellular ATP in human normal and cystic fibrosis airway epithelium. *Br J Pharmacol* **103**:1649, 1991.
403. Massengale AR, Quinn F Jr, Yankaskas J, Weissman D, McClellan WT, Cuff C, Aronoff SC: Reduced interleukin-8 production by cystic fibrosis airway epithelial cells. *Am J Respir Cell Mol Biol* **20**:1073, 1999.

404. Matsui H, Grubb BR, Tarran R, Randell SH, Gatzy JT, Davis CW, Boucher RC: Evidence for periciliary liquid layer depletion, not abnormal ion composition, in the pathogenesis of cystic fibrosis airways disease. *Cell* **95**:1005, 1998.
405. Deleted in proof.
406. Matsui H, Johnson LG, Randell SH, Boucher RC: Loss of binding and entry of liposome-DNA complexes decreases transfection efficiency in differentiated airway epithelial cells. *J Biol Chem* **272**:1117, 1997.
407. Matsushita K, McCray PB, Sigmund RD, Welsh MJ, Stokes JB: Localization of epithelial sodium channel subunit mRNAs in adult rat lung by in situ hybridization. *Am J Physiol* **271**:L332, 1996.
408. Matthews RP, McKnight GS: Characterization of the cAMP response element of the cystic fibrosis transmembrane conductance regulator gene promoter. *J Biol Chem* **271**:31869, 1996.
409. Maurage C, Lenaerts C, Weber A, Brochu P, Yousef I, Roy CC: Meconium ileus and its equivalent as a risk factor for the development of cirrhosis: An autopsy study in cystic fibrosis. *J Pediatr Gastroenterol Nutr* **9**:17, 1989.
410. McCray PB, Bentley L: Human airway epithelia express a β-defensin. *Am J Respir Cell Mol Biol* **16**:343, 1997.
411. McCray PB Jr, Zabner J, Jia HP, Welsh MJ, Thorne PS: Efficient killing of inhaled bacteria in ΔF508 mice: Role of airway surface liquid composition. *Am J Physiol* **277**:L183, 1999.
412. McDonald FJ, Price MP, Snyder PM, Welsh MJ: Cloning and expression of the beta- and gamma-subunits of the human epithelial sodium channel. *Am J Physiol* **268**:C1157, 1995.
413. McDonald FJ, Yang B, Hrstka RF, Drummond HA, Tarr DE, McCray PB Jr, Stokes JB, Welsh MJ, Williamson RA: Disruption of the β subunit of the epithelial Na^+ channel in mice: Hyperkalemia and neonatal death associated with a pseudohypoaldosteronism phenotype. *Proc Natl Acad Sci U S A* **96**:1727, 1999.
414. McDonald RA, Matthews RP, Idzerda RL, McKnight GS: Basal expression of the cystic fibrosis transmembrane conductance regulator gene is dependent on protein kinase A activity. *Proc Natl Acad Sci U S A* **92**:7560, 1995.
415. McIlwaine MP, Davidson AG: Airway clearance techniques in the treatment of cystic fibrosis. *Curr Opin Pulm Med* **2**:447, 1996.
416. McIlwaine PM, Wong LT, Peacock D, Davidson AG: Long-term comparative trial of conventional postural drainage and percussion versus positive expiratory pressure physiotherapy in the treatment of cystic fibrosis. *J Pediatr* **131**:570, 1997.
417. McIntosh JC, Schoumacher RA, Tiller RE: Pancreatic adenocarcinoma in a patient with cystic fibrosis. *Am J Med* **85**:592, 1988.
418. McNicholas CM, Guggino WB, Schwiebert EM, Hebert SC, Giebisch G, Egan ME: Sensitivity of a renal K+ channel (ROMK2) to the inhibitory sulfonylurea compound glibenclamide is enhanced by coexpression with the ATP-binding cassette transporter cystic fibrosis transmembrane regulator. *Proc Natl Acad Sci U S A* **93**:8083, 1996.
419. McNicholas CM, Nason MW Jr, Guggino WB, Schwiebert EM, Hebert SC, Giebisch G, Egan ME: A functional CFTR-NBF1 is required for ROMK2-CFTR interaction. *Am J Physiol* **273**:F843, 1997.
420. Meacham GC, Lu Z, King S, Sorscher E, Tousson A, Cyr DM: The Hdj-2/Hsc70 chaperone pair facilitates early steps in CFTR biogenesis. *EMBO J* **18**:1492, 1999.
421. Mekus F, Ballmann M, Bronsveld I, Dörk T, Bijman J, Tummler B: Cystic-fibrosis-like disease unrelated to the cystic fibrosis transmembrane conductance regulator. *Hum Genet* **102**:582, 1999.
422. Melo CA, Serra C, Stoyanova V, Aguzzoli C, Faraguna D, Tamanini A, Berton G, Cabrini G, Baralle FE: Alternative splicing of a previously unidentified CFTR exon introduces an in-frame stop codon 5′ of the R region. *FEBS Lett* **329**:159, 1993.
423. Mercier B, Lissens W, Audrézet MP, Bonduelle M, Liebaers I, Férec C: Detection of more than 94% cystic fibrosis mutations in a sample of Belgian population and identification of four novel mutations. *Hum Mutat* **2**:16, 1993.
424. Mercier B, Raguenes O, Estivill X, Morral N, Kaplan GC, McClure M, Grebe TA, D Kessler, Pignatti PF, Marigo C, Bombieri C, Andrézet MP, Verlingue C, Férec C: Complete detection of mutations in cystic fibrosis patients of Native American origin. *Hum Genet* **94**:629, 1994.
425. Mickle JE, Macek M Jr, Fulmer-Smentek SB, Egan MM, Schwiebert E, Guggino W, Moss R, Cutting GR: A mutation in the cystic fibrosis transmembrane conductance regulator gene associated with elevated sweat chloride concentrations in the absence of cystic fibrosis. *Hum Mol Genet* **7**:729, 1998.
426. Morales MM, Carroll TP, Morita T, Schwiebert EM, Devuyst O, Wilson PD, Lopes AG, Stanton BA, Dietz HC, Cutting GR, Guggino WB: Both the wild-type and a functional isoform of CFTR are expressed in kidney. *Am J Physiol* **270**:F1038, 1996.
427. Moran A, Doherty L, Wang X, Thomas W: Abnormal glucose metabolism in cystic fibrosis. *J Pediatr* **133**:10, 1998.
428. Moran A, Hardin D, Rodman D, et al: Diagnosis, screening and management of cystic fibrosis related diabetes mellitus: A consensus conference report. *Diabetes Res Clin Pract* **45**:61, 1999.
429. Morral N, Bertranpetit J, Estivill X, Nunes V, Casals T, Giménez J, Reis A, Varon-Mateeva R, Macek M Jr, Kalaydjieva L, Angelicheva D, Dancheva R, Romeo G, Russo MP, Garnerone SRG, Ferrari M, Magnani C, Claustres M, Desgeorges M, Schwartz M, Schwarz M, Dallapiccola D, Novelli G, Ferec C, deArce M, Nemeti M, Kere J, Anvret M, Dahl N, Kadasi L: The origin of the major cystic fibrosis mutation (ΔF508) in European populations. *Nat Genet* **7**:169, 1994.
430. Morral N, Llevadot R, Casals T, Gasparini P, Macek M Jr, Dörk T, Estivill X: Independent origins of cystic fibrosis mutations R334W, R347P, R1162x, and 3849 + 10kbC- → T provide evidence of mutation recurrence in the CFTR gene. *Am J Hum Genet* **55**:890, 1994.
431. Morral N, Nunes V, Casals T, Estivill X: CA/GT microsatellite alleles within the cystic fibrosis transmembrane conductance regulator (CFTR) gene are not generated by unequal crossing over. *Genomics* **10**:692, 1991.
432. Moyer BD, Denton J, Karlson KH, Reynolds D, Wang S, Mickle JE, Milewski M, Cutting GR, Guggino WB, Li M, Stanton BA: A PDZ-interacting domain in CFTR is an apical membrane polarization signal. *J Clin Invest* **104**:1353, 1999.
433. Muller F, Aubry MC, Gasser B, Duchatel F, Boue J, Boue A: Prenatal diagnosis of cystic fibrosis. II. Meconium ileus in affected fetuses. *Prenat Diagn* **5**:109, 1985.
434. Nagel G, Hwang TC, Nastiuk KL, Nairn AC, Gadsby DC: The protein kinase A-regulated cardiac Cl− channel resembles the cystic fibrosis transmembrane conductance regulator. *Nature* **360**:81, 1992.
435. Naren AP, Nelson DJ, Xie W, Jovov B, Pevsner J, Bennett MK, Benos DJ, Quick MW, Kirk KL: Regulation of CFTR chloride channels by cyntaxin and Munc18 isoforms. *Nature* **390**:302, 1997.
436. Naren AP, Quick MW, Collawn JF, Nelson DJ, Kirk KL: Syntaxin 1A inhibits CFTR chloride channels by means of domain-specific protein-protein interactions. *Proc Natl Acad Sci U S A* **95**:10972, 1998.
437. Neglia JP, FitzSimmons SC, Maisonneuve P, Schoni MH, Schoni-Affolter F, Corey M, Lowenfels AB: The risk of cancer among patients with cystic fibrosis. Cystic Fibrosis and Cancer Study Group. *N Engl J Med* **332**:494, 1995.
438. Nepomuceno IB, Esrig S, Moss RB: Allergic bronchopulmonary aspergillosis in cystic fibrosis: Role of atopy and response to itraconazole. *Chest* **115**:364, 1999.
439. Nevin GB, Nevin NC, Redmond AO: Cystic fibrosis in Northern Ireland. *J Med Genet* **16**:122, 1979.
440. Nishioka GJ, Cook PR: Paranasal sinus disease in patients with cystic fibrosis. *Otolaryngol Clin North Am* 29:193-205, 1996.
441. Nixon PA, Orenstein DM, Kelsey SF, Doershuk CF: The prognostic value of exercise testing in patients with cystic fibrosis. *N Engl J Med* **327**:1785, 1992.
442. Noone PG, Bresnihan B: Rheumatic disease in cystic fibrosis, in Yankaskas JR, Knowles MR (eds): *Cystic Fibrosis in Adults*. Philadelphia, Lippincott-Raven, 1999, p 439.
443. Noone PG, Knowles MR: Standard therapy of cystic fibrosis lung disease, in Yankaskas JR, Knowles MR (eds): *Cystic Fibrosis in Adults*. Philadelphia, Lippincott-Raven, 1999, p 145.
444. Nussbaum E, Boat TF, Wood RE, Doershuk CF: Cystic fibrosis with acute hypoelectrolytemia and metabolic alkalosis in infancy. *Am J Dis Child* **133**:965, 1979.
445. O'Connor PJ, Southern KW, Bowler IM, Irving HC, Robinson PJ, Littlewood JM: The role of hepatobiliary scintigraphy in cystic fibrosis. *Hepatology* **23**:281, 1996.
446. O'Neal WK, Hasty P, McCray PB Jr, Casey B, Rivera-Perez J, Welsh MJ, Beaudet AL, Bradley A: A severe phenotype in mice with a duplication of exon 3 in the cystic fibrosis locus. *Hum Mol Genet* **2**:1561, 1993.
447. Ogrinc GB, Kampalath B, Tomashefski JF Jr: Destruction and loss of bronchial cartilage in cystic fibrosis. *Hum Pathol* **29**:65, 1998.
448. Olsen MM, Luck SR, Lloyd-Still J, Raffensperger JG: The spectrum of meconium disease in infancy. *J Pediatr Surg* **17**:479, 1982.
449. Oppenheimer EH, Esterly JR: Pathology of cystic fibrosis review of the literature and comparison with 146 autopsied cases. *Perspect Pediatr Pathol* **2**:241, 1975.
450. Orenstein SR, Orenstein DM: Gastroesophageal reflux and respiratory disease in children. *J Pediatrics* **112**:847, 1988.

451. Ornoy A, Arnon J, Katznelson D, Granat M, Caspi B, Chemke J: Pathological confirmation of cystic fibrosis in the fetus following prenatal diagnosis. *Am J Med Genet* **28**:935, 1987.
452. Osborne LR, Lynch M, Middleton PG, Alton EW, Geddes DM, Pryor JP, Hodson ME, Santis GK: Nasal epithelial ion transport and genetic analysis of infertile men with congenital bilateral absence of the vas deferens. *Hum Mol Genet* **2**:1605, 1993.
453. Ostedgaard LS, Zeiher B, Welsh MJ: Processing of CFTR bearing the P574H mutation differs from wild-type and ΔF508-CFTR. *J Cell Sci* **112**:2091, 1999.
454. Ott SM, Aitken ML: Osteoporosis in patients with cystic fibrosis. *Clin Chest Med* **19**:555, 1998.
455. Paradowski LJ, Egan TM: Lung transplantation for cystic fibrosis, in Yankaskas JR, Knowles MR (eds): *Cystic Fibrosis in Adults*. Philadelphia, Lippincott-Raven, 1999, p 195.
456. Pasque MK, Cooper JD, Kaiser LR, Haydock DA, Triantafillou A, Trulock EP: Improved technique for bilateral lung transplantation: Rationale and initial clinical experience. *Ann Thorac Surg* **49**:785, 1990.
457. Pasyk EA, Foskett JK: Cystic fibrosis transmembrane conductance regulator-associated ATP and adenosine 3′-phosphate 5′ phosphosulfate channels in endoplasmic reticulum and plasma membranes. *J Biol Chem* **272**:7746, 1997.
458. Pasyk EA, Morin XK, Zeman P, Garami E, Galley K, Huan LJ, Wang Y, Bear CE: A conserved region of the R domain of cystic fibrosis transmembrane conductance regulator is important in processing and function. *J Biol Chem* **273**:31759, 1998.
459. Pattishall EN: Longitudinal response of pulmonary function to bronchodilators in cystic fibrosis. *Pediatr Pulmonol* **9**:80, 1990.
460. Pederzini F, Armani P, Barbato A, Borgo G: Newborn screening for cystic fibrosis. Two methods compared on 229,626 newborns tested in 8 years in the Veneto region. *Ital J Pediatr* **9**:445, 1983.
461. Perales JC, Ferkol T, Beegen H, Ratnoff OD, Hanson RW: Gene transfer *in vivo*: Sustained expression and regulation of genes introduced into the liver by receptor-targeted uptake. *Proc Natl Acad Sci U S A* **91**:4086, 1994.
462. Peters KW, Qi J: Syntaxin 1A inhibits regulated CFTR trafficking in xenopus oocytes. *Am J Physiol* **277**:C174, 1999.
463. Phillipson G: Cystic fibrosis and reproduction. *Reprod Fertil Dev* **10**:113, 1998.
464. Picciotto MR, Cohn JA, Bertuzzi G, Greengard P, Nairn AC: Phosphorylation of the cystic fibrosis transmembrane conductance regulator. *J Biol Chem* **267**:12742, 1992.
465. Pickles RJ, McCarty D, Matsui H, Hart PJ, Randell SH, Boucher RC: Limited entry of adenovirus vectors into well-differentiated airway epithelium is responsible for inefficient gene transfer. *J Virol* **72**:6014, 1998.
466. Piedra PA, Grace S, Jewell A, Spinelli S, Bunting D, Hogerman DA, Malinoski F, Hiatt PW: Purified fusion protein vaccine protects against lower respiratory tract illness during respiratory syncytial virus season in children with cystic fibrosis. *Pediatr Infect Dis J* **15**:23, 1996.
467. Pier GB, Grout M, Zaidi TS: Cystic fibrosis transmembrane conductance regulator is an epithelial cell receptor for clearance of *Pseudomonas aeruginosa* from the lung. *Proc Natl Acad Sci U S A* **94**:12088, 1997.
468. Pier GB, Grout M, Zaidi TS, Olsen JC, Johnson LG, Yankaskas JR, Goldberg JB: Role of mutant CFTR in hypersusceptibility of cystic fibrosis patients to lung infections. *Science* **271**:64, 1996.
469. Pilewski JM, Frizzell RA: Role of CFTR in airway disease. *Physiol Rev* **79**:S215, 1999.
470. Piper AJ, Parker S, Torzillo PJ, Sullivan CE, Bye PT: Nocturnal nasal IPPV stabilizes patients with cystic fibrosis and hypercapnic respiratory failure. *Chest* **102**:846, 1992.
471. Pittman N, Shue G, LeLeiko NS, Walsh MJ: Transcription of cystic fibrosis transmembrane conductance regulator requires a CCAAT-like element for both basal and cAMP-mediated regulation. *J Biol Chem* **270**:28848, 1995.
472. Plopper CG, Hill LL, Mariassy AT: Ultrastructure of the nonciliated bronchiolar epithelial (Clara) cell of mammalian lung III. A study of man with comparison of 15 mammalian species. *Exp Lung Res* **1**:171, 1980.
473. Plotkowski MC, de Bentzmann S, Pereira SHM, Zahm J-M, Bajolet-Laudinat O, Roger P, Puchelle E: Pseudomonas aeruginosa internalization by human epithelial respiratory cells depends on cell differentiation, polarity, and junctional complex integrity. *Am J Respir Cell Mol Biol* **20**:880, 1999.
474. Pollard CE, Harris A, Coleman L, Argent BE: Chloride channels on epithelial cells cultured from human fetal epididymis. *J Membr Biol* **124**:275, 1991.
475. Prat AG, Reisin IL, Ausiello DA, Cantiello HF: Cellular ATP release by the cystic fibrosis transmembrane conductance regulator. *Am J Physiol* **270**:C538, 1996.
476. Prince LS, Launspach JL, Zabner J, Welsh MJ: Absence of amiloride-sensitive sodium absorption in the airway of an infant with pseudohypoaldosteronism. *J Pediatrics* **135**:786, 1999.
477. Prince LS, Peter K, Hatton SR, Zaliauskiene L, Cotlin LF, Clancy JP, Marchase RB, Collawn JF: Efficient endocytosis of the cystic fibrosis transmembrane conductance regulator requires a tyrosine-based signal. *J Biol Chem* **274**:3602, 1999.
478. Pritchard DJ: Cystic fibrosis allele frequency, sex ratio anomalies and fertility: A new theory for the dissemination of mutant alleles. *Hum Genet* **87**:671, 1991.
479. Pugh RJ, Pickup JD: Cystic fibrosis in Leeds region: Incidence and life expectancy. *Arch Dis Child* **42**:544, 1967.
480. Qu B-H, Strickland EH, Thomas PJ: Localization and suppression of a kinetic defect in cystic fibrosis transmembrane conductance regulator folding. *J Biol Chem* **272**:15739, 1997.
481. Qu B-H, Thomas PJ: Alteration of the cystic fibrosis transmembrane conductance regulator folding pathway. *J Biol Chem* **271**:7261, 1996.
482. Quinton P: Physiological basis of cystic fibrosis: A historical perspective. *Physiol Rev* **79**:S3, 1999.
483. Quinton PM: Chloride impermeability in cystic fibrosis. *Nature* **301**:421, 1983.
484. Quinton PM: Cystic fibrosis: A disease in electrolyte transport. *FASEB J* **4**:2709, 1990.
485. Quinton PM, Bijman J: Higher bioelectric potentials due to decreased chloride absorption in the sweat glands of patients with cystic fibrosis. *N Engl J Med* **308**:1185, 1983.
486. Ram SJ, Weaver ML, Kirk KL: Regulation of Cl− permeability in normal and cystic fibrosis sweat duct cells. *Am J Physiol* **259**:C842, 1990.
487. Ramsey BW: Management of pulmonary disease in patients with cystic fibrosis. *N Engl J Med* **335**:179, 1996.
488. Ramsey BW: What is the role of upper airway bacterial cultures in patients with cystic fibrosis? *Pediatr Pulmonol* **21**:265, 1996.
489. Ramsey BW, Boat TF: Outcome measures for clinical trials in cystic fibrosis. Summary of a Cystic Fibrosis Foundation consensus conference. *J Pediatr* **124**:177, 1994.
490. Ramsey BW, Farrell PM, Pencharz P: Nutritional assessment and management in cystic fibrosis: A consensus report. The Consensus Committee. *Am J Clin Nutr* **55**:108, 1992.
491. Ramsey BW, Pepe MS, Quan JM, Otto KL, Montgomery AB, Williams-Warren J, Vasiljev K, Borowitz D, Bowman CM, Marshall BC, Marshall S, Smith AL: Intermittent administration of inhaled tobramycin in patients with cystic fibrosis. Cystic Fibrosis Inhaled Tobramycin Study Group. *N Engl J Med* **340**:23, 1999.
492. Randak C, Neth P, Auerswald EA, Eckerskorn C, Assfalg-Machleidt I, Machleidt W: A recombinant polypeptide model of the second nucleotide-binding fold of the cystic fibrosis transmembrane conductance regulator functions as an active ATPase, GTPase and adenylate kinase. *FEBS Lett* **410**:180, 1997.
493. Ratcliff R, Evans MJ, Cuthbert AW, MacVinish LJ, Foster D, Anderson JR, Colledge WH: Production of a severe cystic fibrosis mutations in mice by gene targeting. *Nat Genet* **4**:35, 1993.
494. Rave-Harel N, Kerem E, Nissim-Rafinia M, Madjar I, Goshen R, Augarten A, Rahat A, Hurwitz A, Darvasi A, Kerem B: The molecular basis of partial penetrance of splicing mutations in cystic fibrosis. *Am J Hum Genet* **60**:87, 1997.
495. Reddy MM, Light MJ, Quinton PM: Activation of the epithelial Na^+ channel (ENaC) requires CFTR Cl^- channel function. *Nature* **402**:301, 1999.
496. Reddy MM, Quinton PM: cAMP activation of CF-affected Cl^- conductance in both cell membranes of an absorptive epithelium. *J Membr Biol* **130**:49, 1992.
497. Reddy MM, Quinton PM: Deactivation of CFTR-Cl conductance by endogenous phosphatases in the native sweat duct. *Am J Physiol* **270**:C474, 1996.
498. Reddy MM, Quinton PM, Haws C, Wine JJ, Grygorczyk R, Tabcharani JA, Hanrahan JW, Gunderson KL, Kopito RR: Failure of the cystic fibrosis transmembrane conductance regulator to conduct ATP. *Science* **271**:1876, 1996.
499. Rees DD, Rogers RA, Cooley J, Mandle RJ, Kenney DM, Remold-O'Donnell E: Recombinant human monocyte/neutrophil elastase

inhibitor protects rat lungs against injury from cystic fibrosis airway secretions. *Am J Respir Cell Mol Biol* **20**:69, 1999.
500. Regelmann WE, Elliott GR, Warwick WJ, Clawson CC: Reduction of sputum *Pseudomonas aeruginosa* density by antibiotics improves lung function in cystic fibrosis more than do bronchodilators and chest physiotherapy alone. *Am Rev Respir Dis* **141**:914, 1990.
501. Regelmann, WE, Skubitz KM, Herron JM: Increased monocyte oxidase activity in cystic fibrosis heterozygotes and homozygotes. *Am J Respir Cell Mol Biol* **5**:27, 1991.
502. Regnis JA, Robinson M, Bailey DL, Cook P, Hooper P, Chan HK, Gonda I, Bautovich G, Bye PT: Mucociliary clearance in patients with cystic fibrosis and in normal subjects. *Am J Respir Crit Care Med* **150**:66, 1994.
503. Reid L, de Haller R: The bronchial mucous glands—Their hypertrophy and change in intracellular mucus. *Mod Probl Pediatr* **10**:195, 1966.
504. Reiss J, Cooper DN, Bal J, Slomski R, Cutting GR, Krawczak M: Discrimination between recurrent mutation and identity by descent: Application to point mutations in exon 11 of the CFTR gene. *Hum Genet* **87**:457, 1991.
505. Rich DP, Anderson MP, Gregory RJ, Cheng SH, Paul S, Jefferson DM, McCann JD, Klinger KW, Smith AE, Welsh MJ: Expression of cystic fibrosis transmembrane conductance regulator corrects defective chloride channel regulation in cystic fibrosis airway epithelial cells. *Nature* **347**:358, 1990.
506. Rich DP, Berger HA, Cheng SH, Travis SM, Saxena M, Smith AE, Welsh MJ: Regulation of the cystic fibrosis transmembrane conductance regulator Cl^- channel by negative charge in the R domain. *J Biol Chem* **268**:20259, 1993.
507. Rich DP, Gregory RJ, Anderson MP, Manavalan P, Smith AE, Welsh MJ: Effect of deleting the R domain on CFTR-generated chloride channels. *Science* **253**:205, 1991.
508. Rich DP, Gregory RJ, Cheng SH, Smith AE, Welsh MJ: Effect of deletion mutations on the function of CFTR chloride channels. *Receptors Channels* **1**:221, 1993.
509. Riordan JR, Rommens JM, Kerem B-S, Alon N, Rozmahel R, Grzelczak Z, Zielenski J, Lok S, Plavsic N, Chou J-L, Drumm ML, Iannuzzi MC, Collins FS, Tsui L-C: Identification of the cystic fibrosis gene: Cloning and characterization of complementary DNA. *Science* **245**:1066, 1989.
510. Roberts HE, Cragan JD, Cono J, Khoury MJ, Weatherly MR, Moore CA: Increased frequency of cystic fibrosis among infants with jejunoileal atresia. *Am J Med Genet* **78**:446, 1998.
511. Romanczuk H, Galer CE, Zabner J, Barsomian G, Wadsworth SC, O'Riordan CR: Modification of an adenoviral vector with biologically selected peptides: A novel strategy for gene delivery to cells of choice. *Hum Gene Ther* **10**:2615, 1999.
512. Romeo G, McKusick VA: Phenotypic diversity, allelic series and modifier genes. *Nat Genet* **7**:451, 1994.
513. Rommens JM, Iannuzzi MC, Kerem B-S, Drumm ML, Melmer G, Dean M, Rozmahel R, Cole JL, Kennedy D, Hidaka N, Zsiga M, Buchwald M, Riordan JR, Tsui L-C, Collins FS: Identification of the cystic fibrosis gene: Chromosome walking and jumping. *Science* **245**:1059, 1989.
514. Rosenfeld M, Casey S, Pepe M, Ramsey BW: Nutritional effects of long-term gastrostomy feedings in children with cystic fibrosis. *J Am Diet Assoc* **99**:191, 1999.
515. Rosenfeld M, Emerson J, Accurso F, Armstrong D, Castile R, Grimwood K, Hiatt P, McCoy K, McNamara S, Ramsey B, Wagener J: Diagnostic accuracy of oropharyngeal cultures in infants and young children with cystic fibrosis. *Pediatr Pulmonol* **28**:321, 1999.
516. Rosenstein BJ, Cutting GR: The diagnosis of cystic fibrosis: A consensus statement. *J Pediatr* **132**:589, 1998.
517. Rothbaum RJ: Gastrointestinal complications, in Orenstein DM, Stern RC (eds): *Treatment of the hospitalized cystic fibrosis patient*. New York, Marcel Dekker, 1998, p 135.
518. Roum JH, Buhl R, McElvaney NG, Borok Z, Crystal RG: Systemic deficiency of glutathione in cystic fibrosis. *J Appl Physiol* **75**:2419, 1993.
519. Rozen R, Schwartz RH, Hilman BC, Stanislovitis P, Horn GT, Klinger K, Daigneault J, DeBrackeleer M, Kerem B, Tsui L, et al: Cystic fibrosis mutations in North American populations of French ancestry: Analysis of Quebec French-Canadian and Louisiana Acadian families. *Am J Hum Genet* **47**:606, 1990.
520. Rozmahel R, Wilschanski M, Matin A, Plyte S, Oliver M, Auerbach W, Moore A, Forstner J, Durie P, Nadeau J, Bear C, Tsui L-C: Modulation of disease severity in cystic fibrosis transmembrane conductance regulator-deficient mice by a secondary genetic factor. *Nat Genet* **12**:280, 1996.
521. Rubenstein RC, Egan ME, Zeitlin PL: In vitro pharmacologic restoration of CFTR-mediated chloride transport with sodium 4-phenylbutyrate in cystic fibrosis epithelial cells containing deltaF508-CFTR. *J Clin Invest* **100**:2457, 1997.
522. Rubenstein RC, Zeitlin PL: A pilot clinical trial of oral sodium 4-phenylbutyrate (buphenyl) in deltaF508-homozygous cystic fibrosis patients: partial restoration of nasal epithelial CFTR function. *Am J Respir Crit Care Med* **157**:484, 1998.
523. Rubin BK: Exposure of children with cystic fibrosis to environmental tobacco smoke. *N Engl J Med* **323**:782, 1990.
524. Rubinstein S, Moss R, Lewiston N: Constipation and meconium ileus equivalent in patients with cystic fibrosis. *Pediatrics* **78**:473, 1986.
525. Saiman L, Mehar F, Niu WW, Neu HC, Shaw KJ, Miller G, Prince A: Antibiotic susceptibility of multiply resistant *Pseudomonas aeruginosa* isolated from patients with cystic fibrosis, including candidates for transplantation. *Clin Infect Dis* **23**:532, 1996.
526. Saiman L, Prince A: *Pseudomonas aeruginosa* pili bind to asialoGM1 which is increased on the surface of cystic fibrosis epithelial cells. *J Clin Invest* **92**:1875, 1993.
527. Sanchez I, De Koster J, Holbrow J, Chernick V: The effect of high doses of inhaled salbutamol and ipratropium bromide in patients with stable cystic fibrosis. *Chest* **104**:842, 1993.
528. Santis G: Pulmonary disease and genotypes. *Pediatr Pulm* **8(Suppl)**:140, 1992.
529. Santis G, Osborne L, Knight R, Smith M, Davison T, Hodson M: Genotype-phenotype relationship in cystic fibrosis: Results from the study of monozygotic and dizygotic twins with cystic fibrosis. *Ped Pulm* **8(Suppl)**:239, 1992.
530. Santis G, Osborne L, Knight RA, Hodson ME: Independent genetic determinants of pancreatic and pulmonary status in cystic fibrosis. *Lancet* **336**:1081, 1990.
531. Sato K, Saga K, Sato F: Membrane transport and intracellular events in control and cystic fibrosis eccrine sweat glands, in Mastella G, Quinton PM (eds): *Cellular and Molecular Basis of Cystic Fibrosis*. San Francisco, San Francisco Press, 1988, p 171.
532. Sato K, Sato F: Defective beta-adrenergic response of cystic fibrosis sweat glands *in vivo* and *in vitro*. *J Clin Invest* **73**:1763, 1984.
533. Sato K, Sato F: Variable reduction in beta-adrenergic sweat secretion in cystic fibrosis heterozygotes. *J Lab Clin Med* **111**:511, 1988.
534. Scharfman A, Van Brussel E, Houdret N, Lamblin G, Roussel P: Interactions between glycoconjugates from human respiratory airways and *Pseudomonas aeruginosa*. *Am J Respir Crit Care Med* **154**:S163, 1996.
535. Schidlow DV, Taussig LM, Knowles MR: Cystic Fibrosis Foundation Consensus Conference Report on Pulmonary Complications of Cystic Fibrosis. *Pediatr Pulmonol* **15**:187, 1993.
536. Schroeder SA, Gaughan DM, Swift M: Protection against bronchial asthma by CFTR delta F508 mutation: A heterozygote advantage in cystic fibrosis. *Nat Med* **1**:703, 1995.
537. Schultz BD, Singh AK, Devor DC, Bridges RJ: Pharmacology of CFTR chloride channel activity. *Physiol Rev* **79**:S109, 1999.
538. Schwiebert EM, Benos DJ, Egan ME, Stutts J, Guggino WB: CFTR is a conductance regulator as well as a chloride channel. *Physiol Rev* **79**:S145, 1999.
539. Schwiebert EM, Benos DJ, Egan ME, Stutts MJ, Guggino WB: CFTR is a conductance regulator as well as a chloride channel. *Physiol Rev* **79**:S145, 1999.
540. Scott-Jupp R, Lama M, Tanner MS: Prevalence of liver disease in cystic fibrosis. *Arch Dis Child* **66**:698, 1991.
541. Scully BE, Nakatomi M, Ores C, Davidson S, Neu HC: Ciprofloxacin therapy in cystic fibrosis. *Am J Med* 82:196, 1987.
542. Seibert FS, Tabcharani JA, Chang XB, Dulhanty AM, Mathews C, Hanrahan JW, Riordan JR: cAMP-dependent protein kinase-mediated phosphorylation of cystic fibrosis transmembrane conductance regulator residue Ser-753 and its role in channel activation. *J Biol Chem* **270**:2158, 1995.
543. Seksek O, Biwersi J, Verkman AS: Evidence against defective *trans*-Golgi acidification in cystic fibrosis. *J Biol Chem* **271**:15542, 1996.
544. Selander P: The frequency of cystic fibrosis of the pancreas in Sweden. *Acta Paediatr* **51**:65, 1962.
545. Senecal JJ, Toury CR: Deux cas de fibrose kystrique de pancreas chez l'enfant Africain realisant le syndrome du kwashiorkor. *Bull Med L'Afrique Occidentale Franc* **11**:95, 1954.

546. Sereth H, Shoshani T, Bashan N, Kerem BS: Extended haplotype analysis of cystic fibrosis mutations and its implications for the selective advantage hypothesis. *Hum Genet* **92**:289, 1993.
547. Serre JL, Bouy-Simon B, Mornet E, Jaume-Roig B, Balassopoulou A, Schwartz M, Taillandier A, Boue J, Boue A: Studies of RFLP closely linked to the cystic fibrosis locus throughout Europe lead to new considerations in populations genetics. *Hum Genet* **84**:449, 1990.
548. Shane E, Silverberg SJ, Donovan D, Papadopoulos A, Staron RB, Addesso V, Jorgesen B, McGregor C, Schulman L: Osteoporosis in lung transplantation candidates with end-stage pulmonary disease. *Am J Med* **101**:262, 1996.
549. Sharer N, Schwarz M, Malone G, Howarth A, Painter J, Super M, Braganza J: Mutations of the cystic fibrosis gene in patients with chronic pancreatitis. *N Engl J Med* **339**:645, 1998.
550. Sheppard DN, Rich DP, Ostedgaard LS, Gregory RJ, Smith AE, Welsh MJ: Mutations in CFTR associated with mild disease form Cl^- channels with altered pore properties. *Nature* **362**:160, 1993.
551. Sheppard DN, Welsh MJ: Structure and function of the CFTR chloride channel. *Physiol Rev* **79**:S23, 1999.
552. Shimkets RA, Warnock DG, Bositis CM, Nelson-Williams C, Hansson JH, Schambelan M, Gill JR Jr, Ulick S, Milora RV, Findling JW, et al: Liddle's syndrome: Heritable human hypertension caused by mutations in the beta subunit of the epithelial sodium channel. *Cell* **79**:407, 1994.
553. Short DB, Trotter KW, Reczek D, Kreda SM, Bretscher A, Boucher RC, Stutts MJ, Milgram SL: An apical PDZ protein anchors the cystic fibrosis transmembrane conductance regulator to the cytoskeleton. *J Biol Chem* **273**:19797, 1998.
554. Shoshani T, Augarten A, Gazit E, Bashan N, Yahav Y, Rivlin Y, Tal A, Seret H, Yaar L, Kerem E, Kerem B-S: Association of a nonsense mutation (W1282X), the most common mutation in the Ashkenazi Jewish cystic fibrosis patients in Israel, with presentation of severe disease. *Am J Hum Genet* **50**:222, 1992.
555. Silber SJ, Nagy ZP, Liu J, Godoy H, Devroey P, Van Steirteghern AC: Conventional in-vitro fertilization versus intracytoplasmic sperm injection for patients requiring microsurgical sperm aspiration. *Hum Reprod* **9**:1705, 1994.
556. Sims DE, Horne MM: Heterogeneity of the composition and thickness of tracheal mucus in rats. *Am J Physiol* **273**:L1036, 1997.
557. Singh PK, Jia HVP, Wiles K, Hesselberth J, Liu L, Conway BD, Greenberg EP, Valore E, Welsh MJ, Ganz T, Tack BF, McCray PB Jr: Production of β-defensins by human airway epithelia. *Proc Natl Acad Sci U S A* **95**:14961, 1998.
558. Slotnick RN, Abuhamad AZ: Prognostic implications of fetal echogenic bowel. *Lancet* **347**:85, 1996.
559. Smith AL, Cohen M, Ramsey BW: Pharmacotherapy, in Yankaskas JR, Knowles MR (eds): *Cystic Fibrosis in Adults*. Philadelphia, Lippincott-Raven, 1999, p 345.
560. Smith AN, Barth ML, McDowell TL, Moulin DS, Nuthall HN, Hollingsworth MA, Harris A: A regulatory element in intron 1 of the cystic fibrosis transmembrane conductance regulator gene. *J Biol Chem* **271**:9947, 1996.
561. Smith JJ, Karp PH, Welsh MJ: Defective fluid transport by cystic fibrosis airway epithelia. *J Clin Invest* **93**:1307, 1994.
562. Smith JJ, Travis SM, Greenberg EP, Welsh MJ: Cystic fibrosis airway epithelia fail to kill bacteria because of abnormal airway surface fluid. *Cell* **85**:229, 1996.
563. Smith JJ, Welsh MJ: Fluid and electrolyte transport by cultured human airway epithelia. *J Clin Invest* **91**:1590, 1993.
564. Smyth A, O'Hea U, Williams G, Smyth R, Heaf D: Passive smoking and impaired lung function in cystic fibrosis. *Arch Dis Child* **71**:353, 1994.
565. Smyth RL, Van Velzen D, Smyth AR, Lloyd DA, Heaf DP: Strictures of ascending colon in cystic fibrosis and high-strength pancreatic enzymes. *Lancet* **343**:85, 1994.
566. Snouwaert JN, Brigman KK, Latour AM, Malouf AM, Boucher RC, Smithies O, Koller BH: An animal model for cystic fibrosis made by gene targeting. *Science* **257**:1083, 1992.
567. Snyder PM, Price MP, McDonald FJ, Adams CM, Volk KA, Zeiher BG, Stokes JB, Welsh MJ: Mechanism by which Liddle's syndrome mutations increase activity of a human epithelial Na+ channel. *Cell* **83**:969, 1995.
568. Sobonya RE, Taussig LM: Quantitative aspects of lung pathology in cystic fibrosis. *Am Rev Respir Dis* **134**:290, 1986.
569. Sohma Y, Gray MA, Imai Y, Argent BE: A mathematical model of the pancreatic ductal epithelium. *J Membr Biol* **154**:53, 1996.
570. Sokol RJ, Durie PR: Recommendations for management of liver and biliary tract disease in cystic fibrosis. Cystic Fibrosis Foundation Hepatobiliary Disease Consensus Group. *J Pediatr Gastroenterol Nutr* **28(Suppl 1)**:S1, 1999.
571. Sokol RJ, Reardon MC, Accurso FJ, Stall C, Narkewicz MR, Abman SH, Hammond KB: Fat-soluble vitamins in infants identified by cystic fibrosis newborn screening. *Pediatr Pulmonol Suppl* **7**:52, 1991.
572. Sordelli DO, Macri CN, Maillie AJ, McCerquetti MC: A preliminary study on the effect of anti-inflammatory treatment in cystic fibrosis patients with *Pseudomonas aeruginosa* lung infection. *Int J Immunopathol Pharmacol* **7**:109, 1994.
573. Spector ML, Stern RC: Pneumothorax in cystic fibrosis: A 26-year experience. *Ann Thorac Surg* **47**:204, 1989.
574. Spence JE, Perciaccante RG, Greig GM, Willard HF, Ledbetter DH, Hejtmancik JF, Pollack MS, O'Brien WE, Beaudet AL: Uniparental disomy as a mechanism for human genetic disease. *Am J Hum Genet* **42**:217, 1988.
575. Spicer SS, Briggman JV, Baron DA: Morphological and cytochemical correlates of transport in sweat glands of normal and cystic fibrosis subjects, in Quinton PM, Martinez JR, Hofer U (eds): *Fluid and Electrolyte Abnormalities in Cystic Fibrosis*. San Francisco, San Francisco Press, 1982, p 11.
576. Stark LJ, Powers SW, Jelalian E, Rape RN, Miller DL: Modifying problematic mealtime interactions of children with cystic fibrosis and their parents via behavioral parent training. *J Pediatr Psychol* **19**:751, 1994.
577. Stead RJ, Hodson ME, Batten JC, Adams J, Jacobs HS: Amenorrhoea in cystic fibrosis. *Clin Endocrinol (Oxf)* **26**:187, 1987.
578. Stern RC: Cystic fibrosis and the reproductive system, in Davis PB (ed): *Cystic Fibrosis*. New York, Marcel Dekker, 1993, p 381.
579. Stern RC: The diagnosis of cystic fibrosis. *N Engl J Med* **336**:487, 1997.
580. Stern RC: Cystic fibrosis and the GI tract, in Stern RC D (ed): *Cystic Fibrosis*. New York, Marcel Dekker, 1999, p 401.
581. Stern RC: Inpatient treatment of cystic fibrosis pulmonary disease, in Orenstein DM, Stern RC (eds): *Lung biology in health and disease*. New York, Marcel Dekker, 1999, p 79.
582. Stern RC, Izant RJ Jr, Boat TF, Wood RE, Matthews LW, Doershuk CF: Treatment and prognosis of rectal prolapse in cystic fibrosis. *Gastroenterology* **82**:707, 1982.
583. Stern RC, Rothstein FC, Doershuk CF: Treatment and prognosis of symptomatic gallbladder disease in patients with cystic fibrosis. *J Pediatr Gastroenterol Nutr* **5**:35, 1986.
584. Stevenson AC: The load of hereditary defect in human populations. *Radiat Res Suppl* **1**:306, 1959.
585. Stewart B, Zabner J, Shuber AP, Welsh MJ, McCray PB Jr: Normal sweat chloride values do not exclude the diagnosis of cystic fibrosis. *Am J Respir Crit Care Med* **151**:899, 1995.
586. Sturgess J, Imrie J: Quantitative evaluation of the development of tracheal submucosal glands in infants with cystic fibrosis and control infants. *Am J Pathol* **106**:303, 1982.
587. Sturgess JM: Structural and developmental abnormalities of the exocrine pancreas in cystic fibrosis. *J Pediatr Gastroenterol Nutr* **3(Suppl 1)**:S55, 1984.
588. Stutts MJ, Canessa CM, Olsen JC, Hamrick M, Cohn JA, Rossier BC, Boucher RC: CFTR as a cAMP-dependent regulator of sodium channels. *Science* **269**:847, 1995.
589. Sullivan MM, Denning CR: Diabetic microangiopathy in patients with cystic fibrosis. *Pediatrics* **84**:642, 1989.
590. Summerford C, Samulski RJ: Membrane-associated heparan sulfate proteoglycan is a receptor for adeno-associated virus type 2 virions. *J Virol* **72**:1438, 1998.
591. Super M: Cystic fibrosis in the South West African Afrikaner. *S Afr Med J* **49**:818, 1975.
592. Super M: Factors influencing the frequency of cystic fibrosis in southwest Africa. *Monogr Paediat* **10**:106, 1979.
593. Szaff M, Hoiby N, Flensborg EW: Frequent antibiotic therapy improves survival of cystic fibrosis patients with chronic *Pseudomonas aeruginosa* infection. *Acta Paediatr Scand* **72**:651, 1983.
594. Tabcharani JA, Linsdell P, Hanrahan JW: Halide permeation in wild-type and mutant cystic fibrosis transmembrane conductance regulator chloride channels. *J Gen Physiol* **110**:341, 1997.
595. Takahashi A, Watkins SC, Howard M, Frizzell RA: CFTR-dependent membrane insertion is linked to stimulation of the CFTR chloride conductance. *Am J Physiol* **271**:C1887, 1996.
596. Takahashi T, Matsushita K, Welsh MJ, Stokes JB: Effect of cAMP on intracellular and extracellular ATP content of Cl^--secreting epithelia and 3T3 fibroblasts. *J Biol Chem* **269**:17853, 1994.

597. Taylor CJ, Baxter PS, Hardcastle J, Hardcastle PT: Failure to induce secretion in jejunal biopsies from children with cystic fibrosis. *Gut* **29**:957, 1988.
598. Teem JL, Berger HA, Ostedgaard LS, Rich DP, Tsui L-C, Welsh MJ: Identification of revertants for the cystic fibrosis ΔF508 mutation using STE6-CFTR chimeras in yeast. *Cell* **73**:335, 1993.
599. Teem JL, Carson MR, Welsh MJ: Mutation of R555 in CFTR-ΔF508 enhances function and partially corrects defective processing. *Receptors Channels* **4**:63, 1996.
600. Teng H, Jorissen M, Poppel H, Legius E, Cassiman JJ, Cuppens H: Increased proportion of exon 9 alternatively spliced CFTR transcripts in vas deferens compared with nasal epithelial cells. *Hum Mol Genet* **6**:85, 1997.
601. Tepper RS: Assessment of the respiratory status of infants and toddlers with cystic fibrosis. *J Pediatr* **132**:380, 1998.
602. Tepper RS, Eigen H: Airway reactivity in cystic fibrosis. *Clin Rev Allergy* **9**:159, 1991.
603. Tepper RS, Eigen H, Stevens J, Angelicchio C, Kisling J, Ambrosius W, Heilman D: Lower respiratory illness in infants and young children with cystic fibrosis: Evaluation of treatment with intravenous hydrocortisone. *Pediatr Pulmonol* **24**:48, 1997.
604. Teune TM, Timmers-Reker AJ, Bouquet J, Bijman J, DeJonge HR, Sinaasappel M: In vivo measurement of chloride and water secretion in the jejunum of cystic fibrosis patients. *Pediatr Res* **40**:522, 1996.
605. The Cystic Fibrosis Genotype-Phenotype Consortium. Correlation between genotype and phenotype in patients with cystic fibrosis. *N Engl J Med* **329**:1308, 1993.
606. The IMpact-RSV Study Group: Palivizumab, a humanized respiratory syncytial virus monoclonal antibody, reduces hospitalization from respiratory syncytial virus infection in high-risk infants. *Pediatrics* **102**:531, 1998.
607. Thomassen MJ, Demko C, Doershuk CF, Stern RC, Klinger JD: Pseudomonas cepacia: Decrease in colonization in patients with cystic fibrosis. *Am Rev Respir Dis* **134**:669, 1986.
608. Thomson G: The effect of a selected locus on linked neutral loci. *Genetics* **85**:753, 1977.
609. Tizzano EF, Chitayat D, Buchwald M: Cell-specific localization of CFTR mRNA shows developmentally regulated expression in human fetal tissues. *Hum Mol Genet* **2**:219, 1993.
610. Tomashefski JF Jr, Abramowsky CR, Dahms BB: The pathology of cystic fibrosis, in Davis PB (ed): *Cystic Fibrosis*. New York, Marcel Dekker, 1993, p 469.
611. Tomashefski JF Jr, Bruce M, Stern RC, Dearborn DG, Dahms B: Pulmonary air cysts in cystic fibrosis: Relation of pathologic features to radiologic findings and history of pneumothorax. *Hum Pathol* **16**:253, 1985.
612. Tosi MF, Zakem-Cloud H, Demko CA, Schreiber JR, Stern RC, Konstan MW, Berger M: Cross-sectional and longitudinal studies of naturally occurring antibodies to *Pseudomonas aeruginosa* in cystic fibrosis indicate absence of antibody-mediated protection and decline in opsonic quality after infection. *J Infect Dis* **172**:453, 1995.
613. Townsend RR, Lipniunas PH, Tulk BM, Verkman AS: Identification of protein kinase A phosphorylation sites on NBD1 and R domains of CFTR using electrospray mass spectrometry with selective phosphate ion monitoring. *Protein Sci* **5**:1865, 1996.
614. Travis SM, Berger HA, Welsh MJ: Protein phosphatase 2C dephosphorylates and inactivates cystic fibrosis transmembrane conductance regulator. *Proc Natl Acad Sci U S A* **94**:11055, 1997.
615. Travis SM, Conway BD, Zabner J, Smith JJ, Anderson AM, Singh PK, Greenberg EP, Welsh MJ: Activity of abundant antimicrobials of the human airway. *Am J Respir Crit Care Med* **20**:872, 1999.
616. Trezise AEO, Buchwald M: In vivo cell-specific expression of the cystic fibrosis transmembrane conductance regulator. *Nature* **353**:434, 1991.
617. Triglia JM, Nicollas R: Nasal and sinus polyposis in children. *Laryngoscope* **107**:963, 1997.
618. Trulock EP: Management of lung transplant rejection. *Chest* **103**:1566, 1993.
619. Tsui L, Buchwald M, Barker D, Braman JC, Knowlton R, Schumm JW, Eiberg H, Mohr J, Kennedy D, Plavsic N, Zsiga M, Markiewicz D, Akots G, Brown V, Helms C, Gravius T, Parker C, Rediker K, Donis-Keller H: Cystic fibrosis locus defined by a genetically linked polymorphic DNA marker. *Science* **29**:1054, 1985.
620. Tsui L-C, Buchwald M: Biochemical and molecular genetics of cystic fibrosis, in Harris H, Hirschhorn K (eds): *Advances in Human Genetics*. New York, Plenum, 1991, p 153.
621. Turner DJ, Lanteri CJ, LeSouef PN, Sly PD: Improved detection of abnormal respiratory function using forced expiration from raised lung volume in infants with cystic fibrosis. *Eur Respir J* **7**:1995, 1994.
622. Turpin SV, Knowles MR: Treatment of pulmonary disease in patients with cystic fibrosis, in Davis PB (ed): *Cystic Fibrosis*. New York, Marcel Dekker, 1993, p 277.
623. Ulrich M, Herbert S, Berger J, Bellon G, Louis D, Munker G, Doring G: Localization of *Staphylococcus aureus* in infected airways of patients with cystic fibrosis and in a cell culture model of S. aureus adherence. *Am J Respir Cell Mol Biol* **19**:83, 1998.
624. Uyekubo SN, Fischer H, Maminishkis A, Illek B, Miller SS, Widdicombe JH: cAMP-dependent absorption of chloride across airway epithelium. *Am J Physiol* **275**:L1219, 1998.
625. Vaandrager AB, Smolenski A, Tilly BC, Houtsmuller AB, Ehlert EM, Bot AG, Edixhoven M, Boomaars WE, Lohmann SM, De Jonge HR: Membrane targeting of cGMP-dependent protein kinase is required for CFTR-Cl^- channel activation. *Proc Natl Acad Sci U S A* **95**:1466, 1998.
626. van Heeckeren A, Walenga R, Konstan MW, Bonfield T, Davis PB, Ferkol T: Excessive inflammatory response of cystic fibrosis mice to bronchopulmonary infection with *Pseudomonas aeruginosa*. *J Clin Invest* **100**:2810, 1997.
627. VanDoorninck JH, French PJ, Verbeek E, Peters RHPC, Morreau H, Bijman J, Scholte BJ: A mouse model for the cystic fibrosis delta F508 mutation. *EMBO J* **14**:4403, 1995.
628. Varon R, Magdorf K, Staab D, Wahn U, Krawczak M, Sperling K, Reis A: Recurrent nasal polyps as a monosymptomatic form of cystic fibrosis associated with a novel in-frame deletion (591del18) in the CFTR gene. *Hum Mol Genet* **4**:1463, 1995.
629. Veeze HJ, Sinaasappel M, Bijman J, Bouquet J, de-Jonge HR: Ion transport abnormalities in rectal suction biopsies from children with cystic fibrosis. *Gastroenterology* **101**:398, 1991.
630. Verlingue C, Vuillaumier S, Mercier B, Le Gac M, Elion J, Ferec C, Denamur E: Absence of mutations in the interspecies conserved regions of the CFTR promoter region in cystic fibrosis (CF) and CF related patients. *J Med Genet* **35**:137, 1998.
631. Vic P, Ategbo S, Turck D, Husson MO, Tassin E, Loeuille GA, Deschildre A, Druon D, Elian JC, Arrouet-Lagandre C, Farriaux JP: Tolerance, pharmacokinetics and efficacy of once daily amikacin for treatment of *Pseudomonas aeruginosa* pulmonary exacerbations in cystic fibrosis patients. *Eur J Pediatr* **155**:948, 1996.
632. Vigne E, Mahfouz I, Dedieu JF, Brie A, Perricaudet M, Yeh P: RGD inclusion in the hexon monomer provides adenovirus type 5-based vectors with a fiber knob-independent pathway for infection. *J Virol* **73**:5156, 1999.
633. Vivell VO, Jacobi H, Munchbach K: Zur mucoviscidosis im kidesalter. *Monatsschr Kinderhellkd* **111**:62, 1963.
634. Voss R, Ben-Simon E, Avital A, Godfrey S, Zlotogora J, Dagan JJ, Tikochinski Y, Hillel J: Isodisomy of chromosome 7 in a patient with cystic fibrosis: Could uniparental disomy by common in humans? *Am J Hum Genet* **45**:373, 1989.
635. Vuillaumier S, Dixmeras I, Messai H, Lapoumeroulie C, Lallemand D, Gekas J, Chehab FF, Perret C, Elion J, Denamur E: Cross-species characterization of the promoter region of the cystic fibrosis transmembrane conductance regulator gene reveals multiple levels of regulation. *Biochem J* **327**:651, 1997.
636. Wagener DK, Cavalli-Sforza LL: Ethnic variation in genetic disease: Possible roles of hitchhiking and epistasis. *Am J Med Genet* **27**:348, 1975.
637. Wainwright BJ, Scambler PJ, Schmidtke J, Watson EA, Law H, Farrall M, Cooke HJ, Eiberg H, Williamson R: Localization of cystic fibrosis locus to human chromosome 7een-q22. *Nature* **318**:384, 1985.
638. Walters RW, Grunst T, Bergelson JM, Finberg RW, Welsh MJ, Zabner J: Basolateral localization of fiber receptors limits adenovirus infection from the apical surface of airway epithelia. *J Biol Chem* **274**:10219, 1999.
639. Wang G, Davidson BL, Melchert P, Slepushkin VA, van Es HH, Bodner M, Jolly DJ, McCray PB Jr: Influence of cell polarity on retrovirus-mediated gene transfer to differentiated human airway epithelia. *J Virol* **72**:9818, 1998.
640. Wang S, Raab RW, Schatz PJ, Guggino WB, Li M: Peptide binding consensus of the NHE-RF-PDZ1 domain matches the C-terminal sequence of cystic fibrosis transmembrane conductance regulator (CFTR). *FEBS Lett* **427**:103, 1998.
641. Warburton D (ed): Uniparental disomy: A rare consequence of the high rate of aneuploidy in human gametes. *Am J Hum Genet* **42**:215, 1988.

642. Ward CL, RR Kopito: Intracellular turnover of cystic fibrosis transmembrane conductance regulator. Inefficient processing and rapid degradation of wild-type and mutant proteins. *J Biol Chem* **269**:25710, 1994.
643. Ward CL, Omura S, Kopito RR: Degradation of CFTR by the ubiquitin-proteasome pathway. *Cell* **83**:121, 1995.
644. Wayne CPNTC, National Committee for Clinical Laboratory Standards. Sweat testing: Sample collection and quantitative analysis-approved guideline. *Document C34-A* 1994.
645. Weatherly MR, Palmer CG, Peters ME, Green CG, Fryback D, Langhough R, Farrell PM: Wisconsin cystic fibrosis chest radiograph scoring system. *Pediatrics* **91**:488, 1993.
646. Wei L, Vankeerberghen A, Cuppens H, Droogmans G, Cassiman J-J, Nilius B: Phosphorylation site independent single R-domain mutations affect CFTR channel activity. *FEBS Lett* **439**:121, 1998.
647. Weiyuan M, Korngreen A, Uzlaner N, Priel Z, Silberberg SD: Extracellular sodium regulates airway ciliary motility by inhibiting a P2X receptor. *Nature* **400**:894, 1999.
648. Welsh MJ: Electrolyte transport by airway epithelia. *Physiol Rev* **67**:1143, 1987.
649. Welsh MJ: Gene transfer for cystic fibrosis. *J Clin Invest* **104**:1165, 1999.
650. Welsh MJ, Ostedgaard LS: Cystic fibrosis problem probed by proteolysis. *Nat Struct Biol* **5**:167, 1998.
651. Welsh MJ, Ramsey BW: Research on cystic fibrosis: A journey from the heart house. *Am J Respir Crit Care Med* **157**:S148, 1998.
652. Welsh MJ, Robertson AD, Ostedgaard LS: The ABC of a versatile engine. *Nature* **396**:623, 1998.
653. Welsh MJ, Smith AE: Molecular mechanisms of CFTR chloride channel dysfunction in cystic fibrosis. *Cell* **73**:1251, 1993.
654. White MB, Leppert M, Nielsen D, Zielenski J, Gerrard B, Stewart C, Dean M: A *de novo* cystic fibrosis mutation: CGA (Arg) to TGA (stop) at codon 851 of the CFTR gene. *Genomics* **11**:778, 1991.
655. White NL, Higgins CF, Trezise AEO: Tissue-specific *in vivo* transcription start sites of the human and murine cystic fibrosis genes. *Hum Mol Genet* **7**:363, 1998.
656. White R, Woodward S, Leppert M, O'Connell P, Hoff M, Herbst J, Lalouel JM, Dean M, Vande Woude G: A closely linked genetic marker for cystic fibrosis. *Nature* **318**:382, 1985.
657. Wickham TJ, Roelvink PW, Brough DE, Kovesdi I: Adenovirus targeted to heparan-containing receptors increases its gene delivery efficiency to multiple cell types. *Nat Biotech* **14**:1570, 1996.
658. Widdicombe JH: Cystic fibrosis and beta-adrenergic response of airway epithelial cell cultures. *Am J Physiol* **251**:R818, 1986.
659. Widdicombe JH: Altered NaCl concentration of airway surface liquid in cystic fibrosis. *News Physiol Sci* **14**:126, 1999.
660. Widdicombe JH, Fischer H, Lee CY-C, Uyekubo SN, Miller SS: Elemental composition of airway surface liquid. *Pediatric Pulmonol* **14(Suppl)**:74, 1997.
661. Widdicombe JH, Welsh MJ, Finkbeiner WE: Cystic fibrosis decreases the apical membrane chloride permeability of monolayers cultured from cells of tracheal epithelium. *Proc Natl Acad Sci U S A* **82**:6167, 1985.
662. Wiesemann HG, Steinkamp G, Ratjen F, Bauernfeind A, Przyklenk B, Doring G, von der Hardt H: Placebo-controlled, double-blind, randomized study of aerosolized tobramycin for early treatment of *Pseudomonas aeruginosa* colonization in cystic fibrosis. *Pediatr Pulmonol* **25**:88, 1998.
663. Wilcken B: Newborn screening for cystic fibrosis: Its evolution and a review of the current situation. *Screening* **2**:43, 1993.
664. Wilfond BS, Farrell PM, Laxova A, Mischler E: Severe hemolytic anemia associated with vitamin E deficiency in infants with cystic fibrosis. Implications for neonatal screening. *Clin Pediatr (Phila)* **33**:2, 1994.
665. Will K, Stuhrmann M, Dean M, Schmidtke J: Alternative splicing in the first nucleotide binding fold of CFTR. *Hum Mol Genet* **2**:231, 1993.
666. Williamson R: Universal community carrier screening for cystic fibrosis? *Nat Genet* **3**:195, 1993.
667. Wills PJ, Hall RL, Chan W, Cole PJ: Sodium chloride increases the ciliary transportability of cystic fibrosi and bronchiectasis sputum on the mucus-depleted bovine trachea. *J Clin Invest* **99**:9, 1997.
668. Willumsen NJ, Boucher RC: Transcellular sodium transport in cultured cystic fibrosis human nasal epithelium. *Am J Physiol* **261**:C332, 1991.
669. Wilmott RW, Amin RS, Colin AA, DeVault A, Dozor AJ, Eigen H, Johnson C, Lester LA, McCoy K, McKean LP, Moss R, Nash ML, Jue CP, Regelmann W, Stokes DC, Fuchs HJ: Aerosolized recombinant human DNase in hospitalized cystic fibrosis patients with acute pulmonary exacerbations. *Am J Respir Crit Care Med* **153**:1914, 1996.
670. Wilschanski M, Corey M, Durie P, Tullis E, Bain J, Asch M, Ginzburg B, Jarvi K, Buckspan M, Hartwick W: Diversity of reproductive tract abnormalities in men with cystic fibrosis. *JAMA* **276**:607, 1996.
671. Wilschanski M, Zielenski J, Markiewicz D, Tsui L-C, Corey M, Levison H, Durie PR: Correlation of sweat chloride concentration with classes of the cystic fibrosis transmembrane conductance regulator gene mutations. *J Pediatr* **127**:705, 1995.
672. Wilson DC, Ellis L, Zielenski J, Corey M, Ip WF, Tsui L-C, Tullis E, Knowles MR, Durie PR: Uncertainty in the diagnosis of cystic fibrosis: Possible role of *in vivo* nasal potential difference measurements. *J Pediatr* **132**:596, 1998.
673. Wilson DC, Pencharz PB: Nutrition and cystic fibrosis. *Nutrition* **14**:792, 1998.
674. Wilson JM: Adenovirus as gene-delivery vehicles. *N Engl J Med* **334**:1185, 1996.
675. Winnie GB, Cowan RG, Wade NA: Intravenous immune globulin treatment of pulmonary exacerbations in cystic fibrosis. *J Pediatr* **114**:309, 1989.
676. Winter MC, Sheppard DN, Carson MR, Welsh MJ: Effect of ATP concentration on CFTR $^{Cl-}$ channels: A kinetic analysis of channel regulation. *Biophys J* **66**:1398, 1994.
677. Winter MC, Welsh MJ: Stimulation of CFTR activity by its phosphorylated R domain. *Nature* **389**:294, 1997.
678. Wolter JM, Bowler SD, Nolan PJ, McCormack JG: Home intravenous therapy in cystic fibrosis: A prospective randomized trial examining clinical, quality of life and cost aspects. *Eur Respir J* **10**:896, 1997.
679. Wong PY: Abnormal fluid transport by the epididymis as a cause of obstructive azoospermia. *Reprod Fertil Dev* **2**:115, 1990.
680. Wong PY: CFTR gene and male fertility. *Mol Hum Reprod* **4**:107, 1998.
681. Worgall S, Singh R, Worgall T, Crystal RG: Free cholesterol enhances adenoviral vector gene transfer to CAR-deficient cells in vitro. *American Society of Gene Therapy Program of 2nd Annual Meeting* 131a, 1999.
682. Xie J, Drumm ML, Zhao J, Ma J, Davis PB: Human epithelial cystic fibrosis transmembrane conductance regulator without exon 5 maintains partial chloride channel function in intracellular membranes. *Biophys J* **71**:3148, 1996.
683. Xiong X, Bragin A, Widdicombe JH, Cohn J, Skach WR: Structural cues involved in endoplasmic reticulum degradation of G85E and G91R mutant cystic fibrosis transmembrane conductance regulator. *J Clin Invest* **100**:1079, 1997.
684. Yankaskas JR, Egan TM, Mauro MA: Major complications, in Yankaskas JR, Knowles MR (eds): *Cystic Fibrosis in Adults*. Philadelphia, Lippincott-Raven, 1999, p 175.
685. Yankaskas JR, Mallory GB Jr: Lung transplantation in cystic fibrosis: Consensus conference statement. *Chest* **113**:217, 1998.
686. Yoneda K: Mucous blanket of rat bronchus: An ultrastructural study. *Am Rev Respir Dis* **114**:837, 1976.
687. Yoshimura K, Nakamura H, Trapnell BC, Chu CS, Dalemans W, Pavirani A, Lecocq JP, Crystal RG: Expression of the cystic fibrosis transmembrane conductance regulator gene in cells of non-epithelial origin. *Nucleic Acids Res* **19**:5417, 1991.
688. Yoshimura K, Nakamura H, Trapnell BC, Dalemans W, Pavirani A, Lecocq JP, Crystal RG: The cystic fibrosis gene has a "housekeeping"-type promoter and is expressed at low levels in cells of epithelial origin. *J Biol Chem* **265**:9140, 1991.
689. Zabner J, Fasbender AJ, Moninger T, Poellinger KA, Welsh MJ: Cellular and molecular barriers to gene transfer by a cationic lipid. *J Biol Chem* **270**:18997, 1995.
690. Zabner J, Smith JJ, Karp PH, Widdicombe JH, Welsh MJ: Loss of CFTR chloride channels alters salt absorption by cystic fibrosis airway epithelia *in vitro*. *Mol Cell* **2**:397. 98.
691. Zabner J, Smith JJ, Widdicombe JH, Welsh MJ: Loss of CFTR chloride channels produces airway surface liquid with an increased sodium chloride concentration in cystic fibrosis. *Mol Cell* **2**:397, 1998.
692. Zeiher BG, Eichwald E, Zabner J, Smith JJ, Puga AP, McCray PB Jr, Capecchi MR, Welsh MJ, Thomas KR: A mouse model for the ΔF508 allele of cystic fibrosis. *J Clin Invest* **96**:2051, 1995.
693. Zhang Y, Doranz B, Yankaskas JR, Engelhardt JF: Genotypic analysis of respiratory mucous sulfation defects in cystic fibrosis. *J Clin Invest* **96**:2997, 1995.
694. Zhang, Y, Engelhardt JF: Airway surface fluid volume and Cl content in cystic fibrosis and normal bronchial xenografts. *Am J Physiol* **276**:469, 1999.

695. Zhao C, Wang I, Lehrer RI: Widespread expression of beta-defensin hBD-1 in human secretory glands and epithelial cells. *FEBS Lett* **396**:319, 1996.
696. Zheng W, Lee MG, Yan M, Diaz J, Benjamin I, Marino CR, Kopito R, Freedman S, Cotton C, Muallem S, Thomas P: Immuno and functional characterization of CFTR in submandibular and pancreatic acinar and duct cells. *Am J Physiol* **273**:C442, 1997.
697. Zhou L, Dey CR, Wert SE, DuVall MD, Frizzell RA, Whitsett JA: Correction of lethal intestinal defect in a mouse model of cystic fibrosis by human CFTR. *Science* **266**:1705, 1994.
698. Zielenski I, Corey M, Rozmahel R, Markiewicz D, Aznarez I, Casals T, Larriba S, Mercier B, Cutting GR, Krebsova A, Macek M Jr, Langfelder-Schwind E, Marshall BC, DeCelie-Germana J, Claustres M, Palacio A, Bal J, Nowakowska A, Ferec C, Estivill X, Durie P, Tsui L-C: Detection of a cystic fibrosis modifier locus for meconium ileus on human chromosome 19q13. *Nat Genet* **22**:128, 1999.
699. Zielenski J, Bozon D, Kerem BS, Markiewicz D, Durie P, Rommens JM, Tsui LC: Identification of mutations in exons 1 through 8 of the cystic fibrosis transmembrane conductance regulator (CFTR) gene. *Genomics* **10**:229, 1991.
700. Zielenski J, Markiewicz D, Lin S, Huang F, Yang-Feng TL, Tsui L-C: Skipping of exon 12 as a consequence of a point mutation (1898+5G → %) in the cystic fibrosis transmembrane conductance regulator gene found in a consanguineous Chinese family. *Clin Genet* **47**:125, 1995.
701. Zielenski J, Patrizio P, Corey M, Handelin B, Markiewicz D, Asch R, Tsui L-C: CFTR gene variant for patients with congenital absence of vas deferens. *Am J Hum Genet* **57**:958, 1995.
702. Zielenski J, Rozmahel R, Bozon D, Kerem B-S, Grzelczak Z, Riordan JR, Rommens J, Tsui L-C: Genomic DNA sequence of the cystic fibrosis transmembrane conductance regulator (CFTR) gene. *Genomics* **10**:214, 1991.
703. Zipf W: Cystic fibrosis-related diabetes mellitus, in Orenstein DM, Stern RC (eds): *Treatment of the Hospitalized Cystic Fibrosis Patient: Lung Biology in Health and Disease*. New York, Marcel Dekker, 1998, p 213.
704. Zuelzer WW, Newton WAJ: The pathogenesis of fibrocystic disease of the pancreas. A study of 36 cases with special reference to the pulmonary lesions. *Pediatrics* **4**:53, 1949.

CHAPTER 202

Defects in Sulfate Metabolism and Skeletal Dysplasias

Andrea Superti-Furga

1. Sulfate groups can be found in several different species of organic molecules. In vertebrates, the highest density of sulfate groups is found in the proteoglycans, a broad category of macromolecules characterized by a core protein to which one to several hundred glycosaminoglycan side chains, composed of repeating units of sulfated disaccharides, are attached. Proteoglycans are present in most membranes and cell organelles, but they are particularly abundant in the extracellular matrix of connective tissues.

2. Biologic sulfation is performed by transferring sulfate from a universal high-energy sulfate donor, phosphoadenosine phosphosulfate (PAPS), to an acceptor substrate. Sulfation reactions are catalyzed by substrate-specific sulfotransferases. The availability of PAPS is rate-limiting in most sulfotransferase reactions. PAPS is synthesized in the cytoplasm from inorganic sulfate and ATP by a two-step reaction with adenosine phosphosulfate (APS) as an intermediate product.

3. Inorganic sulfate in the cytoplasm may be either imported from the extracellular fluid in exchange for chloride or produced within the cells by the oxidation of sulfur amino acids and other thiols. Cells with a high rate of proteoglycan synthesis, such as chondrocytes, depend on extracellular sulfate to replenish their cytoplasmic sulfate pool.

4. Deficiencies in specific sulfohydrolases responsible for the lysosomal degradation of sulfated proteoglycans and lipids produce genetic diseases classified under the mucopolysaccharidoses or leukodystrophies (see Chaps. 136 and 148). Genetic defects in the transmembrane transport or the metabolic activation of sulfate affect the synthesis rather than the degradation of proteoglycans and have been associated so far with skeletal dysplasias.

5. Mutations in a sulfate/chloride antiporter of the cell membrane, called *diastrophic dysplasia sulfate transporter* (DTDST), result in a family of skeletal dysplasias that comprises two lethal conditions, achondrogenesis 1B (ACG1B) (MIM 600972) and atelosteogenesis 2 (AO2), as well as two nonlethal conditions, diastrophic dysplasia (MIM 222600) and multiple epiphyseal dysplasia (MIM 226900). The inheritance of all these conditions is recessive. The cartilage of affected individuals contains proteoglycans with insufficient sulfation. Fibroblast and chondrocyte cultures of such individuals exhibit a defect in the uptake and incorporation of exogenous sulfate. The impairment in sulfate uptake in chondrocytes apparently leads to depletion of cytoplasmic sulfate and PAPS and to the synthesis of undersulfated proteoglycans.

6. A mutation in the *ATPSK2* gene coding for the bifunctional enzyme ATP sulfurylase-APS kinase has been observed in several members of one family affected by recessively inherited spondyloepimetaphyseal dysplasia (SEMD).

7. A well-studied spontaneous mouse mutant called *brachymorphic* for the reduced length of its body and limbs is characterized by reduced sulfation of cartilage proteoglycans and by defective PAPS synthesis. The recently defined molecular basis is a missense mutation in the mouse *ATPSK2* gene; *brachymorphic* is thus homologous to human *ATPSK2*-deficient SEMD.

The role of sulfate in metabolism is manifold. Conjugation of xenobiotics with sulfate in the liver allows their detoxification and excretion with the bile. Sulfate groups are also found as structural features on various types of biologic molecules, such as proteins, lipids, and polysaccharides. The highest density of sulfate groups is found in the proteoglycans, a broad category of macromolecules characterized by a core protein to which one to several hundred glycosaminoglycan side chains are attached.[1] The glycosaminoglycan side chains are composed of repeated disaccharide-sulfate units. Proteoglycans are present in the cell nucleus, the cytoplasm, and the cell membrane, but they are particularly abundant in the extracellular matrix of connective tissues.[2]

Sulfate metabolism has been the object of study by toxicologists and hepatologists, as well as by biologists and physicians with an interest in connective tissue, bone, and cartilage. Several heritable disorders involving the biosynthesis and catabolism of sulfated compounds are known. This chapter deals with disorders of sulfate metabolism associated mainly with abnormal development of the skeleton.

THE CELLULAR METABOLISM OF SULFATE

Biologic sulfation involves such diverse molecules as proteoglycans, membrane lipids, plasma proteins, and xenobiotics detoxified in the liver.[3,4] Early studies on sulfation of phenol in liver extracts showed that ATP could accelerate the sulfation reaction significantly (reviewed in reference 3). This observation led to the hypothesis that, in analogy to the phosphate donor ATP, there may be a "universal" sulfate donor that could serve for different substrate-specific sulfotransferases.[3] Studies in yeast, liver tissue,

A list of standard abbreviations is located immediately preceding the index in each volume. Nonstandard abbreviations used in this chapter include: PAPS = phosphoadenosine phosphosulfate; CHO = Chinese hamster ovary; DTDST = diastrophic dysplasia sulfate transporter; APS = adenosine phosphosulfate; DTD = diastrophic dysplasia; ACG2 = achondrogenesis type 2; ACG1B = achondrogenesis type 1B; AO2 = atelosteogenesis type 2; MED = multiple epiphyseal dysplasia; SEMD = spondyloepimetaphyseal dysplasia.

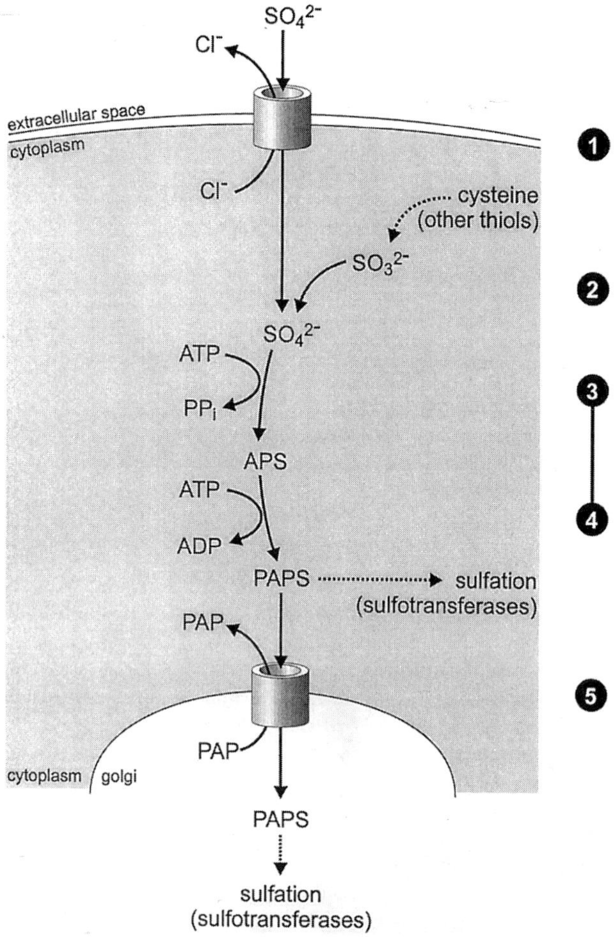

Fig. 202-1 Schematic representation of the cellular metabolism of sulfate. The numbers on the right refer to the following steps: (1) Sulfate/chloride exchange by DTDST. The stoichiometry has not been determined directly, but since the transporter is not ATP-dependent and electrogenic, it is assumed to be two chloride ions for one sulfate ion. (2) Sulfite oxidase, catalyzing final oxidation of thiol-derived sulfite to sulfate (see Chap. 88 & 128). (3, 4) Metabolic activation of inorganic sulfate by the bifunctional enzyme ATP sulfurylase-APS kinase (ATPSK). (5) Translocation of PAPS into the endoplasmic reticulum by a putative PAPS/PAP antiporter.

and cartilage tissue have confirmed this hypothesis by showing that the postulated "universal" high-energy sulfate donor for sulfotransferase reactions exists in the form of phosphoadenosine-phosphosulfate (PAPS). Investigations on the biosynthesis of the high-energy sulfate donor PAPS lead to recognition of the metabolic pathway called the *metabolic activation of sulfate*.[3,4]

The Origin of Intracellular Sulfate

Inorganic sulfate anions in the cytoplasm may either be derived from extracellular fluid or formed in the cytoplasm by catabolism of sulfur-containing amino acids and other thiol compounds with production of sulfite, which is oxidized to sulfate (Fig. 202-1) (see also Chap. 88). The transit of sulfate ions across cell membranes and epithelial tissues is mediated by carrier proteins. Sulfate transport mechanisms have been identified in the intestinal epithelium,[5] renal tubule epithelium,[6,7] basolateral and apical membranes of liver cells,[8–10] fibroblasts,[11] smooth muscle cells, and Chinese hamster ovary (CHO) cells.[12] These transporters function either as sulfate/chloride antiporters (or anion exchangers, since other anions may be transported by some of them) or as sodium/sulfate cotransporters. A coordinated model of the role and importance of each of these transport systems in whole-body sulfate homeostasis in humans has not emerged yet.[13]

Plasma sulfate concentrations in humans span a broad range (250–400 μM; higher values may be seen during pregnancy[14]), and the mechanisms by which plasma sulfate is regulated are still not clear.

Cytoplasmic Sulfate and Proteoglycan Synthesis

Studies on the synthesis and sulfation of proteoglycans in cultured chondrocytes, fibroblasts, endothelial cells and CHO cells have shown that sulfate groups on proteoglycans may be derived both from the intracellular catabolism of cysteine and other thiols and from the extracellular fluid. The relative contribution of the two pathways to the pool of intracellular sulfate apparently varies from one cell type to another. Ion uptake and inhibition studies have indicated that in fibroblasts and chondrocytes, sulfate ions are taken up by an anion-exchange mechanism driven by the chloride gradient; intracellular chloride ions are released, while sulfate ions are taken up by the cell.[11,15] The molecule responsible for this exchange appears to be the chloride/sulfate antiporter designated *diastrophic dysplasia sulfate transporter* (DTDST) (see below). The availability of extracellular sulfate to cultured cells can be curtailed by reducing its concentration in the culture medium, by competing with chlorate, or by inhibiting its uptake with 4,4′-diisothiocyanostilbene-2,2′-disulfonic acid.[15,19] Under these conditions, some cell types synthesize proteoglycans that are undersulfated.[15–22] Chondrocytes appear to be mostly dependent on extracellular sulfate for proteoglycan sulfation,[18,19] whereas CHO cells appear to make more extensive use of cysteine-derived sulfate,[12] and in fibroblasts, both pathways are used.[12,15,22] Thus a high rate of synthesis of proteoglycans seems to correlate with dependence on the uptake of extracellular sulfate.[12] These indirect conclusions have been confirmed by studies in cells from patients with *DTDST* mutations[23] (see below).

The Metabolic Activation of Sulfate

Cytoplasmic sulfate is activated in two steps catalyzed by two distinct enzymes in lower organisms and plants[3,4,24] (see Fig. 202-1). ATP sulfurylase catalyzes the synthesis of adenosine phosphosulfate (APS) from sulfate and ATP. APS kinase cataylzes the synthesis of PAPS from APS and ATP.[4] In the marine worm *Urechis caupo*,[25] in *Drosophila*,[26] and in mice, rats, and humans, a single bifunctional enzyme exists with two activities, ATP sulfurylase and APS kinase,[27–29] contained in the C- and N-terminal segments of the protein, respectively[30,31] (see below). Studies on the bifunctional enzyme of rat chondrosarcoma and mouse cartilage have shown that the substrate of the second reaction is much more likely to come directly from the first active site of the enzyme than from the surrounding fluid; i.e., there is "channeling" of substrate from one active site to the other.[32,33] This is consistent with the observation that the equilibrium for the first reaction is shifted toward inorganic sulfate. Channeling of APS toward the second reaction removes product and facilitates the first reaction. Once formed, PAPS is relatively stable. It is the sulfate donor for sulfation in the cytoplasm. For the sulfation of most membrane-bound and secreted molecules (such as most proteoglycans), PAPS must be transferred to the endoplasmic reticulum and/or the Golgi.[1,34] Earlier suggestions of a nucleoside sulfate/nucleoside exchange system in Golgi membranes[35] have been modified in part by newer studies that have suggested a PAPS/PAP (phosphoadenosine-phosphate) antiporter activity residing in a 230-kDa protein.[36,37] The role of a further PAPS translocase activity from rat liver Golgi associated with a 70-kDa protein present as a dimer is unclear.[38] Studies on the sulfation of xenobiotics have shown that PAPS availability is the rate-limiting factor in many sulfotransferase reactions.[34]

SULFATE METABOLISM AND HUMAN GENETIC DISEASE

Deficiencies in specific sulfohydrolases responsible for the lysosomal degradation of sulfated proteoglycans and lipids result in lysosomal storage disorders classified under the mucopolysaccharidoses (see Chap. 136) or leukodystrophies (see Chap. 148). Mutations in a neutral arylsulfatase, ARSE, have been implied in the pathogenesis of one form of chondrodysplasia punctata (see Chap. 210), whereas mutations in a steroid sulfatase gene are responsible for X-linked ichthyosis (see Chap. 166). Defects involving the cellular uptake and metabolic activation of sulfate, caused by mutations in the *DTDST* and *ATPSK2* genes, have been identified in patients with skeletal dysplasias and are described below.

The *DTDST* Sulfate Transporter Gene

The isolation of a human sulfate/chloride antiporter gene was the end result of a long-term project aimed at elucidating the molecular basis of diastrophic dysplasia (DTD), a skeletal dysplasia particularly frequent in the Finnish population. The locus responsible for this disorder was mapped initially to chromosome 5,[39] with refinement using linkage disequilibrium with polymorphic markers on chromosome 5 in the Finnish population[40] (as well as data obtained later during the cloning of the Treacher-Collins gene; see MIM 154500) to 5q32-q33.1. A candidate cDNA encloned by a gene from that region[41] was noted to have homology with *sat-1*, a rat hepatocyte sulfate transporter.[10] The hypothesis that DTD was associated with impaired sulfate transport was confirmed by the demonstration of reduced sulfate uptake in cultured fibroblasts from patients with DTD and by the demonstration of mutations in the candidate gene in such individuals.[41] Recognition that the gene responsible for DTD encoded a sulfate transporter was a surprise because there was no preceding experimental evidence of abnormal sulfate or proteoglycan metabolism in this disorder.

The coding sequence of *DTDST* is organized in two exons separated by an intron of approximately 1.6 kb and predicts a protein of 739 amino acids that, by hydrophobicity analysis and analogy with *sat-1*, was predicted to have 12 transmembrane domains as well as a terminal hydrophobic domain that may be membrane-associated rather than membrane-spanning (see Fig. 202-2).[41] Northern blot analysis showed that DTDST is expressed in many tissues, but human cartilage was not studied (compare with rat DTDST expression, below). The size of the predominant mRNA species is greater than 8 kb, indicating that there are significant untranslated sequences.[41]

Following characterization of human *DTDST*, rat and mouse orthologues have been cloned. The rat gene has five exons with the coding sequence distributed in two exons separated by an intron positioned at the same position as in human *DTDST*[42]; the rat protein is composed like the human protein of 739 amino acids. Expression of DTDST in rat is widespread but highest in cartilage and intestine. Ion uptake and inhibition studies using *Xenopus* oocytes transfected with rat DTDST mRNA confirmed its function as a sulfate/chloride antiporter.[42]

A mouse cDNA orthologous to human *DTDST* was cloned during an effort to identify genes induced by bone morphogenic protein 2 (BMP-2) and thus associated with osteoblastic differentiation.[43,44] The mouse protein also has 739 amino acids with 81 percent identity with human DTDST.

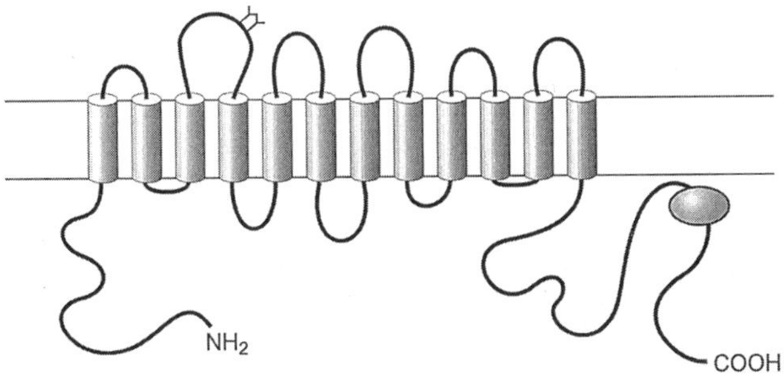

Fig. 202-2 Schematic representation of the DTDST protein. (*Redrawn from Hastbacka et al.*[41])

Clinical Phenotypes Associated with *DTDST* Mutations. There are currently four distinct phenotypes associated with *DTDST* mutations (see below). The division into these four categories is useful for differential diagnosis and prognosis but has no biologic basis, since the spectrum of disease as judged by both clinical and radiologic criteria is continuous. This phenotypic spectrum ranges from a severe disturbance in embryonic morphogenesis as seen in achondrogenesis type 1B to a relatively benign condition such as multiple epiphyseal dysplasia. Genotype-phenotype correlations can be drawn, but it appears that the nature of the *DTDST* mutation is not the only factor in determining phenotypic severity. Phenotypic differences have been observed between unrelated and even first-degree relatives with the same *DTDST* mutation.

Achondrogenesis Type 1B (Fig. 202-3). The name *achondrogenesis* (Greek for "not producing cartilage") was given in 1952 by Fraccaro[45] to the condition he observed in a stillborn female with severe micromelia and marked histologic abnormalities of cartilage. The condition, described shortly thereafter and also designated as *achondrogenesis* by Grebe,[46] was different although superficially similar to Fraccaro's achondrogenesis because of limb shortening and later became known as *Grebe chondrodysplasia* or *Grebe syndrome* (MIM 200700).

Achondrogenesis is one of the most severe forms of chondrodysplasia in humans, invariably lethal before or shortly after birth. Exact figures on the incidence of achondrogenesis are not available, but it is not exceedingly rare. Reviews with large patient numbers have been published.[47,48] In the 1970s, the heterogeneity of achondrogenesis was recognized. By a combination of radiologic and histologic criteria, achondrogenesis type 1 (ACG1) (then also called *Fraccaro-Houston-Harris type*) and achondrogenesis type 2 (ACG2) (called *Langer-Saldino type*) were distinguished.[49,50] In 1976, it was found that chondrocytes of some (though not all) ACG 1 patients contained cytoplasmic inclusions.[51] In the late 1980s, ACG2 was shown to be caused by structural mutations in collagen type 2 and thus represented the severe end of the spectrum of the collagen 2 chondrodysplasias.[52–54] Borochowitz *et al.*[55] and others[56] provided histologic criteria for the subdivision of ACG1 into achondrogenesis type 1A (ACG1A), with apparently normal cartilage matrix but inclusions in chondrocytes, and achondrogenesis type 1B (ACG1B), with abnormal cartilage matrix). Using these criteria, some cases from the earlier literature can be diagnosed unequivocally as ACG1B and others as ACG1A.[57] In 1994, before the *DTDST* gene was cloned, biochemical evidence of a defect in sulfate metabolism in ACG1B was obtained. Cartilage extracted from a newborn with ACG1B was found to stain poorly with toluidine blue after gel electrophoresis, and cultured fibroblasts synthesized proteoglycans that could be marked with radiolabeled glycine or methionine but not with sulfate.[58,59] Furthermore, fibroblasts pulsed with $^{35}SO_4^{2}$ failed to synthesize APS and PAPS. The original interpretation as a sulfate activation defect[58,59] analogous to that seen in the brachymorphic mouse (see below) proved to be wrong, since cocultivation studies with DTD fibroblasts, sulfate uptake studies, and *DTDST* mutation analysis showed that the primary defect in ACG1B was a sulfate uptake defect caused by *DTDST* mutations.[60]

A fetus with ACG1B is frequently in breech position and is immediately perceived as abnormal at birth. There is abundant soft tissue relative to the short skeleton, giving the infant a fat or hydropic appearance, and there is misproportion between the head, which is of normal or near-normal size, and the length, which is much shorter than normal. The face is flat, the neck short, and the soft tissue of the neck thickened. The thorax is narrow, and the abdomen is protuberant. Umbilical and inguinal hernias are frequent. The limbs are severely shortened. The fingers and toes are similarly short and stubby. The feet and toes are rotated inward

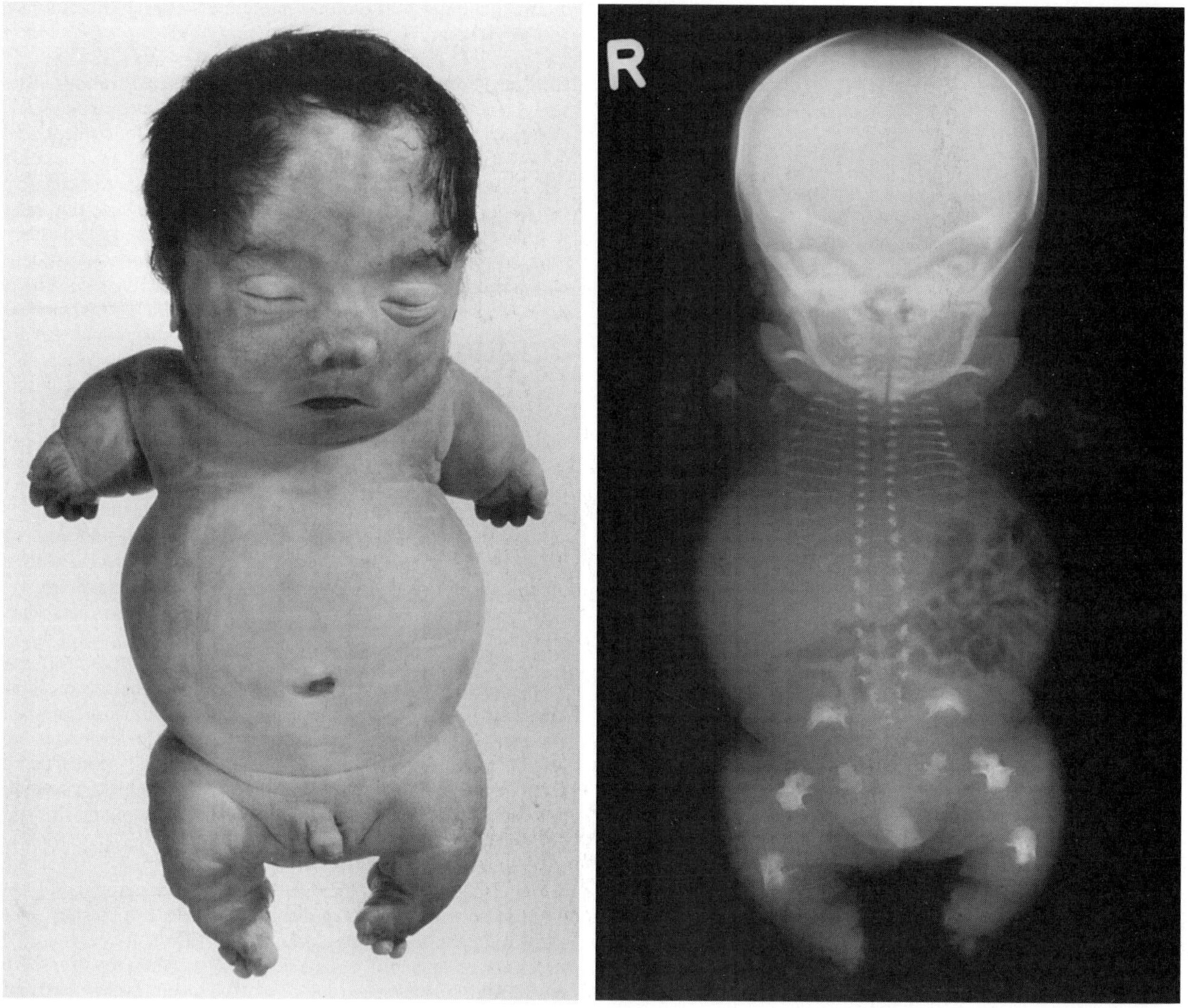

Fig. 202-3 (*Left*) Characteristic appearance of a newborn with achondrogenesis type 1B, born at week 34 and deceased 25 minutes after birth. Note the flat face, the narrow thorax with protuberant abdomen, and the severe micromelia with short, stubby fingers and toes. This patient was homozygous for the *DTDST V340* mutation. (*Right*) X-ray of the same newborn. Following the resuscitation attempts, there is air in the stomach and intestine but not in the lungs. Note the skeletal changes: hypoplasia of the rib cage and severe shortening of the long bones of the limbs. (*Reprinted with permission from Superti-Furga.*[59])

in a fashion reminiscent of DTD. The external genitalia are unremarkable. ACG1B infants may die before birth for reasons that are not understood. Even when heart action is present at birth, respiratory insufficiency and death follow shortly.

The differential diagnosis with other forms of achondrogenesis and other lethal chondrodysplasias requires analysis of radiographic features, histologic study of chondroosseous tissue, and biochemical and molecular studies (reviewed in reference 57; also see below).

Atelosteogenesis Type 2. Sillence[61] first applied this name in 1987 to a group of fetuses or newborns that had been considered previously to have severe DTD but with some radiologic features (e.g., a peculiar tapering of the distal humeri) that resembled those seen in another disorder, atelosteogenesis type 1. Atelosteogenesis type 2 (AO2) is intermediate in severity between ACG1B and DTD. Affected newborns or fetuses present with short limbs, adducted feet, and the "hitchhiker" thumb characteristic of DTD (see below). The disorder is usually lethal, although survival for several months has been known to occur. Several patients classified as having "severe" or "lethal" DTD prior to 1987 would be diagnosed as having AO2 today.[62–64] Radiologic features are similar to those of DTD, with tapering of the distal humerus, as observed with an anteroposterior-projection radiograph, being more pronounced in AO2. Cartilage histology usually shows changes similar to those of DTD.[65–67]

Additionally, a familial severe skeletal dysplasia known as *de la Chapelle dysplasia* may be related to DTD and AO2. It seems likely that some patients reported as having de la Chapelle dysplasia had AO2,[65] but the original patients may have had a similar but different disorder.[68] Yet another lethal chondrodysplasia, called *McAlister dysplasia*,[69] appears to be identical to AO2.[70] These uncertainties show how insecure radiologic nosology may be without additional histologic, biochemical, and molecular data.

Diastrophic Dysplasia (Fig. 202-4). This condition was delineated in 1960 by Lamy and Maroteaux and referred to as "bone anomalies that simulate achondroplasia during the first years of life but show a quite different evolution."[71] The name *diastrophic dwarfism* refers to the "twisted" body shape of affected individuals.[71] DTD is a severe, though usually nonlethal form of skeletal dysplasia with marked short stature (both the trunk and the limbs are shortened, but the limbs more severely so), bilateral clubfoot, cleft palate, characteristic hand deformities, changes of the ear pinnae, progressive kyphoscoliosis of the spine, and joint stiffness. The clinical features of DTD are well reviewed.[72,73]

The newborn with DTD has a normal-sized head, a slightly shortened trunk, and more markedly shortened extremities. There

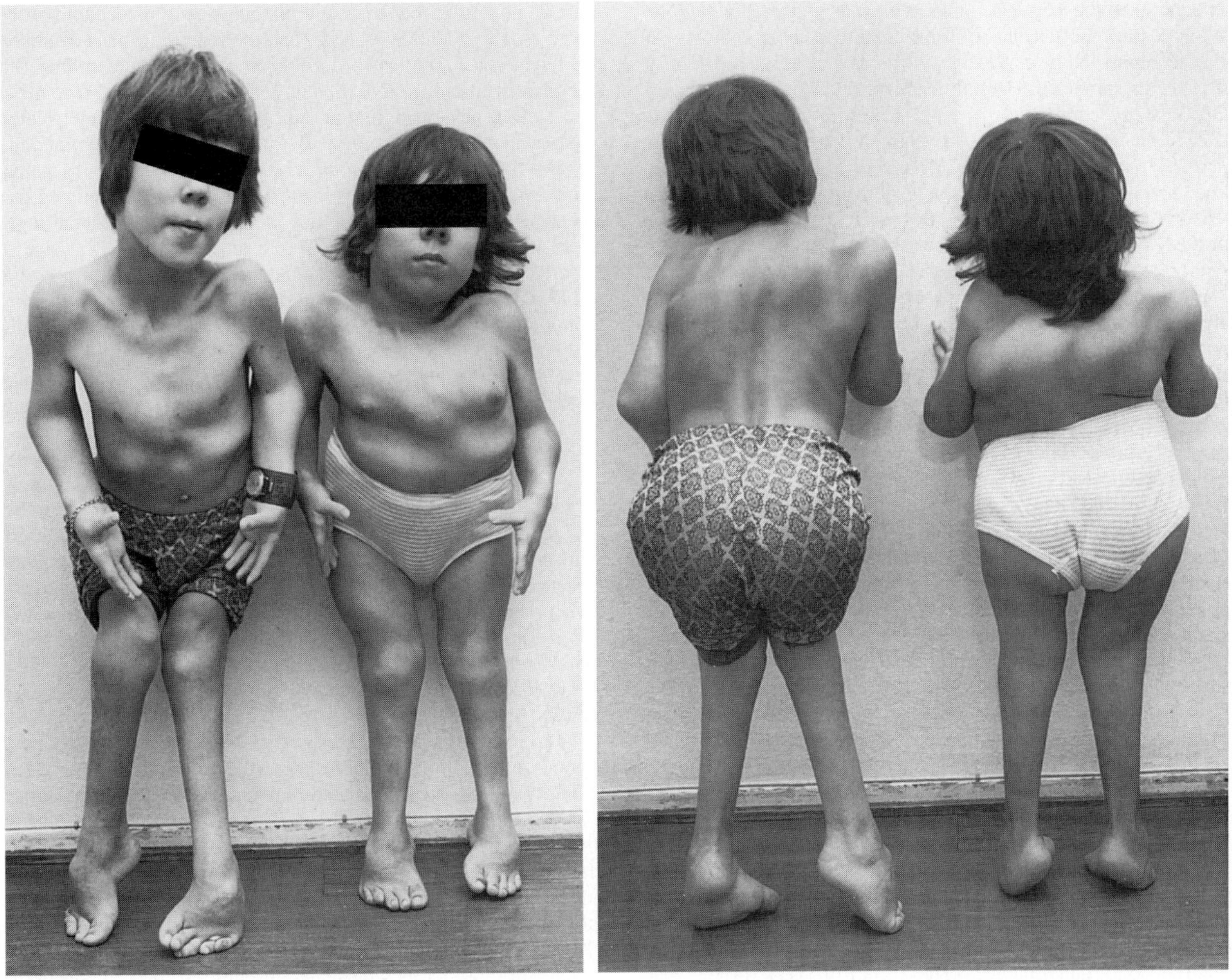

Fig. 202-4 A 14-year-old girl and her 11-year-old brother with diastrophic dysplasia. Note short stature and the following characteristic changes: equinovarus adductus deformity of the feet, muscular hypoplasia of the legs and thighs, flexion contractures of the hips leading to anterior tilting of the pelvis and pronounced lumbar lordosis, limitation of elbow extension, stiff fingers, and the so-called hitchhiker thumbs. The patients, now adults, are physically handicapped but professionally active at academic level. (*Photographs courtesy of Dr. I. Kaitila, Helsinki, Finland, with permission of the patients.*)

may be contractures at the hip, elbow, and knee joints. The fingers are short, and the thumb is both proximally placed and deviated to the radial side (the so-called hitchhiker thumb). The metatarsals are usually markedly adducted (the great toe stands out as a "hitchhiker toe"), and there is equinovarus deformity of the feet not dissimilar to that produced by primary neurologic disorders. The "hitchhiker" thumbs and toes have been observed as early as in the fifteenth and sixteenth weeks of pregnancy (reference 74, and unpublished observations), indicating an early developmental anomaly rather than a deformation.

The face may be slightly flattened and the forehead may be broad, but these changes are not consistent. Flat hemangiomas on the forehead are common. In more than half of DTD newborns, a peculiar process affects the ear pinnae. Within the first weeks of life, the pinnae develop acute inflammation and swelling, with fluctuation or cystic changes on palpation. Inflammation subsides within weeks, leaving a thickened and sometimes deformed pinnae that eventually may calcify.[71,72] When present, these changes are a valuable diagnostic clue; their pathogenesis is obscure. Posterior palatal clefting occurs in approximately one-half of cases. Neonatal adaptation may be troubled by respiratory insufficiency because of the small rib cage and tracheal instability and collapsibility, and mechanical ventilation is required in a significant proportion of cases. Mortality in the first months of life is increased, mainly because of respiratory complications such as pneumonia and sometimes aspiration pneumonia.[72,75]

In the newborn period, DTD appears to involve not only the skeleton but also the tendons, ligaments, and joint capsules, which are usually tighter and shorter than normal, causing restricted joint mobility. The pathogenesis of this ligamentous involvement is not understood. Pretibial dimples may be present, possibly a consequence of reduced intrauterine movements.

DTD is progressive. Degenerative arthrosis of the hip is common in young adults (pain and anterior tilting of the pelvis are the consequences), and the spine may develop excessive lumbar lordosis, thoracolumbar kyphosis, and scoliosis. In addition to brachydactyly, there may be ulnar deviation, phalangeal synostosis, and ankylosis of the finger, with significant disability. Correction of the clubfoot, which appears to be caused by a primary shortening of the Achilles tendon, is difficult to achieve by casting, and even with surgical intervention, there is a high recurrence rate. Most individuals with DTD are unable to bring their heels on the ground and thus stand solely on their metatarsals and toes. The appearance of an adult individual with clubfoot, marked lumbar lordosis, and thoracal kyphoscoliosis is quite typical; this "twisted" appearance originally prompted the name *diastrophic*. Based on the characteristic body posture and hand changes, DTD has been diagnosed retrospectively in "historical" patients.[76]

In addition to the skeletal abnormalities, a mild degree of muscular hypoplasia of the thighs and legs is common. Neurologic complications may occur, particularly in the cervical region.

Broadening of the cervical spine, with a characteristic "cobra-like" appearance, often can be seen on anteroposterior radiographs and is accompanied by cervical kyphosis. Severe cervical kyphosis may lead to spinal cord compression spontaneously and during intubation procedures.[77–81] Severe neuronal degeneration and gliosis of the cervical spinal cord, acquired before birth, have been described in a DTD infant with severe cervical kyphosis who died immediately after birth with respiratory insufficiency.[62]

Hearing loss is unusual, and vision defects are seldom observed, although a tendency toward myopia has been reported.[82] Mental development and intelligence are not affected.

Adult stature was found to range between 100 and 140 cm in an early review of American and European patients.[73] A 1982 study reported a mean adult height of 118 cm,[83] whereas a recent study of Finnish DTD patients (who are genetically homogeneous at the *DTDST* locus) gave a mean adult height of 136 cm for males and 129 cm for females.[84] Growth curves have been produced that can be used for monitoring of DTD patients.[83,84] Discrepancy between the older studies and the recent Finnish study may be due to allelic heterogeneity but also may reflect bias toward more severely affected patients in the older studies.

Based on the experience with Finnish DTD individuals, the Helsinki group has systematically reviewed several clinical features of DTD such as cleft palate,[85] anomalies of dentition,[86] and changes in the spine,[87] hip joint,[88] patellofemoral joint,[89] and foot.[90] A characteristic metacarpophalangeal length pattern has been described.[91]

Variability in DTD. It has long been appreciated that the DTD phenotype may be more variable than in the patients originally described by Maroteaux and Lamy. Affected infants dying during the perinatal period previously were diagnosed as having "severe DTD" but now would be assigned to the AO2 category (see above). Individuals with milder expression of DTD, particularly having only mild statural deficit, previously were designated as having "DTD variant," but more recent studies have shown that the differences between classic DTD and the so-called diastrophic variant are only quantitative.[73] The "death of DTD variant" has been decreed.[92] The molecular studies have confirmed this pronouncement. In addition to interfamilial variability, several authors have observed marked differences between affected siblings.[73,92,93] These observations suggest that other genetic or epigenetic factors influence the phenotype.

Recessively Inherited Multiple Epiphyseal Dysplasia. A single patient has been identified who had clubfoot and hip dysplasia at birth but had no palatal clefting, "hitchhiker" thumb, or ear swelling and who grew normally (adult height, 180 cm). He developed hip pain and digital deformations around puberty and was diagnosed as having multiple epiphyseal dysplasia (MED) with double-layered patella.[94] He was shown to be homozygous (and each parent heterozygous) for the *R279W* allele (see below), and his fibroblasts exhibited a sulfate-incorporation defect similar to that of other DTD patients.[94] Although the radiologic changes and the presence of clubfoot are reminiscent of DTD, the absence of spinal deformity and the relatively tall stature of this individual do not fit the DTD spectrum and justify a separate category. The incidence of this mild variant of DTDST chondrodysplasia remains to be determined. Because it is associated with the most common *DTDST* mutation, it may be more frequent than hitherto recognized.

Diagnosis and Differential Diagnosis of DTDST Skeletal Dysplasias. The differential diagnosis of DTDST-associated chondrodysplasias usually is made within the context of other chondrodysplasias of similar severity and radiographic appearance. ACG1B should be differentiated from other types of achondrogenesis, fibrochondrogenesis, dyssegmental dysplasia, and even thanatophoric dysplasia or severe osteogenesis imperfecta.[57,95] There are subtle radiographic signs suggesting the correct diagnosis, but cartilage histology and histochemistry can more reliably identify ACG1B, and the final diagnosis should rest on biochemical studies in fibroblast or chondrocyte cultures and the identification of *DTDST* mutations. Since prenatal recognition and pregnancy termination of fetuses affected by skeletal dysplasias (including ACG1B) are increasingly common, a diagnostic protocol is of great importance to provide the parents with accurate information.[57,96] AO2 should be differentiated from other severe chondrodysplasias, as mentioned for achondrogenesis, and from other forms of atelosteogenesis[65–67,95]; since the disorder is usually lethal, the same considerations made above for ACG1B apply. DTD is usually diagnosed by radiographic abnormalities and the presence of clinical abnormalities, including cleft palate, clubfoot, "hitchhiker" thumb and first toes, and the development of painful swelling of the external ear cartilage days to weeks after birth. The latter signs, however, are not always present, and their absence does not rule out DTD. Cartilage tissue is not routinely available. Diagnostic confirmation can be obtained by analysis of sulfate uptake and incorporation in cultured fibroblasts or by mutation analysis (see below). In milder cases, the diagnosis may be difficult.[93,94] The association of clubfoot with skeletal changes suggestive of bone dysplasia, even in the absence of typical hand or ear changes or cleft palate, should alert the physician to the possibility of a DTDST disorder. The condition known as *pseudodiastrophic dysplasia*[97] is, despite the name, relatively easy to distinguish from true DTD. There is no DTDST defect in this disorder (reference 98, and unpublished results, 1998).

The biochemical diagnosis can be made in fibroblast or chondrocyte cultures. When these cells from ACG1B, AO2, or DTD patients are incubated in culture medium containing $Na_2{}^{35}SO_4$, they exhibit a characteristic defect in the incorporation of $^{35}SO_4$ into macromolecules. ^3H-labeled glycine or glucosamine can be used as internal reference.[59,60,99] Direct assay of sulfate uptake is technically difficult and thus less suitable for diagnostic purposes.[23] Mutation detection has been successful, and the *DTDST* gene is small. This provides an alternative to biochemical studies in those cases where no cell cultures are available. When the clinical and radiologic features are typical, mutations on both alleles have been found in over 90 percent of cases (see below).

Prenatal diagnosis of ACG1B, AO2, and DTD is frequently requested by families in which a previous child (or pregnancy) has been affected. When molecular studies are not available, ultrasonography may be used. Achondrogenesis can be recognized as early as weeks 13 to 15,[96,100] AO2 and DTD a few weeks later.[74,101,102] DTD has been diagnosed (or excluded) by analysis of chromosome 5 markers linked to the disorder.[103] Identification of the mutations segregating in a given family has allowed direct prenatal diagnosis in several families at risk for ACG1B, AO2, and DTD (A Superti-Furga and A Rossi, unpublished data 1997-1999). The possibility of biochemical diagnosis by sulfate incorporation and/or uptake studies in chorionic villus biopsies or cells cultured from such biopsies has not been explored, but the need for such a diagnostic modality is limited when the molecular defects are known.

Spectrum of *DTDST* Mutations. The mutations identified so far in patients and families with DTDST chondrodysplasias are shown in Table 202-1. Except for 418C > T, which has been shown to cause reduced mRNA levels,[104] formal proof of their pathogenicity is lacking. Assumption of pathogenicity is justified in that some predict a more or less severely truncated polypeptide chain, and others affect amino acids that are located in transmembrane domains or which are conserved in humans, mice, and rats (with the only exception of N77H, where both mice and rats have serine). The *R279W* (862C > T) mutation appears to be the most common mutant allele in non-Finns. The ethnic distribution observed so far for *R279W* would be compatible with a central European origin, but its frequency also may be explained by

Table 202-1 Overview on Pathogenic Mutations in the *DTDST* Gene

Mutation	Predicted Protein Change		Associated Phenotypes	Remarks	Original Description
IVS1+2T>C	mis-splicing	—	DTD, AO2	"Finnish" founder mutation, giving reduced mRNA levels with intact coding sequence	Ref. 105a
74C>G	S16X	First cytoplasmic domain	DTD		Rossi and Cetta, unpublished
82G>T	G19X	First cytoplasmic domain	DTD		McGill and Superti-Furga, unpublished
256A>C	N77H	First cytoplasmic domain	DTD	Observed in a mild DTD variant; mouse and rat genes have serine at this position	LeMerrer and Superti-Furga, unpublished
418T del	FS/stop	—	AO2		Ref. 104
422T>C	L132P	First transmembrane domain	ACG1B	ACG1B variant with proximally pointed femurs	Unger, Chitayat, and Superti-Furga, unpublished
430C>A	Q135R	First extracellular loop	DTD		Plauchu and Superti-Furga, unpublished
476T del	FS/stop	—	ACG1B		Ref. 60
523G>A	G166R	Third transmembrane domain	DTD		Schinzel and Superti -Furga, unpublished
558C>T	R178X	Truncation in third transmembrane domain		Multiple patients	Superti-Furga et al., 1996a
IVS2+1G>C	Mis-splicing?	—	DTD	Multiple patients	Ref. 41
731–737GATGGGC del	FS/stop	—	DTD		Cohn and Superti-Furga, unpublished
791G>A	G255E	Fifth transmembrane domain	AO2, DTD		Ref. 99
803G>T	G259V	Fifth transmembrane domain	AO2	Multiple patients; in one case severe AO2, borderline to ACG1B	Meinecke and Superti-Furga, unpublished
862C>T	R279W	Extracellular loop between fifth and sixth transmembrane domains	AO2, DTD, MED	Most frequent mutation outside Finland; when homozygous, results in mild DTD or MED	Refs. 94, 99, and 104
933–934CT del	FS/stop	—	DTD		Rossi, Bonaventure, and Superti-Furga, unpublished
1045–1047GTT del	*Del* V340	Seventh transmembrane domain	ACG1B, DTD	Recurrent mutation (see text)	Refs. 60 and 105
1221A del	FS/stop	—	ACG1B		Ref. 60
1269–1272AAAC del	FS/stop	—	DTD		Freisinger and Superti-Furga, unpublished
1300A>G	N425D	Ninth transmembrane domain	ACG1B, AO2	Recurrent mutation	Ref. 60
1388A>C	Q454P	Tenth transmembrane domain	DTD	Nonlethal, severe variant DTD with broad bones	Megarbane and Superti-Furga, unpublished
1421T del	FS/stop	—	DTD	Severe variant	Verloes and Superti-Furga, unpublished
1475T>C	L483P	Eleventh transmembrane domain	ACG1B		Ref. 112
1501C>T	R492W	Extracellular loop between eleventh and twelfth transmembrane domains	DTD	Multiple patients	Riconda, Kubas, and Superti-Furga, unpublished
1751A del	FS/stop	—	ACG1B, AO2, DTD	Multiple patients	Ref. 41
1984T>A	C653S	Hydrophobic domain of cytoplasmic tail	DTD		Rossi, Plauchu, and Superti-Furga, unpublished
2010A del	FS/stop	—	DTD		Ref. 41
2021A>C	H665P	Cytoplasmic tail	AO2		Siu and Superti-Furga, unpublished
2060G>T	G678V	Cytoplasmic tail	ACG1B		Ref. 60
2171C>T	A715V	Cytoplasmic tail	AO2		Ref. 99

NOTE: Numbering of nucleotides and amino acids follows ref. 41.

independent recurrences, since it involves a CpG dinucleotide. The ΔV340 (1045–1047Δgtt) mutation has been observed in patients of Turkish,[60] Hispanic,[60] and Japanese origin. This observation and its occurrence at a short direct triplet repeat suggest that it also may be a recurrent mutation. A mutant allele, *S689T* (2092A >T), has been observed.[41] The conservative nature of this substitution, the presence of a serine in the corresponding position of the mouse[43] and rat genes,[42] and the observation of the mutation in several healthy individuals with no apparent relationship to DTDST dysplasias (reference 105, and J Hästbacka and A Superti-Furga, unpublished observations 1996) All suggest that it is a neutral mutation not found infrequently. The Finnish founder mutation has been identified recently.[105a] All suggest that it is a neutral mutation not found infrequently.

The results of mutation analysis in affected individuals obtained so far suggest that (1) most mutations are in the coding region and cause structural changes in the transporter, (2) there is extensive allelic heterogeneity, with only a few common mutations, (3) there is a paucity of polymorphisms both at the genomic and protein levels, implying high selective pressure, and (4) the high rate of mutation detection implies that there is no evidence for a second locus producing skeletal dysplasias mistaken for the DTDST chondrodysplasias. Correlation of the clinical phenotypes with the causation mutations suggests the following[94]: (1) homozygosity or compound heterozygosity for mutations predicting premature truncation of the protein or amino acid substitutions within transmembrane domains usually results in the more severe phenotype, ACG1B; (2) amino acid substitutions within extracellular loops or within the N- or C-terminal cytoplasmic domains may have less severe consequences on the transporter protein and, when compounded with a severe mutation, can rescue the phenotype from ACG1B to AO2 or DTD; (3) although originally identified in a patient with AO2[99], the *R279W* allele is associated with nonlethal dysplasias. In our experience, when homozygous, it results in mild DTD or MED (ref. 94, and unpublished observations, 1998)

Pathogenesis of DTDST Skeletal Dysplasias. Investigations on the pathology and pathogenesis of DTDST chondrodysplasias have focused almost exclusively on the skeletal system. The clinical phenotype points to an involvement of the tendons and joint capsules, but unfortunately, no data are available yet on these tissues.

There are at least two ways by which impairment of DTDST function may result in skeletal dysplasia. The first involves changes in the composition, architecture, and mechanical properties of the extracellular matrix in cartilage; the second, still somewhat hypothetical, may involve secondary changes in the fibroblast growth factor signaling pathway in chondrocytes that depends in part on heparan sulfate proteoglycans.

Chemistry and Pathology of Cartilage. On dissection, ACG1B cartilage is brownish, translucent, and friable rather than white, firm, and elastic as normal cartilage. Its consistency is similar to that of a cooked apple, and it can be cut through easily.[57] In this respect, it resembles cartilage from severe collagen type 2 disorders such as ACG2 or Kniest dysplasia. Light microscopy of cartilage of patients with ACG1B, AO2, and DTD reveals marked changes. In the patient described by Fraccaro, the cartilage looked so different from normal cartilage tissue that the name *achondrogenesis*, meant as failure of cartilage to differentiate properly, was coined (reference 45, and Fraccaro personal communication, 1997). The changes are generalized in ACG1B, resemble those in AO2 and DTD, but are less pronounced, and highly abnormal areas may alternate with those less severely disturbed. There is a reduction in the volume of the extracellular matrix with a corresponding increase in cell density. There is a dearth of ground substance in the matrix, corresponding to the deficiency in sulfated proteoglycans, which leads to the "unmasking" of collagen fibers. These become abnormally coarse and thus visible under the light microscope. In ACG1B, condensation of collagen fibrils around chondrocytes gives a "collagen ring" appearance.[55,57,59] In DTD, the pericellular space may be spared and the changes confined to the matrix of interterritorial spaces.[62,107] Secondarily, there is a disorganization of the growth plate, the organized transition zone between cartilage and bone tissue where cartilage growth and bone calcification take place. The coarse collagen fibers have led investigators on the false track of a collagen defect. An early report on a presumed structural abnormality of collagen type 2 in DTD[108] was disproved by more accurate studies[109] and by exclusion of linkage to the *COL2A1* locus.[110] The observation of a structural anomaly of collagen type 9 in another DTD patient[111] may be explained by the fact that collagen type 9 carries a chondroitin sulfate chain and also may be affected by undersulfation (see below).

Weak or absent metachromasia with cationic blue dyes such as toluidine or Alcian blue of cartilage tissue in DTDST disorders is a consequence of the deficiency in sulfated proteoglycans. Rimoin *et al.*[112] in 1974 studied DTD cartilage histology and suggested an "enzymatic deficiency in chondrocyte mucopolysaccharide metabolism," and Scheck *et al.*[113] reached similar conclusions. Van der Harten *et al.*[56] studied ACG1B cartilage matrix by semi-quantitative histochemical techniques, including a pH-dependent staining with Alcian blue, and postulated a "specific defect in the synthesis of sulfated proteoglycans." Proteoglycans extracted from ACG1B cartilage migrate more slowly on electrophoresis because of reduced negative charges and are poorly stained by cationic dyes.[59,114] The sulfate content of cartilage hydrolysate is markedly reduced in ACG1B[60] and moderately reduced in AO2 and DTD (A Superti-Furga and I Kaitila, unpublished results, 1997), while the glycosaminoglycan content is only mildly reduced.

Chondrocytes from a patients with ACG1B synthesized GAG chains that were of normal length but markedly sulfate-deficient.[115] The disaccharide composition of cartilage proteoglycans in patients with ACG1B, AO2, and DTD has been studied. While nonsulfated disaccharides account for 2 to 10 percent of total disaccharides in controls, they range from 11 to 77 percent in patients (being lower in DTD and highest in ACG1B).[23] These data prove that functional impairment of DTDST results in deficient sulfation of proteoglycans in cartilage. The mechanisms by which the characteristic coarsening of collagen fibers is produced probably involves regulation of collagen fibril diameter by sulfated proteoglycans that can bind to the surface of the collagen fibrils.[116]

The observation of significantly undersulfated proteoglycans in cartilage of patients with *DTDST* mutations implies that DTDST is a major sulfate transporter in chondrocytes. The observation of high DTDST mRNA expression in rat cartilage[42] is compatible with this notion. It is not clear yet why cartilage is the only tissue showing overt changes in the presence of *DTDST* mutations, whereas other proteoglycan-rich tissues (e.g., cornea) do not show overt changes. One possibility is that other sulfate transporters may mediate sulfate uptake in other tissues and cell types. Sulfate levels in plasma and urine of adult DTD patients are within normal ranges, excluding a significant impact of *DTDST* mutations on intestinal absorption or renal tubular secretion or resorption (A Superti-Furga and I Kaitila, unpublished results, 1998) and suggesting the presence of other transport mechanisms.[13]

A further modulating factor in phenotypic expression of *DTDST* mutations is sulfate production from the oxidation of cysteine (and perhaps other thiols). Rossi *et al.*[23] have found that despite their defect in the incorporation of exogenous sulfate, patients' fibroblasts synthesize proteoglycans that are extensively sulfated, almost to the extent of proteoglycans from control fibroblasts.[23] In some cell types, such as CHO cells[12] and mouse fibroblasts,[22] intracellular sulfate may be derived from cysteine rather than taken up from the extracellular medium. Indeed, cysteine-derived sulfate is incorporated at highly increased rates in *DTDST*-mutant fibroblasts and chondrocytes in vitro.[70] Alternative sulfate-producing pathways probably explain the ability of patients' fibroblasts to achieve reasonably good sulfation despite the defect in sulfate uptake. It has not been shown yet that this occurs in vivo and thus may modulate the tissue specificity of the phenotype.

Proteoglycans and Fibroblast Growth Factor Signaling. The notions that fibroblast growth factors (FGFs) require heparin sulfate for efficient signal transmission[117] and that mutations in FGF receptors led to abnormal skeletal development (see Chap. 210) have led to the hypothesis that malfunction of the FGF signaling pathways in chondrocytes may contribute to the development of skeletal dysplasia in presence of *DTDST* mutations.[41,118] It has not yet been shown that heparin sulfate proteoglycans, which are less abundant than chondroitin sulfate proteoglycans and largely cell-associated rather than in the extracellular matrix, are undersulfated in DTDST dysplasias; the sulfotransferase for heparan has a lower K_m for the sulfate donor, PAPS, than that for chondroitin, and therefore, heparin sulfation may remain normal even when chondroitin sulfation is impaired.[20,21] Moreover, the function of the various FGF/FGF receptor (FGFR) systems with respect to chondrocyte proliferation and differentiation is still poorly understood. A mouse model in which the *FGFR-3* gene had been disrupted was longer than control mice rather than dwarfed.[119] Considering these uncertainties, the clinical significance of the recent observation of subnormal proliferation response to FGF stimulation in chondrocytes in which sulfation was inhibited by treatment with chlorate[42] is uncertain.

The ATP Sulfurylase-APS Kinase Genes

Murine and human cDNA and genes coding for ATP sulfurylase-APS kinase have been characterized by several groups.[29–31,120] Recent studies on the brachymorphic mouse and human spondyloepimetaphyseal dysplasia (SEMD) revealed there are at least two *ATPSK* genes, *ATPSK1* and *ATPSK2*, present in both mouse and humans. *ATPSK1* is on human chromosome 4, whereas *ATPSK2* is on human chromosome 10 and mouse chromosome 19[121,122] (where the brachymorphic locus had been mapped[141]). There are preliminary indications of a different expression pattern of the two genes[121,122] (see below).

Human SEMD Associated with a Mutation in *ATPSK2*. Ahmad *et al.*[123] have described a large family from Pakistan in which SEMD segregated as a recessive trait. The clinical phenotype includes short stature, short and bowed lower limbs with enlarged knee joints, kyphoscoliosis, and mild brachydactyly. Radiographs showed platyspondyly, delayed ossification of the epiphyses, and osteoarthritic changes. Corneal changes were not reported (although slit-lamp examination was not performed), and intelligence was normal. Cohn's group showed cosegregation of the disorder with chromosome 10q, in a region syntenic with the brachymorphic locus on mouse chromosome 19.[122] Two pairs of genes coding for ATP sulfurylase-APS kinase were isolated from a homologous chromosomal region in humans and mice, respectively; *ATPSK1* was excluded as the locus for human SEMD and mouse brachymorphism, whereas a stop codon mutation in human *ATPSK2* cosegregated with human SEMD[122] and a missense mutation in mouse *ATPSK2* cosegregated with brachymorphism — the same mutation identified slightly earlier by Schwartz and her group[121] (see below).

Spondylar Dysplasia/Brachyolmia: A Possible Defect in Proteoglycan Sulfation. In 1973, Mourao *et al.*[124] described siblings with isolated, generalized platyspondyly (a condition also named *brachyolmia*, meaning "short trunk") and reported that these siblings excreted undersulfated chondroitin sulfate C in their urine. In a later report on the same family, peripheral corneal opacities were noted,[125] and in 1981, experiments with patients' sera were reported that suggested a defect in PAPS-chondroitin sulfotransferase was suggested.[126] Sewell *et al.*[127] reported on another patient with short stature and brachyolmia. When her urine glycosaminoglycans were digested with chondroitinase, the resulting disaccharides showed an abnormal mobility on electrophoresis consistent with a lack of sulfation. A similar observation was reported (but not shown) in yet another patient.[128] Horton *et al.*[129] have reported three siblings with a recessive condition they designated as "brachyolmia, Hobaek type" that may be the same condition; no biochemical studies were done, but cartilage histology showed glycosaminoglycan deficiency and condensation of collagen fibers, findings that may well fit with a proteoglycan defect. Shohat *et al.*[130] reported patients with similar findings, again without biochemical studies. In summary, it is possible that one form of generalized platyspondyly exists that is associated with undersulfation of cartilage proteoglycans,[131] but the biochemical and molecular bases remain to be characterized.

ANIMAL MODEL: THE BRACHYMORPHIC MOUSE

Brachymorphic (*bm*) is a spontaneously occurring, recessively inherited mouse mutation described by Lane and Dickie in 1968.[132] The phenotype of homozygous *bm/bm* mice becomes apparent a few days after birth and consists of a dome-shaped skull and an abnormally short and thick tail. Their growth rate is retarded, but adult weight is close to normal. The limb bones are shorter than normal, but their width is normal.

The *bm* mouse has considerably stimulated research into proteoglycan and sulfate metabolism and for a long time was the only model for abnormal proteoglycan synthesis. Orkin *et al.*[133] first observed ultrastructural changes in cartilage suggestive of defective proteoglycan synthesis and then showed, by DEAE chromatography and cellulose acetate electrophoresis of cartilage glycosaminoglycans, that chondroitin sulfate was undersulfated.[134] Schwartz *et al.*[135] demonstrated that in *bm* cartilage, $^{35}SO_4^{2}$ incorporation was reduced when inorganic sulfate was offered but normal when PAPS was used and suggested that the defect may be impaired PAPS synthesis. Sugahara and Schwartz[136] went on to show that the activities of ATP sulfurylase and APS kinase were moderately and markedly reduced, respectively, in brachymorphic cartilage. Subsequently, it was shown that the biochemical defect was expressed in cartilage and liver but not in skin or brain.[137–139] Copurification of the two enzymatic activities from rat chondrosarcoma and mouse cartilage indicated that they resided in a single protein molecule, and it could be shown that the bifunctional enzyme from *bm* cartilage was defective in the "channeling" of the product of the first reaction (APS) to the second reaction.[33] The quest for the ATP sulfurylase-APS kinase gene yielded two closely related genes, termed *SK1* and *SK2;* their expression is tissue-specific, and a mutation in the kinase domain of *SK2* causes the brachymorphic phenotype.[121] Expression of the mutated *SK2* in liver (and possibly other tissues) probably explains abnormalities in hepatic sulfate conjugation and in blood clotting seen in brachymorphic mice.[140,141]

OPEN QUESTIONS AND RESEARCH DIRECTIONS

Insight into the biochemical and molecular basis of skeletal dysplasias associated with impaired sulfation of cartilage proteoglycans has highlighted the importance of proteoglycans in cartilage homeostasis and skeletal growth and development and at the same time revealed new aspects on sulfate metabolism. As stated earlier, a unifying model of whole-body sulfate metabolism and the role of the different organs and tissues therein is still missing. The observation that fibroblasts of patients with *DTDST* mutations make extensive use of cysteine-derived sulfate would indicate a possible therapeutic avenue, but the task of delivering micro-to millimolar concentrations of thiols to the chondrocyte by the oral route appears extremely arduous at present.

Genetic defects in one of several sulfotransferase activities[142] can be expected to produce clinical phenotypes, according to substrate specificity and tissue-specific expression, including skeletal phenotypes. A genetic deficiency of the core protein of aggrecan, the major chondroitin sulfate proteoglycan in cartilage, causes severe chondrodysplasia in chickens (nanomelia)[143] and in mice (cartilage matrix deficient)[144]; the human counterpart remains to be identified. Cloning of the gene responsible for Pendred syndrome[145] (MIM 274600; see Chap. 158), a form of heritable deafness associated with thyroid gland dysfunction, has revealed homology with *DRA1*, a chloride transporter (mutations in which cause congenital chloride diarrhea[146]), and indirectly with *DTDST*, leading to speculation on its possible role as a sulfate transporter. Although proof that the main role of pendredin is indeed sulfate transport is lacking (it is possible that chloride, rather than sulfate, transport is its main function), elucidation of the pathogenesis of this disorder may yield further insights into cell-specific aspects of sulfate metabolism.

ACKNOWLEDGMENTS

I am very much indebted to Dr. Johanna Hästbacka (Helsinki), Dr. Ilkka Kaitila (Helsinki), and Dr. Antonio Rossi (Pavia) for sharing of unpublished data and for helpful comments and to the Swiss National Foundation (32-36387.92, 32-45401.95, 32-55898.98) for continuous support.

REFERENCES

1. Rodén L: Structure and metabolism of proteoglycans, in Lennarz WJ (ed): *The Biochemistry of Glycoproteins and Proteoglycans*. New York, Plenum Press, 1980, pp 267–371.
2. Heinegard D, Paulsson M: Structure and metabolism of proteoglycans, in Piez KA, Reddi AH (eds): *Extracellular Matrix Biochemistry*. New York, Elsevier, 1984, pp 277–328.
3. Lipmann F: Biological sulfate activation and transfer. *Science* **128**:575, 1958.
4. Leyh TS: The physical biochemistry and molecular genetics of sulfate activation. *Crit Rev Biochem Mol Biol* **28**:515, 1993.
5. Norbis F, Perego C, Markovich D, Stange G, Verri T, Murer H: cDNA cloning of a rat small-intestinal Na^+/SO_4^2 cotransporter. *Pflugers Arch* **428**:217, 1994.
6. Markovich D, Forgo J, Stange G, Biber J, Murer H: Expression cloning of rat renal Na^+/SO_4^2 cotransport. *Proc Natl Acad Sci USA* **90**:8073, 1993.
7. Markovich D, Bissig M, Sorribas V, Hagenbuch B, Meirer PJ, Murer H: Expression of rat renal sulfate transport systems in *Xenopus laevis* oocytes: Functional characterization and molecular identification. *J Biol Chem* **269**:3022, 1994.
8. Hugentobler G, Meier P: Multispecific anion exchange in basolateral (sinusoidal) rat liver plasma membrane vesicles. *Am J Physiol* **251**:G656, 1986.
9. Meier PJ, Valantinas J, Hugentobler G, Rahm I: Bicarbonate sulfate exchange in canalicular rat liver plasma membranes. *Am J Physiol* **253**:G461, 1987.
10. Bissig M, Hagenbuch B, Stieger R, Koller T, Meirer PJ: Functional expression cloning of the canalicular sulfate transport system of rat hepatocytes. *J Biol Chem* **269**:3017, 1994.
11. Elgavish A, Smith JB, Pillion DJ, Meezan E: Sulfate transport in human lung fibroblasts (IMR-90). *J Cell Physiol* **125**:243, 1985.
12. Esko JD, Elgavish A, Prasthofer T, Taylor EH, Weinke JL: Sulfate transport-deficient mutants of Chinese hamster ovary cells. *J Biol Chem* **261**:15725, 1986.
13. Murer H, Markovich D, Biber J: Renal and small intestinal sodium-dependent symporters of phosphate and sulphate. *J Exp Biol* **196**:167, 1994.
14. Cole DE, Baldwin LS, Stirk LJ: Increased renal reabsorption of inorganic sulfate in third-trimester high-risk pregnancies. *Obstet Gynecol* **66**:485, 1985.
15. Elgavish A, Meezan E: Sulfation by human lung fibroblasts: SO_4^{-2} and sulfur-containing amino acids as sources for macromolecular sulfation. *Am J Physiol* **260**:L450,1991.
16. Humphries DE, Sugumaran G, Silbert JE: Decreasing sulfation of proteoglycans produced by cultured cells. *Methods Enzymol* **179**:428, 1989.
17. Sobue M, Takeuchi J, Ito K, Kimata K, Suzuki S: Effect of environmental sulfate concentration on the synthesis of low and high sulfated chondroitin sulfates by chick embryo cartilage. *J Biol Chem* **253**:6190, 1978.
18. Ito K, Kimata K, Sonue M, Suzuki S: altered proteoglycan synthesis by epihyseal cartilages in culture at low SO_4^2 concentration. *J Biol Chem* **257**:917, 1982.
19. van der Kraan PM, de Vries BJ, Vitters EL, van den Berg WB, van de Putte LBA: The effect of low sulfate concentrations on the glycosaminoglycan synthesis in anatomically intact articular cartilage of the mouse. *J Orthop Res* **7**:645, 1989.
20. Humphries DE, Silbert CK, Silbert JE: Glycosaminoglycan production by bovine aortic endothelial cells cultured in sulfate-depleted medium. *J Biol Chem* **261**:9122, 1986.
21. Humphries DE, Silbert CK, Silbert JE: Sulphation by cultured cells: Cysteine, cysteinesulphinic acid and sulphite as sources for proteoglycan sulphate. *Biochem J* **252**:305, 1988.
22. Keller JM, Keller KM: Amino acid sulfur as a source of sulfate for sulfated proteoglycans produced by Swiss mouse 3T3 cells. *Biochim Biophys Acta* **926**:139, 1987.
23. Rossi A, Kaitila I, Wilcox WR, Rimoin DL, Steinmann B, Cetta G, Superti-Furga A: In vivo and in vitro proteoglycan sulfation in sulfate transporter chondrodyplasias. *Matrix Biol* **17**:361, 1998.
24. Schwartz NB, Lyle S, Ozeran JD, Li H, Deyrup A, Ng K, Westley J: Sulfate activation and trasport in mammals: System components and mechanisms. *Chem Biol Interact* **109**(1–3):143, 1998.
25. Rosenthal E, Leustek T: A multifunctional *Urechis caupo* protein, PAPS synthetase, has both ATP sulfurylase and APS kinase activities. *Gene* **165**:243, 1995.
26. Jullien D, Crozatier M, Kas E: cDNA sequence and expression pattern of the *Drosophila melanogaster* PAPS synthetase gene: A new salivary gland marker. *Mech Dev* **68**:179, 1997.
27. Geller DH, Henry JG, Belch J, Schwartz NB: Co-purification and characterization of ATP-sulfurylase and adenosine-5′-phosphosulfate kinase from rat chondrosarcoma. *J Biol Chem* **262**:7374, 1987.
28. Lyle S, Stanczak J, Ng K, Schwartz NB: Rat chondrosarcoma ATP sulfurylase and adenosine 5′-phosphosulfate kinase reside on a single bifunctional protein. *Biochemistry* **33**:5920, 1994.
29. Li H, Deyrup A, Mensch JR, Domowicz M, Konstantinidis AK, Schwartz NB: The isolation and characterization of cDNA encoding the mouse bifunctional ATP sulfurylase-adenosine 5′-phosphosulfate kinase. *J Biol Chem* **270**:29453, 1995.
30. Venkatachalam KV, Akita H, Strott CA: Molecular cloning, expression, and characterization of human bifunctional 3′-phosphoadenosine 5′-phosphosulfate synthase and ist functional domains. *J Biol Chem* **273**:19311, 1998.
31. Yanagisawa K, Sakakibara Y, Suiko M, Takami Y, Nakayama T, Nakajima H, Takayanagi K, Natori Y, Liu MC: cDNA cloning, expression, and characterization of the human bifunctional ATP sulfurylase/adenosine 5′-phosphosulfate kinase enzyme. *Biosci Biotechnol Biochem* **62**(5):1037, 1998.
32. Lyle S, Ozeran JD, Stanczak J, Westley J, Schwartz NB: Intermediate channeling between ATP sulfurylase and adenosine 5′-phosphosulfate kinase from rat chondrosarcoma. *Biochemistry* **33**:6822, 1994.
33. Lyle S, Stanczak JD, Westley J, Schwartz NB: Sulfate-activating enzymes in normal and brachymorphic mice: Evidence for a channeling defect. *Biochemistry* **34**:940, 1995.
34. Klaassen CD, Boles JW: Sulfation and sulfotransferase 5: The importance of 3′-phosphoadenosine 5′-phosphosulfate (PAPS) in the regulation of sulfation. *FASEB J* **11**:404, 1997.
35. Capasso JM, Hirschberg CB: Mechanisms of glycosylation and sulfation in the Golgi apparatus: Evidence for nucleotide sugar/nucleoside monophosphate and nucleotide sulfate/nucleoside monophosphate antiports in the Golgi apparatus membrane. *Proc Natl Acad Sci USA* **81**:7051, 1984.
36. Ozeran JD, Westley J, Schwartz NB: Kinetics of PAPS translocase: Evidence for an antiport mechanism. *Biochemistry* **35**:3685, 1996.
37. Ozeran JD, Westley J, Schwartz NB: Identification and partial purification of PAPS translocase. *Biochemistry* **35**:3695, 1996.
38. Mandon EC, Milla ME, Kempner E, Hirschberg CB: Purification of the Golgi adenosine 3′-phosphate 5′-phosphosulfate transporter, homodimer within the membrane. *Proc Natl Acad Sci USA* **91**:10707, 1994.
39. Hästbacka J, Kaitila I, Sistonen P, de la Chapelle A: Diastrophic dysplasia gene maps to the distal long arm of chromosome 5. *Proc Natl Acad Sci USA* **87**:8056, 1990.

40. Hästbacka J, de la Chapelle A, Kaitila I, Sistonen P, Weaver A, Lander ES: Linkage disequilibrium mapping in isolated founder populations: Diastrophic dysplasia in Finland. *Nature Genet* **2**:204, 1992.
41. Hastbacka J, de la Chapelle A, Mahtani MM, Clines G, Reeve-Daly MP, Daly M, Hamilton BA, Kusumi K, Trivedi B, Weaver A, Coloma A, Lovett M, Buckler A, Kaitila I, Lander ES: The diastrophic dysplasia gene encodes a novel sulfate transporter: Positional cloning by fine-structure linkage disequilibrium mapping. *Cell* **78**:1073, 1994.
42. Satoh H, Susaki M, Shukunami C, Iyama K, Negoro T, Hiraki Y: Functional analysis of diastrophic dysplasia sufate transporter: Its involvement in growth regulation of chondrocytes mediated by sulfated proteoglycans. *J Biol Chem* **273**:12307, 1998.
43. Kobayashi T, Sugimoto T, Saijoh K, Fukase M, Chihara K: Cloning of mouse diastrophic dysplasia sulfate transporter gene induced during osteoblast differentiation by bone morphogenetic protein-2. *Gene* **198**:341, 1997.
44. Kobayashi T, Sugimoto T, Saijoh K, Fujii M, Chihara K: Cloning and characterization of the 5′-flanking region of the mouse diastrophic dysplasia sulfate transporter gene. *Biochem Biophys Res Commun* **238**:738, 1997.
45. Fraccaro M: Contributo allo studio del mesenchima osteopoietico-l'acondrogenesi. *Folia Hered Pathol* **1**:190, 1952.
46. Grebe H: Die Achondrogenesis: ein einfach-rezessives *Erbmerkmal. Folia Hered Pathol (Milano)* **2**:23, 1952 (followed by several illustrations).
47. Wiedemann HR, Remagen W, Hienz HA, Gorlin RJ, Maroteaux P: Achondrogenesis within the scope of connately manifested generalized skeletal dysplasias. *Z Kinderheilk* **116**:223, 1974.
48. Schulte MJ, Lenz W, Vogel M: Letale Achondrogenesis: eine Übersicht über 56 Fälle. *Klin Paediatr* **191**:327, 1978.
49. Yang SS, Brough AJ, Garewal GS, Bernstein J: Two types of heritable lethal achondrogenesis. *J Pediatr* **85**:796, 1974.
50. Spranger J, Langer LO, Wiedemann HR: *Bone Dysplasias: An Atlas of Constitutional Disorders of Skeletal Development.* Stuttgart, Gustav Fischer Verlag, 1974.
51. Yang SS, Heidelberger KP, Bernstein J: Intracytoplasmic inclusion bodies in the chondrocytes of type I lethal achondrogenesis. *Hum Pathol* **7**:667, 1976.
52. Eyre DR, Upton MP, Shapiro FD, Wilkinson RH, Vawter GF: Nonexpression of cartilage type II collagen in a case of Langer-Saldino achondrogenesis. *Am J Hum Genet* **39**:52, 1986.
53. Godfrey M, Hollister DW: Type II achondrogenesis-hypochondrogenesis: Identification of abnormal type II collagen. *Am J Hum Genet* **43**:904, 1988.
54. Spranger J, Winterpacht A, Zabel B: The type II collagenopathies: A spectrum of chondrodysplasias. *Eur J Paediatr* **153**:56, 1994.
55. Borochowitz Z, Lachman R, Adornian GE, Spear G, Jones K, Rimoin DL: Achondrogenesis type I: Delineation of further heterogeneity and identification of two distinct subgroups. *J Pediatr* **112**:23, 1988.
56. van der Harten HJ, Brons JTJ, Dijkstra PF, Niermeyer MF, Meijer CJLM, van Giejn HP, Arts NFT: Achondrogenesis-hypochondrogenesis: The spectrum of chondrogenesis imperfecta. *Pediatr Pathol* **8**:571, 1988.
57. Superti-Furga A: Achondrogenesis type 1B. *J Med Genet* **33**:957, 1996.
58. Superti-Furga A: Achondrogenesis type 1B: A defect in the metabolic activation of sulfate leading to the synthesis of non-sulfated proteoglycans in cartilage and cultured fibroblasts (Abstract). *Am J Hum Genet* **55**(suppl):A344, 1994.
59. Superti-Furga A: A defect in the metabolic activation of sulfate in a patient with achondrogenesis type 1B. *Am J Hum Genet* **55**:1137, 1994.
60. Superti-Furga A, Hästbacka J, Wilcox WR, Cohn DH, van der Harten JJ, Rossi A, Blau N, Rimoin DL, Steinmann B, Lander ES, Gitzelmann R: Achondrogenesis type IB is caused by mutations in the diastrophic dysplasia sulphate transporter gene. *Nature Genet* **12**:100, 1996.
61. Sillence DO, Kozlowsky K, Rogers JG, Sprague PL, Cullity GJ, Osborn RA: Atelosteogenesis: Evidence for heterogeneity. *Pediatr Radiol* **17**:112, 1987.
62. Briner J, Brandner M: Pathologisch-anatomische und radiologische Untersuchungen bei zwei frühgeborenen Geschwistern mit diastrophischem Zwergwuchs und ausgeprägten Wirbelsäulenveränderungen. *Virchows Arch [A]* **364**:165, 1974.
63. Freedman SI, Taber P, Hollister DW, Rimoin DL: A lethal form of diastrophic dwarfism. *Birth Defects* **10**:43, 1974.
64. Gustavson KH, Holmgren G, Jagell S, Jorulf H: Lethal and non-lethal diastrophic dysplasia. *Clin Genet* **28**:321, 1985.
65. Schrander-Stumpel C, Havenith M, Linden EV, Maertzdorf W, Offermans J, van der Harten JJ: De la Chapelle dysplasia (atelosteogenesis type II): Case report and review of the literature. *Clin Dysmorphol* **3**:318, 1994.
66. Newbury-Ecob R: Atelosteogenesis type 2. *J Med Genet* **35**:49, 1998.
67. Sillence D, Worthington S, Dixon J, Osborn R, Kozlowski K: Atelosteogenesis syndromes: A review, with comments on their pathogenesis. *Pediatr Radiol* **27**:388, 1997.
68. De la Chapelle A, Maroteaux P, Havu N, Granroth G: Une rare dysplasie osseuse lethale de transmission recessive autosomique. *Arch Fr Pediatr* **29**:759, 1972.
69. McAlister WH, Crane JP, Bucy RP, Craig RB: A new neonatal short limbed dwarfism. *Skeletal Radiol* **13**:271, 1985.
70. Rossi A, Bonaventure J, Delezoide AL, Superti-Furga A, Cetta G: Undersulfation of cartilage proteoglycans ex vivo and increased contribution of amino acid sulfur to sulfation in vitro in McAlister dysplasia/atelosteogenesis type 2. *Eur J Biochem* **248**:741, 1997.
71. Lamy M, Maroteaux P: Le nanisme diastrophique. *Presse Med* **68**:1976, 1960.
72. Walker BA, Scott CI, Hall JG, Murdoch JL, McKusick VA: Diastrophic dwarfism. *Medicine* **51**:41, 1972.
73. Horton WA, Rimoin DL, Lachmann RS, Skovby F, Hollister DW, Spranger J, Scott CI, Hall JG: The phenotypic variability of diastrophic dysplasia. *J Pediatr* **93**:609, 1978.
74. Gollop TR, Eigier A: Prenatal ultrasound diagnosis of diastrophic dysplasia at 16 weeks. *Am J Med Genet* **27**:321, 1987.
75. Salle B, Picot C, Vauzelle JL, Deffrenne P, Monnet P, Francois R, Robert J-M: Le nanisme diastrophique — a propos de trois observations chez le nouveau-né. *Pediatrie* **21**:311, 1966.
76. Lapunzina P, Arberas C, Fernandez MC, Tello AM: Diastrophic dysplasia diagnosed in a case published 100 years ago. *Am J Med Genet* **77**:334, 1998.
77. Kash IJ, Sane SM, Samaha FJ, Briner J: Cervical cord compression in diastrophic dwarfism. *J Pediatr* **94**:862, 1974.
78. Kozlowski K, Barylak A: Diastrophic dwarfism. *Aust Radiol* **18**:398, 1974.
79. Krecak J, Starshak RJ: Cervical kyphosis in diastrophic dwarfism: CT and MR findings. *Pediatr Radiol* **17**:321, 1987.
80. Forese LL, Berdon WE, Harcke HAT, Wagner ML, Lachman R, Chorney GS, Roye DP: Severe mid-cervical kyphosis with cord compression in Larsen's syndrome and diastrophic dysplasia: Unrelated syndromes with similar radiologic findings and neurosurgical implications. *Pediatr Radiol* **25**:136, 1995.
81. Lachman RS: The cervical spine in the skeletal dysplasias and associated disorders. *Pediatr Radiol* **27**:402, 1997.
82. Griffin JR, Ault JE, Sillence DO, Rimoin DL: Optometric screening in achondroplasia, diastrophic dysplasia, and spondyloepiphyseal dysplasia congenita. *Am J Optometry Physiol Optics* **57**:118, 1980.
83. Horton WA, Hall JG, Scott CI, Pyeritz RE, Rimoin DL: Growth curves for height for diastrophic dysplasia, spondyloepiphyseal dysplasia congenita, and pseudoachondroplasia. *Am J Dis Child* **136**:316, 1982.
84. Mäkitie O, Kaitila M: Growth in diastrophic dysplasia. *J Pediatr* **130**:641, 1997.
85. Rintala A, Marttinen E, Rantala SL, Kaitila I: Cleft palate in diastrophic dysplasia: Morphology, results of treatment and complications. *Scand J Plast Reconstr Surg* **20**:45, 1986.
86. Karlstedt E, Kaitila I, Pirinen S: Phenotypic features of dentition in diastrophic dysplasia. *J Craniofac Genet Dev Biol* **16**:164, 1996.
87. Poussa M, Merikanto J, Ryoppy S, Marttinen E, Kaitila I: The spine in diastrophic dysplasia. *Spine* **16**:881, 1991.
88. Vaara P, Peltonen J, Poussa M, Merikanto J, Nurminen M, Kaitila I, Ryoppy S: Development of the hip in diastrophic dysplasia. *J Bone Joint Surg* **80B**:315, 1998.
89. Vaara P, Martinen E, Peltonen J: Ultrasonography of the patellofemoral joint in diastrophic dysplasia. *J Pediatr Orthop* **17**:512, 1997.
90. Ryoppy S, Poussa M, Merikanto J, Marttinen E, Kaitila I: Foot deformities in diastrophic dysplasia: An analysis of 102 patients. *J Bone Joint Surg* **74B**:441, 1992.
91. Butler MG, Gale DD, Meaney FJ: Metacarpophalangeal pattern profile analysis in diastrophic dysplasia. *Am J Med Genet* **28**:685, 1987.

92. Lachman R, Sillence D, Rimoin D, Horton W, Hall J, Scott C, Spranger J, Langer L: Diastrophic dysplasia: The death of a variant. *Radiology* **140**:79, 1981.
93. Hall BD: Diastrophic dysplasia: Extreme variability within a sibship. *Am J Med Genet* **63**:28, 1996.
94. Superti-Furga A, Neumann L, Riebel T, Eich G, Steinmann B, Spranger J, Kunze J: Recessively inherited multiple epiphyseal dysplasia with normal stature, clubfoot and double-layered patella caused by a DTDST mutation. *J Med Genet* **36**:621, 1999.
95. Spranger J, Maroteaux P: The lethal osteochondrodysplasias. *Adv Hum Genet* **19**:1, 1990.
96. Tretter AE, Saunders RC, Meyers CM, Dungan JS, Grumbach K, Sun CC, Campbell AB, Wulfsberg EA: Antenatal diagnosis of lethal skeletal dysplasias. *Am J Med Genet* **75**:518, 1998.
97. Eteson DJ, Beluffi GD, Burgio GR, Belloni C, Lachman RS, Rimoin DL: Pseudodiastrophic dysplasia: A distinct newborn skeletal dysplasia. *J Pediatr* **109**:635, 1986.
98. Cetta G, Rossi A, Burgio GR, Beluffi G: Diastrophic dysplasia sulfate transporter (*DTDST*) gene is not involved in pseudodiastrophic dysplasia. *Am J Med Genet* **73**(4):493, 1997.
99. Hästbacka J, Superti-Furga A, Wilcox WR, Rimoin DL, Cohn DH, Lander ES: Atelosteogenesis type II is caused by mutations in the diastrophic dysplasia sulphate transporter gene (*DTDST*): Evidence for a phenotypic series involving three chondrodysplasias. *Am J Hum Genet* **58**:255, 1996.
100. Gordienko IY, Grechanina EYa, Sopko NI, Tarapurova EN, Mikchailets LP: Prenatal diagnosis of osteochondrodysplasias in high risk pregnancy. *Am J Med Genet* **63**:90, 1996.
101. Kaitila I, Ammala P, Karjalainen O, Liukkonen S, Rapola J: Early prenatal detection of diastrophic dysplasia. *Prenat Diagn* **3**:237, 1983.
102. Gembruch U, Niesen M, Kehrberg H, Hansmann M: Diastrophic dysplasia: A specific prenatal diagnosis by ultrasound. *Prenat Diagn* **8**:539, 1988.
103. Hastbacka J, Salonen R, Laurila P, de la Chapelle A, Kaitila I: Prenatal diagnosis of diastrophic dysplasia with polymorphic DNA markers. *J Med Genet* **30**:265, 1993.
104. Rossi A, van der Harten HJ, Beemer FA, Kleijer WJ, Gitzelmann R, Steinmann B, Superti-Furga A: Phenotypic and genotypic overlap between atelosteogenesis type 2 and diastrophic dysplasia. *Hum Genet* **98**:657, 1996.
105. Cai G, Nakayama N, Hiraki Y, Ozone K: Mutational analysis of the *DTDST* gene in a fetus with achondrogenesis type 1B. *Am J Med Genet* **78**:58, 1998.
105a. Hastbacka J, Kerrebrock A, Mokkala K, Clines G, Lovett M, Kaitila I, de la Chapella A, Lander ES: Identification of the Finnish founder mutation for diastrophic dysplasia (DTD). *Eur J Hum Genet* **7**:664, 1999.
106. Superti-Furga A, Rossi A, Steinmann B, Gitzelmann R: A chondrodysplasia family produced by mutations in the diastrophic dysplasia sulfate transporter gene: Genotype/phenotype correlations. *Am J Med Genet* **63**:144, 1996.
107. Shapiro F: Light and electron microscopic abnormalities in diastrophic dysplasia cartilage. *Calcif Tissue Int* **51**:324, 1992.
108. Stanescu R, Stanescu V, Maroteaux P: Abnormal pattern of segment long spacing (SLS) cartilage collagen in diastrophic dysplasia. *Coll Relat Res* **2**:111, 1982.
109. Murray LW, Hollister DW, Rimoin DL: Diastrophic dysplasia: Evidence against a defect of type II collagen. *Matrix* **9**:459, 1989.
110. Elima K, Kaitila I, Mikonoja L, Elonsalo U, Peltonen L, Vuorio E: Exclusion of the *COL2A1* gene as the mutation site in diastrophic dysplasia. *J Med Genet* **26**:314, 1989.
111. Diab M, Wu JJ, Shapiro F, Eyre D: Abnormality of type IX collagen in a patient with diastrophic dysplasia. *Am J Med Genet* **49**:402, 1994.
112. Rimoin DL, Hollister DW, Lachman RS, Kaufman RL, McAlister WH, Rosenthal RE, Hughes GNF: Histologic studies in the chondrodystrophies. *Birth Defects* **10**:275, 1974.
113. Scheck M, Parker J, Daentl D: Hyaline cartilage changes in diastrophic dwarsfism. *Virchows Arch [A]* **378**(4):347, 1978.
114. Kuijer R, van de Stadt RJ, De Koning MH, van Campen GP, van der Korst JK: Influence of cartilage proteoglycans on type II collagen fibrillogenesis. *Connect Tissue Res* **17**:83, 1988.
115. Rossi A, Bonaventure J, Delezoide AL, Cetta G, Superti-Furga A: Undersulphation of proteoglycans synthesized by chondrocytes from a patient with achondrogenesis type 1B homozygous for a Leu483Pro substitution in the diastrophic dysplasia sulphate transporter. *J Biol Chem* **271**:18456, 1996.
116. Hedlund H, Mengarelli-Widholm S, Heinegard D, Reinholt FP, Svensson O: Fibromodulin distribution and association with collagen. *Matrix Biol* **14**:227, 1994.
117. Gallagher JT: Heparan sulphates as membrane receptors for the fibroblast growth factors. *Eur J Clin Chem Clin Biochem* **32**:239, 1994.
118. Wallis GA: Cartilage disorders: The importance of being sulphated. *Curr Biol* **5**:225, 1995.
119. Colvin JS, Bohne BA, Harding GW, McEwen DG, Ornitz DM: Skeletal overgrowth and deafness in mice lacking fibroblast growth factor receptor 3. *Nature Genet* **12**:390, 1996.
120. Girard JP, Baekkevold ES, Amalric F: Sulfation in high endothelial venules: Cloning and expression of the human PAPS synthetase. *FASEB J* **12**:603, 1998.
121. Kurima K, Warman ML, Srinivasan K, Domowicz M, Krueger RC Jr, Deyrup A, Schwartz NB: A member of a family of sulfate-activating enzymes causes murine brachymorphism. *Proc Natl Acad Sci USA* **95**:8681, 1998.
122. Ul Haque MF, King LM, Krakow D, Cantor RM, Rusiniak ME, Swank RT, Superti-Furga A, Haq S, Abbas H, Ahmad W, Ahmad M, Cohn DH: Mutations in novel ATP sulfurylase/APS kinase orthologues in human spondyloepipmetaphyseal dysplasia and the brachymorphic mouse. *Nature Genet* **20**:157, 1998.
123. Ahmad M, Ul Haque MF, Ahmad W, Abbas H, Haque S, Krakow D, Rimoin DL, Lachman RS, Cohn DH: Distinct, autosomal recessive form of spondyloepimetaphyseal dysplasia segregating in an inbred Pakistani kindred. *Am J Med Genet* **78**:468, 1998.
124. Mourao PAS, Toledo SPA, Nader HB, Dietrich CP: Excretion of chondroitin sulfate C with low sulfate content by patients with generalized platyspondyly (brachyolmia). *Biochem Med* **7**:415, 1973.
125. Toledo SPA, Mourao PAS, Lamego C, Alves CAR, Dietrich CP, Assis LM, Mattar E: Recessively inherited, late onset, spondylar dysplasia and peripheral corneal opacity with anomalies in urinary mucopolysaccharides: A possible error of chondroitin-6-sulfate synthesis. *Am J Med Genet* **2**:385, 1978.
126. Mourao PAS, Kato S, Donnelly PV: Spondyloepiphyseal dysplasia, chondroitin sulfate type: A possible defect of PAPS-chondroitin sulfate sulfotransferase in humans. *Biochem Biophys Res Commun* **98**:388, 1981.
127. Sewell AC, Wern C, Pontz BF: Brachyolmia: A skeletal dysplasia with an altered mucopolysaccharide excretion. *Clin Genet* **40**:312, 1991.
128. Grain L, Duke O, Thompson G, Davies EG: Toledo type brachyolmia. *Arch Dis Child* **71**:448, 1994.
129. Horton WA, Langer LO, Collins DL, Dwyer C: Brachyolmia, recessive type (Hobaek): A clinical, radiographic, and histochemical study. *Am J Med Genet* **16**:201, 1983.
130. Shohat M, Lachman R, Gruber HE, Rimoin DL: Brachyolmia: Radiographic and genetic evidence of heterogeneity. *Am J Med Genet* **33**(2):209, 1989.
131. Toledo SPA: Spondylar dysplasia (SD)/brachyolmia (BO), type I: Search for qualitative anomalies in glycosaminoglycans. *Clin Genet* **42**:213, 1992.
132. Lane PW, Dickie MM: Three recessive mutations producing disproportionate dwarfism in mice: Achondroplasia, brachymorphic, and stubby. *J Hered* **59**:300, 1968.
133. Orkin RW, Williams BR, Cranley RE, Poppke DC, Brown KS: Defects in the cartilaginous growth plates of brachymorphic mice. *J Cell Biol* **73**:287, 1977.
134. Orkin RW, Pratt RM, Martin GR: Undersulfated chondroitin sulfate in the cartilage matrix of brachymorphic mice. *Dev Biol* **50**:82, 1976.
135. Schwartz NB, Ostrowsky V, Brown KS, Pratt RM: Defective PAPS-synthesis in epiphyseal cartilage from brachymorphic mice. *Biochem Biophys Res Commun* **82**:173, 1978.
136. Sugahara K, Schwartz NB: Defect in 3′-phosphoadenosine 5′-phosphosulfate formation in brachymorphic mice. *Proc Natl Acad Sci USA* **76**:6615, 1979.
137. Pennypacker JP, Kimata K, Brown KS: Brachymorphic mice (*bm/bm*): A generalized biochemical defect expressed primarily cartilage. *Dev Biol* **81**:280, 1981.
138. Sugahara K, Schwartz NB: Defect in 3′-phosphoadenosine 5′-phosphosulfate synthesis in brachymorphic mice: I. Characterization of the defect. *Arch Biochem Biophys* **214**:589, 1982.
139. Sugahara K, Schwartz NB: Defect in 3′-phosphoadenosine 5′-phosphosulfate synthesis in brachymorphic mice: II. Tissue distribution of the defect. *Arch Biochem Biophys* **214**:602, 1982.

140. Lyman SD, Poland A: Effect of the brachymorphic trait in mice on xenobiotic sulfate ester formation. *Biochem Pharmacol* **32**:3345, 1983.
141. Rusiniak ME, O'Brien EP, Novak EK, Barone SM, McGarry MP, Reddington M, Swank RT: Molecular markers near the mouse brachymorphic (*bm*) gene, which affects connective tissues and bleeding time. *Mamm Genome* **7**:98, 1996.
142. Weinshilboum RM, Otterness DM, Aksoy IA, Wood TC, Her C, Raftogianis RB: Sulfotransferase molecular biology: cDNAs and genes. *FASEB J* **11**:3, 1997.
143. Li H, Schwartz NB, Vertel BM: cDNA cloning of chick cartilage chondroitin sulfate (aggrecan) core protein and identification of a stop codon in the aggrecan gene associated with the chondrodystrophy, nanomelia. *J Biol Chem* **268**:23504, 1993.
144. Watanabe H, Kimata K, Line S, Strong D, Gao L, Kozak CA, Yamada Y: Mouse cartilage matrix deficiency (cmd) caused by a 7 bp deletion in the aggrecan gene. *Nature Genet* **7**:154, 1994.
145. Everett L A,Glaser B, Beck JC, Idol JR, Buchs A, Heyman M, Adawi F, Hazani E, Nassir E, Baxevanis AD, Sheffield VC, Green ED: Pendred syndrome is caused by mutations in a putative sulphate transporter gene (*PDS*). *Nature Genet* **17**:411, 1997.
146. Hoglund P, Haila S, Socha J, Tomaszewski L, Saarialho-Kere U, Karjalainen-Lindsberg ML, Airola K, Holmberg C, de la Chapelle A, Kere J: Mutations of the down-regulated in adenoma (*DRA*) gene cause congenital chloride diarrhoea. *Nature Genet* **14**:316, 1996.

CHAPTER 203

Familial Cardiac Arrhythmias

Mark T. Keating ▪ Michael C. Sanguinetti

1. **Long QT syndrome is characterized clinically by (a) recurrent syncope; (b) sudden death and aborted sudden death; (c) episodic ventricular tachyarrhythmias such as *torsade de pointes* and ventricular fibrillation; and (d) prolongation of the QT interval on surface electrocardiogram. In some cases, long QT syndrome is associated with simple syndactyly. This disorder is inherited as an autosomal dominant trait (Romano-Ward syndrome; MIM 192500, 152427, 600163, 600919, 601005, and 176261). Long QT syndrome can be associated with congenital deafness in the Jervell and Lange-Nielsen syndrome (MIM 220400). In this disorder, congenital deafness is inherited as an autosomal recessive trait. Prolongation of the QT interval and arrhythmia susceptibility is inherited as an autosomal semidominant trait—that is, homozygotes are more severely affected than heterozygotes.**
2. **The frequency of heterozygotes for all dominant long QT syndromes is estimated to be 1 in 10,000 persons. Risk of sudden death in heterozygotes is approximately 0.5 percent per year.**
3. **Homozygotes are rare. They have profound prolongation of the QT interval and risk of arrhythmia. Untreated, most homozygotes die in childhood.**
4. **Idiopathic ventricular fibrillation (MIM 600163) is characterized clinically by (a) sudden death and aborted sudden death; (b) episodic ventricular fibrillation; and (c) variable electrocardiographic findings including prolongation of the QRS complex with a right bundle branch block pattern (Brugada syndrome). This disorder is inherited as an autosomal dominant trait. Prevalence is not known.**
5. **The primary defect in long QT syndrome and idiopathic ventricular fibrillation is a mutation in a gene encoding a cardiac myocyte ion channel. Genes identified to date include *KVLQT1* (GenBank U89364), *KCNE1* or minK (GenBank L33815), and *HERG* (GenBank U04270), which encode potassium channel subunits, and *SCN5A* (GenBank M77235), which encodes the cardiac sodium channel. These proteins are located on the surface of cardiac myocytes and regulate configuration of the cardiac action potential.**
6. ***KVLQT1* is located on the short arm of chromosomal 11. It comprises 16 exons that span 400 kb. The gene encodes a protein of 676 amino acids. More than 78 different mutant alleles have been identified, which represents 45 percent of the arrhythmia-associated mutations discovered.**
7. ***HERG* is located on the long arm of chromosome 7. It comprises 16 exons that span 55 kb. The gene encodes a protein of 1159 amino acids. More than 81 mutations of HERG have been identified thus far. This represents 45 percent of the long QT-associated mutations.**
8. ***SCN5A* is located on the short arm of chromosome 3. It comprises 28 exons that span 80 kb. The gene encodes a single protein that contains 2016 amino acids. Thirteen distinct *SCN5A* mutations have been associated with long QT syndrome. Several *SCN5A* mutations have been associated with idiopathic ventricular fibrillation.**
9. ***KCNE1* encoding minK is located on the short arm of chromosome 21. It comprises 3 exons that span 4 kb. The gene encodes a protein that contains 129 amino acids. Three missense mutations of minK have been associated with long QT syndrome.**
10. **A fifth long QT syndrome locus (LQT4) has been localized to chromosome 4. The gene for this form of long QT syndrome has not been identified.**
11. **Additional locus heterogeneity for long QT syndrome has been defined.**
12. ***SCN5A* encodes the cardiac sodium channel. This gene is expressed in cardiac myocytes and initiates the action potential. *KVLQT1* encodes a voltage-gated potassium channel α subunit. This gene is expressed in cardiac myocytes. KvLQT1 α subunits coassemble with minK β subunits to form cardiac I_{Ks} potassium channels. *HERG* is expressed in cardiac myocytes and encodes α subunits that form cardiac I_{Kr} potassium channels. I_{Kr} and I_{Ks} potassium channels terminate the cardiac action potential.**
13. **Long QT syndrome-associated mutations of *KVLQT1*, *KCNE1*, and *HERG* result in loss of channel function. In most cases, these are missense mutations that result in dominant-negative suppression of channel function. The extent of this dominant-negative effect is variable. As a result, channel function (I_{Kr} or I_{Ks}) is reduced by 50 to 90 percent. This results in prolongation of action potential duration in individual cardiac myocytes, abnormal inhomogeneity of repolarization in the myocardium, and a substrate for arrhythmia.**
14. **Long QT syndrome-associated mutations of *SCN5A* result in a gain-of-channel function. Normally, individual sodium channels open to initiate the action potential, close, and**

A list of standard abbreviations is located immediately preceding the index in each volume. Additional abbreviations used in this chapter include: DI-DIV = domains I-IV; *erg1, erg2, erg3* = symbols for *ether-a-go-go*-related genes in rat; *HERG*/HERG = gene symbol/protein for human *ether-a-go-go*-related gene; I_{Kr} = rapid activating delayed rectifier potassium current; I_{Ks} = slow activating delayed rectifier potassium current; *KCNE1* = gene symbol for potassium voltage-gated channel I_{SK}-related subfamily member 1 encoding minK; *KVLQT1*/KvLQT1=gene symbol/protein for potassium voltage-gated channel KQT-like subfamily, member 1; minK = minimal potassium channel; PAS = protein domain based on homology to *Per, AhR,* and *Arnt* proteins; QTc = corrected QT interval in seconds; S1-S6 = membrane spanning segments 1 to 6; *SCN5A*/SCN5A = gene symbol/protein for sodium channel voltage-gated, type V, α protein. See Table 203-4 for relationships of phenotypic symbols, gene symbols, and proteins.

remain closed for the remainder of the action potential. Long QT syndrome-associated mutations of the cardiac sodium channel destabilize the inactivation gate, resulting in repetitive reopening of a few sodium channels during the plateau phase of the action potential. This prolongs action potential duration in individual cardiac myocytes, resulting in an abnormal inhomogeneity of repolarization and a substrate for arrhythmia.

15. ***SCN5A*** **mutations associated with idiopathic ventricular fibrillation result in a loss-of-channel function. This results in an abnormal inhomogeneity of cardiac conduction and a substrate for ventricular fibrillation.**
16. **KVLQT1 and minK are also expressed in the inner ear. Here the channel functions to conduct potassium ions into the inner ear, creating the potassium-rich fluid endolymph. Individuals harboring two loss-of-function mutations of KvLQT1 or minK have inadequate endolymph production, resulting in degeneration of the organ of Corti and congenital neural deafness.**
17. **Treatment for long QT syndrome includes: (a) β adrenergic blockers that appear to reduce the incidence of arrhythmia in susceptible individuals, but do not eliminate the substrate for arrhythmia; (b) potassium therapy to maintain a high normal serum potassium concentration; (c) placement of an automatic internal defibrillator; and (d) avoidance of drugs that induce long QT syndrome, such as erythromycin, terfenadine, and class III antiarrhythmic agents.**

CLINICAL FEATURES

Familial Cardiac Arrhythmias Cause Syncope and Sudden Death

Cardiac arrhythmias are a leading cause of morbidity and mortality throughout the world. It is estimated that more than 300,000 individuals in the United States die suddenly every year, and in most cases, it is assumed that the underlying cause of sudden death is ventricular tachyarrhythmias.[1,2] Despite the frequency and consequences of cardiac arrhythmias, the ability to predict, prevent, and treat these disorders remains poor.

The familial occurrence of virtually every arrhythmia and conduction abnormality has been reported.[3] In most cases, however, the mode of inheritance is not clear and the molecular basis of the disorder has not been elucidated. However, significant progress has been made into the basis of two disorders that cause life-threatening ventricular arrhythmias: long QT syndrome and idiopathic ventricular fibrillation.

A case report of an individual with a recessively inherited form of long QT syndrome provides insight into these disorders.[4] A 25-year-old woman of Scottish descent presented to her obstetrician for routine evaluation. She was in her 35th week of gestation in an otherwise normal pregnancy. During physical examination, the obstetrician noted that the fetus' heart rate was low at 70 to 80 beats per minute, about half the normal rate. This was of concern, but an ultrasonic evaluation indicated normal fetal development. A decision was made to allow the pregnancy to come to term with periodic examinations. At 36 weeks, the heart rate continued to be slow. A second ultrasound study confirmed normal development, bradycardia, and regular rhythm. The infant was born without complications by normal vaginal delivery at 39 weeks gestation.

The slow heart rate persisted after birth. Mother and child were well until the first bottle feeding when the child experienced a cyanotic episode. The child was rushed to the pediatric intensive care unit where a battery of tests were performed, including blood count, blood cultures, urine analysis, urine cultures, serum electrolytes, chest x-ray, and electrocardiogram. All were normal except the electrocardiogram, which showed sinus bradycardia with a heart rate of 82 beats per minute and a corrected QT interval of 0.61 sec. A pediatric cardiologist was consulted; the cardiologist noted prolongation of the QT interval on the electrocardiogram. The cardiologist also thought that the child might be deaf and made a tentative diagnosis of Jervell and Lange-Nielsen syndrome, an autosomal recessive form of long QT syndrome associated with deafness (Table 203-1). The child was placed on β-blockers and monitored for several days. On the eighth day, audiograms indicated bilateral sensory deafness. A neurologic evaluation was otherwise unremarkable.

Table 203-1 Familial Disorders of Cardiac Rhythm and Conduction

Familial disorders of cardiac conduction
sinoatrial node dysfunction
atrial ventricular node block
bundle branch blocks
Familial arrhythmias
Atrial
Familial atrial fibrillation
Ventricular
Long QT syndrome
Romano-Ward syndrome
Jervell and Lange-Nielsen syndrome
Idiopathic ventricular fibrillation

On day 10, the infant was sent home with an apnea monitor. At the age of 4 weeks, serial audiograms revealed no responses to auditory stimuli. There was no evidence of infection, meningitis, or temporal bone fractures, and no history of treatment with toxic drugs. Because Jervell and Lange-Nielsen syndrome was thought to be a purely recessive disorder, phenotypic evaluation was not performed on the child's parents or other family members. Seven months after delivery of the proband, her mother had a cardiac arrest and died. At the time, she was under a great deal of stress; her husband had recently lost his job and the child's apnea monitor had kept her awake all night. She died when she rose from bed after the alarm clock sounded.

Long QT Syndrome and Idiopathic Ventricular Fibrillation Are Disorders of Episodic Cardiac Arrhythmia

Long QT syndrome is a general term that describes a number of disorders that increase the risk of sudden death from cardiac arrhythmia. These disorders are grouped together because many people with the problem have a subtle electrocardiographic abnormality known as a prolonged QT interval[5] (Fig. 203-1). This interval measures the time of cardiac repolarization, normally about 0.40 sec. With the exception of this electrocardiographic abnormality, most individuals with long QT syndrome appear healthy and normal. However, these individuals are at increased risk for a ventricular tachyarrhythmia known as *torsade de pointes*, which means twisting around the point, an allusion to the alternating axis of the main QRS complex around the isoelectric line during the arrhythmia[6–8] (Fig. 203-2). *Torsade de pointes* can degenerate to ventricular fibrillation, which is the likely cause of death in this disorder.

As electrocardiograms are not routinely performed on young, healthy individuals, affected people often present with syncope (sudden loss of consciousness) or aborted sudden death. In some cases, syncope is associated with seizures and a false diagnosis of epilepsy may be made.[9,10]

Several different forms of long QT syndrome have been defined on clinical grounds (Table 203-2). The first was reported by Jervell and Lange-Nielsen in 1957 and is often referred to as the Jervell and Lange-Nielsen syndrome.[11] The earliest case of recessive long QT syndrome was likely reported by Meissner in 1856.[12] Meissner's report describes a family with a young, congenitally

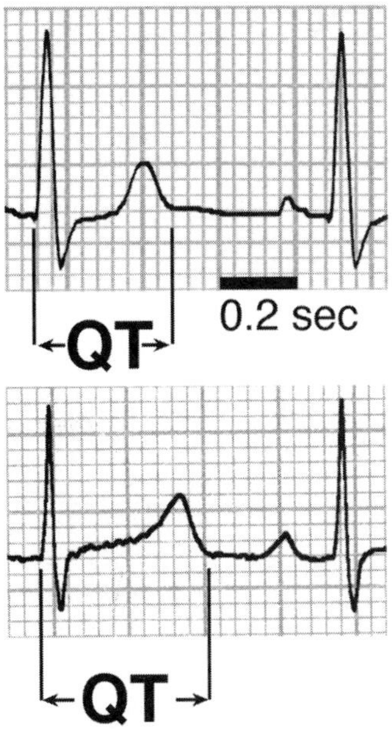

Fig. 203-1 Prolongation of the QT interval on surface electrocardiogram. Normal (top panel) and prolonged QT intervals (lower panel) are shown. The QT interval is measured from the beginning of the Q wave, which represents the onset of ventricular depolarization, to the end of the T wave (the end of ventricular repolarization). (*Adapted, with permission from Donald L. Atkinson, Howard Hughes Medical Institute, 1998.*)

deaf female who died suddenly after being scolded by a teacher. Evaluation of the family revealed that two additional siblings had died under similar circumstances. Additional earlier reports of recessive long QT syndrome are provided by Latham and Munro who described a small family with deafness and syncope, and by Moller, in 1953, who reported a male with deafness, syncope, and prolongation of the QT interval on an electrocardiogram.[13,14]

Jervell and Lange-Neilsen syndrome (MIM 220400) is associated with congenital neural deafness that is inherited as an autosomal recessive trait. Affected individuals show marked prolongation of the QT interval and frequent ventricular tachyarrhythmias, usually resulting in death during childhood. In the initial report, affected children had multiple syncopal episodes and three died suddenly at ages 4, 5, and 9 years. Since then, many other examples of long QT syndrome associated with deafness have been described.[15–17] Parents of affected individuals and some other family members who are heterozygous carriers of the mutant allele have apparently normal hearing. Recent studies indicate that heterozygotes may have a prolonged QT interval on electrocardiogram. As can be seen from the case report described above, heterozygotes such as the proband's mother are also at increased risk for cardiac arrhythmia, but the risk is lower than in homozygotes.

A second form of long QT syndrome was described separately by Romano and Ward in 1963, and is often referred to as the Romano-Ward or Ward-Romano syndrome. This disorder is

Table 203-2 Long QT Syndromes

Familial
Autosomal dominant: Romano-Ward syndrome
Autosomal recessive: Jervell and Lange-Nielsen syndrome
Acquired
Drug-induced
Metabolic abnormalities: hypokalemia; hypocalcemia
Intracranial hemorrhage or surgery
Hypothermia
Anorexa nervosa and rapid weight loss
Sinus bradycardia or pause
Cardiomyopathy

inherited as an autosomal dominant trait and includes prolongation of the QT interval of varying extent and increased risk of ventricular tachyarrhythmia. No other phenotypic abnormalities are definitely associated with this disorder.

A third form of long QT syndrome associated with bilateral cutaneous syndactyly was described in 1995[18] (Fig. 203-3). This form is sporadic, rare, and associated with marked prolongation of the QT interval and frequent arrhythmias, generally leading to death early in childhood. Structural heart disease, especially patent ductus arteriosus, was present in some individuals.[18–20] Analysis of electrocardiograms showed marked prolongation of the QT interval with rate-corrected intervals of greater than 0.66 sec. Several of the children died despite treatment with β-adrenergic blocking agents and permanent pacing.

The most common cause of long QT syndrome is the acquired form of the disorder. The most common acquired cause is drug-induced (Table 203-3). Ironically, many antiarrhythmic medications, such as quinidine and sotalol, can cause prolongation of the QT interval and *torsade de pointes* ventricular tachycardia. Many other medications are associated with long QT syndrome, including the antibiotic erythromycin and the antihistamine terfenadine (Seldane).[21–33] Metabolic abnormalities, particularly hypokalemia and hypocalcemia, can cause prolongation of the QT interval and arrhythmia susceptibility.[34] Anorexia nervosa and severe weight loss, which can cause hypokalemia, are associated with long QT syndrome.[35] Disorders of the central nervous system are implicated in acquired long QT syndrome, particularly intracranial surgery and subarachnoid hemorrhage.[36] Diabetes mellitus is associated with QT interval prolongation and arrhythmia,[37–39] possibly because of a secondary autonomic neuropathy.[40–42] Some cardiac abnormalities, particularly cardiomyopathy, may be associated with prolongation of the QT interval and arrhythmia.[43] Prolongation of the QT interval has also been associated with sudden infant death syndrome (SIDS)[44] and increased risk of death in the general population.[45,46]

Ventricular fibrillation is a common cause of sudden death, accounting for approximately 250,000 to 300,000 sudden deaths per year in the United States. When it occurs, there is no cardiac output. Permanent brain damage and death are imminent unless the arrhythmia is controlled. There are no demonstrable cardiac or noncardiac causes for ventricular fibrillation in approximately 10

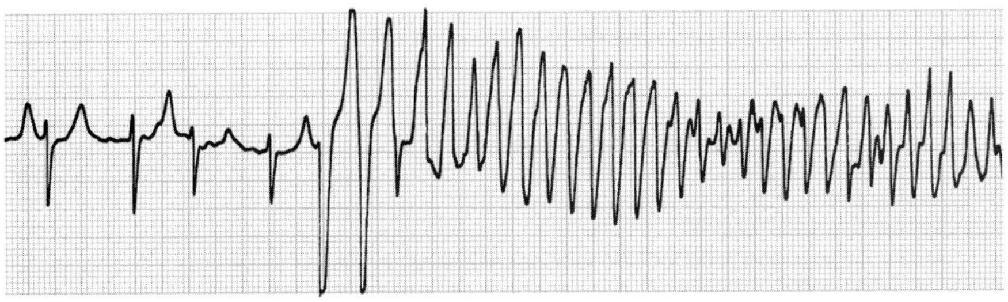

Fig. 203-2 ***Torsade de pointes ventricular tachycardia associated with long QT syndrome.***

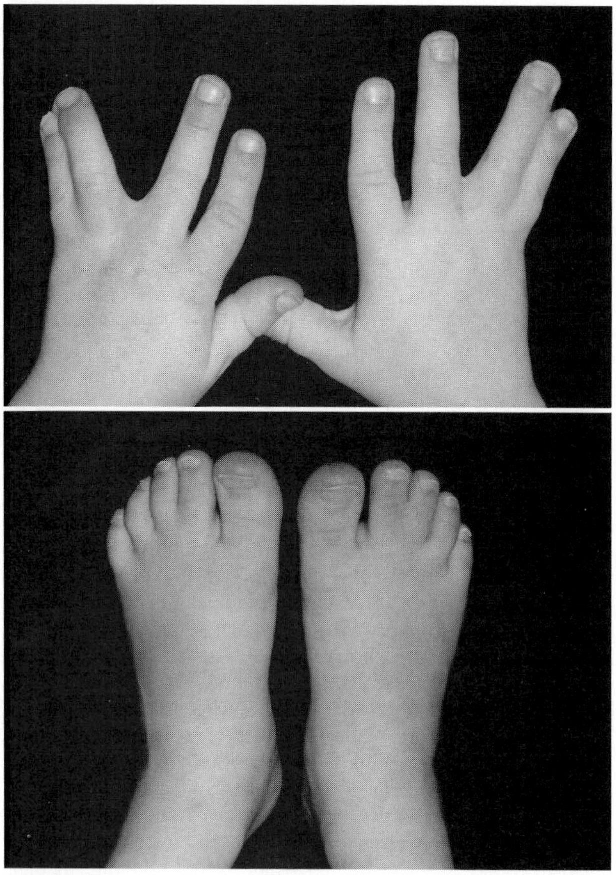

Fig. 203-3 Simple syndactyly associated with long QT syndrome.

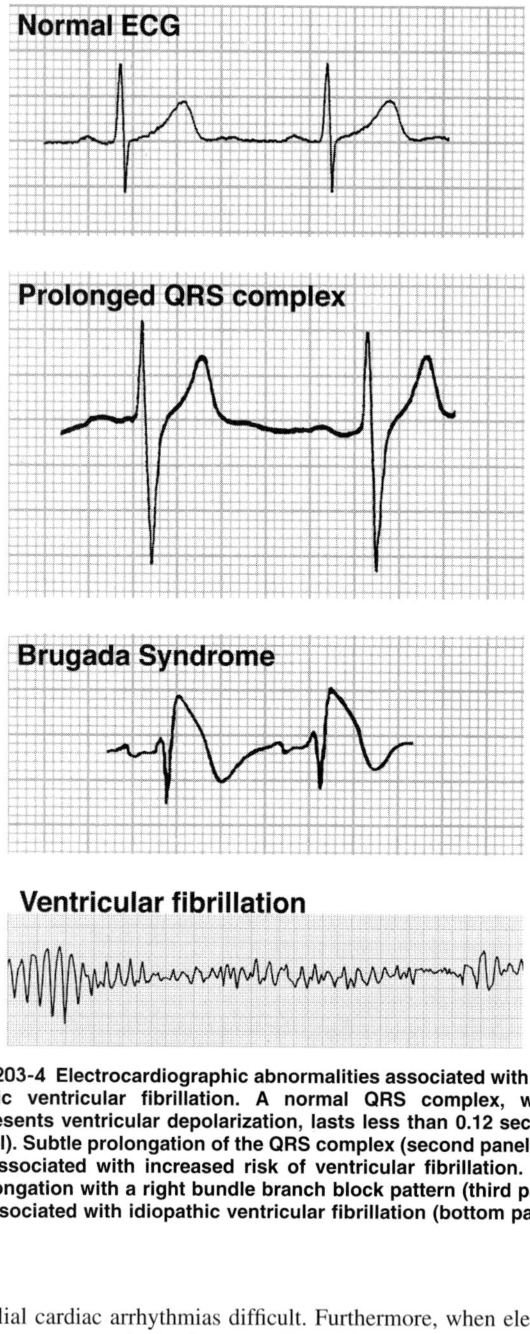

Fig. 203-4 Electrocardiographic abnormalities associated with idiopathic ventricular fibrillation. A normal QRS complex, which represents ventricular depolarization, lasts less than 0.12 sec (top panel). Subtle prolongation of the QRS complex (second panel) can be associated with increased risk of ventricular fibrillation. QRS prolongation with a right bundle branch block pattern (third panel) is associated with idiopathic ventricular fibrillation (bottom panel).

percent of cases. These cases are classified as idiopathic ventricular fibrillation.[1,2,47–50] As in individuals with long QT syndrome, people with idiopathic ventricular fibrillation often appear healthy. Electrocardiographic evaluation of these individuals shows no evidence of QT interval prolongation. In some cases, subtle prolongation of the QRS complex may be demonstrated (Fig. 203-4). A distinct electrocardiographic feature of elevation of the ST segment in leads V1 through V3, with or without right bundle branch block, has been described for some patients with idiopathic ventricular fibrillation.[51–59] This disorder is often referred to as the Brugada syndrome. In all cases, these individuals are at increased risk for episodic ventricular fibrillation that may lead to sudden death.

Presymptomatic Diagnosis of Arrhythmia Susceptibility Is Essential but Difficult

Electrocardiograms are usually not performed on apparently healthy, young individuals, making presymptomatic diagnosis of familial cardiac arrhythmias difficult. Furthermore, when electrocardiograms are obtained, many affected individuals show either subtle or no apparent electrocardiographic abnormalities.[60] For long QT syndrome, even a definition of QT prolongation is challenging. The QT interval varies in duration in a given individual over time depending on a number of factors, including heart rate, gender, autonomic tone, metabolic status, and medications.[61–65] As a result, the spectrum of QT intervals at any given moment varies widely in a normal population. In an effort to make measurement of the QT interval more accurate, most investigators correct the QT interval for heart rate using a formula derived by Bazette in 1939.[66] Using this formula, the corrected QT interval (QTc) is equal to the QT interval in seconds divided by the square root of the RR interval. In the past, a corrected QT interval greater than 0.44 sec was considered abnormal and diagnostic of long QT syndrome. Analysis of a large population of long QT syndrome gene carriers, however, indicated that these criteria were inadequate. The mean corrected QT interval was 0.42 sec in a normal population and 0.49 sec in a population carrying one mutant *KVLQT1* allele with the autosomal dominantly inherited form of long QT syndrome.[60] As Fig. 203-5

Table 203-3 Some Drugs Associated with LQT

Erythromycin
Disopyramide
Amiodarone
Antihistamines
Quinidine
D-Sotalol
Bepridil
Prenylamine
Tricyclic antidepressants
Phenothiazines
Diuretics (hypokalemia)

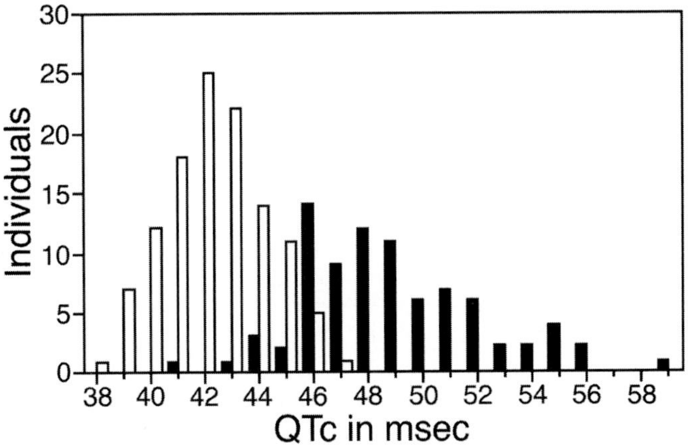

Fig. 203-5 Spectrum of corrected QT intervals (QTc) in long QT and control populations. Open bars indicate normals; black bars indicate affected individuals. Note that there is considerable overlap between these populations, making definitive diagnosis difficult. (*Copyright (c)1992 Massachusetts Medical Society. Vincent et al.*[197] *Adapted with permission.*)

illustrates, there is a great deal of overlap between these two populations, making definitive diagnosis difficult. The corrected QT interval of *KVLQT1* gene carriers ranged from 0.41 to 0.59 sec. By contrast, the corrected QT intervals of noncarriers ranged from 0.38 to 0.47 sec. On average, carriers of the gene for long QT syndrome had longer corrected QT intervals than noncarriers, but there was substantial overlap in 126 of the 199 individuals studied (63 percent). Use of a corrected QT interval above 0.44 sec as a diagnostic cut-off resulted in 22 misclassifications among the 199 family members (11 percent). Corrected QT intervals of 0.47 sec or longer in males and 0.48 sec or longer in females were completely predictive, but resulted in false negative diagnosis in 40 percent of the males and 20 percent of the females. Diagnosis may be improved using exercise electrocardiography, which shows a relative lack of shortening of the QT interval with increasing heart rate during exercise.[67] However, this test is also neither completely sensitive nor specific. Similar results were found when individuals with other forms of long QT syndrome were evaluated.[60,68]

Long QT Syndrome Genotypes Influence the Clinical Course of the Disease

As described below, at least six genes are implicated in long QT syndrome. By carefully examining the electrocardiographic patterns of individuals with different forms of long QT syndrome, distinct patterns have emerged.[69,70] These electrocardiographic patterns are shown in Fig. 203-6.

The spectrum of symptoms of individuals with long QT syndrome is also quite variable. Individuals harboring two mutant copies of long QT syndrome alleles have frequent arrhythmias and usually die during childhood unless treated.[4] Heterozygous individuals, by contrast, have relatively few syncopal events. The incidence of syncope, aborted sudden death, and sudden death was higher in individuals with *KVLQT1* mutations (63 percent) and *HERG* mutations (46 percent) than in *SCN5A* (18 percent).[71] The cumulative mortality through age 40 in all three genotypes was similar, but lethality of cardiac events was higher in individuals harboring *SCN5A* mutations than for *HERG* and *KVLQT1* (20 percent vs. 4 percent respectively). Individuals with *SCN5A* mutations had significantly longer mean corrected QT intervals than individuals with *KVLQT1* and *HERG* mutations. In general, increased symptoms are associated with exercise or excitement.[72] Diving into a pool on a hot day after exercise or at the start of a race as a trigger for arrhythmia is a recurrent story.[73] Pregnancy and delivery also appear to be associated with increased risk of arrhythmia in long QT syndrome.[74]

GENETICS

Arrhythmia susceptibility syndromes can be inherited as autosomal dominant or autosomal recessive traits; sporadic and acquired cases also occur. Autosomal dominant long QT syndrome is often referred to as Romano-Ward syndrome. The incidence of this disorder is not known, but has been estimated at 1 in 10,000 live births. Penetrance is incomplete and phenotypic expression variable.

Autosomal recessive long QT syndrome is often referred to as Jervell and Lange-Nielsen syndrome. In addition to arrhythmia susceptibility, this disorder is characterized by congenital neural deafness. Penetrance is very high and arrhythmia susceptibility is severe. The incidence of this disorder is not known, but has been estimated at 1.6 to 6 cases per million.[75] Autosomal recessive long QT syndrome is most often seen in the setting of a consanguineous

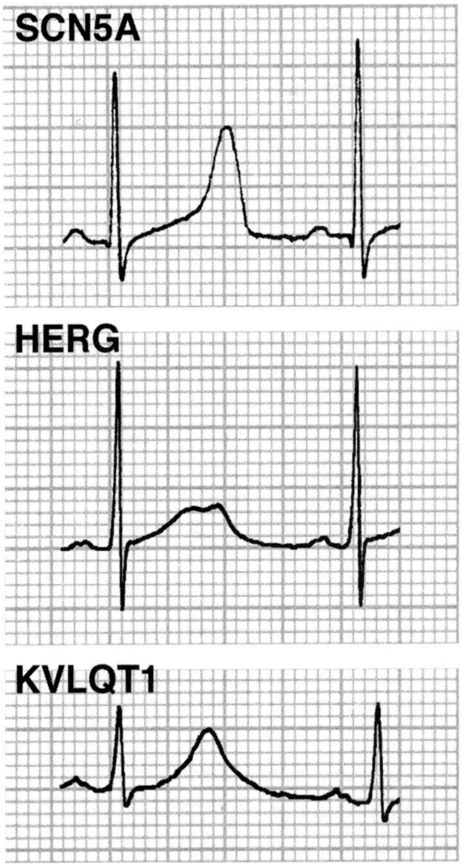

Fig. 203-6 Characteristic electrocardiographic patterns observed in three distinct forms of long QT syndrome resulting from mutations in *KVLQT1*, HERG, and *SCN5A*.

Table 203-4 Arrhythmia Genes

Phenotype Symbol	Map location	Gene symbol	Alternate symbols	Protein	GenBank	MIM
LQT1	11P15.5	*KVLQT1*	*KCNQ1*	KvLQT1	U89364	19250
LQT2	7q35-q36	*HERG*	*KCNH2*	HERG	U04270	152427
LQT3	3p24-p21	*SCNA5*	—	SCNA5	M77235	600163
LQT4	4q25-q27	Unknown	—	Unknown	—	600919
LQT5	21q22.1-q22.2	*KCNE1*	—	minK	L33815	176261
*LQT6**	Unknown	Unknown	—	Unknown	—	601005

* LQT with syndactyly

mating. By definition, parents and other family members who are heterozygous carriers have a form of autosomal dominant long QT syndrome and are at increased risk of cardiac arrhythmia.[4] These individuals appear to have normal hearing. The frequency of QT interval prolongation among deaf children is approximately 1 percent.

Long QT syndrome is most often observed as a sporadic trait. Because of the highly variable expression of the phenotype in individuals with autosomal dominant long QT syndrome, an individual may appear to have sporadic disease when, in fact, a subtle form of the disease is being inherited as an autosomal dominant trait. Environmental and other genetic factors may play a role in the phenotypic expression. A clearly defined sporadic syndrome is long QT syndrome associated with simple syndactyly. New mutation dominant, autosomal recessive, and contiguous gene syndrome are possibilities for this disorder.

Acquired long QT syndrome is the most common form of the disorder. The incidence of acquired long QT syndrome is not known. Individuals harboring long QT syndrome-associated mutations are much more susceptible to arrhythmia in the setting of certain environmental influences, particularly hypokalemia, sinus pause, and drugs. It is not yet clear, however, what percentage of individuals with acquired long QT syndrome harbor genetic variants that make them more susceptible to environmental influences. It is clear that long QT syndrome can be induced in virtually anyone with the right combination of drug, hypokalemia, and bradycardia/sinus pause.

Idiopathic ventricular fibrillation is inherited as an autosomal dominant trait or acquired. One form of autosomal dominant idiopathic ventricular fibrillation is referred to as the Brugada syndrome.

Arrhythmia Susceptibility Genes Encode Cardiac Ion Channels

Five loci have been mapped for arrhythmia susceptibility, and the genes for four of the five loci have been identified[76] (Table 203-4). These include *KVLQT1* on chromosome 11p15.5,[77,78] human *ether-a-go-go*-related gene (*HERG*) on chromosome 7q35-q36, *SCN5A* on chromosome 3p21-p24,[79] *KCNE1* encoding minK on chromosome 21q22.1-q22.2,[80] and a gene that has not yet been identified on chromosome 4.[81] Additional locus heterogeneity also has been identified.[82]

The first long QT syndrome locus was mapped to chromosome 11.p15.5 in 1991.[83] Genetic linkage analysis was performed using restriction fragment length polymorphisms and Southern blot analysis in a large Utah family (Fig. 203-7). The story of this family is illustrative of linkage studies of the time. This family originated in the mid-nineteenth century when two brothers emigrated from Scandinavia to Brigham City, Utah. Relatively little is known about the two brothers other than that they were not allowed to participate in the family profession of fishing because of health concerns. The immigration of these brothers was separated by 10 years. By the time the second brother immigrated to Brigham City, the first brother had moved to southern Utah, so

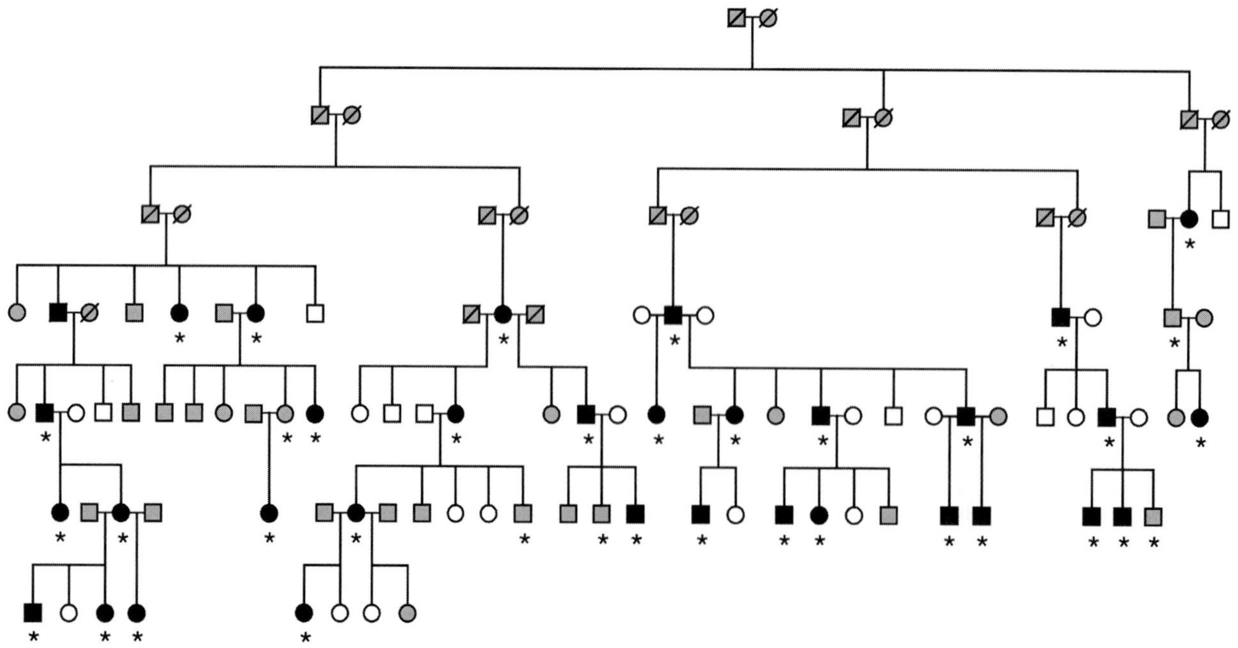

Fig. 203-7 A large pedigree showing autosomal dominant inheritance of long QT syndrome. Males are represented by squares; females by circles. Open signifies unaffected phenotype, grey uncertain, and black affected. Star denotes gene carrier.

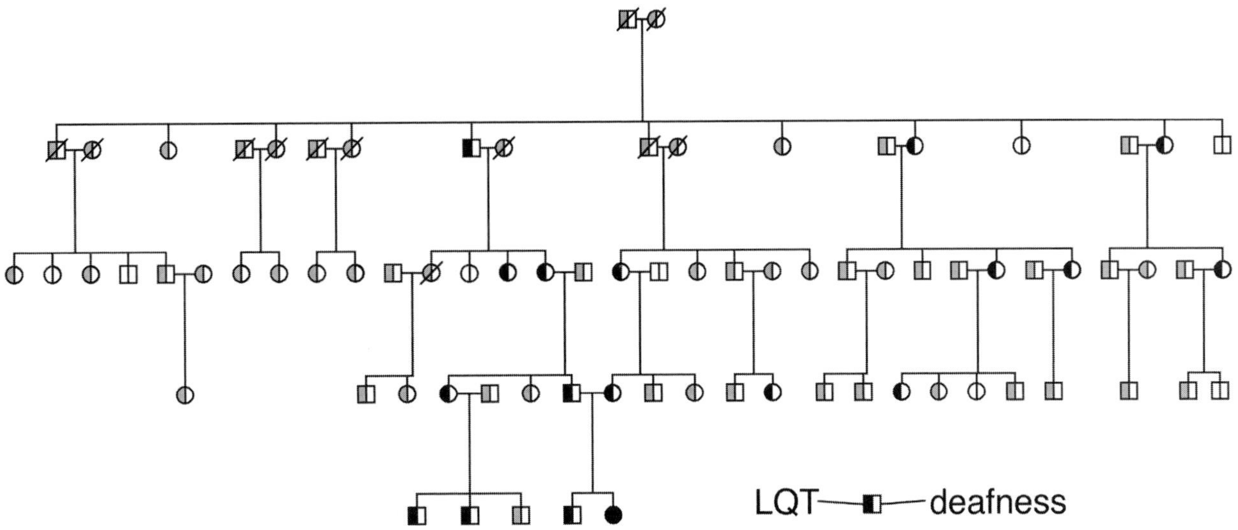

Fig. 203-8 Jervell and Lange-Nielsen syndrome pedigree. The proband (filled circle) shows severe prolongation of the QT interval, frequent arrhythmias, and congenital neural deafness. Ascertainment and phenotypic evaluation of the extended family reveals subtler prolongation of the QT interval and arrhythmia susceptibility in heterozygous carriers. Squares represent males and circles represent females. The left side of the symbol indicates LQT phenotype and the right side indicates deafness. Open signifies unaffected, grey uncertain, and black affected.

the two branches of the family were unaware of their counterparts. Over time, these brothers had offspring that led to a family that now numbers in the thousands, living throughout the western United States. Five distinct branches of the family emerged. Through genealogic studies, however, these groups were merged into one.

Careful phenotypic evaluation indicated that certain branches of the family had a history of syncope and aborted sudden death. Documentation of arrhythmias, however, was rare, as was sudden death. Syncope is a difficult symptom in that there are many causes that are not related to arrhythmia. Approximately 7 percent of the population have experienced at least one syncopal episode. In most cases, these are not due to ventricular tachycardia, but to increased vagal tone, bradycardia, and transient hypotension. In addition, it is difficult to distinguish between true syncope and lightheadedness.

Fortunately, long QT syndrome heterozygotes often demonstrate subtle prolongation of the QT interval on electrocardiogram. Although there was clear overlap of QT intervals in this family (Fig. 203-5), two distinct populations could be identified.[84] Because of the size of the family, it was possible to use very stringent criteria for phenotypic classification. Individuals were classified as affected if they had a corrected QT interval of $\geq$0.47 sec and classified as unaffected if they had a corrected QT interval of $\leq$0.41 sec. Asymptomatic individuals with corrected QT intervals from 0.42 sec to 0.46 sec were classified as phenotypically uncertain. As Fig. 203-7 shows, prolongation of the QT interval on electrocardiogram was inherited as an autosomal dominant trait with incomplete penetrance. However, the number of phenotypically affected and unaffected individuals was suitable for linkage analysis. Initial linkage was discovered using polymorphic markers at the Harvey *ras*-1 locus with a lod score greater than 16.44 at a recombination fraction of 0, indicating odds favoring linkage of more than 10^{16} to 1.[83] Linkage to chromosome 11 was then confirmed in additional families,[85] and locus heterogeneity was discovered.[86–88] Subsequent linkage studies were done using short tandem repeat polymorphisms and the polymerase chain reaction in much smaller families.[85,89] These led to the identification of loci on chromosome 7q35-q36 and 3p21-p24.[89]

Jervell and Lange-Nielsen syndrome was generally thought to be a purely recessive trait consisting of QT interval prolongation, arrhythmia susceptibility, and congenital neural deafness. Recent studies, however, indicate that only one feature, deafness, is truly recessive. The pedigree of the case reported at the beginning of this chapter is shown in Fig. 203-8. After the mother's death, the family was referred for genetic evaluation. Phenotypic evaluation revealed that 14 family members had prolonged corrected QT intervals ranging from 0.47 to 0.53 sec. Thirty-two family members had borderline corrected QT intervals ranging from 0.42 to 0.46 sec. Six family members reported a history of syncope. None of the family members reported hearing deficits. By inspection, it is apparent that the phenotype of QT interval prolongation is inherited as an autosomal dominant trait with incomplete penetrance (Fig. 203-8). Prolongation of the QT interval and arrhythmia susceptibility is inherited as a semi-autosomal dominant trait; that is, homozygotes are more severely affected than heterozygotes. It is important to note that the parents (and other family members) of individuals with Jervell and Lange-Nielsen syndrome are obligate heterozygotes (or at-risk) for long QT-associated mutations and are at increased risk for arrhythmia. It is essential, therefore, to phenotypically characterize members of families with the Jervell and Lange-Nielsen syndrome.

HERG Encodes a Cardiac Potassium Channel

The first long QT syndrome gene identified was *HERG* on chromosome 7q35-q36.[77] After mapping a long QT locus to chromosome 7q35-q36,[89] candidate genes were mapped to the region. One of these was *HERG*, a gene-encoding putative potassium channel that was originally cloned from a brain cDNA library.[90] This channel is also expressed in neural-crest-derived neurons,[91] microglia,[92] and a wide variety of tumor cell lines.[93] In one neuronal cell line, these channels were shown to modulate spike-frequency adaptation.[94] To date, two additional *erg* channel genes have been identified. *Erg2* and *erg3* are expressed exclusively in the nervous system in the rat.[95] The physiological roles of HERG (erg1), erg2, and erg3 in noncardiac cells of mammals is still largely undefined.

Northern analysis indicates that expression of this gene predominates in the heart.[77] Multiple different mutations of *HERG* that cosegregated with the disease in linked families were identified, and the ultimate identification of de novo *HERG* mutations associated with long QT syndrome confirmed the causative relationship.[77] Many different types of *HERG* mutations have been associated with long QT syndrome.[96–101] *HERG* consists of 16 exons and spans 55 kb. Primers have been designed

Table 203-5 Ion Channel Genes Associate with Long QT Syndrome

Type of mutation	Gene				
	KVLQT1	*HERG*	*SCN5A*	*KCNE1*	All
Missense	62	52	7	3	124
Nonsense	6	6	0	0	12
aa Deletion	2	2	6	0	10
Frameshift	1	16	0	0	17
Splice	7	5	0	0	12
Total	78	81	13	3	175

to screen for mutations in all the coding regions of *HERG*.[102] With the genomic structure in hand, 81 mutations of *HERG* have been defined[98] (Table 203-5). These represent 46 percent of the total number of long QT syndrome mutations found to date.[102]

The predicted topology of HERG protein is shown in Fig. 203-9. HERG is thought to encode a typical Shaker-like potassium channel α subunit with six putative membrane-spanning domains, a putative voltage sensor in the 4th membrane-spanning domain (S4), and a potassium-selective pore loop between the 5th and 6th membrane-spanning domains (S5 and S6). HERG has extensive intracellular N-terminal and C-terminal segments. A region in the C-terminal domain of HERG has sequence similarity to nucleotide-binding domains. The first 135 amino acids of HERG is called the eag domain and is conserved in *erg, elk* (*ether-a-go-go*-like), and *eag* (*ether-a-go-go*-gene) channels of other species. The structure of the N-terminal domain has been solved and has structural similarity to PAS domains previously identified in a diverse family of eukaryotic and prokaryotic proteins[103] (Fig. 203-10). Proteins with PAS domains are frequently involved in signal transduction; however, the only function associated with this domain in HERG is modulation of the rate of channel deactivation.[104–107]

Arrhythmia-associated mutations of *HERG* have been identified throughout the coding region, particularly the membrane-spanning domains and the pore region.[98] *HERG* is unusual, however, in that a

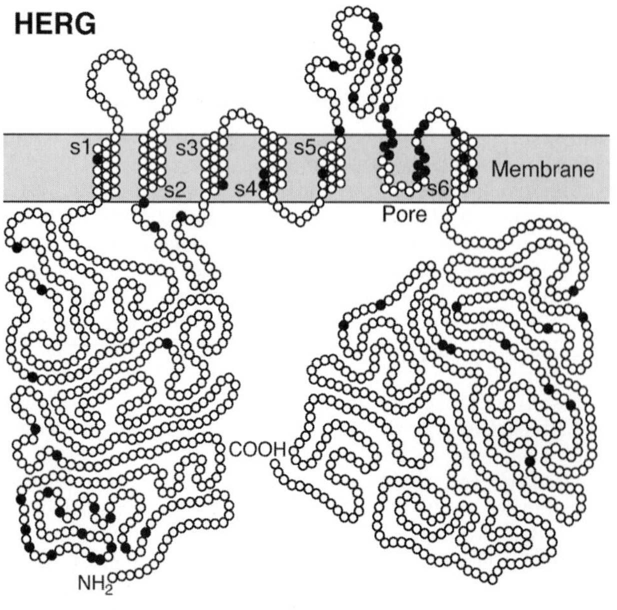

Fig. 203-9 Predicted topology of HERG protein. The relative location of long QT syndrome-associated missense mutations are indicated as filled circles.

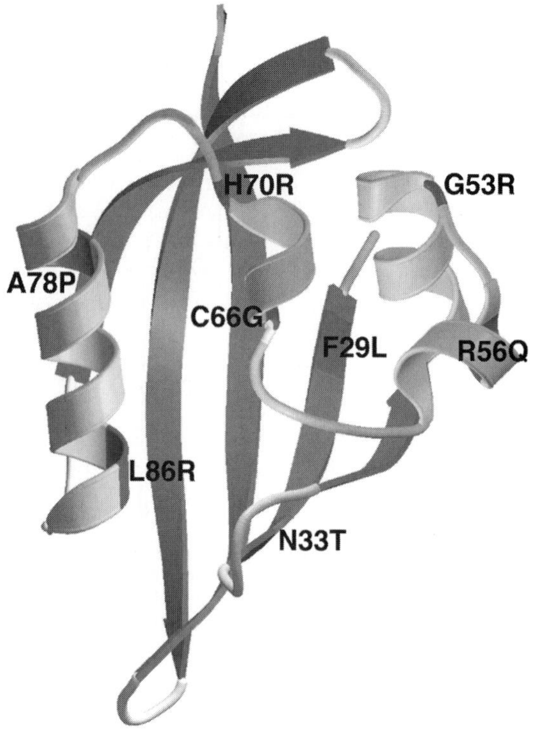

Fig. 203-10 The crystal structure of HERG N-terminal eag domain. Long QT syndrome-associated mutations of this PAS domain are indicated. Supplied by J.H. Morais Cabral.

large number of mutations have also been identified in the intracellular N- and C-terminal domains (Fig. 203-9).

KVLQT1 Encodes a Cardiac Potassium Channel

KVLQT1 was discovered by positional cloning in 1996.[78] This gene is located on chromosome 11p15.5 in the vicinity of the insulin, insulin-like growth factor 2 (IGF2), tyrosine hydroxylase genes, and a region associated with Beckwith-Wiedemann syndrome (see Chaps. 15 and 65).[83,85] Some rearrangements that cause Beckwith-Wiedemann syndrome also disrupt *KVLQT1*.[108] One would predict that these individuals could have arrhythmia susceptibility, but this has not yet been documented. *IGF2* and other genes in the region are subject to genomic imprinting. *KVLQT1* is imprinted with paternal silencing in most tissues, but not in the heart (see Chap. 15).[108–110] Northern analysis indicates that *KVLQT1* is expressed in the heart, placenta, lung, kidney, inner ear, and pancreas.[78] Two homologs of *KVLQT1* have been cloned from human brain. Mutations in either of these genes (*KCNQ2, KCNQ3*) cause benign familial neonatal convulsions, another episodic disorder of excitability (see Chap. 230).[111–113]

Like HERG, KvLQT1 protein is predicted to have a topology similar to a Shaker-like potassium channel (Fig. 203-11). It has six putative membrane-spanning domains, including a putative voltage sensor (S4) and a potassium channel pore signature sequence between S5 and S6. Unlike HERG, the intracellular N-terminal segment of KvLQT1 is short. The genomic structure of *KVLQT1* has been determined.[102] The gene consists of 16 exons and spans approximately 400 kb. Mutational analysis revealed 78 mutations that span *KVLQT1* coding sequences (Table 203-5).[7,97,98,114–118] This represents 45 percent of known arrhythmia-associated mutations discovered to date. Similar to mutations involving *HERG*, many *KVLQT1* mutations have been identified in the membrane-spanning regions as well as in the pore region. However, mutations involving the N-terminal intracellular domain of KvLQT1 are relatively uncommon. Mutations of one *KVLQT1* allele lead to autosomal dominant long QT syndrome,

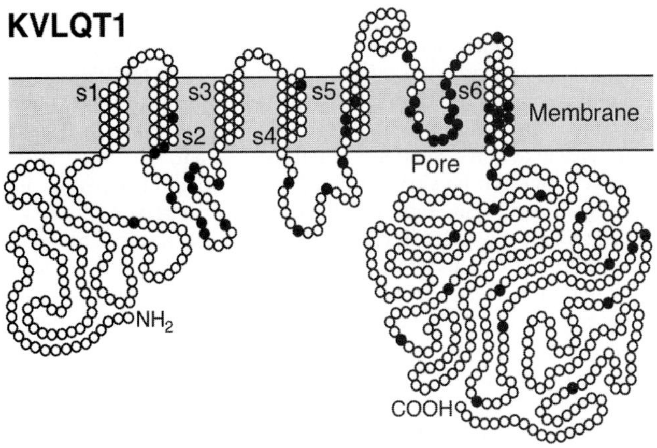

Fig. 203-11 Predicted topology of KvLQT1 protein. Long QT syndrome-associated missense mutations of *KVLQT1* are indicated as filled circles.

whereas two mutant copies of *KVLQT1* lead to congenital neural deafness, marked prolongation of the QT interval, and severe arrhythmia susceptibility in the Jervell and Lange-Nielsen syndrome.[4,119]

KCNE1 Encodes minK, a Cardiac Potassium Channel β Subunit

KCNE1 was defined in 1997 as a long QT syndrome gene by using a candidate gene approach.[80] The gene is located on chromosome 21 and consists of 3 exons that span approximately 40 kb.[102] The minK protein is predicted to have one membrane-spanning domain with small extracellular and intracellular regions (Fig. 203-12). Three arrhythmia-associated mutations of *KCNE1* have been discovered (Table 203-5).[98] The three mutations represent approximately 2 percent of the long QT syndrome mutations defined to date. Individuals with one mutant *KCNE1* allele have QT interval prolongations of variable extent (generally moderate) and moderate arrhythmia susceptibility. Individuals harboring two mutant alleles have congenital neural deafness, marked QT interval prolongation, and severe arrhythmia susceptibility in the Jervell and Lange-Nielsen syndrome.[8,121,122]

SCN5A Encodes the Cardiac Sodium Channel

SCN5A was identified as a long QT syndrome gene in 1995 using a positional cloning/candidate gene approach.[79] This gene is located on chromosome 3p21-p24[123] and consists of 28 exons that span 80 kb.[124] *SCN5A* encodes a protein that is predicted to have a structure with four major domains, DI through DIV (Fig. 203-13). Each of these domains is thought to have a topology similar to a Shaker-like potassium channel with six putative membrane-spanning domains and pore domains located between S5 and S6. This constitutes a sodium channel α subunit that can, by itself,

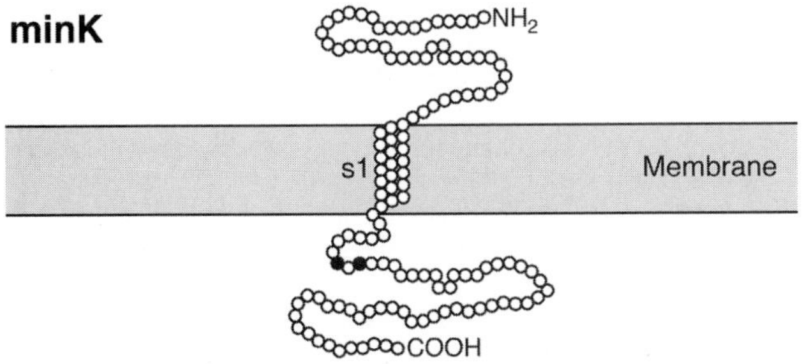

Fig. 203-12 Predicted topology of minK protein. Long QT syndrome-associated missense mutations are indicated as filled circles.

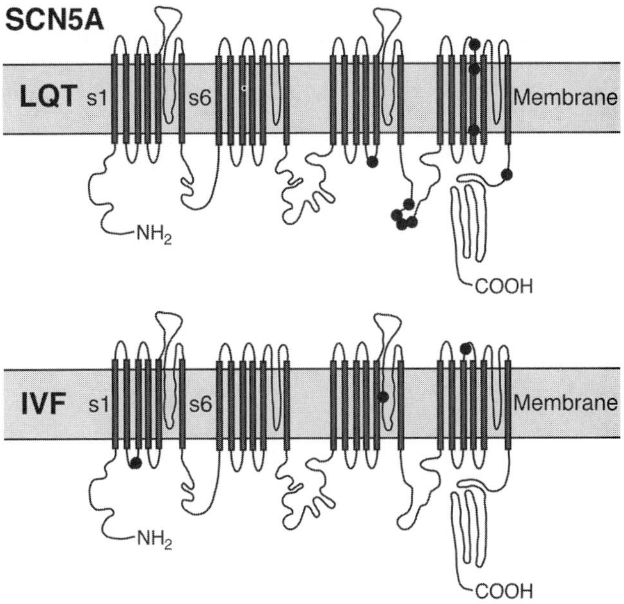

Fig. 203-13 Predicted topology of SCN5A protein. Long QT syndrome-associated mutations of *SCN5A* are indicated as filled circles at top. Mutations associated with idiopathic ventricular fibrillation (IVF) are shown similarly at bottom.

form functional channels. Potassium channel α subunits, by contrast, require four subunits that coassemble to form functional potassium channels. Mutational analysis has revealed 13 distinct mutations that have been associated with long QT syndrome (Table 203-5)[98,125–128].

SCN5A Mutations Also Cause Idiopathic Ventricular Fibrillation

Several *SCN5A* mutations have been associated with idiopathic ventricular fibrillation in families and sporadic cases[129] (Table 203-5). In one family, the insertion of two nucleotides disrupted the splice-donor sequence of intron 7. In a second, a deletion of a single nucleotide at codon 1397 resulted in an in-frame stop codon that eliminates DIII-S6, DIV-S1-S6, and the C-terminal portion of the channel. Two missense mutations were associated with familial forms of idiopathic ventricular fibrillation.

Additional Arrhythmia Susceptibility Genes Await Identification

A fifth long QT syndrome locus (*LQT4*) has been located on chromosome 4q25-q27.[81] The gene for this form of long QT syndrome has not been yet identified. Thus far, this locus has only been identified in a single family in France. Several unlinked families with long QT syndrome have been identified.[89] Thus, at least two additional long QT syndrome genes remain to be identified.

PATHOGENIC MECHANISMS

Arrhythmia Susceptibility Results From Cardiac Ion Channel Dysfunction

Like other excitable cells, cardiac myocyte excitability results from action potentials. Similar to action potentials in neurons, skeletal muscle, and smooth muscle, the action potential in cardiac myocytes is mediated by ion currents through membrane-bound channel proteins. The cardiac myocyte action potential, however, is distinctive in its duration, which is approximately 300 milliseconds. By contrast, the action potential in neurons occurs in a few milliseconds.

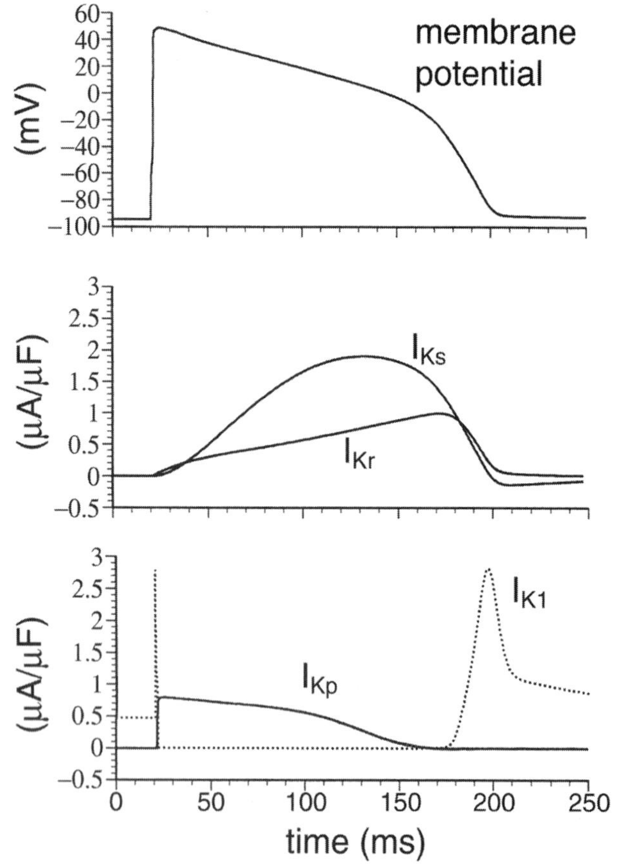

Fig. 203-14 Cardiac action potential and underlying potassium currents that mediate repolarization. (*From Zeng et al.*[198] *Adapted with permission.*)

Figure 203-14 is a stylized ventricular action potential and correlates molecular events with the electrocardiographic findings. The action potential consists of five phases termed 0 to 4. Phase 0 corresponds to depolarization of the myocyte. This phase is initiated by the rapid opening (activation) of voltage-gated sodium channels encoded by *SCN5A*. On the electrocardiogram, depolarization of the ventricle is seen as the QRS complex. Phase 1 of the action potential occurs at the end of rapid depolarization, recognized as a partial repolarization of the membrane. This effect is primarily due to closure (inactivation) of cardiac sodium channels, and activation of a transient outward potassium current and, in some species, a calcium-activated chloride current. Phase 2 is the plateau phase. The relatively long duration of this phase is unique to ventricular and Purkinje fiber myocytes, and is maintained primarily by inward calcium currents through L-type calcium channels and gradually increasing outward potassium currents. The total amount of current during the plateau phase of the cardiac action potential is small. As a result, this phase of the action potential is very susceptible to small changes in ion currents, which can substantially shorten or lengthen the action potential. At this point in the cardiac cycle, the electrocardiogram has returned to the baseline. Phase 3 of the cardiac action potential is a period of cellular repolarization. Repolarization is caused by outward flow of potassium mediated by several different potassium channels. The repolarization phase correlates with the T wave on surface electrocardiogram. Thus, the duration of the QT interval is related directly to the length of ventricular action potentials. The final phase of the action potential is Phase 4, in which the membrane potential has returned to its baseline near −85 mV and correlates with ventricular diastole.

Physiological and pharmacologic studies have defined two main repolarizing potassium currents, I_{Kr} and I_{Ks} (Fig. 203-14). I_{Kr} is the rapidly activating delayed rectifier potassium current that is specifically blocked by methanesulfonamide drugs. When these drugs block the I_{Kr} current, I_{Ks}, the slowly activating delayed rectifier potassium current, remains.

Reduced Cardiac Repolarizing Currents Cause Long QT Syndrome

***HERG* Encodes I_{Kr} Channels.** Expression of *HERG* in heterologous systems led to the discovery that this gene encodes α subunits that form cardiac I_{Kr} potassium channels (Table 203-6). The characteristic biophysical properties of cardiac I_{Kr} were reproduced by expression of this gene in heterologous systems[130,131] (Fig. 203-15). These properties include pronounced rectification of the current-voltage relationship and block by specific antiarrhythmic drugs. Rectification refers to the property whereby the whole-cell conductance decreases as the membrane is strongly depolarized, resulting in a bell-shaped relationship when current magnitude is plotted as a function of membrane voltage (Fig. 203-15). The rectification of I_{Kr} permits the plateau phase of cardiac myocytes to be very long, and explains the prominent role of this current during phase 3 repolarization of the action potential.

The unusual rectification properties of HERG channels result from rapid inactivation and slow deactivation. HERG channels inactivate (close) much more rapidly than they activate (open). These properties vary at different membrane potentials, but the net result is that most HERG channels are inactivated during the depolarization and plateau phases (Phases 0 through 2) of the cardiac action potential. However, during repolarization the channels rapidly recover from the inactivate state to an open state. The subsequent transition from the open state to the closed state

Table 203-6 Molecular and Cellular Mechanisms of Cardiac Arrhythmias

Disease	Inheritance	Gene	Protein	Function	Mechanism
Long QT syndrome	Autosomal dominant	*KVLQT1*	KvLQT1	I_{Ks} channel α subunit	loss of function
		HERG	HERG	I_{Kr} channel α subunit	loss of function
		SCN5A	SCN5A	sodium channel α subunit	gain of function
		LQT4	unknown	?	?
		KCNE1	minK	I_{Ks} channel β subunit	loss of function
		LQT6	unknown	?	?
	Autosomal recessive	*KVLQT1*	KvLQT1	I_{Ks} channel α subunit	loss of function
		KCNE1	minK	I_{Ks} channel β subunit	loss of function
	Syndactyl-associated	?	unknown	?	
	Acquired*	*HERG*		I_{Kr} channel α subunit	acquired loss of function
Idiopathic ventricular fibrillation		*SCN5A*		sodium channel α subunit	loss of function

* No mutation in *HERG*

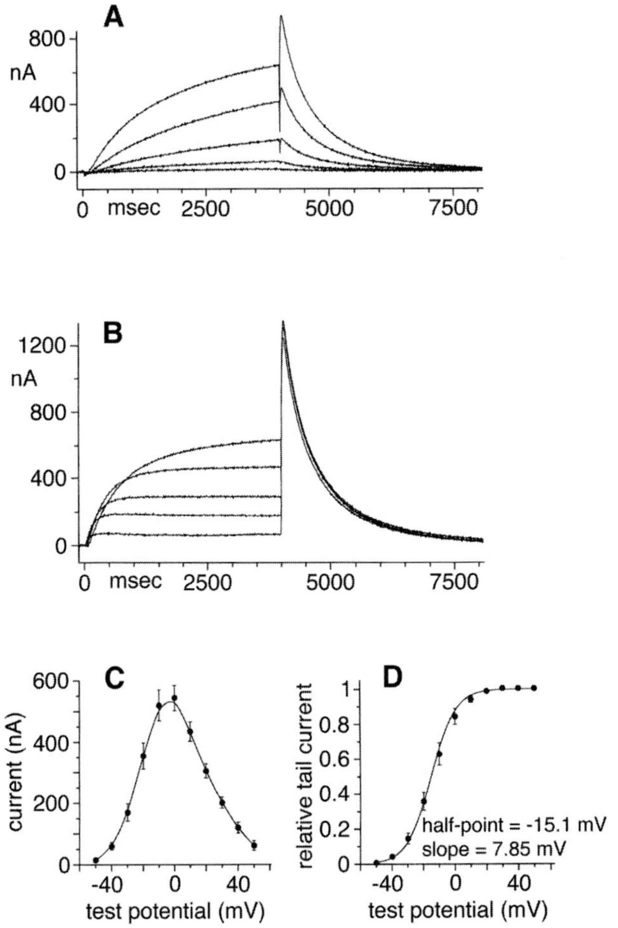

Fig. 203-15 ***HERG*** **encodes I_{Kr}.** ***A,*** **HERG currents recorded from** ***Xenopus*** **oocyte at potentials of −50 to −10 mV, applied in 10 mV steps.** ***B,*** **Currents recorded at potentials of 0 mV (largest) to +40 mV (smallest). Bottom panels show current-voltage relationship (C) and voltage dependence of channel activation (D). (*****From Sanguinetti, et al.*****[130]** ***Adapted, with permission.*****)**

(deactivation) is much slower. As the membrane potential returns to its resting level, the current conducted by HERG channels actually increases, reaching a maximum near −50 mV.

Considerable progress has been made in determining the structural features of HERG channels that are responsible for rapid inactivation. Two distinct mechanisms have been described for inactivation of voltage-gated potassium channels. N-type inactivation is caused by binding of the N-terminal region of the protein to the mouth of the pore. This type of inactivation can be eliminated by removal of the N-terminus. However, this procedure has no effect on inactivation of HERG channels. C-type inactivation involves residues in the pore-loop of the channel and may be caused by collapse of the ion permeation pathway near the outer mouth of the channel. This type of inactivation can be eliminated by mutation of key residues near the outer mouth of the channel. Inactivation of HERG has properties most similar to C-type inactivation as it can be eliminated by mutation of two amino acids (G628C/S631C) in the pore-forming region of the channel.[132] The current-voltage relationship of this mutant HERG channel is linear rather than rectifying, indicating the loss of fast inactivation. Moreover, the inactivation properties of HERG can be transferred to eag channels (which normally do not inactivate) by inserting the pore-loop and half of the S6 transmembrane domain of HERG into eag.[133]

The crystal structure of the eag domain in the N-terminus of HERG channels has been determined.[134] This work demonstrates that the eag domain has a hydrophobic face that binds directly to an intracellular channel region, tentatively identified as the region that links the S4 and S5 transmembrane domains. The interaction of the eag domain with the S4-S5 linker slows the rate of channel deactivation. Removal of the N-terminal region, or mutation of specific residues in the S4-S5 linker, causes the channel to deactivate much faster than normal. The physiological relevance of this interaction is suggested by the finding that alternative splicing of HERG creates an isoform with a shortened N-terminal region. Channels formed by assembly of these subunits alone, or by coassembly with full length HERG subunits, produce a channel that deactivates much faster than those formed by homotetrameric assembly of full-length subunits.[106,107]

Many different types of *HERG* mutations have been identified in association with long QT syndrome. These mutations include large deletions, small deletions, frameshift mutations, and splice-site mutations. The most common *HERG* mutations identified thus far are missense mutations.[77,96–99,101,135,136] As noted above, these mutations span the entire *HERG* coding region, but tend to be clustered in the pore domains, the membrane-spanning domains, and the intracellular N- and C-terminal domains. *HERG* is unusual in that there are many mutations in the intracellular N- and C-terminal domains, presumably due to the unusual properties of these domains in HERG.

At least two distinct molecular mechanisms account for reduced HERG function in the long QT syndrome. In the first, long QT syndrome-associated intragenic deletions of the *HERG* allele can result in the synthesis of aberrant subunits that do not coassemble with normal subunits into the functional tetrameric form. The net effect is a 50 percent reduction in a number of functional channels; that is, haploinsufficiency. In the second mechanism, missense mutations lead to the synthesis of HERG subunits with single amino acid substitutions. Channels formed from the coassembly of normal and mutant subunits have reduced or no function. The result is a greater than 50 percent reduction in HERG channel function, a dominant-negative effect (Fig. 203-16). The severity of dominant-negative effect of a specific mutation varies considerably. In some cases, the dominant-negative effect is relatively small. In others, the effect is complete, leading to marked reduction of I_{Kr} even in the heterozygous state. It is likely that the severity of the dominant-negative effect has an impact on the phenotype of an individual. However, there are many other factors that also impact on the phenotype, so an extensive study is required. Mutations in the pore region (e.g., G628S) lead to complete loss of function and a strong dominant-negative effect,[137,138] presumably because the channel is processed normally[139] and the pore of the channel has been destroyed. As expected, I_{Kr} was absent in a transgenic mouse model expressing high levels of G628S HERG.[140] Mutations in other regions of the channel, however, have less pronounced effects. For example, mutations of the eag domain in the N-terminus of HERG generally disrupt slow deactivation.[140a] As a result, deactivation is accelerated, leading to reduced repolarizing potassium current. Some mutations (e.g., Y611H and V822M) cause defects in biosynthetic processing, resulting in retention of protein in the endoplasmic reticulum.[139] Other mutations (e.g., N470D and T474I) form functional channels but alter gating properties.[137,138] Three mutations in HERG (T474I, A614V, and V630L) cause loss of channel function, but when coexpressed with wild-type subunits, shift the voltage dependence of channel inactivation to more negative potentials and enhance inward rectification, thereby suppressing channel function.[141]

Acquired Long QT Syndrome Results from Block of HERG Channels. Dysfunction of HERG channels and reduced I_{Kr} are also the mechanisms of acquired long QT syndrome. For reasons that are not yet clear, many drugs, including many class III antiarrhythmics, antihistaminics, and some antibiotics, are very potent blockers of HERG channels.[32,120,142–150] Block of I_{Kr} delays cardiac repolarization, lengthens QTc interval, and may induce *torsade de pointes.*[151]

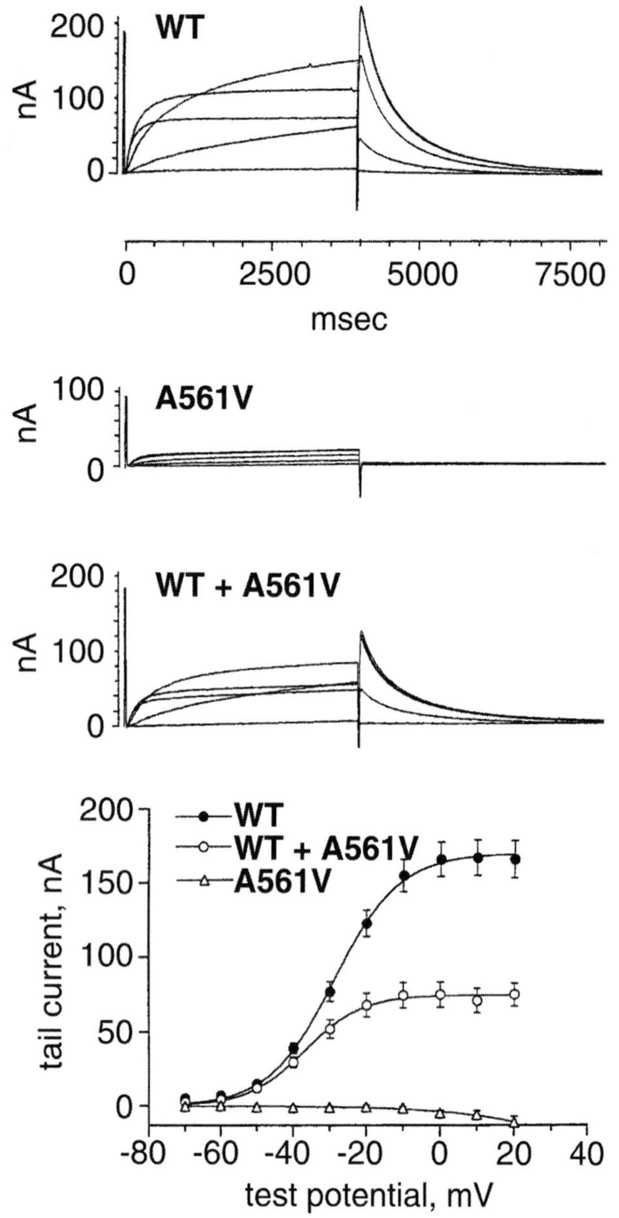

Fig. 203-16 Dominant-negative mutation of *HERG*. Top three panels show currents recorded from a *Xenopus* oocyte expressing wild-type (WT) HERG channels, A561V HERG channels, or a combination of the two channel types. Bottom panel is a plot of currents as a function of voltage for the three conditions. (*From Sanguinetti et al.*[137] *Adapted with permission.*)

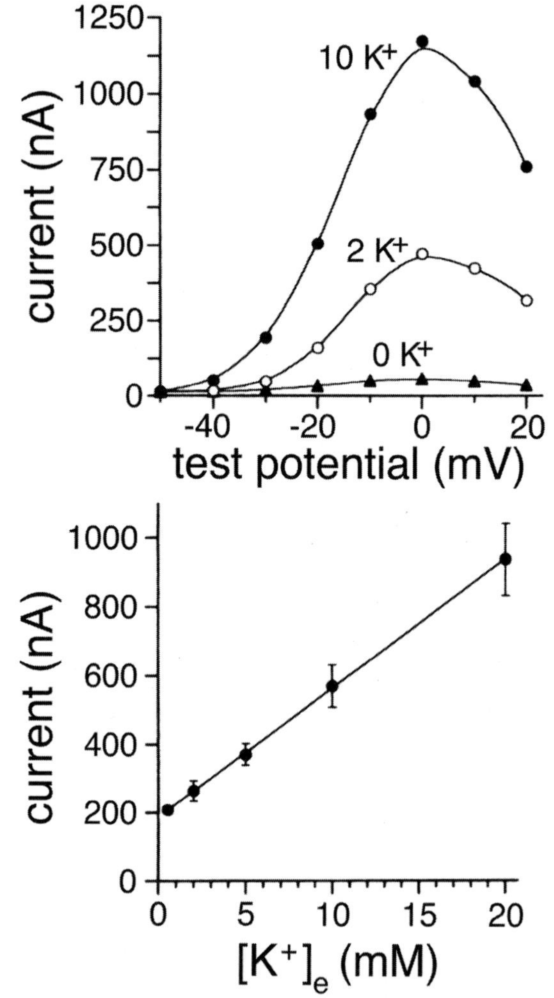

Fig. 203-17 Potassium modulates magnitude of HERG channel function. Top panel shows current-voltage relationship for HERG for different external potassium concentrations. Bottom panel shows relationship between HERG magnitude and external potassium concentration. (*From Sanguinetti, et al*[130] *Adapted with permission.*)

HERG channels are also paradoxically sensitive to extracellular potassium.[130,152] Increasing the extracellular concentration of potassium actually increases outward potassium current, in opposition to the decreased chemical driving force (Fig. 203-17). The mechanism underlying this effect is not precisely known, but it is associated with a slowing[153] and a positive shift in the voltage dependence of HERG inactivation.[154] This shift reduces the degree of channel rectification and increases the magnitude of outward current within the voltage range traversed by a typical cardiac action potential. This effect is observed within the physiological range of serum potassium concentrations. For example, reducing extracellular potassium from 5 mM to 2 mM reduces HERG current by ~35 percent.[130] This may explain the well-documented clinical association between hypokalemia, QT interval prolongation, and arrhythmia susceptibility.[155]

Several new drugs that block I_{Ks} have been described.[156–159] These compounds prolong action potential, but it is unclear whether they will cause *torsade de pointes*.

KvLQT1 Subunits Coassemble with minK Subunits to Form Cardiac I_{Ks} Channels. Heterologous expression of the *KVLQT1* gene in mammalian cells and *Xenopus* oocytes confirm that this gene encodes α subunits that form voltage-gated potassium channels (Fig. 203-18). However, the biophysical properties of KvLQT1 channels were unlike known potassium channels recorded from cardiac myocytes. This led to the hypothesis that KvLQT1 α subunits might coassemble with other subunits to form potassium channels with recognizable biophysical characteristics.

MinK, the minimal potassium channel subunit, was initially cloned by functional expression in *Xenopus* oocytes in 1988.[160] The biophysical properties of the current induced by expression of minK in *Xenopus* oocytes was similar to cardiac I_{Ks}. However, there were several problems. First, the structure of minK was unusual. As noted above, minK is 130 amino acids in length and is thought to contain only one membrane-spanning domain. The typical voltage-gated potassium channel subunit has six membrane-spanning domains, and four subunits are required for coassembly and formation of functional channels. Thus,

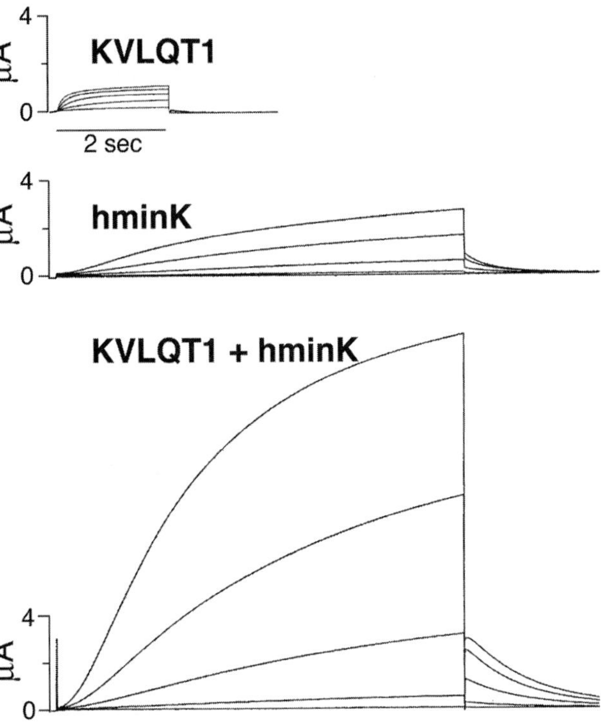

Fig. 203-18 KvLQT1 and minK coassemble to form cardiac I_{Ks} channels. (*From Sanguinetti et al.*[199] *Adapted with permission.*)

investigators hypothesized that many minK subunits might be required to form functional channels, perhaps by aggregating in response to membrane depolarization. Although some experimental evidence supported this hypothesis, other evidence indicated that only two or four minK subunits were required for functional channels[161] and that the channel was more likely a heteromultimeric complex.[162] A second problem with minK was experimental; physiological studies indicated that heterologous expression of minK in *Xenopus* oocytes induced a functional potassium channel, but in most cases (except that described in reference 163), expression in mammalian cells failed to induce a current. The third problem with minK was the observation of saturability; that is, injection of increasing amounts of *KCNE1* cRNA into *Xenopus* oocytes did not lead to increasing current. These data all led to the hypothesis that minK might be a βsubunit that coassembled with another α subunit to form I_{Ks} channels.[164,165] Heterologous expression of KvLQT1 subunits with minK subunits strongly support this hypothesis. As seen in Fig. 203-18, heterologous expression of minK alone in mammalian cells induced no current. However, heterologous expression of KvLQT1 and minK together in mammalian cells led to a large potassium current with the biophysical properties of cardiac I_{Ks}. Thus, KvLQT1 and minK coassemble to form cardiac I_{Ks} channels. Although the stoichiometry of coassembly is not yet known, it is likely that four KvLQT1 α subunits coassemble with four minK subunits to form these channels.

Mutations of *KVLQT1* tend to cluster around the membrane-spanning domains and the pore region. In most cases, these mutations lead to a loss-of-channel function. Most often, missense mutations have a potential to a cause a dominant-negative effect. As with *HERG*, there is a spectrum of dominant-negative suppression of KvLQT1 function. For example, missense mutations (e.g., G306R, T312I, G314S, and D317N) in the pore region or elsewhere (e.g., A178P and L273F) of KvLQT1 are associated with dominant long QT syndrome and cause loss-of-function and a pronounced dominant-negative effect when coexpressed with wild-type KvLQT1 and minK.[166,167] In general, mutations associated with recessive long QT syndrome, such as truncation of the C-terminus of KvLQT1,[166] or missense mutations (e.g., W305S) cause loss-of-function and little or no dominant-negative effect.[168] It should be noted, however, that these same mutations can be found in autosomal dominant long QT syndrome.

Two distinct isoforms of KvLQT1 have been characterized. One is the full-length clone that in heterologous systems coassembles with minK to form cardiac I_{Ks} channels. The other is a truncated form of KvLQT1.[169,170] When coexpressed in vitro with full-length KvLQT1, this isoform has a dominant-negative effect on I_{Ks} channel function. The significance of this finding in vivo, however, is not known.

The findings that mutation of *KVLQT1* caused long QT syndrome and that KvLQT1 coassembles with minK made it likely that mutation of *KCNE1* would also cause long QT syndrome. This was confirmed using single-strand conformation polymorphism (SSCP) analyses of genomic DNA from affected members of a few small families.[80] Two mutations in *KCNE1* have been characterized by heterologous expression in *Xenopus* oocytes. These mutations (S74L and D76N) are located in the putative intracellular domain of the minK protein. Both mutations shift the voltage dependence of activation gating of minK channels to more positive potentials and increase the rate of channel deactivation. These changes in gating reduce the magnitude of outward current during the plateau and repolarizing phases of the action potential. In addition, D76N has a dominant-negative effect on I_{Ks}. That LQT-associated mutations of *KCNE1* alter gating kinetics of I_{Ks} provides compelling evidence that minK forms an integral part of the I_{Ks} channel rather than simply serving as a chaperone, as was once hypothesized. *KCNE1* mutations also lead to a loss-of-function; in some cases, to a dominant-negative loss-of-function.

Gain-of-Function Mutations in *SCN5A* Cause Long QT Syndrome. As noted earlier, a spike of sodium current initiates the cardiac action potential. Cardiac sodium channels open for a very brief time in response to membrane depolarization (Fig. 203-19). Soon after opening, the channels inactivate and remain closed for the remainder of the action potential. An intracellular domain located between DIII and DIV mediates inactivation of the sodium channel. This is often referred to as the inactivation gate and is thought to physically occlude the inner mouth of the channel pore. *SCN5A* mutations associated with long QT syndrome were identified in this region.[79] These mutations included an in-frame deletion of nine base pairs causing deletion of three amino acids (ΔKPQ). Physiological characterization of this mutant led to the discovery that the mutation destabilized the inactivation gate.[75] That is, activation of these sodium channels is normal and the initial current at the whole-cell level appears normal. At the whole-cell level, the rate of inactivation of the ΔKPQ mutant appears a little faster than normal. However, a percentage of mutant sodium channels remain open, resulting in a small steady-state current during a long depolarization (Fig. 203-19). The net effect is a small, maintained, inward current during the plateau of the action potential. Recall that the plateau phase of the action potential is particularly susceptible to small changes in current. Maintained depolarizing sodium current during the plateau phase stalls the process of repolarization and lengthens action potential duration. Three missense mutations of *SCN5A* that cause long QT syndrome have also been characterized. N1325S and R1644H sodium channels exhibit dispersed reopenings after the usual initial opening, whereas ΔKPQ caused both dispersed reopenings and long-lasting bursts after membrane depolarization.[171] Another missense mutation (R1623Q) in the S4 segment of domain IV, caused only minor abnormalities in channel activation, but significantly delayed inactivation. Single-channel recordings showed that mutant channels had prolonged open times with persistent bursting behavior.[172]

Loss-of-Function Mutation in the Cardiac Sodium Channel can Cause Idiopathic Ventricular Fibrillation. *SCN5A*

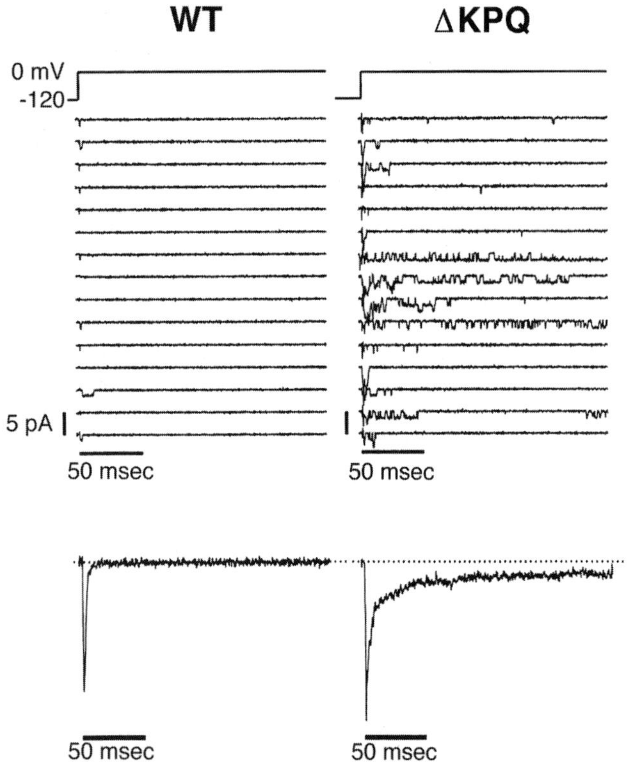

Fig. 203-19 Long QT syndrome-associated mutation in *SCN5A* (ΔKPQ) alters single channel properties. Wild-type (WT) sodium channels open briefly upon membrane depolarization (left panel). Mutant channels (ΔKPQ) repetitively open, indicating dysfunctional inactivation gating (right panel). Lower panels show ensemble averages of single channel traces. (*From Bennett et al.*[75] *Adapted with permission.*)

mutations have been associated with idiopathic ventricular fibrillation. In some cases, these mutations are clearly loss-of-function. For example, a nonsense mutation of *SCN5A* has been associated with idiopathic ventricular fibrillation in an otherwise healthy individual who has borderline corrected QT interval prolongation and no other electrocardiographic abnormality.[129] The functional consequences of the splicing mutation are not known, but are most likely loss-of-function.

Other mutations associated with prolongation of the QRS complex with a right-bundle-branch block pattern are less clear-cut in terms of physiological consequences. Unlike *SCN5A* mutations associated with long QT syndrome, no persistent inactivation-resistant current was observed in missense mutations. Biophysical analysis of the two missense mutations in *SCN5A* showed a shift in the voltage dependence of steady state inactivation toward more positive potentials, associated with an acceleration in recovery time from inactivation.[129] It is not yet clear whether these biophysical properties are responsible for increased risk of idiopathic ventricular fibrillation in these individuals.

Nor is it clear how a reduction in the total number of functional sodium channels and expression of heterogeneous population of sodium channels leads to arrhythmia susceptibility. Inhibition of sodium channel current can cause heterogeneous action potentials in the right ventricular epicardium, leading to marked dispersion of repolarization and refractoriness.[173,174] This creates a substrate for the development of reentrant arrhythmia. It is likely that a premature beat initiates ventricular tachycardia and fibrillation in this substrate, possibly through Phase 2 reentry produced by the underlying substrate.

The Mechanism of Arrhythmia at the Organ Level: Unidirectional Block and Reentry. Multiple molecular mechanisms for arrhythmia susceptibility have been defined and more await discovery. Five loci and four genes are associated with long QT syndrome, and mutations in one gene are associated with idiopathic ventricular fibrillation. Gain-of-function mutations in the cardiac sodium channel, and loss-of-function mutations in cardiac potassium channels, lead to long QT syndrome by prolonging action potential duration in individual cardiac myocytes. Loss-of-function mutations in cardiac sodium channels can cause conduction abnormalities, increasing the risk of unidirectional block. As one might expect, these genes are not expressed uniformly throughout the myocardium but are instead differentially expressed. As a result, the effect of mutations varies from one region to another. Abnormal regional repolarization or conduction can lead to a substrate for arrhythmia. Under certain circumstances, the substrate can become critical when areas of unidirectional block are created (Fig. 203-20). Although necessary, this substrate is not sufficient for arrhythmogenesis. A trigger is still required. Many different triggers have been identified. In long QT syndrome, a common trigger is exercise or excitement, but rest and sleep have also been associated the syndrome.[175] These triggers are thought to be mediated through autonomic tone. Increased autonomic tone increases cyclic AMP-mediated enhancement of calcium channel function, spontaneous secondary depolarizations resulting from reopening of calcium channels. These depolarizations can trigger an arrhythmia.

Several models have been developed to define the mechanism of arrhythmia at the level of the heart. For example, *torsade de pointes* tachyarrhythmias can be mimicked by administering anthopleurin A to dogs.[176,177] This neurotoxin slows inactivation of sodium channels, roughly similar to the effect of mutations in *SCN5A* that cause long QT syndrome. Analysis of tridimensional activation patterns showed that the initial beat of toxin-induced tachyarrhythmia arose as focal activity from a subendocardial site. Subsequent reentrant excitation was due to infringement of a focal activity on the spatial dispersion of repolarization, resulting in functional conduction block and circulating wave fronts. Changing the site of origin of focal activity caused the resulting twisting pattern of the QRS configuration. The development of a functional

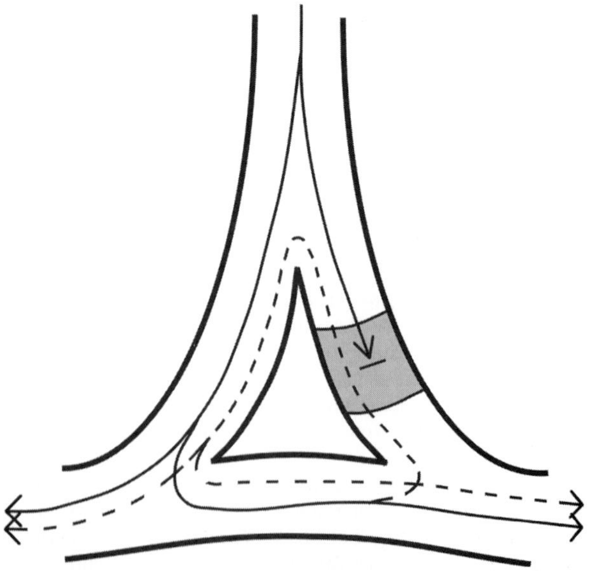

Fig. 203-20 Unidirectional block and reentry. The mechanism of arrhythmia at the organ level involves unidirectional block of conduction through refractive or damaged tissue and development of a reentrant circuit of electrical activity. Solid lines represent normal conduction pathway in a bifurcated Purkinje fiber. Conduction is blocked in an area of refractory tissue (stippled area). If conduction velocity is slowed (dashed line), then reentry through area of refractory tissue can occur.

block between the anterior and posterior right ventricular free wall and septum was responsible for initiating a bifurcation in a rotating scroll into two separate scrolls in each ventricle. The development of multiple reentry circuits within the heart is the likely cause of ventricular fibrillation and sudden death.

Deafness in Jervell and Lange-Nielsen Syndrome Results from Complete Loss of I_{Ks} Channel Function in the Inner Ear. Individuals with Jervell and Lange-Nielsen syndrome carry two mutant copies of either *KVLQT1* or *KCNE1* (see Chap. 254). These mutations lead to complete loss of I_{Ks} function. The result in the heart is substantial prolongation of the QT interval and marked arrhythmia susceptibility. Most individuals with two mutant copies of *KVLQT1* or *KCNE1* die in childhood unless treated. *KVLQT1* and *KCNE1* are also expressed in the inner ear. Here, the channel conducts potassium across the apical membrane of strial marginal cells into the lumen of the vestibular labyrinth of the inner ear.[178] This generates the K^+-rich fluid, endolymph. In the absence of I_{Ks} channels, inadequate endolymph is produced. As a result, Reisner's membrane, a thin membrane that covers the inner ear, collapses. This leads to degeneration of the organ of Corti, the organ that contains hair cells that sense movement of the endolymph, the mechanism responsible for hearing. As a result, individuals harboring these mutations have congenital neural deafness. This mechanism has been demonstrated in mice lacking minK.[179]

TREATMENT

An important goal for the future is prediction and prevention of life-threatening arrhythmias. The ability to detect susceptible populations is extremely important because measures for the prevention of sudden death exist now. The most likely method for early detection is genetic screening. Several things need to be accomplished before genetic screening can be effective. First, all the genes that cause arrhythmia susceptibility in humans must be identified and characterized. Second, mutations and other variants that cause arrhythmia susceptibility must be distinguished from benign polymorphisms that exist in populations but do not cause increased risk. This information must be catalogued and readily accessible. Finally, simple, reliable, and inexpensive devices must be developed for rapidly screening individuals for arrhythmia-associated DNA variants. Although much work remains to be done, the prospect for improved prevention of life-threatening arrhythmias is very good.

Beta-Blockers May Reduce the Incidence of Arrhythmia in Susceptible Populations

Experiments performed in the 1970s in dogs indicated that manipulation of the autonomic nervous system could cause prolongation of the QT interval and *torsade de pointes* ventricular tachycardia. This led to the hypothesis that inherited abnormalities of the autonomic nervous system were responsible for familial long QT syndrome. Although this hypothesis has not been experimentally disproved, it is now clear that most inherited long QT syndromes result from primary dysfunction of cardiac ion channels. However, this dysfunction creates a substrate for arrhythmia that is necessary, but not sufficient, for the arrhythmia. A trigger is still required. In many cases, the trigger is autonomic tone.[180] Arrhythmias in long QT syndrome are often associated with exercise or excitement. A common story is a young healthy child running around on a hot summer day and diving into a pool. This induces a diving reflex, which has a profound influence on parasympathetic tone. Arrhythmias in long QT syndrome are also associated with bradycardia and sleep. Thus, dramatic swings in autonomic tone can trigger arrhythmias in susceptible individuals.

Considerable anecdotal evidence supports the hypothesis that blocking the sympathetic nervous system is beneficial in susceptible populations.[181] Cervical sympathectomy was quite common in the United States a decade ago and is still performed occasionally in Europe.[182–184] Allotransplantation of the heart and complete denervation was completed in one patient, but this did not correct the underlying disorder.[185] By contrast, heart transplantation did correct the underlying repolarization abnormality in one patient.[186] In many cases, however, medical therapy with β-blockers is used in individuals with long QT syndrome. In most cases, this appears to be beneficial, reducing the instances of arrhythmia. The effect of β-blockers on the occurrence of cardiac events was examined in individuals harboring *KVLQT1* and *HERG* mutations. The mean cardiac event rate per patient per year decreased significantly after β-blockers were administered to individuals in these two groups.[71] However, β-blockers do not affect the substrate for arrhythmia, so individuals are still at increased risk. In some cases, β-blockers seem to exacerbate the problem. This may be related to bradycardia and sinus pauses, which can also act as triggers of arrhythmias in susceptible populations. A randomized, controlled study of β-blockers in long QT syndrome has not been done.

As noted earlier, gain-of-function mutations of the cardiac sodium channel can cause a relatively uncommon form of long QT syndrome.[75,79] The physiological consequences of the mutations are destabilization of the channel's inactivation gate. Thus, a percentage of channels open and close repetitively during the plateau phase of the action potential. Sodium channel blockers, like mexiletine and lidocaine, preferentially block sodium channels in the open conformation. Thus, these drugs preferentially block mutant sodium channels.[187] As a result, treatment of individuals with gain-of-function mutations in the cardiac sodium channel with mexiletine or lidocaine can reduce the substrate for arrhythmia. Early evidence supports the hypothesis that this therapy will be effective in specific populations.[44,188–190] However, loss-of-function mutations of the cardiac sodium channel also increase the risk of idiopathic ventricular fibrillation.[129] Thus, continuous therapy with mexiletine may reduce the risk of arrhythmia from repolarization abnormalities, but increase the risk of arrhythmia from conduction abnormalities.

Potassium Supplementation is Prudent Antiarrhythmic Therapy

Most long QT syndrome results from loss-of-function of cardiac potassium channels. This leads to reduced repolarizing current, action potential prolongation, and a substrate for arrhythmia. Potassium channel openers should reverse this process, reducing the substrate for arrhythmia.[191,192] However, commercially available potassium channel openers are not specific and also affect smooth muscle, leading to hypotension. While specific potassium channel openers still hold promise for individuals with long QT syndrome, including individuals with sodium channel mutations, development of these drugs is generally thought to be too expensive at this time. However, another simple and inexpensive therapy is available now.

HERG channels are paradoxically sensitive to extracellular concentrations of potassium.[130] In the physiological range, an increased concentration of potassium increases outward potassium current through HERG channels, whereas decreasing serum potassium concentration decreases outward potassium current through these channels. Increasing serum potassium concentrations in individuals with long QT syndrome should reduce the substrate for arrhythmia.

Evidence supporting this hypothesis has been demonstrated in individuals with *HERG* mutations.[193] Administration of potassium led to a 24 percent reduction in the resting corrected QT interval (from 617 ± 92 to 469 ± 23 milliseconds) compared with a 4 percent reduction in the control group (425 ± 25 to 410 ± 45 msec). QT dispersion became normal in individuals with mutations but did not change in controls. T-wave morphology, which had been biphasic in affected individuals, improved after potassium therapy. In theory, the effect should be even greater in individuals with *KVLQT1*, *KCNE1*, or *SCN5A* mutations, as these individuals will have more functional HERG channels. A combination of potassium and β-blocker therapy might prove highly effective in susceptible populations. A corollary of this finding is also true: it is dangerous to allow individuals who are at increased risk for arrhythmia to have low serum potassium concentrations. Even genetically insusceptible populations can be induced to have arrhythmia with the right combination of ypokalemia, bradycardia, and potassium channel blocking drugs.

The Future of Arrhythmia Therapy May Be Devices with Supplemental Pharmacologic Therapy

The consequence of molecular genetic and physiological studies of long QT syndrome and idiopathic ventricular fibrillation has been to discourage antiarrhythmic drug development. In the short-term, at least, this may be sensible and may save hundreds of millions of dollars in drug development. As loss-of-function mutations of cardiac sodium channels and loss of function mutations of cardiac potassium channels both lead to arrhythmia susceptibility, drugs that block cardiac sodium and potassium channels would be expected to increase arrhythmia susceptibility. Although prolonging action potential duration effectively reduces the risk of reentrant ventricular tachyarrhythmias, this also increases the risk of acquired long QT syndrome and *torsade de pointes* ventricular tachycardia. Thus, pharmacologic therapy may be effective in the short-term, but when taken over years, such therapy may slightly increase the risk of a second type of arrhythmia. To date the only effective and commercially successful pharmacologic antiarrhythmic agents are not directly related to cardiac ion channels (β-blockers) or nonspecific cardiac ion channel modulators (amiodarone).

Antiarrhythmic devices hold great promise for the future. These devices are getting smaller, more reliable, and smarter. Atrial pacing is effective therapy for reducing the instance of arrhythmia in neonates with long QT syndrome.[194] This therapy has been used to treat neonates while they grow large enough for the implantation of an automatic defibrillator.[195] An ideal device might be one that is capable of measuring cardiac conduction and repolarization and rhythm, and can deliver appropriate doses of specific pharmacologic agents to modulate the electrophysiology of the heart, while providing a safety net in the form of an automatic internal defibrillator. Development of these devices is an important goal for the future.

REFERENCES

1. Kannel W, Cupples A, D'Agostino R: Sudden death risk in overt coronary heart diseases: The Framingham study. *Am Heart J* **113**:799, 1987.
2. Willich S, Levy D, Rocco M, Tofler G, Stone P, Muller J: Circadian variation in the incidence of sudden cardiac death in the Framingham heart study population. *Am J Cardiol* **60**:801, 1987.
3. Manolis AS, Katsaros C, Kokkinos DV: Electrophysiological and electropharmacological studies in preexcitation syndromes: Results with propafenone therapy and isoproterenol infusion testing. *Eur Heart J* **13**:1489, 1992.
4. Splawski I, Timothy KW, Vincent GM, Atkinson DL, Keating MT: Molecular basis of the long-QT syndrome associated with deafness. *N Engl J Med* **336**:1562, 1997.
5. Benhorin J, Medina A: Images in clinical medicine. Congenital long-QT syndrome. *N Engl J Med* **336**:1568, 1997.
6. Lazzara R: Twisting of the points. *J Am Coll Cardiol* **29**:843, 1997.
7. Donger C, Denjoy I, Berthet M, Neyroud N, Cruaud C, Bennaceur M, Chivoret G, et al: KVLQT1 C-terminal missense mutation causes a forme fruste long-QT syndrome. *Circulation* **96**:2778, 1997.
8. Duggal P, Vesely MR, Wattanasirichaigoon D, Villafane J, Kaushik V, Beggs AH: Mutation of the gene for IsK associated with both Jervell and Lange-Nielsen and Romano-Ward forms of Long-QT syndrome. *Circulation* **97**:142, 1998.
9. Pacia SV: The prolonged QT syndrome presenting as epilepsy: A report of two cases and literature review. *Neurology* **44**:1408, 1994.
10. Gatto EM: Prolonged QT syndrome presenting as epilepsy. *Neurology* **46**:1188, 1996.
11. Jervell A, Lange-Nielsen F: Congenital deaf-mutism, functional heart disease with prolongation of the QT interval, and sudden death. *Am Heart J* **54**:59, 1957.
12. Meissner FL: Taubstummheit und Taubstummenbildung, in. Leipzig and Heidelberg1856, p 119.
13. Latham AD, Munro TA: Familial myoclonus epilepsy associated with deaf mutism in a family showing other psychobiological abnormalities. *Ann Eugenics London* **8**:166, 1937.
14. Moller T, Herrlin KM: A case of cardiac syncope. *Acta Paediatrica* **42**:391, 1953.
15. Fraser GR, Froggatt P, James TN: Congenital deafness associated with electrocardiographic abnormalities, fainting attacks and sudden death. *Quart J Med* **33**:361, 1964.
16. Jervell A, Thingstad R, Endsjo T: Three new cases of congenital deafness with syncopal attacks and Q-T prolongation in the electrocardiogram. *Am Heart J* **72**:582, 1966.
17. Tesson F, Donger C, Denjoy I, Berthet M, Bennaceur M, Petit C, Coumel P, et al: Exclusion of KCNE1 (IsK) as a candidate gene for Jervell and Lange-Nielsen Syndrome. *J Mol Cell Cardiol* **28**:2051, 1996.
18. Marks M, Whisler S, Clericuzio C, Keating M: A new form of long QT syndrome associated with syndactyly. *J Am Coll Cardiol* **25**:59, 1995.
19. Marks M: Long QT syndrome associated with syndactyly identified in females. *Am J Cardiol* **76**:744, 1995.
20. Levin S: Long QT syndrome associated with syndactyly in a female. *Am J Cardiol* **78**:380, 1996.
21. Schrem SS, Belsky P, Schwartzman D, Slater W: Cocaine-induced torsades de pointes in a patient with the idiopathic long QT syndrome. *Am Heart J* **120**:980, 1990.
22. Nattel S: Erythromycin-induced long QT syndrome: Concordance with quinidine and underlying cellular electrophysiologic mechanism. *Am J Med* **89**:235, 1990.
23. Ohya Y: Factors related to QT interval prolongation during probucol treatment. *Eur J Clin Pharmacol* **45**:47, 1993.
24. Brandriss MW, Richardson WS, Barold SS: Erythromycin-induced QT prolongation and polymorphic ventricular tachycardia (torsades de pointes): Case report and review. *Clin Infect Dis* **18**:995, 1994.
25. Celiker A: Adenosine-induced torsades de pointes in a child with congenital long QT syndrome. *Pacing Clin Electrophysiol* **17**:1814, 1994.
26. Conti C: The nonsedating antihistamine scare. *Clin Cardiol* **17**:1, 1994.
27. Koh K: Torsade de pointes induced by terfenadine in a patient with long QT syndrome. *J Electrocardiol* **27**:343, 1994.
28. Chvilicek J, Hurlbert B, Hill G: Diuretic-induced hypokalaemia inducing torsades de pointes. *Can J Anaesth* **42**:1137, 1995.
29. Johnson A: ECG changes in pediatric patients on tricyclic antidepressants, desipramine, and imipramine. *Can J Psychiatry* **41**:102, 1996.
30. Wysowski DK, Bacsanyi J: Cisapride and fatal arrhythmia. *N Engl J Med* **335**:290, 1996.
31. Bedu A, Lupoglazoff JM, Faure C, Denjoy I, Casasoprana A, Aujard Y: Cisapride high dosage and long QT interval. *J Pediatr* **130**:164, 1997.
32. Mohammad S, Zhou Z, Gong Q, January CT: Blockage of the HERG human cardiac K^+ channel by the gastrointestinal prokinetic agent cisapride. *Am J Physiol* **273**:H2534, 1997.
33. Vogt A: Long Q-T syndrome associated with oral erythromycin used in preoperative bowel preparation. *Anesth Analg* **85**:1011, 1997.
34. Akiyama T: Hypocalcemic Torsades de Pointes. *J Electrocardiol* **22**:89, 1989.
35. Cooke RA, Chambers JB, Singh R, Todd GJ, Smeeton NC, Treasure J, Treasure T: QT interval in anorexia nervosa. *Br Heart J* **72**:69, 1994.
36. Oka H: Prolongation of QTc interval in patients with Parkinson's disease. *Eur Neurol* **37**:186, 1997.
37. Abo K: Torsade de pointes in NIDDM with long QT intervals. *Diabetes Care* **19**:1010, 1996.
38. Sawicki PT, Dahne R, Bender R, Berger M: Prolonged QT interval as a predictor of mortality in diabetic nephropathy. *Diabetologia* **39**:77, 1996.
39. Sivieri R: Prevalence of QT prolongation in a type 1 diabetic population and its association with autonomic neuropathy. The Neuropathy Study Group of the Italian Society for the Study of Diabetes. *Diabet Med* **10**:920, 1993.

40. Kempler P: Prolongation of the QTc-interval reflects the severity of autonomic neuropathy in primary biliary cirrhosis and in other non-alcoholic liver diseases. *Z Gastroenterol* **31**:96, 1993.
41. Kihara H, Terai H, Kihara Y, Takahashi H, Kosuda A, et al: Pheochromocytoma of the left retroperitoneal paraganglion associated with torsade de pointes: A case report. *J Cardiol* **30**:37–44, 1997.
42. Pripp C: Epiglottitis and torsade de pointes tachycardia. *Br Heart J* **72**:205, 1994.
43. Rodney E, Parente T, Vasavada BC, Sacchi TJ: Life-threatening ventricular arrhythmias in patients with silent myocardial ischemia due to coronary-artery spasm. *N Engl J Med* **327**:956, 1992.
44. Schwartz PJ, Stramba-Badiale M, Segantini A, Austoni P, Bosi G, Giorgetti R, Grancini F, et al: Prolongation of the QT interval and the sudden infant death syndrome. *N Engl J Med* **338**:1709, 1998.
45. Algra A, Tijssen JGP, Roelandt J, Pool J, Lubsen J: QTc prolongation measured by standard 12-lead electrocardiography is an independent risk factor for sudden death due to cardiac arrest. *Circulation* **83**:1888, 1991.
46. Dekker JM, Schouten EG, Klootwijk P, Pool J, Kromhout D: Association between QT interval and coronary heart disease in middle-aged and elderly men. The Zutphen Study. *Circulation* **90**:779, 1994.
47. Trappe HJ, Brugada P, Talajic M, Della Bella P, Lezaun R, Mulleneers R, Wellens HJ: Prognosis of patients with ventricular tachycardia and ventricular fibrillation: Role of the underlying etiology. *J Am Coll Cardiol* **12**:166, 1988.
48. Viskin S, Belhassen B: Idiopathic ventricular fibrillation. *Am Heart J* **120**:661, 1990.
49. Wichter T, Breithardt G, Borggrefe M: Mechanism, diagnosis and management, in Podrid P, Kowey P (eds): *Cardiac Arrhythmia*. Baltimore, MD, Williams & Wilkins, 1995, p 1219.
50. Martini B: Ventricular fibrillation without apparent heart disease: Description of six cases. *Am Heart J* **118**:1203, 1989.
51. Brugada J, Brugada R, Brugada P: Right bundle branch block, ST segment elevation in leads V1-V3: A marker for sudden death in patients without demonstrable structural heart disease. *Circulation* **96**:1151, 1997.
52. Brugada P, Brugada J: Right bundle branch block, persistent ST segment elevation and sudden cardiac death: A distinct clinical and electrocardiographic syndrome. A multicenter report. *J Am Coll Cardiol* **20**:1391, 1992.
53. Brugada P, Brugada J: Further characterization of the syndrome of right bundle branch block, ST segment elevation, and sudden cardiac death. *J Cardiovasc Electrophysiol* **8**:325, 1997.
54. Brugada J, Brugada P, Brugada R: Ajmaline unmasks right branch block-like and ST segment elevation in V1-V3 in patients with idiopathic ventricular fibrillation. *PACE* **19**:599, 1996.
55. Miyanuma H, Sakurai M, Odaka H: Two cases of idiopathic ventricular fibrillation with interesting electrocardiographic findings. *Kokyu To Junkan* **41**:287, 1993.
56. Aizawa Y, Tamura M, Chinushi M, Naitoh N, Uchiyama H, Kusano Y, Hosono H, Hosono H, et al: Idiopathic ventricular fibrillation and bradycardia-dependent intraventricular block. *Am Heart J* **126**:1473, 1993.
57. Sumiyoshi M, Nakata Y, Hisaoka T, Ogura S, Nakazato Y, Kawai S, Okada R, et al: A case of idiopathic ventricular fibrillation with incomplete right bundle branch block and persistent ST segment elevation. *Jpn Heart J* **34**:661, 1993.
58. Bjerregaard P, Gussak I, Kotar SL, Gessler JE, Janosik D: Recurrent syncope in a patient with prominent J wave. *Am Heart J* **127**:1426, 1994.
59. Miyazaki T: Autonomic and antiarrhythmic drug modulation of ST segment elevation in patients with Brugada syndrome. *J Am Coll Cardiol* **2**:1061, 1996.
60. Vincent GM, Timothy K, Leppert M, Keating M: The spectrum of symptoms and QT intervals in carriers of the gene for the long QT syndrome. *N Engl J Med* **327**:846, 1992.
61. Schwartz P, Moss A, Vincent G, Crampton R: Diagnostic criteria for the long QT syndrome. *Circulation* **88**:782, 1993.
62. Lehmann MH, Suzuki F, Fromm BS, Frankovich D, Elko P, Steinman RT, Fresard J, et al: T wave "humps" as a potential electrocardiographic marker of the long QT syndrome. *J Am Coll Cardiol* **1994**:746, 1994.
63. Reardon M, Malik M: QT interval change with age in an overtly healthy older population. *Clin Cardiol* **19**:949, 1996.
64. Lehmann MH, Timothy KW, Frankovich D, Fromm BS, Keating M, Locati EH, Taggart RT, et al: Age-gender influence on the rate-corrected QT interval and the QT-heart rate relations in families with genotypically characterized long QT syndrome. *J Am Coll Cardiol* **29**:93, 1997.
65. Locati EH, Zareba W, Moss AJ, Schwartz PJ, Vincent GM, Lehmann MH, Towbin JA, et al: Age and sex-related differences in clinical manifestations in patients with congenital long-QT syndrome: Findings from the International LQTS Registry. *Circulation* **97**:2237, 1998.
66. Bazette H: An analysis of the time-relations of electrocardiograms. *Heart* **7**:353, 1920.
67. Katagiri-Kawade M: Abnormal response to exercise, face immersion, and isoproterenol in children with the long QT syndrome. *Pacing Clin Electrophysiol* **18**:2128, 1995.
68. Vincent GM, Jaiswal D, Timothy KW: Effects of exercise on heart rate, QT, QTc and QT/QS2 in the Romano-Ward inherited long QT syndrome. *Am J Cardiol* **68**:498, 1991.
69. Moss A: ECG T-wave patterns in genetically distinct forms of the hereditary long QT syndrome. *Circulation* **92**:2929, 1995.
70. Schulze-Bahr E, Haverkamp W, Breithardt G, Funke H, Wiebusch H, Assmann G: ECG repolarization patterns in chromosome 7-linked QT syndrome. *Circulation* **94**:2318, 1996.
71. Zareba W, Moss A, Schwartz P, Vincent G, Robinson J, Priori S, Benhorin J, et al: Influence of the genotype on the clinical course of the long-QT syndrome. *N Engl J Med* **339**:960, 1998.
72. Josephson M: Athletes and arrhythmias: Clinical considerations and perspectives. *Eur Heart J* **17**:498, 1996.
73. Ackerman M: A novel mutation in KVLQT1 is the molecular basis of inherited long QT syndrome in a near-drowning patient's family. *Pediatr Res* **1998**:148, 1998.
74. McCurdy CJ: Syncope and sudden arrhythmic death complicating pregnancy. A case report of Romano-Ward syndrome. *J Reprod Med* **38**:233, 1993.
75. Bennett PB, Yazawa K, Makita N, George AL: Molecular mechanism for an inherited cardiac arrhythmia. *Nature* **376**:683, 1995.
76. Keating M, Sanguinetti M: Molecular genetic insights into cardiovascular disease. *Science* **272**:681, 1996.
77. Curran ME, Splawski I, Timothy KW, Vincent GM, Green ED, Keating MT: A molecular basis for cardiac arrhythmia: *HERG* mutations cause long QT syndrome. *Cell* **80**:795, 1995.
78. Wang Q, Curran ME, Splawski I, Burn TC, Millholland JM, VanRaay TJ, Shen J, et al: Positional cloning of a novel potassium channel gene: KVLQT1 mutations cause cardiac arrhythmias. *Nat Genet* **12**:17, 1996.
79. Wang Q, Shen J, Splawski I, Atkinson D, Zhizhong L, Robinson J, Moss A, et al: *SCN5A* mutations associated with an inherited cardiac arrhythmia, long QT syndrome. *Cell* **80**:805, 1995.
80. Splawski I, Tristani-Firouzi M, Lehmann MH, Sanguinetti MC, Keating MT: Mutations in the hminK gene cause long QT syndrome and suppress IKs function. *Nat Genet* **17**:338, 1997.
81. Schott J, Charpentier F, Peltier S, Foley P, Drouin E, Bouhour J, Donnelly P, et al: Mapping of a gene for long QT syndrome to chromosome 4q25-27. *Am J Hum Genet* **57**:1114, 1995.
82. Jiang C, Atkinson D, Towbin JA, Splawski I, Lehmann MH, Li H, Timothy K, et al: Two long QT syndrome loci map to chromosomes 3 and 7 with evidence for further heterogeneity. *Nat Genet* **8**:141, 1994.
83. Keating M, Atkinson D, Dunn C, Timothy K, Vincent GM, Leppert M: Linkage of a cardiac arrhythmia, the long QT syndrome, and the Harvey *ras*-1 gene. *Science* **252**:704, 1991.
84. Keating M: Risk, genotype, and cardiovascular disease. *Circulation* **86**:688, 1992.
85. Keating M, Dunn C, Atkinson D, Timothy K, Vincent GM, Leppert M: Consistent linkage of the long QT syndrome to the Harvey *ras*-1 locus on chromosome 11. *Am J Hum Genet* **49**:1335, 1991.
86. Benhorin J, Kalman YM, Medina A, Towbin J, Rave-Harel N, Dyer TD, Blangero J, et al: Evidence of genetic heterogeneity in the long QT syndrome. *Science* **260**:1960, 1993.
87. Curran M, Atkinson D, Timothy K, G V, Moss A, Leppert M, Keating M: Locus heterogeneity of autosomal dominant long QT syndrome. *J Clin Invest* **92**:799, 1993.
88. Towbin JA, Hejtmancik JF, Brink P, Gelb BD, Zhu XM, Chamberlain JS, McCabe ERB, et al: X-linked dilated cardiomyopathy (XLCM): Molecular genetic evidence of linkage to the Duchenne muscular dystrophy gene at the Xp21 locus. *Circulation* **87**:1854, 1993.

89. Jiang C, Atkinson D, Towbin J, Splawski I, Lehmann M, Li H, Timothy K, et al: Two long QT syndrome loci map to chromosome 3 and 7 with evidence for further heterogeneity. *Nat Genet* **8**:141, 1994.
90. Warmke J, Ganetzky B: A family of potassium channel genes related to *eag* in *Drosophila* and mammals. *Proc Natl Acad Sci U S A* **91**:3438, 1994.
91. Arcangeli A, Rosati B, Cherubini A, Crociani O, Fontana L, Ziller C, Wanke E, et al: HERG- and IRK-like inward rectifier currents are sequentially expressed during neuronal development of neural crest cells and their derivatives. *Eur J Neurosci* **9**:2596, 1997.
92. Pennefather PS, Zhou W, DeCoursey TE: Idiosyncratic gating of HERG-like K^+ channels in microglia. *J Gen Physiol* **111**:795, 1998.
93. Bianchi L, Wible B, Arcangeli A, Taglialatela M, Morra F, Castaldo P, Crociani O, et al: HERG encodes a K^+ current highly conserved in tumors of different histogenesis: A selective advantage for cancer cells? *Cancer Res* **58**:815, 1998.
94. Chiesa N, Rosati B, Arcangeli A, Olivotto M, Wanke E: A novel role for HERG K^+ channels: Spike-frequency adaptation [published erratum appears in *J Physiol (Lond)* **502(Pt 3)**:715, 1997]. *J Physiol (Lond)* **501**:313, 1997.
95. Shi W, Wymore RS, Wang HS, Pan Z, Cohen IS, McKinnon D, Dixon JE: Identification of two nervous system-specific members of the erg potassium channel gene family. *J Neurosci* **17**:9423, 1997.
96. Benson DW, MacRae CA, Vesely MR, Walsh EP, Seidman JG, Seidman CE, Satler CA: Missense mutation in the pore region of *HERG* causes familial long QT syndrome. *Circulation* **93**:1791, 1996.
97. Tanaka T, Nagai R, Tomoike H, Takata S, Yano K, Yabuta K, Haneda N, et al: Four novel KVLQT1 and four novel HERG mutations in familial long-QT syndrome. *Circulation* **95**:565, 1997.
98. Splawski I, Shen J, Timothy KW, Lehmann MH, Priori S, Robinson JL, Moss AJ, et al: Spectrum of mutations in long-QT syndrome genes. KVLQT1, HERG, SCN5A, KCNE1, and KCNE2. *Circulation* **102**:1178, 2000.
99. Akimoto K, Furutani M, Imamura S, Furutani Y, Kasanuki H, Takao A, Momma K, et al: Novel missense mutation (G601S) of HERG in a Japanese long QT syndrome family. *Hum Mutat* **1**:S184, 1998.
100. Itoh T, Tanaka T, Nagai R, Kamiya T, Sawayama T, Nakayama T, Tomoike H, et al: Genomic organization and mutational analysis of HERG, a gene responsible for familial long QT syndrome. *Hum Genet* **102**:435, 1998.
101. Satler CA, Vesely MR, Duggal P, Ginsburg GS, Beggs AH: Multiple different missense mutations in the pore region of HERG in patients with long QT syndrome. *Hum Genet* **102**:265, 1998.
102. Splawski I, Shen J, Timothy KW, Vincent GM, Lehmann MH, Keating MT: Genomic structure of three long QT syndrome genes: KVLQT1, HERG and KCNE1. *Genomics* **51**:86, 1998.
103. Morais JH, Lee A, Cohen SL, Chait BT, Li M, MacKinnon R: Crystal structure and functional analysis of the HERG potassium channel N terminus: A eukaryotic PAS domain. *Cell* **95**:649, 1998.
104. Schonherr R, Heinemann SH: Molecular determinants for activation and inactivation of HERG, a human inward rectifier potassium channel. *J Physiol* **493**:635, 1996.
105. Spector PS, Curran ME, Zou A, Keating MT, Sanguinetti MC: Fast inactivation causes rectification of the IKr channel. *J Gen Physiol* **107**:611, 1996.
106. Lees-Miller JP, Kondo C, Wang L, Duff HJ: Electrophysiological characterization of an alternatively processed ERG K^+ channel in mouse and human hearts. *Circ Res* **81**:719, 1997.
107. London B, Trudeau MC, Newton KP, Beyer AK, Copeland NG, Gilbert DJ, Jenkins NA, et al: Two isoforms of the mouse ether-a-go-go-related gene coassemble to form channels with properties similar to the rapidly activating component of the cardiac delayed rectifier K^+ current. *Circ Res* **81**:870, 1997.
108. Lee MP, Hu R-J, Johnson LA, Feinberg AP: Human *KVLQT1* gene shows tissue-specific imprinting and encompasses Beckwith-Wiedemann syndrome chromosomal rearrangements. *Nat Genet* **15**:181, 1997.
109. Gould T, Pfeifer K: Imprinting of mouse Kvlqt1 is developmentally regulated. *Hum Mol Genet* **7**:483, 1998.
110. Paulsen M, Davies K, Bowden L, Villar A, Franck O, Fuermann M, Dean W, et al: Syntenic organization of the mouse distal chromosome 7 imprinting cluster and the Beckwith-Wiedemann syndrome region in chromosome 11p15.5. *Hum Mol Genet* **7**:1149, 1998.
111. Yang WP, Levesque PC, Little WA, Conder ML, Ramakrishnan P, Neubauer MG, Blanar MA: Functional expression of two KvLQT1-related potassium channels responsible for an inherited idiopathic epilepsy. *J Biol Chem* **273**:19419, 1998.
112. Charlier C, Singh NA, Ryan SG, Lewis TB, Reus BE, Leach RJ, Leppert M: A pore mutation in a novel KQT-like potassium channel gene in an idiopathic epilepsy family. *Nat Genet* **18**:53, 1998.
113. Singh NA, Charlier C, Stauffer D, DuPont BR, Leach RJ, Melis R, Ronen GM, et al: A novel potassium channel gene, KCNQ2, is mutated in an inherited epilepsy of newborns. *Nat Genet* **18**:25, 1998.
114. Russell MW, Dick M, Collins FS, Brody LC: KVLQT1 mutations in three families with familial or sporadic long QT syndrome. *Hum Mol Genet* **5**:1319, 1996.
115. de Jager T, Corbett CH, Badenhorst JC, Brink PA, Corfield VA: Evidence of a long QT founder gene with varying phenotypic expression in South African families. *J Med Genet* **33**:567, 1996.
116. van den Berg MH, Wilde AA, Robles de Medina EO, Meyer H, Geelen JL, Jongbloed RJ, Wellens HJ, et al: The long QT syndrome: A novel missense mutation in the S6 region of the KVLQT1 gene. *Hum Genet* **100**:356, 1997.
117. Kanters J: Novel donor splice site mutation in the KVLQT1 gene is associated with long QT syndrome. *J Cardiovasc Electrophysiol* **9**:620, 1998.
118. Li H, et al: New mutations in the KVLQT1 potasium channel that cause long-QT syndrome. *Circulation* **97**:1264, 1998.
119. Neyroud N, Tesson F, Denjoy I, Leibovici M, Donger C, Barhanin J, Faure S, et al: A novel mutation in the potassium channel gene *KVLQT1* causes the Jervell and Lange-Nielsen cardioauditory syndrome. *Nat Genet* **15**:186, 1997.
120. Taglialatela M: Molecular basis for the lack of HERG K^+ channel block-related cardiotoxicity by the H1 receptor blocker cetirizine compared with other second-generation antihistamines. *Mol Pharmacol* **54**:113, 1998.
121. Schulze-Bahr E, Wang Q, Wedekind H, Haverkamp W, Chen Q, Sun Y, Rubie C, et al: *KCNE1* mutations cause Jervell and Lange-Nielsen syndrome. *Nat Genet* **17**:267, 1997.
122. Tyson J, Tranebjaerg L, Bellman S, Wren C, Taylor JFN, Bathen J, Aslaksen B, et al: IsK and KvLQT1: Mutation in either of the two subunits of the slow component of the delayed rectifier potassium channel can cause Jervell and Lange-Nielsen syndrome. *Hum Mol Genet* **6**:2179, 1997.
123. George A, Varkony T, Drabkin H, Han J, Knops J, Finley W, Brown G, et al: Assignment of the human heart tetrodotoxin-resistant voltage-gated Na^+ channel α-subunit gene (SCN5A) to band 3p21. *Cytogenet Cell Genet* **68**:67, 1995.
124. Wang Q: Genomic organization of the human SCN5A gene encoding the cardiac sodium channel. *Genomics* **34**:9, 1996.
125. Wang W, Shen J, Li Z, Timothy K, Vincent G, Priori S, Schwartz P, et al: Cardiac sodium channel mutations in patients with long QT syndrome, an inherited cardiac arrhythmia. *Hum Mol Genet* **4**:1603, 1995.
126. An R: Novel LQT-3 mutation affects Na^+ channel activity through interactions between alpha- and beta 1-subunits. *Circ Res* **83**:141, 1998.
127. Kambouris NG, Nuss HB, Johns DC, Tomaselli GF, Marban E, Balser JR: Phenotypic characterization of a novel long-QT syndrome mutation (R1623Q) in the cardiac sodium channel. *Circulation* **97**:640, 1998.
128. Makita N, Shirai N, Nagashima N, Matsuoka R, Yamada Y, Tohse N, Kitabatake A: A de novo missense mutation of human cardiac Na^+ channel exhibiting novel molecular mechanisms of long QT syndrome. *FEBS Lett* **423**:5, 1998.
129. Chen Q, Kirsch GE, Zhang D, Brugada R, Brugada J, Brugada P, Potenza D, et al: Genetic basis and molecular mechanism for idiopathic ventricular fibrillation. *Nature* **392**:293, 1998.
130. Sanguinetti MC, Jiang C, Curran ME, Keating MT: A mechanistic link between an inherited and an acquired cardiac arrhythmia: HERG encodes the IKr potassium channel. *Cell* **81**:299, 1995.
131. Trudeau MC, Warmke JW, Ganetzky B, Robertson GA: HERG, a human inward rectifier in the voltage-gated potassium channel family. *Science* **269**:92, 1995.
132. Smith PL, Baukrowitz T, Yellen G: The inward rectification mechanism of the HERG cardiac potassium channel. *Nature* **379**:833, 1996.
133. Herzberg IM, Trudeau MC, Robertson GA: Transfer of rapid inactivation and sensitivity to the class III antiarrhythmic drug E-4031 from HERG to M-eag channels. *J Physiol (Lond)* **511**:3, 1998.
134. Morais JH, Lee A, Cohen SL, Chait BT, Li M, Mackinnon R: Crystal structure and functional analysis of the HERG potassium channel N terminus: A eukaryotic PAS domain. *Cell* **95**:649, 1998.

135. Dausse E, Berthet M, Denjoy I, Andre-Fouet X, Cruaud C, Bennaceur M, Faure S, et al: A mutation in HERG associated with notched T waves in long QT syndrome. *J Mol Cell Cardiol* **28**:1609, 1996.
136. Satler CA, Walsh EP, Vesely MR, Plummer MH, Ginsburg GS, Jacob HJ: Novel missense mutation in the cyclic nucleotide-binding domain of HERG causes long QT syndrome. *Am J Med Genet* **65**:27, 1996.
137. Sanguinetti MC, Curran ME, Spector PS, Keating MT: Spectrum of HERG K^+ channel dysfunction in an inherited cardiac arrhythmia. *Proc Natl Acad Sci U S A* **93**:2208, 1996.
138. Zhou Z, Gong Q, Epstein ML, January CT: HERG channel dysfunction in human long QT syndrome. Intracellular transport and functional defects. *J Biol Chem* **273**:21061, 1998.
139. Zhou Z, Gong Q, Epstein ML, January CT: HERG channel dysfunction in human long QT syndrome. Intracellular transport and functional defects. *J Biol Chem* **273**:21061, 1998.
140. Babij P, Askew GR, Nieuwenhuijsen B, Su CM, Bridal TR, Jow B, Argentieri TM, et al: Inhibition of cardiac delayed rectifier K^+ current by overexpression of the long-QT syndrome HERG G628S mutation in transgenic mice. *Circ Res* **83**:668, 1998.
140a. Chen J, Zou A, Splawski I, Keating MT, Sanguinetti, MC: Long QT syndrome-associated mutations in the Per-Arnt-Sim (PAS) domain of HERG potassium channels accelerate channel deactivation. *J Biol Chem* **274**:10113, 1999.
141. Nakajima T, Furukawa T, Tanaka T, Katayama Y, Nagai R, Nakamura Y, Hiraoka M: Novel mechanism of HERG current suppression in LQT2: Shift in voltage dependence of HERG inactivation. *Circ Res* **83**:415, 1998.
142. Snyders D, Chaudhary A: High affinity open channel block by dofetilide of HERG expressed in a human cell line. *Mol Pharmacol* **49**:949, 1996.
143. Dumaine R: Blockade of HERG and kv1.5 by ketoconazole. *J Pharmacol Exp Ther* **286**:727, 1998.
144. Ficker E: Molecular determinants of dofetilide block of HERG K^+ channels. *Circ Res* **82**:386, 1998.
145. Rampe D: A mechanism for the proarrhythmic effects of cisapride (Propulsid): High affinity blockade of the human cardiac potassium channel HERG. *FEBS Lett* **417**:28, 1997.
146. Suessbrich H: Blockade of HERG channels expressed in *Xenopus* oocytes by the histamine receptor antagonists terfenadine and astemizole. *FEBS Lett* **385**:77, 1996.
147. Spector PS, et al: Class III antiarrhythmic drugs block HERG, a human cardiac delayed rectifier K^+ channel. Open-channel block by methanesulfonamides. *Circ Res* **78**:499, 1996.
148. Suessbrich H, Schonherr R, Heinemann SH, Lang F, Busch AE: Specific block of cloned HERG channels by clofilium and its tertiary analog LY97241. *FEBS Lett* **414**:435, 1997.
149. Suessbrich H, Schonherr R, Heinemann SH, Attali B, Lang F, Busch AE: The inhibitory effect of the antipsychotic drug haloperidol on HERG potassium channels expressed in *Xenopus* oocytes. *Br J Pharmacol* **120**:968, 1997.
150. Taglialatela M, Castaldo P, Pannaccione A, Giorgio G, Annunziato L: Human ether-a-go-go related gene (HERG) K^+ channels as pharmacological targets: Present and future implications. *Biochem Pharmacol* **55**:1741, 1998.
151. Roden DM: A practical approach to torsade de pointes. *Clin Cardiol* **20**:285, 1997.
152. Sanguinetti MC, Jurkiewicz NK: Role of external Ca^{2+} and K^+ in gating of cardiac delayed rectifier K^+ currents. *Pflugers Arch* **420**:180, 1992.
153. Yang T: Rapid inactivation determines the rectification and $[K^+]_o$ dependence of the rapid component of the delayed rectifier K^+ current in cardiac cells. *Circ Res* **80**:782, 1997.
154. Zou A, Xu Q, Sanguinetti MC: A mutation in the pore region of HERG K^+ channels expressed in *Xenopus* oocytes reduces rectification by shifting the voltage dependence of inactivation. *J Physiol* **509**:129, 1998.
155. Roden DM, Lazzara R, Rosen M, Schwartz PJ, Towbin J, Vincent GM: Multiple mechanisms in the long-QT syndrome. Current knowledge, gaps, and future directions. The SADS Foundation Task Force on LQTS. *Circulation* **94**:1996, 1996.
156. Bosch RF, Gaspo R, Busch AE, Lang HJ, Li GR, Nattel S: Effects of the chromanol 293B, a selective blocker of the slow, component of the delayed rectifier K^+ current, on repolarization in human and guinea pig ventricular myocytes. *Cardiovasc Res* **38**:441, 1998.
157. Fiset C, Drolet B, Hamelin BA, Turgeon J: Block of IKs by the diuretic agent indapamide modulates cardiac electrophysiological effects of the class III antiarrhythmic drug dl-sotalol. *J Pharmacol Exp Ther* **283**:148, 1997.
158. Gintant GA: Azimilide causes reverse rate-dependent block while reducing both components of delayed-rectifier current in canine ventricular myocytes. *J Cardiovasc Pharmacol* **31**:945, 1998.
159. Selnick HG, Liverton NJ, Baldwin JJ, Butcher JW, Claremon DA, Elliott JM, Freidinger RM, et al: Class III antiarrhythmic activity in vivo by selective blockade of the slowly activating cardiac delayed rectifier potassium current IKs by (R)-2-(2,4-trifluoromethyl)-N-[2-oxo-5-phenyl-1-(2,2,2-trifluoroethyl)-2,3-dihydro-1H-benzo[e][1,4]-diazepin-3-yl]acetamide. *J Med Chem* **40**:3865, 1997.
160. Takumi T, Ohkubo H, Nakanishi S: Cloning of a membrane protein that induces a slow voltage-gated potassium current. *Science* **242**:1042, 1988.
161. Wang K, Goldstein S: Subunit composition of minK potassium channels. *Neuron* **14**:1303, 1995.
162. Tai KK, Wang K-W, Goldstein SAN: MinK potassium channels are heteromultimeric complexes. *J Biol Chem* **272**:1654, 1997.
163. Freeman LC, Kass RS: Expression of a minimal K^+ channel protein in mammalian cells and immunolocalization in guinea pig heart. *Circ Res* **73**:968, 1993.
164. Attali B, Guillemare E, Lesage F, Honore E, Romey G, Lazdunski M, Barhanin J: The protein IsK is a dual activator of K^+ and Cl^- channels. *Nature* **365**:850, 1993.
165. Tai KK, Wang KW, Goldstein SA: MinK potassium channels are heteromultimeric complexes. *J Biol Chem* **272**:1654, 1997.
166. Wollnik B, Schroeder BC, Kubisch C, Esperer HD, Wieacker P, Jentsch TJ: Pathophysiological mechanisms of dominant and recessive KVLQT1 K^+ channel mutations found in inherited cardiac arrhythmias. *Hum Mol Genet* **6**:1943, 1997.
167. Shalaby FY, Levesque PC, Yang WP, Little WA, Conder ML, Jenkins-West T, Blanar MA: Dominant-negative KvLQT1 mutations underlie the LQT1 form of long QT syndrome. *Circulation* **96**:1733, 1997.
168. Chouabe C, Neyroud N, Guicheney P, Lazdunski M, Romey G, Barhanin J: Properties of KvLQT1 K^+ channel mutations in Romano-Ward and Jervell and Lange-Nielsen inherited cardiac arrhythmias. *EMBO J* **16**:5472, 1997.
169. Demolombe S, Baro I, Pereon Y, Bliek J, Mohammad-Panah R, Pollard H, Morid S, et al: A dominant negative isoform of the long QT syndrome 1 gene product. *J Biol Chem* **273**:6837, 1998.
170. Jiang M, Tseng-Crank J, Tseng GN: Suppression of slow delayed rectifier current by a truncated isoform of KvLQT1 cloned from normal human heart. *J Biol Chem* **272**:24109, 1997.
171. Dumaine R, Wang Q, Keating MT, Hartmann HA, Schwartz PJ, Brown AM, Kirsch GE: Multiple mechanisms of sodium channel-linked long QT syndrome. *Circ Res* **78**:916, 1996.
172. Makita N, Shirai N, Nagashima M, Matsuoka R, Yamada Y, Tohse N, Kitabatake A: A de novo missense mutation of human cardiac Na^+ channel exhibiting novel molecular mechanisms of long QT syndrome. *FEBS Lett* **423**:5, 1998.
173. Krishnan SC, Antzelevitch C: Sodium channel block produces opposite electrophysiological effects in canine ventricular epicardium and endocardium. *Circ Res* **69**:277, 1991.
174. Krishnan SC, Antzelevitch C: Flecainide-induced arrhythmia in canine ventricular epicardium. Phase 2 reentry? *Circulation* **87**:562, 1992.
175. Zareba W, Moss AJ, Schwartz PJ, Vincent GM, Robinson JL, Priori SG, Benhorin J, et al: Influence of genotype on the clinical course of the long-QT syndrome. International Long-QT Syndrome Registry Research Group. *N Engl J Med* **339**:960, 1998.
176. El-Sherif N, Caref EB, Yin H, Restivo M: The electrophysiological mechanism of ventricular arrhythmias in the long QT syndrome. Tridimensional mapping of activation and recovery patterns. *Circ Res* **79**:474, 1996.
177. El-Sherif N: Electrophysiological mechanism of the characteristic electrocardiographic morphology of torsade de pointes tachyarrhythmias in the long-QT syndrome: Detailed analysis of ventricular tridimensional activation patterns. *Circulation* **96**:4392, 1997.
178. Marcus DC, Shen Z: Slowly activating voltage-dependent K^+ conductance is apical pathway for K^+ secretion in vestibular dark cells. *Am J Physiol* **267**:C857, 1994.
179. Vetter DE, Mann JR, Wangemann P, Liu J, McLaughlin KJ, Lesage F, Marcus DC, et al: Inner ear defects induced by null mutation of the isk gene. *Neuron* **17**:1251, 1996.

180. Drouin E: α1-Adrenergic stimulation induces early afterdepolarizations in ferret Purkinje fibers. *J Cardiovasc Pharmacol* **27**:320, 1996.
181. Moss A: Clinical management of patients with the long QT syndrome: Drugs, devices and gene-specific therapy. *Pacing Clin Electrophysiol* **20**:2058, 1997.
182. Mesa A: Dysrhythmias controlled with stellate ganglion block in a child with diabetes and a variant of long QT syndrome. *Reg Anesth* **18**:60, 1993.
183. Cheng TO: Left cardiac sympathetic denervation for long QT syndrome. *Int J Cardiol* **62**:281.
184. Stramba-Badiale M, Goulene K, Schwartz PJ: Effects of beta-adrenergic blockade on dispersion of ventricular repolarization in newborn infants with prolonged QT interval. *Am Heart J* **134**:406, 1997.
185. Shenasa M, Borggrefe M, Haverkamp W, Hindricks G and Breithardt G: Ventricular tachycardia. *Lancet* **341**:512, 1993.
186. Klein HO: Congenital long-QT syndrome: Deleterious effect of long-term high-rate ventricular pacing and definitive treatment by cardiac transplantation. *Am Heart J* **132**:1079, 1996.
187. Wang DW, Yazawa K, Makita N, George AL, Bennett PB: Pharmacological targeting of long QT mutant sodium channels. *J Clin Invest* **99**:1714, 1997.
188. Schwartz K, Carrier L, Guicheney P, Komajda M: Molecular basis of familial cardiomyopathies. *Circulation* **91**:533, 1995.
189. Shimizu W, Antzelevitch C: Sodium channel block with mexiletine is effective in reducing dispersion of repolarization and preventing torsade de pointes in LQT2 and LQT3 models of the long-QT syndrome. *Circulation* **96**:2038, 1997.
190. Sicouri S: Effects of sodium channel block with mexiletine to reverse action potential prolongation in vitro models of the long term QT syndrome. *J Cardiovasc Electrophysiol* **8**:1280, 1997.
191. Sato T, Hata Y, Yamamoto M, Morita H, Mizuo K, Yamanari H, Saito D, et al: Early afterdepolarization abolished by potassium channel opener in a patient with idiopathic long QT syndrome. *J Cardiovasc Electrophysiol* **6**:279, 1995.
192. Shimizu W, Kurita T, Matsuo K, Suyama K, Aihara N, Kamakura S, Towbin JA, et al: Improvement of repolarization abnormalities by a K^+ channel opener in the LQT1 form of congenital long-QT syndrome. *Circulation* **97**:1581, 1998.
193. Compton SJ, Lux RL, Ramsey MR, Strelich KR, Sanguinetti MC, Green LS, Keating MT, et al: Gene derived therapy in inherited long QT syndrome: Correction of abnormal repolarization by potassium. *Circulation* **94**:1018, 1996.
194. Tanel RE, Triedman JK, Walsh EP, Epstein MR, DeLucca JM, Mayer JE Jr, Fishberger SB, et al: High-rate atrial pacing as an innovative bridging therapy in a neonate with congenital long QT syndrome. *J Cardiovasc Electrophysiol* **8**:812, 1997.
195. Moss A: Update on MADIT: The Multicenter Automatic Defibrillator Implantation Trial. The long QT interval syndrome. *Am J Cardiol* **79**:16, 1997.
196. Barinaga M: Tracking down mutations that can stop the heart. *Science* **281**:32, 1998.
197. Vincent GM, Timothy KW, Leppert M, Keating M: The spectrum of symptoms and QT intervals in carriers of the gene for the long-QT syndrome. *N Engl J Med* **327**:846, 1992.
198. Zeng J, Laurita KR, Rosenbaum DS, Rudy Y: Two components of the delayed rectifier K^+ current in ventricular myocytes of the guinea pig type. Theoretical formulations and their role in repolarization. *Circ Res* **77**:140, 1995.
199. Sanguinetti MC, Curran ME, Zou A, Shen J, Spector PS, Atkinson DL, Keating MT: Coassembly of KVLQT1 and minK (IsK) proteins to form cardiac I_{Ks} potassium channel. *Nature* **384**:80, 1996.

CHAPTER 204

Channelopathies: Episodic Disorders of the Nervous System

Joanna Jen ▪ Louis Ptáček

1. **Ion channels are membrane proteins that allow rapid, passive, but selective passage of ions. The dynamic interaction of ion channels is critical for the regulation of membrane excitability and the function of excitable cells, such as nerve and muscle. Indeed, modern molecular techniques have led to the successful identification of mutations in genes encoding both voltage-gated and ligand-gated ion channels in numerous human neuromuscular disorders, collectively termed *channelopathies*. Channelopathies include periodic paralysis, episodic ataxia, congenital myasthenic syndromes, hereditary hyperekplexia, rare epilepsies, cardiac arrhythmias, and migraine syndromes that share similarities in their episodic nature, precipitating factors, therapeutic responses, and long-term degenerative features. Understanding the phenotypic expression of these rare, monogenic channelopathies may shed light on similar mechanisms in the more common, likely polygenic and multifactorial, paroxysmal neurologic disorders, such as migraine and epilepsy. See Table 204-1 for MIM and GenBank numbers.**
2. **Familial periodic paralyses are the prototypical channelopathies. These are autosomal dominant disorders characterized by episodes of weakness or by paralysis precipitated by stress or fatigue, with residual myopathy. Some patients respond well to acetazolamide, a carbonic anhydrase inhibitor. Hyperkalemic periodic paralysis, so named because an oral potassium load can precipitate an attack, is associated with muscle sodium channel mutations. Paramyotonia congenita, characterized by myotonia paradoxically worsened by repeated muscle action, is also associated with muscle sodium channel mutations. Hypokalemic periodic paralysis, characterized by episodic weakness without myotonia precipitated by lowering of serum potassium, is associated with muscle calcium channel mutations. Myotonia congenita, with prominent muscle hyperexcitability inherited dominantly or recessively, is another group of muscle disorders associated with ion channel mutations, specifically muscle chloride channels.**
3. **Episodic ataxia is an autosomal dominant disorder characterized by attacks of gait imbalance and clumsiness precipitated by stress and fatigue and often dramatically responsive to acetazolamide. While most patients have no interictal neurologic deficits, some may experience a slow decline in baseline function with evidence of cerebellar atrophy. Episodic ataxia type 1 (with myokymia) is associated with mutations in a potassium channel gene widely expressed in the nervous system. Episodic ataxia type 2 (with interictal nystagmus) is associated with mutations in a calcium channel gene prominently expressed in the cerebellum and the neuromuscular junction. Other mutations in the same calcium channel gene may cause hemiplegic migraine or severe progressive ataxia in addition to attacks of imbalance.**
4. **Congenital myasthenic syndromes are nonimmune mediated disorders of neuromuscular transmission characterized by weakness, fatigability, and progressive muscle atrophy. Mutations in the α, β, or ε subunit of the nicotinic acetylcholine receptor channel resulting in abnormal channel kinetics or assembly appear to be the cause in many cases of congenital myasthenic syndromes. Slow channel congenital myasthenic syndrome is an autosomal dominant disorder caused by mutations that prolong nicotinic acetylcholine receptor channel opening, which contributes to inappropriate endplate depolarization and potential excitotoxicity. Heteroallelic mutations in the ε subunit gene cause congenital myasthenic syndromes through two different mechanisms: lack of ε subunit leading to deficiency of acetylcholine receptor channels (with partial phenotypic rescue by the expression of the fetal γ subunit), or altered agonist binding and channel kinetics resulting in the low-affinity fast channel syndrome.**
5. **Hereditary hyperekplexia, characterized by an exaggerated startle response and hypertonia, is an autosomal dominant condition associated with mutations in a glycine receptor channel gene. The role of the inhibitory glycine receptors in the brainstem and spinal cord is not completely understood. Benzodiazepines markedly reduce the severity of startle-induced spasms in some individuals.**
6. **Other paroxysmal neurologic disorders share features with known channelopathies. Mutations in ion channels or**

A list of standard abbreviations is located immediately preceding the text in each volume. Additional abbreviations used in this chapter include: ACh = acetylcholine; AChE = acetylcholinesterase; *CACNA1A* = gene encoding the α_{1A} subunit of P/Q type voltage-gated calcium channel; *CACNA1S* = gene encoding the 1S subunit of the muscle L-type voltage-gated calcium channel; *CHRNA, CHRNB, CHRNC* = genes for nicotinic cholinergic receptor α, β, or ε subunits; *CLCN1* = chloride channel 1, skeletal muscle; DI, DII, etc. = domain I, domain II, etc; EA1, EA2 = episodic ataxia type 1 and type 2; FHM = familial hemiplegic migraine; *GLRA1* = glycine receptor α1 subunit; *KCNA1* = gene for voltage-gated potassium channel α1 subunit; Kv1.1 = voltage-gated potassium channel type 1.1; M1, M2, etc. = transmembrane segments for ligand gated channels; nAChR = nicotinic acetylcholine receptor; P – region or p loop = pore region; S1, S2, etc. = transmembrane segments of voltage-gated cation channels; SCA6 = spinocerebellar ataxia type 6; SCCMS = slow-channel congenital myasthenic syndrome; *SCN4A* = gene symbol for voltage-gated sodium channel type IV α subunit.

related proteins likely underlie familial dystonias, migraine, and epilepsy. Indeed, mutations in both ligand- and voltage-gated channels have been identified in several pedigrees with rare, monogenic epilepsies.

CHANNELOPATHIES: EPISODIC DISORDERS OF THE NERVOUS SYSTEM

The field of channelopathies is a newly recognized group of disorders named for the site of the molecular defects: voltage- and ligand-gated ion channels. Although voltage-gated ion channel mutants have been recognized for some time in organisms such as *Drosophila*,[1] the first channelopathy in humans was first reported within the last decade.[2] The recognition of this group of disorders began with definition of the molecular basis of a group of unusual muscle disorders called the periodic paralyses and nondystrophic myotonias.[3] Interestingly, this group of muscle disorders share some phenotypic features with a number of seemingly disparate human diseases that involve skeletal muscle, as well as brain and heart.[4,5] Some similarities that exist among these different disorders include their episodic nature, factors that precipitate attacks, therapeutic agents that can help to treat or prevent attacks, and, in some cases, a degenerative component that arises in addition to the episodic attacks. Channelopathies of skeletal muscle, the neuromuscular junction, and neurons are considered here, while channelopathies causing cardiac arrhythmia or epilepsy are included in other chapters (Table 204-1).

PERIODIC PARALYSES AND NONDYSTROPHIC MYOTONIAS

The process of motor neuron excitation leading to skeletal muscle contraction illustrates the importance of sequential activation and inactivation of voltage- and ligand-gated ion channels with distinct biophysical/pharmacologic properties and subcellular localization. Mutations in genes encoding many components of this complex cascade of events cause neuromuscular dysfunction (Fig. 204-1). Specifically, mutations in genes encoding voltage-gated ion channels in muscle result in periodic paralyses and nondystrophic myotonic syndromes.

Voltage-gated ion channels are proteins critical for the establishment of the resting membrane potential in muscle and nerve, and for the ability of these membranes to generate action potentials, while ligand-gated ion channels mediate intercellular communication via neurotransmitters.[6] Voltage-gated opening of sodium (Na) channels results in the genesis of "all-or-none" action potentials. The action potential propagates along the motor nerve through the activation of neuronal voltage-gated sodium channels, which lets Na enter the cell to depolarize the membrane potential. These channels close (inactivate) over the course of a few milliseconds. A simultaneous effect of membrane depolarization (albeit on a slower time scale) is the opening of voltage-gated potassium channels. Along with the inactivation of the voltage-gated Na channels, the movement of positive potassium ions out of the cell through voltage-gated potassium (K) channels leads to a relatively rapid repolarization of the membrane potential. On reaching the nerve terminal, the action potential activates presynaptic voltage-gated calcium (Ca) channels (including P/Q- and N-type channels, see below). The entry of Ca through these channels triggers the release of acetylcholine (ACh) stored in nearby vesicles in the nerve terminal. The released ACh molecules bind to postsynaptic ligand-gated ion channels nicotinic acetylcholine receptors (nAChRs) to let cations (sodium being the most abundant) into the muscle cell to activate muscle voltage-gated Na channels to spread muscle membrane depolarization. The nAChRs inactivate when ACh molecules become unbound and cleared by acetylcholinesterase in the synaptic cleft. The spread of depolarization activates muscle voltage-gated L-type calcium channels in the transverse (T) tubules. The voltage-gated L-type Ca channel in skeletal muscle, also known as the dihydropyridine receptor because dihydropyridines block this channel, allows conductance of calcium into the cell. It is likely that this calcium is important for effecting other downstream changes of the muscle membrane through signaling pathways, but the calcium conductance itself is not directly important to the depolarization of the muscle membrane. Interestingly, this voltage-gated calcium channel is known to serve as a voltage sensor for excitation-contraction coupling. Depolarization of the muscle membrane leads to changes in the calcium channel protein, which, in turn, interacts with the ryanodine receptor to open slow release calcium channels in the sarcoplasmic reticulum. It is these slow-release channels and the sarcoplasmic reticular calcium stores that lead to elevations in cytosolic calcium that result in the ultimate contraction of muscle. Voltage-gated chloride (Cl) channels are responsible for a majority of the polarity of resting membranes. The activation of these channels coupled with the inactivation of the muscle voltage-gated sodium channels return the muscle membrane potential to the resting level.

Ion Channel Structure

Potassium channels are membrane-bound tetrameric protein complexes.[7] Each subunit is a polypeptide with six putative transmembrane segments (usually denoted S1 to S6) (Fig. 204-2). Four identical subunits may associate to form a homomeric K channel. Alternatively, different subunits may assemble to form a heteromeric K channel. Mutagenesis studies have identified several critical functional domains in K channels. The S4 segments with positively charged arginine and lysine residues at every third position appear important in voltage sensing. The pore (P) region or loop-linking putative membrane-spanning S5 and S6 contains the K channel signature sequence that is highly conserved and critical for K selectivity of the channel pore.[7,8]

Table 204-1 Channelopathies

Disease	Gene	Ion channel	MIM	GenBank
Hyperkalemic periodic paralysis	*SCN4A*	Sodium channel	170500	4506806
Paramyotonia congenita	*SCN4A*	Sodium channel	170500	4506806
Hypokalemic periodic paralysis	*CACNA1S*	Calcium channel	114208	4557400
Myotonia congenita	*CLCN1*	Chloride channel	160800	4502866
Episodic ataxia with myokymia (type 1)	*KCNA1*	Potassium channel	160120	4557684
Episodic ataxia with nystagmus (type 2)	*CACNA1A*	Calcium channel	601011	4557398
Familial hemiplegic migraine	*CACNA1A*	Calcium channel	601011	4557398
Spinocerebellar ataxia type 6 (Chap. 226)	*CACNA1A*	Calcium channel	601011	4557398
Congenital myasthenic syndrome	*CHRNA,B,E*	Acetylcholine receptor	601462	4557456,4557458,4557462
Hereditary hyperekplexia	*GLRA1*	Glycine receptor	138491	4504018
Long QT syndromes (Chap. 203)	Multiple			
Hereditary epilepsies (Chap. 230)	Multiple			

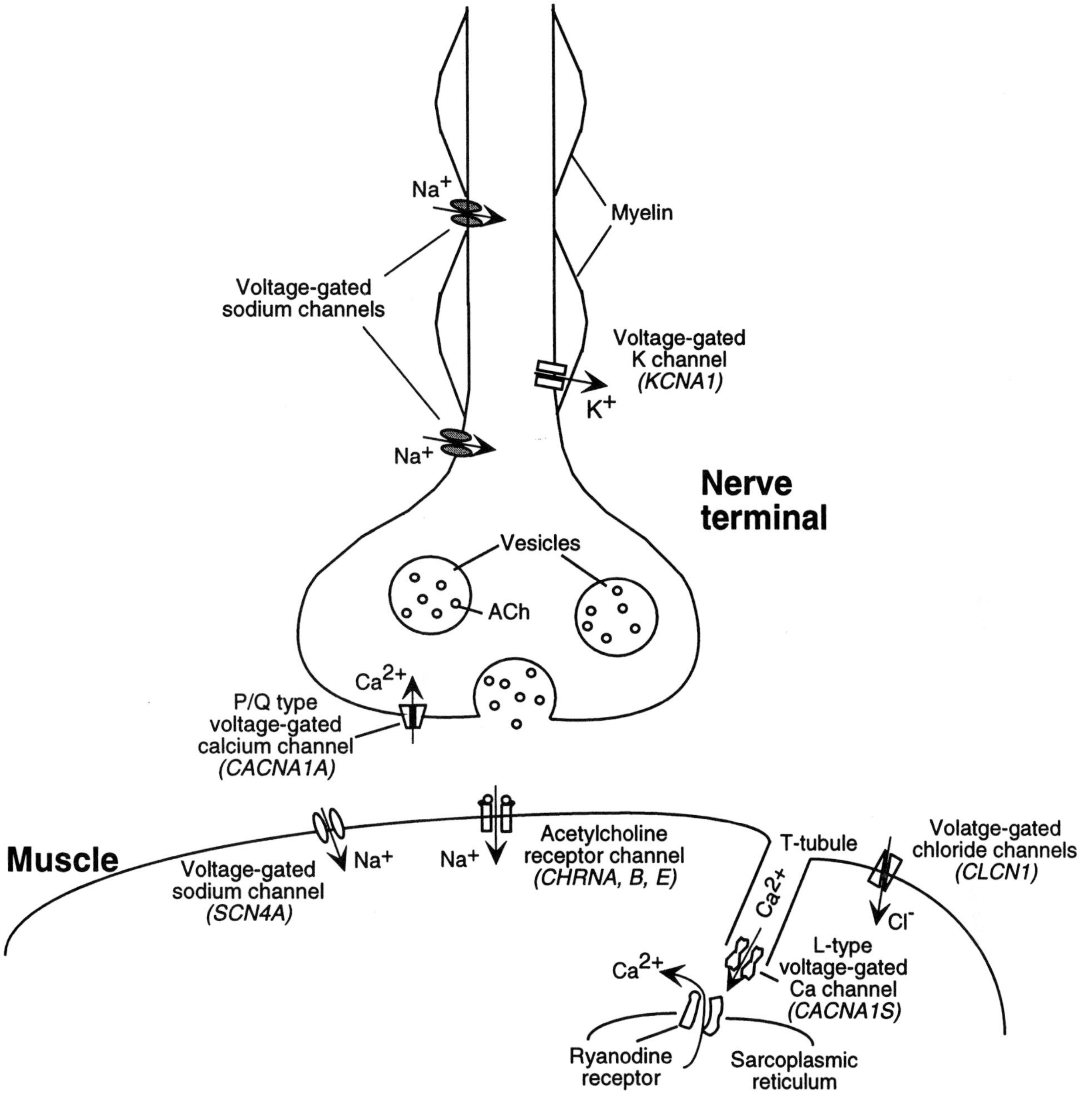

Fig. 204-1 Diagram of the neuromuscular junction with emphasis on components with known mutations causing neuromuscular dysfunction in humans. Gene symbols are italicized. See text for detail.

The voltage-dependent sodium and calcium channels are a large group of homologous genes that are also homologous to the voltage-gated potassium channel genes. Unlike the potassium channel proteins where four subunits must come together to form a homo- or heterotetrameric functional channel, sodium and calcium channel α subunits have evolved to include four domains (I to IV) in tandem in a single transcript; each domain has six transmembrane segments (usually denoted S1 to S6) homologous to voltage-gated potassium channel genes (Fig. 204-3). It is thought that this phenomenon resulted from the duplication of a progenitor 'potassium-like' channel that duplicated and then reduplicated in the genome. The large, pore-forming α subunit alone is sufficient for cation permeability, pharmacologic specificity, gating, and voltage sensitivity. The auxiliary subunits modulate channel biophysical properties and biosynthesis. Voltage-dependent sodium channels are composed of a pore-forming, voltage-sensing α•subunit and a transmembrane β subunit. Voltage-dependent calcium channels are heteromeric complexes composed of a pore-forming α_1 subunit, a disulfide-linked membrane-anchored extracellular α_2-δ subunit, an intracellular β subunit, and a membrane-spanning γ subunit.[9,10]

Voltage-gated chloride channels have been discovered more recently and much less is known about their structure. These proteins have 13 hydrophobic segments but more recent biochemical and immunologic data suggest that not all of these traverse the membrane. It appears that voltage-gated chloride channels form multimeric functional units, but the exact stoichiometry of these channels is not clear. There are no recognized auxiliary subunits of the voltage-gated chloride channels at this time.

Clinical Manifestations

Periodic paralyses and nondystrophic myotonias include a number of distinct clinical entities as well as some intermediate forms of the various disorders.

Myotonia congenita (MIM 118425) is a group of muscle disorders named for the prominent muscle hyperexcitability or myotonia that is seen in these patients. This myotonia is classical myotonia with the phenomenon of "warm-up." These patients

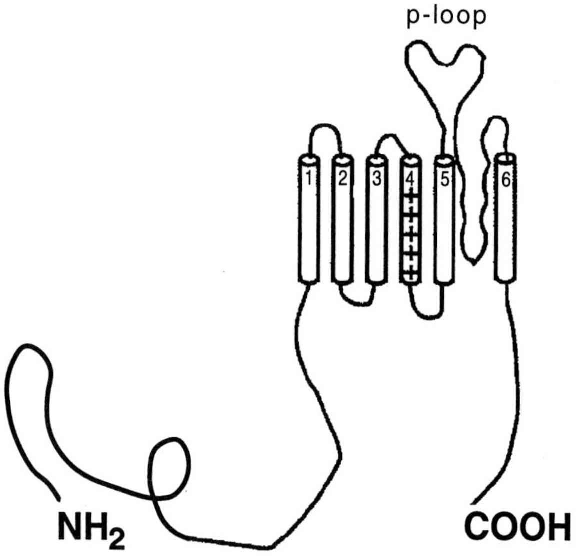

Fig. 204-2 Diagram of a voltage-dependent potassium channel subunit, with an intracellular N-terminus, six transmembrane segments (S1 to S6), and an intracellular C-terminus. The S4 segments with positively charged arginine and lysine residues at every third position are important in voltage sensing. Putative membrane-spanning S5 and S6 and the p loop (pore region) linking the two segments line the channel pore. Four subunits come together to form a potassium channel.

experience extreme muscle stiffness due to delayed relaxation from repetitive electrical activities in muscle, but this myotonia subsides as their muscles warm up with use. Onset of symptoms is generally in childhood through early adult life. These patients often have hypertrophy of their muscles and a Herculean appearance as a result of their myotonia. Two distinct forms of myotonia congenita are recognized. The first, named for Julius Thomsen who described the disease, is an autosomal dominant form of myotonia congenita.[11] These patients do not develop degeneration of their muscles even after years of having the disease. An autosomal recessive form of myotonia congenita was described by Becker.[11] These patients have myotonia with warm-up phenomenon, may have transient bouts of weakness after periods of disuse, and sometimes develop myopathy as part of their disease.

Hyperkalemic periodic paralysis (MIM 170500) is a disorder with myotonia similar to that seen in the above-described disorders. These patients can also have a transition of their muscle membrane hyperexcitability to inexcitability in the form of episodic weakness. This weakness may be so dense as to cause a transient flaccid quadriparesis. However, the disorder does not affect the diaphragm, and patients are able to continue breathing. First described in 1951 by Tyler,[12] this disorder is named because of the ability to precipitate attacks in patients by administrating a sufficient dose of oral potassium. During spontaneous attacks, patients may have elevated potassium, although it is frequently in the normal range. Attacks of weakness can be precipitated by foods high in potassium, rest after vigorous exercise, and with stress and fatigue. The disease is transmitted as an autosomal dominant trait, although sporadic cases are sometimes encountered. Percussion myotonia and action myotonia are frequently elicited clinically and prominent myotonia can be noted on an electromyographic exam. Patients benefit dramatically from treatment with carbonic anhydrase inhibitors.

Paramyotonia congenita (MIM 170500) is yet another disorder in which myotonia is present, although the myotonia is somewhat different as it does not show the classical warm-up phenomenon; instead, it is paradoxical. That is, patients frequently have worsening of their myotonia with repeated muscle action. This can be most prominently seen in the orbicularis oris muscles, when patients forcefully close their eyes repeatedly, and upon such a maneuver the myotonia of these muscles becomes increasingly severe to the point where patients might have difficulty opening their eyes altogether. Of interest, this disorder is a temperature-sensitive mutant of humans. With cooling of their muscles, these patients have worsening of their myotonia and then transition of the hyperexcitability into paralysis. This can be measured quantitatively using electrodiagnostic maneuvers.[13] Paramyotonia congenita is transmitted as an autosomal dominant trait, and like hyperkalemic periodic paralysis, these patients have worsening of their symptoms with stress, fatigue, and rest after vigorous exercise. Patients may be hypo-, normo-, or hyperkalemic during attacks. The classical paramyotonia congenital patients are generally hypokalemic during attacks; those with hyperkalemia seem to represent a clinical entity somewhere in the spectrum between classical paramyotonia congenita and hyperkalemic periodic paralysis. Like the hyperkalemic periodic paralysis patients, these patients benefit dramatically from treatment with carbonic anhydrase inhibitors.

Potassium-activated myotonia (MIM 170500) is a disorder in which patients clinically appear to have myotonia congenita. But their myotonia fluctuates, worsens when potassium is administered, and improves with carbonic anhydrase inhibitors.[14] Interestingly, these patients do not develop attacks of weakness. This disorder is transmitted as an autosomal dominant trait.

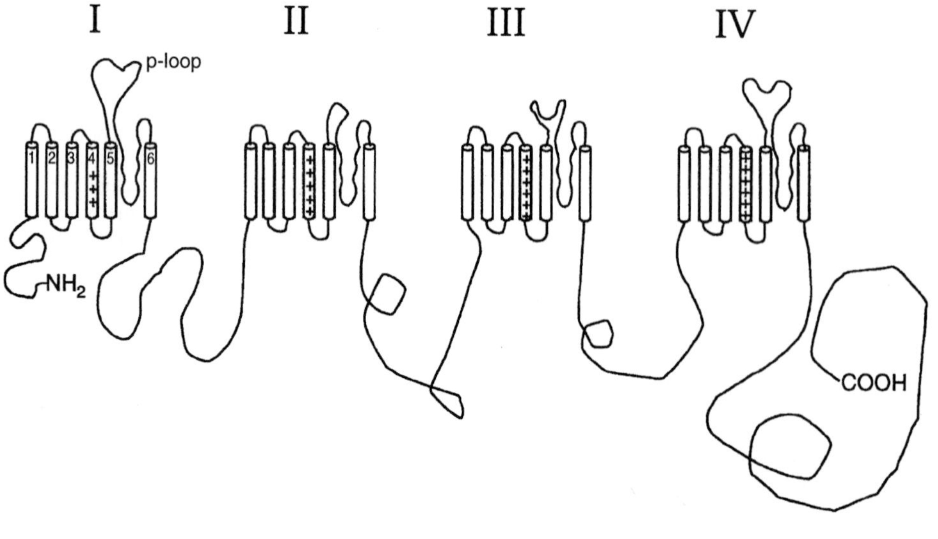

Fig. 204-3 Diagram of an α subunit of a sodium channel or α_1 subunit of a calcium channel with four homologous domains, each with six transmembrane segments.

Hypokalemic periodic paralysis (MIM 114208) is a disorder of episodic weakness in which a myotonia is not seen. These patients are generally hypokalemic during an attack, and lowering potassium with administration of glucose and insulin can precipitate attacks. Furthermore, stress, fatigue, and rest can precipitate attacks after vigorous exercise. Dietary precipitants include high carbohydrate meals and salt load. Hypokalemic periodic paralysis is transmitted as an autosomal dominant trait, although sporadic cases are frequent. Potassium levels during hypokalemia generally remain above 2 mM. Potassium levels below 2 mM during an attack of weakness in a sporadic case raises the possibility of thyrotoxic hypokalemic periodic paralysis, a non-Mendelian form of the disorder that is seen only during periods of thyrotoxicosis.[15] The episodic weakness in patients with hyperkalemic periodic paralysis, paramyotonia congenita, and hypokalemic periodic paralysis all benefit from treatment with the carbonic anhydrase inhibitors acetazolamide (Diamox) and dichlorphenamide (Daranide).

Genetics

Linkage analysis in large pedigrees with hyperkalemic periodic paralysis established that the gene for this disorder resided on chromosome 17q.[16,17] Mapping data showed that the paramyotonia congenita and the potassium-activated myotonia phenotypes also mapped to the same locus.[18,19] Subsequently, a sodium channel gene in this region of chromosome 17q was cloned, characterized, and shown to be the site of mutations in hyperkalemic periodic paralysis,[2,20] paramyotonia congenita,[21,22] and potassium-activated myotonia.[23] The data supporting that sodium-channel gene *SCN4A* was the disease-causing gene included: (a) mutations segregated with the phenotype; (b) the mutations involved highly conserved amino acid residues; (c) these mutations were not found in control individuals; and (d) some of the mutations occurred as de novo mutations in patients with sporadic disease. A large number of sodium channel mutations (MIM 170500) have been identified in patients with hyperkalemic periodic paralysis, paramyotonia congenita, and potassium-aggravated myotonia (Table 204-2).

Similar molecular approaches led to mapping of the hypokalemic periodic paralysis locus to chromosome 1q.[24,25] Subsequently, a voltage-gated calcium channel at this chromosome 1 locus was cloned. This calcium-channel gene *CACNA1S* (MIM 114208) encodes the α1S subunit of an L-type calcium channel, and three patient-specific mutations have been identified.[25,26] The mutations occur at highly conserved residues in the S4 segments of either domain II or domain IV. The domain IV mutations occur at analogous position to the most common paramyotonia congenita mutations in the homologous SCN4A sodium channel.[22]

Genetic linkage analysis in families segregating alleles for both recessive and dominant forms of myotonia congenita showed that both of these phenotypes were linked to a locus on chromosome 7q.[27,28] Subsequent work identified *CLCN1*, a voltage-gated chloride channel at this locus, to be the site of defects in myotonia congenita.[28,29] Subsequently, a long list of mutations in this channel gene were shown to cause dominant and recessive forms of myotonia congenita (MIM 118425; see Table 204-3).[30–37] Interestingly, some of these mutations are recognized to cause both dominant and recessive forms.[36] While it is likely that this is a result of polymorphisms in the chloride-channel gene itself that may modulate the effect of such mutations, no data are available to substantiate this hypothesis. Many of these chloride-channel mutants have been expressed in vitro (either in oocytes or by transfection of mammalian cells growing in culture) and the physiological abnormalities in myotonia congenita are being characterized. The mutations that are currently recognized and physiological data from those that have been studied are outlined in Table 204-3.

Pathophysiology

The large number of sodium-channel mutations described to date share the common feature of altering the inactivation kinetics of the sodium channel, although a number of differences exist among the physiological consequences of various mutations. Discussion of the details of the physiological characterization is beyond the scope of this chapter, but all appear to affect the channel function in a way that leads ultimately to excessive sodium-channel conduction with resultant hyperexcitability of the muscle membranes.[38] The details of potassium sensitivity, temperature sensitivity, and the transition from hyperexcitability to flaccid paralysis are not well understood. Similarly, the basis of response

Table 204-2 Periodic Paralyses Associated with Mutations in a Sodium-Channel Gene *SCN4A*

Mutations[Ref]	Location*	Phenotype†	Physiological Consequences
V445M[117]	I		Unknown
I693T[118]	I	PC	Voltage-dependence of activation shifted −9 mV[118]
T704M[2]	II S5	hyperKPP	Slowed inactivation and voltage-dependence of activation shifted −10 to −15 mV[119]
S804F	II S6	PC	Slowed fast inactivation[120]
A1156T	III S4-S5 loop		Slowed inactivation[121]
I1160V[23]	III S4-S5 loop	PAM	↓Voltage-dependence of steady-state inactivation; slowed deactivation[122]
V1293I[123]	III S6		Slowed fast inactivation, voltage-dependence of activation shifted −6 mV[120]
G1306A	III-IV	PAM	
G1306E	III-IV	PAM	
G1306V[21]	III-IV		
T1313M[21]	III-IV	PC	Slowed inactivation[121]
M1360V[124]	IV S1	PC/hyperKPP	Steady state inactivation curve shifted −13 mV; ↑recovery from inactivation[124]
F1419L[125]	IV S3	hyperKPP	
L1433R[126]	IV S3	PC	Slowed inactivation[121]
R1448C[22]	IV S4	PC	Slowed inactivation[121]
R1448H[22]	IV S4	PC	Slowed inactivation[121]
R1448P[127]	IV S4	PC	
V1458F	IV S4		
F1473S[128]	IV S4-S5 loop	PC	Slows fast inactivation, accelerates recovery from inactivation[128]
V1589M[129]	IV S6		
M1592V[20]	IV S6	hyperKPP	Slowed inactivation[130]

*I, II, etc. = Domain I, domain II, etc; S = putative transmembrane segment
†PC = Paramyotonia congenita; hyperKPP = hyperkalemic periodic paralysis; PAM = potassium aggravated myotonia.

Table 204-3 Myotonia Congenita Associated with Mutations in CLCN1

Mutation	Mode of Transmission*	Physiologic consequences*
G200R	AD[37]	Shift open probability to less negative potentials[131]
G230E	AD or AR[29,36]	Increased pore conductance of sodium[40]
I290M	AD[132]	Shift open probability to less negative potentials[133]
R317Q	AD[32]	Shift open probability to less negative potentials[133]
P480L	AD[30]	Abolishes current with strong dominant negative effect[133]
Q552R	AD[31]	Shift open probability to less negative potentials in heterozygotes; abolishes current when homozygous[133]
R105C	AR[32]	
D136G	AR[33]	Profound changes in channel gating; slowed activation upon hyperpolarization[134]
Y150C	AR[37]	No difference compared to wild-type[131]
V165G	AR[32]	
F167L	AR[34]	
Y261C	AR[37]	No difference compared to wild-type[131]
E291K	AR[32]	No effect when coexpressed with wild-type; abolished current when expressed alone[133]
I329T	AR[32]	
R338Q	AD or AR[34,36]	
F413C	AR[28]	
A415V	AR[37]	
G482R	AR[32]	
G485V	AR[32]	Drastic reduction of macroscopic current and single-channel conductance[131]
R496S	AR[35]	No effect when coexpressed with wild-type; abolished current when expressed alone[35]
Q68X	AR[36]	
Q74X	AR[37]	
R300X	AR[34]	
R894X	AR[34]	Reduced channel conductance to 15% of wild-type level[32]
1095del2	AR[32]	
1278del4	AR[33]	
1437del4	AR[135]	
1962insC	AR[32]	

*Reference numbers in superscript.

to available therapeutic agents (see "Treatment" below) is also not well understood.

Interestingly, the three calcium-channel mutations that have been identified in hypokalemic periodic paralysis patients occur at two specific amino acid residues. Both residues are arginines in the S4 segment of domains 2 and 4, respectively. The D4 arginine residue (R1239), which is mutated to a glycine in a single family and to a histidine in many families, occurs at an analogous position to the most common paramyotonia congenita mutations identified in the sodium channel domain 4. Physiological study of the calcium channel mutations has not shed light on understanding of the pathophysiology of this disorder. The best available data show only a decrease in the calcium current amplitude through these channels when the R528H mutation was expressed in vitro.[39] Understanding of the pathophysiological basis of hypokalemic periodic paralysis caused by calcium channel mutations awaits further study.

Physiological characterization of CLCN1 mutations in myotonia congenita is beginning to elucidate the molecular and physiological basis of these diseases (see Table 204-3). G230E, a dominant mutation, results in alterations of selectivity of the ion-conducting pore. In this mutant, the channel is allowed to pass sodium ions, which has the effect of depolarizing the cell rather than the normal repolarizing function of this channel.[40] This fits nicely with the autosomal dominant transmission known to occur in this mutation in which a single copy of the mutant channel can lead to increased sodium conductance and result in hyperexcitability of the skeletal muscle membrane. Some of the nonsense mutations, insertion mutations, and deletion mutations lead to significantly truncated proteins and are likely to cause recessive phenotype by loss in a single mutation of approximately 50 percent of the chloride channels in the muscle, while some missense mutations exert a dominant negative effect in poisoning function of a large majority of the multimeric functional units.

Treatment

Acetazolamide (Diamox), a carbonic anhydrase inhibitor was for some time recognized anecdotally as beneficial to patients with periodic paralysis.[15] Only recently has a double-blind controlled trial been performed in which patients were classified based on their specific molecular alterations.[23,41] In this trial, a related carbonic anhydrase inhibitor, dichlorphenamide (Daranide), was shown to be effective in preventing attacks of weakness in these patients. The treatment strategies for episodic weakness in this group of disorders are summarized in Table 204-4.

If the patient's primary complaint is that of myotonia (in hyperkalemic periodic paralysis or paramyotonia congenita), then a different strategy of treatment must be undertaken. In these patients, mexiletine is often of benefit. The myotonia of Thomsen myotonia congenita can be treated with quinine, procainamide (Procan), or phenytoin (Dilantin), while the myotonia in Becker myotonia congenita most frequently benefits from mexiletine (Mexitil) or tocainide (Tonocard).

EPISODIC ATAXIA: K CHANNEL AND Ca CHANNEL

Clinical Manifestations

Episodic ataxia is a rare, inherited syndrome of intermittent ataxia of early onset that is to be distinguished from inborn errors of

Table 204-4 Summary of Therapeutic Options for Periodic Paralysis

Disorder	Response to acetazolamide	Other medications	Dietary precipitants
Hyperkalemic periodic paralysis	Yes	Thiazide diuretics	High potassium
Paramyotonia congenita	Yes		
Hypokalemic periodic paralysis	Yes	Spironolactone, triamterene	High carbohydrate, high sodium
Chloride channel periodic paralysis	Yes	Mexiletine	
Thyrotoxic periodic paralysis	No	β-Blockade	

metabolism such as amino acid or organic acid disorders. There are two distinct forms, both with episodic attacks of ataxia responsive to acetazolamide, and features reminiscent of periodic paralysis and suggestive of underlying ion channel abnormalities.[41]

Episodic ataxia type 1 (EA1; MIM 176260), an autosomal dominant disorder involving both the central and the peripheral nervous system, is characterized by attacks of ataxia and persistent myokymia. Episodes of ataxia, with gait imbalance and slurring of speech, occur spontaneously or can be precipitated by sudden movement, excitement, or exercise. The attacks generally last from seconds to several minutes at a time and may recur many times a day. Myokymia, or muscle rippling resulting from motor nerve hyperexcitability, may be observed particularly around the eyes or in the small hand muscles. Subclinical rhythmic muscle activity may be demonstrated by electromyography. Acetazolamide (Diamox), a carbonic anhydrase inhibitor, may be effective in preventing attacks of ataxia.[42,43] The age of onset, frequency of attacks, and severity may vary widely among family members.

Episodic ataxia type 2 (EA2; MIM 601011) is an autosomal dominant disorder with episodes of markedly impaired truncal ataxia lasting hours to days with interictal eye movement abnormalities. Exertion and stress commonly precipitate the episodes. Often, the episodes of ataxia respond to acetazolamide.[44] In some individuals, there may be a gradual baseline ataxia with evidence of cerebellar atrophy. Affected patients may also have migraine; some even complain of basilar migraine.[45]

Genetics

Linkage analysis of several large pedigrees with EA1 mapped the disease locus to 12p13, near a cluster of three K channel genes: *KCNA1*, *KCNA5*, and *KCNA6*.[46] Based on the clinical phenotype and its analogy to episodic disorders of muscle, ion-channel genes were considered good candidate genes for EA1. Browne and colleagues[47] serendipitously focused on *KCNA1*; the individual who led these investigators to exclude *KCNA5* and *KCNA6* later turned out to represent a phenocopy. *KCNA1*, which encodes Kv1.1, a delayed rectifier K channel, has no intervening introns in its 1488-bp sequence. Analysis of the single exon in *KCNA1* identified point mutations in four unrelated EA1 pedigrees.[47] These mutations fulfilled several criteria for disease-causing mutations, as they segregated with the phenotype, involved highly conserved amino acid residues in the potassium-channel gene product, and were not found in controls. Additional mutations in the same gene were subsequently identified in other EA1 pedigrees.[48–50] There is no animal model for episodic ataxia type 1 with missense mutations in *KCNA1*. Smart and colleagues[51] generated Kv1.1 null mice that suffer from frequent spontaneous seizures but display no evidence of ataxia.

The disease locus in EA2 in several pedigrees was localized to chromosome 19p.[52–55] Earlier, the disease locus of half of the pedigrees with familial hemiplegic migraine (FHM) was mapped to the same locus.[56–59] FHM is a dominantly inherited subtype of migraine with aura, characterized by recurrent attacks of migrainous headache with ictal hemiparesis. Recovery is generally complete, with a normal interictal physical examination. The onset is often early in life. Overlap in symptoms between hemiplegic migraine and basilar migraine suggests that hemiplegic migraine may be a form of basilar migraine.[60]

A calcium-channel subunit gene mapping to 19p was an ideal candidate gene for EA2 and FHM. Ophoff and colleagues[59] first defined the complex gene structure of *CACNA1A*, which spans 300,000 bp and consists of 47 exons that encodes the α_{1A} subunit with 2261 amino acids. These investigators then analyzed the exons and flanking introns of *CACNA1A* and identified missense mutations in pedigrees affected with FHM and point mutations, including nonsense and splicing defects in EA2 families.[59] Additional mutations in this gene were subsequently identified in numerous European pedigrees with FHM or EA2.[61,62] The identification of a de novo nonsense mutation in a patient with episodic ataxia but no family history provided further evidence supporting *CACNA1A* as the disease-causing gene in episodic ataxia.[63]

In addition to EA2 and FHM, mutations in *CACNA1A* caused another phenotype. Small expansions of a polymorphic CAG repeat in the same gene were identified in some ataxic patients with a condition since designated SCA6, a dominantly inherited progressive cerebellar ataxia that is clinically indistinguishable from other dominant ataxic syndromes[64] (see Chap. 226).

EA2, FHM, and SCA6 have overlapping clinical features. FHM patients can develop progressive ataxia, similar to SCA6. EA2 patients can have migraine with hemiplegic episodes, as in FHM. Some SCA6 patients experience fluctuating symptoms, similar to episodic ataxia.[65,66] A missense mutation caused severe progressive ataxia and superimposed episodes of vertigo and ataxia.[67]

Of note, mutations in genes encoding calcium-channel subunits have been identified in a number of recessive mouse mutants with ataxia. Homozygous point mutation in the α_{1A} gene (P1802L, domain II P− region) causes epilepsy and ataxia in mutant mouse tottering (*tg*).[68] Novel sequences in the intracellular C-terminus of the α_{1A} subunit also resulted in a mutant mouse phenotype, leaner (tg^{la}), with ataxia and epilepsy.[68] Calcium channel β_4 subunit gene mutation with a predicted deletion of a highly conserved α_1-binding motif caused seizures and ataxia in mutant mouse lethargic (*lh*).[69] Characterization of the genetic defect in the stargazer (*stg*) mutant led to the identification of a putative neuronal calcium channel γ subunit.[10]

Pathophysiology

The voltage-dependent potassium channels display an impressive diversity in channel kinetics, voltage dependence, pharmacology, and cellular distribution. They are important in regulating the overall excitability of neurons and muscles.[6]

Sequencing of the *Shaker* locus encoding a potassium channel in *Drosophila* led to the identification of a large and growing number of homologous genes. *KCNA1* involved in EA1 is a *Shaker* homolog in human. *KCNA1* encodes a subunit of delayed rectifier K channel Kv1.1. The delayed rectifier K channels are a family of K channels that allow sustained K efflux with a delay after membrane depolarization. The outflow of K ions rapidly repolarizes the membrane. Kv1.1 is widely expressed in both the central and the peripheral nervous system in rodents and is present in synaptic zones and along axons in paranodal clusters concealed by myelin[70–72] (Fig. 204-1). Thus, Kv1.1 channels may play a role in neurotransmitter release, action potential generation, as well as in axonal impulse conduction.

Distinct mutations in *KCNA1* have been identified in several pedigrees with EA1. The study of the biophysical properties of these mutant channels expressed in *Xenopus* oocytes or cell lines demonstrated the physiological consequences of genetic mutations and helped define functional domains of the channel complex (Table 204-5).

Recent physiological data provide some explanation of how missense mutations in *KCNA1* may lead to episodes of ataxia and myokymia. In the central nervous system, mutant mice lacking Kv1.1 suffered from seizures.[51] Peripherally, Kv1.1 null mice exhibit abnormal neuromuscular transmission.[72] At the single-channel level, the V408A and E325D mutations cause decreased outward flow of potassium, which prevents proper repolarization of the cell membrane potential after depolarization. Impaired repolarization may lead to prolonged depolarization and continued calcium influx. Inappropriate, prolonged calcium-dependent neurotransmitter release in the cerebellum, as well as in the peripheral nervous system, may cause attacks of ataxia. Furthermore, increased excitability may result in spontaneous or repetitive neuronal discharge, manifesting as myokymia.

Voltage-dependent calcium channels are heteromeric complexes that allow calcium entry in response to membrane depolarization. The influx of calcium ions into the cell through calcium channels serve as a ubiquitous second messenger critical

Table 204-5 Mutations in Potassium Channel Gene *KCNA1* Causing Episodic Ataxia Type 1 (with Myokymia)

	Mutation	Mode of transmission*	Location	Physiological consequences
Human	V174F	AD[47]	S1	↓Amplitude; shift in v-dependence
	I176R	AD[50]	S1	
	F184C	AD[48]	S1	↓Amplitude; shift in v-dependence
	T226S	AD[49]	S2	
	T226A	AD[50]	S2	
	R239S	AD[47]	S2-S3	No detectable current or protein
	F249I	AD[47]	S2-S3	↓Amplitude; ↓protein level
	E325D	AD[48]	S5	↓Open probability
	V404I	AD[50]	S6	
	V408A	AD[47]	S6	Accelerated channel activation/ inact kinetics
Mouse	knockout	AR[51]	null	Epilepsy
Fly		*Shaker*[1]		

*References in superscript.

in many cellular functions, ranging from membrane excitability, neurotransmitter release, and excitation-contraction coupling to migration, gene regulation, and cell death.[6] *CACNA1A* involved in EA2 encodes the α_{1A} subunit, which likely forms the endogenous P/Q channels abundant in Purkinje cells and granule cells in the cerebellum.[73–75] The precise oligomeric structure of voltage-dependent calcium channels in specific cell types remains largely unknown. Although many different α_1-β•combinations may be possible, the β_4 subunit likely associate predominantly with the α_{1A} subunit in the cerebellum.[76] The significance of a short form of the α_{1A} subunit associated with P/Q-type Ca channels is not clear.[77] Other factors that further modulate calcium channel activities include differential but overlapping expression of subunit isoforms, differential subcellular distribution, combination with auxiliary subunits, association with G proteins, and differential phosphorylation.

There is much overlap in clinical symptoms and signs among pedigrees with different mutations in *CACNA1A*. SCA6 with CAG repeat expansions has acetazolamide-responsive episodic ataxia that overlaps with EA2, suggesting that the incorporation of additional glutamines in the C-terminus of the calcium channel subunit may alter the channel function in a way similar to that of point mutations. Point mutations also have features that overlap with CAG repeat expansions in progressive ataxia. For example, G293R, a missense mutation resulting in a change in a highly conserved amino acid residue in the putative P region in domain I, is associated with a progressive ataxic syndrome with superimposed episodic exacerbation. There are also differences in the clinical manifestations of similar mutations. For example, although both mutations involve the putative P region, the missense mutation T666M in domain II causes FHM with a normal baseline, yet another missense mutation G293R in domain I causes early-onset, severe, progressive ataxia.

There have been few reports on the physiological consequences of *CACNA1A* mutations causing EA2, SCA6, or FHM (Table 204-6).[78,79] FHM mutations expressed in nonneuronal cells have been associated with both increased and decreased calcium channel availability.[78,79] CAG repeat expansions in *CACNA1A* expressed in cell lines demonstrated altered voltage dependence of inactivation, likely leading to decreased calcium channel availability.[80]

Treatment

Acetazolamide (Diamox) is effective in preventing attacks of ataxia in some EA1 patients. This is another feature that episodic ataxia shares with the periodic paralyses. The mechanism of action of acetazolamide (Diamox) in preventing attacks is not known.

The clinical benefit of acetazolamide (Diamox) in EA2 and related disorders is presumably mediated by increasing the extracellular concentration of free protons in the cerebellum.[81] Proton block, or alterations in calcium-channel conductance and gating in response to changes in extracellular pH, appears to involve the same region governing calcium permeability within the pore.[82,83]

CONGENITAL MYASTHENIC SYNDROMES AND NICOTINIC ACETYLCHOLINE RECEPTORS

Congenital myasthenic syndromes are a group of rare, hereditary, nonimmune-mediated disorders of neuromuscular transmission. (Fig. 204-1) Briefly, depolarization of the motor neuron activates presynaptic voltage-gated calcium channels to allow calcium ion influx to trigger the release of vesicles containing acetylcholine (ACh). ACh released into the synapse binds to nicotinic ACh receptors (nAChRs) clustered in endplate on the postsynaptic muscle surface membrane. The entry of cations through the activated nAChRs leads to depolarization (endplate potential), thus activating voltage-gated sodium channels and, ultimately, muscle contraction. ACh is cleared from the synaptic cleft by acetylcholinesterase (AChE).

Defects involving the presynaptic, synaptic, and postsynaptic components of the neuromuscular junction have been identified in different pedigrees affected with myasthenic symptoms. Postsynaptic dysfunction accounts for the majority of congenital myasthenic syndromes. A wealth of detailed studies of the physiological, pharmacologic, and molecular properties of nAChR greatly facilitated the clinical characterization and subsequent identification of nAChR dysfunction causing congenital myasthenia. In particular, in two pedigrees with congenital myasthenic syndrome, Engel and colleagues performed electrophysiological studies to demonstrate markedly prolonged muscle endplate potential, which led to the hypothesis that mutations in one or more nAChR channel subunit could underlie the abnormal kinetics observed. This hypothesis was subsequently confirmed by the identification of specific mutations in genes encoding different subunits of the nAChR in slow-channel congenital myasthenic syndrome (SCCMS). In addition, other mutations in nAChR subunit genes were associated with fast-channel syndrome and nAChR deficiency.

Nicotinic Acetylcholine Receptors

The nicotinic acetylcholine receptor (nAChR) complexes are ligand-gated channels expressed in skeletal muscles and brain.[6] Five different classes of subunits exist: α1-α9, β1-β-4, γ, δ, and ε. Different genes on different chromosomes encode these subunits. They are homologous, each with a large N-terminal extracellular domain, four transmembrane regions (usually denoted M1 through M4), with a large intracellular loop between M3 and M4 (Fig. 204-4).

The subunit composition at the neuromuscular junction is fixed: $(\alpha 1)_2(\beta 1)\delta\gamma$ in the fetal form and $(\alpha 1)_2(\beta 1)\delta\varepsilon$ in the adult form.[84] M2 from each subunit lines the channel pore. A leucine residue at homologous locations in each M2 segment forms a hydrophobic ring critical for channel gating. There are two binding sites for ACh, located at the interface between N-terminal hydrophilic domains of α-δ and α-ε or α-γ. The snake neurotoxin α-bungarotoxin irreversibly blocks these binding sites and is useful in labeling and counting nAChR.

Table 204-6 Mutations in Calcium Channel α_{1A} Subunit Gene CACNA1A Causing Hemiplegic Migraine, Episodic Ataxia, and Progressive Ataxia

	Mutation	Mode of transmission*	Location	Phenotype	Physiological consequences*
Human		AD[59]	Nonsense mutation (stop)	EA2	
		AD[59]	Aberrant splicing	EA2	
	R192Q	AD[59]	I S4	FHM	
	T666M	AD[59,62]	II S5-S6	FHM±progressive ataxia	Slowed recovery from inactivation
	V714A	AD[59]	II S6	FHM	Accelerated recovery from inactivation
	D715E	AD[62]	II S6	FHM±progressive ataxia	
	I1811L	AD[59]	IV S6	FHM±progressive ataxia	Accelerated recovery from inactivation
	Polyglutamine tract	AD[64]	C-terminus	SCA6±EA2	Altered voltage dependence of inactivation[80]
	G293R	AD[67]	I S5-S6	EA2	
	2259del2	AD[61]	II S6	EA2	
	3797delC	AD[61]	III S1	EA2	
	R1279X	de novo[63]	III S1-S2	EA2	
	R1547X	AD[61]	IV S1	EA2±hemiplegia	
Mouse	P601L	AR[68]	II S5-S6	*Tottering*: ataxia + epilepsy	Decreased P-type current[136]
	Insertion	AR[68]	Splicing error, altered C-term	*Leaner*: ataxia + epilepsy	Decreased P-type current[136–138]
	Allelic; mutation unidentified	AR		*Rolling nagoya*: ataxia	
	Splicing error in *Cacnb4*	AR[69]	Deletion of α_1 binding site on β_4 subunit	*Lethargic*: ataxia + epilepsy	
	Early transposon insertion in *Cacng2*	AR[10]	Early stop or splicing error in γ_2 subunit	*Stargazer*: ataxia + epilepsy +?vestibulopathy	

*References in superscript.

Binding of two ACh molecules induces conformational changes of the channel complex to an open state to allow mostly sodium, but also calcium, to enter the cell. The channel may undergo further voltage-dependent conformational changes before it closes, and ACh dissociates from the receptor channel complex.

Clinical Features

Slow-channel congenital myasthenic syndrome (SCCMS; MIM 601462) is an autosomal dominant hereditary condition characterized clinically by weakness, fatigability, and progressive muscle atrophy.[85] Patients generally present early, with poor head control and weak suck during infancy. Weakness of skeletal muscles, particularly bulbar, cervical, and hand extensor muscles, may be present since birth. The age of onset and severity may vary among family members. Laboratory testing reveals no presence of anti-AChR antibodies. Morphologic studies at the light microscopic level show focal endplate myopathy. Ultrastructural studies reveal degenerative changes in the basement membrane, postsynaptic membrane, and the synaptic organelles of the neuromuscular junction. Electrophysiological testing demonstrates many abnormalities. At a normal neuromuscular junction, a single stimulus should elicit a single compound-muscle action potential. In contrast, a single stimulus in SCCMS may elicit multiple potentials with decremental response, in addition to the initial compound-muscle action potential. On repetitive stimulation of motor nerves, there is decremental electromyographic response. Intracellular recordings of biopsied muscles show prolonged decay of endplate potentials. Single-channel recordings demonstrate increased channel opening compared to control.

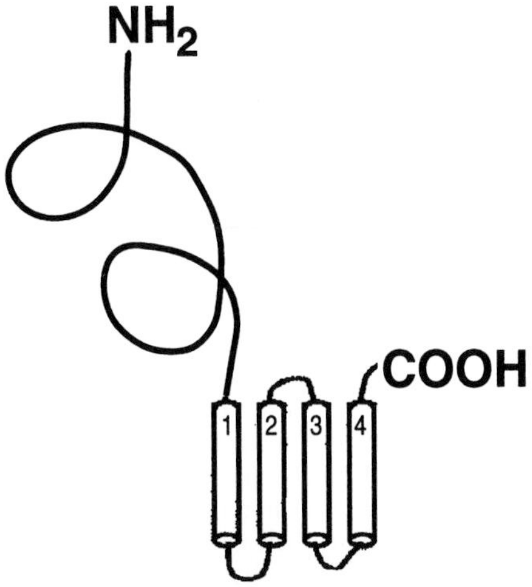

Fig. 204-4 Diagram of a subunit of nicotinic acetylcholine receptor channel or inhibitory glycine receptor channel with a large extracellular N-terminus and four transmembrane segments (M1 to M4).

Deficiency of nAChR is an autosomal recessive disorder causing congenital myasthenic syndrome with generalized weakness of early onset. The most striking abnormality in laboratory studies is the marked reduction in nAChR in motor endplate measured by α-bungarotoxin labeling. The patients usually respond favorably to AChE inhibitors. Immunocytochemical studies using labeled antibodies directed against the γ subunit have successfully demonstrated the presence of the immature subunit at the neuromuscular junction. There may be increased number of small endplates distributed over an increased span of muscle fiber surface. Electrophysiological studies showed evidence of AChR with small conductance and slow kinetics

Table 204-7 Mutations in nAChR Subunit Genes Causing Congenital Myasthenic Syndromes

Gene	Protein	Mutation	Mode of transmission*	Location	Phenotype	Physiological consequences*
CHRNA	$\alpha 1$	G153S	AD[139]	N-terminus	Slow channel	Slows agonist dissociation
		V156M	AD[139]	N-terminus	Slow channel	
		N217K	AD[140]	M1	Slow channel	↓Rate of channel closure; ↑ACh apparent affinity; ↓desensitization
		V249F	AD[141]	M2	Slow channel	↑Channel opening; ↑desensitization
		T254I	AD[139]	M2	Slow channel	Longer channel openings
		S269I	AD[139]	M2-M3	Slow channel	Longer channel openings (in a region not previously identified as being involved in ACh binding or gating)
CHRNB	$\beta 1$	L263M	AD[142]	M2; conserved Leu ring	Slow channel	↑↑Channel open time; profound ultrastructural changes
		V266M	AD[140]	M2	Slow channel	↓Rate of channel closure; +spontaneous opening
CHRNE	ϵ	R147L	AD		Slow channel	
		T264P	AD[140]		Slow channel	+Spontaneous opening
		L269F	AD[143]	M2	Slow channel	↓Rate of channel closure; +spontaneous opening; ↑desensitization. Multiple abnormalities in mutant mouse[144]
		P121L; null	AR[87]	N-term	Fast channel	↓Agonist binding affinity; ↓channel opening transition with fewer, shorter channel opening
		null; R311W	AR[145]	M3-M4	Fast channel	↓Burst open duration (↓channel opening; ↑ACh dissociation) much reduced expression
		C>T in promoter	AR[146]		nAChR def	
		Null;	AR[147]	N-terminus	nAChR def	
		R64X;	AR[145]	N-terminus	nAChR def	Null: impair assembly; single-channel conductance 46pS; missense; normal kinetics
		R147L		N-terminus		
		70insG	AR[148]	N-terminus frameshift	nAChR def	
		C128S; 1254ins18	AR[149]	Null; M3-M4	nAChR def	Abnormal kinetics including decreased open time
		LNG to PHX; P245L	AR[145]	M1	nAChR def	No aberrant splicing; prolonged bursts (↓ rate of channel closure)
		1101insT; 1293insG	AR[140]	M3-M4	nAChR def	
		1206ins19	AR[148]	M3-M4 frameshift	nAChR def	
		1267delG	AR[150]	M3-M4 frameshift	nAChR def	

*References in superscript.

characteristic of γ-containing rather than ε-containing channel complex.

The low-affinity fast channel syndrome is a rare, recessive condition where patients generally present with moderately severe myasthenic symptoms since birth.[86,87] Electrophysiological studies reveal decremental compound-muscle action potential and very small muscle endplate potentials. Single-channel recordings from biopsied muscle endplate show infrequent, abnormally brief openings in response to ACh. Morphologic studies demonstrate normal endplate structure, with normal number of AChR and no evidence of myopathy.

Genetics

The abnormal "slow channel" kinetics suggests abnormal channels, which could result from mutations in one or more subunit of the nAChR. Patients with electrophysiologically confirmed slow-channel phenotype were screened for mutations in genes encoding the $\alpha 1$ (MIM 100690), $\beta 1$ (MIM 100710), δ (MIM 100720), and ε (MIM 100725) subunits. Single-strand conformation polymorphism analysis of PCR-amplified exons and flanking introns of all subunits of nAChR was performed. Direct sequencing of aberrant bands successfully identified mutations in different subunit genes (Table 204-7).

Several groups have reported recessive, heteroallelic mutations in the ε subunit gene in patients with nAChR deficiency or the low-affinity fast channel syndrome.

Pathophysiology

In vitro expression studies helped elucidate the biophysical consequences of these genetic mutations. Furthermore, the expression studies helped identify new functional domains within each subunit. Multiple molecular mechanisms—for example, increased agonist-binding affinity, increased channel open rate, and decreased channel closed rate—could all lead to "slow channel." The slow-channel congenital myasthenic syndrome is caused by mutations that prolong nAChR channel opening through different mechanisms. Some other mutations decrease desensitization, thus shortening the absolute refractory period and contribute to increased channel activity. Some mutations causing spontaneous channel openings in the absence of ACh further contribute to inappropriate endplate depolarization and potential excitotoxicity. All these mutations contribute to prolonged channel opening, allowing excess cation influx. Increased calcium entry likely leads to excitotoxicity, causing endplate myopathy and secondary anatomic change in synaptic structures.

Table 204-8 Mutations in Glycine Receptor Channel Subunit Gene *GLRA1* Causing Hereditary Hyperekplexia

	Mutation	Mode of transmission*	Location	Physiological consequences*
Human				
	R271L	AD[99]	M2-M3	Uncoupling of agonist binding from channel activation in HEK293 cells[151]
	R271Q			
	I244D	AR[152]		Unknown
	Q266H	AD[153]	M2	Unknown
	Del exons 1-6	AR[154]	Null	Unknown
	K276E	AR[155,156]	M2-M3	Decreased channel opening in heteromeric ($\alpha_1\beta$) receptors expressed in *Xenopus* oocytes[157]
	Y279C		M2-M3	
Mouse				
Spasmodic	G494T in *Glra*	AR[102]	Ala52Ser (N-terminus)	Decreased agonist sensitivity in homomeric α_1 glycine receptors in HEK293 cells
Spastic	Intronic LINE-1 element insertion in *Glrb*	AR[158]	Aberrant splicing	Marked reduction in glycine receptors due to impaired receptor assembly
Oscillator	Frameshift mutation in *Glra*	AR[159]	—	No demonstrable channel formation

*References in superscript.

Impaired synaptic transmission could be due to loss of AChR associated with the destruction of the junctional folds. Muscle dysfunction may also be due to the prolonged endplate potentials leading to persistent depolarization of the endplate and inactivation of perijunctional sodium channels, thus resulting in depolarization block.

The recessive mutations in nAChR deficiency result in markedly reduced AChR in the membrane. There is evidence suggesting phenotypic rescue by the expression of γ subunit. Increased presynaptic quantal release in some cases of nAChR deficiency could be a compensatory response.

The missense mutation ε P121L in the setting of a compound heterozygotic nonsense mutation caused a decrease in ACh affinity and marked slowing of channel opening, correlating with infrequent and brief channel openings in the end plate.[87] Decreased channel activation accounts for diminished muscle endplate potential.

Treatment

Therapeutic intervention in SCCMS should be directed at normalizing channel kinetics and preventing progressive muscle atrophy/endplate myopathy. The first example of such an attempt is the use of quinidine sulfate, an antagonist of nAChR in the open state, which was effective in reducing abnormally prolonged open duration of slow-channel myasthenic mutant nAChR expressed in vitro.[88] Contraindicated in other myasthenic syndrome, quinidine sulfate may normalize the kinetic abnormality of mutant channels in SCCMS. Harper and Engel treated six patients with known mutations in nAChR subunit genes and electrophysiologically characterized slow-channel syndrome with quinidine sulfate.[89] In all who tolerated the medication, they found beneficial effects in improved muscle strength testing, lessened decremental response to repetitive stimulation, and decreased number and amplitude of abnormal repetitive compound muscle action potential in response to a single stimulus. In addition to the immediate benefits, which correlated with peak serum concentrations of quinidine sulfate, all patients demonstrated continued improvement during 8 to 14 months of follow-up. This is suggestive of a protective effect of quinidine sulfate in normalizing the open duration, thereby reducing the cationic overload that may lead to endplate myopathy.

AChE inhibitors, which are not likely to be useful in treating myasthenic patients with kinetically abnormal nAChR, have been important in treating nAChR deficiency.

Medications that increase the availability of ACh would predict a favorable clinical response in patients with low-affinity fast-channel congenital myasthenic syndrome. AChE inhibitors, which slow ACh hydrolysis, theoretically would be beneficial. Of note, 3,4-diaminopyridine, a K channel blocker that increases presynaptic ACh release, did lead to significant clinical improvement in one patient.[87]

HEREDITARY HYPEREKPLEXIA: GLYCINE RECEPTOR CHANNEL

Clinical Manifestations

Hereditary hyperekplexia, or startle disease, is a rare, highly penetrant autosomal dominant disorder characterized by an exaggerated startle response and hypertonia. The normal startle reflex is a primitive reflex with a complex, stereotyped pattern of motor behavior in response to unexpected sensory stimuli. The motor response generally consists of blinking, grimacing, flexion of neck and arms, and delayed abduction of the hand muscles. Patients with startle syndromes due to various neuropathologic conditions may present with abnormally exquisite sensitivity or abnormally violent motor response to sudden stimuli. In particular, studying hereditary hyperekplexia has helped elucidate the pathophysiological and genetic basis of abnormal startle response.

A small kindred with "emotionally precipitated drop seizures," described by Kirstein and Silfverskiold in 1958, was perhaps the first case report of hereditary hyperekplexia.[90] Suhren et al. subsequently described a major form and a minor form of excessive response to sudden stimuli in a large Dutch pedigree spanning five generations.[91] The symptoms that characterize the major form consisted of transient hypertonia during infancy, an exaggerated startle response with generalized stiffening causing falls but no loss of consciousness, repetitive limb jerking particularly at night, hyperreflexia, and hesitant gait. Excessive startle without any associated symptoms characterizes the minor form.

Symptoms of the major form of hereditary hyperekplexia could present early, as in two unrelated patients who had unusual fetal movements during gestation, with sudden forceful jerking lasting from seconds to minutes that increased in severity in response to external stimuli.[92] Shortly after birth, both exhibited rigidity, nocturnal limb jerking, and an exaggerated startle response, which are typical findings in the neonatal period in patients with hereditary hyperekplexia. Unexpected stimuli, such as noises or normal handling, could precipitate massive, generalized spasms of skeletal muscles causing apnea, cyanosis, or even death during infancy.[93] Often mistaken for spastic quadriplegia, neonatal stiffness improves in early childhood.[94] Delay in motor development is common because any sudden sound, touch, or movement could cause patients to stiffen and fall. Diffuse stiffness renders the patients completely powerless in breaking their fall. There is no loss of consciousness. Patients may develop an awkward, slow, wide-based gait because of fear of falling. Inguinal and abdominal hernia, as well as generalized seizures independent of startle in patients with hyperekplexia, have also been reported.[91,93] Anxiety, stress, fear, sleep deprivation, and menstruation exacerbate the symptoms.

Physical examination usually reveals diffusely increased muscle tone during infancy that normalizes with age. Tapping of the forehead results in excessive head retraction. Deep tendon reflexes are generally hyperactive. The preservation of consciousness and the absence of epileptiform discharges on EEG distinguish hyperekplexia from startle epilepsy.[94]

Analysis of the electromyographic studies as well as evoked responses demonstrated the same startle pattern in control subjects as in patients with hyperekplexia, regardless of etiology.[95,96] The acoustic startle pathway is not completely understood but is thought to involve mainly the caudal brainstem. Lesion and stimulation studies identified a circuitry, with signals traveling from the auditory nerve to the ventral cochlear nucleus, nuclei of the lateral lemniscus, nucleus reticularis pontis caudalis, reticulospinal tract, spinal interneurons, and, finally, the lower motor neurons to innervate skeletal muscles.[97] Lesions involving the startle circuit spanning the caudal brainstem and the spinal cord could lead to decreased startle. Excessive startle indicates increased excitatory or decreased inhibitory input to the startle circuit.

Genetics

Linkage studies in several unrelated kindreds with autosomal dominant inheritance of hereditary hyperekplexia localized the disease gene to the distal portion of the long arm of chromosome 5.[98] This region contained genes encoding subunits of GABA receptor, glycine receptor, adrenergic receptor, and glutamate receptor. Radiation hybrid mapping analysis demonstrated that only the gene *GLRA1* (MIM 138491) encoding the α_1 subunit of the inhibitory glycine receptor was within the disease gene region.[99] *GLRA1* was a good candidate gene for hyperekplexia because glycinergic transmission mediates recurrent inhibition of pontomedullary reticular neurons as well as spinal motor neurons. Screening by denaturing gradient gel electrophoresis combined with direct sequencing uncovered two different missense mutations in exon 6 of *GLRA1* in affected members from four families, substituting an uncharged amino acid (leucine or glutamine) for arginine, a charged residue. Additional mutations in *GLRA1* were subsequently identified in other hereditary and sporadic cases of hyperekplexia (Table 204-8).

Mice are excellent animal models for studying hereditary hyperekplexia in humans. When given sublethal doses of strychnine, which is a competitive glycine receptor antagonist, normal mice display hypertonia and an exaggerated startle reflex, reminiscent of the cardinal features of hyperekplexia in humans. Furthermore, two autosomal recessive mouse mutants, *spastic* (*spa*) and *spasmodic* (*spd*), exhibit identical phenotypes with striking similarities to hereditary hyperekplexia in humans. Phenotypically normal at birth, the affected animals develop rigidity and fall in response to sudden tactile or acoustic stimuli after the second postnatal week. A lethal mutant, *oscillator* (*ot*), displays more severe symptoms and may be allelic to *spd*.

The phenotypic similarities between *spd* and hereditary hyperekplexia suggest that mutations in glycine receptor gene may be responsible for the *spd* phenotype. The disease locus of *spd* mapped to a small region on mouse chromosome 11 that was homologous to the *GLRA1*-containing region on human chromosome 5q.[100,101] Direct sequencing showed that *spd* indeed was the mouse homologue of hyperekplexia and a specific missense mutation (534G > T) was identified in *spd*, which would result in an A52S substitution in the mouse glycine receptor α_1 subunit, sharing 99 percent peptide sequence homology with the adult human orthologue.[102] Of note, the expression of glycine receptor isoforms is developmentally regulated, switching from the neonatal to the adult isoform around the second postnatal week in mice. The neonatal isoform of the glycine receptor contains α_2 subunits only, while the adult isoform appears to be composed of three α_1 subunits and two β subunits. That *spd* mice are phenotypically normal until after the second postnatal week is consistent with the expression of the mutation-containing $\alpha 1$ subunit gene of the adult isoform of glycine receptor.

Pathophysiology

The inhibitory glycine receptor is a heteropentameric ligand-gated chloride channel composed of strychnine-binding α subunits and the nonstrychnine-binding β subunits. The transmembrane topology of the α subunit is similar to that of the α subunits of the nicotinic acetylcholine receptor, with four putative transmembrane domains M1 to M4 (Fig. 204-4).[103]

There have been some preliminary studies on the physiological consequences of mutations in *GLRA1* that identified functional domains important for biosynthesis, agonist binding, and channel opening (Table 204-7).

Treatment

No medication has been identified that counters the observed kinetic defects in heterologously expressed mutant glycine receptor channels. Empirically, benzodiazepines reduce neonatal hypertonia and markedly decrease the frequency and severity of the startle-induced spasms in some affected individuals.[94,98] That these agonists of $GABA_A$ receptors may compensate for glycinergic dysfunction suggests that GABA-mediated inhibition must play a role in the brainstem and spinal cord. Indeed, spinal interneurons were recently discovered to release both glycine and GABA.[104]

OTHER PAROXYSMAL NEUROLOGIC DISORDERS

A growing list of paroxysmal neurologic disorders has been shown to result from mutations in ion channels. The identification of specific mutations has made diagnosis and patient classification possible. Physiological characterization of mutant channels will continue to reveal new functional domains. The finding that mutations in the auxiliary subunits may have the same clinical manifestations as mutations in the main, pore-forming channel subunits indicates that defects in any component (upstream or downstream) with which the channel protein interacts can lead to dysfunction. That mutations in distinct proteins may produce similar phenotypes provides insight to the functional role of the different channel proteins that must be carefully coordinated to carry out proper neurologic activities. In the case of congenital myasthenic syndromes, defects involving the presynaptic, synaptic, or postsynaptic components of the neuromuscular junction may interfere with normal neuromuscular transmission. It is intriguing that different mutations in the same gene produce different phenotypes (although with some overlap), as illustrated by the allelic disorders involving mutations in *SCN4A* and *CACNA1A*. Phenotypic variability among individuals within the same pedigree or different pedigrees with the same mutation suggests that other genetic and/or environmental factors must contribute to the phenotypic expression.

Understanding the phenotypic expression of the rare, monogenic channelopathies presented in this chapter may help elucidate similar mechanisms in other paroxysmal neurologic disorders, such as familial paroxysmal dyskinesia, migraine, and epilepsy. Familial paroxysmal dyskinesia is a rare group of disorders characterized by episodic involuntary hyperkinetic movement.[105] A familial paroxysmal choreoathetosis syndrome associated with progressive spasticity mapped to chromosome 1p,[106] while paroxysmal dystonic choreoathetosis not associated with spasticity mapped to chromosome 2q34 in several pedigrees.[107–111] Ion channels are candidate genes for these episodic movement disorders.

Because migraine shares many features with known channelopathies, ion channels are likely sites of genetic defects in this heterogeneous and possibly polygenic disorder. In addition to *CACNA1A* mutations discussed in this chapter, two other loci on chromosome 1q have been identified in other pedigrees with familial hemiplegic migraine, which is a rare form of migraine with aura.[112,113]

Epilepsy also shares many features with known channelopathies; indeed, mutations have been identified in both ligand-gated and voltage-gated ion channel genes in different pedigrees with epilepsy[114–116] (see Chap. 230).

With the Human Genome Project and the development of DNA chip technology well under way, we soon will be able to easily identify genes and mutations. Phenotypic variability among individuals in the same pedigree suggests that environmental, metabolic, and other genetic factors must contribute to the phenotypic expression of the mutation in any of the rare monogenic disorders discussed in this chapter. That different genetic mutations can lead to similar clinical symptoms or genetic heterogeneity is not surprising. As exemplified by the neuromuscular junction (Fig. 204-1), disturbance of any component of this temporally and spatially tightly regulated cascade of events can result in neuromuscular dysfunction. One challenge that we face is to understand how these ion channel mutations are translated into paroxysmal neurologic disturbances as well as fixed neurologic deficits. Studying the biophysical properties of individual ion channels is a good start. Other processes, such as gene expression, alternative splicing, assembly, subcellular localization, modulation by protein kinases/phosphatases, interaction with synaptic machinery and cytoskeletal elements, and excitotoxicity, are incompletely understood but clearly important in elucidating the underlying disease-causing mechanism and developing rational treatment.

ACKNOWLEDGMENTS

Funded by NIH (L. P., J. J.) and MDA (L. P.).

REFERENCES

1. Papazian DM, Schwarz TL, Tempel BL, Jan YN, Jan LY: Cloning of genomic and complementary DNA from Shaker, a putative potassium channel gene from *Drosophila*. *Science* **237**:749, 1987.
2. Ptacek LJ, George AL Jr, Griggs RC, Tawil R, Kallen RG, Barchi RL, Robertson M, et al: Identification of a mutation in the gene causing hyperkalemic periodic paralysis. *Cell* **67**:1021, 1991.
3. Ptacek LJ: The familial periodic paralyses and non-dystrophic myotonias. *Am J Med* **105**:58, 1998.
4. Ptacek LJ: Channelopathies: Ion channel disorders of muscle as a paradigm for paroxysmal disorders of the nervous system. *Neuromuscul Disord* **7**:250, 1997.
5. Ptacek LJ: Channelopathies: Ion channels and paroxysomal disorders of the nervous system, in Genton P (ed): *Genetics of Focal Epilepsies*. London, John Libbey, 1998, pp. 203–214.
6. Hille B: *Ionic Channels of Excitable Membranes*. Sunderland, MA, Sinauer Associates, 1992.
7. Doyle DA, Cabral JM, Pfuetzner RA, Kuo A, Gulbis JM, Cohen SL, Chait BT, et al: The structure of the potassium channel: Molecular basis of K^+ conduction and selectivity [see comments]. *Science* **280**:69, 1998.
8. Heginbotham L, Lu Z, Abramson T, MacKinnon R: Mutations in the K^+ channel signature sequence. *Biophys J* **66**:1061, 1994.
9. Walker D, De Waard M: Subunit interaction sites in voltage-dependent Ca^{2+} channels: role in channel function. *Trends Neurosci* **21**:148, 1998.
10. Letts VA, Felix R, Biddlecome GH, Arikkath J, Mahaffey CL, Valenzuela A, Bartlett FS 2d, et al: The mouse stargazer gene encodes a neuronal Ca^{2+}-channel gamma subunit [see comments]. *Nat Genet* **19**:340, 1998.
11. Ptacek LJ, Johnson KJ, Griggs RC: Genetics and physiology of the myotonic muscle disorders. *N Engl J Med* **328**:482, 1993.
12. Tyler FH, Stephens FE, Gunn FD, Perkoff GT: Studies in disorders of muscle VII. Clinical manifestations and inheritance of a type of periodic paralysis without hypopotassemia. *J Clin Invest* **30**:492, 1951.
13. Jackson CE, Barohn RJ, Ptacek LJ: Paramyotonia congenita: abnormal short exercise test, and improvement after mexiletine therapy. *Muscle Nerve* **17**:763, 1994.
14. Trudell RG, Kaiser KK, Griggs RC: Acetazolamide-responsive myotonia congenita. *Neurology* **37**:488, 1987.
15. Ptacek LJ, Griggs RC: Familial periodic paralysis, in Andreoli T (ed): *The Molecular Biology of Membrane Transport Disorders*. New York, Plenum, 1996, pp 625–642.
16. Fontaine B, Khurana TS, Hoffman EP, Bruns GA, Haines JL, Trofatter JA, Hanson MP, et al: Hyperkalemic periodic paralysis and the adult muscle sodium channel alpha-subunit gene. *Science* **250**:1000, 1990.
17. Ptacek LJ, Tyler F, Trimmer JS, Agnew WS, Leppert M: Analysis in a large hyperkalemic periodic paralysis pedigree supports tight linkage to a sodium channel locus. *Am J Hum Genet* **49**:378, 1991.
18. Ptacek LJ, Trimmer JS, Agnew WS, Roberts JW, Petajan JH, Leppert M: Paramyotonia congenita and hyperkalemic periodic paralysis map to the same sodium-channel gene locus. *Am J Hum Genet* **49**:851, 1991.
19. Ptacek LJ, Tawil R, Griggs RC, Storvick D, Leppert M: Linkage of atypical myotonia congenita to a sodium channel locus. *Neurology* **42**:431, 1992.
20. Rojas CV, Wang JZ, Schwartz LS, Hoffman EP, Powell BR, Brown RH Jr: A Met-to-Val mutation in the skeletal muscle Na^+ channel alpha-subunit in hyperkalaemic periodic paralysis. *Nature* **354**:387, 1991.
21. McClatchey AI, Van den Bergh P, Pericak Vance MA, Raskind W, Verellen C, McKenna Yasek D, Rao K, et al: Temperature-sensitive mutations in the III-IV cytoplasmic loop region of the skeletal muscle sodium channel gene in paramyotonia congenita. *Cell* **68**:769, 1992.
22. Ptacek LJ, George AL Jr, Barchi RL, Griggs RC, Riggs JE, Robertson M, Leppert MF: Mutations in an S4 segment of the adult skeletal muscle sodium channel cause paramyotonia congenita. *Neuron* **8**:891, 1992.
23. Ptacek LJ, Tawil R, Griggs RC, Meola G, McManis P, Barohn RJ, Mendell JR, et al: Sodium channel mutations in acetazolamide-responsive myotonia congenita, paramyotonia congenita, and hyperkalemic periodic paralysis. *Neurology* **44**:1500, 1994.
24. Fontaine B, Vale Santos J, Jurkat Rott K, Reboul J, Plassart E, Rime CS, Elbaz A, et al: Mapping of the hypokalaemic periodic paralysis (HypoPP) locus to chromosome 1q31-32 in three European families. *Nat Genet* **6**:267, 1994.
25. Ptacek LJ, Tawil R, Griggs RC, Engel AG, Layzer RB, Kwiecinski H, McManis PG, et al: Dihydropyridine receptor mutations cause hypokalemic periodic paralysis. *Cell* **77**:863, 1994.
26. Fouad G, Dalakas M, Servedei S, Mendell JR, Van den Bergh P, Angelini C, Alderson K, et al: Genotype-phenotype correlations of DHP receptor alpha-1 gene mutations causing hypokalemic periodic paralysis. *Neuromuscul Disord* **7**:33, 1997.
27. Abdalla JA, Casley WL, Cousin HK, Hudson AJ, Murphy EG, Cornelis FC, Hashimoto L, et al: Linkage of Thomsen disease to the T-cell-receptor beta (TCRB) locus on chromosome 7q35. *Am J Hum Genet* **51**:579, 1992.
28. Koch MC, Steinmeyer K, Lorenz C, Ricker K, Wolf F, Otto M, Zoll B, et al: The skeletal muscle chloride channel in dominant and recessive human myotonia. *Science* **257**:797, 1992.
29. George AL Jr, Crackower MA, Abdalla JA, Hudson AJ, Ebers GC: Molecular basis of Thomsen's disease (autosomal dominant myotonia congenita). *Nat Genet* **3**:305, 1993.
30. Steinmeyer K, Lorenz C, Pusch M, Koch MC, Jentsch TJ: Multimeric structure of ClC-1 chloride channel revealed by mutations in dominant myotonia congenita (Thomsen). *Embo J* **13**:737, 1994.

31. Lehmann Horn F, Mailander V, Heine R, George AL: Myotonia levior is a chloride channel disorder. *Hum Mol Genet* **4**:1397, 1995.
32. Meyer Kleine C, Steinmeyer K, Ricker K, Jentsch TJ, Koch MC: Spectrum of mutations in the major human skeletal muscle chloride channel gene (CLCN1) leading to myotonia. *Am J Hum Genet* **57**:1325, 1995.
33. Heine R, George AL Jr, Pika U, Deymeer F, Rudel R, Lehmann Horn F: Proof of a non-functional muscle chloride channel in recessive myotonia congenita (Becker) by detection of a 4-base pair deletion. *Hum Mol Genet* **3**:1123, 1994.
34. George AL Jr, Sloan Brown K, Fenichel GM, Mitchell GA, Spiegel R, Pascuzzi RM: Nonsense and missense mutations of the muscle chloride channel gene in patients with myotonia congenita. *Hum Mol Genet* **3**:2071, 1994.
35. Lorenz C, Meyer Kleine C, Steinmeyer K, Koch MC, Jentsch TJ: Genomic organization of the human muscle chloride channel CIC-1 and analysis of novel mutations leading to Becker-type myotonia. *Hum Mol Genet* **3**:941, 1994.
36. Zhang J, George AL Jr, Griggs RC, Fouad GT, Roberts J, Kwiecinski H, Connolly AM, et al: Mutations in the human skeletal muscle chloride channel gene (CLCN1) associated with dominant and recessive myotonia congenita. *Neurology* **47**:993, 1996.
37. Mailander V, Heine R, Deymeer F, Lehmann Horn F: Novel muscle chloride channel mutations and their effects on heterozygous carriers. *Am J Hum Genet* **58**:317, 1996.
38. Cannon SC: From mutation to myotonia in sodium channel disorders. *Neuromuscul Disord* **7**:241, 1997.
39. Lapie P, Goudet C, Nargeot J, Fontaine B, Lory P: Electrophysiological properties of the hypokalaemic periodic paralysis mutation (R528H) of the skeletal muscle alpha 1s subunit as expressed in mouse L cells. *FEBS Lett* **382**:244, 1996.
40. Fahlke C, Beck CL, George AL Jr: A mutation in autosomal dominant myotonia congenita affects pore properties of the muscle chloride channel. *Proc Natl Acad Sci U S A* **94**:2729, 1997.
41. Griggs RC, Nutt JG: Episodic ataxias as channelopathies [Editorial; Comment]. *Ann Neurol* **37**:285, 1995.
42. Griggs RC, Moxley RT, Lafrance RA, McQuillen J: Hereditary paroxysmal ataxia: Response to acetazolamide. *Neurology* **28**:1259, 1978.
43. Lubbers WJ, Brunt ER, Scheffer H, Litt M, Stulp R, Browne DL, van Weerden TW: Hereditary myokymia and paroxysmal ataxia linked to chromosome 12 is responsive to acetazolamide. *J Neurol Neurosurg Psychiatry* **59**:400, 1995.
44. Griggs RC, Moxley RTd, Lafrance RA, McQuillen J: Hereditary paroxysmal ataxia: Response to acetazolamide. *Neurology* **28**:1259, 1978.
45. Baloh RW, Yue Q, Furman JM, Nelson SF: Familial episodic ataxia: Clinical heterogeneity in four families linked to chromosome 19p [see comments]. *Ann Neurol* **41**:8, 1997.
46. Litt M, Kramer P, Browne D, Gancher S, Brunt ER, Root D, Phromchotikul T, et al: A gene for episodic ataxia/myokymia maps to chromosome 12p13. *Am J Hum Genet* **55**:702, 1994.
47. Browne DL, Gancher ST, Nutt JG, Brunt ER, Smith EA, Kramer P, Litt M: Episodic ataxia/myokymia syndrome is associated with point mutations in the human potassium channel gene, KCNA1 [see comments]. *Nat Genet* **8**:136, 1994.
48. Browne DL, Brunt ER, Griggs RC, Nutt JG, Gancher ST, Smith EA, Litt M: Identification of two new KCNA1 mutations in episodic ataxia/myokymia families. *Hum Mol Genet* **4**:1671, 1995.
49. Comu S, Giuliani M, Narayanan V: Episodic ataxia and myokymia syndrome: A new mutation of potassium channel gene Kv1.1. *Ann Neurol* **40**:684, 1996.
50. Scheffer H, Brunt ER, Mol GJ, van der Vlies P, Stulp RP, Verlind E, Mantel G, et al: Three novel KCNA1 mutations in episodic ataxia type I families. *Hum Genet* **102**:464, 1998.
51. Smart SL, Lopantsev V, Zhang CL, Robbins CA, Wang H, Chiu SY, Schwartzkroin PA, et al: Deletion of the K(V)1.1 potassium channel causes epilepsy in mice. *Neuron* **20**:809, 1998.
52. Kramer PL, Yue Q, Gancher ST, Nutt JG, Baloh R, Smith E, Browne D, et al: A locus for the nystagmus-associated form of episodic ataxia maps to an 11-cM region on chromosome 19p [Letter]. *Am J Hum Genet* **57**:182, 1995.
53. Teh BT, Silburn P, Lindblad K, Betz R, Boyle R, Schalling M, Larsson C: Familial periodic cerebellar ataxia without myokymia maps to a 19-cM region on 19p13. *Am J Hum Genet* **56**:1443, 1995.
54. Vahedi K, Joutel A, Van Bogaert P, Ducros A, Maciazeck J, Bach JF, Bousser MG, et al: A gene for hereditary paroxysmal cerebellar ataxia maps to chromosome 19p [see comments]. *Ann Neurol* **37**:289, 1995.
55. von Brederlow B, Hahn AF, Koopman WJ, Ebers GC, Bulman DE: Mapping the gene for acetazolamide responsive hereditary paroxysmal cerebellar ataxia to chromosome 19p. *Hum Mol Genet* **4**:279, 1995.
56. Joutel A, Bousser MG, Biousse V, Labauge P, Chabriat H, Nibbio A, Maciazek J, et al: A gene for familial hemiplegic migraine maps to chromosome 19. *Nat Genet* **5**:40, 1993.
57. Joutel A, Ducros A, Vahedi K, Labauge P, Delrieu O, Pinsard N, Mancini J, et al: Genetic heterogeneity of familial hemiplegic migraine. *Am J Hum Genet* **55**:1166, 1994.
58. Ophoff RA, van Eijk R, Sandkuijl LA, Terwindt GM, Grubben CPM, Haan J, Lindhout D, et al: Genetic heterogeneity of familial hemiplegic migraine. *Genomics* **22**:21, 1994.
59. Ophoff RA, M. TG, Vergouwe MN, van Eijk R, Oefner PJ, Hoffman SMG, Lamerdin JE, et al: Familial hemiplegic migraine and episodic ataxia type-2 are caused by mutations in the Ca^{2+} gene CACNL1A4. *Cell* **87**:543, 1996.
60. Haan J, Terwindt GM, Ophoff RA, Bos PL, Frants RR, Ferrari MD, Krommenhoek T, et al: Is familial hemiplegic migraine a hereditary form of basilar migraine [see comments]? *Cephalalgia* **15**:477, 1995.
61. Denier C, Ducros A, Vahedi K, Joutel A, Thierry P, Castelnovo G, Deonna T, et al: High prevalence of CACNA1A truncating mutations and broader clinical spectrum in Episodic Ataxia type 2. *Neurology* **52**:1816, 1999.
62. Ducros A, Denier C, Joutel A, Vahedi K, Michel A, Darcel F, Madigand M, et al: Recurrence of the T666M calcium channel CACNA1A gene mutation in familial hemiplegic migraine with progressive cerebellar ataxia. *Am J Hum Genet* **64**:89, 1999.
63. Yue Q, Jen JC, Thwe MM, Nelson SF, Baloh RW: De novo mutation in CACNA1A caused acetazolamide-responsive episodic ataxia. *Am J Med Genet* **77**:298, 1998.
64. Zhuchenko O, Bailey J, Bonnen P, Ashizawa T, Stockton DW, Amos C, Dobyns WB, et al: Autosomal dominant cerebellar ataxia (SCA6) associated with small polyglutamine expansions in the alpha 1A-voltage-dependent calcium channel. *Nat Genet* **15**:62, 1997.
65. Jodice C, Mantuano E, Veneziano L, Trettel F, Sabbadini G, Calandriello L, Francia A, et al: Episodic ataxia type 2 (EA2) and spinocerebellar ataxia type 6 (SCA6) due to CAG repeat expansion in the CACNA1A gene on chromosome 19p. *Hum Mol Genet* **6**:1973, 1997.
66. Jen JC, Yue Q, Karrim J, Nelson SF, Baloh RW: Spinocerebellar ataxia type 6 with positional vertigo and acetazolamide responsive episodic ataxia. *J Neurol Neurosurg Psychiatry* **65**:565, 1998.
67. Yue Q, Jen JC, Nelson SF, Baloh RW: Progressive ataxia due to a missense mutation in a calcium-channel gene. *Am J Hum Genet* **61**:1078, 1997.
68. Fletcher CF, Lutz CM, TN OS, Shaughnessy JD Jr, Hawkes R, Frankel WN, Copeland NG, et al: Absence epilepsy in tottering mutant mice is associated with calcium channel defects. *Cell* **87**:607, 1996.
69. Burgess DL, Jones JM, Meisler MH, Noebels JL: Mutation of the Ca^2 channel beta subunit gene Cchb4 is associated with ataxia and seizures in the lethargic (lh) mouse. *Cell* **88**:385, 1997.
70. Beckh S, Pongs O: Members of the RCK potassium channel family are differentially expressed in the rat nervous system. *Embo J* **9**:777, 1990.
71. Wang H, Kunkel DD, Schwartzkroin PA, Tempel BL: Localization of Kv1.1 and Kv1.2, two K channel proteins, to synaptic terminals, somata, and dendrites in the mouse brain. *J Neurosci* **14**:4588, 1994.
72. Zhou L, Zhang CL, Messing A, Chiu SY: Temperature-sensitive neuromuscular transmission in Kv1.1 null mice: Role of potassium channels under the myelin sheath in young nerves. *J Neurosci* **18**:7200, 1998.
73. Sather WA, Tanabe T, Zhang JF, Mori Y, Adams ME, Tsien RW: Distinctive biophysical and pharmacological properties of class A (BI) calcium channel alpha 1 subunits. *Neuron* **11**:291, 1993.
74. Stea A, Tomlinson WJ, Soong TW, Bourinet E, Dubel SJ, Vincent SR, Snutch TP: Localization and functional properties of a rat brain alpha 1A calcium channel reflect similarities to neuronal Q- and P-type channels. *Proc Natl Acad Sci U S A* **91**:10576, 1994.
75. Volsen SG, Day NC, McCormack AL, Smith W, Craig PJ, Beattie R, Ince PG, et al: The expression of neuronal voltage-dependent calcium channels in human cerebellum. *Brain Res Mol Brain Res* **34**:271, 1995.
76. Ludwig A, Flockerzi V, Hofmann F: Regional expression and cellular localization of the alpha1 and beta subunit of high voltage-activated calcium channels in rat brain. *J Neurosci* **17**:1339, 1997.
77. Scott VE, Felix R, Arikkath J, Campbell KP: Evidence for a 95 kDa short form of the alpha1A subunit associated with the omega-conotoxin MVIIC receptor of the P/Q-type Ca^{2+} channels. *J Neurosci* **18**:641, 1998.

78. Kraus RL, Sinnegger MJ, Glossmann H, Hering S, Striessnig J: Familial hemiplegic migraine mutations change alpha1A Ca^{2+} channel kinetics. *J Biol Chem* **273**:5586, 1998.
79. Hans M, Luvisetto S, Williams ME, Spagnolo M, Urrutia A, Tottene A, Brust PF, et al: Functional consequences of mutations in the human alpha1A calcium channel subunit linked to familial hemiplegic migraine. *J Neurosci* **19**:1610, 1999.
80. Matsuyama Z, Wakamori M, Mori Y, Kawakami H, Nakamura S, Imoto K: Direct alteration of the P/Q-type Ca^{2+} channel property by polyglutamine expansion in spinocerebellar ataxia 6. *J Neurosci* **19**:RC14, 1999.
81. Bain PG, MD OB, Keevil SF, Porter DA: Familial periodic cerebellar ataxia: a problem of cerebellar intracellular pH homeostasis. *Ann Neurol* **31**:147, 1992.
82. Prod'hom B, Pietrobon D, Hess P: Direct measurement of proton transfer rates to a group controlling the dihydropyridine-sensitive Ca^{2+} channel. *Nature* **329**:243, 1987.
83. Chen XH, Bezprozvanny I, Tsien RW: Molecular basis of proton block of L-type Ca^{2+} channels. *J Gen Physiol* 108: 363, 1996.
84. Mishina M, Takai T, Imoto K, Noda M, Takahashi T, Numa S, Methfessel C, et al: Molecular distinction between fetal and adult forms of muscle acetylcholine receptor. *Nature* **321**:406, 1986.
85. Engel AG, Lambert EH, Mulder DM, Torres CF, Sahashi K, Bertorini TE, Whitaker JN: A newly recognized congenital myasthenic syndrome attributed to a prolonged open time of the acetylcholine-induced ion channel. *Ann Neurol* **11**:553, 1982.
86. Uchitel O, Engel AG, Walls TJ, Nagel A, Atassi MZ, Bril V: Congenital myasthenic syndromes: II. Syndrome attributed to abnormal interaction of acetylcholine with its receptor. *Muscle Nerve* **16**:1293, 1993.
87. Ohno K, Wang HL, Milone M, Bren N, Brengman JM, Nakano S, Quiram P, et al: Congenital myasthenic syndrome caused by decreased agonist binding affinity due to a mutation in the acetylcholine receptor epsilon subunit. *Neuron* **17**:157, 1996.
88. Fukudome T, Ohno K, Brengman JM, Engel AG: AChR channel blockade by quinidine sulfate reduces channel open duration in the slow-channel congenital myasthenic syndrome. *Ann N Y Acad Sci* **841**:199, 1998.
89. Harper CM, Engel AG: Quinidine sulfate therapy for the slow-channel congenital myasthenic syndrome. *Ann Neurol* **43**:480, 1998.
90. Kirstein L, Silfverskiold B: A family with emotionally precipitated "drop seizures." *Acta Psychiatr Neurol Scand* **33**:471, 1958.
91. Suhren O, Brruyn G, Tuynman J: Hyperekplexia: a hereditary startle syndrome. *J Neurol Sci* **3**:577, 1966.
92. Leventer RJ, Hopkins IJ, Shield LK: Hyperekplexia as cause of abnormal intrauterine movements [Letter]. *Lancet* **345**:461, 1995.
93. Kurczynski TW: Hyperekplexia. *Arch Neurol* **40**:246, 1983.
94. Andermann F, Keene DL, Andermann E, Quesney LF: Startle disease or hyperekplexia: Further delineation of the syndrome. *Brain* **103**:985, 1980.
95. Brown P, Rothwell JC, Thompson PD, Britton TC, Day BL, Marsden CD: The hyperekplexias and their relationship to the normal startle reflex. *Brain* **114**:1903, 1991.
96. Matsumoto J, Fuhr P, Nigro M, Hallett M: Physiological abnormalities in hereditary hyperekplexia. *Ann Neurol* **32**:41, 1992.
97. Davis M, Gendelman DS, Tischler MD, Gendelman PM: A primary acoustic startle circuit: lesion and stimulation studies. *J Neurosci* **2**:791, 1982.
98. Ryan SG, Sherman SL, Terry JC, Sparkes RS, Torres MC, Mackey RW: Startle disease, or hyperekplexia: Response to clonazepam and assignment of the gene (STHE) to chromosome 5q by linkage analysis. *Ann Neurol* **31**:663, 1992.
99. Shiang R, Ryan SG, Zhu YZ, Hahn AF, O'Connell P, Wasmuth JJ: Mutations in the alpha 1 subunit of the inhibitory glycine receptor cause the dominant neurologic disorder, hyperekplexia. *Nat Genet* **5**:351, 1993.
100. Lane PW, Ganser AL, Kerner AL, White WF: Spasmodic, a mutation on chromosome 11 in the mouse. *J Hered* **78**:353, 1987.
101. Buckwalter MS, Testa CM, Noebels JL, Camper SA: Genetic mapping and evaluation of candidate genes for spasmodic, a neurological mouse mutation with abnormal startle response. *Genomics* **17**:279, 1993.
102. Ryan SG, Buckwalter MS, Lynch JW, Handford CA, Segura L, Shiang R, Wasmuth JJ, et al: A missense mutation in the gene encoding the alpha 1 subunit of the inhibitory glycine receptor in the spasmodic mouse. *Nat Genet* **7**:131, 1994.
103. Grenningloh G, Rienitz A, Schmitt B, Methfessel C, Zensen M, Beyreuther K, Gundelfinger ED, et al: The strychnine-binding subunit of the glycine receptor shows homology with nicotinic acetylcholine receptors. *Nature* **328**:215, 1987.
104. Jonas P, Bischofberger J, Sandkuhler J: Corelease of two fast neurotransmitters at a central synapse [see comments]. *Science* **281**:419, 1998.
105. Demirkiran M, Jankovic J: Paroxysmal dyskinesias: Clinical features and classification. *Ann Neurol* **38**:571, 1995.
106. Auburger G, Ratzlaff T, Lunkes A, Nelles H, Leube B, Binkofski F, Kugel H, et al: A gene for autosomal dominant paroxysmal choreoathetosis/spasticity (CSE) maps to the vicinity of a potassium channel gene cluster on chromosome 1p, probable within 2 cM between D1S443 and D1S197. *Genomics* **31**:90, 1996.
107. Fouad GT, Servidei S, Durcan S, Bertini E, Ptacek LJ: A gene for familial paroxysmal dyskinesia (FPD1) maps to chromosome 2q. *Am J Hum Genet* **59**:135, 1996.
108. Fink JK, Rainer S, Wilkowski J, Jones SM, Kume A, Hedera P, Albin R, et al: Paroxysmal dystonic choreoathetosis: tight linkage to chromosome 2q. *Am J Hum Genet* **59**:140, 1996.
109. Hofele K, Benecke R, Auburger G: Gene locus FPD1 of the dystonic Mount-Reback type of autosomal-dominant paroxysmal choreoathetosis. *Neurology* **49**:1252, 1997.
110. Fink JK, Hedera P, Mathay JG, Albin RL: Paroxysmal dystonic choreoathetosis linked to chromosome 2q: Clinical analysis and proposed pathophysiology. *Neurology* **49**:177, 1997.
111. Raskind WH, Bolin T, Wolff J, Fink J, Matsushita M, Litt M, Lipe H, et al: Further localization of a gene for paroxysmal dystonic choreoathetosis to a 5-cM region on chromosome 2q34. *Hum Genet* **102**:93, 1998.
112. Gardner K, Barmada MM, Ptacek LJ, Hoffman EP: A new locus for hemiplegic migraine maps to chromosome 1q31 [see comments]. *Neurology* **49**:1231, 1997.
113. Ducros A, Joutel A, Vahedi K, Cecillon M, Ferreira A, Bernard E, Verier A, et al: Mapping of a second locus for familial hemiplegic migraine to 1q21-q23 and evidence of further heterogeneity. *Ann Neurol* **42**:885, 1997.
114. Steinlein OK, Mulley JC, Propping P, Wallace RH, Phillips HA, Sutherland GR, Scheffer IE, et al: A missense mutation in the neuronal nicotinic acetylcholine receptor alpha 4 subunit is associated with autosomal dominant nocturnal frontal lobe epilepsy. *Nat Genet* **11**:201, 1995.
115. Steinlein OK, Magnusson A, Stoodt J, Bertrand S, Weiland S, Berkovic SF, Nakken KO, et al: An insertion mutation of the CHRNA4 gene in a family with autosomal dominant nocturnal frontal lobe epilepsy. *Hum Mol Genet* **6**:943, 1997.
116. Biervert C, Schroeder BC, Kubisch C, Berkovic SF, Propping P, Jentsch TJ, Steinlein OK: A potassium channel mutation in neonatal human epilepsy. *Science* **279**:403, 1998.
117. Rosenfeld J, Sloan-Brown K, George AL Jr: A novel muscle sodium channel mutation causes painful congenital myotonia. *Ann Neurol* **42**:811, 1997.
118. Plassart-Schiess E, Lhuillier L, George AL Jr, Fontaine B, Tabti N: Functional expression of the Ile693Thr Na^{+} channel mutation associated with paramyotonia congenita in a human cell line. *J Physiol (Lond)* **507**:721, 1998.
119. Cummins TR, Zhou J, Sigworth FJ, Ukomadu C, Stephan M, Ptacek LJ, Agnew WS: Functional consequences of a Na^{+} channel mutation causing hyperkalemic periodic paralysis. *Neuron* **10**:667, 1993.
120. Green DS, George AL Jr, Cannon SC: Human sodium channel gating defects caused by missense mutations in S6 segments associated with myotonia: S804F and V1293I. *J Physiol (Lond)* **510**:685, 1998.
121. Yang N, Ji S, Zhou M, Ptacek LJ, Barchi RL, Horn R, George AL Jr: Sodium channel mutations in paramyotonia congenita exhibit similar biophysical phenotypes in vitro. *Proc Natl Acad Sci U S A* **91**:12785, 1994.
122. Richmond JE, VanDeCarr D, Featherstone DE, George AL Jr., Ruben PC: Defective fast inactivation recovery and deactivation account for sodium channel myotonia in the I1160V mutant. *Biophys J* **73**:1896, 1997.
123. Koch MC, Baumbach K, George AL, Ricker K: Paramyotonia congenita without paralysis on exposure to cold: A novel mutation in the SCN4A gene (Val1293Ile). *Neuroreport* **6**:2001, 1995.
124. Wagner S, Lerche H, Mitrovic N, Heine R, George AL, Lehmann-Horn F: A novel sodium channel mutation causing a hyperkalemic paralytic and paramyotonic syndrome with variable clinical expressivity. *Neurology* **49**:1018, 1997.

125. Rudolph JA, Spier SJ, Byrns G, Rojas CV, Bernoco D, Hoffman EP: Periodic paralysis in quarter horses: A sodium channel mutation disseminated by selective breeding. *Nat Genet* **2**:144, 1992.
126. Ptacek LJ, Gouw L, Kwiecinski H, McManis P, Mendell JR, Barohn RJ, George AL Jr, et al: Sodium channel mutations in paramyotonia congenita and hyperkalemic periodic paralysis. *Ann Neurol* **33**:300, 1993.
127. Wang J, Dubowitz V, Lehmann Horn F, Ricker K, Ptacek L, Hoffman EP: In vivo sodium channel structure/function studies: Consecutive Arg1448 changes to Cys, His, and Pro at the extracellular surface of IVS4. *Soc Gen Physiol Ser* **50**:77, 1995.
128. Mitrovic N, Lerche H, Heine R, Fleischhauer R, Pika-Hartlaub U, Hartlaub U, George AL Jr, et al: Role in fast inactivation of conserved amino acids in the IV/S4-S5 loop of the human muscle Na^+ channel. *Neurosci Lett* **214**:9, 1996.
129. Heine R, Pika U, Lehmann Horn F: A novel SCN4A mutation causing myotonia aggravated by cold and potassium. *Hum Mol Genet* **2**:1349, 1993.
130. Cannon SC, Strittmatter SM: Functional expression of sodium channel mutations identified in families with periodic paralysis. *Neuron* **10**:317, 1993.
131. Wollnik B, Kubisch C, Steinmeyer K, Pusch M: Identification of functionally important regions of the muscular chloride channel CIC-1 by analysis of recessive and dominant myotonic mutations. *Hum Mol Genet* **6**:805, 1997.
132. Koty PP, Pegoraro E, Hobson G, Marks HG, Turel A, Flagler D, Cadaldini M, et al: Myotonia and the muscle chloride channel: Dominant mutations show variable penetrance and founder effect. *Neurology* **47**:963, 1996.
133. Pusch M, Steinmeyer K, Koch MC, Jentsch TJ: Mutations in dominant human myotonia congenita drastically alter the voltage dependence of the CIC-1 chloride channel. *Neuron* **15**:1455, 1995.
134. Fahlke C, Knittle T, Gurnett CA, Campbell KP, George AL Jr: Subunit stoichiometry of human muscle chloride channels. *J Gen Physiol* **109**:93, 1997.
135. Meyer Kleine C, Ricker K, Otto M, Koch MC: A recurrent 14 bp deletion in the CLCN1 gene associated with generalized myotonia (Becker). *Hum Mol Genet* **3**:1015, 1994.
136. Wakamori M, Yamazaki K, Matsunodaira H, Teramoto T, Tanaka I, Niidome T, Sawada K, et al: Single tottering mutations responsible for the neuropathic phenotype of the P-type calcium channel. *J Biol Chem* **273**:34857, 1998.
137. Lorenzon NM, Lutz CM, Frankel WN, Beam KG: Altered calcium channel currents in Purkinje cells of the neurological mutant mouse leaner. *J Neurosci* **18**:4482, 1998.
138. Dove LS, Abbott LC, Griffith WH: Whole-cell and single-channel analysis of P-type calcium currents in cerebellar Purkinje cells of leaner mutant mice. *J Neurosci* **18**:7687, 1998.
139. Croxen R, Newland C, Beeson D, Oosterhuis H, Chauplannaz G, Vincent A, Newsom-Davis J: Mutations in different functional domains of the human muscle acetylcholine receptor alpha subunit in patients with the slow-channel congenital myasthenic syndrome. *Hum Mol Genet* **6**:767, 1997.
140. Engel AG, Ohno K, Milone M, Wang HL, Nakano S, Bouzat C, Pruitt JN, 2d, et al: New mutations in acetylcholine receptor subunit genes reveal heterogeneity in the slow-channel congenital myasthenic syndrome. *Hum Mol Genet* **5**:1217, 1996.
141. Milone M, Wang HL, Ohno K, Fukudome T, Pruitt JN, Bren N, Sine SM, et al: Slow-channel myasthenic syndrome caused by enhanced activation, desensitization, and agonist binding affinity attributable to mutation in the M2 domain of the acetylcholine receptor alpha subunit. *J Neurosci* **17**:5651, 1997.
142. Gomez CM, Maselli R, Gammack J, Lasalde J, Tamamizu S, Cornblath DR, Lehar M, et al: A beta-subunit mutation in the acetylcholine receptor channel gate causes severe slow-channel syndrome. *Ann Neurol* **39**:712, 1996.
143. Gomez CM, Gammack JT: A leucine-to-phenylalanine substitution in the acetylcholine receptor ion channel in a family with the slow-channel syndrome. *Neurology* **45**:982, 1995.
144. Gomez CM, Maselli R, Williams JM, Bhattacharyya BB, Wollmann RL, Day JW: Genetic manipulation of AChR responses suggests multiple causes of weakness in slow-channel syndrome. *Ann N Y Acad Sci* **841**:167, 1998.
145. Ohno K, Quiram PA, Milone M, Wang HL, Harper MC, Pruitt JN 2d, Brengman JM, et al: Congenital myasthenic syndromes due to heteroallelic nonsense/missense mutations in the acetylcholine receptor epsilon subunit gene: Identification and functional characterization of six new mutations. *Hum Mol Genet* **6**:753, 1997.
146. Nichols P, Croxen R, Vincent A, Rutter R, Hutchinson M, Newsom-Davis J, Beeson D: Mutation of the acetylcholine receptor epsilon-subunit promoter in congenital myasthenic syndrome. *Ann Neurol* **45**:439, 1999.
147. Milone M, Wang HL, Ohno K, Prince R, Fukudome T, Shen XM, Brengman JM, et al: Mode switching kinetics produced by a naturally occurring mutation in the cytoplasmic loop of the human acetylcholine receptor epsilon subunit. *Neuron* **20**:575, 1998.
148. Ohno K, Anlar B, Ozdirim E, Brengman JM, Engel AG: Frameshifting and splice-site mutations in the acetylcholine receptor epsilon subunit gene in three Turkish kinships with congenital myasthenic syndromes. *Ann N Y Acad Sci* **841**:189, 1998.
149. Milone M, Ohno K, Fukudome T, Shen XM, Brengman J, Griggs RC, Engel AG: Congenital myasthenic syndrome caused by novel loss-of-function mutations in the human AChR epsilon subunit gene. *Ann N Y Acad Sci* **841**:184, 1998.
150. Croxen R, Beeson D, Newland C, Betty M, Vincent A, Newsom-Davis J: A single nucleotide deletion in the epsilon subunit of the acetylcholine receptor (AChR) in five congenital myasthenic syndrome patients with AChR deficiency. *Ann N Y Acad Sci* **841**:195, 1998.
151. Rajendra S, Lynch JW, Pierce KD, French CR, Barry PH, Schofield PR: Startle disease mutations reduce the agonist sensitivity of the human inhibitory glycine receptor. *J Biol Chem* **269**:18739, 1994.
152. Rees MI, Andrew M, Jawad S, Owen MJ: Evidence for recessive as well as dominant forms of startle disease (hyperekplexia) caused by mutations in the alpha 1 subunit of the inhibitory glycine receptor. *Hum Mol Genet* **3**:2175, 1994.
153. Milani N, Dalpra L, del Prete A, Zanini R, Larizza L: A novel mutation (Gln266 → His) in the alpha 1 subunit of the inhibitory glycine-receptor gene (GLRA1) in hereditary hyperekplexia [Letter]. *Am J Hum Genet* **58**:420, 1996.
154. Brune W, Weber RG, Saul B, von Knebel Doeberitz M, Grond-Ginsbach C, Kellerman K, Meinck HM, et al: A GLRA1 null mutation in recessive hyperekplexia challenges the functional role of glycine receptors. *Am J Hum Genet* **58**:989, 1996.
155. Elmslie FV, Hutchings SM, Spencer V, Curtis A, Covanis T, Gardiner RM, Rees M: Analysis of GLRA1 in hereditary and sporadic hyperekplexia: A novel mutation in a family cosegregating for hyperekplexia and spastic paraparesis. *J Med Genet* **33**:435, 1996.
156. Baxter P, Connolly S, Curtis A, Spencer V, Ravindranath C, Burn J, Gardner-Medwin D: Co-dominant inheritance of hyperekplexia and spastic paraparesis. *Dev Med Child Neurol* **38**:739, 1996.
157. Lewis TM, Sivilotti LG, Colquhoun D, Gardiner RM, Schoepfer R, Rees M: Properties of human glycine receptors containing the hyperekplexia mutation alpha1 (K276E), expressed in *Xenopus* oocytes. *J Physiol (Lond)* **507**:25, 1998.
158. Kingsmore SF, Giros B, Suh D, Bieniarz M, Caron MG, Seldin MF: Glycine receptor beta-subunit gene mutation in spastic mouse associated with LINE-1 element insertion. *Nat Genet* **7**:136, 1994.
159. Kling C, Koch M, Saul B, Becker CM: The frameshift mutation oscillator (Glra1(spd-ot)) produces a complete loss of glycine receptor alpha 1-polypeptide in mouse central nervous system. *Neuroscience* **78**:411, 1997.

STANDARD ABBREVIATIONS

Abbreviation	Name
ACTH	corticotropin (adrenocorticotropin, adrenocorticotropic hormone)
ADA	adenosine deaminase
AdoMet	s-adenosylmethionine
Ag	antigen
AIDS	acquired immunodeficiency syndrome
ALT	alanine aminotransferase
AMP, ADP, and ATP*	adenosine 5′-mono-, di-, and triphosphates
AP1, AP2	activator protein 1, 2; transcription factors
apo A-I	apolipoprotein A-I
apo A-II	apolipoprotein A-II
apo A-III	apolipoprotein A-III
apo B	apolipoprotein B
apo C-I	apolipoprotein C-I
apo C-II	apolipoprotein C-II
apo C-III	apolipoprotein C-III
apo D	apolipoprotein D
apo E	apolipoprotein E
APRT	adenine phosphoribosyltransferase
ASO	allele-specific oligonucleotide
AST	aspartate aminotransferase
ATPase	adenosine triphosphate
α_1AT	α_1-antitrypsin
B cell	B lymphocyte
BAC	bacterial artificial chromosome
cAMP, cGMP, etc.	cyclic AMP (adenosine 3′: 5′-monophosphate), etc.
CAT	chloramphenicol acetyltransferase
CD	cluster of differentiation or cluster determinant (e.g., CD34)
cDNA	complementary DNA
CHO cells	Chinese hamster ovary cells
CoA (or CoASH)	coenzyme A
CoASAc	acetyl coenzyme A
cM	centimorgan
Cm-cellulose	O-(carboxymethyl)cellulose
CMP, CDP, and CTP*	cytidine 5′-mono-, di-, and triphosphates
CNS	central nervous system
COS cells	CV-I origin, SV40; cells widely used for transfection studies
CPK	creatine phosphokinase
CRM, CRM$^+$, CRM$^-$	cross-reacting material, CRM positive, CRM negative
CT	computerized tomography
CVS	chorionic villus sampling
DEAE-cellulose	O-(diethylaminoethyl)cellulose
DNA	deoxyribonucleic acid
DNase	deoxyribonuclease
DOPA	3,4-dihydroxyphenylalanine
DPN, DPN$^+$, DPNH$^+$	diphosphopyridine nucleotide and its oxidized and reduced forms
DPT	diphtheria, pertussis, tetanus vaccine
dTMP, dTDP, and dTTP*	thymidine 5′-mono-, di-, and triphosphates
DTT	dithiothreitol
EBV	Epstein-Barr virus
EDTA	ethylenediaminetetraacetate
EEG	electroencephalogram
EGF	epidermal growth factor
EGTA	[ethylenebis(oxyethylenenitrilo)] tetraacetic acid
EKG	electrocardiogram
ELISA	enzyme-linked immunosorbent assay
EM	electron microscopy or microscopic

Abbreviation	Name
ER	endoplasmic reticulum
ES cells	embryonic stem cells
FAD and FADH$_2$	flavin-adenine dinucleotide and its fully reduced form
FISH	fluorescence *in situ* hybridization
FITC	fluorescein isothiocyanate
FMN	riboflavin 5′-phosphate
G, G$_i$, G$_s$	guanine nucleotide binding protein, inhibitory form, stimulatory form
G-6-PD	glucose 6-phosphate dehydrogenase
GABA	γ-aminobutyric acid
GC	gas chromatography
GC/MS	gas chromatography/mass spectroscopy
GERL	Golgi endoplasmic reticulum-like
GFR	glomerular filtration rate
GMP, GDP, and GTP*	guanosine 5′-mono-, di-, and triphosphates
GSH and GSSG	glutathione and its oxidized form
Hb, HbCO, HbO$_2$	hemoglobin, carbon monoxide hemoglobin, oxyhemoglobin
HDL	high density lipoprotein
HEPES	4-(2-hydroxyethyl)-1-piperazine ethanesulfonic acid
Hep G2	hepatocellular carcinoma human cell line
HIV	human immunodeficiency virus
HLA	human leukocyte antigens
HMG-CoA	3-hydroxy-3-methylglutaryl-coenzyme A
HPLC	high performance (or pressure) liquid chromotography
HPRT	hypoxanthine-guanine phosphoribosyltransferase
IDDM	insulin-dependent diabetes mellitus
IFN	interferon
Ig	immunoglobulin
IgA	gamma A immunoglobulin
IgG	gamma G immunoglobulin
IgM	gamma M immunoglobulin
IL	interleukin, including IL-1, IL-2, etc.
IM or i.m.	intramuscular
IMP, IDP, and ITP*	inosine 5′-mono-, di, and triphosphates
LDH	lactate dehydrogenase
LDL	low density lipoproteins
LINE	long interspersed repeat element
lod	logarithm of the odds
MCH	erythrocyte mean corpuscular hemoglobin
MCHC	erythrocyte mean corpuscular hemoglobin concentration
MCV	erythrocyte mean corpuscular volume
MHC	histocompatibility complex
MPS	mucopolysaccharide or mucopolysaccharidosis
MRI	magnetic resonance imaging
mRNA	messenger RNA
MS	mass spectrometry
mtDNA, mtRNA	mitochondrial DNA, RNA
Myc	oncogene homologous to avian myelocytomatosis virus including c-*myc*, N-*myc*, and L-*myc*
NAD, NAD$^+$, and NADH†	nicotinamide adenine dinucleotide and its oxidized and reduced forms
NADP, NADP$^+$, and NADPH†	nicotinamide adenine dinucleotide phosphate and its oxidized and reduced forms
NIDDM	non-insulin-dependent diabetes mellitus

(Continues)

STANDARD ABBREVIATIONS (*Cont.*)

Abbreviation	Name	Abbreviation	Name
NK cells	natural killer cells	SE	standard error
NMN	nicotinamide mononucleotide	SEM	standard error of mean
NMR	nuclear magnetic resonance	SER	smooth endoplasmic reticulum
p	probability	SH1, SH2, SH3	Src homology domains 1, 2, 3
p_i	inorganic phosphate	SNP	single nucleotide polymorphism
PAC	P1-derived artificial chromosome	*src*	oncogene homologous to Rous sarcoma virus
PAS	periodic acid Schiff	SSCP	single strand conformational polymorphism
PCR	polymerase chain reaction	STR	short tandem repeat
PEG	polyethylene glycol	SV40	Simian virus 40
PFGE	pulsed-field gel electrophoresis	T_3	triiodothyronine
PKA	protein kinase A	T_4	thyroxine
PKC	protein kinase C	T cell	T lymphocyte
PKU	phenylketonuria	TMP, TDP, and TTP*	ribosylthymine 5′-mono-, di-, and triphosphates
PP_i	inorganic pyrophosphate	TNF	tumor necrosis factor (e.g. TNF-1)
PP-ribose-P	phosphoribosylpyrophosphate	TPN, TPN^+, TPNH†	triphosphopyridine nucleotide and its oxidized and reduced forms
ras	oncogenes homologous to sarcoma retroviruses including HRAS, KRAS, and NRAS, H-*ras*, K-*ras*, and N-*ras*	Tris	tris(hydroxymethyl)aminomethane
RER	rough endoplasmic reticulum	tRNA	transfer RNA
RFLP	restriction fragment length polymorphism	UDP-Gal	uridine diphosphogalactose
RIA	radioimmunoassay	UDP-Glc	uridine diphosphoglucose
rRNA	ribosomal RNA	UMP, UDP, and UTP*	uridine 5′-mono-, di-, and triphosphates
RNase	ribonuclease	UV	ultraviolet light
RT-PCR	reverse transcription-polymerase chain reaction	VLDL	very low density lipoprotein
SD	standard deviation	VNTR	variable number tandem repeat
SDS	sodium dodecyl sulfate	YAC	yeast artificial chromosome
SDS-PAGE	sodium dodecyl sulfate polyacrylamide gel electrophoresis		

*The d prefix may be used to represent the corresponding deoxyribonucleoside phosphates, e.g., dADP.
†Note that DPN = NAD and TPN = NADP.

AMINO ACID SYMBOLS

Name	Symbols		Name	Symbols	
alanine	Ala	A	leucine	Leu	L
arginine	Arg	R	lysine	Lys	K
asparagine	Asn	N	methionine	Met	M
aspartic acid	Asp	D	phenylalanine	Phe	F
cysteine	Cys	C	proline	Pro	P
glutamic acid	Glu	E	serine	Ser	S
glutamine	Gln	Q	threonine	Thr	T
glycine	Gly	G	tryptophan	Trp	W
histidine	His	H	tyrosine	Tyr	Y
isoleucine	Ile	I	valine	Val	V

CARBOHYDRATE SYMBOLS

Name	Symbols	Name	Symbols
fructose	Fru	N-acetylgalactosamine	GalNAc
fucose	Fuc	N-acetylglucosamine	GlcNAc
galactose	Gal	N-acetylneuraminic acid	NeuAc
glucosamine	GlcN	ribose	Rib
glucose	Glc	sialic acid	Sia
glucuronic acid	GlcA	xylose	Xyl
mannose	Man		

INDEX

Page numbers followed by an "f" indicate figures; numbers followed by a "t" indicate tables.

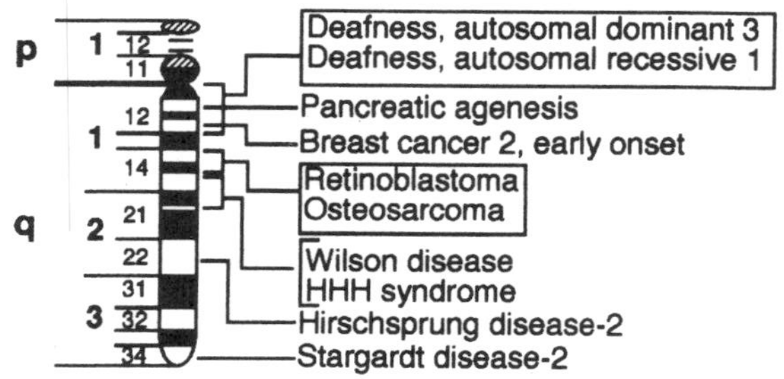

13

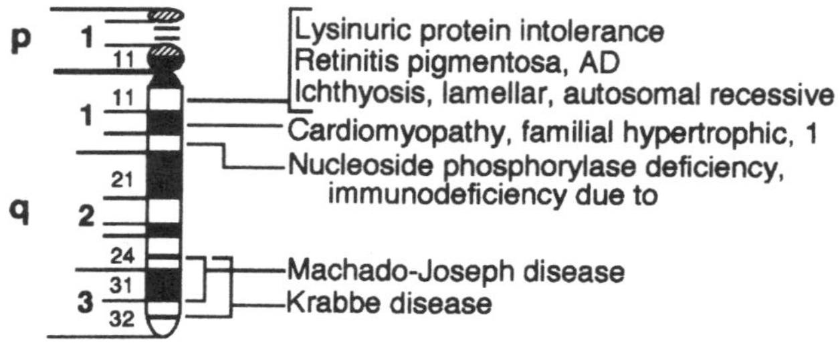

14

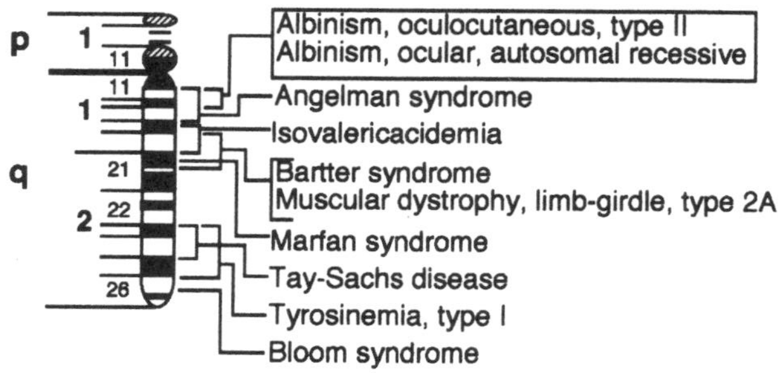

15

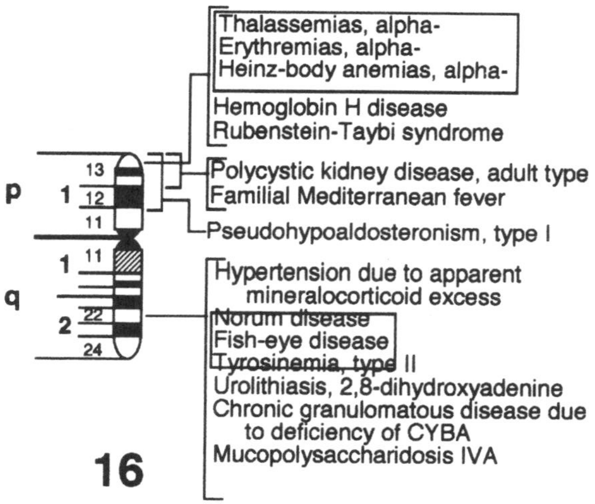

16

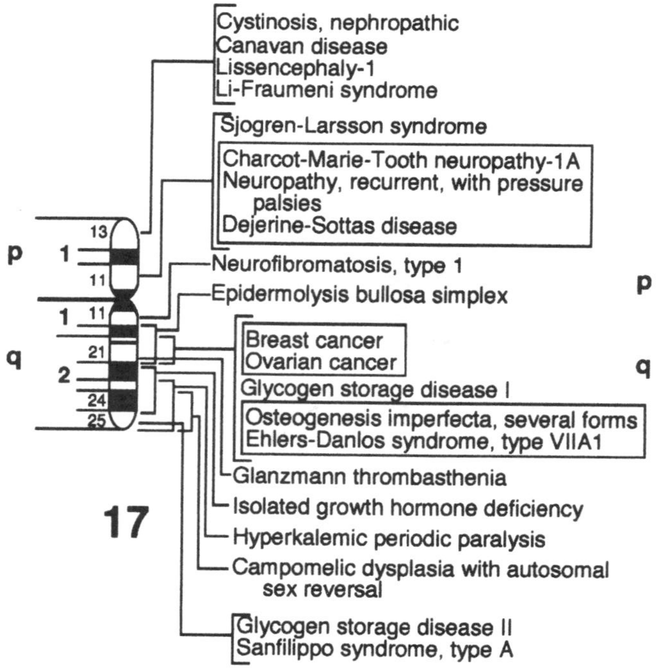

17

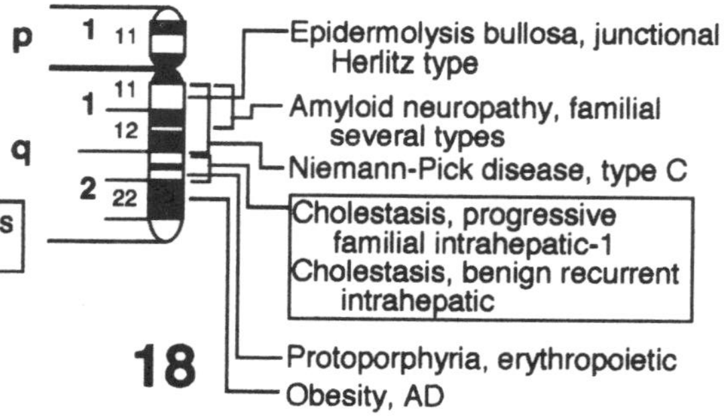

18